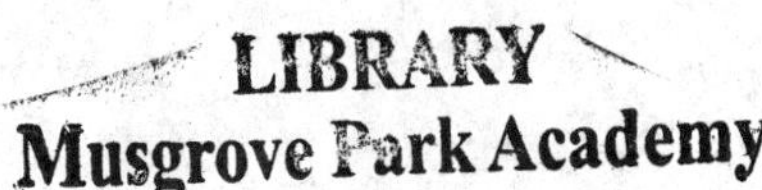

NELSON TEXTBOOK OF PEDIATRICS

*N*ELSON TEXTBOOK OF PEDIATRICS

18th EDITION

Robert M. Kliegman, MD
Professor and Chair
Department of Pediatrics
Medical College of Wisconsin
Pediatrician-in-Chief
Pamela and Leslie Muma Chair in Pediatrics
Children's Hospital of Wisconsin
Executive Vice President
Children's Research Institute
Milwaukee, Wisconsin

Richard E. Behrman, MD
Clinical Professor, Department of Pediatrics
University of California, San Francisco
San Francisco, California
George Washington University,
Washington, DC

Hal B. Jenson, MD
Chief Academic Officer
Baystate Health
Dean of the Western Campus of Tufts University School of Medicine
Springfield, Massachusetts

Bonita F. Stanton, MD
Professor and Schotanus Family Endowed Chair
Carman and Ann Adams Department of Pediatrics
Wayne State University
Pediatrician-in-Chief
Children's Hospital of Michigan
Detroit Medical Center
Detroit, Michigan

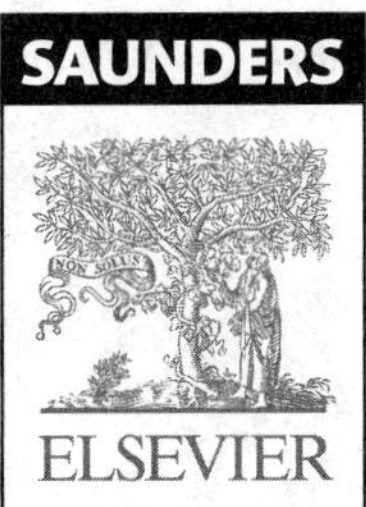

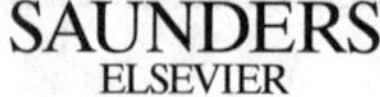

1600 John F. Kennedy Blvd.
Ste 1800
Philadelphia, PA 19103-2899

NELSON TEXTBOOK OF PEDIATRICS, 18/E ISBN: 978-1-4160-2450-7
International Edition ISBN: 978-0-8089-2365-7

Notice

Knowledge and best practice in this field are constantly changing. As new research and experience broaden our knowledge, changes in practice, treatment and drug therapy may become necessary or appropriate. Readers are advised to check the most current information provided (i) on procedures featured or (ii) by the manufacturer of each product to be administered, to verify the recommended dose or formula, the method and duration of administration, and contraindications. It is the responsibility of the practitioner, relying on their own experience and knowledge of the patient, to make diagnoses, to determine dosages and the best treatment for each individual patient, and to take all appropriate safety precautions. To the fullest extent of the law, neither the Publisher nor the Editors assumes any liability for any injury and/or damage to persons or property arising out or related to any use of the material contained in this book.

The Publisher

Previous editions copyrighted 2004, 2000, 1996, 1992, 1987, 1983, 1979, 1975, 1969, 1964, 1959

Library of Congress Cataloging-in-Publication Data
Nelson textbook of pediatrics.—18th ed./[edited by] Robert M. Kliegman . . . [et al.].
p. ; cm.
Includes bibliographical references and index.
ISBN-13: 978-1-4160-2450-7
1. Pediatrics. I. Kliegman, Robert. II. Nelson, Waldo E. (Waldo Emerson), 1898—Textbook of pediatrics. III. Title: Textbook of pediatrics.
[DNLM: 1. Pediatrics. WS 100 N423 2007]
RJ45.N4 2007
618.92–dc22
2006037517

Acquisitions Editor: Judith Fletcher
Developmental Editor: Jennifer Shreiner
Publishing Services Manager: Joan Sinclair

Printed in the United States of America

Last digit is the print number: 9 8 7 6 5 4 3 2

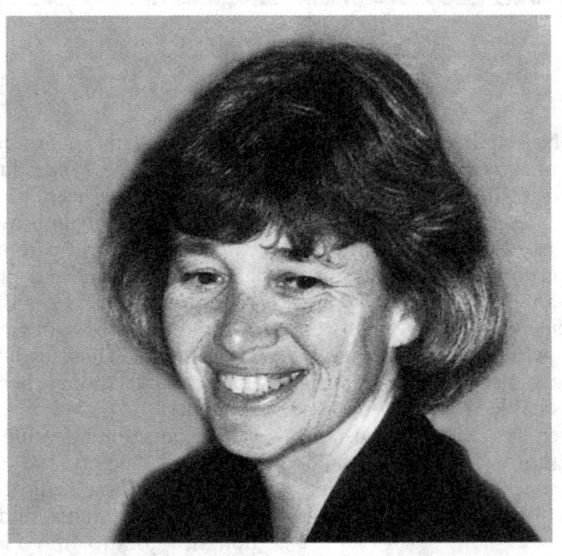

This edition is dedicated to the life of Ann Nelson Behrman, who will live in our hearts forever as a loving and devoted wife, mother, grandmother, educator, and friend. Ann has been intimately associated with many editions of Nelson Textbook of Pediatrics and will be remembered for her insatiable love of life, intellectual curiosity, gracious style, and genuine concern for all children. Her kindness and warmth radiated not only to her family but also to the countless students, residents, and faculty she welcomed into her home, and yes even "to the birds." We all miss her dearly.

Preface

The publication of this 18th Edition of Nelson Textbook of Pediatrics combines an important synthesis of clinical pediatrics with the rapid advances in genomics, diagnosis, imaging, and therapeutics. The 18th edition continues to represent the "state of the art" on the care of the normal and ill neonate, child, or adolescent by presenting both evidence-based medicine as well as astute clinical experiences from leading international authors.

The promise that translational medicine will improve the lives of all children is greater than ever. Knowledge of human development, behavior, and diseases from the molecular to sociologic levels is increasing at fantastic rates. This has led to greater understanding of health and illness in children as well as to substantial improvements in health quality for those who have access to health care. These exciting scientific advances also provide hope to effectively address new and emerging diseases threatening children and their families.

Unfortunately, many children throughout the world have not benefited from the significant advances in the prevention and treatment of health-related problems, primarily because of a lack of political will and misplaced priorities. Additionally, many children are at substantial risk from the adverse effects of poverty, war, and bioterrorism. In order for our increasing knowledge to benefit all children and youth, medical advances and good clinical practice must always be coupled with effective advocacy.

This new edition of Nelson Textbook of Pediatrics attempts to provide the essential information that practitioners, house staff, medical students, and other care providers involved in pediatric health care need to understand to effectively address the enormous range of biologic, psychologic, and social problems that our children and youth may face. Our goal is to be comprehensive, yet concise and reader friendly, embracing both the new advances in science as well as the time-honored art of pediatric practice.

The 18th Edition is substantially reorganized and revised from the previous edition. There are the additions of new diseases and new chapters, as well as substantial expansion or significant modification of others. In addition many more tables, photographs, imaging studies and illustrative figures, as well as up-to-date references have been added. Every subject has been scrutinized for updating and improvement in its exposition and usefulness to pediatric health care providers. Although, to an ill child and his or her family and physician, even the rarest disorder is of central importance, all health problems cannot possibly be covered with the same degree of detail in one general textbook of pediatrics. Thus, leading articles and subspecialty texts are referenced and should be consulted when more information is desired.

The outstanding value of the 18th Edition of the Textbook is due to its expert and authoritative contributors. We are all indebted to these dedicated authors for their hard work, knowledge, thoughtfulness, and good judgment. Our sincere appreciation also goes to Judy Fletcher and Jennifer Shreiner at Elsevier and to Carolyn Redman at the Pediatric Department of the Medical College of Wisconsin. We have all worked hard to produce an edition that will be helpful to those who provide care for children and youth and to those desiring to know more about children's health worldwide.

In this edition we have had informal assistance from many faculty and house staff of the departments of pediatrics at the Medical College of Wisconsin and Wayne State University School of Medicine. The help of these individuals and of the many practicing pediatricians from around the world who have taken the time to offer thoughtful feedback and suggestions is always greatly appreciated and helpful.

Last and certainly not least, we especially wish to thank our families for their patience and understanding without which this textbook would not have been possible.

Robert M. Kliegman, MD
Richard E. Behrman, MD
Hal B. Jenson, MD
Bonita F. Stanton, MD

Contributors

Amy C. Abraham, PhD
Volunteer Clinical Faculty, Department of Psychiatry, Tulane University Health Sciences Center, School of Medicine; Clinical Psychologist, Lafayette Psychotherapy Group, New Orleans, Louisiana
Eating Disorders

Jon S. Abramson, MD
Professor and Chair of Pediatrics, Wake Forest University School of Medicine, Winston-Salem, North Carolina
Streptococcus Pneumoniae (Pneumococcus)

Mark J. Abzug, MD
Professor of Pediatrics (Pediatric Infectious Diseases), University of Colorado School of Medicine; The Children's Hospital, Denver, Colorado
Nonpolio Enteroviruses

James D. Acton, MD
Assistant Professor, Department of Pediatrics, University of Cincinnati College of Medicine; Director, Cystic Fibrosis Center, Division of Pulmonary Medicine, Cincinnati Children's Hospital Medical Center, Cincinnati, Ohio
Cystic Fibrosis

Ira Adams-Chapman, MD
Assistant Professor of Pediatrics, Department of Pediatrics, Division of Nematology, Emory University School of Medicine; Medical Director, Developmental Progress Clinic, Emory University School of Medicine, Atlanta, Georgia
The Fetus; The High-Risk Infant; Nervous System Disorders; Delivery Room Emergencies

Hoover Adger, Jr., MD, MPH
Professor of Pediatrics, Johns Hopkins University School of Medicine; Professor of Pediatrics, Johns Hopkins Hospital, Baltimore, Maryland
Substance Abuse

John Aiken, MD
Associate Professor of Surgery, Medical College of Wisconsin, Milwaukee, Wisconsin
Acute Appendicitis; Inguinal Hernias; Epigastric Hernia

Hassan H. A-Kader, MD
Associate Professor of Pediatrics; Chief, Division of Gastroenterology, Hepatology, and Nutrition, University of Arizona, Tucson, Arizona
Cholestasis

Ramin Alemzadeh, MD
Professor of Pediatrics, Section of Endocrinology and Diabetes, Medical College of Wisconsin; Director, Diabetes Program, Children's Hospital of Wisconsin, Milwaukee, Wisconsin
Diabetes Mellitus

Karl E. Anderson, MD
Professor, Department of Preventive Medicine and Community Health, Internal Medicine, and Pharmacology and Toxicology; Staff, University of Texas Medical Branch, Galveston, Texas
The Porphyrias

Alia Antoon, MD
Assistant Clinical Professor, Harvard Medical School; Chief of Pediatrics, Shriners Hospital for Children, Shriners Burns Hospital, Boston, Massachusetts
Burn Injuries; Cold Injuries

Jacob V. Aranda, MD, PhD, FRCPC, FAAP
Professor, Department of Pediatrics, Pharmacology and Pharmaceutical Sciences, Wayne State University School of Medicine and College of Pharmacy and Allied Health; Director, Clinical Pharmacology and Toxicology and the Pediatric Pharmacology Research Unit Network (PPRU), Children's Hospital of Michigan, Detroit, Michigan
Pharmacogenetics, Pharmacogenomics, and Pharmacoproteomics

Carola A.S. Arndt, MD
Associate Professor of Pediatric and Adolescent Medicine, Chair, Division of Pediatric Hematology/Oncology, Mayo Clinic, Rochester, Minnesota
Soft Tissue Sarcomas; Neoplasms of Bone

Stephen S. Arnon, MD
Founder and Chief, Infant Botulism Treatment and Prevention Program, California Department of Health Services, Richmond, California
Botulism *(Clostridium Botulinum)*; Tetanus *(Clostridium Tetani)*

Stephen C. Aronoff, MD, MBA
Professor and Chairman of Pediatrics, Temple University School of Medicine; Temple University Children's Medical Center, Philadelphia, Pennsylvania
Candida; Cryptococcus Neoformans; Aspergillus; Histoplasmosis *(Histoplasma Capsulatum);* Blastomycosis *(Blastomyces Dermatiditis); Paracoccidioides Brasiliensis;* Sporotrichosis *(Sorothrix Schenckii);* Zygomycosis (Mucormycosis); Primary Amebic Meningoencephalitis; Nonbacterial Food Poisoning

David M. Asher, MD
Chief, Laboratory of Bacterial, Parasitic and Unconventional Agents, Division of Emerging and Transfusion-Transmitted Diseases, Office of Blood Research and Review, Center for Biologics Evaluation and Research, U.S. Food and Drug Administration, Kensington, Maryland
Transmissible Spongiform Encephalopathies

Joann L. Ater, MD
Professor of Pediatrics, University of Texas M.D. Anderson Cancer Center; Professor of Pediatrics, Children's Cancer Hospital, University of Texas M.D. Anderson Cancer Center, Houston, Texas
Brain Tumors in Childhood; Neuroblastoma

Dan Atkins, MD
Assistant Professor of Pediatrics, University of Colorado Health Sciences Center; Professor of Pediatrics, Director, Ambulatory Pediatrics, National Jewish Medical and Research Center, Denver, Colorado
Diagnosis of Allergic Disease; Principles of Treatment of Allergic Disease

Marilyn Augustyn, MD
Associate Professor, Boston University; Assistant Director, Division of Developmental and Behavioral Pediatrics, Boston Medical Center, Boston, Massachusetts
Impact of Violence on Children; Bullying and School Violence

Ellis D. Avner, MD
Associate Dean for Research and Professor of Pediatrics (Nephrology), Medical College of Wisconsin; Director, Children's Research Institute, Children's Hospital Health System of Wisconsin, Milwaukee, Wisconsin
Introduction to Glomerular Diseases; Clinical Evaluation of the Child with Hematuria; Isolated Glomerular Disease with Recurrent Gross Hematuria; Glomerulonephritis Associated with Infections; Membranous Glomerulopathy (Glomerulonephritis); Membranoproliferative (Mesagniocapillary) Glomerulonephritis; Glomerulonephritis Associated with Systemic Lupus Erythematosus; Henoch-Schönlein Purpura Nephritis; Rapidly Progressive (Crescentic) Glomerulonephritis; Goodpasture Disease; Hemolytic-Uremic Syndrome; Upper Urinary Tract Causes of Hematuria; Hematologic Diseases Causing Hematuria; Anatomic Abnormalities Associated with Hematuria; Lower Urinary Tract Causes of Hematuria; Introduction to the Child with Proteinuria; Transient Proteinuria; Orthostatic (Postural) Proteinuria; Fixed Proteinuria; Nephrotic Syndrome; Tubular Function; Renal Tubular Acidosis; Nephrogenic Diabetes Insipidus; Bartter/Gitelman Syndromes and Other Tubular Transport Abnormalities; Tubulointerstitial Nephritis; Toxic Nephropathy; Cortical Necrosis; Renal Failure

Parvin H. Azimi, MD
Clinical Professor of Pediatrics, University of California, San Francisco, San Francisco, California; Director of Children's Hospital and Research Center at Oakland, Oakland, California
Chancroid *(Haemophilus Ducreyi)*; Syphilis *(Treponema Pallidum)*; Nonvenereal Treponemal Infections; Leptospira; Relapsing Fever *(Borrelia)*

Thomas Bahk, MD
Assistant Professor, Department of Pediatrics, Loma Linda University Medical Center, Loma Linda, California
Pulmonary Edema

William F. Balistreri, MD
Medical Director, Pediatric Liver Care Center; Associate Chair for Subspecialty Training, Department of Pediatrics, Cincinnati Children's Hospital Medical Center, Cincinnati, Ohio
Morphogenesis of the Liver and Biliary System; Manifestations of Liver Disease; Cholestasis; Metabolic Diseases of the Liver; Viral Hepatitis; Liver Abscess; Liver Disease Associated with Systemic Disorders, Mitochondrial Hepatopathies

Robert S. Baltimore, MD, FAAP
Professor of Pediatrics and Epidemiology, Departments of Pediatrics and of Epidemiology and Public Health, Yale University School of Medicine; Attending Physician, Pediatrics, Yale-New Haven Children's Hospital, New Haven, Connecticut
Listeria monocytogenes; Pseudomonas, Burkholderia, and *Stenotrophomonas*

Shahida Baqar, PhD
Infectious Diseases Directorate, Enteric Diseases Department, Naval Medical Research Center, Silver Spring, Maryland
Campylobacter

Fred F. Barrett, MD
Professor of Pediatrics (Retired), University of Tennessee Health Science Center; Medical Director, LeBonheur Children's Medical Center, Memphis, Tennessee
Infection Associated with Medical Devices

Christine E. Barron, MD
Assistant Professor of Pediatrics, Brown Medical School; Clinical Director, Child Protection Program, Hasbro Children's Hospital, Providence, Rhode Island
Adolescent Rape

Dorsey M. Bass, MD
Associate Professor of Pediatrics, Stanford University; Attending Physician, Gastroenterology, Lucile Salter Packard Children's Hospital, Stanford, California
Rotaviruses, Caliciviruses, and Astrovirus

Michael D. Bates, MD, PhD
Assistant Professor, Department of Pediatrics, University of Cincinnati College of Medicine; Division of Gastroenterology, Hepatology and Nutrition; Division of Developmental Biology, Cincinnati Children's Hospital Medical Center, Cincinnati, Ohio
Morphogenesis of the Liver and Biliary System

Mark Batshaw, MD
Professor and Chair of Pediatrics, George Washington University; Chief Academic Officer, Children's Hospital National Medical Center, Washington, District of Columbia
Mental Retardation (Intellectual Disability)

Howard Bauchner, MD
Boston University School of Medicine; Boston Medical Center, Boston, Massachusetts
Failure to Thrive

Richard E. Behrman, MD
Clinical Professor of Pediatrics, University of California, San Francisco, San Francisco, California; George Washington University, Washington, District of Columbia; Stanford University, Stanford, California; Lucile Salter Packard Children's Hospital, Palo Alto, California; Executive Chair, Federation of Pediatric Organizations, Pediatric Education Steering Committee, Menlo Park, California
Overview of Pediatrics

Michael J. Bennett, PhD
Professor of Pathology and Laboratory Medicine, University of Pennsylvania; Director, Metabolic Disease Laboratory, Children's Hospital of Philadelphia, Philadelphia, Pennsylvania
Disorders of Mitochondrial Fatty Acid β-Oxidation

Daniel Bernstein, MD
Alfred Woodley Salter and Mabel G. Salter Endowed Professor, Chief, Division of Pediatric Cardiology, Stanford University; Co-Director Children's Heart Center, Lucile Salter Packard Children's Hospital, Palo Alto, California
Cardiac Development; The Fetal to Neonatal Circulatory Transition; History and Physical Examination; Laboratory Evaluation; Epidemiology and Genetic Basis of Congenital Heart Disease; Evaluation of the Infant or Child with Congenital Heart Disease; Acyanotic Congenital Heart Disease: The Left-to-Right Shunt Lesions; Acyanotic Congenital Heart Disease: The Obstructive Lesions; Acyanotic Congenital Heart Disease: Regurgitant Lesions; Cyanotic Congenital Heart Disease: Evaluation of the Critically Ill Neonate with Cyanosis and Respiratory Distress; Cyanotic Congenital Heart Lesions: Lesions Associated with Decreased Pulmonary Blood Flow; Cyanotic Congenital Heart Disease: Lesions Associated with Increased Pulmonary Blood Flow; Other Congenital Heart and Vascular Malformations; Pulmonary Hypertension; General Principles of Treatment of Congenital Heart Disease; Infective Endocarditis; Rheumatic Heart Disease; Diseases of the Myocardium; Diseases of the Pericardium; Tumors of the Heart; Heart Failure; Pediatric Heart and Heart-Lung Transplantation; Disease of the Blood Vessels (Aneurysms and Fistulas); Systemic Hypertension

Michelle Bestic, PharmD
Instructor of Pediatrics, Case Western Reserve University; Division of Pediatric Clinical Pharmacology and Toxicology, Rainbow Babies and Children's Hospital, Cleveland, Ohio
Poisonings

Zulfiqar Ahmed Bhutta, MB, FRCP, FRCPCH, FCPS, PhD
Husein Lalji Dewraj Professor and Chairman of Pediatrics and Child Health, Aga Khan University, Karachi, Pakistan
Salmonella; Acute Gastroenteritis in Children

Leslie G. Biesecker, MD
Adjunct Associate Professor, Johns Hopkins University School of Public Health; Chief, Genetic Disease Research Branch, National Human Genome Research Institute, National Institutes of Health; NIH Clinical Center, National Institutes of Health, Bethesda, Maryland
Dysmorphology

Ari Bitnum, MD, MSc, FRCPC
Assistant Professor of Pediatrics, University of Toronto; Staff Physician, Pediatrics (Division of Infectious Diseases) Hospital for Sick Children, Toronto, Ontario, Canada
Coronaviruses

Samra S. Blanchard, MD
Associate Professor of Pediatrics, Division of Pediatric Gastroenterology, University of Maryland School of Medicine, Baltimore, Maryland
Peptic Ulcer Disease in Children

Ronald Blanton, MD, MSc
Center for Global Health and Disease, Case Western Reserve Institute; Attending Physician, Wade Park Veterans' Administration Hospital, Cleveland, Ohio
Adult Tapeworm Infections; Cysticercosis; Echinococcosis *(Echinococcus Granulosus* and *Echinococcus Multilocularis)*

Archie Bleyer, MD
Professor and Mosbacher Chair of Pediatrics, University of Texas; Director, Community Clinical Oncology Program, University of Texas M.D. Anderson Cancer Center, Houston, Texas
Principles of Diagnosis; Principles of Treatment; The Leukemias

Lynell Boamah, MD
Fellow, Pediatric Gastroenterology, Hepatology, and Nutrition, Cincinnati Children's Hospital Medical Center, Cincinnati, Ohio
Manifestations of Liver Disease

Steven R. Boas, MD
Associate Professor of Pediatrics, Northwestern University, Feinberg School of Medicine; Pediatric Pulmonologist, Evanston Hospital, Evanston, Illinois, Children's Memorial Hospital, Chicago, Illinois
Emphysema and Overinflation; α1-Antitrypsin Deficiency and Emphysema; Other Distal Airway Diseases; Skeketal Diseases Influencing Pulmonary Function

Thomas F. Boat, MD
Professor and Chair, Department of Pediatrics, University of Cincinnati College of Medicine; Chair, Department of Pediatrics, Director, Cincinnati Children's Research Foundation, Cincinnati Children's Hospital Medical Center, Cincinnati, Ohio
Cystic Fibrosis; Chronic or Recurrent Respiratory Symptoms

Mark Boguniewicz, MD
Professor, Division of Pediatric Allergy-Immunology, Department of Pediatrics, National Jewish Medical and Research Center and University of Colorado School of Medicine, Denver, Colorado
Ocular Allergies; Adverse Reactions to Drugs

Robert A. Bonomo, MD
Associate Professor of Medicine, Pharmacology, and Molecular Biology and Microbiology, Case Western Reserve School of Medicine; Section Chief, Infectious Diseases, Louis Stokes Cleveland Veterans' Affairs Medical Center, Cleveland, Ohio
African Trypanosomiasis (Sleeping Sickness, *Trypanosoma Brucei* complex); American Trypanosomiasis (Chagas Disease, *Trypanosoma Cruzi*)

Neil W. Boris, MD
Associate Professor, Community Health Sciences, Tulane University School of Public Health and Tropical Medicine; Associate Professor of Psychiatry and Neurology, Tulane University Health Sciences Center, New Orleans, Louisiana
Assessment and Interviewing; Psychologic Treatment of Children and Adolescents; Psychosomatic Illness; Vegetative Disorders; Habit and Tic Disorders; Anxiety Disorders; Mood Disorders; Suicide and Attempted Suicide; Disruptive Behavioral Disorders; Pervasive Developmental Disorders and Childhood Psychosis

Christopher M. Borrillo, MD
Assistant Professor of Child and Adolescent Psychiatry, Tulane University School of Medicine; Southeast Louisiana Hospital, Youth Services, Mandeville, Louisiana, Jefferson Parish Human Services Authority, Division of Child and Family Services, Metairie, Louisiana
Mood Disorders

Laurence A. Boxer, MD
Professor and Director, Division of Pediatric Hematology/Oncology, Vice-Chair, Department of Pediatrics, Henry and Mala Dorfman Family Professor in Pediatric Hematology/Oncology, University of Michigan; Director, Pediatric Hematology/Oncology, C.S. Mott Children's Hospital, Ann Arbor, Michigan
Neutrophils; Eosinophils; Disorders of Phagocyte Function; Leukopenia; Leukocytosis

Mary Brigid Bradley, MD
Associate Professor of Clinic Pediatrics, Columbia University; Assistant Attending Pediatrician, Morgan Stanley Children's Hospital of New York Presbyterian, New York, New York
Lymphoma

David Branski, MD
Professor of Pediatrics, Hebrew University Medical School; Professor and Chair of Pediatric Departments, Hadassah University Hospitals, Jerusalem, Israel
Probiotics in Gastrointestinal Disorders

David T. Breault, MD, PhD
Instructor in Pediatrics, Harvard Medical School; Assistant in Medicine, Division of Endocrinology, Children's Hospital Boston, Boston, Massachusetts
Diabetes Insipidus; Other Abnormalities of Arginine Vasopressin Metabolism and Action

W. Ted Brown, MD, PhD
Chair, Department of Human Genetics, Director, George A. Jervis Clinic; Director, New York State Institute for Basic Research in Developmental Disabilities, Staten Island, New York
Progeria

Rebecca H. Buckley, MD
J. Buren Sidbury Professor of Pediatrics, Professor of Immunology, Duke University Medical Center, Durham, North Carolina
Evaluation of Suspected Immunodeficiency; T Lymphocytes, B Lymphocytes, and Natural Killer Cells; Primary Defects of Antibody Production; Treatment of B-Cell Defects; Primary Defects of Cellular Immunity; Primary Combined Antibody and Cellular Immunodeficiencies

Cynthia Budek, MS
Pediatric Nurse Practitioner, Children's Memorial Hospital, Chicago, Illinois
Chronic Severe Respiratory Insufficiency

E. Stephen Buescher, MD
Professor of Pediatrics, Eastern Virginia Medical School, Norfolk, Virginia
Diphtheria *(Corynebacterium diphtheriae)*

Karen Burns, MD, MS
Assistant Professor of Clinical Pediatrics, Department of Hematology and Oncology, Cincinnati Children's Hospital Medical Center, Cincinnati, Ohio
Primary Polycythemia (Polycythemia Rubra Vera); Secondary Polycythemia

Mitchell S. Cairo
Professor of Pediatric Medicine and Pathology, Columbia University; Division Head, Pediatrics, Morgan Stanley Children's Hospital of New York Presbyterian, New York, New York
Lymphoma

Bruce M. Camitta, MD
Rebecca Jean Slye Professor of Pediatrics, Medical College of Wisconsin; Director, Midwest Children's Cancer Center, Pediatrics (Hematology and Oncology), Children's Hospital of Wisconsin, Milwaukee, Wisconsin
Primary Polycythemia (Polycythemia Rubra Vara); Secondary Polycythemia; Anatomy and Function of the Spleen; Splenomegaly; Hyposplenism, Splenic Trauma, and Splenectomy; Anatomy and Function of the Lymphatic System; Abnormalities of Lymphatic Vessels; Lymphadenopathy

Rebecca G. Carey, MD
Fellow, Pediatric Gastroenterology, Hepatology and Nutrition, University of Cincinnati; Fellow, Pediatric Gastroenterology, Hepatology and Nutrition, Cincinnati Children's Hospital Medical Center, Cincinnati, Ohio
Metabolic Diseases of the Liver; Mitochondrial Hepatopathies

Andrew J. Carroll, III, PhD
Professor of Genetics, University of Alabama at Birmingham, Birmingham, Alabama
Cytogenetics

James T. Cassidy, MD
Professor Emeritus, Child Health—Pediatric Rheumatology, University of Missouri Health Care, Columbia, Missouri
Treatment of Rheumatic Diseases; Juvenile Rheumatoid Arthritis; Reactive Arthritis

Ellen Gould Chadwick, MD
Professor of Pediatrics, Northwestern University, Feinberg School of Medicine; Associate Director, Section of Pediatric, Adolescent, and Maternal HIV Infection, Division of Infectious Diseases, Children's Memorial Hospital, Chicago, Illinois
Acquired Immunodeficiency Syndrome (Human Immunodeficiency Virus)

Sharon F. Chen, MD, MS
Department of Pediatric Infectious Diseases, Stanford University; Attending Physician, Department of Pediatric Infectious Diseases, Lucile Packard Children's Hospital, Stanford University Medical Center, Stanford, California
Principles of Antiviral Therapy; Principles of Antiparasitic Therapy

Yuan-Tsong Chen, MD, PhD
Professor of Pediatrics and Genetics, Duke University; Duke University Medical Center, Durham, North Carolina
Defects in Metabolism of Carbohydrates; Glycogen Storage Diseases; Defects in Galactose Metabolism; Defects in Fructose Metabolism; Defects in Intermediary Carbohydrate Metabolism Associated with Lactic Acidosis; Defects in Pentose Metabolism

Wanda L. Chenoweth, PhD, RD
Professor Emeritus, Department of Food Science and Human Nutrition, Michigan State University, East Lansing, Michigan
Vitamin B Complex Deficiency and Excess; Vitamin C Ascorbic Acid

Russell W. Chesney, MD
Le Bonheur Professor and Chair, Department of Pediatrics, University of Tennessee Health Science Center; Vice President for Academic Affairs, Le Bonheur Children's Medical Center, Memphis, Tennessee
Rickets Associated with Renal Tubular Acidosis; Bone Structure, Growth, and Hormonal Regulation; Primary Chondrodystrophy (Metaphyseal Dysplasia); Hypophosphatasia; Hyperphosphatasia; Osteoporosis

Robert D. Christensen, MD
Director of Research, Department of Neonatology, Intermountain Healthcare, Inc.; Medical Director, Department of Neonatology, Urban North Area, Intermountain Healthcare, Inc., Ogden, Utah
Development of the Hematopoietic System

Theodore J. Cieslak, MD
Clinical Professor of Pediatrics, University of Texas Health Science Center at San Antonio, San Antonio, Texas; Clinical Associate Professor of Pediatrics, Uniformed Services University of the Health Sciences, Bethesda, Maryland; Chairman, San Antonio Military Pediatric Center, Fort Sam Houston, Texas
Biologic and Chemical Terrorism

Thomas G. Cleary, MD
Professor of Pediatrics, University of Texas Medical School, Houston, Houston, Texas
Shigella; *Escherichia Coli*

Pinchas Cohen, MD
Professor of Pediatrics, David Geffen School of Medicine at University of California, Los Angeles; Chief, Endocrinology, Mattel Children's Hospital at University of California, Los Angeles
Hyperpituitarism, Tall Stature, and Overgrowth Syndromes

F. Sessions Cole, MD
Park J. White, MD, Professor of Pediatrics, Assistant Vice Chancellor for Children's Health, Washington University School of Medicine; Director, Division of Newborn Medicine, Chief Medical Officer Pediatrics, St. Louis Children's Hospital, St. Louis, Missouri
Pulmonary Alveolar Proteinosis; Inherited Disorders of Surfactant Metabolism

John L. Colombo, MD
Professor of Pediatrics, University of Nebraska College of Medicine; Chief, Pediatric Pulmonology, University of Nebraska, Omaha, Nebraska
Aspiration Syndromes; Chronic Recurrent Aspiration

Anne Comi, MD
Assistant Professor, Neurology and Pediatrics, Kennedy Krieger Institute, Johns Hopkins University School of Medicine; Faculty, Neurology and Developmental Medicine, Kennedy Krieger Institute, Baltimore, Maryland
Acute Stroke Syndromes

Tania Condurache, MD
Resident in Pediatrics, University of Louisville School of Medicine, Louisville, Kentucky
Poisonings

Arnold Coran, MD
Professor of Surgery, Section of Pediatric Surgery, University of Michigan, Ann Arbor, Michigan
Diaphragmatic Hernia; Foramen of Morgagni Hernia; Paraesophageal Hernia; Eventration

Roger Cornwall, MD
Assistant Professor of Orthopaedic Surgery, University of Pennsylvania School of Medicine; Attending Pediatric Hand and Upper Extremity Surgeon, Children's Hospital of Philadelphia, Philadelphia, Pennsylvania
The Upper Limb

Ronina A. Covar, MD
Assistant Professor of Pediatrics, University of Colorado Health Sciences Center; Assistant Professor of Pediatrics, National Jewish Medical and Research Center, Denver, Colorado
Childhood Asthma

Kenneth L. Cox, MD
Professor, Pediatrics; Division Chief, Division of Pediatric Gastroenterology, Hepatology, and Nutrition, Lucile Salter Packard Children's Hospital, Palo Alto, California
Liver Transplantation

Susan E. Crawford, MD
Research Associate, Pediatric Infectious Diseases, University of Chicago; Clinical Instructor, General Academic Pediatrics, Children's Memorial Hospital, Chicago, Illinois
Haemophilus Influenzae

James E. Crowe, Jr., MD
Ingraham Professor of Pediatrics, Microbiology, and Immunology, Vanderbilt University Medical Center, Nashville, Tennessee
Human Metapneumovirus

Steven J. Czinn, MD
Professor and Chair of Pediatrics, University of Maryland School of Medicine; Chief of Pediatrics, University of Maryland Hospital for Children, Baltimore, Maryland
Peptic Ulcer Disease in Children

Richard Dalton, MD
Professor of Child/Adolescent Psychiatry, Tulane University Health Sciences Center; Clinical Professor of Pediatrics, Tulane University Health Sciences Center, New Orleans, Louisiana
The Development of Sexual Behavior; Psychologic Treatment of Children and Adolescents; Psychosomatic Illness; Vegetative Disorders; Habit and Tic Disorders; Anxiety Disorders; Suicide and Attempted Suicide; Disruptive Behavioral Disorders; Pervasive Developmental Disorders and Childhood Psychosis

Jorge H. Daruna, PhD
LA-YES—Louisiana Youth Enhanced Services, Office of Mental Health, State of Louisiana
Psychosomatic Illness

Toni Darville, MD
Professor of Pediatrics and Microbiology/Immunology, University of Arkansas for Medical Sciences, Little Rock, Arkansas
Neisseria Gonorrhoeae (Gonococcus)

Robert S. Daum, MD
Professor of Pediatrics, University of Chicago, Chicago, Illinois
Haemophilus Influenzae

Richard S. Davidson, MD
Associate Professor of Orthopaedic Surgery, University of Pennsylvania School of Medicine; Associate Professor of Orthopaedic Surgery, Children's Hospital of Philadelphia, Philadelphia, Pennsylvania
The Foot and Toes

Ira D. Davis, MD, MS
Associate Professor of Pediatrics, Case Western Reserve University School of Medicine; Chief, Division of Pediatric Nephrology, Rainbow Babies and Children's Hospital, Cleveland Ohio
Introduction to Glomerular Diseases; Clinical Evaluation of the Child with Hematuria; Isolated Glomerular Disease with Recurrent Gross Hematuria; Glomerulonephritis Associated with Infections; Membranous Glomerulopathy (Glomerulonephritis); Membranoproliferative (Mesagniocapillary) Glomerulonephritis; Glomerulonephritis Associated with Systemic Lupus Erythematosus; Henoch-Schönlein Purpura Nephritis; Rapidly Progressive (Crescentic) Glomerulonephritis; Goodpasture Disease; Hemolytic-Uremic Syndrome; Upper Urinary Tract Causes of Hematuria; Hematologic Diseases Causing Hematuria; Anatomic Abnormalities Associated with Hematuria; Lower Urinary Tract Causes of Hematuria

Peter S. Dayan, MD
Associate Professor of Clinical Pediatrics, Columbia University College of Physicians and Surgeons; Associate Director, Division of Pediatric Emergency Medicine, The Children's Hospital of New York Presbyterian, New York, New York
Acute Care of the Multiple Trauma Victim

Michael R. DeBaun, MD, MPH
Associate Professor of Pediatrics, Biostatistics, and Neurology, Washington University School of Medicine; Pediatrics, St. Louis Children's Hospital, St. Louis, Missouri
Hemoglobinopathies

Jacqueline L. Deen, MD, MSc
Research Scientist, International Vaccine Institute, Seoul, Korea
Cholera *(Vibrio Cholerae)*

Katherine MacRae Dell, MD
Assistant Professor of Pediatrics, Case Western Reserve University School of Medicine; Attending Pediatric Nephrologist, Rainbow Babies and Children's Hospital, Cleveland, Ohio
Tubular Function; Renal Tubular Acidosis; Nephrogenic Diabetes Insipidus; Bartter/Gitelman Syndromes and Other Inherited Tubular Transport Abnormalities; Tubulointerstitial Nephritis

Arlene E. Dent
Instructor, Center for Global Health and Diseases, Case Western Reserve University; Instructor, Department of Pediatrics, Pediatric Infectious Diseases and Rheumatology Division, Rainbow Babies and Children's Hospital, Cleveland, Ohio
Ascariasis *(Ascaris Lumbricoides)*; Trichuriasis *(Trichuris Trichiura)*; Enterobiasis *(Enterobius Vermicularis)*; Strongyloidiasis *(Strongyloides Stercoralis)*; Lymphatic Filariasis *(Brugia Malayi, Brugia Timori, Wuchereria bancrofti)*; Other Tissue Nematodes; *Toxocariasis* (Visceral and Ocular Larva Migrans); *Trichinosis (Trichinella Spiralis)*

Marie Descartes, MD
Associate Professor of Pediatrics and Genetics, University of Alabama, at Birmingham, Birmingham, Alabama
Cytogenetics

Robert Desnick, MD, PhD
Professor and Chairman of Human Genetics, Mount Sinai School of Medicine; Attending Physician, Pediatrics, Mount Sinai Hospital, New York, New York
Lipidoses; Mucolipidoses; Disorders of Glycoprotein Degradation and Structure; The Porphyrias

Joseph DiCarlo, MD
Assistant Professor, Department of Pediatrics, Stanford University, Palo Alto, California
Scoring Systems and Predictors of Mortality; Nutritional Stabilization

Angelo M. DiGeorge, MD
Emeritus Professor of Pediatrics, Temple University School of Medicine, Philadelphia, Pennsylvania
Hormones and Peptides of Calcium Homeostasis and Bone Metabolism; Hypoparathyroidism; Pseudohypoparathyroidism (Albright Hereditary Osteodystrophy); Hyperparathyroidism

Mary K. Donovan, RN, MS, PNP
Manager of Nurse Practitioners, Care Coordination, and Outpatient Department, Shriners Burns Hospital, Boston, Massachusetts
Burn Injuries; Cold Injuries

John P. Dormans, MD, FACS
Professor of Orthopaedic Surgery, University of Pennsylvania School of Medicine; Chief, Division of Orthopaedic Surgery, Children's Hospital of Philadelphia, Philadelphia, Pennsylvania
The Hip; The Spine; The Neck

M. Denise Dowd, MD, MPH
Professor, Department of Pediatrics, University of Missouri–Kansas City; Chief, Section of Injury Prevention, The Children's Mercy Hospital, Kansas City, Missouri
Emergency Medical Services for Children

Daniel A. Doyle, MD
Assistant Professor of Pediatrics, Thomas Jefferson University, Philadelphia, Pennsylvania; Staff, Endocrinology Division, A.I. Dupont Hospital for Children, Wilmington, Delaware
Hormones and Peptides of Calcium Homeostasis and Bone Metabolism; Hypoparathyroidism; Pseudohypoparathyroidism (Albright Hereditary Osteodystrophy); Hyperparathyroidism

Stephen Dreskin, MD, PhD
Professor of Medicine, Division of Allergy and Immunology, University of Colorado Health Sciences Center, Denver, Colorado; Director, Allergy, Immunology, and Rheumatology Practices, University of Colorado Hospital, Aurora, Colorado
Uticaria (Hives) and Angioderma

Denis S. Drummond, MD
Professor Emeritus, University of Pennsylvania School of Medicine; Emeritus Chief of Pediatric Orthopaedic Surgery, Children's Hospital of Philadelphia, Philadelphia, Pennsylvania
The Neck; Arthrogryposis

Anne M. Dubin, MD
Associate Professor of Pediatrics, Stanford University, Stanford, California; Director of Pediatric Electrophysiology Laboratory, Pediatrics Cardiology, Lucile Salter Packard Children's Hospital, Palo Alto, California
Disturbances of the Rate and Rhythm of the Heart; Sudden Death

Golde Dudell, MD
Associate Professor of Pediatrics, Emory University; Attending Physician, Children's Healthcare at Atlanta, Emory Cranford Long, Grady Memorial Hospital, Atlanta, Georgia
Respiratory Tract Disorders

J. Stephen Dumler, MD
Professor, Department of Pathology, Division of Medical Microbiology, Johns Hopkins University School of Medicine, Professor, Department of Molecular Microbiology and Immunology, Johns Hopkins University Bloomberg School of Public Health; Associate Director, Division of Medical Microbiology, Director, Parasitology Laboratory, Department of Pathology, Division of Medical Microbiology, Johns Hopkins Hospital, Baltimore, Maryland
Spotted Fever Group *Rickettsioses;* Scrub Typhus *(Orientia Tsutsugamushi);* Typhus Group Rickettsioses; Ehrlichioses; Q Fever *(Coxiella Burnetii)*

Paula M. Duncan, MD
Professor of Pediatrics, University of Vermont College of Medicine, Burlington, Vermont
Maximizing Children's Health: Screening, Anticipatory Guidance, and Counseling

Peter F. Ehrlich, MD
Associate Professor of Surgery, Section of Pediatric Surgery, University of Michigan, Ann Arbor, Michigan
Diaphragmatic Hernia; Foramen of Morgagni Hernia; Paraesophageal Hernia; Eventration

Jack S. Elder, MD
Carter Kissell Professor of Urology, Professor of Pediatrics, Vice Chairman, Department of Urology, Case Western Reserve University School of Medicine; Director of Pediatric Urology, Rainbow Babies and Children's Hospital, Cleveland, Ohio
Congenital Anomalies and Dysgenesis of the Kidneys; Urinary Tract Infections; Vesicoureteral Reflux; Obstructions of the Urinary Tract; Anomalies of the Bladder; Neuropathic Bladder; Voiding Dysfunction; Anomalies of the Penis and Urethra; Disorders and Anomalies of the Scrotal Contents; Trauma to the Genitourinary Tract; Urinary Lithiasis

Dianne S. Elfenbein, MD
Associate Professor of Pediatrics, Division of Adolescent Medicine, University of Massachusetts Medical School; Medical Director, Teen-Tot Program, University of Massachusetts Memorial Health Care, Worcester, Massachusetts
Adolescent Pregnancy

Maria Enrione, MD
Assistant Professor, Neoucom; Pediatric Intensivist, Children's Hospital Medical Center of Akron, Akron, Ohio
Sepsis, Septic Shock, and Systemic Inflammatory Response Syndrome

Susan Feigelman, MD
Associate Professor of Pediatrics, University of Maryland School of Medicine, Baltimore, Maryland
Overview and Assessment of Variability; Assessment of Fetal Growth and Development; The First Year; The Second Year; The Preschool Years; Middle Childhood

Marianne E. Felice, MD
Professor and Chair, Department of Pediatrics, University of Massachusetts Medical School; Physician-in-Chief, University of Massachusetts Memorial Children's Medical Center, Worcester, Massachusetts
Adolescent Pregnancy; Adolescent Rape

Eric I. Felner, MD
Assistant Professor of Pediatrics, Department of Pediatrics, Division of Endocrindogy, Emory University School of Medicine, Atlanta, Georgia
Hormones of the Hypothalamus and Pituitary; Hypopituitarism

Patricia Ferrieri, MD
Chairman's Fund Endowed Chair in Laboratory Medicine and Pathology; Professor, Department of Pediatrics, Division of Infectious Diseases, University of Minnesota Medical School; Director, Clinical Microbiology Laboratory, University of Minnesota Medical Center, Fairview, Minneapolis, Minnesota
Principles of Antifungal Therapy

Jonathan D. Finder, MD
Associate Professor of Pediatrics, University of Pittsburgh School of Medicine; Attending Pulmonologist, Children's Hospital of Pittsburgh, Pittsburgh, Pennsylvania
Congenital Disorders of the Lung

Margaret C. Fisher, MD
Professor of Pediatrics, Drexel University College of Medicine, Philadelphia, Pennsylvania; Medical Director, The Children's Hospital at Monmouth Medical Center, Long Branch, New Jersey
Infection Control and Prophylaxis; Pseudomembranous Colitis *(Clostridium Difficile);* Other Anaerobic Infections

Emily Fitzpatrick, MD
Pediatric Resident, Department of Pediatrics, Eastern Virginia Medical School; Pediatric Resident, Department of Pediatrics, Children's Hospital of the Kings Daughters, Norfolk, Virginia
Marfan Syndrome

David M. Fleece, MD
Assistant Professor of Pediatrics, Temple University School of Medicine, Philadelphia, Pennsylvania
Blastomycosis *(Blastomyces Dermatitidis);* Sporotrichosis *(Sporothrix Scherckii)*

Robert G. Flood, MD
Director, Pediatric Emergency Medicine; Assistant Professor, Department of Pediatrics, Temple University School of Medicine/Temple University Children's Medical Center, Philadelphia, Pennsylvania
Eryptococcus Neoformans

Patricia M. Flynn, MD
Professor of Pediatrics and Preventive Medicine, University of Tennessee Health Science Center; Member, Department of Infectious Diseases, St. Jude Children's Research Hospital, Memphis, Tennessee
Infection Associated with Medical Devices; *Cryptosporidium, Isospora, Cyclospora,* and *Microsporidia*

Joel A. Forman, MD
Associate Professor of Pediatrics, Mount Sinai School of Medicine; Vice Chair for Medical Education, Department of Pediatrics, Mount Sinai Hospital, New York, New York
Chemical Pollutants

Norman Fost MD, MPH
Professor, Director, Program in Bioethics, Department of Pediatrics, Medical History and Bioethics, University of Wisconsin Medical School; Pediatrician, University of Wisconsin Hospital and Clinics, Madison, Wisconsin

Lorry R. Frankel, MD, MBA
Associate Professor, Pediatrics, Stanford University School of Medicine; Director, Critical Care Services, Lucile Salter Packard Children's Hospital, Palo Alto, California
Organ Transplantation; Interfacility Transfer of the Critically Ill Infant and Child; Monitoring Techniques for the Critically Ill Infant and Child; Scoring Systems and Predictors of Mortality; Pediatric Emergencies and Resuscitation; Neurologic Emergencies and Stabiliization; Brain Death; Shock; Respiratory Distress and Failure; Mechanical Ventilation; Long-Term Mechanical Ventilation

Melvin H. Freedman, MD, FRCPC, FAAP
Professor Emeritus of Pediatrics, University of Toronto Faculty of Medicine; Senior Scientist Emeritus, Research Institute, Hospital for Sick Children, Toronto, Ontario, Canada
The Constitutional Pancytopenias

Madelyn Freundlich, MSW, MPH, JD, LL.M
Excal Consulting Partners LLC, New York, New York
Adoption; Foster Care

Jared E. Friedman, BA
Clinical Research Coordinator, Division of Orthopaedic Surgery, The Children's Hospital of Philadelphia, Philadelphia, Pennsylvania
The Hip

Peter Gal, PharmD, BCPS, FCCP, FASHP
Clinical Professor, Division of Pharmacotherapy and Experimental Therapeutics, School of Pharmacy, University of North Carolina, Chapel Hill, Chapel Hill, North Carolina; Neonatal Pharmacotherapy Specialist, Department of Neonatology, Women's Hospital, Moses Cone Health System, Greensboro, North Carolina; Director, Graduate Pharmacy Education, Greensboro Area Health Education Center, Greensboro, North Carolina
Principles of Drug Therapy; Poisonings

Paula Gardiner, MD, MPH
Clinical Research Fellow, Division for Research and Education in Complementary and Integrative Medical Therapies, Osher Institute, Harvard Medical School, Boston Massachusetts
Herbal Medicines

Luigi Garibaldi, MD
Professor of Pediatrics, Division of Pediatric Endocrinology, University of Pittsburgh School of Medicine; Clinical Director, Division of Pediatric Endocrinology, Children's Hospital of Pediatric Endocrinology, Children's Hospital of Pittsburgh, Pittsburgh, Pennsylvania
Physiology of Puberty; Disorders of Pubertal Development

Abraham Gedalia, MD
Professor of Pediatrics and Head, Division of Pediatric Rheumatology, Louisiana State University Health Sciences Center; Head, Department of Rheumatology, Children's Hospital, New Orleans, Louisiana
Behçet Disease; Sjögren Syndrome; Hereditary Periodic Fever Syndromes; Amyloidosis

Michael A. Gerber, MD
Professor of Pediatrics, University of Cincinnati College of Medicine; Attending Physician, Division of Infectious Disease, Cincinnati Children's Hospital Medical Center, Cincinnati, Ohio
Group A *Streptococcus;* Non-Group A or B *Streptococci*

Fayez K. Ghishan, MD
Horace W. Steele Endowed Chair in Pediatric Research, Head, Department of Pediatrics, Director, Steele Children's Research Center, University of Arizona College of Medicine; Faculty Member, Department of Pediatrics, The University of Arizona College of Medicine, Tucson, Arizona
Chronic Diarrhea

Purushottam A. Gholve, MD, MBMS, MRCS
Research Fellow, The Children's Hospital of Philadelphia, Philadelphia, Pennsylvania
Torsional and Angular Deformities; Leg Length Discrepancy; Common Fractures

Francis Gigliotti, MD
Professor of Pediatrics, Microbiology, and Immunology, Chief, Pediatric Infectious Diseases, Associate Chair for Academic Affairs, Department of Pediatrics, University of Rochester School of Medicine and Dentistry; Attending Physician, Pediatrics, Golisano Children's Hospital at Strong, Rochester, New York
Pneumocystis Carinii (Pneumocystis Jirovecii)

William S. Gilliam, PhD
Assistant Professor of Child Psychiatry and Psychology, Child Study Center, Yale University School of Medicine, Director, Edward Zigler Center in Child Development and Social Policy, Yale University; Yale-New Haven Children's Hospital, New Haven, Connecticut
Child Care

Charles M. Ginsburg, MD
Marilyn R. Corrigan Distinguished Chair of Pediatric Research, Associate Dean for Academic Affairs, University of Texas Southwestern Medical Center at Dallas, Dallas, Texas
Animal and Human Bites

Bertil Glader, MD, PhD
Professor of Pediatrics and Pathology, Stanford University School of Medicine, Palo Alto, California; Division of Hematology-Oncology, Lucile Salter Packard Children's Hospital, Palo Alto, California
The Anemias; Congenital Hypoplastic Anemia (Diamond-Blackfan Anemia); Pearson Marrow-Pancreas Syndrome; Acquired Pure Red Blood Cell Anemias; Anemia of Chronic Disease and Renal Disease; Congenital Dyserythropoietic Anemias; Physiologic Anemia of Infancy; Megaloblastic Anemias; Iron Deficiency Anemia; Other Microcytic Anemias

Frances Page Glascoe, PhD
Adjunct Professor of Pediatrics, Vanderbilt University, Nashville, Tennessee
Developmental Screening and Surveillance

Mary Margaret Gleason, MD
Clinical Assistant Professor, Brown Medical School, Providence Rhode Island; Clinical Assistant Professor, Tulane University School of Medicine, New Orleans, Louisiana
Assessment and Interviewing; Habit and Tic Disorders

Donald Goldman, MD
Professor of Pediatrics, Children's Hospital, Harvard Medical School; Senior Associate in Infectious Diseases, Children's Hospital Boston, Boston, Massachusetts
Diagnostic Microbiology

Denise M. Goodman, MD
Associate Professor, Pediatric Critical Care Medicine, Northwestern University, Feinberg School of Medicine;

Attending Physician, Pediatric Intensive Care Unit, Children's Memorial Hospital, Chicago, Illinois
Wheezing in Infants: Bronchiolotis; Bronchitis

David Gozal, MD
Children's Foundation Chair of Pediatric Research, Professor of Pediatrics, Pharmacology and Toxicology, Psychology and Brain Sciences, University of Louisville; Director, Rosair Children's Hospital Sleep Medicine and Apnea Center, Louisville, Kentucky
Neuromuscular Diseases with Respiratory Dysfunction

Michael Green, MD, MPH
Professor of Pediatrics and Surgery, University of Pittsburgh School of Medicine; Division of Infectious Diseases, Children's Hospital of Pittsburgh, Pittsburgh, Pennsylvania
Infections in Immunocompromised Persons

Thomas P. Green, MD
Professor and Chairman of Pediatrics, Northwestern University, Feinberg School of Medicine; Children's Memorial Hospital, Chicago, Illinois
Diagnostic Approach to Respiratory Disease; Chronic or Recurrent Respiratory Symptoms; Pulmonary Edema

Larry A. Greenbaum, MD, PhD
Director, Division of Pediatric Nephrology, Emory University School of Medicine; Medical Director of Dialysis, Children's Healthcare of Atlanta, Atlanta, Georgia
Rickets and Hypervitaminosis D; Vitamin E Deficiency; Vitamin K Deficiency; Micronutrient Mineral Deficiencies; Electrolyte and Acid-Base Disorders; Maintenance and Replacement Therapy; Deficit Therapy; Fluids and Electrolyte Treatment of Specific Disorders

David Grossman, MD, MPH
Professor of Pediatrics, University of Washington; Director, Harborview Injury Prevention and Research Center, Seattle, Washington
Injury Control

Gabriel G. Haddad, MD
Professor of Pediatrics and Neuroscience, Chairman, Department of Pediatrics, University of California, San Diego; Physician-in-Chief, Rady Children's Hospital of San Diego, San Diego, California
Congenital Central Hypoventilation Syndrome (Ondine Curse); Diagnostic Approach to Respiratory Disease; Primary Ciliary Dyskinesia (Immotile Cilia Syndrome)

Joseph Haddad, Jr., MD
Professor and Vice Chairman, Otolaryngology/Head and Neck Surgery, Columbia University College of Physicians and Surgeons; Lawrence Savetsky Chair and Director, Pediatric Otolaryngology/Head and Neck Surgery, Morgan Stanley Children's Hospital of New York, New York
Congenital Disorders of the Nose; Acquired Disorders of the Nose; General Considerations and Evaluation; Nasal Polyps; Hearing Loss; Congenital Malformations; External Otitis (Otitis Externa); The Inner Ear and Diseases of the Bony Labyrinth; Traumatic Injuries of the Ear and Temporal Bone; Tumors of the Ear and Temporal Bone

Joseph F. Hagan, Jr., MD, FAAP
Clinical Professor of Pediatrics, University of Vermont College of Medicine; Attending Physician in Pediatrics, Fletcher Allen Health Care, Burlington, Vermont
Maximizing Children's Health: Screening, Anticipatory Guidance, and Counseling

Scott B. Halstead, MD
Adjunct Professor, Preventive Medicine and Biometrics, Uniformed Services University of the Health Sciences, Bethesda, Maryland; Director, Research Department, Pediatric Dengue Vaccine Initiative, International Vaccine Institute, Seoul, Korea
Arboviral Encephalitis in North America; Arboviral Encephalitis Outside North America; Dengue Fever and Dengue Hemorrhagic Fever; Yellow Fever; Other Viral Hemorrhagic Fevers; Hantavirus Pulmonary Syndrome

Margaret R. Hammerschlag, MD
Professor of Pediatrics and Medicine; Director, Division of Pediatric Infectious Diseases, State University of New York Downstate Medical Center, Brooklyn, New York
Chlamydophila Pneumoniae; Chlamydia Trachomatis; Psittarosis *(Chlamydophila Psittaci)*

Aaron Hamvas, MD
Professor of Pediatrics, Washington University School of Medicine; Medical Director, Neonatal Intensive Care Unit, St. Louis Children's Hospital, St. Louis, Missouri
Pulmonary Alveolar Proteinosis; Inherited Disorders of Surfactant Metabolism

James C. Harris, MD
Professor of Psychiatry and Behavioral Sciences, Pediatrics, and Mental Hygiene, Johns Hopkins University School of Medicine; Director, Developmental Neuropsychiatry, Johns Hopkins Hospital, Baltimore, Maryland
Disorders of Purine and Pyrimidine Metabolism

David B. Haslam, MD
Associate Professor, Pediatrics and Molecular Microbiology, Washington University School of Medicine; Attending Physician, Pediatric Infectious Diseases, St. Louis Children's Hospital, St. Louis, Missouri
Enterococcus

Robert H.A. Haslam, MD, FAAP, FRCP(C)
Emeritus Professor and Chairman, Department of Pediatrics and Professor of Medicine (Neurology), University of Toronto; Emeritus Pediatrician-in-Chief, Hospital for Sick Children, Toronto, Canada
Neurologic Evaluation; Headaches; Neurocutaneous Syndromes; Brain Abscess; Pseudotumor Cerebri; Spinal Cord Disorders

Fern R. Hauck, MD, MS
Associate Professor of Family Medicine and Public Health Sciences, University of Virginia School of Medicine; Attending Physician, Family Medicine, University of Virginia Health System, Charlottesville, Virginia
Sudden Infant Death Syndrome

Gregory F. Hayden, MD
Professor of Pediatrics, University of Virginia School of Medicine; Attending Pediatrician, University of Virginia Children's Hospital, Charlottesville, Virginia
The Common Cold; Acute Pharyngitis

Jacqueline T. Hecht, PhD
Professor of Pediatrics, Vice-Chair for Research, Department of Pediatrics, University of Texas-Houston; Active Scientific Staff, Clinical Genetics Consultant, Houston Unit, Shriners Hospital for Children, Houston, Texas
General Considerations; Disorders of Involving Cartilage Matrix Proteins; Disorders Involving Transmembrane Receptors; Disorders Involving Ion Transporter; Disorders Involving Transcription Factors; Disorders Involving Defective Bone Resorption; Disorders for Which Defects Are Poorly Understood or Unknown

Sabrina M. Heidemann, MD
Associate Professor, Pediatrics, Wayne State University School of Medicine; Pediatric Intensivist, Children's Hospital of Michigan, Detroit, Michigan
Respiratory Pathophysiology and Regulation

William C. Heird, MD
Professor of Pediatrics, Baylor College of Medicine, Houston, Texas
Nutritional Needs; The Feeding of Infants and Children; Food Insecurity, Hunger, and Undernutrition

J. Owen Hendley, MD
Professor of Pediatrics, University of Virginia School of Medicine, Charlottesville, Virginia
Sinusitis; Retropharyngeal Abscess, Lateral Pharyngeal (Parapharyngeal) Abscess, and Peritonsillar Cellulitis/Abscess

Fred M. Henretig, MD
Professor of Pediatrics and Emergency Medicine, University of Pennsylvania School of Medicine; Director, Section of Clinical Toxicology, Division of Emergency Medicine, The Children's Hospital of Philadelphia, Philadelphia, Pennsylvania
Biologic and Chemical Terrorism

Gloria P. Heresi, MD
Associate Professor of Pediatrics, Pediatric Infectious Diseases Division, University of Texas Health Science Center at Houston; Pediatrics, Memorial Herrmann Children's Hospital, Houston, Texas
Campylobacter; Yersinia; Aeromonas and Plesiomonas

Cynthia E. Herzog, MD
Associate Professor of Pediatrics, University of Texas M.D. Anderson Cancer Center, Houston, Texas
Retinoblastoma; Gonadal and Germ Cell Neoplasms; Neoplasms of the Liver; Benign Vascular Tumors; Rare Tumors

Lauren D. Holinger, MD
Professor, Otolaryngology—Head and Neck Surgery, Northwestern University Feinberg School of Medicine; Head, Division of Pediatric Otolaryngology, Children's Memorial Hospital, Chicago, Illinois
Congenital Anomalies of the Larynx, Trachea, and Bronchi; Foreign Bodies of the Airway; Laryngotracheal Stenosis, Subglottic Stenosis; Neoplasms of the Larynx, Trachea, and Bronchi

Steve Holve, MD
Clinical Instructor, Johns Hopkins University School of Medicine, Baltimore, Maryland; Chief of Pediatrics, Tuba City Regional Healthcare Corporation, Tuba City, Arizona
Envenomations

Jeffrey D. Hord, MD
Associate Professor of Pediatrics, Northeastern Ohio Universities College of Medicine, Rootstown, Ohio; Director, Pediatric Hematology/Oncology, Children's Hospital Medical Center of Akron, Akron, Ohio
The Acquired Pancytopenias

B. David Horn, MD
Assistant Professor, Orthopaedic Surgery, University of Pennsylvania; Division of Orthopaedic Surgery, The Children's Hospital of Philadelphia, Philadelphia, Pennsylvania
The Hip

William A. Horton, MD
Professor of Molecular and Medical Genetics, Oregon Health and Science University; Director of Research, Shriners Hospitals for Children, Portland, Oregon
General Considerations; Disorders Involving Cartilage Matrix Proteins; Disorders Involving Transmembrane Receptors; Disorders Involving Ion Transporter; Disorders Involving Transcription Factors; Disorders Involving Defective Bone Resorption; Disorders for Which Defects Are Poorly Understood or Unknown

Harish S. Hosalkar, MD, MBMS(Orth), FCPS(Orth), DNB(Orth)
Clinical Instructor, Department of Orthopaedic Surgery, University of Pennsylvania School of Medicine; Editor-in-Chief, University of Pennsylvania Orthopedic Journal, University of Pennsylvania School of Medicine, Philadelphia, Pennsylvania
Growth and Development, Evaluation of the Child; The Foot and Toes; Torsional and Angular Deformities; Leg Length Discrepancy; The Knee; The Hip; The Spine; The Neck; Arthrogryposis; Common Fractures

Peter J. Hotez, MD, PhD, FAAP
Walter G. Ross Professor and Chair, Department of Microbiology, Immunology and Tropical Medicine, The George Washington University; President, The Sabin Vaccine Institute, Washington, District of Columbia
Hookworms *(Necator Americanus* and *Ancylostoma)*

Michele S. Howenstine, MD
Professor of Clinical Pediatrics, Indiana University School of Medicine; Pediatric Pulmonologist, Section of Pediatric Pulmonology, James Whitcomb Riley Hospital for Children, Indiana University, Indianapolis, Indiana
Interstitial Lung Diseases

Vicki Huff, PhD
Associate Professor, Department of Cancer Genetics, University of Texas M.D. Anderson Cancer Center, Houston, Texas
Neoplasms of the Kidney

Denise Hug, MD
Assistant Professor, Departments of Ophthalmology and Pediatrics, University of Missouri–Kansas City School of Medicine; Children's Mercy Hospitals and Clinics, Kansas City, Missouri
Growth and Development; Examination of the Eye; Abnormalities of Refraction and Accommodation; Disorders of Vision; Abnormalities of Pupil and Iris; Disorders of Eye Movement and Alignment; Abnormalities of the Lids; Disorders of the Lacrimal System; Disorders of the Conjunctiva; Abnormalities of the Cornea; Abnormalities of the Lens; Disorders of the Uveal Tract; Disorders of the Retina and Vitreous; Abnormalities of the Optic Nerve; Childhood Glaucoma; Orbital Abnormalities; Orbital Infections; Injuries to the Eye

Carl E. Hunt, MD
Adjunct Professor of Pediatrics, Uniformed Services University of the Health Sciences; National Heart, Lung, and Blood Institute, National Institutes of Health, Bethesda, Maryland
Sudden Infant Death Syndrome

Melissa Hurwitz, MD
Assistant Professor of Pediatrics; Attending Physician, Division of Pediatric Gastroenterology, Hepatology, and Nutrition, Lucile Salter Packard Children's Hospital, Palo Alto, California
Liver Transplantation

Sunny Zaheed Hussain, MD, MRCP
Director, Division of Pediatric Gastroenterology and Nutrition, Christus-Schumpert Sutton Children's Hospital, Shreveport, Louisiana
Embryology, Anatomy, and Function of the Esophagus; Congenital Anomalies: Esophageal Atresia and Tracheoesophageal Fistula; Obstructing and Motility Disorders of the Ecophagus; Dismotility; Hiatal Hernia; Gastroesophageal Reflux Disease (GERD); Eosinophilic Esophagitis and Non-GERD Esophagitis; Esophageal Perforation

Elias S. Hyams, MD
Resident in Urology, New York University School of Medicine, New York, New York
Inflammatory Bowel Disease; Chronic Ulcerative Colitis; Crohn Disease (Regional Enteritis, Regional Ileitis, Granulomatous Colitis); Behcet Syndrome; Food Allergy (Food Hypersensitivity) and Eosinophilic Gastroenteritis; Malformations; Ascites; Peritonitis

Jeffrey S. Hyams, MD
Professor of Pediatrics, University of Connecticut School of Medicine, Farmington, Connecticut; Head, Division of Digestive Diseases, Hepatology, and Nutrition, Connecticut Children's Medial Center, Hartford, Connecticut
Inflammatory Bowel Disease; Food Allergy (Food Hypersensitivity); Malformations; Ascites; Peritonitis

Richard F. Jacobs, MD, FAAP
Horace C. Cabe Professor, Department of Pediatrics, University of Arkansas for Medical Sciences; President, Arkansas Children's Hospital Research Institute, Little Rock, Arkansas
Actinomyces; Nocardia; Tularemia *(Francisella Tularensis); Brucella*

Norman Jaffe, MD, DipPaed, DSc
Professor of Pediatrics, University of Texas; Pediatric Oncologist, University of Texas M.D. Anderson Cancer Center, Houston, Texas
Neoplasms of the Kidney

Renée R. Jenkins, MD
Professor and Chair, Department of Pediatrics and Child Health, Howard University; Adjunct Professor, Department of Pediatrics, George Washington University; Chair, Department of Pediatrics and Child Health, Howard University Hospital, Washington, District of Columbia
The Epidemiology of Adolescent Health Problems; Delivery of Health Care to Adolescents; Violent Behavior; Substance Abuse; The Breast; Menstrual Problems; Contraception; Adolescent Pregnancy; Sexually Transmitted Infections

Peter S. Jensen, MD
Ruane Professor of Child Psychiatry and Director, Center for the Advancement of Children's Mental Health, Department of Psychiatry, Columbia University, New York, New York
Attention Deficit Hyperactivity Disorder

Hal B. Jenson, MD
Professor of Pediatrics and Dean of the Western Campus of Tufts University School of Medicine; Chief Academic Officer, Baystate Health, Springfield, Massachusetts
Chronic Fatigue Syndrome; Epstein-Barr Virus; Lymphocytic Choriomeningitis Virus (LCMV); Polyomaviruses (JC Virus and BK Virus); Human T-Cell Lymphotrophic Viruses Type I and II

Chandy C. John, MD
Associate Professor of Pediatrics and Medicine, Director, Global Pediatrics Program, University of Minnesota Medical School; Attending Physician, University of Minnesota Children's Hospital, Fairview, Minneapolis, Minnesota
Health Advice for Children Traveling Internationally; Amebiasis; Giardiasis and Balantidiasis; Trichomoniasis *(Trichomonas Vaginalis)*

Charles F. Johnson, MD
Emeritus Professor of Pediatrics, The Ohio State University College of Medicine and Public Health, Columbus, Ohio
Abuse and Neglect of Children

Michael V. Johnston, MD
Departments of Neurology, Pediatrics, and Physical Medicine and Rehabilitation, Johns Hopkins University School of Medicine, Baltimore, Maryland; Chief Medical Officer, Kennedy Krieger Institute, Baltimore, Maryland
Congenital Anomalies of the Central Nervous System; Seizures in Childhood; Conditions that Mimic Seizures; Movement Disorders; Encephalopathies; Neurodegenerative Disorders of Childhood; Demyelinating Disorder of the CNS; Acute Stroke Syndromes

Richard B. Johnston, Jr., MD
Professor of Pediatrics, University of Colorado School of Medicine; Associate Dean for Research Development, University of Colorado School of Medicine; Executive Vice President for Academic Affairs, National Jewish Medical and Research Center, Denver, Colorado
Monocytes, Macrophages, and Dendritic Cells; The Complement System; Disorders of the Complement System

James F. Jones, MD
Research Medical Officer, Chronic Viral Diseases Branch, Division of Viral and Rickettsial Diseases, National Center for Zoonotic, Vectorborne, and Enteric Diseases, Coordinating Center for Infectious Diseases, Centers for Disease Control and Prevention, Atlanta, Georgia
Chronic Fatigue Syndrome

Saraswati Kache, MD
Clinical Assistant Professor of Pediatrics, Stanford University School of Medicine; Attending Physician, Pediatric Intensive Care Unit, Lucile Salter Packard Children's Hospital, Palo Alto, California
Shock; Mechanical Ventilation; Long-Term Mechanical Ventilation

Nina S. Kaddan-Lottick, MD, MSPH
Assistant Professor of Pediatrics, Yale University School of Medicine; Medical Director, HERO's Clinic for Survivors of Childhood Cancer, Yale–New Haven Hospital, New Haven, Connecticut
Epidemiology of Childhood and Adolescent Cancer

Harry J. Kallas, MD
Associate Clinical Professor, Department of Pediatrics, University of California, San Francisco at Fresno, Fresno; Chair, Pharmacy, Therapeutics, and Utilization Committee, Department of Anesthesia and Critical Care, Children's Hospital, Central California, Madera, California
Drowning and Submersion Injury

Michael Kashgarian, MD
Professor of Pathology and Molecular, Cellular, and Developmental Biology, Yale University School of Medicine; Attending Pathologist, Yale-New Haven Hospital; Director, Diagnostic Electron Microscopy, Yale-New Haven Hospital, New Haven, Connecticut
Primary Ciliary Dyskinesia (Immotile Cilia Syndrome)

Alessandra N. Kazura, MD
Assistant Professor, Department of Psychiatry and Human Behavior, Brown Medical School; Assistant Professor, Hasbro Children's Research Center, Rhode Island Hospital, Providence, Rhode Island
Psychosomatic Illness

James Kazura, MD
Professor, Center for Global Health and disease, Case Western Reserve University School of Medicine; Professor, Medicine and Pathology Departments, University Hospitals of Cleveland, Cleveland, Ohio
Ascarias *(Ascaris Lumbricoides)*; Trichuriasis *(Trichuris Trichuria)*; Enterobiasis *(Enterobius Vermicularis)* Strongyloidiasis *(Strongyloides Stercoralis)*; Lymphatic Filariasis *(Brugia Malayi, Brugia Timori,* and *Wuchereria Bancrofti)*; Other Tissue Nematodes; Toxocariasis (Visceral and Ocular Larva Migrans); Trichinosis *(Trichinella Spiralis)*

Virginia Keane, MD
Associate Professor of Pediatrics, University of Maryland School of Medicine
Assessment of Growth

Desmond P. Kelly, MB, Ch.B
GHS Professor of Clinical Pediatrics, University of South Carolina School of Medicine; Medical Director, Division of Developmental-Behavioral Pediatrics, Donald A. Gardner Center for Developing Minds; Children's Hospital, Greenville Hospital System, Greenville, South Carolina
Patterns of Development and Function in the School-Aged Child

Kathi J. Kemper, MD, MPH
Caryl J. Guth Chair for Holistic and Integrative Medicine, Professor of Pediatrics and Public Health Sciences, Wake Forest University Baptist Medical Center; Staff, Department of Pediatrics, North Carolina Baptist Hospital, Winston-Salem, North Carolina
Herbal Medicines

Eitan Kerem, MD
Professor, Department of Pediatrics, Hebrew University; Director, Department of Pediatrics, Mount Scopus Campus, Hadassah University Hospital, Jerusalem, Israel
Effect of War on Children

Joseph E. Kershner, MD, FACS, FAAP
Chief, Pediatric Otolaryngology and Academic Vice Chairman, Department of Otolaryngology and Communication Sciences, Senior Associate Dean of Clinical Affairs, Medical College of Wisconsin; Medical Director, Pediatric Otolaryngology, Children's Hospital of Wisconsin, CEO, Children's Specialty Group, Children's Hospital of Wisconsin and Medical College of Wisconsin, Milwaukee, Wisconsin
Otitis Media

Seema Khan, MBBS
Associate Professor, Department of Pediatrics, Thomas Jefferson University Medical College, Philadelphia, Pennsylvania; Department of Pediatric Gastroenterology, Alfred I. du Pont Hospital for Children, Wilmington, Delaware
Embryology, Anatomy, and Function of the Esophagus; Congenital Anomalies: Esophageal Atresia and Tracheoesophageal Fistula; Obstructing and Motility Disorders of the Esophagus; Dysmotility; Hiatal Hernia; Gastroesophageal Reflux Disease (GERD); Eosinophilic Esophagitis and Non-GERD Esophagitis; Esophageal Perforation

Leila Kheirandish, MD
Assistant Professor of Pediatrics, Division of Pediatric Sleep Medicine, University of Louisville, Kentucky
Neuromuscular Diseases with Respiratory Dysfunction

Charles H. King, MD
Center for Global Health and Diseases, Case Western Reserve University School of Medicine, Cleveland, Ohio
Schistosomiasis *(Schistosoma)*; Flukes (Liver, Lung, and Intestinal)

Stephen L. Kinsman, MD
Associate Professor of Pediatrics and Neurology, University of Maryland School of Medicine; Pediatric Neurologist, University of Maryland Hospital for Children; Consulting Neurologist, Kennedy Krieger Institute, Baltimore, Maryland
Congenital Anomalies of the Central Nervous System

Priya S. Kishnani, MD
Associate Professor of Pediatrics, Division of Medical Genetics, Duke University; Associate Professor of Pediatrics, Interim Division Chief, Division of Medical Genetics, Duke University Medical Center, Durham, North Carolina
Defects in Metabolism of Carbohydrates; Glycogen Storage Disease; Defects in Galactose Metabolism; Defects in Fructose Metabolism; Defects in Intermediary Carbohydrate Metabolism Associated with Lactic Acidosis; Defects in Pentose Metabolism

Bruce L. Klein, MD
Associate Professor, Pediatrics and Emergency Medicine, The George Washington University School of Medicine and Health Sciences; Chief, Division of Transport Medicine, Children's National Medical Center, Washington, District of Columbia
Acute Care of the Victim of Multiple Trauma

Michael D. Klein, MD
Arvin I. Philippart III, MD Chair and Professor of Surgery, Wayne State University School of Medicine; Surgeon-in-Chief at Children's Hospital of Michigan, Detroit, Michigan
Surgical Conditions of the Anus, Rectum, and Colon

Marisa S. Klein-Gitelman, MD, MPH
Associate Professor, Northwestern University, Feinberg School of Medicine; Children's Memorial Hospital, Chicago, Illinois
Systemic Lupus Erythematosus

Robert M. Kliegman, MD
Professor and Chair, Department of Pediatrics, Medical College of Wisconsin; Pediatrician-in-Chief, Pamela and Leslie Muma Chair in Pediatrics, Children's Hospital of Wisconsin; Executive Vice President, Children's Research Institute, Milwaukee, Wisconsin
Grief and Bereavement; Infections in International Adoptees

William C. Koch, MD
Associate Professor of Pediatrics, Division of Infectious Diseases, Virginia Commonwealth University School of Medicine; Attending Physician, Pediatrics, Division of Infectious Diseases, Medical College of Virginia Hospitals, Richmond, Virginia
Parvovirus B19

Gideon Koren, MD, FRCPC
Professor, Department of Pediatrics, Pharmacology, Pharmacy, Medical Genetics, University of Toronto, University of Western Ontario; Department of Pediatrics, The Hospital for Sick Children, Toronto, Ontario, Canada
Pharmacogenetics, Pharmacogenomics, and Pharmacoproteomics

Bruce R. Korf, MD, PhD
Wayne H. and Sara Crews Finley Professor and Chair, Department of Genetics, University of Alabama at Birmingham, Birmingham, Alabama
The Genetic Approach in Pediatric Medicine; The Human Genome; Genetics of Common Disorders; Integration of Genetics into Pediatric Practice

Peter J. Krause, MD
Professor of Pediatrics, University of Connecticut School of Medicine, Farmington, Connecticut; Director of Infectious Diseases, Department of Pediatrics, Connecticut Children's Medical Center, Hartford, Connecticut
Malaria *(Plasmodium)*; Babesiosis *(Babesia)*

Heather Krell, MD, MPH
Voluntary Clinical Associate Professor, Department of Psychiatry and Biobehavioral Sciences, Los Angeles, California
Pediatric Pain Management

John Kuttesch, Jr., MD, PhD
Ingraham Associate Professor of Cancer Research, Department of Pediatrics, Vanderbilt University; Director, Brain Tumor Program, Associate Professor, Hematology and Oncology, Monroe Carell Jr. Children's Hospital at Vanderbilt; Ingraham Associate Professor of Cancer Research, Pediatric Hematology and Oncology, Vanderbilt-Ingraham Cancer Center, Nashville, Tennessee
Brain Tumors in Childhood

Catherine S. Lachenauer, MD
Assistant Professor of Pediatrics, Harvard Medical School; Attending Physician, Division of Infectious Diseases, Children's Hospital, Boston, Massachusetts
Group B *Streptococcus*

Stephan Ladisch, MD
Professor and Vice Chairman of Pediatrics, George Washington University; Director, Center for Cancer and Immunology Research, Children's Research Institute, Children's National Medical Center, Washington, District of Columbia
Histiocytosis Syndromes of Childhood

Stephen LaFranchi, MD
Professor of Pediatrics, Oregon Health and Science University; Staff Physician, Doernbecher Children's Hospital, Portland, Oregon
Thyroid Development and Physiology; Defects of Thyroxine-Binding Globulin; Hypothyroidism; Thyroiditis; Goiter; Hyperthyroidism; Carcinoma of the Thyroid

Richard Lampe, MD
Professor and Chairman, Department of Pediatrics, Texas Tech University Health Sciences Center, Lubbock, Texas
Osteomyelitis; Suppurative Arthritis (Septic Arthritis)

Philip J. Landrigan, MD, MSc
Professor and Chairman, Department of Community and Preventive Medicine; Professor of Pediatrics, Mount Sinai School of Medicine, New York, New York
Chemical Pollutants

Gregory L. Landry, MD
Professor of Pediatrics, University of Wisconsin School of Medicine and Public Health; Team Physician, University of Wisconsin-Madison Athletic Teams, Madison, Wisconsin
Epidemiology and Prevention of Injuries; Management of Musculoskeletal Injury; Head and Neck Injuries; Heat Injuries; Female Athletes: Menstrual Problems and Risk for Osteopenia; Ergogenic Aids; Specific Sports and Associated Injuries

Carole Lannon, MD, MPH
Professor, Department of Pediatrics, University of Cincinnati; Co-Director, Center for Health Care Quality, Cincinnati Children's Hospital Medical Center, Cincinnati, Chio
Quality and Safety in Health Care for Children

Philip LaRussa, MD
Professor of Clinical Pediatrics, Columbia University, New York, New York
Varicella-Zoster Virus

Oren Lakser
Assistant Professor of Pediatrics, University of Chicago; Director, Fellowship Program in Pediatric Pulmonary; Director, Pediatric Flexible Fiberoptic Bronchoscopy Services, Section of Pediatric Pulmonary Medicine, University of Chicago, Chicago, Illinois
Parenchymal Disease with Prominent Hypersensitivity, Eosinophilic Infiltration, or Toxin-Mediated Injury; Bronchiectasis; Pulmonary Abscess

Charles T. Leach, MD
Professor of Pediatrics, University of Texas Health Science Center at San Antonio; Staff, University Hospital; Staff, Christus Santa Rosa Children's Hospital, San Antonio, Texas
Roseola (Human Herpesviruses 6 and 7); Human Herspesvirus 8

Chul Lee, PhD
Associate Professor, University of Texas Medical Branch, Galveston, Texas
The Porphyrias

J. Steven Leeder, PharmD, PhD
Professor of Pediatrics and Pharmacology, Schools of Medicine and Pharmacy, University of Missouri-Kansas City; Marion Merrell Dow Chair in Pediatric Pharmacogenomics, Section of Developmental Pharmacology and Experimental Therapeutics, Children's Mercy Hospitals and Clinics, Kansas City, Missouri
Pharmacogenetics, Pharmacogenomics, and Pharmacoproteomics

Margaret W. Leigh, MD
Professor of Pediatrics, University of North Carolina, Chapel Hill; Attending Physician, North Carolina Children's Hospital, Chapel Hill, North Carolina
Sarcoidosis

Steven Lestrud, MD
Instructor of Pediatrics, Northwestern University, Feinberg School of Medicine; Attending Physician, Children's Memorial Hospital, Chicago, Illinois
Bronchopulmonary Dysplasia

Donald Y.M. Leung, MD, PhD
Professor of Pediatrics, University of Colorado Medical School; Head of Pediatric Allergy-Immunology Division, National Jewish Medical and Research Center, Denver, Colorado
Allergy and the Immunologic Basis of Atopic Disease; Diagnosis of Allergic Disease; Principles of Treatment of Allergic Disease; Allergic Rhinitis; Childhood Asthma; Atopic Dermatitis (Atopic Eczema); Insect Allergy; Ocular Allergies; Urticaria (Hives) and Angioedema; Anaphylaxis; Serum Sickness; Adverse Reactions to Foods; Adverse Reactions to Drugs

Stephen Liben, MD
Associate Professor of Pediatrics, McGill University; Director, Palliative Care Program, Department of Pediatrics, The Montreal Children's Hospital of the McGill University Health Center, Montreal, Québec, Canada
The Care of Children with Life-Limiting Illness

Andrew H. Liu, MD
Associate Professor, Division of Allergy and Clinical Immunology, Department of Pediatrics, National Jewish Medical and Research Center; Associate Professor of Pediatrics, University of Colorado Health Sciences Center, Denver, Colorado
Childhood Asthma

Franco Locatelli, MD
Associate Professor of Pediatrics, Pavia University School of Medicine, Pavia, Italy; Head of Pediatric Hematology/Oncology Division, IRCCS Policlinico San Matteo, Pavia, Italy
Principles and Clinical Indications; HSCT from Alternative Sources and Donors; Graft Versus Host Disease (GVHD) and Rejection; Infectious Complications of HSCT; Late Effects of HSCT

Kelsey Logan, MD
Assistant Professor, Connecticut Children's Medical Center; Staff Physician, Elite Sports Medicine, Hartford, Connecticut
Epidemiology and Prevention of Injuries

Sarah S. Long, MD
Section of Infectious Diseases, St. Christopher's Hospital for Children, Philadelphia, Pennsylvania
Pertussis (Bordetella Pertussis and Bordatella Parapertussis)

Daniel J. Lovell, MD, MPH
Joseph E. Levinson Professor of Pediatrics, University of Cincinnati Medical Center; Associate Director, Division of Rheumatology, Cincinnati Children's Hospital Medical Center, Cincinnati, Ohio
Treatment of Rheumatic Diseases

G. Reid Lyon, PhD
Senior Research Professor, Whitney International University and the American College of Education, Dallas, Texas
Dyslexia

Helen N. Lyon, MD, SM
Instructor, Department of Pediatrics, Harvard Medical School; Staff Physician, Division of Genetics/Program in Genomics, Children's Hospital Boston, Boston, Massachusetts
Genetics of Common Disorders

Prashant V. Mahajan, MD, MPH, MBA
Associate Professor of Pediatrics and Emergency Medicine, Vice-Chief and Research Director of Pediatric Emergency Medicine, Carman and Ann Adams Department of Pediatrics, Wayne State University; Children's Hospital of Michigan, Detroit, Michigan
Heavy Metal Intoxication

Joseph A. Majzoub, MD
Thomas Morgan Rotch Professor of Pediatrics, Harvard Medical School; Chief, Division of Endocrinology, Department of Medicine, Children's Hospital Boston, Boston, Massachusetts
Diabetes Insipidus; Other Abnormalities of Arginine Vasopressin Metabolism and Action

Arik V. Marcell, MD, MPH
Assistant Professor of Pediatrics, University of Maryland, School of Medicine, Baltimore, Maryland
Adolescence

Joan C. Marini, MD, PhD
Branch Chief, Bone and Extracellular Matrix Branch, National Institute of Child Health, National Institutes of Health, Bethesda, Maryland
Osteogenesis Imperfecta

Morri Markowitz, MD
Professor of Pediatrics, Albert Einstein College of Medicine; Interim Chief, Division of Pediatric Endocrinology and Member, Division of Pediatric Environmental Sciences, Children's Hospital at Montefiore Hospital, Bronx, New York
Lead Poisoning

Stacene R. Maroushek, MD, PhD
Pediatric Infectious Diseases and General Pediatrics, Division of Pediatrics Infectious Diseases, University of Minnesota and Hannepin County Medical Center, Minneapolis, Minnesota
Principles of Antimycobacterial Therapy

Wilbert Mason, MD, MPH
Professor of Clinical Pediatrics, Keck School of Medicine of the University of Southern California; Head, Division of Infectious Disease, Department of Pediatrics, Children's Hospital Los Angeles, Los Angeles, California
Measles; Rubella; Mumps

Reuben Matalon, MD, PhD
Professor of Pediatrics, University of Texas Medical Branch, Children's Hospital, Galveston, Texas
Aspartic Acid (Canavan Disease)

Lawrence H. Mathers, Jr., MD, PhD
Associate Professor of Pediatrics and Surgery, Stanford University School of Medicine; Attending Physician, Pediatric Intensive Care Unit, Lucile Salter Packard Children's Hospital, Palo Alto California
Organ Transplantation; Pediatric Emergencies and Resuscitation; Brain Death

Robert Mazor, MD
Assistant Professor of Pediatrics, University of Washington; Attending Pediatric Cardiac Intensivist, Pediatric Critical Care Medicine, Children's Hospital and Regional Medical Care, Seattle, Washington
Pulmonary Edema

Paul L. McCarthy, MD
Professor of Pediatrics, Yale School of Medicine; Head, Division of General Pediatrics and Director of Patient

Services, Children's Hospital at Yale-New Haven, New Haven, Connecticut
Evaluation of the Sick Child in the Office and Clinic

Susannah A. McColley, MD
Associate Professor of Pediatrics, Northwestern University, Feinberg School of Medicine; Division Head, Pulmonary Medicine, Director, Cystic Fibrosis Center, Children's Memorial Hospital, Chicago, Illinois
Pulmonary Tumors; Extrapulmonary Diseases with Pulmonary Manifestations

Andrea C.S. McCoy, MD
Associate Professor of Pediatrics, Temple University School of Medicine; Associate Professor of Pediatrics, Temple University Children's Medical Center, Philadelphia, Pennsylvania
Histoplasmosis *(Histoplasma Capsulalum); Paracoccidioides Brasiliensis*

Margaret M. McGovern, MD, PhD
Professor of Human Genetics and Pediatrics, Mount Sinai School of Medicine; Attending Physician, Mount Sinai Hospital, New York, New York
Lipidoses; Mucolipidoses; Disorders of Glycoprotein Degradation and Structure

Kenneth McIntosh, MD
Professor of Pediatrics, Harvard Medical School; Emeritus Chief, Division of Infectious Diseases, Children's Hospital Boston, Boston, Massachusetts
Respiratory Syncytial Virus; Adenoviruses; Rhinoviruses

Rima McLeod, MD
Professor, Ophthalmology and Visual Sciences, Pedriatrics (Infectious Diseases) and the Committees on Molecular Medicine, Immunology, and Genetics and The College, The University of Chicago; Attending Physician, Department of Medicine and Pediatrics, Hospitals of the University of Chicago, Michael Reese Hospital and Medical Center, Chicago, Illinois
Toxoplasmosis *(Toxoplasma Gondii)*

Peter C. Melby, MD
Professor, Department of Medicine, Division of Infectious Diseases, University of Texas Health Science Center at San Antonio; Associate Chief of Staff for Research and Development, Research Service, South Texas Veterans' Health Care System, San Antonio, Texas
Leishmaniasis *(Leishmania)*

Marian G. Michaels, MD, MPH
Professor of Pediatrics and Surgery, University of Pittsburgh School of Medicine; Division of Infectious Disease, Children's Hospital of Pittsburgh, Pittsburgh, Pennsylvania
Infections in Immunocompromised Persons

Peter H. Michelson, MD
Assistant Professor of Pediatrics, Duke University School of Medicine, Durham, North Carolina
Congenital Disorders of the Lung

Henry Milgrom, MD
Professor of Pediatrics and Professor of Clinical Science, University of Colorado Health Sciences Center; Professor of Pediatrics, National Jewish Medical and Research Center, Denver Colorado
Allergic Rhinitis

Michael L. Miller, MD
Associate Professor of Pediatrics, Northwestern University, Feinberg School of Medicine; Attending Physician, Children's Memorial Hospital, Chicago, Illinois
Evaluation of Suspected Rheumatic Disease; Treatment of Rheumatic Diseases; Juvenile Rheumatoid Arthritis; Ankylosing Spondylitis and Other Spondyloarthropathies; Reactive Arthritis; Systemic Lupus Erythematosus; Scleroderma and Raynaud Phenomenon; Vasculitis Syndromes; Musculoskeletal Pain Syndromes; Miscellaneous Conditions Associated with Arthritis

Grant A. Mitchell, MD
Professor of Pediatrics, Division of Medical Genetics, Department of Pediatrics, Centre Hospitalier Universitaire Sainte-Justine, Montreal, Quebec, Canada
Tyrosine

Robert R. Montgomery, MD
Professor of Pediatric Hematology, Medical College of Wisconsin; Attending Physician, Pediatric Hematology, Oncology and Transplant, Children's Hospital of Wisconsin; Senior Investigator, Blood Research Institute, Blood Center of Wisconsin, Milwaukee, Wisconsin
Hemostasis; Hereditary Clotting Factor Deficiencies (Bleeding Disorders); von Willebrand Disease; Hereditary Predisposition to Thrombosis; Acquired Thrombotic Disorders; Postneonatal Vitamin K Deficiency; Liver Disease; Acquired Inhibitors of Coagulation; Disseminated Intravascular Coagulation; Platelet and Blood Vessel Disorders

Joseph G. Morelli, MD
Professor of Dermatology and Pediatrics, University of Colorado School of Medicine; Section Head, Pediatric Dermatology, The Children's Hospital, Denver, Colorado
Morphology of the Skin; Evaluation of the Patient; Principles of Therapy; Diseases of the Neonate; Cutaneous Defects; Ectodermal Dysplasias; Vascular Disorders; Cutaneous Nevi; Hyperpigmented Lesions; Hypopigmented Lesions; Vesiculobullous Disorders; Eczematous Disorders; Photosensitivity; Diseases of the Epidermis; Disorders of Keratinization; Diseases of the Dermis; Diseases of Subcutaneous Tissue; Disorders of the Sweat Glands; Disorders of Hair; Disorders of the Nails; Disorders of the Mucous Membranes; Cutaneous Bacterial Infections; Cutaneous Fungal Infections; Cutaneous Viral Infections; Arthropod Bites and Infestations; Acne; Tumors of the Skin; Nutritional Dermatoses

Anna-Barbara Moscicki, MD
Professor of Pediatrics, University of California, San Francisco, San Francisco, California
Human Papillomaviruses

Hugo W. Moser, MD
Professor of Neurology and Pediatrics, Johns Hopkins University; Director of Neurogenetics Research, Kennedy Krieger Institute, Johns Hopkins University School of Medicine, Baltimore, Maryland
Disorders of Very Long Chain Fatty Acids

Flor M. Munoz, MD
Assistant Professor of Pediatrics and Molecular Virology and Microbiology, Baylor School of Medicine; Attending Physician for Pediatric (Infectious Diseases), Texas Children's Hospital, Houston, Texas
Tuberculosis *(Mycobacterium Tuberculosis)*

Daniel J. Murphy, Jr., MD
Associate Professor of Pediatrics (Cardiology), Stanford University; Associate Chief, Pediatric Cardiology, Lucile

Salter Packard Children's Hospital, Director, Adult Congenital Heart Clinic, Stanford University Hospital, Palo Alto, California
The Adult with Congenital Heart Disease

James R. Murphy, PhD
Research Professor in Pediatrics, University of Texas Medical School, Houston, Houston, Texas
Campylobacter; Yersinia; Aeromonas and Plesiomonas

Martin G. Myers, MD
Professor of Pediatrics and Preventive Medicine, University of Texas Medical Branch; Executive Director, National Network for Immunization Information, Galveston, Texas
Varicella-Zoster Virus

William A. Neal, MD
Professor of Pediatrics, West Virginia University; Director, Preventive Cardiology, West Virginia University Children's Hospital, Morgantown, West Virginia
Disorders of Lipoprotein Metabolism and Transport

Robert M. Nelson, MD, PhD
Associate Professor of Anesthesiology, Critical, Care, and Pediatrics, University of Pennsylvania School of Medicine; Director, Center for Research Integrity, The Children's Hospital of Philadelphia, Philadelphia, Pennsylvania
Ethics in Pediatric Care

Mary A. Nevin, MD, FAAP
Assistant Professor of Pediatrics, Northwestern University Feinberg School of Medicine; Attending Physician, Pulmonary Medicine, Children's Memorial Hospital, Chicago, Illinois
Pulmonary Hemosiderosis; Pulmonary Embolism, Infarction, and Hemorrhage

Zehava Noah, MD
Associate Professor of Pediatrics, Northwestern University, Feinberg School of Medicine; Attending Physician, Pediatric Critical Care, Children's Memorial Hospital, Chicago, Illinois
Chronic Severe Respiratory Insufficiency

Lawrence M. Nogee, MD
Associate Professor of Pediatrics, Division of Neonatalogy, Johns Hopkins University School of Medicine; Attending Neonatalogist, Johns Hopkins Hospital, Baltimore, Maryland
Pulmonary Alveolar Proteinosis; Inherited Disorders of Surfactant Metabolism

Theresa J. Ochoa, MD
Assistant Professor, Center for Infectious Diseases, University of Texas-Houston Health Science Center, Houston, Texas
Shigella

Robin K. Ohls, MD
Professor of Pediatrics, University of New Mexico; Director, Neonatal-Perinatal Fellowship Program, Department of Pediatrics, University of New Mexico, Albuquerque, New Mexico
Development of the Hematopoietic System

Keith T. Oldham, MD
Professor and Chief, Department of Pediatric Surgery, Medical College of Wisconsin; Marie Z. Uihlein Chair and Surgeon-in-Chief, Children's Hospital of Wisconsin, Milwaukee, Wisconsin
Acute Appendicitis; Inguinal Hernias, Epigastric Hernia

Scott Olitsky, MD
Professor of Ophthalmology and Pediatrics, University of Missouri, Kansas City School of Missouri; Children's Mercy Hospitals and Clinics, Kansas City, Missouri
Growth and Development; Examination of the Eye; Abnormalities of Refraction and Accommodation; Disorders of Vision; Abnormalities of Pupil and Iris; Disorders of Eye Movement and Alignment; Abnormalities of the Lids; Disorders of the Lacrimal System; Disorders of the Conjunctiva; Abnormalities of the Cornea; Abnormalities of the Lens; Disorders of the Uveal Tract; Disorders of the Retina and Vitreous; Abnormalities of the Optic Nerve; Childhood Glaucoma; Orbital Abnormalities; Orbital Infections; Injuries to the Eye

John Olsson, MD
Associate Professor, East Carolina University, Brody School of Medicine; Staff, Pitt County Memorial Hospital, Greenville, North Carolina
The Newborn

Susan Orenstein, MD
Professor of Pediatric Gastroenterology, University of Pittsburgh School of Medicine, Pittsburgh, Pennsylvania
Embryology, Anatomy, and Function, of the Esophagus; Congenital Anomalies; Esophageal Atresia and Tracheoesophageal Fistula; Obstructing and Motility Disorders of the Esophagus; Dysmotility; Hiatal Hernia; Gastroesophageal Reflux Disease (GERD); Eosinophilic Esophagitis and Ingestions; Non-GERD Esophagitis; Esophageal Perforation; Esophageal Varices

Walter A. Orenstein, MD
Professor of Medicine and Pediatrics, Emory University School of Medicine; Associate Director, Emory Vaccine Center, Atlanta, Georgia
Immunization Practices

Gary D. Overturf, MD
Professor of Pediatrics and Pathology, University of New Mexico School of Medicine; Director, Pediatric Infectious Diseases, Department of Pediatrics, Children's Hospital of New Mexico; Medical Director, Infectious Diseases Section, TriCore Reference Laboratories, Albuquerque, New Mexico
Streptococcus Pneumoniae (Pneumococcus)

Judith A. Owens, MD, MPH
Associate Professor of Pediatrics, Brown University Medical School; Director, Pediatric Sleep Disorders Clinic, Director, Learning, Attention, and Behavior Clinic, Hasbro Children's Hospital, Providence, Rhode Island
Sleep Medicine

Lauren M. Pachman, MD
Professor of Pediatrics, Northwestern University Feinberg School of Medicine; Director, Molecular and Cellular Pathobiology, Children's Memorial Institute of Education and Research (CMIER); Professor, Department of Rheumatology, The Children's Memorial Hospital, Chicago, Illinois
Juvenile Dermatomyositis; Vasculitis Syndromes

Demosthenes Pappagianis, MD, PhD
Professor of Medical Microbiology and Immunology, University of California School of Medicine, Davis, Davis, California
Coccidioidomycosis *(Coccidioides)*

John S. Parks, MD, PhD
Professor of Pediatrics, Director of Pediatric Endocrinology, Emory University School of Medicine; Attending Physician, Pediatrics Department, Children's Healthcare of Atlanta, Atlanta, Georgia
Hormones of the Hypothalamus and Pituitary; Hypopituitarism

Diane E. Pappas, MD
Associate Professor of Pediatrics, University of Virginia School of Medicine, Charlottesville, Virginia
Sinusitis; Retropharyngeal Abscess, Lateral Pharyngeal (Parapharyngeal) Abscess, and Peritonsillar Cellulitis/Abscess

Ligia Peralta, MD, FAAP
Associate Professor, Department of Pediatrics and Epidemiology, University of Maryland Medical School; Chief, Division of Adolescent and Young Adult Medicine, Department of Pediatrics, University of Maryland Medical School, Baltimore, Maryland
Gender Identity Disorder (GID)

Norma Pérez, DO
Pediatric Infectious Disease Fellow, University of Texas Health Science Center at Houston, Houston, Texas
Aeromonas and Plesiomonas

Michael A. Pesce, Phd
Clinical Professor of Pathology, Columbia University, College of Physicians and Surgeons; Director of the Specialty Laboratory, New York Presbyterian Hospital, Columbia University Medical Center, New York, New York
Laboratory Testing in Infants and Children; Reference Ranges for Laboratory Tests and Procedures

John Peters, DO
Director, Division of Pediatric Gastroenterology, Janet Weis Children's Hospital, Geisinger Medical Center, Danville, Pennsylvania
Embryology, Anatomy, and Function of the Esophagus; Congenital Anomalies: Esophageal Atresia and Tracheoesophageal Fistula; Obstructing and Motility Disorders of the Esophagus; Dysmotility; Hiatal Hernia; Gastroesophageal Reflux Disease (GERD); Eosinophilic Esophagitis and Non-GERD Esophagitis; Esophageal Perforation

Ross E. Petty, MD, PhD
Professor Emeritus, Department of Pediatrics, University of British Columbia and British Columbia's Children's Hospital, Vancouver, British Columbia, Canada
Ankylosing Spondylitis and Other Spondyloarthropathies

Anthony J. Piazza, MD
Assistant Professor of Pediatrics, Emory University School of Medicine, Division of Neonatal-Perinatal Medicine, Atlanta, Georgia
Digestive System Disorders

Larry K. Pickering, MD, FAAP
Professor of Pediatrics, Emory University School of Medicine; Senior Advisor to the Director, National Center for Immunization and Respiratory Diseases, Atlanta, Georgia
Immunization Practices

Dwight A. Powell, MD
Professor of Pediatrics, Ohio State University College of Medicine; Chief, Section of Infectious Diseases, Pediatrics Department, Children's Hospital, Columbus, Ohio
Hansen Disease *(Mycobacterium Leprae);* Nontuberculous Mycobacteria; *Mycoplasma Pneumoniae;* Genital Mycoplasmas *(Mycoplasma Hominis* and *Ureaplasma Urealyticum)*

Keith R. Powell, MD
Professor and Chair, Department of Pediatrics, Northeastern Ohio Universities College of Medicine; Vice President and Dr. Noah Miller Chair of Medicine, Akron Children's Hospital, Akron, Ohio
Fever; Fever Without a Focus; Sepsis, Septic Shock, and Systemic Inflammatory Response Syndrome

Charles G. Prober, MD
Professor of Pediatrics, Medicine, Microbiology, and Immunology; Senior Associate Dean of Education, Stanford University School of Medicine, Stanford, California
Pneumonia; Central Nervous System Infections

Natoshia Raishevich
Research Associate, Department of Psychiatry, Columbia University College of Physicians and Surgeons, New York, New York
Attention-Deficit/Hyperactivity Disorder

Robert Rapaport, MD
Professor of Pediatrics, Director of Division of Pediatric Endocrinology and Diabetes, Mount Sinai Medical Center, New York, New York
Development and Function of the Gonads; Hypofunction of the Testes; Pseudoprecocity Resulting from Tumors of the Testes; Gynecomastia; Hypofunction of the Ovaries; Pseudoprecocity due to Lesions of the Ovary; Disorders of Sex Development (Intersex)

Stanley E. Read, MD, PhD, FRCPC, FAAP
Professor of Pediatrics, University of Toronto; Professor of Pediatrics, Infectious Disease Consultant, Hospital for Sick Children, Toronto, Ontario, Canada
Coronaviruses

Michael Reed, PharmD, FCCP, FCP
Professor of Pediatrics, Case Western Reserve University School of Medicine; Director, Pediatric Clinical Pharmacology and Toxicology, Pediatrics Department, Rainbow Babies and Children's Hospital, Cleveland, Ohio
Principles of Drug Therapy; Poisonings

Gary Remafedi, MD, MPH
Professor, University of Minnesota, Minneapolis, Minnesota; Executive Director, University of Minnesota Youth and AIDS Projects, Minneapolis, Minnesota
Adolescent Homosexuality

Jack S. Remington, MD
Professor Emeritus, Department of Medicine, Division of Infectious Diseases and Geographic Medicine, Stanford University School of Medicine, Stanford, California; Marcus A. Krupp Research Chair and Chairman, Department of Immunology and Infectious Diseases, Research Institute, Palo Alto Medical Foundation, Palo Alto, California
Toxoplasmosis *(Toxoplasma Gondii)*

Jorge Reyes, MD
Professor of Surgery, University of Washington School of Medicine; Division Chief, Transplant Surgery, University of Washington Medical Center, Seattle, Washington
Intestinal Transplantation in Children

Iraj Rezvani, MD
Emeritus Professor of Pediatrics, Temple University; Chief, Section for Endocrine, Diabetes, and Metabolic Disorders, Temple University Children's Medical Center, Philadelphia, Pennsylvania
An Approach to Inborn Errors of Metabolism; Phenylalanine; Tyrosine; Methionine; Cysteine/Cystine; Tryptophan; Valine, Leucine, Isoleucine, and Related Organic Acidemias; Glycine; Serine; Proline; Glutamic Acid; Urea Cycle and Hyperammonemia (Arginine, Citrulline, Ornithine); Histidine; Lysine

Frederick P. Rivara, MD, MPH
George Adkins Professor of Pediatrics, University of Washington, Seattle, Washington
Injury Control; Emergency Medical Services for Children

Nathaniel H. Robin, MD
Associate Professor of Genetics, University of Alabama at Birmingham; University Hospital, University of Alabama at Birmingham, Children's Hospital, Birmingham, Alabama
Patterns of Genetic Transmission

Luther K. Robinson, MD, AB
Associate Professor of Pediatrics, State University of New York at Buffalo School of Medicine and Biomedical Sciences; Director, Dysmorphology and Clinical Genetics, Women and Children's Hospital of Buffalo, Buffalo, New York
Marfan Syndrome

George C. Rodgers, Jr., MD, PhD
Professor of Pediatrics and Pharmacology/Toxicology, Department of Pediatrics, University of Louisville; Associate Medical Director, Kentucky Regional Poison Center, Koasir Childrens Hospital, Louisville, Kentucky
Poisonings

Genie E. Roosevelt, MD, MPH
Assistant Professor of Pediatrics, University of Colorado School of Medicine; Attending Physician, The Children's Hospital, Denver, Colorado
Acute Inflammatory Upper Airway Obstruction (Croup, Epiglottitis, Laryngitis, and Bacterial Tracheitis)

David S. Rosenblatt, MD
Professor and Chairman, Department of Human Genetics, McGill University; Director, Division of Medical Genetics, Department of Medicine, McGill University Health Centre; Chief, Department of Medical Genetics, Sir Mortimer B. Davis Jewish General Hospital, Montreal, Quebec, Canada
Methionine

Anne H. Rowley, MD
Professor of Pediatrics and of Microbiology/Immunology, Northwestern University, Feinberg School of Medicine; Attending Physician, Division of Infectious Diseases, Children's Memorial Hospital, Chicago, Illinois
Kawasaki Disease

Ranna Rozenfeld, MD
Associate Professor of Pediatrics, Northwestern University, Feinberg School of Medicine; Attending Physician, Pediatric Critical Care Medicine, Children's Memorial Hospital, Chicago, Illinois
Atelectasis

Colin D. Rudolph, MD, PhD
Professor and Chief, Pediatric Gastroenterology and Nutrition, Medical College of Wisconsin; Children's Hospital of Wisconsin, Milwaukee, Wisconsin
Overweight and Obesity

Robert A. Salata, MD
Professor of Medicine, Epidemiology/Biostatistics, and International Health, Case Western Reserve University School of Medicine; Attending Physician, Chief, Division of Infectious Diseases and HIV Medicine, University Hospitals Case Medical Center, Cleveland, Ohio
Health Advice for Children Traveling Internationally; Amebiasis; Trichomoniasis *(Trichomonas Vaginalis)* African Trypanosomiasis (Sleeping Sickness, *Trypanosoma Brucei* complex); American Trypanosomiasis (Chagas Disease; *Trypanosoma Cruzi*)

Denise A. Salerno, MD
Associate Professor of Pediatrics, Temple University School of Medicine; Associate Professor of Pediatrics, Temple University Children's Medical Center, Philadelphia, Pennsylvania
Nonbacterial Food Poisoning

Hugh Sampson, MD
Professor of Pediatrics and Immunobiology, Mount Sinai School of Medicine; Attending Physician, Mount Sinai Hospital, New York, New York
Anaphylaxis; Adverse Reactions to Foods

Joseph M. Sanfilippo, MD, MBA
Professor of Obstetrics, Gynecology, and Reproductive Sciences, University of Pittsburgh School of Medicine; Staff, Magee-Women's Hospital, Pittsburgh, Pennsylvania
History and Physical Examination; Vulvovaginitis; Bleeding; Breast Disorders; Hirsutism and Polycystic Ovarian Syndrome; Neoplasms and Abnormal Pap Smear Management; Vulvovaginal and Müllerian Anomalies; Special Gynecologic Needs, Gynecologic Imaging

Ashok P. Sarnaik, MD
Professor of Pediatrics, Wayne State University School of Medicine; Division Chief, Pediatric Critical Care Medicine, Children's Hospital of Michigan, Detroit, Michigan
Respiratory Pathophysiology and Regulation

Harvey B. Sarnat, MD, FRCPC
Professor of Paediatrics, Pathology (Neuropathology), and Clinical Neuroscience, University of Calgary Faculty of Medicine; Head, Division of Paediatric Neurology, Alberta Children's Hospital, Calgary, Alberta, Canada
Evaluation and Investigation; Developmental Disorders of Muscle; Muscular Dystrophies; Endocrine and Toxic Myopathies; Metabolic Myopathies; Disorders of Neuromuscular Transmission and of Motor Neurons; Hereditary Motor-Sensory Neuropathies; Toxic Neuropathies; Autonomic Neuropathies; Guillain-Barré Syndrome; Bell Palsy

Mark R. Schleiss, MD
Professor, Director of Pediatric Infectious Diseases, American Legion Chair of Pediatrics, Co-Director for the Center for Infectious Diseases and Microbiology Translational Research, and Associate Chair for Research, Pediatrics, University of Minnesota; Attending Physician, Pediatrics Department, University of Minnesota Medical Center, Fairview; Attending

Physician, Pediatrics Department, University of Minnesota Children's Hospital, Fairview, Minneapolis, Minnesota; Consulting Physician, Pediatrics Department, Children's Hospitals and Clinics of Minnesota, Minneapolis and St. Paul, Minnesota
Principles of Antibacterial Therapy; Principles of Antimycobacterial Therapy; Principles of Antifungal Therapy; Principles of Antiviral Therapy

Robert L. Schum, PhD
Associate Professor of Pediatrics, Medical College of Wisconsin; Clinical Psychologist, Child Development Center, Children's Hospital of Wisconsin, Milwaukee, Wisconsin
Language Development and Communication Disorders

Gordon G. Schutze, MD
Professor of Pediatrics and Pathology, University of Arkansas for Medical Sciences, College of Medicine; Arkansas Children's Hospital, Little Rock, Arkansas
Actinomyces; Nocardia; Tularemia *(Francisella Tularensis); Brucella*

J. Paul Scott, MD
Professor of Pediatrics, Medical College of Wisconsin; Attending Hematologist/Director, Wisconsin Sickle Cell Center, Department of Pediatrics, Hematology, Oncology, and Transplant, Children's Hospital of Wisconsin; Investigator, Hemostasis Research Section, Blood Research Institute, Blood Center of Wisconsin, Milwaukee, Wisconsin
Hemostasis; Hereditary Clotting Factor Deficiencies (Bleeding Disorders); von Willebrand Disease; Hereditary Predisposition to Thrombosis; Acquired Thrombotic Disorders; Postneonatal Vitamin K Deficiency; Liver Disease; Acquired Inhibitors of Coagulation; Disseminated Intravascular Coagulation; Platelet and Blood Vessel Disorders

Theodore C. Sectish, MD
Associate Professor, Stanford University School of Medicine; Director, Residency Training Program, Lucile Salter Packard Children's Hospital, Palo Alto, California
Pneumonia

George B. Segel, MD
Professor of Pediatrics and Medicine, University of Rochester School of Medicine; Golisano Children's Hospital, Rochester, New York
Definitions and Classification of Hemolytic Anemias; Hereditary Spherocytosis; Hereditary Elliptocytosis; Hereditary Stomacytosis; Other Membrane Defects; Enzymatic Defects; Glucose-6-Phosphate Dehydrogenase (G6PD) and Related Deficiences; Hemolytic Anemias Resulting from Extracellular Factors; Hemolytic Anemias Secondary to Other Extracellular Factors

Janet R. Serwint, MD
Professor of Pediatrics, Johns Hopkins University School of Medicine; Professor of Pediatrics, Director, Pediatric Resident Education, Johns Hopkins Hospital, Baltimore, Maryland
Separation, Loss, and Bereavement

Jane Seward, MBBS, MPH
Acting Deputy Director, Division of Viral Diseases, National Center for Immunizations and Respiratory Diseases, Centers for Disease Control and Prevention, Atlanta, Georgia
Varicella-Zoster Virus

Prachi E. Shah, MD
Associate Professor of Pediatrics, Baylor College of Medicine; Developmental and Behavioral Pediatrician: Meyer Center for Developmental Pediatrics, Texas Children's Hospital, Houston Texas
Assessment and Interviewing; Pervasive Developmental Disorders and Childhood Psychosis

Bruce K. Shapiro, MD
Associate Professor of Pediatrics and Arnold Cepute, MD, MPH Chair in Neurodevelopmental Disabilities, Johns Hopkins University School of Medicine; Vice President, Training, Kennedy Krieger Institute, Johns Hopkins University School of Medicine, Baltimore, Maryland
Mental Retardation (Intellectual Disability)

Eugene D. Shapiro, MD
Professor, Department of Pediatrics, Epidemiology and Public Health, and Investigative Medicine, Yale University; Attending Physician, Pediatrics Department, Children's Hospital of Yale-New Haven
Lyme Disease *(Borrelia Burgdorferi)*

Bennett A. Shaywitz, MD
Professor of Pediatrics and Neurology; Co-Director, Yale Center for the Study of Learning, Reading, and Attention, Department of Pediatrics, New Haven, Connecticut
Dyslexia

Sally E. Shaywitz, MD
Professor of Pediatrics; Co-Director, Yale Center for the Study of Learning, Reading, and Attention, Department of Pediatrics, New Haven, Connecticut
Dyslexia

Joel Shilyanski, MD, FACS, FAAP
Associate Professor, Department of Surgery, University of Iowa; Director of Pediatric Surgery, University of Iowa Hospitals and Clinics, Iowa City, Iowa
Diarrhea from Hormone-Secreting Tumors; Tumors of the Digestive Tract

Melanie Shim, MD
Adjunct Assistant Professor, Department of Pediatric Endocrinology, University of California at Los Angeles; Adjunct Assistant Professor, Department of Pediatric Endocrinology, University of California at Los Angeles, Los Angeles, California; Partner Physician, Department of Pediatric Endocrinology, Kaiser Permanente, Harbor City, California
Hyperpituitarism, Tall Stature, and Overgrowth Syndromes

Benjamin L. Shneider, MD
Professor of Pediatrics, Mount Sinai School of Medicine; Attending Physician, Mount Sinai Medical Center, New York, New York
Autoimmune and Chronic Hepatitis

Stanford T. Shulman, MD
Professor of Pediatrics, Northwestern University, Feinberg School of Medicine; Chief, Division of Infectious Diseases, Children's Memorial Hospital, Chicago, Illinois
Kawasaki Disease

George K. Siberry, MD, MPH
Assistant Professor, Department of Pediatrics, Johns Hopkins University School of Medicine; Medical Director, Harriet Lane Clinic, Department of Pediatrics, Johns Hopkins Hospital, Baltimore, Maryland

Spotted Fever Group *Rickettsioses;* Scrub Typhus (Orientia Tsutsugamushi), Typhus Group Rickettsioses; Ehrlichioses and Anaplasmosis; Q Fever *(Coxiella Burnetii)*

Scott H. Sicherer, MD
Associate Professor of Pediatrics, Jaffe Food Allergy Institute, Division of Pediatric Allergy and Immunology, Mount Sinai School of Medicine, New York, New York
Insect Allergy; Serum Sickness

Mark D. Simms, MD, MPH
Professor of Pediatrics and Chief, Section of Developmental Pediatrics, Medical College of Wisconsin; Medical Director, Child Development Center, Children's Hospital of Wisconsin, Milwaukee, Wisconsin
Language Development and Communication Disorders; Adoption; Foster Care

Eric F. Simoes, MD, DCH
Professor of Pediatrics, Section of Infectious Diseases, University of Colorado at Denver and Health Sciences Center; Professor of Pediatrics, Section of Infectious Diseases, The Children's Hospital, Denver, Colorado
Polioviruses

Joseph A. Skelton, MD
Assistant Professor of Pediatrics, Medical College of Wisconsin; Director, NEW (Nutrition, Exercise, and Weight management) Kids Program™, Children's Hospital of Wisconsin, Milwaukee, Wisconsin
Overweight and Obesity

Thomas L. Slovis, MD
Professor of Radiology and Pediatrics, Wayne State University School of Medicine; Professor of Radiology and Pediatrics, Staff Radiologist, Children's Hospital of Michigan, Detroit, Michigan
Biologic Effects of Radiation on Children

Laura P. Smith, MD
Associate Professor of Ophthalmology and Pediatrics, University of Missouri, Kansas City School of Medicine; Staff, Children's Mercy Hospitals and Clinics, Kansas City, Missouri
Growth and Development; Examination of the Eye; Abnormalities of Refraction and Accommodation; Disorders of Vision; Abnormalities of Pupil and Iris; Disorders of Eye Movement and Alignment; Abnormalities of the Lids; Disorders of the Lacrimal System; Disorders of the Conjunctiva; Abnormalities of the Cornea; Abnormalities of the Lens; Disorders of the Uveal Tract; Disorders of the Retina and Vitreous; Abnormalities of the Optic Nerve; Childhood Glaucoma; Orbital Abnormalities; Orbital Infections; Injuries to the Eye

Manu Sood, MD, MRCP, MBBS
Associate Professor, Medical College of Wisconsin; Director of Gastrointestinal Motility, Children's Hospital of Wisconsin, Milwaukee, Wisconsin
Disorders of Malabsorption

Joseph D. Spahn, MD
Associate Professor of Pediatrics, Division of Allergy, Immunology, and Rheumatology; Director, Immunopharmacology Lab, Division of Clinical Pharmacology; Director, Pediatric Allergy Immunology Fellowship Program, National Jewish Medical and Research Center, Denver, Colorado
Childhood Asthma

Mark A. Sperling, MD
Professor, Department of Pediatrics, University of Pittsburgh; Professor, Division of Pediatric Endocrinology, Diabetes, and Metabolism, Children's Hospital of Pittsburgh, Pittsburgh, Pennsylvania
Hypoglycemia

David A. Spiegel, MD
Assistant Professor of Orthopaedic Surgery, University of Pennsylvania School of Medicine; Orthopaedic Surgeon, The Children's Hospital of Philadelphia, Philadelphia, Pennsylvania
The Foot and Toes; Leg Length Discrepancy; The Neck

Jürgen Spranger, MD
Professor Emeritus of Pediatrics, University of Mainz, Germany; Formerly Head of Children's Hospital, Mainz, Germany
Mucopolysaccharidoses

Brian Stafford, MD, MPH
Assistant Professor of Psychiatry and Pediatrics, University of Colorado Health Sciences Center; Consult-Liaison Psychiatrist, Department of Psychiatry/Behavioral Sciences, The Children's Hospital; Medical Director, Post-partum Depression Intervention Program, Kempe Center, Denver, Colorado
Anxiety Disorders; Eating Disorders

Sergio Stagno, MD
Professor and Chairman, Department of Pediatrics, The University of Alabama at Birmingham; Physician-in-Chief, Children's Hospital of Alabama, Birmingham, Alabama
Cytomegalovirus

Lawrence R. Stanberry, MD, PhD
John Sealy Distinguished Chair and Professor, Department of Pediatrics, University of Texas Medical Branch; Director, Sealy Center for Vaccine Development, University of Texas Medical Branch, Galveston, Texas
Herpes Simplex Virus

Charles A. Stanley, MD
Professor of Pediatrics, University of Pennsylvania School of Medicine; Chief, Division of Endocrinology, The Children's Hospital of Philadelphia, Philadelphia, Pennsylvania
Disorders of Mitochondrial Fatty Acid β-Oxidation

Bonita F. Stanton, MD
Schotanus Professor and Chair, Department of Pediatrics, Wayne State University School of Medicine; Pediatrician-in-Chief, Carman and Ann Adams Department of Pediatrics, Children's Hospital of Michigan, Detroit, Michigan
Overview of Pediatrics; Cultural Issiues in Pediatric Care

Jeffrey R. Starke, MD
Professor and Vice Chairman, Department of Pediatrics, Baylor College of Medicine; Chief of Pediatrics, Ben Taub General Hospital; Infection Control Officer, Texas Children's Hospital, Houston, Texas
Tuberculosis *(Mycobacterium Tuberculosis)*

Barbara W. Stechenberg, MD
Professor of Pediatrics, Tufts University School of Medicine; Director, Pediatric Infectious Diseases, Vice Chairman, Pediatrics Department, Baystate Children's Hospital, Springfield, Massachusetts
Bartonella

Barbara J. Stoll, MD
George W. Brumley, Jr., Professor and Chair, Department of Pediatrics, Emory University School of Medicine, Atlanta, Georgia
Overview of Mortality and Morbidity; The Newborn High-Risk Pregnancies; The Fetus; The High-Risk Infant; Clinical Manifestations of Diseases in the Newborn Period; Nervous System Disorders; Delivery Room Emergencies; Respiratory Tract Disorders; Digestive System Disorders; Blood Disorders; Genitourinary System; The Umbilicus; Metabolic Disturbances; The Endocrine System; Infections of the Neonatal Infant

Laura Stout Sosinsky, PhD
Postdoctoral Associate, Yale Child Study Center, Yale University School of Medicine, New Haven, Connecticut
Child Care

Ronald G. Strauss, MD
Professor of Pathology and Pediatrics, University of Iowa College of Medicine; DeGowin Blood Center Faculty, Department of Pathology, University of Iowa Hospitals and Clinics, Iowa City, Iowa
Red Blood Cell Transfusions and Erythropoietin Therapy; Platelet Transfusions; Neutrophil (Granulocyte) Transfusions; Fresh Frozen Plasma Transfusions; Risks of Blood Transfusions

Frederick J. Suchy, MD
Professor and Chair of Pediatrics, Mount Sinai School of Medicine; Pediatrician-in-Chief, Mount Sinai Hospital, New York, New York
Autoimmune and Chronic Hepatitis; Drug and Toxin-Induced Liver Injury; Fulminant Hepatic Failure; Cystic Diseases of the Biliary Tract and Liver; Diseases of the Gallbladder; Portal Hypertension and Varices

Stuart C. Sweet, MD, PhD
Associate Professor, Department of Pediatrics, Washington University in St. Louis, St. Louis, Missouri
Pulmonary Alveolar Proteinosis; Inherited Disorders of Surfactant Metabolism

Robert P. Thomas, MD
Clinical Assistant Professor, University of Texas Health Science Center; Methodists Children's Hospital and Christus Santa Rosa Children's Hospital, San Antonio, Texas
Surgical Conditions of the Anus, Rectum, and Colon

Norman Tinanoff, DDS, MS
Professor and Chair, Department of Health Promotion and Policy, University of Maryland Dental School, Baltimore, Maryland
Development and Developmental Abnormalities of the Teeth; Disorders of the Oral Cavity Associated with Other Conditions; Malocclusion; Cleft Lip and Palate; Syndromes with Oral Manifestations; Dental Caries; Periodontal Diseases; Dental Trauma; Common Lesions of the Oral Soft Tissues; Diseases of the Salivary Glands and Jaws; Diagnostic Radiology in Dental Assessment

James K. Todd, MD
Professor of Pediatrics, Microbiology, and Preventive Medicine/Biometrics, University of Colorado School of Medicine; Director of Epidemiology, Clinical Microbiology and Clinical Outcomes, Department of Epidemiology and Community Pediatrics, The Children's Hospital, Denver, Colorado
Staphylococcus

Philip Toltzis, MD
Associate Professor of Pediatrics, Case Western Reserve University School of Medicine; Attending Physician, Division of Pharmacology and Critical Care, Rainbow Babies and Children's Hospital, Cleveland, Ohio
Rabies

Lucy Tompkins, MD
Lucy Becker Professor of Medicine, Professor of Microbiology and Immunology, Chief, Division of Infectious Diseases and Geographic Medicine, Stanford University School of Medicine; Medical Director, Hospital Epidemiology and Infection Control, Stanford Hospitals and Clinics, Stanford, California
Legionella

David G. Tubergen, MD
Medical Director, M.D. Anderson Physicians Network, University of Texas M.D. Anderson Cancer Center, Houston, Texas
The Leukemias

Ronald B. Turner, MD
Professor of Pediatrics, University of Virginia School of Medicine, Charlottesville, Virginia
The Common Cold; Acute Pharyngitis

MacDara Tynan, MD, FAAP
Adjunct Clinical Associate Professor, Department of Pediatrics, University of North Carolina, Chapel Hill, North Carolina; Director of Hospitalist Group, Department of Pediatrics, Levine Children's Hospital, Charlotte, North Carolina
Aspergillus; Zygomycosis *(Mucormycosis)*

Rodrigo E. Urizar, MD (Retired)
Professor of Pediatrics, Nephrology, Director of Pediatric Dialysis Services, Albany Medical College, Union University; Attending Pediatric Nephrologist, Children's Hospital, Albany Medical Center, Albany, New York
Renal Transplantation

Douglas Vanderbilt, MD
Assistant Professor of Pediatrics, Boston University School of Medicine; Staff, Division of Developmental and Behavioral Pediatrics, Boston Medical Center, Boston, Massachusetts
Bullying and School Violence

Andrea Velardi, MD
Professor of Hematology, Perugia University School of Medicine, Perugia, Italy
Principles and Clinical Indications; HSCT from Alternative Sources and Donors; Graft Versus Host Disease (GVHD) and Rejection; Infectious Complications of HSCT; Late Effects of HSCT

Elliott Vichinsky, MD
Medical Director, Hematology/Oncology, Children's Hospital and Research Center, Oakland, California
Hemoglobinopathies

Beth A. Vogt, MD
Associate Professor, Case Western Reserve University; Staff Physician, Rainbow Babies and Children's Hospital, Cleveland, Ohio
Introduction to the Child with Proteinuria; Transient Proteinuria; Orthostatic (Postural) Proteinuria; Fixed Proteinuria; Nephrotic Syndrome; Toxic Nephropathy; Cortical Necrosis; Renal Failure

Linda A. Waggoner-Fountain, MD
Associate Professor of Pediatrics, University of Virginia School of Medicine, Charlottesville, Virginia
Child Care and Communicable Diseases

Kimberly Danieli Watts, MD
Fellow, Pediatric Pulmonary Medicine, Northwestern University, Feinberg School of Medicine; Children's Memorial Hospital, Chicago, Illinois
Wheezing in Infants: Bronchiolotis

Martin E. Weisse, MD
Professor of Pediatrics, West Virginia University School of Medicine; Chief, Department of Infectious Diseases, Director, Pediatric Residency Program, West Virginia University School of Medicine, Morgantown, West Virginia
Candida; Malassezia; Primary Amebic Meningoencephalitis

Lawrence Wells, MD
Assistant Professor, Orthopaedic Surgery, University of Pennsylvania School of Medicine; Attending Surgeon, The Children's Hospital of Philadelphia, Philadelphia, Pennsylvania
Growth and Development; Evaluation of the Child; Torsional and Angular Deformities; The Knee; Common Fractures

Steven L. Werlin, MD
Professor of Pediatrics, Medical College of Wisconsin; Children's Hospital of Wisconsin, Milwaukee, Wisconsin
Embryology, Anatomy, and Physiology; Pancreatic Function Tests; Disorders of the Exocrine Pancreas; Treatment of Pancreatic Insufficiency; Pancreatitis; Chronic Pancreatitis; Pseudocyst of the Pancreas; Pancreatic Tumors

Michael Wessels, MD
Professor of Pediatrics and Medicine (Microbiology and Molecular Genetics), Harvard Medical School; Chief, Division of Infectious Diseases, Children's Hospital, Boston, Massachusetts
Group B *Streptococcus*

Ralph Wetmore, MD
Professor of Otorhinolaryngology, University of Pennsylvania School of Medicine; Senior Surgeon, Division of Pediatric Otolaryngology, Children's Hospital of Philadelphia, Philadelphia, Pennsylvania
Tonsils and Adenoids

Randall Wetzel, MD
Professor of Pediatrics and Anesthesiology, Keck School of Medicine; Chairman, Anesthesiology Critical Care Medicine, The Children's Hospital, Los Angeles, California
Anesthesia and Perioperative Care

Isaiah D. Wexler, MD, PhD
Attending Pediatrician, Department of Pediatrics, Mount Scopus Campus, Hadassah University Hospital, Jerusalem, Israel
Effects of War on Children

Perrin C. White, MD
Professor of Pediatrics, University of Texas Southwestern Medical Center; Chief, Endocrinology, Children's Medical Center, Dallas, Texas
Physiology of the Adrenal Gland; Adrenocortical Insufficiency; Congenital Adrenal Hyperplasia and Related Disorders; Cushing Syndrome; Primary Aldosteronism; Adrenal Tumors; Pheochromocytoma; Adrenal Masses

Michael Wilschanski, MBBS
Director, Pediatric Gastroenterology Unit, Hadassah University Hospitals; Senior Lecturer, Division of Pediatrics, Hebrew University, Jerusalem, Israel
Probiotics in Gastrointestinal Disorders

Glenna B. Winnie, MD
Associate Professor of Pediatrics, George Washington University; Chief, Division of Allergy, Pulmonary, and Sleep Medicine, Children's National Medical Center, Washington, District of Columbia
Emphysema and Overinflation; α1-Antitrypsin Deficiency and Emphysema; Pleurisy, Pleural Effusions, and Empyema; Pneumothorax; Pneumomediastinum; Hydrothorax; Hemothorax; Chylothorax

Paul H. Wise, MD, MPH
Professor of Pediatrics, Richard E. Behrman Professor of Child Health and Society, Stanford University School of Medicine; Director, Center for Policy, Outcomes and Prevention, Department of Pediatrics, Lucile Salter Packard Children's Hospital, Palo Alto, California
Developmental Disabilities and Chronic Illness; Chronic Illness in Childhood

Charles R. Woods, MD
Associate Professor of Pediatrics, Wake Forest University School of Medicine; Brenner Children's Hospital, Winston-Salem, North Carolina
Neisseria Meningitidis (Meningococcus)

Laura Worth, MD, PhD
Associate Professor of Pediatrics, Medical Director, Cell Therapy, University of Texas M.D. Anderson Cancer Center; Assistant Professor, University of Texas Health Science Center, Memorial Hermann Hospital, Houston, Texas
Molecular and Cellular Biology of Cancer

Peter Wright, MD
Shedd Chair in Pediatric Infectious Diseases; Professor of Pediatrics, Pathology and Microbiology & Immunology; Chief, Division of Pediatric Infectious Diseases, Vanderbilt University School of Medicine, Nashville, Tennessee
Influenza Viruses; Parainfluenza Viruses

Terry W. Wright, PhD
Associate Professor of Pediatrics and Microbiology & Immunology, University of Rochester School of Medicine, Rochester, New York
Pneumocystis Carinii (Pneumocystis Jiroveci)

David T. Wyatt, MD
Professor of Pediatrics, Section of Endocrinology and Diabetes, Medical College of Wisconsin; Chief, Pediatric Endocrinology, Children's Hospital of Wisconsin, Milwaukee, Wisconsin
Diabetes Mellitus

Robert Wyllie, MD
Chairman, Division of Pediatrics; Physician-in-Chief, Cleveland Clinic Children's Hospital, Cleveland, Ohio
Normal Digestive Tract Phenomena; Major Symptoms and Signs of Digestive Tract Disorders; Normal Development, Structure, and Function; Pyloric Stenosis and Other Congenital Anomalies of the Stomach; Intestinal Atresia, Stenosis, and Malrotation; Intestinal Duplications, Meckel Diverticulum, and Other Remnants of the Omphalomesenteric Duct; Motility Disorders and Hirschsprung Disease; Ileus, Adhesions, Intussusception, and Closed-Loop Obstructions; Foreign Bodies and Bezoars; Recurrent Abdominal Pain of Childhood

Anthony Wynshaw-Boris, MD
Professor of Pediatrics and Medicine Department, Director, Center for Human Genetics and Genomics, Chief, Division

of Genetics, Department of Pediatrics, University of California, San Diego School of Medicine; Rady Children's Hospital, San Diego, California
Dysmorphology

Stavra A. Xanthakos, MD, MS
Assistant Professor of Pediatrics, Department of Pediatrics, Division of Gastroenterology, Hepatology, and Nutrition, Cincinnati Children's Hospital Medical Center, Cincinnati, Ohio
Liver Abscess; Liver Disease Associated with Systemic Disorders

Nada Yazigi, MD
Assistant Professor of Clinical Pediatrics, University of Cincinnati Medical School; Assistant Professor of Clinical Pediatrics, Division of Gastroenterology, Hepatology, and Nutrition, Cincinnati Children's Hospital Medical Center, Cincinnati, Ohio
Viral Hepatitis

Ram Yogev, MD
Professor of Pediatrics, Northwestern University; Director, Section of Pediatric, Addescent, and Maternal HIV Infection, Department of Pediatrics, Children's Memorial Hospital, Chicago, Illinois
Acquired Immunodeficiency Syndrome (Human Immunodeficiency Virus)

Nader Youssef, MD, MBA
Assistant Professor of Pediatrics, University of Medicine & Dentistry of New Jersey—The New Jersey Medical School; Director, Center for Pediatric Irritable Bowel & Motility Disorders, Goryeb Children's Hospital at Atlantic Health, Morristown, New Jersey
Embryology, Anatomy, and Function of the Esophagus; Congenital Anomalies: Esophageal Atresia and Tracheoesophageal Fistula; Obstructing and Motility Disorders of the Esophagus; Dysmotility; Hiatal Hernia; Gastroesophageal Reflux Disease (GERD); Eosinophilic Esophagitis and Non-GERD Esophagitis; Esophageal Perforation

Anita K.M. Zaidi, MBBS, SM
Associate Professor of Pediatrics and Microbiology, Aga Khan University; Pediatric Infectious Diseases Consultant, Aga Khan University Hospital, Karachi, Pakistan
Diagnostic Microbiology

Lonnie K. Zeltzer, MD
Professor of Pediatrics, Anesthesiology, Psychiatry, and Biobehavioral Sciences, David Geffen School of Medicine; Director, Pediatric Pain Program; Mattel Children's Hospital at University of California, Los Angeles, California
Pediatric Pain Management

Maija H. Zile, PhD
Professor of Food Science and Human Nutrition, Michigan State University, East Lansing, Michigan
Vitamin A Deficiencies and Excess; Vitamin B Complex Deficiency and Excess; Thiamin (Vitamin B-1); Riboflavin (Vitamin B-2); Vitamin B-6 (Pyridoxine); Biotin; Folate; Vitamin B-12 (Cobalamine); Vitamin C Deficiency (Ascorbic Acid)

Barry S. Zuckerman, MD
The Joel and Barbara Alpert Professor and Chair of Pediatrics, Boston University School of Medicine, Professor of Public Health, Boston University School of Public Health; Chief, Pediatrics, Boston Medical Center, Boston, Massachusetts
Impact of Violence on Children

Contents

Part I ▪ The Field of Pediatrics

Chapter 1 ▪ Overview of Pediatrics

Bonita Stanton and Richard E. Behrman

Pediatrics is concerned with the health of infants, children, and adolescents; their growth and development; and their opportunity to achieve full potential as adults. Pediatricians must be concerned not only with particular organ systems and biologic processes, but also with environmental and social influences, which have a major impact on the physical, emotional, and mental health and social well-being of children and their families.

Pediatricians should also serve as advocates for all children, irrespective of culture, religion, gender, race, or ethnicity or of local, state, or national boundaries. Children cannot advocate for themselves. The more politically, economically, or socially disenfranchised a population or a nation, the greater the need for advocacy for children by the profession whose entire purpose is to advance the well-being of children. The young are often among the most vulnerable or disadvantaged in society and, thus, their needs require special attention. As artificial divides between nations blur through advanced transportation and communication, through globalization of the economy, and through modern means of warfare and as the categorization of countries into "developed" or "industrialized" and "developing" or "low income" break down due to uneven advances within and across countries, a global perspective for the field of pediatrics becomes both a reality and a necessity.

The number of births in the United States has been increasing since 1976 and is expected to continue to increase at 1–2% annually. Despite increases in the numbers of births, the proportion of children relative to the adult population is decreasing whereas the proportion of older adults relative to younger adults is increasing (Fig. 1-1). Currently, children younger than age 18 constitute approximately $^1/_4$ of the U.S. population.

Worldwide, children represent a higher proportion of the population, with children younger than age 15 accounting for 1.8 billion (28%) of the world's 6.4 billion persons. In 2003, there were an estimated 133 million births worldwide, 120 million (90%) of which were in developing countries. Four million (3%) of these births were in the United States.

SCOPE AND HISTORY OF PEDIATRICS AND VITAL STATISTICS

More than a century ago, pediatrics emerged as a medical specialty in response to increasing awareness that the health problems of children differ from those of adults and that a child's response to illness and stress varies with age. In 1959, the United Nations issued the Declaration of the Rights of the Child, articulating the universal presumption that children everywhere have fundamental needs and rights. Virtually all nations have practicing pediatricians and most medical schools across the globe have departments of pediatrics or child health.

The health problems of children and youth vary widely between and within populations in the nations of the world depending on a number of often interrelated factors. These factors include (1) economic considerations (economic disparities); (2) educational, social, and cultural considerations; (3) the prevalence and ecology of infectious agents and their hosts; (4) climate and geography; (5) agricultural resources and practices (nutritional resources); (6) stage of industrialization and urbanization; (7) the gene frequencies for some disorders; and (8) the health and social welfare infrastructure available within these countries. Health problems are not restricted to single nations and are not limited by country boundaries; the interrelation of health issues across the globe has achieved widespread recognition in the wake of the SARS (severe acute respiratory syndrome) and AIDS epidemics, expansions in the pandemics of cholera and West Nile virus, war and bioterrorism, and the tsunami of 2004.

Child health priorities must reflect local politics, resources, and needs. The state of health of any community must be defined by the incidence of illness and by data from studies that show the changes that occur with time and in response to programs of prevention, case finding, therapy, and surveillance. Accordingly, with time, the relative importance of the various causes of childhood morbidity and mortality may undergo major changes.

Resources also vary greatly by nation, with 78 nations enjoying a per capita income >$9,386/yr (27 >$20,000/yr) and 61 nations struggling with per capita incomes <$765/yr (20 <$300/yr). Likewise, nations expend differently; in the United States, >$5,000 is spent per citizen per year in health care compared to $3 per person in the world's 41 poorest countries, most of which are in sub-Saharan Africa. While there is a strong correlation between per capita income and child health outcomes (and between child health outcomes and expenditure for health), this relationship is not absolute. Singapore enjoys the lowest infant and child mortality rates in the world; the per capita income ranks ≈29th worldwide.

HISTORY OF INFANT AND CHILD HEALTH

INFANT HEALTH. In the late 19th century in the United States, 200 of every 1,000 children born alive died before the age of 1 yr of conditions such as dysentery, pneumonia, diphtheria, and whooping cough. The efforts of pediatricians, scientists, and pioneers in public health have led to a better understanding of the origin and management of diseases of childhood such that, in the past half century, the infant mortality rate in the United States has decreased from around 75/1,000 live births in 1925 to ≈6.8/1,000 in 2001. Although this rate had held steady or improved every year since 1958, the 2003 rate was 6.85/1,000.

Both neonatal (<1 mo) and postneonatal (1–11 mo) mortality have had major reductions. Most of the decline in infant mortality since 1970 is attributable to a decrease in the birthweight-specific infant mortality rate related to neonatal intensive care, not to the prevention of low-birthweight births (see Chapter 93). The majority of deaths of infants younger than 1 yr of age occur in the 1st 28 days of life, most of these in the 1st 7 days; moreover, a large proportion of the deaths in the 1st 7 days occur on the 1st day. An increasing number of severely ill infants born at very low birthweight survive the neonatal period, however, and die later in infancy of neonatal disease, its sequelae, or its complications (Tables 1-1, 1-2, and 1-3).

The preponderance of under-5 mortality (children dying before the age of 5 yr) occurring in the 1st year of life is also applicable to industrialized countries overall, with an infant mortality of 5/1,000 representing >80% of the under-5 mortality rate of 6/1,000 in 2004. In the least developed countries, the infant mortality rate of 98/1,000 accounts for 63% of the under-5 mortal-

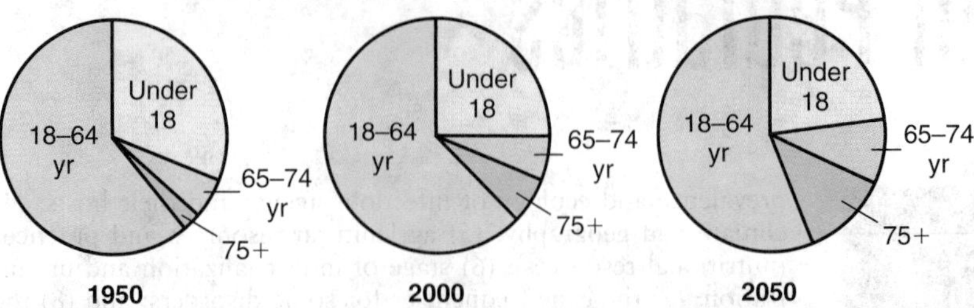

Figure 1-1. Percent of population in 4 age groups: United States, 1950, 2000, and 2050. (From Centers for Disease Control and Prevention, National Center for Health Statistics: *Health, United States, 2004*. DHSS Publication No. 2004–1232.)

TABLE 1-1. Death Rates* for All Causes, According to Sex, Race, and Age: United States, Selected Years, 1960–1999+

	1960		1970		1980		1990		2003	
	White	Black	White	Black	White	Black	White	Black	White	Black
MALE										
<1 yr	2,694	5,307	2,113	4,299	1,230	2,587	896	2,112	659	1,410
1–4 yr	105	209	84	151	66	111	46	86	32	54
5–14 yr	53	75	48	67	35	47	26	41	18	27
15–24 yr	144	212	171	321	167	209	131	252	109	171
FEMALE										
<1 yr	2,008	4,162	1,615	3,369	963	2,124	690	1,736	521	1,132
1–4 yr	85	173	66	129	49	84	36	68	26	40
5–14 yr	35	54	30	44	23	31	18	28	13	19
15–24 yr	55	108	62	112	56	71	46	69	43	54

Death rates per 100,000 population.
+Adapted from *Statistical Abstract of United States 1993*, 113th ed. Lanham, MD, Berman Press, 1993, table 119; Hoyert DL, Arias E, Smith BL, et al: Deaths: Final data for 1999. *Natl Vital Stat Rep* 2001;49:1–113; National Center for Health Statistics: *Health, United States 2005*, DHSS Publication No. 2005-1232, table 35.

ity rate of 155/1,000, indicating a somewhat greater proportion of deaths occurring among children after infancy in these very high risk countries (Table 1-4). Worldwide, 3.9 million of the 10.8 million deaths of children younger than 5 yr occur in the 1st 28 days of life. In populations with the highest child mortality rates, however, just over 20% of all child deaths occurred in the neonatal period, but in countries with mortality rates <35/1,000 livebirths, >50% of child deaths were in neonates (Fig. 1-2). Across the globe, there are significant variations in infant mortality rates by nation, by region, by economic status, and by level of industrial development, the categorizations employed by the World Bank and the United Nations (see Table 1-4). Among the nations categorized as industrialized, in 2004, the infant mortality rate was 5/1,000, whereas among nations categorized as developing, it was 59/1,000, with the poorest rate in sub-Saharan Africa (102/1,000 live births). The U.S. rate in 2004 of 7/1,000 compared unfavorably to that of 40 other nations (including developing countries such as Cuba with a rate of 6/1,000); Finland with a rate of 2/1,000, had the lowest infant mortality in the world.

Causes of death vary by developmental status of the nation. In the United States, the 3 leading causes of death among infants were congenital anomalies, disorders related to gestation and low birthweight, and sudden infant death (Table 1-5). By contrast, in developing countries, the majority of infant deaths result from infectious diseases; even in the neonatal period, 24% of deaths

TABLE 1-2. Deaths Rates for All Causes Among Children and Young Adults According to Sex, Race, Hispanic origin, and Age: 2002

	UNDER 1 YR	1–4 YR	5–14 YR	15–24 YR
	DEATHS PER 100,000 RESIDENT POPULATION			
All persons	695.0	31.2	17.4	81.4
Male	761.5	35.2	20.0	117.3
Female	625.3	27.0	14.7	43.7
MALES				
White	650.9	31.5	18.4	109.7
Black male (African-American)	1,351.5	54.4	28.9	172.6
American Indian or Alaska Native	896.8	48.3	22.0	145.1
Asian or Pacific Islander	461.9	27.1	14.4	58.6
Hispanic or Latino	644.0	34.2	17.4	114.4
White not Hispanic or Latino	643.5	30.3	18.3	106.7
FEMALES				
White	519.4	24.5	13.7	42.4
Black (African-American)	1,172.0	39.5	19.9	54.4
American Indian or Alaska Native	744.1	42.0	21.2	61.7
Asian or Pacific Islander	391.4	19.6	10.4	23.8
Hispanic or Latino	539.1	25.3	13.5	34.1
White not Hispanic or Latino	504.8	23.8	13.6	43.8

TABLE 1-3. Infant, Neonatal, and Postnatal Deaths and Mortality Rates by Specified Race or Origin of Mother: United States, 2002

		MORTALITY RATE PER 1,000 LIVEBIRTHS		
RACE OF MOTHER	LIVEBIRTHS	INFANT	NEONATAL	POSTNATAL
All Races	4,021,726	7.0	4.7	2.3
White	3,174,760	5.8	3.9	1.9
Black or African-American	593,691	13.8	9.3	4.5
American Indian or Alaska Native	42,368	8.6	4.6	4.0
Asian or Pacific Islander	210,907	4.8	3.4	1.4
Chinese	33,673	3.0	2.4	0.7
Japanese	9,264	4.9	3.7	
Filipino	33,016	5.7	4.1	1.7
Hawaiian	6,772	9.6	5.6	4.0
Other Asian or Pacific Islander	128,182	4.7	3.3	1.4
Hispanic or Latino	876,642	5.6	3.8	1.8
Mexican	627,505	5.4	3.6	1.8
Puerto Rican	57,465	8.2	5.8	2.4
Cuban	14,232	3.7	3.2	
Central and South American	125,981	5.1	3.5	1.6
Other and unknown Hispanic or Latino	51,459	7.1	5.1	2.0
Not Hispanic or Latino				
White	2,298,156	5.8	3.9	1.9
Black or African American	578,335	13.9	9.3	4.6

TABLE 1-4. Child Health Indicators Worldwide by Region

	MORTALITY RATE BY YR PER 1,000 LIVEBIRTHS				Per CAPITA INCOME US$	LIFE EXPECTANCY AT BIRTH IN YR	% PRIMARY SCHOOL ATTENDANCE
	UNDER-5		INFANT				
YR	1960	2004	1960	2004	2004	2004	1996–2004
Sub-Saharan Africa	278	171	185	102	611	46	60
Middle East/North Africa	249	56	157	44	2,308	68	79
South Asia	244	92	148	67	600	63	74
East Asia/Pacific	208	36	137	29	1,686	71	96
Latin America/Caribbean	153	31	102	26	3,649	72	93
CEE/OS	112	38	83	32	2,667	67	88
Industrialized countries	39	6	32	5	32,232	79	95
Developing countries	224	87	142	59	1,524	65	80
Least developed countries	278	155	171	98	345	52	60
World	198	79	127	54	6,298	67	82

From UNICEF: The state of the world's children 2005, table 1, page 108.

are caused by severe infections and 7% by tetanus. In developing countries, 29% of neonatal deaths are due to birth asphyxia and 24% due to complications of prematurity.

In the majority of countries, the most robust predictor of infant mortality is a poor level of maternal education. Other maternal risk characteristics, such as unmarried status, adolescence, and high parity, correlate with increased risk of postneonatal mortality and morbidity and low birthweight.

HEALTH AMONG POSTINFANCY CHILDREN. A profound improvement in child health occurred in the 20th century with the introduction of antibacterial disinfectants, antibiotic agents, and vaccines. Early in the 20th century in industrialized nations, efforts to control infectious diseases were complemented by better understanding of nutrition. In the United States, Canada, and parts of Europe, new and continuing discoveries in these areas led to establishment of public well child clinics for low-income families. Although the timing of control of infectious disease was uneven around the globe, this focus on control was accompanied by significant decreases in morbidity and mortality in all countries. The smallpox eradication program of the 1970s resulted in the global eradication of smallpox in 1977. The introduction in the 1970s of the Expanded Program of Immunizations (universal vaccination against polio, diphtheria, measles, tuberculosis, tetanus, and pertussis) by the World Health Organization (WHO) and United Nations' Children's Fund (UNICEF) has resulted in an estimated annual reduction of 2 million deaths per year globally. Recognizing the importance of prevention of infectious diseases to the health of children, several countries ranked by the

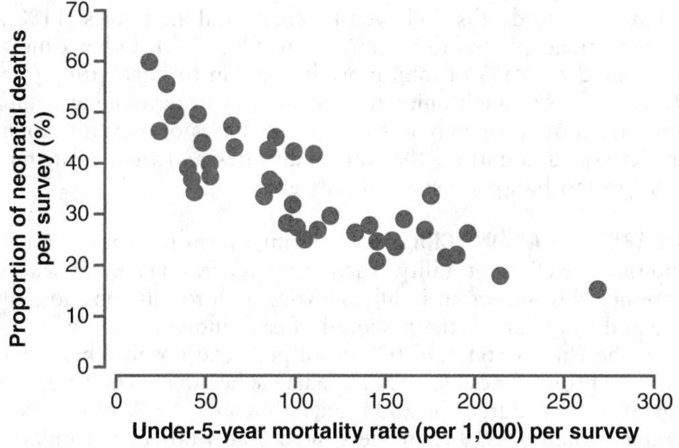

Figure 1-2. Relationship between under-5 year mortality rate and percentage of deaths in neonatal period. (From Black E, Morris S, Bryce J: Where and why are 10 million children dying every year? *Lancet* 2003;361:2226–2234.)

TABLE 1-5. Leading Causes of Death and Numbers of Deaths, According to Age : United States, 2002

AGE AND RANK ORDER	CAUSE OF DEATH	DEATHS
Under 1 yr	All causes	28,034
	Congenital malformation, deformations, and chromosomal abnormalities	5,623
	Disorders related to short gestation and low birthweight, not elsewhere classified	4,637
	Sudden infant death syndrome	2,295
	Newborn affected by maternal complications of pregnancy	1,708
	Newborn affected by complications of placenta, cord, and membranes	1,028
	Unintentional injuries	946
	Respiratory distress of newborn	943
	Bacterial sepsis of newborn	749
	Diseases of circulatory system	667
	Intrauterine hypoxia and birth asphyxia	583
1–4 yr	All causes	4,858
	Unintentional injuries	1,641
	Congenital malformations, deformations, and chromosomal abnormalities	530
	Homicide	423
	Malignant neoplasms	402
	Diseases of heart	165
	Influenza and pneumonia	110
	Septicemia	79
	Chronic lower respiratory diseases	65
	Certain conditions originating in the perinatal period	65
	In situ neoplasms, benign neoplasms, and neoplasms of uncertain or unknown behavior	60
5–14 yr	All causes	7,150
	Unintentional injuries	2,718
	Malignant neoplasms	1,072
	Congenital malformations, deformations, and chromosomal abnormalities	417
	Homicide	356
	Suicide	264
	Diseases of the heart	255
	Chronic lower respiratory diseases	136
	Septicemia	95
	Cerebrovascular diseases	91
	Influenza and pneumonia	91
15–24 yr	All causes	33,046
	Unintentional injuries	15,412
	Homicide	5,219
	Suicide	4,010
	Malignant neoplasms	1,730
	Diseases of the heart	1,022
	Congenital malformations, deformations, and chromosomal abnormalities	492
	Chronic lower respiratory diseases	192
	HIV disease	178
	Diabetes mellitus	171
	Cerebrovascular diseases	171

Adapted from National Center for Health Statistics: *Health, United States 2004*, DHSS Publication No. 2004-1232, table 32, p 158.

World Bank as among the 61 poorest nations (per capita income <$766/yr) have invested heavily in infectious disease control through the development of internal vaccine production capability. Vietnam (per capita income $480/yr), the world's 3rd nation to produce polio vaccine, is now self-sufficient for vaccine production of 2 of the vaccines used in its vaccination program. As diarrheal diseases continued through the mid-1970s to account for ≈25% of infant and childhood deaths in the nonindustrialized countries (4.6 million deaths per year), attention turned to the development and utilization of oral resuscitation fluids to sustain children through potentially life-threatening episodes of acute diarrheal diseases. Oral rehydration solutions are largely credited with the current reduction of diarrheal deaths annually to 1.5 million. This simple medical treatment serves as an important example of "reverse technology" in which a major medical innovation was initially utilized in developing nations and subsequently introduced in the industrialized world (see Chapter 55).

In the later 20th century, with improved control of infectious diseases (including the elimination of polio in the Western hemisphere) through both prevention and treatment, pediatric medicine in industrialized nations increasingly turned its attention to a broad spectrum of conditions. These included both potentially lethal conditions and temporarily or permanently handicapping conditions; among these disorders were leukemia, cystic fibrosis, diseases of the newborn infant, congenital heart disease, mental retardation, genetic defects, rheumatic diseases, renal diseases, and metabolic and endocrine disorders. Thus, in industrialized nations, the last 2 decades of the 20th century were marked by accelerated understanding of new approaches to the management of many disorders as a consequence of advances in molecular biology, genetics, and immunology.

Increasing attention has also been given to behavioral and social aspects of child health, ranging from re-examination of child-rearing practices to creation of major programs aimed at prevention and management of abuse and neglect of infants and children. Developmental psychologists, child psychiatrists, neuroscientists, sociologists, anthropologists, ethnologists, and others have brought us new insights into human potential, including new views of the importance of the environmental circumstances during pregnancy, surrounding birth, and in the early years of child rearing. The later 20th century witnessed the beginning of nearly universal acceptance by pediatric professional societies of attention to normal development, child-rearing, and psychosocial disorders across the continents. In the last decade, irrespective of level of industrialization, nations have developed programs addressing not only causes of mortality and physical morbidity (such as infectious diseases and protein-calorie malnutrition), but also factors leading to decreased cognition and thwarted psychosocial development, including punitive child-rearing practices, child labor, undernutrition, war, and poor schooling. Obesity is recognized as a major health risk. Progress at the turn of the 21st century in unraveling the human genome offers for the 1st time the realization that significant genetic screening, individualized pharmacotherapy, and genetic manipulation will be a part of routine pediatric treatment and prevention practices in the future. The prevention implications of the genome project give rise to the possibility of reducing costs for the care of illness but increase privacy issues (see Chapter 3).

Although local famines and disasters, and regional and national wars have periodically disrupted the general trend for global improvement in child health indices, it was not until the advent of the AIDS epidemic in the later 20th century that the 1st substantial global erosion of progress in child health outcomes occurred. This erosion has resulted in ever-widening gaps between childhood health indices in sub-Saharan Africa compared to the rest of the world. From 1990 to 2002, life expectancy in sub-Saharan Africa decreased from 50 yr to 46 yr; 13 nations have experienced declining life expectancies. Until the WHO's global "3 by 5" campaign (three retroviral agents for 20% of global HIV victims by the year 2005), antiretroviral drugs were essentially unavailable to most developing countries, including all of those hardest hit by the HIV epidemic. Increasing rates of tuberculosis and continued problems with pandemics such as cholera further challenge many of these nations. Strains of drug-resistant malaria are also a major concern in isolated areas around the world, but 90% of malarial deaths (the majority among children) are occurring in sub-Saharan Africa. Diseases once confined to limited geographic niches, including West Nile virus, and diseases previously uncommon among humans, such as SARS and the avian flu virus, increased awareness of the interconnectedness of health around the world. Formerly perceived as a problem of industrialized nations, motor vehicle crashes are now a major cause of mortality in developing countries as well.

Enormous disparities exist in childhood mortality rates across the globe (see Table 1-4). Among the 10.8 million childhood deaths occurring worldwide each year, ≈41% occur in sub-Saharan Africa, home to <10% of the world's population. Fifty percent of the world's childhood deaths are occurring in 6 nations; 90% of childhood deaths are occurring in only 42 of the world's 192 nations. In 2004, the United States had an under-5 mortality rate of 8/1,000 livebirths. Thirty-five nations had under-5 mortality rates lower than that of the United States, with Singapore having the lowest rate at 3/1,000. The comparable child mortality rate in sub-Saharan Africa was 171/1,000 livebirths. Sierra Leone has the highest under-5 mortality rate at 283/1,000 livebirths, followed by Angola at 260, Afghanistan at 257, Liberia at 235, Somalia at 225, and Mali at 219. In 1990, Sierra Leone and Niger had rates in excess of 300/1,000 lives births; their current rates do represent progress. Of the 51 nations with under-5 mortality rates in excess of 200 in the year 1990, in 2003, 18 showed no improvement or a worsening, and 3 nations whose under-5 morality rate had been at <100/1,000 livebirths in 1990 were in excess of 100.

Causes of under-5 mortality differ markedly between developed and developing nations. In developing countries, 66% of all deaths resulted from infectious and parasitic diseases. Among the 42 countries having 90% of childhood deaths, diarrheal disease accounted for 22% of deaths, pneumonia 21%, malaria 9%, AIDS 3%, and measles 1%. Neonatal causes contributed to 33%. The contribution for AIDS varies greatly by country, being responsible for a substantial proportion of deaths in some countries and negligible amounts in others. Likewise, there is substantial co-occurrence of infections; a child may die with HIV, malaria, measles, and pneumonia. Infectious diseases are still responsible for much of the mortality in developing countries. In the United States, pneumonia (and influenza) accounted for only 2% of under-5 deaths, with only negligible contributions from diarrhea and malaria. Unintentional injury is the most common cause of death among U.S. children ages 1–5 yr, accounting for about 33% of deaths, followed by congenital anomalies (11%), malignant neoplasms (8%), and homicides (7%). Other causes accounted for <5% of total mortality within this age group (see Table 1-5). Although unintentional injuries in developing countries are proportionately less important causes of mortality than in developed countries, their absolute rates and their contributions to morbidity are substantially greater.

MORBIDITIES AMONG CHILDREN. It is important to examine morbidities as well as mortality. Adequately addressing special health care needs is important in all countries both to minimize loss of life and to maximize the potential of each individual.

In the United States, ≈70% of all pediatric hospital bed days are for chronic illnesses; 80% of pediatric health expenditures are for 20% of children. In 2004, an estimated 12.8% of children younger than age 18 yr in the United States (about 9.4 million children) have special health care needs. One fifth of U.S. households with children have 1 or more children with special health care needs (see Chapter 38). Significantly more poor children and minority children have special health care needs. Although there are multiple chronic conditions and the prevalence of these disorders vary by population, 2 of these morbidities—obesity and asthma—have a substantial and increasing presence worldwide and are associated with substantial health consequences and costs.

In the United States, ≈25% of children and adolescents are overweight, representing a 2.3- to 3.3-fold increase over the past 25 yr. Similar profiles have been reported from Australia and multiple countries in Europe (see also Chapter 44). Also increasing in prevalence among industrialized nations and in middle- and low-income nations with substantial urbanization are rates of asthma. In the mid-1990s, the United States reported an annual prevalence rate of wheezing of 57.8/1,000 among children ages 0 to 4 yr and 74.4/1,000 among youth ages 5 to 15 yr, approximately twofold higher than comparable prevalence rates in 1980. The International Study of Asthma and Allergies has conducted a systematic review of asthma prevalence, with compelling evidence for a substantial global burden of childhood asthma, although rates vary substantially between and within countries. The highest annual prevalence rates are in the United Kingdom, Australia, New Zealand, and Ireland, with the lowest rates in Eastern European countries, Indonesia, China, Taiwan, India, and Ethiopia. Although there was a tendency for poorer countries to have lower asthma rates, this relationship was not absolute (see Chapter 143).

Chronic cognitive morbidities represent another substantial problem. Although different diagnostic criteria have been applied, attention-deficit/hyperactivity disorder (ADHD) is identified in >10% of children in many countries, including the United States, New Zealand, Australia, Spain, Italy, Colombia, and Great Britain. Variations in cultural tolerance and/or differences in screening approaches or tools may account for some of the differences in prevalence of the disorder by country, but genetic and gene-environmental interactions may also play a role. Despite variations in rate, the condition is universal. Beyond the personal and familial stress caused by the disorder, costs to the educational system are considerable. In the United States in 1995, an estimated $3 billion additional dollars were expended by public school systems on children with ADHD. In developing countries without resources for special education, these children are unlikely to fulfill their academic potential (see Chapter 31).

Mental retardation affects ≈1–3% of children in the United States, with 75% of these children having mild retardation. Rates are severalfold higher among very low birthweight infants, affecting between 20 and 40% of such children born in the mid-1990s. In the United States, there is substantial variation in rates of mild retardation by socioeconomic status (ninefold higher in the lowest compared to the highest socioeconomic stratum) but relatively equivalent rates of severe retardation. A similar income-related distribution is found in other countries, including some of the most impoverished countries such as Bangladesh. Lower overall rates have been reported in some countries, including countries ranging from Saudi Arabia to Sweden to China; the difference is primarily in the prevalence of mild retardation (see Chapter 38).

The prevalence of post-traumatic stress disorder (PTSD) varies considerably around the globe, but in children with substantial exposure to violence, the rates may be very high. After the attacks on the World Trade Center towers and the Pentagon in 2001, 33% of U.S. children had experienced one or more symptoms of PTSD. One half of Palestinian children experience at least 1 significant lifetime trauma and >33% (66% of those experiencing trauma) meet the criteria of PTSD. Natural disasters such as the tsunami of 2004; war, including those in Afghanistan, Sudan, and Iraq; and urban violence all leave their indelible marks on the minds of children. From 1990 to 2003, there were 59 major armed conflicts worldwide, only 4 of which were wars between nations; the majority of these internal conflicts are ethnically based. Approximately 90% of the deaths resulting from these conflicts have been among civilians, 80% among women and children. Sixteen of the world's poorest 20 countries have endured a civil war in the past 15 yr (see Chapter 35).

SPECIAL RISK POPULATIONS

In addition to the enormous differences in infant and child health between regions and nations, within countries there are substantial variations in morbidity and mortality rates by socioeconomic class and ethnicity. Most children at special risk need a nurturing environment but have had their futures compromised by actions or policies arising from their families, schools, communities, nations, or the international community. These problems have several causes, whether the end result is homeless children, runaway children, children in foster care, or children in other disadvantaged groups. The most effective preventive approach involves alleviation of poverty, inadequate parenting, discrimination, violence, poor housing, and poor education. Optimal care of these children requires reducing barriers to health care with organized programs, multidiscipline teams, and special financing.

CHILDREN IN POVERTY. Family income is central to the health and well-being of children. Children living in poor families, especially those located in poor communities, are much more likely than children living in upper- or middle-class families to experience material deprivation and poor health, die during childhood, score lower on standardized tests, be retained in a grade or drop out of school, have out-of-wedlock births, experience violent crime, end up as poor adults, and suffer other undesirable outcomes. In 2003, 17% of U.S. children lived in poverty (defined as income <$18,400/yr for a family of four), a rate among the highest of developed countries. Seven percent lived in extreme poverty. The poverty rates are higher for children than adults and are highest for infants and toddlers. Children who are poor have higher than average rates of death and illness from almost all causes (exceptions being suicide and motor vehicle crashes, which are most common among white, non-poor children). Many factors associated with poverty are responsible for these illnesses; crowding, poor hygiene and health care, poor diet, environmental pollution, poor education, and stress.

Similar poverty-linked disparities may exist in countries with very high infant mortality rates (sub-Saharan Africa). In the low-income developing countries, the rate of infant mortality among the poorest quintile of the population is more than twice that of the wealthiest quintile (Fig. 1-3).

Poverty and economic loss diminish the capacity of parents to be supportive, consistent, and involved with their children. Clinicians need to be especially alert to the development and behavior of children whose parents have lost their jobs or who live in permanent poverty. Fathers who become unemployed frequently develop psychosomatic symptoms, and their children often develop similar symptoms. Young children who grew up in the Great Depression in the United States and whose parents were subject to acute poverty suffered more than older children, especially if the older ones were able to take on responsibilities for helping the family economically. Such responsibilities during adolescence seem to give purpose and direction to an adolescent's life. The younger children, faced with parental depression and unable to do anything to help, suffered a higher frequency of illness and a diminished capacity to lead productive lives even as adults.

Pediatricians and other child health workers have a responsibility both to mitigate the effects of poverty on their patients and to contribute to efforts to reduce the number of children living in poverty. Clinicians should ask parents about their economic resources, adverse changes in their financial situation, and the family's attempts to cope. Encouraging concrete methods of

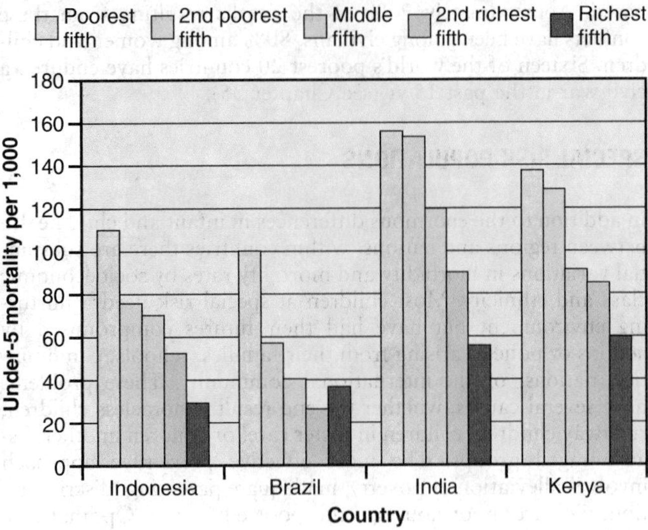

Figure 1-3. Under-5 mortality rates by socioeconomic quintile of the household in selected countries. (From Victora CG, Wagstaff A, Schellenberg JA, et al: Applying an equity lens to child health and mortality: More of the same is not enough. *Lancet* 2003;362:233–241.)

coping, suggesting ways to reduce stressful social circumstances while increasing social networks that are supportive, and referring patients and their families to appropriate welfare, job training, and family agencies can significantly improve the health and functioning of children at risk when their families live in poverty. In many cases, special services, especially social services, need to be added to the traditional medical services; outreach is required to find and encourage parents to use health services and bring their children into the health care system. Pediatricians also have the responsibility to contribute to and advocate for safety net services for impoverished children within and outside the boundaries of their own country. An increasing number of programs are available to help children of greatest need worldwide, such as Project Smile, CARE, Project Hope, and Doctors Without Borders.

CHILDREN OF IMMIGRANTS AND RACIAL MINORITY GROUPS INCLUDING U.S. NATIVE AMERICANS. Eleven percent of the U.S. population is foreign-born; 1 of every 5 children lives in an immigrant family. The United States is experiencing a wave of immigration larger than that occurring in the early 20th century. There has been an increase in immigration from China, India, Southeast Asia, Mexico, the Dominican Republic, and the former Soviet Union nations. Until the mid-20th century, emigrants to the United States were primarily white and from Europe. Such individuals now represent only about 10% of immigrants; the remainder are overwhelmingly of color and from throughout the world. Although immigrants in the United States have faced discrimination and oppression throughout history, the potential for such discrimination is compounded by the racial differences represented in the current immigrant pool. In the United States, about 240,000 children legally immigrate each year, and an estimated 50,000/yr enter the country illegally. Immigrants now comprise >15% of the population in >50 countries, including many Western European countries.

The immigrant population constitutes a substantial proportion of the low-wage labor market. Immigrants represent 14% of all U.S. workers but 20% of low-wage workers. Immigrants are twice as likely as U.S.-born citizens to earn less than minimum wage. The poverty rate of children in immigrant families is 50% greater than in U.S.-born families, with 50% of immigrant children compared to 33% of children in U.S.-born families being below the 200% poverty level. Contributing to the lack of access to higher salaried jobs is the lack of proficiency in English (≈66% of immigrants) and the lack of education (40% have not completed high school). Immigrant fathers are as likely as U.S.-born fathers to work full-time (80%) but are 33–50% less likely to receive social welfare benefits. This gap exists for cultural reasons (many immigrants feeling it inappropriate to accept social support or fearing contact with governmental authorities), logistical complications (especially problematic given limited language skills), and reduced eligibility since the Welfare Reform Act of 1996. In the past decade, about 9 million immigrants attained permanent residency status. There may be 850,000–1,000,000 illegal immigrant children.

Families of different origins obviously bring different health problems and different cultural backgrounds, which influence health practices and use of medical care. To provide appropriate services, clinicians need to understand these influences (see Chapter 4). For example, the high prevalence of hepatitis among women from Southeast Asia makes use of hepatitis B vaccine essential for their newborns. Children from Southeast Asia and South America have growth patterns that are generally below the norms established for children of Western European origin, as well as high rates of hepatitis, parasitic diseases, and nutritional deficiencies and high degrees of psychosocial stress. Foreign-born children may surpass American-born children in many health outcomes, but their health deteriorates as they become acculturated (see Chapter 4).

Refugee children who escape from war or political violence and whose families have been subjected to extreme stress represent a subset of immigrant children who have faced severe trauma. These children have a particularly high incidence of mental and behavioral problems (see Chapter 24).

"Linguistically isolated households," in which no one older than 14 yr of age speaks English, often present significant obstacles to providing quality health care to children because of difficulties in understanding and communicating basic concerns and instructions, avoiding compromising privacy and confidentiality interests, and obtaining informed consent (see Chapter 4).

The United States is home to multiple minority populations, including the 2 largest groups, Latinos and African Americans. The nonwhite minority groups will constitute >50% of the U.S. population by 2050 (see Chapter 4). Nonwhite children in the United States disproportionately experience adverse child health outcomes (see Tables 1-1, 1-2, and 1-3). Infants born to African-American mothers experience low-birthweight and infant mortality rates twice those with white mothers (see Chapter 93). Rates of these 2 adverse health outcomes are also substantially higher among Hispanic infants and children, although there is great variation by country of origin. The rates are particularly high among those of Puerto Rican descent (≈1.5 times the rates for white infants). In 2002, the infant mortality rate for white infants was 5.8/1,000, whereas that for African-America infants was 12.5; for Native Americans, 8.1; and for Hispanics, 5.9 (Table 1-6). Latino, Native American, and African-American children are substantially more likely to live in poverty than are white children.

There are ≈2.5 million Native Americans (4.1 in combination with other races/ethnicities) and 558 federally recognized tribes. With 840,000 children (1.4 million in combination), the Native American population has a much higher proportion of children (34%) than does the remainder of the U.S. population (26%). About 60% of Native Americans live in urban areas, not on or near native lands. Like their minority immigrant counterparts, they have faced social and economic discrimination. The unemployment and poverty levels of Native Americans are, respectively, threefold and fourfold that of the white population, and far fewer Native Americans graduate from high school or go to college. The rate of low birthweight among Native Americans is more than the white rate but less than the black rate. The neona-

TABLE 1-6. Incidence of Low Birthweight and Infant Mortality Among Selected Groups of Native-Born vs Foreign-Born Mothers

	LOW BIRTHWEIGHT (PERCENT)		INFANT MORTALITY (RATE PER 1,000 BIRTHS)	
Racial/Ethnic/ Immigrant Group	Native-Born Mother	Foreign-Born Mother	Native-Born Mother	Foreign-Born Mother
White	4.5	3.9	5.8	4.6
African American	11.8	8.0	12.9	10.5
Mexican	5.4	4.1	6.6	5.3
Puerto Rican	7.9	7.5	7.8	7.0
Cuban	4.7	4.4	5.3	4.7
Central/South American	5.2	4.8	5.2	5.0
Chinese	4.8	3.8	4.6	4.3
Filipino	6.9	6.1	6.8	4.8
Japanese	5.0	5.0	3.7	3.7
Other Asian	5.3	5.7	6.2	5.3

From Landale NS, Oropesa RS, Gorman BK: Immigrants and infant health: Birth outcomes of immigrant and native-born women. In Hernandez DJ (ed): *Children of Immigrants: Health, Adjustment, and Public Assistance.* Washington, DC, National Academy Press, 1999, pp 244–285.

tal and the postneonatal mortality rates are higher for Native Americans living in urban areas than for urban white Americans. Deaths in the 1st yr of life due to sudden infant death syndrome, pneumonia, and influenza are higher than the average in the United States, whereas deaths due to congenital anomalies, respiratory distress syndrome, and disorders relating to short gestation and low birthweight are similar.

Unintended injury deaths among Native Americans occur at twice the rate for other U.S. populations; deaths due to malignant neoplasms are lower. During adolescence and young adulthood, suicide and homicide are the 2nd and 3rd causes of death in this population and occur at about twice the rates of the rest of the population. There may be significant underreporting of deaths of Native American children.

As many as 75% of Native American children have recurrent otitis media and high rates of hearing loss, resulting in learning problems. Tuberculosis and gastroenteritis, formerly much more common among Native Americans, now occur at about the national average. Psychosocial problems are more prevalent in these populations than in the general population: depression, alcoholism, drug abuse, out-of-wedlock teenage pregnancy, school failure and dropout, and child abuse and neglect.

Most other nations have indigenous populations who are subjected to discrimination, social and economic sanctions, and/or physical maltreatment and who demonstrate the poorest child health outcomes. An estimated 300 million indigenous persons live in 70 countries (50% in Asia) and speak ≈4,000 languages. Such children endure lower vaccination rates, lower school entry and higher dropout rates, higher rates of poverty, and lower access to justice. Indigenous children in Latin America account for 66% of the deaths of children younger than age 2 yr.

In the United States, existing programs for meeting child health problems are not available to all families in need, with gaps between eligibility for public support and parents' ability to pay for services. Needed services for immigrants are often either nonexistent or fragmented among programs, agencies, or policies. Programs are often poorly coordinated, and the data collection is inadequate.

CHILDREN OF MIGRANT WORKERS. Families facing economic, social, or political hardship have been forced to leave their land and homes in search of better opportunities; such migrations are often within a country or between neighboring countries. Both industrialized and developing countries experience these migrations.

In the United States, there are an estimated 3–5 million migrant and seasonal farmworkers and their families. The eastern migration is primarily from Florida, whereas the western migration comes from Texas, other border states, and Mexico. Many children travel with their parents and experience poor housing, frequent moves, and a socioeconomic system controlled by a crew boss who arranges the jobs, provides transportation, and often, together with the farm owners, provides food, alcohol, and drugs under a "company store" system that leaves migrant families with little money or in debt. Children often go without schooling; medical care is usually limited.

The medical problems of children of migrant farmworkers are similar to those of children of homeless families: increased frequency of infections (including HIV), trauma, poor nutrition, poor dental care, low immunization rates, exposures to animals and toxic chemicals, anemia, and developmental delays.

Among the most substantial migrant populations in the world is China's "floating population," an estimated 100 million (almost 10% of China's population) of rural to urban migrants. The rapidly growing urban versus rural income gradient and a relaxation of restrictions on movement in the country has fueled this influx of rural residents who arrive in China's urban areas without health, education, or employment benefits for themselves or their children. Similar patterns are seen in many countries in Asia, Africa, and South America. In most of these countries there are few legal or social programs to aid the families or their children, spawning massive squatter settlements without provisions for water, sanitation, education, or basic health needs. Government policies vary worldwide, but frequently their response to such communities is to bulldoze the settlements and imprison or deport the residents.

HOMELESS CHILDREN. Families with children are the fastest growing segment of the homeless population in the United States. Children make up about 25% of the homeless population, with an estimated 100,000 children living in shelters on a given night and about 500,000 homeless each year. Many homeless are not in shelters (living in the street or with extended families), and thus these figures are low estimates. The population of homeless children has been increasing as a consequence of more families with children living in poverty or near poverty, fewer available affordable dwellings for these families, decreasing public assistance programs for the non-elderly poor, and the rising prevalence of substance abuse.

Homeless children have an increased frequency of illness, including intestinal infections, anemia, neurologic disorders, seizures, behavioral disorders, mental illness, and dental problems, as well as increased frequency of trauma and substance abuse. Homeless children are admitted to U.S. hospitals at a much higher rate than the national average. They have higher school failure rates, and the likelihood of their being victims of abuse and neglect is much higher. In one study, 50% of such children were found to have psychosocial problems, such as developmental delays, severe depression, or learning disorders. The increased frequency of maternal psychosocial problems, especially depression, in homeless households has a significant untoward impact on the mental and physical health of these children. Because families tend to break apart under the strain of poverty and homelessness, many homeless children end up in foster care. If their families remain intact, frequent moves make it very difficult for them to receive continuity of medical care.

Homelessness exists worldwide. There are an estimated 3 million people in the 15 countries of the European Union who do not have a permanent home. In Toronto, Canada, 6,500 people stayed in emergency shelters on a typical night in late 1997, a 66% increase over the previous year. In some nations in Latin America, Asia, and Africa, the distinction between rural-to-urban migrants and homelessness is blurred.

Provision of adequate housing, job retraining for the parents, and mental health and social services are necessary to prevent homelessness from occurring. Physicians can have an important role in motivating society to adopt the social policies that will prevent homelessness from occurring by educating policy-makers that these homeless children are at greater risk of becoming burdens both to themselves and to society if their special health needs are not met.

RUNAWAY AND THROWN-AWAY CHILDREN. The number of runaway and thrown-away children and youths in the United States is estimated at about 500,000; several hundred thousand of these children have no secure and safe place to stay. Teenagers make up most of both groups. The usual definition of a runaway is a youth younger than 18 yr who is gone for at least 1 night from his or her home without parental permission. Most runaways leave home only once, stay overnight with friends, and have no contact with the police or other agencies. This group is no different from their "healthy" peers in psychologic status. A smaller but unknown number become multiple or permanent "runners" and are significantly different from the one-time runners.

Thrown-aways include children told directly to leave the household, children who have been away from home and are not allowed to return, abandoned or deserted children, and children who run away but whose caretakers make no effort to recover them or do not appear to care if they return. The same constellation of causes common to many of the other special-risk groups is characteristic of permanent runaways, including environmental problems (family dysfunction, abuse, poverty) and personal problems of the young person (poor impulse control, psychopathology, substance abuse, or school failure). Thrown-aways experience more violence and conflicts in their families.

In the United States, it is a minority of runaway youths who become homeless street people. These youths have a high frequency of problem behaviors, with 75% engaging in some type of criminal activity and 50% engaging in prostitution. A majority of permanent runaways have serious mental problems; more than 33% are the product of families who engage in repeated physical and sexual abuse (see Chapter 36). These children also have a high frequency of medical problems, including hepatitis, sexually transmitted infections, and drug abuse. Although runaways often distrust most social agencies, they will come to and use medical services. Medical care may become the point of re-entry into mainstream society and the path to needed services. U.S. parents who seek a physician's advice about a runaway child should be asked about the child's history of running away, the presence of family dysfunction, and personal aspects of the child's development. If the youth contacts the physician, the latter should examine the youth and assess his or her health status, as well as willingness to return home. If it is not feasible for the youth to return home, foster care, a group home, or an independent living arrangement should be sought by referral to a social worker or a social agency. Although legal considerations involved in the treatment of homeless minor adolescents may be significant, most states, through their "Good Samaritan" laws and definitions of emancipated minors, authorize treatment of homeless youths. Legal barriers should not be used as an excuse to refuse medical care to runaway or thrown-away youths.

The issue of runaway youths is very complex in many developing nations, where in many instances the youth may be orphaned and/or leaving situations of forced sex or other abusive situations. In 2003, there were an estimated 15 million HIV orphans in Africa, an increase of 3.5 million in 2 yr. This number is estimated to grow to 18 million by 2010. With school attendance <50% in many parts of sub-Saharan Africa, children who are orphaned are 17% less likely to attend school. Humanitarian and international organizations have begun to focus on this very vulnerable group of youths across the globe. Rates are often uncertain, and in many countries, these children have not even been recognized as an at-risk group, so great is the social chaos and so massive are the unmet needs.

INHERENT STRENGTHS IN VULNERABLE CHILDREN AND INTERVENTIONS. By age 20–30 yr, many children in the United States and other developed countries who were at special risk will have made moderate successes of their lives. Teenage mothers and children who were born prematurely or in poverty demonstrate that, by this age, the majority have made the transition to stable marriages and jobs and are accepted by their communities as responsible citizens. As the numbers of risk factors increases for an individual, however, the odds for a successful adulthood decline.

Certain biologic characteristics are associated with success, such as being born with an accepting temperament. Avoidance of additional social risks is even more important. Premature infants or preadolescent boys with conduct disorders and poor reading skills, who must also face a broken family, poverty, frequent moves, and family violence, are at much greater risk than children with only 1 of these risks. Perhaps most important are the protective buffers that have been found to enhance children's resilience because these can be aided by an effective health care system and community. Children generally do better if they can gain social support, either from family members or from a nonjudgmental adult outside the family, especially an older mentor or peer. Providers of medical services should develop ways to "prescribe" supportive "other" persons for children who are at risk. Promotion of self-esteem and self-efficacy is a central factor in protection against risks. It is essential to promote competence in some area of these children's lives. Prediction of the consequences of risk is never 100% accurate. However, the confidence that, even without aid, many such children will achieve a good outcome by age 30 yr does not justify ignoring or withholding services from them in early life.

A team is needed because it is rare for 1 individual to be able to provide the multiple services needed for high-risk children. Successful programs are characterized by at least 1 caring person who can make personal contact with these children and their families. Most successful programs are relatively small (or are large programs divided into small units) and nonbureaucratic but are intensive, comprehensive, and flexible. They work not only with the individual, but also with the family, school, community, and at broader societal levels. Generally, the earlier the programs are started, in terms of the age of the children involved, the better is the chance of success. It is also important for services to be continued over a long period.

THE CHALLENGE TO PEDIATRICIANS. Concerns about the aforementioned problems of children throughout the world have generated 3 sets of goals. The *1st set* includes that all families have access to adequate perinatal, preschool, and family-planning services; that international and national governmental activities be effectively coordinated at the global, regional, national, and local levels; that services be so organized that they reach populations at special risk; that there be no insurmountable or inequitable financial barriers to adequate care; that the health care of children have continuity from prenatal through adolescent age periods; and that every family ultimately have access to all necessary services, including developmental, dental, genetic, and mental health services. A *2nd set* of goals addresses the need for reducing unintended injuries and environmental risks, for meeting nutritional needs, and for health education aimed at fostering health-promoting lifestyles. A *3rd set* of goals covers the need for research in biomedical and behavioral science, in fundamentals of bioscience and human biology, and in the particular problems of mothers and children.

The unfinished business in the quest for physical, mental, and social health in the community is illustrated by the disparities with which deaths due to disease, injuries, and violence are distributed among white, black, and Hispanic children in the United States and between and within nations. Homicide is a major cause of adolescent deaths and has increased in rate among the very young, in whom the increase may, in part, represent the more accurate identification of child abuse (see Chapter 36). Among adolescents, homicide may reflect unresolved social tensions, substance abuse (cocaine, crack), and an unhealthy preoccupation with violence in our society (see Part III and Chapters 35, 112, and 113).

PATTERNS OF HEALTH CARE

In 2002, children younger than 18 yr made ≈232 million patient visits to U.S. physicians' offices and hospital outpatient departments. This represents 320 visits per 100 children per year, up from 275 in 1995. Pediatricians report an average of 50 preventive care visits per week, 33% for infants. The visits average 17 to 20 min, increasing in length as children become adolescents. The principal diagnoses, accounting for ≈40% of these visits, are well child visits (15%), middle-ear infections (12%), and injuries (10%). Ambulatory visits by children and youth decrease with age. The opposite occurs with adults. Nonwhite children are more likely than white children to use hospital facilities (including the emergency room) for their ambulatory care; the number of well child visits annually is almost 80% higher among white infants than black infants. Children with private insurance are more likely than children with public insurance who, in turn, are more likely than uninsured children to receive non–emergency room care. Insurance coverage increases outpatient utilization and receipt of preventive care by approximately 1 visit per year for children.

In 2002, there were 80 hospitalizations per 1,000 children, down from 1997 (91/1,000 children), but up from 2000 (76 per 1,000 children). White children are less likely to be hospitalized than black or Hispanic children, but more likely than Asian children. Poor children are nearly twice as likely as non-poor children to be hospitalized. Insurance coverage also appears to reduce hospital admissions that are potentially manageable in an ambulatory setting.

Health care utilization differs significantly among nations. In most countries, however, hospitals are sources of both routine and intensive child care, with medical and surgical services that may range from immunization and developmental counseling to open heart surgery and renal transplantation. In most countries, clinical conditions and procedures requiring intensive care are also likely to be clustered in university-affiliated centers serving as regional resources—if these resources exist.

In the United States, the hospitalization rates for children (excluding newborn infants) are less than those of adults younger than 65 yr of age, except in the 1st yr of life. The rate of hospitalization and lengths of hospital stay have declined significantly for children and adults in the past decade. Children represent <8% of the total acute hospital discharges; in children's hospitals, ≈70% of admissions are for chronic conditions. Ten to 12% of pediatric hospitalizations are related to birth defects and genetic diseases.

Patterns of health care vary widely around the globe, reflecting differences in the geography and wealth of the country, the priority placed on health care vs other competing needs and interests, philosophy regarding prevention vs curative care, and the balance between child health and adult health care needs. The significant declines in infant and child mortality enjoyed in many of the developing countries in the past 3 decades have occurred in the context of support from international agencies like UNICEF, WHO, and the World Bank, bilateral donors (the aid provided from one country to another), and nongovernmental agencies to develop integrated, universal primary pediatric care with an emphasis on primary (vaccination) and selected secondary (oral rehydration solution [ORS], treatment of pneumonia and malaria) prevention strategies.

PLANNING AND IMPLEMENTING A SYSTEM OF CARE

Through much of the 20th century, pediatricians were primarily focused on the treatment and prevention of physical illness and disorders. Currently, physicians caring for children, especially those in developed countries, have been increasingly called on to advise in the management of disturbed behavior of children and adolescents or problematic relationships between child and parent, child and school, or child and community. They are increasingly concerned with problems of mental, social, and societal health. The medical problems of children are often intimately related to problems of mental and social health. There is also an increasing concern about disparities in how the benefits of what we know about child health reach various groups of children. In both developed and developing nations, the health of children lags far behind what it could be if the means and will to apply current knowledge were focused on the health of children. The children most at risk are disproportionately represented among ethnic minority groups. Pediatricians have a responsibility to address these problems aggressively.

Linked with these views of the broad scope of pediatric concern is the concept that access to at least a basic level of quality services to promote health and treat illness is a right of every person. Among children in the United States, having health insurance is strongly associated with access to primary care. The failure of health services and health benefits to reach all children who need them has led to re-examination of the design of health care systems in many countries, but unresolved problems remain in most health care systems, such as the maldistribution of physicians, institutional unresponsiveness to the perceived needs of the individual, failure of medical services to adjust to the need and convenience of patients, and deficiencies in health education. Efforts to make the delivery of health care more efficient and effective have led imaginative pediatricians to create new categories of health care providers, such as pediatric nurse practitioners in industrialized nations and trained birth attendants in developing countries, and to participate in new organizations for providing care to children, such as various managed care arrangements.

New insights into the needs of children have reshaped the child health care system in other ways. Growing understanding of the need of infants for certain qualities of stimulation and care has led to revision of the care of newborn infants (see Chapters 7 and 94) and of procedures leading to an adoption or to placement with foster families (see Chapters 33 and 34). For handicapped children, the massive centralized institutions of past years are being replaced by community-centered arrangements offering a better opportunity for these children to achieve their maximum potential.

HEALTH SERVICES FOR AT-RISK POPULATIONS. Adverse health outcomes are not evenly distributed among all children, but are concentrated in certain high-risk populations. At-risk populations may require additional, targeted, or special programs designed to be effective with unique populations. All nations, regardless of wealth and level of industrialization, have subgroups of children at particular risk, requiring additional services.

In the United States, the largest vulnerable group is children living in poverty, representing about 14% of U.S. children. Substantial proportions of children in other industrialized countries are also living in poverty. The approach to addressing the needs of this group in the United States has been the establishment of a targeted insurance program, Medicaid, which became law in 1965 as a jointly funded cooperative venture between the federal and state governments to assist states in the provision of adequate medical care to eligible needy persons. The federal statute identifies >25 different eligibility categories for which federal funds are available. These statutory categories can be classified into 5 broad coverage groups: children, pregnant women, adults in families with dependent children, individuals with disabilities, and individuals ≥65 yr old. Pediatric care in the United States is highly dependent on Medicaid; however, only a relatively small proportion of the Medicaid funds actually go to child health, with the remainder serving older adults. Following broad national guidelines, each state establishes its own eligibility standards; determines the type, amount, duration, and scope of services; sets the rate of payment for services; and administers its own program. Although Medicaid has made great strides in enrolling low-income children, significant numbers of children remain uninsured. From 1988 to 1998, the proportion of children insured through Medicaid increased from 15.6% to 19.8%, but the percentage of children without health insurance increased from 13.1% to 15.4%. Minority children were disproportionately among those without insurance. The Balanced Budget Act of 1997 created a new children's health insurance program called the State Children's Health Insurance Program (SCHIP). This program gave each state permission to offer health insurance for children, up to age 19 yr, who are not already insured. SCHIP is a state-administered program and each state sets its own guidelines regarding eligibility and services. There is great variation by state, but in many states, the SCHIP program has begun to reduce racial inequities in access to health care for children.

Many industrialized nations have adapted different "safety net" systems to assure adequate coverage of all youth. Many of these programs provide health insurance for all children, regardless of income, hoping to avoid problems with children losing insurance coverage and access to health care due to changes in eligibility by providing a single form of insurance that all providers accept. The response of developing countries to the issue of universal access to care for children has been uneven, with some providing no safety net, but many having limited universal or safety net services.

To address the special needs of Native Americans in the United States, the Indian Health Service, established in 1954, has been the responsibility of the Public Health Service, but the 1975 Indian Self-Determination Act gave tribes the option of managing Native American health services in their communities. The Indian Health Service is managed through local administrative units, and some tribes contract outside the Indian Health Service for health care. Much of the emphasis is on adult services: treatment for alcoholism, nutrition and dietetic counseling, and public health nursing services. There are also >40 urban programs for Native Americans, with an emphasis on increasing access of this population to existing health services, providing special social services, and developing self-help groups. In an effort to accommodate traditional Western medical, psychologic, and social services to the Native American cultures, such programs include the "Talking Circle," the "Sweat Lodge," and other interventions based on Native American culture (see Chapter 4). The efficacy of any of these programs, especially those to prevent and treat the sociopsychologic problems particular to Native Americans, has not been determined.

Recognizing the health needs of migrants in the United States, the U.S. Public Health Service initiated in 1964 the Migrant Health Program to provide funds for local groups to organize medical care for migrant families. Many migrant health projects, which were staffed initially by part-time providers and were open for only part of the year, have been transformed into community health care centers that provide services not only for migrants, but also for other local residents. In 2001, the ≈400 Migrant Health Centers served >650,000 migrant and seasonal farmworkers; >85% were people of color. Health services for migrant farmworkers often need to be organized separately from existing primary care programs because the families are migratory. Special record-keeping systems that link the health care provided during winter months in the south with the care provided during the migratory season in the north are difficult to maintain in ordinary group practices or individual physicians' offices. Outreach programs that take medical care to the often remote farm sites are necessary, and specially organized Head Start, early education, and remedial education programs should also be provided. Approaches in other countries have also focused on business initiatives for migrant populations to enable them to overcome the cycle of financial dependency on their migratory lifestyle.

The United States has spent >$10 billion through the 1987 McKinney Act to provide emergency food, shelter, and health care; to finance help for young runaways; to aid homeless people in making their way back into the housing market; and to place homeless children in school. Mobile vans, with a team consisting of a physician, nurse, social worker, and welfare worker, have been shown to provide effective comprehensive care, ensure delivery of immunizations, link the children to school health services, and bring the children and their families into a stable relationship with the conventional medical system. Special record-keeping systems have been introduced to enhance continuity and to provide a record of care once the family has moved to a permanent location. Because of the high frequency of developmental delays in this group, linkage of preschool homeless children to Head Start programs is an especially important service. The Runaway Youth Act, Title III of the Juvenile Justice and Delinquency Prevention Act of 1974 (Public Law 93-414) and its amended version (Public Law 95-509) have supported shelters and provide a toll-free 24 hr telephone number (1-800-621-4000) for youths who wish to contact their parents or request help after having run away.

In Belgium, Finland, the Netherlands, Portugal, and Spain, the right to housing has been incorporated into the national constitutions. The Finnish government has devised a multifaceted response to the problem, including house building, social welfare and health care services, and the obligation to provide a home of minimum standards for every homeless person. The number of homeless in Finland has been reduced by 50%.

COSTS OF HEALTH CARE

The growth of high technology, the increasing number of people older than 65 yr, the redesign of health institutions (particularly with respect to the needs for and the uses of personnel), the public's demand for medical services, the increase in administrative bureaucracies, and the manner in which the costs of health care are paid have driven the costs of health care in the United States up to a point at which they represent a significant proportion of the gross national product. Although children (0–18 yr) represent about 25% of the population, they account for only about 12% of the health care expenditures, or about 60% of adult per capita expenditures. Efforts to contain costs have led to revisions of the way in which physicians and hospitals are paid for services. Limits have been set on the fees for some services, capitated prepayment and various managed care systems flourish, a program of reimbursement (diagnosis-related groups [DRGs]) based on the diagnosis rather than on the particular services rendered to an individual patient has been implemented, and a relative value scale for varying rates of payment among different physician services has been instituted. These and other changes in the system of financing health services raise important ethical, quality of care, and professional issues for pediatricians to address (see Chapter 3).

Health care costs have been better contained in most other industrialized nations, the majority of which also enjoy lower childhood mortality rates than does the United States.

EVALUATION OF HEALTH CARE

The shaping of health care systems to meet the needs of children and their families requires accurate statistical data and difficult decisions in setting priorities. Along with growing concerns about the design and cost of health care systems and the ability to distribute health services equitably has come increasing concern about the quality of health care and about its efficiency and effectiveness. There are large local and regional variations among similar populations of children in the rates of use of procedures and technology and of hospital admissions. These variations require continuing evaluation and explanation in terms of the actual impact of medical and surgical services on health status and the outcome of illness.

The Institute of Medicine (IOM) issued a report, "Crossing the quality chasm: A new health system for the 21st century" in 2001. This report, challenging American physicians to renew efforts to focus not just on access and cost, but also on quality of care, has been furthered in several pediatric initiatives, including but not limited to: specific initiatives for monitoring child health outlined in the IOM report "Children's Health, the Nation's Wealth," challenge/demonstration grants funded by the Robert Wood Johnson Foundation, the National Initiative for Children's Healthcare Quality, and training initiatives by the Federation of Pediatric Organizations. Importantly, each of these initiatives is calling for the establishment of measurable standards for assessment of quality of care and for the establishment of routine plans for periodic reassessment thereof. Efforts have been initiated at some medical centers to establish evidence-based clinical pathways for disorders (such as asthma) where there exists sound evidence to advise these guidelines. Pediatricians have developed tools to evaluate the content and delivery of pediatric preventive "anticipatory guidance," the cornerstone of modern pediatrics (see Chapter 5).

Increased attention has been focused during residency training and as part of continuing education on the importance of providing pediatricians with the skills to communicate effectively with parents and patients. These efforts are having an impact, with evidence that 66% of children are receiving good or excellent preventive care with no disparities according to race or income level. The increased focus on quality improvement in pediatric practice is reflected in the pediatric residency training competency requirements of practice-based learning and improvement- and system-based practice.

ORGANIZATION OF THE PROFESSION AND THE GROWTH OF SPECIALIZATION

The 20th century witnessed the formation of professional societies of pediatricians around the globe. Some of these societies, such as the American Board of Pediatrics (ABP), are concerned with education and the awarding of credentials certifying competence as a pediatrician and/or a pediatric subspecialist. At the beginning of 2004, the ABP reported that there were ≈79,000 board-certified pediatricians. Among those presenting for 1st time certification to the ABP in 2003, 80% were American Medical Graduates (20% were International Medical Graduates) and 63% were women. Other societies are primarily concerned with organizing members of the profession in their country or region to dedicate their efforts and resources toward children. In the United States, the American Academy of Pediatrics (AAP), formed in 1930, currently has a membership of ≈60,000 child health specialists in both academic and private practice. Most general pediatricians in the United States enter private practice; ≈66% are in group practices, 5% enter solo practice, and 5% work in a health maintenance organization. The AAP provides a variety of continuing educational services to pediatricians in multiple national and regional settings and tracks the professional activities and practices of its members. A comparable group in India, the Indian Academy of Pediatrics, was formed in 1963, and now has >13,000 members and 16 subspecialty chapters. Likewise, the Pakistani Pediatrics Association is >35 years old, the Malaysian Pediatric Association was started about 25 years ago, and the Canadian Pediatric Society was founded in 1922. These societies represent but a few of the many national and regional pediatric professional organizations around the world.

The amount of information relevant to child health care is rapidly expanding, and no person can become master of it all. Physicians are increasingly dependent on one another for the highest quality of care for their patients. About 25% of pediatricians in the United States claim an area of special knowledge and skill, including 15,000 who have board certification in 1 of the 13 pediatric subspecialties with board certification. Each year about 10% of the ≈3,000 pediatric residents training in the United States are enrolled in a dual residency training program that will lead to eligibility for board certification in both pediatrics and internal medicine.

The growth of specialization within pediatrics has taken a number of different forms: interests in problems of age groups of children have created neonatology and adolescent medicine; interests in organ systems have created pediatric cardiology, neurology, child development, allergy, hematology, nephrology, gastroenterology, child psychiatry, pulmonology, endocrinology, and specialization in metabolism and genetics; interests in the health care system have created pediatricians devoted to ambulatory care, emergency care, and intensive care; and, finally, multidisciplinary subspecialties have grown up around the problems of handicapped children, to which pediatrics, neurology, psychiatry, psychology, nursing, physical and occupational therapy, special education, speech therapy, audiology, and nutrition all make essential contributions. This growth of specialization has been most conspicuous in university-affiliated departments of pediatrics and medical centers for children.

In the United States, most subspecialists practice in academic settings or children's hospitals. Likewise, specialists are growing in number in other industrialized countries and in developing nations that are becoming industrialized.

NEED FOR CONTINUING SELF-EDUCATION

The explosion of information has also created new challenges for continuing education. In earlier years, new information in any field of medicine was easily accessible through a relatively small number of journals, texts, or monographs. Today, relevant information is so widely dispersed among the many journals that elaborate electronic data systems are necessary to make it accessible. The Internet has dramatically improved access to information by physicians and patients, but judgment about the quality, clinical significance, accuracy, bias, and appropriate use of such information is a challenge. In 2002, 95% of pediatricians surveyed reported using a computer in the office; 50% reported accessing the Internet daily, most for medical information. One third used a personal digital assistant, most frequently for scheduling and for access to pharmacology references. Only 14% reported using email to communicate with patients, although about 50% would accept prescription refill requests by email. The American Board of Pediatrics and the American Academy of Pediatrics have arranged for close linkage of continuing education of pediatricians to recertification in pediatrics.

Whereas the Internet is important in the United States, it is revolutionizing access to medical knowledge in developing and transitional countries. Previously, medical schools in these settings were highly dependent on slow and often unpredictable mail systems to connect them with medical advances, new directions in medical practice, and medical colleagues in general. Now, many of the same schools have immediate access to hundreds of journals and their professional counterparts across the globe.

There is no touchstone through which physicians can ensure that the process of their own continuing education will keep them abreast of advancing knowledge in the field, but they must find a way to base their decisions on the best available scientific evidence if they are to discharge their responsibility to their patients. An essential element of this process may be for physicians to take an active role, such as participating in medical student and resident education. Efforts in continuing self-education will also be fostered if clinical problems can be made a stimulus for a review of standard literature, alone or in consultation with an appropriate colleague or consultant. This continuing review will do much to identify those inconsistencies or contradictions that will indicate, in the ultimate best interest of patients, that things are not what they seem or have been said to be. Physicians still learn most from their patients, but this will not be the case if they fall into the easy habit of accepting their patients' problems casually or at face value because the problems appear to be simple.

The tools that physicians must use in dealing with the problems of children and their families fall into three main categories: *cognitive* (up-to-date factual information about diagnostic and therapeutic issues, available on recall or easily found in readily accessible sources, and the ability to relate this information to the pathophysiology of their patients in the context of individual biologic variability); *interpersonal or manual* (the ability to carry out a productive interview, execute a reliable physical examination, perform a deft venipuncture, or manage cardiac arrest or resuscitation of a depressed newborn infant); and *attitudinal* (the physician's unselfish commitment to the fullest possible implementation of knowledge and skills on behalf of children and their families in an atmosphere of empathic sensitivity and concern). With regard to this last category, it is important that children participate with their families in informed decision-making about their own health care in a manner appropriate to their stage of development and the nature of the particular health problem.

The workaday needs of professional persons for knowledge and skills in care of children vary widely. Primary care physicians need depth in developmental concepts and in the ability to organize an effective system for achieving quality and continuity in assessing and planning for health care during the entire period of growth. They may often have little or no need for immediate recall of esoterica. On the other hand, consultants or subspecialists not only need a comfortable grasp of both common and uncommon facts within their field and perhaps within related fields, but also must be able to cope with controversial issues with flexibility that will permit adaptation of various points of view to the best interest of their unique patient.

At whatever level of care (primary, secondary, or tertiary) or in whatever position (student, pediatric nurse practitioner, resident pediatrician, practitioner of pediatrics or family medicine, or pediatric or other subspecialists), professional persons dealing with children must be able to identify their roles of the moment and their levels of engagement with a child's problem; each must determine whether his or her experience and other resources at hand are adequate to deal with this problem and must be ready to seek other help when they are not. Among the necessary resources are general textbooks, more detailed monographs in subspecialty areas, selected journals, access to Internet materials, audiovisual aids, and, above all, colleagues with exceptional or complementary experience and expertise. The intercommunication of all these levels of engagement with medical and health problems of children offers the best hope of bringing us closer to the goal of providing the opportunity for all children to achieve their maximum potential.

Annie E. Casey Foundation: *African-American Children: State-Level Measures of Child Well-Being from the 2000 Census: Kids Count 2003*. Baltimore, Annie E. Casey Foundation, 2004.

Anell A, Willis M: International comparison of health care systems using resource profiles. *Bull World Health Organ* 2000;78:770–778.

Black E, Morris S, Bryce J: Where and why are 10 million children dying every year? *Lancet* 2003;361:2226–2234.

Dwivedi KN, Banhattie RG: Attention deficit/hyperactivity disorder and ethnicity. *Arch Dis Child* 2005;90:i10–i12.

Ebbeling CB, Pawlak DB, Ludwig DS: Childhood obesity: Public-health crisis, common sense cure. *Lancet* 2002;360:473–482.

Haskins R, Greenberg M, Fremstad S: Federal policy for immigrant children: Room for common ground? *Future Child* 2004;14:1–6.

Horton R: Indigenous peoples: Time to act now for equity and health. *Lancet* 2006;367:1705–1707.

Khamis V: Post-traumatic stress disorder among school age Palestinian children. *Child Abuse Negl* 2005;29:81–95.

Kochanek K, Smith B: Deaths: Preliminary data for 2002. *Natl Vital Stat Rep* 2004;52:1–47.

Lancet: Getting it right for children: a review of UNICEF joint health and nutrition strategy for 2006–2015. *Lancet* 2006;368:817–818.

Laraque D, Boscarino JA, Battista A, et al: Reactions and needs of tristate-area pediatricians after the events of September 11th: Implications for children's mental health services. *Pediatrics* 2004;113:1357–1366.

Marmot M: Social determinants of health inequalities. *Lancet* 2006;365: 1099–1104.

Navarro V, Muntaner C, Borrell C, et al: Politics and health outcomes. *Lancet* 2006;368:1033–1037.

Oberg CN, Rinaldi M: Pediatric health disparities. *Current Problems in Pediatric and Adolescent Health Care.* 2006;36:245–276.

Okie S: Global health: The Gates-Buffett effect. *N Engl J Med* 2006;355: 1084–1088.

Pearson HA, Anunziato D, Baker JP, et al: Committee report: American pediatrics: Milestones at the millennium. *Pediatrics* 2001;107:1482–1491.

Santos Pais M, Bissell S: Overview and implementation of the UN convention on the rights of the child. *Lancet* 2006;367:689–701.

Srivastava R, Norlin C, James BC, et al: Community and hospital-based physicians' attitudes regarding pediatric hospitalist systems. *Pediatrics* 2005;115: 34–38.

United Nation's Children's Fund (UNICEF): Children in jeopardy: The challenge of freeing poor nations from the shackles of debt. New York, UNICEF, 1999.

United Nation's Children's Fund (UNICEF): The state of the world's children 2005. New York, UNICEF, 2004.

US Census Bureau: Income, poverty, and health insurance coverage in the United States: 2003. Washington DC, US Census Bureau, 2004.

US Department of Health and Human Services, National Center for Health Statistics: *Health, United States, 2004. Trends in the Health of American Chartbook*. Washington, DC, US Department of Health and Human Services, 2004.

Woolf SH, Johnson RE, Geiger HJ: The rising prevalence of severe poverty in America—a growing threat to public health. *Am J Prev Med* 2006;31: 332–341.

Zuckerman B, Stevens GD, Inkelas M, Halfon N: Prevalence and correlates of high-quality basic pediatric preventive care. *Pediatrics* 2004;114: 1522–1529.

Chapter 2 ■ Quality and Safety in Health Care for Children

Carole Lannon

THE QUALITY GAP

Some care, for some children, some of the time is excellent: evidence-based, responsive to child and family needs, and resulting in superb outcomes. Advances in public health, management of infectious and other diseases, and technology in the past century have greatly improved the health of children and families. Despite concerted efforts by physicians and dedicated clinical teams, a large gap exists between knowledge and practice. These are significant variations in the outcomes of care across providers and communities, in the utilization of appropriate care, in disparities of care for ethnic and minority children, and in the safety and quality of care for all children:

- **One quarter of young children are not up-to-date on immunizations**
- **One third of parents of young children are not asked about their child's speech and language development**
- **Less than half of adolescents discuss health behaviors with their clinician**
- **Up to three quarters of sexually active adolescents do not receive chlamydia screening**
- **One third of children with persistent asthma do not receive a prescription for long-acting medications to control their asthma.**
- **Across cystic fibrosis centers, patient life expectancy varies by as much as 14 yr**

The Institute of Medicine (IOM) highlighted this gap between knowledge and practice. "At no time in the history of medicine has the growth in knowledge and technologies been so profound . . . As medical science and technology have advanced at a rapid pace, however, the healthcare system has floundered in its ability to provide consistently high-quality care to all Americans."

WHAT IS "QUALITY CARE"?

Avedis Donabedian posited that "the balance of health benefits and harm is the essential core of a definition of quality." An IOM report defined quality of care as "the degree to which healthcare services for individuals and populations increase the likelihood of desired health outcomes and are consistent with current professional knowledge."

The IOM described quality in a goal-oriented manner and established 6 aims for the 21st century health care system: safe, effective, patient-centered, timely, efficient, and equitable (Table 2-1). Implicit in these definitions is the idea that quality components can be *measured* and *improved.*

HOW DO WE MEASURE QUALITY?

A **quality measure** attempts to quantify the nature of the care currently being provided and what that care would be like if based on the current best evidence as determined by pre-established criteria (www.ahrq.gov/qual/measurix.htm). Three different components to assess the quality of health care are: *structure, process, and outcome.*

Structure refers to the resources and organizational characteristics that are in place to deliver care. Examples of organizational characteristics include the type of care provided (primary, specialty), the supports to provide care (number of nurses staffing a pediatric intensive care unit, the percentage of board-certified pediatricians at a facility), and the use of specific systems for improving care (an electronic health record or registry). Accreditation by recognized national organizations, such as the Joint Commission on Accreditation of Healthcare Organizations, is based in part on assessment of structural characteristics.

Process measures address how care and services are provided (assessment, evaluation, diagnosis, treatment). The frequency of use of a structured assessment to appropriately diagnose a child with attention-deficit/hyperactivity disorder (ADHD) is a *process* measure. Similarly, the proportion of families of children with asthma that receive a written asthma management plan is a process measure. Process measures are the usual targets of quality improvement interventions, as making changes in practice involves addressing particular clinical processes.

Outcome measures describe how the care delivered affects the patient's health, health status, or function. Emergency department (ED) visits or hospitalizations due to asthma exacerbations are considered outcome measures. Health outcomes may occur infrequently and are often influenced by a variety of factors. Improvement efforts often focus on structural or process measures that have been proven to be associated with health outcomes. Research has shown that the use of an asthma management plan (a process measure) results in decreased hospitalizations and ED visits (outcome measures).

Quality measures describe an *observed* level of performance (percentage of hospitalized children with bloodstream infections related to central lines) but do not address *why* the result is at a certain level or the factors that contribute to it. Multiple factors have been shown to affect the rate of central line infections, including handwashing protocols, barrier protection during insertion, and antiseptic preparation.

Quality measures can be influenced by a variety of factors, including data availability, data accuracy and completeness, and patient characteristics. Although measures should be adjusted for patient characteristics ("case mix," "severity adjustment"), these differences can highlight important factors in variation such as disparities in care between races. Further, patient characteristics are not limited to biologic considerations but also include personal, social, and cultural issues. Quality of care can be described as the best possible science in the context of what the patient wants and needs (patient-centered care).

TABLE 2-1. Crossing the Quality Chasm

- **Safe:** avoiding injuries to patients from the care that is intended to help them
- **Effective:** providing services based on scientific knowledge to all who could benefit and refraining from providing services to those not likely to benefit
- **Patient-centered:** providing care that is respectful of and responsive to individual patient preferences, needs, and values and ensuring that patient values guide all clinical decisions
- **Timely:** reducing waits and sometimes harmful delays for both those who receive and those who give care
- **Efficient:** avoiding waste, including waste of equipment, supplies, ideas, and energy
- **Equitable:** providing care that does not vary in quality because of personal characteristics such as gender, ethnicity, geographic location, and socioeconomic status

From Institute of Medicine: Committee on Quality Health Care in America, *Crossing the Quality Chasm: A New Health System for the 21st Century.* Washington, DC, National Academy Press, 2001. Reprinted with permission from the National Academies Press, Copyright 2001, National Academy of Sciences.

THE USE OF MEASURES

Measurement for continuous quality improvement can be used to help a practice or organization understand its own care processes as well as understand how its performance compares to others. A practice or organization can use data to compare its performance: (1) against itself over time, (2) against other organizations collecting data in the same way and using the same measures, and (3) to industry leaders or exemplary performing organizations. This is benchmarking: Initial steps in improvement efforts involve the use of measures to document performance gaps as well as identify and learn from high functioning organizations.

The IOM has outlined uses of quality measures that involve accountability as well as improvement: (1) ensuring the rapid translation of clinical research into practice; (2) holding providers accountable for delivering high-quality care; (3) setting standards of participation in federally sponsored programs including Medicaid, SCHIP, Title V, and community health centers; (4) helping parents and purchasers make choices; (5) establishing benchmarks to stimulate quality improvement; and (6) conducting ongoing national surveillance on trends in quality. These applications have the potential to involve a variety of users, including patients, providers, purchasers, payers, business coalitions, accrediting organizations, and government.

Multiple measures of quality that assess various components of a specific aspect of health care may be selected to give a more complete picture of overall performance and increase the reliability of the result. A state agency may choose to use several parental perception measures as well as several measures of the delivery of preventive care to assess the quality of a health plan or program in delivering health care to enrolled children. By identifying variations in care, opportunities for improvement and best practices can be identified (www.ahrq.gov/qual/measurix.htm).

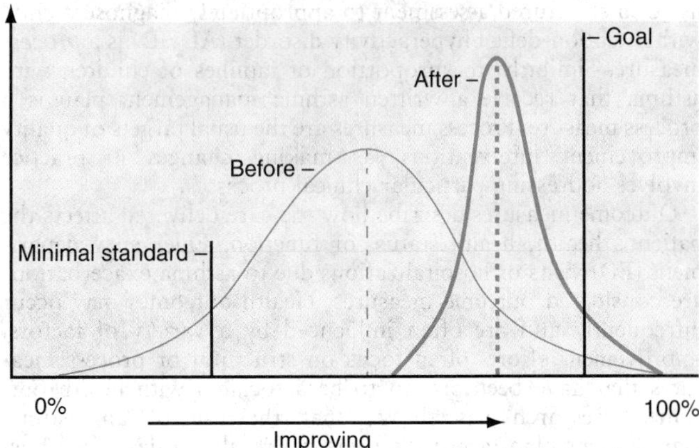

Figure 2-1. Improving quality by reducing variation and shifting the mean. This is illustrated in an example from the End-Stage Renal Disease Registry (see Fig. 2-4).

With enough available data, a quality measure is likely to have a normal distribution curve (Fig. 2-1). Quality improvement methods aim to standardize the process of care and improve outcomes by narrowing the distribution and shifting the curve to the right.

Table 2-2 provides a framework for achieving the IOM 6 aims or goals for the 21st century health care (see Table 2-1).

TABLE 2-2. The Chain of Effect in Improving Healthcare Quality

I. Environmental context
II. Macro-organization (health care organizations)
III. Microsystem of care delivery (practice)
IV. Patient and the community

A THEORETICAL FRAMEWORK FOR IMPROVING QUALITY OF CARE IN THE HEALTH SYSTEM

This framework recognizes that multiple layers of the health care system influence the ability to improve care for the child and family: the experience of patients and families (patient and the community); the functioning of small units of care delivery (microsystems); the functioning of the organizations that house or otherwise support microsystems (macrosystems); and the environment (policy, payment, regulation) that shapes the behavior, interests, and opportunities of the organizations. Efforts at each of the different levels of the health care system *and the interactions between them* can influence the ability to achieve patient safety and quality of care objectives.

Strategies to improve care must be targeted at all four levels in order to close the gap between current knowledge and practices. It is not surprising that multiple studies of strategies used to change practice demonstrate that the passive provision of information, as in traditional didactic continuing medical education, rarely achieves its intended goal. Knowledge is essential but not sufficient to produce behavior change. Successful efforts to improve care recognize that multiple layers of the health care system must work together to achieve better outcomes. This may be why multifaceted interventions based on assessment of potential barriers at all levels of the health care system are more likely to be effective than interventions that only focus on addressing barriers related to individual levels of the health care system. Guidelines can be most effectively translated into standard practice through active learning opportunities, learning delivered in a longitudinal or sequenced manner, and the provision of methods to facilitate implementation in the practice setting (tools and resources).

One example of an effort to effect change by understanding and addressing gaps at all four levels of health care and their interaction is the development of a multifaceted American Academy of Pediatrics (AAP) program, "From Policy to Practice: Improving care for Children with Attention Deficit Hyperactivity Disorder (ADHD)," which translates guidelines for the diagnosis and treatment of ADHD into clinical practice. The ADHD effort consists of a several-year program of coordinated activities targeting the various levels of the health care system. It includes advocacy efforts to dismantle financial and organizational obstacles to promote timely access to care in the medical home setting (environment). Structured educational opportunities support improved care in AAP chapters and residency programs (macrosystem). These opportunities provide clinicians with practical tools as well as a web-based continuing medical education/quality improvement program (the AAP's Education for Quality Improvement in Pediatric Practice, www.eqipp.org) [microsystem]. AAP also developed multiple resources for children and families, such as a parent education brochure, a full-length book, a video, and patient education materials for teens (patient and community). A key component of this effort has been supporting the development of systems for improvement at the AAP state chapter level for clinicians, families, and schools. AAP's effort demonstrates how a theoretical framework can aid in the design and implementation of improvement efforts, including the use by clinicians and in practices of improvement science to implement successful strategies for change at the microsystem level.

PRACTICAL STRATEGIES FOR IMPROVEMENT: THE FOUNDATIONS OF IMPROVEMENT SCIENCE

The foundation of improvement science consists of the interplay among theories of systems, variation, psychology, and knowledge. A system is described as "a network of interdependent components that work together to try to accomplish the aim of the system." Systems theory suggests that the success of an organization will depend on its ability to integrate and align the various components that make up its system. Variation occurs in *all* systems. The application of QI methods can decrease unintended variation. This is important because standardization of care provides the necessary base in which new approaches can be tested and evaluated more rapidly. In addition, it is essential that those leading improvement efforts acknowledge that making changes to established patterns is difficult. It is useful to learn techniques to establish buy-in, overcome resistance, and facilitate helpful interactions among team members. The scientific method of testing hypotheses is illustrated in the following section.

THE MODEL FOR IMPROVEMENT. This model contains three fundamental questions that form the basis of improvement science (Fig. 2-2). The initial step is to develop the aim, a written statement that specifies what measurable improvements the team will accomplish and in what time frame. Next, measures are selected that will help the teams assess progress. After considering what changes can be made to improve care, the clinician next must determine *how* to implement and test whether the changes have resulted in improvement. This can be done using a framework for rapid cycle improvement known as the Plan-Do-Study-Act (PDSA, PDCA, or Shewhart) Cycle (Fig. 2-3). Recognizing that not all changes result in improvement, but that all improvement requires change, the cycle begins with a plan and ends with action based on the learning from the cycle. This approach has 4 distinct phases for developing a change, testing the change, implementing it, and then studying its results. A series of these small-scale tests can build knowledge sequentially and yield useful information quickly. In the microsystems in which care is delivered (a newborn nursery, an office practice, a pediatric inten-

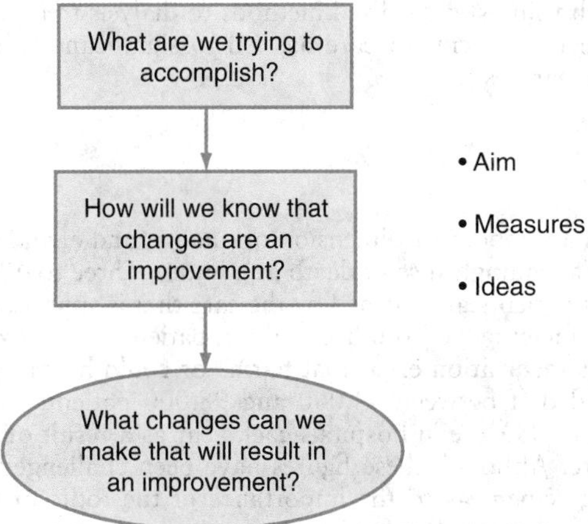

Figure 2-2. Model for Improvement. (From Langley GJ: *The Improvement Guide: A Practical Guide to Enhancing Organizational Performance.* San Francisco, Jossey-Bass, 1996. © 1996 by Gerald J. Langley, Kevin M. Nolan, Thomas W. Nolan, L. Norman, and Lloyd P. Provost. Reprinted with permission of John Wiley & Sons, Inc.)

sive care unit), a series of PDSA tests linked with simple tracking of data for improvement can be helpful in determining whether a change has resulted in improvement.

The Vermont Oxford Network (VON) has used the Model for Improvement to make significant improvements in the quality of neonatal care. VON is a voluntary collaboration of health professionals whose mission is to improve the quality and safety of medical care for newborn infants and their families. VON maintains a database for very low birthweight infants at its >500 member hospitals across the United States and in other countries. In an effort to integrate research into daily practice, VON has used this database for clinical trials, cohort studies, outcomes research, and quality improvement collaborative efforts. The network undertook a program to reduce rates of chronic lung disease in extremely low birthweight infants. Based on evidence review, expert consensus, and network experience, a series of key changes were identified involving the use of surfactant for premature infants. Participating clinical teams assessed their current

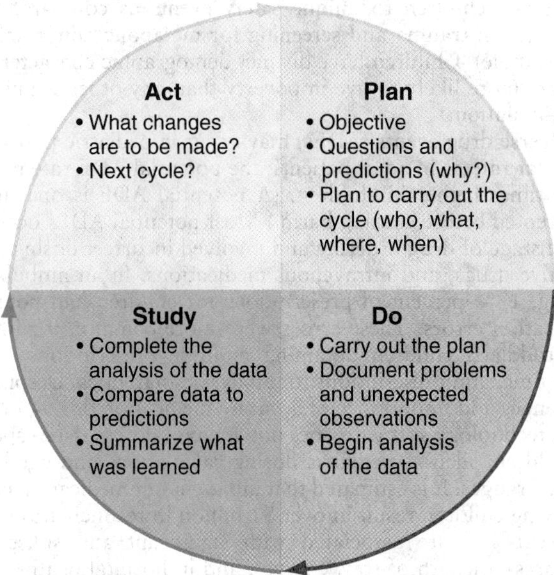

Figure 2-3. The Plan-Do-Study-Act Cycle. (From Langley GJ: *The Improvement Guide: A Practical Guide to Enhancing Organizational Performance.* San Francisco, Jossey-Bass, 1996. © 1996 by Gerald J. Langley, Kevin M. Nolan, Thomas W. Nolan, L. Norman, and Lloyd P. Provost. Reprinted with permission of John Wiley & Sons, Inc.)

TABLE 2-3. An Example of Using the Model for Improvement

AIM	Intubation and surfactant administration to all infants <29 wk gestation in the delivery room within 10 min of birth
MEASURES	Time to administration of surfactant after birth
IDEAS	1. Make the surfactant available in the delivery room. 2. Eliminate need for a chest radiograph to confirm endotracheal tube position (waiting for a chest x-ray delays administration of surfactant). 3. Have discussions with the other physicians and nurse practitioners in group to get everyone to agree to the practice change.

practice using special reports from the VON database, reviewed the evidence with faculty experts, and then set measurable improvement goals. Each team set its own aims based on their assessment of the evidence and of the tradeoffs involved with changing practice. The teams received quality improvement (QI) training and ongoing support through conference calls and email for a 12 mo period. VON achieved a 37% increase in early surfactant administration for preterm infants, one of the largest effects seen in the literature for changing the behavior of health professionals and promoting evidence-based practice (Table 2-3).

Performance measurement, collaboration among clinical teams, and quality improvement support are common elements in successful improvement efforts. Quality measurement and improvement efforts such as those of VON are facilitated through the use of an integrated data system, quality improvement toolkits, workshops, and technical assistance. The Vermont Child Health Improvement Program (VCHIP) and the California Perinatal Quality Care Collaborative (CPQCC) are additional examples of organizational programs that collaborate with multiple health care partners to provide quality improvement training and data feedback that support improvements in care at a statewide level.

CREATING AN ENVIRONMENT THAT REQUIRES AND SUPPORTS QUALITY IMPROVEMENT

Several efforts in the policy arena work to create an environment that is conducive to quality improvement throughout the health care system.

CERTIFICATION OF INDIVIDUAL PHYSICIANS AND TRAINING PROGRAMS. Specialty certification in medicine was once based solely on individual knowledge (passing an examination) rather than actual performance in practice. Beyond individual state requirements for continuing medical education, no further evidence of competency needed to be demonstrated. There is significant variation in care, even among board-certified physicians, indicating that medical knowledge is necessary but not sufficient for the delivery of quality care. In response to evolving evidence about the limited effectiveness of knowledge-based approaches alone in ensuring the quality of care, the American Board of Medical Specialties (ABMS) and its member boards, including the American Board of Pediatrics (ABP), have created a more continuous process of recertification in which physicians will be required to document performance measurement, practice improvement, and systems thinking as a part of Maintenance of Certification (MOC) in addition to periodically passing a test of knowledge. Of particular relevance is Part IV of MOC of the ABP, the Practice Performance component, which will require demonstration of the assessment of quality of care and implementation of systematic improvement strategies.

The ABMS actions have built on the competencies for residency training programs developed by the Accreditation Council for Graduate Medical Education (ACGME). The ACGME now requires Common Program Requirements that mandate that certified residency training programs ensure that residents demonstrate "practice-based learning and improvement" involving assimilation of scientific evidence and systems-based practice (www.acgme.org) in addition to other competencies (knowledge, patient care, communication skills, professionalism).

POLICY AND REGULATORY EFFORTS TO INDUCE IMPROVEMENT EFFORTS. Public and private organizations have attempted to influence quality of care through policy. In the late 1990s, policy-makers and payer organizations began to develop programs that reward high-quality care in an effort to improve quality in the U.S. health care system. The programs use provider performance measures as quality indicators. These programs are called pay-for-performance (P4P). An IOM report has called for "purchasing strategies that encourage the adoption of best practices through the release of public domain comparative quality data and the provision of financial and other rewards to achieve high levels of quality." Although there is little research to date regarding the effectiveness of reward programs on quality, supporters of P4P programs believe that these incentive efforts will lead to significant improvements in the quality of care.

Other organizations have attempted to provide practices with guidance for effective measurement and reporting of quality data. The National Quality Forum (NQF) was created in 1999 with the intent of improving American health care through the endorsement of consensus-based national standards for measurement and public reporting of health care performance data that provide meaningful information about whether care meets the six IOM dimensions of quality (see Table 2-1). The congressionally mandated National Healthcare Quality and Disparities Report, published annually by the Agency for Healthcare Research and Quality, includes a broad set of performance and outcome indicators to monitor the nation's progress toward improved health care quality.

QUALITY IMPROVEMENT AS A MEANS OF ADDRESSING DISPARITIES IN CARE

Advances in quality can help to minimize racial, ethnic, and socioeconomic disparities in health outcomes that result, at least partially, from differential quality of care. As a result, the quality curve not only shifts to the right (denoting improvement), but it also narrows, demonstrating a reduction in the variation of outcomes among different populations (see Fig. 2-1). An excellent example of this is the End-Stage Renal Disease Network. The management of end-stage renal disease has shown significant improvement in quality of care (effectiveness of dialysis; Fig. 2-4) with the use of a national database and a collaborative approach using standardized methods to dialysis treatment. This focus on the systems of care has led to significant reduction in racial disparities.

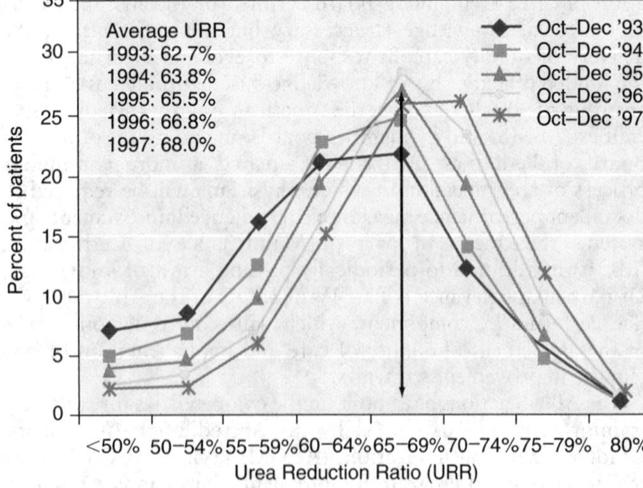

Figure 2-4. Improving renal function. An example from the End-Stage Renal Disease registry.

SAFETY

Safety is an important dimension of quality, and errors in health care are a leading cause of death and injury. Three to 4% of hospitalized patients are harmed by the care that is supposed to help them. On average, of 100 hospitalized patients, 7 are exposed to a serious medication error that harms or could harm them. It is estimated that between 44,000 and 98,000 patients of all ages within the USA die in hospitals each year as a result of errors in their care. Although these figures have been challenged, there is no disagreement as to the importance of the topic or the existence of substantial safety concerns in health care. Multiple factors contribute to errors: an increasingly complex health care system with diffuse accountability; a culture of attributing errors to individuals, which overlooks problematic systems; lack of allegiance between physicians and hospitals, which detracts from patient-centered practices; and reimbursement policies that frequently discourage safety measures. The ABMS has stated, "The ability to assess and systematically improve the safety of medical practice is an essential competency of every certified physician."

Medical Errors in Children's Health Care. Few epidemiologic data are available regarding medication errors in the pediatric setting, although Woods and colleagues found that rates of preventable adverse events in neonates and infants were 0.53% and in children <12 yr of age 0.22%. The *potential* for pediatric inpatient medical errors is substantial. This may be due, in part, to the fact that children have unique clinical experiences that are prone to error. These unique risk factors or safety issues, the "4 D's," are: developmental change, dependence on adults, different disease epidemiology, and demographic characteristics. Developmental change might refer to the unique susceptibility of neonates to infections or the need for weight-based dosing with growth. Children's dependence on adults also puts them at heightened risk for experiencing medical errors because children do not usually manage their own treatments, have the insight to question their own care, or provide their own medical history. Different disease epidemiology refers to the unique illnesses and medical needs that predispose children to unique safety events as compared with adults (birth trauma and screening for metabolic abnormalities, for example). Children have distinct demographic characteristics and are more likely to live in poverty than any other segment of the population.

Adverse drug events (ADEs) may occur in pediatric patients at a similar rate as in adult patients; the potential ADE rate may be three times higher in children. (A potential ADE is one that is intercepted before causing harm.) Most potential ADEs occurred at the stage of drug ordering and involved incorrect dosing, anti-infective drugs, and intravenous medications. In an ambulatory setting, 13% percent of prescriptions for children had potential medication errors. These errors were more common for infants and toddlers, children obtaining multiple prescriptions at the same time, and prescriptions for analgesics/narcotics. Despite the challenges and importance of accurate medication dosing in children, technology software does not always address issues specific to children, such as pediatric dosing calculations and age-based normal ranges. It is estimated that inpatient nonmedication errors involving children result in over $1 billion in reconciliation costs per year and are associated with significant and substantial increases in length of stay, charges, and in-hospital deaths.

Key Issues in Patient Safety. Making care safer requires the identification and control of things that could cause harm to patients. Several key concepts regarding patient safety are summarized in the following sections and are available in curriculum overviews at www.patientsafety.gov, www.npsf.org, and www.va.gov.

SYSTEMS APPROACH. One of the most significant changes resulting from the emphasis on patient safety is the recognition that the majority of health care errors result from faults intrinsic to the processes by which health care is delivered, rather than individual mistakes. This systems approach compels organizations to respond to adverse events not by blaming individuals, but rather by endeavoring to improve the conditions under which individuals work. An error is viewed as a symptom of trouble in a process that offers an opportunity for improvement and the potential to implement safeguards.

DEVELOPING A CULTURE OF SAFETY. The biggest challenge in making the health system safer is changing the culture from one of treating errors as personal failures to one of treating errors as opportunities to improve the system. Organizations need to foster a culture of learning in which each individual will feel accountable for ensuring a safe and quality program, communication is open, and teamwork is valued. Reporting of errors should be valued, reports of adverse events handled confidentially, and those who report errors protected from discovery. In addition, developing a culture of learning involves the compassionate and appropriate disclosure of system failures and medical errors to patients and families.

Communication. Good communication among the health care team is essential for patient safety. Health care involves the safe transfer of responsibility for patient care and the transfer of patient information. Poor communication or miscommunication creates the opportunity for incorrect or incomplete transfer of vital information during the transfer of responsibility for patient care from one provider to another, thus placing the patient at risk for serious medical error. The potential for harm is increased when the health care team and the patient do not share a native language. Errors in medical interpretation are common, with omissions being the most frequent. Ad hoc interpreters are significantly more likely to commit errors with harmful clinical consequences than are hospital interpreters.

Teamwork and Authority Gradients. Ensuring a systems approach to health care safety involves a paradigm shift. Health care has tended to be a hierarchical endeavor, with physicians in leadership roles that allowed significant amounts of autonomy. This authority gradient can predispose to communication failures: junior team members may be hesitant to speak up and senior members may resist feedback. A medical student or nursing assistant may be hesitant to inform an attending physician of a potential error. In contrast, in a culture of safety, team members with different positions of authority must interact to facilitate optimal patient care; all are empowered to voice a safety concern. The composition of the teams may vary day to day because of shifting schedules. Senior leaders must be able to engender trust rapidly among team members, accept that human error is inevitable, and encourage behaviors that prevent or mitigate the harm that results from errors.

Human Factors Engineering (HFE). This is a discipline concerned with the design of tools, machines, and systems that takes into account human capabilities, limitations, and characteristics. It builds on ergonomics and utilizes what is known about human performance and system interaction. HFE can play an important role in the optimal design of equipment, the development of effective processes, monitoring for unintended consequences, and the planning for and introduction of new technologies. HFE techniques used to identify hazards or areas for improving safety can be proactive (addressing complex areas of health care before implementing an intervention) or reactive (reviewing reports of "close calls" or injuries). An example of an application of HFE in health care is development and implementation of computerized physician order entry, which has been shown to decrease the rate of medication errors in pediatric inpatient settings.

Reliability. Reliability in health care is defined as the measurable capability of a process, procedure, or health service to perform its intended function in the required time under commonly occurring conditions (i.e., providing intended care on a consistent basis). Most health care organizations currently perform at **Level 1 reliability** which means that processes are performed with only an 80–90% success rate. To achieve **Level 2 performance** (≤5 failures/100 opportunities), process must be *intentionally designed* with tools and concepts based on the principles of human factors engineering. Performance at **Level 3** (≤5 failures/1000 opportunities), requires a well-designed system with low variation and cooperative relationships and a state of what has been called "mindfulness," where attention is paid to processes, structure, and their relationship to outcomes. For example, Cincinnati Children's Hospital Medical Center used reliability science and The Model for Improvement to institute a ventilator-associated pneumonia (VAP) protocol that has led to an 87% reduction in VAPs per 1000 ventilator days (from a fiscal year average of 7.5 to an average of only 0.95 for the year ending September 2006).

ONGOING AND FUTURE SAFETY MEASURES. The Joint Commission on Accreditation of Healthcare Organizations (JCAHO) includes safety measures in their requirements and the ACGME has instituted hour limitations in residency training to minimize errors related to fatigue. Future efforts to make care safer for children will involve a focus on appropriate information technology, including the development and implementation of electronic medical records appropriate for use in pediatrics (e.g., the inclusion of pediatric dosing calculations, age-based normal ranges, ability to calculate age in intervals less than a year, and adolescent confidentiality issues). Efficient dissemination of information regarding best practices and providing safety training to health care professionals are also needed. Continued and significant efforts are required to ensure a safe health care system for children. Safety must be viewed, however, as one component of a broader commitment to providing optimal health care for children.

Brilli RJ, Wells D, Shaw J: Implementation of a pediatric specific VAP bundle results in near elimination of ventilator-associated pneumonia at a tertiary pediatric ICU. *Chest.* 2006;130:138S.

Chassin MR, Galvin RW: The urgent need to improve health care quality: Institute of Medicine National Roundtable on Health Care Quality. *JAMA* 1998;280:1000–1005.

Donabedian A: Evaluating the quality of medical care. *Milbank Q* 1966;44:166–203.

Flores G, Laws MB, Mayo SJ, et al: Errors in medical interpretation and their potential clinical consequences in pediatric encounters. *Pediatrics* 2003;111:6–14.

Forrest CF, Shipman SA, Dougherty D, et al: Outcomes research in pediatric settings: Recent trends and future directions. *Pediatrics* 2003;111:171–178.

Horbar JD, Carpenter JH, Buzas J, et al: Collaborative quality improvement to promote evidence based surfactant for preterm infants: A cluster randomised trial. *Br Med J* 2004;329:1004.

Institute of Medicine: *Leadership by Example: Coordinating Government Roles in Improving Healthcare Quality.* Washington, DC, National Academy Press, 2002.

Institute of Medicine Committee on Quality of Health Care in America: *Crossing the Quality Chasm: A New Health System for the 21st Century.* Washington, DC, National Academy Press, 2001.

Institute of Medicine Committee on Quality of Health Care in America: *To Err Is Human: Building a Safer Health System.* Washington, DC, National Academy Press, 1999.

Kaushal R, Bates DW, Landrigan C, et al: Medication errors and adverse drug events in pediatric inpatients. *JAMA* 2001;285:2114–2120.

King, WJ, Paice N, Rangrej J, et al: The effect of computerized physician order entry on medication errors and adverse drug events in pediatric inpatients. *Pediatrics* 2003;112:506–509.

Leape LL, Berwick DM: Five years after To Err Is Human: What have we learned? *JAMA* 2005;293:2384–2390.

Leatherman S, McCarthy D: *Quality of Care for Children and Adolescents: A Chartbook.* Commonwealth Fund, 2004. www.cmwf.org.

Lohr KN (ed): *Medicare: A Strategy for Quality Assurance,* vol I. Washington, DC: Institute of Medicine, National Academy Press, 1990.

Longo DR, Hewett JE, Ge B, Schubert S: The long road to patient safety. *JAMA* 2005;294:2858–2865.

Lurie N: Health disparities—less talk, more action. *N Engl J Med* 2005;353:727–729.

Marmot M: Social determinants of health inequalities. *Lancet* 2005;365:1099–1104.

Mazmanian PE, Davis DA: Continuing medical education and the physician as a learner: Guide to the evidence. *JAMA* 2002;288:1057–1060

Miller MR, Elixhauser A, Zhan C: Patient safety events during pediatric hospitalizations. *Pediatrics* 2003;111:1358–1366.

Miller MR, Zhan C: Pediatric patient safety in hospitals: A national picture in 2000. *Pediatrics* 2004;113:1741–1746.

Papadakis MA, Teherani A, Banach MA, et al: Disciplinary action by medical boards and prior behavior in medical school. *N Engl J Med* 2005;353:2673–2682.

Psaty BM, Burke SP: Institute of medicine on drug safety. *N Engl J Med* 2006;355:1753–1755.

Scott JT, Rundall TG, Vogt TM, Hsu J: Kaiser Permanente's experience of implementing an electronic medical record: A qualitative study. *Br Med J* 2005;331:1313–1316.

Sehgal AR: Impact of quality improvement efforts on race and sex disparities in hemodialysis. *JAMA* 2003;289:996–1000.

Simpson LA, Dougherty D: Measuring the quality of children's health care: A prerequisite to action. *Pediatrics* 2004;113:185–198.

Trivedi AN, Zaslavsky AM, Schneider EC, et al: Trends in the quality of care and racial disparities in medicare managed care. *N Engl J Med* 2005;353:692–700.

US Department of Health & Human Services: Highlights from the 1998 ESRD Core Indicators Project, September 1998. Available at http://www.cms.hhs.gov/esrd/4r.pdf.

Woods D, Thomas E, Holl J, et al: Adverse events and preventable adverse events in children. *Pediatrics* 2005;115;1–155.

Wright AA, Katz IT: Bar coding for patient safety. *N Engl J Med* 2005;353:329–331.

Chapter 3 ■ Ethics in Pediatric Care

Robert M. Nelson

The proper scope of parental decision-making is bounded by the concept of a child's best interest and by the emerging desire and capacity for autonomy or self-determination of an older child or adolescent. The pediatric clinician also has an independent professional obligation to act in a child's "best interest," thus creating the possibility of conflict among child, parent, and clinician. The approach to the ethical issues that arise in pediatric practice must include respect for both a parent's responsibility for the life and health of a child and a child's developing capacity and autonomy. Further complexity is added by the varying social, cultural, and religious views of the role of family, parental authority, appropriate methods for disciplining a child, age of majority, and alternative approaches to health care.

INFORMED CONSENT, PARENTAL PERMISSION, AND CHILD ASSENT

A competent adult patient has the right to decide, after consultation with a physician, which medical interventions he or she will or will not accept. This right of **self-determination** (or **autonomy**) based on personal preferences and values is reflected in the doctrine of voluntary and informed consent. This doctrine, however, has limited direct application to children and adolescents who lack the decisional capacity or legal empowerment to give informed consent to medical care. The capacity for informed decision-making in health care is thought to involve the ability to understand and communicate, to reason and deliberate, and to analyze conflicting elements of a decision using a set of personal values. The age at which a competent patient may legally exercise voluntary and informed consent for medical care varies from state to state and may be limited to specific conditions (sexually transmitted infections, family planning, drug or alcohol abuse).

In contrast to decisions about one's own care, a parent's right to direct a child's medical care is more limited. It is constrained both by the child's best interest and the independent obligation of clinicians to act in the child's best interest, even if this places them in conflict with a parent. The concept of parental permission (rather than consent) reflects this shared decision-making involved in pediatric health care. In any given instance, the decision of what is or is not in a child's best interest may be difficult, especially given the diverse views of acceptable child rearing and child welfare. Parents are (and should be) granted wide discretion in raising their children. Nevertheless, in cases involving a substantial risk of harm, the moral focus should be on **what is best for the child**, not on a parental right to decide.

Respect for children must account for both a child's vulnerability and developing capacity. Thus, this respect encompasses both the protective role of parental permission and the developmental role of **child assent** (the child's affirmative agreement). At times, respect for a child requires overriding a child's dissent when a proposed intervention is essential to his or her welfare. Otherwise, assent should be obtained and dissent honored. In seeking younger children's assent, a clinician should help them understand their condition, tell them what they can expect, assess their understanding and whether they feel pressured to assent, and solicit their willingness to participate. Older children or adolescents may have the cognitive and emotional capacity to fully participate in health care decisions, especially if they are living with a chronic illness. If so, the adolescent should be provided with the same information as would be given to an adult patient. The adolescent's parent still remains in a guiding and protective role. The process of communication and negotiation will be more complex should disagreement arise between the parent and adolescent (see the later section "Adolescent Health Care").

TREATMENT OF CRITICALLY ILL CHILDREN

Most children who are critically ill recover and are able to return to an acceptable quality of life. Some children either respond partially or fail to respond to life-sustaining medical treatment (LSMT), progressing toward death over a time span ranging from minutes to years. Most children who die in an intensive care unit (ICU) do so after a decision has been made to either limit or withdraw (forgo) some form of LSMT. Under these circumstances, a number of questions arise. Should one initiate or continue LSMT? How does one arrive at this decision? What treatments should be provided as part of palliative care? Is there any difference between starting and stopping a medical intervention? What about specific interventions such as cardiopulmonary resuscitation or artificially provided hydration and nutrition? Should newborn infants and older children be treated differently when considering LSMT?

TRANSITIONING FROM "CURE" TO "CARE." The provision of LSMT assumes that the burden of treatment is justified by the anticipated benefit of returning to or sustaining an acceptable quality of life. As the anticipated quality of the outcome deteriorates or becomes increasingly unlikely, or as the burden of treatment becomes intolerable, the family and the health care team ask whether continued LSMT makes sense. Answering this question is difficult, involving a range of possible outcomes, complex estimates of probabilities, differing values of each outcome, and dealing with uncertainty and hope. Medical technology and other treatments should only be used when the benefits for the child outweigh the burdens, especially for children living with life-threatening or terminal conditions.

The concept of **futility** has been invoked in support of the unilateral forgoing of LSMT by health care professionals over the objections of patients and family. Although it seems self-evident that clinicians should not provide futile (or useless) interventions, the application of this principle is problematic if used to justify unilateral professional action based on values that are not shared by the affected patient or family. The concept of futility should be reserved for those interventions that will not, in fact, achieve a given physiologic outcome. The appeal to futility should not be used to short-circuit the collaborative process by which medical interventions are seen to be disproportionately burdensome.

Effective **communication** empowers parents and children to be involved in decisions about their medical care. Approaching a child's parents to initiate a discussion about forgoing LSMT can be difficult. A reasonable starting point is to explore a parent's hopes, fears, and expectations about possible outcomes; the anticipated burden of treatment in attempting to achieve an acceptable outcome; and the degree of uncertainty in predicting a child's response to treatment. Parents often prefer to hear difficult information from a familiar clinician who knows the family and can communicate truthfully, clearly, and compassionately.

The disclosure of "bad news" such as a life-altering diagnosis or life-threatening complication is often poorly communicated. Parents and children may perceive a clinician to be uncaring and insensitive, resulting in emotional distress. Insufficient training, lack of experience, and feelings of inadequacy about communicating with parents and children over the transition to palliative care and other end-of-life issues may distress clinicians and affect the quality of care. Clinicians who feel less competent may distance themselves emotionally in distressing situations. Inadequate support for clinicians caring for dying children can lead to depression, emotional withdrawal, and other symptoms.

LIFE-SUSTAINING MEDICAL TREATMENT OR PALLIATIVE CARE? A rigid distinction between LSMT and palliative care may be difficult to draw in any given instance, and their integration is often desirable (see Chapter 40). LSMT can be broadly defined as any intervention that may prolong the life of a patient or alter substantially the expected progression toward death. Examples of LSMT include cardiopulmonary resuscitation, organ transplantation, ventilator therapy, dialysis, and treatment with vasoactive medications, or more mundane interventions such as antibiotics, chemotherapy, and artificially provided nutrition and hydration. Palliative care interventions focus on the relief of symptoms and conditions that may detract from a child's (and family's) quality of life regardless of the impact on a child's underlying disease process (see Chapter 40). The control of pain and other symptoms, as well as concern for the psychologic or spiritual problems associated with life-threatening or terminal disease, are usually considered palliative and are often appropriate during LSMT. Certain LSMT may also be appropriate in the palliative management of the dying child.

WITHHOLDING AND WITHDRAWING LIFE-SUSTAINING TREATMENT. A palliative care plan involves the assessment of available diagnostic and therapeutic interventions based on the goal of improving a child's quality of life while living with a life-threatening or terminal disease. Some interventions that are currently being provided may be withdrawn. Other interventions that are not being provided may be withheld. Although the prevailing view is that there is no moral distinction between withholding or withdrawing interventions that are not medically indicated, the uncertainty inherent in predicting a child's response to treatment suggests that withdrawing treatment based on a child's failure to respond is morally preferable to withholding that same treatment. In addition, withholding treatment out of concern that the withdrawal of that same treatment in the future would be more difficult risks undertreating some children who would, in fact, respond favorably to that treatment. The withdrawal of LSMT may be psychologically more stressful than withholding LSMT, and may add complexity as the moral values associated with treatment of any given child may shift over time. This alleged symmetry between the decision to withhold or to withdraw LSMT assumes that the technology itself is morally neutral and that other changes that may occur over time are not morally relevant. Both assumptions may not be appropriate, especially when transitioning to technologies such as a tracheostomy or gastrostomy tube.

The decision not to attempt **cardiopulmonary resuscitation** is often the initial focus of discussion with parents of children living with life-threatening or terminal conditions. Obtaining a "do not attempt resuscitation" (DNAR) order may become a symbol of a clinician's success at negotiating limits to LSMT with a child's parents and eclipse other interventions that should be considered in providing for a child's comfort. Clinicians may assume inappropriately that a DNAR order reflects a desire not to pursue other interventions. The decision for a DNAR order does not imply a decision to withhold or withdraw other aspects of providing medical treatment, such as oxygen, suctioning, pain medications, and so forth. The value of specific resuscitative interventions may vary depending on the patient's clinical condition and anticipated outcome. Thus, DNAR orders should address separately the provision of mechanical ventilation with or without endotracheal intubation, the use of cardiac medications, chest compressions, and cardioversion. In addition, a DNAR decision is not irrevocable. Clinicians may assume that the absence of a DNAR order obligates them to perform a prolonged resuscitation. If the futility of resuscitative efforts is based on a lack of physiologic response, a physician should tailor resuscitative efforts to a child's clinical condition.

Advance Directives. A DNAR order is a specific form of a more general advance directive (AD), which allows patients and/or appropriate surrogates to designate the desired medical interventions under applicable circumstances. A DNAR order should be part of a comprehensive plan of care that is periodically reviewed and that should be respected in all aspects of a child's care, including schooling. The extension of DNAR orders for children to the out-of-hospital setting can be an important component of providing comprehensive care. Mechanisms and laws should be in place for DNAR orders to be respected in schools and the prehospital emergency medical system.

The 1991 federal Patient Self-Determination Act requires that health care institutions ask adult (>18 yr) patients whether they have completed an AD and, if not, inform them of their right to do so. Many states have implemented a "prehospital AD" by which adults may indicate their desire not to be resuscitated by emergency personnel. The use of an AD in pediatrics has generally been limited to inpatient settings for at least two reasons: (1) the availability of parents and (2) the lack of a standardized process to facilitate the identification, validation, and interpretation of an outpatient AD. Some institutions have established local policies and procedures by which an appropriately executed outpatient AD can be honored upon a child's arrival in the emergency department. Key features include a standardized format, attending physician involvement, educational programming, and administration by the institution's palliative care service. Although advocated by some, an AD has not been used for delivery room resuscitation given the uncertainty in predicting an infant's postnatal prognosis based on prenatal information except under extreme circumstances. An adolescent with a chronic and/or life-threatening condition should be supported in developing an AD as part of a comprehensive plan for end-of-life care.

Artificial Hydration and Nutrition. One of the more difficult issues in withholding or withdrawing LSMT is the provision of artificial hydration and nutrition. Any person sufficiently dependent on the care of others will die as a result of not receiving hydration and nutrition. Some contend that the artificiality of some methods of providing hydration and nutrition (such as the use of a gastrostomy tube or intravenous hyperalimentation) indicates that they may be withheld or withdrawn as with any LSMT. Another argument is that nutrition and hydration are not in a particular child's best interest regardless of the method of administration. Some states require "clear and convincing evidence" of a patient's prior wishes in order to withdraw such LSMT from patients who are either incompetent or in a permanent vegetative state. This "substituted judgment" is not possible in young children or in patients who became incompetent before expressing such wishes. Although there are legal cases that have allowed the removal of artificial nutrition and hydration based on a patient's "best interests," the rulings are generally in regard to adult patients and are thus of uncertain pediatric applicability. Forgoing nutrition and hydration under the appropriate circumstances may be ethically defensible. Such a decision should be made by a child's parents after due consideration of the moral and legal implications.

Causing Death? The decision to withhold or withdraw LSMT does not necessarily imply an intent or choice to hasten a child's death. One can choose how to live while dying without choosing death, even when death is the anticipated outcome of one's choice. The provision of adequate sedation and analgesia to relieve rapidly progressive symptoms such as pain and dyspnea need not be interpreted as causing a child's death. The primary relief of pain and agitation under these circumstances is a moral good of such magnitude that the secondary effect of hastening death is an acceptable (albeit unintended) consequence (see Chapter 40). Two key features of this so-called "doctrine of double effect" (DDE) are worth noting: (1) the unintended outcome (i.e., death) should not be the means of achieving the intended outcome (relief of pain); and (2) intentionality is not a psychologic state, but an objective feature of the act itself (choice of medication, dose, timing, route of administration). The DDE provides a moral framework for clinicians who desire to provide compassionate end-of-life care without intending or causing the death of their patients.

If a decision has been made that continued survival is not in a patient's best interest, it would seem irrelevant to some clinicians whether he or she died by forgoing LSMT or the administration of a drug. Indeed, the administration of a lethal drug might be preferable because of the opportunity to minimize suffering. The reasons for opposition to such decisions are only partly related to concerns for the interests of patients. The objections are based, in part, on the swiftness and irreversibility of action, precluding the possibility of changing course if it is discovered that the decision was wrong. The greater concern, however, has been for "slippery slope" effects: the claim that lowering the barrier against killing will make it easier for physicians to kill others, that boundaries will become less distinct, and that patients without a clear interest in dying will be harmed. In addition, the backlash against physician-assisted suicide may render the appropriate provision of palliative care more difficult through fear of legal prosecution based simply on the dose of sedatives or narcotics administered.

DISABLED NEWBORNS AND LSMT

In 1982, an infant with Down syndrome and esophageal atresia was allowed to die at 6 days of age at the parents' request. The case was similar to many others that had occurred during the preceding decade, particularly involving undertreatment of newborns with Down syndrome and spina bifida. Many of these children appeared to have excellent prospects for long, happy lives, suggesting that the decisions were not being made in the best interests of the children. In two large surveys, most pediatricians supported parental control of such decisions; some pediatricians stated that they considered their duty was not to serve the interests of their patient but rather to serve the interests of the family. These problems were compounded by the fact that decisions were often based on erroneous medical assumptions, including inappropriately pessimistic prognoses about quality of life.

As a consequence of concern about this issue in the United States, regulations were eventually promulgated under the authority of a federal child abuse law that prohibited withholding medically beneficial treatment from disabled infants except under certain conditions. These conditions are permanent unconsciousness, "futile" treatment, and "virtually futile" treatment that imposes excessive burdens on an infant. This rule seemed to disqualify one of the most common justifications for forgoing LSMT in children, namely, the likelihood that continued biologic existence would not serve the patients' interests precisely because the child would be so disabled that the burden of treatment would be greater than the benefit. One unintended consequence of this rule was an apparent shift from undertreatment to widespread overtreatment, defined as life-prolonging treatment that, in the opinion of the physician, does not serve the interests of the child. The regulations address state eligibility for federal child abuse funding and, absent the incorporation of similar language in state statutes, do not dictate the proper scope of medical interventions. A subsequent case involving an infant with spina bifida and other abnormalities upheld the right of a parent to decide to forgo LSMT for their child. The application of these federal (and related state) regulations (referred to as "Baby Doe" rules) to parental decisions about the provision of LSMT to critically ill newborns and infants is incompatible with compassionate end-of-life care based on the best interests of the individual child.

DECLARING DEATH AND ORGAN DONATION

Organ donation can occur after a patient is declared dead based on either irreversible cessation of neurologic function of the brain and brainstem ("brain death") or a predetermined period of cardiac asystole ("non-heart-beating donor" or NHBD) [see Chapter 67.1]. The request for organ donation should be separated from the clinical discussion of either brain death or withdrawal of LSMT. Although parents and other family members may ask questions of the clinicians, the discussion of organ donation should be done by other individuals who are specifically trained for this purpose. The decoupling of clinical decision-making from a request for organ donation by trained individuals improves donation rates, and avoids an apparent conflict of interest on the part of clinicians caring for the patient.

BRAIN DEATH. Diagnostic guidelines for establishing brain death in children of different ages have been established, with infants and younger children requiring a longer period of observation than older children or adolescents (see Chapter 67.1). The period of observation may be shortened through the use of confirmatory tests such as an electroencephalogram (demonstrating electrical cerebral silence) or cerebral perfusion study (demonstrating absent blood flow to the whole brain). Given documented variability in the clinical determination of brain death (including failure to perform a complete neurologic examination), many institutions (and some states) have established policies stipulating the required examinations, tests, and observation periods. Observing a skilled clinician perform a complete "brain death" examination including an apnea test may help parents who are having difficulty with the use of neurologic criteria to determine a child's death. The clinician should have performed the complete examination previously so as not to be surprised by unexpected findings, such as vigorous spinal reflexes.

Currently two states (New York and New Jersey) allow families to object on religious grounds to the declaration of death using "brain death" criteria. In effect, the clinical determination of the cessation of cortical and brainstem activity sets the stage for a discussion of forgoing LSMT, rather than the death of the patient. A unilateral decision not to initiate new or escalate existing interventions is reasonable under these circumstances. A unilateral decision to withdraw existing interventions may be inappropriate absent the need to triage scarce pediatric ICU resources. Institutional procedures for conflict resolution, including involvement of the courts if necessary, should be followed. Absent applicable state law, ongoing third party reimbursement for the cost of continued LSMT for a "brain dead" patient may need to be addressed.

CARDIAC DEATH. NHBD protocols have been developed to allow for organ procurement after cardiac asystole. Organ procurement from NHBD can occur under either controlled (after planned withdrawal of LSMT) or uncontrolled (after failed CPR) circumstances. The routine use of NHBD protocols in pediatrics following planned withdrawal of LSMT may significantly increase the number of organs available for transplantation. The number of potential donors depends somewhat on the choice of an acceptable time period for asystole to occur after the withdrawal of LSMT and before organ procurement (generally in the range of 1–2 hr).

Ethical concerns about the development of NHBD protocols focus on two principles that have served as the basis for organ donation: (1) the "dead donor rule" limiting the donation of vital organs to those who are irreversibly dead, and (2) the absence of conflict of interest between clinical care and organ procurement. With NHBD protocols, irreversibility is limited to spontaneous return of circulation after forgoing CPR, rather than failure to restore neurologic function in spite of any possible intervention. The waiting time after cardiac asystole to the start of organ procurement varies among NHBD protocols, with some arguing for a uniform 5 min interval. There are rare case reports of spontaneous return of cardiac function after more than 5 min of asystole, and uncertainty remains whether the generally accepted neurologic criteria for death are satisfied after 5 min of asystole. On this basis, some argue for extending the time period between asystole and organ procurement to 10 min. The clinical finding of asystole does not define the patient's death absent a prior moral decision to forgo CPR. Proponents of NHBD protocols point out that the use of neurologic criteria to determine death also involves moral and religious values.

Some clinicians are concerned about the appearance of a conflict of interest when families are approached about organ donation after a decision to withdraw LSMT. Also, the initiation of organ preservation procedures before death may create a conflict of interest between the ongoing care of the dying patient and actions taken to preserve the viability of transplantable organs. Will families assume that the recommendation to withdraw LSMT was for the purpose of obtaining the child's organs? To avoid this interpretation, some argue that any discussion about NHBD organ procurement after forgoing LSMT should be only in response to a family-initiated question about organ donation. Also, the location and process of withdrawing LSMT should also be considered carefully. Some institutions withdraw LSMT in the operating room after the child has been prepared for organ procurement. As a result, there may be considerable pressure exerted on the clinicians managing the child to hasten death so that organ procurement can take place within the predetermined time limit.

INSTITUTIONAL (HOSPITAL) ETHICS COMMITTEES

The controversy over forgoing LSMT of disabled newborn infants led to the formation of the "infant bioethics committee" as a pediatric forerunner of today's institutional ethics committee (IEC). An IEC usually provides voluntary consultation, which may involve enhanced communication or conflict resolution. For the vast majority of decisions involving the medical treatment of children (including forgoing LSMT), pediatric clinicians and parents are usually in agreement about the desirability of the proposed intervention. The views of a child should also be given considerable weight, especially when the burden of treatment is great and the potential benefit uncertain or remote.

An IEC typically performs at least three different functions: (1) the drafting and review of institutional policy on such issues as DNAR orders and forgoing LSMT; (2) the education of health care professionals, patients, and families about ethical issues in health care; and (3) case consultation and conflict resolution. Although the process of case consultation may vary, ideally the IEC should adopt a collaborative approach that uncovers all the readily available and relevant facts, takes into account the feelings of those involved, and balances the vested interests, while arriving at a recommendation based on a consistent ethical analysis. The Joint Commission on Accreditation of Hospitals requires these committees, or an appropriate alternative; the committee often plays a consultative role when parents and medical staff cannot agree on the proper course of action. IECs have acquired considerable influence and are increasingly recognized by state courts as an important aid in decision-making. The membership, policies, and procedures of an IEC should conform to accepted professional standards.

SCREENING AND GENETIC TESTING

Screening is the search for asymptomatic illness in a defined population; it is usually performed for the purpose of treatment, but it is sometimes done for counseling or research. Several programs, such as newborn screening for inborn errors of metabolism (phenylketonuria [PKU] and hypothyroidism), are counted among the triumphs of contemporary pediatrics. The success of such programs sometimes obscures serious ethical issues that continue to arise in proposals to screen for other conditions for which the benefits, risks, and costs have not been clearly established. Advances in genetics have led to exponential growth in the number of conditions for which screening tests are available, with insufficient opportunity to study each proposed testing program.

The introduction of screening tests should be done in a carefully controlled manner that allows for the evaluation of the costs (financial, medical, and psychologic) and benefits of screening, including the effectiveness of follow-up and treatment protocols. New programs should be considered experimental until the risks and benefits are demonstrated. Screening tests that identify candidates for treatment need to have demonstrated sensitivity, specificity, and high predictive value, lest individuals be falsely labeled and subject to possibly toxic treatments or to psychosocial risks. As these tests are being developed, parents should generally be given the opportunity to exercise informed consent or refusal. These safeguards have not always been systematically applied to screening programs, often resulting in serious harm to many children, without compensating benefits. Familiar examples include routine fetal monitoring, which contributed to the rising rate of cesarean sections with little benefit for many infants, and the screening of premature infants for acidosis, resulting in administration of toxic amounts of sodium bicarbonate before its risks were adequately studied.

A persistent ethical issue is whether screening should be voluntary ("opt in"); routine, with the ability to "opt out" or refuse; or mandatory. A voluntary approach entails an informed decision by parents before screening. Concern is often expressed that seeking informed consent is ethically inappropriate for tests of clear benefit, such as PKU screening, because refusal would constitute neglect. Routine testing with an "opt out" approach requires an explicit refusal of screening by parents who object to this intervention. The principal ethical justification for mandatory screening is the claim that society's obligation to promote child welfare through early detection and treatment of selected conditions supersedes any parental right to refuse this simple medical intervention. Obtaining informed consent for newborn screening may allow for more prompt and efficient responses to positive results and for incorporating experimental tests into established screening programs. Although more research is necessary, one study showed that a reasonable attempt at consent could be made on a statewide basis without excessive time or cost and without undue effects on compliance.

These same two ethical principles of demonstrated benefit justifying the risks of screening and informed consent can be applied to genetic testing for late-onset disorders. The knowledge of increased risk status may lead to lifestyle changes that can reduce morbidity and the risk of mortality, or may precipitate adverse emotional and psychologic responses and discrimination. Because many adults choose not to be tested for late-onset disorders, we cannot assume that a child would want or will benefit from similar testing. Genetic testing of children and adolescents for late-onset disorders is generally inappropriate unless such testing will result in interventions that have been shown to reduce morbidity and mortality when initiated in childhood. Otherwise, such testing should be deferred until the child has the capacity to make an informed and voluntary choice.

ADOLESCENT HEALTH CARE

ADOLESCENT ASSENT AND CONSENT. Many adolescents resemble adults more than they do children in their competence to consent to health care (see Chapters 12 and 111). Competence is not a global quality: Teenagers may not be able to support themselves, yet they may still be competent to consent to health care. In addition to competence, there are public health reasons for allowing adolescents to consent to their own health care with regard to reproductive decisions, such as contraception, abortion, and treatment of sexually transmitted infections. Strict requirements for parental consent may deter many adolescents from seeking health care, with serious implications for their health and other community interests.

Weighed against these arguments are the legitimate interests of parents in maintaining responsibility and authority for child rearing, including the opportunity to influence the sexual attitudes and practices of their children. Another claim is that public support for access to such treatment, particularly contraception and abortion, implicitly endorses and encourages sexual activity, aggravating rather than ameliorating the problems. Similar concerns underlie the objection to providing sterile needles for intravenous drug abusers for the purpose of reducing the risk of acquiring hepatitis or HIV. Critics complain that such programs give children the message that illegal drug use is supported by the state as long as it is done safely, even though it is now generally accepted that access to sterile needles results in a decrease in new cases of AIDS. The pediatrician's role and behavior in these disputes will be influenced by his or her own moral beliefs and by assessments of the competing facts and arguments. Physicians need to consider the possibility that a moralistic position may deter adolescents from seeking health care or counseling.

CHRONIC ILLNESS. The normal process of adolescent development involves gradually separating from parents, establishing self-confidence, asserting individuality, and focusing on peer relationships and the ability to function independently outside the family. Under parental supervision, an adolescent should take on increasing autonomy in health care decisions, a process that may be accelerated for children who are experienced in living with a chronic disease. A chronically ill and/or dying adolescent may fail to achieve other normal developmental milestones due to a lack of peer interaction or acceptance and an ongoing need for parental support. While valuing parental expertise and involvement, clinicians should support adolescents in expressing their wishes about medical treatment. The development of self-management skills depends on the capacity for self-determination. Adolescents >14 yr old should be provided the freedom to make their own health care decisions with the guidance of their parents and clinicians.

DECISIONS IN TERMINALLY ILL ADOLESCENTS. The presumption that an adolescent >14 yr old has the capacity to make binding medical decisions should be extended to the provision of LSMT (and other end-of-life issues) for a dying adolescent. Most adolescents want to share end-of-life decision-making with other family members, highlighting the importance of open communication and flexibility about treatment preferences regardless of legal status. The development of an advance directive may clarify the perspective and wishes of the dying adolescent, with implementation emerging out of this collaborative process as responsible parents (and others) support the adolescent's insights, values, and autonomy. From the time of diagnosis of a life-threatening condition, clinicians should include the child in a developmentally appropriate process of communication that enables an increasing level of involvement in medical decisions up to and including palliative care. Such an approach builds a foundation of mutual respect and trust, which will minimize the potential for future conflict as the adolescent's condition deteriorates.

RESEARCH

The central ethical distinction between research and standard clinical practice is researchers' commitment to generating knowledge, perhaps to the benefit of future patients or society, in addition to their responsibility for patients who are the human subjects of the investigation. Research is defined in the federal regulations as "a systematic investigation designed to develop or contribute to generalizable knowledge." For any research to be performed, the risks should be minimized and reasonable with respect to any anticipated benefits to the subjects and the importance of the resulting knowledge. Because children generally cannot give voluntary and informed consent to their own research participation, there are further restrictions on the research risks to which a child may be exposed. These restrictions specify the conditions under which a parent has the moral and legal authority to permit a child to participate in research.

In **nontherapeutic research,** there is no expected direct benefit for the subject; therefore, any risk may present an unfavorable risk:benefit ratio. Some argue that children, along with other nonconsenting subjects, should never be used in nontherapeutic research, as a person should never be used solely as a means to an end. The more widely held opinion is that children may be exposed to at least minimal risks, although the reasons for this exception are disputed. Some argue that children have a duty to contribute to the social welfare, although the federal regulations do not allow competent adults to be used as research subjects for this justification without their consent. Others argue that participation in research can provide a benefit by fostering a sense of altruism or citizenship through a child's assent. The federal regulations allow healthy children to participate in minimal-risk research based on an analogy to parental authority to make decisions about risk exposure in everyday life. The regulations also state that children with a condition can be exposed to slightly more than minimal risk in nontherapeutic research if the child's experience is similar to everyday life with that condition and the anticipated knowledge is of vital importance for understanding or benefiting that condition. This "minor increase over minimal risk" category is the most controversial.

Much of the controversy over nontherapeutic research stems from the wide variability in the interpretation of minimal risk. The federal regulations define minimal risks as the risks that are "ordinarily encountered in daily life or during the performance of routine physical or psychologic examinations or tests." Some interpret this to include procedures similar to those done in primary care office visits, but others claim that an invasive procedure such as a liver biopsy may be done if the risks, in the hands of a particular investigator, are empirically no higher than those of a routine office visit or if the procedure is routine for a visit to a specialist. When originally proposed, the definition of minimal risk referred to the life of a healthy child. The regulations omitted this phrase out of concern that research would be hindered, thus contributing to the wide range of interpretation. Many advocate restoring the phrase "of healthy children" to the definition of minimal risk because valuable research on a condition may still proceed under the "minor increase over minimal risk" category. As originally proposed, the concept of minimal risk serves a moral purpose in limiting a parent's authority to permit nontherapeutic research on a healthy child. To define minimal risk using only statistical considerations (such as the product of probability and magnitude) may overlook this moral purpose. The risks of each intervention or procedure in the research need to be considered separately and balanced against any direct benefit to the subject or knowledge to be gained.

The term **therapeutic research** is misleading in that not all interventions or procedures included in a research study may offer the prospect of direct benefit to the subject. There are likely to be nontherapeutic aspects of the research, such as an extra blood test or chest radiograph. The nontherapeutic parts of the research need to be no more than a "minor increase over minimal risk" and cannot be justified by the anticipated benefit of other parts of the overall research study. The risks of interventions that offer direct benefit can be more than minimal. The risks must be justified by the anticipated benefit, and the balance of anticipated benefit to the risk should be at least as favorable as that presented by available alternatives. Being enrolled in a research study should not disadvantage a child.

Innovative therapy is defined as a new and unproven intervention done primarily for the benefit of the patient, with no intent to gather new information. Such innovations may be more hazardous and ethically more problematic than research, in part because they are not subject to peer review and because toxicity is not being systematically assessed. This kind of therapy is also subject to abuse because its definition is a matter of intent, and thus difficult for others to disprove. Although innovative medical and surgical interventions are not subject to research regulations, some argue that clinicians have a moral obligation to submit innovative therapies to formal evaluation. Others express concern that the institutional system for review of research protocols lacks the timeliness and expertise needed to evaluate innovative treatments.

The regulations in the United States for the protection of human research subjects rest on two foundations: (1) voluntary and informed consent, and (2) the independent review of the research risks. An ethical and responsible researcher is often added as the 3rd foundation needed for the protection of human research subjects. The standard for informed consent in a research setting is higher than for clinical care because the risks and benefits are typically less clear, the investigator has a conflict of interest, and humans have historically been subjected to unauthorized risks when strict requirements for consent were not respected.

Adolescents who are competent may sometimes consent to be research subjects. It is also generally acknowledged that children should be given the opportunity to dissent, particularly for nontherapeutic research, when there cannot be a claim that participation is in the child's interest. In the United States, national regulations require that reasonable efforts be made at least to inform children who are capable of understanding that participation is not part of their care and that, therefore, they are free to refuse to participate. The regulations do not require child assent but only parental permission if the research offers a direct benefit to the child that would not otherwise be available. For some research, parental permission may not be required if an appropriate mechanism for protecting the children enrolled in the research is established. This provision does not apply to research conducted under the jurisdiction of the Food and Drug Administration (FDA).

In addition to the protection that informed consent is intended to provide, virtually all research involving human subjects in the United States is reviewed by an **institutional review board** (IRB), required by federal regulations for institutions receiving federal research funds and for FDA-regulated drug research. It is uncertain whether such review is legally required for research that is not federally funded or for research in settings that receive no federal funds, such as private clinics. The principles of ethical decision-making that led to the involvement of ethics committees in clinical decisions argue for a similar review of research involving children, regardless of the source of funding. For research that does not meet criteria for local IRB approval, there is a process for federal review of research that "presents a reasonable opportunity to further the understanding, prevention, or alleviation of a serious problem affecting the health or welfare of children."

A general ethical principle is that individuals who are capable of voluntary and informed consent be approached 1st about research participation. In addition, children should not be included in research unless scientifically necessary. An unintended result is that the majority of marketed medications are not labeled for use in children. Pediatricians are left with a difficult choice of using medications "off label" and risking increased toxicity or decreased efficacy, or not using a medication and potentially denying a child an important therapeutic advance. To ameliorate this problem, the United States has granted 6 mo patent extensions for the performance of requested pediatric studies, resulting in new pediatric labeling for many important drugs. New drug applications must include studies of children unless granted a specific waiver. In addition, grants submitted to the National Institutes of Health must include children in the absence of scientific or ethical reasons to the contrary.

FETAL WELL-BEING AND TREATMENT

As our knowledge of factors influencing fetal development and well-being expands, there is increasing discussion about the proper balancing of maternal and fetal interests when a pregnant woman's behavior affects the well-being of her fetus. Interventions can now be directed primarily toward specific medical and surgical conditions of the fetus, rather than toward the general health of the pregnant woman with a secondary impact on the fetus. As a result, questions arise about a clinician's responsibility when the interests of the pregnant woman and her fetus appear to conflict. There are two particularly controversial areas in which this question arises: the provision of fetal medical or surgical treatment, and the reporting of pregnant women for drug and alcohol use.

The most dramatic of these conflicts arises when a pregnant woman refuses standard, effective treatment essential for the benefit of a fetus/infant who is at high risk of death or serious disability, such as refusal of cesarean section for placenta previa in a voluntary pregnancy near term involving a presumably normal fetus/infant. Courts in the United States have sometimes decided that a woman can be required to undergo such a procedure when the benefit to the emergent child is clear. A federal court decided that such an order was inappropriate in a case involving a 26 wk old fetus and, by implication, other cases in which the benefit of intervention was in doubt. In general, a clinician should not oppose a pregnant woman's refusal of a recommended intervention unless (1) the risk to the pregnant woman is negligible, (2) the intervention has been shown effective, and (3) the harm to the fetus is certain, substantial, and irrevocable. When these three conditions exist, a clinician may try to persuade and, if unsuccessful, seek some other avenue of conflict resolution (such as through an IEC). Rarely, and only as a last resort, should a clinician seek judicial authorization to override a pregnant woman's dissent.

Child abuse statutes have also been invoked in attempts to modify the behavior of women who ingest alcohol or illicit drugs during pregnancy and expose the fetus/infant to harm. Pediatricians considering reporting such cases must consider the likelihood of benefit from reporting, the harm to the child as well as to the mother if criminal charges or custody changes are sought, and the possible effects that reporting may have on driving pregnant women away from the health care system, particularly from prenatal care. The U.S. Supreme Court has held that drug testing of pregnant women without consent was in direct violation of the Fourth Amendment, which provides protection from unreasonable searches.

ACCESS TO HEALTH CARE: RATIONING (DISTRIBUTIVE JUSTICE)

The most serious ethical problem in health care in the U.S. may be the inequality in access to health care. No other major industrial country rations basic health care on the basis of ability to pay. Comprising nearly one of every five uninsured persons, more than nine million children and adolescents lack basic health care coverage. This lack of adequate and affordable health care has serious consequences in terms of death, disability, and suffering. The central ethical principle at stake is fair opportunity to participate in the benefits of society; preventable death and disability undermine the claim that the society is one of equal opportunity. Another aspect of the claim of unfairness is that the present system is maintained by those who are already advantaged because of financial or social status, thereby aggravating existing inequalities.

Rationing of health care can be defined as limiting access to wanted and needed services of known benefit. It is increasingly recognized that no society can provide all beneficial services to all its citizens; rationing is therefore unavoidable. The question is not whether to ration health care services but how to do so fairly. Apart from ability to pay, other ways of rationing could be based on cost:benefit analysis, age, or likely effects on quality of life. Even universal systems of health care coverage effectively ration through limited availability, with the option of purchasing additional desired services using private resources. Some argue that such a multitiered system is fair as long as the basic health care package is appropriately defined and sufficiently funded.

American Academy of Pediatrics, Committee on Bioethics: Institutional ethics committees. *Pediatrics* 2001;107:205–209.

American Academy of Pediatrics, Committee on Bioethics: Fetal therapy—Ethical considerations. *Pediatrics* 1999;103:1061–1063.

American Academy of Pediatrics, Committee on Bioethics: Religious objections to medical care. *Pediatrics* 1997;99:279–281.

American Academy of Pediatrics, Committee on Bioethics: Ethics and the care of critically ill infants and children. *Pediatrics* 1996;98:149–152.

American Academy of Pediatrics, Committee on Bioethics: Informed consent, parental permission, and assent in pediatric practice. *Pediatrics* 1995;95:314–317.

American Academy of Pediatrics, Committee on Bioethics and Committee on Hospital Care: Palliative care for children. *Pediatrics* 2000;106:351–357.

Ashcroft RE: Reforming research ethics committees. *Br Med J* 2005;331:587–588.

Bell MD: Non-heart beating organ donation: Old procurement strategy—New ethical problems. *J Med Ethics* 2003;29:176–181.

Brown SD, Truog RD, Johnson JA, Ecker JL: Do differences in the American Academy of Pediatrics and the American College of Obstetricians and Gynecologists position on the ethics of maternal-fetal interventions reflect subtly divergent professional sensitivities to pregnant women and fetuses? *Pediatrics* 2006;117:1382–1387.

Caldwell PHY, Murphy SB, Butow PN, Craig JC: Clinical trials in children. *Lancet* 2004;364:803–811.

Casarett D, Kapo J, Caplan A: Appropriate use of artificial nutrition and hydration—Fundamental principles and recommendations. *N Engl J Med* 2005;353:2607–2612.

Committee on Hospital Care and Section on Surgery, American Academy of Pediatrics: Pediatric Organ Donation and Transplantation: Policy statement: Organizational principles to guide and define the child health care system and/or improve the health of all children. *Pediatrics* 2002;109:982–984.

Committee on School Health and Committee on Bioethics, American Academy of Pediatrics: Do not resuscitate orders in schools. *Pediatrics* 2000;105:878–879.

Fallat ME, Deshpande JK, Section on Surgery, Anesthesia, and Pain Medicine, Committee on Bioethics: Do-not-resuscitate orders for pediatric patients who require anesthesia and surgery. *Pediatrics* 2004;114:1686–1692.

Field MJ, Behrman RE (eds): *Ethical Conduct of Clinical Research Involving Children.* Washington, DC, National Academy Press, 2004.

Freyer DR: Care of the dying adolescent: Special considerations. *Pediatrics* 2004;113:381–388.

Hall DMB: Children, rights, and responsibilities. *Arch Dis Child* 2005;90:171–173.

Kopelman LM: Are the 21-year-old Baby Doe rules misunderstood or mistaken? *Pediatrics* 2005;115:797–802.

Lazar NM, Shemie S, Webster GC, et al: Bioethics for clinicians: 24. Brain death. *CMAJ* 2001;164:833–836.

Leask K: The role of the courts in clinical decision-making. *Arch Dis Child* 2005;90:1256–1258.

Lo B, Rubenfeld G: Palliative sedation in dying patients. *JAMA* 2005;294:1810–1816.

Msall ME: The limits of viability and the uncertainty of neuroprotection: Challenges in optimizing outcomes in extreme prematurity. *Pediatrics* 2007;119:158–160.

Nelson RM, Botkjin JR, Kodish ED, et al; Committee on Bioethics: Ethical issues with genetic testing in pediatrics. *Pediatrics* 2001;107:1451–1455.

Provoost V, Mortier F, Bilsen J, et al: Medical end-of-life decisions in neonates and infants in Flanders. *Lancet* 2005;365:1315–1320.

Solomon MZ, Sellers DE, Heller KS, et al: New and lingering controversies in pediatric end-of-life care. *Pediatrics* 2005;116:872–883.

Tripp J, McGregor D: Withholding and withdrawing of life sustaining treatment in the newborn. *Arch Dis Child Fetal Neonatal Ed* 2006;91:F67–F71.

Truog RD, Christ G, Browning DM, Meyer EC: Sudden traumatic death in children. *JAMA* 2006;295:2646–2654.

Vince T, Petros A: Should children's autonomy be respected by telling them of their imminent death? *J Med Ethics* 2006;32:21–23.

Vrakking AM, van der Heide A, Onwuteaka-Philipsen BD, et al: Medical end-of-life decisions made for neonates and infants in the Netherlands, 1995–2001. *Lancet* 2005;365:1329–1331.

Walsh-Kelly CM, Lang KR, Chevako J, et al: Advance directives in a pediatric emergency department. *Pediatrics* 1999;103:826–830.

Wendler D, Belsky L, Thompson KM, Emmanuel EJ: Quantifying the federal minimal risk standard. *JAMA* 2005;294:826–832.

Woolley S: Children of Jehovah's Witnesses and adolescent Jehovah's Witnesses: What are their rights? *Arch Dis Child* 2005;90:715–719.

Chapter 4 ■ Cultural Issues in Pediatric Care

Bonita Stanton

Pediatricians live and work in a multicultural world. Among the world's 6 billion people residing in >200 countries, >6,000 languages are spoken. In virtually all countries, there is greater ethnic and economic diversity as the global population becomes more mobile and integrated; from 1970 to 2000, the foreign-born population in the United States increased threefold. According to the 2000 census, 25 to 30% of Americans self-identify as belonging to an ethnic or racial minority group. Since 1990, the number of children in immigrant families has expanded sevenfold more rapidly than the number of children in families with U.S.-born parents such that currently 1 of every 5 children lives in an immigrant family. Whereas in 1920, 97% of immigrant families in the United States were from Europe or Canada, in 2000, 84% of U.S. immigrant children were from Latin America or Asia. Nonwhite children are projected to outnumber white children in the United States by the year 2030. Increased migration and diversity in the migrant pool is not limited to the United States; immigrants account for over 15% of the population in >50 nations.

Physicians are not limiting their professional exposure to a single country. The number of medical schools in the United States offering electives abroad has increased severalfold in the past decade, with most schools indicating an interest in continuing or expanding these opportunities. With increased globalization of the economy, more physicians will have the opportunity to practice outside their homeland.

THE IMPORTANCE OF CULTURE TO MEDICAL PRACTICE. Culture is a community's or a society's shared history, beliefs, and values, including frameworks for learning, understanding events and history, and defining concepts such as prosperity, success, knowledge, and health. Cultures are dynamic and interactive, so that even as individuals act within a culture, those actions effect changes in that culture. Although culture is not synonymous with language, race, ethnicity, nationality, or socioeconomic status, groups with similar backgrounds with respect to these characteristics often share cultural norms.

Tables 4-1 and 4-2 display some cultural values associated with four minority populations in the United States: Latinos, Muslims, Native Americans, and African-Americans, illustrating both areas of significant overlap and great variation that are relevant to health perceptions and health seeking. Latinos may subscribe to the importance of "personalismo," placing great importance on politeness in the face of stress and adversity and thus expect a display of warmth from their physician, including physical touching such as handshakes, hands on the shoulder, and occasionally

TABLE 4-1. Cultural Values* Relevant to Health and Health-Seeking Behavior

	RELEVANT CULTURAL NORMS	
CULTURAL GROUP	DESCRIPTION OF NORM	CONSEQUENCES OF FAILURE TO APPRECIATE
Latino	*Fatalismo:* Fate is predetermined, reducing belief in the importance of screening and prevention	Less preventive screening
	Simpatia: Politeness/kindness in the face of adversity—expectation that the physician should be polite and pleasant, not detached	Nonadherence to therapy, failure to make follow-up visits
	Personalismo: Expectation of developing a warm, personal relationship with the clinician, including introductory touching	Refusal to divulge important parts of medical history, dissatisfaction with treatment
	Respecto: Deferential behavior on the basis of age, social stature, and economic position, including reluctance to ask questions	Mistaking a deferential nod of the head/not asking questions for understanding; anger at not receiving due signs of respect
	Familismo: Needs of the extended family outrank those of the individual, and thus family may need to be consulted in medical decision-making	Unnecessary conflict, inability to reach a decision
Muslim	*Fasting* during the holy month of Ramadan: Fasting from sunrise to sundown, beginning during the teen years. Women are exempted during pregnancy, lactation, and menstruation and exemptions for illness, but may be associated with a sense of personal failure.	Inappropriate therapy; will not take medicines during daytime misinterpreted as noncompliance; misdiagnosed
	Modesty: Women's body including hair, body, arms, and legs not to be seen by men other than in immediate family. Female chaperone and/or husband must be present during exam and only that part of the body being examined should be uncovered.	Deep personal outrage, seeking alternative care
	Touch: Forbidden to touch members of the opposite sex other than close family. Even a handshake may be inappropriate.	Patient discomfort, seeking care elsewhere
	After death, body belongs to God: Postmortem exam will not be permitted unless required by law, family may wish to perform after-death care	Unnecessary intensification of grief and loss.
	Cleanliness essential before prayer: Individual must perform ritual ablutions before prayer, especially elimination of urine and stool. Nurse may need to assist in cleaning if patient is incapable.	Affront to religious beliefs.
	God's will: God causes all to happen for a reason and only God can bring about healing.	Allopathic medicine will be rejected if it conflicts with religious beliefs, family may not seek health care
	Patriarchal, extended family: Older male typically is head of household and family may defer to him for decision-making.	Child's mother or even both parents may not be able to make decisions about child's care; emergency decisions may require additional time.
	Halal (permitted) vs *harem* (forbidden) foods and medications: Foods and medicine containing alcohol (some cough and cold syrups) or pork (some gelatin-coated pills) are not permitted.	Refusal of medication, religious effrontery
Native American	*Nature* provides the spiritual, emotional, physical, social, and biologic means for human life; by caring for the earth, Native Americans will be provided for. Harmonious living is important.	Spiritual living is required of Native Americans; if treatments do not reflect this view, they are likely not to be followed
	Passive forbearance or right of the individual to chose his/her path: Another family member cannot intervene.	Mother's failure to intervene in a child's behavior and/or use of noncoercive disciplinary techniques may be mistaken for neglect
	Natural unfolding of the individual: Parents further the development of their children by limiting direct interventions and viewing their natural unfolding.	Many pediatric preventive practices will run counter to this philosophy
	Talking circle format to decision-making: Interactive learning format including diverse tribal members	Lecturing, excluding the views of elders is likely to result in advice that will be disregarded
African-American	Great heterogeneity in beliefs and culture among African-Americans	Risk of stereotyping and/or making assumptions that do not apply to a specific patient or family
	Extended family and variations in family size and child care arrangements are common; matriarchal decision-making regarding health care	Advice/instructions given only to the parent and not to others involved in health decision-making may not be effective
	Parenting style often involves stricter adherence to rules than seen in some other cultures	Advice regarding discipline may be disregarded if it is inconsistent with perceived norms; other parenting styles may not be effective
	History-based widespread mistrust of medical profession and strong orientation toward culturally specific alternative/complementary medicine	In patient noncompliance, physicians will be consulted as a last resort
	Greater orientation toward others; the role of an individual is emphasized as it relates to others within a social network	Compliance may be difficult if the needs of one individual are stressed above the needs of the group
	Spirituality/religiosity important; church attendance central in most African-American families	Loss of opportunity to work with the church as an ally in health care

*Adherence to these or other beliefs will vary among members of a cultural group based on nation of origin, specific religious sect, degree of acculturation, age of patient, etc.

TABLE 4-2. Examples of Disease Beliefs or Practices

CULTURAL GROUP	EXAMPLES
Latino	Use of traditional medicines (nopales or cooked prickly pear cactus as a hypoglycemic agent) along with allopathic medicine
	Recognition of disorders not recognized in Western allopathic medicine (*empacho*, in which food adheres to the intestines or stomach), which are treated with folk remedies but also brought to the pediatrician
	Cultural interpretation of disease (*caida de mollera* or fallen fontanel) as a cultural interpretation of severe dehydration in infants
Muslim	Female genital mutilation: Practiced in some Muslim countries, the majority do not practice it and it is not a direct teaching of the Koran
	Koranic faith healers: Utilize verses from the Koran, holy water, and specific foods to bring about recovery
Native American	Traditional "interpreters" or "healers" interpret signs and answers to prayers. Their advice may be sought in addition or instead of allopathic medicine.
	Dreams are believed to provide guidance; messages in the dream will be followed
African-American	Congregation may be asked to pray for the health of a child
	Specific practices such as using catnip or covering the child's head to reduce colic may be seen in some parts of the country
	Herbs, home remedies may be used alone or in conjunction with allopathic medicines

hugging. By contrast, in the Muslim culture, for a person to touch the body of a member of the opposite gender, including on the arm or a pat on the shoulder, is considered highly inappropriate. Other values may be shared across disparate cultural groups. Multiple ethnic groups including Latinos and Muslims as well as Sudanese and Bengalis share a cultural belief of fatalism, which has similar implications for health-seeking behavior although it emerges from differing belief systems. Despite the existence of shared values within a defined population group, there may be substantial variations within subgroups, such as the Latino national subgroups (Cuban, Mexican, and so on), resulting in great variation in specific health-seeking behaviors. Likewise, within an overarching culture ("American"), persons who are economically and/or politically disenfranchised may utilize resistance, inverting the values of the dominant socioeconomic group. Such a reaction may include distrust of recommendations regarding health care from members of the perceived dominant or controlling group. Immunizations have been viewed with distrust among the poor in countries around the globe, as they were believed to be a form of birth control or sterilization and were often offered through institutions associated with "Western" and postcolonial rule. There are often significant generational differences between foreign-born parents and their children, particularly as these children go through adolescence. With each generation, assimilation moves the group further into the new country's "culture."

NEWLY RECOGNIZED CULTURAL GROUPS. Groups such as adolescents, gay, lesbian, or transgender youth, and deaf youth who may not traditionally be recognized as cultural groups may have shared values with implications for health and health seeking. Failure on the part of the pediatrician to recognize accepted language and frame of reference of these groups may result in the unintentional use of offensive terminology or assumptions, leading to loss of the physician's credibility or noncompliance from the patient.

THE CULTURE OF THE MEDICAL PROFESSION. The profession of medicine also has a distinct culture. Like other cultural groups, physicians share a common history, admiring the same role models, sharing the same preparatory courses that must be mastered for entrance into training for the profession, and subscribing to a common meaning of "competence" in medical practice. Physicians learn a new way to describe health and illness, requiring a new vocabulary and a prescribed pattern to the narrative history, which is not shared by those outside medicine. Physician reliance on "evidence-based practice" carries the implication that it is synonymous with truth or real knowledge. Of particular importance in the relationship with patients has been the lack of physician insight into the existence of a physician culture and the potential biases that may be inherent to that culture. While physicians around the world recognize the great strides that have been made in child survival through the use of oral rehydration therapy in the treatment of dehydrating diarrheal diseases, parents are often anxious because the treatment does not stop the diarrhea. Physicians may be dependent on a particular style of communication and they may miss information from patients utilizing alternative narrative styles. Likewise, the physician-researcher forms questions through the prism of his or her own beliefs and literature, thereby reducing the likelihood of exploring alternative explanations or questions. While vast segments of the world's population understand disease as an imbalance of "hot" and "cold," this belief system has not been well represented in contemporary medical research.

CULTURAL COMPETENCE. Recognizing that physicians and patients bring to their interaction personal and professional values from multiple cultural systems, which have significant implications for the delivery of health care, has lead to recognition of the need for physician "cultural competence." Among the proposed frameworks for cultural competence, Campinha-Bacote's model is the most frequently cited: (1) learning to value and understand other cultures, in part through self-awareness of one's own cultural values ("cultural awareness"); (2) learning basic fundamentals about other cultures, particularly those of the patients with whom the physician will interact ("cultural knowledge"); (3) developing the ability to apply cultural knowledge in patient encounters ("cultural skills"); (4) seeking exposure to cross-cultural interactions ("cultural encounters"); and (5) being motivated to achieve all of the previous ("cultural desire"). This framework provides an important guide to pediatric education and practice and, thus, will serve as the outline for the remainder of this chapter.

Cultural Awareness. Recognition of the importance of differing cultural expectations and explanations is critical to a pediatrician's successful interactions with patients. For example, in the Muslim culture kinship is of great importance and decision-making may involve the extended family. Likewise, failure on the part of the pediatrician to realize that a mother may not feel comfortable or competent to make a decision about the health of her child may result in an apparent noncompliance on the part of the mother.

Cultural Knowledge. Physicians and patients have differing definitions of health and illness and differing concepts of the origins of disease and therapeutic responses. Understanding the patient perspective will both increase the likelihood of correct diagnosis and patient adherence to therapy and decrease the possibility of misdiagnosis. The belief that becoming chilled causes dysentery is common among rural Chinese and medical advice that directly challenges or runs contrary to this belief may be disregarded. Likewise, diarrhea among Bangladeshi children during teething may be regarded as normal and would not be identified as a health issue. Thus, asking the parent if the child has been ill might not reveal the presence of diarrhea. Rubbing a coin against a child's skin is thought by some parents in Asia to reduce fever. Failure by the pediatrician to recognize the practice of "coining" could lead to the erroneous diagnosis of a rash or child abuse.

Cultural Skill. Describing a diagnostic or therapeutic course of action that respects cultural beliefs but is consistent with good medical practice can be challenging. Common among many Latino groups is the belief of *empacho*, a condition wherein food is "stuck" to the stomach or intestinal wall, resulting in obstruction. The condition is believed to cause nausea, vomiting, diarrhea, and anorexia. Although most Latino parents would take a child with *empacho* to the physician for treatment, in Western settings, a pediatrician diagnosing the condition as viral gastroenteritis might only advise supportive management, leaving the parents perplexed and with no option but to seek independent treatment from a folk healer. A culturally skilled pediatrician might suggest partnering with the traditional healer in such a situation. Likewise, in response to parents subscribing to a belief in fatalism and, consequently, a notion that preventive medicine or screening is not necessary, a skilled pediatrician might suggest that screening is the mechanism through which their destiny is intended to be reached.

Central to "cultural skill" is the employment of language fully comprehended by the child's parents. This goal is best realized if the pediatrician is conversant, if not fluent, in the parent's language, and thus a requirement for a second language is a reasonable goal for physicians. Familiarity with a language should not be confused with fluency or even competency. Professional interpreters should be available and accessed to overcome the language barriers. Ad hoc use of individuals at the workplace who are known to possess skill in the indicated language and/or use of telephone interpreter services may suffice if a professional interpreter is not available. A genuinely bilingual family member or friend may be helpful, but issues of confidentiality, disruption of social roles, and uncertain or inaccurate translation of medical terms may pose serious problems. Medical errors occur at a significantly higher rate among non-English speaking patients when nonprofessional (e.g., family members) translators are used to obtain a history or give medical advice.

Cultural Encounters. While cultural knowledge may be acquired through didactic training, the development of cultural skills requires experience that can only be gained through repeated "cultural encounters." Studies have confirmed that, after controlling for relevant variables, clinicians provide lower quality of care to Latino and African-American patients, with these children being less likely to receive analgesia and/or nebulizers for asthma. Latino mothers have reported clinician attitudes as a major barrier to seeking care for their children. Another study among physicians revealed that participation in diverse medical educational settings and experience in community clinics predicted cultural knowledge. Cultural knowledge and participation in diverse educational settings, as well as Latino ethnicity and bilingual skills, predicted cultural awareness. Only cultural awareness predicted culturally competent actions. Consistent with observations that cultural competence may not be valued in the traditional medical culture is the observation that *higher* specialty training (e.g., subspecialty training among internists compared to general physicians, family medicine, or internal medicine generalists) predicted *less* cultural awareness. In another study among children, two thirds of whom had persistent asthma, patients receiving care from practice sites with the highest cultural competence scores were less likely to underutilize preventive asthma medications.

Cultural Desire. Cultural competence is not something that can be achieved and retained in the absence of continued effort. The recognition that culture is integral to health and healing, and to disease and sickness, is central to the concept of "cultural competence." Understanding of the role of culture in health outcomes is nascent, however. Although speculation abounds, it is not yet known why less acculturated Latinos in the United States demonstrate significantly lower rates of low birthweight, depression, tobacco use, illicit drug use, and older age at 1st intercourse compared to those who are more acculturated. Likewise, less acculturation among Asian children is associated with lower prevalence of chronic illness. Perhaps environment more than gene type may represent a significant influence on the phenotype of acculturated individuals.

Eschiti VS: Holistic approach to resolving American Indian/Alaska native health care disparities. *J Holist Nurs* 2004;22:201–208.

Flores G: Culture, ethnicity, and linguistic issues in pediatric care: Urgent priorities and unanswered questions. *Ambul Pediatr* 2004;4:276–282.

Flores G: Culture and the patient-physician relationship: Achieving cultural competency in health care. *J Pediatr* 2000;136:14.

Hernandez DJ: Changing demographics: Past and future demands for early childhood programs. *Future Child* 1995;5:145–160.

Kirk-Smith MD, Stretch DD: The influence of medical professionalism on scientific practice. *J Eval Clin Pract* 2003;9:417–422.

Lawrence P, Rozmus C: Culturally sensitive care of the Muslim patient. *J Transcult Nurs* 2001;12:228–233.

Lieu TA, Finkelstein JA, Lozano P, et al: Cultural competence policies and other predictors of asthma care quality for Medicaid-insured children. *Pediatrics* 2004;114:e102–e110.

Pachter LM: Culture and clinical care: Folk illness beliefs and behaviors and their implications for health care delivery. *JAMA* 1994;271:690–694.

Reimann JO, Talavera GA, Salmon M, et al: Cultural competence among physicians treating Mexican Americans who have diabetes: A structural model. *Soc Sci Med* 2004;59:2195–2205.

Smitherman LC, Janisse J, Mathur A: The use of folk remedies among children in an urban black community: remedies for fever, colic and teething. *Pediatrics* 2005;115:297–304.

Taylor JS: Confronting "culture" in medicine's "culture of no culture." *Acad Med* 2003;78:555–559.

Chapter 5 ■ Maximizing Children's Health Screening, Anticipatory Guidance, and Counseling

Joseph F. Hagan Jr and Paula M. Duncan

The health supervision encounter with the well child is the keystone to the care of the infant, child, and adolescent in the United States. No other nation's health care system places such emphasis on periodic and regular preventive health care, and although preventive services are also recommended for adults, the constantly changing tableau of a child's development lends added value to these encounters between children and their families and practitioners of pediatric health care.

The evolution of this preventive health care approach is derived from the long-standing view that the science of pediatrics is a science of health and development. To assure the optimal health of the developing child, pediatric care in this country evolved into regularly scheduled visits to assure adequate nutrition, detect and immunize against infectious diseases, and observe the child's development. Immunization, nutrition assessment, and developmental assessment remain essential elements of the well child health supervision visit, but changes in the population's health have led to the addition of other components to the content of today's well child encounter.

PERIODICITY. The frequency and content for well child care activities are derived from expert consensus, both from federal agencies and professional organizations such as the American Academy of Pediatrics (AAP), and from evidence-based practice, when available. The Periodicity Schedule (Table 5-1) is a compilation of recommendations listed by age-based visits (Table 5-2). It is intended to guide practitioners of pediatric primary care to perform certain services and make observations at age-specific visits.

GUIDELINES. Several organizations have compiled recommendations or guidelines for how the care of well children should be accomplished. These comprehensive guides are based on the Periodicity Schedule, but they expand it further and recommend how

TABLE 5-1. Bright Futures Periodicity Schedule

INFANCY PERIODICITY SCHEDULE
Initial Visit
Newborn
In the 1st wk
1 mo
2 mo
4 mo
6 mo
9 mo
EARLY CHILDHOOD PERIODICITY SCHEDULE
1 yr
15 mo
18 mo
2 yr
3 yr
4 yr
MIDDLE CHILDHOOD PERIODICITY SCHEDULE
5 yr
6 yr
8 yr
10 yr
ADOLESCENCE PERIODICITY SCHEDULE
11 yr
12 yr
13 yr
14 yr
15 yr
16 yr
17 yr
18 yr
19 yr
20 yr
21 yr

From Green M, Palfrey JS (editors): *Bright Futures: Guidelines for Health Supervision of Infants, Children, and Adolescents*, 2nd ed, rev. Arlington, VA, National Center for Education in Maternal and Child Health, 2002.

practitioners might accomplish the tasks outlined in the Periodicity Schedule. In addition to numerous recommendations developed by individual communities or local health care systems, three major sources of guidelines have been: *Bright Futures,* from the Maternal Child Health Bureau of the U.S. Department of Health and Human Services, the American Academy of Pediatrics' *Guidelines for Health Supervision,* and the American Medical Association's *Guidelines for Adolescent Preventive Services (GAPS).* Under the leadership of the Maternal Child Health Bureau, these organizations, the National Association of Pediatric Nurse Practitioners, the American Academy of Family Physicians, and others have developed the *Bright Futures Guidelines, 3rd Edition.* This subsumes previous guidelines and is consistent with the AAP Periodic Schedule. See Table 5-1.

TASKS OF WELL CHILD CARE. The well child encounter has unique contributions for promoting the physical and emotional well-being of children and youth. Child health professionals, including pediatricians, family medicine physicians, nurse practitioners, and physician assistants, take advantage of the opportunity the well child visits provide to elicit parental questions and concerns, gather relevant family and individual health information, perform a physical examination, and initiate screening tests.

The tasks of each well child visit include:

- Disease detection
- Disease prevention
- Health promotion
- Anticipatory guidance

To achieve these outcomes, health care professionals employ techniques to screen for disease, screen for risk of disease, and provide advice about healthy behaviors. These activities lead to the formulation of appropriate anticipatory guidance and health advice.

Clinical detection of disease in the well child encounter is accomplished by both surveillance and screening. In well child care surveillance occurs in every health encounter and is enhanced by the opportunity for repeated visits and observations with advancing developmental stages. It relies on the experience of a skilled clinician over time. Screening is a more formal process utilizing some form of tool, which has been validated and has known sensitivity and specificity. For example, anemia surveillance is accomplished through taking a dietary history and seeking signs of anemia in the physical examination. Anemia screening is by hematocrit or hemoglobin tests. Developmental surveillance relies on the observations of parents and the watchful eyes of providers of pediatric health care who are experienced in child development. Developmental screening utilizes a structured developmental screening tool or approach by personnel trained in its use or in the scoring and interpretation of parent report questionnaires.

The 2nd essential action of the well child encounter, *disease prevention,* may include both *primary prevention* activities applied to a whole population and *secondary prevention* activities aimed at patients with specific factors of risk. For example, counseling about reducing fat intake is appropriate for all children and families. Counseling is intensified in the presence of a family history of hyperlipidemia and its sequellae. The child and adolescent health care professional needs to individualize disease prevention strategies to the community, as well as the specific family and patient.

Health promotion and **anticipatory guidance** activities distinguish the well child health supervision visit from all other encounters with the health care system. Disease detection and disease prevention activities are germane to all interactions of children with physicians and other health care providers, but health promotion and anticipatory guidance shift the focus to wellness and to the strengths of the family, for example, what is being done well and how this might be improved. This approach is an opportunity to help the family address relationship issues, to broach important safety topics, to access community services, and to engage with extended family, school, neighborhood, and church.

It is not possible to cover all the topics suggested by comprehensive guidelines such as *Bright Futures* in the average 18 min well child visit. Child health professionals must prioritize the most important topics to cover. Consideration should be given to a discussion of:

- The topics where evidence suggests counseling is effective in behavioral change
- The topics where there is a clear rationale for the issue's critical importance to health, for example, "back to sleep" to prevent SIDS, physical activity
- A summary of the child's progress in emotional and social development, physical growth, and strengths
- Issues that address the questions, concerns, or specific health problems relevant to the individual family
- Community-specific problems that could significantly impact the child's health, for example, bike paths that promote activity or neighborhood violence from which children need protection

It is important to note that this approach is directed at all children, including those with special health needs (see Chapter 38). Children with special health needs are no different from other children in their need for guidance about healthy nutrition, physical activity, progress in school, connection with friends, a healthy sense of self-efficacy, and avoidance of risk-taking behaviors. The coordination of specialty consultation, medication monitoring, and functional assessment, which should occur in their periodic visits, needs to be balanced with a discussion of the child's unique ways of accomplishing the emotional, social, and developmental tasks of childhood and adolescence.

TABLE 5-2. Recommendations for Preventive Pediatric Health Care (RE9535)

COMMITTEE ON PRACTICE AND AMBULATORY MEDICINE

Each child and family is unique; therefore, these **Recommendations for Preventive Pediatric Health Care** are designed for the care of children who are receiving competent parenting, have no manifestations of any important health problems, and are growing and developing in satisfactory fashion. **Additional visits may become necessary** if circumstances suggest variations from normal.

These guidelines represent a consensus by the Committee on Practice and Ambulatory Medicine in consultation with national committees and sections of the American Academy of Pediatrics. The Committee emphasizes the great importance of **continuity of care** in comprehensive health supervision and the need to avoid **fragmentation of care**.

	INFANCY[4]									EARLY CHILDHOOD[4]					MIDDLE CHILDHOOD[4]				ADOLESCENCE[4]										
AGE[5]	PRENATAL[1]	NEWBORN[2]	2–4d[3]	By 1 mo	2 mo	4 mo	6 mo	9 mo	12 mo	15 mo	18 mo	24 mo	3 y	4 y	5 y	6 y	8 y	10 y	11 y	12 y	13 y	14 y	15 y	16 y	17 y	18 y	19 y	20 y	21 y
HISTORY																													
Initial/Interval	•	•	•	•	•	•	•	•	•	•	•	•	•	•	•	•	•	•	•	•	•	•	•	•	•	•	•	•	•
MEASUREMENTS																													
Height and Weight		•	•	•	•	•	•	•	•	•	•	•	•	•	•	•	•	•	•	•	•	•	•	•	•	•	•	•	•
Head Circumference		•	•	•	•	•	•	•	•	•	•	•																	
Blood Pressure													•	•	•	•	•	•	•	•	•	•	•	•	•	•	•	•	•
SENSORY SCREENING																													
Vision		S	S	S	S	S	S	S	S	S	S	S	O[6]	O	O	O	O	O	S	O	S	S	O	S	S	O	S	S	S
Hearing		O[7]	S	S	S	S	S	S	S	S	S	S	S	O	O	O	O	O	S	O	S	S	O	S	S	O	S	S	S
DEVELOPMENTAL/BEHAVIORAL ASSESSMENT[8]		•	•	•	•	•	•	•	•	•	•	•	•	•	•	•	•	•	•	•	•	•	•	•	•	•	•	•	•
PHYSICAL EXAMINATION[9]		•	•	•	•	•	•	•	•	•	•	•	•	•	•	•	•	•	•	•	•	•	•	•	•	•	•	•	•
PROCEDURES-GENERAL[10]																													
Hereditary/Metabolic Screening[11]		←	•	→																									
Immunization[12]		•	•	•	•	•	•	•	•	•	•	•	•	•	•	•	•	•	•	•	•	•	•	•	•	•	•	•	•
Hematocrit or Hemoglobin[13]								• →	→	★ →	→	→	→	→	→				←	→	•[14]	→	→	→	→	→	→	→	→
Urinalysis															•				←	→	→	→	→	•[15]	→	→	→	→	→
PROCEDURES-PATIENTS AT RISK																													
Lead Screening[16]								★ →	→			★																	
Tuberculin Test[17]									★	★	★	★	★	★	★	★	★	★	★	★	★	★	★	★	★	★	★	★	★
Cholesterol Screening[18]												★	★	★	★	★	★	★	★	★	★	★	★	★	★	★	★	★	★
STD Screening[19]																			★	★	★	★	★	★	★	★	★	★	★
Pelvic Exam[20]																			★	★	★	★	★	★	★	★ ←	•[20]	★ →	★
ANTICIPATORY GUIDANCE[21]	•	•	•	•	•	•	•	•	•	•	•	•	•	•	•	•	•	•	•	•	•	•	•	•	•	•	•	•	•
Injury Prevention[22]	•	•	•	•	•	•	•	•	•	•	•	•	•	•	•	•	•	•	•	•	•	•	•	•	•	•	•	•	•
Violence Prevention[23]	•	•	•	•	•	•	•	•	•	•	•	•	•	•	•	•	•	•	•	•	•	•	•	•	•	•	•	•	•
Sleep Positioning Counseling[24]	•	•	•	•	•	•	•																						
Nutrition Counseling[25]	•	•	•	•	•	•	•	•	•	•	•	•	•	•	•	•	•	•	•	•	•	•	•	•	•	•	•	•	•
DENTAL REFERRAL[26]									←	←	←	←	•																

1. A prenatal visit is recommended for parents who are at high risk, for first-time parents, and for those who request a conference. The prenatal visit should include anticipatory guidance, pertinent medical history, and a discussion of benefits of breastfeeding and planned method of feeding per AAP statement "The Prenatal Visit" (1996).
2. Every infant should have a newborn evaluation after birth. Breastfeeding should be encouraged and instruction and support offered. Every breastfeeding infant should have an evaluation 48–72 hours after discharge from the hospital to include weight, formal breastfeeding evaluation, encouragement, and instruction as recommended in the AAP statement "Breastfeeding and the Use of Human Milk" (1997).
3. For newborns discharged in less than 48 hours after delivery per AAP statement "Hospital Stay for Healthy Term Newborns" (1995).
4. Developmental, psychosocial, and chronic disease issues for children and adolescents may require frequent counseling and treatment visits separate from preventive care visits.
5. If a child comes under care for the first time at any point on the schedule, or if any items are not accomplished at the suggested age, the schedule should be brought up to date at the earliest possible time.
6. If the patient is uncooperative, rescreen within 6 months.
7. All newborns should be screened per the AAP Task Force on Newborn and Infant Hearing statement, "Newborn and Infant Hearing Loss: Detection and Intervention" (1999).
8. By history and appropriate physical examination: if suspicious, by specific objective developmental testing. Parenting skills should be fostered at every visit.
9. At each visit, a complete physical examination is essential, with infant totally unclothed, older child undressed and suitably draped.
10. These may be modified, depending upon entry point into schedule and individual need.
11. Metabolic screening (e.g., thyroid, hemoglobinopathies, PKU, galactosemia) should be done according to state law.
12. Schedule(s) per the Committee on Infectious Diseases, published annually in the January edition of *Pediatrics*. Every visit should be an opportunity to update and complete a child's immunizations.
13. See AAP *Pediatric Nutrition Handbook* (1998) for a discussion of universal and selective screening options. Consider earlier screening for high-risk infants (e.g., premature infants and low birth weight infants). See also "Recommendations to Prevent and Control Iron Deficiency in the United States." *MMWR* 1998;47(RR-3):1–29.
14. All menstruating adolescents should be screened annually.
15. Conduct dipstick urinalysis for leukocytes annually for sexually active male and female adolescents.
16. For children at risk of lead exposure, consult the AAP statement "Screening for Elevated Blood Levels" (1998). Additionally, screening should be done in accordance with state law where applicable.
17. TB testing per recommendations of the Committee on Infectious Diseases, published in the current edition of *Red Book: Report of the Committee on Infectious Diseases*. Testing should be done upon recognition of high-risk factors.
18. Cholesterol screening for high-risk patients per APP statement "Cholesterol in Childhood" (1998). If family history cannot be ascertained and other risk factors are present, screening should be at the discretion of the physician.
19. All sexually active patients should be screened for sexually transmitted diseases (STDs).
20. All sexually active females should have a pelvic examination. A pelvic examination and routine Pap smear should be offered as part of preventive health maintenance between the ages of 18 and 21 years.
21. Age-appropriate discussion and counseling should be an integral part of each visit for care per the AAP *Guidelines for Health Supervision III* (1998).
22. From birth to age 12, refer to the AAP injury prevention program (TIPP) as described in *A Guide to Safety Counseling in Office Practice* (1994).
23. Violence prevention and management for all patients per AAP Statement "The Role of the Pediatrician in Youth Violence Prevention in Clinical Practice and at the Community Level" (1999).
24. Parents and caregivers should be advised to place healthy infants on their backs when putting them to sleep. Side positioning is a reasonable alternative but carries a slightly higher risk of SIDS. Consult the AAP statement "Positioning and Sudden Infant Death Syndrome (SIDS): Update" (1996).
25. Age-appropriate nutrition counseling should be an integral part of each visit per the AAP *Handbook of Nutrition* (1998).
26. Earlier initial dental examinations may be appropriate for some children. Subsequent examinations as prescribed by dentist.

Key: ● = to be performed ★ = to be performed for patients at risk
S = subjective, by history O = objective, by a standard testing method
←●→ = the range during which a service may be provided, with the dot indicating the preferred age.

NB: Special chemical, Immunologic, and endocrine testing is usually carried out upon specific indications. Testing other than newborn (e.g., inborn errors of metabolism, sickle disease, etc.) is discretionary with the physician.

The recommendations in this statement do not indicate an exclusive course of treatment or standard of medical care. Variations, taking into account individual circumstances, may be appropriate. American Academy of Pediatrics, Committee on Practice and Ambulatory Medicine. Policy Statement: Recommendations for Preventive Pediatric Health Care. *Pediatrics* 2000;105(3):645–646.

INFANCY AND EARLY CHILDHOOD. Nutrition, physical activity, sleep, safety, and emotional, social, and physical growth along with parental well-being are critical for all children. For each well child visit, there are topics that are specific to individual children based on their age, family situation, chronic health condition, or a parental concern, for example, "back to sleep," activities to lose weight, and fences around swimming pools. Attention should also be focused on the family milieu, for example, screening for maternal depression (especially postpartum depression) and other mental illness, family violence, substance abuse, nutritional inadequacy, or lack of housing. These issues are essential to the care of young children.

Answering parents' questions is one of the most important priorities of the well child visit. Promoting family-centered care and partnership with parents increases the ability to elicit parent concerns, especially about their child's development, learning, and behavior. It is important to identify children with developmental disorders as early as possible. Developmental surveillance at every visit combined with a structured developmental screening at some visits is a way to improve diagnosis, especially of some of the more subtle language delays.

MIDDLE CHILDHOOD AND ADOLESCENCE. As the child enters school-aged years, additional considerations emerge. The six health behaviors that are most important in adolescent and adult morbidity and mortality are: nutrition, physical activity, sexuality related behavior, tobacco, alcohol and other drug use, behaviors that contribute to unintentional and intentional injuries, and violence. Emotional well-being with attention to the developmental tasks of adolescence (competence at school and other activities, connection to friends and family, autonomy, empathy, and a sense of self-worth), as well as early diagnosis and treatment of mental health problems, are of equal importance.

OFFICE INTERVENTION FOR BEHAVIORAL AND MENTAL HEALTH ISSUES. Twenty percent of primary care encounters with children are for a behavioral or mental health problem, or are sickness visits complicated by a mental health issue. Pediatricians need increased knowledge for diagnosis, treatment, and referral criteria for attention-deficit/hyperactivity disorder (ADHD), depression, anxiety, and conduct disorder, as well as an understanding of the pharmacology of the frequently prescribed psychotropic medications. Encouragement of behavioral change is also an important responsibility of the clinician. Motivational interviewing provides a structured approach that has been designed to help patients and parents identify the discrepancy between their desire for health and their behavioral choices. It also allows the clinician to use proven strategies that lead to a patient-initiated plan for change.

STRENGTH-BASED APPROACHES AND FRAMEWORK. Questions about school or extracurricular accomplishments or competent personal characteristics should be integrated into the content of the well child visit. This often sets a positive context for the visit, deepens the partnership with the family, and acknowledges the child's healthy development. This facilitates discussing social-emotional development with children and their parents. There is a strong relationship between appropriate social-emotional development (e.g., children's strong connection to their family, social friends, and mentors; competence, empathy, and appropriate autonomy) and decreased participation in all the risk behaviors of adolescence (related to drugs, sex, and violence). An organized approach to the identification and encouragement of a child's strengths during health supervision visits provides both the child and parent with an understanding of how to promote healthy achievement of the developmental tasks of childhood and adolescence. Children with special health needs often have a different timetable, but they have an equal need to be encouraged to develop strong family and peer connections, competence in a variety of arenas, ways to do things for others, and appropriate independent decision-making.

OFFICE SYSTEM CHANGE FOR QUALITY IMPROVEMENT. Some of the office strategies to improve the preventive services delivered to children and youth include screening schedules and parent handouts, flow sheets, registries, and the use of parent and youth previsit questionnaires. These efforts are part of a larger national effort that is built on a coordinated team approach in the office setting and the use of continuous measurement for improvement.

EVIDENCE. The clinical encounter with the well child is guideline and recommendation driven and requires the integration of clinician goals, family needs, and community realities in seeking better health for the child. Few well child care activities have been evaluated for efficacy, yet these activities are highly valued; lack of evidence is not the same as lack of benefit. The rationale for well child care activities is a balance of evidence from research, clinical practice guidelines, professional recommendations, expert opinion, experience, habit, intuition, and preferences or values. Clinical or counseling decisions and recommendations may also be based on legislation (seatbelts), on common sense measures not likely to be studied experimentally (lowering water heater temperatures), or on the basis of relational evidence (television watching associated with violent behavior in young children). Most important, sound clinical and counseling decisions are responsive to family needs and desires, and support "patient-centered decision-making."

CARING FOR THE CHILD AND YOUTH IN THE CONTEXT OF THE FAMILY AND COMMUNITY. A successful primary care practice for children incorporates families, is family centered, and embraces the concept of the medical home. A medical home is defined by the AAP as primary care that is accessible, continuous, comprehensive, family centered, coordinated, compassionate, and culturally effective. In a medical home, a pediatrician works in partnership with the family and patient to assure that all medical and non-medical needs of the child are met. Through this partnership, the child health care professional helps the family/patient access and coordinate specialty care, educational services, out-of-home care, family support, and other public and private community services that are important to the overall health of the child and family.

Ideally, health promotion activities occur not only in the medical home, but also in partnership with community members and other health and education professionals. This rests on a clear understanding of the important role that the community plays in supporting healthy behaviors among families. Communities where children and families feel safe and valued, and have access to positive activities and relationships, provide the important base that the health care professional can build on and refer to for needed services that support health but are outside the realm of the health care system or primary care pediatric office. It is important for the medical home and community agencies to identify mutual resources, communicate well with families and each other, and partner in designing service delivery systems. This interaction is the practice of community pediatrics, whose unique feature is its concern for all of the population: those who remain well but need preventive services, those who have symptoms but do not receive effective care, and those who do seek medical care either in a physician's office or in a hospital.

American Academy of Pediatrics, Committee on Community Health Services: The pediatrician's role in community pediatrics. *Pediatrics* 1999;103:1304–1307.

American Academy of Pediatrics, Committee on Practice and Ambulatory Medicine. Recommendations for preventive pediatric health care. *Pediatrics* 2000;105(3):645–646.

American Academy of Pediatrics, Division of Health Policy Research. Periodic Survey of Fellows #56: Executive Summary, *Pediatricians' Provision of Preventive Care and Use of Health Supervision Guidelines,* May 2004.

American Medical Association: *Guidelines for Preventive Health Services (GAPS) Recommendations.* Chicago, American Medical Association, 1997.

Bordley WC, Margolis PA, Stuart J, et al: Improving preventive service delivery through office systems. *Pediatrics* 2001;108:E41.

Green M, Palfrey JS (eds): *Bright Futures Guidelines for Health Supervision of Infants, Children, and Adolescents,* 2nd ed. Arlington, VA, National Center for Education in Maternal Child Health, 2000.

Haggerty RJ: Community pediatrics: Past and present. *Pediatr Ann* 1994;23:657–658, 661–663.

Kelleher KJ, McInerney TK, Gardner WP, et al: Increasing identification of psychosocial problems: 1979–1996. *Pediatrics* 2000;105:1313–1321.

Medical Home Initiatives for Children with Special Needs Project Advisory Committee, American Academy of Pediatrics: The medical home. *Pediatrics* 2002;110:184–186.

Moore K, Halle T: Preventing problems vs. promoting the positive: what do we want for our children? *Child Trends Research Brief* www.childtrends.org. May 2000.

Murphey DM, Hale K, Carney J, et al: Relationships of a brief measure of youth assets to health promoting and risk behaviors. *J Adolesc Health* 2004;34:184–191.

Resnick MD: Resilience and protective factors in the lives of adolescents. *J Adolesc Health* 2000;27(1):1–2.

Resnicow KD, DiIorio C, Soet JE, et al: Motivational interviewing in health promotion: It sounds like something is changing. *Health Psychol* 2002;21:444–451.

Stein MT, Wolraich MI, Cohen GJ, et al: *Guidelines for Health Supervision III.* Elk Grove Village, IL, American Academy of Pediatrics, 2002.

Part II ■ Growth, Development, and Behavior

Chapter 6 ■ Overview and Assessment of Variability

Susan Feigelman

The goal of pediatric care is to maximize each child's potential. Pediatricians need to understand normal growth, development, and behavior in order to monitor children's progress, to identify delays or abnormalities in development, and to counsel parents. In addition to clinical experience and personal knowledge, effective practice requires familiarity with major theoretical perspectives and evidence-based strategies for optimizing growth and development. To target factors that increase or decrease risk, pediatricians need to understand how biologic and social forces interact within the parent-child relationship, within the family, and between the family and the larger society. Growth is an indicator for overall well-being, chronic disease, and interpersonal and psychologic stress. By monitoring children and families over time, pediatricians can observe the interrelationships between physical growth and cognitive, motor, and emotional development. At the same time, observation is enhanced by familiarity with developmental theory. Understanding developmental models will help explain normal patterns of behavior and help with prevention of behavior problems.

BIOPSYCHOSOCIAL MODELS OF DEVELOPMENT

Development, the individual level of functioning a child is capable of as a result of maturation of the nervous system and psychologic reactions, is not determined solely by either genetics (nature) or the environment (nurture), but rather by a combination of both. Height is a function of a child's genetic endowment (biologic), personal eating habits (psychologic), and access to nutritious food (social).

The **biopsychosocial model** was developed in response to the failures of the biomedical model. The biomedical model was predicated on a dualism: the patient as provider of disease manifestations, and the physician, who was focused on diseases of the body. This model neglects the psychologic aspect of a person who exists in the larger realm of the family and society. In the biopsychosocial model, physicians needed to consider higher-level systems simultaneously with the lower-level systems that make up the person and the person's environment (Fig. 6-1). A patient's symptoms are examined and explained in the context of the patient's existence. This basic model can be used to understand health and both acute and chronic disease.

Research demonstrating the profound impact of early experience on the development of the brain (**neural plasticity**) has illuminated the interaction of nature and nurture. The brain comprises 100 billion neurons at birth, with each neuron developing on average 15,000 synapses by 3 yr of age. The number of synapses stays roughly constant through the first decade of life as the number of neurons declines. Synapses in frequently used pathways are preserved, whereas less-used ones atrophy. Thus, experience (nurture) has a direct effect on the physical properties of the brain (nature). Children with different talents and temperaments (nature) also elicit different stimuli from their environment (nurture).

Early experience is particularly important because learning proceeds more efficiently along established synaptic pathways. Sensory deprivation has profound effects. Traumatic experiences also create enduring alterations in the neurotransmitter and endocrine systems that mediate the stress response, with effects noted later in life. But experiences, positive or negative, rarely determine the total outcome. Rather, they shift the probabilities one way or another, by influencing the child's ability to respond adaptively to future stimuli. The plasticity of the brain continues into adolescence, with further development of the prefrontal cortex, which is important in decision-making, future planning, and emotional control.

Although biologic, psychologic, and social factors combine to shape development, it is helpful to consider each class of influence separately.

BIOLOGIC INFLUENCES. Biologic influences on development include genetics, in utero exposure to teratogens, postnatal illnesses, exposure to hazardous substances, and maturation. Adoption and twin studies consistently show that heredity accounts for approximately ½ of the variance in IQ and in other personality traits, such as sociability and desire for novelty. The specific genes underlying these traits have begun to be identified. The effects on development of prenatal exposure to teratogens, such as mercury and alcohol, and of postnatal insults, such as meningitis and traumatic brain injury, have been extensively studied. Any chronic illness can affect growth and development, either directly or through changes in nutrition, parenting, or peer interactions.

Physical and neurologic maturation propels children forward and sets lower limits for the emergence of most abilities. The age at which children walk independently is similar around the world, despite great variability in child-rearing practices. The attainment of other skills, such as the use of complex sentences, is less tightly bound to a maturational schedule. Maturational changes also generate behavioral challenges at predictable times. Decrements in growth rate and sleep requirements around 2 yr of age often generate concern about poor appetite and refusal to nap. Although it is possible to accelerate many developmental milestones (toilet training a 12 mo old or teaching a 3 yr old to read), the long-term benefits of such precocious accomplishments are questionable.

In addition to physical changes in size, body proportions, and strength, maturation brings about hormonal changes. Sexual differentiation, both somatic and neurologic, begins in utero. Behavioral effects of testosterone may be evident even in young children and continue to be salient throughout life. Correlations between testosterone and such traits as aggression or novelty seeking have not been consistently demonstrated.

A biologic influence of particular clinical importance is **temperament.** Temperament refers to a child's characteristic behavioral responses to internal and external stimuli. The classic theory

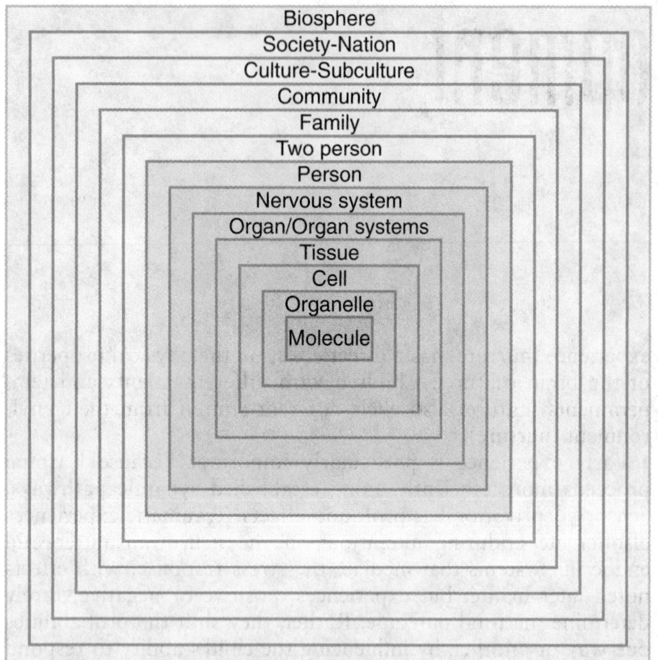

Figure 6-1. Continuum and hierarchy of natural systems in the biopsychosocial model. (From Engel GL: The clinical application of the biopsychosocial model. *Am J Psych* 1980;137:535–544.)

of Thomas and Chess proposes 9 dimensions of temperament (Table 6-1). These characteristics lead to 3 common constellations: (1) the easy, highly adaptable child, who has regular biologic cycles; (2) the difficult child, who withdraws from new stimuli and is easily frustrated; and (3) the slow-to-warm-up child, who needs extra time to adapt to new circumstances. Various combinations of these clusters also occur. Temperament is intrinsic to a child and relatively resistant to modification by parenting practices. Stability of temperamental characteristics over time improves as the child ages into middle childhood.

The concept of temperament is clinically useful in 2 ways. First, it can help parents understand and accept the characteristics of their children without feeling responsible for having caused them. Children who have difficulty adjusting to change may have behavior problems when a new baby arrives or at the time of school entry. Second, pointing out the child's temperament may allow for adjustment in parenting styles. Behavioral and emotional problems may develop when the temperamental characteristics of children and parents conflict.

PSYCHOLOGIC INFLUENCES: ATTACHMENT AND CONTINGENCY. The influence of the child-rearing environment dominates most current models of development. Infants in hospitals and orphanages, devoid of opportunities for attachment, have severe developmental deficits. *Attachment* refers to a biologically determined tendency of a young child to seek proximity to the parent during times of stress and also to the relationship that allows securely attached children to use their parents to re-establish a sense of well-being after a stressful experience. Insecure attachment may be predictive of later behavioral and learning problems.

At all stages of development, children progress optimally when they have adult caregivers who pay attention to their verbal and nonverbal cues and respond accordingly. In early infancy, such contingent responsiveness to signs of overarousal or underarousal helps maintain infants in a state of quiet alertness and fosters autonomic self-regulation. **Contingent responses** (reinforcement depending on the behavior of the other) to nonverbal gestures create the groundwork for the shared attention and reciprocity that are critical for later language and social development. Children learn best when new challenges are just slightly harder than what they have already mastered, a degree of difficulty dubbed the "zone of proximal development." Psychologic forces, such as attention problems or mood disorders, will have profound effects on the older child's other activities.

SOCIAL FACTORS: FAMILY SYSTEMS AND THE ECOLOGIC MODEL. Contemporary models of child development recognize the critical importance of influences outside of the mother-child dyad. Increasingly, fathers are recognized as playing critical roles, both in their direct relationships with their children and in supporting mothers. As traditional "nuclear" families become less dominant, the influence of other family members (grandparents, foster and adoptive parents, same-sex partners) becomes increasingly important. In addition, children are increasingly raised by non-related caregivers while parents work.

Families function as systems, with internal and external boundaries, subsystems, roles, and rules for interaction. In families with rigidly defined parental subsystems, children may be denied any decision-making at all, exacerbating rebelliousness. In families with relatively porous parent-child boundaries, children may be required to take on responsibilities beyond their years, or may be recruited to play a spousal role.

Individuals within systems adopt implicit roles. For example, one child may be the "troublemaker," whereas another is the "negotiator" and another is "quiet." Birth order may have profound effects on personality development, through its influence on family roles and patterns of interaction. Families are also dynamic. Changes in one person's behavior affect every other member of the system; roles shift until a new equilibrium is found. The birth of a new child, attainment of developmental milestones such as independent walking, the onset of nighttime

TABLE 6-1. Temperamental Characteristics: Descriptions and Examples**

CHARACTERISTIC	DESCRIPTION	EXAMPLES*
Activity level	Amount of gross motor movement	"She's constantly on the move." "He would rather sit still than run around."
Rhythmicity	Regularity of biologic cycles	"He's never hungry at the same time each day." "You could set a watch by her nap."
Approach and withdrawal	Initial response to new stimuli	"She rejects every new food at first." "He sleeps well in any place."
Adaptability	Ease of adaptation to novel stimulus	"Changes upset him." "She adjusts to new people quickly."
Threshold of responsiveness	Intensity of stimuli needed to evoke a response (e.g., touch, sound, light)	"He notices all the lumps in his food and objects to them." "She will eat anything, wear anything, do anything."
Intensity of reaction	Energy level of response	"She shouts when she is happy and wails when she is sad." "He never cries much."
Quality of mood	Usual disposition (e.g., pleasant, glum)	"He does not laugh much." "It seems like she is always happy."
Distractibility	How easily diverted from ongoing activity	"She is distracted at mealtime when other children are playing." "He doesn't even hear me when he is playing."
Attention span and persistence	How long a child pays attention and sticks with difficult tasks	"He goes from toy to toy every minute." "She will keep at a puzzle until she has mastered it."

*Typical statements of parents, reflecting the range for each characteristic from very little to very much.
**Based on Chess S, Thomas A: *Temperament in Clinical Practice.* New York, NY, Guilford, 1986.

fears, and the death of a grandparent are all changes that require renegotiation of roles within the family and have the potential for healthy adaptation or dysfunction.

The family system, in turn, functions within the larger systems of extended family, subculture, culture, and society. Bronfenbrenner's ecologic model depicts these relationships as concentric circles, with the parent-child dyad at the center (with associated risks and protective factors) and the larger society at the periphery. Changes at any level are reflected in the levels above and below. The shift from an industrial economy to one based on service and information is an obvious example of societal change with profound effects on families and children.

UNIFYING CONCEPTS: THE TRANSACTIONAL MODEL, RISK, AND RESILIENCE. The transactional model proposes that a child's status at any point in time is a function of the interaction between biologic and social influences. The influences are bidirectional: Biologic factors, such as temperament and health status, both affect the child-rearing environment and are affected by it. A premature infant may cry little and sleep for long periods; the infant's depressed parent may welcome this "good" behavior, setting up a cycle that leads to poor nutrition and inadequate growth. The child's failure to thrive may reinforce the parent's sense of failure as a parent. At a later stage, impulsivity and inattention associated with early, prolonged undernutrition may lead to aggressive behavior. The "cause" of the aggression in this case is not the prematurity, the undernutrition, or the maternal depression, but the interaction of all these factors (Fig. 6-2). Conversely, children with biologic risk factors may nevertheless do well developmentally if the child-rearing environment is supportive. Premature infants with electroencephalographic evidence of neurologic immaturity may be at increased risk for cognitive delay. However, this risk may only be realized when the quality of parent-child interaction is poor. When parent-child interactions are optimal, prematurity carries a reduced risk of developmental disability.

Children growing up in poverty are in double developmental jeopardy, because of increased exposure to biologic risk factors, such as environmental lead and undernutrition, lack of stimulation in the home, and decreased access to interventional education and therapeutic experiences. Children of adolescent mothers are also at risk. When early intervention programs provide timely, intensive, comprehensive, and prolonged services, at-risk children show marked and sustained upswings in their developmental trajectory. Early identification of children at developmental risk, along with early intervention to support parenting, is critically important.

An estimate of developmental risk can begin with a tally of risk factors, such as low income, limited parental education, and exposure to community violence. There may be a nearly linear relationship between developmental outcome at age 13 yr and the number of social and family risk factors at age 4 yr (Fig. 6-3). Protective (resilience) factors must also be considered. These factors, like risk factors, may be either biologic (temperamental persistence, athletic talent) or social. The personal histories of children who overcome poverty often include at least 1 trusted adult (parent, grandparent, teacher) with whom the child has a special, supportive, close relationship.

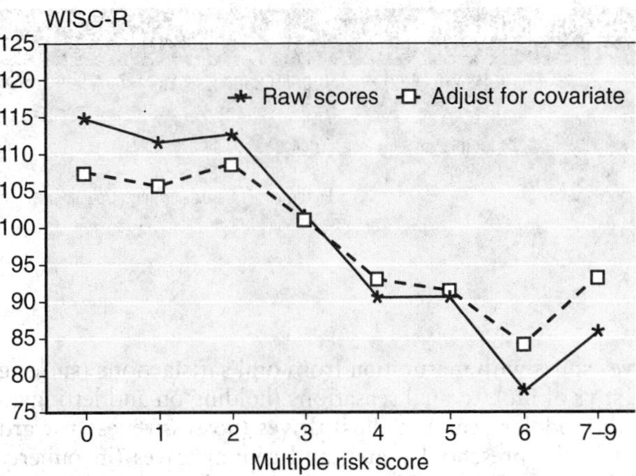

Figure 6-3. Relationship between mean IQ scores at 13 yr (both raw and adjusted for covariation of mother's IQ), as related to the number of risk factors. *WISC-R*, Wechstler Intelligence Scale-Revised (From Sameroff AJ, Seifer R, Baldwin A, et al: Stability of intelligence from preschool to adolescence; the influence of social and family risk factors. *Child Develop* 1993;64:80–97.)

DEVELOPMENTAL DOMAINS AND THEORIES OF EMOTION AND COGNITION. Child development can also be tracked by the child's developmental progress in particular domains, such as gross motor, fine motor, social, emotional, language, and cognition. Within each of these categories are developmental lines, or sequences of changes leading up to particular attainments. Developmental lines in the gross motor domain, leading from rolling to creeping to independent walking, are obvious. Others, such as the line leading to the development of conscience, are subtler.

The concept of a developmental line implies that a child passes though successive stages. Several psychoanalytic theories are based on stages as qualitatively different epochs in the development of emotion and cognition (Table 6-2). In contrast, behavioral theories rely less on qualitative change and more on the gradual modification of behavior and accumulation of competence.

Psychoanalytic Theories. At the core of freudian theory is the idea of body-centered (or, broadly, "sexual") drives. The focus of

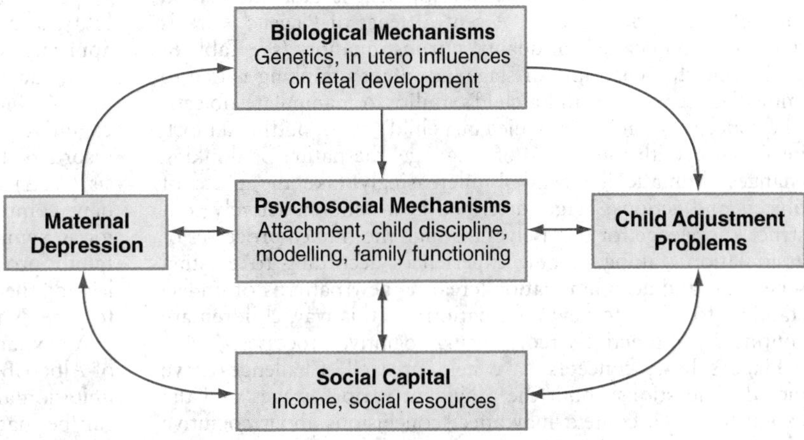

Figure 6-2. Theoretical model of mutual influences on maternal depression and child adjustment. (From Elgar FJ, McGrath PJ, Waschbusch DA, et al: Mutual influences on maternal depression and child adjustment problems. *Clin Psychol Rev* 2004;24:441–459.)

TABLE 6-2. Classic Stage Theories

	INFANCY (0–1 YR)	TODDLERHOOD (2–3 YR)	PRESCHOOL (3–6 YR)	SCHOOL AGE (6–12 YR)	ADOLESCENCE (12–20 YR)
Freud: psychosexual	Oral	Anal	Phallic/oedipal	Latency	Genital
Erikson: psychosocial	Basic trust vs mistrust	Autonomy vs shame and doubt	Initiative vs guilt	Industry vs inferiority	Identity vs role diffusion
Piaget: cognitive	Sensorimotor	Sensorimotor	Preoperational	Concrete operations	Formal operations
Kohlberg: moral	—	Preconventional: avoid punishment/obtain rewards (stages 1 and 2)	Conventional: conformity (stage 3)	Conventional: law and order (stage 4)	Postconventional: moral principles

the drives shifts with maturation from oral satisfactions (sucking in the 1st yr of life), to anal sensations (holding on and letting go during the toddler years), oedipal drives (possessiveness toward a parent in the preschool years), and genital drives (in puberty and beyond) [see Table 6-2]. At each stage, the child's drive can potentially conflict with the rules of society. Infants may want to suck longer than the mother wants to nurse, or toddlers may decide that they like making a mess. The emotional health of both the child and the adult depends on adequate resolution of these conflicts. Freud saw middle childhood as a period of latency, when the sexual drive is redirected (sublimated) to the achievement of social or external goals.

Freudian ideas have been challenged. Few believe that the manner of toilet training permanently shapes personality, and middle childhood is no longer seen as conflict-free. Moreover, the effectiveness of psychoanalytic therapy has been difficult to demonstrate empirically. Nonetheless, the freudian legacy includes concepts that are central to an understanding of emotional development: the importance of a child's inner life and sexuality, the normative existence of emotional conflict during childhood, and the possibility that emotional disturbance can have early roots.

Erikson's chief contribution was to recast Freud's stages in terms of the emerging personality (see Table 6-2). The child's sense of basic trust develops through the successful negotiation of infantile needs, corresponding to Freud's oral period. As children progress through these psychosocial stages, different issues become salient. Thus, it is predictable that a toddler will be preoccupied with establishing a sense of autonomy, whereas a late adolescent may be more focused on establishing meaningful relationships and an occupational identity. Erikson recognized that these stages arise in the context of Western European societal expectations; in other cultures, the salient issues may be quite different.

Erikson's work calls attention to the intrapersonal challenges facing children at different ages in a way that facilitates professional intervention. Knowing that the salient issue for school-aged children is industry vs inferiority, pediatricians know to inquire about a child's experiences of mastery and failure and (if necessary) suggest ways to ensure adequate successes.

Cognitive Theories. Cognitive development is best understood through the work of Piaget. A central tenet of Piaget's work is that cognition changes in quality, not just quantity (see Table 6-2). During the sensorimotor stage, an infant's thinking is tied to immediate sensations and a child's ability to manipulate objects. The concept of "in" is embodied in a child's act of putting a block into a cup. With the arrival of language, the nature of thinking changes dramatically; symbols increasingly take the place of objects and actions. Piaget described how children actively construct knowledge for themselves through the linked processes of assimilation (taking in new experiences according to existing schemata) and accommodation (creating new patterns of understanding to adapt to new information). In this way, children are continually and actively reorganizing cognitive processes.

Piaget's basic concepts have held up well. Challenges have included questions about the timing of various stages and the extent to which context may affect conclusions about cognitive stage. Children's understanding of cause and effect may be considerably more advanced in the context of sibling relationships than in the context of inanimate objects (various machines); in many children, logical thinking appears well before puberty, the age postulated by Piaget. Of undeniable importance are Piaget's focus on cognition as a subject of empirical study, the universality of the progression of cognitive stages, and the image of a child as actively and creatively interpreting the world.

Piaget's work is of special importance to pediatricians for 3 reasons: (1) It helps make sense of many puzzling behaviors of infancy, such as the common exacerbation of sleep problems at 9 and 18 mo of age. (2) Piaget's observations often lend themselves to quick replication in the office, with little special equipment. (3) Open-ended questioning, based on Piaget's work, can provide insights into children's understanding of illness and hospitalization.

Based on cognitive development, **Kohlberg** developed a theory of moral development in 6 stages from early childhood through adulthood. Preschoolers' earliest sense of right and wrong is egocentric, motivated by externally applied controls. In later stages, children perceive equality, fairness, and reciprocity in their understanding of interpersonal interactions through perspective-taking. Most youth will reach stage 4, conventional morality, by mid to late adolescence. The basic theory has been modified to distinguish morality from social conventions. Whereas moral thinking considers interpersonal interactions, justice, and human welfare, social conventions are the agreed-on standards of behavior particular to a social or cultural group. Within each stage of development, children are guided by the basic precepts of moral behavior, but also may take into account local standards, such as dress code, classroom behavior, and dating expectations.

Behavioral Theory. This theoretical perspective distinguishes itself by its lack of concern with a child's inner experience. Its sole focus is on observable behaviors and measurable factors that either increase or decrease the frequency with which these behaviors occur. No stages are implied: Children, adults, and indeed animals all respond in the same way. In its simplest form, the behaviorist orientation asserts that behaviors that are positively reinforced occur more frequently; behaviors that are negatively reinforced or ignored occur less frequently.

The strengths of this position are its simplicity, wide applicability, and conduciveness to scientific verification. A behavioral approach lends itself to interventions for various common problems, such as temper tantrums and aggressive preschool behavior, in which behaviors are broken down into discrete units. In cognitively limited children and children with autism spectrum disorders, behavioral interventions using applied behavior analysis (ABA) approaches have demonstrated their ability to teach new, complex behaviors. However, in cases in which misbehavior is symptomatic of an underlying emotional, perceptual, or family problem, an exclusive reliance on behavior therapy risks leaving the cause untreated. Behavioral approaches can be taught to parents to apply at home.

An expansion of behavioral theory is the social learning theory of Albert Bandura and others, in which social reinforcement and imitation are driving forces in changing behavior. Reinforcement can be material or emotional. The models for behavior are ini-

TABLE 6-3. Relationship Between SD and Normal Range for Normally Distributed Quantities

OBSERVATIONS INCLUDED IN THE NORMAL RANGE		PROBABILITY OF A "NORMAL" MEASUREMENT DEVIATING FROM THE MEAN BY THIS AMOUNT	
SD	%	*SD*	%
±1	68.3	≥1	16.0
±2	95.4	≥2	2.3
±3	99.7	≥3	0.13

SD, standard deviation.

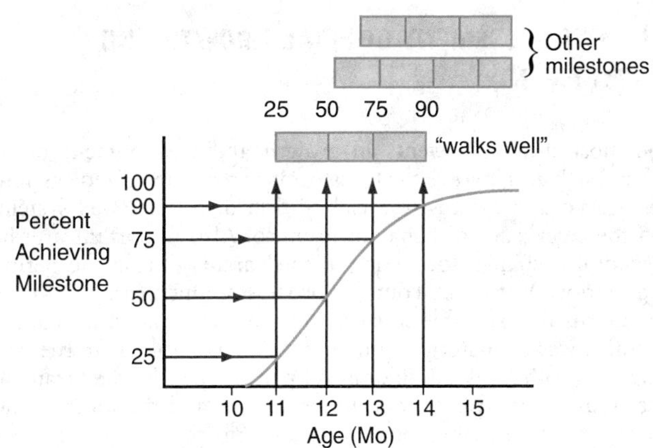

Figure 6-5. Method of presenting percentiles for developmental milestones.

tially the parents. As children develop, they seek models from the peer group and other outside networks.

STATISTICS USED IN DESCRIBING GROWTH AND DEVELOPMENT (SEE ALSO CHAPTERS 14 AND 15). In everyday use, the term *normal* is synonymous with *healthy*. In a statistical sense, *normal* means that a set of values generates a normal (bell-shaped, or gaussian) distribution. This is the case with anthropometric quantities, such as height and weight, and with many developmental milestones, such as the age of independent standing. For a **normally distributed measurement,** a histogram with the quantity (height, age) on the *x*-axis and the frequency (the number of children of that height, or the number who stand on their own at that age) on the *y*-axis generates a bell-shaped curve. In an ideal bell-shaped curve, the peak corresponds to the arithmetic mean (average) of the sample and to the median and the mode as well. The **median** is the value above and below which 50% of the observations lie; the mode is the value having the highest number of observations. Distributions are termed *skewed* if the mean, median, and mode are not the same number.

The extent to which observed values cluster near the mean determines the width of the bell and can be described mathematically by the **standard deviation (SD).** In the ideal normal curve, a range of values extending from 1 SD below the mean to 1 SD above the mean includes approximately 68% of the values, and each "tail" above and below that range contains 16% of the values. A range encompassing ±2 SD includes 95% of the values (with the upper and lower tails each comprising approximately 2.5% of the values), and ±3 SD encompasses 99.7% of the values (Table 6-3 and Fig. 6-4).

For any single measurement, its distance away from the mean can be expressed in terms of the number of SDs (also called a *z score*); one can then consult a table of the normal distribution to find out what percentage of measurements fall within that distance from the mean. Software to convert anthropometric data into z scores for epidemiologic purposes is available. A measurement that falls "outside the normal range"—arbitrarily defined as 2, or sometimes 3, SDs on either side of the mean—is atypical, but not necessarily indicative of illness. The further a measurement (say, height, weight, or IQ) falls from the mean, the greater the probability that it represents not simply normal variation, but rather a different, potentially pathologic, condition.

Another way of relating an individual to a group uses percentiles. The **percentile** is the percentage of individuals in the group who have achieved a certain measured quantity (a height of 95 cm) or developmental milestone. For anthropometric data, the percentile cutoffs can be calculated from the mean and SD. The 5th, 10th, and 25th percentiles correspond to −1.65 SD, −1.3 SD, and −0.7 SD, respectively. Figure 6-4 demonstrates how frequency distributions of a particular parameter (height) at different ages relate to the percentile lines on the growth curve. For developmental milestones, the percentiles are often displayed in boxes, derived from graphs plotting age (*x*-axis) against the percentage of subjects achieving the particular milestone (*y*-axis), as shown in Figure 6-5.

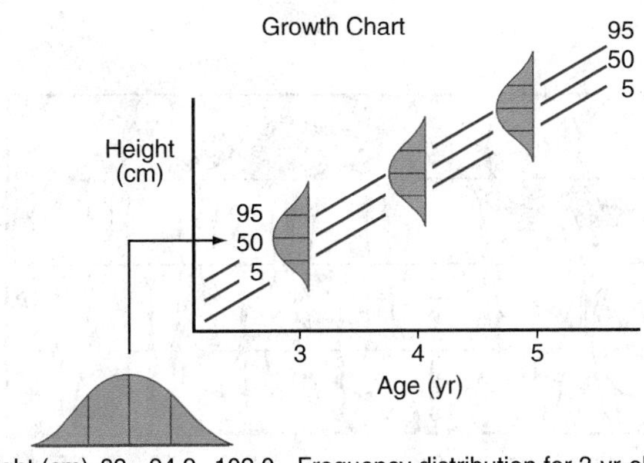

Figure 6-4. Relationship between percentile lines on the growth curve and frequency distributions of height at different ages.

Allmond B, Tanner J: *The Family Is the Patient.* Baltimore, Williams & Wilkins, 1999.

Bandura A: *Social Learning Theory.* Englewood Cliffs, NJ: Prentice-Hall, 1977, pp 2–13.

Bronfenbrenner U: *The Ecology of Human Development.* Cambridge, MA, Harvard University Press, 1979.

Carey WB: Teaching parents about infant temperament. *Pediatrics* 1998; 102:1311.

Evans GW: The environment of childhood poverty. *American Psychologist* 2004;59:77–92.

Keverne EB: Understanding well-being in the evolutionary context of brain development. *Phil Trans R Soc Lond* 2004;359:1349–1358.

Letourneau NL, Stewart MJ, Barnfather AK: Adolescent mothers: Support needs, resources, and support-education interventions. *J Adolesc Health* 2004;35:509–525.

Rutter M: Nature, nurture and development: From evangelism through science toward policy and practice. *Child Dev* 2002;73:1–21.

Shonkoff J, Phillips D: National Research Council and Institute of Medicine: *From Neurons to Neighborhoods: The Science of Early Childhood Development.* Washington, DC, National Academy Press, 2000.

Werner EE: The children of Kauai: Resiliency and recovery in adolescence and adulthood. *J Adolesc Health* 1992;13:262–268.

6.1 • Assessment of Fetal Growth and Development

The most dramatic events in growth and development occur before birth and involve the transformation of a fertilized egg into an embryo and a fetus, the elaboration of the nervous system, and the emergence of behavior in utero. Also important are the psychologic changes occurring in the parents during the period of gestation. With such complex processes, much can go wrong. The uterus is permeable to such adverse social and environmental influences as maternal undernutrition; alcohol, cigarette, and drug use (both legal and illicit); and perhaps psychologic trauma. The complex interplay between these forces and the somatic and neurologic transformations occurring in the fetus influence infants' behavior at birth and may affect parent-child interactions throughout infancy.

SOMATIC DEVELOPMENT

EMBRYONIC PERIOD. Milestones of prenatal development are presented in Table 6-4. By 6 days postconceptual age, as implantation begins, the embryo consists of a spherical mass of cells with a central cavity (the blastocyst). By 2 wk, implantation is complete and the uteroplacental circulation has begun; the embryo has 2 distinct layers, endoderm and ectoderm, and the amnion has begun to form. By 3 wk, the 3rd primary germ layer (mesoderm) has appeared, along with a primitive neural tube and blood vessels. Paired heart tubes have begun to pump.

During wk 4–8, lateral folding of the embryologic plate, followed by growth at the cranial and caudal ends and the budding of arms and legs, produces a human-like shape. Precursors of skeletal muscle and vertebrae (somites) appear, along with the branchial arches that will form the mandible, maxilla, palate, external ear, and other head and neck structures. Lens placodes appear, marking the site of future eyes; the brain grows rapidly. By the end of wk 8, as the embryonic period closes, the rudiments of all major organ systems have developed; the average embryo weighs 9 g and has a crown-rump length of 5 cm.

FETAL PERIOD. From the 9th wk on (fetal period), somatic changes consist of increases in cell number and size and structural remodeling of several organ systems. Changes in body proportion are depicted in Figure 6-6. By 10 wk, the face is recognizably human. The midgut returns from the umbilical cord into the abdomen, rotating counterclockwise to bring the stomach, small intestine, and large intestine into their normal positions. By 12 wk, the gender of the external genitals becomes clearly distinguishable. Lung development proceeds, with the budding of bronchi, bronchioles, and successively smaller divisions. By 20–24 wk, primitive alveoli have formed and surfactant production has begun; before that time, the absence of alveoli renders the lungs useless as organs of gas exchange.

During the 3rd trimester, weight triples and length doubles as body stores of protein, fat, iron, and calcium increase.

NEUROLOGIC DEVELOPMENT

During the 3rd wk, a neural plate appears on the ectodermal surface of the trilaminar embryo. Infolding produces a neural tube that will become the central nervous system (CNS) and a neural crest that will become the peripheral nervous system. Neuroectodermal cells differentiate into neurons, astrocytes, oligodendrocytes, and ependymal cells, whereas microglial cells are derived from mesoderm. By the 5th wk, the 3 main subdivisions of forebrain, midbrain, and hindbrain are evident. The dorsal and ventral horns of the spinal cord have begun to form, along with the peripheral motor and sensory nerves. Myelinization begins at midgestation and continues throughout the 1st 2 yr of life.

By the end of the embryonic period (wk 8), the gross structure of the nervous system has been established. On a cellular level, neurons migrate outward to form the 6 cortical layers. Migration is complete by the 6th mo, but differentiation continues. Axons and dendrites form synaptic connections at a rapid pace, making the CNS vulnerable to teratogenic or hypoxic influences throughout gestation. Rates of increase in DNA (a marker of cell number), overall brain weight, and cholesterol (a marker of myelinization) are shown in Figure 6-7. The prenatal and postnatal peaks of DNA probably represent rapid growth of neurons and glia, respectively. By the time of birth, the structure of the brain is complete. Synapses will be pruned back substantially and new connections will be made, largely as a result of experience.

BEHAVIORAL DEVELOPMENT

Muscle contractions first appear around 8 wk, soon followed by lateral flexion movements. By 13–14 wk, breathing and swallowing motions appear and tactile stimulation elicits graceful movements. The grasp reflex appears at 17 wk and is well developed by 27 wk. Eye opening occurs around 26 wk. By midgestation, the full range of neonatal movements can be observed.

During the 3rd trimester, fetuses respond to external stimuli with heart rate elevation and body movements (see Chapter 96). As with infants in the postnatal period, reactivity to auditory

TABLE 6-4. Milestones of Prenatal Development

WK	DEVELOPMENTAL EVENTS
1	Fertilization and implantation; beginning of embryonic period
2	Endoderm and ectoderm appear (bilaminar embryo)
3	First missed menstrual period; mesoderm appears (trilaminar embryo); somites begin to form
4	Neural folds fuse; folding of embryo into human-like shape; arm and leg buds appear; crown-rump length 4–5 mm
5	Lens placodes, primitive mouth, digital rays on hands
6	Primitive nose, philtrum, primary palate; crown-rump length 21–23 mm
7	Eyelids begin
8	Ovaries and testes distinguishable
9	*Fetal* period begins; crown-rump length 5 cm; weight 9 g
10	External genitals distinguishable
20	Usual lower limit of viability; weight 460 g; length 19 cm
25	Third trimester begins; weight 900 g; length 25 cm
28	Eyes open; fetus turns head down; weight 1,000 g
38	Term

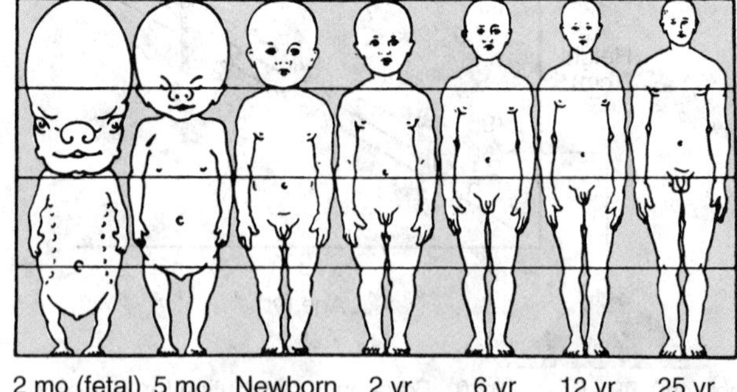

Figure 6-6. Changes in body proportions form the 2nd fetal mo to adulthood. (From Robbins WJ, Brody S, Hogan AG, et al: *Growth*. New Haven, Yale University Press, 1928.)

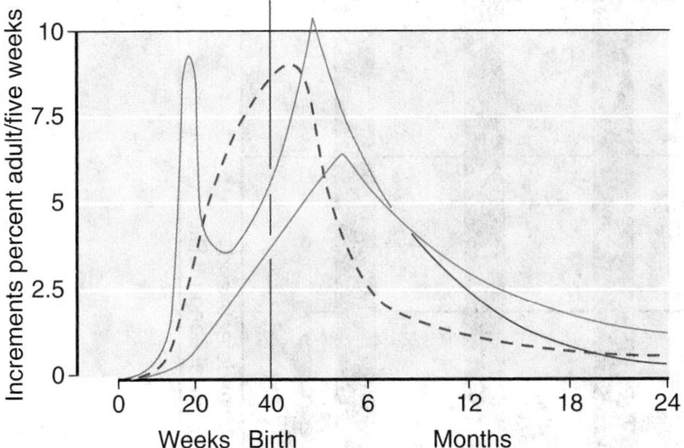

Figure 6-7. Velocity curves of the various components of human brain growth. *Solid line with two peaks*, DNA; *dashed line*, brain weight; *solid line with a single peak*, cholesterol. (From Brasel JA, Gruen RK: In Falkner F, Tanner JM [editors]: *Human Growth: A Comprehensive Treatise*. New York, Plenum Press, 1986, pp 78–95.)

(vibroacoustic) and visual (bright light) stimuli vary depending on their behavioral state, which can be characterized as quiet sleep, active sleep, or awake. Individual differences in the level of fetal activity are commonly noted by mothers and have been observed ultrasonographically. Fetal behavior is affected by maternal medications and diet, increasing after ingestion of caffeine; behavior may be entrained to the mother's diurnal rhythms.

Fetal movement increases in response to a sudden auditory tone, but decreases after several repetitions (habituation). If the tone changes in pitch, the movement increases again, evidence that the fetus distinguishes between a familiar, repeated tone and a novel one. The ability to habituate to repeated stimuli, a form of learning, is diminished in neurologically impaired or physically stressed fetuses. Similar responses to visual and tactile stimuli have been observed.

PSYCHOLOGIC CHANGES IN PARENTS

The psychologic changes during pregnancy fall roughly into 3 stages. Stage 1 begins when a woman first learns that she is pregnant. Ambivalent feelings are the norm, whether or not the pregnancy was planned. Elation at the thought of producing a baby and the wish to be the perfect parent compete with fears of inadequacy and of the lifestyle changes that mothering will impose. Old conflicts may resurface as a woman psychologically identifies with her own mother and with herself as a child. The father-to-be faces similar mixed feelings, and problems in the parental relationship may intensify.

Stage 2 begins with awareness of fetal movements, or quickening, at approximately 20 wk, or earlier with ultrasonic visualization. This palpable evidence that a fetus exists as a separate being often heightens a woman's feelings, both positive and negative. Parents worry about the fetus's healthy development and mentally rehearse what they will do if the child is malformed. Reassurances based on ultrasound examinations or amniocentesis may not completely allay these fears. During stage 3, toward the end of pregnancy, a woman becomes aware of patterns of fetal activity and reactivity and begins to ascribe to her fetus an individual personality and an ability to survive independently. Appreciation of the psychologic vulnerability of the expectant mother and father and of the powerful contribution of fetal behavior facilitates supportive clinical intervention.

THREATS TO FETAL DEVELOPMENT

Mortality and morbidity are highest during the prenatal period (see Chapter 93). Some 30% of pregnancies end in spontaneous abortion, most often during the 1st trimester as a result of chromosomal or other abnormalities. Major congenital malformations requiring neonatal surgical intervention occur in approximately 2% of live births. Teratogens associated with gross physical and mental abnormalities include various infectious agents (toxoplasmosis, rubella, syphilis), chemical agents (mercury, thalidomide, antiepileptic medications, ethanol), high temperature, and radiation (see Chapters 96 and 706). Most of the variation in birth weight is due to the in utero environment.

For any potential teratogen, the extent and nature of its effects are determined by characteristics of the host as well as the dose and timing of the exposure. Inherited differences in the metabolism of ethanol may predispose certain individuals or groups to fetal alcohol syndrome, for example. Organ systems are most vulnerable during periods of maximum growth and differentiation, generally during the first trimester (organogenesis). Figure 6-8 depicts sensitive periods during gestation for various organ systems.

Teratogenic effects may include not only gross physical malformation but also decreased growth and cognitive or behavioral deficits that only become apparent later in life. Prenatal exposure to cigarette smoke is associated with lower birthweight, shorter length, and smaller head circumference, as well as decreased IQ and increased rates of learning disabilities. The effects of prenatal exposure to cocaine remain controversial and may be less dramatic than popularly believed. The effects include direct neurotoxic effects and effects mediated by reduced placental blood flow; associated risk factors include other prenatal exposures (alcohol and cigarettes used in large amounts by many cocaine-addicted women) as well as "toxic" postnatal environments frequently characterized by instability, multiple caregivers, and abuse and neglect (see Chapter 36). Severe maternal starvation will lead to lower birthweight. High levels of psychologic stress during pregnancy may also adversely affect fetal development.

The wide range of outcomes observed reflects the complex interactions among biologic and social risk and protective factors.

Brazelton TB, Cramer BG: *The Earliest Relationship*. Reading, MA, Addison-Wesley, 1990.

Buitelaar JK, Huizink AC, Mulder EJ, et al: Prenatal stress and cognitive development and temperament in infants. *Neurobiol Aging* 2003;24 (Suppl 1):S5360.

Frank DA, Augustyn M, Knight WG, et al: Growth, development, and behavior in early childhood following prenatal cocaine exposure: A systematic review. *JAMA* 2001;285:1613–1625.

Kiuchi M, Nagata N, Ikeno S, et al: The relationship between the response to external light stimulation and behavioral states in the human fetus: How it differs from vibroacoustic stimulation. *Early Hum Dev* 2000;58:153–165.

Krageloh-Mann I: Imaging of early brain injury and cortical plasticity. *Exp Neurol* 2004:190 (Suppl 1):S84–S90.

Moore KL: *Before We Are Born: Basic Embryology and Birth Defects,* 5th ed. Philadelphia, WB Saunders, 1998.

Relier JP: Influence of maternal stress on fetal behavior and brain development. *Biol Neonate* 2001;79:168–171.

Thadani PV, Strauss JF 3rd, Dey SK, et al: National Institute on Drug Abuse Conference report on placental proteins, drug transport, and fetal development. *Am J Obstet Gynecol* 2004;191:1858–1862.

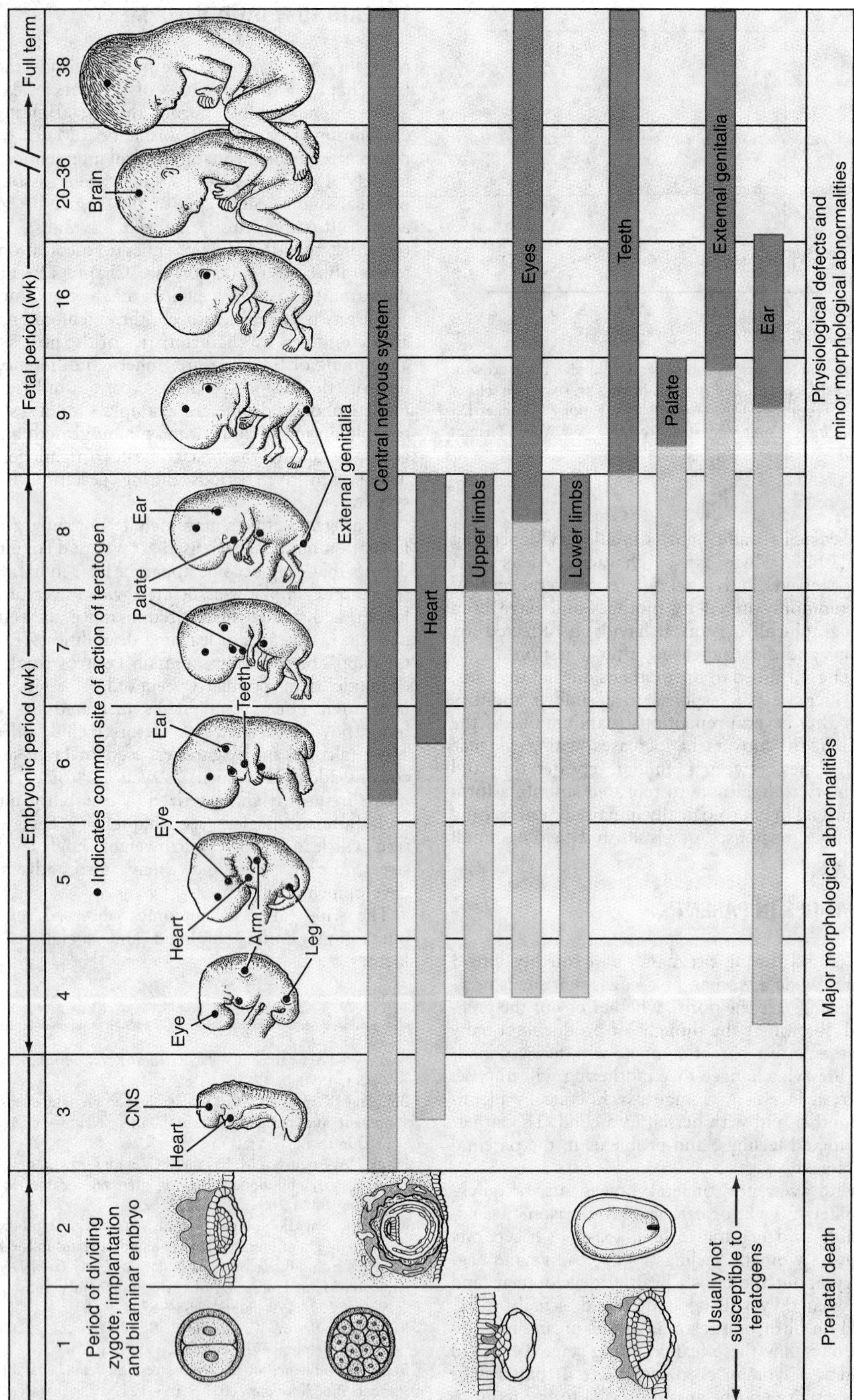

Figure 6-8. Schematic illustration of the sensitive or critical periods in prenatal development. *Dark boxes* denote highly sensitive periods; *light boxes* indicate states that are less sensitive to teratogens. (From Moore KL: *Before We Are Born: Basic Embryology and Birth Defects*, 2nd ed. Philadelphia, WB Saunders, 1977.)

Chapter 7 ■ The Newborn John Olsson

The **newborn (neonatal) period** begins at birth and includes the 1st mo of life. During this time, marked physiologic transitions occur in all organ systems and the infant learns to respond to many forms of external stimuli. Infants thrive physically and psychologically only in the context of their social relationships. Therefore, any description of the newborn's developmental status has to include consideration of the parents' role as well.

PARENTAL ROLE IN MATERNAL-INFANT ATTACHMENT

Parenting a newborn infant requires dedication because a newborn's needs are urgent, continuous, and often unclear. Parents must attend to an infant's signals and respond empathically. Many factors influence parents' ability to assume this role.

PRENATAL FACTORS. Pregnancy is a period of psychologic preparation for the profound demands of parenting. Women may experience ambivalence, particularly (but not exclusively) if the pregnancy was unplanned. If financial worries, physical illness, prior miscarriages or stillbirths, or other crises interfere with psychologic preparation, the neonate may not be welcomed. For adolescent mothers, the demand that they relinquish their own developmental agenda, such as an active social life, may be especially burdensome.

The early experience of being mothered may establish unconsciously held expectations about nurturing relationships that permit mothers to "tune in" to their infants. These expectations are linked with the quality of later infant-parent interactions. Mothers whose early childhoods were marked by traumatic separations, abuse, or neglect may find it especially difficult to provide consistent, responsive care. Instead, they may reenact their childhood experiences with their own infants as if unable to conceive of the mother-child relationship in any other way. Bonding may be adversely affected by several risk factors during pregnancy and in the postpartum period, which undermine the mother-child relationship and may threaten the infant's cognitive and emotional development (Table 7-1).

Social support during pregnancy, particularly support from the father and close family members, is also important. Conversely, conflict with or abandonment by the father during pregnancy may diminish the mother's ability to become absorbed with her infant. Anticipation of an early return to work may make some women reluctant to fall in love with their babies due to anticipated separation. Returning to work should be delayed at least until after 6 wk, when feeding and basic behavioral adjustments have been established.

Many decisions have to be made by parents in anticipation of the birth of their child. The most important choice is that of how the infant will be nourished. Among the important benefits of breast-feeding is the role of promoting bonding. Providing breast-feeding education for the parents at the prenatal visit by the pediatrician and by the obstetrician during prenatal care can increase maternal confidence in breast-feeding after delivery and reduce stress during the newborn period (see Chapter 42).

PERIPARTUM AND POSTPARTUM INFLUENCES. The continuous presence during labor of a woman trained to offer friendly support and encouragement (a **doula**) results in shorter labor, fewer obstetric complications (including cesarean section), and reduced postpartum hospital stays. Early skin-to-skin contact between mothers and infants immediately after birth may correlate with an increased rate and longer duration of breast-feeding.

TABLE 7-1. Prenatal Risk Factors for Attachment

Recent death of a loved one
Previous loss of or serious illness in another child
Prior removal of a child
History of depression or serious mental illness
History of infertility or pregnancy loss
Troubled relationship with parents
Financial stress or job loss
Marital discord or poor relationship with the other parent
Recent move or no community ties
No friends or social network
Unwanted pregnancy
No good parenting model
Experience of poor parenting
Drug and/or alcohol abuse
Extreme immaturity

From Dixon SD, Stein MT: *Encounters with Children: Pediatric Behavior and Development*, 3rd ed. St. Louis, Mosby, 2000, p 74.

Most new parents value even a brief period of uninterrupted time in which to get to know their new infant, and increased mother-infant contact over the first days of life may improve long-term mother-child interactions. Nonetheless, early separation, although predictably very stressful, does not inevitably impair a mother's ability to bond with her infant. Early discharge home from the maternity ward may undermine bonding, particularly when a new mother is required to resume full responsibility for a busy household.

THE INFANT'S ROLE IN MATERNAL-INFANT ATTACHMENT

The in utero environment contributes greatly but not completely to the future growth and development of the fetus. Abnormalities in maternal-fetal placental circulation and maternal glucose metabolism or the presence of maternal infection can result in abnormal fetal growth. Infants may be small or large for gestational age as a result. These abnormal growth patterns not only predispose infants to an increased requirement for medical intervention but also may affect their ability to respond behaviorally to their parents.

PHYSICAL EXAMINATION. Examination of the newborn should include an evaluation of growth and an observation of behavior. The average term newborn weighs approximately 3.4 kg (7½ lb); boys are slightly heavier than girls are. The average length and head circumference are about 50 cm (20 in) and 35 cm (14 in), respectively, in term infants. Each newborn's growth parameters should be plotted on growth curves specific for that infant's gestational age to determine the appropriateness of size. The infant's response to being examined may be useful in assessing its vigor, alertness, and tone. Observing how the parents handle their infant, their comfort and affection, is also important. The order of the physical examination should be from the least to the most intrusive maneuver. Assessing visual tracking and response to sound and noting changes of tone with level of activity and alertness are very helpful. Performing this examination and sharing impression with parents is an important opportunity to facilitate bonding (see Chapter 94).

INTERACTIONAL ABILITIES. Soon after birth, neonates are alert and ready to interact and nurse. This first alert-awake period may be affected by maternal analgesics and anesthetics or fetal hypoxia. Nearsighted neonates have a fixed focal length of 8–12 in, approximately the distance from the breast to the mother's face, as well as an inborn visual preference for faces. Hearing is well developed, and infants preferentially turn toward a female voice. These innate abilities and predilections increase the likelihood that when a mother gazes at her newborn, the baby will gaze back. The initial period of social interaction, usually lasting about 40 min, is followed by a period of somnolence. After that, briefer periods of alertness or excitation alternate with sleep. If a mother misses her baby's first alert-awake period, she may not experience as long a period of social interaction for several days.

MODULATION OF AROUSAL. Adaptation to extrauterine life requires rapid and profound physiologic changes, including aeration of the lungs, rerouting of the circulation, and activation of the intestinal tract. The necessary behavioral changes are no less profound. To obtain nourishment, to avoid hypo- and hyperthermia, and to ensure safety, neonates must react appropriately to an expanded range of sensory stimuli. Infants must become aroused in response to stimulation, but not so overaroused that their behavior becomes disorganized. Underaroused infants are not able to feed and interact; overaroused infants show signs of **autonomic instability,** including flushing or mottling, perioral pallor, hiccupping, vomiting, uncontrolled limb movements, and inconsolable crying.

BEHAVIORAL STATES. The organization of infant behavior into discrete behavioral states may reflect an infant's inborn ability to regulate arousal. Six states have been described: quiet sleep, active sleep, drowsy, alert, fussy, and crying. In the **alert state,** infants visually fixate on objects or faces and follow them horizontally and (within a month) vertically; they also reliably turn toward a novel sound, as if searching for its source. When overstimulated, they may calm themselves by looking away, yawning, or sucking on their lips or hands, thereby increasing parasympathetic activity and reducing sympathetic nervous activity. The behavioral state determines an infant's muscle tone, spontaneous movement, electroencephalogram pattern, and response to stimuli. In **active sleep,** an infant may show progressively less reaction to a repeated heel stick (habituation), whereas in the **drowsy state,** the same stimulus may push a child into fussing or crying.

MUTUAL REGULATION. Parents actively participate in an infant's state regulation, alternately stimulating and soothing. In turn, they are regulated by the infant's signals, responding to cries of hunger with a letdown of milk (or with a bottle). Such interactions constitute a system directed toward furthering the infant's physiologic homeostasis and physical growth. At the same time, they form the basis for the emerging psychologic relationship between parent and child. Infants come to associate the presence of the parent with the pleasurable reduction of tension (as in feeding) and show this preference by calming more quickly for their mother than for a stranger. This response, in turn, strengthens a mother's sense of efficacy and her connection with her baby.

IMPLICATIONS FOR THE PEDIATRICIAN

The pediatrician can support healthy newborn development in several ways.

OPTIMAL PRACTICES. A prenatal pediatric visit allows pediatricians to assess potential threats to bonding (a tense spousal relationship) and sources of social support. Supportive hospital policies include the use of birthing rooms rather than operating suites and delivery rooms; encouragement for the father or a trusted relative or friend to remain with the mother during labor or the provision of a professional doula; the practice of giving the newborn infant to the mother immediately after drying and a brief assessment; placement of the newborn in the mother's room rather than in a central nursery; and avoiding in-hospital distribution of infant formula. Such policies (Baby Friendly Hospital) have been shown to significantly increase breast-feeding rates (see Chapter 94). After discharge, home visits by nurses and lactation counselors can reduce early feeding problems and identify emerging medical conditions in either mother or baby. Infants requiring transport to another hospital should be brought to see the mother first, if at all possible. On discharge home, fathers can shield mothers from unnecessary visits and calls and take over household duties, allowing mothers and infants time to get to know each other without distractions. The first office visit should occur during the first 2 wk after discharge to determine how smoothly the mother and infant are making the transition to life at home. Babies who are discharged early, those who are breast-feeding, and those who are at risk for jaundice should be seen 2 to 5 days after discharge.

ASSESSING PARENT-INFANT INTERACTIONS. During a feeding or when infants are alert and face-to-face with their parents, it is normal for them to appear absorbed in one another. Infants who become overstimulated by the mother's voice or activity may turn away or close their eyes, leading to a premature termination of the encounter. Alternatively, the infant may be ready to interact, whereas the mother may appear preoccupied. Asking a new mother about her own emotional state, and inquiring specifically about a history of depression, facilitates referral for therapy, which may provide long-term benefits to the child. Pediatricians may detect **postpartum depression** using the Edinburgh Postnatal Depression Scale (EPDS) at well child visits during the first year (Table 7-2).

TEACHING ABOUT INDIVIDUAL COMPETENCIES. The Newborn Behavior Assessment Scale (NBAS) provides a formal measure of an infant's neurodevelopmental competencies, including state control, autonomic reactivity, reflexes, habituation, and orientation toward auditory and visual stimuli. This examination can also be used to demonstrate to parents an infant's capabilities and vulnerabilities. Parents might learn that they need to undress their infant to increase the level of arousal or to swaddle the infant to reduce overstimulation by containing random arm movements. The NBAS can be used to support the development of positive early parent-infant relationships. Demonstration of the NBAS to parents in the 1st wk of life has been shown to correlate with improvements in the caretaking environment months later.

Brazelton TB, Nugent JK: *The Neonatal Behavioral Assessment Scale,* 3rd ed. London, MacKeith Press, 1995.

Crockenberg S, Leerkes E: Infant social and emotional development in family context. In Zeanah CH (editor): *Handbook of Infant Mental Health,* 2nd ed. New York, Guilford Press, 2000, pp 60–91.

Currie ML, Rademacher R: The pediatrician's role in recognizing and intervening in postpartum depression. *Pediatr Clin North Am* 2004;51:785–801.

Hodnett ED: Caregiver support for women during childbirth. *Cochrane Database Syst Rev* 2002:CD000199.

Kennell JH, Klaus MH: Bonding: Recent observations that alter perinatal care. *Pediatr Rev* 1998;19:4–12.

Chaudron LH, Szilagyi PG, Kitzman HJ, et al: Detection of postpartum depressive symptoms by screening at well-child visits. *Pediatrics* 2004; 113(3):551–558.

Philipp BL, Merewood A: The baby friendly way: the best breastfeeding start. *Pediatr Clin N Am* 2004;51:761–783.

Section on Breastfeeding, American Academy of Pediatrics: Breastfeeding and the use of human milk. *Pediatrics* 2005;115:496–506.

TABLE 7-2. Edinburgh Postnatal Depression Scale

INSTRUCTIONS FOR USERS

1. The mother is asked to underline the response that comes closest to how she has been feeling in the previous 7 days.
2. All 10 items must be completed.
3. Care should be taken to avoid the possibility of the mother discussing her answers with others.
4. The mother should complete the scale herself, unless she has limited English or has difficulty with reading.
5. The Edinburgh Postnatal Depression Scale may be used at 6–8 weeks to screen postnatal women. The child health clinic, a postnatal checkup, or a home visit may provide a suitable opportunity for its completion.

Edinburgh Postnatal Depression Scale
Name:
Address:
Baby's age:

Because you have recently had a baby, we would like to know how you are feeling. Please underline the answer that comes closest to how you have felt in the past 7 days, not just how you feel today.

Here is an example, already completed.
I have felt happy:
Yes, all the time
Yes, most of the time
No, not very often
No, not at all
This would mean: "I have felt happy most of the time" during the past week. Please complete the other questions in the same way.

In the past 7 days:

1. I have been able to laugh and see the funny side of things
   As much as I always could
   Not quite so much now
   Definitely not so much now
   Not at all
2. I have looked forward with enjoyment to things
   As much as I ever did
   Rather less than I used to
   Definitely less than I used to
   Hardly at all

*3. I have blamed myself unnecessarily when things went wrong
   Yes, most of the time
   Yes, some of the time
   Not very often
   No, never

4. I have been anxious or worried for no good reason
   No, not at all
   Hardly ever
   Yes, sometimes
   Yes, very often

*5. I have felt scared or panicky for no very good reason
   Yes, quite a lot
   Yes, sometimes
   No, not much
   No, not at all

*6. Things have been getting on top of me
   Yes, most of the time I haven't been able to cope at all
   Yes, sometimes I haven't been coping as well as usual
   No, most of the time I have coped quite well
   No, I have been coping as well as ever

*7. I have been so unhappy that I have had difficulty sleeping
   Yes, most of the time
   Yes, sometimes
   Not very often
   No, not at all

*8. I have felt sad or miserable
   Yes, most of the time
   Yes, quite often
   Not very often
   No, not at all

*9. I have been so unhappy that I have been crying
   Yes, most of the time
   Yes, quite often
   Only occasionally
   No, never

*10. The thought of harming myself has occurred to me
   Yes, quite often
   Sometimes
   Hardly ever
   Never

Response categories are scored 0, 1, 2, and 3 according to increased severity of the symptom. Items marked with an asterisk (*) are reverse scored (i.e., 3, 2, 1, and 0). The total score is calculated by adding the scores for each of the 10 items. Users may reproduce the scale without further permission providing they respect copyright (which remains with the *British Journal of Psychiatry*) by quoting the names of the authors, the title, and the source of the paper in all reproduced copies.
From Currie ML, Rademacher R: The pediatrician's role in recognizing and intervening in postpartum depression. *Pediatr Clin North Am* 2004;51:785–801.

Chapter 8 ■ The First Year

Susan Feigelman

The 1st yr of life is marked by physical growth, maturation, acquisition of competence, and psychologic reorganization. These changes qualitatively change a child's behavior and social relationships. Children acquire new competences in all developmental domains. The concept of developmental trajectories highlights how more complex skills build on simpler ones; it is also important to realize how development in each domain affects functioning in all of the others. Physical growth parameters and normal ranges for attainable weight, length, and head circumference are found in the Centers for Disease Control growth charts (see Figs. 9-1 and 9-2). Table 8-1 presents an overview of key milestones by domain; Table 8-2 presents similar information arranged by age.

AGE 0–2 MONTHS

In this period, the infant experiences tremendous growth. Physiologic changes allow the establishment of effective feeding routines and a predictable sleep-wake cycle. The social interactions that occur as parents and infants accomplish these tasks lay the foundation for cognitive and emotional development.

PHYSICAL DEVELOPMENT. A newborn's weight may decrease 10% below birthweight in the 1st wk as a result of excretion of excess extravascular fluid and limited intake. Nutrition improves as

TABLE 8-1. Developmental Milestones in the First 2 Yr of Life

MILESTONE	AVERAGE AGE OF ATTAINMENT (MO)	DEVELOPMENTAL IMPLICATIONS
GROSS MOTOR		
Holds head steady while sitting	2	Allows more visual interaction
Pulls to sit, with no head lag	3	Muscle tone
Brings hands together in midline	3	Self-discovery of hands
Asymmetric tonic neck reflex gone	4	Can inspect hands in midline
Sits without support	6	Increasing exploration
Rolls back to stomach	6.5	Truncal flexion, risk of falls
Walks alone	12	Exploration, control of proximity to parents
Runs	16	Supervision more difficult
FINE MOTOR		
Grasps rattle	3.5	Object use
Reaches for objects	4	Visuomotor coordination
Palmar grasp gone	4	Voluntary release
Transfers object hand to hand	5.5	Comparison of objects
Thumb-finger grasp	8	Able to explore small objects
Turns pages of book	12	Increasing autonomy during book time
Scribbles	13	Visuomotor coordination
Builds tower of 2 cubes	15	Uses objects in combination
Builds tower of 6 cubes	22	Requires visual, gross, and fine motor coordination
COMMUNICATION AND LANGUAGE		
Smiles in response to face, voice	1.5	More active social participant
Monosyllabic babble	6	Experimentation with sound, tactile sense
Inhibits to "no"	7	Response to tone (nonverbal)
Follows one-step command with gesture	7	Nonverbal communication
Follows one-step command without gesture	10	Verbal receptive language (e.g., "Give it to me")
Says "mama" or "dada"	10	Expressive language
Points to objects	10	Interactive communication
Speaks first real word	12	Beginning of labeling
Speaks 4–6 words	15	Acquisition of object and personal names
Speaks 10–15 words	18	Acquisition of object and personal names
Speaks 2-word sentences (e.g., "Mommy shoe")	19	Beginning grammaticization, corresponds with 50+ word vocabulary
COGNITIVE		
Stares momentarily at spot where object disappeared	2	Lack of object permanence (out of sight, out of mind) [e.g., yarn ball dropped]
Stares at own hand	4	Self-discovery, cause and effect
Bangs 2 cubes	8	Active comparison of objects
Uncovers toy (after seeing it hidden)	8	Object permanence
Egocentric symbolic play (e.g., pretends to drink from cup)	12	Beginning symbolic thought
Uses stick to reach toy	17	Able to link actions to solve problems
Pretend play with doll (e.g., gives doll bottle)	17	Symbolic thought

colostrum is replaced by higher-fat breast milk, as infants learn to latch on and suck more efficiently, and as mothers become more comfortable with feeding techniques. Infants regain or exceed birth weight by 2 wk of age and should grow at approximately 30 g (1 oz)/day during the 1st mo (see Table 14-1). This is the period of fastest postnatal growth. Limb movements consist largely of uncontrolled writhing, with apparently purposeless opening and closing of the hands. Smiling occurs involuntarily. Eye gaze, head turning, and sucking are under better control and thus can be used to demonstrate infant perception and cognition. An infant's preferential turning toward the mother's voice is evidence of recognition memory.

Six behavioral states have been described (see Chapter 7). Initially, sleep and wakefulness are evenly distributed throughout the 24 hr day (Fig. 8-1). Neurologic maturation accounts for the consolidation of sleep into blocks of 5 or 6 hr at night, with brief awake, feeding periods. Learning also occurs; infants whose parents are consistently more interactive and stimulating during the day learn to concentrate their sleeping during the night.

COGNITIVE DEVELOPMENT. Caretaking activities provide visual, tactile, olfactory, and auditory stimuli; all of these support the development of cognition. Infants habituate to the familiar, attending less and less to repeated stimuli and increasing their attention when the stimulus changes. Infants can differentiate among patterns, colors, and consonants. They can recognize facial expressions (smiles) as similar, even when they appear on different faces. They also can match abstract properties of stimuli, such as contour, intensity, or temporal pattern, across sensory modalities. For example, infants at 2 mo of age can discriminate rhythmic patterns in native vs. non-native language. Infants appear to seek stimuli actively, as though satisfying an innate need to make sense of the world. These phenomena point to the integration of sensory inputs in the central nervous system.

EMOTIONAL DEVELOPMENT. The infant is dependent on the environment to meet his or her needs. The consistent availability of a trusted adult to meet the infant's urgent needs creates the conditions for secure attachment. Basic trust vs mistrust, the first of Erikson's psychosocial stages, depends on attachment and reciprocal maternal bonding. Crying occurs in response to stimuli that may be obvious (a soiled diaper), but are often obscure. Infants who are consistently picked up and held in response to distress cry less at 1 yr and show less aggressive behavior at 2 yr. Cross-cultural studies show that in societies in which infants are carried close to the mother, babies cry less than in societies in which babies are only periodically carried. Crying normally peaks at

TABLE 8-2. Emerging Patterns of Behavior During the 1st Year of Life*

NEONATAL PERIOD (1ST 4 WK)	
Prone:	Lies in flexed attitude; turns head from side to side; head sags on ventral suspension
Supine:	Generally flexed and a little stiff
Visual:	May fixate face on light in line of vision; "doll's-eye" movement of eyes on turning of the body
Reflex:	Moro response active; stepping and placing reflexes; grasp reflex active
Social:	Visual preference for human face
AT 1 MO	
Prone:	Legs more extended; holds chin up; turns head; head lifted momentarily to plane of body on ventral suspension
Supine:	Tonic neck posture predominates; supple and relaxed; head lags when pulled to sitting position
Visual:	Watches person; follows moving object
Social:	Body movements in cadence with voice of other in social contact; beginning to smile
AT 2 MO	
Prone:	Raises head slightly farther; head sustained in plane of body on ventral suspension
Supine:	Tonic neck posture predominates; head lags when pulled to sitting position
Visual:	Follows moving object 180 degrees
Social:	Smiles on social contact; listens to voice and coos
AT 3 MO	
Prone:	Lifts head and chest with arms extended; head above plane of body on ventral suspension
Supine:	Tonic neck posture predominates; reaches toward and misses objects; waves at toy
Sitting:	Head lag partially compensated when pulled to sitting position; early head control with bobbing motion; back rounded
Reflex:	Typical Moro response has not persisted; makes defensive movements or selective withdrawal reactions
Social:	Sustained social contact; listens to music; says "aah, ngah"
AT 4 MO	
Prone:	Lifts head and chest, with head in approximately vertical axis; legs extended
Supine:	Symmetric posture predominates, hands in midline; reaches and grasps objects and brings them to mouth
Sitting:	No head lag when pulled to sitting position; head steady, tipped forward; enjoys sitting with full truncal support
Standing:	When held erect, pushes with feet
Adaptive:	Sees pellet, but makes no move to reach for it
Social:	Laughs out loud; may show displeasure if social contact is broken; excited at sight of food
AT 7 MO	
Prone:	Rolls over; pivots; crawls or creep-crawls (Knobloch)
Supine:	Lifts head; rolls over; squirms
Sitting:	Sits briefly, with support of pelvis; leans forward on hands; back rounded
Standing:	May support most of weight; bounces actively
Adaptive:	Reaches out for and grasps large object; transfers objects from hand to hand; grasp uses radial palm; rakes at pellet
Language:	Forms polysyllabic vowel sounds
Social:	Prefers mother; babbles; enjoys mirror; responds to changes in emotional content of social contact
AT 10 MO	
Sitting:	Sits up alone and indefinitely without support, with back straight
Standing:	Pulls to standing position; "cruises" or walks holding on to furniture
Motor:	Creeps or crawls
Adaptive:	Grasps objects with thumb and forefinger; pokes at things with forefinger; picks up pellet with assisted pincer movement; uncovers hidden toy; attempts to retrieve dropped object; releases object grasped by other person
Language:	Repetitive consonant sounds ("mama," "dada")
Social:	Responds to sound of name; plays peek-a-boo or pat-a-cake; waves bye-bye
AT 1 YR	
Motor:	Walks with one hand held (48 wk); rises independently, takes several steps (Knobloch)
Adaptive:	Picks up pellet with unassisted pincer movement of forefinger and thumb; releases object to other person on request or gesture
Language:	Says a few words besides "mama," "dada"
Social:	Plays simple ball game; makes postural adjustment to dressing

*Data are derived from those of Gesell (as revised by Knobloch), Shirley, Provence, Wolf, Bailey, and others.
Knobloch H, Stevens F, Malone AF: *Manual of Developmental Diagnosis.* Hagerstown, MD, Harper + Row, 1980.

about 6 wk of age, when healthy infants cry up to 3 hr/day, then decreases to 1 hr or less by 3 mo.

The emotional significance of any experience depends on both the individual child's temperament and the parent's responses (see Table 6-1). Consider the impact of different feeding schedules. Hunger generates increasing tension; as the urgency peaks, the infant cries, the parent offers the bottle or breast, and the tension dissipates. Infants fed "on demand" consistently experience this link between their distress, the arrival of the parent, and relief from hunger. Most infants fed on a fixed schedule quickly adapt their hunger cycle to the schedule. Those who cannot because they are temperamentally prone to irregular biologic rhythms experience periods of unrelieved hunger as well as unwanted feedings when they already feel full. Similarly, infants fed at the parents' convenience, with neither attention to the infant's hunger cues nor a fixed schedule, may not consistently experience feeding as the pleasurable reduction of tension. These infants often show increased irritability and physiologic instability (spitting, diarrhea, poor weight gain) as well as later behavioral problems.

IMPLICATIONS FOR PARENTS AND PEDIATRICIANS. Success or failure in establishing feeding and sleep cycles determines parents' feelings of efficacy. When things go well, the parents' anxiety and ambivalence, as well as the exhaustion of the early weeks, decrease. Infant issues (colic) or familial conflict will prevent this from occurring. With physical recovery from delivery and endocrinologic normalization, the mild postpartum depression that affects many mothers passes. If the mother continues to feel sad, overwhelmed, and anxious, the possibility of moderate to severe postpartum depression, found in 10% of postpartum women, needs to be considered. Major **depression** that arises during pregnancy or in the postpartum period threatens the mother-child relationship and is a risk factor for later cognitive and behavioral problems. The pediatrician may be the first professional to encounter the depressed mother and should be instrumental in assisting her in seeking treatment (see Chapter 7).

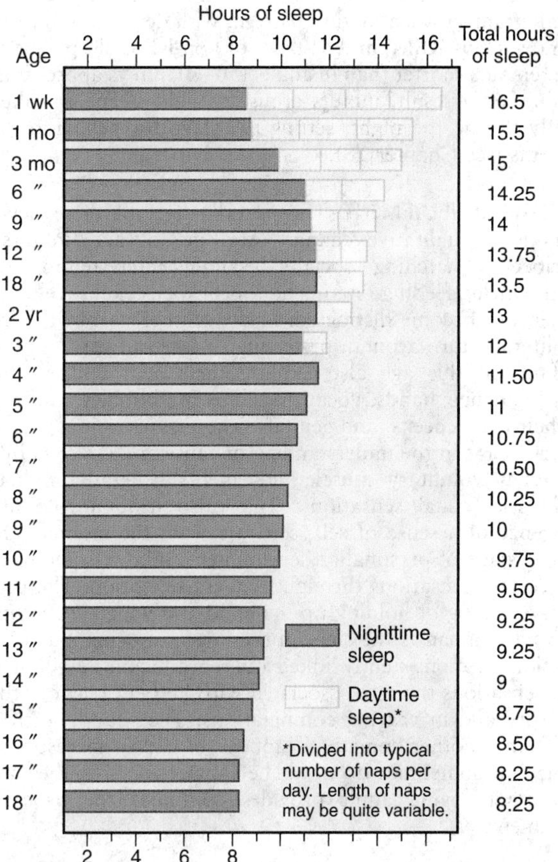

Figure 8-1. Typical sleep requirements in children. (From Ferber R: *Solve Your Child's Sleep Problems.* New York, Simon & Schuster, 1985.)

AGE 2–6 MONTHS

At about 2 mo, the emergence of voluntary (social) smiles and increasing eye contact mark a change in the parent-child relationship, heightening the parents' sense of being loved back. During the next months, an infant's range of motor and social control and cognitive engagement increases dramatically. Mutual regulation takes the form of complex social interchanges, resulting in strong mutual attachment and enjoyment. Parents are less fatigued.

PHYSICAL DEVELOPMENT. Between 3 and 4 mo of age, the rate of growth slows to approximately 20 g/day (see Table 14-1 and Figs. 9-1 and 9-2). By 4 mo, birth weight is doubled. Early reflexes that limited voluntary movement recede. Disappearance of the asymmetric tonic neck reflex means that infants can begin to examine objects in the midline and manipulate them with both hands (see Chapter 591). Waning of the early grasp reflex allows infants both to hold objects and to let them go voluntarily. A novel object may elicit purposeful, although inefficient, reaching. The quality of spontaneous movements also changes, from larger writhing to smaller, circular movements that have been described as "fidgety." Abnormal or absent fidgety movements may constitute a risk factor for later neurologic abnormalities.

Increasing control of truncal flexion makes intentional rolling possible. Once infants can hold their heads steady while sitting, they can gaze across at things rather than merely looking up at them, and can begin taking food from a spoon. At the same time, maturation of the visual system allows greater depth perception.

In this period, infants achieve stable state regulation and regular sleep-wake cycles. Total sleep requirements are approximately 14–16 hr/24 hr, with about 9–10 hr concentrated at night and 2 naps/day. About 70% of infants sleep for a 6–8 hr stretch by age 6 mo (see Fig. 8-1). By 4–6 mo, the sleep electroencephalogram shows a mature pattern, with demarcation of rapid eye movement (REM) and 4 stages of non-REM sleep. The sleep cycle remains shorter than in adults (50–60 min vs approximately 90 min). As a result, infants arouse to light sleep or wake frequently during the night, setting the stage for behavioral sleep problems (see Chapter 18).

COGNITIVE DEVELOPMENT. The overall effect of these developments is a qualitative change. At 4 mo of age, infants are described as "hatching" socially, becoming interested in a wider world. During feeding, infants no longer focus exclusively on the mother, but become distracted. In the mother's arms, the infant may literally turn around, preferring to face outward.

Infants at this age also explore their own bodies, staring intently at their hands, vocalizing, blowing bubbles, and touching their ears, cheeks, and genitals. These explorations represent an early stage in the understanding of cause and effect as infants learn that voluntary muscle movements generate predictable tactile and visual sensations. They also have a role in the emergence of a sense of self, separate from the mother. This is the first stage of personality development. Infants come to associate certain sensations through frequent repetition. The proprioceptive feeling of holding up the hand and wiggling the fingers always accompanies the sight of the fingers moving. Such "self" sensations are consistently linked and reproducible at will. In contrast, sensations that are associated with "other" occur with less regularity and in varying combinations. The sound, smell, and feel of the mother sometimes appear promptly in response to crying, but sometimes do not. The satisfaction that the mother or another loving adult provides continues the process of attachment.

EMOTIONAL DEVELOPMENT AND COMMUNICATION. Babies interact with increasing sophistication and range. The primary emotions of anger, joy, interest, fear, disgust, and surprise appear in appropriate contexts as distinct facial expressions. When face-to-face, the infant and a trusted adult match affective expressions (smiling or surprise) about 30% of the time. Initiating "games" (facial imitation, singing, hand games) increases social development. Such face-to-face behavior reveals the infant's ability to share emotional states, the first step in the development of communication. Infants of depressed parents show a different pattern, spending less time in coordinated movement with their parents and making fewer efforts to re-engage. Rather than anger, they show sadness and a loss of energy when the parents continue to be unavailable.

IMPLICATIONS FOR PARENTS AND PEDIATRICIANS. Motor and sensory maturation makes infants at 3–6 mo exciting and interactive. Some parents experience their 4 mo old child's outward turning as a rejection, secretly fearing that their infants no longer love them. For most parents, however, this is a happy period. Most parents excitedly report that they can hold "conversations" with their infants, taking turns vocalizing and listening. Pediatricians share in the enjoyment, as the baby coos, makes eye contact, and moves rhythmically. If this visit does not feel joyful and relaxed, causes such as social stress, family dysfunction, parental mental illness, or problems in the infant-parent relationship should be considered. Parents can be reassured that responding to an infant's emotional needs cannot "spoil" him or her. Giving vaccines and drawing blood while the child is seated on the parent's lap increases pain tolerance.

AGE 6–12 MONTHS

With achievement of the sitting position, increased mobility, and new skills to explore the world around them, 6–12 mo old infants show advances in cognitive understanding and communicative competence, and there are new tensions around the themes of attachment and separation. Infants develop will and intentions, characteristics that most parents welcome, but still find challenging to manage.

PHYSICAL DEVELOPMENT. Growth slows more (see Table 14-1 and Figs. 9-1 and 9-2). By the 1st birthday, birthweight has tripled, length has increased by 50%, and head circumference has increased by 10 cm. The ability to sit unsupported (6–7 mo) and to pivot while sitting (around 9–10 mo) provides increasing opportunities to manipulate several objects at a time and to experiment with novel combinations of objects. These explorations are aided by the emergence of a thumb-finger grasp (8–9 mo) and a neat pincer grasp by 12 mo. Many infants begin crawling and pulling to stand around 8 mo, followed by cruising. Some walk by 1 yr. Motor achievements correlate with increasing myelinization and cerebellar growth. These gross motor skills expand infants' exploratory range and create new physical dangers as well as opportunities for learning. Tooth eruption occurs, usually starting with the mandibular central incisors (Table 8-3). Tooth development reflects skeletal maturation and bone age, although there is wide individual variation (Table 8-4).

COGNITIVE DEVELOPMENT. The 6 mo old infant has discovered his hands and will soon learn to manipulate objects. At first, everything goes into the mouth. In time, novel objects are picked up, inspected, passed from hand to hand, banged, dropped, and then mouthed. Each action represents a nonverbal idea about what things are for (in Piagetian terms, a *schema*). The complexity of an infant's play, how many different schemata are brought to bear, is a useful index of cognitive development at this age. The pleasure, persistence, and energy with which infants tackle these challenges suggest the existence of an intrinsic drive or mastery

TABLE 8–3. Chronology of Human Dentition of Primary or Deciduous and Secondary or Permanent Teeth

	CALCIFICATION		AGE AT ERUPTION		AGE AT SHEDDING	
	Begins At	Complete At	Maxillary	Mandibular	Maxillary	Mandibular
PRIMARY TEETH						
Central incisors	5th fetal mo	18–24 mo	6–8 mo	5–7 mo	7–8 yr	6–7 yr
Lateral incisors	5th fetal mo	18–24 mo	8–11 mo	7–10 mo	8–9 yr	7–8 yr
Cuspids (canines)	6th fetal mo	30–36 mo	16–20 mo	16–20 mo	11–12 yr	9–11 yr
First molars	5th fetal mo	24–30 mo	10–16 mo	10–16 mo	10–12 yr	10–12 yr
Second molars	6th fetal mo	36 mo	20–30 mo	20–30 mo	10–12 yr	11–13 yr
SECONDARY TEETH						
Central incisors	3–4 mo	9–10 yr	7–8 yr	6–7 yr		
Lateral incisors	Max, 10–12 mo Mand, 3–4 mo	10–11 yr	8–9 yr	7–8 yr		
Cuspids (canines)	4–5 mo	12–15 yr	11–12 yr	9–11 yr		
First premolars (bicuspids)	18–21 mo	12–13 yr	10–11 yr	10–12 yr		
Second premolars (bicuspids)	24–30 mo	12–14 yr	10–12 yr	11–13 yr		
First molars	Birth	9–10 yr	6–7 yr	6–7 yr		
Second molars	30–36 mo	14–16 yr	12–13 yr	12–13 yr		
Third molars	Max, 7–9 yr Mand, 8–10 yr	18–25 yr	17–22 yr	17–22 yr		

Adapted from chart prepared by P.K. Losch, Harvard School of Dental Medicine, who provided the data for this table.
Mand, mandibular; Max, maxillary.

motivation. Mastery behavior occurs when infants feel secure; those with less secure attachments show limited experimentation and less competence.

A major milestone is the achievement at about 9 mo of **object permanence** (constancy), the understanding that objects continue to exist, even when not seen. At 4–7 mo of age, infants look down for a yarn ball that has been dropped, but quickly give up if it is not seen. With object constancy, infants persist in searching, finding objects hidden under a cloth or behind the examiner's back. Peek-a-boo brings unlimited pleasure as the child magically brings back the other player. Events seem to occur as a result of the child's own activities.

EMOTIONAL DEVELOPMENT. The advent of object permanence corresponds with qualitative changes in social and communicative development. Infants look back and forth between an approaching stranger and a parent, and may cling or cry anxiously, demonstrating "*stranger anxiety*." Separations often become more difficult. Infants who have been sleeping through the night for months begin to awaken regularly and cry, as though remembering that the parents are in the next room.

A new demand for autonomy also emerges. Poor weight gain at this age often reflects a struggle between an infant's emerging independence and parent's control of the feeding situation. Use of the 2-spoon method of feeding (1 for the child and 1 for the parent), finger foods, and a high chair with a tray table can avert potential problems. Tantrums make their first appearance as the drives for autonomy and mastery come in conflict with parental controls and the infants' still-limited abilities.

COMMUNICATION. Infants at 7 mo of age are adept at nonverbal communication, expressing a range of emotions and responding to vocal tone and facial expressions. Around 9 mo of age, infants become aware that emotions can be shared between people; they show parents toys as a way of sharing their happy feelings. Between 8 and 10 mo of age, babbling takes on a new complexity, with many syllables ("ba-da-ma") and inflections that mimic the native language. Infants now lose the ability to distinguish between vocal sounds that are undifferentiated in their native language. Social interaction (attentive adults taking turns vocalizing with the infant) profoundly influences the acquisition and production of new sounds. The first true word (i.e., a sound used consistently to refer to a specific object or person) appears in concert with an infant's discovery of object permanence. Picture books now provide an ideal context for verbal language acquisition. With a familiar book as a shared focus of attention, a parent and child engage in repeated cycles of pointing and labeling, with elaboration and feedback by the parent.

IMPLICATIONS FOR PARENTS AND PEDIATRICIANS. With the developmental reorganization that occurs around 9 mo of age, previously resolved issues of feeding and sleeping re-emerge. Pediatricians can prepare parents at the 6 mo visit so that these problems can be understood as the result of developmental progress and not regression. Parents should be encouraged to plan ahead for necessary, and inevitable, separations (e.g., baby sitter, daycare). Routine preparations may make these separations easier. Introduction of a **"transitional object"** may allow the infant to self-comfort in the parents' absence.

Infants' wariness of strangers often makes the 9 mo examination difficult, particularly if the infant is temperamentally prone to react negatively to unfamiliar situations. Initially, the pediatrician should avoid direct eye contact with the child. Time spent talking with the parent and introducing the child to a small, washable toy will be rewarded with more cooperation. The examination can be continued on the parent's lap when feasible.

Brazelton TB: *Touchpoints: The Essential Reference.* Reading, MA, Addison-Wesley, 1992.

Hunziker UA, Barr RG: Increased carrying reduces infant crying: A randomized controlled trial. *Pediatrics* 1986;77:641–648.

Jusczyk PW: Chunking language input to find patterns. In Rakison DH, Oakes LM (editors): *Early Category and Concept Development: Making Sense of the Blooming, Buzzing Confusion.* New York, Oxford, 2003.

Kuhl PK: Human speech and birdsong: Communication and the social brain. *Proc Natl Acad Sci* 2003:100;9645.

McLearn KT, Minkovitz CS, Strobino DM, Marks E, Hou W: The timing of maternal depressive symptoms and mothers' parenting practices with young children: implications for pediatric practice. *Pediatrics* 2006:118;e174–e182.

Stern D: *The Interpersonal World of the Infant.* New York, Basic Books, 1985.

Zuckerman BS, Frank DA, Augustyn M: Infancy and toddler years. In Levine MD, Carey WB, Crocker AC (editors): *Developmental-Behavioral Pediatrics,* 3rd ed. Philadelphia, WB Saunders, 1999, pp 24–37.

TABLE 8–4. Time of Appearance in Roentgenograms of Centers of Ossification in Infancy and Childhood

BOYS—AGE AT APPEARANCE*	BONES AND EPIPHYSEAL CENTERS	GIRLS—AGE AT APPEARANCE*
HUMERUS, HEAD		
3 wk		3 wk
CARPAL BONES		
2 mo ± 2 mo	Capitate	2 mo ± 2 mo
3 mo ± 2 mo	Hamate	2 mo ± 2 mo
30 mo ± 16 mo	Triangular†	21 mo ± 14 mo
42 mo ± 19 mo	Lunate†	34 mo ± 13 mo
67 mo ± 19 mo	Trapezium†	47 mo ± 14 mo
69 mo ± 15 mo	Trapezoid†	49 mo ± 12 mo
66 mo ± 15 mo	Scaphoid†	51 mo ± 12 mo
No standards available	Pisiform†	No standards available
METACARPAL BONES		
18 mo ± 5 mo	II	12 mo ± 3 mo
20 mo ± 5 mo	III	13 mo ± 3 mo
23 mo ± 6 mo	IV	15 mo ± 4 mo
26 mo ± 7 mo	V	16 mo ± 5 mo
32 mo ± 9 mo	I	18 mo ± 5 mo
FINGERS (EPIPHYSES)		
16 mo ± 4 mo	Proximal phalanx, 3rd finger	10 mo ± 3 mo
16 mo ± 4 mo	Proximal phalanx, 2nd finger	11 mo ± 3 mo
17 mo ± 5 mo	Proximal phalanx, 4th finger	11 mo ± 3 mo
19 mo ± 7 mo	Distal phalanx, 1st finger	12 mo ± 4 mo
21 mo ± 5 mo	Proximal phalanx, 5th finger	14 mo ± 4 mo
24 mo ± 6 mo	Middle phalanx, 3rd finger	15 mo ± 5 mo
24 mo ± 6 mo	Middle phalanx, 4th finger	15 mo ± 5 mo
26 mo ± 6 mo	Middle phalanx, 2nd finger	16 mo ± 5 mo
28 mo ± 6 mo	Distal phalanx, 3rd finger	18 mo ± 4 mo
28 mo ± 6 mo	Distal phalanx, 4th finger	18 mo ± 5 mo
32 mo ± 7 mo	Proximal phalanx, 1st finger	20 mo ± 5 mo
37 mo ± 9 mo	Distal phalanx, 5th finger	23 mo ± 6 mo
37 mo ± 8 mo	Distal phalanx, 2nd finger	23 mo ± 6 mo
39 mo ± 10 mo	Middle phalanx, 5th finger	22 mo ± 7 mo
152 mo ± 18 mo	Sesamoid (adductor pollicis)	121 mo ± 13 mo
HIP AND KNEE		
Usually present at birth	Femur, distal	Usually present at birth
Usually present at birth	Tibia, proximal	Usually present at birth
4 mo ± 2 mo	Femur, head	4 mo ± 2 mo
46 mo ± 11 mo	Patella	29 mo ± 7 mo
FOOT AND ANKLE‡		

Values represent mean ± standard deviation, when applicable.
*To nearest month.
†Except for the capitate and hamate bones, the variability of carpal centers is too great to make them very useful clinically.
‡Standards for the foot are available, but normal variation is wide, including some familial variants, so this area is of little clinical use.
The norms present a composite of published data from the Fels Research Institute, Yellow Springs, OH (Pyle SI, Sontag L: *Am J Roentgenol* 1943; 49:102), and unpublished data from the Brush Foundation, Case Western Reserve University, Cleveland, OH, and the Harvard School of Public Health, Boston, MA. Compiled by Lieb, Buehl, and Pyle.

Chapter 9 ■ The Second Year

Susan Feigelman

The skills emerging in the 2nd yr of life shape the child's sense of self and others. The child has a newly found independence; the ability to walk allows separation, yet the child continues to need secure attachment to the parents. At approximately 18 mo of age, the emergence of symbolic thought and language causes a reorganization of behavior, with implications across many developmental domains.

AGE 12–18 MONTHS

PHYSICAL DEVELOPMENT. The growth rate slows further in the 2nd yr of life (see Table 14-1) and appetite declines. Toddlers have relatively short legs and long torsos, with exaggerated lumbar lordosis and protruding abdomens. Brain growth, with continuing myelinization, results in an increase in head circumference of 2 cm over the year.

Most children begin to walk independently near their 1st birthday; some do not walk until 15 mo of age. Early walking is not associated with advanced development in other domains. Infants initially toddle with a wide-based gait, with the knees bent and the arms flexed at the elbow; the entire torso rotates with each stride; the toes may point in or out, and the feet strike the floor flat. The appearance is that of genu varus (bowleg). Subsequent refinement leads to greater steadiness and energy efficiency. After several months of practice, the center of gravity shifts back and the torso stays more stable, while the knees extend and the arms swing at the sides for balance. The feet are held in better alignment, and the child is able to stop, pivot, and stoop without toppling over (see Chapters 671 and 672).

COGNITIVE DEVELOPMENT. Exploration of the environment increases in parallel with improved dexterity (reaching, grasping, releasing) and mobility. Learning follows the precepts of Piaget's sensory-motor stage. Toddlers manipulate objects in novel ways to create interesting effects, such as stacking blocks or putting things into a computer disk drive. Playthings are also more likely to be used for their intended purposes (combs for hair, cups for drinking). Imitation of parents and older children is an important mode of learning. Make-believe (symbolic) play centers on the child's own body (pretending to drink from an empty cup) [Table 9-1; see Table 8-1].

EMOTIONAL DEVELOPMENT. Infants who are approaching the developmental milestone of taking their first steps may be irritable. Once they start walking, their predominant mood changes markedly. Toddlers are described as "intoxicated" or "giddy" with their new ability and with the power to control the distance between themselves and their parents. Exploring toddlers orbit around their parents, moving away and then returning for a reassuring touch before moving away again. A securely attached child will use the parent as a secure base from which to explore independently. Proud of her or his accomplishments, the child illustrates Erikson's stage of autonomy and separation. The toddler who is overly controlled and discouraged from active exploration will feel doubt, shame, anger, and insecurity. All children will experience tantrums, reflecting their inability to delay gratification, suppress or displace anger, or verbally communicate their emotional states. The quality of the maternal-child relationship may moderate negative effects of child care arrangements when parents work.

LINGUISTIC DEVELOPMENT. Receptive language precedes expressive language. By the time infants speak their first words around 12 mo of age, they already respond appropriately to several simple statements, such as "no," "bye-bye," and "give me." By 15 mo, the average child points to major body parts and uses 4–6 words spontaneously and correctly. Toddlers also enjoy **polysyllabic** jargoning (see Tables 8-1 and 9-1), but do not seem upset that no one understands. Most communication of wants and ideas continues to be nonverbal.

IMPLICATIONS FOR PARENTS AND PEDIATRICIANS. Parents may express concern about poor intake as growth slows. The growth chart should provide reassurance. Parents who cannot recall any other milestone tend to remember when their child began to walk, perhaps because of the symbolic significance of walking as an act of independence. All toddlers should be encouraged to explore their environments; a child's ability to wander out of sight also increases the risks of injury and the need for supervision.

TABLE 9-1. Emerging Patterns of Behavior from 1 to 5 Yr of Age*

15 MO	
Motor:	Walks alone; crawls up stairs
Adaptive:	Makes tower of 3 cubes; makes a line with crayon; inserts raisin in bottle
Language:	Jargon; follows simple commands; may name a familiar object (e.g., ball)
Social:	Indicates some desires or needs by pointing; hugs parents
18 MO	
Motor:	Runs stiffly; sits on small chair; walks up stairs with one hand held; explores drawers and wastebaskets
Adaptive:	Makes tower of 4 cubes; imitates scribbling; imitates vertical stroke; dumps raisin from bottle
Language:	10 words (average); names pictures; identifies one or more parts of body
Social:	Feeds self; seeks help when in trouble; may complain when wet or soiled; kisses parent with pucker
24 MO	
Motor:	Runs well, walks up and down stairs, one step at a time; opens doors; climbs on furniture; jumps
Adaptive:	Makes tower of 7 cubes (6 at 21 mo); scribbles in circular pattern; imitates horizontal stroke; folds paper once imitatively
Language:	Puts 3 words together (subject, verb, object)
Social:	Handles spoon well; often tells about immediate experiences; helps to undress; listens to stories when shown pictures
30 MO	
Motor:	Goes up stairs alternating feet
Adaptive:	Makes tower of 9 cubes; makes vertical and horizontal strokes, but generally will not join them to make cross; imitates circular stroke, forming closed figure
Language:	Refers to self by pronoun "I"; knows full name
Social:	Helps put things away; pretends in play
36 MO	
Motor:	Rides tricycle; stands momentarily on one foot
Adaptive:	Makes tower of 10 cubes; imitates construction of "bridge" of 3 cubes; copies circle; imitates cross
Language:	Knows age and sex; counts 3 objects correctly; repeats 3 numbers or a sentence of 6 syllables
Social:	Plays simple games (in "parallel" with other children); helps in dressing (unbuttons clothing and puts on shoes); washes hands
48 MO	
Motor:	Hops on one foot; throws ball overhand; uses scissors to cut out pictures; climbs well
Adaptive:	Copies bridge from model; imitates construction of "gate" of 5 cubes; copies cross and square; draws man with 2 to 4 parts besides head; identifies longer of 2 lines
Language:	Counts 4 pennies accurately; tells story
Social:	Plays with several children, with beginning of social interaction and role-playing; goes to toilet alone
60 MO	
Motor:	Skips
Adaptive:	Draws triangle from copy; names heavier of 2 weights
Language:	Names 4 colors; repeats sentence of 10 syllables; counts 10 pennies correctly
Social:	Dresses and undresses; asks questions about meaning of words; engages in domestic role-playing

*Data derived from those of Gesell (as revised by Knobloch), Shirley, Provence, Wolf, Bailey, and others. After 5 yr, the Stanford-Binet, Wechsler-Bellevue, and other scales offer the most precise estimates of developmental level. To have their greatest value, they should be administered only by an experienced and qualified person.

In the office setting, many toddlers are comfortable exploring the examination room, but cling to the parents under the stress of the examination. Performing most of the physical examination in the parent's lap may help allay fears of separation. Infants who become more, not less, distressed in their parents' arms or who avoid their parents at times of stress may be insecurely attached. Young children who, when distressed, turn to strangers rather than parents for comfort are particularly worrisome. The conflicts between independence and security manifest in issues of discipline, temper tantrums, toilet training, and changing feeding behaviors. Parents should be counseled on these matters within the framework of normal development.

AGE 18–24 MONTHS

PHYSICAL DEVELOPMENT. Motor development is incremental at this age, with improvements in balance and agility and the emergence of running and stair climbing. Height and weight increase at a steady rate during this year, with a gain of 5 in and 5 lb. By 24 mo, children are about ½ of their ultimate adult height. Head growth slows slightly (Figs. 9-1 and 9-2; see also Table 14-1). Ninety percent of adult head circumference is achieved by age 2 yr, with just an additional 5 cm gain over the next few years.

COGNITIVE DEVELOPMENT. At approximately 18 mo of age, several cognitive changes come together to mark the conclusion of the sensory-motor period. These can be observed during self-initiated play. Object permanence is firmly established; toddlers anticipate where an object will end up, even though the object was not visible while it was being moved. Cause and effect are better understood, and toddlers demonstrate flexibility in problem solving (e.g., using a stick to obtain a toy that is out of reach, figuring out how to wind a mechanical toy). Symbolic transformations in play are no longer tied to the toddler's own body, so that a doll can be "fed" from an empty plate. Like the reorganization that occurs at 9 mo, the cognitive changes at 18 mo correlate with important changes in the emotional and linguistic domains (see Table 9-1).

EMOTIONAL DEVELOPMENT. In many children, the relative independence of the preceding period gives way to increased clinginess around 18 mo. This stage, described as "rapprochement," may be a reaction to growing awareness of the possibility of separation. Many parents report that they cannot go anywhere without having a small child attached to them. **Separation anxiety** will be manifest at bedtime. Many children use a special blanket or stuffed toy as a **transitional object,** which functions as a symbol of the absent parent. The transitional object remains important until the transition to symbolic thought has been completed and the symbolic presence of the parent has been fully internalized. Despite the attachment to the parent, the child's use of "no" is a way of declaring independence. Individual differences in temperament, in both the child and the parents, play a critical role in determining the balance of conflict vs cooperation in the parent-child relationship. As effective language emerges, conflicts become less frequent.

Self-conscious awareness and internalized standards of behavior first appear at this age. Toddlers looking in a mirror will, for the first time, reach for their own face rather than the mirror image if they notice something unusual on their nose. They begin to recognize when toys are broken and may hand them to their parents to fix. When tempted to touch a forbidden object, they may tell themselves "no, no." Language becomes a means of impulse control, early reasoning, and connection between ideas. This is the very beginning of the formation of a conscience. The fact that they often go on to touch the object anyway demonstrates the relative weakness of internalized inhibitions at this stage.

LINGUISTIC DEVELOPMENT. Perhaps the most dramatic developments in this period are linguistic. Labeling of objects coincides with the advent of symbolic thought. After the realization that words can stand for things occurs, a child's vocabulary balloons from 10–15 words at 18 mo to between 50 and 100 at 2 yr. After acquiring a vocabulary of about 50 words, toddlers begin to combine them to make simple sentences, the beginning of grammar. At this stage, toddlers understand **2-step commands,** such as "Give me the ball and then get your shoes." Language also gives the toddler a sense of control over the surroundings, as in "night-night" or "bye-bye." The emergence of verbal language marks the end of the sensory-motor period. As toddlers learn to use symbols to express ideas and solve problems, the need for cognition based on direct sensation and motor manipulation wanes.

IMPLICATIONS FOR PARENTS AND PEDIATRICIANS. With children's increasing mobility, physical limits on their explorations become

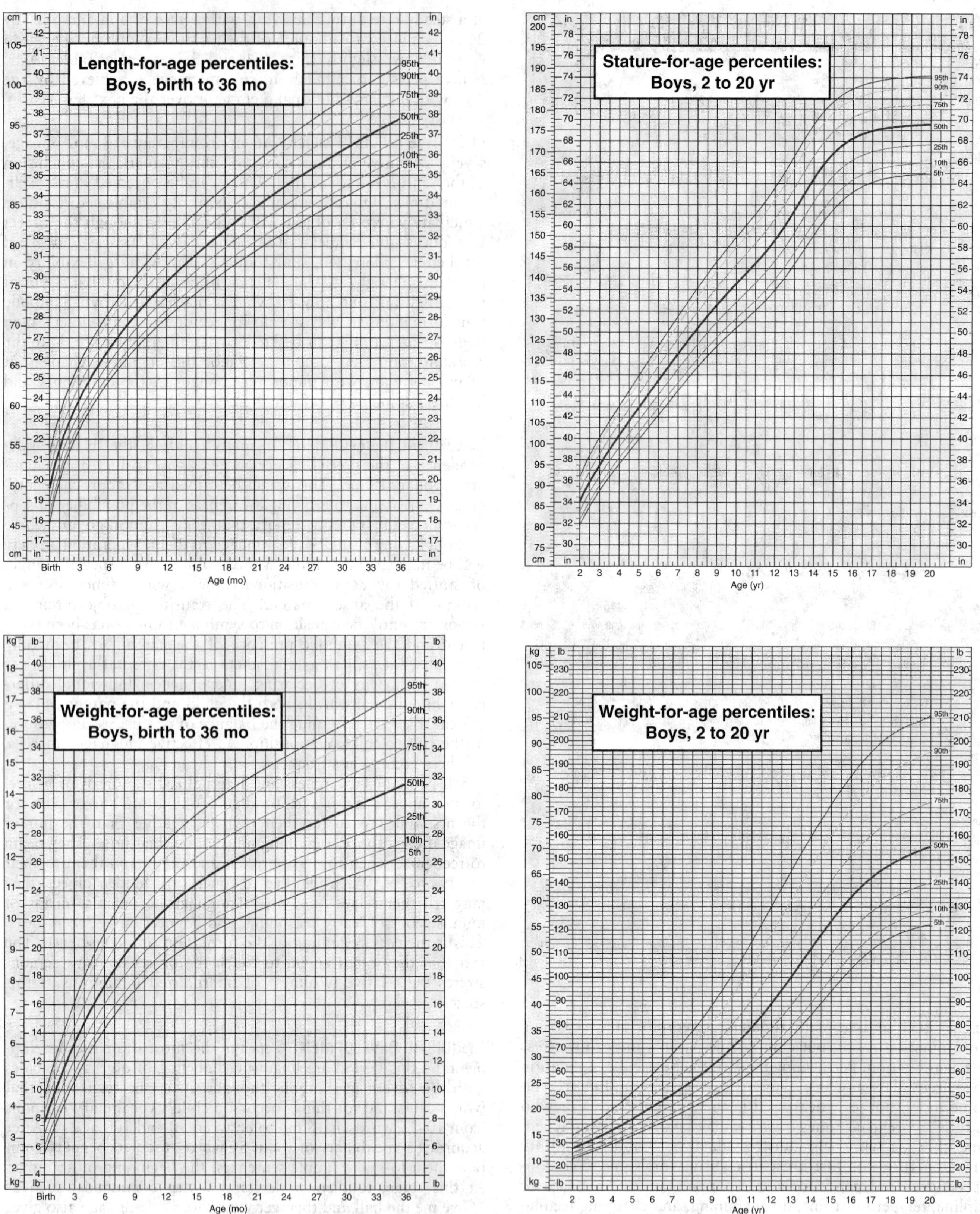

Figure 9-1. Percentile curves for weight and length/stature by age for boys *(A)* and girls *(B)* birth to 20 yr of age. (Official 2000 Centers for Disease Control [CDC] growth charts, created by the National Center for Health Statistics [NCHS; see Chapter 14]. Infant length was measured lying; older children's stature was measured standing. Additional information and technical reports available at *www.cdc.gov/nchs.*)

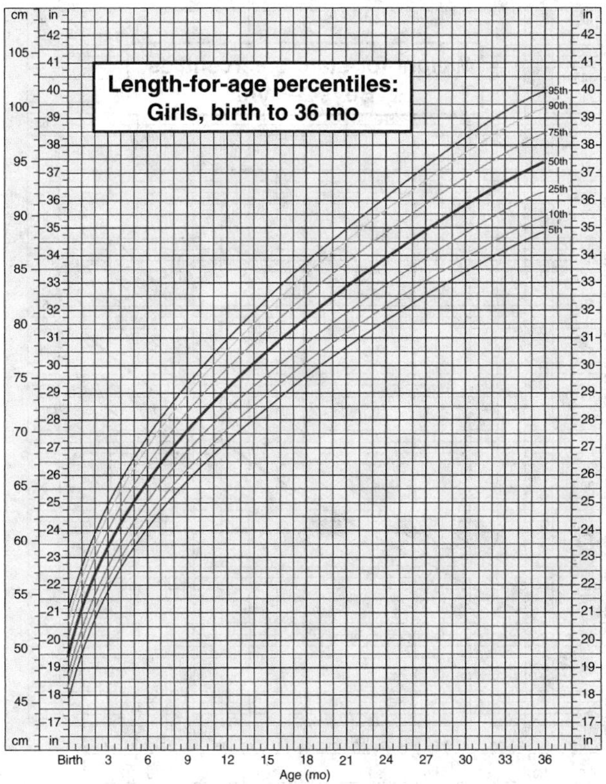

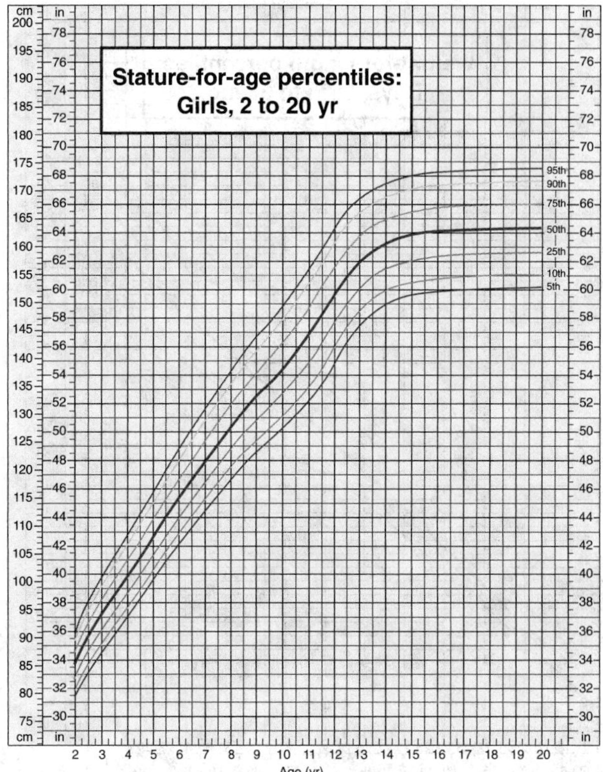

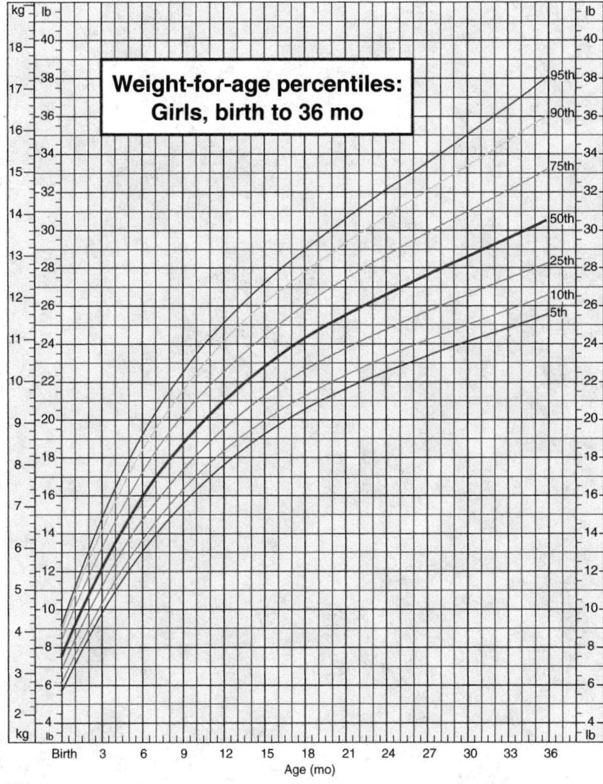

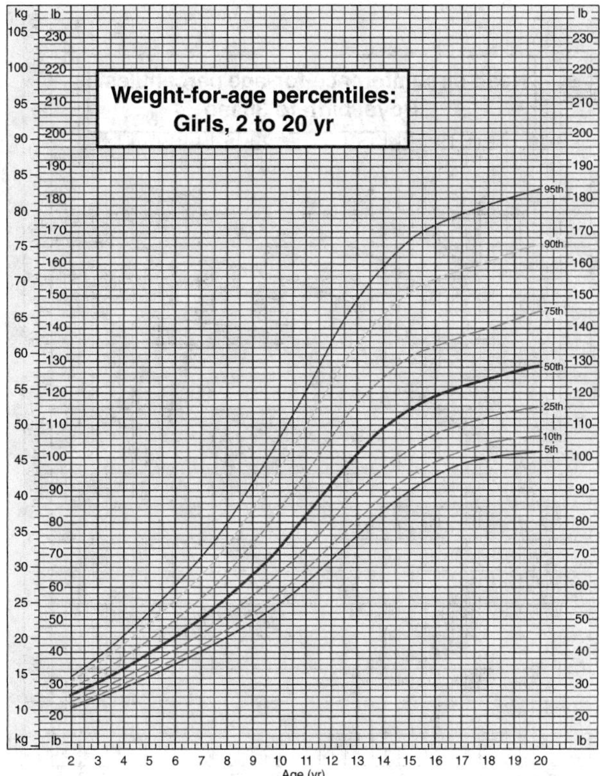

B

Figure 9-1. *Continued*

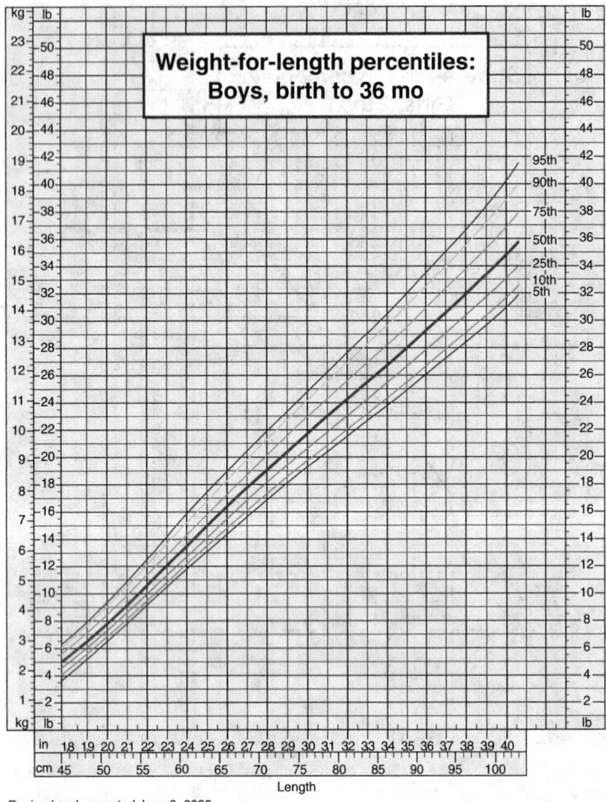

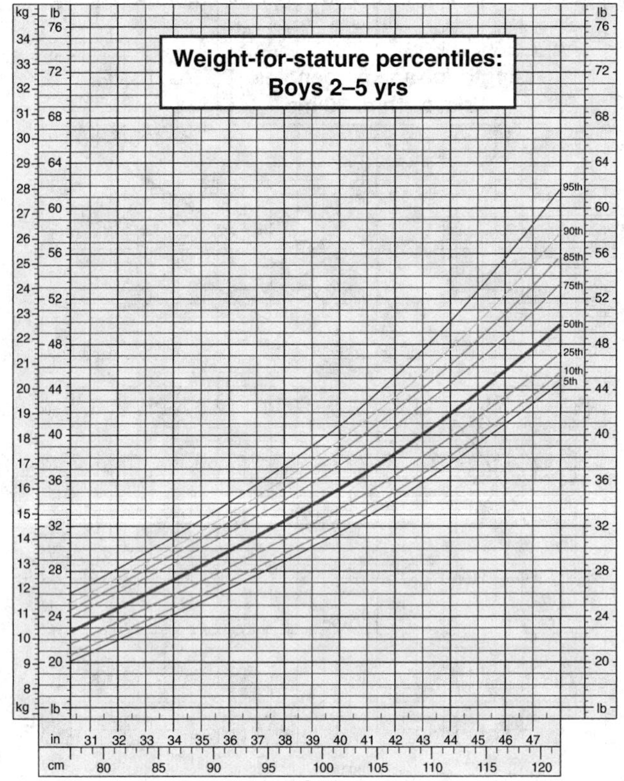

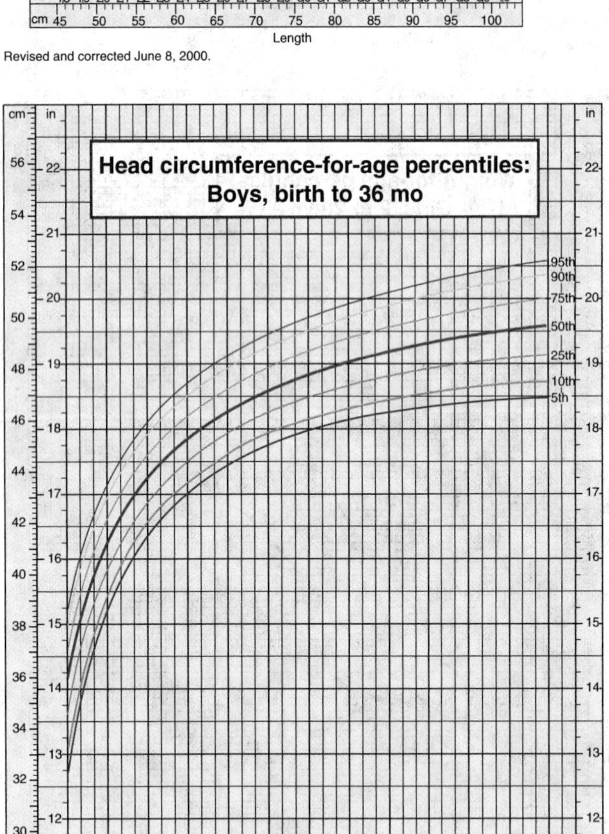

A

Figure 9-2. Head circumference and length/stature by weight for boys *(A)* and girls *(B)*. (Official 2000 Centers for Disease Control [CDC] growth charts, created by the National Center for Health Statistics [NCHS; see Chapter 14]. Additional information and technical reports are available at *www.cdc.gov/nchs*.)

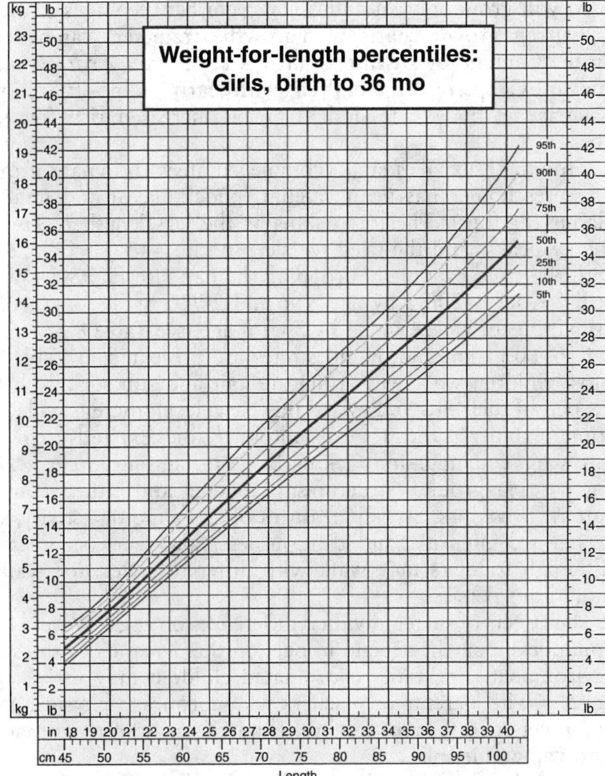

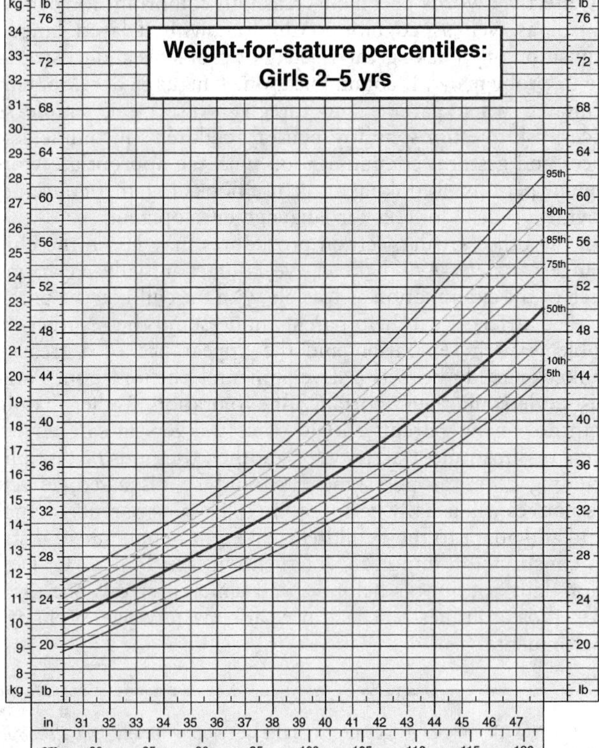

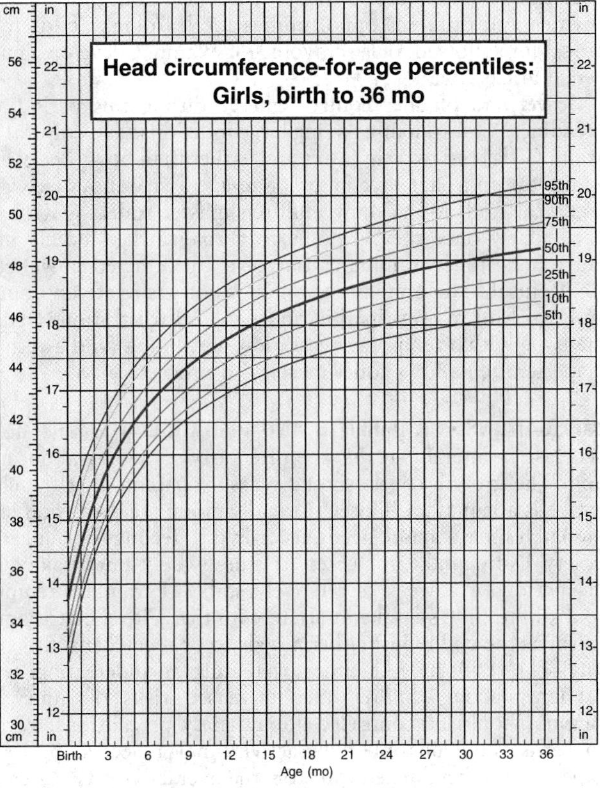

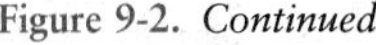

Figure 9-2. *Continued*

less effective; words become increasingly important for behavior control as well as cognition. Children with delayed language acquisition often have greater behavior problems and frustrations due to problems with communication. Language development is facilitated when parents and caregivers use clear, simple sentences; ask questions; and respond to children's incomplete sentences and gestural communication with the appropriate words. Regular periods of looking at picture books together continue to provide an ideal context for language development.

In the office setting, certain procedures may lessen the child's **stranger anxiety.** Avoid direct eye contact initially. Perform as much of the examination as feasible with the child on the parent's lap. Pediatricians can help parents understand the resurgence of problems with separation and the appearance of a treasured blanket or teddy bear as a developmental phenomenon. Parents must understand the importance of exploration. Rather than limiting movement, parents should place toddlers in safe environments or substitute 1 activity for another. Methods of discipline, including corporal punishment, should be discussed; effective alternatives will usually be appreciated. Helping parents to understand and adapt to their children's different temperamental styles can constitute an important intervention (see Table 6-1). Developing daily routines is helpful to all children at this age. Rigidity in those routines reflects a need for mastery over a changing environment.

Bates E, Dick F: Language, gesture, and the developing brain. *Dev Psychobiol* 2002;40:293–310.

Dixon SD, Hennessy MJ: One year: One giant step forward. In Dixon SD, Stein MT (editors): *Encounters with Children: Pediatric Behavior and Development*. St. Louis, Mosby, 2000, pp 247–276.

Fraiberg S: *The Magic Years*. New York: Scribner's, 1959.

Lieberman A: *The Emotional Life of the Toddler.* New York, Free Press, 1993.

Mahler MS, Pine S, Bergman A: *The Psychological Birth of the Infant.* London, Hutchinson, 1975.

National Institute of Child Health and Human Development Early Child Care Research Network: Families matter—even for kids in child care. *J Dev Behav Pediatr* 2003;24:58–62.

Chapter 10 ■ The Preschool Years

Susan Feigelman

The ages between 2 and 5 yr are governed by the emergence of language and exposure of children to an expanding social sphere. As toddlers, children learn to walk away and come back to the secure adult or parent. As preschoolers, they explore emotional separation, alternating between stubborn opposition and cheerful compliance, between bold exploration and clinging dependence. Increasing time spent in classrooms and playgrounds challenges a child's ability to adapt to new rules and relationships. Preschool children know that they can do more than ever before, but they are also very aware of the constraints imposed on them by the adult world and their own limited abilities.

PHYSICAL DEVELOPMENT

By the end of the 2nd year, somatic and brain growth slows, with corresponding decreases in nutritional requirements and appetite, and the emergence of "picky" eating habits (see Table 14-1). Expect a gain of approximately 2 kg (4–5 lb) in weight and 7–8 cm (2–3 in) in height per year. Birthweight quadruples by 2½ yr of age. An average 4 yr old weighs 40 lb and is 40 in tall. The head will grow only an additional 5 cm between ages 3 and 18 yr. Current growth charts, with growth parameters, can be found on the Centers for Disease Control website *(www.cdc.gov/nchs)* and in Chapter 14. Children with early adiposity rebound (increase in body mass index) are at increased risk for adult obesity.

Growth of sexual organs is commensurate with somatic growth. The preschooler has genu valgum (knock-knees) and mild pes planus (flatfoot). The torso slims as the legs lengthen. Physical energy peaks, and the need for sleep declines to 11–13 hr/24 hr, with the child eventually dropping the nap (see Fig. 8-1). Visual acuity reaches 20/30 by age 3 yr and 20/20 by age 4 yr. All 20 primary teeth have erupted by 3 yr of age (see Table 8-3).

Gross and fine motor milestones are presented in Table 9-1. Most children walk with a mature gait and run steadily before the end of their 3rd yr. Beyond this basic level, there is wide variation in ability as the range of motor activities expands to include throwing, catching, and kicking balls; riding on bicycles; climbing on playground structures; dancing; and other complex pattern behaviors. Stylistic features of gross motor activity, such as tempo, intensity, and cautiousness, also vary significantly. Although toddlers may walk with different styles, toe walking should not persist.

The effects of such individual differences on cognitive and emotional development depend in part on the demands of the social environment. Energetic, coordinated children may thrive emotionally with parents or teachers who encourage physical activity; lower-energy, more cerebral children may thrive with adults who value quiet play.

Handedness is usually established by the 3rd yr. Frustration may result from attempts to change children's hand preference. Variations in fine motor development reflect both individual proclivities and different opportunities for learning. Children who are seldom allowed to use crayons, for example, develop a mature pencil grasp later.

Bowel and bladder control emerge during this period, with "readiness" for toileting having large individual and cultural variation. Girls tend to train faster and earlier than boys. Bed-wetting is normal up to age 4 yr in girls and age 5 yr in boys (see Chapters 22.3 and 543). Many children master toileting with ease, particularly once they are able to verbalize their bodily needs. For others, toilet training can involve a protracted power struggle. Refusal to defecate in the toilet or potty is relatively common and can lead to constipation and parental frustration. Defusing the issue with a temporary cessation of training (and a return to diapers) often allows toilet mastery to proceed.

IMPLICATIONS FOR PARENTS AND PEDIATRICIANS. The normal decrease in appetite at this age often arouses worry about nutrition. The growth charts should reassure parents that the child's intake is adequate. Children normally modulate their food intake to match their somatic needs according to feelings of hunger and satiety. Daily intake fluctuates, at times widely, but intake during the period of a week is relatively stable. Parental attempts to control the child's intake interfere with this self-regulatory mechanism as the child must either accede to or rebel against the pressure. The result may be either overeating or undereating.

Highly active children face increased risks of injury, and parents should be counseled about safety precautions. Parental concerns about possible hyperactivity may reflect inappropriate expectations, heightened fears, or true overactivity. Children who engage in reckless, uncontrollable activity with no apparent regard for personal safety should be evaluated further.

LANGUAGE, COGNITION, AND PLAY

These three domains all involve symbolic function, a mode of dealing with the world that emerges during the preschool period.

LANGUAGE. Language development occurs most rapidly between 2 and 5 yr of age. Vocabulary increases from 50–100 words to more than 2,000. Sentence structure advances from telegraphic phrases ("Baby cry") to sentences incorporating all of the major grammatical components. As a rule of thumb, between the ages of 2 and 5 yr, the number of words in a typical sentence equals the child's age (2 by age 2 yr, 3 by age 3 yr, and so on.) By 21 mo to 2 yr, most children are using possessives ("My ball"), progressives (the "-ing" construction, as in "I playing"), questions, and negatives. By 4 yr of age, most children can count to 4 and use the past tense; by 5 yr of age, they can use the future tense. Children do not use figurative speech; they will only comprehend the literal meaning of words. For example, referring to an object as "light as a feather" may produce a quizzical look on a child.

It is important to distinguish between *speech* (the production of intelligible sounds) and *language,* which refers to the underlying mental act. Language includes both expressive and receptive functions. Receptive language (understanding) varies less in its rate of acquisition than does expressive language; therefore, it has greater prognostic importance (see Chapters 15 and 32).

Language acquisition depends critically on environmental input. Key determinants include the amount and variety of speech directed toward children and the frequency with which adults ask questions and encourage verbalization. Children raised in poverty perform lower on measures of language development compared to children from economically advantaged families.

Although experience influences the rate of language development, many linguists believe that the basic mechanism for language learning is "hard-wired" in the brain. Children do not simply imitate adult speech. Rather, they abstract the complex rules of grammar from the ambient language, generating implicit hypotheses. Evidence for the existence of such implicit rules comes from analysis of grammatical errors, such as the overgeneralized use of "-s" to signify the plural and "-ed" to signify the past ("We seed lots of mouses.").

Language is linked to both cognitive and emotional development. Language delays may be the first indication that a child has mental retardation, has an autism spectrum disorder, or has been maltreated. Language plays a critical part in the regulation of behavior through internalized "private speech" in which a child repeats adult prohibitions, first audibly and then mentally. Language also allows children to express feelings, such as anger or frustration, without acting them out; consequently, language-delayed children show higher rates of tantrums and other externalizing behaviors.

Preschool language development lays the foundation for later success in school. Approximately 35% of USA children may enter school lacking the language skills that are the prerequisites for acquiring literacy. Children from socially and economically disadvantaged backgrounds have an increased risk of school problems, making early detection, along with referral and enrichment, important. Although children typically learn to read and write in elementary school, critical foundations for literacy are established during the preschool years. Through repeated early exposure to written words, children learn about the uses of writing (telling stories or sending messages) and about its form (left to right, top to bottom). Early errors in writing, like errors in speaking, reveal that literacy acquisition is an active process involving the generation and revision of hypotheses.

Picture books have a special role not only in familiarizing young children with the printed word but also in the development of verbal language. Children's vocabulary and receptive language improve when their parents consistently read to them. Reading aloud with a young child is an interactive process in which a parent repeatedly focuses the child's attention on a particular picture, asks questions, and then gives the child feedback. The elements of shared attention, active participation, immediate feedback, repetition, and graduated difficulty make such routines ideal for language learning. Programs in which physicians provide books to preschool children, especially among disadvantaged populations, have shown improvement in language skills among the children.

The period of rapid language acquisition is also when **developmental dysfluency** and **stuttering** are most likely to emerge; these can be traced to activation of the cortical motor, sensory, and cerebellar areas. Common difficulties include pauses and repetitions of initial sounds. Stress or excitement exacerbates these difficulties, which generally resolve on their own. Although it is common in preschool children, about 1% of children continue to have significant stuttering after age 8 yr. Children with stuttering should be referred for evaluation if it is severe, persistent, or associated with anxiety, or if parental concern is elicited. **Treatment** includes guidance to parents to reduce pressures associated with speaking.

COGNITION. The preschool period corresponds to Piaget's preoperational (prelogical) stage, characterized by magical thinking, egocentrism, and thinking that is dominated by perception, not abstraction (see Table 6-2). Magical thinking includes confusing coincidence with causality, animism (attributing motivations to inanimate objects and events), and unrealistic beliefs about the power of wishes. A child might believe that people cause it to rain by carrying umbrellas, that the sun goes down because it is tired, or that feeling resentment toward a sibling can actually make that sibling sick. Egocentrism refers to a child's inability to take another's point of view and does not connote selfishness. A child might try to comfort an adult who is upset by bringing him or her a favorite stuffed animal. After 2 yr of age, the child develops a concept of herself or himself as an individual and senses the need to feel "whole."

Piaget demonstrated the dominance of perception over logic. In one experiment, water is poured back and forth between a tall, thin vase and a low, wide dish, and children are asked which container has more water. Invariably, they choose the one that looks larger (usually the tall vase), even when the examiner points out that no water has been added or taken away. Such misunderstandings reflect young children's developing hypotheses about the nature of the world as well as their difficulty in attending simultaneously to multiple aspects of a situation.

PLAY. Maria Montessori considered play to be the work of childhood; however, she did not lend credence to the importance of fantasy and imagination (symbolic play). Play involves learning, physical activity, socialization with peers, and practicing adult roles. Play increases in complexity and imagination, from simple imitation of common experiences, such as shopping and putting baby to bed (2 or 3 yr of age), to more extended scenarios involving singular events, such as going to the zoo or going on a trip (3 or 4 yr of age), to the creation of scenarios that have only been imagined, such as flying to the moon (4 or 5 yr of age). By age 3 yr, cooperative play is seen in activities such as building a tower of blocks together; later, more structured role-play activity, as in playing house, is seen. Play also becomes increasingly governed by rules, from early rules about asking (rather than taking) and sharing (2 or 3 yr of age), to rules that change from moment to moment, according to the desires of the players (4 and 5 yr of age), to the beginning of the recognition of rules as relatively immutable (5 yr of age and beyond).

Play also allows for resolution of conflicts and anxiety and for creative outlets. Children can vent anger safely (spanking a doll), take on superpowers (dinosaur and superhero play), and obtain things that are denied in real life (a make-believe friend or stuffed animal). Creativity is particularly apparent in drawing, painting, and other artistic activities. Themes and emotions that emerge in a child's drawings often reflect the emotional issues of greatest importance for the child.

Difficulty distinguishing fantasy from reality colors a child's perception of what he or she views in the media, through programming and advertising. One fourth of young children have a television set in their bedroom and watch many hours of television per week, and much of what they view is violent. Attitudes about violence are formed early, and early exposure has been associated with later behavior problems.

IMPLICATIONS FOR PARENTS AND PEDIATRICIANS. The significance of language as a target for assessment and intervention cannot be overestimated because of its central role as an indicator of cognitive and emotional development and a key factor in behavioral regulation and later school success. As language emerges, parents can support emotional development by using words that describe the child's feeling states ("You sound angry right now.") and urging the child to use words to express, rather than act out, feelings. Active imaginations will come into play when children offer explanations for misbehavior. A parent's best way of dealing with untruths is to address the event, not the child, and have the child participate in making things right.

Parents should have a regular time each day for reading or looking at books with their children. Programs in which pediatricians give out picture books along with appropriate guidance during primary care visits have been effective in increasing reading aloud and thereby promoting language development, particularly in lower-income families. Television and similar media should be limited to 2 hr/day of quality programming, and parents should be watching the programs with their children and debriefing their young children afterward. At-risk children, particularly those living in poverty, can better meet future school challenges if they have early high-quality experiences, such as Head Start.

Preoperational thinking constrains how children understand experiences of illness and treatment. Children begin to understand that bodies have "insides" and "outsides." Children should be given simple, concrete explanations for medical procedures and given some control over procedures if possible. Children should be reassured that they are not to blame when receiving a vaccine or venipuncture. An adhesive bandage will help to make the body whole again in a child's mind.

The active imagination that fuels play and the magical, animist thinking characteristic of preoperational cognition can also generate intense fears. More than 80% of parents report at least 1 fear in their preschool children. Refusal to take baths or to sit on the toilet may arise from the fear of being washed or flushed away, reflecting a child's immature appreciation of relative size. Attempts to demonstrate rationally that there are no monsters in the closet often fail, inasmuch as the fear arises from prerational thinking. However, this same thinking allows parents to be endowed with magical powers that can banish the monsters with "monster spray" or a night light. Parents should acknowledge the fears, offer reassurance and a sense of security, and give the child some sense of control over the situation. Use of the Draw-a-Person, in which a child is asked to draw the best person he or she can, may help explain a child's viewpoint.

EMOTIONAL AND MORAL DEVELOPMENT

Emotional challenges facing preschool children include accepting limits while maintaining a sense of self-direction, reining in aggressive and sexual impulses, and interacting with a widening circle of adults and peers. At 2 yr of age, behavioral limits are predominantly external; by 5 yr of age, these controls need to be internalized if a child is to function in a typical classroom. Success in achieving this goal relies on prior emotional development, particularly the ability to use internalized images of trusted adults to provide a secure environment in times of stress. The love a child feels for important adults is the main incentive for the development of self-control.

Children learn what behaviors are acceptable and how much power they wield vis-à-vis important adults by testing limits. Testing increases when it elicits attention, even though that attention is often negative, and when limits are inconsistent. Testing often arouses parental anger or inappropriate solicitude as a child struggles to separate, and it gives rise to a corresponding parental challenge: letting go. Excessively tight limits can undermine a child's sense of initiative, whereas overly loose limits can provoke anxiety in a child who feels that no one is in control.

Control is a central issue. Young children cannot control many aspects of their lives, including where they go, how long they stay, and what they take home from the store. They are also prone to lose internal control, that is, to have temper tantrums. Fear, overtiredness, inconsistent expectations, or physical discomfort can also evoke tantrums. Tantrums normally appear toward the end of the 1st yr of life and peak in prevalence between 2 and 4 yr of age. Tantrums lasting more than 15 min or regularly occurring more than 3 times/day may reflect underlying medical, emotional, or social problems.

Preschool children normally experience complicated feelings toward their parents that can include strong attachment and possessiveness toward the parent of the opposite sex, jealousy and resentment of the other parent, and fear that these negative feelings might lead to abandonment. These emotions, most of which are beyond a child's ability to comprehend or verbalize, often find expression in highly labile moods. The resolution of this crisis (a process extending over years) involves a child's unspoken decision to identify with the parents rather than compete with them. Play and language foster the development of emotional controls by allowing children to express emotions and role-play.

Curiosity about genitals and adult sexual organs is normal, as is masturbation. Excessive masturbation interfering with normal activity, acting out sexual intercourse, extreme modesty, or mimicry of adult seductive behavior all suggests the possibility of sexual abuse or inappropriate exposure. Modesty appears gradually between 4 and 6 yr of age, with wide variations among cultures and families. Parents should begin to teach children about "private" areas before school entry.

Moral thinking is constrained by a child's cognitive level and language abilities, but develops as the child continues her or his identity with the parents. Beginning before the 2nd birthday, the child's sense of right and wrong stems from the desire to earn approval from the parents and avoid negative consequences. The child's impulses are tempered by external forces; she or he has not yet internalized societal rules or a sense of justice and fairness. Over time, as the child internalizes parental admonitions, words are substituted for aggressive behaviors. Finally, the child accepts personal responsibility. Actions will be viewed by damage caused, not by intent. Empathic responses to others' distress arise during the 2nd yr of life, but the ability to consider another child's point of view remains limited throughout this period. In keeping with a child's inability to focus on more than 1 aspect of a situation at a time, fairness is taken to mean equal treatment, regardless of circumstance. A 4 yr old will acknowledge the importance of taking turns, but will complain if he didn't get enough time. Rules tend to be absolute, with guilt assigned for bad outcomes, regardless of intentions.

IMPLICATIONS FOR PARENTS AND PEDIATRICIANS. The importance of the preschooler's sense of control over his or her body and surroundings has implications for practice. Preparing the patient by letting the child know how the visit will proceed is reassuring. Tell the child what will happen, but don't ask permission unless you are willing to deal with a "no" answer.

The visit of the 4 or 5 yr old should be entertaining, due to the child's ability to communicate, as well as his or her natural curiosity. Physicians should realize that all children are occasionally difficult. Guidance emphasizing appropriate expectations for behavioral and emotional development and acknowledging normal parental feelings of anger, guilt, and confusion should be part of all visits at this time. Parents should be queried about daily routines and their expectations of child behavior. Providing children with choices (all options being acceptable to the parent) and encouraging independence in self-care activities (feeding, dressing, bathing) will reduce conflicts.

Corporal punishment is inappropriate in the modern context in which most families live. Parents usually claim that they do not like spanking, and many acknowledge that it is not very effective. As children habituate to repeated spanking, parents have to spank ever harder to get the desired response, increasing the risk of serious injury. Sufficiently harsh punishment may inhibit undesired behaviors, but at great psychologic cost. Children mimic the corporal punishment that they receive, and it is common for preschool children to strike their parents or other children. Whereas spanking is the use of force, externally applied, to produce behavior change, **discipline** is a method that allows the child to internalize controls on behavior. Alternative discipline strategies should be offered, such as the "countdown," consistent limit setting, clear communication of rules, and frequent approval. Discipline should be immediate, specific to the behavior, and time-limited. Time-out for approximately 1 min/yr of age is very effective.

Anderson LM, Shinn C, Fullilove MT, et al: The effectiveness of early childhood development programs: A systematic review. *Am J Prev Med* 2003:24(3S):32–46.

Brazelton TB, Christophersen ER, Frauman AC, et al: Instruction, timeliness, and medical influences affecting toilet training. *Pediatrics* 1999;103: 1353–1358.

Dietz WH: Overweight in childhood and adolescence. *N Engl J Med* 2004;350:855–857.

Dixon SD: Two years: Language emerges. In Dixon SD, Stein MT (editors): *Encounters with Children: Pediatric Behavior and Development.* St Louis, Mosby, 2000, pp 300–326.

Faber A, Mazlish E: *How to Talk So Kids Will Listen & Listen So Kids Will Talk,* revised. New York, Avon, 1999.

Fraiberg, S: *The Magic Years.* New York, Scribner's, 1959.

Gordon N: Stuttering: Incidence and causes. *Dev Med Child Neurol* 2002;44:278–282.

National Institute of Child Health and Human Development Early Child Care Research Network: Duration and developmental timing of poverty and children's cognitive and social development from birth through third grade. *Child Development* 2005;76:795–810

Needlman R, Silverstein M: Pediatric interventions to support reading aloud: How good is the evidence? *Dev Behav Pediatr* 2004;25:352.

Schickedanz JA: *Much More than the ABCs: The Early Stages of Reading and Writing.* Washington, DC, National Association for the Education of Young Children (NAEYC), 1999.

Chapter 11 ■ Middle Childhood

Susan Feigelman

During middle childhood (6–11 yr of age), children increasingly separate from parents and seek acceptance from teachers, other adults, and peers. Self-esteem becomes a central issue, as children develop the cognitive ability to consider their own self-evaluations and their perception of how others see them. For the first time, they are judged according to their ability to produce socially valued outputs, such as getting good grades, playing a musical instrument, or hitting home runs. Children are under pressure to conform to the style and ideals of the peer group.

PHYSICAL DEVELOPMENT

Growth during the period averages 3–3.5 kg (7 lb) and 6–7 cm (2.5 in) per year (see Figs. 9-1 and 9-2). Growth occurs **discontinuously,** in 3–6 irregularly timed spurts each year, with each growth spurt lasting, on average, 8 wk. The head grows only 2–3 cm in circumference throughout the entire period, reflecting a slowing of brain growth. Myelinization is complete by 7 yr of age. Body habitus is more erect than previously, with long legs compared with the torso.

Growth of the midface and lower face occurs gradually. Loss of deciduous (baby) teeth is a more dramatic sign of maturation, beginning after eruption of the 1st molars around 6 yr of age. Replacement with adult teeth occurs at a rate of about 4 per year, so that by age 9 yr, children will have 8 permanent incisors and 4 permanent molars. Premolars erupt by 11–12 yr of age. Lymphoid tissues hypertrophy, often giving rise to impressive tonsils and adenoids.

Muscular strength, coordination, and stamina increase progressively, as does the ability to perform complex movements, such as dancing or shooting baskets. Such higher-order motor skills are the result of both maturation and training; the degree of accomplishment reflects wide variability in innate skill, interest, and opportunity.

There has been a general decline in physical fitness among school-aged children. Sedentary habits at this age are associated with increased lifetime risk of obesity and cardiovascular disease. The number of overweight children and the degree of overweight are both increasing. Most youth do not participate in any organized physical activity outside of school; ¼ do not engage in any free-time physical activity.

Prior to puberty, the sensitivity of the hypothalamus and the pituitary changes, leading to increased gonadotropin synthesis. For most children, the sexual organs remain physically immature, but interest in gender differences and sexual behavior remains active in many children and increases progressively until puberty. Although this is a period when sexual drives are limited, masturbation is common, and children may be interested in differences between genders.

Puberty may be occurring at younger ages. Early-developing girls may feel uncomfortable, particularly if expected to behave as an older child would. Girls may worry that they are overweight, and many engage in unhealthy dieting to achieve an abnormally thin cultural ideal.

IMPLICATIONS FOR PARENTS AND PEDIATRICIANS. Middle childhood is generally a time of excellent health. However, children have variable sizes, shapes, and abilities. Children of this age compare themselves with others, eliciting feelings about their physical attributes and abilities. Fears of being "defective" can lead to avoidance of situations in which physical differences might be revealed, such as gym class or medical examinations. Children with actual physical disabilities may face special stresses. Medical, social, and psychologic risks tend to occur together.

Children should be asked about regular physical activity. Participation in organized sports or other organized activities can foster skill, teamwork, and fitness, as well as a sense of accomplishment, but pressure to compete when the activity is no longer enjoyable has negative effects. Prepubertal children should not engage in high-stress, high-impact sports, such as power lifting or football, because skeletal immaturity increases the risk of injury.

COGNITIVE DEVELOPMENT

The thinking of early elementary school-aged children differs qualitatively from that of preschool children. In place of magical, egocentric, and perception-bound cognition, school-aged children increasingly apply rules based on observable phenomena, factor in multiple dimensions and points of view, and interpret their perceptions using physical laws. Piaget documented this shift from *"preoperational"* to *"concrete logical operations."* When 5 yr olds watch a ball of clay being rolled into a snake, they might insist that the snake has "more" because it is longer. In contrast, 7 yr olds typically reply that the ball and the snake must weigh the same because nothing has been added or taken away or because the snake is both longer and thinner. This cognitive reorganization occurs at different rates in different contexts. In the context of social interactions with siblings, young children often demonstrate an ability to understand alternate points of view long before they demonstrate that ability in their thinking about the physical world. Understanding time and space constructs occurs in the later part of this period.

The concept of **"school readiness"** is controversial. There is no consensus on whether there is a defined set of skills needed for success on school entry, and whether certain skills predict later achievement. By age 5 yr, most children have the ability to learn in a school setting, as long as the setting is sufficiently flexible to support children with a variety of developmental achievements. Delaying entry may not improve ultimate school success and may be associated with behavior problems, especially in adolescence. Separation anxiety, or school refusal, is common in the early school years.

School makes increasing cognitive demands on the child. Mastery of the elementary curriculum requires that a large number of perceptual, cognitive, and language processes work efficiently (Table 11-1), and children are expected to attend to many inputs at once. The first 2 to 3 yr of elementary school are devoted to acquiring the fundamentals: reading, writing, and basic mathematics skills. By 3rd grade, children need to be able to sustain attention through a 45 min period and the curriculum requires more complex tasks. The goal of reading a paragraph is no longer to decode the words, but to understand the content; the goal of writing is no longer spelling or penmanship, but composition. The volume of work increases along with the complexity.

Cognitive abilities interact with a wide array of attitudinal and emotional factors in determining classroom performance. These factors include external rewards (eagerness to please adults and approval from peers) and internal rewards (competitiveness, willingness to work for a delayed reward, belief in one's abilities, and ability to risk trying when success is not ensured). Success predisposes to success, whereas failure impacts self-esteem and reduces self-efficacy, diminishing a child's ability to take future risks.

Children's intellectual activity extends beyond the classroom. Beginning in the 3rd or 4th grade, children increasingly enjoy strategy games and wordplay (puns and insults) that exercise their growing cognitive and linguistic mastery. Many become experts on subjects of their own choosing, such as sports trivia, or develop hobbies, such as special card collections. Others become avid readers or take on artistic pursuits. Whereas board and card games were once the usual leisure time activity of youth, video and computer games currently fill this need.

IMPLICATIONS FOR PARENTS AND PEDIATRICIANS. Concrete operations allow children to understand simple explanations for illnesses and necessary treatments, although they may revert to prelogical thinking when under stress. A child with pneumonia may be able to explain about white cells fighting the "germs" in the lungs, but still secretly harbors the belief that the sickness is a punishment for disobedience.

Academic and classroom behavior problems are important areas for the pediatrician to assess and manage. Referrals may be made to the school for remediation or to community resources (medical or psychologic) when appropriate. The causes may be one or more of the following: deficits in perception (vision and hearing); specific learning disabilities; global cognitive delay (mental retardation); primary attention deficit; and attention deficits secondary to family dysfunction, depression, anxiety, or chronic illness (see Chapters 15 and 30). Children whose learning style does not fit the classroom culture may have academic difficulties and need attention before failure sets in. Simply having a child repeat a failed grade rarely has any beneficial effect and often seriously undercuts the child's self-esteem. In addition to

TABLE 11-1. Selected Perceptual, Cognitive, and Language Processes Required for Elementary School Success

PROCESS	DESCRIPTION	ASSOCIATED PROBLEMS
PERCEPTUAL		
Visual analysis	Ability to break a complex figure into components and understand their spatial relationships	Persistent letter confusion (e.g., between *b*, *d*, and *g*); difficulty with basic reading and writing and limited "sight" vocabulary
Proprioception and motor control	Ability to obtain information about body position by feel and unconsciously program complex movements	Poor handwriting, requiring inordinate effort, often with overly tight pencil grasp; special difficulty with timed tasks
Phonologic processing	Ability to perceive differences between similar sounding words and to break down words into constituent sounds	Delayed receptive language skill; attention and behavior problems secondary to not understanding directions; delayed acquisition of letter-sound correlations (phonetics)
COGNITIVE		
Long-term memory, both storage and recall	Ability to acquire skills that are "automatic" (i.e., accessible without conscious thought)	Delayed mastery of the alphabet (reading and writing letters); slow handwriting; inability to progress beyond basic mathematics
Selective attention	Ability to attend to important stimuli and ignore distractions	Difficulty following multistep instructions, completing assignments, and behaving well; problems with peer interaction
Sequencing	Ability to remember things in order; facility with time concepts	Difficulty organizing assignments, planning, spelling, and telling time
LANGUAGE		
Receptive language	Ability to comprehend complex constructions, function words (e.g., if, when, only, except), nuances of speech, and extended blocks of language (e.g., paragraphs)	Difficulty following directions; wandering attention during lessons and stories; problems with reading comprehension; problems with peer relationships
Expressive language	Ability to recall required words effortlessly (word finding), control meanings by varying position and word endings, and construct meaningful paragraphs and stories	Difficulty expressing feelings and using words for self-defense, with resulting frustration and physical acting out; struggling during "circle time" and in language-based subjects (e.g., English)

finding the problem areas, assessing and acknowledging each child's strengths is important. Educational approaches that value a wide range of talents ("multiple intelligences") beyond the traditional ones of reading, writing, and mathematics may allow more children to succeed.

The change in cognition allows the child to understand "if/when" clauses. Increased responsibilities and expectations accompany increased rights and privileges. Discipline strategies should move toward negotiation and a clear understanding of consequences, including removal of privileges for infringements.

SOCIAL, EMOTIONAL, AND MORAL DEVELOPMENT

SOCIAL AND EMOTIONAL DEVELOPMENT. In this period, previously referred to as *"latency,"* energy is directed toward creativity and productivity. The central Ericksonian psychosocial issue, the crisis between industry and inferiority, guides social and emotional development. Changes occur in three spheres: the home, the school, and the neighborhood. Of these, the home and family remain the most influential. Increasing independence is marked by the 1st sleepover at a friend's house and the 1st time at overnight camp. Parents should make demands for effort in school and extracurricular activities, celebrate successes, and offer unconditional acceptance when failures occur. Regular chores, associated with an allowance, provide an opportunity for children to contribute to family functioning and learn the value of money. These responsibilities may be a testing ground for psychologic separation, leading to conflict. Siblings have critical roles as competitors, loyal supporters, and role models.

The beginning of school coincides with a child's further separation from the family and the increasing importance of teacher and peer relationships. Social groups tend to be same-sex, with frequent changing of membership, contributing to a child's growing social development and competence. Popularity, a central ingredient of self-esteem, may be won through possessions (having the latest electronic gadgets or the right clothes) as well as through personal attractiveness, accomplishments, and actual social skills.

Some children conform readily to the peer norms and enjoy easy social success. Those who adopt individualistic styles or have visible differences may be teased. Such children may be painfully aware that they are different, or they may be puzzled by their lack of popularity. Children with deficits in social skills may go to extreme lengths to win acceptance, only to meet with repeated failure. Attributions conferred by peers, such as funny, stupid, bad, or scary, may become incorporated into a child's self-image and affect the child's personality. Parents may have their greatest effect indirectly, through actions that change the peer group (moving to a new community or insisting on involvement in structured after-school activities).

In the neighborhood, real dangers, such as busy streets, bullies, and strangers, tax school-aged children's common sense and resourcefulness. Interactions with peers without close adult supervision call on increasing conflict resolution or pugilistic skills. Media exposure to adult materialism, sexuality, and violence may be frightening, reinforcing children's feeling of powerlessness in the larger world. Compensatory fantasies of being powerful may fuel the fascination with heroes and superheroes. A balance between fantasy and an appropriate ability to negotiate real-world challenges indicates healthy emotional development.

MORAL DEVELOPMENT. By the age of 5 or 6 yr, the child has developed a conscience, meaning that he or she has internalized the rules of the society. She or he can distinguish right from wrong, but may take context and motivation into account. Children will adopt family and community values, seeking approval of peers, parents, and other adult role models. Social conventions are important, even though the reason behind some rules may not be understood. Initially, children have a rigid sense of morality, relying on clear rules for themselves and others. By age 10 yr, most children understand fairness as reciprocity (treat others as you wish to be treated).

IMPLICATIONS FOR PARENTS AND PEDIATRICIANS. Children need unconditional support as well as realistic demands as they venture into a world that is often frightening. A daily query from parents over the dinner table or at bedtime about the good and bad things that happened during the child's day may uncover problems early. Parents may have difficulty allowing the child independence or may exert excessive pressure on their children to achieve academic or competitive success. Children who struggle to meet such expectations may have behavior problems or psychosomatic complaints.

Many children face stressors that exceed the normal challenges of separation and success in school and the neighborhood. Divorce affects nearly 50% of children. Domestic violence, parental substance abuse, and other mental health problems may also impair a child's ability to use home as a secure base for refueling emotional energies. In many neighborhoods, random violence makes the normal development of independence extremely dangerous. Older children may join gangs as a means of self-protection and a way to appropriate power and belong to a cohesive group. Children who bully others, or are victims of bullying, should be evaluated, since this behavior is associated with mood disorders, family problems, and school adjustment problems. Parents should reduce exposure to hazards where possible. Due to the risk of unintentional firearm injuries to children, parents should be encouraged to ask parents of playmates whether a gun is kept in their home and, if so, how it is secured. The high prevalence of adjustment disorders among school-aged children attests to the effects of such overwhelming stressors on development.

Pediatrician visits are infrequent in this period; therefore, each visit is an opportunity to assess children's functioning in all contexts (home, school, neighborhood). Maladaptive behaviors, both internalizing and externalizing, occur when stress in any of these environments overwhelms the child's coping responses. Due to continuous exposure and the strong influence of media (programming and advertisements) on children's beliefs and attitudes, parents must be alert to exposures from the television and Internet. An average American youth spends 4–6 hr/day with a variety of media, and over ½ of these children have a television in their bedrooms. Parents should be advised to remove the television from their children's rooms, limit viewing to 2 hr/day, and monitor what programs children watch. The Draw-a-Person (for ages 3–10 yr, with instructions to "draw a complete person") and Kinetic Family Drawing (beginning at age 5, with instructions to "draw a picture of everyone in your family doing something") are useful office tools to assess a child's functioning.

American Academy of Pediatrics, Committee on Nutrition: Prevention of pediatric overweight and obesity. *Pediatrics* 2003;112:424–430.

American Academy of Pediatrics, Committee on Sports Medicine and Fitness and Committee on School Health: Organized sports for children and preadolescents. *Pediatrics* 2001;107:1459–1462.

Boyce WT, Essex MJ, Woodward HR, et al: The confluence of mental, physical, social, and academic difficulties in middle childhood: I. Exploring the head waters of early life morbidities. *J Am Acad Child Adolesc Psychiatry* 2002;41:580–587.

Centers for Disease Control and Prevention: Physical activity levels among children aged 9–13 years—United States, 2002. *MMWR* 2003;52:785–788.

Datar A, Sturm R: Childhood overweight and elementary school outcomes. *Int J Obes (Lond)* 2006;14:[epub ahead of print].

Dake JA, Price JH, Telljohann SK: The nature and extent of bullying at school. *J School Health* 2003;73:173–180.

Elkind D: *The Hurried Child: Growing Up Too Fast Too Soon*, 3rd ed. Cambridge, MA: Da Capo Press, 2001.
Levine M: *A Mind at a Time*. New York: Simon & Schuster, 2002.
Rideout V, Roberts DF, Foehr UG: *Generation M: Media in the lives of 8–18 year-olds*. The Henry J. Kaiser Family Foundation, March 2005. Available at http://www.kff.org/entmedia/7250.cfm.
Strasburger VC: Children, adolescents, and the media. *Curr Probl Pediatr Adolesc Health Care* 2004;34:54–113.
Wells RD, Stein MT: Seven to ten years: The world of middle childhood. In Dixon SD, Stein MT (editors): *Encounters with Children: Pediatric Behavior and Development*. St Louis, Mosby, 2000, pp 402–425.

Chapter 12 ■ Adolescence

Arik V. Marcell

See also Part XII and Chapters 562 and 563.

Between 10 and 20 yr of age, young people undergo rapid changes in body structure and physiologic, psychologic, and social functioning. Hormones set this developmental agenda together with social structures designed to foster the transition from childhood to adulthood. Adolescence proceeds across three distinct periods—early, middle, and late—each marked by a characteristic set of salient biologic, psychologic, and social issues (Table 12-1). Specifically, pubertal changes follow a predictable sequence. Individual variation is substantial, in both the timing of somatic changes and the quality of the experience. Gender and subculture profoundly affect the developmental course, as do physical and social stressors.

EARLY ADOLESCENCE

BIOLOGIC DEVELOPMENT. While adolescence is defined as a period of development, puberty is the biologic process in which a child becomes an adult. These changes include appearance of the secondary sexual characteristics, increase to adult size, and development of reproductive capacity. Adrenal production of androgen (chiefly dehydroepiandrosterone sulfate [DHEAS]) may occur as early as 6 yr of age, with development of underarm odor and faint genital hair (adrenarche). Levels of luteinizing hormone (LH) and follicle-stimulating hormone (FSH) rise progressively throughout middle childhood without dramatic effect. Rapid pubertal changes begin with increased sensitivity of the pituitary to gonadotropin-releasing hormone (GnRH); pulsatile release of GnRH, LH, and FSH during sleep; and corresponding increases in gonadal androgens and estrogens. The triggers for these changes are incompletely understood, but may involve ongoing neuronal development throughout middle childhood and adolescence. Contemporary children in the United States may enter puberty earlier than the published norms (although reports of dramatically earlier puberty are controversial), perhaps related to increased weight and adiposity (see Chapters 563 and 564). The resulting sequence of somatic and physiologic changes gives rise to the sexual maturity rating (SMR), or Tanner stages. Figures 12-1 and 12-2 depict the somatic changes used in the SMR scale; Tables 12-2 and 12-3 describe these changes in words. Table 12-4 lists mean ages and normal ranges for stages of pubic hair, breast, and genital development. Note that the SMR stages are not perfectly synchronized (e.g., SMR2 genital development may

TABLE 12-2. Classification of Sex Maturity States in Girls

SMR STAGE	PUBIC HAIR	BREASTS
1	Preadolescent	Preadolescent
2	Sparse, lightly pigmented, straight, medial border of labia	Breast and papilla elevated as small mound; diameter of areola increased
3	Darker, beginning to curl, increased amount	Breast and areola enlarged, no contour separation
4	Coarse, curly, abundant, but less than in adult	Areola and papilla form secondary mound
5	Adult feminine triangle, spread to medial surface of thighs	Mature, nipple projects, areola part of general breast contour

From Tanner JM: *Growth at Adolescence*, 2nd ed. Oxford, England, Blackwell Scientific Publications, 1962.
SMR, sexual maturity rating.

TABLE 12-1. Central Issues in Early, Middle, and Late Adolescence

VARIABLE	EARLY ADOLESCENCE	MIDDLE ADOLESCENCE	LATE ADOLESCENCE
Age (yr)	10–13	14–16	17–20 and beyond
Sexual maturity rating*	1–2	3–5	5
Somatic	Secondary sex characteristics Beginning of rapid growth Awkward appearance	Height growth peaks Body shape and composition change Acne and odor Menarche/spermarche	Physically mature Slower growth
Cognitive and moral	Concrete operations Unable to perceive long-term outcome of current decision-making Conventional morality	Emergence of abstract thought (formal operations) May perceive future implications, but may not apply in decision-making Questioning mores	Future-oriented with sense of perspective Idealism; absolutism Able to think things through independently
Self-concept/identity formation	Preoccupied with changing body Self-consciousness about appearance and attractiveness Fantasy and present-oriented	Concern with attractiveness Increasing introspection "Stereotypical adolescent"	More stable body image Attractiveness may still be of concern Emancipation complete Firmer identity
Family	Increased need for privacy Increased bid for independence	Conflicts over control and independence Struggle for acceptance of greater autonomy	Emotional and physical separation from family Increased autonomy
Peers	Seeks same-sex peer affiliation to counter instability	Intense peer group involvement Preoccupation with peer culture Peers provide behavioral example	Peer group and values recede in importance Intimacy/possible commitment takes precedence
Sexual	Increased interest in sexual anatomy Anxieties and questions about genital changes, size Limited dating and intimacy	Testing ability to attract partner Initiation of relationships and sexual activity Questions of sexual orientation	Consolidation of sexual identity Focus on intimacy and formation of stable relationships Planning for future and commitment
Relationship to society	Middle school adjustment	Gauging skills and opportunities	Career decisions (e.g., college, work)

*See text and Figures 12-1 and 12-2.

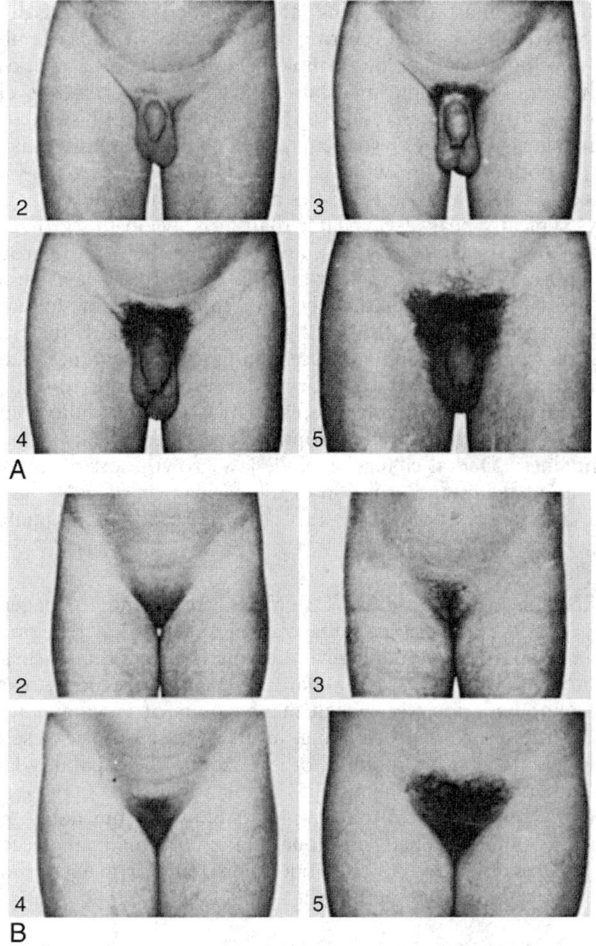

Figure 12-1. Sex maturity ratings (2 to 5) of pubic hair changes in adolescent boys *(A)* and girls *(B)* (see Tables 12–2 and 12–3). (Courtesy of J. M. Tanner, MD, Institute of Child Health, Department for Growth and Development, University of London, London, England.)

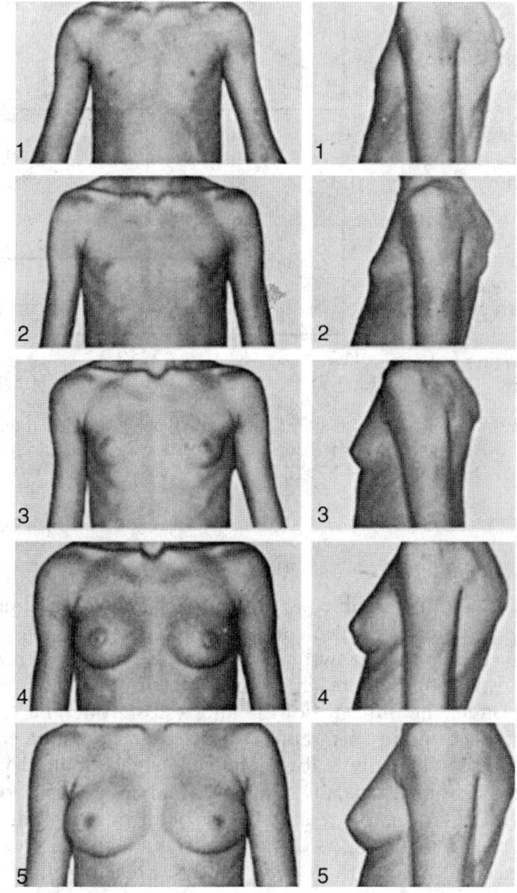

Figure 12-2. Sex maturity ratings (1 to 5) of breast changes in adolescent girls. (Courtesy of J. M. Tanner, MD, Institute of Child Health, Department for Growth and Development, University of London, London, England.)

precede SMR2 pubic hair development). Figures 12-3 and 12-4 depict the typical sequence of pubertal changes in boys and girls, respectively. The range of normal progress through sexual maturation is wide.

In girls, the first visible sign of puberty and the hallmark of SMR2 is the appearance of breast buds, between 8 and 12 yr of age. Menses typically begins 2–2½ yr later, during SMR3–4 (median age, 12 yr; normal range, 9–16 yr), around the peak height velocity (see Fig. 12-4). Less obvious changes include enlargement of the ovaries, uterus, labia, and clitoris, and thickening of the endometrium and vaginal mucosa.

TABLE 12-3. Classification of Sex Maturity States in Boys

SMR STAGE	PUBIC HAIR	PENIS	TESTES
1	None	Preadolescent	Preadolescent
2	Scanty, long, slightly pigmented	Minimal change/ enlargement	Enlarged scrotum, pink, texture altered
3	Darker, starting to curl, small amount	Lengthens	Larger
4	Resembles adult type, but less quantity; coarse, curly	Larger; glans and breadth increase in size	Larger, scrotum dark
5	Adult distribution, spread to medial surface of thighs	Adult size	Adult size

From Tanner JM: *Growth at Adolescence*, 2nd ed. Oxford, England, Blackwell Scientific Publications, 1962.
SMR, sexual maturity rating.

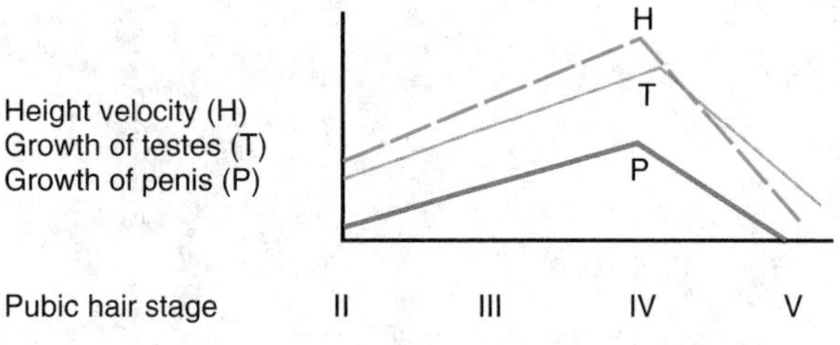

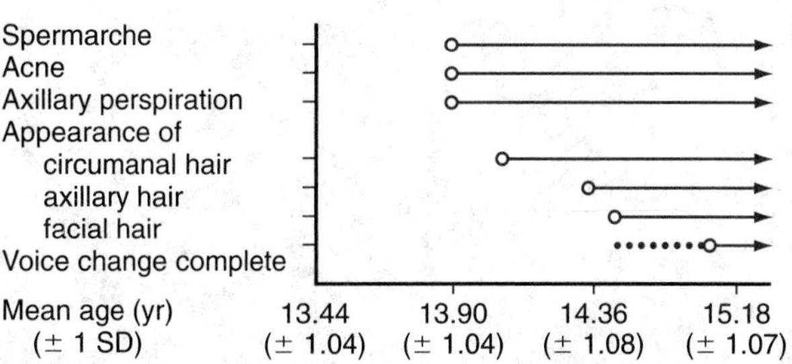

Figure 12-3. Sequence of maturational events in boys. (Adapted from Marshall WA, Tanner JM: Variations in the pattern of pubertal changes in boys. *Arch Dis Child* 1970;45:13.)

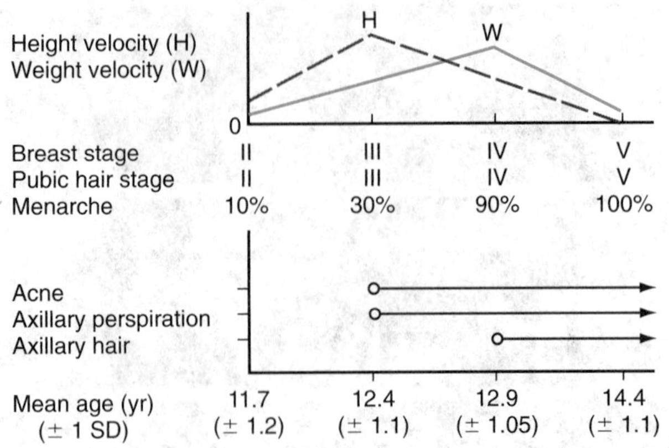

Figure 12-4. Sequence of maturational events in girls. (Adapted from Marshall WA, Tanner JM: Variations in the pattern of pubertal changes in boys. *Arch Dis Child* 1970;44:291.)

In boys, the first visible sign of puberty and the hallmark of SMR2 is testicular enlargement, beginning as early as 9½ yr. This is followed by penile growth during SMR3. Peak growth occurs when testis volumes reach approximately 9–10 cm^3 during SMR4. Under the influence of LH and testosterone, the seminiferous tubules, epididymis, seminal vesicles, and prostate enlarge. The left testis normally is lower than the right. Some degree of breast hypertrophy, typically bilateral, occurs in 40–65% of boys during SMR2–3 due to a relative excess of estrogenic stimulation. Gynecomastia sufficient to cause embarrassment and social disability occurs in fewer than 10% of boys. Breast swelling <4 cm in diameter has a 90% chance of spontaneous resolution within 3 yr. Gynecomastia presenting later in puberty, occurring in the prepubertal period, or occurring in the absence of signs of pubertal development may be pathologic and requires a work-up, including a thorough medication (e.g., H_2-blockers, psychotropics), drug (e.g., anabolic steroids), and medical history (e.g., Klinefelter syndrome, testicular failure, thyroid disease, tumor).

For both sexes, growth acceleration begins in early adolescence, but peak growth velocities are not reached until SMR3–4. Boys typically peak 2–3 yr later than girls, begin this growth at a later SMR stage (Fig. 12-5), and continue their linear growth for approximately 2–3 yr after girls have stopped. The asymmetric growth spurt begins distally, with enlargement of the hands and feet, followed by the arms and legs, and finally, the trunk and chest, giving young adolescents a gawky appearance. Rapid enlargement of the larynx, pharynx, and lungs leads to changes in vocal quality, typically preceded by vocal instability (voice cracking). Elongation of the optic globe often results in nearsightedness. Dental changes include jaw growth, loss of the final deciduous teeth, and eruption of the permanent cuspids, premolars, and finally, molars (see Table 8-3). Orthodontic appliances may be needed.

COGNITIVE AND MORAL DEVELOPMENT. According to Piagetian theory, adolescence marks the transition from concrete operational thinking to formal **logical thinking (abstract thought).** This includes the ability to manipulate algebraic expressions, reason from known principles, weigh many points of view, and think about the process of thinking itself. Some early adolescents demonstrate abstract thought, others acquire the capability later, and others never fully acquire it. Young adolescents may be able to apply formal logical thinking to schoolwork, but not to personal dilemmas. When emotional stakes are high, adolescents may regress to more concrete operational and/or magical thinking. This can interfere with higher-order cognition and ultimately

TABLE 12-4. Mean Age in Years and SE for Sexual Maturation Stage in Girls (Pubic Hair and Breast Development) and Boys (Pubic Hair and Genital Development) by Race

	AGE IN STAGE					
	NON-HISPANIC WHITE		NON-HISPANIC BLACK		MEXICAN-AMERICAN	
STAGE	Mean	SE	Mean	SE	Mean	SE
GIRLS						
Pubic Hair						
PH2	10.96*	0.23	10.25*	0.15	11.17*	0.21
PH3	12.41*	0.19	11.37*	0.23	12.84*	0.18
PH4	15.11*	0.18	13.69*	0.31	14.61*	0.26
PH5	16.53*	0.17	16.05*	0.14	16.61*	0.12
Breast Development						
B2	11.05*	0.18	10.25*	0.20	10.70	0.21
B3	12.80*	0.19	11.94*	0.22	12.61*	0.20
B4	15.16*	0.32	13.61*	0.34	14.03*	0.27
B5	16.25*	0.18	15.78*	0.14	16.21*	0.12
BOYS						
Pubic Hair						
PH2	11.81	0.16	11.48*	0.13	12.20*	0.24
PH3	13.03	0.27	12.79*	0.19	13.44*	0.26
PH4	14.89	0.18	15.21	0.26	15.25	0.16
PH5	16.84	0.13	16.67*	0.08	17.14*	0.10
Genital Development						
G2	11.08	0.18	10.79	0.13	11.09	0.17
G3	12.55	0.29	12.03*	0.28	12.97*	0.28
G4	15.29	0.19	15.07	0.33	15.38	0.19
G5	16.64	0.15	16.42*	0.09	16.85*	0.13

*Significant pair-wise racial difference, $p < 0.05$.
Adapted from Tables 3 and 5 in Sun SS: National estimates of the timing of sexual maturation and racial differences among US children. *Pediatrics*, 2002; 110(5):911–919.
Note: For sample sizes, refer to tables in original article.
SE, standard error.

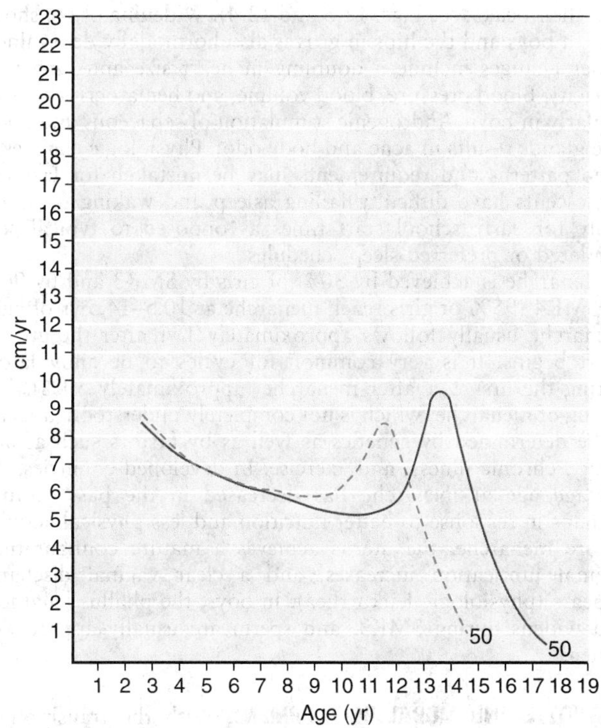

Figure 12-5. Height velocity curves for American boys *(solid line)* and girls *(dashed line)* who have their peak height velocity at the average age (i.e., average growth tempo). (From Tanner JM, Davies PSW: Clinical longitudinal standards for height and height velocity for North American children. *J Pediatr* 1985;107:317.)

affect the ability to perceive long-term outcomes of current decision-making.

Some theorists argue that the transition from concrete to formal operations follows from quantitative increases in knowledge, experience, and cognitive efficiency rather than from a qualitative reorganization of thinking. Consistent with this view are data showing a steady rise in cognitive processing speed from late childhood through early adulthood, associated with a reduction in synaptic number (pruning of less-used pathways) and continued myelination of neurons. Adolescents also experience the development of the dorsolateral prefrontal cortex and the superior temporal gyrus, areas responsible for higher-order associations, including the ability to inhibit impulses, weigh the consequences of decisions, prioritize, and strategize. It is unclear whether the hormonal changes of puberty directly affect cognitive development. Related to neurobehavioral maturation, adolescents may experience an increased intensity of emotion and/or greater inclination to seek experiences that create such high-intensity emotions. Cognitive development also differs by gender, with girls developing at earlier ages than boys.

The development of **moral thinking** roughly parallels cognitive development. Whereas younger children view relationships with adults in terms of power and fear of punishment, preadolescents begin to perceive right and wrong as absolute and unquestionable. Punishments and rewards must be fair; otherwise, the adolescent may complain or become angry.

SELF-CONCEPT. Self-consciousness increases exponentially in response to the somatic transformations of puberty. Self-awareness at this age centers on external characteristics, in contrast to the introspection of later adolescence. It is normal for early adolescents to be preoccupied with their body changes, scrutinize their appearance, and feel that everyone else is staring at them (Elkind's imaginary audience).

The media, with its overrepresentation of sex, violence, and substance use, has a profound influence on cultural norms and an adolescents' sense of identity. Adolescents use, on average, 7 hr of media per day (e.g., television, Internet). Half of all high school students have a television in their bedrooms, 70% live in homes with a personal computer, and the proportion with Internet access is approximately 75%.

This exposure may cause girls to develop a distorted sense of femininity, and they may be at risk for viewing themselves as overweight, leading to eating disorders and depression (Chapter 27). Similarly, boys may have difficulties with self-image. Images of masculinity may be confusing, leading to self-doubt, insecurity, and misleading conceptions about male behavior. Adolescents who develop earlier than their peers, especially girls, may have higher rates of school difficulty, body dissatisfaction, and depression. These adolescents look like adults and may have adult expectations placed on them, but are not cognitively or psychologically mature.

RELATIONSHIPS WITH FAMILY, PEERS, AND SOCIETY. In early adolescence, young teens become less interested in parental activities and more interested in the peer group, typically with peers of the same sex. A symbolic expression of this shift is to renounce family norms of dress and grooming in favor of the peer group "uniform," such as hair, clothes, and body ornamentation. Such stylistic changes may spark conflicts that are truly about power or difficulty accepting separation. Adolescents also seek more privacy, which may contribute to family discord.

The trend toward separation from family often involves selecting adults outside of the family as role models and developing close relationships with particular teachers or the parents of other children. Organizations such as scouting or sports teams can also provide an important sense of extrafamilial belonging.

Early adolescents often socialize in same-sex peer groups. Scatological jokes, teasing directed against the other gender, and rumor mongering about who likes whom attest to burgeoning sexual interest. Belonging is all important. In one-to-one friendships, boys and girls differ in important ways. Female friendships may center on sharing confidences, whereas male relationships may focus more on shared activities and competition.

An early adolescent's relationship to society centers on school. The shift from elementary school to middle school or junior high school entails giving up the protection of the homeroom in exchange for the additional stimulation and responsibility involved in moving from class to class. This change in school structure mirrors and reinforces the changes involved in separating from the family.

SEXUALITY. Sexuality includes not only sexual behaviors but also interest and fantasies, sexual orientation, attitudes toward sex, and awareness of socially defined roles and mores. Anxiety and interest in sex and sexual anatomy increase during early puberty. It is normal for young adolescents to compare themselves with others. In boys, ejaculation occurs for the first time, usually during masturbation and later as nocturnal emissions, and may be a cause of anxiety. Early adolescents sometimes masturbate together; mutual sexual exploration is not necessarily a sign of homosexuality. Sexual behavior, other than masturbation, is less common in early puberty, although 31% of an urban sample reported sexual intercourse before 14 yr of age. The relationship between hormonal changes and sexual interest and activity is controversial; no consistent links between hormones and sexual arousal, age of first intercourse, or frequency of intercourse have been found.

IMPLICATIONS FOR PEDIATRICIANS AND PARENTS. Parents may have concerns that they are hesitant to discuss. Parents can be interviewed before the adolescent to avoid undermining the adolescent's trust. When interviewing and examining an adolescent, health care providers should keep in mind that physical maturation correlates with sexual maturity, whereas psychosocial development correlates more closely with chronological age. Early adolescents typically need reassurance that the somatic changes they are experiencing are common and normal.

The pediatrician needs to help parents differentiate between the normal discomforts of the age and truly concerning behaviors. Bids for autonomy, such as avoiding family activities, demanding privacy, and increasing argumentativeness, are normal; extreme withdrawal or antagonism may be dysfunctional. Bewilderment and dysphoria at the start of junior high school are normal; continued failure to adapt several weeks to months later suggests a more serious problem. Risk-taking is limited in early adolescence; escalation of risk-taking behaviors is problematic. Parents must adapt discipline measures to the changing abilities of the adolescent, who can think through problems, assess consequences, and problem solve. Thus, the development of negotiation strategies is critical. Children and adolescents raised by parents who use negotiating as part of child rearing have more positive outcomes than those raised by parents who use more authoritarian or permissive styles.

MIDDLE ADOLESCENCE

BIOLOGIC DEVELOPMENT. In middle adolescence, growth accelerates above the prepubertal rate of 6–7 cm (3 in) per year. In the average girl, the growth spurt peaks at 11.5 yr at a top velocity of 8.3 cm (3.8 in) per year and then slows to a stop at 16 yr (see Fig. 12-4). In the average boy, the growth spurt starts later, peaks at 13.5 yr at 9.5 cm (4.3 in) per year, and then slows to a stop at 18 yr. Weight gain parallels linear growth, with a delay of several months, so that adolescents seem first to stretch and then to fill out. Muscle mass also increases, followed approximately 6 months later by an increase in strength; boys show greater gains in both. Lean body mass, approximately 80% in the average prepubertal child, increases to 90% in boys and decreases to 75% in girls as subcutaneous fat accumulates.

Bone maturation correlates closely with SMR because epiphyseal closure is under androgenic control (Table 12-5). Boys with SMR3 pubic hair and SMR4 genitals normally have their peak growth spurts ahead of them; girls at the same SMR are usually past their peaks (see Figs. 12-3 and 12-4). Widening of the shoulders in boys and the hips in girls is also hormonally determined. Other changes include a doubling in heart size and lung vital capacity. Blood pressure, blood volume, and hematocrit rise, particularly in boys. Androgenic stimulation of sebaceous and apocrine glands results in acne and body odor. Physiologic changes in sleep patterns and requirements may be mistaken for laziness; adolescents have difficulty falling asleep and waking up, especially for early school start times as opposed to typical self-regulated or preferred sleep schedules.

Menarche is achieved by 30% of girls by SMR3 and by 90% by SMR4 (95% of girls reach menarche at 10.5–14.5 yr of age). Menarche usually follows approximately 1 yr after the growth spurt begins. It is very common for cycles to be anovulatory during the first 2 yr after menarche (approximately 50%). The timing of menarche, which is not completely understood, appears to be determined by genetics as well as by factors such as adiposity, chronic illness, and exercise. In developed countries, the average age at menarche has decreased in the past century, perhaps in response to better nutrition and less physical activity. Before menarche, the uterus achieves a mature configuration, vaginal lubrication increases, and a clear vaginal discharge appears (physiologic leukorrhea). In boys, the phallus lengthens and widens during SMR3, and sperm are usually apparent in semen.

TABLE 12-5. Modal Age at Onset and Completion of Fusion in Skeletal Areas in Adolescence

BOYS MODAL AGE BETWEEN (Yr)	AREA	GIRLS MODAL AGE BETWEEN (Yr)
ELBOW		
13.0–13.5	Onset in humerus	11.0–11.5
15.0–15.5	Complete in ulna	12.5–13.0
FOOT AND ANKLE		
14.0–14.5	Onset in great toe	12.5–13.0
15.5–16.0	Complete in tibia, fibula	14.0–14.5
HAND AND WRIST		
15.0–15.5	Onset in distal phalanges	13.0–13.5
17.5–18.0	Complete in radius	16.0–16.5
KNEE		
15.0–15.5	Onset in tibial tuberosity	13.5–14.0
17.5–18.0	Complete in fibula	16.0–16.5
HIP AND PELVIS		
15.5–16.0	Onset in greater trochanter	14.0–14.5
After 18.0	Complete in symphysis	17.5–18.0
SHOULDER AND CLAVICLE		
15.5–16.0	Onset in greater tubercle of humerus	14.0–14.5
After 18.0	Complete in clavicle	17.5–18.0

COGNITIVE AND MORAL DEVELOPMENT. With the transition to formal logical thinking, middle adolescents start to question and analyze extensively. Young people now have the cognitive ability to understand the intricacy of the world they live in, to see beyond themselves, and to begin to understand their own actions in a moral and legal context. Questioning of moral conventions fosters the development of personal codes of ethics, which may be similar to or different from those of their parents. An adolescent's new flexibility of thought can have pervasive effects on relationships with the self and others.

SELF-CONCEPT. Middle adolescents are more accepting of their own body changes and become preoccupied with idealism in exploring future options. Affiliation with a peer group is an important step in confirming one's identity and self-image. It is normal for middle adolescents to experiment with different personas, changing styles of dress, groups of friends, and interests from month to month. Many philosophize about the meaning of life and wonder, "Who am I?" and "Why am I here?" Intense feelings of inner turmoil and misery are common. Girls may tend to characterize themselves and their peers according to interpersonal relationships ("I am a girl with close friends."), whereas boys may focus on abilities ("I am good at sports."). Adolescents of both genders, but especially boys, who develop later than their peers may experience poorer self-image and have higher rates of difficulty in school.

RELATIONSHIPS WITH FAMILY, PEERS, AND SOCIETY. Middle adolescence refers to "stereotypical adolescence." Relationships with parents become more strained and distant due to redirected energies toward peer relationships and separation from the family. Dating can become a lightning rod for parent-child battles, in which the real issue may be the separation from parents rather than the particulars of "with whom" or "how late." The majority of teenagers progress through adolescence with minimal difficulties rather than experiencing the stereotypical "storm and stress." It is the large minority of adolescents (approximately 20–30%) who *do* experience stress and struggle through this period who require support. Adolescents with visible differences are also at risk for problems, such as not developing adequate social skills and confidence and having more difficulty establishing satisfying relationships.

As part of middle adolescents' exploration of future options, they begin to think seriously about what they want to do as adults, a question that formerly had been comfortably hypothetical. The process involves self-assessment and exploration of available opportunities. The presence or absence of realistic role models, as opposed to the idealized ones of earlier periods, can be crucial.

SEXUALITY. Dating becomes a normative activity as middle adolescents assess their ability to attract others. The degree of sexual activity and its onset vary widely. At age 16 yr, approximately 33% of girls and 42% of boys report having oral or vaginal sex. Most adolescents have kissed by age 14 yr (71%). French kissing is more common by age 15 yr, and petting is more common among teen boys at age 16 yr (75%), but it catches up with teen girls by age 17 yr (76%). Homosexual experimentation is common and does not necessarily reflect a child's ultimate sexual orientation. Many adolescents worry that they might be homosexual and dread being found out. Homosexual adolescents face an increased risk of isolation and depression. Fear of stigmatization may keep them from discussing their concerns with pediatricians or other potentially helpful adults (see Chapter 13).

In addition to sexual orientation, middle adolescents begin to sort out other important aspects of sexual identity, including beliefs about love, honesty, and propriety. Relationships at this age are often superficial and emphasize attractiveness and sexual experimentation rather than intimacy. Adolescents tend to choose one of three sexual paths: celibacy, monogamy, or polygamous experimentation. Most have some knowledge of the risks of pregnancy, HIV, and other sexually transmitted diseases, but knowledge does not consistently control behavior. Fewer than 70% of adolescents consistently use condoms, and approximately 26% of girls do not use any method of contraception at their first intercourse.

IMPLICATIONS FOR PEDIATRICIANS AND PARENTS. Middle adolescence is a time when the opportunity to talk confidentially with a nonjudgmental, informed adult can be particularly appreciated and helpful in the midst of significant psychologic and biologic change.

Adolescents vary greatly in their rate of physical and social progress and in the resolution of central conflicts about autonomy and self-esteem. Questions about family and peer relationships can help locate a child along the developmental continuum and facilitate individualized counseling. Early- and late-maturing adolescents are at risk for psychologic problems. Anticipatory guidance with parents or guardians and appropriate referral to mental health professionals of these adolescents may be warranted.

In asking about dating and sex, do not assume heterosexuality; this approach increases the likelihood that concerns about sexual orientation will surface. Intention to have sex and whether close friends are sexually active are good indications that a youth may be initiating sexual activity shortly. Parental connectedness and close supervision or monitoring of the youth's activities and peer group can be protective against early onset of sexual activity and involvement in other risk-taking behaviors, and can foster positive youth development. Parents should also assume an active role in their adolescent's transition to adulthood to ensure that their child receives appropriate preventive health services.

LATE ADOLESCENCE

BIOLOGIC DEVELOPMENT. The somatic changes in this period are modest by comparison to earlier periods. The final stages of breast, penile, and pubic hair development occur by 17–18 yr of age in 95% of males and females. Minor changes in hair distribution often continue for several years in males, including the growth of facial and chest hair and the onset of male pattern baldness in a few. Acne occurs in the majority of adolescents, particularly males.

PSYCHOSOCIAL DEVELOPMENT. Slowing physical changes permit the emergence of a more stable body image. Cognition tends to be less self-centered, with increasing thoughts about concepts such as justice, patriotism, and history. Older adolescents are more future-oriented and able to act on long-term plans, delay gratification, compromise, set limits, and think independently. Older adolescents are often idealistic, but may also be absolutist and intolerant of opposing views. Religious or political groups that promise answers to complex questions may hold great appeal.

With emancipation complete, older adolescents begin the transition to adult roles in work and their relationships.

They also have more constancy in their emotions. The peer group and peer values recede in importance. Individual, particularly intimate relationships take precedence, providing an important component of identity for many older adolescents. In contrast to the often superficial dating relationships of middle adolescence, these relationships increasingly involve love and commitment. Career decisions become pressing because an adolescent's self-concept is increasingly bound up in his or her emerging role in society.

IMPLICATIONS FOR PEDIATRICIANS AND PARENTS. Erikson identified the crucial task of adolescence as the establishment of a stable sense of identity, including emotional and physical separation from the family of origin, initiation of intimacy, and realistic planning for economic independence. The relationship changes from one of parent-child to an adult-adult model. Continued difficulty in any of these areas may constitute an indication for referral for counseling. Adolescents who become parents may have the added difficulty of achieving appropriate developmental milestones prior to assuming adult responsibilities.

Dahl RE: Adolescent brain development: Vulnerabilities and opportunities. *Ann N Y Acad Sci* 2004;1021:1–22.

Delemarre-van de Waal HA: Regulation of puberty. *Best Pract Res Clin Endocrinol Metab* 2002;16:1–12.

Felice M, Maehr J: Eleven to thirteen years: Early adolescence—age of rapid changes. Fourteen to sixteen years: Mid-adolescence—dating game. In Dixon SD, Stein MT (editors): *Encounters with Children: Pediatric Behavior and Development.* St Louis, Mosby, 2000, pp 426–476.

Ford CA, Coleman WL: Adolescent development and behavior: Implications for the primary care physician. In Levine MD, Carey WB, Crocker AC (editors): *Developmental-Behavioral Pediatrics,* 3rd ed. Philadelphia, WB Saunders, 1999, pp 69–80.

Joffe A, Blythe M (editors): Handbook of Adolescent Medicine. *State of the Art Reviews: Adolescent Medicine* 2003;14:231–262.

Strasburger VC, Donnerstein E: Children, adolescents, and the media in the 21st century. *Adolescent Medicine: State of the Art Reviews* 2000;11:51–68.

Chapter 13 ■ Sexual Behavior

13.1 • The Development of Sexual Behavior •

Richard Dalton

Knowledge about emerging sexual behavior and its many variations is very important when assessing and treating children and adolescents. Knowing what is expected behavior and what behavior is a sign of a different orientation is fundamental to working effectively with children and adolescents. The inclusion of patient data about sexual development, gender development, and sexual behavior is essential to a complete clinical evaluation and the opportunity to intervene meaningfully.

Gender identity needs to be distinguished from *gender role.* The former refers to an individual's sense of self as a male or a female, while the latter refers to those public behaviors commonly thought (within a culture) to be associated with maleness or femaleness. Children identify themselves as boys or girls by about 18 mo of age (establishment of gender identity). Between 18 and 30 mo of age, children establish **gender stability,** the concept that boys become men and girls become women. By 30 mo, gender constancy, the immutability of one's gender, is firmly established and resistant to change. Although there are numerous theories suggesting which environmental and biologic factors are most important to the establishment of a firm gender identity, we still do not understand in a way that has treatment implications which factors are most important in any given child.

Children are naturally curious about their bodies. Parents should provide information to children about sexual development in accordance with their ability to learn. The 2 yr old child ought to be taught the proper names for the parts of the body, including the genitals. Parents should provide uncomplicated and straightforward answers to their school-aged children's questions about sexual issues. Parents should monitor adolescent sexual behavior and should provide useful and helpful information about both romance and sexual issues.

Reasonable and expected sexual behaviors by children under 12 yr of age include conversations about genitals and reproduction, playing "doctor," occasional masturbation, and using dirty words and telling dirty jokes. Behaviors that should cause concern include sexually explicit talk, precocious sexual knowledge, simulating foreplay, attempting to expose others' genitals, and preoccupation with masturbation. Problem behaviors include touching another person's genitals, threats of force, sexually explicit proposals, exposing one's genitals, sexually explicit talk with significantly younger children, and compulsive masturbation. Absolute problem behaviors include forced exposure of others' genitals, simulating intercourse with peers (without clothes), and any genital injury not explained by accidental cause.

Adolescent sexual behavior has changed through the years. Expected reasonable behaviors include sexually explicit conversation and jokes, solitary masturbation, hugging, kissing, holding hands, and fondling. Behaviors that should concern parents include interest in pornography, promiscuity, violation of others' body space, and sexually aggressive and obscene actions. Clearly inappropriate behaviors include sexually explicit threats, degrading and humiliating oneself or others with sexual themes, attempting to expose others' genitals, and explicit conversations about sex with significantly younger children. Illegal sexual behaviors include sexual abuse (any inappropriate sexual contact between an adult and a minor or between two minors if one is ≥3 yr younger than the other), forced sexual contact, bestiality, and genital injury to others.

The number of adolescents who have engaged in sexual intercourse has decreased: 54% in 1991 compared with 47% in 2003. The changing patterns of adolescent dating and sexual behavior confound the interpretation of these data. *Hooking up,* the practice of engaging in oral sex with opposite sex friends (often referred to as *friends with benefits*), has become more popular with some adolescents than traditional dating. One teen website started in 1990 and used for "hooking up" had over 40 million members in 2000. In a college survey, 60% of respondents said that their high school sexual partners were friends, not romantic partners. Increased communication and greater mobility have provided today's adolescents with increased opportunities for both casual and anonymous sexual encounters and have contributed to changing patterns of sexual behavior.

In addition to the usual sexual behaviors, clinicians must know about the many variations of sexual behavior. Clinicians should be cautious about interpreting variant behavior as pathologic and should not let the usual social opprobriums about sexual behavior influence clinical decision-making. Sexual variations are pathologic when they lead directly to aggressive or self-destructive behavior.

Transsexualism is the conviction by a person who is biologically a member of one gender that he or she is a member of the other gender. Transsexual adolescents (transpersons) feel discomfort and a sense of inappropriateness about their assigned sex (see Chapter 13.2). Transsexuals usually have a difficult time with social and occupational functioning. Concurrent psychopathologic conditions and depression are common, as is societal consternation. The natural history of transsexualism is not well understood. A preponderance of adult transsexuals had gender identity disorders as children and adolescents (see Chapter 13.2). Extreme femininity in boys is a predisposing factor. Some remember being confused about gender identity as early as 2 yr of age. Which particular effeminate boys will later show transsexual behavior cannot be accurately predicted.

Treatment of transsexualism has taken two directions. Many transsexual adults have opted for hormonal and surgical therapies to produce primary and secondary sexual characteristics of the gender with which they identify (see Chapter 13.2). Follow-up studies reveal that the outcome of these treatments is variable. Long-term dynamic and behavioral therapies also have been tried. Although there are anecdotal reports of successful re-identification with the given biologic sex, without statistical controls, it is impossible to know whether this represents a response to therapy or a spontaneous change that would have occurred without it.

Transvestism, or cross-dressing, may occur transiently in preschool boys who dress up in their mothers' clothing, or it may occur chronically in preschool and school-aged boys who feel genuinely excited when dressed in women's clothing. Cross-dressing in girls is rarely an identified problem. Chronic cross-dressing rarely represents underlying transsexualism. Transvestism usually indicates that other gender roles may also be unsatisfying for the individual. A cross-dressing man finds relief in wearing women's clothing; he often obtains sexual arousal and may masturbate or engage in other sexual activity.

Physicians consulted by parents should investigate other areas of gender identification and gender behavior. Does the child verbalize a preference to be the opposite sex? Does the child deny or disparage his or her own sexual anatomy or assert that the anatomic structures of the opposite sex will develop? Approximately 3–6% of school-aged boys and 10–12% of school-aged girls often behave like the opposite sex, but fewer than 2% of boys and 2–4% of girls actually wish to be the opposite sex.

Denizet B: Friends, friends with benefits, and benefits of the local mail. *New York Times* May 30, 2004.

Duncan P, Dixon R, Carlson J: Childhood and adolescent sexuality. *Pediatr Clin North Am* 2003;50:765–780.

13.2 • Gender Identity Disorder • Ligia Peralta

Gender identity disorder (GID) is defined as a strong, persistent discomfort (dysphoria) with one's anatomic gender coupled with persistent cross-gender identification. An anatomic male (or female) believes that he (or she) is the wrong gender and seeks to relieve this tension by re-assignment to the opposite, more personality congruent sex. The diagnosis is made if the child or adolescent has evidence of clinically significant distress or impairment in social, occupational, or other important areas of psychologic functioning. The diagnosis of GID does not apply to an individual with a concurrent physical intersex medical condition. In addition, it should be distinguished from gender-atypical behaviors, especially when observed in male children compatible with gay identity in adulthood without evidence of GID. Patients who identify themselves with transsexualism are known as *transpeople*, either *transmen* (born female) or *transwomen* (born male). After hormonal and surgical intervention, a transperson usually prefers to be called a man or a woman.

EPIDEMIOLOGY AND ETIOLOGY. While there are no epidemiologic studies to provide data on the prevalence of GID in children, some authors have stated that its prevalence in adolescents is similar to that in adults. European studies based on adult males and females seeking re-assignment surgery have shown the prevalence of GID to be approximately 1/30,000 adult males and 1/100,000 adult females. The difference may be due to underreporting by females.

Psychosocial mechanisms might include social enforcement, prenatal sex preference, and mother-child and father-child relationships. These have been explored more thoroughly in boys than in girls, but a causal link has not been established. Another hypothesis involves neurodevelopmental alterations of sexually dimorphic hypothalamic nuclei during fetal life. The area of the limbic nucleus is a strong possibility. In the absence of sex hormone therapy, the brains of male-to-female transpersons have a female pattern.

CLINICAL MANIFESTATIONS AND DIAGNOSIS. For children referred with GID, symptoms usually have started between 2 and 4 yr of age. Although only a small number of children with cross-gender interests and activities continue to display symptoms during adolescence, those children with persistent symptoms are usually traditionally referred around the time they enter primary school. In adolescents, the clinical presentation commonly includes a history of GID during childhood, and about 75% of boys report homosexual orientation by late adolescence. Nonetheless, the sexual orientation (the sex that is erotically attractive) of transpersons may be heterosexual, homosexual, or bisexual. The ratio of these choices is not different than in non-transpersons; most are heterosexual after hormonal and surgical sex re-assignment.

The diagnostic criteria for GID in children and adolescents are presented in Table 13-1. Although this version is clinically useful, it is controversial because it is based on diagnostic criteria for which reliability or validity has not been established. The *Diagnostic and Statistical Manual of Mental Disorders,* 4th edition, text revision, diagnostic criteria for GID include: (1) a strong, persistent cross-gender identification (not merely a desire for any perceived cultural advantages of being the other sex); (2) persistent discomfort with his or her sex or sense of inappropriateness in the gender role of that sex; (3) the disturbance is not concurrent with physical intersex condition; and (4) the disturbance causes clinically significant distress or impairment in social, occupational, or other important areas of functioning.

The **medical evaluation** of children with GID involves a full history and physical examination. For children, there are several well-validated psychometric assessment instruments that can be used in the office setting and easily administered during a clinic visit. These instruments include a Parent-Report Gender Identity Questionnaire, the Draw-a-Person Test, and the Gender Identity Interview for Children. For adolescents, clinical indicators include a history of strong and persistent cross-gender identification and persistent discomfort with one's gender. Transient feelings or behaviors related to sexual orientation are not symptoms of GID. Additional laboratory tests, such as karyotype or sex hormone assays, are not necessary in the presence of normal findings on patient history and physical examination.

TABLE 13-1. DSM-IV TR* Gender Identity Disorder Diagnostic Criteria

A. A strong persistent cross-gender identification (not merely a desire for any perceived cultural advantages of being the other sex). In children, four or more of the following are manifestations of the disturbance:
1. Repeatedly stated desire to be, or insistence that he or she is, the other sex.
2. In boys, preference for cross-dressing or simulating female attire; in girls, insistence on wearing only stereotypically masculine clothing.
3. Strong and persistent preferences for cross-sex roles in make believe play or persistent fantasies of being the other sex.
4. Intense desire to participate in the stereotypical games and pastimes of the other sex.
5. Strong preference for playmates of the other sex.

In adolescents and adults, the disturbance is manifested by symptoms such as a stated desire to be the other sex, frequent passing as the other sex, desire to live or be treated as the other sex, or the conviction that he or she has the typical feelings and reactions of the other sex.

B. Persistent discomfort with his or her sex or sense of inappropriateness in the gender role of that sex. In children, the disturbance is manifested by any of the following:

In boys, assertion that his penis or testes are disgusting or will disappear or the assertion that it would be better not to have a penis, or aversion toward rough-and-tumble play and rejection of male stereotypical toys, games and activities.

In girls, rejection of urinating in a sitting position, assertion that she has or will grow a penis, or assertion that she does not want to grow breasts or menstruate or marked aversion toward normative feminine clothing.

In adolescents and adults, the disturbance is manifested by symptoms such as preoccupation with getting rid or primary and secondary sex characteristics (e.g., request for hormones, surgery, or other procedures to physically alter sexual characteristics to simulate the other sex) or belief that he or she was born the wrong sex.

C. The disturbance is not concurrent with physical intersex condition.

D. The disturbance causes clinically significant distress or impairment in social, occupational, or other important areas of functioning.

*Adapted from American Psychiatric Association: *Diagnostic and Statistical Manual of Mental Disorders*, 4th ed., text revision, (DSM-IV TR) Washington, DC, American Psychiatric Associations, 2000.

Disorders associated and coexisting with this condition include separation anxiety disorder, generalized anxiety disorder, and symptoms of depression, particularly in adolescents. These children and youth also become victims of social isolation and ostracism, which may contribute to school aversion or dropping out of school. In addition, they may suffer from psychologic and sexual abuse. Prostitution, HIV, suicide attempts, and substance abuse may be associated with GID, but many believe that they are consequences of discrimination and undeserved shame. Genital mutilation and suicide are additional problems.

DIFFERENTIAL DIAGNOSIS. Gender identity and sexual orientation are different developmental constructs. As a protective mechanism, a child or youth who self-identifies as homosexual may be successful at hiding his or her sexual orientation. However, a youth with GID feels trapped inside the body of his or her biologic gender and has difficulty hiding the desire to be a member of the opposite gender. GID should also be distinguished from nonconformity to stereotypical sex role behavior and also from transvestic fetishism that occurs in heterosexual or bisexual males for whom the cross-dressing behavior is for the purpose of sexual excitement. GID may also occur in individuals with a coexisting congenital intersex condition, such as androgen insensitivity syndrome or congenital adrenal hyperplasia, who experience discomfort with their assigned gender.

TREATMENT. The treatment of GID implies controversial and complex social and ethical issues related to future sexual orientation. Many clinicians emphasize that the primary goal of the treatment of children who have GID is to resolve the conflicts that are associated with the disorder, regardless of the child's eventual sexual orientation. Youth with GID may experience a great deal of suffering; many of them are preoccupied with gender identity issues, are subjected to social ostracism and feel alienation, and have other psychiatric and behavioral difficulties. Most clinicians believe that therapy designed to reduce the gender dysphoria will lessen the degree of social ostracism and reduce the psychiatric comorbidity.

It is important for a clinician who provides care to a patient with GID to share with the family that there are no studies demonstrating that therapeutic intervention in childhood alters the developmental path toward either transsexualism or homosexuality and that there are no randomized clinical trials to guide the treatment. However, some clinicians believe that psychosocial treatments, such as behavior therapy, psychodynamic therapy, parental counseling, and group therapy, are effective in reducing gender dysphoria. Individual therapy includes uncovering the factors that contribute to one's desire to be the opposite sex. Parent counseling in this instance focuses on helping the child to feel more comfortable about being a boy or a girl. Other clinicians believe that the focus of medical treatment should be to relieve the distress of gender dysphoria and not to attempt to change one's gender identity.

If hormonal and surgical re-assignment is proposed (usually in adulthood), the transperson should have opportunities to consolidate his or her chosen gender by living functionally as that gender in real-life experiences or with psychotherapy. After a minimum of 1 yr of supervision with successful functional real-life experiences as a member of the chosen gender and compliance with hormonal therapy, surgical interventions should begin to be discussed. Transmen may undergo hysterectomy, oophorectomy, mastectomy, and creation of a scrotum and penis. Transwomen require removal of the penis and testes, creation of a clitoris and vagina, breast augmentation, and cosmetic surgery of the nose and cricothyroid cartilage.

Younger age (as an adult), excellent psychologic preparation, good social support (family, friends), and surgical expertise all contribute to the prognosis for re-assignment.

American Psychiatric Association: *Diagnostic and Statistical Manual of Mental Disorders,* 4th ed., text revision, Washington, DC, American Psychiatric Association, 2000.

Bradley SJ, Zucker KJ: Gender identity disorder: A review of the past 10 years. *J Am Acad Child Adolesc Psychiatry* 1997;36(7):72–80.

Cohen-Kettenis PT, Owen A, Kaijser VG, et al: Demographic characteristics, social competence, and behavior problems in children with gender identity disorder: A cross-national, cross-clinic comparative analysis. *J Abnorm Child Psychol* 2003;31(1):41–53.

Harry Benjamin International Gender Dysphoria Association's Standards of Care for Gender Identity Disorders: http://www.hbigda.org. Sixth version, February 2001.

Hepp U, Kraemer B, Schnyder U, et al: Psychiatric comorbidity in gender identity disorder. *J Psychosom Res* 2005;58(3):59–61.

Johnson LL, Bradley SJ, Birkenfeld-Adams AS, et al: A parent-report gender identity questionnaire for children. *Arch Sex Behav* 2004;33(2):5–16.

Swaab DF: Sexual differentiation of the human brain: Relevance for gender identity, transsexualism and sexual orientation. *Gynecol Endocrinol* 2004;19(6):1–12.

Wylie K: Gender related disorders. *BMJ* 2004;329:615–617.

Zucker KJ: Gender identity development and issues. *Child Adolesc Psychiatr Clin North Am* 2004;13(3):551–568.

Zucker KJ, Beaulieu N, Bradley SJ, et al: Handedness in boys with gender identity disorder. *J Child Psychol Psychiatry* 2001;42(6):767–776.

Zucker KJ, Bradley SJ, Lowry Sullivan CB: Traits of separation anxiety in boys with gender identity disorder. *J Am Acad Child Adolesc Psychiatry* 1996;5(6):791–798.

13.3 • Adolescent Homosexuality •

Gary Remafedi

Sexual orientation is a persistent pattern of physical and/or emotional attraction to members of the same or the opposite sex. It encompasses different aspects of sexuality, including sexual fantasy, emotional attraction, sexual behavior, self-identification, and cultural affiliation. The heterosexual or homosexual direction of these different dimensions may be inconsistent, defying the simple categorization of individuals as heterosexual, homosexual, or bisexual. Sexual orientation can be viewed as a continuum between absolute heterosexuality and homosexuality. **Homosexuality** refers to a persistent pattern of same-sex arousal, accompanied by weak or absent heterosexual arousal; and **bisexuality** refers to attractions for both genders. Most homosexual people today refer to themselves as **gay** men and **lesbian** women. In this chapter, *homosexual* refers to both males and females, whereas the term *gay* applies specifically to men and *lesbian,* to women.

EPIDEMIOLOGY. Homosexuality has existed in all societies and cultures and in all times. Prevalence estimates vary according to the time, place, and definitions used in the research. A sizable proportion of youths begin adolescence unsure of their sexual orientation; uncertainty generally resolves with advancing age and sexual experience. Reported homosexual attractions (4.5%) may exceed fantasies, the latter being more common in girls (3.1%) than in boys (2.2%). Overall, 1.1% of students describe themselves as predominantly homosexual or bisexual. The prevalence of reported homosexual experiences remained constant (0.9%) among girls, but increases from 0.4–2.8% in boys between the ages of 12 and 18 yr. Only about ⅓ of the teens reporting homosexual experiences or fantasies identified themselves as homosexual or bisexual.

ETIOLOGY. Ample evidence points to fundamental biologic differences between heterosexual and homosexual people. The clustering of homosexuality within some families has long been recognized. Compared with dizygotic twins, the greater concordance of homosexuality in monozygotic twins highlights the role of genetic constitution; a putative gene locus associated with male homosexuality has been identified. Although heterosexual and homosexual adults have comparable levels of circulating sex steroids, it has been proposed that perinatal hormones organize and activate key areas of the brain early in life. This might contribute to the eventual development of neuroanatomic and neuropsychological functional differences related to sexual orientation.

Less well understood is the way that biology interacts with environment and experience in shaping the expression of sexual orientation. Well-designed studies have not found differences in the familial and social backgrounds of homosexual and heterosexual men and women, nor any evidence that homosexuality is related to abnormal parenting, sexual abuse, or other traumatic events. However, the environment may potentially modulate the expression of fundamental biologic predisposition by influencing the social behavior and visibility of homosexual people.

DEVELOPMENT OF A HOMOSEXUAL IDENTITY. Several models that describe the process of homosexual identity development have been reconstructed from adults' recollections of childhood. Most of these theories describe initial stages of sensitization and confusion about sexual orientation, followed by understanding and acceptance of homosexuality, disclosure to others, and eventual integration of the sexual identity into a comprehensive sense of self. In contrast to adolescents with transgender issues, most gay and lesbian children are not readily identified by public behavior or styles.

Initially, individuals might experience a vague feeling of being different from their peers in childhood or early adolescence, not necessarily related to sexuality. During early or middle adolescence, a perception of actual sexual difference can arise from awareness of same-sex arousal, the absence of heterosexual arousal, and possibly same-sex experiences. Misinformation and stigma can lead to significant inner turmoil and anxiety. Identity assumption, the personal acknowledgment of homosexuality, typically evolves from extended interaction with other homosexual people. Volitional disclosure usually starts with close friends before parents, and with mothers before fathers. Disclosure can happen unwittingly or prematurely, creating considerable distress. The developmental process seldom is direct and easy. Successful resolution, characterized by personal acceptance and healthy intimate relationships, depends on many factors, such as maturity, access to accurate information, positive role models, and social support.

IMPLICATIONS FOR HEALTH

HOMOPHOBIA. The common occurrence of psychosocial problems among gay and lesbian youths is best understood in the context of homophobia. *Homophobia* is an irrational fear, hatred, or otherwise distorted perception of homosexuality that can manifest in personal discomfort, stereotypes, prejudice, and violence. At a time in life when peers play a critical role in healthy personal and social development, isolation and stigma can be highly traumatic. Compared with classmates, homosexual students are more likely to fear for their safety and to be attacked and injured. With repeated exposure, homosexual youths might internalize negative stereotypes and engage in self-defeating behaviors.

SOCIAL ISSUES. Academic underachievement, truancy, and dropping out are common consequences of abuse and violence at school. Some parents are unable to adopt a supportive attitude, and a substantial number of homosexual children run away or are evicted. Homosexual young people are overrepresented in homeless and runaway populations across the USA. Life on the streets exposes them to drugs and sexual abuse and promotes illegal conduct for survival.

MENTAL HEALTH ISSUES. Substance abuse, anxiety, depression, disordered eating behaviors, and attempted suicide are prevalent. Compared with heterosexual peers, homosexual youths initiate tobacco use at younger ages and are more likely to smoke regularly. In a study of 13–21 year old gay and bisexual male adolescents, frequent (>40 times/yr) alcohol use was reported by 24.5% of participants; frequent marijuana use, by 8.4%; and frequent cocaine or crack use, by 2.4%. More than 4% had used intravenous drugs in the previous year.

Rates of attempted suicide among homosexual youths, especially males, are consistently higher than expected in the general population of adolescents, ranging from 20–42%. Suicide attempts often occur in proximity to "identity assumption" and may be associated with family conflict. Identified risk factors include young age at first awareness of homosexuality, experience of rejection based on sexual orientation, substance use, and perceived gender non-conformity.

Data on eating disorders are sparse and somewhat conflicting. Twenty-five percent of gay youths report a poor body image, and about 10% diet frequently or purge. Compared with heterosexual males, all indicators of eating problems are more prevalent in gay youths. By contrast, lesbian adolescents report a better body image than heterosexual females, without significant differences in eating-disordered behaviors.

MEDICAL THREATS TO HEALTH. Homosexual adolescents generally have the same medical concerns as heterosexual youths. **Risky sexual behaviors,** not sexual orientation, can endanger health. The most common and serious sexually related conditions arise from unprotected anal intercourse. The epithelial surfaces of the fragile rectal mucosa are easily damaged during sex, facilitating the transmission of pathogens. Rectal intercourse has been shown to be the most efficient route of infection by hepatitis B, cytomegalovirus, and HIV. Oral-anal or digital-anal contact can transmit enteric pathogens, such as the hepatitis A virus. Unprotected oral sex also can lead to oropharyngeal disease in the receptive partner as well as gonococcal and non-gonococcal urethritis for the insertive partner. Certain sexually transmitted infections (STIs), particularly ulcerative diseases, such as syphilis and herpes simplex virus infection, can facilitate the spread of HIV.

Although possible, female-to-female sexual transmission of HIV is inefficient, and women who only engage in same-sex behavior are less likely than other youths to acquire STIs in general. High-risk sexual behavior and HIV infection among young men who have sex with men (MSM) remains unfortunately common for various reasons, including misinformation, non-communication with partners about risk reduction, potentially false assumptions about partners' serostatus, substance use, and impaired reasoning and judgment.

RECOMMENDATIONS FOR CARE

The American Academy of Pediatrics recognizes the physician's responsibility to provide comprehensive, nonjudgmental health care and guidance to gay and lesbian adolescents as well as to young people struggling with issues of sexual orientation. As with all adolescents, the goals of care are to promote normal adolescent development, social and emotional well-being, and physical health.

If they have personal barriers to providing nonjudgmental care and information, clinicians should refer patients to more appropriate resources. A trusting, mutual relationship between the patient and the physician is the basis of effective communication. Waiting room materials addressing sexual orientation, information about support groups, and other community resources indicate that the staff is open to discussing homosexuality. Interviewing the teen with and without parents present, giving explicit assurance of confidentiality, and setting limits are important elements of good communication. For some teens, multiple visits might be necessary to complete an evaluation sensitively. Caution should be exercised when recording sensitive information in accessible parts of the medical chart.

EVALUATION. Providers should be aware of the various threats to the medical and psychosocial health of homosexual teenagers and screen for them appropriately. Classifying the adolescent's sexual orientation usually is unnecessary, but assessing specific sexual practices can help determine risks and direct further evaluation. Sexual history taking should avoid heterosexual assumptions, with the clinician inquiring sensitively about the direction of romantic interests and the gender of partners. The basic physical examination and laboratory evaluation are the same for all sexually active teenagers, with additional work-up guided by the sexual risk assessment. Voluntary HIV antibody counseling and testing should be routinely offered to adolescents who have engaged in unprotected sex.

PREVENTION, TREATMENT, AND REFERRALS. Special emphasis should be placed on education and counseling to prevent the spread of HIV and STIs through safer sexual behavior, including limiting the numbers of sexual partners, avoiding anal intercourse, staying sober in sexual situations, and consistently using condoms. The use of dental dams or plastic wrap during oral sex and the use of latex condoms for sexual appliances are recommended for lesbians. Given the fact that some homosexual adolescents might engage in sex with the opposite sex, pregnancy prevention should be addressed. Hepatitis A vaccine is recommended for MSM (see Chapter 355). For treatment of STIs, see Chapters 119, 191, 215, and 223. Complicated STIs and HIV infection warrant referral to medical subspecialists.

Many minor psychosocial problems can be handled by referral to social support groups, sometimes known as gay–straight alliances. In many localities, specialized social service agencies can help with social, educational, and other unmet needs. Adolescents with severe psychiatric symptoms, such as suicidal ideation, depression, and chemical dependency, should be referred to mental health specialists who have experience treating homosexual adolescents. Individual or family therapy might be indicated for personal, family, or environmental adjustment difficulties. So-called "reparative therapy," aiming to change sexual orientation, is not only ineffective but also contraindicated because of its potential to heighten guilt and anxiety.

Well-informed professionals can help adolescents and their parents to explore their feelings and learn about topics related to homosexuality and its etiology, psychologic normalcy, spiritual and cultural implications, disclosure to a significant other, preventive care, and community resources. With appropriate support from families, school, and communities, homosexual youths have the same potential as others to lead happy, healthy, and productive lives.

Frankowski BL and the Committee on Adolescence: Sexual orientation and adolescents. *Pediatrics* 2004;113(6):1827–1832.

French SA, Story M, Remafedi G, et al: Sexual orientation and prevalence of body dissatisfaction and eating disordered behaviors: A population-based study of adolescents. *Int J Eat Disord* 1996;19(2):119–126.

Remafedi G: Sexual orientation and youth suicide. *JAMA* 1999;282: 1291–1292.

Remafedi G, Resnick M, Blum R, et al: Demography of sexual orientation in adolescents. *Pediatrics* 1992;89(4):714–721.

Russell ST, Franz BT, Driscoll AK: Same-sex romantic attraction and experiences of violence in adolescence. *Am J Public Health* 2001;91:903–906.

Stronski-Huwiler SM, Remafedi G: Adolescent homosexuality. *Adv Pediatr* 1998;5:107–144.

Valleroy LA, MacKellar DA, Karon JM, et al: HIV prevalence and associated risks in young men who have sex with men. *JAMA* 2000;84(2):198–204.

Winters KC, Remafedi G, Chan BY: Assessing drug abuse among gay-bisexual young men. *Psychol Addict Behav* 1996;10(4):228–236.

Chapter 14 ■ Assessment of Growth

Virginia Keane

Growth assessment is an essential component of pediatric health surveillance. Many biophysiologic and psychosocial problems can adversely affect growth, and aberrant growth may be the first sign of an underlying problem. The most powerful tool in growth assessment is the growth chart (see Figs. 9-1 and 9-2) used in combination with accurate measurements of height, weight, and head circumference.

PROCEDURES FOR ACCURATE MEASUREMENT

Accurate measurement is a key component of assessing growth. Weight, in pounds or kilograms, must be determined using an accurate scale. For infants, weight, length, and head circumference are obtained. Head circumference is determined using a flexible tape measure run from the supraorbital ridge to the occiput in the path that leads to the largest possible measurement. Length is most accurately measured by two examiners (one to position the child), with the child supine on a measuring board. For older children, the measure is stature or height, taken using a stadiometer. Measurements obtained in alternative manners, such as marking examination paper at the foot and head of a supine infant, or using a simple wall growth chart with a book or ruler on the head, can lead to inaccuracy that may render the measurement useless. It is essential to compare measurements with previous growth trends and repeat any that are inconsistent.

DERIVATION AND INTERPRETATION OF GROWTH CHARTS

In 2000, the Centers for Disease Control and Prevention (CDC) published revised growth charts. These charts contain data from five national surveys conducted between 1963 and 1994. Data are representative of the USA population, both demographically and in terms of breast-feeding prevalence. Excluded from the charts are data from very low birthweight children and the latest data set for children 6 yr of age and younger, so the recent increase in the prevalence of obesity does not unduly raise the upper limits of normal. Several deficiencies of the older charts have been corrected, such as the over-representation of bottle-fed infants and the reliance on a local data set for the infant charts. The disjunction between length and height, when moving from the infant curves to those for older children, no longer exists. The new standard provides body mass index (BMI) curves through age 20 yr, facilitating identification of obesity.

The data are presented in 5 standard gender-specific charts: (1) weight for age; (2) height (length and stature) for age; (3) head circumference for age; (4) weight for height (length and stature) for infants; and (5) BMI for children over 2 yr of age (see Figs. 9-1 and 9-2 and Fig. 14-1). Charts with lines for the 3rd and 97th percentiles are available.

Each chart is composed of 7 or 8 percentile curves, representing the distribution of weight, length, stature, or head circumference values at each age. The percentile curve indicates the percentage of children at a given age on the *x*-axis whose measured value falls below the corresponding value on the *y*-axis. On the weight chart for boys 0–36 mo of age (see Fig. 9-1*A*), the 9 mo age line intersects the 25th percentile curve at 8.6 kg, indicating that 25% of the 9 mo old boys in the National Center for Health Statistics sample weigh less than 8.6 kg (75% weigh more). Similarly, a 9 mo old boy weighing more than 11.2 kg is heavier than 95% of his peers. The median, or 50th percentile (see Fig. 6-5), is also termed the *standard value,* in the sense that the standard height for a 7 mo old girl is 67 cm (see Fig. 9-1*B*). The weight-for-height charts (Fig. 9-2) are constructed in an analogous fashion, with length or stature in place of age on the *x*-axis; the median or standard weight for a girl measuring 110 cm is 18.6 kg.

For infants, it is important to realize that the revised charts represent observed but not necessarily optimal growth because they still incorporate data from many bottle-fed infants. Since 1970, only about ½ of all infants have been breast-fed, with 30% breast-fed for 3 mo or more. Compared with current standards, an exclusively breast-fed infant would be expected to plot higher for weight in the 1st 6 mo, but relatively lower in the 2nd half of the 1st year. Awareness of this growth difference should avoid overidentification of growth problems in breast-fed infants.

In an effort to set an internationally usable standard for optimal growth in young children, the World Health Organization is conducting the Multicenter Growth Reference Study (MGRS) to develop growth curves that can be used for assessing early growth among children from around the world. Rather than describing the growth of typical children, the MGRS describes the growth of children who are raised under optimal conditions, following recommended health practices, such as environments that support exclusive breast-feeding, Baby-Friendly Hospitals, and mothers who agree to breast-feed their infants. Six study sites represent 5 continents in the major regions of the world: United States, Brazil, Norway, Ghana, Oman, and India. The MGRS

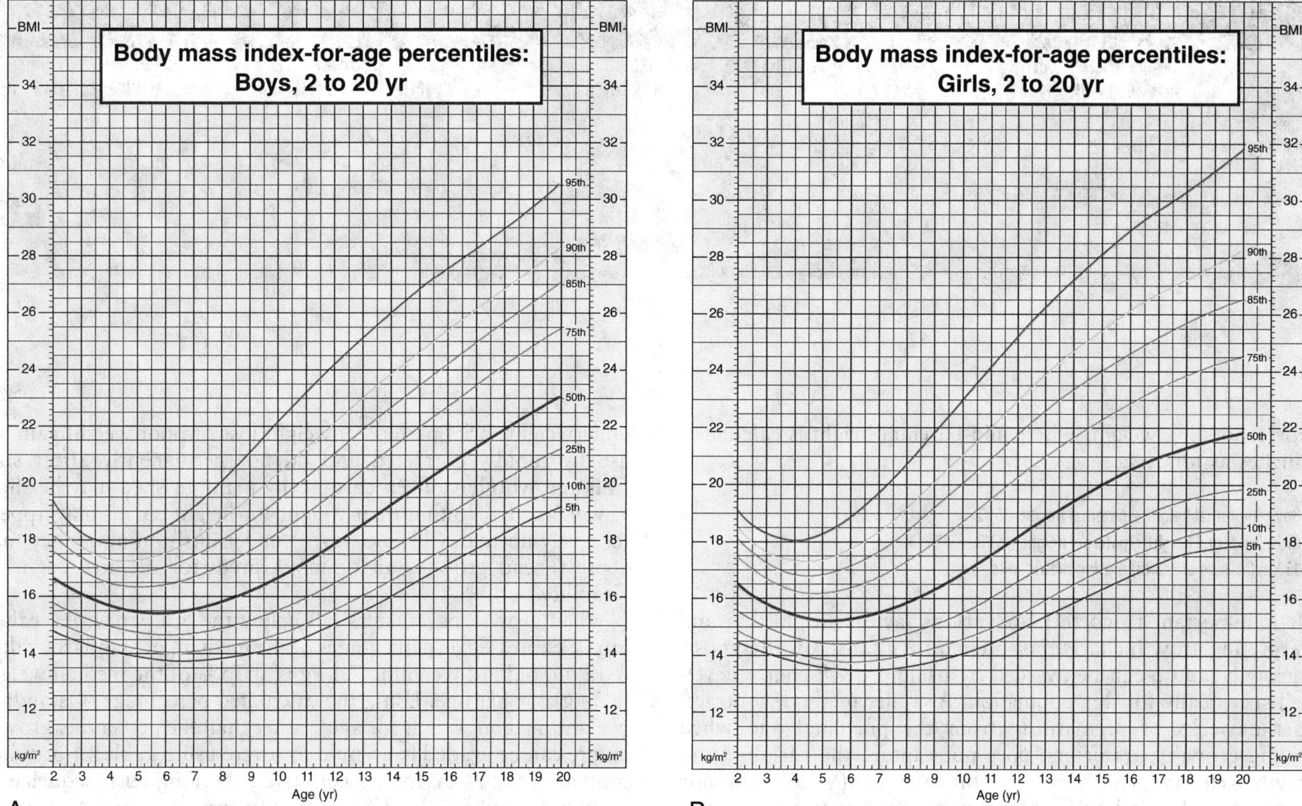

Figure 14-1. Body mass index (BMI) percentiles for boys *(A)* and girls *(B)* age 2–20 yr. (Official Centers for Disease Control [CDC] growth charts, as described in this chapter. The 85th to 95th percentile is at risk for overweight; >95th percentile is overweight; <5th percentile is underweight. Technical information and interpretation and management guides are available at *www.cdc.gov/nchs*.)

references will serve as normative standards that represent early growth under optimal conditions. Charts are available at www.who.int/childgrowth/mgrs/en/.

For adolescents, caution must be used in applying cross-sectional charts. Growth during adolescence is linked temporally to the onset of puberty, which varies widely. By using cross-sectional data based on chronological age, the charts combine youth who are at different stages of maturation. Normal variations in the timing of the growth spurt can lead to misdiagnosis of growth abnormalities. The data for 12 yr old boys include both early-maturing boys who are at the peak of their growth spurts and late-maturing ones who are still growing at their prepubertal rate. The net result is to artificially level off the growth peak, making it appear that adolescents grow more gradually and for a longer period than they do. When additional precision is necessary, growth charts derived from longitudinal data, such as the height velocity charts of Tanner and colleagues, are recommended.

Specialized charts have been developed for USA children with various conditions, including very low birthweight and prematurity; Down, Turner, and Klinefelter syndromes, and achondroplasia. In addition, growth charts for children of distinct ethnic groups or nationalities may be found on the World Wide Web.

Body mass index (BMI) is added to the standard growth charts for children over 2 yr of age. BMI can be calculated as weight in kilograms/(height in meters)^2 or weight in pounds/(height in inches)$^2 \times 703$, with fractions of pounds and inches expressed as decimals. Values may be plotted on standard BMI charts; (see Fig. 14-1). These calculations can be easily performed electronically using a variety of desktop and hand-held devices. BMI percentile varies with age over childhood: a 6 yr old girl with a BMI of 21 is overweight, while a 16 yr old girl with the same BMI is just above the 50th percentile.

ANALYSIS OF GROWTH PATTERNS

Growth is a process rather than a static quality. An infant at the 5th percentile of weight for age may be growing normally, may be failing to grow, or may be recovering from growth failure, depending on the trajectory of the growth curve. Infants may lose up to 10% of their birthweight in the 1st wk of life and regain it by the end of the 2nd wk. They will then gain steadily at a rate of 20–30 g/day for the first 3 mo. Table 14-1 gives typical growth and calorie requirements for children through age 6 yr. Table 14-2 helps estimate growth at different ages, given the birthweight and length.

Despite the facts that the National Center for Health Statistics (NCHS) tables represent cross-sectional rather than longitudinal data, and that children tend to grow in spurts, most children tend to track along a percentile, referred to as "following the curve." A normal exception commonly occurs during the first 2 yr of life. For full-term infants, size at birth reflects the influence of the uterine environment; however, size at age 2 yr correlates with mean parental height, reflecting the influence of genes. Between 6 and 18 mo of age, infants may shift percentiles upward or downward toward their genetic potential. Thereafter, most children will track along a growth percentile, with variation within two large percentile bands (a small infant might track between the 5th and 25th percentiles, a large one between the 75th and 95th). This tracking often represents the mid-parental height and

TABLE 14-1. Growth and Caloric Requirements

AGE	APPROXIMATE DAILY WEIGHT GAIN (g)	APPROXIMATE MONTHLY WEIGHT GAIN	GROWTH IN LENGTH (cm/mo)	GROWTH IN HEAD CIRCUMFERENCE (cm/mo)	RECOMMENDED DAILY ALLOWANCE (Kcal/kg/day)
0–3 mo	30	2 lb	3.5	2.00	115
3–6 mo	20	1.25 lb	2.0	1.00	110
6–9 mo	15	1 lb	1.5	0.50	100
9–12 mo	12	13 oz	1.2	0.50	100
1–3 yr	8	8 oz	1.0	0.25	100
4–6 yr	6	6 oz	3 cm/yr	1 cm/yr	90–100

Adapted from National Research Council, Food and Nutrition Board: *Recommended Daily Allowances.* Washington, DC, National Academy of Sciences, 1989; Frank D, Silva M, Needlman R: Failure to thrive: Myth and method. *Contemp Pediatr* 1993;10:114.

a corresponding weight, where **mid-parental height** is calculated in inches as follows:

- **Boys: (maternal height + paternal height + 5)/2**
- **Girls: (maternal height + paternal height − 5)/2**
- **13 cm (instead of ± 5 in) if using metric units**

It is important to correct for various factors in plotting and interpreting growth charts. For premature infants, overdiagnosis of growth failure can be avoided by using growth charts developed specifically for this population. A cruder method, subtracting the weeks of prematurity from the postnatal age when plotting growth parameters, does not capture the variability in growth velocity that very low birthweight (VLBW) infants demonstrate. While VLBW infants may continue to show catch-up growth through early school age, most achieve weight catch-up during the second year and height catch-up by 2.5 yr of age, barring medical complications (see Chapter 97). For children with particularly tall or short parents, there is a risk of overdiagnosing growth disorders if parental height is not taken into account or, conversely, of underdiagnosing growth disorders if parental height is accepted uncritically as the explanation.

The analysis of growth patterns and the detection of aberrant growth patterns provide critical information for the detection of pathologic conditions. Calculation of daily and monthly growth, such as weight gain in grams/day (see Table 14-1), allows more precise comparison of growth rate to the norm. Weight loss, or failure to gain normally, is often the first sign of pathology.

The diagnosis of failure to thrive (see Chapter 37), usually a diagnosis of children under 3 yr of age, is considered if a child's weight is below the 5th percentile, if it drops down more than two major percentile lines, or if weight for height is less than the 5th percentile. Weight for height below the 5th percentile remains the single best growth chart indicator of acute undernutrition. A BMI less than the 5th percentile also indicates that a child is underweight. Brief periods of weight loss or poor weight gain are usually rapidly corrected and do not permanently affect size. Children who have been chronically malnourished may be short as well as thin, so that their weight-for-height curves may appear relatively normal. Chronic, severe undernutrition in infancy may depress head growth, an ominous predictor of later cognitive disability.

When growth parameters fall below the 5th percentile, values can be expressed as percentages of the median, or standard, value. A 12 mo old girl weighing 7.1 kg is at 75% of the median weight (9.5 kg) for her age. Using the calculated percentage of standard (weight/median weight for age) rather than the percentile, growth failure can be graded from mild to severe using Table 14-3. When compared with developing countries, the long-term sequelae of growth failure in the USA are less certain. Another way to describe designations correlates with the risk of mortality in developing countries; extremes of growth and growth retardation are expressed in terms of height (or weight) age, the age at which the standard (median) height (or weight) equals the child's current height (or weight). A 30 mo old child who is as tall (or heavy) as an average 13 mo old has a height (or weight) age of 13 mo.

Linear growth problems are more likely to be due to congenital, constitutional, familial, or endocrine causes than to nutritional deficiency (see also Chapter 43). In endocrine disorders, length or height declines first or at the same time as weight; weight for height is normal or elevated. In nutritional insufficiency, weight declines before length and weight for height is low (unless there has been chronic stunting). Figure 14-2 depicts typical growth curves for four classes of decreased linear growth. In congenital pathologic short stature, an infant is born small and growth gradually tapers off throughout infancy. Causes include chromosomal abnormalities (Turner syndrome, trisomy 21), perinatal infection (TORCH), teratogens (phenytoin, alcohol), and extreme prematurity. In constitutional growth delay, weight and height decrease near the end of infancy, parallel the norm through

TABLE 14-2. Formulas for Approximate Average Height and Weight of Normal Infants and Children

WEIGHT	KILOGRAMS	(POUNDS)
At birth	3.25	(7)
3–12 mo	$\frac{\text{Age (mo)} + 9}{2}$	(age [mo] + 11)
1–6 yr	Age (yr) × 2 + 8	(age [yr] × 5 + 17)
7–12 yr	$\frac{\text{Age (yr)} \times 7 - 5}{2}$	(age [yr] × 7 + 5)
HEIGHT	**CENTIMETERS**	**(INCHES)**
At birth	50	(20)
At 1 yr	75	(30)
2–12 yr	age (yr) × 6 + 77	(age [yr] × 2½ + 30)

TABLE 14-3. Severity of Malnutrition: Stunting and Wasting

GRADE OF MALNUTRITION	WEIGHT FOR AGE* (WASTING)	HEIGHT FOR AGE† (STUNTING)	WEIGHT FOR HEIGHT‡
0, normal	>90	>95	>90
1, mild	75–90	90–95	81–90
2, moderate	60–74	85–89	70–80
3, severe	<60	<85	<70

Values represent percentage of median for age.
*Data from Gomez F, Galvan RR, Frank S, et al: Mortality in second- and third-degree malnutrition. *J Trop Pediatr* 1956;2:77.
†Data from Waterlow JC: Evolution of kwashiorkor and marasmus. *Lancet* 1974;2:712.
‡Data from Waterlow JC: Classification and definition of protein-calorie malnutrition. *BMJ* 1972;3:566.

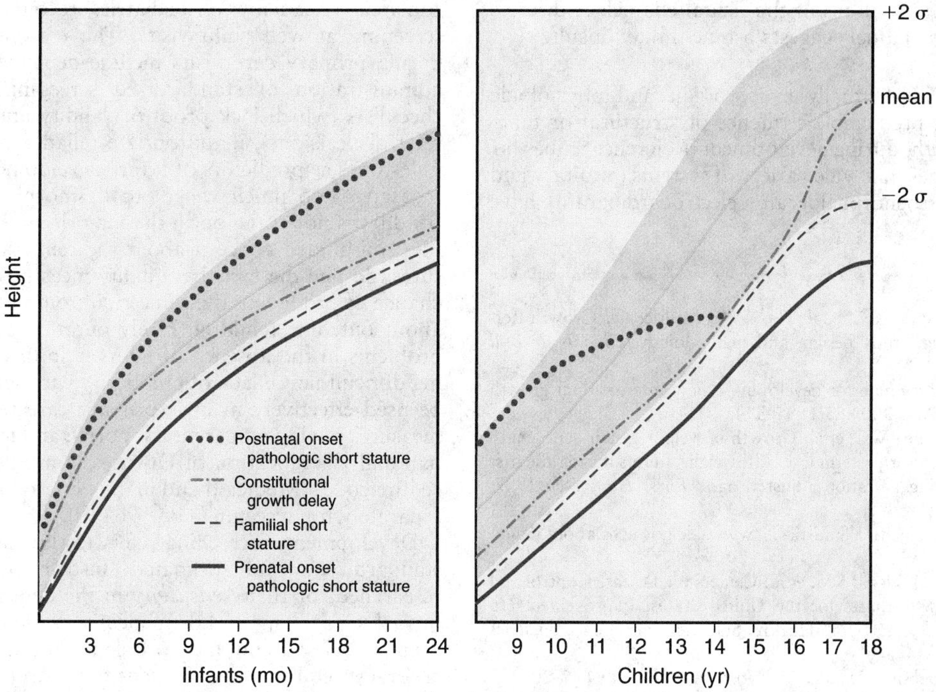

Figure 14-2. Height-for-age curves of the four general causes of proportional short stature: postnatal onset pathologic short stature, constitutional growth delay, familial short stature, and prenatal onset short stature. (From Mahoney CP: Evaluating the child with short stature. *Pediatr Clin North Am* 1987;34:825.)

middle childhood, and accelerate toward the end of adolescence. Adult size is normal. In familial short stature, both the infant and the parents are small; growth runs parallel to and just below the normal curves.

Obesity affects large numbers of children. Growth charts can confirm an impression of obesity if the weight for height exceeds 120% of the standard (median) weight for height. According to the CDC, a BMI over the 95th percentile indicates "overweight" and a BMI between the 85th and 95th percentiles indicates "risk of overweight." Although widely accepted as the best clinical measure of under- and overweight, BMI may not provide an accurate index of adiposity, because it does not differentiate lean tissue and bone from fat. Measurement of the triceps, subscapular, and suprailiac skinfold thickness can be used to estimate adiposity; considerable experience is needed for accuracy. The *American Academy of Pediatrics Nutrition Handbook,* 5th edition, questions the use of fat folds to estimate total body fat, noting that the method has not been validated in young children and that basic assumptions of the method, that subcutaneous fat is a marker of total fat and that measured sites represent average skin fat thickness, are not true. Other methods of measuring fat, such as hydrodensitometry, bioelectrical impedance, and total body water measurement are used in research, but not in clinical evaluation.

OTHER INDICES OF GROWTH

BODY PROPORTIONS. Body proportions follow a predictable sequence of changes with development (see Table 14-2). The head and trunk are relatively large at birth, with progressive lengthening of the limbs throughout development, particularly during puberty. The **lower body segment** is defined as the length from the symphysis pubis to the floor, and the **upper body segment** is the height minus the lower body segment. The ratio of upper body segment divided by lower body segment (U/L ratio) equals approximately 1.7 at birth, 1.3 at 3 yr of age, and 1.0 after 7 yr of age. Higher U/L ratios are characteristic of short-limb dwarfism or bone disorders, such as rickets.

SKELETAL MATURATION. Reference standards for bone maturation facilitate estimation of bone age (see Tables 8-4 and 12-5). Bone age correlates well with stage of pubertal development and can be helpful in predicting adult height in early- or late-maturing adolescents. In familial short stature, the bone age is normal (comparable to chronological age). In constitutional delay, endocrinologic short stature, and undernutrition, the bone age is low and comparable to the height age. Skeletal maturation is linked more closely to sexual maturity rating than to chronological age. It is more rapid and less variable in girls than in boys.

DENTAL DEVELOPMENT. Dental development includes mineralization, eruption, and exfoliation (see Table 8-3). Initial mineralization begins as early as the 2nd trimester (mean age for central incisors, 14 wk) and continues through 3 yr of age for the primary (deciduous) teeth and 25 yr of age for the permanent teeth. Mineralization begins at the crown and progresses toward the root. Eruption begins with the central incisors and progresses laterally. Exfoliation begins at about 6 yr of age and continues through 12 yr of age. Eruption of the permanent teeth may follow exfoliation immediately or may lag by 4–5 mo. The timing of dental development is poorly correlated with other processes of growth and maturation. **Delayed eruption** is usually considered when there are no teeth by approximately 13 mo of age (mean + 3 standard deviations). Common causes include hypothyroid, hypoparathyroid, familial, and (the most common) idiopathic. Individual teeth may fail to erupt because of mechanical blockage (crowding, gum fibrosis). Causes of **early exfoliation** include histiocytosis X, cyclic neutropenia, leukemia, trauma, and idiopathic factors. Nutritional and metabolic disturbances, prolonged illness, and certain medications (tetracycline) commonly result in discoloration or malformations of the dental enamel. A discrete line of pitting on the enamel suggests a time-limited insult.

STRUCTURAL GROWTH. Virtually every organ and physiologic process undergoes a predictable sequence of structural or functional changes, or both, during development. Reference values for developmental changes in a wide variety of systems (pituitary and renal function, electroencephalogram, electrocardiogram) have been published.

De Onis M, Garza C, Victora CG, et al: The WHO Multicenter Growth Reference Study: Planning, study design, and methodology. *Food Nutr Bull* 2004;25(1):S15–S26.

Garza C, De Onis M: Rationale for developing a new international growth reference. *Food Nutr Bull* 2004;25(1):S5–S14.

Guo SS, Roche AF, Chumlea WC, et al: Growth in weight, recumbent length and head circumference for preterm low birthweight infants during the first three years of life using gestation adjusted ages. *Early Hum Dev* 1997; 47:305–325.

National Center for Health Statistics: www.cdc.gov.nchs.about.major.nhanes.growthcharts.

Ogden CL, Kuczmarski RJ, Flegal KM, et al: Centers for Disease Control and Prevention 2000 growth charts for the United States: Improvements to the 1977 National Center for Health Statistics version. *Pediatrics* 2002;109:45–60.

Strauss RS: Childhood obesity. *Pediatr Clin North Am* 2002;49:175–201.

Tanner JM, Davies PSW: Clinical longitudinal standards for height and height velocity for North American children. *J Pediatr* 1985;107:317.

Tanner JM, Whitehouse RH, Cameron N, et al: *Assessment of Skeletal Maturity and Prediction of Adult Height (TW2 Method)*. London, Academic Press, 1983.

Tillmann V, Thalange NK, Foster PJ, et al: The relationship between stature, growth, and short-term changes in height and weight in normal prepubertal children. *Pediatr Res* 1998;44:882–886.

World Health Organization: The WHO growth standards. www.who.int/childgrowth/mgrs/en.

Wright C: Growth charts for babies. *BMJ* 2005;330:1399–1400.

Chapter 15 ■ Developmental Screening and Surveillance

Frances Page Glascoe

The Individuals with Disabilities Education Act (IDEA) provides a national system to locate and treat children, beginning at birth, who are deemed at risk for developmental problems or have established delays (see Chapter 16). These conditions, such as speech-language impairment, learning disabilities, autism spectrum disorders, mild to moderate mental retardation, and psychosocial problems, are common (see Chapters 28–32). Together with school failure and high school drop-out rates, they affect approximately 1 : 4 to 1 : 5 children. Some of these problems are preventable, and others may be ameliorated by interventions, especially when instituted prior to school entrance. These problems are often not identified until kindergarten entrance, at which point some children have lost opportunities for early intervention, which is known to increase school success and reduce subsequent high school drop-out rates, teen pregnancy, delinquency, and unemployment.

Because only 30% of children with developmental and behavioral problems are identified by their primary care providers, the American Academy of Pediatrics recommends developmental screening at well child visits. The reasons for underdetection during primary care visits include dependence on nonstandard administration of standardized screening tests and informal checklists (which lack proof of validity and criteria for making referral decisions); inappropriate reliance on prior development milestones as predictors of future development; clinical judgment that gives too much weight to dysmorphology and organicity, conditions not common in the majority of children with disabilities; misguided concern about the reliability of screening measures, despite the fact that quality measures usually have a 90% chance of producing the same result on retesting; false optimism about outcome (children rarely outgrow serious developmental problems in the absence of intervention); discomfort at delivering difficult news; lack of familiarity with screening tools that can be used effectively in busy primary care settings (e.g., accurate measures relying on parental reports); and ineffective use of International Classification of Diseases, ninth revision (ICD-9), procedure codes (Medicaid and many private carriers now reimburse separately for screening code 96110).

Developmental screening refers to the administration of brief, standardized, and validated instruments that have been researched for their *sensitivity* in the detection of children with probable problems and their *specificity* in determining when children probably do not have problems. Standards for screening test accuracy require 70–80% sensitivity and specificity. Although these figures are low compared with standards for most medical screens, developmental problems develop over time, and repeated screening usually compensates for this underdetection. Over-referrals are of less concern because research shows that most children with false-positive screening tests, while ineligible for special education services under IDEA, are nevertheless in need of remedial programs (Head Start, after-school tutoring, summer school, quality preschool or daycare), due to psychosocial risk factors (e.g., poverty, limited maternal education) and below-average performance in the predictors of school success (language, intelligence, and academic/pre-academic skills).

Table 15-1 lists a range of tools useful for early detection of developmental and behavioral problems. During a primary care visit, children may be recalcitrant, ill, hungry, sleepy, or frightened; these are not ideal states for demonstrating developmental accomplishments. Well child visits are brief and have large agendas, including physical examinations, immunizations, anticipatory guidance, safety and injury prevention counseling, and developmental promotion. Thus, developmental screens that rely on information from parents are ideal because they can be completed in advance of appointments, on-line or in waiting or examination rooms.

In addition to repeated developmental screening, physicians are encouraged to practice developmental surveillance at each well child visit. **Developmental surveillance** provides a context for screening results and involves scrutinizing family functioning, observing child behavior and developmental skills, longitudinally eliciting and attending to parents' concerns, and using the knowledge obtained from a child's medical history (Fig. 15-1). Information obtained through surveillance should not be used to override a positive screening test result, but it can be used to elevate suspicions about negative screening test results. Surveillance is essential for making judgments about referrals, determining service needs, and selecting optimal methods to help parents promote positive development (through written materials, hands-on parent training, or social work services). Table 15-2 presents a practice algorithm that combines screening and surveillance, and Table 15-3 provides related resources.

Once a possible disability has been detected, children should be referred for more comprehensive assessment and intervention. A general pediatrician may initiate the evaluation by following

TABLE 15-1. Tools for Developmental Screening and Surveillance*

DEVELOPMENTAL SCREENS RELYING ON INFORMATION FROM PARENTS	AGE RANGE	DESCRIPTION	SCORING	ACCURACY	TIME FRAME/COSTS
Parents' Evaluations of Developmental Status (PEDS) [1997]. Ellsworth & Vandermeer Press, P.O. Box 68164, Nashville, TN 37206; 615-226-4460; fax: 615-227-0411; $30.00 http://www.pedstest.com Online at *www.forepath.org*	Birth–9 yr	10 questions eliciting parents' concerns in English, Spanish, Vietnamese, and other languages. Written at the 4th–5th grade level. Also serves as a surveillance and triage tool and determines when to refer, provide a second screen, provide patient education, or monitor developmental, behavior/emotional, and academic progress. Also available online, together with the Modified Checklist of Autism in Toddlers for electronic medical records.	Identifies children as low, moderate, or high risk for various kinds of disabilities and delays, and indicates the optimal course of action	Sensitivity ranging from 74–79% and specificity ranging from 70–80% across age levels	About 2 min (if interview needed) Print materials ~$0.31 Administration ~$0.88 Total ~$1.19
PEDS-Developmental Milestones (PEDS-DM (October, 2006) Ellsworth & Vandermeer Press, Ltd. 1013 Austin Court, Nolensville, TN 37136 Phone: 615-776-4121; fax: 615-776-4119 http://www.pedstest.com, to be online at www.forepath.org	0–8 years	PEDS-DM is a validated checklist of milestones, consisting of 6–8 items at each age level (spanning the well visit schedule). Each item taps a different domain (fine/gross motor, self-help, academics, expressive/receptive language, social-emotional). It can be used to complement PEDS or stand alone. Administered by parent report or directly.	Cutoffs tied to performance above and below the 16th percentile for each item and its domain.	Sensitivity (0.75–0.87): specficity (0.71–0.88) to performance in each domain. Sensitivity (0.70–0.94); specificity (0.77–0.93) across age	About 3 minutes Materials ~$.20 Admin. ~$1.00 Total ~$1.20
Ages and Stages Questionnaire (formerly Infant Monitoring System) [1994]. Paul H. Brookes Publishers, P.O. Box 10624, Baltimore, MD 21285; 1-800-638-3775; $190.00 *http://www.pbrookes.com/*	4–60 mo	Parents indicate children's developmental skills on 25–35 items (4–5 pages) using a different form for each well visit. Reading level varies across items from 3rd–12th grade. Can be used in mass mailings for child-find programs. In English, Spanish, and French.	Single pass/fail score for developmental status	Sensitivity ranged from 70–90% at all ages except the 4-mo level; specificity ranged from 76–91%	About 15 min (if interview needed) Materials ~$0.40 Administration ~$4.20 Total ~$4.60
BEHAVIORAL/EMOTIONAL SCREENS RELYING ON INFORMATION FROM PARENTS					
Pediatric Symptom Checklist. Jellinek MS, Murphy JM, Robinson J, et al: Pediatric Symptom Checklist: Screening school age children for academic and psychosocial dysfunction. *J Pediatr* 1988;112:201–209 (the test is included in the article) Also can be freely downloaded at *http://psc.partners.org/* or with factor scores at *www.pedstest.com*	4–16 yr	35 short statements of problem behaviors, including both externalizing (conduct) and internalizing (depression, anxiety, adjustment, etc.). Ratings of never, sometimes, or often are assigned a value of 0, 1, or 2, respectively. Scores totaling 28 or more suggest referrals. Factor scores identify attentional, internalizing, and externalizing problems. Factor scoring is available for download at: http://www.pedstest.com/links/resources.html	Single refer/nonrefer score	All but 1 study showed high sensitivity (80–95%) but somewhat scattered specificity (68–100%)	About 7 min (if interview needed) Materials ~$0.10 Administration ~$2.38 Total ~$2.48
Ages & Stages Questionnaires: Social-Emotional (ASQ:SE). Paul H. Brookes, Publishers. P.O. Box 10624, Baltimore, MD 21285; 1-800-638-3775; $125.00 *http://www.pbrookes.com/*	6–60 mo	Designed to supplement the ASQ, the ASQ:SE consists of 30-item forms (4–5 pages long) for each of 8 visits between 6 and 60 months. Items focus on self-regulation, compliance, communication, adaptive functioning, autonomy, affect, and interaction with people.	Single cutoff score indicating when a referral is needed	Sensitivity ranged from 71–85%; specificity from 90–98%	10–15 min (if interview needed) Materials ~$0.40 Administration ~$4.20 Total ~$4.40
Brief-Infant-Toddler Social-Emotional Assessment (BITSEA). 19500 Bulverde Road, San Antonio, TX 78259; 1-800-211-8378; $99.00 *http://harcourtassessment.com/*	12–36 mo	42-item parent-report measure for identifying social-emotional/behavioral problems and delays in competence. Items were drawn from the assessment level measure, the ITSEA. Written at the 4th–6th grade level. Available in Spanish, French, Dutch, and Hebrew.	Cut-points based on child age and sex show presence/absence of problems and competence	Sensitivity (80–85%) in detecting children with social-emotional/behavioral problems; specificity 75–80%	7–10 min Materials ~$4.00 Administration ~$2.38 Total ~$6.38 (Note: publisher has not yet listed price of protocols apart from test manual so material costs may drop.)
Modified Checklist for Autism in Toddlers (M-CHAT) [1997]. Free download at the First Signs website: http://www.firstsigns.org/downloads/m-chat.PDF. Online for parents and electronic records at *www.forepath.org*	24 mo	Second-stage screen recommended for use if children have difficulty with measures such as the ASQ or PEDS. It presents parents with 23 questions written at a 4th–6th grade reading level. Available in English and Spanish. Uses telephone follow-up for concerns. The M-CHAT is copyrighted, but remains free for use on the First Signs Web site. The full text article appeared in the April 2001 issue of the *Journal of Autism and Developmental Disorders.*	Cutoff based on 2 of 3 critical items or any 3 from checklist	Initial study shows sensitivity at 90%; specificity at 99%; over-referrals tend to be of children with substantial language or intellectual disabilities.	About 5 min Print materials ~$0.10 Administration ~$0.88 Total ~$0.98
Eyberg Child Behavior Inventory/ Sutter-Eyberg Student Behavior Inventory. Psychological Assessment Resources, P.O. Box 998, Odessa, FL 33556; 1-800-331-8378; $120.00 *http://www.parinc.com/*	2–16 yr	36–38 short statements of common behavior problems. A score of more than 16 suggests a referral for behavioral interventions. A lower score enables the measure to function as a problem list for planning in-office counseling and selecting handouts. The tools are helpful in monitoring behavioral progress.	Single refer/nonrefer score for externalizing problems: conduct, attention, aggression, etc.	Sensitivity 80%, specificity 86% for disruptive behavior problems	About 7 min (if interview needed) Materials ~$0.30 Administration ~$2.38 Total ~$2.68

TABLE 15-1. Tools for Developmental Screening and Surveillance*—Continued

DEVELOPMENTAL SCREENS RELYING ON INFORMATION FROM PARENTS	AGE RANGE	DESCRIPTION	SCORING	ACCURACY	TIME FRAME/COSTS
Connors Rating Scale-Revised (CRS-R). Multi-Health Systems P.O. Box 950, North Tonawanda, NY 14120-0950; 1-800-456-3003 or 1-416-492-2627; Fax 1-888-540-4484 or 1-416-492-3343; $193.00 *http://www.mhs.com/*	3–17 yr	Three versions are used for diagnosis: teacher report, parent report, and youth self-report. 7 factor scores: Cognitive Problems/Inattention, Hyperactivity, Oppositional, Anxious-Shy, Perfectionism, Social Problems, and, Psychosomatic. Several subscales specific to ADHD are also included: DSM-IV symptom subscales (Inattentive, Hyperactive/Impulsive, and Total); Global Indices [GI] (Restless-Impulsive, Emotional Lability, and Total), and an ADHD Index. The GI is useful for treatment monitoring. Also available in French.	Cutoff tied to the 93rd percentile for each factor	Sensitivity 78–92% Specificity 84–94%	About 20 min Materials ~$2.25 Administration ~$20.15 Total ~$22.40
FAMILY SCREENS					
Family Psychosocial Screening. Kemper KJ, Kelleher KJ: Family psychosocial screening: instruments and techniques. *Ambulatory Child Health* 1996;4:325–339 (measures are included in article) Also downloadable at *http://www.pedstest.com*	Screens parents and best used along with above screens	2-page clinic intake form that identifies psychosocial risk factors associated with developmental problems, including a 4-item measure of parental history of physical abuse as a child; (2) a 6-item measure of parental substance abuse; and (3) a 3-item measure of maternal depression.	Refer/nonrefer scores for each risk factor; also has guides to referring and resource lists	All studies showed sensitivity and specificity to larger inventories >90%	About 15 min (if interview needed) Materials ~$0.20 Administration ~$4.20 Total ~$4.40
DEVELOPMENTAL SCREENS RELYING ON ELICITING SKILLS DIRECTLY FROM CHILDREN					
Brigance Screens-II (2005). Curriculum Associates, Inc., 153 Rangeway Road, N. Billerica, MA 01862; 1-800-225-0248; $1,029.95 *http://www.curriculumassociates.com/*	0–90 mo	7 separate forms, 1 for each 12-mo age range. Tape, for all ages, speech-language, motor, readiness, general knowledge, self-help, and play skills, and also reading and math at older ages. Uses direct elicitation and observation. At 0–2 yr, can be administered by parent report.	Cutoff, quotients, percentiles, age equivalent scores in various domains and overall	Sensitivity and specificity to giftedness and to developmental and academic problems 70–82% across ages	10–15 min Materials ~$1.53 Administration ~$10.15 Total ~$11.68
Bayley Infant Neurodevelomental Screen (BINS) [1995]. The Psychological Corporation, 555 Academic Court, San Antonio, TX 78204; 1-800-228-0752; $299.00 *http://www.psychcorp.com*	3–24 mo	Uses 10–13 directly elicited items per 3–6 mo age range to assess neurologic processes (reflexes and tone); neurodevelopmental skills (movement and symmetry), and developmental accomplishments (object permanence, imitation, and language).	Categorizes performance into low, moderate, or high risk via cut scores; provides subtest cut scores for each domain	Specificity and sensitivity 75–86% across ages	10–15 min Materials ~$0.30 Administration ~$10.15 Total ~$10.45
SCHOOL PERFORMANCE SCREENS					
Comprehensive Inventory of Basic Skills-Revised Screener (CIBS-R Screener) [1985]. Curriculum Associates, 153 Rangeway Road, N. Billerica, MA 01862; 1-800-225-0248; $224.00 *http://www.curriculumassociates.com/*	Grade 1–6	Involves 1 or more of 3 subtests (reading comprehension, math computation, and sentence writing). Timing performance also enables an assessment of information processing skills, especially rate.	Computerized or hand scoring produces percentiles, quotients, cutoffs	70–80% accuracy across all grades	Takes 10–15 min Materials ~$0.53 Administration ~$10.15 Total ~$10.68
Safety Word Inventory and Literacy Screener (SWILS). Glascoe FP, Clinical Pediatrics in press. Items courtesy of Curriculum Associates, Inc. The SWILS can be freely downloaded at: *http://www.pedstest.com/*	6–14 yr	Children are asked to read 29 common safety words (e.g., High Voltage, Wait, Poison) aloud. The number of correctly read words is compared to a cutoff score. Results predict performance in math, written language and a range of reading skills. Test content may serve as a springboard to injury prevention counseling.	Single cutoff score indicating the need for a referral	78–84% sensitivity and specificity across all ages	About 7 min (if interview needed) Materials ~$0.30 Administration ~$2.38 Total ~$2.68

*This chart is a list of measures that correctly identify, at all ages, at least 70–80% of children with disabilities and at least 70–80% of children without disabilities. All listed measures were standardized on national samples, proven to be reliable, and validated against a range of diagnostic measures and diagnosed conditions.

The first column provides publication information and the cost of purchasing a specimen set. The "Description" column provides information on alternative ways, if available, to administer measures (e.g., waiting rooms). The "Accuracy" column shows the percentage of patients with and without problems identified correctly. The "Time Frame/Costs" column shows the cost of materials per visit along with the cost of professional time (using an average salary of $50/hr) needed to administer each measure, but does not include the time needed for generating referral letters. For parent report tools, administration time reflects not only scoring of test results, but also the relationship between each test's reading level and the percentage of parents with less than a high school education (who may or may not be able to complete measures in waiting rooms due to literacy problems and thus will need interview administration).

Not included are measures, such as the Denver-II, that fail to meet the 70–80% standard of accuracy, measures not fully tested for accuracy (e.g., Battelle Developmental Inventory Screening Test-2, DIAL-3), or narrow-band measures of single developmental domains (e.g., just language or motor skills).

Updated in 2005 from Glascoe FP. *Collaborating with Parents.* Nashville, Tennessee: Ellsworth & Vandermeer Press, Ltd, 1998. Permission is granted for reproduction of this table.

ADHD, Attention-deficit/hyperactivity disorder; DSM-IV, *Diagnostic and Statistical Manual of Mental Disorders, 4th ed.*

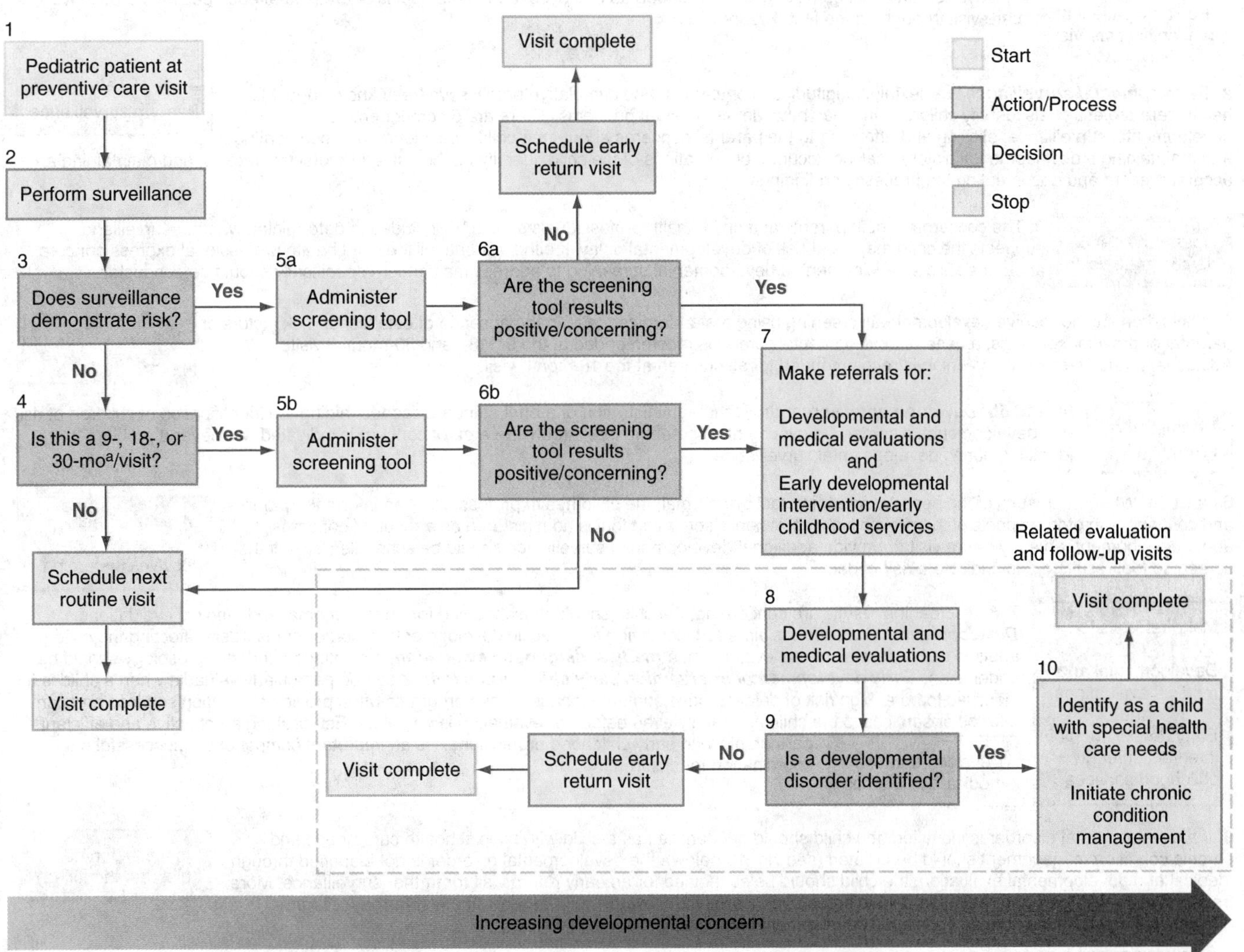

[a]Because the 30-month visit is not yet a part of the preventive care system and is often not reimbursable by third party payers at this time, developmental screening can be performed at 24 months of age.

Figure 15-1. Developmental surveillance and screening algorithm within a pediatric care visit.[a] Because the 30-month visit is not yet a part of the preventive care system and is often not reimbursable by third-party payers at this time, developmental screening can be performed at 24 months of age. (From AAP Policy Statement: Identifying infants and young children with developmental disorders in the medical home: an algorithm for developmental surveillance and screening. *Pediatrics* 2006;118:405–420.)

Pediatric patient at preventive care visit

1. Developmental concerns should be included as one of several health topics addressed at each pediatric preventive care visit throughout the first 5 years of life.

2. *Developmental surveillance* is a flexible, longitudinal, continuous, and cumulative process whereby knowledgeable health care professionals identify children who may have developmental problems. There are 5 components of developmental surveillance: eliciting and attending to the parents' concerns about their child's development, documenting and maintaining a developmental history, making accurate observations of the child, identifying the risk and protective factors, and maintaining an accurate record and documenting the process and findings.

Perform surveillance

Does surveillance demonstrate risk?

3. The concerns of both parents and child health professionals should be included in determining whether surveillance suggests the child may be at risk of developmental delay. If either parents or the child health professional express concern about the child's development, a developmental screening to address the concern specifically should be conducted.

4. All children should receive developmental screening using a standardized test. In the absence of established risk factors or parental or provider concerns, a general developmental screen is recommended at the 9-, 18-, and 30-month[a] visits. Additionally, autism-specific screening is recommended for all children at the 18-month visit.

Is this a 9-, 18-, or 30-mo[a]/visit?

Administer screening tool

5a and 5b. *Developmental screening* is the administration of a brief standardized tool aiding the identification of children at risk of a developmental disorder. Developmental screening that targets the area of concern is indicated whenever a problem is identified during developmental surveillance.

6a and 6b. When the results of the periodic screening tool are normal, the child health professional can inform the parents and continue with other aspects of the preventive visit. When a screening tool is administered as a result of concerns about development, an early return visit to provide additional developmental surveillance should be scheduled even if the screening tool results do not indicate a risk of delay.

Are the screening tool results positive/concerning?

Make referrals for:

Developmental and medical evaluations and Early developmental intervention/early childhood services

7–8. If screening results are concerning, the child should be scheduled for developmental and medical evaluations. ***Developmental evaluation*** is aimed at identifying the specific developmental disorder or disorders affecting the child. In addition to the developmental evaluation, a ***medical diagnostic evaluation*** to identify an underlying etiology should be undertaken. ***Early developmental intervention/early childhood services*** can be particularly valuable when a child is first identified to be at high risk of delayed development, because these programs often provide evaluation services and can offer other services to the child and family even before an evaluation is complete. Establishing an effective and efficient partnership with early childhood professionals is an important component of successful care coordination for children.

Developmental and medical evaluations

9. If a developmental disorder is identified, the child should be identified as a child with special health care needs and chronic condition management should be initiated (see No. 10 below). If a developmental disorder is not identified through medical and developmental evaluation, the child should be scheduled for an early return visit for further surveillance. More frequent visits, with particular attention paid to areas of concern, will allow the child to be promptly referred for further evaluation if any further evidence of delayed development or a specific disorder emerges.

Is a developmental disorder identified?

Identify as a child with special health care needs

Initiate chronic condition management

10. When a child is discovered to have a significant developmental disorder, that child becomes a child with special health care needs, even if that child does not have a specific disease etiology identified. Such a child should be identified by the medical home for appropriate chronic condition management and regular monitoring and entered into the practice's children and youth with special health care needs registry.

Figure 15-1. *Continued*

TABLE 15-2. Combining Screening and Surveillance: A Practice Algorithm

1. **REVIEW MEDICAL CHART FOR HEALTH RISK FACTORS.**
Consider potential teratogenic exposures, including radiation or medications, infectious illnesses, fever, addictive substances, trauma, and results of neonatal screens, including phenylketonuria, hypothyroidism, and other metabolic conditions. The perinatal history includes birthweight, gestational age, Apgar scores, and any medical complications (see Chapter 94.1). Postnatal medical factors that are sometimes overlooked include chronic respiratory or allergic illness, recurrent otitis, head trauma, and sleep problems (particularly signs of obstructive sleep apnea [Chapter 18]).
2. **DETERMINE PRESENCE OF PSYCHOSOCIAL RISK FACTORS.**
This includes parents with less than a high school education, parental mental health or substance abuse problems, 4 or more children in the home, single parent, poverty, frequent household moves, limited social support, parental history of abuse as a child, and ethnic minority. Four or more risk factors tend to reduce developmental status into the below average range and suggest the need for enrichment or remedial programs, regardless of screening results. An intake measure, such as the Family Psychosocial Screen (see **Table 15-1**), is often helpful for capturing psychosocial risk factors.
3. **ELICIT PARENTS' CONCERNS.**
This may be accomplished informally, although careful attention to wording is essential. The American Academy of Pediatrics (AAP)'s Bright Futures guidelines contain helpful trigger questions. An alternative is to use a measure, such as Parents' Evaluations of Developmental Status (see **Table 15-1**), which has empirically tested wording and offers a way to weight the types of concerns parents raise, assign levels of risk, and identify optimal responses.
4. **PROVIDE PHYSICAL EXAMINATION.**
Points of particular importance include growth parameters and head shape and circumference, facial and other body dysmorphology, eye findings (e.g., cataracts in various inborn errors of metabolism), vascular markings and signs of neurocutaneous disorders (café-au-lait spots in neurofibromatosis, hypopigmented macules in tuberous sclerosis). Vision and hearing screenings are essential.
5. **ADMINISTER/SCORE DEVELOPMENTAL SCREENING TESTS.**
Use of parent report measures, before the visit or in the waiting/examination room reduces the amount of time needed for screening. Positive results should be followed by additional screens of social-emotional functioning (e.g., Ages + Stages Questionnaire: Social-Emotional, Modified Checklist for Autism in Toddlers) to identify the areas of delay and types of services needed.
6. **RESPOND TO POSITIVE SCREENING TEST RESULTS WITH ADDITIONAL MEDICAL SCREENS.**
This includes screens for iron deficiency and lead toxicity because these are common contributors to developmental delays and are easily detected. Electroencephalograms and neuroimaging are not routinely indicated, but should be used if there is clinical suspicion of seizure or encephalopathy or in cases of microcephaly or rapidly expanding head circumference. Neurologic evaluation (see Chapter 591) is also warranted, along with metabolic screens for ammonia, and organic and amino acids. Human immunodeficiency virus must be considered (Chapter 273) with progressive loss of milestones, especially if there is associated growth delay.
7. **EXPLAIN RESULTS TO PARENTS.**
Results should be presented in person by the primary medical provider, with positive regard for available services and improved outcome. It is advisable to use euphemistic terms for diagnosis, since the specific condition will not be known (e.g., developmental delay, "behind other children," "having difficulties with . . ."). Offers to re-explain findings to other family members are helpful. At this time, it is wise to ask the parents if they know any families with children who have developmental differences. This may be helpful in understanding any strong reaction to the information being presented.
8. **MAKE REFERRALS FOR SUBSPECIALTY MEDICAL SERVICES.**
If records review and physical examination suggest the need, referral for further evaluation should be offered (e.g., to developmental-behavioral or neurodevelopmental pediatricians, geneticists, endocrinologists, neurologists, psychiatrists, audiologists, occupational or physical therapists.).
9. **MAKE REFERRALS FOR NONMEDICAL INTERVENTIONS.**
This should include, in the case of positive screens, IDEA programs (www.nectac.org). They do not charge families and generally provide high-quality therapies and evaluations. Other options include remediation programs and high-quality preschool for those with psychosocial risk factors (or when further evaluation reveals that screening results were false-positive). Referral letters are helpful (as are requests to parents and to IDEA programs for copies of their evaluation report). Letters should include suggestions for the types of evaluations needed (e.g., speech-language therapy, occupational and physical therapy, social-emotional assessment, intelligence, academics). And documentation of hearing and vision status because IDEA programs require this information before evaluations are provided.
10. **PROVIDE DEVELOPMENTAL PROMOTION.**
Helping parents encourage language and preacademic/academic development is critical. This can be accomplished via written patient education materials, by encouraging parents to visit websites with quality information, or by parent training classes, group well visits, or social work services. In any case, a well-organized system for filing and retrieving parent-focused materials is essential. A list of helpful resources is included in Table 15-3.
11. **ENSURE A MEDICAL HOME.**
Children with developmental and behavioral problems or special health care needs use health care services at more than twice the rate of other patients. Their visits are often complex due to the need to make referrals, locate information from prior visits and services, make follow-up appointments, and coordinate with other providers. The AAP's Medical Home model (*www.medicalhomeinfo.org*) is an essential guide to organizing practices to ensure continuity of care and to best meet the needs of children with disabilities and their families.

TABLE 15-3. Resources for Screening, Nonmedical Referral, and Developmental Promotion

Parker S, Zuckerman B: *Behavioral and Developmental Pediatrics: A Handbook for Primary Care*, 2nd ed. Baltimore, Lippincott Williams & Wilkins, 2005.

Dixon SD, Stein MT: *Encounters with Children: Pediatric Behavior and Development*, 4th ed. St. Louis, Mosby, 2005.

Schmitt BD, Fletcher J: *Instructions for Pediatric Patients*, 2nd ed. Philadelphia, Elsevier, 1998. This text consists of 1–2 page photocopyable handouts on a range of medical and nonmedical topics, including behavior and development.

The American Academy of Pediatrics Section on Developmental and Behavioral Pediatrics (*www.dbpeds.org*) has a website devoted to developmental screening and surveillance. This includes tutorials on implementation, working with office staff, rationale for tool use, information on billing and coding for services provided, guidelines for delivering difficult news, and online discussion groups for general and developmental-behavioral pediatricians.

Links to services, such as local Head Start centers, links to parent training programs, quality day care, and patient education materials may be found through the parent and professional links pages at *www.pedstest.com* This site also offers links to quality parenting information Web sites, such as the Nemours Foundation, and houses several screens, especially for adolescents. Several of these measures can be downloaded without charge.

American Academy of Pediatrics: *Bright Futures: Guidelines for Health Supervision of Infants, Toddlers and Adolescents*, 2nd ed. Chicago, AAP, 2000. *http://www.brightfutures.org/*.

Reach Out and Read is a pediatrician-designed initiative to encourage parents to read to children, a process known to promote early language development and build preacademic skills. Materials and information and training dates are available at *http://www.reachoutandread.org/*.

practice parameters (Fig. 15-2) or identifying clues from the history and physical examination and laboratory tests (Table 15-4). Developmental assessment or evaluation is also provided without charge by IDEA-funded programs (see Chapter 16). In children 0–3 yr of age, IDEA Part C programs provide assessment and intervention. For older children, referrals are best made through local school boards, departments of psychology, or special education programs. Private, multidisciplinary evaluations should be reserved for second opinions when needed. Information on how to make referrals is available on-line through the National Early Childhood Technical Assistance Center (*www.nectac.org*). A medical diagnosis is not essential for enrollment in early intervention, and most children are served while they remain on waiting lists for comprehensive evaluations. IDEA programs provide an assessment that is sufficiently detailed to define strengths and weaknesses, determine the current level of delays, measure progress, and generate an individual educational plan. However, by age 8 yr, for continued special education enrollment, school systems are required to diagnose the general type of disability.

In addition to referrals for IDEA services, pediatricians may want to refer to developmental-behavioral pediatricians, neurodevelopmental pediatricians, developmental or clinical

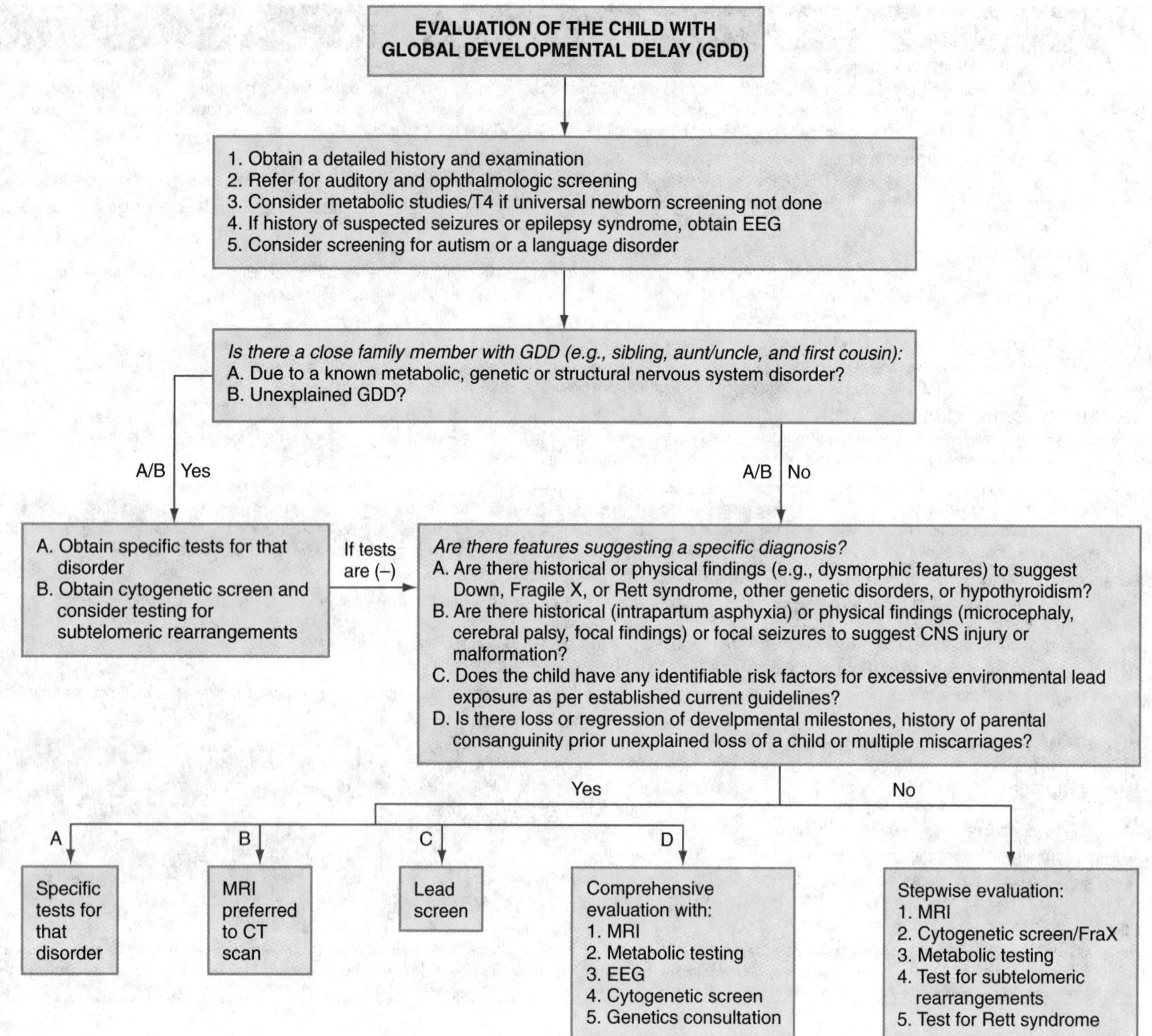

EVALUATION OF THE CHILD WITH GLOBAL DEVELOPMENTAL DELAY (GDD)
1. Obtain a detailed history and examination
2. Refer for auditory and ophthalmologic screening
3. Consider metabolic studies/T4 if universal newborn screening not done
4. If history of suspected seizures or epilepsy syndrome, obtain EEG
5. Consider screening for autism or a language disorder
Is there a close family member with GDD (e.g., sibling, aunt/uncle, and first cousin):
A. Due to a known metabolic, genetic or structural nervous system disorder?
B. Unexplained GDD?
A/B Yes
A/B No
A. Obtain specific tests for that disorder
B. Obtain cytogenetic screen and consider testing for subtelomeric rearrangements
If tests are (–)
Are there features suggesting a specific diagnosis?
A. Are there historical or physical findings (e.g., dysmorphic features) to suggest Down, Fragile X, or Rett syndrome, other genetic disorders, or hypothyroidism?
B. Are there historical (intrapartum asphyxia) or physical findings (microcephaly, cerebral palsy, focal findings) or focal seizures to suggest CNS injury or malformation?
C. Does the child have any identifiable risk factors for excessive environmental lead exposure as per established current guidelines?
D. Is there loss or regression of develpmental milestones, history of parental consanguinity prior unexplained loss of a child or multiple miscarriages?
Yes
No
A
B
C
D
Specific tests for that disorder
MRI preferred to CT scan
Lead screen
Comprehensive evaluation with:
1. MRI
2. Metabolic testing
3. EEG
4. Cytogenetic screen
5. Genetics consultation
Stepwise evaluation:
1. MRI
2. Cytogenetic screen/FraX
3. Metabolic testing
4. Test for subtelomeric rearrangements
5. Test for Rett syndrome

Figure 15-2. Algorithm for the evaluation of the child with developmental delay. Audiologic and ophthalmologic screening is recommended in all children with global developmental delay. Metabolic studies usually consist of obtaining a urine organic acid screen, quantitative serum amino acids, serum lactate and ammonia levels, capillary or arterial blood gas levels, and thyroid function studies. CNS, central nervous system; CT, computed tomography; EEG, electroencephalogram; MRI, magnetic resonance imaging; T_4, thyroxine. (From Shevell M, Ashwal S, Donley D, et al: Practice parameter: Evaluation of the child with global developmental delay. *Neurology* 2003;60:367–380.)

psychologists, or developmental evaluation centers for comprehensive assistance with diagnosis, medication management, child and family intervention, and so on. In the case of children suspected of having autism spectrum disorders, referrals should also be made to a child psychiatrist or psychologist. Finally, children who do not qualify for special education services are often those at continuing risk due to adverse psychosocial factors (e.g., parents with limited education, language barriers, poverty). These children need both careful monitoring and referral to Head Start, quality daycare, or remedial programs.

American Academy of Pediatrics: Developmental surveillance and screening of infants and young children (RE0062). *Pediatrics* 2001;108:192

American Academy of Pediatrics: Council on children with disabilities, section on developmental behavioral pediatrics, bright futures steering committee, medical home initiative for children with special needs project advisory committee, identifying infants and young children with developmental disorders in the medical home: an algorithim for developmental surveillance and screening. *Pediatrics* 2006;118:405–420.

Busari JO, Weggelaar NM: How to investigate and manage the child who is slow to speak. *BMJ* 2004;328:272–276.

Dworkin PE, Glascoe FP: Developmental surveillance and developmental screening: An either/or proposition? www.dbpeds.org. *AAP SODBP Newsletter* April 2005.

Filipek PA, Accardo PJ, Ashwal S, et al: Practice parameter: Screening and diagnosis of autism. Report of the Quality Standards Subcommittee of the American Academy of Neurology and the Child Neurology Society. *Neurology* 2000;55:468–479.

Gillberg C, Soderstrom H: Learning disability. *Lancet* 2003;362:811–821.

Glascoe FP: Are over-referrals on developmental screening tests really a problem? *Arch Pediatr Adolesc Med* 2001;155:54.

Glascoe FP: Early detection of developmental and behavioral problems. *Pediatr Rev* 2000;21:272–279, quiz 280.

Glascoe FP, Macias MM: Implementing the AAP's new policy on developmental and behavioral screening. *Contemp Pediatr* 2003;4:85.

TABLE 15-4. Diagnostic Work-Up in Learning Disability

NEUROPSYCHOLOGICAL TEST ASSESSMENTS	RELEVANT CLINICAL QUESTIONS AND POSSIBLE CONDITIONS TARGETED BY THE METHOD
Wechsler scales (WPPSI, WISC-III, WAIS-R) or Vineland	General level, verbal-visuospatial differences, specific peaks or troughs
CLINICAL EXAMINATION	
Hight, weight, hyper/hypogenitalism	Sex chromosome aneuploidies, Prader-Willi syndrome
Head circumference	Autism, Sotos syndrome, microcephaly, Rett syndrome
Minor physical anomalies	Chromosomal aberrations
Skin (including Wood light)	Tuberous sclerosis, Ito hypomelanosis, neurofibromatosis, Sturge-Weber syndrome
Scoliosis/kyphosis	Rett syndrome
Heart murmur	Williams syndrome, 22q11 deletion, Down syndrome
Eyesight (including fundus), hearing	Fetal alcohol syndrome, intrauterine infections such as toxoplasmosis, Spielmeyer-Vogt syndrome, homocysteinuria, cytomegalovirus, rubella embryopathy
Hand and overall motor function, tonus, and neurologic aberrations	Rett syndrome, Prader-Willi syndrome, neuromuscular disorders, frontal lobe dysfunctions, central nervous system immaturity
AUTISM SCREENING	
Dysfunction in social interaction, communication, and flexibility, assessed according to the DSM-IV, ICD-10, or by use of a specific rating scale	Autism spectrum disorders
BEHAVIORAL CHARACTERIZATION	
Gaze avoidance, turning away on greeting	Fragile X syndrome
Overeating, skin-picking, temper tantrums	Prader-Willi syndrome
Social chatting, garrulousness, anxiety	Williams syndrome
Aggression	Y chromosome aneuploidies
BASIC LABORATORY ASSESSMENTS (ALL NEWLY DIAGNOSED CASES)	
Thyroid hormones	Hypothyroidism
Hematologic and electrolytic markers	Vitamin or other nutrition deficiencies, endocrine disorders
Karyotype	All sorts of aneuploidies, translocations, deletions, rearrangements
SPECIAL LABORATORY ASSESSMENTS (AS INDICATED BY BASIC WORK-UP)	
Sexual steroids	Inborn errors in sexual hormone metabolism
Parathyroid hormone	Hypoparathyroidism
HIV	AIDS or AIDS-related complex, including cognitive dysfunction and dementia
Polymerase chain reaction/DNA tests	Fragile X, Angelman, Prader-Willi, 22q11 deletion, Williams syndrome
MRI	Malformations, scarring, enlargement of ventricle system, cortical atrophy, white matter changes, migration disturbances, tuberous sclerosis
Electroencephalogram	Slow waves or epileptiform activity
Auditory brainstem responses	Deafness
Metabolic screen, blood/urine	Inborn errors of metabolism, e.g., Sanfilippo syndrome and other mucopolysaccharidoses
Lumbar puncture; protein electrophoresis, gangliosides, amino acids, monoamine metabolites, tau protein, growth-associated protein-43, glial fibrillary acidic protein	Nonketotic hyperglycinemia, infections, nerve cell degeneration, synaptic degeneration and regeneration

From Gillberg C, Soderstrom H: Learning disability. *Lancet* 2003;362:811–821.
DSM-IV, Diagnostic and Statistical Manual of Mental Disorders IV; ICD, international classification of disease.

Schor EL: Rethinking well-child care. *Pediatrics* 2004;114:210–216.

Shevell M, Ashwal S, Donley D, et al: Practice parameter: Evaluation of the child with global developmental delay. *Neurology* 2003;60:367–380.

Shevell MI, Majnemer A, Rosenbaum P, et al: Etiologic yield of subspecialists' evaluation of young children with global developmental delay. *J Pediatr* 2000;136:593–598.

Shonkoff JP, Phillips D (editors): *From Neurons to Neighborhoods: The Science of Early Childhood Development*. Washington, DC, National Academies Press, 2000.

Chapter 16 ■ Child Care

Laura Stout Sosinsky and Walter S. Gilliam

HOW PEDIATRICIANS CAN SUPPORT CHILDREN AND FAMILIES

Child care is a primary developmental context for millions of young children, with important implications for child and family well-being. Second only to the time that young children spend with their families at home is the time that they spend in child care, and child-care providers play a major role in the day-to-day safety, health, and developmental well-being of young children. Given the large number of young children in child-care settings, child-care providers are an important potential ally to parents and pediatricians. The provision of child care in America, however, is complex. Pediatricians need to understand how child care is structured and utilized, the challenges parents face in finding and accessing high-quality child-care arrangements, and the challenges child-care providers face in maintaining a physically and developmentally healthy environment, in order to maximize their effectiveness across all of the environments in which young children grow and develop.

THE PROVISION AND REGULATION OF CHILD CARE IN AMERICA

USAGE OF CHILD CARE. About 10.7 million young children are regularly in care by someone other than their parents, largely due to the vast increase in employment of mothers of young children in recent decades. Eighty percent of 5 yr old children and 75% of children 4 yr old and younger with employed parents are in regular child care, attending an average of 40 hr/week. The largest increase has been in the use of child care by infants and toddlers, with 41% of infants and 53% of toddlers in child care.

CHILD-CARE SETTINGS. Child-care settings vary widely and fall into 4 broad categories, from the least to the most formal: relative care, in-home nonrelative care (nannies, au pairs), family daycare, and center-based care. Parents more often utilize home-based care for infants and toddlers, due in part to preference, greater flexibility and availability, and sometimes lower cost. Almost 30% of infants and toddlers in care are in family daycare homes. Family daycare providers typically provide care in their homes for up to 6 young children, often of mixed ages. The use of center-based child care, provided in nonresidential facilities, typically for 13 or more children, is greater among preschoolers. Early education settings for preschoolers (Head Start, prekindergarten, nursery school) technically are not considered child care (they may have a greater focus on educational activities and are often part-day programs), but the health and safety issues involved with child participation in early education programs are similar to those presented by other group child-care settings, and these programs may also play an important role in caring for young children of working parents. Child-care centers and early education programs are administered by a wide array of businesses and organizations, including for-profit independent companies and chains, religious organizations, public and private schools, community organizations, cooperatives, and public agencies.

Sick children are typically excluded from out-of-home arrangements; settings under state licensure are required to exclude children with certain conditions, described in the next section and in Table 16-1. Most families need to make arrangements to keep sick children at home (staying home from work). Alternative care arrangements outside the home for sick children are relatively rare, but include care in the child's own center, with special provisions designed for the care of ill children (sometimes called the *infirmary model* or *sick daycare*), and care in a center that serves only children with illness or temporary health conditions. Although it is important that such arrangements emphasize preventing further spread of disease, one study found no occurrence of additional transmission of communicable disease in children attending a sick center. The impact of group care of ill children on their subsequent health and on the health of their families and the community is unknown.

LICENSING, REGULATION, AND ACCREDITATION OF CHILD CARE. Most child-care centers and preschools and many family daycare providers are subject to state licensing and regulation. Licensing and regulatory requirements for the most part mandate basic health and safety standards, such as sanitary practices, child vaccinations, access to a health care professional, and safety of facilities and equipment, as well as basic structural and caregiver characteristics, such as the ratio of children to staff, group sizes, and minimum education and training requirements for caregivers. Guidelines for health and safety in out-of-home care from the American Academy of Pediatrics, the American Public Health Association, and the National Resource Center for Health and Safety in Child Care offer recommendations regarding the conditions under which sick children should and should not be excluded from group programs (Table 16-2), including fever, vomiting, and diarrhea, as well as certain parasitic conditions. State laws typically mirror these guidelines, but may be stricter in some states.

Many providers are exempt from licensing requirements (programs operated by a religious organization or a public school), many others are out of compliance, and an unknown proportion of family daycare homes are unregulated and "underground." Health and safety conditions may be unsatisfactory in unlicensed settings. Furthermore, in most states, licensing and regulatory standards are inadequate to promote optimal child development, and in many states, standards are so low as to endanger child health and safety. Therefore, even licensed providers may be providing care at levels far below professional recommendations. Many states legally allow infant-to-staff ratios of 5–6 : 1, whereas professional organizations such as the National Association for the Education of Young Children (NAEYC; *www.naeyc.org*) and the National Association for Family Child Care (NAFCC; *www.nafcc.org*) recommend infant-to-staff ratios of 3 : 1.

A small portion of providers become accredited by NAEYC, NAFCC, or other organizations by voluntarily meeting high-quality, developmentally appropriate, professionally recommended standards. The accreditation process goes beyond health and safety practices and structural and caregiver characteristics to examine the quality of child-caregiver interactions, which are crucial for child development, as described in the next section. Indeed, research indicates that child-care programs that complete voluntary accreditation through NAEYC improve in quality and provide an environment that better facilitates children's overall development. However, fewer than 8% of providers are accredited; this is due in part to a lack of knowledge, resources, and incentives for providers to improve quality, but it is also due in part to expenses providers incur in the process as well as to insufficient capacity of accrediting organizations.

THE ROLE OF CHILD CARE IN CHILD HEALTH AND DEVELOPMENT

CHARACTERISTICS OF CHILD CARE AND CHILD DEVELOPMENTAL OUTCOMES. High-quality child care is characterized by warm, responsive, and stimulating interactions between children and caregivers. In high-quality interactions, caregivers express positive feelings in interactions with children, are emotionally involved, engaged, and aware of the child's needs and sensitive and responsive to their initiations, speak directly with children in a manner that is elaborative and stimulating while being age-appropriate, and ask questions and encourage children's ideas and verbalizations. Structural quality features of the setting,

TABLE 16-1. Child Care Resources

ORGANIZATION	SPONSOR	WEBSITE AND CONTACT INFORMATION
Child Care Aware	National Association of Child Care Resource and Referral Agencies	*http://www.childcareaware.org/*800-424-2246
Healthy Child Care America	American Academy of Pediatrics (AAP)	*www.healthychildcare.org*
National Association for Family Child Care		*www.nafcc.org*
National Association for Sick Child Daycare (NASCD)		*www.nascd.com*
National Association for the Education of Young Children (NAEYC)		*www.naeyc.org*
National Child Care Information Center	U.S. Department of Health and Human Services, Administration for Children & Families Child Care Bureau	*http://www.nccic.org/*
National Resource Center for Health and Safety in Child Care (NRC)		*http://nrc.uchsc.edu* 800-598-KIDS (5437) For the 2002 report from the AAP, APHA & NRC, *Caring for Our Children: National Health and Safety Performance Standards: Guidelines for Out-of-Home Child Care: Second Edition.* go to: *http://nrc.uchsc.edu/CFOC/index.html*

TABLE 16-2. Conditions That May or May Not Require Exclusion From Group Child Care Settings

CONDITIONS THAT REQUIRE EXCLUSION	COMMENTS
Illness preventing the child from participating comfortably in activities as determined by the child care provider	Providers should specify in their policies, approved by the facilities' health care consultant, what severity level of illness the facility can manage and how much and what types of illness will be addressed. Severity level 1 consists of children whose health condition is accompanied by high interest and complete involvement in activity associated with an absence of symptoms of illness (such as children recovering from pinkeye, rash, or chickenpox), but who need further recuperation time. Severity level 2 encompasses children whose health condition is accompanied by a medium activity level because of symptoms (such as children with low-grade fever, children at the beginning of an illness, and children in the early recovery period of an illness). Severity level 3 is composed of children whose health condition is accompanied by a low activity level because of symptoms that preclude much involvement.
Illness resulting in a greater need for care than the child care staff can provide without compromising the health and safety of the other children as determined by the child care provider	
Fever	Accompanied by behavior changes or other signs or symptoms of illness until medical professional evaluation finds the child able to be included at the facility
Symptoms and signs of possibly severe illness, including lethargy, uncontrolled coughing, inexplicable irritability or persistent crying, difficult breathing, wheezing, or other unusual signs for the child	Until evaluation by a medical professional finds the child able to be included at the facility
Diarrhea	Children whose stools remain loose but who otherwise seem well and whose stool cultures are negative need not be excluded. Children with diarrheal illness of infectious origin generally may be allowed to return to child care once the diarrhea resolves, except children with positive cultures for *Salmonella typhi* (3 negative stool cultures required for inclusion), *Shigella*, or *Escherichia coli 0157:H7* (2 negative stool cultures required for inclusion)
Blood in stool	Not explained by dietary change, medication, or hard stools
Vomiting	2 or more episodes of vomiting in the previous 24 hours until vomiting resolves or until a health care provider determines that the cause of the vomiting is not contagious and the child is not in danger of dehydration
Abdominal pain	Persistent (continues more than 2 hours) or intermittent associated with fever or other signs or symptoms
Mouth sores with drooling	Unless a health care professional or health department official determines that the child is noninfectious
Rash with fever or behavior changes	Until a physician determines that these symptoms do not indicate a communicable disease
Purulent conjunctivitis	Defined as pink or red conjunctiva with white or yellow eye discharge, until after treatment has been initiated
Pediculosis (head lice)	Exclusion at the end of the day is appropriate
Scabies	Until after treatment has been completed
Tuberculosis	Until a health care provider or health official states that the child is on appropriate therapy and can attend child care
Impetigo	Until 24 hours after treatment has been initiated
Strep throat	Or other streptococcal infection until 24 hours after initial antibiotic treatment and cessation of fever
Varicella-Zoster (chickenpox)	Until all sores have dried and crusted (usually 6 days)
Pertussis	Until 5 days of appropriate antibiotic treatment (currently erythromycin, which is given for 14 consecutive days) has been completed
Mumps	Until 9 days after onset of parotid gland swelling
Hepatitis A virus	Until 1 week after onset of illness, jaundice, or as directed by the health department when passive immunoprophylaxis (currently, immune serum globulin) has been administered to appropriate children and staff members
Measles	Until 4 days after onset of rash
Rubella	Until 6 days after onset of rash
Unspecified respiratory tract illness	
Shingles (herpes zoster)	
Herpes simplex	
CONDITIONS THAT DO NOT REQUIRE EXCLUSION	**COMMENTS**
Presence of bacteria or viruses in urine or feces in the absence of illness symptoms, like diarrhea	Exceptions include children infected with highly contagious organisms capable of causing serious illness
Nonpurulent conjunctivitis	Pink conjunctiva with a clear, watery eye discharge and without fever, eye pain, or eyelid redness
Rash without fever and without behavioral changes	
CMV infection	
Hepatitis B virus carrier state	Provided that children who carry HBV chronically have no behavioral or medical risk factors, such as unusually aggressive behavior (biting, frequent scratching), generalized dermatitis, or bleeding problems
HIV infection	Provided that the health, neurologic development, behavior, and immune status of an HIV-infected child are appropriate as determined on a case-by-case basis by qualified health professionals, including the child's health care provider, who are able to evaluate whether the child will receive optimal care in the specific facility being considered and whether that child poses a potential threat to others
Parvovirus B19 infection	In a person with a normal immune system

Adapted from American Academy of Pediatrics, American Public Health Association, National Resource Center for Health and Safety in Child Care. *Caring for Our Children: National Health and Safety Performance Standards: Guidelines for Out-of-Home Child Care:* Second Edition. Elk Grove Village, IL: American Academy of Pediatrics, American Public Health Association, and National Resource Center for Health and Safety in Child Care; 2002, pp. 124–129. *http://nrc.uchsc.edu/CFOC/index.html*

including ratio of children to adults, group size, and caregiver education and training, act indirectly on child outcomes by facilitating high-quality child-caregiver interactions. It would be difficult for even the most sensitive and stimulating provider to provide high-quality interactions with each child if he or she was the sole caregiver of 10 toddlers.

The quality, as well as the quantity and type, of child care experienced by young children contributes to child development. Child's experience of child care *per se* is not related to better or worse outcomes for children compared to child's experience of exclusive maternal care. Child care use by itself does not affect maternal-child attachment. Only when combined with low maternal sensitivity and responsiveness does poor-quality child care, larger quantities of child care, or multiple child care arrangements predict greater likelihood of insecure attachment.

Adjusting for family factors (parental income, education, race/ethnicity, family structure, parental sensitivity) child care quality is a consistent and modest predictor of child outcomes across most domains of development, child care quantity is a consistent, modest predictor of social behavior, and type of child care setting is an inconsistent, modest predictor of cognitive and social outcomes. Specifically in regards to quality, children who experience higher-quality child care perform better than other children on cognitive, language, and academic skill tests and, at some points in early childhood, show more prosocial skills and fewer behavior problems and negative peer interactions. Compared to these effects, which are relatively consistent and modest in magnitude, the effects of parenting quality on the same outcomes are consistent and strong, being about twice as strong as the effects of child care quality.

The magnitudes of the effects of quantity and type of child care are less strong and consistent. Quantity of child care is related only to social outcomes. Children who spend more time in any kind of child care are rated or observed at some points in the preschool period to display more problem behaviors, more teacher–child conflict, and more negative behaviors in interactions with friends. The magnitudes of these effects of child care hours on social outcomes are modest. Type of care shows mixed associations with child outcomes. Although findings vary across age, children who experience more center care have stronger cognitive, language, and memory skills and display more positive behaviors in interactions with a friend, but also show fewer prosocial skills and more behavior problems. These effects of center-based care on child outcomes are less consistent and modest compared to other reported effects.

Despite the importance of high-quality child care for child development, several studies have found that most child care is of "poor to mediocre" quality. In one study, only 14% of centers (8% of center-based infant care) were found to provide developmentally appropriate care, while 12% scored at minimal levels that compromised health and safety (40% for infant care). Similarly, in another study, 58% of family day care homes provided adequate or custodial care, and only 8% provided good care. Children with the greatest amount of family risk may be the most likely to receive child care that is substandard in quality. Many children from lower-risk families also receive lower-quality care, and despite advantages at home, these children may not be protected from the negative effects of poor-quality care.

Affordable, accessible, high-quality child care is hard to find. Middle-class families spend about 6% of their annual income on child care expenses, while poor families spend about 33% (on par with housing expenses). Infant and toddler care is particularly expensive with fewer available slots. In addition to the stress of meeting such a high expense, many parents worry that their child will feel unhappy in group settings, will suffer from separation from the parents, or will even be subjected to neglect or abuse. This worry is especially likely among low-income parents with more risk factors, fewer resources, and fewer high-quality options available. Parents are the purchasers but not the recipients of care, and are not in the best position to judge its quality. Many parents are 1st time purchasers of child care with little experience and very immediate needs, selecting care in a market that does little to provide them with useful information about child care arrangements. To inform their care decisions, parents may turn to their child's pediatrician as the only professional with expertise in child development with whom they have regular and convenient contact. Pediatricians can best aid parents with this major decision if armed with straightforward understanding of child care and knowledge of key research findings on its quality and effects on child development.

CHILD CARE AND CHILD HEALTH (SEE ALSO CHAPTER 172). Child care has specific implications for child health. First, a disproportionate number of sudden infant death syndrome (SIDS) deaths occur in child-care centers or family-based child-care homes (approximately 20%). Infants who are back-sleepers at home, but are put to sleep on the abdomen in child-care settings, have a higher risk of SIDS. Providers and parents should be made aware of the importance of placing infants on their backs to sleep.

Second, children enrolled in child care are of an age that places them at increased risk for acquiring infectious diseases. Participation in group settings elevates exposure. Children enrolled in such settings have a higher incidence of illness, especially in the preschool years (upper respiratory tract infections, otitis media, diarrhea, hepatitis A infections, skin conditions, and asthma) than those cared for at home. Child-care providers who follow guidelines for handwashing, diapering, food handling, and managing child illness appropriately can reduce communicable illnesses.

There is debate about whether exposure to child care serves as a risk or a protective factor for asthma. One cross-sectional study found that preschoolers in child care had increased risk of the common cold and otitis media, and children who began child care before the age of 2 yr had increased risk of recurrent otitis media and asthma. However, a longitudinal study found that children who were exposed to older children at home or to other children at child care during the first 6 mo of life were less likely to have frequent wheezing from age 6–13 yr, suggesting that child care exposure protects against the development of asthma and frequent wheezing later in childhood. Other factors may also be relevant to this issue (children in child care may be exposed to less passive smoking than children at home).

CHILD CARE AND CHILDREN WITH SPECIAL NEEDS (SEE ALSO CHAPTER 38). The needs of children with mental, physical, or emotional disabilities who, because of their chronic illness, require special care and instruction may require particular attention when it comes to participation in most child-care settings. Guiding principles of services for children with disabilities advocate supporting children in natural environments, including child care. Furthermore, the Americans with Disabilities Act and Section 504 of the Rehabilitation Act of 1973 prohibit discrimination against children and adults with disabilities by requiring equal access to offered programs and services.

Although many child-care providers and settings are unprepared to identify or administer services to children with special needs, child care could be utilized for delivery of support services to these children and/or for linking families to services, such as early intervention and physician referrals. Furthermore, pediatricians can draw on child-care providers to help provide important evaluative data regarding a child's well-being, since these providers have extensive daily contact with the child and may have a broad, professional understanding of normative child development. For example, a child-care provider may be the first to identify a child's potential language delay. Child-care providers are also necessary and valuable partners in the development and administration of early intervention service plans.

Children with special needs may be eligible for services under the Individuals with Disabilities Education Act (IDEA). The purpose of this law is to provide "free appropriate public education," regardless of disability or chronic illness, to all eligible children aged birth to 21 yr in a natural and/or least restrictive environment. Eligible children include those with mental, physical, or emotional disabilities who, because of their disability or chronic illness, require special instruction in order to learn. As a part of these services, a formal plan of intervention is to be developed by the service providers, the children's families, and the children's health care providers. Federal funds are available to implement a collaborative early intervention system of services for eligible infants and toddlers between the ages of birth and 3 yr and their families. These services include screening, assessment, service coordination, and collaborative development of an **individualized family service plan (IFSP)**. The IFSP describes early intervention services for the infant or toddler and the family, including family support and the child's health, therapeutic, and educational needs. An understanding of the child's routines and real-life opportunities and activities, such as eating, playing, interaction with others, and working on developmental skills, is crucial to enhancing a child's ability to achieve the functional goals of the IFSP. Therefore, it is critical that child-care providers be involved in IFSP development or revision, with parental consent. Child-care providers should also become familiar with the child's IFSP and understand the providers' role and the resources available to support the family and child-care provider.

In addition, IDEA provides support for eligible preschool children to receive services through the local school district. These services include development of a written **individualized education program (IEP)**, with implementation being the responsibility of the local education agency in either a public or a private preschool setting. As with IFSPs, child-care providers should become familiar with the preschooler's special needs as identified in the IEP and may become involved, with parental consent, in IEP development and review meetings. In cases where children may have or may be at risk for developmental delays, a diagnosis is important for obtaining and coordinating services and further evaluation. Pediatricians can partner with child-care providers to screen and monitor children's behavior and development.

THE ROLE OF PEDIATRIC PROVIDERS IN CHILD CARE

Pediatricians can promote successful child-care experiences for their young patients in several ways, including helping parents understand child-care issues, helping children with disabilities and their families have successful child-care experiences, and consulting with child-care or early intervention and education providers.

ADVISING PARENTS ON CHILD CARE SELECTION. Little organized professional guidance in choosing child care is available, and pediatricians may be many parents' only source of professional consultation regarding their child. Pediatricians can help parents understand the importance for their child's development of high-quality care, describe how it looks, and provide referrals and tips on how to find and select high-quality child care (see Table 16-1). In addition, pediatricians can help parents determine how to adjust child-care arrangements to best meet their child's specific needs (e.g., allergies, eating and sleeping habits). For most parents, finding child care that they can afford, access, manage, and accept as a good environment for their child is a very difficult process and one that many parents find distressing. Many parents are also worried about how their child will fare in child care (e.g., Will the child feel distressed by group settings, suffer from separation from the parents, or even be subjected to neglect or abuse?). These worries are especially likely among low-income parents with fewer family and community resources. A few parents may think of child care only as baby sitting, and may not consider consequences for their child's development so long as the child is safe and warm. These parents are less likely to select a high-quality child-care arrangement, which is especially problematic if the family is facing socioeconomic challenges that already place them at risk for receiving lower-quality care for their children. For these parents, it is vital to stress the importance of high-quality child care and its implications for their child's cognitive, language, and behavioral development and school readiness.

ADVISING PARENTS ON CHILD CARE HEALTH ISSUES. First, parents of infants should be advised to ensure that child-care providers put infants on their backs to sleep to prevent SIDS. Second, when children are ill, parents should be advised to follow guidelines for inclusion and exclusion (see Table 16-2). Parents may disagree with child-care staff about whether a child meets or does not meet the exclusion criteria. However, professional guidelines state that "if the reason for exclusion relates to the child's ability to participate or the caregiver's ability to provide care for the other children, the child-care provider is entitled to make this decision and cannot be forced by a parent to accept responsibility for the care of an ill child. If the reason for exclusion relates to a decision about whether the child has a communicable disease that poses a risk to the other children in the group, different health care professionals in the community might give conflicting opinions. In these cases, the health department has the legal authority to make a determination." Third, pediatricians should emphasize the importance of following vaccination schedules; most states require compliance for children to participate in licensed group child-care settings.

HELPING CHILDREN WITH SPECIAL NEEDS. Pediatricians should work with parents and communicate with other service providers and early intervention staff to identify problems, remove access barriers, and coordinate service delivery for children with special needs. They should also encourage the involvement of parents and child-care providers in IFSP or IEP development.

CONSULTATION AND PARTNERING WITH CHILD-CARE PROVIDERS. Pediatricians can provide consultation to child-care providers about measures to protect and maintain the health and safety of children and staff. This may include proper practices to prevent SIDS; prevent and reduce the spread of communicable diseases; reduce allergen, toxin, and parasite exposure; ensure vaccinations for children and staff; remove environmental hazards; and prevent injuries. Most state regulations mandate that licensed programs have a formal relationship with a health care provider.

American Academy of Pediatrics, American Public Health Association, National Resource Center for Health and Safety in Child Care: *Caring for Our Children: National Health and Safety Performance Standards: Guidelines for Out-of-Home Child Care,* 2nd ed. Elk Grove Village, IL, American Academy of Pediatrics, American Public Health Association, and National Resource Center for Health and Safety in Child Care, 2002.

Ball TM, Castro-Rodriguez JA, Griffith KA, et al: Siblings, day-care attendance, and the risk of asthma and wheezing during childhood. *N Engl J Med* 2000;343:538–543.

Belsky J, Rovine MJ: Nonmaternal care in the first year of life and the security of infant-parent attachment. *Child Dev* 1988;59:157–167.

Dompeling E, Jobsis R, van Schayck O: Siblings, day-care attendance, and the risk of asthma and wheezing. [comment]. *N Engl J Med* 2000;343:1967; author reply 1968.

Farkas S, Duffet A, Johnson J: *Necessary compromises: How parents, employers, and children's advocates view child care today.* Washington, DC, Public Agenda, 2000.

Gilliam WS, Meisels SJ, Mayes LC: Screening and surveillance in early intervention systems. In: Guralnick MJ, ed. *The developmental systems approach to early intervention.* Baltimore, MD, Paul H. Brookes, 2005.

Helburn SW, ed: *Cost, quality, and child outcomes in child care centers, Public report, second edition.* Denver, CO: Department of Economics, Center for Research in Economic and Social Policy, University of Colorado; 1995.

Helburn SW: Preface. *Ann Am Acad Pol and Soc Sci* 1999;563:8–19.

Kontos S, Howes C, Shinn M, Galinsky E: *Quality in family child care and relative care.* New York, Teachers College Press, 1995.

Lombardi J: *Time to care: Redesigning child care to promote education, support families, and build communities.* Philadelphia, Temple University Press, 2003.

Nafstad P, Hagen JA, Oie L, Magnus P, Jaakkola JJ: Day care centers and respiratory health. *Pediatrics* 1999;103:753–758.

NICHD Early Child Care Research Network: The effects of infant child care on infant-mother attachment security: Results of the NICHD study of early child care. *Child Dev* 1997;68:860–879.

NICHD Early Child Care Research Network: *Child care and child development: Results from the NICHD Study of Early Child Care and Youth Development.* New York, The Guilford Press, 2005.

NICHD Early Child Care Research Network: Child-care effect sizes for the NICHD Study of Early Child Care and Youth Development. *Am Psychol* 2006;61:99–116.

Peisner-Feinberg ES, Burchinal MR: Relations between preschool children's child-care experiences and concurrent development: The Cost, Quality, and Outcomes Study. *Merrill-Palmer Quarterly* 1997;43:451–477.

Shonkoff JP, Phillips DA: *From Neurons to Neighborhoods: The Science of Early Childhood Development.* Washington, DC, National Academy Press, 2000.

Sosinsky LS: *Parental selection of child care quality: Income, demographic risk, and beliefs about harm of maternal employment to children* [Dissertation]. New Haven, CT, Department of Psychology, Yale University, 2005.

Whitebook M, Sakai L, Howes C: *NAEYC Accreditation as a Strategy for Improving Child Care Quality.* Washington, DC, National Center for the Early Childhood Workforce, 1999.

Young KT, Marsland KW, Zigler EF: The regulatory status of center-based infant and toddler child care. *Am J of Orthopsychiatry* 1997;67:535–544.

Chapter 17 ■ Separation, Loss, and Bereavement

Janet R. Serwint

Children may experience involuntary separation from loved ones, think about death, and encounter death in their personal lives. Parents and children often turn to their pediatrician and other health care professionals for help following various types of personal losses. Relatively brief separations of children from their parents, such as vacations, usually produce minor transient effects, but more enduring and frequent separation may cause sequelae. The potential impact of each event must be considered in light of the age and stage of development of the child, the particular relationship with the absent person, and the nature of the situation. As a trustworthy, familiar resource, pediatricians are uniquely positioned to offer information, support, and guidance, and to facilitate coping.

SEPARATION AND LOSS. Separations may occur for a variety of reasons. These may be due to temporary causes, such as vacations, parental job restrictions, natural disasters, or parental or sibling illness requiring hospitalization. More long-term separations occur due to divorce, placement in foster care, or adoption, while permanent separation may occur due to death. The initial reaction of young children to separation of any duration may involve crying, either of a tantrum-like, protesting type or of a quieter, sadder type. Children's behavior may be subdued, withdrawn, fussy, moody, or resistant to authority. Specific problems may include poor appetite, behavior issues such as acting against caregiver requests, reluctance to go to bed, sleep problems, or regressive behavior such as requesting a bottle or bet-wetting. School-aged children may experience impaired cognitive functioning and poor performance in school. While some children may repeatedly ask for the absent parent and question when he or she will return, other children may not refer to parental absence at all. The child may go to the window or door or out into the neighborhood to look for the absent parent; a few may even leave home or their place of temporary placement to search for their parents.

A child's response to **reunion** may surprise or alarm an unprepared parent. A parent who joyfully returns to the family may be met by wary or cautious children. After a brief interchange of affection, children may seem indifferent to the parent's return. This response may indicate anger at being left and wariness that the event will happen again, or the child may feel as if he or she caused the parent's departure due to magical thinking. If the mother who frequently says "Stop it, or you'll give me a headache" is hospitalized, the child may feel unrealistically at fault and guilty. As a result of these feelings, children may seem to be more closely attached to the other present parent than to the absent one, or even to the grandparent or baby sitter who cared for them during their parent's absence. Immediately after the reunion or after a few days, some children, particularly younger ones, may become more clinging and dependent than they were before the separation, while continuing any regressive behavior that occurred during the separation. Such behavior may engage the returned parent more closely and help to re-establish the bond that the child felt was broken. Such reactions are usually transient; within 1–2 wk, children will have recovered their usual behavior and equilibrium. Recurrent separations may tend to make children more wary and guarded about re-establishing the relationship with the repeatedly absent parent, and these traits may affect other personal relationships. Parents should not try to ameliorate a child's behavior by threatening to leave.

DIVORCE. Experiences of loss, such as divorce or placement in foster care, can give rise to the same kinds of reactions noted earlier, but they are more intense and possibly more lasting. Currently, as many as 40% of marriages end in divorce. Divorce has been found to be associated with negative parent functioning such as parental depression and feelings of incompetence, negative child behavior such as noncompliance and whining, and negative parent-child interaction such as inconsistent discipline, decreased communication, and decreased affection. Greater childhood distress is associated with greater parental distress. Continued parental conflict and loss of contact with the noncustodial parent, usually the father, is common. Two of the most important factors that contribute to morbidity of the children in a divorce include parental psychopathology and disrupted parenting before the separation. While the year following the divorce is the period when problems are most apparent, these problems tend to dissipate over the next 2 yr. In some children, depression is present 5 yr later, and educational or occupational decline may occur 10 yr later. It is difficult to sort out all of the confounding factors. Children may suffer when exposed to parental conflict that may not end after divorce, and in some cases may escalate. The degree of inter-parental conflict may be the most important factor associated with child morbidity. A continued relationship with the non-custodial parent, as long as there is minimal inter-parental conflict, was a factor associated with more positive outcomes.

School-aged children may respond with evident depression, may seem indifferent, or may be markedly angry. Other children appear to deny or avoid the issue, behaviorally or verbally. Most children cling to the hope or fantasy that the actual placement or separation is not real and is only temporary. The child may experience guilt by feeling that the loss, separation, or placement represents rejection and perhaps punishment for misbehavior. Children may protect a parent and assume guilt, believing that their own "badness" caused the parent to depart. Outwardly blaming parents may be perceived by a child as fairly risky; parents who discover that a child harbors resentment might punish him or her further for these thoughts or feelings. Children who feel that their misbehavior caused their parents to separate or become divorced have the fantasy that their own trivial or recurrent behavioral patterns caused their parents to become angry with each other. Some children have behavioral or psychosomatic symptoms and unwittingly adopt a "sick" role as a strategy for reuniting their parents.

In response to separation and divorce of parents, older children and adolescents commonly show intense anger. Five years after the breakup, about ⅓ of the children are "consciously and intensely unhappy and dissatisfied with their life in the post-divorce family." Another ⅓ show clear evidence of a satisfactory adjustment, and the remaining ⅓ demonstrate a mixed picture, with good achievement in some areas and faltering achievement in others. After 10 yr, 45% do well, but 41% may have academic, social, and/or emotional problems. As adults, some are reluctant to form intimate relationships, fearful of repeating their parents' experience. Parental divorce has a moderate long-term negative impact on the adult mental health status of children who had experienced it, even after controlling for changes in economic status and problems before divorce. Good adjustment of children after a divorce is related to ongoing involvement with 2 psychologically healthy parents who minimize conflict, and to the siblings and other relatives as a positive support system. Divorcing parents should be encouraged to avoid the adversarial process and to use a trained mediator to resolve disputes. Joint custody arrangements may reduce ongoing parental conflict, but children in joint custody may feel overburdened by the demands of maintaining a strong presence in 2 homes.

The primary care provider may provide an important role for divorcing and divorced parents and their children. When asked about the effects of divorce, parents should be informed that different children may have different reactions, but that the parents' behavior and the way they interact with each other will have a major effect on the child's adjustment. The continued presence of both parents in the child's life, provided it doesn't cause continued inter-parental conflict, is most beneficial to the child.

MOVE/FAMILY RELOCATION. Another version of a separation experience occurs when a child's family moves. A significant proportion of the population of the USA changes residence each year. The effects of this movement on children and families are frequently overlooked; for children, the move is essentially involuntary and out of their control. When such changes in family structure as divorce or death precipitate moves, children face the stresses created by both the precipitating events and the move itself. Parental sadness surrounding the move may transmit unhappiness to the children. Children who move lose their old friends, the comfort of a familiar bedroom and house, and their ties to school and community. They not only must sever old relationships but also are faced with developing new ones in new neighborhoods and new schools. Children may enter neighborhoods with new and different customs and values, and because academic standards and curricula vary among communities, children who have performed well in one school may find themselves struggling in a new one. Frequent moves during the school years are likely to have adverse consequences on social and academic performance.

Migrant children and children who move from other countries present with special circumstances. These children not only need to adjust to a new house, school, and community but also need to adjust to a new culture and, in many cases, a new language. Because children have faster language acquisition than adults, they may function as translators for the adults in their families. This powerful position may lead to role reversal and potential conflict within the family. In the evaluation of migrant children and families, it is also important to ask about the circumstances of the migration, including legal status, violence or threat of violence, conflict of loyalties, and moral, ethical, and religious differences.

Parents should prepare children well in advance of any move and allow them to express any unhappy feelings or misgivings. Parents should acknowledge their own mixed feelings and agree that they will miss their old home while looking forward to a new one. Visits to the new home in advance are often useful preludes to the actual move. Transient periods of regressive behavior may be noted in preschool children after moving, and these should be understood and accepted. Parents should assist the entry of their children into the new community, and whenever possible, exchanges of letters and visits with old friends should be encouraged.

SEPARATION DUE TO HOSPITALIZATION. Potential challenges for hospitalized children include coping with separation, adapting to a new environment, adjusting to multiple caregivers, seeing very sick children, and sometimes experiencing the disorientation of intensive care, anesthesia, and surgery. To help mitigate potential problems, a preadmission visit to the hospital is important to allow the child to meet the people who will be offering care and ask questions about what will happen. For children younger than 5–6 yr of age, parents should room with the child if feasible. Creative and active recreational or socialization programs, with liberal visiting hours (including visits from siblings), and chances to act out feared procedures in play with dolls or mannequins all are helpful. Sensitive, sympathetic, and accepting attitudes toward children and parents by the hospital staff are very important. An underlying tension may exist between the hospital caregivers and the parent, often exacerbated by hospital routines and schedules. Guilt and anger can result, unnecessarily complicating an already difficult situation.

The psychologic aspects of illness should be evaluated from the outset, and physicians should act as a model for parents and children by showing interest in a child's feelings and demonstrating that it is possible and appropriate to communicate discomfort in verbal, symbolic language. Continuity of medical personnel may be reassuring to the child and family.

PARENTAL/SIBLING DEATH. Approximately 5–8% of USA children will experience parental death; rates are much higher in other parts of the world more directly affected by war, AIDS, and natural disasters. Children from homes where a parent has died may display fewer long-term problem behaviors than children from homes where parents have divorced. Anticipated deaths due to chronic illness may place a significant strain on a family, with frequent bouts of illness, hospitalization, disruption of normal home life, absence of the ill parent, and perhaps more responsibilities placed on the child. Additional strains include changes in daily routines, financial pressures, and the need to cope with aggressive treatment options.

Children can and should continue to be involved with the sick parent or sibling, but they need to be prepared for what they will see in the home or hospital setting. The stresses that a child will face include visualizing the physical deterioration of the family member, helplessness, and emotional lability. Forewarning the child that the family member may demonstrate physical changes, such as appearing thinner or losing hair, will help the child to adjust. These warnings, combined with simple yet specific explanations of the need for equipment such as a nasogastric tube for nutrition, an oxygen mask, or a ventilator, will help lessen the child's fear. The primary care provider can be of great help in addressing these issues. Children should be honestly informed of what is happening, in language they can understand, allowing them choices, but with parental involvement in decision-making. They should be encouraged, but not forced to see their ill family member. Parents who are caring for a dying spouse or child may be too emotionally depleted to be able to tend to their healthy child's needs or to continue regular routines. Children of a dying parent may suffer the loss of security and belief in the world as a safe place, and the surviving parent may be inclined to impose his or her own need for support and comfort onto the child. However, the well parent and caring relatives must keep in mind that children need to be allowed to remain children, with appropriate support and attention.

GRIEF AND BEREAVEMENT. Grief is a personal, emotional state of bereavement or an anticipated response to loss. Common reactions include sadness, anger, guilt, fear, and at times, relief. The normality of these reactions needs to be emphasized. Most bereaved families remain socially connected and expect that life will return to some new, albeit different, sense of normalcy. However, the pain and suffering imposed by grief should never be automatically deemed "normal" and thus neglected or ignored. In uncomplicated grief reactions, the steadfast concern of the pediatrician can help promote the family's sense of well-being. In more distressing reactions (such as those seen in traumatic grief), the pediatrician may be a major, first-line force in helping children and families address their loss.

Participation in the care of a child with a life-threatening or terminal illness is a profound experience. See Chapter 40 for a discussion of palliative and end-of-life care. Parents experience much anxiety and worry during the final stages of their child's life. Forty-five percent of children dying from cancer died in the pediatric intensive care unit, and parents report that 89% of their children suffered "a lot" or "a great deal" during the last month of life. Physicians consistently underreport children's symptoms in comparison to parents' reports. We need to find ways to better provide for dying children, to allow them comfort, and to arrange for them to die at home if that is their desire. Only then can parents be truly supported and find some peace at the time of their child's anticipated death.

The practice of withholding information from children and parents and parents regarding a child's diagnosis and prognosis has generally been abandoned as physicians have learned that protecting parents and patients from the seriousness of their child's condition does not alleviate concerns and anxieties. Even very young children may have a real understanding of their illness. Children who have serious diseases and are undergoing aggressive treatments or medication regimens, but are told by their parents that they are okay, are not reassured by their parents. These children understand that something serious is happening to them, and they are often forced to suffer in silence and isolation because the message they have been given by their parents is not to discuss it and to maintain a cheerful demeanor. Children have the right to know their diagnosis and should be informed early in their treatment. The content and depth of the discussion needs to be tailored to the child's personality and developmental level of understanding. Parents have choices as to how to orchestrate the disclosure. Parents may want to be the ones to inform the child themselves, may choose for the pediatric health care provider to do so, or may do it in partnership with the pediatrician.

A death, especially the **death of a family member,** is the most difficult loss for a child. Many changes in normal patterns of functioning may occur, including loss of love and support from the deceased family member, a change in income, the possible need to relocate, less emotional support from surviving family members, altering of routines, and a possible change in status from sibling to only child. Relationships between family members may become strained, and children may blame themselves or other family members for the death of a parent or sibling. Bereaved children may exhibit many of the emotions discussed earlier, in addition to behaviors of withdrawal into their own world, sleep disturbances, nightmares, and symptoms such as headache, abdominal pains, or possibly symptoms similar to those of the family member who has died. Children 3–5 yr of age who have experienced a family bereavement, compared with children who have not, are more likely to demonstrate nausea, skin rash, and bed-wetting. In children 6–11 yr old, symptoms include nonspecific pains, headaches, nausea, eye problems, skin rash, stomachache, vomiting, and daytime wetting, while in children 12–18 yr old, symptoms include exacerbation of asthma, nonspecific aches and pains, headaches, nausea, skin rash, and stomachaches. The presence of secure and stable adults who can meet the child's needs and who permit discussion about the loss is most important in helping a child to grieve. The pediatrician should help the family understand this necessary presence and encourage the protective functioning of the family unit.

Death, separation, and loss as a result of natural catastrophes and man-made disasters have become increasingly common events in children's lives. Exposure to such disasters occurs either directly or indirectly, where the event is experienced through the media. Examples of indirect exposure include televised scenes of hurricanes, tsunamis, and the terrorist attacks in the USA on 9/11/01, with the subsequent news stories about anthrax and heightened states of alert. Children who experience personal loss in disasters tend to watch more television coverage than children who do not. However, children without a personal loss watch as a way of participating in the event and may thus experience repetitive exposure to traumatic scenes and stories. The loss and devastation for a child who personally lives through a disaster is significant; the effect of the simultaneous occurrence of disaster and personal loss complicates the bereavement process as grief reactions become interwoven with post-traumatic stress symptoms (see Chapter 24). After a death that occurs as a result of aggressive or traumatic circumstances, access to expert help may be required. Under conditions of threat and fear, children seek proximity to safe, stable, protective figures.

It is important for parents to grieve with their children. Some parents feel they want to protect their children from their grief, so they put on an outwardly brave front or don't talk about the deceased family member. Instead of the desired protective effect, however, the child receives the message that demonstrating grief or talking about death is wrong, leading him or her to feel isolated, to grieve privately, or to delay grieving. The child may also conclude that the parents didn't really care about the deceased since they have forgotten him or her so easily or demonstrate no emotion. In addition, the parents' efforts to avoid talking about the death may cause them to isolate themselves from their children at a time when they are most needed. Children need to know that their parents love them and will continue to protect them. Children need opportunities to talk about their relative's death and associated memories. This is much easier to do if parents also feel comfortable with these discussions.

A **surviving sibling** may feel guilty simply because he or she has survived, especially if the death was due to an accident that involved both children. Siblings' grief, especially when compounded by feelings of guilt, may be manifested by regressive behavior or anger. Parents should be informed of this possibility and encouraged to discuss the possibility with their children.

DEVELOPMENTAL PERSPECTIVE. Children's responses to death reflect the family's current culture, their past heritage, and the sociopolitical environment. Personal experience with terminal illness and dying may also facilitate children's comprehension of death and familiarity with mourning. Developmental differences in children's efforts to make sense of and master the concept and reality of death do exist and profoundly influence their grief reactions.

Children younger than 3 yr of age have little or no understanding of the concept of death. Despair, separation anxiety, and detachment may occur at the withdrawal of nurturing caretakers. Young children may respond in reaction to observing distress in others, such as a parent or sibling who is crying, withdrawn, or angry. Young children also express signs and symptoms of grief in their emotional states, such as irritability or lethargy. If the reaction is severe, failure to thrive may occur.

Preschool children are in the preoperational cognitive stage, in which communication takes place through play and fantasy. They do not show well-established cause-and-effect reasoning. They feel that death is reversible, analogous to someone going away. In attempts to master the finality and permanence of death, preschoolers frequently ask unrelenting, repeated questions about when the person who died will be returning. This makes it difficult for parents, who may become frustrated because they don't understand why the child keeps asking and don't like the constant reminders of the person's death. The primary care provider has a very important role in helping families understand the child's ability to comprehend death. Preschool children typically express magical explanations of death events, sometimes resulting in guilt and self-blame ("He died because I wouldn't play with him." "She died because I was mad at her."). Some children have these thoughts, but do not express them verbally due to embarrassment or guilt. Parents and primary care providers need to be aware of magical thinking and must reassure preschool children that their thoughts had nothing to do with the outcome. Children this age are often frightened by prolonged, powerful expressions of grief by others. Children conceptualize events in the context of their own experiential reality, and therefore consider death in terms of sleep, separation, and injury. Young children express grief intermittently and show marked affective shifts over brief periods. Regression, accompanied by longing, sadness, and anger, may accompany grief.

Younger school-aged children think concretely, recognize that death is irreversible but feel it won't happen to them or affect them, and begin to understand biologic processes of the human body ("You'll die if your body stops working."). Information gathered from the media, peers, and parents forms lasting impressions. Consequently, they may ask candid questions about death that adults will have difficulty addressing ("He must have been blown to pieces, huh?").

Children 9 yr of age and older do understand that death is irreversible and that it may involve them or their families. These children tend to experience more anxiety, more overt symptoms of depression, and more somatic complaints than do younger children. School-aged children are often left with anger focused on the loved one, those who could not save the deceased, or those presumed responsible for the death. Contact with the pediatrician may provide great reassurance, especially for the child with somatic symptoms, and particularly when the death followed a medical illness. School and learning problems may also occur, and these reactions are often linked to difficulty concentrating or preoccupation with the death. Close collaboration with the child's school may provide important diagnostic information and offer opportunities to mobilize intervention or support.

At **12–14 yr** of age, children begin to use symbolic thinking, reason abstractly, and analyze hypothetical, or "what if," scenarios systematically. Death and the end of life become concepts, rather than events. Teenagers are often ambivalent about dependence and independence and may withdraw emotionally from surviving family members, only to mourn in isolation. Adolescents begin to understand complex physiologic systems in relationship to death. Since they are often egocentric, they may be more concerned about the impact of the death on themselves than about the deceased or other family members. Fascination with dramatic, sensational, or romantic death sometimes occurs and may find expression in copycat behavior (cluster suicides) as well as competitive behavior to forge emotional links to the deceased person ("He was my best friend."). Somatic expression of grief may revolve around highly complex syndromes (eating disorders or conversion reactions) as well as symptoms limited to the more immediate perceptions, as with younger children (stomachaches). Quality of life takes on meaning, and the teenager develops a focus on the future. Depression, resentment, mood swings, rage, and risk-taking behaviors can emerge as the adolescent seeks answers to questions of values, safety, evil, and fairness. Alternately, the adolescent may seek philosophical or spiritual explanations ("being at peace") to ease their sense of loss. Death of a peer may be especially traumatic.

Families often struggle with how to inform their children of the death of a family member. The answer depends on the child's developmental level. It is best to avoid misleading euphemisms and metaphor. A child who is told that the relative who died "went to sleep" may become frightened of falling asleep, resulting in sleep problems or nightmares. Children can be told that the person is "no longer living" or "no longer moving or feeling." Using examples of pets that have died sometimes can help children gain a more realistic idea of the meaning of death. Parents who have religious beliefs may comfort their children with explanations, such as "Your sister's soul is in heaven" or "Grandfather is now with God," provided those beliefs are honestly held. If these are not religious beliefs that the parents share, children will sense the insincerity and experience anxiety rather than the hoped-for reassurance. Children's books about death can provide an important source of information, and when read together, these books may help the parent to find the right words, while addressing the child's needs.

ROLE OF THE PEDIATRICIAN IN GRIEF. The pediatrician has an important role in helping grieving families, because death has become an uncommon experience in our society. Whereas in earlier times, parents could turn to other family members or friends who had had a similar experience, bereaved parents are now more likely to turn to their physician, hospital staff, or medical home staff for support. The pediatric health care provider who has had a longitudinal relationship with the family will be an important source of support in the disclosure of bad news and critical decision-making, during both the dying process and the bereavement period.

The involvement of the health care provider may include being present at the hospital at the time of death, being available to the family by phone during the bereavement period, sending a sympathy card, attending the funeral, and/or scheduling a follow-up visit. Attendance at the funeral sends a strong message that the family and the child are important and can also help the pediatric health care provider to grieve and reach personal closure about the death. A family meeting 1–3 mo later may be helpful since parents may not be able to formulate their questions at the time of death. This meeting allows the family time to ask questions, share concerns, and review autopsy findings (if one was performed), and allows the health care provider to determine how the parents and family are adjusting to the death.

Instead of leaving the family feeling abandoned by a health care system that they have counted on, this visit allows them to have continued support. This is even more important when the health care provider will be continuing to provide care for surviving siblings. The visit can be used to determine how the mourning process is progressing, detect evidence of marital discord, and evaluate how well surviving siblings are coping. This is also an opportunity to evaluate whether referrals to support groups or mental health providers may be of benefit. Continuing to recognize the child who has died is important. Families very much appreciate the receipt of a card on their child's birthday or the anniversary of their child's death.

The health care provider needs to be an educator about disease, death, and grief. The pediatrician can offer a safe environment for the family to talk about painful emotions, express fears, and share memories. By giving families permission to talk and modeling how to address children's concerns, the pediatrician demystifies death. Parents often request practical help. The health care provider can offer families resources, such as literature (both fiction and nonfiction), referrals to therapeutic services, and tools to help them learn about illness, loss, and grief. In this way, the physician reinforces the sense that other people understand what they are going through and helps to normalize their distressing emotions. The pediatrician can also facilitate and demystify the grief process by sharing basic tenets of grief therapy. There is no single right or wrong way to grieve. Everyone grieves differently; mothers may grieve differently than fathers, and children mourn differently than adults. Helping family members to respect these differences and reach out to support each other is critical. Grief is not something to "get over," but a lifelong process of adapting, readjusting, and reconnecting.

Parents may need help in knowing what constitutes normal grieving. Hearing, seeing, or feeling their child's presence may be a normal response. Vivid memories or dreams may occur. The pediatrician can help parents to learn that, although their pain and sadness may seem intolerable, other parents have survived similar experiences, and their pain will lessen over time. The support of the pediatrician, medical home staff, support groups, or individual counselors may be needed during this time.

Pediatricians are often asked whether children should attend the funeral of a parent or sibling. These rituals allow the family to begin their mourning process. Children older than 4 yr of age should be given a choice. If the child chooses to attend, he or she should have a designated, trusted adult, who is not part of the immediate family, to stay with the child, offer comfort, and be willing to leave with the child if the experience proves to be overwhelming. If the child chooses not to attend, he or she should be offered additional opportunities to share in a ritual, go to the cemetery to view the grave, tell stories about the deceased, or obtain a keepsake object from the deceased family member as a remembrance.

In the current era of tertiary care medicine, it is common for the primary care provider and medical home staff not to be informed when one of their patients dies in the hospital. Yet, this communication is critically important. Because of their longitudinal relationship with the family, primary care providers may offer much needed support. There are practical issues, such as the need to cancel previously made appointments and the need to alert office and nursing staff so that they are prepared should the family return for a follow-up visit or for ongoing health maintenance care with the surviving siblings. In addition, even minor illnesses in the surviving siblings may frighten children. Parents may contribute to this anxiety since their inability to protect the child who has died may leave them with a sense of guilt or helplessness. They may seek medical attention sooner or may be hypervigilant in the care of the siblings because of guilt over the other child's death, concern about their judgment, or the need for continued reassurance. A visit to the pediatrician can do a lot to allay their fears.

Clinicians must remain vigilant for risk factors in each family member and in the family unit as a whole. Primary care providers, who care for families over time, know bereft patients' premorbid functioning and can identify those at current or future risk for physical and psychiatric morbidity. Providers must focus on symptoms that interfere with a patient's normal activities and compromise a child's attainment of developmental tasks. Symptom duration, intensity, and severity, in context with the family's culture, can help identify complicated grief reactions in need of therapeutic attention. Descriptive words, such as "unrelenting," "intense," "intrusive," or "prolonged," should raise concern. Total absence of signs of mourning, specifically, an inability to discuss the loss or express sadness, also suggests potential problems.

No specific sign, symptom, or cluster of behaviors identifies the child or family in need of help. However, further assessment is indicated if the following occur: (1) persistent somatic or psychosomatic complaints of undetermined origin (headache, stomachache, eating and sleeping disorders, conversion symptoms, symptoms related to the deceased's condition, hypochondriasis); (2) unusual circumstances of death or loss (sudden, violent, or traumatic death; inexplicable, unbelievable, or particularly senseless death; prolonged, complicated illness; unexpected separation); (3) school or work difficulties (declining grades or school performance, social withdrawal, aggression); (4) changes in home or family functioning (multiple family stresses, lack of social support, unavailable or ineffective functioning of caretakers, multiple disruptions in routines, lack of safety); (5) concerning psychologic factors (persistent guilt or blame, desire to die or talk of suicide, severe separation distress, disturbing hallucinations, self-abuse, risk-taking behaviors, symptoms of trauma such as hyperarousal or severe flashbacks, grief from previous or multiple deaths).

TREATMENT. Suggesting interventions outside the natural support network of family and friends can often prove useful to grieving families. Bereavement counseling should be readily offered if needed or requested by the family. Interventions that enhance or promote attachments and security, as well as give the family a means of expressing and understanding death, help to reduce the likelihood of future or prolonged disturbance, especially in children. Collaboration between pediatric and mental health professionals can help determine the timing and appropriateness of services.

Interventions for children and families who are struggling to cope with a loss in the community include gestures such as sending a card or offering food to the relatives of the deceased and teaching children the etiquette of behaviors and rituals around bereavement and mutual support. Performing community service or joining charitable organizations, such as fund-raising in memory of the deceased, may be useful. In the wake of a disaster, parents and older siblings can give blood or volunteer in search and recovery efforts. When a loss does not involve an actual death (e.g., parental divorce or geographic relocation), empowering the child to join or start a "divorced kids' club" in school or planning a "new kids in town" party may help. Participating in a constructive activity helps move the family away from a sense of helplessness and hopelessness and helps them to find meaning in their loss.

Psychotherapeutic services may benefit the entire family or individual members. Many support or self-help groups focus on specific types of losses (sudden infant death syndrome, suicide, widow/widowers, or AIDS) and provide an opportunity to talk with other people who have experienced similar losses. Family, couple, or individual counseling may be useful, depending on the nature of the residual coping issues. Combinations of approaches may work well for children or parents with evolving needs. A child may participate in family therapy to deal with the loss of a sibling and use individual treatment to address issues of personal ambivalence and guilt related to the death.

The question of **pharmacologic** intervention for grief reactions often arises in the pediatrician's office. Explaining that medication does not cure grief and often does not reduce the intensity of some symptoms (separation distress) can help. Although medication can blunt reactions, the psychologic work of grieving still must occur. The pediatrician must consider the patient's premorbid psychiatric vulnerability, current level of functioning, other available supports, and the use of additional therapeutic interventions. Medication, as a first line of defense, rarely proves useful in normal or uncomplicated grief reactions. In certain situations (severe sleep disruption, incapacitating anxiety, or intense hyperarousal), use of an anxiolytic or antidepressant medication for symptom relief and to provide the patient with the emotional energy to mourn may help. Medication used in conjunction with some form of psychotherapy, and in consultation with a psychopharmacologist, has optimal results (see Chapter 20).

SPIRITUAL ISSUES. Responding to patients' and families' spiritual beliefs can help in comforting them during family tragedies. Offering to call members of pastoral care teams or their own spiritual leader can be a real support to them and aid in decision-making. Families have found it important to have their beliefs and their need for hope acknowledged in end-of-life care. The majority of patients report welcoming discussions on spirituality. Spirituality may help individual patients cope with illness, disease, dying, and death. In addressing spirituality, physicians need to follow certain guidelines, including maintaining respect for the patient's beliefs, following the patient's lead in exploring how spirituality affects his or her decision-making, acknowledging the limits of their own expertise and role in spirituality, and maintaining their own integrity by not saying or doing anything that violates their own spiritual or religious views. Health care providers should not impose their own religious or antireligious beliefs on patients, but rather should listen respectfully to their patients. By responding to spiritual needs, physicians may better aid their patients and families in end-of-life care and bereavement and take on the role of healers.

SELF-CARE OF THE HEALTH CARE PROVIDER. Just as the death of a child is very stressful for the family, it is also stressful for health care providers. Since the death of a child is contrary to everything for which a pediatrician strives, the death of a patient can cause a grief reaction in physicians that is comparable to the death of a loved one, resulting in emotions of sadness, anger, guilt, and occasionally, relief. We must create a medical culture where health care providers acknowledge their own grief and mourning and select ways to address it in order to prevent burnout. It is also important to practice regular self-care. Possibilities include attending the memorial service or funeral, participating in a debriefing with colleagues within the hospital or medical home, and creating opportunities to both mourn the patient's death and celebrate the patient's life. Getting exercise, maintaining good nutrition, getting adequate sleep, meditating, spending time with family and friends, participating in hobbies, and taking vacations are all examples of self-care. Health care providers have difficult, but rewarding jobs. They need to maintain their inner strength and resilience in order to be effective in their profession. The way that a health care professional integrates the death of a child can change this experience from a very tragic and stressful one, leading to burnout, to a rewarding and memorable experience, in which he or she functions as a true healer to a family.

FUTURE CONSIDERATIONS. The field of bereavement intervention has faced new challenges, for which scant research and experience exist as guides. One such area involves helping children and families cope in the aftermath of horrific, inexplicable deaths and losses, such as terrorist attacks on civilians. The effects of chronic exposure to massive death and destruction, the lack of a "geographic safety zone" in which to feel secure, and the identification and management of long-term traumatic grief reactions in children to such attacks are unknown. Another understudied area involves helping children and families cope with grief in nontraditional ways. Health care providers must develop increased sensitivity and cultural awareness of attitudes about death and the rituals surrounding mourning in families of different ethnic and religious beliefs.

American Academy of Child and Adolescent Psychiatry (2001): How to Help Children after a Disaster. From www.aacp.org/publications/facts-fam/disaster/htm.

American Academy of Pediatrics, Committee on Psychosocial Aspects of Child and Family Health: How pediatricians can respond to the psychosocial implications of disasters. *Pediatrics* 1999;103:521–523.

Birenbaum LK: Assessing children's and teenagers' bereavement when a sibling dies from cancer: A secondary analysis. *Child Care Health Dev* 2000;26(5):381–400.

Cerel J, Fristad MA, Verducci J, Weller RA, Weller EB: Childhood bereavement: psychopathology in the 2 years post parental death. *J Am Acad Child Adolesc Psychiatry* 2006;45:681–690.

Christ GH, Siegel K, Christ AE: Adolescent grief: "It never really hit me . . . until it actually happened." *JAMA* 2002; 288(1):1269–1278.

Field MJ, Behrman RE (editors): *When Children Die: Improving Palliative and End-of-Life Care for Children and Their Families.* Washington, DC, National Academies Press, 2003.

Lo B, Ruston D, Kates LW, et al: For the Working Group on Religious and Spiritual Issues at the End of Life. *JAMA* 2002;287(6):749–754.

Monroe-Blum H, Boyle M, Offord D, et al: Immigrant children: Psychiatric disorder, school performance and service utilization. *Am J Orthopsychiatry* 1989;59:510.

Radziewicz RM: Self-care for the caregiver. *Nurs Clin North Am* 2001;36(4):855–869.

Saldinger A, Cain A, Porterfield K: Managing traumatic stress in children anticipating parental death. *Psychiatry* 2003;66(2):168–181.

Seecharan GA, Andresen EM, Norris K, et al: Parents' assessment of quality of care and grief following a child's death. *Arch Pediatr Adolesc Med* 2004;158:515–520.

Serwint JR, Nellis ME: Deaths of pediatric patients: Relevance to their medical home, an urban primary care clinic. *Pediatrics* 2005;115(1):57–63.

Tennant C: Parental loss in childhood: Its effect in adult life. *Arch Gen Psychiatry* 1988;45:1045–1050.

Wallerstein JS: The long-term effects of divorce on children: A review. *J Am Acad Child Adolesc Psychiatry* 1991;30:349.

Wolfe J, Grier HE, Klar N, et al: Symptoms and suffering at the end of life in children with cancer. *N Engl J Med* 2000;342:326–333.

Wood K, Chase E, Aggleton P: 'Telling the truth is the best thing': teenage orphans' experience of parental AIDS: related illness and bereavement in Zimbabwe. *Soc Sci Med* 2006; epub ahead of print.

Chapter 18 ■ Sleep Medicine

Judith A. Owens

GENERAL CONSIDERATIONS

To evaluate sleep problems, it is important first to have an understanding of what constitutes "normal" sleep in children and adolescents. Sleep disturbances, as well as many characteristics of sleep itself, have some distinctly different features in children from sleep and sleep disorders in adults. Sleep architecture and sleep patterns and behaviors change significantly across the age spectrum from infancy to preschool to adolescence. As children mature, they assume more adult sleep patterns (shorter sleep duration, longer sleep cycles, less daytime sleep); there is a dramatic decline in daytime sleep (scheduled napping) between 18 mo and 5 yr, and a less marked and more gradual continued decrease in nocturnal sleep amounts into late adolescence. Sleep-wake patterns also become increasingly irregular, with larger discrepancies between school night and non-school night bedtimes and wake times from middle childhood through adolescence; there is a gradual shift to a later bedtime and a later sleep onset time that begins in middle childhood and accelerates in early to mid-adolescence. Finally, there are significant changes in sleep architecture, including a dramatic decrease in the proportion of rapid eye movement (REM) sleep from birth (50% of sleep) through early childhood and into adulthood (25–30%). In addition, the initial predominance of slow-wave sleep (SWS), which peaks in early childhood, has an abrupt drop-off after puberty, and then declines over the lifespan. A summary of some of the more important normal developmental changes in children's sleep is found in Table 18-1.

Although sleep patterns and the types of sleep disorders most commonly found in adolescents share features with those of both younger children and adults, the physiologic changes that occur during puberty and the developmental challenges of adolescence contribute to a number of unique characteristics of adolescent sleep. To appreciate the impact of these physiologic and psychologic changes, it is important first to consider them in the context of human sleep regulation and some of the basic principles that govern sleep and wakefulness. The first principle relates to those mechanisms that determine the relative level of sleepiness or alertness occurring throughout a given 24 hr period; these include both the intrinsic circadian sleep-wake rhythm ("circadian clock") and the homeostatic sleep drive (dependent on the time awake since the last sleep period as well as the duration and quality of previous sleep). There are 2 periods of clock-dependent maximum sleepiness ("circadian troughs") and maximum alertness that occur during the course of a 24 hr day. The degree of sleepiness experienced during a given circadian period is also influenced by the relative sleep need existing at the time (is increased in the sleep-deprived individual). Intrinsic circadian rhythms, which govern many physiologic processes in addition to sleep-wake rhythms, are in turn affected to a degree by exter-

TABLE 18-1. Normal Developmental Changes in Children's Sleep

AGE CATEGORY	AVERAGE SLEEP DURATION (24 HR)	SLEEP PATTERNS	ADDITIONAL VARIABLES IMPACTING ON SLEEP	SLEEP DISORDERS
Newborn (0–3 mo)	16–20 hr	1–4 hr sleep periods followed by 1–2 hr awake periods Amount daytime sleep = amount nighttime sleep	Prematurity: few differences in sleep development Birth trauma associated with sleep disruption Breast-fed: shorter sleep periods	Colic Apnea of infancy
Infant (3–12 mo)	14–15 hr total at 4 mo; 13–14 hr total at 6 mo (11 hr/night; 3 hr in 2 naps/day) Nap for 2–4 hr/day at 9–12 mo	Sleep periods 3–4 hr first 3 mo; 6–8 hr periods at 4–6 mo; day/night differentiation develops at 6 wk to 3 mo 70–80% "settle" (sleep through the night) at 9 mo	Self-smoothing skills develop starting at 3 mo; may "signal" night wakings (crying) to parents Settling and night wakings influenced by parenting, feeding practices Co-sleeping common	Sleep onset association disorder/night wakings Rhythmic movement disorders (head banging, body rocking)
Toddler (1–3 yr)	12–14 hr total Nap 1.5–3.5 hr (1 nap/day)	Night wakings often resume	Nighttime fears develop; transitional objects, bedtime routines important	Sleep onset association disorder Limit-setting sleep disorder/bedtime resistance
Preschool (3–6 yr)	11–12 yr Napping declines; most stop by age 5 yr	Night waking in about 20%	Napping patterns influenced by parental, school practices Sleep problems may become chronic	Limit-setting sleep disorder Sleepwalking Sleep terrors Obstructive sleep apnea
Middle childhood (6–12 hr)	10 hr	Low levels of daytime sleepiness Increased discrepancy between amount of sleep on school vs non-school nights	School and behavior problems may be related to sleep problems Stressful events affect sleep; poor sleep affects coping skills	Nightmares Anxiety-related sleep onset delay Insufficient sleep
Adolescence (>12 yr)	9 hr ideal; 7 hr actual	Often irregular; influence of lifestyle; later bedtimes/earlier rise times	Phase delay at puberty; daytime alertness decreases at midpuberty	Insufficient sleep Delayed sleep phase Narcolepsy Restless legs syndrome/periodic limb movement disorder

nal time cues, or "zeitgebers" (timing of meals, alarm clocks), but they are most sensitive to light-darkness signals, which switch the production of the hormone melatonin by the pineal gland off (light) or on (dark).

A second important principle of sleep regulation relates to the consequences of the failure to meet basic sleep needs. Individual sleep needs are dependent on a number of factors, including age and the amount of sleep obtained in the preceding period. Inadequate sleep on a chronic basis results in what is called a *sleep debt*. If the sleep debt becomes large enough and is not voluntarily paid back, the body may respond by overriding voluntary control of wakefulness, resulting in periods of decreased alertness, dozing off, and napping. In addition, the sleep-deprived individual may experience very brief (several seconds) repeated daytime microsleeps of which he or she may be completely unaware, but which nonetheless may result in significant lapses in attention and vigilance. This becomes a particularly problematic issue in adolescents, who may be operating motor vehicles ("drowsy driving").

Adolescent sleep needs are not dramatically different from the sleep needs of preadolescents, about 9 hr/night. Most adolescents obtain on the order of 7–7½ hr of sleep/night, which results in a considerable sleep debt over time. Part of the reason for this insufficient sleep relates to pubertal influences on melatonin and circadian sleep-wake cycles, which cause a relative phase delay (later sleep onset and wake times). Adolescents are less likely than younger children to fall asleep early, and the start time of many high schools precludes a corresponding later wake time. Many adolescents have highly irregular sleep-wake patterns from weekday to weekend; when coupled with a physiologic tendency toward decreased daytime alertness in mid- to late puberty, the result is a considerable increase in sleepiness levels and consequent impairment in mood, attention, memory, behavioral control, and academic performance. Adolescents may also suffer from a number of sleep disorders. Studies have suggested that the prevalence of significant sleep problems in adolescents is high (at least 20%), and particular groups of adolescents, such as those with chronic medical or psychiatric problems, may be at increased risk.

Finally, as in adults, both insufficient quantity and poor quality of sleep in children and adolescents usually result in excessive daytime sleepiness and decreased daytime alertness levels. Sleepiness, especially in young children, may not be immediately recognizable as drowsiness, yawning, and the other "classic" manifestations of sleepiness that occur in adults. Instead, it often takes the form of mood disturbances, behavioral problems such as hyperactivity and poor impulse control, and neurocognitive dysfunction, including inattention, impaired vigilance, and compromised "executive" higher level cognitive skills. Over time, these deficits may ultimately result in significant social, school, and learning problems.

COMMON SLEEP DISORDERS

Most sleep problems in children may be broadly conceptualized as resulting from either inadequate duration of sleep for age and sleep needs (**insufficient sleep quantity**) or disruption and fragmentation of sleep (**poor sleep quality**). Insufficient sleep is usually the result of difficulty initiating (**delayed sleep onset**) and/or maintaining sleep (**prolonged night wakings**), whereas sleep fragmentation most often results from frequent, repetitive, and brief arousals during sleep. Inadequate sleep duration, especially in older children and adolescents, may also represent a conscious lifestyle decision to sacrifice sleep in favor of competing priorities, such as homework and social activities. The underlying causes of sleep onset delay/prolonged night wakings or sleep fragmentation may in turn be related to primarily behavioral factors (bedtime resistance resulting in shortened sleep duration) and/or medical causes (obstructive sleep apnea causing frequent, brief arousals). A listing of recognizable sleep disorders is noted in Table 18-2.

Certain pediatric populations are relatively more vulnerable to acute or chronic sleep problems. These include children with

TABLE 18-2. Sleep Disorders in Children

SLEEP DISORDER (ALTERNATE OR OTHER COMMONLY USED NAME)
INSOMNIA: PROBLEMS FALLING ASLEEP AND STAYING ASLEEP
Psychophysiological Insomnia (conditioned insomnia)
Adjustment Sleep Disorder (transient insomnia)
Inadequate Sleep Hygiene
Idiopathic Insomnia (childhood onset insomnia)
Behavioral Insomnia of Childhood (sleep onset association and limit-setting subtypes)
Insomnia Due to Other Known Condition
Insomnia Due to Substance Abuse
Insomnia Due to Adverse Drug Effect
Insomnia Due to Psychiatric/Behavioral or Medical Condition
SLEEP-RELATED BREATHING DISORDER: EDS AND/OR RESTLESS SLEEP
Primary Central Sleep Apnea
Primary Sleep Apnea of Infancy (infant sleep apnea)
Obstructive Sleep Apnea, Pediatric
Sleep-related Breathing Disorder Due to Cardiorespiratory Disease
Congenital Central Alveolar Hypoventilation Syndrome
HYPERSOMNIA NOT DUE TO A SLEEP-RELATED BREATHING DISORDER: EDS
Narcolepsy with Cataplexy
Narcolepsy Without Cataplexy
Recurrent Hypersomnia (Kleine-Levin syndrome)
Idiopathic Hypersomnia with Long Sleep Time
Idiopathic Hypersomnia Without Long Sleep Time
Behaviorally-induced Insufficient Sleep Syndrome
Other Hypersomnia Due to Substance Abuse
Other Hypersomnia Due to the Adverse Effects of a Drug
Hypersomnia Due to Psychiatric/Behavioral or Medical Condition
CIRCADIAN RHYTHM SLEEP DISORDER: EDS AND/OR PROBLEMS FALLING ASLEEP AND STAYING ASLEEP
Primary
Delayed Sleep Phase Type (delayed sleep phase syndrome)
Advanced Sleep Phase Type (advanced sleep phase syndrome)
Irregular Sleep-wake Type
Non-entrained Type
Other Primary Circadian Rhythm Sleep Disorder Due to a Known Physiological Condition
Behaviorally Induced
Jet-lag Type
Shift-work Type
Circadian Rhythm Disorders Due to Substance Abuse
Circadian Rhythm Sleep Disorders Due to Adverse Drug Effect
PARASOMNIA: HISTORY OF ABNORMAL SLEEP-RELATED BEHAVIOR
Confusional Arousals
Sleepwalking
Sleep Terrors
REM Sleep Behavior Disorder, including Parasomnia Overlap Disorder
Recurrent Isolated Sleep Paralysis
Nightmare Disorder
Sleep-related Enuresis
Parasomnia Due to Substance Abuse
Parasomnia Due to Psychiatric Disorders
SLEEP-RELATED MOVEMENT DISORDER: PROBLEMS INITIATING OR MAINTAINING SLEEP, EXCESSIVE SLEEP MOVEMENTS, OR EDS
Restless Legs Syndrome
Periodic Limb Movement Disorder
Sleep-related Leg Cramps
Sleep-related Bruxism
Sleep-related Rhythmic Movement Disorder (body rocking, head banging)
ISOLATED SYMPTOMS, APPARENTLY NORMAL VARIANTS, AND UNRESOLVED ISSUES
Long Sleeper
Short Sleeper
Snoring
Sleeptalking
Sleep Starts, Hypnagogic Jerks
Benign Sleep Myoclonus of Infancy

Modified from Sheldon SH, Ferber R, Kryger MH: *Principles and Practice of Pediatric Sleep Medicine*. Philadelphia, Elsevier/Saunders, 2005, p 18–19.
EDS, excessive daytime sleepiness; REM, rapid eye movement.

medical problems, including chronic illnesses, such as cystic fibrosis, asthma, and rheumatoid arthritis, and acute illnesses, such as otitis media; children taking medications that have stimulant (methylphenidate), sleep-disrupting (some asthma medications), or daytime sedating (some anticonvulsants, α-agonists) effects; hospitalized children; and children with a variety of psychiatric disorders, including attention-deficit/hyperactivity disorder (ADHD) (Chapter 31), depression, bipolar disorder (Chapter 25), and anxiety disorders (Chapter 24). Children with neurologic disorders may be more prone to nocturnal seizures, as well as other sleep disruptions, and children with blindness, severe mental retardation, some chromosomal syndromes (Smith-Magenis, fragile X), and autism spectrum disorders are at increased risk for severe sleep onset difficulty and night wakings, as well as circadian rhythm disturbances.

BEHAVIORALLY BASED SLEEP DISORDERS

BEHAVIORAL INSOMNIA OF CHILDHOOD. Sleep problems, like many behavioral issues in children, are often primarily defined by parental concerns rather than by objective criteria. Many of the behaviorally based sleep disorders are the result of the interaction between normal developmental sleep changes, as outlined earlier, and parental response to those changes. One of the most common sleep disorders found in infants and toddlers is **sleep onset association disorder.** In this disorder, the child learns to fall asleep only under certain conditions or associations, such as being rocked or fed, and does not develop the ability to self-soothe. During the night, when the child experiences the type of brief arousal that normally occurs at the end of a sleep cycle (every 60–90 min in infants) or awakens for other reasons, he or she is not able to get back to sleep without those same conditions being present. The infant then "signals" the parent by crying (or coming into the parents' bedroom, if the child is no longer in a crib) until the necessary associations are provided. Thus, the problem is one of prolonged night waking resulting in insufficient sleep (for both child and parent).

The ***treatment*** approach to sleep onset association disorder typically involves a program of rapid withdrawal (extinction) or more gradual withdrawal (graduated extinction) of parental assistance at sleep onset and during the night. Graduated extinction involves weaning the child from dependence on parental presence with periodic "checks" by the parents at successively longer intervals during the sleep-wake transition. In older infants, the introduction of more appropriate sleep associations that will be readily available to the child during the night (transitional objects, such as a blanket or toy), in addition to positive reinforcement (stickers for remaining in bed), is often beneficial. The goal is to allow the infant or child to develop skills in self-soothing during the night, as well as at bedtime. Other behavioral management strategies that have empirical support include bedtime fading (temporarily setting the bedtime closer to the actual sleep onset time and then gradually advancing the bedtime to the target bedtime) and positive bedtime routines. If the child has become habituated to awaken for nighttime feedings ("learned hunger"), then these feedings should be slowly eliminated. Parents must be consistent in applying behavioral programs to avoid inadvertent, intermittent reinforcement of night wakings; they should also be forewarned that crying behavior often temporarily escalates at the beginning of treatment ("post-extinction burst").

In contrast, **limit setting sleep disorder,** a disorder most common in preschool-aged and older children, is characterized by difficulty falling asleep and bedtime resistance ("curtain calls") rather than by night wakings. The prolonged sleep onset delay results in inadequate sleep duration. Most commonly, this disorder is caused by a parent's inability or unwillingness to set consistent bedtime rules and enforce a regular bedtime, and it is often

TABLE 18-3. Basic Principles of Sleep Hygiene for Children

1. **Have a set bedtime and bedtime routine** for your child.
2. **Bedtime and wake-up time should be about the same time on school nights and non-school nights.** There should not be more than about an hour difference from one day to another.
3. **Make the hour before bed shared quiet time.** Avoid high-energy activities, such as rough play, and stimulating activities, such as watching television or playing computer games, just before bed.
4. **Don't send your child to bed hungry.** A *light* snack (such as milk and cookies) before bed is a good idea. Heavy meals within an hour or two of bedtime, however, may interfere with sleep.
5. **Avoid products containing caffeine for at least several hours before bedtime.** These include caffeinated sodas, coffee, tea, and chocolate.
6. **Make sure your child spends time outside every day** whenever possible and is involved in regular exercise.
7. **Keep your child's bedroom quiet and dark.** A low-level night light is acceptable for children who find completely dark rooms frightening.
8. **Keep your child's bedroom at a comfortable temperature** during the night (<75°).
9. **Don't use your child's bedroom for time-out or punishment.**
10. **Keep the television set out of your child's bedroom.** Children can easily develop the bad habit of "needing" the television to fall asleep. It's also much more difficult to control your child's viewing if the set is in the bedroom.

exacerbated by the child's oppositional behavior. In some cases, however, the child's resistance at bedtime is due to an underlying problem in falling asleep that is caused by other factors (medical conditions, such as asthma or medication use; a sleep disorder, such as restless legs syndrome; or anxiety) or a mismatch between the child's intrinsic circadian rhythm ("night owl") and parental expectations.

Successful ***treatment*** of limit setting sleep disorder generally involves a combination of parent education regarding appropriate limit setting, decreased parental attention for bedtime-delaying behavior, establishment of bedtime routines, and positive reinforcement (sticker charts) for appropriate behavior at bedtime. Older children may benefit from being taught relaxation techniques to help themselves fall asleep more readily. Following the principles of sleep hygiene for children is essential (Table 18-3).

PSYCHOPHYSIOLOGIC INSOMNIA. This sleep disorder occurs largely in adolescents and is unusual in younger children. In this disorder, the individual has conditioned anxiety around difficulty falling or staying asleep, which leads to heightened physiologic arousal and further compromises the ability to sleep. Treatment usually involves educating the adolescent about the principles of sleep hygiene (Table 18-4), instructing him or her to use the bed for sleep only and to get out of bed if he or she is unable to fall asleep (stimulus control), restricting time in bed to the actual time asleep (sleep restriction), and teaching relaxation techniques to reduce anxiety. Hypnotic medications are rarely needed.

MEDICALLY BASED SLEEP DISORDERS

OBSTRUCTIVE SLEEP APNEA (OSA). OSA is characterized by brief, repeated episodes of airflow obstruction at the nose and mouth that occur during sleep. These periods of complete airflow cessation (apnea) or partial airflow obstruction (hypopnea) result in both frequent, transient reductions in oxygen (hypoxia) and increases in carbon dioxide levels (hypercapnia) that are associated with partial awakenings or arousals throughout the night. OSA is part of the spectrum of sleep-disordered breathing (SDB) that also includes the following:

PRIMARY SNORING. Primary snoring is not accompanied by ventilatory abnormalities, such as hypoxia and hypercapnia. A number of different epidemiologic studies suggest that about 10% of children habitually snore. It was once thought that snoring alone in both children and adults was relatively benign. However, in addition to being a relative risk factor for the later development of OSA, there may be a link between snoring, with or without associated breathing problems, and poor school performance.

UPPER AIRWAY RESISTANCE SYNDROME (UARS). UARS is used to describe ventilatory abnormalities associated with intrathoracic pressure swings during partially obstructed breathing. The risk factors for UARS are similar to those for OSA (enlarged tonsils and adenoids). Symptoms of UARS include snoring, often accompanied by paradoxical breathing (paradoxical movement of the chest and abdominal muscles during inspiration) and frequent arousals, resulting in sleep disruption and daytime sleepiness. UARS is not captured on a standard polysomnogram (PSG) recording; intraesophageal pressure monitoring (balloon manometry) is required to make the diagnosis. Since this is a relatively invasive technique, it is only available in a few pediatric sleep laboratories.

OBSTRUCTIVE HYPOVENTILATION (HYPOPNEAS). Hypopneas are the most common form of SDB in children. Hypopneas represent a 50% reduction in airflow. From a clinical standpoint, this means that frank apneic pauses (complete cessation of airflow) are relatively less common in children than in adults. Even though they are less severe, repeated hypopneas throughout the night have consequences (oxygen desaturation, disrupted sleep) similar to those of frequent apneas.

SLEEP APNEA. Apnea represents the complete cessation of airflow through the nose and mouth for a duration that is determined by age-appropriate norms. Apnea is divided further into **central sleep apnea,** which is lack of airflow through the nose and mouth *without* accompanying respiratory effort and **obstructive sleep apnea,** which is cessation of airflow *despite* respiratory effort and movement. **Mixed apneas** have evidence of both obstructive and central components during an event.

About 20% of children occasionally snore at night, while 10% snore almost every night. OSA occurs in about 1–3% of children of preschool age; more than 300,000 children in the USA are affected by OSA. Unfortunately, there is little information on how common OSA is in other age groups. There is approximately equal male : female preponderance in prepubertal children.

TABLE 18-4. Basic Principles of Sleep Hygiene for Adolescents

1. **Wake up and go to bed at about the same time** every night. Bedtime and wake-up time should not differ from school to non-school nights by more than approximately an hour.
2. **Avoid sleeping in on weekends** to "catch up" on sleep. This makes it more likely that you will have problems falling asleep.
3. If you take **naps,** they should be **short** (no more than an hour) and **scheduled in the early to midafternoon.** However, if you have a problem with falling asleep at night, **napping** during the day may make it worse and should be avoided.
4. **Spend time outside** every day. Exposure to sunlight helps to keep your body's internal clock on track.
5. **Exercise regularly.** Exercise may help you fall asleep and sleep more deeply.
6. **Use your bed for sleeping only.** Don't study, read, listen to music, watch television, etc., on your bed.
7. Make the 30–60 minutes before a **quiet or wind-down time.** Relaxing, calm, enjoyable activities, such as reading a book or listening to calm music, help your body and mind slow down enough to let you get to sleep. Don't study, watch exciting/scary movies, exercise, or get involved in "energizing" activities just before bed.
8. Eat regular meals and **don't go to bed hungry.** A light snack before bed is a good idea; eating a full meal in the hour before bed is not.
9. **Avoid** eating or drinking products containing **caffeine** from dinner time on. These include caffeinated sodas, coffee, tea, and chocolate.
10. **Do not use alcohol.** Alcohol disrupts sleep and may cause you to awaken throughout the night.
11. **Smoking disturbs sleep.** Don't smoke at least one hour before bed (and preferably, not at all!).
12. Don't use **sleeping pills, melatonin,** or other **over-the-counter sleep aids** to help you sleep unless specifically recommended by your doctor. These can be dangerous, and the sleep problems often return when you stop taking the medicine.

TABLE 18-5. Clinical History of Obstructive Sleep Apnea Syndrome

SLEEP	WAKEFULNESS
Snoring	Poor school performance
Witnessed apnea	Aggressive behavior
Choking noises	Hyperactivity
Increased work of breathing	Attention deficit disorder
Paradoxical breathing	Excessive daytime sleepiness
Enuresis	Morning headaches
Restless sleep	
Diaphoresis	
Hyperextended neck	
Frequent awakenings	
Dry mouth	

CLINICAL MANIFESTATIONS. The clinical manifestations of OSA may be divided into sleep-related and daytime symptoms (Table 18-5). The most common nocturnal manifestations of OSA in children and adolescents are loud, frequent, and disruptive snoring, breathing pauses, choking or gasping arousals, restless sleep, and nocturnal diaphoresis. Many children who snore do not have OSA, but very few children with OSA do not snore. Most children, like adults, tend to have more frequent and more severe obstructive events in REM sleep and when sleeping in the supine position. Children with OSA may adopt unusual sleeping positions, keeping their necks hyperextended, for example, in order to maintain airway patency. Frequent arousals associated with obstruction may result in nocturnal awakenings, but are more likely to cause fragmented sleep.

Daytime symptoms of OSA include morning headaches resulting from CO_2 retention, dry mouth, chronic mouth breathing and nasal congestion, and nasal speech. In more severe cases, poor appetite and even frank failure to thrive may be noted. Children with OSA may have secondary enuresis, most likely as a result of the disruption of the normal nocturnal pattern of antidiuretic hormone secretion. Partial arousals parasomnias (sleepwalking and sleep terrors) may occur more frequently in children with OSA, related to the frequent associated arousals and an increased percentage of delta sleep, or SWS.

Although less is known about the neurobehavioral consequences of OSA in children than in adults, most pediatric studies have supported a similar range of deficits in attention, memory, and executive functions, as well as an increase in subjective sleepiness and mood disturbance. The neurobehavioral consequences of OSA in children range from profound daytime sleepiness with drowsiness, difficulty in morning waking, and unplanned napping or dozing off during activities, to more subtle signs of sleepiness, such as inattention, behavioral disinhibition, and mood lability. Behavioral manifestations of OSA also include increased distractibility, low frustration tolerance, hyperactivity, behavioral impulsivity, aggressive behavior, social withdrawal, learning problems, and compromised academic performance. Many of these symptoms overlap with other childhood conditions, most notably ADHD. Studies that have looked at changes in behavior and neuropsychological functioning in children following treatment (usually adenotonsillectomy) for OSA or SDB have documented significant improvement in daytime sleepiness, behavior, and academic performance, and objective improvements in neuropsychological measurements of attention, vigilance, and reaction time, and cognitive functions. In addition, studies that have examined the prevalence of SDB signs and/or symptoms in children with identified behavioral and academic problems have found an increased prevalence of snoring in children with behavioral problems and in children being evaluated for or diagnosed with ADHD.

TABLE 18-6. Anatomic Factors that Predispose to Obstructive Sleep Apnea and Hypoventilation in Children

NOSE
Anterior nasal stenosis
Choanal stenosis/atresia
Deviated nasal septum
Seasonal or perennial rhinitis
Nasal polyps, foreign body, hematoma, mass lesion
NASOPHARYNGEAL AND OROPHARYNGEAL
Adenotonsillar hypertrophy
Macroglossia
Cystic hygroma
Velopharyngeal flap repair
Cleft palate repair
Pharyngeal mass lesion
CRANIOFACIAL
Micrognathia/retrognathia
Midface hypoplasia (e.g., trisomy 21, Crouzon, Apert syndrome)
Mandibular hypoplasia (Pierre Robin sequence, Treacher Collins, Cornelia de Lange)
Craniofacial trauma
Skeletal and storage diseases
Achondroplasia
Glycogen storage disease (e.g., Hunter, Hurler syndrome)

The risk factors for OSA in children relate to the underlying pathophysiology of the disorder; they increase the obstructive component, result in narrowing of the upper airway, and/or decrease airway patency by means of decreased muscle tone in the upper airway dilators (Tables 18-6 and 18-7). The most common risk factor for childhood OSA is **adenotonsillar hypertrophy.** However, it should be noted that the degree of hypertrophy does not necessarily correlate with the degree of obstruction and, thus, the severity of symptoms. Children with seasonal and environmental allergies, asthma, and/or frequent sinus infections may also be at increased risk for OSA due to increased resistance in the upper and lower airways. Gastroesophageal reflux may also result in posterior pharyngeal irritation, edema, and obstruction. Any chronic condition characterized by relative muscle hypotonia (muscular dystrophies) or midface hypoplasia (achondroplasia) increases the risk of OSA. Individuals with Down syndrome, by virtue of their facial anatomy, hypotonia, macroglossia, and central adiposity, as well as the increased incidence of hypothyroidism, are at particularly high risk for OSA, with some estimates of as great as 70% prevalence. African-

TABLE 18-7. Functional Factors That Predispose to Obstructive Sleep Apnea and Hypoventilation in Children

- Rapid eye movement sleep–related pharyngeal hypotonia
- Abnormal neural control
  - Generalized hypotonia (e.g., trisomy 21)
  - Global CNS injury (e.g., birth asphyxia, cerebral palsy)
  - Brainstem dysfunction
    - Chiari malformation (II or I)
    - Foramen magnum stenosis (e.g., achondroplasia)
    - Injury (e.g., anoxia, tumor, infection)
- Drugs
  - Sedative: chloral hydrate, benzodiazepines, phenothiazines
  - Anesthetics
  - Narcotics
- Other
  - Autonomic dysfunction
  - Dysphagia
  - Excess oral secretions
  - Obesity
  - Prematurity

American and Asian children may have a higher risk of OSA due to anatomic features of the upper airway. Children with a repaired cleft palate (velopharyngeal flap) have a greater incidence of upper airway obstruction. Finally, children with a positive family history of OSA are increased risk for the condition.

Obesity is the major risk factor for OSA in adults, and it appears to be one risk factor for childhood OSA as well. This is obviously concerning, given the alarming increase in childhood obesity over the past several decades. The relationship between obesity and OSA is most likely a multifactorial one that includes increased adipose tissue deposits in the upper airway that result in airway narrowing, increased resistance to thoracic excursion during inspiration, and abnormal central respiratory control in some cases. Children with congenital syndromes that have obesity as a prominent feature, such as Prader-Willi syndrome (PWS), are at particularly high risk. Independent of the SDB component, children with PWS also have a higher incidence of excessive daytime sleepiness that may reflect a fundamental abnormality of hypothalamic function.

There are no **physical examination** findings that are pathognomonic for OSA, and most healthy children with OSA appear normal; however, certain physical examination findings may suggest OSA (Table 18-8). Growth parameters may be abnormal (obesity or failure to thrive), and there may be evidence of nasal obstruction (hyponasal speech, "adenoidal facies") or mouth breathing, as well as signs of atopic disease. Oropharyngeal examination may reveal enlarged tonsils, excess soft tissue, and a narrowed posterior pharyngeal space. Any abnormalities of the facial structure, such as retrognathia and/or micrognathia, midfacial hypoplasia, even in the absence of adenotonsillar hypertrophy, increase the likelihood of OSA and should be noted. In very severe cases, there may be evidence of pulmonary hypertension, right-sided heart failure, and cor pulmonale; systemic hypertension, unlike in adults, is relatively uncommon.

DIAGNOSIS. The American Academy of Pediatrics clinical practice guidelines provide excellent information for the evaluation of uncomplicated childhood OSA. Because no combination of clinical history and physical findings can accurately predict which children with snoring have OSA, the gold standard for diagnosing OSA is an overnight **polysomnogram.** An overnight PSG is a technician-supervised, monitored electrographic study that documents physiologic variables during sleep, including sleep stages (limited electroencephalogram montage), muscle tone (electromyogram of the chin and leg), eye movements, airflow (nasal/oral thermistor, pressure transducer, end-tidal CO_2), oxygen saturation, and heart rate, with or without transcutaneous CO_2 and O_2. The scoring criteria used for pediatric studies, which are different from those used for adults, are outlined in the American Thoracic Society consensus statement, although it should be noted that there is no consensus on the polysomnographic predictors of morbidity or the cutoff points for clinical significance. Ancillary tests that may be helpful in select cases include a lateral neck radiograph to evaluate the size of the adenoids, because direct visualization is only possible with endoscopy; a complete blood count to detect polycythemia suggestive of chronic hypoxemia; and measurement of electrolytes to detect an elevated bicarbonate level suggestive of compensation for hypoventilation. Chest radiograph, electrocardiogram, and echocardiogram may reveal evidence of cor pulmonale or right ventricular hypertrophy in severe cases.

TABLE 18-8. Physical Examination in Obstructive Sleep Apnea Syndrome

GENERAL
Sleepiness
Obesity
Failure to thrive
HEAD
Swollen mucous membranes
Deviated septum
Adenoidal facies
Infraorbital darkening
Elongated face
Mouth breathing
Tonsillar hypertrophy
High arched palate
Overbite
Crowded oropharynx
Macroglossia
Glossoptosis
Midfacial hypoplasia
Micrognathia/retrognathia
CARDIOVASCULAR
Hypertension
Loud P2 (heart sound)
EXTREMITIES
Edema
Clubbing (rare)

From Sheldon SH, Ferber R, Kryger MH: *Principles and Practice of Pediatric Sleep Medicine.* Philadelphia, Elsevier/Saunders, 2005, p 199.

TABLE 18-9. Treatment of Obstructive Sleep Apnea and Hypoventilation in Childhood

Adenotonsillectomy
Medical therapies
Nasopharyngeal airway
Continuous positive airway pressure via nasal mask
Supplemental oxygen to minimize hypoxemia
Pharmacologic
Topical nasal steroids
Antibiotics
Nasal decongestants (short-term only)
Weight loss
Other surgical therapies
Craniofacial surgical procedures
Mandibular distraction osteogenesis
Mandibular/maxillary plastic surgical procedures
Stenting procedures for nasal stenosis/atresia
Cleft palate revision procedures
Uvulopalatopharyngoplasty
Correction of deviated septum, nasal polypectomy
Tracheostomy

TREATMENT. In the majority of cases of pediatric OSA, adenotonsillectomy is the first line of treatment (Table 18-9). It is important to note that adenoidectomy alone may not be curative, because adenoids may "grow back" as a result of continued hypertrophy of residual adenoidal tissue postoperatively. Reported cure rates post-adenotonsillectomy range from 75–100% in normal healthy children. Although cure rates in obese children may not be as high, most obese children also benefit from adenotonsillectomy. The age of the child (<2 yr), the presence of additional risk factors (obesity, hypotonia, craniofacial anomalies), and the severity of the OSA (more clinical sequelae present) may increase the risk of perioperative complications and may affect the timing of the surgery and postoperative care. High-risk patients may warrant additional testing (PSG) to ensure resolution of symptoms or determine if further therapy is warranted.

Additional treatment measures that may be appropriate include weight loss, positional therapy (attaching a firm object, such as a tennis ball, to the back of a sleep garment to prevent the child

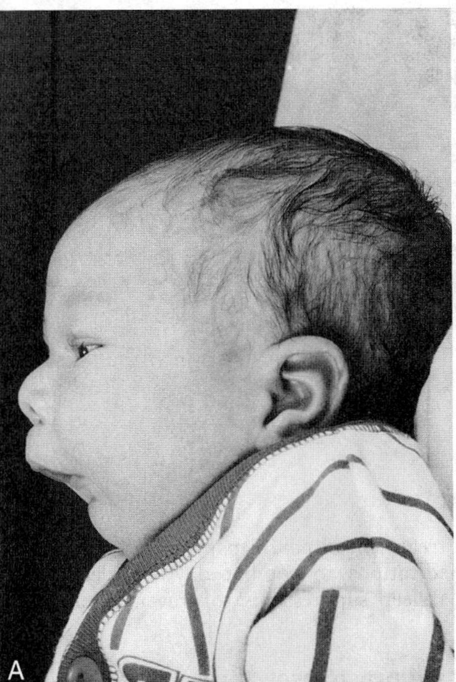

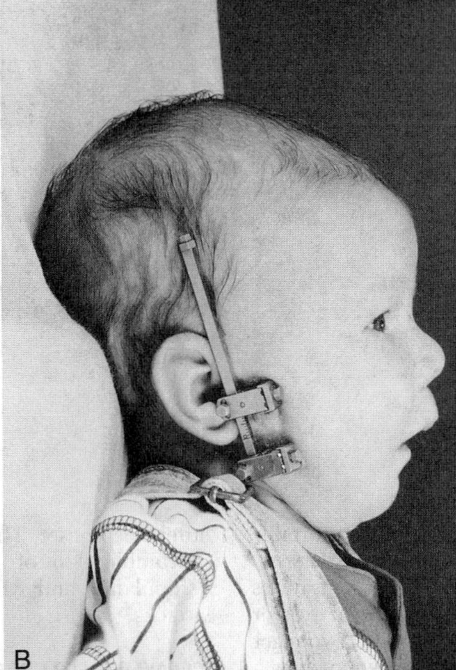

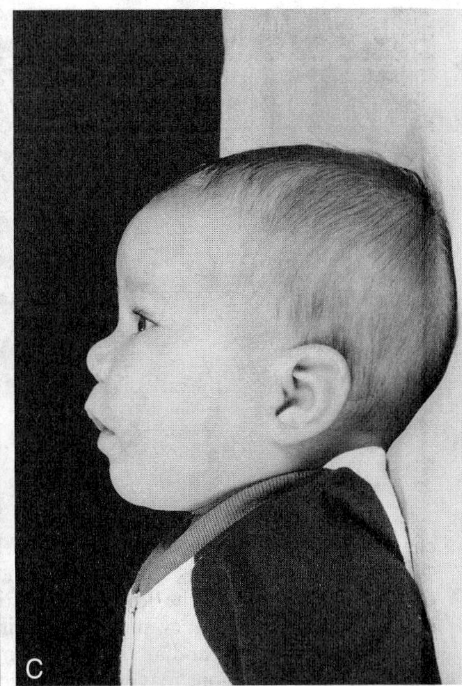

Figure 18-1. An infant with Robin sequence at 10 days of age *(A)*. At 21 days of age, with right mandibular distraction in place *(B)*. At 3 mo of age, 6 wk after mandibular distraction was removed *(C)*. (From Denny A, Kalantarian B: Mandibular distraction in neonates: A strategy to avoid tracheostomy. *Plast Reconstr Surg* 2002;109:896–904.)

from sleeping in the supine position), and aggressive treatment of additional risk factors when present, such as asthma, seasonal allergies, and gastroesophageal reflux. There are no controlled data to suggest that nasal dilators or nasal steroids are effective in treating childhood OSA. Oral appliances and uvulopharygoplasty (UPPP) are commonly used in adults, but have little supporting data in children. Continuous or bilevel positive airway pressure (nasal CPAP or BiPAP) is the most common treatment for OSA in adults and can be used successfully in children and adolescents. CPAP delivers humidified, warmed air through an interface (mask, nasal pillows) that, under pressure, effectively "splints" the upper airway open. CPAP may be recommended if removing the adenoids and tonsils is not indicated, if there is residual disease following adenotonsillectomy, or if there are major risk factors that are not amenable to treatment with surgery (obesity, hypotonia). Surgery may also be indicated for patients with velopharyngeal insufficiency and those with severe micrognathia. Mandibular distraction has been used to treat micrognathia in older patients, but is also used to treat neonates with conditions such as Robin sequence (Chapter 308) [Fig. 18-1].

PARASOMNIAS. Parasomnias are defined as episodic nocturnal behaviors that often involve cognitive disorientation and autonomic and skeletal muscle disturbance. Many of the parasomnias are associated with relative central nervous system immaturity and tend to be more common in children than in adults; they may abate with age. The partial arousal parasomnias, which include **sleepwalking** and **sleep terrors,** have several features in common. Because they typically occur at the transition out of stage 4 sleep, or SWS, partial arousal parasomnias have clinical features of both the awake (ambulation, vocalizations) and the sleeping (high arousal threshold, unresponsiveness to the environment) states; there is usually amnesia for the events. They are more common in preschool and school-aged children because of the relatively higher percentage of SWS in younger children. Furthermore, any factor that is associated with an increase in the relative percentage of SWS (certain medications, previous sleep deprivation) may increase the frequency of events in a predisposed child. The typical timing of partial arousal parasomnias during the first 2 hr of sleep is related to the predominance of SWS in the first third of the night. There appears to be a genetic predisposition for both sleepwalking and night terrors.

In contrast, **nightmares,** which are much more common than the partial arousal parasomnias, but are often confused with them, are concentrated in the last third of the night, when REM sleep is most prominent. Partial arousal parasomnias may also be difficult to distinguish from nocturnal seizures. Table 18-10 summarizes similarities and differences among these four nocturnal arousal events.

The treatment of partial arousal parasomnias involves parental education and reassurance; avoidance of exacerbating factors, such as sleep deprivation; and particularly in the case of sleepwalking, institution of safety precautions. Pharmacotherapy or psychotherapy is rarely indicated. Frequent and persistent nightmares in a child warrant further investigation regarding possible trauma, such as sexual abuse, and/or evaluation for a more global anxiety disorder.

Rhythmic movement disorders, including body rocking and head banging, are parasomnias that are much more common in the 1st yr of life and usually disappear by 4 yr of age. They occur largely during sleep-wake transition and are characterized by repetitive, stereotypical movements involving large muscle groups. Although occasionally associated with developmental delay, most of the time they occur in normal children and do not result in physical injury to the child. Treatment is generally parental reassurance.

RESTLESS LEGS SYNDROME (RLS)/PERIODIC LIMB MOVEMENT DISORDER (PLMD). RLS is a neuromotor sleep disorder that is

TABLE 18-10. Differentiation of Episodic Nocturnal Phenomena

CHARACTERISTICS	SLEEPWALKING	SLEEP TERRORS	NIGHTMARES	NOCTURNAL SEIZURES
Timing during night	First third	First third	Last third	Variable; often at sleep-wake transition
Sleep stage	SWS	SWS	REM	Non-REM > REM
Clinical description				
Displacement from bed	Usual during event	May occur during event	Occasional after event	Unusual
Autonomic arousal/agitation	Low to mild	High to extreme	Mild to high	Variable
Stereotypic/repetitive behavior	Variable; complex behaviors	Variable	None; little motor behavior	Common
Arousal threshold	High; agitated if awakened	High; agitated if awakened	Low; awake and agitated after event	High; awake and confused after event
Associated daytime sleepiness	None	None	Yes, if night waking prolonged	Probable
Recall of event	None or fragmentary	None or fragmentary	Frequent, vivid	None
Incidence	Common (20% at least one episode; 1–6% chronic)	Rare (1–6%); 10% of sleepwalkers	Very common	Infrequent
Family history	Common	Common	No	Variable

REM, rapid eye movement; SWS, slow-wave sleep.

characterized by what is often described as uncomfortable "creeping" or "crawling" sensations and motor restlessness occurring primarily in the lower extremities. These sensations typically increase in the evening and during periods of rest or inactivity (sleep onset) and are relieved by movement. In younger children, these sensations may be manifested as "growing pains." The symptoms often result in significantly delayed sleep onset. RLS appears to have a genetic basis, and exacerbating factors include increased caffeine intake, iron deficiency (especially low ferritin), and pregnancy. Although the prevalence of RLS in adolescents is unknown, approximately 10% of adults have the disorder. RLS may be related to decreased dopaminergic activity; pharmacologic treatment generally involves dopaminergic precursors (carbidopa, levodopa) and agonists (pramipexole, ropinirole, pergolide), and occasionally opiates, benzodiazepines, and anticonvulsants. Approximately 80% of patients with RLS also have repetitive rhythmic kicking movements of the lower extremities during sleep called **periodic limb movements.** The sleeper is usually unaware of the leg movements and the resulting sleep fragmentation. Both RLS and PLMD may result in significant daytime sleepiness, including inattention and hyperactivity. RLS is a clinical diagnosis; the diagnosis of PLMD requires a PSG to detect the characteristic rhythmic movements of the anterior tibialis muscle group and the frequent arousals.

NARCOLEPSY. Narcolepsy is a primary disorder of excessive daytime sleepiness that affects an estimated 0.05% of Americans. Narcolepsy often presents with symptoms in adolescence, but usually goes unrecognized and undiagnosed until adulthood. In about 25% of cases, there is a family history of narcolepsy; secondary narcolepsy following brain injury or in association with other medical illnesses may also occur. The cardinal and usual initial presenting feature of narcolepsy is repetitive episodes of profound sleepiness that may occur both at rest and during periods of activity (talking, eating). These **sleep attacks** may be very brief (microsleeps), resulting primarily in lapses in attention and in mood disturbances. Thus, patients with narcolepsy may be initially misdiagnosed with a psychiatric disorder, such as ADHD or depression. Other features that may occur in narcolepsy include **cataplexy** (sudden loss of partial or total body muscle tone, usually in response to an emotional stimulus); **hypnagogic** (at sleep onset) and/or **hypnopompic** (on waking) visual, auditory, or tactile **hallucinations;** and **sleep paralysis** (temporary loss of voluntary muscle control) at sleep onset or offset. The "gold standard" of diagnosis is an overnight PSG followed by a multiple sleep latency test. This test involves a series of 4–5 opportunities to nap (20 min long) during which narcoleptics demonstrate a pathologically shortened sleep onset latency as well as periods of REM sleep occurring immediately after sleep onset. The treatment of narcolepsy generally involves a combination of medications to combat daytime sleepiness (stimulants) and REM sleep suppressants to prevent cataleptic attacks.

DELAYED SLEEP PHASE SYNDROME (DSPS). DSPS is most common in adolescents, and it represents a more severe form of the normal puberty-mediated sleep-wake phase delay. In this disorder, the quantity and quality of sleep are generally normal, but the timing of the sleep is problematic. In individuals with DSPS, the preferred bedtime and wake time are much later than normal (sleep onset is typically at 2 A.M. or later), and they conflict with scheduled daytime activities, such as school. DSPS may be successfully treated with a combination of a gradual advance of bedtime in the evening and the use of bright light therapy in the morning to help "reset" the clock. Teenagers with a severely delayed sleep phase (sleep onset >3 to 4 hr later than the desired bedtime) may benefit from a technique called **chronotherapy,** in which the sleep onset and wake times are successively delayed over time until the new sleep onset time coincides with the desired bedtime.

HEALTH SUPERVISION. Sleep disturbances are common issues raised by parents during health supervision; it is estimated that up to 25% of children experience a significant sleep problem at some point during childhood. Although many sleep problems in infants and children are transient and self-limited, certain intrinsic and extrinsic risk factors (difficult temperament, acute or chronic illness, maternal depression, family stress) predispose a child to more chronic sleep disturbance. Inadequate or poor sleep in children may have negative consequences on a host of functional domains, including mood, behavior, learning, and health. The impact of childhood sleep problems is intensified by their direct effect on parents' sleep, resulting in daytime fatigue, mood disturbances, and a decreased level of effective parenting.

Therefore, it is especially important for pediatricians to both screen for and recognize sleep disorders in children and adolescents during health encounters. The well child visit is an opportunity to educate parents about normal sleep in children and to teach strategies to prevent sleep problems from developing (primary prevention) or from becoming chronic, if problems already exist (secondary prevention). Developmentally appropriate screening for sleep disturbances should take place in the context of every well child visit and should include a range of potential sleep problems; one simple sleep screening algorithm, the "BEARS," is outlined in Table 18-11. Because parents may not always be aware of sleep problems, especially in older children and adolescents, it is also important to question the child directly about sleep concerns. The recognition and evaluation of

TABLE 18-11. BEARS Sleep Screening Algorithm

The BEARS instrument is divided into 5 major sleep domains, providing a comprehensive screen for the major sleep disorders affecting children 2–18 years old. Each sleep domain has a set of age-appropriate "trigger questions" for use in the clinical interview.
B = Bedtime problems
E = Excessive daytime sleepiness
A = Awakenings during the night
R = Regularity and duration of sleep
S = Snoring

EXAMPLES OF DEVELOPMENTALLY APPROPRIATE TRIGGER QUESTIONS

	Toddler/Preschool Child (2–5 yr)	School-aged Child (6–12 yr)	Adolescent (13–18 yr)
1. **B**edtime problems	Does your child have any problems going to bed? Falling asleep?	Does your child have any problems at bedtime? (P) Do you have any problems going to bed? (C)	Do you have any problems falling asleep at bedtime? (C)
2. **E**xcessive daytime sleepiness	Does your child seem overtired or sleepy a lot during the day? Does she still take naps?	Does your child have difficulty waking in the morning, seem sleepy during the day, or take naps? (P) Do you feel tired a lot? (C)	Do you feel sleepy a lot during the day? In school? While driving? (C)
3. **A**wakenings during the night	Does your child wake up a lot at night?	Does your child seem to wake up a lot at night? Any sleepwalking or nightmares? (P) Do you wake up a lot at night? Do you have trouble getting back to sleep? (C)	Do you wake up a lot at night? Do you have trouble getting back to sleep? (C)
4. **R**egularity and duration of sleep	Does your child have a regular bedtime and wake time? What are they?	What time does your child go to bed and get up on school days? Weekends? Do you think he is getting enough sleep? (P)	What time do you usually go to bed on school nights? Weekends? How much sleep do you usually get? (C)
5. **S**noring	Does your child snore a lot or have difficulty breathing at night?	Does your child have loud or nightly snoring or any breathing difficulties at night? (P)	Does your teenager snore loudly or nightly? (P)

C, child; P, Parent.

sleep problems in children requires both an understanding of the association between sleep disturbances and daytime consequences, such as irritability, inattention, and poor impulse control, and familiarity with the developmentally appropriate differential diagnoses of common presenting sleep complaints (difficulty initiating and maintaining sleep, episodic nocturnal events). An assessment of sleep patterns and possible sleep problems should be part of the initial evaluation of every child presenting with behavioral and/or academic problems, especially ADHD.

Effective preventive measures include educating parents of newborns about normal sleep amounts and patterns. The ability to regulate sleep, or control internal states of arousal to fall asleep at bedtime and to fall back asleep during the night, begins to develop in the first 12 wk of life. Thus, it is important to recommend that parents put their 2–4 mo old infants to bed "drowsy but awake" to avoid dependence on parental presence at sleep onset and to foster the infants' ability to "self-soothe." Other important sleep issues include discussing the importance of regular bedtimes, bedtime routines, and transitional objects for toddlers, and providing parents and children with basic information about good "sleep hygiene" (see Tables 18-3 and 18-4) and adequate sleep amounts.

The cultural and family context within which sleep problems in children occur should be considered. Co-sleeping of infants and parents is a common and accepted practice in many ethnic groups, including African-Americans, Hispanics, and Southeast Asians. The goal of independent "self-soothing" in young infants may not be shared by these families. On the other hand, the institution of co-sleeping by parents as an attempt to address a child's underlying sleep problem, rather than as a lifestyle choice, is likely to yield only a temporary respite from the problem and may set the stage for more significant sleep issues.

EVALUATION OF PEDIATRIC SLEEP PROBLEMS. The clinical evaluation of a child presenting with a sleep problem involves obtaining a careful medical history to assess for potential medical causes of sleep disturbances, such as allergies, concomitant medications, and acute or chronic pain conditions. A developmental history is important because of the aforementioned frequent association of sleep problems with developmental delays and autism spectrum disorders. Assessment of the child's current level of functioning (school, home) is a key part of evaluating possible mood, behavioral, and neurocognitive sequelae of sleep problems. Current sleep patterns, including the usual sleep duration and sleep-wake schedule, are often best assessed with a sleep diary, in which parents record daily sleep behaviors for an extended period. A review of sleep habits, such as bedtime routines, daily caffeine intake, and the sleeping environment (e.g., temperature, noise level) may reveal environmental factors that contribute to the sleep problems. Nocturnal symptoms that may be indicative of a medically based sleep disorder, such as OSA (loud snoring, choking or gasping, sweating) or periodic limb movements (restless sleep, repetitive kicking movements), should be elicited. An overnight sleep study is seldom warranted in the evaluation of a child with sleep problems unless there are symptoms suggestive of OSA or periodic leg movements, unusual features of episodic nocturnal events, or daytime sleepiness that is unexplained.

AAP Clinical practice guideline: Diagnosis and management of childhood obstructive sleep apnea. *Pediatrics* 2002;9(4):704–712.

Carskadon MA, Ed: *Adolescent Sleep Patterns: Biological, Social, and Psychological Influences.* New York, Cambridge University Press, 2002.

Hiscosk H, Wake M: Randomised controlled trial of behavioural infant sleep interventions to improve infant sleep and maternal mood. *BMJ* 2002;324:1062–1065.

Jenni OG, O'Connor BB: Children's sleep: An interplay between culture and biology. *Pediatrics* 2005;115:204–216.

Lipton AJ, Gozal D: Treatment of obstructive sleep apnea in children: Do we really know how? *Sleep Med Rev* 2003;7(1):61–80.

Millman R, Kaplan D, Carskadon M, et al: Excessive sleepiness in adolescents and young adults: causes, consequences, and treatment strategies. *Pediatrics* 2005;115(6):1774–1786.

Mindell J, Owens J: *A Clinical Guide to Pediatric Sleep: Diagnosis and Management of Sleep Problems in Children and Adolescents.* Philadelphia, Lippincott Williams & Wilkins, 2003.

Owens J, Witmans M: Sleep problems. *Curr Probl Pediatr Adolesc Health Care* 2004;34(4):154–179.

Owens J, Babcock D, Blumer J, et al: The use of pharmacotherapy in the treatment of pediatric insomnia in primary care: Rational approaches. A Consensus Meeting Summary. *J Clin Sleep Med* 2005;1(1):49–59.

Pelayo R, Chen W, Monzon S, Guilleminault C: Pediatric sleep pharmacology: You want to give my kid sleeping pills? *Pediatr Clin N Am* 2004;51: 117–134.

Rosen CL: Obstructive sleep apnea syndrome in children: Controversies in diagnosis and treatment. *Pediatr Clin North Am* 2004;51:153–167.

Schecter M: AAP Technical report: Diagnosis and management of childhood obstructive sleep apnea. *Pediatrics* 2002;109(4):1–20.

Sheldon SH: Parasomnias in childhood. *Pediatr Clin North Am* 2004;51:69–88.

Sheldon SH, Ferber R, Kryger MH (editors): *Principles and Practices of Pediatric Sleep Medicine.* Philadelphia, Elsevier, 2005.

Whiteford L, Fleming P, Henderson AJ: Who should have a sleep study for sleep related breathing disorders? *Arch Dis Child* 2004;89:851–855.

Part III ▪ Psychologic Disorders

Chapter 19 ▪ Assessment and Interviewing

The Clinical Interview •

Mary Margaret Gleason, Prachi Shah, and Neil W. Boris

The clinical interview is a major means of diagnosis and an important way to engage patients and their families in active management of their care (see Chapter 5). Most pediatricians are comfortable interviewing children and parents about signs and symptoms, medical history, and a review of systems related to physical illness. Other aspects of a patient's life, such as psychosocial functioning, receive less attention in patient interactions. There is a significant effect of emotional, behavioral, and social problems on the course of disease, compliance with treatment recommendations, and use of medical resources. Parents expect their pediatrician to ask about psychosocial issues, although parents are often reluctant to present psychosocial concerns themselves.

Pediatricians can use clinical interviews to enhance their relationship with the patient and family, assess the emotional state of patients, and uncover suggestions of psychosocial distress or disturbance within the family context. Successful interviewing is maximized by using a developmental approach and some principles of family assessment (see Chapter 5).

GENERAL PRINCIPLES OF THE CLINICAL INTERVIEW

The assessment of a child's emotional state or of family functioning requires specific skills. Some general principles regarding interviewing and assessment are useful to consider. Efficient communication requires unbroken attention; keeping the door closed and avoiding interruptions can promote efficiency. Privacy will increase the amount of information shared during an interview and is especially important when sensitive psychosocial issues are being discussed. In situations in which privacy cannot be easily attained (an open ward), pediatricians must always be aware that a patient (or the family) may not be comfortable enough to share relevant information. Equally important is the need to explicitly address issues of confidentiality with patients and parents before clinical assessment.

Setting aside adequate time for an interview is important. The 1st goal is to build rapport with both family and child. Developmentally appropriate overtures to the child often start this process. Examples include playing peek-a-boo with a toddler and commenting on sports with a child who is wearing a baseball cap. After an overture with the child, it is useful to allow the accompanying caregiver an opportunity to present his or her concerns. *Family-centered interviewing* refers to the method of guiding patients or their parents through the interview by explicitly allowing them to present their most significant concerns. With practice, it takes no longer to focus on the concerns of the patient and/or parent than to "lead" the interview. Centering the dialogue on the patient's or family's agenda often results in fewer misunderstandings. Both caregivers and children (particularly adolescents) often seek medical care to discuss a **hidden agenda.** Such hidden agendas may relate to psychosocial issues, which the patient may not discuss unless he or she perceives that the physician has provided an appropriate opportunity during the visit. Using a family-centered approach increases this opportunity. A primary determinant of malpractice claims is poor physician-patient (or physician-family) communication; from the patient's perspective, "not being heard" is the central communication problem. Family-centered interviewing improves data-gathering and increases patient satisfaction, which in turn, improves compliance.

Much interview data can also be gathered through careful attention to nonverbal cues. Scanning for nonverbal cues and commenting on them is part of effective interviewing. An adolescent who is expressionless and averts his or her eyes is obviously uncomfortable. If the physician notes this and inquires gently about what might be bothering the patient, he or she creates an opportunity to reach the adolescent. Patients with psychosocial issues that are not addressed may return repeatedly or seek care elsewhere.

An interview is a reciprocal interaction, and the way that a physician provides information can influence medical outcomes. Patients respond to both verbal and nonverbal cues. Language should be clear, and trained interpreters should be used whenever there is a chance that a language difference will impair communication in either direction. Although it is often tempting to use a child as an interpreter, this practice is strongly discouraged because parents may not be able to express their concerns comfortably and children may edit the information that is transmitted (see Chapter 4). It is useful to check in with parents when providing feedback to ensure comprehension. Courtesies such as sitting down to talk with the parent or patient can demonstrate that the pediatrician values the interaction and the relationship with the patient and family. Maintaining eye contact and using a positive tone of voice when detailing a medication regimen will increase the likelihood that the patient or parent will understand the information. Providing legibly written instructions, a clear explanation of why the intervention is being used, and instructions for follow-up will further increase compliance.

Although most pediatricians do not have the time or training to perform an in-depth psychiatric interview, they spend much of their time addressing concerns about children's behavior. Familiarity with and use of available screening instruments allows the practitioner to follow up on impressions regarding psychosocial concerns by getting more in-depth data. The Bright Futures in Practice: Mental Health website *(http://brightfutures.aap.org/web/)* provides developmentally specific checklists that can provide structure for these screenings. The **Pediatric Symptom Checklist** is a 35-item parent and child report questionnaire about psychosocial functioning that can be a useful adjunct to the clinical interview (Fig. 19-1). For children with clear symptoms, the **Child Behavior Checklist** helps to cluster symptoms. Teacher reports can also be useful if there is concern that parental perception may differ from the child's experiences at school. These checklists do not provide diagnoses, but can help to determine what intervention or referral might be most appropriate. Even children who do not seem to have a specific disorder, but who are experiencing distress in the context of parental discord or peer relationships, may require extra support or even referral for counseling.

BRIGHT FUTURES TOOL FOR PROFESSIONALS

Pediatric Symptom Checklist (PSC)

Emotional and physical health go together in children. Because parents are often the first to notice a problem with their child's behavior, emotions, or learning, you may help your child get the best care possible by answering these questions. Please indicate which statement best describes your child.

Please mark under the heading that best decribes your child:

		Never	Sometimes	Often
1. Complains of aches and pains	1	____	____	____
2. Spends more time alone	2	____	____	____
3. Tires easily, has little energy	3	____	____	____
4. Fidgety, unable to sit still	4	____	____	____
5. Has trouble with teacher	5	____	____	____
6. Less interested in school	6	____	____	____
7. Acts as if driven by a motor	7	____	____	____
8. Daydreams too much	8	____	____	____
9. Distracted easily	9	____	____	____
10. Is afraid of new situations	10	____	____	____
11. Feels sad, unhappy	11	____	____	____
12. Is irritable, angry	12	____	____	____
13. Feels hopeless	13	____	____	____
14. Has trouble concentrating	14	____	____	____
15. Less interested in friends	15	____	____	____
16. Fights with other children	16	____	____	____
17. Absent from school	17	____	____	____
18. School grades dropping	18	____	____	____
19. Is down on him- or herself	19	____	____	____
20. Visits the doctor with doctor finding nothing wrong	20	____	____	____
21. Has trouble sleeping	21	____	____	____
22. Worries a lot	22	____	____	____
23. Wants to be with you more than before	23	____	____	____
24. Feels he or she is bad	24	____	____	____
25. Takes unnecessary risks	25	____	____	____
26. Gets hurt frequently	26	____	____	____
27. Seems to be having less fun	27	____	____	____
28. Acts younger than children his or her age	28	____	____	____
29. Dose not listen to rules	29	____	____	____
30. Does not show feelings	30	____	____	____
31. Does not understand other people's feelings	31	____	____	____
32. Teases others	32	____	____	____
33. Blames others for his or her troubles	33	____	____	____
34. Takes things that do not belong to him or her	34	____	____	____
35. Refuses to share	35	____	____	____

Total score____________

Does your child have any emotional or behavioral problems for which she or he needs help? ( ) N ( ) Y

Are there any services that you would like your child to receive for these problems? ( ) N ( ) Y

If yes, what services?____

Figure 19-1. Pediatric Symptom Checklist. (From Green M, Palfrey JS [editors]: *Bright Futures: Guidelines of the Health Supervision of Infants, Children, and Adolescents,* 2nd ed, revised. Arlington, VA, National Center for Education in Maternal and Child Health, 2002.)

TOPICS FOR ALL AGES

Emotional and behavioral well-being should be assessed at every well child visit, beginning with the 1st visit. Even prenatal appointments can be useful in understanding a family's expectations, coping strategies, and level of stress. Setting basic ground rules for when and how to call for help is reassuring to parents. As the child develops, **anticipatory guidance** about common stress points for parents is critical. Routine provision of web-based or written parent resources is highly valued by most parents.

Using family-centered interviewing does not mean that the pediatrician should eliminate an agenda for a given visit. The pediatrician should screen for maternal depression, a disease that significantly affects young children's emotional development and medical outcomes. The developmental effects of maternal depression can be seen in the 1st week of life, when infants of depressed mothers show altered physiologic responsiveness and changes in electroencephalographic activation. Maternal depression is associated with poor maternal responsiveness to the infant and, in time, with insecure child attachment. Primary care physicians are in the optimal position to screen for postpartum depression because mothers do not return to see their obstetrician until 6 wk postpartum. Postpartum screening about mood and functioning can be done by using the U.S. Public Health 2-Question screen ("Have you been feeling down, depressed, or hopeless?" and "Have you had little interest or pleasure in doing things?"). It is important to remember that **"baby blues"** last only 10 days; mood symptoms that persistent beyond 10 days should be further evaluated. It is useful to have copies of formal screening measures, such as the Edinburgh Postnatal Depression Scale or the Beck Depression Inventory, in the office to assist with deciding which caregivers need referral for treatment. The majority of depressed parents will readily fill out a screening questionnaire, and most are relieved to be able to discuss their difficulties. The pediatrician who recognizes parental depression and completes a referral may significantly improve the developmental course of the affected child.

Family violence is another common problem that is associated with developmental consequences for children (see Chapter 35). There are no simple demographic indicators of families at greatest risk for domestic violence: Partner violence cuts across socioeconomic groups. Many practitioners feel anxious inquiring about family violence, but a query about family discourse easily leads to pertinent follow-up questions. First stating "I always ask about how a child's parents are handling their stress. How are you doing in this regard?" suggests that family concerns are also the concern of the pediatrician. A follow-up question might be, "You know, an issue that really affects children is parental fighting, especially physical fights. Has this ever been a problem in your home?" Data suggest that, when asked, both victims and victimizers will offer details about family violence. Because parents are usually more comfortable talking about these issues outside the child's presence, the pediatrician should offer this option.

When the pediatrician hears about physical fighting in the home, he or she should ask about the current situation and **assess family safety** directly, including the child's physical and emotional safety. Parents affected by partner violence should be given information about domestic violence resources in the community, especially local shelters. Telephone hotlines, such as the National Domestic Violence Hotline (1-800-799-SAFE), are useful to parents involved in violent relationships. Women living in violent relationships rarely move out the 1st time a professional raises the issue; this delay, however, should not be interpreted as noncompliance. Close follow-up with families after discussions of violence is critical, and parents should be repeatedly encouraged to consider their safety and that of their family. It is imperative that screening for child maltreatment, commonly associated with family violence, be undertaken any time a caregiver reports family violence (see Chapter 36).

There is much evidence that children are adversely affected by ongoing family violence. However, there is no clear clinical profile of an affected child. Common symptoms associated with family violence include aggression, behavioral dysregulation, school failure, and anxiety and mood symptoms. Structured checklists, such as the Child Behavior Checklist, are useful in screening for highly symptomatic children; obtaining data from >1 source (parent, teacher) is important. An assessment of children's behavioral functioning should 1st consider the child's developmental stage. The pediatrician who keenly observes the parent-child interaction and deftly interviews children will identify those with psychosocial problems early. Early identification of children with psychosocial problems, when coupled with appropriate intervention, is associated with improved developmental outcomes.

USING A DEVELOPMENTAL APPROACH TO INTERVIEWING CHILDREN

INFANCY AND TODDLERHOOD. Infants and toddlers have tremendous capacity for forming memories, although they do not have language available to describe them. This means that the frequent office or clinic visits before 3 yr of age can collectively provide a "positive memory bank" for an individual child, which can then become the building blocks for a positive and meaningful physician relationship with the child and his or her family. Children at this stage of development are learning through sensory experiences. A soft tone of voice and gentle handling of the infant are important means of helping the infant develop a sense of trust and comfort with the practitioner. The practitioner who actively engages, even briefly, with young children will create these positive relationship building blocks. Furthermore, paying this kind of direct attention to the young child is almost always comforting to parents; infants and young children are highly adept at sensing parental anxiety.

Toward the end of the 1st year of life, the child begins to show focused attachment behavior toward his primary caregiver. By 10 mo of age, the child will explore unfamiliar environments, but return to the caregiver for emotional support when distressed. If by 18 mo, the distressed child displays uncertainty in accessing support from the primary caregiver, the pediatrician should be concerned about the quality of the parent-child attachment. The watchful practitioner can assess the developing attachment relationship because the typical health supervision visit is enough of a stressor for the toddler to yield important information about how he or she seeks comfort from the caregiver. The Infant-Toddler Social and Emotional Assessment questionnaire is a well-validated parent report screening device that is particularly useful when the pediatrician has concerns about a given child's social or emotional development. The Checklist for Autism in Toddlers is also useful for children who make limited verbal and nonverbal social contact with their caregivers.

PRESCHOOL CHILDREN. The verbal and cognitive capacities of preschoolers mean that they may anticipate physician visits with some anxiety. At this age, children commonly interpret medical procedures, such as needlesticks, as punishments for being bad. The use of stickers and other small gifts may help to counteract this natural way of thinking and enrich the relationship with the preschool patient.

The preschool visit should also be used to address issues of emotional health and well-being. Although most children with mild behavioral difficulties do not have significant psychiatric disorders, 1 in 10 preschoolers has a clinically significant emotional or behavioral disorder, including attention-deficit/hyperactivity disorder (ADHD), depression, and anxiety disorders. Using a color-coded sticker in the chart when the parent notes behavioral, sleep, or eating difficulties allows the physician to inquire at a return visit if a suggested behavioral intervention was effective.

When basic interventions, such as teaching the time-out technique, do not seem effective, it is important to explore the symptoms further, reassess the diagnosis, and reconsider the plan, possibly including a mental health referral. Reports of expulsions or suspensions in child-care or preschool settings should not be dismissed. Early aggression (even before age 3 yr) is quite stable over time and is predictive of an evolving mental health problem. Family-based interventions are effective, although the longer the pattern of aggression and defiance persists, the more difficult it is to treat. Another notable symptom is **anhedonia,** which is limited enjoyment of activities, often accompanied by high levels of irritability. Anhedonia is the most specific predictor of clinically significant depression in preschoolers, whereas **excessive crying** is the most sensitive predictor. Persistent anxiety symptoms, such as fear of separation from the caregiver, also require further evaluation, especially when the child's anxiety impairs the family's functioning (associated with parents missing work or the child's missing school).

SCHOOL-AGED CHILDREN. As children reach school age, it is important to ask (in developmentally appropriate language) about their interests directly at the outset of any interaction. It can be helpful to document specific interests or activities in the patient chart to allow for follow-up queries at subsequent visits. School-aged children look up to medical providers, and the pediatrician who personalizes the visit by remembering the child's interests will strengthen the physician-patient relationship. This effort will be rewarded in the teen years, when the typical suspicion of adult authority is moderated by the teen's sense of the provider as interested and caring.

A complete health maintenance visit includes a review of the child's emotional functioning. In the school-aged child, the most common psychiatric disorders are attention-deficit/hyperactivity disorder (ADHD; see Chapter 31), major depression (see Chapter 25), anxiety disorders (see Chapter 24), and learning disorders (see Chapter 32).

Asking children and their parents about school achievement, peer relationships, and family functioning is an appropriate entry into the subject of emotional functioning. Attentional problems, learning disorders, and sometimes anxiety disorders can be identified in a discussion of school problems. Peer problems can indicate developmental delays and/or social skill deficits. The increasing incidence of **pervasive developmental disorders** requires the pediatrician to be familiar with this diagnostic category (see Chapter 29). Family functioning can provide clues about parental discord, child emotional or behavioral difficulties, parental mental health problems, or the effect of family stressors, such as poverty, community violence, or domestic violence. During the clinical interview, careful tracking of the child's affect, or facial expression of emotion, will provide information about his or her internal state. When children are sad or anxious, noting this by inquiring directly about what makes them feel sad or anxious is important.

Although the hyperactive form of ADHD presents by the school-age years, the inattentive type is under-recognized, especially in girls. Children who are reported to have school difficulties should be screened for ADHD using readily available checklists, such as the Conner Rating Scale for ADHD. Parents who describe irritability or opposition may be alerting the pediatrician to a mood disorder, especially if there is a family history of mood disorders. The age at which children begin using illegal drugs has been decreasing over the last decade. In 2004, 21.5% of 8th graders reported a lifetime use of illicit substances (see Chapter 113). It is therefore important to discuss substance use with children in the prepubertal years.

ADOLESCENTS. A key developmental milestone for adolescents is gaining autonomy from their parents or caretakers (see Part XII). Pediatricians can support this autonomy by structuring the patient interaction to include time spent with the patient alone without the parent. This practice affords the adolescent a sense of privacy and increases the chance of gaining insight into issues that would not be discussed in front of parents. Confidentiality, and the limits thereof, should be discussed with both the patient and the parent together, before the parent leaves the room. Not all practitioners ask parents to leave the room during health maintenance visits, although adolescents value this time and such interactions enhance the quality of information obtained and care provided. Physical examinations of adolescents should also be conducted without the parents present, unless the patient requests otherwise.

Although adolescence has been traditionally viewed as a period of storm and stress, most adolescents do not experience more stress at this developmental stage than at others. Risk-taking behavior (use of alcohol, tobacco, or drugs; sexual activity) is common among adolescents, and most adolescents report peer pressure to take risks. Adolescence is also a period when the incidence of several major mental illnesses increases dramatically. Major depression, bipolar disorder, panic disorder, and schizophrenia are chronic conditions that frequently present during adolescence; early stabilization of these illnesses may improve long-term outcome. Rates of depression in teens are equivalent to those in adults, and suicide is the 3rd most common cause of death in adolescence. Adolescence is a stage during which consolidation of sexual orientation generally occurs, and this process, especially for many youth who self-identify as homosexual, is associated with considerable stress, elevated levels of risk-taking, and higher rates of suicide attempts (see Chapter 13).

Each adolescent visit requires a careful social history. The use of a structured format for briefly assessing risk-taking behaviors, social stressors, sexual identity and orientation, substance abuse, and emotional adjustment is recommended to ensure that all topics are covered in the interview. A commonly used format for adolescent interviewing is the **Home, Health, Education, Employment, Activities, Drugs, Depression, Safety, Sexuality (HEADDSS) Screen** (see Table 111-3). Using an adolescent report questionnaire and having a provider form that prompts the provider to ask about these topics enhances screening in the primary care setting. Positive reinforcement for healthy behaviors should always be included in the interaction. If mental illness is suspected, a psychiatric review of symptoms should be part of the clinical interview. As part of such an assessment, suicidal ideation (see Chapter 26) should also be discussed. Inquiring about suicide does not promote suicidal ideation. **Suicidal ideation** can be described as **active** (reflecting a thought to harm oneself) or **passive** (a desire to be dead without a plan). Having referral resources and a plan of action can make asking this question easier for the clinician.

With practice, an interview that begins with open-ended questions about social functioning and finishes with an inquiry about suicidal ideation should be possible in a 15-min visit with an adolescent. Good eye contact, a practiced transition statement ("Now I'd like to ask about some issues that I ask all teens about"), and the use of reflection and encouragement can help to put most adolescents at ease. Creating an atmosphere in which the adolescent has permission to discuss his or her most private concerns is critical. Even if the adolescent denies current suicidal ideation, substance abuse, or relationship violence, asking about these topics shows that the physician is willing to talk about sensitive issues.

For the parent, caring for an adolescent can be challenging. Maintaining open communication between parents and their teenage children promotes positive adjustment for the adolescent. However, parents sometimes feel disconnected from their adolescents, in part because peer influence becomes more and more important during adolescence, resulting in a degree of withdrawal from the parents. The pediatrician can play the role of parenting coach effectively at this developmental stage by modeling behavior (asking to meet with the adolescent alone to talk about teen issues) and suggesting that the parent routinely do the same. Again, addressing parents' specific concerns is important, and there are a number of web-based and print resources that can provide backup information for the busy physician (www.aap.org/parents.html). Parents typically value being pointed in the direction of good parenting books and resources.

When basic interventions involving the parents, the child, and school personnel do not lead to improved functioning, referral to a mental health professional is indicated. It is important that pediatricians avoid communicating that mental health referral is a last resort. The need for mental health consultation should be expressed in terms of the joint need of the family and the physician for help in areas where the mental health provider has special expertise, with the understanding that the collaboration of the physician and the family in the management of the other health care needs of the child remains intact. To be most effective, referral should begin with a call to the mental health provider after written permission to exchange health information is obtained from the parent. Results from parent- or teacher-reported screening instruments discussed in this section might be helpful to the receiving clinician.

PSYCHIATRIC CONSULTATION. A psychiatric consultation may be a valuable part of the assessment of a child's symptoms (including physical symptoms) or family stress or discord. The physician should inform both the parent and the child what the psychiatric consultation is intended to assess. The child's consent is helpful and is usually easily obtained when the reasons for the referral are explained and the child is given some idea of what to expect. Helpful information on psychiatric assessment is available to both the physician and the parents. Standardized guidelines for psychiatric assessment of infants, children, and adolescents have been published by the American Academy of Child and Adolescent Psychiatry, and free, printable "Facts for Families" sheets on various psychiatric symptoms are available on the web (www.aap.org; see resources for families) or by telephone. The need for a psychiatric consultation or referral can be expressed in terms of the joint need of the family and the physician for help in areas where the psychiatrist has special expertise, with the understanding that the collaboration of the physician and the family in the management of the other health care needs of the child will remain intact.

Briggs-Gowan MJ, Carter AS, Irwin JR, et al: Brief infant-toddler social and emotional assessment: Screening for social-emotional problems and delays in competence. *J Pediatr Psychol* 2004;29:143–155.

Carlat DJ: The psychiatric review of symptoms: A screening tool for family physicians. *Am Fam Physician* 1998;58:1617–1624.

Ellingson KD, Briggs-Gowan MJ, Carter AS, et al: Parent identification of early emerging child behavior problems: Predictors of sharing parental concern with health providers. *Arch Pediatr Adolesc Med* 2004;158: 766–772.

Kim-Cohen J, Moffit TE, Taylor A, et al: Maternal depression and children's antisocial behavior. *Arch Gen Psychiatry* 2005;62:173–181.

McLennan JD, Kotelchuck M, Cho H: Prevalence, persistence, and correlates of depressive symptoms in a national sample of mothers of toddlers. *J Am Acad Child Adolesc Psychiatry* 2001;40:1316–1323.

Ozer EM, Adams SH, Lustig JL, et al: Increasing the screening and counseling of adolescents for risky healthy behaviors: A primary care intervention. *Pediatrics* 2005;115:960–968.

Smith RC, Marshall-Dorsey AA, Osborn GG, et al: Evidence-based guidelines for teaching patient-centered interviewing. *Patient Educ Couns* 2000;39:27.

Stein MT, Coleman WL, Epstein RM: "We've tried everything and nothing works": Family-centered pediatrics and clinical problem-solving. *J Dev Behav Pediatr* 2001;22:S55–S60.

Virshup BB, Oppenberg AA, Coleman MM: Strategic risk management: Reducing malpractice claims through more effective patient-doctor communication. *Am J Med Qual* 1999:14:153–159.

Weissman MM, Pilowski DJ, Wickramaratne PJ, et al: Remissions in maternal depression and child psychopathology. *JAMA* 2006;295:1389–1398.

Zuckerman B, Parker S, Kaplan-Sanoff M, et al: Healthy steps: A case study of innovation in pediatric practice. *Pediatrics* 2004;114:820–826.

Chapter 20 ■ Psychologic Treatment of Children and Adolescents

Richard Dalton and Neil W. Boris

20.1 • Illness and Death

Physicians should focus on patients' discomfort rather than on a categorization of clinical manifestations as either organically or psychologically determined. All clinical phenomena relate to various organizational levels: molecular, anatomic, physiologic, intrapsychic, interpersonal, familial, and social. The psychologic aspects of illness should be evaluated from the outset, and physicians should act as a model for parents and children by showing interest in a child's feelings and demonstrating that it is possible and appropriate to communicate discomfort with words.

For **hospitalized children**, potential challenges include: coping with separation; adapting to a new environment; adjusting to multiple caregivers; associating with other sick children; undergoing uncomfortable or scary procedures; and sometimes experiencing the disorientation of intensive care, anesthesia, and surgery. To help mitigate potential problems, a preadmission visit to the hospital is often important to meet the people who will be offering care and to ask questions about what will happen. For most children, particularly those younger than age 5–6 yr, parents should room with the child if feasible. Creative and active recreational or socialization programs, with liberal visiting hours (including visits from siblings and friends), parental rooming-in, and chances to act out feared procedures in play with dolls are helpful. Sensitive, sympathetic, and accepting attitudes toward children and parents by the hospital staff are very important. There is often an underlying tension between hospital caregivers and parents. Hospital routines and schedules often complicate the relationship between parents and hospital workers. Guilt and anger can result, unnecessarily complicating an already difficult situation.

Ambulatory care in clinics or offices where patients receive discontinuous care from a series of physicians whose intercommunication is often limited may create a problem. Parents often become confused and unable to verbalize major concerns about their children. Recommendations for care may become inappropriate or irrelevant, and compliance with advice or directions becomes poor. At the end of any initial diagnostic or management activity, physicians should habitually ask whether there are other things the parents or children wish to talk about during this visit. In busy emergency rooms, conflicting expectations between how the professional staff expects the emergency room to be used and what patients actually need can lead to confusion. When these different expectations are critically examined, ways may be found to deal more effectively with the patterns of use of emergency services.

With **chronically or fatally ill children,** patients and parents experience every symptom as a threat to the child's physical integrity and life. The more serious the clinical state, the greater the intensity of the emotions aroused. By age 9 yr, children begin to conceive of death as meaning more than just going away. By adolescence, they think of death in philosophic terms, much as adults do, albeit with limited experience (see Chapters 38 and 40).

When a child has a chronic illness that shortens life, the parents need physicians' early support in developing a relatively guilt-free understanding of the disease and how to manage it. They need guidance to help them comfortably answer their child's questions about the disease. Young children take most cues from their parents. With older children, especially adolescents, parents must be prepared to deal with the child's anger because of his or her fate. Children need both the parents' psychologic strengths and resources and the physician's availability and objectivity. The siblings of an ill child require information about the disease and the support and attention of the parents for their own needs.

The physician must offer hope and relief of discomfort, ready to help parents and children avoid emotionally crippling psychologic handicaps. Parents must be encouraged to meet their own needs, even when this requires temporary and perhaps recurrent separation from their child; at times, this may help a child to learn to tolerate frustration. Parents of critically or fatally ill children may support each other creatively in group meetings under the professional guidance of physicians, psychologists, or social workers.

In potentially **fulminant lethal processes,** the intensity of parental anxiety, guilt, and despair may be greater than it is with more chronic illnesses. With most children older than 9–10 yr, it is most helpful to discuss the illness factually with the child, as far as diagnosis and prognosis are concerned, but always to offer realistic hope. Children do not usually ask a physician if and when they are going to die, although they may reveal their fears to others in the hospital. Young children primarily want to be reassured that their parents will not desert them and that they are loved. A hospital team approach representing medical, nursing, psychologic, and social work disciplines, among others, should provide support. The primary physician needs to stay involved and close to the child and the clinical situation.

After **the death of a child,** the parents need opportunities to talk about their feelings with the physician, one of whose goals should be to help them avoid psychologically encapsulating the lost child in an unmourned state. Many parents can be helped and comforted by being with and holding the dying infant or child or seeing and touching him or her after death. Physicians need the patience to listen (to both the stated and the implied questions and misconceptions), to answer questions, and to help families with funeral arrangements.

20.2 • Psychopharmacology

The effects of pharmacotherapy on behavior are influenced by the maturity of the central nervous system, by intrapsychic and psychosocial factors, by pharmacogenetics (see Chapter 56) and drug interactions (see Chapter 57), by the personality of the physician prescribing them, by the problem itself, and by the milieu (patient, parents, time of day given) [Table 20-1]. Although they are often helpful, psychiatric medications may cause serious side effects. Even though some guidelines are offered in Table 20-1 for their use, only clinicians with appropriate training and experience should prescribe antipsychotics, mood stabilizers, and tricyclic antidepressants. There is a rapidly expanding pool of data regarding psychopharmacologic interventions in children; on the other hand, rigorous trials are rare and off-label prescribing is common.

Antipsychotics are appropriately used for hallucinations, delusions, thought disorders, and severe agitation. They are primarily indicated for children and adolescents with schizophrenic disorders, mood-congruent and mood-incongruent psychotic reactions associated with major affective disorders, autism presenting with stereotypical and withdrawal symptoms and self-abuse, and pediatric bipolar disorder. Although the **neuroleptics** are the class of drugs with the longest track record of use in children, their significant side effects and relatively narrow therapeutic windows have led to increased use of **atypical antipsychotics.** Atypical antipsychotics are now far more commonly used in most practices, although they are associated with metabolic syndromes, particularly weight gain and hyperprolactinemia.

Neuroleptics can be rather sedating, producing numerous anticholinergic side effects and extrapyramidal symptoms. The most worrisome side effect is the development of **tardive dyskinesia.** This is characterized by choreoathetoid movements of the trunk, limbs, and facial musculature; these movements develop in approximately 20–30% of children who receive long-term treatment with neuroleptics. **Extrapyramidal symptoms,** which cause a Parkinson-like syndrome (akathisia, bradykinesia, torticollis, drooling, involuntary hand movements), occur in at least 25% of children treated with neuroleptics. This syndrome can be treated by decreasing the dose of the neuroleptic or adding an anticholinergic agent (trihexyphenidyl HCl [Artane], benztropine mesylate [Cogentin]). **Neuroleptic malignant syndrome,** a rare side effect of neuroleptic use, can be fatal. Its development is heralded by a high fever, metabolic acidosis, and "lead pipe" stiffness of the extremities. The creatinine phosphokinase level is also markedly elevated. Immediate discontinuation of the drug and supportive care are necessary during the early part of the syndrome (see Chapters 76 and 174).

Atypical antipsychotics are better tolerated than neuroleptics: they are less sedating, are not strongly associated with anticholinergic symptoms, and are far less likely to cause extrapyramidal symptoms. Atypical antipsychotics are associated with weight gain over time as well as with hyperprolactinemia. Case reports of glucose dysregulation and dyslipidemia associated with the use of atypical antipsychotics have been published. Whether atypical antipsychotic use is associated with type II diabetes mellitus is controversial.

Stimulant medications are used to treat the signs and symptoms of attention-deficit/hyperactivity disorder (ADHD) [see Chapter 31] and oppositional-defiant disorder (see Chapter 28). Stimulants increase children's attention, improve classroom behavior, and increase social acceptance of affected children in various situations. Stimulants have a long track record and are safe if used as prescribed. Mild elevation in blood pressure with the use of stimulants is common; blood pressure should be monitored. Stimulants are associated with appetite suppression and insomnia, although these side effects can usually be managed by changing the time of administration or dosing. There is no evidence that nongeneric stimulants are more effective, better tolerated, or safer than methylphenidate or dextroamphetamine. Stimulants have some potential for abuse, although a small proportion of adolescents use them recreationally. Boys with ADHD are less likely to have substance abuse disorders when treated with stimulants.

Serotonin reuptake inhibitors (SSRIs), especially fluoxetine (Prozac), sertraline (Zoloft), and paroxetine (Paxil) are effective in adolescents and adults with mild depressive symptoms, anxiety, and compulsions. Because the few rigorous studies conducted in children have also shown positive effects and because SSRIs have a better side effect profile and a much less narrow therapeutic window, SSRIs have replaced tricyclic antidepressants for the treatment of depressive and/or anxiety disorders. In 2004, the U.S. Food and Drug Administration (FDA) directed pharmaceutical companies to issue a warning about the increased risk of suicidal thinking and behavior (suicidality) in children and adolescents with major depressive disorder undergoing treatment with antidepressants. The FDA did not prohibit the use of antidepressants in children and adolescents, but recommended that physicians and families closely monitor children and adolescents who are taking the medications for worsening symptoms of depression or unusual changes in behavior, especially during the early phases of treatment. Careful review of these data suggests that the association more likely reflects the long-established link

TABLE 20-1. Psychopharmacology

MEDICATION CLASS	USE	DOSAGE	SIDE EFFECTS/TOXICITY/CAUTION	PRETREATMENT WORK-UP
ANTIPSYCHOTICS—TRADITIONAL				
	All: Severe agitation; psychosis; mania; stereotypic movements; self-abuse; extreme aggressiveness; Tourette syndrome		**All classes:** Sedation, weight gain, anticholinergic effects (dry mouth, blurred vision; constipation); hypersensitivity reactions (hepatic, skin); blood dyscrasias; parkinsonism; neuroleptic malignant syndrome; orthostatic hypotension; agranulocytosis and seizures (especially with clozapine) **N.B.:** Thioridazine (Mellaril) is no longer recommended because of hepatotoxicity **N.B.:** Tardive dyskinesia is a potential side effect	CBC with differential, blood chemistry panel (including hepatic enzymes) Pregnancy test; height and weight measures
Low-Potency/High-Dosage				
Chlorpromazine (Thorazine)		Initial: 10–30 mg/24 hr in single or divided doses; maintenance: 100–900 mg/24 hr in divided doses		
Mid-Potency/Mid-Dosage				
Mesoridazine (Serentil)		10–75 mg/24 hr in divided doses		
High-Potency/Low-Dosage				
Haloperidol (Haldol)		Initial: 0.5–1 mg/24 hr in single or divided doses		
Trifluoperazine (Stelazine)				
Thiothixine (Navane)				
ANTIPSYCHOTICS—NOVEL (ATYPICAL)				
			Same general side effects as traditional antipsychotics treatment emergent diabetes; hyperlipidemia	**All:** Cardiovascular history; ECG; Comprehensive metabolic panel; electrolytes; pregnancy tests: weight and height measures
Clozapine (Clozaril)		Initial: 12.5–25 mg/24 hr; increased by 25–50 mg/24 hr; maintenance: 250–500 mg/24 hr in divided doses	Seizures, agranulocytosis, weight gain	History of seizures; CBC/differential
Risperidone (Risperdal)		Initial: 0.5 mg bid; increased by 0.5 mg each 3–4 days to 2–4 mg/24 hr	Weight gian, mild EPS, increase in prolactin levels, prolongation of QTc	
Quetiapine (Seroquel)		Initial: 25 mg bid; increased by 50–100 mg every 2–3 days to 50–500 mg/24 hr	Sedation, weight gain	Ophthalmologic examination
Olanzapine (Zyperxa)		Initial: 2.5–5.0 mg hs; if necessary, increased 2.5 mg every 3–4 days to 5–15 mg/24 hr	Sedation, weight gian, prolongation of QTc	
Ziprasidone (Geodon)		40–80 mg/24 hr in divided doses	Prolongation of QTc	
Aripiprazole (Ability)		Initial and maintenance: 10–15 mg/24 hr	Slight weight gain, headache	
STIMULANTS	**All drugs:** ADHD (with and without behavioral acting out): narcolepsy (methylphenidate, dextroamphetamine)		Lower seizure threshold; insomnia, decreased appetite, possible weight loss; irritability and tearfulness; abdominal pain, headache; elevated systolic blood pressure; development and worsening of tics; possible subnormal height and weight growth. Possible precipitation of hypomania in bipolar patients; possible cardiovascular effects include myocardial infarction; pemoline (Cylert) is no longer recommended because of hepatotoxicity	Medical history, heart rate, blood pressure, CBC with differential (with prolonged use)
Methylphenidate (Ritalin, Concerta, Metadate ER, Flocalin)		Ritalin: 0.3–1.0 mg/kg/24 hr in divided doses Concerta: 18 mg in single dose; increased to 36 mg if necessary Metadate ER: 10 mg increased to 60 mg/24 hr if necessary Flocalin: ½ of Ritalin dose		
Dextroamphetamine (Dexedrine, Adderall, Adderall XR)		Dexedrine: 0.2–0.6 mg/kg/24 hr in divided doses Adderall: Initial: 2.5–5 mg; increased by 2.5–5.0 mg/24 hr to 60 mg/24 hr (narcolepsy) Adderall XR: Initial: 10–20 mg/24 hr; increase weekly to 0.5–1.0 mg/kg/24 hr		
Presynaptic Norepinephrine Transport Inhibitor				
Atomoxetine (Strattera)	ADHD symptoms (with or without comorbid depression and anxiety)	Initial: 18–25 mg/24 hr; increased every 4–7 days to 1.2–1.8 mg/kg/24 hr	Decreased appetite and weight; slight increase in blood pressure and pulse rate	

TABLE 20-1.—*Cont'd.* Psychopharmacology

MEDICATION CLASS	USE	DOSAGE	SIDE EFFECTS/TOXICITY/CAUTION	PRETREATMENT WORK-UP
ANTIDEPRESSANTS				
Tricyclics				
Desipramine (Norpramin)	Major depressive disorder in mid to late adolescence; ADHD (12 yr and older); separation anxiety disorder	For major depression disorder and separation anxiety disorder, 2–3 mg/kg/24 hr in divided doses. (therapeutic blood level, 100–250 mg/mL)	Possible sudden death in doses >3.5–5.0 mg/kg; hypertension, orthostatic hypotension, cardiac arrhythmia, lengthening of P-R or QRS interval on ECG; overdose leading to death	Thorough individual and family history for cardiologic problems; 12-lead ECG; blood pressure monitoring. Plasma blood levels indicated after therapy has begun only if clinical response is poor
Imipramine (Tofranil)	As above; enuresis	As above, for enuresis, usually 25–50 mg qhs (continued for at least 4–6 mo after remission of enuresis)	As above	As above
Clomipramine (Anafranil)	OCD	Initial: 25 mg, increased slowly (2–3 wk) to either 100 mg or 3 mg/kg (whichever is smaller) in divided doses; thereafter, increased to a maximum of 250–300 mg	Seizures; overdose leading to death; ST-T wave changes on ECG, conduction abnormalities; psychiatric changes including mania and confusion; weight gain; hyperthermia; vertigo; constipation	As above
Selective Serotonin Reuptake Inhibitors				
			N.B.: Evidence suggests that SSRIs increase suicidal ideation and parasuicidal behavior in children and adolescents (but not suicide)	**N.B.:** Thorough individual and family history of suicidal behavior and the risk factors for suicide
Fluoxetine (Prozac)	Mild–moderate depression, anxiety, OCD	10–20 mg/24 hr (possibly higher for OCD)	Fluoxetine and its principal metabolite have a long half-life (1–4 days). Can inhibit its own metabolism; thus, an increase in dose may result in a disproportionate increase in side effects. Drug interactions with compounds metabolized by several isoenzymes of the cytochrome P450 system (especially terfenadine, astemizole, cisapride); gastrointestinal difficulties (nausea, diarrhea, vomiting); CNS effects (agitation, disinhibition, jitteriness, headache, insomnia); tremor; serotonin syndrome (fever, myoclonus, confusion, tachycardia, rigidity) when taken with MAO inhibitors or L-tryptophan; mania; self-injurious behavior and behavioral activation and dyscontrol	
Paroxetine (Paxil)	As above	10–30 mg/24 hr	As above, except shorter half-life (24 hr); withdrawal symptoms if stopped abruptly	
Sertraline (Zoloft)	As above	25–50 mg/24 hr with meals	Similar to paroxetine; fairly inactive metabolite has longer half-life; exhibits linear relationship between dose and side effects	
Fluvoxamine (Luvox)	OCD	Initial: 25–50 mg each night; increased slowly to no more than 300 mg/24 hr in divided doses	Similar to sertraline; less interference with cytochrome P450 system	
Venlafaxine (Effexor)	Depression	Initial: 37.5 mg/24 hr; increased by no more than 37.5–75.0 mg/24 hr to a maximum of 225 mg/24 hr in divided doses, with meals	As above, except little interference with cytochrome P450 system	
Citalopram (Celexa, Lexapro)		Initial: 10–20 mg/24 hr; increase weekly by 10–20 mg/24 hr to a maximum of 20–60 mg/24 hr in divided doses		
Aminoketone				
Bupropion (Wellbutrin)	Depression, ADHD	Initial: 75–100 mg/24 hr; increased slowly to 200–300 mg/24 hr (bid dosing); total daily dose should not exceed 450 mg	Seizures, restlessness, agitation, weight loss, rashes, nocturia, mania, flu-like symptoms	
MOOD STABILIZERS				
Lithium carbonate	Bipolar cycling typical of older adolescents and adults, some cases of unipolar illness, affective type of aggression	Initial: 300–600 mg/day increased to 600–1,200 mg/24 hr (therapeutic blood level: 0.6–1.2 mEq/L)	Gastrointestinal disturbance, tremor, ataxia, confusion, coma, death; hypothyroidism. Once discontinued, lithium is often not as effective when restarted. Overdose leading to death	Creatinine clearance, thyroid studies, ECG, electrolytes, calcium, phosphorus, comprehensive metabolic panel, pregnancy test, CBC with differential
Carbamazepine (Tegretol)	Bipolar cycling, including rapid cycling; aggressive behavior in organically impaired patients	Initial: 100–200 mg/24 hr; increased to 400–1,000 mg/24 hr (therapeutic blood level: 8–12 μg/mL)	Fever, sore throat, hematologic problems (white cell decrease), dizziness, drowsiness, neuromuscular disturbance, blurred vision; overdose leading to death	Physical examination, medical history, CBC with differential, BUN, hepatic enzymes; ECG; pregnancy test
Valproic acid (Depakene)	Rapid cycling bipolar disorder, aggression	Initial: 125–250 mg/24 hr or 10–15 mg/kg; increased by 5–10 mg/kg/24 hr up to 20–30 mg/kg/24 hr in divided doses (therapeutic blood level: 50–120 μg/mL)	Hepatic failure (usually in the first few mo of treatment); younger children (under 10 yr, especially under 2 yr), patients with prior hepatic disease history, those on multiple anticonvulsants, those with severe seizure history plus mental retardation, and those with congenital metabolic disorders are especially vulnerable. Obesity, birth defects in pregnancy; possible clotting problems; depression; nausea, vomiting, indigestion (at intiation of therapy), rashes; overdose leading to coma and possibly death; pancreatitis; polycystic ovary syndrome	Physical examination, medical history, hepatic enzymes; amylase; comprehensive metabolic panel; CBC with differential; ECG; FSH/LH for girls

TABLE 20-1.—*Cont'd.* Psychopharmacology

MEDICATION CLASS	USE	DOSAGE	SIDE EFFECTS/TOXICITY/CAUTION	PRETREATMENT WORK-UP
Lamotrigine (Lamictil)	Bipolar depression, especially eipolar II depression; dysphoric mania, rapid cycling bipolar II disorder	Initial: 25 mg/24 hr during first 2 wk; if necessary, increased by 50 mg/24 hr each wk to a maximum of 300–400 mg/24 hr **N.B.:** NOT yet recommended for patients under 18 yr	Sedation, nausea, headache; Rash in 10% of patients (risk of Stevens-Johnson reaction); concurrent use with valproic acid doubles the lamotrigine blood level	Same as with other mood stabilizers
Gabapentin (Neurontin)	Mood stabilization; anxiety and insomnia	Initial: 100–200 mg bid; maintenance: 1600–2400 mg/24 hr	Increased cycling in 4–7% of patients	BUN, creatinine
Topiramate (Topamax)	Mood stabilization	Initial: 25 mg/24 hr; increased weekly by 25 mg/24 hr to a maximum dose of 50–300 mg/24 hr	Nephrolithiasis in 1–2% of patients; somnolence, fatigue, anorexia	
ANTIHYPERTENSIVES				
Clonidine (Catapres)	Hyperactivity; aggression associated with ADHD; secondary use in tic disorder	Initial dose 0.05–0.1 mg increased only if no ↓BP or sedation to 0.1–0.25 mg/24 hr	Sedating bradycardia, hypotension; withdrawal symptoms; sudden death reported when used with stimulants	Physical examination, medical history, blood pressure, ECG
Guanfacine (Tenex)	Aggression associated with ADHD; tic disorder	0.5–1.0 mg qhs	Sedation, headaches (less hypotension than clonidine)	Blood pressure

ADHD, attention-deficit/hyperactivity disorder; BUN, blood urea nitrogen; CBC, complete blood count; CNS, central nervous system; ECG, electrocardiogram; EPS, extrapyramidal symptoms; FSH, follicle-stimulating hormone; LH, luteinizing hormone; MAO, monoamine oxidase; OCD, obsessive-compulsive disorder.

between depression and suicide, although clearly, all patients taking SSRIs should be monitored frequently. Children with mild or moderate depressive symptoms can often be referred for psychotherapy before the initiation of pharmacologic intervention; only when symptoms worsen or therapy is deemed ineffective is pharmacologic intervention for these children necessary.

Mood stabilizers, including lithium, carbamazepine, and valproate, have efficacy in pediatric bipolar disorder. A pretreatment lithium evaluation includes thyroid studies, renal function tests, and electrolyte determinations. Lithium blood levels should also be determined while patients are taking the medication. Prolonged use of lithium may cause hypothyroidism. Carbamazepine and valproic acid are associated with liver damage, and pretreatment liver function tests and regular (twice yearly) monitoring of liver function are indicated. Patients (and their parents) should be warned that these drugs should be discontinued if a new rash is apparent. Because the management of pediatric bipolar disorder is often complex, consultation with a child psychiatrist is indicated.

Some parents are adamantly opposed to the use of psychotropic medications. If drugs are used, they should be used for as short a time as possible. Physicians should avoid using several medications at the same time and should not shift back and forth from one medication to another when no immediate response occurs. Because psychotropic medications have significant biochemical effects on developing children, it is important for physicians to give an appropriate explanation to parents and children about the rationale for medication. Parents and children must have an opportunity to discuss their feelings and thoughts about psychotropic medication use in general and about the specific drug that is ordered. Even with thought disorders, in which pharmaco-therapy has a firmly established place, medication is rarely, if ever, the sole treatment indicated. The complexity of emotional conditions demands an integrated approach involving various therapies and the use of resources in the family, school, and community. These factors must be knowledgeably selected, judiciously coordinated, and skillfully applied to ensure maximal benefit.

20.3 • Psychotherapy

When it has been determined that psychopathology exists in a child or within a family and that it requires intervention, a pediatrician may develop and implement the therapeutic plan or may refer the patient for a more specialized level of care within the community. The choice of treatment should be left to the consultant, with the referring physician reassuring the family and patient that he or she will maintain close communication with the consultant. The primary physician should continue to evaluate the child's progress throughout the treatment process and also provide medical care for the patient.

There are many types of individual psychotherapy. Most involve the development of an alliance with patients that provides an opportunity to look at the problems precipitating therapy. Younger children often express their concerns and developmental issues in **play therapy,** a specific modality designed to foster symbolic and metaphoric individual expression. Older children and adolescents are more likely to participate in talking during therapy. **Dynamic therapy** is designed to understand the psychologic motivations for a child's problems and to develop a therapeutic process based on that understanding. **Behavior therapy** and **cognitive-behavioral therapy** are especially useful in treating anxiety, depression, and some behavioral problems. Cognitive-behavioral therapy has amassed the strongest evidence base of all psychotherapeutic interventions.

There are several types of **family therapy:** directive, structural, strategic, and object-relations. In each type, the therapist works primarily with the family to impart understanding or to help organize change. A particular directive approach, **parent management training,** is very useful in treating conduct disorder. This approach involves training parents to respond in specific and consistent ways to a child's behavior.

Group therapy is especially useful for children with poorly developed social skills. Group therapy for preadolescents tends to emphasize structured activities through which both therapist and children can discover how they relate to each other and find ways to change. It is an especially profitable approach for treating the social problems of adolescents.

Barriers to involving the generalist or pediatrician in psychotherapeutic activities with children include a presumed lack of time and lack of an adequate conceptual background. Although psychotherapy primarily emphasizes listening and interviewing, two skills important to all fields of medicine, experience is an important and necessary asset for psychotherapists.

20.4 • Psychiatric Hospitalization

Psychiatric hospitalization of a child in a general, pediatric, or psychiatric hospital is at times necessary, and it may serve a number of functions. In children with psychosomatic disorders or in a suicidal or drugged adolescent, medical clearance is essential before the patient can be admitted to a psychiatric facility. Indications for psychiatric admission include thought, behavior, and affect that are harmful to the self or to others. Some children are admitted for psychiatric treatment if their condition is not responsive to less restrictive therapy. Indications for admission include complex psychiatric problems that require skilled medical and nursing care, extremely disturbed family interactions that contribute to problematic behavior or interfere with needed care, and dangerous behavior that cannot otherwise be managed. Admission to residential treatment reflects the family's decompensation as often as the child's.

Baldessarini RJ, Pompili M, Tondo L: Suicidal risk in antidepressant drug trials. *Arch Gen Psychiatry* 2006;63:246–248.

Beck MH, Cataldo M, Slifer KJ, et al: Teaching children with attention deficit hyperactivity disorder (ADHD) and autistic disorder (AD) how to swallow pills. *Clin Pediatr* 2005;44:515–526.

Bostwick JM: Do SSRIs cause suicide in children? The evidence is underwhelming. *J Clin Psychol* 2006;62:235–241.

Davis JM: The choice of drugs for schizophrenia. *N Engl J Med* 2006;354: 518–520.

Emslie GJ, Mayes TL: Mood disorders in children and adolescents: Psychopharmacological treatment. *Biol Psychiatry* 2001;49:1082–1090.

Fedorowicz VJ, Fombonne E: Metabolic side effects of atypical antipsychotics in children: A literature review. *J Psychopharmacol* 2005;19:533–550.

Hall WD: How have the SSRI antidepressants affected suicide risk? *Lancet* 2006;367:1959–1962.

Hammerness PG, Vivas FM, Geller DA: Selective serotonin reuptake inhibitors in pediatric psychopharmacology: A review of the evidence. *J Pediatr* 2006;148:158–165.

Isbister GK, Balit CR, Kilham HA: Antipsychotic poisoning in young children: A systematic review. *Drug Saf* 2005;28:1029–1044.

Jureidini JN, Doecke CJ, Mansfield PR, et al: Efficacy and safety of antidepressants for children and adolescents. *BMJ* 2004;328:879–883.

Katusic SK, Barbaresi WJ, Colligan RC, et al: Psychostimulant treatment and risk for substance abuse among young adults with a history of attention-deficit/hyperactivity disorder: A population-based, birth cohort study. *J Child Adolesc Psychopharmacol* 2005;15:764–776.

Pappadopulos EA, Tate Guelzow B, Wong C, et al: A review of the growing evidence base for pediatric psychopharmacology. *Child Adolesc Psychiatr Clin N Am* 2004;13:817–855.

Ruths S, Steiner H: Psychopharmacologic treatment of aggression in children and adolescents. *Pediatr Ann* 2004;33:318–327.

Weisz JR, McCarty CA, Valeri SM: Effects of psychotherapy for depression in children and adolescents: A meta-analysis. *Psychol Bull* 2006;132:132–149.

Williams J, Klinepeter K, Palmes G, et al: Diagnosis and treatment of behavioral health disorders in pediatric practice. *Pediatrics* 2004;114:601–606.

Wong IC, Besag FM, Santosh PJ, et al: Use of selective serotonin reuptake inhibitors in children and adolescents. *Drug Saf* 2004;27:991–1000.

Chapter 21 ■ Psychosomatic Illness

Jorge H. Daruna, Alessandra N. Kazura, Neil W. Boris, and Richard Dalton

The idea that mental activity can cause illness has a long history in medicine. The psychosomatic approach, as exemplified by Engel's biopsychosocial model of disease, is grounded in integrative scientific disciplines, such as psychoneuroimmunology. *Somatoform* and *factitious* disorders have prominent psychologic factors.

Somatoform disorders present with somatic symptoms and/or dysfunction, which the patient actually experiences, but for which physical findings are absent or insufficient to explain the symptoms (Tables 21-1 to 21-3). Subsumed under this category are *body dysmorphic disorder, conversion disorder, hypochondriasis, somatization disorder,* and *somatoform pain disorder.*

TABLE 21-1. Features of Somatoform Disorders of Children and Adolescents

PSYCHOPHYSIOLOGIC DISORDER
Presenting complaint is a physical symptom
Physical symptom is caused by a known physiologic mechanism
Physical symptom is stress-induced
Patient may recognize an association between the symptom and stress
Symptom responds to medication, biofeedback, and stress reduction
CONVERSION REACTION
Presenting complaint is physical (loss of function, pain, or both)
Physical symptom is not caused by a known physiologic mechanism
Physical symptom is related to an unconscious idea, fantasy, or conflict
Patient does not recognize an association between the symptom and the unconscious
Symptom responds slowly to resolution of unconscious factors
SOMATIZATION DISORDER
Presenting complaint is >13 physical symptoms in girls, >11 in boys
Physical symptoms are not caused by a known physiologic or pathologic mechanism
Physical symptoms are related to the need to maintain the sick role
Patient is convinced that the symptoms are unrelated to psychologic factors
Symptoms tend either to persist or to change character despite treatment
HYPOCHONDRIASIS
Presenting complaint is a physical sign or symptom
Physical sign or symptom is normal
Patient interprets the physical symptom to indicate disease
Conviction regarding illness may be related to depression or anxiety
Symptom does not respond to reassurance; medication directed at underlying psychologic problems often helps
MALINGERING
Presenting complaint is a physical symptom
Physical symptom is under voluntary control
Physical symptom is used to gain reward (e.g., money, avoidance of military service)
Patient consciously recognizes the symptom as factitious
Symptom may not lessen when the reward is attained (need to retain reward)
FACTITIOUS DISORDER (E.G., MUNCHAUSEN SYNDROME)
Presenting complaint is a symptom complex mimicking a known syndrome
Symptom complex is under voluntary control
Symptom complex is used to attain medical treatment (including surgery)
Patient consciously recognizes the symptom complex as factitious, but is often psychologically disturbed so that unconscious factors also are operating
Symptom complex often results in multiple diagnoses and multiple operations

*From Kliegman RM, Marcdante KJ, Jenson HB, et al (editors): *Nelson Essentials of Pediatrics,* 5th ed. Philadelphia, Elsevier/Saunders, 2006, p 82.

Body dysmorphic disorder is characterized by extreme preoccupation with perceived abnormalities in appearance when the perception is not reflective of the actual physical features. The anxious obsession with physical appearance that defines body dysmorphic disorder is often associated with social limitations and dysphoria. The prevalence of this disorder in children and adolescents is not known, although studies in adults with this diagnosis indicate that the onset of symptoms frequently occurs during adolescence (see Chapter 27).

Conversion disorder is the loss or alteration of physical functioning without demonstrable organic pathology (Table 21-4). Typically, it presents in adolescence or adulthood, although numerous childhood cases have been reported. Conversion reactions usually start suddenly, can often be traced to a precipitating environmental event, and may end abruptly after a short duration. Voluntary musculature and organs of special sense are the most frequent target sites for expressions of conversion reactions. Such reactions may take the form of blindness, paralysis, diplopia, and postural or gait disturbances. Pseudoseizures are a common manifestation of a conversion disorder. Physical examination frequently does not show objective abnormalities. The history may show a close relationship with someone who exhib-

TABLE 21-2. Somatoform Symptoms

PAIN SYMPTOMS (SITE OR FUNCTION)
Head
Back
Joints
Chest
Rectum
Abdomen
Extremities
Menstruation
Urination
Sexual intercourse

GASTROINTESTINAL SYMPTOMS
Nausea
Bloating
Food intolerance
Vomiting
Diarrhea

SEXUAL SYMPTOMS
Sexual indifference
Erectile dysfunction
Vomiting throughout pregnancy
Irregular menses
Ejaculatory dysfunction
Excessive menstrual bleeding

PSEUDONEUROLOGIC SYMPTOMS
Difficulty swallowing
Loss of touch or pain sensation
Hallucinations
Aphonia
Seizures
Double vision
Blindness
Deafness
Urinary retention
Loss of consciousness
Dissociative symptoms (e.g., amnesia)
Impaired coordination or balance
Paralysis or localized weakness

*From Kliegman RM, Marcdante KJ, Jenson HB, et al (editors): *Nelson Essentials of Pediatrics,* 5th ed. Philadelphia, Elsevier/Saunders, 2006, p 83.

TABLE 21-3. Criteria for Diagnosis of Somatization Disorder

Each of the following criteria must have been met, with individual symptoms occurring at any time during the course of disturbance

1. **Four pain symptoms:** a history of pain related to at least 4 different sites or functions (e.g., head, abdomen, back, joints, extremities, chest, rectum, during menstruation, during sexual intercourse, or during urination)
2. **Two gastrointestinal symptoms:** a history of at least 2 gastrointestinal symptoms other than pain (e.g., nausea, bloating, vomiting other than during pregnancy, diarrhea, or intolerance of several different foods)
3. **One sexual symptom:** a history of at least 1 sexual or reproductive symptom other than pain (e.g., sexual indifference, erectile or ejaculatory dysfunction, irregular menses, excessive menstrual bleeding, vomiting throughout pregnancy)
4. **One pseudoneurologic symptom:** a history of at least 1 symptom or deficit suggesting a neurologic condition not limited to pain (conversion symptoms such as impaired coordination or balance, paralysis or localized weakness, difficulty swallowing or lump in throat, aphonia, urinary retention, hallucinations, loss of touch or pain sensation, double vision, blindness, deafness, seizures; dissociative symptoms such as amnesia; or loss of consciousness other than fainting)

Either (1) or (2)

1. After appropriate investigation, each of the symptoms from the above criteria cannot be fully explained by a known general medical condition or the direct effects of a substance (e.g., drug of abuse, medication)
2. When there is a related general medical condition, the physical complaints or resulting social or occupational impairment are in excess of what would be expected from the history, physical examination, or laboratory findings

*From Kliegman RM, Marcdante KJ, Jenson HB, et al (editors): *Nelson Essentials of Pediatrics,* 5th ed. Philadelphia, Elsevier/Saunders, 2006, p 83.

TABLE 21-4. Criteria for the Diagnosis of Conversion Disorder

A. One or more symptoms or deficits affecting voluntary motor or sensory function that suggest a neurologic or other general medical condition
B. Psychologic factors are judged to be associated with the symptom or deficit because the initiation or exacerbation of the symptom or deficit is preceded by conflicts or other stressors
C. The symptom or deficit is not intentionally produced or feigned (factitious disorder or malingering)
D. After appropriate investigation, the symptom or deficit cannot be fully explained by a general medical condition, by the direct effects of a substance, or as a culturally sanctioned behavior or experience
E. The symptom or deficit causes clinically significant distress or impairment in social, occupational, or other important areas of functioning or warrants medical evaluation
F. The symptom or deficit is not limited to pain or sexual dysfunction, does not occur exclusively during the course of somatization disorder, and is not better accounted for by another mental disorder

SPECIFY TYPE OF SYMPTOM OR DEFICIT
With motors symptom or deficit
With sensory symptom or deficit
With seizures or convulsions
With mixed presentation

*From Kliegman RM, Marcdante KJ, Jenson JB, et al (editors): *Nelson Essentials of Pediatrics,* 5th ed. Philadelphia, Elsevier/Saunders, 2006, p 84.

ited similar symptoms or had a recent episode of acute illness. Findings inconsistent with organic pathology are often seen. Deep tendon reflexes can be elicited in a paralyzed limb, or pupillary responses to light may be seen in patients who report blindness. Decreased cortical activation is noted in the contralateral brain region corresponding to the muscle groups affected by dissociative paralysis. Videoelectroencephalography and postictal serum prolactin levels (elevated in true seizures) are useful in diagnosing pseudoseizures. **Astasia-abasia** is a conversion disorder manifest as an inability to stand or walk. Vulnerability to conversion disorder is not clearly linked to any specific cause, although anxiety and family disturbance can be factors. Children with conversion disorder are highly suggestible, which often helps in treatment. Cultural background affects how illness and distress are expressed and should be considered before conversion disorder is diagnosed. Follow-up studies indicate that approximately ⅓ of children diagnosed with conversion disorder are later found to have a medical disorder that can explain the original symptoms.

Hypochondriasis is a preoccupation with the frightening idea of having a serious illness (Table 21-5). *Somatization disorder* is a condition in which multiple somatic symptoms are evident in association with generalized anxiety. In **somatoform pain disorder,** pain is the primary physical symptom (Table 21-6). These disorders are characterized by recurrence. Prevalence studies suggest that 11% of boys and 15% of girls have ongoing somatic symptoms. Recurrent abdominal pain accounts for 2–4% of all pediatric visits, and headaches account for an additional 1–2%. Most of these children do not have any positive clinical findings.

TABLE 21-5. Criteria for Diagnosis of Hypochondriasis

A. Preoccupation with fears of having, or the idea that one had, a serious disease based on the person's misinterpretation of bodily symptoms
B. The preoccupation persists despite appropriate medical evaluation and reassurance
C. The belief in criterion A is not of delusional intensity (as in delusional disorder, somatic type) and is not restricted to a circumscribed concern about appearance (as in body dysmorphic disorder)
D. The preoccupation causes clinically significant distress or impairment in social, occupational, or other important areas of functioning
E. The duration of the disturbance is at least 6 mo
F. The preoccupation is not better accounted for by generalized anxiety disorder, obsessive-compulsive disorder, panic disorder, major depressive episode, separation anxiety, or another somatoform disorder

SPECIFY IF
With poor insight: if, for most of the time during the current episode, the person does not recognize that the concern about having a serious illness is excessive or unreasonable

*From Kliegman RM, Marcdante KJ, Jenson HB, et al (editors): *Nelson Essentials of Pediatrics,* 5th ed. Philadelphia, Elsevier/Saunders, 2006, p 85.

TABLE 21-6. Criteria for Diagnosis of Pain Disorder

A. Pain in ≥1 anatomic sites is the predominant focus of the clinical presentation and is of sufficient severity to warrant clinical attention
B. The pain causes clinically significant distress or impairment in social, occupational, or other important areas of functioning
C. Psychologic factors are judged to have an important role in the onset, severity, exacerbation, or maintenance of the pain
D. The symptom or deficit is not intentionally produced or feigned (as in factitious disorder or malingering)
E. The pain is not better accounted for by a mood, anxiety, or psychotic disorder and does not meet the criteria for dyspareunia

CODE AS FOLLOWS

Pain disorder associated with psychologic factors: psychologic factors are judged to have a major role in the onset, severity, exacerbation, or maintenance of the pain. (If a general medical condition is present, it does not have a major role in the onset, severity, exacerbation, or maintenance of the pain.) This type of pain disorder is not diagnosed if criteria also are met for somatization disorder

SPECIFY IF

Acute: duration <6 mo
Chronic: duration ≥6 mo

Pain disorder associated with psychological factors and a general medical condition: psychologic factors and a general medical condition are judged to have important roles in the onsets, severity, exacerbation, or maintenance of the pain

SPECIFY IF

Acute: duration <6 mo
Chronic: duration ≥6 mo

Note: The following is not considered to be a mental disorder and is included here to facilitate differential diagnosis

Pain disorder associated with a general medical condition: a general medical condition has a major role in the onset, severity, exacerbation, or maintenance of the pain. (If psychologic factors are present, they are not judged to have a major role in the onset, severity, exacerbation, or maintenance of the pain.) The diagnostic code for the pain is selected based on the associated general medical condition if 1 has been established or on the anatomic location of the pain if the underlying general medical condition is not yet clearly established (e.g., low back, joint, bone, abdominal, breast, renal, ear, eye, throat, tooth, urinary)

*From Kliegman RM, Marcdante KJ, Jenson HB, et al (editors): *Nelson Essentials of Pediatrics,* 5th ed. Philadelphia, Elsevier/Saunders, 2006, p 85.

Factitious disorders cause somatic and/or psychologic symptoms that are deliberately fabricated in the absence of any potential gain to the patient, other than the benefit of assuming the sick role (Table 21-7). If there is clear potential for gain (financial compensation), then the diagnosis of *malingering* should be made. *Munchausen syndrome* is an example of a chronic factitious disorder, typically seen in adults who persist in seeking medical treatments, including surgery, despite the lack of any real disease. *Munchausen syndrome by proxy* is a variant in which parents induce physical symptoms in their children to assume the sick role by proxy (see Chapter 36.2). In such cases, infants and young children may present with fractures, poisonings, persistent episodes of apnea, and other unusual ailments. It is considered a form of child abuse, which can be lethal, and it must be reported to the appropriate authorities.

TABLE 21-7. Criteria for Disgnosis of Factitious Disorder

A. Intentional production or feigning of physical or psychologic signs or symptoms
B. The motivation for the behavior is to assume the sick role
C. External incentives for the behavior (e.g., economic gain, avoiding legal responsibility, or improving physical well-being, as in malingering) are absent

CODE BASED ON TYPE

With predominantly psychological signs and symptoms: if psychologic signs and symptoms predominate in the clinical presentation

With predominantly physical signs and symptoms: if physical signs and symptoms predominate in the clinical presentation

With combined psychological and physical signs and symptoms: if psychologic and physical signs and symptoms are present, but neither predominates in the clinical persentation

*From Kliegman RM, Marcdante KJ, Jenson HB, et al (editors): *Nelson Essentials of Pediatrics,* 5th ed. Philadelphia, Elsevier/Saunders, 2006, p 84.

Psychologic factors affecting medical conditions is a very broad diagnostic category that essentially acknowledges the potential influence of psychologic factors (anxiety, hostility) on the onset and course of any illness. This category also encompasses psychologic and behavioral characteristics that hinder treatment adherence or increase the risk of complications, although the latter are modes of influence not traditionally within the realm of psychosomatics. This diagnosis requires physical findings of disease (asthma, diabetes) and clear evidence that psychologic factors are temporally related to the appearance or exacerbation of physical symptoms. However, the psychologic influence would not be expected to be evident in all patients with the particular medical condition.

MANAGEMENT. Pediatric management should routinely incorporate the influence of psychologic factors across the board and not simply when physical findings are not sufficiently evident. Clinical assessment should routinely include questions about the patient's social circumstances and psychologic characteristics as well as the life events that make up the patient's history. It is also important to ask whether others in the family have had similar symptoms, not only to ascertain genetic risk, but also because the child may simply be emulating what he or she has seen. It is essential to explore whether there is any gain that may result from the sick role (avoidance of school, extra parental attention). In cases where physical findings are not sufficient to explain the symptoms, it is best to avoid treatments that may have adverse effects. Response to placebo is not a reliable method for differentiating somatoform disorders from those with detectable physical pathology. Interventions that address psychologic factors in both the child and the family by educational approaches, including psychotherapy, may prove quite beneficial. There are instances in which parental treatment is necessary to ensure a favorable outcome. Symptoms of somatoform disorders are actually experienced by the patient; even when they are intentionally fabricated, as in factitious disorders, they are still unconsciously motivated. Therefore, attempting to talk the patient out of the symptoms or confronting the patient with the lack of a physical basis for the symptoms is not productive. Rather, emphasis should be placed on early return to normal activities, including school, recreation, and socialization with peers. Parents should be informed that some children unconsciously use their symptoms to avoid situations or to maintain excessive dependence, and that firm, gentle insistence on the fullest possible range of activities for the child is indicated. Ideally, parents and children should understand the psychologic origin of symptoms; however, functional improvement may be achieved without full insight. Psychoactive medications may be useful in cases where symptoms of anxiety or depression appear prominent.

American Psychiatric Association: *Diagnostic and Statistical Manual of Mental Disorders,* 4th ed, text revision. Washington, DC, American Psychiatric Publishing, 2000.

Burgmer M, Konrad C, Jansen A, et al: Abnormal brain activation during movement observation in patients with conversion paralysis. *Neuroimage* 2006;29:1336–1343.

Campo JV, Fritsch SL: Somatization disorder in children and adolescents. *J Am Acad Child Adolesc Psychiatry* 1994;33:1223.

Dyl J, Kittler J, Phillips KA, et al: Body dysmorphic disorder and other clinically significant body image concerns in adolescent psychiatric inpatients: prevalence and clinical characteristics. *Child Psychiatry Hum Dev* 2006;36:369–382.

Daruna JH: *Introduction to Psychoneuroimmunology.* San Diego, CA, Elsevier/Academic Press, 2004.

Engel G: The clinical application of the biopsychosocial model. *Am J Psychiatry* 1980;137:535.

Fritz GK, Fritsch SL, Hagino O: Somatoform disorders in children and adolescents: A review of the past 10 years. *J Am Acad Child Adolesc Psychiatry* 1997;36:1329.

Levenson JL (editor): *Textbook of Psychosomatic Medicine*. Washington, DC, American Psychiatric Publishing, 2005.
Stickler GB, Cheung-Patton A: Astasia-abasia: A conversion reaction. *Clin Pediatr* 1989;28:12–16.
Vencovsky J, Huizinga TWJ: Somatisation: A joint responsibility of a doctor and patient. *Lancet* 2006;367:452.

Chapter 22 ■ Vegetative Disorders

Neil W. Boris and Richard Dalton

Eating Disorders

22.1 • Rumination Disorder

(See also Chapter 27.) The hallmark of rumination disorder is weight loss or failure to gain at the expected level because of repeated regurgitation of food without nausea or associated gastrointestinal illness. This rare disorder occurs more commonly in males and usually appears at 3–14 mo of age. It is potentially fatal; some reports indicate that up to ¼ of affected children die. There are psychogenic and self-stimulating ruminators. Psychogenic rumination occurs in infants with otherwise normal development, although there is often a disturbed parent-child relationship and the child may fail to thrive. The self-stimulating type is usually seen in mentally retarded individuals of any age, and it often occurs even in the presence of nurturing parents. The differential diagnosis includes congenital anomalies that affect the development of the gastrointestinal system, pyloric stenosis, increased intracranial pressure, adrenogenital syndrome, and inborn errors of metabolism.

TREATMENT. Behavioral treatment is directed toward positively reinforcing correct eating behavior and negatively reinforcing rumination. Adverse conditioning is often used. Parent counseling and family therapy are often necessary to manage underlying conflicts and to help educate the parents about appropriate approaches toward the child and the problem.

22.2 • Pica

Pica involves repeated or chronic ingestion of non-nutritive substances, which may include plaster, charcoal, clay, wool, ashes, paint, and earth. Although tasting or mouthing of objects is normal in infants and toddlers, pica after the 2nd yr of life needs investigation. Mental retardation and lack of parental nurturing (psychologic, nutritional) are predisposing factors; pica appears to be more common in children with autism and other brain-behavior disorders, such as **Kleine-Levin syndrome.** Persistent pica is also often associated with family disorganization, poor supervision, and psychologic neglect. Pica appears to be more prevalent in lower socioeconomic groups. It usually remits in childhood, but can continue into adolescence and adulthood. In particular, **geophagia** (eating of earth) is associated with pregnancy and is not seen as abnormal in some cultures. Children with pica are at increased risk for lead poisoning (see Chapter 709), iron-deficiency anemia (see Chapter 455), and parasitic infections (see Part XVI, Sections 15 and 16).

TREATMENT. Screening for lead intoxication, iron-deficiency anemia, and parasitic infestation is indicated. Ingestion of hair (most common in children with trichotillomania) may lead to a bezoar and require surgical intervention.

Elimination Disorders

22.3 • Enuresis (Bed-Wetting)

Enuresis is defined as the voluntary or involuntary repeated discharge of urine into clothes or bed after a developmental age when bladder control should be established. Most children with a mental age of 5 yr have obtained bladder control during the day and night. The diagnosis of enuresis is made when urine is voided twice a week for at least 3 consecutive months or when clinically significant distress occurs in areas of the child's life as a result of the wetting (see also Chapters 5 and 543). The prevalence of enuresis at age 5 yr is 7% in males and 3% in females. At age 10 yr, it is 3% in males and 2% in females, and at age 18 yr, it is 1% in males and extremely rare in females. Evidence suggests different rates of bed-wetting by ethnicity and culture.

ETIOLOGY. Twin studies show a marked familial pattern, with documented concordance rates of 68% in monozygotic twins and 36% in dizygotic twins. Linkage studies have implicated multiple chromosomes, particularly chromosome 22, with varying patterns of transmission. Beyond genetic factors, the cause of enuresis likely involves a complex web of physiologic and perhaps psychologic factors. Children with nocturnal enuresis may hyposecrete arginine vasopressin (AVP) and also may be less responsive to the lower urine osmolality associated with fluid loading. Tubular sodium-potassium exchange in the kidney, partly influenced by AVP secretion, is associated with nocturnal enuresis. AVP receptor function in the tubule may be a key factor in the pathophysiology of the disorder. There may also be associations between sleep and enuresis. Although enuresis may occur at any stage of sleep, there is some support for a relationship between sleep architecture, diminished capacity to be aroused from sleep, and abnormal bladder function in patients with enuresis.

The relationship between enuresis and psychologic functioning is complex. Older enuretic children have a higher incidence of psychopathology than non-enuretic children, although no single disorder accounts for the group differences. Children with attention-deficit/hyperactivity disorder may be more likely to be enuretic than age-matched comparison children. Delayed maturation of bladder function may account for many cases of primary enuresis. Secondary enuresis is associated with life stress and/or traumatic experiences, particularly in children who were late in first achieving nighttime dryness. The pediatrician should inquire about stressful events with all children who present with secondary enuresis.

Differing rates by culture suggest that child-rearing practices may also play an etiologic role.

CLINICAL MANIFESTATIONS. Bed-wetting may be divided into the **persistent (primary) type,** in which the child has never been dry at night, and the **regressive (secondary) type,** in which a child who has been continent for 6 mo or longer then begins to wet the bed. Primary enuresis represents approximately 90% of all cases. Further classification involves **nocturnal enuresis** (voiding urine at night), and **diurnal enuresis** (voiding urine while awake). Primary nocturnal enuresis is the most common. Diurnal enuresis is more common in girls and rarely occurs after the age of 9 yr. The most common cause of daytime enuresis in the preschool or school-aged child is waiting until the last minute to void urine (**micturition deferral**). In addition to micturition deferral, etiologic factors to consider in diurnal enuresis include urinary tract infection, chemical urethritis, associated constipation, diabetes, and giggle or stress incontinence. Children with both nocturnal and diurnal enuresis, especially in the presence of voiding difficulties, are more likely to have abnormalities of the urinary tract, and ultrasonography or uroflowmetry is indicated. Otherwise, anatomic abnormalities are rarely associated with either nocturnal or diurnal enuresis and invasive or costly studies are contraindicated. Urinalysis and urine culture will rule out both infectious causes and the elevated urine osmolality associated with diabetes.

TREATMENT. Management of the child with enuresis should begin with behavioral treatment. General guidelines for a 1st-line approach would be as follows:

1. It is important to enlist the cooperation of the child to deal with the problem. Rewarding the child for being dry at night is a useful step. The child or parent can chart dry nights, and with each dry night, a small reward can be given. More substantial rewards should be given for increasing success.
2. The child should void before retiring.
3. Waking the child repeatedly to take him or her to the bathroom is not generally useful and may further engender or aggravate anger in the child or parents. Enuretic children may be more difficult to awaken than age-matched peers. However, using an alarm clock to wake the child once 2–3 hr after he or she falls asleep is indicated.
4. Punishment or humiliation of the child by parents or others should be strongly discouraged.

Consistent dry bed training with positive reinforcement has a success rate of 85% or more. The use of conditioning devices (an alarm that rings when the child wets a special sheet) is often helpful in training the child to improve bladder capacity and avoid enuresis. In effect, these devices provide a consistent mode for behavioral retraining. Consent of the child should be a prerequisite for the use of such a device. Bell-and-pad alarm systems have a success rate of approximately 75% across many studies, with relapse rates that are lower than those with pharmacologic intervention. These devices are simple and cost-effective.

Psychotherapy for traumatized children with secondary enuresis may be indicated, especially when behavioral training has failed and traumatic experiences temporally associated with the onset of enuresis are noted. Once the child has successfully learned to stop wetting, overlearning (drinking just before bedtime) may be a useful adjunctive treatment; increasing bladder capacity over time guards against relapse.

Pharmacotherapy for enuresis is 2nd-line treatment and should be reserved for cases in which behavioral treatment is unsuccessful. Comparison of the bell-and-pad system vs imipramine and desmopressin acetate (DDAVP) shows lower relapse rates for the bell-and-pad system, although the initial response rates are similar. Imipramine (Tofranil) at starting doses of 10–25 mg in children >5 yr and maximum doses of 75 mg in adolescents before bedtime has a success rate of approximately 50%, with a relapse rate of 30% or more even after 6 mo of treatment. Imipramine is associated with cardiac conduction disturbances and may be lethal in overdose. DDAVP can be administered orally or intranasally at bedtime. The fast action of DDAVP suggests a role for special occasions (such as overnight visits) when rapid control of enuresis is desired. Unfortunately, the relapse rate on discontinuation of DDAVP is very high, and 1 mo of treatment typically costs as much as a bell-and-pad system (which can be used for several months, as necessary). DDAVP is also associated with rare side effects of hyponatremia and water intoxication, with resulting seizures.

22.4 • Encopresis

Encopresis is the passage of feces into inappropriate places after a chronological age of 4 yr (or the equivalent developmental level). Subtypes include encopresis with constipation and overflow incontinence (retentive encopresis) and encopresis without constipation and overflow incontinence (nonretentive encopresis). Encopresis may persist from infancy onward (primary) or may appear after successful toilet training (secondary). Approximately ⅔ of cases are of the retentive type and are associated with chronic constipation; it is less clear what percentage of cases are primary vs secondary (see Chapter 329). In children younger than 4 yr of age, the male:female ratio for chronic constipation is 1:1. In the school-aged child, encopresis is more common in boys.

CLINICAL MANIFESTATIONS. The first consideration in managing encopresis is assessment of fecal retention. A positive finding on rectal examination is sufficient to document fecal retention, but a negative finding in the presence of encopresis requires plain abdominal roentgenograms. The presence of fecal retention is evidence of chronic constipation, and treatment will require active constipation management (see Chapters 325 and 329).

Many children with encopresis present with abnormal anal sphincter physiology documented by electromyography or difficulty in defecating a rectal balloon. Inability to defecate a balloon at presentation is associated with poorer response to treatment. Abnormal anal sphincter function is a marker for chronic constipation; children with this pathology do not appear to have a higher incidence of behavioral or psychiatric disorders than those without it. Primary encopresis in boys appears to be associated with global developmental delays and enuresis, whereas secondary encopresis is associated with high levels of psychosocial stressors and conduct disorder. Associated behavioral or psychiatric problems obviously may complicate the treatment of encopresis, especially when parents respond to soiling with retaliatory, punitive measures and children become angry, ashamed, and resistant to intervention. School performance and attendance may be secondarily affected, as the child becomes the target of scorn and derision from schoolmates because of the offensive odor.

TREATMENT. The standard treatment approach to encopresis begins with clearance of impacted fecal material and short-term use of mineral oil or laxatives to prevent further constipation (see Chapter 329). Concomitant behavioral management is also indicated. The focus of behavioral treatment should be on compliance with regular postprandial toilet sitting and adoption of a high-fiber diet. In some cases, manual disimpaction is required before treatment can begin; rarely, megacolon is observed and referral to a gastroenterologist is required. Once impacted stool is removed, the combination of constipation management and simple behavior therapy is successful in the majority of cases, although it is often a period of months before soiling stops completely. Compliance may wane, and failure of this standard treatment approach sometimes requires more intensive intervention, with a special emphasis on adherence to a high-fiber diet and family support for behavioral change. From the outset of treatment, parents should be actively encouraged to issue the child rewards for compliance and to avoid power struggles with the child. Keeping records of the child's progress is necessary. In cases where behavioral or psychiatric problems are evident, group or individual psychotherapy may be necessary.

Biofeedback, which is used to train the anal sphincter muscle, has been helpful in some cases, but controlled trials do not suggest higher rates of improvement compared with the standard treatment regimen. Long-term laxative use is contraindicated. Improvement in some children may occur with tricyclic antidepressants, although there are not enough data to warrant regular use of these drugs, particularly given their narrow therapeutic window and association with cardiac dysrhythmias. Furthermore, tricyclic antidepressants often cause or exacerbate constipation and should be avoided in children with retentive encopresis. The few long-term follow-up studies suggest that encopresis eventually resolves in most children, regardless of the treatment approach.

Bernstein SA, Williford SL: Intranasal desmopressin-associated hyponatremia: A case report and literature review. *J Fam Pract* 1997;44:203.

Butler RJ, Golding J, Northstone K: ALSPAC Study Team: Nocturnal enuresis at 7.5 years old. Prevalence and analysis of clinical signs. *BJU Int* 2005;96:404–410.

Foreman DM, Thambirajah MS: Conduct disorder, enuresis and specific developmental delays in two types of encopresis: A case-note study of 63 boys. *Eur Child Adolesc Psychiatry* 1996;5:33.

Glazener CM, Evans JH, Peto RE: Alarm interventions for nocturnal enuresis in children. *Cochrane Database Syst Rev* 2005:CD002911.

Kern L, Starosta K, Adelman BE: Reducing pica by teaching children to exchange inedible items for edibles. *Behav Modif* 2006;30:135–158.

Mellon MW, Whiteside SP, Friedrich WN: The relevance of fecal soiling as an indicator of child sexual abuse: A preliminary analysis. *J Dev Behav Pediatr* 2006;27:25–32.

Mikkelsen EJ: Enuresis and encopresis: Ten years of progress. *J Am Acad Child Adolesc Psychiatry* 2001;40:1146.

Reid H, Bahar RJ: Treatment of encopresis and chronic constipation in young children: Clinical results from interactive parent-child guidance. *Clin Pediatr* 2006;45:157–164.

Rose EA, Porcerelli JH, Neale AV: Pica: Common but commonly missed. *J Am Board Fam Pract* 2000;13:353.

Chapter 23 ■ Habit and Tic Disorders

Mary Margaret Gleason, Neil W. Boris, and Richard Dalton

Habit disorders are a heterogenous group of repetitive behaviors, including thumb or digit sucking, teeth grinding (bruxism), skin picking, hair pulling, and head banging. Involuntary movements or vocalizations (tics) can also be considered habitual behaviors. Whether these behavior patterns are considered disorders that require intervention beyond reassurance depends on the degree to which they interfere with the child's physical, emotional, or social functioning.

The prevalence of habit disorders is not known, although they are common. Parents of preschoolers report that up to 60% of children show 1 or more habitual behaviors. These behaviors are typically related to self-soothing in young children. Sometimes habits can persist without parental reinforcement, occurring when the child is put to bed or is alone; rhythmic movements, such as rocking, seem to provide a kind of sensory solace for the child. Habitual behaviors, such as head banging or self-biting, meet a child's sensory needs and may be related to frustration. Literature on the treatment of head banging is limited, but if the child is safe, it is reasonable to instruct parents to avoid highly emotional responses to the behavior and to consider finding alternative ways to give the child attention for prosocial behaviors.

Certain habit disorders are more common in children with developmental delays, particularly those with pervasive developmental disorders. Self-injurious habits, such as self-biting or head banging, can occur in up to 25% of normally developing toddlers, but are almost invariably associated with developmental delays in children older than 5 yr. Habit disorders in developmentally disabled children are more refractory to treatment than those in typically developing children, and referral to a developmental pediatrician or child psychiatrist for behavioral and/or psychopharmacologic management is often indicated. The pediatrician must also rule out severe neglect, which is associated with repetitive rocking, spinning, or other stereotypies. Institutionalized children have the highest rates of these kinds of stereotypies.

Teeth grinding, or **bruxism**, is common, can begin in the first 5 yr of life, and may be associated with daytime anxiety. Untreated bruxism may create problems with dental occlusion. Helping the child find ways to reduce anxiety may relieve the problem, although studies of psychologic treatment for bruxism are rare. Bedtime can be made more enjoyable and relaxing by reading or talking with the child and allowing the child to discuss fears or concerns. Praise and other emotional support are useful at these times. Persistent bruxism requires referral to a dentist and may present as muscular or temporomandibular joint pain.

Thumb sucking is normal in infancy and toddlerhood. In older children, thumb sucking occasionally affects the alignment of the teeth. Like other rhythmic patterns of behavior, thumb sucking is self-soothing. Intervention to reduce thumb sucking should not be considered until at least age 4–5 yr and then only if it is causing impairment for the child. Basic behavioral management, including encouraging parents to ignore thumb sucking and instead focus on providing the child with praise for substitute behaviors, is often effective. Simple reinforcers, such as giving the child a sticker for each block of time that he or she does not suck the thumb, can also be considered. Although some literature suggests that the use of noxious agents (bitter salves) may be effective in controlling thumb sucking, this approach should rarely be necessary and is considered a 2nd-line approach.

Trichotillomania is the repetitive pulling of hair, often causing patches of alopecia with telltale broken strands of hair. The usual age of onset of trichotillomania is in the prepubertal group, although preschoolers have been described with this disorder. Children with trichotillomania often have other sensory behavior patterns and can be seen "fiddling" with objects as a means of sensory input. The prevalence of trichotillomania in children is not well known, but is believed to be <1%. Although trichotillomania often remits spontaneously, treatment of those whose disorder has been present for >6 mo is more difficult and requires behavioral treatment. The efficacy of psychopharmacologic interventions is not well studied, although selective serotonin reuptake inhibitors, such as fluoxetine and anxiolytics, have been tried with some success.

Tics involve sudden, rapid, repetitive, involuntary movements of muscle groups or vocalizations and represent discharges of tension related to central nervous system electrochemical signals. Parts of the body that are most frequently involved are the muscles of the face, neck, shoulders, trunk, and hands. Simple tics involve only 1 muscle group, as in eye blinking, shoulder shrugging or neck jerking, whereas complex tics may include multiple muscle groups and cause more complex motions. Simple vocalizations include grunting and throat clearing; complex vocalizations include the use of repetitive obscenities (coprolalia). Motor or vocal tics lasting <1 yr are transient; those lasting >1 yr are chronic.

Tics must be distinguished from petit mal or other nongeneralized seizure disorders, which are characterized by both transient inability to interact and amnesia for the event. An electroencephalogram may be necessary in some cases to distinguish tic disorders from seizure disorders. Tics can be distinguished from dyskinetic movements and dystonias by their discontinuation during sleep and because conscious control can be achieved for short periods. It is very difficult to continuously and consciously inhibit tics. Tics are made worse with stress and may improve with moderate physical or mental activity.

Most children with simple motor tics do not require treatment, although some may experience associated problems, including neuropsychologic dysfunction, academic underachievement, or low self-esteem. These associated problems may require psychotherapeutic intervention.

The course of tic disorders is waxing and waning; however, emotional stressors may exacerbate tic triggers, and the triggers are often not identifiable. In some patients, immunologic factors play a role in the exacerbation of symptoms. **Pediatric autoimmune neuropsychiatric disorder associated with streptococcal infection** (PANDAS) is a condition in which antibodies to group A streptococcus (see Chapter 182) cross react with basal ganglia tissue and precipitate symptoms. Data supporting the pathophysiology of PANDAS include: (1) the ability to prevent tic relapses with antibiotic prophylaxis; (2) high rates of cross-reactive antibodies for both group A streptococcus and basal ganglia proteins found in some samples from patients with tics compared with control subjects; and (3) enlargement of the basal ganglia during acute exacerbations of neuropsychiatric symptoms in patients with PANDAS. Five clinical characteristics define the subgroup of patients with PANDAS: (1) the presence of obsessive-compulsive disorder and/or tic disorder; (2) prepubertal age of onset; (3) abrupt onset and relapsing-remitting course; (4) association with neurologic abnormalities (chorea, hyperactivity, tics) during exacerbations; and (5) temporal association between symptom exacerbations and group A streptococcal infection (a positive antistreptolysin O titer). **Treatment** of PANDAS includes acute antistreptococcal antibiotic therapy; prophylactic penicillin or azithromycin may decrease the number of episodes. The role of immunotherapy is controversial, and therapeutic plasma exchange is indicated for severely affected children.

Tourette syndrome is characterized by a history of motor **and** vocal tics (not necessarily present concurrently). Tourette syndrome has a lifetime prevalence rate of 0.5/1,000 individuals and commonly presents in childhood, beginning with simple motor tics, often before age 7 yr. In many cases, multiple tics and complex vocal sounds, such as barking and grunting, develop over time and peak in severity by age 10–12 yr. Shouting obscene words (**coprolalia**) is characteristic, but is seen in only 10% of affected patients. Tourette syndrome is more common in 1st-degree relatives of patients with Tourette syndrome than in the general population, and it affects boys 3–4 times more often than girls. In some families, it is an autosomal dominant disorder with greater penetrance in males. Criteria for the diagnosis include:

1. **Multiple motor and vocal tics lasting >1 yr, with no tic-free interval lasting >3 mo**
2. **Onset before age 18 yr**
3. **No medical causes (drugs, central nervous system disease)**

Children with Tourette syndrome often have behavioral, emotional, and academic problems. In particular, these children have higher rates of obsessive-compulsive disorder (see Chapter 24), attention-deficit/hyperactivity disorder (see Chapter 31), and oppositional-defiant disorder (see Chapter 28). The fact that Tourette syndrome is highly comorbid with these specific psychiatric disorders suggests dysfunction in particular regions of the brain. Although the etiology of Tourette syndrome is uncertain, interplay among genetic, neurobiologic, psychologic, and environmental factors is likely. Neuroimaging studies suggest that there is a lack of normal asymmetry within the striatum and a decrease in the size of the cavum septum pellucidum. Single-photon emission computed tomography scan data implicate dysfunction in dopamine receptor binding in severely affected children. Studies have also implicated systemic and local cytokine responses in Tourette syndrome and in the exacerbation of symptoms. Lyme disease may rarely present with clinical manifestations of Tourette syndrome (see Chapter 219). Many environmental factors are emotional stressors, which may also precipitate or increase tics. Laboratory studies are nonspecific; up to 80% of patients with Tourette syndrome have nonspecific abnormal electroencephalographic findings. Abnormal amounts of various neurotransmitter metabolites and lower scores on verbal subscales of psychometric tests have been reported.

Treatment for Tourette syndrome should only occur after careful consideration of the functional limitations associated with the child's symptoms, any associated symptoms, and the risks and benefits of pharmacotherapy. In many cases, supportive management is all that is indicated. Many children with Tourette syndrome require medication for obsessive-compulsive symptoms or attention and impulsivity problems. There was once concern about stimulants unmasking tics, but studies have not substantiated this concern. The recommendation is that tic disorders should not be considered a contraindication to the judicious use of stimulants. Pharmacotherapy, targeting the tics themselves, is indicated when tics interfere with social development or classroom function. For 1st-line treatment, neuroleptics have the strongest track record in controlled trials. Haloperidol and pimozide, dopaminergic antagonists, have been shown to reduce the severity of tics by 65%. Because potentially severe side effects are associated with traditional neuroleptics, most clinicians recommend risperidone. Risperidone is equivalent to clonidine in reducing tics. Clonidine, an α_2 agonist, is effective; sedation and low blood pressure are common side effects of clonidine and require careful monitoring. The role of guanfacine (Tenex), which is a less sedating α_2 agonist, has not been firmly established (see Table 20.1). Botulinum toxin has been shown to be effective for motor tics.

Affected children and their families should be encouraged to be active participants in the management of Tourette syndrome. Support from organizations such as the Tourette Syndrome Association, which has a user-friendly website (www.tsa-usa.org), is often very beneficial to affected families. The natural course of Tourette syndrome includes a significant diminution or remission in symptoms in adolescence and early adulthood in approximately ⅔ of cases. It is difficult to predict which patients will experience fewer symptoms over time.

Obsessive-compulsive symptoms may persist into adulthood.

Bloch MH, Peterson BS, Scahill L, et al: Adulthood outcome of tic and obsessive-compulsive symptom severity in children with Tourette syndrome. *Arch Pediatr Adolesc Med* 2006;160:65–69.

Cheifetz AT, Osganian SK, Allred EN, et al: Prevalence of bruxism and associated correlates in children as reported by parents. *J Dent Child (Chic)* 2005;72:67–73.

Coffey BJ, Biederman J, Geller DA, et al: The course of Tourette's disorder: A literature review. *Harv Rev Psychiatry* 2000;8:192–198.

Foster LG: Nervous habits and stereotyped behaviors in preschool children. *J Am Acad Child Adolesc Psychiatry* 1998;37:711–717.

Mahalski PA, Stanton WR: The relationship between digit sucking and behaviour problems: A longitudinal study over 10 years. *J Child Psychol Psychiatry* 1992;33:913–923.

March JS, Leonard HL: Obsessive-compulsive disorder in children and adolescents: A review of the past 10 years. *J Am Acad Child Adolesc Psychiatry* 1996;35:1265–1273.

Scahill L, Chappell PB, King RA, et al: Pharmacologic treatment of tic disorders. *Child Adolesc Psychiatr Clin North Am* 2000;9:99–117.

Scahill L, Sukhodolsky DG, Bearss K, et al: Randomized trial of parent management training in children with tic disorders and disruptive behavior. *J Child Neur* 2006;21:650–656.

Snider LA, Lougee L, Slattery M, et al: Antibiotic prophylaxis with azithromycin or penicillin for childhood-onset neuropsychiatric disorders. *Biol Psychiatry* 2005;57:788–792.

Snider LA, Swedo SE: PANDAS: Current status and directions for research. *Mol Psychiatry* 2004;9:900–907.

Swedo SE, Leonard HL, Rapoport JL: The pediatric autoimmune neuropsychiatric disorders associated with streptococcal infection (PANDAS) subgroup: Separating fact from fiction. *Pediatrics* 2004;113:907–911.

Tourette's Syndrome Study Group: Treatment of ADHD in children with tics: A randomized controlled trial *Neurology* 2004;58:527–536.

Chapter 24 ■ Anxiety Disorders

Brian Stafford, Neil W. Boris, and Richard Dalton

Anxiety is a normal phenomenon that has evolutionary value. Anxiety has both a physiologic component, mediated by the autonomic nervous system, and a cognitive and behavioral component, expressed in worrying and wariness. When anxiety becomes disabling, interfering with social interactions and development, a diagnosis should be made and intervention initiated. Separation anxiety disorder (SAD), childhood-onset social phobia, generalized anxiety disorder (GAD), obsessive-compulsive disorder (OCD), phobias, post-traumatic stress disorder (PTSD), and panic disorder are all defined by the occurrence of either diffuse or specific anxiety, often related to predictable situations or cues. Anxiety disorders are the most common psychiatric disorders of childhood: epidemiologic data suggest that they occur in 5–18% of all children and adolescents. Anxiety disorders are often comorbid with other psychiatric disorders (including a 2nd anxiety disorder); significant impairment in day-to-day functioning is common.

Because anxiety is both a normal phenomenon and, when highly activated, strongly associated with impairment, the pediatrician will be required to differentiate normal anxiety from abnormal anxiety across development. Anxiety has an identifiable developmental progression for most children; most infants exhibit stranger wariness or anxiety beginning at 7–9 mo of age. Behavioral inhibition to the unfamiliar (withdrawal or fearfulness to novel stimuli associated with physiologic arousal) is evident in approximately 10–15% of the population at 12 mo of age, and is moderately stable. Most children who show behavioral inhibition do not eventually have impairing levels of anxiety. However, data from a cohort of behaviorally inhibited infants who were followed longitudinally showed that both a family history of anxiety disorders and maternal overinvolvement or enmeshment predicted later clinically significant anxiety. The infant who is excessively clingy and difficult to calm during pediatric visits should be followed for signs of increasing levels of anxiety.

Preschoolers typically have specific fears related to the dark, animals, and imaginary situations. Preoccupation with orderliness and routines ("just right" phenomena) also often takes on an anxious quality for preschool children. Parental reassurance is usually sufficient to help the child through this period. Although most school-aged children abandon the imaginary fears of early childhood, some replace them with fears of bodily harm or other worries (Table 24-1). In adolescence, both social anxiety and general worrying (about school, friends, or family) are common.

Genetic or temperamental factors contribute more to the development of some anxiety disorders, whereas environmental factors are closely linked to the cause of others. Specifically, behavioral inhibition appears to be a heritable tendency and is linked with social phobia, generalized anxiety, and selective mutism. OCD and other disorders associated with OCD-like behaviors, such as Tourette syndrome and other tic disorders, tend to have high genetic risk as well (see Chapter 597.4). Environmental factors, such as parent-infant attachment and exposure to trauma, contribute more to SAD and PTSD.

Separation anxiety disorder is characterized by unrealistic and persistent worries of possible harm befalling the affected child or his or her primary caregivers, reluctance to go to school or to sleep without being near the parents, persistent avoidance of being alone, nightmares involving themes of separation, numerous somatic symptoms, and complaints of subjective distress. The 1st clinical sign may not appear until 3rd or 4th grade, typically after a holiday or a period where the child has been home because of illness, or when the stability of the family structure has been threatened by illness, divorce, or another calamity. Parents are often unable to be assertive in returning the child to school. Mothers of children with SAD are likely to have a history of an anxiety disorder. In these cases, the pediatrician should screen for parental depression or anxiety. Often referral for parental treatment or family therapy is necessary before SAD and concomitant school refusal can be successfully treated.

A large percentage of children with SAD have feelings of panic when they are coerced to separate from their parents. Children with SAD are 3 times as likely as children without SAD to develop panic disorder in adolescence. When a child reports recurring acute severe anxiety, antidepressant or anxiolytic medication is often necessary. Controlled studies of tricyclic antidepressants (imipramine) and benzodiazepines (clonazepam) show that these agents are not generally effective. Data support the use of selective serotonin reuptake inhibitors (SSRIs) [see Table 20-1]. Cognitive behavioral therapy benefits children with SAD, especially when the parents are involved in treatment.

Childhood-onset social phobia is characterized by excessive anxiety in social settings (including school), leading to social isolation (Table 24-2). These children and adolescents often maintain the desire for involvement with family and familiar peers. The long-term course is variable, although good longitudinal studies are lacking. However, some children are very distressed by their inability to engage in meaningful relationships with peers and seek treatment. A family history of social phobia or extreme shyness is common. SSRIs are considered the treatment of choice (see Table 20-1). There is some evidence to suggest that adolescents with social phobia who are treated with SSRIs improve, primarily in school performance. Antianxiety agents are not effective.

School refusal, which occurs in approximately 1–2% of children, is associated with anxiety in 40–50% of cases, depression in 50–60% of cases, and oppositional behavior in 50% of cases. Younger anxious children who refuse to attend school are more likely to have SAD, whereas older anxious children usually refuse

TABLE 24-1. Criteria for Diagnosis of Specific Phobia

A. Marked and persistent fear that is excessive or unreasonable, cued by the presence or anticipation of a specific object or situation (e.g., flying, heights, animals, receiving an injection, seeing blood)
B. Exposure to the phobic stimulus almost invariably provokes an immediate anxiety response, which may take the form of a situationally bound or situationally predisposed panic attack. **Note:** In children, the anxiety may be expressed by crying, tantrums, freezing, or clinging
C. The person recognizes that the fear is excessive or unreasonable. **Note:** In children, this feature may be absent
D. The phobic situation is avoided or else is endured with intense anxiety or distress
E. The avoidance, anxious anticipation, or distress in the feared situation interferes significantly with the person's normal routine, occupational (or academic) functioning, or social activities or relationships, or there is marked distress about having the phobia
F. In children <18 yr, the duration is ≥6 mo
G. The anxiety, panic attacks, or phobic avoidance associated with the specific object or situation is not better accounted for by another mental disorder, such as obsessive-compulsive disorder (e.g., fear of dirt in someone with an obsession about contamination), post-traumatic stress disorder (e.g., avoidance of stimuli associated with a severe stressor), separation anxiety disorder (e.g., avoidance of school), social phobia (e.g., avoidance of social situations because of fear of embarrassment), panic disorder with agoraphobia, or agoraphobia without a history of panic disorder

SPECIFY TYPE:

Animal type is fear elicited by animals or insects
Natural environment type (e.g., heights, storms, water)
Blood/injection/injury type is fear related to seeing blood, injuries, or injections, or having an invasive medical procedure
Situational type is fear caused by specific situations (e.g., airplanes, elevators, enclosed places)
Other type (e.g., fear of choking, vomiting, or contracting an illness; in children, fear of loud sounds or costumed characters)

From Kliegman RM, Marcdante KJ, Jenson HB, et al (editors): *Nelson Essentials of Pediatrics;* 5th ed. Philadelphia, Elsevier/Saunders, 2006, p 92.

TABLE 24-2. Criteria for Diagnosis of Social Phobia

A. A marked and persistent fear of $\geq$1 social or performance situations in which the person is exposed to unfamiliar people or to possible scrutiny by others. The individual fears that he or she will act in a way (or show anxiety symptoms) that will be humiliating or embarrassing. **Note:** In children, there must be evidence of the capacity of age-appropriate social relationships with familiar people, and the anxiety must occur in peer settings, not just in interactions with adults

B. Exposure to the feared social situation almost invariably provokes anxiety, which may take the form of a situationally bound or situartionally predisposed panic attack. **Note:** In children, the anxiety may be expressed by crying, tantrums, freezing, or shrinking from social situations or unfamiliar people

C. The person recognizes that the fear is excessive or unreasonable. **Note:** In children, this feature may be absent

D. The feared social or performance situations are avoided or else are endured with intense anxiety or distress

E. The avoidance, anxious anticipation, or distress in the feared social or performance situation interferes significantly with the person's normal routine, occupational (academic) functioning, or social activities or relationships, or there is marked distress about having the phobia

F. In children <18 yr, the duration is $\geq$6 mo

G. The fear or avoidance is not due to the direct physiologic effects of a drug of abuse, a medication, or a general medical condition and is not better accounted for by another mental disorder (e.g., panic disorder with or without agoraphobia, separation anxiety disorder, body dysmorphic disorder, pervasive developmental disorder, or schizoid personality disorder)

H. If a general medical condition or another mental disorder is present, the fear in criterion A is unrelated to it (e.g., the fear is not of stuttering, trembling in Parkinson's disease, or exhibiting abnormal eating behavior in anorexia nervosa or bulimia nervosa)

SPECIFY IF

Generalized: if the fears include most social situations (e.g., initiating or maintaining conversations, participating in small groups, dating, speaking to authority figures, attending parties). **Note:** Also consider the additional diagnosis of avoidant personality disorder

From Kliegman RM, Marcdante KJ, Jenson HB, et al (editors): *Nelson Essentials of Pediatrics,* 5th ed. Philadelphia, Elsevier/Saunders, 2006, p 93.

TABLE 24-4. Criteria for Diagnosis of a Panic Attack

A discrete period of intense fear or discomfort, in which $\geq$4 of the following symptoms developed abruptly and reached a peak within 10 min

Palpitations, pounding heart, or accelerated heart rate
Sweating
Trembling or shaking
Sensations of shortness of breath or being smothered
Feeling of chocking
Chest pain or discomfort
Nausea or abdominal distress
Feeling dizzy, unsteady, light-headed, or faint
Derealization (feelings of unreality) or depersonalization (being detached from oneself)
Fear of losing control or going crazy
Paresthesias (numbness or tingling sensations)
Chills or hot flashes

From Kliegman RM, Marcdante KJ, Jenson HB, et al (editors): *Nelson Essentials of Pediatrics,* 5th ed. Philadelphia, Elsevier/Saunders, 2006, p 87.

to attend school because of social phobia. Somatic symptoms, especially abdominal pain and/or headaches, are common. There may be increasing tension in the parent-child relationship or other indicators of family disruption (domestic violence, divorce, or other major stressors) contributing to school refusal. Management of school refusal typically requires parent management or even family therapy. Working with school personnel is always indicated; anxious children often require special attention from teachers, counselors, or school nurses. Parents who are coached to calmly send the child to school and to reward the child for each completed day of school are usually successful. In cases of ongoing school refusal, referral to a child psychiatrist is indicated. Young children with affective symptoms have a good prognosis, whereas adolescents with more insidious onset or with significant somatic complaints have a more guarded prognosis.

Selective mutism (previously classified as *elective mutism*) is conceptualized as a disorder that overlaps with social phobia. Children with selective mutism talk almost exclusively at home, although they are reticent to do so in other settings, such as school, daycare, or even relatives' homes. Often, one or more stressors, such as a new classroom or parental or sibling conflict, will drive an already shy child to become reluctant to speak. Fluoxetine in combination with behavioral therapy has been shown to be effective for children whose school performance is severely limited by their symptoms (see also Chapter 32).

Panic disorder is a syndrome of recurrent, discrete episodes of marked fear or discomfort in which individuals experience abrupt onset of physical and psychologic symptoms (Tables 24-3 and 24-4). Physical symptoms can include palpitations, sweating, shaking, shortness of breath, dizziness, chest pain, and nausea. Children may present with acute respiratory distress, but without fever, wheezing, or stridor. The associated psychologic symptoms include fear of death, impending doom, and loss of control. Panic disorder is uncommon before adolescence, with the peak age of onset at 15–19 yr of age. The postadolescence prevalence of panic disorder is 1–2%. A predisposition to react to autonomic arousal with anxiety may be a specific risk factor leading to panic disorder. Twin studies suggest that 30–40% of the variance is attributed to genetics. The increasing rates of panic attack are also directly related to earlier sexual maturity. Some adolescents with panic disorder also may have **agoraphobia,** a subsequent fear that a panic attack may occur in a place where help or escape may be unavailable (Table 24-5). SSRIs have shown effectiveness in the treatment of adolescents (see Table 20-1). The recovery rate is approximately 70%.

Generalized anxiety disorder occurs in children who frequently experience unrealistic worries about future events or about the

TABLE 24-3. Criteria for Diagnosis of Panic Disorder

A. Both (1) and (2)
   1. Recurrent unexpected panic attacks
   2. At least 1 of the attacks has been followed by $\geq$1 mo of $\geq$1 of the following:
      a. Persistent concern about having additional attacks
      b. Worry about the implications of the attack or its consequences (e.g., losing control, having a heart attack, "going crazy")
      c. A significant change in behavior related to the attacks

B. The presence or absence of agoraphobia

C. The panic attacks are not due to the direct physiologic effects of a drug of abuse or a medication or a general medical condition (e.g., hyperthyroidism)

D. The panic attacks are not better accounted for by another mental disorder, such as social phobia (e.g., occurring on exposure to feared social situations), specific phobia (e.g., on exposure to a specific phobic situation), obsessive-compulsive disorder (e.g., on exposure to dirt in someone with an obsession about contamination), post-traumatic stress disorder (e.g., in response to stimuli associated with a severe stressor), or separation anxiety disorder (e.g., in response to being away from home or close relatives)

From Kliegman RM, Marcdante KJ, Jenson HB, et al (editors): *Nelson Essentials of Pediatrics,* 5th ed. Philadelphia, Elsevier/Saunders, 2006, p 87.

TABLE 24-5. Criteria for Diagnosis of Agoraphobia

Anxiety about being in places or situations from which escape might be difficult (or embarrassing) or in which help may not be available in the event of having an unexpected or situationally predisposed panic attack or panic-like symptoms

Agoraphobic fears typically involve characteristic clusters of situations that include being outside the home alone; being in a crowd or standing in line; being on a bridge; and traveling in a bus, train, plane, or automobile

Note: Consider the diagnosis of specific phobia if the avoidance is limited to 1 or only a few specific situations or social phobia if the avoidance is limited to social situations in general

The anxiety or phobic avoidance is not better accounted for by another mental disorder, such as social phobia (e.g., avoidance limited to social situations because of fear of embarrassment), specific phobia (e.g., avoidance limited to a single situation, such as elevators), obsessive-compulsive disorder (e.g., avoidance of dirt in someone with an obsession about contamination), post-traumatic stress disorder (e.g., avoidance of stimuli associated with a severe stressor), or separation anxiety disorder (e.g., avoidance of leaving home or relatives)

From Kliegman RM, Marcdante KJ, Jenson HB, et al (editors): *Nelson Essentials of Pediatrics,* 5th ed. Philadelphia, Elsevier/Saunders, 2006, p 88.

TABLE 24-6. Criteria for Diagnosis of Generalized Anxiety Disorder

A. Excessive anxiety and worry (apprehensive expectation), occurring more days than not for ≥6 mo, about numerous events or activities (e.g., work or school performance)
B. The person finds it difficult to control the worry
C. The anxiety and worry are associated with ≥3 of the following 6 symptoms (with at least some symptoms present for more days than not for the past 6 mo).
Note: Only 1 symptom is required in children
1. Restlessness or felling keyed up or on edge
2. being easily fatigued
3. Difficulty concentrating or mind going blank
4. Irritability
5. Muscle tension
6. Sleep disturbance (difficulty falling or staying asleep or restless, unsatisfying sleep)

D. The focus of the anxiety and worry is not confined to features of a disorder (e.g., the anxiety or worry is not about having a panic attack, as in panic disorder; being embarrassed in public, as in social phobia; being contaminated, as in obsessive-compulsive disorder; being away from home or close relatives, as in separation anxiety disorder; gaining weight, as in anorexia nervosa; having multiple physical complaints, as in somatization disorder; or having a serious illness, as in hypochondriasis), and the anxiety and worry do not occur exclusively during post-traumatic stress disorder
E. The anxiety, worry, or physical symptoms cause clinically significant distress or impairment in social, occupational, or other important areas of functioning
F. The disturbance is not due to the direct physiologic effects of a drug (e.g., a drug of abuse or a medication) or a general medical condition (e.g., hyperthyroidism) and does not occur exclusively during a mood disorder, a psychotic disorder, or a pervasive developmental disorder

From Kliegman RM, Marcdante KJ, Jenson HB, et al (editors): *Nelson Essentials of Pediatrics*, 5th ed. Philadelphia, Elsevier/Saunders, 2006, p 89.

TABLE 24-7. Criteria for Diagnosis of Obsessive-Compulsive Disorder

A. Either obsessions or compulsions
Obsessions are defined by (1), (2), (3), and (4)
1. Recurrent and persistent thoughts, impulses, or images that are experienced, at some time during the disturbance, as intrusive and inappropriate and that cause marked anxiety or distress
2. The thoughts, impulses, or images are not simply excessive worries about real-life problems
3. The person attempts to ignore or suppress such thoughts, impulses, or images or to neutralize them with some other thought or action
4. The person recognizes that the obsessional thoughts, impulses, or images are a product of his or her own mind (not imposed from without, as in thought insertion)

Compulsions are defined by (1) and (2)
1. Repetitive behaviors (e.g., handwashing, ordering, checking) or mental acts (e.g., praying, counting, repeating words silently) that the person feels driven to perform in response to an obsession or according to rules that must be applied rigidly
2. The behaviors or mental acts are aimed at preventing or reducing distress or preventing some dreaded event or situation; however, these behaviors or mental acts either are not connected in a realistic way with what they are designed to neutralize or prevent or are clearly excessive

B. At some point during the course of the disorder, the person has recognized that the obsessions or compulsions are excessive or unreasonable. **Note:** This does not apply to children
C. The obsessions or compulsions cause marked distress; are time-consuming (taking >1 hr/day); or significantly interfere with the person's normal routine, occupational (or academic) functioning, or usual social activities or relationships
D. If another Axis I disorder is present, the content of the obsessions or compulsions is not restricted to it (e.g., preoccupation with food in the presence of an eating disorder, hair pulling in the presence of trichotillomania, concern with appearance in the presence of body dysmorphic disorder, preoccupation with drugs in the presence of a substance use disorder, preoccupation with having a serious illness in the presence of hypochondriasis, preoccupation with sexual urges or fantasies in the presence of a paraphilia, or guilty ruminations in the presence of major depressive disorder)
E. The disturbance is not due to the direct physiologic effects of a drug of abuse, a medication, or a general medical condition

SPECIFY IF
With poor insight: if, for most of the time during the current episode, the person does not recognize that the obsessions and compulsions are excessive or unreasonable

From Kliegman RM, Marcdante KJ, Jenson HB, et al (editors): *Nelson Essentials of Pediatrics*, 5th ed. Philadelphia, Elsevier/Saunders, 2006, p 98.

appropriateness of past behavior and their own competence (Table 24-6). They frequently present with somatic symptoms, are markedly self-conscious, and have other anxiety disorders, such as simple phobia and panic disorder. Onset may be gradual or sudden, although GAD does not often become manifest until puberty. Boys and girls are equally affected, and the prevalence in adolescence is 2.4%. GAD is characteristically seen in middle-class and upper-middle-class white children. Children with GAD are generally good candidates for cognitive-behavioral therapy (CBT), although a trial of buspirone or an SSRI may be indicated when symptoms are particularly limiting (see Table 20-1). The recovery rate is approximately 80%.

It is important to distinguish children with GAD from those who present with specific repetitive thoughts that invade consciousness (**obsessions**) or repetitive rituals or movements that are driven by anxiety (**compulsions**). The most common obsessions are concerned with bodily wastes and secretions, the fear that something calamitous will happen, or the need for sameness. The most common compulsions are handwashing, continual checking of locks, and touching. At times of stress (bedtime, preparing for school), some children touch certain objects, say certain words, or wash their hands repeatedly. **Obsessive-compulsive disorder (OCD)** is diagnosed when the thoughts or rituals cause distress, consume time, or interfere with occupational or social functioning (Table 24-7). The Children's Yale-Brown Obsessive-Compulsive Scale (C-YBOCS) and the Anxiety Disorders Interview Schedule for Children (ADIS-C) are reliable and valid methods for discriminating individuals with OCD from those without the disorder. The C-YBOCS is also very helpful in following the progression of symptoms with treatment. Neuroimaging studies of individuals with OCD have documented abnormalities in the frontal lobes, the basal ganglia, and their associated pathways. OCD may present in preschoolers or may appear suddenly later in development. Both pharmacotherapy and CBT are effective therapies for OCD. Fifty percent of children who receive combined treatment (CBT plus SSRI) experience a remission, compared with 39% who receive only CBT and 21% who are treated only with SSRIs. Referral of patients with OCD to a mental health professional is always indicated.

In 10% of children with OCD, symptoms are triggered or exacerbated by group A β-hemolytic streptococcal infection (GABHS) [see Chapter 23]. GABHS bacteria trigger antineuronal antibodies that cross react with caudate neural tissue in genetically susceptible hosts, leading to swelling of this region and resultant obsessions and compulsions. This subtype of OCD, called **pediatric autoimmune neuropsychiatric disorders associated with streptococcal infection (PANDAS)**, is characterized by sudden and dramatic onset or exacerbation of OCD or tic symptoms, associated neurologic findings, and a recent streptococcal infection. The pediatrician should be aware of the infectious cause of some cases of tic disorders and OCD and follow management guidelines (see Chapter 23).

Children with **phobias** avoid specific objects or situations that reliably trigger physiologic arousal (dogs or spiders) [see Table 24-1]. Neither obsessions nor compulsions are associated with the fear response; phobias only rarely interfere with social, educational, or interpersonal functioning. The parents of phobic children should remain calm in the face of the child's anxiety or panic. Parents who become anxious themselves may reinforce their children's anxiety, and the pediatrician can usefully interrupt this cycle by calmly noting that phobias are not unusual and rarely cause impairment. The prevalence of specific phobias in childhood is 0.5–2.0%. Systematic desensitization is a form of behavior therapy that gradually exposes the individual to the fear-inducing situation or object while simultaneously teaching relaxation techniques for anxiety management. Successful repeated exposure leads to extinguishing anxiety for that stimulus.

Post-traumatic stress disorder is an anxiety disorder resulting from the long- and short-term effects of trauma that cause behavioral and physiologic sequelae in toddlers, children, and adolescents (Table 24-8). A new diagnostic category, *acute stress disorder,* has been added to the nosology, reflecting the fact that traumatic events often cause acute symptoms that may or may

TABLE 24-8. Criteria for Diagnosis of Post-Traumatic Stress Disorder

A. The person has been exposed to a traumatic event in which both of the following were present:
   1. The person experienced, witnessed, or was confronted with an event or events that involved actual or threatened death or serious injury or a threat to the physical integrity of self or others
   2. The person's response involved intense fear, helplessness, or horror. **Note:** In children, this may be expressed instead by disorganized or agitated behavior

B. The traumatic event is persistently re-experienced in ≥1 of the following ways:
   1. Recurrent and intrusive distressing recollections of the event, including images, thoughts, or perceptions. **Note:** In young children, repetitive play may occur in which themes or aspects of the trauma are expressed
   2. Recurrent distressing dreams of the event. **Note:** In children, there may be frightening dreams without recognizable content
   3. Acting or feeling as if the traumatic event were recurring (includes a sense of reliving the experience, illusions, hallucinations, and dissociative flashback episodes, including flashbacks that occur on awakening or when intoxicated). **Note:** In young children, trauma-specific reenactment may occur
   4. Intense psychologic distress on exposure to internal or external cues that symbolize or resemble an aspect of the traumatic event
   5. Physiologic reactivity on exposure to internal or external cues that symbolize or resemble an aspect of the traumatic event

C. Persistent avoidance of stimuli associated with the trauma and numbing of general responsiveness (not present before the trauma), as indicated by ≥3 of the following:
   1. Efforts to avoid thoughts, feelings, or conversations associated with the trauma
   2. Efforts to avoid activities, places, or people that arouse recollections of the trauma
   3. Inability to recall an important aspect of the trauma
   4. Markedly diminished interest or participation in significant activities
   5. Feeling of detachment or estrangement from others
   6. Restricted range of affect (e.g., unable to have loving feelings)
   7. Sense of a foreshortened future (e.g., does not expect to have a career, marriage, children, or a normal life span)

D. Persistent symptoms of increased arousal (not present before the trauma), as indicated by ≥2 of the following:
   1. Difficulty falling or staying asleep
   2. Irritability or outbursts of anger
   3. Difficulty concentrating
   4. Hypervigilance
   5. Exaggerated startle response

E. Duration of the disturbance (symptoms in criteria B, C, and D) is >1 mo

F. The disturbance causes clinically significant distress or impairment in social, occupational, or other important areas of functioning

SPECIFY IF

Acute: if duration of symptoms is <3 mo

Chronic: if duration of symptoms is ≥3 mo

SPECIFY IF

With delayed onset: if onset of symptoms is ≥6 mo after the stressor

From Kliegman RM, Marcdante KJ, Jenson HB, et al (editors): *Nelson Essentials of Pediatrics,* 5th ed. Philadelphia, Elsevier/Saunders, 2006, p 90.

not resolve. Previous trauma exposure, a history of other psychopathology, and parental symptoms of PTSD predict childhood-onset PTSD. Many adolescent and adult psychopathologic conditions, such as conduct disorder, depression, and some personality disorders, relate to previous trauma. PTSD also is linked to mood disorders, disruptive behavior, and other diagnoses in childhood. Epidemiologic studies have placed the lifetime prevalence of PTSD by age 18 yr at 6% in a community sample. Up to 40% may show symptoms, but do not fulfill the diagnostic criteria (see Chapter 35).

Life-threatening events that pose harm to the child or the caregiver and that produce considerable stress or fear are required to make the diagnosis of PTSD. Three clusters of symptoms are also essential for diagnosis: re-experiencing, avoidance, and hyperarousal. Persistent re-experiencing of the stressor through intrusive recollections, nightmares, and reenactment in play are typical responses in children. Persistent avoidance of reminders and numbing of emotional responsiveness, such as isolation, amnesia, and avoidance, constitute the 2nd cluster of behaviors. Symptoms of hyperarousal, such as hypervigilance, poor concentration, extreme startle responses, agitation, and sleep problems, complete the symptom profile of PTSD. Occasionally, children regress in some of their developmental milestones after a traumatic event. Avoidance symptoms are commonly observable in younger children, whereas older children may be more able to describe re-experiencing and hyperarousal symptoms. Repetitive play involving the event, psychosomatic symptoms, and nightmares may also be observed.

Initial interventions after a trauma should focus on reunification with a parent and attending to the child's physical needs in a safe place. Aggressive treatment of pain may decrease the likelihood of PTSD, and facilitating a return to comforting routines, including regular sleep, is indicated. Long-term treatment may include individual, group, school-based, or family therapy as well as pharmacotherapy in selected cases. Individual treatment involves transforming the child's concept of himself or herself as victim to that of survivor, and can occur through play therapy, psychodynamic therapy, or CBT. Group work is also helpful for identifying which children may need more intensive assistance. Goals of family work include helping the child establish a sense of security, validating his or her emotions, and anticipating situations when the child will need more support from the family. Clonidine or guanfacine may be helpful for sleep disturbance, persistent arousal, and exaggerated startle response. Comorbid depression and affective numbing may respond to an SSRI, such as sertraline, paroxetine, or nefazodone (see Table 20-1). Tricyclic antidepressants may also be effective agents in adolescents, although their efficacy in younger children is questionable.

Compton S, March J, Brent D, et al: Cognitive-behavioral psychotherapy for anxiety and depressive disorders in children and adolescents: An evidence-based medicine review. *J Am Acad Child Adolesc Psychiatry* 2004;43:930–959.

Crawford AM, Manassis K: Familial predictors of treatment outcome in childhood anxiety disorders. *J Am Acad Child Adolesc Psychiatry* 2001;40:1182–1189.

Geller D, Biederman J, Stewart SE, et al: Which SSRI? A meta-analysis of pharmacotherapy trials in pediatric obsessive-compulsive disorder. *Am J Psychiatry* 2003;160:1919–1928.

Hayward C, Wilson KA, Lagle K, et al: Parent-reported predictors of adolescent panic attacks. *J Am Acad Child Adolesc Psychiatry* 2004;43:613–620.

Heyman I, Mataix-Cols D, Fineberg NA: Obsessive-compulsive disorder. *BMJ* 2006;333:424–429.

Kanton WJ: Panic disorder. *N Engl J Med* 2006;354:2360–2367.

Kendall PC, Brady EU, Verduin TL: Comorbidity in childhood anxiety disorders and treatment outcome. *J Am Acad Child Adolesc Psychiatry* 2001;40:787–794.

Kennedy JA, Spence SH, Macleod AC: Screening for posttraumatic stress disorder in children after accidental injury. *Pediatrics* 2006;118:1002–1009.

King NJ, Bernstein GA: School refusal in children and adolescents: A review of the past 10 years. *J Am Acad Child Adolesc Psychiatry* 2001;40:197–205.

Labellarte MJ, Ginsburg GS, Walkup JT, et al: The treatment of anxiety disorders in children and adolescents. *Biol Psychiatry* 1999;46:1567–1578.

McClure EB, Adlen A, Monk CS, et al: fMRI predictors of treatment outcome in pediatric anxiety disorders. *Psychopharmacology* 2006 (EPub ahead of print).

POTS (Pediatric OCD Study Team): Cognitive-behavioral therapy, sertraline, and their combination for children and adolescents with obsessive-compulsive disorder. *J Am Med Assoc* 2004;292:1–8.

Rapoport JL, Inoff-Germain G: Treatment of obsessive-compulsive disorder in children and adolescents. *J Child Psychol Psychiatry* 2000;41:419–431.

Roy-Byrne PP, Craske MG, Stein MB: Panic disorder. *Lancet* 2006;368:1023.

Schneier FR: Social anxiety disorder. *N Engl J Med* 2006;355:1029–1036.

Szeszko PR, Ardekani BA, Ashtari M, et al: White matter abnormalities in obsessive-compulsive disorder. *Arch Gen Psychiatry* 2005;62:782–790.

Taylor CB: Panic disorder. *BMJ* 2006;332:951–955.

Zahn-Waxler C, Klimes-Dougan B, Slattery MJ: Internalizing problems of childhood and adolescence: Prospects, pitfalls, and progress in understanding the development of anxiety and depression. *Dev Psychopathol* 2000;12:443–456.

Zatzick D: Post-traumatic stress and its effect in health outcomes in children. *J Pediatr* 2005;146:309–310.

Chapter 25 ■ Mood Disorders

Christopher M. Borrillo and Neil W. Boris

Major depressive disorder, dysthymic disorder, and bipolar disorder are the 3 major types of affective, or mood, disorders seen in children and adolescents.

25.1 • Major Depression

Major depression is characterized by persistent sadness (which in children may present as irritability) and an obvious loss of interest and pleasure in usual activities (Table 25-1). Diagnostic symptoms also include decreased or increased food intake (sometimes associated with weight change), insomnia or hypersomnia, psychomotor agitation or retardation, fatigue or loss of energy on most days, feelings of worthlessness and excessive guilt, diminished ability to concentrate, and recurrent thoughts of death, with or without suicidal ideation.

EPIDEMIOLOGY. The prevalence of depression varies. Studies report rates of 0.4–2.5% in childhood and 0.4–8.3% in adolescence. There is compelling evidence that some preschool children have depression. The lifetime prevalence of depression is 15–20%, underscoring the fact that depression is a common disorder. Depression is considered a chronic, recurring disorder marked by discrete episodes of dysfunction. At least twice as many girls as boys meet the criteria for depression during adolescence; prepubertal depression is equally common among the sexes. Depression is undertreated across the life span, despite available and effective treatments shown to counter the high cost of lost productivity (school failure in adolescence) associated with ongoing depression.

TABLE 25-1. Criteria for Diagnosis of Major Depressive Episode

A. Five or more of the following symptoms have been present during the same 2-wk period and represent a change from previous functioning; at least 1 of the symptoms is either (1) depressed mood or (2) loss of interest or pleasure. **Note:** Do not include symptoms that are clearly due to a general medical condition or mood-incongruent delusions or hallucinations
   1. Depressed mood most of the day, nearly every day, as indicated by either subjective report (e.g., feels sad or empty) or observation made by others (e.g., appears tearful). **Note:** In children and adolescents, mood can be irritable
   2. Markedly diminished interest or pleasure in all, or almost all, activities most of the day, nearly every day (as indicated by either subjective account or observation made by others)
   3. Significant weight loss when not dieting or weight gain (e.g., a change of >5% of body weight in 1 mo) or decrease or increase in appetite nearly every day. **Note:** In children, consider failure to make expected weight gains
   4. Insomnia or hypersomnia nearly every day
   5. Psychomotor agitation or retardation nearly every day (observable by others, not merely subjective feelings of restlessness or being slowed down)
   6. Fatigue or loss of energy nearly every day
   7. Feelings of worthlessness or excessive or inappropriate guilt (which may be delusional) nearly every day (not merely self-reproach or guilt about being sick)
   8. Diminished ability to think or concentrate or indecisiveness nearly every day (either by subjective account or as observed by others)
   9. Recurrent thoughts of death (not just fear of dying), recurrent suicidal ideation without a specific plan, or a suicide attempt or a specific plan for committing suicide

B. The symptoms do not meet the criteria for a mixed manic episode

C. The symptoms cause clinically significant distress or impairment in social, occupational, or other important areas of functioning

D. The symptoms are not due to the direct physiologic effects of a drug of abuse, a medication, or a general medical condition (e.g., hypothyroidism)

E. The symptoms are not better accounted for by bereavement (i.e., after the loss of a loved one), and the symptoms persist >2 mo or are characterized by marked functional impairment, morbid preoccupation with worthlessness, suicidal ideation, psychotic symptoms, or psychomotor retardation

From Kliegman RM, Marcdante KJ, Jenson HB, et al (editors): *Nelson Essentials of Pediatrics*, 5th ed. Philadelphia, Elsevier/Saunders, 2006, p 94.

ETIOLOGY. Many factors contribute to depression. There is strong evidence of a genetic basis for major depressive disorders in all age groups. Individuals at increased genetic risk are more sensitive to the effects of adverse environmental conditions. Twin studies have shown a 76% concordance rate for depression among monozygotic twins reared together and a rate of 67% in monozygotic twins reared apart, compared with 19% in dizygotic twins reared together. There is also an increased rate of depression (3–6 times greater) in 1st-degree relatives of patients with a major affective disorder. Low functional levels of norepinephrine and serotonin are believed to be important genetic markers for depression. Positron emission tomography scans show altered metabolic activity in specific brain regions associated with mood, sleep, and appetite regulation. Neuroimaging data are reinforced by the fact that antidepressants that block presynaptic reuptake of serotonin are effective in treating depression. The development of hopelessness and helplessness secondary to an actual loss or the perception of loss suggests that cognitive factors play a role in the onset and maintenance of depression. Adverse life events have a role in causing depression.

CLINICAL MANIFESTATIONS. Depressive symptoms vary according to age and developmental level. Observational studies of institutionalized infants document withdrawal, apathy, hypotonia, lethargy, and sad facial expressions. These infants often cry silently, and when picked up, they may cling to a stranger, although they are usually inconsolable. In young children, irritability, crying spells, and lack of interest or pleasure in activities are key symptoms. Affected young children may also have separation anxiety and somatic symptoms, such as headache or abdominal pain. Postpubertal children often describe pervasive sadness and neurovegetative symptoms, such as sleep disturbance and appetite changes. The hallmark of psychotic depression in children is the occurrence of **hallucinations;** delusions are more common in adolescents and adults.

The symptoms of a major depressive episode usually develop over a period of many days or wk. The duration of each episode of depression is variable, although symptoms often persist for 7–9 mo without treatment; 6–10% of episodes are more protracted. Children and adolescents who are depressed are at risk for later episodes of depression. Within 2 yr of the 1st major depressive episode, 40% of children experience a relapse; depression should be considered a chronic disease marked by periods of normal mood. Within 3–4 yr of discharge, 20–40% of teenagers hospitalized with major depression have a manic episode. Three predictors of later mania in depressed adolescents are: (1) a depressive symptom cluster characterized by rapid onset, psychomotor retardation, and mood-congruent psychotic features; (2) a family history of bipolar illness or other affective illness; and (3) induction of hypomania by antidepressant medication. Depression is further complicated by the fact that comorbidities commonly occur: 20–50% of depressed children have 2 or more diagnoses, including an anxiety disorder (30–80%), a disruptive behavior disorder (10–80%), dysthymic disorder (30–80%), or a substance abuse disorder (20–30%).

DIAGNOSIS. A clinical interview with the child and multiple adults familiar with the child remains the gold standard (see Table 25-1). The Children's Depression Inventory, Children's Depression Scale, Depression Self-Rating Scale, and Center for Epidemiological Studies—Depression Scale have all been shown to be helpful to clinicians in diagnosing depression in children and adolescents. There are no biologic tests specific for depression, although various biologic markers have been studied. During major depressive episodes, some children have been shown to hyposecrete growth hormone in response to insulin-induced hypoglycemia, whereas others produce higher growth hormone peaks during sleep. No test has sufficient sensitivity or specificity to assist in diagnostic assessment.

TREATMENT. Both psychotherapy and pharmacotherapy are effective in treating depression in childhood and adolescence. Psychotherapy is especially important for patients with multiple diagnoses or precipitants related to family disruption or conflict, although these children tend to have more refractory disease. Cognitive-behavioral therapy (12–16 wk) is effective in approximately 40–50% of cases of adolescent depression. Combination therapy with fluoxetine and cognitive-behavioral therapy results in significant clinical improvement in 71% of depressed adolescent patients. This improvement rate exceeds that of other approaches, such as treatment with fluoxetine alone (61%) or cognitive-behavioral therapy alone (43%).

The lack of efficacy and the poor side effect profile of tricyclic antidepressants (TCAs) has made selective serotonin reuptake inhibitors (SSRIs) the primary class of antidepressants used for pharmacologic therapy (see Table 20-1). Only 1 of 12 controlled studies of TCAs has demonstrated efficacy, and these agents, which have a narrow therapeutic window and serious side effects, are rarely indicated for depression in childhood. Because depression is strongly associated with suicidal ideation and attempts and TCAs are deadly in overdose, the pediatrician should avoid using these drugs for depression.

In approximately 70% of cases, SSRIs reduce depressive symptoms. The possibility that SSRIs might be associated with an increased risk of suicidal behaviors in children and adolescents with major depressive disorder has been raised. In 2004, the U.S. Food and Drug Administration (FDA) directed pharmaceutical companies to warn about the increased risk of suicidal thinking and behavior in children and adolescents with major depressive disorder undergoing treatment with any antidepressants. The FDA did not prohibit the use of antidepressants in children and adolescents, but recommended that physicians and families closely monitor youth taking the medications for worsening symptoms of depression or unusual changes in behavior, especially during the early phases of treatment. The FDA reviewed 23 clinical trials involving the treatment of depressed children and adolescents with antidepressants. No suicides occurred in any of these studies. In addition, the suicide rate for children 10–19 yr old has significantly decreased since SSRIs were 1st introduced in the late 1980s. Although there are multiple risk factors to consider in assessing the complex nature of suicidal behavior, none of these factors is linked specifically to the use of antidepressants by children and adolescents. Antidepressants continue to be an important part of the comprehensive treatment of pediatric mental disorders. Adults with refractory depression have been treated experimentally with deep brain stimulation.

Prevention is the new frontier in the management of depression. Mood disorders (both depression and bipolar disorder) are associated with later substance abuse. Pediatricians should inform families about the relationship between mood disorders and substance abuse and screen adolescents who have had 1 or more episodes of depression for substance abuse at each visit (see Chapter 113). There is also evidence that family-based interventions can prevent the onset of depression in offspring of depressed parents. Pediatricians should routinely screen for peripartum depression. When the pediatrician identifies parental depression or the child's family history includes depression in a 1st-degree relative, preventive intervention is indicated. Most mental health clinicians who work with family units can provide short (typically 8 sessions), focused interventions that may significantly reduce the likelihood that the preadolescent child will have a mood disorder.

25.2 • Dysthymic Disorder

Compared with major depression, dysthymic disorder is a less severe, but more protracted syndrome involving depressed mood for at least 1 yr. Poor appetite, sleep problems, decreased energy and self-esteem, and feelings of hopelessness are characteristic of dysthymia. Dysphoria is less intense, but more chronic, with only brief periods of normal mood.

ETIOLOGY. Although the genetic basis for major depression has been demonstrated, the data regarding the genetic basis for dysthymic disorder are less firm. Dysthymia may be a partial phenotypic expression of an underlying genetic disorder or a different syndrome that has certain symptom clusters in common with major depression. The prevalence is 0.6–1.7% in childhood and 1.6–8.0% in adolescence.

CLINICAL MANIFESTATIONS. With the exception of hallucinations and delusions, other symptoms of major depression may be present, although severe sleep disturbance, appetite loss, or anhedonia suggests evolving major depression. Children who have dysthymia have had frequent disruptions of important relationships, often beginning as early as infancy. There is often a history of depressive illness in both parents. Affected children show more general emotional and social maladjustment. They often present as helpless, passive, clinging, dependent, and lonely children. Others relate in a more hardened, aloof, negativistic manner, and are reluctant to invest emotion or trust in relationships. Untreated dysthymic disorder is generally chronic and is associated with increased risk of the subsequent development of major depression (70%), bipolar disorder (13%), and substance abuse disorder (15%). Frequently, children with dysthymia have a co-occurring 2nd psychiatric disorder.

TREATMENT. Antidepressant pharmacotherapy is useful in the treatment of dysthymic patients, although there are few good studies of dysthymia in children (see Table 20-1). Antidepressants are especially helpful for those who show vegetative symptoms of depression. When dysthymic symptoms are associated with a 2nd condition (anorexia, somatization disorder, substance abuse disorder, physical illness), both conditions require intervention. Often a full spectrum of therapies, including alliance building and dynamic psychotherapy, family therapy, parent management training, liaison work with the child's school, and pharmacotherapy, is indicated.

25.3 • Bipolar Disorder

Bipolar disorder is characterized by either alternating depression and mania (a typical adult presentation) or rapid cycling of mood, which may appear as irritable depression and dysregulation of affect. The rapid-cycling, mixed variant is more common in children and young adolescents. Of adult patients with bipolar disorder, 1% report that their symptoms began in early childhood; approximately 10% report that their symptoms began in early adolescence. Epidemiologic studies suggest that the prevalence rate during childhood and adolescence is 1%, although differing diagnostic standards have led to varying estimates.

ETIOLOGY. Bipolar disorder is in part genetic: a concordance rate of 65% in monozygotic twins and >20% in dizygotic twins supports this hypothesis. Further, 1st-degree relatives of individuals with bipolar disorder are much more likely than the general population to have a mood disorder. Of adolescents presenting with major depressive symptoms, >20% have manic episodes

TABLE 25-2. Mania Symptoms

A. A distinct period of abnormally and persistently elevated, expansive, or irritable mood, lasting at least 1 wk (or any duration, if hospitalization is necessary)
B. During the period of mood disturbance, ≥3 of the following symptoms have persisted (4 if the mood is only irritable) and have been present to a significant degree
   1. Inflated self-esteem or grandiosity
   2. Decreased need for sleep (e.g., feels rested after only 3 hr of sleep)
   3. More talkative than usual or pressure to keep talking
   4. Flight of ideas or subjective experience that thoughts are racing
   5. Distractibility (i.e., attention too easily drawn to unimportant or irrelevant external stimuli)
   6. Increased goal-directed activity (socially, at work or school, or sexually) or psychomotor agitation
   7. Excessive involvement in pleasurable activities that have a high potential for painful consequences (e.g., engaging in unrestrained buying sprees, sexual indiscretions, or foolish business investments)
C. The symptoms do not meet the criteria for a mixed episode
D. The mood disturbance is sufficiently severe to cause marked impairment in occupational functioning or in usual social activities or relationships with others or to necessitate hospitalization to prevent harm to self or others, or there are psychotic features
E. The symptoms are not due to the direct physiologic effects of a substance (e.g., a drug of abuse, a medication, or other treatment) or a general medical condition (e.g., hyperthyroidism). **Note:** Manic-like episodes that are clearly caused by somatic antidepressant treatment (e.g., medication, electroconvulsive therapy, light therapy) should not count toward a diagnosis of bipolar I disorder

From Kliegman RM, Marcdante KJ, Jenson HB, et al (editors): *Nelson Essentials of Pediatrics*, 5th ed. Philadelphia, Elsevier/Saunders, 2006, p 96.

later. Bipolar disorder may follow childhood traumatic stress, such as child abuse (physical or sexual).

CLINICAL MANIFESTATIONS. The clinical manifestations of bipolar disorder may be different for prepubertal children and early adolescents compared with older adolescents and adults. Defined episodes of depression alternating with euphoria, grandiose thoughts, high activity levels, pressured speech, distractibility, hypersexuality, hyper-religiosity, overspending, and hallucinations and delusions are characteristic of classic bipolar disorder, and represent the typical mid to late adolescent or adult pattern of symptoms (Table 25-2). In 70% of these cases, a careful history shows that at least 1 episode of depression preceded the manic symptoms. Some children and adolescents present with irritability, grandiosity, explosive aggression, hyperactivity, rapid thinking, and cognitive impairment. These children, who often do not fully meet the current American Psychiatric Association's *Diagnostic and Statistical Manual,* 4th edition, criteria for bipolar disorder, clearly have symptoms that impair their functioning and require intervention. Rarely, symptoms are evident as early as the preschool period. Because some studies suggest that children with early-onset symptoms are more likely to have 1st-degree relatives with a mood disorder, these children are considered to have pediatric bipolar disorder. They may also fulfill the criteria for 1 or more disruptive behavioral disorders, particularly attention-deficit/hyperactivity disorder and/or conduct disorder. There is considerable controversy about the prevalence and diagnostic features of this early-onset form of bipolar disorder. Severe early mood instability is associated with high levels of school failure, poor peer relations, and high levels of risk-taking behaviors and substance abuse in early adolescence.

TREATMENT. Therapy for bipolar disorder typically requires the use of mood-stabilizing medications; the use of a 2nd adjunctive medication is often indicated (see Table 20-1). Psychotherapy alone is usually ineffective for bipolar disorder, although therapies such as parent training can be very useful adjuncts to pharmacotherapy. Pharmacologic management of bipolar disorder is generally best left to child psychiatrists, except in unusual circumstances. The 2 best-studied mood stabilizers used in pediatric bipolar disorder are lithium carbonate and divalproic acid. **Lithium carbonate** is effective in the treatment of bipolar disorder and manic symptoms in >½ of cases. Lithium is administered orally, followed by measurement of blood levels. The ideal therapeutic range for the initial treatment of acute symptoms is a blood level of 1.0–1.2 mEq/L, and the recommended blood level for maintenance therapy is 0.5–0.8 mEq/L. Lithium is associated with renal impairment and hypothyroidism; baseline and follow-up renal and thyroid function tests are imperative. The side effects are the major reason why lithium is not always useful for maintenance therapy. The antiepileptic **valproic acid** is also commonly used and may be especially effective in rapid-cycling bipolar disorder. Most pediatric patients tolerate valproate, although it is potentially toxic to the liver; baseline and follow-up liver function tests are imperative.

Carbamazepine is another antiepileptic used for mood stabilization; like valproate, carbamazepine requires monitoring of liver function. Carbamazepine may also rarely lead to leukopenia and even agranulocytosis; it is also associated with Stevens-Johnson syndrome. **Lamotrigine** is a promising drug, especially for depression associated with bipolar disorder. Approximately 10% of children and adolescents taking lamotrigine have a rash; because a high percentage of these rashes evolve into Stevens-Johnson syndrome, the drug should be discontinued when the rash is 1st noted.

Open-label trials suggest that risperidone and olanzapine may be helpful adjuncts to mood stabilizers both in the management of acute mania and in maintenance therapy. Addition of an antipsychotic agent may be especially useful in children from chaotic families who cannot be relied on to comply with difficult dosing requirements and frequent laboratory visits. Weight gain is common with this class of drugs.

Early onset of symptoms and high levels of aggression appear to be related to treatment failure. There is consensus that early recognition of bipolar disorder, particularly in the prodromal phase, is key to long-term management. The pediatrician should carefully monitor the behavior of children who have 1 or more parents with bipolar disorder. Those with bilineal pedigrees are particularly likely to show early symptoms. Children with prepubertal depression or early mood instability and a family history of bipolar disorder should be referred for psychiatric management. Those who are irritable, are sensitive to rejection, are stubborn, have attention difficulties, or are particularly anxious should be carefully monitored and referred early.

American Academy of Child and Adolescent Psychiatry: Practice parameters for the assessment and treatment of children and adolescents with depressive disorders. *J Am Acad Child Adolesc Psychiatry* 1998;37(Suppl):63S–83S.

Beardslee WR, Gladstone TR, Wright EJ, et al: A family-based approach to the prevention of depressive symptoms in children at risk: Evidence of parental and child change. *Pediatrics* 2003;112:e119–e131.

Bostwick JM: Do SSRIs cause suicide in children? The evidence is underwhelming. *J Clin Psychol* 2006;62:235–241.

Coyle JT, Pine DS, Charney DS, et al: Depression and Bipolar Support Alliance Consensus Development Panel: Depression and Bipolar Support Alliance Consensus Statement on the Unmet Needs in Diagnosis and Treatment of Mood Disorders in Children and Adolescents. *J Am Acad Child Adolesc Psychiatry* 2003;42:1494–1503.

Ebmeier KP, Donaghey C, Steele JD: Recent developments and current controversies in depression. *Lancet* 2006;367:153–167.

Emslie GJ, Mayes TL: Mood disorders in children and adolescents: Psychopharmacological treatment. *Biol Psychiatry* 2001;49:1082–1090.

Friedrich MJ: Molecular studies probe bipolar disorder. *JAMA* 2005;293:535–536.

Geller B, Tillman R, Craney JL, et al: Four-year prospective outcome and natural history of mania in children with a prepubertal and early adolescent bipolar disorder phenotype. *Arch Gen Psychiatry* 2004;61:459–467.

Geller B, Williams M, Zimerman B, et al: Prepubertal and early adolescent bipolarity differentiate from ADHD by manic symptoms, grandiose delusions, ultra-rapid or ultradian cycling. *J Affective Disord* 1998;51:81–91.

Kowatch RA, Fristad M, Birmaher B, et al: Treatment guidelines for children and adolescents with bipolar disorder. *J Am Acad Child Adolesc Psychiatry* 2005;44:213–235.
Leverich GS, Post RM: Course of bipolar illness after history of childhood trauma. *Lancet* 2006;367:1040–1042.
Luby JL, Heffelfinger AK, Mrakotsky C, et al: The clinical picture of depression in preschool children. *J Am Acad Child Adolesc Psychiatry* 2003; 42:340–348.
Lundahl B, Risser HJ, Lovejoy MC: A meta-analysis of parent training: Moderators and follow-up effects. *Clin Psychol Rev* 2006;26:86–104.
Pavuluri MN, Birmaher B, Naylor MW: Pediatric bipolar disorder: A review of the past 10 years. *J Am Acad Child Adolesc Psychiatry* 2005;44:846–871.
Rappaport N, Bostic JQ, Prince JB, Jellinek M: Treating pediatric depression in primary care: coping with the patients' blue mood and the FDA's black box. *J Pediatr* 2006;148:567–568.
Rush AJ, Trivedi MH, Wisniewski SR, et al: Bupropion-SR, sertraline, or venlafaxine-XR after failure of SSRIs for depression. *N Engl J Med* 2006;354:1231–1242.
Ryan ND: Treatment of depression in children and adolescents. *Lancet* 2005;366:933–940.
Schlaepfer TE, Lieb K: Deep brain stimulation for treatment of refractory depression. *Lancet* 2005;366:1420–1422.
Wagner KD, Ambrosini P, Rynn M, et al: Efficacy of sertraline in the treatment of children and adolescents with major depressive disorder. *JAMA* 2003;290:1033–1041.
Weissman MM, Wickramaratne P, Warner V, et al: Offspring of depressed parents: 20 years later. *Am J Psychiatry* 2006;163:1001–1008.
Wilens TE, Biederman J, Kwon A, et al: Risk of substance use disorders in adolescents with bipolar disorder. *J Am Acad Child Adolesc Psychiatry* 2004;43:1380–1386.

Chapter 26 ■ Suicide and Attempted Suicide

Neil W. Boris and Richard Dalton

Globally, an estimated 4 million adolescents attempt suicide annually, resulting in approximately 100,000 deaths. Suicide is the 3rd leading cause of death among adolescents in the U.S., where the rate of completed suicide for males has increased dramatically over the last 4 decades. The vast majority of children and adolescents who complete suicide have some form of psychiatric illness. Pediatricians and primary care providers should ask about depression and suicidal ideation at each adolescent visit and must be comfortable assessing suicide risk and knowing when to refer children and adolescents for mental health care.

EPIDEMIOLOGY. Suicide is extremely rare before puberty. Rates of completed suicide increase steadily across the teen years and into young adulthood, peaking in the early 20s. Yearly in the U.S., approximately 2,000 13–19 yr olds are reported to complete suicide; underreporting of suicide has been documented. As age increases from prepuberty to late adolescence, the male : female ratio for completed suicide rises from 3 : 1 to approximately 4.5 : 1. It is estimated that there are 5–45 suicide attempts for each completed suicide, and in some samples, as many as 25% of all adolescents admit to suicidal ideation. Approximately 3 times as many females attempt suicide as males. Most female suicide attempts involve ingestion or superficial cutting, whereas males use more lethal means (hanging, firearms) [Fig. 26-1]. The increase in suicide rates has been greater in black youth than in white youth, and as a result, the rate of suicide among black teens approaches that of white teens, especially in late adolescence; 3–5 times as many black males complete suicide as black females.

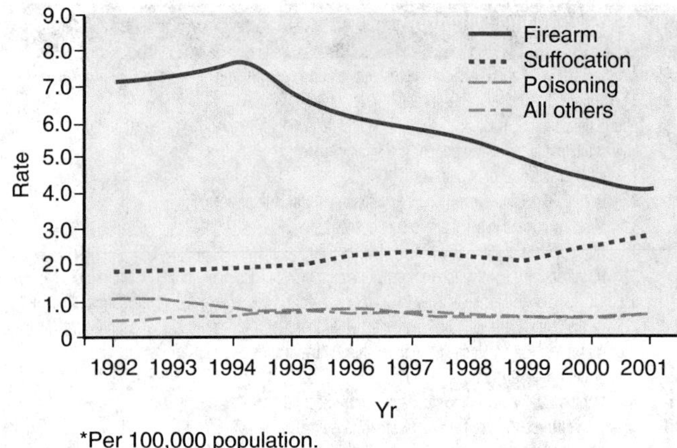

Figure 26-1. Annual suicide rates among persons aged 15–19 yr, by year and method, United States, 1992–2001. (From Centers for Disease Control) Methods of suicide among persons aged 10–19 years, United States, 1992–2001. *MMWR* 2004;53:471–474.)

RISK FACTORS. The origins of suicidal behavior can be understood using a biopsychosocial framework. Twin studies that control for life events known to be related to suicidal behavior show that suicidal ideation and suicide attempts are significantly more common among monozygotic twin pairs than among dizygotic twin pairs. Pedigree analyses further support the influence of genetic factors on suicidal behavior. Heritable alterations in the serotonin system are associated with suicide completion. The serotonin system is important in regulating impulsivity, aggression, and mood, and these 3 factors are related to both psychiatric diagnosis and sex. Although adolescent females are more at risk for depression compared with males, males are generally more aggressive and impulsive than females. There is a strong association between mood disorders and both suicide attempts and suicide completion in both sexes. For males, the addition of conduct disorder or chronic anxiety is also associated with completed suicide, especially when combined with alcohol abuse (which is associated with impulsivity). In females, chronic anxiety, especially panic disorder, is associated with suicide completion. Children and adolescents with a history of previous suicide attempts are at higher risk for suicide completion, regardless of their psychiatric status. These data suggest that several interconnected risks, probably mediated primarily by biologic and genetic factors, predict suicide.

Psychologic and social factors must also be considered to obtain a more complete picture of suicidal behavior. Of children and adolescents who attempt suicide, ⅔ can name a precipitating event for their action. A remote or recent history of child maltreatment or sexual assault is associated with suicide. There is a more general association between family conflict and suicide attempts; this association is strongest in children and early adolescents. In older adolescents, life events, such as relationship breakups, are commonly associated with suicide attempts. Adolescents who identify themselves as homosexual are at increased risk for suicide; those with gender dysphoria appear also to be at high risk. When a feeling of hopelessness is associated with an adolescent's current psychologic state, then suicide risk increases. For some recent immigrants, suicidal ideation is associated with high levels of acculturative stress, especially in the context of family dysfunction and the perception of limited options.

A major factor predicting death from suicide is the lethality of the means used by the suicidal child or adolescent. "Violent" suicides, those completed by means of firearms or hanging, account for the increased suicide rate among adolescent males. The use of carbon monoxide poisoning in adolescent suicide is uncommon, but deadly. Overdoses are common, but do not often kill. Preadolescents most commonly attempt suicide by jumping from heights; self-poisoning, hanging, stabbing, and running into traffic are less common. Episodes of self-poisoning that occur after age 6 yr are less likely to be accidental and should be treated as a potential suicide attempt or a possible case of child abuse and neglect.

ASSESSMENT AND MANAGEMENT. Assessment of suicidal ideation should be a part of each health visit in adolescence (see Chapter 111). There is no evidence that discussing suicide with patients increases the likelihood that they will harm themselves. There is evidence that suicidal persons who seek medical care do not discuss suicidal thoughts, symptoms of depression, or patterns of drug use unless specifically asked. Given that suicide is a leading cause of death in adolescence, the physician can prevent more deaths by asking about suicide than by auscultation of the lungs.

The 1st principle of **suicide assessment** is that suicidal ideation should be taken seriously. Physicians, parents, and others must scrupulously avoid sarcasm, kidding, daring, or belittling the individual who reveals thoughts of suicide. If a suicidal threat is labeled manipulative, power or control becomes a major issue influencing behavior, and the risk of suicide may increase. In the case of the child or adolescent who is seen after a suicide attempt, a thorough history regarding ingestion is necessary, and aggressive management of poisoning must be implemented as indicated. Alcohol or drug intoxication is common and may require acute management (see Chapter 113).

The 2nd principle of suicide assessment is that the child or adolescent must be understood within the biopsychosocial framework (Table 26-1). The child's or adolescent's psychiatric status is a primary concern. A careful psychiatric history and a mental status examination are necessary to assess the risk of suicide completion. Physicians who are uncomfortable with psychiatric assessment should seek immediate consultation with a mental health professional. Signs and symptoms of mood disorders, conduct problems, chronic anxiety, or substance abuse suggest the need for intervention and indicate a risk of eventual suicide completion. Previous suicide attempts should also be documented. To identify precipitating events, the physician should carefully explore, in detail, the child's life during the 48–72 hr before either the threat or the suicide attempt. The degree of premeditation or impulsivity should be assessed. In most instances, children and adolescents will openly discuss how intent they were on harming themselves, their reasons for attempting suicide, and whether they remain suicidal. Furthermore, the physician should be able to evaluate the response of the immediate family to the suicide attempt and to assess the degree of ongoing family conflict.

When a suicidal patient has been seen in the physician's office, the physician should enter into a **no-suicide contract** with the patient. The parents should be notified, and a psychiatric consultation should be obtained. Because 50% of those who attempt suicide do not attend even 1 outpatient psychiatric session, the physician should schedule an appointment within 1–2 days. If possible, the patient and family should meet the therapist immediately after the examination by the physician. In most cases, suicide attempters who are seen in the emergency room should be admitted to the hospital for 1 day or more so that an adequate evaluation can be made of the patient's frame of mind and the family or environmental circumstances. Such admissions usually require 2–3 days, unless the patient's medical needs require a longer stay or if a serious psychiatric disorder, such as depression or psychosis, is found. If social service and psychiatric assessments are adequate and arrangements for appropriate follow-up care can be made, disposition can be made fairly rapidly. The physician must pay careful attention to how the family and friends have responded to the patient's act. A hostile and angry family, as is frequently seen, necessitates a different disposition or resolution than a supportive, sympathetic, and understanding family. The latter situation supports a decision for the patient to return home. Some families may completely deny the seriousness of the behavior; this can be discouraging and provocative to the patient, whose act has been an attempt to compel a different response. Family members should be helped to examine their roles in the interactions that preceded the attempt, without being made to feel overly guilty. Psychiatric hospitalization is indicated when the individual continues to be actively suicidal, when he or she is found to have a major psychiatric disorder, or when major family problems complicate his or her ongoing protection.

A body of literature indicates that suicide may be preventable, and school-based programs appear to hold promise. Pediatricians working in school-based settings should encourage further trials of such preventive interventions (Fig. 26-2).

TABLE 26-1. Checklists for Assessing Child or Adolescent Suicide Attempters in an Emergency Room or Crisis Center

ATTEMPTERS AT GREATER RISK FOR SUICIDE

Suicidal history
- Still thinking of suicide
- Have made a prior suicide attempt

Demographics
- Male
- Live alone

Mental state
- Depressed, manic, hypomanic, severely anxious, or a mixture of these states
- Substance abuse alone or in association with a mood disorder
- Irritable, agitated, threatening violence to others, delusional, or hallucinating

Do not discharge such patients without psychiatric evaluation.

Look for signs of clinical depression:
- Depressed mood most of the time
- Loss of interest or pleasure in usual activities
- Weight loss or gain
- Can't sleep or sleeps too much
- Restless or slowed down
- Fatigue, loss of energy
- Feelings of worthlessness or guilt
- Low self-esteem, disappointed with self
- Feelings of hopelessness about the future
- Can't concentrate, indecisive
- Recurring thoughts of death
- Irritable, upset by little things

Look for signs of mania or hypomania:
- Depressed mood most of the time
- Elated, expansive, or irritable mood
- Inflated self-esteem, grandiosity
- Decreased need for sleep
- More talkative than usual, pressured speech
- Racing thoughts
- Abrupt topic changes when talking
- Distractible
- Excessive participation in multiple activities
- Agitated or restless
- Hypersexual, spends foolishly, uninhibited remarks

From American Foundation for Suicide Prevention: Today's suicide attempter could be tomorrow's suicide (poster). New York, American Foundation for Suicide Prevention, 1999, 1-888-333-AFSP.

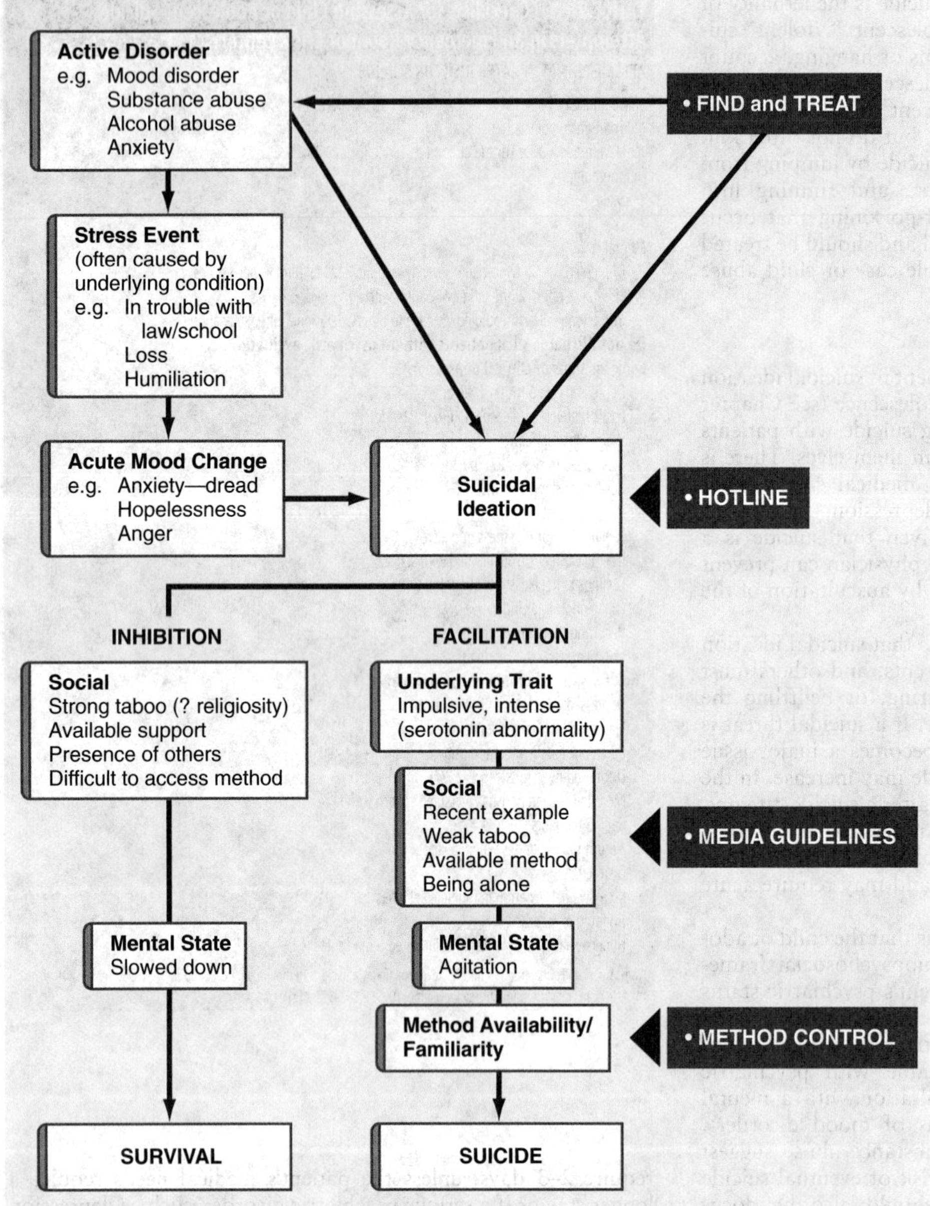

Figure 26-2. This model shows how suicide occurs and highlights types of targeted preventive interventions. (From American Academy of Child and Adolescent Psychiatry) Practice parameter for the assessment and treatment of children and adolescents with suicidal behavior. *J Am Acad Child Adolesc Psychiatry* 2001;40[Suppl]:24S–51S.)

American Academy of Child and Adolescent Psychiatry: Practice parameter for the assessment and treatment of children and adolescents with suicidal behavior. *J Am Acad Child Adolesc Psychiatry* 2001;40(Suppl):24S–51S.

Aseltine RH, DeMartino R: An outcome evaluation of the SOS Suicide Prevention Program. *Am J Public Health* 2004;94:446–451.

Bostwick JM: Do SSRIs cause suicide in children? The evidence is underwhelming. *J Clin Psychol* 2006;62:235–241.

Brent D, Baugher M, Bridge B, et al: Age- and sex-related risk factors for adolescent suicide. *J Am Acad Child Adolesc Psychiatry* 1999;38:1497–1505.

Centers for Disease Control: Methods of suicide among persons aged 10–19 years, United States, 1992–2001. *MMWR* 2004;53:471–474.

Centers for Disease Control: Suicide among black youths—United States, 1980–1995. *MMWR* 1998;47:193–195.

Hammad TA, Laughren T, Racoosin: Suicidality in pediatric patients treated with antidepressant drugs. *Arch Gen Psychiatry* 2006;63:332–339.

Kessler RC, Berglund P, Borges G, et al: Trends in suicide ideation, plans, gestures, and attempts in the United States, 1990–1992 to 2001–2003. *JAMA* 2005;293:2487–2495.

Kim WJ, Singh T: Trends and dynamics of youth suicides in developing countries. *Lancet* 2004;363:1090.

Levine LJ, Schwarz DF, Argon J, et al: Discharge disposition of adolescents admitted to medical hospitals after attempting suicide. *Arch Pediatr Adolesc Med* 2005;159:860–866.

Mann JJ, Apter A, Bertolote J, et al: Suicide prevention strategies. *JAMA* 2005;294:2064–2074.

Mann JJ, Brent DA, Arango V: The neurobiology and genetics of suicide and attempted suicide: A focus on the serotonergic system. *Neuropsychopharmacology* 2001;24:467–477.

Mittendorfer-Rutz E, Rasmussen F, Wasserman D: Restricted fetal growth and adverse maternal psychosocial and socioeconomic conditions as risk factors for suicidal behavior in offspring: a cohort study. *Lancet* 2004;364:1135–1140.

Russell ST, Joyner K: Adolescent sexual orientation and suicide risk: Evidence from a national study. *Am J Public Health* 2001;91:1276–1281.

Sequeira A, Gwadry FG, French-Mullen JMH, et al: Implication of SSAT by gene expression and genetic variation in suicide and major depression. *Arch Gen Psychiatry* 2006;63:35–48.

Shaffer D, Scott M, Wilcox H, et al: The Columbia Suicides Screen: Validity and reliability of a screen for youth suicide and depression. *J Am Acad Child Adolesc Psychiatry* 2004;43:71–79.

Chapter 27 ■ Eating Disorders

Amy Abraham and Brian Stafford

ANOREXIA, BULIMIA, AND BINGE EATING

DEFINITIONS. **Anorexia nervosa (AN) and bulimia nervosa (BN)** are common psychiatric disorders in adolescents and young adults, and they have the highest rates of morbidity and mortality of any psychologic condition. A central feature of both disorders is an intense fear of becoming overweight. AN is a condition of self-produced weight loss, usually seen in adolescent girls and young women, and less frequently in children or middle-aged adults. AN involves an intense preoccupation with weight and shape, behaviors aimed at a relentless pursuit of thinness, and the resulting physical consequences of these behaviors. BN is more common than AN, and is marked by long-term dietary restraint interrupted by episodes of reactive hyperphagia and compensatory behaviors, such as vomiting and laxative abuse. Unlike in AN, where patients are emaciated, BN patients' weight fluctuates, usually within the normal range. Bulimic episodes are often planned, and the binge-purge behavior is often concealed from others. **Binge eating disorder (BED)**, which involves episodes of severe overeating without the compensatory behaviors of BN, has also been identified as an eating disorder in need of clinical intervention, although its diagnostic status is the subject of debate. Obesity is not listed as a disorder in the American Psychiatric Association's *Diagnostic and Statistical Manual of Mental Disorders,* 4th edition (DSM-IV), although 10–20% of individuals with BED are obese (see Chapter 44).

EPIDEMIOLOGY. The incidence of AN and BN has increased over the last 2 decades. Eating disorders are more prevalent in females than in males, by approximately 8:1, although reported cases of eating disorders in males are also increasing. It is estimated that, in the U.S., 1 in every 100 females 16–18 yr old has AN. A bimodal distribution occurs, with 1 peak at 14.5 yr and the other at 18 yr; 25% may be younger than the age of 13 yr. The reported lifetime prevalence of AN among women is 0.5–3.7%. Initially reported only in middle and upper socioeconomic groups, AN occurs in lower socioeconomic levels and in a variety of ethnic and racial groups as well as in both developed and developing countries.

Even more common than AN is BN. The reported lifetime prevalence of BN among women in the U.S. ranges from 1.1–4.2%. The condition is found throughout the world, although the rates vary by location and over time. The incidence of BED is estimated to be 2–3% in the general U.S. population and 8% in the obese population. BED is also common in men and minority groups. Many prevalence studies do not include the category of eating disorder not otherwise specified, which may add approximately 50% more cases to current prevalence estimates.

ETIOLOGY. An individual's unique sense of self, biologic and genetic makeup, developmental stage, family constellation, and culture all contribute to the development of pathology. Eating disorders commonly begin as innocent dieting behavior, not unlike that seen in many other adolescent girls; however, girls and women with AN gradually progress to profound weight loss with emaciation. Dieting may also leave individuals vulnerable to an eating disorder by creating a biochemical imbalance of serotonin. Even short-term dieting can alter the function of serotonin, an important neurotransmitter involved in the regulation of mood, sleep, and food intake; reduced levels of serotonin are linked to eating disorders. Eating disorders may run in families, with both AN and BN occurring in 1st-degree family members of probands with either disorder.

Anorexia Nervosa. Premorbid psychiatric characteristics of patients with AN may include excessive dependence, developmental immaturity, and isolation. Their families have been described as having difficulty with problem solving and as being intrusive and overprotective. Eating disorders have been conceptualized as a defense against emerging sexuality, a problem with identity development, a disorder of mood, obsessionality and compulsiveness with associated neurotransmitter abnormalities, and a cultural-bound syndrome. All of these theories are partially true, and the field awaits a synthesis of these perspectives.

Bulimia Nervosa. Risk factors for BN include familial factors such as parental obesity, alcohol abuse, and affective disorders, as well as criticism by family members about body weight or eating habits. The incidence of BN is 3.7 times as high in the relatives of probands with BN as in the relatives of normal controls, suggesting a familial origin. There may be a genetic susceptibility to BN, although it is difficult to distinguish a biologic predisposition from environmental influences, given that existing twin studies have produced inconsistent results, with estimates of heritability for BN ranging from 30–83%.

Binge Eating Disorder. Individuals with BED typically have disorganized eating patterns that differ from those of patients with BN and those of obese individuals who do not binge eat. They have low levels of dietary restraint, unlike individuals with BN, who alternate binge eating with high levels of dietary restriction. BED is associated with obesity, but this relationship is not invariable, and nonobese individuals can meet the criteria for BED. Childhood obesity and parental obesity are specific risk factors for BED, and BED is associated with a rare genetic cause of obesity related to mutations of the gene for the melanocortin 4 receptor.

DIAGNOSIS

Anorexia Nervosa. The DSM-IV criteria for the diagnosis of AN include: (1) intense fear of becoming obese, which does not diminish as weight loss progresses; (2) disturbance in the way in which one's body weight, size, or shape is experienced (claiming to "feel fat," even when one is emaciated, or believing that 1 area of the body is "too fat," even when one is obviously underweight); (3) refusal to maintain body weight over a minimal normal weight for age and height (weight loss leading to maintenance of body weight of 15% < expected weight; failure to make expected weight gain during a period of growth, leading to body weight of 15% < expected weight); and (4) in females, absence of at least 3 consecutive menstrual cycles when otherwise expected to occur (primary or secondary amenorrhea). In patients older than 17 yr, a body mass index of <17.5 is also suggestive. AN is characterized further by excessive physical activity in the face of apparent inanition; denial of hunger; preoccupation with food preparation, frequently accompanied by bizarre eating behaviors; and often studiousness and academic success. Many are described as having been model children before the onset of the illness. Patients who have AN are subdivided into **restrictor** and **BN** subgroups, according to their method of caloric reduction. Restrictors severely limit their intake of carbohydrate- and fat-containing foods, whereas bulimics tend to eat in binges and then to purge themselves of food by self-induced vomiting or the use of cathartics.

Bulimia Nervosa. The DSM-IV separates BN from AN as a diagnostic entity, defining BN as follows: (1) recurrent episodes of binge eating (rapid consumption of a large amount of food in a discrete period, usually <2 hr); (2) during the eating binges, a fear of not being able to stop eating; (3) regularly engaging in self-induced vomiting, use of laxatives, or rigorous dieting or fasting to counteract the effects of binge eating; (4) a minimum average of 2 binge eating episodes/wk for at least 3 mo; and (5) self-evaluation is unduly influenced by body weight and shape, but the disturbance does not occur exclusively during episodes of AN. The binge-purge pattern may occur in children who are of normal weight or are slightly obese.

Binge Eating Disorder. Research criteria for BED include the following: (1) recurrent episodes of binge eating similar to BN; (2) binge eating episodes are associated with eating more rapidly than normal, eating until uncomfortably full, eating large amounts of food when not feeling physically hungry, eating alone because of being embarrassed by how much one is eating, and/or feeling disgusted with oneself, depressed, or very guilty after eating; (3) marked distress regarding binge eating; (4) binge eating occurs on average at least 2 days/wk for 6 mo; and (5) the binge eating is not associated with the regular use of inappropriate compensatory behaviors, and does not occur exclusively during the course of AN or BN.

Patients with eating disorders frequently present with a combination of symptoms that do not meet the classification for a specific eating disorder. Patients who initially meet the diagnostic criteria for 1 disorder may also have symptoms of the other disorder. Fifty percent of patients with AN have symptoms of BN. The **eating disorder not otherwise specified** diagnosis is applied to the many patients who have a variety of eating disorder behaviors that cannot be classified as either AN or BN. Many adolescents fall into this category.

SCREENING. Many patients with eating disorders are secretive about their behavior and do not seek assistance from designated eating disorder or psychiatric specialists. Primary care or emergency physicians may be the 1st health care professionals to come into contact with these patients. Frequent, vague complaints from patients with eating disorders include fatigue, anxiety, stress, depression, and headaches, or concerns about hair loss, brittle nails, or cold intolerance. Patients may also be seen for fractures resulting from osteoporosis. To obtain an accurate history of dietary restraint and medical details, physicians must question patients carefully in a compassionate and nonjudgmental manner. Questionnaires that may be used to screen for disordered eating behaviors and cognitions include the Eating Attitudes Test, the Bulimia Test, and the Eating Disorder Inventory, although these self-report measures may not be reliable, given the self-denial and minimization of symptoms inherent in eating disorders. Implementing educational and early prevention programs in school systems may be beneficial in increasing recognition of disordered eating behaviors in children and adolescents.

CLINICAL MANIFESTATIONS.

Anorexia Nervosa. Anorexia nervosa has the highest mortality rate of any psychiatric disorder (a 21-yr follow-up study found a mortality rate of 15.6%), usually caused by severe electrolyte disturbance, cardiac arrhythmia, or congestive heart failure in the recovery phase. **Physical complications** include disturbances in almost every organ system, most of which are believed to result from severe malnutrition or rapid fluctuations in electrolytes during starvation, bingeing, purging, or refeeding. Individuals may have palpitations, weakness, dizziness, shortness of breath, and chest pains. Physical signs such as an irregular, weak pulse and peripheral vasoconstriction are found, along with bradycardia, postural hypotension, and other electrocardiographic arrhythmias. Pulse rates can be as low as 20 beats/min, and a variety of electrocardiographic abnormalities are common, including low voltage, T-wave inversion and flattening, and ST depression, as well as supraventricular and ventricular dysrhythmias, some preceded by a prolonged QTc interval. Decreased cardiac output and mitral valve prolapse may result from myofibrillar atrophy. Patients who have abused ipecac may have myocarditis. Death from congestive heart failure is a late event and may result from unduly rapid rehydration and refeeding. Cardiovascular and peripheral vascular functioning usually improve with nutritional therapy.

Disorders of the hypothalamic-pituitary-ovarian axis are manifested as arrested psychosexual maturation, loss of libido, and amenorrhea associated with immature patterns of secretion of luteinizing hormone. These findings may represent a primary hypothalamic defect rather than being secondary to weight loss (which also causes amenorrhea); amenorrhea antedates weight loss in ⅓ to ½ of patients with AN, and a similar proportion of patients do not resume menses when normal weight is restored. One fourth of patients may be amenorrheic for 10 or more yr, despite weight rehabilitation. Many have problems becoming pregnant and maintaining a pregnancy.

Other metabolic symptoms, such as fatigue, lassitude, and cold intolerance, may be due to hypothalamic-pituitary-adrenal axis dysfunction. **Laboratory findings** include increased secretion of cortisol, loss of diurnal variation in its secretion, and failure of dexamethasone to suppress it. The last finding may also occur in starvation; abnormal results of dexamethasone suppression tests have persisted after weight rehabilitation in nearly ½ of cases. Growth hormone secretion is abnormally high in these patients, and the level of somatomedin C is low. Thyroid-stimulating hormone levels are normal, thyroxine and triiodothyronine levels are low, and the reverse triiodothyronine level is elevated, presumably in adaptation to a lowered basal metabolic rate as a result of malnutrition and carbohydrate deprivation. Problems with thermal regulation, particularly hypothermia, are common. Hypothermia also occurs in patients with BN who are of normal weight. In some patients, peripheral edema in the absence of congestive heart failure or hypoproteinemia has been attributed to inappropriate secretion of antidiuretic hormone.

Elevations of the blood urea nitrogen level may occur, reflecting dehydration and a decreased glomerular filtration rate, but normal levels may be found under these same conditions because of low protein intake, even in the dehydrated patient. Mild proteinuria, hematuria, and pyuria, with negative findings on urine cultures, generally resolve with proper rehydration, although pitting edema may occur. Pseudoproteinuria is often found because the alkalinity of the urine gives a false-positive reaction to albumin on the dipstick.

Bone density may be abnormally low, resulting in bone pain during exercise and an associated risk of stress fractures, but osteopenia appears to improve with weight gain. A number of possible mechanisms have been suggested to explain this finding, including low levels of estrogen and calcium and elevated cortisol levels. Bone marrow hypoplasia is common in AN and may also contribute to fatigue and cold intolerance. Leukopenia, anemia, and (rarely) thrombocytopenia can be found in combination with low erythrocyte sedimentation rates, perhaps reflecting low fibrinogen production secondary to malnutrition. Patients with AN appear to be remarkably resistant to infection. The fact that protein intake is relatively good in these otherwise malnourished persons may contribute to this finding. Delayed gastric emptying is a common complication in AN, and may lead to vomiting, abdominal pain, obstipation, and constipation. Esophagitis is common in those who vomit. Decreased gastrointestinal tract motility may be a cause of perforation after nasogastric tube insertion. Elevations in amylase levels may be associated with **bilateral parotid swelling** or with pancreatitis. Electrolyte imbalance (in addition to hypophosphatemia in refeeding) results from vomiting, "water loading" (a practice of surreptitiously drinking large amounts of water to achieve an agreed-on weight gain), or abuse of diuretics or laxatives. Potassium depletion, associated with a hypochloremic alkalosis, is common. Abnormalities of calcium, magnesium, and phosphorus metabolism may result from laxative abuse, either secondary to malabsorption or resulting from the use of preparations containing phosphate. Paradoxically, cholesterol levels are often elevated in AN.

The skin of patients with AN is dry, and lanugo hair is often seen. Hair loss often occurs in the refeeding phase. Scarring on the dorsum of the knuckles and enamel erosions are signs of self-induced vomiting.

Psychologic symptoms seen in patients with AN include social isolation, depression, anxiety, and obsessional symptoms, perfectionistic traits, and rigid cognitive styles. Other psychologic symptoms of AN include loss of sexual libido, reduced alertness and concentration, and dysphoria. Introversion, poor peer relations, and low self-esteem are premorbid psychologic correlates of AN. Patients typically react to efforts to alter their eating behavior with anger, deception, and manipulation, because resuming normal eating conflicts with their behavioral standards. In chronic cases, patients with AN can become absorbed by their illness, resulting in dependence on family and therapists, regression, invalidism, and social isolation.

Bulimia Nervosa. **Physical complications** of BN include weakness and irritability as a side effect of dehydration, gastrointestinal distress and dysmotility as a result of vomiting and laxative abuse, irregular menses and fertility problems, dental decay and parotid gland swelling, and cardiac problems as the result of ipecac abuse. **Psychologically,** young women with BN frequently have depressive, anxious, and obsessional symptoms, as well as a sense of shame associated with their behavior that prevents early treatment-seeking. **Depression** is the most commonly diagnosed co-occurring psychologic disorder in patients with BN, and it may precede or follow the disordered eating. Anxiety disorders, specifically generalized anxiety disorder and social phobia, also often co-occur with BN. Anxiety has been theorized to be central to both the etiology and the maintenance of BN in that bingeing and purging serve to decrease anxiety in the individual. Other co-occurring psychiatric disorders include obsessive-compulsive disorder, substance abuse, and to a lesser extent, bipolar disorder. Sexual conflicts and intimacy difficulties are also common in BN. Childhood sexual abuse is also reported more often by women with eating disorders than by women in the general population, and it is more common in patients with BN than in those with restricting AN. Patients with BN have a variety of deficits in impulse regulation, including self-injury, substance abuse, **suicidality,** and sexual promiscuity. Interpersonal problems are also common in BN, including poor social adjustment and peer relationships, sensitivity to criticism, excessive social dependence, inadequate social support, and an intense desire to please others. Personality disorders are also prevalent in BN (specifically, borderline and avoidant personality disorders), and are more common among patients with the binge eating and purging subtype of AN than in those with the restricting subtype or in patients with BN who are of normal weight. Patients with both BN and personality disorders are also more likely than patients with eating disorders but no personality disorders to have co-occurring mood or substance abuse disorders.

Binge Eating Disorder. **Physical complications** of BED include weight gain and, rarely, gastric rupture. BED is also associated with psychologic traits of negative self-esteem, impaired social functioning, and distress. Most studies have documented higher rates of **psychologic** difficulties in patients with BED than in non-patient control subjects or in persons with obesity who do not binge eat, although these rates are lower than for persons with BN. Major depressive disorder is the most common comorbid diagnosis, but rates of alcohol abuse and anxiety disorders are also elevated.

TREATMENT. A thoughtful pretreatment evaluation to determine the initial level of care is required. A successful treatment regimen includes assessment and treatment by a multdisciplinary team that integrates physiologic monitoring, psychotherapy (individual and family), behavior modification techniques, nutritional rehabilitation, and occasionally, pharmacologic therapy.

Anorexia Nervosa. **Inpatient medical hospitalization** is indicated in many cases. Indications for hospitalization include the constellation of risks listed in Table 27-1. **Psychiatric residential treatment** is indicated if the patient is medically stable to the extent that intravenous fluids, nasogastric feeding, and daily laboratory tests are not required, but structured supervision is still required during meal and bathroom times. **Day treatment** is indicated if the patient is medically stable, but needs structure to gain weight and avoid compulsive exercising and purging. **Intensive outpatient psychiatric treatment** is indicated if the patient can be self-sufficient in eating, is able to avoid compulsive exercising, accepts support from other individuals, and is highly motivated to recover. Because AN is a complex, serious, chronic, and potentially fatal condition, multiple treatment modalities are used at different stages of illness and recovery. **Nutritional counseling** can help to determine a healthy target weight and provide patients and their families with appropriate educational information about diet, levels of exercise, and the short- and long-term risks of disordered eating. **Psychotherapeutic intervention** to address psychodynamic conflicts and defenses, cognitive distortions, family roles, and obsessionality may be very helpful if integrated with other aspects of treatment. Psychotherapy alone is rarely helpful in severely malnourished individuals and is usually required for a minimum of 1 yr. Due to the enduring nature of many features that contribute to AN, treatment usually requires 5–6 yr of ongoing support and monitoring. **Medications** have a limited role in the integrated treatment of AN. If the patient has comorbid depression or obsessive-compulsive disorder, initiation of a selective serotonin reuptake inhibitor (SSRI) is indicated. The role of SSRIs in preventing relapse among weight-restored patients has not been determined.

TABLE 27-1. Indications for In-patient Medical Hospitalization of Patients with Anorexia Nervosa

PHYSICAL/LABORATORY
Heart rate <45 beats/min
Other cardiac rhythm disturbances
Blood pressure <80/50 mm Hg
Postural hypotension resulting in a >10 mm Hg drop or a >20 beats/min increase
Hypokalemia
Hypophosphatemia
Hypoglycemia
Dehydration
Body temperature <97°F
<75% healthy body weight
Hepatic, cardiac, or renal compromise
PSYCHIATRIC
Suicidal intent and plan
Very poor motivation to recover (in family and patient)
Preoccupation with ego-syntonic thoughts
Coexisting psychiatric disorders
MISCELLANEOUS
Requires supervision after meals and while using the restroom
Failed day treatment

Bulimia Nervosa. For BN, **inpatient medical hospitalization** is indicated when the patient has severe symptoms that do not respond to outpatient treatment, general medical problems (metabolic abnormalities, hematemesis, vital sign changes, uncontrolled vomiting), suicidality, psychiatric disturbances independent of the eating disorder that require hospitalization, or severe co-occurring substance abuse. The decision to hospitalize a patient with BN in a psychiatric or medical hospital depends on the patient's general medical status, the skills and abilities of the staff to manage the patient, and the availability of appropriate outpatient, partial, and aftercare programs to meet the patient's medical and psychiatric needs. Most patients with uncomplicated BN may be seen in **intensive outpatient psychiatric treatment.** Treatment goals include restoring the patient to a healthy weight, treating the physical complications, increasing the patient's motivation to change, educating the patient about healthy nutrition and eating patterns, modifying dysfunctional thoughts and feelings associated with the eating disorder, addressing co-occurring psychologic symptoms (mood disturbance, self-esteem), engaging the family and providing family therapy where appropriate, and developing relapse prevention skills. BN has been treated with a variety of psychotherapeutic approaches, including cognitive-behavioral therapy (CBT), behavioral therapy, psychodynamic therapy, family therapy, experiential therapy, and an addiction model. **Psychodynamic therapy** may be helpful once binge eating and purging behaviors are improved, and family therapy may be considered for adolescents who are still living at home or for older patients who are still struggling with family conflicts. Behavioral strategies include stimulus control procedures and exposure with response prevention. The most widely used and most empirically supported treatment for BN is CBT. Remission rates and long-term outcomes are also favorable after CBT. CBT also appears to affect both the specific and the general psychopathology associated with BN, such as depression, self-esteem, social functioning, and personality disturbance. **Interpersonal therapy (IPT)**, which focuses on relationship stressors that contribute to the eating disorder, is another empirically supported therapy for BN that is relatively equal in effectiveness to CBT at long-term follow-up. Working on the patient's motivation for change before initiating other therapies has also recently been found to improve treatment response. Patients with co-occurring symptoms of AN or with personality disorders may be helped by extended psychotherapy. **Nutritional counseling** in BN is also warranted to decrease the behaviors associated with the eating disorder, such as decreasing food restriction, increasing the variety of foods eaten (especially high-protein foods), and encouraging healthy exercise behaviors. **Pharmacologic therapy,** primarily with antidepressants, has also been used to correct hypothesized serotonin deficits that may be linked to BN. Both tricyclics and fluoxetine have been reported to be significantly more effective than placebo (see Table 20-1). Treatments that integrate both CBT and antidepressants are more effective than either treatment individually. SSRIs are beneficial for patients with significant depressive, anxious, or impulsive symptoms or for patients with minimal response to psychotherapy. Antidepressant medications can also reduce binge eating and purging behavior, and may assist in preventing relapse. A combination of psychotherapy and medication may improve remission rates.

Binge Eating Disorder. The two most intensively studied **psychologic treatments** for BED are CBT and IPT. CBT for BED uses cognitive and behavioral techniques similar to those used with CBT for BN, but with an emphasis on moderation of food intake; modification of critical, stereotyped views of overweight; some acceptance of body size; and encouragement of weight control behavior. CBT has been demonstrated to result in abstinence from binge eating in 50% of patients at post-treatment and in 60% of patients at 1 yr follow-up. CBT also has short- and long-term beneficial effects on reducing dietary restraint, changing distorted attitudes about weight and body shape, and improving psychiatric symptoms. IPT is also effective in treating BED by helping patients to identify and change the interpersonal context of the eating disorder. IPT for BED is similar to IPT for BN, but also encourages patients to examine the effect of their weight status on their relationships. IPT is equal to CBT in short- and long-term positive outcomes in BED. **Behavioral weight loss treatment (BWL)** is another treatment for BED that reduces both binge eating and weight. BWL treatments attempt to modify weight through caloric restriction, improved nutrition (especially protein intake), and physical activity, and appear to reduce both binge eating and body weight in the short term. Studies of **self-help** treatment approaches (guided and unguided books) have also reported reductions in binge eating and associated psychopathology. **Pharmacologic treatment** of BED with antidepressants appears similar to medical management of BN. Treatment with SSRIs is associated with a short-term reduction of 60–90% in binge frequency, as well as improvement in depressive symptoms. Medication alone may not be effective in the long term for most patients with BED, and combining medication with BWL or psychologic therapies may reduce relapse rates.

PROGNOSIS

Anorexia Nervosa. Mortality is a substantial risk in individuals with AN, and it results from suicide or the physical complications of the chronic eating disorder. The mortality risk has declined over the last 25 yr with improved identification and treatment of AN. The majority of patients with AN recover from their initial illness. Approximately 25% of patients with AN remain symptomatic, and a considerable minority have chronic AN. The recovery process usually occurs within 2 yr of the onset of AN and is atypical >5 yr after onset. In some cases, AN evolves from another eating disorder, such as BN, which is less easily detected by family members and physicians. A strong risk factor for the development of BN is "recovery" from AN.

Bulimia Nervosa. Community samples report modest spontaneous improvement in reducing symptoms of BN over 1–2 yr. Patients who received psychologic treatment or medications report a short-term success rate of 50–70%. Relapse rates for patients with BN after 6 mo–6 yr range from 30–50%, although slow improvement has been reported as follow-up studies extend to 10–15 yr. Patients who are functioning well and have milder symptoms at the beginning of treatment have a more favorable prognosis, as do outpatients compared with hospitalized inpatients with severe symptoms. Some studies have reported that a higher frequency of pretreatment vomiting is predictive of poorer outcomes.

Binge Eating Disorder. BED has a high remission rate, even without treatment. There appears to be no tendency for BED to develop into any other eating disorder.

American Psychiatric Association: Practice Guideline for the Treatment of Patients with Eating Disorders, 2nd ed. Available at www.psych.org.

Branson R, Potoczna N, Kral JG, et al: Binge eating as a major phenotype of melanocortin 4 receptor gene mutations. *N Engl J Med* 2003;348:1096–1103.

Bulik CM, Sullivan PF, Tozzi F, et al: Prevalence, heritability, and prospective risk factors for anorexia nervosa. *Arch Gen Psychiatry* 2006;63:305–312.

Crow SJ: Fluoxetine treatment of anorexia nervosa. *JAMA* 2006;295:2659–2660.

Hudson JI, Lalonde JK, Berry JM, et al: Binge-eating disorder as a distinct familial phenotype in obese individuals. *Arch Gen Psychiatry* 2006;63:313–319.

Latner JD, Wilson GT: Binge eating and satiety in bulimia nervosa and binge eating disorder: Effects of macronutrient intake. *Int J Eat Disord* 2004;402–415.

Lock J, Agras WS, Bryson S, et al: A comparison of short- and long-term family therapy for adolescent anorexia nervosa. *J Am Acad Child Adolesc Psychiatry* 2005;44:632–639.

Lock J, Couturier J, Agras WS: Comparison of long-term outcomes in adolescents with anorexia nervosa treated with family therapy. *J Am Acad Child Adolesc Psychiatry* 2006;45:666–672.

Mitchell JE, de Zwaan M, Roerig JL: Drug therapy for patients with eating disorders. *Curr Drug Targets CNS Neurol Disord* 2003;2:17–29.

Nicholls D, Viner R: Eating disorders and weight problems. *BMJ* 2005;330:950–953.

Russell J: Management of anorexia nervosa revisited. *BMJ* 2004;328:479–480.

Sysko R, Walsh BT, Schebendach J, et al: Eating behavior among women with anorexia nervosa. *Am J Clin Nutr* 2005;82:296–301.

Ulger Z, Gurses D, Ozyurek AR, et al: Follow-up of cardiac abnormalities in female adolescents with anorexia nervosa after refeeding. *Acta Cardiol* 2006;61:43–49.

Walsh BT, Kaplan AS, Attia E, et al: Fluoxetine after weight restoration in anorexia nervosa. *JAMA* 2006;295:2605–2612.

Wilson G, Fairburn, C: The treatment of binge eating disorders. *Eur Eat Disord Rev* 2000;8:351–354.
Wilson GT, Shafran R: Eating disorders guidelines from NICE. *Lancet* 2005; 365:79–81.
Yager J, Anderson AE: Anorexia nervosa. *N Engl J Med* 2005;353:1481–1488.

Chapter 28 ■ Disruptive Behavioral Disorders

Neil W. Boris and Richard Dalton

Disruptive behaviors should be considered from both a developmental and a biopsychosocial framework. Disruptive behaviors at 18 mo–4 yr of age, when symptoms such as temper tantrums and breath holding present, may reflect toddlers' typical struggles for autonomy and independence. Managing toddlers can be very challenging for parents; approximately ½ of preschoolers in the United States are brought to the attention of physicians because of destructive and disobedient behaviors. As children age, oppositional and defiant behavior may continue and result in children having persisting conflicts with adults and peers at home and at school. Some studies suggest that antisocial behaviors, such as stealing and truancy, are intermittently committed by almost 50% of adolescents.

Although disruptive behaviors are common across developmental stages, the pediatric maxim of watching and waiting may be detrimental from the biopsychosocial perspective. **Persistent aggression**, even among preschoolers, is a very strong predictor of the development of psychopathology. Although the causes and correlates of aggression are many, aggressive behavior appears to be quite stable (particularly among boys) and is heritable. Families often develop coercive strategies for managing aggressive behavior that only serve to worsen its course. Early intervention with parents and their young children is clearly most effective for managing ongoing aggression; the cost to families and society of waiting to intervene with aggressive children until adolescence is exorbitant in part because aggressive behavior among adolescents is less amenable to intervention.

INFANCY AND TODDLERHOOD. *Oppositionalism, temper tantrums,* and *breath holding spells* are not unusual during the 1st years of life and are age-typical expressions of frustration or anger. Parental and caregiver response to these behaviors is very important. Caregivers who respond to toddler defiance with punitive anger run the risk of reinforcing the defiance. Parents are best advised to attempt to avert angry responses by giving the child choices; once the child has begun a tantrum, turning away briefly is the only effective course of action. It is useful to advise parents to tell their child, once he or she is calm, that the reasons for frustration are understandable, but that oppositional behavior is not acceptable.

Parents are often particularly concerned about **breath holding spells.** Although some children hold their breath until they lose consciousness, sometimes leading to a seizure, there is no increased risk of seizure disorders in children who have had a seizure during a breath holding spell. As with other types of tantrums, parents are best advised to ignore breath holding once it has started. Without sufficient reinforcement, breath holding most often disappears. In most toddlers, this is not a voluntary act of "defiance."

The first key to the office management of oppositionalism ("terrible 2s"), temper tantrums, and breath holding spells is to help parents to intercede before the child is highly distressed. The pediatrician should advise parents to look for early signs of oppositional behavior and then to calmly place the child in time-out for 2–3 min. When breath holding does not respond to parent coaching or is accompanied by head banging or high levels of aggression, referral for developmental evaluation or family counseling is indicated.

If behavioral measures such as time-out fail, physicians must assess how the parents handle anger before making further recommendations about how to approach the child's problems. Children are often frightened by the strength and intensity of their own angry feelings and by the intensity of the angry feelings they arouse in their parents. It is therefore of prime importance that parents model the anger control that they wish their children to exhibit. Some parents are unable to see that they sometimes lose control themselves; this denial does not help their children to internalize controls. Advising parents to calmly provide simple choices will help the child to feel more in control and to develop a sense of autonomy. Providing the child with options also typically helps reduce the child's feelings of anger and shame. Such negative, internalized feelings may later have adverse effects on interpersonal relationships, intimacy, and personality development.

Lying is often used by 2–4 yr olds as a method of playing with the language. By observing the reactions of parents and caregivers, preschoolers learn about expectations for honesty in communication. Lying is also a form of fantasy for children, who describe things as they wish them to be rather than as they are. To avoid an unpleasant confrontation, a child who has not done something that a parent wanted may say that it has been done. The child's sense of time and reason does not permit the realization that this only postpones an even angrier confrontation.

CHILDHOOD AND ADOLESCENCE. In **school-aged children,** lying most often is an effort to cover up something that the child does not want to accept in his or her own behavior. The lie is invented to achieve a temporary good feeling and to protect the child against a loss of self-esteem. Although lying is common in childhood, children with low self-esteem are more prone to lie habitually. In many cases, habitual lying is also promoted by poor adult modeling. When mothers and fathers accuse each other frequently of lying, the child, drawn into a loyalty conflict, is likely to become distressed and increase defensive lying. Many adolescents lie to avoid parental disapproval. As with other antisocial behaviors, lying may be used as a method of rebellion.

Regardless of age or developmental level, when lying becomes a frequent way of managing conflict and anxiety, intervention is warranted. Initially, the parents should confront the child to give a clear message of what is acceptable. At the same time, sensitivity and support are necessary for a successful intervention, because children and adolescents may react to their shame and embarrassment with angry denial and acting out. If the situation cannot be resolved through parental understanding of the situation and the child's understanding that lying is not a reasonable alternative, professional intervention is indicated. In some cases, chronic lying occurs in combination with several other antisocial behaviors and is a sign of an underlying psychopathology or family dysfunction.

Almost all children **steal** something at some point in their lives. When preschoolers and school-aged children steal more than once or twice, the behavior may be a response to a sense of internal loss. These children frequently feel neglected and are, in fact, emotionally deprived. Their stealing is impulsive, but the gratification derived does not satisfy the underlying need. In children and adolescents, stealing can sometimes be an expression of anger or revenge for real or imagined frustrations by the parents. In many instances, stealing becomes one way in which the child or adolescent can manipulate and attempt to control interactions with parents. Like lying, stealing can be learned from adults. Parents who boast about outwitting tax laws or exceeding speed limits are implicitly condoning rule breaking as an acceptable behavior.

It is important for parents to help the child undo the theft by returning the stolen articles or by rendering their equivalent either in money that the child can earn or in services. When stealing is part of a pattern of conduct problems, referral to a child psychiatrist is warranted. Both problematic peer influence and lack of parental supervision may exacerbate stealing and other conduct problems. Interventions as simple as getting a child a Big Brother or Big Sister have been shown to improve school function and diminish conduct problems. In some cases, more intensive intervention may be necessary.

Truancy and run-away behavior are never developmentally appropriate. Approximately ½ of school refusal incidents result from child and adolescent behavioral problems; the other ½ of incidents are related to mood and anxiety symptoms. Often, truancy represents disorganization within the home, developing personality problems, or both. Whereas younger children often threaten to run away out of frustration or a desire to get back at parents, children who run away with nowhere to go are almost always expressing a serious underlying problem. During middle childhood, most runaways are escaping abuse and neglect within the home. In adolescence, disagreements with the parents, developing personality problems, and abuse and neglect all must be considered as possible precipitants. Adolescent runaways are at extremely high risk for substance abuse, intimate partner violence, and other risk-taking behaviors.

Although interest in fire is ubiquitous in early childhood, unsupervised **fire setting** is always inappropriate. Early school-aged children tend to set fires because of both curiosity and latent hostility secondary to deprivation within a disorganized and neglectful family. These young children set fires by themselves within their homes. In adolescence, fire setting is a sign of delinquency; again, traumatic experiences, often associated with family conflict, are common. Teenagers often set fires in small groups, seeking revenge on school and community authorities.

Fire setting always requires intervention by the parents and generally also by mental health professionals. A combination of family therapy, alliance-building individual therapy, parent management training, and community involvement is often necessary to effect a reasonable change. The recidivistic young fire setter is very difficult to manage. Many adult arsonists were childhood fire setters.

Although there is no totally satisfactory theory about the nature and cause of antisocial behavior, risk factors within the individual and the family have been identified. Adoption and twin studies strongly suggest that both genetic factors and child-rearing practices contribute to the development of aggressive behaviors. Adopted children with antisocial biological fathers presented later in life with more antisocial behaviors than did those with antisocial adoptive fathers. Children with both antisocial biological fathers and antisocial adoptive fathers were the most antisocial in later life. Sociocultural factors, temperament, some psychiatric conditions, and cognitive limitations can also predispose individuals to antisocial acting out.

Aggression is a serious symptom and is associated with significant morbidity and mortality in childhood. Data suggest that aggression is often stable over time. Children may not "grow out" of this behavior; early intervention is indicated for persistent aggressive behavior. Aggressive tendencies are heritable, although environmental factors may promote aggression in susceptible children. Both enduring and temporary risk conditions affecting a family may increase aggressive behavior in children. Aggression in childhood is correlated with family unemployment, discord, criminality, and psychiatric disorders as well as births to teenage or unmarried mothers. Boys are almost universally reported to be more aggressive than girls. A difficult temperament and later aggressiveness have been shown to be related, although there is evidence that these children may elicit punitive caregiving within the family environment, setting up a cycle of increasing aggression. Aggressive children often misperceive social cues and react with inappropriate hostility toward both peers and parents. Nonetheless, marital discord and aggression within the home certainly contribute to aggression by children.

Clinically, it is important to differentiate the causes and motives for childhood aggression. Intentional aggression may be primarily instrumental, to achieve an end, or primarily hostile, to inflict physical or psychologic pain. Children who are callous and not empathetic and who are frequently aggressive require mental health intervention. These children are at high risk for suspension from school and eventual school failure. Learning disorders are common, and aggressive children should be screened. Other forms of psychopathology are not uncommon; in particular, aggressive children with attention-deficit/hyperactivity disorder (ADHD; see Chapter 31) may have oppositional-defiant disorder and/or conduct disorder. Some aggressive, impulsive children may instead have bipolar disorder; a family history of mood disorders, grandiosity, and cyclic mood disturbance may be evident in the history of these children.

Aggressive behavior in boys is relatively consistent from the preschool period through adolescence; a boy with a high level of aggressive behavior at 3–6 yr of age has a high probability of carrying this behavior into adolescence, especially without effective family-focused intervention. The developmental progression of aggression among girls is less well studied. There are clearly fewer girls with physically aggressive behavior in early childhood; interpersonal coercive behavior, especially in peer relationships, is not uncommon among girls and appears to be related to the development of more physical aggression in adolescence (fighting, stealing).

Children exposed to aggressive models on television or in play show more aggressive behavior compared with children not exposed to these models (see Chapter 35). Parental anger and aggressive or harsh punishment model behavior that children may imitate when they are physically or psychologically hurt. Parental abuse may be transmitted to the next generation by several modes: children imitate aggression that they have witnessed, abuse can cause brain injury (which itself predisposes the child to violence), and internalized rage often results from abuse.

Conduct disorder is a distinct clinical entity manifested by several different antisocial behaviors: stealing, lying, fire setting, truancy, property destruction (vandalism), cruelty to animals, rape, use of a weapon while fighting, armed robbery, physical cruelty to others, and repeated attempts to run away from home. A pattern of such behaviors that has existed for at least 6 mo warrants the diagnosis of conduct disorder. Between ⅓ and ½ of patients treated at adolescent psychiatric clinics present with symptoms of conduct disorder. **Oppositional-defiant disorder** is defined by less severe behavior than conduct disorder: loss of temper, continuous arguing with authority figures, defiance of rules, continual blaming of others, angry and resentful affect, spiteful and vindictive behavior, and frequent use of obscene language. Some children may present with symptoms of all 3 disruptive behavior disorders (ADHD, oppositional-defiant disorder, and conduct disorder). Approximately ⅓ of children and adolescents with psychiatric diagnoses seen in community-based clinics are considered oppositional, and children with ADHD are significantly more likely to meet the criteria for oppositional-defiant disorder than those with other presenting problems. Still, the majority of children diagnosed with a disruptive behavior disorder meet the criteria only for that disorder. The risk factors (from the child, parent, or environment) associated with the development of conduct disorder are very similar to those mentioned in association with the development of specific antisocial and aggressive behaviors. Aggressive behavior is stable across generations within families. Inconsistent parenting practices and overly punitive disciplinary measures have been associated with conduct disorder in children. Parents of children with conduct disorder are less accepting of their children and show them less warmth and support compared with parents of unaffected children. However, only approximately ⅓ of children with conduct disorder go on to have antisocial personality disorder in adulthood. Adult criminality is predicted by an early age of onset of conduct disorder symptoms, numerous episodes and varieties of antisocial behaviors, parental criminality, and marital discord.

In many children, oppositional behavior may appear in the form of **passive-aggressive behaviors.** Prevalence rates of 16–22% have been noted. Children with passive-aggressive behavior express hostility indirectly as procrastination, stubbornness, or resistance. Parents often complain that such children do not hear them and do not respond to repeated requests. Academic underachievement is common. Children may unconsciously adopt passive-aggressive strategies for a variety of motives: to gain independence while maintaining dependence, to counter underlying low self-esteem, to maintain control and autonomy when threatened by anxiety, and to get revenge. These children are fearful of direct expression of assertiveness, aggression, and hostility. The child-rearing styles of their parents are often intimidating, critical, and inconsistent, or on the other hand, indulgent and permissive.

TREATMENT. Many different approaches have been used in the treatment of children and adolescents with aggressive behavior, conduct disorder, and oppositional-defiant disorder. Individual treatment focusing on alliance building and conflict resolution is sometimes useful in establishing the basic trust necessary for a positive therapeutic outcome. Individual therapy is not always effective in ameliorating behavioral problems. **Group therapy** has shown some promise in treating adolescents with behavioral difficulties; anger management therapy has demonstrated some positive results with younger children. Training in problem-solving skills involves modeling, role-playing, and practicing to help children deal more successfully with interpersonal relationships; it is somewhat effective in modifying maladaptive styles of relating and behaving. Effective results have been obtained with parent management training, in which parents are trained directly to promote prosocial behaviors within the home and to place reasonable limits on unwanted, destructive behaviors. In the case of passive-aggressive behavior, for instance, parents would be encouraged to set firm limits and expectations for the child and to reach agreement with the child on his or her important tasks and responsibilities. Compliance and age-appropriate assertiveness and independence are then promoted and rewarded. **Multisystemic therapy,** an in-home treatment involving the identified patient, parents, siblings, and peers as well as school, neighborhood, and other environmental forces, has been shown to be effective with aggressive children and adolescents who have conduct disorder. This multilevel approach is informed by data on the varying ecologic risks related to conduct disorder.

Pharmacotherapy for aggression or disruptive and antisocial behavior is generally used as an adjunct to family-based therapy, parent training, or multisystemic therapy. There are few data suggesting that pharmacotherapy alone is effective in reducing persistent aggression, oppositional behavior, or antisocial behavior. Children with an underlying biologic vulnerability (intermittent psychotic disorders, attention deficit disorder) may benefit from judicious use of appropriate medication. There are no medications specifically intended for the treatment of antisocial behaviors. Lithium, antipsychotics, anticonvulsants such as valproate, and α_2 agonists such as clonidine may diminish aggressive acting out in selected individuals, although these medications may also have significant side effects (see Chapter 20.1). Some children present with such severe behavioral problems that residential treatment or psychiatric hospitalization is necessary for a successful outcome.

American Academy of Child and Adolescent Psychiatry: Practice parameters for the assessment and treatment of children and adolescents with conduct disorder. *J Am Acad Child Adolesc Psychiatry* 1997;36(Suppl):122S–139S.

DiMario FJ Jr: Prospective study of children with cyanotic and pallid breath-holding spells. *Pediatrics* 2001;107:265–269.

Henneggler SW, Schoenwald SK, Pickrel SAG: *Multisystemic Treatment of Antisocial Behavior in Children and Adolescents.* New York, Guilford, 1998.

Hicks BM, Krueger RF, Lacono WG, et al: Family transmission and heritability of externalizing disorders: A twin-family study. *Arch Gen Psychiatry* 2004;61:922–928.

Kazdin AE: Treatments for aggressive and antisocial children. *Child Adolesc Clin N Am* 2000;9:841–858.

Leiberman AF: *The Emotional Life of the Toddler.* New York, Simon and Schuster, 2000.

McMahon RJ, Frick PJ: Evidence-based assessment of conduct problems in children and adolescents. *J Clin Child Adolesc Psychol* 2005;34:477–505.

Renaud J, Brent DA, Birmaher B, et al: Suicide in adolescents with disruptive disorders. *J Am Acad Child Adolesc Psychiatry* 1999;38:846–851.

Speltz ML, McClellan J, DeKlyen M, et al: Preschool boys with oppositional defiant disorder: Clinical presentation and diagnostic change. *J Am Acad Child Adolesc Psychiatry* 1999;38:838–845.

Webster-Stratton C, Hammond M: Treating children with early-onset conduct problems: A comparison of child and parent training interventions. *J Consult Clin Psychol* 1997;65:93–109.

Chapter 29 ■ Pervasive Developmental Disorders and Childhood Psychosis

Prachi E. Shah, Richard Dalton, and Neil W. Boris

Pervasive developmental disorders include autistic disorder, Asperger disorder, childhood disintegrative disorder, and Rett disorder (Table 29-1).

29.1 • Autistic Disorder

Autism is a neurodevelopmental disorder of unknown etiology, but with a strong genetic basis. It develops and is typically diagnosed before 36 mo of age. It is characterized by a behavioral phenotype that includes qualitative impairment in the areas of language development or communication skills, social interactions and reciprocity, and imagination and play (Table 29-2).

CLINICAL FEATURES. Autism is a neurodevelopmental disorder in which the clinical presentation can vary with the severity of the impairment. Despite the variability in the clinical pattern, all children with autism manifest some degree of impairment in the areas of reciprocal social interaction, communication, and restrictive and repetitive stereotypical patterns of behavior, interests, or activities. Although there is no pathognomonic symptom or behavior seen in all children with autism, most children have some impairment in joint attention or pretend play. **Joint attention** is the ability to use eye contact and pointing for the purposes of sharing experiences with others. It is a skill that typically develops by 18 mo. Other precursor skills to joint attention that are often absent in children with autism are **protoimperative pointing** (the use of pointing to obtain an object of desire) and **protodeclarative pointing** (the use of pointing to an object of interest simply to have another share in the interest with him or her). The symptoms of autism can vary in the severity of their presentation.

TABLE 29-1. Pervasive Developmental Disorders/Autism Spectrum Disorders

KEY FEATURES				
AUTISM	ASPERGER SYNDROME	RETT SYNDROME	CHILDHOOD DISINTEGRATIVE DISORDER	PERVASIVE DEVELOPMENTAL DISORDER—NOT OTHERWISE SPECIFIED
Delayed and disordered communication	Similar to autism except language skills relatively intact	Almost always affects girls	Clinically significant regression in skills (language, social skills, bowel, bladder control, play motor skills) before 10 yr of age	Features of 1 of the other autism spectrum disorders, but insufficient for a diagnosis of autism specifically
Atypical social interaction		Regression in skills between 6 and 18 mo of age		
Restricted range of interests	Usually not congnitively delayed	Repetitive hand movements		
Onset before 3 yr of age				

From Manning-Courtney P, Brown J, Molloy CA, et al: Diagnosis and treatment of autism spectrum disorders. *Curr Probl Pediatr Adolesc Health Care* 2003; 33: 283–312.

Some children with autism may make no eye contact and seem totally aloof, whereas others may show intermittent engagement with their environment and may make inconsistent eye contact, smile, and hug. These social behaviors often come on the child's own terms, and are difficult to elicit from another person. Children with autism may also present with varying verbal abilities. They can range from being nonverbal to having advanced speech, capable of imitating songs, rhymes, or television commercials. What is most notable in children with autism is the quality of their speech and language. The speech may have an odd prosody or intonation and may be characterized by echolalia, pronoun reversal, nonsense rhyming, and other idiosyncratic language forms. Intellectual functioning can vary from mental retardation to superior intellectual functioning in select areas. Some children with autism show typical development in certain skills and may even show areas of strength in specific areas, such as puzzles, art, or music. Play skills in children with autism are typically aberrant, characterized by little symbolic play, ritualistic rigidity, and preoccupation with parts of objects. **Stereotypical body movements,** a marked need for **sameness,** and a very narrow range of interests are also common. The autistic child is often withdrawn and spends hours in solitary play. Ritualistic behavior prevails, reflecting the child's need to maintain a consistent, predictable environment. Tantrum-like rages may accompany disruptions of routine. Eye contact is typically minimal or absent. Visual scanning of hand and finger movements, mouthing of objects, and rubbing of surfaces may indicate a heightened awareness of and sensitivity to some stimuli, whereas diminished responses to pain and lack of startle responses to sudden loud noises reflect lowered sensitivity to other stimuli.

EPIDEMIOLOGY. The prevalence rate of all pervasive developmental disorders appears to be 58.7 per 10,000 children. This prevalence rate includes autism (22/10,000), Asperger syndrome (11/10,000), Pervasive Developmental Disorder not otherwise specified (24.8/10,000), and child disintegrative disorder (0.9/10,000). This is consistent with previous research that identified the prevalence of all pervasive developmental disorders as 60/10,000. The incidence of the *diagnosis* of autism may have increased. There is evidence that the increase in the number of children identified with autism is likely related to changes in the definition of and diagnostic criteria for autism, as well as improvements in the recognition of autism at younger ages. An increase in the availability of diagnostic services, treatment facilities, and professionals trained in childhood development disorders has greatly increased the capacity of the health care system to identify and treat children with autistic spectrum disorders at younger ages.

ETIOLOGY. The exact cause of autism is unknown, but is believed to be multifactorial, with a strong genetic influence. There is a 60–90% concordance rate for monozygotic twins and a 0% concordance rate for dizygotic twins. There is a 92% concordance rate for monozygotic twins and a 30% concordance rate for dizygotic twins for the broader spectrum of social and communication difficulties. The genetic component of autism is believed to

TABLE 29-2. Diagnostic Criteria for Autism

AUTISTIC DISORDER*

A. A total of 6 (or more) items from (1), (2), and (3), with at least 2 from (1) and 1 each from (2) and (3):
   1. Qualitative impairment in social interaction, as manifested by at least 2 of the following:
      a. Marked impairment in the use of multiple nonverbal behaviors, such as eye-to-eye gaze, facial expression, body postures, and gestures to regulate social interaction
      b. Failure to develop peer relationships appropriate to developmental level
      c. Lack of spontaneous seeking to share enjoyment, interests, or achievements with other people (e.g., by a lack of showing, bringing, or pointing out objects of interest)
      d. Lack of social or emotional reciprocity
   2. Qualitative impairments in communication, as manifested by at least 1 of the following:
      a. Delay in, or total lack of, development of spoken language (not accompanied by an attempt to compensate through alternative modes of communication, such as gesture or mime)
      b. In individuals with adequate speech, marked impairment in ability to initiate or sustain a conversation with others
      c. Stereotyped and repetitive use of language or idiosyncratic language
      d. Lack of varied, spontaneous make-believe play or social imitative play appropriate to developmental level
   3. Restricted, repetitive, and stereotyped patterns of behavior, interests, and activities, as manifested by at least 1 of the following:
      a. Encompassing preoccupation with ≥1 stereotyped and restricted pattern of interest that is abnormal in either intensity or focus
      b. Apparently inflexible adherence to specific, nonfunctional routines or rituals
      c. Stereotyped and repetitive motor mannerisms (e.g., hand or finger flapping or twisting or complex whole body movements)
      d. Persistent precoccupation with parts of objects

B. Delay or abnormal functioning in at least 1 of the following areas, with onset < age 3 yr: (1) social interaction, (2) language as used in social communication, or (3) symbolic or imaginative play

C. The disturbance is not better accounted for by Rett disorder or childhood disintegrative disorder

*Autistic disorder is 1 of 3 autism spectrum disorders categorized within the 5 pervasive developmental disorders included in DSM-IV-TR, 2000. The other 2 autism spectrum disorders are Asperger disorder and pervasive developmental disorder—not otherwise specified. The 2 remaining pervasive developmental disorders are Rett disorder and childhood disintegrative disorder.

From Parental report of diagnosed autism in children aged 4–17 years—United States, 2003–2004. *MMWR* 2006; 55: 481.

American Psychiatric Association: *Diagnostic and Statistical Manual of Mental Disorders*, 4th ed., text revision (DSM-IV-TR, 2000). Arlington, VA, American Psychiatric Association, 2000.

be heterogeneous, attributed to as many as 100 genes, and genetic abnormalities in autism have been identified in mitochondrial genes and in all chromosomes except 14 and 20. It is believed that multiple genes interact with varied environmental causes to produce the disorder, and that the causative genes may vary from one population to another. Because of the complex heterogeneity and the variable behavioral phenotype of autism, linkage studies have not identified specific chromosomal regions that are universally believed to harbor the genes causing autism. Compared with other disorders of a similar behavioral phenotype, certain genes are believed to be more strongly implicated in the heritability of autism, including chromosome 7q (seen in the similar behavioral phenotype of specific language impairment disorder), chromosome 2q, and chromosome 15q11–13 (seen in Prader-Willi syndrome [see Chapter 108] and Angelman syndrome [see Chapter 81], both of which manifest traits of rigidity and stereotypical behaviors). Autism and Asperger disorder are 4 and 8 times more prevalent in males than in females, respectively, suggesting a strong X-linked component. Autism has also been linked with other neurodevelopmental disorders, including seizure disorder, fragile X syndrome (see Chapter 81), and tuberous sclerosis (see Chapter 596.2). Various environmental factors have been explored as causative agents in autism. Despite previously held notions, autism is not associated with certain emotionally distant parenting styles ("refrigerator mothers"). Many excellent epidemiologic studies have established that **there is no association** between the administration of the measles-mumps-rubella vaccine and the development of autism.

NEUROANATOMIC FINDINGS. The first 2 yr of life are crucial in early brain development, and this period is characterized by tremendous neuronal and axonal growth, synapse formation, and myelination. Retrospective analysis of head circumference in children with autism, in conjunction with MRI studies, has shown differences in the brain structure of children with autism compared with children without autism. The head circumference of children with autism is normal or slightly smaller than normal at birth until 2 mo of age. Longitudinal studies of children with autism showed an abnormally rapid increase in head circumference from 6–14 mo of age, which was largely concluded by the end of the 2nd yr of life. MRI studies done at 2–4 yr of age show that autistic toddlers have increased brain volume characterized by increased volume of the cerebellum, cerebrum, and amygdala compared with normal volumes. The abnormal growth in the first 2 yr is most marked in the frontal, temporal, cerebellar, and limbic regions of the brain, the areas of the brain responsible for higher-order cognitive, language, emotional, and social functions, which are most impaired in autism. It is believed that the early abnormal growth processes in the brain in the first 2 yr of life underlie the emergence of preclinical behavioral abnormalities seen in autism. This period of early, accelerated brain growth appears to stop early in childhood and is followed by abnormally slow or arrested growth, resulting in areas of underdeveloped and abnormal circuitry in parts of the brain. It is hypothesized that the postnatal growth of the brain is in response to adverse prenatal events; this association remains speculative.

Additional studies of neuroanatomy in children with autism have demonstrated anatomic changes in the anterior cingulate gyrus, an area of the brain associated with decision-making and the ascription of feelings and thoughts. Deficits in the reticular activating system, structural cerebellar changes, forebrain hippocampal lesions, and neuroradiologic abnormalities in the prefrontal and temporal lobe areas have been documented, and abnormal neurochemical findings have also been associated with autism; in addition, the dopamine, catecholamine, and serotonin levels or pathways have been implicated.

DIAGNOSIS. Aberrant social skill development is the hallmark of autism spectrum disorders (ASDs), and early social skill deficits may include abnormal eye contact, failure to orient to name, failure to use gestures to point or show, a lack of interactive play, failure to smile, lack of sharing, and lack of interest in other children. Combined language and social delays and regression in language or social milestones are important early red flags for an ASD, and should prompt an immediate evaluation. **Early signs** include unusual use of language or loss of language skills, nonfunctional rituals, inability to adapt to new settings, lack of imitation, and absence of imaginary play. Retrospective analysis of home videos shows that deviations in social and emotional development, such as decreased eye contact, failure to orient to name, and lack of joint attention, are often detected by 1 yr of age. The absence of expected social, communication, and play behaviors often precedes the emergence of odd or stereotypical behaviors or the unusual language usage that is seen in autism in the later years.

Several screening tools have been developed to aid in the early detection of children with ASDs. **The Checklist for Autism in Toddlers (CHAT)** is a screening tool designed for use with 18 mo old children in primary care settings. The CHAT combines parent responses to a brief interview with direct observation in the clinic setting. Although its positive predictive value was high, it showed low sensitivity. **The Modified Checklist for Autism in Toddlers (M-CHAT)** is a 23-item parent questionnaire modified from the CHAT. It has shown good sensitivity and specificity (0.87% and 0.99%, respectively), which suggests its utility as a screening tool. **The Pervasive Developmental Disorders Screening Test (PDDST)** is a parent-completed survey that targets children from birth–3 yr of age and incorporates a 3-tiered approach: 1 for the primary care clinic, 1 for the developmental clinic, and 1 for the multidisciplinary autism clinic. All 3 tiers contain items that measure various aspects of language, social skills, pretend play, attachment, sensory responses, and motor stereotypies.

In children with ASDs, intelligence, as measured by conventional psychologic testing, usually falls in the functionally retarded range; the deficits in language and socialization make it difficult to obtain an accurate estimate of the autistic child's intellectual potential. Some autistic children perform adequately in nonverbal tests, and those with developed speech may show adequate intellectual capacity. Autistic children also show deficits in their understanding of what the other person might be feeling or thinking, a so-called lack of a **theory of mind.** On some psychologic tests, children with autism pay more attention to specific details while overlooking the entire gestalt of the object, demonstrating a **lack of central coherence.**

A comprehensive evaluation should always include a thorough physical examination, with special attention paid to head circumference. Twenty-five percent of children with an ASD can have **macrocephaly,** but enlarged head size may not be apparent until after the 2nd yr of life. In the absence of dysmorphic features or focal neurologic signs, additional neuroimaging for investigation of the macrocephaly is not usually indicated. The presence of other physical stigmata should be noted, and examination of the skin with a Wood lamp should be performed to look for hypopigmented lesions that can be seen in tuberous sclerosis. Special attention should be paid to identify the dysmorphic features of fragile X syndrome (long face, large ears, large testes) and Angelman syndrome (ataxic gait, broad mouth). An audiologic evaluation and a comprehensive speech and language evaluation should be undertaken in any child with language delays. The lead level should be checked if the child shows signs of pica or lives in a high-risk environment. Chromosomal analysis should be performed if the child has evidence of mental retardation and dysmorphic features; an electroencephalogram should be performed in children with ASDs who have symptoms of developmental regression or suspicion of seizures.

TREATMENT. There is compelling evidence that intensive behavioral therapy, beginning before 3 yr of age and targeted toward speech and language development, is successful in improving both language capacity and later social functioning. Controlled studies of early intensive interventions involving 40 hr/wk of intensive 1:1 behavioral training (**applied behavioral analysis**) with young children for 2 yr have shown significant cognitive and behavioral gains. The training method focuses on the acquisition of compliance behavior, imitation activities, language acquisition, and integration with peers. Treatment is most successful when geared toward the individual's particular behavior patterns and language function. Parent education, training, and support are always indicated, and pharmacotherapy for certain target symptoms may be helpful.

Working with the family of an autistic child is vital to the child's overall care. Children with autism require alternate educational approaches, even when language capacity is near normal. Such services in general have not yet been sufficiently developed to provide adequate support and continuity of care. One successful educational model is the program for the Treatment and Education of Autistic and Related Communication Handicapped Children (TEACCH). The following treatment principles are emphasized: use of objective measures, such as the Childhood **Autism Rating Scale (CARS)**, to measure behavior and behavioral change; enhancement of skills and acceptance by the environment of autism-related deficits; use of interventions based on cognitive and behavioral theories; use of visual structures for optimal education; and multidisciplinary training for all professionals working with autistic children. Educational programming should begin as early as possible, preferably by age 2–4 yr.

Older children and adolescents with relatively higher intelligence, but with poor social skills and psychiatric symptoms (depression, anxiety, obsessive-compulsive disorder) may require psychotherapy, behavioral or cognitive behavioral therapy, and pharmacotherapy. Typically, behavior modification is a major part of the overall treatment for older children with autism. These procedures include enhancement (rewards emphasizing appropriate choice) and reduction (extinction, time-out, punishment). Ethical concerns about vigorous aversive therapy approaches have led to specific guidelines. Social skill training is also currently used as a treatment modality, and it appears effective, especially in a group format.

Unfortunately, there are unfounded claims of beneficial results from many unproven therapies for autism, almost all of which have not been subjected to scientific study. Those studies that have been done have discredited the technique of facilitated communication and have shown that auditory integration therapy has no positive effect. Claims of beneficial results from the use of secretin, a peptide hormone that stimulates pancreatic secretion, have not been substantiated. Similarly, the dietary supplement *N,N*-dimethylglycine has no benefit.

Because a subgroup of autistic children presents with psychiatric symptoms, pharmacotherapy is sometimes used to ameliorate target behaviors. The behaviors include hyperactivity, tantrums, physical aggression, self-injurious behavior, stereotypies, and anxiety symptoms, especially obsessive-compulsive behaviors. The older neuroleptics were limited in their usefulness because of their tendency to produce extrapyramidal symptoms and tardive dyskinesia. Open-label trials of atypical neuroleptics (risperidone, olanzapine) have shown effectiveness in treating these behaviors, and in some instances, have also improved social relatedness (see Chapter 20.1).

Naltrexone, an opiate antagonist, was also originally touted as useful, especially for self-injurious behavior, but its utility has not yet been proven. Clomipramine, a tricyclic antidepressant that inhibits serotonin reuptake, has demonstrated usefulness in reducing compulsions and stereotypies in autistic children. However, it does lower the seizure threshold, can cause agranulocytosis, and has cardiotoxic and behavior toxicity effects. Other medications used to treat psychiatric symptoms in autistic children include stimulants, selective serotonin reuptake inhibitors (SSRIs), and clonidine. The SSRIs, in particular, appear to be somewhat effective in diminishing hyperactive, agitated, and obsessive-compulsive behaviors, although there have not yet been sufficient, controlled studies regarding their utility (see Chapter 20.1).

PROGNOSIS. Some children, especially those with speech, may grow up to live self-sufficient, employed, albeit isolated, lives in the community. Many others remain dependent on their family for their everyday lives or require placement in facilities outside the home. Because early, intensive therapy may improve language and social function, delayed diagnosis may lead to a poor outcome. There is no increased risk of schizophrenia in adulthood, but the cost of delayed diagnosis across the life span is high. A better prognosis is associated with higher intelligence, functional speech, and less bizarre symptoms and behavior. The symptom profile for some children may change as they grow older and seizures or self-injurious behavior becomes more common.

29.2 • Asperger Disorder

Children with Asperger disorder have a qualitative impairment in the development of reciprocal social interaction, often showing repetitive behaviors and restricted, obsessional, idiosyncratic interests. They have deficits in nonverbal and pragmatic aspects of communication (facial expressions, gestures). They do not have the severe language impairments that characterize autism. Although they are somewhat socially aware, these children appear to others to be peculiar or eccentric. They are awkward and clumsy and have unusual postures and gait. To meet the diagnostic criteria for Asperger syndrome, a child must manifest impairments in social interactions and show restrictive, repetitive patterns of behavior, interests, or achievements with other people; these disturbances must cause significant impairments in social or occupational functioning. Unlike children with autism, those diagnosed with Asperger syndrome have a history of normal language milestones, with single words used by age 2 yr and communicative phrases used by age 3 yr. There are often similar traits in family members. Prevalence is estimated to be approximately 11/10,000 children. This disorder may represent a form of high-functioning autism (children with autism who do not have cognitive impairment), although this distinction remains controversial. Group social skill training is the hallmark of intervention, although children with Asperger disorder appear to be at high risk for other psychiatric disorders, particularly oppositional-defiant disorder and mood disorders. Cognitive-behavioral therapy has been useful in patients with associated anxiety, whereas risperidone may improve negative symptoms similar to those seen in schizophrenia.

29.3 • Childhood Disintegrative Disorder

This disorder, also known as **Heller dementia**, is a rare condition of unknown cause. It is characterized by normal development up to 2–4 yr of age, followed by severe deterioration of mental and social functioning, with regression to a very impaired "autistic" state before age 10 yr. Language, social skills, and imagination are profoundly affected; bowel and bladder control may be lost; and motor stereotypies and seizures are often present. Although this condition may be the result of an underlying neurologic illness, none has been identified. The prognosis is always poor.

29.4 • Rett Disorder

Rett disorder is a neurodevelopmental disorder resulting from a genetic mutation of the *MECP2* gene. It is an X-linked dominant disorder affecting predominantly girls and few boys. It has a prevalence of 1/10,000. Development is initially normal, but then rapidly regresses in the latter ½ of the 1st year of life. Children with Rett syndrome initially have normal prenatal and perinatal development, with normal head circumference and normal psychomotor development until 5 mo of age. After this period of normal development, all of the following are observed: deceleration of head growth at 5–48 mo, with development of microcephaly; loss of previously acquired purposeful hand skills at 5–30 mo, with subsequent development of stereotyped hand movements (hand-wringing); loss of social engagement; poorly coordinated gait or trunk movements; and severely impaired receptive and expressive language development, with severe psychomotor retardation. These girls present with midline, stereotypical hand-wringing; ataxia; breathing dysfunction; bruxism; scoliosis; and profound intellectual handicap. Autistic behaviors are typical, but over time, social relatedness may improve. Lower limb involvement may progress, leading to wheelchair dependence. Postmortem examinations have revealed greatly reduced brain size and weight as well as a reduced number of synapses. Abnormalities on electroencephalogram are detected in almost all children with Rett syndrome.

29.5 • Childhood Schizophrenia

Psychotic reactions in older children tend to more closely resemble the psychoses of adulthood, and the same diagnostic criteria apply (Table 29-3). Psychosis associated with a mood disorder, such as bipolar illness, is discussed in Chapter 25.

CLINICAL MANIFESTATIONS. In childhood schizophrenia, prominent symptoms include thought disorder, disorganized speech, delusions, and hallucinations. The latter 2 symptoms, in addition to later onset, higher intelligence scores, and fewer perinatal complications, differentiate schizophrenia from autism. As the symptoms imply, schizophrenic children are typically severely impaired. They may have paranoid delusions, aggressive behavior, hebephrenic silliness, social withdrawal, and alternating moods not apparently related to environmental stimuli.

The prevalence of adult schizophrenia is 1%. The typical age of onset is late adolescence to early adulthood. Early-onset schizophrenia (before puberty or in early adolescence) is rare. As infants, ½ of schizophrenic children have had abnormally delayed development and unusual sensory sensitivity. Schizophrenic children show significant premorbid maladjustments, including social withdrawal, disruptive behaviors, developmental delays, and speech and language problems. The onset of the disorder is usually insidious. Auditory hallucinations are seen in 80% of schizophrenic children. Delusions and formal thought disorders usually do not present until midadolescence. Children with early-onset schizophrenia show preliminary evidence of progressive ventricular enlargement, a decrease in total cerebral volume, and a decline in intellectual functioning. The prognosis is poor. The symptoms in childhood that most strongly predict psychotic adult psychopathology are affective blunting and disturbed interpersonal relationships, as opposed to delusions and hallucinations. In schizophrenic children, initial presenting symptoms cluster around violent aggression and school problems. Psychotic symptoms are 1st recognized at 2–11 yr, followed 2 yr later by a diagnosis of schizophrenia. Before diagnosis, patients are often treated with stimulants, antidepressants, low-dose neuroleptics, mood stabilizers, and alternative treatments. Before diagnosis, children with schizophrenia often have a prodromal period characterized by deficits in attention, impaired language and verbal memory, poor gross motor skills, and impaired coordination. Most children receive a psychiatric diagnosis before the development of psychosis, with the most common diagnoses being pervasive developmental disorder, attention-deficit/hyperactivity disorder, and depression. In the premorbid period before the diagnosis of schizophrenia, affected children showed higher rates of social withdrawal and greater global impairment, and had fewer friends.

Individuals with various psychotic processes are often misdiagnosed as having schizophrenia. In a National Institute of Mental Health study of childhood-onset schizophrenia, >1,300 children were referred with a putative diagnosis of childhood-onset schizophrenia. After various screening and evaluation procedures, approximately 5% were actually diagnosed as having childhood-onset schizophrenia and accepted into the research program. The majority of misdiagnosed patients were later noted

TABLE 29-3. Criteria for Diagnosis of Schizophrenia

A. *Characteristic symptoms:* ≥2 of the following, each present for a significant portion of time during a 1-mo period (or less, if successfully treated)
   1. Delusions
   2. Hallucinations
   3. Disorganized speech (e.g., frequent derailment or incoherence)
   4. Grossly disorganized or catatonic behavior
   5. Negative symptoms (i.e., affective flattening, alogia, or avolition)

   Note: Only 1 criterion A symptom is required if delusions are bizarre or if hallucinations consist of a voice keeping up a running commentary on the person's behavior or thoughts or ≥2 voices conversing with each other

B. *Social/occupational dysfunction:* For a significant portion of the time since the onset of the disturbance, ≥1 major areas of functioning, such as work, interpersonal relations, or self-care, are markedly below the level achieved before the onset (or when the onset is in childhood or adolescence, failure to achieve expected level of interpersonal, academic, or occupational achievement)

C. *Duration:* Continuous signs of the disturbance persist for at least 6 mo. This 6-mo period must include at least 1 mo of symptoms (or less, if successfully treated) that meet criterion A (i.e., active-phase symptoms) and may include periods of prodromal or residual symptoms. During these prodromal or residual periods, signs of disturbance may be manifested by only negative symptoms or ≥2 symptoms listed in criterion A present in an attenuated form (e.g., odd beliefs, unusual perceptual experiences)

D. *Schizoaffective and mood disorder exclusion:* Schizoaffective disorder and mood disorder with psychotic features have been ruled out because either (1) no major depressive, manic, or mixed episodes have occurred concurrently with the active-phase symptoms or (2) if mood episodes have occurred during active-phase symptoms, their total duration has been brief relative to the duration of the active and residual periods

E. *Substance/general medical condition exclusion:* The disturbance is not due to the direct physiologic effects of a drug of abuse, a medication, or a general medical condition

F. *Relationship to a pervasive developmental disorder:* If there is a history of autistic disorder or another pervasive development disorder, the additional diagnosis of schizophrenia is made only if prominent delusions or hallucinations also are present for at least 1 mo (or less, if successfully treated)

CLASSIFICATION OF LONGITUDINAL COURSE (can be applied only after at ≥1 yr has elapsed since the initial onset of active-phase symptoms)

Episodic with interepisode residual symptoms (episodes are defined by the re-emergence of prominent psychotic symptoms); *also specify if:* **with prominent negative symptoms**

Episodic with no interepisode residual symptoms

Continuous (prominent psychotic symptoms are present throughout the period of observation) *also specify if:* **with prominent negative symptoms**

From Kliegman RM, Marcdante KJ, Jenson HB, et al (editors): *Nelson Essentials of Pediatrics,* 5th ed. Philadelphia, Elsevier/Saunders, 2004, p 101.

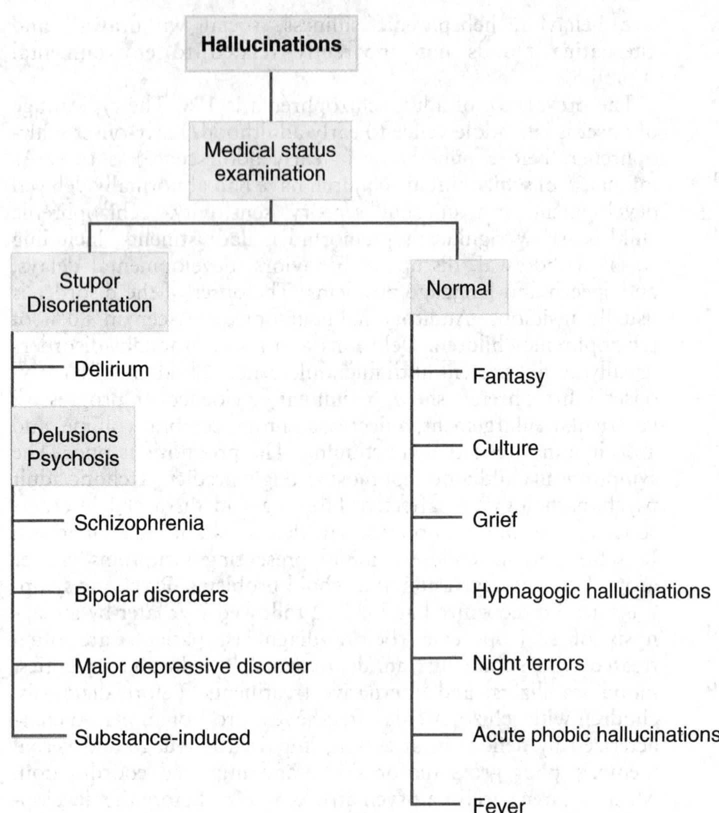

Figure 29-1. Evaluation of hallucinations. (From Kliegman RM, Greenbaum LA, Lyle PS: *Practical Strategies in Pediatric Diagnosis and Therapy,* 2nd ed. Philadelphia, Elsevier/Saunders, 2004, p 601.)

to have bipolar disorder, major depressive disorder with psychosis, or psychosis not otherwise specified.

TREATMENT. A multimodal therapeutic approach is necessary to manage this illness. Parent training is necessary to teach effective techniques to modify the schizophrenic child's behavior to improve social functioning. Individual therapy designed to build a positive alliance is also very important. School and community liaison work can establish and maintain a day-to-day schedule for the patient. Neuroleptic therapy is often effective in managing hallucinations and psychotic delusions. The use of haloperidol has largely been replaced by newer atypical antipsychotics, such as risperidone and olanzapine. These medications appear to have lower risks of extrapyramidal symptoms and tardive dyskinesia. However, weight gain is common with atypical neuroleptics. Clozapine appears to be the most effective antipsychotic medication for refractory cases, but the risk of agranulocytosis and seizures limits its use (see Chapter 20.1).

29.6 • Acute Phobic Hallucinations

Hallucinations are disturbing to the patient and parents, and they often signify a serious disorder that requires immediate attention, especially in children with altered levels of consciousness, delusions, confusion, or any abnormalities on mental status examination (Fig. 29-1).

Acute phobic hallucinations are benign and common and occur in previously healthy preschool children. The hallucinations are often visual or tactile, last 10–60 min, and occur at any time, but most often at night. The child is quite frightened and may complain that bugs or snakes are crawling over him or her and attempt to remove them. The cause is unknown. The **differential diagnosis** includes drug overdose or poisoning, high fever, encephalitis, and psychosis.

The child's fear is not alleviated by reassurance by the parent or physician, and the child is not amenable to reason. Findings on physical and mental status examinations are otherwise normal. Symptoms may persist for 1–3 days, slowly abating over 1–2 wk. Treatment with benzodiazepines may be beneficial.

American Academy of Child and Adolescent Psychiatry: Practice parameters for the assessment and treatment of children and adolescents with schizophrenia. *J Am Acad Child Adolesc Psychiatry* 2001;40(Suppl):4S–23S.

American Academy of Child and Adolescent Psychiatry: Practice parameters for the assessment and treatment of children, adolescents, and adults with autism and other pervasive developmental disorders. *J Am Acad Child Adolesc Psychiatry* 1999;38(Suppl):32S–54S.

American Academy of Neurology: Practice parameter: Screening and diagnosis of autism. *Neurology* 2000;55:468–479.

Badawi N, Dixon G, Felix JF, et al: Autism following a history of newborn encephalopathy: More than a coincidence? *Dev Med Child Neurol* 2006;48:85–89.

Baird G, Cass H, Slonims V: Diagnosis of autism. *BMJ* 2003;327:488–493.

Baird G, Simonoff E, Pickles A, et al: Prevalence of disorders of the autism spectrum in a population cohort of children in South Thames: the Special Needs and Autism Projects (SNAP). *Lancet* 2006;368:210–215.

Barbaresi WJ, Katusic SK, Colligan RC, et al: The incidence of autism in Olmstead County, Minnesota, 1976–1997. *Arch Pediatr Adolesc Med* 2005;159:37–44.

Baron-Cohen S: Two new theories of autism: Hyper-systemising and assortative mating. *Arch Dis Child* 2006;91:5–7.

Cederlund M: One hundred males with Asperger syndrome: A clinical study of background and associated factors. *Dev Med Child Neurol* 2004;46:652–660.

Centers for Disease Control and Prevention: Parental report of diagnosed autism in children aged 4–17 years, United States, 2003–2004. *MMWR* 2006;55:481–486.

Chakrabarti S, Fombonne E: Pervasive developmental disorders in preschool children: Confirmation of high prevalence. *Am J Psychiatry* 2005;162:1133–1141.

Dumont-Mathieu T, Fein D: Screening for autism in young children: The Modified Checklist for Autism in Toddlers (M-CHAT) and other measures. *Ment Retard Dev Disabil Res Rev* 2005;11:253–262.
Eliez S, Reiss AL: MRI neuroimaging of childhood psychiatric disorders: A selective review. *J Child Psychol Psychiatry* 2000;41:679–694.
Foster B, King BH: Asperger syndrome: To be or not to be? *Curr Opin Pediatr* 2003;15:491–494.
Frohna JG: Toward better evidence for parent training programs for autism spectrum disorder. *J Pediatr* 2005;147:283–284.
Goodlin-Jones BL, Tassone F, Gane LW, et al: Autistic spectrum disorder and the fragile X permutation. *J Dev Behav Pediatr* 2004;25:392–398.
Harrison MJ, O'Hare AE, Campbell H, et al: Prevalence of autistic spectrum disorders in Lothian, Scotland: An estimate using the "capture-recapture" technique. *Arch Dis Child* 2006;91:16–19.
Honda H, Shimizu Y, Rutter M: No effect of MMR withdrawal on the incidence of autism: A total population study. *J Child Psychol Psychiatry* 2005;46:572–579.
King BH, Bostic JQ: An update on pharmacologic treatments for autism spectrum disorders. *Child Adolesc Psychiatr Clin N Am* 2006;15:161–175.
Kuehn BM: Studies probe autism anatomy, genetics. *JAMA* 2006;295:19–20.
Kurita H: Disorders of the autism spectrum. *Lancet* 2006;368:179–181.
Landa R, Garrett-Mayer E: Development in infants with autism spectrum disorders: a prospective study. *J Child Psych Psychiatry* 2006;47:629–638.
Lawler CP, Croen LA, Grether JK, et al: Identifying environmental contributions to autism: Provocative clues and false leads. *MMRD Res Rev* 2004;10:292–302.
Lieberman JA, Stroup TS, McEvoy JP, et al: Effectiveness of antipsychotic drugs in patients with chronic schizophrenia. *N Engl J Med* 2005;353:1209–1223.
Manning-Courtney P, Brown J, Molloy CA, et al: Diagnosis and treatment of autism spectrum disorders. *Curr Probl Pediatr Adolesc Health Care* 2003;33:277–312.
McClellan J, Breiger D, McCurry C, et al: Premorbid functioning in early-onset psychotic disorders. *J Am Acad Child Adolesc Psychiatry* 2003;42:666–672.
Murch S: Diet, immunity, and autistic spectrum disorders. *J Pediatr* 2005;146:582–584.
Pao M, Lohman C, Gracey D, et al: Visual, tactile, and phobic hallucinations: Recognition and management in the emergency department. *Pediatr Emerg Care* 2004;20:30–34.
Polleux F, Lauder JM: Toward a developmental neurobiology of autism. *MMRD Res Rev* 2004;10:303–317.
Pons R, Andreu AL, Checcarelli N, et al: Mitochondrial DNA abnormalities and autistic spectrum disorders. *J Pediatr* 2004;144:81–85.
Posserud MB, Lundervold AJ, Gillberg C: Autistic features in a total population of 7–9-year-old children assessed by the ASSQ (Autism Spectrum Screening Questionnaire). *J Child Psychol Psychiatry* 2006;47:167–175.
Rapoport JL, Inoff-Germain G: Update on childhood-onset schizophrenia. *Curr Psychiatry Rep* 2000;2:410–415.
Rausch JL, Sirota EL, Londino DL, et al: Open-label risperidone for Asperger's disorder: Negative symptom spectrum response. *J Clin Psychiatry* 2005;66:1592–1597.
Research units on Pediatric Psychopharmacology Autism Network: Risperidone treatment of autistic disorder: Longer-term benefits and blinded discontinuation after 6 months. *Am J Psychiatry* 2005;162:1361–1369.
Reichenberg A, Weiser M, Rapp MA, et al: Elaboration on premorbid intellectual performance in schizophrenia. *Arch Gen Psychiatry* 2005;62:1297–1304.
Rogers SJ: Interventions that facilitate socialization in children with autism. *J Autism Dev Disord* 2000;30:399–409.
Scheffer J, Ross R: Childhood onset schizophrenia: Premorbid and prodromal diagnostic and treatment histories. *J Am Acad Child Adolesc Psychiatry* 2002;41:538.
Sigman M, Dijamco A, Gratier M, et al: Early detection of core deficits in autism. *MMRD Res Rev* 2004;10:221–233.
Smeeth L, Cook C, Fombonne E, et al: MMR vaccination and pervasive developmental disorders: A case-control study. *Lancet* 2004;364:963–969.
Sofronoff K, Attwood T, Hinton S: A randomized controlled trial of a CBT intervention for anxiety in children with Asperger syndrome. *J Child Psychol Psychiatry* 2005;46:1152–1160.
St. Clair D, Xu M, Wang P, et al: Rates of adult schizophrenia following prenatal exposure to the Chinese famine of 1959–1961. *JAMA* 2005;294:557–562.
Technical report: The pediatrician's role in the diagnosis and management of autistic spectrum disorder in children. *Pediatrics* 2001;107:1–18.
Toren P, Ratner S, Laor N, et al: Benefit-risk assessment of atypical antipsychotics in the treatment of schizophrenia and comorbid disorders in children and adolescents. *Drug Saf* 2004;27:1135–1156.
Wallace GL, Treffert DA: Head size and autism. *Lancet* 2004;363:1003–1004.
Wassink TH, Brzustowicz LM, Bartlett CW, et al: The search for autism disease genes. *MMRD Res Rev* 2004;10:272–283.
Werner E, Dawson G: Validation of the phenomenon of autistic regression using home videotapes. *Arch Gen Psychiatry* 2005;62:889–895.
Williams JG, Higgins JPT, Brayne CEG: Systematic review of prevalence studies of autism spectrum disorders. *Arch Dis Child* 2006;91:8–15.
Wong V, Stella LH, Lee WC, et al: A modified screening tool for autism (checklist for autism in toddlers [CHAT-23]) for Chinese children. *Pediatrics* 2004;114:e166–e176.

Chapter 30 ■ Patterns of Development and Function in the School-aged Child

Desmond P. Kelly

A **neurodevelopmental function** is a basic brain process that may be needed for learning and productivity. **Neurodevelopmental variation** refers to the differences in neurodevelopmental strengths and weaknesses that exist between individuals and that can change over time. Wide variations exist among individuals, and these differences need not represent pathology or abnormality. **Neurodevelopmental dysfunctions** reflect disruptions of neuroanatomic structure or psychophysiologic function and may be associated with academic underachievement, behavioral difficulties, and problems with social adjustment.

ETIOLOGY. Multiple factors underlie neurodevelopmental dysfunctions. These include genetic, medical, environmental, and sociocultural influences. Some of the genes that contribute to these dysfunctions have been identified. It is well established that reading disorders can be both familial and heritable; studies have linked some reading disabilities to specific gene loci on chromosomes 6 and 15. Chromosomal abnormalities can lead to unique patterns of dysfunction, such as visual-spatial difficulties in girls with Turner syndrome or language deficits in individuals with fragile X syndrome (see Chapter 81). Perinatal risk factors that have been associated with subsequent academic problems include very low birthweight, severe intrauterine growth restriction, perinatal hypoxic-ischemia encephalopathy, and prenatal exposure to alcohol or other drugs. Increased risk of disorders of learning and attention is associated with environmental toxins, including lead (see Chapter 709); infections, such as meningitis and AIDS; and brain injury as a result of intraventricular hemorrhage or head trauma. There have been conflicting reports regarding the contribution of persistent otitis media with effusion and associated conductive hearing loss to subsequent language problems. Environmental and sociocultural deprivation can lead to, or potentiate, neurodevelopmental dysfunction. In the child with a learning disorder there is frequently a combination of etiologic factors, and a single definite cause is seldom ascertained.

PATHOGENESIS. Functional magnetic resonance imaging has indicated decreased left temporoparietal cortical activity during a phonologic task of rhyming and decreased occipitoparietal extrastriate activity during an orthographic task of letter matching in children with **reading disorder (dyslexia)** compared with children with normal reading abilities. Studies of children with attention deficits have noted structural changes involving the frontal/striatal system, and intra- and interhemispheric white matter projections and near-infrared spectroscopy studies have indicated prefrontal cortical hypometabolism in children with **attention-deficit/hyperactivity disorder.** Quantitative electroencephalograms have been reported to be abnormal in 25–45% of children with learning disorders. The heterogeneity of study populations impedes generalization of these findings or clinical application for individual students.

EPIDEMIOLOGY. Estimates of the prevalence of learning disabilities range from 3–10%, whereas attention deficits have been reported in 4–12% of school-aged children. These estimates are beset by differences in the definitions and criteria used for classification and diagnosis and depend on the method of assessment. Medical classification systems include the American Psychiatric Association *Diagnostic and Statistical Manual of Mental Disorders,* 4th edition (DSM-IV) and the *International Classification of Diseases* (ICD) of the World Health Organization. The DSM-IV differentiates learning disorders (reading disorder, mathematics disorder, disorder of written expression) from motor skills disorder and communication disorders. Neurologists favor diagnostic terms, such as **dyslexia** (reading disorder), **dyscalculia** (mathematics disorder), or **dysgraphia** (writing disorder). Within the educational system, specific learning disabilities are defined by discrepancies between scores on tests of intelligence (ability) and tests of academic achievement that are used to determine eligibility for special education services.

CLINICAL MANIFESTATIONS. School-aged children with neurodevelopmental dysfunctions vary widely with regard to clinical symptoms. Their specific patterns of academic performance and behavior represent final common pathways, the convergence of many forces, including interacting cognitive strengths and deficits, environmental or cultural factors, temperament, educational experience, and intrinsic resilience. Symptoms of learning disorders differ with age. Early signs of a reading disorder might include difficulty appreciating the concept of rhyming or delayed abilities in naming letters and their associated sounds. Children with early signs of a mathematics disability might have difficulty with concepts of quantity or difficulty adding or subtracting without using concrete materials, such as their fingers, past 7 yr of age. Some neurodevelopmental dysfunctions do not manifest until later in school, when they are uncovered by increasing academic demands.

Neurodevelopmental functions that are critical for academic function fall within the following domains.

Attention. Attention subsumes a series of control mechanisms mediated by neural systems in the frontal cortex, brainstem, and elsewhere through which the brain regulates behavior and learning. Children with attentional dysfunction comprise a widely heterogeneous group who show various patterns of impairment of these controls (also see Chapter 31). The resulting symptoms may affect learning, behavior, or social interactions. Components of attention include:

1. **Mental energy related to central nervous system (CNS) arousal and the mobilization and distribution of mental effort:** Children with diminished alertness and arousal are likely to exhibit signs of mental fatigue in a classroom. They often yawn, stretch, fidget, and daydream. They sometimes become overactive in an effort to attain a higher level of arousal. They may have difficulty falling asleep or awakening on time. They are apt to have difficulty allocating and sustaining their concentration, and their efforts at work may be erratic and unpredictable, with extreme performance inconsistency.
2. **Processing and regulation of incoming stimuli:** These children may have difficulty discriminating between important and unimportant information (also known as **selective attention**). Such weaknesses of saliency determination result in focusing on the wrong stimuli at home and in school and impede the ability to take notes, summarize information, or know what to study for a test. More overt forms of weak processing controls result in various types of **distractibility,** which may take the form of listening to extraneous noises instead of a teacher, staring out the window, or constantly thinking about the future. These children often show evidence of superficial concentration, not focusing with sufficient intensity to capture specific information. As a result, directions and explanations may have to be repeated or details, such as changes in operational signs in mathematics, may be missed. These children may exhibit difficulties with cognitive activation, passively processing and not linking information with prior knowledge and experience, or over-relying on prior experience. Many of these children display insatiability and are often restless, are bored easily, and require constant high levels of stimulation or excitement.
3. **Production, or the output of work, behavior, and social activity:** Children with attention difficulties have a tendency to perform without previewing a likely outcome or thinking through what they are about to do. The consequent impulsivity can lead to careless mistakes in academic work and unintended misbehavior. They may show hyperactivity and have difficulty pacing, or doing tasks at the appropriate speed. Such children have difficulty with self-monitoring, not knowing how they are doing during and right after an academic endeavor or a behavior. As a result, they can get into trouble without realizing it. These children commonly are under-responsive to punishment and reward.

There is considerable overlap between attention abilities and **executive functions.** The concept of *executive functions* has been proposed to describe the loosely related cognitive processes that reside in the prefrontal region and enable self-regulation, problem-solving, and goal-oriented actions. Components of executive functions have been postulated to include inhibition, flexibility (ability to shift between activities or thoughts), emotional control, working memory, and monitoring.

It is important to appreciate that most children with attentional dysfunction also harbor other forms of neurodevelopmental dysfunction. The DSM-IV uses the term *attention-deficit/hyperactivity disorder* (ADHD) and makes a distinction between individuals who have trouble predominantly with inattention and those who predominantly exhibit hyperactivity and impulsivity (see Chapter 31). Although ADHD is not classified as a specific learning disability, children with ADHD frequently have associated learning disorders (with some estimates suggesting up to 60% comorbidity).

Memory. As children proceed through school, demand for the efficient use of memory progressively increases. Students are expected to be selective, systematic, and strategic in entering new procedures and factual data in memory. They must become proficient in their use of both long- and short-term memory to file and retrieve rules, facts, concepts, and skills. By secondary school, rapid and precise recall is heavily emphasized.

Some children have difficulty with the initial registration of information in **short-term memory.** They have trouble quickly determining whether new information is relevant and transforming it to fit into short-term memory by condensing or shortening it. In some cases, children with attention deficits have problems being selective and sufficiently alert to register salient information in memory. Others have difficulty registering newly introduced information at the level or depth needed to retain it. **Registration weaknesses** can be highly specific. Some students may have trouble with registering visual-spatial data in memory, whereas others may be deficient in the registration of language. Still others have a problem putting linear chunks or sequences of data in short-term memory.

Many children experience problems with **active working memory.** They are ineffective at temporarily suspending information in memory while they are working on it. Normally, active working memory enables a student to keep in mind all of the different components of a task, such as a mathematics problem, while completing it. A student with an active working memory dysfunction might carry a number and then forget what it was that he or she intended to do after carrying that number. Active working memory during reading enables children to remember the beginning of a paragraph when they arrive at the end of it. It lets them remember what they intend to express in writing while they are attempting to remember where to place a comma or how to spell a particular word. It also enables the linkage between new incoming information that is held in short-term memory with prior knowledge or skills held in long-term memory.

Other children experience frustration in their efforts at consolidating information in **long-term memory.** They are ineffective when filing data for later access. Ordinarily, consolidation in long-term memory is accomplished in 1 or more of 4 ways: (1) pairing 2 bits of information (such as a group of letters and the English sound it represents); (2) storing procedures (consolidating new skills, such as the steps in solving mathematics problems); (3) classifying data in categories (filing all insects together in memory); and (4) linking new information to established rules, patterns, or systems of organization (rule-based learning).

Some children can register and consolidate facts and procedures in memory, but seem to have inordinate difficulty accessing or **retrieving** these items when they need them. They may have difficulty remembering ½ of a paired association, such as matching a name with a face or a historical event with a date. They are likely to encounter difficulty with simultaneous recall, which is the frequent need to retrieve several facts or procedures at once. Some students exhibit **delayed automatization.** Not enough of what they have learned in the past is accessible to them instantaneously and with no expenditure of effort. Such skills as letter formation, the mastery of mathematic facts, and word decoding must ultimately become automatic if students are to make good academic progress.

Language. All of the basic academic skills are conveyed largely through language, and it is not surprising that children with language dysfunctions usually have troubled educational careers. Up to 80% of children with learning disabilities have problems that are language-based.

Language disorder has many forms. Some children have particular problems with phonology (see Chapter 32). They experience unclear reception of English language sounds and are said to have difficulty with phonologic awareness. They may have trouble discriminating between, and forming associations with, the sounds of their native language. Language sounds are most often composed of >1 acoustic signal. In English, there are stop consonants, such as *puh* and *kuh*. For the brain to process these language sounds, it must accommodate the very rapid transition (≈30 msec in duration) from the sound *k* to the *uh* in *kuh*. In some cases, affected students may have trouble processing these acoustic signals within language sounds rapidly enough. Commonly, a weak phonologic sense has a negative effect on reading. A student with a poor appreciation of language sounds is likely to form unstable associative linkages between those sounds and visual symbols (letter combinations). It can be hard for these students to conceptualize words as made up of language sound segments (phonemes); thus, their ability to break words down into their constituent sounds and then reblend them into pronounceable words is impeded. They may also have problems manipulating language sounds in their minds and blending them to form a word.

Semantic deficits are also common. Affected children have trouble learning the meaning of new words and using them appropriately. It is especially hard for them to develop a strong enough sense of how the meanings of words relate to each other. Other common language deficiencies include difficulty with syntax (word order), problems with discourse (paragraphs and passages), an underdeveloped sense of how language works (metalinguistics), and trouble with drawing appropriate inferences (supplying missing information) from language. Difficulty with the social application of language (pragmatics) can be another significant impediment. Many adolescents do not develop higher language functions. They have problems dealing with abstract and symbolic language, highly technical vocabulary, verbal concepts, densely packed verbal information in textbooks, foreign languages, and figures of speech (including metaphors and similes).

It is important to distinguish between **receptive language dysfunctions** (those affecting understanding) and **expressive language dysfunctions** (those impeding production or communication). Children with primarily receptive language problems may have difficulty following instructions in the classroom, understanding verbal explanations, and interpreting what they have read. Expressive weaknesses can result from problems with speech as well as language. Speech difficulties include oromotor problems affecting articulation and verbal fluency. Some students experience difficulty with sound sequencing within words. Others find it hard to regulate the rhythm or prosody of their language. Their speech may be disfluent, hesitant, and inappropriate in its tone. Problems with word retrieval can also thwart expressive language fluency. Despite an adequate vocabulary, affected children have problems in finding exact words when they need them (as in a class discussion). They may show marked hesitation and keep substituting definitions for words (circumlocution). Still others with expressive impediments have trouble formulating sentences, using grammar acceptably, and organizing spoken (and possibly written) narrative. Some studies have linked expressive language dysfunction to delinquent behavior. This is especially true when an expressive language disorder occurs in a context of environmental deprivation or turmoil.

Students with strong language abilities may make use of their linguistic facility to overcome other learning problems. It may be possible to verbalize one's way through a mathematics curriculum, thereby circumventing a tendency to be confused by predominantly nonverbal concepts (ratio, equation, diameter).

Visual-spatial Ordering. Visual processing abilities entail the appreciation of spatial attributes. Awareness of shape and position and perception of relative size, foreground and background relationships, and form constancy are among the constituents of spatial ordering. Children with visual-spatial weaknesses may encounter some initial problems with letter and word recognition. Spelling may emerge as a weakness because these children commonly have trouble recalling the precise visual configurations of words. In mathematics, they may have difficulty lining up digits accurately in columns and mastering geometric concepts. Children who are confused about spatial attributes are unlikely to have long-standing or serious academic problems unless their visual-spatial weaknesses are complicated by additional academically relevant neurodevelopmental dysfunctions. Visual-spatial processing dysfunctions are not a common cause of chronic reading disabilities.

Children with visual-spatial weaknesses may be late in discriminating between left and right. They may also show signs of gross motor clumsiness because they may be poor at making use of visual-spatial data to program motor responses, or they may have difficulty drawing and engaging in crafts activities.

Temporal-sequential Ordering. Awareness of time and sequence is an important neurodevelopmental function. Students in school need to be able to manage time, process and produce multistep explanations and procedures, and develop memory capacity for extended sequences. The latter includes preservation of serial order in motor procedures, narratives, and various mathematical algorithms.

Children who have difficulties with temporal-sequential ordering may be delayed in learning to tell time. They may have great difficulty in following multistep commands, performing acts that necessitate a sequence of steps in the proper order, mastering the months of the year, or organizing narrative works. Affected children may also have trouble managing time. They may be frustrated in adhering to schedules, learning the order of their classes in school, or meeting deadlines.

Neuromotor Function. There are 3 distinct, yet related, forms of neuromotor ability relating to function in school: fine motor dexterity, graphomotor function, and gross motor coordination.

Problems with **fine motor function** can affect a child's ability to excel in artistic and crafts activities. These problems may also interfere with learning a musical instrument or mastering a computer keyboard. Eye-hand incoordination may be prominent because the child has trouble with the rapid and precise integration of visual inputs with specific motor plans for hand movements. Other children may have difficulty remembering fine motor procedures, such as tying shoelaces or playing a musical instrument. The term *dyspraxia* in general relates to difficulty in developing an ideomotor plan and activating coordinated motor actions to complete a task or solve a motor problem, such as assembling a model.

Graphomotor function refers to the specific motor aspects of written output. Several subtypes of graphomotor dysfunction significantly impede writing. Some students harbor weaknesses of visualization during writing. They have trouble picturing the configurations of letters and words as they write. Their written output tends to be poorly legible, with inconsistent spacing between words. Others have weaknesses in graphomotor memory, the ability to recall letter and number forms rapidly and accurately. They labor over individual letters and much prefer printing (manuscript) to cursive writing. Some of them exhibit signs of finger agnosia or difficulty with graphomotor feedback; they have trouble localizing their fingers while they write. As a result, they need to keep their eyes very close to the page and tend to apply excessive pressure to the pencil. Others struggle with graphomotor production deficits. Such students have trouble producing the highly coordinated motor sequences needed for writing and have difficulty assigning writing roles to specific muscle groups in their hands. This phenomenon has also been described as **dyspraxic dysgraphia.** It is important to emphasize that a child may show excellent fine motor dexterity (as revealed in mechanical or artistic domains), but very poor graphomotor fluency (with labored or poorly legible writing).

Some children exhibit **gross motor incoordination.** They may have problems in processing "outer spatial" information to guide gross motor actions; affected children are inept at catching or throwing a ball because they cannot form accurate judgments about trajectories in space. Still others demonstrate diminished body position sense. They do not efficiently receive or interpret proprioceptive and kinesthetic feedback from peripheral joints and muscles. They are likely to be impaired when activities demand balance and ongoing tracking of body movement. Others are unable to satisfy the motor praxis demands of certain gross motor activities. It is hard for them to recall or plan complex motor procedures (such as those needed for dancing, gymnastics, or swimming). Children with gross motor problems may incur considerable embarrassment in physical education classes. Gross motor weaknesses can lead to social rejection, withdrawal, and generalized feelings of inadequacy.

Higher-order Cognition. This series of functions consists of various sophisticated thinking skills. Included are the formation of concepts, critical thinking, problem-solving skills, understanding and formulation of rules, brainstorming and creativity, and metacognition (the ability to think about thinking).

Children vary considerably in their capacity to understand the conceptual bases of skills and content areas (**critical thinking**). As students progress through their education, concepts become increasingly abstract and complex. New concepts are likely to contain previously encountered concepts. Some of these children have a pervasive weak grasp of concepts, whereas others have difficulty only with concepts in highly specific domains (mathematics, social studies, science). Some students prefer to conceptualize verbally, whereas others are more comfortable in forming concepts without the interposition of language (perhaps using visual imagery). Many of the best students try to solidify concepts both linguistically and nonverbally.

Problem-solving skills are an important part of mathematics and virtually every other subject in school. Children with good problem-solving skills are good strategists. They are excellent at previewing or estimating answers, coming up with several alternative techniques to meet challenges, selecting the best techniques, and monitoring what they are doing so that they can use alternative strategies as needed. Poor problem solvers, on the other hand, tend to be rigid or impulsive and fail to undertake challenges in a stepwise fashion. They may then encounter significant difficulties in coursework that requires methodical strategy deployment and flexible problem solving.

Brainstorming skills are needed to develop a topic for a report, think about the best way to undertake a project, and deal with various other open-ended academic challenges. Some students cannot generate original ideas. They prefer to be told exactly what to do. They balk at having to devise a topic, use imagination, develop an argument, or think freely and independently.

Critical thinking skills represent another higher cognitive ability acquired during childhood. Successful students often display a keen ability to evaluate statements, products, and people using objective criteria. They are able to tease out their own personal biases and appreciate the viewpoints of others.

Metacognitive ability is the capacity to think about thinking. Children with good metacognition are able to observe themselves thinking or studying. They can thereby develop an understanding of thought processes, enabling them to enhance their personal learning strategies and become more efficient and active learners. Children who lack metacognition tend to perform intellectual tasks the hard way. They are unlikely to appropriate effective techniques to study for a test, write a report, or meet other complex academic challenges. Weaknesses of higher-order cognition can manifest in a variety of forms. Students whose overall intelligence falls in the below-average range (1–2 SD below the mean) are sometimes referred to as *slow learners* and encounter many of the difficulties described in this section.

Social Cognition. A student's social abilities are stringently tested throughout the school day and in the neighborhood after school. Increasing evidence shows that social cognition exists as a discrete area of neurodevelopmental function. There are multiple subskills within social cognition. These include the ability to enter smoothly into new relationships, the capacity to time and stage interactions effectively, sensitivity to social feedback cues, knowledge of how to resolve social conflict without aggression, the adaptive use of language in social contexts (**verbal pragmatics**), the ability to establish truly reciprocal (**sharing**) relationships with others (especially peers), and the inclination to overcome one's innate egocentricity to praise or nurture others. In addition to these skills, students need to be conscious of their own image development and to be adept at marketing themselves to peers and adults. Some children have no idea of how adversely they are affecting others. Social skill deficits can exert an enduring negative effect on behavioral adjustment, mental health, and ultimately, success in a career.

ACADEMIC EFFECTS. Neurodevelopmental dysfunctions are likely to occur in varying clusters within individual children. Combinations of dysfunctions commonly result in academic delays, frequently affecting the acquisition of basic skills and subskills in reading, spelling, writing, and mathematics.

Reading. (See Chapter 32.) Reading disabilities, also termed **dyslexia,** may stem from many neurodevelopmental factors. Most commonly, language dysfunctions are present in children with significant reading delays. Initially, such children are likely to show poor phonologic awareness, as observed in their difficulty appreciating and manipulating language sounds (discussed earlier). They may then have problems in forming associations in memory between English language sounds and combinations of letters. This gap results in deficiencies at the level of decoding individual words. Affected children may be slow to acquire a sight vocabulary (a repertoire of words they can identify instantly). When decoding skills are delayed or overly laborious, reading comprehension is subsequently seriously compromised. Students with visual-spatial dysfunctions may also have trouble learning to read, but this is a relatively rare cause of reading difficulty. Children with weaknesses of temporal-sequential ordering or active working memory may experience difficulty in breaking down words into their component sounds (phonemes) and reblending them into correct sequences. Memory difficulties can cause problems with reading recall and summarization, with associative memory for sounds and symbols, and with the acquisition of vocabulary. Some children with higher-order cognitive deficiencies have trouble understanding what they read because they lack a strong grasp of the concepts in a text.

Children with reading difficulties commonly avoid reading. Thus, it is not unusual for a child whose reading is deficient to superimpose on this problem a lack of reading practice. Consequently, a delay in reading proficiency becomes increasingly pronounced over time. Early identification of reading difficulties, with appropriate instructional interventions, can minimize the long-term effects of reading disability. Phonologically based reading programs have been shown to significantly improve reading and result in changes in the function of brain regions that are critical for reading fluency.

SPELLING. Impairments in spelling ability take various forms. Those with language disorders may have difficulty applying knowledge of phonology to spelling. They may overuse their visual (configurational) sense of words; thus, their attempts at spelling are phonetically poor approximations, yet visually comparable to the actual word (*faght* for *fight*). Other youngsters seem to have the opposite problem, trouble with revisualization, or the recall of word configurations. When their phonologic abilities are adequate, their spelling efforts are often phonetically correct, but visually far afield (*fite* for *fight*). Some children lack a sense of the morphology of language, the sense that certain letter combinations impart certain meanings within words. They may be insensitive to suffixes, prefixes, and word roots. This can be reflected in their spelling patterns. A child may spell the word *played* as *plade.*

Children with certain memory disorders can spell words adequately during a spelling bee or on a spelling list, but misspell the same words when writing a paragraph. They appear to have a memory problem that leads to difficulty in sustaining several different operations simultaneously.

Some students commit mixed spelling errors, many of which are orthographically illegal (they use letter combinations never found in English). Such children have the worst prognoses with regard to spelling proficiency. Overall, the analysis of a child's spelling errors can provide valuable insights into the nature of his or her overall neurodevelopmental profile.

Writing. As children proceed through school, demands for large amounts of well-organized written output increase. Writing difficulties have been classified as disorder of written expression, or **dysgraphia.** In many cases, writing is laborious because of an underlying graphomotor dysfunction. In such instances, a child's graphomotor fluency does not keep pace with ideation and language production. Thoughts may also be forgotten or underdeveloped during writing because the mechanical effort is so taxing.

Just as students with active working memory deficiencies experience difficulty with spelling in paragraphs, they are also prone to serious problems with writing in general. Their written output is often inconsistent in its legibility, ideation, and use of rules (of punctuation, capitalization, or grammar). Children with sequential ordering problems may have difficulty in organizing their ideas effectively when they write. Those with expressive language dysfunctions may not be able to use language effectively on paper. Students with active working memory dysfunctions have difficulty getting the ideas in a paragraph to cohere because they keep forgetting what they wish to express. Students with attention deficits may find it hard to mobilize and sustain the mental effort, pacing, and self-monitoring demands of writing. Writing difficulties are the most frequently encountered academic problems among these children.

Mathematics. Delays in mathematical ability, known as *mathematics disorder* or **developmental dyscalculia,** can be especially refractory to correction. In a school-based study, it was found that no student who was delayed >6 mo in mathematics in 6th grade ever caught up, and another study has shown persistence of severe arithmetic disorder in ½ of affected preteen children. Factors associated with persistence of difficulties included severe disorder and similar problems in siblings of the probands. Significant mathematical weaknesses can become virtually insurmountable because the subject is so highly cumulative in its structure. Various forms of mathematical disability plague students.

Some children experience mathematics failure because of discrete higher-order cognitive weaknesses. They cannot grasp arithmetic concepts. It may be hard for them to apply concepts effectively or to be systematic in solving word problems or when confronted with practical situations. Good mathematicians are able to use both verbal and nonverbal conceptual abilities to understand such concepts as fractions, percentages, equations, and proportion.

Some children show circumscribed semantic memory weaknesses that compromise mathematical ability. Some have trouble automatizing mathematical facts (such as the multiplication tables). Others have difficulty recalling appropriate procedural sequences or algorithms (such as the steps involved in solving a long division problem). Still others have weak active working memory; thus, when they focus on 1 portion of a mathematical problem, they are likely to forget other components of the same problem.

Some students with language dysfunctions have difficulty in mathematics because they have trouble understanding their teachers' verbal explanations of quantitative concepts and operations. Such students are likely to experience frustration in solving word problems and in processing the vast network of technical vocabulary in this subject area. Many students with attention deficits falter in mathematics classes because they are poor at focusing on fine detail (such as operational signs). They may take an impulsive approach to mathematical problem solving and engage in little or no self-monitoring, committing frequent careless errors. Mathematics involves a degree of visualization. Children who have difficulty forming and recalling visual imagery to enhance learning may be at a disadvantage in acquiring mathematical skills. It may be hard, for example, for them to picture geometric shapes or to think about fractions. Visual-spatial difficulties can result in problems writing numbers correctly and difficulty with place value location and alignment of mathematical equations.

It is not unusual for individuals with mathematical disabilities to have superimposed mathematical phobias. Anxiety over mathematics can be especially disheartening and can aggravate an underlying skill delay.

Content Area Subjects. Children with neurodevelopmental dysfunctions may experience difficulty in a wide range of academic content areas. The sciences may be a special problem, especially because they necessitate the processing of dense verbal material in textbooks and the rapid convergent recall of facts. Social studies courses often entail the use of sophisticated language and mastery of verbal abstract concepts (democracy, liberalism, and taxation without representation). Students with higher cognitive weaknesses may not grasp such concepts.

Learning foreign languages can be a serious problem for students with language disorders or memory gaps. In particular, those with even mild trouble with phonologic awareness, semantics, or syntax in their 1st language may have serious problems adding a 2nd language. Some adolescents require foreign language waivers to graduate from high school and enter college. Younger children with learning problems often need to postpone foreign language learning until well into their high school years.

Some students harbor incapacitating organizational problems (involving deficits in executive functions) that adversely affect performance in content area subjects. They often lack effective learning strategies. Some are too impulsive to make use of techniques to facilitate studying and work output. Others struggle because they are unable to maintain a systematized notebook, keep track of assignments, get to places on time, meet deadlines, find things, organize a locker, and remember what books to take home from school. Many disorganized students also have trouble studying for tests. They do not seem to know how and what to study and for how long. They frequently lack self-testing skills.

NONACADEMIC AND EMOTIONAL EFFECTS. Neurodevelopmental dysfunctions commonly have effects that extend far beyond school. Some nonacademic effects are closely related to the dysfunctions themselves, whereas other sequelae are secondary to persistent failure and frustration. The impulsivity and lack of effective self-monitoring of children with attention deficits may lead to unacceptable actions that were unintentional. In some cases, children with neurodevelopmental dysfunctions have excessive performance anxiety or clinical depression. Sadness, self-deprecatory comments, declining self-esteem, chronic fatigue, loss of interests, and even suicidal ideation may ensue. Some children lose motivation. They tend to give up and exhibit learned helplessness, a sense that they have no personal control over their destiny. Therefore, they feel no need to exert effort. This perspective ultimately can promote depression, pessimism, and a loss of ambition.

DIAGNOSIS (ASSESSMENT). The primary care pediatrician has a critical role in the identification and evaluation of the child with a learning disorder. A system of screening and surveillance should be incorporated into routine office visits to promote early identification of learning difficulties. This could include standard screening questionnaires or direct questioning of parents regarding possible concerns about their child's school performance. If problems emerge, the pediatrician should rule out medical causes and can participate in the assessment process. He or she can advise and assist parents in obtaining necessary evaluations through the school or by referral to independent clinicians.

A child who is functioning poorly during the school years requires a multidisciplinary evaluation, including a pediatrician, a psychologist or psychiatrist, and a psychoeducational specialist (sometimes called an *educational diagnostician*). The latter is a clinician (usually a special educator or an educational psychologist) who can undertake a detailed analysis of academic skills and subskills. Other professionals should become involved, as needed, in individual cases, such as a speech-language pathologist, an occupational therapist, a neurologist, and a social worker.

Many children undergo evaluations in school. Such assessments are guaranteed in the United States under Public Law 101-476, the Individuals with Disabilities Education Act (IDEA). In addition, children found to have attentional dysfunction and other disorders may qualify for educational accommodations under Section 504 of the Rehabilitation Act of 1973.

Multidisciplinary evaluations conducted in schools are usually very helpful, but they are focused primarily on determination of whether a student meets the eligibility criteria for special education services. School budgeting constraints or lack of personnel may also affect the quality of evaluations and the extent of recommended services. Because of such limitations, demand for independent evaluations and for second opinions outside of the school setting is growing. Many pediatricians become involved in such outside assessments.

Pediatricians can be helpful in gathering and organizing data on a child with neurodevelopmental dysfunctions. They can obtain such data through the use of questionnaires completed by the parents, the school, and (if old enough) the child. These questionnaires can provide up-to-date information about behavioral adjustment, patterns of academic performance, and traits associated with specific developmental dysfunctions. In addition, questionnaires can elicit relevant data about a child's health history, family background, and demographic variables relevant to a learning difficulty. Standardized behavioral checklists, including the Child Behavior Checklist (CBCL) and the Behavior Assessment System for Children (BASC) can aid in evaluation.

Evaluation of a child with suspected neurodevelopmental dysfunctions should include complete physical, neurologic, and sensory examinations to rule out underlying or associated conditions that could be exacerbating learning difficulties. A physician may also perform an extended neurologic and developmental assessment. Available pediatric neurodevelopmental examination instruments that facilitate direct sampling of various neurodevelopmental functions, such as attention, memory, and language, include the Pediatric Early Elementary Examination (PEEX II) and the Pediatric Examination of Educational Readiness at Middle Childhood (PEERAMID II). Examinations of this type also include direct behavioral observations and assessment of minor neurologic indicators (sometimes called *soft signs*). The latter include various associated movements and other phenomena frequently associated with neurodevelopmental dysfunction.

An evaluation commonly includes intelligence testing that provides an overall IQ. This testing can be useful in relating specific subtest scores to other diagnostic data. Such comparisons can uncover patterns suggestive of specific neurodevelopmental dysfunctions.

Psychoeducational tests yield relevant data, especially when such assessments include careful analyses that pinpoint where breakdowns are occurring in the processes of reading, spelling, writing, and mathematics. Input from multiple sources can be used in formulating specific recommendations for regular and special educational teachers and for interventions that can be implemented at home.

A mental health specialist can be valuable in identifying family-based issues or psychiatric disorders that may be complicating or aggravating neurodevelopmental dysfunctions.

TREATMENT. Management of children with neurodevelopmental dysfunctions often also needs to be multidisciplinary. Most children require several of the following forms of intervention.

Demystification. Many children with neurodevelopmental dysfunctions have little or no understanding of the nature or sources of their learning difficulties. Once an appropriate descriptive assessment has been performed, it is important to explain to the child the nature of the dysfunction while delineating his or her strengths. This explanation should be provided in nontechnical language, communicating a sense of optimism and a desire to be helpful and supportive.

Bypass Strategies (Accommodations). Numerous techniques can enable a child to circumvent neurodevelopmental dysfunctions. Such bypass strategies are ordinarily used in the regular classroom; individual forms of intervention in other settings are aimed at strengthening deficient functions. Examples of bypass strategies include using a calculator while solving mathematical problems, writing essays with a word processor, presenting oral instead of written reports, solving fewer mathematical problems, being seated near the teacher to minimize distraction, presenting correctly solved mathematical problems visually, and taking the Scholastic Aptitude Test untimed. These bypass strategies do not cure neurodevelopmental dysfunctions, but they minimize their academic and nonacademic effects and can provide a scaffold for more successful learning and achievement.

Interventions (Remediation of Skills). Interventions can be used at home and in school to strengthen the weak links in the learning process. Reading specialists, mathematical tutors, and other such professionals can use diagnostic data to select techniques that use a student's neurodevelopmental strengths in an effort to improve decoding skills, writing ability, or mathematical computation skills. Remediation need not focus exclusively on specific academic areas. Many students need assistance in acquiring study skills, cognitive strategies, and productive organizational habits.

Remediation may take place in a resource room or learning center at school. To qualify for these services in school, students may need to be classified as learning disabled. To be so designated, testing must document a substantial discrepancy between the child's IQ and his or her academic skill. Unfortunately, some needy students with significant neurodevelopmental dysfunctions do not display such a discrepancy. Fortunately, increasing numbers of schools and regulatory agencies are giving up these arbitrary criteria and providing help to all children who have an academic delay.

Interventions that can be implemented at home could include drills to aid the automatization of subskills, such as arithmetic facts or letter formations, or the use of phonologically based reading programs.

Developmental Therapy. Controversy exists about the efficacy of treatments to enhance weak developmental functions. It has not been convincingly demonstrated that it is possible to improve substantially a child's fine motor skills, memory, problem-solving proficiency, or temporal-sequential ordering abilities. Nevertheless, some forms of developmental therapy are widely accepted. Speech-language pathologists commonly offer intervention for children with various forms of language disability. Occupational therapists strive to improve the motor skills of certain students with writing problems or gross motor clumsiness.

Curriculum Modifications. Many children with neurodevelopmental dysfunctions require alterations in the school curriculum to succeed, especially as they progress through secondary school. Students with memory weaknesses may need to have their courses selected for them so that they do not have an inordinate cumulative memory load in any 1 semester. The timing of foreign language learning, the selection of a mathematical curriculum, and the choice of science courses are critical issues for many of these struggling adolescents.

Strengthening of Strengths. Affected children need to have their affinities, potentials, and talents identified clearly and exploited widely. It is as important to strengthen strengths as it is to attempt to remedy deficiencies. Athletic skills, artistic inclinations, creative talents, and mechanical abilities are among the potential assets of certain students who are underachieving academically. Parents and school personnel need to create opportunities for such students to build on these assets and to achieve respect and praise for their efforts. These well-developed personal assets can ultimately have implications for the transition into young adulthood, including career or college selection.

Individual and Family Counseling. When learning difficulties are complicated by family problems or identifiable psychiatric disorders, psychotherapy may be indicated. Clinical psychologists or child psychiatrists may offer long- or short-term therapy. Such intervention may involve the child alone or the entire family. Cognitive-behavioral therapy is a technique that is increasingly popular. It is essential, however, that the therapist have a firm understanding of the nature of a child's neurodevelopmental dysfunctions.

Controversial Therapies. A variety of treatment methods for neurodevelopmental dysfunctions have been proposed that have no known scientific proof of efficacy. This list includes dietary interventions (vitamins, fatty acids, or elimination of food additives or potential allergens), neuromotor programs or medications to address vestibular dysfunction, eye exercises, filters, tinted lenses, biofeedback, and other technologic devices. Parents should be cautioned against expending the excessive amounts of time and financial resources usually demanded by these remedies. In many cases, it is difficult to distinguish the nonspecific beneficial effects of increased support and attention paid to the child from the supposed target effects of the intervention.

Medication. Psychopharmacologic agents may be especially helpful in lessening the toll of neurodevelopmental dysfunctions (see Chapters 20, 24, 25, 28, and 31). Most commonly, stimulant medications are used in the treatment of children with attention deficits. They are not a panacea because most children with attention deficits have other associated dysfunctions (such as language disorders, memory problems, motor weaknesses, or social skill deficits). Nevertheless, medications such as methylphenidate (Ritalin, Concerta, Metadate), dextroamphetamine (Dexedrine, Adderall), and atomoxetine (Strattera) can be important adjuncts to treatment because they seem to help some children focus more selectively and control their impulsivity. These medications, including their indications, administration, and complications, are described in Chapter 31. When depression or excessive anxiety is a significant component of the clinical picture, antidepressants or antianxiety drugs may be helpful (see Chapters 24 and 25). Other drugs may improve behavioral control (see Chapter 28). Children receiving medication need regular follow-up visits that include a history to check for side effects, a review of current behavioral checklists, a complete physical examination, and appropriate modifications of the medication dose. Periodic trials off medication are recommended to establish whether the medication is still necessary.

ROLE OF THE PEDIATRICIAN. The pediatrician's longitudinal contact with the child and family enables him or her to critically assess the medical, family, and developmental history to identify children at risk. Pediatricians are well positioned to assess whether early perturbations in developmental progression represent normal variations or warning signs of future learning problems. Regular contact over the course of the school years provides the opportunity to identify and participate in the assessment of learning difficulties, coordinate their management, and function as a counselor and advocate.

The pediatrician needs to maintain an accurate base of knowledge regarding the clinical manifestations of neurodevelopmental dysfunction, methods of diagnosis and management, the resources available within the school system and from other clinicians in the region, and the public laws that entitle eligible students to modifications, accommodations, and interventions. Assistance should be provided in the interpretation of the findings of evaluations by other specialists, ensuring appropriate demystification of the child and coordination of care if other medical specialists are involved. Pediatricians can also play a critical role when children require medication as a component of a management plan.

Drawing on their relationship with the child and parents, pediatricians can provide helpful advice and counseling in dealing with the stresses associated with learning challenges, such as confrontations about homework, and ensuring that students are afforded regular opportunities to pursue their affinities. Children with neurodevelopmental dysfunctions and associated learning disorders require informed advocacy. They need to have their rights upheld in school and the community. Pediatricians can be especially helpful in advocating for children in school. Some children, for example, are devastated by being held back a grade, and the likelihood of benefit may be minimal, especially if the child does not receive accommodations or interventions to address his or her learning difficulties. A physician may need to represent the rights of the child in opposing such grade retention and may need to argue strongly for a child to receive services in school or to benefit from modifications in the curriculum. Pediatricians can also perform advocacy within their communities. In serving on a school board, for example, a physician can exert a major influence on local policy and on the allocation of resources to schoolchildren with special educational needs.

All children with learning disorders can benefit from the support and guidance of a case manager or mentor, a professional who can offer advice in a continuing manner and be available to monitor function through the years. Pediatricians may be the ideal professionals to assume this responsibility. With time, new questions inevitably emerge as a child's neurodevelopmental dysfunctions evolve and academic expectations undergo progressive changes. Because children with learning disorders represent an extremely heterogeneous group, no two children require the same management plan, nor is it possible to predict with certainty at age 7 yr the needs of a child at age 14 yr. Consequently, affected children and their families require vigilant follow-up and individualized objective advice throughout their academic careers.

American Academy of Pediatrics, Committee on Children with Disabilities: The pediatrician's role in development and implementation of an Individual Education Plan (IEP) and/or an Individual Family Service Plan (IFSP). *Pediatrics* 1999;104:124–127.

American Academy of Pediatrics, Committee on Quality Improvement and Subcommittee on Attention-Deficit/Hyperactivity Disorder: Diagnosis and evaluation of the child with attention-deficit/hyperactivity disorder. *Pediatrics* 2000;105:1158–1170.

Chabot RJ, di Michele F, Prichep L, et al: The clinical role of computerized EEG in the evaluation and treatment of learning and attention disorders in children and adolescents. *J Neuropsychiatry Clin Neurosci* 2001;13:171–186.

Kelly DP, Aylward GP: Identifying school performance problems in the pediatric office. *Pediatr Ann* 2005;34:288–298.

Kucian K, Loenneker T, Dietrich T, et al: Impaired neural networks for approximate calculation in dyscalculic children: a functional MRI study. *Behav Brain Func* 2006;31(E pub ahead of print).

Levine MD: *Developmental Variation and Learning Disorders,* 2nd ed. Cambridge, MA, Educators Publishing Service, 1999.

Messer D, Dockrell JE: Children's naming and word-finding difficulties: descriptions and explanations. *J Speech Lang Hear Res* 2006;49:309–324.

Shalev RS: Developmental dyscalculia. *J Child Neurol* 2004;19:765–771.

Shaywitz BA, Shaywitz S, Blachman BA, et al: Development of left occipitotemporal systems for skilled reading in children after a phonologically based intervention. *Biol Psychiatry* 2004;55:926–933.

Temple E, Poldrack R, Salidis J, et al: Disrupted neural responses to phonological and orthographic processing in dyslexic children: An fMRI study. *Neuroreport* 2001;12:299–307.

Weber P, Lutschg J, Fahnenstich H: Cerebral hemodynamic changes in response to an executive function task in children with attention-deficit hyperactivity disorder measured by near-infrared spectroscopy. *J Dev Behav Pediatr* 2005;26:105–111.

Whitmore K, Hart H, Willems G (editors): *A Neurodevelopmental Approach to Specific Learning Disorders.* Cambridge, UK, MacKeith Press, 1999.

Chapter 31 ■ Attention-deficit/Hyperactivity Disorder

Natoshia Raishevich and Peter Jensen

Attention-deficit/hyperactivity disorder (ADHD) is the most common neurobehavioral disorder of childhood, 1 of the most prevalent chronic health conditions affecting school-aged children, and the most extensively studied mental disorder of childhood. According to the 4th edition of the American Psychiatric Association's *Diagnostic and Statistical Manual* (DSM-IV), ADHD is characterized by: (1) inattention, including increased distractibility and difficulty sustaining attention; (2) poor impulse control and decreased self-inhibitory capacity; and (3) motor overactivity and motor restlessness (Table 31-1). Definitions may vary in Europe (Table 31-2). Affected children commonly experience academic underachievement, problems with interpersonal relationships with family members and peers, and low self-esteem. ADHD frequently co-occurs with other emotional, behavioral, language, and learning disorders (Table 31-3). A variety of safe and effective pharmacologic therapies are available to treat the major symptoms of ADHD. Research shows the importance of carefully titrating medications to increase treatment efficacy. There are also effective psychosocial and behavioral treatments that may be beneficial in children with ADHD.

ETIOLOGY. Evidence suggests that there is no single factor that determines the expression of ADHD. The emergence of ADHD is best viewed as a final common pathway for a variety of complex brain developmental processes. Multiple factors have been implicated in the etiology of ADHD. Mothers of children with ADHD are more likely to experience birth complications, such as toxemia, lengthy labor, and complicated delivery. Maternal drug use has also been identified as a risk factor in the development of ADHD. Maternal smoking and alcohol use during pregnancy are commonly linked to attentional difficulties associated with the development of ADHD.

There appears to be a strong genetic component to ADHD, with heritability estimates purported to be as high as 0.80. Genetic studies have primarily implicated 2 candidate genes, the dopamine transporter gene *(DAT1)* and a particular form of the dopamine 4 receptor gene *(DRD4),* in the development of ADHD. Additional genes that may contribute to ADHD include *DOCK2* associated with a pericentric inversion 46N inv(3)(p14:q21) involved in cytokine regulation, a sodium-hydrogen exchange gene, and *DRD5, SLC6A3, DBH, SNAP25, SLC6A4,* and *HTR1B.*

Exposure to toxins, such as maternal smoking or alcohol use and postnatal exposure to lead, has also traditionally been correlated with ADHD.

Abnormal brain structures are linked to an increased risk of ADHD, because ⅕ of children with severe traumatic brain injury are reported to have subsequent onset of substantial symptoms of impulsivity and inattention. Structural (functional) abnormalities have been identified in children with ADHD without preexisting identifiable brain injury. These include dysregulation of the frontal subcortical circuits; small cortical volumes in this region; widespread, small-volume reduction throughout the brain; and abnormalities of the cerebellum.

Psychosocial family stressors may also contribute to or exacerbate the symptoms of ADHD.

EPIDEMIOLOGY. Studies of the prevalence of ADHD across the globe have generally reported that 5–10% of school-aged children are affected, although rates vary considerably by country, perhaps in part due to differing sampling and testing techniques. Rates may be higher if symptoms (inattention, impulsivity, hyperactivity) are considered in the absence of functional impairment. The prevalence rate in adolescent samples is 2–6%. Approximately 2% of adults have ADHD. ADHD is often underdiagnosed in children and adolescents. Youth with ADHD are often undertreated with respect to what is known about the needed and appropriate doses of medications. Many children with ADHD also present with comorbid psychiatric diagnoses, including oppositional-defiant disorder, conduct disorder, learning disabilities, and anxiety disorders (see Table 31-3).

PATHOGENESIS. In children with ADHD, MRI studies indicate a loss of normal asymmetry in the brain, in addition to smaller brain volumes of specific structures, such as the prefrontal cortex and basal ganglia. Children with ADHD have approximately a 5–10% reduction in these brain structures. Functional MRI findings suggest low blood flow to the striatum. The prefrontal cortex and basal ganglia are rich in dopamine receptors. This knowledge, plus data about the dopaminergic mechanisms of action of medication treatment for ADHD, has led to the **dopamine hypothesis,** which postulates that disturbances in the dopamine system may be related to the onset of ADHD. Fluorodopa positron emission tomography scans have also supported the dopamine hypothesis through the identification of low levels of dopamine activity in adults.

CLINICAL MANIFESTATIONS. Development of the DSM-IV criteria leading to the diagnosis of ADHD has occurred mainly in field trials with children 5–12 yr of age (see Table 31-1). The current DSM-IV criteria state that the behavior must be developmentally

TABLE 31-1. DSM-IV Diagnostic Criteria for Attention-Deficit/Hyperactivity Disorder

A. **Either 1 or 2**

1. Six (or more) of the following symptoms of inattention have persisted for ≥6 mo to a degree that is maladaptive and inconsistent with development level:

Inattention

a. Often fails to give close attention to details or makes careless mistakes in schoolwork, work, or other activities
b. Often has difficulty sustaining attention in tasks or play activities
c. Often does not seem to listen when spoken to directly
d. Often does not follow through on instructions and fails to finish schoolwork, chores, or duties in the workplace (not due to oppositional behavior or failure to understand instructions)
e. Often has difficulty organizing tasks and activities
f. Often avoids, dislikes, or is reluctant to engage in tasks that require sustained mental effort (such as schoolwork or homework)
g. Often loses things necessary for tasks or activities (e.g., toys, school assignments, pencils, books, tools)
h. Is often easily distracted by extraneous stimuli
i. Is often forgetful in daily activities

2. Six (or more) of the following symptoms of hyperactivity-impulsivity have persisted for ≥6 mo to a degree that is maladaptive and inconsistent with developmental level:

Hyperactivity

a. Often fidgets with hands or feet or squirms in seat
b. Often leaves seat in classroom or in other situations in which remaining seated is expected
c. Often runs about or climbs excessively in situations in which it is inappropriate (in adolescents or adults, may be limited to subjective feelings of restlessness)
d. Often has difficulty playing or engaging in leisure activities quietly
e. Is often "on the go" or often acts as if "driven by a motor"
f. Often talks excessively

Impulsivity

g. Often blurts out answers before questions have been completed
h. Often has difficulty awaiting turn
i. Often interrupts or intrudes on others (e.g., butts into conversations or games)

B. Some hyperactive-impulsive or inattentive symptoms that caused impairment were present before 7 yr of age
C. Some impairment from the symptoms is present in 2 or more settings (e.g., at school [or work] or at home)
D. There must be clear evidence of clinically significant impairment in social, academic, or occupational functioning
E. Symptoms do not occur exclusively during the course of a pervasive developmental disorder, schizophrenia, or other psychotic disorder, and are not better accounted for by another mental disorder (e.g., mood disorder, anxiety disorder, dissociative disorder, personality disorder)

CODE BASED ON TYPE

314.01 Attention-deficit/hyperactivity disorder, combined type: if both criteria A1 and A2 are met for the past 6 mo
314.00 Attention-deficit/hyperactivity disorder, predominantly inattentive type: if criterion A1 is met but criterion A2 is not met for the past 6 mo
314.01 Attention-deficit/hyperactivity disorder, predominantly hyperactive-impulsive type: if criterion A2 is met but criterion A1 is not met for the past 6 mo

Reprinted with permission from the *Diagnostic and Statistical Manual of Mental Disorders*, 4th ed., text revision. Washington, DC, American Psychiatric Association, 2000. Copyright 2000 American Psychiatric Association.
DSM-IV, *Diagnostic and Statistical Manual of Mental Disorders*, 4th ed.

inappropriate (substantially different from that of other children of the same age and developmental level), must begin before age 7 yr, must be present for at least 6 mo, must be present in 2 or more settings, and must not be secondary to another disorder. There are 3 subtypes of ADHD that are identified in the DSM-IV. The 1st subtype, *attention-deficit/hyperactivity disorder, predominantly inattentive type,* often includes cognitive impairment and is more common in females. The other 2 subtypes, *attention-deficit/hyperactivity disorder, predominantly hyperactive-impulsive type,* and *attention deficit/hyperactivity disorder, combined type,* are more commonly diagnosed in males. Clinical manifestations of ADHD may change with age. The symptoms may vary from motor restlessness and aggressive and disruptive behavior, which are common in preschool children, to disorganized, distractible, and inattentive symptoms, which are more typical in older adolescents and adults. ADHD is often difficult to diagnose in preschoolers because distractibility and inattention are often considered developmental norms during this period.

TABLE 31-2. Differences Between U.S. and European Criteria for ADHD or HKD

	DSM-IV ADHD	ICD-10 HKD
Symptoms	Either or both of following: At least 6 of 9 inattentive symptoms At least 6 of 9 hyperactive or impulsive symptoms	All of following: At least 6 of 8 inattentive symptoms At least 3 of 5 hyperactive symptoms At least 1 of 4 impulsive symptoms
Pervasiveness	Some impairment from symptoms is present in >1 setting	Criteria are met for >1 setting

From Biederman J, Faraone S: Attention-deficit hyperactivity disorder. *Lancet* 2005; 366: 237–248.
ADHD, *attention-deficit/hyperactivity disorder;* DSM-IV, *Diagnostic and Statistical Manual of Mental Disorders,* 4th ed.; HKD, *hyperkinetic disorder;* ICD-10, *International Classification of Diseases.*

TABLE 31-3. Differential Diagnosis of Attention-Deficit/Hyperactivity Disorder (Including Coexisting Disorders)

DIMENSIONAL FACTORS	COEXISTING CONDITIONS WITH POSSIBLE ATTENTION-DEFICIT/HYPERACTIVITY DISORDER PRESENTATION
Behaviors are within the spectrum of normal	Oppositional-defiant disorder
Behaviors are problematic, but fall short of meeting the full criteria for diagnosis	Anxiety disorders
	Conduct disorder
	Depressive disorders
	Learning disorders
	Language disorders
PSYCHOSOCIAL	**DIAGNOSES WITH ASSOCIATED ATTENTION-DEFICIT/HYPERACTIVITY DISORDER BEHAVIORS**
Response to physical or sexual abuse	Fragile X syndrome
Response to inappropriate parenting practices	Fetal alcohol syndrome
Response to parental psychopathology	Pervasive developmental disorders
Response to acculturation	Obsessive–compulsive disorder
Response to inappropriate classroom setting	Tourette syndrome
	Attachment disorder
	Psychosis or schizophrenia
	Adjustment disorder with mixed emotions and conduct
MEDICAL	**NEUROLOGIC**
Thyroid disorders (including general resistance to thyroid hormone)	Auditory and visual processing disorders
	Seizure disorder
Heavy metal poisoning (including lead)	Neurodegenerative disorder
Adverse effects of medications	Post-traumatic head injury
Effects of abused substances	Postencephalitic disorder
Sensory deficits (hearing and vision)	

From Reiff MI, Stein MT: Attention-deficit/hyperactivity disorder evaluation and diagnosis: A practical approach in office practice. *Pediatr Clin North Am* 2003;50:1019–1048. Adapted from Reiff MI: Attention-deficit/hyperactivity disorders. In Bergman AB (editor): *20 Common Problems in Pediatrics.* New York, McGraw-Hill, 2001, p 273.

DIAGNOSIS AND DIFFERENTIAL DIAGNOSIS. A diagnosis of ADHD is made primarily in clinical settings after a thorough evaluation, including a careful history and clinical interview to rule in or to identify other causes or contributing factors; completion of behavior rating scales; a physical examination; and any necessary or indicated laboratory tests. It is important to systematically gather and evaluate information from a variety of sources, including the child, parents, teachers, physicians, and when appropriate, other caretakers.

Clinical Interview and History. The clinical interview allows for a comprehensive understanding of whether the symptoms meet the diagnostic criteria for ADHD. During the interview, the clinician should gather information pertaining to the history of the presenting problems, the child's overall health and development, and the social and family history. The interview should emphasize factors that might affect the development or integrity of the central nervous system or reveal chronic illness, sensory impairments, or medication use that might affect the child's functioning. Disruptive social factors, such as family discord, situational stress, and abuse or neglect, may result in hyperactive or anxious behaviors. A family history of 1st-degree relatives with ADHD, mood or anxiety disorders, learning disability, antisocial disorder, or alcohol or substance abuse may indicate an increased risk of ADHD and/or comorbid conditions.

Behavior Rating Scales. Behavior rating scales are useful in establishing the magnitude and pervasiveness of the symptoms, but are not sufficient alone to make a diagnosis of ADHD. There are a variety of well-established behavior rating scales that have obtained good results in discriminating between children with ADHD and control subjects. These measures include, but are not limited to, the Conner Rating Scale; the ADHD Index; the Swanson, Nolan, and Pelham Checklist (SNAP); and the ADD-H: Comprehensive Teacher Rating Scale (AcTERS). Other broad-band checklists, such as the Achenbach Child Behavior Checklist (CBCL), are useful, particularly in instances where the child may be experiencing co-occurring problems in other areas (anxiety, depression, conduct problems).

Physical Examination and Laboratory Findings. There are no laboratory tests available to identify ADHD in children. The presence of hypertension, ataxia, or a thyroid disorder should prompt further diagnostic evaluation. Impaired fine motor movement and poor coordination and other **soft signs** (finger tapping, alternating movements, finger-to-nose, skipping, tracing a maze, cutting out paper) are common, but are not sufficiently specific to contribute to a diagnosis of ADHD. The clinician should also identify any possible vision or hearing problems. The clinician should consider testing for elevated lead levels in children who present with some or all of the diagnostic criteria, if these children are exposed to environmental factors that may put them at risk (substandard housing, old paint). Behavior in the structured laboratory setting may not reflect the child's typical behavior in the home or school environment. Therefore, reliance on observed behavior in a physician's office may result in an incorrect diagnosis. Computerized attentional tasks and electroencephalographic assessments are not needed to make the diagnosis.

Differential Diagnosis. Chronic illnesses (migraine headaches, absence seizures, asthma and allergies, hematologic disorders, diabetes, childhood cancer) affect up to 20% of children in the U.S. and may impair children's attention and school performance, either because of the disease itself or because of the medications used to treat or control the underlying illness (medications for asthma, steroids, anticonvulsants, antihistamines) [see Table 31-3]. In older children and adolescents, **substance abuse** may result in declining school performance and inattentive behavior.

Sleep disorders, including those secondary to chronic upper airway obstruction from enlarged tonsils and adenoids, frequently result in behavioral and emotional symptoms, although such problems are not likely to be principal contributing causes of ADHD (see Chapter 18). Behavioral and emotional disorders may cause disrupted sleep patterns.

Depression and anxiety disorders (see Chapters 24 and 25) may cause many of the same symptoms as ADHD (inattention, restlessness, inability to focus and concentrate on work, poor organization, forgetfulness), but may also be comorbid conditions. Obsessive-compulsive disorder may mimic ADHD, particularly when recurrent and persistent thoughts, impulses, or images are intrusive and interfere with normal daily activities. Adjustment disorders secondary to major life stresses (death of a close family member, parental divorce, family violence, parental substance abuse, a move) or parent-child relationship disorders involving conflicts over discipline, overt child abuse and/or neglect, or overprotection may result in symptoms similar to those of ADHD.

Although ADHD is believed to be due to primary impairment of attention, impulse control, and motor activity, there is also a high prevalence of comorbidity with other psychiatric disorders (see Table 31-3). The National Institute of Mental Health reported that 15–25% of children with ADHD also have learning disabilities; 30–35% also have language disorders; 15–20% are also diagnosed with mood disorders; 20–25% have coexisting anxiety disorders; and children diagnosed with ADHD may also have co-occurring diagnoses of sleep disorders, memory impairment, and decreased motor skill function.

TREATMENT

Psychosocial Treatments. Once the diagnosis of ADHD has been established, the parents and child should be educated with regard to the ways in which ADHD can affect learning, behavior, self-esteem, social skills, and family function. The clinician should set goals for the family to improve the child's interpersonal relationships, develop study skills, and decrease disruptive behaviors.

Behaviorally Oriented Treatments. Treatments geared toward behavioral management often occur in the time frame of 8–12 sessions. The goal of such treatment is for the clinician to identify targeted behaviors that cause impairment in the child's life (disruptive behavior, difficulty in completing homework, failure to obey home or school rules) and for the child to work on progressively improving his or her skill in these areas. The clinician should guide the parents and teachers in implementing rules, consequences, and rewards to encourage desired behaviors. In short-term comparison trials, stimulants have been more effective than behavioral treatments used alone; behavioral interventions are only modestly successful at improving behavior, but may be particularly useful for children with complex comorbidities and family stressors, when combined with medication.

Medications. The most widely researched medications used in the treatment of ADHD are the psychostimulant medications, including methylphenidate (Ritalin, Concerta, Metadate), amphetamine, and/or various dextroamphetamine preparations (Dexedrine, Adderall) [Table 31-4]. Longer-acting, once-daily forms of each of the major types of stimulant medications are available and facilitate compliance with treatment. The clinician should prescribe a stimulant treatment, either methylphenidate or an amphetamine compound. If a full range of methylphenidate doses are used, approximately ¼ of patients will have an optimal response on a low (<20 mg/day), medium (20–40 mg/day), or high (>40 mg/day) daily dose; another ¼ will be unresponsive or will have side effects, making that drug particularly unpalatable for the family. Over the first 4 wk, the physician should increase the medication dose as tolerated (keeping side effects minimal to absent) to achieve maximum benefit. If this strategy does not yield satisfactory results, or if side effects prevent further dose adjustment in the presence of persisting symptoms, the clinician should

TABLE 31-4. Medications Used in the Treatment of Attention-Deficit/Hyperactivity Disorder

GENERIC NAME	BRAND NAME	DURATION	DOSAGE RANGE	SIDE EFFECTS
METHYLPHENIDATE				
Immediate-release	Ritalin, Methylin	3–4 hr	5, 10, and 20 mg tablets	Moderate appetite suppression, mild sleep disturbances, transient weight loss, irritability, emergence of tics
Extended-release	Metadate ER, Methylin ER,	4–6 hr	10 and 20 mg extended-release tablets	Moderate appetite suppression, mild sleep disturbances,
	Metadate-CD	8–10 hr	10, 20, and 30 mg extended-release capsules	transient weight loss, irritability, emergence of tics
	Ritalin LA	8–10 hr	20, 30, and 40 mg capsules	
	Concerta	10–12 hr	18, 27, 36, and 54 mg capsules	Moderate appetite suppression, mild sleep disturbances, transient weight loss, irritability, emergence of tics
Sustained-release	Ritalin SR, Methylphenidate SR	4–6 hr	20 mg sustained release tablets	Moderate appetite suppression, mild sleep disturbances, transient weight loss, irritability, emergence of tics
DEXMETHYLPHENIDATE				
	Focalin	4–6 hr	2.5, 5, and 10 mg tablets	Moderate appetite suppression, mild sleep disturbances, transient weight loss, irritability, emergence of tics
Extended-release	Focalin XR	6–8 hr		Moderate appetite suppression, mild sleep disturbances, transient weight loss, irritability, emergence of tics
DEXTROAMPHETAMINE				
Short-acting	Dexedrine, DextroStat	4–6 hr	5, 10, and 15 mg tablets	Moderate appetite suppression, mild sleep disturbances, transient weight loss, irritability, emergence of tics
Intermediate-acting	Dexedrine Spansule	6–8 hr	5, 10, and 20 mg tablets	Same as for short-acting dextroamphetamine
MIXED AMPHETAMINE SALTS				
Intermediate-acting	Adderall	4–6 hr	5, 10, and 20 mg tablets	Same as for methylphenidate
Extended-release	Adderall XR	8–12 hr	5, 10, 15, 20, 25, and 30 mg capsules	Same as for methylphenidate
ATOMOXETINE				
Extended-release	Strattera	12 hr	10, 18, 25, 40, and 60 mg capsules	Nervousness, sleep problems, fatigue, stomach upset, dizziness, dry mouth; may lead in rare cases to severe liver injury or to suicidal ideation
Bupropion	Wellbutrin,	4–5 hr	100 and 150 mg tablets	Difficulty sleeping, headache, seizures
	Wellbutrin SR, Wellbutrin XL		100, 150, and 200 mg tablets	
TRICYCLIC ANTIDEPRESSANTS				
Imipramine	Tofranil	Variable	See Table 20-1	Nervousness, sleep problems, fatigue, stomach upset, dizziness, dry mouth, accelerated heart rate
Desipramine*	Norpramin			
Nortriptyline	Aventyl, Pamelor			
ALPHA AGONIST				
	Clonidine	6–12 hr	3–10 μg/kg/day bid–qid	Sedation, depression, dry mouth, rebound hypertension on discontinuing, confusion

*Has been associated with deaths due to cardiac problems. Not recommended for children.

use an alternative class of stimulants that was not used previously. If a methylphenidate compound is unsuccessful, the clinician should switch to an amphetamine product. If satisfactory treatment results are not obtained with the 2nd stimulant, clinicians may choose to prescribe atomoxetine, a noradrenergic reuptake inhibitor that is superior to placebo in the treatment of ADHD in children, adolescents, and adults, and that has been approved by the U.S Food and Drug Administration (FDA) for this indication. Atomoxetine should be initiated at a dose of 0.3 mg/kg/day and titrated over 1–3 wk to a maximum dose of 1.2–1.8 mg/kg/day.

The clinician should consider careful monitoring of medication a necessary component of treatment in children with ADHD. When physicians prescribe medications for the treatment of ADHD, they tend to use lower than optimal doses. Optimal treatment usually requires somewhat higher doses than tend to be found in routine practice settings. All-day preparations are also useful to maximize positive effects and minimize side effects, and regular medication follow-up visits should be offered (4 or more times/yr) vs the twice-yearly medication visits often used in standard community care settings.

It should be noted that medication alone is not always sufficient to treat ADHD in children, particularly in instances where children have multiple psychiatric disorders or stressed home environments. When children do not respond to medication, it may be appropriate to refer them to a mental health specialist. Consultation with a child psychiatrist or psychologist may also be beneficial to determine the next steps for treatment, including adding other components and supports to the overall treatment program. Nonetheless, evidence suggests that children who receive careful medication management, accompanied by frequent treatment follow-up, all within the context of an educative, supportive relationship with the primary care provider, are likely to experience behavioral gains for up to 24 mo.

Stimulant drugs used to treat ADHD may be associated with an increased risk of adverse cardiovascular events, including sudden cardiac death, myocardial infarction, and stroke in adults and rarely in children. In some of the reported cases, the patient had an underlying disorder, such as hypertrophic obstructive cardiomyopathy, which is made worse by sympathomimetic agents. These events are rare, but nonetheless warrant consideration before initiation and during monitoring of treatment with stimulant medications. A pediatric drug advisory committee to the FDA recommended that the drug package insert warn about these risks in children with underlying heart disease and urged follow-up, with monitoring of blood pressure, heart rate, and growth.

PROGNOSIS. A childhood diagnosis of ADHD often leads to persistent ADHD throughout the life span. From 60–80% of children diagnosed with ADHD continue to experience symptoms in adolescence, and up to 40–60% of adolescents exhibit ADHD symptoms into adulthood. In children diagnosed with ADHD, a reduction in hyperactive behavior often occurs with age. However, other symptoms associated with ADHD can become more prominent with age, such as inattention, impulsivity, and disorganization, and these exact a heavy toll on young adult functioning. A variety of risk factors can affect children with untreated ADHD as they become adults. These risk factors include engaging in risk-taking behaviors (sexual activity, delinquent behaviors, substance use), educational underachievement or employment difficulties, and relationship difficulties. With proper treatment, the risks associated with the disorder can be significantly reduced.

American Academy of Child and Adolescent Psychiatry: Summary of the practice parameter for the use of stimulant medications in the treatment of children, adolescents, and adults. *J Am Acad Child Adolesc Psychiatry* 2001;40:1352–1355.

American Academy of Pediatrics, Committee on Quality Improvement, Subcommittee on Attention-Deficit/Hyperactivity Disorder: Clinical practice guideline: Diagnosis and evaluation of the child with attention-deficit/hyperactivity disorder. *Pediatrics* 2000;105:1158–1170.

American Academy of Pediatrics, Committee on Quality Improvement, Subcommittee on Attention-Deficit/Hyperactivity Disorder: Clinical practice guideline: Treatment of the school-aged child with attention-deficit/hyperactivity disorder. *Pediatrics* 2001;108:1033–1044.

Barkley RA, Fischer M, Smallish L, et al: Young adult outcome of hyperactive children: Adaptive functioning in major life activities. *J Am Child Adolesc Psychiatry* 2006;45:192–202.

Biederman J, Faraone SV: Attention-deficit hyperactivity disorder. *Lancet* 2005;366:237–248.

Biederman J, Wilens T, Mick E, et al: Pharmacotherapy of attention-deficit/hyperactivity disorder reduces risk for substance use disorder. *Pediatrics* 1999;104:e20.

Brookes KJ, Mill J, Guindalini C, et al: A common haplotype of the dopamine transporter gene associated with attention-deficit/hyperactivity disorder and interacting with maternal use of alcohol during pregnancy. *Arch Gen Psychiatry* 2006;63:74–81.

Centers for Disease Control and Prevention: Mental health in the United States: Prevalence of diagnosis and medication treatment for attention-deficit/hyperactivity disorder—United States, 2003. *MMWR* 2005;54: 842–847.

De Silva MG, Elliott K, Dahl HH, et al: Disruption of a novel member of a sodium/hydrogen exchanger family and *DOCK3* is associated with an attention deficit hyperactivity disorder-like phenotype. *J Med Genet* 2003;40:733–740.

Dwivedi KN, Banhatti RG: Attention deficit/hyperactivity disorder and ethnicity. *Arch Dis Child* 2005;90(Suppl):i10–i12.

Jensen PS, Hinshaw SP, Swanson JM, et al: Findings from the NIMH Multimodal Treatment Study of ADHD (MTA): Implications and applications for primary care providers. *J Dev Behav Pediatr* 2001;22:1–14.

Kratochvil CJ, Heiligenstein JH, Dittmann R, et al: Atomoxetine and methylphenidate treatment in children with ADHD: A prospective, randomized, open-label trial. *J Am Child Adolesc Psychiatry* 2002;41:776–784.

MTA Cooperative Group: A 14-month randomized clinical trial of treatment strategies for attention-deficit/hyperactivity disorder. *Arch Gen Psychiatry* 1999;56:1073–1086.

Nissen SE: ADHD drugs and cardiovascular risk. *N Engl J Med* 2006; 354:1445–1448.

Okie S: ADHD in adults. *N Engl J Med* 2006;354:2637–2641.

Pliszka SR, Greenhill LL, Crismon ML, et al: The Texas Children's Medication Algorithm Project: Report of the Texas consensus conference panel on medication treatment of childhood attention-deficit/hyperactivity disorder. Part I. Attention-deficit/hyperactivity disorder. *J Am Acad Child Adolesc Psychiatry* 2000;39:908–919.

Pliszka SR, Greenhill LL, Crismon ML, et al: The Texas Children's Medication Algorithm Project: Report of the Texas consensus conference panel on medication treatment of childhood attention-deficit/hyperactivity disorder. Part II. Tactics. *J Am Acad Child Adolesc Psychiatry* 2000;39: 920–927.

Sowell ER, Thompson PM, Welcome SE, et al: Cortical abnormalities in children and adolescents with attention-deficit disorder. *Lancet* 2003;362:1699–1707.

Spencer TJ: ADHD and comorbidity in childhood. *J Clin Psychiatry* 2006;67 supp. 8:27–31.

Wilens TE, Prince JB, Spencer TJ, Biederman J: Stimulants and sudden death: what is a physician to do? *Pediatrics* 2006;118:1215–1219.

Chapter 32 ■ Specific Language and Learning Disabilities

32.1 • Dyslexia • G. Reid Lyon, Sally E. Shaywitz, and Bennett A. Shaywitz

Dyslexia is characterized by an unexpected difficulty in reading in children and adults who otherwise possess the intelligence, motivation, and opportunities to learn considered necessary for accurate and fluent reading. Dyslexia is the most common and most comprehensively studied of the **learning disabilities,** affecting at least 80% of children identified as manifesting learning disabilities. When asked to read aloud, most children and adults with dyslexia display an effortful approach to decoding and recognizing single words, an approach in children characterized by hesitations, mispronunciations, and repeated attempts to sound out unfamiliar words. In contrast to the difficulties they experience in decoding single words, individuals with dyslexia typically possess the vocabulary, syntax, and other higher-level abilities involved in comprehension.

ETIOLOGY. There are numerous theories regarding the etiology of dyslexia, including those implicating deficits in the temporal processing of auditory and visual stimuli and those that hypothesize language-specific impairments. The latter category posits that at a cognitive-linguistic level, dyslexia reflects deficits within a specific component of the language system, the phonologic module, which is engaged in processing the sounds of speech. As predicted by this model, dyslexic individuals have difficulty developing an awareness that words, both spoken and written, can be segmented into smaller elemental units of sound (**phonemes**)—an essential ability given that reading an alphabetic language (English) requires that the reader map or link printed symbols to sound. The linguistic abilities related to learning to read involve phonology, with deficits in phonologic awareness a strong predictor of dyslexia.

Dyslexia is both familial and heritable. Family history is one of the most important risk factors; approximately ½ of children who have a parent with dyslexia, ½ of the siblings of dyslexic individuals, and ½ of the parents of dyslexics may have the disorder. Replicated linkage studies of dyslexia implicate loci on chromosomes 1, 2, 3, 6, 15, and 18 for the transmission of phonologic awareness deficits and subsequent reading problems. The gene *DCDC2,* which may be involved with cortical neuronal migration, is a possible susceptibility gene for dyslexia. Dyslexia is more common in males.

EPIDEMIOLOGY. Dyslexia may be the most common neurobehavioral disorder affecting children, with prevalence rates ranging from 5–10% in clinic- and school-identified samples to 17.5% in unselected population-based samples in the U.S. and other countries. Dyslexia fits a dimensional model in which reading ability and disability occur along a continuum, with dyslexia representing the lower tail of a normal distribution of reading ability. Both prospective and retrospective longitudinal studies indicate that dyslexia is a persistent, chronic condition rather than a transient developmental lag. Although dyslexic and poor readers maintain their relative positions along the distribution of reading ability, approaches using focused, early, and intensive intervention provide indications that these trends can be modified.

PATHOGENESIS. A range of neurobiologic investigations using postmortem brain specimens and brain morphometry as well as diffusion tensor MRI imaging suggests that there are differences

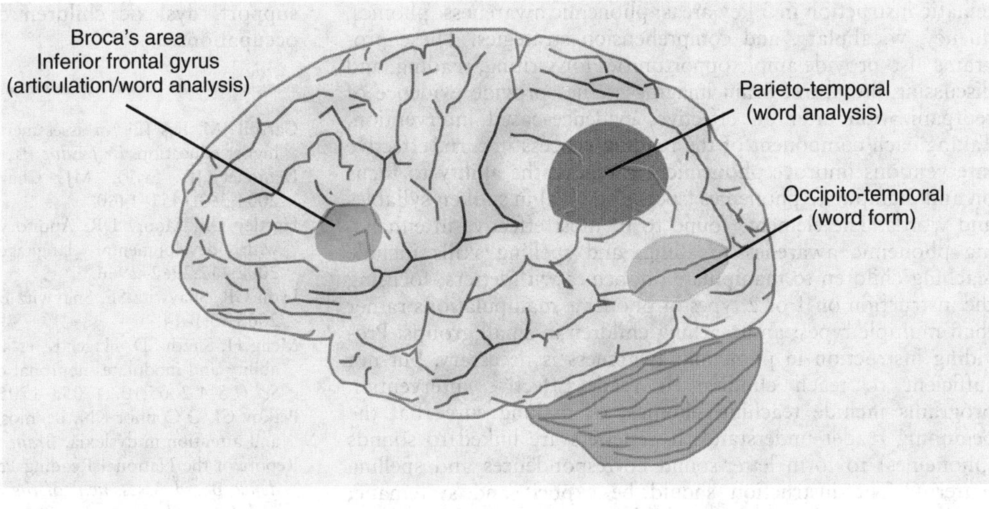

Figure 32-1. Left lateral image of the brain indicating the 3 major reading systems, including 1 anterior (inferior frontal gyrus) and 2 posterior (parietotemporal and occipitotemporal) systems. The occipitotemporal system is also called the *word-form* area. (From Shaywitz SE: *Overcoming Dyslexia: A New and Complete Science-Based Program for Reading Problems at Any Level.* New York, Alfred A. Knopf, 2003.)

in the *left temporo-parieto-occipital brain regions* between dyslexic and nonimpaired readers. Functional brain imaging in both children with dyslexia and adult dyslexic readers demonstrates a failure of the left hemisphere posterior brain systems to function properly during reading, with increased activation in the frontal regions. These data suggest that rather than the smoothly functioning and integrated reading systems observed in nonimpaired children (Fig. 32-1), disruption of the posterior reading systems results in dyslexic children attempting to compensate by shifting to other, ancillary systems, for example, anterior sites, such as the inferior frontal gyrus and right hemisphere sites. In dyslexic readers, a disruption of the posterior reading systems underlies the failure of skilled reading to develop, whereas a shift to ancillary systems supports accurate, but not automatic word reading.

CLINICAL MANIFESTATIONS. Difficulties in decoding and word recognition may vary according to age and developmental level. The cardinal signs of dyslexia observed in school-aged children and adults are a labored approach to decoding, word recognition, and text reading. Listening comprehension is typically robust. Older children have been found to improve reading accuracy over time, albeit without commensurate gains in reading fluency; they remain slow readers. Difficulties in spelling typically reflect the phonologically based difficulties observed in oral reading. A parental history frequently identifies early subtle language difficulties in dyslexic children. During the preschool and kindergarten years, at-risk children display difficulties playing rhyming games and learning the names for letters and numbers. Kindergarten assessments of these language skills are predictive of later reading skill. Parents also frequently report that although their child enjoys being read to, he or she may resist reading aloud to the parent or reading independently. Dyslexia may co-occur with attention-deficit/hyperactivity disorder (see Chapter 31). Although this comorbidity has been documented in both referred samples (40% comorbidity) and nonreferred samples (15% comorbidity), the 2 disorders are distinct.

DIAGNOSIS. Dyslexia is a clinical diagnosis. The clinician seeks to determine through history, observation, and psychometric assessment, if there are: (1) unexpected difficulties in reading (based on the person's cognitive capacity as shown by age, intelligence, or level of education or professional status) and (2) associated linguistic problems at the level of phonologic processing. There is no single test score that is pathognomonic of dyslexia. The diagnosis of dyslexia should reflect a thoughtful synthesis of all clinical data available. Dyslexia is distinguished from other disorders that may prominently feature reading difficulties by the unique, circumscribed nature of the phonologic deficit, one that does not intrude into other linguistic or cognitive domains. Family history, teacher and classroom observation, and tests of language (particularly phonology), reading, and spelling represent a core assessment for the diagnosis of dyslexia in children; additional tests of intellectual ability, attention, memory, general language skills, and mathematics may be administered as part of a more comprehensive evaluation of cognitive, linguistic, and academic function.

For informal screening, the primary care physician in an office setting can listen to the child read aloud from his or her own grade-level reader. Keeping a set of graded readers available in the office serves the same purpose and eliminates the need for the child to bring in schoolbooks. Oral reading is a sensitive measure of reading accuracy and fluency. The most consistent and telling sign of a reading disability in an accomplished young adult is slow and laborious reading and writing. It must be emphasized that the failure either to recognize or to measure the lack of fluency in reading is perhaps the most common error in the diagnosis of dyslexia in older children and accomplished young adults. Simple word identification tasks will not detect dyslexia in a person who is accomplished enough to be in honors high school classes or to graduate from college or obtain a graduate degree. Tests relying on the accuracy of word identification alone are inappropriate to use to diagnose dyslexia in accomplished young adults; tests of word identification show little to nothing of the struggle to read. It is important to recognize that, because they assess reading accuracy but not automaticity (speed), the kinds of reading tests commonly used for school-aged children may provide misleading data on bright adolescents and young adults. The most critical tests are those that are timed; they are the most sensitive in detecting a phonologic deficit in a bright adult. There are few standardized tests for young adult readers that are administered under timed and untimed conditions; the Nelson-Denny Reading Test is an exception. Any scores obtained on testing must be considered relative to peers with the same degree of education or professional training.

TREATMENT. The management of dyslexia demands a life-span perspective; early on, the focus is on remediation of the reading problem. Application of knowledge of the importance of early language and phonologic skills leads to significant improvements in children's reading, even in predisposed children. As a child matures and enters the more time-demanding setting of secondary school, the emphasis shifts to the important role of providing accommodations. Based on the work of the National Reading Panel, evidence-based reading intervention methods and programs are identified. Effective intervention programs provide systematic instruction in 5 key areas: phonemic awareness, phonics, fluency, vocabulary, and comprehension strategies. These programs also provide ample opportunities for writing, reading, and discussing literature. Brain imaging studies provide evidence of reorganization after an effective, evidence-based intervention. Taking each component of the reading process in turn, effective interventions improve **phonemic awareness:** the ability to focus on and manipulate phonemes (speech sounds) in **spoken** syllables and words. The elements found to be most effective in enhancing phonemic awareness, reading, and spelling skills include teaching children to manipulate phonemes with letters; focusing the instruction on 1 or 2 types of phoneme manipulations rather than multiple types; and teaching children in small groups. Providing instruction in phonemic awareness is necessary, but not sufficient to teach children to read. Effective intervention programs include teaching phonics, or making sure that the beginning reader understands how letters are linked to sounds (phonemes) to form letter-sound correspondences and spelling patterns. The instruction should be explicit and systematic; phonics instruction enhances children's success in learning to read, and systematic phonics instruction is more effective than instruction that teaches little or no phonics or teaches phonics haphazardly or with a "by-the-way" approach.

Fluency is of critical importance because it allows for the automatic, attention-free recognition of words, thus permitting these attentional resources to be directed to comprehension. Although it is generally recognized that fluency is an important component of skilled reading, it is often neglected in the classroom. The most effective method to build reading fluency is a procedure referred to as **guided repeated oral reading:** the teacher models reading a passage aloud, and the student rereads the passage repeatedly to the teacher, another adult, or a peer, receiving feedback until he or she is able to read the passage correctly. Evidence indicates that guided repeated oral reading has a clear and positive effect on word recognition, fluency, and comprehension at a variety of grade levels and for all students—good readers as well as those experiencing reading difficulties. The evidence is less clear for programs for struggling readers that encourage large amounts of independent reading, that is, silent reading without any feedback to the student. Thus, even though independent silent reading is intuitively appealing, at this time, the evidence is insufficient to support the notion that, in struggling readers, reading fluency improves. In contrast to teaching phonemic awareness, phonics, and fluency, interventions for reading comprehension are not as well established. The most effective methods to teach reading comprehension involve teaching vocabulary and strategies that encourage active interaction between the reader and the text.

The treatment of dyslexia in students in high school, college, and graduate school is typically based on accommodation rather than remediation. College students with a childhood history of dyslexia require extra time in reading and writing assignments as well as examinations. Many adolescent and adult students have been able to improve their reading accuracy, but without commensurate gains in reading speed. Other helpful accommodations include the use of laptop computers with spelling checkers, tape recorders in the classroom, recorded books, access to lecture notes, tutorial services, alternatives to multiple-choice tests, and a separate quiet room for taking tests.

PROGNOSIS. Application of evidence-based methods to young children (kindergarten–grade 3), provided with sufficient intensity and duration, can result in significant improvements in reading accuracy and fluency. In older children and adults, interventions result in improved accuracy, but not fluency. In the future, this may change with the development of more effective interventions for adolescents. For those who have not had the benefit of early, effective interventions, accommodations are critical in allowing the dyslexic child to demonstrate his or her knowledge. Parents should be informed that, with proper support, dyslexic children can succeed in a range of future occupations.

Carroll JM, Iles JE: An assessment of anxiety levels in dyslexic students in higher education. *Br J Educ Psychol* 2006;76:651–662.

Demonet JF, Taylor MJ, Chaix Y: Developmental dyslexia. *Lancet* 2004;363:1451–1460.

Hartley DE, Moore DR: Auditory processing efficiency deficits in children with developmental language impairments. *J Acoust Soc Am* 2002;112:2962–2966.

Lyon GR, Shaywitz SE, Shaywitz BA: A definition of dyslexia. *Ann Dyslexia* 2003;53:1–14.

Meng H, Smith SD, Hager K, et al: *DCDC2* is associated with reading disability and modulates neuronal development in the brain. *Proc Natl Acad Sci U S A* 2005;102:17053–17058.

Petkov CI, O'Connor KN, Benmoshe G, et al: Auditory perceptual grouping and attention in dyslexia. *Brain Res Cogn Brain Res* 2005;24:343–354.

Report of the National Reading Panel: *Teaching Children to Read: An Evidence Based Assessment of the Scientific Research Literature on Reading and Its Implications for Reading Instruction* (NIH Pub. No. 00-4754). Bethesda, MD, U.S. Department of Health and Human Services, Public Health Service, National Institutes of Health, National Institute of Child Health and Human Development, 2000.

Roongpraiwan R, Ruangdaraganon N, Visudhiphan P, et al: Prevalence and clinical characteristics of dyslexia in primary school students. *J Med Assoc Thai* 2002;85(Suppl 4):S1097–S1103.

Rutter M, Caspi A, Fergusson D, et al: Sex differences in developmental reading disability. *JAMA* 2004;291:2007–2012.

Schumacher J, Anthoni H, Dahdouh F, et al: Strong genetic evidence of DCDC2 as a susceptibility gene for dyslexia. *Am J Hum Genet* 2006; 78:52–62.

Shaywitz BA, Lyon GR, Shaywitz SE: The role of functional magnetic resonance imaging in understanding reading and dyslexia. *Dev Neuropsychol* 2006;30:613–632.

Shaywitz BA, Shaywitz SE, Blachman BA, et al: Development of left occipitotemporal systems for skilled reading in children after a phonologically-based intervention. *Biol Psychiatry* 2004;55:926–933.

Shaywitz S: *Overcoming Dyslexia: A New and Complete Science-Based Program for Reading Problems at Any Level.* New York, Alfred A. Knopf, 2003.

Shaywitz S, Shaywitz B: Dyslexia (specific reading disability). *Biol Psychiatry* 2005;57:1301–1309.

32.2 • Language Development and Communication Disorders • Mark D. Simms and Robert L. Schum

For most children, learning to communicate in their native language is a naturally acquired skill, whose potential is present at birth. No specific instruction is required, although children must be exposed to a language-rich environment. Normal development of speech and language is predicated on the infant's ability to hear, see, comprehend, and remember. Equally important are sufficient motor skills to imitate oral motor movements and the social ability to interact with others.

NORMAL LANGUAGE DEVELOPMENT. For the purposes of analysis, language is subdivided into several essential components. **Communication** consists of a wide range of behaviors and skills. At the level of basic verbal ability, **phonology** refers to the correct use of speech sounds to form words, **semantics** refers to the correct use of words, and **syntax** refers to the appropriate use of grammar to make sentences. At a more abstract level, verbal skills include the ability to link thoughts in a coherent fashion and to maintain a topic of conversation. **Pragmatic** abilities include verbal and nonverbal skills that facilitate the exchange of ideas, including the appropriate choice of language for the situation and circumstance and the appropriate use of body language (posture, eye contact, gestures). Social pragmatic and behavioral skills also play an important role in effective interactions with communication partners (engaging, responding, maintaining reciprocal exchanges).

It is customary to divide language skills into **receptive** (hearing and understanding) and **expressive** (talking) abilities. Language development usually follows a fairly predictable pattern and parallels general intellectual development (Table 32-1).

Receptive Language Development. From birth, newborns show preferential response to human voices over inanimate sounds. The infant will alert and turn toward the direction of an adult who speaks in a soft, high-pitched voice. Over the 1st 3 mo, infants appear to recognize their parent's voice and will quiet if crying. Between 4 and 6 mo, infants will visually search for the source of sounds, again showing a preference for the human voice over other environmental sounds. By 5 mo, infants can passively follow the adult's line of visual regard, resulting in a "joint reference" to the same objects and events in the environment. The ability to share the same experience is critical to the development of further language, social, and cognitive skills. By 8 mo, the infant can actively show, give, and point to objects. Comprehension of words often becomes apparent by 9 mo, when the infant selectively responds to his or her name and appears to comprehend the word *no*. Social games, such as "peek-a-boo," "so big," and waving "bye-bye" can be elicited by simply mentioning the words. At 12 mo, many children can follow a simple, 1-step request without a gesture ("Give it to me"). Between 1 and 2 yr, comprehension of language accelerates rapidly. Toddlers can point to body parts on command, identify pictures in books when named, and respond to simple questions ("Where's your shoe?"). The 2 yr old is able to follow a 2-step command involving unrelated tasks ("Take off your shoes, then go sit at the table") and can point to objects described by their use ("Give me the one we drink from"). By 3 yr of age, children typically understand simple *wh-* question forms (who, what, where, why). By 4 yr of age, most children can follow adult conversation. They can listen to a short story and answer simple questions about it. Typically, 5 yr olds have a receptive vocabulary of >2,000 words and can follow 3- to 4-step commands.

Expressive Language Development. Cooing noises are established by 4–6 wk of age. Over the 1st 3 mo of life, parents may distinguish their infant's different vocal sounds for pleasure, pain, fussing, or tiredness. Many 3 mo old infants vocalize in a reciprocal fashion with an adult to maintain a social interaction ("vocal tennis"). By 4 mo, infants begin to make bilabial ("raspberry") sounds, and by 5 mo, monosyllables and laughing are noticeable. At 6–8 mo, polysyllabic babbling ("lalala," "mamama") is heard and the infant may begin to communicate

TABLE 32-1. Normal Language Milestones

HEARING AND UNDERSTANDING	TALKING
BIRTH–3 MO	
Startles to loud sounds Quiets or smiles when spoken to Seems to recognize your voice and quiets if crying Increases or decreases sucking behavior in response to sound	Makes pleasure sounds (cooing, gooing) Cries differently for different needs Smiles when sees you
4–6 MO	
Moves eyes in direction of sounds Responds to changes in tone of your voice Notices toys that make sounds Pays attention to music	Babbling sounds more speech-like, with many different sounds, including *p, b,* and *m* Vocalizes excitement and displeasure Makes gurgling sounds when left alone and when playing with you
7 MO–1 YR	
Enjoys games such as peekaboo and pat-a-cake Turns and looks in direction of sounds Listens when spoken to Recognizes words for common items, such as *cup, shoe,* and *juice* Begins to respond to requests (*Come here. Want more?*)	Babbling has both long and short groups of sounds, such as *tata upup bibibibi.* Uses speech or noncrying sounds to get and keep attention Imitates different speech sounds Has 1 or 2 words (*bye-bye, Dada, Mama*), although they may not be clear
1–2 YR	
Points to a few body parts when asked Follows simple commands and understands simple questions (*Roll the ball. Kiss the baby. Where's your shoe?*) Listens to simple stories, songs, and rhymes Points to pictures in a book when named	Says more words every month Uses some 1–2 word questions (*Where kitty? Go bye-bye? What's that?*) Puts 2 words together (*more cookie, no juice, mommy book*) Uses many different consonant sounds at the beginning of words
2–3 YR	
Understands differences in meaning (e.g., go-stop, in-on, big-little, up-down) Follows 2-step requests (*Get the book and put it on the table.*)	Has a word for almost everything Uses 2–3 word "sentences" to talk about and ask for things Speech is understood by familiar listeners most of the time Often asks for or directs attention to objects by naming them
3–4 YR	
Hears you when you call from another room Hears television or radio at the same loudness level as other family members Understands simple *who, what, where, why* questions	Talks about activities at school or at friends' homes Usually understood by people outside the family Uses a lot of sentences that have ≥4 words Usually talks easily without repeating syllables or words
4–5 YR	
Pays attention to a short story and answers simple questions about it Hears and understands most of what is said at home and in school	Voice sounds as clear as other children's Uses sentences that include details (*I like to read my books.*) Tells stories that stick to a topic Communicates easily with other children and adults Says most sounds correctly except a few, such as *l, s, r, v, z, ch, sh,* and *th* Uses the same grammar as the rest of the family

From: American Speech-Language-Hearing Association, 2005; http://professional.asha.org.

with gestures. At 8–10 mo, babbling makes a phonologic shift toward the particular sound patterns of the child's native language (the child produces more native sounds than non-native sounds). At 9–10 mo, babbling becomes truncated into specific words ("mama," "dada") for their parents.

Over the next several months, infants learn 1 or 2 words for common objects and begin to imitate words presented by an adult. These words may appear to come and go from the child's repertoire until a stable group of 10 or more words is established. The rate of acquisition of new words is approximately 1/wk at 12 mo, but accelerates to approximately 1/day by 2 yr. The first words to appear are used primarily to label objects (nouns) or to ask for objects and people (requests). By 18–20 mo, toddlers should use a minimum of 20 words and produce jargon (strings of wordlike sounds) with language-like inflection patterns (rising and falling speech patterns). This jargon usually contains some embedded true words. Spontaneous 2-word phrases (pivotal speech), consisting of the flexible juxtaposition of words with clear intention ("Want juice!," "Me down!") are characteristic of a 2 yr old and reflect the emergence of grammatical ability (syntax). Two-word, combinational phrases do not usually emerge until the child has acquired a lexicon of 50–100 words. Thereafter, the acquisition of new words accelerates rapidly. As knowledge of grammar increases, there is a proportional increase in the use of verbs, adjectives, and other words that serve to define the relationship between objects and people (predicates). By 3 yr, sentence length increases and the child uses pronouns and simple present tense verb forms. These 3–5 word sentences typically have a subject and verb, but lack conjunctions, articles, and complex verb forms. The *Sesame Street* character Cookie Monster ("Me want cookie!") typifies the "telegraphic" nature of 3 yr old sentences. By 4 to 5 yr, children should be able to carry on conversations using adult-like grammatical forms and to use sentences that provide details ("I like to read my books").

VARIATIONS OF NORMAL. Language milestones have been found to be largely universal across languages and cultures, with some variations, depending on the complexity of the grammatical structure of individual languages. In Italian (where verbs often occupy a prominent position at the beginning or end of sentences), 14 mo olds produce a greater proportion of verbs compared with English-speaking infants. Within a given language, development usually follows a fairly predictable pattern, paralleling general cognitive development. Although the sequences are predictable, the exact timing of achievement is not. There are marked variations among normal children in the rate of development of babbling, comprehension of words, production of single words, and use of combinational forms within the first 2–3 yr of life.

Two basic patterns of language learning have been identified: analytic and holistic. The analytic pattern is the most common and reflects the mastery of increasingly larger units of language forms. As reflected in the earlier discussion of milestones, the child's analytic skills proceed from simple to more complex and lengthy forms. Children who follow a holistic, or "gestalt," learning pattern may start by using relatively large chunks of speech in familiar contexts. They may memorize familiar phrases or dialog from movies or stories and repeat them in an overgeneralized fashion. Their sentences often have a formulaic pattern, reflecting inadequate mastery of the use of grammar to flexibly and spontaneously combine words appropriately in the child's own unique utterance. Over time, these children gradually break down the meaning of phrases and sentences into their component parts, and they learn to analyze the linguistic units of these memorized forms. As this occurs, more original speech productions emerge and the child is able to assemble thoughts in a more flexible manner. Both analytic and holistic learning processes are necessary for normal language development to occur.

LANGUAGE AND COMMUNICATION DISORDERS

EPIDEMIOLOGY. Disorders of speech and language affect up to 8% of preschool children. Nearly 20% of 2 yr olds are thought to have delayed onset of speech. By age 5 yr, 19% of children are identified as having a speech and language disorder (6.4% speech impairment, 4.6% speech and language impairment, and 8% language impairment). Developmental stuttering occurs in 4–5% of 3–5 yr olds and 1% of adolescents. Boys are nearly twice as likely as girls to have an identified speech or language impairment.

ETIOLOGY. Normal language ability is a complex function that is widely distributed across the brain through interconnected neural networks that are synchronized for specific activities. Although early researchers in language disorders, noting what appeared to be clinical parallels between acquired aphasia in adults and childhood language disorders, expected to find similar lesions in the brains of affected children, for the most part, unilateral, focal lesions acquired in early life do not seem to have the same effects in children as in adults. Risk factors for neurologic injury are absent in the majority of children with language impairment. Genetic factors appear to play a major role in influencing how children learn to talk. Language disorders appear to cluster in families. A careful family history may identify current or past speech or language problems in up to 30% of 1st-degree relatives of proband children. Children who are exposed to parents with language difficulty might be expected to experience poor language stimulation and inappropriate language modeling. Studies of twins have shown the concordance rate for low language test scores and/or a history of speech therapy to be approximately 50% in dizygotic pairs, increasing to >90% in monozygotic pairs. A number of potential gene loci have been identified, but no consistent genetic markers have been established. The most plausible genetic mechanism involves a disruption in the timing of early prenatal neurodevelopmental events affecting migration of nerve cells from the germinal matrix to the cerebral cortex.

Severe expressive language delay is rarely associated with a **duplication** of the locus for Williams syndrome. **Microdeletions,** in contrast, cause Williams syndrome, which leads to normal articulation and fluent expressive language in affected patients.

PATHOGENESIS. Language disorders are associated with a fundamental deficit in the brain's capacity to process complex information rapidly. Simultaneous evaluation of words (semantics), sentences (syntax), prosody (tone of voice), and social cues may overtax the child's ability to comprehend and respond appropriately in a verbal setting. Limitations in the amount of information that can be stored in verbal working memory may further limit the rate at which language information is processed. Electrophysiologic studies show abnormal latency in the early phase of auditory processing in children with language disorders. Neuroimaging studies have identified an array of anatomic abnormalities in regions of the brain that are central to language processing. MRI scans in children with **specific language impairment** (SLI) may show white matter lesions, white matter volume loss, ventricular enlargement, focal gray matter heterotopia within the right and left parietotemporal white matter, abnormal morphology of the inferior frontal gyrus, atypical patterns of asymmetry of the language cortex, or increased thickness of the corpus callosum. Postmortem studies of children with language disorders have found evidence of atypical symmetry in the plana temporale and cortical dysplasia in the region of the sylvian fissure. Some researchers have identified a high incidence of paroxysmal electroencephalogram (EEG) anomalies during sleep in children with SLI. Although these findings may represent a mild variant of **Landau-Kleffner syndrome** (acquired verbal auditory agnosia), they likely represent an epiphenomenon in which paroxysmal activity is related to architectural dysplasia. In support of a genetic mechanism affecting cerebral development, a high rate of atypical perisylvian asymmetries has also been documented in parents of children with SLI.

CLINICAL MANIFESTATIONS. Primary disorders of speech and language development are frequently found in the absence of broader cognitive or motor dysfunction. Disorders of communication are the most common comorbid condition in individuals with generalized cognitive disorders (autism or mental retardation; see Chapters 29 and 38), structural anomalies of the organs of speech (velopharyngeal insufficiency from cleft palate), and neuromotor conditions affecting oral motor coordination (dysarthria from cerebral palsy or other neuromuscular disorders).

Classification. There is no universally accepted classification of childhood communication disorders. Each professional discipline has adopted a somewhat different classification system, based on cluster patterns of symptoms. One of the simplest classifications is that adopted by the American Psychiatric Association's *Diagnostic and Statistical Manual of Mental Disorders* (DSM-IV). This system recognizes 4 types of communication disorders: expressive language disorder, mixed receptive-expressive language disorder, phonologic disorder, and stuttering (Table 32-2). In clinical practice, childhood speech and language disorders occur as a number of distinct entities.

Specific Language Impairment (SLI). Also referred to as **developmental dysphasia** or **developmental language disorder,** SLI is characterized by a significant discrepancy between the child's overall cognitive level (typically nonverbal measures of intelligence) and functional language level. These children follow an atypical pattern of language acquisition and use. Closer examination of the child's skills may show deficits in the understanding and use of word knowledge (semantics) and grammatical understanding (syntax). Children with SLI are often delayed in starting to talk and usually have difficulty understanding spoken language. The problem may stem from insufficient understanding of single words or from the inability to deconstruct and analyze the meaning of sentences. Many affected children show a "holistic" pattern of language development, repeating memorized phrases or dialog from movies or stories (echolalia). In contrast to their difficulty with spoken language, children with SLI appear to learn visually and demonstrate their ability on nonverbal tests of intelligence. Although they have difficulty interacting with peers who are more verbally adept, many children with SLI play appropriately with younger or older children. Despite their communication impairment, they engage in pretend play, show imagination, share emotions (affective reciprocity), and demonstrate joint referencing behaviors appropriate to their age. There is a high incidence of difficulty with fine motor coordination in these children. A combination of increased joint mobility and mild muscular hypotonia often results in motor clumsiness. Although children with SLI respond to therapeutic and educational interventions and show a trend toward improvement of communication skills, adults with a history of childhood language disorder continue to show evidence of impaired language ability, even when surface features of the communication difficulty may have improved considerably. This suggests that many individuals find successful ways of adapting to their impairment.

TABLE 32-2. DSM-IV Diagnostic Criteria for Communication Disorders

EXPRESSIVE LANGUAGE DISORDER

A. The scores obtained from standardized individually administered measures of expressive language development are substantially below those obtained from standardized measures of both nonverbal intellectual capacity and receptive language development. The disturbance may be manifest clinically by symptoms that include having a markedly limited vocabulary, making errors in tense, or having difficulty recalling words or producing sentences with developmentally appropriate length or complexity
B. The difficulties with expressive language interfere with academic or occupational achievement or with social communication
C. Criteria are not met for mixed receptive-expressive language disorder or a pervasive developmental disorder
D. If mental retardation, a speech-motor or sensory deficit, or environmental deprivation is present, the language difficulties are in excess of those usually associated with these problems
Coding note: If a speech-motor or sensory deficit or a neurologic condition is present, code the condition on Axis III

MIXED RECEPTIVE-EXPRESSIVE LANGUAGE DISORDER

A. The scores obtained from a battery of standardized individually administered measures of both receptive and expressive language development are substantially below those obtained from standardized measures of nonverbal intellectual capacity. Symptoms include those for expressive language disorder as well as difficulty understanding words, sentences, or specific types of words, such as spatial terms
B. The difficulties with receptive and expressive language significantly interfere with academic or occupational achievement or with social communication
C. Criteria are not met for a pervasive developmental disorder
D. If mental retardation, a speech-motor or sensory deficit, or environmental deprivation is present, the language difficulties are in excess of those usually associated with these problems
Coding note: If a speech-motor or sensory deficit or a neurologic condition is present, code the condition on Axis III

PHONOLOGICAL DISORDER

A. Failure to use developmentally expected speech sounds that are appropriate for age and dialect (e.g., errors in sound production, use, representation, or organization such as, but not limited to, substitutions of 1 sound for another [use of /t/ for target /k/ sound] or omissions of sounds such as final consonants)
B. The difficulties in speech sound production interfere with academic or occupational achievement or with social communication
C. If mental retardation, a speech-motor or sensory deficit, or environmental deprivation is present, the speech difficulties are in excess of those usually associated with these problems
Coding note: If a speech-motor a sensory deficit or a neurologic condition is present, code the condition on Axis III

STUTTERING

A. Disturbance in the normal fluency and time patterning of speech (inappropriate for the individual's age), characterized by frequent occurrences of ≥1 of the following:
 1. Sound and syllable repetitions
 2. Sound prolongations
 3. Interjections
 4. Broken words (e.g., pauses within a word)
 5. Audible or silent blocking (filled or unfilled pauses in speech)
 6. Circumlocutions (word substitutions to avoid problematic words)
 7. Words produced with an excess of physical tension
 8. Monosyllabic whole-word repetitions (e.g., *I-I-I-I see him*)
B. The disturbance in fluency interferes with academic or occupational achievement or with social communication
C. If a speech-motor or sensory deficit is present, the speech difficulties are in excess of those usually associated with these problems
Coding note: If a speech-motor or sensory deficit or a neurologic condition is present, code the condition on Axis III

COMMUNICATION DISORDER NOT OTHERWISE SPECIFIED

This category is for disorders in communication that do not meet the criteria for any specific communication disorder; for example, a voice disorder (i.e., an abnormality of vocal pitch, loudness, quality, tone, or resonance)

Many children with SLI show difficulties with social interaction, particularly with same-aged peers. Social interaction is mediated by oral communication, and a child deficient in communication is at a distinct social disadvantage. Children with SLI tend to be more dependent on older children or adults, who can adapt their communication to match the child's level of function. At times, these children may gravitate toward younger children who communicate at a level they can comprehend. Generally, social interaction skills are more closely correlated with language level than with nonverbal cognitive level; a developmental progression of increasingly sophisticated social interaction is usually seen as the child's language abilities improve. In this context, social ineptitude is not necessarily a sign of asocial distancing (autism), but rather a delay in the ability to negotiate social interactions.

Pragmatic Language Disorder. The ability to communicate effectively with others depends on mastery of a range of skills that go beyond basic understanding of words and rules of grammar. These higher-order abilities include knowledge of the conversational partner, knowledge of the social context in which the conversation is taking place, and general knowledge of the world. Social and linguistic aspects of communication are often difficult to tease apart, and individuals who have trouble interpreting these relatively abstract aspects of communication typically have difficulty forming and maintaining relationships. Symptoms of pragmatic difficulty include extreme literalness and inappropriate verbal and social interactions. Proper use and understanding of humor, slang, and sarcasm depend on correct interpretation of both the meaning and the context of language and the ability to draw proper inferences. Failure to provide a sufficient referential base to one's conversational partner—to take the perspective of another person—results in the appearance of talking or behaving randomly or incoherently. Pragmatic language impairment often occurs in the context of specific language impairment, but it has been recognized as a symptom of a wide range of disorders, including damage to the right hemisphere of the brain, autism, Asperger syndrome, Williams syndrome, and nonverbal learning disabilities.

Mental Retardation. (See Chapter 38.) Most children with a mild degree of mental retardation learn to talk at a slower than normal rate, although they follow a normal sequence of language acquisition and eventually master basic communication skills. Difficulties may be encountered with higher-level language concepts and usage. Individuals with moderate to severe degrees of cognitive retardation may have great difficulty in acquisition of basic communication skills. Approximately ½ of individuals with IQ <50 are able to communicate using single words or simple phrases; the rest are typically nonverbal.

Autism and Pervasive Developmental Disorders. (See Chapter 29.) A disordered pattern of language development is one of the core features of autism and other pervasive developmental disorders. The language profile of children with autism is indistinguishable from that of children with specific language impairments. The key points of distinction between these conditions are the lack of reciprocal social relationships that characterizes individuals with autism; limitation in the ability to develop functional, symbolic, or pretend play; and an obsessive need for sameness and resistance to change. Approximately 75–80% of children with autism are also mentally retarded, and this may limit their ability to develop functional communication skills. Language abilities may range from absent to grammatically intact, but with limited pragmatic features and/or odd prosody patterns. Some autistic individuals have highly specialized, but isolated, "savant" skills, such as calendar calculations and hyperlexia (the precocious ability to recognize written words beyond expectation based on general intellectual ability). Regression in language and social skills (autistic regression) occurs in approximately 30% of children with autism, usually before 2 yr of age. No explanation for this phenomenon has been identified. Once the regression has "stabilized," recovery of function does not usually occur (Fig. 32-2). Other causes of language regression include acquired brain lesions, neurodegenerative disorders, disintegrative disorders (autistic behavior, cognitive deficit seen in older children), or acquired epileptic aphasia (Landau-Kleffner syndrome).

Asperger Disorder. (See Chapter 29.2.) Although sharing many characteristics of autism (deficits in social relatedness, restricted range of interests), individuals with Asperger syndrome typically show normal early language development (syntax, semantics). As they mature, higher-order social and language pragmatic impairments become prominent. These children have an unusually circumscribed range of interests that are all-absorbing and that interfere with learning other skills and social adaptation. They may engage in long-winded, verbose monologues about their topics of special interest, with little regard to the reaction of others. Their inflection pattern (prosody) may be inappropriate to the content of their conversation, and they may not adjust their rate of speech or vocal volume to the setting.

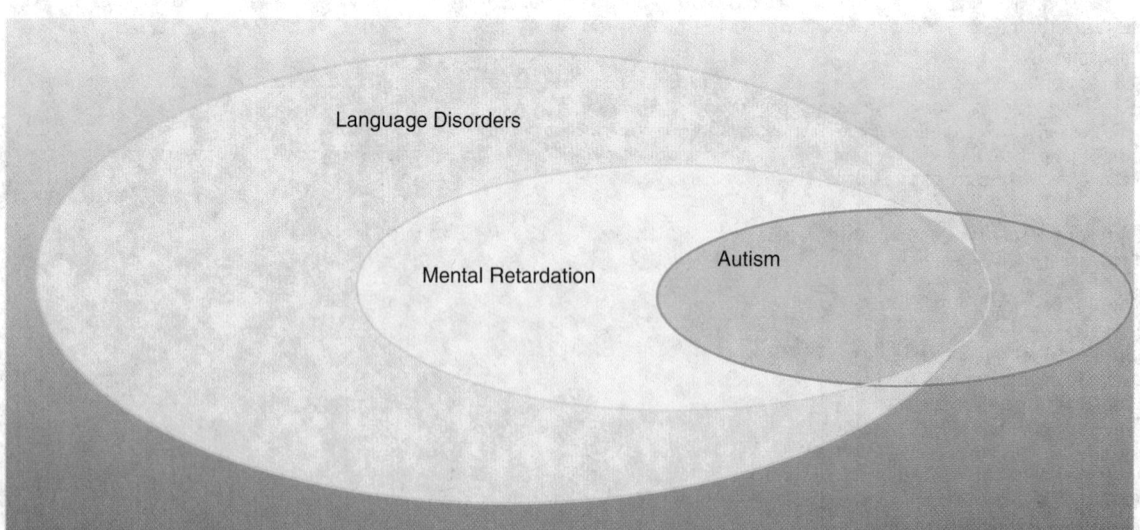

Figure 32-2. Relationship of autism, language disorders, and mental retardation. (From Simms MD, Schum RL: Preschool children who have atypical patterns of development. *Pediatr Rev* 2000; 21:147–158.)

Selective Mutism. (See Chapter 24.) *Selective mutism* is defined as a failure to speak in specific social situations, despite speaking in other situations; it is typically a symptom of an underlying anxiety disorder. Children with selective mutism can speak normally in certain settings, such as within their home or when they are alone with their parents, but do not speak in other social settings, such as at school or at other places outside their home. Other symptoms associated with selective mutism can include excessive shyness, withdrawal, dependency on parents, and oppositional behavior. Most cases of selective mutism are not the result of a single traumatic event, but rather are the manifestation of a chronic pattern of anxiety. Mutism is not passive-aggressive behavior. Mute children report that they want to speak in social settings, but are afraid to do so. It is important to emphasize that the underlying anxiety disorder is the likely origin of selective mutism. Often, one or both parents of a child with selective mutism have a history of anxiety symptoms, including childhood shyness, social anxiety, or panic attacks. This suggests that the child's anxiety represents a familial trait. For an unknown reason, the child converts the anxiety into mutism. The mutism is highly functional for the child in that it reduces anxiety and protects the child from the perceived challenge of social interaction. Treatment of selective mutism should focus on reduction of the general anxiety, rather than focusing only on the mute behaviors. Selective mutism reflects a difficulty with social interaction and not a disorder of language processing.

Isolated Expressive Language Disorder. More commonly seen in boys than in girls, isolated expressive language disorder (**late talker syndrome**) is a diagnosis best made in retrospect. These children have age-appropriate receptive language and social ability. Once they start talking, their speech is clear. There is no increased risk of language or learning disability as they progress through school. A family history of other males with a similar developmental pattern is often reported. This pattern of language development likely reflects a variation of normal.

MOTOR SPEECH DISORDERS.

Dysarthria. Motor speech disorders may originate from neuromotor disorders, such as cerebral palsy, muscular dystrophy, myopathy, or facial palsy. The resulting dysarthria affects both speech and nonspeech functions (smiling, chewing). Lack of strength and muscular control manifests as slurring of words and distortion of vowels. Speech patterns are often slow and labored. Poor velopharyngeal function may result in mixed nasal resonance (hyper- or hyponasal speech). In many cases, feeding difficulty, drooling, an open-mouth posture, and a protruding tongue accompany the dysarthric speech.

Verbal Apraxia. Difficulty in planning and coordinating movements for speech production may result in inconsistent distortion of speech sounds. The same word may be pronounced differently each time. Intelligibility tends to decrease as the length and complexity of the child's speech increase. Consonants may be deleted and sounds transposed. As they try to talk spontaneously or imitate another's speech, children with verbal apraxia may display oral groping or struggling behaviors. Children with verbal apraxia often have a history of early feeding difficulty, limited sound production as infants, and delayed onset of spoken words. They may point, grunt, or develop an elaborate gestural communication system in an attempt to overcome their verbal difficulty. Apraxia may be limited to oral-motor function, or it may be a more generalized problem affecting fine and/or gross motor coordination.

Phonologic Disorder. Children with phonologic speech disorder are frequently unintelligible, even to their parents. Articulation errors are not the result of neuromotor impairment, but seem to reflect an inability to process correctly the words they hear. As a result, they lack understanding of how to fit sounds together properly to create words. In contrast to children with apraxia, those with phonologic disorder are fluent—although unintelligible—and produce a consistent, highly predictable pattern of articulation errors. Children with phonologic speech disorder are at high risk for later reading and learning disability.

Hearing Impairment. Hearing loss can be a major cause of delayed or disordered language development. Approximately 16–30/1,000 children have mild to severe hearing loss that is significant enough to affect educational progress (see Chapter 636). An additional 1/1,000 children are deaf (profound bilateral hearing loss). Hearing loss can be present at birth or acquired postnatally. Newborn screening programs can identify many forms of congenital hearing loss, but progressive hearing loss or acquired deafness may develop after birth.

The most common types of hearing loss are due to a conductive (middle ear) or sensorineural deficit. Although it is not possible to predict accurately the effect of hearing loss on a child's language development, the type and degree of hearing loss, the age of onset, and the duration of the auditory impairment clearly play important roles. Children with significant hearing impairment frequently have problems developing facility with language and often have related academic difficulties. Presumably, the language impairment is caused by lack of exposure to fluent language models starting in infancy.

Approximately 30% of hearing impaired children have at least 1 other disability that often affects the development of speech and language (mental retardation, cerebral palsy, craniofacial anomalies). Accordingly, any child who shows developmental warning signs of a speech and language problem should have a hearing assessment by an audiologist and an examination by a geneticist as part of a comprehensive evaluation.

Hydrocephalus. Some children with hydrocephalus are described as having "cocktail party syndrome." Although they may use sophisticated words, their comprehension of abstract concepts may be limited, and their pragmatic conversational skills may be weak, resulting in superficial discussion of topics or the appearance of a monologue.

Dysfluency (Stuttering).* Fluent speech requires timely synchronization of phonatory and articulatory muscle groups. There is also an important interaction between speech and language skills. Stuttering involves involuntary frequent repetitions, lengthenings (prolongations) or arrests (blocks, pauses) of syllables, or sounds that are exacerbated by emotionally or syntactically demanding speech. The World Health Organization's definition of *stuttering* is a disorder in the rhythm of speech in which the individual knows precisely what he/she wishes to say, but at the same time may have difficulty saying it because of an involuntary repetition, prolongation, or cessation of sound. Stuttering often leads to frustration and avoidance of speaking situations.

EPIDEMIOLOGY/ETIOLOGY. Stuttering usually begins at 3–4 yr of age and is seen more often in males (4:1). Approximately 3–5% of preschool children stutter to some degree; only 0.7–1% of young adults stutter. Stuttering is common in families. Females and those with a history of recovery in the family are most likely to have spontaneous recovery by adolescence. This recovery is not related to the severity of the stuttering.

Stuttering may be due to impaired timing between areas of the brain involved in language preparation and execution. Adults who stutter and those with fluent speech activate similar areas of the brain. In addition, adults who stutter overactivate parts of the motor cortex and cerebellar vermis, show right-sided laterality, and have no auditory activation on hearing their own speech.

DIAGNOSIS. Stuttering must be differentiated from the normal developmental dysfluency of preschool children (Tables 32-3 and 32-4). Developmental dysfluency is characterized by brief periods of stuttering that resolve by school age, and it usually involves whole words, with <10 dysfluences/100 words. The DSM-IV diagnostic criteria for stuttering are noted in Table 32-2. Stuttering that persists and is associated with tics may be

*R.M. Kliegman contributed to this topic.

TABLE 32-3. Differences Between Stuttering and Developmental Dysfluency

BEHAVIOR	STUTTERING	DEVELOPMENTAL DYSFLUENCY
Frequency of syllable repetition per word	≥2	≤1
Tempo	Faster than normal	Normal
Airflow	Often interrupted	Rarely interrupted
Vocal tension	Often apparent	Absent
Frequency of prolongations per 100 words	≥2	≤1
Duration of prolongation	≥2 sec	≤1 sec
Tension	Often present	Absent
Silent pauses within a word	May be present	Absent
Silent pauses before a speech attempt	Unusually long	Not marked
Silent pauses after the dysfluency	May be present	Absent
Articulating postures	May be inappropriate	Appropriate
Reaction to stress	More broken words	No change in dysfluency
Frustration	May be present	Absent
Eye contact	May waver	Normal

Adapted with permission from Van Riper C: *The Nature of Stuttering.* Englewood Cliffs, NJ, Prentice-Hall, 1971, p 28. From Lawrence M, Barclay DM III: Stuttering: A brief review. *Am Family Physician* 1998;57:2175–2178. http://www.aafp.org/afp/980501ap/lawrence.html.

a manifestation of **Tourette syndrome** (see Chapters 24 and 597.4).

TREATMENT. Preschool children with developmental dysfluency (see Table 32-3) can be observed with parental education and reassurance. Parents should not reprimand the child or create undue anxiety. Preschool or older children with stuttering should be referred to a speech pathologist. Therapy is most effective if started during the preschool period. In addition to the risks noted in Table 32-3, indications for referral include 3 or more dysfluencies/100 syllables *(b-b-but; th-th-the; you, you, you);* avoidances or escapes (pauses, head nod, blinking); discomfort or anxiety while speaking; and suspicion of an associated neurologic or psychotic disorder.

Most preschool children respond to interventions taught by speech pathologists and to behavioral feedback by parents. Parents shouldn't yell at the child, but should calmly praise periods of fluency ("That was smooth") or nonjudgmentally note episodes of stuttering ("That was a bit bumpy"). The child can be involved with self-correction and respond to requests ("Can you say that again?") made by a calm parent.

Older children, adolescents, and adults have also been treated with risperidone or olanzapine with varying but usually positive results if behavioral speech therapy is unsuccessful.

RARE CAUSES OF LANGUAGE IMPAIRMENT

Hyperlexia. Hyperlexia is the precocious development of reading single words that spontaneously occurs in some young children (2–5 yr of age) without specific instruction. It is typically associated with developmental disorders such as **pervasive developmental disorder (PDD)** or SLI. It stands in contrast to *precocious reading development* in young children who do not have any other developmental disorders. Although hyperlexia has been considered a rare and peculiar symptom associated with autism, it is recognized as a variation seen in young children with disordered language who do not have the social deficits or restricted or repetitive behaviors associated with autism. A typical manifestation is for a child with SLI to read single words orally or to match pictures with single words. Although hyperlexic children show early and well-developed word decoding skills, they usually have no precocious ability for comprehension of text. Rather, text comprehension is closely intertwined with oral comprehension, and children who have difficulty decoding the syntax of language are also at risk for reading comprehension problems.

Landau-Kleffner Syndrome (Verbal Auditory Agnosia). Children with Landau-Kleffner syndrome have a history of normal language development until they experience a regression in their ability to comprehend spoken language (verbal auditory agnosia). The regression may be sudden or gradual, and it usually occurs at 3–7 yr of age. Expressive language skills typically deteriorate, and some children may become mute. Despite their language regression, these children typically retain appropriate play patterns and the ability to interact in a socially appropriate manner. An EEG may show a distinct pattern of status epilepticus in sleep (continuous spike wave in slow-wave sleep); up to 80% of children with this condition eventually have clinical seizures. A number of treatment approaches have been reported, including antiepileptic medication, steroids, and intravenous gamma globulin, with varying results. The prognosis for return of normal language ability is uncertain, even with resolution of the EEG abnormality, which may represent an epiphenomenon of an underlying brain abnormality.

Metabolic and Neurodegenerative Disorders. (See Part X.) Regression of language development may accompany loss of neuromotor function at the outset of a number of metabolic diseases, including lysosomal storage disorders (metachromatic leukodystrophy), peroxisomal disorders (adrenal leukodystrophy), ceroid lipofuscinosis (Batten disease), and mucopolysaccharidosis (Hunter disease, Hurler disease). Recently, creatine transporter deficiency was identified as an X-linked disorder that presents with language delay in boys and mild learning disability in female carriers.

SCREENING. At each well child visit, developmental surveillance should include specific questions about normal language developmental milestones and observations of the child's behavior. Clinical judgment, defined as eliciting and responding to parental concerns, can detect the majority of speech and language problems. Many clinicians use standardized developmental screening questionnaires and observation checklists designed for use in a pediatric setting (see Chapter 15). All general developmental screening instruments include items about language development (Denver Developmental Screening Test II [DDST-II], Child Development Inventory [CDI], Ages and Stages Questionnaire [ASQ], Parents' Evaluations of Developmental Status [PEDS]). Specific language screening tools are also available, such as the Early Language Milestone (ELM) Scale and the Clinical Linguistic and Auditory Milestone Scale (CLAMS). Because of the high prevalence of speech and language disorders in the general population, referral to a speech and language pathologist for further evaluation and treatment should be made whenever there is suspicion of delay. Specific warning signs that should always prompt referral for comprehensive multidisciplinary developmental evaluation are shown in Table 32-5.

NONCAUSES OF LANGUAGE DELAY. Twinning, birth order, "laziness," exposure to multiple languages (bilingualism), tongue-tie, and otitis media are not adequate explanations for significant language delay. Normal twins learn to talk at the same age as normal single-born children, and effects of birth order on language development have not been consistently found. The drive to communicate and the rewards for successful verbal interaction are so strong that children who let others talk for them usually cannot

TABLE 32-4. Examples of Normal Dysfluency in Preschoolers

TYPE OF DYSFLUENCY	EXAMPLES
Voiced repetitions	Occasionally 2 word parts (*mi . . . milk*)
	Single-syllable words (*I . . . I see you*)
	Multisyllabic words (*Barney . . . Barney is coming!*)
	Phrases (*I want . . . I want Elmo.*)
Interjections	*We went to the . . . uh . . . cottage.*
Revisions: incomplete phrases	*I lost my. . . . Where is Daddy going?*
Prologations	*I am Toooommy Baker.*
Tense pauses	Lips together, no sound produced

From Costa D, Kroll R: Stuttering: An update for physicians. *CMAJ* 2000; 162:1849–1855.

TABLE 32-5. Warning Signs of Language Problems

Not babbling, pointing, or gesturing by 10–12 mo
Not understanding simple commands by 18 mo
Not using any words by 18–21 mo
No word combinations by 24 mo
Speech is difficult for parents to understand by 24–36 mo
Speech is difficult for others to understand by 36–48 mo
Child avoids talking situations
Stuttering of more than tension-free, whole-word repetition
Any regression in language or social skills at any age

talk for themselves and are not "lazy." Toddlers who are exposed to >1 language may show a mild delay in starting to talk, and they may initially mix elements (vocabulary and syntax) of the different languages they are learning (code switching). However, they learn to segregate the languages by 24–30 mo and are equal to their monolingual peers by 3 yr of age. An extremely tight lingual frenulum *(tongue-tie)* may affect feeding and speech articulation, but will not prevent the acquisition of language abilities. Frequent ear infections and/or serous otitis media in early childhood do not result in language disorder.

DIAGNOSTIC EVALUATION. It is important to distinguish developmental delay (abnormal timing) from developmental disorder (abnormal patterns or sequences). A child's language and communication skills must also be interpreted within the context of his or her overall cognitive and physical abilities. It is important to evaluate the child's use of language to communicate with others in the broadest sense (communicative intent). Thus, a multidisciplinary evaluation is often warranted. At a minimum, this should include psychologic evaluation, neurologic assessment, and speech and language examination.

Psychologic Evaluation. There are 2 main goals for the psychologic evaluation of a young child with a communication disorder. Nonverbal cognitive ability must be assessed to determine if the child is mentally retarded, and the child's social behaviors must be assessed to determine whether autism or a form of PDD is present. Additional diagnostic considerations may include emotional disorders such as anxiety, depression, mood disorders, obsessive-compulsive disorder, academic learning disorders, and attention-deficit/hyperactivity disorder.

COGNITIVE ASSESSMENT. *Mental retardation* is defined as retardation in the development of cognitive abilities and adaptive behaviors. Children with mental retardation show delayed development of communication skills; delayed communication does not necessarily signal mental retardation. Therefore, a broad-based cognitive assessment is an important component of the evaluation of children with language delays, including evaluation of both verbal and nonverbal skills. If a child has mental retardation, both verbal and nonverbal scores will be low compared with norms (≤2nd percentile). In contrast, a typical cognitive profile for a child with SLI will include a significant difference between nonverbal and verbal abilities, with nonverbal IQ > verbal IQ and the nonverbal score within the average range.

EVALUATION OF SOCIAL BEHAVIORS. Social interest is the key difference between children with a primary language disorder (e.g., SLI) and those with a communication disorder secondary to autism or PDD. Children with SLI have an interest in social interaction, but may have difficulty acting on this interest because of their limitations to communication. In contrast, autistic children show little social interest. Four key nonverbal behaviors that are often shown by children with SLI—but not autistic children (especially toddlers and preschoolers)—are joint attention, affective reciprocity, pretend play, and direct imitation.

RELATIONSHIP OF LANGUAGE AND SOCIAL BEHAVIORS TO MENTAL AGE. Cognitive assessment provides a mental age for the child, and the child's behavior must be evaluated in that context. Whereas most 4 yr old children engage peers in interactive play, most 2 yr olds are playful, but primarily focused on interactions with adult caretakers. A 4 yr old with mild to moderate mental retardation and a mental age of 2 yr may not play with peers; however, this is because of cognitive limitation, not a lack of desire for social interaction.

Speech and Language Evaluation. A certified speech-language pathologist should perform a speech and language evaluation. A typical evaluation includes assessment of language, speech, and the physical mechanisms associated with speech production. Both expressive and receptive language is assessed by a combination of standardized measures and informal interactions and observations. All components of language are assessed, including syntax, semantics, pragmatics, and fluency. Speech assessment similarly uses a combination of standardized measures and informal observations. Assessment of physical structures includes oral structures and function, respiratory function, and vocal quality. A speech-language pathologist often works with an audiologist, who can perform an appropriate hearing evaluation. If an audiologist is not available in that setting, then a separate referral should be made. No child is too young for a speech-language or hearing evaluation. A referral for evaluation is appropriate whenever language impairment is suspected.

Medical Evaluation. A careful history and physical examination should focus on the identification of potential contributors to the child's language and communication difficulties. A family history of delay in talking, the need for speech and language therapy, or academic difficulty may suggest a genetic predisposition to language disorders. Pregnancy history may show risk factors for prenatal developmental anomalies, such as polyhydramnios or decreased fetal movement patterns. Speech and language difficulty is more likely to occur in a child who is small-for-gestational-age at birth, who has symptoms of neonatal encephalopathy, or who has early and persistent oral-motor feeding difficulty. The developmental history should focus both on the age at which various language skills were mastered and on the sequences and patterns of milestone acquisition. Regression or loss of acquired skills should raise immediate concern. **Physical examination** should include measurement of height (length), weight, and head circumference. The skin should be examined for lesions consistent with phakomatosis (tuberous sclerosis, neurofibromatosis, Sturge-Weber syndrome) and other disruptions of pigment (hypomelanosis of Ito). Anomalies of the head and neck, such as white forelock and hypertelorism (Waardenburg syndrome), ear malformations (Goldenhar syndrome), facial and cardiac anomalies (Williams syndrome, velocardiofacial syndrome), retrognathism of the chin (Pierre-Robin anomaly), or cleft lip and/or palate, are associated with hearing and speech abnormalities. Neurologic examination may show muscular hypertonia or hypotonia, both of which may affect neuromuscular control of speech. Generalized muscular hypotonia, with increased range of motion of the joints, is commonly seen in children with SLI. The reason for this association is not clear, but it may account for the fine and gross motor clumsiness often seen in these children. Mild hypotonia is not a sufficient explanation for the impairments of expressive and receptive language.

No routine diagnostic studies are indicated for SLI or isolated language disorders. When language delay is part of a generalized cognitive or physical disorder, referral for further genetic evaluation, chromosome testing (including fragile X testing), neuroimaging studies, and EEG may be considered, if clinically indicated.

TREATMENT. The federal IDEA laws (**Individuals with Disabilities Education Act**) require that schools provide special education services to children who have learning difficulties. This includes children with speech and language disorders. Services are provided to children from birth through 21 yr of age. Each state has various methods for providing services, and for young children, these can include birth–3, early childhood, and early learning programs. These programs provide speech-language therapy as part of public education, in conjunction with other special education resources. Children can also receive therapy from nonprofit service agencies, hospital and rehabilitation centers, and speech pathologists in private practice.

Speech-language therapy includes a variety of goals. Sometimes both speech and language activities are incorporated into therapy. Speech goals focus on the development of more intelligible speech. Language goals can focus on expanding vocabulary (lexicon) and understanding of the meaning of words (semantics), improving syntax by using proper forms or learning to expand single words into sentences, and social use of language (pragmatics). Therapy can include individual sessions, group sessions, and mainstream classroom integration. Individual sessions may use either drill activities for older children or play activities for younger children, to target specific goals. Group sessions can include several children with similar language goals to help them practice peer communication activities and bridge the gap into more naturalistic communication situations. Classroom integration may include the therapist team-teaching or consulting with the teacher to facilitate the child's use of language in common academic situations.

For children with severe language impairment, alternative methods of communication are often included in therapy. These may include the use of manual sign language or the use of pictures (**Picture Exchange Communication System [PECS]**). Often the ultimate goal is to achieve better spoken language. Early use of sign language or pictures can help the child to establish better functional communication and understand the symbolic nature of words to facilitate the language process. There is no evidence that the use of signs or pictures will interfere with the development of oral language if the child has the capacity to speak. Furthermore, many clinicians believe that these alternative methods accelerate the learning of language. They also reduce the frustration of parents and children who cannot communicate for basic needs.

Parents can consult with their child's speech-language therapist about home activities to enhance language development and extend therapy activities through appropriate language stimulation activities and recreational reading. Parent language activities should focus on emerging communication skills that are within the child's repertoire, rather than teaching the child new skills. The speech pathologist can guide parents in effective modeling and eliciting communication from their child.

Recreational reading focuses on expanding the child's comprehension of language. Sometimes the child's avoidance of reading is a sign that the parent is presenting material that is too complex. The speech-language therapist can guide the parent in selecting an appropriate level of reading material.

PROGNOSIS. Although the majority of children improve their communication ability with time, 50–80% of preschoolers with language delay and normal nonverbal intelligence continue to show language difficulties up to 20 yr beyond the initial diagnosis. Early language difficulty is strongly related to later reading disorders. Approximately 50% of children with early language difficulty later have a reading disorder, and 55% of children with a reading disorder have a history of impaired early oral language development. Children who eventually manifest a specific reading disorder produced fewer words per utterance, expressed less complicated sentences, and showed more pronunciation difficulties at 2–3 yr of age compared with non–reading-disordered peers. By 5 yr of age, verbal sentence complexity has little predictive power, but expressive vocabulary and phonologic awareness of words (the ability to manipulate the component sounds of words) are highly correlated with later reading achievement.

Comorbid Psychiatric Disorders. Early language disorders, particularly difficulty with auditory comprehension, appear to be a specific risk factor for later emotional dysfunction. Boys and girls with language disorders have a higher than expected rate of anxiety disorders (**principally social phobia**). Boys with language disorders are more likely to have symptoms of attention-deficit/hyperactivity disorder, conduct disorder, and antisocial personality disorder compared with normally developing peers. Language disorders are common in children referred for psychiatric services, but they are frequently underdiagnosed and their effect on children's behavior and emotional development is often overlooked.

Preschoolers with language difficulty commonly express their frustration through anxious, socially withdrawn, or aggressive behaviors. As their ability to communicate improves, parallel improvements are usually noted in their behavior, suggesting a cause and effect relationship between language and behavior. However, the persistence of emotional and behavioral problems over the life span of individuals with early language disability is suggestive of a strong biologic or genetic connection between language development and subsequent emotional disorders.

ROLE OF PEDIATRICIANS. Evaluation of children's language development should be an important component of every well child supervision visit. All children who appear to have delayed speech or language should be referred for further assessment and treatment.

Children with symptoms of mental retardation, birth defect syndromes, or neuromotor impairment should be referred for comprehensive multidisciplinary evaluation to identify a specific etiology for their developmental disorder. The child with speech and language disorder may experience social and behavioral difficulties interacting with peers. These difficulties should be evaluated in the context of the child's functional language and mental age. Anxiety disorders may require behavioral and/or psychopharmacologic interventions. Throughout the school years, children should be monitored for evidence of reading disorders.

Most children with language disorders can improve their communication ability through a process of educational programs and speech-language therapy. The physician can help the parents to understand that improvement is a long developmental process guided by teachers and therapists. Many parents question if the child will catch up to his or her peers. Sometimes that occurs, but not all the time. Although most children show significant improvement in communication ability as they grow, language disorders appear to persist over the life span in the majority of affected individuals.

Beitchman JH, Nair B, Clegg M, et al: Prevalence of psychiatric disorders in children with speech and language disorders. *J Am Acad Child Psychiatry* 1986;25:528–535.

Bernstein Rattner N: Clinicians deserve better: Observations on a clinical forum titled "What Child Language Research May Contribute to the Understanding and Treatment of Stuttering" (2004). *Lang Speech Hear Serv Sch* 2005;36:152–159.

Brown S, Ingham RJ, Ingham JC, et al: Stuttered and fluent speech production: An ALE meta-analysis of functional neuroimaging studies. *Hum Brain Mapp* 2005;25:105–117.

Costa D, Kroll R: Stuttering: An update for physicians. *CMAJ* 2000;162: 1849–1855.

Craig A, Hancock K, Chang E, et al: A controlled clinical trial for stuttering in persons aged 9 to 14 years. *J Speech Hear Res* 1996;39:808–826.

De Fosse L, Hodge SM, Makris N, et al: Language-association cortex asymmetry in autism and specific language impairment. *Ann Neurol* 2004;56:757–766.

Feldman HM: Evaluation and management of language and speech disorders in preschool children. *Pediatr Rev* 2005;26:131–141.

Fisher SE: On genes, speech, and language. *N Engl J Med* 2005; 353:1655–1657.

Giddan JJ, Milling L, Campbell NB: Unrecognized language and speech deficits in preadolescent psychiatric inpatients. *Am J Orthopsychiatry* 1996;66:85–92.

Grizzle KL, Simms MD: Early language development and language learning disabilities. *Pediatr Rev* 2005;26:274–283.

Herbert MR, Ziegler DA, Deutsch CK, et al: Brain asymmetries in autism and developmental language disorder: A nested whole-brain analysis. *Brain* 2005;128:213–226.

Hill EL: A dyspraxic deficit in specific language impairment and developmental coordination disorder? Evidence from hand and arm movements. *Dev Med Child Neurol* 1998;40:388–395.

Johnson CJ, Beitchman JH, Young A, et al: Fourteen-year follow-up of children with and without speech/language impairments: Speech/language stability and outcomes. *J Speech Lang Hear Res* 1999;42:744–760.

Jones M, Onslow M, Packman A, et al: Randomised controlled trial of the Lidcombe programme of early stuttering intervention. *BMJ* 2005;331:659.

Lawrence M, Barclay DM III: Stuttering: A brief review. *Am Fam Physician* 2005; http://www.aafp.org/afp/980501ap/lawrence.html.

Maguire GA, Yu BP, Franklin DL, et al: Alleviating stuttering with pharmacological interventions. *Expert Opin Pharmacother* 2004;5:1565–1571.

Plexico L, Manning WH, DiLollo A: A phenomenological understanding of successful stuttering management. *J Fluency Disord* 2005;30:1–22.

Rapin I: Practitioner review: Developmental language disorders. A clinical update. *J Child Psychol Psychiatry* 1996;37:643–655.

Rapin I, Dunn M: Update on the language disorders of individuals on the autistic spectrum. *Brain Dev* 2003;25:166–172.

Rescorla L, Mirak J: Normal language acquisition. *Semin Pediatr Neurol* 1997;4:70–76.

Rinaldi W: Pragmatic comprehension in secondary school-aged students with specific developmental language disorder. *Int J Lang Commun Disord* 2000;35:1–29.

Roberts JE, Rosenfeld RM, Zeisel SA: Otitis media and speech and language: A meta-analysis of prospective studies. *Pediatrics* 2004;113:e238–e248.

Shevell MI, Majnemer A, Webster RI, et al: Outcomes at school age of preschool children with developmental language impairment. *Pediatr Neurol* 2005;32:264–269.

Simms MD, Schum RL: Preschool children who have atypical patterns of development. *Pediatr Rev* 2000; 21:147–158.

Somerville MJ, Mervic CB, Young EJ, et al: Severe expressive-language delay related to duplication of the Williams-Beuren locus. *N Engl J Med* 2005;353(16):1694–1700.

Sommer M, Koch MA, Paulus W, et al: Disconnection of speech-relevant brain areas in persistent developmental stuttering. *Lancet* 2002;360:380–383.

Spinath FM, Price TS, Dale PS, et al: The genetic and environmental origins of language disability and ability. *Child Dev* 2004;75:445–454.

Toppelberg CO, Shapiro T: Language disorders: A 10-year research update review. *J Am Acad Child Adolesc Psychiatry* 2000;39:143–152.

Trauner D, Wulfeck B, Tallal P, et al: Neurological and MRI profiles of children with developmental language impairment. *Dev Med Child Neurol* 2000;42:470–475.

Venkatagiri HS: Recent advances in the treatment of stuttering: A theoretical perspective. *J Commun Disord* 2005;38:375–393.

Webster RI, Majnemer A, Platt RW, et al: Motor function at school age in children with a preschool diagnosis of developmental language impairment. *J Pediatr* 2005;146:80–85.

Webster RI, Shevell MI: Neurobiology of specific language impairment. *J Child Neurol* 2004;19:471–481.

Wilson S, Djukic A, Shinnar S, et al: Clinical characteristics of language regression in children. *Dev Med Child Neurol* 2003;45:508–514.

Part IV ■ Children with Special Needs

Chapter 33 ■ Adoption

Mark D. Simms and Madelyn Freundlich

Adoption is a social, emotional, and legal process that provides a new family for children when the birth family is unable or unwilling to parent. Approximately 1 million children living in the United States are adopted; 2–4% of all American families have adopted. About 127,000 children are adopted annually. Of these, ≈40% were stepparent or relative adoptions, 40% were adoptions of children in foster care, and 15% were adoptions of children from other countries adopted by U.S. families. Private agencies or independent practitioners, such as lawyers, handled approximately one third of adoptions. In Britain, the number of adopted children peaked in 1968, with 25,000 adoptions.

There have been significant increases in the number of children adopted from the foster care system in the United States as well as in the number of children adopted from other countries by U.S. families. Changes in federal law in 1997 require that children in foster care who cannot be safely returned to their families within a reasonable period of time be placed with adoptive families. With the implementation of the Adoption and Safe Families Act, the number of adoptions of children in foster care grew from what previously had been about 18,000 adoptions of children in foster care each yr. In 1997, some 31,000 children were adopted and, by 2002, ≈53,000 children in foster care had been adopted. The number of children in foster care who need adoptive families has also grown dramatically. In September 2002, an estimated 126,000 children in foster care were waiting to be adopted (see Chapter 34). Many children in foster care who are waiting to be adopted have "special needs" because they are of school age, are part of a sibling group, are members of ethnic or racial minority groups, or have physical, emotional, or developmental needs (HIV/AIDS infection or prenatal exposure to illicit substances). Federal adoption subsidies, tax credits, special minority recruitment efforts, increased postplacement services, and approval of adoptions by "nontraditional" families (particularly single adults and older couples) are aimed at increasing the adoption opportunities for these children.

INTERNATIONAL ADOPTIONS

The AIDS epidemic, wars, and natural disasters have produced increasing numbers of orphans worldwide (see Chapter 1). Asia has an estimated 87 million orphans and sub-Saharan Africa has ≈44 million orphans from all causes. International adoptions have correspondingly increased in many nations in the past decade. In 2003, families in the United States adopted 21,616 children from other countries (compared to 7,093 in 1990). Of the ≈220,000 children adopted in the United States from other countries since 1986, China, Russia, Guatemala, and South Korea are the primary sending countries. There have been 1,800–2,200 international adoptions per yr by Canadian families since the mid-1990s; nearly half have been from China.

Most children placed for international adoption have histories of poverty and social hardship in their home countries, and many are adopted from orphanages and other institutional settings. Children who are adopted internationally may be healthy infants but also may be older children with "special needs" that are similar to the needs of children in the U.S. foster care system. Under a federal law implementing the **Hague Convention on Intercountry Adoption,** agencies in the United States that arrange international adoptions must make efforts to obtain accurate and complete health histories on children whom families are considering for adoption.

ROLE OF PEDIATRICIANS

PREADOPTION MEDICAL RECORD REVIEWS. Pediatricians can help prospective adoptive parents evaluate the health and developmental history of a child and available background information from birth families to assess actual and potential problems or risks that children may have. Although it is likely that more background information will be available in domestic adoptions than in international adoptions, pediatricians can assist adoptive families in understanding and evaluating the information that is available about the child's background and current condition. The nature and quality of preadoption medical records of children living outside the United States vary widely. Poor translation and use of medical terminology that is unfamiliar to U.S. trained physicians are common. Review of the child's medical records may raise more questions than provide answers. Each medical diagnosis should be considered carefully before being rejected or accepted. Specifically, use of country-specific growth curves should be avoided as they may be inaccurate or reflect a general level of poor health and nutrition in the country of origin. Serial growth data should be plotted on U.S. standard growth curves; this may reveal a pattern of poor growth due to malnutrition or other chronic illness. Photographs or videotapes may provide the only objective data regarding a child's health status. Full-face photographs may reveal dysmorphic features consistent with fetal alcohol syndrome or findings suggestive of other congenital disorders.

Frank interpretations of available information should be shared with the prospective adoptive parents. The American Academy of Pediatrics Committee on Early Childhood, Adoption and Dependent Care has noted, "It is not the pediatrician's role to judge the advisability of a proposed adoption, but it is appropriate and necessary that the prospective parents and any involved agency be apprised clearly and honestly of any special health needs detected now or anticipated in the future."

POSTADOPTION CARE. After the child is settled in the new home, pediatricians should encourage adoptive parents to seek a comprehensive assessment of the child's health and development. A significant number of internationally adopted children have acute or chronic medical problems, including growth deficiencies, anemia, fetal alcohol syndrome, hepatitis B and C infection, tuberculosis, intestinal parasites, elevated blood lead, dental decay, strabismus, birth defects, developmental delay, feeding and sensory difficulty, and attachment disorders. All children with symptoms of an acute illness should receive immediate medical care. Routine screening for infectious diseases and disorders of growth and development are recommended for all children arriving in the United States (Table 33-1) (Chapter 173.1). Immunizations are frequently inadequate; at least 35% of entering children are not up-to-date in their immunizations. Despite adequate vaccination histories, as many as 30–60% of international adoptees from China and Russia and other eastern European countries may not have protective immunity to tetanus and diph-

TABLE 33-1. Recommended Screening Tests for Newly Arriving Adoptees

INFECTIOUS DISEASE SCREENING
Screening for hepatitis B surface antigen, surface antibody, and core antibody
Screening for hepatitis C virus
HIV ELISA (also consider PCR if the child is <6 months of age)
Mantoux test
Rapid plasma reagin (consider *Treponema pallidum* particle agglutination or fluorescent treponemal antibody absorption also)
Stool culture for ova, parasites, and *Giardia* antigen; repeat if later symptoms warrant
Assess presence of antibodies to verify immunity from administered vaccines (if necessary)
OTHER SCREENING TESTS
Complete blood cell count
Determination of lead levels
Urinalysis
Thyroxine and thyroid-stimulating hormone
Determination of aspartate aminotransferase, alanine aminotransferase, bilirubin, and alkaline phosphatase levels
Vision and hearing screening
Developmental testing
OTHER SCREENING TESTS TO CONSIDER BASED ON CLINICAL FINDINGS AND AGE OF THE CHILD
Detection of *Helicobacter pylori* antibody or ^{13}C-urea breath test
Stool cultures for bacterial pathogens
Newborn screen to State Board of Health (usually includes hemoglobin electrophoresis)
Glucose-6-phosphate dehydrogenase deficiency screening

ELISA, enzyme-linked immunosorbent assay; PCR, polymerase chain reaction.
From Miller LC: International adoption: Infectious diseases issues. *Clin Infect Dis* 2005;40:286–293. Reprinted by permission of the publisher, University of Chicago Press.

theria. Current recommendations for management of immunizations of international adoptees (summarized on the Advisory Committee on Immunization Practices website: *http://www.cdc.gov/mmwr/preview/mmwrhtml/rr5102a1.htm*) are that antibody levels should be measured to verify immunity, or the child should be revaccinated. Refugee children who are adopted from areas of international conflict may have specific psychologic disorders (Table 33-2).

Adoptive parents may need guidance regarding all aspects of infant and child care and may need extra assistance during the early adjustment period. Young children often learn their new language at a remarkable rate and adapt to their new surroundings without difficulty. Older children, however, may be disoriented by disruption in their familiar routines, new foods, a new bed, a new language, and different weather. Dramatic catch-up growth in height, weight, and head circumference is common in the 1st 6–12 mo following the adoption. Over time, developmental delays and behavioral problems may emerge, indicating the need for further psychologic and educational intervention.

TABLE 33-2. Summary of Common Presenting Symptoms of Psychologic Disorders in Refugee Children

POST-TRAUMATIC STRESS DISORDER
Persistent avoidance of stimuli: specific fears, fear of being alone, withdrawal
Re-experiencing aspects of the trauma: nightmares, visual images, feelings of fear and helplessness
Persistent symptoms of increased arousal: easily aroused, disorganized and agitated behavior, lack of concentration
OTHER ANXIETY SYMPTOMS
Marked anxiety and worry: irritability, restlessness
Other sleep disorders
Somatic symptoms including headaches and abdominal pain
DEPRESSION
Low mood
LOSS OF INTEREST OR PLEASURE
Declining school performance
CONDUCT DISORDERS

From Fazel M, Stein A: The mental health of refugee children. *Arch Dis Child* 2002;87:366–370.

Families should be encouraged to speak freely and repeatedly about adoption with the child, beginning in the toddler years and continuing through adolescence. Pediatricians may need to respond to a number of concerns and questions on the part of adoptive parents or adopted adolescents when the adoptee's health and genetic history is incomplete or unknown.

Most adopted children and families adjust well and lead healthy, productive lives. In one study conducted in Great Britain, 2% of adoptive displacement had disrupted. Disruption rates are higher among children adopted from foster care, which may be associated with their older ages at time of adoption and a history of multiple placements prior to their adoptions. As a result of a greater understanding of the needs of families who adopt children from foster care, agencies are placing greater emphasis on the preparation of adoptive parents and ensuring the availability of a full range of postadoption services, including physical health, mental health, and developmental services for their adopted children.

American Academy of Pediatrics, Committee on Early Childhood, Adoption and Dependent Care: Families and adoption: The pediatrician's role in supporting communication. *AAP News,* February 1992.

———. Initial medical evaluation of an adopted child. *Pediatrics* 1991;88:642–644.

Aronson J: Medical evaluation and infectious considerations on arrival. *Pediatr Ann* 2000;29:218–223.

Bledsoe JM, Johnston BD: Preparing families for international adoption. *Pediatr Rev* 2004;25:242–250.

Fazel M, Stein A: The mental health of refugee children. *Arch Dis Child* 2002;87:366–370.

Holloway JS: Outcome in placements for adoption or long-term fostering. *Arch Dis Child* 1997;76:227–230.

Howard JA, Smith SL: *After Adoption: The Needs of Adopted Youth.* Washington, DC, CWLA Press, 2003.

Juffer F, van Ijzendoorn MH: Behavior problems and mental health referrals of international adoptees. *JAMA* 2005;293:2501–2515.

Kim WJ: Benefits and risks of intercountry adoption. *Lancet* 2002;360:423–425.

Landgren M, Grönlund MA, Elfstrand PO, et al: Health before and after adoption from Eastern Europe. *Acta Paediatrics* 2006;95:720–725.

Miller LC: International adoption: Infectious diseases issues. *Clin Infect Dis* 2005;40:286–293.

———. Initial assessment of growth, development, and the effects of institutionalization in internationally adopted children. *Ann Pediatr* 2000; 29:224–232.

———. Caring for internationally adopted children. *N Engl J Med* 1999;341:1539–1540.

Saiman L, Aronson J, Zhou J, et al: Prevalence of infectious diseases among internationally adopted children. *Pediatrics* 2001;108:608–612.

Chapter 34 ■ Foster Care Mark D. Simms and Madelyn Freundlich

Approximately 532,000 children were in state-supported foster care in the United States in 2002, compared to 262,000 children in 1982. In the past two decades, efforts to reduce the number of children in foster care have been unsuccessful, although there has been a slight yearly decline in the foster population in the past six yr.

Developed as a temporary measure to assist families in crisis, the foster care system became overwhelmed in the 1960s and 1970s as the number of children determined to be abused or neglected and in need of foster care increased dramatically. By the late 1970s, it had become apparent that far too many children were remaining in foster care for extended periods of time without clear plans for their futures. In 1980, the Adoption Assistance and Child Welfare Act (P.L. 96-272) changed the emphasis of public policy by requiring states to make "reasonable efforts" to prevent children from entering foster care and to reunify children in foster care with their families. The act advanced permanency planning as a process to prevent children from remaining in foster care for indefinite periods of time. It required that children in foster care have clearly defined permanency goals (return home, placement with relatives, or adoption) no later than 18 mo from the time they entered foster care and that there be periodic court reviews of children's placements and progress toward achieving their permanency goals. Although some progress was realized through the mid-1980s, the illegal drug epidemic (cocaine) that began in the late 1980s set the stage for a new influx of children into foster care. The population of children in foster care remained at >500,000 children in the subsequent decade. In 1997, a federal law, the Adoption and Safe Families Act (P.L. 105-89), was enacted in an effort to prompt more timely permanency planning for children in foster care. Under this law, a permanency plan must be made for a child in foster care no later than 12 mo from the child's entry into care and a petition to terminate parental rights must be filed to free the child for adoption when a child has been in foster care for 15 of the most recent 22 mo (with some exceptions). Adoption (see Chapter 33) is viewed as an important option for children in foster care.

In 2002, there were 2.6 million reports of child abuse and neglect; of these reports, 790,400 were substantiated (see Chapter 36). The vast majority of children in foster care have histories of abuse or neglect. Far fewer children are in care because of the child's own physical or mental health problems or because parents, as a result of a personal or family emergency, voluntarily place their child in foster care. Although foster care has narrowed so that most children and their families can gain access to help only if the child is abused or significantly neglected, federal programs have been developed to assist families prior to crises involving child abuse or serious neglect. The Promoting Safe and Stable Families program (under Title IV-B of the Social Security Act), in particular, funds a range of family support and family preservation programs. Although foster care payments under Title IV-E of the Social Security Act continue to far exceed funding for child and family services programs under Title IV-B, greater efforts are being made to address the issues that are associated with child abuse and neglect and the need for children to be placed in foster care: parental substance abuse, domestic violence, inadequate housing and homelessness, lack of parenting skills, unemployment and underemployment, mental and physical health problems, and parental incarceration.

A large number of children entering foster care are young; 40% of children entering foster care in 2002 were under the age of 5 yr. The majority of these children were white (46%); significant percentages were black (28%) and Latino (17%). Children continue to remain in care for significant periods of time; the average for children who entered foster care in September 2002 was 18 mo. Importantly, about 44% of the children in foster care had been in foster care for ≥2 yr.

Children who enter foster care have high rates of medical, developmental, and mental health problems (Table 34-1). The majority have behavioral and adjustment problems. Nearly 60% of preschoolers in foster care are developmentally delayed, and more than half of the school-aged children lag behind their peers academically. A disproportionate number of children in foster care have chronic medical conditions (35%), physical growth failure (25%), and congenital abnormalities (15%). Many are children with special health care needs (see Chapter 38). Children in foster care have high utilizations rates for all types of care (especially inpatient hospitalization and outpatient mental health services); as a group, they incur high health care costs. Both the chances of entering foster care and the likelihood of longer stays in care are associated with the presence of mental health problems, physical disabilities, and developmental delays. Nonetheless, when children receive needed services, they experience significant improvements in overall health status, stabilization of chronic conditions, and growth and development.

TABLE 34-1. Health Problems of Children Enrolled in Foster Care

GROWTH
Failure to thrive
Short stature
PERINATAL
In utero illegal drug exposure
Perinatal acquired HIV
Sequelae of prematurity
Congenital anomalies
Cerebral palsy
ADOLESCENT RISK-TAKING BEHAVIOR
Illegal drug use
Early sexual activity
Sexual or IV drug use associated HIV
MENTAL/DEVELOPMENTAL HEALTH
Manifestations of abuse and neglect
School failure
Learning disorders
Conduct disorders
Attention-deficit/hyperactivity disorder
Aggressive behavior
Depression
CHRONIC HEALTH PROBLEMS
Poor vision or hearing
Asthma
Dental caries
Delayed immunizations
Lack of medical home

In 1988, the Child Welfare League of America, in collaboration with the American Academy of Pediatrics, published *Standards for Health Care Services for Children in Out-of-Home Care* to serve as a blueprint for the effective delivery of services to children in foster care. These standards, in general, have not been implemented. Moreover, despite the availability of comprehensive diagnostic and treatment services under the Medicaid program known as EPSDT (Early Periodic Screening, Diagnosis and Treatment), which is mandatory in all states, the majority of children in foster care do not receive these services.

A variety of factors act as barriers to the health care of children in foster care. Most public and private child welfare agencies do not have formal policies or arrangements to provide health care services and, instead, rely on local physicians and/or health clinics funded by Medicaid. It is often difficult to obtain complete information on the health histories of children who enter foster care as they often have had erratic contact with various health care providers before they enter foster care and social workers are not always able to obtain detailed information from biologic parents at the time children enter care. Once children enter foster care, there is often a diffusion of responsibility regarding obtaining health care services for children. Foster parents often are given very little information about the health care needs of the children for whom they are caring, but they typically are expected to decide when and where children receive health care services. In some cases, social workers may oversee the health care of children in foster care, but coordination with health care providers is often lacking. Uncertainty as to who may make health care treatment decisions for children may further delay health care or result in the denial of health care services.

The majority of children in foster care for relatively short periods have only one or two placements while they are in care (84.3% of the children who are in care for <12 mo). For children in care for longer periods of time, a much smaller percentage has only one or two placements. In many states, for example, more than half of the children in foster care for ≥4 yr have had three or more placements. Changes in caregivers and residences are associated with poorer psychologic and developmental outcomes for children and, often, multiple changes in health care providers. Irrespective of whether children's placements change, children's social workers often change (primarily because of high turnover rates) and, as a result, key aspects of health care planning and coordinating may be disrupted.

The health care of poor children, in general, and of children in foster care, in particular, continues to be a key policy issue. The traditional "safety net" previously provided by federal and state programs for economically distressed families (as represented in the past by the Aid to Families with Dependent Children [AFDC] program, Supplemental Security Income [SSI] program, and food stamps) has been substantially dismantled or replaced by new time-limited, benefit-limited programs. Welfare reform replaced AFDC with the Temporary Assistance for Needy Families (TANF) program and significantly narrowed the eligibility of children with disabilities under the SSI program. The cumulative impact of these policy and program changes may result in even more children needing foster care placement unless careful attention is paid to meeting the range of needs of vulnerable children and families.

American Academy of Pediatrics, Committee on Early Childhood, Adoption and Dependent Care: Developmental issues for young children in foster care. *Pediatrics* 2000;106:1145–1150.

Chamberlain P, Price JM, Reid JB, et al: Who disrupts from placement in foster and kinship care? *Child Abuse and Neglect* 2006;30:409–424.

Child Welfare League of America: *Standards for Health Care Services for Children in Out-of-Home Care.* Washington, DC, Child Welfare League of America, 1988.

Diaz A, Edwards S, Neal WP, et al: Foster children with special needs: The Children's Aid Society experience. *Mt Sinai J Med* 2004;71:166–169.

Hansen RL, Mawjee FL, Barton K, et al: Comparing the health status of low-income children in and out of foster care. *Child Welfare* 2004;83:367–380.

Horwitz SM, Balestracci KMB, Simms MD: Foster care placement improves children's functioning. *Arch Pediatr Adolesc Med* 2001;155:1255–1260.

Horwitz SM, Owens PM, Simms MD: Specialized assessment for children in foster care. *Pediatrics* 2000;106:59–66.

Kendall-Tacket KA (editor): *Health Consequences of Abuse in the Family: A Clinical Guide for Evidence-Based Practice.* Washington, DC, American Psychological Association, 2004.

Leslie LK, Hurlburt MS, Landsverk J, et al: Outpatient mental health services for children in foster care: A national perspective. *Child Abuse Negl* 2004;28:699–714.

Leslie LK, Hurlburt MS, Landsverk J, et al: Comprehensive assessments for children entering foster care: A national perspective. *Pediatrics* 2003;112:134–142.

Rubin DM, Alessandrini EA, Feudtner C, et al: Placement changes and emergency department visits in the first year of foster care. *Pediatrics* 2004;114:e354–e360.

Simms MD, Dubowitz H, Szilagyi M: Health care needs of children in the foster care system. *Pediatrics* 2000;106:909–918.

Wyatt DT, Simms MD, Horwitz SM: Widespread growth retardation and variable growth recovery in foster children in the first year after initial placement. *Arch Pediatr Adolesc Med* 1997;151:813–816.

Chapter 35 ■ Impact of Violence on Children

Marilyn Augustyn and Barry Zuckerman

Violence is a major public health problem throughout the world, affecting victim, witness, and perpetrator (see Chapter 1). The focus of pediatrics should not be limited to the traditional care of violence-related injury. Exposure to violence disrupts the healthy development of children; pediatricians need to be aware of this threat. Pediatric providers also have a wider responsibility to advocate on local, state, national, and international levels for safer environments in which all children can grow and thrive.

Witnessing violence is detrimental to children. Because their scars as bystanders are emotional and not physical, the pediatric clinician may not fully appreciate their distress and thereby miss an opportunity to provide needed interventions. For children not living in war zones, the source of 1st exposure to violence is often **domestic violence.** The World Health Organization (WHO) reports that, in every nation studied, 10–50% of women describe having been physically abused by an intimate partner in their lifetime. Each year in the United States, as many as 324,000 pregnant women experience intimate partner violence; pregnancy is one of the highest risk times for domestic violence to a woman. Slightly more than half of female victims of intimate violence live in households with children <12 yr of age; family violence is most likely to be perpetrated by those between the age of 18 and 30 yr ("the child-rearing years"). The majority of children in these homes have witnessed violence; by some estimates, up to three million children per yr. In a national survey, 50% of the men who frequently assaulted their wives also frequently abused their children. Most of the children were injured when they intervened to protect their mother from her partner (see Chapter 36).

Another source of witnessed violence is **community violence.** More than one third of New Orleans school-aged children had witnessed severe violence; 40% had seen a dead body. In inner city Boston, 10% of children <6 yr of age had seen a knifing or shooting. In Los Angeles County, the sheriff's office estimates that children witness 20% of all murders. Young children living in high crime and violence areas observe death more frequently and at younger ages than children growing up in more secure surroundings.

The most ubiquitous source of witnessing violence for children in the United States is **television violence.** The average child 2–5 yr of age watches 20 to 30 hr of television a week, hours that are increasingly filled with scenes of violence. More than 3,500 research studies have examined the association between media violence and violent behavior; all but 18 have shown a positive relationship. Perhaps the most significant event that brought home the power and significance of media exposure in regard to children is September 11, 2001. Children watched TV coverage of the attacks for a mean of 3 hr on September 11; only 34% of parents reported that they restricted their children's television viewing. Although exposure to media violence cannot be equated to exposure to "real-life" violence, many studies confirm that media violence desensitizes children to the meaning and impact of violent behavior. In the case of September 11, among children whose parents did not try to restrict television viewing, there was an association between the number of hours of television viewing and the number of reported stress symptoms. Not all children are equally affected by television violence. Children most at risk from viewing television violence may be children who are also exposed regularly to real-life violence in their homes and communities. Interventions to reduce exposure to media violence are noted in Table 35-1.

TABLE 35-1. Public Health Recommendations to Reduce Effects of Media Violence on Children and Adolescents

Parents should:
- Be made aware of the risks associated with children viewing violent imagery, as it promotes aggressive attitudes, antisocial behavior, fear, and desensitization
- Review the nature, extent, and context of violence in media available to their children before children view
- Assist children's understanding of violent imagery appropriate to their developmental level

Professionals should:
- Offer support and advice to parents who allow their children unsupervised access to extreme violent imagery as this could be seen as a form of emotional abuse and neglect
- Educate all young people in critical film appraisal, in terms of realism, justification, and consequences
- Exercise greater control over access to inappropriate violent media entertainment by young people in secure institutions
- Use violent film material in anger management programs under guidance

Media producers should:
- Reduce violent content and promote antiviolence themes and publicity campaigns
- Ensure that when violence is presented it is in context and associated with remorse, criticism, and penalty
- Ensure that violent action is not justified or its consequences understated

Policy makers should:
- Monitor the nature, extent, and context of violence in all forms of media and implement appropriate guidelines, standards, and penalties
- Ensure that education in media awareness is a priority and a part of school curricula

From Browne KD, Hamilton-Giachritsis C: The influence of violent media on children and adolescents: A public-health approach. *Lancet* 2005;365:702–710.

IMPACTS OF VIOLENCE

The violence children experience and witness also has a profound impact on health and development. In a cross-sectional analysis of a Head Start preschool age cohort, being abused, exposed to domestic violence, and having a mother using substances were associated with a higher number of health problems. Beyond injuries, violence affects children psychologically and behaviorally; it may influence how they view the world and their place in it. Children can come to see the world as a dangerous and unpredictable place. This fear may thwart their exploration of the environment, which is essential to learning in childhood. Children may experience overwhelming terror, helplessness, and fear even if they are not immediately in danger. Preschoolers are most vulnerable to threats that involve the safety (or perceived safety) of their caretakers. High exposure to violence in older children correlates with poorer performances in school, symptoms of anxiety and depression, and lower self-esteem. Violence, particularly domestic violence, can also teach children especially powerful early lessons about the role of violence in relationships. Violence may change the way that children view their future; they may believe that they could die at an early age and thus take more risks, such as drinking alcohol, abusing drugs, not wearing a seatbelt, and not taking prescribed medication.

Some children exposed to severe and/or chronic violence may suffer from post-traumatic stress disorder (PTSD), exhibiting constricted emotions, difficulty concentrating, autonomic disturbances, and re-enactment of the trauma through play or action (see Chapters 1 and 24). Although young children may not fully meet these criteria, certain behavioral changes are commonly associated with exposure to trauma, such as sleep disturbances, aggressive behavior, new fears, and increased anxiety about separations ("clinginess"). A particular challenge in treating and diagnosing pediatric PTSD is that a child's caregiver exposed to the same trauma may be suffering from it as well.

DIAGNOSIS AND FOLLOW-UP. The simplest way to recognize whether violence has become a problem in a family is to question both children (after ≈8 yr of age, depending on the child) and parents on a regular basis. This is particularly important during pregnancy and the immediate postpartum period when women may be at highest risk for being abused. It is important to assure families that they are not being singled out but that all families are asked about their exposure to violence. A direct approach may be useful: "Violence is a major problem in our world today and one that impacts everyone in our society. Thus I have started asking all my patients and families about violence that they are experiencing in their lives. . . ." In other cases, beginning with general questions and then moving to the specific may be helpful. "Do you feel safe in your home and neighborhood? Has anyone ever hurt you or your child?" When violence has impacted the child, it is important to gather details about symptoms and behaviors.

The pediatrician can effectively counsel many parents and children who have been exposed to violence. Regardless of the type of violence to which the child has been exposed, the following components are part of the guidance: careful review of the facts and details of the event, gaining access to support services, providing information about the symptoms and behaviors common in children exposed to violence, assistance in restoring a sense of stability to the family in order to enhance the child's feelings of safety, and helping parents talk to their children about the event. When the symptoms are chronic (>6 mo in duration) or not improving, if the violent event involved the death or departure of a parent, if the caregivers are unable to empathize with the child, or if the ongoing safety of the child is a concern, it is important that the family be referred to mental health professionals for additional treatment.

American Academy of Pediatrics, Committee on Public Education: Media violence. *Pediatrics* 2001;108:1222–1226.

Augustyn M, Groves B, et al: If we don't ask they aren't going to tell: Screening for domestic vidence. *Contemp Pediatr* 2005;22:43–52.

Bickham DS, Rich M: Is television viewing associated with social isolation? Roles of exposure time, viewing context, and violent content. *Arch Pediatr Adolesc Med* 2006;160(4):387–392.

Browne KD, Hamilton-Giachritsis C: The influence of violent media on children and adolescents: A public-health approach. *Lancet* 2005;365:702–710.

Buka SL, Stichick TL, Birdhistle I, et al: Youth exposure to violence: Prevalence, risks, and consequences. *Am J Orthopsychiatry* 2001;71:298–310.

Davies P, Lee L, Fox A, et al: Could nursery rhymes cause violent behaviour? A comparison with television viewing. *Arch Dis Child* 2004;89:1103–1105.

Eisenstat SA, Bancroft L: Domestic violence. *N Engl J Med* 1999;341:886–892.

Gazmararian JA, Petersen R, Spitz AM, et al: Violence and reproductive health; current knowledge and future research directions. *Matern Child Health J* 2000;4:79–84.

Graham-Bermann SA, Seng J: Violence exposure and traumatic stress symptoms as additional predictors of health problems in high-risk children. *J Pediatr* 2005;146:309–310.

Groves B: Witness to violence. In Parker S, Zuckerman B, Augustyn M (editors): *Handbook of Developmental and Behavioral Pediatrics,* 2nd ed. Baltimore, Lippincott Williams & Wilkins, 2005, pp 370–372.

Hurt H, Malmud E, Brodky NL, et al: Exposure to violence. *Arch Pediatr Adolesc Med* 2001;155:1351–1356.

Martin SL, Mackie L, Kupper LL, et al: Physical abuse of women before, during, and after pregnancy. *JAMA* 2001;285:1581–1584.

Nansel TR, Overpeck M, Pilla RS, et al: Bullying behaviors among US youth: Prevalence and association with psychosocial adjustment. *JAMA* 2001;285:2094–2100.

Roy E, Haley N, Leelere P, et al: Mortality in a cohort of street youth in Montreal. *JAMA* 2004;292:569–574.

Schuster MA, Stein BD, Jaycox LH, et al: A national survey of stress reactions after the September 11, 2001 terrorist attacks. *N Engl J Med* 2001;345:1507–1512.

Stringham P: Violent youth. In Parker S, Zuckerman B, Augustyn M (editors): *Handbook of Developmental and Behavioral Pediatrics,* 2nd ed. Baltimore, Lippincott Williams & Wilkins, 2005, pp 361–365.

U.S. Department of Justice: Violence by Intimates: Analysis of Data on Crimes by Current or Former Spouses, Boyfriends, and Girlfriends, March 1998.

World Health Organizations: Violence against women. *http://www.who.int/mediacentre/factsheets.*

35.1 • Bullying and School Violence •

Douglas Vanderbilt and Marilyn Augustyn

BULLYING

DEFINITION. Bullying affects a large number of children and lays the groundwork for ongoing depression, suicidality, conduct problems, and psychosomatic concerns seen in children. Bullying is the assertion of power through aggression that involves a bully repeatedly and intentionally targeting a weaker victim through social, emotional, or physical means. Children can move between being a bully, victim, bully-victim (both a bully and a victim at different times), or bystander. Bullying can be **direct**, involving physical aggression such as hitting, stealing, and threatening with a weapon or verbal aggression such as name-calling, public humiliation, and intimidation, or it can be **indirect,** involving relational aggression such as spreading rumors, social rejection, exclusion from peer groups, and ignoring. Bullying occurs most frequently at school when there is minimal supervision during breaks, recess, and lunch at playgrounds, in hallways, and en route to and from school. The Internet is another venue for this behavior and takes place through mass emailing, chat rooms, and message boards.

EPIDEMIOLOGY. Bullying is a common occurrence for schoolchildren. Bullying occurs in all countries, affecting 9% to 54% of youth. In the United States, 30% of middle and upper school students report moderate or frequent involvement with bullying as a victim, perpetrator, or bully-victim. National studies have found 7% of children aged 12–18 yr self-report being bullied while at school, with higher rates seen among rural and public schools and in lower grades. Older children are less likely to talk about their victimization, with only 50% of all children confiding in anyone. Boys are twice as likely as girls to be bullies, more than three times as likely to be bully-victims, and twice as likely to be victims.

HEALTH STATUS. Involvement in bullying is associated with poorer psychosocial adjustment; bullies, victims, and bully-victims report greater health problems and poorer emotional and social adjustment. Victims tend to be either physically weak and emotionally vulnerable or provocative, with attention or conduct problems. Overall, **both** victim groups are anxious, insecure, lonely, and lack social skills; their external characteristics do not necessarily set them apart from others. Victims can have lower social status and higher social marginalization and isolation. They have more depression, psychosomatic complaints, and suicidality. Long-term consequences in adulthood of being bullied as a child include depression, poor self-esteem, and abusive relationships.

Bullies have higher rates of both conduct disorders and social standing. They have the lowest rates of adjustment problems because of their higher social status, but peers avoid them. Bullies have higher rates of depression and psychological distress as compared to those who deny their bullying behavior. They have higher negative attitudes toward school and more use drugs. Childhood bullies have a fourfold increase in criminal behavior by their mid twenties and are at higher risk of dropping out of school. The bully-victim has problems with peer relationships and high rates of depression, loneliness, alcohol use, and weapon carrying.

SCHOOL VIOLENCE

EPIDEMIOLOGY. Bullying may be an important precursor to more serious school violence; it is not a normative aspect of development. School violence and weapon carrying occur throughout the United States and other sites worldwide. In Great Britain, about 30% of 11–15 yr old males and 10% of females report having taken a weapon to school once; 3% of Norwegian 12–14 yr old respondents report having been involved in a fight using a weapon at least once in the past year; and 11% of Swiss adolescents brought a weapon to school during their lifetime. Whereas urban schools experience more episodes of violence, the episodes of "rampage" gun violence in rural and suburban schools demonstrate that no region is immune to lethal violence.

RISK FACTORS. Nonlethal violence, serious bullying, carrying illegal guns, mental health problems, student attacks on teachers, and the effects of rapid economic change in communities can all lead to school violence. Additional risk factors for violence include early childbearing, low intelligence, poor academic performance, early aggression, victimization as a child, weak family bonding, substance abuse, poverty, and racism. In one study, the homicide perpetrators in school-associated violent deaths were twice as likely to have been bullied as compared to the homicide victims.

There is more school violence in areas with higher crime rates and more street gangs, with little improvement with additional security measures. These risks take away students' ability to learn in a safe environment and leave many children with traumatic stress and grief reactions.

TREATMENT AND PREVENTION OF BULLYING AND SCHOOL VIOLENCE

Pediatricians are in a unique position to screen, treat, and advocate for reducing the impact of school violence by treating those affected and seeking to prevent further occurrences. **Signs** of a child being bullied include physical complaints such as insomnia, stomachaches, headaches, and new onset enuresis. **Psychologic symptoms** such as depression, loneliness, anxiety, and suicidal ideation may occur. **Behavioral changes** such as irritability, poor concentration, school avoidance, and substance abuse are common. **School problems** such as academic failure, social problems, and lack of friends can also occur. Additional vigilance must be made for those children with chronic medical illnesses, obesity, or physical deformities, and students in special education who may be potential targets. A bully may be more difficult to identify due to the bully's desire to obscure the behavior. Children who are aggressive, overly confident, lacking in empathy, and having conduct problems may need careful screening. The physical, behavioral, psychologic, and school symptoms of bullying may overlap with other conditions such as medical illness, learning problems, and psychologic disorders.

Management of bullying involves interventions with parents, victims, bullies, and the school. Interventions should include supporting families, victims, and bullies; referring those children in need of further mental health services; and expecting behavioral change from the bully and social change from the school environment. The clinician should listen empathetically to the child to help empower and reassure him or her. The clinician should not blame the victim or trivialize the child's concern. Suggestions should include having the child seek social support from teachers and friends and avoid situations where the bullying may occur. Role-playing an encounter can be helpful for the child. Extracurricular activities like drama clubs and sports can be used to help to bolster the child's self-esteem. The clinician should identify safety issues such as suicidal ideation and plans, substance abuse, and other high-risk behaviors.

Once a bully is identified and appropriate screening for risk factors is completed, the clinician should educate the parents and child about the seriousness of the behavior and its potential consequences. The clinician should label the behavior as the problem and help the family and child to acknowledge the behavior as hurtful. For example: "Do you feel bad when other children hurt your feelings?" "Bullying hurts other children's feelings." The school and parents should ensure accountability for the child's subsequent behavior.

School violence prevention programs focus on many pathways to aggressive behavior. One group of programs addresses problem solving, basic interpersonal skill building, and nonviolent conflict resolution. These programs have been found to be effective in the short-term studies. More broad-based strategies, which involve parents and community organizations with the school, can reduce violence by increasing rewards for academic achievement. Addressing access to firearms, the sensitivity of youth's fragile self-esteem, and the gap between youth and adults are important in creating a safe school climate.

American Medical Association's Council on Scientific Affairs (CSA): CSA: Report 11 of the Council on Scientific Affairs (I-99) Full Text: School Violence, available at http://www.ama-assn.org/ama/pub/category/13596.html, accessed 4/20/05.

American Medical Association's Council on Scientific Affairs (CSA): Featured CSA Report: Bullying Behaviors Among Children and Adolescents (A-02) Full Text, available at http://www.ama-assn.org/ama/pub/category/14312.html, accessed 4/20/05.

Department of Health and Human Services: Take a stand! Lend a hand! Stop bullying now! available at http://stopbullyingnow.hrsa.gov/index.asp, accessed.

Fekkes M, Pijpers FI, Verloove-Vanhorick SP: Effects of antibullying school program on bullying and health complaints. *Arch Pediatr Adolesc Med* 2006;160(6):638–644.

Kuntsche EN, Klingemann HK: Weapon-carrying at Swiss schools? A gender-specific typology in context of victim and offender related violence. *J Adolesc* 2004;27:381–393.

Moore M, Petrie C, Braga A, McLaughlin B (editors): *Deadly Lessons: Understanding Lethal School Violence.* National Research Council 2003, available at http://www.nap.edu/books/0309084121/html/1.html, accessed 4/20/05.

Nansel TR, Craig W, Overpeck MD, et al: Cross-national consistency in the relationship between bullying behaviors and psychosocial adjustment. *Arch Pediatr Adolesc Med* 2004;158:730–736.

National Center for Education Statistics: Indicators of School Crime and Safety: 2004, available at http://nces.ed.gov/pubs2005/crime_safe04/index.asp, accessed 4/20/05.

Juvonen J, Graham S, Schuster M: Bullying among young adolescents: The strong, the weak, and the troubled. *Pediatrics* 2003;112:1231–1237.

Nansel TR, Overpeck M, Pilla RS, et al: Bullying behaviors among US youth: Prevalence and association with psychosocial adjustment. *JAMA* 2001;285:2094–2100.

Vanderbilt D: Bullying. In Parker S, Zuckerman B, Augustyn M (editors): *Behavioral and Developmental Pediatrics: A Handbook for Primary Care.* Lippincott Williams & Wilkins 2004, pp 141–144.

35.2 • Effects of War on Children •

Isaiah D. Wexler and Eitan Kerem

The impact of war is devastating, and its effects can last for decades after hostilities have ceased. Based on the most recent statistics accrued by the United Nations Children's Fund (UNICEF), of the 3.6 million people killed as a result of military conflict between the years 1990 and 2003, 90% were civilian and 50% were children. During the violent civil war in Rwanda, 300,000 children were killed over a 90 day period.

Mortality and morbidity related to the long-term effects of war and civil strife are often higher than that occurring during actual fighting. War and violence are not listed as leading causes of childhood mortality. Nonetheless, the regions with the highest levels of child mortality, especially among children <5 yr of age, are the same locations involved in military conflicts. Nations, especially the least developed, devote substantial portions of their budgets to military expenditures at the expense of the health care infrastructure.

TABLE 35-2. Impact of War on Children

PHYSICAL
Death
Rape
Injuries
Amputations and fractures
Head trauma
Ballistic wounds
Blast injuries
Burns
Chemical and biologic induced
Malnutrition and starvation
Infectious disease
Displacement
PSYCHOSOCIAL
Loss of caregivers and family members
Separation from community
Lack of education
Inappropriate socialization
Acute stress reaction
Post-traumatic stress disorder
Depression
Maladaptive behavior
EXPLOITATION
Conscription as soldiers
Coerced involvement in terrorist activities
Prostitution
Slavery
Forced adoption

The morbidity of children exposed to conflicts is significant (Table 35-2). Many more children are physically harmed than killed. The number of children who have suffered serious injuries in the past decade is estimated to be six million; over 20 million children have been displaced from their homes as a result of war and associated human rights violations. Children bear the psychological scars of war resulting from exposure to violent events, loss of primary caregivers, and forced removal from their homes. During periods of war, children are more susceptible to exploitation in the forms of forced conscription as soldiers, sexual exploitation, and slavery. There are ≈300,000 soldiers under the age of 18 yr who are actively participating in military conflicts worldwide. Lacking the appropriate education and socialization, the moral compass of these children is often misaligned. They are not capable of understanding the sources of conflict or why they have been targeted. Their thought processes are more concrete; it is easier for them to dehumanize their adversaries. Children, who themselves are exposed to violence and cruelty, often become the worst perpetrators of atrocities.

After cessation of hostilities, children are still at risk for life-endangering injuries from landmines and unexploded ordnance. The International Campaign to Ban Landmines estimates that there are up to 20,000 landmine and unexploded ordnance casualties per yr; a significant proportion are children. The U.S. Centers for Disease Control and Prevention (CDC) reported that in a 5 yr period ending in 2002, the proportion of children injured by landmines and unexploded ordnance was 2.3 times higher than adults in Afghanistan.

SUSCEPTIBILITY OF CHILDREN IN TIMES OF WAR

Children do not have the physical or intellectual capabilities to defend themselves. It is easier for adults to victimize children rather than other adults. Older children's curiosity, desire for adventure, and imperfect assessment of risk often lead them to participate in risky behavior. Younger children, because of their small size and immature physiology, are more susceptible to disease and starvation, and are more likely to sustain fatal injuries from ballistic projectiles and explosive devices such as mines.

During times of war, there is a breakdown of social inhibitions and cultural norms. Aberrant behavior such as rape, torture, and pillaging, which would be nearly inconceivable in times of peace, is common during war. Children may be attacked or used as human shields. Instincts such as parents' desires to protect their children are often extinguished.

The changing nature of war has adversely affected children. Conventional warfare in which armies of professional soldiers representing different countries battle each other has become less common. Intrastate conflicts in the form of civil war are more frequent. Of the 190 armed conflicts occurring after World War II, 75% of them were intrastate. These conflicts are often rooted in ethnic or religious differences, and the participants are frequently nonprofessional "irregulars" who lack discipline and accountability to higher echelons. Quite often, the military resources of the antagonists are disproportionate, leading the weaker protagonist to develop compensatory tactics that can include guerrilla and terrorist activities. Low-intensity conflicts have become more common. These types of conflicts are often characterized by military activities targeting civilian populations with the goal of disrupting normal routines and generating publicity for the perpetrators. Children are often victims, as this serves to maximize the impact of terrorist activity. A particularly tragic example was the takeover of a public school in Beslan, Russia, in 2004; more than 800 children, together with their teachers and parents, were taken hostage and many of them were subsequently killed.

Terrorism is designed to coerce and/or intimidate both individuals and entire societies. The destruction of the New York City World Trade Center Towers in 2001 and the nearly 3,000 fatalities showed that highly organized and motivated terrorists have few inhibitions and can strike anywhere. Biological and chemical terrorism has also been realized with nerve gas attacks on subways in Japan and the release of anthrax spores in the United States. Children are more susceptible to chemical and biological toxins because of their higher respiratory rates, more permeable skin, and other developmental vulnerabilities. Heavier-than-air gases such as sarin and chlorine cling to the ground and are more likely to be inhaled by children, who are relatively short (see also chapter 712).

The media has had a significant role in exacerbating the effects of war on children. Media coverage of war and terrorist events is extensive and graphic. Children, who are more impressionable than adults, often view this material in an uncontrolled fashion (see Table 35-1). Uncensored pictures of victims, unbridled violence, people in shock, or family members searching through ruins for relatives may either traumatize children or encourage inappropriate behavior. Overt broadcast propaganda glorifying war and violence may sway children to participate in militaristic or antisocial activities.

PSYCHOLOGICAL IMPACT OF WAR

Exposure to war and violence can have a significant impact on a child's psychosocial development. Displacement, loss of caregivers, physical suffering, and the lack of appropriate socialization all contribute to abnormal child development (see Table 35-2). Often the reactions are age-specific (Table 35-3). Preschoolers may have an increase in somatic complaints and sleep disturbances, and have acting-out behavior such as tantrums or excessively clinging behavior. School-aged children will show regressive behavior such as enuresis and thumb sucking. They too have an increase in somatic complaints; there is often a negative impact on school performance. For teenagers, psychological withdrawal and depression are common. Adolescents often exhibit trauma-stimulated acting-out behavior. Motivated by the desire for revenge, they may be quick to join in the violence and contribute to the continuation of conflict.

TABLE 35-3. Manifestations of Stress Reactions in Children and Adolescents Exposed to War and Terrorism

CHILDREN ≤5 YEARS
Excessive fear of separation
Clinging behavior
Uncontrollable crying or screaming
Freezing (persistent immobility)
Sleep disorders
Terrified affect
Regressive behavior
CHILDREN 6–11 YEARS
Decline in school performance
Truancy
Sleep disorders
Somatization
Depressive affect
Abnormally aggressive or violent behavior
Irrational fears
Regressive and childish behavior
ADOLESCENTS 12–17 YEARS
Decline in school performance
Sleep disturbances
Flashbacks
Emotional numbness
Antisocial behavior
Substance abuse
Revenge fantasies
Suicidal ideation
Withdrawal

There is an increased incidence of both acute stress reactions and PTSD (see Chapter 24). The true incidence is difficult to assess because of the heterogeneous nature of war, degree of exposure to violence, and methodologic challenges. The incidence of PTSD increased from 2% to 10.5% among New York City metropolitan area school-aged children and adolescents after the destruction of the World Trade Center. Risk factors for having a more serious psychologic response to a violent event include severity of the incident, personal involvement (physical injury, proximity, loss of a relative), prior history of exposure to traumatic events, female gender, and a dysfunctional parental response to the same event.

The manifestations of PTSD in children differ from those of adults, and include anxiety, disorganized and agitated behavior (hypervigilance, hyperactivity), autonomic hypersensitivity, somatization, depression, and sleep disturbances. The onset of PTSD symptomatology can be delayed; it is not unusual for children to develop PTSD many years after the traumatic event. Children do not have to be directly exposed to violent activity, and media coverage of terrorist events may be sufficient to trigger PTSD.

EFFORTS TO PROTECT CHILDREN FROM THE EFFECTS OF WAR

INTERNATIONAL CONVENTIONS. War and terror violate the human rights of children, including the right to life, the right to be nurtured and protected, the right to develop appropriately, the right to be with family and community, and the right to a healthy existence. Several international treaties and conventions have been ratified beginning with the **4th Geneva Convention** (1949) that set forth guidelines regarding appropriate treatment of children in times of war. The **United Nations Convention on the Rights of the Child (1990)** delineated specific human rights inherent to every child (defined as any individual younger than the age of

18 yr). **The Rome Statute of the International Criminal Court** that was enacted in 2002 declared that the conscription or enlistment of children younger than the age of 15 yr is a prosecutable war crime.

Although these treaties and conventions define the extent of protection afforded to children, the means of enforcement available to the international community is limited. Individuals, motivated by religious fervor, nationalistic zeal, or ethnic xenophobia, are unlikely to curb their activities because of fear of prosecution. These treaties better serve in heightening awareness regarding the protected status of children in wartime, and perhaps deter high-ranking leaders who fear being held accountable for war crimes.

HUMANITARIAN EFFORTS. Several organizations, either nongovernmental or under the auspices of the United Nations, are involved in mitigating the effects of war on children. These organizations, which include the International Red Cross, UNICEF, United Nations Refugee Agency (UNCHR), World Health Organization, and Medicins Sans Frontieres (Doctors Without Borders) have had a significant impact on reducing violence-related casualties in war-torn regions. The infusion of humanitarian aid into developing countries often improves overall mortality and morbidity by increasing the level of medical and social services available to the general population. Other organizations such as Amnesty International, Stockholm International Peace Research Institute, and Physicians for Human Rights actively monitor human rights abuses involving children and other civilian groups. In 2005, the United Nations Security Council approved the establishment of a monitoring and reporting system designed to protect children exposed to war. United Nations–led task forces will conduct active surveillance in regions of conflict and monitor the killing or injuring of children, recruitment of child soldiers, attacks directed against schools or hospitals, sexual violence against children, abduction of children, and denial of humanitarian access for children.

THE ROLE OF PEDIATRICIANS AND ALLIED HEALTH PROFESSIONALS

War is a chronic condition and health providers need to be prepared to treat childhood casualties resulting from military or terrorist activity as well as caring for children suffering from the aftermath of war or related violence. Community and hospital pediatricians need to be involved in community disaster planning. Quite often, general disaster planning ignores the unique needs and requirements of children; in planning for a possible chemical attack, appropriate resuscitation equipment suitable for children needs to be stockpiled. The signs of biological infection or chemical intoxication are different for children, and pediatricians and emergency personnel need to be aware of these differences (see Chapter 711). Professional organizations such as the American Academy of Pediatrics (AAP) and the CDC have published position papers; there is a special section in the AAP *Red Book* that presents guidelines for treating specific pathogens likely to be utilized in biological warfare. In regions where violent terrorist activity is likely, pediatricians, nurses, and rescue personnel should consider becoming certified in the Red Cross Basic and Advanced Trauma Life Support.

Pediatricians need to be cognizant of the effects that war and terror can have on parents and children. Parents, who themselves are under tremendous strain, may not be sensitive to the effects that the same stressors have on their children. Pediatricians should draw out both parents and children, and encourage them to talk freely about their feelings. Child health care providers can be instrumental in educating parents to be more aware of inappropriate responses by children to war and violence. When necessary, pediatricians can serve their families by referring them to appropriate support services.

In day-to-day patient interactions, a pediatrician is most likely to confront situations related to stress reactions such as PTSD. Recognition of PTSD is essential so that early treatment can be initiated. Clues to the presence of PTSD include changes in behavior, school performance, affect, and sleep patterns, and an increase in somatic complaints. The fact that the triggering event is neither temporally nor physically proximate should not dissuade the pediatrician from making an appropriate referral to mental health professionals expert in childhood stress disorders. There are several brief and easy to administer psychologic instruments based on the *Diagnostic and Statistical Manual of Mental Disorders, 4th Edition* (DSM-IV) criteria for PTSD such as the Trauma Symptom Checklist for Children and the Impact of Events Scale—8 items for children (IES-8). Many are available on the internet (http://www.ncptsd.va.gov).

It is not to be expected that health care personnel remain neutral in times of war. Pediatricians, similar to other individuals, are motivated by patriotism, nationalistic pride, political ideologies, and religious fervor. They often serve as military physicians and may be active participants in military campaigns. Medical profession standards, however, demand from each physician that he or she treat all patients equitably without regard to their background. Both international law and professional medical societies ban physicians from actively participating in torture or other activities that infringe on human rights, including those of children. It is difficult to countenance any situation in which a health professional, even acting as a representative of his or her country, might directly or indirectly injure a minor.

Barenbaum J, Ruchkin V, Schwab-Stone M: The psychosocial aspects of children exposed to war: Practice and policy initiatives. *J Child Psychol Psychiatry* 2004;45:41–62.

Bellamy C: *The State of the World's Children 2005*. New York, United Nations Children's Fund, 2004.

Fremont WP: Childhood reactions to terrorism-induced trauma: A review of the past 10 years. *J Am Acad Child Adolesc Psychiatry* 2004;43:381–392.

Hagan JF Jr; American Academy of Pediatrics Committee on Psychosocial Aspects of Child and Family Health; Task Force on Terrorism: Psychosocial implications of disaster or terrorism on children: A guide for the pediatrician. *Pediatrics* 2005;116:787–795.

Joshi PT, O'Donnell DA: Consequences of child exposure to war and terrorism. *Clin Child Fam Psychol Rev* 2003;6:275–292.

Krug EG, Dahlberg LL, Mercy JA, et al (editors): *World Report on Violence and Health*. Geneva, World Health Organization, 2002.

[no authors listed]: Chemical-biological terrorism and its impact on children: A subject review. American Academy of Pediatrics. Committee on Environmental Health and Committee on Infectious Diseases. *Pediatrics* 2000;105:662–670.

Pfefferbaum B, Seale TW, Brandt EN Jr, et al: Media exposure in children one hundred miles from a terrorist bombing. *Ann Clin Psychiatry* 2003;15:1–8.

Seaman J, Maguire S: The special needs of children and women. *Br Med J* 2005;331:34–36.

Wexler ID, Branski D, Kerem E: Treatment of sick children during low-intensity conflict. *Lancet* 2005;365:1278–1279.

Wiesel E: Without conscience. *N Engl J Med* 2005;352:1511–1513.

Chapter 36 ■ Abuse and Neglect of Children

Charles F. Johnson

Child maltreatment encompasses a spectrum of abusive actions, or acts of **commission**, and lack of action, or acts of **omission**, that result in morbidity or death (Fig. 36-1). Acts of omission and commission before birth, such as maternal drug abuse and failure to seek appropriate health care during pregnancy, may also have adverse effects on the child. **Physical abuse** may be narrowly

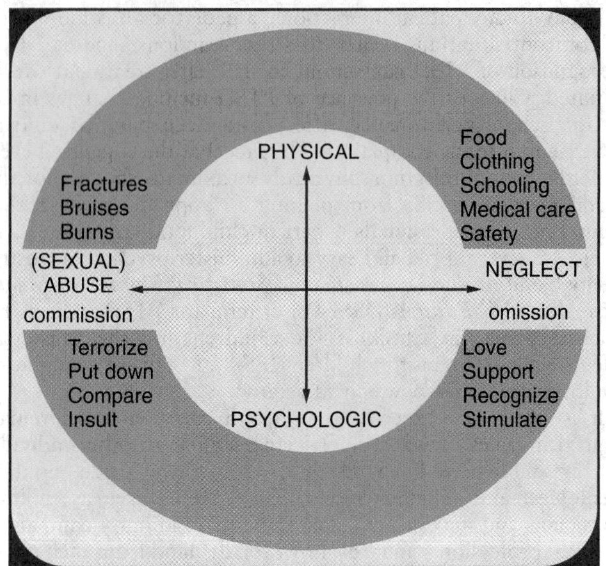

Figure 36-1. The spectrum of child maltreatment. Child maltreatment encompasses acts of commission, abuse, and acts of omission or neglect by a caretaker that adversely affect children. The act can be physical or psychologic. The boundaries between these areas are indistinct and psychologic; physical abuse and neglect overlap and may exist at the same time or various times in a child's life. Sexual abuse may be considered a specific type of physical abuse that has strong emotional components. Physical abuse and neglect invariably have short- and long-term psychologic consequences. Psychologic consequences may persist long after the physical wounds heal.

defined as intentional injuries to a child by a caregiver that result in bruises, burns, fractures, lacerations, punctures, or solid organ damage. A broader definition would include short- and long-term emotional consequences, which can be more debilitating and longer lasting than the physical effects. **Physical neglect** and other acts of omission may result in failure to thrive, developmental or education delays, and increased susceptibility to infection. **Nutritional neglect** is the most common cause of poor weight gain in infancy and may account for more than half the cases of failure to thrive (see Chapter 37). Physicians are most likely to identify medical neglect that results from the failure of a parent to provide appropriate medical care, whereas failure to provide shelter, schooling, adequate clothing, and protection from environmental hazards tends to be observed by neighbors, relatives, teachers, home visiting nurses, and social workers. **Medical neglect** of a child with an acute or chronic disease may result in worsening of the condition and death.

Parents may refuse to allow recommended medical treatments because of personal or religious beliefs. The determination of whether this constitutes neglect and, if so, what the appropriate action for a physician to take is a difficult decision (see Chapter 4). Neglect of appropriate precautions by caregivers to ensure a child's safety may also involve difficult matters of judgment. Children may be injured despite a variety of protective actions by well-meaning parents. Parenting practices regarding physical punishment vary widely according to different religious and cultural beliefs. Spanking (with an open hand) is one of the most commonly practiced forms of discipline, with over 90% of families in the United States reporting the use of spanking at some time to discipline their children.

Psychologic maltreatment includes intentional verbal or behavioral acts or omissions that result in adverse emotional or physical consequences. A caregiver may intentionally fail to provide nurturing verbal and behavioral actions that are necessary for healthy development. Psychologic maltreatment of a child by a caregiver includes spurning, exploiting/corrupting, withholding emotional responsiveness, isolating, or terrorizing. Psychologic maltreatment may be difficult to document when psychiatric, physical, or emotional consequences are delayed. **Sexual abuse** refers to any act intended for the sexual gratification of an adult. Sexual abuse may be perpetrated by family members (incest), acquaintances, or, least often, strangers. (See also Chapter 118.)

Medications, toxins, and other substances may be given to poison a child intentionally. When this or any other deceptive action is undertaken to simulate a disorder, it is referred to as **Munchausen syndrome by proxy.** The induced symptoms and signs may lead to unnecessary medical investigation, hospital admissions, or treatment; death occurs in as many as 10% of these cases.

Legal definitions of what constitutes abuse and neglect vary from state to state in the United States and between nations. Physicians and other providers of care to children are required by law in all 50 states in the United States to report **suspected** child abuse or neglect. These laws afford protection from lawsuits to mandated reporters who report in good faith; they also allow for clinical and laboratory evaluations and photo documentation without the parent's or guardian's permission. Failure to report suspected child abuse may result in a penalty. It may also result in a malpractice claim for damages incurred as a result of failure to report, which might have protected the child from further injury. At least seven nations—Austria, Denmark, Finland, Germany, Iceland, Norway, and Sweden—have laws that specifically prohibit physical punishment of children.

EPIDEMIOLOGY

U.S. STATISTICS. After mandated reporting began in the United States in the 1960s, the number of reports to Children's Protective Services (CPS) and law enforcement agencies in the county in which the alleged abuse or neglect occurred steadily increased. In 1976, there were 669,000 *reports* of child maltreatment. This number reached three million in 1995 (1 in every 25 children). The increase in reports has been attributed to improved case finding and reporting. From 1993 to 1999, victimization rates per 1,000 children gradually declined from 15.3 to 11.8. They gradually rose to 12.3/1,000 in 2002. The Child Maltreatment 2000 report indicated an estimated 896,000 victims in 2002. Of the victims, 60% experienced neglect, 10% were sexually abused, and 7% suffered psychologic maltreatment. The highest victimization rate of 16/1,000 was among children from birth to 3 yr of age. The highest rates of victimization were among American Indian or Alaska Native (21.7/1,000) and African-American (20.2/1,000) children in comparison to white children (10.7/1,000).

The National Child Abuse and Neglect Data System (NCANDS) indicated that neglect, physical abuse, sexual abuse, and psychologic maltreatment constituted 60%, 20%, 10%, and 7%, respectively, of *confirmed* cases. The rate of maltreatment declined with advancing age of the child. Of perpetrators, 80% were parents; 58% were female. Males were the most common perpetrators of sexual abuse. Of 2.6 million referrals to CPS involving 4.5 million children, 65% (≈1.8 million) were accepted for investigation. Of the reports, 30% were substantiated as maltreatment and, of those, 59% received services. An estimated 1,400 children or 1.98 per 100,000 died of abuse in 2002. Children <1 yr old accounted for 41% of the fatalities; 76% were <4 yr old. Neglect was the most common cause of death (38.2%), followed by abuse (30%) and multiple maltreatment (29%). With the advent of child death review teams, it is expected that more child abuse deaths will be ascertained. Studies in Colorado and North Carolina indicate that 50–60% of child maltreatment deaths are not recorded.

The prevalence of abuse is unknown. A survey of families with children aged 3–18 yr indicated that 140/1,000 (14%) were kicked, bitten, punched, hit with an object, beaten up, or threatened with a knife or gun in 1 yr. A 1995 Gallup telephone survey indicated that 49 of every 1,000 children (5%) may have been physically abused. The spectrum of child victimization is quite broad and the services are fragmented. A survey of parents and children conducted between December 2002 and February 2003 of the experiences of 2,030 children aged 2–17 yr indicated that more than half of the children had experienced an assault in that period, with 10% suffering an injury. Of the assault perpetrators, 54% were family members, including siblings. One in 12 experienced sexual victimization. Child maltreatment occurred to approximately one in 7 children. In a study of adverse childhood experiences (ACEs), the prevalence of sexual abuse, physical abuse, and witnessing maternal battering during childhood was 22%, 21%, and 14%, respectively. Approximately 10% of injuries to children <5 yr old that are seen in emergency departments are due to abuse; 15% of children admitted for burns and 50% of children <1 yr of age with fractures have been abused.

GLOBAL STATISTICS. In its 5th edition of the Innocenti Report Card, a series of analyses of child health and welfare in the 30 nations in the Organization for Economic Cooperation and Development, the nations producing two thirds of the world's services and goods, the United Nations Children's Fund (UNICEF) estimates that 3,500 children die annually from child abuse occurring in developed nations. Death rates due to abuse range from 0.1 per 100,000 children in Spain to 2.4 in the United States and Mexico (Table 36-1). When deaths of "undetermined intent" are included, the rates remain the same in Spain but increase among several nations including the United States, Mexico, and Portugal where the adjusted rates are, respectively, 2.4, 3.0, and 3.7 deaths per 100,000 children. Among the 23 nations for which longitudinal data are available, 14 demonstrate a decline in child maltreatment death rates from the 1970s through the 1990s, while four are static and five show an increase. Those countries with the lowest child maltreatment death rates also have the lowest adult homicide rates; those with the highest child maltreatment death rates also have the highest adult homicide rates. Recognizing that data from much of the world are uncertain, UNICEF estimates that, globally, 40 million children aged <15 yr suffer from abuse and neglect. An estimated two million children are involved in pornography or prostitution and 300,000 serve as soldiers in armed conflict.

TABLE 36-1. Child Maltreatment Deaths by Nation

Country	Deaths per 100,000 children*
Spain	0.1
Greece	0.2
Italy	0.2
Ireland	0.3
Norway	0.3
Netherlands	0.6
Sweden	0.6
Korea	0.8
Australia	0.8
Germany	0.8
Denmark	0.8
Finland	0.8
Poland	0.9
UK	0.9
Swizerland	0.9
Canada	1.0
Austria	1.0
Japan	1.0
Slovak Republic	1.0
Belgium	1.1
Czech Republic	1.2
New Zealand	1.3
Hungary	1.3
France	1.4
USA	2.4
Mexico	3.0
Portugal	3.7

*Deaths include obvious maltreatment and those of undermined intent.
From UNICEF: A league table of child maltreatment deaths in rich nations. *Inocenti Report Card* No 5, September 2003, UNICEF Innocenti Research Centre, Florence. Figure 1b, page 4.

PHYSICAL ABUSE. Although varying definitions and reporting requirements prevent detailed comparisons, parents who abuse their children have been reported from most ethnic, geographic, religious, educational, occupational, and socioeconomic groups. Groups living in poverty have increased reports of physical abuse because of the increased number of crises in their lives (unemployment or overcrowding); limited access to economic or social resources for support in times of stress; the increased violence in the communities where they live; an association of poverty with other risk factors, such as teenaged and single parenthood and substance abuse; and the possibility of more scrutiny by community agencies and neighbors. Likewise, an increased incidence of physical abuse has been noted on military bases. This may be due to increased surveillance as well as increased risk factors. The presence of spouse abuse increases the likelihood of child abuse (see Chapter 35). Substance abuse is a common finding in families with abused children. Approximately 10–40% of abusive parents have experienced physical abuse as children.

Physical abuse is most likely to occur when a high-risk parent responsible for the care of a high-risk child undergoes stress and reacts to stress with violence. More than 90% of abusing parents have neither psychotic nor criminal personalities. They tend to be lonely, unhappy, angry, young, single parents who do not plan their closely spaced pregnancies, have little or no knowledge of child development and child health, and have **unrealistic expectations** for child behavior. Mentally retarded children are more at risk for abuse and neglect. Their parents may injure them in anger after being provoked by what they consider a misbehavior that is actually related to a handicap. Associated neuromuscular problems may increase the likelihood of nonaccidental trauma. Other high-risk children include premature infants, infants with chronic medical conditions, colicky babies, and children with learning and behavior problems. The child may be normal but misperceived by an inexperienced parent as difficult, unusual, or abnormal. Behaviors such as crying, wetting, soiling, and spilling may cause the parent to lose control and injure a child. A family crisis may precipitate the abuse: loss of a job or home, marital strife, death of a sibling, physical exhaustion, or development of an acute or chronic physical or mental illness in the parent or child. Determination of risk factors for abuse and neglect should begin during pregnancy and continue through childhood as part of the routine well baby care and in all cases of childhood injury. Risk factors in parents or child may increase the suspicion of abuse. Even when abuse cannot be documented, significant risk factors should necessitate referral to CPS for support, education, treatment, and preventive services.

CLINICAL MANIFESTATIONS. Physical abuse is suspected when an injury is unexplained, unexplainable, or implausible. If an injury is incompatible with the history given or with the child's development, **suspected abuse** should be reported. Diagnostic certainty of physical abuse is not required to file a report. The ultimate determination of maltreatment (**substantiation**) is made by CPS and the legal system. When children are hurt, it is expected that parents will bring them immediately for examination. A delay in seeking medical help should increase suspicion of abuse or neglect. A delay may also be due to a lack of transportation or ignorance about the significance of disease or injury. Before reporting suspected medical neglect, the physician should determine whether the parents have an understanding of disease processes and the intellectual, emotional, economic, and physical

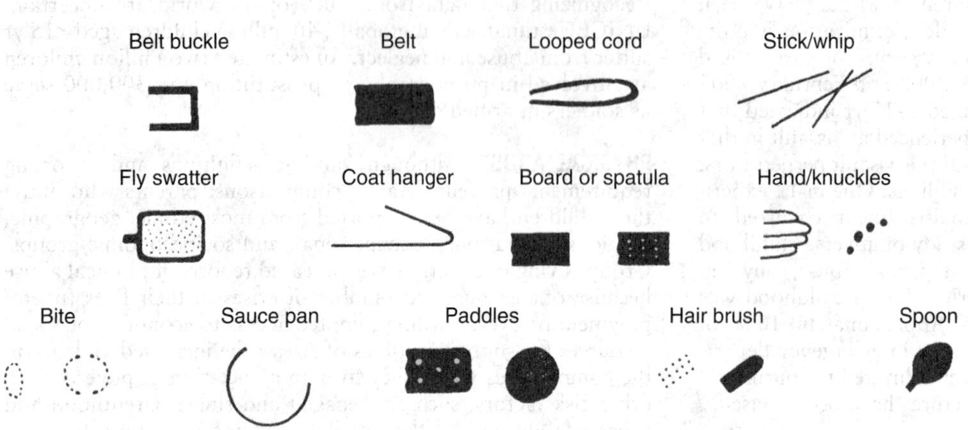

Figure 36-2. A variety of instruments may be used to inflict injury on a child. Often the choice of an instrument is a matter of convenience. Marks tend to silhouette or outline the shape of the instrument. The possibility of intentional trauma should prompt a high degree of suspicion when injuries to a child are geometric, paired, mirrored, of various ages or types, or on relatively protected parts of the body. Early recognition of intentional trauma is important to provide therapy and prevent escalation to more serious injury.

resources needed to provide for their children. The goal of a report of suspected neglect is to bring needed services.

Bruises are the most common manifestation of child abuse and may be found on any body surface. Nonintentional bruises, from impact trauma, are most commonly found on the thin leading surfaces overlying bone edges, such as the shins, forearms, chin, and brows. Bruises to the buttocks, back, genitals, ears, and back of the hands are less likely to be due to an accident. Children may be poisoned, struck, thrown, burned, bitten, lacerated, or punctured. The shape, depth, and type of the injury should suggest the object used. Paddles, belts, hands, and other instruments leave specific marks (Fig. 36-2). The most commonly used "instrument" to inflict trauma is the open or fisted hand. Bilateral, symmetric, or geometric injuries, especially on soft parts, the back, head, or neck and in immobile infants, should raise suspicion of child abuse. Although the color of a bruise is influenced by the age of the injury and depth of injury, the body surface involved, and the skin color, the dating of a bruise is inexact. A new bruise generally appears blue or red-purple. A bruise is older if it is yellow, green, or brown. Bruises of different colors on the same body surface are generally not compatible with a single event. Dark skin masks bruises.

Wrenching or pulling an extremity of an infant may result in a corner chip or "bucket-handle" fracture of the metaphysis. **Inflicted fractures** of the bone shaft are more likely to be spiral from twisting rather than transverse from impact. Spiral fractures of the femur after the age of walking or toddler fractures are usually nonintentional and associated with running and falling. Cardiopulmonary resuscitation or accidental impact rarely causes rib fractures or retinal hemorrhages in children; both are highly suspicious of physical abuse (Fig. 36-3). Bruises, burns, scars, internal organ damage, and fractures in various stages of healing should suggest the battered child syndrome. The earliest manifestation of fracture healing, callus formation, occurs around 7–10 days. Skull fractures cannot be dated. Dating of subdural bleeding may be confused by sedimentation of blood.

Hair that is pulled causes alopecia in which the hairs are broken at various lengths. Infants who are left to lie on their backs from neglect or to prevent sudden infant death syndrome (SIDS) may have a flattened occiput with an overlying area of thin or missing hair (see Chapter 372). Frequent injury also may be due to safety neglect.

Petechiae of the face and shoulders from intense retching, coughing, crying, or straining to evacuate stool may be mistaken for abuse, as may a variety of conditions such as mongolian spots, capillary hemangiomas, pigmented nevi, and other congenital, allergic, self-inflicted, and infectious skin conditions. A single 1 cm, rounded lesion of impetigo may be difficult to differentiate from a cigarette burn that has become infected. Blood dyscrasias, vascular fragility, and coagulopathies can result in petechiae and readier bruising; however, the bruise generally results from some form of trauma and is rarely "spontaneous." Old and new fractures can be seen in Wilson disease (see Chapter 354.2), Schmid-like metaphyseal chondrodysplasia (see Chapter 693), biliary atresia (see Chapter 353), and osteogenesis imperfecta (OI) [see Chapter 699]. OI should be suspected in the presence of blue sclera, osteopenia, short stature, bowing of bones, wormian bones, or a positive family history. Severe monilia of the diaper area may resemble an immersion burn. Metaphyseal lesions may follow cephalic version and cesarean section.

Approximately 10% of cases of physical abuse involve **burns** (see Chapter 74). The shape or pattern of a burn may be diagnostic when it reflects the pattern of an object or method of injury. Cigarette burns produce circular, punched-out lesions of uniform size (Fig. 36-4). An immersion burn occurs when a child is placed in hot water intentionally or unintentionally (Fig. 36-5). Immersion in 147°F water for 1 sec can result in a 2nd-degree burn. Extremity immersions result in glove or stocking burn patterns. When a child's body is placed in hot water, the level of burn demarcation is uniform and distinct. Flexion creases may be spared when the child protectively flexes the extremities. Depending on how the child is held when immersed, the hands and feet may be spared and splash burns may not be seen. The immersion burn pattern is incompatible with falling into a tub or the child turning on the hot water while in the bathtub. It is necessary to ascertain the developmental skills of the child, water temperature over time, tub height, and knob type in the investigation of scald burns. Children <24 mo of age are usually unable to turn a rotary knob. Immersion burns are most common in infants. If a toddler does enter a tub, it is generally sideways or head first. Intentional burns may be associated with frustration over toilet training failure.

The **most common cause of death** from physical abuse is intentional head trauma (IHT) in the form of suffocation, acceleration-deceleration, or impact. Twenty-nine per cent of child abuse reports from a children's hospital recorded injuries to the head, face, or cranial contents. More than 95% of serious intracranial injuries in the 1st yr of life are the result of IHT. If an infant presents with coma, convulsions, apnea, or increased intracranial pressure, intentional head injury should be considered. A CT scan may reveal intracranial bleeding (Fig. 36-6). An eye exam may reveal retinal hemorrhage (RH). Retinal hemorrhages are seen in 85% of infants who are shaken. They occur commonly with normal birth with resolution in 2–6 wk, and are rarely seen with coagulopathies, blood dyscrasias, meningitis, endocarditis, severe hypertension, cardiopulmonary resuscitation, or impact trauma

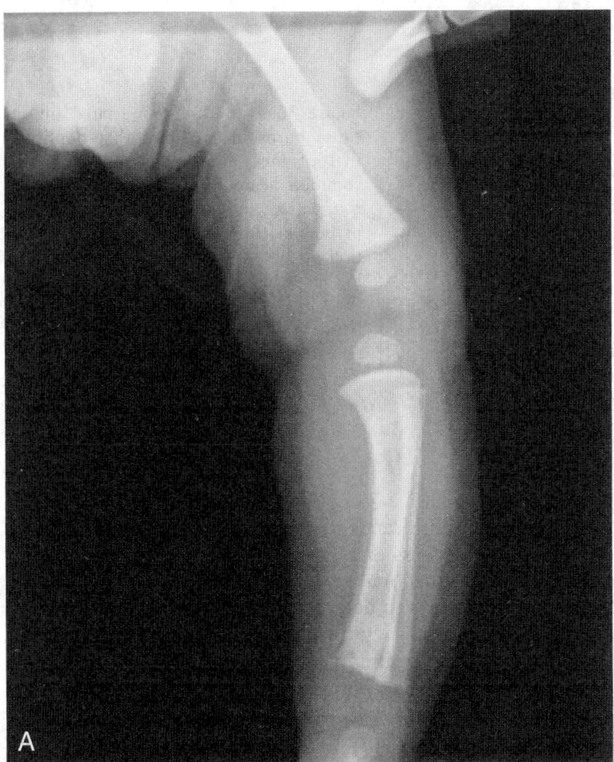

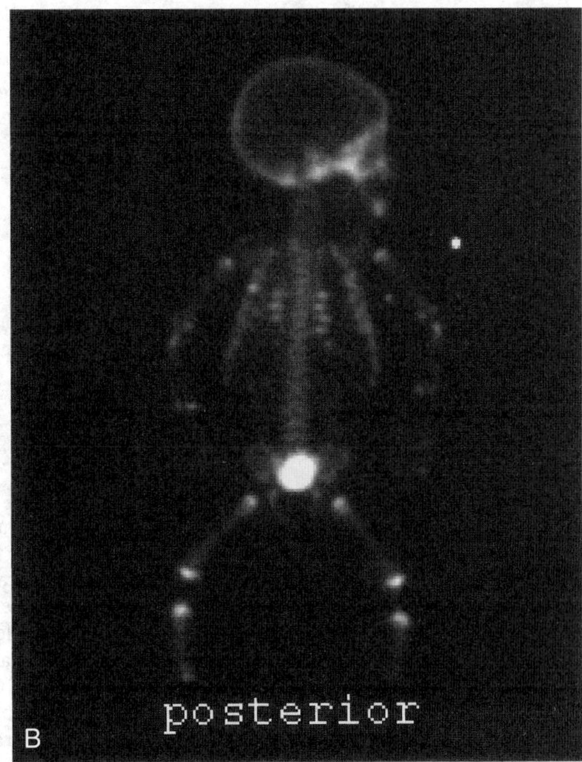

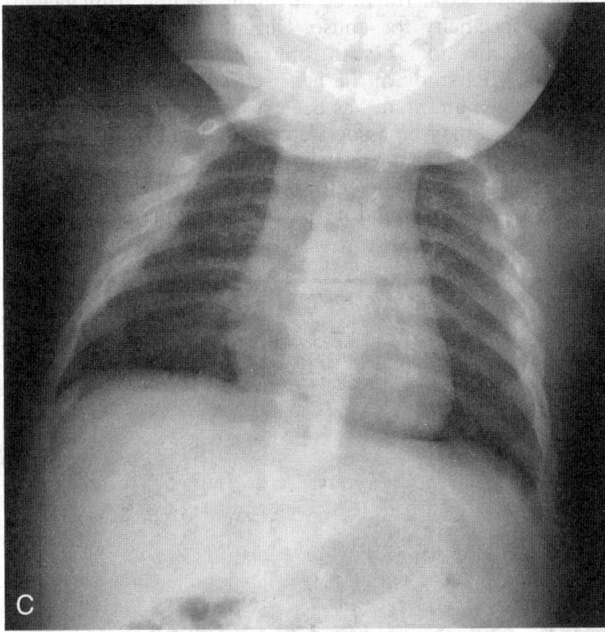

Figure 36-3. *A*, Metaphyseal fracture of the distal tibia in a 3 mo old infant admitted to the hospital with severe head injury. There is also periosteal new bone formation of the tibia, perhaps from previous injury. *B*, Bone scan of same infant. Initial chest x-ray showed a single fracture of the right posterior 4th rib. A radionuclide bone scan performed 2 days later revealed multiple previously unrecognized fractures of the posterior and lateral ribs. *C*, Follow-up radiographs 2 wk later showed multiple healing rib fractures. This pattern of fracture is highly specific for child abuse. The mechanism of these injuries is usually violent squeezing of the chest.

(Fig. 36-7). In abuse, retinal hemorrhages are often bilateral, include preretinal structures and the macular, and have associated alterations of mental status and seizures. More subtle symptoms of central nervous system (CNS) injury, such as vomiting, irritability, or lethargy, may be misdiagnosed as due to other causes. A missed diagnosis of IHT can lead to further injury, morbidity, and mortality. A bloody spinal tap may not be from the procedure, particularly if xanthochromia is present. Subdural hematomas (SDHs) seen on CT or MRI (see Fig. 36-6) in which there are no scalp marks or skull fractures may result from a blow from a hand or being thrown against a wall or onto a bed. The source of injury may be revealed at autopsy when a subgaleal handprint is found. Although grab marks or metaphyseal fractures and rib fractures have been described in association with shaking (acceleration-deceleration) and slamming the head against an object, there are often no external marks or fractures. The term IHT is preferred to shaken-impact syndrome. There is controversy about acceleration-deceleration causing serious head injury. Confessions and biomechanical models support acceleration-deceleration as a cause of SDH and RH.

Intra-abdominal injuries from impacts are the second most common cause of death in battered children. Affected children may present with recurrent vomiting, abdominal distention, absent bowel sounds, localized tenderness, or shock. Because the

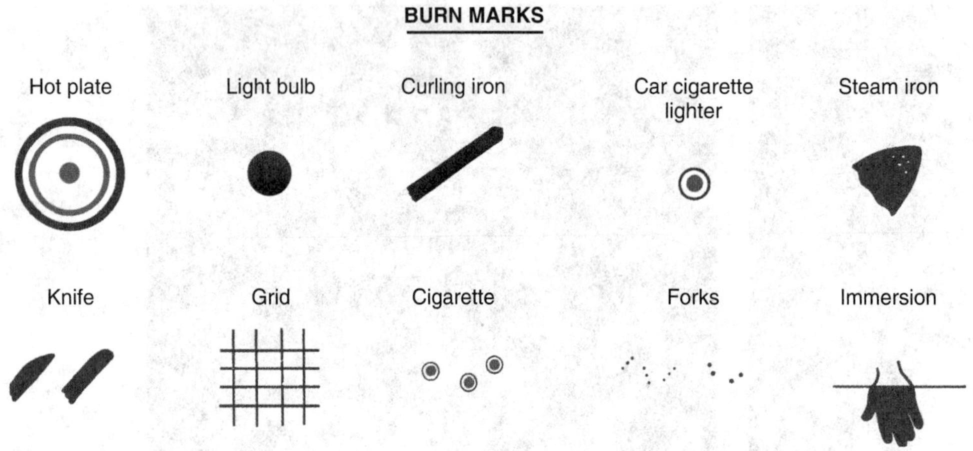

BURN MARKS

Hot plate
Light bulb
Curling iron
Car cigarette lighter
Steam iron
Knife
Grid
Cigarette
Forks
Immersion

Figure 36-4. Marks from heated objects cause burns in a pattern that duplicates that of the object. Familiarity with the common heated objects that are used to traumatize children facilitates recognition of possible intentional injuries. The location of the burn is important in determining its cause. Children tend to explore surfaces with the palmar surface of the hand and rarely touch a heated object repeatedly or for a long time.

abdominal wall is flexible, the overlying skin may be free of bruises. If the child is struck with a fist, a row of three to four 1 cm teardrop-shaped bruises in a slight curve may be seen on the abdomen wall. The blows may result in a ruptured liver or spleen (with or without overlying rib fractures) or a perforation or laceration of the small intestine at sites of ligamental support, such as the duodenum and proximal jejunum. Intramural hematomas of the intestines can lead to obstruction. Chylous ascites and pseudocyst of the pancreas also have been reported from intentional injury.

LABORATORY FINDINGS. Screening tests should be obtained in all cases of bruising to rule out a bleeding diathesis. These tests include a prothrombin time, partial thromboplastin time, and platelet count. In some cases, such as Von Willebrand disease, a hematology consultant may suggest further testing (see Chapter 477). Abnormal coagulation study results may follow intracranial bleeding. It is important to remember that children with a hematologic condition may also be abused.

When physical abuse is suspected in a child <2 yr old, a radiographic bone survey consisting of multiple views of the skull, thorax, long bones, hands, feet, pelvis, and spine is necessary. These films should be repeated in 7–10 days to reveal healing fractures not seen on the initial films. Bone scans may be complementary to the skeletal survey in detecting new fractures of the hands, feet, or ribs, but are not valuable in detecting skull fractures. For older children, radiographs need be obtained only if there is bone tenderness or a limited range of motion on physical examination. If films of a tender site are negative, they should be repeated in 7–10 days to detect any calcification, subperiosteal bleeding, or nondisplaced epiphyseal separations that were initially undetected. Bone trauma is found in 10–20% of physically abused children. Fractures considered highly specific for child abuse include metaphyseal, rib, scapular, distal clavicular, vertebral, and phalangeal and femoral in preambulating children; fractures of different ages; bilateral fractures; and complex skull fractures. Midclavicular, simple linear, and single diaphyseal fractures and simple skull fractures in infants falling from heights have a low specificity for abuse. Despite an absence of CNS abnormalities, a head CT scan, ophthalmologic exam, and, if indicated, an MRI study of the head, chest, and abdomen must be obtained when an infant has been severely injured. Fractures, burns, or bruises may be associated with an old or a new head injury. Liver and pancreatic enzyme studies or an abdominal CT scan may reveal occult damage to these organs. Urine and stool should be screened for blood if abdominal trauma is suspected.

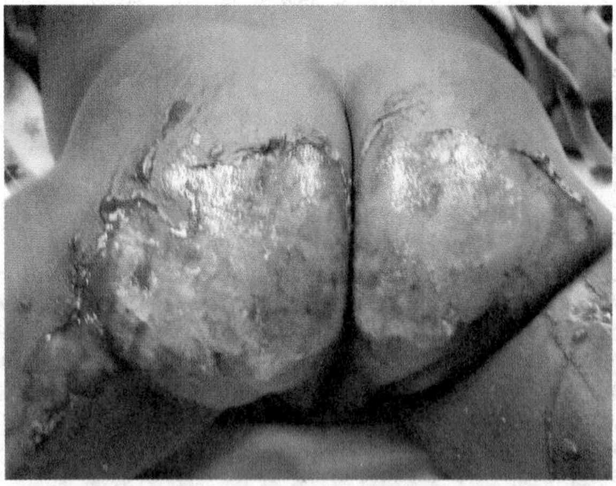

Figure 36-5. A 1 yr old child brought to a hospital with a history that she sat on a hot radiator. Suspicious injuries such as this require a full medical and social investigation including a skeletal survey to look for occult skeletal injuries and a child welfare evaluation.

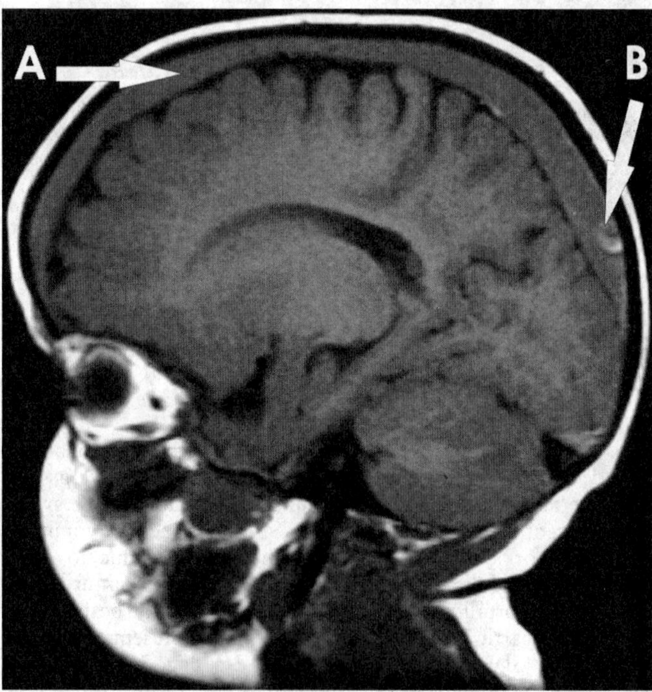

Figure 36-6. CT scan indicating intracranial bleeding. *A,* Older blood. *B,* New blood.

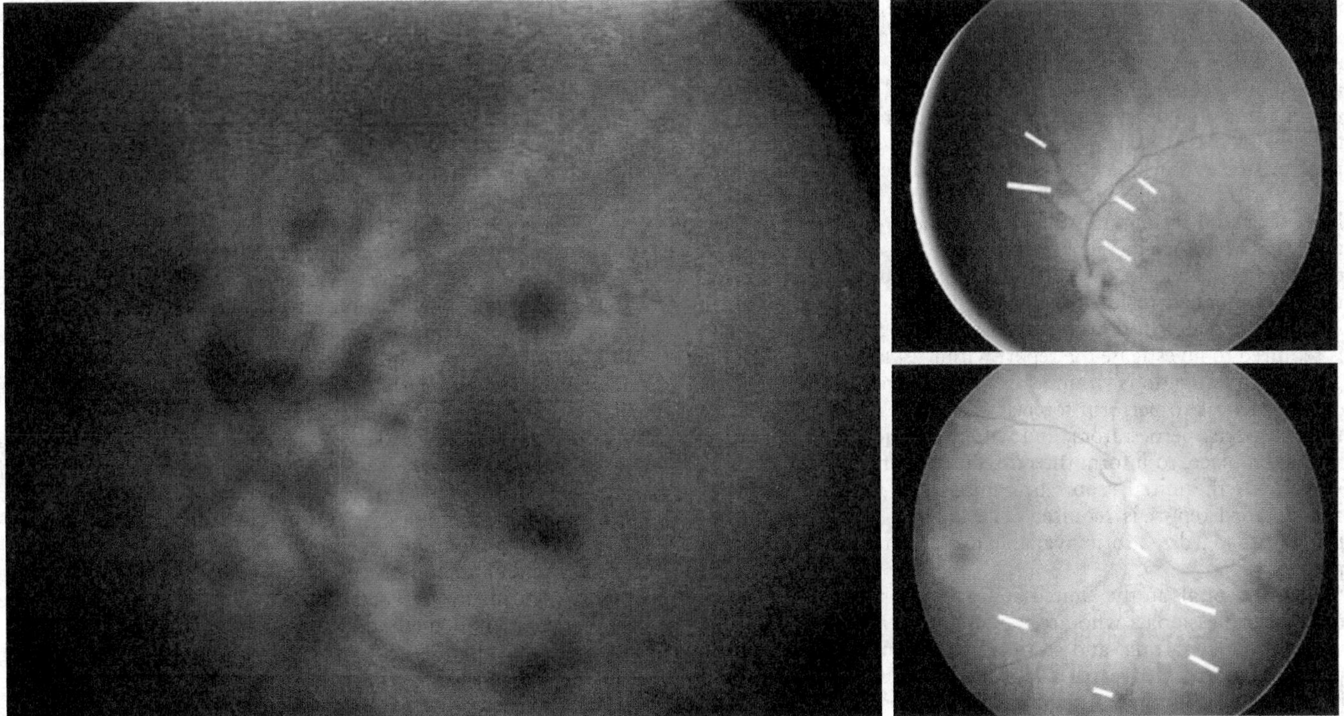

Figure 36-7. Retinal hemorrhages. Lines point to hemorrhages of various sizes.

DIAGNOSIS. Suspicion of physical abuse or neglect is based on a detailed history with a time line that is not in keeping with physical findings or the child's developmental stage. All information should be legibly recorded. This is best done when typed or printed on a standardized form that includes all needed information. All visible lesions should be photographed with a quality analog or digital camera. A color chart, patient identification, and measuring scales should be included in the field. An analysis of the circumstances of the injury is critical. The consequences of a fall depend on **child variables,** such as age, size, motor skills, motor tone, clothing, pre-existing medical conditions, and momentum, and **environmental variables,** such as distance traveled and physical qualities (soft, hard, padded, sharp, dull) of contact surfaces. Data from studies of witnessed falls from hospital beds, bunk beds, windows, and school yard equipment help estimate the force required to cause brain damage and fractures. A fall from 3 ft rarely results in a simple linear fracture of the skull or clavicle. Falls from 6 ft rarely result in concussions, subdural hemorrhages, or lacerations. There are no reports of death or severe brain injury from witnessed falls of <10 ft. Falls down stairs have not been reported to be fatal.

After separation from caretakers, a child older than aged 3 yr may be able to tell a sensitive and skillful interviewer that a particular adult hurt him or her. Children may not give a history of intentional injury if they are concerned about retribution from the perpetrator or separation from their home, school, siblings, friends, or nonoffending parent.

The differential diagnosis depends on the particular injuries. Roentgenograms of bones in scurvy (see Chapter 47) and syphilis (see Chapter 215) and normally growing bone shafts of infants may resemble nonaccidental bone trauma. The bony changes in these conditions are often symmetric. Children with osteogenesis imperfecta, severe osteomalacia, or sensory deficits (myelomeningocele, paraplegia) have an increased incidence of pathologic fractures, but rarely of the metaphysis. Biochemical and genetic analysis can facilitate the diagnosis of osteogenesis imperfecta (see Chapter 699). Bone density studies, at this time, cannot predict easy spontaneous fracturing. The theorized condition of transient bone fragility has not been proven.

Hospital admission is indicated for children whose medical or surgical condition requires inpatient management, in whom the diagnosis is unclear, and when no alternative safe place for custody is immediately available. If the safety of the child is in doubt, the physician, agency, and court should err on the side of protecting the child. If the parents refuse hospitalization or treatment, an emergency court order must be obtained. Efforts must be made to keep the child from being removed against medical advice. The parents should be told by the physician: why an inflicted injury is suspected; that the physician is legally obligated to report the circumstance; that the referral is being made to protect the child and to provide the family with services; and that a CPS social worker and law enforcement officer will be involved in the investigation. Siblings and all other children baby sat by suspected abusers should have full examinations within 24 hr of the recognition of child abuse. Approximately 20% of them will be found to have signs of physical abuse. Children younger than 2 yr should have skeletal surveys, which are repeated in 2 wk.

Professionals may experience anger and threats from abusing or neglectful caretakers; however, returning anger in response to this behavior damages rapport, increases caretaker defensiveness, and makes their cooperation less likely. Repeated interrogations, confrontations, and accusations may be avoided by involving CPS workers and law enforcement as a team during the investigation. If the child is hospitalized, the **supervised** parents should be encouraged to visit, and the hospital staff must be counseled to be courteous, helpful, and observant. The primary physician should maintain contact with the parents. An evaluation by hospital social services and pastoral care when indicated should be obtained to determine existing problems, needs, supports, and strengths in the family. An agency caseworker and, when a site investigation is needed, a police officer should visit the home. A psychiatric evaluation of the parents and siblings may be indicated.

TREATMENT. Appropriate medical, surgical, and psychiatric treatment should be promptly initiated. The law requires that a child in the United States suspected of being abused or neglected be reported immediately to CPS. Children with suspected abuse should not be discharged from the clinic or office without consulting the county CPS agency. The caseworker confers with the physician to determine whether the child will be safe if released to a parent or whether the child should be taken to an agency office with a safe escort. A caseworker should come to the hospital or office to evaluate the situation and determine the child's future safety and the need for crisis services. Children and siblings at risk for serious abuse should be placed in homes of appropriate relatives or emergency receiving homes. CPS workers are expected to provide a case plan, which delineates those services that are intended to lead to the safe return of the child to the home if the plan is followed and desired changes take place. CPS is required to investigate the report within 24 hr and should complete its investigation within a reasonable time. The role of law enforcement is to perform forensic scene investigations, to interview suspects, perpetrators, and witnesses, and, if a criminal act has taken place, to inform the prosecutor's office. In most states, 48 hr after the initial report by a mandated reporter, a written and detailed report is required. The latter is best accomplished using a standardized form available in some states or from abuse programs.

Most hospitals in the United States caring for children have a team of professionals who are trained and skilled in child abuse recognition, reporting, and services. This team should include a pediatrician knowledgeable and skilled in child maltreatment, a hospital social worker, a pediatric nurse, a psychologist or psychiatrist, and a data coordinator. The role of each team member as well as that of the public agencies involved should be formalized in hospital protocols and a community plan. Legal and medical specialty consultants should be available and experienced in child maltreatment. When evaluations are completed, the team should meet with the child's primary care physician, ward nurse, CPS representative, and, as appropriate, a law enforcement officer, prosecutor, or any other member of the community agencies involved with the family to share information, clarify medical and social findings, and plan immediate and long-range goals and therapies.

It is important for the pediatrician to coordinate the health care of the abused child. Abused and neglected children require more intensive surveillance and well child care than do nonabused children. A prior history of abuse is a major risk factor for re-abuse. Placement in foster care may complicate preventive care and treatment of acute and chronic illnesses. Because of the number of difficulties experienced by abusive families, no single agency or discipline can provide all the needed services. Services may include economic support, parent aides, homemakers, Parents Anonymous groups, telephone hotlines, environmental crisis therapy, substance abuse treatment, Big Brothers and Big Sisters, "foster" grandparents, anger management, and child-rearing and child development training. Traditional psychotherapy, in isolation, may be ineffective.

PREVENTION. The pediatrician's role in primary abuse prevention includes identifying parents and children at high risk. High-risk parents may be unable or unwilling to accept, love, properly discipline, or care for their offspring. The history obtained from all parents should include information about pregnancy planning, the pregnancy itself, emotional and physical health, domestic violence, attitudes about the child, knowledge of child health and development, and child-rearing experiences and techniques. Parental risks include a history of family violence or child abuse, drug addiction, depression, lack of support, socioeconomic problems, serious psychiatric illness, mental retardation, young parental age, closely spaced pregnancies, single-parent status of the mother, negative parental comments about the newborn infant, lack of evidence of maternal attachment, infrequent visits to a new infant whose discharge is delayed because of prematurity or illness, inappropriate anger toward or spanking of an infant younger than 18 mo or a handicapped child, and neglect of infant hygiene.

The use of an instrument to inflict injury on any part of the body, a bruise from corporal punishment, or striking any part of the body aside from the hands or buttocks should be considered inappropriate and reportable. Child risks include mental or physical handicap, chronic illness, prematurity, being a twin, and learning or behavior problems. Abuse and serious neglect may be prevented when at-risk families receive intensive training and support during pregnancy and after delivery. Prevention efforts should include early and frequent contact between mother and baby in the delivery room, rooming-in, increased parental contact with premature infants, extra help calming the crying or "difficult" infant, more frequent office visits for at-risk infants, ongoing counseling regarding discipline and the use of nonphysical responses to unwanted behaviors, rewards for desired behaviors, public health nurse visits or trained home visitors, parenting classes, stress and anger management classes, close follow-up of acute and chronic illnesses, telephone hotlines, arrangement for child care or preschool, respite for stressed parents, and assistance in family planning. Even though it recognizes that spanking is common and endorsed by some cultures and religions, the American Academy of Pediatrics recommends that parents be encouraged to find methods other than spanking to discipline their child because: (1) to be effective the intensity of spanking needs to be increased over time; (2) repeated spanking may cause agitated, aggressive behavior on the part of the child; (3) spanking models aggressive behavior as a solution to conflict; and (4) spanking has been associated with higher rates of physical aggression, substance use, and crime and violence.

PROGNOSIS. Early studies of abused children in the United States returned to their parents without any intervention indicate that about 5% are subsequently killed and that 25% are seriously re-injured. With comprehensive, intensive family treatment, 80–90% of families involved in child maltreatment may be rehabilitated to provide adequate care for their children. Approximately 10–15% of maltreating families, especially those with a history of substance abuse, will require an indefinite continuation of supporting services, which may include drug monitoring, until their children are old enough to leave home. Termination of parental rights or continued foster placement is required in 2–3% of cases (see Chapter 34). If a parent is unable to respond to a treatment plan, this should be documented as soon as possible to afford the child the opportunity to develop in a healthy and permanent home.

Children with injuries to the CNS may develop mental retardation, learning problems, behavior problems, blindness, deafness, motor problems, organic brain syndrome, seizures, hydrocephalus, and ataxia. Experiencing violence affects brain growth and behavior. Common emotional traits of abused children include fearfulness, aggression, hypervigilance, denial, projection, post-traumatic stress disorder (see Chapter 35), lack of trust, low self-esteem, juvenile delinquency, substance abuse, and hyperactivity. Unsuccessful treatment may result in children who become bullies, juvenile delinquents, violent and antisocial adults, spouse and elder abusers, and the next generation of child abusers.

36.1 • Sexual Abuse (see also Rape, Chapter 118)

Sexual abuse includes any activity with a child, before the age of legal consent, that is for the sexual gratification of an adult or a significantly older child. Sexual abuse includes oral-genital, genital-genital, genital-rectal, hand-genital, hand-rectal, or hand-breast contact; exposure of sexual anatomy; encouraged or forced viewing of sexual anatomy; and showing of pornography to a child or using a child in the production of pornography. **Sexual intercourse** includes vaginal, oral, or rectal penetration. Penetration denotes entry into an orifice with an object with or without tissue injury. Adolescent perpetrators tend to have younger victims but are more likely to have intercourse with older victims. Sex acts perpetrated by young children are learned behaviors and are associated with experiencing sexual abuse or exposure to adult sex or pornography. Without detection and intervention, sexual abuse may progress from viewing pornography to touching to intercourse. **Sexual play** is defined as viewing or touching of the genitals, buttocks, or chest by preadolescent children separated by not more than 4 yr, in which there has been no force, coercion, or power difference. See Chapter 13 for a discussion of the development of sexual identity and behavior.

Sexual mistreatment of children by family members (incest) and nonrelatives known to the child is the most common type of sexual abuse. The least common offender is a stranger. Intrafamilial sexual abuse is difficult to document and manage. The child may be coerced into not revealing the abuse or into denying the abuse. The child victim must be protected from additional abuse while attempts are made to preserve the family unit. Children may also be coerced to recant accusations of abuse by relatives, or they may decide to recant the abuse for fear of ridicule or teasing, retaliation, attendance in court, guilt, or loss of contact with needed or loved relatives and friends.

EPIDEMIOLOGY. Most of the increase in child abuse reports in the United States through 1992 was due to increased reporting of sexual abuse. The rate of sexual abuse, estimated by the American Association for Protecting Children, went from 1.4/10,000 to 17/10,000 children between 1976 and 1984. Surveys of adult women indicate that 12–38% were sexually abused by the age of 18 yr. The results of one study indicated that the likelihood of extrafamilial and intrafamilial sexual abuse being reported were 8% and 2%, respectively. The incidence of sexual abuse of males ranges from 3 to 9%, accounting for up to 20% of reports. Because fixed pedophiles show a predilection for boys, the number of males who are sexually abused is probably higher. Furthermore, boys may refrain from reporting what they might interpret as a homosexual action or a consequence of their failure to protect themselves from assault.

In 1997, 679 reports (71% of all abuse reports) from a children's hospital were for sexual abuse. Of 744 patients referred to a diagnostic clinic for suspected sexual abuse, 230 (31%) were reported. A lack of substantiation may be due to a child's young age and inability to give a detailed history or a lack of significant physical or laboratory findings. Caregivers may mistake genital erythema, enuresis, masturbation, or fear of an individual or place as being due to sexual abuse. Suspicion may be increased during divorce proceedings due to mutual distrust and changes in the child's behavior caused by the divorce process. Approximately 30% of sexual abuse victims are <6 yr of age, 30% are 6–12 yr of age, and the rest are 12–18 yr of age. Reported offenders are 97% male. Females are more often perpetrators in child-care settings, including baby sitting. The number of female perpetrators may actually be higher than reported because younger children may confuse sexual abuse by a female with normal hygiene care, and adolescent males may not be trained to recognize sexual activity with an older female as a form of abuse. Sexual abuse by stepfathers is nearly five times higher than by natural fathers. Incest is described in most cultures and is seen at all socioeconomic levels to a greater degree than are physical abuse and neglect. Unsuspecting poor, single mothers may bring sexual abusers into their home for economic and emotional support and perpetrators may seek out these situations.

ETIOLOGY. The abuse of daughters by fathers and stepfathers is the most common form of reported incest, although brother-sister incest is considered to be the most common type. Studies of incarcerated adult perpetrators state that sexual abuse begins with selection of vulnerable and available victims, innocent physical contact, and seduction through gifts and attention. The propensity for pedophiles to become sexually involved with children often appears in their adolescence. Pedophiles have indicated that they seek positions and opportunities where they can be in contact with potential victims. The vulnerable children they described include those with mental and physical handicaps, unloved and unwanted children, previously abused children, children in single-parent families, children of drug abusers, their own children, and children with low self-esteem and poor achievement. Pornography may be used to initiate sexual activity with a child. Threats, bribes, and injury may be used to entice children and to keep them from telling. Boys and girls may be told that they are at fault and will be punished because they did not protect themselves. Care must be exercised when evaluating data from incarcerated perpetrators or perpetrators in therapy because they may be different from other perpetrators. A father's desire for sexual gratification and a daughter's need for affection and nurturing and a desire to maintain the family unit may lead to incest when the mother is unavailable due to work or physical or emotional illness. These incestuous fathers have been described as rigid, patriarchal, and emotionally immature. They are unlikely to engage in extramarital relationships, and there is a high incidence of alcoholism. The mothers have been described as chronically depressed, unavailable to their husbands because of work or illness, and often the victims of childhood sexual abuse. The child victim tends to be pseudomature and to have taken on many of the adult roles, including housekeeping. The tendency for some of these families to be closely knit and socially isolated prevents detection.

Violence is not common in sexual abuse; its incidence increases with the age and size of the victim and specific traits in the perpetrator. Violence is more likely to occur in association with a single incident by a stranger. In cases of violent incest, the father has been described as sociopathic, with sexual abuse extending outside the family circle. Sexually abused children may also be physically abused and vice versa.

CLINICAL MANIFESTATIONS. A child may 1st disclose sexual abuse to the mother and be brought to a physician at that time. If the mother does not believe the child, they may not see a physician and the child may delay further comment. Later, the child may tell a friend, relative, friend's mother, teacher, or school counselor. Children, given the opportunity, may disclose their abuse to a physician in a private interview or physical examination. Sexual abuse should be considered as the cause of physical symptoms such as vaginal, penile, or rectal pain; discharge, bruising, erythema, or bleeding; chronic dysuria, enuresis, constipation, or encopresis; and, rarely, premature puberty in a female. Certain behaviors, although more likely to be associated with sexual abuse, have not been found to be diagnostic. They include sexualized activity with peers, animals, or objects; seductive be-havior; and age-inappropriate sexual knowledge and curiosity. Nonspecific behaviors include suicide gestures, fear of an individual or place, nightmares, sleep disorders, regression, aggression, withdrawn behavior, post-traumatic stress disorder, low self-esteem, depression, poor school performance, running away, self-mutilation, anxiety, fire setting, multiple personalities, somatization, phobias, trauma, prostitution, drug abuse, eating disorders, dysmenorrhea, and dyspareunia. Because of secrecy, a desire to protect the abuser or family, or threats by the abuser, the cause of symptoms, medical findings, or abuse behaviors may be denied by the child. When the perpetrator is a breadwinner or is violent, the abuse may also be denied by the nonoffending and dependent parent.

Investigating the possibility of sexual abuse requires skilled, supportive, sensitive, and detailed history taking. Because of variance in the type of abuse, the ages of the victim and perpetrator, and the time since abuse, <5% of cases yield physical or laboratory findings. Ideally, the recorded forensic interview, which uses open-ended, nonleading questions, should be conducted on one occasion by one or two experienced interviewers in the presence of law enforcement, prosecutors, and social service workers who observe via closed-circuit television. This obviates the need for repeated interviews in most instances and possible further trauma to the child. After an initial interview, children who gain trust and comfort may experience a decrease in guilt and fear of reprisal or loss of love and give more detailed information in subsequent interviews. Interviewing should proceed at the child's pace and level of development. It should begin with discussion of general topics, naming of body parts including "private" parts, and differentiation of good and bad touch, and proceed to details about each incident. The sophistication of the information that can be obtained from the child varies with the development of the child and the skill of the interviewer. Anatomic pictures may help clarify the names of body parts and aid in describing the abuse. With young children, skilled professionals may use anatomically correct dolls.

Physical Examination. Older female and male victims may prefer that a physician of the same sex examine them; when possible, their desires should be queried and respected. A thorough and complete physical examination should be conducted, with special attention to the neck and mouth. The mouth should be examined for redness, abrasions, or purpura that may be due to recent trauma. If present, bite marks should be measured, and wax impressions and wiping for saliva should be done to aid in identification of the perpetrator. The abdominal examination should assess the possibility of pregnancy. The rectum should be examined for signs of trauma. A thorough examination will also help rule out associated physical abuse.

A young female who is resistant to the genital-rectal examination, despite preparation, may be examined while sitting on the parent's lap. Occasionally, the child will be able to separate the labia or buttocks herself. The examination should be explained to the girl; anxiety can be reduced by distracting her. She can be asked to blow on a pinwheel, sing, or count. A female child is most easily examined in the supine frog leg position. The hymen is exposed by separation of the labia laterally or by grasping the labia majora with the gloved thumbs and forefingers and gently tugging the labia toward the examiner (Fig. 36-8). This labial traction is best accomplished by an assistant, while the genitals are viewed in good lighting and with magnification, optimally with a colposcope that also allows photo documentation. If abnormalities are found on supine examination, the child should be re-examined in the prone knee-chest position. In that position, gravity may allow better visualization of the hymen anatomy and confirmation of suspected abnormalities. There are several normal shapes to the hymen. In the infant or prepubertal child, flaps or tabs on the hymen may obscure the opening. This is rectified when drops of sterile saline are used to "float" the tabs, to reveal the opening. Maternal hormones thicken the newborn's hymen in a manner similar to the effects of endogenous hormones in adolescence. As this hormone effect wanes, by 1 yr the hymen becomes thin, in some cases to the point of transparency with visible vascularity. As the hymen thickens in adolescence (Fig. 36-9), it folds on itself. This undulation makes the hymen more distensible and the examination of the hymen rim more difficult. A moist cotton swab, a swab covered with a rubber balloon or, less commonly, a Foley catheter may assist in the examination. The Foley is inserted through the hymen opening and then inflated with saline before being drawn against the inner hymen wall. Opening size of the hymen is not considered of diagnostic value; however, the width of the hymenal rim can be. The examination of the hymen should include inspection of the labia, fourchette, introitus, vestibule, urethra, edge of the hymen, and anus. A speculum examination of the vagina with collection of specimens is indicated when the victim is postpubertal or when nonmenstrual vaginal bleeding or major trauma of the external genitals is present. No child should be forced to have an examination. General anesthesia or sedation may be required if the examination is deemed necessary or if there is bleeding from the rectum or vagina.

Drawings of trauma should be supplemented with photographs or video recordings using the colposcope or photos from a handheld analog or digital camera with a macro lens. Diagnostic findings in keeping with a history of sexual abuse include: a hymen with new or healed lacerations or transections (Fig. 36-10), absence, or remnants; posterior fourchette lacerations; vaginal

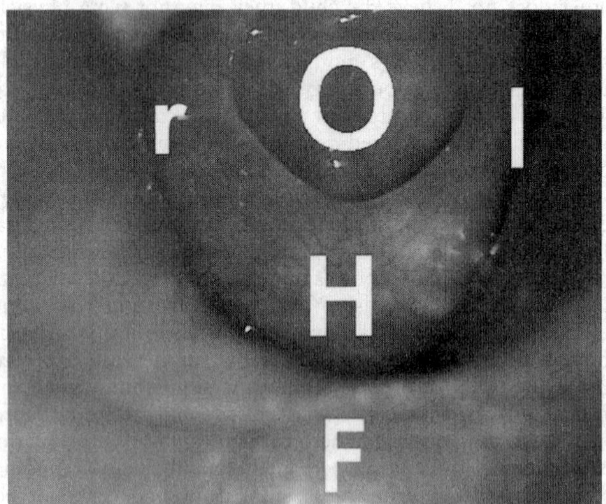

Figure 36-8. Normal hymen. This is the hymen of an 8 yr old. The hymen opening *(O)* has a delicate and almost transparent edge. There is a right *(r)* and left *(l)* wall, which may vary in size from 1 to 3 mm. The base of the hymen *(H)* may vary from 1 to 4 mm. The term *attenuation* is applied to the base when it is <1 mm wide. The fourchette *(F)* is the joining of the labia minora posteriorly. It may be injured from trauma. The vestibule, or space anterior to the hymen, which is surrounded by the labia minora, may be penetrated without damage to the hymen.

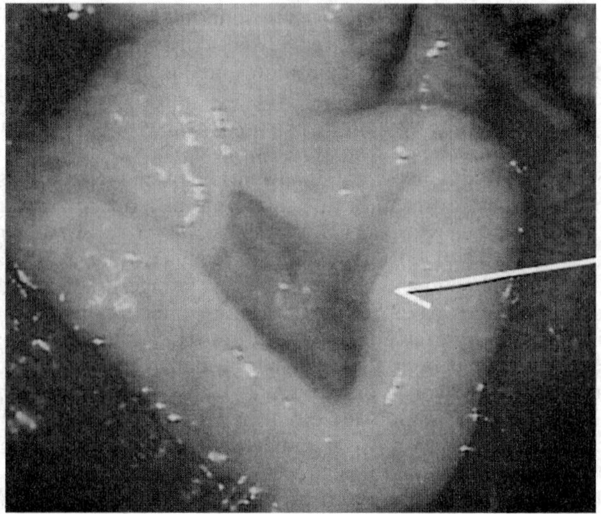

Figure 36-9. Hymen with estrogen effects and wart. With the onset of puberty, the hymen becomes thickened, paler in color, and redundant. The resulting folds make it difficult to determine whether there are abnormalities of the edge of the hymen. The *arrow* points to a glistening bump on the left hymen wall. This is a venereal wart. The appearance of these warts varies with location. Other warts on the skin surface were dark in color with an irregular "cauliflower-like" appearance.

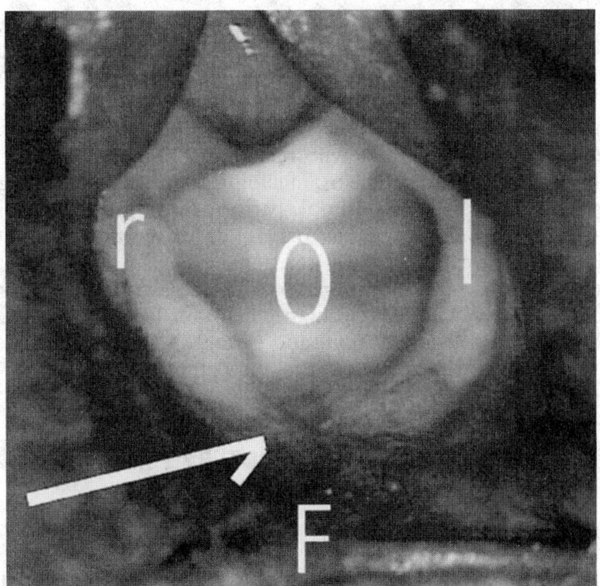

Figure 36-10. Hymen tear. The base *(arrow)* of the hymen has been torn to the floor of the vagina. The injury, from finger insertion to an 8 yr old patient, is bleeding. The fourchette *(F)* has escaped injury. Careful observation may reveal complete healing of the injury over time. The tear may also heal with a V-shaped notch, or remain separated. O, hymen opening; r, right wall of hymen; l, left wall of hymen.

wall tears; and perianal lacerations. Healed tears may heal as shallow or deep notches. These findings and attenuation are less likely to be considered diagnostic. The presence of sperm, semen, and pregnancy (in a child prior to the age of consent) are also diagnostic of sexual abuse. Suggestive findings include bite marks on the genitals or inner thigh or scarring or tears of the labia minora. Straddle injuries usually result in trauma to the labia and clitoris and rarely involve the relatively protected hymen. Accidental penetration of the hymen is unusual and is associated with penetration of underclothing and possibly the wall of the vagina.

Abnormal anal findings, even with a history of repeated anal penetration, are unusual. A fissure can result from the insertion of an object larger than the child's normal stool. The use of lubrication may minimize penetration damage. Frequent passage or insertion of a dilating object can result in decreased anal tone and changes in the appearance of anal folds. Examination by an experienced professional, with photo documentation, is necessary if there are any questions about anogenital findings. If immediate dilation of the anus reveals an anterior-posterior diameter >20 mm, with no stool present in the rectal ampulla, that is a marker for possible abuse. Scar formation, even following an episode of forceful sodomy, is unusual. There are two common, naturally occurring, midline entities that may be confused with scar tissue in the perianal region. The 1st is a smooth, wedged-shaped area known as diastasis ani. This can be found either anterior or posterior to the anus. The 2nd finding is an extension of the median or perineal raphe that has a taglike appearance on the anterior side of the anus. Anal fissures, decreased anal tone, or disruption of folds must be interpreted with caution, because they can be the result of chronic constipation or underlying disease, such as Crohn disease.

Injuries to the male genitals are usually the result of an accident or physical abuse. A bite mark may be found which must be differentiated from a laceration from a zipper. The forceful retraction of the foreskin may result in a dehiscence of the tissues. Injury from a sexual assault most likely causes a nonspecific, transitory redness of the penis. Routine examination of the genitals of males and females facilitates recognition of normal findings and helps guarantee future cooperation from the child. Follow-up studies of anal and genital trauma attest to the rapid and complete healing of trauma, especially of anal fissures. In one study of 37 cases with hymenal injury, two transactions healed after surgery and 15 persisted unchanged. Partial tears, hymenal abrasions, or hematomas healed completely or with minor or nonspecific changes. Of 47 injuries to the posterior fourchette, 22 healed completely. Of 31 cases of anal trauma, 29 healed completely.

LABORATORY FINDINGS. The extent of laboratory investigation depends on the history and the time elapsed since injury. When a victim is seen within 72 hr of sexual abuse, a rape kit is completed (see Chapter 118). Clothing and skin are swabbed with a moist cotton applicator. A variety of substances, including semen and urine, fluoresce under a Wood lamp. In addition, specimens of possible offender blood and hair and the victim's nail clippings and clothing should be collected. Tests for rectal blood may be indicated. In the vagina, motile sperm can be found for 6 hr; nonmotile sperm, which may be difficult to identify, may exist for >72 hr. Acid phosphatase is present for 24 hr. Sperm and semen may also be recovered from the mouth, rectum, and clothing. Semen may be detected for an indefinite period on unwashed fabric. Although the presence of semen substantiates the victim's history of vaginal intercourse, the absence of semen does not contradict it. If there is a history of contact with the perpetrator's genitals, gonorrhea and chlamydia cultures should be obtained from the mouth, anus, and genitals. Less than 5% of victims have positive cultures for gonorrhea or chlamydia. Symptomatic victims, those with positive cultures for other sexually transmitted infections, and children with a history of contact with the perpetrator's genitals should also be tested for syphilis, HIV, and hepatitis B. All specimens should be transferred to the forensic laboratory in sealed, signed, and dated envelopes to ensure an official chain of evidence.

DIAGNOSIS. It is most common for the diagnosis of suspected sexual abuse to depend on the history offered by the victim. False accusations are rare except in unusual cases involving adolescents, emotionally disturbed patients, or patients in custody disputes. Abuse may be revealed during a custody dispute because the child has been separated from an offender and is able to communicate without fear of retaliation or further abuse. The genitals and rectum may heal completely after extensive trauma; minor trauma, such as abrasions, may heal in 3–4 days. The tear may remain separated, heal to the point where the hymen cannot be easily differentiated from normal, or heal with a V-shaped notch of varying depth (see Fig. 36-10). Healing depends on the degree of trauma; however, even the most severe trauma, requiring surgical repair, may appear normal after a year or less. There may be no observable physical trauma in as many as 95% of children who report sexual abuse. The anus or vagina may not be penetrated, although there is pain experienced. Superficial injuries such as abrasions or erythema heal in days with no lasting signs. Certain types of sexual abuse such as oral or digital stimulation or labial intercourse may not result in tissue damage. If an inserted object is smaller than the expanded size of an opening, no tissue damage would be expected. The data from an interview by a professional trained and experienced in forensic interviewing techniques should not be minimized because there are no physical findings. In one study of 18 victims whose abusers confessed to vaginal penetration, seven children had normal genital examination findings. Abnormal physical or laboratory findings should be reported even if no history is available.

Laboratory findings of pregnancy, sperm, semen, and nonpregnancy- or delivery-related syphilis, gonorrhea, chlamydia, herpes type II (genital), and HIV may be considered diagnostic of sexual abuse and reported. Condyloma acuminatum appearing after 3 yr of age and *Trichomonas vaginalis* are considered "probably diagnostic." Herpes type I and nonvenereal warts may be autoinoculated to the genitorectal area or transmitted by a perpetrator's mouth or hand. The significance of bacterial vaginosis and genital mycoplasma infection is uncertain. DNA typing of blood, semen, sperm, or tissue may positively identify the perpetrator.

TREATMENT. Sexual abuse is a criminal offense and is investigated by the police. All victims of sexual abuse require psychologic support. Parents, relatives, and siblings may deny the accusation and rebuke or punish the child for reporting the incident. The consequences and appropriate therapy of sexual abuse vary, depending on the type of abuse, the age and other physical and emotional factors in the victim, the frequency of abuse, and the identity of the abuser. Victims of a single nonviolent episode of touching or exposure by a stranger may require reassurance and a chance to express feelings about the event in one or two therapy sessions. Victims may be less distressed by the incident than their parents. In contrast, a single episode of family-related sexual abuse may cause serious, long-term emotional distress and require prolonged individual and group treatment. The therapist may recommend that the victim of incest be returned home if the perpetrator is out of the home or has confessed and is in therapy. The child victim should be placed in foster care if this is his or her desire; if the nonoffending parent is not protective of the child, does not believe the child's story, or is likely to encourage the child to recant; and if family life is chaotic or collection of evidence is not yet complete. Medication to prevent pregnancy may be given to postmenarchal girls in midcycle who have experienced vaginal intercourse in the previous 72 hr. Treatment with antibiotics (and antiretroviral agents if indicated) is initiated to prevent sexually transmitted infection if the perpetrator is known to be infected, if the victim has signs of infection, or if the likelihood of follow-up is poor (see Chapter 118). All victims should revisit their primary care physicians within 2 wk to ensure that recommended services have been implemented.

Incest offenders may respond to treatment, but success requires a coordinated, multifaceted, multidisciplinary approach. The offending parent and spouse should be referred for psychiatric or psychologic evaluation. The police should investigate offenders, and criminal prosecution should be supported. There is evidence, especially in pedophilia, that incarceration may ensure access to, and efficacy of, simultaneous treatment. Incarceration of a breadwinner may have serious adverse consequences for the family. The behavior of chronic sexual offenders may be resistant to a variety of therapies. All juvenile and prejuvenile offenders should receive therapy to prevent recurrences. In one diagnostic center, 17% of offenders were <17 yr of age.

PREVENTION. The primary prevention of sexual abuse is related, in part, to normal developmental education and sexual behavior (see Chapter 13). Teaching children the proper names of all body parts, including the names, function, and significance of "private parts" (nipples, genitals, rectum), should begin in the home and continue in the pediatrician's office and school. Children should be taught to say "no" to any action, by any person, that makes them uncomfortable, but especially actions directed to their "private" areas. They should be given the opportunity to report to a trusted adult any of these actions. Caregivers, including baby sitters and their companions and the boyfriends of single mothers, should be carefully screened. Written permission should be obtained from any caregiver to allow a police screening for offenses. Victim therapy should decrease the potential for re-abuse and reactive abuse. Routine family and classroom discussions of uncomfortable events in the lives of children may reveal unsuspected abuse. To improve diagnostic skills, physicians should examine the genitals and rectum routinely, record their findings, become familiar with normal rectal and genital anatomy and the consequences of trauma, listen to and seriously consider what children tell them, and be willing to report and testify when abuse is suspected.

PROGNOSIS. With early and adequate intervention, victims may lead normal adult lives. Even with intervention, however, certain adolescent victims may run away from home (see Chapter 1) and fall prey to adolescent prostitution, violence (see Chapter 112), substance abuse (see Chapter 113), and unprepared parenthood (see Chapter 117). Others who remain at home may manifest a variety of emotional problems, including depression, suicidal gestures, deterioration in school performance, and conversion reactions. As adults, victims may have difficulties with close relationships; enter abusive relationships; have a variety of somatic complaints of the genitourinary, gastrointestinal, and other systems; and need psychiatric help for depression, anxiety, substance abuse, dissociation, and eating disorders. The risk of untoward effects is greatest for incest victims.

36.2 • Munchausen Syndrome by Proxy (MSBP)

The term *Munchausen syndrome* is used to describe situations in which adults falsify their own symptoms. In MSBP, a parent, typically the mother, simulates or causes disease in a child. The parent may fabricate a medical history; cause symptoms by repeatedly exposing the child to a toxin, medication, infectious agent, or physical trauma, including smothering; or alter laboratory samples or temperature measurements. Depending on the parent's sophistication and secrecy, a variety of convincing, novel, and exotic diseases may be simulated or created. The parent may deny any involvement and, in instances of intentional poisoning, smothering, or trauma, may continue the action while the child is hospitalized. Parents of children hospitalized for evaluation of **acute life-threatening events** have been videotaped in the process of smothering their children. MSBP is inflicted on children who are either unable or unwilling to identify the true offense and offender. Abusing caregivers gain attention from the relationships formed with health care providers or their own families as a result of the problems created.

CLINICAL MANIFESTATIONS. The child's symptoms, their pattern, or the response to treatment may not be compatible with a recognized disease. They may involve any organ system and suggest a panoply of disease processes. Although generally reported in preverbal children, cases have been recognized in children up to 16 yr of age. There may be a history of actual disease in which symptoms persist beyond the time when cure is anticipated. Symptoms in younger children are always associated with the proximity of the mother to the child. The mother may have a background in health care, may be supported by the father who may be unavailable, and may present as a devoted and model parent who forms close relationships with members of the health care team. She may have a history of Munchausen syndrome (MS) and seem relatively unconcerned about the severity of the child's illness.

Apnea and **seizures** are two common manifestations of MSBP. The observation may be falsified or may be created by partial suffocation. Toxins, medications, water, and salts can also create symptoms. Recognition of MSBP requires familiarity with those substances available to families and the wide array of consequences from misuse of these substances. The clinical pattern is variable, depending on the agent. It includes forced ingestion of medications such as ipecac to cause chronic vomiting or laxatives to cause diarrhea, or injection of insulin with consequent seizures. The skin, which is more easily accessible to the perpetrator, may be burned, dyed, tattooed, lacerated, or punctured to simulate acute or chronic skin conditions. Infectious or toxic agents may be administered into any available orifice. Provision of intravenous lines during hospitalization may provide an opportunity for injection of infectious agents from feces, toxins, and pharmacologic agents. Urine and blood samples may be contaminated with foreign blood or stool. Older children may become convinced that they have an illness and subsequently become dependent on the increased attention associated with the situation. This may lead to the child feigning symptoms.

DIAGNOSIS. Investigations should be based on a high index of suspicion of this diagnosis so that unpleasant, dangerous, or unnecessary tests are not undertaken on the child. Specimens that are carefully collected and documented through a chain of evidence should be analyzed for potentially harmful agents and for "foreign" blood. All steps in the investigation should be carefully documented. Records from other hospitals for the index child and siblings should be obtained and carefully reviewed. Hospitalized children should be under constant surveillance. This may include hidden television monitoring in coordination with law enforcement. Frequent staff meetings with detailed minutes are necessary to ensure that all information is gathered and recorded in a planned and forensic manner. This will facilitate the credibility of the diagnosis, which has already become controversial in England, and the protection of the child.

TREATMENT. After all laboratory information is collected and the diagnosis is established, the offending parent should be confronted by a nonaccusatory physician and staff who offer help. Any approach may be met with resistance, denial, and threats. All cases should be reported promptly and with careful documentation to CPS. The consequences of MSBP include persistence of abuse, emotional problems, chronic disability in 8% of cases, and death. Other siblings may be, or may have been, at risk; there is an association of this syndrome with unexplained infant deaths.

General

American Academy of Pediatrics: Guidance for Effective Discipline. *Pediatrics* 1998;101:723–728.

American Humane Association, Children's Division, 63 Inverness Drive East, Englewood, CO 80112-5117; http://www.amerhumane.org.

American Professional Society Against Child Abuse, 407 South Dearborn, Suite 1300, Chicago, IL 60605; http://www.apsac.org.

Block RW: Child abuse—Controversies and imposters. *Curr Probl Pediatr* 1999;29:249–272.

Committee on Child Abuse and Neglect, 2nd Committee on Children with Disabilities: Assessment of maltreatment of children with disabilities. *Pediatrics* 2001;108:508–511.

Drum PD, Cummings P, Krauss MR, et al: Identified spouse abuse as a risk factor for child abuse. *Child Abuse Negl* 2000;24:1375–1381.

Edwards VJ, Holden GW, Felitti VJ, et al: Relationship between multiple forms of childhood maltreatment and adult mental health in community respondents: Results from the Adverse Childhood Experiences Study. *Am J Psychiatry* 2003;160:1453–1460.

Finkelhor D, Omrod R, Turner H, et al: The victimization of children and youth: A comprehensive, national survey. *Child Maltreat* 2005;10:5–25.

Giardino A, Alexandor R (eds): *Child Maltreatment: A Clinical Guide and Reference,* 3rd edition. St Louis, GW Medical Publishing, 2005.

Meyers JEB, Berliner L, Briere J, et al (editors): *The APSAC Handbook on Child Maltreatment,* 2nd ed. Thousand Oaks, CA, Sage Publications, 2002.

National Clearinghouse on Child Abuse and Neglect, 330 C Street SW, Washington, DC 20477; (800) 394-3366; http.//nccanch.acf.hhs.gov.

Reece RM, Ludwig S (editors): *Child Abuse: Medical Diagnosis and Management.* Baltimore, Lippincott Williams & Wilkins, 2001.

Teicher MH, Samson JA, Polcari A, McGreenery CE: Sticks, stones, and hurtful words: relative effects of various forms of childhood maltreatment. *Am J Psychiatry* 2006;163(6):993–1000.

UNICEF: *A League Table of Child Maltreatment Deaths in Rich Nations. Innocenti Report Card No. 5.* New York, UNICEF, September 2003.

Physical Abuse

American Academy of Pediatrics Committee on Child Abuse and Neglect: Shaken baby syndrome: Rotational cranial injuries—technical report. *Pediatrics* 2001;108:206–210.

Barlow J, Stewart-Brown S: Child abuse and neglect. *Lancet* 2005;365:1750–1752.

Barnes PM, Norton CM, Dunstan FD, et al: Abdominal injury due to child abuse. *Lancet* 2005;366:234–235.

Bechtel K, Stoessel K, Leventhal JM, et al: Characteristics that distinguish accidental from abusive injury in hospitalized young children with head trauma. *Pediatrics* 2004;114:165–168.

Block RW, Krebs NF, Committee on Child Abuse and Neglect, and the Committee on Nutrition: Failure to thrive as a manifestation of child neglect. *Pediatrics* 2005;116:1234–1237.

Boos SC: Constrictive asphyxia: A recognizable form of fatal child abuse. *Child Abuse Negl* 2000;24:1503–1507.

Cabinum-Foeller E, Fraiser L: Bruising in children. *Lancet* 2005;365:1369–1370.

Carty HM: Fractures caused by child abuse. *J Bone Joint Surg Br* 1993;75:849–857.

Geddes JF, Plunkett J: The evidence base for shaken baby syndrome. *Br Med J* 2004;328:719–720.

Golden MH, Samuels MP, Southall DP: How to distinguish between neglect and deprivational abuse. *Arch Dis Child* 2003;88:105–107.

Hobbs CJ: Abdominal injury due to child abuse. *Lancet* 2005;366:187–188.

Kemp AM, Stoodley N, Cobley C, et al: Apnoea and brain swelling in non-accidental head injury. *Arch Dis Child* 2003;88:472–476.

Labbe J, Cauette G: Recent skin injuries in normal children. *Pediatrics* 2001;108:271–276.

Lantz PE, Sinal SH, Stanton CA, et al: Perimacular retinal folds from childhood head trauma. *Br Med J* 2004;328:754–756.

Laskey AL, Holsti M, Runyan DK, et al: Occult head trauma in young suspected victims of physical abuse. *J Pediatr* 2004;144:719–722.

Levene S, Bacon CJ: Sudden unexpected death and covert homicide in infancy. *Arch Dis Child* 2004;89:443–447.

MacMillan HL, Thomas BH, Jamison E, et al: Effectiveness of home visitation by public-health nurses in prevention of the recurrence of child physical abuse and neglect: A randomized controlled trial. *Lancet* 2005;365:1786–1792.

Maguire S, Mann MK, Sibert J, Kemp A: Are there patterns of bruising in childhood which are diagnostic or suggestive of abuse? A systematic review. *Arch Dis Child* 2005;90:182–186.

Maguire S, Mann MK, Sibert J, Kemp A: Can you age bruises accurately in children? A systematic review. *Arch Dis Child* 2005;90:187–189.

Mandelstam SA, Cook D, Fitzgerald M, et al: Complementary use of radiological skeletal survey and bone scintigraphy in detection of bony injuries in suspected child abuse. *Arch Dis Child* 2003;88:387–390.

Marlowe A, Pepin MG, Byers PH: Testing for osteogenesis imperfecta in cases of suspected non-accidental injury. *J Med Genet* 2002;39:382–386.

Mei-Zahav M, Uziel Y, Raz J, et al: Convulsions and retinal haemorrhage: Should we look further? *Arch Dis Child* 2002;86:334–335.

Miola J: Non-accidental injury in children: Making sense of the courts. *Lancet* 2004;364:228–230.

Nashelsky MB, Dix JD: The time interval between lethal infant shaking and onset of symptoms: A review of the shaken baby syndrome literature. *Am J Forensic Med Pathol* 1995;16:154–157.

Raiha NK, Soma D: Victims of child abuse and neglect in the U.S. Army. *Child Abuse Negl* 1997;21:759–768.

Reijneveld SA, van der Wal MF, Brugman E, et al: Infant crying and abuse. *Lancet* 2004;364:1340–1342.

Southall DP, Samuels MP, Golden MH: Classification of child abuse by motive and degree rather than type of injury. *Arch Dis Child* 2003;88:101–104.

Vinchon M, Noule N, Tchofo PJ, et al: Imaging of head injuries in infants: Temporal correlates and forensic implications for the diagnosis of child abuse. *J Neurosurg* 2004;101(1 Suppl):44–52.

Sexual Abuse

Almroth L, Elmusharaf S, El Hadi N, et al: Primary infertility after genital mutilation in girlhood in Sudan: A case-control study. *Lancet* 2005;366:385–391.

Bays J, Chadwick D: Medical diagnosis of the sexually abused child. *Child Abuse Negl* 1993;17:91–110.

Berenson AB, Chacko MR, Wiemann CM, et al: A case-control study of anatomic changes resulting from sexual abuse. *Am J Obstet Gynecol* 2000;182:820–831.

Christian C, Lavelle J, Dejong JL, et al: Forensic evidence findings in prepubertal victims of sexual assault. *Pediatrics* 2000;106:100–104.

Drach KM, Wientzen J, Ricci LR: The diagnostic utility of sexual behavior problems in diagnosing sexual abuse in a forensic child abuse clinic. *Child Abuse Negl* 2001;25:489–503.

Heger A, Emans SJ, Muram D (editors): *Evaluation of the Sexually Abused Child.* New York, Oxford University Press, 2000.
Heppenstall-Heger A, McConnell G, Ticson L, et al: Healing patterns in anogenital injuries: A longitudinal study of injuries associated with sexual abuse, accidental injuries, or genital surgery in the preadolescent child. *Pediatrics* 2003;112:829–837.
Holmes WC, Slap GB: Sexual abuse of boys. *JAMA* 1998;280:1855–1862.
Ingram DM, Everett VD, Ingram DL: The relationship between the transverse hymenal orifice diameter by the separation technique and other possible markers of sex abuse. *Child Abuse Negl* 2001;25:1109–1120.
Johnson CF: Child sexual abuse. *Lancet* 2004;364:462–470.
Jones LM, Finkelhor D, Kopiec K: Why is sexual abuse declining? A survey of state protection administrators, 2001. *Child Abuse Negl* 2001;25:1139–1158.
Kellogg N, American Academy of Pediatrics Committee on Child Abuse and Neglect: The evaluation of sexual abuse in children. *Pediatrics* 2005;116:506–512.
Leder MR, Knight JR, Emans SJ: Sexual abuse: Management strategies and legal issues, 2001. *Contemp Pediatr* 1;5:77–92.
McCann J, Voris J, Simon M, et al: Perianal findings in prepubertal children selected for nonabuse: A descriptive study. *Child Abuse Negl* 1989;13:179–193.
Swanston HY, Tebbutt JS, O'Toole BI, et al: Sexually abused children 5 years after presentation: A case controlled study. *Pediatrics* 1997;100:600–608.

Munchausen Syndrome by Proxy

Craft AW, Hall DMB: Munchausen syndrome by proxy and sudden infant death. *Br Med J* 2004;328:1309–1312.
Foreman DM: Detecting fabricated or induced illness in children. *Br Med J* 2005;331:978–979.
Hall DE, Eubanks L, Meyyazhagen S, et al: Evaluation of covert video surveillance in the diagnosis of Munchausen syndrome by proxy: Lessons from 41 cases. *Pediatrics* 2000;105:1305–1312.
Rosenberg DA: Munchausen syndrome by proxy: Medical diagnostic criteria. *Child Abuse Negl* 2003:27:421–430.
Schreier H: Munchausen by proxy. *Curr Probl Pediatr Adolesc Health Care* 2004;34:121–148.
Sheridan MS: The deceit continues: An updated literature review of Munchausen syndrome by proxy. *Child Abuse Negl* 2003;27:431–451.
Turner J, Reid S: Munchausen's syndrome. *Lancet* 2002;339:346–349.

Chapter 37 ■ Failure to Thrive

Howard Bauchner

Failure to thrive (FTT) is diagnosed in an infant or child whose physical growth is significantly less than that of his or her peers; it may be associated with poor developmental and cognitive functioning. FTT usually refers to growth below the 3rd or 5th percentile or a change in growth that has crossed two major growth percentiles (from above the 75th percentile to below the 25th) in a short time. **Organic FTT** is marked by an underlying medical condition; **nonorganic or psychosocial FTT** occurs in a child who is usually <5 yr old and has no known medical condition that causes poor growth.

EPIDEMIOLOGY AND ETIOLOGY. The prevalence of FTT depends on the population sampled. From 5 to 10% of premature infants and children living in poverty in developed countries may have FTT; the prevalence is much higher in developing countries with high rates of malnutrition and/or HIV infection. Family dysfunction, maternal deprivation, neonatal problems in addition to low birthweight, and maternal depression are associated with FTT. In developed countries, psychosocial FTT is far more common than organic FTT.

The causes of organic FTT are numerous (Table 37-1). Every organ system is represented. Psychosocial FTT usually occurs in

TABLE 37-1. Failure to Thrive: Differential Diagnosis by System

PSYCHOSOCIAL/BEHAVIORAL
Inadequate diet because of poverty/food insufficiency, errors in food preparation
Poor parenting skills (lack of knowledge of sufficient diet)
Child/parent interaction problems (autonomy struggles, coercive feeding, maternal depression)
Food refusal
Rumination
Parental cognitive or mental health problems
Child abuse or neglect; emotional deprivation
NEUROLOGIC
Cerebral palsy
Hypothalamic and other CNS tumors
Neuromuscular disorders
Neurodegenerative disorders
RENAL
Urinary tract infection
Renal tubular acidosis
Renal failure
ENDOCRINE
Diabetes mellitus
Diabetes insipidus
Hypothyroidism/hyperthyroidism
Growth hormone deficiency
Adrenal insufficiency
GENETIC/METABOLIC/CONGENITAL
Sickle cell disease
Inborn errors of metabolism (organic acidosis, hyperammonemia, storage disease)
Fetal alcohol syndrome
Skeletal dysplasias
Chromosomal disorders
Multiple congenital anomaly syndromes (VATER, CHARGE)
GASTROINTESTINAL
Pyloric stenosis
Gastroesophageal reflux
Repair of tracheoesophageal fistula
Malrotation
Malabsorption syndromes
Celiac disease
Milk intolerance: lactose, protein
Pancreatic insufficiency syndromes (cystic fibrosis)
Chronic cholestasis
Inflammatory bowel disease
Chronic congenital diarrhea states
Short bowel syndrome
Pseudo-obstruction
Hirschsprung disease
Food allergy
CARDIAC
Cyanotic heart lesions
Congestive heart failure
Vascular rings
PULMONARY/RESPIRATORY
Severe asthma
Cystic fibrosis; bronchiectasis
Chronic respiratory failure
Bronchopulmonary dysplasia
Adenoid/tonsillar hypertrophy
Obstructive sleep apnea
MISCELLANEOUS
Collagen-vascular disease
Malignancy
Primary immunodeficiency
Transplantation
INFECTIONS
Perinatal infection (TORCH)
Occult/chronic infections
Parasitic infestation
Tuberculosis
HIV

CHARGE, coloboma, heart disease, atresia choanae, retarded growth and retarded development and/or central nervous system anomalies, genital hypoplasia, and ear anomalies and/or deafness; TORCH, toxoplasma, other, rubella, cytomegalovirus, herpes simplex; VATER, vertebral defects, imperforate anus, tracheoesophageal fistula, and radial and renal dysplasia.

TABLE 37-2. Common Causes of Malnutrition in Early Life

NEONATE
Failed breastfeeding
Improper formula preparation
Psychosocial failure to thrive
Congenital syndromes
Prenatal infections
Teratogenic exposures
EARLY INFANCY
Psychosocial failure to thrive
Maternal depression
Improper formula preparation
Congenital heart disease
Cystic fibrosis
Neurologic abnormalities
Child neglect
Recurrent infections
LATER INFANCY
Celiac disease
Food intolerance
Child neglect
Delayed introduction of age-appropriate foods
Recurrent infections
Food allergy
AFTER INFANCY
Acquired chronic diseases
Highly distractible child
Inappropriate mealtime environment
Inappropriate diet
Recurrent infections

the setting of poverty or poor child-parent interaction. It occasionally occurs with severe family stress such as child or spousal abuse. Organic and nonorganic etiologic factors may also occur together, in children who are victims of abuse and neglect, temperamentally difficult premature infants, or HIV orphans who themselves are infected with HIV.

CLINICAL MANIFESTATIONS. The clinical presentation of FTT ranges from failure to meet expected age norms for height and weight to alopecia, loss of subcutaneous fat, reduced muscle mass, dermatitis, recurrent infections, and malnutrition (marasmus, kwashiorkor; see Chapter 43) [Table 37-2]. In developed countries, the most common presentation is poor growth detected in an ambulatory setting; in developing countries, recurrent infections, marasmus, and kwashiorkor are more common presentations.

Depending on severity, the infant with FTT may exhibit thin extremities, a narrow face, prominent ribs, and wasted buttocks. Neglect of hygiene may be evidenced by diaper rash, unwashed skin, untreated impetigo, uncut and dirty fingernails, or unwashed clothing (see Chapter 36). A flattened occiput with hair loss may indicate that the child has been lying on his or her back. This flattening may be due to being unattended for prolonged periods or positioning to prevent sudden infant death syndrome (SIDS) [see Chapter 372]. Delays in social and speech development are common. Other findings may include an avoidance of eye contact, an expressionless face, hypotonia, and the absence of a cuddling response.

The degree of FTT is usually measured by calculating each growth parameter (weight, height, and weight/height ratio) as a percentage of the median value for age based on appropriate growth charts. Appropriate growth charts are often not available for children with specific medical problems; serial measurements are especially important for these children. For premature infants, correction must be made for the extent of prematurity. Corrected age, rather than chronologic age, should be used in calculations of their growth percentiles until 1–2 yr of corrected age.

TABLE 37-3. Approach of Failure to Thrive Based on Signs and Symptoms

HISTORY/PHYSICAL EXAMINATION	DIAGNOSTIC CONSIDERATION
Spitting, vomiting, food refusal	Gastroesophageal reflux, chronic tonsillitis, food allergies
Diarrhea, fatty stools	Malabsorption, intestinal parasites, milk protein intolerance
Snoring, mouth breathing, enlarged tonsils	Adenoid hypertrophy, obstructive sleep apnea
Recurrent wheezing, pulmonary infections	Asthma, aspiration, food allergy
Recurrent infections	HIV or congenital immunodeficiency diseases
Travel to/from developing countries	Parasitic or bacterial infections of the gastrointestinal tract

Adapted from Frank D, Silva M: Failure to thrive: Myth and method. *Contemp Pediatr* 1993;10:114–133.

For weight, mild, moderate, and severe FTT is equivalent to 75–90%, 60–74%, and <60% of standard, respectively. For height, the corresponding values are 90–95%, 85–89%, and <85%. For the weight/height ratio, the values are 81–90%, 70–80%, and <70%. The weight for age percent of the standard value traditionally decreases early in the course of FTT, followed by a decrement of height for age. Children with chronic malnutrition often have a normal weight for height because both their weight and height are reduced.

DIAGNOSIS. The history, physical examination, and observation of the parent-child interaction usually suggest the diagnosis (Fig. 37-1). The latter observation, especially with feeding, is often critical to the diagnosis of psychosocial FTT.

The causes of insufficient growth include (1) failure of a parent to offer adequate calories, (2) failure of the child to take sufficient calories, and (3) failure of the child to retain sufficient calories. Reasons why parents or other caregivers may not offer appropriate or sufficient foods include lack of knowledge, parental depression, unusual dietary beliefs, or lack of food. The dietary history in infants with nutritional neglect may not be adequate because the parent misinforms the physician that the baby is receiving adequate calories. With young infants, it is particularly important to obtain a detailed dietary history, including what the diet consists of, how often the infant is fed, and how the parents respond when the child cries or sleeps for prolonged periods. Children may have difficulty swallowing if they have oral-motor dysfunction, anatomic abnormalities, cardiopulmonary dysfunction, or enlarged and recurrently infected tonsils and adenoids. Vomiting, diarrhea, and malabsorption are general causes of inadequate caloric absorption. It may be helpful to approach the diagnosis in terms of age (see Table 37-2) or signs and symptoms (Table 37-3).

Observation of the mother and infant may be helpful. In psychosocial FTT, the amount of time the mother spends holding, playing with, or talking to her child is usually reduced or inappropriate. An angry or depressed mother may feed her baby with unnecessary force (possibly resulting in a torn frenulum and aversion to feeding) or apathy, establishing no eye contact or positive interaction.

The laboratory evaluation of children with FTT is not always helpful and should be used judiciously. A complete blood count, lead level, and urinalysis represent a reasonable initial screen. Bone age is often helpful in distinguishing familial short stature (bone age equivalent to chronological age) from endocrine or nutritional abnormalities (bone age is less than chronological age). A skeletal survey is indicated in children <2 yr old who have evidence of possible physical abuse. Other tests, such as for thyroid function, gastroesophageal reflux and malabsorption, organic and amino acids, HIV and other infectious etiologies, or cystic fibrosis (sweat test), should be performed if indicated by the history or physical examination (see Fig. 37-1). Clinicians should be aware that celiac disease is more prevalent than once thought, and should be considered in infants and children with FTT and/or short stature. In addition, because of the possibility of allergic disease and availability of quantitative RAST testing, assessment for food allergy should be considered.

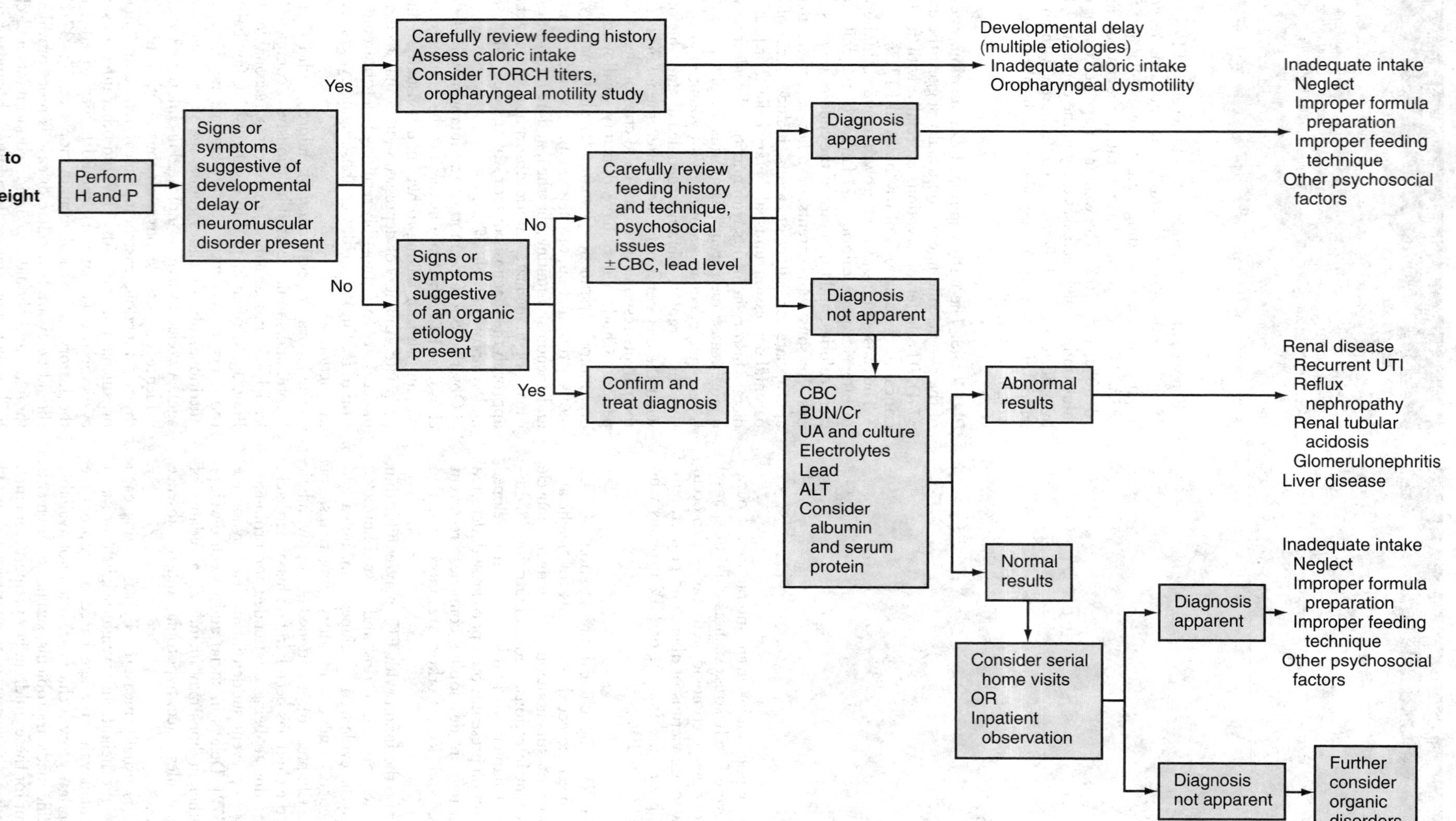

Figure 37-1. Flow chart for the stepwise evaluation of a child with failure to thrive (and weight loss). TORCH, toxoplasma, other, rubella, cytomegalovirus, herpes simplex; UTI, urinary tract infection. (Modified from Pomeranz AJ, Busey SL, Sabnis S, et al [editors]: *Pediatric Decision-Making Strategies to Accompany Nelson Textbook of Pediatrics*. Philadelphia, WB Saunders, p 313.)

Indications for **hospitalization** include severe malnutrition, further diagnostic and laboratory evaluation, lack of catch-up growth, and evaluation of the parent-child feeding interaction. Parents of children with organic FTT should be comfortable with the diagnosis and treatment before discharge. Children with suspected psychosocial FTT generally should be hospitalized and given an age-appropriate unlimited diet for ≈1 wk, usually approaching 150 kcal/kg (ideal weight) per 24 hr. The goals of hospitalization are to obtain sustained catch-up growth (generally >30 g/day for the 1st wk in young infants) and to educate parents about appropriate foods and feeding styles. A nursing plan should include careful charting of intake, weight, and observations of the mother's feeding style and interactions with the child. Staff should instruct the mother how to improve behaviors that may be deprivational, including instructions on how to hold the baby close during feeding.

For both organic and psychosocial FTT, the approach to feeding in the hospital should mimic the anticipated treatment at home before discharge.

TREATMENT. The treatment of FTT requires an understanding of all the elements that contribute to a child's growth: a child's health and nutritional status, family issues, and the parent-child interaction. Regardless of cause, an appropriate feeding atmosphere at home is important. Children with severe malnutrition must be re-fed carefully.

For children with organic FTT, the underlying medical condition should be treated. The type of caloric supplementation must be based on the severity of FTT and the underlying medical condition. The amount of protein in the diet must be carefully monitored in children with renal failure. The response to caloric supplementation depends on the specific diagnosis, medical treatment, and severity of FTT.

For older infants and young children with psychosocial FTT, mealtimes should be ≈20–30 min, solid foods should be offered before liquids, environmental distractions should be minimized, and children should eat with other people and not be force-fed. The intake of water, juice, soda, and low-calorie beverages should be limited. High-calorie foods, such as peanut butter, whole milk, cheese, and dried fruits, should be emphasized. The rule of 3's is quite helpful—3 meals, 3 snacks, and 3 choices. High-calorie supplementation such as Duocal or Polycose, high-calorie liquids such as Carnation Instant Breakfast with whole milk, or formulas containing >20 calories/oz (PediaSure, Ensure, Resource) are sometimes necessary. Weight gain in response to adequate caloric feedings usually establishes the diagnosis of psychosocial FTT.

PROGNOSIS. FTT in the 1st yr of life, regardless of cause, is particularly ominous. Maximal postnatal brain growth occurs in the 1st 6 mo of life. The brain grows as much in the 1st yr of life as in the rest of a child's life. Approximately ⅓ of children with psychosocial FTT are developmentally delayed and have social and emotional problems. The prognosis for children with organic FTT is more variable, depending on the specific diagnosis and severity of FTT. Ongoing assessment and monitoring of cognitive and emotional development, with appropriate intervention, is necessary for all children with FTT.

Alaimo K, Olson CM, Frongillo EA Jr: Food insufficiency and American school-aged children's cognitive, academic, and psychosocial development. *Pediatrics* 2001;108:44–53.

Fleisher DR: Comprehensive management of infants with gastroesophageal reflux and failure to thrive. *Curr Probl Pediatr* 1995;25:247–253.

Frank D, Silva M: Failure to thrive: Myth and method. *Contemp Pediatr* 1993;10:114–133.

Jolley CD: Failure to thrive. *Curr Probl Pediatr Adolesc Health Care* 2003;33:183–206.

Kelleher KJ, Casey PH, Bradley RH, et al: Risk factors and outcomes for failure to thrive in low birth weight preterm infants. *Pediatrics* 1993;91:941–948.

Maggioni A, Lifshitz F: Nutritional management of failure to thrive. *Pediatr Clin North Am* 1995;42:791–810.

National Institutes for Health: Consensus Development Conference on Celiac Disease. Available at http://consensus.nih.gov/cons/118/118cdc_intro.htm Accessed June 22, 2006.

Olson AL, Dietrich AJ, Prazar G, et al: Two approaches to maternal depression screening during well child visits. *J Dev Behav Pediatr* 2005;26:169–176.

Tanner EM, Finn-Stevenson M: Nutrition and brain development: Social policy implications. *Am J Orthopsychiatry* 2002;72:182–193.

Wilson TA, Rose SR, Cohen P, et al: Update of guidelines for the use of growth hormone in children: The Lawson Wilkins Pediatric Endocrinology Society Drug and Therapeutics Committee. *J Pediatr* 2003;143:415–421.

Chapter 38 ■ Developmental Disabilities and Chronic Illness

Paul H. Wise

Developmental disabilities and chronic illness represent a larger portion of childhood morbidity and mortality than ever before. This growing importance is due to the dramatic reduction in serious, acute infectious diseases in children coupled with a moderate rise in the prevalence of chronic conditions in the past several decades. This changing epidemiology presents clinicians who care for children with challenges and opportunities that will increasingly redefine the nature and scope of pediatric practice and child health policy.

OVERVIEW

DEFINITIONS. Chronic illness is defined by its duration, generally as a health condition that persists longer than 3 mo. It is also important to consider certain diseases as chronic based on their nature and expected duration. Certain categories of illness such as eczema, attention-deficit/hyperactivity disorder (ADHD), cerebral palsy, leukemia, and arthritis are often designated as chronic illnesses based on the diagnosis alone. Because the nature and seriousness of these categorically defined conditions can vary profoundly, some measure of severity or impact on daily life must also be utilized in assessing chronic illness in children. The specific impact on function that a condition generates is labeled a **functional limitation.** A **disability** generally refers to the social impact of a condition on a child's daily life, and is commonly assessed by measuring limitations in a child's ability to participate in expected activities, such as school attendance, age-appropriate play and sports, or community functions or rituals. **Children with special health care needs** (CSHCN) is a designation for children who have a risk for or the presence of a chronic physical, developmental, behavioral, or emotional condition and who also require health and related services of a type or amount beyond that required by children generally.

DEVELOPMENT AND CHRONIC ILLNESS AND DEVELOPMENTAL DISABILITIES IN CHILDREN

For children, the nature and cadence of developmental change will shape and reshape the ultimate impact of chronic illness on daily life. In **infancy,** chronic disorders can affect both growth and development. **Failure to thrive** is a common manifestation, as chronic illness can affect feeding and metabolic demands (see Chapter 37). Infants with chronic illnesses can also be easily fatigued and may not be as responsive to caretakers or their surroundings as healthy infants are. Disorders in this period may also have lasting effects as they can influence developmental processes in critical periods of system maturation, such as for vision and hearing. In the **toddler period,** chronic illness can alter normal developmental progressions, including measured milestones, speech, and children's exploration of their surroundings. Frequent illness episodes and hospitalizations can also alter normal parental relationships with their children and may leave a parent with a lasting sense that the child is highly vulnerable even if, with time, all real danger has passed. In the **preschool years,** children tend to relate their illness to the consequences of their own behavior, particularly if they have disobeyed parental rules: *disease as punishment* for behavioral transgressions. Later, in the **mid elementary school years,** children begin to frame disease as a result of external agents, such as germs, entering the body: *disease as combat,* in which germs and the body are engaged in ongoing battle. **Preteens and teens** develop a more abstract sense of disease causation, principally as the interaction of inheritance, organ functions, and the external environment: *disease as feeling bad,* with the confluence of symptoms into broader somatic and emotional states. This developmental progression should help guide the clinician in addressing children's concerns and in shaping educational materials directed at children with specific chronic conditions.

Many children with chronic illness become highly sophisticated in the medical jargon and treatment routines associated with their condition. This may obscure a poor understanding of the causes and implications of their illness and mask health-related beliefs and fears that are typical of children of their age and developmental stage. A child's cognitive level may not translate into enhanced compliance with medical recommendations. Rebellious behavior may be greatest and compliance with risk-reduction advice and medication regimens may be poorest among adolescents, despite the fact that they possess the most advanced cognitive abilities to understand their illness and its consequences.

Clinicians should be particularly attentive to child and family needs during several critical, **developmental transitions.** Discharge from the hospital is often a time of critical need, particularly if the hospitalization was prolonged, the child's diagnosis was 1st ascertained, or major home care tasks will be required. Establishing close follow-up by primary care providers is essential after hospital discharge, as acute exacerbations can occur and medical regimens arranged by hospital staff may encounter unforeseen obstacles as time passes. A 2nd period of difficult transition is when the parent or other caretaker with primary responsibility for the daily care of the child becomes employed. Primary health care providers may be asked to assist families in finding appropriate child care arrangements and to convey necessary medical information and advice to the child care facility. A 3rd special transition occurs with school entry. Health providers will often help ensure that school programs are responsive to the child's needs and that school personnel have prepared for possible emergencies and can administer any medications or services that need to be provided in the school setting. A 4th transition is at adolescence. Chronic conditions may complicate the usual difficulties facing adolescents and their families, including risk taking, drug and alcohol use, peer relationships and developing sexuality. The 5th, and often the most difficult, transition is the passage from adolescence to adulthood. In addition to the aging of their parents, young adults with a chronic illness often become ineligible for the public programs they long utilized as children and adolescents, which can complicate the already complex task of seeking personal and economic independence.

PUBLIC PROGRAMS OF IMPORTANCE TO CHILDREN WITH CHRONIC ILLNESS AND DISABILITIES

There are public programs in the United States that can provide assistance to families of children with chronic illness. Several provide health insurance coverage. **Medicaid,** Title XIX of the Social Security Act, is the principal public health insurance program for poor children. Eligibility is based on family income and wealth. Federal mandates require that children <6 yr of age be eligible if their income falls below the federal poverty line, which for 2005 was $19,350 of annual income for a family of four. For older children and adolescents, the income requirements generally become more stringent but can vary considerably by state. A range of services is covered in all states, including immunizations, screening, physician services, hospitalizations, and most medications. Considerable variation among the states may exist in coverage for dental care, eyewear, equipment such as wheelchairs or monitoring devices, and home-based and other support services. The **State Children's Health Insurance Program (SCHIP)** is directed at assisting families whose income is too high for Medicaid eligibility but too low to reasonably expect that they will be able to acquire coverage in the private market. SCHIP provides the states considerable autonomy in determining covered services, which in most states are far more limited than those covered by Medicaid. The **Supplemental Security Income (SSI)** program provides cash assistance and Medicaid coverage for families whose children have severe physical, mental, or developmental disabilities. The states also administer federal funds for maternal and child health services from **Title V** of the Social Security Act. These programs provide a variety of coordinating and clinical services for children who have chronic illnesses and developmental disabilities. The **Individuals with Disability Education Act (IDEA)** mandates that all children with disabilities receive an appropriate education in the least restrictive environment and funds a variety of early intervention and special education programs. **Early Intervention (EI)** programs provide a range of direct services for children <3 years of age with chronic illness or developmental needs. These services are directed at enhancing the developmental progress of participating children and generally offer important family-centered support and education services.

38.1 • Chronic Illness in Childhood

• Paul H. Wise

EPIDEMIOLOGY. Patterns of chronic illness in childhood are both complex and dynamic. Unlike chronic disease in adults, serious chronic illness in children is relatively rare and widely heterogeneous. This has profound implications for the organization of children's health services, as pediatricians have the difficult task of identifying and caring for children with unusual and varied conditions. Accordingly, child health services have become far more reliant on standardized screening programs and formal systems of referral to regional specialty care programs than are health care systems for adults. Pediatrics has been characterized by rapid progress in preventing serious acute illnesses and in extending the lives of children who previously would have succumbed to their illness early in life. These factors have made the epidemiology of childhood far more dynamic than that of the adult world.

National survey data suggest that ≈30% of all children have some form of chronic health condition. If allergies, eczema, minor visual impairments, and other conditions not likely to generate serious consequences are excluded, then between 15 and 20% of all children have a chronic physical, learning, or developmental disorder. Boys have higher rates of chronic illness than do girls. There is considerable variation in the nature and severity of chronic illnesses in children (Table 38-1). The most common serious chronic condition is asthma, with >12% of children having received a diagnosis of asthma at some time in their lives; half of these children were reported to have experienced asthma symptoms in the prior 12 mo (see Chapter 143). Approximately 6% of children are reported to have a diagnosis of ADHD (see Chapter 31). Overweight is not usually included as a chronic health condition; however, nearly 17% of all children aged 6

TABLE 38-1. Prevalence and Activity Limitation for Selected Chronic Diseases in Children <18 Years of Age: United States, 2000–2003

CONDITION	NUMBER (IN THOUSANDS)	PREVALENCE (PER 100,000 CHILDREN)	ACTIVITY LIMITATION* (% OF CHILDREN WITH CONDITION)
Asthma	9,017	12,419	6.9
ADHD/ADD	4,034	6,078	5.5
Developmental delay	2,061	3,145	16.7
Congenital and other heart conditions	957	1,318	9.76
Mental retardation	447	677	27.7
Cerebral palsy	273	375	36.24
Autism	234	322	18.2
Sickle cell anemia	151	209	23.91
Diabetes	120	166	4.8
Down syndrome	104	141	23.9
Arthritis	73	101	37.11
Muscular dystrophy	35	48	81.3
Cystic fibrosis	29	40	33.9

*Presence of an impairment or health problem that limits the ability to crawl, walk, run, or play.
Figures based on weighted and age-adjusted national sample. ADD, attention-deficit disorder; ADHD, attention-deficit/hyperactivity disorder.
Data from National Health Interview Survey, 2000–2003. National Center for Health Statistics, Centers for Disease Control.

through 19 have a body mass index above the 95th percentile (see Chapter 44). Reliable national data on major childhood depression are not currently available; some estimates suggest prevalence among 9 to 17 yr olds of ≈5% (see Chapter 25).

The severity and impact of chronic illnesses can vary significantly (see Table 38-1). Approximately 8% of all children have activity limitations due to one or more chronic illnesses. Of these children, ≈40% have developmental or learning disorders, 35% have chronic physical conditions, and 25% report chronic mental health disorders. Approximately 2% of children have chronic conditions and activity limitation severe enough to meet eligibility criteria for the SSI program. Approximately 13% of all children meet the chronic illness and elevated service needs of the CSHCN definition.

These current prevalence figures represent a substantial increase in childhood chronic illness in the past several decades. While ≈8% of children were reported to have a chronic health condition that limited their activities in 2003, the comparable figure in 1960 was only 2%. Although the increase in childhood chronic illness is likely due in part to changes in survey methodologies, improvements in diagnosis, and expanded public awareness of behavioral and developmental disorders, there is strong evidence that the prevalence of certain important chronic child health conditions has increased. Asthma rates rose from <4% in 1980 to ≈13% in 2003. The prevalence of ADHD and autism has also increased considerably. Although improvements in the survival of infants and young children from prematurity, congenital anomalies, and genetic disorders have also contributed to the rising prevalence rates, this source accounts for only a small portion of all chronic illness in childhood.

Chronic illness accounts for a growing portion of serious illness, hospitalizations, and deaths among children in the United States. Children with a chronic illness are hospitalized approximately four times more often and spend more than seven times as many days in the hospital as children without a chronic illness. Estimates suggest that chronic illness accounts for the majority of all nontraumatic hospitalizations for children, a figure that has more than doubled in the past four decades. Multiple admissions in any given year have also risen substantially. The majority of all non–trauma related deaths in children are now due to chronic disorders. This historical shift in the distribution of pediatric hospitalization and mortality reflects not only the rise in the prevalence of childhood chronic illness, but also marked reductions in the incidence of serious acute pediatric illness.

Chronic illness is also contributing more profoundly to **social disparities** in child health. There are somewhat conflicting data on the association of poverty and the prevalence of chronic disorders in children, although most studies suggest a moderate elevation among poor children. Poor and African-American children have greater limitations in activity due to chronic conditions. Children enrolled in welfare cash assistance programs are more likely to have a chronic illness than in previous years. Although prematurity and homicide remain the largest contributors to elevated mortality among African-American children in the United States, chronic conditions have become the fastest growing contributor in the past two decades.

ENHANCED NEEDS OF CHILDREN WITH CHRONIC ILLNESS AND THEIR FAMILIES

Although the nature and severity of chronic illness in children is quite heterogeneous, there are important clinical considerations that are common to virtually all such conditions regardless of their specific diagnosis or specialty group.

FINANCIAL COSTS. The care required by children with serious chronic illnesses is usually associated with high financial costs. Most states have some mechanism to facilitate health insurance coverage for children, although the nature and scope of these programs can vary considerably. A growing number of private and public health insurance plans require deductibles and co-payments, which can accumulate rapidly for a child with a chronic illness. Some plans offer coverage up to a designated cost, period of hospitalization, or for a certain number of specialty visits. Once this cap has been reached, a larger portion or all of the costs may be borne by the family. Of great importance for children with serious chronic disorders, many new procedures, medications, or therapeutic regimens may be considered "experimental" by some insurers and not covered. Insurance coverage policies often generate strong incentives for hospital rather than outpatient care, even if the latter is indicated. Frequent medical visits and hospitalizations can interfere with parental employment and undermine job performance and security.

COMPLEX CLINICAL MANAGEMENT. Children with serious chronic disorders usually require intense clinical management both in community and hospital settings. Close surveillance of disease progression, symptoms and functioning, and adverse medication effects often necessitates frequent communication and office visits. Managing hospital admissions and discharge planning may also prove complex and involve a variety of clinicians and community resources. As pressure to reduce hospitalization has grown, the burden on outpatient systems has increased accordingly. An uncoordinated approach to the multitude of required clinical visits can prove highly burdensome to the family and can undermine even the most committed family's attempts to comply.

Pain. Many chronic illnesses are characterized by constant or episodic bouts of severe pain that can alter a child's affect and interfere with most daily activities, including school, social activities, and sleeping patterns (see Chapter 77). Assessing pain in young children or those with developmental disorders can be difficult; parents or other caretakers often have significant insight into the location and severity of pain in their children. Because serious, chronic pain is relatively unusual in children, many child health practitioners may be inexperienced with pain management and require the involvement of specialty providers or regional programs with expertise in this area. The emotional toll on parents of children experiencing chronic pain can also be profound and require close attention by medical personnel.

Behavioral and Adjustment Issues. Although chronic illness in children elevates the likelihood that they will experience psychologic and behavioral problems, most children with chronic illness will experience the same level of psychologic and behavioral issues as other children their age. Behavioral and adjustment problems are more likely to occur the earlier the onset of the illness, particularly if it emerges in infancy. The risk of psychologic and behavioral problems does not appear to be associated with the severity of the chronic illness per se. These effects can occur across all diagnoses, although are more profound for disorders that affect the central nervous system, including cerebral palsy, head trauma, and treatment-related complications that affect the brain, such as chemotherapy for cancer. Children with higher levels of cognitive ability appear to be less likely to develop serious behavioral or adjustment problems. Familial strife and mental illness, particularly depression in the mother, have been associated with an enhanced risk for psychologic and behavioral consequences.

Impact on Families. Like all children, a child with a chronic illness usually brings a mix of challenges and joy to a family. The presence of a chronic illness can add extra burdens, which can be expressed in a variety of forms. First, the daily requirements of care should never be underestimated, particularly when the child is unable to perform tasks such as bathing, dressing, toilet use, and feeding. Second, the care required by the child with chronic illness may divert needed attention from siblings and strain normal family dynamics. Third, the ultimate burden faced by families of children with a chronic illness is the emotional toll exacted by the daily struggles, pain, and, occasionally, early death that chronic illness can imply. Fourth, among the most difficult attributes of childhood chronic illness is the inherent unpredictability of its course and ultimate impact. Clinicians should be sensitive to how difficult it can be living with a child whose condition can worsen at any moment and without apparent cause. Fifth, children with serious chronic illness and their parents may harbor powerful hopes for new breakthroughs or divine intervention. Clinicians should understand the importance of these hopes for the families under their care and should explore related hopes for lesser, more incremental steps, such as attending school, playing sports, or taking a special trip.

Comprehensive Care and the Medical Home. All children require a clinician who takes responsibility for their comprehensive health care needs. To meet this responsibility, the coordinated implementation of a series of essential practice components, often termed the **medical home,** is recommended. While essential for all children, these practice elements take on special importance for children with chronic disorders and are outlined as follows.

Preventive Services. Primary care is an essential component of health care for children with chronic disease. This requirement can easily be overlooked in addressing the more specialized needs of these patients. Children with chronic disorders are commonly less well immunized than their healthy counterparts. Well child care may be disrupted by visits for acute exacerbations of the chronic disorder and clinicians may postpone immunizations due to generally inappropriate fears that the chronic illness or its symptoms are contraindications to immunization. A family's reliance on specialty services can be so great that the need for primary care is overlooked. Special effort may be required to ensure the provision of high quality primary care to children with chronic illness.

Continuity of Care. Children with chronic illnesses are particularly dependent on a stable, ongoing relationship with clinicians and the health care system. The duration and complexity of chronic illness in children require that the clinician responsible for coordinating the child's care have a good understanding of the child's clinical history, including patterns of exacerbation and response to medications and other interventions. Continuity of care also serves as a basis for building trust and effective communication between affected families and clinicians, a prerequisite for high quality care. Practice structures, therefore, should ensure the identification of a principal clinical provider and facilitate the provider's involvement in all necessary care.

Access to Urgent Care. Clinicians should expect that children with chronic illness will have enhanced requirements for urgent consultation, emergency care, and hospitalization. Practice mechanisms that ensure rapid access to medical consultation both by telephone and office visitation are essential. Procedures for urgent referral to appropriate facilities for emergency evaluation and hospitalization should also be established. This is particularly important in managed care systems that may require primary care referral or approval for care at referral sites.

Access to Specialty Care. Children with chronic illness commonly require specialized care. The need for specialty referral is particularly important in pediatrics because serious disorders are relatively rare in children. Regional systems of specialty referral and hospitalization have been formalized in the past several decades, particularly for perinatal care, pediatric trauma, and children with serious chronic illness. These systems of "regionalized" specialty care have been shown to reduce dramatically morbidity and mortality among affected children. The heavy reliance on specialty care referral enhances the importance of the medical home. Responsive communication between primary care practices and specialty programs is essential, particularly in conveying the reasons for referral, patient history, the nature and findings of the specialty evaluation, hospital course, and the collaborative development of a follow-up management plan.

Enhanced Information Systems. Children with chronic illness often require careful monitoring of their clinical status and the rapid evaluation of exacerbations. On-call and related coverage systems must include immediate access to up-to-date medical record information for children with complex histories and management regimens. Electronic medical records and systems that permit parent or other caretakers routine access to computerized medical record information may also prove useful.

Linkage to Schools, Support Groups, and Community Services. Children with chronic illnesses often have special educational needs and may require the active participation of teachers and school health personnel in medical care plans. Special mechanisms should be established to ensure close coordination with schools, including provisions for collaborative evaluations of needs, monitoring of educational performance and social interactions, and the ongoing refinement of medical and educational management regimens. Clinicians can prevent the isolation many families feel by connecting them to support and advocacy groups comprised of other parents with similarly affected children. Such connections have been facilitated by use of the Internet, which can link children and families over wide geographic areas.

Logistic Access. The difficulties that families can experience in transporting children with serious physical or behavioral disorders should never be underestimated. Particularly for older children or those requiring wheelchairs or other equipment, urban public transportation systems may be seriously impractical. In suburban and rural areas, transportation may involve traveling over great distances. For parents who have daytime employment, extended clinic hours may be required. Many communities have implemented innovative transportation programs for families in need of health and social services, particularly when available means of travel to clinical facilities is deemed unsafe or if it requires specially equipped vehicles or the assistance of trained personnel. In a growing number of areas, specially designed telephone, radio, or Internet communication systems have greatly enhanced access to primary and specialty care consultation.

Cultural and Language Competency (see also Chapter 4). Clinicians must possess a basic understanding of the meaning of illness and traditions of healing in the communities they serve. While such cultural competence of individual providers is important, access also depends on creating clinical programs that respond to local perceptions and social institutions. Cultural competence not only reduces the likelihood of misunderstandings and medical errors, but also helps ensure that clinical programs can take full advantage of the many strengths that exist in culturally defined communities.

The most basic element of communication between clinicians and families of children with a chronic illness is that they share a common language. Clinicians should not overestimate their own or a parent's basic command of a language and must ensure that conveyed information is well understood. Children should not be used as interpreters despite the fact that they often have a better command of English than do their parents. Given the complex issues chronic illness can generate, it is far more useful to integrate trained interpreters into programs for chronically ill children in locations characterized by diverse language groups.

Nondiscrimination in Access and Clinical Decision-Making. Clinicians who care for children with chronic illness must recognize the power of social status to define access to care. A history of inadequate service provision or different levels of service for distinct social groups can generate deep resentment and distrust for the medical system. Many studies have suggested that even when patients have adequate health insurance, poor and minority patients are less likely to be offered recommended diagnostic and therapeutic interventions. While the precise reasons for these observations remain unclear, it is important that provider preconceptions do not replace a careful consideration of the true desires and capabilities of families, particularly in association with new, specialized, or home-based interventions. Strategies to confront these issues include the training and recruitment of minority health providers, educational programs for clinicians, and the active assessment of clinical decision-making and family experiences at clinical facilities.

American Academy of Pediatrics, Committee on Children with Disabilities: The role of the pediatrician in transitioning children and adolescents with developmental disabilities and chronic illnesses from school to work or college. *Pediatrics* 2000;106:854–856.

Kastner TA; American Academy of Pediatrics, Committee on Children with Disabilities: Managed care and children with special health care needs. *Pediatrics* 2004;114:1693–1698.

Medical Home Initiatives for Children with Special Needs Project Advisory Committee, American Academy of Pediatrics: The medical home. *Pediatrics* 2002;110:184–186.

Newacheck PW, Kim SE: A national profile of health care utilization and expenditures for children with special health care needs. *Arch Pediatr Adolesc Med* 2005;159:10–17.

Palfrey JS, Sofis LA, Davidson EJ, et al: The pediatric alliance of coordinated care: Evaluation of a medical home model. *Pediatrics* 2004;113:1507–1516.

Perrin EC, Gerrity PS: There's a demon in your belly: Children's understanding of illness. *Pediatrics* 1981;67:841–848.

Perrin JM, Shayne MW, Bloom SR: *Home and Community Care for Chronically Ill Children.* New York, Oxford University Press, 1993.

Stein REK (ed): *Caring for Children with Chronic Illness.* New York, Springer, 1989.

Strickland B, McPherson M, Weissman G, et al: Access to the medical home: Results of the National Survey of Children with Special Health Care Needs. *Pediatrics* 2004;113:1485–1492.

Wise PH: The transformation of child health in the United States. *Health Aff (Millwood)* 2004;23:9–25.

38.2 • Mental Retardation (Intellectual Disability) • Bruce K. Shapiro and Mark L. Batshaw

Mental retardation refers to a group of disorders that have in common deficits of adaptive and intellectual function and an age of onset before maturity is reached.

DEFINITION. The most commonly used definition of mental retardation comes from the U.S. special education law, the Individuals with Disabilities Education Act (IDEA). It defines mental retardation as "significantly sub-average general intellectual functioning, existing concurrently with deficits in adaptive behavior and manifested during the developmental period, that adversely affects a child's educational performance" [34 Code of Federal Regulations §300.7(c)(6)]. The most commonly used medical diagnostic criteria for mental retardation are those contained in the American Psychiatric Association's (APA's) *Diagnostic and Statistical Manual of Mental Disorders, Fourth Edition, Text Revision (DSM-IV-TR)* [Table 38-2]. The classification of mental retardation that results from these definitions has been criticized for depending on IQ test performance rather than adaptive behavior, not taking the standard error of measurement into account, and not being predictive of outcomes for individuals. The American Association on Mental Retardation (AAMR) has proposed a different classification system. Instead of defining degrees of deficit (mild to profound), the AAMR definition substitutes levels of support required (intermittent, limited, extensive, or pervasive) in areas of adaptive function. The reliability of this approach has been challenged, and it blurs the distinction between mental retardation and other developmental disorders (communication disorder, autism, specific learning disabilities). The AAMR and APA classifications of mental retardation use different definitions of significantly sub-average intellectual function. The AAMR definition increases the IQ threshold for mental retardation from 70 to 75 to reflect the standard error of IQ measurement. This definition doubles the prevalence of mental retardation.

TABLE 38-2. Diagnostic Criteria for Mental Retardation

A. Significantly sub-average intellectual functioning: an IQ score of ≈70 or below on an individually administered IQ test (for infants, a clinical judgment of significantly sub-average intellectual functioning).
B. Concurrent deficits or impairments in present adaptive functioning (i.e., the person's effectiveness in meeting the standards expected for his or her age by his or her cultural group) in at least two of the following areas: communication, self-care, home living, social/interpersonal skills, use of community resources, self-direction, functional academic skills, work, leisure, health, and safety.
C. The onset is before age 18 years.

Code based on degree of severity reflecting level of intellectual impairment:

317	Mild Mental Retardation:	IQ level 50–55 to ≈70
318.0	Moderate Mental Retardation:	IQ level 35–40 to 50–55
318.1	Severe Mental Retardation:	IQ level 20–25 to 35–40
318.2	Profound Mental Retardation:	IQ level below 20–25
319	Mental Retardation, Severity Unspecified:	when there is a strong presumption of mental retardation but the person's intelligence is untestable by standard tests

From American Psychiatric Association: *Diagnostic and Statistical Manual of Mental Disorders, Fourth Edition, Text Revision.* Washington, DC, American Psychiatric Association 2000, p 49, reprinted by permission.

The term **mental retardation** itself has been challenged because it is stigmatizing, has been used to limit the achievements of the individual, and has not met its initial objective of providing assistance to people with the disorder. The term **intellectual disability** has not been universally adopted because intellectual disability may refer to other conditions besides mental retardation and existing laws and their attendant entitlements use the term mental retardation. In Europe, the term **learning disability** is often used to describe intellectual disability. **Global developmental delay** is a term often used to describe young children whose limitations have not yet resulted in a formal diagnosis of mental retardation; it is often inappropriately used beyond the point when it is clear the child has mental retardation.

ETIOLOGY. There appear to be two overlapping populations of children with intellectual disability: mild mental retardation (IQ >50), which is more associated with environmental influences; and severe mental retardation (IQ <50), which is more frequently linked to biologic causes (see Chapter 1). Mild mental retardation is four times more likely to be found in the offspring of women who have not completed high school than in women who have graduated. This is presumably a consequence of both genetic (children may inherit an intellectual impairment) and socioeconomic (poverty, undernutrition) factors. The specific causes of mild mental retardation are currently identifiable in <50% of affected individuals. The most common biologic causes of mild mental retardation include genetic syndromes with multiple minor congenital anomalies, fetal deprivation, prematurity, perinatal insults, intrauterine exposure to drugs of abuse, and sex chromosomal abnormalities. Familial clustering is frequent.

In children with severe mental retardation, a biologic cause (most commonly prenatal) can be identified in >75% of cases. Causes include chromosomal (Down syndrome) and other genetic syndromes (fragile X syndrome), abnormalities of brain development (lissencephaly), and inborn errors of metabolism/neurodegenerative disorders (mucopolysaccharidoses) [Table 38-3]. Consistent with finding that disorders that affect early embryogenesis are the most common and severe, the earlier the problem occurs in development, the more severe its consequences tend to be.

EPIDEMIOLOGY. The prevalence of mental retardation depends on the definition, the method of ascertainment, and the population. According to statistics (based on the APA definition), 2.5% of the population should have mental retardation, and 85% of these individuals should fall into the range of mild mental retardation. In 2001–2002, ≈592,000 or 1.2% of school-aged children received services for mental retardation in federally supported school programs in the United States. For several reasons, fewer children than predicted are identified as having mild mental retardation. Because it is more difficult to diagnose mild mental retardation than the more severe forms, professionals may defer the diagnosis of mental retardation and "give the benefit of the doubt" to the child. Some instruments (Stanford-Binet, 4th edition) under-identify young children with mild mental retardation

Young children may show cognitive limitations without significant delays in adaptive behavior. As a result, new cases of mild mental retardation continue to be diagnosed among children up to ≈9 yr of age. Children with mental retardation may be incorporated into another diagnosis (autism, cerebral palsy). It is possible that the number of children with mild mental retardation is actually decreasing as a result of public health measures. While this may be true, the number of school children who receive services for mental retardation has not changed appreciably since 1997.

Unlike mild mental retardation, the prevalence of severe mental retardation has not changed appreciably since the 1940s and is ≈0.3–0.5% of the population. Many of the causes of severe mental retardation involve genetic or congenital brain malformations that can neither be anticipated nor treated at present. In addition, new populations with severe intellectual disability have offset the decreases in the prevalence of severe mental retardation that resulted from improved health care. Although prenatal diagnosis has been associated with a decreased prevalence of Down syndrome (see Chapter 81) and early intervention has helped to reduce mental retardation caused by phenylketonuria and congenital hypothyroidism, the increased prevalence of prenatal drugs of abuse (see Chapter 96.4) and improved survival of "micro" premature infants have increased the prevalence of mental retardation.

Overall, mental retardation occurs more frequently in boys than in girls: 2:1 in mild mental retardation and 1.5 : 1 in severe mental retardation. In part this may be a consequence of the many X-linked disorders associated with intellectual disability, the most prominent being fragile X syndrome.

TABLE 38-3. Identification of Cause in Children with Severe Mental Retardation

CAUSE	EXAMPLES	PERCENT OF TOTAL
Chromosomal disorder	Trisomies 21, 18, 13, Klinefelter syndrome	22
Genetic syndrome	Fragile X, Prader-Willi syndrome	21
Developmental brain abnormality	Hydrocephalus ± meningomyelocele, lissencephaly	9
Inborn errors of metabolism/ neurodegenerative disorder	PKU, Tay-Sachs	8
Congenital infections	HIV, toxoplasmosis, rubella, CMV, syphilis, herpes simplex	4
Familial retardation	Environment, syndromic, or genetic	6
Perinatal causes	HIE, meningitis, IVH, PVL, fetal alcohol syndrome	4
Postnatal causes	Trauma, meningitis, hypothyroidism	5
Unknown	Cerebral palsy	21
Total		100

CMV, cytomegalovirus; HIE, hypoxic ischemic encephalopathy; HIV, human immunodeficiency virus; IVH, intraventricular hemorrhage; PKU, phenylketonuria; PVL, periventricular leukomalacia.

Modified from Stromme P, Hayberg G: Aetiology in severe and mild mental retardation: A population based study of Norwegian children. *Dev Med Child Neurol* 2000;42:76–86.

PATHOLOGY/PATHOGENESIS. The limitations in our knowledge of the neuropathology of intellectual disability are exemplified by the fact that 10–20% of brains of individuals with severe mental retardation appear entirely normal by standard neuropathologic study. The majority of brains of these individuals show only mild, nonspecific changes that correlate poorly with the degree of intellectual disability. These changes include microcephaly, gray matter heterotopias in the subcortical white matter, unusually regular columnar arrangement of the cortex, and neurons that are more tightly packed than usual. Only a minority of the brain shows more specific changes in dendritic and synaptic organization, with dysgenesis of dendritic spines or cortical pyramidal neurons, or impaired growth of dendritic trees.

The programming of the central nervous system (CNS) involves a process of induction; CNS maturation is defined in terms of genetic, molecular, autocrine, paracrine, and endocrine influences. Receptors, signaling molecules, and genes are critical to brain development. The maintenance of different neuronal phenotypes in the adult brain involves the same genetic transcripts that play a crucial role during fetal development with activation of similar intracellular signal transduction mechanisms. Several syndromes that were thought to involve complex chromosomal abnormalities are caused by single gene mutations involving induction. Rubinstein-Taybi syndrome (see Chapter 81), a disorder marked clinically by broad thumbs and great toes, characteristic facies, and severe mental retardation, has been shown to result from a mutation in the gene encoding for the transcrip-

TABLE 38-4. Common Presentations of Mental Retardation by Age

AGE	AREA OF CONCERN
Newborn	Dysmorphic syndromes, microcephaly Major organ system dysfunction (e.g., feeding and breathing)
Early infancy (2–4 mo)	Failure to interact with the environment Concerns about vision and hearing impairments
Later infancy (6–18 mo)	Gross motor delay
Toddlers (2–3 yr)	Language delays or difficulties
Preschool (3–5 yr)	Language difficulties or delays Behavior difficulties, including play Delays in fine motor skills: cutting, coloring, drawing
School age (>5 yr)	Academic underachievement Behavior difficulties (attention, anxiety, mood, conduct, and so on)

tional co-activator CREB binding protein (CBP), a factor important in the control of gene expression in early embryogenesis.

CLINICAL MANIFESTATIONS. Early diagnosis of mental retardation facilitates earlier intervention, realistic goal setting, easing of parental anxiety, and greater acceptance of the child in the community. Most children with intellectual disability 1st come to the pediatrician's attention in infancy because of dysmorphisms, associated dysfunctions, or failure to meet age-appropriate developmental milestones. There are no specific physical characteristics of intellectual disability, but dysmorphisms are the earliest signs that bring children to the attention of the pediatrician. They may comprise a genetic syndrome such as Down syndrome or be isolated, as in microcephaly. Associated dysfunctions are neurologic disorders (seizures, cerebral palsy, autism) that are seen more frequently in conjunction with mental retardation than in the general population.

Most children with intellectual disability do not keep up with their peers and fail to meet age-expected norms. In early infancy, failure to meet age-appropriate expectations may include a lack of visual or auditory responsiveness, unusual muscle tone (hypo- or hypertonia) or posture, and feeding difficulties. Between 6 and 18 mo of age, motor delay (lack of sitting, crawling, walking) is the most common complaint. Language delay and behavior problems are common concerns after 18 mo (Table 38-4). Earlier identification of atypical development is likely to occur with more severe impairments; mental retardation is usually identifiable by age 3 yr.

LABORATORY FINDINGS. The most commonly used medical diagnostic testing for children with mental retardation include neuroimaging; metabolic, genetic, and chromosomal blood testing; and electroencephalography (EEG). These tests should not be used as screening tools for all children with an intellectual disability. In some children, there is a reasonable yield for testing whereas in others the yield of <1% does not support its use. Decisions on diagnostic testing should be based on the medical/family history, physical examination, testing by other disciplines, and the family's wishes (Fig. 38-1). Table 38-5 summarizes clinical practice parameters that have been published to assist in the evaluation of the child with global developmental delay/mental retardation. Karyotyping particularly focusing on the number of chromosomes, duplications, deletions, or chromosomal translocations and the **subtelomeric region** (a "hot" spot) is indicated in children with multiple anomalies or a positive family history. Molecular genetic testing for fragile X syndrome is appropriate for a male with moderate mental retardation, unusual physical features, and/or a family history of mental retardation; or a female with more subtle cognitive deficits associated with severe shyness and a relevant family history. A child with a progressive neurologic disorder or acute behavioral changes will need metabolic investigation (urinary organic acids, plasma amino acids, blood lactate, lysosomal enzymes in lymphocytes); a child with

TABLE 38-5. Suggested Evaluation of the Child with Mental Retardation/Global Developmental Delay

TEST	YIELD	COMMENT
In-depth history		Includes pre-, peri- and postnatal events (including seizures); developmental attainments; and 3-generation pedigree in family history
Physical examination		Particular attention to minor/subtle abnormalites; neurologic examination for focality and skull abnormalities Behavioral phenotype
Vision/hearing evaluation		
Karyotype	3.7%	
Fragile X screen	2.6%	Preselection on clinical grounds may increase yield to 7.6%
Neuroimaging	40–55%	MRI preferred. Positives increased by abnormalities of skull contour or size, or focal neurologic examination. Identification of specific etiologies is rare. Most conditions that are found do not alter treatment plan. Need to weigh risk of sedation against possible yield.
Thyroid (T4, TSH)	≈4%	Near 0% in settings with universal newborn screening program
Serum lead	?	If there are identifiable risk factors for excessive environmental lead exposure
Metabolic testing	≈1%	Urine organic acids, plasma amino acids, ammonia, lactate, and a capillary blood gas. Focused testing based on clinical findings warranted.
Subtelomeric deletion	6.6	Obtain in the presence of dysmorphisms but with a normal karyotype and fragile X DNA study. Higher in severe mental retardation.
MECP2 for Rett syndrome	?	Females with severe mental retardation
EEG	≈1%	May be deferred in absence of history of seizures
Repeated history and physical examination		May give time for maturation of physical and behavioral phenotype. New technology may be available for evaluation.

Based on Curry et al, 1997; Shevell et al, 2003; Shapiro BK, Batshaw ML: Mental retardation. In Burg FD, Ingelfinger JR, Polin RA, Gershon AA: *Gellis and Kagan's Current Pediatric Therapy*, 18th ed. Philadelphia, WB Saunders, 2005, used with permission.

seizure-like episodes should have an EEG performed. Finally, children with abnormal head growth or asymmetric and new or focal neurologic findings should have a neuroimaging procedure.

Some children with more subtle physical or neurologic findings can also have determinable biologic causes of their intellectual disability. About 6% of unexplained mental retardation can be accounted for by "micro" chromosomal abnormalities that can be identified by high-resolution chromosomal banding, fluorescent in situ hybridization (FISH), or chromosome painting for subtelomeric rearrangements. Magnetic resonance imaging scans identify a significant number of subtle markers of cerebral dysgenesis in children with intellectual disability. Formes frustes of amino acid and organic acid disorders are associated with mental retardation in the absence of the more commonly associated manifestations of behavior change, lethargy, and coma.

How intensively one investigates the cause of a child's intellectual disability is based on a number of factors:

(1) WHAT IS THE DEGREE OF INTELLECTUAL DISABILITY? One is less likely to find a biologic cause in a child with mild mental retardation than in a child with a severe intellectual disability.

(2) IS THERE A SPECIFIC DIAGNOSTIC PATH TO FOLLOW? If there is a medical history, a family history, or physical findings pointing to a specific disorder, a diagnosis is more likely to be made. In the absence of these indicators, it is difficult to choose specific tests to perform.

(3) ARE THE PARENTS PLANNING ON HAVING ADDITIONAL CHILDREN? If so, one would be more likely to intensively seek disorders for which prenatal diagnosis or a specific early treatment option is available.

(4) WHAT ARE THE PARENTS' WISHES? Some parents have little interest in searching for the cause of the intellectual disability and focus exclusively on treatment. Others will be so focused on obtaining a diagnosis that they will have difficulty following through on interventions until a cause has been found. Both extremes must be respected, but supportive guidance should be provided in the context of parent education.

DIFFERENTIAL DIAGNOSIS. One of the important roles of pediatricians is the early recognition and diagnosis of cognitive deficits.

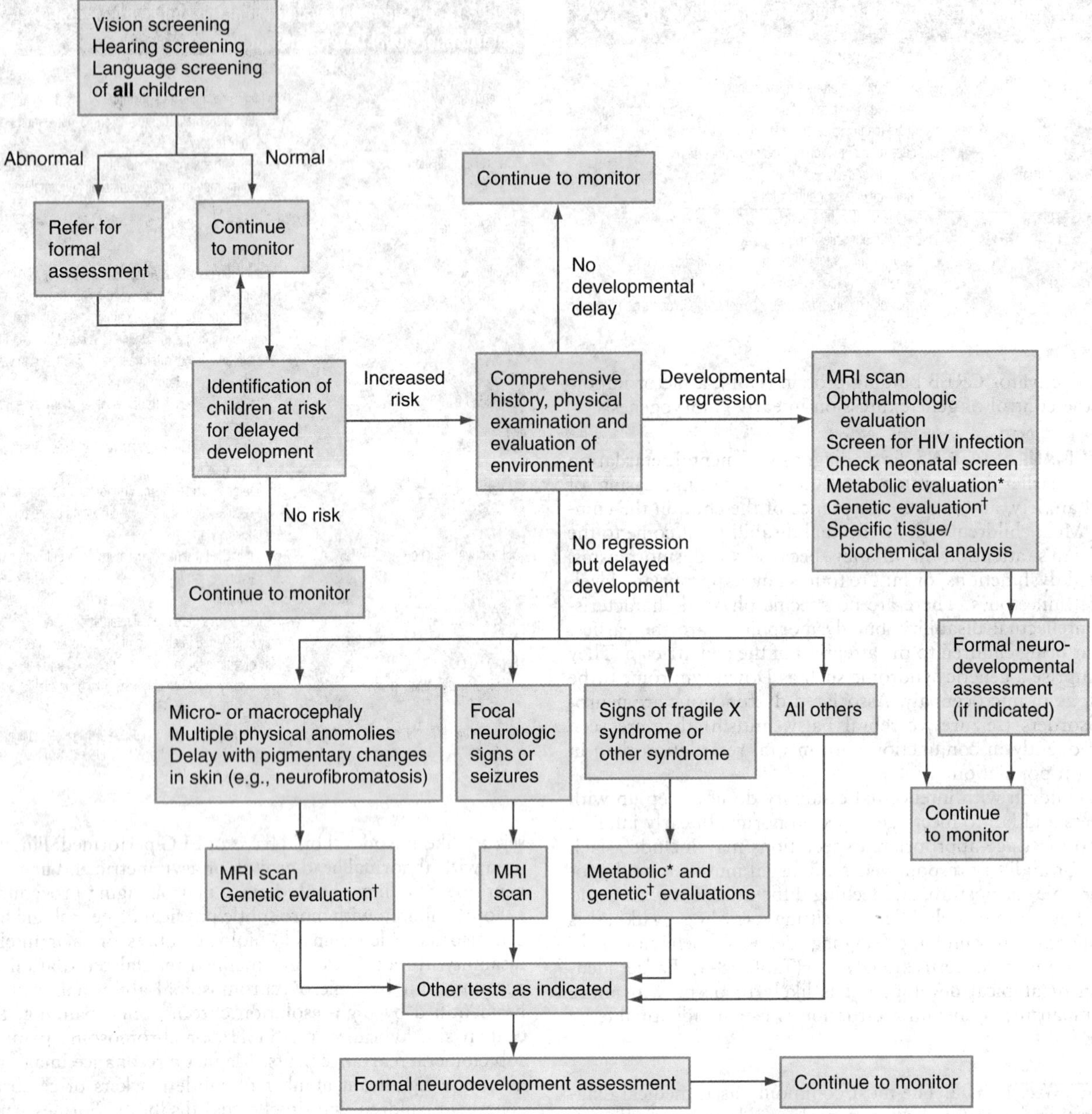

Figure 38-1. Diagnostic strategy for identifying and assessing individuals with developmental delay. *Metabolic evaluation includes serum amino acids, serum and urine organic acids, serum lactate, and ammonia. †Genetic evaluation includes karyotype, cytogenetics, specific gene probes, and dysmorphology consultation if indicated. (From Kliegman RM, Greenbaum LA, Lye PS: *Practical Strategies in Pediatric Diagnosis and Therapy,* 2nd ed. Philadelphia, Elsevier/Saunders, 2004, p 553.)

The developmental surveillance approach to early diagnosis of intellectual disability must be multifaceted. Parental concerns and observations about their child's development should be listened to carefully, because their observations have been found to be as accurate as developmental screening tests. Medical, genetic, and environmental risk factors should be recognized. Infants at high risk (prematurity, maternal substance abuse, perinatal insult) should be registered in newborn follow-up programs in which they are evaluated periodically for developmental lags in the 1st 2 yr of life; they should be referred to early intervention programs as appropriate. Developmental milestones should be recorded routinely during health care maintenance visits. Whether developmental surveillance is a more effective technique for identification than recognition of failure to meet age-appropriate milestones (see earlier discussion) has not been clearly established.

Before making the diagnosis of mental retardation, other disorders that affect cognitive abilities and adaptive behavior should be considered. There include conditions that mimic mental retardation and others that involve intellectual disability as an associated impairment. Sensory deficits (severe hearing and vision loss), communication disorders, and poorly controlled seizure disorders may mimic mental retardation; certain progressive neurologic disorders may appear as mental retardation before regression is appreciated. More than half of children with cerebral palsy (see Chapter 598.1) or autism (see Chapter 29.1) also have mental retardation as an associated deficit. Differentiation of isolated **cerebral palsy** from mental retardation relies on motor skills being more affected than cognitive skills and on the presence of pathologic reflexes and tone changes. In **autism,** language and social adaptive skills are more affected than nonverbal reasoning skills, whereas in mental retardation there are usually more equivalent deficits in social, motor, adaptive, and cognitive skills.

DIAGNOSIS. The formal diagnosis of mental retardation requires the administration of individual tests of intelligence and adaptive functioning.

The **Bayley Scales of Infant Development (BSID-II)**, the most commonly utilized infant intelligence scale, assesses language, visual problem-solving skills, behavior, fine motor skills, and gross motor skills in children between 1 mo and 3 yr of age. A Mental Developmental Index (MDI) and a Psychomotor Development Index score (PDI, a measure of motor competence) are derived from the results. This test permits the differentiation of infants with severe mental retardation from typically developing infants, but is less helpful in distinguishing between a typical child and one with mild mental retardation.

The most commonly used psychologic tests for children >3 yr of age are the **Wechsler Scales** (see Chapter 15). The Wechsler Preschool and Primary Scale of Intelligence–revised (WPPSI-III) is used for children with mental ages of 2.5–7.3 yr. The Wechsler Intelligence Scale for Children–4th edition (WISC-IV) is used for children who function above a 6 yr mental age. Both scales contain a number of subtests in the areas of verbal and performance skills. Although children with mental retardation usually score below average on all subscale scores, they occasionally score in the average range in one or more performance areas.

The most commonly used test of adaptive behavior is the **Vineland Adaptive Behavior Scale** (VABS), which involves parental and/or caregiver/teacher semistructured interviews that assess adaptive behavior in four domains: communication, daily living skills, socialization, and motor skills. Other tests of adaptive behavior include the Woodcock-Johnson Scales of Independent Behavior and the American Association on Mental Retardation Adaptive Behavior Scale (ABS). There is usually (but not always) a good correlation between scores on the intelligence and adaptive scales. Basic adaptive abilities (feeding, dressing, hygiene) are more responsive to remedial efforts than is the IQ score. Adaptive abilities are also more variable, which may relate to the underlying condition and to environmental expectations. While individuals with Prader-Willi syndrome (see Chapter 108) have stability of adaptive skills through adulthood, individuals with fragile X syndrome (see Chapter 81) may have increasing deficits over time.

COMPLICATIONS. Children with mental retardation have higher rates of vision, hearing, orthopedic, and behavioral/emotional disorders than do typically developing children. These other problems are identified later in children with mental retardation. If untreated, the associated impairments can potentially adversely affect the individual's outcome more than the intellectual disability does.

The most common associated deficits are motor impairments, behavioral/emotional disorders, medical complications, and seizures. The more severe the retardation, the greater are the number and severity of associated impairments. Knowing the cause of the mental retardation can help predict which associated impairments are most likely to occur. Fragile X syndrome and fetal alcohol syndrome (see Chapter 106.2) are associated with a high rate of behavioral disorders; Down syndrome has many medical complications (hypothyroidism, celiac disease, congenital heart disease, atlantoaxial subluxation). If there are associated impairments, they may require ongoing physical therapy, occupational therapy, speech-language therapy, adaptive equipment, glasses, hearing aids, and medication. Failure to identify and treat these impairments adequately may hinder successful habilitation and result in difficulties in the school, home, and/or neighborhood environment.

PREVENTION. Examples of primary prevention programs include:

(1) Increasing the public's awareness of the adverse effects of alcohol and other drugs of abuse on the fetus
(2) Preventing teen pregnancy and promoting early prenatal care
(3) Preventing traumatic injury: encouraging the use of guards and railings to prevent falls and other avoidable injuries in the home; using appropriate seat restraints when driving and the wearing of a safety helmet when biking/skateboarding; teaching firearms safety
(4) Preventing poisonings: teaching parents about locking up medications and potential poisons
(5) Encouraging safe sexual practices to prevent the transmission of diseases
(6) Implementing immunization programs to reduce the risk of intellectual disability due to encephalitis, meningitis, and congenital infections.

Presymptomatic detection of certain disorders can result in treatment that prevents adverse consequences. State newborn screening for metabolic disorders (phenylketonuria [PKU], hypothyroidism), newborn hearing screening, and preschool lead poisoning prevention programs are examples. Radiologic screening for atlantoaxial subluxation in a child with Down syndrome is an example of presymptomatic testing in a disorder associated with mental retardation.

TREATMENT. Although mental retardation is not treatable, many associated impairments are amenable to intervention and, therefore, benefit from early identification. Most children with an intellectual disability do not have a behavioral or emotional disorder as an associated impairment, but challenging behaviors (aggression, self-injury, oppositional-defiant behavior) and mental illness (mood and anxiety disorders) occur with greater frequency in this population than among children with typical intelligence. These behavioral/emotional disorders are the primary cause for out-of-home placements, reduced employment prospects, and decreased opportunities for social integration. Some behavioral and emotional disorders are difficult to diagnose in children with more severe mental retardation because of the individual's limited abilities to understand, communicate, interpret, or generalize. Other disorders are masked by the mental retardation. The detection of ADHD [see Chapter 31] in the presence of moderate to severe mental retardation may be difficult, as may be discerning a thought disorder (psychosis) in someone with autism and mental retardation.

Although mental illness is generally of biologic origin and responds to medication, behavioral disorders may result from a mismatch between the child's abilities and the demands of the situation, organic problems, and/or family difficulties. They may represent attempts by the child to communicate, gain attention, or avoid frustration. In assessing the challenging behavior, one must also consider whether it is inappropriate for the child's *mental age,* rather than the *chronological age.* When intervention is needed, an environmental change, such as a more appropriate classroom setting, may improve certain behavior problems. Behavior management techniques are useful; psychopharmacologic agents may be appropriate in certain situations.

Medication is not useful in treating the core symptoms of mental retardation; no agent has been found to improve intellectual function. Medication may be helpful in treating associated behavioral and psychiatric disorders. **Psychopharmacology** is generally directed at specific symptom complexes including ADHD (stimulant medication), self-injurious behavior and aggression (neuroleptics), and anxiety and depression (selective serotonin reuptake inhibitors). Before long-term therapy with any psychopharmacologic agent is initiated, a short trial should be conducted. Even if a medication proves successful, its use should be re-evaluated at least yearly to assess the need for continued treatment.

SUPPORTIVE CARE AND MANAGEMENT. Each child with mental retardation needs a medical home with a pediatrician who is readily accessible to the family to answer questions, help coordinate care, and discuss concerns. The role of the pediatrician includes involvement in prevention efforts, early diagnosis, identification of associated deficits, interdisciplinary management, provision of primary care, and advocacy for the child and family. The management strategies for children with an intellectual disability should be multimodal, with efforts directed at all aspects of the child's life: health, education, social and recreational activities, behavior problems, and associated impairments. Support for parents and siblings should also be provided.

Primary Care. For children with an intellectual disability, primary care has a number of important components:

(1) Provision of the same primary care received by all other children of similar chronological age (see Chapter 5)
(2) Anticipatory guidance relevant to the child's level of function: feeding, toileting, school, accident prevention, sexuality education
(3) Assessment of issues that are specifically relevant to that child's disorder: examination of the teeth in children who exhibit bruxism, thyroid function in children with Down syndrome, cardiac function in Williams syndrome (see Chapter 108).

The American Academy of Pediatrics has published a series of guidelines for children with specific genetic disorders associated with mental retardation (Down syndrome, fragile X syndrome, and Williams syndrome). Goals should be considered and programs adjusted as needed during the primary care visit. Decisions should also be made about what additional information is required for future planning or to explain why the child is not meeting expectations. Other evaluations, such as formal psychologic or educational testing, may need to be scheduled.

Interdisciplinary Management. The pediatrician has the responsibility for consulting with other disciplines to make the diagnosis of mental retardation and coordinate treatment services. Consultant services may include psychology, speech/language pathology, physical therapy, occupational therapy, audiology, nutrition, nursing, and/or social work, as well as medical specialties such as neurodevelopmental disabilities, neurology, genetics, psychiatry, and/or surgical specialties. Contact with early intervention/school personnel is equally important to help prepare the child's **Individual Family Service Plan (IFSP).** The family should be an integral part of the planning and direction of this process. Care should be family centered and culturally sensitive; for older children, their participation in planning and decision-making should be promoted to whatever extent possible.

Periodic Re-Evaluation. The child's abilities and the family's needs change over time. As the child grows, more information must be provided to the child and parents, goals must be reassessed, and programming needs adjusted. A periodic review should include information about the child's health status as well as his or her functioning at home, school, and in other community settings. Other information, such as formal psychologic or educational testing, may be helpful. Re-evaluation should be undertaken at routine intervals (6–12 mo during early childhood), at any time the child is not meeting expectations, or when he or she is moving from one service delivery system to another. This is especially true during the transition to adulthood, beginning at age 14 yr as mandated by the Individuals with Disabilities Education Act Amendments of 2004. This transitioning should include the transfer of care to the adult health care system by age 21.

Educational Services. Education is the single most important discipline involved in the treatment of children with an intellectual disability. The educational program must be relevant to the child's needs and address the child's individual strengths and weaknesses. The child's developmental level, his or her requirements for support, and goals for independence provide a basis for establishing an **Individualized Education Program (IEP)** for school-aged children, as mandated by federal legislation.

Leisure and Recreational Activities. The child's social and recreational needs should be addressed. Although young children with mental retardation are generally included in play activities with children who have typical development, adolescents with intellectual disability frequently do not have opportunities for appropriate social interactions. Participation in sports should be encouraged even if the child is not competitive because it offers many benefits, including weight management, development of physical coordination, maintenance of cardiovascular fitness, and improvement of self-image. Social activities are equally important, including dances, trips, dating, and other typical social and recreational events.

Family Counseling. Many families adapt well to having a child with mental retardation, but some have emotional/social difficulties. The risks of parental depression and child abuse and neglect are higher in this group of children than in the general population. Among the factors that have been associated with good family coping and parenting skills are stability of the marriage, good parental self-esteem, limited number of siblings, higher socioeconomic status, lower degree of disability/associated impairments, appropriate parental expectations and acceptance of the diagnosis, supportive extended family members, and availability of community programs and respite care services. In those families in which the emotional burden of having a child with mental retardation is great, family counseling, parent support groups, respite care, and home health services should be an integral part of the treatment plan.

Advocacy. The pediatrician can play a number of advocacy roles: maintaining close contact with the department of health/local school district to advocate for an appropriate IFSP/IEP; identifying eligibility for financial supports through Supplemental Security Income (SSI) from Social Security; assessing the impact of the Americans with Disabilities Act (ADA) on the adolescent's access to jobs and community activities; referring families to appropriate parental support groups or websites for their specific disorder/syndrome; assuring adequate respite care services for the family; becoming involved in the community to help develop educational, recreational, and leisure programs for children with disabilities; and advocating for improved health care coverage by both private and governmental insurers.

PROGNOSIS. In children with severe mental retardation, the prognosis is often evident by early childhood. Mild mental retardation may not always be a lifelong disorder. Children may meet criteria for mental retardation at an early age but later evolve into a more specific developmental disorder (communication disorder, autism, slow learner–borderline normal intelligence). Others who are diagnosed with mild mental retardation during their school years may develop sufficient adaptive behavior skills so that they no longer fit the diagnosis as adolescents, or the effects of maturation and plasticity may result in children moving from one diagnostic category to another (from moderate to mild retardation). Some children who are diagnosed with a specific learning disability or communication disorder may not maintain their rate of cognitive growth and fall into the range of mental retardation over time. By adolescence, the diagnosis has generally stabilized.

The long-term outcome of individuals with mental retardation depends on the underlying cause, the degree of cognitive and adaptive deficits, the presence of associated medical and developmental impairments, the capabilities of the families, and the school/community supports, services, and training provided to the child and family (Table 38-6). As adults, many individuals with mild mental retardation are capable of gaining economic and social independence with functional literacy. They may need periodic supervision, especially when under social or economic stress. Most live successfully in the community, either independently or in supervised settings. Life expectancy is not adversely affected by mental retardation itself.

For individuals with moderate mental retardation, the goals of education are to enhance adaptive abilities and "survival" academic and vocational skills so they are better able to live in the adult world (see Table 38-6). The concept of supported employment has been very beneficial to these individuals; the person is

TABLE 38-6. Severity of Mental Retardation and Adult Age Functioning

LEVEL	MENTAL AGE AS ADULT*	ADULT ADAPTATION
Mild	9–11 yr	Reads at 4th–5th grade level; simple multiplication/division; writes simple letter, lists; completes job application; basic independent job skills (arrive on time, stay at task, interact with coworkers); uses public transportation, may qualify for driver's license; keeps house, cooks using recipes
Moderate	6–8 yr	Sight-word reading; copies information, e.g., address from card to job application; matches written number to number of items; recognizes time on clock; communicates; some independence in self-care; housekeeping with supervision or cue cards; meal preparation, can follow picture recipe cards; job skills learned with much repetition; uses public transportation with some supervision
Severe	3–5 yr	Needs continuous support and supervision; may communicate wants and needs, sometimes with augmentative communication techniques
Profound	<3 yr	Limitations of self-care, continence, communication, and mobility; may need complete custodial or nursing care

*International Statistical Classification of Diseases and Related Health Problems, 10th revision (World Health Organization).
From Dr. Robert L. Schum, Grand Rounds Presentation at Children's Hospital of Wisconsin, 2003.

trained by a coach to do a specific job in the setting in which the person is to work. This bypasses the need for a sheltered workshop experience and has resulted in successful work adaptation in the community for many people with an intellectual disability. These individuals generally live at home or in a supervised setting in the community.

As adults, people with severe-profound mental retardation usually require extensive to pervasive supports (see Table 38-6). These individuals may have associated impairments, such as cerebral palsy, behavioral disorders, epilepsy, or sensory impairments, that further limit their adaptive functioning. They may perform simple tasks in supervised settings, and most people with this level of mental retardation are able to live in the community with appropriate supports.

American Academy of Pediatrics, Committee on Children with Disabilities: Pediatrician's role in the development and implementation of an Individualized Education Plan (IEP) and/or an Individual Family Service Plan (IFSP). *Pediatrics* 1999;104:124–127.

American Psychiatric Association: *Diagnostic and Statistical Manual of Mental Disorders, 4th Edition (DSM-IV, Text Revision)*. Washington, DC, American Psychiatric Association, 2000.

Batshaw ML, Shapiro BK: Developmental delay and intellectual disability. In Batshaw ML: *Children with Disabilities,* 6th ed. Baltimore, Brookes Publishing, in press.

Curry CJ, Stevenson RE, Aughton D, et al: Evaluation of mental retardation: Recommendations of a consensus conference. *Am J Med Genet* 1997;72:468–477.

Roeleveld N, Zielhuis GA, Gabreëls F: The prevalence of mental retardation: A critical review of recent literature. *Dev Med Child Neurol* 1997;39:125–132.

Shapiro BK, Batshaw ML: Mental Retardation. In Burg FD, Ingelfinger JR, Polin RA, Gershon AA: *Gellis and Kagan's Current Pediatric Therapy,* 18th ed. Philadelphia, WB Saunders, 2005.

Shevell M, Ashwal S, Donley D, et al: Practice parameter: Evaluation of the child with global developmental delay. *Neurology* 2003;60:367–380.

Strømme P, Hagberg G: Aetiology in severe and mild mental retardation: A population-based study of Norwegian children. *Dev Med Child Neurol* 2000;42:76–86.

Wilson-Costello, Friedman H, Minich N, et al. Improved survival rates with increased neurodevelopmental disability for extremely low birth weight infants in the 1990s. *Pediatrics* 2005;115:997–1003.

Yeargin-Allsopp M, Boyle C: The epidemiology of neurodevelopmental disorders. *Ment Retard Dev Disabil Res Rev* 2002;8:113–211.

Chapter 39 ■ Organ Transplantation

Lawrence H. Mathers and
Lorry R. Frankel

Pediatric organ transplantation continues to develop as more organs become available and the expertise to care for the patient from both medical and surgical perspectives becomes more universal. The care of transplant patients falls on a wide range of health care providers, including those responsible for: identification of potential recipients, care and support of recipients awaiting transplant, the system that identifies and makes available appropriate donor organs, the process of organ procurement, transplantation, immediate postoperative care in the intensive care unit, and the extended post-transplant care required to ensure success of the transplant and to monitor for complications. In the post-transplant phase of the recipient's life, consistent monitoring and evaluation by the outpatient care providers are crucial to identifying and combating the complications to which the recipient is vulnerable, including organ rejection, infections related to chronic immunosuppression, and issues of patient compliance in the taking of medications meant to suppress rejection. This challenge requires the efforts of pediatricians (in both the pre- and post-transplant stages), transplant surgeons, intensive care specialists, hospitalists, organ-specific pediatric subspecialists, and a variety of consultants including immunologists, infectious disease specialists, and child mental health providers.

Approximately 2,000 pediatric renal transplants, 275 heart transplants, and 525 liver transplants are performed annually in the United States. Although there are many potential recipients waiting for a transplant, many die before an organ becomes available. Survival rates have improved due to better pretransplant care, improvement in the technical skills in those centers performing significant numbers of transplants, and refinements in post-transplant immunosuppression and monitoring for complications.

In addition to transplants of kidney, heart, and liver, other transplants of solid organs occur, in much smaller numbers. These include lung transplants, small bowel transplants, pancreatic transplants, and combination transplants such as liver–small bowel and heart-lung. These procedures are performed at a smaller number of medical centers, and statistics regarding their effectiveness are less meaningful.

Donors include living donors (kidney, split liver) and those who donate after death (nonliving donor: heart, heart-lung, lung, liver, kidney, liver–small bowel). Living donors include those who donate a dispensable tissue such as cartilage, skin, or bone marrow as well as those who donate a part or all of one of their vital organs (kidney, partial or split liver, or lung). Acquiring an organ from nonliving donors requires that there be a determination of brain death (see Chapter 67.1) and that the vital organs remain perfused and oxygenated (Table 39-1). In the United States, ≈20% of nonliving donors are children. While the potential to donate is much greater than actual donation, the number of patients currently on waiting lists exceeds by a factor of 10 the number of needed organs that are being donated.

RENAL TRANSPLANTATION

Most pediatric renal transplants occur in teenaged patients (≈70%). Male recipients outnumber females by a 60 : 40 ratio. The most common diagnoses leading to transplantation are obstructive uropathy, congenital abnormalities, and a variety of glomerulonephropathies that have deteriorated to end-stage renal disease (ESRD) [see Chapter 536]. Despite growing numbers of

TABLE 39-1. Contraindications to Organ Donation

ORGAN	RELATIVELY ABSOLUTE CONTRAINDICATIONS	ABSOLUTELY RELATIVE CONTRAINDICATIONS	COMMENTS
General	Infection: HIV (incl. high-risk groups and hemophiliacs); hepatitis B, antigen-positive; untreated infections	Hepatitis C, CMV, CNS infection, treated infection	Preferably test viral load, p24-antigen; seek to match donor and recipient for CMV
	Malignancies: all except some CNS and nonmelanotic skin tumors	Some CNS tumors	
	SLE and other collagen vascular disease, congenital metabolic disorders, hemoglobinopathies	Hypertension under treatment, diabetes mellitus, sustained hypotension, high-dose inotropes or pressors	
Kidney	Renal disease or trauma amyloidosis, dysproteinemias	Established acute renal failure	Elevated creatinine caused by dehydration is not a contraindication
Liver	Liver disease or trauma, peritonitis	Advanced cardiovascular disease, alcoholism, drug overdose, moderately elevated liver tests	Drug overdose is only a relative contraindication even if paracetamol
Pancreas	Diabetes mellitus, acute or chronic pancreatitis	Previous duodenal or pancreatic surgery	
Heart	Heart disease: valvular, ischemic, cardiomyopathy	Severe chest trauma, prolonged cardiac arrest, varying limits of MAP, CVP, PCWP, ejection fraction, ECG abnormalities	
Lung	History of chronic lung disease, tuberculosis, significant acute lung disease, aspiration, severe chest trauma or previous surgery	Smoking >20 pack-years, minor opacities on radiography, Pa_{O_2} <300 mm Hg at Fi_{O_2} = 1 and PEEP = 5 mm Hg, positive sputum culture (even yeasts), purulent secretions	Judge both lungs as two separate organs

CMV, cytomegalovirus; CVP, central venous pressure; MAP, mean arterial pressure; PCWP, pulmonary capillary wedge pressure; PEEP, positive end-expiratory pressure; SLE, systemic lupus erythematosus.
From Lutz-Dettinger N, de Jaeger A, Kerremans I: Care of the potential pediatric organ donor. *Pediatr Clin North Am* 2001;48:715–749.

transplants, almost ½ of the children waiting for a transplant in a given year do not receive an organ, and are forced to undergo treatment with dialysis or to survive in a state of significant renal insufficiency. In the United States, about 50% of the organs transplanted into children are from living related donors (LRD). The rest are cadaveric transplants (CAD).

The most urgent considerations after transplant are patency of the vascular anastomoses and support of graft kidney function. Strict regulation of the patient's position in bed (to prevent kinking of the vascular pedicle of the kidney) and anticoagulant measures (although the maintenance of relatively high blood pressures in recipients may obviate the need for anticoagulants) are important concerns. Ultrasonography is an effective and simple way of assessing blood flow in the transplanted kidney. At most centers, the transplanted kidney is encouraged, through the supply of sometimes prodigious amounts of intravenous fluids, to produce urine at rates many times the normal level of urine output. This is especially important if the transplanted kidney has come from a donor who is significantly larger and/or older than the recipient (encountered when a parent or other adult is the donor).

In the past, acute rejection occurred in about 50% of organ graft failures. Today, with improved surgical techniques, more effective immunosuppression, and better monitoring, the number is closer to 30%, and in some centers has dropped below 10%. In addition, the success in defeating acute rejection has improved to >65%. Regularly scheduled biopsies help to detect and confirm early rejection, even in those patients for whom there are no clinical signs of rejection.

LIVER TRANSPLANTATION

The most common indication for pediatric liver transplantation is biliary atresia (see Chapter 365). Hepatitis C infection and hepatocellular carcinoma are increasingly frequent indications for liver transplantation. Additional indications include other congenital causes of cirrhosis, several inborn errors of metabolism (tyrosinemia, Wilson disease), ingestion of toxic substances (acetaminophen overdose, mushroom poisoning), various forms of acute and chronic hepatitis, certain isolated nonmetastatic liver malignancies, and liver trauma. Hepatic failure results in various life-threatening conditions, including acidosis, coagulopathy, hyperammonemia and hepatic coma, hypoalbuminemia and anasarca, and portal hypertension with varices. Hyperammonemic hepatic coma may accelerate the consideration of transplant because it produces unconsciousness and apnea.

Liver transplantation involves anastomosis of the donor's and recipient's hepatic arteries, hepatic veins/inferior vena cava, portal veins, and biliary ducts. Patency of these anatomoses is among the most urgent concerns immediately after transplant and is monitored closely with ultrasonic studies. Liver recipients are routinely treated with antiplatelet aggregation therapies (aspirin, persantine, dextran) and some patients are treated with heparin to reduce clot formation. Liver transplants are increasingly performed with liver segments from living related donors, usually relatives. Most frequently, the left lateral segment of the donor liver is transplanted into the child.

The liver graft is subject to an array of potential problems after transplantation. Hyperacute graft rejection is very rare but may occur within minutes of revascularization of a transplanted organ. The organ must be removed and replaced. Acute rejection can occur in the 1st 5–7 days after transplant and is manifested by rising levels of liver enzymes, worsening coagulopathy, and hepatic encephalopathy. It can be treated by increasing the dosage of steroids, cyclosporine, or tacrolimus and, if these fail, antithymocyte antibody preparations. Vascular anastomosis breakdown produces hemorrhage and requires surgical re-exploration. Thrombus formation deprives the liver of blood flow and also requires surgery. Intestinal perforations, especially if infection is present, may occur and can be detected by observation of free air in the abdomen. Various abscesses and other fluid accumulations may need surgical exploration.

At the time of transplantation, children typically receive corticosteroids and either cyclosporine or tacrolimus. In some centers, small doses of antithymocyte globulin (ATG) or muromonab-CD[3] (OKT3) are given as well. The early phase of immunosuppression extends for 2–3 wk postoperatively, and most patients continue taking steroids at a low dosage for life. Because of concerns about the long-term growth of the child, there is increasing interest in and employment of protocols that severely limit (or even eliminate) the use of steroids. Interleukin-2 receptor monoclonal antibodies such as basilixumab and daclizumab are also being studied as a means of controlling rejection with less overall immunosuppression and other long-term toxicities of current drug regimens. An ultimate goal is to induce tolerance of the new organ or segment by the recipient, which will involve some means of eliminating or inactivating clones of T cells capable of attacking the transplanted organ.

With increasing long-term survival, interest in the long-term complications of transplantation increases. Post-transplant hepatitis can lead to increasing fibrosis and organ failure. Prolonged use of the calcineurin inhibitors (cyclosporine, tacrolimus) can lead to renal injury, often involving hypertension. Use of immunosuppressives also increases the risk of post-transplant lymphoproliferative disorders (PTLDs). These are usually B-cell proliferations, and may be driven by Epstein-Barr virus or cytomegalovirus reactivation in these immunosuppressed recipients.

Donor shortage remains one of the most serious problems in the area of liver transplantation. Studies continue in developing minimal use of immunosuppressives and it is to be hoped that even complete avoidance of steroid use will lead to improved survival and quality of life; at the same time, late-term complications will become more common and will require further study and understanding.

LIVER AND INTESTINAL TRANSPLANTATION

A subgroup of patients with irreversible liver failure also have short bowel syndrome (see Chapter 336). They are maintained on parenteral nutrition almost exclusively. The continued use of parenteral nutrition may produce liver dysfunction and necessitate dual organ transplant in the hopes of allowing patients to receive their nutrition enterally and for the new liver to restore normal liver function. These transplants are performed at fewer institutions than are liver transplants alone. Often, these patients require significant pretransplant care and may benefit from a bowel rehabilitation program.

HEART TRANSPLANTATION

Heart transplantation becomes a valid treatment option in children who are born with certain congenital heart malformations and in children who suffer acquired heart disease, usually a cardiomyopathy (see Chapter 443). This acquired injury to the heart may be of viral origin, may result from treatment with anthracyclines for a previous malignancy, or may be idiopathic. The decision to seek transplantation depends on the severity of the illness in the patient and the likelihood that the patient's projected survival is no more than 2 yr. Many children referred for transplant for congenital heart disease have already undergone one or more complex heart surgeries, adding to the technical challenge of implanting the transplanted heart.

Although many patients listed for heart transplant are in the hospital and severely ill, some are managed very well as outpatients and only come to the hospital for routine follow-up and the eventual transplant. The children who are critically ill may require extensive support in the intensive care unit (ICU); this may include vasoactive administration, mechanical ventilatory support, and, on occasion, circulatory assistance as a bridge to transplantation. Despite this, the waiting time for receiving a transplant ranges from 2 to 6 mo, and many potential recipients die before an organ becomes available.

Once the transplant is performed, a combination of immunosuppressive agents are used: calcineurin inhibitors (cyclosporine, tacrolimus), steroids, and azothioprine. There is increasing use of interleukin-2 receptor monoclonal antibodies such as daclizumab, and some protocols substitute mycophenolate mofetil (CellCept) for azathioprene. Weaning of steroids typically begins after 3–6 mo of treatment. Frequent biopsies of the heart are required to assist in determining whether any clinical signs of rejection are present. These biopsies are performed in the catheterization laboratory; catheters are threaded through the femoral vein to the right ventricle where biopsies are then obtained. Most heart transplant recipients experience at least one episode of acute rejection in the 1st 3 yr after transplant, most often in the 1st 3 to 6 mo. The biopsy-proven severity of the rejection and the presence or absence of inflammatory cellular infiltrates dictate the treatment elected. The most severe rejection warrants hospital admission and treatment with intravenous high-dose steroids and antilymphocyte therapies (OKT3, ATG, or total lymphoid irradiation).

Pediatric heart transplantation offers hope of a long and active life. Evidence indicates that the transplanted heart will grow along with the whole child, and scars or strictures at the sites of vascular anastomosis during the transplant are rare. After 5–10 yr, the coronary arteries may develop a reactive vasculitis that results in narrowing of the arteries, decreased substrate delivery to the myocardium, and eventual myocardial damage. These patients may need another heart transplant. Among the most serious risks as the recipient approaches puberty and adolescence is the growing incidence of noncompliance with medication regimens. Evidence shows that complications can set in rapidly even many years after transplant if the drug regimen is not followed. This is a unique group of patients that requires medication adjustments and, often, psychiatric support. It is hoped that protocols emphasizing minimal steroid use will encourage teenagers to continue their post-transplant treatment into adulthood.

LUNG TRANSPLANTATION

Pediatric lung transplants are less common than transplants of other organs; approximately 1,300 have been performed to date in children (see Chapter 443). Indications for lung transplants in children include cystic fibrosis, chronic interstitial disease, and irreversible pulmonary hypertension. Transplantable organs are particularly rare, and great attention is paid to selecting recipients who will abide by treatment regimens. Single lung transplantation is common in adults but rarely used in children. Bilateral lung transplant is indicated in situations such as cystic fibrosis, in which the continuing illness and infection of the remaining native lung would jeopardize the single transplanted lung.

Surgery in the mediastinum predisposes the recurrent laryngeal and phrenic nerves to injury, which can lead to vocal cord paralysis or diaphragmatic paralysis. If the lung transplant recipient has a history of previous thoracic surgery or has undergone pleurodesis, then the technical challenge of transplanting a lung increases considerably. The postoperative immunosuppressive regimen is similar to that for other solid organ transplants. Immediate post-transplant treatment often includes bronchoscopy to inspect the site of the bronchial anastomoses. Transbronchial biopsies are used to diagnose infections or inflammatory conditions in the transplanted lungs.

Bronchiolitis obliterans is a significant threat to long-term survival. This disease involves progressive focal fibrosis and, eventually, obstruction of small airways, lymphocyte infiltration, and deposits of fibrous tissue in various parts of the lung. It is present in more than half of all lung transplant recipients (adults and children) but occurs less in children. A reliable treatment has not been developed, though increased doses of immunosuppressives may have some beneficial effect.

HEART-LUNG TRANSPLANTS

More than 400 heart-lung transplants have been performed in children, with 1 and 5 yr survival at 75% and 45%, respectively. Initially, one of the major problems in heart-lung transplant in advanced pulmonary disease was the high rate of complications (strictures, scars) with the anastomosis of main stem bronchi. In the past decade, the risk for this complication was greatly diminished and the number of pediatric heart-lung transplants increased. Another initial concern for heart-lung transplant was the belief that right-sided cardiac hypertrophy (cor pulmonale) would make a lung transplant ineffective, but it has been found that the right-sided cardiac abnormalities often resolve after lung transplantation alone.

Alonso EM: Long-term renal function in pediatric liver and heart recipients. *Pediatr Transplant* 2004;8:381–385.

Baum M, Freier MC, Chinnock R: Neurodevelopmental outcome of solid organ transplantation in children. *Pediatr Clin North Am* 2003;50:1493–1503.

Cescon M, Spada M, Colledan M, et al: Split-liver transplantation with pediatric donors: A multicenter experience. *Transplantation* 2005;79:1148–1153.

Feinstein S, Keich R, Becker-Cohen R, et al: Is noncompliance among adolescent renal transplant recipients inevitable? *Pediatrics* 2005;115:969–973.

Fine R, Kelly D, Webber S: Pediatric solid organ transplantation. *Pediatr Clin North Am* 2003;50:6.

Freier MC, Babikian T, Pivonka J, et al: A longitudinal perspective on neurodevelopmental outcome after infant cardiac transplantation. *J Heart Lung Transplant* 2004;23:857–864.

Grant D, Abu-Elmagd K, Reyes J, et al: 2003 report of the Intestine Transplant Registry: A new era has dawned. *Ann Surg* 2005;241:607–613.

Green M, Webber S: Posttransplantation lymphoproliferative disorders. *Pediatr Clin North Am* 2003;50:1471–1491.

Harmon WE, McDonald RA, Reyes JD, et al: Pediatric transplantation, 1994–2003. *Am J Transplant* 2005;5:887–903.

Keough WL, Michaels MG: Infectious complications in pediatric solid organ transplantation. *Pediatr Clin North Am* 2003;50:1451–1469.

Kirklin JK, McGiffin DC, Pinderski LJ, et al: Selection of patients and techniques of heart transplantation. *Surg Clin North Am* 2004;84:257–287.

Lopez MJ, Thomas S: Immunization of children after solid organ transplantation. *Pediatr Clin North Am* 2003;50:1435–1449.

Magee JC, Bucuvalas JC, Farmer DG, et al: Pediatric transplantation. *Am J Transplant* 2004;4:954–971.

Mallory GB, Spray TL: Paediatric lung transplantation. *Eur Respir J* 2004;24:839–845.

Qvist E, Jalanko H, Holmberg C: Psychosocial adaptation after solid organ transplantation in children. *Pediatr Clin North Am* 2003;50:1505–1519.

Rostaing L, Cantarovich D, Mourad G, et al: Corticosteroid-free immunosuppression with tacrolimus, mycophenolate mofetil, and daclizumab induction in renal transplantation. *Transplantation* 2005;79:807–814.

Smith JM, Nemeth TL, McDonald RA: Current immunosuppressive agents: Efficacy, side effects, and utilization. *Pediatr Clin North Am* 2003;50:1283–1300.

Woo MS: An overview of paediatric lung transplantation. *Paediatr Respir Rev* 2004;5:249–254.

Chapter 40 ■ Pediatric Palliative Care

The Care of Children with Life-Limiting Illness • Stephen Liben

In the United States, ≈55,000 children die annually; 50% of these deaths occur in acute-care hospitals. Although 30% of these deaths are from chronic conditions known to be life-threatening, the majority of these children also die in hospitals. Among children dying from cancer, about 50–60% die in the hospital and 50% at home; approximately 65% of childhood AIDS deaths occur in the hospital. Pediatric deaths from chronic illnesses in Canada and Australia generally occur in the hospital. In many developing countries, the majority of pediatric deaths occur at home, with or without palliative care. Some countries, such as Great Britain, make greater use of home and hospice facilities. Global partnerships, such as the Children's International Project on Palliative/Hospice Services, share existing clinical and scientific knowledge in an attempt to establish international standards for palliative care.

The World Health Organization defines palliative care as "an approach that improves the quality of life of patients and their families facing the problem associated with life-threatening illness, through the prevention and relief of suffering by means of early identification and impeccable assessment and treatment of pain and other problems, physical, psychosocial and spiritual." Palliative care is provided in hospitals (some with specialized palliative care units), in the home whenever possible and desired, and in hospices. **Hospices** provide a structured model of how to finance, maintain, and coordinate a range of palliative care services, often in a freestanding facility. In some countries, specialized pediatric hospices provide an important bridge between hospital care and home care.

The mandate of pediatricians to oversee children's physical, mental, and emotional health and development from conception to maturity includes the practice of palliative medicine for those children in their care who live with a significant possibility of death before reaching adulthood (Table 40-1). Many pediatric subspecialties have a responsibility for a unique population of children with life-threatening or life-shortening illnesses at high risk for dying. Acquiring the basic knowledge, attitudes, and skills of palliative medicine is integral to the education of both the generalist and subspecialist pediatrician (Table 40-2). Such training has the added benefit of improving skills in other areas of care such as communication and symptom control.

Compared with adult end-of-life care, pediatric palliative care has:

1. **Smaller numbers of dying children.** Even professionals specializing in the care of children may only rarely encounter the death of a child.
2. **A broad spectrum of illnesses,** including many rare diseases, that often requires involvement of a number of disciplines (see Table 40-1). In pediatrics, the wide range of often poorly understood disorders limits the ability to generalize from any one disease-specific research study to another.
3. **Unpredictable illness trajectories** with significant prognostic uncertainty. It is difficult to predict accurately the progression of illness for many life-threatening illnesses in pediatrics. This leads to child and family distress from uncertainty coupled with problems of funding and sustaining pediatric palliative care programs that may need to provide varied amounts of services for years. Palliative care for these children may necessarily involve some overlap with chronic curative care, with palliative care becoming more prominent as the child progresses from being chronically to terminally ill.
4. **More uncertainty about whether treatments are supportive/palliative** vs those that primarily cure or prolong life. Deciding whether a specific treatment is palliative or life-prolonging is not always possible with emerging technologies such as noninvasive respiratory ventilation.

TABLE 40-1. Conditions Appropriate for Pediatric Palliative Care*

Conditions for which curative treatment is possible but may fail
Advanced or progressive cancer or cancer with a poor prognosis
Complex and severe congenital or acquired heart disease
Conditions requiring intensive long-term treatment aimed at maintaining the quality of life
Human immunodeficiency virus infection
Cystic fibrosis
Severe gastrointestinal disorders or malformations such as gastroschisis
Severe epidermolysis bullosa
Severe immunodeficiencies
Renal failure in cases in which dialysis, transplantation, or both are not available or indicated
Chronic or severe respiratory failure
Muscular dystrophy
Progressive conditions in which treatment is exclusively palliative after diagnosis
Progressive metabolic disorders
Certain chromosomal abnormalities such as trisomy 13 or trisomy 18
Severe forms of osteogenesis imperfecta
Conditions involving severe, nonprogressive disability, causing extreme vulnerability to health complications
Severe cerebral palsy with recurrent infection or difficult-to-control symptoms
Extreme prematurity
Severe neurologic sequelae of infectious disease
Hypoxic or anoxic brain injury
Holoprosencephaly or other severe brain malformations

*Premature death is likely or expected with many of these conditions.

From Himelstein BP, Hilden JM, Boldt AM, Weissman D: Pediatric palliative care. *N Engl J Med* 2004;350:1752–1762.

TABLE 40-2. Common Goals and Examples of Pediatric Palliative Care

GOAL	EXAMPLES OF CARE
Physical comfort	Using medications and behavioral interventions to prevent or relieve a child's pain, fatigue, or other symptoms
	Providing physical therapy to improve function and relieve pain
Emotional comfort	Providing psychotherapy including verbal and play techniques
	Arranging art, music, or other expressive therapies
	Encouraging visits from family and friends
Normal life	Informing the child and involving him or her in decisions (consistent with intellectual and emotional maturity)
	Planning with teachers and administrators for a child's return to school
	Organizing travel or camp experiences
Family functioning	Helping parents make special time for siblings
	Arranging respite for parents
Cultural or spiritual values	Accommodating religious rituals and traditional customs
	Encouraging continuation or adaptation of family holiday traditions
Preparing for death	Planning for parents, siblings, and others to be with the child at and after death
	Planning for remembrances or legacies of the child's life including pictures, videos, locks of hair, and handprints or handmolds
	Funeral arrangements

From Field MJ, Behrman RE (editors): *When Children Die: Improving Palliative and End-of-Life Care for Children and Their Families.* Washington, DC, Institute of Medicine, 2003.

Advances in pediatric medicine have resulted in an increase in the number of children who live longer, often with significant dependence on new (and expensive) technologies. These children have complex chronic conditions across the spectrum of congenital and acquired life-threatening disorders (see Chapter 38). Children with complex chronic conditions require a combination of palliative and curative treatments. These children, who may survive frequent near-death crises followed by the renewed need for rehabilitative and life-prolonging treatments, are best served by a system that is flexible and responsive to changing needs. Palliative care for all patients must address specific practice that focuses on physical, psychosocial, and spiritual concerns as well as advanced care planning and the realities of care (see Table 40-2).

CARE PLANNING. Although it may not be possible to determine accurately how long a child may live, there is often a delay between the time that a terminal prognosis is first recognized by physicians and when the prognosis is understood by parents. This time delay may impede informed decision-making about how these children spend the end of their lives. Given the inherent prognostic uncertainty of a life-limiting diagnosis, the time when the physician recognizes a significant possibility of patient mortality is probably the best time to initiate discussions concerning resuscitation, symptom control, and end-of-life care planning. Patients and families may be most comfortable continuing with physicians and other care providers with whom they have an established relationship; in most cases, the services of a palliative care specialist or hospice program can be consultative to the primary or subspecialty care physician and team. Physician discomfort in discussing end-of-life care should not result in the discussion being deferred to others or to a later time. Physician feelings of discomfort are to be expected given the difficult nature and highly charged atmosphere of a child facing death, and physicians may need varying levels of support themselves as they map out a care plan with the child and parents. The populations of children who die before reaching adulthood include a disproportionate number of nonverbal and preverbal children who are developmentally unable to make autonomous care decisions. Although some adolescents may be capable of such decision-making, currently, only one state in the United States recognizes an advance directive signed by a child. Parents are, therefore, legally the primary decision-maker in most situations in the United States, but children should be as fully involved in discussions and decisions about their care as appropriate for their developmental status.

Home care of the dying child requires 24 hr per day accessibility to experts in pediatric palliative care, a team approach, and an identified coordinator who serves as a link between hospitals, the community, and specialists and can arrange for hospital admissions and respite care, as needed. Provision of respite services is especially important to families caring for children with complex chronic conditions over prolonged periods of time. Such care may involve temporary placement of a child with another family or in an institution such as a hospital or hospice. It is important to plan a respite admission before the family caring for the child feels overwhelmed. The family should be reassured that taking respite is not a personal failure. Although children, when given the choice, prefer to remain at home, a child may need to return periodically to the hospital or hospice even when there is comprehensive home support.

Good end-of-life care can be effectively carried out in a hospital setting when institutions are flexible enough to modify protocols that may present unnecessary obstacles to the care of dying patients. In tertiary care hospitals, the neonatal and pediatric intensive care units (ICUs) are the locations where most children die. Many of the children in ICUs die after discussions that lead to the limitation or withdrawal of therapy (see Chapter 3). Improving the care of these hospitalized children and their families involves liberalizing visiting policies and respecting privacy, as well as removing some of the obstacles inherent in intensive care settings, such as routine testing and monitoring of vital signs. The philosophy of palliative care can be successfully implemented in a hospital setting when the focus of care is maintained on comfort and quality of life. All interventions that affect the child and family need to be assessed in relation to these goals. This proactive approach asks the question "What can we offer that will improve the quality of this child's life?" instead of "What therapies are we no longer going to offer this patient?" Staff who are comfortable and supportive of this approach need to be carefully chosen with consideration given to the fact that pediatric palliative care, like other types of intensive care, is not a skill with which everyone is comfortable. Comprehensive palliative care also requires a multidisciplinary approach that may include nurses, physicians, psychologists, psychiatrists, social workers, religious counselors, child-life specialists, and trained volunteers.

COMMUNICATION ISSUES AND ANTICIPATORY GUIDANCE

THE PARENTS. Parents need to know that their physician will not abandon them as the goals of care shift primarily from cure to comfort. Physicians should recognize the important role they have in continuing to care for the child and family as the primary goal of treatment changes from prolongation of life to quality of life. Regular meetings between caregivers and the family are essential in order to reassess and manage symptoms, explore the impact of illness on immediate family members, and provide anticipatory guidance. At these meetings, important issues include finding an appropriate physical setting for the meeting, reviewing what was previously discussed, listening to concerns and issues as they are revealed, having parents repeat back what was said to ensure clarity, and responding with honest, factual answers in areas of uncertainty. Parents may blame themselves for their child's illness even when logic dictates that they had nothing to do with what is happening to their child ("If only I had taken him to the doctor sooner") and may spend considerable energy and resources looking for "miracle cures." The physician should be sensitive to these possible and not necessarily easily expressed parental concerns. There is potential for physicians to provide much needed support to parents at these times by engaging in active listening while validating the range of concerns that parents may have. Parents also need to know about the availability of home care, respite services, educational books and videotapes, and support groups. It is important to discuss how parents envision their child's death and to address myths surrounding pain control and the benefit of involving siblings.

In communications with the child and family, the physician should avoid giving estimates of survival length, even when the child or family explicitly asks for them. These predictions are invariably inaccurate because population-based statistics do not predict the course for individual patients. A more honest approach may be to explore ranges of time in general terms ("weeks to months," "months to years"). The physician can also ask parents what they might do differently if they knew how long their child would live and then assist them in thinking through the options relating to their specific concerns (suggest celebrating upcoming holidays/important events earlier in order to take advantage of times when the child may be feeling better). It is generally wise to suggest that relatives who wish to visit might do so earlier rather than later, given the unpredictability of the time course of many illnesses. For the child and family, the integration of bad news is a process, not an event. The physician should expect that some issues previously discussed may not be fully resolved for the child and parents (do-not-resuscitate orders, artificial feedings) and may need to be revisited over time. Parents of a chronically ill child may reject the reality of an impending death because past predictions may not have been accurate. Parents of a child dying from an acute fulminant disease or accident may experience great anxiety, guilt, or despair.

THE CHILD. Responding in a developmentally appropriate fashion (Table 40-3) to children's questions about death, such as "What's happening to me? Am I dying?" requires a careful exploration of what is already known by the child, what is really being asked (the question behind the question), and why the question is being asked at this particular time and in this setting. A child's perception of death depends on his or her concepts of universality (the recognition that all things inevitably die), irreversibility (the ability to understand that dead people cannot come back to life), nonfunctionality (the understanding that being dead means that all biologic functions cease), and causality (the ability to understand the objective causes of death). (See Chapter 17.) Children's fears of death are centered on the concrete fear of being separated from parents and other loved ones, rather than on the existential consequences of an afterlife common to adults. This fear of separation may be responded to in different ways, with some families giving reassurance that loving relatives will be waiting, and others using religious figures or referring to an eternal spiritual connection ("I will always be there for you"). Many children are concerned with what will happen to their parents rather than themselves.

A child's expressed question may have different levels of meaning. A child asking, "Am I dying?" may really be testing the honesty of the person being asked. The child asking, "Why is this happening to me?" may be signaling a need to be with someone who is comfortable listening to such unanswerable questions. Many children find nonverbal expression much easier than talking; art, play therapy, and storytelling may be more helpful than direct conversation. Parents have an instinctive duty to protect their children from harm. When facing the death of their child, many parents attempt to keep the reality of impending death hidden from their children with the hope that their child can be "protected" from the harsh reality. Although it is important to respect parental wishes to avoid the subject of death with their children, it is also true that many young children already know what is happening to them even when it has been purposely left unspoken. Perpetuating the myth that "everything is going to be all right" takes away the chance to explore fears and provide reassurance. Children may blame themselves for their illness and the hardships that it causes for their loved ones. Open, honest communication that takes into account the child's developmental stage and unique lived experience can help to address their guilt.

THE SIBLINGS. Brothers and sisters are at special risk both during their sibling's illness and after their death. Because of the extraordinary demands placed on parents to meet the needs of their ill child, healthy siblings may feel that their own needs are not being acknowledged. These feelings of neglect may then trigger guilt about their own good health and resentment toward their parents and ill sibling. Younger siblings may react to the stress by becoming seemingly oblivious to the turmoil around them. Some younger siblings may feel guilty as a result of "wishing" the affected child would die so they could get their parents back ("magical thinking"). Parents need to know that this is a normal response, and siblings should be encouraged to maintain the

TABLE 40-3. Development of Death Concepts and Spirituality in Children

AGE RANGE	CHARACTERISTICS	PREDOMINANT CONCEPTS OF DEATH	SPIRITUAL DEVELOPMENT	INTERVENTIONS
0–2 yr	Has sensory and motor relationship with environment Has limited language skills Achieves object permanence May sense that something is wrong	None	Faith reflects trust and hope in others Need for sense of self-worth and love	Provide maximal physical comfort, familiar persons and transitional objects (favorite toys), and consistency Use simple physical communication
>2–6 yr	Uses magical and animistic thinking Is egocentric Engages in symbolic play Developing language skills	Believes death is temporary and reversible, like sleep Does not personalize death Believes death can be caused by thoughts	Faith is magical and imaginative Participation in ritual becomes important Need for courage	Minimize separation from parents Correct perceptions of illness as punishment Evaluate for sense of guilt and assuage if present Use precise language (dying, dead)
>6–12 yr	Has concrete thoughts	Development of adult concepts of death Understands that death can be personal Interested in physiology and details of death	Faith concerns right and wrong May accept external interpretations as the truth Connects ritual with personal identity	Evaluate child's fears of abandonment Be truthful Provide concrete details if requested Support child's efforts to achieve control and mastery Maintain access to peers Allow child to participate in decision-making
>12–18 yr	Generality of thinking Reality becomes objective Capable of self-reflection Body image and self-esteem paramount	Explores nonphysical explanations of death	Begins to accept internal interpretations as the truth Evolution of relationship with God or higher power Searches for meaning, purpose, hope, and value of life	Reinforce child's self-esteem Allow child to express strong feelings Allow child privacy Promote child's independence Promote access to peers Be truthful Allow child to participate in decision-making

From Himelstein BP, Hilden JM, Boldt AM, Weissman D: Pediatric palliative care. *N Engl J Med* 2004;350:1752–1762.

normal routines of daily living. Siblings who are most involved with their sick brothers or sisters before death usually adjust better both at the time of and after the death. Acknowledging and validating sibling feelings, being honest and open, and appropriately involving them in the life of their sick sibling provide a good foundation for coping with loss.

THE STAFF. Studies indicate that inadequate support for the staff providing end-of-life care can result in depression, emotional withdrawal, and other symptoms. Staff need to be able to discuss their grief and their experiences. Staff forums that support and facilitate examination assist staff to be better able to assist parents and families through their grief.

DECISION-MAKING. In the course of a child's life-limiting illness, a series of difficult decisions need to be made in relation to truth telling and disclosure, location of care, medications with risks and benefits (steroids), the principle of double effect in the beneficent use of narcotic analgesics, withholding and or withdrawing life-prolonging technologies, experimental treatments in research protocols, and the use of "alternative" therapies (see Chapter 3). Decision-making should remain focused on the goals of therapy rather than on specific limitations of care; "This is what we can offer" instead of "This is what we can no longer do." Instead of meeting specifically to discuss a do-not-resuscitate order, a more general discussion centered on the goals of therapy will naturally lead to considering which interventions are in the **child's best interests.** Unclear terms used in doctor's orders in the chart such as "withholding heroic or extraordinary measures" are best replaced by reference to specific interventions that are then documented in a care plan ("suction airway secretions prn" rather than "do not do lab tests"). It is important to support parents in the decision-making process rather than to make them feel that it is up to them alone to choose what is best. Rather than asking parents if they want to forgo cardiopulmonary resuscitation for their child (placing the full burden of decision-making on them), it might be preferable to discuss why deciding against resuscitation attempts is a reasonable course of action. Once the goals of therapy are agreed on, the physician may draft a letter that outlines the end-of-life care plan for the child. The letter should be as detailed as possible, including suggestions for medications and the telephone numbers of caregivers who know the patient best. Such a letter, given to the parents, with copies to involved caregivers and institutions, can be a useful aid in communication, especially in times of crisis.

Conflicts in decision-making can occur within families, within health care teams, between the child and family, and between the family and professional caregivers. For children who are developmentally unable to provide guidance in decision-making (neonates, very young children, neurologically impaired children), parents and health care professionals may come to different conclusions as to what is in the child's best interests. In some families and cultures, truth telling and autonomy are much less valued when compared with family integrity (see Chapter 4). Although frequently encountered, differences in opinion are often manageable for all involved when lines of communication are kept open and the main goals of care, to provide comfort and quality of life, are agreed on. Decision-making with adolescents presents specific challenges given the shifting boundary that separates childhood from adulthood (see Chapters 12 and 111).

Euthanasia is the intentional, active intervention to terminate a life. The withdrawal of treatments with burdens that outweigh benefits is not euthanasia (see Chapter 3). Providing sufficient analgesia to relieve pain, even if it may have the unintentional effect of shortening life (the principle of double effect), is not the same as intentionally terminating a life. The American Academy of Pediatrics (AAP) statement on palliative care for children specifically recommends that the practice of euthanasia or physician-assisted suicide for children should not be supported.

TABLE 40-4. Pain and Symptom Management

Establish realistic goals of treatment—maintaining comfort is a priority.
Anticipate and plan for symptoms before they occur.
Utilize a stepwise approach to pain management (see Fig. 77-1).
Choose the least invasive route for medications—by mouth whenever possible.
Prescribe regular (not prn) medications for constant pain.
Consider the use of adjuvant drugs:
- Antidepressants and anticonvulsants for neuropathic pain
- Neuroleptics for nausea and agitation
- Sedatives and hypnotics for anxiety and muscle spasm
- Steroids for resistant, severe pain
- Stimulants for opioid-induced somnolence

Consider anesthetic blocks for regional pain. Use topical local anesthetics when possible (see Chapters 76 and 77).
Always include cognitive (guided imagery, distraction), physical (TENS, physiotherapy, massage), and behavioral (biofeedback, behavior modification) techniques.

TENS, transcutaneous electrical nerve stimulation.

SYMPTOM MANAGEMENT (TABLE 40-4). Pain control is of paramount importance in reducing the suffering of the child, family, and caregivers, but many dying children do not have their pain successfully treated. (See Chapters 77 and 494 for effective management of pain.) In 1998, the World Health Organization stated: "Nothing would have a greater impact on the quality of life of children with cancer than the dissemination and implementation of the current principles of palliative care, including pain relief and symptom control."

Pain is a complex sensation influenced by tissue damage as well as by situational factors, including cognitive, behavioral, emotional, social, and cultural issues that are unique to each person. In end-of-life care, it is important to form and initiate a pain treatment plan even when the diagnosis is unclear, the prognosis uncertain, and the ability of the child to communicate limited. Many children with life-limiting illness are unable to verbalize their symptoms and instead communicate their discomfort nonverbally. Presumptive therapy should be initiated promptly, and treatment plans can then be modified based on the response. For the dying child, in whom accurate assessment of the cause of pain may be difficult, it is important to reassess therapy frequently and to inform parents honestly that it may take several dose and medication adjustments in order to determine optimal analgesic requirements. Guidelines for the treatment of pain and the use of opioids are summarized in Tables 40-4 to 40-7.

Dying children have a multitude of symptoms, in addition to pain, for significant periods before their death (see Tables 40-6 and 40-7). Respiratory symptoms such as **dyspnea** (the subjective sensation of shortness of breath) are common because many children with chronic illnesses have difficulty swallowing and handling their airway secretions. Excessive airway secretions and salivation owing to poor swallowing may sometimes

TABLE 40-5. Opioid Use Guidelines

Clarify the differences between tolerance vs physical dependence vs addiction.
Dispel the myth that strong medications should be saved for last.
Anticipate and treat/prevent common side effects (constipation, pruritus, nausea, dysphoria, somnolence).
Always start constipation treatment when starting opioids.
Begin with weak opioids for mild pain (e.g., codeine). Replace with strong opioids (e.g., morphine) for unresponsive or persisting pain (see Fig. 77-1).
Start with short-acting opioids at regular intervals then convert to long-acting only when dose requirements have stabilized.
Consider switching to a different opioid when limited by side effects (e.g., myoclonus).
Consider subcutaneous infusions when oral/rectal routes are no longer possible.

TABLE 40-6. Medications Used for Common Symptoms in Pediatric Palliative Care

INDICATION	MEDICATION	INITIAL REGIMEN
Pain or dyspnea	Morphine	0.3 mg/kg of body weight orally, SL, or PR every 3–4 hr*
Agitation	Lorazepam	0.05 mg/kg orally, SL, or PR every 4–6 hr
	Haloperidol	0.01–0.02 mg/kg orally, SL, or PR every 8–12 hr
Pruritus	Diphenhydramine	0.5–1.0 mg/kg orally every 6–8 hr
Nausea and vomiting	Prochlorperazine	0.1–0.15 mg/kg orally or PR every 6–8 hr
	Ondansetron	0.15 mg/kg orally or IV every 6–8 hr
Seizures	Diazepam	0.3–0.5 mg/kg PR every 2–4 hr
Secretions	Hyoscyamine†	0.0625–0.125 mg orally or SL every 4 hr for children 2–12 yr
		0.125–0.25 mg orally or SL every 4 hr for children >12 yr

*Infants <6 mo of age should receive one third to one half of this dose.

†The regimen for infants is provided in Taketomo CK, Hodding JH, Kraus DM: *Pediatric Dosage Handbook*, 8th ed. Cleveland, Lexi-Comp, 2001.

IV, intravenous; PR, per rectum; SL, sublingual.

From Himelstein BP, Hilden JM, Morstad Boldt A, Weissman D: Pediatric palliative care. *N Engl J Med* 2004;350:1752–1762.

be helped by treatment with oral glycopyrrolate (oral dose 40–100 μg/kg/dose 3–4 times/day. As death approaches, a buildup of secretions may result in noisy respiration sometimes referred to as a death rattle. Patients at this stage are usually unconscious, and noisy respirations are often more distressing for others than for the child. It may be helpful to point out the child's lack of distress and to use an anticholinergic drug, such as hyoscine. Pneumonia is a frequent complication in dying children. Dyspnea (vs tachypnea, which may not be associated with feelings of distress) can be relieved with the use of regularly scheduled plus as-needed doses of opioids. Oxygen may be helpful in certain cases to relieve hypoxemia-related headaches. Giving oxygen to the cyanotic child who is otherwise quiet and relaxed may relieve staff discomfort while having no impact on patient distress.

Neurologic symptoms include **seizures** that are often part of the antecedent illness but may increase in frequency and severity

TABLE 40-7. Common Symptoms Experienced by Children with Life-Threatening Illness and Management Options

SYMPTOM	APPROACH TO MANAGEMENT
Pain	Assess quality, frequency, duration, and intensity of pain; reassess efficacy of interventions
	Prevent pain when possible by limiting unnecessary painful procedures, giving pre-emptive treatment prior to a procedure (e.g., including sucrose for procedures in neonates)
	Treat underlying cause if possible, weighing benefits vs risks to treatment
	Consider/treat coincident anxiety and lack of control
	Medications: opioids (morphine, hydromorphone, fentanyl, methadone, hydrocodone, oxycodone, codeine), nonopioid analgesics and NSAIDs (acetaminophen, ibuprofen, ketorolac, naproxen, etc.), adjuvants, and other medications (tricyclic antidepressants at low doses [eg, amitriptyline, nortriptyline] trazodone, antiepileptics (gabapentin, carbamazepine, topiramate), local anesthetics (lidocaine, prilocaine, bupivacaine), ketamine, baclofen, cyclobenzaprine
	Nonpharmacologic strategies: guided imagery, relaxation, hypnosis, art/pet/play therapy, acupuncture/acupressure, biofeedback, massage, heat/cold, hydrotherapy, stretching, yoga, transcutaneous electric nerve stimulation, encourage enjoyable recreation/activities, distraction, routine/structure
Dyspnea or air hunger	Suction of secretions if present, positioning, comfortable loose clothing, fan to circulate air
	Educate/reassure family about "death rattle," uneven, irregular, and deep respirations near end of life
	Limit volume of IV fluids, consider diuretics if fluid overload/pulmonary edema present
	Antibiotics (if pneumonia present)
	Consider treating anemia if present
	Oxygen via non/least distressing delivery mechanism
	Behavioral strategies including breathing exercises, guided imagery, relaxation, music
	Medications: opioids (as above), sedatives/anxiolytics (benzodiazepines), antimuscarinics (atropine, glycopyrrolate), expectorants (guaifenasin)
Fatigue	Sleep hygiene
	Medications: stimulants (dexedrine, dextroamphetamine), short-acting medications to restore sleep cycle (zolpidem, zaleplon)
Nausea/vomiting	Limit causative medications if possible
	Consider dietary modifications (bland, soft, adjust timing/volume of foods or feeds)
	Aromatherapy: peppermint, lavender
	Acupuncture/acupressure
	Medications: ondansetron, granisetron, metoclopramide, scopolamine, dexamethasone, promethazine, lorazepam, diphenhydramine, dronabinol
Constipation	Increase fiber in diet, encourage fluids
Oral lesions/dysphagia	Oral hygiene and appropriate liquid, solid and oral medication formulation (texture, taste, fluidity). Treat infections, complications (mucositis, pharyngitis, dental abscess, esophagitis). Orophayngeal motility study and speech (feeding team) consultation.
Anorexia-cachexia syndrome	Manage treatable lesions causing oral pain, dysphagia, anorexia. Support caloric intake during phase of illness when anorexia is reversible. Acknowledge that anorexia/cachexia is intrinsic to the dying process and at some point is not reversible.
	Prevent: start stimulant + softener whenever starting constipating medications such as opiates
	Medications: polyethylene glycol-electrolyte solution, docusate, senna, glycerin, bisacodyl, milk of magnesia, magnesium, citrate, mineral oil, sodium phosphate enema
Pruritis	Consider cause, opiate rotate if severe/related to opiate
	Moisturize skin
	Trim child's nails to prevent excoriation
	Try specialized anti-itch lotions
	Counterstimulation, distraction, relaxation
	Medications: sedating and nonsedating antihistamines (diphenhydramine, hydroxyzine, cetirizine, loratadine, fexofenadine), nalbuphine if opioid related
Diarrhea	Evaluate/treat if obstipation
	Assess and treat infection
	Medications: loperamide, diphenoxylate and atropine, bismuth
Depression	Psychotherapy, behavioral techniques
	Medications: selective serotonin reuptake inhibitors (fluoxetine, sertraline, paroxetine, citalopram), buproprion, venlafaxine
Anxiety	Psychotherapy (individual and family), behavioral techniques
	Medications: anxiolytics (clonazepam), antidepressants (see those listed under depression)
Agitation/terminal restlessness	Evaluate for organic or drug causes
	Educate family
	Lighten or deepen sedating medications based on child's need for control
	Medications: benzodiazepines (lorazepam, midazolam, diazepam), haloperidol, phenobarbital
Seizures	Position patient for safety during involuntary movements
	Benzodiazepines (lorazepam, diazepam), antiepileptics (phenytoin, phenobarbital, valproic acid)

From Sourkes B, Frankel L, Brown M, et al: Food, toys, and love: Pediatric palliative care. *Curr Probl Pediatr Adolesc Health Care* 2005;35:345–392.

toward the end of life. Anticonvulsants should be administered, and parents can be taught to use rectal diazepam at home. Increased irritability accompanies some neurodegenerative disorders; it may be particularly disruptive because of the resultant break in normal sleep-wake patterns and the difficulty in finding respite facilities for children who have prolonged crying. Judicious use of sedatives in the daytime (benzodiazepines) combined with hypnotics at night (chloral hydrate) may achieve a balance that can dramatically improve the quality of life for both child and caregivers.

Feeding and hydration issues raise ethical questions that include the use of nasogastric and gastrostomy feedings for the child who can no longer feed by mouth (see also Chapter 3). These complex questions require evaluating the risks and benefits of artificial feedings and taking into consideration the child's functional level and prognosis. At times, it may be appropriate to initiate a trial of tube feedings with the understanding that they may be discontinued at a later stage of the illness. A commonly held but unsubstantiated belief is that hydration is a "comfort measure," which may result in well-meaning but disruptive and invasive attempts to administer intravenous fluids to a dying child. Studies of dying adults show that the sensation of thirst may be alleviated by careful efforts to keep the mouth moist and clean. There may also be deleterious side effects to artificial hydration in the form of increased secretions, need for frequent urination, and exacerbation of dyspnea.

Nausea demands prompt treatment after a search for common causes (drug effects, constipation, primary disease, metabolic disturbance). Drugs such as metoclopramide, phenothiazines, ondansetron, and steroids may be used, depending on the cause and desired secondary effects (if sedation is desired, a sedating phenothiazine may be used). **Vomiting** may accompany nausea but may also occur without nausea in the presence of bowel obstruction. **Constipation** is common in neurologic disorders, and the 1st step is to assess stool frequency and quantity. Children with minimal solid food intake may be comfortable with bowel movements as infrequent as weekly. Children on regular opioids should routinely be placed on stool softeners (docusate) and may also need the addition of laxative agents (senna derivatives, lactulose). **Diarrhea** may be particularly difficult for the child and family and may be treated with loperamide and opioids. Paradoxical diarrhea, a result of overflow resulting from constipation, must also be considered.

Hematologic issues include consideration of transfusions for anemia and thrombocytopenia. Most children in the palliative phase may be managed by intermittent red cell and platelet transfusions for bleeding that interferes with the quality of life. Serious bleeding is disturbing for all concerned, and a plan involving the use of fast-acting sedatives should be prepared in advance.

Skin care issues include the prevention of problems such as bedsores by the early use of inexpensive egg-crate type foam mattresses and careful attention to positioning. Pruritus may be secondary to systemic disorders or drug therapy. Treatment includes avoiding excessive use of soap, using moisturizers, trimming fingernails, and wearing loose-fitting clothing, in addition to administering topical or systemic steroids. Oral antihistamines and other specific therapies may also be indicated (cholestyramine in biliary disease).

When discussing possible therapies or interventions with adolescent patients or with the parents of any ill child, it is important to raise the issue of complementary or alternative medicine because it has been shown that many patients use some form of alternative medicine therapy but are reluctant to bring it up with their physician (see Chapters 4 and 59). Although mostly unproven, some therapies are inexpensive and provide relief to individual patients. Other therapies may be expensive, painful, intrusive, and even toxic. By initiating conversation and inviting discussion in a nonjudgmental way, the physician can offer advice on the safety of different therapies and may help avoid expensive and dangerous interventions.

THE TERMINAL PHASE. As death approaches, the major tasks of the physician are to help prepare the child and family for expected problems and issues and to continue to stay involved in care. If the child is at home, regular phone calls should be made to help manage new symptoms as they occur (airway secretions, seizures, irritability, myoclonus, vomiting). Legal issues such as who will perform the declaration of death may be addressed, and the necessary documents can be partially filled out and left in a sealed envelope in the child's home. For children in the hospital, the care plan should be clear to all involved professionals and should include an understanding of the specific needs and requests of the child and family.

Initiating a discussion of the options for funeral arrangements may be appropriate inasmuch as some parents prefer to settle these practical issues before the child's death. Attendance of young siblings at the funeral should be discussed and sibling participation encouraged. Excluding siblings from the funeral deprives them of an opportunity for partial closure and may devalue their need to grieve.

In an intensive care setting, where technology can put distance between the child and parent, the physician should discontinue the use of unneeded equipment. While still in the ICU, even children on ventilators can be placed in their parents' arms. Parents who may not have held their infant since birth may be afraid to ask permission to hold their child but will be relieved to be offered the opportunity when it is presented. Hearing and the ability to sense touch is often present until death. Siblings and family members should be encouraged to talk to and touch the child, even if he or she seems unresponsive. It seems that many children who live with prolonged illness die only after their parents have begun the process of "letting go." Some children appear to wait for "permission to die," and their parents' acceptance of the inevitable may play a role in the timing of their death.

For the family, the moment of death is an event that is recalled in detail for years to come. After death, they should be given the option of remaining with their child for as long as they would like. During this time, physicians and other professionals do best by not trying to "do and say too much." Quietly sitting with the family and asking whether they would consider holding the infant may be appropriate in some cultures. Different ethnic and cultural practices should be taken into consideration and facilitated. In some traditions, it is important to have the family take the child directly to the place of worship instead of passing through the hospital morgue. Arranging this and other details in advance will help avoid some stress for both family and staff.

The physician should discuss the option of an autopsy and organ donation, answering questions that parents may be reluctant to ask ("Will the face be disturbed?"). Parents might also be reminded that they may have questions later that can be answered by an autopsy ("Will present and future siblings and grandchildren be affected?"). The parents can also be offered genetic counseling when appropriate.

The physician's decision to attend the funeral is a personal one. It may serve the dual purpose of showing respect as well as helping him or her cope with a personal sense of loss.

THE PEDIATRICIAN. Care for children with life-limiting illness places unique and at times intense demands on the pediatrician. The ability to care effectively for dying children and their families is not a skill shared by all. Most pediatricians have had little, if any, formal palliative care education and limited clinical experience in how to care for a dying child. For most physicians, however, the duty to care for their patients through the illness spectrum including the terminal phase is a commitment that reaches to the core of their professional identity. Most physicians have had training that emphasized their role as conquerors of disease. This notion, coupled with limited training in psychosocial care, in communication skills, and in pain and symptom management may promote a feeling of personal and professional failure when facing the death of a patient. Pediatricians caring for dying children and their families may require supervision from other trained professionals in examining their personal feelings, values, and attitudes about the meaning and goals of their work.

40.1 • Grief and Bereavement*

• Robert M. Kliegman

Grief is a personal, emotional state of bereavement or an anticipated response to loss. Not all children and families require professional intervention during or after a loss event; the presence of symptoms such as sadness and loneliness are understandable and predictable. Most bereaved families remain socially connected and expect that life will return to some new, albeit different, sense of normalcy.

Many secondary losses also occur as a result of a family death (change in income, possible need to relocate, less emotional support from surviving family members, altering of routines, change in status from sibling to only child). The presence of secure and stable adults who can meet the needs of a surviving sibling and who permit discussion about the loss is most important in helping a child grieve.

DEVELOPMENTAL PERSPECTIVE. When a death occurs in a family, children's responses reflect the family's current culture, past heritage, and sociopolitical environment. Personal experience with terminal illness and dying may also facilitate children's comprehension of death and familiarity with mourning. Developmental differences in children's efforts to make sense of and master the concept and reality of death do exist and profoundly influence their grief reactions.

Infants and toddlers do not understand all dimensions of death, especially its permanence (see Table 40-3). Primitive protest, despair, separation anxiety, and detachment may, however, occur at withdrawal of nurturing caretakers. Very young children also respond to observing distress in others. Young children may express signs and symptoms of grief such as irritability or lethargy. In severe cases of grief, failure to thrive may occur.

The thinking process of **preschool years** is prelogical and egocentric (see Table 40-3). **Preschool children** do not show well-established cause and effect reasoning. They typically express magical explanations of death events, sometimes resulting in guilt and self-blame ("He died because I wouldn't play with him"). Children conceptualize events in the context of their own experiential reality, and therefore consider death in terms of sleep, separation, and injury. In attempts to master the finality and permanence of death, preschoolers frequently ask unrelenting, repeated questions such as "After he finishes getting dead, will Johnny go on vacation with us?" or "When will they put the plane that crashed back together, so Mommy can fly home to make dinner?" Young children will express grief intermittently and show marked affective shifts over brief periods of time. Regression, sadness, and anger may accompany grief.

School-aged children think more concretely, recognize the permanence of death, and begin to understand biologic processes of the human body ("You'll die if your body stops working") [see Table 40-3]. Information gathered from the media, peers, and parents form lasting impressions. Consequently, they may ask candid questions about death that adults will have difficulty addressing ("He must have been blown to pieces, huh?"). Those in middle childhood, the elementary school years, tend to experience more anxiety, more overt symptoms of depression, and more somatic complaints than do younger children. School-aged children are often left with anger focused on the loved one, those who could not save the deceased, or those presumed responsible for the death. Contact with the pediatrician may provide great reassurance, especially for the child with somatic symptoms, and particularly when the death followed medical illness. School and learning problems, which are often linked to concentration difficulties or preoccupation with the death, may also occur. Close collaboration with the child's school can provide important diagnostic information and offer opportunities to mobilize intervention or support.

Around the age of 12 yr, children begin to use symbolic thinking, reason abstractly, and analyze hypothetical or "what if" scenarios systematically. Death and end of life become concepts, rather than events. **Teenagers** begin to understand complex physiologic systems in relationship to death. Fascination with dramatic, sensational, or romantic death sometimes occurs and may find expression in copycat behavior (cluster suicides) as well as competitive behavior to forge emotional links to the deceased person ("He was my best friend"). Somatic expression of grief may revolve around highly complex syndromes (eating disorders or conversion reactions) as well as symptoms limited to the more immediate reactions, as with younger children (stomachaches). Quality of life takes on meaning, and the teenager develops a focus on the future. Depression, resentment, mood swings, rage, and risk-taking behaviors can emerge as the adolescent seeks answers to questions of values, safety, evil, and fairness. Alternately, the adolescent may seek philosophic or spiritual explanations ("being at peace") to ease the sense of loss. Death of a peer may be especially traumatic.

ROLE OF THE PEDIATRICIAN IN GRIEF. Children often demonstrate that open discussion of their grief provides relief, and they readily share their story with others. School-aged children often attempt to cope with traumatic loss by seeking out and acquiring information on their own. As a source of accurate and reliable information, the pediatrician should reserve time to meet with the child, parents, and/or entire family to discuss concerns and assess the level of functioning. The pediatrician can perform several preventive roles in such meetings.

The 1st role is to be an educator about disease, death, and grief. The pediatrician should prepare to address questions such as "Can this happen to me (or someone else I care about)?" or "Did she suffer?" Truthful accounts presented in understandable language help considerably. Even for very young children, clear and honest explanation of what has happened enhances coping. For example, "Dad's heart stopped beating forever because it was damaged in the automobile accident. He doesn't breathe, eat, or move anymore. When those things happen, you are dead. Dad can never be alive again." In attempting to make sense of their loss, children and parents often become angry with health care professionals for "letting" their loved one die. School-aged children often concretely believe in the omnipotence of physicians and may also have been told "Dr. Jones will make Mommy better." Questions such as "Why didn't you . . ." should be answered in a responsive manner and without defensiveness. For example, "We did everything we could for your Mom. Sometimes it's hard to understand why someone we love has to die and leave us."

The pediatrician can also offer a safe environment to talk about painful emotions, express fears, and share memories. By giving families permission to talk and by modeling how to address children's concerns, the pediatrician demystifies death. Parents often request practical help. By providing resources, such as literature (both fiction and nonfiction) or referrals to therapeutic services,

* Edited from L. Sayler Gudas and G. P. Koocher, 17th ed.

and offering families tools to learn about illness, loss, and grief, the physician reinforces the sense that other people understand what they are going through and helps normalize their distressing emotions. The pediatrician can also facilitate and demystify the grief process by sharing basic tenets of grief therapy. There is no single right or wrong way to grieve. Everyone grieves differently, and children mourn differently from adults. Grief is not something to "get over" but is a lifelong process of adapting, readjusting, and reconnecting.

In addition, the pediatrician should assess routine health and life skills in families affected by loss and coach the family toward a sense of cohesion, moving gradually toward normalcy. Parents and children often report feeling so overwhelmed by grief that they cannot organize and manage such daily tasks as meal preparation or homework. Children cope best with grief in homes where caretakers provide safe, consistent, and predictable routines and life patterns.

The pediatrician's knowledge and understanding of child development can assist in planning age-appropriate solutions and, in a nonauthoritarian manner, help families reach decisions about such questions as "How do we tell the children?" "Does he know he's dying?" "Will I get cancer?" "Do I have to tell the kids at school?" "Should Sarah watch TV coverage of the scary event?" "When will things be normal?" "Should Johnny go to the funeral?" The pediatrician might 1st help parents identify important data to assist in the decision ("What would Johnny prefer?" "What do you believe you should do?" "What will help him feel most safe and emotionally connected to others at this sad time?"). Second, a review of what might happen and what to tell Johnny might occur ("There will be a lot of people at the funeral. Some will be crying because they are sad and miss the dead person. A box called a casket will have the body in it."). Finally, adaptive alternatives could be presented to the family ("Could Johnny have a private showing with just the family present?" "Would Johnny prefer finding ways to remember his brother without attending the service?").

Clinicians must remain vigilant for risk factors in each family member and in the family unit as a whole. Primary care providers, who care for families over time, know bereft patients' premorbid functioning and can identify those at current or future risk for physical and psychiatric morbidity. Providers must focus on symptoms that interfere with a patient's normal activities and compromise a child's attainment of developmental tasks. Symptom duration, intensity, and severity, in the context of the family's culture, can help identify complicated grief reactions in need of therapeutic attention. Descriptive words such as unrelenting, intense, intrusive, or prolonged should raise concern. Total absence of mourning signs, specifically an inability to discuss the loss or express sadness, should also suggest potential problems.

No specific grief sign, symptom, or cluster of behaviors identifies the child or family in need of help. Further assessment is indicated if the following occur: (1) persistent somatic or psychosomatic complaints of undetermined origin (headache, stomachache, eating and sleeping disorders, conversion symptoms, symptoms related to the deceased's condition, hypochondriasis); (2) unusual circumstances of death or loss (sudden, violent, or traumatic death; inexplicable, unbelievable, or particularly senseless death; prolonged, complicated illness; unexpected separation); (3) school/academic/work difficulties (declining grades or school performance, social withdrawal, aggression); (4) changes in home/family functioning (multiple family stresses, lack of social support, unavailable or ineffective functioning of caretakers, multiple disruptions in routines, lack of safety); and (5) concerning psychologic factors (persistent guilt or blame, desire to die or talk of suicide, severe separation distress, disturbing hallucinations, self-abuse, risk-taking, symptoms of trauma such as hyperarousal or severe flashbacks, grief from previous or multiple deaths).

TREATMENT. Suggesting interventions outside the natural support network of family and friends can often prove useful to grieving families. Interventions that enhance or promote attachments and security, as well as give means of expressing and understanding death, help to reduce the likelihood of future or prolonged disturbance, especially in children. Collaboration between pediatric and mental health professionals can help determine timing and appropriateness of services.

Often overlooked interventions for children and families struggling to cope with a loss in the community include positive activities enabling conversation about or active coping with their grief. Sending a card or offering food to relatives of the deceased can help children learn the etiquette of behaviors and rituals around bereavement and mutual support. Performing community service or joining charitable organizations, such as fund-raising in memory of the deceased, often prove useful. In the wake of a disaster, parents and older siblings can give blood or volunteer in search and recovery efforts. Bereavement support groups include the Compassionate Friends and Candlelighters/Lamplighters. Many children's hospitals have their own support groups and counselors. Participating in constructive activity helps move the family away from a sense of helplessness and hopelessness and facilitates meaning in their loss.

Psychotherapeutic services may benefit the entire family or individual members. Many support or self-help groups focus on specific types of losses (sudden infant death syndrome, suicide, widow/widowers, or AIDS) and provide an opportunity to talk with other people who have experienced similar losses. Family, couple, or individual counseling may be useful depending on the nature of the residual coping issues. Combinations of approaches may work well for children or parents with evolving needs. A child may participate in family therapy to deal with the loss of a sibling and use individual treatment to address issues of personal ambivalence and guilt feelings related to the death.

The question of pharmacologic intervention for grief reactions often arises in the pediatrician's office. Explaining that medication does not cure grief and often does not reduce the intensity of some symptoms can help. Although medication can blunt reactions, the psychologic work of grieving must still occur. The pediatrician must consider the patient's premorbid psychiatric vulnerability, current level of functioning, other available supports, and the use of additional therapeutic interventions. Medication, as a 1st line of defense, rarely proves useful in normal or uncomplicated grief reactions. In certain situations (severe sleep disruption, incapacitating anxiety, or intense hyperarousal), use of an anxiolytic or antidepressant medication for symptom relief and to provide the patient with the emotional energy to mourn may help. Medication used in conjunction with some form of psychotherapy, and in consultation with a psychopharmacologist, has optimal results.

American Academy of Pediatrics: Palliative care for children. *Pediatrics* 2000;106:351–357.

Contro NA, Larson J, Scofield S, et al: Hospital staff and family: Perspectives regarding quality of pediatric palliative care. *Pediatrics* 2004;114:1248–1252.

Eccleston C, Malleson P: Managing chronic pain in children and adolescents. *Br Med J* 2003;326:1408–1409.

Field MJ, Behrman RE (editors): *When Children Die: Improving Palliative and End-of-Life Care for Children and Their Families.* Washington, DC, National Academies Press, 2003.

Friedrichsdorf SJ, Menke A, Brun S, et al: Status quo of palliative care in pediatric oncology—a nationwide survey in Germany. *J Pain Symptom Manage* 2005;29:156–164.

Himelstein BP, Hilden JM, Boldt AM, Weissman D: Pediatric palliative care. *N Engl J Med* 2004;350:1752–1762.

Kolarik RC, Walker G, Arnold RM: Pediatric resident education in palliative care: a needs assessment. *Pediatrics* 2006;117:1949–1954.

Murray SA, Boyd S, Sheikh: Palliative care in chronic illness. *Br Med J* 2005;330:611–612.

Sourkes B, Frankel L, Brown M, et al: Food, toys, and love: Pediatric palliative care. *Curr Probl Pediatr Adolesc Health Care* 2005;35:345–392.

Taketomo CK, Hodding JH, Kraus DM: *Pediatric Dosage Handbook,* 8th ed. Cleveland, Lexi-Comp, 2001.

Tan GH, Totaplly BR, Torbati D, Wolfsdorf J: End-of-life decisions and palliative care in a children's hospital. *J Palliat Med* 2006;9:332–342.

Wolfe J, Grier HE, Klar N, et al: Symptoms and suffering at the end of life in children with cancer. *N Engl J Med* 2000;342:326–333.

Wolfe J, Klar N, Grier HE, et al: Understanding of prognosis among parents of children who died of cancer. *JAMA* 2000;284:2469–2475.

World Health Organization: Cancer *Pain Relief and Palliative Care in Children.* Geneva, WHO, 1998.

Part V ■ Nutrition

Chapter 41 ■ Nutritional Needs

William C. Heird

The dramatic growth of infants during the 1st yr of life (a 3-fold increase in weight; a 50% increase in length) and continued growth, albeit at lower rates, from 1 yr of age through adolescence impose unique nutritional needs (see Chapters 7–12). The needs for growth are superimposed on relatively high maintenance needs incident to the higher metabolic and nutrient turnover rates of infants and children compared with adults. Because the rapid rates of growth are accompanied by marked developmental changes in organ function and composition, failure to provide sufficient nutrients during this time is likely to have adverse effects on development as well as growth. Provision of these special nutrient needs, particularly during early life, is complicated by the young infant's lack of teeth, immature digestive and metabolic processes, and dependence on caregivers.

Reference intakes of most nutrients have been established, and these appear to support normal growth of the infant and young child. The recommendations of the Food and Nutrition Board, National Academy of Sciences, for infants, children, and adolescents are summarized in Tables 41-1 to 41-3.

REQUIREMENT VS RECOMMENDED INTAKE VS REFERENCE INTAKE

The **estimated average requirement (EAR)** of a specific nutrient is the amount of that nutrient that results in some predetermined physiologic end-point. In infants and children, this end-point is usually maintenance of satisfactory rates of growth and development and/or prevention of specific nutritional deficiencies. The EAR is usually defined experimentally, often over a relatively short period and in a relatively small study population. The EAR meets the needs of roughly half the population in which it was established, but not those of the other half. For some, it may be excessive, but for others, it may be inadequate.

The **recommended daily allowance (RDA)** of a specific nutrient is the intake deemed to meet the "requirement" for that nutrient by most healthy members of a population. If the EAR of a specific nutrient is known and is normally distributed within the population in which it was established, the RDA for that nutrient usually is set at the mean requirement (the EAR) plus 2 standard deviations. Because the requirements for many nutrients are not normally distributed, other considerations of population variability frequently are necessary. If the "requirement" appears to be adequate for most of the study population, the RDA may be less than the EAR plus 2 standard deviations. RDAs are useful for assessing the nutrient intakes of individuals or groups, but not for ascertaining the adequacy, inadequacy, or excess of an individual subject's intake of a specific nutrient.

Since the mean requirement for many nutrients is not known with certainty, it is often difficult to establish an RDA. This is particularly true for infants. In recognition of the lack of a valid EAR for most nutrients and the uncertainty of an RDA based on limited information, the recommendations of the Food and Nutrition Board, National Academy of Sciences, are termed **dietary reference intakes (DRIs)**. These include RDAs for those nutrients for which an EAR has been established and for which an RDA can reliably be established, as well as other "reference intakes." These latter include **adequate intake (AI)** and **tolerable upper intake level (UL)**.

The **AI** of a specific nutrient is the observed or approximated daily intake of that nutrient by a group of healthy individuals. It is used when an RDA cannot be established, but it is not synonymous with an RDA. The content of a specific nutrient in the average volume of milk consumed by healthy, normally growing, breast-fed infants is considered an adequate intake of that nutrient for infants younger than 6 mo of age. This definition is consistent with national and international recommendations for exclusive breast-feeding for the 1st 4–6 mo of life. The AI for most nutrients for the 7–12 mo old infant is set at the amount of the nutrient in the average volume of human milk plus the average amount of complementary foods consumed by healthy, normally growing 7–12 mo old infants. The EARs for a few nutrients have been established for older children, either directly or by extrapolation from data obtained in adults and/or older children. For these nutrients, an RDA can be established. This is impossible for most nutrients, and for these, an AI based on the mean intake of apparently "normal" infants and/or children has been established.

The **UL** is the highest daily intake of a specific nutrient that is likely to pose no risk. It is not a recommended level of intake, but rather, an aid for avoiding excessive intake and adverse effects secondary to such intake.

DIETARY REFERENCE INTAKES OF SELECTED NUTRIENTS

ENERGY. Because an energy intake that is adequate for all or almost all individuals will result in excessive weight gain by individuals with a low or an average requirement, the reference energy intakes reflect the **estimated energy requirement (EER)** for each population: the dietary energy intake predicted to maintain energy balance in a healthy individual of a defined age, sex, weight, height (length), and level of physical activity. The EERs are based on predictive equations for normal-weight individuals that include daily energy expenditure measured by the doubly labeled water method plus an allowance for energy deposition. Because an RDA, by definition, will exceed the EER for many individuals and result in excessive weight gain, setting an RDA for energy would undoubtedly contribute to the growing prevalence of overweight and obesity. Similarly, a UL for energy is not appropriate because any intake above the EER will result in excessive weight gain.

Expressed per unit of body weight, the EER of the normal infant is approximately twice that of the normal adult. The greater energy requirement of the infant reflects primarily the higher metabolic rate of infants and children and their special needs for growth and development. The inefficient intestinal absorption of the neonate compared with the adult contributes only minimally to the higher energy requirement of infants fed human milk or modern infant formula.

There is no evidence that either carbohydrate or fat is a superior source of energy. Sufficient carbohydrate to prevent ketosis and/or hypoglycemia is necessary (≈5.0 g/kg/24 hr), as is enough fat to provide essential fatty acid requirements (0.5–1.0 g/kg/24 hr of linoleic acid plus a smaller amount of α-linolenic acid) [see Table 41-1]. There is concern that infants also require long-chain, polyunsaturated fatty acids (LC-PUFA). These fatty acids

TABLE 41-1. Dietary Reference Intakes (DRIs): Recommended Intakes for Individuals, Macronutrients (Food and Nutrition Board, Institute of Medicine, National Academies)*

LIFE STAGE GROUP	TOTAL WATER[†] (L/day)	CARBOHYDRATE (g/day)	TOTAL FIBER (g/day)	FAT (g/day)	LINOLEIC ACID (g/day)	α-LINOLENIC ACID (g/day)	PROTEIN[‡] (g/day)
INFANTS							
0–6 mo	0.7*	60*	ND	31*	4.4*	0.5*	9.1*
7–12 mo	0.8*	95*	ND	30*	4.6*	0.5*	**11.0**
CHILDREN							
1–3 yr	1.3*	**130**	19*	ND	7*	0.7*	**13**
4–8 yr	1.7*	**130**	25*	ND	10*	0.9*	**19**
MALES							
9–13 yr	2.4*	**130**	31*	ND	12*	1.2*	**34**
14–18 yr	3.3*	**130**	38*	ND	16*	1.6*	**52**
19–30 yr	3.7*	**130**	38*	ND	17*	1.6*	**56**
FEMALES							
9–13 yr	2.1*	**130**	26*	ND	10*	1.0*	**34**
14–18 yr	2.3*	**130**	26*	ND*	11*	1.1*	**46**
19–30 yr	2.7*	**130**	25*	ND	12*	1.1*	**46**
PREGNANCY							
14–18 yr	3.0*	**175**	28*	ND	13*	1.4*	**71**
19–30 yr	3.0*	**175**	28*	ND	13*	1.4*	**71**
LACTATION							
14–18 yr	3.8*	**210**	29*	ND	13*	1.3*	**71**
19–30 yr	3.8*	**210**	29*	ND	13*	1.3*	**71**

*This table presents recommended dietary allowances (RDAs) in **bold type** and adequate intakes (AIs) in ordinary type followed by an asterisk (*). RDAs and AIs may both be used as goals for individual intake. RDAs are set to meet the needs of almost all (97–98%) individuals in a group. For healthy infants fed human milk, the AI is the mean intake. The AI for other groups in believed to cover the needs of all individuals in the group, but because of lack of data or uncertainty in the data it is not possible to specify with confidence the percentage of individuals covered by this intake.

[†]*Total* water includes all water contained in food, beverages, and drinking water.

[‡]Based on 0.8 g/kg body weight for the reference body weight.

ND, not determined.

TABLE 41-3. Dietary Reference Intakes (DRIs): Recommended Intakes for Individuals, Elements (Food and Nutrition Board, Institute of Medicine, National Academies)*

LIFE STAGE GROUP	CALCIUM (mg/day)	CHROMIUM (μg/day)	COPPER (μg/day)	FLUORIDE (mg/day)	IODINE (μg/day)	IRON (mg/day)	MAGNESIUM (mg/day)
INFANTS							
0–6 mo	210*	0.2*	200*	0.01*	110*	0.27*	30*
7–12 mo	270*	5.5*	220*	0.5*	130*	**11**	75*
CHILDREN							
1–3 yr	500*	11*	**340**	0.7*	**90**	**7**	**80**
4–8 yr	800*	15*	**440**	1*	**90**	**10**	**130**
MALES							
9–13 yr	1,300*	25*	**700**	2*	**120**	**8**	**240**
14–18 yr	1,300*	35*	**890**	3*	**150**	**11**	**410**
19–30 yr	1,000*	35*	**900**	4*	**150**	**8**	**400**
FEMALES							
9–13 yr	1,300*	21*	**700**	2*	**120**	**8**	**240**
14–18 yr	1,300*	24*	**890**	3*	**150**	**15**	**360**
19–30 yr	1,000*	25*	**900**	3*	**150**	**18**	**310**
PREGNANCY							
14–18 yr	1,300*	29*	**1,000**	3*	**220**	**27**	**400**
19–30 yr	1,000*	30*	**1,000**	3*	**220**	**27**	**350**
LACTATION							
14–18 yr	1,300*	44*	**1,300**	3*	**290**	**10**	**360**
19–30 yr	1,000*	45*	**1,300**	3*	**290**	**9**	**310**

*This table presents recommended dietary allowances (RDAs) in **bold type** and adequate intakes (AIs) in ordinary type followed by an asterisk (*). RDAs and AIs may both be used as goals for individual intake. RDAs are set to meet the needs of almost all (97–98%) individuals in a group. For healthy breast-fed infants, the AI is the mean intake. The AI for other groups is believed to cover the needs of all individuals in the group, but because of lack of data or uncertainty in the data it is not possible to specify with confidence the percentage of individuals covered by this intake.

SOURCES: *Dietary Reference Intakes for Calcium, Phosphorous, Magnesium, Vitamin D, and Fluoride* (1977); *Dietary Reference Intakes for Thiamin, Riboflavin, Niacin, Vitamin B_6, Folate, Vitamin B_{12}, Pantothenic Acid, Biotin, and Choline* (1988); *Dietary Reference Intakes for Vitamin C, Vitamin E, Selenium, and Carotenoids* (2000); *Dietary Reference Intakes for Vitamin A, Vitamin K, Arsenic, Boron, Chromium, Copper, Iodine, Iron, Manganese, Molybdenum, Nickel, Silicon, Vanadium, and Zinc* (2001); and *Dietary Reference Intakes for Water, Potassium, Sodium, Chloride, and Sulfate* (2004). These reports may be accessed at *http://www.nap.edu.*

TABLE 41-2. Dietary Reference Intakes (DRIs): Recommended Intakes for Individuals, Vitamins (Food and Nutrition Board, Institute of Medicine, National Academies)*

LIFE STAGE GROUP	VITAMIN A (μg/day)[†]	VITAMIN C (mg/day)	VITAMIN D (μg/day)[‡§]	VITAMIN E (mg/day)[‖]	VITAMIN K (μg/day)	THIAMIN (mg/day)	RIBOFLAVIN (mg/day)	NIACIN (mg/day)[¶]	VITAMIN B_6 (mg/day)	FOLATE (μg/day)[#]	VITAMIN B_{12} (μg/day)	PANTOTHENIC ACID (mg/day)	BIOTIN (μg/day)	CHOLINE** (mg/day)
INFANTS														
0–6 mo	400*	40*	5*	4*	2.0*	0.2*	0.3*	2*	0.1*	65*	0.4*	1.7*	5*	125*
7–12 mo	500*	50*	5*	5*	2.5*	0.3*	0.4*	4*	0.3*	80*	0.5*	1.8*	6*	150*
CHILDREN														
1–3 yr	**300**	**15**	5*	**6**	30*	**0.5**	**0.5**	**6**	**0.5**	**150**	**0.9**	2*	8*	200*
4–8 yr	**400**	**25**	5*	**7**	55*	**0.6**	**0.6**	**8**	**0.6**	**200**	**1.2**	3*	12*	250*
MALES														
9–13 yr	**600**	**45**	5*	**11**	60*	**0.9**	**0.9**	**12**	**1.0**	**300**	**1.8**	4*	20*	375*
14–18 yr	**900**	**75**	5*	**15**	75*	**1.2**	**1.3**	**16**	**1.3**	**400**	**2.4**	5*	25*	550*
19–30 yr	**900**	**90**	5*	**15**	120*	**1.2**	**1.3**	**16**	**1.3**	**400**	**2.4**	5*	30*	550*
FEMALES														
9–13 yr	**600**	**45**	5*	**11**	60*	**0.9**	**0.9**	**12**	**1.0**	**300**	**1.8**	4*	20*	375*
14–18 yr	**700**	**65**	5*	**15**	75*	**1.0**	**1.0**	**14**	**1.2**	**400**[††]	**2.4**	5*	25*	400*
19–30 yr	**700**	**75**	5*	**15**	90*	**1.1**	**1.1**	**14**	**1.3**	**400**[††]	**2.4**	5*	30*	425*
PREGNANCY														
14–18 yr	**750**	**80**	5*	**15**	75*	**1.4**	**1.4**	**18**	**1.9**	**600**[††]	**2.6**	6*	30*	450*
19–30 yr	**770**	**85**	5*	**15**	90*	**1.4**	**1.4**	**18**	**1.9**	**600**[‡‡]	**2.6**	6*	30*	450*
LACTATION														
14–18 yr	**1,200**	**115**	5*	**19**	75*	**1.4**	**1.6**	**17**	**2.0**	**500**	**2.8**	7*	35*	550*
19–30 yr	**1,300**	**120**	5*	**19**	90*	**1.4**	**1.6**	**17**	**2.0**	**500**	**2.8**	7*	35*	550*

*This table (taken from the DRI reports, see *www.nap.edu*) presents recommended dietary allowances (RDAs) in **bold type** and adequate intakes (AIs) in ordinary type followed by an asterisk (*). RDAs and AIs may both be used as goals for individual intake. RDAs are set to meet the needs of almost all (97–98%) individuals in a group. For healthy breast-fed infants, the AI is the mean intake. The AI for other groups is believed to cover the needs of all individuals in the group, but because of lack of data or uncertainty in the data it is not possible to specify with confidence the percentage of individuals covered by this intake.

[†]As retinol activity equivalents (RAEs). 1 RAE = 1 μg retinol, 12 μg β-carotene, 24 μg α-carotene, or 24 μg β-cryptoxanthin. The RAE for dietary provitamin A carotenoids is 2-fold greater than retinol equivalents (RE), whereas the RAE for preformed vitamin A is the same as RE.

[‡]As cholecalciferol. 1 μg cholecalciferol = 40 IU vitamin D.

[§]In the absence of adequate exposure to sunlight.

[‖]As α-tocopherol. α-Tocopherol includes *RRR*-α-tocopherol, the only form of α-tocopherol that occurs naturally in foods, and the *2R*-stereoisomeric forms of α-tocopherol (*RRR-*, *RSR-*, *RRS-*, and *RSS*-α-tocopherol) that occur in fortified foods and supplements. It does not include the *2S*-stereoisomeric forms of α-tocopherol (*SRR-*, *SSR-*, *SRS-*, and *SSS*-α-tocopherol), also found in fortified foods and supplements.

[¶]As niacin equivalents (NE). 1 mg of niacin = 60 mg of tryptophan; 0–6 mo = preformed niacin (not NE).

[#]As dietary folate equivalents (DFE). 1 DFE = 1 μg food folate = 0.6 μg of folic acid from fortified food or as a supplement consumed with food = 0.5 μg of a supplement taken on an empty stomach.

**Although AIs have been set for choline, there are few data to assess whether a dietary supply of choline is needed at all stages of the life cycle, and it may be that the choline requirement can be met by endogenous synthesis at some of these stages.

[††]In view of evidence linking folate intake with neural tube defects in the fetus, it is recommended that all women capable of becoming pregnant consume 400 μg from supplements or fortified foods in addition to intake of food folate from a varied diet.

[‡‡]It is assumed that women will continue consuming 400 μg from supplements or fortified food until their pregnancy is confirmed and they enter prenatal care, which ordinarily occurs after the end of the periconceptional period—the critical time for formation of the neural tube.

MANGANESE (mg/day)	MOLYBDENUM (μg/day)	PHOSPHORUS (mg/day)	SELENIUM (μg/day)	ZINC (mg/day)	POTASSIUM (g/day)	SODIUM (g/day)	CHLORIDE (g/day)
0.003*	2*	100*	15*	2*	0.4*	0.12*	0.18*
0.6*	3*	275*	20*	**3**	0.7*	0.37*	0.57*
1.2*	**17**	**460**	**20**	**3**	3.0*	1.0*	1.5*
1.5*	**22**	**500**	**30**	**5**	3.8*	1.2*	1.9*
1.9*	**34**	**1,250**	**40**	**8**	4.5*	1.5*	2.3*
2.2*	**43**	**1,250**	**55**	**11**	4.7*	1.5*	2.3*
2.3*	**45**	**700**	**55**	**11**	4.7*	1.5*	2.3*
1.6*	**34**	**1,250**	**40**	**8**	4.5*	1.5*	2.3*
1.6*	**43**	**1,250**	**55**	**9**	4.7*	1.5*	2.3*
1.8*	**45**	**700**	**55**	**8**	4.7*	1.5*	2.3*
2.0*	**50**	**1,250**	**60**	**12**	4.7*	1.5*	2.3*
2.0*	**50**	**700**	**60**	**11**	4.7*	1.5*	2.3*
2.6*	**50**	**1,250**	**70**	**13**	5.1*	1.5*	2.3*
2.6*	**50**	**700**	**70**	**12**	5.1*	1.5*	2.3*

are more than 18 carbons in length and have 2 or more double bonds. Those that are most relevant to infant nutrition are arachidonic acid (ARA; 20:4ω6) and docosahexaenoic (DHA; 22:6ω3) acid. By convention, the 1st number indicates the length of the carbon chain, the number after the colon indicates the number of double bonds, and the designations ω6 and ω3 indicate the site of the 1st double bond from the noncarboxyl (ω) end of the molecule. These 2 fatty acids are the most prevalent ω6 and ω3 fatty acids, respectively, in the central nervous system, and the latter accounts for up to 40% of the fatty acid content of the retinal photoreceptor membranes. Both are synthesized by the same series of desaturation and elongation reactions from the essential fatty acids linoleic acid (LA; 18:2ω6) and α-linolenic acid (ALA; 18:3ω3).

Although infants can convert LA and ALA, respectively, to ARA and DHA, the contents of ARA and, particularly, DHA in the plasma and erythrocyte lipids of formula-fed infants are lower than the contents in breast-fed infants. Autopsy studies show that the low erythrocyte lipid content of DHA, but not ARA, is accompanied by a lower concentration in the brain. These differences are assumed to reflect the presence of LC-PUFA in human milk, but not in formula, suggesting that the synthetic pathway, although intact, does not synthesize enough LC-PUFA. The better visual and, particularly, cognitive development of breast-fed compared with formula-fed infants also has been attributed to the presence of LC-PUFA in human milk, but not in formula.

Because human milk contains a number of factors other than LC-PUFA that might be important for development, the specific role of LC-PUFA in the visual and cognitive development of infants cannot be determined by studies of formula-fed vs breast-fed infants. There are major psychosocial and socioeconomic differences between mothers who choose breast-feeding and those who choose formula-feeding. Thus, over the last decade, many studies have addressed differences in the visual function and/or neurodevelopmental status of infants fed LC-PUFA–supplemented vs unsupplemented formulas. Some of these studies have shown distinct advantages of supplementation, but others have not, and the reasons for the different findings are not clear. When advantages for visual function are detected, the magnitude of the advantage equates to approximately 1 line on a Snellen chart. Data concerning the neurodevelopmental outcomes of infants fed supplemented vs unsupplemented formulas also are quite variable. Some studies have shown advantages, but others have not.

Although a report prepared by the Life Sciences Research Office to advise the U.S. Food and Drug Administration concerning desirable nutrient contents of term infant formulas marketed in the USA did not recommend the inclusion of LC-PUFA, similar groups in other countries have advised supplementation. Formulas containing ARA and DHA have been available for some time in many parts of the world and are available in the USA. These formulas appear to be safe, and in theory, they may confer developmental advantages for some infants.

The minimal needs for carbohydrate and fat, including LC-PUFA, amount to no more than 30 kcal (125.5 kJ)/kg/24 hr, or only about ⅓ of the total energy need. Whether the remainder should be composed predominantly of carbohydrate, fat, or equicaloric amounts of each is not known. Human milk and most available formulas contain roughly equicaloric amounts of each. Because a higher percentage of energy as carbohydrate, depending on which carbohydrate is used, may increase osmolality and a higher percentage as fat may exceed the somewhat limited ability of the infant to digest and absorb fat, providing roughly equicaloric amounts of each seems appropriate.

PROTEIN. The normal infant also requires more protein per unit of body weight than the adult (see Table 41-1). It is believed that the infant requires a higher proportion of essential amino acids than the adult. These include the amino acids recognized as essential (or indispensable) for the adult (leucine, isoleucine, valine, threonine, methionine, phenylalanine, tryptophan, lysine, histidine) as well as cysteine, tyrosine, and perhaps arginine. The need for cysteine is believed to be secondary to delayed development of hepatic cystathionase activity; this key enzyme in the conversion of methionine to cysteine does not reach adult levels until approximately 4 mo of age. The reason for the infant's apparent need for tyrosine is not clear; the hepatic activity of phenylalanine hydroxylase, the rate-limiting enzyme for the conversion of phenylalanine to tyrosine, is at or near adult levels early in gestation. It also appears that even preterm infants can convert phenylalanine to tyrosine.

Human milk protein and all proteins used in infant formulas contain adequate amounts of all essential amino acids, including cysteine, tyrosine, and arginine. The sum of the highest estimates of the necessary intake of each essential amino acid is considerably less than the total protein requirement. However, the necessary intake of a specific protein depends on its quality, which is usually defined as how closely its amino acid pattern resembles the pattern of human milk. The overall quality of a specific protein can be improved by supplementing it with the essential amino acid or acids that result in its quality being low, the limiting amino acid. Native soy protein has insufficient methionine, but when it is fortified with methionine, its quality approaches that of bovine milk protein.

The AI for protein established by the Food and Nutrition Board, National Academy of Science, for the 0–6 mo old infant, 9.3 g/24 hr, or approximately 1.5 g/kg/24 hr (assuming a mean weight of 6 kg), is based on the observed mean protein intake of 0–6 mo old infants fed principally with human milk. EARs for protein were established for the 7–12 mo old infant as well as for the 1–3 yr old child and the 4–8 yr old child. These are based on maintenance protein needs plus the additional need for protein deposition, as determined by measurements of the body composition of normally growing infants and children, assuming an efficiency of deposition of dietary protein intake of 56%. The EAR for the 7–12 mo old infant is 0.98 g/kg/24 hr. That for the 1–3 yr old child is 0.86 g/kg/24 hr, and that for the 4–8 yr old child is 0.76 g/kg/24 hr. Because the calculated coefficient of variation is approximately 12%, RDAs are 1.24 times the EAR: 1.2 g/kg/24 hr for the 7–12 mo old, 1.05 g/kg/24 hr for the 1–3 yr old, and 0.95 g/kg/24 hr for the 4–8 yr old.

The AIs for the essential amino acids for the 0–6 mo old infant are set at the amounts of each in the amount of human milk protein equal to the AI for protein. For the 7–12 mo old, 1–3 yr old, and 4–8 yr old, EARs for the essential amino acids are based on the pattern of these amino acids in body protein and the EAR for protein. The AIs for the essential amino acids for the 0–6 mo old infant and the EARs for the older infant and young child are shown in Table 41-4.

ELECTROLYTES, MINERALS, AND VITAMINS. Intakes of electrolytes by the breast-fed and formula-fed infant as well as by children 1–8 yr of age appear to approximate the DRIs for each (see Tables 41-2 and 41-3).

TABLE 41-4. Dietary Reference Intakes of Essential Amino Acids by Infants and Children

AMINO ACID	0–6 MO	7–12 MO	1–3 YR	4–8 YR
Aromatic amino acids (mg/kg/24 hr)	120	61	46	38
Isoleucine (mg/kg/24 hr)	78	36	28	25
Leucine (mg/kg/24 hr)	139	71	56	47
Lysine (mg/kg/24 hr)	95	66	51	43
Sulfur amino acids (mg/kg/24 hr)	52	32	25	21
Threonine (mg/kg/24 hr)	65	36	27	22
Tryptophan (mg/kg/24 hr)	25	10	7	6
Valine (mg/kg/24 hr)	77	42	32	27

The normal newborn infant is believed to have sufficient stores of iron to meet the requirements for 4–6 mo. Iron stores at birth as well as the absorption of iron are quite variable. Thus, iron deficiency is common during infancy (see Chapter 455). Although human milk contains considerably less iron than modern formulas, iron deficiency is less common in breast-fed infants. Nonetheless, to prevent iron deficiency, routine iron supplementation of breast-fed infants and the use of iron-fortified formulas for formula-fed infants are recommended. The use of iron-fortified formulas is believed to be a major factor in the dramatic decrease in the prevalence of iron deficiency.

If protein intake is adequate, vitamin deficiencies are rare; if not, deficiencies of nicotinic acid and choline, which are synthesized, respectively, from tryptophan and methionine, may develop. In contrast, if bovine milk and infant formulas were not supplemented with vitamin D, hypovitaminosis D would be endemic among formula-fed infants, particularly those with limited exposure to sunlight. Breast-fed infants are even more susceptible than formula-fed infants to the development of vitamin D deficiency; routine vitamin D supplementation of breast-fed infants as well as supplementation of formulas is recommended. Reports of rickets in both breast-fed and formula-fed, dark-skinned infants and infants consistently protected from sunlight have led to recommendations for routine vitamin D supplementation for all infants.

Routine perinatal administration of vitamin K is recommended as prophylaxis against hemorrhagic disease of the newborn (see Chapters 94, 103, and 480). Thereafter, deficiency of this vitamin is uncommon except in infants and children receiving prolonged antibiotic therapy and in individuals with conditions associated with fat malabsorption.

WATER. The normal infant's absolute requirement for water probably is 75–100 mL/kg/24 hr. However, because of higher obligate renal, pulmonary, and dermal water losses as well as a higher overall metabolic rate, the young infant is more susceptible to the development of dehydration, particularly with vomiting and/or diarrhea or if solute intake is high. This is one of the major reasons that intake of bovine milk before 1 yr of age is discouraged. The DRIs for water are 700 mL/24 hr, 800 mL/24 hr, 1,300 ml/24 hr, and 1,700 mL/24 hr for the 0–6 mo old infant, the 7–12 mo old infant, the 1–3 yr old child, and the 4–8 yr old child, respectively (see Table 41-1). These are based on the mean fluid intake of infants and children from human milk (87% water), human milk plus complementary foods or the usual food, and fluid intake of children older than 1 yr of age. The typical breast-fed or formula-fed infant usually consumes at least this amount for the 1st several weeks to months of life and **does not** need additional water. After 1 yr of age, milk is continued; children will also need drinking water as well as a limited intake of juices and other beverages.

THE CHILD OLDER THAN 1 YR

After 1 yr of age, the child's rate of growth and, hence, the nutrient needs for growth decrease. The rate of growth remains appreciable, and activity increases. Thus, on a body weight basis, nutrient needs after the 1st year of life are only minimally less than those during the 1st year of life (see Tables 41-1 and 41-3).

The Food and Nutrition Board, National Academy of Sciences, provides separate reference intakes for all nutrients for the 1–3 yr old child and the 4–8 yr old child. The major physiologic reason for separating the 2 age groups is the somewhat greater rate of increase in height at 1–3 yr of age compared with 4–8 yr of age. In contrast, there are many practical reasons for differentiating these 2 periods. Children enter school at approximately 4 yr of age, and the availability of reference intakes for the 4–8 yr old child makes it easier for school systems to design meals. Separation of the 2 age groups also makes it easier to assess the intake of individual children. A reasonable amount of data on which to establish EARs is available for the 4–8 yr old group. Ending this period at 8 (or 9) yr of age, of course, circumvents the need to consider the effect of endocrine changes associated with puberty on nutrient needs.

TABLE 41-5. Servings From Each Food Group Generated by My Pyramid for Moderately Active 6 Yr Old Children

	AMOUNT/DAY	
FOOD GROUP	BOYS	GIRLS
Calories	1,600	1,400
Grain*	5 oz (½ whole grain)	5 oz*
Vegetables	2 cups	1.5 cups
Fruit	1.5 cups	1.5 cups
Milk	3 cups	2 cups
Meat†	5 oz	5 oz
Discretionary calories (sugar, oils)	130	170

*1 oz = 1 slice bread; 1 cup breakfast cereal; ½ cup cooked rice/pasta.

†1 oz = 1 oz lean meat, poultry, or fish; 1 tbs peanut butter; ½ oz nuts; ¼ cup dry beans.

After 1–2 yr of age, most children are eating the same foods as the rest of the family. At this time, a diet based on an appropriate number of servings from the various food groups will provide adequate amounts of most nutrients. Table 41-5 summarizes the recommended number of servings from each food group as well as the size of a serving for moderately active 6 yr olds, as calculated by the My Pyramid Plan. Guidelines for 2–6 yr old children are not yet available. According to the older guidelines, 2–3 yr old children should receive the same number of servings from each food group, but each serving should be only approximately ⅔ the size of that recommended for the 6 yr old child.

USING THE DIETARY REFERENCE INTAKES

The DRIs are useful for assessing the nutrient intake of individuals as well as groups. For the individual, the EAR can be used to examine the possibility that the reported intake of a specific nutrient is adequate or inadequate. A reported intake below the EAR suggests inadequacy. However, because individual requirements vary, such an intake may or may not be inadequate for an individual subject. Similarly, an intake of a specific nutrient that is greater than the EAR suggests that the intake is adequate or perhaps excessive, but because of individual differences in requirements, it may not be. In contrast, the EAR can be used to estimate the prevalence of inadequate intake in a group (the percentage of the group that has an intake below the EAR).

Assessment of a reported intake against the AI or RDA is likely to be more useful, particularly for assessing the adequacy of a reported intake. An intake equal to or greater than the AI or RDA is likely to be adequate. However, an intake below the AI or RDA also may be adequate for many individuals. Mean intake of a group at the AI, on the other hand, implies a low prevalence of inadequate intake.

Individual or mean group intakes approaching or exceeding the UL suggest the risk of adverse effects for both the individual and the group.

For planning purposes, for either an individual or a group, the aim should be to achieve intakes equal to the AI or the RDA and to avoid intakes above the UL. This helps ensure adequate intakes of all nutrients, with minimal risk of adverse effects due to excessive intakes. Using the reference intakes as described requires an accurate assessment of the usual intake. For individuals, this is best obtained from a food diary maintained over a period of several days. Any reasonable, statistically valid estimate of the mean intake of groups can be used.

Food and Nutrition Board, Institute of Medicine: *Dietary Reference Intakes for Water, Potassium, Sodium, Chloride, and Sulfate.* Washington, DC, National Academy Press, 2004.

Heird WC: Infant Nutrition. In Bowman BA, Russell RM (editors): *Present Knowledge in Nutrition,* 9th ed. Washington, DC, International Life Sciences Institute (ILSI) Press, in press.

Heird WC, Cooper A: Nutritional requirements during infancy and childhood. In Shils ME, Shike M, Ross AC, et al. (editors): *Modern Nutrition in Health and Disease,* 10th ed. Baltimore, Lippincott Williams & Wilkins, 2006; pp 797–817.

Heird WC, Lapillonne A: The role of essential fatty acids in development. *Annu Rev Nutr* 2005; 2005;25:549–571.

Panel on Dietary Antioxidants and Related Compounds, Subcommittees on Upper Reference Levels of Nutrients and Interpretation and Uses of Dietary Reference Intakes, and the Standing Committee on the Scientific Evaluation of Dietary Reference Intakes, Food and Nutrition Board, Institute of Medicine: *Dietary Reference Intakes for Vitamin C, Vitamin E, Selenium and Carotenoids.* Washington, DC, National Academy Press, 2000.

Panel on Macronutrients, Subcommittees on Upper Reference Levels of Nutrients and of Interpretation and Use of Dietary Reference Intakes, and the Standing Committee on the Scientific Evaluation of Dietary Reference Intakes, Food and Nutrition Board, Institute of Medicine: *Dietary Reference Intakes for Energy, Carbohydrate, Fiber, Fat, Fatty Acids, Cholesterol, Protein and Amino Acids.* Washington, DC, National Academy Press, 2002.

Panel on Micronutrients, Subcommittees on Upper Reference Levels of Nutrients and of Interpretation and Use of Dietary Reference Intakes, and the Standing Committee on the Scientific Evaluation of Dietary Reference Intakes, Food and Nutrition Board, Institute of Medicine: *Dietary Reference Intakes for Vitamin A, Vitamin K, Arsenic, Boron, Chromium, Copper, Iodine, Iron, Manganese, Molybdenum, Nickel, Silicon, Vanadium, and Zinc.* Washington, DC, National Academy Press, 2001.

Standing Committee on the Scientific Evaluation of Dietary Reference Intakes and Its Panel on Folate, Other B Vitamins and Choline and Subcommittee on Upper Reference Levels of Nutrients, Food and Nutrition Board, Institute of Medicine: *Dietary Reference Intakes for Thiamin, Riboflavin, Niacin, Vitamin B_6, Folate, Vitamin B_{12}, Pantothenic Acid, Biotin and Choline.* Washington, DC, National Academy Press, 1998.

Standing Committee on the Scientific Evaluation of Dietary Reference Intakes, Food and Nutrition Board, Institute of Medicine: *Dietary Reference Intakes for Calcium, Phosphorus, Magnesium, Vitamin D and Fluoride.* Washington, DC, National Academy Press, 1997.

Chapter 42 ■ The Feeding of Infants and Children

William C. Heird

The establishment of feeding practices that are comfortable and satisfying for both the parents and the infant is crucial not only for the emotional well-being of both but also for ensuring adequate nutrient intakes for the infant. Maternal feelings are readily transmitted to the infant and are a major determinant of the emotional setting in which feeding takes place. Mothers who are anxious or emotionally labile are more likely to experience a difficult feeding relationship. Appropriate guidance and support from an empathetic and experienced relative, friend, or health professional can increase such a mother's confidence, which in turn, allows her to relax and increases the likelihood of establishing successful feeding practices during infancy as well as throughout childhood and beyond.

FEEDING DURING THE 1ST 6 MO OF LIFE

Feedings should be initiated as soon after birth as possible, depending on the infant's ability to tolerate enteral nutrition. This helps maintain normal metabolism during the transition from fetal to extrauterine life and also promotes bonding between the mother and infant. Most infants can start breast-feeding immediately after birth, almost always within 1–4 hr. Mothers who wish to initiate breast-feeding in the delivery room should be supported in doing so, provided there is no question about the infant's tolerance of enteral feeding. If so, feedings should be withheld until the infant is carefully evaluated. It if appears that feedings must be withheld for some time, parenteral fluids should be administered.

The successful feeding of infants requires practical interpretation of specific nutritional needs and the wide variability among normal infants in appetite and behavior regarding food. The time required for an infant's stomach to empty may vary from 1–4 hr or more during a single day. Thus, the infant's desire for food will vary at different times of the day. Ideally, the feeding schedule established should be based on this reasonable "self-regulation" by the infant. However, this "self-regulation" is not established immediately; considerable variation in the time between feedings and in the amount taken per feeding is to be expected during the 1st few weeks of life. Most infants will have established a suitable and reasonably regular schedule by 1 mo of age.

By the end of the 1st wk of life, most healthy infants will be taking 60–90 mL/feeding and want 6–9 feedings/24 hr. Some will take enough at 1 feeding to be satisfied for as long as 4 hr, but others will want to be fed as often as every 2–3 hr. Breast-fed infants prefer shorter feeding intervals than formula-fed infants. Feeding can be considered to have progressed satisfactorily if the infant is no longer losing weight by the end of the 1st wk of life and is gaining weight by the end of the 2nd wk. Most infants will wake for a middle-of-the-night feeding until 3–6 wk of age; some never desire this feeding, and others continue it beyond 3–6 wk of age. Between 4–8 mo of age, many infants will lose interest in the late evening feeding and, by 9–12 mo of age, most will be satisfied with 3 meals/day plus snacks. *All infants do not conform to these general guidelines.*

Infants cry for reasons other than hunger; hence, they do not need to be fed every time they cry. Those who wake and cry consistently at short intervals may not be receiving enough milk or may have discomfort from some cause other than hunger (too much clothing; soiled, wet, or uncomfortable diapers; swallowed air ["gas"]; an uncomfortably hot or cold environment). Some infants cry to gain sufficient or additional attention, whereas others become indifferent to lack of attention. Some cry because they simply want to be held. Those who stop crying as soon as they are picked up or held usually do not want or need food. Those who continue to cry when held and when food is offered should be carefully evaluated for other causes of distress. The habit of offering frequent, small feedings or holding and feeding to pacify all crying should be avoided. On the other hand, satisfying the infant's true hunger as it is expressed is important. This allows physiologic requirements to be met promptly, and it helps prevent the infant's associating prolonged crying and discomfort with feeding. It also helps prevent eating practices such as gulping an entire feeding or taking small amounts too frequently.

Most infants establish a regular feeding schedule that permits the family to resume normal functioning within a few weeks after birth. If not, individual feedings or the whole day's schedule can be moved ahead or delayed sufficiently to avoid conflicts with necessary family activities. Some mothers will not understand the goals of infant "self-regulation." Others will misinterpret the physician's instructions or may be unable to adjust to the infant's regimen. These, as well as overanxious and compulsive parents, may do better with more specific feeding instructions.

The postpartum period is a time of great anxiety and insecurity, particularly for the 1st-time mother, who may be temporarily overwhelmed by the responsibilities of motherhood. Thus, it is important for the physician to set aside sufficient time shortly after birth to address the questions and concerns of inexperienced or uncertain mothers. Ideally, these anticipatory guidance sessions should include fathers and other household members.

Knowing the personalities and expectations of both parents is invaluable in helping avert physical and psychologic problems centered on feeding. Also, because parental misconceptions and confusion about the dietary and satiety needs of infants are often the basis for abnormal parent-child relations, appropriate counseling can help avoid these problems.

BREAST-FEEDING

One of the 1st decisions a new or expectant mother must make—ideally, some time before the infant is born—is whether the infant will be breast-fed or formula-fed. Human milk is uniquely adapted to the infant's needs and is the most appropriate milk for the human infant. Breast-feeding has practical and psychologic advantages. Thus, all mothers should be encouraged to breast-feed their babies, but they should not be coerced to do so.

ADVANTAGES OF BREAST-FEEDING. Breast milk is the natural food for full-term infants and is the appropriate milk for the 1st year of life. It is always available at the proper temperature and requires no preparation time. It is fresh and free of contaminating bacteria, thereby reducing the chances of gastrointestinal disturbances. Although there is little, if any, difference in mortality rates between breast-fed and formula-fed infants receiving good care, the protective effects of breast milk against enteric and other pathogens result in less morbidity. These effects are particularly important in developing countries or any locality without a safe supply of potable water and effective methods for disposal of human waste.

Breast-feeding is associated with fewer feeding difficulties incident to allergy and/or intolerance to bovine milk. These include diarrhea, intestinal bleeding, occult melena, "spitting up," colic, and atopic eczema. Breast-fed infants also appear to have a lower frequency of certain allergic and chronic diseases in later life than formula-fed infants.

Human milk contains bacterial and viral antibodies, including relatively high concentrations of secretory immunoglobulin A, that prevent microorganisms from adhering to the intestinal mucosa. It also contains substances that inhibit the growth of many common viruses as well as specific antibodies that are thought to provide local gastrointestinal immunity against organisms entering the body via this route. These factors probably account, at least partially, for the lower prevalence of diarrhea, otitis media, pneumonia, bacteremia, and meningitis during the 1st year of life in infants who are breast-fed exclusively compared with those who are formula-fed for the 1st 4 mo of life.

Macrophages in human milk may synthesize complement, lysozyme, and lactoferrin. In addition, breast milk contains lactoferrin, an iron-binding whey protein that is normally approximately ⅓ saturated with iron and has an inhibitory effect on the growth of *Escherichia coli* in the intestine. Further, the lower pH of the stool of breast-fed infants is thought to contribute to the favorable intestinal flora of infants fed human milk compared with formula (more bifidobacteria and lactobacilli; fewer *Escherichia coli*), and this helps protect against infections caused by some species of *E. coli*. Human milk also contains bile salt-stimulated lipase, which kills *Giardia lamblia* and *Entamoeba histolytica*. Transfer of tuberculin responsiveness by breast milk suggests passive transfer of T-cell immunity.

Milk from the mother whose diet is sufficient and properly balanced will supply all the necessary nutrients except fluoride and vitamin D. If the water supply is not adequately fluoridated (≤0.3 ppm), the breast-fed infant should receive at least 10 μg of fluoride daily for the 1st 6 mo of life; thereafter, the fluoride intake should approximate the adequate intake (see Table 41-3). The vitamin D intake should be 200 IU/day, starting at 2 mo of age for all breast-fed infants. The iron content of human milk is low, but most normal term infants have sufficient iron stores for the 1st 4–6 mo of life. Human milk iron is well absorbed. Nonetheless, by 4–6 mo of age, the breast-fed infant's diet should be supplemented with iron-fortified complementary foods and/or a ferrous iron preparation.

The vitamin K content of human milk also is low and may contribute to hemorrhagic disease of the newborn. Parenteral administration of 1 mg of vitamin K_1 at birth is recommended for all infants, and this is especially important for those who will be breast-fed.

The psychologic advantages of breast-feeding for both mother and infant are well recognized. The mother is personally involved in nurturing of her infant, and this results in both a feeling of being essential and a sense of accomplishment. At the same time, the infant develops a close and comfortable physical relationship with the mother.

The resumption of menstruation should not deter continued breast-feeding. Pregnancy does not necessitate immediate cessation of nursing, but the combined demands of supplying milk to the infant and supplying nutrients to the developing fetus are formidable, necessitating special attention to maternal nutrition.

Transmission of **HIV** by breast-feeding is well documented (see Chapter 273). Thus, if safe alternatives are available, breast-feeding by HIV-infected mothers is not recommended. However, in many developing countries, breast-feeding may be crucial for infant survival; the risk of HIV transmission by breast-feeding may be less than the risk of other feeding methods. The World Health Organization (WHO) recommends that breast-feeding be continued, even in areas of high endemic rates of HIV infection, unless safe infant formula is readily available. This reflects the belief that the risk of formula-feeding in many developing countries is significantly greater than the risk of HIV infection with breast-feeding.

Cytomegalovirus (CMV), human T-cell lymphotropic virus type 1, rubella virus, hepatitis B virus, and herpes simplex virus have also been demonstrated in breast milk. Approximately ⅔ of CMV-seronegative breast-fed infants may become infected with CMV. In term infants, this appears to occur without symptoms or sequelae, but the risk of more serious infection in preterm infants may be greater. Thus, the use of fresh donor milk for feeding preterm infants is contraindicated unless the milk is known to be CMV-negative.

Evidence of breast milk transmission of other viruses is rare. However, vesicles have been noted in the mouths of infants whose mothers' milk contained herpes simplex virus. Thus, nursing women with active herpes simplex lesions should observe scrupulous handwashing technique and should avoid nursing if there are active lesions on or near the nipple.

Although hepatitis B virus has been isolated from human milk, the predominant means of mother-infant transmission of this virus appears to be through delivery. Active immunization of the infant within the 1st 24 hr of life, coupled with administration of specific high-titer hepatitis B immune globulin and a follow-up active vaccination, should permit the mother who is infected with hepatitis B to nurse with minimal risk to the infant. If a nursing mother acquires hepatitis B, the infant should receive the accelerated protocol of immunization (see Chapter 170).

PREPARATION OF THE MOTHER FOR BREAST-FEEDING. Most women, if encouraged, educated, and protected from discouraging experiences and comments while milk secretion is becoming established, can successfully breast-feed their infants. The physician who is interested in helping the prospective mother breast-feed successfully should discuss the advantages of breast-feeding with her as early as the mid-trimester of pregnancy or whenever the mother begins planning for her infant (see Chapter 94). Many mothers who are ambivalent toward breast-feeding are able to nurse successfully if reassured and supported. Training of maternity staff and adoption of the Baby-Friendly Hospital Initiative,

TABLE 42-1. Steps to Encourage Breast-Feeding in the Hospital: UNICEF/WHO Baby-Friendly

HOSPITAL INITIATIVES
Provide all pregnant women with information and counseling.
Document the desire to breast-feed in the medical record.
Document the method of feeding in the infant's record.
Place the newborn and mother skin-to-skin, and initiate breast-feeding within 1 hr of birth.
Continue skin-to-skin contact at other times and encourage rooming in.
Assess breast-feeding and continue encouragement and teaching on each shift.
MOTHERS TO LEARN
Proper position and latch on
Nutritive sucking and swallowing
Milk production and release
Frequency and feeding cues
Expression of milk if needed
Assessment of the infant's nutritional status
When to contact the clinician
ADDITIONAL INSTRUCTIONS
Refer to lactation consultation if any concerns arise.
Infants should go to the breast at least 8–12 times/24 hr, day and night.
Avoid time limits on the breasts; offer both breasts at each feeding.
Do not give sterile water, glucose, or formula unless indicated.
If supplements are given, use cup feeding, a Haberman feeder, fingers, or syringe feedings.
Avoid pacifiers in the newborn nursery except during painful procedures.
Avoid antilactation drugs.

as recommended by WHO, are successful interventions to encourage breast-feeding (see Chapter 94) [Table 42-1].

Factors that are conducive to successful breast-feeding include good nutritional health, a proper balance of rest and exercise, freedom from worry, early and sufficient treatment of any intercurrent disease, and adequate nutrition. Retracted and/or inverted nipples are detractions but not contraindications to breast-feeding. Retracted nipples usually benefit from daily manual breast-pump suction during the latter weeks of pregnancy, and truly inverted nipples may be helped by the use of milk cups, starting as early as the 3rd month of pregnancy.

If the mother's diet is adequate, she need not gain or lose weight while breast-feeding. Nursing will help the uterus return to its normal size sooner and also may help the mother return to her pre-pregnancy weight sooner. Many women must be reassured that breast tone will be preserved by the use of a properly fitted brassiere to support the breasts, especially before delivery and during the nursing period. Breast-feeding has no long-term adverse cosmetic effects on the breast appearance.

ESTABLISHING AND MAINTAINING THE MILK SUPPLY. The most satisfactory stimulus to the secretion of human milk is regular and complete emptying of the breasts. Efforts should be directed toward the early establishment of normal, vigorous nursing, even during the 1st few days after birth, when there appears to be little, if any, milk. Breast-feeding should begin as soon after delivery as the conditions of the mother and the infant permit. Infants should room in with the mother and should not be offered other milks or water supplements. Infants who can't be fed on demand should be brought to the mother for feeding approximately every 3 hr during the day and night. Once lactation is well established, most mothers are capable of producing more milk than their infant needs.

Appropriate care for tender or sore nipples should be instituted before severe pain from abrasions and cracking develops. Exposing the nipples to air, applying pure lanolin, avoiding soap and other drying agents, changing disposable nursing pads frequently, nursing more often, manually expressing milk, nursing in different positions, and keeping the breast dry between feedings are recommended. If nipple tenderness is sufficient to make the mother apprehensive, the milk-ejection reflex may be delayed. This leads to frustration of the infant and increasingly vigorous nursing, which further injures the nipple and areolar area. Nipple shields may be helpful in some such situations.

The 1st 2 wk after birth are crucial for establishing breast-feeding. Daily weight gains of the infant, although important for ascertaining the volume of milk produced, should **not** be overly emphasized during this time. Supplemental bottle-feedings to achieve weight gain should be limited because these may compromise attempts at breast-feeding.

Although the difference between breast and bottle nipples may confuse the infant, this is usually not a serious problem. It is perfectly satisfactory to have the mother pump her breasts and feed the infant breast milk via a bottle for the 1st 1–2 wk. Then, when she is relaxed and less anxious, she can attempt breast-feeding 1 or 2 times daily until she and the infant have achieved a successful nursing routine. The additional pumping will usually increase milk production, thereby helping to ensure an adequate supply. Even after nursing is well established, it may be appropriate for the mother to pump extra milk and store it (in a home freezer for up to 1 mo or in a refrigerator for up to 24 hr) for use when she is not available. This allows the mother some freedom and, at the same time, allows the father or other caregivers to be more involved in the infant's feeding and care.

Lactation usually is not well established before the mother is discharged from the hospital, and the excitement of going home may impede an initially successful in-hospital nursing experience. It is wise to anticipate this possibility and discuss it with the mother. Providing her with enough formula for a few feedings may prevent discouragement that might prejudice further nursing.

No factor is more important for successful breast-feeding than the mother's happy, relaxed state of mind. Mothers may worry that their infants are abnormal when they cry, are drowsy, sneeze, or regurgitate milk. They are often upset by any suggestion that their milk may be lacking in quantity or quality, and they may be disturbed by the scanty supply of colostrum, nipple tenderness, and the fullness of the breasts on the 4th or 5th day after delivery. Many mothers do not feel comfortable when trying to nurse in an open ward, or even with another person in the room. Many also may worry about what is going on at home while they are in the hospital or what is going to happen when they return home. An alert physician recognizes and appreciates these worries, particularly if the infant is a firstborn, and provides tactful reassurance and explanations that minimize worry and enhance the likelihood of successful breast-feeding. The support plan for individual mothers, of course, must include consideration of social and cultural factors.

HYGIENE. Proper hygiene will help prevent irritation and infection of the nipples caused by prolonged initial nursing, maceration from wetness of the nipple, or rubbing of clothing.

The breasts should be washed at least once a day. If soap appears to dry the nipple and areolar area, a milder, non-drying soap should be substituted or the use of soap should be temporarily discontinued. The nipple area should be kept as dry as possible.

Many mothers are more comfortable wearing a properly fitted brassiere day and night. If this is done, plastic liners should be removed and a commercially available absorbent pad or clean cloth should be placed inside the brassiere to absorb any leaked milk.

MATERNAL DIET AND OTHER FACTORS. The breast-feeding mother's diet should contain enough calories and other nutrients to compensate for those secreted in the milk as well as for those required to produce it. A varied diet sufficient to maintain weight and generous in fluid, vitamins, and minerals is important. Weight-reducing diets should be avoided, particularly while the infant is exclusively breast-fed. Milk is an important component of the mother's diet, but it should not replace other essential foods. If the mother is allergic to milk or dislikes it, her diet should be supplemented with 1 g calcium daily. Daily fluid intake should approximate 3 qt.

Ingestion of some foods (berries, tomatoes, onions, members of the cabbage family, chocolate, spices, condiments) by the mother may occasionally cause the infant to have gastric distress or loose stools. However, no food need be withheld from the mother unless it is known to cause, or is strongly suspected to cause, distress to the infant.

Nursing mothers should not take drugs unless they are absolutely necessary (see Chapter 94). Many preparations are harmful to the neonate; many have not been evaluated. Antithyroid medications, lithium, anticancer agents, isoniazid, recreational drugs, and phenindione are contraindicated for the breast-feeding mother. If the mother requires any of these agents, diagnostic radiopharmaceuticals, chloramphenicol, metronidazole, sulfonamides, and/or anthraquinone-derivative laxatives, temporary cessation of breast-feeding should be considered. Nursing mothers should limit intake of fish from waters contaminated with polychlorinated biphenyls or other substances (mercury). Smoking cigarettes and drinking alcoholic beverages should be discouraged during breast-feeding. It is important for the breast-feeding mother to avoid fatigue. She should exercise sufficiently to promote her sense of physical well-being.

TECHNIQUE OF BREAST-FEEDING. Breast-feeding sometimes becomes impossible because the attending physician fails to recognize that the difficulties are in the feeding technique. It is important to review the technical aspects of breast-feeding with the mother, particularly the mother who has not breast-fed before (see Chapter 94).

At feeding time, the infant should be hungry, dry, and neither too cold nor too warm. He or she should be held in a comfortable, semi-sitting position to prevent vomiting with eructation. The mother, too, should be comfortable and completely at ease. A moderately low chair with an armrest is preferable, and a low stool for resting her foot and raising her knee on the nursing side is helpful. The infant should be supported comfortably with the face held close to the mother's breast by 1 arm and hand while the other hand supports the breast, making the nipple easily accessible to the infant's mouth without obstructing nasal breathing. The infant's lips should engage considerable areola as well as nipple.

Success in breast-feeding depends, in large part, on the adjustments made during the 1st few days of life. Difficulties often result from attempts to adapt the infant to a nursing procedure rather than designing a procedure that satisfies the infant. Most problems can be avoided by conforming to the infant's spontaneous pattern. If the infant is breast-fed when hungry and his or her appetite is satisfied, the fundamental requirements are met.

Several reflexes or behavior patterns that facilitate breast-feeding are present at birth. These include the rooting, sucking, swallowing, and satiety reflexes. The **rooting reflex** is the 1st to come into play. When the infant smells milk, he or she moves the head in an attempt to find the source of the smell. If the cheek is touched by a smooth object (the mother's breast), the infant will turn toward that object and open his or her mouth in anticipation of grasping the nipple (rooting with the mouth for the nipple). The infant's rooting reflex brings the entire areolar area into the infant's mouth and contact of the nipple against the infant's palate and posterior tongue elicits sucking, while the buccal fat pads help keep the nipple in place. This sucking reflex is a process of squeezing the sinuses of the areola rather than simply sucking on the nipple, as is required for bottle-feeding. Finally, milk in the infant's mouth triggers the swallowing reflex.

The breast-feeding infant's sucking results in afferent impulses to the mother's hypothalamus and then to both the anterior and the posterior pituitary. Prolactin release from the anterior pituitary stimulates milk secretion by the cuboidal cells in the acini or alveoli of the breast, whereas secretion of oxytocin by the posterior pituitary results in contraction of the myoepithelial cells surrounding the alveoli deep in the breast. This, in turn, "squeezes" milk into the larger ducts, where it is more easily available to the sucking infant. When this "let down" or milk ejection reflex functions well, milk flows from the opposite breast as the infant begins to nurse. The reflex is often absent or erratic during periods of pain, fatigue, or emotional distress. This is thought to be a common cause of milk retention in women who are unsuccessful at breast-feeding.

Mothers should know that the infant who is not hungry will not search for the nipple or suck. Most infants are usually sleepy for several days after birth; hence, they are not avid suckers. By the 3rd day of life, when there has been some weight loss, many mothers become anxious if the infant seems uninterested in nursing. It reassures them to learn that most healthy infants "wake up" and become good nursers by the 4th or 5th day of life. Infants whose mothers were sedated during labor usually suck at lower rates and pressures and also consume less milk than infants of non-sedated mothers.

Some infants will empty a breast in 5 min; others will nurse at a more leisurely pace, sometimes for 20 min or longer. Most of the milk is obtained early in the feeding (50% in the 1st 2 min and 80–90% in the 1st 4 min). Unless the mother has sore nipples, the infant should be allowed to suck until satisfied. If the infant does not "unlatch" from the breast after a reasonable period, a finger can be inserted into the corner of his or her mouth to decrease suction and facilitate removal. The infant should not be pulled from the breast.

At the end of the nursing period, the infant should be held erect over the mother's shoulder or on her lap, with or without gentle rubbing or patting of the back to assist in expelling swallowed air. This "burping" procedure often is necessary 1 or more times during the feeding as well as 5–10 min after the infant has been returned to the crib. It is an essential procedure during the early months of life, but should not be overdone.

The infant should empty at least 1 breast at each feeding; otherwise, the breast will not be stimulated sufficiently to refill. Both breasts should be used at each feeding during the early weeks to encourage maximal milk production. After the milk supply is established, the breasts may be alternated at successive feedings. The infant will usually be satisfied with the amount obtained from 1 breast. If milk secretion becomes too great, both breasts may be offered at each feeding but incompletely emptied, thereby decreasing milk production.

DETERMINING THE ADEQUACY OF MILK SUPPLY. If the infant is satisfied after each nursing period, sleeps 2–4 hr between feedings, and gains weight adequately, the milk supply is sufficient. Infants who are "light sleepers" usually require considerable body contact with the mother during the 1st months of life; hence, it should not be assumed automatically that mothers of such infants have a poor milk supply. On the other hand, if the infant nurses avidly and completely empties both breasts, but appears unsatisfied afterward (does not go to sleep after nursing or sleeps fitfully and awakens after 1–2 hr) and fails to gain weight satisfactorily, the milk supply is probably inadequate. The **La Leche League,** which establishes close relationships between successful nursing mothers and mothers needing assistance with nursing, is often helpful in such circumstances.

In general, weighing the infant before and after every nursing to judge the adequacy of the milk supply is neither necessary nor desirable. The amount of milk an infant takes at a single feeding ranges from 1 to several oz throughout a 24 hr period and, hence, is usually unimportant with respect to daily intake. Small gains may worry the mother and, in turn, may diminish her milk supply. In addition, she may give the infant a bottle to reassure herself that the infant is getting enough to eat, and the better result with the "test bottle" may discourage breast-feeding, even if she has an adequate milk supply.

Three possibilities should be excluded before assuming that a mother cannot produce sufficient milk: (1) errors in the feeding technique; (2) remediable maternal factors related to diet, rest, or emotional distress; (3) physical disturbances of the infant that interfere with nursing or weight gain. Infrequently, infants who seem to be nursing well may not thrive because of inadequate milk supply. In such cases, more frequent feedings may be indicated. However, nursing more often than every 2 hr may inhibit prolactin secretion and further decrease milk production. This usually is not a problem with feeding at 2 hr intervals. Other aids include stimulation of prolactin secretion by small doses of chlorpromazine for a few days and the use of feeding tube devices attached to the nipple, such as the **Lact-Aid**, which supplement the infant's intake.

EXPRESSION OF BREAST MILK. Expression of breast milk is useful to relieve engorgement of the breasts. Although convenient and more effective than manual expression, battery-operated and electric breast pumps may be prohibitively expensive for many mothers. Nonetheless, pumping increases milk production. It also relieves sore nipples because it does not cause as much nipple irritation as suckling. Pumped breast milk can be safely stored in the freezer or refrigerator and used for feeding the infant at a later time.

SUPPLEMENTAL FEEDINGS. Most mothers who are returning to work plan to pump enough milk while at work to feed their infant while they are at work. However, because of stress and time constraints at work and at home, this often is impossible. These mothers should be reassured that it is acceptable to feed the infant a commercial formula during the day and to continue nursing in the evening. Breast milk production will gradually decrease so that the mother is not plagued by engorged, leaking breasts, but most will continue to produce enough milk for 2–3 feedings/day for several months.

If formula or stored breast milk is to be given after the infant has completed a breast-feeding, the bottle containing the milk should be available so that it can be offered immediately after the infant has been "burped." The holes in the nipples should not be so large that the infant gets this portion of food without effort; if this happens, he or she may quickly abandon any efforts to nurse adequately at the mother's breast. Some employers provide child care at the workplace or provide convenient facilities for pumping. These enable mothers to continue nursing successfully and, hence, should be commended and encouraged.

WEANING FROM BREAST-FEEDING

Between 6 and 12 mo of age, after they become accustomed to solid foods and liquids by bottle and/or cup, most infants decrease the volume and frequency of breast-feeding (Table 42-2). As the infant demands less milk, the mother's supply gradually diminishes without causing discomfort from engorgement. Weaning can be initiated when mutually desired by the mother and infant by substituting formula by bottle or cup for part and, subsequently, all of a breast-feeding. Breast-feeding is eventually replaced with formula-feeding, at which time the infant is weaned completely. Occasionally, an infant takes a cup as readily as a bottle. If so, the intermediate transfer from breast to bottle before transferring from bottle to cup can be avoided. These changes should be made gradually and should be a pleasant experience, not a conflict, for both the mother and the infant.

When cessation of nursing is necessary at an early age, use of a tight breast binder and application of ice bags may help decrease milk production. Restriction of the mother's fluid intake and small doses of estrogen for 1–2 days also may help decrease milk production.

TABLE 42-2. Important Principles for Weaning

Begin at ≈ 6 mo of age
Avoid foods with high allergenic potential (cow's milk, eggs, fish, nuts, soybeans).
At the proper age, encourage a cup rather than a bottle.
Introduce 1 food at a time.
Energy density should exceed that of breast milk.
Iron-containing foods (meat, iron-supplemented cereals) are required.
Zinc intake should be encouraged with foods such as meat, dairy products, wheat, and rice.
Phytate intake should be low to enhance mineral absorption.
Breast milk should continue to 12 mo; formula or cow's milk is then substituted. **Give no more than 24 oz/day of cow's milk.**
Fluids other than breast milk, formula, and water should be discouraged. **Give no more than 4–6 oz/day of fruit juices. No soda.**

CONTRAINDICATIONS TO BREAST-FEEDING. Provided the mother's milk supply is ample, her diet is adequate, and she is not infected with HIV, there are no disadvantages of breast-feeding for the healthy term infant (see Chapter 94). Allergens to which the infant is sensitized can be conveyed in the milk, but the presence of such allergens is rarely a valid reason to stop breast-feeding. Rather, an attempt should be made to identify the allergen and remove it from the mother's diet.

There also are few maternal contraindications to breast-feeding. Markedly inverted nipples may be troublesome, as may fissuring or cracking of the nipples, but the latter can usually be avoided by preventing engorgement. **Mastitis** usually can be alleviated by continued and frequent nursing on the affected breast to keep it from becoming engorged, but local heat applications and antibiotics may occasionally be necessary. Acute maternal infection may contraindicate breast-feeding if the infant does not have the same infection; otherwise, there is no need to stop nursing unless the condition of either the mother or the infant necessitates it. When the infant is unaffected, the breast may be emptied and the milk given to the infant by bottle or cup. Mothers with septicemia, active tuberculosis, typhoid fever, breast cancer, or malaria should not breast-feed. Substance abuse and severe neuroses or psychoses also are contraindications to breast-feeding. Infants with galactosemia should not be breast-fed, but should receive a non–lactose-containing formula.

FORMULA-FEEDING

Objective nutritional studies of growing infants younger than 4–6 mo of age (e.g., rate of growth in weight and length, normality of various constituents in blood, performance in metabolic studies, body composition) differ minimally, if at all, between breast-fed infants and infants fed modern infant formulas. Although such investigations may not allow the detection of small but important variations and/or differences, they attest to the ability of modern infant formulas to support normal growth and development. Thus, the mother who cannot or does not wish to nurse her infant need have no less sense of accomplishment or of affection for her infant than the nursing mother. Moreover, the quality of attachment and mothering and the degree of security and affection provided the breast-fed infant need not be different with formula-feeding.

TECHNIQUE OF FORMULA-FEEDING. The setting for formula-feeding should be similar to that for breast-feeding, with the mother or caregiver and the infant in a comfortable position, unhurried, and free from distractions. The infant should be hungry, fully awake, warm, and dry. He or she should be held as though being breast-fed. The nipple holes should be of a size that allows the milk to drip slowly, and the bottle should be held so that milk, not air, channels through the nipple. Bottle propping, even with a "safe" holder, should be avoided; this not only deprives the infant of the physical contact and security of being held, but also may be dangerous, particularly for small infants, who may aspirate if unattended. In addition, otitis media is more common in infants fed with a propped bottle.

The bottle of formula is usually warmed to body temperature. This may be tested by dropping milk onto the wrist. However, no harmful effects from feeding formula at room or even refrigerator temperature have been demonstrated.

Eructation of air swallowed during feeding is important for avoiding regurgitation and abdominal discomfort, especially during the 1st 6–7 mo of life. The technique of "burping" should be the same as described for the breast-fed infant. A few infants relieve themselves best after being returned to the crib. All infants occasionally regurgitate or "spit up" a small amount of milk after feeding, a fact that the mother should know. Spitting up seems to occur more often in the formula-fed than in the breast-fed infant.

A feeding may last from 5–25 min, depending on the age and the vigor of the infant. Because the infant's appetite varies from 1 feeding to another, each bottle should contain more than the average amount taken per feeding, but in no case should the infant be urged to take more than desired. Excess formula should be discarded.

COMPOSITION OF INFANT FORMULAS. The nutrient content of infant formulas marketed in the USA is regulated by the Food and Drug Administration (FDA) according to the Infant Formula Act, and most industrialized as well as many developing countries have similar regulations. All marketed formulas must contain minimum amounts of all nutrients known or thought to be required by infants, and increasing emphasis is being placed on not exceeding a reasonable maximum content of each nutrient. The most recent recommendations for the minimum and maximum nutrient contents of infant formulas marketed in the USA are shown in Table 42-3. These recommendations were made by a committee appointed by the Life Sciences Research Organization to advise the FDA. Note that the minimum recommended amount of each nutrient is greater than the amount of that nutrient in human milk and, hence, greater than the most recent dietary reference intake (DRI) for that nutrient (see Tables 41-1 and 41-3). This, most likely, reflects the perceived lower bioavailability of nutrients in formula compared with human milk.

Manufacturers of infant formulas are responsible for assuring the FDA that each formula contains the minimum recommended amount and no more than the maximum recommended amount of each nutrient for the intended shelf life of the formula and also that the formula was manufactured safely and hygienically. Each batch of manufactured formula is assayed continually over the shelf life of the product. Manufacturers also are responsible for assuring the FDA that each marketed formula, as the infant's source of nutrition, supports normal growth and development for at least the 1st 4 mo of life. This is usually done by conducting growth studies during all or part of the 1st 4 mo, but at least 2 mo of life, in a sufficient number of infants to detect a 3 g/24 hr difference in rate of weight gain between infants fed the "new formula" compared with a standard formula or human milk. The efficacy and safety of substituting alternative sources of various nutrients also must be demonstrated by appropriate studies.

Most infant formulas contain a protein source, usually a mixture of bovine milk proteins, but also soy protein or a variety of hydrolyzed proteins; lactose and/or other sugars; a mixture of vegetable oils; mineral salts; and vitamins. The composition of selected formulas available in the USA is shown in Table 42-4. Most are available in powder, concentrated liquid (intended to be diluted 1 : 1 with water), and ready-to-feed forms. Similarities to bovine milk from which they evolved are virtually nonexistent.

TABLE 42-3. Recommended Minimum and Maximum Contents of Various Nutrients for Infant Formula Manufactured in the United States*

	MINIMUM	MAXIMUM
ENERGY (Kcal/dl)	63	71
Fat (g)	4.4	6.4
Linoleic acid (% of fatty acids)	8	35
α-Linolenic acid (% of fatty acids)	1.75	4
Carbohydrate (g)	9	13
Protein (g)	1.7	3.4
ELECTROLYTES AND MINERALS		
Calcium (mg)	50	140
Phosphorus (mg)	20	70
Magnesium (mg)	4	17
Sodium (mg)	25	50
Chloride (mg)	50	160
Potassium (mg)	60	160
Iron (mg)	0.2	1.65
Zinc (mg)	0.4	1.0
Copper (μg)	60	160
Iodine (μg)	8	35
Selenium (μg)	1.5	5
Manganese (μg)	1.0	100
Fluoride (μg)	0	60
VITAMINS		
Vitamin A (IU)	200	500
Vitamin D (IU)	40	100
Vitamin E (mg α-TE)	0.5	5.0
Vitamin K (μg)	1	25
Vitamin C (mg)	6	15
Thiamine (μg)	30	200
Riboflavin (μg)	80	300
Niacin (μg)	550	2,000
Vitamin B_6 (μg)	30	130
Folate (μg)	11	40
Vitamin B_{12} (μg)	0.08	0.7
Biotin (μg)	1	15
Pantothenic acid (μg)	300	1,200
OTHER INGREDIENTS		
Carnitine (mg)	1.2	2.0
Taurine (mg)	0	12
Myoinositol (mg)	4	40
Choline (mg)	7	30

*Amounts/100 kcal, unless otherwise indicated.

NUMBER OF FEEDINGS DAILY. The number of feedings required daily decreases throughout the 1st year of life from 8 or more shortly after birth to only 3 or 4 at 1 yr of age. The desired interval between feedings differs considerably among infants, but in general, ranges from 3–5 hr during the 1st year of life, averaging approximately 4 hr. For the 1st 1–2 mo, feedings are taken throughout the 24 hr period; thereafter, as the quantity of milk consumed at each feeding increases and the infant adjusts his or her demand to the family pattern of daytime activities, the infant usually sleeps for longer periods at night. As the infant develops psychologically and the relationship between the parent and the infant evolves, demand feeding should gradually be replaced by a feeding regimen that accommodates the needs of the rest of the family as well as those of the infant.

QUANTITY OF FORMULA. The quantity of formula taken at a feeding varies among infants of the same age and within infants at different feedings. Rarely will an infant want more than 7–8 oz at a single feeding. The desire for formula (or breast milk) is somewhat less during the 1st 2 wk of life than during the following 5–6 mo. After 6 mo of age, formula (or breast milk) is

TABLE 42-4. Composition of Standard Formulas for Normal Infants*

Component	Similac[†]	Enfamil[‡]	Good Start[§]	Isomil[†‖]	Prosobee[‡]
Protein (g)	2.07 (cow's milk whey)	2.1 (cow's milk, whey)	2.4 (whey)	2.45 (soy protein isolate, L-methionine)	2.5 (soy protein isolate, L-methionine)
Fat (g)	5.4 (high-oleic safflower, coconut, and soy oils)	5.3 (palmolein, soy, coconut, and high-oleic sunflower oils)	5.1 (palmolein, soy, coconut, and high-oleic safflower oils)	5.3 (soy, high-oleic safflower, coconut oils)	5.3 (palmolein, soy, coconut and high-oleic sunflower oils)
Carbohydrate (g)	10.8 (lactose)	10.7 (lactose)	11.0 (lactose, corn maltodextrin)	10.3 (corn syrup, sucrose)	10.6 (corn syrup solids)
ELECTROLYTES AND MINERALS					
Calcium (mg)	78	78	64	105	104
Phosphorus (mg)	42	53	36	75	82
Magnesium (mg)	6.1	8	7.1	7.5	11
Iron (mg)	1.8	1.8	1.5	1.8	1.8
Zinc (mg)	0.75	1	0.8	0.75	1.2
Manganese (μg)	5	15	7.1	25	25
Copper (μg)	90	75	80.5	75	75
Iodine (μg)	6.1	10	12	15	15
Selenium (μg)					
Sodium (mg)	24	27	24	44	35
Potassium (mg)	105	107	101	108	120
Chloride (mg)	65	63	65.5	62	80
VITAMINS					
Vitamin A (IU)	300	2,094	302	300	294
Vitamin D (IU)	60	60	60	60	60
Vitamin E (IU)	1.5	2	2	1.5	2
Vitamin K (μg)	8	8	8.0	11	8
Thiamine (μg)	100	80	60	60	80
Riboflavin (μg)	150	140	141	90	90
Vitamin B_6 (μg)	60	60	75	60	60
Vitamin B_{12} (μg)	0.25	0.3	0.25	0.45	0.3
Niacin (μg)	1,050	1,000	750	1,350	1,000
Folic acid (μg)	15	16	15	15	16
Pantothenic acid (μg)	450	500	453	754	500
Biotin (μg)	4.4	3	2.2	4.5	3
Vitamin C (mg)	9	12	9	9	12
Choline (mg)	16	12	12	8	8
Inositol (mg)	4.7	6	18	5	6

*Amount/100 kcal.
[†]Ross Laboratories, Columbus, OH.
[‡]Mead-Johnson Nutritionals, Evansville, IN.
[§]Carnation Nutritional Products, Glendale, CA.
[‖]Isomil-SF (sucrose-free) has similar composition except that glucose polymers are substituted for corn syrup and sucrose.

rarely the sole source of the infant's nutrient intake. However, it remains an important source of many nutrients (calcium).

It is rarely necessary to feed more than 1 qt (960 mL) of formula/day. Ingesting more than this volume has no advantages and may displace intake of other essential foods. By the time the infant is taking this amount, other foods should be added to the diet.

INFANT FORMULA VS BOVINE MILK. Although current recommendations are to avoid intake of bovine milk, particularly low-fat or skim milk, before 1 yr of age, surveys suggest that a number of infants between 6 and 12 mo of age are fed homogenized bovine milk rather than infant formula, and a number of these are fed low-fat or skim milk, often on the inappropriate advice of their physician.

The consequences of these practices are not known with certainty. However, infants fed bovine milk, on average, ingest roughly 3 times the DRI of protein and 2 or more times the DRI of sodium, but only approximately ⅔ of the DRI of iron and only ½ of the DRI of linoleic acid. Ingestion of bovine milk also increases intestinal blood loss and, hence, further contributes to the development of iron-deficiency anemia.

The protein and sodium intakes of infants fed skim rather than whole bovine milk are even higher, the iron intake is equally low, and the intake of linoleic acid is very low. Interestingly, although the most common reason for substituting low-fat or skim milk for whole milk or formula is to reduce fat and energy intakes, the total energy intake of infants fed skim milk is not necessarily lower than that of infants fed whole milk or formula. This suggests that infants compensate for the lower energy density of low-fat or skim milk by taking more of it and/or increasing intake of other foods.

Whether the high protein and sodium intakes of infants fed whole or skim milk are problematic is not known with certainty. The low iron intake, clearly, is undesirable, but medicinal iron supplementation should prevent the development of deficiency. The low intake of linoleic acid may be more problematic. Whereas signs and/or symptoms of linoleic acid deficiency appear to be uncommon in infants fed either whole or skim milk, an exhaustive search for such symptoms has not been made. Biochemical evidence of essential fatty acid deficiency without overt signs and symptoms occurs in both younger and older infants fed formulas with a low content of linoleic acid; thus, an exhaustive search, including biochemical indices, is likely to reveal a reasonably high incidence of essential fatty acid deficiency. On the other hand, infants who were breast-fed or fed formulas with high linoleic acid content earlier in life may have sufficient body stores to limit the consequences of low intake later. Essential fatty acid deficiency in animals is associated with long-term deleterious effects on development; it is not wise to assume that biochemical essential fatty acid deficiency without clinically detectable symptoms is without consequences.

Resolving the issues concerning the use of bovine milk in feeding the infant is important for economic as well as health reasons. Because the cost of bovine milk is considerably less than that of infant formula, replacing formula with homogenized bovine milk obviously has important economic advantages for most families, particularly those with limited income. If the federal food assistance programs could provide homogenized bovine milk rather than formula to infants, even infants older than 6 mo of age, the program's current funds would permit expansion of benefits to many more needy infants (see Chapter 43).

FEEDING DURING THE 2ND 6 MO OF LIFE

By 4–6 mo of age, the infant's capacity to digest and absorb a variety of dietary components as well as to metabolize, use, and excrete the absorbed products of digestion is near the capacity of the adult. Moreover, teeth are beginning to erupt, and the infant is more active and beginning to explore his or her surroundings. With the eruption of teeth, the role of dietary carbohydrate in the development of dental caries must be considered as well as the long-term effects of inadequate or excessive intakes during infancy and the psychosocial role of foods during development. These considerations, rather than concerns about delivery of adequate amounts of nutrients, are major factors underlying the feeding practices advocated during the 2nd 6 mo of life.

It is clear that all nutrient needs during the 2nd 6 mo of life can be met with a reasonable amount of currently available infant formulas. In contrast, the volume of milk produced by some women may not be adequate to meet all nutrient needs of the breast-fed infant beyond approximately 4–6 mo of age. This is particularly true for iron. Thus, for breast-fed infants, complementary foods are an important source of nutrients. They also have important psychosocial roles for both the breast-fed and the formula-fed infant.

Complementary foods (additional foods, including formula, given to the breast-fed infant) or replacement foods (foods other than formula given to formula-fed infants) should be introduced in a stepwise fashion to both breast-fed and formula-fed infants, beginning about the time the infant is able to sit unassisted, usually at 4–6 mo of age (see Table 42-2). Cereals, a good source of iron, are usually introduced 1st, followed by vegetables and fruits, then meats, and finally, eggs. However, the order in which these foods are introduced is not crucial, but only 1 new food should be introduced at a time and additional new foods should be spaced by at least 3–4 days to allow detection of any adverse reaction(s) to each newly introduced food. This is particularly important if there is a family history of food and/or other allergies.

Either home-prepared or manufactured complementary or replacement foods can be used. The latter are convenient, and many contain supplemental nutrients (iron). These foods also are available in different consistencies to match the infant's ability to tolerate larger size particles as he or she matures.

Prepared dinners and soups containing meat and 1 or more vegetables are quite popular. However, the protein content of these products is not as high as that of strained meat. Puddings and desserts also are popular items, but aside from their milk and egg content, they are poor sources of nutrients other than energy; thus, intakes of these should be limited. Moreover, intake of egg-containing products generally should be delayed, especially if there is a family history of food and/or other allergies, until after the infant has demonstrated tolerance to eggs (either a mashed hard boiled egg yolk or a commercial egg yolk preparation).

Aside from the association of bottle-feeding with dental caries after teeth have erupted, little is known about either the potential hazards or the non-nutritional role of diet during the latter half of the 1st year of life. Thus, feeding practices during this period vary widely. Nonetheless, recent surveys indicate that infants fed according to current practices receive adequate intake of most nutrients.

FEEDING PROBLEMS DURING THE 1ST YEAR OF LIFE

UNDERFEEDING. Underfeeding is suggested by restlessness and crying as well as by failure to gain weight adequately. It may also result from the infant's failure to take a sufficient quantity of food, even when offered. In these cases, the frequency of feedings, the mechanics of feeding, the size of the holes in the nipple, the adequacy of eructation of air, the possibility of abnormal mother-infant "bonding," and possible systemic disease in the infant should be considered.

The extent and duration of underfeeding determine the clinical manifestations. Constipation, failure to sleep, irritability, and excessive crying are to be expected. Weight gain may be slow, or there may be an actual loss of weight. In the latter case, the skin becomes dry and wrinkled, subcutaneous tissue disappears, and the infant assumes the appearance of an "old man." Deficiencies of vitamins A, B, C, and D as well as of iron and protein may be responsible for the characteristic clinical manifestations (see Chapters 45–50).

Treatment of underfeeding includes increasing nutrient intake, correcting any deficiencies of vitamins and/or minerals, and instructing the caregiver in the art and practice of infant feeding. If an underlying systemic disease, child abuse or neglect, or a psychologic problem is responsible, specific management of that disorder is necessary (see Chapters 36 and 37).

OVERFEEDING. As a rule, postprandial discomfort from excessive intake limits the amount of food an infant voluntarily ingests, but there are exceptions. If intake is excessive, regurgitation and vomiting are the most frequent symptoms. Diets that are too high in fat delay gastric emptying, cause abdominal distention and discomfort, and may cause excessive weight gain. Diets that are too high in carbohydrate are likely to cause undue fermentation in the intestine, resulting in distention and flatulence as well as more rapid weight gain than desirable. Because neither breast milk nor formula contains either excessive fat or excessive carbohydrate, excessive intakes usually result from supplementation. This practice also tends to dilute the protein, vitamin, and mineral contents of formula and, hence, should be avoided (also see Chapter 44).

REGURGITATION AND VOMITING. *Regurgitation* refers to the return of small amounts of swallowed food during or shortly after eating. Vomiting, on the other hand, is the more complete emptying of the stomach, often occurring some time after feeding. Within limits, regurgitation is a natural occurrence, especially during the 1st several months of life. It can be reduced to a negligible amount by adequate eructation of swallowed air during and after eating, by gentle handling, by avoiding emotional conflicts, and by placing the infant on the right side for a short time immediately after eating (but not for napping or sleeping). The head should not be lower than the rest of the body to help avoid gastroesophageal reflux, which is common during the 1st 4–6 mo of life.

Vomiting is one of the most common symptoms in infancy and may be associated with a variety of disturbances both trivial and serious. Its cause should always be investigated.

LOOSE OR DIARRHEAL STOOLS. The stool of the breast-fed infant is naturally softer than that of the formula-fed infant. From about the 4th to the 6th day of life, the stools of the breast-fed infant go through a transitional stage of being loose, greenish-yellow in color and containing mucus to the typical "milk stool." Subsequently, the use of laxatives or the ingestion of certain foods by the mother may be temporarily responsible for a breast-fed infant's loose stools. Excessive intake of breast milk may also increase the frequency and water content of the stool. Actual diarrhea from overfeeding, however, is unusual; thus, diarrhea should be considered infectious until proven otherwise.

Although the stools of formula-fed infants tend to be firmer than those of breast-fed infants, loose stools also may result from artificial feeding. Overfeeding may cause loose, frequent stools, particularly during the 1st 2 wk or so of life. Later, formulas that are too concentrated or too high in sugar content, especially in lactose, may result in loose, frequent stools. However, as noted earlier, this is unlikely unless sugar has been added to the formula. Many diarrheal disturbances in formula-fed infants result from contaminants that would not disturb an older child. These usually are not serious enough to cause prolonged difficulty for the infant. The ease with which formula-fed infants acquire diarrheal disturbances and their potential seriousness are strong arguments for extreme care in preparation and storage to assure that the formula or food is free of pathogenic bacteria and remains that way until it is fed to the infant.

Mild diarrheal disturbances caused by overfeeding respond quickly to a temporary decrease or cessation of feeding. Withholding all solid food as well as 1 or several feedings and substituting boiled water or a balanced electrolyte solution is usually all that is required.

CONSTIPATION (SEE CHAPTERS 22.4 AND 329.2). Constipation is practically unknown in breast-fed infants receiving an adequate amount of milk and is rare in formula-fed infants receiving an adequate intake. The consistency of the stool, not its frequency, is the basis for diagnosis. Most infants have 1 or more stools daily, but some occasionally have a stool of normal consistency at intervals of up to 36–48 hr.

Whenever constipation or obstipation is present from birth or shortly after birth, a rectal examination should be performed. Tight or spastic anal sphincters may occasionally be responsible for obstipation, and finger dilation is frequently corrective. Anal fissures or cracks may also cause constipation. If irritation is alleviated, healing usually occurs quickly. Aganglionic megacolon may be manifested by constipation in early infancy; the absence of stool in the rectum on digital examination suggests this possibility, but further diagnostic work-up is indicated (see Chapter 329).

Constipation may be caused by an insufficient amount of food or fluid. In some cases, it may result from diets that are too high in protein or deficient in bulk. Simply increasing the amount of fluid or sugar in the formula may be corrective during the 1st few months of life. After this age, better results are obtained by adding or increasing the intakes of cereal, vegetables, and fruits. Prune juice (½–1 oz) may be helpful, but adding foods with some bulk is usually more effective. Milk of magnesia may be given in doses of 1–2 tsp, but should be reserved for unresponsive or severe constipation.

Enemas and suppositories should never be more than temporary measures.

COLIC. Colic is a symptom complex of paroxysmal abdominal pain, presumably of intestinal origin, and severe crying (see Chapter 303). It usually occurs in infants younger than 3 mo of age. The clinical manifestations are characteristic. The attack usually begins suddenly, with a loud, sometimes continuous cry. The paroxysms may persist for several hours. The infant's face may be flushed, or there may be circumoral pallor. The abdomen is usually distended and tense. The legs may be extended for short periods, but are usually drawn up on the abdomen. The feet are often cold, and the hands are usually clenched. The attack may not terminate until the infant is completely exhausted. Sometimes, however, the passage of feces or flatus appears to provide relief.

Some infants seem to be particularly susceptible to colic. The etiology usually is not apparent, but in some infants, the attacks seem to be associated with hunger or with swallowed air that has passed into the intestine. Overfeeding may cause discomfort and distention, and some foods, especially those with high carbohydrate content, may result in excessive intestinal fermentation. However, a change of diet rarely prevents further colic attacks.

Crying with intestinal discomfort occurs in infants with intestinal allergy, but colic is not limited to this group. Colic may mimic intestinal obstruction or peritoneal infection. Attacks commonly occur in the late afternoon or early evening, suggesting that events in the household routine may be involved. Worry, fear, anger, or excitement may cause vomiting in an older child and may cause colic in an infant, but no single factor consistently accounts for colic and no treatment consistently provides satisfactory relief. Careful physical examination is important to eliminate the possibility of intussusception, strangulated hernia, or other serious causes of abdominal pain.

Holding the infant upright or prone across the lap or on a hot water bottle or heating pad occasionally helps. Passage of flatus or fecal material spontaneously or with expulsion of a suppository or enema sometimes affords relief. Carminatives before feedings are ineffective in preventing the attacks. Sedation is occasionally indicated for a prolonged attack. If other measures fail, both the child and the parent may be sedated for a period. In extreme cases, temporary hospitalization of the infant, often with no more than a change in the feeding routine and a period of rest for the parent, may help. Prevention of attacks should be sought by improving feeding techniques, including "burping," providing a stable emotional environment, identifying possibly allergenic foods in the infant's or nursing mother's diet, and avoiding underfeeding or overfeeding. Although it is not serious, colic can be particularly disturbing for the parents as well as the infant. Thus, a supportive and sympathetic physician can be particularly helpful, even if attacks do not resolve immediately. The fact that the condition rarely persists beyond 3 mo of age should be reassuring.

FEEDING DURING THE 2ND YEAR OF LIFE

By the end of the 1st year of life, most infants will have adapted to a schedule of 3 meals/day plus 2 or 3 snacks. Although considerable latitude in the diet of each infant should be permitted to allow for personal idiosyncrasies and family habits, the caregiver should be given an outline of the basic daily dietary needs. Equally important, the caregiver should be aware of what to expect in terms of eating behavior as the child matures.

REDUCED FOOD INTAKE. The rate of growth decreases toward the end of the 1st year of life, and the child's intake, accordingly, also decreases or fails to increase as rapidly as it did during the 1st year of life. It is not unusual for the child to have temporary periods during which he or she is not interested in certain foods or, indeed, in any food. Failure to expect and recognize these changes in eating behavior often results in attempts to force-feed. The child naturally rebels, and feeding problems ensue. Because preventing problems is easier and more effective than correcting them, the changing pattern of food habits during the 2nd year of life should be explained to the parents before it is apparent. The parents should be reassured that the lack of interest in food is probably temporary and that attempts to force-feed not only are futile but also are likely to result in more severe feeding problems.

SELF-SELECTION OF DIET. Children's strong likes or dislikes of particular foods become apparent after approximately 1 yr of age, and if possible and practicable, they should be respected. For example, the virtues of some foods (spinach) that are nonessential have been overemphasized, and conflicts about such foods should not be allowed to occur. Often a food that is refused when it is first offered will be accepted when it is offered again a few days or weeks later. On the other hand, if basic staples, such as milk and cereal, are consistently rejected, food allergy should be considered. If this is not a problem, alternative forms of these basic staples (cheese, yogurt, breads) should be offered.

Children tend to select diets that, over several days, are well balanced. Thus, the child may be permitted a wide choice of foods as long as he or she eats adequately over the longer term. Normally, the child determines how much of a given food or an entire meal to eat. At this age, eating habits, particularly food likes and dislikes, also may be influenced by older children in the family. Because eating patterns and habits developed in the 1st 2 yr of life usually persist for several years, such influences should be monitored closely.

SELF-FEEDING BY INFANTS. Infants should be allowed to feed themselves as soon as they seem physically able to do so, usually long before 1 yr of age. By approximately 6 mo of age, infants can hold a bottle, and within another 2–3 mo, they can hold a cup. Zwieback, crackers, bagels, or other hand-held foods can be introduced by the age of 7–8 mo. The infant may be allowed to use a spoon as soon as he or she can hold it and direct it to the mouth, usually between 10 and 12 mo of age. Mothers often inhibit this important learning process because of its messiness, but it is an important aspect of the infant's overall development and should be encouraged. By the end of the 2nd year of life, infants should be largely responsible for feeding themselves. However, because the risk of aspiration is reasonably high until approximately 4 yr of age, younger infants should not be given foods that are easily aspirated (grapes, nuts, chunks of cheese, meat) unless a responsible adult is present.

BASIC DAILY DIET. Parents should be given a basic daily diet plan for the child from which the family menu can be prepared. Daily selection from each of the food groups (grains, fruits, vegetables, meats, and dairy products) provides a balanced diet with sufficient macronutrients and micronutrients. The quantity of intake after the basic requirements have been met can usually be determined by the healthy growing child. The child's dietary history is essential for evaluating the nutrient intake, but unless an accurate dietary diary is kept for several days, such histories are often unreliable. Correcting the diet can be much more effective if reliable information is available.

The older child should learn the content of a basic well-balanced diet and understand its importance to proper growth and good health. However, this information should never be presented as a threat to enforce rigid feeding practices.

EATING HABITS. Eating habits formed in the 1st and 2nd yr of life distinctly affect those of the subsequent years. Feeding difficulties frequently result from excessive parental insistence on eating and subsequent anxiety of the parents and the child if the child fails to heed this insistence. The child's negative reactions often result from undue mealtime stress, the correction of which requires improvement in parent-child relations. Other factors that disturb eating are too much confusion at mealtime, insufficient time for eating on the part of either the adults and older children of the household or the child, food dislikes of other members of the family, and poorly prepared and/or unattractively served food. Mealtimes should be happy, with conversation concerning subjects of interest to the entire family. A comfortable chair of proper height with a footrest is important for the smaller child's ease at the table.

The child's appetite should be respected; if his or her desire for food is below average at times, there should be no persuasion to eat more. Adults should realize that eating habits are taught better by example than by formal explanation.

SNACKS BETWEEN MEALS. During the 2nd year of life and for several years thereafter, milk, fruit juice, and/or a cracker may be given at either or both of the between-meal periods. However, the amount of food given as a snack should not be enough to interfere with intake at mealtimes. Snacks served in child-care facilities should be as nutritious as those served at home.

VEGETARIAN DIETS. Vegetarian diets can supply all necessary nutrients, but to do so, the vegetables and grains that make up the diet must be selected from different classes. Vegetables are high in fiber content, vitamins, and minerals. Because of their higher fiber intake, vegetarians usually have faster gastrointestinal transit time, bulkier stools, and lower serum cholesterol levels; as adults, they may be less likely to have diverticulitis and appendicitis than meat eaters. Vegetarians who consume eggs (ovovegetarians) and/or milk (lactovegetarians) obviously have more choices for constructing a well-balanced diet than those who consume only vegetables (vegans). Vegans may have vitamin B_{12} deficiency, and because of their high fiber intake, also may have trace mineral deficiencies. Nursing vegan mothers must be given supplemental vitamin B_{12} to prevent vitamin B_{12} deficiency in their breast-fed infants. There also is some concern that vegetarian infants may not grow as rapidly as omnivores during the 1st 2 yr of life.

FEEDING DURING LATER CHILDHOOD

A child's diet after 2 yr of age should not differ from that of the rest of the family. All known required nutrients are supplied by a varied diet selected according to the current guidelines. These guidelines, with emphasis on grains, fruits, and vegetables, are consistent with the recommendations of the National Cholesterol Education Program (restriction of dietary fat to approximately 30% of the total daily energy intake, saturated fatty acids to <10% of energy, and cholesterol to no more than 100 mg/1,000 kcal, with polyunsaturated fatty acids supplying 7–8% of energy and monounsaturated fatty acids supplying 12–13%). This diet, the American Heart Association Step I Diet, is recommended to decrease atherosclerotic heart disease in adulthood and may also be effective in limiting the development of obesity. Except for children with a strong family history of atherosclerotic heart disease, there is some argument about the importance of such a diet before adolescence. However, such diets support normal growth of children as young as 1 yr of age, and implementing them after approximately 2 yr of age may be easier than doing so at adolescence.

The Food Guide Pyramid incorporates current dietary guidelines that have a strong focus on activity. "My Pyramid" reflects the fact that a single food guide is not appropriate for all individuals; rather, nutrient needs vary as a function of age, sex, weight, height, and level of activity (Fig. 42-1). Each individual can access his or her pyramid at the website *MyPyramid.gov.* The program provides the appropriate daily amounts of each food group for that individual. My Pyramid has not yet been adapted for 2–6 yr old children but can be used for those as young as 6 yr of age.

The daily amounts of each food group needed by a relatively inactive (<30 min of vigorous activity/day), a moderately active (30–60 min of vigorous activity/day), and a very active 6 yr old boy are shown in Table 42-5. The needs of 6 yr old girls with the same levels of activity are approximately 200 kcal/day fewer. The goal of the guideline is to support normal rates of weight gain without excessive fat deposition. Most children, if not forced to

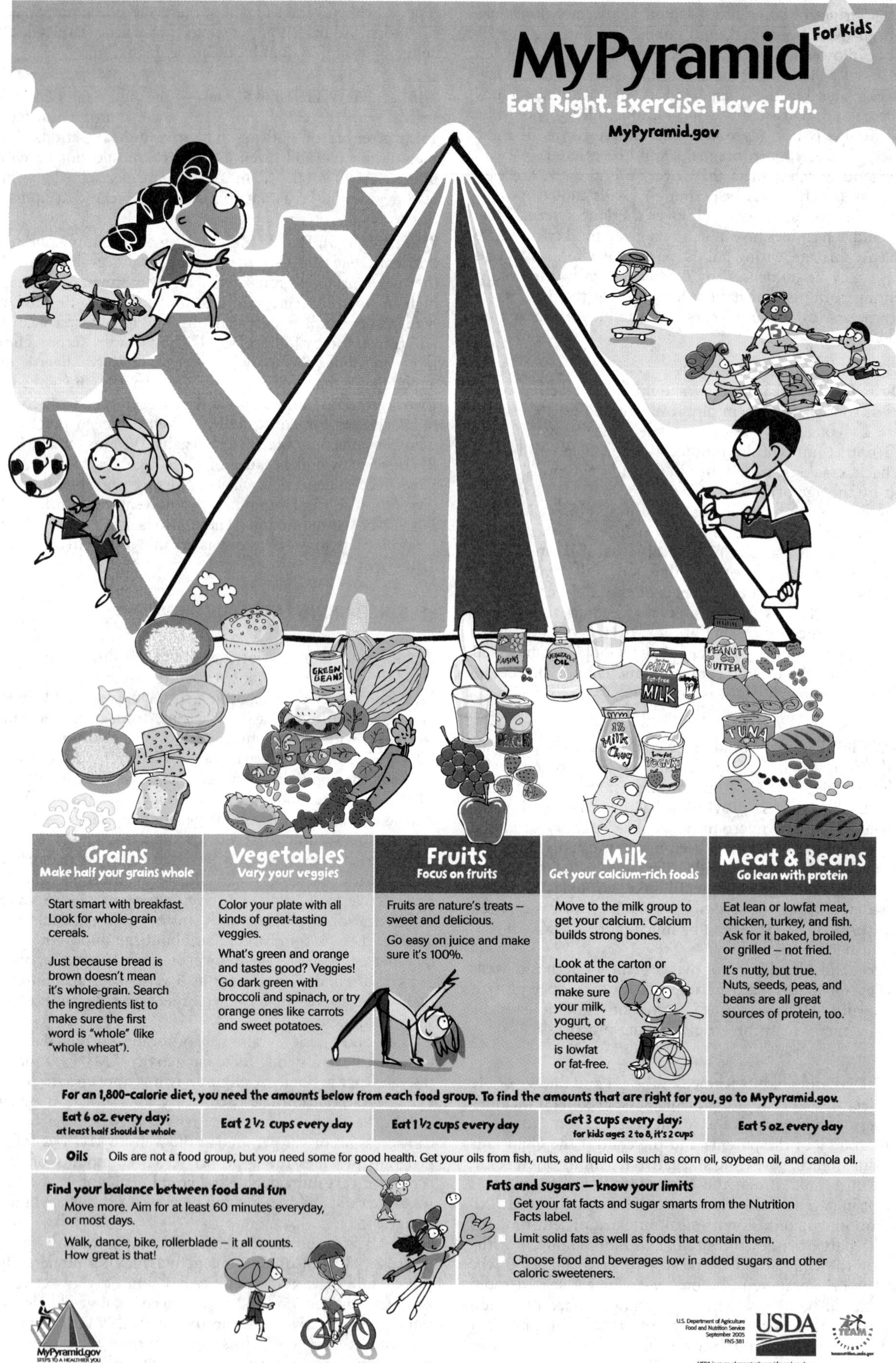

Figure 42-1. Food guide pyramid. (From *MyPyramid.gov.*)

TABLE 42-5. Daily Intakes of Each Food Group Needed by an Inactive, a Moderately Active, and a Very Active 6 yr Old Boy*

FOOD GROUP	INACTIVE	MODERATELY ACTIVE	VERY ACTIVE
Energy (kcal/day)	1,400	1,600	1,800
Grains (oz/day)	5	5	6
Vegetables (cups/day)	1.5	2	2.5
Fruits (cups/day)	1.5	1.5	1.5
Milk (cups/day)	2	3	3
Meat, beans (oz/day)	4	5	5

*From *MyPyramid.gov*.

eat more, will adjust intake to achieve this goal. Helpful hints are also provided.

As children become more independent, they eat an increasing number of meals away from home, often at "fast food" restaurants, where adherence to a healthy diet is difficult, perhaps impossible. An obvious solution is to limit such occasions to once or, at most, twice per week. However, this is often resisted by the child. Moreover, with the increasing number of mothers in the workforce, many family meals are either eaten at similar restaurants or purchased there for consumption at home. Perhaps the most a pediatrician or nutritionist can expect is that the parents understand the importance of a well-balanced diet and how best to achieve it without undue hardship for themselves or their children.

American Academy of Pediatrics: Dietary recommendations for children and adolescents: A guide for practitioners. *Pediatrics* 2006;117:544–559.

American Academy of Pediatrics Policy Statement: Breastfeeding and the use of human milk. *Pediatrics* 2005;115:496–506.

American Academy of Pediatrics Policy Statement: The use and misuse of fruit juice in pediatrics. *Pediatrics* 2001;107:1210–1213.

Bouwstra H, Boersma ER, Boehm DAJ, et al: Exclusive breastfeeding of healthy term infants for at least 6 weeks improves neurological condition. *J Nutr* 2003;133:4243–4245.

Center for Nutrition Policy and Promotion: *Tips for Using the Food Guide Pyramid for Young Children 2 to 6 Years Old.* United States Department of Agriculture, Program Aid 1647, March 1999.

Coutinho SB, Cabral de Lira PI, de Carvalho Lima M, et al: Comparison of the effect of two systems for the promotion of exclusive breastfeeding. *Lancet* 2005;366:1094–1100.

Foote KD, Marriott LD: Weaning of infants. *Arch Dis Child* 2003;88:488–492.

Greer FR, Krebs NF, Committee on Nutrition: Optimizing bone health and calcium intakes of infants, children, and adolescents. *Pediatrics* 2006; 117:578–585.

La Leche League International: *The Womanly Art of Breast Feeding.* Franklin Park, IL, La Leche League International, 1976.

Lawrence RA, Lawrence RM: *Breast Feeding, a Guide for the Medical Profession,* 6th ed. Philadelphia, Elsevier, 2005.

Lozoff B: Do breast-fed babies benefit from iron before 6 months? *J Pediatr* 2003;143:554–556.

Ostrea EM Jr, Mantaring JB III, Silvestre MA: Drugs that affect the fetus and newborn infant via the placenta or breast milk. *Pediatr Clin N Am* 2004;51:539–579.

Philipp BL, Merewood A: The baby-friendly way: The best breastfeeding start. *Pediatr Clin N Am* 2004;51:761–783.

Polhamus B, Dalenius K, Thompson D, et al: *Pediatric Nutrition Surveillance 2003 Report.* Atlanta: U.S. Department of Health and Human Services, Centers for Disease Control and Prevention, 2004.

Raiten DJ, Talbot JM, Waters JH: Assessment of nutrient requirements for infant formulas. *J Nutr* 1998;128:2059S–2293S.

Chapter 43 ■ Food Insecurity, Hunger, and Undernutrition

William C. Heird

Food insecurity, hunger, and undernutrition are viewed as a continuum, with food insecurity resulting in hunger, and ultimately, if sufficiently severe and/or of sufficient duration, in undernutrition. **Food insecurity** indicates inadequate access to food for whatever reason, **hunger** is the immediate physiologic manifestation of inadequate food intake, and **undernutrition** describes the biochemical and/or physical consequences of long-term inadequate intake. This continuum from food insecurity to hunger and ultimately to undernutrition affects many children, particularly in developing countries; however, not all food-insecure children experience hunger, and not all undernourished children experience food insecurity before becoming undernourished. Each condition, not only undernutrition, has consequences for the individual, the family, and society. Thus, viewing them as an inevitable continuum distorts estimates of the prevalence, causes, and consequences of each condition. It also may lead to inappropriate policy responses as well as to inappropriate treatment and/or failure to recognize and remedy conditions other than overt undernutrition. Instead, it is important to understand the nature of each of these problems as well as their relationships to each other.

FOOD INSECURITY

The broadest generally accepted definition of food insecurity is, "limited or uncertain availability of nutritionally adequate and safe foods in socially acceptable form and by socially acceptable ways." This definition encompasses concepts of the certainty of both short-term and long-term availability of and access to food; concerns about the sufficiency, nutritional quality, and safety of food; and the cultural and social acceptability of accessible food as well as the means by which this food is acquired.

The concept of food security differs depending on whether it is viewed from a global, a national, a household, or an individual perspective. Globally, food security concerns the overall availability of sufficient food to feed the population of the world. Food security, from a national perspective, also concerns the availability of food; however, the national issue is not whether enough food is produced globally to feed the population of the world, but whether enough food is produced and/or imported to feed the population of the country. From a household perspective, food security concerns the availability of and access to adequate food from household production, local purchase, or some combination of production and purchase. Food security, from an individual perspective, concerns the amount and quality of food available for consumption by the individual. This is a function of the availability of and access to food by the household and the distribution of food within the household.

In some developing countries, food insecurity results from the lack of sufficient food to feed the entire population of the country. This often is a result of war, famine, or some other disaster, but it also can result from a lack of resources to assure adequate production, importation, storage, and/or distribution of food. However, the consequences of food insecurity in such countries as well as in food-rich countries are experienced primarily at the household and individual levels. At the household level, the consequences usually result from a managed process in which inadequate means to obtain food, either because it is not available or because resources are limited, leads to anxiety about the supply of food; this anxiety, in turn, results in a variety of coping tactics (stretching food money). If these coping tactics are not successful, intake eventually is restricted, resulting in both nutritional and emotional consequences for the household as well as the individual members of the household. The anxiety over the availability of food usually leads first to lower intakes of food or to intake of foods of lower nutritional quality by women, then to a lower quantity and/or quality of the overall household food supply, and eventually, to lower quantity and/or quality of children's intakes.

Food insecurity in both developing and developed countries is a form of deprivation, either deprivation per se or the feeling of deprivation. The subjective experience of food insecurity at the individual level is central. Thus, the relevant assessment of food security is that perceived by the household or individual rather than what is decided by researchers or policymakers. If individuals do not believe that their food supply is secure, then food insecurity is a problem. Moreover, this problem is a multilevel and multidimensional one that has implications for how food security is assessed and for the efforts made to improve food security.

MEASUREMENT OF FOOD INSECURITY. Estimates of global and national levels of food insecurity are made by estimating the number of people whose intake does not provide enough energy to meet basic energy requirements. This is often equated to the number of undernourished individuals. However, this definition reflects only national food availability, not an individual's ability to access food. Thus, whereas the number of undernourished individuals is a direct measure of food security at the global or national level, it does not reflect access to and use of food by individuals. Hence, it is not a measure of food security at the household or individual level.

Although a number of instruments are available to measure food security, none is without problems. Certainly, food insecurity affects intake and, ultimately, nutritional status. Furthermore, measuring intakes of individuals, either directly or indirectly, by the number of undernourished individuals, assesses some aspects of food security (energy adequacy). However, it does not fully assess the cognitive and affective components of the uncertainty of food security; nor does it assess the unacceptability and unsustainability of food insecurity. Food insecurity exists if there is anxiety that the food supply, although currently sufficient, may become inadequate. Not only does growth status, per se, not assess many components of food security, it is also an indirect outcome that depends on health and care as well as intake. Thus, in assessing food insecurity, it is important to measure not only the availability of and access to food but also the experience of food insecurity (how individuals feel about the security of their food supply).

The questionnaires that have been used to assess food insecurity in developed countries (the United States Food Security Survey Module [US FSSM]) include questions on the availability of food, concern about the availability of food, and whether lack of availability is associated with hunger. The scores, as expected, are related to income, indicating that food insecurity is more prevalent among families with incomes close to the poverty level. Scores on these questionnaires defining food insecurity also are in agreement with data on weekly food expenditures.

PREVALENCE OF FOOD INSECURITY. Food insecurity is much more prevalent in developing countries than in developed countries. Approximately18% of all individuals in developing countries are undernourished. Estimates of prevalence vary throughout the world, ranging from approximately 33% of all individuals in most parts of Africa and approximately 17% of all individuals in Asia and the Pacific to much lower percentages in most other parts of the world. Because these estimates are based on the number of undernourished individuals, they obviously include only those individuals whose intakes are sufficiently low to result in undernutrition. Hence, the prevalence of food insecurity, as defined more broadly, is considerably greater. On the other hand, these estimates equate food insecurity with undernutrition that results from some combination of inadequate nutrient intake and inadequate care.

Based on responses to the US FSSM, food insecurity affected >10% of all households in the USA in 2003. The prevalence of food insecurity without hunger was approximately 8% of all households, and the prevalence of food insecurity with hunger was 3.5% of all households. This prevalence of food insecurity suggests that >30 million Americans live in food-insecure households. The prevalence of food insecurity is higher in central city and rural areas than in suburban areas. It also is much higher among African-American and Hispanic households as well as in households headed by single women. The prevalence of food insecurity without hunger in these households is estimated at 20–30%.

A typical food-insecure household in the USA is not necessarily one in which there is no working member. Rather, at least 1 member of the household is likely to be employed, albeit in a job that pays barely enough to enable the family to "get by." In such households, food becomes expendable when the available resources are needed to meet expenses, such as rent and/or utilities, transportation to continue employment, medical care, and/or other basic needs.

CONSEQUENCES OF FOOD INSECURITY. Biologic consequences of food insecurity are secondary to inadequate intake. However, the social and behavioral consequences can be secondary to the other aspects of food insecurity experienced at the household or individual level in addition to the biologic consequences. Food insecurity among women of sufficient severity to result in nutrient insufficiency and, hence, undernutrition leads to a higher prevalence of low birthweight infants and may affect breast milk production adversely. These effects, in turn, result in impaired cognitive and neurologic development of the offspring, lower educational achievement and, hence, a lower likelihood of finding productive work as adults. The more severely affected individuals may also have a limited capacity to work, further decreasing their ability to achieve food security. This vicious cycle may continue from one generation to the next and perpetuate both the biologic consequences of food insecurity and the consequences secondary to psychologic and behavioral responses to food insecurity.

Even food insecurity that does not result in overt undernutrition may be associated with a low intake of foods such as fresh fruits and vegetables and, hence, a low intake of several essential nutrients (vitamins A, E, C, and B_6 as well as magnesium, potassium, zinc, and/or fiber). Women from food-insecure households may be more likely to have a high body mass index and to be obese than women from food-secure households (see Chapter 44). Plausible mechanisms include the lower cost and, hence, overconsumption of energy-dense foods; overeating when food is available; metabolic changes resulting in more efficient use of energy; fear of food restriction; preoccupation with eating; and a variety of environmental cues. The relationship between high body mass index and obesity is not linear; neither the incidence of obesity nor the body mass index of women from households with more severe problems (childhood hunger) differs from those of women from food-secure households.

CLINICAL MANIFESTATIONS AND TREATMENT OF FOOD INSECURITY. Unless food insecurity is of sufficient severity to result in food insufficiency and undernutrition, it is not associated with obvious manifestations. Thus, it is not likely to be recognized by physicians and other health care workers. Furthermore, even if food insecurity is suspected, a physician can do little except offer understanding, support, and referral to social services and entitlement programs. Considering the apparent prevalence of food insecurity among low-income families, physicians caring for these families are likely to encounter children from food-insecure households. If food insecurity is suspected, further inquiries should be made both to confirm the food insecurity and to assess its severity. These assessments should include information about the child's diet.

A food frequency interview, which provides such information as the number of servings per week of each major food group (see Fig. 42-1), is a reasonable place to start. Should this suggest an imbalanced diet (low intake of any of the food groups), the next step is to have the caregiver complete a 3–5 day food diary. If obtained and analyzed appropriately, this can provide quantitative information about dietary intake, including estimates of the intake of specific nutrients. This can be done by the physician, a nutritionist, or a dietitian.

If intake of any nutrient is less than the dietary reference intake for that nutrient, appropriate dietary advice should be given and/or appropriate supplements prescribed (see Tables 41-1 to 41-3). Some food-insecure children may benefit from a multivitamin supplement, but few are likely to require macronutrient supplements. If no specific deficiencies are identified, the family may benefit from nutritional counseling. This should include the desired number of servings from each food group as well as the most economical source(s) of these foods. The physician should also ensure that the family is aware of the federal, state, and/or local resources available for assistance.

HUNGER

Hunger is the unpleasant sensation that results from lack of food. It is a potential, although not inevitable, consequence of food insecurity. The concept of hunger differs among individuals, even individuals with similar dietary intakes. Thus, it is even more difficult to define and assess than is food insecurity.

PREVALENCE OF HUNGER. A questionnaire developed by the Community Childhood Hunger Identification Project reliably categorizes families as "hungry," "at risk for hunger," or "not hungry" on the basis of answers to 8 standardized questions about child and family experiences of food insecurity or insufficiency attributable to constrained resources. Using this measure of food insufficiency as the principal indicator of hunger, the project estimates that, in the USA, 8% of poor children younger than age 12 yr experience hunger from time to time and an additional 21% are "at risk for hunger." Hunger is even more prevalent in children from families with the lowest incomes. Among these families, as many as 21% of children may be hungry and an additional 50% may be "at risk for hunger." This suggests that almost 75% of the poorest children in the USA may experience food insecurity or insufficiency. It also suggests that hunger is an issue for many of these children and is a serious problem for some. These children do not always experience food insecurity and hunger of sufficient severity to result in undernutrition.

Psychosocial problems, like food insecurity and hunger, also are common among children from low-income families. The prevalence of such problems in these children is estimated at 10–30%; estimates of the prevalence of such problems among children from more advantaged families are considerably lower. There also is a relationship between hunger and the prevalence of other psychosocial problems among low-income families. In one study, 29% of "hungry" children, 15% of "at risk for hunger" children, and 14% of "not hungry" children were receiving special education services. In the same study, 21% of "hungry" children and 12% of children "at risk for hunger," but only 5% of "not hungry" children had a history of mental health counseling. "Hungry" children were also more likely to have a history of academic failure and to demonstrate anxious, irritable, aggressive, and/or oppositional behaviors than their low-income, but "not hungry," peers. These findings are similar to the behavioral findings associated with more severe, chronic undernutrition in developing countries.

These estimates are based on correlations that do not necessarily prove a cause-and-effect relationship. Although it is possible that hunger causes the types of behavior problems noted, it also is possible that hunger is a correlate of yet another variable and is not the direct cause of the problems. Parents who are emotionally drained by chronic illness and/or the constant struggle to make ends meet are less likely to be able to plan nutritious and economic food purchases. In other words, hunger may be more prevalent in such families, but the other problems affecting the families may play an equal or a larger role in determining how well the children function.

CLINICAL MANIFESTATIONS AND TREATMENT OF HUNGER. The vague nature of hunger makes it difficult to recognize. Moreover, because the perception of hunger varies considerably among individuals, even individuals ingesting the same diet, as well as within the same individual from day to day, asking the child if he or she is ever hungry or questioning the parent may not be helpful.

If hunger is suspected, use of the parental questionnaire developed by the Community Childhood Hunger Identification Project or a similar questionnaire may be useful. Children identified by this instrument as "hungry" or "at risk for hunger" should be evaluated for the possibility of nutrient deficiencies. If present, these should be treated with either supplements or dietary advice, and the parents should be referred to the appropriate agency for assistance.

In some cases, a change in meal patterns without an increase in overall intake may be useful. If entire meals are missed to stretch the available food money, it might help to decrease the quantity of other meals to provide an appropriate number of meals per day.

UNDERNUTRITION

Investigators have searched unsuccessfully for a single cause or a specific set of causes of undernutrition and the appropriate intervention strategies to correct that cause or set of causes. Attention has shifted from inadequate protein to inadequate energy to inadequate micronutrients, with accompanying shifts of focus concerning appropriate intervention and treatment strategies. Problems and causes of undernutrition that are debated include growth faltering, low birthweight, maternal undernutrition, deficiencies of specific nutrients (iodine, vitamin A, iron, zinc), diarrhea, HIV infection and other infectious diseases, chronic illness, inadequate infant and child feeding practices, time constraints, limited household income, limited agricultural production, food insecurity, environmental degradation, and urbanization. A wide array of solutions to these problems also is debated. These include growth monitoring, promotion of more optimal breast-feeding and complementary feeding practices, nutrition education, oral rehydration programs, child spacing, food fortification, supplementation of specific or multiple nutrients (vitamin A, iron, and/or zinc), income generation, food aid, home gardening, and agricultural intensification. To a great extent, this shifting illustrates the poor understanding of many aspects of the major worldwide problem of undernutrition.

The problem of undernutrition is multifaceted, and solving it at a national level requires understanding, trust, and cooperation among diverse governmental agencies accustomed to dealing solely with health, agriculture, education, or finance issues. The frequent shifting of focus has not generated a coherent and understandable approach to the problem, but rather, has helped create the perception among many national policymakers and planners that the nutrition problem is "too complicated." This, in turn, has delayed coordination of efforts across international and local governmental agencies. Equally important, it has failed to generate a consensus within the nutrition community about priority problems and the actions and strategies needed to solve them.

In response to this situation, the United Nations International Children's Emergency Fund (UNICEF) has developed and is promoting an inclusive conceptual framework for organizing scientific knowledge and experience concerning undernutrition (or malnutrition), fostering a common understanding, and developing coherent strategies for addressing the problem. A key feature of this framework is the recognition that undernutrition is a biologic manifestation of the combined effects of inadequate dietary intake and disease, both of which are closely related to social and economic development. Thus, malnutrition cannot be viewed as distinct from other development problems, but rather, as a reflection of these other problems.

Another feature of this framework is that the assumptions underlying various approaches to malnutrition should be stated explicitly so that they can be questioned and debated rather than assuming implicitly that malnutrition is due solely to a specific cause (lack of food, inadequate health care, limited education, poor breast-feeding practices, inadequate agricultural production). Another key feature of the UNICEF framework is that the relative importance of the underlying causes of malnutrition (inadequate food and health care) must be recognized widely across households, communities, and countries. This implies that universal causes and solutions do not exist and that constraints in providing adequate food and health care must be assessed and acted on in each setting. Rather than imposed national or global solutions, a highly decentralized approach to assessment, analysis, and action is required.

MEASUREMENT OF UNDERNUTRITION. The traditional approach to nutritional assessment measures only the physical manifestations of the problem (clinical, anthropometric, biochemical indicators) and perhaps some of the immediate causes related to dietary intake. These indicators may be adequate for estimating the magnitude of the problem, but additional approaches are needed to assess the broader nutrition situation. These approaches include consideration not only of dietary intake but also of health care and control of resources at the household, community, and national levels.

Despite the need for additional approaches, a number of anthropometric indices have been used successfully for many years to estimate the prevalence of undernutrition among preschool-aged children. These include height-for-age, weight-for-age, and weight-for-height. The 1st is an index of the cumulative effects of undernutrition during the life of the child, the 2nd reflects the combined effects of both recent and longer-term levels of nutrition, and the last reflects recent nutritional experiences. Values <80–90% of expected are considered abnormally low.

These indices are reasonably sensitive indicators of the immediate and underlying general causes of undernutrition, but they are not specific for any particular cause. They do not reveal the relative importance of dietary intake, infectious diseases, food insecurity, inadequate health/environmental services, low birthweight, suboptimal childcare practices, income constraints, or disparities in control of resources. These factors are part of the assessment of the overall nutrition situation and are distinct from the biochemical and/or anthropometric indicators that reflect the severity and extent of the problem, its distribution across geographic and social groups, and trends over time.

PREVALENCE OF UNDERNUTRITION. In 2000, 26.7% of preschoolers in the developing world were estimated to be underweight, as reflected by a low weight-for-age and 32.5% were estimated to be stunted based on a low height-for-age. Compared with estimates in 1980, these estimates are approximately 11% and approximately 15% lower, respectively, suggesting considerable improvement, at least in some regions, over these 2 decades. However, the population of the developing world increased during this time; thus, the total number of underweight children and children with stunted growth has not changed dramatically since 1980.

Data from the USA and other developed countries indicate that the prevalence of undernutrition, as manifested by a low weight-for-age or height-for-age measure, is very low. Data from the United States National Health and Nutrition Examination Survey (NHANES) III (1988–1994) indicate that the prevalence of low height-for-age measure (<5th percentile) was 4–5% among children from 2 mo to 11 yr of age, approximately the same prevalence noted by NHANES I (1971–1974) 2 decades earlier. The NHANES III data also show that populations with a high prevalence of poverty do not have a higher prevalence of undernutrition than the general population, emphasizing the importance not only of adequate intake but also of adequate care, as defined in the framework of UNICEF.

In contrast to the low prevalence of undernutrition among the general population of children in the USA and other developed countries, the prevalence among hospitalized children is often as high as that in developing countries.

CONSEQUENCES OF UNDERNUTRITION. The cumulative evidence suggests that undernutrition has pervasive effects on immediate health and survival as well as on subsequent performance. These include not only acute effects on morbidity and mortality but also longer-term effects on cognitive and social development, physical work capacity, productivity, and economic growth. The magnitude of both the acute and the longer-term effects is considerable. Prospective studies suggest that severely underweight children (<60% of reference weight for age) have more than an 8-fold greater risk of mortality than normally nourished children, that moderately underweight children (60–69% of reference weight for age) have a 4- to 5-fold greater risk, and that even mildly underweight children (70–79% of reference weight for age) have a 2- to 3-fold greater risk. The high prevalence of mortality, even in children with mild and moderate undernutrition, suggests that >50% of child deaths may be caused directly or indirectly by undernutrition. Moreover, 83% of these deaths result from mild to moderate forms of undernutrition. A major factor is the potentiation of infectious diseases by undernutrition.

Survivors of childhood undernutrition frequently have deficits in height and weight that persist beyond adolescence into adulthood. These deficits are often accompanied by deficits in frame size as well as muscle circumference and strength. The implications of these deficits with respect to the work capacity of both men and women and to women's reproductive performance are obvious. Survivors of childhood malnutrition also have deficits in cognitive function and school performance relative to normally nourished children from the same environment. Mean deficits in scores on standard tests of cognition range from 5–15 points. The fact that severely undernourished children, as assessed by low length-for-age measures, have greater deficits in cognitive performance than children with mild or moderate undernutrition strongly suggests that the intellectual deficits are related to the severity of undernutrition.

The extent to which intellectual deficits can be decreased by dietary intervention alone is not clear. However, these deficits can be decreased by a combination of dietary and behavioral interventions, coupled with improvements in the overall quality of the home and/or school environment. Such interventions appear to be much more effective if instituted in early life.

PREVENTION OF UNDERNUTRITION. Food insecurity and undernutrition are the behavioral and biologic manifestations, respectively, of problems that are rooted in the social world from the level of individuals and households to the community, national, and international levels. Thus, a wide range of scientific disciplines must be drawn on to maximize the possibility of effective, sustainable solutions. An intervention as simple as supplementing the population with vitamin A requires an understanding of the behavior of households, communities, clinical workers, program managers, and policymakers.

The evolution of thought about food insecurity and undernutrition in developed and developing countries has some commonalities with significant policy implications. The major commonality is the recognition that the causes of these problems, although strongly related globally to poverty, are highly contextual and, hence, easily misunderstood. In most developed countries, for example, not all food-insecure individuals live in poverty, and not all those living in poverty have food insecurity. Similarly, in developing countries, child malnutrition secondary to suboptimal health conditions or caring practices is common, even among households with ample food resources. Thus, food insecurity and undernutrition arise from a variety of social, economic, and ecologic situations that vary from time to time and from place to place. Therefore, the coping strategies and behaviors of individuals and households as well as communities and nations are highly responsive to a variety of micro contextual factors. Moreover, these coping strategies and behaviors are strongly influenced by the ways in which food-insecure and undernourished individuals experience reality. The risk-avoidance and risk-management strategies of poor households often discourage them from adopting new crop varieties or making other changes in their livelihood strategy, despite the fact that such changes appear desirable and rational to outsiders.

Many policies and programs have been ineffective because they do not adequately assess, anticipate, and embrace the coping strategies and likely responses of the population. Some programs that do so have been initiated in communities throughout the developing world and are currently being evaluated. The results of these efforts should suggest strategies to improve the total nutrition situation and reduce the high prevalence of childhood undernutrition worldwide.

CLINICAL MANIFESTATIONS AND TREATMENT OF UNDERNUTRITION. Undernutrition ranges from a lower than desired intake of 1 or more nutrients, with either no symptoms or only vague symptoms, to severe malnutrition (discussed later). The approach to treating mild undernutrition is the same as that suggested for food insecurity of sufficient severity to result in low intake of specific nutrients. Treatment of vitamin deficiencies is discussed in Chapters 45–50, and treatment of the most severe form of undernutrition is discussed in the next section of this chapter.

SEVERE CHILDHOOD UNDERNUTRITION (PROTEIN-ENERGY MALNUTRITION)

Deficiency of a single nutrient is an example of undernutrition or malnutrition, but deficiency of a single nutrient usually is accompanied by a deficiency of several other nutrients. Protein-energy malnutrition (PEM) is manifested primarily by inadequate dietary intakes of protein and energy, either because the dietary intakes of these 2 nutrients are less than required for normal growth or because the needs for growth are greater than can be supplied by what otherwise would be adequate intakes. However, PEM is almost always accompanied by deficiencies of other nutrients. For this reason, the term *severe childhood undernutrition,* which more accurately describes the condition, is preferred.

The terms *primary malnutrition* and *secondary malnutrition* refer, respectively, to malnutrition resulting from inadequate food intake and malnutrition resulting from increased nutrient needs, decreased nutrient absorption, and/or increased nutrient losses. Both primary and secondary malnutrition occur in developing as well as developed countries; malnourished children often present with gastroenteritis or pneumonia.

Severe childhood undernutrition (SCU), whether primary or secondary, is a spectrum ranging from mild undernutrition resulting in some decrease in length-for-age and/or weight-for-age through severe forms of undernutrition resulting in more marked deficits in weight-for-age and length-for-age as well as wasting (a low weight-for-length measure). Historically, the most severe forms of SCU, **marasmus** (non-edematous SCU with severe wasting) and **kwashiorkor** (edematous SCU), were considered distinct disorders. Non-edematous SCU was believed to result primarily from inadequate energy intake or inadequate intakes of both energy and protein, whereas edematous SCU was believed to result primarily from inadequate protein intake. A third disorder, **marasmic kwashiorkor,** has features of both disorders (wasting and edema). The 3 conditions have distinct clinical and metabolic features, but they also have a number of overlapping features. A low plasma albumin concentration, often believed to be a manifestation of edematous SCU, is common in children with both edematous and non-edematous SCU. In addition, the underlying causes of this spectrum of conditions are quite similar. Among these are social and economic factors such as poverty and ignorance, social factors such as food taboos, biologic factors such as maternal malnutrition and inadequate intakes of breast milk and other foods, and environmental factors such as overcrowded and unsanitary living conditions.

In the USA, SCU has been reported in families who use unusual and inadequate foods to feed infants whom the parents believe to be at risk for milk allergies and also in families who believe in fad diets. Many cases are associated with rice milk diets, a product that is very low in protein content.

In addition, SCU has been noted in chronically ill patients in neonatal or pediatric intensive care units as well as among patients with burns, HIV, cystic fibrosis, failure to thrive, chronic diarrhea syndromes, malignancies, bone marrow transplantation, and inborn errors of metabolism.

CLINICAL MANIFESTATIONS OF SCU. **Non-edematous SCU (marasmus)** is characterized by failure to gain weight and irritability, followed by weight loss and listlessness until emaciation results. The skin loses turgor and becomes wrinkled and loose as subcutaneous fat disappears. Loss of fat from the sucking pads of the cheeks often occurs late in the course of the disease; thus, the infant's face may retain a relatively normal appearance compared with the rest of the body, but this, too, eventually becomes shrunken and wizened. Infants are often constipated, but may have starvation diarrhea, with frequent, small stools containing mucus. The abdomen may be distended or flat, with the intestinal pattern readily visible. There is muscle atrophy and resultant hypotonia. As the condition progresses, the temperature usually becomes subnormal and the pulse slows.

Edematous SCU (kwashiorkor) may initially present as vague manifestations that include lethargy, apathy, and/or irritability. When advanced, there is lack of growth, lack of stamina, loss of muscle tissue, increased susceptibility to infections, vomiting, diarrhea, anorexia, flabby subcutaneous tissues, and edema. The edema usually develops early and may mask the failure to gain weight. It is often present in internal organs before it is recognized in the face and limbs. Liver enlargement may occur early or late in the course of disease. Dermatitis is common, with darkening of the skin in irritated areas, but in contrast to pellagra (see Chapter 46), not in areas exposed to sunlight. Depigmentation may occur after desquamation in these areas, or it may be generalized (Figs. 43-1, 43-2, and 43-3). The hair is sparse and thin, and in dark-haired children, it may become streaky red or gray. Eventually, there is stupor, coma, and death.

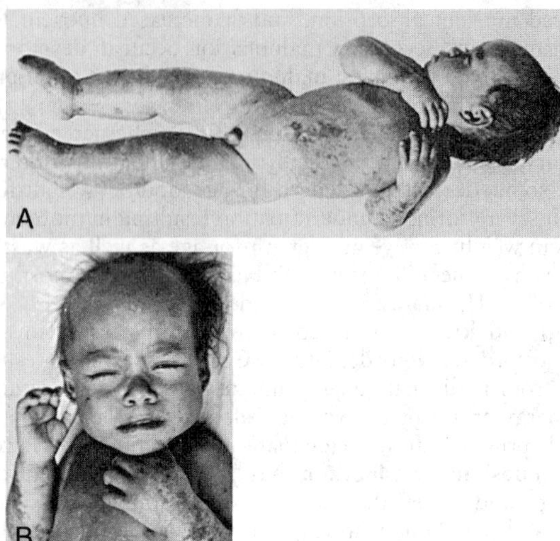

Figure 43-1. *A,* Kwashiorkor in a 2 yr old boy. Note the generalized edema, the typical skin lesions, and the state of prostration. *B,* Close-up view of the same child showing the hair changes and psychic alterations (apathy and misery); the edema of the face and skin lesions can be seen more clearly. (Photographs made available by the Institute of Nutrition of Central Panama, Guatemala, courtesy of Moises Behar, MD.)

Noma is a chronic necrotizing ulceration of the gingiva and the cheek (Fig. 43-4). It is associated with malnutrition and is often preceded by a debilitating illness (measles, malaria, tuberculosis, diarrhea, ulcerative gingivitis) in a nutritionally compromised host. Noma presents with fever, malodorous breath, anemia, leukocytosis, and signs of malnutrition. If untreated, it produces sever disfiguration. Polymicrobial infection with *Fusobacterium necrophorum* and *Prevotella intermedia* may be inciting agents.

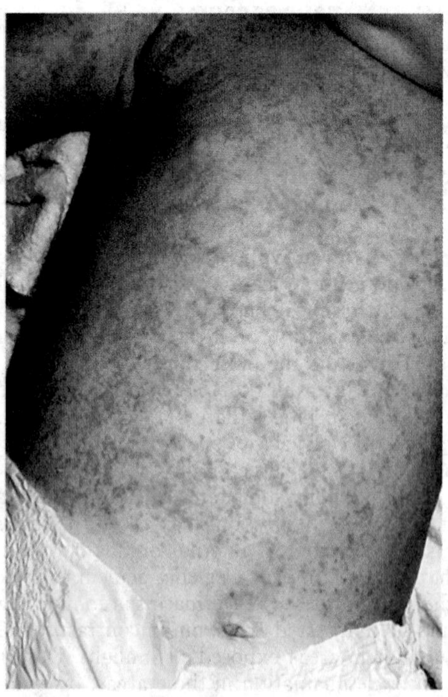

Figure 43-2. Diffuse fine scale in a reticulated pattern over the abdomen. (From Liu T, Howard RM, Mancini AJ, et al: Kwashiorkor in the United States. *Arch Dermatol* 2001;137:630–636.)

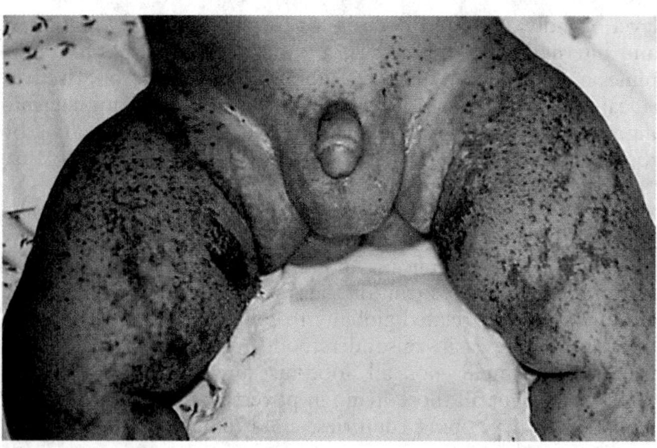

Figure 43-3. "Flaky paint" dermatosis on the thighs. (From Liu T, Howard RM, Mancini AJ, et al: Kwashiorkor in the United States. *Arch Dermatol* 2001;137:630–636.)

Treatment includes local wound care, penicillin, and metronidazole as well as therapy for the underlying predisposing condition.

PATHOPHYSIOLOGY OF SCU. Many of the manifestations of SCU represent adaptive responses to inadequate energy and/or protein intakes. In the face of inadequate intakes, activity and energy expenditure decrease. However, despite this adaptive response, fat stores are mobilized to meet the ongoing, albeit lower, energy requirement. Once these stores are depleted, protein catabolism must provide the ongoing substrates for maintaining basal metabolism.

Why edematous SCU develops in some children and non-edematous SCU develops in others is unknown. Although no specific factor has been identified, a number have been suggested. One concerns the variability among infants in nutrient requirements and in body composition at the time the dietary deficit is incurred. It also has been proposed that giving excess carbohydrate to a child with non-edematous SCU reverses the adaptive

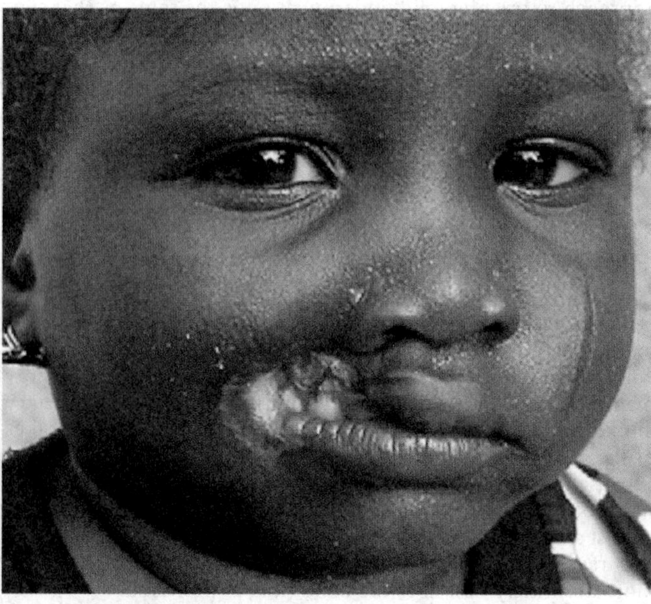

Figure 43-4. Noma lesion. (From Baratti-Mayer D, Pittet B, Montandon D, et al for the Geneva Study Group on Noma [GESNOMA]: Noma: An infectious disease of unknown aetiology. *Lancet Infect Dis* 2003;3:419–431.)

TABLE 43-1. Time Frame for the Management of a Child with Severe Malnutrition*

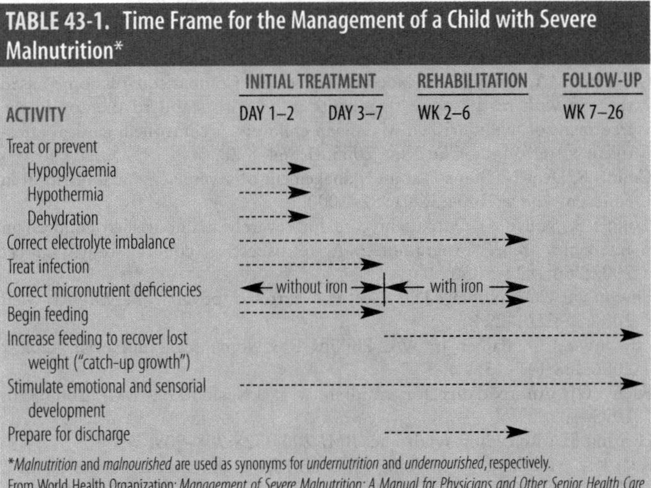

	INITIAL TREATMENT		REHABILITATION	FOLLOW-UP
ACTIVITY	DAY 1–2	DAY 3–7	WK 2–6	WK 7–26
Treat or prevent				
Hypoglycaemia	------→			
Hypothermia	------→			
Dehydration	------→			
Correct electrolyte imbalance	--------	--------	-------→	
Treat infection	--------	-------→		
Correct micronutrient deficiencies	← without iron	→	← with iron →	
Begin feeding	--------	-------→		
Increase feeding to recover lost weight ("catch-up growth")			--------	-------→
Stimulate emotional and sensorial development	--------	--------	--------	-------→
Prepare for discharge			-------→	

*Malnutrition and malnourished are used as synonyms for undernutrition and undernourished, respectively.
From World Health Organization: *Management of Severe Malnutrition: A Manual for Physicians and Other Senior Health Care Workers*. Geneva, WHO, 1999.

TABLE 43-3. Composition of F75 and F100 Diets

	AMOUNT-100 mL	
CONSTITUENT	F75	F100
Energy	75 $kcal_{th}$ (315 kJ)	100 $kcal_{th}$ (420 kJ)
Protein	0.9 g	2.9 g
Lactose	1.3 g	4.2 g
Potassium	3.6 mmol	5.9 mmol
Sodium	0.6 mmol	1.9 mmol
Magnesium	0.43 mmol	0.73 mmol
Zinc	2.0 mg	2.3 mg
Copper	0.25 mg	0.25 mg
Percentage of energy from:		
Protein	5%	12%
Fat	32%	53%
Osmolarity	333 mOsmol/L	419 mOsmol/L

From World Health Organization: *Management of Severe Malnutrition: A Manual for Physicians and Other Senior Health Care Workers*. Geneva, WHO, 1999.

responses to low protein intake, resulting in mobilization of body protein stores. Eventually, albumin synthesis decreases, resulting in hypoalbuminemia with edema. Fatty liver also develops secondary, perhaps, to lipogenesis from the excess carbohydrate intake and reduced apolipoprotein synthesis. Other causes of edematous SCU are aflatoxin poisoning as well as diarrhea, impaired renal function and decreased Na^+ K^+ ATPase activity. Finally, free radical damage has been proposed as an important factor in the development of edematous SCU. This proposal is supported by low plasma concentrations of methionine, a dietary precursor of cysteine, which is needed for synthesis of the major antioxidant factor, glutathione. This possibility also is supported by lower rates of glutathione synthesis in children with edematous compared with non-edematous SCU.

TREATMENT OF SCU. The usual approach to the treatment of SCU includes 3 phases (Table 43-1). The initial phase (1–7 days) is a stabilization phase. During this phase, dehydration, if present, is corrected and antibiotic therapy is initiated to control bacterial or parasitic infection. Because of the difficulty of estimating hydration, **oral rehydration** therapy is preferred (see Chapters 55 and 337). If intravenous therapy is necessary, estimates of dehydration should be reconsidered frequently, particularly during the first 24 hr of therapy. Oral feedings are also started with specialized high-calorie formula (Tables 43-2 and 43-3), proposed by the World Health Organization, that can be made with simple ingredients. The initial phase of oral treatment is with the F75 diet (75 kcal or 315 kg/100 mL). The rehabilitation diet is with the F100 diet (100 kcal or 420 kg/100 mL). Feedings are initiated with higher frequency and smaller volumes; over time, the frequency is reduced from 12 to 8 to 6 feedings/24 hr. The initial caloric intake is estimated at 80–100 kcal/kg/day. In developed countries, 24–27 calorie/oz infant formulas may be initiated with the same daily caloric goals. If diarrhea starts or fails to resolve and lactose intolerance is suspected, a non–lactose-containing formula should be substituted. If milk protein intolerance is suspected, a soy protein hydrolysate formula can be used.

Laboratory evaluation (Table 43-4) and ongoing monitoring (Table 43-5), when available, help guide therapy and prevent complications. Fluid status must be monitored very carefully in anemic patients, who may require a packed red blood cell transfusion.

The second rehabilitation phase (wk 2–6) may include continued antibiotic therapy with appropriate changes, if the initial combination was not effective, and introduction of the F100 diet (see Tables 43-2 and 43-3), with a goal of at least

TABLE 43-2. Preparation of F75 and F100 Diets

	AMOUNT	
INGREDIENT	F75*	F100†
Dried skim milk	25 g	80 g
Sugar	70 g	50 g
Cereal flour	35 g	
Vegetable oil	27 g	60 g
Mineral mix‡	20 mL	20 mL
Vitamin mix‡	140 mg	140 mg
Water to make	1,000 mL	1,000 mL

*To prepare the F75 diet, add the dried skim milk, sugar, cereal flour, and oil to some water and mix. Boil for 5–7 min. Allow to cool, then add the mineral mix and vitamin mix, and mix again. Make up the volume to 1,000 mL with water.
A comparable formula can be made from 35 g of whole dried milk, 70 g of sugar, 35 g of cereal flour, 17 g of oil, 20 mL of mineral mix, 140 mg of vitamin mix, and water to make 1,000 mL. Alternatively, use 300 mL of fresh cow's milk, 70 g of sugar, 35 g of cereal flour, 17 g of oil, 20 mL of mineral mix, 140 mg of vitamin mix, and water to make 1,000 mL.
Isotonic versions of F75 (280 mOsmol/L), which contain maltodextrins instead of cereal flour and some of the sugar and which include all the necessary micronutrients, are available commercially.
If cereal flour is not available or there are no cooking facilities, a comparable formula can be made from 25 g of dried skim milk, 100 g of sugar, 27 g of oil, 20 mL of mineral mix, 140 mg of vitamin mix, and water to make 1,000 mL. However, this formula has a high osmolarity (415 mOsmol/L) and may not be well tolerated by all children, especially those with diarrhea.
†To prepare the F100 diet, add the dried skim milk, sugar, and oil to some warm boiled water and mix. Add the mineral mix and vitamin mix, and mix again. Make up the volume to 1,000 mL with water.
A comparable formula can be made from 110 g of whole dried milk, 50 g of sugar, 30 g of oil, 20 mL of mineral mix, 140 mg of vitamin mix, and water to make 1,000 mL. Alternatively, use 880 mL of fresh cow's milk, 75 g of sugar, 20 g of oil, 20 mL of mineral mix, 140 mg of vitamin mix, and water to make 1,000 mL.
‡If only small amounts of feed are being prepared, it will not be feasible to prepare the vitamin mix because of the small amounts involved. In this case, give a proprietary multivitamin supplement. Alternatively, a combined mineral and vitamin mix for malnourished children is available commercially and can be used in these diets.
From World Health Organization: *Management of Severe Malnutrition: A Manual for Physicians and Other Senior Health Care Workers*. Geneva, WHO, 1999.

TABLE 43-4. Laboratory Features of Severe Malnutrition

BLOOD OR PLASMA VARIABLES	INFORMATION DERIVED
Hemoglobin, hematocrit, erythrocyte count, mean corpuscular volume	Degree of dehydration and anemia; type of anemia (iron/folate and vitamin B_{12} deficiency, hemolysis, malaria)
Glucose	Hypoglycemia
Electrolytes and alkalinity	
Sodium	Hyponatremia, type of dehydration
Potassium	Hypokalemia
Chloride, pH, bicarbonate	Metabolic alkalosis or acidosis
Total protein, transferrin, (pre-)albumin	Degree of protein deficiency
Creatinine	Renal function
C-reactive protein, lymphocyte count, serology, thick and thin blood films	Presence of bacterial or viral infection or malaria
Stool examination	Presence of parasites

From Müller O, Krawinkel M: Malnutrition and health in developing countries. *CMAJ* 5; 173(3):279–286. © 2005 Canadian Medical Association. Reprinted with permission of the publisher.

TABLE 43-5. Elements in the Management of Severe Protein-Energy Malnutrition

PROBLEM	MANAGEMENT
Hypothermia	Warm patient up; maintain and monitor body temperature
Hypoglycemia	Monitor blood glucose; provide oral (or intravenous) glucose
Dehydration	Rehydrate carefully with oral solution containing less sodium and more potassium than standard mix
Micronutrients	Provide copper, zinc, iron, folate, multivitamins
Infections	Administer antibiotic and antimalarial therapy, even in the absence of typical symptoms
Electrolytes	Supply plenty of potassium and magnesium
Starter nutrition	Keep protein and volume load low
Tissue-building nutrition	Furnish a rich diet dense in energy, protein, and all essential nutrients that is easy to swallow and digest
Stimulation	Prevent permanent psychosocial effects of starvation with psychomotor stimulation
Prevention of relapse	Start early to identify causes of protein-energy malnutrition in each case; involve the family and the community in prevention

From Müller O, Krawinkel M: Malnutrition and health in developing countries. *CMAJ* 5; 173(3):279–286. © 2005 Canadian Medical Association. Reprinted with permission of the publisher.

100 kcal/kg/day. This phase usually lasts an additional 4 wk. At any time, if the infant is unable to take the feedings from a cup, syringe, or dropper, administration by a nasogastric tube rather than by the parenteral route is preferred. Bottles may be contaminated in certain locales, and their use is discouraged unless cleanliness is assured. Once ad libitum feedings are allowed, intakes of both energy and protein are often substantial. Iron therapy usually is not started until this phase of treatment; iron may interfere with the protein's host defense mechanisms. There also is concern that free iron during the early phase of treatment may exacerbate oxidant damage, precipitating infections (malaria), clinical kwashiorkor, or marasmic kwashiorkor in a child with clinical marasmus. Some recommend treatment with antioxidants.

By the end of the 2nd phase, any edema that was present has usually been mobilized, infections are under control, the child is becoming more interested in his or her surroundings, and his or her appetite is returning. The child is then ready for the final follow-up phase, which consists of feeding to cover catch-up growth as well as the provision of emotional and sensory stimulation. The child should be fed ad libitum.

In developing countries, this final phase is often carried out at home. In all phases, parental education is crucial for continued effective treatment as well as prevention of additional episodes.

Refeeding syndrome may complicate the acute nutritional rehabilitation of children who are undernourished from any cause. The hallmark of refeeding syndrome is the development of severe hypophosphatemia after the cellular uptake of phosphate during the 1st week of starting to refeed. Serum phosphate levels of ≤0.5 mmol/L can produce weakness, rhabdomyolysis, neutrophil dysfunction, cardiorespiratory failure, arrhythmias, seizures, altered level of consciousness, or sudden death. Phosphate levels should be monitored during refeeding, and if low, phosphate should be administered during refeeding to treat severe hypophosphatemia (see Chapter 52.6).

Baqui AH, Ahmed T: Diarrhoea and malnutrition in children. *BMJ* 2006;332:378.

Berkley J, Mwangi I, Griffiths K, et al: Assessment of severe malnutrition among hospitalized children in rural Kenya. *JAMA* 2005;294:591–597.

Carvalho NF, Kenney RD, Carrington PH, et al: Severe nutritional deficiencies in toddlers resulting from health food milk alternatives. *Pediatrics* 2001;107:e46.

Caufield LE, de Onis M, Blössner M, et al: Undernutrition as an underlying cause of child deaths associated with diarrhea, pneumonia, malaria, and measles. *Am J Clin Nutr* 2004;80:193–198.

Centers for Disease Control and Prevention: Nutritional and health status of children during a food crisis—Niger, September 17–October 14, 2005. *MMWR* 2006;55:1172–1176.

Ciliberto MA, Sandige H, Ndekha MJ, et al: Comparison of home-based therapy with ready-to-use therapeutic food with standard therapy in the treatment of malnourished Malawian children: A controlled, clinical effectiveness trial. *Am J Clin Nutr* 2005;81:864–870.

Collins S, Dent N, Binns P, et al: Management of severe acute malnutrition in children. *Lancet* 2006;368:1992–2000.

Collins S, Sadler K: Outpatient care for severely malnourished children in emergency relief programmes: A retrospective cohort study. *Lancet* 2002;360:1824–1830.

Enwonwu CO: Noma: The ulcer of extreme poverty. *N Engl J Med* 2006;354:221–224.

Enwonwu CO, Falker Jr. WA, Phillips RS: Noma (cancrum oris). *Lancet* 2006;368:147–156.

Fuchs GJ: Antioxidants for children with kwashiorkor. *BMJ* 2005;330: 1095–1096.

Hearing SD: Refeeding syndrome. *BMJ* 2004;328:908–909.

Katz KA, Mahlberg MH, Honig PJ, et al: Rice nightmare: Kwashiorkor in 2 Philadelphia-area infants fed Rice Dream beverage. *J Am Acad Dermatol* 2005;52:S69–S72.

Lancet: Global childhood malnutrition. *Lancet* 2006;367:1459.

Liu T, Howard RM, Mancini AJ, et al: Kwashiorkor in the United States. *Arch Dermatol* 2001;137:630–636.

Müller O, Krawinkel M: Malnutrition and health in developing countries. *JAMC* 2005;173:279–286.

Nord M, Andrews M, Carlson S: *Household Food Insecurity in U.S. Households, 1995–99. Food and Rural Economics Division, Economic Research Service, U.S. Department of Agriculture, Food Assistance and Nutrition Research Report No. 35,* Washington, DC, 2003, pp 1–58.

Pelletier DL, Olson CM, Frongillo EA Jr: Food insecurity, hunger, and undernutrition. In Bowman BA, Russell RM (editors): *Present Knowledge in Nutrition,* 8th ed. Washington, DC, ILSI Press, 2001, pp 701–713.

Penny ME, Creed-Kanashiro HM, Rober RC, et al: Effectiveness of an educational intervention delivered through the health services to improve nutrition in young children: a cluster-randomised controlled trial. *Lancet* 2005;365:1863–1872.

Rivera JA, Sotres-Alvarez D, Habicht JP, et al: Impact of the Mexican program for education, health, and nutrition (Progresa) on rates of growth and anemia in infants and young children. *JAMA* 2004;291:2563–2570.

World Health Organization: *Management of Severe Malnutrition: A Manual for Physicians and Other Senior Health Care Workers.* Geneva, 1999.

Chapter 44 ■ Overweight and Obesity

Joseph A. Skelton and Colin D. Rudolph

Obesity and *overweight* are terms that are commonly used interchangeably in children, with *overweight* being the preferred term. As the prevalence of overweight has increased in children and adolescents, complications of overweight are now well recognized in children. Therefore, the prevention and treatment of overweight have emerged as a challenge to the pediatric practitioner.

EPIDEMIOLOGY

The National Health and Nutrition Examination Survey (NHANES) IV, 1999–2002, documents that 16% of children are overweight and 31% are at risk for becoming overweight or are already overweight, representing a nearly 300% increase since the 1960s and a 45% increase since the last complete NHANES survey for 1988–94. African-American girls and Hispanic boys and girls have the highest rates of overweight.

The first predictor of overweight is high birthweight, probably linked to maternal obesity or maternal diabetes. Paradoxically, lower birthweight appears to place people at risk for later central obesity. Children who are overweight are more likely to be overweight as adults, with the likelihood increasing as the age of the overweight child increases. The strongest predictor of childhood overweight, as well as later adult obesity, is parental obesity. Parental obesity doubles the risk of adult obesity among children younger than 10 yr of age, regardless of current weight.

PATHOGENESIS

Overweight results from a dysregulation of caloric intake and energy expenditure. A complex interplay between each individual's genetic predispositions and the environment affects an intricate system that controls appetite and energy expenditure. Prehistoric ancestors of humans experienced long periods of food scarcity, so energy conservation and storage during times of food availability had a survival advantage. There was a selection for a "thrifty genotype" that maximized energy storage in adipose tissue, improving survival during periodic famines. Even in relatively recent history, overabundant food supplies remained uncommon and food acquisition required substantial physical effort. In industrialized countries, improved food technologies have assured a more plentiful, safe food supply, causing the thrifty genotype to become detrimental instead of beneficial. The excess caloric intake is stored in adipose tissue, but for most individuals in these countries, there are no longer prolonged periods of reduced caloric intake, leading to a net increase in adipose tissue deposition over time.

ENVIRONMENTAL CHANGES. The type and cost of food has dramatically changed over the last several decades. The food industry in developed countries supports sophisticated advertising that encourages people to eat convenience foods, which are relatively inexpensive and have high levels of calories, fat, simple carbohydrates, and sodium, and low levels of fiber and micronutrients. Snacking in between meals has risen steadily over the last 2 decades, with many snacks being high in fat, sugar, or both. The convenience of fast food, the increase in dual working parents and single-parent households, and the common practice of overscheduling children have led to fast food being a staple of the diets of many families in the USA. One-third of children in the USA eat fast food daily; a typical single meal can contain 2,000 kcal, 84 g of fat, and only 12 g of fiber. Many children consume excessive calories, with the intake of large amounts of sweetened beverages, including soda, juice, and sport drinks. Sweetened beverages have been linked to higher weight, increased risk of obesity, and increased caloric intake, because children who drink high amounts of sugar do not eat significantly less at meals. The average adult may gain 0.8 kg/yr, which is the equivalent of an excess caloric intake of only 20–50 calories/day (a can of soda has ≈ 140 calories).

An increase in sedentary activity and a lack of exercise also contribute to an increase in the prevalence of overweight. Budget constraints have led many school systems in the USA to reduce or eliminate physical education classes. Children may watch as much as 20 hr/wk of television, which decreases their physical activity, exposes them to food advertising, and increases caloric intake. Other "screen time," such as video games, Internet computer use, telephone use, and home viewing of movies all may reduce childhood physical activity. A school-based intervention that focuses only on reducing the time spent watching television and movies and playing video games can decrease the body mass index (BMI).

ENDOGENOUS WEIGHT CONTROL MECHANISMS. Monitoring of "stored fuel" and short-term control of food intake (appetite and satiety) occur through neuroendocrine feedback from adipose tissue and the gastrointestinal tract to the central nervous system (Fig. 44-1). Gastrointestinal hormones, including cholecystokinin, glucagon-like peptide-1, and peptide YY, and vagal neuronal feedback promote satiety, whereas ghrelin stimulates appetite. Adipose tissue provides feedback regarding energy storage levels to the brain through hormonal release of leptin and adiponectin. These hormones act on the arcuate nucleus in the hypothalamus and on the solitary tract nucleus in the brainstem and, in turn, activate distinct neuronal networks. Numerous neuropeptides in the brain, including neuropeptide Y, agouti gene-related peptide, and orexin appear to be involved in appetite stimulation, whereas melanocortins and α-melanocortin-stimulating hormone are involved in satiety. The neuroendocrine control of appetite and weight is in a negative feedback system, balanced between short-term control of appetite (ghrelin, PYY) and long-term control of adiposity (leptin).

The important role of genetics in weight regulation is demonstrated by studies of identical twins who are reared apart. The weights of the twins are similar, despite variations in their environments or adoptive parental weights, indicating that environmental factors play less of a role than genetic factors. Genes appear to determine a "weight set point" that can also be considered as the protected level of stored fuel that satisfies that individual. Genetic defects in this control system manifest early-onset obesity; even in early-onset obesity, genetic abnormalities are uncommon (Table 44-1). Mutations in the leptin gene and a resultant leptin deficiency result in severe obesity and hyperphagia accompanied by hyperinsulinism, hypothyroidism, and immune dysfunction. Treatment with subcutaneous recombinant leptin replacement improves all symptoms. Deficiency of pro-opiomelanocortin (POMC) causes early-onset obesity, adrenal insufficiency, and red hair. By 2004, only 173 cases of obesity in humans due to single-gene mutations had been reported. In another study, 4% of children who were severely overweight before age 10 yr had a defect in the melanocortin-4 receptor. Genes also control resting energy expenditure (REE), which varies with ethnicity, being higher in white compared with African-American children.

TABLE 44-1. Diseases Associated with Childhood Obesity*

SYNDROME	MANIFESTATION
Alström syndrome	Hypogonadism, retinal degeneration, deafness, diabetes mellitus
Bardet-Biedl syndrome	Retinal degeneration, syndactyly, polydactyly, hypogonadism, mental retardation, autosomal recessive
Carpenter syndrome	Polydactyly, syndactyly, cranial synostosis, mental retardation
Cohen syndrome	Midchildhood-onset obesity, short stature, prominent maxillary incisors, hypotonia, mental retardation, microcephaly, decreased visual activity
Cushing syndrome	Adrenal hyperplasia or pituitary tumor
Deletion 9q 34	Early-onset obesity, mental retardation, brachycephaly, synophrys, prognathism, behavior and sleep disturbances
ENPP1 gene mutations	Insulin resistance, childhood obesity, chromosome 6q
Fröhlich syndrome	Hypothalamic tumor
Hyperinsulinism	Nesidioblastosis, pancreatic adenoma, hypoglycemia, Mauriac syndrome (poor diabetic control)
Leptin or leptin receptor gene mutation	Early-onset severe obesity, infertility (hypogonadotropic hypogonadism); uncommon; leptin deficiency treatable with recombinant leptin
Melanocortin 4 receptor gene mutation	Early-onset severe obesity, increased linear growth, hyperphagia, hyperinsulinemia; homozygous worse than heterozygous; common genetic cause of obesity
Muscular dystrophy	Late-onset obesity due in part to inactivity
Myelodysplasia	Spina bifida due in part to inactivity
Prader-Willi syndrome	Neonatal hypotonia, normal growth immediately after birth, small hands and feet, mental retardation, hypogonadism; some have partial deletion of chromosome 15 and loss of paternally expressed genes; hyperphagia leading to severe childhood obesity; ghrelin paradoxically elevated
Pro-opiomelanocortin deficiency	Obesity, red hair, adrenal insufficiency, hyperproinsulinemia
Pseudohypoparathyroidism	Variable hypocalcemia, cutaneous calcifications
Turner syndrome	Ovarian dysgenesis, lymphedema, web neck, XO chromosome

*These diseases represent <5% of cases of childhood obesity.

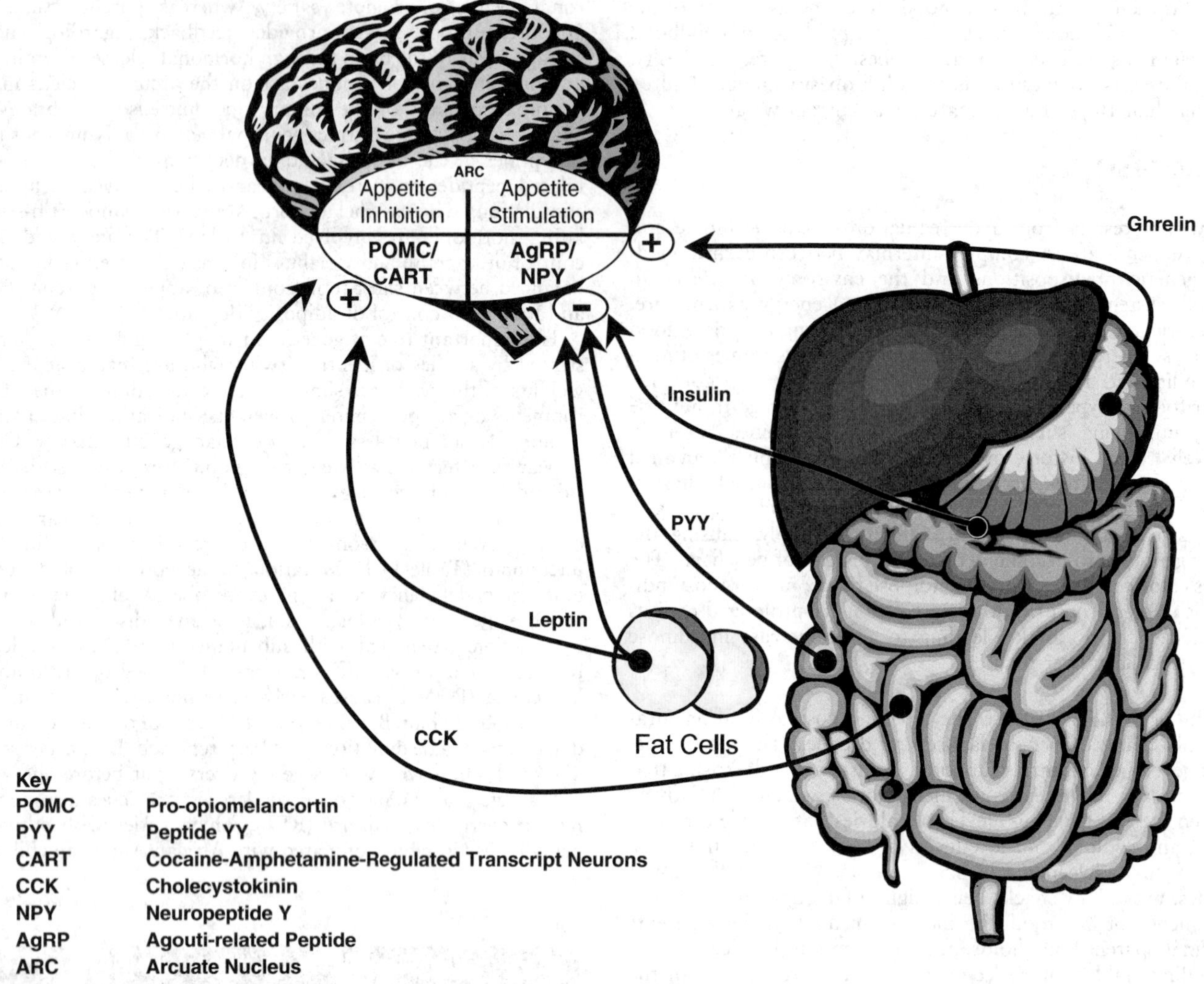

Figure 44-1. Control of appetite.

These differences may be due to varied genotypes of mitochondrial uncoupling proteins. More than 600 genes, markers, and chromosomal regions have been associated with obesity in humans.

DIAGNOSTIC CRITERIA FOR OVERWEIGHT

The diagnosis of obesity in adults is based on calculation of the BMI by dividing the weight in kilograms by the height in meters squared (kg/m^2). The calculated BMI can overestimate adiposity in trained athletes or muscular children, but it is generally recognized as the most reliable method to determine healthy and unhealthy adiposity. Other methods of determining adiposity are useful, but are either too expensive to be of practical use in a clinical setting (ultrasound, CT, MRI, DEXA, total body conductivity, air displacement plethysmography), require specialized training (skinfold thickness), have poor reproducibility (waist-hip ratios), or lack extensive normative data in children (bioelectric impedance analysis). Therefore, BMI in combination with clinical assessment is sufficient to make the diagnosis. Absolute numbers for BMI in adults determine adiposity (Table 44-2). Given changing adiposity during childhood, the BMI percentile is used for classification (Table 44-3 and Fig. 44-2). Children's adiposity rises in the 1st year of life, reaches a nadir around 5–6 yr of age, and then increases again throughout childhood. This is called the *adiposity rebound*. The 95th percentile BMI for a 4 yr old is approximately 19, but it is 25 in a 13 yr old. Consistent use of the BMI growth chart aids in early identification of children at risk for later obesity; an earlier adiposity rebound (increase in BMI younger than 5 yr of age) coincides with later obesity.

TABLE 44-2. Body Mass Index (BMI) Classification of Adults

BMI (kg/m^2)	WEIGHT STATUS
<18.5	Underweight
18.5–24.9	Normal weight
25–29.9	Overweight
30–34.9	Obese
35–39.9	Moderately obese
40–49.9	Morbid obesity
≥50	Super morbid obesity

TABLE 44-3. Body Mass Index (BMI) Classification of Children and Adolescents

BMI PERCENTILE FOR AGE	WEIGHT STATUS
<5th percentile	Underweight
5th–84th percentile	Normal weight
85th–94th percentile	At risk for overweight
≥95th percentile	Overweight

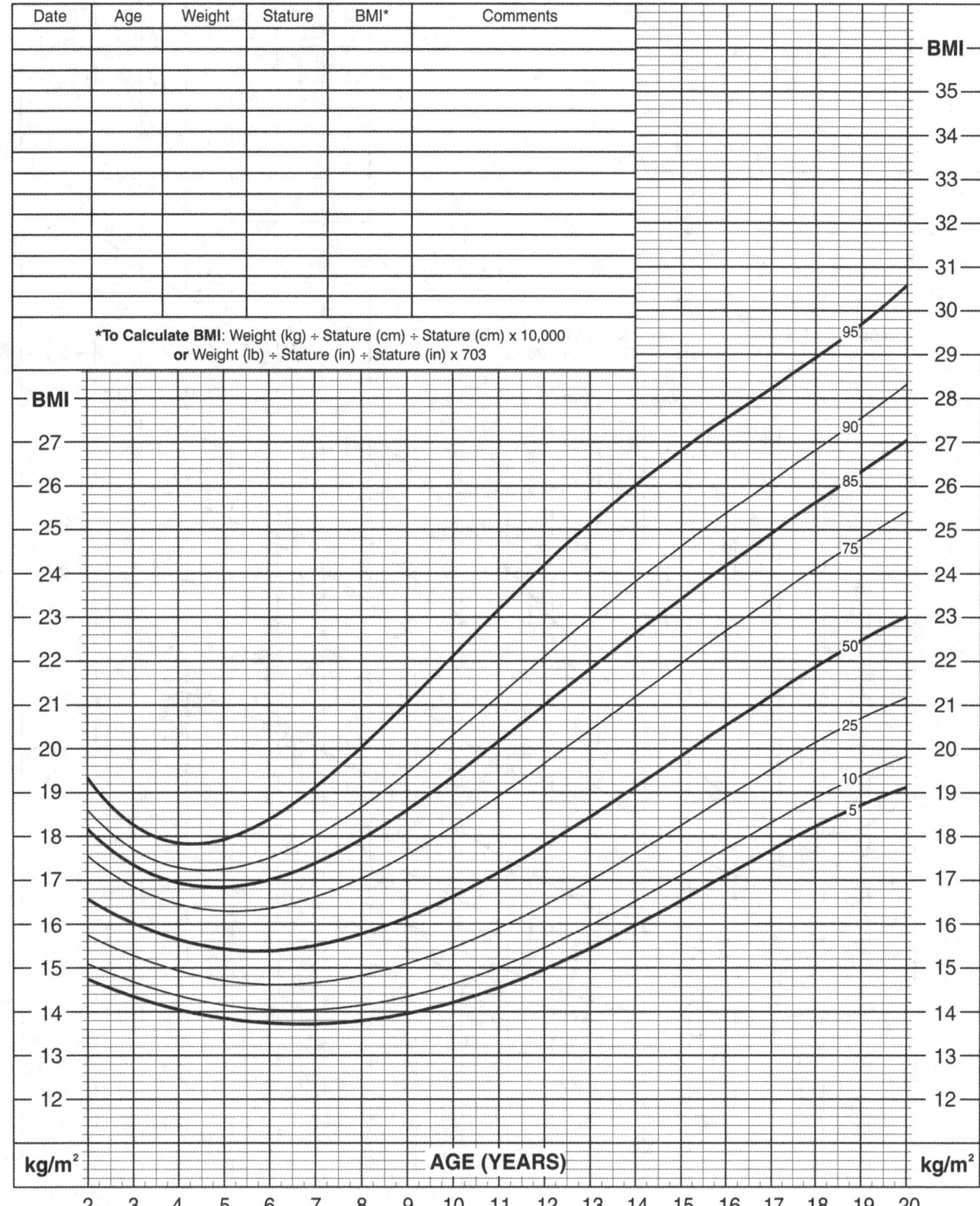

2 to 20 years: Boys
Body mass index-for-age percentiles

Date	Age	Weight	Stature	BMI*	Comments

***To Calculate BMI**: Weight (kg) ÷ Stature (cm) ÷ Stature (cm) x 10,000
or Weight (lb) ÷ Stature (in) ÷ Stature (in) x 703

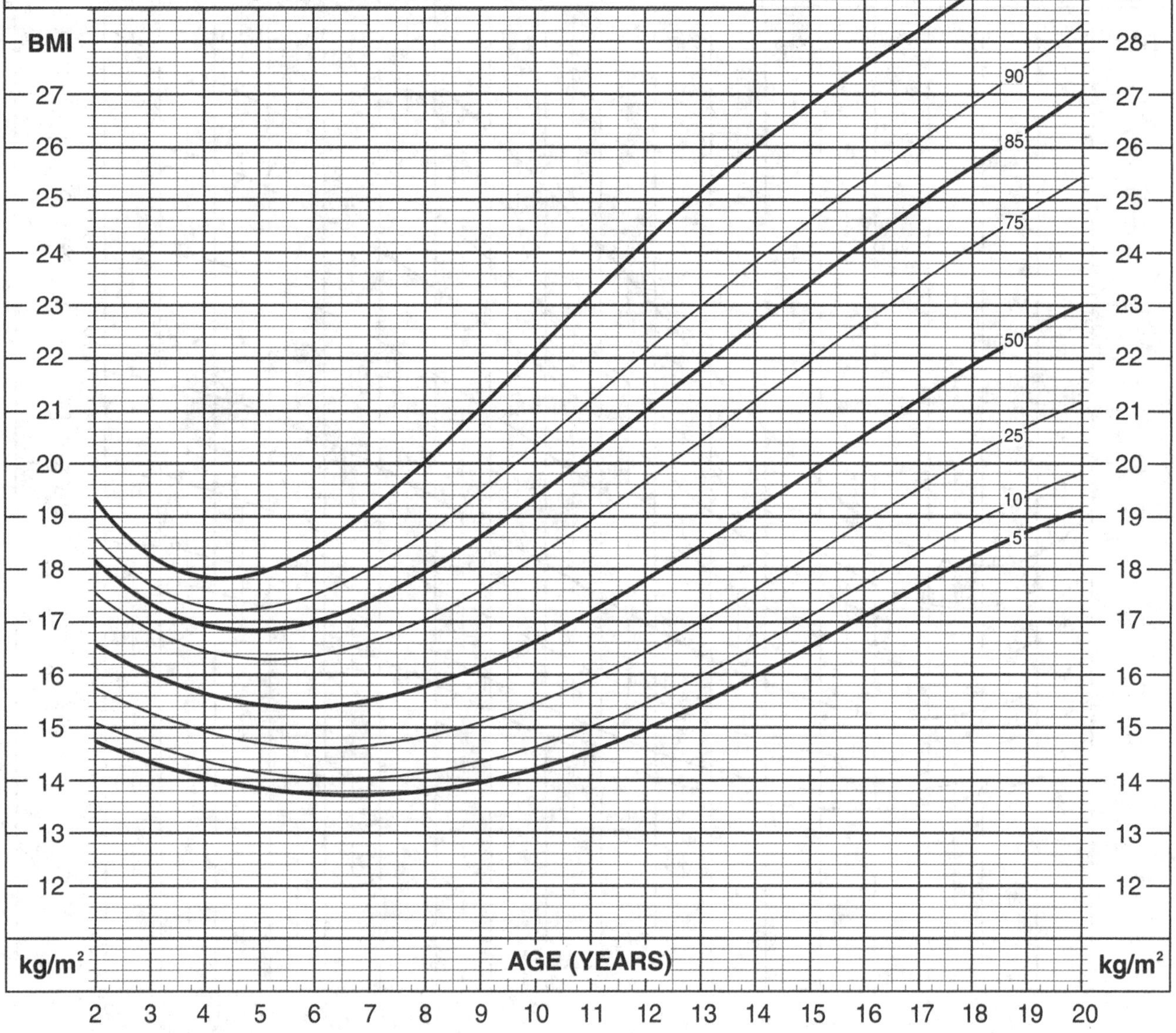

BMI

35
34
33
32
31
30
29
28
27
26
25
24
23
22
21
20
19
18
17
16
15
14
13
12

kg/m²

95
90
85
75
50
25
10
5

AGE (YEARS)

2 3 4 5 6 7 8 9 10 11 12 13 14 15 16 17 18 19 20

Published May 30, 2000 (modified 10/16/00).

SOURCE: Developed by the National Center for Health Statistics in collaboration with the National Center for Chronic Disease Prevention and Health Promotion (2000).
http://www.cdc.gov/growthcharts

CDC
SAFER • HEALTHIER • PEOPLE™

A

Figure 44-2. Body mass index (BMI)-for-age profiles for boys and men *(A)* and girls and women *(B)*. (Continued)

2 to 20 years: Girls
Body mass index-for-age percentiles

NAME ____________________

RECORD # ____________

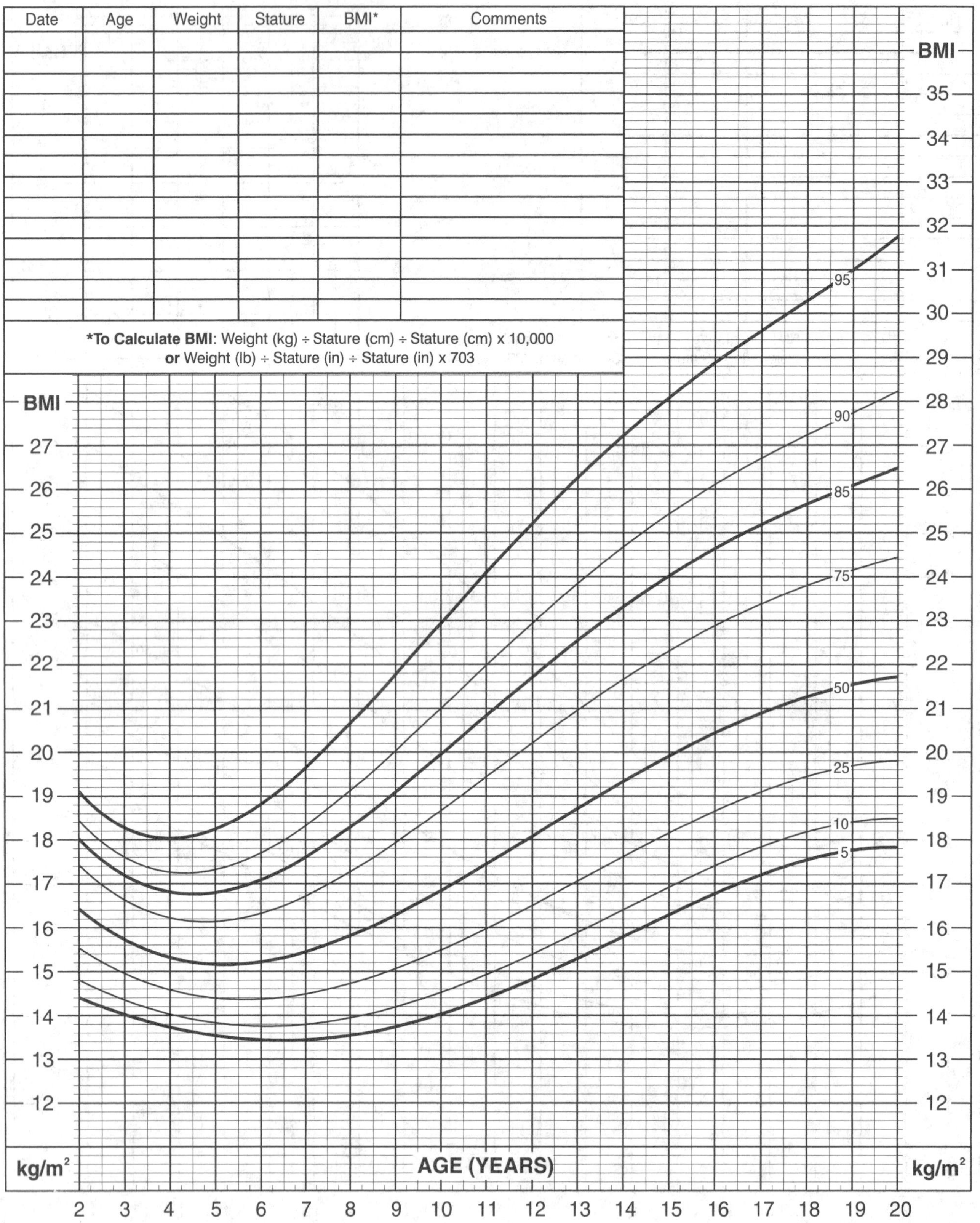

Date	Age	Weight	Stature	BMI*	Comments

***To Calculate BMI**: Weight (kg) ÷ Stature (cm) ÷ Stature (cm) x 10,000
or Weight (lb) ÷ Stature (in) ÷ Stature (in) x 703

Published May 30, 2000 (modified 10/16/00).
SOURCE: Developed by the National Center for Health Statistics in collaboration with the National Center for Chronic Disease Prevention and Health Promotion (2000).
http://www.cdc.gov/growthcharts

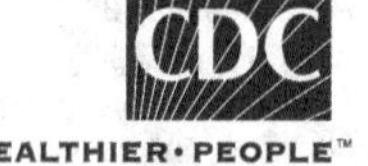

B

Figure 44-2. *Cont'd.* 2–20 yr of age. (Developed by the National Center for Health Statistics in collaboration with the National Center for Chronic Disease Prevention and Health Promotion [2000]. *http://www.cdc.gov/growthcharts*).

EVALUATION OF THE OVERWEIGHT CHILD. Evaluation of overweight children and their families requires sensitivity and compassion, because the general public often perceives overweight individuals as unhealthy, unintelligent, unhygienic, and lazy. Overweight children often have decreased self-esteem, and their overweight parents may have similar psychosocial issues due to the stigma of being overweight. Obesity is a chronic medical problem that requires management in a manner similar to that of other chronic disorders. Explaining this construct to the family in an objective and nonjudgmental manner helps in building a trusting relationship that is important for successful treatment. The initial evaluation is focused on exploring dietary practices, family structure, and habits because alteration of these factors is usually the basis of successful treatment. It is also important to determine if there may be an underlying secondary cause of obesity or if there are current comorbidities from being overweight.

DIFFERENTIAL DIAGNOSIS. The vast majority of overweight children do not have an underlying secondary treatable cause of increased weight (see Table 44-1). Evaluation of the child's growth chart and historical features and the physical examination provide important clues that may trigger further evaluation for endocrine (hypothyroid, Cushing syndrome) or genetic disorders. In children with excessive weight gain or BMI during the infant and toddler years, associated genetic syndromes, such as Prader-Willi, Bardet-Biedl, Alström, Beckwith-Wiedemann and other causes of hyperinsulinism, Cohen, and Lawrence-Moon-Biedl, should be considered. Each is associated with some combination of dysmorphic features, developmental delay, vision and hearing abnormality, or poor linear growth. Other specific genetic disorders associated with leptin deficiency or with other abnormalities of weight control mechanisms are noted in Table 44-1. Only leptin deficiency is currently treatable with specific therapy. Hypothyroidism can be associated with obesity, but usually weight gain is modest, because appetite is often reduced and problems of poor linear growth, delayed skeletal development, and delayed puberty are more prominent features. The onset of relatively rapid weight gain, an increase in BMI percentiles, and central obesity in a child or adolescent may occur with Cushing syndrome, but other symptoms or findings, such as muscle weakness, ecchymoses, unexplained osteoporosis, and hypokalemia may be present.

Normal linear growth alone generally precludes the diagnosis of endocrinologic diseases.

Therefore, studies to rule out secondary causes of overweight are unnecessary unless there has been a rapid alteration in the rate of weight gain, the child has poor linear growth, or syndromic features are present. A family history of endocrinopathies increases the risk in a child. Overweight children who are below the 50th percentile for height for age should be screened for an endocrinologic abnormality. Free thyroxine and thyroid-stimulating hormone levels are helpful in evaluating hypothyroidism, and the 24 hr urinary free cortisol level is used to diagnose hypercortisolism (Cushing syndrome). In children with early-onset obesity, evaluation by a geneticist may be helpful, and in those without a recognized syndrome, leptin levels should be considered.

COMORBITIES OF OVERWEIGHT. Complications of being overweight may affect children, but the major concern is focused on long-term consequences. The Harvard Growth Study showed a doubling of the death rate from cardiovascular disease in males who were overweight during adolescence. The Bogalusa Heart Study observed that children with a BMI above the 85th percentile were more likely to have hypercholesterolemia, hypertriglyceridemia, or hypertension than other children. Comorbidities observed during childhood and adolescence include insulin resistance, Type 2 diabetes, hypercholesterolemia, hypertriglyceridemia, metabolic syndrome, hypertension, orthopedic and musculoskeletal complications, asthma, sleep apnea, polycystic ovary syndrome, and psychosocial disorders (Table 44-4). Higher blood pressures and a higher prevalence of hypertension occur in overweight children, independent of race, sex, and age. The **metabolic syndrome** (hypertension, glucose intolerance, hypertriglyceridemia, decreased high-density lipoprotein level, abdominal central obesity) confers an excessively high risk of cardiovascular disease, with an overall prevalence of 4% in adolescents and approximately 30% in overweight adolescents. Orthopedic complications include Blount disease, characterized by an overgrowth of the medial aspect of the proximal tibial metaphysis, leading to bowing of the legs (see Chapter 674) and slipped capital femoral epiphysis, where the epiphysis of the proximal femur slips off the metaphysis posteriorly and medially due to increased weight on the cartilaginous growth plate of the hip

TABLE 44-4. Comorbidities of Obesity: Evaluation and Testing

COMORBIDITY	FINDING ON HISTORY AND PHYSICAL	TESTING
Asthma	Shortness of breath, wheezing, coughing, exercise intolerance	Pulmonary function tests, peak flow
Insulin resistance, Type 2 diabetes mellitus	Acanthosis nigricans, family history, polyuria, polydipsia, unintentional weight loss	Fasting glucose, hemoglobin A_{1c}, insulin level, C-peptide, oral glucose tolerance test
Dyslipidemia	Family history (high cholesterol, early-onset heart disease), xanthomas	Fasting total cholesterol, HDL, LDL, triglycerides
Gallstones	Abdominal pain, vomiting, jaundice	Ultrasound
Hypertension	Elevated blood pressure >95th percentile for age, sex, and height	Serial testing, urinalysis, electrolytes, blood urea nitrogen, creatinine
Musculoskeletal problems (Blount disease, slipped capital femoral epiphysis)	Back pain, joint pain, frequent strains/sprains, limp, hip pain, groin pain, leg bowing	X-rays
Nonalcoholic fatty liver disease, nonalcoholic steatohepatitis	Hepatomegaly, abdominal pain, dependent edema	AST, ALT, ultrasound, CT, or MRI
Obstructive sleep apnea	Snoring, disturbed sleep pattern, daytime somnolence, enuresis (daytime and nocturnal)	Polysomnography, hypoxia, electrolytes (respiratory acidosis with metabolic alkalosis)
Polycystic ovary syndrome	Dysmenorrhea, hirsutism, acne, acanthosis nigricans, hair loss, central obesity, history of insulin resistance, infertility	Pelvic ultrasound, testosterone, free testosterone, luteinizing hormone, follicle-stimulating hormone
Behavioral complications	Disordered eating, signs of depression, worsening school performance, social isolation, low self-esteem, bullying, being bullied	Child Behavior Checklist, Children's Depression Inventory, PEDS QL, Eating Disorder Inventory 2, subjective ratings of stress/depression, Behavior Assessment/System for Children Pediatric Symptom Checklist
Pseudotumor cerebri	Headache, dizziness, diplopia, unsteady gate, papilledema	Cerebrospinal fluid opening pressure, CT, MRI
Slipped capital femoral epiphysis	Hip pain, limp	Hip x-rays
Blount disease	Knee pain, limp, bowing of legs	Knee x-rays

ALT, alanine aminotransferase; AST, aspartate aminotransferase; HDL, high-density lipoprotein; LDL, low-density lipoprotein; PEDS QL, Pediatric Quality of Life Inventory.

TABLE 44-5. Simplified Laboratory Norms for Assessing Overweight Children

Laboratory Test	Normal Value
Glucose	<110 mg/dL
Insulin	<15 mU/L
Hemoglobin A_{1c}	<6.0%
AST 2–8 yr	<58 U/L
9–15 yr	<46 U/L
15–18 yr	<35 U/L
ALT	<35 U/L
Total cholesterol	<170 mg/dL
LDL	<110 mg/dL
HDL	<35 mg/dL
Triglycerides	
2–15 yr	<100 mg/dL
15–19 yr	<125 mg/dL

From the NEW Kids Program™, Children's Hospital of Wisconsin, http://www/chw.org/newkids
AST, aspartate aminotransferase; ALT, alanine aminotransferase; LDL, low-density lipoprotein; HDL, high-density lipoprotein.

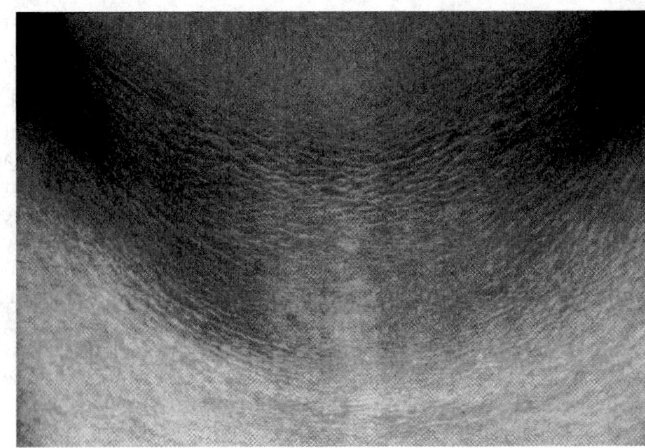

Figure 44-3. Acanthosis nigricans. (From Gagagan S: Child and adolescent obesity. *Curr Probl Pediatr Adolesc Health Care* 2004;34:6–43.)

(see Chapter 677.4). Some prospective studies suggest a causal link between obesity and asthma, but it is unclear what role this plays in childhood. Obstructive sleep apnea is more common in overweight children and may contribute to problems such as hypertension, daytime fatigue, and pulmonary hypertension (see Chapter 18). Nonalcoholic fatty liver disease (NAFLD) has been reported in 10–25% of very overweight adolescents (see Chapter 354.6). NAFLD is characterized by a mild increase in transaminases, a hyperechoic liver on ultrasound, and evidence of steatosis and periportal fibrosis on histologic examination. Progression to liver cirrhosis may occur with time. Proteinuria caused by focal segmental glomerulosclerosis has been reported in severely obese African-American adolescents. In addition to these complications that may present in adolescents, obesity in adults is associated with increased risk of malignancies and osteoarthritis.

Screening for these complications of overweight is accomplished from the history, physical examination, and selected use of screening laboratory tests (Table 44-5). Recognition of these complications at the time of diagnosis is important so that treatment for the specific condition (which may include weight control) is initiated and because conditions such as severe hypertension, asthma, or orthopedic problems may require treatment before an exercise regimen can be prescribed as a part of the treatment approach for promoting weight control.

HISTORY. A family history of Type 2 diabetes, a high-risk ethnicity (African-American, Hispanic, Native American), and central adiposity increase the risk of hyperinsulinism or Type 2 diabetes. Symptoms of polyuria, nocturia, polydipsia, and unexplained rapid weight loss are all associated with the onset of Type 2 diabetes. A history of maternal diabetes or obesity and being large or small for gestational age increase the risk of metabolic syndrome. Snoring, episodes of nighttime coughing fits, or excessive daytime sleepiness can be due to obstructive sleep apnea, which warrants further investigation with referral to a sleep laboratory for polysomnography. A history of wheezing, shortness of breath, or coughing can be due to asthma. Hip, knee, or leg pain is often present due to orthopedic complications. Asthma and orthopedic problems may require treatment and/or alterations in prescribed exercise programs, so identification of these problems during the initial evaluation is important. Irregular menses occur in overweight females with polycystic ovary syndrome.

PHYSICAL FINDINGS AND LABORATORY SCREENING. Careful screening for hypertension using an appropriately sized blood pressure cuff is important. Acanthosis nigricans suggests insulin resistance (Fig. 44-3). Tanner staging is useful to identify premature adrenarche. Hirsutism, male pattern baldness, and severe acne are noted with polycystic ovary syndrome. Laboratory screening tests recommended during the initial evaluation of the overweight child are listed in Table 44-5. Findings from the history and physical examination and tests associated with comorbidities are listed in Table 44-4.

TREATMENT. Successful treatment of obesity is challenging, and treatment goals vary, depending on the age of the child and the severity of complications from being overweight. Children are still growing, so severe caloric restriction and weight loss may be detrimental. Weight maintenance rather than weight loss is frequently a reasonable initial goal. As children grow in stature, BMI decreases. Weight loss should be attempted only in skeletally mature children or in those with serious complications from obesity. Weight loss should be slow (1 lb or 0.5 kg or less/wk), because more rapid weight loss requires overly restrictive dieting. An initial goal of a 10% reduction in weight is reasonable because this amount of weight loss has been shown to significantly improve overall health. Once achieved, the new weight should be maintained for 6 mo before further weight loss is attempted.

Successful long-term weight loss in adults is uncommon, despite the wide variety of diet plans and commercial products. There is a propensity to regain weight and adapt unhealthy behaviors with recurrent fad dieting. The most successful approach to weight maintenance or weight loss requires substantial lifestyle changes that include increased physical activity and altered eating habits. Similar approaches are used to prevent weight gain in children who are at risk for overweight and to promote weight maintenance or weight loss in overweight children. Therapies often combine diet, exercise, behavior modification, medications, and rarely, surgery. There is no clear and universally accepted treatment approach, but there are some generally accepted principles.

OFFICE-BASED MANAGEMENT. Prevention and treatment of childhood overweight should be part of the anticipatory guidance provided during routine health supervision visits, particularly in families with children at risk for overweight (Table 44-6). Calculating and plotting the BMI yearly will identify children experiencing rapid weight gain or early adiposity rebound. Anticipatory guidance includes discussion of the benefits of increased physical activity and decreased sedentary activity, and the promotion of healthy eating habits. Identifying particular parenting styles can alter the management approach to an overweight child. Rigid, controlling styles of feeding may decrease a child's preference for healthier foods. Alternatively, if parents

TABLE 44-6. Anticipatory Guidance: Establishing Healthy Eating Habits in Children

Do not punish a child during mealtimes with regard to eating. The emotional atmosphere of a meal is very important. Interactions during meals should be pleasant and happy.
Do not use foods as rewards.
Parents, siblings, and peers should model healthy eating, tasting new foods, and eating a well-balanced meal.
Children should be exposed to a wide range of foods, tastes, and textures.
Foods should be offered multiple times. Repeated exposure to initially disliked foods will break down resistance.
Offering a range of foods with low energy density helps children balance energy intake.
Restricting access to foods will increase rather than decrease a child's preference for that food.
Forcing a child to eat a certain food will decrease his or her preference for that food. Children's wariness of new foods is normal and should be expected.
Children tend to be more aware of satiety than adults, so allow children to respond to satiety, and let that dictate servings. Do not force children to "clean their plate."

Adapted from Benton D: Role of parents in the determination of food preferences of children and the development of obesity. *Int J Obes Relat Metab Disord* 2004;28:858–869. Copyright 2004. Reprinted by permission from Macmillan Publishers Ltd.

avoid conflict by allowing the child to dictate all choices, the result may be poor nutritional choices. In the overweight child, the principles elucidated during anticipatory guidance need to be reinforced as being central to the child's success in achieving weight loss. Behavioral change within the entire family will need to focus on decreasing sedentary activity, increasing physical activity, improving nutrition, addressing unhealthy eating practices (fast food, skipped meals), and improving family interactions. Helpful measures in this educational process include the use of food and activity logs, which give the physician insight into eating practices as well as busy family schedules and provide opportunities to educate the family on portion sizes and sweetened beverage intake. By identifying obstacles to care, goal-setting can be more focused. For example, instead of a goal of "eat out less," the goal can be "find a meal that the family can prepare together and freeze for later in the week." Recognition of a lack of resources for obtaining healthy foods may allow referral of the family to a food pantry or co-op that can provide healthier alternatives for less expense. Many parents lack any knowledge of food preparation or have inadequate parenting skills. Others live in unsafe communities, where access to playgrounds or recreational activities is limited due to concerns about safety. Enlistment of community resources that can overcome these barriers is of utmost importance in the overall management strategy. Identification of small, achievable goals is useful to promote success and subsequent compliance. Regular follow-up with the patient and family, with reassessment of the goals and identification of any barriers to compliance with the plan, is important. Unfortunately, office-based management is rarely successful due to the frequency of follow-up visits required and the lack of payment for services. Multidisciplinary and community-based approaches to overweight management may be more successful in promoting family change.

MULTIDISCIPLINARY AND COMMUNITY-BASED MANAGEMENT. Community-based programs to inform families regarding age-appropriate healthy eating choices, meal and portion size planning, decreasing "screen time," and approaches to increasing physical activity provide an important service for families with children at risk for becoming overweight or mildly to moderately overweight without comorbidities. Severely overweight children and adolescents with complications from obesity are best managed by a multidisciplinary team. The treatment models used in most pediatric centers feature family-based behavioral treatment, which is the only approach shown to have long-term efficacy. Teams may include a physician, a psychologist, a dietitian, an exercise specialist (physical therapist, exercise physiologist, educator), a nurse, and counselors. Management consists of dietary counseling, exercise therapy, and behavioral management. Psychologists screen families for underlying problems that have led to a child's overweight, problems arising from health complications of overweight, and barriers to successful adaptation of a healthier lifestyle. Once problems are identified, psychologists and counselors can use cognitive behavioral and family therapy to address such issues. Methods used include positive reinforcement, changes in the home and family environment, self-monitoring, goal-setting, contracting, and parenting skills training. Comorbid conditions, such as eating disorders, depression, and anxiety, can be more effectively treated in the multidisciplinary setting. Exercise specialists can help overweight children exercise in age-appropriate, fun ways, as well as compensate for deficiencies arising from being overweight, such as deconditioning, orthopedic conditions (Blount disease, slipped capital femoral epiphysis), or muscular weakness. Formal rehabilitative therapy is sometimes required in very overweight patients due to years of inactivity with muscle deconditioning combined with orthopedic problems.

At a societal level, obesity must also be addressed in schools, by industry, and by the government (Table 44-7).

DIETARY COUNSELING. Recommendations for healthy eating should be age-specific and flexible enough to accommodate family and ethnic food preferences (see also Chapters 41 and 42). In toddlers, limiting sweetened beverages is usually the most useful initial strategy. The American Academy of Pediatrics (AAP) recommends a maximum intake of 4–6 oz of fruit juice/day for children ages 1–6 yr and 8–12 oz for 7–18 yr olds. Other simple interventions include changing to skim milk in children older than the age of 2 yr and assuring exposure to a wide variety of foods, including less calorie-dense food choices and limitation of between-meal snacking. For preschool-aged children, sweetened beverages should be limited and parents should continue to offer healthy foods. The parents should be educated about approaches to dealing with food refusals as diets are modified. It often requires more than 10 repeated exposures to a new food before a child will regularly accept it as part of the regular diet. As children reach school age, busy schedules and exposure to food advertisements often increase fast food intake. Education regarding meal planning and the value of family mealtimes in maintaining family structures can decrease the number of meals eaten away from home. Including children in meal choices and food preparation helps them to learn healthy eating patterns. Adolescents also fall victim to busy schedules, and given their increasing independence, they are more likely to develop unhealthy eating patterns, such as skipping meals and following fad diets. Encouraging children to eat breakfast, decreasing their intake of sweetened beverages, and teaching them the principles of balanced nutrition (eating from all food groups) are useful strategies for the overweight adolescent.

More severe dietary restriction should be used only in a supervised program. Some centers have reported success with specific dietary interventions, such as a protein-sparing modified fast, which is usually managed in an inpatient setting or in a closely supervised outpatient clinic. An extremely low-calorie diet (≈800 kcal/24 hr) is used for children with severe obesity needing rapid weight loss. Low-carbohydrate or controlled-carbohydrate diets show superior weight loss compared with low-fat diets in adolescents. Adult studies show similar weight loss between this approach and other diets, so the benefit is uncertain. Nutrition plans based on the glycemic index of foods has shown great promise in overweight children. The **glycemic index** is based on the insulin response to a carbohydrate, with simple carbohydrates having a higher, and therefore less desirable, glycemic index compared with complex carbohydrates, such as non-starchy vegetables and whole grains. Multidisciplinary teams and dietitians usually focus on identifying problem areas in a child's and family's regular diet and then teach them about healthier alter-

TABLE 44-7. Proposed Suggestions for the Prevention of Obesity

PREGNANCY
Normalize body mass index before pregnancy.
Do not smoke.
Maintain moderate exercise as tolerated.
In gestational diabetics, provide meticulous glucose control.

POSTPARTUM AND INFANCY
Breast-feeding is preferred for a minimum of 3 mo.
Postpone the introduction of solid foods and sweet liquids.

FAMILIES
Eat meals as a family in a fixed place and time.
Do not skip meals, especially breakfast.
No television during meals.
Use small plates, and keep serving dishes away from the table.
Avoid unnecessary sweet or fatty foods and soft drinks.
Remove televisions from children's bedrooms; restrict times for television viewing and video games.

SCHOOLS
Eliminate fundraisers with candy and cookie sales.
Review the contents of vending machines and replace with healthier choices.
Install water fountains.
Educate teachers, especially physical education and science faculty, about basic nutrition and the benefits of physical activity.
Educate children from preschool through high school on appropriate diet and lifestyle.
Mandate minimum standards for physical education, including 30–45 min of strenuous exercise 2–3 times weekly.
Encourage "the walking schoolbus": Groups of children walking to school with an adult.

COMMUNITIES
Increase family-friendly exercise and play facilities for children of all ages.
Discourage the use of elevators and moving walkways.
Provide information on how to shop and prepare healthier versions of culture-specific foods.

HEALTH CARE PROVIDERS
Explain the biologic and genetic contributions to obesity.
Give age-appropriate expectations for body weight in children.
Work toward classifying obesity as a disease to promote recognition, reimbursement for care, and willingness and ability to provide treatment.

INDUSTRY
Mandate age-appropriate nutrition labeling for products aimed at children (e.g., red light/green light foods, with portion sizes).
Encourage marketing of interactive video games in which children must exercise in order to play.
Use celebrity advertising directed at children for healthful foods to promote breakfast and regular meals.

GOVERNMENT AND REGULATORY AGENCIES
Classify obesity as a legitimate disease.
Find novel ways to fund healthy lifestyle programs, (i.e., with revenues from food/drink taxes).
Subsidize government-sponsored programs to promote the consumption of fresh fruits and vegetables.
Provide financial incentives to industry to develop more healthful products and to educate the consumer on product content.
Provide financial incentives to schools that initiate innovative physical activity and nutrition programs.
Allow tax deductions for the cost of weight loss and exercise programs.
Provide urban planners with funding to establish bicycle, jogging, and walking paths.
Ban advertising of fast foods directed at preschool children, and restrict advertising to school-aged children.

From Speiser PW, Rudolf MCJ, Anhalt H, et al: Consensus statement: Childhood obesity. *J Clin Endocrinol Metabol* 2005;90:1871–1887.

natives and eating patterns. This approach creates sustainable, lifelong change, which is more useful than restrictive diets, which are usually not maintained, with resultant weight gain. A successful approach used in preschool and preadolescent children is the *traffic light* or *stoplight* diet. Foods are grouped by nutrient and caloric density, with the color indicating the frequency of recommended consumption (Table 44-8). It is designed to limit calories, yet achieve good nutrient balance and is easily adaptable to fit particular ethnicities and nutrition plans, such as low-carbohydrate or glycemic index diets.

PHYSICAL ACTIVITY. Decreasing sedentary activity is essential for achieving weight control. Increased activity not only increases calorie use but also appears to decrease appetite. In children younger than 2 yr of age, the AAP recommends avoiding television and computers. Children 2–18 yr of age should have <2 hr/day of "screen time" (television, video games, computer), and televisions should be removed from children's bedrooms. Enforcing this behavior change is difficult unless the entire family decreases sedentary activity and screen time. Children use computers for homework, and this must be taken into account when giving recommendations. Although prescribed exercise regimens can be useful, an office setting gives little opportunity to provide such guidance. Simple measures, such as daily walks, can be discussed. In the severely overweight child, problems of exercise tolerance may warrant referral to an experienced physical or exercise therapist to provide a safe and graded exercise regimen. Identifying opportunities in the community for increased physical activity can be of great importance to some families.

TABLE 44-8. Stoplight Diet Plan

COLOR	GREEN LIGHT FOOD	YELLOW LIGHT FOODS	RED LIGHT FOODS
Quality	Low-calorie, high-fiber, low-fat, nutrient-dense	Nutrient-dense, but higher in calories and fat	High in calories, sugar, and fat
Types of food	Fruits, vegetables	Lean meats, dairy, starches, grains	Fatty meats, sugar, fried foods
Quantity	Unlimited	Limited	Infrequent or avoided

MEDICATIONS. Pharmacologic treatment is sometimes indicated as an adjunct to diet and physical activity in overweight adults with obesity-related complications (Table 44-9). Medication of overweight children and adolescents is reserved for those with severe medical complications. The use of sibutramine, a norepinephrine and serotonin reuptake inhibitor, is not recommended in children younger than 16 yr of age. Orlistat, an intestinal lipase inhibitor, has been effective in adolescents older than 12 yr of age, but gastrointestinal side effects of diarrhea and abdominal pain are common, and the potential effects on fat-soluble vitamin and mineral absorption in growing adolescents are a concern. Topiramate, an anti-epileptic, has marked anorectic effects. It is now used frequently in adult populations for weight loss and may have potential for selected pediatric populations. Metformin is being studied in adult patients and appears to promote weight loss and prevent the development of metabolic syndrome. Although met-

TABLE 44-9. Medications Used for Weight Loss in Adults

DRUG	MECHANISM OF ACTION	SIDE EFFECTS
Sibutramine*†	Appetite suppressant: combined norepinephrine and serotonin reuptake inhibitor	Modest increases in heart rate and blood pressure, nervousness, insomnia
Phentermine*†	Appetite suppressant: sympathomimetic amine	Cardiovascular, gastrointestinal
Diethylpropion*†	Appetite suppressant: sympathomimetic amine	Palpitations, tachycardia, insomnia, gastrointestinal
Orlistat*	Lipase inhibitor: decreased absorption of fat	Diarrhea, flatulence, bloating, abdominal pain, dyspepsia
Bupropion	Appetite suppressant: mechanism unknown	Paresthesia, insomnia, central nervous system effects
Fluoxetine	Appetite suppressant: selective serotonin reuptake inhibitor	Agitation, nervousness, gastrointestinal
Sertraline	Appetite suppressant: selective serotonin reuptake inhibitor	Agitation, nervousness, gastrointestinal
Topiramate	Mechanism unknown	Paresthesia, changes in taste
Zonisamide	Mechanism unknown	Somnolence, dizziness, nausea

*Approved by the U.S. Food and Drug Administration for weight loss.
†Drug Enforcement Administration schedule IV.
From Snow V, Barry P, Fitterman N, et al: Pharmacologic and surgical management of obesity in primary care: A clinical practice guideline from the American Collge of Physicians. *Ann Intern Med* 2005;142:525–531.

formin does appear to have some efficacy in promoting weight loss and lifestyle changes, octreotide has shown promise for weight control in children with hypothalamic obesity. Rimonabant, a cannabinoid type 1 receptor antagonist, has been effective in obese adults in reducing weight and ameliorating abnormal metabolic parameters. At this time, the use of pharmacologic agents for the treatment of overweight children and adolescents is of marginal value, with unclear risks, and it is best reserved for use in clinical trials.

Dietary supplements and herbal therapies are heavily marketed for weight loss. Therefore, discussion of the risks and benefits should be part of patient education and counseling. Adolescents are particularly prone to use over-the-counter or herbal agents and also to engage in unsafe activities, such as purging. There is some evidence of modest weight loss secondary to ephedra-caffeine ingestion, but the risk of psychiatric, autonomic, or gastrointestinal adverse events, seizures, and heart palpitations has led to its removal from the USA market. Other popular agents include chromium, linoleic acid, ginseng, glucomannan, green tea, hydroxycitric acid, L-carnitine, psyllium, pyruvate, and St. John's wort, but there is inadequate evidence regarding their efficacy or safety.

BARIATRIC SURGERY. There is some efficacy of bariatric surgery in adolescents; the long-term safety has not been adequately studied. In the USA, the Roux-en-Y gastric bypass is one approach for weight control surgery. This procedure consists of gastric stapling to restrict the volume of food comfortably ingested combined with anastomosis of a loop of jejunum to the stomach, which results in malabsorption. Weight loss that approaches 60–70% of excess body weight is often achieved. The procedure has been shown to be safe and effective in selected pediatric populations, but it is a permanent operation and requires a substantial change in lifestyle and eating habits. Furthermore, monitoring for nutritional complications is mandatory because deficiencies of iron, vitamin B_{12}, folate, thiamine, vitamin D, and calcium have been reported. Cases of Wernicke encephalopathy have occurred in some patients who have not complied with the recommended dietary supplements after surgery. There have also been pediatric reports of dry beriberi after bariatric surgery. For adolescent girls planning on future childbearing, the risks of folate deficiency are of particular concern. The American Pediatric Surgical Association Guidelines recommend that surgery be considered only in children with a BMI > 40 and a medical complication of obesity after they have failed 6 mo of a multidisciplinary weight management program. Evaluation, surgery, and care should be provided at a tertiary care center with experience in caring for overweight children and their families. Less invasive procedures than the Roux-en-Y gastric bypass are available and include the **adjustable gastric band** that functions only by extrinsic gastric restriction. In European and Australian trials, weight loss approaching 40–50% of excess body weight has been achieved. One benefit is the band can be removed.

Alberti KGMM, Zimmet P, Shaw J, et al: The metabolic syndrome: A new worldwide definition. *Lancet* 2005;366:1059–1062.

American Academy of Pediatrics: The use and misuse of fruit juice in pediatrics. *Pediatrics* 2001;107:1210–1213.

American Academy of Pediatrics Committee on Nutrition: Prevention of pediatric overweight and obesity. *Pediatrics* 2003;112:424–430.

Centers for Disease Control and Prevention: Overweight among students in grades K–12—Arkansas, 2003–04 and 2004–05 school years. *MMWR* 2006;55:5–8.

Centers for Disease Control and Prevention National Health and Nutrition Examination Survey: *http://www.cdc.gov/nchs/about/major/nhanes/growthcharts/clinical_charts.htm.*

Chanoine JP, Hampl S, Jensen C, et al: Effect of orlistat on weight and body composition in obese adults. *JAMA* 2005;293:2873–2883.

Cook S: The metabolic syndrome: Antecedent of adult cardiovascular disease in pediatrics. *J Pediatr* 2004;145:427–430.

Cormier-Daire V, Molinari F, Rio M, et al: Cryptic terminal deletion of chromosome 9q34: A novel cause of syndromic obesity in childhood? *J Med Genet* 2003;40:300–303.

Department of Health and Human Services Centers for Disease Control and Prevention: Public health strategies for preventing and controlling overweight and obesity in school and worksite settings. *MMWR* 2005;54:1–12.

Dietz WH: Physical activity recommendations: Where do we go from here? *J Pediatr* 2005;146:719–720.

Dietz WH, Robinson TN: Overweight children and adolescents. *N Engl J Med* 2005;352:2100–2109.

Ebbeling CB, Feldman HA, Osganian SK, et al: Effects of decreasing sugar-sweetened beverage consumption on body weight in adolescents: a randomized, controlled pilot study. *Pediatrics* 2006;117:673–680.

Ebbeling CB, Sinclair KB, Pereira MA, et al: Compensation for energy intake from fast food among overweight and lean adolescents. *JAMA* 2004;291: 2828–2832.

Farooqi IS, Keogh JM, Yoe GSH, et al: Clinical spectrum of obesity and mutations in the melanocortin 4 receptor gene. *N Engl J Med* 2003;348: 1085–1094.

Gagagan S: Child and adolescent obesity. *Curr Probl Pediatr Adolesc Health Care* 2004;34:1–48.

Graham TE, Yang Q, Blüher M, et al: Retinol-binding protein 4 and insulin resistance in lean, obese, and diabetic subjects. *N Engl J Med* 2006;354:2552–2562.

Guo SS, Wu W, Chumlea WC, et al: Predicting overweight and obesity in adulthood from body mass index values in childhood and adolescence. *Am J Clin Nutr* 2002;76:653–658.

Hallal PC, Wells JCK, Reichert FF, et al: Early determinants of physical activity in adolescence: prospective birth cohort Study. *BMJ* 2006;332:1002–1005.

Herbert A, Gerry NP, McQueen MB, et al: A common genetic variant is associated with adult and childhood obesity. *Science* 2006;312:279–283.

Inge TH, Krebs NF, Garcia VF, et al: Bariatric surgery for severely overweight adolescents: Concerns and recommendations. *Pediatrics* 2004;114: 217–223.

Lancet: Carbohydrates: how low can you go? *Lancet* 2006;367:880–881.

Lancet: Curbing the obesity epidemic. *Lancet* 2006;367:1549.

Lawson ML, Kirk S, Mitchell T, et al: One-year outcomes of Roux-en-Y gastric bypass for morbidly obese adolescents: a multicenter study from the Pediatric Bariatric Study Group. *J Pediatr Surg* 2006;41:137–143.

Lean M, Finer N: ABC of obesity. Management: part II—drugs. *BMJ* 2006; 333:794–797.

McGarvey E, Keller A, Forrester M, et al: Feasibility and benefits of a parent-focused preschool child obesity intervention. *Am J Public Health* 2004; 94:1490–1495.

Meyre D, Bouatia-Naji N, Tounian A, et al: Variants of *ENPP1* are associated with childhood and adult obesity and increase the risk of glucose intolerance and type 2 diabetes. *Nat Genet* 2005;37:863–867.

Miech RA, Kumanyika SK, Stettler N, et al: Trends in the association of poverty with overweight among US adolescents, 1971–2004. *JAMA* 2006;295:2385–2393.

Owen CG, Martin RM, Whincup PH, et al: Effect of infant feeding on the risk of obesity across the life course: A quantitative review of published evidence. *Pediatrics* 2005;115:1367–1377.

Pagotto U, Pasquali R: Fighting obesity and associated risk factors by antagonizing cannabinoid type 1 receptors. *Lancet* 2005;365:1363–1364.

Pereira MA, Swain J, Goldfine AB, et al: Effects of a low-glycemic load diet on resting energy expenditure and heart disease risk factors during weight loss. *JAMA* 2004;292:2482–2490.

Perusse L, Rankinen T, Zuberi A, et al: The human obesity gene map: The 2004 update. *Obesity Res* 2005;13:381–481.

Pi-Sunyer FX, Aronne LJ, Heshmati HM, et al: Effect of rimonabant, a cannabinoid-1 receptor blocker, on weight and cardiometabolic risk factors in overweight or obese patients. *JAMA* 2006;295:761–775.

Quattrin T, Liu E, Shaw N, et al: Obese children who are referred to the pediatric endocrinologist: Characteristics and outcome. *Pediatrics* 2005;115:348–351.

Reilly JJ: Physical activity and obesity in childhood and adolescence. *Lancet* 2005;366:268–269.

Riley MR, Bass NM, Rosenthal P, et al: Underdiagnosis of pediatric obesity and under screening for fatty liver disease and metabolic syndrome by pediatricians and pediatric subspecialists. *J Pediatr* 2005;147:839–842.

Snow V, Barry P, Fitterman N, et al: Pharmacologic and surgical management of obesity in primary care: A clinical practice guideline from the American College of Physicians. *Ann Intern Med* 2005;142:525–531.

Speiser PW, Rudolf MCJ, Anhalt H, et al: Consensus statement: Childhood obesity. *J Clin Endocrinol Metabol* 2005;90:1871–1887.

Washington R: One way to decrease an obesogenic environment. *J Pediatr* 2005;147:417–418.

Weiss R, Dziura J, Burgert TS, et al: Obesity and the metabolic syndrome in children and adolescents. *N Engl J Med* 2004;350:2362–2374.

Zeller M, Daniels S: The obesity epidemic: Family matters. *J Pediatr* 2004;145:3–4.

Chapter 45 ■ Vitamin A Deficiencies and Excess

Maija Zile

OVERVIEW OF VITAMINS. Vitamins are essential organic compounds that are required in very small amounts (micronutrients) and are involved in fundamental functions in the body, such as growth, maintenance of health, and metabolism. A vitamin may have several functions. Because our bodies cannot biosynthesize vitamins, they must be supplied by the diet or as supplements. The dietary reference intakes (DRIs) for infants and children are summarized in Table 41-2. Vitamins are not chemically similar. Based on their chemical properties, they are classified as either water-soluble or fat-soluble; these two groups are handled differently by the body. The water-soluble vitamins (except vitamin C) are members of the B-complex. Deficiency states in developed countries are rare, except in some impoverished populations (see Chapter 43) or after mistakes in food preparation, but are common in many developing countries and are often associated with global malnutrition (see Chapter 43). In the clinical setting, vitamin deficiencies may also occur as complications in children with various chronic disorders or diseases. Information obtained in the medical history related to dietary habits can be important in identifying the possibility of such nutritional problems. Except for vitamins A and D, toxicity from excess intake of vitamins is rare. The food sources, functions, and deficiency and excess symptoms of the vitamins are summarized in Tables 45-1 and 48-1.

VITAMIN A. Vitamin A is an essential micronutrient because it cannot be biogenerated de novo by animals. It must be obtained from plants in the form of provitamin-A carotenoids: α-, β-, and γ-carotenes; and β-cryptoxanthin. These substances can be converted to vitamin A compounds in the body.

The term *vitamin A* refers to *all-trans*-retinol, the alcohol form of the vitamin. The storage form of vitamin A is retinyl palmitate; the aldehyde form of vitamin A, retinal, functions in vision. The physiologically most important vitamin A metabolite is the acid derivative, retinoic acid. Retinoic acid functions at the gene level as a ligand for specific nuclear transcription factors; thus, the retinoid receptors regulate many genes involved in fundamental biologic activities of the cell. The term *retinoids* includes both natural and synthetic compounds with vitamin A activity and is most often used in the context of vitamin A action at the gene level.

Absorption, Transport, Metabolism, Storage. The body acquires vitamin A either as preformed vitamin A (usually as esters) or as provitamin-A carotenoids. In the USA, grains and vegetables supply approximately 55% of vitamin A intake from food, and dairy and meat products supply approximately 30%. Vitamin A as well as the provitamins-A are fat-soluble, and their absorption depends on the presence of adequate lipid and protein within the meal. Chronic intestinal disorders or lipid malabsorption syndromes may result in vitamin A deficiency. Ingested and absorbed provitamins-A are bioconverted to vitamin A molecules in the small intestine by the carotene cleavage enzyme dioxygenase; β-carotene provides twice the vitamin A activity of the other provitamins-A. Further processing in the enterocyte involves the esterification of vitamin A to retinyl palmitate and its incorporation into chylomicrons, which are released into lymph and transported via the circulation for storage to the liver or delivered to other tissues. At birth, the vitamin A content in the liver is low, but normally, it increases 60-fold during the first 6 mo of life. If the growing child has a well-balanced diet and obtains vitamin A from various foods that are rich in vitamin A or provitamin-A (see Table 45-1), the risk of vitamin A deficiency is small. However, even subclinical vitamin A deficiency may have serious consequences.

Stored vitamin A is released from the liver into the circulation as retinol bound to its specific transport protein, retinol-binding protein (RBP), which binds to the thyroid hormone transport protein, transthyretin; this complex delivers retinol (as well as the thyroid hormone) to tissues. Normal plasma levels of retinol are 20–50 μg/dL in infants and 30–225 μg/dL in older children and adults. Uncleaved provitamin-A carotenoids in the intestine are also incorporated into chylomicrons and delivered to various tissues. Malnutrition, particularly protein deficiency, can cause vitamin A deficiency by the impaired synthesis of retinol transport protein. However, if dietary vitamin A is provided, in the absence of RBP, vitamin A is transported to the tissues via chylomicrons and almost completely alleviates the symptoms of vitamin A deficiency. In developing countries, subclinical or clinical zinc deficiency may increase the risk of vitamin A deficiency. There is also some evidence of marginal zinc intakes in children in the USA.

Function and Mechanism of Action. Vitamin A is required throughout the life cycle, beginning with embryogenesis. Except for its role in vision, the pleiotropic actions of this micronutrient include many systemic functions that are mediated at the gene level by *all-trans*-retinoic acid (RA), which is a ligand for specific nuclear transcription factors, the retinoid receptors RARs and RXRs. When activated by the presence of RA, retinoid receptors bind to target genes that have specific recognition sites. Thus, vitamin A, via its active form, retinoic acid, regulates many genes that are involved in the fundamental biologic activities of cells, such as cell division, cell death, and cell differentiation. Thus, it affects many physiologic processes, including reproduction, growth, embryonic and fetal development, and bone development, in addition to respiratory, gastrointestinal, hematopoietic, and immune functions. The role in immune function and host defense is particularly important in developing countries, where vitamin A supplementation or therapy reduces the morbidity and mortality rates of various diseases, such as measles (see Chapter 122). Retinoic acid is among the most important signaling molecules in vertebrate ontogenesis.

The best understood function of vitamin A is its nongenomic role in vision. The human retina has two distinct photoreceptor systems: the rods, containing rhodopsin, which can detect low-intensity light, and the cones, containing iodopsin, which can detect different colors. The aldehyde form of vitamin A, retinal, is the prosthetic group on both visual proteins. The mechanism of vitamin A action in vision is based on the ability of the vitamin A molecule to photoisomerize (change shape when exposed to light). Thus, in the dark, low-intensity light isomerizes the rhodopsin prosthetic group, *11-cis* retinal, to *all-trans*-retinal; this generates an electrical signal that is transmitted via the optic nerve to the brain, resulting in visual sensation.

VITAMIN A DEFICIENCY

Clinical Manifestations. The most obvious symptoms of vitamin A deficiency are associated with the requirement of this vitamin for the maintenance of epithelial functions. In intestine, a normal, mucus-secreting epithelium is an effective barrier against a path-

TABLE 45-1. Vitamins A, B Complex, and C

NAMES AND SYNONYMS	CHARACTERISTICS	BIOCHEMICAL ACTION	EFFECTS OF DEFICIENCY	EFFECTS OF EXCESS	SOURCES
VITAMIN A					
Retinol (vitamin A_1); 1 μg retinol = 3.3 IU vitamin A = 1 RAE. Provitamins A: the plant pigments α-, β-, and γ-carotenes and cryptoxanthin have partial retinol activity: 12 μg β-carotene, or 24 μg of other provitamin A carotenoids = 1 μg retinol	Fat-soluble; heat-stable; destroyed by oxidation, drying; bile necessary for absorption; stored in liver; protected by vitamin E	In vision, as retinal, for synthesis of the visual pigments rhodopsin and iodopsin; in growth, reproduction, embryonic and fetal development, bone growth, immune and epithelial functions, via retinoic acid as a ligand for specific nuclear transcription factors, regulating genes involved in many fundamental cellular processes	Nyctalopia; photophobia, xerophthalmia, Bitot spots, conjunctivitis, keratomalacia leading to blindness; faulty epiphyseal bone formation; defective tooth enamel; keratinization of mucous membranes and skin; retarded growth; impaired resistance to infection, anemia, reproductive failure, fetal abnormalities	Anorexia, slow growth, drying and cracking of skin, enlargement of liver and spleen, swelling and pain of long bones, bone fragility, increased intracranial pressure, alopecia, carotenemia; fetal abnormalities	Liver, fish liver oils, dairy products, except skim milk; egg yolk, fortified margarines and fortified skim milk; carotenoids from plants: green vegetables, yellow fruits and vegetables
VITAMIN B COMPLEX					
Thiamin: vitamin B_1; (antiberiberi vitamin)	Water and alcohol soluble; fat-insoluble; stable in slightly acid solution; labile to heat, alkali, sulfites	Component of thiamine pyrophosphate involved in oxidative decarboxylation of α-keto acids, such as pyruvate, and in transketolation reactions	Beriberi, fatigue, irritability, anorexia, constipation, headache, insomnia, tachycardia, polyneuritis, cardiac failure, edema, elevated pyruvic acid in blood	None from oral intake	Meat, especially pork; whole-grain or enriched cereals; legumes; nuts, wheat germ; liver
Riboflavin: vitamin B_2	Sparingly soluble in water; sensitive to light and alkali; stable to heat, alkali, oxidation, acid	Constituent of flavoprotein enzymes important in oxidation-reduction reactions: amino acid, fatty acid, and carbohyrate metabolism and cellular respiration	Ariboflavinosis; photophobia blurred vision, burning and itching of eyes, corneal vascularization, poor growth, cheilosis	Not harmful	Milk, cheese; whole-grain or enriched grains; meat, fish; eggs; green leafy vegetables; liver and other organ meats
Niacin: nicotinamide; nicotinc acid (antipellagra vitamin)	Water- and alcohol-soluble; stable to acid, alkali, light, heat, oxidation	Constituent of NAD and NADP, coenzymes in numerous oxidation-reduction reactions	Pellagra, multiple B-vitamin deficiency syndrome, diarrhea, dementia, dermatitis	Nicotinic acid (not the amide) is vasodilator; skin flushing and itching; hepatopathy	Meat, fish, poultry; whole-grain and enriched cereals; green vegetables; peanuts; liver; also from conversion of trytophan to niacin
Vitamin B_6 active forms: pyridoxine, pyridoxal, pyridoxamine	Water-soluble; destroyed by ultraviolet light and by heat	Constituent of coenzymes for decarboxylation, transamination, trans-sulfuration; fatty acid metabolism; heme synthesis; homocysteine metabolism	Irritability, convulsions, hypochromic anemia; peripheral neuritis in patients receiving isoniazid; oxaluria	Sensory neuropathy (from high-dose supplements, not food)	Meat, fish, poultry; whole-grain and fortified cereals; soybeans; nuts; potatoes; noncitrus fruits; liver and kidney
Biotin	Crystallized from yeast; soluble in water	Coenzyme carboxylases; involved in CO_2 transfer	Dermatitis, seborrhea; inactivated by avidin in raw egg white	Unknown	Widely distributed in foods; animal products, yeast, liver
Pantothenic acid	Limited data on stability during cooking and food processing	Component of coenzyme A and acyl carrier protein involved in fatty acid metabolism	Experimentally produced deficiency in humans: irritability, fatigue, gastric complaints, numbness, paresthesias, muscle cramps	Unknown	Widely distributed in foods; beef, poultry, whole grains, liver and kidney, yeast, egg yolks
Folate: folic acid, folacin; a group of related compounds containing pteridine ring, para-amino benzoic acid, and glutamic acid; pteroylglutamic acid	Slightly soluble in water: labile to heat, light, acid	Concerned with formation and metabolism of 1-carbon units; participates in synthesis of purines, pyrimidines, nucleoproteins, homocysteine metabolism	Megaloblastic anemia (infancy, pregnancy) usually secondary to malabsorption disease, glossitis, pharyngeal ulcers, impaired immunity	Unknown	Green vegetables, enriched grain products, oranges and other fruits, legumes, nuts, liver, yeast
Vitamin B_{12}: cyanocobalamin	Slightly soluble in water; stable to heat in neutral solution; labile in acid or alkaline ones; destroyed by light; castle intrinsic factor of the stomach required for absorption	Transfer of 1-carbon units in purine and labile methyl group metabolism; essential for maturation of red blood cells in bone marrow; metabolism of nervous tissue; homocysteine metabolism; Adenosylcobalamin is coenzyme for methylmalonyl coenzyme A mutase	Pernicious anemia due to defect in absorption rather than dietary lack; also secondary to gastrectomy, celiac disease, inflammatory lesions of small bowel, long-term drug therapy (PAS, neomycin); methylmalonic aciduria; homocystinuria	Unknown	Animal foods: muscle and organ meats, fish; eggs; milk; cheese; fortified cereal products; fortified soy products
VITAMIN C					
Ascorbic acid, antiscorbutic vitamin	Water-soluble; easily oxidized, accelerated by heat, light, alkali, oxidative enzymes, traces of copper or iron	As an antioxidant, maintains Fe and Cu ions in reduced state in hydroxylases involved in collagen synthesis, metabolism of cholesterol and neurotransmitters; may be needed to maintain folate in a reduced form; facilitates non-heme Fe absorption and Fe transfer from tansferritin to ferritin	Scurvy: poor wound healing, bleeding gums, petechiae, ecchymoses, follicular hyperkeratosis, arthralgia	Adverse effects usually not serious; may include osmotic diarrhea, other gastrointestinal symptoms; oxaluria	Citrus fruits, tomatoes, berries, cantaloupe, cabbage, broccoli, cauliflower, spinach, potatoes; cooking has destructive effect

NAD(P), Nicotinamide adenine dinucleotide (phosphate); PAS, para-aminosalicylic acid

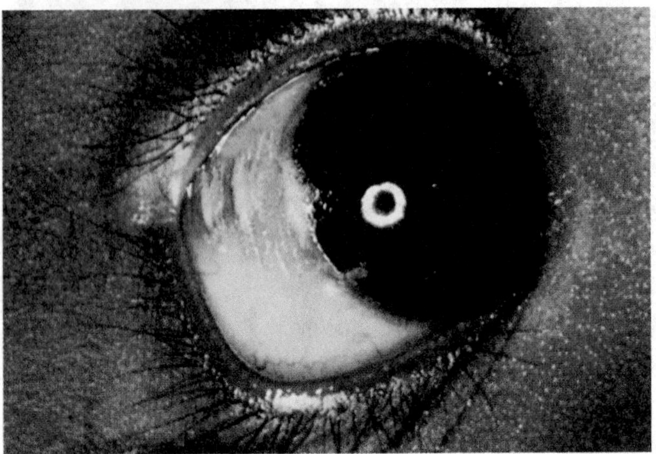

Figure 45-1. Bitot spots with hyperpigmentation seen in a 10 mo old Indonesian boy. (Oomen HAPC: Vitamin A deficiency, xerophthalmia and blindness. *Nutr Rev* 1974;6:161–166.)

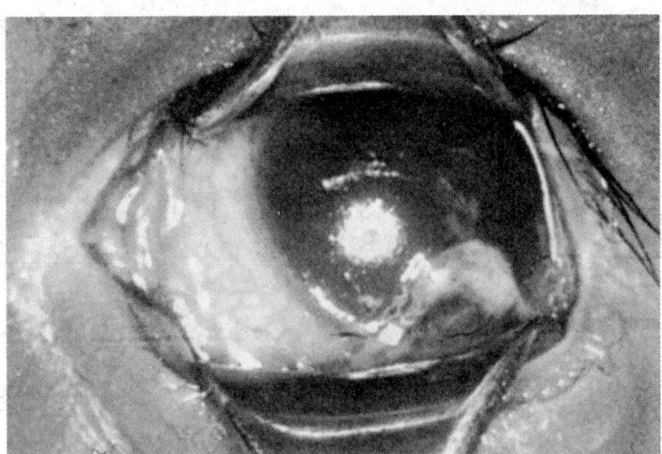

Figure 45-2. Advanced xerophthalmia with an opaque, dull cornea and some damage to the iris in a 1 yr old boy. (Oomen HAPC: Vitamin A deficiency, xerophthalmia and blindness. *Nutr Rev* 1974;6:161–166.)

ogenic attack that can cause diarrhea. Similarly, in the respiratory tract, a mucus-secreting epithelium is essential for the disposal of inhaled pathogens and toxicants. Epithelial changes in the respiratory system can result in bronchial obstruction. Characteristic changes due to vitamin A deficiency in the epithelia include a proliferation of basal cells, hyperkeratosis, and the formation of stratified, cornified squamous epithelium. Squamous metaplasia of the renal pelves, ureters, vaginal epithelium, and the pancreatic and salivary ducts may lead to increased infections in these areas. In the urinary bladder, loss of epithelial integrity may result in pyuria and hematuria. Epithelial changes in the skin due to vitamin A deficiency are manifested as dry, scaly, hyperkeratotic patches, commonly on the arms, legs, shoulders, and buttocks. The combination of defective epithelial barriers to infection, low immune response, and lowered response to inflammatory stress, all due to insufficient vitamin A, can cause poor growth and serious health problems in children. The most characteristic and specific signs of vitamin A deficiency are eye lesions. Lesions due to vitamin A deficiency develop insidiously and rarely occur before 2 yr of age. An early symptom is delayed adaptation to the dark; later when vitamin A deficiency is more advanced, it leads to **night blindness** due to the absence of retinal in the visual pigment, rhodopsin, of the retina. Photophobia is a common symptom. As vitamin A deficiency progresses, the epithelial tissues of the eye become severely altered.

The cornea protects the eye from the environment and is also important in light refraction. In early vitamin A deficiency, the cornea keratinizes, becomes opaque, is susceptible to infection, and forms dry, scaly layers of cells (**xerophthalmia**). In later stages, infection occurs, lymphocytes infiltrate, and the cornea becomes wrinkled; it degenerates irreversibly (keratomalacia), resulting in blindness. The conjunctiva keratinizes and develops plaques (**Bitot spots** [Fig. 45-1]), it becomes dry (**conjunctival xerosis**), and the lacrimal glands keratinize. The pigment epithelium, the structural element of the retina, keratinizes. When it degenerates, the rods and cones have no support, so they break down and blindness results. Advanced xerophthalmia is shown in Figure 45-2; xerophthalmia with permanent damage to the eye is shown in Figure 45-3. These eye lesions are primarily diseases of the young and are a major cause of blindness in developing countries. Other clinical signs of vitamin A deficiency may include poor overall growth, diarrhea, susceptibility to infections, anemia, apathy, mental retardation, and increased intracranial pressure with wide separation of the cranial bones at the sutures. There may be vision problems due to bone overgrowth causing pressure on the optic nerve.

Diagnosis. Dark adaptation tests can be used to assess early-stage vitamin A deficiency. Although Bitot spots develop early, those related to active vitamin A deficiency are usually confined to preschool-aged children. Xerophthalmia is a very characteristic lesion of vitamin A deficiency. Caution must be exercised to exclude other, similar eye abnormalities from those associated with vitamin A deficiency. To detect marginal vitamin A status, there are 3 useful indicators: conjunctival impression cytology, relative dose response, and modified relative dose response. There is a relatively high prevalence of marginal vitamin A state among pregnant and lactating women. The plasma retinol level is not an accurate indicator of vitamin A status unless the deficiency is severe and liver stores are depleted.

The range of normal vitamin A levels is 20–60 µg/dL; a level <20 µg/dL occurs in deficiency.

Prevention. The daily recommended dietary allowance (RDA) is expressed as retinol activity equivalents (RAEs; 1 RAE = 1 µg *all-trans*-retinol; equivalents for provitamin-A in foods = 12 µg β-carotene, 24 µg α-carotene, or 24 µg β-cryptoxanthin). The

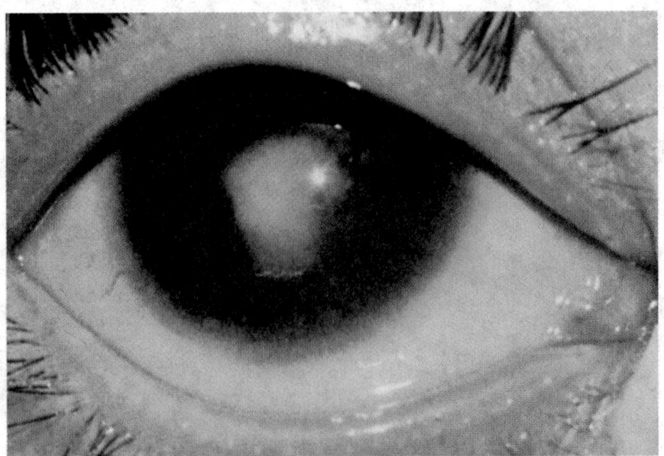

Figure 45-3. Recovery from xerophthalmia, showing a permanent eye lesion. (From Bloch CE: Blindness and other diseases arising from deficient nutrition [lack of fat soluble A factor]. *Am J Dis Child* 1924;27:139.)

RAE for infants 0–1 yr of age is 400–500 µg; for children 3 yr of age, 300 µg; for children 4–8 yr of age, 400 µg; for children 9–13 yr of age, 600 µg; for boys 14–18 yr of age and men, 900 µg; and for girls 14–18 of age and women, 700 µg (also see Table 41-2). During pregnancy, the RDA is 750–770 µg, whereas during lactation, it is increased to 1200–1300 µg to ensure sufficient vitamin A content during breast-feeding. A daily tolerable upper level of vitamin A for adults is 3,000 µg of preformed vitamin A. Approximately 80% of dietary vitamin A is absorbed as long as the meal contains some fat (>10 g). Low-fat diets may need to be supplemented with vitamin A. In disorders with poor fat absorption or increased excretion of vitamin A, water-miscible preparations should be administered in amounts higher than the RDAs. Premature infants have poor lipid absorption; thus, they should receive water-miscible vitamin A and should be monitored closely.

Epidemiology, Public Health Issues. Vitamin A deficiency and xerophthalmia occur throughout much of the developing world and are linked to undernourishment and complicated by illness. More than 350,000 cases of childhood blindness are reported annually due to severe vitamin A deficiency. Because maternal vitamin A status is reflected in the vitamin A content of breast milk, intervention trials are ongoing with mothers of breast-fed infants living in regions where vitamin A deficiency is common. In these trials, 2 doses of 200,000 IU (60 mg) each of vitamin A are given to the mother immediately postpartum, and their infants are given 3 doses of 25, 000 IU (1.2 mg) each of vitamin A at 1–3 mo of age. (Note: 1 IU = 0.3 µg retinol).

Treatment. The safety and efficacy of vitamin A supplementation depend on the individual's state of health and the regimens of other treatments. A daily supplement of 1,500 µg of vitamin A is sufficient for treating latent vitamin A deficiency. In children without overt vitamin A deficiency, morbidity and mortality rates from viral infections such as measles can be lowered by daily administration of 1,500–3,000 µg of vitamin A, under careful monitoring to avoid toxicity associated with excess vitamin A. Xerophthalmia is treated by giving 1,500 µg/kg body weight orally for 5 days followed by intramuscular injection of 7,500 µg of vitamin A in oil, until recovery.

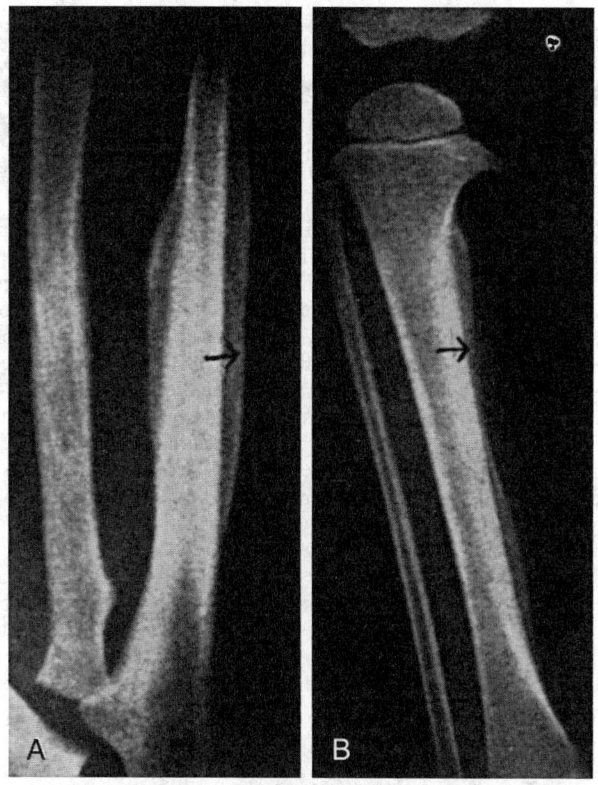

Figure 45-4. Hyperostosis of the ulna and tibia in an infant 21 mo of age, resulting from vitamin A positioning. *A*, Long, wavy cortical hyperostosis of the ulna *(arrow)*. *B*, Long, wavy cortical hyperostosis of the right tibia *(arrow)*, with a striking absence of metaphyseal changes, (From Caffey J: *Pediatric X-ray Diagnosis*, 5th ed. Chicago, Year Book, 1967, p 994.)

HYPERVITAMINOSIS A. Chronic hypervitaminosis A results from excessive ingestion of vitamin A for several weeks or months. Toxicity can be induced in adults and children with chronic daily intakes of 15,000 µg and 6,000 µg, respectively. Symptoms subside rapidly on withdrawal of the vitamin. Signs of subacute or chronic toxicity may include headache; vomiting; anorexia; dry, itchy desquamating skin; seborrheic cutaneous lesions; fissuring at the corners of the mouth; alopecia and /or coarsening of the hair; bone abnormalities; swelling of the bones; enlargement of the liver and spleen; diplopia; increased intracranial pressure; irritability; stupor; limited motion; and dryness of the mucous membranes. In addition, desquamation of the palms and the soles of the feet is common. Radiographs show **hyperostosis** affecting several long bones, especially in the middle of the shafts (Fig. 45-4). Serum levels of vitamin A are elevated. Hypercalcemia and/or liver cirrhosis may be present. Hypervitaminosis A is distinct from cortical hyperostosis (see Chapter 698).

In young children, toxicity is associated with vomiting and bulging fontanelles. An affected child has anorexia, pruritus, and a lack of weight gain. Acute hypervitaminosis A toxicity has occurred in infants in developing countries after ingestion of very high amounts of vitamin A during vaccine administration. Symptoms include nausea, vomiting, and drowsiness; less common symptoms include diplopia, papilledema, cranial nerve palsies, and other symptoms suggestive of **pseudotumor cerebri.** Severe congenital malformations occur in infants of mothers who consumed therapeutic doses (0.5–1.5 mg/kg) of oral 13-*cis*-retinoic acid during the 1st trimester of pregnancy for treatment of acne or cancer. This results in a high incidence (>20%) of spontaneous abortions and birth defects.

Excessive intake of carotenoids is not associated with toxicity, but may cause yellow coloration of the skin that disappears when intake is reduced; this disorder (carotenemia) is especially likely to occur in children with liver disease, diabetes mellitus, or hypothyroidism, and in those who do not have enzymes that metabolize carotenoids.

Benn CS, Martins C, Rodrigues A, et al: Randomized study of effect of different doses of vitamin A on childhood morbidity and mortality. *BMJ* 2005;331:1428–1430.

Erhardt J: Biochemical methods for the measurement of vitamin A deficiency disorders (VADD). *Sight and Life* 2003;2:5–7.

Gropper SS, Smith JL, Groff JL (editors): *Advanced Nutrition and Human Metabolism,* 4th ed. Belmont, CA, Thomson Wadsworth, 2005.

Labadarios D, Randal P: Presentation highlights: Vitamin A and the common agenda for micronutrients. XXII IVACG meeting, 15–17 November 2004, Lima, Peru. *Sight and Life* 2005;1:9–17.

Sommer A, West, KP Jr: Treatment of vitamin A deficiency and xerophthalmia. In *Vitamin A Deficiency: Health Survival and Vision.* New York, Oxford University Press, 1996.

Sporn MB, Roberts AB, Goodman DS (editors): *The Retinoids: Biology, Chemistry and Medicine,* 2nd ed. New York, Raven Press, 1994.

Chapter 46 ■ Vitamin B Complex Deficiency and Excess

Wanda L. Chenoweth

All of the water-soluble vitamins are included as part of the vitamin B complex except vitamin C. These essential nutrients include thiamine, riboflavin, niacin, vitamin B_6, folate, vitamin B_{12}, biotin, and pantothenic acid. Choline and inositol, also considered part of the B complex, are important for normal body functions. However, specific deficiency syndromes have not been attributed to a lack of these factors in the diet.

B-complex vitamins serve as coenzymes in many metabolic pathways that are functionally closely related. Consequently, a lack of 1 of the vitamins has the potential to interrupt a chain of chemical processes, including reactions that are dependent on other vitamins, and ultimately may produce diverse clinical manifestations.

Because diets deficient in any 1 of the B-complex vitamins are frequently poor sources of other B vitamins, manifestations of several vitamin B deficiencies usually can be observed in the same person. It is advisable to treat a patient with evidence of deficiency of a specific B vitamin with the entire complex of B vitamins.

46.1 • Thiamine (Vitamin B_1)

Thiamine (vitamin B_1) provides the functional group for the coenzyme thiamine pyrophosphate, which is involved in decarboxylation of pyruvate and α-ketoglutarate and, thus, is important in the release of energy from carbohydrates. It also participates in the hexose monophosphate shunt that generates nicotinamide adenine dinucleotide phosphate and pentose.

Thiamine also is required for the synthesis of acetylcholine, and deficiency results in impaired nerve conduction.

Good sources of thiamine include meat (especially lean pork), legumes, and cereals. Unless enriched, refined cereals and flours have a much lower content of thiamine than whole grains. The vitamin is easily destroyed by heat, particularly in alkaline media, and significant amounts are lost in discarded cooking water. The breast milk of a well-nourished mother provides adequate thiamine; breast-fed infants of thiamine-deficient mothers, however, are at risk for deficiency. Most infants and older children obtain an adequate intake of thiamine from food and do not require supplements.

Thiamine is absorbed efficiently in the gastrointestinal tract, but may be decreased in persons with gastrointestinal or liver disease. **Deficiency (beriberi)** has been reported in adolescents after gastric bypass surgery. Intakes in excess of tissue needs are excreted in the urine. Fever and/or stress may increase the requirement for thiamine and unmask marginal thiamine sufficiency, but these factors are unlikely to cause deficiency. **Thiamine dependence** has been described in a child with megaloblastic anemia and in an infant with otherwise typical maple syrup urine disease. In addition, the urine of children with Leigh encephalomyelopathy as well as that of their parents inhibits the formation of thiamine pyrophosphate, and large doses of thiamine improve some of the abnormalities associated with the disease.

THIAMINE DEFICIENCY

CLINICAL MANIFESTATIONS. Early manifestations of thiamine deficiency include fatigue, apathy, irritability, depression, drowsiness, poor mental concentration, anorexia, nausea, and abdominal discomfort (see Table 45-1). As the condition progresses, other manifestations include peripheral neuritis, with tingling, burning, and paresthesias of the toes and feet; decreased deep tendon reflexes; loss of vibration sense; tenderness and cramping of the leg muscles; congestive heart failure; and psychic disturbances. Patients may have ptosis of the eyelids and atrophy of the optic nerve. Hoarseness or aphonia caused by paralysis of the laryngeal nerve is a characteristic sign. Muscle atrophy and tenderness of the nerve trunks are followed by ataxia, loss of coordination, and loss of deep sensation. Later signs include increased intracranial pressure, meningismus, and coma.

An epidemic of life-threatening thiamine deficiency was seen in infants fed a defective soy-based formula that had undetectable thiamine levels. Manifestations included emesis, lethargy, restlessness, ophthalmoplegia, abdominal distention, developmental delay, failure to thrive, lactic acidosis, nystagmus, diarrhea, apnea, and seizures. Intercurrent illnesses that resembled Wernicke encephalopathy often precipitated the symptoms.

A severe deficiency of thiamine leads to the deficiency disease **beriberi.** Two forms exist, wet beriberi and dry beriberi. The child with wet beriberi is undernourished, pale, and edematous; has dyspnea, vomiting, and tachycardia; and has waxy skin. The urine often contains albumin and casts. The child with dry beriberi appears plump, but is pale, flabby, and listless, with dyspnea, tachycardia, and hepatomegaly.

Death from thiamine deficiency usually is secondary to cardiac involvement. The initial signs are slight cyanosis and dyspnea, but tachycardia, enlargement of the liver, loss of consciousness, and convulsions may develop rapidly. The heart, especially the right side, is enlarged. The electrocardiogram shows an increased Q-T interval, inverted T waves, and low voltage. These changes as well as the cardiomegaly rapidly revert to normal with treatment, but without prompt treatment, cardiac failure can develop rapidly and result in death. In fatal cases of beriberi, lesions are located principally in the heart, peripheral nerves, subcutaneous tissue, and serous cavities. The heart is dilated, and fatty degeneration of the myocardium is common. Generalized edema or edema of the legs, serous effusions, and venous engorgement are often present. Degeneration of myelin and axon cylinders of the peripheral nerves, with wallerian degeneration beginning in the distal locations, also is common, particularly in the lower extremities. Lesions in the brain include vascular dilation and hemorrhage.

DIAGNOSIS. The early symptoms of thiamine deficiency are nonspecific and of limited value in establishing a diagnosis. Low red blood cell transketolase activity is the best indicator of deficiency of thiamine in body tissues. Urinary excretion of thiamine or its metabolites, thiazole or pyrimidine, after an oral loading dose of thiamine may be measured to help identify the deficiency state. High blood or urinary glyoxylate levels also may be used as diagnostic indicators. Clinical response to administration of thiamine is the best test for thiamine deficiency, but does not necessarily rule out the coexistence of other B vitamin deficiencies.

PREVENTION. A maternal diet containing sufficient amounts of thiamine prevents thiamine deficiency in breast-fed infants, and infant formulas marketed in all developed countries provide recommended levels of intake. After a period of exclusive breastfeeding or formula-feeding, adequate thiamine intake can be achieved with a varied diet that includes meat and enriched or whole-grain cereals. Thiamine requirements are higher if the carbohydrate content of the diet is high, but this is rarely a problem, except possibly in patients maintained on parenteral feedings with a high glucose content.

TREATMENT. If beriberi develops in a breast-fed infant, both the mother and the child should be treated with thiamine. The daily dose for children and adults, respectively, is 10 mg and 50 mg. In the absence of gastrointestinal disturbances, oral administration is effective. Children with cardiac failure should be given thiamine intramuscularly or intravenously. Dramatic improvement usually occurs, but complete cure requires several weeks of treatment. The heart is not permanently damaged. Patients with beriberi often have other B-complex vitamin deficiencies; therefore, all other B-complex vitamins also should be administered.

TOXICITY. There are no reports of adverse effects from consumption of excess thiamine by ingestion of food or supplements. A few isolated cases of pruritus and anaphylaxis have been reported in patients after parenteral administration of the vitamin.

46.2 • Riboflavin (Vitamin B_2)

Riboflavin is part of the structure of the coenzymes flavin adenine dinucleotide (FAD) and flavin mononucleotide, which provide the functional groups for several enzymes important in electron transport. Riboflavin is essential for growth and tissue respiration. It also may play a role in light adaptation, and it is required for conversion of pyridoxine to pyridoxal phosphate. Riboflavin is stable to heat, but is destroyed by light. In the USA adult population, the major sources of riboflavin are milk and milk drinks, followed by enriched and fortified cereals and bread products. Other sources of riboflavin are eggs, legumes, meat, dark green vegetables, organ meats, and brewer's yeast.

RIBOFLAVIN DEFICIENCY

A single deficiency of riboflavin is rare, but deficiency symptoms frequently are present in deficiencies of other B-complex vitamins (see Table 45-1). Inadequate intake is the most common cause of deficiency, but faulty absorption may contribute in patients with biliary atresia or hepatitis as well as in those receiving probenecid, phenothiazine, or oral contraceptives. Increased destruction of riboflavin has been reported in infants with neonatal jaundice who were treated with phototherapy.

CLINICAL MANIFESTATIONS. Signs and/or symptoms of riboflavin deficiency include cheilosis (perlèche), glossitis, keratitis, conjunctivitis, photophobia, lacrimation, marked corneal vascularization, and seborrheic dermatitis. Cheilosis begins with pallor at the angles of the mouth and progresses to thinning and maceration of the epithelium. Superficial fissures, often covered by yellow crusts, develop in the angles of the mouth and extend radially into the skin for distances of 1–2 cm. With glossitis, the tongue is smooth, with loss of papillary structure. There is evidence that poor riboflavin status interferes with iron handling, which may explain the anemia that is common in riboflavin deficiency, especially when iron intakes are low.

DIAGNOSIS. The signs and symptoms of riboflavin deficiency are too nonspecific to make a definitive diagnosis. A functional test of riboflavin status is done by measuring the activity of erythrocyte glutathione reductase (EGR), with and without the addition of FAD. An EGR activity coefficient (ratio of EGR activity with added FAD to EGR activity without FAD) of >1.4 is used as an indicator of deficiency. Urinary excretion of riboflavin <30 µg/24 hr suggests low or deficient intakes.

PREVENTION. Reference daily intakes of riboflavin for children up to 8 yr of age are presented in Table 41-1. The recommended dietary allowance (RDA) for children 9–13 yr of age is 0.9 mg/day; for adolescents 14–18 yr of age, it increases to 1.0 mg/day (females) and 1.3 mg/day (males). Deficiency is unlikely if diets contain adequate amounts of milk, eggs, enriched or fortified cereal products, meats, and dark green vegetables.

TREATMENT. Treatment includes oral administration of 3–10 mg/day of riboflavin. If no response occurs within a few days, intramuscular injections of 2 mg of riboflavin in saline may be given as often as 3 times/day. The child should also be given a well-balanced diet, including, at least temporarily, generous supplements of other B-complex vitamins.

TOXICITY. No adverse effects associated with riboflavin intakes from food or supplements have been reported.

46.3 • Niacin

The term *niacin* refers to nicotinamide (niacinamide), nicotinic acid, and derivatives that show the same biologic activity as nicotinamide. Nicotinamide forms part of 2 cofactors, nicotinamide adenine dinucleotide and nicotinamide adenine dinucleotide phosphate, which are important in electron transfer and glycolysis. Dietary tryptophan can be converted to niacin, but the amount is insufficient to meet the total needs for the vitamin. Major food sources of niacin in the diet are meat, fish, and poultry. Enriched and whole-grain bread and bread products as well as fortified cereal products and legumes also are major contributors to niacin intake. Milk and eggs contain little niacin, but are good sources of tryptophan, which can be converted to nicotinamide adenine dinucleotide (60 mg tryptophan = 1 mg niacin).

NIACIN DEFICIENCY

Pellagra, the deficiency disease caused by a lack of niacin, affects all tissues of the body. It occurs chiefly in countries where corn (maize), a poor source of tryptophan, is the major foodstuff (Table 45-1).

CLINICAL MANIFESTATIONS. The early symptoms of pellagra are vague: anorexia, lassitude, weakness, burning sensations, numbness, and dizziness. After a long period of deficiency, the classic triad of dermatitis, diarrhea, and dementia appears. Manifestations in children with parasites or chronic disorders may be especially severe.

Dermatitis, the most characteristic manifestation of pellagra, may develop suddenly or insidiously and may be elicited by irritants, including intense sunlight. The lesions first appear as symmetric areas of erythema on exposed surfaces, resembling sunburn. Thus, in mild cases, the dermatitis may not be recognized. The lesions are usually sharply demarcated from the healthy skin around them, and their distribution may change frequently. The lesions on the hands often have the appearance of a glove (Fig. 46-1). Similar demarcations may also occur on the foot and leg (pellagrous boot) or around the neck (Casal necklace) [Fig. 46-2]. In some cases, vesicles and bullae develop (wet type). In others, there may be suppuration beneath the scaly, crusted epidermis, and in still others, the swelling may disappear after a short time, followed by desquamation (Fig. 46-3). The healed parts of the skin may remain pigmented. The cutaneous lesions may be preceded by or accompanied by stomatitis, glossitis, vomiting, and/or diarrhea. Swelling and redness of the tip of the tongue and its lateral margins is often followed by intense redness, even ulceration, of the entire tongue and the papillae. Nervous symptoms include depression, disorientation, insomnia, and delirium.

The classic symptoms of pellagra usually are not well developed in infants and young children, but anorexia, irritability,

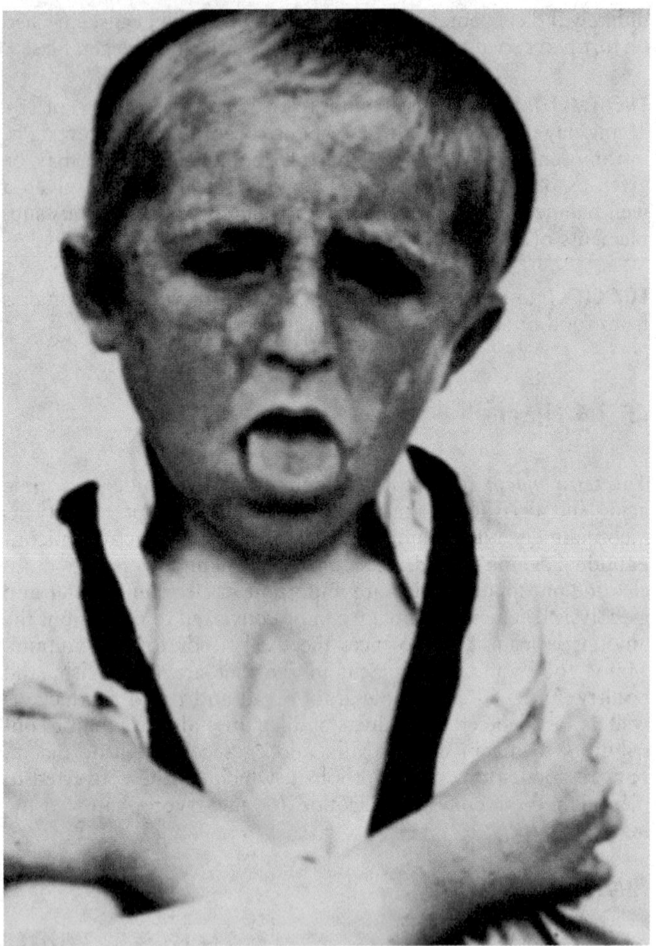

Figure 46-1. Boy with pellagra showing characteristic skin lesions on areas of the skin exposed to sunlight. (From *Nutrition Today Teaching Aid YP30. Vitamins, Minerals, and Water,* 1979. Slide 13.)

anxiety, and apathy are common. They may also have sore tongues and lips, and their skin is usually dry and scaly. Diarrhea and constipation may alternate, and a moderate secondary anemia may occur. Children who have pellagra often have evidence of other nutritional deficiency diseases.

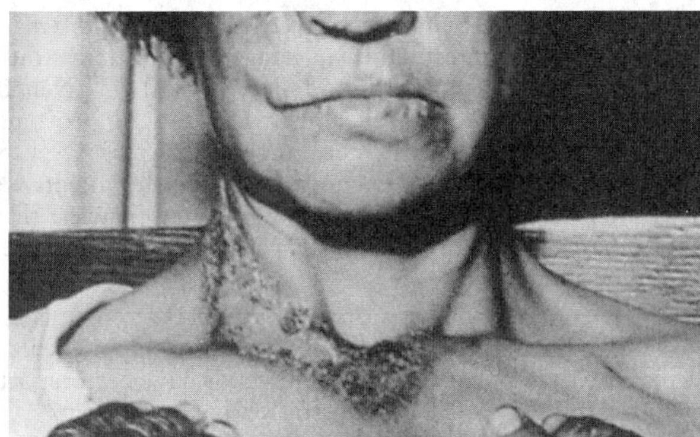

Figure 46-2. Pellagra showing an early lesion on the neck (Casal necklace).

PATHOLOGY. Histologically, there is edema and degeneration of the superficial collagen of the dermis. The papillary vessels are engorged, and there is perivascular lymphocytic infiltration. The epidermis is hyperkeratotic and later becomes atrophic. Changes similar to those in the skin also are present in the tongue, buccal mucous membranes, and vagina. These may be associated with secondary infection and ulceration.

The walls of the colon are thickened and inflamed, with patches of pseudomembrane and usually mucosal atrophy. Changes in the nervous system occur relatively late in the disease. These include patchy areas of demyelination and degeneration of ganglion cells; demyelination of both the posterior and the lateral columns may be seen in the spinal cord.

DIAGNOSIS. Because of lack of a good functional test to evaluate niacin status, the diagnosis of deficiency is usually made from the physical signs of glossitis, gastrointestinal symptoms, and a symmetric dermatitis. Rapid clinical response to niacin is an important confirming test. A decrease in the concentration and/or a change in the proportion of the niacin metabolites N^1-methylnicotinamide and 2-pyridone in the urine provide biochemical evidence of deficiency and can be seen before the appearance of overt signs of deficiency.

PREVENTION. Adequate intakes of niacin are easily met by consumption of a diet that consists of a variety of foods and includes meat, eggs, milk, and enriched or fortified cereal products. Sup-

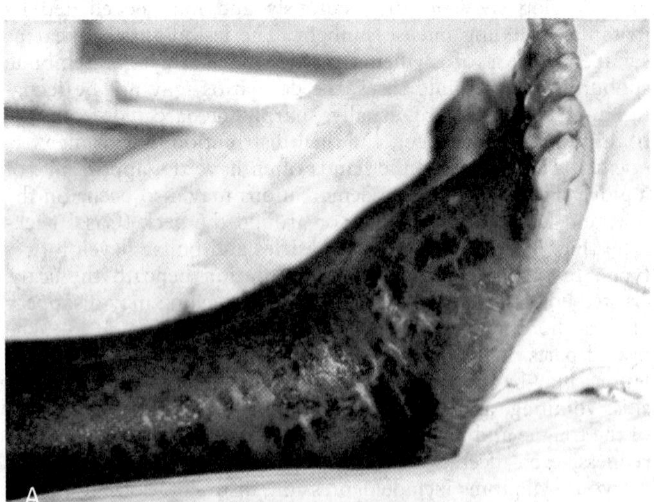

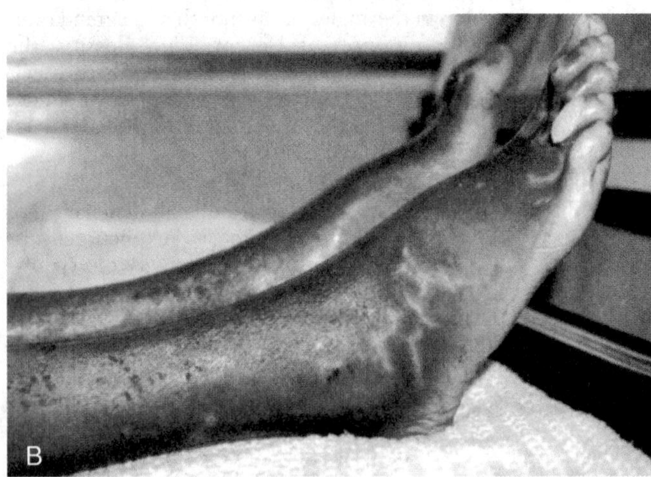

Figure 46-3. Clinical manifestations of niacin deficiency before *(A)* and after *(B)* therapy. (From Weinsier RL, Morgan SL: *Fundamentals of Clinical Nutrition.* St. Louis; Mosby, 1993, p 99.)

plements of niacin are necessary only in breast-fed infants whose mothers have pellagra or in children consuming very restricted diets.

TREATMENT. Children usually respond rapidly to treatment. A liberal and varied diet should be supplemented with 50–300/day of niacin; in severe cases or in cases of poor intestinal absorption, 100 mg may be given intravenously. The diet also should be supplemented with other vitamins, especially other B-complex vitamins. Sun exposure should be avoided during the active phase of pellagra, and the skin lesions may be covered with soothing applications. Hypochromic anemia, if present, should be treated with iron. Even after successful treatment, the diet should continue to be monitored to prevent recurrence.

TOXICITY. There are no toxic effects associated with the intake of naturally occurring niacin in foods. However, shortly after the ingestion of large doses of nicotinic acid taken as a supplement or a pharmacologic agent, a person often experiences a burning, tingling, and itching sensation as well as a reddened flush on the face, arms, and chest. These adverse effects are not produced by niacinamide. Large doses of niacin also may have nonspecific gastrointestinal effects and may cause cholestatic jaundice or hepatotoxicity. Tolerable upper intake levels for children are approximately double the recommended dietary allowance.

46.4 • Vitamin B_6 (Pyridoxine)

Vitamin B_6 includes a group of interchangeable compounds: pyridoxine, pyridoxal, and pyridoxamine, and their 5′-phosphate derivatives. Pyridoxal 5′-phosphate (PLP) and, to a lesser extent, pyridoxamine phosphate, function as coenzymes for many enzymes involved in amino acid metabolism, including aminotransferases, decarboxylases, racemases, and dehydratases. PLP-dependent reactions are involved in the synthesis of many essential compounds: neurotransmitters, such as serotonin (from 5-hydroxytryptophan), γ-amino butyric acid (from glutamate), and dopamine; histamine; heme; and porphyrins. Other roles of vitamin B_6 include participation in the metabolism of glycogen, conversion of tryptophan to niacin, synthesis of cysteine from methionine, active transport of amino acids across cell membranes, chelation of metals, and synthesis of arachidonic and docosahexaenoic acids from linoleic and linolenic acids, respectively. If vitamin B_6 is lacking, glycine metabolism may lead to oxaluria. The major excretory product in the urine is 4-pyridoxic acid.

The vitamin B_6 content of human milk and infant formulas is adequate. Good food sources of the vitamin include fortified ready-to-eat cereals, meat, fish, poultry, liver, and certain vegetables. Large losses of the vitamin may occur during high-temperature processing of foods or milling of cereals. Recommended intakes of vitamin B_6 are given in Table 41-1. Because of the importance of the vitamin in amino acid metabolism, high protein intakes may increase the requirement for vitamin B_6; however, the RDAs are sufficient to cover the expected range of protein intakes in the population. The risk of deficiency is increased in persons receiving drug therapies that inhibit the activity of vitamin B_6 (isoniazid, penicillamine, corticosteroids, anticonvulsants), in young women taking oral progesterone-estrogen contraceptives, and in patients receiving maintenance dialysis.

PYRIDOXINE DEFICIENCY

CLINICAL MANIFESTATIONS. Several types of vitamin B_6 **dependence syndromes,** presumably due to errors in enzyme structure or function, respond to very large amounts of pyridoxine (see Table 45-1). These syndromes include vitamin B_6–dependent convulsions, a vitamin B_6–responsive anemia, xanthurenic aciduria, cystathioninuria, and homocystinuria (see Chapters 85, 451, and 593).

Signs and symptoms of vitamin B_6 deficiency observed in patients with one of the vitamin B_6 dependence syndromes or in individuals with low dietary intakes include convulsions in infants, peripheral neuritis, dermatitis, and anemia. Infants fed a formula deficient in vitamin B_6 for 1–6 mo exhibit irritability and generalized seizures. Electroencephalogram (EEG) abnormalities have been reported in infants as well as in young adult subjects in controlled depletion studies. Gastrointestinal distress and an aggravated startle response also are common. Peripheral neuropathy may occur during treatment of tuberculosis with isonicotinic acid hydrazide. The neuropathy responds to the administration of pyridoxine or to a decrease in the dose of the drug. Skin lesions include cheilosis, glossitis, and seborrheic dermatitis around the eyes, nose, and mouth. Microcytic anemia, although not common in infants, may occur. Oxaluria, oxalic acid bladder stones, hyperglycinemia, lymphopenia, decreased antibody formation, and infections also have been associated with vitamin B_6 deficiency.

DIAGNOSIS. The activity of the erythrocyte transaminases glutamic oxaloacetic transaminase and glutamic pyruvic transaminase is low in vitamin B_6 deficiency; thus, tests measuring the activity of these enzymes before and after the addition of PLP may be useful as indicators of vitamin B_6 status. Abnormally high xanthurenic acid excretion after tryptophan ingestion also provides evidence of deficiency. Plasma PLP assays are being used more frequently, but factors other than deficiency may influence the results. All infants with seizures should be suspected of having vitamin B_6 deficiency or dependence. If more common causes of infantile seizures (e.g., hypocalcemia, hypoglycemia, infection) are eliminated, 100 mg of pyridoxine should be injected. If the seizure stops, vitamin B_6 deficiency should be suspected. In older children, 100 mg of pyridoxine may be injected intramuscularly while the EEG is being recorded; a favorable response of the EEG suggests pyridoxine deficiency.

PREVENTION. Deficiency is unlikely in children consuming diets that meet their energy needs and contain a variety of foods. Low intakes may occur with vegetarian diets. RDA of vitamin B_6 range from 0.3 mg for older infants to 1.2 mg and 1.3 mg for adolescent females and males, respectively. Infants whose mothers have received large doses of pyridoxine during pregnancy are at increased risk for seizures from pyridoxine dependence, and supplements during the 1st few weeks of life should be considered. Any child receiving a pyridoxine antagonist, such as isoniazid, should be carefully observed for neurologic manifestations; if these develop, vitamin B_6 should be administered or the dose of the antagonist should be decreased.

TREATMENT. Intramuscular administration of 100 mg of pyridoxine is used to treat convulsions due to vitamin B_6 deficiency. One dose should be sufficient if adequate dietary intake follows. For pyridoxine-dependent children, daily doses of 2–10 mg intramuscularly or 10–100 mg orally may be necessary.

TOXICITY. Adverse effects have not been associated with high intakes of vitamin B_6 from food sources. However, ataxia and sensory neuropathy have been reported with dosages as low as 100 mg/day in adults taking vitamin B_6 supplements for several months.

46.5 • BIOTIN

Biotin is used as a cofactor for enzymes involved in carboxylation reactions. In humans, there are 5 biotin-dependent carboxylases that catalyze key reactions in gluconeogenesis, fatty acid metabolism, and amino acid catabolism. There is limited information on the biotin content of foods; however, it is believed to be widely distributed, thus making a deficiency unlikely. Avidin found in raw egg whites acts as a biotin antagonist. Signs of biotin deficiency have been demonstrated in individuals who consume large amounts of raw egg whites over long periods. Deficiency also has been described in infants and children receiving parenteral nutrition infusates not containing biotin. The clinical findings of biotin deficiency include dermatitis, conjunctivitis, alopecia, and central nervous system abnormalities (see Table 45-1). Conditions involving deficiencies in the enzymes holocarboxylase synthetase and biotinidase that respond to treatment with biotin are described in Chapter 85.6.

46.6 • FOLATE

Folate exists in a number of different chemical forms. Folic acid (pteroylglutamic acid) is the synthetic form used in fortified foods and supplements. Naturally occurring folates in foods (pteroylpolyglutamate) are not used as well as folic acid. Folate coenzymes are involved in a variety of reactions, including synthesis of deoxyribonucleic acid and purine, amino acid interconversion, and conversion of homocysteine to methionine. Because of its role in protein synthesis, the risk of deficiency is increased during periods of rapid growth or increased cellular metabolism. Impaired folate status may be associated with long-term drug treatment of various non-neoplastic diseases, including the use of high-dose nonsteroidal anti-inflammatory drugs; the anticonvulsants diphenylhydantoin and phenobarbital; and methotrexate used in the treatment of rheumatoid arthritis, psoriasis, asthma, and inflammatory bowel disease. The hematologic effects of folate deficiency are discussed in Chapter 454.1.

Maternal folic acid status is known to be protective for neural tube defects, primarily spina bifida and anencephaly. To prevent such birth defects, it is recommended that women of childbearing age consume 400 μg of folic acid from supplements or fortified foods in addition to intake of food folate from a varied diet. A significant reduction in the incidence of neural tube defects and improved folic acid status in women have been reported since folic acid fortification of enriched cereal grain products became mandatory in the USA in 1998.

DEFICIENCY. Folate deficiency may result from poor nutrient intake or poorly prepared foods (see Table 45-1); malabsorption (hereditary folate malabsorption, celiac disease, inflammatory bowel disease, alcoholism); diseases with a high cell turnover rate (sickle cell anemia, psoriasis); inborn errors of folate metabolism (methylene tetrahydrofolate reductase, methionine synthase reductase, glutamate formiminotransferase deficiencies) [see Chapter 85]; or autoantibodies against the cerebral folate receptor in the choroid plexus.

Hereditary folate malabsorption presents within 1–3 mo of age with recurrent or chronic diarrhea, failure to thrive, oral ulcerations, neurologic deterioration, and megaloblastic anemia. Neurologic outcome is poor once central nervous system manifestations are present. It is not possible to achieve the normal cerebrospinal fluid (CSF)-serum folate ratio of 3:1 despite normalization of serum levels. Children with this disorder also have depressed immunity and are susceptible to opportunistic infections.

Treatment of hereditary folate malabsorption may be possible with intramuscular folinic acid; some patients may respond to high-dose oral folinic acid therapy.

Cerebral folate deficiency presents within 4–6 mo of age with irritability, microcephaly, developmental delay, cerebellar ataxia, pyramidal tract signs, choreoathetosis, ballismus, and seizures. Subsequently, blindness due to optic atrophy develops. Serum and red blood cell 5-methyltetrahydrofolate levels are normal, but markedly low in the CSF. A high-affinity blocking autoantibody against the membrane-bound folate receptor in the choroid plexus may be the cause of the infantile cerebral folate deficiency.

Treatment with oral folinic acid corrects the low CSF folate levels and improves the clinical manifestations.

TOXICITY. No adverse effects of folate have been associated with the consumption of amounts normally found in fortified foods. Excessive intakes of folate supplements may obscure or mask and potentially delay the diagnosis of vitamin B_{12} deficiency.

46.7 • VITAMIN B_{12} (COBALAMIN)

Vitamin B_{12} functions as a cofactor for an enzyme that catalyzes the isomerization of methylmalonyl coenzyme A to succinyl coenzyme A, an essential reaction in lipid and carbohydrate metabolism. Vitamin B_{12} also is essential in folate metabolism, and the interaction of the 2 vitamins is essential for the conversion of homocysteine to methionine, for protein biosynthesis, for synthesis of purines and pyramides, for methylation reactions, and for the maintenance of cellular levels of folate.

Vitamin B_{12} in the diet is obtained almost exclusively from animal foods (muscle meats, eggs, dairy products). Certain fermented foods, such as tempeh and nori, contain vitamin B_{12}, but the amounts are variable and some of the vitamin may be in a form that is not absorbed or used. Fortified ready-to-eat cereals can be an important source of the vitamin in children and adolescents.

Vitamin B_{12} deficiency due to inadequate dietary intake occurs primarily in individuals consuming strict vegetarian diets (vegan, macrobiotic). A vegan diet, undiagnosed pernicious anemia, or another malabsorption syndrome in the mother will result in breast milk that is deficient in the vitamin. With the increase of exclusive breast-feeding in developed countries, reports of severely affected vitamin B_{12}–deficient infants are not uncommon. The hematologic and neurologic manifestations of vitamin B_{12} deficiency are discussed in Chapters 335.12 and 454.2.

TOXICITY. High doses of vitamin B_{12} have not been associated with any toxic effects. However, individuals who are at risk for Leber optic atrophy and are deficient in vitamin B_{12} should not be treated with the cyanocobalamin form of the vitamin.

Bailey LB: Folate and vitamin B12 recommended intakes and status in the United States. *Nutr Rev* 2004;62(Part 2):S14–S20.

Department of Health and Human Services Centers for Disease Control and Prevention: Neurologic Impairment in Children Associated with Maternal Dietary Deficiency of Cobalamin, Georgia, 2001. *MMWR* 2003;52:61–64.

Fattal-Valevski A, Kesler A, Sela BA, et al: Outbreak of life-threatening deficiency in infants in Israel caused by a defective soy-based formula. *Pediatrics* 2005;115:e233–e238.

Geller J, Kronn D, Jayabose S, et al: Hereditary folate malabsorption. *Medicine* 2002;81:51–68.

Green NS: Folic acid supplementation and prevention of birth defects. *J Nutr* 2002;132(8 Suppl):2356S–2360S.

Gropper SS, Smith JL, Groff JL (editors): *Advanced Nutrition and Human Metabolism,* 4th ed. Belmont, CA, Thomson Wadsworth, 2005.

Hoffman TL, Simon EM, Ficicioglu C: Biotinidase deficiency: The importance of adequate follow-up for an inconclusive newborn screening result. *Eur J Pediatr* 2005;164:298–301.

Powers HJ: Riboflavin (vitamin B-2) and health. *Am J Clin Nutr* 2003;77:1352–1360.

Prousky JE: Pellagra may be a rare secondary complication of anorexia nervosa: A systematic review of the literature. *Altern Med Rev* 2003;8:180–185.

Ramaekers VT, Rothenberg SP, Sequeira JM, et al: Autoantibodies to folate receptors in the cerebral folate deficiency syndrome. *N Engl J Med* 2005;352:1985–1990.

Schwartz RS: Autoimmune folate deficiency and the rise and fall of "horror autotoxicus." *N Engl J Med* 2005;352:1948–1950.

Siega-Riz AM, Savitz DA, Zeisel SH, et al: Second trimester folate status and preterm birth. *Am J Obstet Gynecol* 2004;191:1851–1857.

Stabler SP, Allen RH: Vitamin B12 deficiency as a worldwide problem. *Annu Rev Nutr* 2004;24:299–326.

Stover PJ: Physiology of folate and vitamin B12 in health and disease. *Nutr Rev* 2004;62(6 Pt 2):S3–S12.

Towin A, Inge TH, Garcia VF, et al: Beriberi after gastric bypass surgery in adolescence. *J Pediatr* 2004;145:263–267.

Chapter 47 ■ Vitamin C (Ascorbic Acid)

Maija Zile and Wanda Chenoweth

Although most animals are able to synthesize ascorbic acid, humans lack the enzyme gulonolactone oxidase and thus depend on dietary sources of the vitamin. Certain vegetables and fruits, especially citrus, are the best food sources of vitamin C (see Table 45-1). Absorption of the vitamin occurs in the small intestine by an active process or by simple diffusion when large amounts are ingested. The oxidized form of vitamin C, dehydroascorbate, is absorbed passively or by a glucose transporter. Dehydroascorbate is rapidly reduced to ascorbate, which is the plasma transport form of vitamin C. Vitamin C is not stored in the body, but is taken up by all tissues; the highest levels are found in the pituitary and adrenal glands. When a mother's intake of vitamin C during pregnancy and lactation is adequate, the newborn will have adequate tissue levels of vitamin C, subsequently maintained by the vitamin C in breast milk or commercial infant formulas. Cow's milk and evaporated milk have little vitamin C, and supplements need to be provided if these are the major foods in the diet of infants.

FUNCTION, MECHANISM OF ACTION, PHYSIOLOGY

Vitamin C is essential for the hydroxylation of lysine and proline in collagen formation; it is involved in the conversion of dopamine to norepinephrine, tryptophan to serotonin (neurotransmitter metabolism), and cholesterol to steroids, and for the biosynthesis of carnitine. In these reactions, vitamin C functions to maintain the iron and copper atoms, cofactors of the metalloenzymes, in a reduced (active) state (see Table 45-1). Vitamin C is an important antioxidant (electron donor) in the aqueous milieu of the body. Vitamin C enhances non-heme iron absorption, the transfer of iron from transferrin to ferritin, and the formation of tetrahydrofolic acid, and thus may affect the functions of the hematopoietic system (immune response, leukocytes, macrophages, red blood cells).

DIETARY NEEDS

The recommended dietary intakes for vitamin C for infants and children up to age 8 yr are given in Table 41-2. The recommended daily intake for children 9–13 yr of age is 45 mg and increases to 65 mg and 75 mg for females and males, respectively, at ages 14–18 yr. To ensure adequate body stores of the vitamin in the newborn and in breast milk, the RDAs during pregnancy and lactation are 85 and 120 mg/day, respectively.

CLINICAL MANIFESTATIONS

Very low intake of vitamin C over time may lead to the deficiency disease **scurvy.** In infants and young children, the usual age of onset of clinical manifestations of scurvy is 6–24 mo. The early symptoms are rather general and include low-grade fever, irritability, tachypnea, digestive disturbances, loss of appetite, and generalized tenderness, particularly in the legs, which is noticeable when the diaper is changed. The pain results in pseudoparalysis, with the hips and knees semi-flexed and the feet rotated outward (Fig. 47-1). Edematous swelling along the shafts of the legs may be present; in some cases, there is subperiosteal hemorrhage at the end of the femur (Fig. 47-2). A "rosary" at the costochondral junctions and depression of the sternum are other typical features (Fig. 47-3). The angulation of scorbutic beads is usually sharper than that of a rachitic rosary. Changes in the gums are most noticeable after teeth have erupted and are manifested as bluish purple, spongy swellings of the mucous membrane, especially over the upper incisors (Fig. 47-4). Anemia, which is seen primarily in infants and young children, may be related to impaired ability to use iron or folate (see Chapters 454 and 455). Patients may present with the sicca syndrome of Sjögren, consisting of xerostomia, keratoconjunctivitis sicca, and enlarged salivary glands (see Chapter 161). Other clinical manifestations seen in infants as well as in older children and adolescents include swollen joints, purpura and ecchymoses, poor wound and fracture healing, petechiae, perifollicular hemorrhages (Fig. 47-5), hyperkeratosis of hair follicles, arthralgia, and muscle weakness. Endochondral bone formation may not proceed because osteoblasts cannot form osteoid. Bony trabeculae that have been formed become brittle and fracture easily. Irritability and other psychologic manifestations are likely due to impaired neurotransmitter metabolism. Severe vitamin C deficiency may result in degeneration of skeletal muscles, cardiac hypertrophy, bone marrow depletion, and adrenal atrophy.

Scurvy now is rare in the USA, although it formerly had been observed in infants fed exclusively cow's milk. Occasional cases of scurvy are reported in children and adolescents with self-imposed restricted dietary habits. Toddlers who are "picky" eaters may refuse foods containing vitamin C. The requirement for vitamin C may be increased by febrile illnesses, especially during infectious and diarrheal diseases.

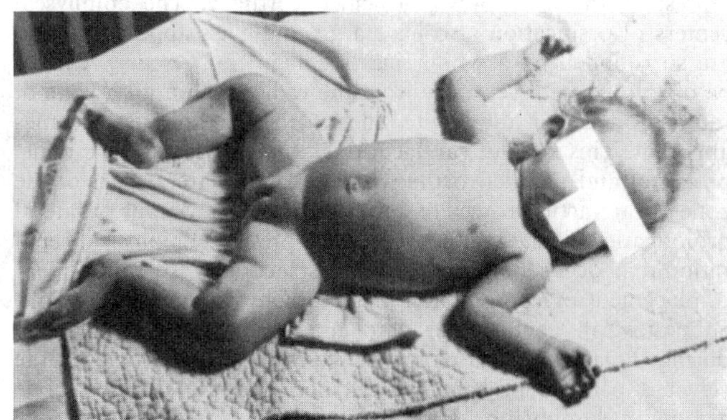

Figure 47-1. An infant with scurvy characteristically lies with the legs flexed at the knees and the hips partially flexed and externally rotated. (From *Nutrition*, 4th ed. Kalamazoo, MI, The Upjohn Company, 1980, p 42. Used with permission of Pfizer, Inc.)

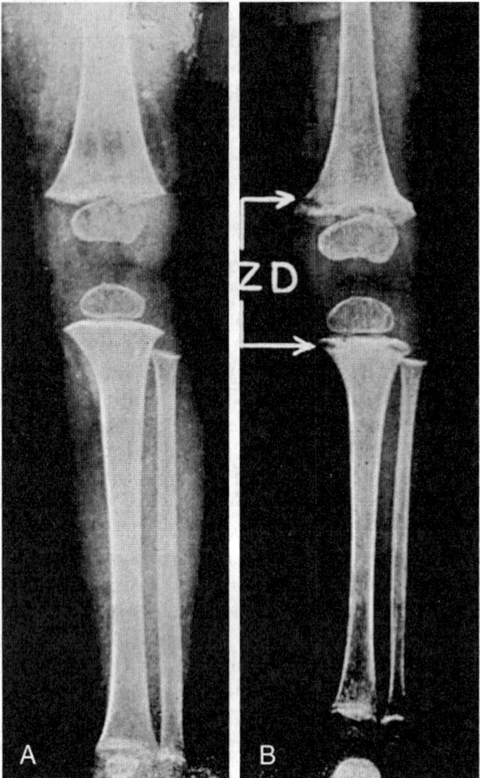

Figure 47-2. Radiographs of a leg. *A,* An early scurvy "white line" is visible on the ends of the shafts of the tibia and fibula; rings are shown around the epiphyses of the femur and tibia. *B,* More advanced scorbutic changes; zones of destruction (ZD) are evident in the femur and tibia.

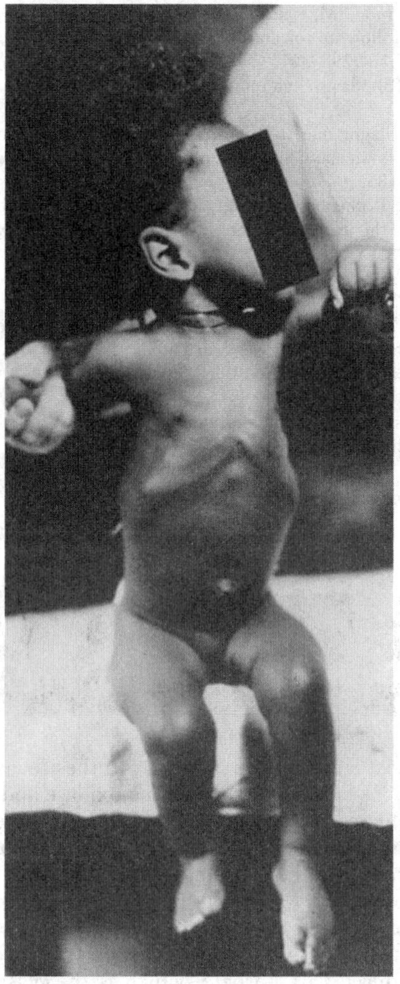

Figure 47-3. Scorbutic rosary and depression of scurvy.

DIAGNOSIS

Diagnosis of vitamin C deficiency is usually based on the characteristic clinical picture, the radiographic appearance of the long bones, and a history of poor vitamin C intake. The typical radiographic changes occur at the distal ends of the long bones; these are particularly common at the knee. In the early stages of deficiency, the appearance resembles that of simple bone atrophy. The trabeculae of the shaft cannot be discerned, and the bone has a ground-glass appearance. The cortex is quite thin, and the epiphyseal ends of the bones are sharply outlined. The white line of Fraenkel, an irregular but thickened white line at the metaphysis, represents the zone of well-calcified cartilage. The epiphyseal centers of ossification also have a ground-glass appearance and are surrounded by a white ring (see Fig. 47-2). Scurvy cannot be diagnosed with certainty from the radiograph until a zone of rarefaction under the white line at the metaphysis becomes apparent. This zone of rarefaction is a linear break in the bone, proximal and parallel to the white line. The lateral part of the zone of rarefaction is seen as a triangular defect. A spur or lateral prolongation of the white line may be present. Epiphyseal separation may occur along the line of destruction, with either linear displacement or compression of the epiphysis against the shaft. Subperiosteal hemorrhages are not visible radiographically during the active phase of scurvy. During healing, however, the elevated periosteum becomes calcified and the affected bone assumes a dumbbell or club shape.

Plasma and serum vitamin C concentrations respond to changes in dietary vitamin C intake and thus can be used to assess recent vitamin C intake, but are poor indicators of tissue levels of the vitamin. A plasma ascorbate concentration of <0.2 mg/dL usually is considered deficient. Leukocyte concentration of vitamin C is a better indicator of body stores, but this measurement is technically more difficult to perform. Leukocyte concentrations of $\leq 10\ \mu g/10^8$ WBC are considered deficient and indicate latent scurvy, even in the absence of clinical signs of deficiency. Saturation of the tissues with vitamin C can be estimated from the urinary excretion of the vitamin after a test dose of ascorbic acid. In healthy children, 80% of the test dose appears in the urine within 3–5 hr after parenteral administration. Generalized

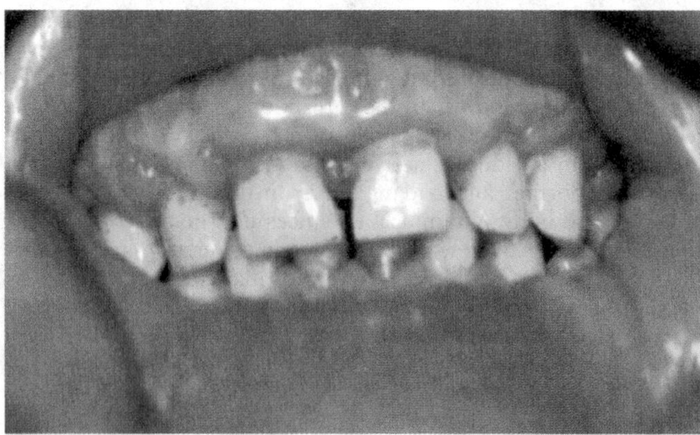

Figure 47-4. Gingival lesions in advanced scurvy. (From *Nutrition,* 4th ed. Kalamazoo, MI, The Upjohn Company, 1980, p 80. Used with permission of Pfizer, Inc.)

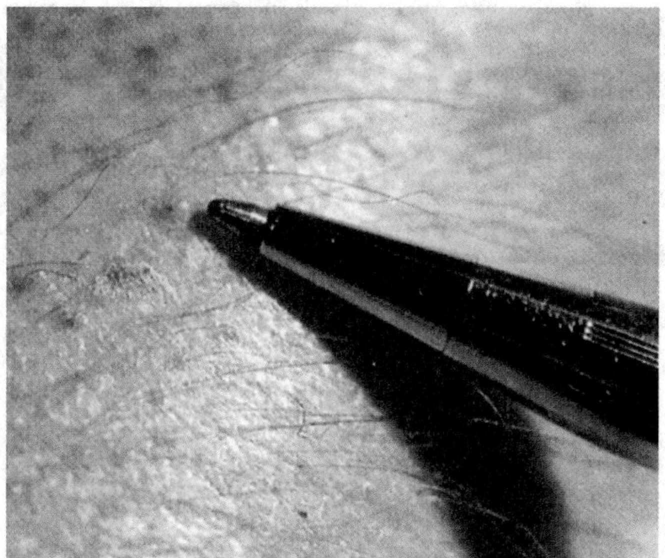

Figure 47-5. Perifollicular petechiae in scurvy. (From Weinsier RL, Morgan SL: *Fundamentals of Clinical Nutrition.* St. Louis, Mosby, 1993, p 85.)

nonspecific aminoaciduria is common in scurvy, whereas plasma amino acid levels remain normal.

Scurvy is often misdiagnosed as arthritis or acrodynia. Copper deficiency also results in a radiographic picture that is very similar to that of scurvy. Henoch-Schönlein purpura, thrombocytopenic purpura, leukemia, meningitis, or nephritis may also be suspected.

TREATMENT

Daily intake of 3–4 oz of orange or tomato juice produces healing in children with scurvy. Vitamin C supplements of 100–200 mg orally or parenterally are preferable to ensure more rapid and complete cure. With proper treatment, recovery, including resumption of normal growth, is rapid, although the swelling associated with subperiosteal hemorrhage may not subside for several months.

TOXICITY

Daily intakes of <2 g of vitamin C are generally without adverse effects in adults. Larger doses may cause gastrointestinal problems, such as abdominal pain and osmotic diarrhea. In populations at risk for calcium oxalate, uric acid nephrolithiasis, or iron toxicity (hemochromatosis, thalassemia, sideroblastic anemia) intake of >2 g of vitamin C is unsafe. Limited data exist on vitamin C toxicity in children. The following values for tolerable upper intake levels were extrapolated from data for adults based on body weight differences: for children 1–3 yr, 400 mg; 4–8 yr, 650 mg; 9–13 yr, 1200 mg, and 14–18 yr, 1800 mg.

Bingham AC, Kimura Y, Imundo L: A 16-year-old boy with purpura and leg pain. *J Pediatr* 2003;142:560–563.

Food and Nutrition Board: *Dietary Reference Intakes for Vitamin C, Vitamin E, Selenium, and Carotenoids.* Washington, DC, National Academy Press, 2000.

Gropper SS, Smith JL, Groff JL (editors): *Advanced Nutrition and Human Metabolism,* 4th ed. Belmont, CA, Thomson Wadsworth, 2005.

Hampl JS, Taylor CA, Johnston CS: Vitamin C deficiency and depletion in the United States: The Third National Health and Nutrition Examination Survey, 1988 to 1994. *Am J Public Health* 2004;94:870–875.

Naidu KA: Vitamin C in human health and disease is still a mystery? An overview. *Nutr J* 2003;2:7.

Tamura Y, Welch DC, Zic JA, et al: Scurvy presenting as painful gait with bruising in a young boy. *Arch Pediatr Adolesc Med* 2000;154:732–735.

Chapter 48 ■ Rickets and Hypervitaminosis D

Larry A. Greenbaum

RICKETS

General. Bone consists of a protein matrix called *osteoid* and a mineral phase, principally composed of calcium and phosphate, mostly in the form of hydroxyapatite. **Osteomalacia** is present when there is inadequate mineralization of bone osteoid; it occurs in children or adults. **Rickets,** a disease of growing bone, occurs in children only before fusion of the epiphyses, and is due to unmineralized matrix at the growth plates. Because growth plate cartilage and osteoid continue to expand, but mineralization is inadequate, the growth plate thickens. There is also an increase in the circumference of the growth plate and the metaphysis. This increases bone width at the location of the growth plates, causing some of the classic clinical manifestations, such as widening of the wrists and ankles. There is a general softening of the bones that causes them to bend easily when subject to forces such as weight bearing or muscle pull. This leads to a variety of bone deformities.

Rickets, principally due to vitamin D deficiency (Table 48-1), was rampant in northern Europe and the United States during the early years of the 20th century. Although this problem was largely corrected through public health measures that provided children with adequate vitamin D, rickets remains a persistent problem in developed countries, with many cases still secondary to preventable nutritional vitamin D deficiency. In developing countries it remains a significant problem, with some community-based and general hospital-based surveys among children in Africa finding the prevalence of rickets to exceed 10%. UNICEF has estimated that up to 25% of children in China have some evidence of rickets.

Etiology. There are many causes of rickets (Table 48-2), including vitamin D disorders, calcium deficiency, phosphorous deficiency, and distal renal tubular acidosis.

Clinical Manifestations. Most manifestations of rickets are due to skeletal changes (Table 48-3). **Craniotabes,** a softening of the cranial bones, can be detected by applying pressure at the occiput or over the parietal bones. The sensation is similar to the feel of pressing into a Ping-Pong ball and then releasing. Craniotabes may also be secondary to osteogenesis imperfecta, hydrocephalus, and syphilis. It is a normal finding in many newborns, especially near the suture lines, but it typically disappears within a few months of birth. Widening of the costochondral junctions results in a **rachitic rosary;** this feels like the beads of a rosary as the examiner's fingers move along the costochondral junctions from rib to rib (Fig. 48-1). **Growth plate** widening is also responsible for the enlargement at the wrists and ankles. The horizontal depression along the lower anterior chest known as **Harrison groove** occurs due to pulling of the softened ribs by the diaphragm during inspiration (Fig. 48-2). Softening of the ribs also impairs air movement and predisposes patients to atelectasis. The risk of pneumonia appears to be elevated in children with rickets; in Ethiopia, there may be a 13-fold higher incidence of rickets among children with pneumonia.

There is some variation in the clinical presentation of rickets based on the etiology. Changes in the lower extremities tend to

TABLE 48.1. Physical and Metabolic Properties and Food Sources of the Vitamins (D, E, and K)

NAMES AND SYNONYMS	CHARACTERISTICS	BIOCHEMICAL ACTION	EFFECTS OF DEFICIENCY	EFFECTS OF EXCESS	SOURCES
VITAMIN D					
Vitamin D_3 (3-cholecalciferol), which is synthesized in the skin, and vitamin D_2 (from plants or yeast) are biologically equivalent; 1 μg = 40 IU vitamin D	Fat-soluble, stable to heat, acid alkali, and oxidation; bile necessary for absorption; hydroxylation in the liver and kidney necessary for biologic activity	Necessary for gastrointestinal absorption of calcium; also increases absorption of phosphate; direct actions on bone, including mediating resorption	Rickets in growing children; osteomalacia; hypocalcemia may cause tetany and seizures	Hypercalcemia, which may cause emesis, anorexia, pancreatitis, hypertension, arrhythmias, central nervous system effects, polyuria, nephrolithiasis, and renal failure	Exposure to sunlight (ultraviolet light); fish oils, fatty fish, egg yolks, and vitamin D–fortified formula, milk, cereals, and bread
VITAMIN E					
Group of related compounds with similar biologic activities; α-tocopherol is the most potent and the most common form	Fat-soluble; readily oxidized by oxygen, iron, rancid fats; bile acids necessary for absorption	Antioxidant; protection of cell membranes from lipid peroxidation and formation of free radicals	Red cell hemolysis in premature infants; posterior column and cerebellar dysfunction; pigmentary retinopathy	Unknown	Vegetable oils, seeds, nuts, green leafy vegetables, and margarine
VITAMIN K					
Group of naphthoquinones with similar biologic activities; K_1 (phylloquinone) from diet; K_2 (menaquinones) from intestinal bacteria	Natural compounds are fat-soluble; stable to heat and reducing agents; labile to oxidizing agent, strong acids, alkali, light; bile salts necessary for intestinal absorption	Vitamin K–dependent proteins include coagulation factors II, VII, IX, and X; proteins C, S, Z; matrix Gla protein, osteocalcin	Hemorrhagic manifestations; long-term bone and vascular health	Not established; analogues (no longer used) caused hemolytic anemia, jaundice, kernicterus, and death	Green leafy vegetables, liver, and certain legumes and plant oils; widely distributed

be the dominant feature in X-linked hypophosphatemic rickets. Symptoms secondary to hypocalcemia occur only in those forms of rickets associated with decreased serum calcium (Table 48-4).

The chief complaint in a child with rickets is quite variable. Many children present because of skeletal deformities, whereas others may have difficulty walking due to a combination of deformity and weakness. Other common presenting complaints include failure to thrive and symptomatic hypocalcemia (see Chapter 572).

Radiology. Rachitic changes are most easily visualized on posteroanterior radiographs of the wrist, although characteristic rachitic changes can be seen at other growth plates (Figs. 48-3 and 48-4). Decreased calcification leads to thickening of the growth plate. The edge of the metaphysis loses its sharp border,

TABLE 48-2. Causes of Rickets

VITAMIN D DISORDERS
Nutritional vitamin D deficiency
Congenital vitamin D deficiency
Secondary vitamin D deficiency
Malabsorption
Increased degradation
Decreased liver 25-hydroxylase
Vitamin D–dependent rickets type 1
Vitamin D–dependent rickets type 2
Chronic renal failure
CALCIUM DEFICIENCY
Low intake
Diet
Premature infants (rickets of prematurity)
Malabsorption
Primary disease
Dietary inhibitors of calcium absorption
PHOSPHORUS DEFICIENCY
Inadequate intake
Premature infants (rickets of prematurity)
Aluminum-containing antacids
RENAL LOSSES
X-linked hypophosphatemic rickets*
Autosomal dominant hypophosphatemic rickets*
Hereditary hypophosphatemic rickets with hypercalciuria
Overproduction of phosphatonin
Tumor-induced rickets*
McCune-Albright syndrome*
Epidermal nevus syndrome*
Neurofibromatosis*
Fanconi syndrome
Dent disease
DISTAL RENAL TUBULAR ACIDOSIS

*Disorders secondary to excess phosphatonin.

TABLE 48-3. Clinical Features of Rickets

GENERAL
Failure to thrive
Listlessness
Protuding abdomen
Muscle weakness (especially proximal)
Fractures
HEAD
Craniotabes
Frontal bossing
Delayed fontanelle closure
Delayed dentition; caries
Craniosynostosis
CHEST
Rachitic rosary
Harrison groove
Respiratory infections and atelectasis*
BACK
Scoliosis
Kyphosis
Lordosis
EXTREMITIES
Enlargement of wrists and ankles
Valgus or varus deformities
Windswept deformity (combination of valgus deformity of 1 leg with varus deformity of the other leg)
Anterior bowing of the tibia and femur
Coxa vara
Leg pain
HYPOCALCEMIC SYMPTOMS†
Tetany
Seizures
Stridor due to laryngeal spasm

*These features are most commonly associated with the vitamin D deficiency disorders.
†These symptoms develop only in children with disorders that produce hypocalcemia (see Table 48-4).

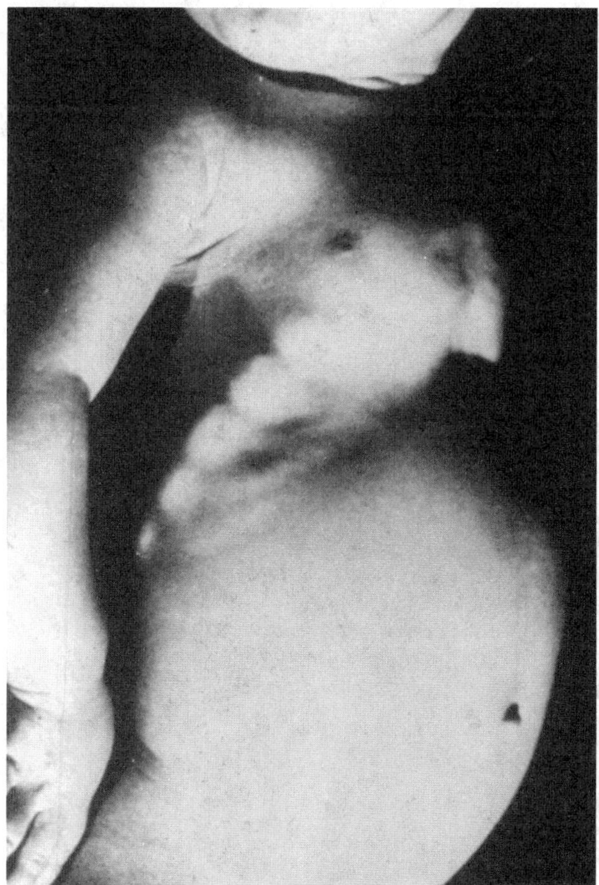

Figure 48-1. Rachitic rosary in a young infant.

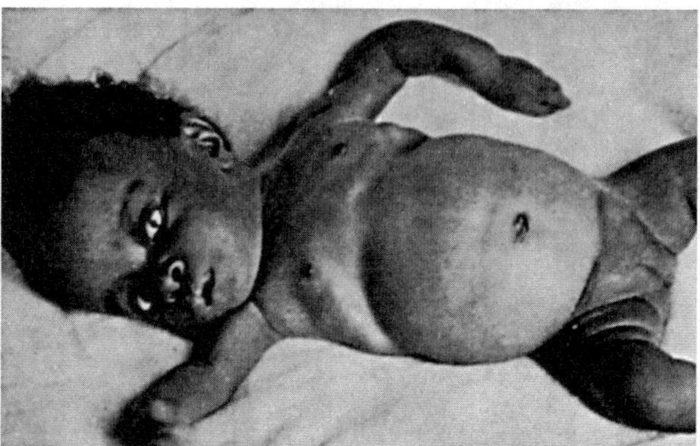

Figure 48-2. Deformities in rickets showing curvature of the limbs, potbelly, and Harrison groove.

which is described as fraying. In addition, the edge of the metaphysis changes from a convex or flat surface to a more concave surface. This is termed *cupping,* and is most easily seen at the distal ends of the radius, ulna, and fibula. There is widening of the distal end of the metaphysis, corresponding to the clinical observation of thickened wrists and ankles, as well as the rachitic rosary. Other radiologic features include coarse trabeculation of the diaphysis and generalized rarefaction.

Diagnosis. Most cases of rickets are diagnosed based on the presence of classic radiographic abnormalities. The diagnosis is supported by physical examination findings (see Table 48-3) and a history and laboratory test results that are consistent with a specific etiology.

Clinical Evaluation. Because the majority of children with rickets have a nutritional deficiency, the initial evaluation should focus on a dietary history, emphasizing intake of vitamin D and calcium. Most children in industrialized nations receive vitamin D from formula, fortified milk, or vitamin supplements. Along with the amount, the exact composition of the formula or milk is pertinent because rickets has occurred in children given products that are called *milk* (soy milk), but are deficient in vitamin D and/or minerals.

Cutaneous synthesis mediated by sunlight exposure is an important source of vitamin D. It is important to ask about time spent outside, sunscreen use, and clothing, especially if there may be a cultural reason for increased covering of the skin. Because winter sunlight is ineffective at stimulating cutaneous synthesis of vitamin D, the season is an additional consideration. Children with increased skin pigmentation are at increased risk for vitamin D deficiency because of decreased cutaneous synthesis.

The presence of **maternal risk** factors for nutritional vitamin D deficiency, including diet and sun exposure, is an important consideration when a neonate or young infant has rachitic findings, especially if the infant is breast-fed. Determining a child's intake of dairy products, the main dietary source of calcium, provides a general sense of calcium intake. High dietary fiber may interfere with calcium absorption.

The child's **medication** use is relevant because certain medications, such as the anticonvulsants phenobarbital and phenytoin, increase degradation of vitamin D, and aluminum-containing antacids interfere with the absorption of phosphate.

Malabsorption of vitamin D is suggested by a history of liver or intestinal disease. Undiagnosed liver or intestinal disease should be suspected if the child has gastrointestinal symptoms,

TABLE 48-4. Laboratory Findings in Disorders Causing Rickets

DISORDER	Ca	Pi	PTH	25-OHD	$1,25\text{-}(OH)_2D$	ALK PHOS	URINE Ca	URINE Pi
Vitamin D deficiency	N, ↓	↓	↑	↓	↓, N, ↑	↑	↓	↑
VDDR, type 1	N, ↓	↓	↑	N	↓	↑	↓	↑
VDDR, type 2	N, ↓	↓	↑	N	↑↑	↑	↓	↑
Chronic renal failure	N, ↓	↑	↑	N	↓	↑	N, ↓	↓
Dietary Pi deficiency	N	↓	N, ↓	N	↑	↑	↑	↓
XLH	N	↓	N	N	RD	↑	↓	↑
ADHR	N	↓	N	N	RD	↑	↓	↑
HHRH	N	↓	N, ↓	N	RD	↑	↑	↑
Tumor-induced rickets	N	↓	N	N	RD	↑	↓	↑
Fanconi syndrome	N	↓	N	N	RD or ↑	↑	↓ or ↑	↑
Dietary Ca deficiency	N, ↓	↓	↑	N	↑	↑	↓	↑

ADHR, autosomal dominant hypophosphatemic rickets; Alk Phos, alkaline phosphatase; Ca, calcium; HHRH, hereditary hypophosphatemic rickets with hypercalciuria; N, normal; Pi, phosphorus; PTH, parathyroid hormone; RD, relatively decreased (because it should be increased given the concurrent hypophosphatemia); VDDR, vitamin D–dependent rickets; XLH, X-linked hypophosphatemic rickets; $1,25\text{-}(OH)_2D$, 1,25-dihydroxyvitamin D; 25-OHD, 25-hydroxyvitamin D; ↓, decreased; ↑, increased; ↑↑, extremely increased.

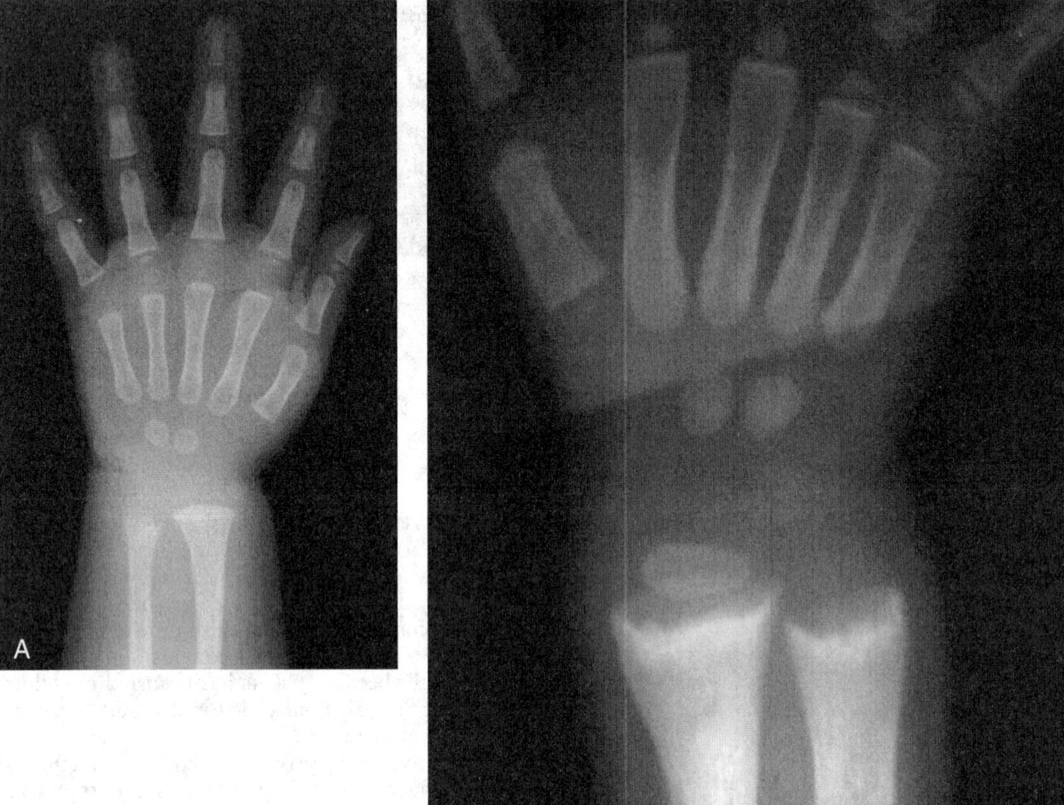

Figure 48-3. Wrist x-rays in a normal child *(A)* and a child with rickets *(B)*. The child with rickets has metaphyseal fraying and cupping of the distal radius and ulna.

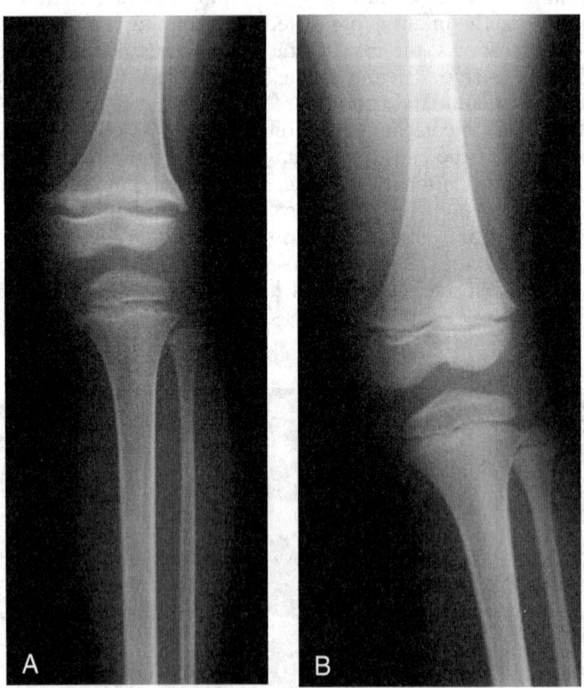

Figure 48-4. X-rays of the knees in a 7 yr old girl with distal renal tubular acidosis and rickets. *A,* At initial presentation, there is widening of the growth plate and metaphyseal fraying. *B,* Dramatic improvement after 4 mo of therapy with alkali.

although occasionally, rickets may be the presenting complaint. Fat malabsorption is often associated with diarrhea or oily stools, and there may be signs or symptoms suggestive of deficiencies of other fat-soluble vitamins (A, E, and K; Chapters 45, 49, and 50).

A history of **renal disease** (proteinuria, hematuria, urinary tract infections) is an additional significant consideration, given the importance of chronic renal failure as a cause of rickets. Polyuria may occur in children with chronic renal failure or Fanconi syndrome.

Children with rickets may have a history of dental caries, poor growth, delayed walking, waddling gait, pneumonia, and hypocalcemic symptoms.

The family history is critical, given the large number of **genetic causes** of rickets, although most are rare. Along with bone disease, it is important to inquire about leg deformities, difficulties with walking, or unexplained short stature because some parents may be unaware of their diagnosis. An undiagnosed mother is not unusual in X-linked hypophosphatemia. A history of a unexplained sibling death during infancy may be present in the child with cystinosis, the most common cause of Fanconi syndrome in children.

The physical examination focuses on detecting manifestations of rickets (see Table 48-3). It is important to observe the child's gait, auscultate the lungs to detect atelectasis or pneumonia, and plot the patient's growth. Alopecia suggests vitamin D–dependent rickets type 2.

The **initial laboratory** tests in a child with rickets should include serum calcium; phosphorus; alkaline phosphatase; parathyroid hormone (PTH); 25-hydroxyvitamin D; 1,25-dihydroxyvitamin D_3; creatinine; and electrolytes (see Table

48-4 for interpretation). Urinalysis is useful for detecting the glycosuria and aminoaciduria (positive dipstick for protein) seen with Fanconi syndrome. Evaluation of urinary excretion of calcium (24 hr collection for calcium or calcium-creatinine ratio) is helpful if hereditary hypophosphatemic rickets with hypercalciuria or Fanconi syndrome is suspected. Direct measurement of other fat-soluble vitamins (A, E, and K) or indirect assessment of deficiency (prothrombin time for vitamin K deficiency) is appropriate if malabsorption is a consideration.

VITAMIN D DISORDERS

VITAMIN D PHYSIOLOGY. Vitamin D can be synthesized in skin epithelial cells and therefore technically is not a vitamin. Cutaneous synthesis, which is normally the most important source of vitamin D, depends on the conversion of 7-dehydrochlesterol to vitamin D_3 (3-cholecalciferol) by ultraviolet B radiation from the sun. The efficiency of this process is decreased by melanin; hence, more sun exposure is necessary for vitamin D synthesis in people with increased skin pigmentation. Measures to decrease sun exposure, such as covering the skin with clothing or applying sunscreen, also decrease vitamin D synthesis. Children who spend less time outside have reduced vitamin D synthesis. The winter sun away from the equator is ineffective at mediating vitamin D synthesis.

There are few natural dietary sources of vitamin D. Fish liver oils have a high vitamin D content. Other good dietary sources include fatty fish and egg yolks. Most children in industrialized countries receive vitamin D via fortified foods, especially formula and milk (both of which contain 400 IU/L) and some breakfast cereals and breads. Supplemental vitamin D may be vitamin D_2 (which comes from plants or yeast) or vitamin D_3; they are biologically equivalent. Breast milk has a low vitamin D content, approximately 12–60 IU/L.

Vitamin D is transported bound to vitamin D–binding protein to the liver, where 25-hydroxlase converts vitamin D into 25-hydroxyvitamin D (25-D), the most abundant circulating form of vitamin D. Because there is little regulation of this liver hydroxylation step, measurement of 25-D is the standard method for determining a patient's vitamin D status. The final step in activation occurs in the kidney, where 1α-hydroxylase adds a second hydroxyl group, resulting in 1,25-dihydroxyvitamin D (1,25-D). The 1α-hydroxylase is upregulated by PTH and hypophosphatemia; hyperphosphatemia and 1,25-D inhibit this enzyme. Most 1,25-D circulates bound to vitamin D–binding protein.

1,25-D acts by binding to an intracellular receptor, and the complex affects gene expression by interacting with vitamin D–response elements. In the intestine, this results in a marked increase in calcium absorption, which is highly dependent on 1,25-D. There is also an increase in phosphorus absorption, but this is less significant because most dietary phosphorus absorption is vitamin D–independent. 1,25-D also has direct effects on bone, including mediating resorption. 1,25-D directly suppresses PTH secretion by the parathyroid gland, thus completing a negative feedback loop. PTH secretion is also suppressed by the increase in serum calcium mediated by 1,25-D. 1,25-D inhibits its own synthesis in the kidney and increases the synthesis of inactive metabolites.

NUTRITIONAL VITAMIN D DEFICIENCY. Vitamin D deficiency remains the most common cause of rickets globally and is prevalent, even in industrialized countries. Because vitamin D can be obtained from dietary sources or from cutaneous synthesis, most patients in industrialized countries have a combination of risk factors that lead to vitamin D deficiency.

Etiology. Vitamin D deficiency most commonly occurs in infancy due to a combination of poor intake and inadequate cutaneous synthesis. Transplacental transport of vitamin D, mostly 25-D, typically provides enough vitamin D for the 1st 2 mo of life unless there is severe maternal vitamin D deficiency. Infants who receive formula receive adequate vitamin D, even without cutaneous synthesis. Breast-fed infants, because of the low vitamin D content of breast milk, rely on cutaneous synthesis or vitamin supplements. Cutaneous synthesis can be limited due to the ineffectiveness of the winter sun in stimulating vitamin D synthesis; avoidance of sunlight due to concerns about cancer, neighborhood safety, or cultural practices; and decreased cutaneous synthesis because of increased skin pigmentation.

The effect of skin pigmentation explains why most cases of nutritional rickets in the USA and northern Europe occur in breast-fed children of African descent or other dark-pigmented populations. The additional impact of the winter sun is supported by the fact that such infants more commonly present in the late winter or spring. In some groups, complete covering of infants or the practice of not taking infants outside has a significant role, explaining the occurrence of rickets in infants living in areas of abundant sunshine, such as the Middle East. Because the mothers of some infants may have the same risk factors, decreased maternal vitamin D may also contribute, both by leading to reduced vitamin D content in breast milk and by lessening transplacental delivery of vitamin D. Rickets caused by vitamin D deficiency may also be secondary to unconventional dietary practices, such as vegan diets that use unfortified soy milk or rice milk.

Clinical Manifestations. The clinical features are typical of rickets (see Table 48-3), with a significant minority presenting with symptoms of hypocalcemia; prolonged laryngospasm is occasionally fatal. In addition, these children have an increased risk of pneumonia and muscle weakness, leading to a delay in motor development.

Laboratory Findings. Table 48-4 summarizes the principal laboratory findings. Hypocalcemia is a variable finding due to the actions of the elevated PTH to increase the serum calcium concentration. The hypophosphatemia is due to PTH-induced renal losses of phosphate, combined with a decrease in intestinal absorption.

The wide variation in 1,25-D levels (low, normal, or high) is secondary to the upregulation of renal 1α-hydroxylase due to concomitant hypophosphatemia and hyperparathyroidism. Because serum levels of 1,25-D are normally much lower than the levels of 25-D, even with low levels of 25-D there is still often enough 25-D present to act as a precursor for 1,25-D synthesis in the presence of an upregulated 1α-hydroxylase. The level of 1,25-D is only low when there is severe vitamin D deficiency.

Some patients have a metabolic acidosis secondary to PTH-induced renal bicarbonate-wasting. There may also be generalized aminoaciduria.

Diagnosis and Differential Diagnosis. The diagnosis of nutritional vitamin D deficiency is based on the combination of a history of poor vitamin D intake and risk factors for decreased cutaneous synthesis, radiographic changes consistent with rickets, and typical laboratory findings (see Table 48-4). A normal PTH level almost never occurs with vitamin D deficiency and suggests a primary phosphate disorder. Calcium deficiency may occur with or without vitamin D deficiency. A normal level of 25-D and a dietary history of poor calcium intake support a diagnosis of isolated calcium deficiency.

Treatment. Children with nutritional vitamin D deficiency should receive vitamin D and adequate nutritional intake of calcium and phosphorus. There are 2 strategies for administration of vitamin D. With stoss therapy, 300,000–600,000 IU of vitamin D are administered orally or intramuscularly as 2–4 doses over 1 day. Because the doses are observed, stoss therapy is ideal in situations where adherence to therapy is questionable. The alternative is daily, high-dose vitamin D, with doses ranging from 2,000–5,000 IU/day over 4–6 wk. Either strategy should be followed by daily vitamin D intake of 400 IU/day, typically given as a multivitamin. It is important to ensure that children receive adequate dietary calcium and phosphorus; this is usually provided by milk, formula, and other dairy products.

Children who have symptomatic hypocalcemia may need intravenous calcium acutely, followed by oral calcium supplements, which typically can be tapered over 2–6 wk in children who receive adequate dietary calcium. Transient use of intravenous or oral 1,25-D (calcitriol) is often helpful in reversing hypocalcemia in the acute phase by providing active vitamin D during the delay as supplemental vitamin D is converted to active vitamin D. Calcitriol doses are typically 0.05 μg/kg/day. Intravenous calcium is initially given as an acute bolus for symptomatic hypocalcemia (20 mg/kg of calcium chloride or 100 mg/kg of calcium gluconate). Some patients require a continuous intravenous calcium drip, titrated to maintain the desired serum calcium level. These patients should transition to enteral calcium, with most infants requiring approximately 1,000 mg of elemental calcium.

Prognosis. Most children have an excellent response to treatment, with radiologic healing occurring within a few months. Laboratory test results should also normalize rapidly. Many of the bone malformations improve dramatically, but children with severe disease may have permanent deformities. Short stature does not resolve in some children. Rarely, patients may benefit from orthopedic intervention for leg deformities, although this is generally not done until the metabolic bone disease has healed, there is clear evidence that the deformity will not self-resolve, and the deformity is causing functional problems.

Prevention. Most cases of nutritional rickets can be prevented by universal administration of a daily multivitamin containing 200–400 IU of vitamin D to children who are breast-fed. For other children, the diet should be reviewed to ensure that there is a source of vitamin D.

CONGENITAL VITAMIN D DEFICIENCY. **Congenital rickets,** which is quite rare in industrialized countries, occurs when there is severe maternal vitamin D deficiency during pregnancy. Maternal risk factors include poor dietary intake of vitamin D, lack of adequate sun exposure, and closely spaced pregnancies. These newborns may have symptomatic hypocalcemia, intrauterine growth retardation, and decreased bone ossification, along with classic rachitic changes. Subtler maternal vitamin D deficiency may have an adverse effect on neonatal bone density and birthweight, cause a defect in dental enamel, and predispose infants to neonatal hypocalcemic tetany. Treatment of congenital rickets includes vitamin D supplementation and adequate intake of calcium and phosphorus. Use of prenatal vitamins containing vitamin D prevents this entity.

SECONDARY VITAMIN D DEFICIENCY.

Etiology. Along with inadequate intake, vitamin D deficiency can develop due to inadequate absorption, decreased hydroxylation in the liver, and increased degradation. Because vitamin D is fat-soluble, its absorption may be decreased in patients with a variety of liver and gastrointestinal diseases, including cholestatic liver disease, defects in bile acid metabolism, cystic fibrosis and other causes of pancreatic dysfunction, celiac disease, and Crohn disease. Malabsorption of vitamin D can also occur with intestinal lymphangiectasia and after intestinal resection.

Severe liver disease, which is usually also associated with malabsorption, can cause a decrease in 25-D formation due to insufficient enzyme activity. Because of the large reserve of 25-hydroxlase activity in the liver, this usually requires a loss of >90% of liver function. A variety of medications, by inducing the P450 system, increase the degradation of vitamin D. Rickets due to vitamin D deficiency can develop in children receiving anticonvulsants, such as phenobarbital or phenytoin; the antituberculosis medications isoniazid and rifampin may also have a deleterious effect on vitamin D levels.

Treatment. Treatment of vitamin D deficiency due to malabsorption requires high doses of vitamin D. Because of its better absorption, 25-D (25–50 μg/day or 5–7 μg/kg/day) is superior to vitamin D_3. The dose is adjusted based on monitoring of serum levels of 25-D. Alternatively, patients may be treated with 1,25-D, which also is better absorbed in the presence of fat malabsorption, or with parenteral vitamin D. Children with rickets due to increased degradation of vitamin D by the P450 system require the same acute therapy as indicated for nutritional deficiency (discussed earlier), followed by long-term administration of high doses of vitamin D (e.g., 1,000 IU/day), with dosing titrated based on serum levels of 25-D. Some patients require as much as 4,000 IU/day.

VITAMIN D–DEPENDENT RICKETS, TYPE 1. Children with vitamin D–dependent rickets type 1, an autosomal recessive disorder, have mutations in the gene encoding renal 1α-hydroxylase, preventing conversion of 25-D into 1,25-D. These patients, who normally present during the 1st 2 yr of life, can have any of the classic features of rickets (see Table 48-3), including symptomatic hypocalcemia. They have normal levels of 25-D, but low levels of 1,25-D (see Table 48-4). Occasionally, 1,25-D levels may be at the lower limit of normal, but this is inappropriate, given the high PTH and low serum phosphorus levels, both of which should increase the activity of renal 1α-hydroxylase and cause elevated levels of 1,25-D. As in nutritional vitamin D deficiency, renal tubular dysfunction may cause a metabolic acidosis and generalized aminoaciduria.

Treatment. These patients respond to long-term treatment with 1,25-D (calcitriol). Initial doses are 0.25–2 μg/day, with lower doses used once the rickets has healed. Especially during initial therapy, it is important to ensure adequate intake of calcium. The dose of calcitriol is adjusted to maintain a low-normal serum calcium level, a normal serum phosphorus level, and a high-normal serum PTH level. Targeting a low-normal calcium concentration and a high-normal PTH level avoids excessive dosing of calcitriol, which can cause hypercalciuria and nephrocalcinosis. Hence, patient monitoring includes periodic assessment of urinary calcium excretion, with a target of <4 mg/kg/day.

VITAMIN D–DEPENDENT RICKETS, TYPE 2. Patients with vitamin D–dependent rickets type 2 have mutations in the gene encoding the vitamin D receptor, preventing a normal physiologic response to 1,25-D. Levels of 1,25-D are extremely elevated in this autosomal recessive disorder (see Table 48-4). Most patients present during infancy, although less severely affected patients may not be diagnosed until adulthood. Less severe disease is associated with a partially functional vitamin D receptor. Approximately 50–70% of children have **alopecia,** which tends to be associated with a more severe form of the disease. It can range from alopecia areata to alopecia totalis. Epidermal cysts are a less common manifestation.

Treatment. Some patients, especially those without alopecia, respond to extremely high doses of vitamin D_2, 25-D, or 1,25-D. This response is due to a partially functional vitamin D receptor. All patients with this disorder should be given a 3–6 month trial of high-dose vitamin D and oral calcium. The initial dose of 1,25-D should be 2 μg/day, but some patients require doses as high as 50–60 μg/day. Calcium doses range from 1,000–3,000 mg/day. Patients who do not respond to high-dose vitamin D may be treated with long-term intravenous calcium, with possible transition to very high-dose oral calcium supplements. Treatment of patients who do not respond to vitamin D is difficult.

CHRONIC RENAL FAILURE (SEE CHAPTER 535.2). With chronic renal failure, there is decreased activity of 1α-hydroxylase in the kidney, leading to diminished production of 1,25-D. In chronic renal failure, unlike the other causes of vitamin D deficiency, patients have hyperphosphatemia as a result of decreased renal excretion (see Table 48-4). Along with inadequate calcium absorption and secondary hyperparathyroidism, the rickets may be worsened by the metabolic acidosis of chronic renal failure. In addition, failure to thrive and growth retardation may be accentuated because of the direct effect of chronic renal failure on the growth hormone axis.

Treatment. Therapy requires the use of a form of vitamin D that can act without 1-hydroxylation by the kidney (calcitriol), which both permits adequate absorption of calcium and directly suppresses the parathyroid gland. Because hyperphosphatemia is a stimulus for PTH secretion, normalization of the serum phosphorus level, via a combination of dietary phosphorus restriction and the use of oral phosphate binders, is as important as the use of activated vitamin D. In addition, the chronic metabolic acidosis should be corrected with alkali.

CALCIUM DEFICIENCY

Pathophysiology. Rickets secondary to inadequate dietary calcium is a significant problem in some countries in Africa, although there are cases in other regions of the world, including industrialized countries. Because breast milk and formula are excellent sources of calcium, this form of rickets develops after children have been weaned from breast milk or formula, and it is more likely to occur in children who are weaned early. Rickets develops because the diet has low calcium content, typically <200 mg/day. There is little intake of dairy products or other sources of calcium. In addition, the diet, because of reliance on grains and green leafy vegetables, may be high in phytate, oxalate, and phosphate, which decrease absorption of dietary calcium. In industrialized countries, rickets due to calcium deficiency may occur in children who consume an unconventional diet. Examples include children with milk allergy who have low dietary calcium and children who transition from formula or breast milk to juice, soda, or a calcium-poor soy drink, without an alternative source of dietary calcium.

This type of rickets can develop in children who receive intravenous nutrition without adequate calcium. Malabsorption of calcium can occur in celiac disease, intestinal abetalipoproteinemia, and after small bowel resection. There may be concurrent malabsorption of vitamin D.

Clinical Manifestations. Children have the classic signs and symptoms of rickets (see Table 48-3). Presentation may occur during infancy or early childhood, although some cases are diagnosed in teenagers. Because calcium deficiency occurs after the cessation of breast-feeding, it tends to occur later than the nutritional vitamin D deficiency that is associated with breast-feeding. In Nigeria, nutritional vitamin D deficiency is most common at 4–15 mo of age, whereas calcium-deficiency rickets typically presents at 15–25 mo of age.

Diagnosis. Laboratory findings include increased levels of alkaline phosphatase, PTH, and 1,25-D (see Table 48-4). Calcium levels may be normal or low, although symptomatic hypocalcemia is uncommon. There is decreased urinary excretion of calcium, and serum phosphorus levels may be low due to renal wasting of phosphate from secondary hyperparathyroidism, which may also cause aminoaciduria. In some children, there is coexisting nutritional vitamin D deficiency; 25-D levels would then be low.

Treatment. Treatment focuses on providing adequate calcium, typically as a dietary supplement (doses of 350–1,000 mg/day of elemental calcium are effective). Vitamin D supplementation is necessary if there is concurrent vitamin D deficiency (discussed earlier). Prevention strategies include discouraging early cessation of breast-feeding and increasing dietary sources of calcium. In countries such as Kenya, where many children have diets high in cereal with negligible intake of cow's milk, school-based milk programs have been effective in reducing the prevalence of rickets.

PHOSPHOROUS DEFICIENCY

INADEQUATE INTAKE. With the exception of starvation or severe anorexia, it is almost impossible to have a diet that is deficient in phosphorus because phosphorus is present in most foods. Decreased phosphorus absorption can occur in diseases associated with malabsorption (celiac disease, cystic fibrosis, cholestatic liver disease), but if rickets develops, the primary problem is usually malabsorption of vitamin D and/or calcium.

Isolated malabsorption of phosphorus occurs in patients with long-term use of aluminum-containing antacids. These compounds are very effective at chelating phosphate in the gastrointestinal tract, leading to decreased absorption. This results in hypophosphatemia with secondary osteomalacia in adults and rickets in children. This entity responds to discontinuation of the antacid and short-term phosphorus supplementation.

PHOSPHATONIN. Phosphatonin is a humoral mediator that decreases renal tubular reabsorption of phosphate and therefore decreases serum phosphorus. Phosphatonin also decreases the activity of renal 1α-hydroxylase, resulting in a decrease in the production of 1,25-D. Fibroblast growth factor-23 (FGF-23) is the most well characterized phosphatonin, but there are a number of other putative phosphatonins (discussed later). Increased levels of phosphatonin cause many of the phosphate-wasting diseases (see Table 48-2).

X-LINKED HYPOPHOSPHATEMIC RICKETS. Among the genetic disorders causing rickets due to hypophosphatemia, X-linked hypophosphatemic rickets (XLH) is the most common, with a prevalence of 1/20,000. The defective gene is on the X chromosome, but female carriers are affected, so it is an X-linked dominant disorder.

Pathophysiology. The defective gene is called *PHEX* because it is a PHosphate-regulating gene with homology to Endopeptidases on the X chromosome. The product of this gene appears to have either a direct or an indirect role in inactivating a phosphatonin or phosphatonins. FGF-23 may be the target phosphatonin. In the absence of *PHEX*, there is decreased degradation of phosphatonin. Because the actions of phosphatonin include inhibition of phosphate reabsorption in the proximal tubule, there is increased phosphate excretion. Phosphatonin also inhibits renal 1α-hydroxylase, leading to decreased production of 1,25-D.

Clinical Manifestations. These patients have rickets, but abnormalities of the lower extremities and poor growth are the dominant features. Delayed dentition and tooth abscesses are also common. Some patients have hypophosphatemia and short stature without clinically evident bone disease.

Laboratory Findings. Patients have high renal excretion of phosphate, hypophosphatemia, and increased alkaline phosphatase; PTH and serum calcium levels are normal (see Table 48-4). Hypophosphatemia, because it normally upregulates renal 1α-hydroxylase, should lead to an increase in 1,25-D, but these patients have low or inappropriately normal levels.

Treatment. Patients respond well to a combination of oral phosphorus and 1,25-D (calcitriol). The daily need for phosphorus supplementation is 1–3 g of elemental phosphorus divided into 4–5 doses. Frequent dosing helps to prevent prolonged decrements in serum phosphorus because there is a rapid decline after each dose. In addition, frequent dosing decreases diarrhea, a complication of high-dose oral phosphorus. Calcitrol is administered 30–70 ng/kg/day divided into 2 doses.

Complications of treatment occur when there is not an adequate balance between phosphorus supplementation and calcitriol. Excess phosphorus, by decreasing enteral calcium absorption, leads to secondary hyperparathyroidism, with worsening of the bone lesions. In contrast, excess calcitriol causes hypercalciuria and nephrocalcinosis; it may even cause hypercalcemia. Hence, laboratory monitoring of treatment includes serum calcium, phosphorus, alkaline phosphatase, PTH, and urinary calcium, as well as periodic renal ultrasounds to evaluate patients for nephrocalcinosis. Because of variation in the serum phosphorus level and the importance of avoiding excessive phosphorus dosing, normalization of alkaline phosphatase levels is a more useful method of assessing the therapeutic response than measuring serum phosphorus. For children with significant short stature, growth hormone is an effective option. Children with severe deformities may need osteotomies, but this should be done only when treatment has led to resolution of the bone disease.

Prognosis. The response to therapy is usually good, although frequent dosing may lead to problems with compliance. Girls generally have less severe disease than boys, probably due to the X-linked inheritance. Short stature may persist despite healing of the rickets. Adults generally do well with less aggressive treatment, with some receiving calcitriol alone. Adults with bone pain or other symptoms improve with oral phosphorus supplementation and calcitriol.

AUTOSOMAL DOMINANT HYPOPHOSPHATEMIC RICKETS. This disorder is much less common than XLH. There is incomplete penetrance and variable age of onset. Patients with autosomal dominant hypophosphatemic rickets (ADHR) have a mutation in the gene encoding FGF-23. The mutation prevents degradation of FGF-23 by proteases, leading to increased levels of this phosphatonin. The actions of FGF-23 include decreased reabsorption of phosphate in the renal proximal tubule, which results in hypophosphatemia, and inhibition of the 1α-hydroxylase in the kidney, causing a decrease in 1,25-D synthesis.

In ADHR, as in XLH, abnormal laboratory findings are hypophosphatemia, an elevated alkaline phosphatase level, and a low or inappropriately normal 1,25-D level (see Table 48-4). Treatment is similar to the approach used in XLH.

HEREDITARY HYPOPHOSPHATEMIC RICKETS WITH HYPERCALCIURIA. Hereditary hypophosphatemic rickets with hypercalciuria (HHRH) is a rare disorder that is mainly described in the Middle East.

Pathophysiology. The primary problem is a renal phosphate leak that causes hypophosphatemia, which then stimulates production of 1,25-D. The high level of 1,25-D increases intestinal absorption of calcium, suppressing PTH. Hypercalciuria ensues due to the high absorption of calcium and the low level of PTH, which normally decreases renal excretion of calcium. The genetic features of this disorder are unclear. Inheritance appears to be autosomal recessive, but with variable manifestations in heterozygous individuals.

Clinical Manifestations. The dominant symptoms are rachitic leg abnormalities (see Table 48-3), muscle weakness, and bone pain. Patients may have short stature, with a disproportionate decrease in the length of the lower extremities. The severity of the disease varies, and some family members have no evidence of rickets, but have kidney stones secondary to hypercalciuria.

Laboratory Findings. Laboratory findings include hypophosphatemia, renal phosphate wasting, elevated serum alkaline phosphatase levels, and elevated 1,25-D levels. PTH levels are low (see Table 48-4). The laboratory abnormalities are less severe, but still present, in the patients with nephrolithiasis but no rachitic changes.

Treatment. Therapy relies on oral phosphorus replacement (1–2.5 g/day of elemental phosphorus in 5 divided oral doses). Treatment of the hypophosphatemia decreases serum levels of 1,25-D and corrects the hypercalciuria. The response to therapy is usually excellent, with resolution of pain, weakness, and radiographic evidence of rickets. There is also an increase in growth.

OVERPRODUCTION OF PHOSPHATONIN. **Tumor-induced osteomalacia** is more common in adults than in children. When this entity does occur in children, it may produce classic rachitic findings. Most tumors are mesenchymal in origin. The tumors are usually benign, small, and located in bone. These tumors secrete a number of different putative phosphatonins (FGF-23; frizzled-related protein 4, and matrix extracellular phosphoglycoprotein), with different tumors secreting different phosphatonins or combinations of phosphatonins. These phosphatonins produce a biochemical phenotype that is similar to XLH and ADHR, including urinary phosphate wasting, hypophosphatemia, elevated alkaline phosphatase levels, and low or inappropriately normal 1,25-D levels (see Table 48-4). Curative treatment is excision of the tumor. If the tumor cannot be removed, treatment is identical to that used for XLH.

Renal phosphate wasting leading to hypophosphatemia and rickets (or osteomalacia in adults) is a potential complication in **McCune-Albright syndrome,** an entity that includes the triad of polyostotic fibrous dysplasia, hyperpigmented macules, and polyendocrinopathy (see Chapter 563.6). Affected patients have inappropriately low levels of 1,25-D and elevated levels of alkaline phosphatase. The renal phosphate wasting and inhibition of 1,25-D synthesis are related to the polyostotic fibrous dysplasia. Patients have elevated levels of the phosphatonin FGF-23, presumably produced by the dysplastic bone. Hypophosphatemic rickets can also occur in children with isolated polyostotic fibrous dysplasia. Although it is rarely possible, removal of the abnormal bone can cure this disorder in children with McCune-Albright syndrome. Most patients receive the same treatment as children with XLH. In addition, bisphosphonate treatment decreases the pain and fracture risk associated with the bone lesions. It also decreases the elevated alkaline phosphatase level.

Rickets is an unusual complication of **epidermal nevus syndrome,** a rare, sporadic disorder consisting of congential epidermal nevi associated with anomalies of other organ systems, especially the skeleton and central nervous system (see Chapter 652). Some patients also have abnormalities of the eyes, heart, or genitourinary system. Patients have hypophosphatemic rickets due to renal phosphate wasting; they also have an inappropriately normal or low level of 1,25-D. The putative mechanism is excessive production of a phosphatonin. The timing of presentation with rickets varies from infancy to early adolescence. Resolution of hypophosphatemia and rickets has occurred after excision of the epidermal nevi in some patients, but not in others. In most cases, the skins lesions are too extensive to be removed, necessitating treatment with phosphorus supplementation and 1,25-D. Rickets due to phosphate wasting is an extremely rare complication in children with **neurofibromatosis** (see Chapter 596.1), again presumably due to the production of a phosphatonin.

FANCONI SYNDROME

Pathogenesis. Fanconi syndrome is secondary to generalized dysfunction of the renal proximal tubule (see Chapter 529.4). There are renal losses of phosphate, amino acids, bicarbonate, glucose, urate, and other molecules that are normally reabsorbed in the proximal tubule. Some patients may have partial dysfunction, with less generalized losses. The most clinically relevant consequences are hypophosphatemia due to phosphate losses and proximal renal tubular acidosis due to bicarbonate losses. The findings of aminoaciduria, glucosuria, and a low serum uric acid level are helpful diagnostically.

Fanconi syndrome in children is often secondary to an underlying genetic disorder. Cystinosis is the most common genetic etiology; other causes include Wilson disease, Lowe syndrome, and tyrosinemia. Primary familial Fanconi syndrome is extremely rare. Fanconi syndrome may also be secondary to heavy metal exposure or drug toxicity (ifosfamide, valproate, aminoglycosides).

Clinical Manifestations. Clinically, patients have rickets as a result of hypophosphatemia, with exacerbation from the chronic metabolic acidosis, which causes bone dissolution. Failure to thrive is a consequence of both rickets and renal tubular acidosis. In addition, patients usually have polyuria and polydipsia.

Laboratory Findings. Along with hypophosphatemia and metabolic acidosis, patients may have hypokalemia and hyponatremia. Most patients also have impaired synthesis of 1,25-D; levels are inappropriately low, given the presence of hypophosphatemia, which normally upregulates renal 1α-hydroxylase. In a few cases, patients have appropriately increased levels of 1,25-D; this increases calcium absorption, leading to hypercalciuria.

Treatment. In a child with Fanconi syndrome, the etiology must be determined because it dictates part of the management. Heavy metal exposure must be eliminated; chelation therapy may be curative. Toxic drugs should be discontinued if possible. Although many genetic disorders have specific therapies (cysteamine in cystinosis; avoidance of tyrosine in tyrosinemia), Fanconi syndrome may persist because the tubular damage may be irreversible. Treatment includes bicarbonate and phosphorus supplementation to correct acidosis and hypophosphatemia, respectively. In addition, oral 1,25-D (calcitriol) is usually a necessary adjunct because of the underlying defect in its synthesis and the negative effect of phosphorus supplementation on calcium absorption. In cases in which 1,25-D levels are increased, phosphorus supplementation alone is sufficient; it leads to a decrease in 1,25-D levels and a resolution of hypercalciuria (analogous to the situation in HHRH).

DENT DISEASE (SEE CHAPTER 531.3). Dent disease is an X-linked disorder due to mutations in the gene encoding a chloride channel that is expressed in the kidney. Affected males have variable manifestations, including hematuria, nephrolithiasis, nephrocalcinosis, rickets, and chronic renal failure. Almost all patients have low molecular weight proteinuria and hypercalciuria. Other, less universal abnormalities are aminoaciduria, glycosuria, hypophosphatemia, and hypokalemia. Rickets occurs in approximately 25% of patients, and it responds to oral phosphorus supplements. Some patients may also need 1,25-D, but this should be used cautiously because it may worsen the hypercalciuria.

RICKETS OF PREMATURITY (SEE CHAPTER 106). Rickets in very low birthweight infants has become a significant problem as the survival rate for this group of infants increased.

Pathogenesis. The transfer of calcium and phosphorus from mother to fetus occurs throughout pregnancy, but 80% occurs during the 3rd trimester. Premature birth interrupts this process, with rickets developing when the premature infant does not have an adequate supply of calcium and phosphorus to support mineralization of the growing skeleton.

Most cases of rickets of prematurity occur in infants with a birthweight <1,000 g. It is more likely to develop in infants with lower birthweight and younger gestational age. Rickets occurs because unsupplemented breast milk and standard infant formula do not contain enough calcium and phosphorus to supply the needs of the premature infant. Other risk factors include cholestatic jaundice, a complicated neonatal course, prolonged use of parenteral nutrition, the use of soy formula, and medications such as diuretics and corticosteroids.

Clinical Manifestations. Rickets of prematurity presents 1–4 mo after birth. Infants may have nontraumatic fractures, especially of the legs, arms, and ribs. Most fractures are not suspected clinically. Because fractures and softening of the ribs lead to decreased chest compliance, some infants have respiratory distress due to atelectasis and poor ventilation. This rachitic respiratory distress usually develops >5 weeks after birth, distinguishing it from the early-onset respiratory disease of premature infants. These infants have poor linear growth, with negative effects on growth persisting beyond 1 yr of age. An additional long-term effect is enamel hypoplasia. Poor bone mineralization may contribute to dolichocephaly. There may be classic rachitic findings, such as frontal bossing, rachitic rosary, craniotabes, and widened wrists and ankles (see Table 48-3). Most infants with rickets of prematurity have no clinical manifestations, with the diagnosis based on radiographic and laboratory findings.

Laboratory Findings. Due to inadequate intake, the serum phosphorus level is low or low-normal in rickets of prematurity. The renal response is appropriate, with conservation of phosphate leading to a low urine phosphate level; the tubular reabsorption of phosphate is >95%. Most patients have normal levels of 25-D, unless there has been inadequate intake or poor absorption (discussed earlier). The hypophosphatemia stimulates renal 1α-hydroxylase, so levels of 1,25-D are high or high-normal. These high levels may contribute to bone demineralization because 1,25-D stimulates bone resorption. Serum levels of calcium are low, normal, or high, and patients often have hypercalciuria. Elevated serum calcium levels and hypercalciuria are secondary to increased intestinal absorption and bone dissolution due to elevation of 1,25-D levels and the inability to deposit calcium in bone because of an inadequate phosphorus supply. The hypercalciuria indicates that phosphorus is the limiting nutrient for bone mineralization, although increased provision of phosphorus alone is frequently unable to correct the mineralization defect; increased calcium is also necessary. Hence, there is an inadequate supply of calcium and phosphorus, but the deficiency in phosphorus is greater.

Alkaline phosphatase levels are often elevated, but some affected infants have normal levels. In some instances, normal alkaline phosphatase levels may be secondary to resolution of the bone demineralization because of an adequate mineral supply despite the continued presence of radiologic changes, which take longer to resolve. However, alkaline phosphatase levels may be normal despite active disease. No single blood test is 100% sensitive for the diagnosis of rickets. The diagnosis should be suspected in infants with an alkaline phosphatase level that is more than 5–6 times the upper limit of normal for adults (unless there is concomitant liver disease) or a phosphorus level <5.6 mg/dL. The diagnosis is confirmed by radiologic evidence of rickets, which is best seen on films of the wrists and ankles. Films of the arms and legs may reveal fractures. The rachitic rosary may be visible on chest x-ray. Unfortunately, x-rays are not able to detect early demineralization of bone because changes are not evident until there is >20–30% reduction in the bone mineral content.

Diagnosis. Because many premature infants have no overt clinical manifestations of rickets, screening tests are recommended. These should include weekly measurements of calcium, phosphorus, and alkaline phosphatase. Periodic measurement of the serum bicarbonate concentration is also important because metabolic acidosis causes dissolution of bone. At least 1 screening x-ray for rickets at 6–8 wk of age is appropriate in infants who are at high risk for rickets; additional films may be indicated in very high-risk infants.

Prevention. Provision of adequate amounts of calcium, phosphorus, and vitamin D significantly decreases the risk of rickets of prematurity. Parenteral nutrition is often necessary initially in very premature infants. In the past, adequate parenteral calcium and phosphorus delivery was difficult because of limits secondary to insolubility of these ions when their concentrations were increased. Current amino acid preparations allow for higher concentrations of calcium and phosphate; this decreases the risk of rickets. Early transition to enteral feedings is also helpful. These infants should receive either human milk fortified with calcium and phosphorus or preterm infant formula, which has higher concentrations of calcium and phosphorus than standard formula. Soy formula should be avoided because there is decreased bioavailability of calcium and phosphorus. Increased mineral feedings should continue until the infant weighs 3–3.5 kg. These infants should also receive approximately 400 IU/day of vitamin D via formula and vitamin supplements.

Treatment. Therapy for rickets of prematurity focuses on ensuring adequate delivery of calcium, phosphorus, and vitamin D. If mineral delivery has been good and there is no evidence of healing, then it is important to screen for vitamin D deficiency by measuring serum 25-D. Measurement of PTH, 1,25-D, and urinary calcium and phosphorus may be helpful in some cases.

DISTAL RENAL TUBULAR ACIDOSIS (SEE CHAPTER 529)

Distal renal tubular acidosis usually presents with failure to thrive. Patients have a metabolic acidosis with an inability to acidify the urine appropriately. Hypercalciuria and nephrocalcinosis are typically present. There are many possible etiologies, including autosomal recessive and autosomal dominant forms. Rickets is variable, and it responds to alkali therapy (see Fig. 48-4).

HYPERVITAMINOSIS D

Etiology. Hypervitaminosis D is secondary to excessive intake of vitamin D. It may occur with long-term high intake or with a substantial, acute ingestion (see Table 48-1). Most cases are secondary to misuse of prescribed or over-the-counter vitamin D supplements, but other cases have been secondary to accidental overfortification of milk, contamination of table sugar, and inadvertent use of vitamin D supplements as a cooking oil. The recommended upper limits for long-term vitamin D intake are 1,000 IU for children younger than 1 year old and 2,000 IU for older children and adults. Hypervitaminosis D can also result from excessive intake of synthetic vitamin D analogs (25-D, 1,25-D) Vitamin D intoxication is never secondary to excessive exposure to sunlight, probably because ultraviolet irradiation can transform vitamin D_3 and its precursor into inactive metabolites.

Pathogenesis. Although vitamin D increases intestinal absorption of calcium, the dominant mechanism of the hypercalcemia is excessive bone resorption.

Clinical Manifestations. The signs and symptoms of vitamin D intoxication are secondary to hypercalcemia. Gastrointestinal manifestations include nausea, vomiting, poor feeding, constipation, abdominal pain, and pancreatitis. Possible cardiac findings are hypertension, decreased Q-T interval, and arrhythmias. The central nervous system effects of hypercalcemia include lethargy, hypotonia, confusion, disorientation, depression, psychosis, hallucinations, and coma. Hypercalcemia impairs renal concentrating mechanisms, which may lead to polyuria, dehydration, and hypernatremia. Hypercalcemia can also lead to acute renal failure, nephrolithiasis, and nephrocalcinosis, which may result in chronic renal insufficiency. Deaths are usually associated with arrhythmias or dehydration.

Laboratory Findings. The classic findings in vitamin D intoxication are hypercalcemia and extremely elevated levels of 25-D (>150 ng/mL). Hyperphosphatemia is also common. PTH levels are appropriately decreased due to hypercalcemia. Hypercalciuria is universally present and may lead to nephrocalcinosis, which is visible on renal ultrasound. Hypercalcemia and nephrocalcinosis may lead to renal insufficiency; monitoring of renal function is critical.

Surprisingly, levels of 1,25-D are usually normal. This may be due to downregulation of renal 1α-hydroxylase by the combination of low PTH, hyperphosphatemia, and a direct effect of 1,25-D. There is evidence indicating that the level of free 1,25-D may be high due to displacement from vitamin D–binding proteins by 25-D. Nephrocalcinosis is often visible on ultrasound or CT scan. Anemia is sometimes present; the mechanism is unknown.

Diagnosis and Differential Diagnosis. The diagnosis is based on the presence of hypercalcemia and an elevated serum 25-D level, although children with excess intake of 1,25-D or another synthetic vitamin D preparation have normal levels of 25-D. With careful sleuthing, there is usually a history of excess intake of vitamin D, although in some situations (overfortification of milk by a dairy), the patient and family may be unaware.

The **differential diagnosis** of vitamin D intoxication focuses on other causes of hypercalcemia. **Hyperparathyroidism** produces hypophosphatemia, whereas vitamin D intoxication usually causes hyperphosphatemia. **Williams syndrome** is often suggested by phenotypic features and accompanying cardiac disease. **Subcutaneous fat necrosis** is a common cause of hypercalcemia in young infants; skin findings are usually present. The hypercalcemia of **familial benign hypocalciuric hypercalcemia** is mild, asymptomatic, and associated with hypocalciuria. Hypercalcemia of **malignancy** is an important consideration. High intake of calcium, especially in the presence of renal insufficiency, can also cause hypercalcemia. Questioning about calcium intake should be part of the history in a patient with hypercalcemia. Occasionally, patients are intentionally taking high doses of calcium and vitamin D.

Treatment. The treatment of vitamin D intoxication focuses on control of hypercalcemia. Many patients with hypercalcemia are dehydrated as a result of polyuria from nephrogenic diabetes insipidus, poor oral intake, and vomiting. Rehydration lowers the serum calcium level via dilution and corrects prerenal azotemia. The resultant increased urine output increases urinary calcium excretion. Urinary calcium excretion is also increased by high urinary sodium excretion. The mainstay of the initial treatment is aggressive therapy with normal saline, often in conjunction with a loop diuretic to further increase calcium excretion.

Normal saline, with or without a loop diuretic, is often adequate for treating mild or moderate hypercalcemia. More significant hypercalcemia usually requires other therapies. Glucocorticoids decrease intestinal absorption of calcium by blocking the action of 1,25-D. There is also a decrease in the levels of 25-D and 1,25-D. The usual dose of prednisone is 1–2 mg/kg/24 hr.

Calcitonin, which lowers calcium by inhibiting bone resorption, is a useful adjunct, but its effect is usually not dramatic. There is an excellent response to intravenous or oral bisphosphonates in vitamin D intoxication. Bisphosphonates inhibit bone resorption through their effects on osteoclasts. Hemodialysis, using a low or 0 dialysate calcium, can rapidly lower serum calcium in patients with severe hypercalcemia that is refractory to other measures.

Along with controlling hypercalcemia, it is imperative to eliminate the source of excess vitamin D. Additional sources of vitamin D, such as multivitamins and fortified foods, should be eliminated or reduced. Avoidance of sun exposure, including the use of sunscreen, is prudent. The patient should also restrict calcium intake.

Prognosis. Most children make a full recovery, but hypervitaminosis D can be fatal or may lead to chronic renal failure. Because vitamin D is stored in fat, levels may remain elevated for months, necessitating regular monitoring of 25-D, serum calcium, and urine calcium.

Barrueto F Jr, Wang-Flores HH, Howland MA, et al: Acute vitamin D intoxication in a child. *Pediatrics* 2005;116:e453–e456.

Bereket A, Erdogan T: Oral bisphosphonate therapy for vitamin D intoxication of the infant. *Pediatrics* 2003;111:899–901.

Bishop N: Don't ignore vitamin D. *Arch Dis Child* 2006;91:549–550.

Dawodu A, Agarwal M, Sankarankutty M, et al: Higher prevalence of vitamin D deficiency in mothers of rachitic than nonrachitic children. *J Pediatr* 2005;147:109–111.

Ezgu FS, Buyan N, Gunduz M, et al: Vitamin D intoxication and hypercalcaemia in an infant treated with pamidronate infusions. *Eur J Pediatr* 2004;163:163–165.

Gartner LM, Greer FR, Section on Breastfeeding, Committee on Nutrition, American Academy of Pediatrics: Prevention of rickets and vitamin D deficiency: New guidelines for vitamin D intake. *Pediatrics* 2003;111:908–910.
Hatun S, Islam O, Cizmecioglu F, et al: Subclinical vitamin D deficiency is increased in adolescent girls who wear concealing clothing. *J Nutr* 2005;135:218–222.
Jonsson KB, Zahradnik R, Larsson T, et al: Fibroblast growth factor 23 in oncogenic osteomalacia and x-linked hypophosphatemia. *N Engl J Med* 2003;348:1656–1663.
Ladhani S, Srinivasa L, Buchanan C, et al: Presentation of vitamin D deficiency. *Arch Dis Child* 2004;89:781–784.
Lanon AJ: Bone health in children. *BMJ* 2006;333:763–764.
Mylott BM, Kump T, Bolton ML, et al: Rickets in the dairy state. *WMJ* 2004;103:84–87.
Oginni LM, Sharp CA, Badru OS, et al: Radiological and biochemical resolution of nutritional rickets with calcium. *Arch Dis Child* 2003;88:812–817.
Pettifor JM: Nutritional rickets: Deficiency of vitamin D, calcium, or both? *Am J Clin Nutr* 2004;80(suppl):1725S–1729S.
Rajakumar K, Thomas SB: Reemerging nutritional rickets. *Arch Pediatr Adolesc Med* 2005;159:335–341.
Robinson PD, Högler W, Craig ME, et al: The re-emerging burden of rickets: a decade of experience from Sydney. *Arch Dis Child* 2006;91:564–568.
Tenenhouse HS, Murer H: Disorders of renal tubular phosphate transport. *J Am Soc Nephrol* 2003;14:240–248.
Yamamoto T, Imanishi Y, Kinoshita E, et al: The role of fibroblast growth factor 23 for hypophosphatemia and abnormal regulation of vitamin D metabolism in patients with McCune-Albright syndrome. *J Bone Miner Metab* 2005;23:231–237.

Chapter 49 ■ Vitamin E Deficiency

Larry A. Greenbaum

Vitamin E functions as an antioxidant, but its precise biochemical functions are not known. Vitamin E deficiency, which may cause hemolysis or neurologic manifestations, occurs in premature infants, in patients with malabsorption, and in an autosomal recessive disorder affecting vitamin E transport. Because of its role as an antioxidant, there is considerable research on the potential role of vitamin E supplementation in chronic illnesses.

PATHOGENESIS. The term *vitamin E* denotes a group of 8 compounds with similar structures and antioxidant activity. The most potent member of these compounds is α-tocopherol, which is also the main form in humans. The best dietary sources of vitamin E are vegetable oils, seeds, nuts, green leafy vegetables, and margarine (Table 48-1).

The majority of vitamin E is located within cell membranes, where it prevents lipid peroxidation and the formation of free radicals. Other antioxidants, such as ascorbic acid, enhance the antioxidant activity of vitamin E. The importance of other functions of vitamin E is still being delineated.

Premature infants are particularly susceptible to vitamin E deficiency because there is significant transfer of vitamin E during the last trimester of pregnancy. Vitamin E deficiency in premature infants causes thrombocytosis, edema, and hemolysis potentially causing anemia. The risk of symptomatic vitamin E deficiency was increased by the use of formulas for premature infants that had a high content of polyunsaturated fatty acids. This led to a high content of polyunsaturated fatty acids in red blood cell membranes, making them more susceptible to oxidative stress, which could be ameliorated by vitamin E. Oxidative stress was augmented by aggressive use of iron supplementation; iron increases the production of oxygen radicals. The incidence of hemolysis due to vitamin E deficiency in premature infants decreased secondary to the use of formulas with a lower content of polyunsaturated fatty acids, less aggressive use of iron, and provision of adequate vitamin E.

Because vitamin E is plentiful in common foods, primary dietary deficiency is rare except in premature infants and in severe, generalized malnutrition. Vitamin E deficiency does occur in children with fat malabsorption secondary to the need for bile acid for vitamin E absorption. Although symptomatic disease is most common in children with cholestatic liver disease, it may occur in patients with cystic fibrosis, celiac disease, short-bowel syndrome, or Crohn disease. The autosomal recessive disorder **abetalipoproteinemia** (see Chapter 86) causes fat malabsorption, and vitamin E deficiency is a frequent complication.

In **ataxia with isolated vitamin E deficiency** (AVED), a rare autosomal recessive disorder, there are mutations in the gene for α-tocopherol transfer protein. These patients are unable to incorporate vitamin E into lipoproteins before their release from the liver. This leads to reduced serum levels of vitamin E. There is no associated fat malabsorption, and absorption of vitamin E from the intestine occurs normally.

CLINICAL MANIFESTATIONS. A severe, progressive neurologic disorder occurs in patients with prolonged vitamin E deficiency. Clinical manifestations do not appear until after 1 yr of age, even in children with cholestasis since birth. Patients may have cerebellar disease, posterior column dysfunction, and retinal disease. Loss of deep tendon reflexes is usually the initial finding. Subsequent manifestations include limb ataxia (intention tremor, dysdiadochokinesia), truncal ataxia (wide-based, unsteady gait), dysarthria, ophthalmoplegia (limited upward gaze), nystagmus, decreased proprioception (positive Romberg test), decreased vibratory sensation, and dysarthria. Some patients have pigmentary retinopathy. Visual field constriction may progress to blindness. Cognition and behavior may also be affected. Myopathy and cardiac arrhythmias are less common findings.

In premature infants, hemolysis due to vitamin E deficiency typically develops during the 2nd month of life. Edema may also be present.

LABORATORY FINDINGS. Serum vitamin E levels increase in the presence of high serum lipid levels, even when vitamin E deficiency is present. Hence, vitamin E status is best determined by measuring the ratio of vitamin E to serum lipids; a ratio <0.8 mg/g is abnormal. Premature infants with hemolysis due to vitamin E deficiency also often have elevated platelet counts.

Neurologic involvement may cause abnormal somatosensory evoked potentials and nerve conduction studies. Abnormalities on electroretinography may precede physical examination findings in patients with retinal involvement.

DIAGNOSIS AND DIFFERENTIAL DIAGNOSIS. Premature infants with unexplained hemolytic anemia after the 1st month of life, especially if thrombocytosis is present, either should be empirically treated with vitamin E or should have serum vitamin E and lipid levels measured. Children with neurologic findings and a disease that causes fat malabsorption should have their vitamin E status evaluated.

Because children with AVED do not have symptoms of malabsorption, a correct diagnosis requires a high index of suspicion. Some patients have been misdiagnosed with **Friedreich ataxia** (Chapter 597.1). Children with unexplained ataxia should be screened for vitamin E deficiency.

TREATMENT. For correction of deficiency in neonates, the dose of vitamin E is 25–50 units/day for 1 wk, followed by adequate dietary intake. α-Tocopheryl polyethylene glycol succinate (TPGS) is a water-soluble preparation of vitamin E that is absorbed in the absence of bile salts. Unlike conventional fat-soluble vitamin E preparations, TPGS is effective in children with vitamin E deficiency secondary to severe malabsorption. Typical doses are 20–25 units/kg/day, with adjustment based on the ratio of vitamin E to serum lipids. TPGS enhances absorption of the other fat-soluble vitamins (A, D, and K) and a variety of medications. Children with milder malabsorption can receive conventional vitamin E preparations. Children with AVED normalize their serum vitamin E levels with high doses of vitamin E; they do not need to receive TPGS because there is not a defect in gastrointestinal absorption.

PROGNOSIS. The hemolytic anemia in infants resolves with correction of the vitamin E deficiency. Some neurologic manifestations of vitamin E deficiency may be reversible with early treatment, but many patients have little or no improvement. Treatment prevents progression.

PREVENTION. Premature infants should receive sufficient vitamin E and formula without a high content of polyunsaturated fatty acids. Children at risk for vitamin E deficiency due to malabsorption should be screened for deficiency and given adequate vitamin E supplementation. Vitamin preparations with high content of all of the fat-soluble vitamins are available.

Brion LP, Bell EF, Raghuveer TS: Variability in the dose of intravenous vitamin E given to very low birth weight infants. *J Perinatol* 2005;25:139–142.

Chow CK: Biological functions and metabolic fate of vitamin E revisited. *J Biomed Sci* 2004;11:295–302.

Gabsi S, Gouider-Khouja N, Belal S, et al: Effect of vitamin E supplementation in patients with ataxia with vitamin E deficiency. *Eur J Neurol* 2001;8:477–481.

Horwitt MK: Critique of the requirement for vitamin E. *Am J Clin Nutr* 2001;73:1003–1005.

Kayden HJ: The genetic basis of vitamin E deficiency in humans. *Nutrition* 2001;17:797–798.

Owen AJ, Batterham MJ, Probst YC, et al: Low plasma vitamin E levels in major depression: Diet or disease? *Eur J Clin Nutr* 2005;59:304–306.

Traber MG: Vitamin E: Too much or not enough? *Am J Clin Nutr* 2001;73:997–998.

Chapter 50 ■ Vitamin K Deficiency

Larry A. Greenbaum

Deficiency of vitamin K, which is necessary for the synthesis of clotting factors II, VII, IX, and X, may result in clinically significant bleeding. This typically affects infants, who experience a transient deficiency related to inadequate intake, or patients of any age who have decreased vitamin K absorption. Mild vitamin K deficiency may affect long-term bone and vascular health (see Chapters 103.4 and 480).

PATHOGENESIS. Vitamin K is a group of compounds that have a common naphthoquinone ring structure. Phylloquinone, called *vitamin K_1*, is present in a variety of dietary sources, with green leafy vegetables, liver, and certain legumes and plant oils having the highest content. Vitamin K_1 is the form used to fortify foods and as a medication in the USA. Vitamin K_2 is a group of compounds called *menaquinones,* which are produced by intestinal bacteria. There is uncertainty regarding the relative importance of intestinally produced vitamin K_2. Menaquinones are also present in meat, especially liver, and cheese. A menaquinone is used pharmacologically in some countries.

Vitamin K is a cofactor for γ-glutamyl carboxylase, an enzyme that performs post-translational carboxylation, converting glutamate residues in proteins to γ-carboxyglutamate (Gla). The Gla residues, by facilitating calcium binding, are necessary for protein function.

The classic Gla-containing proteins involved in blood coagulation that are decreased in vitamin K deficiency are factors II (prothrombin), VII, IX, and X. In addition, vitamin K deficiency causes a decrease in proteins C and S, which inhibit blood coagulation, and protein Z, which also has a role in coagulation. All of these proteins are made only in the liver, except for protein S, a product of various tissues.

Gla-containing proteins are also involved in bone biology (e.g., osteocalcin and protein S) and vascular biology (matrix Gla protein and protein S). Based on the presence of reduced levels of Gla, these proteins appear more sensitive to subtle vitamin K deficiency than the coagulation proteins. There is evidence suggesting that mild vitamin K deficiency may have a deleterious effect on long-term bone strength and vascular health.

Because it is fat-soluble, vitamin K requires the presence of bile salts for its absorption. Unlike other fat-soluble vitamins, there are limited body stores of vitamin K. In addition, there is high turnover of vitamin K and the vitamin K-dependent clotting factors have a short half-life. Hence, symptomatic vitamin K deficiency may develop within weeks when there is inadequate supply due to low intake or malabsorption.

There are 3 forms of **vitamin K–deficiency bleeding (VKDB)** of the newborn (see Chapter 103.4). Early VKDB, formerly called *classic hemorrhagic disease of the newborn,* occurs at 1–14 days of age. Early VKDB is secondary to low stores of vitamin K at birth due to the poor transfer of vitamin K across the placenta and inadequate intake during the 1st few days of life. In addition, there is no intestinal synthesis of vitamin K_2 because the newborn gut is sterile. Early VKDB occurs mostly in breast-fed infants due to the low vitamin K content of breast milk (formula is fortified). Delayed feeding is an additional risk factor.

Late VKDB most commonly occurs at 2–12 wk of age, although cases can occur up to 6 mo after birth. Almost all cases are in breast-fed infants due to the low vitamin K content of breast milk. An additional risk factor is occult malabsorption of vitamin K, such as occurs in children with undiagnosed cystic fibrosis or cholestatic liver disease (e.g., biliary atresia, α_1-antitrypsin deficiency). Without vitamin K prophylaxis, the incidence is 4–10/100,000 newborns.

The 3rd form of VKDB of the newborn occurs at birth or shortly thereafter. It is secondary to maternal intake of medications (warfarin, phenobarbital, phenytoin) that cross the placenta and interfere with vitamin K function.

Vitamin K–deficiency bleeding due to fat malabsorption may occur in children of any age. Potential etiologies include cholestatic liver disease, pancreatic disease, and intestinal disorders (celiac sprue, inflammatory bowel disease, short-bowel syndrome). Prolonged diarrhea, especially in breast-fed infants, may cause vitamin K deficiency. Children with cystic fibrosis are most likely to have vitamin K deficiency if they have pancreatic insufficiency and liver disease.

Beyond infancy, low dietary intake by itself never causes vitamin K deficiency. However, the combination of poor intake and the use of broad-spectrum antibiotics that eliminate the intestine's vitamin K_2–producing bacteria can cause vitamin K deficiency. This is especially common in the intensive care unit. Vitamin K deficiency may also occur in patients who receive total parenteral nutrition without vitamin K supplementation.

CLINICAL MANIFESTATIONS. In early VKDB, the most common sites of bleeding are the gastrointestinal tract, mucosal and cutaneous tissue, the umbilical stump, and the post-circumcision site;

intracranial bleeding is less common. Gastrointestinal blood loss can be severe enough to require a transfusion. In contrast, the most frequent site of bleeding in late VKDB is intracranial, although cutaneous and gastrointestinal bleeding may be the initial manifestation. Intracranial bleeding may cause convulsions, permanent neurologic sequelae, or death. In some cases of late VKDB, the presence of an underlying disorder may be suggested by jaundice or failure to thrive. Older children with vitamin K deficiency may present with bruising, mucocutaneous bleeding, or more serious bleeding.

LABORATORY FINDINGS. In patients with bleeding due to vitamin K deficiency, the prothrombin time (PT) is prolonged. The PT must be interpreted based on the patient's age because it is normally prolonged in newborns (see Chapter 475.2). The partial thromboplastin time (PTT) is usually prolonged, but may be normal in early deficiency because factor VII has the shortest half-life of the coagulation factors (isolated factor VII deficiency does not affect the PTT). The platelet count and fibrinogen level are normal.

When there is mild vitamin K deficiency, the PT is normal, but there are elevated levels of the undercarboxylated forms of the proteins that are normally carboxylated in the presence of vitamin K. These undercarboxylated proteins are called *proteins induced by vitamin K absence* (PIVKA). Measurement of undercarboxylated factor II (PIVKA-II) can be used to detect mild vitamin K deficiency. Determination of blood vitamin K levels is less useful because of significant variation based on recent dietary intake; levels are not always reflective of tissue stores.

DIAGNOSIS AND DIFFERENTIAL DIAGNOSIS. The diagnosis is established by the presence of a prolonged PT that corrects rapidly after administration of vitamin K. This also stops the active bleeding. Other possible causes of bleeding and a prolonged PT include **disseminated intravascular coagulation** (DIC), liver failure, and rare hereditary deficiencies of clotting factors. DIC, which is most commonly secondary to sepsis, is associated with thrombocytopenia, low fibrinogen, and elevated D-dimers. In addition, most patients have hemodynamic instability that does not correct with restoration of blood volume. Severe liver disease results in decreased production of clotting factors; the PT does not fully correct with administration of vitamin K. Children with a hereditary disorder have a deficiency in a specific clotting factor (I, II, V, VII, X).

Coumarin derivatives inhibit the action of vitamin K by preventing its recycling to an active form after it functions as a cofactor for γ-glutamyl carboxylase. Bleeding can occur with overdosage of the commonly used anticoagulant warfarin or with ingestion of rodent poison, which contains a coumarin derivative. High doses of salicylates also inhibit vitamin K regeneration, potentially leading to a prolonged PT and clinical bleeding.

TREATMENT. Infants with VKDB should receive 1 mg of parenteral vitamin K. The PT should decrease within 6 hr and normalize within 24 hr. For rapid correction in adolescents, the parenteral dose is 2.5–10 mg. In addition to vitamin K, a patient with severe, life-threatening bleeding should receive an infusion of fresh frozen plasma, which corrects the coagulopathy rapidly. Children with vitamin K deficiency due to malabsorption require chronic administration of high doses of oral vitamin K (2.5 mg twice/wk–5 mg/day). Parenteral vitamin K may be necessary if oral vitamin K is ineffective.

PREVENTION. Administration of either oral or parenteral vitamin K soon after birth prevents early VKDB of the newborn. In contrast, a single dose of oral vitamin K does not prevent a substantial number of cases of late VKDB. However, a single intramuscular injection of vitamin K (1 mg), the current practice in the USA, is almost universally effective, except in children with severe malabsorption. This increased efficacy of the intramuscular form is believed to be due to a depot effect. Concerns about an association between parenteral vitamin K at birth and the later development of malignancy are unsubstantiated.

Discontinuing the offending medications before delivery can prevent VKDB due to maternal medications. If this is not possible, administration of vitamin K to the mother may be helpful. In addition, the neonate should receive parenteral vitamin K immediately after birth. If this does not correct the coagulopathy rapidly, then the child should receive fresh frozen plasma.

Children at high risk for malabsorption of vitamin K should receive supplemental vitamin K and periodic measurement of the PT.

American Academy of Pediatrics Committee on Fetus and Newborn: Controversies concerning vitamin K and the newborn. *Pediatrics* 2003;112:191–192.

Conway SP, Wolfe SP, Brownlee KG, et al: Vitamin K status among children with cystic fibrosis and its relationship to bone mineral density and bone turnover. *Pediatrics* 2005;115:1325–1331.

Hey E: Vitamin K: What, why, and when. *Arch Dis Child Fetal Neonatal Ed* 2003;88:F80–F83.

Puckett RM, Offringa M: Prophylactic vitamin K for vitamin K deficiency bleeding in neonates. *Cochrane Database Syst Rev* 2000:CD002776.

Sutor AH: New aspects of vitamin K prophylaxis. *Semin Thromb Hemost* 2003;29:373–376.

Chapter 51 ■ Micronutrient Mineral Deficiencies

Larry A. Greenbaum

Micronutrients include vitamins (see Chapters 45–50) and trace elements. By definition, a trace element is <0.01% of the body weight. Trace elements have a variety of essential functions (Table 51-1). With the exception of iron deficiency, trace element deficiency (see Table 51-1) is uncommon in developed countries, but some deficiencies (iodine, zinc, selenium) are important public health problems in a number of developing countries. Because of low nutritional requirements and plentiful supply, deficiencies of some of the trace elements are extremely rare in humans, and are only rarely described, typically in patients receiving unusual diets or prolonged total parenteral nutrition without adequate delivery of a specific trace element. Excess intake of trace elements (see Table 51-1) is uncommon, but it may occur due to environmental exposure or overuse of supplements.

For a number of reasons, children are especially susceptible to trace element deficiency. First, growth creates an increased demand for most trace elements. Second, some organs are more likely to sustain permanent damage due to trace element deficiency during childhood. The developing brain is particularly vulnerable to the consequences of certain deficiency states (iron, iodide). Similarly, adequate fluoride is most critical for dental health during childhood. Third, children, especially in the developing world, are more prone to gastrointestinal disorders that may cause trace element deficiencies due to malabsorption.

A normal diet provides adequate intake of most trace elements. However, the intake of certain trace elements varies significantly in different geographic locations. Iodide-containing food is plentiful near the ocean, but inland areas often have inadequate sources, leading to goiter and **hypothyroidism.** This is not a problem in the USA because of the widespread use of iodized salt;

TABLE 51-1. Trace Elements

ELEMENT	PHYSIOLOGY	EFFECTS OF DEFICIENCY	EFFECTS OF EXCESS	DIETARY SOURCES
Chromium	Potentiates the action of insulin	Impaired glucose tolerance, peripheral neuropathy and encephalopathy	Unknown	Meat, brewer's yeast
Copper	Absorbed via specific intestinal transporter; circulates bound to ceruloplasmin; enzyme cofactor (superoxide dismutase, cytochrome oxidase, and enzymes involved in iron metabolism and connective tissue formation)	Microytic anemia, osteoporosis, neutropenia, neurologic symptoms, depigmentation of hair and skin	Acute: nausea, emesis, abdominal pain, coma, and hepatic necrosis; chronic toxicity (liver and brain injury) occurs in Wilson disease and another genetic disorder (see Chapters 354.2 and 354.3) and secondary to excess intake (see Chapter 354.4)	Oysters, nuts, liver, margarine, legumes, corn oil
Fluoride	Incorporated into bone	Dental caries (see Chapter 309)	Chronic: dental fluorosis water (see Chapter 304)	Toothpaste, fluoridated water
Iodine	Component of thyroid hormone (see Chapter 565)	Hypothyroidism (see Chapters 567 and 569.2)	Hypothyroidism and goiter (see Chapters 566 and 568); maternal excess may cause congenital hypothyroidism and goiter (see Chapter 569.1)	Saltwater fish, iodized salt
Iron	Component of hemoglobin, myoglobin, cytochromes, and other enzymes	Anemia (see Chapter 455), decreased alertness, impaired learning	Acute (see Chapter 58): nausea, vomiting, diarrhea, abdominal pain, and hypotension; chronic excess usually secondary to hereditary disorders (see Chapter 462.9 and 354.5); causes organ dysfunction	Deficiency may also result from blood loss (hookworm infestation, menorrhagia)
Manganese	Enzyme cofactor	Hypercholesterolemia, weight loss, decreased clotting proteins*	Neurologic manifestations, cholestatic jaundice	Nuts, grains, tea
Molybdenum	Enzyme cofactor (xanthine oxidase and others)	Tachycardia, tachypnea, night blindness, irritability, coma*	Hyperuricemia and increased risk of gout	Legumes, grains, liver
Selenium	Enzyme cofactor (prevents oxidative damage)	Cardiomyopathy (Keshan disease), myopathy	Nausea, diarrhea, neurologic manifestations, nail and hair changes, garlic odor	Meat, seafood, whole grains, garlic
Zinc	Enzyme cofactor; constituent of zinc finger proteins, which regulate gene transcription	Decreased growth, dermatitis of extremities and around orifices, impaired immunity, poor wound healing, hypogonadism, diarrhea; supplements beneficial in diarrhea and improve neurodevelopmental outcomes	Abdominal pain, diarrhea, vomiting; may worsen copper deficiency	Meat, shellfish, whole grains, legumes, cheese

*These deficiency states have been reported only in case reports associated with parenteral nutrition or highly unusual diets.

however, symptomatic iodine deficiency (goiter and hypothyroidism) is common in many developing countries. Selenium content of the soil, and consequently of food, is also quite variable. Dietary selenium deficiency (associated with cardiomyopathy) occurs in certain locations, such as some parts of China.

The consequences of severe, isolated trace mineral deficiency are illustrated in certain genetic disorders. The manifestations of **Menkes disease** (see Chapter 600) are due to a mutation in the gene coding for a protein that facilitates intestinal copper absorption. This results in severe copper deficiency; subcutaneous copper is an effective treatment. The recessive disorder **acrodermatitis enteropathica** (see Chapter 670) is secondary to malabsorption of zinc. These patients respond dramatically to zinc supplementation.

Children may have apparently asymptomatic deficiencies of certain trace elements, but still benefit from supplementation. This is dramatically illustrated by the effective use of zinc in treating children before or during diarrheal illnesses in the developing world.

Zinc deficiency is quite common in the developing word and is often associated with malnutrition or other micronutrient deficiencies (iron). Chronic zinc deficiency is associated with dwarfism, hypogonadism, dermatitis, and T-cell immunodeficiency. Diets rich in phytates bind zinc, impairing its absorption. Zinc supplementation of at-risk children reduces the incidence and severity of diarrhea, pneumonia, and possibly malaria. Children with diarrhea in developing countries have been treated with zinc (20 mg/day orally for 14 days), with improved morbidity and mortality rates.

Angermayr L, Clar C: Iodine supplementation for preventing iodine deficiency disorders in children. *Cochrane Database Syst Rev* 2004:CD003819.

Baqui AH, Black RE, Arifeen SE, et al: Effect of zinc supplementation started during diarrhoea on morbidity and mortality in Bangladeshi children: Community randomized trial. *BMJ* 2002;325:1059–1062.

Bergqvist AG, Chee CM, Lutchka L, et al: Selenium deficiency associated with cardiomyopathy: A complication of the ketogenic diet. *Epilepsia* 2003;44:618–620.

Brooks WA, Santosham M, Roy SK, et al: Efficacy of zinc in young infants with acute watery diarrhea. *Am J Clin Nutr* 2005;82:605–610.

Darlow BA, Austin NC: Selenium supplementation to prevent short-term morbidity in preterm neonates. *Cochrane Database Syst Rev* 2003:CD003312.

Fok TF, Chui KK, Cheung R, et al: Manganese intake and cholestatic jaundice in neonates receiving parenteral nutrition: A randomized controlled study. *Acta Paediatr* 2001;90:1009–1015.

Prasad AS: Zinc deficiency. *BMJ* 2003;326:409–410.

Robberstad B, Strand T, Black RE, et al: Cost-effectiveness of zinc as adjunct therapy for acute childhood diarrhoea in developing countries. *Bull World Health Organ* 2004;82:523–531.

Ryan GJ, Wanko NS, Redman AR, et al: Chromium as adjunctive treatment for type 2 diabetes. *Ann Pharmacother* 2003;37:876–885.

Shrimpton R, Gross R, Darnton-Hill I, Young M: Zinc deficiency: What are the most appropriate interventions? *BMJ* 2005;330:347–350.

Taneja S, Bhandari N, Bahl R, et al: Impact of zinc supplementation on mental and psychomotor scores of children aged 12 to 18 months: A randomized, double-blind trial. *J Pediatr* 2005;146:506–511.

Tomkins A: Improving iron status in children in poor environments. *BMJ* 2002;325:1125.

Zlotkin S: Another small step in the path to controlling micronutrient deficiencies . . . but we still have a long way to go. *J Pediatr* 2004;145:4–6.

Part VI ▪ Pathophysiology of Body Fluids and Fluid Therapy

Chapter 52 ▪ Electrolyte and Acid-Base Disorders Larry A. Greenbaum

52.1 • Composition of Body Fluids

TOTAL BODY WATER. Water is the most plentiful constituent of the human body. Total body water (TBW) as a percentage of body weight varies with age (Fig. 52-1). The fetus has very high TBW, which gradually decreases to approximately 75% of birthweight for a term infant. Premature infants have higher TBW than term infants. During the 1st yr of life, TBW decreases to approximately 60% of body weight and basically remains at this level until puberty. At puberty, the fat content of females increases more than that of males, who acquire more muscle mass than females. Because fat has very low water content and muscle has high water content, by the end of puberty, TBW in males remains at 60%, but TBW in females decreases to approximately 50% of body weight. The high fat content in overweight children causes a decrease in TBW as a percentage of body weight. During dehydration, TBW decreases and, thus, is a smaller percentage of body weight.

FLUID COMPARTMENTS. TBW is divided between 2 main compartments: intracellular fluid (ICF) and extracellular fluid (ECF). In the fetus and newborn, the ECF volume is larger than the ICF volume (see Fig. 52-1). The normal postnatal diuresis causes an immediate decrease in the ECF volume. This is followed by continued expansion of the ICF volume, which results from cellular growth. By 1 yr of age, the ratio of the ICF volume to the ECF volume approaches adult levels. The ECF volume is approximately 20–25% of body weight and the ICF volume is approximately 30–40% of body weight, close to twice the ECF volume (Fig. 52-2). With puberty, the increased muscle mass of males causes them to have a higher ICF volume than females. There is no significant difference in the ECF volume between postpubertal females and males.

The ECF is further divided into the plasma water and the interstitial fluid (see Fig. 52-2). The plasma water is 5% of body weight. The blood volume, given a hematocrit of 40%, is usually 8% of body weight, although it is higher in newborns and young infants. In premature newborns, it is approximately 10% of body weight. The volume of plasma water can be altered by pathologic conditions, including dehydration, anemia, polycythemia, heart failure, abnormal plasma osmolality, and hypoalbuminemia. The interstitial fluid, normally 15% of body weight, can increase dramatically in diseases associated with edema, such as heart failure, protein-losing enteropathy, liver failure, nephrotic syndrome, and sepsis. An increase in interstitial fluid also occurs in patients with ascites or pleural effusions.

There is normally a delicate equilibrium between the intravascular fluid and the interstitial fluid. The balance between hydrostatic and oncotic forces regulates the intravascular volume, which is critical for proper tissue perfusion. The intravascular fluid has a higher concentration of albumin than the interstitial fluid, and the consequent oncotic force draws water into the intravascular space. The maintenance of this gradient depends on the limited permeability of albumin across the capillaries. The hydrostatic pressure of the intravascular space, which is due to the pumping action of the heart, drives fluid out of the intravascular space. These forces favor movement into the interstitial space at the arterial ends of the capillaries. The decreased hydrostatic forces and increased oncotic forces, which result from the dilutional increase in albumin concentration, cause movement of fluid into the venous ends of the capillaries. Overall, there is usually a net movement of fluid out of the intravascular space, but this fluid is returned to the circulation via the **lymphatics.** An imbalance in these forces may cause expansion of the interstitial volume at the expense of the intravascular volume. In children with hypoalbuminemia, the decreased oncotic pressure of the intravascular fluid contributes to the development of **edema.** Loss of fluid from the intravascular space may compromise the intravascular volume, placing the child at risk for inadequate blood flow to vital organs. This is especially likely in diseases in which capillary leak occurs because the loss of albumin from the intravascular space is associated with an increase in the albumin concentration in the interstitial space, further compromising the oncotic forces that normally maintain intravascular volume. In contrast, with **heart failure,** there is an increase in venous hydrostatic pressure from expansion of the intravascular volume, which is caused by impaired pumping by the heart, and the increase in venous pressure causes fluid to move from the intravascular space to the interstitial space. Expansion of the intravascular volume and increased intravascular pressure also cause the edema that occurs with acute glomerulonephritis.

ELECTROLYTE COMPOSITION. The composition of the solutes in the ICF and ECF are very different (Fig. 52-3). Sodium and chloride are the dominant cation and anion, respectively, in the ECF. The sodium and chloride concentrations in the ICF are much lower. Potassium is the most abundant cation in the ICF, and its concentration within the cells is approximately 30 times higher than in the ECF. Proteins, organic anions, and phosphate are the most plentiful anions in the ICF. The dissimilarity between the anions in the ICF and the ECF is largely determined by the presence of intracellular molecules that do not cross the cell membrane, the barrier separating the ECF and the ICF. In contrast, the difference in the distribution of cations—sodium and potassium—is due to the activity of the Na^+, K^+-ATPase pump, which uses cellular energy to actively extrude sodium from cells and move potassium into cells. The chemical gradient between the intracellular potassium concentration and the extracellular potassium concentration creates the electrical gradient across the cell membrane. The concentration-dependent movement of potassium out of the cell makes the intracellular space negative relative to the extracellular space.

The difference in the electrolyte compositions of the ECF and the ICF has important ramifications in the evaluation and treatment of electrolyte disorders. The serum concentration of an

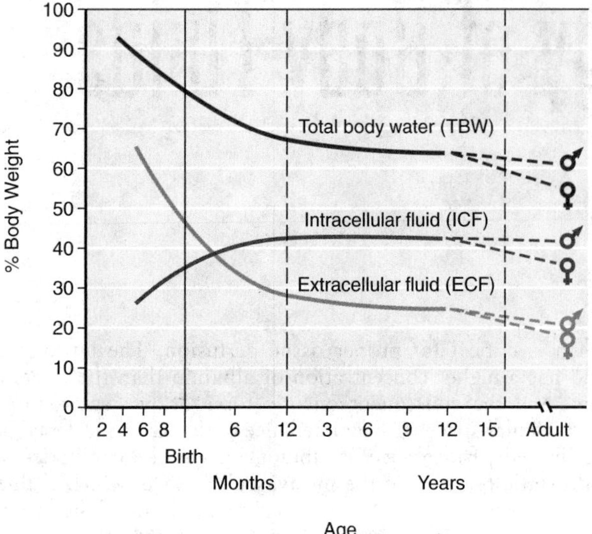

Figure 52-1. Total body water, intracellular fluid, and extracellular fluid as a percentage of body weight and a function of age. (From Winters RW: Water and electrolyte regulation. In Winters RW [editor]: *The Body Fluids in Pediatrics*. Boston, Little, Brown, 1973.)

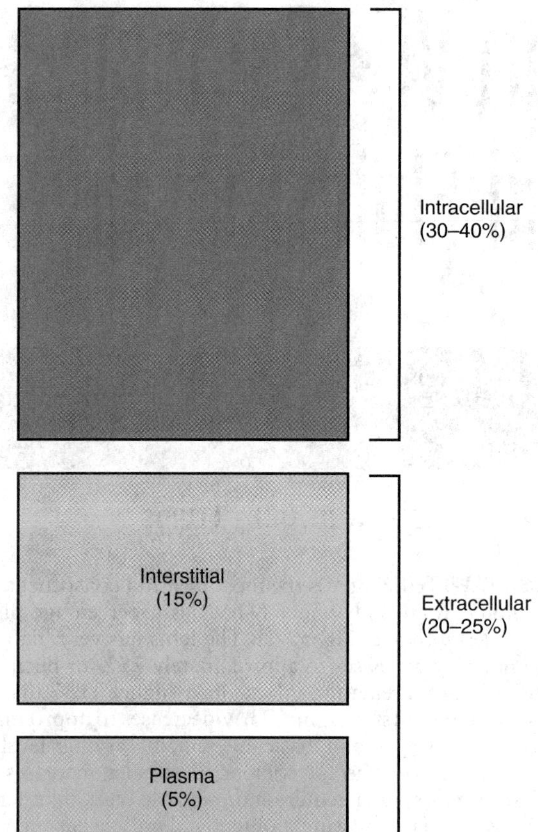

Figure 52-2. Compartments of total body water, expressed as a percentage of body weight, in an older child or adult.

electrolyte, which is measured clinically, does not always reflect the body content. This is due to the larger volume of the ICF compared with the ECF and the variation in electrolyte concentrations between these 2 compartments. For example, the intracellular potassium concentration is much higher than the serum concentration. A shift of potassium from the intracellular space can maintain a normal or even an elevated serum potassium concentration, despite massive losses of potassium from the intracellular space. This is dramatically seen in diabetic ketoacidosis, in which a state of significant potassium depletion is often masked because of a transmembrane shift of potassium from the ICF to the ECF. For potassium and phosphorus, electrolytes with a high intracellular concentration, the serum level may not reflect total body content. Similarly, the serum calcium concentration does not predict the body content of calcium, which is largely in bone.

OSMOLALITY. The ICF and the ECF are in **osmotic equilibrium** because the cell membrane is permeable to water. If the osmolal-

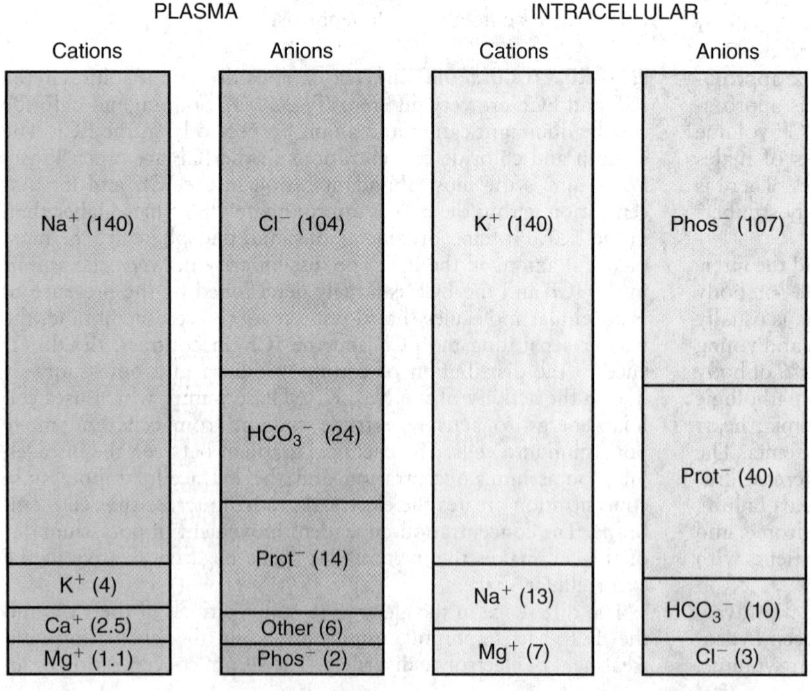

Figure 52-3. The concentrations of the major cations and anions in the intracellular space and the plasma, expressed in mEq/L.

ity in 1 compartment changes, then water movement leads to a rapid equalization of osmolality. This can lead to significant shifts of water between the intracellular space and the extracellular space. Clinically, the primary process is usually a change in the osmolality of the ECF, with a resultant shift of water into the ICF if the ECF osmolality decreases or a shift of water out of the ICF if the ECF osmolality increases. The osmolality of the ECF can be determined, and this usually equals the ICF osmolality. The plasma osmolality is normally 285–295 mOsm/kg, and it is measured by the degree of freezing point depression. The plasma osmolality can also be estimated by a calculation based on the following formula:

$$\text{Osmolality} = 2 \times [\text{Na}] + [\text{glucose}]/18 + [\text{BUN}]/2.8$$

Glucose and blood urea nitrogen (BUN) are measured in mg/dL. Division of these values by 18 and 2.8, as shown, converts the units into mmol/L. Multiplication of the sodium value by 2 accounts for its accompanying anions, principally chloride and bicarbonate. The calculated osmolality is usually slightly lower than the measured osmolality.

Glucose and urea usually contribute little to the plasma osmolality; multiplication of the sodium value by 2 provides an approximation of the osmolality. Urea is not confined to the extracellular space because it readily crosses the cell membrane and its intracellular concentration approximately equals its extracellular concentration. Whereas an elevated sodium concentration causes a shift of water from the intracellular space, with uremia, there is no osmolar gradient between the 2 compartments and consequently, no movement of water. The only exception is during **hemodialysis,** when the decrease in extracellular urea is so rapid that the intracellular urea does not have time to equilibrate. This may lead to the **disequilibrium syndrome,** in which water shifts into brain cells, potentially causing severe symptoms. Ethanol, because it freely crosses cell membranes, is another ineffective osmole. The effective osmolality can be calculated as follows:

$$\text{Effective osmolality} = 2 \times [\text{Na}] + [\text{glucose}]/18$$

The effective osmolality (also called the *tonicity*) determines the osmotic force that is mediating the shift of water between the ECF and the ICF.

Hyperglycemia causes an increase in the plasma osmolality because it is not in equilibrium with the intracellular space. During hyperglycemia there is a shift of water from the intracellular space to the extracellular space. This is clinically important in children with hyperglycemia during diabetic ketoacidosis. The shift of water causes dilution of the sodium in the extracellular space, causing hyponatremia despite an elevated plasma osmolality. The magnitude of this effect can be calculated as follows:

$$[\text{Na}]_{\text{corrected}} = [\text{Na}]_{\text{measured}} + 1.6 \times ([\text{glucose}] - 100\,\text{mg/dL})/100$$

where $[\text{Na}]_{\text{measured}}$ = sodium concentration measured by the clinical laboratory and $[\text{Na}]_{\text{corrected}}$ = corrected sodium concentration (the sodium concentration if the glucose concentration were normal and its accompanying water moved back into the cells). The $[\text{Na}]_{\text{corrected}}$ is the more reliable indicator of the patient's true ratio of total body sodium to TBW, the normal determinant of the sodium concentration.

Normally, the measured osmolality and the calculated osmolality are within 10 mOsm/kg. However, there are some clinical situations in which this does not occur. The presence of **"unmeasured osmoles"** causes the measured osmolality to be significantly elevated when compared with the calculated osmolality. This difference is the **osmolal gap,** which is present when the measured osmolality exceeds the calculated osmolality by >10 mOsm/kg. Examples of unmeasured osmoles include ethanol, ethylene glycol, methanol, and mannitol. These substances increase the measured osmolality, but are not part of the equation for calculating osmolality. The presence of an osmolal gap is a clinical clue to the presence of unmeasured osmoles and may be diagnostically useful when there is clinical suspicion of poisoning with methanol or ethylene glycol.

Pseudohyponatremia is a 2nd situation in which there is discordance between the measured osmolality and the calculated osmolality. Lipids and proteins are the solids of the serum. In patients with elevated serum lipids or proteins, the water content of the serum decreases because water is displaced by the increased amount of solids. Some clinical laboratories measure sodium concentration by determining the amount of sodium per liter of serum, including the solid component. When the solid component increases, there is a decrease in the sodium concentration per liter of serum, despite a normal concentration of sodium when based on the amount of sodium per liter of serum water. It is the concentration of sodium in serum water that is physiologically relevant. In such situations, the plasma osmolality is normal despite the presence of pseudohyponatremia because the method for measuring osmolality is not appreciably influenced by the percentage of serum that is composed of lipids and proteins. Pseudohyponatremia is diagnosed by finding a normal measured plasma osmolality despite hyponatremia. This laboratory artifact does not occur if the sodium concentration in water is measured directly with an ion-specific electrode, the technique that is increasingly used in clinical laboratories.

When there are no unmeasured osmoles and pseudohyponatremia is not a concern, the calculated osmolality provides an accurate estimate of the plasma osmolality. Measurement of plasma osmolality is useful for detecting or monitoring unmeasured osmoles and confirming the presence of true hyponatremia. Whereas many children with high plasma osmolality are dehydrated—as seen with hypernatremic dehydration or diabetic ketoacidosis—high osmolality does not always equate with dehydration. A child with **salt poisoning** or **uremia** has an elevated plasma osmolality, but may be volume overloaded. In many situations, it is best to focus on the components of the plasma osmolality and to analyze them individually to reach a correct clinical conclusion.

Olhager E, Flinke E, Hannerstad U, et al: Studies on human body composition during the first 4 months of life using magnetic resonance imaging and isotope dilution. *Pediatr Res* 2003;54:906–912.

Steinberger BA, Ford SM, Coleman TA: Intravenous immunoglobulin therapy results in post-infusional hyperproteinemia, increased serum viscosity, and pseudohyponatremia. *Am J Hematol* 2003;73:97–100.

Turchin A, Seifter JL, Seely EW: Clinical problem-solving: Mind the gap. *N Engl J Med* 2003;349:1465–1469.

52.2 • Regulation of Osmolality and Volume

The regulation of plasma osmolality and the intravascular volume are controlled by independent systems for water balance, which determines osmolality, and sodium balance, which determines volume status. Maintenance of normal osmolality depends on control of water balance. Control of volume status depends on regulation of sodium balance. When volume depletion is present, this takes precedence over regulation of osmolality, and retention of water contributes to the maintenance of intravascular volume.

REGULATION OF OSMOLALITY. The plasma osmolality is tightly regulated and maintained at 285–295 mOsm/kg. Modification of water intake and excretion maintains normal plasma osmolality.

In the steady state, the combination of water intake and water produced by the body from oxidation balances water losses from the skin, lungs, urine, and gastrointestinal tract. Only water intake and urinary losses can be regulated.

Osmoreceptors in the hypothalamus sense the plasma osmolality (see Chapter 559). An elevated effective osmolality leads to secretion of antidiuretic hormone (ADH) by neurons in the supraoptic and paraventricular nuclei in the hypothalamus. The axons of these neurons terminate in the posterior pituitary. Circulating ADH binds to its V_2 receptors in the collecting duct cells of the kidney, and, via the generation of cyclic adenosine monophosphate, causes insertion of water channels (aquaporin-2) into the renal collecting ducts. This produces increased permeability to water, permitting resorption of water into the hypertonic renal medulla. The end result is that the urine concentration increases and water excretion decreases. Urinary water losses cannot be completely eliminated because there is obligatory excretion of urinary solutes, such as urea and sodium. The regulation of ADH secretion is tightly linked to plasma osmolality, with responses detectable with a 1% change in the osmolality. ADH secretion virtually disappears when the plasma osmolality is low, allowing excretion of maximally dilute urine. The consequent loss of **free water** (water without sodium) corrects the plasma osmolality. ADH secretion is not an "all or nothing" response; there is a graded adjustment as the osmolality changes.

Production of concentrated urine under the control of ADH requires a hypertonic renal medulla. The countercurrent multiplier, produced by the loop of Henle and the vasa recta, generates this hypertonicity. ADH stimulates sodium transport in the loop of Henle, helping to maintain this gradient when water retention is necessary.

Water intake is regulated by hypothalamic osmoreceptors, although these are different from the osmoreceptors that determine ADH secretion. These osmoreceptors, by linking to the cerebral cortex, stimulate thirst when the serum osmolality increases. Thirst occurs with a small increase in the serum osmolality.

Control of osmolality is subordinate to maintenance of an adequate intravascular volume. When volume depletion is present, both ADH secretion and thirst are stimulated, regardless of the plasma osmolality. The sensation of thirst requires moderate volume depletion, but only a 1–2% change in the plasma osmolality. Although all of the mechanisms are not clear, angiotensin II, which is increased during volume depletion, is known to stimulate thirst. Baroreceptors, when sensing volume depletion, may also stimulate thirst.

A number of conditions can limit the kidney's ability to excrete adequate water to correct low plasma osmolality. In the **syndrome of inappropriate antidiuretic hormone (SIADH)**, ADH continues to be produced despite a low plasma osmolality. In the presence of ADH, urinary dilution does not occur, and sufficient water is not excreted (see Chapters 52.3 and 560).

The glomerular filtration rate (GFR) affects the kidney's ability to eliminate water. With a decrease in the GFR, less water is delivered to the collecting duct, limiting the amount of water that can be excreted. The impairment in the GFR must be quite significant to limit the kidney's ability to respond to an excess of water.

The **minimum urine osmolality** is approximately 30–50 mOsm/kg. This places an upper limit on the kidney's ability to excrete water; there must be sufficient solute present to permit water loss. Massive water intoxication may exceed this limit, whereas a lesser amount of water is necessary in the child with a diet that has very little solute. This is occasionally seen and can produce severe hyponatremia in children who receive little salt and have little urea production as a result of inadequate protein intake. Volume depletion is an extremely important cause of decreased water loss by the kidney despite a low plasma osmolality. This "appropriate" secretion of ADH occurs because volume depletion takes precedence over the osmolality in the regulation of ADH.

The normal response to an increased plasma osmolality is conservation of water by the kidney. In **central diabetes insipidus,** this does not occur because of an absence of ADH secretion (see Chapter 559.1). Patients with **nephrogenic diabetes insipidus** have an inability to respond to ADH and produce dilute urine despite an increase in plasma osmolality (see Chapters 52.3, 530, and 559).

The **maximum urine osmolality** is about 1,200 mOsm/kg. The obligatory solute losses dictate the minimum volume of urine that must be produced, even when maximally concentrated. Obligatory water losses increase in patients with high salt intake or high urea losses, as may occur after relief of a urinary obstruction or during recovery from acute tubular necrosis. An increase in urinary solute and, consequently, water losses occurs with an **osmotic diuresis,** classically seen due to glycosuria in diabetes mellitus, and iatrogenically after mannitol administration. There are developmental changes in the kidney's ability to concentrate the urine. The maximum urine osmolality in a newborn, especially a premature newborn, is less than that in an older infant or child. This limits the ability to conserve water and makes these patients more vulnerable to hypernatremic dehydration. Very high fluid intake, as seen with **psychogenic polydipsia,** can dilute the high osmolality in the renal medulla, which is necessary for maximal urinary concentration. If fluid intake is restricted in these patients, there may be some impairment in the kidney's ability to concentrate the urine, although this defect corrects after a few days without polydipsia. This may also occur during the initial treatment of central diabetes insipidus with desmopressin acetate; the renal medulla takes time to achieve its normal maximum osmolality. Loop diuretics, such as furosemide, by inhibiting sodium resorption in the ascending limb of the loop of Henle, decrease medullary hypertonicity, preventing excretion of maximally concentrated urine.

REGULATION OF VOLUME. An appropriate intravascular volume is critical for survival; both volume depletion and volume overload may cause significant morbidity and mortality. Because sodium is the principal extracellular cation and it is restricted to the ECF, adequate body sodium is necessary for maintenance of intravascular volume. The principal extracellular anion, chloride, is also necessary, but for simplicity, sodium balance is considered the main regulator of volume status because body content of sodium and that of chloride usually change proportionally, given the need for equal numbers of cations and anions. In some situations, chloride depletion is considered the dominant derangement causing volume depletion (metabolic alkalosis with volume depletion). In other situations, such as volume depletion with metabolic acidosis, sodium depletion may exceed chloride depletion.

The kidney determines sodium balance because there is little homeostatic control of sodium intake, even though salt craving does occasionally occur, typically in children with chronic renal salt loss. The kidney regulates sodium balance by altering the percentage of filtered sodium that is resorbed along the nephron. Normally, the kidney excretes <1% of the sodium filtered at the glomerulus. In the absence of disease, extrarenal losses and urinary output match intake, with the kidney having the capacity to adapt to large variations in sodium intake. When necessary, urinary sodium excretion can be reduced to virtually undetectable levels or increased dramatically.

Urinary sodium excretion is regulated by both intrarenal and extrarenal mechanisms. The most important determinant of renal sodium excretion is the volume status of the child; it is the *effective* intravascular volume that influences urinary sodium excretion. The effective intravascular volume is the volume status that is sensed by the body's regulatory mechanisms. Congestive heart failure is a state of volume overload, but the effective intravascular volume is low because poor cardiac function prevents adequate perfusion of the kidneys and other organs. This explains the avid renal sodium retention that is often present in such patients.

Sodium resorption occurs throughout the nephron (see Chapter 528). Whereas the majority of filtered sodium is resorbed in the proximal tubule and the loop of Henle, the distal tubule and the collecting duct are the main sites for precise regulation of sodium balance. Approximately 65% of the filtered sodium is reclaimed in the proximal tubule, which is the major site for resorption of bicarbonate, glucose, phosphate, amino acids, and other substances that are filtered by the glomerulus. The transport of all these substances is linked to sodium resorption by co-transporters or a sodium-hydrogen exchanger in the case of bicarbonate. This is clinically important for bicarbonate and phosphate because their resorption parallels sodium resorption. In patients with metabolic alkalosis and volume depletion, correction of the metabolic alkalosis requires urinary loss of bicarbonate, but the volume depletion stimulates sodium and bicarbonate retention, preventing correction of the alkalosis. Volume expansion causes increased urinary losses of phosphate, even when there is phosphate depletion. Resorption of uric acid and urea occurs in the proximal tubule and increases when sodium retention increases. This accounts for the elevated uric acid and BUN measurements that often accompany dehydration, which is a stimulus for sodium retention in the proximal tubule. The cells of the proximal tubule are permeable to water; thus, water resorption in this segment parallels sodium resorption.

The loop of Henle is, in terms of absolute amount, the 2nd most important site of sodium resorption along the nephron. The Na^+, K^+, $2Cl^-$ co-transporter on the luminal side of the membrane reclaims filtered sodium and chloride, whereas most of the potassium is recycled back into the lumen. This is the transporter that is inhibited by furosemide and other loop diuretics, which are highly effective at increasing sodium excretion. The ascending limb of the loop of Henle is not permeable to water, permitting sodium retention without water. ADH stimulates sodium retention in this segment; this helps to create a more hypertonic medulla, which maximizes water conservation when ADH acts in the medullary collecting duct. Because loop diuretics inhibit sodium retention in this segment, their use causes a less hypertonic medulla, and this prevents excretion of maximally concentrated urine in the presence of ADH.

Sodium retention in the distal tubule is mediated by the thiazide-sensitive Na^+, Cl^- co-transporter. This segment of the nephron is relatively impermeable to water and, along with sodium and chloride retention, the distal tubule is important for delivery of fluid with a low sodium concentration to the collecting duct. This allows for excretion of water without sodium in patients who stop secreting ADH due to low plasma osmolality. Thiazide diuretics, by inhibiting sodium and chloride retention in this segment, prevent the excretion of water without electrolytes. This is a partial explanation for the severe hyponatremia that occasionally develops in patients receiving chronic thiazide diuretics.

The collecting duct, the final segment of the nephron, is important for the regulation of excretion of water, potassium, acid, and sodium. Even though the amount of sodium resorbed in this segment is less than in any other segment, this is the critical site for the regulation of sodium balance. Sodium resorption occurs via a sodium channel that is regulated by aldosterone. When these channels are open under the influence of aldosterone, almost all of the sodium can be resorbed. The uptake of sodium creates a negative charge in the lumen of the collecting duct, which facilitates the secretion of potassium and hydrogen ions. The potassium-sparing diuretics amiloride and triamterene block these sodium channels, and the inhibition of sodium uptake decreases potassium excretion. The potassium-sparing diuretic spironolactone blocks the binding of aldosterone to its receptor; thus, it indirectly decreases the activity of the sodium channels. The collecting duct is important for the regulation of water balance because it responds to ADH by inserting water channels that increase the permeability to water, and the hypertonicity of the renal medulla allows for maximal concentration of the urine.

A number of systems are involved in the regulation of renal sodium excretion. The amount of sodium filtered at the glomerulus is directly proportional to the GFR. If sodium resorption in the nephron were constant, this would lead to complete resorption of sodium with a small decrease in the GFR and significant renal sodium wasting with a small increase. This does not occur, however, because sodium resorption in the nephron is proportional to sodium delivery, a principle called **glomerular tubular balance.**

The **renin-angiotensin system** is an important regulator of renal sodium excretion. The juxtaglomerular apparatus produces renin in response to decreased effective intravascular volume. Specific stimuli for renin release are decreased perfusion pressure in the afferent arteriole of the glomerulus, decreased delivery of sodium to the distal nephron, and β_1-adrenergic agonists, which increase in response to intravascular volume depletion. Renin, a proteolytic enzyme, cleaves angiotensinogen, producing angiotensin I. Angiotensin-converting enzyme (ACE) converts angiotensin I into angiotensin II. The actions of angiotensin II include direct stimulation of the proximal tubule to increase sodium resorption and stimulation of the adrenal gland to increase aldosterone secretion. Through its actions in the distal nephron, specifically, the late distal convoluted tubule and the collecting duct, aldosterone increases sodium resorption. Aldosterone also stimulates potassium excretion, causing increased urinary losses. Along with decreasing urinary loss of sodium, angiotensin II acts as a vasoconstrictor, which helps to maintain adequate blood pressure in the presence of volume depletion.

Volume expansion stimulates the synthesis of atrial natriuretic peptide, which is produced by the atria in response to atrial wall distention. Along with increasing the GFR, atrial natriuretic peptide inhibits sodium resorption in the medullary portion of the collecting duct, facilitating an increase in urinary sodium excretion.

Volume overload occurs when sodium intake exceeds output. In children with kidney failure, there is an impaired ability to excrete sodium. This tends to be proportional to the decrease in the GFR, although in some kidney diseases, such as renal dysplasia or juvenile nephronophthisis, damaged tubules cause significant sodium loss until the GFR is quite low. In general, as the GFR decreases, restriction of sodium intake becomes increasingly necessary. The GFR is low at birth, which limits a newborn's ability to excrete a sodium load. In other situations, there is a loss of the appropriate regulation of renal sodium excretion. This occurs in patients with excessive aldosterone, as is seen in primary hyperaldosteronism or renal artery stenosis, wherein excess renin production leads to high aldosterone levels. In acute glomerulonephritis, even without a significantly reduced GFR, the normal intrarenal mechanisms that regulate sodium excretion malfunction, causing excessive renal retention of sodium and volume overload.

Renal retention of sodium occurs during volume depletion, but this appropriate response causes the severe excess in total body sodium that is present in congestive heart failure, liver failure, nephrotic syndrome, and other causes of hypoalbuminemia. In these diseases, the effective intravascular volume is decreased, causing the kidney and the various regulatory systems to respond, leading to renal sodium retention and edema formation.

Volume depletion usually occurs when sodium losses exceed intake. The most common etiology in children is gastroenteritis. Excessive losses of sodium may also occur from the skin in children with burns, in sweat from patients with cystic fibrosis, or after vigorous exercise. Inadequate intake of sodium is uncommon except in neglect, in famine, or with an inappropriate choice of liquid diet in a child who cannot take solids. Urinary sodium wasting may occur in a range of renal diseases, from renal dysplasia to tubular disorders, such as Bartter syndrome. The neonate, especially if premature, has a mild impairment in the ability to conserve sodium. Iatrogenic renal sodium wasting takes place during diuretic therapy. Renal sodium loss occurs as a result of derangement in the normal regulatory systems. An absence of aldosterone, seen most commonly in children with **congenital adrenal hyperplasia** due to 21-hydroxylase deficiency, causes sodium wasting (Chapter 577). In **cerebral salt wasting,** there may be a brain natriuretic peptide that produces volume depletion secondary to renal sodium loss.

Isolated disorders of water balance can affect volume status and sodium balance. Because the cell membrane is permeable to water, changes in TBW influence both the extracellular volume and the intracellular volume. In isolated water loss, as occurs in diabetes insipidus, the impact is greater on the intracellular space because of its higher volume compared with the extracellular space. This is why, compared with other types of dehydration, hypernatremic dehydration has less impact on plasma volume; most of the fluid loss comes from the intracellular space. Yet, significant water loss eventually affects intravascular volume and will stimulate renal sodium retention, even if total body sodium content is normal. Similarly, with acute water intoxication or SIADH, there is an excess of TBW, but most is in the intracellular space. However, there is some impact on the intravascular volume, and this causes renal excretion of sodium. Children with SIADH or water intoxication have high urine sodium concentrations, despite hyponatremia. This reinforces the concept that there are independent control systems for water and sodium, yet the 2 systems interact when pathophysiologic processes dictate, and control of effective intravascular volume always takes precedence over control of osmolality.

Ishikawa SE, Schrier RW: Pathophysiological roles of arginine vasopressin and aquaporin-2 in impaired water excretion. *Clin Endocrinol (Oxf)* 2003;58:1–17.

Schafer JA: Renal water reabsorption: A physiologic retrospective in a molecular era. *Kidney Int Suppl* 2004:S20–S27.

52.3 • Sodium

SODIUM METABOLISM

BODY CONTENT AND PHYSIOLOGIC FUNCTION. Sodium is the dominant cation of the ECF (see Fig. 52-3), and it is the principal determinant of extracellular osmolality. Sodium is therefore necessary for the maintenance of intravascular volume. Less than 3% of sodium is intracellular. More than 40% of total body sodium is in bone; the remainder is in the interstitial and intravascular spaces. The low intracellular sodium concentration, approximately 10 mEq/L, is maintained by Na^+, K^+-ATPase, which exchanges intracellular sodium for extracellular potassium.

INTAKE. A child's diet determines the amount of sodium ingested—a predominantly cultural determination in older children. An occasional child has salt craving due to an underlying salt-wasting renal or endocrine disease. Children in the United States tend to have very high sodium intakes because their diets include a large amount of "junk food" or "fast food." Infants receive sodium from breast milk (≈7 mEq/L) and formula (7–13 mEq/L for 20 calorie/oz formula).

Sodium is readily absorbed throughout the gastrointestinal tract. Mineralocorticoids increase sodium transport into the body, although this has limited clinical significance. The presence of glucose enhances sodium absorption due to the presence of a co-transport system. This is the rationale for including sodium and glucose in oral rehydration solutions (Chapter 55.1).

EXCRETION. Sodium excretion occurs in stool and sweat, but the kidney regulates sodium balance and is the principal site of sodium excretion. There is some sodium loss in stool, but this is minimal unless diarrhea is present. Normally, sweat has 5–40 mEq/L of sodium. There is increased sweat sodium concentration in children with cystic fibrosis, aldosterone deficiency, or pseudohypoaldosteronism. The higher sweat losses in these conditions may cause or contribute to sodium depletion.

Sodium is unique among electrolytes because water balance, not sodium balance, usually determines its concentration. When the sodium concentration increases, the resultant higher plasma osmolality causes increased thirst and increased secretion of ADH, which leads to renal conservation of water. Both of these mechanisms increase the water content of the body, and the sodium concentration returns to normal. During hyponatremia, the decrease in plasma osmolality stops ADH secretion, and consequent renal water excretion leads to an increase in the sodium concentration. Even though water balance is usually regulated by osmolality, volume depletion does stimulate thirst, ADH secretion, and renal conservation of water. Volume depletion takes precedence over osmolality; volume depletion stimulates ADH secretion, even if a patient has hyponatremia.

The excretion of sodium by the kidney is *not* regulated by the plasma osmolality. The patient's effective plasma volume determines the amount of sodium in the urine. This is mediated by a variety of regulatory systems, including the renin-angiotensin-aldosterone system and intrarenal mechanisms. In hyponatremia or hypernatremia, the underlying pathophysiology determines the amount of urinary sodium, not the serum sodium concentration.

HYPERNATREMIA

Hypernatremia is a sodium concentration >145 mEq/L, although it is sometimes defined as >150 mEq/L. Mild hypernatremia is fairly common in children, especially among infants with gastroenteritis. Hypernatremia in hospitalized patients may be iatrogenic, caused by inadequate water administration or, less often, by excessive sodium administration. Moderate or severe hypernatremia has significant morbidity, including the result of underlying disease, the effects of hypernatremia on the brain, and the risks of overly rapid correction.

ETIOLOGY AND PATHOPHYSIOLOGY. There are 3 basic mechanisms of hypernatremia (Table 52-1). Sodium intoxication is frequently iatrogenic in a hospital setting as a result of correction of metabolic acidosis with sodium bicarbonate. Baking soda, a putative home remedy for upset stomach, is another source of sodium bicarbonate; the hypernatremia is accompanied by a profound metabolic alkalosis. In hyperaldosteronism, there is renal retention of sodium and resultant hypertension; the hypernatremia is usually mild.

The classic causes of hypernatremia from a water deficit are **nephrogenic** and **central diabetes insipidus** (see Chapters 530 and 559). Hypernatremia in diabetes insipidus develops only if the patient does not have access to water or cannot drink adequately because of immaturity, neurologic impairment, emesis, or anorexia. Infants are at high risk because of their inability to control their own water intake. Central diabetes insipidus and the genetic forms of nephrogenic diabetes insipidus typically cause massive urinary water losses and very dilute urine. The water losses are less dramatic, and the urine often has the same osmolality as plasma when nephrogenic diabetes insipidus is secondary to disease (obstructive uropathy, renal dysplasia, sickle cell disease).

TABLE 52-1. Causes of Hypernatremia

EXCESSIVE SODIUM
Improperly mixed formula
Excess sodium bicarbonate
Ingestion of seawater or sodium chloride
Intentional salt poisoning (child abuse or Münchausen syndrome by proxy)
Intravenous hypertonic saline
Hyperaldosteronism
WATER DEFICIT
Nephrogenic diabetes insipidus
Acquired
X-linked (MIM 304800)
Autosomal recessive (MIM 222000)
Autosomal dominant (MIM 125800)
Central Diabetes Insipidus
Acquired
Autosomal recessive (MIM 125700)
Autosomal dominant (MIM 125700)
Wolfram syndrome (MIM 222300)
Increased insensible losses
Premature infants
Radiant warmers
Phototherapy
Inadequate intake
Ineffective breast-feeding
Child neglect or abuse
Adipsia (lack of thirst)
WATER AND SODIUM DEFICITS
Gastrointestinal losses
Diarrhea
Emesis/nasogastric suction
Osmotic cathartics (lactulose)
Cutaneous losses
Burns
Excessive sweating
Renal losses
Osmotic diuretics (mannitol)
Diabetes mellitus
Chronic kidney disease (dysplasia and obstructive uropathy)
Polyuric phase of acute tubular necrosis
Postobstructive diuresis

MIM, database number from the Mendelian Inheritance in Man (*http://www3.ncbi.nlm.nih.gov/Omim/*).

The other causes of a water deficit are also secondary to an imbalance between losses and intake. Newborns, especially if premature, have high insensible water losses. Losses are further increased if the infant is placed under a radiant warmer or with the use of phototherapy for hyperbilirubinemia. The renal concentrating mechanisms are not optimal at birth, providing an additional source of water loss. Ineffective breast-feeding, often in a primiparous mother, can cause severe hypernatremic dehydration. Adipsia, the absence of thirst, is usually secondary to damage to the hypothalamus, such as from trauma, tumor, hydrocephalus, or histiocytosis. Primary adipsia is rare.

When hypernatremia occurs in conditions with deficits of sodium and water, the water deficit exceeds the sodium deficit. This occurs only if the patient is unable to ingest adequate water. Diarrhea results in depletion of both sodium and water. Because diarrhea is hypotonic—typical sodium concentration of 35–65 mEq/L—water losses are in excess of sodium losses, potentially leading to hypernatremia. Most children with gastroenteritis do not have hypernatremia because they drink enough hypotonic fluid to compensate for stool water losses (see Chapter 337). Fluids such as water, juice, and formula are more hypotonic than the stool losses, allowing correction of the water deficit, and potentially even causing hyponatremia. Hypernatremia is most likely to occur in the child with diarrhea who has inadequate intake due to emesis, lack of access to water, or anorexia.

Osmotic agents, including mannitol or glucose in diabetes mellitus, lead to excessive renal losses of water and sodium. Because the urine is hypotonic—sodium concentration of approximately 50 mEq/L—during an osmotic diuresis, water loss exceeds sodium loss, and hypernatremia may occur if water intake is inadequate. Certain chronic kidney diseases, such as renal dysplasia and obstructive uropathy, are associated with tubular dysfunction, leading to excessive losses of water and sodium. Many such children have disproportionate water loss and are at risk for hypernatremic dehydration, especially if gastroenteritis supervenes. Similar mechanisms occur during the polyuric phase of acute tubular necrosis and after relief of urinary obstruction (postobstructive diuresis). These patients may have an osmotic diuresis from urinary losses of urea and an inability to conserve water because of tubular dysfunction.

CLINICAL MANIFESTATIONS. Most children with hypernatremia are dehydrated and show the typical clinical signs and symptoms (see Chapter 54). Children with hypernatremic dehydration tend to have better preservation of intravascular volume because of the shift of water from the intracellular space to the extracellular space. This maintains blood pressure and urine output, and allows hypernatremic infants to be less symptomatic initially and potentially to become more dehydrated before medical attention is sought. Breast-fed infants with hypernatremia are often profoundly dehydrated, with failure to thrive. Probably because of intracellular water loss, the pinched abdominal skin of a dehydrated, hypernatremic infant has a "doughy" feel.

Hypernatremia, even without dehydration, causes central nervous system symptoms that tend to parallel the degree of sodium elevation and the acuity of the increase. Patients are irritable, restless, weak, and lethargic. Some infants have a high-pitched cry and hyperpnea. Alert patients are very thirsty, even though nausea may be present. Hypernatremia may cause fever, although many patients have an underlying process that contributes to the fever. Hypernatremia is associated with hyperglycemia and mild hypocalcemia; the mechanisms are unknown. Beyond the sequelae of dehydration, there is no clear direct effect of hypernatremia on other organs or tissues, except the brain.

Brain hemorrhage is the most devastating consequence of hypernatremia. As the extracellular osmolality increases, water moves out of brain cells, resulting in a decrease in brain volume. This can result in tearing of intracerebral veins and bridging blood vessels as the brain moves away from the skull and the meninges. Patients may have subarachnoid, subdural, and parenchymal hemorrhage. Seizures and coma are possible sequelae of the hemorrhage, although seizures are more common during correction of hypernatremia. The cerebrospinal fluid protein is often elevated in infants with significant hypernatremia, probably due to leakage from damaged blood vessels. Neonates, especially if premature, seem especially vulnerable to hypernatremia and excessive sodium intake. There is an association between rapid or hyperosmolar sodium bicarbonate administration and the development of intraventricular hemorrhages in neonates. Even though central pontine myelinolysis (CPM) is classically associated with overly rapid correction of hyponatremia, both CPM and extrapontine myelinolysis can occur in children with hypernatremia. Thrombotic complications occur in severe hypernatremic dehydration and include stroke, dural sinus thrombosis, peripheral thrombosis, and renal vein thrombosis. This is secondary to dehydration and possibly hypercoagulability associated with hypernatremia.

DIAGNOSIS. The etiology of hypernatremia is usually apparent from the history. Hypernatremia resulting from water loss occurs only if the patient does not have access to water or is unable to drink. In the absence of dehydration, it is important to ask about sodium intake. Children with excess sodium intake do not have signs of dehydration, unless another process is present. Severe sodium intoxication causes signs of volume overload, such as pulmonary edema and weight gain. **Salt poisoning** is associated with an elevated fractional excretion of sodium, whereas hypernatremic dehydration causes a low fractional excretion of sodium. In hyperaldosteronism, hypernatremia is usually mild or absent and is associated with edema, hypertension, hypokalemia, and metabolic alkalosis.

When there is isolated water loss, the signs of volume depletion are usually less severe initially because much of the loss is from the intracellular space. When pure water loss causes signs of dehydration, the hypernatremia and water deficit are usually severe. In the child with renal water loss, either central or nephrogenic diabetes insipidus, the urine is inappropriately dilute and urine volume is not low. The urine is maximally concentrated and urine volume is low if the losses are extrarenal or due to inadequate intake. With extrarenal causes of loss of water, the urine osmolality should be >1,000 mOsm/kg. When diabetes insipidus is suspected, the evaluation may include measurement of ADH and a water deprivation test, including a trial of desmopressin acetate (synthetic ADH analog) to differentiate between nephrogenic and central diabetes insipidus (see Chapter 559.1). A water deprivation test is unnecessary if the patient has simultaneous documentation of hypernatremia and poorly concentrated urine (osmolality lower than that of plasma). In children with central diabetes insipidus, administration of desmopressin acetate increases the urine osmolality above the plasma osmolality, although maximum osmolality does not occur immediately because of the decreased osmolality of the renal medulla from the chronic lack of ADH. In children with central diabetes insipidus, urine is concentrated when desmopressin acetate is given, but in children with nephrogenic diabetes insipidus, there is no such response.

With combined sodium and water deficits, analysis of the urine differentiates between renal and nonrenal etiologies. When the losses are extrarenal, the kidney responds to volume depletion with low urine volume, concentrated urine, and sodium retention (urine sodium <20 mEq/L, fractional excretion of sodium <1–2%). With renal causes, the urine volume is not appropriately low, the urine is not maximally concentrated, and the urine sodium may be inappropriately elevated.

TREATMENT. As hypernatremia develops, the brain generates **idiogenic osmoles** to increase the intracellular osmolality and prevent the loss of brain water. This mechanism is not instantaneous and is most prominent when hypernatremia has developed gradually. If the serum sodium concentration is lowered rapidly, there is movement of water from the serum into the brain cells to equalize the osmolality in the 2 compartments (Fig. 52-4). The resultant brain swelling manifests as seizures or coma.

Because of the associated dangers, hypernatremia should not be corrected rapidly. The goal is to decrease the serum sodium by <12 mEq/L every 24 hr, a rate of 0.5 mEq/L/hr. The most important component of correcting moderate or severe hypernatremia is frequent monitoring of the serum sodium so that fluid therapy can be adjusted to provide adequate correction, neither too slow nor too fast. If a child has seizures as a result of brain edema secondary to rapid correction, administration of hypotonic fluid should be stopped. An infusion of 3% saline can acutely increase the serum sodium, reversing the cerebral edema.

In the child with hypernatremic dehydration, as in any child with dehydration, the **1st priority is restoration of intravascular volume** with isotonic fluid (see Chapter 54). Normal saline is preferable to lactated Ringer solution because the lower sodium concentration of the lactated Ringer solution can cause the serum sodium to decrease too rapidly, especially if multiple fluid boluses are given. Repeated boluses of normal saline (10–20 mL/kg) may be required to treat hypotension, tachycardia, and signs of poor perfusion (peripheral pulses, capillary refill time) [see Chapters 54 and 68].

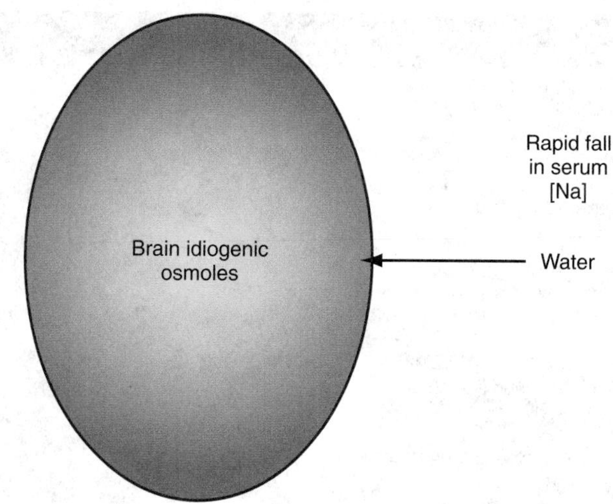

Figure 52-4. Mechanism of brain edema during correction of hypernatremia. A rapid decrease of the serum concentration during treatment of hypernatremia causes movement of water into brain cells, leading to cerebral edema. The presence of idiogenic osmoles in brain cells is responsible for the osmotic gradient.

The sodium concentration of the deficit replacement fluid, the rate of fluid administration, and the presence of continued water losses determine the rate of decrease of the sodium concentration. The following formula is often cited for calculating the water deficit:

$$\text{Water deficit} = \text{Body weight} \times 0.6\,(1 - 145/[\text{current sodium}])$$

This is equivalent to 3–4 mL of water/kg for each 1 mEq that the current sodium level exceeds 145 mEq. The utility of such formulas has never been proven in clinical practice. Most patients with hypernatremic dehydration do well with a fluid sodium concentration of approximately ½ normal saline (NS), but with a fluid rate that is only 20–30% greater than maintenance. This prevents excessive delivery of free water and too rapid a decrease in the serum sodium level. Patients with pure water loss may require a more hypotonic fluid (0.2 NS). Excessive water and sodium losses may also need to be replaced. If signs or symptoms of volume depletion develop, the patient receives additional boluses of isotonic saline. Monitoring of the rate of decrease of the serum sodium concentration permits adjustment in the rate and sodium concentration of the fluid that the patient is receiving, avoiding overly rapid correction of the hypernatremia. Many patients with mild to moderate hypernatremic dehydration due to gastroenteritis can be managed with oral rehydration (see Chapter 55).

Acute, severe hypernatremia, usually secondary to sodium administration, can be corrected more rapidly because idiogenic osmoles have not had time to accumulate. This balances the high morbidity and mortality rates associated with hypernatremia with the dangers of overly rapid correction. When hypernatremia is severe and is due to sodium intoxication, it may be impossible to administer enough water to correct the hypernatremia rapidly without worsening the volume overload. In this situation, peritoneal dialysis allows for removal of the excess sodium. This requires dialysis fluid with a high glucose concentration and a low sodium concentration. In less severe cases, the addition of a loop diuretic increases the removal of excess sodium and water, decreasing the risk of volume overload. With sodium overload, hypernatremia is corrected with sodium-free intravenous fluid (D5W).

Hyperglycemia from hypernatremia is not usually treated with insulin because the acute decrease in glucose may precipitate cerebral edema by lowering plasma osmolality. Rather, the glucose concentration of intravenous fluids should be reduced (from D5W to D2.5W). The secondary hypocalcemia is treated as needed.

It is important to address the underlying cause of the hypernatremia, if possible. The child with central diabetes insipidus should receive desmopressin acetate. Because this reduces renal excretion of water, excessive intake of water must consequently be avoided to prevent overly rapid correction of the hypernatremia or the development of hyponatremia. Over the long term, reduced sodium intake and the use of medications can somewhat ameliorate the water losses in nephrogenic diabetes insipidus (see Chapter 530). The daily water intake of a child who is receiving tube feeding may need to be increased to compensate for high losses. The patient with significant ongoing losses, such as diarrhea, may need supplemental water and electrolytes (see Chapter 53). Sodium intake is reduced if it contributed to the hypernatremia.

HYPONATREMIA

Hyponatremia, a very common electrolyte abnormality in hospitalized patients, is a serum sodium level <135 mEq/L. Both total body sodium and TBW determine the serum sodium concentration. Hyponatremia exists when the ratio of water to sodium is increased. This can occur with low, normal, or high levels of body sodium. Similarly, body water can be low, normal, or high.

ETIOLOGY AND PATHOPHYSIOLOGY. The causes of hyponatremia are listed in Table 52-2. Pseudohyponatremia is a laboratory artifact that is present when the plasma contains very high concentrations of protein (multiple myeloma, intravenous immunoglobulin infusion) or lipid (hypertriglyceridemia, hypercholesterolemia). It does not occur when a direct ion-selective electrode determines the sodium concentration, a technique that is increasingly used in clinical laboratories. In true hyponatremia, the measured osmolality is low, whereas it is normal in pseudohyponatremia. Hyperosmolality due to mannitol or glucose causes a low serum sodium concentration because water moves down its osmotic gradient from the intracellular space into the extracellular space, diluting the sodium concentration. However, because the manifestations of hyponatremia are due to the low plasma osmolality, patients with hyponatremia resulting from hyperosmolality do not have symptoms of hyponatremia. When the etiology of the hyperosmolality resolves, such as hyperglycemia in diabetes mellitus, water moves back into the cells and the sodium concentration increases to its “true” value.

Classification of hyponatremia is based on the patient’s volume status. In **hypovolemic hyponatremia,** the child has lost sodium from the body. The water balance may be positive or negative, but sodium loss has been higher than water loss. The pathogenesis of the hyponatremia is usually a combination of sodium loss and water retention to compensate for the volume depletion. The patient has a pathologic increase in fluid loss, and this fluid contains sodium. Most fluid that is lost has a lower sodium concentration than that of plasma. Viral diarrhea fluid has, on average, a sodium concentration of 50 mEq/L. Replacing diarrheal fluid, which has a sodium concentration of 50 mEq/L, with formula, which has only approximately 10 mEq/L of sodium, reduces the sodium concentration. Intravascular volume depletion interferes with renal water excretion, the body’s usual mechanism for preventing hyponatremia. The volume depletion stimulates ADH synthesis, resulting in renal water retention in the collecting duct. Volume depletion also decreases the GFR and enhances water resorption in the proximal tubule, which reduces water delivery to the collecting duct.

Diarrhea due to gastroenteritis is the most common cause of **hypovolemic hyponatremia** in children. Emesis causes hyponatremia if the patient takes in hypotonic fluid, either intravenously or enterally, despite the emesis. Most patients with emesis have either a normal sodium concentration or hypernatremia. Burns may cause massive losses of isotonic fluid and resultant volume depletion. Hyponatremia develops if the patient receives hypotonic fluid. Losses of sodium from sweat are especially high in children with cystic fibrosis, aldosterone deficiency, or pseudohypoaldosteronism, although high losses can occur simply due to a hot climate. Third space losses are isotonic and can cause significant volume depletion, leading to ADH production and water retention, which can cause hyponatremia if the patient receives hypotonic fluid. In diseases that cause volume depletion due to extrarenal sodium loss, the urine sodium level should be low (<10 mEq/L) as part of the renal response to maintain the intravascular volume. The only exceptions are diseases that cause both extrarenal and renal sodium losses: adrenal insufficiency and pseudohypoaldosteronism.

Renal sodium loss may occur in a variety of situations. In some situations, the urine sodium concentration is >140 mEq/L; thus,

TABLE 52-2. Causes of Hyponatremia

PSEUDOHYPONATREMIA

HYPEROSMOLALITY
- Hyperglycemia
- Mannitol

HYPOVOLEMIC HYPONATREMIA
- Extrarenal losses
  - Gastrointestinal (emesis, diarrhea)
  - Skin (sweating or burns)
  - (Third space losses)
- Renal losses
  - Thiazide or loop diuretics
  - Osmotic diuresis
  - Postobstructive diuresis
  - Polyuric phase of acute tubular necrosis
  - Juvenile nephronophthisis (MIM 256100/606966/602088/604387)
  - Autosomal recessive polycystic kidney disease (MIM 263200)
  - Tubulointerstitial nephritis
  - Obstructive uropathy
  - Cerebral salt wasting
  - Proximal (type II) renal tubular acidosis (MIM 604278)*
  - Lack of aldosterone effect (high serum potassium)
    - Absent aldosterone (e.g., 21-hydroxylase deficiency [MIM 201910])
    - Pseudohypoaldosteronism type I (MIM 264350 and 177735)
    - Urinary tract obstruction and/or infection

EUVOLEMIC HYPONATREMIA
- Syndrome of inappropriate antidiuretic hormone
- Nephrogenic syndrome of inappropriate antidiuresis (MIM 304800)
- Desmopressin acetate
- Glucocorticoid deficiency
- Hypothyroidism
- Water intoxication
  - Iatrogenic (excess hypotonic intravenous fluids)
  - Feeding infants excessive water products
  - Swimming lessons
  - Tap water enema
  - Child abuse
  - Psychogenic polydipsia
  - Diluted formula
  - Marathon running with excessive water intake
  - Beer potomania

HYPERVOLEMIC HYPONATREMIA
- Congestive heart failure
- Cirrhosis
- Nephrotic syndrome
- Renal failure
- Capillary leak due to sepsis
- Hypoalbuminemia due to gastrointestinal disease (protein-losing enteropathy)

MIM, database number from the Mendelian Inheritance in Man (*http://www3.ncbi.nlm.nih.gov/Omim/*).
*Most cases of proximal renal tubular acidosis are not due to this primary genetic disorder. Proximal renal tubular acidosis is usually part of Fanconi syndrome, which has multiple etiologies.

hyponatremia may occur without any fluid intake. In many cases, the urine sodium level is less than the serum concentration; thus, the intake of hypotonic fluid is necessary for hyponatremia to develop. In diseases associated with urinary sodium loss, the urine sodium level is >20 mEq/L despite volume depletion. This may not be true if the urinary sodium loss is no longer occurring, as is frequently the case if diuretics are discontinued. Because loop diuretics prevent generation of a maximally hypertonic renal medulla, patients can neither maximally dilute nor concentrate the urine. The inability to maximally retain water provides some protection against severe hyponatremia. Patients receiving thiazide diuretics can concentrate the urine and are at higher risk for severe hyponatremia. Osmotic diuretics, such as glucose, during diabetic ketoacidosis, cause loss of both water and sodium. Urea accumulates during renal failure and then acts as an osmotic diuretic after relief of urinary tract obstruction and during the polyuric phase of acute tubular necrosis. Transient tubular damage in these conditions further impairs sodium conservation. The serum sodium concentration in these conditions is dependent on the sodium concentration of the fluid used to replace the losses. Hyponatremia develops when the fluid is hypotonic relative to the urinary losses.

Renal salt wasting occurs in hereditary kidney diseases, such as juvenile nephronophthisis and autosomal recessive polycystic kidney disease. Obstructive uropathy, most commonly a consequence of posterior urethral valves, produces salt wasting, but these patients may also have hypernatremia due to impaired ability to concentrate urine and high water loss. Acquired tubulointerstitial nephritis, usually secondary to either medications or infections, may cause salt wasting, along with other evidence of tubular dysfunction. Central nervous system injury may produce cerebral salt wasting, which appears to be mediated by the production of a natriuretic peptide that causes renal salt wasting. In type II renal tubular acidosis (RTA), usually associated with Fanconi syndrome (see Chapter 529), there is increased excretion of sodium and bicarbonate in the urine. Patients with Fanconi syndrome also have glycosuria, aminoaciduria, and hypophosphatemia due to renal phosphate wasting.

Aldosterone is necessary for renal sodium retention and for the excretion of potassium and acid. In congenital adrenal hyperplasia due to 21-hydroxylase deficiency, the absence of aldosterone produces hyponatremia, hyperkalemia, and metabolic acidosis. In pseudohypoaldosteronism, aldosterone levels are elevated, but there is no response because of either a defective sodium channel or a lack of aldosterone receptors. A lack of tubular response to aldosterone may occur in children with urinary tract obstruction, especially during an acute urinary tract infection.

In **hypervolemic hyponatremia,** there is an excess of TBW and sodium, although the increase in water is greater than the increase in sodium. In most of the conditions that cause hypervolemic hyponatremia, there is a decrease in the effective blood volume, due to either 3rd space fluid loss or poor cardiac output. The regulatory systems sense a decrease in effective blood volume and attempt to retain water and sodium to correct the problem. ADH causes renal water retention and the kidney, under the influence of aldosterone and other intrarenal mechanisms, retains sodium. The patient's sodium concentration decreases because water intake exceeds sodium intake, and ADH prevents the normal loss of excess water.

In these disorders, there is a low urine sodium concentration (<10 mEq/L) and an excess of both total body water and sodium. The only exception is the patient with renal failure and hyponatremia. These patients have an expanded intravascular volume, and hyponatremia can therefore appropriately suppress ADH production. Water cannot be excreted because very little urine is being made. Serum sodium is diluted by ingesting water. Because of renal dysfunction, the urine sodium concentration may be elevated, but urine volume is so low that urine sodium excretion has not kept up with sodium intake, leading to sodium overload. The urine sodium concentration in renal failure varies. In acute glomerulonephritis, because it does not affect the tubules, the urine sodium level is usually low, whereas in patients with acute tubular necrosis, it is elevated due to tubular dysfunction.

Patients with hyponatremia and no evidence of volume overload or volume depletion have **euvolemic hyponatremia.** These patients typically have an excess of TBW and a slight decrease in total body sodium. Some of these patients have an increase in weight, implying that they are volume-overloaded. Nevertheless, from a clinical standpoint, they usually appear normal or have subtle signs of fluid overload.

In SIADH, the secretion of ADH is not inhibited by either low serum osmolality or expanded intravascular volume (see Chapter 560). The result is that the child with SIADH is unable to excrete water. This results in dilution of the serum sodium and hyponatremia. The expansion of the extracellular volume due to the retained water causes a mild increase in intravascular volume. The kidney increases sodium excretion in an effort to decrease intravascular volume to normal; thus, these patients have a mild decrease in body sodium. SIADH most commonly occurs with disorders of the central nervous system, but lung disease and tumors are other potential causes. A variety of medications may cause SIADH. Recreational use of 3,4-methylenedioxymethylamphetamine (MDMA, or "ecstasy") may cause SIADH and life-threatening hyponatremia. The diagnosis of SIADH is one of exclusion, because other causes of hyponatremia must be eliminated (Table 52-3). Because SIADH is a state of intravascular volume expansion, low serum uric acid and BUN levels are supportive of the diagnosis.

A rare gain of function mutation in the renal ADH receptor causes **nephrogenic syndrome of inappropriate antidiuresis.** Patients with this autosomal recessive disorder appear to have SIADH, but have undetectable levels of ADH.

Hyponatremia in hospitalized patients is frequently due to inappropriate production of ADH and administration of hypotonic intravenous fluids. Causes of inappropriate ADH production include stress, medications such as narcotics or anesthetics, nausea, and respiratory illness. The synthetic analog of ADH, desmopressin acetate, causes water retention and may cause hyponatremia if fluid intake is not appropriately limited. The main uses of desmopressin acetate in children are for the management of central diabetes insipidus and nocturnal enuresis.

Excess water ingestion can produce hyponatremia. In these cases, the sodium concentration decreases as a result of dilution. This suppresses ADH secretion, and there is a marked water diuresis by the kidney. Hyponatremia develops only because the intake of water exceeds the kidney's ability to eliminate water. This is more likely to occur in infants because their lower GFR limits their ability to excrete water. In some situations, the water intoxication causes acute hyponatremia and is due to a massive acute water load. Examples include infant swimming lessons, inappropriate use of hypotonic intravenous fluids, water enemas, and forced water intake as a form of child abuse. Chronic hyponatremia occurs in children who receive water, but limited sodium and protein. The minimum urine osmolality is approximately 50 mOsm/kg, so the kidney can excrete 1 L of water only if there is enough solute ingested to produce 50 mOsm for urinary

TABLE 52-3. Diagnostic Criteria for Syndrome of Inappropriate Antidiuretic Hormone

Absence of:
Renal, adrenal, or thyroid insufficiency
Congestive heart failure, nephrotic syndrome, or cirrhosis
Diuretic ingestion
Dehydration
Urine osmolality > 100 (usually > plasma)
Serum osmolality < 280 and serum sodium < 135
Urine sodium > 25

excretion. Because sodium and urea—a breakdown product of protein—are the principal urinary solutes, a lack of intake of sodium and protein prevents adequate water excretion. This occurs with the use of diluted formula or other inappropriate diets. Subsistence on beer, a poor source of sodium and protein, causes hyponatremia resulting from the inability to excrete the high water load ("beer potomania").

The pathogenesis of the hyponatremia in glucocorticoid deficiency or hypothyroidism is incompletely understood. There is an inappropriate retention of water by the kidney, but the precise mechanisms are not clearly elucidated.

CLINICAL MANIFESTATIONS. Hyponatremia causes a decrease in the osmolality of the extracellular space. Because the intracellular space then has a higher osmolality, water inevitably moves from the extracellular space to the intracellular space to maintain osmotic equilibrium. The increase in intracellular water causes cells to swell. Although cell swelling is not problematic in most tissues, it is potentially dangerous in the brain because it is contained in a fixed shell, the skull. As brain cells swell, there is an increase in intracranial pressure. Acute, severe hyponatremia can cause brainstem herniation and apnea; respiratory support is often necessary. Brain cell swelling is responsible for most of the symptoms of hyponatremia. Neurologic symptoms of hyponatremia include anorexia, nausea, emesis, malaise, lethargy, confusion, agitation, headache, seizures, coma, and decreased reflexes. Patients may have hypothermia and Cheyne-Stokes respirations. Hyponatremia can cause muscle cramps and weakness.

The symptoms of hyponatremia are mostly due to the decrease in extracellular osmolality and the resulting movement of water down its osmotic gradient into the intracellular space. Brain swelling can be significantly obviated if the hyponatremia develops gradually because the brain adapts to the decreased extracellular osmolality by decreasing its internal osmolality. Initially, this is mostly through loss of sodium, potassium, and chloride. More chronically, there is loss of intracellular osmoles, such as amino acids. This explains why the range of symptoms in hyponatremia is related to both the serum sodium level and its rate of decrease. A patient with chronic hyponatremia may be asymptomatic with a serum sodium level of 110 mEq/L, but another patient may have seizures due to an acute decline from 140 to 125 mEq/L.

Patients with hyponatremic dehydration have more manifestations of intravascular volume depletion than patients who have equivalent water loss but normal or increased sodium concentrations. During hyponatremia, there is movement of water into the cells, which depletes the water of the extracellular space, including the plasma volume.

DIAGNOSIS. The history usually points to a likely etiology of the hyponatremia. Most patients with hyponatremia have a history of volume depletion. Diarrhea and diuretic use are very common etiologies of hyponatremia in children. A history of polyuria, perhaps with enuresis, and/or salt craving is present in children with primary kidney diseases or absence of aldosterone effect. Children may have signs or symptoms suggesting a diagnosis of hypothyroidism or adrenal insufficiency (see Chapters 566 and 577). Brain injury raises the possibility of SIADH or cerebral salt wasting. Liver disease, nephrotic syndrome, renal failure, or congestive heart failure may be acute or chronic. The history should include a review of the patient's intake, both intravenous and enteral, with careful attention to the amount of water, sodium, and protein.

The traditional 1st step in the diagnostic process is determination of the plasma osmolality. This is done because some patients with a low serum sodium value do not have a low osmolality. The clinical effects of hyponatremia are secondary to the associated low osmolality. Without a low osmolality, there is no movement of water into the intracellular space.

A patient with hyponatremia can have a low, normal, or high osmolality. A normal osmolality in combination with hyponatremia occurs in pseudohyponatremia. Children with an elevated serum glucose concentration or another effective osmole (mannitol) have a high plasma osmolality and hyponatremia. The presence of a low osmolality indicates "true" hyponatremia. These patients are at risk for neurologic symptoms and require further evaluation to determine the etiology of their hyponatremia.

In some situations, true hyponatremia is present despite a normal or elevated plasma osmolality. The presence of an ineffective osmole, most commonly urea, increases the plasma osmolality, but because it has the same concentration in the intracellular space, it does not cause fluid to move into the extracellular space. There is no dilution of the serum sodium by water, and the sodium concentration remains unchanged if the ineffective osmole is eliminated. Most importantly, the ineffective osmole does not protect the brain from edema as a result of hyponatremia. Hence, a patient may have symptoms of hyponatremia despite a normal or increased osmolality caused by uremia.

In patients with true hyponatremia, the next step in the diagnostic process is to clinically evaluate the patient's volume status. Patients with hyponatremia can be hypovolemic, hypervolemic, or euvolemic. The diagnosis of volume depletion relies on the usual findings with dehydration (see Chapter 54). Children with hypervolemia are **edematous** on physical examination. They may have ascites, pulmonary edema, pleural effusion, or hypertension.

Hypovolemic hyponatremia can have renal or nonrenal causes. The urine sodium is very useful in differentiating between renal and nonrenal causes. When the losses are nonrenal and the kidney is working properly, there is renal retention of sodium, a normal homeostatic response to volume depletion. Thus, the urinary sodium concentration is low, typically <10 mEq/L, although sodium conservation in neonates is less avid. When the kidney is the cause of the sodium loss, the urine will have a sodium concentration of >20 mEq/L, reflecting the defect in renal sodium retention. The interpretation of the urine sodium level is challenging with diuretics because it is high when diuretics are being used but low after the diuretic effect is gone. This becomes an issue only when diuretic use is surreptitious. The urine sodium is not useful if a metabolic alkalosis is present; the urine chloride must be used instead (see Chapter 52.7).

Differentiating among the nonrenal causes of hypovolemic hyponatremia is usually facilitated by the history. Although the renal causes are more challenging to distinguish, a high serum potassium concentration is associated with disorders in which the sodium wasting is due to absent or ineffective aldosterone.

In the patient with hypervolemic hyponatremia, the urine sodium concentration is a helpful parameter. It is usually <10 mEq/L, except in the patient with renal failure. An elevated urine sodium concentration is a useful indication that a child may have acute tubular necrosis superimposed on 1 of the other causes of hypervolemic hyponatremia.

TREATMENT. The management of hyponatremia is based on the pathophysiology of the specific etiology. The management of all causes requires judicious monitoring and avoidance of an overly quick normalization of the serum sodium concentration. A patient with severe symptoms (shock or seizures), no matter the etiology, should be given a bolus of hypertonic saline to produce a small, rapid increase in serum sodium.

With all causes of hyponatremia, it is important to avoid "overly rapid" correction. This is because rapid correction of hyponatremia may cause **central pontine myelinolysis** (CPM). This syndrome produces neurologic symptoms, including confusion, agitation, flaccid or spastic quadriparesis, and death. There are usually characteristic pathologic and radiologic changes in the brain, especially in the pons.

Central pontine myelinolysis is more common in patients who are treated for chronic hyponatremia than in those treated for acute hyponatremia. Presumably, this is based on the adaptation of brain cells to the hyponatremia. The reduced intracellular osmolality that is an adaptive mechanism for chronic hyponatremia makes brain cells susceptible to dehydration during rapid correction of the hyponatremia, and this may be the mechanism of CPM. Even though CPM is rare in pediatric patients, it is advisable to avoid correcting the serum sodium by >12 mEq/L/day. This guideline does not apply to acute hyponatremia, as may occur with water intoxication, because the hyponatremia is more often symptomatic and there has not been time for the adaptive decrease in brain osmolality to occur. The consequences of brain edema in acute hyponatremia exceed the small risk of CPM.

Patients with hyponatremia can have severe neurologic symptoms, such as seizures and coma. The seizures associated with hyponatremia are generally poorly responsive to anticonvulsants. The child with hyponatremia and severe symptoms needs to receive treatment that will quickly reduce cerebral edema. This is best accomplished by increasing the extracellular osmolality so that water moves down its osmolar gradient from the intracellular space to the extracellular space.

Intravenous hypertonic saline rapidly increases serum sodium, and the effect on serum osmolality leads to a decrease in brain edema. Each mL/kg of 3% sodium chloride increases the serum sodium by approximately 1 mEq/L. A child with active symptoms often improves after receiving 4–6 mL/kg of 3% sodium chloride.

The child with **hypovolemic hyponatremia** has a deficiency in sodium and may have a deficiency in water. The cornerstone of therapy is to replace the sodium deficit and any water deficit that is present. The 1st step in treating any dehydrated patient is to restore the intravascular volume with isotonic saline. This is frequently needed in hyponatremic dehydration because the low serum osmolality causes water to move intracellularly, further depleting the intravascular volume. Ultimately, complete restoration of intravascular volume suppresses ADH production, which permits excretion of the excess water. Chapter 54 discusses the management of hyponatremic dehydration.

The management of **hypervolemic hyponatremia** is difficult. These patients have an excess of both water and sodium. Administration of sodium leads to worsening volume overload and edema. In addition, these patients are retaining water and sodium because of their ineffective intravascular volume or renal insufficiency. The cornerstone of therapy is water and sodium restriction because these patients are volume-overloaded. Diuretics may help by causing excretion of both sodium and water. Patients with low albumin due to nephrotic syndrome have a better response to diuretics after an infusion of albumin; the sodium concentration often normalizes due to expansion of the intravascular volume. A child with congestive heart failure may have an increase in renal water and sodium excretion if there is an improvement in cardiac output. This will "turn off" the regulatory hormones that are causing renal water (ADH) and sodium (aldosterone) retention. The patient with renal failure cannot respond to any of these therapies except fluid restriction. Insensible fluid losses eventually result in an increase in the sodium concentration as long as insensible and urinary losses are greater than intake. A more definitive approach in children with renal failure is to perform dialysis, which removes water and sodium.

In **isovolumic hyponatremia,** there is usually an excess of water and a mild sodium deficit. Therapy is directed at eliminating the excess water. The child with excessive water intake loses water in the urine because ADH production is turned off as a result of the low plasma osmolality. It takes time to eliminate the excess water, and limiting water intake allows this process to occur more quickly. For acute, symptomatic hyponatremia due to water intoxication, hypertonic saline may be needed to reverse cerebral edema. For chronic hyponatremia as a result of poor solute intake, the child needs to receive an appropriate formula, and excess water intake should be eliminated. Families who feed their infants excessive amounts of commercially available baby waters have induced acute normovolemic hyponatremia. Despite the dramatic presentation, these infants may correct their hyponatremia spontaneously over 3–6 hr.

Children with iatrogenic hyponatremia due to the administration of hypotonic intravenous fluids should receive 3% saline if they are symptomatic. Subsequent management is dictated by the patient's volume status. The hypovolemic child should receive isotonic intravenous fluids. The child with nonphysiologic stimuli for ADH production should be fluid restricted. Prevention of this iatrogenic complication requires judicious use of intravenous fluids (see Chapter 53).

Specific hormone replacement is the cornerstone of therapy for the hyponatremia of hypothyroidism or cortisol deficiency. Correction of the underlying defect permits appropriate elimination of the excess water. SIADH is a condition of excess water, with limited ability of the kidney to excrete water. The mainstay of therapy is fluid restriction. The sodium concentration will increase as long as intake of water is less than insensible loss. Fluid restriction obviously requires time; thus, there is a temptation to treat these patients with normal or hypertonic saline. Therapy with saline can create problems in children with SIADH. Infusions of saline temporarily increase the sodium concentration, but increase the child's blood pressure. This causes the kidneys to eliminate almost all of the sodium, eliminating any benefit from the therapy. The water contained in the saline is retained; thus, the hyponatremia may actually worsen.

Furosemide is more successful in the patient with SIADH and severe hyponatremia. Even in a patient with SIADH, furosemide causes an increase in water and sodium excretion. The loss of sodium is somewhat counterproductive, but this sodium can be replaced with hypertonic saline. Because the patient has a net loss of water and the urinary losses of sodium have been replaced, there is an increase in the sodium concentration, but no significant increase in blood pressure.

Treatment of chronic SIADH is challenging. Fluid restriction in children is difficult for nutritional and behavioral reasons. The mainstays of adult therapy, demeclocycline and lithium, which blunt the effect of ADH, are problematic in children because of their potential toxicity. Another option is chronic furosemide therapy with sodium supplementation.

Conivaptan, a V_2-receptor antagonist, decreases the permeability of the collecting duct to water producing an aquaresis. It is approved for short-term treatment of euvolemic patients with hyponatremia (usually SIADH). Thirst is a complication. Future uses may include treatment of patients with hypervolemic hyponatremia (heart failure, cirrhosis).

Alam NH, Yunus M, Faruque ASG, et al: Symptomatic hyponatremia during treatment of dehydrating diarrheal disease with reduced osmolarity oral rehydration solution. *JAMA* 2006;296:567–573.

Budisavljevic MN, Stewart L, Sahn SA, et al: Hyponatremia associated with 3,4-methylenedioxymethylamphetamine ("ecstasy") abuse. *Am J Med Sci* 2003;326:89–93.

Coulthard MG, Haycock GB: Distinguishing between salt poisoning and hypernatraemic dehydration in children. *BMJ* 2003;326:157–160.

Feldman BJ, Rosenthal SM, Vargas GA, et al: Nephrogenic syndrome of inappropriate antidiuresis. *N Engl J Med* 2005;352:1884–1890.

Gross P: Treatment of severe hyponatremia. *Kidney Int* 2001;60:2417–2427.

Halberthal M, Halperin ML, Bohn D: Acute hyponatremia in children admitted to hospital: Retrospective analysis of factors contributing to its development and resolution. *BMJ* 2001;322:780–782.

Hanna S, Tibby SM, Durward A, et al: Incidence of hyponatraemia and hyponatraemic seizures in severe respiratory syncytial virus bronchiolitis. *Acta Paediatr* 2003;92:430–434.

Haycock GB: Hypernatraemia: diagnosis and management. *Arch Dis Child Educ Pract Ed* 2006;91:ep8–ep13.

Haycock GB: Hyponatraemia: diagnosis and management. *Arch Dis Child Educ Pract Ed* 2006;91:ep37–ep41.

Hoorn EJ, Geary D, Robb M, et al: Acute hyponatremia related to intravenous fluid administration in hospitalized children: An observational study. *Pediatrics* 2004;113:1279–1284.
Laing IA, Wong CM: Hyponatraemia in the first few days: Is the incidence rising? *Arch Dis Child Fetal Neonatal Ed* 2002;87:F158–F162.
Manganaro R, Mami C, Marrone T, et al: Incidence of dehydration and hypernatremia in exclusively breast-fed infants. *J Pediatr* 2001;139: 673–675.
The Medical Letter: Conivaptan (*Vaprisol*) for hyponatremia. *Med Lett* 2006;48:51–52.
Moritz ML, Ayus JC: Hospital-acquired hyponatremia: Why are there still deaths? *Pediatrics* 2004;113:1395–1396.
Moritz ML, Ayus JC: Disorders of water metabolism in children: Hyponatremia and hypernatremia. *Pediatr Rev* 2002;23:371–380.
Neville KA, Verge CF, Rosenberg AR, et al: Isotonic is better than hypotonic saline for intravenous rehydration of children with gastroenteritis: a prospective randomized study. *Arch Dis Chil* 2006;91:226–232.
Reynolds RM, Padfield PL, Seckl JR: Disorders of sodium imbalance. *BMJ* 2006;332:702–705.
Schwaderer AL, Schwartz GJ: Treating hypernatremic dehydration. *Pediatr Rev* 2005;26:148–150.
Singh S, Bohn D, Carlotti AP, et al: Cerebral salt wasting: Truths, fallacies, theories, and challenges. *Crit Care Med* 2002;30:2575–2579.

52.4 • Potassium

POTASSIUM METABOLISM

BODY CONTENT AND PHYSIOLOGIC FUNCTION. The intracellular concentration of potassium, approximately 150 mEq/L, is much higher than the plasma concentration (see Fig. 52-3). The majority of body potassium is contained in muscle. As muscle mass increases, there is an increase in body potassium. There is thus an increase in body potassium during puberty, and it is more significant in males. The majority of extracellular potassium is in bone; <1% of total body potassium is in plasma.

Because most potassium is intracellular, the plasma concentration does not always reflect the total body potassium content. A variety of conditions alter the distribution of potassium between the intracellular and extracellular compartments. The Na^+, K^+-ATPase maintains the high intracellular potassium concentration by pumping sodium out of the cell and potassium into the cell. This balances the normal leak of potassium out of cells via potassium channels that is driven by the favorable chemical gradient. Insulin increases potassium movement into cells by activating the Na^+, K^+-ATPase. Because hyperkalemia stimulates insulin secretion, this may have a protective effect during hyperkalemia. Acid-base status affects potassium distribution, probably via potassium channels and the Na^+, K^+- ATPase. A decrease in pH drives potassium extracellularly; an increase in pH has the opposite effect. β-Adrenergic agonists stimulate the Na^+, K^+-ATPase, increasing cellular uptake of potassium. This may also be protective in that hyperkalemia stimulates adrenal release of catecholamines. α-Adrenergic agonists and exercise cause a net movement of potassium out of the intracellular space. An increase in plasma osmolality, as with mannitol infusion, leads to water movement out of the cells, and potassium follows as a result of solvent drag. The serum potassium concentration increases by approximately 0.6 mEq/L with each 10-mOsm increase in plasma osmolality. This occurs in diabetic ketoacidosis as a result of the increase in osmolality from hyperglycemia. Hyperglycemia in patients without insulin deficiency does not increase the plasma potassium concentration because the secondary insulin production causes potassium to move intracellularly.

The high intracellular concentration of potassium, the principal intracellular cation, is maintained via the Na^+, K^+-ATPase. The resulting chemical gradient is used to produce the resting membrane potential of cells. Potassium is necessary for the electrical responsiveness of nerve and muscle cells and for the contractility of cardiac, skeletal, and smooth muscle. The changes in membrane polarization that occur during muscle contraction or nerve conduction make these cells susceptible to changes in serum potassium levels. The ratio of intracellular to extracellular potassium determines the threshold for a cell to generate an action potential and the rate of cellular repolarization. The intracellular potassium concentration affects cellular enzymes and intracellular pH. Low intracellular potassium raises the pH, whereas high intracellular potassium lowers the pH. These acid-base changes modify cell functions. Potassium is necessary for maintaining cell volume because of its important contribution to intracellular osmolality.

INTAKE. Potassium is plentiful in food. Dietary consumption varies considerably, even though 1–2 mEq/kg is the recommended intake. The intestines normally absorb approximately 90% of ingested potassium. Most absorption occurs in the small intestine, whereas the colon exchanges body potassium for luminal sodium. Regulation of intestinal losses normally has a minimal role in maintaining potassium homeostasis, although renal failure, aldosterone, and glucocorticoids increase colonic secretion of potassium. The increase in intestinal losses in the setting of renal failure and hyperkalemia, which stimulates aldosterone production, is clinically significant, helping to protect against hyperkalemia. Colonic secretion is important after an acute potassium load. Patients with kidney failure who have constipation or receive an ACE inhibitor, an indirect inhibitor of aldosterone production, may have less colonic secretion; therefore, hyperkalemia occurs. Colonic secretion is never more than a small part of overall potassium excretion.

EXCRETION. There is some loss of potassium in sweat, but this is normally minimal. The colon has the ability to eliminate some potassium. In addition, after an acute potassium load, much of the potassium, >40%, moves intracellularly, through the actions of epinephrine and insulin, which are produced in response to hyperkalemia. This provides transient protection from hyperkalemia, but most ingested potassium is eventually excreted in the urine. The kidneys principally regulate chronic potassium balance, and they alter excretion in response to a variety of signals. Potassium is freely filtered at the glomerulus, but 90% is resorbed before the distal tubule and collecting duct, the principal sites of potassium regulation. The distal tubule and the collecting duct have the ability to absorb and secrete potassium. It is the amount of tubular secretion that regulates the amount of potassium that appears in the urine. The plasma potassium concentration directly influences secretion in the distal nephron. As the potassium concentration increases, secretion increases.

The principal hormone regulating potassium secretion is aldosterone, which is released by the adrenal cortex in response to increased plasma potassium. Its main site of action is the cortical collecting duct, where aldosterone stimulates sodium movement from the tubule into the cells. This creates a negative charge in the tubular lumen, facilitating potassium excretion. In addition, the increased intracellular sodium stimulates the basolateral Na^+, K^+-ATPase, causing more potassium to move into the cells lining the cortical collecting duct. Glucocorticoids, ADH, a high urinary flow rate, and high sodium delivery to the distal nephron also increase urinary potassium excretion. Potassium excretion is decreased by insulin, catecholamines, and urinary ammonia. Loop and thiazide diuretics increase potassium secretion by increasing sodium delivery to the distal nephron and increasing the urinary flow rate in the distal nephron. Whereas ADH increases potassium secretion, it also causes water resorption, decreasing urinary flow. The net effect is that ADH has little overall impact on potassium balance. Alkalosis causes potassium to move into cells, including the cells lining the collecting duct.

This increases potassium secretion, and because acidosis has the opposite effect, it decreases potassium secretion.

The kidney can dramatically vary potassium excretion in response to changes in intake. Normally, approximately 10–15% of the filtered load is excreted. In an adult, excretion of potassium can vary from 5–1,000 mEq/day.

HYPERKALEMIA

Hyperkalemia—because of the potential for lethal arrhythmias—is 1 of the most alarming electrolyte abnormalities.

ETIOLOGY AND PATHOPHYSIOLOGY. There are 3 basic mechanisms that cause hyperkalemia (Table 52-4). In the individual patient, the etiology is sometimes multifactorial.

Fictitious hyperkalemia is very common in children because of the difficulties in obtaining blood specimens. This is usually due to hemolysis during a heelstick or phlebotomy, but it can be the result of prolonged tourniquet application or fist clenching because these cause local potassium release from muscle.

The serum potassium level is normally 0.4 mEq/L higher than the plasma value, secondary to release from cells during clot formation. This phenomenon is exaggerated with thrombocytosis because of potassium release from platelets. For every 100,000/m^3 increase in the platelet count, the serum potassium level increases by approximately 0.15 mEq/L. This also occurs with the marked white blood cell count elevations sometimes seen with leukemia. Elevated white blood cell counts, typically >200,000/m^3, can cause a dramatic elevation in the serum potassium concentration. Analysis of a plasma sample usually provides an accurate result. It is important to analyze the sample promptly to avoid potassium release from cells. This occurs if the sample is stored in the cold, whereas storage at room temperature can lead to cellular uptake of potassium and spurious hypokalemia.

Because of the kidney's ability to excrete potassium, it is unusual for excessive intake, by itself, to cause hyperkalemia. This can occur in a patient who is receiving large quantities of intravenous or oral potassium as a result of excessive losses that are no longer present. Frequent or rapid blood transfusions can acutely increase the potassium level because of the potassium content of blood, which is variably elevated. Increased intake may precipitate hyperkalemia if there is an underlying defect in potassium excretion.

The intracellular space has a very high potassium concentration, so a shift of potassium from the intracellular space to the extracellular space can have a significant impact on the plasma potassium level. This occurs with metabolic acidosis, but the effect is minimal with an organic acid (lactic acidosis, ketoacidosis). A respiratory acidosis has less impact than a metabolic acidosis. Cell destruction, as seen with rhabdomyolysis, tumor lysis syndrome, tissue necrosis, or hemolysis, releases potassium into the extracellular milieu. The potassium released from red blood cells in internal bleeding, such as hematomas, is resorbed and enters the extracellular space.

Normal doses of succinylcholine or β-blockers and fluoride or digitalis intoxication all cause a shift of potassium out of the intracellular compartment. Succinylcholine should not be used during anesthesia in patients at risk for hyperkalemia. β-Blockers prevent the normal cellular uptake of potassium mediated by binding of β-agonists to the β_2-adrenergic receptors. Potassium release from muscle cells occurs during exercise, and levels can increase by 1–2 mEq/L with high activity. With an increased plasma osmolality, water moves from the intracellular space and potassium follows. This occurs with hyperglycemia, although in nondiabetic patients, the resultant increase in insulin causes potassium to move intracellularly. In diabetic ketoacidosis, the absence of insulin causes potassium to leave the intracellular space, and this is compounded by the hyperosmolality. The effect of hyperosmolality causes a transcellular shift of potassium into the extracellular space after mannitol or hypertonic saline infusions. **Malignant hyperthermia,** which is triggered by some inhaled anesthetics, causes muscle release of potassium (see Chapter 610.2). **Hyperkalemic periodic paralysis** is an autosomal dominant disorder caused by a mutated sodium channel. It results in episodic cellular release of potassium and attacks of paralysis (see Chapter 610.1).

The kidneys excrete most of the daily potassium intake, so a decrease in kidney function can cause hyperkalemia. The decrease in potassium excretion and the risk of hyperkalemia are proportional to the degree of renal insufficiency. Newborn infants in general, and especially premature infants, have decreased kidney

TABLE 52-4. Causes of Hyperkalemia

SPURIOUS LABORATORY VALUE
Hemolysis
Tissue ischemia during blood drawing
Thrombocytosis
Leukocytosis
INCREASED INTAKE
Intravenous or oral
Blood transfusions
TRANSCELLULAR SHIFTS
Acidosis
Rhabdomyolysis
Tumor lysis syndrome
Tissue necrosis
Hemolysis/hematomas/gastrointestinal bleeding
Succinylcholine
Digitalis intoxication
Fluoride intoxication
β-Adrenergic blockers
Exercise
Hyperosmolality
Insulin deficiency
Malignant hyperthermia (MIM 145600)
Hyperkalemic periodic paralysis (MIM 170500)
DECREASED EXCRETION
Renal failure
Primary adrenal disease
Acquired Addison disease
21-hydroxylase deficiency (MIM 201910)
3β-hydroxysteroid dehydrogenase deficiency (MIM 201810)
Lipoid congenital adrenal hyperplasia (MIM 201710)
Adrenal hypoplasia congenita (MIM 300200)
Aldosterone synthase deficiency (MIM 203400)
Adrenoleukodystrophy (MIM 300100)
Hyporeninemic hypoaldosteronism
Urinary tract obstruction
Sickle cell disease (MIM 603903)
Kidney transplant
Lupus nephritis
Renal tubular disease
Pseudohypoaldosteronism type I (MIM 264350 and 177735)
Pseudohypoaldosteronism type II (MIM 145260)
Urinary tract obstruction
Sickle cell disease
Kidney transplant
Medications
Angiotensin-converting enzyme inhibitors
Angiotensin II blockers
Potassium-sparing diuretics
Calcineurin inhibitors
Nonsteroidal anti-inflammatory drugs
Trimethoprim
Heparin
Drug-induced potassium channel syndrome

MIM, database number from the Mendelian Inheritance in Man (*http://www3.ncbi.nlm.nih.gov/Omim/*).

function at birth and thus are at increased risk for hyperkalemia, despite an absence of intrinsic renal disease.

A wide range of primary **adrenal disorders,** both hereditary and acquired, can cause decreased production of aldosterone, with secondary hyperkalemia (see Chapters 577 and 578). These patients typically have metabolic acidosis and salt wasting with hyponatremia. Children with more subtle adrenal insufficiency may have electrolyte problems only during acute illnesses. With less severe adrenal insufficiency, hyponatremia may be the only electrolyte abnormality. Causes of acquired adrenal dysfunction include hemorrhage (Waterhouse-Friderichsen syndrome in meningococcemia), tuberculous, and autoimmune disease. The most common form of **congenital adrenal hyperplasia,** 21-hydroxylase deficiency, typically presents in male infants with hyperkalemia, metabolic acidosis, hyponatremia, and volume depletion. Females with this disorder usually are diagnosed as newborns because of their ambiguous genitalia; treatment prevents the development of electrolyte problems.

Renin, via angiotensin II, stimulates aldosterone production. A deficiency in renin, a result of kidney damage, can lead to decreased aldosterone production. Hyporeninemia occurs in many kidney diseases, with some of the more common pediatric causes listed in Table 52-4. These patients typically have hyperkalemia and a metabolic acidosis, without hyponatremia. Some of these patients have impaired renal function, partially accounting for the hyperkalemia, but the impairment in potassium excretion is more extreme than expected for the degree of renal insufficiency.

A variety of **renal tubular disorders** impair renal excretion of potassium. Children with **pseudohypoaldosteronism type 1** have hyperkalemia, metabolic acidosis, and salt wasting leading to hyponatremia and volume depletion; aldosterone levels are elevated. In the autosomal recessive variant, there is a defect in the renal sodium channel that is normally activated by aldosterone. These patients have severe symptoms, beginning in infancy. In the autosomal dominant form, patients have a defect in the aldosterone receptor, and the disease is milder, often remitting in adulthood. **Pseudohypoaldosteronism type 2,** also called **Gordon syndrome,** is an autosomal dominant disorder characterized by hypertension due to salt retention and impaired excretion of potassium and acid, leading to hyperkalemia and metabolic acidosis. Activating mutations in either WNK1 or WNK4, both serine-threonine kinases located in the distal nephron, cause Gordon syndrome.

Acquired renal tubular dysfunction, with an impaired ability to excrete potassium, occurs in a number of conditions. These disorders, all characterized by tubulointerstitial disease, are often associated with impaired acid secretion and a secondary metabolic acidosis. In some children, the metabolic acidosis is the dominant feature, although a high potassium intake may unmask the defect in potassium handling. The tubular dysfunction can cause renal salt wasting, potentially leading to hyponatremia. A defect in water handling, secondary nephrogenic diabetes insipidus, takes place in some children. This predisposes them to dehydration and may lead to hypernatremia. Among children with the disorders listed in Table 52-4, those with obstructive uropathy, usually secondary to posterior urethral valves, are at risk for the most significant tubular dysfunction. Because of the tubulointerstitial damage, these conditions may also cause hyperkalemia as a result of hyporeninemic hypoaldosteronism.

The risk of hyperkalemia resulting from medications is greatest in patients with underlying renal insufficiency. The predominant mechanism of medication-induced hyperkalemia is impaired renal excretion, although ACE inhibitors may worsen hyperkalemia in anuric patients, probably by inhibiting gastrointestinal potassium loss, which is normally upregulated in renal insufficiency. The hyperkalemia caused by trimethoprim generally occurs only at the very high doses used to treat *Pneumocystis jiroveci* pneumonia in patients with AIDS. Potassium-sparing diuretics may easily cause hyperkalemia, especially because they are often used in patients who are receiving oral potassium supplements. Hyperkalemia has been reported in critically ill patients receiving drugs that open a potassium channel. It is reversed by glyburide, a potassium channel inhibitor.

CLINICAL MANIFESTATIONS. The most important effects of hyperkalemia are due to the role of potassium in membrane polarization. The cardiac conduction system is usually the dominant concern. Electrocardiographic (ECG) changes begin with peaking of the T waves. This is followed, as the potassium level increases, by an increased P-R interval, flattening of the P wave, and widening of the QRS complex. This can eventually progress to ventricular fibrillation. Asystole may also occur. Some patients have paresthesias, weakness, and tingling, but cardiac toxicity usually precedes these clinical symptoms, emphasizing the danger of assuming that an absence of symptoms implies an absence of danger.

DIAGNOSIS. The etiology of hyperkalemia is often readily apparent. Spurious hyperkalemia is very common in children, so obtaining a repeat potassium level is often appropriate. If there is a significant elevation of the white blood cell or platelet count, then the repeat sample should be obtained from plasma that is evaluated promptly. The history should initially focus on potassium intake, risk factors for transcellular shifts of potassium, medications that cause hyperkalemia, and the presence of signs of renal insufficiency, such as oliguria or abnormal findings on urinalysis. Initial **laboratory evaluation** should include creatinine, BUN, and assessment of the acid-base status. Many etiologies of hyperkalemia cause a metabolic acidosis; a metabolic acidosis worsens hyperkalemia by the transcellular shift of potassium out of cells. Renal insufficiency is a common cause of the combination of metabolic acidosis and hyperkalemia. This association is also seen in diseases associated with aldosterone insufficiency or aldosterone resistance. Children with absent or ineffective aldosterone often have hyponatremia and volume depletion due to salt wasting. Genetic diseases, such as congenital adrenal hyperplasia and pseudohypoaldosteronism, usually present in infancy and should be strongly considered in the infant with hyperkalemia and metabolic acidosis, especially if hyponatremia is present. It is important to consider the various etiologies of a transcellular shift of potassium. In some of these disorders, the potassium level continues to increase, despite the elimination of all potassium intake, especially when there is concurrent renal insufficiency. This is potentially seen in tumor lysis syndrome, hemolysis, rhabdomyolysis, and other causes of cell death. All of these entities can cause concomitant hyperphosphatemia and hyperuricemia. Rhabdomyolysis produces an elevated creatinine phosphokinase (CPK) level and hypocalcemia, whereas children with hemolysis have hemoglobinuria and a decreasing hematocrit. For the child with diabetes, an elevated blood glucose level suggests a transcellular shift of potassium.

When there is no clear etiology of hyperkalemia, the diagnostic approach should focus on differentiating decreased potassium excretion from the other etiologies. Measuring urinary potassium assesses renal excretion of potassium. The transtubular potassium gradient (TTKG) is a useful method to evaluate the renal response to hyperkalemia:

$$\text{TTKG} = [K]_{urine}/[K]_{plasma} \times (\text{plasma osmolality/urine osmolality})$$

where $[K]_{urine}$ = urine potassium concentration and $[K]_{plasma}$ = plasma potassium concentration. The urine osmolality must be greater than the serum osmolality for the result to be valid. The TTKG normally varies widely, ranging from 5–15. The TTKG should be >10 in the setting of hyperkalemia, assuming normal renal excretion of potassium. A TTKG of <8 during hyperkalemia suggests a defect in renal potassium excretion, which is usually due to lack of aldosterone or an inability to respond to aldosterone. Measurement of aldosterone is useful for differentiating these possible mechanisms. Patients with a lack of aldosterone respond to fludrocortisone, an oral mineralocorticoid, by increasing urinary potassium and decreasing serum potassium. An appropriate TTKG with normal kidney function argues for a nonrenal cause of hyperkalemia.

TREATMENT. The plasma potassium level, the ECG, and the risk of the problem worsening determine the aggressiveness of the therapeutic approach. High serum potassium levels and the presence of ECG changes require vigorous treatment. An additional source of concern is the patient with increasing plasma potassium levels, despite minimal intake. This can happen if there is cellular release of potassium (tumor lysis syndrome), especially in the setting of diminished excretion (renal failure).

The 1st action in a child with a concerning elevation of plasma potassium is to stop all sources of additional potassium (oral, intravenous) [see Chapter 535]. Washed red blood cells can be used for patients who require blood transfusions. If the potassium level is >6.0–6.5 mEq/L, an ECG should be obtained to help assess the urgency of the situation. The treatment of hyperkalemia has 2 basic goals: (1) to stabilize the heart to prevent life-threatening arrhythmias and (2) to remove potassium from the body. The treatments that acutely prevent arrhythmias all have the advantage of working quickly (within minutes), but do not remove potassium from the body. Calcium stabilizes the cell membrane of heart cells, preventing arrhythmias. It is given intravenously over a few minutes, and its action is almost immediate. Calcium should be given over 30 minutes in a patient receiving digitalis because it may cause arrhythmias. Bicarbonate causes potassium to move intracellularly, lowering the plasma potassium level. It is most efficacious in a patient with a metabolic acidosis. Insulin causes potassium to move intracellularly, but it must be given with glucose to avoid hypoglycemia. The combination of insulin and glucose works within 30 min. Nebulized albuterol, by stimulation of β_1-receptors, leads to rapid intracellular movement of potassium. This has the advantage of not requiring an intravenous route of administration, allowing it to be given concurrently with the other measures.

It is critical to begin measures that remove potassium from the body. Because none of these work quickly, it is important to start them as soon as possible. In patients who are not anuric, a loop diuretic increases renal excretion of potassium. A high dose may be required in a patient with significant renal insufficiency. Sodium polystyrene sulfonate (Kayexalate) is an exchange resin that is given either rectally or orally. Sodium in the resin is exchanged for body potassium, and the potassium-containing resin is then excreted from the body. Some patients require dialysis for acute potassium removal. Dialysis is often necessary if there is severe renal failure or if there is an especially high rate of endogenous potassium release, as is sometimes present with tumor lysis syndrome or rhabdomyolysis. Hemodialysis rapidly lowers plasma potassium levels. Peritoneal dialysis is not nearly as quick or reliable, but it is usually adequate as long as the acute problem can be managed with medications and if the endogenous release of potassium is not extremely high.

Chronic management of hyperkalemia includes reducing intake via dietary changes and eliminating or reducing medications that cause hyperkalemia (see Chapter 535). Some patients require medications to increase potassium excretion. These include sodium polystyrene sulfonate and loop or thiazide diuretics. Some infants with chronic renal failure may need to start dialysis to allow adequate caloric intake without hyperkalemia. It is unusual for an older child to require dialysis principally to control chronic hyperkalemia. The disorders that are due to a deficiency in aldosterone respond to replacement therapy with fludrocortisone.

HYPOKALEMIA

Hypokalemia is common in children, with most cases related to gastroenteritis.

ETIOLOGY AND PATHOPHYSIOLOGY. There are 4 basic mechanisms of hypokalemia (Table 52-5). Spurious hypokalemia occurs in patients with leukemia and very elevated white blood cell counts if plasma for analysis is left at room temperature permitting the white cells to take up potassium from the plasma. With a transcellular shift, there is no change in total body potassium, although there may be concomitant potassium depletion resulting from other factors. Decreased intake, extrarenal losses,

TABLE 52-5. Causes of Hypokalemia
SPURIOUS
High white blood cell count
TRANSCELLULAR SHIFTS
Alkalemia
Insulin
β-Adrenergic agonists
Drugs/toxins (theophylline, barium, toluene, cesium chloride)
Hypokalemic periodic paralysis (MIM 170400)
Thyrotoxic period paralysis
DECREASED INTAKE
Anorexia nervosa
EXTRARENAL LOSSES
Diarrhea
Laxative abuse
Sweating
Sodium polystyrene sulfonate (Kayexalate) or clay ingestion
RENAL LOSSES
With metabolic acidosis
Distal rental tubular acidosis (MIM 179800/602722/267300)
Proximal renal tubular acidosis (MIM 604278)*
Ureterosigmoidostomy
Diabetic ketoacidosis
Without specific acid-base disturbance
Tubular toxins: amphotericin, cisplatin, aminoglycosides
Interstitial nephritis
Diuretic phase of acute tubular necrosis
Postobstructive diuresis
Hypomagnesemia
High urine anions (e.g., penicillin or penicillin derivatives)
With metabolic alkalosis
Low urine chloride
Emesis nasogastric suction
Chloride-losing diarrhea (MIM 214700)
Cystic fibrosis (MIM 219700)
Low-chloride formula
Posthypercapnia
Previous loop or thiazide diuretic use
High urine chloride and normal blood pressure
Gitelman syndrome (MIM 263800)
Bartter syndrome (MIM 602023/607364/602522/241200/601678)
Autosomal dominant hypoparathyroidism (MIM 146200)
Loop and thiazide diuretics
High urine chloride and high blood pressure
Adrenal adenoma or hyperplasia
Glucocorticoid-remedial aldosteronism (MIM 103900)
Renovascular disease
Renin-secreting tumor
17α-hydroxylase deficiency (MIM 202110)
11β-hydroxylase deficiency (MIM 202010)
Cushing syndrome
11β-hydroxysteroid dehydrogenase deficiency (MIM 218030)
Licorice ingestion
Liddle syndrome (MIM 177200)

MIM, database number from the Mendelian Inheritance in Man *(http://www3.ncbi.nlm.nih.gov/Omim/)*.

*Most cases of proximal renal tubular acidosis are not due to this primary genetic disorder. Proximal renal tubular acidosis is usually part of Fanconi syndrome, which has multiple etiologies.

and renal losses are all associated with total body potassium depletion.

Because the intracellular potassium concentration is much higher than the plasma level, a significant amount of potassium can move into cells without markedly changing the intracellular potassium concentration. Alkalemia is 1 of the more common causes of a transcellular shift. The effect is much greater with a metabolic alkalosis than with a respiratory alkalosis. The impact of exogenous insulin on potassium movement into the cells is substantial in patients with diabetic ketoacidosis. Endogenous insulin may be the cause when a patient is given a bolus of glucose. Both endogenous (epinephrine in stress) and exogenous (albuterol) β-adrenergic agonists stimulate cellular uptake of potassium. Theophylline overdose, barium intoxication, cesium chloride (a homeopathic cancer remedy), and toluene intoxication from paint or glue sniffing cause a transcellular shift hypokalemia, often with severe clinical manifestations. Children with **hypokalemic periodic paralysis,** a rare autosomal dominant disorder, have acute cellular uptake of potassium (see Chapter 610). **Thyrotoxic periodic paralysis,** which is more common in Asians, is an unusual initial manifestation of hyperthyroidism. Patients have dramatic hypokalemia due to a transcellular shift of potassium.

Inadequate potassium intake occurs in **anorexia nervosa;** accompanying bulimia and laxative or diuretic abuse exacerbates the potassium deficiency. Sweat losses of potassium can be significant during vigorous exercise in a hot climate. Associated volume depletion and hyperaldosteronism increase renal losses of potassium (discussed later). Diarrhea has a high concentration of potassium, and the resulting hypokalemia is usually associated with a metabolic acidosis resulting from stool losses of bicarbonate. In contrast, a normal acid-base balance or a mild metabolic alkalosis is seen with laxative abuse. Intake of sodium polystyrene sulfonate or ingestion of clay due to pica increases stool losses of potassium

Urinary potassium wasting may be accompanied by a metabolic acidosis (proximal or distal renal tubular acidosis [RTA]). In diabetic ketoacidosis, although often associated with normal plasma potassium caused by transcellular shifts, there is significant total body potassium depletion from urinary losses due to the osmotic diuresis, and the potassium level may decrease dramatically with insulin therapy (see Chapter 590). Both the polyuric phase of acute tubular necrosis and postobstructive diuresis cause transient, highly variable potassium wasting and may be associated with a metabolic acidosis. Tubular damage, either directly from medications or secondary to interstitial nephritis, is often accompanied by other tubular losses, including magnesium, sodium, and water. Such tubular damage may cause a secondary RTA with a metabolic acidosis. Isolated magnesium deficiency causes renal potassium wasting. Penicillin is an anion that is excreted in the urine, resulting in increased potassium excretion because the penicillin anion must be accompanied by a cation. Hypokalemia from penicillin occurs only with the sodium salt of penicillin, not with the potassium salt.

Urinary potassium wasting is often accompanied by a metabolic alkalosis. This is usually associated with increased aldosterone, which increases urinary potassium and acid losses, contributing to the hypokalemia and the metabolic alkalosis. Other mechanisms often contribute to both the potassium losses and the metabolic alkalosis. With emesis or nasogastric suction, there is gastric loss of potassium, but this is fairly minimal, given the low potassium content of gastric fluid (≈10 mEq/L). More important is the gastric loss of HCl, leading to a metabolic alkalosis and a state of volume depletion. The kidney compensates for the metabolic alkalosis by excreting bicarbonate in the urine, but there is obligate loss of potassium and sodium with the bicarbonate. The volume depletion increases aldosterone levels, which prevents correction of the metabolic alkalosis and hypokalemia until the volume depletion is corrected. Urinary chloride is low as a response to the volume depletion. Because the volume depletion is secondary to chloride loss, this is a state of chloride deficiency. There were cases of chloride deficiency resulting from infant formula deficient in chloride, which caused a metabolic alkalosis with hypokalemia and low urine chloride levels. Current infant formula is not deficient in chloride. A similar mechanism occurs in cystic fibrosis because of chloride loss in sweat. In congenital chloride-losing diarrhea, an autosomal recessive disorder, there is high stool loss of chloride, leading to metabolic alkalosis, an unusual sequela of diarrhea. Because of stool potassium losses, chloride deficiency, and metabolic alkalosis, these patients have hypokalemia. During respiratory acidosis, there is renal compensation, with retention of bicarbonate and excretion of chloride. After the respiratory acidosis is corrected, patients have chloride deficiency and post-hypercapnic alkalosis with secondary hypokalemia. Patients with chloride deficiency, metabolic alkalosis, and hypokalemia have a urinary chloride level of <10 mEq/L. Loop and thiazide diuretics lead to hypokalemia, metabolic alkalosis, and chloride deficiency. During treatment, these patients have high urine chloride levels resulting from the effect of the diuretic. However, after the diuretics are discontinued, there is residual chloride deficiency, the urinary chloride level is appropriately low, and neither the hypokalemia nor the alkalosis resolves until the chloride deficiency is corrected.

The combination of metabolic alkalosis, hypokalemia, a high urine chloride level, and normal blood pressure is characteristic of **Bartter syndrome, Gitelman syndrome,** and **current diuretic use.** These patients have high urinary losses of potassium and chloride, despite a state of relative volume depletion with secondary hyperaldosteronism. Bartter and Gitelman syndromes are autosomal recessive disorders caused by defects in tubular transporters (see Chapter 531). Bartter syndrome is usually associated with hypercalciuria, often with nephrocalcinosis, whereas children with Gitelman syndrome have low urinary calcium losses, but hypomagnesemia due to urinary magnesium losses. Some patients with hypoparathyroidism and hypocalcemia due to an activating mutation of the calcium-sensing receptor (autosomal dominant hypoparathyroidism) have hypokalemia, hypomagnesemia, and metabolic alkalosis. This is because activation of the calcium-sensing receptor in the loop of Henle impairs tubular resorption of sodium and chloride, causing volume depletion and secondary hyperaldosteronism.

In the presence of high aldosterone, there is urinary loss of potassium, hypokalemia, metabolic alkalosis, and an elevated urinary chloride level. There is also renal retention of sodium, leading to hypertension. Primary hyperaldosteronism caused by adenoma or hyperplasia is much less common in children than in adults (see Chapter 579). Glucocorticoid-remedial aldosteronism, an autosomal dominant disorder that leads to high levels of aldosterone, is often diagnosed in childhood.

Increased aldosterone levels may be secondary to increased renin production. Renal artery stenosis leads to hypertension from increased renin and secondary hyperaldosteronism. The increased aldosterone can cause hypokalemia and metabolic alkalosis, although most patients have normal electrolyte levels. Renin-producing tumors, which are extremely rare, can cause hypokalemia.

A variety of disorders cause hypertension and hypokalemia without increased aldosterone. Some are due to increased levels of mineralocorticoids other than aldosterone. This occurs in 2 forms of **congenital adrenal hyperplasia** (see Chapter 577). In 11β-hydroxylase deficiency, which is associated with virilization, the level of 11-deoxycorticosterone (DOC) is elevated, which causes variable hypertension and hypokalemia. A similar mechanism, increased DOC, occurs in 17α hydroxylase deficiency, but these patients are more uniformly hypertensive and hypokalemic, and they have a defect in sex hormone production. Cushing syndrome, frequently associated with hypertension, less commonly causes metabolic alkalosis and hypokalemia. This is secondary to the mineralocorticoid activity of cortisol. In 11β-hydroxysteroid dehydrogenase deficiency, an autosomal recessive disorder, the enzymatic defect prevents the conversion of cortisol to cortisone in the kidney. Because cortisol binds and activates the aldosterone receptor, these children have all of the features of excessive mineralocorticoids, including hypertension, hypokalemia, and metabolic alkalosis. Patients with this disorder, which is also called *apparent mineralocorticoid excess,* respond to spironolactone therapy, which blocks the mineralocorticoid receptor. An acquired form of 11β-hydroxysteroid dehydrogenase deficiency occurs from the ingestion of substances that inhibit this enzyme. A classic example is glycyrrhizic acid, which is found in natural licorice. **Liddle syndrome** is an autosomal dominant disorder that results from an activating mutation of the distal nephron sodium channel that is normally upregulated by aldosterone. Patients have the characteristics of hyperaldosteronism—hypertension, hypokalemia, and alkalosis—but low serum aldosterone levels. These patients respond to the potassium-sparing diuretics (triamterene and amiloride) that inhibit this sodium channel (Chapter 531.3).

CLINICAL MANIFESTATIONS. The heart and skeletal muscle are especially vulnerable to hypokalemia. ECG changes include a flattened T wave, a depressed ST segment, and the appearance of a U wave, which is located between the T wave (if still visible) and the P wave. Ventricular fibrillation and torsades de pointes may occur, although usually only in the context of underlying heart disease. Hypokalemia makes the heart especially susceptible to digitalis-induced arrhythmias, such as supraventricular tachycardia, ventricular tachycardia, and heart block (see Chapter 435).

The clinical consequences in skeletal muscle include muscle weakness and cramps. Paralysis is a possible complication, generally only at levels <2.5 mEq/L. This usually starts with the legs, followed by the arms. Respiratory paralysis may require mechanical ventilation. Some patients have rhabdomyolysis; the risk increases with exercise. Hypokalemia slows gastrointestinal motility. This manifests as constipation or, with levels <2.5 mEq/L, an ileus may occur. Hypokalemia impairs bladder function, potentially leading to urinary retention.

Hypokalemia causes **polyuria** and **polydipsia** by 2 mechanisms: primary polydipsia and impaired urinary concentrating ability, producing a nephrogenic diabetes insipidus. Hypokalemia stimulates renal ammonia production, which is clinically significant if hepatic failure is present because the liver cannot metabolize the ammonia. Hypokalemia may therefore worsen hepatic encephalopathy.

Chronic hypokalemia may cause kidney damage, including interstitial nephritis and renal cysts. In children, chronic hypokalemia, as in Bartter syndrome, leads to poor linear growth.

DIAGNOSIS. Most causes of hypokalemia are readily apparent from the history. It is important to review the child's diet, gastrointestinal losses, and medications. Both emesis and diuretic use can be surreptitious. The presence of hypertension suggests excess mineralocorticoids. Concomitant electrolyte abnormalities are useful clues. The combination of hypokalemia and metabolic acidosis is characteristic of diarrhea and of distal and proximal RTA. A concurrent metabolic alkalosis is characteristic of emesis or nasogastric losses, aldosterone excess, use of diuretics, and Bartter and Gitelman syndromes.

If a clear etiology is not apparent, the measurement of urinary potassium distinguishes between renal and extrarenal losses. The kidneys should conserve potassium in the presence of extrarenal losses. Urinary potassium losses can be assessed with a 24-hr urine collection, a spot potassium-creatinine ratio, a fractional excretion of potassium, or calculation of the TTKG, which is the most widely used approach in children:

$$\text{TTKG} = [\text{K}]_{\text{urine}}/[\text{K}]_{\text{plasma}} \times (\text{plasma osmolality}/\text{urine osmolality})$$

where $[K]_{urine}$ = urine potassium concentration and $[K]_{plasma}$ = plasma potassium concentration.

The urine osmolality must be greater than the serum osmolality for the result to be valid. A TTKG of >4 in the presence of hypokalemia suggests excessive urinary losses of potassium. The urinary potassium excretion can be misleading if the stimulus for renal loss, such as a diuretic, is no longer present.

TREATMENT. Factors that influence the treatment of hypokalemia include the potassium level, clinical symptoms, renal function, the presence of transcellular shifts of potassium, ongoing losses, and the patient's ability to tolerate oral potassium. Severe, symptomatic hypokalemia requires aggressive treatment. Supplementation is more cautious if renal function is decreased because of the kidney's limited ability to excrete excessive potassium. The plasma potassium level does not always provide an accurate estimation of the total body potassium deficit. This is because there may be shifts of potassium from the intracellular space to the plasma. Clinically, this occurs most commonly with metabolic acidosis and the insulin deficiency of diabetic ketoacidosis; the plasma potassium underestimates the degree of total body potassium depletion. When these problems are corrected, potassium moves into the intracellular space, so these patients require more potassium supplementation to correct their hypokalemia. Likewise, the presence of a transcellular shift of potassium into the cells indicates that the total body potassium depletion is less severe. In an isolated transcellular shift, as occurs in hypokalemic periodic paralysis, potassium supplementation should be used cautiously, given the risk of hyperkalemia when the transcellular shift resolves. This is especially true in thyrotoxic periodic paralysis, which responds dramatically to propranolol, with correction of weakness and hypokalemia. Patients who have ongoing losses of potassium need correction of their deficit and replacement of the ongoing losses.

Because of the risk of hyperkalemia, intravenous potassium should be used very cautiously. Oral potassium is safer, albeit not as rapid in urgent situations. The dose of intravenous potassium is 0.5–1 mEq/kg, usually given over 1 hr. The adult maximum dose is 40 mEq. Conservative dosing is generally preferred. Potassium chloride is the usual choice for supplementation, although the presence of concurrent electrolyte abnormalities may dictate other options. Patients with acidosis and hypokalemia can receive potassium acetate or potassium citrate. If hypophosphatemia is present, then some of the potassium deficit can be replaced with potassium phosphate. It is sometimes possible to decrease ongoing losses of potassium. For patients with excessive urinary losses, potassium-sparing diuretics are effective, but they need to be used cautiously in patients with renal insufficiency. If hypokalemia, metabolic alkalosis, and volume depletion are present (with gastric losses), then restoration of intravascular volume with adequate sodium chloride will decrease urinary potassium losses. Disease-specific therapy is effective in many of the genetic tubular disorders.

Kim GH, Han JS: Therapeutic approach to hypokalemia. *Nephron* 2002;92(Suppl 1):28–32.

Loke YK: The potassium-channel syndrome: Does it exist? *Lancet* 2005;365:1834–1836.

Palmer BF: Managing hyperkalemia caused by inhibitors of the renin-angiotensin-aldosterone system. *N Engl J Med* 2004;351:585–592.

Rastegar A, Soleimani M: Hypokalaemia and hyperkalaemia. *Postgrad Med J* 2001;77:759–764.

Schoen EJ, Bhatia S, Ray GT, et al: Transient pseudohypoaldosteronism with hyponatremia-hyperkalemia in infant urinary tract infection. *J Urol* 2002;167:680–682.

Singer M, Coluzzi F, O'Brien A, et al: Reversal of life-threatening, drug-related potassium-channel syndrome by glibenclamide. *Lancet* 2005;365: 1873–1875.

Welfare W, Sasi P: Challenges in managing profound hypokalemia. *BMJ* 2002;324:269–270.
Wilson FH, Disse-Nicodeme S, Choate KA, et al: Human hypertension caused by mutations in WNK kinases. *Science* 2001;293:1107–1112.
Zelikovic I: Hypokalaemic salt-losing tubulopathies: An evolving story. *Nephrol Dial Transplant* 2003;18:1696–1700.

52.5 • MAGNESIUM

MAGNESIUM METABOLISM

BODY CONTENT AND PHYSIOLOGIC FUNCTION. Magnesium is the 4th most common cation in the body and the 3rd most common intracellular cation (see Fig. 52-3). Between 50% and 60% of body magnesium is in bone, where it serves as a reservoir because 30% is exchangeable, allowing movement to the extracellular space. Most intracellular magnesium is bound to proteins; only approximately 25% is exchangeable. Because cells with higher metabolic rates have higher magnesium concentrations, most intracellular magnesium is present in muscle and liver.

The normal plasma magnesium concentration is 1.5–2.3 mg/dL (1.2–1.9 mEq/L; 0.62–0.94 mmol/L), with some variation between clinical laboratories. In the USA, serum magnesium is reported as mg/dL (Table 52-6). Infants have slightly higher plasma magnesium concentrations than older children and adults. Only 1% of body magnesium is extracellular (60% ionized; 15% complexed; 25% protein bound).

Magnesium is a necessary cofactor for hundreds of enzymes. It is important for membrane stabilization and nerve conduction. Adenosine triphosphate (ATP) and guanosine triphosphate need associated magnesium when they are used by ATPases, cyclases, and kinases.

INTAKE. Between 30% and 50% of dietary magnesium is absorbed. Good dietary sources include green vegetables, cereals, nuts, meats, and hard water, although many foods contain magnesium. Human milk contains approximately 35 mg/L of magnesium; formula contains 40–70 mg/L. The small intestine is the major site of magnesium absorption, but the regulation of magnesium absorption is poorly understood. There is passive absorption, which permits high absorption in the presence of excessive intake. This probably occurs via a paracellular mechanism. Absorption is diminished in the presence of substances that complex with magnesium (free fatty acids, fiber, phytate, phosphate, oxalate); increased intestinal motility and calcium also decrease magnesium absorption. Vitamin D and parathyroid hormone (PTH) may enhance absorption, although this effect is limited. Intestinal absorption does increase when intake is decreased, possibly via a saturable active transport system. If there is no oral intake of magnesium, obligatory secretory losses prevent the complete elimination of intestinal losses.

TABLE 52-6. Conversion Factors for Calcium, Magnesium, and Phosphorus

	UNIT	CONVERSION FACTOR	UNIT
Calcium	mg/dL	0.25	mmol/L
	mEq/L	0.5	mmol/L
	mg/dL	0.5	mEq/L
Magnesium	mg/dL	0.411	mmol/L
	mEq/L	0.5	mmol/L
	mg/dL	0.822	mEq/L
Phosphorus	mg/dL	0.32	mmol/L

Values in the left unit column are converted into the right unit column via multiplying by the conversion factor (e.g., calcium of 10 mg/dL × 0.25 = 2.5 mmol/L). Division of the right unit column by the conversion factor converts to the units of the left unit column.

EXCRETION. Renal excretion is the principal regulator of magnesium balance. There is no defined hormonal regulatory system, although PTH may increase tubular resorption. Approximately 15% of resorption occurs in the proximal tubule and 70% in the thick ascending limb (TAL) of the loop of Henle. Proximal resorption may be higher in neonates. High serum magnesium levels inhibit resorption in the TAL, suggesting that active transport is involved. Approximately 5–10% of filtered magnesium is resorbed in the distal tubule. Hypomagnesemia increases absorption in the TAL and the distal tubule.

HYPOMAGNESEMIA

Hypomagnesemia is relatively common in hospitalized patients, although most cases are asymptomatic. Detection requires a high index of suspicion because magnesium is not measured in most basic metabolic panels.

ETIOLOGY AND PATHOPHYSIOLOGY. Gastrointestinal or renal losses are the major causes of hypomagnesemia (Table 52-7). Diarrhea has up to 200 mg/L of magnesium; gastric contents have only approximately 15 mg/L, but high losses can cause depletion. Steatorrhea causes magnesium loss as a result of the formation of magnesium-lipid salts; restriction of dietary fat can decrease losses.

TABLE 52-7. Causes of Hypomagnesemia

GASTROINTESTINAL DISORDERS
Diarrhea
Nasogastric suction or emesis
Inflammatory bowel disease
Celiac disease
Cystic fibrosis
Intestinal lymphangiectasia
Small bowel resection or bypass
Pancreatitis
Protein-calorie malnutrition
Hypomagnesemia with secondary hypocalcemia (MIM 602014)*

RENAL DISORDERS
Medications: amphotericin, cisplatin, cyclosporin, loop diuretics, mannitol, pentamidine, aminoglycosides, thiazide diuretics
Diabetes
Acute tubular necrosis (recovery phase)
Postobstructive nephropathy
Chronic kidney diseases: interstitial nephritis, glomerulonephritis, postrenal transplant
Hypercalcemia
Intravenous fluids
Primary aldosteronism
Genetic diseases
- Gitelman syndrome (MIM 263800)
- Bartter syndrome (MIM 602023/607364/602522/241200/601678)
- Familial hypomagnesemia with hypercalciuria and nephrocalcinosis (MIM 248250)
- Autosomal recessive renal magnesium wasting (MIM 248250)
- Autosomal dominant renal magnesium wasting (MIM 154020)
- Autosomal dominant hypoparathyroidism (MIM 146200)
- Mitochondrial disorders (MIM 500005)

MISCELLANEOUS CAUSES
Poor intake
Hungry bone syndrome
Insulin administration
Pancreatitis
Intrauterine growth retardation
Infants of diabetic mothers
Exchange transfusion

MIM, database number from the Mendelian Inheritance in Man (*http://www3.ncbi.nlm.nih.gov/Omim/*).
*This disorder is also associated with renal magnesium wasting.

Hypomagnesemia with secondary hypocalcemia, a rare autosomal recessive disorder, is due to decreased intestinal absorption of magnesium and renal magnesium wasting. These patients have mutations in a gene *(TRPM6)* that is expressed in intestine and kidney. *TRPM6* codes for a transient receptor potential cation channel. The patients have seizures, tetany, tremor, or restlessness at 2–8 wk of life due to severe hypomagnesemia (0.2–0.8 mg/dL) and secondary hypocalcemia.

Renal losses may occur due to medications that are direct tubular toxins. Amphotericin frequently causes significant magnesium wasting and is typically associated with other tubular defects (especially potassium wasting). Cisplatin produces dramatic renal magnesium losses. Diuretics affect tubular handling of magnesium. Loop diuretics cause a mild increase in magnesium excretion, and thiazide diuretics have even less effect. Potassium-sparing diuretics reduce magnesium losses. Osmotic agents, such as mannitol, glucose in diabetes mellitus, or urea in the recovery phase of acute tubular necrosis, increase urinary magnesium losses. Intravenous fluid, by expanding the intravascular volume, decreases renal resorption of sodium and water, which impairs magnesium resorption. Hypercalcemia inhibits magnesium resorption in the loop of Henle, although this does not occur in hypercalcemia due to familial hypercalcemic hypocalciuria or lithium.

There are a number of rare genetic diseases that cause renal magnesium loss. **Gitelman and Bartter syndromes,** both autosomal recessive disorders, are the most common entities (see Chapter 531). Gitelman syndrome, which is due to a defect in the thiazide-sensitive Na-Cl co-transporter in the distal tubule, is usually associated with hypomagnesemia. In Bartter syndrome, which can be caused by mutations in at least 4 different genes, hypomagnesemia is uncommon; when it does occur, it is usually associated with a defect in the basolateral chloride channel. In both disorders, there is hypokalemic metabolic alkalosis, but in Gitelman syndrome, there is hypocalciuria, and patients with Bartter syndrome frequently have hypercalciuria and secondary nephrocalcinosis. In these disorders, hypomagnesemia is typically not severe and is asymptomatic, although tetany due to hypomagnesemia occasionally occurs.

Familial hypomagnesemia with hypercalciuria and nephrocalcinosis (Michelis-Castrillo syndrome), an autosomal recessive disorder, is due to mutations in the gene for paracellin-1, which is located in the tight junctions of the thick ascending limb of the loop of Henle. Patients have severe renal wasting of magnesium and calcium with secondary hypomagnesemia and nephrocalcinosis; serum calcium levels are normal. Chronic renal failure frequently occurs during childhood. Other features include kidney stones, urinary tract infections, hematuria, increased PTH levels, tetany, seizures, incomplete distal renal tubular acidosis, hyperuricemia, ocular abnormalities, polyuria, and polydipsia. Autosomal recessive renal magnesium wasting without hypercalciuria is less commonly described, and the genetic basis is unknown.

Autosomal dominant renal magnesium wasting is usually due to a dominant-negative mutation in the gene encoding the Na^+, K^+-ATPase γ subunit and is associated with hypomagnesemia, increased urinary magnesium losses, hypocalciuria, and normocalcemia. There are families without genetic linkage to this locus. Patients may present with seizures; most are asymptomatic, despite serum magnesium levels of 0.8–1.5 mg/dL. **Autosomal dominant hypoparathyroidism** is caused by an activating mutation in the calcium-sensing receptor, which also senses magnesium levels in the kidney (Chapter 572). The mutated receptor inappropriately perceives that magnesium and calcium levels are elevated, leading to urinary wasting of both cations. Hypomagnesemia, if present, is usually mild. A mutation in a mitochondrially encoded transfer RNA is associated with hypomagnesemia, hypertension, and hypercholesterolemia. Hypomagnesemia is occasionally present in children with other mitochondrial disorders.

Poor intake is an unusual cause of hypomagnesemia, although it can be seen in children who are hospitalized and receive only intravenous fluids without magnesium. In **hungry bone syndrome,** which most frequently occurs after parathyroidectomy in patients with hyperparathyroidism, magnesium moves into bone as a result of accelerated bone formation. These patients usually have hypocalcemia and hypophosphatemia via the same mechanism. A similar mechanism can occur during the **refeeding phase of protein-calorie malnutrition** in children, with high magnesium use during cell growth depleting the patient's limited reserves. Insulin therapy stimulates uptake of magnesium by cells, and in diabetic ketoacidosis, in which total body magnesium is low because of osmotic losses, hypomagnesemia frequently occurs. In **pancreatitis,** there is saponification of magnesium and calcium in necrotic fat, causing both hypomagnesemia and hypocalcemia.

Transient hypomagnesemia in newborns, which is sometimes idiopathic, is more commonly seen in infants of diabetic mothers, presumably due to maternal depletion from osmotic losses. Other maternal diseases that cause magnesium losses predispose infants to hypomagnesemia. Hypomagnesemia is more common in infants with intrauterine growth restriction. Hypomagnesemia may develop in newborn infants who require exchange transfusions because of magnesium removal by the citrate in banked blood (see Chapter 106).

CLINICAL MANIFESTATIONS. Hypomagnesemia causes secondary hypocalcemia by impairing the release of PTH by the parathyroid gland and through blunting the tissue response to PTH. Thus, hypomagnesemia is part of the differential diagnosis of hypocalcemia (see Chapter 572). This usually occurs only at magnesium levels <0.7 mg/dL. The dominant manifestations of hypomagnesemia are due to hypocalcemia: tetany, positive Chvostek and Trousseau signs, and seizures. However, with severe hypomagnesemia, these same signs and symptoms may be present despite normocalcemia. Persistent hypocalcemia due to hypomagnesemia is a rare cause of rickets.

Many causes of hypomagnesemia also result in hypokalemia. Hypomagnesemia may produce renal potassium wasting and hypokalemia that corrects only with magnesium therapy. ECG changes with hypomagnesemia include flattening of the T wave and lengthening of the ST segment. Arrhythmias may occur, almost always in the setting of underlying heart disease.

DIAGNOSIS. The etiology of hypomagnesemia is often readily apparent from the clinical situation. The child should be assessed for gastrointestinal disease, adequate intake, and kidney disease, with close attention paid to medications that may cause renal magnesium wasting. When the diagnosis is uncertain, an evaluation of urinary magnesium losses distinguishes between renal and nonrenal causes. The fractional excretion of magnesium is calculated via the following formula:

$$FE_{Mg} = (U_{Mg} \times P_{Cr})/([0.7 \times P_{Mg}] \times U_{Cr}) \times 100$$

where FE_{Mg} = fractional excretion of magnesium, U_{Mg} = urinary magnesium concentration, P_{Cr} = plasma creatinine concentration, P_{Mg} = plasma magnesium concentration, and U_{Cr} = urinary magnesium concentration. The plasma magnesium concentration is multiplied by 0.7 because approximately 30% is bound to albumin and not filtered at the glomerulus.

The fractional excretion of magnesium does not vary with age, but it does change based on the serum magnesium concentration. The fractional excretion ranges from 1–8% in children with normal magnesium levels. In the presence of hypomagnesemia due to extrarenal causes, it should be low due to renal conservation, typically <2%. The fractional excretion of magnesium is inappropriately elevated in the setting of renal magnesium wasting; values are usually >4% and frequently are >10%. The measurement should not be evaluated during a magnesium infusion because the acute increase in serum magnesium increases urinary magnesium. Other approaches for evaluating urinary magnesium losses include calculation of 24-hr urinary magnesium losses and the ratio of urine magnesium to urine creatinine, both of which vary with age.

The genetic causes of renal magnesium loss are distinguished based on the measurement of other serum and urinary electrolytes. Children with Gitelman and Bartter syndromes have hypokalemia and metabolic alkalosis.

TREATMENT. Severe hypomagnesemia is treated with parenteral magnesium. Magnesium sulfate is given at a dose of 25–50 mg/kg (0.05–0.1 mL/kg of a 50% solution; 2.5–5.0 mg/kg of elemental magnesium). This is administered as a slow intravenous infusion, although it may be given intramuscularly in neonates. The rate of intravenous infusion should be slowed if a patient experiences diaphoresis, flushing, or a warm sensation. The dose is often repeated every 6 hr (every 8–12 hr in neonates), for a total of 2–3 doses, before the plasma magnesium concentration is rechecked. Lower doses are used in children with renal insufficiency.

Long-term therapy is usually given orally. Preparations include magnesium gluconate (5.4 mg elemental magnesium/100 mg), magnesium oxide (60 mg elemental magnesium/100 mg), and magnesium sulfate (10 mg elemental magnesium/100 mg). There are sustained-released preparations, such as Slow-Mag (60 mg elemental magnesium/tablet) and Mag-Tab SR (84 mg elemental magnesium/tablet). Oral magnesium dosing should be divided to decrease cathartic side effects. Alternatives to oral magnesium are intramuscular injections and nighttime nasogastric infusion, both designed to minimize diarrhea. Magnesium supplementation must be used cautiously in the context of renal insufficiency.

HYPERMAGNESEMIA

Clinically significant hypermagnesemia is almost always secondary to excessive intake. It is unusual, except in neonates born to mothers who are receiving intravenous magnesium for preeclampsia or eclampsia (see Chapter 106).

ETIOLOGY AND PATHOPHYSIOLOGY. There is no feedback mechanism to prevent magnesium absorption from the gastrointestinal tract. Magnesium is present in high amounts in certain laxatives, enemas, cathartics used to treat drug overdoses, and antacids. It is also usually present in total parenteral nutrition, and neonates may receive high amounts transplacentally if maternal levels are elevated. Usually the kidneys excrete excessive magnesium, but this ability is diminished in patients with chronic renal failure. In addition, neonates and young infants are vulnerable to excessive magnesium ingestion because of their reduced GFR. Most pediatric cases not related to maternal hypermagnesemia occur in infants as a result of excessive use of antacids or laxatives. Mild hypermagnesemia may occur in chronic renal failure, familial hypocalciuric hypercalcemia, diabetic ketoacidosis, lithium ingestion, milk alkali syndrome, and tumor lysis syndrome. The hypermagnesemia in diabetic ketoacidosis occurs despite significant intracellular magnesium depletion due to urinary losses; hypomagnesemia often occurs after insulin treatment.

CLINICAL MANIFESTATIONS. Symptoms usually do not appear until the plasma magnesium level is >4.5 mg/dL. Hypermagnesemia inhibits acetylcholine release at the neuromuscular junction, producing hypotonia, hyporeflexia, and weakness; paralysis occurs at high concentrations. The neuromuscular effects may be exacerbated by aminoglycoside antibiotics. Direct central nervous system depression causes lethargy and sleepiness; infants have a poor suck. Elevated magnesium levels are associated with hypotension because of vascular dilation, which also causes flushing. Hypotension can be profound at higher concentrations due to a direct effect on cardiac function. ECG changes include prolonged P-R, QRS, and Q-T intervals. Severe hypermagnesemia (>15 mg/dL) causes complete heart block and cardiac arrest. Other manifestations of hypermagnesemia include nausea, vomiting, and hypocalcemia.

DIAGNOSIS. Except for the case of the neonate with transplacental exposure, a high index of suspicion and a good history are necessary to make the diagnosis. Prevention is essential; magnesium-containing compounds should be used judiciously in children with renal insufficiency.

TREATMENT. Most patients with normal renal function rapidly clear excessive magnesium. Intravenous hydration and loop diuretics can accelerate this process. In severe cases, especially with underlying renal insufficiency, dialysis may be necessary. Hemodialysis works faster than peritoneal dialysis. Exchange transfusion is another option in newborn infants. Supportive care includes monitoring of cardiorespiratory status, provision of fluids, monitoring of electrolyte levels, and the use of pressors for hypotension. In acute emergencies, especially in the context of severe neurologic or cardiac manifestations, 100 mg/kg of intravenous calcium gluconate is transiently effective.

Ali A, Walentik C, Mantych GJ, et al: Iatrogenic acute hypermagnesemia after total parenteral nutrition infusion mimicking septic shock syndrome: Two case reports. *Pediatrics* 2003;112:e70–e72.

Schlingmann KP, Konrad M, Seyberth HW: Genetics of hereditary disorders of magnesium homeostasis. *Pediatr Nephrol* 2004;19:13–25.

Walder RY, Landau D, Meyer P, et al: Mutation of trpm6 causes familial hypomagnesemia with secondary hypocalcemia. *Nat Genet* 2002;31:171–174.

Wilson FH, Hariri A, Farhi A, et al: A cluster of metabolic defects caused by mutation in a mitochondrial tRNA. *Science* 2004;306:1190–1194.

52.6 • PHOSPHORUS

Approximately 65% of plasma phosphorus is in phospholipids, but these compounds are insoluble in acid and are not measured by clinical laboratories. It is the phosphorus content of plasma phosphate that is determined. The result is reported as either phosphate or phosphorus, although even when the term *phosphate* is used, it is actually the phosphorus concentration that is measured and reported. The result is that the terms *phosphate* and *phosphorus* are often used interchangeably. The term *phosphorus* is preferred when referring to the plasma concentration. Conversion from the units used in the USA (mg/dL) to mmol/L is straightforward (see Table 52-6).

PHOSPHORUS METABOLISM

BODY CONTENT AND PHYSIOLOGIC FUNCTION. Most phosphorus is in bone or is intracellular, with < 1% in plasma. At a physiologic pH, there are monovalent and divalent forms of phosphate because the pK of these forms is 6.8. Approximately 80% is divalent, and the remainder is monovalent at a pH of 7.4. A small percentage of plasma phosphate, approximately 15%, is protein bound. The remainder can be filtered by the glomerulus, with most existing as free phosphate and a small percentage complexed with calcium, magnesium, or sodium. Phosphate is the most plentiful intracellular anion, although the majority is part of a larger compound (ATP).

TABLE 52-8. Serum Phosphorus During Childhood

AGE	PHOSPHORUS
0–5 day	4.8–8.2 mg/dL
1–3 yr	3.8–6.5 mg/dL
4–11 yr	3.7–5.6 mg/dL
12–15 yr	2.9–5.4 mg/dL
16–19 yr	2.7–4.7 mg/dL

More than any other electrolyte, the phosphorus concentration varies with age (Table 52-8). The teleologic explanation for the high concentration during childhood is the need for phosphorus to facilitate growth. There is diurnal variation in the plasma phosphorus concentration, with the peak during sleep.

Phosphorus, as a component of ATP and other trinucleotides, is critical for cellular energy metabolism. It is necessary for nucleic acid synthesis, and it is a component of cell membranes and other structures. Along with calcium, phosphorus is an essential component of bone, and it is necessary for skeletal mineralization. There is a significant need for a net positive phosphorus balance during growth, with the growing skeleton especially vulnerable to deficiency.

INTAKE. Phosphorus is readily available in food. Milk and milk products are the best sources of phosphorus; high concentrations are present in meat and fish. Vegetables have more phosphorus than fruits and grains. Gastrointestinal absorption is fairly proportional to intake, with approximately 65% of intake being absorbed, including a small amount that is secreted. Absorption, almost exclusively in the small intestine, occurs via a paracellular diffusive process and a vitamin D–regulated transcellular pathway. However, the impact of the change in phosphorus absorption caused by vitamin D is relatively small compared with the effect of variations in phosphorus intake.

EXCRETION. Despite the wide variation in phosphorus absorption dictated by oral intake, excretion matches intake, except for the needs for growth. The kidney regulates phosphorus balance, which is determined by intrarenal mechanisms and hormonal actions on the nephron.

Approximately 90% of plasma phosphate is filtered at the glomerulus, although there is some variation based on plasma phosphate and calcium concentrations. There is no significant secretion of phosphate along the nephron. Resorption of phosphate occurs mostly in the proximal tubule, even though a small amount can be resorbed in the distal tubule. Normally, approximately 85% of the filtered load is resorbed. The transport of phosphate from the tubular lumen into the cells of the proximal tubule is coupled with the transport of sodium down its chemical gradient. A sodium-phosphate co-transporter mediates the uptake of phosphate into the cells of the proximal tubule.

The dietary phosphorus determines the amount of phosphate resorbed by the nephron. There are both acute and chronic changes in phosphate resorption based on intake. Many of these changes appear to be mediated by intrarenal mechanisms that are independent of regulatory hormones. PTH, which is secreted in response to low plasma calcium, decreases resorption of phosphate, increasing urinary phosphate. This appears to have a minimal effect during normal physiologic variation in PTH levels. However, it does have an impact in the setting of pathologic changes in PTH synthesis.

Low plasma phosphorus stimulates the 1α-hydroxylase in the kidney that converts 25-hydroxyvitamin D to 1,25-dihydroxyvitamin D (calcitriol). Calcitriol increases intestinal absorption of phosphorus and is necessary for maximal renal resorption of phosphate. The effect of a change in calcitriol on urinary phosphate is significant only when the level of calcitriol was initially low, arguing against a role for calcitriol in nonpathologic conditions.

A humoral mediator called *phosphatonin* inhibits renal resorption of phosphorus, causing both phosphaturia and hypophosphatemia in a variety of pathologic conditions. Phosphatonin also inhibits synthesis of calcitriol in the kidney by decreasing 1α-hydroxylase activity. In autosomal dominant hypophosphatemic rickets, fibroblast growth factor type 23 has been identified as the phosphatonin that causes the disease. Other putative phosphatonins include frizzled-related protein 4 and matrix extracellular phosphoglycoprotein. The role of phosphatonins in normal physiology is not clear.

HYPOPHOSPHATEMIA

Because of the wide variation in normal plasma phosphorus levels, the definition of hypophosphatemia is age-dependent (see Table 52-8). The normal range reported by a laboratory may be based on adult normal values and, therefore, may be misleading in children. A serum phosphorus level of 3 mg/dL, a normal value in an adult, indicates clinically significant hypophosphatemia in an infant.

The plasma phosphorus level does not always reflect the total body stores because only 1% of phosphorus is extracellular. Thus, a child may have significant phosphorus deficiency despite a normal plasma phosphorus concentration. This is especially common in conditions in which there is a shift of phosphorus from the intracellular space.

ETIOLOGY AND PATHOPHYSIOLOGY. A variety of mechanisms cause hypophosphatemia (Table 52-9). A transcellular shift of phosphorus into cells occurs with processes that stimulate cellular usage of phosphorus (glycolysis). Usually, this causes only a minor, transient decrease in plasma phosphorus, but if intracellular phosphorus deficiency is present, the plasma phosphorus level can decrease significantly, producing symptoms of acute hypophosphatemia. Glucose infusion stimulates insulin release, which leads to entry of glucose and phosphorus into the cells. Phosphorus is then used during glycolysis and other metabolic processes. A similar phenomenon can occur during the treatment of diabetic ketoacidosis, and these patients are typically phosphorus-depleted due to urinary phosphorus losses. **Refeeding** of patients with protein-calorie malnutrition causes anabolism, which leads to significant cellular demand for phosphorus. The increased phosphorus uptake for incorporation into newly synthesized compounds containing phosphorus leads to hypophosphatemia, which can be severe and symptomatic. Refeeding hypophosphatemia occurs frequently during treatment of severe anorexia nervosa. It can occur during treatment of children with malnutrition due to any cause, including cystic fibrosis, Crohn disease, burns, neglect, chronic infection, or famine. Hypophosphatemia usually occurs within the 1st 5 days of refeeding, and is prevented by a gradual increase in nutrition with appropriate phosphorus supplementation (see Chapter 43). Total parenteral nutrition without adequate phosphorus can cause hypophosphatemia.

Phosphorus moves into the intracellular space during a respiratory alkalosis and during recovery from a respiratory acidosis. An acute decrease in the carbon dioxide concentration, by increasing the intracellular pH, stimulates glycolysis, leading to intracellular use of phosphorus and hypophosphatemia. Because a metabolic alkalosis has less effect on the intracellular pH (carbon dioxide diffuses across cell membranes much faster than bicarbonate), there is minimal transcellular phosphorus movement with a metabolic alkalosis.

Tumors that grow rapidly, such as leukemia and lymphoma, may use large amounts of phosphorus, leading to hypo-

TABLE 52-9. Causes of Hypophosphatemia

TRANSCELLULAR SHIFTS
Glucose infusion
Insulin
Refeeding
Total parenteral nutrition
Respiratory alkalosis
Tumor growth
Bone marrow transplantation
Hungry bone syndrome
DECREASED INTAKE
Nutritional
Premature infants
Low phosphorus formula
Antacids and other phosphate binders
RENAL LOSSES
Hyperparathyroidism
Parathyroid hormone–related peptide
X-linked hypophosphatemic rickets (MIM 307800)
Tumor-induced osteomalacia
Autosomal dominant hypophosphatemic rickets (MIM 193100)
Fanconi syndrome
Dent disease (MIM 300009)
Hypophosphatemic rickets with hypercalciuria (MIM 241530)
Hypophosphatemia due to mutations in the sodium-phosphate cotransporter (MIM 182309)
Volume expansion and intravenous fluids
Metabolic acidosis
Diuretics
Glycosuria
Glucocorticoids
Kidney transplantation
MULTIFACTORIAL
Vitamin D deficiency
Vitamin D–dependent rickets type 1 (MIM 264700)
Vitamin D–dependent rickets type 2 (MIM 277440)
Alcoholism
Sepsis
Dialysis

MIM, database number from the Mendelian Inheritance in Man *(http://www3.ncbi.nlm.nih.gov/Omim/)*.

phosphatemia. A similar phenomenon may occur during the hematopoietic reconstitution that follows bone marrow transplantation. In **hungry bone syndrome,** there is avid bone uptake of phosphorus, along with calcium and magnesium, which can produce plasma deficiency of all 3 ions. Hungry bone syndrome is most common after parathyroidectomy for hyperparathyroidism because the stimulus for bone dissolution is acutely removed, but bone synthesis continues.

Nutritional phosphorus deficiency is unusual because most foods contain phosphorus. However, infants are especially susceptible because of their high demand for phosphorus to support growth, especially of the skeleton. Very low birthweight infants have particularly rapid skeletal growth, and phosphorus deficiency and rickets may develop if they are fed human milk or formula for term infants. There is also a relative deficiency of calcium. The provision of additional calcium and phosphorus, using breast milk fortifier or special premature infant formula, prevents this complication. Phosphorus deficiency, sometimes with concomitant calcium and vitamin D deficiency, occurs in infants who are not given enough milk or who receive a milk substitute that is nutritionally inadequate.

Antacids containing aluminum hydroxide, such as Maalox and Mylanta, bind dietary phosphorus and secreted phosphorus, preventing absorption. This can cause phosphorus deficiency and rickets in growing children. A similar mechanism causes hypophosphatemia in patients who are overtreated for hyperphosphatemia with phosphorus binders. In children with kidney failure, the addition of dialysis to phosphorus binders increases the risk of iatrogenic hypophosphatemia in these normally hyperphosphatemic patients. This complication, which is more common in infants, can worsen renal osteodystrophy.

Excessive renal losses of phosphorus occur in a variety of inherited and acquired disorders. Because PTH inhibits the resorption of phosphorus in the proximal tubule, **hyperparathyroidism** causes hypophosphatemia (see Chapter 574). The dominant clinical manifestation, however, is hypercalcemia, and the hypophosphatemia is usually asymptomatic. The phosphorus level in hyperparathyroidism is not extremely low, and there is no continued loss of phosphorus because a new steady state is achieved at the lower plasma phosphorus level. Renal excretion, therefore, does not chronically exceed intake. There are occasional malignancies that produce PTH-related peptide, which has the same actions as PTH and causes hypophosphatemia and hypercalcemia.

In **X-linked hypophosphatemic rickets,** there is urinary wasting of phosphorus and hypophosphatemia (see Chapter 48). **Tumor-induced osteomalacia** is a rare disorder that clinically resembles X-linked hypophosphatemic rickets, except that it is not hereditary. Tumor resection is curative. This condition has occasionally been seen in patients with epidermal nevus syndrome, neurofibromatosis, and fibrous dysplasia. **Autosomal dominant hypophosphatemic rickets** is due to a mutation that prevents the degradation of fibroblast growth factor type 23. High levels of this phosphatonin lead to renal phosphorus wasting, hypophosphatemia, inappropriately normal 1,25-diydroxyvitamin D levels, and rickets.

Fanconi syndrome is a generalized defect in the proximal tubule leading to urinary wasting of bicarbonate, phosphorus, amino acids, uric acid, and glucose (see Chapter 529). The clinical sequelae are due to the metabolic acidosis and hypophosphatemia. In children, an underlying genetic disease, most commonly cystinosis, often causes Fanconi syndrome, but it can be secondary to a variety of toxins and acquired diseases. Some patients have incomplete Fanconi syndrome, and phosphorus wasting may be 1 of the manifestations. The hypophosphatemia of Fanconi syndrome is generally associated with rickets and does not usually cause symptomatic acute hypophosphatemia.

Dent disease, an X-linked disorder resulting from a defective chloride channel, can cause renal phosphorus wasting and hypophosphatemia, although this is not present in most cases. Other possible manifestations of Dent disease include tubular proteinuria, hypercalciuria, nephrolithiasis, rickets, and chronic renal failure. **Hypophosphatemic rickets with hypercalciuria** is a rare disorder, principally described in kindreds from the Middle East. Mutations in the sodium-phosphate co-transporter cause hypophosphatemia, and complications may include nephrolithiasis and osteoporosis; the disorder is autosomal dominant.

Metabolic acidosis inhibits resorption of phosphorus in the proximal tubule. In addition, metabolic acidosis causes a transcellular shift of phosphorus out of cells because of intracellular catabolism. This released phosphorus is subsequently lost in the urine, leading to significant phosphorus depletion, even though the plasma phosphorus level may be normal. This classically occurs in diabetic ketoacidosis in which renal phosphorus loss is further increased by the osmotic diuresis. With correction of the metabolic acidosis and the administration of insulin, both of which cause a transcellular movement of phosphorus into the cells, there is a marked decrease in the plasma phosphorus level.

Volume expansion from any cause, such as hyperaldosteronism or SIADH, inhibits resorption of phosphorus in the proximal tubule. This also occurs with high rates of intravenous fluids. Thiazide and loop diuretics can increase renal phosphorus excretion, but this is seldom clinically significant. Glycosuria and glucocorticoids inhibit renal conservation of phosphorus. Hypophosphatemia is common after kidney transplantation due to urinary phosphorus losses. Possible explanations include pre-existing secondary hyperparathyroidism from chronic renal failure, glucocorticoid therapy, and upregulation of phosphatonins before transplantation. The hypophosphatemia usually resolves in a few months.

Both acquired and genetic causes of **vitamin D deficiency** are associated with hypophosphatemia (see Chapter 48). The pathogenesis is multifactorial. Vitamin D deficiency, by impairing intestinal calcium absorption, causes secondary hyperparathyroidism that leads to increased urinary phosphorus wasting. An absence of vitamin D decreases intestinal absorption of phosphorus and directly decreases renal resorption of phosphorus. The dominant clinical manifestation is rickets, although some patients have muscle weakness that may be related to phosphorus deficiency.

Alcoholism is the most common cause of severe hypophosphatemia in adults. Fortunately, many of the risk factors that predispose adult alcoholics to hypophosphatemia are not usually present in adolescents (malnutrition, antacid abuse, recurrent episodes of diabetic ketoacidosis). Hypophosphatemia often occurs in sepsis, but the mechanism is not clear. Aggressive, protracted hemodialysis, as might be used for the treatment of methanol or ethylene glycol ingestion, can cause hypophosphatemia.

CLINICAL MANIFESTATIONS. There are acute and chronic manifestations of hypophosphatemia. Rickets occurs in children with long-term phosphorus deficiency. The clinical features of rickets are described in Chapter 48.

Severe hypophosphatemia, typically at levels <1–1.5 mg/dL, may affect every organ in the body because phosphorus has a critical role in maintaining adequate cellular energy. Phosphorus is a component of ATP and is necessary for glycolysis. With inadequate phosphorus, red blood cell 2,3-diphosphoglycerate levels decrease, impairing release of oxygen to the tissues. Severe hypophosphatemia can cause hemolysis and dysfunction of white blood cells. Chronic hypophosphatemia causes proximal muscle weakness and atrophy. In the intensive care unit, phosphorus deficiency may slow weaning from the ventilator or cause acute respiratory failure. **Rhabdomyolysis** is the most common complication of acute hypophosphatemia, usually in the setting of an acute transcellular shift of phosphorus into cells in a child with chronic phosphorus depletion (anorexia nervosa). The rhabdomyolysis is actually somewhat protective in that there is cellular release of phosphorus. Other manifestations of severe hypophosphatemia include cardiac dysfunction and neurologic symptoms, such as tremor, paresthesia, ataxia, seizures, delirium, and coma.

DIAGNOSIS. The history and basic laboratory evaluation often suggest the etiology of hypophosphatemia. The history should investigate nutrition, medications, and familial disease. Hypophosphatemia and rickets in an otherwise healthy young child suggests a genetic defect in renal phosphorus conservation, Fanconi syndrome, inappropriate use of antacids, poor nutrition, vitamin D deficiency, or a genetic defect in vitamin D metabolism. In Fanconi syndrome, there is usually a metabolic acidosis, glycosuria, aminoaciduria, and a low plasma uric acid. Measurement of 25-hydroxyvitamin D and 1,25-dihydroxyvitamin D, calcium, and PTH differentiates among the various vitamin D deficiency disorders and X-linked hypophosphatemic rickets. Hyperparathyroidism is easily distinguished by the presence of elevated plasma PTH and calcium levels.

TREATMENT. The plasma phosphorus level, the presence of symptoms, the likelihood of chronic depletion, and the presence of ongoing losses dictate the approach to therapy. Mild hypophosphatemia does not require treatment unless the clinical situation suggests that chronic phosphorus depletion is present or that ongoing losses are occurring. Oral phosphorus can cause diarrhea, so the doses should be divided. Intravenous therapy is effective in patients who have severe deficiency or who cannot tolerate oral medications. Intravenous phosphorus is available as either sodium phosphate or potassium phosphate, with the choice usually based on the patient's plasma potassium level. Starting doses are 0.08–0.16 mmol/kg over 6 hr. The oral preparations of phosphorus are available with various ratios of sodium and potassium. This is an important consideration because some patients may not tolerate the potassium load, whereas supplemental potassium may be helpful in some diseases, such as Fanconi syndrome or malnutrition. Oral maintenance doses are 2–3 mmol/kg/day in divided doses.

Increasing dietary phosphorus is the only intervention needed in infants with inadequate intake. Other patients may also benefit from increased dietary phosphorus, usually dairy products. Phosphorus-binding antacids should be discontinued in patients with hypophosphatemia. Certain diseases require specific therapy. Vitamin D supplementation, not phosphorus, is the principal therapy in nutritional vitamin D deficiency. X-linked hypophosphatemic rickets is usually treated with a combination of 1,25-dihydroxyvitamin D and oral phosphorus.

HYPERPHOSPHATEMIA

ETIOLOGY AND PATHOPHYSIOLOGY. Renal insufficiency is the most common cause of hyperphosphatemia, with the severity proportional to the degree of kidney impairment (see Chapter 535). This occurs because gastrointestinal absorption of the large dietary intake of phosphorus is unregulated, and the kidneys normally excrete this phosphorus. As renal function deteriorates, increased excretion of phosphorus, partially mediated by increased PTH levels, is able to compensate. When kidney function is <30% of normal, hyperphosphatemia usually develops, although this may vary considerably based on dietary phosphorus absorption. Many of the other causes of hyperphosphatemia are more likely to develop in the setting of renal insufficiency (Table 52-10).

Cellular content of phosphorus is high relative to plasma phosphorus, and cell lysis can release substantial phosphorus. This is the etiology of hyperphosphatemia in **tumor lysis syndrome, rhabdomyolysis,** and **acute hemolysis.** These disorders cause concomitant potassium release and the risk of hyperkalemia. Additional features of tumor lysis and rhabdomyolysis are hyperuricemia and hypocalcemia, whereas indirect hyperbilirubinemia and elevated lactate dehydrogenase levels are often present with hemolysis. An elevated CPK level is suggestive of rhabdomyolysis. During lactic acidosis or diabetic ketoacidosis, there is decreased usage of phosphorus by cells and phosphorus shifts into the extracellular space. This problem reverses when the underlying problem is corrected, and especially with diabetic

TABLE 52-10. Causes of Hyperphosphatemia

TRANSCELLULAR SHIFTS
Tumor lysis syndrome
Rhabdomyolysis
Acute hemolysis
Diabetic ketoacidosis and lactic acidosis
INCREASED INTAKE
Enemas and laxatives
Cow's milk in infants
Treatment of hypophosphatemia
Vitamin D intoxication
DECREASED EXCRETION
Renal failure
Hypoparathyroidism or pseudohypoparathyroidism (MIM 146200/603233/103580/241410/203330)
Acromegaly
Hyperthyroidism
Tumoral calcinosis with hyperphosphatemia (MIM 211900)

MIM, database number from the Mendelian Inheritance in Man (*http://www3.ncbi.nlm.nih.gov/Omim/*).

ketoacidosis, patients subsequently become hypophosphatemic as a result of previous renal phosphorus loss.

Excessive intake of phosphorus is especially dangerous in children with renal insufficiency. Neonates are at risk because renal function is normally reduced during the 1st few months of life. In addition, they may erroneously be given doses of phosphorus that are meant for an older child or adult. In infants fed cow's milk, which has higher phosphorus content than breast milk or formula, hyperphosphatemia may develop. **Fleet enemas** have a high amount of phosphorus that can be absorbed, especially if there is an ileus. Infants and children with Hirschsprung disease are especially vulnerable. There is often associated hypernatremia due to sodium absorption and water loss from diarrhea. Sodium phosphorus laxatives may cause hyperphosphatemia if the dose is excessive or if renal insufficiency is present. Hyperphosphatemia occurs in children who receive overly aggressive treatment for hypophosphatemia. Vitamin D intoxication causes excessive gastrointestinal absorption of both calcium and phosphorus, and the suppression of PTH by hypercalcemia decreases renal phosphorus excretion.

The absence of PTH in **hypoparathyroidism** or PTH responsiveness in **pseudohypoparathyroidism** causes hyperphosphatemia because of increased resorption of phosphorus in the proximal tubule of the kidney (see Chapters 573 and 574). The associated hypocalcemia is responsible for the clinical symptoms. The hyperphosphatemia in hyperthyroidism or acromegaly is usually minor. It is secondary to increased resorption of phosphorus in the proximal tubule due to the actions of thyroxine or growth hormone. Excessive thyroxine can also cause bone resorption, which may contribute to the hyperphosphatemia and cause hypercalcemia. Patients with **familial tumoral calcinosis,** a rare autosomal recessive disorder, have hyperphosphatemia due to decreased renal phosphate excretion and heterotopic calcifications. The disease may be secondary to mutations in the genes for a glycosyltransferase or the phosphatonin fibroblast growth factor 23.

CLINICAL MANIFESTATIONS. The principal clinical consequences of hyperphosphatemia are hypocalcemia and systemic calcification. The hypocalcemia is probably due to tissue deposition of calcium-phosphorus salt, inhibition of 1,25-dihydroxyvitamin D production, and decreased bone resorption. Symptomatic hypocalcemia is most likely to occur when the phosphorus increases rapidly or when diseases predisposing to hypocalcemia are present (chronic renal failure, rhabdomyolysis). Systemic calcification occurs because the solubility of phosphorus and calcium in the plasma is exceeded. This is believed to happen when plasma calcium × plasma phosphorus, both measured in mg/dL, is more than 70. Clinically, this is often apparent in the conjunctiva, where it manifests as a foreign body feeling, erythema, and injection. More ominous manifestations are hypoxia from pulmonary calcification and renal failure from nephrocalcinosis.

DIAGNOSIS. The plasma creatinine and BUN should be assessed in any patient with hyperphosphatemia. The history should focus on intake of phosphorus and the presence of chronic diseases that may cause hyperphosphatemia. Measurement of potassium, uric acid, calcium, lactate dehydrogenase, bilirubin, and CPK may be indicated if rhabdomyolysis, tumor lysis, or hemolysis is suspected. With mild hyperphosphatemia and significant hypocalcemia, measurement of the serum PTH level distinguishes between hypoparathyroidism and pseudohypoparathyroidism.

TREATMENT. The treatment of acute hyperphosphatemia depends on its severity and etiology. Mild hyperphosphatemia in a patient with reasonable renal function spontaneously resolves; this can be accelerated by dietary phosphorus restriction. If kidney function is not impaired, then intravenous fluids can enhance renal phosphorus excretion. For more significant hyperphosphatemia or a situation such as tumor lysis or rhabdomyolysis, in which endogenous phosphorus generation is likely to continue, addition of an oral phosphorus binder prevents absorption of dietary phosphorus and can remove phosphorus from the body by binding what is normally secreted and absorbed by the gastrointestinal tract. Phosphorus binders are most effective when given with food. Binders containing aluminum hydroxide are especially efficient, but calcium carbonate is an effective alternative and may be preferred if there is a need to treat concomitant hypocalcemia. Preservation of renal function, for example with high urine flow in rhabdomyolysis or tumor lysis, is an important adjunct because this will permit continued excretion of phosphorus. If the hyperphosphatemia is not responding to conservative management, especially if renal insufficiency is supervening, then dialysis may be necessary to increase phosphorus removal.

Dietary phosphorus restriction is necessary for diseases causing chronic hyperphosphatemia. However, such diets are often difficult to follow, given the abundance of phosphorus in a variety of foods. Dietary restriction is often sufficient in conditions such as hypoparathyroidism or mild renal insufficiency. For more problematic hyperphosphatemia, such as with moderate renal insufficiency and end-stage renal disease, phosphorus binders are usually necessary. These include calcium carbonate, calcium acetate, and sevelamer hydrochloride. Aluminum-containing phosphorus binders are no longer used in chronic renal insufficiency because of the risk of aluminum toxicity. The risk is especially high if the patient is also taking oral citrate, which increases gastrointestinal absorption of aluminum. Dialysis directly removes phosphorus from the blood in end-stage renal disease, but it is only an adjunct to dietary restriction and phosphorus binders in that elimination of phosphorus by dialysis is not efficient enough to keep up with normal dietary intake.

Benet-Pages A, Orlik P, Strom TM, et al: An fgf23 missense mutation causes familial tumoral calcinosis with hyperphosphatemia. *Hum Mol Genet* 2005;14:385–390.

Blumsohn A: What have we learnt about the regulation of phosphate metabolism? *Curr Opin Nephrol Hypertens* 2004;13:397–401.

Jonsson KB, Zahradnik R, Larsson T, et al: Fibroblast growth factor 23 in oncogenic osteomalacia and x-linked hypophosphatemia. *N Engl J Med* 2003;348:1656–1663.

Ornstein RM, Golden NH, Jacobson MS, et al: Hypophosphatemia during nutritional rehabilitation in anorexia nervosa: Implications for refeeding and monitoring. *J Adolesc Health* 2003;32:83–88.

Schiavi SC, Kumar R: The phosphatonin pathway: New insights in phosphate homeostasis. *Kidney Int* 2004;65:1–14.

Tenenhouse HS, Murer H: Disorders of renal tubular phosphate transport. *J Am Soc Nephrol* 2003;14:240–248.

Topaz O, Shurman DL, Bergman R, et al: Mutations in GALNT3, encoding a protein involved in O-linked glycosylation, cause familial tumoral calcinosis. *Nat Genet* 2004;36:579–581.

Uckan D, Cetin M, Dida A, et al: Hypophosphatemia and hypouricemia in pediatric allogeneic bone marrow transplant recipients. *Pediatr Transplant* 2003;7:98–101.

52.7 • Acid-Base Balance

ACID-BASE PHYSIOLOGY

INTRODUCTION AND TERMINOLOGY. Close regulation of pH is necessary for cellular enzymes and other metabolic processes, which function optimally at the normal pH. Chronic, mild derangements in acid-base status may interfere with normal growth and development, whereas acute, severe changes in pH can be fatal. Control of acid-base balance depends on the kidneys, the lungs, and intracellular and extracellular buffers.

A normal pH is 7.35–7.45. There is an inverse relationship between the pH and the hydrogen ion concentration. When the hydrogen ion concentration decreases, the pH increases, and when the hydrogen ion concentration increases, the pH decreases. At a pH of 7.40, the hydrogen ion concentration is 40 nmol/L. A normal serum sodium concentration, 140 mEq/L, is >1 million times higher. Maintaining a normal pH is necessary because hydrogen ions are highly reactive and are especially likely to combine with proteins, altering their function.

An **acid** is a substance that releases ("donates") a hydrogen ion (H^+). A base is a substance that accepts a hydrogen ion. An acid (HA) can dissociate into a hydrogen ion and a conjugate base (A^-):

$$HA \leftrightarrow H^+ + A^-$$

A strong acid is highly dissociated, so in this reaction, there is little HA. A weak acid is poorly dissociated; not all of the hydrogen ions are released from HA. A^- acts as a base when the reaction moves to the left. These reactions are in equilibrium. When HA is added to the system, there is dissociation of some HA until the concentrations of H^+ and A^- increase enough that a new equilibrium is reached. Addition of hydrogen ions causes a decrease in A^- and an increase in HA. Addition of A^- causes a decrease in hydrogen ions and an increase in HA.

Buffers are substances that attenuate the change in pH that occurs when acids or bases are added to the body. Given the extremely low concentration of hydrogen ions in the body at physiologic pH, without buffers, a small amount of hydrogen ions could cause a dramatic decline in the pH. Buffers prevent the decrease in pH by binding the added hydrogen ions:

$$A^- + H^+ \rightarrow HA$$

The increase in hydrogen ion concentration drives this reaction to the right. Similarly, when base is added to the body, buffers prevent the pH from increasing by releasing hydrogen ions:

$$HA \rightarrow A^- + H^+$$

The best buffers are weak acids and bases. This is because a buffer works best when it is 50% dissociated (half HA and half A^-). The pH at which a buffer is 50% dissociated is its pK. The best physiologic buffers have a pK close to 7.40. The concentration of a buffer and its pK determine the buffer's effectiveness (buffering capacity). When the pH is lower than the pK of a buffer, there is more HA than A^-. When the pH is higher than the pK, there is more A^- than HA.

PHYSIOLOGIC BUFFERS. The bicarbonate and non-bicarbonate buffers protect the body against major changes in pH. The **bicarbonate buffer system** is routinely monitored clinically. The bicarbonate buffer system is based on the relationship between carbon dioxide (CO_2) and bicarbonate (HCO_3^-):

$$CO_2 + H_2O \leftrightarrow H^+ + HCO_3^-$$

Carbon dioxide acts as an acid in that, after combining with water, it releases a hydrogen ion; bicarbonate acts as its conjugate base in that it accepts a hydrogen ion. The pK of this reaction is 6.1. The Henderson-Hasselbalch equation expresses the relationship between pH, pK, and the concentrations of an acid and its conjugate base. This relationship is valid for any buffer. The Henderson-Hasselbalch equation for bicarbonate and carbon dioxide is:

$$pH = 6.1 + \log [HCO_3^-]/[CO_2]$$

The Henderson-Hasselbalch equation for the bicarbonate buffer system has 3 variables: pH, [HCO_3^-], and [CO_2]. Thus, if any 2 of these variables is known, it is possible to calculate the 3rd. In using the Henderson-Hasselbalch equation, it is important that carbon dioxide and bicarbonate have the same units. Carbon dioxide is reported clinically as mm Hg and must be multiplied by its solubility constant, 0.03 mmol/L/mm Hg, before the Henderson-Hasselbalch equation can be used. Mathematical manipulation of the Henderson-Hasselbalch equation produces the following relationship:

$$[H^+] = 24 \times PCO_2/[HCO_3^-]$$

At a normal hydrogen ion concentration of 40 nmol (pH 7.40), the PCO_2, which is expressed as mm Hg in this equation, is 40 when the bicarbonate concentration is 24 mEq/L. This equation emphasizes that the hydrogen ion concentration, and hence pH, can be determined by the ratio of PCO_2 and the bicarbonate concentration.

The bicarbonate buffer system is very effective as a result of the high concentration of bicarbonate in the body (24 mEq/L) and the fact that it is an open system. The remaining body buffers are in a closed system. The bicarbonate buffer system is an open system because the lungs increase carbon dioxide excretion when the blood carbon dioxide concentration increases. When acid is added to the body, the following reaction occurs:

$$H^+ + HCO_3^- \rightarrow CO_2 + H_2O$$

In a closed system, the CO_2 would increase. The higher CO_2 concentration would lead to an increase in the reverse reaction:

$$CO_2 + H_2O \rightarrow H^+ + HCO_3^-$$

This would increase the concentration of hydrogen ions, limiting the buffering capacity of bicarbonate. However, because the lungs excrete the excess carbon dioxide, the reverse reaction does not increase; this enhances the buffering capacity of bicarbonate. The same principle holds with the addition of base because the lungs decrease carbon dioxide excretion and prevent the level of carbon dioxide from falling. The lack of change in carbon dioxide concentration dramatically increases the buffering capacity of bicarbonate.

The **non-bicarbonate buffers** include proteins, phosphate, and bone. Protein buffers consist of extracellular proteins, mostly albumin and intracellular proteins, including hemoglobin. Proteins are effective buffers, largely due to the presence of the amino acid histidine, which has a side chain that can bind or release hydrogen ions. The pK of histidine varies slightly, depending on its position in the protein molecule, but its average pK is approximately 6.5. This is close enough to a normal pH (7.4) to make histidine an effective buffer. Hemoglobin and albumin have 34 and 16 histidine molecules, respectively.

Phosphate can bind up to 3 hydrogen molecules, so it can exist as PO_4^{3-}, HPO_4^{2-}, $H_2PO_4^{1-}$, or H_3PO_4. However, at a physiologic pH, most phosphate exists as either HPO_4^{2-} or $H_2PO_4^{1-}$. $H_2PO_4^{1-}$ is an acid, and HPO_4^{2-} is its conjugate base:

$$H_2PO_4^{1-} \leftrightarrow H^+ + HPO_4^{2-}$$

The pK of this reaction is 6.8, making phosphate an effective buffer. The concentration of phosphate in the extracellular space is relatively low, which limits the overall buffering capacity of phosphate; it is less important than albumin. However, phosphate is found at a much higher concentration in the urine, where it is an important buffer. In the intracellular space, most phosphate is covalently bound to organic molecules (ATP), but it still serves as an effective buffer.

Bone is an important buffer. Bone is basic—it is composed of compounds such as sodium bicarbonate and calcium carbonate—and thus, dissolution of bone releases base. This can buffer an acid load, although at the expense of bone density, if this occurs over an extended period. In contrast, bone formation, by consuming base, helps to buffer excess base.

Clinically, we measure the extracellular pH, but it is the intracellular pH that affects cell function. Measurement of the intracellular pH is unnecessary because changes in the intracellular pH parallel the changes in the extracellular pH. However, the change in the intracellular pH tends to be less than the change in the extracellular pH because of the increased buffering capacity in the intracellular space.

NORMAL ACID-BASE BALANCE

The lungs and kidneys maintain a normal acid-base balance. Carbon dioxide generated during normal metabolism is a weak acid. The lungs prevent an increase in the partial pressure of CO_2 (PCO_2) in the blood by excreting the CO_2 that the body produces. CO_2 production varies depending on the body's metabolic needs, increasing with physical activity. The rapid pulmonary response to changes in the CO_2 concentration occurs via central sensing of the PCO_2 and a subsequent increase or decrease in ventilation to maintain a normal PCO_2 (35–45 mm Hg). An increase in ventilation decreases the PCO_2, and a decrease in ventilation increases the PCO_2.

The kidneys excrete endogenous acid. An adult normally produces approximately 1–2 mEq/kg/24 hr of hydrogen ions. Children normally produce 2–3 mEq/kg/24 hr of hydrogen ions. The 3 principal sources of hydrogen ions are dietary protein metabolism, incomplete metabolism of carbohydrates and fat, and stool losses of bicarbonate. Because metabolism of protein generates hydrogen ions, endogenous acid production varies with protein intake. The complete oxidation of carbohydrates or fats to carbon dioxide and water does not generate hydrogen ions; the lungs remove the carbon dioxide. However, incomplete metabolism of carbohydrates or fats produces hydrogen ions. Incomplete glucose metabolism can produce lactic acid, and incomplete triglyceride metabolism can produce keto acids, such as β-hydroxybutyric acid or acetoacetic acid. There is always some baseline incomplete metabolism that contributes to endogenous acid production. This increases in pathologic conditions, such as lactic acidosis or diabetic ketoacidosis. Stool loss of bicarbonate is the 3rd major source of endogenous acid production. The stomach secretes hydrogen ions, but most of the remainder of the gastrointestinal tract secretes bicarbonate, and the net effect is a loss of bicarbonate from the body. To secrete bicarbonate, the cells of the intestine produce hydrogen ions that are released into the bloodstream. For each bicarbonate molecule lost in the stool, the body gains 1 hydrogen ion. This source of endogenous acid production is normally minimal, but may increase dramatically in a patient with diarrhea.

The hydrogen ions formed from endogenous acid production are neutralized by bicarbonate, potentially causing the bicarbonate concentration to decrease. The kidneys regenerate this bicarbonate by secreting hydrogen ions. The lungs cannot regenerate bicarbonate, even though loss of carbon dioxide lowers the hydrogen ion concentration:

$$H^+ + HCO_3^- \rightarrow CO_2 + H_2O$$

A decrease in carbon dioxide concentration causes the reaction to move to the right, which decreases the hydrogen ion concentration, but it also lowers the bicarbonate concentration. During a metabolic acidosis, hyperventilation can lower the carbon dioxide concentration, decrease the hydrogen ion concentration, and thus increase the pH. The underlying metabolic acidosis is still present. Similarly, the kidneys cannot correct an abnormally high carbon dioxide concentration:

$$H^+ + HCO_3^- \rightarrow CO_2 + H_2O$$

An increase in the bicarbonate concentration also causes the reaction to move to the right, which increases the carbon dioxide concentration while simultaneously decreasing the hydrogen ion concentration. During a respiratory acidosis, increased renal generation of bicarbonate can decrease the hydrogen ion concentration and increase the pH, but cannot repair the respiratory acidosis. Both the lungs and the kidneys can affect the hydrogen ion concentration and hence the pH. However, only the lungs can regulate the carbon dioxide concentration, and only the kidneys can regulate the bicarbonate concentration.

RENAL MECHANISMS. The kidneys regulate the serum bicarbonate concentration by modifying acid excretion in the urine. This requires a 2-step process. First, the renal tubules resorb the bicarbonate that is filtered at the glomerulus. Second, there is tubular secretion of hydrogen ions. The urinary excretion of hydrogen ions generates bicarbonate that neutralizes endogenous acid production. The tubular actions necessary for renal acid excretion occur throughout the nephron (Fig. 52-5).

The resorption of filtered bicarbonate is a necessary 1st step in renal regulation of the acid-base balance. A normal adult has a GFR of approximately 180 L/24 hr. This fluid enters Bowman's space with a bicarbonate concentration that is essentially identical to the plasma concentration, normally 24 mEq/L. Multiplying 180 L × 24 mEq/L indicates that >4,000 mEq of bicarbonate enters Bowman's space each day. This bicarbonate, if not reclaimed along the nephron, would be lost in the urine and would cause a profound metabolic acidosis.

The proximal tubule reclaims approximately 85% of the filtered bicarbonate. The final 15% is reclaimed beyond the proximal tubule, mostly in the ascending limb of the loop of Henle (Fig. 52-6). Bicarbonate molecules are not transported from the tubular fluid into the cells of the proximal tubule. Rather, hydrogen ions are secreted into the tubular fluid, leading to conversion of filtered bicarbonate into carbon dioxide and water. The secretion of hydrogen ions by the cells of the proximal tubule is coupled to generation of intracellular bicarbonate, which is transported across the basolateral membrane of the proximal tubule cell and enters the capillaries. The bicarbonate produced in the cell replaces the bicarbonate filtered at the glomerulus.

Increased bicarbonate resorption by the cells of the proximal tubule—the result of increased hydrogen ion secretion—occurs in a variety of clinical situations. Volume depletion increases bicarbonate resorption. This is partially mediated by activation of the renin-angiotensin system; angiotensin II increases bicarbonate resorption. Increased bicarbonate resorption in the proximal tubule is 1 of the mechanisms that accounts for the metabolic alkalosis that may occur in some patients with volume depletion. Other stimuli that increase bicarbonate resorption include hypokalemia and an increased PCO_2. This partially explains the observations that hypokalemia causes a metabolic alkalosis and that a respiratory acidosis leads to a compensatory increase in serum bicarbonate concentration.

Stimuli that decrease bicarbonate resorption in the proximal tubule may cause a decrease in the serum bicarbonate concentration. A decrease in the PCO_2 (respiratory alkalosis) decreases proximal tubule bicarbonate resorption, partially mediating the decrease in the serum bicarbonate concentration that compensates for a respiratory alkalosis. PTH decreases proximal tubule bicarbonate resorption; hyperparathyroidism may cause a mild metabolic acidosis. A variety of medications and diseases cause a metabolic acidosis by impairing bicarbonate resorption in

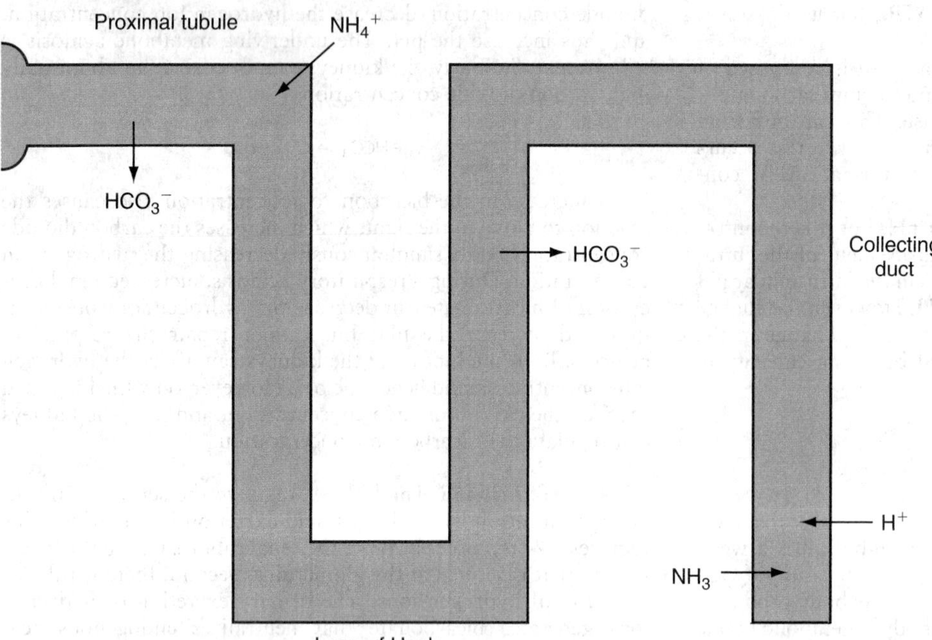

Figure 52-5. Tubular sites involved in acid-base balance. The proximal tubule is the site where most filtered bicarbonate is reclaimed, even though other sites along the nephron, especially the thick ascending limb of the loop of Henle, resorb some of the filtered bicarbonate. The collecting duct is the principal location for the hydrogen ion secretion that acidifies the urine. The proximal tubule generates the ammonia that serves as a urinary buffer in the collecting duct.

the proximal tubule. Examples include the medication acetazolamide, which directly inhibits carbonic anhydrase, and the many disorders that cause a proximal RTA (see Chapter 529).

After reclaiming filtered bicarbonate, the kidneys perform the 2nd step in renal acid-base handling, the excretion of the acid created by endogenous acid production. Excretion of acid occurs mostly in the collecting duct, with a small role for the distal tubule.

Along with secretion of hydrogen ions by the tubular cells lining the collecting duct, adequate excretion of endogenous acid requires the presence of urinary buffers. The hydrogen pumps in the collecting duct cannot lower the urine pH below 4.5. The hydrogen ion concentration at pH 4.5 is <0.04 mEq/L; it would require >25 L of water with a pH of 4.5 to excrete 1 mEq of hydrogen ions. A 10-kg child, with an endogenous acid production of 20 mEq of hydrogen ions each day, would need to have a daily urinary output of >500 L without the presence of urinary buffers. As in the blood, buffers in the urine attenuate the decrease in pH that occurs with the addition of hydrogen ions. The 2 principal urinary buffers are phosphate and ammonia.

Urinary phosphate is proportional to dietary intake. Whereas most of the phosphate filtered at the glomerulus is resorbed in the proximal tubule, the urinary phosphate concentration is usually much greater than the serum phosphate concentration. This allows phosphate to serve as an effective buffer via the following reaction:

$$H^+ + HPO_4^{2-} \rightarrow H_2PO_4^{1-}$$

The pK of this reaction is 6.8, making phosphate an effective buffer as the urinary pH decreases from 7.0 to 5.0 within the collecting duct. Whereas phosphate is an effective buffer, its buffering capacity is limited by its concentration; there is no mechanism for increasing urinary phosphate excretion in response to changes in acid-base status.

In contrast, ammonia production can be modified, allowing for regulation of acid excretion. The buffering capacity of ammonia is based on the reaction of ammonia with hydrogen ions to form ammonium:

$$NH_3 + H^+ \rightarrow NH_4^+$$

The cells of the proximal tubule are the source of the excreted ammonia, mostly through metabolism of glutamine via the following reactions:

$$\text{Glutamine} \rightarrow NH_4^+ + \text{glutamate}^-$$

$$\text{Glutamate}^- \rightarrow NH_4^+ + \alpha\text{-ketoglutarate}^{2-}$$

The metabolism of glutamine generates 2 ammonium ions. In addition, the metabolism of α-ketoglutarate generates 2 bicarbonate molecules. The ammonium ions are secreted into the lumen of the proximal tubule, whereas the bicarbonate molecules exit the proximal tubule cells via the basolateral Na^+, $3HCO_3^-$ co-transporter (see Fig. 52-6). This would seem to accomplish the goal of excreting hydrogen ions (as NH_4^+) and regenerating bicarbonate molecules. However, the ammonium ions secreted in the proximal tubule do not remain within the tubular lumen. Cells of the thick ascending limb of the loop of Henle resorb the ammonium ions. The result is that there is a high medullary interstitial concentration of ammonia, but the tubular fluid entering the collecting duct does not have significant amounts of ammonium ions. Moreover, the hydrogen ions that were secreted with ammonia, as ammonium ions, in the proximal tubule enter the bloodstream, canceling the effect of the bicarbonate generated in the proximal tubule. The excretion of ammonium ions, and hence hydrogen ions, is dependent on the cells of the collecting duct.

The cells of the collecting duct secrete hydrogen ions and regenerate bicarbonate, which is returned to the bloodstream (Fig. 52-7). This bicarbonate neutralizes endogenous acid production. Phosphate and ammonia buffer the hydrogen ions secreted by the collecting duct. Ammonia is an effective buffer because of the high concentrations in the medullary interstitium and because the cells of the collecting duct are permeable to ammonia, but not permeable to ammonium. As ammonia diffuses into the lumen of the collecting duct, the low urine pH causes almost all of the ammonia to be converted into ammonium. This maintains a low luminal ammonia concentration. Because the luminal pH is lower than the pH in the medullary interstitium, there is a higher concentration of ammonia within the medullary interstitium than in the tubular lumen, favoring movement of ammonia into the tubular lumen. Even though the concentration of ammonium in the tubular lumen is higher than in the interstitium, the cells of the collecting duct are impermeable to ammonium, preventing back-diffusion of ammonium out of the tubular lumen. This permits ammonia to be an effective buffer.

The kidneys adjust hydrogen ion excretion based on physiologic needs. There is variation in endogenous acid production, largely due to diet and to pathophysiologic stresses, such as diarrheal losses of bicarbonate, which increase the need for acid excretion. Hydrogen excretion is increased by upregulating hydrogen ion secretion in the collecting duct. This causes the pH of the urine to decrease. This response is fairly prompt, occurring within hours of an acid load, but it is limited by the buffering capacity of the urine; the hydrogen pumps in the collecting duct cannot lower the pH to <4.5. A more significant increase in acid excretion requires upregulation of ammonia production by the proximal tubule so that there is more ammonia available to serve as a buffer in the tubular lumen of the collecting duct. This response to a low serum pH reaches its maximum within 5–6 days; ammonia excretion can increase approximately 10-fold from baseline.

Acid excretion by the collecting duct increases in a number of different clinical situations. The extracellular pH is the most important regulator of renal acid excretion. A decrease in the extracellular pH from either a respiratory or a metabolic acidosis causes an increase in renal acid excretion. Aldosterone stimulates hydrogen ion excretion in the collecting duct, causing an increase in the serum bicarbonate concentration. This explains the metabolic alkalosis that occurs with primary hyperaldosteronism or secondary hyperaldosteronism due to volume depletion. Hypokalemia increases acid secretion, by both stimulating ammonia production in the proximal tubule and increasing hydrogen ion secretion in the collecting duct. Hypokalemia therefore tends to produce a metabolic alkalosis. Hyperkalemia causes the opposite effects, which may cause a metabolic acidosis.

In patients with an increased pH, the kidney has 2 principal mechanisms for correcting the problem. First, less bicarbonate is resorbed in the proximal tubule, leading to an increase in urinary bicarbonate losses. Second, in a limited number of specialized cells, the process for secretion of hydrogen ions by the collecting duct (see Fig. 52-7) can be reversed, leading to secretion of bicarbonate into the tubular lumen and secretion of hydrogen ions into the peritubular fluid, where they enter the bloodstream.

CLINICAL ASSESSMENT OF ACID-BASE DISORDERS

The following equation, a rearrangement of the Henderson-Hasselbalch equation, emphasizes the relationship between the PCO_2, the bicarbonate concentration, and the hydrogen ion concentration:

$$[H^+] = 24 \times PCO/[HCO_3^-]$$

An increase in the PCO_2 or a decrease in the bicarbonate concentration increases the hydrogen ion concentration; the pH

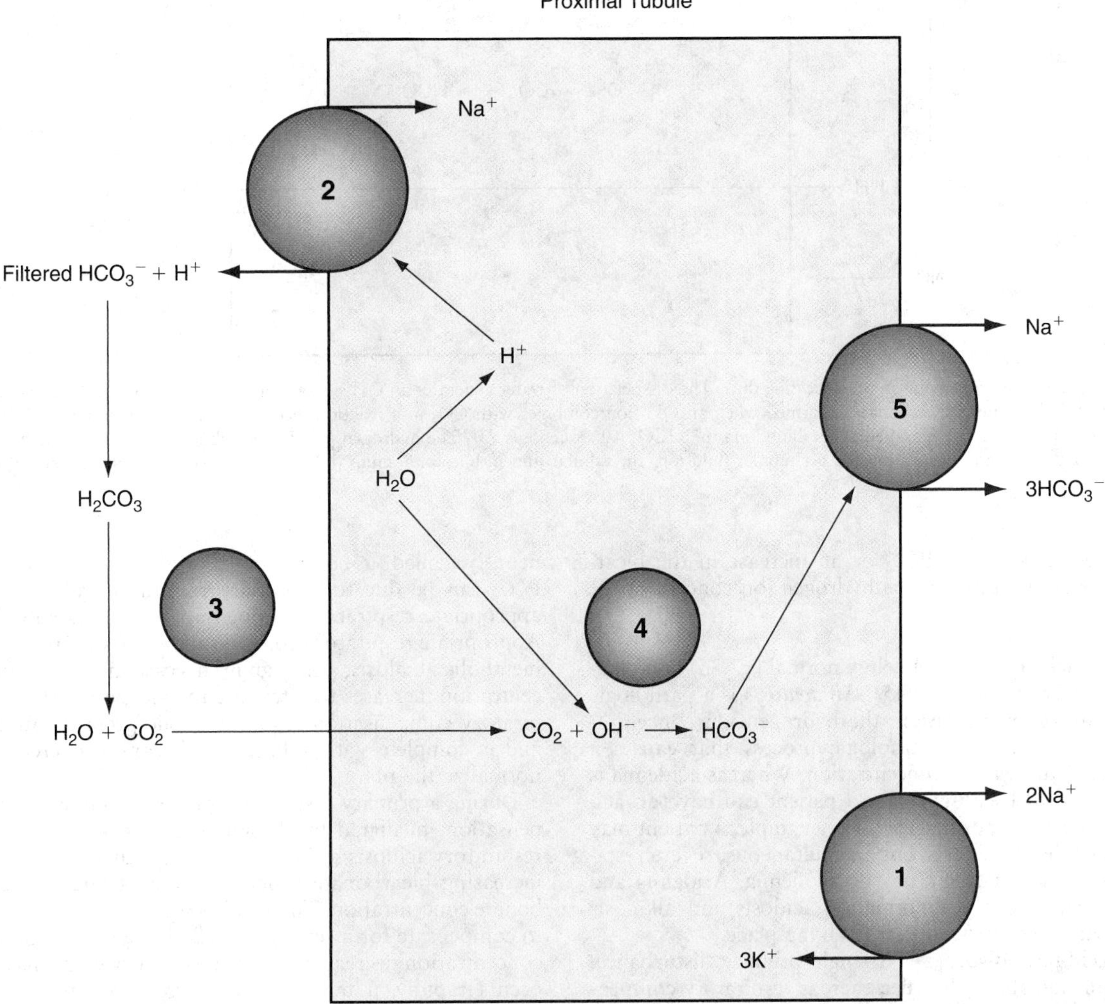

Figure 52-6. Resorption of filtered bicarbonate in the proximal tubule. The Na^+, K^+-ATPase *(1)* excretes sodium across the basolateral cell membrane, maintaining a low intracellular sodium concentration. The low intracellular sodium concentration provides the energy for the Na^+, H^+ antiporter *(2)*, which exchanges sodium from the tubular lumen for intracellular hydrogen ions. The hydrogen ions that are secreted into the tubular lumen then combine with filtered bicarbonate to generate carbonic acid. CO_2 and water are produced from carbonic acid (H_2CO_3). This reaction is catalyzed by luminal carbonic anhydrase *(3)*. CO_2 diffuses into the cell and combines with OH^- ions to generate bicarbonate. This reaction is catalyzed by an intracellular carbonic anhydrase *(4)*. The dissociation of water generates an OH^- ion and an H^+ ion. The Na^+, H^+ *(2)* antiporter secretes the hydrogen ions. Bicarbonate ions cross the basolateral membrane and enter the blood via the $3HCO_3^-/1Na^+$ co-transporter *(5)*. The energy for the $3HCO_3^-/1Na^+$ co-transporter comes from the negatively charged cell interior, which makes it electrically favorable to transport a net negative charge (i.e., 3 bicarbonates and only 1 sodium) out of the cell.

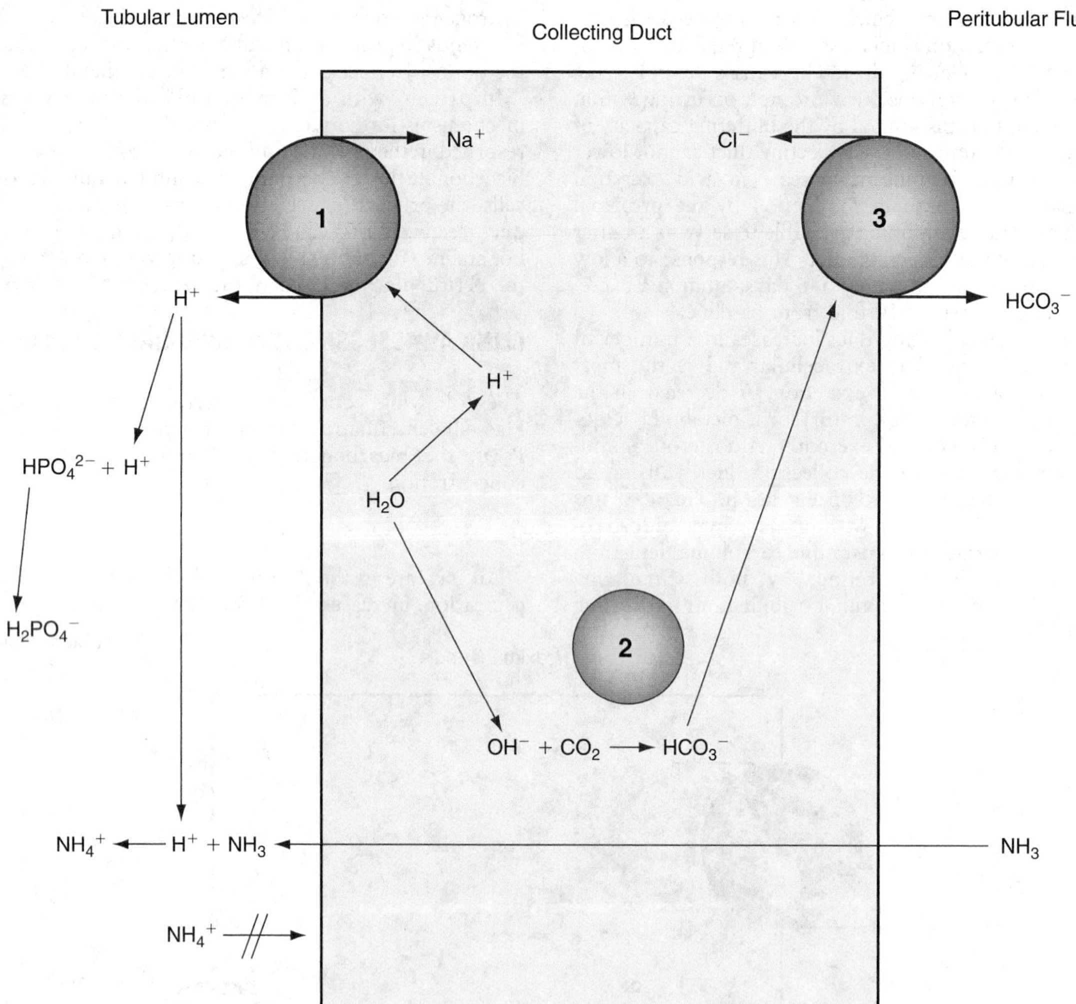

Figure 52-7. Secretion of hydrogen ions in the collecting duct. The dissociation of water generates an OH^- ion and an H^+ ion. The H^+-ATPase *(1)* secretes hydrogen ions into the tubular lumen. Bicarbonate is formed when an OH^- ion combines with CO_2 in a reaction mediated by carbonic anhydrase *(2)*. Bicarbonate ions cross the basolateral membrane and enter the blood via the HCO_3^-/Cl^- exchanger *(3)*. The hydrogen ions in the tubular lumen are buffered by phosphate and ammonia (NH_3). NH_3 can diffuse from the peritubular fluid into the tubular lumen, but ammonium (NH_4^+) cannot pass through the cells of the collecting duct.

decreases. A decrease in the P_{CO_2} or an increase in the bicarbonate concentration decreases the hydrogen ion concentration; the pH increases.

TERMINOLOGY. **Acidemia** is a pH below normal (<7.35) and **alkalemia** is a pH above normal (>7.45). An *acidosis* is a pathologic process that causes an increase in the hydrogen ion concentration, and an *alkalosis* is a pathologic process that causes a decrease in the hydrogen ion concentration. Whereas acidemia is always accompanied by an acidosis, a patient can have an acidosis and a low, normal, or high pH. For example, a patient may have a mild metabolic acidosis, but a simultaneous, severe respiratory alkalosis; the net result may be alkalemia. Acidemia and alkalemia indicate the pH abnormality; acidosis and alkalosis indicate the pathologic process that is taking place.

A **simple acid-base disorder** is a single primary disturbance. During a simple metabolic disorder, there is respiratory compensation. With a metabolic acidosis, the decrease in the pH increases the ventilatory drive, causing a decrease in the P_{CO_2}. The decrease in the carbon dioxide concentration leads to an increase in the pH. This appropriate respiratory compensation is expected with a primary metabolic acidosis. Despite the decrease in the carbon dioxide concentration, appropriate respiratory compensation is not a respiratory alkalosis, even though it is sometimes erroneously called a *compensatory respiratory alkalosis.* A low P_{CO_2} can be due to a primary respiratory alkalosis or due to appropriate respiratory compensation for a metabolic acidosis. Appropriate respiratory compensation also occurs with a primary metabolic alkalosis, although in this case the carbon dioxide concentration increases to attenuate the increase in the pH. The respiratory compensation for a metabolic process happens quickly and is complete within 12–24 hr; it cannot overcompensate or normalize the pH.

During a primary respiratory process, there is metabolic compensation, mediated by the kidneys. The kidneys respond to a respiratory acidosis by increasing hydrogen ion excretion, thereby increasing bicarbonate generation and raising the serum bicarbonate concentration. The kidneys increase bicarbonate excretion to compensate for a respiratory alkalosis; the serum bicarbonate concentration decreases. Unlike respiratory compensation, which occurs rapidly, it takes 3–4 days for the kidneys to complete appropriate metabolic compensation. There is, however, a small and rapid compensatory change in the bicarbonate concentration during a primary respiratory process. The expected appropriate metabolic compensation for a respiratory disorder is dependent on whether the process is acute or chronic.

A **mixed acid-base disorder** is present when there is more than 1 primary acid-base disturbance. An infant with bronchopul-

TABLE 52-11. Appropriate Compensation During Simple Acid-Base Disorders

DISORDER	EXPECTED COMPENSATION
Metabolic acidosis	$P_{CO_2} = 1.5 \times [HCO_3^-] + 8 \pm 2$
Metabolic alkalosis	P_{CO_2} increases by 7 mm Hg for each 10 mEq/L increase in serum $[HCO_3^-]$
Respiratory acidosis	
Acute	$[HCO_3^-]$ increases by 1 for each 10-mm Hg increase in P_{CO_2}
Chronic	$[HCO_3^-]$ increases by 3.5 for each 10-mm Hg increase in P_{CO_2}
Respiratory alkalosis	
Acute	$[HCO_3^-]$ falls by 2 for each 10-mm Hg decrease in P_{CO_2}
Chronic	$[HCO_3^-]$ falls by 4 for each 10-mm Hg decrease in P_{CO_2}

monary dysplasia may have a respiratory acidosis from chronic lung disease and a metabolic alkalosis from the furosemide used to treat the chronic lung disease. More dramatically, a child with pneumonia and sepsis may have severe acidemia due to a combined metabolic acidosis caused by lactic acid and respiratory acidosis caused by ventilatory failure.

There are formulas for calculating the appropriate metabolic or respiratory compensation for the 6 primary simple acid-base disorders (Table 52-11). The appropriate compensation is expected in a simple disorder; it is not optional. If a patient does not have the appropriate compensation, then a mixed acid-base disorder is present. A patient has a primary metabolic acidosis with a serum bicarbonate concentration of 10 mEq/L. The expected respiratory compensation is a carbon dioxide concentration of 23 mm Hg ± 2 ($1.5 \times 10 + 8 \pm 2 = 23 \pm 2$; see Table 52-11). If the patient's carbon dioxide concentration is >25 mm Hg, a concurrent respiratory acidosis is present; the carbon dioxide concentration is higher than expected. A patient may have a respiratory acidosis despite a carbon dioxide level below the "normal" value of 35–45 mm Hg. In this example, a carbon dioxide concentration <21 mm Hg indicates a concurrent respiratory alkalosis; the carbon dioxide concentration is lower than expected.

TABLE 52-12. Normal Values of Arterial Blood Gas

pH	7.35–7.45
$[HCO_3^-]$	20–28 mEq/L
P_{CO_2}	35–45 mm Hg

DIAGNOSIS. A systematic evaluation of an arterial blood gas sample, combined with the clinical history, can usually explain the patient's acid-base disturbance. Assessment of an arterial blood gas sample requires knowledge of normal values (Table 52-12). In most cases, this is accomplished via a 3-step process (Fig. 52-8):

- **Determine whether acidemia or alkalemia is present.**
- **Determine a cause of the acidemia or alkalemia.**
- **Determine whether a mixed disorder is present.**

Most patients with an acid-base disturbance have an abnormal pH, although there are 2 exceptions. The 1st exception is in the patient with a mixed disorder, wherein the 2 processes have opposite effects on pH (a metabolic acidosis and a respiratory alkalosis) and cause changes in the hydrogen ion concentration that are comparable in magnitude, albeit opposite. The 2nd exception is in the patient with a simple chronic respiratory alkalosis; in some instances, the appropriate metabolic compensation is enough to normalize the pH. In both of these situations, the presence of an acid-base disturbance is deduced because of the abnormal carbon

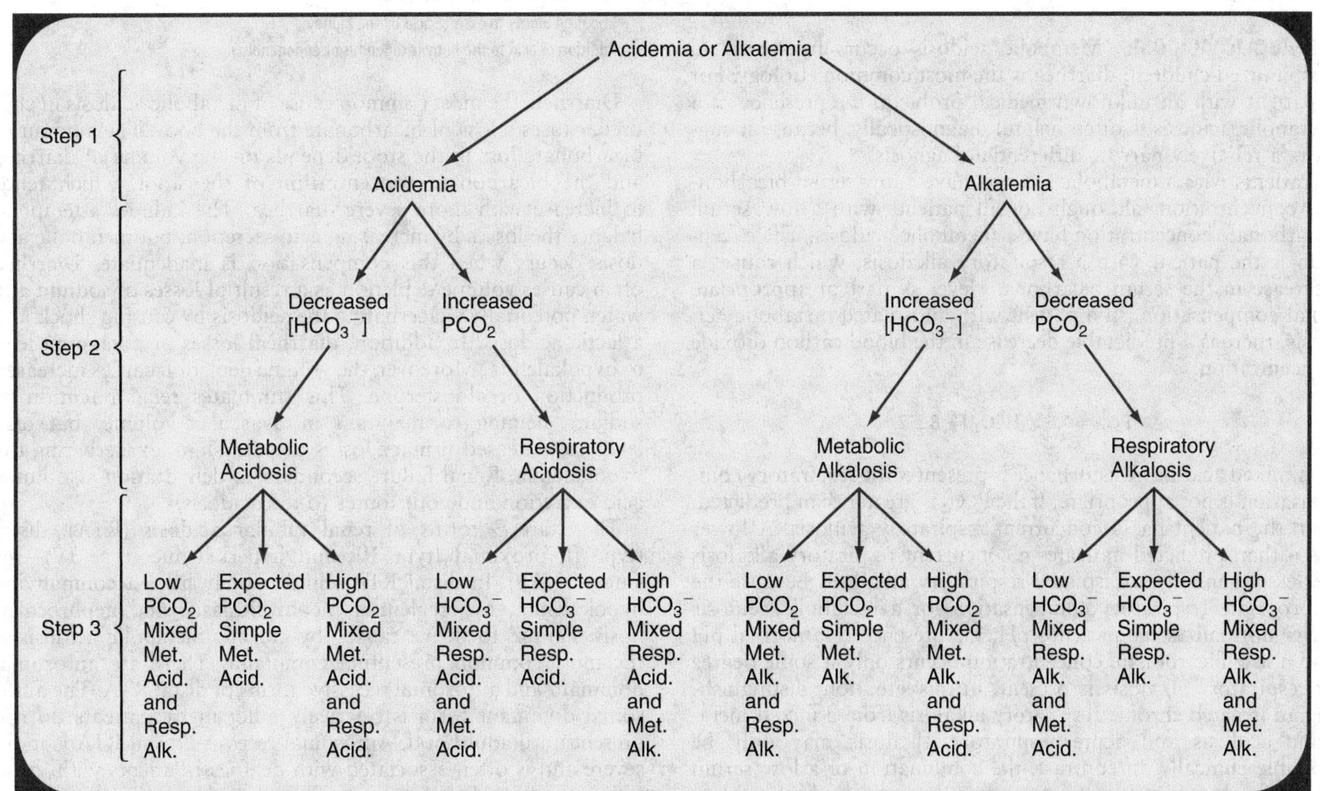

Figure 52-8. Three-step process for interpreting acid-base disturbances. In step 1, determine whether the pH is low (acidemia) or high (alkalemia). In step 2, establish an explanation for the acidemia or alkalemia. In step 3, calculate the expected compensation (see Table 52-11) and determine whether a mixed disturbance is present. Met. alk., metabolic alkalosis; met. acid., metabolic acidosis; resp. alk., respiratory alkalosis; resp. acid., respiratory acidosis.

dioxide and/or bicarbonate levels. Determining the acid-base disturbance in these situations requires proceeding to the 3rd step of this process (discussed later).

The 2nd step requires inspection of the serum bicarbonate and carbon dioxide concentrations to determine a cause of the abnormal pH (see Fig. 52-8). In most cases, there is only 1 obvious explanation for the abnormal pH. In some mixed disorders, however, there may be 2 possibilities (a high P_{CO_2} and a low $[HCO_3^-]$ in a patient with acidemia). In such cases, the patient has 2 causes of the abnormal pH (a metabolic acidosis and a respiratory acidosis, in this instance), and it is unnecessary to proceed to the 3rd step.

The 3rd step requires determining whether the patient's compensation is appropriate. The patient is assumed to have the primary disorder diagnosed in the 2nd step, and the expected compensation is calculated (see Table 52-11). If the compensation is appropriate, then a simple acid-base disorder is present. If the compensation is not appropriate, then a mixed disorder is present. The identity of the 2nd disorder is determined by deciding whether the compensation is too little or too much compared with what was expected (see Fig. 52-8).

The history is always useful in evaluating and diagnosing patients with acid-base disturbances. This is especially true with a respiratory process. The expected metabolic compensation for a respiratory process changes based on whether the process is acute or chronic. This can be deduced only by the history. The metabolic compensation for a patient with an acute respiratory acidosis is less than that for a chronic respiratory acidosis. In a patient with a respiratory acidosis, a small increase in the bicarbonate concentration would be consistent with a simple acute respiratory acidosis or a mixed disorder (a chronic respiratory acidosis and a metabolic acidosis). Only the history can differentiate among the possibilities. Knowledge of the length of the respiratory process and the presence or absence of a risk factor for a metabolic acidosis (diarrhea) allows the correct conclusion to be reached.

METABOLIC ACIDOSIS. Metabolic acidosis occurs frequently in hospitalized children; diarrhea is the most common etiology. For a patient with an unknown medical problem, the presence of a metabolic acidosis is often helpful diagnostically, because it suggests a relatively narrow differential diagnosis.

Patients with a metabolic acidosis have a low serum bicarbonate concentration, although not all patients with a low serum bicarbonate concentration have a metabolic acidosis. The exception is the patient with a respiratory alkalosis, which causes a decrease in the serum bicarbonate level as part of appropriate renal compensation. In a patient with an isolated metabolic acidosis, there is a predictable decrease in the blood carbon dioxide concentration:

$$P_{CO_2} = 1.5 \times [HCO_3^-] + 8 \pm 2$$

A mixed acid-base disturbance is present if the respiratory compensation is not appropriate. If the P_{CO_2} is greater than predicted, then the patient has a concurrent respiratory acidosis. A lower P_{CO_2} than predicted indicates a concurrent respiratory alkalosis or, less commonly, an isolated respiratory alkalosis. Because the appropriate respiratory compensation for a metabolic acidosis **never normalizes** the patient's pH, the presence of a normal pH and a low bicarbonate concentration occurs only if some degree of respiratory alkalosis is present. In this situation, distinguishing an isolated chronic respiratory alkalosis from a mixed metabolic acidosis and acute respiratory alkalosis may only be possible clinically. In contrast, the combination of a low serum pH and a low bicarbonate concentration occurs only if a metabolic acidosis is present.

Etiology and Pathophysiology. There are many causes of a metabolic acidosis (Table 52-13), which occur via 3 basic mechanisms:

TABLE 52-13. Causes of Metabolic Acidosis

NORMAL ANION GAP
Diarrhea
Renal tubular acidosis (RTA)
Distal (type I) RTA (MIM 179800/602722/267300)*
Proximal (type II) RTA (MIM 604278)[†]
Hyperkalemic (type IV) RTA (MIM 201910/264350/177735/145260)[‡]
Urinary tract diversions
Posthypocapnia
Ammonium chloride intake
INCREASED ANION GAP
Lactic acidosis
Tissue hypoxia (shock, hypoxemia, severe anemia)
Liver failure
Malignancy
Intestinal bacterial overgrowth
Inborn errors of metabolism
Medications (nucleoside analogues, metformin)
Ketoacidosis
Diabetic ketoacidosis
Starvation ketoacidosis
Alcoholic ketoacidosis
Kidney failure
Poisoning
Ethylene glycol
Methanol
Salicylate
Toluene
Paraldehyde
Inborn errors of metabolism

MIM, database number from the Mendelian Inheritance in Man (*http://www3.ncbi.nlm.nih.gov/Omim/*).
*Along with these genetic disorders, distal renal tubular acidosis (RTA) may be secondary to renal disease or medications.
[†]Most cases of proximal RTA are not due to this primary genetic disorder. Proximal RTA is usually part of Fanconi syndrome, which has multiple etiologies.
[‡]Hyperkalemic RTA can be secondary to a genetic disorder (some of the more common are listed) or other etiologies.

- **Loss of bicarbonate from the body**
- **Impaired ability to excrete acid by the kidney**
- **Addition of acid to the body (exogenous or endogenous)**

Diarrhea, the most common cause of metabolic acidosis in children, causes a loss of bicarbonate from the body. The amount of bicarbonate lost in the stool depends on the volume of diarrhea and the bicarbonate concentration of the stool, which tends to increase with more severe diarrhea. The kidneys attempt to balance the losses by increasing acid secretion, but metabolic acidosis occurs when this compensation is inadequate. Diarrhea often causes volume depletion as a result of losses of sodium and water, potentially exacerbating the acidosis by causing shock and a lactic acidosis. In addition, diarrheal losses of potassium lead to hypokalemia. Moreover, the volume depletion causes increased production of aldosterone. This stimulates renal retention of sodium, helping to maintain intravascular volume, but also leads to increased urinary losses of potassium, exacerbating the hypokalemia. Renal failure secondary to dehydration also limits acid excretion and contributes to the acidosis.

There are 3 forms of **renal tubular acidosis** (RTA): distal (type I), proximal (type II), and hyperkalemic (type IV) [see Chapter 529]. In distal RTA, children may have accompanying hypokalemia, hypercalciuria, nephrolithiasis, and nephrocalcinosis. Failure to thrive caused by chronic metabolic acidosis is the most common presenting complaint. There are autosomal dominant and autosomal recessive forms of distal RTA. The autosomal dominant form is relatively mild; many patients do not present until adulthood. Autosomal recessive distal RTA is more severe and is often associated with deafness. Patients with distal RTA cannot acidify their urine and, thus, have a urine pH >5.5 despite a metabolic acidosis.

Proximal RTA is rarely present in isolation. In most patients, proximal RTA is part of Fanconi syndrome, a generalized dysfunction of the proximal tubule. This leads to glycosuria, aminoaciduria, and excessive urinary losses of phosphate and uric acid. The presence of a low serum uric acid level, glycosuria, and aminoaciduria is helpful diagnostically. Chronic hypophosphatemia leads to rickets in children (see Chapter 48). Rickets and/or failure to thrive may be the presenting complaint. The ability to acidify the urine is intact in proximal RTA; thus, untreated patients have a urine pH <5.5. However, bicarbonate therapy increases bicarbonate losses in the urine, and the urine pH increases.

In hyperkalemic RTA, renal excretion of acid and potassium is impaired. Hyperkalemic RTA is due to either an absence of aldosterone or an inability of the kidney to respond to aldosterone. In severe aldosterone deficiency, as occurs with congenital adrenal hyperplasia due to 21α-hydroxylase deficiency, the hyperkalemia and metabolic acidosis are accompanied by hyponatremia and volume depletion from renal salt wasting. Incomplete aldosterone deficiency causes less severe electrolyte disturbances; children may have isolated hyperkalemic RTA, hyperkalemia without acidosis, or isolated hyponatremia. Patients may have aldosterone deficiency due to decreased renin production by the kidney; renin normally stimulates aldosterone synthesis. Children with hyporeninemic hypoaldosteronism usually have either isolated hyperkalemia or hyperkalemic RTA. The manifestations of aldosterone resistance depend on the severity of the resistance. In the autosomal recessive form of pseudohypoaldosteronism type I, which is due to an absence of the sodium channel that normally responds to aldosterone, there is often severe salt wasting and hyponatremia. In contrast, the aldosterone resistance in kidney transplant patients usually produces either isolated hyperkalemia or hyperkalemic RTA; hyponatremia is unusual. Similarly, the medications that cause hyperkalemic RTA do not cause hyponatremia. Pseudohypoaldosteronism type II, an autosomal recessive disorder also known as **Gordon syndrome,** is a unique cause of hyperkalemic RTA because the genetic defect causes volume expansion and hypertension.

Children with **abnormal urinary tracts,** usually secondary to congenital malformations, may require diversion of urine through intestinal segments. Ureterosigmoidostomy, anastomosis of a ureter to the sigmoid colon, almost always produces a metabolic acidosis and hypokalemia. Consequently, ileal conduits are now the more commonly used procedure, although there is still a risk of a metabolic acidosis.

The **appropriate metabolic compensation for a chronic respiratory alkalosis** is a decrease in renal acid excretion. The resultant decrease in the serum bicarbonate concentration lessens the alkalemia caused by the respiratory alkalosis. If the respiratory alkalosis resolves quickly, the patient continues to have a decreased serum bicarbonate concentration, causing acidemia due to a metabolic acidosis. This resolves over 1–2 days via increased acid excretion by the kidneys.

Lactic acidosis most commonly occurs when inadequate oxygen delivery to the tissues leads to anaerobic metabolism and excess production of lactic acid. Lactic acidosis may be secondary to shock, severe anemia, or hypoxemia. When the underlying cause of the lactic acidosis is alleviated, the liver is able to metabolize the accumulated lactate into bicarbonate, correcting the metabolic acidosis. There is normally some tissue production of lactate that is metabolized by the liver. In children with severe liver dysfunction, impairment in lactate metabolism may produce a lactic acidosis. Rarely, a metabolically active malignancy grows so fast that its blood supply becomes inadequate, with resultant anaerobic metabolism and lactic acidosis. Patients who have short bowel syndrome due to small bowel resection can have bacterial overgrowth. In these patients, excessive bacterial metabolism of glucose into D-lactic acid can cause a lactic acidosis. Lactic acidosis occurs in a variety of inborn errors of metabolism, especially those affecting mitochondrial oxidation (see Chapter 87.4). Finally, medications can cause lactic acidosis. Nucleoside reverse transcriptase inhibitors that are used to treat HIV infection inhibit mitochondrial replication; lactic acidosis is a rare complication, although elevated serum lactate levels without acidosis are quite common. Metformin, commonly used for treating type 2 diabetes mellitus, is most likely to cause a lactic acidosis in patients with renal insufficiency.

In **insulin-dependent diabetes mellitus,** inadequate insulin leads to hyperglycemia and diabetic ketoacidosis (see Chapter 590). Production of acetoacetic acid and β-hydroxybutyric acid causes the metabolic acidosis. Administration of insulin corrects the underlying metabolic problem and permits conversion of acetoacetate and β-hydroxybutyrate into bicarbonate, which helps to correct the metabolic acidosis. However, in some patients, urinary losses of acetoacetate and β-hydroxybutyrate may be substantial, preventing rapid regeneration of bicarbonate. In these patients, full correction of the metabolic acidosis requires renal regeneration of bicarbonate, a slower process. The characteristic odor of the breath in diabetic ketoacidosis is caused by the conversion of some acetoacetic acid into acetone, a volatile ketone that leaves the blood via the lungs. The hyperglycemia causes an osmotic diuresis, usually producing volume depletion, along with substantial losses of potassium, sodium, and phosphate. Despite severe total body potassium depletion, the serum potassium level initially may be normal as a result of a shift of potassium from the intracellular space into the extracellular space because of the lack of insulin and the metabolic acidosis. Hypokalemia develops with insulin therapy unless the patient receives adequate potassium.

In **starvation ketoacidosis,** the lack of glucose leads to keto acid production. This can produce a metabolic acidosis, although it is usually mild as a result of increased acid secretion by the kidney. In alcoholic ketoacidosis, which is much less common in children than in adults, the acidosis usually follows a combination of an alcoholic binge with vomiting and poor intake of food. The acidosis is potentially more severe than with isolated starvation, and the blood glucose level may be low, normal, or high. Hypoglycemia and acidosis also suggest an inborn error of metabolism.

Renal failure causes a metabolic acidosis because of the need for the kidneys to excrete the acid produced by normal metabolism. With mild or moderate renal insufficiency, the remaining nephrons are usually able to compensate by increasing acid excretion. When the GFR is <20–30% of normal, the compensation is inadequate and a metabolic acidosis develops. In some children, especially those with chronic renal failure due to tubular damage, the acidosis develops at a higher GFR because of a concurrent defect in acid secretion by the distal tubule (a distal RTA).

A variety of **toxic ingestions** (see Chapter 710) can cause a metabolic acidosis. Salicylate intoxication is much less common since aspirin is no longer recommended for fever control in children. Acute salicylate intoxication occurs after a large overdose. Chronic salicylate intoxication is possible with gradual buildup of the drug. Especially in adults, respiratory alkalosis may be the dominant acid-base disturbance. In children, the metabolic acidosis is usually the more significant finding. Other symptoms of salicylate intoxication include fever, seizures, lethargy, and coma. Hyperventilation may be particularly marked. Tinnitus, vertigo, and hearing impairment are more likely with chronic salicylate intoxication.

Ethylene glycol, a component of antifreeze, is converted in the liver to glyoxylic and oxalic acids, causing a severe metabolic acidosis. Excessive oxalate excretion causes calcium oxalate crystals to appear in the urine, and calcium oxalate precipitation in the kidney tubules can cause renal failure. The toxicity of methanol ingestion is also dependent on liver metabolism; formic acid is the toxic end product that causes the metabolic acidosis and other sequelae, which include damage to the optic nerve and central nervous system. Symptoms may include nausea, emesis, visual impairment, and altered mental status. Toluene inhalation and paraldehyde ingestion are other potential causes of a metabolic acidosis.

Many **inborn errors of metabolism** cause a metabolic acidosis (see Chapters 84–87). The metabolic acidosis may be due to excessive production of keto acids, lactic acid, and/or other organic anions. Some patients have accompanying hypoglycemia or hyperammonemia. In most patients, the acidosis occurs episodically, only during acute decompensations, which may be precipitated by ingestion of specific dietary substrates, the stress of a mild illness, or poor compliance with dietary or medical therapy. In a few inborn errors of metabolism, patients have a chronic metabolic acidosis.

Clinical Manifestations. The underlying disorder usually produces most of the signs and symptoms in children with a mild or moderate metabolic acidosis. The clinical manifestations of the acidosis are related to the degree of acidemia; patients with appropriate respiratory compensation and less severe acidemia have fewer manifestations than those with a concomitant respiratory acidosis. At a serum pH <7.20, there may be impaired cardiac contractility and an increased risk of arrhythmias, especially if underlying heart disease or other predisposing electrolyte disorders are present. With acidemia, there may be a decrease in the cardiovascular response to catecholamines, potentially exacerbating hypotension in children with volume depletion or shock. Acidemia causes vasoconstriction of the pulmonary vasculature, which is especially problematic in newborn infants with persistent pulmonary hypertension (see Chapter 101.8).

The normal respiratory response to metabolic acidosis—compensatory hyperventilation—may be subtle with mild metabolic acidosis, but it causes discernible increased respiratory effort with worsening acidemia. The acute metabolic effects of acidemia include insulin resistance, increased protein degradation, and reduced ATP synthesis. Chronic metabolic acidosis causes failure to thrive in children. Acidemia causes potassium to move from the intracellular space to the extracellular space, thereby increasing the serum potassium concentration. Severe acidemia impairs brain metabolism, eventually resulting in lethargy and coma.

Diagnosis. The etiology of a metabolic acidosis is often apparent from the history and physical examination. Acutely, diarrhea and shock are common causes of a metabolic acidosis. Shock, which causes a lactic acidosis, is usually apparent on physical examination and can be secondary to dehydration, acute blood loss, sepsis, or heart disease. Failure to thrive suggests a chronic metabolic acidosis, as happens with renal insufficiency or RTA. New onset of polyuria occurs in children with undiagnosed diabetes mellitus and diabetic ketoacidosis. Metabolic acidosis with seizures and/or a depressed sensorium, especially in an infant, warrants consideration of an inborn error of metabolism. Meningitis and sepsis with lactic acidosis are more common explanations for metabolic acidosis with neurologic signs and symptoms. Identification of toxic ingestions, such as ethylene glycol or methanol, is especially important because of the potential excellent response to specific therapy. A variety of medications can cause a metabolic acidosis; they may be prescribed or accidentally ingested. Hepatomegaly and metabolic acidosis may occur in children with sepsis, congenital or acquired heart disease, hepatic failure, or inborn errors of metabolism.

Basic laboratory tests in a child with a metabolic acidosis should include BUN, creatinine, serum glucose, urinalysis, and electrolytes. Elevated BUN and creatinine values are present in renal insufficiency, whereas an elevated BUN : creatinine ratio (>20 : 1) supports a diagnosis of prerenal azotemia and the possibility of poor perfusion with lactic acidosis. Metabolic acidosis, hyperglycemia, glycosuria, and ketonuria support a diagnosis of diabetic ketoacidosis. Starvation causes ketosis, but the metabolic acidosis, if present, is usually mild (HCO_3^- >18). Most children with ketosis due to poor intake and metabolic acidosis have a concomitant disorder, such as gastroenteritis with diarrhea, as an explanation for the metabolic acidosis. Alternatively, metabolic acidosis with or without ketosis occurs in inborn errors of metabolism; these patients may have hyperglycemia, normoglycemia, or hypoglycemia. Adrenal insufficiency may cause metabolic acidosis and hypoglycemia. Metabolic acidosis with hypoglycemia also occurs with liver failure. Metabolic acidosis, normoglycemia, and glycosuria occur in children when type II RTA is part of Fanconi syndrome; the defect in resorption of glucose by the proximal tubule of the kidney causes the glycosuria.

The serum potassium level is often abnormal in children with a metabolic acidosis. Even though a metabolic acidosis causes potassium to move from the intracellular space to the extracellular space, many patients with a metabolic acidosis have a low serum potassium level due to excessive body losses of potassium. With diarrhea, there are high stool losses of potassium and often secondary renal losses of potassium, whereas in type I or type II RTA, there are increased urinary losses of potassium. In diabetic ketoacidosis, urinary losses of potassium are high, but the shift of potassium out of cells due to lack of insulin and metabolic acidosis is especially significant. Consequently, the initial serum potassium level can be low, normal, or high, even though total body potassium is almost always decreased. The serum potassium level is usually increased in patients with acidosis due to renal insufficiency; urinary potassium excretion is impaired. The combination of metabolic acidosis, hyperkalemia, and hyponatremia occurs in patients with severe aldosterone deficiency (adrenogenital syndrome) or aldosterone resistance. Patients with less severe type IV RTA often have only hyperkalemia and metabolic acidosis. Very ill children with metabolic acidosis may have an elevated serum potassium level as a result of a combination of renal insufficiency, tissue breakdown, and a shift of potassium from the intracellular space to the extracellular space secondary to the metabolic acidosis.

The **plasma anion gap** is useful for evaluating patients with a metabolic acidosis. It divides patients into 2 diagnostic groups: normal anion gap and increased anion gap. The following formula determines the anion gap:

$$\text{Anion gap} = [Na^+] - [Cl^-] - [HCO_3^-]$$

A normal anion gap is 4–11. The number of serum anions must equal the number of serum cations to maintain electrical neutrality (Fig. 52-9). The anion gap is the difference between the measured cation (sodium) and the measured anions (chloride + bicarbonate). The anion gap is also the difference between the unmeasured cations (potassium, magnesium, calcium) and the unmeasured anions (albumin, phosphate, urate, sulfate). An increased anion gap occurs when there is an increase in unmeasured anions. With a lactic acidosis, there is endogenous production of lactic acid, which is composed of positively charged hydrogen ions and negatively charged lactate anions. The hydrogen ions are largely buffered by serum bicarbonate, resulting in a decrease in the bicarbonate concentration. The hydrogen ions that are not buffered by bicarbonate cause the serum pH to decrease. The lactate anions remain, and this causes the increase in the anion gap.

An increase in unmeasured anions, along with hydrogen ion generation, is present in all causes of an increased gap metabolic acidosis (see Table 52-13). In diabetic ketoacidosis, the keto acids β-hydroxybutyrate and acetoacetate are the unmeasured anions. In renal failure, there is retention of unmeasured anions, including phosphate, urate, and sulfate. The increase in unmeasured anions in renal failure is usually less than the decrease in the bicarbonate concentration. Renal failure is thus a mix of an increased gap and a normal gap metabolic acidosis. The normal gap metabolic acidosis is especially prominent in children with renal failure due to tubular damage, as occurs with renal dysplasia or obstructive uropathy, because these patients actually

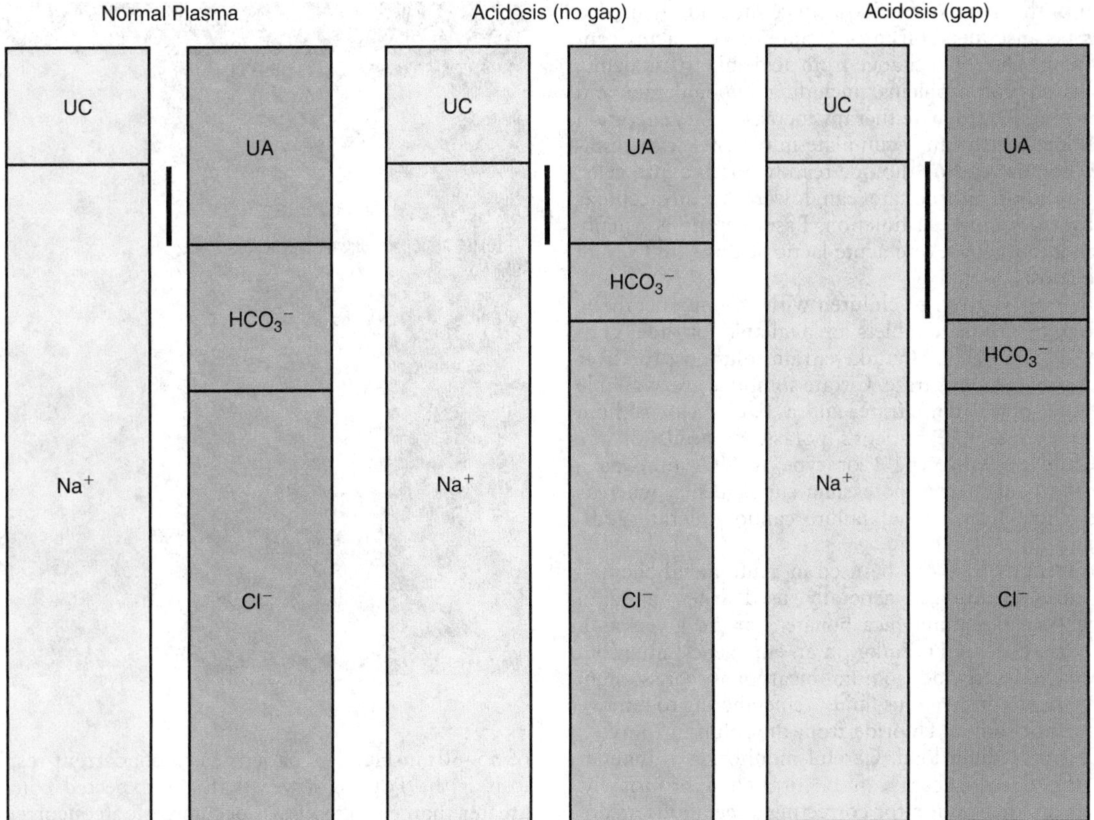

Figure 52-9. The anion gap, which is the difference between the sodium concentration and the combined concentrations of chloride and bicarbonate *(vertical line)*. In both a gap and a non-gap metabolic acidosis, there is a decrease in the bicarbonate concentration. There is an increase in unmeasured anions (UA) in patients with a gap metabolic acidosis. In a non-gap metabolic acidosis, there is an increase in the serum chloride concentration. UC, unmeasured cations.

have a concurrent RTA. The unmeasured anions in toxic ingestions vary: formate in methanol intoxication, glycolate in ethylene glycol intoxication, and lactate and keto acids in salicylate intoxication. In inborn errors of metabolism, the unmeasured anions depend on the specific etiology and may include keto acids, lactate, and other organic anions. In a few inborn errors of metabolism, the acidosis occurs without generation of unmeasured anions; thus, the anion gap is normal.

A **normal anion gap** metabolic acidosis occurs when there is a decrease in the bicarbonate concentration without an increase in the unmeasured anions. With diarrhea, there is a loss of bicarbonate in the stool, causing a decrease in the serum pH and bicarbonate concentration; the serum chloride concentration increases to maintain electrical neutrality (see Fig. 52-9). Hyperchloremic metabolic acidosis is an alternative term for a normal anion gap metabolic acidosis. Calculation of the anion gap is more precise than using the chloride concentration to differentiate between a normal and an increased gap metabolic acidosis in that the anion gap directly determines the presence of unmeasured anions. Electrical neutrality dictates that the chloride concentration increases or decreases depending on the serum sodium concentration, making the chloride concentration a less reliable predictor of unmeasured anions than the more direct measure, the anion gap.

Approximately 11 mEq of the anion gap is normally secondary to albumin. A 1-g/dL decrease in the albumin concentration decreases the anion gap by roughly 2.5 mEq/L. Similarly, an increase in unmeasured cations, such as calcium, potassium, or magnesium, decreases the anion gap. Conversely, a decrease in unmeasured cations is a very unusual cause of an increased anion gap. Because of these variables, the broad range of a normal anion gap, and other variables, the presence of a normal or an increased anion gap is not always reliable in differentiating among the causes of a metabolic acidosis, especially when the metabolic acidosis is mild. Some patients have more than 1 explanation for their metabolic acidosis, such as the child with diarrhea and lactic acidosis due to poor perfusion. The anion gap should not be interpreted in dogmatic isolation; consideration of other laboratory abnormalities and the clinical history improves its diagnostic utility.

Treatment. The most effective therapeutic approach for patients with a metabolic acidosis is repair of the underlying disorder, if possible. The administration of insulin in diabetic ketoacidosis and the restoration of adequate perfusion in lactic acidosis eventually result in normalization of the acid-base balance. In other diseases, the use of bicarbonate therapy is indicated because the underlying disorder is irreparable. Children with metabolic acidosis due to RTA or chronic renal failure require long-term base therapy. Patients with acute renal failure and metabolic acidosis need base therapy until their kidneys' ability to excrete hydrogen normalizes. In other disorders, the cause of the metabolic acidosis eventually resolves, but base therapy is necessary during the acute illness. In salicylate poisoning, for example, alkali administration increases renal clearance of salicylate and decreases the amount of salicylate in brain cells. Short-term base therapy is often necessary in other poisonings (ethylene glycol, methanol) and inborn errors of metabolism (pyruvate carboxylase deficiency, propionic acidemia). Some inborn errors of metabolism require long-term base therapy.

The use of base therapy in diabetic ketoacidosis and lactic acidosis is controversial, with little evidence that it improves patient outcome and a variety of potential side effects. The risks of giving sodium bicarbonate include the possibility of causing hypernatremia or volume overload. Furthermore, the patient may have overcorrection of the metabolic acidosis once the underlying disorder resolves because metabolism of lactate or keto acids generates bicarbonate. The rapid change from acidemia to alkalemia can cause a variety of problems, including hypokalemia and hypophosphatemia. Bicarbonate therapy increases the generation of carbon dioxide, which can accumulate in patients with respiratory failure. Because carbon dioxide readily diffuses into cells, the administration of bicarbonate can lower the intracellular pH, potentially worsening cell function. Base therapy is usually reserved for children with severe acute lactic acidosis and severe diabetic ketoacidosis.

Oral base therapy is given to children with chronic metabolic acidosis. Sodium bicarbonate tablets are available for older children. Younger children generally take citrate solutions; the liver generates bicarbonate from citrate. Citrate solutions are available as sodium citrate, potassium citrate, and a 1:1 mix of sodium and potassium citrate. The patient's potassium needs dictate the choice. Children with type I or type II RTA may have hypokalemia and benefit from potassium supplements, whereas most children with chronic renal failure cannot tolerate additional potassium.

Oral or intravenous base can be used in acute metabolic acidosis; intravenous therapy is generally used when a rapid response is necessary. Sodium bicarbonate may be given as a bolus, usually at a dose of 1 mEq/kg, in an emergency situation. Another approach is to add sodium bicarbonate or sodium acetate to the patient's intravenous fluids, remembering to remove an equal amount of sodium chloride from the solution to avoid giving an excessive sodium load. Careful monitoring is mandatory so that the dose of base can be titrated appropriately. Hemodialysis is another option for correcting a metabolic acidosis, and it is an appropriate choice in patients with renal insufficiency, especially if significant uremia or hyperkalemia is also present. Hemodialysis is advantageous for correcting the metabolic acidosis due to methanol or ethylene glycol intoxication because hemodialysis removes the offending toxin. In addition, these patients often have a severe metabolic acidosis that does not respond easily to intravenous bicarbonate therapy. Peritoneal dialysis is another option for correcting the metabolic acidosis due to renal insufficiency, although, because it relies on lactate as the source of base, it may not correct the metabolic acidosis in patients with concomitant renal failure and lactic acidosis.

Many causes of metabolic acidosis require specific therapy. Administration of a glucocorticoid and a mineralocorticoid is necessary in patients with adrenal insufficiency. Patients with diabetic ketoacidosis require insulin therapy, whereas patients with lactic acidosis respond to measures that alleviate tissue hypoxia. Along with correction of acidosis, patients with methanol or ethylene glycol ingestion should receive an agent that prevents the breakdown of these agents to their toxic metabolites. Traditionally, this has been done with an ethanol infusion, but fomepizole is an effective alternative with fewer side effects. Both agents work by inhibiting alcohol dehydrogenase, the enzyme that performs the 1st step in the metabolism of ethylene glycol or methanol. There are a variety of disease-specific therapies for patients with a metabolic acidosis due to an inborn error of metabolism.

METABOLIC ALKALOSIS. Metabolic alkalosis in children is most commonly secondary to emesis or diuretic use. The serum bicarbonate concentration is increased with a metabolic alkalosis, although a respiratory acidosis also leads to a compensatory elevation of the serum bicarbonate concentration. With a simple metabolic alkalosis, however, the pH is elevated; alkalemia is present. Patients with a respiratory acidosis are acidemic. A metabolic alkalosis, by decreasing ventilation, causes appropriate respiratory compensation. PCO_2 increases by 7 mm Hg for each 10-mEq/L increase in the serum bicarbonate concentration. Appropriate respiratory compensation never exceeds a PCO_2 of 55–60 mm Hg. The patient has a concurrent respiratory alkalosis if the PCO_2 is lower than the expected compensation. A greater than expected PCO_2 occurs with a concurrent respiratory acidosis.

TABLE 52-14. Causes of Metabolic Alkalosis

CHLORIDE RESPONSIVE (URINARY CHLORIDE < 15 mEq/L)
Gastric losses (emesis or nasogastric suction)
Diuretics (loop or thiazide)
Chloride-losing diarrhea (MIM 214700)
Chloride-deficient formula
Cystic fibrosis (MIM 219700)
Post-hypercapnia
CHLORIDE RESISTANT (URINARY CHLORIDE > 20 mEq/L)
High blood pressure
Adrenal adenoma or hyperplasia
Glucocorticoid-remedial aldosteronism (MIM 103900)
Renovascular disease
Renin-secreting tumor
17α-hydroxylase deficiency (MIM 202110)
11β-hydroxylase deficiency (MIM 202010)
Cushing syndrome
11β-hydroxysteroid dehydrogenase deficiency (MIM 218030)
Licorice ingestion
Liddle syndrome (MIM 177200)
Normal blood pressure
Gitelman syndrome (MIM 263800)
Bartter syndrome (MIM 602023/607364/602522/241200/601678)
Autosomal dominant hypoparathyroidism (MIM 146200)
Base administration

MIM, database number from the Mendelian Inheritance in Man (*http://www3.ncbi.nlm.nih.gov/Omim/*).

Etiology and Pathophysiology. The kidneys normally respond promptly to a metabolic alkalosis by increasing base excretion. Two processes are therefore usually present to produce a metabolic alkalosis. The 1st process is the generation of the metabolic alkalosis. This requires the addition of base to the body. The 2nd process is the maintenance of the metabolic alkalosis. This requires impairment in the kidney's ability to excrete base.

The etiologies of a metabolic alkalosis are divided into 2 categories, based on the urinary chloride level (Table 52-14). The alkalosis in patients with a **low urinary chloride** level is maintained by **volume depletion;** thus, volume repletion is necessary for correction of the alkalosis. The volume depletion in these patients is due to losses of sodium and potassium, but the loss of chloride is usually greater than that of sodium and potassium combined. Because chloride losses are the dominant cause of the volume depletion, these patients require chloride to correct their volume depletion and metabolic alkalosis; they are called **chloride responsive.** In contrast, the patients with an elevated urinary chloride level do not respond to volume repletion; they are called **chloride resistant.**

Emesis or nasogastric suction results in **loss of gastric fluid,** which has a high content of HCl. Generation of hydrogen ions by the gastric mucosa causes simultaneous release of bicarbonate into the bloodstream. Normally, the hydrogen ions in gastric fluid are reclaimed in the small intestine (by neutralizing secreted bicarbonate). Thus, there is no net loss of acid. With loss of gastric fluid, this does not occur and a metabolic alkalosis develops. This is the generation phase of the metabolic alkalosis.

The maintenance phase of the metabolic alkalosis from gastric losses is due to the volume depletion ("chloride depletion" from gastric loss of HCl). Volume depletion interferes with urinary loss of bicarbonate, the normal renal response to a metabolic alkalosis. During volume depletion, several mechanisms prevent renal bicarbonate loss. First, there is a reduction in the GFR, so less bicarbonate is filtered. Second, volume depletion increases resorption of sodium and bicarbonate in the proximal tubule, limiting the amount of bicarbonate that can be excreted in the urine. This effect is mediated by angiotensin II and by adrenergic stimulation of the kidney, which are both increased in response to volume depletion. Third, the increase in aldosterone during volume depletion increases bicarbonate resorption and hydrogen ion secretion in the collecting duct.

In addition to volume depletion, gastric losses are usually associated with hypokalemia as a result of both gastric loss of potassium and, most importantly, increased urinary potassium losses. The increased urinary losses of potassium are mediated by aldosterone, due to volume depletion, and by the increase in intracellular potassium secondary to the metabolic alkalosis, which causes potassium to move into the cells of the kidney, causing increased potassium excretion. Hypokalemia contributes to the maintenance of the metabolic alkalosis by decreasing bicarbonate loss. Hypokalemia increases hydrogen ion secretion in the distal nephron and stimulates ammonia production in the proximal tubule. Ammonia production enhances renal excretion of hydrogen ions.

A metabolic alkalosis can develop in patients receiving **loop or thiazide diuretics.** Diuretic use leads to volume depletion, which increases angiotensin II, aldosterone, and adrenergic stimulation of the kidney. Diuretics increase the delivery of sodium to the distal nephron, further enhancing acid excretion. Moreover, these diuretics cause hypokalemia, which increases acid excretion by the kidney. The increase in renal acid excretion generates the metabolic alkalosis, and the decrease in bicarbonate loss maintains the metabolic alkalosis. In addition, patients who are receiving diuretics have a "contraction alkalosis." Diuretic use causes fluid loss without bicarbonate; thus, the remaining body bicarbonate is contained in a smaller total body fluid compartment. The bicarbonate concentration increases, helping to generate the metabolic alkalosis.

Diuretics are often used in patients with edema, such as in patients with nephrotic syndrome, heart failure, or liver failure. In many of these patients, metabolic alkalosis resulting from diuretic use develops despite the continued presence of edema. This is because the effective intravascular volume is low, and it is the effective intravascular volume that stimulates the compensatory mechanisms that cause and maintain a metabolic alkalosis. Many of these patients have a decreased effective intravascular volume before they begin diuretic therapy, increasing the likelihood of diuretic-induced metabolic alkalosis.

Diuretic use increases chloride excretion in the urine. Consequently, while a patient is receiving diuretics, the urine chloride level is typically high (>20 mEq/L). After the diuretic effect has worn off, the urinary chloride level is low (<15 mEq/L) due to appropriate renal chloride retention in response to volume depletion. Thus, categorization of diuretics based on the urinary chloride level depends on the timing of the measurement. However, the metabolic alkalosis from diuretics is clearly chloride responsive; it corrects only after adequate volume repletion. This is the rationale for including it among the chloride-responsive causes of a metabolic alkalosis.

Most patients with diarrhea have a metabolic acidosis due to stool losses of bicarbonate. In **chloride-losing diarrhea,** an autosomal recessive disorder, there is a defect in the normal intestinal exchange of bicarbonate for chloride, causing excessive stool losses of chloride (see Chapter 335). In addition, stool losses of hydrogen ions and potassium cause metabolic alkalosis and hypokalemia, both of which are exacerbated by increased renal hydrogen and potassium losses due to volume depletion. Treatment is with oral supplements of potassium and sodium chloride. Use of a gastric proton pump inhibitor, by decreasing gastric HCl production, reduces the volume of diarrhea and decreases the need for electrolyte supplementation.

An infant formula with an extremely low chloride content has led to chloride deficiency and volume depletion. The infants fed this formula, which is no longer available, had a metabolic alkalosis and hypokalemia. **Cystic fibrosis** can cause metabolic alkalosis, hypokalemia, and hyponatremia due to excessive losses of sodium chloride in sweat (see Chapter 400). The volume depletion causes the metabolic alkalosis and hypokalemia through increased urinary losses, whereas the hyponatremia, a less common finding, is secondary to sodium loss combined with renal water conservation in an effort to protect the intravascular volume ("appropriate" ADH production).

A **post-hypercapnic metabolic alkalosis** occurs after the correction of a chronic respiratory acidosis. This is typically seen in patients with chronic lung disease who are placed on a ventilator. During chronic respiratory acidosis, appropriate renal compensation leads to an increase in the serum bicarbonate concentration. This elevated bicarbonate concentration, because it is still present after acute correction of the respiratory acidosis, causes a metabolic alkalosis. The metabolic alkalosis persists because the patient with a chronic respiratory acidosis is intravascularly depleted due to chloride loss that occurred during the initial metabolic compensation for the primary respiratory acidosis. In addition, many children with a chronic respiratory acidosis receive diuretics, further decreasing the intravascular volume. The metabolic alkalosis responds to correction of the intravascular volume deficit.

The **chloride-resistant** causes of metabolic alkalosis can be subdivided based on blood pressure. Patients with **hypertension** either have increased aldosterone or act as if they have increased aldosterone. Aldosterone levels are elevated in children with adrenal adenomas or hyperplasia. Aldosterone causes renal retention of sodium, with resultant hypertension. Metabolic alkalosis and hypokalemia result from aldosterone-mediated renal excretion of hydrogen ions and potassium. The urinary chloride level is not low because these patients are volume-overloaded, not volume-depleted. The volume expansion and hypertension allow normal excretion of sodium and chloride despite the presence of aldosterone. This is known as the *mineralocorticoid escape phenomenon.*

In **glucocorticoid-remedial aldosteronism,** an autosomal dominant disorder, there is excess production of aldosterone due to the presence of an aldosterone synthase gene that is regulated by adrenocorticotropic hormone (ACTH) [see Chapter 577.7]. Glucocorticoids effectively treat this disorder by inhibiting ACTH production by the pituitary, downregulating the inappropriate aldosterone production. Renovascular disease and renin-secreting tumors both cause excessive renin, leading to an increase in aldosterone, although hypokalemia and metabolic alkalosis are less common findings than hypertension. In 2 forms of **congenital adrenal hyperplasia,** 11β-hydroxylase deficiency and 17α-hydroxylase deficiency, there is excessive production of the mineralocorticoid 11-deoxycorticosterone (see Chapters 577.2 and 577.4). Hypertension, hypokalemia, and metabolic alkalosis are more likely in 17α-hydroxylase deficiency than in 11β-hydroxylase deficiency. These patients respond to glucocorticoids because the excess production of 11-deoxycorticosterone is under the control of ACTH.

Cushing syndrome frequently causes hypertension. Cortisol has some mineralocorticoid activity, and high levels can produce hypokalemia and metabolic alkalosis in patients with Cushing syndrome.

Cortisol can bind to the mineralocorticoid receptors in the kidney and function as a mineralocorticoid. This normally does not occur because 11β-hydroxysteroid dehydrogenase in the kidney converts cortisol to cortisone, which does not bind to the mineralocorticoid receptor. In 11β-hydroxysteroid dehydrogenase deficiency, also called **apparent mineralocorticoid excess,** cortisol is not converted in the kidney to cortisone. Cortisol is therefore available to bind to the mineralocorticoid receptor in the kidney and act as a mineralocorticoid. These patients, despite low levels of aldosterone, are hypertensive and hypokalemic, and they have a metabolic alkalosis. The same phenomenon can occur with excessive intake of natural licorice because a component of natural licorice, glycyrrhizic acid, inhibits 11β-hydroxysteroid dehydrogenase. The autosomal dominant disorder **Liddle syndrome** is secondary to an activating mutation of the sodium channel in the distal nephron (see Chapter 531.3). Upregulation of this sodium channel is 1 of the principal actions of aldosterone. Because this sodium channel is continuously open, these children have the features of hyperaldosteronism, including hypertension, hypokalemia, and metabolic alkalosis, but low serum levels of aldosterone.

Bartter syndrome and **Gitelman syndrome** are autosomal recessive disorders associated with **normal blood pressure,** elevated urinary chloride levels, metabolic alkalosis, and hypokalemia (see Chapter 531). In Bartter syndrome, patients have a defect in sodium and chloride resorption in the loop of Henle. This leads to excessive urinary losses of sodium and chloride, and as in patients receiving loop diuretics, volume depletion and secondary hyperaldosteronism occur, causing hypokalemia and metabolic alkalosis. Gitelman syndrome is usually milder than Bartter syndrome. Patients have renal sodium and chloride wasting with volume depletion due to an absence of the thiazide-sensitive sodium-chloride transporter in the distal tubule. As in patients receiving a thiazide diuretic, affected patients have volume depletion and secondary hyperaldosteronism with hypokalemia and metabolic alkalosis. Children with Gitelman syndrome have hypocalciuria and hypomagnesemia. Some patients with autosomal dominant hypoparathyroidism have hypokalemia and metabolic alkalosis due to impaired sodium and chloride resorption in the loop of Henle.

Excessive base intake can cause a metabolic alkalosis. These patients do not have a low urine chloride level, unless there is associated volume depletion. In the absence of volume depletion, excess base is rapidly corrected via renal excretion of bicarbonate. Rarely, massive base intake can cause a metabolic alkalosis by overwhelming the kidney's ability to excrete bicarbonate. This may occur in infants who are given baking soda as a "home remedy" for colic or stomach upset. Each teaspoon of baking soda has 42 mEq of sodium bicarbonate. Infants have increased vulnerability due to a lower GFR, limiting the rate of compensatory renal bicarbonate excretion. A metabolic alkalosis may also occur in patients who receive a large amount of sodium bicarbonate during cardiopulmonary resuscitation. Blood products are anticoagulated with citrate, which is converted into bicarbonate by the liver. Patients who receive large amounts of blood products may have a metabolic alkalosis. Iatrogenic metabolic alkalosis can occur as a result of acetate in total parenteral nutrition. Aggressive use of bicarbonate therapy in a child with a lactic acidosis or diabetic ketoacidosis may cause a metabolic alkalosis. This is especially likely in a patient in whom the underlying cause of the lactic acidosis is successfully corrected (restoration of intravascular volume in a patient with severe dehydration). Once the cause of the lactic acidosis resolves, lactate can be converted by the liver into bicarbonate, and when combined with infused bicarbonate, this can create a metabolic alkalosis. A similar phenomenon can occur in a child with diabetic ketoacidosis because the administration of insulin allows keto acids to be metabolized, producing bicarbonate. However, this rarely occurs because of judicious use of bicarbonate therapy in diabetic ketoacidosis and because there are usually significant pretreatment losses of keto acids in the urine, preventing massive regeneration of bicarbonate. Base administration is most likely to cause a metabolic alkalosis in patients who have an impaired ability to excrete bicarbonate in the urine. This occurs in patients with concurrent volume depletion or renal insufficiency.

Clinical Manifestations. The symptoms in patients with a metabolic alkalosis are often related to the underlying disease and associated electrolyte disturbances. Children with chloride-responsive causes of metabolic alkalosis often have symptoms related to volume depletion, such as thirst and lethargy. In contrast, children with chloride-unresponsive causes may have symptoms related to hypertension.

Alkalemia causes potassium to shift into the intracellular space, producing a decrease in the extracellular potassium concentration. Alkalemia leads to increased urinary losses of potassium. Increased potassium losses are present in many of the conditions that cause a metabolic alkalosis. Therefore, most patients with a metabolic alkalosis have hypokalemia, and symptoms may be related to the hypokalemia (see Chapter 52.4).

The symptoms of a metabolic alkalosis are due to the associated alkalemia. The magnitude of the alkalemia is related to the severity of the metabolic alkalosis and the presence of concurrent respiratory acid-base disturbances. During alkalemia, the ionized calcium concentration decreases as a result of increased binding of calcium to albumin. The decrease in the ionized calcium concentration may cause symptoms of **tetany** (carpopedal spasm).

Arrhythmias are a potential complication of a metabolic alkalosis, and this risk increases if there is concomitant hypokalemia. Alkalemia increases the risk of digoxin toxicity, and antiarrhythmic medications are less effective in the presence of alkalemia. In addition, alkalemia may decrease cardiac output. A metabolic alkalosis causes a compensatory increase in the P_{CO_2} by decreasing ventilation. In patients with underlying lung disease, the decrease in ventilatory drive can cause hypoxia. The hypoventilation in patients with severe metabolic alkalosis can cause hypoxia in patients with normal lungs.

Diagnosis. Measurement of the urinary chloride concentration is the most helpful test in differentiating among the causes of a metabolic alkalosis. The urine chloride level is low in patients with a metabolic alkalosis resulting from volume depletion, unless there is a defect in renal handling of chloride. The urine chloride level is superior to the urine sodium level in assessing volume status in patients with a metabolic alkalosis because the normal renal response to a metabolic alkalosis is to excrete bicarbonate. Because bicarbonate is negatively charged, it can be excreted only with a cation, usually sodium and potassium. Hence, a patient with a metabolic alkalosis may excrete sodium in the urine despite the presence of volume depletion, which normally causes avid sodium retention. The urine chloride level is usually a good indicator of volume status, and it differentiates among the chloride-resistant and chloride-responsive causes of a metabolic alkalosis.

Diuretics and gastric losses are the most common causes of metabolic alkalosis and are usually readily apparent from the patient history. Occasionally, metabolic alkalosis, usually with hypokalemia, may be a clue to the presence of bulimia or surreptitious diuretic use (see Chapter 27). Patients with bulimia have a low urine chloride level, indicating that they have volume depletion as a result of an extrarenal etiology, but there is no alternative explanation for their volume depletion. Surreptitious diuretic use may be diagnosed by obtaining a urine toxicology screen for diuretics. The urine chloride level is increased while diuretics are being used, but is low when the patient stops taking diuretics. Rarely, children with mild Bartter syndrome or Gitelman syndrome are misdiagnosed as having bulimia or abusing diuretics. The urine chloride level is always elevated in Bartter syndrome and Gitelman syndrome, and the urine toxicology screen for diuretics is negative. Metabolic alkalosis and hypokalemia is occasionally the initial manifestation of cystic fibrosis. An elevated sweat chloride finding is diagnostic.

Patients with a metabolic alkalosis and a high urinary chloride level are separated based on blood pressure. Children with normal blood pressure may have Bartter syndrome or Gitelman syndrome. Excess base administration is another diagnostic possibility, but this is usually apparent from the history. In patients with sodium bicarbonate ingestion (baking soda), which may be unreported by the parent, the metabolic alkalosis usually occurs with significant hypernatremia. In addition, unless volume depletion is superimposed, the metabolic alkalosis from base ingestion self-resolves once the source of base is eliminated.

Measuring serum concentrations of renin and aldosterone differentiates children with a metabolic alkalosis, a high urinary chloride level, and elevated blood pressure. Both renin and aldosterone are elevated in children with either renovascular disease or a renin-secreting tumor. Aldosterone is high and renin is low in patients with adrenal adenomas or hyperplasia and glucocorticoid-remediable aldosteronism. Renin and aldosterone are low in children with Cushing syndrome, Liddle syndrome, licorice ingestion, 17α-hydroxylase deficiency, 11β-hydroxylase deficiency, and 11β-hydroxysteroid dehydrogenase deficiency. An elevated 24-hr urine cortisol level is diagnostic of Cushing syndrome, which is suspected by the presence of the other classic features of this disease (see Chapter 578). 11-Deoxycorticosterone levels are elevated in 17α-hydroxylase deficiency and 11β-hydroxylase deficiency.

Treatment. The approach to treatment of metabolic alkalosis depends on the severity of the alkalosis and the underlying etiology. In children with a mild metabolic alkalosis ($[HCO_3^-] < 32$), intervention is often unnecessary, although this depends on the specific circumstances. In a child with congenital heart disease who is receiving a stable dose of a loop diuretic, a mild alkalosis does not require treatment. In contrast, intervention may be appropriate in a child with a worsening mild metabolic alkalosis due to nasogastric suction. The presence of a concurrent respiratory acid-base disturbance also influences therapeutic decision-making. A patient with a concurrent respiratory acidosis should have some increase in bicarbonate due to metabolic compensation; thus, the severity of the pH elevation is more important than the bicarbonate concentration. In contrast, a patient with a respiratory alkalosis and a metabolic alkalosis is at risk for severe alkalemia; treatment may be indicated, even if the increase in bicarbonate is only mild.

Intervention is usually necessary in children with moderate or severe metabolic alkalosis. The most effective approach is to address the underlying etiology. In some children, nasogastric suction may be decreased or discontinued. Alternatively, the addition of a gastric proton pump inhibitor reduces gastric secretion and losses of HCl. Diuretics are an important cause of metabolic alkalosis and, if tolerated, they should be eliminated or the dose reduced. Adequate potassium supplementation or the addition of a potassium-sparing diuretic is also helpful in a child with a metabolic alkalosis caused by diuretics. Potassium-sparing diuretics not only decrease renal potassium losses, but, by blocking the action of aldosterone, also decrease hydrogen ion secretion in the distal nephron, increasing urinary bicarbonate excretion. Many children cannot tolerate discontinuation of diuretic therapy; thus, potassium supplementation and potassium-sparing diuretics are the principal therapeutic approach. Arginine HCl may also be used to treat chloride-responsive metabolic acidosis if sodium or potassium salts are not appropriate. Arginine HCl may raise the serum potassium levels during administration. Rarely, in cases of severe metabolic alkalosis, acetazolamide is an option. Acetazolamide, a carbonic anhydrase inhibitor, decreases resorption of bicarbonate in the proximal tubule, causing significant bicarbonate loss in the urine. The patient must be monitored closely because acetazolamide produces major losses of potassium in the urine and increases fluid losses, potentially necessitating a reduction in other diuretics.

Most children with a metabolic alkalosis have 1 of the chloride-responsive etiologies. In these situations, administration of sufficient sodium chloride and potassium chloride to correct the volume deficit and the potassium deficit is necessary to correct the metabolic alkalosis. This may not be an option in the child who has volume depletion due to diuretics because volume repletion may be contraindicated. Adequate replacement of gastric losses of sodium and potassium in a child with a nasogastric tube can minimize or prevent the development of the metabolic alkalosis. With adequate intravascular volume and a normal serum potassium concentration, the kidney is able to excrete the excess bicarbonate within a couple of days.

In children with the chloride-resistant causes of a metabolic alkalosis that are associated with hypertension, volume repletion is contraindicated because it exacerbates the hypertension and does not repair the metabolic alkalosis. Ideally, treatment focuses on eliminating the excess aldosterone effect. Adrenal adenomas can be resected, licorice intake can be eliminated, and renovascular disease can be repaired. Glucocorticoid-remediable aldosteronism, 17α-hydroxylase deficiency, and 11β-hydroxylase deficiency respond to the administration of glucocorticoids. The mineralocorticoid effect of cortisol in 11β-hydroxysteroid dehydrogenase deficiency can be decreased by using spironolactone, which blocks the mineralocorticoid receptor. In contrast, children with Liddle syndrome do not respond to spironolactone; however, either triamterene or amiloride is effective therapy because these agents block the sodium channel that is constitutively active in Liddle syndrome.

In children with Bartter syndrome and Gitelman syndrome, therapy includes oral potassium supplementation and potassium-sparing diuretics. Children with Gitelman syndrome often require magnesium supplementation, whereas children with severe Bartter syndrome often benefit from indomethacin.

RESPIRATORY ACIDOSIS. A respiratory acidosis is an inappropriate increase in blood carbon dioxide (PCO_2). Carbon dioxide is a byproduct of metabolism, and it is removed from the body by the lungs. During a respiratory acidosis, there is a decrease in the effectiveness of carbon dioxide removal by the lungs. A respiratory acidosis is secondary to either pulmonary disease, such as severe bronchiolitis, or nonpulmonary disease, such as a narcotic overdose. Even though body production of carbon dioxide can vary, normal lungs are able to accommodate this variation; excess production of carbon dioxide is not an isolated cause of a respiratory acidosis. With impaired alveolar ventilation, the rate of body production of carbon dioxide may affect the severity of the respiratory acidosis, but this is usually not a significant factor.

A respiratory acidosis causes a decrease in the blood pH, but there is normally a metabolic response that partially compensates, minimizing the severity of the acidemia. The acute metabolic response to a respiratory alkalosis occurs within minutes. The metabolic compensation for an acute respiratory acidosis is secondary to titration of acid by non-bicarbonate buffers. This buffering of hydrogen ions causes a predictable increase in the serum bicarbonate concentration: Plasma bicarbonate increases by 1 for each 10-mm Hg increase in the PCO_2 (acute compensation).

With a chronic respiratory acidosis, there is more significant metabolic compensation and, thus, less severe acidemia than in an acute respiratory acidosis with the same increase in PCO_2. During a chronic respiratory acidosis, the kidneys increase acid excretion. This response occurs over 3–4 days and causes a predictable increase in the serum bicarbonate concentration: Plasma bicarbonate increases by 3.5 for each 10-mm Hg increase in the PCO_2 (chronic compensation).

The increase of serum bicarbonate during a chronic respiratory acidosis is associated with a decrease in body chloride. After acute correction of a chronic respiratory acidosis, the plasma bicarbonate continues to be increased, and the patient has a metabolic alkalosis. Because of the chloride deficit, this is a chloride-responsive metabolic alkalosis; it corrects once the patient's chloride deficit is replaced.

A mixed disorder is present if the metabolic compensation is inappropriate. A higher than expected bicarbonate value occurs in the setting of a concurrent metabolic alkalosis, and a lower than expected bicarbonate value occurs in the setting of a concurrent metabolic acidosis. Evaluating whether compensation is appropriate during a respiratory acidosis requires clinical knowledge of the acuity of the process, because the expected compensation is different depending on whether the process is acute or chronic.

The P_{CO_2} cannot be interpreted in isolation to determine whether a patient has a respiratory acidosis. A respiratory acidosis is always present if a patient has acidemia and an elevated P_{CO_2}. However, an elevated P_{CO_2} also occurs as appropriate respiratory compensation for a simple metabolic alkalosis. The patient is alkalemic; this is not a respiratory acidosis. During a mixed disturbance, a patient can have a respiratory acidosis and a normal or even a low P_{CO_2}. This may occur in a patient with a metabolic acidosis; a respiratory acidosis is present if the patient does not have appropriate respiratory compensation (the P_{CO_2} is higher than expected, based on the severity of the metabolic acidosis).

Etiology and Pathophysiology. The causes of a respiratory acidosis are either pulmonary or nonpulmonary (Table 52-15). Central nervous system disorders can decrease the activity of the central respiratory center, reducing ventilatory drive. A variety of medications and illicit drugs suppress the respiratory center. The signals from the respiratory center need to be transmitted to the respiratory muscles via the nervous system. Respiratory muscle failure can be secondary to disruption of the signal from the central nervous system in the spinal cord, the phrenic nerve, or the neuromuscular junction. Disorders directly affecting the muscles of respiration can prevent adequate ventilation, causing a respiratory acidosis.

Mild or moderate lung disease often causes a respiratory alkalosis as a result of hyperventilation secondary to hypoxia or stimulation of lung mechanoreceptors or chemoreceptors. Only more severe lung disease causes a respiratory acidosis. Upper airway diseases, by impairing air entry into the lungs, may decrease ventilation, producing a respiratory acidosis.

Increased production of carbon dioxide is never the sole cause of a respiratory acidosis, but can increase the severity of the disease in a patient with decreased ventilation of carbon dioxide. Increased production of carbon dioxide occurs in patients with fever, hyperthyroidism, excess caloric intake, and high levels of physical activity. Increased respiratory muscle work also increases carbon dioxide production.

Clinical Manifestations. Patients with a respiratory acidosis are often tachypneic in an effort to correct the inadequate ventilation. Exceptions include patients with a respiratory acidosis resulting from central nervous system depression and patients who are on the verge of complete respiratory failure secondary to fatigue of the respiratory muscles.

The symptoms of respiratory acidosis are related to the severity of the hypercarbia. Acute respiratory acidosis is usually more symptomatic than chronic respiratory acidosis. Symptoms are also increased by concurrent hypoxia or metabolic acidosis. In a patient breathing room air, hypoxia is always present if a respiratory acidosis is present. The potential central nervous system manifestations of respiratory acidosis include anxiety, dizziness, headache, confusion, asterixis, myoclonic jerks, hallucinations, psychosis, coma, and seizures.

Acidemia, no matter the etiology, affects the cardiovascular system. An arterial pH <7.20 impairs cardiac contractility and the normal response to catecholamines, in both the heart and the peripheral vasculature. Hypercapnia causes vasodilation, most dramatically in the cerebral vasculature, but hypercapnia produces vasoconstriction of the pulmonary circulation. Respiratory acidosis increases the risk of cardiac arrhythmias, especially in a child with underlying cardiac disease.

Diagnosis. The history and physical findings often point to a clear etiology. For the obtunded patient with poor respiratory effort, evaluation of the central nervous system is often indicated. This may include imaging studies (CT or MRI) and, potentially, a lumbar puncture. A toxicology screen for illicit drugs may also be appropriate. A response to naloxone is both diagnostic and

TABLE 52-15. Causes of Respiratory Acidosis

CENTRAL NERVOUS SYSTEM DEPRESSION
Encephalitis
Head trauma
Brain tumor
Central sleep apnea
Primary pulmonary hypoventilation (Ondine curse)
Stroke
Hypoxic brain damage
Obesity-hypoventilation (Pickwickian syndrome)
Increased intracranial pressure
Medications
Narcotics
Barbiturates
Anesthesia
Benzodiazepines
Propofol
Alcohols
DISORDERS OF THE SPINAL CORD, PERIPHERAL NERVES, OR NEUROMUSCULAR JUNCTION
Diaphragmatic paralysis
Guillain-Barré syndrome
Poliomyelitis
Spinal muscular atrophies
Tick paralysis
Botulism
Myasthenia
Multiple sclerosis
Spinal cord injury
Medications
Vecuronium
Aminoglycosides
Organophosphates (pesticides)
RESPIRATORY MUSCLE WEAKNESS
Muscular dystrophy
Hypothyroidism
Malnutrition
Hypokalemia
Hypophosphatemia
Medications
Succinylcholine
Corticosteroids
PULMONARY DISEASE
Pneumonia
Pneumothorax
Asthma
Bronchiolitis
Pulmonary edema
Pulmonary hemorrhage
Adult respiratory distress syndrome
Respiratory distress syndrome, neonatal
Cystic fibrosis
Bronchopulmonary dysplasia
Hypoplastic lungs
Meconium aspiration
Pulmonary thromboembolus
Interstitial fibrosis
UPPER AIRWAY DISEASE
Aspiration
Laryngospasm
Angioedema
Obstructive sleep apnea
Tonsillar hypertrophy
Vocal cord paralysis
Extrinsic tumor
Extrinsic or intrinsic hemangioma
MISCELLANEOUS
Flail chest
Cardiac arrest
Kyphoscoliosis
Decreased diaphragmatic movement due to ascites or peritoneal dialysis

therapeutic. In many of the diseases affecting the respiratory muscles, there is evidence of weakness in other muscles. Stridor is a clue that the child may have upper airway disease. Along with a physical examination, a chest radiograph is often helpful in diagnosing pulmonary disease.

In many patients, respiratory acidosis may be multifactorial. A child with bronchopulmonary dysplasia, an intrinsic lung disease, may worsen due to respiratory muscle dysfunction from severe hypokalemia as a result of chronic diuretic therapy. Conversely, a child with muscular dystrophy, a muscle disease, may worsen because of aspiration pneumonia.

For a patient with respiratory acidosis, calculation of the gradient between the alveolar oxygen concentration and the arterial oxygen concentration, the A-a gradient, is useful for distinguishing between poor respiratory effort and intrinsic lung disease. The A-a gradient is increased if the hypoxemia is due to intrinsic lung disease (see Chapter 370).

Treatment. Respiratory acidosis is best managed by treating the underlying etiology. In some instances, the response is very rapid, such as after the administration of naloxone to a patient with a narcotic overdose. In contrast, the child with pneumonia may require a number of days of antibiotic therapy before the respiratory status improves. In many children with a chronic respiratory acidosis, there is no curative therapy, although an acute respiratory illness superimposed on a chronic respiratory condition is usually reversible.

All patients with an acute respiratory acidosis are hypoxic and therefore need to receive supplemental oxygen. Mechanical ventilation is necessary in some children with a respiratory acidosis. Children with a significant respiratory acidosis due to a central nervous system disease usually require mechanical ventilation because these disorders are unlikely to respond quickly to therapy. In addition, hypercarbia causes cerebral vasodilation, and the increase in intracranial pressure can be dangerous in a child with an underlying central nervous system disease. Readily reversible central nervous system depression, such as from a narcotic overdose, may not require mechanical ventilation. Decisions on mechanical ventilation for other patients depend on a number of factors. Patients with severe hypercarbia—$P_{CO_2} > 75$—usually require mechanical ventilation (see Chapters 69, 70, and 371). The threshold for intubation is lower if there is concomitant metabolic acidosis, a slowly responsive underlying disease, or hypoxia that responds poorly to oxygen, or if the patient appears to be tiring and respiratory arrest seems likely.

In patients with a chronic respiratory acidosis, the respiratory drive is often less responsive to hypercarbia and more responsive to hypoxia. Hence, with chronic respiratory acidosis, excessive use of oxygen can blunt the respiratory drive and therefore increase the P_{CO_2}. In these patients, oxygen must be used cautiously.

When possible, it is best to avoid mechanical ventilation in a patient with a chronic respiratory acidosis because extubation is often difficult. However, an acute illness may necessitate mechanical ventilation in a child with a chronic respiratory acidosis. When intubation is necessary, the P_{CO_2} should be lowered only to the patient's normal baseline, and this should be done gradually. These patients normally have an elevated serum bicarbonate level as a result of metabolic compensation for their respiratory acidosis. A rapid lowering of the P_{CO_2} can cause a severe metabolic alkalosis, potentially leading to complications, including cardiac arrhythmias, decreased cardiac output, and decreased cerebral blood flow. In addition, prolonged mechanical ventilation at a normal P_{CO_2} causes the metabolic compensation to resolve. When the patient is subsequently extubated, the patient will no longer benefit from metabolic compensation, causing a more severe acidemia due to the respiratory acidosis.

RESPIRATORY ALKALOSIS. A respiratory alkalosis is an inappropriate reduction in the blood carbon dioxide concentration. This is usually secondary to hyperventilation, initially causing removal of carbon dioxide to surpass production. Eventually, a new steady state is achieved, with removal equaling production, albeit at a lower carbon dioxide tension (P_{CO_2}). A respiratory alkalosis that is not due to hyperventilation may occur in children receiving extracorporeal membrane oxygenation or hemodialysis, with carbon dioxide lost directly from the blood in the extracorporeal circuit.

With a simple respiratory alkalosis, the pH increases, but there is a normal metabolic response that attenuates some of the change in the blood pH. A metabolic response to an acute respiratory alkalosis occurs within minutes, mediated by hydrogen ion release from non-bicarbonate buffers. The metabolic response to an acute respiratory alkalosis is predictable: Plasma bicarbonate falls by 2 for each 10-mm Hg decrease in the P_{CO_2} (acute compensation).

A chronic respiratory alkalosis leads to more significant metabolic compensation due to the actions of the kidneys, which decrease acid secretion, producing a decrease in the serum bicarbonate concentration. Both the proximal and distal tubules decrease acid secretion. Metabolic compensation for a respiratory alkalosis develops gradually and takes 2–3 days to produce the full effect: Plasma bicarbonate falls by 4 for each 10-mm Hg decrease in the P_{CO_2} (chronic compensation).

A chronic respiratory alkalosis is the only acid-base disturbance wherein appropriate compensation may normalize the pH, albeit >7.40.

A mixed disorder is present if the metabolic compensation is inappropriate. A higher than expected bicarbonate level occurs in the setting of a concurrent metabolic alkalosis, and a lower than expected bicarbonate level occurs in the setting of a concurrent metabolic acidosis. Evaluating whether compensation is appropriate during a respiratory alkalosis requires clinical knowledge of the acuity of the process, because the expected compensation is different depending on whether the process is acute or chronic.

A low P_{CO_2} does not always indicate a respiratory alkalosis. The P_{CO_2} also decreases as part of the appropriate respiratory compensation for a metabolic acidosis; this is not a respiratory alkalosis. A metabolic acidosis is the dominant acid-base disturbance in a patient with acidemia and a low P_{CO_2}, even though there could still be a concurrent respiratory alkalosis. In contrast, a respiratory alkalosis is always present in a patient with alkalemia and a low P_{CO_2}. Even a normal P_{CO_2} may be consistent with a respiratory alkalosis in a patient with a metabolic alkalosis because an elevated P_{CO_2} is expected as part of appropriate respiratory compensation for the metabolic alkalosis.

Etiology and Pathophysiology. A variety of stimuli can increase the ventilatory drive and cause a respiratory alkalosis (Table 52-16). Arterial hypoxemia or tissue hypoxia stimulates peripheral chemoreceptors to signal the central respiratory center in the medulla to increase ventilation. The resultant increased respiratory effort increases the oxygen content of the blood, but depresses the P_{CO_2}. The effect of hypoxemia on ventilation begins when the oxygen saturation decreases to approximately 90% ($P_{O_2} = 60$ mm Hg), and hyperventilation increases as hypoxemia worsens. Acute hypoxia is a more potent stimulus for hyperventilation than chronic hypoxia; thus, chronic hypoxia, as occurs in cyanotic heart disease, causes a much less severe respiratory alkalosis than an equivalent degree of acute hypoxia. There are many causes of hypoxemia or tissue hypoxia, including primary lung disease, severe anemia, and carbon monoxide poisoning.

The lungs contain chemoreceptors and mechanoreceptors that respond to irritants and stretching and send signals to the respiratory center to increase ventilation. Aspiration or pneumonia may stimulate the chemoreceptors, whereas pulmonary edema may stimulate the mechanoreceptors. Most of the diseases that activate these receptors may also cause hypoxemia and can, therefore, potentially lead to hyperventilation via 2 mechanisms.

TABLE 52-16. Causes of Respiratory Alkalosis

HYPOXEMIA OR TISSUE HYPOXIA
Pneumonia
Pulmonary edema
Cyanotic heart disease
Congestive heart failure
Asthma
Severe anemia
High altitude
Laryngospasm
Aspiration
Carbon monoxide poisoning
Pulmonary embolism
Interstitial lung disease
Hypotension
LUNG RECEPTOR STIMULATION
Pneumonia
Pulmonary edema
Asthma
Pulmonary embolism
Hemothorax
Pneumothorax
Respiratory distress syndrome (adult or infant)
CENTRAL STIMULATION
Central nervous system disease
Subarachnoid hemorrhage
Encephalitis or meningitis
Trauma
Brain tumor
Stroke
Fever
Pain
Anxiety (panic attack)
Psychogenic hyperventilation or anxiety
Liver failure
Sepsis
Pregnancy
Medications
Salicylate intoxication
Theophylline
Progesterone
Exogenous catecholamines
Caffeine
Mechanical ventilation
Hyperammonemia
Extracorporeal membrane oxygenation or hemodialysis

Although patients with primary lung disease may initially have a respiratory alkalosis, worsening of the disease, combined with respiratory muscle fatigue, often causes respiratory failure and the development of a respiratory acidosis.

Hyperventilation in the absence of lung disease occurs with direct stimulation of the central respiratory center. This occurs with central nervous system diseases, such as meningitis, hemorrhage, and trauma. Central hyperventilation due to lesions, such as infarcts or tumors near the central respiratory center in the midbrain, increases the rate and depth of the respiratory effort. This respiratory pattern portends a poor prognosis because these midbrain lesions are frequently fatal. Systemic processes may cause centrally mediated hyperventilation. Although the exact mechanisms are not clear, liver disease causes a respiratory alkalosis that is usually proportional to the degree of liver failure. Pregnancy causes a chronic respiratory alkalosis, probably mediated by progesterone acting on the respiratory centers. Salicylates, although often causing a concurrent metabolic acidosis, directly stimulate the respiratory center to produce a respiratory alkalosis. The respiratory alkalosis during sepsis is probably due to cytokine release.

Hyperventilation may be secondary to an underlying disease that causes pain, stress, or anxiety. In psychogenic hyperventilation, there is no disease process accounting for the hyperventilation. This may occur in a child who has had an emotionally stressful experience. Alternatively, it may be part of a panic disorder, especially if there are repeated episodes of hyperventilation. In these patients, the symptoms of acute alkalemia increase anxiety, potentially perpetuating the hyperventilation.

A respiratory alkalosis is quite common in children receiving mechanical ventilation because the respiratory center is not controlling ventilation. In addition, these children may have a decreased metabolic rate and hence less carbon dioxide production because of sedation and paralytic medications. Normally, decreased carbon dioxide production and the resultant hypocapnia decrease ventilation, but this physiologic response cannot occur in a child who cannot reduce his ventilatory effort.

Clinical Manifestations. The disease process that is causing the respiratory alkalosis is usually more concerning than the clinical manifestations of the respiratory alkalosis. Chronic respiratory alkalosis is usually asymptomatic because metabolic compensation decreases the magnitude of the alkalemia.

Acute respiratory alkalosis may cause chest tightness, palpitations, lightheadedness, circumoral numbness, and paresthesias of the extremities. Less common manifestations include tetany, seizures, muscle cramps, and syncope. The lightheadedness and syncope are probably due to the reduction in cerebral blood flow that is caused by hypocapnia. The reduction in cerebral blood flow is the rationale for using hyperventilation to treat children with increased intracranial pressure. The paresthesias, tetany, and seizures may be partially related to the reduction in ionized calcium that occurs because alkalemia causes more calcium to bind to albumin. A respiratory alkalosis also causes a mild reduction in the serum potassium level. Patients with psychogenic hyperventilation tend to be most symptomatic as a result of the respiratory alkalosis, and these symptoms, along with a sensation of breathlessness, exacerbate the hyperventilation.

Diagnosis. In many patients, hyperventilation producing a respiratory alkalosis is not clinically detectable, even with careful observation of the patient's respiratory effort. Metabolic compensation for a respiratory alkalosis causes a low serum bicarbonate concentration. When hyperventilation is not appreciated and only serum electrolytes are evaluated, there is often a presumptive diagnosis of a metabolic acidosis. If a respiratory alkalosis is suspected, only a blood gas determination can make the diagnosis.

Hyperventilation does not always indicate a primary respiratory disorder. In some patients, the hyperventilation is appropriate respiratory compensation for a metabolic acidosis. With a primary metabolic acidosis, acidemia is present and the serum bicarbonate level is usually quite low if there is clinically detectable hyperventilation. In contrast, the serum bicarbonate level never goes below 17 mEq/L as part of the metabolic compensation for acute respiratory alkalosis, and simple acute respiratory alkalosis causes alkalemia.

The etiology of a respiratory alkalosis is often apparent from the physical examination or history, and it may include lung disease, neurologic disease, or cyanotic heart disease. Hypoxemia is a common cause of hyperventilation, and it is important to diagnose because it suggests a significant underlying disease that requires expeditious treatment. Hypoxemia may be detected on physical examination (cyanosis) or by pulse oximetry. However, normal pulse oximetry does not completely eliminate hypoxemia as the etiology of the hyperventilation. There are 2 reasons why pulse oximetry is not adequate for eliminating hypoxemia as a cause of a respiratory alkalosis. First, pulse oximetry is not very sensitive at detecting a mildly low pO_2. Second, the hyperventilation during a respiratory alkalosis causes the pO_2 to increase, possibly to a level that is not identified as abnormal by pulse oximetry. Only an arterial blood gas measurement can completely eliminate hypoxia as an explanation for a respiratory alkalosis. Along with hypoxemia, it is important to consider processes that cause tissue hypoxia without necessarily causing hypoxemia. Examples include carbon monoxide poisoning, severe anemia, and congestive heart failure.

Lung disease without hypoxemia may cause hyperventilation. Although this is often apparent by history or physical examination, a chest radiograph may detect more subtle disease. Patients with a pulmonary embolism may have benign chest x-ray findings, normal pO_2, and isolated respiratory alkalosis, although hypoxia may eventually occur. Diagnosis of a pulmonary embolism requires a high index of suspicion and should be considered in children without another explanation for respiratory alkalosis, especially if risk factors are present, such as prolonged bed rest or a hypercoagulable state (e.g., nephrotic syndrome or lupus anticoagulant).

Treatment. There is seldom a need for specific treatment of respiratory alkalosis. Rather, treatment focuses on the underlying disease. Mechanical ventilator settings are adjusted to correct iatrogenic respiratory alkalosis, unless the hyperventilation has a therapeutic purpose (e.g., treatment of increased intracranial pressure).

For patients with hyperventilation secondary to anxiety, efforts should be undertaken to reassure the child, usually enlisting the parents. Along with reassurance, patients with psychogenic hyperventilation may benefit from benzodiazepines. During an acute episode of psychogenic hyperventilation, rebreathing into a paper bag increases the patient's PCO_2. Using a paper bag, instead of a plastic bag, allows adequate oxygenation, but permits the carbon dioxide concentration in the bag to increase. The resultant increase in the patient's PCO_2 decreases the symptoms of the respiratory alkalosis that tend to perpetuate the hyperventilation. Rebreathing should be done only once other causes of hyperventilation have been eliminated; pulse oximetry during the rebreathing is prudent.

Kraut JA, Kurtz I: Metabolic acidosis of CKD: Diagnosis, clinical characteristics, and treatment. *Am J Kidney Dis* 2005;45:978–993.

Rodriguez Soriano J: Renal tubular acidosis: The clinical entity. *J Am Soc Nephrol* 2002;13:2160–2170.

Schwaderer AL, Schwartz GJ: Back to basics: Acidosis and alkalosis. *Pediatr Rev* 2004;25:350–357.

Shaer AJ: Inherited primary renal tubular hypokalemic alkalosis: A review of Gitelman and Bartter syndromes. *Am J Med Sci* 2001;322:316–332.

Toth HL, Greenbaum LA: Severe acidosis caused by starvation and stress. *Am J Kidney Dis* 2003;42:E16–E19.

Wrong O, Bruce LJ, Unwin RJ, et al: Band 3 mutations, distal renal tubular acidosis, and southeast Asian ovalocytosis. *Kidney Int* 2002;62:10–19.

Chapter 53 ■ Maintenance and Replacement Therapy

Larry Greenbaum

Maintenance intravenous fluids are used in a child who cannot be fed enterally. Along with maintenance fluids, children may require concurrent **replacement fluids** if they have continued excessive losses such as may occur with drainage from a nasogastric (NG) tube or with high urine output due to nephrogenic diabetes insipidus. If dehydration is present, the patient also needs to receive **deficit** replacement (see Chapter 54). A child awaiting surgery may need only maintenance fluids, whereas a child with diarrheal dehydration needs maintenance and deficit therapy and also may require replacement fluids if significant diarrhea continues.

MAINTENANCE THERAPY. Children normally have large variations in their daily intake of water and electrolytes. The only exceptions are patients who receive fixed dietary regimens orally, via a gastric tube, or as intravenous total parenteral nutrition. Healthy children can tolerate significant variations in intake because of the many homeostatic mechanisms that can adjust absorption and excretion of water and electrolytes (see Chapter 52). The calculated water and electrolyte needs that form the basis of maintenance therapy are not absolute requirements. Rather, these calculations provide reasonable guidelines for a starting point to estimate intravenous therapy. Children do not need to be placed on intravenous fluids simply because their intake is being monitored in a hospital and they are not taking "maintenance fluids" orally, unless there is a pathologic process present that necessitates high fluid intake.

Maintenance fluids are most commonly necessary in preoperative and postoperative surgical patients; many nonsurgical patients also require maintenance fluids. It is important to recognize when it is necessary to begin maintenance fluids. A normal teenager who is given nothing by mouth (NPO) overnight for a morning procedure does not require maintenance fluids because a healthy adolescent can easily tolerate 12 or 18 hr without oral intake. In contrast, a 6 mo old child waiting for surgery should begin receiving intravenous fluids within 8 hr of the last feeding. Infants become dehydrated more quickly than older patients. A child with obligatory high urine output from nephrogenic diabetes insipidus should begin receiving intravenous fluids soon after being made NPO.

Maintenance fluids are composed of a solution of water, glucose, sodium, and potassium. This solution has the advantages of simplicity, long shelf life, low cost, and compatibility with peripheral intravenous administration. Such a solution accomplishes the major objectives of maintenance fluids (Table 53-1). Patients lose water, sodium, and potassium in their urine and stool; water is also lost from the skin and lungs. Maintenance fluids replace these losses and therefore avoid the development of dehydration and deficiencies of sodium or potassium.

The glucose in maintenance fluids provides approximately 20% of the normal caloric needs of the patient, prevents the development of starvation ketoacidosis, and diminishes the protein degradation that would occur if the patient received no calories. Glucose also provides added osmoles, thus avoiding the administration of hypotonic fluids that may cause hemolysis.

Maintenance fluids do not provide adequate calories, protein, fat, minerals, or vitamins. This is typically not problematic for a patient receiving intravenous fluids for a few days. A patient receiving maintenance intravenous fluids is receiving inadequate calories and will lose 0.5–1% of weight each day. It is imperative that patients not remain on maintenance therapy indefinitely; total parental nutrition should be used for children who cannot be fed enterally for more than a few days, especially patients with underlying malnutrition (see Chapter 55).

Prototypical maintenance fluid therapy does not provide electrolytes such as calcium, phosphorus, magnesium, or bicarbonate. For most patients, this is not problematic for a few days, although there are patients who will not tolerate this omission, usually because of excessive losses. A child with renal tubular acidosis wastes bicarbonate in urine. Such a patient will rapidly become acidemic unless bicarbonate (or acetate) is added to the maintenance fluids. It is important to remember the limitations of maintenance fluid therapy.

TABLE 53-1. Goals of Maintenance Fluids
Prevent dehydration
Prevent electrolyte disorders
Prevent ketoacidosis
Prevent protein degradation

TABLE 53-2. Body Weight Method for Calculating Daily Maintenance Fluid Volume

BODY WEIGHT	FLUID PER DAY
0–10 kg	100 mL/kg
11–20 kg	1,000 mL + 50 mL/kg for each kg > 10 kg
>20 kg	1,500 mL + 20 mL/kg for each kg > 20 kg*

*The maximum total fluid per day is normally 2,400 mL.

MAINTENANCE WATER. Water is a crucial component of maintenance fluid therapy because of the obligatory daily water losses. These losses are both measurable (urine, stool) and not measurable (insensible losses from the skin and lungs). Failure to replace these losses leads to a thirsty, uncomfortable child and, ultimately, a dehydrated child.

The goal of maintenance water is to provide enough water to replace these losses. Although urinary losses are approximately 60% of the total, the normal kidney has the ability to markedly modify water losses, with daily urine volume potentially varying by more than a factor of 20. Maintenance water is designed to provide enough water so that the kidney does not need to significantly dilute or concentrate the urine. This also provides a margin of safety so that normal homeostatic mechanisms can adjust urinary water losses to prevent overhydration or dehydration. This adaptability obviates the need for absolute precision in determining water requirements. This is important, given the absence of absolute accuracy in the formulas for calculation of water needs. Table 53-2 provides a system for calculating maintenance water based on the patient's weight and emphasizes the high water needs of smaller, less mature patients. This approach is reliable, although calculations based on weight do overestimate the water needs of overweight patients, where it is better to base the calculations on the child's lean body weight, which can be estimated by using the 50th percentile of body weight for the child's height. It is also important to remember that there is an upper limit of 2.4 L/24 hr in adult-sized patients. Intravenous fluids are written as an hourly rate. The formulas in Table 53-3 enable rapid calculation of the rate of maintenance fluids.

INTRAVENOUS SOLUTIONS. The components of the commonly available solutions are shown in Table 53-4. Normal saline (NS) and Ringer lactate (LR) are isotonic solutions; they have approximately the same tonicity as plasma. Isotonic fluids are generally used for the acute correction of intravascular volume depletion (see Chapter 54). The usual choices for maintenance fluid therapy in children are ½ NS and 0.2 NS. These solutions are available with 5% dextrose (D5). In addition, they are available with 20 mEq/L of potassium chloride, 10 mEq/L of potassium chloride, or no potassium. A hospital pharmacy can also prepare custom-made solutions with different concentrations of glucose, sodium, or potassium. In addition, other electrolytes, such as calcium, magnesium, phosphate, acetate, and bicarbonate, can be added to intravenous solutions. Custom-made solutions take time to prepare and are much more expensive than commercial solutions. The use of custom-made solutions is necessary only for patients who have underlying disorders that cause significant electrolyte imbalances. The use of commercial solutions saves both time and expense.

TABLE 53-3. Hourly Maintenance Water Rate

For body weight of 0–10 kg: 4 mL/kg/hr
For body weight of 10–20 kg: 40 mL/hr + 2 mL/kg/hr × (wt − 10 kg)
For body weight of >20 kg: 60 mL/hr + 1 mL/kg/hr × (wt − 20 kg)*

*The maximum fluid rate is normally 100 mL/hr.

TABLE 53-4. Composition of Intravenous Solutions

FLUID	$[Na^+]$	$[Cl^-]$	$[K^+]$	$[Ca^{2+}]$	$[Lactate^-]$
Normal saline (0.9% NaCl)	154	154			
½ normal saline (0.45% NaCl)	77	77			
0.2 normal saline (0.2% NaCl)	34	34			
Ringer lactate	130	109	4	3	28

A normal plasma osmolality is 285–295 mOsm/kg. Infusing an intravenous solution peripherally with a much lower osmolality can cause water to move into red blood cells, causing hemolysis. Thus, intravenous fluids are generally designed to have an osmolality that is either close to 285 or greater (fluids with moderately higher osmolality do not cause problems). Thus, 0.2 NS (osmolality = 68) should not be administered peripherally, but D5 0.2 NS (osmolality = 346) or D5 ½ NS + 20 mEq/L KCl (osmolality = 472) can be administered.

There is controversy about the appropriate sodium content of maintenance fluids, considering the suggestion that excessive amounts of hypotonic fluids may cause hyponatremia, which at times may have serious sequelae. One approach to avoid water intoxication is to reduce the rate of infusion of fluids containing 0.2 NS or ½ NS. The other recommends that normal saline be used as the maintenance fluid; most centers have not adopted the routine use of NS as the initiating maintenance solution.

GLUCOSE. Maintenance fluids usually contain 5% dextrose (D5), which provides 17 calories/100 mL and nearly 20% of the daily caloric needs. This is enough to prevent ketone production and helps to minimize protein degradation, but the child will lose weight on this regimen. This is the principal reason why a patient needs to be started on total parental nutrition after a few days of maintenance fluids if enteral feedings are still not possible. Maintenance fluids are also lacking in such crucial nutrients as protein, fat, vitamins, and minerals.

SELECTION OF MAINTENANCE FLUIDS. After calculation of water and electrolyte needs, children typically receive either D5 ½ NS + 20 mEq/L KCl or D5 0.2 NS + 20 mEq/L KCl. Children weighing less than approximately 10 kg do best with the solution containing 0.2 NS because of their high water needs per kilogram. Larger children and adults may receive the solution with ½ NS. These guidelines assume that there is no disease process present that would require an adjustment in either the volume or the electrolyte composition of maintenance fluids (children with renal insufficiency may be hyperkalemic or unable to excrete potassium and may not tolerate 20 mEq/L of potassium). These solutions work well in children who have normal homeostatic mechanisms for adjusting urinary excretion of water, sodium, and potassium. In children with complicated pathophysiologic derangements, it may be necessary to empirically adjust the electrolyte composition and rate of maintenance fluids based on electrolyte measurements and assessment of fluid balance. **In all children, it is critical to carefully monitor weight, urine output, and electrolytes to determine over- or underhydration, hyponatremia, or other electrolyte disturbances, and to then adjust the rate or composition of the intravenous solution.**

MAINTENANCE FLUIDS AND HYPONATREMIA. Patients who are producing antidiuretic hormone (ADH) may retain water, creating a risk of hyponatremia due to water intoxication. Patients who may be producing ADH due to subtle volume depletion or other mechanisms (respiratory disease, stress, pain, nausea, medications such as narcotics) may be more safely treated with fluids with a higher sodium concentration, a decrease in fluid rate, or a combination of these strategies. Patients with persistent ADH production due to an underlying disease process (syndrome of inappropriate ADH [SIADH], congestive heart failure, nephrotic syndrome, liver disease) should receive less than maintenance fluids. Treatment is individualized, and careful monitoring is critical. Special caution is needed in patients who are known to have low-normal serum sodium concentrations or hyponatremia.

Hyponatremia as a complication of intravenous fluids is particularly a concern in the postoperative patient who is intravascularly volume-depleted from surgical losses, third space losses (discussed later), and venous pooling (due to lying supine and the effects of anesthesia and sedation). Surgical patients typically receive isotonic fluids (NS, LR) during surgery and in the recovery room for 6–8 hr postoperatively; the rate is typically approximately $\frac{2}{3}$ of the calculated maintenance rate. Subsequent maintenance fluids should contain $\frac{1}{2}$ NS, even in smaller patients, unless there is a specific indication to use 0.2 NS. Electrolytes should be measured at least daily.

Patients with other potential causes of ADH production must have careful monitoring of their electrolytes and fluid input and output. Patients with possible subtle volume depletion (see Chapter 54) should receive 20 mL/kg (maximum of 1 L) of isotonic fluid (NS, LR) over 1–2 hr to restore their intravascular volume before maintenance fluids are initiated. The patient can then be switched to D5 $\frac{1}{2}$ NS + 20 mEq/L KCl at a standard maintenance rate. Patients of any weight with possible volume depletion should not routinely receive fluids with 0.2 NS, unless there is a specific indication. Patients who are at risk for producing ADH due to etiologies other than volume depletion may need to receive less than maintenance fluids to avoid hyponatremia.

VARIATIONS IN MAINTENANCE WATER AND ELECTROLYTES. The calculation of maintenance water is based on standard assumptions regarding water losses. There are patients, however, in whom these assumptions are incorrect. To identify such situations, it is helpful to understand the source and magnitude of normal water losses. Table 53-5 lists the 3 sources of normal water loss.

Urine is the most important contributor to normal water loss. Insensible losses represent approximately $\frac{1}{3}$ of total maintenance water (40% in infants and closer to 25% in adolescents and adults). Insensible losses are composed of evaporative losses from the skin and lungs that cannot be quantitated. The evaporative losses from the skin do not include sweat, which would be considered an additional (sensible) source of water loss. Stool normally represents a minor source of water loss.

Maintenance water and electrolyte needs may be increased or decreased, depending on the clinical situation. This may be obvious, in the case of the infant with profuse diarrhea, or subtle, in the case of the patient who has decreased insensible losses while receiving mechanical ventilation. It is helpful to consider the sources of normal water and electrolyte losses and to determine whether any of these sources is being modified in a specific patient. It is then necessary to adjust maintenance water and electrolyte calculations.

Table 53-6 lists a variety of clinical situations that modify normal water and electrolyte losses. The skin can be the source of very significant water loss, particularly in neonates, especially premature infants, who are under radiant warmers or are receiving phototherapy. Very low birthweight infants can have insensible losses of 100–200 mL/kg/24 hr. Burns can result in massive losses of water and electrolytes, and there are specific guidelines for fluid management in children with burns (see Chapter 74). Sweat losses of water and electrolytes, especially in a warm climate, can also be significant. Children with cystic fibrosis have increased sodium losses from the skin. Some children with pseudohypoaldosteronism also have increased cutaneous salt losses.

TABLE 53-5. Sources of Water Loss

Urine: 60%
Insensible losses: ~35% (skin and lungs)
Stool: 5%

Fever increases evaporative losses from the skin. These losses are somewhat predictable, leading to a 10–15% increase in maintenance water needs for each 1°C increase in temperature above 38°C. These guidelines are for a patient with a persistent fever; a 1-hr fever spike does not cause an appreciable increase in water needs.

Tachypnea or a tracheostomy increases evaporative losses from the lungs. A humidified ventilator causes a decrease in insensible losses from the lungs and can even lead to water absorption via the lungs; a ventilated patient has a decrease in maintenance water requirements. It may be difficult to quantify the changes that take place in the individual patient in these situations.

REPLACEMENT FLUIDS. The gastrointestinal (GI) tract is potentially a source of considerable water loss. GI water losses are accompanied by electrolytes and thus may cause disturbances in intravascular volume and electrolyte concentrations. GI losses are often associated with loss of potassium, leading to hypokalemia. Because of the high bicarbonate concentration in stool, children with diarrhea usually have a metabolic acidosis, which may be accentuated if volume depletion causes hypoperfusion and a concurrent lactic acidosis. Emesis or losses from an NG tube can cause a metabolic alkalosis (see Chapter 52).

In the absence of vomiting, diarrhea, or NG drainage, GI losses of water and electrolytes are usually quite small. All GI losses are considered excessive, and the increase in the water requirement is equal to the volume of fluid losses. Because GI water and electrolyte losses can be precisely measured, it is possible to use an appropriate replacement solution.

It is impossible to predict the losses for the next 24 hr; it is better to replace excessive GI losses as they occur. The child should receive an appropriate maintenance fluid that does not consider the GI losses. The losses should then be replaced after they occur, using a solution with the same approximate electrolyte concentration as the GI fluid. The losses are usually replaced every 1–6 hr, depending on the rate of loss, with very rapid losses being replaced more frequently.

Diarrhea is a common cause of fluid loss in children. It can cause dehydration and electrolyte disorders. In the unusual patient with significant diarrhea and a limited ability to take oral fluid, it is important to have a plan for replacing excessive stool losses. The volume of stool should be measured, and an equal volume of replacement solution should be given. The electrolyte

TABLE 53-6. Adjustments in Maintenance Water

SOURCE	CAUSES OF INCREASED WATER NEEDS	CAUSES OF DECREASED WATER NEEDS
Skin	Radiant warmer Phototherapy Fever Sweat Burns	Incubator (premature infant)
Lungs	Tachypnea Tracheostomy	Humidified ventilator
Gastrointestinal tract	Diarrhea Emesis Nasogastric suction	
Renal	Polyuria	Oliguria/anuria
Miscellaneous	Surgical drain Third spacing	Hypothyroidism

TABLE 53-7. Replacement Fluid for Diarrhea

AVERAGE COMPOSITION OF DIARRHEA
Sodium: 55 mEq/L
Potassium: 25 mEq/L
Bicarbonate: 15 mEq/L
APPROACH TO REPLACEMENT OF ONGOING LOSSES
Solution: D5 0.2 normal saline + 20 mEq/L sodium bicarbonate + 20 mEq/L KCl
Replace stool mL/mL every 1–6 hr

TABLE 53-9. Adjusting Fluid Therapy for Altered Renal Output

OLIGURIA/ANURIA
Place patient on insensible fluids (25–40% of maintenance)
Replace urine output mL/mL with ½ normal saline
POLYURIA
Place patient on insensible fluids (25–40% of maintenance)
Measure urine electrolytes
Replace urine output mL/mL with solution based on measured urine electrolytes

composition of a replacement solution is always best determined by measuring the electrolyte content of the fluid that is being replaced. Data are available on the average electrolyte composition of diarrhea in children (Table 53-7). Using this information, it is possible to design an appropriate replacement solution. The solution shown in Table 53-7 replaces stool losses of sodium, potassium, chloride, and bicarbonate. Each 1 mL of stool should be replaced by 1 mL of this solution. The average electrolyte composition of diarrhea is just an average, and there may be considerable variation. It is therefore advisable to consider measuring the electrolyte composition of a patient's diarrhea, particularly if the amount is especially excessive or if the patient's serum electrolytes are problematic.

Loss of gastric fluid, via either emesis or NG suction, is also likely to cause dehydration in that most such patients have impaired oral intake of fluids. Electrolyte disturbances, particularly hypokalemia and metabolic alkalosis, are also common. These complications can be avoided by judicious use of a replacement solution. The composition of gastric fluid shown in Table 53-8 is the basis for designing a replacement solution.

Patients with gastric losses frequently have hypokalemia, although the potassium concentration of gastric fluid is relatively low. The associated urinary loss of potassium is an important cause of hypokalemia in this situation (see Chapter 52). These patients may need additional potassium either in their maintenance fluids or in their replacement fluids to compensate for prior or ongoing urinary losses. Restoration of the patient's intravascular volume, by decreasing aldosterone synthesis, lessens the urinary potassium losses.

Urine output is normally the largest cause of water loss. Diseases such as renal failure and SIADH can lead to a decrease in urine volume. The patient with oliguria or anuria has a decreased need for water and electrolytes; continuation of maintenance fluids produces fluid overload. In contrast, postobstructive diuresis, the polyuric phase of acute tubular necrosis, diabetes mellitus, and diabetes insipidus increase urine production. To prevent dehydration, the patient must receive more than standard maintenance fluids when urine output is excessive. The electrolyte losses in patients with polyuria are variable. In diabetes insipidus, the urine electrolyte concentration is usually low, whereas children with diseases such as juvenile nephronophthisis or obstructive uropathy usually have increased losses of both water and sodium.

The approach to decreased or increased urine output is similar (Table 53-9). The patient receives fluids at a rate to replace insensible losses. This is accomplished by a rate of fluid administration that is 25–40% of the normal maintenance rate, depending on the patient's age. Replacing insensible losses in the anuric child will theoretically maintain an even fluid balance, with the caveat that 25–40% of the normal maintenance rate is only an estimate of insensible losses. In the individual patient, this rate is adjusted based on monitoring of the patient's weight and volume status. Most children with renal insufficiency receive little or no potassium because the kidney is the principal site for potassium excretion.

TABLE 53-8. Replacement Fluid for Emesis or Nasogastric Losses

AVERAGE COMPOSITION OF GASTRIC FLUID
Sodium: 60 mEq/L
Potassium: 10 mEq/L
Chloride: 90 mEq/L
APPROACH TO REPLACEMENT OF ONGOING LOSSES
Solution: normal saline + 10 mEq/L KCl
Replace output mL/mL every 1–6 hr

For the oliguric child, it is important to add a urine replacement solution to prevent dehydration. This is especially important in the patient with acute renal failure because output may increase slowly, which could lead to volume depletion and worsening of renal failure if the patient remains on only insensible fluids. A replacement solution of D5 ½NS is usually appropriate initially, although its composition may need to be adjusted if urine output increases significantly.

Most children with polyuria (except in diabetes mellitus; see Chapter 590) should be placed on insensible fluids plus urine replacement. This avoids the need to attempt to calculate the volume of urine output that is "normal" so that the patient can be given replacement fluid for the excess. In these patients, urine output is, by definition, excessive, and it is important to measure the sodium and potassium concentrations of the urine to help in formulating the urine replacement solution.

Surgical drains and chest tubes can produce measurable fluid output. These losses should be replaced when they are significant. They can be measured and replaced with an appropriate replacement solution. Third space losses manifest with edema and ascites and are due to a shift of fluid from the intravascular space into the intersitial space. Although these losses cannot be quantitated easily, third space losses can be large and may lead to intravascular volume depletion, despite the patient's weight gain. Replacement of third space fluid is empirical, but should be anticipated in patients who are at risk, such as children who have burns or abdominal surgery. Third space losses and chest tube output are isotonic; thus, they usually require replacement with an isotonic fluid, such as NS or LR. Adjustments in the amount of replacement fluid for third space losses are based on continuing assessment of the patient's intravascular volume status. Protein losses from chest tube drainage can be significant, occasionally necessitating that 5% albumin be used as a replacement solution.

Choong K, Kho ME, Menon K, Bohr D: Hypotonic versus isotonic saline in hospitalised children: a systematic review. *Arch Dis Child* 2006;91:828–835.

Friedman AL: Pediatric hydration therapy: Historical review and a new approach. *Kidney Int* 2005;67:380–388.

Grunhagen DJ, de Boer MG, de Beaufort AJ, et al: Transepidermal water loss during halogen spotlight phototherapy in preterm infants. *Pediatr Res* 2002;51:402–405.

Hatherill M: Rubbing salt in the wound: The case against isotonic parenteral maintenance solution. *Arch Dis Child* 2004;89:414–418.

Holliday MA, Friedman AL, Segar WE, et al: Acute hospital-induced hyponatremia in children: A physiologic approach. *J Pediatr* 2004;145:584–587.

Hoorn EJ, Geary D, Robb M, et al: Acute hyponatremia related to intravenous fluid administration in hospitalized children: An observational study. *Pediatrics* 2004;113:1279–1284.

Moritz ML, Ayus JC: Prevention of hospital-acquired hyponatremia: A case for using isotonic saline. *Pediatrics* 2003;111:227–230.

Neville KA, Verge CF, Rosenberg AR, et al: Isotonic is better than hypotonic saline for intravenous rehydration of children with gastroenteritis: a prospective randomised study. *Arch Dis Child* 2006;91:226–232.

Taylor D, Durward A: Pouring salt on troubled waters: The case for isotonic parenteral maintenance solution. *Arch Dis Child* 2004;89:411–414.

Chapter 54 ■ Deficit Therapy

Larry Greenbaum

Dehydration, most often due to gastroenteritis, is a common problem in children. Most cases can be managed with oral rehydration (see Chapters 55 and 337). **Even children with mild to moderate hyponatremic or hypernatremic dehydration can be managed with oral rehydration.** This chapter focuses on the child who requires intravenous therapy, although many of the same principles are used in oral rehydration.

CLINICAL MANIFESTATIONS. The first step in caring for the child with dehydration is to assess the degree of dehydration (Table 54-1). This dictates both the urgency of the situation and the volume of fluid needed for rehydration. The infant with mild dehydration (3–5% of body weight dehydrated) has few clinical signs or symptoms. The infant may be thirsty; the alert parent may notice a decline in urine output. The history is most helpful. The infant with moderate dehydration has clear physical signs and symptoms. Intravascular space depletion is evident by an increased heart rate and reduced urine output. This patient needs fairly prompt intervention. The infant with severe dehydration is gravely ill. The decrease in blood pressure indicates that vital organs may be receiving inadequate perfusion. Immediate and aggressive intervention is necessary. If possible, the child with severe dehydration should initially receive intravenous therapy. For older children and adults, mild, moderate, or severe dehydration represents a lower percentage of body weight lost. This difference occurs because water is a higher percentage of body weight in infants (see Chapter 52).

Clinical assessment of dehydration is only an estimate; thus, the patient must be continually re-evaluated during therapy. The degree of dehydration is underestimated in hypernatremic dehydration because the movement of water from the intracellular space to the extracellular space helps to preserve the intravascular volume. The opposite occurs with hyponatremic dehydration; dangerous intravascular volume depletion can occur with less severe fluid deficits.

The history usually suggests the etiology of the dehydration and may predict whether the patient will have a normal sodium concentration (isotonic dehydration), hyponatremic dehydration, or hypernatremic dehydration. The neonate with dehydration due to poor intake of breast milk often has hypernatremic dehydration. Hypernatremic dehydration is likely in any child with losses of hypotonic fluid and poor water intake, such as may occur with diarrhea, and poor oral intake due to anorexia or emesis. Hyponatremic dehydration occurs in the child with diarrhea who is taking in large quantities of low-salt fluid, such as water or diluted formula.

Some children with dehydration are appropriately thirsty, but in others, the lack of intake is part of the pathophysiology of the dehydration. Even though decreased urine output is present in most children with dehydration, good urine output may be deceptively present if a child has an underlying renal defect, such as diabetes insipidus or a salt-wasting nephropathy, or in infants with hypernatremic dehydration.

Physical examination findings are usually proportional to the degree of dehydration. Parents may be helpful when assessing the child for the presence of sunken eyes because this finding may be subtle. Pinching and gently twisting the skin of the abdominal or thoracic wall detects tenting of the skin (turgor, elasticity). Tented skin remains in a pinched position rather than springing quickly back to normal. It is difficult to properly assess tenting of the skin in premature infants or severely malnourished children. Activation of the sympathetic nervous system causes tachycardia in children with intravascular volume depletion; diaphoresis may also be present. Postural changes in blood pressure are often helpful for evaluating and assessing the response to therapy in children with dehydration. Tachypnea in children with dehydration may be present secondary to a metabolic acidosis from stool losses of bicarbonate or due to lactic acidosis from shock (see Chapter 68).

LABORATORY FINDINGS. Several laboratory findings are useful for evaluating the child with dehydration. The serum sodium concentration determines the type of dehydration. Metabolic acidosis may be due to stool bicarbonate losses in children with diarrhea, secondary renal insufficiency, or lactic acidosis from shock. The anion gap is useful for differentiating among the various causes of a metabolic acidosis (see Chapter 52). Emesis or nasogastric losses usually cause a metabolic alkalosis. The serum potassium concentration may be low as a result of diarrheal losses. In children with dehydration due to emesis, gastric potassium losses, metabolic alkalosis, and urinary potassium losses all contribute to hypokalemia. Metabolic acidosis, which causes a shift of potassium out of cells, and renal insufficiency may lead to hyperkalemia. A combination of mechanisms may be present; thus, it may be difficult to predict the child's acid-base status or serum potassium level by the history alone.

The blood urea nitrogen (BUN) and serum creatinine concentration are useful in assessing the child with dehydration. Volume depletion without parenchymal renal injury may cause a disproportionate increase in the BUN with little or no change in the creatinine concentration. This is secondary to increased passive resorption of urea in the proximal tubule due to appropriate renal conservation of sodium and water. This increase in the BUN with moderate or severe dehydration may be absent or blunted in the child with poor protein intake because urea production is dependent on protein degradation. The BUN may be disproportionately increased in the child with increased urea production, as occurs with a gastrointestinal bleed or with the use of glucocorticoids, which increase catabolism. A significant elevation of the creatinine concentration suggests renal insufficiency, although a small, transient increase can occur with dehydration. **Acute tubular necrosis** (see Chapter 535) due to volume depletion is the most common etiology of renal insufficiency in a child with volume depletion, but occasionally, the child may have previously undetected chronic renal insufficiency or an alternative explanation for the acute renal failure. Renal vein thrombosis is a well-described sequela of severe dehydration in infants; possible

TABLE 54-1. Clinical Evaluation of Dehydration
Mild dehydration (<5% in an infant; <3% in an older child or adult): normal or increased pulse; decreased urine output; thirsty; normal physical findings
Moderate dehydration (5–10% in an infant; 3–6% in an older child or adult): tachycardia; little or no urine output; irritable/lethargic; sunken eyes and fontanel; decreased tears; dry mucous membranes; mild delay in elasticity (skin turgor); delayed capillary refill (>1.5 sec); cool and pale
Severe dehydration (>10% in an infant; >6% in an older child or adult): rapid and weak or absent peripheral pulses; decreased blood pressure; no urine output; very sunken eyes and fontanel; no tears; parched mucous membranes; delayed elasticity (poor skin turgor); very delayed capillary refill (>3 sec); cold and mottled; limp, depressed consciousness

findings include thrombocytopenia and hematuria (see Chapter 519). The baseline normal creatinine concentration increases with age; thus, a normal adult creatinine concentration of 1 mg/dL may indicate significant renal insufficiency in an infant. The BUN and creatinine concentration are dependent on the timing of the disease process. Urea and creatinine are waste products that build up gradually with decreased renal excretion. A child with acute, severe dehydration may have only a minimal elevation of the serum creatinine concentration despite marked renal insufficiency; the creatinine concentration will increase over time.

Urinalysis is most helpful in the measurement of urine specific gravity, which is usually elevated in cases of significant dehydration, but returns to normal after rehydration. Although infants have a reduced ability to concentrate the urine, even those who are a few weeks of age can show a clear elevation in specific gravity with significant dehydration. A specific gravity <1.020 indicates mild or no dehydration or indicates a urinary concentrating defect, as in chronic renal disease or primary or secondary diabetes insipidus. With dehydration, urinalysis may show hyaline and granular casts, a few white cells and red cells, and 30–100 mg/dL of proteinuria. These findings are not usually associated with significant renal pathology, and they remit with therapy.

Hemoconcentration as a result of dehydration causes an increase in hematocrit, hemoglobin, and serum proteins. These values normalize with rehydration. A normal hemoglobin concentration during acute dehydration may mask an underlying anemia. A decreased albumin level in a dehydrated patient suggests a chronic disease, such as malnutrition, nephrotic syndrome, or liver disease, or an acute process, such as capillary leak. An acute or chronic protein-losing enteropathy may also cause a low serum albumin concentration.

CALCULATION OF THE FLUID DEFICIT. Determining the fluid deficit necessitates clinically determining the percent dehydration and multiplying this percentage by the patient's weight; a child who weighs 10 kg and is 10% dehydrated has a fluid deficit of 1 L.

APPROACH TO DEHYDRATION. The child with dehydration requires acute intervention to ensure that there is adequate tissue perfusion. This resuscitation phase requires rapid restoration of the circulating intravascular volume and treatment of shock with an isotonic solution, such as normal saline (NS) or Ringer lactate (LR) [see Chapter 68]. The child is given a fluid bolus, usually 20 mL/kg of the isotonic fluid, over approximately 20 min. The child with severe dehydration may require multiple fluid boluses and may need to receive the boluses as fast as possible. In a child with a known or probable metabolic alkalosis (the child with isolated vomiting), LR should not be used because the lactate will worsen the alkalosis.

Colloids, such as blood, 5% albumin, and plasma, are rarely needed for fluid boluses. A crystalloid solution (NS or LR) is satisfactory, with both less infectious risk and lower cost. Blood is obviously indicated in the child with significant anemia or acute blood loss. Plasma is useful for children with a coagulopathy. The child with hypoalbuminemia may benefit from 5% albumin, although there is evidence that albumin infusions increase mortality in adults. The volume and the infusion rate for colloids are generally modified compared with crystalloids (see Chapters 470 and 473).

The initial resuscitation and rehydration phase is complete when the child has an adequate intravascular volume. Typically, the child shows clinical improvement, including a lower heart rate, normalization of blood pressure, improved perfusion, better urine output, and a more alert affect.

With adequate intravascular volume, it is appropriate to plan the fluid therapy for the next 24 hr. A general approach is outlined in Table 54-2, with the caveat that there are many different approaches to correcting dehydration. In isonatremic or hyponatremic dehydration, the entire fluid deficit is corrected over 24 hr; a slower approach is used for hypernatremic dehydration (discussed later). To assure that the intravascular volume is restored, the patient receives an additional 20-mL/kg bolus of an isotonic fluid over 2 hr. The child's total fluid needs are added together (maintenance + deficit). The volume of isotonic fluids that the patient has received is subtracted from this total. The remaining fluid volume is then administered over 24 hr. The potassium concentration may need to be decreased or, less commonly, increased, depending on the clinical situation. Potassium is not usually included in the intravenous fluids until the patient voids. Children with significant ongoing losses need to receive an appropriate replacement solution (see Chapter 53).

TABLE 54-2. Fluid Management of Dehydration

Restore intravascular volume
Normal saline: 20 mL/kg over 20 min
Repeat as needed
Rapid volume repletion: 20 mL/kg normal saline or Ringer Lactate (maximum = 1 L) over 2 hr
Calculate 24-hr fluid needs: maintenance + deficit volume
Subtract isotonic fluid already administered from 24 hr fluid needs
Administer remaining volume over 24 hr using D5 ½ normal saline + 20 mEq/L KCl
Replace ongoing losses as they occur

MONITORING AND ADJUSTING THERAPY. The formulation of a plan for correcting a child's dehydration is only the beginning of management. **All calculations in fluid therapy are only approximations.** This is especially true with the assessment of percent dehydration. It is equally important to monitor the patient during treatment and to modify therapy based on the clinical situation. The cornerstones of patient monitoring are listed in Table 54-3. The patient's vital signs are useful indicators of intravascular volume status. The child with decreased blood pressure and an increased heart rate will probably benefit from a fluid bolus. Central venous pressure is an excellent indicator of fluid status in the critically ill child with shock.

The patient's intake and output are critically important in the dehydrated child. The child who, after 8 hr of therapy, has more output than input due to continuing diarrhea needs to be placed on a replacement solution. See the guidelines in Chapter 53 for selecting an appropriate replacement solution. Urine output and urine specific gravity are useful for evaluating the success of therapy. Good urine output indicates that rehydration has been successful. This is supported by decreasing urine specific gravity. If urine specific gravity is <1.010 and the patient is clinically well hydrated, it may be appropriate to decrease the intravenous fluid rate.

Signs of dehydration on physical examination suggest the need for continued rehydration. Signs of fluid overload, such as edema or pulmonary congestion, are present in the child who is overhydrated. An accurate daily weight measurement is critical for

TABLE 54-3. Monitoring Therapy

VITAL SIGNS
Pulse
Blood pressure
INTAKE AND OUTPUT
Fluid balance
Urine output and specific gravity
PHYSICAL EXAMINATION
Weight
Clinical signs of depletion or overload
ELECTROLYTES

the management of the dehydrated child. There should be a gain in weight during successful therapy.

Measurement of electrolytes at least daily is appropriate for any child who is receiving intravenous rehydration. These children are at risk for sodium, potassium, and acid-base disorders. It is always important to look at trends. For instance, a sodium value of 144 mEq/L is normal. Yet, if the sodium concentration was 136 mEq/L 12 hr earlier, then there is a distinct risk that the child will be hypernatremic in 12 or 24 hr. It is advisable to be proactive in adjusting fluid therapy.

Both hypokalemia and hyperkalemia are potentially serious (see Chapter 52). Because dehydration can be associated with acute renal failure and hyperkalemia, potassium is withheld from intravenous fluids until the patient has voided. The potassium concentration in the patient's intravenous fluids is not rigidly prescribed. Rather, the patient's serum potassium level and underlying renal function are used to modify potassium delivery. The patient with an elevated creatinine value and a potassium level of 5 mEq/L does not receive any potassium until the serum potassium level decreases. Conversely, the patient with a potassium level of 2.5 mEq/L may require additional potassium.

Metabolic acidosis can be quite severe in dehydrated children. Although normal kidneys eventually correct this problem, a child with renal dysfunction may be unable to correct a metabolic acidosis, and a portion of the patient's intravenous sodium chloride may need to be replaced with sodium bicarbonate or sodium acetate.

The serum potassium level is modified by the patient's acid-base status. Acidosis increases serum potassium by causing intracellular potassium to move into the extracellular space. Thus, as acidosis is corrected, the potassium concentration decreases. Again, it is best to anticipate this problem and to monitor the serum potassium concentration and adjust potassium administration appropriately.

HYPONATREMIC DEHYDRATION. The pathogenesis of hyponatremic dehydration is usually due to a combination of sodium and water loss and water retention to compensate for the volume depletion. The patient has a pathologic increase in fluid loss, and this fluid contains sodium. Most fluid that is lost has a lower sodium concentration, so patients with only fluid loss would have hypernatremia. Diarrhea has, on average, a sodium concentration of 50 mEq/L. By replacing diarrheal fluid with water, which has almost no sodium, there is a reduction in the serum sodium concentration. The volume depletion stimulates synthesis of antidiuretic hormone, resulting in reduced renal water excretion. Hence, the body's usual mechanism for preventing hyponatremia, renal water excretion, is blocked. The risk of hyponatremia is further increased if the volume depletion is due to loss of fluid with a higher sodium concentration, as may occur with renal salt wasting, third space losses, or diarrhea with a high sodium content (cholera).

Hyponatremic dehydration produces more substantial intravascular volume depletion due to the shift of water from the extracellular space into the intracellular space. In addition, some patients have symptoms, predominantly neurologic, as a result of hyponatremia (see Chapter 52).

The initial goal in treating hyponatremia is correction of intravascular volume depletion with isotonic fluid (NS or LR). An overcorrection in the serum sodium concentration (>135 mEq/L) is associated with an increased risk of **central pontine myelinolysis** (CPM). The risk of CPM also increases with overly rapid correction of the serum sodium concentration, so it is best to avoid increasing the sodium by >12 mEq/L each 24 hr. Most patients with hyponatremic dehydration do well with the same basic strategy that is outlined in Table 54-2. Again, potassium delivery is adjusted based on the initial serum potassium level and the patient's renal function. Potassium is not given until the patient voids.

The patient's sodium concentration is monitored closely to ensure appropriate correction, and the sodium concentration of the fluid is adjusted accordingly. Patients with ongoing losses require an appropriate replacement solution (see Chapter 53). Patients with neurologic symptoms (seizures) as a result of hyponatremia need to receive an acute infusion of hypertonic (3%) saline to increase the serum sodium concentration rapidly (see Chapter 52).

HYPERNATREMIC DEHYDRATION. Hypernatremic dehydration is the most dangerous form of dehydration due to complications of hypernatremia and of therapy. Hypernatremia can cause serious neurologic damage, including central nervous system hemorrhages and thrombosis. This appears to be secondary to the movement of water from the brain cells into the hypertonic extracellular fluid, causing brain cell shrinkage and tearing blood vessels within the brain (see Chapter 52).

The movement of water from the intracellular space to the extracellular space during hypernatremic dehydration partially protects the intravascular volume. Thus, children with hypernatremia often appear less ill than children with a similar degree of isotonic dehydration. Urine output may be preserved longer, and there may be less tachycardia. Unfortunately, because the initial manifestations are milder, children with hypernatremic dehydration are often brought for medical attention with more profound dehydration.

Children with hypernatremic dehydration are often lethargic, and they may be irritable when touched. Hypernatremia may cause fever, hypertonicity, and hyperreflexia. More severe neurologic symptoms may develop if cerebral bleeding or thrombosis occurs.

Overly rapid treatment of hypernatremic dehydration may cause significant morbidity and mortality. Idiogenic osmoles are generated within the brain during the development of hypernatremia. These idiogenic osmoles increase the osmolality within the cells of the brain, providing protection against brain cell shrinkage caused by movement of water out of the cells and into the hypertonic extracellular fluid. They dissipate slowly during the correction of hypernatremia. With overly rapid lowering of the extracellular osmolality during the correction of hypernatremia, there may be an osmotic gradient created that causes water movement from the extracellular space into the cells of the brain, producing cerebral edema. Symptoms of the resultant cerebral edema can range from seizures to brain herniation and death.

To minimize the risk of cerebral edema during the correction of hypernatremic dehydration, the serum sodium concentration should not decrease by >12 mEq/L every 24 hr. The deficits in severe hypernatremic dehydration may need to be corrected over 2–4 days (Table 54-4).

The initial resuscitation of hypernatremic dehydration requires restoration of the intravascular volume with NS. LR should not be used because it is more hypotonic than NS and may cause too rapid a decrease in the serum sodium concentration, especially if multiple fluid boluses are necessary.

To avoid cerebral edema when correcting hypernatremic dehydration, the fluid deficit is corrected slowly. The rate of correction depends on the initial sodium concentration (see Table 54-4). There is no general agreement on the choice or the rate of fluid for correcting hypernatremic dehydration. The choice and the rate of fluid administration are not nearly as important as vigilant monitoring of the serum sodium concentration and adjustment of the therapy based on the result (see Table 54-4). The rate of decrease of the serum sodium concentration is roughly related to the "free water" delivery, although there is considerable variation between patients. Free water is water without sodium. NS contains no free water, ½ NS is 50% free water, and water is 100% free water. Smaller patients, to achieve the same decrease in the sodium concentration, tend to need higher amounts of free

TABLE 54-4. Treatment of Hypernatremic Dehydration

RESTORE INTRAVASCULAR VOLUME
Normal saline: 20 mL/kg over 20 min
(Repeat until intravascular volume restored)
DETERMINE TIME FOR CORRECTION BASED ON INITIAL SODIUM CONCENTRATION
[Na]: 145–157 mEq/L: 24 hr
[Na]: 158–170 mEq/L: 48 hr
[Na]: 171–183 mEq/L: 72 hr
[Na]: 184–196 mEq/L: 84 hr
ADMINISTER FLUID AT CONSTANT RATE OVER TIME FOR CORRECTION
Typical fluid: D5 ½ normal saline (with 20 mEq/L KCl unless contraindicated)
Typical rate: 1.25–1.5 times maintenance
FOLLOW SERUM SODIUM CONCENTRATION
ADJUST FLUID BASED ON CLINICAL STATUS AND SERUM SODIUM CONCENTRATION
Signs of volume depletion: administer normal saline (20 mL/kg)
Sodium decreases too rapidly
Increase sodium concentration of intravenous fluid, or
Decrease rate of intravenous fluid
Sodium decreases too slowly
Decrease sodium concentration of intravenous fluid, or
Increase rate of intravenous fluid
REPLACE ONGOING LOSSES AS THEY OCCUR

water delivery per kilogram because of higher insensible fluid losses. D5 ½ NS is usually an appropriate starting solution for a patient with hypernatremic dehydration. Some patients, especially infants with ongoing high insensible water losses, may need to receive D5 0.2 NS. Others require a higher sodium concentration than is present in D5 ½ NS. A child with dehydration due to pure free water loss, as usually occurs with diabetes insipidus, usually needs a more hypotonic fluid than a child with depletion of both sodium and water due to diarrhea.

Adjustment in the sodium concentration of the intravenous fluid is the most common approach for modifying the rate of decrease in the serum concentration (see Table 54-4). For difficult patients with severe hypernatremia, having 2 intravenous solutions (D5 ¼ NS and D5 NS, both with the same concentration of potassium) at the bedside can facilitate this approach by allowing for rapid adjustments of the rates of the 2 fluids. If the serum sodium concentration decreases too rapidly, the rate of D5 NS can be increased and the rate of D5 ½ NS can be decreased by the same amount. Adjustment in the total rate of fluid delivery is another approach for modifying free water delivery. For example, if the serum sodium concentration is decreasing too slowly, the rate of the intravenous fluid can be increased, thereby increasing the delivery of free water. There is limited flexibility in modifying the rate of the intravenous fluid because patients generally should receive 1.25–1.5 times the normal maintenance fluid rate. Nevertheless, in some situations, this can be a helpful adjustment.

Because increasing the rate of the intravenous fluid increases the rate of decline of the sodium concentration, signs of volume depletion are treated with additional isotonic fluid boluses. The serum potassium concentration and the level of renal function dictate the potassium concentration of the intravenous fluid; potassium is held until the patient voids. Patients with hypernatremic dehydration need an appropriate replacement solution if they have ongoing, excessive losses (see Chapter 53).

Seizures are the most common manifestation of **cerebral edema** from an overly rapid decrease of the serum sodium concentration during correction of hypernatremic dehydration. Acutely, increasing the serum concentration via an infusion of 3% sodium chloride can reverse the cerebral edema. Each 1 mL/kg of 3% sodium chloride increases the serum sodium concentration by approximately 1 mEq/L. An infusion of 4–6 mL/kg often results in resolution of the symptoms. This is similar to the strategy used for treating symptomatic hyponatremia (see Chapter 52).

In patients with severe hypernatremia, oral fluids must be used cautiously. Infant formula, because of its low sodium concentration, has a high free water content, and especially if added to intravenous therapy, it may contribute to a rapid decrease in the serum sodium concentration. Less hypotonic fluid, such as an oral rehydration solution, may be more appropriate initially (see Chapter 55). If oral intake is allowed, its contribution to free water delivery must be taken into account, and adjustment in the intravenous fluid is usually appropriate. Judicious monitoring of the serum sodium concentration is critical.

Friedman JN, Goldman RD, Srivastava R, et al: Development of a clinical dehydration scale for use in children between 1 and 36 months of age. *J Pediatr* 2004;145:201–207.

Haspolat S, Duman O, Senol U, et al: Extrapontine myelinolysis in infancy: Report of a case. *J Child Neurol* 2004;19:913–915.

Haycook GB: Hypernatraemia: Diagnosis and management. *Arch Dis Child Educ Pract Ed* 2006;91:ep8–ep13.

Manganaro R, Mami C, Marrone T, et al: Incidence of dehydration and hypernatremia in exclusively breast-fed infants. *J Pediatr* 2001;139: 673–675.

Reynolds RM, Padfield PL, Seckl JR: Disorders of sodium balance. *BMJ* 2006;332:702–705.

Schwaderer AL, Schwartz GJ: Treating hypernatremic dehydration. *Pediatr Rev* 2005;26:148–150.

Steiner MJ, DeWalt DA, Byerley JS: Is this child dehydrated? *JAMA* 2004;291:2746–2754.

Wathen JE, MacKenzie T, Bothner JP: Usefulness of the serum electrolyte panel in the management of pediatric dehydration treated with intravenously administered fluids. *Pediatrics* 2004;114:1227–1234.

Yilmaz K, Karabocuoglu M, Citak A, et al: Evaluation of laboratory tests in dehydrated children with acute gastroenteritis. *J Paediatr Child Health* 2002;38:226–228.

Chapter 55 ■ Fluid and Electrolyte Treatment of Specific Disorders

Larry Greenbaum

55.1 • Acute Diarrhea and Oral Rehydration

Also see Chapter 337.

Diarrhea is a serious problem in many areas of the world and is especially lethal when superimposed on malnutrition. Diarrhea results in large losses of water and electrolytes, especially sodium and potassium, and frequently is complicated by severe systemic acidosis. In approximately 70–80% of patients, the losses of water and sodium are proportionate, with **isotonic dehydration** developing. **Hyponatremic dehydration** is seen in approximately 10–15% of all patients with diarrhea. It occurs when large amounts of electrolytes, especially sodium, are lost in the stool out of proportion to fluid losses. It occurs more frequently with bacillary dysentery or cholera. Hyponatremia may develop or worsen if there is a considerable oral intake of low-electrolyte or electrolyte-free fluids during diarrhea (see Chapter 54).

Disproportionately large net losses of water compared with losses of electrolytes result in **hypernatremic dehydration** (see Chapter 54). It is seen in 10–20% of patients with diarrhea and may occur during the course of diarrhea when oral homemade electrolyte solutions with high concentrations of salt are administered or when infants are fed boiled skim milk, which produces a high renal solute load and increased urinary water losses. The potential for hypernatremia also increases with increased evapo-

TABLE 55-1. Composition of Oral Rehydration Solutions

SOLUTION	GLUCOSE (mmol/L)	Na (mEq/L)	K (mEq/L)	Cl (mEq/L)	BASE (mEq/L)	OSMOLALITY (mOsm/kg)
WHO solution	111	90	20	80	30	311
Rehydralyte	140	75	20	65	30	310
Pedialyte	140	45	20	35	30	250
Pediatric Electrolyte	140	45	20	35	55	250
Infalyte	70*	50	25	45	34	200
Naturalyte	140	45	20	35	55	238

*Rice syrup solids are the carbohydrate source.
WHO, World Health Organization.

rative water loss as a result of fever, high environmental temperatures, and hyperventilation, and with decreased availability of free water.

Mild to moderate dehydration from diarrhea of any cause can be treated effectively in a wide range of age groups using a simple oral glucose-electrolyte solution (Table 55-1) [see Chapter 337]. These solutions rely on the coupled transport of sodium and glucose in the intestine. Oral rehydration therapy is used in many countries and has significantly reduced the morbidity and mortality from acute diarrhea and lessened diarrhea-associated malnutrition. Oral rehydration is underused in developed countries, but it should be attempted for most patients with mild to moderate diarrheal dehydration when adequate supervision is available. Oral rehydration therapy is less expensive than intravenous therapy and has a lower complication rate. Intravenous therapy may be required for patients with severe dehydration (see Chapter 54); those with uncontrollable vomiting; those unable to drink because of extreme fatigue, stupor, or coma; or those with gastric or intestinal distention.

As a guideline for oral rehydration, 50 mL/kg of the oral rehydration solution (ORS) should be given within 4 hr to patients with mild dehydration and 100 mL/kg over 4 hr to those with moderate dehydration (see Chapter 337). Supplementary ORS is given to replace ongoing losses from diarrhea or emesis. An additional 10 mL/kg of ORS is given for each stool. Fluid intake should be decreased if the patient appears fully hydrated earlier than expected or if periorbital edema develops. Breast-feeding should be allowed after rehydration in infants who are breast-fed; in other patients, their usual formula, milk, or feeding should be offered after rehydration. Along with its nutritional benefits, early refeeding decreases the duration of diarrhea. Most children can tolerate a lactose-containing formula, although some children benefit from a lactose-free formula if malabsorption is present.

Vomiting may occur during the first 2 hr of administration of ORS, but it usually does not prevent successful oral rehydration if the ORS is given in small amounts at short intervals (1 tsp every 1–2 min). Emesis usually lessens over time. The volume of ORS can be increased slowly, with an increasing interval between feedings. If sustained and severe vomiting occurs, intravenous therapy should be instituted. The patient's progress should be assessed frequently and changes in body weight monitored, if possible, to determine the degree of rehydration.

When rehydration is complete, maintenance therapy should be started. Patients with mild diarrhea usually can then be treated at home with 100 mL of ORS/kg/24 hr until the diarrhea stops. Breast-feeding or supplemental water intake should be maintained. Patients with more severe diarrhea require continued supervision. The volume of ORS ingested should equal the volume of stool losses. If stool volume cannot be measured, an intake of 10–15 mL of ORS/kg/hr is appropriate.

There is a significant difference in the sodium concentration between the World Health Organization (WHO) solution and the commercially available solutions that are generally used in the USA (see Table 55-1). Low-sodium solutions were advocated because hypernatremia was seen frequently in the USA when oral electrolyte solutions with sodium concentrations of 50 mEq/L or more were used to treat infantile diarrhea. Extensive use of ORS in many developing countries has shown hypernatremia to be a rare complication, probably because ORS has been used primarily for rehydration (previously, oral therapy was used primarily to prevent dehydration or for maintenance); because large amounts of water are ingested in addition to ORS, often a 2:1 ratio of ORS to H_2O; and because ORS has been administered under close supervision by trained personnel. The WHO ORS has also been effective in treating acute diarrheal illnesses in well-nourished children in developed countries. There is a risk of hypernatremia with the WHO ORS if it is used as a maintenance solution without supplemental water or formula. Several commercially available electrolyte solutions for oral use have been reformulated with a sodium concentration of approximately 50 mEq/L. These solutions are effective in the treatment of mild to moderate dehydration. Reduced-osmolality solutions (primarily reduced sodium and glucose) are associated with reduced stool output. Recipes to improve ORS have been developed that include adding substrates for sodium co-transport or substituting complex carbohydrates for the glucose (rice or other cereal-based ORS). Rice-based ORS is particularly effective in treating dehydration due to cholera.

Alam NH, Yunus M, Faruque ASG, et al: Symptomatic hyponatremia during treatment of dehydrating diarrheal disease with reduced osmdarity oral rehydration solution. *JAMA* 2006;296:567–573.

Dutta P, Mitra U, Manna B, et al: Double blind, randomised controlled clinical trial of hypo-osmolar oral rehydration salt solution in dehydrating acute diarrhoea in severely malnourished (marasmic) children. *Arch Dis Child* 2001;84:237–240.

Fonseca BK, Holdgate A, Craig JC: Enteral vs intravenous rehydration therapy for children with gastroenteritis: A meta-analysis of randomized controlled trials. *Arch Pediatr Adolesc Med* 2004;158:483–490.

Guarino A, Albano F, Guandalini S, et al: Oral rehydration: Toward a real solution. *J Pediatr Gastroenterol Nutr* 2001;33:S2–S12.

Hahn S, Kim S, Garner P: Reduced osmolarity oral rehydration solution for treating dehydration caused by acute diarrhoea in children. [Update of *Cochrane Database Syst Rev* 2001;(2):CD002847; PMID: 11406049]. *Cochrane Database Syst Rev* 2002:CD002847.

King CK, Glass R, Duggan C: Managing acute gastroenteritis among children: Oral rehydration, maintenance and nutritional therapy. *MMWR* 2003;52 (RR16):1–16.

Ozuah PO, Avner JR, Stein RE: Oral rehydration, emergency physicians, and practice parameters: A national survey. *Pediatrics* 2002;109:259–261.

Sarker SA, Mahalanabis D, Alam NH, et al: Reduced osmolarity oral rehydration solution for persistent diarrhea in infants: A randomized controlled clinical trial. *J Pediatr* 2001;138:532–538.

Spandorfer PR, Alessandrini EA, Joffe MD, et al: Oral versus intravenous rehydration of moderately dehydrated children: A randomized, controlled trial. *Pediatrics* 2005;115:295–301.

Zaman K, Yunus M, Rahman A, et al: Efficacy of a packaged rice oral rehydration solution among children with cholera and cholera-like illness. *Acta Paediatr* 2001;90:505–510.

55.2 • Diarrhea in Chronically Malnourished Children

Severe malnutrition complicated by diarrheal dehydration is common in tropical and subtropical countries and occurs occasionally in the temperate zones. Many of the signs normally used to assess hydration state and/or shock are unreliable in infants and children with severe malnutrition. Severe malnutrition is frequently accompanied by sepsis; thus, differentiating dehydration from septic shock may be important. In contrast to the finding of severe dehydration (see Table 54-1), children with septic shock may not have diarrhea, thirst, or sunken eyes, but may be hypothermic, hypoglycemic, or febrile. The electrocardiogram (ECG) frequently shows tachycardia, low amplitude, and flat or inverted T waves. Cardiac reserve seems lowered, and heart failure is a common complication.

Despite clinical signs of dehydration and reduced body water, urinary osmolality may be low in the chronically malnourished child. This defect in renal concentration may result from the relative absence of urea to contribute to a hypertonic milieu in the renal papillae, a defect associated with a low dietary protein intake and resulting in a failure of tubular conservation of water. The glomerular filtration rate is low, resulting in a smaller loss of water than would be expected otherwise. Renal concentrating ability returns after several days of high-protein feedings. The renal acidifying ability is also limited in patients with malnutrition.

Therapy should be adapted to meet the specific disturbances in body composition characteristic of the dehydrated *and* malnourished infant, in whom there appears to be overexpansion of the extracellular space accompanied by extracellular and presumably intracellular hypo-osmolality. Serum sodium, potassium, and magnesium levels tend to be low, and tetany occasionally may result from a magnesium or calcium deficiency. Serum protein levels are frequently <3.6 g/dL. The sodium content of all cells is high; the potassium and magnesium contents are low. Overall, these children are deficient in potassium and have elevated sodium levels; thus, they require a special ORS whose composition is described in Table 55-2 and is available commercially (ReSoMal).

Survival of the malnourished infant with diarrhea is limited by caloric deficit to a greater extent than by water and electrolyte deficit. These infants are also at much greater risk for infection, and intravenous therapy should be avoided, if possible. Reparative calories can be given by slow drip through an indwelling nasogastric tube in conjunction with oral or, when necessary, intravenous rehydration. If appetite is poor and vomiting and gastric distention are absent, feeding is begun early (30–40 calories/kg/24 hr), given by slow intragastric drip. Increases to 80–100 calories/kg/24 hr and 1–2 g of protein/kg/24 hr are made as fast as possible (24–48 hr). Ad libitum intake should be permitted in the succeeding days and weeks, up to 250–300 calories/kg/24 hr, and the diet should include an adequate supply of iron and copper.

TABLE 55-2. Composition of Oral Rehydration Salts Solution for Severely Malnourished Children (ReSoMal)

COMPONENT	CONCENTRATION (mmol/l)
Glucose	125
Sodium	45
Potassium	40
Chloride	70
Citrate	7
Magnesium	3
Zinc	0.3
Copper	0.045
Osmolarity	300

From the World Health Organization: *Management of Severe Malnutrition: A Manual for Physicians and Other Senior Health Workers.* 1999, p 11.

Initial parenteral therapy in profound dehydration is designed to improve the circulation and expand extracellular volume. For patients with edema, the quantity of fluid and the rate of administration may need to be readjusted from recommended levels to avoid over hydration and pulmonary edema. Blood should be given if the patient is in shock and severely anemic. Potassium salts can be given early if urine output is good. Clinical and ECG improvement may be more rapid with magnesium therapy. Seizures occurring during recovery from diarrhea complicating severe malnutrition may respond to magnesium.

Alam NH, Hamadani JD, Dewan N, et al: Efficacy and safety of a modified oral rehydration solution (ReSoMal) in the treatment of severely malnourished children with watery diarrhea. *J Pediatr* 2003;143:614–619.

Brown KH: Diarrhea and malnutrition. *J Nutr* 2003;133:328S–332S.

Caulfield LE, de Onis M, Blossner M, et al: Undernutrition as an underlying cause of child deaths associated with diarrhea, pneumonia, malaria, and measles. *Am J Clin Nutr* 2004;80:193–198.

Sharma A, Kumar R: Study on efficacy of WHO-ORS in malnourished children with acute dehydrating diarrhoea. *J Indian Med Assoc* 2003; 101:346.

World Health Organization: *Management of Severe Malnutrition: A Manual for Physicians and Other Senior Health Workers.* Geneva, WHO, 1999.

55.3 • Pyloric Stenosis

Also see Chapter 326.1.

Pyloric stenosis exemplifies the conditions requiring the correction of deficits associated with alkalosis. Therapy differs little from that for other causes of dehydration, except that potassium replacement should begin early, as soon as the child has urinated. These patients have a chloride-responsive metabolic alkalosis (see Chapter 52), and only volume repletion, via administration of sodium chloride and potassium chloride, will allow correction of the metabolic alkalosis. Correction of the hypochloremia and alkalosis by administering ammonium chloride without correcting the potassium deficit is not recommended.

Severe depletion of intracellular potassium results in the increased exchange of hydrogen ions for sodium in the distal nephrons of the kidney. The paradoxical presence of acid urine with systemic alkalosis should be interpreted as signifying a marked potassium deficit and a need to increase the amount of potassium used for repletion.

It is not uncommon for deficits to be replaced and for serum levels of electrolytes to return to normal within 6–12 hr. However, except in the mildly ill infant without signs of dehydration, it is preferable to delay surgery for at least 24–48 hr to achieve optimal readjustment of body functions. During this preparation period, adequate fluid therapy prevents dehydration, and the stomach may be decompressed by gentle suction.

Miozzari HH, Tonz M, von Vigier RO, et al: Fluid resuscitation in infantile hypertrophic pyloric stenosis. *Acta Paediatr* 2001;90:511–514.

Starinsky R, Klin B, Siman-Tov Y, et al: Does dehydration affect thickness of the pyloric muscle? An experimental study. *Ultrasound Med Biol* 2002;28:421–423.

55.4 • Perioperative Fluids

Preoperatively, preparing a patient who has no pre-existing deficit or in whom the deficit has been repaired consists mainly of supplying adequate carbohydrate for sustenance and protein sparing and the usual maintenance requirements of water and electrolytes. Young infants who are not vomiting should receive carbohydrate and electrolyte mixtures by mouth until 3 hr before the operation. Such fluids are readily absorbed from the gastrointestinal tract. Preparing the newborn involves certain unique hazards. Deficits of water and electrolytes from vomiting or from stasis caused by intestinal obstruction should be replaced before the surgery. In cases of intestinal obstruction, conjugated bilirubin may be deglucuronidated by intestinal enzymes; enterohepatic circulation of unconjugated bilirubin can then lead to high serum levels and kernicterus. Hypoprothrombinemia should be prevented by administering 1 mg of vitamin K.

During surgery, blood, plasma, saline, or other volume expanders may be given if blood loss, tissue trauma, third spacing, or excessive evaporative loss occurs. The magnitude of such losses is best judged by the experienced surgeon in the course of the procedure. **The most common error in administering parenteral fluid during and after surgery is excessive administration,** particularly of dextrose in water, rather than the use of isotonic solutions. Under most circumstances, little to no potassium need be administered during this time, because extensive tissue trauma or anoxia may result in the release of large amounts of intracellular potassium, with the potential of causing hyperkalemia. If shock occurs, acute renal failure may ensue, impairing the ability to eliminate through the renal route large amounts of released potassium.

Postoperatively, fluid intake should be limited for 24 hr. Thereafter, the usual maintenance therapy is resumed gradually. The water intake should not exceed 85% of maintenance, because of antidiuresis resulting from trauma, circulatory readjustment, general anesthesia, or narcotic pain relief, unless renal ability to concentrate the urine is limited, as in patients with sickle cell disease, chronic pyelonephritis, or obstructive uropathy. If the intake of water is not limited, whether given parenterally or orally, water intoxication may occur in association with severe hyponatremia and even fatal cerebral edema. This has been reported in post-tonsillectomy patients. Fluid therapy in the postoperative period largely depends on the complex but anticipated response of the body to trauma through modification of water and sodium excretion and the concomitant occurrence of complications from surgery. The patient's clinical condition dictates the final fluid and electrolyte requirements incurred as a result of these processes.

Postoperatively, some children have elevated blood antidiuretic hormone (ADH) levels due to syndrome of inappropriate ADH (SIADH) or to an appropriate response to fluid restriction and resultant volume contraction. If decreasing urine output after surgery is the result of SIADH, the patient is euvolemic and has a normal circulatory status, weight is stable to slightly increased, and urinary sodium excretion is elevated. If a child has oliguria related to third spacing and true depletion of intravascular volume, there is decreased urinary sodium excretion associated with clinical signs of hypovolemia, such as weight loss, tachycardia, changes in skin turgor and peripheral perfusion, and hypotension. Isotonic solutions are indicated in this setting.

Pait O, Lacroix F: Recent developments in the perioperative fluid management for the pediatric patient. *Curr Opin Anaesthesiol* 2006;19:268–277.

Part VII ■ Pediatric Drug Therapy

Chapter 56 ■ Pharmacogenetics, Pharmacogenomics, and Pharmacoproteomics

J. Steven Leeder, Gideon Koren, and Jacob V. Aranda

Interindividual variability in the response, intended or unanticipated, to similar doses of a given drug is an inherent characteristic of drug therapy. The role of genetic factors in drug disposition and response is termed **pharmacogenetics** and is due to variations in human genes that can lead to variability in drug responses in individual patients (Table 56-1). Pharmacogenetic variability contributes to the broad range of drug responses observed in children at any given age or developmental stage; pharmacogenetics will help to identify the right drug for the right patient (Fig. 56-1).

PHARMACOGENETICS, PHARMACOGENOMICS, AND THE CONCEPT OF PERSONALIZED MEDICINE

Certain adverse drug reactions, such as unusually prolonged respiratory muscle paralysis due to succinylcholine, hemolysis associated with antimalarial therapy, and isoniazid-induced neurotoxicity, are a consequence of inherited variations in enzyme activity. **Pharmacogenetics** is the study of genetically determined variations in drug response; the importance of genetic variation in drug disposition is illustrated by observations that the half-lives of several drugs are more similar in monozygotic twins than in dizygotic twins. In addition, environmental factors (diet, smoking status, concomitant drug or toxicant exposure), physiologic variables (age, sex, disease, pregnancy), and patient compliance contribute to variations in drug metabolism and response. **Therapeutic drug monitoring** programs have been the earliest application of personalized medicine; these programs recognize that all patients are unique and that the serum concentration-time data for an individual patient theoretically could be used to optimize pharmacotherapy. Routine therapeutic drug monitoring, however, does not necessarily translate to improved patient outcome in all situations.

The **pharmacokinetic** properties of a drug are determined by the genes that control its disposition in the body (absorption, distribution, metabolism, excretion), with drug-metabolizing enzymes and drug transporters assuming particularly important roles (Table 56-2). The functional consequences of genetic variations in several drug-metabolizing enzymes have been described in subjects representative of different ethnic groups. The most common clinical manifestation of pharmacogenetic variability in drug biotransformation is an increased risk of concentration-dependent toxicity due to reduced clearance and drug accumulation. In addition, the concentration-effect relationship (**pharmacodynamics**) is more relevant for optimizing drug efficacy. The pharmacogenetics of drug receptors and other target proteins involved in signal transduction or disease pathogenesis can also be expected to contribute significantly to interindividual variability in drug response.

Pharmacogenomics represents the marriage of pharmacology and genomics and can be defined as the study of the **genome-wide** response to low molecular weight compounds administered with therapeutic intent; the goal is to find the right drug for the right disease.

DEFINITION OF PHARMACOGENETIC TERMS

All copies of a specific gene present within a population may not have identical nucleotide sequences (**genetic polymorphisms**); these contribute to the variability observed in that population. The presence of different nucleotides at a given position within a gene is a **single-nucleotide polymorphism (SNP)** [see Chapter 82]. **Haplotypes** are collections of SNPs and other allelic variations that are located close to each other and when inherited together create a catalog of haplotypes, or **HapMap.** In genes in which polymorphisms are detected, alternative forms of the gene are called **alleles.** When the alleles at a particular gene locus on both chromosomes are identical, a **homozygous** state exists, whereas the term **heterozygous** refers to the situation in which different alleles are present at the same gene locus. **Genotype** refers to an individual's genetic constitution, whereas the observable characteristics or physical manifestations constitute the **phenotype,** which is the net consequence of genetic and environmental effects (see Chapters 78–83). Pharmacogenetics focuses on the phenotypic consequences of allelic variation in single genes. **Pharmacogenetic polymorphism** is a monogenic trait caused by the presence (in the same population) of >1 allele (at the same locus) and >1 phenotype with regard to drug interaction with the organism. The key elements of pharmacogenetic polymorphisms are heritability, the involvement of a single gene locus, and the fact that distinct phenotypes are observed within the population only after drug challenge. Furthermore, ethnicity is another potential genetic determinant of drug variability. Chinese patients who are HLA-B*1502-positive have an increased risk of carbamazepine-induced Stevens-Johnson syndrome; white patients who are HLA-B*5701-positive have an increased risk of hypersensitivity to abacavir (Table 56-3).

DEVELOPMENTAL OR PEDIATRIC PHARMACOGENETICS AND PHARMACOGENOMICS

Our current understanding of pharmacogenetic principles involves enzymes responsible for drug **biotransformation.** Individuals are classified as being "fast," "rapid," or "extensive" metabolizers at 1 end of the spectrum, and "slow" or "poor" metabolizers at the other end of a continuum that may, depending on the particular enzyme, also include an "intermediate" metabolizer group. Pediatric patients have more complexity because fetuses and newborns may be phenotypically "slow" or "poor" metabolizers for certain drug-metabolizing pathways, acquiring a phenotype consistent with their genotype at some point later in the developmental process as those pathways mature (glucuronidation, some cytochrome P450 [CYP] activities) [see Chapters 57, 96, and 97]. It is apparent that not all infants acquire drug metabolism activity at the same rate due to the interaction between genetics and environmental factors. Interindividual variability in the trajectory (rate and extent) of acquired drug biotransformation capacity may be considered a **developmental phenotype** (Fig. 56-2), and it helps to explain the considerable variability in some CYP activities observed immediately after birth.

TABLE 56-1. Examples of Effects of Gene Polymorphisms on Drug Response

GENE	ENZYME/TARGET	DRUG	CLINICAL RESPONSE
CYP2D6	Cytochrome P450 2D6	Codeine	Individuals homozygous for an inactivating mutation do not metabolize codeine to morphine and thus experience no analgesic effect; rapid metabolizers may experience opiate toxicity
CYP2C9	Cytochrome P450 2C9	Warfarin	Individuals heterozygous for a polymorphism need a lower dose of warfarin to maintain anticoagulation
NAT2	*N*-Acetyltransferase 2	Isoniazid, hydralazine	Individuals homozygous for "slow acetylation" polymorphisms are more susceptible to isoniazid toxicity, or hydralazine-induced systemic lupus erythematosus
TPMT	Thiopurine S-methyltransferase	Azathioprine	Individuals homozygous for an inactivating mutation have severe toxicity if treated with standard doses of azathioprine; rapid metabolism causes undertreatment
ADRB2	β-Adrenergic receptor	Albuterol	Individuals homozygous for a polymorphism get worse with regular use of albuterol
KCNE2	Potassium channel, voltage gated	Erythromycin	Individuals heterozygous for a polymorphism are more susceptible to life-threatening arrhythmias
SUR1	Sulfonylurea receptor 1	Sulfonylureas	Individuals heterozygous for a polymorphism exhibit diminished sensitivity in sulfonylurea-stimulated insulin secretion
F5	Coagulation factor V (Leiden)	Oral contraceptives	Individuals heterozygous for a polymorphism are at increased risk for venous thrombosis
RYR1	Calcium ion release channel	Halothane, succinylcholine	Malignant hyperthermia
BCHE	Butyrylcholinesterase	Succinylcholine	Prolonged paralysis
G6PD	Glucose-6-phosphate dehydrogenase	Primaquine (others)	Hemolysis
CYP3A	Cytochrome P450	Grapefruit juice	Moderate inhibitor of intestinal (presystemic) first pass metabolism of many drugs*
DRD3	Dopamine D_3 receptor	Antipsychotic agents	Tardive dyskinesia
DHFR	Dihydrofolate reductase	Methotrexate	Drug resistance
TOP1	Topoisomerase 1	Anthracycline agents	Drug resistance
EGFR	Epidermal growth factor receptor	Gefitinib	Drug resistance

*Albendazole, benzodiazepines, buspirone, carbamazepine, cyclosporine, fexofenadine, fluoxetine, indinavir, itraconazole, sertraline, sirolimus, tacrolimus, verapamil, warfarin.
Modified from Jorde LB, Carey JC, Bamshad MJ, et al: *Medical Genetics*, 3rd ed. St. Louis, Mosby, 2006, p 157.

TABLE 56-2. Some Important Relationships Between Drugs and Cytochrome P450 (CYP) Enzymes* and P-Glycoprotein (P-gp) Transporter

ENZYME	DRUG SUBSTRATES	INHIBITORS	INDUCERS
CYP1A2	Caffeine, clomipramine (*Anafranil*†), clozapine (*Clozaril*†), theophylline	Cimetidine (*Tagamet*†) Flucoxamine (*Luvox*†) Ciprofloxacin (*Cipro*)	Omeprazole (*Prilosec*†) Tobacco
CYP2C9	Diclofenac (*Voltaren*†), ibuprofen (*Motrin*†), piroxicam (*Feldene*†), losartan (*Cozaar*), irbesartan (*Avapro*), celecoxib (*Celebrex*), tolbutamide (*Orinase*†), warfarin (*Coumadin*†), phenytoin (*Dilantin*)	Fluconazole (*Diflucan*) Fluvastatin (*Lescol*) Amiodarone (*Cordarone*) Zafirlukast (*Accolate*)	Rifampin (*Rifadin*†)
CYP2C19	Omeprazole, lansoprazole (*Prevacid*), pantoprazole (*Protonix*), (S)-mephenytoin, nelfinavir (*Viracept*), diazepam (*Valium*†), voriconazole (*Vfend*)	Cimetidine Fluvoxamine	Rifampin
CYP2D6	**CNS-active agents:** Atomoxetine (*Strattera*), amitriptyline (*Elavil*†), desipramine (*Norpramin*†), imipramine (*Tofranil*†), paroxetine (*Paxil*), haloperidol (*Haldol*†), risperidone (*Risperdal*), thioridazine (*Mellaril*†) **Antiarrhythmic agents:** Mexiletine (*Mexitil*), propafenone (*Rythmol*) **β Blockers:** Propranolol (*Inderal*†), metoprolol (*Lopressor*†), timolol (*Blocadren*†) **Narcotics:** Codeine, dextromethorphan, hydrocodone (*Vicodin*†) Tamoxifen (*Nolvadex*)	Amidoarone (*Cordarone*†) Cimetidine Fluoxetine (*Prozac*†) Terbinafine Paroxetine (*Paxil*) Quinidine (*Quinidex*†) Ritonavir	
CYP3A4	**Calcium channel blockers:** Diltiazem (*Cardizem*†), felodipine (*Plendil*), nimodipine (*Nimotop*), nifedipine (*Adalat*†), nisoldipine (*Sular*), nitrendipine, verapamil (*Calan*†) **Immunosupressive agents:** Cyclosporine A (*Sandimmune, Neoral*†), tacrolimus (*Prograf*) **Steroids:** Budesonide (*Pulmicort*), cortisol, 17β-estradiol, progesterone, testosterone **Macrolide antibiotics:** Clarithromycin (*Biaxin*), erythromycin (*Ertythrocin*†), troleandomycin (*TAO*) **Anticancer agents:** Cyclophosphamide (*Cytoxan*†), gefitinib (*Iressa*), ifosfamide (*Ifex*), tamoxifen, vincristine (*Oncovin*†), vinblastine (*Velban*†), **Benzodiazepines:** Alprazolam (*Xanax*†), midazolam *Versed*†), triazolam (*Halcion*†) **Opioids:** Alfentanyl (*Alfenta*†), fentanyl (*Sublimaze*†), sufentanil (*Sufenta*†) **HMG-CoA reductase inhibitors:** Lovastatin (*Mevacor*†, simvastitin (*Zocor*), atorvastatin (*Lipitor*) **HIV protease inhibitors:** Indinavir (*Crixivan*), nelfinavir, ritonavir (*Norvir*), saquinavir (*Invirase, Fortovase*), amprenavir (*Agenerase*) **Others:** Quinidine (*Quinidex*†), sildenafil (*Viagra*), eletriptan (*Relpax*), ziprasidone (*Geodon*)	Amiodarone Clarithromycin Erythromycin Fluconazole Grapefruit juice Imatinib Itraconazole (*Sporanox*) Ketoconazole (*Nizoral*†) Nefazodone (*Serzone*) Ritonavir‡ Indinavir Troleandomycin	Barbiturates Carbamazepine (*Tegretol*†) Efavirenz (*Sustiva*) Nevirapine (*Viramune*) Phenytoin (*Dilantin*†) Rifampin Ritonavir‡ St. John's wort
P-gp	Aldosterone, amprenavir, atorvastatin, cyclosporine, dexamethasone (*Decadron*†), digoxin (*Lanoxin*†), diltiazem, domperidone (*Motilium*), doxorubicin (*Adriamycin*†), erythromycin, etoposide (*Vepesid*), fexofenadine (*Allegra*), hydrocortisone, indinavir, ivermectin (*Stromectol*), lovastatin loperamide (*Imodium*†), nelfinavir, ondansetron (*Zofran*), paclitaxel (*Taxol*), quinidine, saquinavir, simvastatin, verapamil, vinblastine, vincristine	Amiodarone Carvedilol (*Coreg*) Clarithromycin Cyclosporine Erythromycin Itraconazole Ketoconazole Quinidine Ritonavir‡ Tamoxifen Verapamil	Amprenavir Clotrimazole (*Mycelex*†) Phenothiazine Rifampin Ritonavir‡ St. John's wort

*www.drug-interactions.com.
†Also available generically.
‡Can be both an inhibitor and an inducer.
From *Med Lett* 2003;45:47.
CNS, central nervous system.

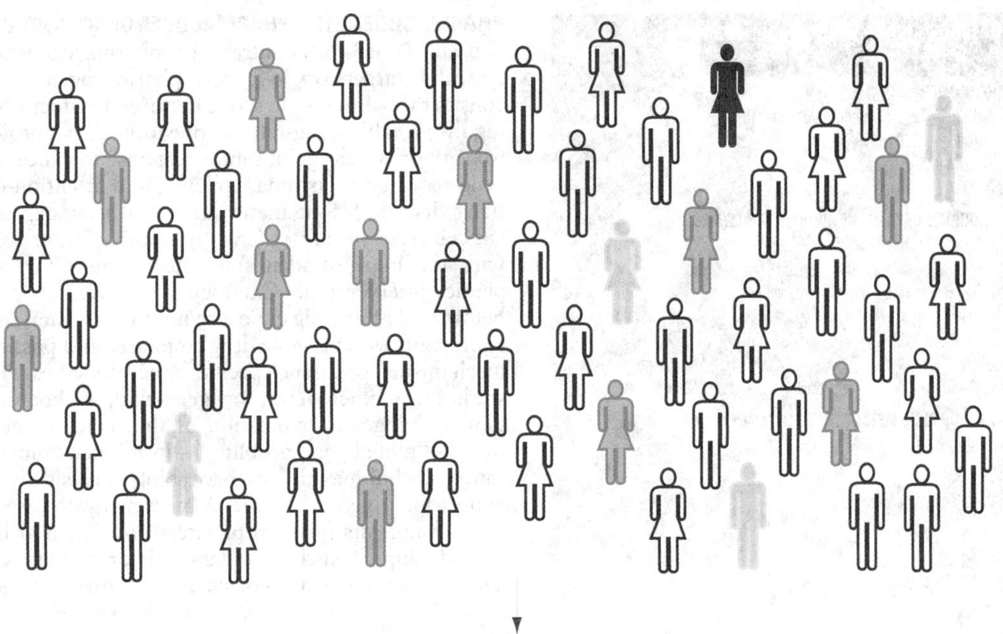

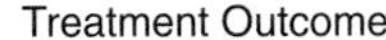

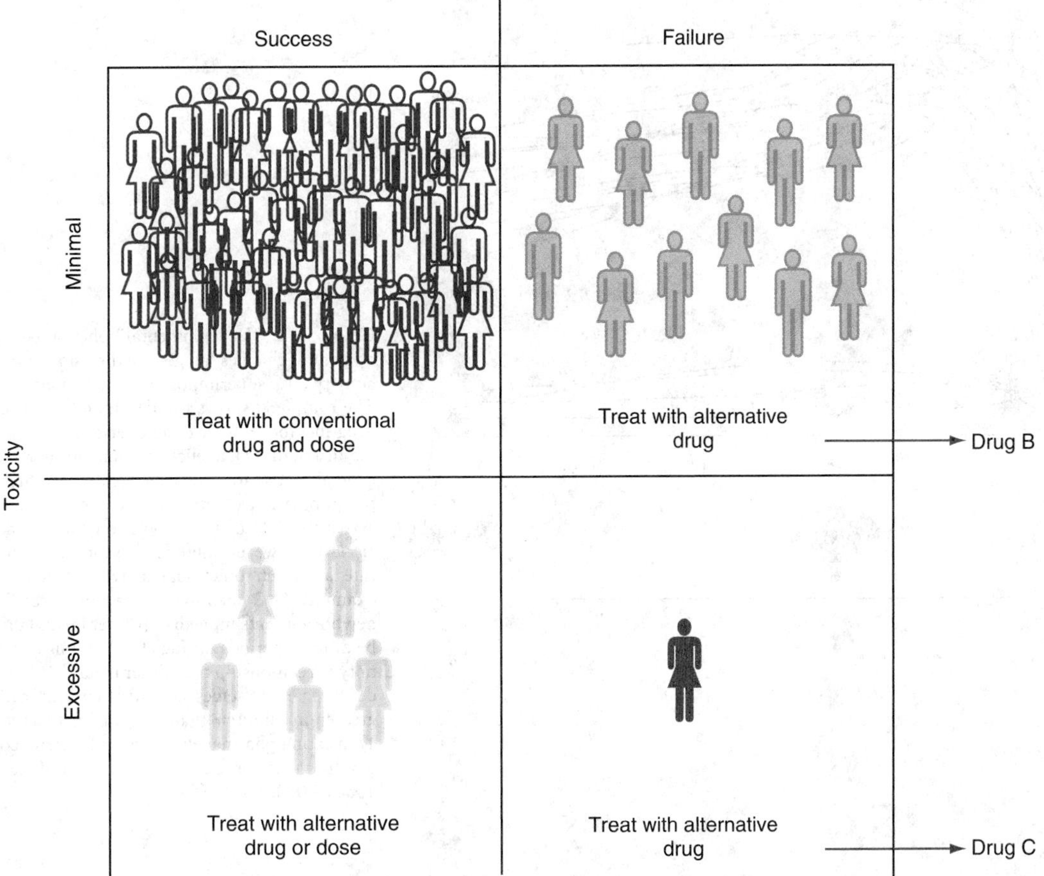

Figure 56-1. The promise of genomic medicine to human health and disease. The goal of personalized medicine will be achieved by identifying subgroups of patients who will respond favorably to a given drug with a minimum of side effects, as well as those who will not respond or who will show excessive toxicity with standard doses. A further benefit of pharmacogenomics will be the ability to select the most appropriate alternative drug for patients who cannot be treated successfully with conventional drugs and doses. (Adapted from Yaffe SJ, Aranda JV: Neonatal and Pediatric Pharmacology, 3/e. Philadelphia: Lippincott Williams & Wilkins, 2004.)

TABLE 56-3. Internet Resources for Pharmacogenetics and Pharmacogenomics*

INTRODUCTION TO PHARMACOGENOMICS	
http://www.ornl.gov/TechResources/Human_Genome/medicine/pharma.html	
http://www.ama-assn.org/ama/pub/category/2306.html	
http://www.ncbi.nlm.nih.gov/About/primer/pharm.html	
http://pubs.acs.org/cen/coverstory/7933/7933pharmacogenomics.html	
PHARMACOGENETICS: ALLELIC VARIANTS OF DRUG METABOLIZING ENZYMES	
CYP2C9	http://www.imm.ki.se/CYPalleles/cyp2c9.htm
CYP2C19	http://www.imm.ki.se/CYPalleles/cyp2c19.htm
CYP2D6	http://www.imm.ki.se/CYPalleles/cyp2d6.htm
CYP3A4	http://www.imm.ki.se/CYPalleles/cyp3a4.htm
CYP3A5	http://www.imm.ki.se/CYPalleles/cyp3a5.htm
UGTs	http://som.flinders.edu.au/FUSA/ClinPharm/UGT/allele_table.html
NAT1 and NAT2	http://www.louisville.edu/medschool/pharmacology/NAT.html
PHARMACOGENETICS: SUBSTRATES OF DRUG METABOLIZING ENZYMES	
http://www.drug-interactions.com	
INTRODUCTION TO PROTEOMICS	
http://www.ama-assn.org/ama/pub/category/3668.html	
http://www.e-proteomics.net	

*All sites were accessible on March 31, 2006.

PHARMACOGENETIC, PHARMACOGENOMIC, AND PHARMACOPROTEOMIC TOOLS. In contrast to pharmacogenetic studies that typically target single genes, pharmacogenomic analyses are considerably broader in scope because they focus on complex and highly variable drug-related phenotypes (valproic acid hepatotoxicity or weight gain; tumor response to cancer chemotherapy; drug response in asthma, epilepsy, and attention-deficit/hyperactivity disorder). Systematic surveys of gene expression in different cell types (tumor cells vs "normal" cells) are often conducted with the hope of identifying new targets for pharmacotherapeutic intervention. Cataloging differential gene expression before and after drug exposure has the potential to correlate gene expression with variable drug responses and possibly uncover the mechanisms of tissue-specific drug toxicities. These types of studies use **microarray,** or **gene-chip, technology** to monitor global changes in expression of thousands of genes simultaneously—"global gene profiling"—in marked contrast to the laboratory technique of Northern blot analysis that studies gene expression 1 gene at a time. A microarray consists of a matrix of DNA fragments (probes) precisely positioned at high density on a solid support, such as a glass slide or a filter (see Chapter 79). The probes serve as molecular detectors for messenger RNA (mRNA) in the sample. Common experimental designs involve

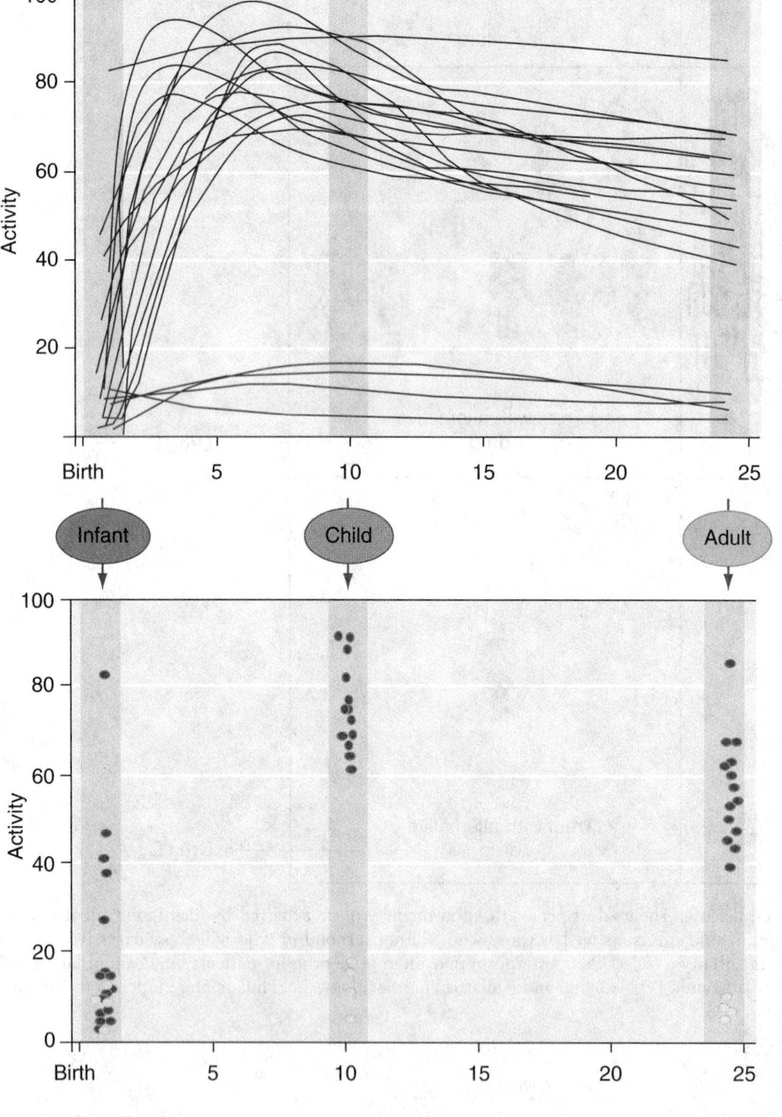

Figure 56-2. "Developmental" phenotypes. Variability in developmental changes in gene expression and functional enzyme activity are superimposed on pharmacogenetic determinants. The *top panel* shows the developmental profile of a theoretical drug-metabolizing enzyme over a 25 yr span in 20 subjects. At maturity (adults), allelic variation within the coding region of the gene gives rise to 2 distinct phenotypes, high activity in 92% of the population ("extensive metabolizers"; *red circles*) and low activity in 8% of the population ("poor metabolizers"; *yellow circles*). However, there is also interindividual variability in the rate at which functional activity is acquired after birth. For example, the 2 phenotypes may not be readily distinguishable in newborn infants immediately after birth. Furthermore, there may be discrete periods during childhood in which the genotype-phenotype relationship may differ from that observed in adults (e.g., developmental stages at which enzyme activity appears to be greater in children than in adults). (Adapted from Leeder JS: Translating pharmacogenetics and pharmacogenomics into drug development for clinical pediatric and beyond. *Drug Discov Today* 2004;9:567–573.)

labeling mRNA (or complementary DNA [cDNA]) from a control sample with 1 fluorescent dye and mRNA or cDNA from the disease or treatment sample with a 2nd fluorescent dye, using an experimental strategy that allows expression to be compared with the sample pair. The expression pattern of thousands of genes can be analyzed in a single sample with the underlying hypothesis that the measured intensity for each arrayed gene represents its relative expression level. DNA chips can also be made that focus on specific polymorphisms in a particular enzyme system. The FDA has approved a chip for the P450 system enzymes CYP2D6 and CYP2C19, which may be responsible for 25% of all drug metabolism in humans. A 2nd expression profiling technique, **serial analysis of gene expression (SAGE)**, overcomes technical limitations of microarrays related to their ability to conduct comparative data analyses and effectively detect low-abundance transcripts.

Proteomic studies use many different techniques to detect, quantify, and identify proteins in a sample (**expression proteomics**), and to characterize protein function in terms of activity and protein-protein or protein–nucleic acid interactions (**functional proteomics**). Two-dimensional electrophoresis (2DE) coupled with mass spectral detection (2DE-MS) is the mainstay of expression proteomics. Protein "spots" of interest are "picked"; digested with a proteolytic enzyme, such as trypsin; and identified by mass spectrometry. The data generated are compared with theoretically derived peptide mass databases for protein identification.

DEVELOPMENTAL PHARMACOGENETICS OF DRUG BIOTRANSFORMATION: APPLICATIONS TO PEDIATRIC DRUG THERAPY PRACTICE

The major consequence of pharmacogenetic polymorphism in drug-metabolizing enzymes is concentration-dependent toxicity due to impaired drug clearance. In certain cases, reduced conversion of prodrug to therapeutically active compounds is also of clinical importance (see Table 56-1). Chemical modification of drugs via biotransformation reactions generally results in termination of biologic activity through decreased affinity for receptors or other cellular targets as well as more rapid elimination from the body. The process of drug biotransformation can be very complex, but is characterized by 3 important features. First is the concept of broad substrate specificity—a single isozyme may metabolize a large variety of chemically diverse compounds. Second, many different enzymes may be involved in the biotransformation of a single drug (enzyme multiplicity). Finally, a given drug may undergo several different reaction types. One example of this product multiplicity is racemic warfarin, where at least 7 hydroxylated metabolites have been identified and are produced by different CYP isoforms.

Drug biotransformation reactions are conveniently classified into 2 main types, phase I and phase II reactions, which occur sequentially (see Chapter 57). Phase I reactions introduce or reveal (by oxidation, reduction, or hydrolysis) a functional group within the substrate drug molecule that serves as a site for a phase II conjugation reaction. Conjugation with endogenous substrates, such as acetate, glucuronic acid, glutathione, glycine, and sulfate, further increases the polarity of an intermediate metabolite and thereby enhances its renal excretion. Interindividual variability in drug biotransformation activity is a consequence of the complex interplay among genetic (genotype, sex, race or ethnic background) and environmental (diet, disease, concurrent medication, other xenobiotic exposure) factors. The pathway and rate of a given compound's biotransformation is a function of each individual's unique phenotype with respect to the forms and amounts of drug-metabolizing enzymes expressed.

The **CYPs**, quantitatively the most important of the **phase I enzymes**, are heme-containing proteins that catalyze the metabolism of many lipophilic endogenous substances (steroids, fatty acids, fat-soluble vitamins, prostaglandins, leukotrienes, thromboxanes) and exogenous compounds, such as drugs. CYP nomenclature is based on evolutionary considerations and uses the root symbol *CYP* for *cytochrome P450*. CYPs that share at least 40% homology are grouped into families denoted by an Arabic number after the *CYP* root. Subfamilies, designated by a letter, appear to represent clusters of highly related genes. Members of the human CYP2 family, for example, have >67% amino acid sequence homology. Individual P450s in a subfamily are numbered sequentially (CYP3A4, CYP3A5). CYPs that have been identified as being important in human drug metabolism are predominantly found in the CYP1, CYP2, and CYP3 gene families. Enzyme activity may be induced or inhibited by various agents (see Table 56-2).

Phase II enzymes include arylamine *N*-acetyltransferases (NAT1, NAT2), glucuronosyl transferases (UGTs), epoxide hydrolase, glutathione *S*-transferases (GSTs), sulfotransferases (SULTs), and methyltransferases (catechol *O*-methyltransferase, thiopurine *S*-methyltransferase, several *N*-methyltransferases). Like the CYPs, UGTs, SULTs, and GSTs are gene families with multiple individual isoforms, each having its own preferred substrates, mode of regulation, and tissue-specific pattern of expression.

For most CYPs, genotype-phenotype relationships are influenced by development in that fetal expression is limited (with the exception of CYP3A7) and functional activity is acquired postnatally in isoform-specific patterns. Clearance of some compounds appears to be greater in children relative to adults, obscuring the correlation between genotype and phenotype in neonatal life through adolescence.

CYP2D6. The *CYP2D6* gene locus is highly polymorphic, with >75 allelic variants identified to date (*http://www.imm.ki.se/CYPalleles/cyp2d6.htm;* see Table 56-2). Individual alleles are designated by the gene name *(CYP2D6)* followed by an asterisk, and an Arabic number; *CYP2D6*1* designates, by convention, the fully functional wild-type allele. Allelic variants are the consequence of point mutations, single base pair deletions or additions, gene rearrangements, or deletion of the entire gene, resulting in a reduction or complete loss of activity. Inheritance of 2 recessive loss-of-function alleles results in the **poor-metabolizer phenotype**, which is found in approximately 5–10% of white subjects and approximately 1–2% of Asian subjects. In white subjects, the *3, *4, *5, and *6 alleles are the most common loss-of-function alleles and account for approximately 98% of poor-metabolizer phenotypes. In contrast, CYP2D6 activity on a population basis tends to be lower in Asian and African-American populations due to a lower frequency of nonfunctional alleles (*3, *4, *5, and *6) **and** a relatively high frequency of population-selective alleles that are associated with decreased activity relative to the wild-type *CYP2D6*1* allele. The *CYP2D6*10* allele occurs at a frequency of approximately 50% in Asians, whereas *CYP2D6*17* and *CYP2D6*29* occur at relatively high frequencies in subjects of black African origin. Homozygosity for the **10* allele is associated with decreased clearance of CYP2D6 substrates, such as metoprolol and nortriptyline.

CYP2D6 is involved in the biotransformation of >40 therapeutic entities, including several β-receptor antagonists, antiarrhythmics, antidepressants, antipsychotics, and morphine derivatives (for an updated list, see *http://medicine.iupui.edu/flockhart;* see Table 56-2). Selective serotonin reuptake inhibitors (SSRIs; fluoxetine, paroxetine, sertraline), atomoxetine, codeine, and dextromethorphan are commonly encountered in pediatrics. Very limited CYP2D6 activity is present in fetal liver in vitro (≈1% of adult values), but CYP2D6 protein is detectable in all samples from newborns. Thereafter, both CYP2D6 protein and catalytic activity progressively increase over the 1st 28 days of life to 20% of activity observed in adult samples. In contrast, in vivo data derived from a longitudinal phenotyping study conducted over the 1st year of life using dextromethorphan as a probe compound suggest that the CYP2D6 phenotype is concordant with genotype by 2 wk of age. Dextromethorphan phenotyping data from older children suggest that CYP2D6 catalytic activity in children is comparable to that in adults by at least 10 yr of age, and probably much earlier. There are insufficient data from pharmacokinetic studies to determine the age at which the clearance of CYP2D6 substrates is comparable to that observed in adults.

One consequence of CYP2D6 developmental pharmacogenetics may be the syndrome of irritability, tachypnea, tremors, jitteriness, increased muscle tone, and temperature instability in neonates born to mothers receiving SSRIs during pregnancy. Controversy currently exists as to whether these symptoms reflect a neonatal withdrawal (hyposerotonergic) state or represent manifestations of serotonin toxicity analogous to the hyperserotonergic state associated with the SSRI-induced serotonin syndrome in adults (see Chapter 106). Delayed expression of CYP2D6 (and CYP3A4) in the 1st few wk of life is consistent with a hyperserotonergic state due to delayed clearance of paroxetine and fluoxetine (CYP2D6) or sertraline (CYP3A4) in neonates exposed to these compounds during pregnancy. Furthermore, decreases in plasma SSRI concentrations and resolution of symptoms would be expected with increasing postnatal age and maturation of these pathways. Given that treatment of a "withdrawal" reaction may include administration of an SSRI, there is considerable potential for increased toxicity in affected neonates. Resolution of the hyperserotonergic vs hyposerotonergic pathogenesis is essential for appropriate management of SSRI-induced neonatal adaptation syndromes. Until further data are available, it would be prudent to consider newborns and infants younger than 28 days of age as CYP2D6 poor metabolizers.

In older children, drug accumulation and resultant concentration-dependent toxicities in CYP2D6 genotypic poor metabolizers should be anticipated as they are in adults due to the risk of significant morbidity and mortality. Experience with paroxetine shows that the risk of drug accumulation is not necessarily limited to the poor-metabolizer phenotype. Although the pharmacokinetics of the CYP2D6 substrates paroxetine and nefazodone correlate with the CYP2D6 phenotype in children and adolescents 7–17 yr of age, chronic dosing of paroxetine may lead to greater than anticipated drug accumulation in children classified as CYP2D6 extensive metabolizers. In depressed children and adolescents as well as in adults, there is a disproportionate increase in peak concentration and area under the serum concentration-time curve at higher dose levels. However, nonlinearity is more prominent in patients who are CYP2D6 extensive metabolizers, especially those with gene duplication events and 3 or more functional alleles. The largest decreases in paroxetine clearance observed with ascending dose are seen in patients who have the greatest clearance at the initial dose level (10 mg/day) and are predicted to have the greatest CYP2D6 activity, based on CYP2D6 genotype. This rather paradoxical effect is best explained in the context of recent data from in vitro studies. One proposed mechanism involves oxidation of paroxetine within the CYP2D6 active site to form a reactive intermediate that is associated with irreversible modification of the CYP2D6 protein in or near the active site. The greater the initial CYP2D6 activity, the greater the burden of reactive metabolite formation and thereby the greater the loss of CYP2D6 catalytic activity. As a consequence, as the paroxetine dose is increased in patients with higher initial drug clearance, the risk of excessive drug accumulation escalates disproportionately.

Theoretically, younger children may experience decreased efficacy or therapeutic failure with drugs such as codeine and tramadol that are dependent on functional CYP2D6 activity for conversion to the pharmacologically active species. Infants and children appear capable of converting codeine to morphine, achieving morphine : codeine ratios comparable to those of adults. However, in one study, morphine and its metabolites were not detected in 36% of children receiving codeine and codeine analgesia was found to be unreliable in the studied pediatric population and not related to the CYP2D6 phenotype. Ultrarapid CYP2D6 metabolism of codeine may result in opiate intoxication. CYP2D6 catalyzes the O-demethylation of codeine to morphine. Ultrarapid metabolism of codeine results in high serum and breast milk concentrations of morphine and may have adverse effects in the breastfed neonate.

CYP2C9. Although several clinically useful compounds are substrates for CYP2C9 *(http://medicine.iupui.edu/flockhart)* [see Table 56-2], the effects of allelic variation are most profound for drugs with a narrow therapeutic index, such as phenytoin, warfarin, and tolbutamide. In vitro studies show a progressive increase in CYP2C9 expression from 1–2% of mature levels in the 1st trimester to approximately 30% at term. Considerable variability (≈35-fold) in expression is apparent over the 1st 5 mo of life, with approximately ½ of the samples exhibiting values equivalent to those observed in adults. One interpretation of these data is broad interindividual variability in the rate at which CYP2C9 expression is acquired after birth, and in general, the ontogeny of CYP2C9 activity in vivo, as inferred from pharmacokinetic studies of phenytoin in newborns, is consistent with the in vitro results. The apparent half-life of phenytoin is prolonged (approximately 75 hr) in preterm infants, but decreases to approximately 20 hr in term newborns during the 1st yr of life. By 2 wk of age, the half-life has further declined to 8 hr. The appearance of concentration-dependent (saturable) metabolism of phenytoin, reflecting the functional acquisition of CYP2C9 activity, does not appear until approximately 10 days of age. The maximal velocity of phenytoin metabolism has been reported to decrease from an average of 14 mg/kg/day in infants to 8 mg/kg/day in adolescents, which may reflect changes in the ratio of liver mass to total body mass observed over this period of development, as has been observed for warfarin.

At least 24 allelic variants of *CYP2C9* have been reported, but not all have been evaluated for their functional consequences. The *CYP2C9*2* allele is associated with approximately 5.5-fold decreased intrinsic clearance for *S*-warfarin relative to the wild-type enzyme. Allelic variations resulting in amino acid changes within the enzyme active site, such as the *CYP2C9*3, CYP2C9*4,* and *CYP2C9*5* alleles, are associated with activities that are approximately 5% of the wild-type protein. Approximately ⅓ of the white population carries a variant *CYP2C9* allele (*2 and *3 alleles, most commonly), whereas the *2 and *3 alleles are virtually nonexistent in African-American, Chinese, Japanese, or Korean populations. In contrast, the *5 allele has been detected in African-Americans, but not in white subjects. The risk of bleeding complications in patients treated with warfarin and with concentration-dependent phenytoin toxicity is most pronounced for individuals with a *CYP2C9*3/*3* genotype. Although the relationship between the *CYP2C9* genotype and warfarin dosing and pharmacokinetics has not been as extensively studied in children, consequences of allelic variation can be expected to be similar to those observed in adults.

CYP2C19. In vitro, CYP2C19 protein and catalytic activity can be detected at levels representing 12–15% of mature values by 8 wk gestation and remain essentially unchanged throughout gestation and at birth. Over the 1st 5 mo of postnatal age, CYP2C19 activity increases linearly. Adult levels are achieved by 10 yr of age, although variability in expression is estimated to be approximately 21-fold between 5 mo and 10 yr of age. The major source of this variability likely is pharmacogenetic in nature. The CYP2C19 poor-metabolizer phenotype (also known as *mephenytoin hydroxylase deficiency*) is present in 3–5% of the white population and 20–25% of Asians. Although 19 variant alleles have been reported to date, the 2 most common variant alleles, *CYP2C19*2* and *CYP2C19*3*, result from single base substitutions that introduce premature stop codons and, consequently, truncated polypeptide chains that possess no functional activity. Despite the increases in CYP2C19 activity observed in vitro over the 1st 5 mo of life, the results of an in vivo phenotyping study with omeprazole in Mexican children implied that 17% of infants younger than 4 mo of age could be classified as poor metabolizers, whereas none were detected beyond that point. In contrast, 20% of children 3–9 mo old were classified as ultrarapid metabolizers compared with 6% of infants 1–3 mo of age. For omeprazole, pharmacokinetic parameters comparable to those observed in adults are achieved by 2 yr of age.

In Japanese adults treated with lansoprazole, amoxicillin, and clarithromycin for *Helicobacter pylori* infection, the eradication rate for CYP2C19 poor metabolizers (97.8%) and heterozygous extensive metabolizers (1 functional *CYP2C19* allele; 92.1%) was significantly greater than that observed in homozygous extensive metabolizers (72.7%). Of the 35 patients in whom initial treatment did not eradicate *H. pylori,* 34 had at least 1 functional *CYP2C19* allele and eradication could be achieved with higher lansoprazole doses in almost all cases. Given that the frequency of the functional *CYP2C19*1* allele is considerably greater in white subjects (≈0.84 [84%]) compared with Japanese subjects (≈0.55 [55%]), eradication failure can be expected to occur more frequently in whites. Because proton pump inhibitors are also widely used clinically in pediatrics, pharmacogenetic as well as developmental considerations should guide dosing strategies in children.

CYP3A4, CYP3A5, AND CYP3A7. The CYP3A subfamily consists of 4 members in humans (CYPs 3A4, 3A5, 3A7, and 3A43) and is quantitatively the most important group of CYPs in terms of human hepatic drug biotransformation. These isoforms catalyze the oxidation of many different therapeutic entities, several of which are of potential importance to pediatric practice (for an updated list, see *http://medicine.iupui.edu/flockhart;* see Table 56-2). CYP3A7 is the predominant CYP isoform in fetal liver and can be detected in embryonic liver as early as 50–60 days' gestation. CYP3A4, the major CYP3A isoform in adults, is essentially absent in fetal liver, but increases gradually throughout childhood. Over the 1st 6 mo of life, CYP3A7 expression exceeds that of CYP3A4, although its catalytic activity toward most CYP3A substrates is rather limited compared with that of CYP3A4. CYP3A4 is also abundantly expressed in intestine, where it contributes significantly to the 1st-pass metabolism of orally administered substrates, such as midazolam. CYP3A5 is polymorphically expressed and is present in approximately 25% of adult liver samples studied in vitro.

Several methods have been proposed to measure CYP3A activity. Using these various phenotyping probes, CYP3A4 activity has been reported to vary widely (up to 50-fold) among individuals, but the population distributions of activity are essentially unimodal and evidence for polymorphic activity has been elusive. Although 20 allelic variants have been identified *(http://www.imm.ki.se/CYPalleles/cyp3a4.htm)*, most occur relatively infrequently and do not appear to be of clinical importance. Of interest to pediatrics is the *CYP3A4*1B* allele present in the *CYP3A4* promoter region. The clinical significance of this allelic variant appears limited with respect to drug biotransformation activity, despite being associated with 2-fold increased activity over the wild-type *CYP3A4*1* allele in in vitro assays. Although there does not appear to be an association between the *CYP3A4*1B* allele and age of menarche, a significant relationship does exist between the number of *CYP3A4*1B* alleles and the age at onset of puberty, as defined by Tanner breast score. In one study, 90% of 9 yr old girls with a *CYP3A4*1B/*1B* genotype had a Tanner breast score of ≥2 compared with 56% of *CYP3A4*1A/*1B* heterozygotes and 40% of girls homozygous for the *CYP3A4*1A* allele. Because CYP3A4 plays an important role in testosterone catabolism, the authors of the latter study proposed that the estradiol : testosterone ratio may be shifted toward higher values in the presence of the *CYP3A4*1B* allele and trigger the hormonal cascade that accompanies puberty. Intestinal CYP3A4 activity is inhibited by grapefruit juice and may result in higher levels of the many drugs metabolized by this enzyme; very large quantities of grapefruit juice may also inhibit the hepatic CYP3A4 enzyme (see Table 56-1).

Polymorphic *CYP3A5* expression is largely due to a SNP in intron 3 that creates a cryptic splice site and gives rise to mRNA splice variants that retain part of intron 3 with a premature stop codon. The truncated mRNA transcripts associated with this allele, *CYP3A5*3,* cannot be translated into a functional protein. Individuals with at least 1 wild-type *CYP3A5*1* allele express functional CYP3A5 protein, whereas those homozygous for *CYP3A5*3 (CYP3A5*3/*3)* do not. Approximately 60% of African-Americans show functional hepatic CYP3A5 activity compared with only 33% of European Americans. Clinically important consequences of *CYP3A5* allelic variation have been reported in children. In pediatric heart transplant patients with a *CYP3A5*1/*3* genotype, tacrolimus concentrations were approximately 50% of those observed in patients with *CYP3A5*3/*3* genotypes, when corrected for dose, 3 mo, 6 mo, and 12 mo after transplant. Thus, larger doses of tacrolimus are required to achieve comparable blood levels to minimize the risk of rejection.

GLUCURONOSYL TRANSFERASES. The UGT gene superfamily catalyzes the conjugation of several drugs used clinically in pediatrics, including morphine, acetaminophen, nonsteroidal anti-inflammatory drugs, and benzodiazepines, with glucuronic acid. The effect of development on glucuronidation capacity is well known to pediatricians in the form of hyperbilirubinemia, **gray baby syndrome** (the cardiovascular collapse associated with high doses of chloramphenicol in newborns), and the 3.5-fold increase in morphine clearance observed in premature neonates at 24–39 wk post-conceptional age. As with the CYPs, there are multiple UGT isoforms, and the acquisition of functional UGT activity appears to be isoform- and substrate-specific.

UGT1A1 is the major UGT gene product responsible for bilirubin glucuronidation, and >60 genetic alterations have been reported, most of which are rare and are more properly considered mutations rather than gene polymorphisms (see Chapters 102 and 354.1). Inheritance of 2 defective alleles is associated with reduced bilirubin-conjugating activity and gives rise to clinical conditions, such as Crigler-Najjar syndrome and Gilbert syndrome. More frequently occurring polymorphisms involve a dinucleotide (TA) repeat in the atypical TATA box of the *UGT1A1* promoter. The wild-type *UGT1A1*1* allele has 6 repeats (TA_6), and the TA_5 *(UGT1A1*33)*, TA_7 *(UGT1A1*28)*, and TA_8 *(UGT1A1*34)* variants are all associated with reduced activity. *UGT1A1*28*, the most frequent variant, is a contributory factor to prolonged neonatal jaundice and is associated with impaired glucuronidation and thus toxicity of the irinotecan active metabolite, SN-38. Allelic variation in *UGT1A7* and *UGT1A9* also has been associated with irinotecan toxicity in adults with colorectal cancer.

The consequences of allelic variation in the *UGT2B* family are less certain. The predominant routes of morphine elimination include biotransformation to the pharmacologically active 6-glucuronide (M6G) and the inactive 3-glucuronide (M3G). M6G formation is almost exclusively catalyzed by UGT2B7, whereas several UGTs in the UGT1A subfamily, as well as UGT2B7, contribute to M3G formation. Increased M6G : morphine ratios have been reported in individuals homozygous for the SNPs constituting the *UGT2B7*2* allele. Although individuals genotyped as *UGT2B7*2/*2* may produce higher than anticipated concentrations of pharmacologically active morphine and its metabolites, prospective pharmacogenetic studies addressing phenotype-genotype correlations and the consequences of morphine analgesia have not been conducted.

Arylamine *N*-Acetyltransferases. One of the earliest discovered and most widely recognized genetic polymorphisms is the NAT2 polymorphism. Approximately 50% of whites and African-Americans in North America are phenotypically slow metabolizers, placing a substantial number of individuals at increased risk for the development of adverse drug effects, such as sulfasalazine-induced hemolysis, hydrazine or arylamine-induced peripheral neuropathy, procainamide- or isoniazid-induced systemic lupus erythematosus, and Stevens-Johnson syndrome or toxic epidermal necrolysis associated with sulfonamide administration. NAT2 function is inherited in an autosomal dominant fashion, with the inheritance of 2 "slow" alleles required for expression of the slow-metabolizer phenotype. The relative proportion of rapid and slow metabolizers varies considerably with ethnic or geographic origin. The percentage of slow acetylators among Canadian Eskimos is 5%, but it approaches 90% in some Mediterranean populations. According to the standardized NAT2 nomenclature, the wild-type and 3 additional "fast" alleles give rise to the rapid acetylator phenotype, whereas 9 "slow" alleles have been described.

In vivo, with the use of caffeine as a phenotyping probe, all infants 0–55 days of age appear to be phenotypically slow acetylators, whereas 50% and 62% of infants 122–224 and 225–342 days of age, respectively, can be characterized as fast acetylators. Several independent studies indicate that maturation of the NAT2 phenotype occurs during the first 4 yr of life. Phenotype-genotype discordance is likely to be most apparent in the first 2–4 mo of life, and drugs that are highly dependent on NAT2 function for their elimination should be used with caution.

Thiopurine *S*-Methyltransferase. Thiopurine *S*-methyltransferase (TPMT) is a cytosolic enzyme that catalyses the *S*-methylation of aromatic and heterocyclic sulfur-containing compounds, such as 6-mercaptopurine (6MP), azathioprine, and 6-thioguanine, used in the treatment of acute lymphoblastic anemia (ALL), inflammatory bowel disease, and juvenile arthritis, and to prevent renal allograft rejection. To exert its cytotoxic effects, 6MP requires metabolism to thioguanine nucleotides by a multistep process that is initiated by hypoxanthine guanine phosphoribosyl transferase. TPMT prevents thioguanine nucleotide production by methylating 6MP (Fig. 56-3*A*). TPMT activity is usually measured in blood, with activity in erythrocytes reflecting that found in other tissues, including liver and leukemic blasts. Although approximately 89% of whites and African-Americans have high TPMT activity and 11% have intermediate activity, 1 in 300 individuals inherits TPMT deficiency as an autosomal recessive trait (Fig. 56-3*B*). In newborn infants, peripheral blood TPMT activity is reported to be 50% greater than in race-matched adults and shows a distribution of activity that is consistent with the polymorphism characterized in adults. There are no data currently to indicate how long this higher activity is maintained, although TPMT activities were comparable to previously reported adult values in a population of Korean schoolchildren aged 7–9 yr. In patients with intermediate or low activity, more drug is shunted toward production of cytotoxic thioguanine nucleotides. TPMT can also methylate 6-thioinosine 5′-monophosphate to generate a methylated metabolite that is capable of inhibiting de novo purine synthesis (Fig. 56-3C). In the small population (i.e., 0.3%) of treated patients with relative TPMT deficiency, severe and potentially life-threatening myelosuppression can develop in those receiving standard doses of thiopurine; starting doses must be reduced to 6–10% of the normal dose.

*TPMT*3A* is the most common mutant allele and is characterized by 2 nucleotide transition mutations, G460A and A719G, that lead to 2 amino acid substitutions Ala154Thr and Tyr240Cys (Fig. 56-3*D*). Although the *3A allele only has a frequency of 0.03% in the general population, it represents 55% of all mutant alleles. Either mutation alone results in loss of functional activity through the production of unstable proteins that are subject to accelerated proteolytic degradation. Less frequent allelic variants involve SNPs that produce amino acid substitutions in the coding region and defective intron-exon splicing. A polymorphic locus has been identified in the promoter region of the *TPMT* gene involving 4–8 repeats of a specific nucleotide sequence in tandem. Although these repeats appear to modulate TPMT activity when expressed in vitro, their role in regulating activity in vivo has not been clearly established.

The relatively few patients with low to absent TPMT activity are at increased risk for **severe myelosuppression** if treated with routine doses of thiopurines; thus, they require a 10–15-fold reduction in dose to minimize this risk. Furthermore, these patients may be at increased risk for relapse as a result of inadequate or absent treatment with thiopurines. Given the expanding use of 6MP and azathioprine in pediatrics to treat inflammatory bowel disease and juvenile arthritis and to prevent renal allograft rejection, TPMT deficiency is not a trivial matter.

Introduction of the TPMT phenotype or genotype determination into pediatric practice will lead to safer, more efficacious treatment in pediatric patient groups. Although most research has been conducted in ALL, the observation that patients classified as having intermediate TPMT activity are more likely to be intolerant of 6MP or azathioprine and to require more frequent dosage reductions in response to drug-induced myelosuppression is equally applicable to other pediatric patient groups treated with this family of drugs.

DEVELOPMENTAL PHARMACOGENETICS OF DRUG TRANSPORTERS

ORGANIC ANION TRANSPORTERS. The organic anion transporter (OAT) family transports a wide variety of xenobiotics, including penicillins, cephalosporins, sulfonamides, loop and thiazide diuretics, barbiturates, salicylates, and ochratoxin A, 2,4-dichlorophenoxyacetic acid, as well as nonsteroidal anti-inflammatory drugs. Located at the basolateral membrane of the tubular cells, the OAT family is capable of removing scores of xenobiotics through active tubular secretion. This transport is tertiary, involving Na^+, K^+-ATPase, which maintains the Na^+ gradient between the blood and tubular cells. The Na^+ gradient drives a Na^+ dicarboxylate cotransporter, sustaining a dicarboxylate gradient that is used by a dicarboxylate/organic anion exchanger to move the substrate into the cell. This cascade allows an organic anion to enter the tubular cell against its concentration gradient and against the electric potential of the cell.

The identification of the gene encoding for the OAT1 transporter led to the discovery of several isoforms, including cOAT2, hOAT3, and hOAT4. The different OATs have substantial overlap in substrate specificity, while maintaining important differences. Para-aminohippurate has high affinity for OAT1 and OAT3, but much lower affinity for OAT2 and OAT4.

The newborn excretes penicillins (renal) at very low rates compared with children and adults, whereas toddlers need a much higher dose per kilogram of body weight compared with adults. Before the maturation of tubular expression and function of the OAT family, neonates exhibit very limited capacity to eliminate renally anionic drugs. This is followed by an overshoot during which toddlers have higher expression and function than adults, subsequently decreasing to levels that are maintained during adulthood. The fact that all members of the OAT family appear to develop in a coordinated fashion suggests that these proteins are controlled by a common signal for expression and/or transcription. Another important phenomenon encountered with the tubular secretion of organic anions is substrate induction, leading to enhanced elimination of organic anions with repeated exposure. This phenomenon is unique, although its biologic pattern has not yet been elucidated.

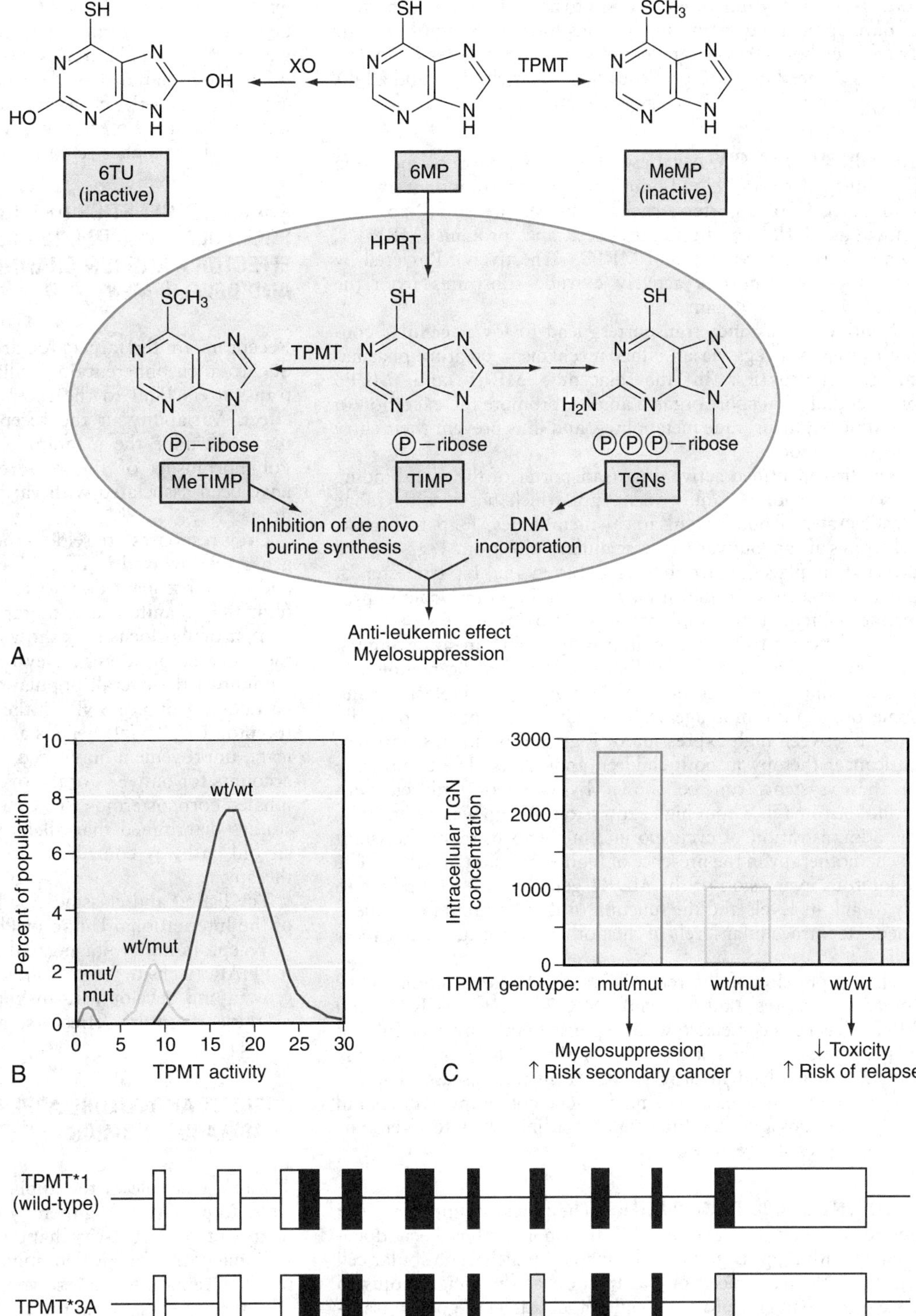

Figure 56-3. Thiopurine *S*-methyltransferase (TPMT) polymorphism. *A,* 6-Mercaptopurine (6MP) undergoes metabolism to thioguanine nucleotides (TGNs) to exert its cytotoxic effects. TPMT and xanthine oxidase reduce the amount of 6MP available for the bioactivation pathway to TGNs. TPMT can also methylate 6-thioinosine 5′-monophosphate (TIMP) to generate a methylated compound capable of inhibiting de novo purine synthesis. *B,* Distribution of TPMT activity in humans. Of the population, 89% has high activity, whereas 11% has intermediate activity. Approximately 1 in 300 individuals homozygous for 2 loss-of-function alleles has very low activity. *C,* Correlation between the TPMT genotype and intracellular TGN concentrations. In TPMT poor metabolizers, more 6MP is available to go down the bioactivation pathway to form TGNs; this situation is associated with an increased risk of myelosuppression. *D,* The most common variant TPMT allele is the result of 2 mutations that give rise to an unstable protein product that undergoes proteolytic degradation. 6TU, 6-thiouric acid; MeMP, 6-methylmercaptopurine; HPRT, 6-thiomethylinosine 5-monophosphate; MeTIMP, hypoxanthine-guanine phosphoribosyl transferase; wt, wild type; mut, mutant. (Modified with permission from Relling MV, Dervieux T: Pharmacogenetics and cancer therapy. *Nat Rev Cancer* 2001;11:99–108; copyright 2001, Macmillan Magazines Ltd [130.])

ORGANIC CATION TRANSPORTERS. An organic cation transport system in the renal tubular cell is responsible for active renal secretion of several cationic drugs.

This secretory process occurs mostly at the proximal tubule. More specifically, the organic cation is located at the brush border membrane, and its function is mediated by an organic cation-proton antiporter. Similar to the OAT family, the organic cation transporter (OCT) plays a critical role in removing a large number of medicinal and other organic cations from the plasma, against the concentration gradient. Most of the transporters that secrete organic cations belong to a single family of transport proteins, the OCT family.

Neonates possess very limited ability to eliminate organic cations. This ability increases rapidly during the 1st few months of life, and when standardized for body weight or surface area, it tends to exceed adult levels during the toddler stage. Subsequently, secretory function decreases to adult levels. This pattern of development has major implications for the dosing of cationic drugs: newborns require reductions in dose, whereas toddlers commonly need much larger doses than older children and adults when corrected for body weight or surface area.

THE ABC SUPERFAMILY. A variety of epithelial barriers, including the kidney, liver, and blood-brain barrier have abundant expression of ABC transporters, such as P-glycoprotein (P-gp; also known as *MDR1*), and multidrug resistance proteins (MRPs) 1, 2, and 3 (MRP1, MRP2, and MRP3, respectively). Powered by ATP, these transporters actively extrude substrates from the respective cell and organ.

Multidrug resistance transporters lead to lower cellular concentrations of drugs via an efflux mechanism, creating pharmacologic sanctuaries. In the placenta, MRP1 and MRP3 preferentially transport organic anions, promote the excretion of glutathione/glucuronide metabolites, and thus prevent their entry into fetal blood.

The first identified active drug transporter of the ATP-binding cassette transporter family was P-gp, which has a wide range of substrates. Abundant in apical membranes, P-gp transports substrates in an outward (extracellular) direction. P-gp can be detected in placental trophoblasts during the 1st trimester of pregnancy, suggesting that it may play an important role in protecting the fetus from amphipathic xenotoxins.

In an attempt to reverse multidrug resistance in solid tumors, the use of cyclosporine, an inhibitor of P-gp, has been shown to increase tumor concentrations of daunorubicin, vinblastine, and some other antitumor agents. Correlation has been repeatedly shown between high expression of P-gp and tumor resistance to anticancer therapy in both children and adults. The complexity of these systems can be shown by cases of children with retinoblastoma in whom high expression of P-gp was reversed by the administration of cyclosporine, but who were still resistant to chemotherapy in the presence of high expression of MRPs. The ubiquitous expression of the *MDR1* gene has led researchers to try to link its levels and the function of P-gp to failure to achieve adequate intracellular levels of chemotherapeutic agents in cancer cells.

High expression of different ABC transporters, including BCRP (breast cancer-resistant protein), MRP2, MRP3, MRP4, and MRP5, has been correlated with response to therapy in childhood acute myeloid leukemia. It appears that MRP3 and possibly MRP2 are involved in drug resistance in this disease. These 2 transport proteins may well predict chemotherapy failure and lead to the possible development of specific drugs to overcome multidrug resistance.

ONTOGENY OF ABC TRANSPORTERS. The potential importance of age-related development of ABC transporters has been documented with P-gp. Digoxin is eliminated by the renal tubular cell by P-gp. Neonates need only a fraction of the weight-adjusted dose of digoxin given to older children or adults. P-gp also transports a variety of other compounds, including vinblastine, verapamil, cyclosporine A, and daunomycin. High expression of P-gp at a young age may lead to a protective mechanism in which both endogenous and exogenous toxins are efficiently excreted from the body. P-gp, MRP1, and MRP2 act synergistically with CYPs to protect the organism against potentially toxic compounds. With each having its own specific age-dependent expression throughout kidney development, they may prevent the body from obtaining the desired therapeutic concentration.

Digoxin serves as an excellent example of the ontogeny of renal elimination by P-gp. The drug is excreted by glomerular filtration, but is also extensively secreted by the tubular cell by P-gp. Young children need 3-fold higher doses of digoxin per kilogram of body weight than adults. This difference could not be explained by changes in the glomerular filtration rate alone, because the glomerular filtration rate per kilogram of body weight in young children is <2-fold higher than in adults. A significant correlation has been demonstrated between renal P-gp expression and the clearance rate of digoxin in developing rats, implying that the ontogeny of P-gp renders young children more likely to have higher renal clearance of P-gp substrates.

PHARMACOGENETICS OF DRUG RESPONSE: POLYMORPHISMS IN DRUG RECEPTORS, EFFECTORS, AND ION CHANNELS DURING GROWTH AND DEVELOPMENT

Receptors are the targets for drugs and endogenous transmitters due to their inherent molecular recognition sites. Drugs and transmitters bind to the receptor to produce a pharmacologic effect. Variability in the receptor protein or the ion channel may determine the magnitude of the pharmacologic response. Polymorphisms of the β_2-adrenergic receptor gene *(ADRB2)* have been associated with variable responses to bronchodilator drugs.

Drug responses are seldom monogenic events because multiple genes are involved in drug binding to the pharmacologic target and the subsequent downstream signal transduction events that ultimately manifest as a therapeutic effect. Although genotypes at a particular locus may show a statistically significant effect on the outcome of interest, they may account for a relatively small amount of the overall population variability in that measure. A particular group of SNPs in the corticotropin-releasing hormone receptor 1 *(CRHR1)* gene is associated with a statistically significant improvement in forced expiratory volume in 1 sec, but accounts for only 6% of the overall variability in the response to inhaled corticosteroids (see Chapter 143). A series of subsequent studies determined that allelic variation in several genes in the steroid pathway contributes to overall response to this form of therapy.

The listing and classification of receptors is a major initiative of the International Union of Pharmacology (IUPHAR). The list of receptors and voltage-gated ion channels is available on the IUPHAR website *(http://www.iuphar-db.org)*. The effect of growth and development on the activities and binding affinities of these receptors, effectors, and ion channels remain to be elucidated.

CURRENT AND FUTURE APPLICATIONS FOR PHARMACOGENOMICS IN PEDIATRICS

The best example of the application of pharmacogenomic principles to pediatric drug therapy is the progress being made in the treatment of ALL (see Chapter 495). Despite improved understanding of the genetic determinants of drug response, many complexities remain to be resolved. Patients with ALL who have 1 wild-type allele and intermediate TPMT activity tend to have a better response to 6MP therapy than patients with 2 wild-type alleles and full activity. Reduced TPMT activity also places patients at risk for irradiation-induced secondary brain tumors and etoposide-induced acute myeloid leukemias. Pharmacogenetic polymorphisms of several additional genes also have the potential to influence successful treatment of ALL. Multiple genetic and treatment-related factors interact to create patient subgroups with varying degrees of risk, and these represent an opportunity for pharmacogenomic approaches to identify subgroups of patients who will tolerate specific treatment regimens and those who will be at risk for short- and long-term toxicities.

The 20% of patient with ALL who do not respond to chemotherapy represent an additional challenge for pharmacogenomic research. Gene expression (microarray) studies in ALL blasts are able to discriminate among phenotypic subtypes and identify some individuals who are at risk for treatment failure. An analysis of acute treatment-induced changes in the gene response of ALL blasts obtained 1 day after the initiation of 6MP and methotrexate as single agents or in combinations of high-dose or low-dose methotrexate and 6MP showed several important insights into the cellular response to these treatment. Changes in gene expression were treatment-specific and could accurately discriminate among the 4 treatments. ALL cells of different molecular subtypes shared common cellular responses to treatment, suggesting that it may be possible to personalize treatment strategies in ALL.

AmpliChip CYP450 test. *Med Lett Drugs Ther* 2005;47:71–72.

Blake MJ, Castro L, Leeder JS, et al: Ontogeny of drug metabolizing enzymes in the neonate. *Semin Fetal Neonatal Med* 2005;10:123–138.

Chen N, Aleksa K, Woodland C, et al: Ontogeny of drug elimination by the human kidney. *Pediatr Nephrol* 2006;21:160–168.

CYP3A and drug interactions. *Med Lett Drugs Ther* 2005;47:54–55.

Drug interactions with grapefruit juice. *Med Lett Drugs Ther* 2004;46:2–4.

Eliasson E: Ethnicity and adverse drug reactions. *BMJ* 2006;332:1163–1164.

Evans WE, McLeod HL: Pharmacogenomics: Drug disposition, drug targets, and side effects. *N Engl J Med* 2003;348:538–549.

Freund CL, Gregory DF, Clayton EW: Evaluating pharmacogenetic tests. *Arch Pediatr Adolesc Med* 2004;158:276–279.

Gasche Y, Daali Y, Fathi M, et al: Codeine intoxication associated with ultra-rapid CYP2D6 metabolism. *N Engl J Med* 2004;351:2827–2830.

Goldstein JA: Clinical relevance of genetic polymorphisms in the human CYP2C subfamily. *Br J Clin Pharmacol* 2001;52:349–355.

Haga SB, Burke W: Using pharmacogenetics to improve drug safety and efficacy. *JAMA* 2004;291:2869–2871.

Hines RN, McCarver DG: The ontogeny of human drug-metabolizing enzymes: Phase I oxidative enzymes. *J Pharmacol Exp Ther* 2002;300:355–360.

Hines RN, McCarver DG: Pharmacogenomics and the future of drug therapy. *Pediatr Clin North Am* 2006;53(4):591–619.

Johnson JA, Lima JJ: Drug receptor/effector polymorphisms and pharmacogenetics: Current status and challenges. *Pharmacogenetics* 2003;13:525–534.

Kim H, Neubert JK, San Miguel A, et al: Genetic influence on variability in human acute experimental pain sensitivity associated with gender, ethnicity and psychological temperament. *Pain* 2004;109:488–496.

Koren G, Cairns J, Chitayat D, et al: Pharmacogenetics of morphine poisoning in a breastfed neonate of a codeine-prescribed mother. *Lancet* 2006;368:704–705.

Leeder JS: Pharmacogenetics and pharmacogenomics. *Pediatr Clin North Am* 2001;48:756–781.

McCarver DG, Hines RN: The ontogeny of human drug metabolizing enzymes: Phase II conjugation enzymes and regulatory mechanisms. *J Pharmacol Exp Ther* 2002;300:361–366.

McLeod HL, Marsh S: Pharmacogenetics goes 3D. *Nat Genet* 2005;37:794–795.

Need AC, Motulsky AG, Goldstein DB: Priorities and standards in pharmacogenetic research. *Nat Genet* 2005;37:671–681.

Shah J: Criteria influencing the clinical uptake of pharmacogenomic strategies. *BMJ* 2004;328:1482–1486.

Tucker G: Pharmacogenetics: Expectations and reality. *BMJ* 2004;329:4–6.

Wall AM, Rubnitz JE: Pharmacogenomic effects on therapy for acute lymphoblastic leukemia in children. *Pharmacogenomics J* 2003;3:128–135.

Weinshilboum R: Inheritance and drug response. *N Engl J Med* 2003;348:529–537.

Weiss ST, Litonjua AA, Lange C, et al: Overview of the pharmacogenetics of asthma treatment. *Pharmacogenomics J* 2006;6:311–326.

Wilkerson GR: Drug metabolism and variability among patients in drug response. *N Engl J Med* 2005;352:2211–2221.

Williams DG, Patel A, Howard RF: Pharmacogenetics of codeine metabolism in an urban population of children and its implications for analgesic reliability. *Br J Anaesth* 2002;89:839–845.

Witzman FA, Grant RA: Pharmacoproteomics in drug development. *Pharmacogenomics J* 2003;3:69–76.

Chapter 57 ■ Principles of Drug Therapy

Peter Gal and Michael D. Reed

The use of drugs requires a clear understanding of the predetermined targeted end-points, the likelihood of achieving the effects sought, and the relative risks of exposing patients to the drug(s) selected. The pediatric population is not well studied for most drug therapies. The need for safe and effective drugs for use in sick neonates, infants, children, and adolescents requires the establishment of thoughtful drug therapy strategies.

Clinical pharmacology incorporates numerous concepts combined to deliver drugs in the correct amount to the desired site to achieve the correct action while avoiding unwanted toxicity. Principles applied include pharmacokinetics, pharmacodynamics, pharmacogenomics, proteomics, chronopharmacology, and pharmacophysiology. **Pharmacokinetics** describes a drug's disposition within the body and is most often characterized by the following pharmacokinetic parameter estimates: systemic bioavailability, distribution, metabolism, and elimination, as well as the factors that influence these processes. Classically, these processes are described by the acronym *ADME: a*bsorption, *d*istribution, *m*etabolism, and *e*xcretion. However, pharmacokinetics is a far more complex process. **Absorption** is one process by which drugs are made bioavailable to the body, and thus is more aptly described as drug delivery to the body through any of multiple processes and routes, including oral, buccal, rectal, percutaneous, intrauterine, inhalation, intranasal, intramuscular, subcutaneous, intraocular, and otic. In the absence of administration of **prodrugs** (pharmacologically inactive parent compounds), the systemic bioavailability of a drug administered in a manner that results in the release of the parent compound after intravenous drug administration equals 100%. **Drug distribution** throughout the body is influenced by a variety of drug-specific physiochemical factors, including the role of drug transporters, blood/tissue protein binding, and blood and tissue pH and perfusion. **Metabolism** involves conversion of drugs in the body to active or inactive compounds that can be more readily excreted either by the kidneys or by other routes (hepatic/bile, exhalation). Most drug metabolism takes place in the liver via hepatic enzymes, although other organ systems are sometimes involved. **Excretion** or secretion of drugs involves not only the kidneys or liver, but also removal of drugs by extracorporeal systems, such as dialysis, hemofiltration, or heart-lung bypass machines.

Pharmacodynamics describes the relationship between drug dose or drug concentration and response. The response may be desirable *(effectiveness)* or untoward *(toxicity)*. Although in clinical practice the response to drugs in different patient populations is often described by a standard dosing or concentration range, response is best described on a continuum. At a lower concentration range, response rates may be quite low, and with gradual increases in drug concentration, a higher proportion of patients achieve the desired response. If this concentration-response curve is plotted in parallel with a concentration-toxicity curve, a sense of the therapeutic index of the drug (i.e., relative efficacy and safety profile) can be obtained (Fig. 57-1). Pharmacodynamic profiles may involve the parent drug, active metabolites, or some combination.

The finding that drug responses can be influenced by the patient's genetic profile has offered great hope for realizing patient-specific targeted pharmacotherapy (see Chapter 56). Studies of single-gene variants and multiple-gene interactions have documented their influence on the manner and extent of drug metabolism, the susceptibility of certain patient groups to drug response or toxicity, and the genetic profiles of patients who benefit most from selected therapies (see Chapter 56). Genetic polymorphisms occur in at least 1% of the population. Impor-

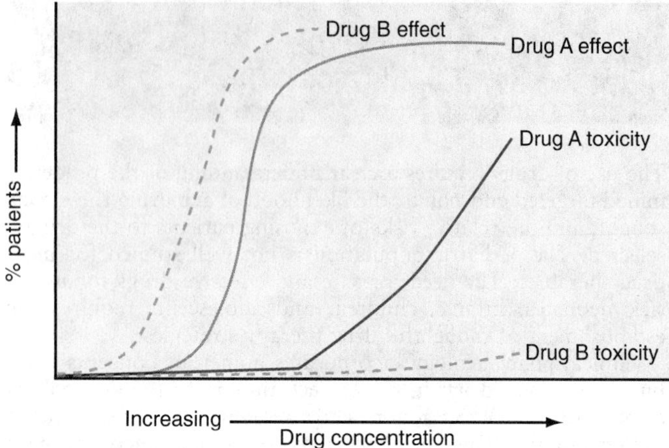

Figure 57-1. Drugs with a narrow therapeutic index (drug A, *solid lines*) vs a wide therapeutic index (drug B, *dashed lines*). Note that a drug with a narrow therapeutic index is more likely to cause toxicity at serum concentrations needed to obtain an adequate therapeutic response, whereas a drug with a wide therapeutic index is unlikely to cause toxicity at concentrations needed for an adequate therapeutic response.

tant cytochrome P450 (CYP) drug-metabolizing enzyme genes associated with drug response include the phase I enzymes CYP1A2, CYP2C9, CYP2C19, CYP2D6, CYP2E1, and CYP3A4, and the phase II enzymes *N*-acetyltransferase, uridine diphosphate glucoronyltransferase, and glucose-6-phosphate dehydrogenase (see Chapter 56). Polymorphisms responsible for clinically important interpatient variability in patient response to drugs metabolized by polymorphically expressed CYP isoenzymes have been described for CYP2C9 and CYP2D6. In addition, some drug transporter proteins control drug efflux from cells (P-glycoprotein, multidrug resistant proteins [MRPs] 1 and 2), impart drug resistance to cancer cells and infectious agents, and influence drug distribution to various parts of the body (placenta, central nervous system [cerebrospinal fluid]).

Chronobiology, chronopharmacology, and **chronotherapeutics** involve the study of circadian rhythms and timing of drug doses on pharmacologic effects. Optimal timing of certain drug doses can affect the efficacy or toxicity of drug therapy. This has been particularly important in asthma, hypertension, H_2 receptor antagonist therapy for peptic ulcer disease, and cancer chemotherapy. Time-sensitive changes are noted in both the pharmacokinetics and the pharmacodynamics of certain drugs. Physiologic changes affect drug disposition; **pharmacophysiology** is the use of a drug's pharmacokinetic profile to help identify a physiologic response. Examples of this application are the use of a large gentamicin volume of distribution to detect clinically silent patent ductus arteriosus and an abrupt reduction in the indomethacin volume of distribution when the patent ductus arteriosus is closed. A common practical approach is to use aminoglycoside clearance as a marker of the patient's glomerular filtration rate.

INFLUENCE OF AGE ON DRUG THERAPY. Pediatrics encompasses a broad range of ages at which certain stages of life profoundly influence drug response and disposition. Dramatic pharmacokinetic, pharmacodynamic, and psychosocial changes occur as preterm infants mature toward term, as infants mature during the 1st few yr of life, and as children reach puberty and adolescence. To meet the needs of these different pediatric groups, different formulations are needed for drug delivery that can influence drug absorption and disposition, and different psychosocial issues influence compliance, timing of drug administration, and reactions to drug use. These additional factors must be considered in conjunction with known pharmacokinetic and pharmacodynamic influences of age when developing an optimal, patient-specific drug therapy strategy.

TABLE 57-1. Physiologic Factors that Influence the Oral Absorption of Medications

PARAMETER	NEONATE	INFANT	CHILD
Gastric acid secretion	Reduced	Normal	Normal
Gastric emptying time	Decreased	Increased	Increased
Intestinal motility	Reduced	Normal	Normal
Biliary function	Reduced	Normal	Normal
Microbial flora	Acquiring	Adult pattern	Adult pattern

DRUG ADMINISTRATION ISSUES AND BIOAVAILABILITY. The administration of drugs can occur via multiple routes, and during acute and chronic illness, the amount of drug that is delivered to the bloodstream (**bioavailability**) or that reaches the intended site of action may vary. Common routes of drug delivery include oral, sublingual, rectal, intravenous, intramuscular, subcutaneous, inhaled, topical, transdermal, intraocular, intranasal, and otic. The success of each of these routes depends on proper adherence to the administration technique and awareness of the limitations and problems that may arise with each route. Because children may resist the administration of drugs that have an unpleasant taste or that cause pain, burning, or other discomfort, strategies for reducing these problems must be addressed. Not all drugs administered by a particular route are administered in the same way. Some oral medications are best taken with food, whereas others require an empty stomach. Some inhaled medications require rapid inspiration for delivery, whereas others require slow and steady inhalation. Because the proper administration technique may affect therapeutic success, it is desirable to advise the patient to review the proper administration technique for all drugs with the dispensing pharmacist. Although certain xenobiotics and nutrients are absorbed by active transport or facilitated diffusion, most drugs are absorbed from the gastrointestinal tract by passive diffusion. A number of important patient variables can affect the rate and extent of gastrointestinal drug absorption, including pH-dependent diffusion; the presence, absence, and type of gastric contents; gastric emptying time; and gastrointestinal motility. These physiologic processes reflect a clear, but highly variable dependence on a patient's age (Tables 57-1 and 57-2). Despite the clear maturational changes observed in the functional capacity of these processes and their importance to intestinal drug absorption, the overall bioavailability of most orally administered medications in neonates, infants, children, and adolescents is adequate. For acid-labile drugs, such as penicillin or ampicillin, oral absorption may actually be increased in premature and newborn infants vs older infants and children with age-appropriate gastric acid concentrations. Other drugs may have slower absorption, with delayed and blunted peak concentrations (phenobarbital). The dosage form may also be important, particularly for infants and younger children, because spitting of foul-tasting medication and accurate measurement of small volumes of liquid medications may influence the accuracy of the drug dosage actually delivered. Solid dosage forms (tablets, capsules) must dissolve into solution

TABLE 57-2. Developmental Aspects of Body Fluid Compartment Sizes

AGE	TOTAL BODY WATER*	EXTRACELLULAR FLUID*	INTRACELLULAR FLUID*
<3 mo fetus	92	65	25
Term gestation	75	35–44	33
4–6 mo	60	23	37
12 mo		26–30	
Puberty	≈60	20	40
Adult	50–60	20	40

*Expressed as percentage of total body weight.

before the drug can cross cell membranes. Most drugs administered to infants and young children are available in a liquid formulation, including some as a suspension. In general, the rate of absorption is faster after administration of a liquid dosing formulation (liquid > suspension) compared with solid formulations (capsule ≥ tablet > sustained/delayed-release tablet). Drug interactions with concurrent medications or dietary intake may markedly alter the bioavailability (especially oral) of selected drugs and should be considered when dosing drugs.

Intravenous drug administration is assumed to be the most dependable and accurate route for drug delivery. However, intravenous drug administration systems have many potential sources of error, resulting in incomplete drug delivery or unintended bolus doses that may lead to serious adverse drug reactions. Many pediatric hospitals use syringe pumps as a means to increase accuracy, but regardless of the system used, drug loss in the intravenous tubing through binding to the tubing or inactivation, delayed drug delivery, unintended bolus infusions, and occlusion of the intravenous catheter confound reliable prediction of the dosage delivered. The frequency and magnitude of errors are increased when pump flow rates are low, especially <1/hr, as is often the case in small infants or fluid-restricted patients. Even with the "smart pumps" designed to reduce drug administration problems, the rates of drug errors may not significantly change due to poor nursing compliance with pump specifications. Drug administration errors must be considered when unexpected adverse drug reactions occur, patient response to drug therapy is unexpectedly poor, or drug concentrations are unexpectedly low.

DRUG DISTRIBUTION. Understanding the distribution characteristics of a drug in the body is important when selecting the dose. Although the **distribution volume** (V_d), or "apparent volume of distribution," for a drug does not denote any real physiologic volume, an estimate of this pharmacokinetic parameter provides insight into the total amount of drug present in the body relative to its concentration in blood and thus the tissue distribution. Knowledge of the V_d of a drug is important when selecting an initial **loading dose** or designing an optimal dosage regimen to attain a preselected **target concentration.** The V_d for a number of drugs is influenced by patient age and can differ markedly among newborns (premature vs full-term), infants, and children compared with adults. These differences are the result of many important age-dependent variables, including the composition and size of body water compartments, protein-binding characteristics, and hemodynamic factors, including cardiac output, regional blood flow, and membrane permeability. The absolute amounts and distribution of body water and fat depend on a child's age and nutritional habits. Obesity is common in children and affects the volume of distribution of various drugs. Changes in body water compartment sizes, blood volume, and water distribution account for the differences observed in the V_d in infants and children.

The extent to which a drug is **bound** to circulating plasma proteins directly influences the drug's distribution characteristics. Only **free,** unbound drug can be distributed from the vascular space into other body fluids and tissues, where it binds to its receptor and stimulates a response. Drug binding to plasma proteins depends on a number of age-related variables, including the absolute amount of proteins available, their respective number of available binding sites, the affinity constant of the drug for the protein, the influence of pathophysiologic conditions, and the presence of endogenous substances, which may compete for protein binding (protein displacement interactions). These and other clinically important variables can affect drug protein binding relative to age. The extent to which a drug is bound to protein markedly influences its V_d and **body clearance** (Cl) as well as the intensity of pharmacologic effects.

Albumin, α_1-acid glycoprotein, and lipoproteins are the most important circulating proteins responsible for drug binding in plasma. The absolute concentration of these proteins is influenced by age, nutrition, and disease. Basic drugs bind mainly to albumin, α_1-acid glycoprotein, and lipoprotein, whereas acidic and neutral compounds bind primarily to albumin. Serum albumin and total protein concentrations are decreased during infancy, approaching adult values by the age of 10–12 mo. A similar pattern of maturation is observed with α_1-acid glycoprotein; concentrations appear to be approximately 3 times lower in neonatal plasma compared with maternal plasma, achieving values comparable to those of adults by 12 mo of age.

Several endogenous substances present in human plasma may bind to plasma proteins and compete for available drug-binding sites. During the neonatal period, free fatty acids, bilirubin, and 2-hydroxybenzoylglycine compete for albumin-binding sites and influence the resultant balance between free and bound drug concentrations. Clinically significant protein-binding displacement reactions occur only when a drug of high potency is >80–90% protein-bound and has a small V_d. The requirement for all 3 of these variables—high potency, extensive degree of protein binding, and a small V_d—for a clinically relevant drug-protein displacement reaction explains why such reactions are unusual in pediatric practice. It is prudent to assess a drug's potential for displacement of bilirubin from protein-binding sites before its administration to premature and newborn infants.

For some drugs in which the unbound portion of the drug may be measured to guide clinical decisions, it is important to consider sample handling, because changes in sample temperature or pH can markedly alter results, affording false values and exaggerating unbound drug concentrations. In addition to protein binding, drug transporters, such as P-glycoprotein, MDR1, and MDR2, (multidrug resistance 1 or 2) play an important role in drug distribution. These drug transporters can markedly influence the extent to which drugs cross membranes in the body and whether drugs can penetrate or are secreted from the target sites (inside cancer cells or microorganisms, or crossing the blood-brain barrier). Thus, **drug resistance** to cancer chemotherapy, antibiotics, or epilepsy may be conferred by these drug transport proteins and their effect on drug distribution.

DRUG METABOLISM. The moment a drug molecule is present within the body, the process of its removal begins. The overall rate of drug removal is described by the **pharmacokinetic parameter clearance (Cl),** or **body** *Cl.* A drug's body Cl is the summation of all clearance mechanisms involved in removing that compound from the body. The primary organ for drug metabolism is the liver, although the kidney, intestine, lung, adrenals, blood (phosphatases, esterases), and skin can also biotransform certain compounds. For most drugs (lipophilic weak acids or weak bases), biotransformation to more polar, water-soluble compounds facilitates their elimination from the body through the bile, kidney, or lung. Although the biotransformation of most drugs results in pharmacologically weaker or inactive compounds, parent compounds may be transformed into active metabolites or intermediates (theophylline to caffeine, carbamazepine to 10,11-carbamazepine epoxide). Conversely, pharmacologically inactive parent compounds, or prodrugs, may be converted to an active moiety (chloramphenicol succinate to active chloramphenicol base, cefuroxime axetil to active cefuroxime) before subsequent biotransformation and body elimination.

Drug metabolism within the hepatocyte involves 2 primary enzymatic processes: **phase I,** or nonsynthetic, and **phase II,** or synthetic, reactions. Phase I reactions include oxidation, reduction, hydrolysis, and hydroxylation reactions, whereas phase II reactions primarily involve conjugation with glycine, glucuronide, or sulfate. Most drug-metabolizing enzymes are located in the smooth endoplasmic reticulum of cells. Of these mixed-function oxidase systems, the CYP450 system has been studied in greatest detail. The CYP450 enzyme system is a supergene family, with at least 16 primary enzymes and a number of isozymes of specific gene families. The specific subfamilies, or isozymes, most responsible for human drug metabolism involve CYP1A2, CYP2C9, CYP2C19, CYP2D6, CYP2E1, and CYP3A4 (see Chapter 56). At birth, the concentration of drug-oxidizing enzymes in fetal liver (corrected for liver weight) appears similar to that in adult liver. The activity of these oxidizing enzyme systems is reduced, which is reflected by prolonged body elimination of drugs that depend on oxidation pathways in newborns (phenytoin, caffeine, diazepam, and many others). Postnatally, the hepatic CYP mono-oxygenase enzymes appear to mature at different rates; for example, CYP1A2 and CYP3A4 mature a few mo before CYP2C9 and CYP2C19 (see Chapter 56). Metabolic activity similar to or in excess of the adult value is achieved by approximately 6–12 mo of age. An understanding of the substrates for specific isozymes and the effects certain drugs may have on isoenzyme activity (induction, inhibition) allows the clinician to predict the possibility of clinically important metabolic-based drug-drug interactions (see Table 56-2). These are so numerous that the potential for significant interactions with current therapies should always be checked in a database before new drugs or diets are recommended for the patient. Most pharmacies use electronic databases that can screen for such interactions, and many electronic drug resources available to prescribers offer a basic list. Commonly prescribed medications in pediatrics linked to the specific CYP isoenzymes responsible for their metabolism with clinically important CYP inducers and inhibitors are shown in Table 56-2.

The activity of certain hydrolytic enzymes, including blood esterases, is also reduced during the neonatal period. Blood esterases are important for the metabolic clearance of cocaine, and the reduced activity of these plasma esterases in the newborn may account for the delayed metabolism of cocaine in neonates.

Because elimination of metabolites is reduced in preterm and full-term infants, accumulation of active metabolites that are not considered clinically relevant in older infants, children, and adults may occur in infants. Such is the case with the *N*-methylation of theophylline to caffeine. This pathway becomes more important in neonates because theophylline is less readily metabolized, making it more available for *N*-methylation. Caffeine itself is normally metabolized before elimination, but in preterm infants with immature liver enzymes, caffeine elimination is primarily by the kidneys. This renal elimination is slow because of the immaturity of renal function in young infants, resulting in the potential for caffeine accumulation, contributing to the possibility that methylxanthine effect or toxicity will be undetected if only theophylline concentrations are monitored.

Understanding the sequence of maturation of processes of drug metabolism is important when developing dosage recommendations for drugs that undergo extensive hepatic metabolism. An example of the consequences of failing to appreciate these processes is the tragedy that occurred after the administration of usual doses of chloramphenicol (75–100 mg/kg/24 hr) to premature and newborn infants (**fatal gray baby syndrome**) and the resultant beneficial use of this compound in the same patient population when the dose was appropriately adjusted (15–50 mg/kg/24 hr) to compensate for the decreased hepatic ability for glucuronidation. Chloramphenicol glucuronide is the primary metabolite of chloramphenicol, which is then excreted through the kidneys.

The ultimate ability of children to metabolize drugs is genetically modulated. Pharmacogenetic predisposition to slow drug metabolism along certain enzymatic pathways can provide important clues to patients who are at risk for drug toxicity. The polymorphic characteristics of the important human drug-metabolizing CYP isoenzymes are shown in Tables 56-1 and 56-2.

DRUG EXCRETION. The amount of drug that is filtered by the glomerulus per unit of time depends on the functional ability of the glomerulus, the integrity of renal blood flow, and the extent of drug-protein binding. The amount of drug filtered is inversely related to the degree of protein binding. Only free drug is filtered by the glomerulus and excreted. Although highly variable, renal blood flow averages 12 mL/min at birth, approaching adult values by 5–12 mo of age (see Chapter 508). The glomerular filtration rate is 2–4 mL/min in full-term infants, increases to 8–20 mL/min by 2–3 days of life, and approaches adult values by 3–5 mo of age. Before 34 wk of gestation, glomerular filtration is markedly reduced and increases more slowly than in term infants.

PHARMACOKINETICS AND DRUG DOSING CONSIDERATIONS

Pharmacokinetic-based methods can be used to predict drug concentration at any time after a dose is administered and can facilitate calculation of a drug dose to achieve a desired concentration. Recognizing that the pharmacologic and toxicologic effects correlate best with a drug's concentration in a biologic fluid (blood, cerebrospinal fluid), rather than the absolute dose administered, is the foundation of applied clinical pharmacokinetics. The biodisposition of most drugs used clinically is best described using the principles of **linear, or 1st-order, pharmacokinetics:** The serum concentration (or the amount of drug in the body) is directly proportional to the dose administered. If the dose of a drug that follows linear pharmacokinetics is doubled, its resultant concentration in blood (at steady state) also doubles. This characteristic of proportionality, combined with appropriate patient monitoring, is often used clinically to make adjustments in drug dosing. In contrast, some drugs, such as phenytoin, salicylate, and alcohol, exhibit **saturation kinetics;** their elimination pathways become saturated, and the resultant drug concentration in the blood changes disproportionately to the dose administered. Under usual clinical conditions, these drugs often exhibit linear (1st-order) elimination characteristics at low doses (low serum concentrations), but as the amount of drug in the body increases with increasing dose, their elimination pathways become saturated. Such drugs are often referred to as following the principles of **zero-order** (or Michaelis-Menten) **kinetics.** The classic principles of elimination half-life ($t_{1/2}$) and Cl do not apply to drugs that exhibit zero-order kinetics.

PHARMACOKINETIC CALCULATIONS AND BOLUS DOSING CONSIDERATIONS. In the event that therapeutic drug monitoring is available, calculation of individualized pharmacokinetic parameters is feasible. When this is not practical, age-appropriate, population-based pharmacokinetic values can be used to design an optimum dosing strategy.

Typically, in the acute setting, a loading dose or bolus dose of drug is provided to achieve effective drug serum (tissue/receptor) concentrations rapidly. To do this effectively, a dose can be calculated using the known relationship between the dose, the drug's volume of distribution (V_d), and the serum concentration achieved. This relationship is described by:

$$\text{Dose (mg/kg)} = (V_d \text{L/kg}) \times \text{change in serum concentration desired (mg/L)}$$

Where population values are known, this is a practical way to determine an appropriate loading dose. If the volume of distribution of caffeine is 1 L/kg and the target concentration is 10 mg/L, then the loading dose of caffeine base is 10 mg/kg:

$$\text{Dose mg/kg} = (1.0\ \text{L/kg}) \times (10\ \text{mg/L}) = 10\ \text{mg/kg}$$

It is important to recognize that this calculated dose represents that of caffeine base. Because caffeine is available as a salt (citrate, benzoate) and only 50% of a caffeine citrate dose is caffeine base, the actual caffeine citrate dose needed to achieve a target serum caffeine concentration of 10 mg/L would be 20 mg/kg.

This same principle can be used to adjust a specific dose regimen to achieve an alternate serum drug concentration. For example, a patient's serum caffeine concentration is 10 mg/L, but the desired target serum concentration is 15 mg/L. Using the same calculation:

$$\text{Dose (mg/kg)} = (1.0\ \text{L/kg}) \times (15 - 10 = 5\ \text{mg/L}) = 5\ \text{mg/kg caffeine base}$$

The V_d can also be applied as a physiologic marker for certain diseases. For example, a gentamicin V_d of >0.7 L/kg has 92% specificity for physiologically significant patent ductus arteriosus, even when it is clinically silent.

It is apparent from the relationship described by the formula relating V_d to dose and drug concentration that drug elimination from the body, or drug clearance (Cl), does not influence the initial or loading dose of a drug. Although a drug may be eliminated from the body only through the kidneys, the **initial dose is the same** for patients with normal renal function as for those with compromised or no renal function. The 1st dose of drug achieves an equilibrium concentration between body fluids and tissues. If a drug dose is administered by a route other than intravenously (oral, rectal, intramuscular, subcutaneous), the bioavailability of the drug must also be taken into account. In that case, the loading dose is calculated as: intravenous loading dose/bioavailability.

MAINTENANCE DOSING CONSIDERATIONS. The **elimination half-life** ($t_{1/2}$) of a drug is the time required for any given concentration in blood (or other biologic fluid) to decrease to ½ of the initial value, or the time required for ½ of the amount of drug present in the fluid to be cleared. The $t_{1/2}$ can be determined as:

$$t_{1/2} = 0.693/Kd$$

where *Kd* is equal to the slope of the terminal portion of the natural log of the linear serum concentration-time curve. The $t_{1/2}$ depends on both the Cl and the V_d of the drug. A more useful formula for $t_{1/2}$, which reflects these important relationships, is:

$$t_{1/2} = \frac{(0.693)(V_d)}{Cl}$$

A change in $t_{1/2}$ does not necessarily reflect a change in the body Cl of a drug. This dependence of $t_{1/2}$ on V_d is exemplified by the influence of extracorporeal membrane oxygenation (ECMO) on drug disposition. For most drugs, ECMO-induced changes are due to an increase in drug V_d (volume present within the apparatus) rather than a change in drug Cl. Despite this important distinction, the $t_{1/2}$ is often used clinically to adjust dosing intervals, primarily because it can easily be calculated in the clinic or at the patient's bedside. The $t_{1/2}$ of a drug can also be used to determine the time necessary to achieve the steady-state concentration, or the point at which the amount of drug administered (dose) is equivalent to the amount of drug cleared from the body. For drugs whose pharmacokinetic characteristics are best described by a linear, or 1st-order, process, 87.5% of the steady-state concentration is achieved after 3 half-lives; after 4 half-lives, it is 93.8%; and after 5 half-lives, it is 100%. When integrated with a target concentration strategy, the $t_{1/2}$ of a drug is often used to determine a drug's dosage interval.

Clearance (Cl) is the pharmacokinetic parameter that estimates the theoretical volume from which a drug is removed per unit of time. The *body Cl* of a drug reflects the amount of drug removed or eliminated from the body per unit of time, whereas *renal Cl* reflects the amount of drug cleared by the kidneys per unit of time. *Total body Cl* is the summation of all Cl mechanisms for a given drug (Cl_{renal}, $Cl_{hepatic}$, Cl_{lung}). The body Cl can be calculated as:

$$Cl = \frac{(0.693)(V_d)}{t_{1/2}}$$

with the preferred mathematical method of: drug dose/plasma drug **area under the concentration-time curve** where the dose is corrected for bioavailability.

Knowledge of a drug's Cl is fundamental and a necessity when determining the dose for a drug and how often its dose must be repeated to maintain a given serum concentration. It is the most important pharmacokinetic parameter for determining the steady-state drug concentration for a given dose rate. Changes in organ function that affect the removal of a drug from the body are reflected as a change in the drug's Cl. A drug's body Cl is influenced by the integrity of blood flow and the functional ability of the organs involved in removing the drug from the body. Diminished drug Cl can be used as an important marker of compromised organ function in situations such as perinatal asphyxia or progressive renal or liver dysfunction, and may be used to prompt other diagnostic tests. When Cl is known and a target **steady-state serum concentration** (C_{ss}) is determined, the maintenance dose (MD) can be calculated by the formula:

$$\text{MD (mg)} = C_{ss}\ (\text{mg/L}) \times (1\ \text{L/hr}) \times \text{dosing interval (hr)}$$

Again, it is important to correct for bioavailability by dividing the calculated MD by bioavailability.

INDIVIDUALIZATION OF DRUG DOSE. The clinical response to an average or usual recommended dose of drug can vary considerably, even when the dose is administered relative to a patient's body weight, surface area, and stage of maturation (see Chapter 56). This variation is a result of interindividual differences in drug pharmacokinetics and pharmacodynamics and a number of biologic variables, including genetic differences in drug metabolism or drug receptors, and concurrent pathophysiology or the presence of enzyme-inhibiting or enzyme-inducing drugs. Individual variability with respect to drug efficacy and possibly toxicity frequently necessitates the adjustment of dosage regimens for specific patients, especially for drugs with a low therapeutic index. For some drugs, the dose may be adjusted according to the patient's immediate and readily quantifiable clinical response. For other drugs, dosage adjustment may be guided more appropriately by combining clinical response with measurement of the concentration of drug in plasma or serum. Such an approach to therapy is often called a **target concentration strategy,** where a drug's pharmacologic or toxicologic response can be directly related to a specific serum concentration range. It is important to recognize that the therapeutic ranges described for drugs reflect a continuum of concentrations along which increasing percentages of patients can be expected to have a clinical response and toxicity (pharmacodynamic curves), and it is the tradeoff between benefit and risk that each clinician must use to decide whether targeting the lower or upper region of the therapeutic range, or even exceeding the therapeutic range, is optimal. Close attention to pharmacologic actions and physiologic responses is necessary for this optimal target concentration strategy.

Reported therapeutic concentration ranges for drugs are usually determined from studies of only a limited number of patients, mostly adults, and these therapeutic ranges represent an average (mean) value; therefore, not all in the population will be encompassed within the 2 standard deviations that surround this mean value. Thus, clinical monitoring of serum drug concentrations serves only as a guide to pharmacologic intervention and dose adjustment. Serum drug concentration values must be interpreted individually. One patient may have a complete clinical response when the serum concentration of drug X is within the "low" portion of the therapeutic range or window. The next patient, with the same disease of similar severity and requiring the same drug X, may require a serum drug concentration above or below the reported therapeutic concentration range to achieve the same degree of positive therapeutic response. Toxicity may limit how much above the therapeutic range the serum drug concentration may safely be raised. Therapeutic ranges for serum drug concentrations serve only as guidelines for therapy. Drug efficacy must be assessed by the clinical response.

Serum drug concentration-time values or profiles may also be compared with previously determined patient-specific values or literature reports to assess patient compliance with a prescribed drug regimen. If drug concentrations are very low at fairly high doses, **poor compliance** or drug delivery problems may be suspected. More commonly, determination of a drug concentration in biologic fluid helps to achieve an optimal therapeutic regimen while reducing the likelihood of drug toxicity. Finally, determination of a drug concentration in a biologic fluid provides a means to assess the influences, if any, of a disease process or drug interaction on a drug's disposition profile.

Therapeutic drug monitoring is not appropriate, necessary, or practical for all drugs. Drugs with well-defined and easily recognizable and monitored pharmacodynamic effects do not warrant routine monitoring (diuresis with diuretics, lowering of blood pressure by an antihypertensive). For therapeutic drug monitoring to be of clinical value, a clear concentration-response or concentration-toxicity relationship should be identifiable. Patient age and the extent or severity of disease can influence the relationships among drug concentration, efficacy, and toxicity. A clear relationship between a specific serum drug concentration and effect is available for only a limited number of drugs in contrast to the large number of drugs with "recommended" therapeutic ranges.

A number of variables should be considered when designing strategies to monitor therapy using a serum drug concentration. When measuring a drug's concentration in blood, the pharmacokinetic characteristics of that drug must be recalled so that blood samples can be obtained at appropriate times in relation to administration of the drug. This permits proper interpretation of drug concentrations and therapeutic effects and helps to avoid serious therapeutic errors. Peak drug concentrations in blood usually do not refer to the highest concentration achieved in blood with that drug, but instead to the postdistribution peak drug concentration. Thus, a lag time often exists between the time of drug administration and the time that is recommended to obtain the peak blood sample. Most clinical determinations of drug concentrations in biologic fluids routinely measure (report) the total drug concentration in that fluid:

Free drug concentration + concentration of drug bound to protein = total drug concentration

This approach assumes a constant ratio of free to bound drug at various concentrations and under differing pathophysiologic conditions, which may not always be true; thus, caution must be exercised in its extrapolation. Clinically important imbalances between free and total drug concentrations have been observed with the drug phenytoin in critically ill trauma patients and in patients with severe renal dysfunction. As a result, many laboratories report both free and total serum concentrations of drugs or have these results available on request. Despite these differences, it is unusual for an imbalance in this ratio to be clinically significant, except for drugs whose protein binding, under normal circumstances, is >90%.

ADDITIONAL CONSIDERATIONS

METHOD OF DRUG ADMINISTRATION. Intravenous administration of a drug is not always rapid or complete. The length of time necessary to infuse the total dose of an intravenously administered drug depends on a number of factors, including the flow rate of the primary intravenous fluid, the dead space of the system into which the drug is injected, and the total volume in which the drug is diluted. Because most standard intravenous fluid delivery systems, including their tubing, are designed for adult use, they contain a large volume per unit of length. This introduces a relatively large dead space factor, which causes substantial infusion delays when operated at the slow flow rates necessary for infants and children. Even intravenous infusion systems designed for pediatric patients can have problems and limitations that may confound drug therapy management and require clinician awareness.

Several steps can be taken to minimize problems with intravenous drug administration to small infants and children, including standardization and documentation of the total administration time; documentation of the volume and content of the solution used to "flush" an intravenous dose; standardization of specific infusion techniques (infusion duration, volumes) for drugs with a narrow therapeutic index; standardization of dilution and infusion volumes for drugs given by intermittent intravenous injection; avoidance of the practice of attaching lines for drug infusion to a central hub with other solutions infused concurrently at widely disparate rates; preferential use of large-gauge cannulas; maintenance of the recommended solution at a specified height above the infusion site for use with a gravity-based controller; and the use of low-volume tubing and the most distal sites for access of the drug into an existing intravenous line.

DRUG-DRUG INTERACTIONS. When 2 or more drugs are administered to the same patient, the pharmacokinetic and pharmacodynamic properties of each agent may be modified by their interaction. Drugs may interact by a number of mechanisms classified on the basis of pharmaceutics, pharmacokinetics, pharmacodynamics, or a combination thereof. These interactions may result in unpredictable clinical effects or toxicologic responses. Pharmaceutic interactions include those resulting in drug inactivation when compounds are mixed together physically before patient administration, as with the use of syringes, infusion tubing, dialysate solutions, or parenteral fluid preparations.

Pharmacokinetic interactions can occur when the disposition characteristics of 1 compound (absorption, distribution, metabolism, excretion, or a combination thereof) are influenced by those of another. This type of interaction may involve 1 or more aspects of the pharmacokinetic profile of the drug. One drug may reduce the rate, but not the overall extent of absorption, or a compound may displace a drug from its protein-binding sites while concomitantly retarding its elimination from the body. Metabolic-based drug-drug interactions can occur whenever 2 compounds compete for the same metabolic site (see Table 56-2).

Drugs may interact pharmacodynamically and compete for the same receptor or physiologic system, thus altering a patient's response to drug therapy. The number of known, clinically important drug interactions, combined with the ever-increasing number of available pharmacologic agents, emphasizes the need to critically assess the possibility of drug-drug and drug-food interactions in any patient receiving multiple drugs (Table 56-3).

DRUGS IN HUMAN MILK. Almost all drugs administered to lactating women are secreted to some extent into their milk and may be ingested by the nursing infant (see Chapter 94). Although drug use should be as minimal as possible during (pregnancy and) lactation, it is not possible or desirable for lactating women to stop taking needed medications. There are very few drug contraindications for maternal use during lactation. Although a drug may distribute or concentrate in breast milk, the actual infant dose

TABLE 57-3. Partial Listing of Drug Interactions of Potential Importance in Pediatric Practice

INTERACTING AGENT	ADVERSE EFFECT
ACETAMINOPHEN	
Alcohol	Hepatotoxicity
Oral anticoagulants	↑ Anticoagulation
Probenecid	↑ Acetaminophen toxicity
Zidovudine	Granulocytopenia
ACYCLOVIR	
Narcotics	↑ Narcotic toxicity?
Zidovudine	Lethargy
ALCOHOL	
Antidepressants (tricyclic)	↑ Toxicity
Barbiturates	↑ CNS depression (acute)
Benzodiazepines	↑ CNS depression
Cephalosporins (not all)	Disulfiram effect
Chloral hydrate	↑ CNS depression
Doxycycline	↓ Antibiotic effect
Isoniazid	↑ Hepatotoxicity
Metronidazole	Disulfiram effect
Phenothiazines	Impaired coordination
Phenytoin	↑ Phenytoin toxicity
ALLOPURINOL	
Aluminum hydroxide	↓ Allopurinol absorption
Ampicillin	Rash
Anticoagulants (oral)	↑ Anticoagulant effect
Azathioprine	↑ Azathioprine toxicity
Captopril	↑ Cutaneous hypersensitivity
Cyclophosphamide	↑ Cyclophosphamide toxicity
Theophylline	↑ Theophylline toxicity
Thiazide diuretics	↑ Allopurinol toxicity
AMINOGLYCOSIDE ANTIBIOTICS	
Amphotericin B	↑ Nephrotoxicity
Bumetanide	↑ Ototoxicity
Cisplatin	↑ Nephrotoxicity
Cyclosporine	↑ Nephrotoxicity
Furosemide	↑ Nephrotoxicity and ototoxicity
Magnesium	↑ Neuromuscular blockade
Neuromuscular blocking agents	↑ Blockade
Vancomycin	↑ Nephrotoxicity?
ANTACIDS	
β-Adrenergic blockers	↓ Absorption
Captopril	↓ Absorption
Cimetidine	↓ Absorption
Corticosteroids	↓ Absorption
Digoxin	↓ Absorption
Iron	↓ Absorption
Isoniazid	↓ Absorption
Ketoconazole	↓ Absorption
Nonsteroidal anti-inflammatory agents	↓ Absorption
Phenytoin	↓ Absorption
Salicylates	↓ Absorption
Tetracycline	↓ Absorption
Theophylline	↑ Toxicity
ASPIRIN	
Anticoagulants (oral)	↑ Bleeding
Captopril	↓ Antihypertensive effect
BARBITURATES	
Anticoagulants (oral)	↓ Anticoagulation
β-Adrenergic blockers	↓ β Blockade
Carbamazepine	↑ Production of carbamazepine epoxide
Chloramphenicol	↑ Barbiturate toxicity
Contraceptives (oral)	↓ Contraception
Corticosteroids	↓ Steroid effect
Influenza vaccine (viral)	↑ Barbiturate toxicity
Rifampin	↓ Barbiturate effect
Theophylline	↓ Theophylline effect
Valproate	↑ Barbiturate toxicity
BLEOMYCIN	
Oxygen	↑ Pulmonary toxicity
CAPTOPRIL	
Allopurinol	↑ Cutaneous hypersensitivity
Aspirin	↓ Antihypertensive effect
Cimetidine	Neuropathy
Nonsteroidal anti-inflammatory agents	↓ Antihypertensive effect
Potassium	Hyperkalemia
Spironolactone	Hyperkalemia
CARBAMAZEPINE	
Anticoagulants (oral)	↓ Anticoagulation
Antidepressants (tricyclic)	↑ Toxicity (both drugs)
Cimetidine	↑ Carbamazepine toxicity
Contraceptives (oral)	↓ Contraception
Corticosteroids	↓ Steroid effect
Cyclosporine	↓ Cyclosporine effect
Erythromycins	↑ Carbamazepine toxicity
Influenza vaccine (viral)	↑ Carbamazepine toxicity
Isoniazid	↑ Toxicity (both drugs)
Phenytoin	↓ Carbamazepine effect
Theophylline	↓ Theophylline effect
Valproate	↓ Valproate effect
CIMETIDINE	
Alcohol	↑ Alcohol effect
Antacids	↓ Cimetidine effect
Anticoagulants (oral)	↑ Anticoagulation
Antidepressants (tricyclic)	↑ Antidepressant toxicity
Benzodiazepines	↑ Benzodiazepine toxicity
β-Adrenergic blocking agents	↑ β-Blockade toxicity
Captopril	Neuropathy
Carbamazepine	↑ Carbamazepine toxicity
Digoxin	↑ Digoxin toxicity
Ketoconazole	↓ Ketoconazole absorption
Metoclopramide	↓ Cimetidine effect
Phenytoin	↑ Phenytoin toxicity
Theophylline	↑ Theophylline toxicity
CONTRACEPTIVES (ORAL)	
Anticoagulants (oral)	↓ Anticoagulation
Antidepressants (tricyclic)	↑ Antidepressant toxicity
Barbiturates	↓ Contraception
Carbamazepine	↓ Contraception
Griseofulvin	↓ Contraception
Penicillins (ampicillin, oxacillin)	↓ Contraception?
Phenytoin	↓ Contraception
Rifampin	↓ Contraception
Theophylline	↑ Theophylline toxicity
CYCLOSPORINE	
Alkylating agents	↑ Nephrotoxicity
Aminoglycosides	↑ Nephrotoxicity
Amphotericin B	↑ Nephrotoxicity
Carbamazepine	↓ Cyclosporine effect
Erythromycins	↑ Cyclosporine toxicity
Furosemide	Gout
Ketoconazole	↑ Nephrotoxicity
Metoclopramide	↑ Cyclosporine toxicity
Nafcillin	↓ Cyclosporine effect
Phenytoin	↓ Cyclosporine effect
Rifampin	↓ Cyclosporine effect
DIGOXIN	
Antacids	↓ Absorption
Anticholinergics	↑ Digoxin toxicity
Cholestyramine	↓ Absorption
Cimetidine	↑ Digoxin toxicity
Diuretics (hypokalemia)	↑ Digoxin toxicity
Phenytoin	↓ Digoxin effect
Quinidine	↑ Digoxin toxicity
Verapamil	↑ Digoxin toxicity
ERYTHROMYCINS	
Anticoagulants (oral)	↑ Anticoagulation
Astemizole (Hismanal)	↑ Astemizole toxicity: arrhythmias
Carbamazepine	↑ Carbamazepine toxicity
Cyclosporine	↑ Cyclosporine toxicity
Phenytoin	↓ Phenytoin effect
Terfenadine (Seldane)	↑ Terfenadine toxicity: arrhythmias
Theophylline	↑ Theophylline toxicity

TABLE 57-3. Partial Listing of Drug Interactions of Potential Importance in Pediatric Practice—cont'd

INTERACTING AGENT	ADVERSE EFFECT
FLUOROQUINOLONES	
Antacids	↓ Antibiotic effect
Theophylline	↑ Theophylline toxicity
GRISEOFULVIN	
Anticoagulants (oral)	↓ Anticoagulants
Contraceptive (oral)	↓ Contraceptive
ISONIAZID	
Alcohol	Hepatitis
Antacids	↓ Isoniazid absorption
Carbamazepine	↑ Toxicity (both)
Ketoconazole	↓ Ketoconazole effect
Phenytoin	↑ Phenytoin toxicity
Rifampin	↑ Hepatotoxicity
Valproate	↑ Hepatic and CNS toxicity
KETOCONAZOLE	
Antacids	↓ Absorption
Anticoagulants (oral)	↑ Anticoagulation
Cimetidine	↓ Ketoconazole effect
Cyclosporine	↑ Nephrotoxicity
Isoniazid	↓ Ketoconazole effect
Phenytoin	Altered metabolism of both drugs
Rifampin	↑ Effects of both drugs
METHOTREXATE	
Blood transfusion	↑ Toxicity
Cisplatin	↑ Methotrexate toxicity
Etretinate	↑ Hepatotoxicity
Nonsteroidal anti-inflammatory drugs	↑ Methotrexate toxicity
Trimethoprim/sulfamethoxazole	Megaloblastic anemia
METOCLOPRAMIDE	
Carbamazepine	Neurotoxicity
Cimetidine	↓ Cimetidine effect
Cyclosporine	↑ Cyclosporine toxicity
Digoxin	↓ Absorption
Narcotics	↑ Sedation
NIFEDIPINE	
β-Adrenergic blockers	Heart failure, atrioventricular block
Cyclosporine	↑ Gingival hyperplasia
Phenytoin	↑ Phenytoin toxicity
Prazosin	Hypotension
Quinidine	↓ Quinidine effect
PHENYTOIN	
Alcohol	↑ Toxicity (acute)
Antacids	↓ Phenytoin effect
Anticoagulants (oral)	↓ Phenytoin toxicity, ↑↓ anticoagulation
Antidepressants (tricyclic)	↑ Phenytoin toxicity
Carbamazepine	↓ Carbamazepine effect
Chloramphenicol	↑ Toxicity (both drugs)
Cimetidine	↑ Phenytoin toxicity
Contraceptives (oral and implant)	↓ Contraception
Corticosteroids	↓ Corticosteroid effect
Cyclosporine	↓ Cyclosporine effect
Digoxin	↓ Digoxin effect
Dopamine	Hypotension
Folic acid	↓ Phenytoin effect
Isoniazid	↑ Phenytoin toxicity
Miconazole	↓ Phenytoin effect
Neuromuscular blocking agents	↓ Blockade
Nifedipine	↑ Phenytoin toxicity
Quinidine	↓ Quinidine effect
Rifampin	↓ Phenytoin effect
Theophylline	↓ Effects (both drugs)
Valproate	↑ Phenytoin toxicity
QUINIDINE	
Amiodarone	↑ Quinidine toxicity
Anticoagulants (oral)	↑ Anticoagulation
Barbiturates	↓ Quinidine effect
Cimetidine	↑ Quinidine toxicity
Digoxin	↑ Digoxin toxicity
Metoclopramide	↓ Quinidine effect
Phenytoin	↓ Quinidine effect
Procainamide	↑ Procainamide toxicity
Rifampin	↓ Quinidine effect
Verapamil	Hypotension
RIFAMPIN	
Anticoagulants (oral)	↓ Anticoagulation
Barbiturates	↓ Barbiturate effect
β-Adrenergic blockers	↓ β Blockade
Chloramphenicol	↓ Chloramphenicol effect
Contraceptives (oral)	↓ Contraception
Corticosteroids	↓ Corticosteroid effect
Cyclosporine	↓ Cyclosporine effect
Isoniazid	↑ Hepatotoxicity
Ketoconazole	↓ Effects (both drugs)
Phenytoin	↓ Phenytoin effect
Quinidine	↓ Quinidine effect
Theophylline	↓ Theophylline effect
Verapamil	↓ Verapamil effect
THEOPHYLLINE	
Barbiturates	↓ Theophylline effect
β-Adrenergic blockers	↑ Theophylline toxicity
Carbamazepine	↓ Theophylline effect
Cimetidine	↑ Theophylline toxicity
Erythromycins	↑ Theophylline toxicity
Fluoroquinolones	↑ Theophylline toxicity
Influenza vaccine (viral)	↑ Theophylline toxicity
Interferon	↑ Toxicity?
Marijuana smoking	↓ Theophylline effect
Phenytoin	↓ Effect (both drugs)
Rifampin	↓ Theophylline effect
Tobacco smoking	↓ Theophylline effect
Troleandomycin	↑ Theophylline toxicity
TRIMETHOPRIM/SULFAMETHOXAZOLE	
Anticoagulants (oral)	↑ Anticoagulation
Antidepressants (tricyclic)	Depression
Mercaptopurine	↓ Antileukemia effect
Methotrexate	Megaloblastic anemia
VALPROATE	
Barbiturates	↑ Phenobarbital toxicity
Benzodiazepines	↑ Diazepam toxicity
Carbamazepines	↓ Valproate effect
Cimetidine	↑ Valproate toxicity?
Ethosuximide	↑ Ethosuximide toxicity?
Phenytoin	↑ Phenytoin toxicity

*When possible, an alternate drug combination should be given. If not possible, drug levels and signs of toxicity must be monitored.
Modified from Rizack M, Hillman C: *The Medical Letter Handbook of Adverse Drug Interactions*. New Rochelle, NY, The Medical Letter, 1989.
CNS, central nervous system; ?, possible effect.

received (volume of milk consumed), combined with the drug's bioavailability (in the infant) and the amount of drug (over the feeding periods), usually negates any clinically relevant effects in the breast-fed infant. If a question exists about the amount of drug a breast-feeding infant may be receiving or about possible drug effects in the infant, a sample of the mother's milk can be analyzed. Up-to-date and specific information about breast milk distribution of medications and the amount a nursing infant would actually receive (absorb) can be obtained by consulting a clinical pharmacy/pharmacology service.

PRESCRIBING MEDICATIONS. Factors such as taste, smell, color, consistency, dosing frequency, and cost affect the degree to which patients comply with their therapeutic drug regimen. Prescribing generically equivalent medications can sometimes reduce the cost of a drug. Such prescribing should be done only when it is clearly known that the generic brand affords equivalent bioavailability, bioeffectiveness, and patient acceptability. Complete bioequivalence data are not available for all drugs; when in doubt, the prescribing physician should consult with the pharmacist.

A prescription issued by the prescribing physician should always direct the dispensing of just enough drug to treat the patient, leaving only a small amount of drug left over after the prescribed course of therapy has been completed. This small residual allows for the loss of some drug in case of doses accidentally spilled, spit out, or lost. Parents should be instructed to discard all remaining doses of a prescribed medication after the completed course of therapy to protect against accidental poisoning or improper self-medication at a later date. Patient medication instructions on the prescription should state the specific number of doses the patient should receive each day and the total duration of therapy (number of days of therapy). The number of times the prescribing physician allows the prescription to be refilled should be noted on the prescription label; if no refills are to be permitted, this should also be specified on the written prescription.

COMPLIANCE WITH THE PRESCRIBED REGIMEN. Little is known about the many factors that determine the degree of compliance with a physician's instructions, but many patients frequently do not take medication consistently or in the manner intended or prescribed. Patients frequently take home remedies or medications that are not recommended or prescribed by their physician. A child's compliance with a prescribed therapeutic regimen is usually only as good as that of the parents. Compliance can be maximized by carefully educating the family about the nature of the child's illness, the action of the medications prescribed, and the importance of following the instructions precisely. Compliance with the therapeutic regimen is improved when the instructions are written down clearly and in detail for the family and when the regimen results in minimal interference with the daily living schedule (particularly parental sleeping habits). Collaboration between the prescribing physician and the dispensing pharmacist can often identify compliance problems and improve compliance through patient education.

Benedetti MS, Baltes E: Drug metabolism and disposition in children. *Fund Clin Pharmacol* 2003;17:281–299.

Björkman S: Prediction of drug disposition in infants and children by means of physiologically based pharmacokinetic (PBPK) modeling: Theophylline and midazolam as model drugs. *Br J Clin Pharmacol* 2004;59:691–704.

Carr RR, Ensom MHH: Drug disposition and therapy in adolescence: The effects of puberty. *J Pediatr Pharmacol Ther* 2003;8:86–96.

Eichelbaum M, Ingelman-Sundberg M, Evans WE: Pharmacogenomics and individualized drug therapy. *Ann Rev Med* 2006;57:11.1–11.19.

Johnson TN: The development of drug metabolising enzymes and their influence on the susceptibility to adverse drug reactions in children. *Toxicology* 2003;192:37–48.

Kearns GL, Abdel-Rahman SM, Alander SW, et al: Developmental pharmacology: Drug disposition, action, and therapy in infants and children. *N Engl J Med* 2003;349:1157–1167.

Paul IM: Advances in pediatric pharmacology, therapeutics, and toxicology. *Adv Pediatr* 2005;52:321–365.

Stephenson T: How children's responses to drugs differ from adults. *Br J Clin Pharmacol* 2005;59:670–673.

Waters MD, Fostel JM: Toxicogenomics and systems toxicology: Aims and prospects. *Nat Rev Genet* 2004;5:936–948.

Chapter 58 ■ Poisonings

George C. Rodgers, Jr., Tania Condurache, Michael D. Reed, Michelle Bestic, and Peter Gal

EPIDEMIOLOGY

Of the >2 million human poisoning exposures reported annually to the Toxic Exposure Surveillance System (TESS) of the American Association of Poison Control Centers (AAPCC), >50% occur in children 5 yr of age or younger. Almost all of these exposures are unintentional and reflect the propensity for children in this age group to put virtually anything in their mouths.

More than 90% of toxic exposures in children occur in the home, and most involve only a single substance. Ingestion is the most common route of poisoning exposure (77% of cases), with the dermal, inhalation, and ophthalmic routes accounting for approximately 7.5%, 6%, and 5% of cases, respectively. Approximately 50% of cases involve nondrug substances, such as common household products (cosmetics, personal care items, cleaning solutions, plants, foreign bodies, hydrocarbons). Pharmaceutical preparations comprise the remainder, with analgesics, cough and cold products, antimicrobial agents, and vitamins the most common categories. These are products that are familiar to young children; in addition, they are usually manufactured in visually appealing and great-tasting formulations. More than 85% of pediatric poisoning exposures can be managed without direct medical intervention, because either the product involved is not inherently very toxic or the quantity of the material involved is not sufficient to produce clinically relevant toxic effects (Table 58-1). Death due to unintentional poisoning in young children is uncommon owing to increased product safety measures (child-resistant packaging), increased poison prevention education, early recognition of exposure, improvements in medical management, and the availability of 24 hr/day, 7 day/wk 800 number access to regionally based poison control centers.

Poison prevention education should be an integral part of all well child visits, even before a child is mobile. Counseling parents and other caregivers about potential poisoning risks, how to "poison-proof" a child's environment, and what to do if a poisoning occurs diminishes the likelihood of serious morbidity or mortality from an exposure. Poison prevention educational materials are available from both the American Academy of Pediatrics and regional poison control centers. A network of poison control centers exists in the U.S., and anyone at any time can contact a regional poison center by calling a toll-free number: **1-800-222-1222.** The ready access to this number should be discussed often during the 1st 2 yr of office visits and annually thereafter. The sharing of this toll-free number with grandparents, relatives, and caregiver programs is also highly desirable.

Poisoning exposures in children 6–12 yr of age are much less common, involving approximately 6% of all pediatric exposures. Toxic exposures in adolescents are primarily intentional (suicide, abuse) or occupational. Pediatricians should be aware of the signs of drug abuse or suicidal ideation in this population and should aggressively intervene. Pediatric fatalities after a poisoning exposure are most common in adolescents, with 6.1% of the 1,261 fatalities reported to the TESS program in 2005 occurring in 13–19 yr old patients compared with 1.9% in children 6 yr old or younger and 1.0% in children 6–12 yr of age.

TABLE 58-1. Common Nontoxic and Minimally Toxic* Products

Abrasives	Ink (black, blue—nonpermanent)
Antacids, non-salicylate-containing	Iodophil disinfectants (unless the individual is allergic)
Antibiotics, topical	Laxatives
Antifungals, topical	Lipstick
Ballpoint pen ink	Lozenges (without anesthetics)
Bathtub floating toys	Lubricating oils (unless aspirated)
Bath oil (unless aspirated)	Magazines
Body conditioners	Markers, porous tip
Bubble bath soap	Makeup
Calamine lotion	Matches
Candles (beeswax or paraffin)	Mineral oil (unless aspirated)
Caps (toy pistols, potassium chlorate)	Modeling compound (Play-Doh)
Chalk (calcium carbonate)	Newspaper (chronic ingestion may result in lead poisoning)
Children's toy cosmetics	Paint, indoor latex, water-based
Clay (modeling)	Paints, watercolor
Oral contraceptives without iron	Pencil lead (graphite, coloring)
Corticosteroids, topical	Petroleum jelly (Vaseline)
Cosmetics	Plant food (no insecticides or herbicides)
Crayons (marked A.P. or C.P., gel)	Polaroid picture coating fluid
Dehumidifying packets (e.g., silica)	Putty
Deodorants, underarm	Rubber cement
Fabric softeners	Shampoo
Fertilizers (no insecticides or herbicides)	Shaving creams and lotions
Detergents, hand, dishwashing	Silica gel
Diaper rash creams/ointments	Soap and soap products (noncaustic)
Fishbowl additives	Spackles
Glow products	Starch
Glues and paste	Sunscreen
Golf ball (core may cause mechanical injury)	Sweetening agents (saccharin, aspartame)
Grease	Toothpaste(with and without fluoride)
Hand lotions and creams	Warfarin rodenticides (<0.5%)
Hydrogen peroxide (medicinal 3%)	Watercolor paints
Incense	Zinc oxide
Indelible markers	

*The potential for toxicity is dependent on the magnitude and amount of exposure. These agents are considered nontoxic or minimally toxic for mild to moderate exposure. The potential for toxicity increases with increased amount of exposure.

APPROACH TO THE POISONED PATIENT

The initial approach to the patient with a documented or suspected poisoning should be no different than that in any other sick child. A detailed history and physical examination serves as the foundation for a thoughtful differential diagnosis and the formation of an initial prognosis (Table 58-2). The history and physical examination should not await the collection of body fluid and the results of a "tox screen." Toxicology laboratory analyses, or "screens," in fact evaluate for only a small fraction of common pediatric exposures and rarely make (vs confirm) the diagnosis.

INITIAL PATIENT EVALUATION

PATIENT HISTORY. Obtaining an accurate problem-oriented history is of paramount importance if a poisoning has occurred or is suspected. The following information should be obtained during the initial assessment.

Description of Toxins. Product names (brand, generic, chemical) and ingredients, along with their concentrations, may be obtained from labels. Because many brand names that sound alike have very different ingredients, it is important to be precise. If the ingredient information is not readily available on the product, consultation with a poison control center can usually provide this information rapidly. Most products used in the home or workplace contain multiple ingredients in varying concentrations, and the poison control center can provide specific information regarding all ingredients in the particular product as well as prioritize possible clinical effects from individual ingredients or a combination of ingredients. Furthermore, most pills and capsules have markings, including letters, numerals, or both, and based on these markings, the poison center may be able to identify the ingredients. Several characteristic toxic syndromes, or "toxidromes," exist for some of the more common exposures and may assist in identifying the offending agent. The more common **"toxidromes"** and other poisoning manifestations categories are shown in Tables 58-3 to 58-5.

Magnitude of Exposure. It is important to attempt to determine as accurately as possible how much of the substance has been ingested. This may be difficult, but is of paramount importance in refining the initial prognosis guiding the initial management plans. Numerous methods can be used to estimate the amounts

TABLE 58-2. Historical and Physical Findings in Poisoning

ODOR	
Bitter almonds	Cyanide
Acetone	Isopropyl alcohol, methanol, paraldehyde, salicylates
Alcohol	Ethanol
Wintergreen	Methyl salicylate
Garlic	Arsenic, thallium, organophosphates
OCULAR SIGNS	
Miosis	Narcotics (except meperidine), organophosphates, muscarinic mushrooms, clonidine, phenothiazines, chloral hydrate, barbiturates (late), PCP
Mydriasis	Atropine, alcohol, cocaine, amphetamines, antihistamines, cyclic antidepressants, cyanide, carbon monoxide
Nystagmus	Phenytoin, barbiturates, ethanol, carbon monoxide
Lacrimation	Organophosphates, irritant gas or vapors
Retinal hyperemia	Methanol
Poor vision	Methanol, botulism, carbon monoxide
CUTANEOUS SIGNS	
Needle tracks	Heroin, PCP, amphetamines
Bullae	Carbon monoxide, barbiturates
Dry, hot skin	Anticholinergic agents, botulism
Diaphoresis	Organophosphates, nitrates, muscarinic mushrooms, aspirin, cocaine
Alopecia	Thallium, arsenic, lead, mercury
Erythema	Boric acid, mercury, cyanide, anticholinergics
ORAL SIGNS	
Salivation	Organophosphates, salicylates, corrosives, strychnine
Dry mouth	Amphetamines, anticholinergics, antihistamine
Burns	Corrosives, oxalate-containing plants
Gum lines	Lead, mercury, arsenic
Dysphagia	Corrosives, botulism
INTESTINAL SIGNS	
Cramps	Arsenic, lead, thallium, organophosphates
Diarrhea	Antimicrobials, arsenic, iron, boric acid
Constipation	Lead, narcotics, botulism
Hematemesis	Aminophylline, corrosives, iron, salicylates
CARDIAC SIGNS	
Tachycardia	Atropine, aspirin, amphetamines, cocaine, cyclic antidepressants, theophylline
Bradycardia	Digitalis, narcotics, mushrooms, clonidine, organophosphates, β blockers, calcium channel blockers
Hypertension	Amphetamines, LSD, cocaine, PCP
Hypotension	Phenothiazines, barbiturates, cyclic antidepressants, iron, β blockers, calcium channel blockers
RESPIRATORY SIGNS	
Depressed respiration	Alcohol, narcotics, barbiturates
Increased respiration	Amphetamines, aspirin, ethylene glycol, carbon monoxide, cyanide
Pulmonary edema	Hydrocarbons, heroin, organophosphates, aspirin
CNS SIGNS	
Ataxia	Alcohol, antidepressants, barbiturates, anticholinergics, phenytoin, narcotics
Coma	Sedatives, narcotics, barbiturates, PCP, organophosphates, salicylates, cyanide, carbon monoxide, cyclic antidepressants, lead
Hyperpyrexia	Anticholinergics, quinine, salicylates, LSD, phenothiazines, amphetamines, cocaine
Muscle fasciculation	Organophosphates, theophylline
Muscle rigidity	Cyclic antidepressants, PCP, phenothiazines, haloperidol
Paresthesia	Cocaine, camphor, PCP, MSG
Peripheral neuropathy	Lead, arsenic, mercury, organophosphates
Altered behavior	LSD, PCP, amphetamines, cocaine, alcohol, anticholinergics, camphor

From Kliegman RM, Marcdante KJ, Jenson HB (editors): *Nelson Essentials of Pediatrics*, 5th ed. Philadelphia, Elsevier, 2006, p 205.
CNS, central nervous system; LSD, lysergic acid diethylamide; MSG, monosodium glutamate; PCP, phencyclidine.

TABLE 58-3. Recognizable Poison Syndromes

POISON SYNDROME	ASSOCIATED SIGNS	POSSIBLE TOXINS
Increased sympathetic nervous system activity	Pyrexia Flushing Tachycardia Hypertension Pupillary constriction Sweating	Cough and decongestant preparations Amphetamines Cocaine Ecstasy Theophylline
Anticholinergic activity	Similar clinical picture to sympathomimetics **Clinical differences** include: pupillary dilation, dry mouth, hot, dry skin	Tricyclic antidepressants Antiparkinsonian drugs Antihistamines Atropine and nightshade Antispasmodics Phenothiazines Mushroom poisoning (*Amanita* species) Cyclopentolate eyedrops
Increased parasympathetic nervous system activity: **cholinergic crisis**	Pupillary constriction Diarrhea Urinary incontinence Sweating Excessive salivation Muscle weakness Fasciculation Paralysis Lacrimation	Organophosphate insecticides Drugs for myasthenia gravis (e.g., pyridostigmine) Nicotine Carbamate insecticides
Metabolic acidosis	Tachyopnea Kussmaul breathing (sighing respiration)	Ethanol Carbon monoxide Antifreeze Iron Diabetic medication Tricyclic antidepressants Salicylates
Chemical pneumonitis	Cough Respiratory distress Central nervous system depression A history of vomiting after ingestion need not be a feature	Stoddard solvent (white spirit) Turpentine Essential oils
Acute ataxia or nystagmus		Antihistamines Alcohol Anticonvulsants (especially phenytoin and carbamazepine) Piperazine Diphenylhydantoin Barbiturates Carbon monoxide Organic solvents Bromides
Methemoglobinemia	Cyanosis resistant to oxygen therapy	Alanine dyes Nitrates Benzocaine Phenacetin Nitrobenzene Chlorates Sulphonamides and metoclopramide (in neonates)
Renal failure	Oliguria or anuria Hematuria Myoglobinuria	Carbon tetrachloride Ethylene glycol Methanol Mushrooms Oxalates
Violent emesis		Aspirin Theophylline Corrosives Fluoride Boric acid Iron
Generalized muscle rigidity	Seizure-like, generalized muscle contractions or painful spasms (neck and limbs) and usually tachycardia and hypertension Intact sensorium	Strychnine
Oropharyngeal pain and ulcerations	Lip, mouth, and pharyngeal ulcerations and burning pain Dyspnea and hemoptysis secondary to pulmonary edema or hemorrhage; can progress to pulmonary fibrosis over days to weeks	Paraquat* Diquat Caustics (i.e., acids and alkalis) Inorganic mercuric salts Mustards (e.g., sulfur)
Cellular hypoxia	Mild: Nausea, vomiting, and headache Severe: Altered mental status, dyspnea, hypotension, seizures, and metabolic acidosis Bitter almond odor† Hypocalcemia or hypokalemia	Cyanide* (e.g., hydrogen cyanide gas or sodium cyanide) Sodium monofluoroacetate (SMFA)* Carbon monoxide Hydrogen sulfide Sodium azide Methemoglobin-causing agents
Peripheral neuropathy and/or neurocognitive effects	Peripheral neuropathy signs and symptoms: Muscle weakness and atrophy, "glove and stocking" sensory loss, and depressed or absent deep tendon reflexes Neurocognitive effects: Memory loss, delirium, ataxia, and/or encephalopathy Visual disturbances, paresthesias, and/or ataxia Delirium and/or peripheral neuropathy Encephalopathy and/or peripheral neuropathy	Mercury (organic)* Arsenic (inorganic)* Thallium Lead Acrylamide
Severe gastrointestinal illness, dehydration	Abdominal pain, vomiting, profuse diarrhea (possibly bloody), and hypotension, possibly followed by multisystem organ failure Inhalation an additional route of exposure; severe respiratory illness possible Hypokalemia common	Arsenic* Ricin* Colchicine Barium
Serotonin	Altered mental status (agitation, confusion, coma), autonomi instability (tachycardia, hyper- or hypotension), hyperkinetic neuromuscular (tremor, clonus, hyperreflexia), mydriasis, diaphoresis, increased bowel motility	SSRIs, antidepressants, some opioids (meperidine), tramadol, St. John's wort, MAOIs
Withdrawal	Abdominal cramps, diarrhea, lacrimation, sweating, "goose flesh," yawning, tachycardia, restlessness, hallucinations	Cessation of alcohol, barbiturates, benzodiazepines, narcotics

*Potential agents for a covert chemical release based on historic use (i.e., intentional or inadvertent use), high toxicity, and/or ease of availability.
†Unreliable sign.

involved; it is better to overestimate than to underestimate. Estimates can often be accomplished by counting the remaining tablets or measuring the remaining volume of liquid. Whatever amount is missing and cannot be definitively accounted for should be assumed to be the amount ("dose") to which the patient was exposed. When >1 child is involved, initial clinical assessments should assume that each child was exposed to the entire amount estimated, even if the child or children state otherwise. These probable overestimates of exposure provide a safety margin early during the clinical assessment. Estimates can be refined as the patient is assessed over time and initial laboratory data become available. Because the toxicity of most agents is dose-related, knowing the age or weight of the child aids in assessment. For inhalation, ocular, or dermal exposures, the concentration of the offending agent and the length of contact time with the material should be determined, in addition to the time course for associated symptoms to occur, their progression, and possible resolution.

Time of Exposure. For some products, toxic manifestations may be delayed for hr or days. Knowing the time lapse between expo-

TABLE 58-4. Screening Laboratory Clues in Toxicologic Diagnosis

METABOLIC ACIDOSIS (MNEMONIC = MUDPIES)
Methanol,* carbon monoxide
Uremia*
Diabetes mellitus*
Paraldehyde,* phenformin
Isoniazid, iron
Ethanol,* ethylene glycol*
Salicylates, starvation, seizures

HYPOGLYCEMIA
Ethanol
Isoniazid
Insulin
Propranolol
Oral hypoglycemic agents
Salicylates

HYPERGLYCEMIA
Salicylates
Isoniazid
Iron
Phenothiazines
Sympathomimetics

HYPOCALCEMIA
Oxalate
Ethylene glycol
Fluoride

RADIOPAQUE SUBSTANCE ON KUB (MNEMONIC = CHIPPED)
Chloral hydrate, calcium carbonate
Heavy metals (lead, zinc, barium, arsenic, lithium, bismuth, as in Pepto-Bismol)
Iron
Phenothiazines
Play-Doh, potassium chloride
Enteric-coated pills
Dental amalgam

*Hyperosmolar condition.
From Kliegman RM, Mascdante KJ, Jenson HB (editors): *Nelson Essentials of Pediatrics*, 5th ed. Philadelphia, Elsevier, p 207.
KUB, kidney-ureter-bladder radiograph.

sure and the onset of symptoms and/or medical evaluation will markedly influence decisions about obtaining certain diagnostic testing as well as therapeutic intervention.

Progression of Symptoms. Knowing the nature and progression of symptoms is very helpful for assessing the need for immediate life support, the prognosis, and the type of intervention that may be needed.

MEDICAL HISTORY. Underlying diseases may make a child more susceptible to the effects of a toxin. Concurrent drug therapy may also increase susceptibility because certain drugs may interact with the toxin. Pregnancy is a common precipitating factor in adolescent suicide attempts and can influence the patient evaluation and treatment plan. At 6 mo of age or younger, it is very unlikely that an infant could become accidentally exposed to a sufficient quantity of a potentially harmful product in the absence of other extraneous factors that require further investigation (social environment).

DEMOGRAPHIC INFORMATION. It is particularly important to obtain demographic information regarding the patient and the caller. Obtaining the caller's telephone number and street address is important for follow-up and also to allow for dispatch of emergency personnel if telephone contact is disrupted.

INITIAL MEDICAL CARE

If the patient is managed at home, follow-up assessment calls should be made at varying times after exposure because any change in the patient's condition may alter the decision to remain at home. The timing of follow-up calls depends on the type and extent of the exposure, combined with a number of clinical variables, including the expectation for when symptoms would begin to occur and progress. Usually, it is advisable to initiate the 1st follow-up call 0.5–1.0 hr after the exposure to detect any symptoms that may manifest if the timing, nature, and/or amount of exposure were different than initially thought; a 2nd follow-up call should be made 1–3 hr after the first. Consultation with a poison control center for assistance in monitoring such patients should be considered. Poison control centers are staffed by nurses, pharmacists, and physicians specially trained to respond

TABLE 58-5. Drugs Associated with Major Modes of Presentation

COMMON TOXIC CAUSES OF CARDIAC ARRHYTHMIA
Amphetamine
Antiarrhythmics
Anticholinergics
Antihistamines
Arsenic
Carbon monoxide
Chloral hydrate
Cocaine
Cyanide
Cyclic antidepressants
Digitalis
Freon
Phenothiazines
Physostigmine
Propranolol
Quinine, quinidine
Theophylline

CAUSES OF COMA
Alcohol
Anticholinergics
Antihistamines
Barbiturates
Carbon monoxide
Clonidine
Cyanide
Cyclic antidepressants
Hypoglycemic agents
Lead
Lithium
Methemoglobinemia*
Methyldopa
Narcotics
Phencyclidine
Phenothiazines
Salicylates

COMMON AGENTS CAUSING SEIZURES (MNEMONIC = CAPS)
Camphor
Carbamazepine
Carbon monoxide
Cocaine
Cyanide
Aminophylline
Amphetamine
Anticholinergics
Antidepressants (cyclic)
Pb (lead) [also lithium]
Pesticide (organophosphate)
Phencyclidine
Phenol
Phenothiazines
Propoxyphene
Salicylates
Strychnine

*Causes of methemoglobinemia: amyl nitrite, aniline dyes, benzocaine, bismuth subnitrate, dapsone, primaquone, quinones, spinach, sulfonamides.
From Kliegman RM, Mascdante KJ, Jenson HB (editors): *Nelson Essentials of Pediatrics*, 5th ed. Philadelphia, Elsevier, 2006, p 208.

TABLE 58-6. Common Antidotes for Poisoning

ANTIDOTE	POISONING	DOSE	ROUTE	ADVERSE EFFECTS/WARNINGS/COMMENTS
N-Acetylcysteine (Mucomyst)	Acetaminophen; carbon tetrachloride and chloroform (experimental)	140 mg/kg loading, followed by 70 mg/kg q4h for 17 doses	PO	Nausea, vomiting
N-Acetylcysteine (Acetodote)	Acetaminophen	150 mg/kg over 30–60 min, followed by 50 mg/kg over 4 hrs, followed by 100 mg/kg over 16 hrs.	IV	Nausea, vomiting, allergic reactions
Atropine	Organophosphate and carbamate pesticides; bradycardia due to atrioventricular conduction defects, β-blocking agents	0.05 mg/kg repeated q5–10min as needed; dilute in 1–2 mL of NS for ET instillation	IV/ET	Tachycardia, dry mouth, blurred vision, urinary retention
BAL in oil (dimercaprol)	Arsenic, mercury, other metals	3–5 mg/kg/dose q4hr, for the 1st day; subsequent dosing depends on the toxin	Deep IM	Local injection site pain and sterile abscess, nausea, vomiting, fever, salivation, nephrotoxicity
Benztropine (Cogentin)	Acute dystonic reactions	0.02–0.05 mg/kg/dose qd or bid (max, 4 mg)	IV/PO	Sedation, blurred vision, dry mouth, tachycardia
Cyanide antidote kit	Cyanide	Amyl nitrite: 1 crushable ampule; inhale 30 sec of each min	Inhalation	Methemoglobinemia
	Hydrogen sulfide (nitrites only)	Sodium nitrite: 0.33 mL/kg of 3% solution if hemoglobin level is not known; otherwise, based on tables with product	IV	Methemoglobinemia
		Sodium thiosulfate: 1.6 mL (400 mg)/kg of 25% solution; may be repeated every 30–60 min to max of 50 mL	IV	
Deferoxamine (Desferal)	Iron	Infusion of 15 mg/kg/hr (max, 6 g/24 hr)	IV(preferred)	Hypotension (minimized by avoiding rapid infusion rates)
		IM: 90 mg/kg/dose q8h (max, 6 g/24 hr)	IM	
Digoxin-specific Fab antibodies (Digibind)	Digitalis glycosides (synthetic or natural)	1 vial binds 0.6 mg of digitalis glycoside; ingested dose may be estimated from the serum level (see table with product)	IV	Allergic reactions (rare), return of condition being treated with digitalis glycoside
Dimercaptosuccinic acid (succimer, DMSA, Chemet)	Lead and probably mercury, arsenic, and perhaps other metals	10 mg/kg/dose q8h for 5 days, then 10 mg/kg q12h for 14 days	PO	Nausea and vomiting; repeated courses may be needed
Diphenhydramine (Benadryl)	Extrapyramidal symptoms, acute dystonic reactions, allergic reactions	5 mg/kg divided q8h; max, 300 mg/24 hr	IV/PO	Sedation or paradoxical agitation, ataxia
EDTA, calcium (calcium disodium, Versenate)	Lead, manganese, nickel, zinc, and perhaps chromium	1–1.5 g/m^2/24 hr in divided doses q12h for 5 days	IV	Nausea, vomiting, fever, hypertension, arthralgias, allergic reactions, local inflammation, nephrotoxicity (maintain adequate hydration)
Ethanol (ethyl alcohol)	Methanol, ethylene glycol	750 mg/kg loading dose followed by 80–150 mg/kg/hr infusion of 5% or 10% ethanol	IV/PO	Nausea, vomiting, sedation, add folate for methanol
Flumazenil (Romazicon)	Benzodiazepines	0.2 mg over 30 sec; if response is inadequate, repeat q1min to 1 mg max	IV	Nausea, vomiting, facial flushing, agitation, headache, dizziness, seizures; do not use for unknown or antidepressant ingestions *Note*: May not reverse respiratory depression
Fomepizole (4-methylpyrazole, Antizole)	Ethylene glycol, methanol	15 mg/kg load; 10 mg/kg q12h for 4 doses; 15 mg/kg q12h until level is <20 mg/dL No specific dose for children	IV	Infuse slowly over 30 min; increase doses to q4h if dialysis is concurrent Thiamine and pyridoxine may be helpful
Glucagon	β Blockers, calcium channel blockers, hypoglycemic agents	0.05 mg/kg bolus followed by infusion of 0.05 mg/kg/hr	IV	Hyperglycemia, nausea, vomiting
Methylene blue	Methemoglobinemia	0.1–0.2 mL/kg of 1% solution by slow infusion; may be repeated q30–60min	IV	Nausea, vomiting, headache, dizziness
Naloxone (Narcan)	Narcotics Clonidine (inconsistent response)	0.01 mg/kg; if no effect, give 0.1 mg/kg; may be repeated as needed; may give continuous infusion	IV	Acute withdrawal symptoms if given to addicted patients
Octreotide	Sulfonylureas	1–2 µg/kg q8hr	IV/SC	Used in addition to high-dose glucose; may add glucagon
Physostigmine (Antilirium)	Anticholinergic agents	0.02 mg/kg by slow push; may repeat q5–10min to 2 mg max	IV/IM	Bradycardia, asystole, seizures, bronchospasm, vomiting, headache *Note*: Do not use with cyclic antidepressants
Pralidoxime (2-PAM, Protopam)	Organophosphate insecticides	25–50 mg/kg over 5–10 min (max, 200 mg/min); can be repeated after 1–2 hr, then q10–12hr as needed	IV/IM	Nausea, dizziness, headache, tachycardia, muscle rigidity, bronchospasm (rapid administration)
Pyridoxine (Vitamin B_6)	Isoniazid, *Gyromitra* mushrooms Ethylene glycol (investigational)	Isoniazid; dose = dose of isoniazid Mushrooms: 25 mg/kg	IV	Uncommon
Oxygen	Carbon monoxide	100%, hyperbaric	Inhalation	Half-life of carboxyhemoglobin is 5 hr in room air, but 1.5 hr in 100% O_2 and 15–30 min in 3 atmospheres hyperbaric
Vitamin K	Coumarin	5–10 mg	IV/SC	Monitor prothrombin time; give fresh frozen plasma for acute bleeding; repeat vitamin K for superwarfarin

BAL, British antilewisite; DMSA, dimercaptosuccinic acid; EDTA, ethylene diamine tetraacetic acid; ET, endotracheal; IM, intramuscular; IV, intravenous; max, maximum; NS, normal saline; PO, Oral.

to and monitor poisoning exposures. If the patient requires hospital treatment, the probability of life-threatening symptoms dictates the mode of transportation used (see Chapter 63). After a decision to transport a patient is made, emergency department personnel should be notified so that they can properly prepare. All product containers related to the exposure should be collected and transported with the patient. If the patient has vomited, the emesis should also be brought to the emergency department for possible toxicologic analysis.

Once the patient has arrived in the appropriate medical care setting, initial attention should focus on life support, with primary emphasis on cardiorespiratory care. Initial treatment of shock, dysrhythmias, and seizures is generally the same as for any other critically ill patient (see Chapter 66). Only a small number of antidotes exist for only a few poisons (Tables 58-6 and 58-7), underscoring the importance of thoughtful, timely institution and maintenance of supportive measures, combined with close, continuous clinical monitoring.

PREVENTING ABSORPTION. Most toxins are rapidly absorbed from the gastrointestinal tract or through inhalation. Many toxins may also be well absorbed on dermal contact (insecticides).

TABLE 58-7. Additional Antidotes

ANTIDOTES	TOXIN/POISON
Latrodectus antivenin	Black widow spider
Botulin antitoxin	Botulism
Glucagon and/or insulin and glucose	Calcium channel antagonists
Diphenhydramine and/or benztropine	Dystonic reactions
Calcium salts	Fluoride, calcium channel blockers
Protamine	Heparin
Folinic acid	Methotrexate, trimethoprim, pyrimethamine
Crotab-specific fab antibodies	Rattlesnake envenomation
Sodium bicarbonate	Sodium channel blockade (tricyclic antidepressants, type 1 antiarrhythmics)

Prompt action to remove the toxin and minimize contact with the absorptive surface is crucial and may prevent the development of major toxicity. Dermal and ocular decontamination can be accomplished by flushing the affected area with tepid water. Flushing for a minimum of 10 min is recommended for ocular exposures, although some chemicals, particularly alkaline corrosives, may require much longer periods of flushing. Effective ocular irrigation can be instituted by positioning the patient's face under a faucet to allow a mild (not forceful) stream of tepid water to hit the side of the nose and stream across the eye and down the cheek. It is probably advisable to prevent the irrigation fluid from flowing from 1 eye across to the other eye. It is better to irrigate 1 eye for 20–30 sec and then to switch to irrigating the other affected eye, and so forth, for approximately 10 min. For dermal exposures, copious irrigation, followed by a mild soap wash, can be used. For inhaled toxins, decontamination is generally accomplished simply by immediately moving the patient to fresh air and, if necessary, administering oxygen. In addition to supportive care, a few specific antidotes are used for some specific inhaled toxins.

Several procedures are used to prevent absorption of an ingested toxin from the stomach and gastrointestinal tract, and each has limitations and risks. The decision to use one particular method over another should be based on whether the technique chosen is likely to be of sufficient value to merit the risk of the procedure. Timing is a limitation because many toxins are rapidly absorbed from the stomach. With the exception of orally administered activated charcoal (see Activated Charcoal), a decontamination procedure instituted after the drug is absorbed poses a risk to the patient with no potential for benefit. Most liquid drug products are almost completely absorbed within 30–45 min of ingestion, and most solid dosage forms are absorbed within 1–2 hr. When a large overdose involves solid dose forms (tablets, powder-filled capsules), complete intestinal absorption can be delayed by as much as 3–6 hr, and for drugs or toxins with anticholinergic (intestinal slowing) properties, absorption can be delayed by up to 8–12 hr. Certain drugs are predisposed to bezoar formation, which must also be considered in the formulation of the patient's initial decontamination and treatment plans (Table 58-8). While bezoars are rare, a bezoar should be suspected in any patient who has symptoms days after apparent complete resolution of the associated symptoms.

Activated Charcoal. An effective means to decrease or prevent the intestinal absorption of a few drugs and toxins as well as enhance the elimination of drugs already absorbed and present within the systemic circulation is oral administration of activated charcoal. Activated charcoal is specially prepared to have a very large adsorptive surface area. Many, but not all, toxins are adsorbed onto its surface, preventing absorption from the gastrointestinal tract. *Some toxins, including heavy metals, iron, lithium, hydrocarbons, cyanide, and low molecular weight alcohols, are not significantly bound to charcoal.*

Usually, a dose of 10–50 g (≈1 g/kg) for a child and 50–100 g for an adolescent or an adult is administered. In practice, the usual dose administered to a child represents the maximum tolerated dose. Airway reflexes must be preserved or the airway protected by endotracheal intubation.

Activated charcoal is commercially available in many forms and is commonly mixed as a slurry in water or a solution of sorbitol, a cathartic. Flavoring may be added to improve palatability, but it rarely improves the acceptance to drinking in younger children. A cathartic should be used only with the 1st charcoal dose to prevent major fluid loss and dehydration. Approximately 25% of patients receiving activated charcoal experience 1 episode of vomiting. Aspiration of activated charcoal into the lungs occurs occasionally. There is no evidence that aspiration of activated charcoal is more serious than aspiration of gastric contents alone. If charcoal is given through a gastric tube, placement of the tube should be carefully confirmed before activated charcoal is given because instillation of charcoal directly into the lungs has disastrous effects.

The use of repeat-dose activated charcoal (a dose every 2–4 hr) is recommended by some toxicologists for the hospitalized poisoned patient at a dose of approximately 0.25–0.50 g/kg every 2–4 hr or hourly at a rate of approximately 0.25 g/kg for 24 hr as long as bowel sounds are present due to the risk of constipation or intestinal impaction. The primary benefit of oral activated charcoal in the treatment of severe poisonings is its effect of increasing the body (systemic) clearance of toxins already present within the body.

A nasogastric tube should be inserted for charcoal instillation if the child will not voluntarily swallow the charcoal slurry or is otherwise unable to protect the airway due to the risk of aspiration. If the patient cannot tolerate a bolus dose of activated charcoal via the nasogastric tube, the charcoal dose can be administered as a slow continuous drip (≈0.25 g/kg/hr).

Cathartics. Cathartics have been used in conjunction with activated charcoal to hasten clearance of the charcoal-toxin complex. There is no evidence demonstrating their value. Cathartics do not need to be administered with each dose of activated charcoal and should only be administered as needed. Commonly used cathartics are sorbitol (maximum dose, 1 g/kg), magnesium sulfate (maximum dose, 250 mg/kg), and magnesium citrate (maximum dose, 250 mL/kg). Cathartics should be used with care in young children because of the risk of dehydration and electrolyte imbalance.

TABLE 58-8. Common Medications Implicated in Bezoar Formation

ANTACIDS
Aluminum hydroxide
BULK-FORMING LAXATIVES
Combination laxatives (e.g., Perdiem)
Psyllium
EXTENDED-RELEASE PRODUCTS
Nifedipine
Procainamide
Verapamil
ION-EXCHANGE RESINS
Sodium polystyrene sulfonate
Calcium polystyrene sulfonate
VITAMIN AND NATURAL PRODUCTS
Ascorbic acid
Ferrous sulfate
Lecithin
OTHER MEDICATIONS
Carbamazepine
Cholestyramine
Enteric-coated aspirin
Lithium
Salicylic acid
Sucralfate

Whole Bowel Irrigation. Whole bowel irrigation involves instilling large volumes (30 mL/kg/hr) of a nonabsorbed polyethylene glycol electrolyte solution (e.g., Colyte, GoLYTELY) into the stomach to flow through the entire length of the bowel to "cleanse" the entire gastrointestinal tract. This technique has been successfully used to remove slowly absorbed products, such as iron or sustained-release preparations, as well as foreign bodies, including drug packets (cocaine packets via body packers). Whole bowel irrigation can be combined with the use of activated charcoal, if appropriate (cocaine body packers). It should be used with caution in young children because of the possibility of fluid and electrolyte imbalance.

Enhancing Elimination. Enhancing excretion is useful for only a few toxins. Dialytic techniques are not useful for drugs that are either highly protein-bound or have a large volume of distribution. These techniques are also invasive and associated with risk. Certain procedures can be used for very specific agents.

Emesis. The emetic used in the past was syrup of ipecac; it contains 2 emetic alkaloids that work both in the central nervous system (CNS) and locally in the gastrointestinal tract to produce vomiting. The onset of emesis is usually 20–30 min after dosing, with vomiting occurring in 90–95% of patients. Several episodes of vomiting usually occur over a 1–2 hr period. The dose is 10 mL for infants 6–12 mo of age, 15–30 mL for children 1–12 yr of age, and 30 mL for older children and adults. Ipecac should not be used in infants younger than 6 mo of age because these infants have a far greater risk of aspiration. Ipecac should be followed by at least 6–8 oz of water or other clear fluid, with the actual final volume age- and child-dependent.

The use of ipecac syrup is not recommended for routine ingestions. Emesis with syrup of ipecac removes approximately ⅓ of the stomach contents. Because of the delay in onset of emesis and the poor yield, it should not be used as a general treatment for ingestions. Ipecac-induced emesis is contraindicated after the ingestion of caustics (acids/bases), hydrocarbons, and agents likely to cause rapid onset of CNS or cardiovascular symptoms. Ipecac abuse and cardiac toxicity is noted in some adolescents with bulimia (see Chapter 27).

Gastric Lavage. This technique involves placing a tube into the stomach to aspirate contents, followed by flushing with aliquots of fluid, usually normal saline. Although gastric lavage was used for many years, objective data do not document or support clinically relevant efficacy, particularly in children, in whom only small-bore tubes often can be used. Lavage is time-consuming, and under the best circumstances, it removes only a fraction of gastric contents. Lavage should only be used in older children and possibly only in select situations (iron, calcium channel blockers, tricyclic antidepressants, lithium). If gastric lavage is to be performed, repeated instillation and removal of small volumes of lavage solution is generally better tolerated, with less risk of aspiration. The airway also needs to be secure.

Diuresis. For most toxins, renal clearance is not proportional to urine volume; thus, diuresis or "forced" diuresis alone does not increase elimination. Increasing the pH of the urine with IV bicarbonate can augment the elimination of weak acids, such as salicylates and phenobarbital. Alternately, acidifying the urine to increase the elimination of weak bases, such as amphetamine and phencyclidine, is rarely clinically useful. Despite the theoretical advantages of such a therapeutic approach, the need to closely monitor fluid balance, combined with the need to alter systemic pH to change the urine pH, restricts the use of this therapeutic maneuver to very rare circumstances.

Dialysis. Hemodialysis and peritoneal dialysis have been used successfully to treat poisonings by select agents. Although hemodialysis is generally more efficient at removing toxins, peritoneal dialysis is often easier to perform in young children, and may be sufficient. Few drugs or toxins are removed by dialysis in amounts sufficient to justify the risks and difficulty of dialysis. Examples of toxins for which dialysis may be useful include the toxic alcohols, methanol, and ethylene glycol as well as large symptomatic ingestions of salicylates, theophylline or lithium.

Hemoperfusion. Hemoperfusion is a dialytic technique in which blood is passed through a column of activated charcoal or resin. It can successfully treat large ingestions of salicylate, theophylline, and a few other selected agents. It is rarely used because of the associated risks.

LABORATORY EVALUATION. For some intoxications (salicylates, anticonvulsants, acetaminophen, iron, digoxin, methanol, lithium, theophylline, ethylene glycol, carbon monoxide), blood concentrations can be integral to confirming the diagnosis and formulating the treatment plan. For most intoxicants, qualitative measurement is not possible or likely to change treatment. Examples include opioid toxicity, in which definitive treatment is based on symptoms, not serum drug concentrations, and cyanide, in which treatment must be started rapidly and would be significantly delayed if the clinician were to wait for laboratory confirmation. Comprehensive, qualitative "drug screens" vary widely in their ability to detect toxins and generally add little information, particularly if the agent is known and the patient's symptoms are consistent with that agent (see Tables 58-3 to 58-5). If a drug screen is ordered, it is important to know the specific drugs that can be identified by the test because the components screened for in the "tox screen" vary from hospital to hospital. Although drug screens can be performed on any body fluid, urine is generally the best fluid to sample because the toxin or metabolite is concentrated in the urine. The best way to use the laboratory is to discuss the case with the poison control center, a medical toxicologist, or a laboratory technologist and to provide appropriate samples and clinical data so that the most appropriate tests can be performed and properly interpreted.

SELECTED COMPOUNDS COMMONLY INVOLVED IN PEDIATRIC POISONINGS

ACETAMINOPHEN. Acetaminophen is the most widely used analgesic and antipyretic in pediatrics, primarily due to the finding of a relationship between Reye syndrome and salicylates. Consequently, acetaminophen, which is available in multiple formulations and different strengths, is commonly available in the home, where it can be unintentionally ingested by young children (good-tasting chewable tablets) or taken in an intentional overdose by adolescents and adults. Acetaminophen intoxication is a common cause of acute liver failure in adolescents and adults.

Pathophysiology. Acetaminophen toxicity results from the formation of a highly reactive intermediate metabolite, *N*-acetyl-p-benzoquinoneimine (NAPQI). When therapeutic doses are administered, only a small amount (≈4%) of a dose is metabolized by the hepatic cytochrome P450 enzyme CYP2E1 to NAPQI, which is immediately conjugated with glutathione to form a harmless mercapturic acid conjugate. When hepatic stores of glutathione are depleted to <70% of normal, the NAPQI metabolite can combine with hepatic macromolecules to produce hepatocellular damage. The acute toxic dose of acetaminophen is generally considered to be >200 mg/kg in children younger than 12 yr of age; a single ingestion of >7.5 g is considered a minimum toxic dose in adolescents and adults. Repeated administration of acetaminophen at doses exceeding those recommended (>60 mg/kg/day for consecutive days) may lead to hepatic injury or failure in some children. Parents should be advised to follow closely the manufacturer's dosing guidelines and should be aware of the availability of sustained-release formulations and the drug's presence in many combination products.

Children younger than 6 yr of age are unlikely to have significant toxicity after a single ingestion of even relatively large doses of acetaminophen. Any child with a history of a significant ingestion should have the plasma acetaminophen concentration mea-

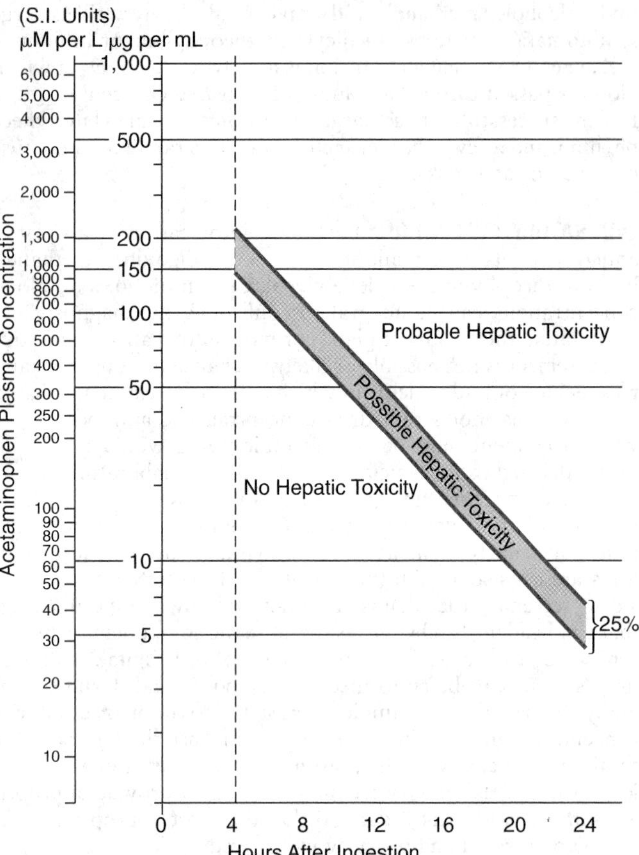

Figure 58-1. Rumack-Matthew nomogram for acetaminophen poisoning, a semilogarithmic plot of plasma acetaminophen concentrations vs time. Cautions for the use of this chart: (1) The time coordinates refer to time after ingestion. (2) Serum concentrations obtained before 4 hr may not represent peak concentrations. (3) The graph should be used only in relation to a single acute ingestion. This nomogram is not useful for chronic exposures, nor has it been validated for use after ingestions involving sustained-release acetaminophen products. (4) The lower *solid line* 25% below the standard nomogram is included to allow for possible errors in acetaminophen plasma assays and estimated time from ingestion of an overdose. (From Rumack BH, Hess AJ [editors]: Poisindex. Denver, Micromedex, 1995. Adapted from Rumack BH, Matthew H: Acetaminophen poisoning and toxicity. *Pediatrics* 1975;55: 871–876.)

sured and receive treatment with *N*-acetylcysteine (NAC) if the plasma concentration falls within the toxic range on the nomogram (Fig. 58-1). In infants whose nutritional intake has been compromised by the concurrent intestinal illness and whose hepatic glutathione stores are suboptimal, the risk may possibly be higher for acetaminophen hepatotoxicity. Adolescents have a higher incidence of toxic plasma concentrations after ingestion than do children, and their exposures are often associated with intentional overdose. Chronic alcohol ingestion increases the risk of acetaminophen hepatotoxicity. Even if a serious case of hepatotoxicity develops, the mortality rate is <0.5%, reflecting the safety and efficacy of NAC antidote therapy. Severely affected patients may require liver transplantation (see Chapter 365).

Clinical and Laboratory Manifestations. If untreated, patients with an acute overdose may pass through the 4 stages of acetaminophen toxicity (Table 58-9). Because early symptoms are nonspecific, physicians may not diagnose the ingestion without a good history or a high index of suspicion. If a toxic ingestion is suspected, the plasma acetaminophen concentration should be measured 4 hr or more after ingestion. Measurement earlier than 4 hr after ingestion may be useful to determine if ingestion has occurred, but it cannot be used to determine the severity of an overdose. The plasma acetaminophen concentration should be plotted on the Rumack-Matthew nomogram (see Fig. 58-1) to determine whether antidotal treatment is indicated. The nomogram should only be used to evaluate the risk after acute exposure to regular-release products. The nomogram's predictive strength does not apply to plasma acetaminophen concentrations obtained after the use of sustained-release formulations, ingestions involving repeated exposures over multiple days. The nomogram's predictive strength may not always extend to patients who are believed to have depleted glutathione stores (malnourishment, prolonged illness). A minimum of 2 plasma acetaminophen concentrations should be obtained from patients who have ingested a sustained-release preparation; the 1st at least 4 hr after the exposure and a 2nd sample 4–6 hr after the 1st. If at any time the plasma acetaminophen concentration exceeds the treatment value of the Rumack-Matthew nomogram, the patient should receive NAC antidote therapy. This approach is conservative, and more data are needed to better define an optimal approach to treating patients ingesting sustained-release formulations as well as those with consecutive days of high-dose ingestion. Weighing the real toxicity associated with acetaminophen intoxication against the definite benefit of treatment with a very safe antidote, a conservative approach dictates treating if toxicity is suspected, despite the plasma concentration plot on the treatment nomogram (see Fig. 58-1). These plasma acetaminophen concentrations are most useful for the asymptomatic patient; symptomatic patients require therapy individualized to their specific requirements. Liver function studies, including hepatic enzymes, bilirubin, and prothrombin time, should be followed daily to every other day in all patients with plasma acetaminophen concentrations falling within the toxic range on the nomogram.

Treatment. After a large acute oral overdose, and when the need for antidotal treatment is determined, treatment should be started as soon as possible, including within 1–2 hr of the ingestion. The antidote for acetaminophen poisoning is NAC, which serves as a precursor for hepatic glutathione synthesis, replenishing glutathione stores and preventing the reaction of NAPQI with hepatocytes. NAC therapy is most effective when initiated early in the course of intoxication (within 8 hr), but may have value even if started 24–36 hr after the ingestion in severe cases. It is important to note that NAC administration has no effect on the plasma acetaminophen concentration or the drug's elimination from the body. In acute large overdoses, particularly patients ingesting sustained-release preparations or co-ingestions with drugs that decrease gastrointestinal transit, oral administration of activated charcoal should be considered. The extent to which activated charcoal may bind to orally administered NAC (≈30%) remains a point of debate, although most authorities administer the same oral NAC dose (140 mg NAC/kg oral loading dose +70 mg oral NAC/kg every 4 hr, for a total of 17 doses), regardless of whether oral activated charcoal has been administered. Oral NAC is unpalatable and can be irritating to the gastrointestinal tract, so it should be diluted to a 5% solution with soda or fruit juice to minimize vomiting. Antiemetics (ondansetron) may be used to control vomiting and/or NAC may be administered directly into

TABLE 58-9. Classic Stages in the Clinical Course of Acetaminophen Toxicity

STAGE	TIME AFTER INGESTION	CHARACTERISTICS
I	0.5–24 hr	Anorexia, nausea, vomiting, malaise, pallor, diaphoresis
II	24–48 hr	Resolution of earlier symptoms; right upper quadrant abdominal pain and tenderness; elevated bilirubin, prothrombin time, hepatic enzymes; oliguria
III	72–96 hr	Peak liver function abnormalities; anorexia, nausea, vomiting, and malaise may reappear
IV	4 days–2 wk	Resolution of hepatic dysfunction or complete liver failure

the stomach or upper intestine by tube. An IV preparation of NAC is also available (Acetadote) and was approved by the U.S. Food and Drug Administration for IV administration within 8–10 hr after ingestion of a potentially hepatotoxic quantity of acetaminophen. For the IV formulation, an initial IV loading dose of 150 mg/kg is infused over 15–60 min, followed by an initial maintenance dose of 50 mg/kg infused over 4 hr, followed by 100 mg/kg infused over 16 hr. Anaphylactoid reactions may be minimized by a 60 min infusion. Clinicians are encouraged to consult with a medical toxicologist or a regional poison control center for cases involving subacute or chronic exposure, extended-release products, or co-ingestions, as stated earlier; the Rumack-Matthew nomogram is not always useful in making treatment decisions under these circumstances.

SALICYLATES. The incidence of salicylate poisoning is low, particularly in young children, because the use of alternative antipyretics has increased in an effort to avoid Reye syndrome. Salicylate toxicity must still be considered in therapeutic situations as well as in cases of acute overdose; the common use of baby aspirin preparations by parents and grandparents for cardiovascular prophylaxis places the drug in many home environments and thus makes it available for accidental poisoning. Methyl salicylate is the active ingredient in oil of wintergreen, a common component in rubefacients. Every 1 g of methyl salicylate contains the equivalent of 1.5 g of salicylate, underscoring the risk of moderate to serious symptoms associated with what might seem a small amount of commonly used over-the-counter rubs or topical sports medicines.

Pathophysiology. Salicylates directly or indirectly affect most organ systems by uncoupling oxidative phosphorylation, inhibiting Krebs cycle enzymes, and inhibiting amino acid synthesis. Various complex metabolic abnormalities result. Salicylates also decrease platelet adhesiveness and increase pulmonary capillary permeability. The acute toxic dose of salicylates is generally considered >150 mg/kg for mild symptoms and >300–500 mg/kg for moderate to severe intoxication.

Clinical and Laboratory Manifestations. The clinical presentation after acute poisoning differs significantly from that of chronic toxicity. Chronic toxicity results in signs and symptoms that are easily attributed to other causes, such as flu or other febrile illness. Young children are more susceptible to toxic effects because they are less able to buffer the acid load produced by salicylates.

After acute salicylate ingestion, nausea and vomiting occur due to gastric irritation. Salicylates directly stimulate the respiratory center, leading to hyperventilation and hyperpnea. An increased respiratory rate results in **respiratory alkalosis** with compensatory alkaluria. Both potassium and sodium bicarbonate are excreted in the urine; however, soon after exposure, the serum potassium concentration may be in the normal range. When sufficient potassium has been lost through the kidneys, an exchange of potassium for hydrogen ion occurs and the urine becomes relatively acidic. This "paradoxical aciduria" occurs in the presence of continued respiratory alkalosis. Dehydration and progressive **metabolic acidosis,** caused by the accumulation of lactic acid and other metabolic acids, eventually develop. Seriously poisoned patients are >5–10% dehydrated. Patients with chronic salicylate poisoning usually present with metabolic acidosis.

Important signs of serious toxicity are CNS changes. Agitation, restlessness, and confusion are common in children. Coma may develop as a result of cerebral edema. Pulmonary edema or hemorrhage may develop in more severe cases. Hyperglycemia (acute) or hypoglycemia (chronic), particularly in infants, has also been observed. Hepatotoxicity occurs after chronic exposure or with very large acute ingestions. Death results from pulmonary edema and respiratory failure, cerebral edema, hemorrhage, severe electrolyte imbalance, or cardiovascular collapse. Hyperpyrexia may also occur.

Serial serum salicylate concentrations (initially at 4 hr postingestion and then every 3–4 hr) should be monitored to evaluate for either continued absorption or impairment of excretion. After acute ingestion, patients with serum salicylate concentrations of >20 mg/dL should undergo continued observation and monitoring. Acute serum concentrations of >70–100 mg/dL may produce life-threatening effects. **Plasma levels do not always correlate with clinical toxicity.** The Done nomogram is of poor value and is no longer used. Patients with chronic salicylate toxicity may have a serum concentration within the usual therapeutic range (10–20 mg/dL). Salicylate disposition is characterized by nonlinear Michaelis-Menten characteristics, where the drug's body elimination is saturable. The disproportionate increase in the serum salicylate concentration, but more importantly, the disproportionality of the drug's slow body clearance, particularly in overdose, should be anticipated and the treatment plan adjusted accordingly.

Urine pH and volume should be measured hourly in all seriously poisoned children. Plasma pH, glucose, potassium, and other electrolytes should be monitored at regular intervals. Clotting studies and liver function tests should also be closely monitored in all severely poisoned patients.

Treatment. Initial treatment should include gastric decontamination, preferably with activated charcoal, if the patient presents soon after an acute ingestion. Salicylate tablets occasionally form into bezoars, which may be suspected if serum salicylate concentrations continue to rise many hr after ingestion or are persistently elevated. Gastric decontamination is typically not useful after chronic exposure.

Initial therapy focuses on aggressive rehydration and correction of electrolyte abnormalities (see Chapter 52). Large quantities of potassium and bicarbonate may be needed if symptoms have been present for some time after an acute ingestion or in the case of chronic salicylate poisoning, because body stores of these electrolytes may be severely depleted.

Urinary excretion of unmetabolized salicylate becomes an important route of elimination in overdose. Urinary clearance of salicylate is affected by urine pH. Because metabolic acidosis produces more acidic urine, a higher percentage of filtered salicylate remains in the un-ionized form, which is effectively reabsorbed. Urinary salicylate elimination can be increased using "ion trapping" by increasing urine pH to convert a greater percentage of salicylate to the ionized form, which is then excreted in the urine. Each 1-unit increase in urine pH increases urinary salicylate clearance 4-fold. Urine pH should be increased to at least 7.0–7.5, using IV bicarbonate. The shift of salicylate to the ionized form also serves to decrease CNS penetration because un-ionized drugs generally cross the blood-brain barrier more efficiently. It may be difficult to alkalize the urine without adequately replenishing tissue stores of potassium. Acetazolamide (Diamox) should not be used in an attempt to achieve urine alkalization.

In severe cases of salicylate intoxication, dialysis may be required both to remove salicylate and to correct electrolyte abnormalities. Indications for extracorporeal removal include serum salicylate concentrations of >90 mg/dL, changes in neurologic status (depressed level of consciousness or difficult to control seizures), respiratory or cardiovascular instability, refractory metabolic acidosis, severe hypokalemia, and renal failure. Hemodialysis is preferred over either peritoneal dialysis or charcoal hemoperfusion. Repeat-dose activated charcoal may aid in enhancing the body clearance of salicylate. Dialysis can be effective in correcting and/or maintaining the patient's fluid and electrolyte balance.

IBUPROFEN AND OTHER NONSTEROIDAL ANTI-INFLAMMATORY DRUGS. Ibuprofen and other nonsteroidal anti-inflammatory drugs (NSAIDs) are often involved in unintentional and intentional overdoses because of their wide distribution and their common use as analgesics; in particular, ibuprofen is used as an antipyretic in pediatric practice. Fortunately, serious effects after NSAID overdose are rare.

Pathophysiology. These drugs inhibit prostaglandin synthesis by inhibiting the activity of cyclo-oxygenase, the primary enzyme responsible for the biosynthesis of prostaglandins and certain other autocoids. This disruption produces the side effects reported with therapeutic use, such as gastrointestinal irritation, reduced renal blood flow, and platelet dysfunction. NSAID analogs have been developed that are more specific for the inducible form of COX (the COX-2 isoform) vs the constitutive form, the COX-1 isoform. These drugs attempt to minimize or reduce the occurrence of therapy-associated adverse effects. Overdose of the more selective COX-2 inhibitors (celecoxib [Celebrex]) is treated no differently than for nonspecific COX inhibitors (ibuprofen) because at higher doses, COX-2 selective agents lose their COX inhibitory selectivity. Ibuprofen, the primary NSAID used in pediatrics, is well tolerated, even after overdose. In children, acute doses of <100 mg/kg rarely cause toxicity, whereas doses of >400 mg/kg are capable of producing more serious effects, including bradycardia, hepatic dysfunction, seizures, and coma.

Clinical and Laboratory Manifestations. Symptoms usually develop within 4–6 hr of NSAID ingestion and resolve within 24 hr. Common initial effects include nausea, vomiting, and epigastric pain, followed by drowsiness, lethargy, and ataxia. Anion gap metabolic acidosis, coma, transient apnea, renal failure, hypotension, and seizures can occur with large overdoses, but are rare. Other reported effects include nystagmus, diplopia, headache, tinnitus, and transient deafness. Renal function studies and acid-base balance should be monitored after ingestion of large doses.

Treatment. Good supportive care is essential in the treatment of acute NSAID overdose or poisoning. There is no specific antidotal therapy for this class of drugs. Emesis is of little benefit, but activated charcoal can be administered. Extracorporeal removal methods have not been adequately evaluated and are not recommended, particularly when considering the extensive degree to which each of these analogs is bound to plasma protein.

ANTIDEPRESSANTS: TRICYCLICS AND SEROTININ-MODULATING DRUGS. Tricyclic antidepressants (TCAs) and selective serotonin-reuptake inhibitors (SSRIs) are the 2 most common classes of antidepressants of toxicologic significance (see Chapter 25). Antidepressants include amitriptyline, nortriptyline, and imipramine, among others. SSRIs include fluoxetine, sertraline, paroxetine, and citalopram. Antidepressants not selective for serotonin, often referred to as *nonselective serotonin-reuptake inhibitors (NSSRIs),* include venlafaxine, bupropion, duloxetine, mirtazapine, and nefazodone.

Tricyclic Antidepressants

PATHOPHYSIOLOGY. Tricyclic antidepressants block the neuronal reuptake of norepinephrine, serotonin, and dopamine in both the central and peripheral nervous systems. They also produce varying degrees of sedation, α-receptor blocking, and anticholinergic effects. Inhibition of fast sodium channels in the myocardium leads to the development of cardiac dysrhythmias and myocardial depression.

CLINICAL AND LABORATORY MANIFESTATIONS. The primary organ systems affected by TCAs are the CNS and cardiovascular system. Symptoms can develop as early as 30 min after ingestion, with serious symptoms usually developing within 6 hr of ingestion. In large ingestions, patient symptoms may be delayed (>6–8+ hr), reflecting the anticholinergic properties of TCAs in slowing gastric emptying and bowel motility. The pattern of toxicity in children is different from that described in adolescents and adults in that CNS effects occur more frequently in children than do cardiovascular effects. Drowsiness, lethargy, or coma is reported in as many as 30% of pediatric cases. Coma, when it occurs, usually resolves in a few hr, but may last >24 hr. Seizures develop in approximately 15% of cases and can occur without warning, but are usually brief and resolve without treatment. Adolescents with comparable blood TCA levels have more significant toxicity than younger children.

Tachycardia, likely attributed to the anticholinergic actions of TCAs, is the most common cardiovascular effect, but does not usually compromise blood pressure. Hypertension may occur soon after ingestion, but rarely requires treatment. Hypotension is uncommon, but is a poor prognostic sign. Other cardiac findings include slowing of myocardial conduction, multifocal premature ventricular contractions, and ventricular tachycardia or fibrillation. In addition to widening of the QRS complex, QT prolongation occurs with T-wave flattening or inversion, ST segment depression, right bundle branch block, and complete heart block.

Hypoventilation with respiratory arrest may occur without warning. Other reported effects include hyperthermia, choreiform movements, agitation, and twitching. Anticholinergic syndrome, including mydriasis, disorientation, hallucinations, urinary retention, and diminished bowel sounds, may be present.

The electrocardiogram (ECG) should be closely monitored for QRS widening and QT and QTc prolongation. QRS duration and axis deviation and the level of consciousness have been suggested as predictors of potential toxicity. ECG changes may not be useful predictors of toxicity in younger children. Plasma TCA concentrations are not helpful in assessing or predicting the severity of exposure, but may aid in establishing a diagnosis or assessing the rate of TCA body clearance with therapy.

TREATMENT. After general life support measures are instituted, including if indicated, endotracheal intubation, efforts should be undertaken to prevent absorption. Emesis is contraindicated because of the danger of aspiration from vomiting after the onset of CNS depression (loss of gag reflex) or seizures. Activated charcoal should be administered. Because of the effects of TCAs on slowing intestinal motility, additional doses of activated charcoal can be administered 4 hr apart, concurrent with a cathartic (sorbitol), if required, based on the patient's bowel motility status. IV sodium bicarbonate in doses sufficient to achieve and maintain a serum pH of 7.45–7.50 should be administered to treat and prevent dysrhythmias. IV sodium bicarbonate is one of the most effective therapies in treating and/or preventing a TCA-induced decrease in cardiac conduction, and it should be considered for all TCA-exposed patients with such abnormalities on ECG. Lidocaine is used to treat dysrhythmias that are unresponsive to serum alkalization. Quinidine and procainamide or similar agents should not be used because they further depress cardiac conduction. Hypotension may respond to standard fluid therapy, although vasopressors, such as norepinephrine, may be required. Severe, unresponsive hypotension is a poor prognostic sign. Hypertension usually is transient and does not require treatment. Seizures, if they require treatment, usually respond to benzodiazepine therapy. Physostigmine, once promoted as an "antidote" for TCA toxicity, is a dangerous agent that can cause seizures and dysrhythmias and should not be used. Because of the large volumes of distribution and the high degree of plasma protein binding of TCAs, extracorporeal removal is of no clinical value. Oral activated charcoal and possibly repeat-dose activated charcoal may be effective in enhancing the body clearance after very large overdoses, although limited data suggest such a strategy.

Asymptomatic children should be observed and the ECG monitored for at least 6 hr after exposure. If any manifestations of toxicity, including a QRS interval of >100 msec, conduction defects, altered mental status, hypotension, or hypoventilation, develop, the patient should be admitted for continued monitoring in an intensive care unit for 24 hr. Only completely asymptomatic children should be discharged after 6 hr of observation.

Selective Serotonin-Reuptake Inhibitors. Selective serotonin-reuptake inhibitors differ from TCAs in that they specifically inhibit reuptake of serotonin in the CNS. They have little or no

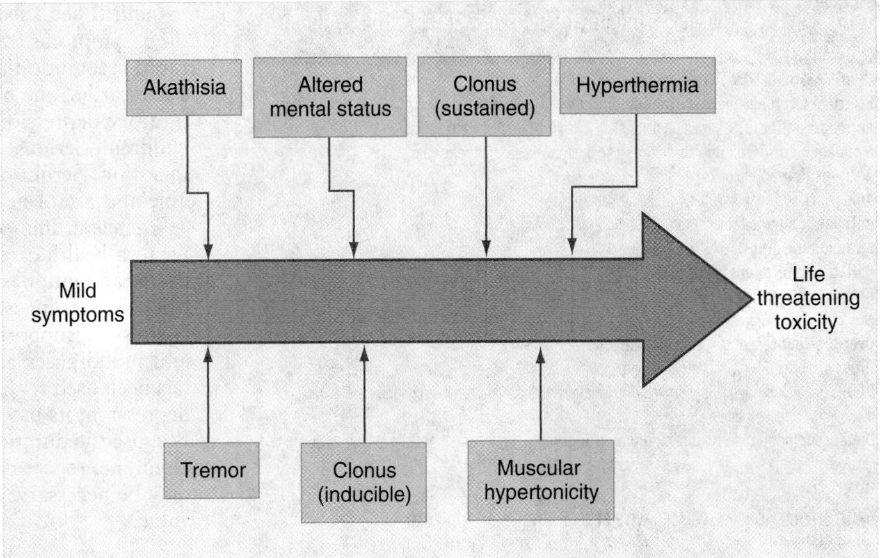

Figure 58-2. Manifestations of the serotonin syndrome range from mild to life-threatening. The *arrows* suggest the approximate point at which each clinical finding initially appears in the spectrum of the disease, but all findings may not be consistently present in a single patient. Severe signs may mask other clinical findings. For example, muscular hypertonicity can overwhelm tremor and hyperreflexia. (From Boyer EW, Shannon M: The serotonin syndrome. *N Engl J Med* 2005;352: 1112–1120.)

effect on norepinephrine or dopamine reuptake and minimal, if any, anticholinergic or α-blocking effects.

CLINICAL MANIFESTATIONS. These drugs have a wide therapeutic index, and toxic effects are usually mild. The usual onset of symptoms is within 3 hr, with resolution of symptoms within 24 hr in treated patients. Most children remain asymptomatic. Drowsiness or hyperactivity, agitation, and tachycardia are the most commonly reported effects. Nausea, vomiting, tremor, dizziness, and abdominal pain are less common. Life-threatening effects, such as seizures, coma, and hyperthermia, are rare, but have been reported after very large ingestions. Cardiac conduction defects are not common. Adolescents have an increased incidence of symptoms, although when they manifest, they are still relatively minor. The toxic dose of these agents is not well defined.

A serotonin syndrome has been well described after overdose of SSRIs as well as after therapeutic use in some patients (see Table 58-3 and Figs. 58-2 and 58-3). Certain drug-drug interactions (meperidine, monoamine oxidase inhibitor) also manifest as serotonin syndrome, which is a predictable reaction that results from excess serotonin agonism of CNS and peripheral serotonin receptors and includes confusion and disorientation, agitation, coma, hyperthermia, myoclonus, hyperreflexia, tremor, and muscle rigidity (Table 58-10).

TREATMENT. Gastrointestinal decontamination with activated charcoal is the preferred treatment of the serotonin syndrome; emesis should not be attempted because of the real potential for CNS depression. Treatment depends on the severity of symptoms, but requires removal of the inciting drugs and prompt provision of supportive care, allowing the severity of the

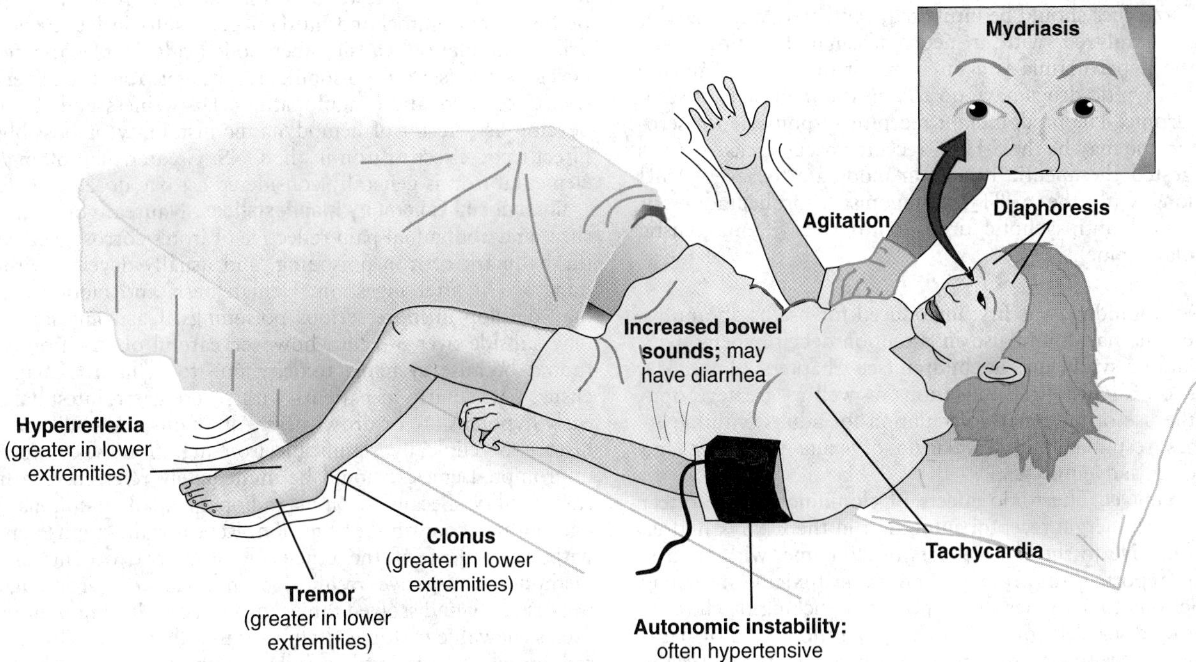

Figure 58-3. Findings in a patient with moderately severe serotonin syndrome. Hyperkinetic neuromuscular findings of tremor or clonus and hyperreflexia should lead the clinician to consider the diagnosis of the serotonin syndrome. (From Boyer EW, Shannon M: The serotonin syndrome. *N Engl J Med* 2005;352:1112–1120.)

TABLE 58-10. Drugs and Drug Interactions Associated with Serotonin Syndrome

DRUGS ASSOCIATED WITH SEROTONIN SYNDROME
Selective serotonin-reuptake inhibitors: Sertraline, fluoxetine, fluvoxamine, paroxetine, citalopram
Antidepressant drugs: Trazodone, nefazodone, buspirone, clomipramine, venlafaxine
Monoamine oxidase inhibitors: Phenelzine, moclobemide, clorgiline, isocarboxazid
Anticonvulsants: Valproate
Analgesics: Meperidine, fentanyl, tramadol, pentazocine
Antiemetic agents: Ondansetron, granisetron, metoclopramide
Antimigraine drugs: Sumatriptan
Bariatric medications: Sibutramine
Antibiotics: Linezolide (a monoamine oxidase inhibitor), ritonavir (through inhibition of cytochrome P450 enzyme isoform 3A4)
Over-the-counter cough and cold remedies: Dextromethorphan
Drugs of abuse: Methylenedioxymethamphetamine (MDMA, or "ecstasy"), lysergic acid diethylamide (LSD), 5-methoxydiisopropyltryptamine ("foxy methoxy"), Syrian rue (contains harmine and harmaline, both monoamine oxidase inhibitors)
Dietary supplements and herbal products: Tryptophan, *Hypericum perforatum* (St. John's wort), *Panax ginseng* (ginseng)
Other: Lithium

DRUG INTERACTIONS ASSOCIATED WITH SEVERE SEROTONIN SYNDROME
Sertraline (Zoloft), fluoxetine (Prozac, Savatem), fluvoxamine (Luvox), paroxetine (Paxil), citalopram (Celexa), trazodone (Desyrel), nefadozone (Serzone), buspirone (Buspar), clomipramine (Anafranil), venlafaxim (Effexor), phenelzine (Navdil), moclobemide (Manerex), isocarboxazid (Marplan), divalproex (Depakote), meperidine (Demerol), flutanyl (Duragesic, Sublimaze), tramadol (Ultram), pentazoicine (Talwin), ondansetron (Zofran), granisetron (Kytril), metoclopramide (Reglan), sumatriptun succinate (Imitrex), sibutramine (Meridia), dexfenfluramine (Redux), fenfluramine (Pondimin), linezolid (Zyvox), ritonavir (Norvir), tranylcypromine (Parnate), imipramine (Tofranil), mirtazapine (Remeron)
Phenelzine and meperidine
Tranylcypromine and imipramine
Phenelzine and selective serotonin-reuptake inhibitors
Paroxetine and buspirone
Linezolide and citalopram
Moclobemide and selective serotonin-reuptake inhibitors
Tramadol, venlafaxine, and mirtazapine

From Bayer EW, Shannon M: The serotonin syndrome. *N Engl J Med* 2005;352:1112–1120.

patient's symptoms to direct specific therapies, including benzodiazepine for control of agitation and hyperreflexia or tremors. All patients with moderate to severe symptoms require continuous cardiac and body temperature monitoring. Patients whose muscle effects and resultant hyperthermia are poorly responsive to benzodiazepines should be intubated, ventilated, and pharmacologically paralyzed with a neuromuscular blocking drug. Because the hyperthermia is a direct result of increased muscle activity, antipyretic drugs have no role in the treatment of serotonin syndrome. The predominant receptor responsible for serotonin syndrome may be the 5-HT_{2A} receptor because case reports have suggested therapeutic benefit in moderate to severe SSRI intoxications with the 5-HT_{2A} antagonist cyproheptadine or newer atypical antipsychotic drugs with 5-HT_{2A} antagonistic activity (olanzapine).

CLONIDINE. Clonidine was first introduced for use as an antihypertensive, but has found use in attention-deficit/hyperactivity disorder and tic syndromes in children (see Chapters 23 and 31). Increased use for pediatric indications as well as greater popularity of the use of the patch formulation for adults with hypertension has resulted in an escalation of acute poisoning and therapeutic misadventures.

Pathophysiology. The toxic effects of clonidine are the direct result of α_2-adrenergic receptor inhibition in the CNS. Children are very sensitive to the toxic effects of clonidine, with as little as 0.1 mg reported to produce significant toxicity in young infants. Serious toxicity has developed after sucking or chewing on a new or discarded topical patch preparation. It is of paramount importance to inform families in which a member uses the clonidine patch that a substantial amount of clonidine remains in the patch on removal and that the used patch should be folded by sealing the adhesive surface and then discarded in the trash.

Clinical and Laboratory Manifestations. In clonidine-naïve children, symptoms frequently develop within 1 hr of ingestion; thus, rapid recognition and intervention is essential. Lethargy, miosis, bradycardia, and hypotension occur in all age groups. Apnea, respiratory depression, and coma are common findings in younger children. Serious symptoms usually resolve within 24 hr of ingestion. Serum clonidine concentrations are not readily available and are of no clinical value.

Treatment. Immediate recognition of an exposure, with transfer to a health care facility, is of paramount importance. Gastric decontamination is usually of little value owing to the small quantities usually ingested and the rapid onset of serious symptoms. Aggressive supportive care is imperative. The ECG, vital signs, and blood gases are monitored as symptoms dictate. Naloxone has been used with mixed success to reverse CNS and respiratory depression; its use should not replace aggressive supportive care. Because the duration of effect of naloxone is shorter than that of clonidine, repeat doses or administration by continuous infusion may be necessary. Extracorporeal removal techniques are not of value.

IRON. Iron is one of the most common causes of childhood poisoning death. Iron-containing products are common in many homes, and iron-containing vitamins, which often resemble candy, are frequently freely given to children by their parents. The potential severity of exposure is based on the amount of elemental iron ingested. The amount of elemental iron ingested is calculated on the basis of the number of tablets ingested and the percentage of elemental iron present in the salt form ingested. The amount of elemental iron is 20% in ferrous sulfate, 12% in ferrous gluconate, and 33% in ferrous fumarate. Most multivitamin products containing iron list on the product label the amount of iron per tablet as the elemental iron content.

Pathophysiology. Iron is corrosive to the gastrointestinal mucosa and may lead to intestinal ulceration, edema, and occasionally melena, hematemesis, and possibly perforation. It also accumulates in the mitochondria and tissues to produce cellular damage and systemic toxicity. Iron causes venodilation and increased capillary permeability, leading to hypotension. Early hypovolemia from intestinal losses, leading to reduced peripheral perfusion and mitochondrial damage, results in lactic and citric acid accumulation, causing metabolic acidosis. Hepatic necrosis develops after serious poisoning, resulting in abnormal liver function test results and coagulopathies. Drowsiness and coma may develop as a result of hemodynamic instability or possibly as a direct toxic effect of iron in the CNS. Greater than 60 mg/kg of elemental iron is generally considered a toxic dose.

Clinical and Laboratory Manifestations. Nausea, vomiting, diarrhea, and abdominal pain reflective of iron's corrosive effects are the hallmark of iron poisoning, and usually develop within 30 min to 6 hr after ingestion. Hematemesis and bloody diarrhea may develop in more serious poisonings. Gastrointestinal signs may subside over 6–12 hr; however, careful observation is warranted because systemic toxicity due to cellular damage may ensue, particularly in patients with severe gastrointestinal signs, early hypotension, or drowsiness. All infants and children with a history of clinically significant iron ingestion who experience unprompted emesis should be immediately referred to a health care facility. Because iron is radiopaque, an abdominal radiograph may confirm the ingestion. Repeat radiographs may help with assessment of the efficiency of gastric decontamination methods. A negative result does not rule out iron ingestion because only undissolved tablets can be seen. Iron present in children's chewable multiple vitamins is usually not visualized on the radiograph because of the low concentration of iron and the rapid dissolution of the chewed tablet. Gastric scarring, pyloric stenosis, and intestinal strictures can develop 2–4 wk after a large ingestion or in instances when iron tablets remain in prolonged contact with the gastrointestinal mucosa. Strictures may be symptomatic and occasionally require surgical intervention.

Serum iron concentrations should be measured and evaluated in the context of symptoms and should be obtained approximately 4 hr after ingestion. Serum iron concentrations of <500 µg/dL, measured 4–8 hr after ingestion, indicate a low risk of significant toxicity. Serum concentrations of >500 µg/dL indicate that significant toxicity is likely. Serum iron concentrations are of greatest prognostic value in the asymptomatic iron-exposed patient. Because of the severe morbidity and mortality associated with iron intoxication and the time-sensitive variability of serum iron values (best obtained 4–6 hr postingestion), symptomatic patients with a history of even mild to moderate exposure should be referred to a health care facility for evaluation and possible chelation therapy. Blood gas levels, the serum glucose concentration, liver function tests, and coagulation studies should be obtained in symptomatic patients and those with serum iron concentrations of >500 µg/dL. Further, the patient's cardiovascular status should be continuously monitored because early and evolving hypovolemia resulting from gastrointestinal losses may culminate in hypovolemic shock. Direct iron toxicity to mitochondria may also produce cardiovascular collapse.

Treatment. Close clinical monitoring, combined with good supportive and symptomatic care, is essential in cases of iron poisoning. Ipecac-induced emesis may be used to remove tablets from the stomach, but appears to be of limited utility once the patient presents to the health care facility. Gastric lavage is not recommended in young children because of its inefficiency, particularly because of the large size of many iron tablets. Activated charcoal does not adsorb iron and should not be used, whereas whole bowel irrigation may be of benefit. In cases in which tablets adhere to the gastric mucosa, removal by endoscopic or surgical intervention (gastrotomy) or aggressive whole bowel irrigation has been attempted with mixed success. Oral bicarbonate, dilute oral saline laxative, and magnesium hydroxide (milk of magnesia) react with iron to form less soluble, poorly absorbed iron salts; this technique is of very questionable clinical benefit and should not be attempted. Complexation of iron in the gastrointestinal tract using oral deferoxamine is expensive, may actually increase iron absorption, and is generally not recommended. Whole bowel irrigation should be used for patients with numerous iron tablets present in the gastrointestinal tract.

Deferoxamine is a specific chelator of iron and is the antidote for moderate to severe iron intoxication (see Table 58-6). Acute, transient hypotension, with or without flushing, may be observed on instituting deferoxamine administration, particularly if a loading dose is given. These effects associated with deferoxamine administration appear to be due to the drug's ability to induce histamine release, which often resolves on slowing of the IV infusion rate. Indications for deferoxamine include a serum iron concentration of >500 µg/dL, regardless of symptoms, or moderate to severe symptoms, regardless of the serum iron concentration. It should be administered as a continuous IV infusion and continued until the patient is symptom-free. Prolonged deferoxamine infusion (>24 hr) has been associated with pulmonary toxicity (adult respiratory distress syndrome) and *Yersinia* sepsis. The deferoxamine-iron complex may color the urine reddish (vin rosé), although this is an unreliable indicator of iron excretion and is rarely observed. Intramuscular deferoxamine administration should be avoided whenever possible because absorption may be erratic, particularly in more severely intoxicated patients with impaired cardiovascular function.

CALCIUM CHANNEL BLOCKERS. Calcium channel blockers (CCBs) encompass a variety of chemical structures that produce various effects on the myocardium and the systemic vasculature. Specific agents include nifedipine, diltiazem, verapamil, amlodipine, and felodipine. They are available as regular-release and sustained-release preparations, as well as in combination with diuretics and other antihypertensives. Their expanding therapeutic use, while making CCBs the most commonly prescribed cardiovascular drugs, has also increased the incidence of poisoning exposure.

Pathophysiology. The toxic effects of these drugs are an extension of their therapeutic effect in that they antagonize L-type calcium channels, inhibiting calcium influx into myocardial and vascular smooth muscle cells; this results in depressed myocardial contractility and conduction as well as peripheral vasodilation, with subsequent hypotension and bradydysrhythmias. Calcium influx is also impaired in the β-islet cells of the pancreas, leading to impaired insulin release and subsequent hyperglycemia. CCBs have a narrow therapeutic index; thus, any dose greater than the usual maximum daily therapeutic dose should be considered potentially toxic.

Clinical and Laboratory Manifestations. The onset of symptoms may occur within minutes of the ingestion of a regular-release product or may be delayed several hr after the ingestion of a sustained-release product. All CCBs invariably cause hypotension, accompanied by bradycardia, normal heart rate, or even tachycardia, depending on the agent. Myocardial depression may lead to shock in severe cases. One clinical characteristic of CCB overdose is profound hypotension with preserved consciousness. Nausea and vomiting are common.

Careful blood pressure and electrocardiographic monitoring is essential. The electrocardiogram may show variable prolongation of the P-R interval with normal QRS width. Hyperglycemia is another characteristic of CCB overdose, so serial serum glucose measurements should be followed. Although these agents block calcium channels, the serum calcium level is not affected. Blood levels of CCBs are not readily available and are not useful in guiding therapy.

Treatment. After appropriate supportive care has been instituted, absorption should be prevented by early administration of activated charcoal. Whole bowel irrigation should be considered if a sustained-release product has been ingested. Pharmacotherapy should be directed at maintaining cardiac output and peripheral vascular tone, both of which are impaired in CCB poisonings. Useful agents include atropine, calcium, insulin, glucagon, fluids, and vasopressors. Atropine is the drug of choice for symptomatic bradycardia; a pacemaker should be considered for refractory cases.

Administration of IV calcium may reverse myocardial depression, impaired conduction, and hypotension, but it is not consistently effective. Calcium chloride is preferred over calcium gluconate because it contains a greater amount of calcium per gram. Because calcium salts have a much shorter duration of action than CCBs, administration by continuous infusion may be necessary (see Table 58-7). Hypercalcemia does not produce clinical effects and is not a concern.

High-dose insulin combined with euglycemic therapy has been successfully used to treat hypotension, especially in verapamil overdoses. Insulin has intrinsic inotropic effects and also improves the use of glucose by the myocardium. Glucagon improves cardiac conduction and contractility by promoting calcium ion influx through calcium channels indirectly (see Table 58-7). Its efficacy in the treatment of CCB overdose is not consistent. Other inotropic agents have also been used with mixed success. Extracorporeal membrane oxygenation and cardiac assist devices have been successfully used to support cardiac function until the drug is cleared from the body. Extracorporeal elimination methods are not useful for removing CCBs.

β-ADRENERGIC RECEPTOR BLOCKERS. Also known as *type II antidysrhythmic agents,* these drugs competitively block the action of catecholamines at the β receptor. They are used for the treatment of a wide variety of cardiac and noncardiac problems. Cardioselective agents, such as metoprolol, atenolol, and esmolol, act selectively at the β_1 receptors, whereas others, such as propranolol, sotalol, timolol, and labetalol, block both β_1 and β_2 receptors.

Pathophysiology. In overdose, β blockers lead to decreased chronotropy, impaired AV conduction, and decreased inotropy, manifested as bradycardia, heart block, and hypotension. Patients with reactive airway disease may have severe bronchospasm as a result of β-blocker toxicity (the β_2-mediated bronchodilation being blocked). β_2-receptor blockers also interfere with glycogenolysis and gluconeogenesis, impairing the ability to recover from hypoglycemia.

Clinical and Laboratory Manifestations. The onset of symptoms usually occurs within 1–3 hr of the ingestion of a regular-release product or may be delayed up to 10 hr with a sustained-release product. The most common features of severe poisoning are bradycardia, hypotension, low-output cardiac failure, and cardiogenic shock due to delayed conduction and poor myocardial contractility. Blood pressure and ECG monitoring are essential. The ECG may show decreased sinoatrial node function with sinus bradycardia, sinus pauses, or sinus arrest, or decreased AV conduction with various degrees of AV block. Respiratory depression is also common, along with bronchospasm, in susceptible patients. Delirium, altered level of consciousness, coma, and seizures occur with more lipophilic agents and with membrane-stabilizing agents. Hypoglycemia is also characteristic of β-blocker overdose, especially in children, and blood glucose should be monitored. Serum levels of β blockers are not readily available for routine clinical use, and are not useful.

Treatment. Supportive care is essential. Gastrointestinal decontamination is very important. Orogastric lavage can be considered in older patients who present within 1 hr of ingestion, but only after atropine administration. Activated charcoal is also recommended, and whole bowel irrigation should be considered after the ingestion of sustained-release preparations. Pharmacologic therapy should be directed at maintaining cardiac output, heart rate, contractility, and blood pressure. Useful agents include atropine, fluid boluses, glucagon, high-dose insulin, and vasopressors. Glucagon is the drug of choice for β-blocker poisonings, given its β_1 agonist effects and the lack of undesirable peripheral vasodilatory effects. If symptomatic bradycardia is refractory to all of the measures described earlier, ventricular pacing should be considered, although it may not improve cardiac output; extracorporeal membrane oxygenation or cardiac assist devices may be necessary for refractory hypotension.

DIGOXIN. Digoxin is a cardiac glycoside extracted from the leaves of *Digitalis lanata;* Digitalis glycosides are also present in *Digitalis purpura* (foxglove), *Nerium oleander* (oleander), *convallaria majalis* (lily of the valley), Siberian ginseng, and some toads' venom *(Bufo bufo)*. As a therapeutic agent, digoxin is used in children for the treatment of heart failure and some supraventricular tachydysrhythmias. Although digoxin was once considered 1 of the most dangerous poisons, the incidence of digoxin toxicity has decreased, due in part to progress in the understanding of its pharmacodynamics and drug interactions and in part to the availability of an effective antidote. Acute overdose may occur from dosing errors (especially in younger children), from accidental or intentional medication ingestion, or from ingestion of plant material containing digitalis glycosides. Chronic overdose occurs most frequently in 1 of the following 3 circumstances: alteration of the digoxin dose, alteration in digoxin clearance due to renal impairment, or drug interactions.

Pathophysiology. Digoxin blocks the Na^+, K^+-ATPase pump, leading to intracellular loss of K^+ and gain of Na^+ and Ca^{2+}, thus increasing the Ca^{2+} available to the contractile myocardium after excitation (positive inotropic effect). The increased intracellular calcium leads to increased myocardial automaticity, with subsequent atrial, nodal, and ventricular ectopy. The impaired Na-K exchange also leads to **dangerously high levels of serum potassium** in these patients. Digoxin also affects the cardiac autonomic system (vagally mediated mechanism), leading to an increased refractory period, decreased sinus node firing, and slowed conduction through the AV node, with sinus bradycardia, AV block, or even sinus arrest. The overall effect of digoxin overdose is a combination of slowed or blocked conduction and increased ectopy. Digoxin has a very narrow therapeutic index; toxicity can develop even from therapeutic doses. The therapeutic plasma concentration is 0.5–2.0 ng/mL, whereas levels >2 ng/mL are considered toxic; a digoxin level of >6 ng/mL is considered potentially lethal. Digoxin interacts with a wide variety of other drugs, by a variety of mechanisms, increasing the potential for toxicity at therapeutic doses.

Clinical and Laboratory Manifestations. Acute toxic effects usually occur within 6 hr of ingestion and include gastrointestinal, cardiovascular, and CNS manifestations. Nausea and vomiting are invariably associated with acute digoxin toxicity and usually represent the presenting symptoms. Cardiovascular manifestations include bradycardia, heart block, and ventricular dysrhythmias. **Bradydysrhythmias** are more common in previously healthy hearts, whereas previously diseased hearts usually respond with **tachydysrhythmias.** Continuous ECG monitoring is crucial for assessing digoxin's effects and guiding therapy. Blood pressure is usually preserved despite significant bradycardia. CNS manifestations include visual changes, headache, fatigue, lethargy, confusion, and hallucinations. Chronic cardiac glycoside toxicity leads to a combination of ventricular dysrhythmias and impaired AV conduction. The serum digoxin level should be assessed at least 6 hr after ingestion and carefully interpreted in the clinical context because the digoxin level alone is not reflective of the severity of intoxication. The serum potassium level should be monitored as a useful marker of severe toxicity: It may be dangerously increased (a poor prognostic sign), although decreased potassium levels may occur with concomitant use of loop diuretics, and hypokalemia enhances digoxin toxicity. Renal function should also be monitored.

Treatment. Initial treatment includes good general supportive care in an intensive care unit and gastric decontamination with activated charcoal if the ingestion was recent. Immediate therapy should aim for early recognition and aggressive treatment of life-threatening effects of digoxin toxicity, including mounting hyperkalemia and ventricular dysrhythmias. Hemodialysis may temporarily attenuate hyperkalemia, but digoxin cannot be eliminated in this way, due to its high tissue binding. An antidote for digoxin, **digoxin-specific Fab antibody fragments (Digibind)** is available (see Table 58-6). Digibind binds free digoxin in both the intravascular and the interstitial spaces and facilitates its renal clearance. Effects of Digibind usually begin within 1 hr of administration. Indications for the use of Digibind include digoxin-related life-threatening dysrhythmias, K^+ value of >5 mEq/L in the setting of acute digoxin overdose, significantly altered mental status, renal failure, serum digoxin level of >10 ng/mL, and ingestion of >4 mg in children or >10 mg in adults. In the absence of Digibind, ventricular ectopy should be treated with phenytoin, which may reverse the digoxin-induced slowed AV conduction and suppress the tachydysrhythmia without diminishing contractility. Atropine is the standard therapy for symptomatic bradycardia associated with digoxin overdose while Digibind is being prepared for administration.

CAUSTICS. Caustics include acids and alkalis as well as a few common oxidizing agents, such as bleach (see Chapter 324.2).

Pathophysiology. Acids coagulate proteins, causing local tissue necrosis, which limits its tissue penetration. Alkalis digest and dissolve proteins, producing transmural liquefaction necrosis, with the risk of perforation if the injury is located in the intestinal tract. The severity of the chemical burn produced depends on the pH, the concentration of the agent, and the length of contact time. Agents with a pH of <2 or >12 are most likely to produce significant injury.

Clinical Manifestations. Ingestion of caustic materials may produce oral burns, visualized as reddened areas or whitish plaques. Symptoms include pain, drooling, vomiting, and difficulty swallowing or refusal to swallow. Circumferential burns of the esophagus are likely to cause strictures on healing, which may require repeated dilation or surgical correction (see Chapter 324.2). Strong acids may sometimes produce scarring around the pylorus, leading to delayed onset of gastric obstruction. Caustics on the skin or in the eye can cause significant tissue damage.

Treatment. Initial treatment of caustic exposure includes thorough removal of the product from the skin or eye by flushing with water. Contaminated clothing should also be removed. Ingested agents should be rinsed from the oral cavity. Emesis and lavage are contraindicated. Activated charcoal should not be used because it does not bind these agents and may predispose the patient to violent vomiting and possible aspiration. Patients should be evaluated for evidence of esophageal burns, and if symptoms are present, oral fluids or solids should be withheld. The absence of visible oral injury does not preclude significant esophageal lesions. Endoscopy should be performed in symptomatic patients or those in whom injury is suspected on the basis of history. The use of corticosteroids and esophageal stents is controversial. Prophylactic antibiotics do not improve outcomes.

METHANOL AND ETHYLENE GLYCOL. Methanol is commonly found in windshield washer fluids, fuel additives, liquid fuel canisters, and industrial solvents. Ethylene glycol is commonly found in car radiator antifreeze. Both solvents are well absorbed via the intestine, through inhalation, or after skin contact; accidental ingestion is the most common route of exposure in children. The pathophysiology, clinical effects, and treatment of both chemicals are similar. Although each parent compound is capable of producing mild toxicity, it is the metabolites of each product that are responsible for the serious clinical effects that can follow exposure. Isopropyl alcohol (rubbing alcohol) also causes intoxication similar to that associated with ethanol; its metabolite is acetone. Its management is similar to that for ethanol (see Chapter 113.1).

Methanol

PATHOPHYSIOLOGY. Methanol is metabolized in the liver by alcohol dehydrogenase to formaldehyde, which is further metabolized to formic acid by aldehyde dehydrogenase. Formic acid is metabolized through folate-dependent pathways to carbon dioxide and water. Toxicity is caused primarily by formic acid, which inhibits mitochondrial respiration. The development of serious toxic effects is delayed while formic acid is generated and accumulates in blood and tissues.

CLINICAL AND LABORATORY MANIFESTATIONS. Drowsiness, mild inebriation, and gastric irritation, including nausea and vomiting, develop early after ingestion. The onset of serious effects, including profound metabolic acidosis and visual disturbances, is often delayed for up to 10–12 hr, and possibly up to 24 hr, as the parent methanol is undergoing metabolic activation to its toxic metabolites. Visual disturbances include blurred or cloudy vision, constricted visual fields, decreased acuity, and the "feeling of being in a snowstorm." Small children may not be able to describe these visual changes. Pupils may be dilated and nonreactive to light; retinal edema and optic disc hyperemia may be noted. Visual disturbances are usually reversible, but in significant poisonings, blindness has occasionally been permanent. An anion gap metabolic acidosis and an osmolar gap develop; thus, serum electrolytes, pH, osmolarity, and acid-base balance should be monitored.

Children are usually discovered with an open container of product soon after an exposure, and determining if a significant exposure has occurred is usually a problem. Methanol blood concentrations are usually available and can rule out an exposure; however, blood concentrations do not correlate well with toxicity. Formic acid concentrations may correlate more closely with toxicity; however, these blood concentration determinations are not routinely available. If methanol blood concentrations are not available, estimation of an osmolar gap has been recommended as a surrogate. Serum osmolarity is measured by the freezing point depression method and compared with a calculated serum osmolarity. The osmolar gap can be used to estimate the serum methanol concentration using the following formula:

$$\text{Osmolar gap} \times 3.2 = \text{estimated methanol blood concentration (mg/dL)}$$

TREATMENT. Treatment is discussed later.

Ethylene Glycol

PATHOPHYSIOLOGY. Ethylene glycol is metabolized by alcohol dehydrogenase in the liver to glycoaldehyde, which is further converted to glycolic acid by aldehyde dehydrogenase. Glycolic acid is metabolized to glyoxylic acid and oxalic acid, which are responsible for most of the observed toxicity. The development of serious toxic effects is delayed while these acids are generated and accumulate in blood and tissues. Oxalic acid combines with serum and tissue calcium, causing hypocalcemia and the formation of calcium oxalate crystals.

CLINICAL AND LABORATORY MANIFESTATIONS. As with acute methanol consumption, early symptoms associated with ethylene glycol exposure occur 1–12 hr after ingestion and include gastric irritation, including nausea and vomiting, and CNS effects, including drowsiness and inebriation. Metabolic acidosis begins to develop. Approximately 12–24 hr after ethylene glycol ingestion, cardiac dysrhythmias, muscle pain, and tetany due to **hypocalcemia** may occur. Later in the clinical course, cardiac failure, seizures, cerebral edema, and renal failure can occur. Renal failure is caused by the deposition of **calcium oxalate crystals** in renal tubules.

Ethylene glycol blood concentrations are often readily available, but as with methanol, the values do not correlate well with toxicity. Glycolic acid and glyoxylic acid concentrations may correlate more closely with ethylene glycol toxicity, but these determinations are not routinely available. Sodium fluorescein is an additive in many commercial antifreeze products. It is renally excreted and may be visualized in urine up to 6 hr after ingestion when illuminated with a Wood lamp. This simple test may be used to confirm ethylene glycol ingestion in children; a negative test result does not preclude a possible ingestion. Ethylene glycol serum concentrations can be estimated from an osmolar gap. Serum osmolarity is measured by the freezing point depression method and compared with a calculated serum osmolarity. The osmolar gap can be used to estimate the serum ethylene glycol concentration using the following formula:

$$\text{Osmolar gap} \times 6.2 = \text{estimated ethylene glycol concentration (mg/dL)}$$

Calcium oxalate crystals are commonly observed in urine on microscopy, but may not be evident early after exposure. Electrolytes, including calcium, should be monitored, as well as ECG and renal function studies.

TREATMENT. Because methanol and ethylene glycol are rapidly absorbed, gastric decontamination is usually not of value. Activated charcoal does not bind either agent and thus should not be used. Metabolic acidosis is treated with IV sodium bicarbonate at doses of 1–2 mEq/kg or, if needed, via extracorporeal hemofiltration. With the prompt institution of effective treatment (discussed later), the need for sodium bicarbonate is often limited. In patients with moderate to severe systemic metabolic imbalance, hemofiltration or dialysis may be far more effective in correcting these abnormalities while concurrently enhancing body elimination of the toxic alcohol and metabolites (discussed later).

Ethanol is considered the classic antidote for both methanol and ethylene glycol poisoning because it is preferentially metabolized over methanol and ethylene glycol by alcohol dehydrogenase, thus minimizing the formation of toxic metabolites (see Table 58-6). The parent compounds are then excreted via the lungs and kidneys. **Fomepizole,** a potent competitive inhibitor of alcohol dehydrogenase, if available, has replaced the use of ethanol because of its ease of administration, lack of CNS and metabolic effects, and overall excellent patient tolerability profile. Indications for fomepizole or ethanol therapy are a serum ethylene glycol concentration of >25 mg/dL or a serum methanol concentration of >20 mg/dL, a significantly symptomatic patient, ingestion of >0.4 mL/kg of 100% ethylene glycol or methanol, and systemic acid-base abnormalities.

Hemodialysis effectively removes ethylene glycol, methanol, the acid metabolites, and any antidote administered (fomeprazole, ethanol). Thus, specific supplemental doses of either antidote are required in patients undergoing hemodialysis. Dialysis is also useful for correcting severe metabolic acidosis. Indications for hemodialysis include methanol or ethylene glycol levels >50 mg/dL refractory metabolic acidosis and renal failure. When treating these patients, it is advisable to consult with a regional poison control center regarding therapy, in particular, supplemental antidote administration in dialyzed patients.

HYDROCARBONS. Hydrocarbons include a wide array of chemical substances found in thousands of commercial products. Many factors determine whether a particular product and exposure will produce systemic toxicity, local toxicity, or both. Nevertheless, aspiration of hydrocarbons into the lung can lead to serious, even life-threatening toxicity, underscoring the need for prompt attention in exposed patients.

Pathophysiology. The most important adverse effect of hydrocarbons is aspiration pneumonitis (see Chapter 394). Aspiration usually occurs at the time of ingestion, when coughing and gagging are common, but can also be secondary to vomiting, which commonly occurs after ingestion. The propensity of a hydrocarbon to cause aspiration pneumonitis is inversely proportional to its viscosity. Compounds with low viscosity, such as mineral spirits, naphtha, kerosene, gasoline, and lamp oil, spread rapidly across surfaces and cover large areas of the lungs when aspirated. Only small quantities (<1 mL) of low-viscosity hydrocarbons need be aspirated to produce significant injury. Pneumonitis does not result from dermal absorption of hydrocarbons or from ingestion in the absence of aspiration. Gasoline and kerosene are poorly absorbed, but often cause considerable gastrointestinal mucosal irritation as they pass through the intestines.

Certain hydrocarbons, most notably, halogen-substituted compounds, can be absorbed after ingestion, inhalation, or dermal contact. Most of these hydrocarbons have anesthetic properties and can cause transient CNS depression. Several chlorinated solvents, most notably, **carbon tetrachloride,** can produce hepatic toxicity. A few hydrocarbons have also been associated with renal and bone marrow toxicity. Benzene is known to cause cancer in humans after long-term exposure. The malignancy most commonly associated with benzene is acute myelogenous leukemia. **Methylene chloride,** found in some paint removers, is metabolized to carbon monoxide. Nitrobenzene, aniline, and related compounds can produce methemoglobinemia. Methemoglobin can be identified in the laboratory; its presence is also suggested if a drop of blood applied to filter paper remains brown as it dries. Methemoglobinemia is treated with the antidote methylene blue (see Table 58-6).

A number of volatile hydrocarbons, including toluene, propellants, refrigerants, and volatile nitrites, are commonly **abused** by inhalation. Some of these substances can sensitize the myocardium to the effects of endogenous catecholamines, with the risk of dysrhythmias and sudden death. Chronic abuse of these agents can lead to cerebral atrophy, neuropsychological changes, peripheral neuropathy, and renal disease (see Chapter 113.4). All volatile hydrocarbons are lipid solvents and can cause defatting of the skin, producing local irritation or, with prolonged exposure, chemical burns.

Clinical and Laboratory Manifestations. Transient, mild CNS depression is common after hydrocarbon ingestion. Aspiration is characterized by coughing, which usually is the first clinical finding. Cough usually begins immediately or within 2–5 min of the aspiration, and persists. Chest radiographs may be normal for as long as 8–12 hr after aspiration, but more often will be positive after 6 hr or longer from the time of exposure. Whenever possible, chest radiograph should be delayed until 6 hr or longer after the hydrocarbon exposure. Respiratory symptoms may remain mild or may progress rapidly to respiratory failure. Patient symptoms often correlate very poorly with abnormalities observed on chest radiograph, underscoring the importance of close clinical monitoring of the patient's respiratory status. Fever occurs and may persist for as long as 10 days after aspiration. Accompanying leukocytosis may be misleading because, in most cases of aspiration pneumonitis, no bacteria are present in the lungs. Chest radiographs may remain abnormal long after the patient is clinically normal, and they should not be used to guide acute treatment. Pneumatoceles may appear on the chest radiograph 2–3 wk after exposure.

Treatment. Emesis is contraindicated because of the risk of aspiration. Likewise, gastric lavage is contraindicated, except under special circumstances of ingestion of highly toxic hydrocarbons (carbon tetrachloride), because of the risk of vomiting and aspiration. If gastric lavage is to be performed, the patient should be intubated with a cuffed tube to protect the airway from further aspiration. Activated charcoal also is not useful because it does not bind the common hydrocarbons. If hydrocarbon-induced pneumonitis develops, respiratory treatment is supportive (see Chapter 394). Corticosteroids should be avoided because they are not effective and may increase the risk of infection. Prophylactic antibiotics should not be given because bacterial pneumonia occurs in only a very small percentage of cases. Respiratory failure has been successfully treated both with standard ventilation and with extracorporeal membrane oxygenation.

CHOLINESTERASE-INHIBITING INSECTICIDES. The most commonly used insecticides are organophosphates and carbamates; both are inhibitors of cholinesterase enzymes. Nerve agents used in warfare are usually organophosphates. Most pediatric poisonings occur as the result of accidental exposure to insecticides in and around the home or farm.

Pathophysiology. Both organophosphates and carbamates bind to cholinesterase enzymes, preventing the degradation of acetylcholine, resulting in its accumulation at nerve synapses. Enzymes affected include acetylcholinesterase or red blood cell cholinesterase, pseudocholinesterase (found in plasma), and neurotoxic esterase (nervous system). If left untreated, organophosphates form a permanent bond to these enzymes, inactivating them. This process, called *aging,* occurs over a variable period, but may occur as soon as 18 hr to 2–3 days after exposure. A period of weeks to months is required to regenerate inactivated enzymes. In contrast, carbamates form a temporary bond to the enzymes, allowing regeneration of the enzymes over several hours.

Clinical and Laboratory Manifestations. Clinical manifestations of organophosphate and carbamate toxicity relate to the accumulation of acetylcholine at peripheral nicotinic and muscarinic synapses and in the CNS (see Table 58-3). Muscarinic signs and symptoms include diaphoresis, emesis, urinary and fecal incontinence, tearing, drooling, bronchorrhea and bronchospasm, miosis, hypotension, and bradycardia. Nicotinic signs and symptoms include muscle weakness, fasciculations, tremors, hypoventilation (diaphragm paralysis), hypertension, tachycardia, and dysrhythmias. CNS effects include malaise, confusion, delirium, seizures, and coma. Symptoms caused by carbamate toxicity are usually less severe than those seen with organophosphates. A commonly used mnemonic for the most common symptoms of cholinergic excess is **DUMB BELS,** which stands for *d*iarrhea/defecation, *u*rination, *m*iosis, *b*ronchorrhea, *b*radycardia, *e*xcitation (muscle)/emesis, *l*acrimation and *s*alivation, and gastrointestinal cramps. Severe manifestations include coma, seizures, shock, arrhythmias, and respiratory failure.

Red blood cell cholinesterase and pseudocholinesterase concentrations can be readily measured in the laboratory. They may be useful in documenting an exposure, but do not correlate well with the magnitude of exposure or symptoms. Significant symptoms do not generally occur until measured enzyme concentrations fall to <25% of normal. Red blood cell cholinesterase, although more difficult to measure, is a better reflection of enzyme activity in the nervous system. Nevertheless, the magnitude and rate of progression of the patient's clinical findings are of greatest importance in determining the patient's disposition. These laboratory acetylcholinesterase determinations are of limited utility in acute exposures, although they may be of value in confirming an exposure or determining the extent of prolonged exposure.

Treatment. Basic decontamination should be performed on exposed persons, including washing all exposed skin with soap and water and immediate removal of all exposed clothing. Activated charcoal can be used for gastric decontamination, but for insecticides, it is of limited value because these highly lipid-soluble agents are rapidly absorbed. Basic supportive care should be provided, including fluid and electrolyte replacement and intubation, with artificial ventilation, if necessary. Two "antidotes" are useful to treat poisoning with cholinesterase inhibitors: atropine and pralidoxime (see Table 58-6). Atropine, which antagonizes the muscarinic acetylcholine receptor, is useful for both organophosphate and carbamate intoxication. Often, large doses of atropine must be administered by intermittent bolus or via continuous infusion. The absolute amount (dose) combined with the frequency of need for atropine can be used to estimate the magnitude of the patient's exposure and the probable time course to resolution. Pralidoxime chemically breaks the bond between the organophosphate and the enzyme, liberating the enzyme and thus enhancing the insecticide's body clearance. Pralidoxime is only effective if used before the bond "ages" and becomes permanent. For most commercially available organophosphate insecticides, this aging process evolves, usually becoming clinically relevant within approximately 18 hr after exposure. In the case of military nerve gases, shorter "aging" times are desired to limit the effectiveness of current antidote therapy. Pralidoxime is not necessary for carbamate poisonings because the bond between the insecticide and the enzyme degrades spontaneously. For significant organophosphate poisonings, both antidotes are used and large doses of atropine may be necessary to achieve adequate reversal of symptoms. Without treatment, symptoms of organophosphate poisoning may persist for weeks, requiring continuous supportive care. Even with treatment, neurologic symptoms may occur and persist.

TOXIC GASES

CARBON MONOXIDE. Although many industrial and naturally occurring gases pose a health risk by inhalation, the most common gas involved in pediatric exposures is carbon monoxide (CO). CO is a colorless, odorless gas produced during the combustion of any carbon-containing fuel. The less efficient the combustion, the greater the amount of CO produced. Wood-burning stoves, old furnaces, and automobiles are potential sources.

Pathophysiology. Toxicity develops through at least 3 mechanisms. First, it binds to hemoglobin, displacing oxygen-forming carboxyhemoglobin (COHb), with an affinity for hemoglobin that is approximately 250 times that of oxygen. Second, CO impairs the ability of hemoglobin to release oxygen to tissues. Finally, CO binds to cytochrome oxidase in tissues, impeding oxygen use. Although the relative contribution of each of these mechanisms to CO toxicity is unclear, the net result is tissue hypoxia.

Clinical and Laboratory Manifestations. Symptoms of CO poisoning are usually proportional to the concentration of COHb in the blood. COHb concentrations can be measured in almost all hospital laboratories. Early symptoms are nonspecific and include headache, malaise, and nausea, which are often confused with the flu. At higher exposure levels, headaches become severe, and dizziness, visual changes, and weakness may be present. Cherry-red mucosal coloring and retinal hemorrhage may also be present. Children may experience syncopal episodes as a first symptom. At high concentrations, coma, seizures, respiratory instability, and death may occur (see Chapter 74). Symptoms usually appear at COHb levels of >15%, toxicity is present at levels of >20%, and severe neurologic effects are universal at levels of >40%.

Treatment. In addition to general supportive care, treatment of CO poisoning requires the administration of 100% oxygen. High concentrations of oxygen shorten the COHb half-life in the blood and tissues. In healthy volunteers, the COHb half-life averages 5–6 hr (range, 2–7 hr), which is dramatically reduced to approximately 40–60 min by the administration of 100% oxygen at normal atmospheric pressures by a non-rebreathing face mask. In more severe and/or chronic exposures, hyperbaric oxygen therapy may be required, which at 2.5–3.0 atm reduces the COHb half-life to approximately 15–30 min. Severely poisoned patients benefit from hyperbaric oxygen therapy. Indications for hyperbaric oxygen include neurologic symptoms compatible with CO poisoning and a COHb level of >25% in children and pregnant women. After a significant exposure, some patients may experience delayed-onset neurotoxicity, which may be permanent. Aggressive early treatment of patients with significant symptoms may diminish the risk of neurologic sequelae.

HYDROGEN CYANIDE

Pathophysiology. Cyanide produces toxicity by interfering with oxygen use in the cytochrome oxidase system, resulting in cellular hypoxia.

Clinical and Laboratory Manifestations. Clinical symptoms occur rapidly after significant exposure and include headache, agitation and confusion, loss of consciousness, convulsions, and cardiac dysrhythmias. Severe metabolic acidosis occurs rapidly, and death may occur. Cyanide levels can be measured in the blood, but tests are not readily available and levels do not correlate well with symptoms. Severe metabolic acidosis in a patient with suspected cyanide exposure (fire victims) should be assumed to be cyanide poisoning.

Treatment. The cornerstone of treatment is rapid administration of high concentrations of oxygen, together with the use of the Lilly cyanide antidote kit. The kit includes nitrites (amyl nitrite and sodium nitrite) used to produce methemoglobin, which reacts with cyanide, forming cyanmethemoglobin. The kit also contains sodium thiosulfate, which is given to hasten the metabolism of cyanmethemoglobin to hemoglobin and the less toxic thiocyanate. Hydroxocobalamin (vitamin B_{12a}), which reacts with cyanide to produce cyanocobalamin (vitamin B_{12}), is an alternative antidote, but is not currently available in the U.S.

PLANTS. Exposure to plants, both inside the home and outside in backyards and fields, is one of the most common causes of unintentional poisoning in children. Ingestion of most plant parts (leaves, seeds, flowers) results in mild, self-limiting effects (Table 58-11). The treatment is symptomatic and supportive. The inherent toxicity of the product is so low that the ingestion of small to moderate quantities of plant material is unlikely to produce toxic symptoms.

The potential toxicity of a particular plant is highly variable, depending on the part of the plant involved (flowers are gener-

TABLE 58-11. Nontoxic and Minimally Toxic Plants*

African violet	Dracaena	Palm
Aluminum plant	Fern species (not asparagus fern)	Peperomia
Aralia, false	Fig	Petunia
Aster	Gardenia	Poinsettia
Barberry	Geranium	Pokeberries
Begonia species	Hen and chicks	Pyracantha
Boston fern	Honeysuckle	Rose
Carnation	Impatiens	Rubber plant
Chinese evergreen	Jade plant	Schefflera
Christmas cactus	Kalanchoe	Snake plant
Coleus	Magnolia	Spider plant
Corn plant	Marigold	Violet
Dandelion	Mother-in-law's tongue	Wandering Jew
Daylily	Nasturtium	Yucca
Dogwood	Norfolk Island pine	

*The potential for toxicity is dependent on the magnitude and amount of exposure. These agents are considered nontoxic or minimally toxic for mild to moderate exposure. The potential for toxicity increases with increased amount of exposure. Further, many plants contain substances that can be irritating to the mucosa (dermal/oroesophageal) and/or may precipitate allergic responses.

ally less toxic than the root or seed), the time of year, growing conditions, and the route of exposure. Assessment of the potential severity after a plant exposure is also complicated by the difficulty in properly identifying the plant. Many plants are known by several common names, which may vary between communities. Poison control centers have access to individuals able to assist in the proper identification of plants. They also keep current on the common poisonous plants in their service area and the seasons in which they are more abundant; thus, consultation with a poison control center is recommended if a potentially toxic plant is involved in the exposure (Table 58-12). Gastrointestinal decontamination for potentially toxic ingestions includes the use of activated charcoal; otherwise, treatment is supportive and symptomatic. Parents and grandparents of young children should be reminded to obtain the botanical and common names for plants that they purchase. In addition, for indoor plants, it is important to label the container (on the underside, for aesthetic acceptance), so that the poison control center can be given the correct name in case of an exposure. Similarly, landscapers or

TABLE 58-12. Commonly Ingested Plants with Significant Toxic Potential

PLANT	POISONOUS PARTS	SYMPTOMS	MANAGEMNT
Laburnum	All parts Seed ingestion is the must common presentation	Vomiting Pallor Dilated pupils Tachycardia Dizziness	Activated charcoal if >5 seeds ingested Observation
Deadly nightshade (*Atropa belladonna*)	All parts are poisonous, but berry ingestion is the most common presentation	Dry mouth Dilated pupils Hallucinations Urinary retention Agitation Ataxia Muscle incoordination Convulsions Coma	Activated charcoal if any plant material has been ingested; additional methods of gastric decontamination if >5 berries ingested; intestinal motility may be impaired and absorption prolonged Treatment is supportive, physostigmine should be reserved for cases where life-threatening symptoms do not respond to adequate supportive measures Symptoms can be delayed for up to 12 hr after ingestion Hospital admission is mandatory
Laurel (*Prunus laurocerasus*)	Leaves and broken seeds of the fruit are the most poisonous parts	Gastrointestinal upset Salivation Flushing Convulsions Coma Arrhythmias	If only the pulp of the berry was eaten, or if stones were swallowed whole, no treatment is required Activated charcoal is given if leaves or broken seeds were eaten Symptoms can be delayed for up to 4 hr
Lupin			Only toxic in large quantities Activated charcoal is given
Yew trees	All parts of the tree are toxic, except the pulp of the berry	Nausea Vomiting Anticholinergic effects Drowsiness Bradycardia Arrhythmia Convulsions	Asymptomatic children should be observed for 4 hr Gastric decontamination does not seem to influence outcome Treatment is supportive Serious cases are very rare
Woody nightshade (*Solanum dulcamara*) "Bittersweet"	All parts of the plant are toxic, particularly unripe fruits	Drowsiness Ataxia Nausea Vomiting Oropharyngeal irritation	Activated charcoal is given if >5 ripe berries or any unripe berries have been consumed Asymptomatic patients should be observed for 8 hr Treatment is supportive
Cuckoo pint (*Arum maculatum*)		Mucosal irritation, edema, and occasionally ulceration Local skin irritation and blistering	Treatment is symptomatic Analgesia and antihistamines Effects appear rapidly; observation of asymptomatic children is unnecessary
Elder (*Sambucus nigra*)	All parts of the plant are mildly toxic, particularly unripe berries	Nausea Vomiting Dizziness Tachycardia Convulsions	Consider gastric decontamination if >10 berries were consumed Treatment is symptomatic
Mistletoe	All parts of the plant are toxic except the flesh of the berry	Nausea Vomiting Diarrhea Muscle weakness Pupil dilation Diuresis Bradycardia can occur	Symptoms are unlikely if <3 berries were consumed Treatment is symptomatic; atropine is given for bradycardia Effects can last for several days
Rhubarb	The leaves contain oxalates and are toxic	Symptoms of gastric irritation predominate Oxalates chelate calcium and hypocalcemia can complicate ingestion	Milk may help to neutralize oxalic acid Treatment is otherwise supportive

From Riordan M, Rylance G, Berry K: Poisoning in Children 4: Household products, plants, and mushrooms. *Arch Dis Child* 2002; 87:403–406.

nurseries can identify outdoor plants surrounding the child's primary living environment.

Acetylcysteine (Acetadote) for acetaminophen overdosage. *Med Lett Drugs Ther* 2005;47:70–71.
American Academy of Clinical Toxicology & European Association of Poisons Centres and Clinical Toxicologists: Position paper: Single-dose activated charcoal. *Clin Toxicol* 2005;43:61–87.
Bailey B: Glucagon in β-blocker and calcium channel blocker overdoses: A systematic review. *J Toxicol Clin Toxicol* 2003;41:595–602.
Barry JD: Diagnosis and management of the poisoned child. *Pediatr Ann* 2005;34:937–946.
Belson MG, Sullivan K, Geller RJ: Beta-adrenergic antagonist exposures in children. *Vet Hum Toxicol* 2001;43:361–365.
Bernal W, Donaldson N, Wyncoll D, et al: Blood lactate as an early predictor of outcome in paracetamol-induced acute liver failure: A cohort study. *Lancet* 2002;359:558–562.
Boyer EW, Duic PA, Evans A: Hyperinsulinemia/euglycemia therapy for calcium channel blocker poisoning. *Pediatr Emerg Care* 2002;18:36–37.
Boyer EW, Shannon M: The serotonin syndrome. *N Engl J Med* 2005; 352:1112–1120.
Bryant S, Singer J: Management of toxic exposure in children. *Emerg Med Clin North Am* 2003;21:101–119.
Centers for Disease Control and Prevention: Nonfatal, unintentional medication exposures among young children, United States, 2001–03. *MMWR* 2006;55:1–5.
Centers for Disease Control and Prevention: Recognition of illness associated with exposure to chemical agents, United States, 2003. *MMWR* 2003; 52:938–940.
De Silva HA, Fonseka MMD, Pathmeswaran A, et al: Multiple-dose activated charcoal for treatment of yellow oleander poisoning: A single-blind, randomized, placebo-controlled trial. *Lancet* 2003;361:1935–1938.
Dugandzic RM, Tierney MG, Dickinson GE, et al: Evaluation of the validity of the Done nomogram in the management of acute salicylate intoxication. *Ann Emerg Med* 1989;18:1186–1190.
Eddleston M, Eyer P, Worek F, et al: Differences between organophosphorus insecticides in human self-poisoning: A prospective cohort study. *Lancet* 2005;36:1452–1459.
Eddleston M, Karalliedde L, Buckley N, et al: Pesticide poisoning in the developing world: A minimum pesticides list. *Lancet* 2002;360:1163–1167.
Eddy O, Howell JM: Are one or two dangerous? Clonidine and topical imidazolines exposure in toddlers. *J Emerg Med* 2003;25:297–302.
Ener RA, Meglathery SB, Van Decker WA, et al: Serotonin syndrome and other serotonergic disorders. *Pain Med* 2003;4:63–74.
Eyal D, Molczan KA, Carroll LS: Digoxin toxicity: Pediatric survival after asystolic arrest. *Clin Toxicol (Phila)* 2005;43:51–54.
Fugh-Berman A: Herb-drug interactions. *Lancet* 2000;355:134–138.
Gleyzer A, Traub S, Hoffman RS: Calcium channel blocker ingestions in children. *Am J Emerg Med* 2001;19:456–457.
Gracia R, Shepherd G: Cyanide poisoning and its treatment. *Pharmacotherapy* 2004;24:1358–1365.
Henry K, Harris CR: Deadly ingestions. *Pediatr Clin North Am* 2006; 53:293–315.
Kanabar D, Volans G: Accidental superwarfarin poisoning in children: Less treatment is better. *Lancet* 2002;360:963.
Klein-Schwarz W: Trends and toxic effects from pediatric clonidine exposures. *Arch Pediatr Adolesc Med* 2002;156:392–396.
Love JN, Enlow B, Howell JM, et al: Electrocardiographic changes associated with beta-blocker toxicity. *Ann Emerg Med* 2002;40:603–610.
Manoguerra AS, Erdman AR, Booze LL, et al: Iron ingestion: An evidence-based consensus guideline for out-of-hospital management. *Clin Toxicol (Phila)* 2005;43:553–570.
Michael JB, Sztajnkrycer MD: Deadly pediatric poisons: Nine common agents that kill at low doses. *Emerg Med Clin North Am* 2004;22:1019–1050.
Ralston ME. This issue: Managing emergencies part 2. *Pediatr Ann* 2005; 34:921–923.
Riordan M, Rylance G, Berry K: Poisoning in children 1: General management. *Arch Dis Child* 2002;87:392–396.
Riordan M, Rylance G, Berry K: Poisoning in children 2: Painkillers. *Arch Dis Child* 2002;87:397–399.
Riordan M, Rylance G, Berry K: Poisoning in children 3: Common medicines. *Arch Dis Child* 2002;87:400–402.
Riordan M, Rylance G, Berry K: Poisoning in children 4: Household products, plants, and mushrooms. *Arch Dis Child* 2002;87:403–406.
Riordan M, Rylance G, Berry K: Poisoning in children 5: Rare and dangerous poisons. *Arch Dis Child* 2002;87:407–410.
Schmidt LE, Knudson TT, Dalhoff K, et al: Effect of acetylcysteine on prothrombin index in paracetamol poisoning without hepatocellular injury. *Lancet* 2002;360:1151–1152.
Sinha Y, Cranswick NE: Clonidine poisoning in children: A recent experience. *J Paediatr Child Health* 2004;40:678–680.
Spiller HA, Klein-Schwarz W, Kolvin JM, et al: Toxic clonidine ingestions in children. *J Pediatr* 2005;146:263–266.
Turrina S, Neri C, De Leo D: Effect of combined exposure to carbon monoxide and cyanides in selected cases. *J Clin Forensic Med* 2004;11:264–267.
Verhulst L, Waggie Z, Hatherhill M, et al: Presentation and outcome of severe anticholinesterase insecticide poisoning. *Arch Dis Child* 2002;86:352–355.
Weaver LK, Hopkins RO, Chan KJ, et al: Hyperbaric oxygen for acute carbon monoxide poisoning. *N Engl J Med* 2002;347:1057–1067.
Woolf A, Litovitz T: Progress in the prevention of childhood iron poisoning. *Arch Pediatr Adolesc Med* 2005;159:593–595.

Chapter 59 ■ Herbal Medicines

Kathi J. Kemper and Paula Gardiner

Herbs and other dietary supplements are the most commonly used complementary therapies for children and adolescents. More than $4 billion is spent on these products each year in the U.S. Use rates are higher among children with chronic, incurable, or recurrent conditions, such as asthma, allergies, arthritis, cancer, chronic or recurrent pain, cystic fibrosis, and inflammatory bowel disease, but even previously healthy children seen in primary care and emergency departments frequently use herbs, home remedies, or supplements. Use is also common among teenagers; 41% of adolescents reported having used herbs and supplements, such as echinacea, ginseng, ginger, *Ginkgo biloba,* green tea, omega-3 fatty acids, soy supplements, St. John's wort, valerian, or zinc. Fewer than ½ of patients who use herbs and supplements have talked with their physician about their use, in part because physicians have not routinely asked patients and families about their use of these products.

Herbal products are widely perceived as being safe because they are natural. They are also frequently considered as having low therapeutic efficacy, owing to a paucity of publications about them in scientific journals. Conventional wisdom may be mistaken, resulting in risks to patients and providers.

Although they are generally safe, herbal products can cause serious toxicity. Acute hepatic toxicity and death may result from ingestion of even small amounts of *Amanita* mushrooms; overdoses of other herbs, such as digitalis, ephedra, and pennyroyal can cause life-threatening complications. Ephedra has significant cardiac toxicity. A widely used anxiolytic herb, kava kava (banned in several countries), has been linked to hepatotoxicity. Chronic use of other herbs, such as *Aristolochia,* coltsfoot, and licorice can cause severe hepatic or renal damage, cancer, or life-threatening electrolyte disturbances. Earl Grey tea causes muscle cramps, paresthesias, and blurred vision, whereas Japanese star anise (often a contaminant of Chinese star anise) is a neurotoxin. Even when an herb is safe when used correctly, it can cause mild or severe toxicity when used incorrectly. Tea tree oil is safe when applied to mild fungal infections of the skin, but can cause stinging and irritation when applied to eczema; if taken orally, it can cause coma in small children. Although peppermint is a commonly used and usually benign gastrointestinal spasmolytic (included in after-dinner mints and teas and increasingly used to ease discomfort during colonoscopy), it can exacerbate gastroesophageal reflux in other patients.

TABLE 59-1. Herbs for Asthma

HERB OR COMBINATION	RCTs	DEMONSTRATED BENEFIT	ADVERSE EFFECTS/DRUG INTERACTIONS	PURPORTED MECHANISM
Coffee/tea	None recently in children	Epidemiologic data suggest fewer symptoms in coffee drinkers	Tachycardia, insomnia, jitteriness, decreased appetite; potential interaction with β agonists	Methylxanthines Increased intracellular cAMP Bronchodilator
Shinpi-to	None in children	Yes, in historical data	Unknown; potential interaction with leukotriene blockers	Blocks 5-lipo-oxygenase and phospholipase A_2
Saiboku-to	Yes, in adults	Yes, corticosteroid-sparing effects in adults	Unknown; potential increase in corticosteroid adverse effects	Inhibits 11 β-hydroxylase (blocks steroid breakdown) Blocks 5-lipo-oxygenase Inhibits platelet-activating factor
Ma huang (*Ephedra sinica*)	Yes	Yes	Cardiovascular and central nervous system toxicity, deaths reported, potential interaction with β agonists	β Agonist Bronchodilator
Licorice (*Glycyrrhize glabra*)	No	Case series suggest corticosteroid-sparing effects	Pseudohyperaldosteronism, hypertension, peripheral edema, potential increase in corticosteroid adverse effects	Inhibits 11 β-hydroxylase and cortisol breakdown
Coleus forskolii	No	Case series in adults	Unknown	Decreased cAMP metabolism Bronchodilator
Tylophora indica	Yes, in adults	Yes	Unknown	Unknown
Ginkgo biloba	No	Yes, in a pilot study	Unknown	Platelet-activating factor antagonist Antioxidant
Onions (*Allium cepa*)	No	In vitro and animal data support use	Hypersensitivity is rare	Blocks leukotriene synthesis
Bee pollen	No	No	Anaphylaxis	Unknown

From Kemper KJ, Lester MR: Alternative asthma therapies: An evidence-based review. *Contemp Pediatr* 1999;16:162–195.
cAMP, cyclic adenosine monophosphate; RCT, randomized controlled trials.

TABLE 59-2. Commonly Used Sedative Herbs

SEDATIVE HERBS	SCIENTIFIC STUDIES	POTENTIAL ADVERSE EFFECTS OR INTERACTIONS	ADULT DOSE
German chamomile	In controlled trials, chamomile and its constituents have positive effects as a mild sedative	**Adverse effects:** Allergic reactions **Pregnancy and lactation:** No known adverse effects in pregnancy, lactation, and childhood **Drug interactions:** None known	**Tea:** 150 mL of boiling water over 3 g fresh flower heads, steep for 5–10 min; 3 × day
Hops (*Humulus lupulus*)	Historical and anecdotal use Controlled trials have used hops/valerian combinations; these show improvements in sleep with the combination	**Adverse effects:** Allergic reactions, skin irritation **Pregnancy and lactation:** No data available **Drug interactions:** Sedative activity increases the sleeping time induced by pentobarbital	**Tea:** 0.5–1.0 g dried hops before bed, typically in combination with valerian
Kava kava (*Piper methysticum*)	Randomized controlled trials in adults show anxiolytic effects	**Adverse effects:** Drowsiness, lethargy; slowed reaction time; withdrawal syndrome; chronic use may lead to yellow, dry skin and red eyes **Pregnancy and lactation:** Insufficient information available **Drug interactions:** May potentiate sedative and anxiolytic effects of other herbs and medications	**Capsules:** 60–120 mg kava lactones, up to 300 mg of kava lactones daily to dried root/rhizome; 1.5–3.0 g/day in divided doses
Lavender (*Lavandula*)	Animal data, adult case series, and controlled trials suggest anticonvulsant and sedative effects	**Adverse effects:** Allergies with topical use; toxic if large doses taken internally **Pregnancy and lactation:** Historically contraindicated during pregnancy owing to possible emmenagogue effects; no documented adverse effects **Drug interactions:** May potentiate sedative and anticonvulsant effects of other drugs	**Massage aromatherapy:** 1–10 mL of the essential oil can be added to 25 mL of a carrier oil **Bath soak:** add ¼–½ cup of dried lavender flowers to hot bath water
Lemon balm (*Melissa officinalis*)	Animal data suggest sedative hypnotic effects All RCTs have examined lemon balm/valerian combinations; most show enhanced sleep quality	**Adverse effects:** Allergic reactions are possible **Pregnancy and lactation:** Insufficient data; generally recognized as safe **Drug interactions:** None known	**Tea:** 2–3 g of dried herb, steeped in water; usually combined with valerian or lavender
Passionflower (*Passiflora alata*)	Case reports and historical use; most often combined with other herbs, such as valerian	**Adverse effects:** Allergic reactions are possible **Pregnancy and lactation:** Insufficient data **Drug interactions:** None known	**Tea:** 0.25–1 g (about 1 tsp of crushed dried flowers/cup of water) **Solid extract:** 150–300 mg (sold in capsules) daily
Valerian (*Valeriana officinalis*)	Randomized double-blind placebo controlled studies in adults show decreased sleep latency and improved sleep quality	**Adverse effects:** Headaches, insomnia **Pregnancy and lactation**: Insufficient data **Drug interactions:** Sedative activity increases the sleeping time induced by pentobarbital	**Tea:** 2–3 g of fresh or dried root/cup; 1–3 × day **Capsules:** 400 mg before bed

From Gardiner P, Kemper KJ: Herbs for sleep problems. *Contemp Pediatr* 2002;19(2):69–87 and Gardiner P, Kemper KJ: Herbs in pediatric and adolescent medicine. *Pediatr Rev* 2000;21:44–57.

Because of natural variability, herbal products may contain widely varying concentrations of active ingredients; variations of 10- to 1,000-fold have been reported for several popular herbs, even across lots produced by the same manufacturer. Labels may not accurately reflect the contents or the concentrations of ingredients. Herbal products may be unintentionally contaminated with pesticides, animal wastes, or the wrong herb that was misidentified during harvesting. Products from developing countries (e.g., Ayurvedic products from South Asia)

TABLE 59-3. Herbs for Skin Conditions

ACTION	HERB/SUPPLEMENT FOR TOPICAL USE
Soothing/emollient	Aloe, calendula
Anti-inflammatory	Aloe, chamomile, evening primrose oil, lemon balm
Antiviral	Aloe vera, calendula, chamomile, lemon balm
Antibacterial	Aloe vera, calendula, chamomile, lavender, lemon balm, tea tree oil
Antifungal	Lavender, tea tree oil

From Gardiner P, Coles D, Kemper KJ: The skinny on herbal remedies for dermatologic disorders. *Contemp Pediatr* 2001;18:103–104, 107–110, 112–114.

TABLE 59-4. Potentially Toxic Herbs

HERB	TOXIC CONSTITUENTS	TYPICAL USES	POTENTIAL ACUTE ADVERSE EFFECTS	HOW TO TREAT OVERDOSE
Aconitum (monkshood, wolfsbane)	**Diester alkaloids:** Hypaconitine and aconitine (aconitine increases permeability for sodium ions and slows down repolarization, leading to paralysis of the nerve)	Facial neuralgia and sciatica Headache and migraines Rheumatic pain, arthritis, gout Pericarditis sicca	Nausea, vomiting, hypersalivation **Central nervous system:** Paresthesias, muscular weakness, dizziness, ataxia, seizures, coma **Cardiac:** Bradycardia, hypotension, rhythm disorders	Supportive care Dioxin-specific antibodies, unless history excludes cardiac glycosides Do not give ipecac Activated charcoal and gastric emptying may help Avoid type 1 antiarrhythmics
Artemisia absinthium (wormwood)	**Thujone and isothujone:** Neurotoxins	Anorexia Dyspeptic conditions Liver and gallbladder disorders	**Mental status changes:** Restlessness, vertigo, tremors, agitation, seizures, headache Vomiting, stomach and intestinal cramps Rhabdomyolysis and renal failure	Supportive care Benzodiazepines
Atropa belladonna (deadly nightshade)	**Alkaloids:** Hyoscyamine (the L-isomer of atropline)	Gastrointestinal symptoms Cardiac insufficiency and arrhythmia Asthma	**Anticholinergic reaction:** Tachycardia, hyperthermia, mydriasis, urinary and bowel retention, restlessness Nervous system and respiratory depression	Gastric lavage Physostigmine given in consultation with a poison specialist External cooling if temperature is >102°F Benzodiazepines Hydration
Ayurvedic herbal remedies	Contaminated with lead, mercury, or arsenic	Traditional medicine from India; many purposes	Acute or chronic heavy metal toxicity	Depends on heavy metal
Digitalis purpurea (foxglove)	**Cardioactive glycosides:** Purpurea glycoside, digitoxin gitoxin	Ulcers, boils, headaches, abscesses, paralysis, cardiac insufficiency	Nausea and vomiting, headache, loss of appetite Cardiac rhythm disorders **Central nervous system:** Stupor, confusion, visual disorders, depression, psychosis, hallucinations	Supportive care Gastric lavage Activated charcoal Treatment of symptoms
Ephedra sinica (ma huang) Common names: Miner's tea Mexican tea Desert herb	**Alkaloids:** Ephedrine, pseudoephedrine (stimulates sympathomimetic receptors and the central nervous system)	Decongestant for upper respiratory infection Asthma Weight loss Stimulant	**Cardiac:** Hypertension, cardiomyopathy, myocardial infarction, arrhythmias **Central nervous system:** Dizziness, restlessness, headaches, anxiety, hallucinations, tremors, seizures, psychosis, strokes Nausea and vomiting Contraindicated in diabetes or hypertension, angle-closure glaucoma, anxiety, prostate adenoma, thyroid disease, pheochromocytoma	Activated charcoal Benzodiazepine for seizures and sedation Vasodilators for hypertension Lidocaine and β blockers for arrhythmias External cooling if temperature is >102°F Hydration therapy
Illicium anisatum (Japanese star anise tea)	Anisatins; block γ-aminobutyric acid	Colic in Latino and Caribbean populations	Seizures, tonic postures, myoclonus, hyperexcitability, irritability	Recovery with supportive care within 48 hr
Lobelia inflata (lobelia)	**Piperidine alkaloid:** L-Lobeline (stimulates nicotinic receptors)	Expectorant Asthma Spasmolytic Emetic To induce mental clarity and a feeling of well-being	**Gastrointestinal:** Nausea and vomiting, abdominal pain, diarrhea **Central nervous system:** Anxiety, headache, dizziness, tremors, seizures, paresthesias, euphoria **Cardiac:** Arrhythmias, bradycardia, transient increase in blood pressure, decreased respiratory rate In overdose, lobeline may cause hypotension Diaphoresis, muscle fasciculations and weakness, tremors, respiratory depression Dermatitis	Supportive care Gastric emptying Activated charcoal Benzodiazepines
Longdan xieganwan	Aristolochic acid	Enhance health	Renal interstitial fibrosis End stage renal failure Renal cell carcinoma	Supportive care
Mentha pulegium (pennyroyal)	Pennyroyal oil has a hepatotoxic effect Acute poisoning is not found with proper administration of the designated therapeutic use of pennyroyal leaf; however, the drug is not recommended owing to hepatotoxicity	Insect repellent Respiratory illness Digestive disorders Emmenagogue Abortifacient Wound treatment Gout	Uterine contractions **Gastrointestinal:** Nausea, vomiting, abdominal pain, hepatitis **Neurotoxin:** Delirium, dizziness, convulsions, seizures, paralysis, encephalopathy, coma Renal failure and hypertension Shock and disseminated Intravascular coagulation Contraindicated in pregnancy	Supportive care *N*-Acetylcysteine
Pausinystalia yohimbe (yohimbe)	Indole alkaloids **Yohimbe:** α_2-Adrenoreceptor antagonist	Sexual disorders Exhaustion Improve muscle function	**Adverse reactions:** Dizziness, headache, anxiety, hypertension, indigestion, rash, insomnia, tachycardia, tremor, vomiting, hallucinations, nervousness, paresthesias, hypothermia, salivation, mydriasis, diarrhea, palpations, tachycardia Contraindicated in kidney and liver disease	Gastric emptying Activated charcoal Antiarrhythmics Hydration
Phytolacca americana (pokeweed, American nightshade)	Triterpene saponins (irritate mucous membranes) Lectins (toxic)	Anti-inflammatory Arthritis Cancer Emetic and cathartic Rheumatism	Dizziness, somnolence, nausea, vomiting, diarrhea, tachycardia, hemorrhagic gastritis, hypotension, lymphocytosis, headache, respiratory depression, seizures	Hydration therapy, electrolyte correction, gastric emptying Activated charcoal Electrolyte replacement Emesis should not be induced if patient is experiencing symptoms of overdose
Stramonium folium (jimsonweed)	**Alkaloids:** Hyoscyamine (the L-isomer of atropine)	Asthma and cough Diseases of the autonomic nervous system	In high doses, leads to restlessness, mania, hallucinations, delirium **Overdose:** Tachycardia, mydriasis, flushing, dry mouth, decreased sweating, miction, constipation	Supportive care Gastric lavage Decreasing temperature Physostigmine Benzodiazepines
Viscum album (mistletoe)	Alkaloids Viscotoxins (*Viscum album*) cause hypotension, bradycardia, and arterial vasoconstriction Lectins	Antineoplastic adjuvant Antihypertensive Nervous disorders: calmative agent Rheumatism Antispasmodic	Fever, headaches, nausea, vomiting, diarrhea, bradycardia, angina, change in blood pressure, seizures, confusion, hallucination, allergic reactions, miosis, mydriasis, chills, coma 2 reported deaths in the last 35 yr; most ingestions lead to mild reactions	Supportive therapy Data inconclusive for inducing emesis Activated charcoal

From Gardiner P, Kemper KJ: Herbs for sleep problems. *Contemp Pediatr* 2002;2:69–87: and Gardiner P, Kemper KJ: Herbs in pediatric and adolescent medicine. *Pediatr Rev* 2000;21:44–57.

may contain toxic levels of mercury, cadmium, arsenic, or lead, either from unintentional contamination during manufacturing or from intentional additions by producers who believe that these metals have therapeutic value. Approximately 30–40% of Asian patent medicines include potent pharmaceuticals, such as analgesics, antibiotics, hypoglycemic agents, or corticosteroids; typically, the labels for these products are not written in English and do not note the inclusion of pharmaceutical agents.

Many families use dietary supplements concurrently with medications, thus posing hazards of interactions. St. John's wort induces CYP3A4 activity of the P450 enzyme system (see Chapter 56) and thus can enhance elimination of digoxin, cyclosporine, protease inhibitors, and numerous antibiotics, leading to **subtherapeutic serum** levels of these important medications. It may also increase the risk of serotonin syndrome in patients taking antidepressant medications. Ginkgo may increase the risk of bleeding in patients taking anticoagulants. Licorice may enhance the anti-inflammatory effects and adverse effects of glucocorticoid medications.

In the U.S., herbal products are not regulated in the same way as medications. The 1994 U.S. Dietary Supplement and Health Education Act (DSHEA) allows herbal products to be marketed without previous testing for efficacy or safety. Products may contain little or none of the herb listed on the label, and they may contain other herbs. Although they may not claim to prevent or treat specific medical conditions, product labels may make "structure-function" claims. A label may claim that a product "promotes a healthy immune system," but it may not claim to cure the common cold. The U.S. Food and Drug Administration (FDA) can only restrict sales of certain products after receiving reports of adverse effects. Adverse reactions should be reported to the FDA's MedWatch program; failure to do so limits the FDA's ability to monitor and manage the clinical and public health risks of these products.

Some widely used products are relatively safe, but do not appear to be effective in the treatment of conditions for which they are promoted. One trial did not show that echinacea reduced the severity or duration of cold symptoms in children. In addition, St. John's wort was equivalent to placebo in the treatment of mild to moderate depression.

Some herbal products may be helpful adjunctive treatments for common childhood problems. Two studies, 1 with fennel and another with an herbal combination (chamomile, fennel, vervain, licorice, balm mint), found that these remedies were helpful for **infant colic.** Ginger has been shown to be an effective antiemetic; herbal eardrops have been shown to provide significant analgesia for children with mild to moderate otitis media. Enteric-coated peppermint oil may be helpful for children with irritable bowel syndrome. Probiotics may help prevent and treat diarrhea in children (see Chapter 337).

Most herbs have undergone far more testing in adult than in pediatric populations. Herbalists recommend that teenagers use adult doses, children 7–12 yr of age use ½ of the adult dose, children 3–6 yr of age use ¼ of the adult dose, and that herbs be used only cautiously, if at all, in children 2 yr of age or younger. Herbs used for common conditions and the toxicity of selected herbs are described in Tables 59-1 through 59-5, and resources for information on herbal medicine are listed in Table 59-6.

TABLE 59-5. Spanish-English Botanical Name Translation Chart*

SPANISH NAME	ENGLISH NAME	BOTANICAL NAME
Ajo	Garlic	*Allium sativum*
Azarcon	Lead tetraoxide	Not a plant
Azogue	Mercury	Not a plant
Cebolla	Onion	*Allium cepa*
Cenela	Cinnamon	*Cinnamomum aromaticum*
Clavo	Cloves	*Eugenia aromatica*
Comino	Cumin	*Cuminum cyminum*
Epasote or Herba Sancti Mariae	Wormseed	*Chenopodium anthelminticum*
Estafiate	Wormwood	*Artemisia absinthium*
Eucalipto	Eucalyptus	*Eucalyptus globulus*
Granada	Pomegranate	*Punica granatum*
Jengibre	Ginger	*Zingiber officinale*
Limon	Lemon	*Citrus limon*
Manzanilla	Chamomile	*Anthemis nobilis* or *Chamomilla recutita* or *Matricaria chamomilla*
Oregano	Oregano	*Origanum vulgare*
Pelos de elote	Corn silk	*Zea mays*
Savila	Aloe vera	*Aloe vera*
Siete jarabes	Mixture of syrup of sweet almond, castor oil, balsam resin, wild cherry, licorice, cocillana bark, honey	
Tomillo	Thyme	*Thymus vulgaris*
Una de gato	Cat's claw	*Uncaria tomentosa*
Valeriana	Valerian	*Valeriana officinalis*
Yerba buena	Spearmint	*Mentha spicata*

*Prepared with assistance from Laura Howell, MD.

TABLE 59-6. Resources

PERIODICALS

Prescribers Letter. Therapeutic Research Center (209-472-2240)
Review of Natural Products. Facts and Comparison (1-800-223-0554)

WEB SITES

Academic

Longwood Herbal Task Force: http://www.mcphs.edu/MCPHSWeb/herbal
Memorial Sloan-Kettering Cancer Center: http://www.mskcc.org/mskcc/html/11570.cfm
University of Texas M. D. Anderson Cancer Center: http://www.mdanderson.org/departments/CIMER/dIndex.cfm?pn=6EB86A59-EBD9-11D4-810100508B603A14
Wake Forest University School of Medicine, BestHealth: http://www.besthealth.com/cam/The_Herbs_Supplements.htm

Government

FDA MEDWATCH, monitoring program for reporting adverse effects: http://www.fda.gov/medwatch (1-800-FDA-1088)
International Bibliographic Information on Dietary Supplements (IBIDS): http://ods.od.nih.gov/databases/ibids.html
National Cancer Institute: http://www.cancer.gov/cam
National Center for Complementary and Alternative Medicine: http://www.nccam.nih.gov/health/bottle
NIG Office of Dietary Supplements: http://odp.od.nih.gov
U.S. Department of Agriculture Food and Nutrition Center: http://www.nal.usda.gov/fnic/etext/000015.html
U.S. Food and Drug Administration Office of Dietary Supplements: http://vm.cfsan.fda.gov/~dms/supplmnt.html

Nonprofit

American Botanical Council: http://www.herbalgram.org
Children's Hospital and Boston Medical Center: www.holistickids.org
The Natural Pharmacist: www.tnp.com

Subscription Products

Micromedex Internet Health Care Series: www.micromedex.com
Natural Medicine Comprehensive Database: http://www.naturaldatabase.com
Natural Standards: www.naturalstandards.com
ConsumerLabs: www.consumerlabs.com

Toxicology Information

Toxicology Information Resource Center: http://www.ornl.gov/TechResources/tirc/hmepg.html
TOXLINE and TOXNET, from the National Library of Medicine: http://sis.nlm.nih.gov/ToxSearch.htm

Alexandrovich I, Rakovitskaya O, Kolmo E, et al: The effect of fennel *(Foeniculum vulgare)* seed oil emulsion in infantile colic: A randomized, placebo-controlled study. *Altern Ther Health Med* 2003;9:58–61.
Ball SD, Kertesz D, Moyer-Mileur LJ: Dietary supplement use is prevalent among children with a chronic illness. *J Am Diet Assoc* 2005;105:78–84.
Centers for Disease Control and Prevention: Suspected moonflower intoxication—Ohio, 2002. *MMWR* 2003;52:788–791.
De Smet PAGM: Herbal remedies. *N Engl J Med* 2002;347:2046–2056.

Finkel RS: Blue cohosh and perinatal stroke. *N Engl J Med* 2004;351: 302–303.

Finsterer J: Earl Grey tea intoxication. *Lancet* 2002;359:1484–1485.

Garrard J, Harms S, Eberly LE, et al: Variations in product choices of frequently purchased herbs. *Arch Intern Med* 2003;163:2290–2295.

Ize-Ludlow D, Ragone S, Bruck IS, et al: Neurotoxicities in infants seen with the consumption of star anise tea. *Pediatrics* 2004;114:e653–e656.

Kline RM, Kline JJ, Di Palma J, et al: Enteric-coated, pH-dependent peppermint oil capsules for the treatment of irritable bowel syndrome in children. *J Pediatr* 2001;138:125–128.

Koretz RL, Rotblatt M: Complementary and alternative medicine in gastroenterology: The good, the bad, and the ugly. *Clin Gastroenterol Hepatol* 2004;2:957–967.

Laing C, Hamour S, Sheaff M, et al: Chinese herbal uropathy and nephropathy. *Lancet* 2006;368:338–339.

Lanski SL, Greenwald M, Perkins A, et al: Herbal therapy use in a pediatric emergency department population: Expect the unexpected. *Pediatrics* 2003;111:981–985.

Markowitz JS, Donovan JL, DeVane CL, et al: Effect of St. John's wort on drug metabolism by induction of cytochrome P450 3A4 enzyme. *JAMA* 2003;290:1500–1504.

McBride BF, Karapanos AK, Krudysz A, et al: Electrocardiographic and hemodynamic effects of a multicomponent dietary supplement containing ephedra and caffeine. *JAMA* 2004;291:216–221.

Mills E, Montori VM, Wu P, et al: Interaction of St. John's wort with conventional drugs: Systematic review of clinical trials. *BMJ* 2004;329:27–30.

Saper RB, Kales SN, Paquin J, et al: Heavy metal content of Ayurvedic herbal medicine products. *JAMA* 2004;292:2868–2873.

Shekelle PG, Hardy ML, Morton SC, et al: Efficacy and safety of ephedra and ephedrine for weight loss and athletic performance. *JAMA* 2003;289: 1537–1544.

Sibinga EM, Ottolini MC, Duggan AK, et al: Parent-pediatrician communication about complementary and alternative medicine use for children. *Clin Pediatr (Phila)* 2004;43:367–373.

Szajewska H, Mrukowicz JZ: Probiotics in the treatment and prevention of acute infectious diarrhea in infants and children: A systematic review of published randomized, double-blind, placebo-controlled trials. *J Pediatr Gastroenterol Nutr* 2001;33:S17–S25.

Taylor JA, Weber W, Standish L, et al: Efficacy and safety of echinacea in treating upper respiratory tract infections in children: A randomized controlled trial. *JAMA* 2003;290:2824–2830.

Turner RB, Bauer R, Woelkart K, et al: An evaluation of *Echinacea angustifolia* in experimental rhinovirus infections. *N Engl J Med* 2005;353: 341–348.

Wilson KM, Klein JD: Adolescents' use of complementary and alternative medicine. *Ambul Pediatr* 2002;2:104–110.

Yussman SM, Ryan SA, Auinger P, et al: Visits to complementary and alternative medicine providers by children and adolescents in the United States. *Ambul Pediatr* 2004;4:429–435.

Part VIII ■ The Acutely Ill Child

Chapter 60 ■ Evaluation of the Sick Child in the Office and Clinic

Paul L. McCarthy

There are many reasons for a sick child visit, but most are due to acute self-limited intercurrent infections; often the child is febrile. When evaluating an acutely ill, febrile child, the pediatrician must be aware of categorical statistics about the probable occurrence of serious illness, because one of the major goals of the sick child visit is to identify the seriously ill child who requires specific therapeutic intervention. The risk for and the cause of serious illness in the acutely febrile child vary, depending on age. The infant in the 1st 3 mo of life is more susceptible to sepsis and meningitis caused by group B streptococci and gram-negative organisms. Infants in the 1st mo of life are at highest risk. Urinary tract infections are more frequent in males; infants in this age group more often have an underlying anatomic abnormality of the urinary tract than do older children with urinary tract infections (see Chapter 538). As the infant matures beyond 3 mo, the bacterial pathogens that usually cause bacteremia, sepsis, and meningitis are *Streptococcus pneumoniae, Haemophilus influenzae* type b (if the child is unimmunized or only partially immunized), and *Neisseria meningitidis.* Immunization against some serotypes of *S. pneumoniae* may reduce the occurrence of occult bacteremia and serious infections caused by that organism, as has immunization against *H. influenzae* type b. After infancy, urinary tract infections are seen more often in females. Immunity develops rapidly to the common bacterial pathogens during the first 3–4 yr of life. *N. meningitidis* is the leading cause of bacterial meningitis. In children older than 36 mo, pharyngitis caused by group A streptococci is a common bacterial infection. *Mycoplasma pneumoniae* assumes increasing importance as a cause of pulmonary infiltrates in children older than 5 yr of age. Table 60-1 shows serious illnesses documented in children in the 1st 3 yr of life who presented with fever and acute illness at a university hospital and private practice. In many studies, urinary tract infections are the most common serious bacterial infections. Soft tissue infections due to streptococcus or staphylococcus may include cellulitis, fasciitis, osteomyelitis, and septic arthritis. Noninfectious, but serious disease should also be considered and include trauma (abuse), midgut volvulus, appendicitis, intussusception, poisoning (salicylates), metabolic disorders (hypoglycemia, hyperammonemia), neurologic disorders (seizures, infant botulism), or inflammatory diseases (Kawasaki disease, juvenile rheumatoid arthritis, Henoch-Schönlein purpura).

The acutely ill child with a serious illness is identified by careful observation, history taking, physical examination, appreciation of age and body temperature as risk factors, and the judicious use of screening laboratory tests. The physician can use the data to make informed decisions about the need for more definitive laboratory tests (urine culture), therapy, and the advisability of hospital admission. Observation, history, and physical examination are integrated when the sick child evaluation is being done; that is, as the child is being observed, historical data are gathered. History taking and observational assessment often continue as the physical examination is performed. If abdominal tenderness is found on examination, additional history about blood in the stool, cramping abdominal pain, and vomiting may be sought.

OBSERVATION

Observation is important in the evaluation of the acutely ill child. The child should be observed for specific evidence of a serious illness, such as grunting, which might indicate pneumonia or sepsis, or a bulging fontanel, which might indicate bacterial meningitis or head trauma. Most observational data that the pediatrician gathers during an acute illness should focus, however, on assessing the child's response to stimuli. How does the crying child respond to the parents' comforting? How quickly does the sleeping child awaken with a stimulus? Does the child smile when the examiner interacts with him or her? Assessing responses to stimuli, while often providing those stimuli, requires knowledge of normal responses for different age groups, the manner in which those normal responses are elicited, and to what degree a response might be impaired.

Sometimes the manner in which the child responds to stimuli is readily apparent. For example, the child may vocalize and smile as the examiner enters the room. At other times, more effort and more stimuli are needed to cause the child to act in a normal manner. Often the fussing, irritable child begins to look around and focus on the examiner when held and walked by the parent. This normal visual behavior is an important indicator of well-being. Thus, during observation, the pediatrician must be both clinically and developmentally oriented.

Six observation items and their scales (Acute Illness Observation Scales) that have reliably and validly identified serious illness in febrile children are shown in Figure 60-1. A normal finding is scored as 1, moderate impairment as 3, and severe impairment as 5. The best possible score is 6 items × 1 = 6; the worst score is 6 items × 5 = 30. The chance of serious illness is 1–2% if the total score is 10 or less; if the score is >10, the risk of serious illness increases by at least 10-fold. It is not clear whether these scales can be used in the first 1–3 mo of life because infants may not have developed the skills required to score some of these items.

HISTORY

History taking is complex. Parents must transmit how a younger child has been "feeling." Parents should also provide information on a specific symptom, such as bloody diarrhea or cyanosis when coughing. The older child's perception of symptoms may reflect a developmentally immature understanding of causation. The examiner pursues the historical information provided by the parents or child to define the symptoms precisely. If the complaint is blood in the stool, additional questions can be asked about other evidence of bowel inflammation, such as watery stools, mucus in the stools, or increased frequency of stooling. If the historical information indicates crying with defecation and streaks of blood on the outer portion of a hard stool, without other changes in the character or frequency of the stool, a diagnosis of a rectal fissure is tenable.

Questions should focus on those entities that are seen most commonly in acute febrile childhood illnesses. The more serious diagnoses are outlined in Table 60-1. Organ-specific questions are helpful, such as those concerning fast breathing, cyanosis, retraction, and wheezing with pneumonia, or pain, swelling, and pseudoparalysis with septic arthritis. Because most acute illnesses in children are caused by minor viral infections, specific questions about the epidemiology of the illness can offer important insights.

6 OBSERVATION ITEMS AND THEIR SCALES

(PLEASE CHECK BOXES THAT DESCRIBE YOUR CHILD'S APPEARANCE AND BEHAVIOR)

OBSERVATION ITEM	NORMAL	MODERATE IMPAIRMENT	SEVERE IMPAIRMENT
1. **QUALITY OF CRY**	STRONG WITH NORMAL TONE ☐ *OR* CONTENT AND NOT CRYING ☐	WHIMPERING ☐ *OR* SOBBING ☐	WEAK ☐ *OR* MOANING ☐ *OR* HIGH-PITCHED ☐
2. **REACTION TO PARENT STIMULATION** (Effect on crying when held, patted on back, jiggled on lap, or carried)	CRIES BRIEFLY, THEN STOPS ☐ *OR* CONTENT AND NOT CRYING ☐	CRIES OFF AND ON ☐	CONTINUAL CRY ☐ *OR* HARDLY RESPONDS ☐
3. **STATE VARIATION** (Going from awake to asleep or asleep to awake)	IF AWAKE, THEN STAYS AWAKE ☐ *OR* IF ASLEEP AND STIMULATED, THEN WAKES UP QUICKLY ☐	EYES CLOSE BRIEFLY, THEN AWAKENS ☐ *OR* AWAKENS WITH PROLONGED STIMULATION ☐	WILL NOT ROUSE ☐ *OR* FALLS TO SLEEP ☐
4. **COLOR**	PINK ☐	PALE HANDS, FEET ☐ *OR* ACROCYANOSIS (BLUE HANDS AND FEET) ☐	PALE ☐ *OR* BLUE ☐ *OR* ASHEN (GRAY) ☐ *OR* MOTTLED ☐
5. **HYDRATION** (Moisture in skin, eyes, mouth)	SKIN NORMAL *AND* EYES, MOUTH MOIST ☐	SKIN, EYES NORMAL *AND* MOUTH SLIGHTLY DRY ☐	SKIN DOUGHY OR TENTED *AND* EYES MAY BE SUNKEN *AND* DRY EYES AND MOUTH ☐
6. **RESPONSE TO SOCIAL OVERTURES** (Being held, kissed, hugged, touched, talked to, comforted)	SMILES ☐ *OR* ALERTS ☐ (2 months or less)	BRIEF SMILE ☐ *OR* ALERTS BRIEFLY ☐ (2 months or less)	NO SMILE, FACE ANXIOUS ☐ *OR* DULL, EXPRESSIONLESS ☐ *OR* NO ALERTING ☐ (2 months or less)

Figure 60-1. Acute illness observational scales for use in clinical evaluation of the well and sick child. (From McCarthy PL, Sharpe MR, Spiesel SZ, et al: Observation scales to identify serious illness in febrile children. *Pediatrics* 1982;70:802, with permission.)

Are there other children in the family with similar symptoms? Has the child had other illness exposures? Finally, it is important to be aware of any underlying chronic problems that might predispose the child to recurring infections or a serious acute illness; for example, the child with sickle cell anemia or AIDS is at increased risk for recurrent episodes of bacteremia. Benign viral illnesses may produce serious secondary consequences, such as dehydration or severe respiratory syncytial virus pneumonia in infants who had bronchopulmonary dysplasia as neonates. Additional questions to assess hydration, such as questions about wet diapers, tears, or awakeness, should be used to assess secondary complications.

TABLE 60-1. Diagnosis of Serious Illnesses During 996 Episodes of Acute Infectious Illness in Febrile Children Younger Than 36 Mo*

	CASES	
DIAGNOSIS	NO.	%
Bacterial meningitis	9	0.9
Aseptic meningitis	12	1.2
Pneumonia	30	3.0
Bacteremia	10	1.0
Focal soft tissue infection†	10	1.0
Urinary tract infection	8	0.8
Bacterial diarrhea	1	0.1
Abnormal electrolytes or blood gases	9	0.9
Total	89	8.9

*Nonserious illness includes benign viral diseases, such as roseola, herpesvirus 6 or 7, enteroviruses, respiratory syncytial virus, influenza, metapneumovirus, parainfluenza, and rotavirus.

†Includes cellulitis, osteomyelitis, and septic arthritis.

From McCarthy PL: Acute infectious illness in children. *Compr Ther* 1988; 14:51.

PHYSICAL EXAM

During physical examination, the pediatrician seeks evidence of illnesses, especially serious illnesses (see Table 60-1), that are causes of acute febrile episodes in children. The portions of the physical examination that require the child to be optimally cooperative are completed first. Initially, it is best to seat the child on the parent's lap; the older child may be seated on the examination table. Vital signs are often overlooked, but are valuable in assessing ill children. The degree of fever, the presence of tachycardia out of proportion to the fever, and the presence of tachypnea and hypotension all suggest a serious infection. In addition to the general level of interaction, color, and hydration, as assessed by the Acute Illness Observation Scales (see Fig. 60-1), the child's respiratory status is evaluated. This evaluation includes determining respiratory rate and noting any evidence of inspiratory stridor, expiratory wheezing, grunting, or coughing. Evidence of increased work of breathing—retraction, nasal flaring, and the use of abdominal musculature—is sought. Because acute infections in children are most often caused by viral infections, the presence of nasal discharge is noted. It is possible at this time to assess the skin for rashes. Frequently, viral infections cause an exanthematous eruption, and many of these eruptions are diagnostic (the reticulated rash and "slapped-cheek" appearance caused by parvovirus infections or the typical appearance of hand-foot-and-mouth disease caused by coxsackieviruses). The skin examination may also yield evidence of more serious infections (bacterial cellulitis or petechiae associated with bacteremia). Cutaneous perfusion should be assessed by warmth and capillary refill time. When the child is seated and is least perturbed, an assessment of fontanel tension can be completed; it can be determined if the fontanel is depressed, flat, or bulging. It is also important to assess the child's willingness to move and ease of movement. Usually, the child with meningitis will hold the neck stiffly and will often cry when any attempt is made to flex the neck, even during cuddling by the parent. This is termed *paradoxic irritability.* The child with cellulitis, osteomyelitis, or septic arthritis in an extremity will resist movement of that limb. The child with peritoneal inflammation will sit quietly and become irritable during movement. It is reassuring to see the child moving about on the parent's lap with ease and without discomfort.

During this initial portion of the physical examination, when the child is most comfortable, the heart and lungs are auscultated. In the acutely febrile child, because of the relatively frequent occurrence of respiratory illnesses, it is important to assess adequacy of air entry into the lungs, equality of breath sounds, and evidence of adventitial breath sounds, especially wheezes, rales, and rhonchi. The coarse sound of air moving through a congested nasal passage is frequently transmitted to the lungs. The examiner can become attuned to these coarse sounds by placing the stethoscope near the child's nose and then compensating for this sound as the chest is auscultated. The cardiac examination is completed next; findings such as pericardial friction rub, loud murmurs, or distant heart sounds may indicate an infectious process involving the heart. The eyes are examined to identify features that might indicate an infectious process. Often, viral infections result in a watery discharge or redness of the bulbar conjunctivae. Bacterial infection, if superficial, results in purulent drainage; if the infection is more deep-seated, tenderness, swelling, and redness of the tissues surrounding the eye are present, as well as proptosis, reduced visual acuity, and altered extraocular movement. The extremities may then be evaluated not only for ease of movement, but also for the possibility of swelling, heat, or tenderness; such abnormalities may indicate focal infections.

The components of the physical examination that are more bothersome to the child are completed last. This is best done with the patient on the examination table. Initially, the neck is examined to assess for areas of swelling, redness, or tenderness, as may be seen in cervical adenitis. The neck is then flexed to evaluate suppleness; resistance to flexion is indicative of meningeal irritation. The Kernig and Brudzinski signs may be sought at this time. In children younger than 18 mo, meningeal signs may not always be present with meningitis; however, if they are present, the diagnostic implications are the same as for the child older than 18 mo. During examination of the abdomen, the diaper is removed. The abdomen is inspected for distention. Auscultation is performed to assess adequacy of bowel sounds, followed by palpation. The child often fusses as the abdomen is auscultated and palpated. Every attempt should be made to quiet the child; if this is not possible, increased fussing as the abdomen is palpated may indicate tenderness, especially if this finding is reproducible. In addition to focal tenderness, palpation may elicit involuntary guarding or rebound tenderness; these findings indicate peritoneal irritation, as is seen in appendicitis. The inguinal area and genitals are then sequentially examined. In the febrile child, inguinal adenitis or a strangulated hernia may be the cause of fever. The child is then placed in the prone position, and abnormalities of the back are sought. The spine and costovertebral angle areas are percussed to elicit any tenderness; such findings may be indicative of osteomyelitis or diskitis and pyelonephritis, respectively.

Examining the ears and throat completes the physical examination. These are usually the most bothersome parts of the examination for the child, and parents frequently can be helpful in minimizing head movement. During the oropharyngeal examination, it is important to document the presence of enanthemas; these may be seen in many infectious processes, such as hand-foot-and-mouth disease caused by coxsackievirus. This portion of the examination is also important in documenting inflammation or exudates on the tonsils, which may be viral or bacterial.

At times, repeating portions of the assessment is indicated. If the child cried continuously during the initial clinical evaluation, the examiner may not be certain if the crying was caused by the high fever, stranger anxiety, or pain, or is indicative of a serious illness. Continual crying also makes portions of the physical examination, such as auscultation of the chest, more difficult. Before a repeat assessment is performed, efforts to make the child as comfortable as possible are indicated. Such efforts include reducing the fever with antipyretics and offering the child a bottle. Because most children with fever do not have serious illnesses, repeated assessments are more likely to document normal findings. If, on the other hand, the child is persistently irritable, the possibility of serious illness increases.

RISK FACTORS

The sensitivity of the carefully performed clinical assessment, observation, history, and physical examination for the presence of serious illness is approximately 90%. Careful data gathering is necessary in the observation, history, and physical examination, because each component of the evaluation is as effective as the others in identifying serious illness. Other data, however, should be sought to improve this sensitivity level. In the child with an acute febrile illness, important supplemental data are age, body temperature, and the results of screening laboratory tests. Febrile children in the first 3 mo of life have yet to achieve immunologic maturity and therefore are more susceptible to severe infections and to infections by unusual organisms. Thus, the febrile infant is at greater risk for serious bacterial infection than the child beyond 3 mo of age (see Chapter 175). In febrile children, the higher the fever, the greater the risk of serious illness. The risk of bacteremia in infants increases as the degree of fever increases. The limit of physiologic thermoregulation is 41.1°C (106°F); fevers in this range and higher indicate bacteremia, but also possible central nervous system infection, pneumonia, or pathologic hyperthermia.

Screening laboratory tests may be helpful in identifying the febrile child at increased risk for selected serious illnesses. *S. pneumoniae* is currently the most common cause of occult bacteremia not associated with a focal soft tissue infection. A total white blood cell count of ≥15,000/mm^3 and/or an absolute neutrophil count of ≥10,000/mm^3, in addition to age 3–36 mo, higher grades of fever, and a more ill appearance, are indicators of increased risk for occult bacteremia caused by *S. pneumoniae.* The incidence of occult pneumococcal bacteremia in febrile children may be declining because of the introduction of conjugated pneumococcal vaccine. Urinalysis and urine culture must be considered when the source of fever is not apparent, especially in the highest-risk groups: females and uncircumcised males younger than 2 yr of age and all boys younger than 1 yr of age. The presence of leukocyte esterase, >5 white blood cells/high-power field on a spun urine specimen, or bacteria by Gram stain on an unspun urine specimen suggests urinary tract infection, but the sensitivity of these indicators is, on average, only 75–85% and urine culture is the definitive test. An elevated C-reactive protein value may also distinguish bacterial from viral infection.

MANAGEMENT

If the febrile child is older than 3 mo and appears well, if the history or physical examination does not suggest a serious illness, and if no age or temperature risk factors are present, the child may be followed expectantly (see also Chapters 109 and 175). If otitis media is present, it should be treated (see Chapter 639). This profile applies to most children with acute infectious illnesses. If, on the other hand, the child appears ill or the history or physical examination suggests a serious illness, definitive laboratory tests appropriate for those findings are indicated (e.g., chest radiograph for a child with grunting). The area of greatest controversy is whether laboratory studies are needed in a febrile child who appears well and has no abnormalities on history and physical examination, but who is younger than 3 mo of age or whose temperature is high. Many would agree that a sepsis work-up is indicated in the febrile child younger than 1 mo and possibly younger than age 3 mo (see Chapters 109 and 175). Obtaining blood cultures in children older than 3 mo with higher grades of fever has gained increased acceptance.

If the physician feels comfortable in following as an outpatient the child in whom no specific diagnosis has been established, a follow-up examination often yields a diagnosis. During the initial visit, or from one visit to the next during the acute illness, the change in symptoms or in the findings on physical examination over time may provide important diagnostic clues. For the child in whom a diagnosis has already been established and who does not require hospitalization, follow-up by telephone or an office visit should be used to monitor the course of the illness and to further educate and support the parents.

Baker MD, McCarthy PL: Fever and occult bacteremia in infants and young children. In Jenson HB, Baltimore RS (editors): *Pediatric Infectious Diseases: Principles and Practice.* Philadelphia, WB Saunders, 2002.

Black S, Shinefield H, Baxter R, et al: Post licensure surveillance for pneumococcal invasive disease after use of heptavalent pneumococcal conjugate vaccine in Northern California Kaiser Permanente. *Pediatr Infect Dis J* 2004;23:485–489.

McCarthy P, Walls T, Cicchetti D, et al: Prediction of resource use during acute pediatric illnesses. *Arch Pediatr Adolesc Med* 2003;157:990–996.

Pantell RH, Newman TB, Bernzweig J, et al: Management and outcome of care of fever in early infancy. *JAMA* 2004;291:1203–1212.

Stoll ML, Rubin LG: Incidence of occult bacteremia among highly febrile young children in the era of the pneumococcal conjugate vaccine. *Arch Pediatr Adolesc Med* 2004;158:671–675.

Whitney CG, Farley MM, Hadler J, et al: Decline in invasive pneumococcal disease after the introduction of protein-polysaccharide conjugate vaccine. *N Engl J Med* 2003;348:1736–1746.

Chapter 61 ■ Injury Control

Frederick P. Rivara and David Grossman

Injuries are the most common cause of death during childhood and adolescence beyond the 1st few mo of life and represent 1 of the most important causes of preventable pediatric morbidity and mortality. The identification of risk factors for injuries has led to the development of successful programs for prevention and control. Strategies for injury prevention and control should be taught by the pediatrician in the office, emergency department, hospital, or community setting.

INJURY CONTROL

The term **accident prevention** has been replaced by **injury control.** The word **accident** implies an event occurring by chance, without pattern or predictability. In fact, most injuries occur under fairly predictable circumstances to high-risk children and families. *Accident* connotes a random event that cannot be prevented. The use of the term **injury** promotes an awareness of a medical condition with defined risk and protective factors that can be used to define prevention strategies.

The reduction of morbidity and mortality from injuries can be accomplished not only through primary prevention (averting the event or injury in the first place), but also through secondary and tertiary prevention. The latter 2 approaches include appropriate emergency medical services for injured children; regionalized trauma care for the child with multiple injuries, severe burns, or head injury; and specialized pediatric rehabilitation services that attempt to return children to their previous level of functioning. This broadened scope of prevention is more properly described by the term *injury control.*

This expanded definition also encompasses intentional injuries (assaults, self-inflicted injuries). These injuries are important in adolescents and young adults, and in some populations, they rank 1st or 2nd as causes of death in these age groups. Many of the same principles of injury control can be applied to these problems; limiting access to firearms may reduce both unintentional shootings and suicides.

SCOPE OF THE PROBLEM

MORTALITY. Injuries cause 44% of deaths among 1–4 yr old children and 3 times more deaths than the next leading cause, congenital anomalies. For the rest of childhood and adolescence up to the age of 19 yr, 65% of deaths are due to injuries, more than all other causes combined. In 2002, injuries caused 17,589 deaths among individuals 19 yr old and younger in the United States (Table 61-1), resulting in more years of potential life lost than any other cause. An international perspective is noted in Figure 61-1.

Motor vehicle injuries lead the list of injury deaths at all ages during childhood and adolescence, even in children younger than 1 yr of age. In children and adults, motor vehicle **occupant** injuries account for the majority of these deaths. During adolescence, occupant injuries are the leading cause of injury death, accounting for >50% of unintentional trauma mortality in this age group.

Drowning ranks 2nd overall as a cause of unintentional trauma deaths, with peaks in the preschool and later teenage years (see Chapter 73). In some areas of the United States, drowning is the leading cause of death from trauma for preschool-aged children. The causes of drowning deaths vary with age and geographic area. In young children, bathtub and swimming pool drowning predominate, whereas in older children and adolescents, drowning occurs predominantly in natural bodies of water while the victim is swimming or boating.

Fire and burn deaths account for nearly 5% of all unintentional trauma deaths and 11% in those younger than 5 yr of age (see Chapter 74). Most of these are due to house fires; deaths are caused by smoke inhalation and asphyxiation rather than severe burns. Children and the elderly are at greatest risk for these deaths because of difficulty in escaping from burning buildings.

Suffocation accounts for approximately 50% of all unintentional deaths in children younger than 1 yr of age. The majority

TABLE 61-1. Injury Deaths in the United States, 2002*

CAUSE OF DEATH	YOUNGER THAN 1 YR	1–4 YR	5–9 YR	10–14 YR	15–19 YR	0–19 YR
ALL CAUSES	**28,034**	**4,858**	**3,018**	**4,132**	**13,812**	**53,854**
ALL INJURIES	**1,350**	**2,121**	**1,346**	**2,063**	**10,709**	**17,589**
All unintentional	946	1,641	1,176	1,542	7,137	12,442
Motor vehicle occupant	71	235	281	416	3,125	4,128
Pedestrian	6	158	149	147	292	752
Other motor vehicle	46	217	234	387	2,217	3,101
Drowning	63	454	159	162	320	1,158
Fire and burn	40	226	153	101	86	606
Poisoning	26	31	15	28	486	586
Bicycle	0	4	37	89	53	183
Firearm	1	11	14	34	107	167
Fall	16	37	18	24	83	178
Suffocation	636	139	40	70	68	953
Other unintentional	41	129	76	84	300	630
All intentional	303	423	144	479	3,429	4,778
Suicide	0	0	4	260	1,513	1,777
Firearm suicide	0	0	0	86	742	828
Homicide	303	423	140	216	1,892	2,974
Firearm homicide	9	49	55	150	1,567	1,830
Undetermined intent	101	57	26	42	143	369

*Injury data from Centers for Disease Control and Prevention. Web-based Injury Statistics Query and Reporting System (WISQARS) [Online]. (2004). National Center for Injury Prevention and Control, Centers for Disease Control and Prevention (producer). Available from: URL: www.cdc.gov/ncipc/wisqars. Accessed April 27, 2005.

of these deaths result from choking on food items, such as hot dogs, candy, grapes, and nuts. Nonfood items that can cause choking include undersized infant pacifiers, small balls, and latex balloons.

Homicide is the 3rd leading cause of injury death in children 1–4 yr of age and the 2nd leading cause of injury death in adolescents (15–19 yr old). Homicide in the pediatric age group falls into 2 patterns: infantile and adolescent. Infantile homicide involves children younger than the age of 5 yr and represents child abuse (see Chapter 36). The perpetrator is usually a caretaker; death is generally the result of blunt trauma to the head and/or abdomen. The adolescent pattern of homicide involves peers and acquaintances and is due to firearms in >80% of cases. The majority of these deaths involve handguns. Children between these 2 age groups experience homicides of both types.

Suicide is rare in children younger than age 10 yr; only 1% of all suicides occur in children younger than age 15 yr. The suicide rate increases markedly after the age of 10 yr, with the result that suicide is now the 3rd leading cause of death for 15–19 yr olds. Native American teenagers are at the highest risk, followed by white males; black females have the lowest rate of suicide in this age group. Approximately ½ of teenage suicides involve firearms (see Chapter 26).

NONFATAL INJURIES. Mortality statistics reflect only a small portion of the effects of childhood injuries. Approximately 20–25% of children and adolescents receive medical care for an injury each year in hospital emergency departments, and at least an equal number are treated in physicians' offices. Of these, 2.5% require inpatient care and 55% have at least short-term temporary disability as a result of their injuries.

The distribution of these nonfatal injuries is very different from that of fatal trauma (Fig. 61-2). Falls are the leading cause of both emergency department visits and hospitalizations. Bicycle-related trauma is the most common type of sports and recreational injury, accounting for approximately 300,000 emergency department visits annually. Nonfatal injuries, such as anoxic encephalopathy from near-drowning, scarring and disfigurement from burns, and persistent neurologic deficits from head injury, may be associated with severe morbidity, leading to substantial changes in the quality of life for victims and their families.

PRINCIPLES OF INJURY CONTROL

Injury prevention once centered on attempts to pinpoint the innate characteristics of a child that result in greater frequency of injury. Most now discount the theory of the *accident-prone child*. Although longitudinal studies have demonstrated an association between hyperactivity and impulsivity and increased rates of injury, the sensitivity and specificity of these traits for injury are extremely low. The concept of *accident proneness* is, in fact, counterproductive in that it shifts attention away from potentially more modifiable factors, such as product design or the environment. It is more appropriate to examine the physical and social environment of children with frequent rates of injury than to try to identify particular personality traits or temperaments, which are difficult to modify. Children at high risk for injury are likely to be relatively poorly supervised, to have disorganized or stressed families, and to live in hazardous environments.

Efforts to control injuries include education or persuasion, changes in product design, and modification of the social and physical environment. Efforts to persuade individuals, particularly parents, to change their behaviors have constituted the greater part of injury control efforts. Speaking with parents specifically about using child car seat restraints and bicycle helmets, installing smoke detectors, and checking the tap water temperature is likely to be more successful than offering well-meaning, but too-general advice about supervising the child closely, being careful, and "childproofing" the home. This information should be geared to the developmental stage of the child and presented in moderate doses in the form of anticipatory guidance at well-child visits. Important topics to discuss at each developmental stage are shown in Table 61-2.

The most successful injury prevention strategies generally are those involving changes in product design, as shown in Table 61-3. These passive interventions protect all individuals in the population, regardless of cooperation or level of skill, and are likely to be more successful than active measures that require repeated behavior change by the parent or child. However, for some types of injuries, effective passive interventions are not available or feasible; we must rely heavily on attempts to change the behavior of individuals. Turning down the water heater temperature, installing smoke detectors, and using child-resistant caps on med-

Rank	0–4 yr	5–14 yr	15–29 yr
1	Lower respiratory infections 2,134,248	Childhood cluster diseases 200,139	HIV/AIDS 855,406
2	Diarrheal diseases 1,315,412	Road traffic injuries 118,212	Road traffic injuries 354,692
3	Childhood cluster diseases 1,108,666	Drowning 113,614	Tuberculosis 238,021
4	Low birthweight 1,025,488	Lower respiratory infections 112,739	Self-inflicted injuries 216,661
5	Malaria 905,838	Diarrheal diseases 88,430	Interpersonal violence 188,451
6	Birth asphyxia and birth trauma 787,179	Malaria 76,257	War injuries 95,015
7	HIV/AIDS 419,480	HIV/AIDS 46,022	Drowning 78,639
8	Congenital heart anomalies 281,751	War injuries 43,761	Lower respiratory infections 65,153
9	Protein-energy malnutrition 172,530	Tuberculosis 36,362	Poisonings 61,865
10	STDs excluding HIV 142,176	Tropical cluster diseases 31,845	Fires 61,341
11	Drowning 115,922	Fires 30,599	Maternal hemorrhage 59,456
12	Anencephaly 85,247	Interpersonal violence 24,688	Rheumatic heart disease 48,062
13	Meningitis 76,870	Leukemia 23,808	Leukemia 44,740
14	Road traffic injuries 75,710	Poisonings 23,293	Nephritis and nephrosis 41,300
15	Tuberculosis 67,372	Self-inflicted injuries 21,967	Diarrheal diseases 40,392

Figure 61-1. Leading causes of death (rank 1–15) worldwide by age. STD, sexually transmitted disease. (Modified from Krug EG: Injury surveillance is key to preventing injuries. *Lancet* 2004;364:1563–1566.)

icines and household products are examples of effective product modifications. Many interventions require both active and passive measures. Smoke detectors provide passive protection when fully functional, but behavior change is required to ensure annual battery changes and proper testing.

Modification of the environment often requires greater changes than individual product modification, but may be very effective in reducing injuries. Safe roadway design, decreased traffic volume and speed limits in neighborhoods, and elimination of guns from households are examples of such interventions. Included in this concept are changes in the social environment through legislation, such as laws mandating child seat restraint and seatbelt use, bicycle helmet use, and graduated motor vehicle licensing laws.

Prevention campaigns combining 2 or more of these approaches have been particularly effective in reducing injuries. The classic example is the combination of legislation and education to increase child seat restraint and seatbelt use; other examples are programs to promote bike helmet use among school-aged children and improvements in occupant protection in motor vehicles.

RISK FACTORS FOR CHILDHOOD INJURIES

Major factors associated with an increased risk of injuries to children include age, sex, race and ethnicity, socioeconomic status, rural-urban location, and the environment.

AGE. Toddlers are at greatest risk for burns, drowning, and falls. As these children acquire mobility and exploratory behavior, poisonings become another risk. Young school-aged children are at greatest risk for pedestrian injuries, bicycle-related injuries (the most serious of which usually involve motor vehicles), motor vehicle occupant injuries, burns, and drowning. During the teenage years, there is a markedly increased risk from motor vehicle occupant trauma, a continued risk from drowning and burns, and the new risk of intentional trauma. Work-related injuries associated with child labor, especially for 14–16 yr olds, are an additional risk.

Injuries occurring at a particular age represent a window of vulnerability during which a child or an adolescent encounters a new task or hazard that he or she may not have the developmental skills to handle successfully. Toddlers do not have the judgment to know that medications can be poisonous or that some houseplants are not to be eaten; they do not understand the hazard presented by a swimming pool or an open 2nd-story window. For young children, parents may inadvertently set up this mismatch between the skills of the child and the demands of the task. A walker converts an infant into a mobile toddler and greatly increases contact with hazards. Many parents expect young school-aged children to walk home from school, the playground, or the local candy store, tasks for which most children are not developmentally ready. Likewise, the lack of skills and experience to handle many tasks during the teenage years contributes to an increased risk of injuries, particularly motor vehicle injuries. The high rate of motor vehicle crashes among 15–17 yr old teens is caused in part by inexperience, but also appears to reflect their level of development and maturity. Alcohol and other drugs often add to these limitations.

Age also influences the severity of injury as well as the risk of long-term disability. Young school-aged children have an incompletely developed pelvis. In a motor vehicle crash, the seatbelt does not anchor onto the pelvis, but rides up onto the abdomen, resulting in the risk of serious abdominal injury. Age also interacts with vehicle characteristics in that most children ride in the rear seat, which in the past was equipped only with lap belts and not with lap-shoulder harnesses. Proper restraint for 4–8 yr old children requires the use of booster seats. Children younger than the age of 2 yr have much poorer outcomes from traumatic brain injuries than do older children and adolescents.

SEX. Beginning at 1–2 yr of age and continuing until the 7th decade of life, males have higher rates of injury than females. During childhood, this does not appear to be due to developmental differences between the sexes, differences in coordination, or differences in muscle strength. Variation in exposure to risk may account for the male predominance in some types of injuries.

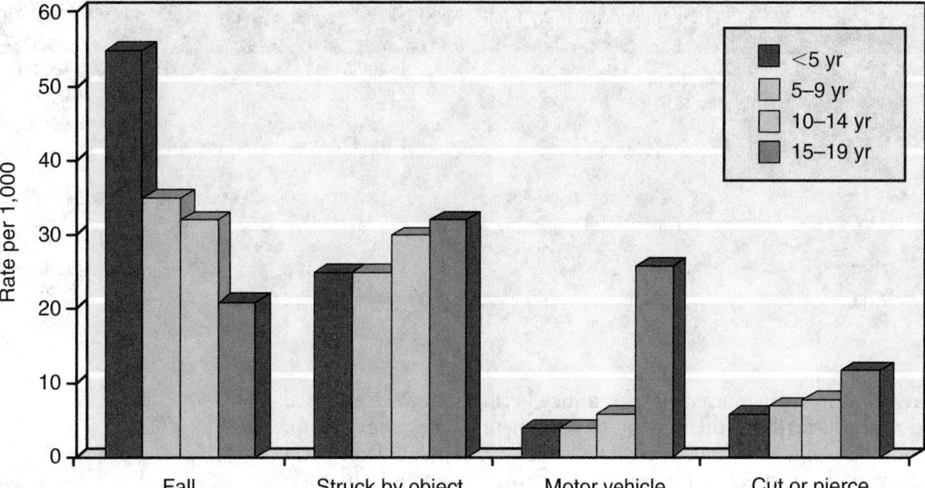

Figure 61-2. Emergency department visit rates for leading 1st-listed causes of injury by age: United States, 1993–1994. (Data from Centers for Disease Control and Prevention, National Center for Health Statistics, and National Hospital Ambulatory Medical Case Survey.)

Although boys in all age groups have higher rates of bicycle-related injuries, adjusting for exposure reduces this excess rate. Boys may have higher rates of injuries because they use bicycles more frequently or for more hours. Sex differences in rates of pedestrian injuries do not appear to be caused by differences in the amount of walking, but rather reflect differences in behavior between young girls and boys. Greater risk-taking behavior, combined with greater frequency of alcohol use, may lead to the disproportionately high rate of motor vehicle crashes among teenage males.

RACE AND ETHNICITY. African-Americans have higher rates of injuries than whites, whereas Asians have lower rates; rates for Hispanics are intermediate between those for African-Americans and those for whites. Native Americans have the highest death rate from unintentional injuries. These discrepancies are even more pronounced for some injuries. The homicide rate for African-Americans age 15–19 yr was 31.4/100,000 in 2002, compared with 5.3/100,000 for whites. The suicide rate for Native American youth is twice the rate for whites and nearly 4-fold greater than that for Asians. The rate of fire and burn deaths in African-American preschool children is more than 3 times higher than that for whites: 3.4/100,000 compared with 1.0/100,000, respectively.

These disparities appear to be primarily related to poverty, the educational status of parents, and the presence of hazardous environments, rather than to race. Homicide rates among African-Americans are nearly equivalent to those among whites, when adjusted for socioeconomic status. It is important to understand racial disparities in injury rates, but inappropriate to ascribe the etiology of these differences to race or ethnicity.

SOCIOECONOMIC STATUS. Poverty is one of the most important risk factors for childhood injury. Mortality from fires, motor vehicle crashes, and drowning is 2–4-fold higher in poor children. Death rates among both African-Americans and whites have an inverse relationship to income level: the higher the income level, the lower the death rate. Native Americans have especially high rates. Other factors are single-parent families, teenage mothers, multiple care providers, family stress, and multiple siblings; these are primarily a function of poverty rather than independent risk factors.

RURAL-URBAN LOCATION. Injury rates are generally higher in rural than in urban areas. Homicide rates are higher in urban areas, as is violent crime in general. Case fatality from injury is generally twice as high in rural areas than in urban areas, reflecting both the increased severity of some injuries (such as motor vehicle crashes occurring at higher speeds) and poorer access to emergency medical services and definitive trauma care in rural areas. Some injuries are unique to rural areas, such as agricultural injuries to children and adolescents.

ENVIRONMENT. Poverty increases the risk of injury to children, at least in part through its effect on the environment. Children who

TABLE 61-2. Injury Prevention Topics for Anticipatory Guidance by the Pediatrician

NEWBORN
Car seats
Tap water temperature
Smoke detectors

INFANT
Car seats
Tap water temperature
Bath safety

TODDLER AND PRESCHOOLER
Car seats
Pedestrian skills training
Water safety
Childproof caps on medicines and household poisons

PRIMARY SCHOOL CHILD
Pedestrian skills training
Water skills training
Seatbelts
Bicycle helmets
Removal of firearms from home

MIDDLE SCHOOL CHILD
Seatbelts
Removal of firearms from home
Pedestrian skills training

HIGH SCHOOL AND OLDER ADOLESCENT
Seatbelts
Alcohol and drug use, especially while driving, boating, and swimming
Occupational injuries
Removal of firearms from home

TABLE 61-3. Injury Control Interventions

PRODUCT MODIFICATION	ENVIRONMENTAL MODIFICATION	EDUCATION
Child-resistant caps	Cabinet locks	Anticipatory guidance
Airbags	Roadway design	Public service announcements
Fire-safe cigarettes	Smoke detectors	School safety programs

TABLE 61-4. Recommended Child Restraint Methods

	INFANTS	TODDLERS	YOUNG CHILDREN
Recommended age/weight requirements	Birth to 1 yr; up to 20–22 lb	Older than 1 yr and 20–40 lb	>40 lb and under 4′ 9″; generally between 4 and 8 years of age, 40–80 lb
Type of seat	Infant only or rear-facing convertible	Convertible/forward-facing harness seat	Belt positioning booster seat
Seat position	Rear-facing only	Can be rear-facing until 30 lb if seat allows; generally forward-facing	Forward-facing
Notes	Children should use rear-facing seat until 1 yr and at least 20 lb	Harness straps should be at or above shoulder level	Belt positioning booster seats must be used with both lap and shoulder belts
	Harness straps should be at or below shoulder level	Most seats require top slot for forward-facing use	Make sure the lap belt fits low and tightly across the lap/upper thigh area and the shoulder belt fits snugly, crossing the chest and shoulder to avoid abdominal injuries

From Ebel BE, Grossman DC: Crash proof kids? An overview of current motor vehicle child occupant safety Strategies. *Curr Probl Pediatr Adolesc Health Care* 2003;33:33–64. Adapted from NHTSA Proper Child Safety Seat Chart (http://www.nhtsa.gov/CPS/UsingItRight2002/generalinfo.htm).

are poor are at increased risk for injury because they are exposed to more hazards in their living environments. They may live in poor housing, which is more likely to be dilapidated and less likely to be protected by smoke detectors. The roads in their neighborhoods are more likely to be major thoroughfares. Their neighborhoods are more likely to experience higher levels of violence, and they are more likely to be victims of assault than are children and adolescents living in the suburbs. The focus on the environment is also important because it directs attention away from relatively immutable factors, such as family dynamics, poverty, and race, and directs efforts toward factors that can be changed through interventions.

MECHANISMS OF INJURY

MOTOR VEHICLE INJURIES. Motor vehicle injuries are the leading cause of serious and fatal injuries for individuals of all ages. Among adolescents, motor vehicle crashes alone account for 38% of all deaths, including deaths from natural causes. Large and sustained reductions in motor vehicle crash injuries can be accomplished by identifiable interventions.

Occupants. Injuries to passenger vehicle occupants are the predominant cause of motor vehicle deaths among children and adolescents, with the exception of the 5–9 yr old group, in whom pedestrian injuries make up the largest proportion. The peak injury and death rate for both males and females in the pediatric age group occurs between 15 and 19 yr of age (see Table 61-1). Proper restraint use in vehicles is the single most effective method for preventing serious or fatal injury. The recommended restraints at different ages are shown in Table 61-4. Examples of car safety seats are noted in Figure 61-3.

Much attention has been given to child occupants younger than 4 yr of age. Use of child restraint devices can be expected to reduce fatalities by 71% and the risk of serious injuries by 67% in this age group. All 50 states and the District of Columbia have laws mandating their use. Handouts given to parents by physicians emphasizing the positive benefits of child seat restraints have been successful in improving parent acceptance. Pediatricians should point out to parents that toddlers who normally ride restrained behave better during car trips than children who ride unrestrained.

Excellent films are available that discuss the advantages of child seat restraints; these can be shown to parents in waiting rooms or to mothers on postpartum hospital floors. Many hospitals and communities have adopted loan programs, renting restraints at low cost. This is especially important for low-income families, who have the lowest rate of restraint use. A list of acceptable devices is available from the American Academy of Pediatrics. Children weighing <20 lb may use an infant seat or be placed in a convertible infant-toddler child restraint device. Infants younger than 1 yr or weighing <20 lb should be placed in the rear seat facing backward; older toddlers and children can be placed in the rear seat in a forward-facing child harness seat. Emphasis must

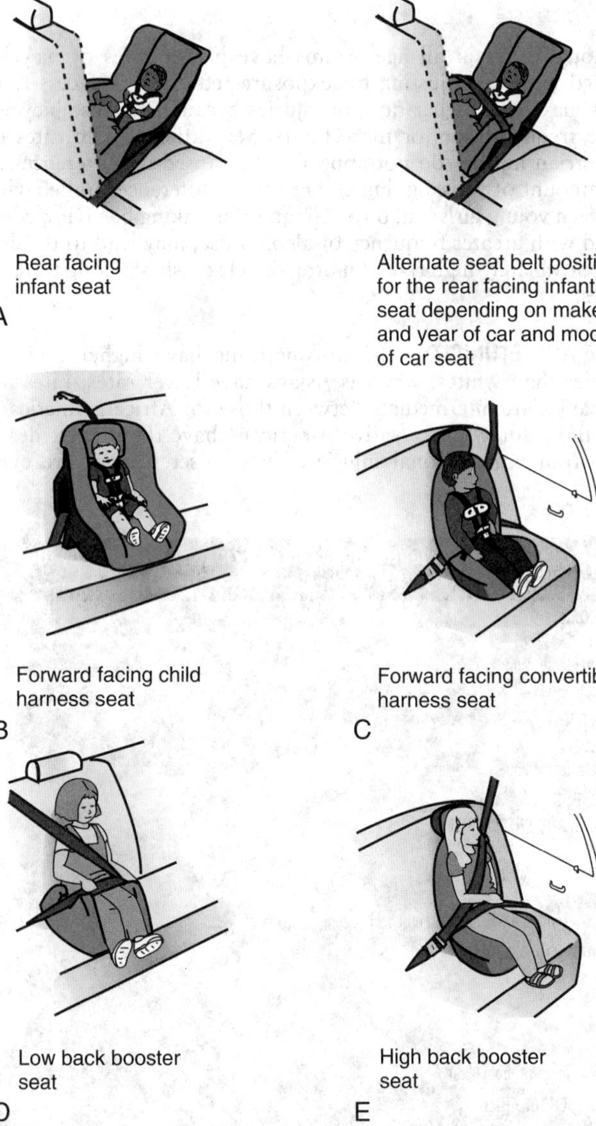

Figure 61-3. Car safety seats. *A*, Rear-facing infant seat; *B*, forward-facing child harness seat; *C*, forward-facing convertible harness seat; *D*, low-back booster seat; *E*, high-back booster seat. (From Ebel BE, Grossman DC: Crash proof kids? An overview of current motor vehicle child occupant safety strategies. *Curr Probl Pediatr Adolesc Health Care* 2003;33:33–64; Source: NHTSA; graphics courtesy of Transportation Safety Training Center, Virginia Commonwealth University [*http://www.nhtsa.dot.gov/people/injury/childps/safetycheck/typeseats/index.htm*].)

be placed on the correct use of these seats, including placing the seat in the right direction, routing the belt properly, and ensuring that the child is buckled into the seat correctly. Government regulations have made the fit between car seats and the car easier, quicker, and less prone to error. Children younger than age 13 yr should never sit in the front seat, especially if an airbag is present. Inflating airbags can be lethal to infants in rear-facing seats and to small children in the front passenger seat.

Older children are often not adequately restrained. Many children ride in the rear seat restrained with lap belts only. Unfortunately, the use of lap belts alone has been associated with a marked rise in seatbelt-related injuries, especially fractures of the lumbar spine and hollow-viscus injuries of the abdomen. These flexion-distraction injuries of the spine are usually accompanied by injuries to the abdominal organs; the presence of cutaneous seatbelt contusions in restrained children should alert the clinician to possible abdominal or spine injury. Booster seats have been shown to decrease the risk of injury by 59%, and should be used by children who are between 40 lb (≈4 yr of age) and 80 lb, are <8 yr of age, and are <4 ft, 9 in tall. Many states have extended their car seat laws to include children of booster seat age as well. Shoulder straps placed behind the child or under the arm do not provide adequate crash protection and may increase the risk of serious injury.

Transportation of premature infants presents special problems. The possibility of oxygen desaturation, sometimes associated with bradycardia, among premature infants while in child seat restraints has led the American Academy of Pediatrics to recommend monitoring of infants born at <37 wk of gestational age in the seat before discharge and the use of oxygen or alternative restraints for infants who experience desaturation or bradycardia, such as seats that can be reclined and used as a car bed. Monitoring in the neonatal intensive care unit should be done for 60–90 min. Car seats should only be used for travel and not as a general use infant seat around the home.

Children riding in the back of pickup trucks are at special risk for injury because of the possibility of ejection from the truck and resultant serious head injury. Children traveling in the back of covered pickup trucks are at risk for carbon monoxide poisoning from faulty exhaust systems.

The rear seat is clearly much safer than the front seat for both children and adults. One study of children younger than the age of 15 yr found that the risk of injury in a crash was 70% lower for children in the rear seat compared with those sitting in the front seat. Frontal airbags appear to offer little protection to children in crashes and also present a risk of serious or fatal injury from the airbag itself. Side airbags also pose a risk for children who are in the front seat and are leaning against the door at the time of a crash. The safest place for children is in the rear seat, properly restrained for their age and size. Educational and legislative interventions to increase the number of children traveling in the rear seat have been successful.

Teenage Drivers. Drivers aged 15–17 yr have > twice the rate of collisions compared with motorists 18 yr of age and older. Formal driver education courses appear to be ineffective as a primary means of decreasing the number of collisions, and in fact can be counterproductive by allowing younger teens to drive. The risk of serious injury and mortality is directly related to the speed at the time of the crash and inversely related to the size of the vehicle. Small, fast cars greatly increase the risk of a fatal outcome in the event of a crash.

The number of passengers traveling with teen drivers influences the risk of a crash. The risk of death for 17 yr old drivers is 50% greater driving with 1 passenger compared with driving alone; this risk is 2.6-fold higher with 2 passengers and 3-fold higher with 3 or more passengers. The risk is also increased if the driver is male and the passengers are younger than age 30 yr.

Teens driving at night are overrepresented in crashes and fatal crashes, with nighttime crashes accounting for >33% of teen motor vehicle fatalities. Almost 50% of fatal crashes involving drivers younger than age 18 yr occur in the 4 hr before or after midnight. Teens are 5–10-fold more likely to be in a fatal crash while driving at night compared with driving during the day. The difficulty of driving at night combined with the inexperience of teen drivers appears to be a deadly combination.

Graduated licensing laws consist of a series of steps over a designated period before a teen can get full, unrestricted driving privileges. These laws usually place initial restrictions on the number of passengers allowed in the vehicle and limit driving during late-night hours. There is a median decrease in the number of accidents of 31% among 16 yr old drivers in the 1st yr using a graduated licensing system. Elements of graduated licensing programs have been adopted by many states.

Alcohol use is a major cause of motor vehicle trauma among adolescents. The combination of inexperience in driving and inexperience with alcohol is particularly dangerous. Approximately 20% of all deaths from motor vehicle crashes in this age group are the result of alcohol intoxication, with impairment of driving seen at blood alcohol concentrations as low as 0.05 g/dL. Approximately 30% of adolescents report riding with a driver who had been drinking. All states have adopted a zero tolerance policy, which defines any measurable alcohol content as legal intoxication, to adolescent drinking while driving. All adolescent motor vehicle injury victims should have their blood alcohol concentration measured in the emergency department and be screened for chronic alcohol use with a standard test (the CAGE or the Short Michigan Alcohol Screening Test) to identify those with alcohol abuse problems (see Chapter 113.1). Individuals who have evidence of alcohol abuse should not leave the emergency department or hospital without plans for appropriate alcohol abuse treatment. Interventions for problem drinking can be effective in decreasing the risk of subsequent motor vehicle crashes. Even brief interventions in the emergency department using motivational interviewing can be successful in decreasing adolescent problem drinking.

BICYCLE INJURIES. Each year in the United States, approximately 200 children and adolescents die of injuries incurred while riding bicycles, and another 300,000 are treated in emergency departments, making bicycle-related injuries 1 of the most common reasons that children with trauma visit emergency departments. The majority of severe and fatal bicycle injuries involve head trauma. A logical step in the prevention of these head injuries is the use of helmets. Helmets are very effective, reducing the risk of head injury by 85% and the risk of brain injury by 88%. Helmets also reduce injuries to the mid and upper face by as much as 65%. Pediatricians can be effective advocates for the use of bicycle helmets and should incorporate this advice into their anticipatory guidance schedules for parents and children. Appropriate helmets are those with a firm polystyrene liner that fit properly on the child's head. Parents should avoid buying a larger helmet to give the child "growing room."

Promotion of helmet use can and should be extended beyond the pediatrician's office. Community education programs spearheaded by coalitions of physicians, educators, bicycle clubs, and community service organizations have been successful in promoting the use of bicycle helmets to children across the socioeconomic spectrum, resulting in helmet use rates of 60% or more with a concomitant reduction in the number of head injuries. Passage of bicycle helmet laws also leads to increased helmet use.

Consideration should also be given to other types of preventive activities, although the evidence supporting their effectiveness is limited. Bicycle paths are a logical method for separating bicycles and motor vehicles.

PEDESTRIAN INJURIES. Pedestrian injuries are 1 of the most common causes of traumatic death for 5–9 yr old children in the United States and in most industrialized countries. Although case fatality rates are <5%, serious nonfatal injuries constitute a much larger problem, resulting in 60,000 emergency department visits annually. Pedestrian injuries are the most important cause of traumatic coma in children and a frequent cause of serious lower extremity fractures, particularly in school-aged children.

Most injuries occur during the day, with a peak in the after-school period. Improved lighting or retroreflective clothing would, therefore, be expected to prevent few injuries. Surprisingly, approximately 30% of pedestrian injuries occur while the individual is in a marked crosswalk, perhaps reflecting a false sense of security and decreased vigilance in these areas. The risk of pedestrian injury is greater in neighborhoods with high traffic volumes, speeds >approximately 25 mph, absence of play space adjacent to the home, household crowding, and low socioeconomic status.

One important risk factor for childhood pedestrian injuries is the developmental level of the child. Children younger than age 5 yr are at risk for being run over in the driveway. Few children younger than 9 or 10 yr of age have the developmental skills to successfully negotiate traffic 100% of the time. Young children have poor ability to judge the distance and speed of traffic and are easily distracted by playmates or other factors in the environment. Many parents are not aware of this potential mismatch between the abilities of the young school-aged child and the skills needed to cross streets safely.

Prevention of pedestrian injuries is difficult, but should consist of a multifaceted approach. Education of the child in pedestrian safety should be initiated at an early age by the parents and continue into the school-age years. Younger children should be taught never to cross streets when alone; older children should be taught (and practice how) to negotiate quiet streets with little traffic. Major streets should not be crossed alone until the child is 10 yr of age or older.

Legislation and police enforcement are important components of any campaign to reduce pedestrian injuries. Right-turn-on-red laws increase the hazard to pedestrians. In many cities, few drivers stop for pedestrians in crosswalks, a special hazard for young children. Engineering changes in roadway design are extremely important as passive prevention measures. Most important are measures to slow the speed of traffic and to route traffic away from schools and residential areas; these efforts are endorsed by parents and can decrease the risk of injuries and death by 10–35%. Other modifications include networks of 1-way streets, proper placement of transit or school bus stops, sidewalks in urban and suburban areas, edge stripping in rural areas to delineate the edge of the road, and curb parking regulations. Comprehensive traffic "calming" schemes using these strategies have been very successful in reducing child pedestrian injuries in Sweden, the Netherlands, Germany, and increasingly, the United States.

FIRE- AND BURN-RELATED INJURIES. See Chapter 74. Fire- and burn-related injuries are the 5th most common cause of unintentional injury death in the United States, with approximately 3,200 fire and burn deaths occurring each year. For both injuries and deaths, the 1st decade of life is the period of highest risk. The likelihood of burn injury is strongly related to low socioeconomic status, with the highest rates among the poor, the less educated, and those living in mobile homes. Burns are much more frequent among males than among females. Among children 10–14 yr of age with burns involving flammable substances, males are burned 8 times more frequently than females.

One of the 1st effective interventions involved using nonflammable fabrics. Flame burns resulting from ignition of clothing were a common, serious burn injury, especially in small children. At least 30% of those injuries involved infant sleepwear. Such burns averaged 30% of the body surface, requiring hospitalization for an average of 70 days. In 1967, the Federal Flammable Fabrics Act was passed, requiring children's sleepwear to be flame-retardant. As a result of this and similar state legislation, clothing ignition burns in small children now account for only a small fraction of burns in children. Parents should not circumvent these protective regulations by using cotton T-shirts for infant and child sleepwear.

Another hazard modification resulting in substantial reduction of injury involves scald burns due to tap water. Scalds account for 40% of burn injuries in children requiring hospitalization, and a substantial proportion of these scald burns involve tap water. Scalds from hot liquids and foods are the most common reason for a burn admission to the hospital in children younger than age 5 yr. Avoiding the use of electric kettles or frying pans with long cords, avoiding the use of baby walkers, avoiding drinking hot tea or coffee while holding an infant, and keeping children away from pots cooking on the stove will help to prevent many of these injuries. Unlike those with flame burns, children with scalds generally do not die; many children have long hospitalizations, multiple surgical procedures, and severe disfigurement. The risk of full-thickness burns increases geometrically at water temperatures >125°F. At 150°F, a full-thickness burn will be produced in adult skin in 2 sec. A simple and effective preventive maneuver is to lower the water heater temperature to 125°F (51.6°C). At this setting, dishwashers and washing machines operate effectively, but the risk of serious scald injury is greatly reduced. New water heaters are usually preset at this lower temperature.

Fireworks are a seasonal injury, and >40% of those injured by fireworks are children younger than 15 yr of age. Community restrictions on certain types of fireworks and adult supervision of the use of all fireworks have been effective in decreasing burns, amputations, and ocular injuries caused by these devices.

More than 80% of all fire deaths in the United States occur in private dwellings. Of these deaths, 60% are caused by smoke asphyxiation and not by flame burns. Smoke detectors are an inexpensive but effective method of preventing the majority of these deaths; photoelectric detectors have a lower rate of false alarms than ionization detectors and may be less likely to be intentionally disabled by families. Physicians can alter parental behavior and increase smoke detector use by offering information on smoke detectors in their offices.

Cigarettes are estimated to cause 45% of all fires and 22–56% of deaths from house fires. The combination of smoking and alcohol use appears to be particularly lethal. Most cigarettes made in the United States contain additives in both the paper and the tobacco that allow them to burn for as long as 28 min, even if left unattended. If fire-safe or self-extinguishing cigarettes replaced the current types, nearly 2,000 deaths and >6,000 burns would be prevented annually.

Some burns result from fire setting by children or adolescents. In young children, this usually represents exploratory play. However, such behavior in older children and adolescents may signify a serious conduct disorder and warrants careful psychiatric and family evaluation. More than 50% of adolescent fire setters will be involved in repeat incidents.

POISONING. See Chapter 58. Deaths caused by unintentional poisoning among children have decreased dramatically over the past 2 decades, particularly among children younger than 5 yr of age. In 1970, 226 poisoning deaths of children younger than age 5 yr occurred, compared with only 57 in 2002. Poisoning prevention demonstrates the effectiveness of passive strategies, including the use of child-resistant packaging and limited doses per container. The Poison Packaging Prevention Act currently includes 28 categories of household products and drugs. This law has been remarkably effective in reducing poisoning deaths and hospitalizations. Nevertheless, ingestions by children younger than 6 yr account for 50% of all calls to poison control centers in the United States. The most common substances ingested by young children are cosmetics, cleaning agents, analgesics, topical medications, and cough and cold preparations. In contrast, tricyclic antidepressants, antipsychotics, quinine derivatives, calcium channel blockers, opioids, and oral hypoglycemics were responsible for 40% of fatal ingestions to toddlers in 1990–2000.

Difficulty using child-resistant containers by adults is an important cause of poisoning in young children today. A survey by the U.S. Centers for Disease Control and Prevention found that 18.5% of households in which poisoning occurred in children younger than 5 yr of age had replaced the child-resistant closure and 65% of the packaging used did not work properly. Nearly 20% of ingestions occur from drugs owned by grandparents, a group that has difficulty using traditional child-resistant containers. There is a need for better child-resistant closures that do not require manual dexterity or strength greater than the capabilities of older adults.

Other poisoning interventions, such as "Mr. Yuk" stickers, are far less effective. They do not deter young children from ingesting labeled medications and may, in fact, be attractive to children younger than 3 yr of age. The most important feature of the Mr. Yuk sticker is the telephone number of the local or regional poison control center. Poison control centers serve as the frontline for managing poisonous ingestions in the United States; efforts to educate parents about the role of poison control centers can increase their use and the cost-effective management of ingestions. Home use of ipecac is no longer recommended.

DROWNING. See Chapter 73. In 2002, 1,158 drownings, primarily associated with recreational activities, occurred among children and adolescents in the United States. Among young children, drowning ranks 2nd only to motor vehicle injury as a cause of traumatic death. It is estimated that an additional 4,453 near-drownings resulted in an emergency department visit in 2003. Diving headfirst into shallow water accounts for the most serious aquatic injuries because of spinal cord damage. Of the estimated 700 spinal cord injuries resulting from aquatic activities each year, the majority result in permanent paralysis.

The proportion of drowning deaths occurring in pools varies by region of the country. In Los Angeles, CA, ½ of all drownings take place in residential pools, a rate similar to that in other areas with large numbers of pools. Children younger than 5 yr of age do not understand the consequences of falling into deep water and usually do not call for help. A majority of child victims drown during lapses in adult supervision. Clearly, the most effective way to prevent childhood pool drowning is through circumferential fencing. To give the greatest protection, these barriers should restrict entry to the pool from the yard and residence, use self-closing and self-latching gates, be at least 5 ft high, and have no vertical openings more than 4 in wide. Ordinances to require appropriate fencing have been demonstrated to be effective. Some people have advocated "water-babies" and other swimming instruction for young children. The efficacy of such techniques is untested. The potential exists for both parent and child to become less vigilant around water, possibly with tragic consequences.

Among adolescents and young adults, alcohol and drug use has been found to be involved in nearly 50% of all drowning deaths. The risk of drowning while boating is increased 10–50-fold with alcohol intoxication, both because of the risk of falling overboard and the increased risk of drowning if drunk while submerged. The restriction of the sale and consumption of alcoholic beverages in boating, pool, harbor, marina, and beach areas may combat this dangerous combination of activities. More restrictive licensing of boat owners should also be considered.

Personal flotation devices (PFDs) are believed to be an important device to protect children from drowning. Although the exact protective effect of PFDs is unknown, a study by the U.S. Coast Guard showed that although only 7% of boats involved in mishaps lacked available PFDs, they accounted for 29% of boating fatalities. All children and adolescents should wear a PFD when boating in open water.

The risk of bathtub drowning is markedly increased in poorly supervised toddlers and in children with a seizure disorder, including older children and adolescents. Older children with seizure disorders should be instructed to shower instead of using a bathtub and younger children need careful, constant supervision while bathing.

FIREARM INJURIES. Injuries to children and adolescents involving firearms occur in 3 different situations: unintentional injury, suicide attempt, and assault. The injury induced may be fatal or may result in permanent sequelae.

Unintentional firearm injuries and deaths have continued to decrease and account for only a small fraction of all firearm injuries among children and adolescents. The majority of these deaths occur to teens during hunting or recreational activities. Suicide is the 3rd most common cause of trauma death in teenage males and the 4th in females. During the period from the 1950s to 1970, suicide rates for children and adolescents more than doubled; firearm suicide rates peaked in 1994 and decreased by >50% in 2002. It remains the most common means of suicide in males of all ages. The difference in the rate of suicide between males and females is related less to the number of attempts than to the method. Women die less often in suicide attempts, partly because they use less lethal means (mainly drugs) and perhaps have a lower degree of intent. The use of firearms in a suicidal act usually converts an attempt into a fatality.

Homicides are 2nd only to motor vehicle crashes among causes of death in teenagers older than the age of 15 yr. In 2002, 2,974 children and adolescents were homicide victims; nonwhite teenagers accounted for 52% of the total, making homicides the most common cause of death among nonwhite teenagers. In 2002, 83% of homicides among males involved firearms, 75% of which are handguns.

In the United States, there are an estimated 210–220 million firearms. During the past 2 decades, >6 million firearms were sold in the United States each year. Handguns account for approximately 20% of the firearms in use today, yet they are involved in 90% of criminal and other firearm misuse. Home ownership of guns increases the risk of adolescent suicide 3–10-fold and the risk of adolescent homicide up to 4-fold. In homes with guns, the risk to the occupants is far greater than the chance that the gun will be used against an intruder; for every death occurring in self-defense, there may be 1.3 unintentional deaths, 4.6 homicides, and 37 suicides.

Of all firearms, handguns pose the greatest risk to children and adolescents. Access to handguns by adolescents is surprisingly common and is not restricted to those involved in gang or criminal activity. Stricter approaches to reduce youth access to handguns, rather than all firearms, would appear to be the most appropriate focus of efforts to reduce shooting injuries in children and adolescents.

Locking and unloading guns as well as storing ammunition locked in a different location substantially reduces the risk of a suicide or unintentional firearm injury. Because up to ½ of homes have at least 1 firearm stored unsafely, 1 potential approach to reducing these injuries could focus on improving firearm storage practices. However, no data yet exist to support the effectiveness of clinic or community programs in decreasing the number of gunshot wounds in children.

There is insufficient evidence to conclude that office counseling of all types of patients about firearm ownership and storage leads to changed family behavior. Adolescents with mental health conditions and alcoholism are at particularly high risk for firearm injury. In the absence of conclusive evidence, physicians should continue to work with families to eliminate access to guns in these households.

FALLS. Falls are the leading cause of nonfatal injury in children up to age 15 yr and the 2nd leading cause of nonfatal injury in

15–19 yr olds. Altogether, there were 2,793,363 nonfatal falls that led to emergency department visits in 2003 alone; approximately 2.5% of these visits led to a hospitalization. Relatively little is known about the epidemiology of falls. One reason is that in the *International Classification of Diseases,* 9th edition, the codes for external cause of injury are relatively nonspecific and do not describe mechanisms with sufficient detail. There have been relatively few in-depth analytic studies of falls, except in particular circumstances, such as playground injuries. Strategies to prevent falls depend on the environmental circumstances and social context in which they occur. Window falls have been successfully prevented with the use of devices that prevent egress, and injuries from playground falls can be mitigated through the use of proper surfacing, such as woodchips or other soft, energy-absorbing materials. Alcohol may also contribute to falls among teenagers, and these injuries can be reduced by general strategies to reduce teen alcohol use.

VIOLENCE. Although the current rates of homicide are much lower than they were at their peak in the late 1980s and early 1990s, the problem of violence is still large. The origins of violence occur during childhood. Adults who commit violent acts usually have a history of violent behavior during childhood or adolescence. Longitudinal studies following groups of individuals from birth have found that aggression occurs among infants and that most children learn to control this aggression early in childhood. Children who later become violent adolescents and adults do not learn to control this aggressive behavior.

The most successful interventions for violence are those occurring early in life. These include home visits by nurses beginning in the prenatal period and continuing for the 1st few years of life to provide support and guidance to parents, especially parents without other resources. Early childhood education starting at age 3 yr has been shown to be effective in improving school success, keeping children in school, and decreasing the chance that the child will be a delinquent adolescent. School-based interventions, including curricula to increase the social skills of children and improve the parenting skills of caregivers, have long-term effects on violence and risk-taking behavior. Early identification of behavior problems by primary care pediatricians can best be accomplished through the routine use of formal screening tools. Interventions in adolescence, such as family therapy, multisystemic therapy, and therapeutic foster care, can decrease problem behavior and a subsequent decline into delinquency and violence.

PSYCHOSOCIAL CONSEQUENCES OF INJURIES

Many children and their parents have substantial psychosocial sequelae from trauma. Studies in adults indicate that 10–40% of hospitalized injured patients will have post-traumatic stress disorder (PTSD). Among injured children involved in motor vehicle crashes, 90% of families will have symptoms of acute stress disorder after the crash, although the diagnosis of acute stress disorder is not predictive of later PTSD. Standardized questionnaires that collect data from the child, the parents, and the medical record at the time of initial injury can serve as useful screening tests for later development of PTSD. Early mental health intervention, with close follow-up, is important for the treatment of PTSD and for minimizing its effect on the child and family.

American Academy of Pediatrics Committee on Injury and Poison Prevention: Children in pickup trucks. *Pediatrics* 2000;106:857–859.

American Academy of Pediatrics Committee on Injury Prevention and Poison Prevention: *Injury Prevention and Control for Children and Youth,* 3rd ed. Elk Grove Village, IL, American Academy of Pediatrics, 1997.

Asher KN, Rivara FP, Felix D, et al: Water safety training as a potential means of reducing the risk of young children's drowning. *Injury Prev* 1995;1:228–233.

Barrios LC, Davis MK, Kann L, et al: School health guidelines to prevent unintentional injuries and violence. *MMWR* 2001;50(Dec 7):1–73.

Bunn F, Colloer T, Frost C, et al: Area-wide traffic calming for preventing traffic related injuries. *Cochrane Database Syst Rev* 2003;(1):CD003110.

Chen LH, Baker SP, Li G: Graduated driver licensing programs and fatal crashes of 16-year-old drivers: a national evaluation. *Pediatrics* 2006; 118:56–62.

Chiavello C, Christoph R, Bond G: Infant walker related injuries: A prospective study of severity and incidence. *Pediatrics* 1994;93:974–976.

Committee on Injury Prevention and Poison Prevention Committee on Community Health Services: Prevention of agricultural injuries among children and adolescents. *Pediatrics* 2001;108:1016–1019.

Committee on Injury, Violence, and Poison Prevention Committee on Adolescence: The teen driver. *Pediatrics* 2006;118:2571–2581.

Committee on Sports Medicine and Fitness and Committee on Injury and Poison Prevention, American Academy of Pediatrics: Swimming programs for infants and toddlers. *Pediatrics* 2000;105:868–870.

Coyne-Beasley T, Schoenbach VJ, Johnson RM: "Love our kids, lock your guns": A community-based firearm safety counseling and gun lock distribution program. *Arch Pediatr Adolesc Med* 2001;155:659–664.

Cummings P, Koepsell TD, Rivara FP, et al: Airbags and passenger fatality according to passenger age and restraint use. *Epidemiology* 2002; 13:525–532.

Dowswell T, Towner E: Social deprivation and the prevention of unintentional injury in childhood: A systematic review. *Health Educ Res* 2002;7:221–237.

Duperrex O, Roberts I, Bunn F: Safety education of pedestrians for injury prevention: A systematic review of randomized controlled trials. *BMJ* 2002;324:1129.

Durbin DR, Elliott MR, Winston FK: Belt-positioning booster seats and reduction in risk of injury among children in vehicle crashes. *JAMA* 2003; 289:2835–2840.

Evans CA Jr, Fielding JE, Brownson RC, et al: Motor vehicle occupant injury: Strategies for increasing use of child safety seats, increasing use of safety belts, and reducing alcohol-impaired driving. *MMWR* 2001;50(May 18): 1–14.

Farrington DP, Loeber R: Epidemiology of juvenile violence. *Child Adolesc Psychiatry Clin North Am* 2000;9:733–748.

Foss RD, Feaganes JR, Rodgman EA: Initial effects of graduated driver licensing on 16-year-old driver crashes in North Carolina. *JAMA* 2001; 286:1588–1592.

Grossman DC, Mueller BA, Riedy C, et al: Gun storage practices and risk of youth suicide and unintentional firearm injuries. *JAMA* 2005;293: 740–741.

Harborview Injury Prevention and Research Center: Reviews of child injury prevention strategies. *http://www.hiprc.org/childinjury.*

Johnston BD, Rivara FP, Drowsch RM, et al: Behavior change counseling in the emergency department to reduce injury risk: A randomized controlled trial. *Pediatrics* 2002;110:267–274.

Kellermann AL, Rivara FP, Somes G, et al: Suicide in the home in relation to gun ownership. *N Engl J Med* 1992;327:467–472.

Krug EG: Injury surveillance is key to preventing injuries. *Lancet* 2004; 364:1563–1566.

Laraque D, Spivak H, Bull M: Serious firearm injury prevention does make sense. *Pediatrics* 2001;107:408–410.

Monti PM, Colby SM, Barnett NP, et al: Brief intervention for harm reduction with alcohol-positive older adolescents in a hospital emergency department. *J Consult Clin Psychol* 1999;67:989–994.

Norton C, Nixon J, Sibert JR: Playground injuries to children. *Arch Dis Child* 2004;89:103–108.

Rivara FP, Thompson DC, Patterson MQ, et al: Prevention of bicycle-related injuries: Helmets, education, and legislation. *Ann Rev Public Health* 1998;19:293–318.

Rogers GB: Effects of state helmet laws on bicycle helmet use by children and adolescents. *Inj Prev* 2002;8:42–46.

Rogers GB: The effectiveness of child-resistant packaging for aspirin. *Arch Pediatr Adolesc Med* 2002;156:929–933.

Shope JT, Molnar LJ, Elliott MR, et al: Graduated driver licensing in Michigan. *JAMA* 2001;286:1593–1598.

Thompson DC, Nunn ME, Thompson RS, et al: Effectiveness of bicycle helmets in preventing serious facial injury. *JAMA* 1996;276:1974–1975.

Tremblay RE, Nagin DS, Seguin JR, et al: Physical aggression during early childhood: Trajectories and predictors. *Pediatrics* 2004;114:e43–50.

Winston FK, Kallan MJ, Elliott MR, et al: Risk of injury to child passengers in compact extended-cab pickup trucks. *JAMA* 2002;287:1147–1152.
Winston FK, Kassam-Adams N, Garcia-Espana F, et al: Screening for risk of persistent posttraumatic stress in injured children and their parents. *JAMA* 2003;290:643–649.

Chapter 62 ■ Emergency Medical Services for Children

M. Denise Dowd and Frederick P. Rivara

Most children who require emergency medical care are seen in physicians' offices, clinics, and community emergency departments (EDs) and not in specialized pediatric EDs. This requires a community-based approach to emergency care of the child. Emergency medical services for children (EMS-C) embody a continuum of care that encompasses prevention, prehospital care and transport, ED and inpatient care, and necessary follow-up, including rehabilitation (Fig. 62-1).

THE ROLE OF THE PRIMARY CARE PHYSICIAN

The primary care physician (PCP) has multiple important roles in EMS-C. As an educator, the PCP's primary goal is prevention. By providing anticipatory guidance, the provider can help shape the attitudes, knowledge, and behaviors of parent and child, with the goal of preventing acute medical events, such as injury or status asthmaticus, and managing them should they occur. As triage officer, the PCP receives calls that necessitate directing families to the appropriate site for emergency care. The PCP frequently serves as an emergency care provider and, as such, must be prepared (with education, equipment, and policies) to deliver initial emergency care for common problems. Because most children are not treated in a children's hospital ED, but are treated in general community hospital EDs or urgent care centers, pediatricians should be consultants to these facilities and assist them in planning and delivering high-quality pediatric emergency care. Only 10% of ambulance calls are for pediatric patients; EMS providers may lack training and experience in caring for children; policies or procedures for caring for children may not exist or may be outdated. The pediatrician can be an advocate for integrating pediatric emergency care within the existing local EMS system.

OFFICE PREPAREDNESS

Providing anticipatory guidance to families regarding injury prevention, prompt recognition and treatment of illness, and accessing emergency care are important roles for the PCP. These may involve providing written materials and developmentally appropriate counseling. Parents and other adult caretakers of medically fragile children should consider learning CPR, and children can be taught to access 911. In addition to teaching the family how to prevent and manage emergencies, the PCP's office should be prepared to handle patients with medical emergencies.

Although the need for full CPR occurs relatively infrequently in an office setting, most practices see children in need of acute intervention or hospitalization on a regular basis. The PCP and staff members may find themselves ill equipped to treat patients with impending shock, respiratory failure, or a seizure. Emergency preparedness in the office requires training and continuing education for staff members, policies and procedures for emergency intervention, ready availability of appropriate resuscitation equipment, knowledge of local resources for EMS response and transport, and a working relationship with area EDs to ensure that children are cared for in facilities with expertise in pediatric emergency care.

STAFF TRAINING AND CONTINUING EDUCATION. Initial recognition by an office staff member that a child requires emergency treatment may occur in the course of a telephone call, in the waiting room, or in an examination room. All office personnel, including those at the front desk, must be capable of recognizing a child with altered mental status, shock, or respiratory distress or failure, and must be aware of an appropriate action plan for rapid intervention.

It is a reasonable expectation that all office staff, including receptionists and medical assistants, be trained in adult and child CPR as well as first aid and that they maintain their certification on an annual basis. In addition to these requirements, nurses and physicians should have training in a systematic approach to pediatric medical and trauma resuscitation. Core knowledge may be

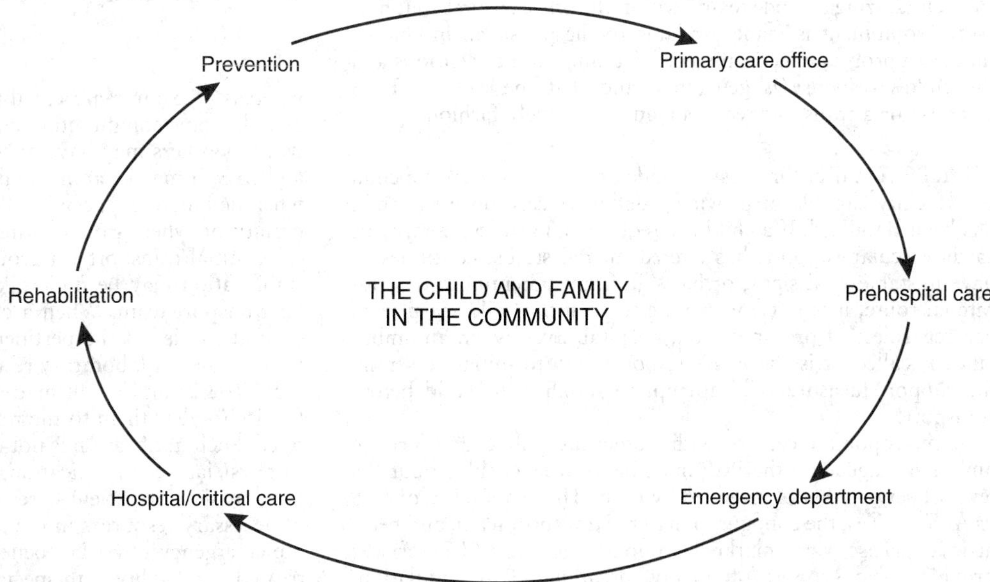

Figure 62-1. The emergency medical services for children (EMS-C) continuum of care: Seriously ill and injured children interface with a large number of health care personnel as they move through the EMS-C system. The system both begins and ends in the community.

obtained through standardized courses in pediatric advanced life support (ALS) offered by national medical and nursing associations. Frequent recertification is important for maintaining knowledge and skill. Examples include the American Heart Association's Pediatric Advanced Life Support (PALS) course, the Advanced Pediatric Life Support (APLS) course sponsored by the American Academy of Pediatrics (AAP) and the American College of Emergency Physicians (ACEP), and the Emergency Nurses Pediatric Course (ENPC), the Neonatal Resuscitation Program (NRP), and the Pediatric Emergency Nursing self-instruction manual sponsored by the Emergency Nurses Association.

POLICIES AND PROCEDURES. Standardized protocols for telephone triage of seriously ill or injured children are essential, especially if non-physician personnel take after-hours calls. When a child's status is in question and prehospital care is available, ambulance transport in the care of trained personnel is always preferable to transport by private car. This avoids the potentially serious medical consequences of relying on unskilled and distraught parents without the ability to provide even basic life support (BLS) measures to transport an unstable child to an ED. Written office policies and procedures for the management of status asthmaticus, upper airway obstruction, seizures, ingestions, shock, sepsis/meningitis, trauma, head injury, anaphylaxis, and cardiopulmonary arrest should be made available to all potentially involved staff members.

RESUSCITATION EQUIPMENT. Availability of necessary equipment is a vital part of an emergency response. Every physician's office should have essential resuscitation equipment and medications packaged in a pediatric resuscitation cart or kit (Table 62-1). This kit should be checked on a regular basis and kept in an accessible location known to all office staff. Outdated medications, a laryngoscope with a failed light source, or an empty oxygen tank represents a catastrophe in a resuscitation setting. Such incidents can be easily avoided if an equipment checklist and maintenance schedule is implemented. Responsible staff should receive routinely scheduled in-service training on equipment location and use, a task that may best be accomplished by a regular schedule of "mock codes" in which all office staff participate. A pediatric kit that includes posters, laminated cards, or resuscitation tapes specifying emergency drug doses and equipment size by age, weight, or height is invaluable in avoiding critical therapeutic errors during resuscitation.

To facilitate emergency response when a child needs rapid intervention in the office, all personnel should have a preassigned role. Organizing a "code team" within the office ensures that necessary equipment is made available to the physician in charge, that an appropriate medical record detailing all interventions and the child's response is generated, and that the call for EMS response or a transport team is made in a timely fashion.

TABLE 62-1. Office Emergency Drugs and Supplies

	PRIORITY
DRUGS	
Albuterol for inhalation	E
Epinephrine (1 : 1,000)	E
Activated charcoal	S
Antibiotics	S
Anticonvulsants (diazepam/lorazepam)	S
Corticosteroids (parenteral/oral)	S
Dextrose (25%)	S
Diphenhydramine (parenteral)	S
Epinephrine (1 : 10,000)	S
Atropine sulfate (0.1 mg/mL)	O
Naloxone (0.4 mg/mL)	O
Sodium bicarbonate (4.2%)	O
IV fluids:	
Normal saline (NS) or lactated Ringer's (500-mL bags)	O
5% dextrose, 0.45 NS (500-mL bags)	O
AIRWAY	
Oxygen and delivery system	E
Bag-valve-mask (450 mL and 1,000 mL)	E
Clear oxygen masks, breather and non-rebreather, with reservoirs	E
Suction device, tonsil tip, bulb syringe	E
Peak flow meter	E
Nebulizer (or metered-dose inhaler with spacer/mask)	E
Oral airways (sizes 00–5)	E
Nasal airways (sizes 12–30F)	S
Magill forceps (pediatric, adult)	S
Suction catheters (sizes 5–14F)	S
Nasogastric tubes (sizes 6–14F)	S
Pulse oximeter	S
Laryngoscope handle (pediatric, adult) with extra batteries, bulbs	S
Laryngoscope blades (straight 0–4; curved 2–3)	S
Endotracheal tubes (uncuffed 2.5–5.5; cuffed 6.0–8.0)	S
Stylets (pediatric, adult)	S
FLUID MANAGEMENT	
Butterfly needles (19–25 gauge)	S
Catheter-over-needle device (14–24 gauge)	S
Arm boards, tape, tourniquet	S
Intraosseous needles (16, 18 gauge)	S
Intravenous tubing, microdrip	S
MISCELLANEOUS EQUIPMENT AND SUPPLIES	
Color-coded tape or preprinted drug doses	E
Cardiac arrest board/backboard	E
Sphygmomanometer (infant, child, adult, thigh cuffs)	E
Splints, sterile dressings	E
Spot glucose test	S
Stiff neck collars (small/large)	S

E, essential; O, optional; S, suggested.

TRANSPORT. A decision must be made on how to transport a child to a facility capable of providing definitive care once the child has been stabilized. If a child has required an artificial airway or cardiovascular support, has altered mental status, continues to have unstable vital signs, or has significant potential to deteriorate en route, it is not appropriate to send the child via private car, regardless of proximity to a hospital. Even when an ambulance is called, it is the PCP's responsibility to initiate essential life support measures and attempt to stabilize the child before transport.

In metropolitan centers with numerous public and private ambulance agencies, the PCP must be knowledgeable about the level of service that is provided by each. The availability of BLS vs ALS services, the configuration of the transport team, and pediatric expertise vary markedly among agencies. BLS services provide basic support of airway, breathing, and circulation, whereas ALS units are capable of providing resuscitation drugs as well. Some communities may have only BLS services available, whereas others may have a 2-tiered system, providing both BLS and ALS. It may be appropriate to consider medical air transport when definitive or specialized care is not available within a community or when ground transport times are prolonged. In that case, initial transport via ground to a local hospital for interval stabilization may be undertaken pending arrival of the medical air transport team. When a child is to be transported by air or ground, copies of the pertinent medical records and any radiologic studies or laboratory results should be sent with the patient (Table 62-2) and a call made to the physicians at the receiving facility to alert them to the referral and any treatments administered. Such notification is not merely a courtesy; direct physician-to-physician communication is essential to ensure adequate transmission of patient care information, to allow mobilization of necessary resources in the ED, and to redirect the transport if the emergency physician believes that the child would be better treated at a facility with specialized services. The referring physi-

TABLE 62-2. Checklist for Patient Transport

Obtain written consent for transfer from the patient's parent or guardian.
Call the receiving physician and document acceptance of transfer on the appropriate form and the patient's medical record, including name of the accepting physician and time of acceptance.
Call and give the report to the appropriate transport agency.
Copy the medical record, including transport consent forms.
Copy all diagnostic tests, including radiographs.
Document the name of the transport agency and the time at which the transport occurred.

cian is legally responsible for patient safety until the patient's care is taken over by the accepting physician.

PEDIATRIC PREHOSPITAL CARE

Prehospital care refers to emergency assistance rendered by trained emergency medical personnel before a child reaches a treating medical facility. Although most communities in the United States have a formalized EMS system, the nature of the emergency medical response depends in part on local demographics and population base. EMS may be provided by volunteers or paid professionals. Key points to recognize in considering the interface between the community physician and the local EMS system include access to the system, provider capability, response and transport times, and destination.

ACCESS TO THE EMS SYSTEM. Most metropolitan and many rural communities in the United States have a 911 telephone system that provides direct access to a dispatcher who coordinates police, fire, and EMS response. Some communities have an enhanced 911 system, in which the location of the caller is automatically provided to the dispatcher, permitting emergency response even if the caller, such as a young child, cannot give an address. The extent of medical training for these dispatchers varies between communities, as do the protocols by which they assign an emergency response (BLS vs ALS). In some smaller communities, no coordinated dispatch exists and emergency medical calls are handled by the local law enforcement agency.

When activating the 911 system, physicians must make clear to the dispatcher the nature of the medical emergency and the condition of the child. In many communities, dispatchers are trained to ask a series of questions per protocol, allowing them to send out EMS personnel with an appropriate level of training.

PROVIDER CAPABILITY. There are many levels of training for prehospital EMS providers, ranging from individuals capable of providing only first aid to those trained and licensed to provide ALS in the field. All EMS personnel, whether emergency medical technicians (EMTs) or paramedics, receive training in pediatric emergencies; however, pediatric cases actually constitute a minority (≈10%) of all EMS cases.

First responders may be law enforcement officers, firefighters, or community volunteers who are dispatched to provide emergency medical assistance. They have approximately 40 hr of training in first aid and CPR. Their role is to provide rapid response and stabilization pending the arrival of more highly trained personnel. In some smaller communities, this is the only prehospital emergency medical response available.

In the United States, the bulk of emergency medical response is provided by EMTs, who may be volunteers or paid professionals. Basic EMTs may staff an ambulance after undergoing an approximately 100-hr training program. They are licensed to provide BLS services, but may receive further training to expand their scope of practice to include intravenous catheter placement and fluid administration, endotracheal intubation, and use of an automatic external defibrillator, under the direction of a physician advisor.

Paramedics, or EMT-Ps, represent the highest level of EMT response, with medical training and supervised field experience of approximately 1,000 hr. They provide ALS services in the prehospital setting, functioning out of an ambulance equipped as a mobile intensive care unit. Paramedic skills may include endotracheal intubation; placement of peripheral, central, or intraosseous lines; intravenous administration of drugs; administration of nebulized aerosols; needle thoracotomy; and cardioversion and defibrillation. Paramedics work under the supervision of a physician advisor.

The configuration of medical air transport teams can vary widely and may include physicians, nurses, respiratory therapists, or paramedics. The amount of pediatric training of team members also varies, and it is important to confirm that an appropriate standard of care can be provided during interfacility transport.

The level of training of the prehospital personnel dispatched to the scene of a medical emergency depends on the condition of the patient, available resources, and local protocols. Training and equipment for pediatric emergency care have historically been given inadequate attention in national certification curricula and by EMS agencies primarily geared toward adult patients. In some communities, the standard of pediatric prehospital care may not match that offered to adult patients in a similar condition. The EMS-C initiative sponsored by the Maternal and Child Health Bureau, U.S. Department of Health and Human Services, has provided program development grants to improve pediatric EMS in all 50 states. This has led to increased awareness of the special needs of acutely ill and injured children and to the development of many programs and products to enhance their care. The American Academy of Pediatrics has taken the lead in developing Pediatric Education for Prehospital Professionals (PEPP), a comprehensive course for EMTs and paramedics in prehospital pediatric care.

A critical aspect of providing quality prehospital care to children in the community is input by pediatricians on EMS policy, protocols, and procedures. Such input is considered under the umbrella term *medical control* and can be either direct or indirect. **Direct medical control** consists of direct contact between a physician (usually in an ED) and an EMS provider. Medical guidance is provided according to established protocols. **Indirect medical control** consists of physicians providing input into the creation of EMS protocols and treatment guidelines. This is usually accomplished through a medical advisory committee or a physician advisor.

RESPONSE AND TRANSPORT TIMES. Depending on the demographics of a community, the location of the incident, and the nature of the EMS available, EMS response times after a call for assistance may range from a few min to >1 hr. Unfortunately, even in communities with relatively rapid response times, individuals may be reluctant to call for help because of a misperception that the 911 system should be activated only for full resuscitations. If a child is physiologically unstable (with marked respiratory distress, cyanosis, signs of early shock, or altered mental status) or has significant potential to deteriorate en route to the ED, or if the parents' ability to comply promptly with recommendations for ED evaluation is in question, then an EMS transport should be initiated. Inherent dangers lie in the attitude that a parent can get to the hospital faster by private car.

DESTINATION. The destination to which a pediatric patient is transported may be defined by parental preference, provider preference, or agency protocol. In communities with an organized trauma system or a system of pediatric designation based on the objective capabilities of the area hospitals, seriously ill or injured children may be triaged by protocol to the highest-level center reachable within a reasonable amount of time. The Pediatric Trauma Score (PTS) or Revised Trauma Score (RTS; see Chapter

71) can be used to assess the severity of injury. Children with a PTS of <8 or an RTS of <11 should be treated in a designated trauma center. In communities that do not have a hospital with the equipment and personnel resources to provide definitive inpatient care, interfacility transport of a child to a regional center should be undertaken after initial stabilization. The PCP may be involved in this decision-making process and must make a critical assessment of the local hospital's capabilities. When interfacility transport is to be undertaken, indications for transfer, parental consent for transfer, and acceptance of the patient by the receiving physician all must be clearly documented in the medical record.

THE EMERGENCY DEPARTMENT. The ability of hospital EDs to respond to the emergency care of children varies and depends on a number of factors, including available equipment and supplies, training and experience of the staff, and availability of pediatric subspecialists. The majority of children who require emergency care are evaluated in community hospitals by physicians or other health care providers with variable degrees of pediatric training and experience. Children account for 25–30% of all ED visits, but only a fraction of them represent true emergencies. Because the volume of critical pediatric cases is low, emergency physicians and nurses working in community hospitals often have limited opportunity to reinforce their knowledge and skills in pediatric resuscitation. Pediatricians from the community may be consulted when a seriously ill or injured child presents to the ED, and they should have a structured approach to the initial evaluation and treatment of an unstable child of any age, regardless of the underlying diagnosis. Early recognition of life-threatening abnormalities in oxygenation, ventilation, perfusion, and central nervous system function and rapid intervention to correct those abnormalities are key to successful pediatric resuscitation.

Because not all EDs are equally capable of treating an ill or injured child, it is the responsibility of the referring physician to be aware of the pediatric capabilities of hospitals in the area. Critically ill and injured patients have an improved outcome when cared for in regional referral centers, such as a pediatric trauma center or an adult trauma center with special qualifications in pediatric care. This is particularly true for neonatal emergencies, major trauma, burns, head injuries, and specific pediatric surgical problems. Thus, although initial stabilization of these patients may take place in a local community hospital, definitive and long-term care should be delivered in major referral centers especially equipped to provide such care.

Minimal standards must be met by community EDs to ensure that children receive the best emergency care possible. Guidelines for the care of children in the ED have been published and are endorsed by both the AAP and the ACEP. These guidelines provide current information on policies, procedures, protocols, quality assurance methods, and equipment and supplies considered essential for managing pediatric emergencies. Specific recommendations on equipment, supplies, and medications for the ED are listed and updates are available on the AAP and ACEP websites. Sample policies and protocols for EDs that treat children are given in Table 62-3.

In addition to the need for individuals skilled in the emergency care of children, the environment of the ED treating children must be respectful of the needs and expectations of children and their families. A child-safe ED is the first priority. Wires and sharps boxes in examination rooms should be out of reach; waste containers should be covered, tall, and stable; and electrical sockets should be covered. Within practical limits, the child must be separated from the frightening sights and sounds that are so common in EDs. Examples of ways to meet this goal include: (1) a separate ambulance entrance; (2) resuscitation rooms that are private; (3) "quiet rooms" for upset family members; and (4) soundproof procedure rooms. Distraction and entertainment go a long way toward helping the child and family waiting for or undergoing treatment in an ED. Televisions, game boards, interactive toys, and crafts can be considered essential tools for emergency care of the child. These techniques are not only comforting to the child and family, but also helpful to the practitioner who is attempting to assess the child. The examination of a calm child is much more reliable than that of a frightened, crying child.

TABLE 62-3. Pediatric-specific Policies and Protocols for the Community Emergency Department

Triage and initial assessment
Child safety
Suspected child abuse or neglect
Family violence
Consent for treatment
Emancipated minors
Sedation and analgesia
Transfer to a higher level of pediatric care
Telephone consultation with pediatric subspecialists
Do not resuscitate
Death of a child
Sudden infant death and apparent life-threatening event
Daily verification of location and functioning of pediatric equipment and supplies
Immunizations
Parental presence during procedures
Ground and air transport procedures

The way in which the family supports the child during a crisis is critical to recovery. Surveys of parents have indicated that the majority of them want to be with their child during invasive procedures and even resuscitation. This has been shown to reduce parental and patient anxiety and does not interfere with the procedure.

THE COMMUNITY

SCHOOLS. Because children spend a great deal of time in schools, schools must be prepared to attend to the emergency needs of normally healthy children as well as children with special health care needs. In 1990, as a result of passage of the Individuals with Disabilities Education Act, more chronically ill and technologically dependent children began to attend regular school; thus, the need for preparation to deal with acute medical problems has increased. Guidelines for emergency medical care in schools have been published by the AAP and include suggested procedures, staff and staff training, documentation, and parental notification.

The range of pediatric emergencies taking place in schools is wide and includes acute emotional or behavioral events (suicide), exacerbation of chronic disease (asthma), injuries, and disclosure of child abuse. School nurses may not be available to assist in the handling of such emergencies, requiring faculty to be prepared to do so. Key factors in determining a school's ability to respond to medical emergencies include comprehensive written policies for managing an emergency; a basic emergency supply kit; training of all school personnel required to respond to an emergency in CPR and basic first aid; familiarity and collaborative relationships with local EMS providers and EDs; communication with parents and caregivers concerning children's medical needs; and incorporation of injury prevention and basic first aid training activities into the educational curriculum.

DISASTER PREPAREDNESS. Natural and manmade disasters are unfortunate but common events that affect children and their families. Children's medical and emotional needs should be addressed specifically in any community's disaster plan. Child health specialists can participate in all areas of the EMS-C response to disaster, including planning, acute management, and aftermath activities. Critical elements of a comprehensive disaster plan include guidelines for plan activation, use of space and procurement of extra supplies, security, delineation of the responsibilities of key personnel, notification of key personnel, care and transfer of nondisaster patients, care of the deceased, critical incident stress debriefing, and plans for disaster drills. Response to threats of bioterrorism is addressed in Chapter 711.

LEGAL ASPECTS OF EMS-C. A physician treating a child for any emergency condition must be aware of the legal aspects of providing such care. There are numerous federal, state, and local laws with which the physician should become familiar, including issues pertaining to consent, requirements of the Emergency Medical Treatment and Active Labor Act (EMTALA), Good Samaritan laws, and child protection issues.

Written policies that conform to local and state laws regarding consent to treat minors should be developed for all practice settings in which children are treated. Parental consent for medical treatment of a minor is required before treatment; however, physicians may proceed with treatment without consent in the event that a delay would endanger the well-being of the child. The definition of which emergencies fit this category varies among jurisdictions and does not merely include life- or limb-threatening events. If parents or legal guardians are not available to give consent, every attempt must be made to reach them and those attempts documented in the child's chart.

In all 50 states, by state law, physicians are mandated to report suspected child abuse to the local child protection service. Penalties for failure to report suspected abuse vary from state to state, but may involve criminal action and substantial fines. Most states provide immunity from civil or criminal litigation for those who report suspected abuse if the report was made in good faith. Definitions of abuse and neglect and reporting procedures vary from state to state (see Chapter 36).

The purpose of EMTALA, which was enacted by Congress in 1986, is to address the concern that hospital EDs were turning away or inappropriately transferring uninsured patients, known as *patient dumping*. This law applies to hospitals with EDs that participate in Medicare or Medicaid and to individual physicians practicing in those hospitals. There are 3 requirements of EMTALA:

1. The hospital must provide an appropriate medical screening to assess if the patient has an emergency medical condition.
2. If an emergency condition exists, the patient's condition must be stabilized, or if such measures exceed the hospital's expertise, the patient must be transferred to a hospital capable of stabilization. This aspect of the law applies to any pediatrician who is on call for consultation to the ED.
3. A hospital may transfer an unstable patient only under limited circumstances. Failure to follow EMTALA requirements can result in penalties imposed by the federal authorities.

Good Samaritan laws vary from state to state and are designed to protect individuals who provide emergency assistance at the scene of an emergency. Good Samaritan laws only apply if the physician providing care did not have a pre-existing duty to render care. These laws will not protect against acts of gross negligence. Some state laws protect only physicians who are licensed in the state where the emergency aid is given. Good Samaritan laws do not apply when giving voluntary medical assistance during air emergencies. Of related importance, medical kits aboard airplanes are not currently required to carry pediatric equipment.

PSYCHOSOCIAL ASPECTS OF EMS-C. Emergencies involving children are undoubtedly stressful for the child, the parent, and the EMS-C providers. The health care system must be responsive to the emotional and mental health needs of all involved. Parents should be given the opportunity to be with their child in the ED during procedures, even during resuscitation, and must be involved in decision-making. The attitude of the individual communicating with the family and the clarity of the information given are crucial, especially when the news is bad. Verbal information should be accompanied by written plans and instructions whenever possible.

Staff should be trained in appropriate coping and calming techniques for parents and for children at different developmental levels. Distraction skills, the use of appropriate language to explain procedures, and methods to support children and parents should be priorities in continuing education programs for staff.

Screening for and addressing mental health needs should occur in the ED. Approximately 60–90% of families in which a child was injured in a motor vehicle crash will be affected by symptoms of acute stress after the crash. These symptoms often occur in conjunction with depression and alcohol use in adolescents or parents. Screening for the risk of post-traumatic stress disorder can be accomplished in the ED with a brief questionnaire and is highly predictive of persistent traumatic stress symptoms in both children and parents. Increasing evidence that post-traumatic stress disorder affects recovery from illness and injury necessitates that patients and families obtain appropriate follow-up services. Screening for substance abuse among adolescents presenting for care, especially with trauma, is as important as treating their injuries. Brief interventions in the ED using motivational interviewing can have a significant effect on problem drinking and later risk of injury.

ADVOCACY FOR EMS-C

Tremendous variation in preparedness and the quality of children's emergency care is evident in the United States. In 1991, the Institute of Medicine convened a 19-member Committee on Pediatric Emergency Medical Services that reviewed the current status of pediatric emergency medical care and published its recommendations in the 1993 Report on Emergency Medical Services for Children. Since then, much progress has been made in education and training, planning, evaluation, research, communication, and funding to achieve those recommendations, but continued improvement is needed.

As the expert in child health care, the pediatrician is a powerful advocate for local EMS-C issues. There are many ways in which to advocate and good resources to turn to for assistance. Advocating for EMS-C can include education of community leaders, including both elected and nonelected officials; direct lobbying; providing pediatric expertise to EMS administrators; and coalition-building. The AAP has produced several speakers' kits to assist advocates in this work. Topics include the importance of EMS-C, injury prevention, child abuse, and motor vehicle occupant safety.

American Academy of Pediatrics, Committee on Pediatric Emergency Medicine: Childhood emergencies in the office, hospital, and community: organizing systems of care. *Pediatrics* 2000;106(2 Pt 1):337–338.

American Academy of Pediatrics, Committee on Pediatric Emergency Medicine: The pediatrician's role in disaster preparedness. *Pediatrics* 1997;99:130–133.

American Academy of Pediatrics, Committee on Pediatric Emergency Medicine, and American College of Emergency Physicians, Pediatric Committee Care of Children in the Emergency Department: Guidelines for preparedness. *Pediatrics* 2001;107:777–781.

American Academy of Pediatrics, Committee on School Health: Guidelines for emergency medical care in school. *Pediatrics* 2001;107:435–436.

American Academy of Pediatrics: *Pediatric Education for Prehospital Professionals (PEPP)*. Sudbury, MA, Jones and Bartlett, 2000.

American Academy of Pediatrics, Section of Emergency Medicine (*www.aap.org/ sections/semed.htm*).

American Academy of Pediatrics Task Force on Inter-hospital Transport: *Guidelines for Air and Ground Transport of Neonatal and Pediatric Patients*. Elk Grove Village, IL, American Academy of Pediatrics, 1999.

American Association of Poison Control Centers *(www.aapcc.org)*.

American College of Emergency Physicians *(www.acep.org)*.

American College of Surgeons, Committee on Trauma: *Advanced Trauma Life Support*. Chicago, American College of Surgeons, 1997.
American Heart Association *(www.amhrt.org)*.
American Heart Association Emergency Cardiac Care Committee and Subcommittees: Guidelines 2000. Conference on Cardiopulmonary Resuscitation and Emergency Cardiac Care VI: Pediatric advanced life support. *Circulation* 2000;102:I-291–I-342.
Bole ET, Moore GP, Brummett C, et al: Do parents want to be present during invasive procedures performed on their children in the emergency department? A survey of 400 parents. *Ann Emerg Med* 1999;34:70–74.
Emergency Medical Services for Children *(www.ems-c.org)*.
Emergency Medical Services for Children: A 10-year retrospective based on the recommendations of the Committee on Pediatric Emergency Medical Services of the National Academy of Sciences Institute of Medicine. *http://www.ems-c.org/Downloads/PDF/EMSCRetrospective.pdf* (accessed April 11, 2005).
Henretig F, Cieslak TJ: Bioterrorism and pediatric emergency medicine. *Clin Pediatr Emerg Med* 2001;2:211–222.
Horowitz L, Kassam-Adams N, Bergstein J: Mental health aspects of emergency medical services for children: Summary of a consensus conference. *Acad Emerg Med* 2001;8:1187–1196.
Institute of Medicine Committee on Pediatric Emergency Medical Services: Durch JS, Lohr KN (editors): *Emergency Medical Services for Children*. Washington, DC, National Academy Press, 1993.
Jurkovich GJ, Pierce B, Pananen L, et al: Giving bad news: The family perspective. *J Trauma* 2000;48:865–873.
Monti PM, Colby SM, Barnett NP, et al: Brief intervention for harm reduction with alcohol-positive older adolescents in a hospital emergency department. *J Consult Clin Psychol* 1999;67:989–994.
Seidel J, Tittle S, Hodge D, et al: Guidelines for pediatric equipment and supplies for emergency departments. *Ann Emerg Med* 1998;31:54–57.
Winston FK, Kassam-Adams N, Garcia-Espana F, et al: Screening for risk of persistent posttraumatic stress in injured children and their parents. *JAMA* 2003;290:643–649.
Zarzick D, Russo J, Grossman D, et al: Posttraumatic stress and depressive symptoms, alcohol use, and recurrent traumatic life events in a representative sample of hospitalized injured adolescents and their parents. *J Pediatr Psychol* 2006;31:377–387.

Chapter 63 ■ Interfacility Transfer of the Critically Ill Infant and Child

Lorry R. Frankel

Specialized transport programs (interfacility transport) take patients from community facilities to regionalized pediatric intensive care units (PICUs). Children are usually taken by an emergency medical services provider or by their parents to the local emergency department, where their condition is assessed to determine the extent of injury, severity of illness, and amount of physiologic instability (see Chapter 62). If the local facility does not have the capabilities to provide comprehensive intensive care, the child must be transported to a PICU. If possible, the child should be stabilized in the referring hospital while awaiting the arrival of the pediatric transport team. Regional pediatric centers have a responsibility not only to transport patients as rapidly and safely as possible, but also to provide community educational programs that enable local health care providers to develop the necessary skills required for physiologic stabilization until the transport team arrives.

The American Academy of Pediatrics, the Association of Air Medical Services, and the Federal Aviation Administration have developed recommendations for pediatric transport programs. The members of the transport team must have the cognitive and technical skills required to meet the needs of pediatric patients and should be supervised by an attending physician (medical control physician [MCP]) who has expertise in either pediatric emergency medicine or pediatric critical care. All transport teams should have a team leader who is able to interact with the MCP during the transport and also manage the airway, provide respiratory support, and obtain vascular access. The team leader should also have basic knowledge of pediatric drug dosing and understand the basic pathophysiology of pediatric disease and the transport environment. The transport program must have a medical director who organizes the overall program and institutes a quality assurance program that reviews transports, the equipment, and the proper use of vehicles.

DISPATCH AND TRANSFER CENTERS. The regional PICU should provide telephone consultation and deploy a team of specialized health care providers to assist in stabilization of patients to transport them in a safe mobile environment to the PICU. Regional centers may develop different protocols for activation of transport or consultation requests. Some encourage direct access to the unit, some go through the emergency department, and others prefer to use a dispatch center or transfer center to screen calls and facilitate the coordination of a transport. Once it has been determined that an ill child must be transported to the regional center, the MCP should be consulted to provide further input into the patient's care and to determine the best team composition and the appropriate vehicle to transport the patient.

MEDICAL CONTROL PHYSICIAN. The MCP may have other clinical responsibilities; however, transport requests and consultations should be prioritized so that the necessary clinical information is obtained, appropriate therapeutic interventions can occur, and undue delays are avoided when transferring critically ill patients. The referring hospital provides some of the initial life-sustaining support required for these patients. It is often necessary for the MCP to provide further input into the patient's care while the patient is in the local facility. The MCP may seek additional medical or surgical consultation from other subspecialists, if necessary. In addition to having the knowledge required to stabilize a critically ill infant or child, the MCP must be familiar with the transport requirements needed, the transport environment, and the pertinent geography. Finally, the MCP must have good interpersonal skills and the ability to maintain collegiality during a potentially difficult and stressful situation for the referring physician and facility. The MCP will assume significant responsibility for a patient who has not yet been seen.

TEAM COMPOSITION. Composition of the team is based on a number of factors, including the severity of the patient's illness, the distance to the referring facility, the referring facility's insistence that certain team members be present (a physician), and the ability of the team members to work together in unfamiliar surroundings. The severity of illness is assessed by the MCP based on the information provided by the referring hospital. Many transports can be staffed by a non-physician team leader with telephone contact with the MCP. In addition to the team leader, a critical care nurse is responsible for providing nursing care, monitoring the patient's condition, and administering medications. If the child requires airway and respiratory support, a respiratory therapist should be included.

Various scoring systems have been developed to predict the need for a physician during transport. It also appears that the team member's experience and skill in caring for critically ill patients is more important than the team member's educational degree. These individuals receive this experience through ongoing didactic sessions, skill training in airway management and vascular access, and case review. The use of physicians as team leaders may provide for both cognitive and decision-making capabilities, but the MCP and a non-physician team leader can manage many situations via telephone contact. The evolution of advanced practice nursing has enabled transport programs to use these professionals as team leaders. Team leaders must have adequate training in the assessment of the critically ill child, including such skills as airway management and vascular access, understanding the basic pathophysiology of pediatric disease, and having knowledge of the transport environment.

VEHICLE SELECTION. The selection of the vehicle is made by the MCP in coordination with the referring hospital and the transport team. Factors to consider are the severity of illness or injury, the distance to the referring hospital, the travel time required, weather conditions, vehicle availability, equipment needs, and expense. Ground ambulance is used for the majority of transports, which are <100 miles. Traffic patterns must be considered in evaluating response time. The major advantages of this mode of transport are the ability to stop en route if the patient's condition worsens and further intervention is required and the ability to take a larger team with more equipment. Fixed-wing aircraft are usually used to reach infants and children who live >100–150 miles from the regional PICU. These vehicles may be able to fly to certain areas when the weather or altitude prevents the use of a helicopter. However, the use of fixed-wing aircraft requires several ambulance transfers. In addition, flying at some altitudes (especially >5,000 feet) can have serious effects on the partial pressure and volume of gases in various body cavities and closed containers. Thus, patients who have respiratory failure and require supplemental oxygen and those with a pneumothorax or an ileus require special care to prevent further deterioration. Helicopters enable a more rapid response, but are expensive; the greatest hazards are poor weather and difficulty landing in poorly visualized or nondesignated landing areas. Helicopters are most useful for transports within a radius of 100–200 miles and for going directly to the site of an injury (to pick up a trauma victim).

All vehicles must have the capability for radio or telephone contact with the MCP or the base station. In addition, each vehicle must be able to provide on-board oxygen, electrical power, and suction, and must have space for adequate supplies and equipment, including oxygen tanks, pharmacy packs, respiratory therapy devices, infusion pumps and solutions, stretchers or incubators, and monitors. Additional space may be needed for advanced technologies, such as extracorporeal membrane oxygenation and inhaled nitric oxide or helium.

COMMUNICATION. Communication is 1 of the most crucial components of a regional transport system. Dealing with a critically ill or injured infant or child is an uncommon event for many community physicians. Therefore, a referring physician needs to know whom, how, and when to call for assistance in the evaluation, stabilization, and transfer of a child. Telephone contact is required at all levels to ensure that physicians talk to physicians and that nurses talk to nurses. A child's condition may change rapidly; the ability to obtain information and provide advice needs to be continuing. Using a dispatch center as the patching system to the MCP and others allows the referring physician or hospital to need only 1 telephone number and to address acute changes that require an immediate response.

The MCP determines if more tests should be done at the referring hospital (various imaging studies) or if various therapeutic interventions should be initiated (elective intubation for progressive respiratory distress, initiation of inotropic support for cardiovascular failure).

Once the transport team arrives at the referring facility, the team leader should reassess the patient's condition, review all of the pertinent laboratory data and medications, and discuss the situation with the parents and referring physicians. If the patient's condition has changed significantly, the team leader should contact the MCP for additional advice. All medical records, including radiographs and scans, should be copied to take to the accepting facility. Before the transport team leaves with the child, the MCP should be consulted again and the PICU contacted to finalize preparations to receive the patient.

The referring physician should provide written documentation of the need to transfer the patient to a facility that can provide a higher level of care than can be provided at the referring hospital. This should include a statement that the risks, benefits, and alternatives have been discussed with the parents and that their informed consent has been obtained to have their child transferred to another hospital with PICU capacity. Medicolegal responsibility is probably shared once communication has begun. It is therefore important to document what has been recommended to the referring facility to better stabilize the patient.

One problem sometimes caused by community facilities is either transferring a critically ill child with a team that does not have the necessary expertise or equipment or using some other system that is equally not prepared to care for the unique needs of a pediatric patient. There may be a misconception that the more rapidly the patient is transported, the better the outcome. Unless there is a surgical emergency, it is preferred to stabilize the child and keep the patient in the referring hospital awaiting the arrival of the trained pediatric team. Regional pediatric centers have a responsibility not only to transport the patient in as rapid and safe a manner as possible, but also to provide educational opportunities for the community so that personnel can develop the necessary skills required for further stabilization until the transport team arrives.

It is also important that both the referring facility and the regional PICU have realistic expectations about the transport team's capabilities. If it is determined that a physician with significant critical care skills is required for the transport, then the PICU has an obligation to provide a team leader with this skill level. The referring hospital should not delay lifesaving interventions while awaiting the arrival of the transport team (intubation of the trachea, initiation of mechanical ventilation, pharmacologic support), especially if recommended by the MCP.

Federal legislation prohibits hospitals from refusing, limiting, or terminating patient care for financial reasons. This originates from the Consolidated Omnibus Budget Reconciliation Act (COBRA) passed in 1986 and revised in 1990. This act requires the hospital to evaluate all patients who arrive with emergent conditions and to stabilize patients before transfer. It also requires that the transferring hospital be responsible for the medical capabilities of the receiving hospital. To facilitate the transfer of critically ill pediatric patients, some regional PICUs have developed transfer agreements with referring hospitals. This ensures that the referring hospital has developed a plan as to where and how to transfer a patient. These relationships ensure that the appropriate and safe transfer of the infant or child with a life-threatening illness occurs as smoothly and safely as possible.

As telecommunication systems improve, it will become possible to provide live video viewing of the patient at the referring hospital. The expansion of telemedicine will enable the MCP to work in conjunction with the referring physicians in the evaluation and stabilization of the critically ill child. This will improve outcomes because it provides the necessary critical care expertise at the bedside of the ill patient.

American Academy of Pediatrics, Committee on Pediatric Emergency Medicine, American College of Critical Care Medicine, Society of Critical Care Medicine: Consensus report for regionalization of services for critically ill or injured children. *Pediatrics* 2000;105:152–155.

Cornette L: Contemporary neonatal transport: Problems and solutions. *Arch Dis Child Fetal Neonatal Ed* 2004;89:F212–F214.

Das UG, Leuthner SR: Preparing the neonate for transport. *Pediatr Clin North Am* 2004;51:581–598.

Leslie A, Stephenson T: Neonatal transfers by advanced neonatal nurse practitioners and paediatric registrars. *Arch Dis Child Fetal Neonatal Ed* 2003;88:F509–F512.

Linden V, Palmer K, Reinhard J, et al: Inter-hospital transportation of patients with severe acute respiratory failure on extracorporeal membrane oxygenation-national and international experience. *Intensive Care Med* 2001;10:1643–1648.

Nieman CT, Merlino JI, Kovach B, et al: Intubated pediatric patients requiring transport: A review of patients, indications, and standards. *Air Med J* 2001;21:22–25.

Woodward GA, Insoft RM, Pearson-Shaver AL, et al: The state of pediatric interfacility transport: Consensus of the second national pediatric and neonatal interfacility transport medicine leadership conference. *Pediatr Emerg Care* 2002;18:38–43.

Chapter 64 ■ Monitoring Techniques for the Critically Ill Infant and Child

Lorry R. Frankel

Monitoring critically ill patients involves obtaining biologic and physiologic data by invasive or noninvasive techniques. Noninvasive monitoring can involve continuous evaluation of heart rate and rhythm and respiratory rate, whereas noncontinuous monitoring measures blood pressure and various laboratory values, such as blood gases. Hemodynamic and respiratory monitoring involves the placement of invasive catheters to continuously determine blood pressure and central venous pressure (CVP) and to obtain intermittent arterial blood gas values. Invasive monitoring requires special expertise in the insertion of catheters and nursing care in their maintenance. This type of monitoring has potential serious complications (infections, thrombosis, air embolism, bleeding). Noninvasive monitoring devices also enable critically ill patients to be monitored continuously with fewer complications, allowing for greater patient comfort at a reduced expense. Invasive monitoring is widely used, particularly in unstable critically ill patients; routine bedside monitoring may also incorporate noninvasive devices that allow for continuous and real-time measurement of physiologic data. The different types of monitoring complement each other and enable the clinician to have a better awareness of minute-to-minute changes.

Monitoring requirements can be divided into hemodynamic, pulmonary, and neurologic; techniques can be classified as invasive or noninvasive (Table 64-1). Both noninvasive and invasive monitors must use age- and disease-specific criteria for setting monitor alarms because normal values for heart rate, blood pressure, and respiratory rate vary with a child's age, whereas acceptable oxygen saturations vary with different cyanotic congenital heart lesions.

HEMODYNAMIC MONITORING. Hemodynamic monitoring is indicated for any patient who is admitted to the pediatric intensive care unit (PICU) and is in shock, has respiratory failure, or has sustained an acute neurologic insult. Hemodynamic monitoring includes heart rate and blood pressure as well as CVP and pulmonary capillary wedge pressure, and occasionally in postoperative cardiovascular patients, right atrial and left atrial pressure. Heart rate can be measured with conventional electrodes placed on the chest, which can also provide rhythm strips, usually in lead II. The lead can be changed if indicated to evaluate for other dysrhythmias, but it should not substitute for a 12-lead electrocardiogram (ECG).

Blood pressure can be measured invasively or noninvasively. The choice is determined by the instability of the patient, the skill level of the physicians, and the ability of the staff to maintain such devices. Noninvasive blood pressure monitoring provides for manual or automatic repeated, but intermittent readings. Whether a conventional sphygmomanometer or an

TABLE 64-1. Monitoring Devices Commonly Used in the PICU

MONITORING DEVICE	SITE	MEASURED VARIABLES	LIMITATIONS/CONCERNS
NONINVASIVE MONITORING TECHNIQUES			
Cardiorespiratory	Chest leads	Heart rate, rhythm, respiratory rate	Only lead II recording; difficulty with dysrhythmia recognition
Pulse oximetry	Digits, palms, ear lobe	Continuous Sa_{O_2}	Patient must be well perfused; abnormal hemoglobins and nail polish may affect results
Transcutaneous oxygen and carbon dioxide	Usually chest wall	O_2 and CO_2	Surface electrodes warm skin to 43°C, can cause thermal injury, must be changed every 3–4 hr, useful in young infants
Near-infrared spectroscopy	Forehead over CNS, back over kidneys	Tissue regional changes in oxygenation	May be difficult to differentiate superficial vs deeper tissue changes in oxygenation and perfusion
Capnography	End of the endotracheal tube	End-tidal CO_2 using breath-by-breath analysis	Capnographic trace is important to determine actual measurement; it is a true end-tidal representation of alveolar CO_2
Blood pressure	Upper arm, thigh, or calf	Cuff that allows for periodic cycling q1–15 min	Similar to cuff pressure; important to have the appropriate cuff size
Electroencephalogram	Scalp surface	Provides for continuous monitoring of cranial electrical activity	Requires a specialized technician to place the electrodes and special training in interpreting the waveforms
INVASIVE MONITORING TECHNIQUES			
Arterial	Radial, dorsalis pedis, posterior tibial, femoral, axillary (rarely brachial)	Continuous determination of blood pressure; ability to measure blood gases and other laboratory tests	Expertise in placement and monitoring needed; may require cutdown technique
Central venous access for pressure measurement (CVP) and infusion	Femoral, subclavian, internal or external jugular, antecubital, or advanced from the saphenous	Allows for CVP determination and administration of vasoactive agents and hypertonic solutions (TPN)	Requires expertise in placement, especially in very young patients; attempt to use multilumen catheters; need chest x-ray film to determine placement
Pulmonary artery catheter	Place through a sheath in the internal or external jugular, femoral, or subclavian	Allows for measurement of cardiac output, Sv_{O_2}, pulmonary artery pressure; can calculate SVR and PVR	Less commonly used in pediatrics; may assist in titration of inotropic support, vasodilators, adjustment of PEEP
ICP	Skull, with a subdural bolt, an epidural fiberoptic device, or an IVC	Measures ICP when CNS pathology is associated with cerebral edema (e.g., head injury, Reye's syndrome, or unexplained GCS score < 8)	Insertion requires a neurosurgeon; may be done at the bedside; increased risk of infection after 5 days; IVC can be used to remove fluid
Jugular bulb catheter	Internal jugular and threaded to the jugular bulb	Measured Sv_{O_2} at the jugular bulb; cerebral oxygen extraction can be calculated	Technically difficult to insert; requires training in the utility of the device and the values obtained; may allow modification of therapy

CNS, central nervous system; CVP, central venous pressure; GCS, Glasgow Coma Scale; ICP, intracranial pressure; IVC, intraventricular catheter; PEEP, positive end-expiratory pressure; PICU, pediatric intensive care unit; PVR, pulmonary vascular resistance; Sa_{O_2}, arterial oxygen saturation; Sv_{O_2}, venous oxygen saturation; SVR, systemic vascular resistance; TPN, total parenteral nutrition.

ultrasonic/Doppler device is used, appropriate cuff sizes are required to obtain an accurate blood pressure measurement. The cuff should encompass approximately ⅔ of the length of the part of the extremity from which the measurement is obtained. The upper arm, lower leg, and upper leg offer the best sites for obtaining noninvasive blood pressure measurements. Besides cuff size, factors that affect peripheral blood flow or pulmonary vascular resistance or produce significant peripheral edema may result in abnormal values for noninvasively measured blood pressure.

Because of the technical limitations of noninvasive monitoring, invasive hemodynamic monitoring may be preferred. Sites commonly used to place catheters in an artery for invasive monitoring include the radial, ulnar, posterior tibial, and dorsalis pedis arteries. Less frequently used are the femoral, axillary, and brachial arteries, and when available, the umbilical artery. Arterial lines may be inserted, either percutaneously or via cutdown, if percutaneous attempts are unsuccessful. Before an attempt is made to insert an arterial line, it is important to ensure that collateral circulation exists, if possible, by performing an **Allen test** (for radial or ulnar lines). Once the catheter is properly inserted, a pressure transducer and pressure tubing are used to connect the catheter to the monitor. A continuous pressure waveform tracing can then be displayed on the monitor screen and should be displayed along with the simultaneous ECG tracing. The arterial waveform may be helpful in diagnosing hypovolemia (very narrowed and blunted dicrotic notch), determining the severity of cardiac dysrhythmias (pulsus alternans), and evaluating the effects of respirations (air trapping) or high pericardial pressure on blood pressure (pulsus paradoxus). Arterial lines also allow for the frequent sampling of blood for various laboratory tests, including arterial blood gases, electrolytes, and coagulation panels, as needed.

Complications from arterial catheterization are rare, but may be very serious and require aggressive therapy. Bleeding and infection are relatively rare. Usually, direct pressure to the insertion site reduces further bleeding. Cutdowns may require resuturing or placing topical clotting material in the incision. Colonization around the insertion site may produce bacteremia and septicemia. The most serious complication is arterial thrombosis. This is seen in patients with low cardiac output states (shock), in patients in whom heparin was not used in the flush solution, and in patients who required prolonged catheter placement. Thrombosis necessitates immediate removal of the catheter. The use of intravenous heparin or thrombolytic therapy or topical nitroglycerin paste is indicated if the extremity continues to have evidence of poor perfusion. Other complications include vascular spasm, cutaneous mottling, arterial tears, pseudoaneurysms, peripheral nerve damage, and arteriovenous fistula formation. Temporal artery sites are associated with retrograde flow into the carotid artery, resulting in cerebrovascular accidents and therefore should be avoided. Decreased flow distal to an extremity site may result in serious necrosis of an extremity. Excellent nursing care is required to evaluate patients on a frequent and regular basis to monitor for complications. Patients with arterial lines may undergo excessive blood testing; in small infants, this may contribute to the development of anemia.

A **central venous catheter** (CVC) is required in many critically ill patients. A CVC provides important information about volume status (CVP) and permits the safe infusion of hypertonic solutions (parenteral nutrition, bicarbonate, calcium chloride, glucose) and vasoactive agents (epinephrine, norepinephrine, dopamine) that can produce severe peripheral soft tissue damage if they extravasate from peripheral lines into local tissues. Rapid infusions of large volumes of fluids or blood products are also possible.

A CVC may be inserted from different sites; the catheter is advanced into the thoracic cavity, with the tip in the inferior or superior vena cava. Sites include the femoral, subclavian, external jugular, internal jugular, antecubital and, rarely, saphenous veins. These catheters may be inserted percutaneously or via cutdown and tunneled under the skin to reduce the risk of infection. Catheter sizes vary with the size and age of the patient. Use of a multilumen catheter is ideal because this provides multiple ports for the various infusions required to care for the patient. Before the procedure, the patient should have ECG leads placed so that heart rate is monitored during the procedure to detect dysrhythmias from inadvertent intracardiac placement. The line should terminate at the atriocaval junction to minimize cardiac perforation and tamponade. An x-ray film ensures that the catheter is in the proper position. The catheter is connected via a transducer to the monitor to allow the waveform to be monitored and CVP to be obtained. A true CVP waveform contains characteristic a, c, and v waves. The presence of these waves ensures appropriate placement in the thoracic cavity, but not necessarily in the appropriate location; therefore, chest x-ray is required. Rarely, an intravenous dye contrast study or fluoroscopy may be needed to confirm placement, because some catheters are not radiopaque. Ultrasonic guidance, via images or sound (Doppler for arteries), is helpful in difficult situations.

Immediate complications of CVCs include dysrhythmias, pneumothorax, hydrothorax, hemothorax, air embolism, shearing of the vessel, intravascular loss of the guide wire, bleeding, apnea, oversedation, and airway obstruction. The patient should be monitored for any of these early complications. Infection usually occurs later and is associated with longer duration of catheter placement and the use of percutaneous vs tunneled catheters. Thrombosis is a concern because of the duration of catheter placement and the potential for associated pulmonary embolic events. The most serious and life-threatening acute or delayed complication is cardiac tamponade. This is usually caused by an intra-atrial catheter. This problem must be immediately recognized and aggressively treated.

Pulmonary artery catheters monitor the patient's hemodynamic status when the filling pressures of the right- and left-sided circulation may vary. This is common in adults after a myocardial infarction in which the left ventricle is more severely affected than the right, resulting in ventricular discordance. These catheters allow monitoring of a number of hemodynamic parameters if a balloon thermodilution catheter is used (Fig. 64-1). One can measure core temperature, CVP as well as pulmonary artery pressure and occlusion pressure, cardiac output, and mixed venous oxygen saturation, and calculate systemic and pulmonary vascular resistance, oxygen delivery, stroke volume, arteriovenous oxygen content differences, oxygen extraction ratios, and shunt fractions.

Pulmonary artery catheters are rarely used in pediatric patients. The most common indications are for cardiogenic shock; for severe distributive shock; for the use of very high ventilator pressures to achieve adequate oxygenation, allowing modulation of therapy in patients with severe pulmonary hypertension; and for perioperative management of patients who have undergone complex cardiac or other major surgery. The limitations to the use of these catheters are predominantly patient size and unfamiliarity with these catheters. The smallest thermodilution catheter is 5 French, although a single-lumen, 4-French catheter exists and is useful for measuring pulmonary artery pressure or obtaining oxygen saturation of central mixed venous blood ($M\text{v}o_2$). The single-lumen catheter does not permit measurement or calculation of the data that can be obtained from the larger catheters. Balloon catheters are able to "float" into the pulmonary artery and wedge into a distal position. This provides the pulmonary artery occlusion pressure or pulmonary capillary wedge pressure, which is usually reflective of left ventricle end-diastolic filling pressure. Once this number is determined, the balloon is deflated and allowed to remain in the pulmonary artery. This minimizes potential complications of pulmonary artery erosion or infarction. Other complications include dys-

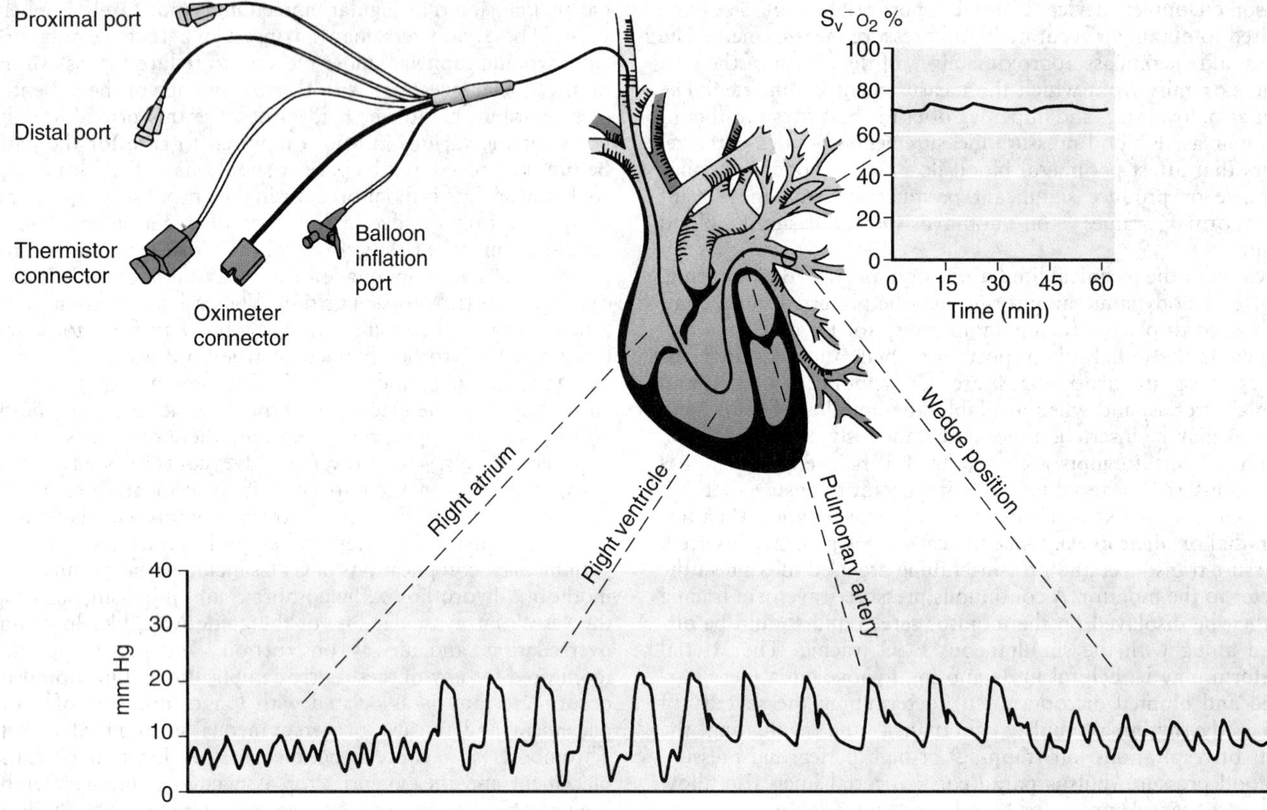

Figure 64-1. Components and functional features of a thermodilution flow-directed balloon flotation pulmonary artery catheter. A flexible multilumen catheter with the balloon at the distal tip inflated is in the wedge position. The proximal ends of the 5 lumens are labeled. The distal port is connected to a pressure measurement system for catheter insertion and subsequent monitoring. When the distal tip is within the central venous circulation, the balloon is inflated to enhance flow direction of the tip through the right atrium into the right ventricle and then to the pulmonary artery. Recorded pressures in the lower part of the figure correspond to these locations, confirming the course of the catheter. The last tracing on the right is that corresponding to the "wedge" position, commonly reflecting the pressure transmitted from the left atrium via the pulmonary veins and fiberoptic monitor available on adult-sized catheters. (Redrawn from Daily EK, Tilkian AG: Hemodynamic monitoring. In Tilkian AG, Daily EK [editors]: *Cardiovascular Procedures, Diagnostic Techniques and Therapeutic Procedures*. St. Louis, CV Mosby, 1986.)

rhythmias, damage to the pulmonic valve, coiling in the right ventricle, balloon rupture, and infection. When these complications occur, the pulmonary artery catheter must be removed.

PULMONARY MONITORING. Monitoring requirements for patients who require significant respiratory support include blood gas determination, from arterial or, less frequently, capillary and venous blood gases. Arterial blood gas sampling requires a special technique similar to inserting an arterial line. Measuring capillary gases usually involves the use of the infant's heel. It must be warmed to "arterialize" the blood. In the laboratory, a blood gas analyzer measures partial pressure of oxygen (Po_2), partial pressure of carbon dioxide $(Pco)_2$, and pH; the bicarbonate value is usually calculated from pH and Po_2. The pH and partial pressure of carbon dioxide (Pco_2) from a capillary or venous sample should closely resemble the arterial blood gas sample. However, capillary Po_2 does not correlate well with arterial partial pressure of oxygen (Pao_2), and when peripheral blood flow is adversely affected, all other parameters obtained from capillary blood gases may not correlate. Capillary and venous blood gas sampling have significant limitations.

Intermittent blood gas sampling is labor-intensive and expensive. However, it provides the most reliable assessment of acid-base and ventilation-oxygenation status in the critically ill patient. When the patient's clinical status requires both continuous blood pressure monitoring and frequent assessments of respiratory status, an indwelling arterial line is indicated. Devices can provide continuous pH, $Paco_2$, and Pao_2 values when the monitoring catheter is placed in an artery; blood flows from the catheter into a closed-loop system, passing the blood gas electrodes. Data are obtained continuously or intermittently. These devices are expensive and require blood vessels of sufficient size to permit the insertion of a large catheter (at least 20-gauge). These devices are useful when placed in central venous lines and used in conjunction with pulse oximetry; this combination shows good correlation of venous pH with arterial pH and of venous Pco_2 with arterial $Paco_2$.

Point-of-care testing in the intensive care environment is more expensive, yet more expedient, and provides valuable information in minutes and at the bedside. Point-of-care testing may be accomplished with a handheld device that is also useful in the transport environment; in areas where the patient is not in the PICU, but must have blood gas analysis performed, such as a radiographic imaging suite; or when the patient's condition is so unstable that an instantaneous analysis is required. These simple devices may perform a number of other analyses, such as measuring serum electrolytes, glucose, creatinine, urea, ionized calcium, and hematocrit.

A variety of noninvasive devices and monitors have improved the care of critically ill children. Transcutaneous instruments permit the simultaneous determination of transcutaneous carbon dioxide tension ($Tcco_2$) and transcutaneous oxygen tension (Tco_2). Bicarbonate levels or pH cannot be measured by transcutaneous monitoring. Other limitations include skin thickness; transcutaneous monitoring is limited to smaller infants. Transcutaneous electrodes must be warmed to 43°C, which may cause burns, and they must be changed every 3–4 hr. The electrodes take 20 min to calibrate; this must be done every 4 hr. Thus, there may be various delays in obtaining important blood gas information. The major advantage of transcutaneous monitoring is the ability to follow $Paco_2$ continuously, permitting more rapid ventilator adjustments and facilitating weaning as well as reducing the costs associated with blood gas analysis.

End-tidal CO_2 ($EtCO_2$) analysis (capnography) measures the Pco_2 in exhaled gas. This technique is used in patients who are intubated and have minimal lung disease without significant intrapulmonary shunting. Capnography is based on the principle that the highest concentration of CO_2 sampled in the respiratory circuit represents the alveolar CO_2 concentration, which should be close to the arterial ($Paco_2$) concentration. Gas is constantly monitored from a side port to the connector from the ventilator to the endotracheal tube. A small amount of gas is diverted from the respiratory circuit and analyzed in a spectrophotometer to determine $Paco_2$. The removal of small amounts of respiratory gas must be accounted for when calculating delivered and exhaled tidal volumes.

In interpreting $Etco_2$ results, it is necessary to evaluate the graphic picture of the exhalation capnographic image to ensure that the alveolar plateau and peak are achieved. Patients who have significant intrapulmonary shunts or are spontaneously breathing may not produce an acceptable capnographic trace, thus invalidating $EtCO_2$ monitoring. This device permits trending and the potential for weaning patients from mechanical ventilation; it does not replace blood gas analysis.

Capnography can also determine if the trachea has been intubated, and it is useful in emergent intubations. Using an analyzer that changes color on exposure to levels of CO_2 permits differentiation between esophageal and tracheal intubations. The CO_2 concentration in the stomach is very low, approaching atmospheric levels of close to zero, whereas that in the lungs is markedly higher. With cardiopulmonary arrest and absent pulmonary blood flow, $Etco_2$ will also be undetectable. Successful reestablishment of the circulation can also be assessed by an elevation of $Etco_2$.

Pulse oximetry is the standard for noninvasive bedside oxygenation monitoring. Pulse oximetry can be used in patients of all ages and does not usually cause tissue damage. Its accuracy is dependent on adequate tissue perfusion; its utility is limited in patients with significant vasoconstriction and poor peripheral perfusion. Pulse oximetry measures oxygen saturation, not the partial pressure of a gas. This is important in interpreting the significance of the value obtained. Normally, arterial oxygen saturation is 95% or more (except in patients with cyanotic congenital heart lesions). Although pulse oximetry does not provide PaO_2, it provides information that is just as good, if not better, regarding real-time oxygen saturation. It permits rapid assessment of oxygenation of a critically ill patient. It requires little, if any, warm-up time and is extremely portable, enabling assessment of oxygenation of patients not only in the PICU, but also during transport (see Chapter 63), during procedures that require conscious sedation, and in various settings outside the ICU, such as the emergency department or office. The information is extremely reliable and relatively inexpensive compared with blood gas analysis. Pulse oximetry does not provide direct measurements of Pco_2, acid-base status, or bicarbonate levels.

NEAR-INFARED SPECTROSCOPY. Light in the near-red spectrum (700–1000 nm) can pass through skin, bone, and other tissues, and can help detect changes in regional oxygenation and perfusion, such as the brain and kidneys. It is most often used to continuously monitor changes in regional perfusion during and after cardiac surgery (Fig. 64-2).

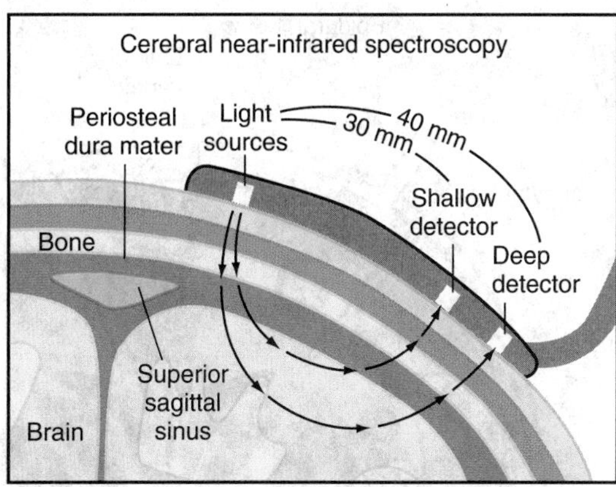

Figure 64-2. Cerebral near-infrared spectroscopy allows detection of potential brain compromise before it occurs or as it is occurring. It uses a small adhesive patch applied across the forehead that reads reflected light waves. (Redrawn courtesy of Children's Hospital of Wisconsin, Milwaukee, Wisconsin.)

NEUROPHYSIOLOGIC MONITORING. Neurologic monitoring involves careful clinical observation accompanied by highly technical noninvasive devices (electroencephalography, evoked potentials, near-infrared spectroscopy), or invasive catheters placed to monitor intracranial pressure (ICP).

Acute neurologic deterioration is the reason for a significant number of PICU admissions. Trauma, tumors, infections, seizures, vascular malformation, strokes, hypoxia, or various metabolic disorders may produce serious neurologic injury. An experienced PICU nurse should be able to perform careful serial clinical neurologic examinations. These frequent examinations are done to evaluate the cranial nerves, especially the pupillary reflexes, and score a modified Glasgow Coma Scale (GCS) for infants and children. The GCS provides a method to quantitate the patient's level of consciousness and ability to respond to painful stimuli in an easy and standard format (see Chapter 66). The scores range from 3–15. Most patients with a score of <12 should be observed in the PICU until they are stable enough to be cared for in less intensely monitored areas.

Advanced techniques in electrophysiologic monitoring enable monitoring of the brain's electrical activity through continuous **electroencephalograms (EEGs)**. Managing a child with severe status epilepticus helps to determine if anticonvulsant drugs are affecting both the electrical and the clinical seizure activity. Patients who have refractory seizures may require a barbiturate coma; monitoring EEG activity facilitates the suppression of seizure activity. Clinical examinations are not useful in patients requiring paralytic agents or heavy sedation; the ability to monitor seizures through continuous EEGs is essential. In interpreting the data, it is important to remember that artifacts can be produced from the various monitors, ventilators, or other electrical equipment commonly found in the ICU setting. Video-EEG permits recording of the electrical changes associated with a seizure and allows the changes to be correlated with the clinical picture.

Evoked potentials enable evaluation of a variety of sensory pathways that include visual evoked responses, brainstem auditory evoked potentials, and somatosensory evoked potentials. These are not affected by sedative medications, which may produce an isoelectric EEG. The brainstem and somatosensory tests are the most commonly performed evoked potential studies. They may serve as an aid in providing prognostic information. Their utility in diagnosing brain death is not well recognized.

The **bispectral index (BIS)** can be used to monitor the neurologic status of both sedated and unsedated critically ill patients. BIS is a statistically derived variable that provides information about the interaction of brain cortical and subcortical regions. The BIS score ranges from 0–100 and is a reliable index of the state of consciousness in normal subjects. Scores >95 indicate full

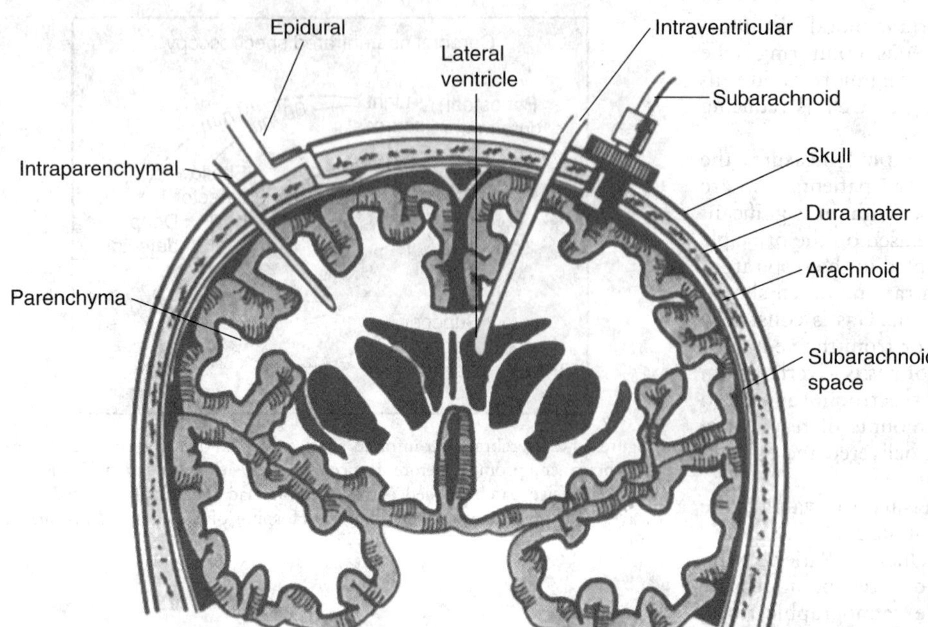

Figure 64-3. Sites for monitoring intracranial pressure. A variety of monitor types are shown. Intraventricular catheters are most often fluid-filled tubes connected by pressure tubing to a pressure transducer. Cerebrospinal fluid (CSF) can be withdrawn through the catheter. Subarachnoid (also subdural) monitors are fluid-filled, hollow devices that can be bolted to the calvaria and connected by pressure tubing to a pressure transducer. CSF cannot be withdrawn. Epidural monitors are wafer-like devices of several types that are placed in the epidural space. They can be used to monitor intraparenchymal pressure, but cannot withdraw CSF. (Redrawn from Lyons MK, Meyer FB: Cerebrospinal fluid physiology and the management of increased intracranial pressure. *Mayo Clin Proc* 1990;65:684.)

consciousness. Of sedated patients, 95% are unconscious if the BIS score is 50. BIS correlates with the depth of sedation of patients who require mechanical ventilation and sedation after surgery or medical illness. BIS has been proposed as a guide to prevent oversedation in the critically ill. Unfortunately, the BIS score may be complicated if the EEG also reflects changes in the neurologic status of the patient that are caused by the illness itself. Another form of neuromonitoring is done using transcranial oxygen saturation. This device is capable of measuring oxygen saturation using infrared technology of the intracranial blood vessels. It is helpful in children undergoing cardiac surgery who require bypass. Monitoring may continue in the immediate postoperative period until the patient emerges from anesthesia. It may have greater application in the management of children with severe central nervous system injuries, where treatment is focused on the delivery of oxygen and substrate to the injured tissue.

Radionuclide imaging is rarely performed in the PICU; it may provide some useful information about cerebral blood flow. A portable gamma camera allows tests to be performed at the bedside. Cerebral blood flow studies allow the confirmation of brain death if there is equivocation. It also permits quantification of cerebral blood flow to injured areas of the brain. The clinical significance of this is unclear.

Invasive neurologic monitoring involves ICP monitoring and jugular bulb catheterization. Indications for ICP monitoring include any acute neurologic deterioration in which elevated ICP may produce further injury to the patient. Usually, acute traumatic events in patients with a GCS score of <8 require a monitoring device inserted either in the operating room or at the bedside in the PICU. The type of device and how it is inserted are usually the responsibility of the neurosurgeon placing the device (Fig. 64-3). Ventriculostomy or intraparenchymal, subdural, or subarachnoid placement of catheters can be used. All but the intraparenchymal catheters are connected to the transducer via a fluid-filled tubing device. Ventriculostomy and intraparenchymal fiberoptic devices are the most reliable and most commonly used devices for monitoring ICP. A ventricular catheter allows not only measurement of ICP, but also removal of fluid, if necessary, thereby providing a therapeutic option. The intraparenchymal fiberoptic system provides a very reliable method for ICP measurement, but does not permit the removal of cerebrospinal fluid. It is not a fluid-filled system, but is easy to use.

The device is connected to a transducer and then to the monitor. It produces a waveform with a numeric value. The ICP should be <20 cm H_2O. When monitoring ICP, it is imperative that systemic arterial blood pressure be determined simultaneously. The difference between the mean arterial pressure and the ICP is the cerebral perfusion pressure. This should be >50 in older patients and slightly less in younger children. Complications associated with ICP monitoring include bleeding (check coagulation factors before insertion), infection if the device is left in for >5 days, injury to the brain parenchyma (usually only intraventricular catheters), and cerebrospinal fluid leak.

Jugular bulb monitoring enables continuous oxygen saturation measurements to be obtained using an indwelling fiberoptic catheter placed in the jugular vein and advanced cephalad to the level of the jugular bulb. The values obtained correlate with the jugular Pa_{O_2} content and do not require blood sampling for actual determination of oxygen saturation. The jugular bulb is located at the base of the skull, just outside the jugular foramen. It is the point of exit of the blood draining most of the cerebral hemispheres. The clinician is provided with information that indicates how well the injured brain is using oxygen. If the saturation of oxygen in the systemic arterial and jugular veins is known, it is possible to calculate the arteriojugular difference for oxygen. This is normally 4–9 mg/dL. Lower levels indicate cerebral hyperemia, and the clinician may select therapies designed to decrease cerebral blood flow. Levels >10 mg/dL may indicate ischemia and necessitate further tests to determine the extent of brain injury. The values obtained for ICP, the arteriojugular difference for oxygen, and cerebral blood flow may help alter therapy to improve outcome.

Gilbert TT, Wagner MR, Halukurike V, et al: Use of bispectral electroencephalogram monitoring to assess neurologic status in unsedated, critically ill patients. *Crit Care Med* 2001;29:1996–2000.

Grindstaff RJ, Tobias JD: Applications of bispectral index monitoring in the pediatric intensive care unit. *J Intensive Car Med* 2004;19:111–116.

The National Heart, Lung, and Blood Institute Acute Respiratory Distress Syndrome (ARDS) Clinical Trials Network: Pulmonary-artery versus central venous catheter toguide treatment of acute lung injury. *N Engl J Med* 2006;354:2213–2224.

Tobias JD, Connors D, Strauser L, et al: Continuous pH and P_{CO_2} monitoring during respiratory failure in children with the Paratrend 7 inserted into the peripheral venous system. *J Pediatr* 2000;136:623–627.

Chapter 65 ■ Scoring Systems and Predictors of Mortality Joseph DiCarlo and Lorry R. Frankel

Scoring systems are useful for making triage decisions and assessing the performance of an intensive care unit (ICU), but they are of limited use in predicting prognosis in individual cases. Various scoring systems are currently used in the pediatric intensive care unit (PICU). These include: (1) **organ-specific** systems, such as the Glasgow Coma Scale (see Chapter 66 and Table 66-5) or the croup score (see Chapter 382); (2) **mechanism-of-injury** systems, such as the Pediatric Trauma Score (see Table 71-2) or Injury Severity Score; and (3) **pediatric** systems, such as the Pediatric Index of Mortality (PIM) and the Pediatric Risk of Mortality (PRISM).

PEDIATRIC RISK OF MORTALITY. This system, a revision of the Physiologic Stability Index (PSI), assesses the severity of illness in a population of pediatric patients. The PRISM, in its 3rd iteration (PRISM III), is used to compare and evaluate performance and resource use among various PICUs. It is based on 17 physiologic variables subdivided into 26 ranges (Fig. 65-1). The patient's medical history is also taken into account, particularly chronic illness and previous PICU days. The PRISM score has a consistently strong relationship between the number of malfunctioning organ systems at 12 and 24 hr and the mortality risk in a given PICU. *PRISM is designed for population assessments and is not valid for decision-making for an individual patient.* PRISM is most useful in assessing case mix adjustments between units and the overall outcomes for a population of patients in a PICU. PRISM can determine if a PICU is performing on a par with standards that are periodically calibrated to a reference population. If performance is below standard, a chart review may show the reasons, such as high secondary infection rates, comorbidity issues, and decisions to withdraw or limit therapy. Changes in the score over time may document improvement or deterioration. As a performance assessment tool, PRISM is applied either periodically or constantly, depending on institutional data-collecting capabilities. PRISM is also useful in research in ensuring that control and experimental groups are similar.

PEDIATRIC INDEX OF MORTALITY. The PIM uses a logistic regression model to predict population mortality risk. It is based on 8 physiologic variables. Its 2nd iteration, PIM2, has been calibrated to a cohort of >20,000 children in 14 ICUs in Australia, New Zealand, and Great Britain. Its algorithm is available at no charge. Its ease of use has made it a relatively popular tool for assessment of both ICU performance and research population comparisons.

PEDIATRIC TRAUMA SCORE. This score takes into account a child's size, the accessibility of the airway, the systolic blood pressure, the level of consciousness, and the presence or absence of wounds and fractures. Below a certain cutoff, transfer to a dedicated trauma center is recommended (see Chapter 71).

OTHER PHYSIOLOGIC SCORING SYSTEMS. Other scoring systems are less useful in pediatrics. The Acute Physiology and Chronic Health Evaluation (APACHE) system is used widely in adult ICUs, but PRISM III is better suited to the physiology of a child. The Therapeutic Intervention Scoring System (TISS) relies on the type and amount of therapy given and therefore may indirectly reflect the severity of illness and directly reflect resource usage. A single calculation, the Oxygenation Index [OI = (FIO_2 × mean airway pressure)/PaO_2] is predictive of survival in many forms of respiratory failure.

Gemke RJ, van Vught J: Scoring systems in pediatric intensive care: PRISM III versus PIM. *Intensive Care Med* 2002;28:2004–2007.

Meyer S, Gottschling S, Biran T, et al: Assessing the risk of mortality in paediatric cancer patients admitted to the paediatric intensive care unit: A novel risk score? *Eur J Pediatr* 2005;164:563–567.

Michel E, Zernikow B: Can PRISM predict length of PICU stay? An analysis of 2000 cases. *Med Inform Internet Med* 2003;28:209–219.

Perondi MBM, Reis AG, Paiva EF, et al: A comparison of high dose and standard dose epinephrine in children with cardiac arrest. *N Engl J Med* 2004;350:1722–1730.

Slater A, Shann F, Pearson G, et al: PIM2: A revised version of the Paediatric Index of Mortality. *Intensive Care Med* 2003;29:278–285.

Chapter 66 ■ Pediatric Emergencies and Resuscitation Lawrence H. Mathers and Lorry R. Frankel

Each year in the United States >150,000 emergencies threaten the lives of children; approximately 10,000 of these children die (of the total of ≈ 55,000 annual pediatric deaths overall), and at least 90,000 survive with permanent disability. These emergencies may need immediate treatment in various settings (home, community, hospital). Bystander rescuers, parents, or health care providers may have to provide immediate resuscitation while simultaneously activating the emergency care system and facilitating patient transport to the nearest appropriate facility. Because of the growing number of children with increased vulnerability to serious illness, such as surviving premature infants and children with chronic disease, it is critical to know how to respond to pediatric emergencies (see Chapter 62).

Pediatric emergencies are of various types: respiratory, cardiac, endocrine, traumatic, and infectious. Most pediatric arrests are respiratory, not cardiac. Sudden, unanticipated, nontraumatic cardiac arrests are uncommon in children, in contrast to the primary nature of cardiac arrest in adults from ischemic heart disease and subsequent ventricular fibrillation or ventricular tachycardia. Cardiac arrests in children may develop in the presence of known (preoperative or postoperative congenital heart disease) or unknown (hypertrophic cardiomyopathy, aberrant coronary arteries, prolonged Q-T syndrome, critical aortic stenosis) lesions during strenuous exercise in adolescents (see Chapter 436).

Respiratory arrests are even more common in children with pre-existing chronic lung disease or those who become acutely ill with shock or airway compromise (Table 66-1). Respiratory failure can become a preterminal event after severe asthma, pneumonia, submersions, trauma, sepsis, and foreign body or gastric content aspiration.

Pediatric cardiopulmonary arrests in a hospital setting are usually initially respiratory arrests and are often predictable. Apnea usually precedes bradycardia with poor perfusion; many patients have a pre-existing chronic life-threatening or life-shortening condition. In the hospital, the 1st recorded electrocardiogram (ECG) is asystole in >50%; pulseless electrical activity in approximately 10%; bradycardia with poor perfusion in 25%; and ventricular fibrillation or pulseless ventricular tachycardia in approximately 15%. The older the patient, the higher the likelihood of ventricular fibrillation or ventricular tachycardia, dys-

PRISM III

CARDIOVASCULAR/NEUROLOGIC VITAL SIGNS (1–6)

Systolic blood pressure (mm Hg)
Measurement ______________

	Score = 3	Score = 7
Neonate	40–55	<40
Infant	45–65	<45
Child	55–75	<55
Adolescent	65–85	<65

Heart rate (beats/min)
Measurement ______________

	Score = 3	Score = 4
Neonate	215–225	>225
Infant	215–225	>225
Child	185–205	>205
Adolescent	145–155	>155

Temperature
Measurement ______________

	Score = 3
All ages	<33°C (91.4°F) or >40.0°C (104.0°F)

Pupillary Reflexes
Measurement ______________

	Score = 7	Score = 11
All ages	One fixed	Both fixed one reactive

Mental status
Measurement ______________

	Score = 5
All ages	Stupor/Coma (GCS <8)

ACID-BASE/BLOOD GASES (1, 2, 7, 8)

Acidosis (Total CO_2 (mmol/L) or pH)
Measurement ______________

	Score = 2	Score = 6
All ages	pH 7.0–7.28	pH <7.0
or total	CO_2 5–16.9	or total CO_2 <5

Total CO_2 (mmol/L)
Measurement ______________

	Score = 4
All ages	>34.0

pH
Measurement ______________

	Score = 2	Score = 3
All ages	7.48–7.55	>7.55

PaO_2 (mm Hg)
Measurement ______________

	Score = 3	Score = 6
All ages	42.0–49.9	<42.0

PCO_2 (mm Hg)
Measurement ______________

	Score = 1	Score = 3
All ages	50.0–75.0	>75.0

CHEMISTRY TESTS (1, 2, 9)

Glucose
Measurement ______________

	Score = 2
All ages	>200 mg/dL or >11.0 mmol/L

Potassium (mmol/L)
Measurement ______________

	Score = 3
All ages	>6.9

Creatinine
Measurement ______________

	Score = 2
Neonate	>0.85 mg/dL or >75 μmol/L
Infant	>0.90 mg/dL or >80 μmol/L
Child	>0.90 mg/dL or >80 μmol/L
Adolescent	>1.30 mg/dL or >115 μmol/L

Blood urea nitrogen (BUN)
Measurement ______________

	Score = 3
Neonate	>11.9 mg/dL or >4.3 mmol/L
All other ages	>14.9 mg/dL or >5.4 mmol/L

HEMATOLOGY TESTS (1, 2)

White blood cell count (cells/mm³)
Measurement ______________

	Score = 4
All ages	<3,000

Prothrombin time (PT) or partial thromboplastin time (PTT) (sec)
Measurement ______________

	Score = 3
Neonate	PT >22.0 or PTT >85.0
All other ages	PT >22.0 or PTT >57.0

Platelet Count (cells/mm³)
Measurement ______________

	Score = 2	Score = 4	Score = 5
All ages	100,000–200,000	50,000–99,999	<50,000

TOTAL PRISM III SCORE __________

OTHER FACTORS (10)

☐ Nonoperative CV disease ☐ Chromosomal anomaly ☐ Cancer ☐ Previous PICU admission
☐ Pre-ICU CPR ☐ Postoperative ☐ Acute diabetes (e.g. DKA) ☐ Admission from inpatient unit (exclude postoperative patients)

Notes:

1. PRISM III mortality risk equations are available for the first 12 hr and the first 24 hr of PICU care.
2. General: Use the highest and/or the lowest values for scoring. When there are both low and high ranges, PRISM III points may be assigned for the low and the high ranges. Readmissions are included as separate patients. Exclude admissions routinely cared for in other hospital locations, staying in the PICU <2 hr; and those admitted in continuous CPR who do not achieve stable vital signs for ≥2 hr. Deaths occurring in the OR are included only if the operation occurred during the PICU stay and was a therapy for the illness requiring PICU care. Terminally ill patients transferred from the PICU for "comfort care" are included as PICU patients for the 24 hr following PICU discharge or, if receiving technologic support, until 24 hr after the technologic support is discontinued. Ages: neonate = 0–<1 month; infant = ≥1 mon–12 mon; child = ≥12–144 mon; adolescent >144 mon.
3. Heart Rate: Do not assess during crying or iatrogenic agitation.
4. Temperature: Use rectal, oral, blood, or axillary temperatures.
5. Pupillary Reflexes: Nonreactive pupils must be >3 mm. Do not assess after iatrogenic pupillary dilatation.
6. Mental Status: Include only patients with known or suspected, acute CNS disease. Do not assess within 2 hours of sedation, paralysis, or anesthesia. If there is constant paralysis and/or sedation, use the time period without sedation, paralysis, or anesthesia closest to the PICU admission for scoring. Stupor/coma is defined as GCS score <8 or stupor/coma using other mental status scales.
7. Acid-Base: Use calculated bicarbonate values from blood gases only if total CO_2 is not measured routinely. PCO_2 and pH may be measured from arterial, capillary, or venous sites.
8. PaO_2: Use arterial measurements only.
9. Whole Blood Corrections: Whole blood measurements should be increased as follows: glucose - 10%; sodium - 3 mmol/L; potassium - 0.4 mmol/L. (Pediatric Reference Ranges, Soldin SJ, Hicks JM eds, AACC Press, Washington, D.C., 1995).
10. Nonoperative CV disease includes acute cardiac and vascular conditions as the primary reasons for admission. Cancer and chromosomal anomalies are acute or chronic. Previous PICU admission and pre-PICU CPR refer to the current hospital admission. CPR requires cardiac massage. Post-operative is the initial 24 hr following an OR surgical procedure. Catheterizations are not post-operative. Acute diabetes includes acute manifestation of diabetes (e.g. DKA) as the primary reason for PICU admission. Admission from routine care area includes all inpatient locations except the operating or recovery rooms.

Figure 65-1. Pediatric Risk of Mortality III (PRISM III) score. Numbers in *parentheses* refer to notes. CNS, central nervous system; CV, cardiovascular; DKA, diabetic ketoacidosis; GCS, Glasgow Coma Scale; ICU, intensive care unit; PaO_2, PCO_2; PICU, pediatric intensive care unit. (Adapted from Pollack MM, Patel KM, Ruttimann UE: PRISM III: An updated pediatric risk of mortality score. *Crit Care Med* 1996;24:743–752.)

TABLE 66-1. Respiratory Emergencies

UPPER AIRWAY OBSTRUCTION

The child usually presents in obvious respiratory distress, with stridor or leaning with the chin forward and drooling.

Do not put instruments into the airway unless prepared to intubate immediately. This is especially risky in presumed epiglottitis and bacterial tracheitis or when a foreign body is present.

A lateral neck radiograph can show an enlarged epiglottis at base of the tongue or possibly a foreign body.

The major challenge is to avoid irritation of the airway, which can precipitate complete airway obstruction.

SMALL AIRWAYS

Usually this is an exacerbation of a previously existing condition, such as asthma, cystic fibrosis, or bronchopulmonary dysplasia. Patients present with wheezing.

Mucus and/or bronchospasm causes air trapping—inspired air enters the alveoli more easily than it leaves them. As a result, the distal airways and alveoli distend with gas, and efficient exchange is impaired. Pneumothorax may also occur.

In extreme cases, status asthmaticus or bronchiolitis can be fatal.

Necessary steps for therapy are oxygen, bronchodilators (aerosols and intravenous), steroids (delayed action), relaxation, and reassurance.

PNEUMONIA

Impaired gas exchange is due to alveolar injury; it usually involves surfactant deficiency, plus fluid in the alveoli.

Therapy includes: oxygen, antibiotics, and mechanical ventilatory support for serious disease.

Parenchymal disease increases the tendency for intrapulmonary shunts, increasing the hypoxia.

Pneumonia becomes life-threatening only when large portions of the lungs are involved.

Sickle cell acute chest syndrome is particularly dangerous.

rhythmias that would be much more common in adults with life-threatening events.

The proper response to each emergency requires an awareness of the mechanisms of disease and the immediate physiologic threats and their proper treatment. A number of factors contribute to the physiologic instability of infants and young children (Table 66-2). Children who are at risk for recurring life-threatening illnesses (seizure disorders, asthma, cardiac dysrhythmias) may be able to take precautions to minimize the risk of such threats. Parental vigilance and anticipation of potential dangers in the home, especially for young children, can prevent many injuries and deaths (see Chapter 61).

Emergency personnel should have an approach that will allow them, in the best interest of the patient, to refrain from initiating or continuing resuscitations when efforts are futile. With many chronically ill children being cared for at home or in care facilities, emergency personnel may be presented with an advance directive or another document indicating the wish that resuscitation not be performed. It may be difficult to interrupt or not to initiate a resuscitative effort on the basis of these documents unless a community-wide means of establishing their credibility is developed.

TABLE 66-2. Factors Contributing to Infant Physiologic Instability

TEMPERATURE

Neonates have thin skin (radiating heat) and underdeveloped hypothalamic control. They lack the efficient neural mechanisms for temperature control (e.g., shivering) and are greatly influenced by environmental temperature.

FLUID REQUIREMENTS

Thin skin allows more evaporation; fluid content in an infant's body is higher than in an adult's (75–80% in newborn); kidneys reabsorb electrolytes inefficiently; infants need proportionately more fluid per unit of weight than adults.

AIRWAY

The airway is small and narrow; resistance to gas flow is inversely proportional to the 4th power of the radius, so small mucous obstructions can seriously threaten air movement; laryngeal and tracheal cartilages are softer than in adults and more easily collapse to obstruct the airway.

CARDIAC OUTPUT

Heart rate is the major mechanism for varying cardiac output.

GLUCOSE METABOLISM

Newborn infants, especially, have only marginal glycogen stores and may mobilize fat poorly; hypoglycemia occurs more readily than in adults, because of dependence on an exogenous supply of glucose.

TABLE 66-3. Vital Signs at Various Ages

AGE	HEART RATE (BEATS/MIN)	BLOOD PRESSURE (MM HG)	RESPIRATORY RATE (BREATHS/MIN)
Premature	120–170*	55–75/35–45†	40–70‡
0–3 mo	100–150*	65–85/45–55	35–55
3–6 mo	90–120	70–90/50–65	30–45
6–12 mo	80–120	80–100/55–65	25–40
1–3 yr	70–110	90–105/55–70	20–30
3–6 yr	65–110	95–110/60–75	20–25
6–12 yr	60–95	100–120/60–75	14–22
12⁺ yr	55–85	110–135/65–85	12–18

*In sleep, infant heart rates may drop significantly lower, but if perfusion is maintained, no intervention is required.

†A blood pressure cuff should cover approximately 2/3 of the arm; too small a cuff yields spuriously high pressure readings, and too large a cuff yields spuriously low pressure readings.

‡Many premature infants require mechanical ventilatory support, making their spontaneous respiratory rate less relevant.

LIFE-THREATENING EMERGENCIES AND PRE-ARREST STATES IN CHILDREN

The most common life-threatening illnesses in children are those involving respiratory (see Chapters 69 and 419), cardiac (see Chapters 434 and 442), or neurologic (see Chapter 67) failure. Acute failure of the liver (see Chapter 361), kidneys (see Chapter 535), or adrenals (see Chapter 576) also places pediatric patients at risk. Identifying the cause of various types of organ failure may take considerable time, but treatment of the physiologically unstable child must begin immediately.

DETECTING AND ASSESSING PHYSIOLOGIC INSTABILITY. A simple and consistent approach is necessary for rapid and efficient evaluation of a pediatric patient who may be in serious distress. Observation begins with determination of the alertness of the patient, including response to stimuli, spontaneous vocalization or movement, and muscle tone. In basic life support, this is assessed by asking, "Are you all right?" This is followed by assessment of the vital signs (Table 66-3) and other basic indicators of the physiologic state.

PULSE AND HEART RATE. The ability to detect a pulse in the compromised patient is unreliable among many lay rescuers. Medical professionals and parents of chronically ill children who were taught to palpate a pulse should do so as part of the initial assessment (Table 66-4). Lay rescuers should check for other physical signs of adequate circulation (breathing, movement, coughing, color), but should not check for a pulse. In children younger than age 8 yr or those with trauma, near-drowning, a drug overdose, or other obvious respiratory causes of an arrest, resuscitation should begin before activation of emergency medical services (EMS; the *phone fast* protocol). In children older than age 8 yr, those with a history of cardiac disease, and those who experience a sudden collapse during exercise, ventricular fibrillation or ventricular tachycardia may be present. This situation creates a more urgent need to activate EMS to be able to initiate defibrillation, if needed, as soon as possible. Therefore, the **phone first proto-**

TABLE 66-4. Chest Compression: Ventilation Relationships

	NEONATE	1–8 YR	>8 YR
Compression rate	120	At least 100	100
*Compression-ventilation ratio**	3 : 1	5 : 1	15 : 2†
Pulse check‡	Umbilical artery	Brachial	Carotid

*Ventilation should be given without interrupting chest compression. It is asynchronous.

†Once intubated, go to 5 : 1.

‡For lay rescuers, no pulse check is necessary; it actually delays cardiopulmonary resuscitation. Lay rescuers should check for signs of circulation: cyanosis, breathing, coughing, and movement.

col with a lone rescuer involves activating EMS before formal resuscitation begins. If 2 rescuers are present, then activation of EMS and resuscitation occur simultaneously. Many community settings (shopping malls, airports, high schools) are equipped with automatic external defibrillators that can be used to rapidly assess the rhythm and to defibrillate (if needed) any child older than 8 yr.

When a child's heart rate lies outside the normal physiologic parameters, cardiac output may be affected. A rapid heart rate (supraventricular tachycardia or ventricular tachycardia) may be associated with a serious reduction in stroke volume, as reflected in poor perfusion (see Chapter 435). Cardiac failure may develop with pulmonary edema (see Chapter 69). Bradycardia may also represent a serious pre-arrest condition (see Chapter 435). Alternatively, the change in heart rate may reflect an appropriate physiologic response (sinus tachycardia) and may not necessarily constitute significant cardiac pathophysiology. Sinus tachycardia may be distinguished from supraventricular tachycardia (SVT) by the history as well as by the presence of upright P waves in sinus tachycardia in leads I and aVF, whereas SVT may show negative P waves in leads II, III, and aVF. Sinus tachycardia has a rate that is usually <220 beats/min in infants and <180 beats/min in children. SVT has an abrupt onset and an abrupt termination and can be terminated by vagal maneuvers (Valsalva maneuver, application of an ice-water bag to the face), intravenous adenosine, or synchronized cardioversion (0.5–1 J/kg).

BLOOD PRESSURE. Blood pressure (BP) is most often measured by auscultation, but automated devices such as the Dinamap (GE Medical Systems) can be set to measure BP repeatedly and at very short intervals (see Chapter 445). To help define poor perfusion, the lower limit of systolic BP should be <60 mm Hg for neonates; <70 mm Hg from 1 mo–1 yr; <70 mm Hg + 2 × age from 1–10 yr; and <90 mm Hg if older than age 10 yr.

ORGAN PERFUSION. Adequate cardiac output is reflected in good perfusion of the skin (central and in distal extremities). Skin perfusion may be assessed by the temperature of the skin or by capillary refill time (the time required for color to return to the skin after pressure blanching is released). Normal capillary refill time is 2 sec or less; however, low environmental temperature may cause peripheral vasoconstriction and lengthening of capillary refill time. Pulse oximetry measures hemoglobin oxygen saturation; because adequate perfusion is required to produce reliable measurements, a strong signal indicates good peripheral perfusion.

The normal temperature range for humans is constant throughout life. Premature infants and small term infants may have difficulty maintaining their appropriate core temperature if they are left uncovered in a cool environment. Infants may not be able to generate an elevated temperature in response to infection (see Chapter 109).

RESPIRATORY EFFORT AND GAS EXCHANGE. Muscle retractions in the chest and neck and flaring of the nostrils at inspiration are signs of an abnormally high level of effort required to move air into the lungs. Grunting is a moaning, crying-like noise at expiration, associated with generation of positive pressure to maintain alveolar patency. A child who is inadequately oxygenated demonstrates cyanosis (blue or dusky color of the skin and mucous membranes) [see Chapters 69 and 371]. Although observations of respiratory effort provide useful information about impending respiratory failure, arterial blood gases provide a more accurate assessment of respiratory gas exchange (see Chapters 69 and 371) and evidence of a lactic acidosis due to poor perfusion.

CARDIAC DYSRHYTHMIAS. See Chapter 435. Disturbances in cardiac rate and rhythm are not rare in children; the majority of these dysrhythmias are transient and have no hemodynamic significance. Life-threatening cardiac emergencies in children are more likely to be bradycardia or asystole than ventricular fibrillation, which is more common in adolescents and adults. The prevalence of pediatric rhythm disturbances is increasing as more children with congenital heart anomalies undergo surgical correction and survive through childhood. Abnormal cardiac rhythms may be manifested as sudden collapse, dyspnea, tachypnea, tachycardia, palpitations (consciousness of skipped or irregular beats), syncope, dizziness, or angina (rarely). Tachyarrhythmias or bradycardias may not pose any danger to a patient initially; but when they affect cardiac output, patients become symptomatic.

The diagnosis and management of specific rhythm disturbances in children are discussed in Chapter 435. Asystole, symptomatic tachycardias, and bradycardia present distinct resuscitative paradigms that require swift recognition and intervention; personnel in offices, clinics, and inpatient areas should be prepared to manage these complicated situations (Figs. 66-1 to 66-4). Electrolyte imbalances also may produce life-threatening dysrhythmias (see Chapter 52). Children who experience significant fluid loss or who are receiving diuretics or digoxin are especially at risk.

ALTERATIONS OF PULMONARY BLOOD FLOW. In various congenital heart conditions and with some physiologic disturbances, blood flow to the lungs meets with resistance, resulting in pulmonary hypertensive crises. These patients are at risk for serious hypoxic/anoxic events (see Chapter 433).

ASSESSING METABOLIC STATUS. Two important acute destabilizing metabolic disorders are acidosis and hypoglycemia. The causes, consequences, and management of respiratory, metabolic, and mixed acidosis are discussed in Chapters 52 and 55. Arterial blood sampling is discussed in Chapter 64. Measurement of the oxygen content of central venous blood (mixed venous oxygen content [Mvo_2]), especially blood from the pulmonary artery (Swan-Ganz) catheter, is helpful in assessing the adequacy of tissue perfusion and increased anaerobic metabolism. Abnormally low oxygen content of venous blood relative to arterial blood suggests that the delivery of blood to tissues is inadequate, resulting in increased extraction of oxygen and metabolic acidosis. If the venous blood oxygen content is abnormally high, either blood is being delivered too rapidly to the tissues (high cardiac output), so that a lower than normal fraction of oxygen is extracted as blood passes through capillary beds, or there is abnormal mixing of venous and arterial blood near the heart and great vessels, or the tissue is no longer viable. Assaying a patient's blood and urine for specific organic acids if an inborn error is suspected may be helpful in diagnosing an underlying metabolic abnormality.

Current guidelines for resuscitation emphasize the importance of establishing airway and ventilation, heart rate, and adequate peripheral perfusion before $NaHCO_3$ or another buffering agent is administered. Sodium bicarbonate is indicated for symptomatic hyperkalemia, hypermagnesemia, and some tricyclic antidepressant drug intoxications, and with adverse events due to sodium channel blocking agents. Routine administration during CPR is discouraged because it may worsen acidosis if the patient is not ventilated well. Sodium bicarbonate use should be considered in the presence of a severe metabolic acidosis, as documented by arterial blood gas analysis, and during prolonged resuscitation, when it may be given every 10 min during the arrest.

Hypoglycemia is defined as a low blood glucose level that destabilizes energy production (see Chapter 92). The brain is dependent on an adequate level of circulating glucose and requires a constant supply to support energy-consuming cerebral activities. Hypoglycemia produces weakness and lethargy and can

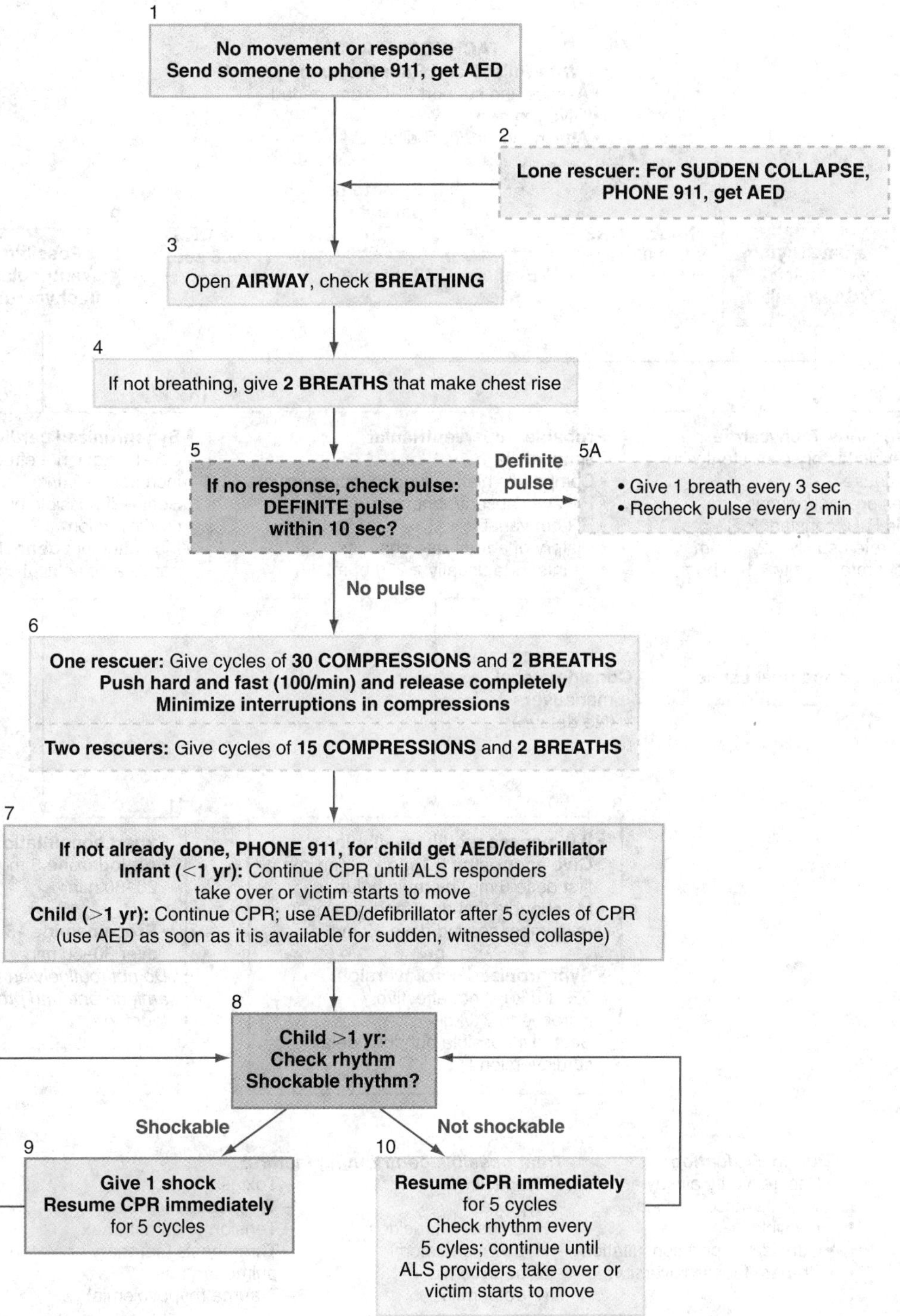

Figure 66-1. Pediatric health care provider basic life support algorithm. The boxes bordered by *dotted lines* are performed by health care providers and not by lay rescuers. AED, automated external defibrillator; ALS, advanced life support. (From American Heart Association Guidelines for Cardiopulmonary Resuscitation and Emergency Cardiovascular Care. *Circulation* 2005;112:IV-156–IV-166.)

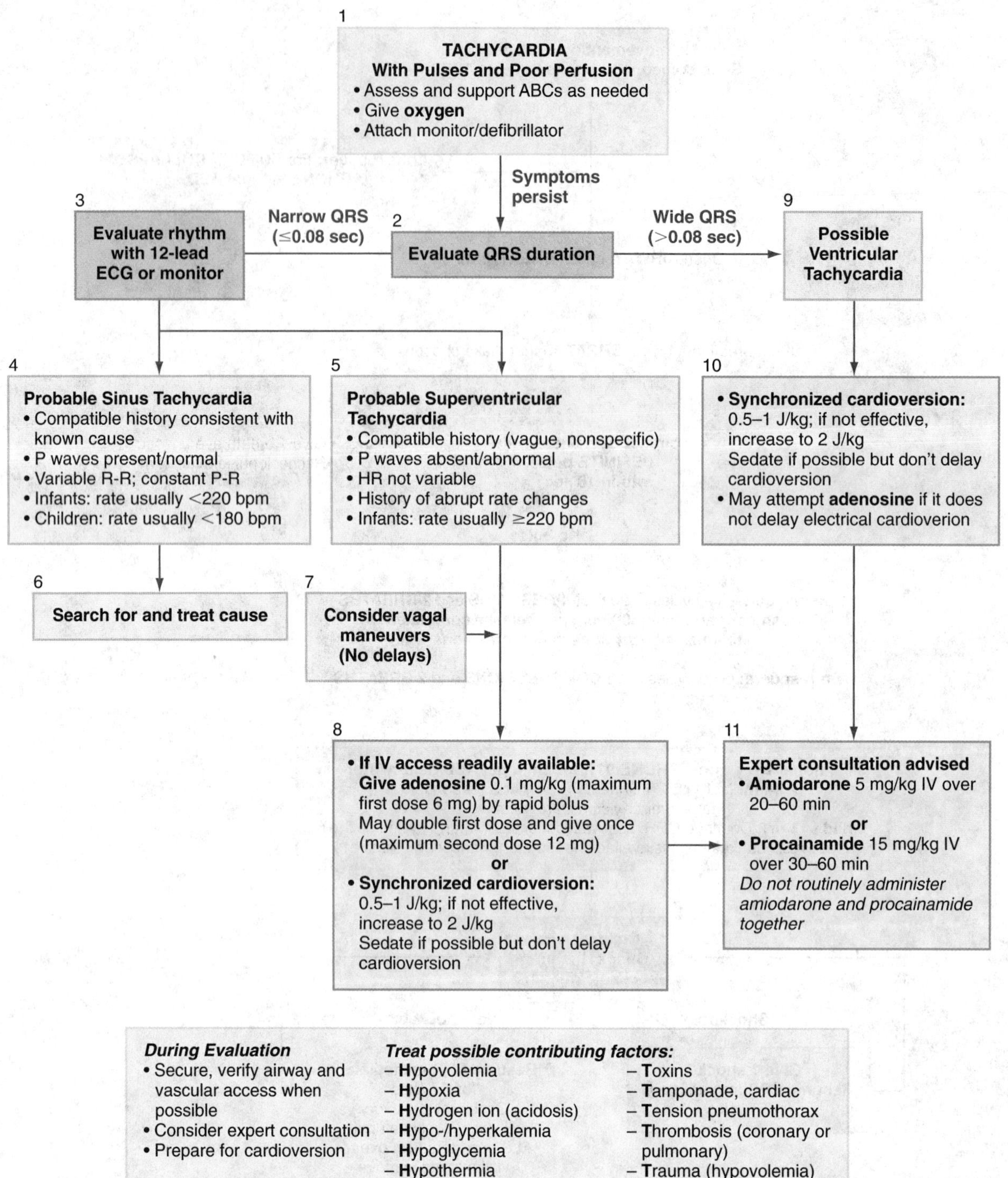

Figure 66-2. Pediatric advanced life support tachycardia algorithm. ABC, airway, breathing, and circulation; ECG, electrocardiogram. (From American Heart Association Guidelines for Cardiopulmonary Resuscitation and Emergency Cardiovascular Care. *Circulation* 2005;112:IV-167–IV-187.)

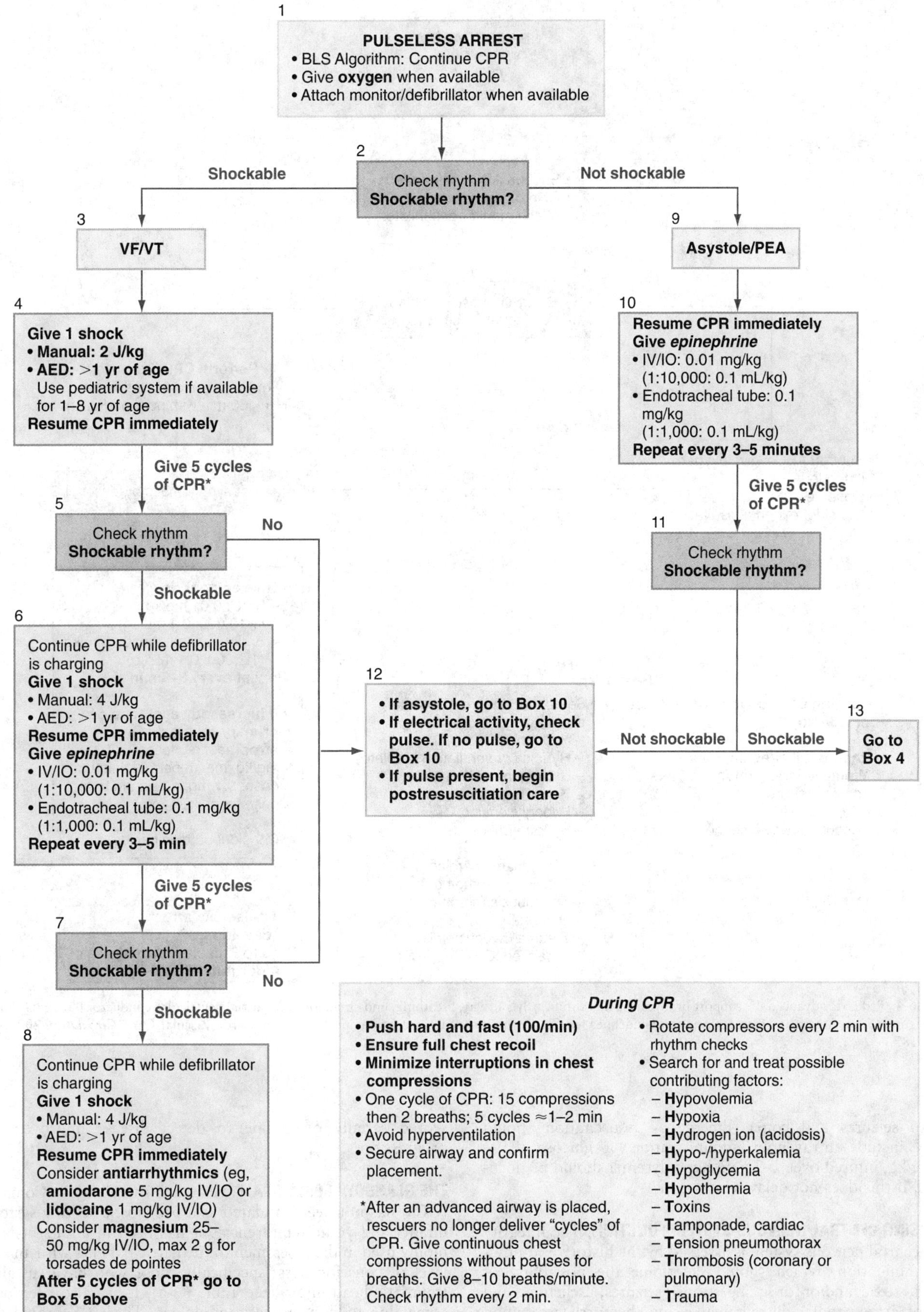

Figure 66-3. Pediatric advanced life support pulseless arrest algorithm. AED, automated external defibrillator; BLS, basic life support; PEA, pulseless electrical activity; VF, ventricular fibrillation; VT, ventricular tachycardia. (From American Heart Association Guidelines for Cardiopulmonary Resuscitation and Emergency Cardiovascular Care. *Circulation* 2005;112:IV-167–IV-187.)

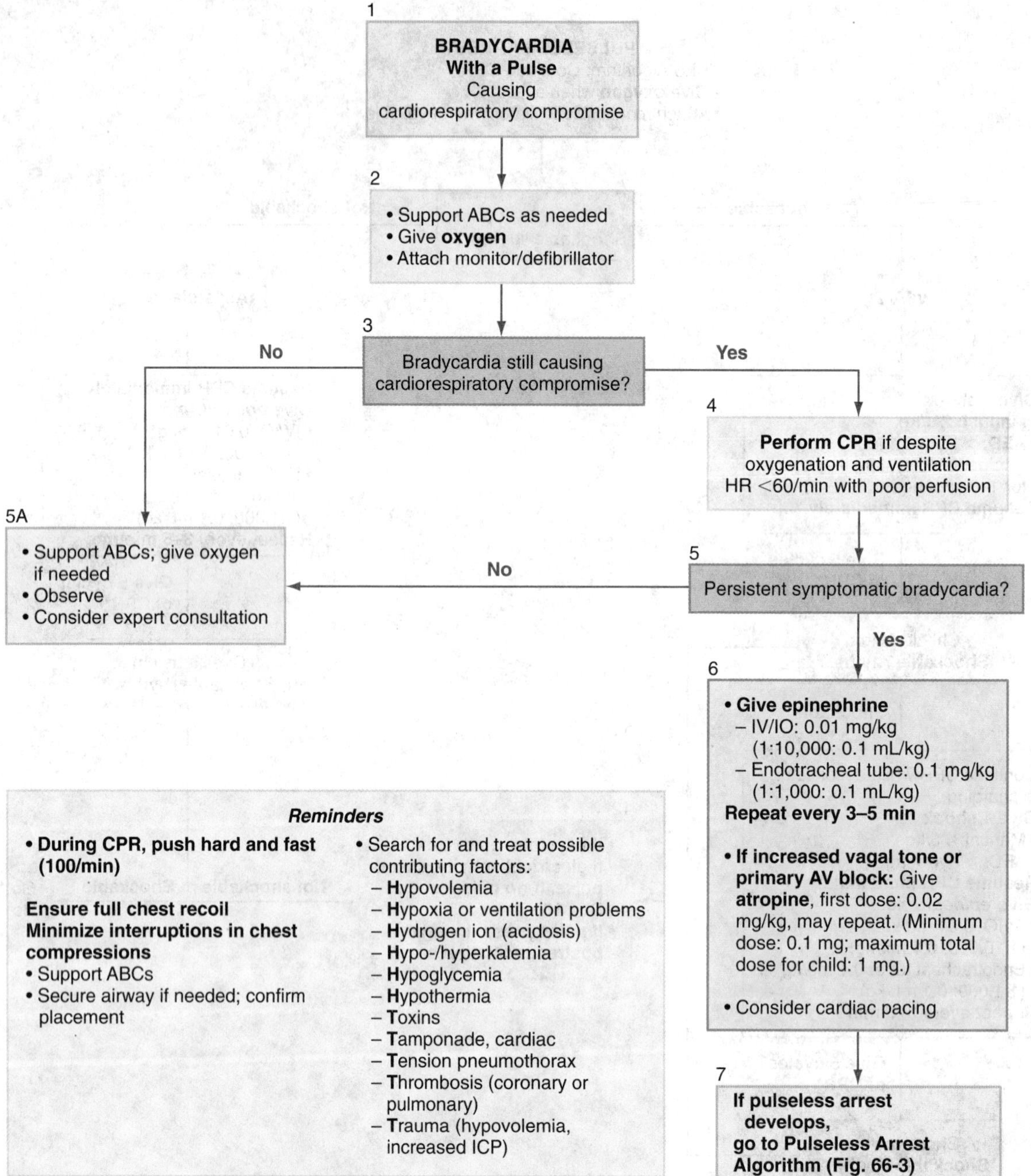

Figure 66-4. Pediatric advanced life support bradycardia algorithm. ABC, airway, breathing, and circulation; AV, atrial ventricular conductor block; ICP, intracranial pressure. (From American Heart Association Guidelines for Cardiopulmonary Resuscitation and Emergency Cardiovascular Care. *Circulation* 2005;112:IV-167–IV-187.)

lead to seizures and coma. Emergency resuscitation should usually include intravenous administration of glucose (250–500 mg/kg, infused over 1–2 min; hypoglycemia should be documented if this does not delay treatment).

ASSESSING CENTRAL NERVOUS SYSTEM FUNCTION. The integrity of the central nervous system is assessed by the history and physical examination, which should determine the possibility of trauma, toxic and/or drug ingestions, seizures, ischemia, and signs of an expanding intracranial lesion (hemorrhage, tumor, abscess, vascular malformation). Tables 66-5 and 66-6 are examples of important scoring or staging criteria that are universally used to assess neurologic status. These criteria should be scored serially over time to detect disease improvement or progression.

THE GLASGOW COMA SCALE. Although the Glasgow Coma Scale (GCS) has not been validated as a prognostic scoring system for infants and young children, as it has been in adults, it is commonly used in the assessment of pediatric patients with an altered level of consciousness, specifically those who have sustained a traumatic head injury (see Table 66-5). It has also been used in coma due to nontraumatic etiologies. The GCS provides very rapid assessment of cerebrocortical function. Patients with a GCS score of 8 or less may require aggressive management, including mechanical ventilation and intracranial pressure monitoring.

TABLE 66-5. Glasgow Coma Scale

EYE OPENING (TOTAL POINTS 4)			
Spontaneous	4		
To voice	3		
To pain	2		
None	1		
VERBAL RESPONSE (TOTAL POINTS 5)			
Older Children		**Infants and Young Children**	
Oriented	5	Appropriate words; smiles, fixes, and follows	5
Confused	4	Consolable crying	4
Inappropriate	3	Persistently irritable	3
Incomprehensible	2	Restless, agitated	2
None	1	None	1
MOTOR RESPONSE (TOTAL POINTS 6)			
Obeys	6		
Localizes pain	5		
Withdraws	4		
Flexion	3		
Extension	2		
None	1		

Adapted and modified from Teasdale G, Jennett B: Assessment of coma and impaired consciousness: A practical scale. *Lancet* 1974;2:81.

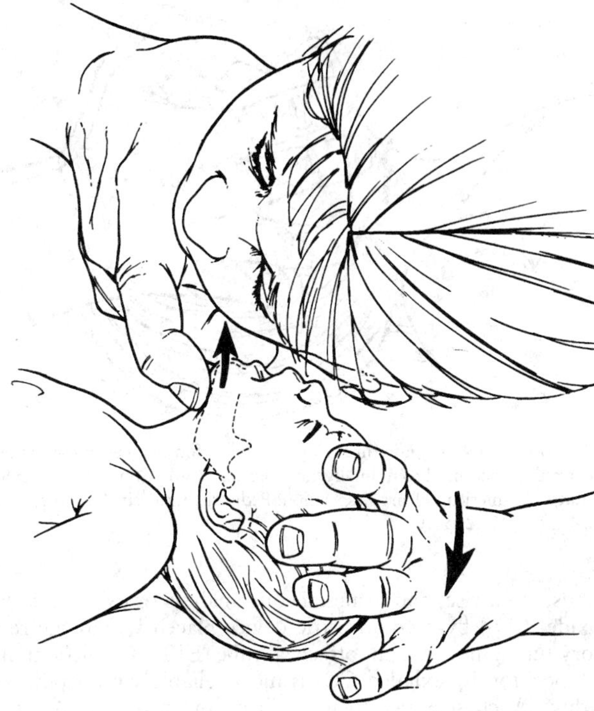

Figure 66-5. Opening the airway with the head-tilt/chin-lift maneuver. One hand is used to tilt the head, extending the neck. The index finger of the rescuer's other hand lifts the mandible outward by lifting the chin. Head-tilt should not be performed if a cervical spine injury is suspected. (From Emergency Cardiac Care Committee and Subcommittees, American Heart Association: Pediatric Basic Life Support, part 5. *JAMA* 1992;268:2251.)

RESUSCITATION

The goal in pediatric resuscitation is to maintain adequate oxygenation and perfusion of blood throughout the body while steps are taken to stabilize the child and establish long-term homeostasis. An orderly sequence of events should be instituted, beginning with the *ABCs: airway, breathing,* and *circulation* (see Chapter 62 and Fig. 66-1). In addition to *airway, A* represents *assessment of responsiveness* ("Are you all right?"), *activation of EMS,* and *anticipation of high-risk situations,* such as trauma, respiratory distress, or exacerbations of chronic life-shortening conditions. Anticipation is the key to the prevention of cardiopulmonary arrest.

Many pediatric patients undergoing resuscitation recover to a substantial degree. Hospitalized children with acute life-threatening conditions often recover spontaneous circulation after an arrest. Children with a respiratory arrest, a short duration of CPR, and a pulse present at the time of apnea have the best chance of survival. The majority of survivors have no change in neurologic function compared with their pre-arrest status. If a patient is asystolic on arrival at the hospital or is in the advanced stages of a chronic disease process before receiving acute medical care, the chances of a successful resuscitation decline dramatically.

RESPIRATORY SUPPORT. If no obstruction by a foreign body is found and if a child has no spontaneous respirations, steps should be immediately taken to breathe for the child. A common cause of airway obstruction in an unresponsive child is the tongue occluding the airway. Assessment includes (1) opening the airway (head-tilt/chin-lift or jaw-thrust, if the cervical spine is unstable); (2) looking for the rise and fall of the chest, listening at the nose and mouth for breathing, and (3) feeling air exiting the child's airways (Figs. 66-5 and 66-6). This should be done in <10 sec. If a foreign body is seen, it should be removed; health care workers should perform a tongue/jaw-lift if a foreign body is suspected, but not initially visualized. If the patient resumes adequate spontaneous ventilation, the patient's body is turned on its side to the recovery position, with the head to the side (if in the field).

Rescue breathing should be done by mouth-to-mouth or mouth-to-nose breathing, a mask over the patient's nose and mouth and mouth-to-mask breathing, or bag-mask respirations (Figs. 66-7 and 66-8). Successful rescue breathing will provide good chest motion and relief of deep cyanosis. Exhaled air is 16–17% oxygen, which corresponds to an alveolar oxygen pressure of 80 mm Hg in the patient. If these measures do not facilitate adequate air entry, recheck that the airway is patent and that the seal is tight; if so, endotracheal intubation is indicated. **Indicators for endotracheal intubation** include apnea, loss of central nervous system control of respirations, airway obstruction unrelieved by airway-opening maneuvers, increased work of breathing that may lead to fatigue, the need for positive end-expiratory pressure or a high peak inspiratory pressure, poor airway-protective reflexes, sedation, or the need for paralysis. Once the patient is intubated, proper tube placement is assessed by breath

TABLE 66-6. Clinical Staging of Encephalopathy

CLINICAL STAGE				
1	2	3	4	5
Lethargic	Combative	Comatose	Comatose	Comatose
Follows commands	Inconsistent following of commands	Occasional response to commands	Responds only to pain	No response to pain
Reactive pupils	Sluggish pupils	Eyes may deviate	Weak pupillary response	No pupillary response
Normal breathing	May hyperventilate	Irregular breathing	Very irregular breathing	Requires mechanical ventilation
Normal muscle tone	Inconsistent reflexes	Decorticate posturing	Decerebrate posturing	Tendon reflexes absent—flaccid

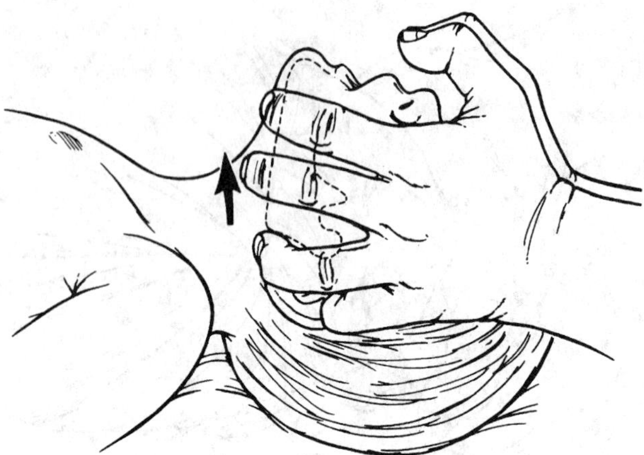

Figure 66-6. Combined jaw-thrust/spine stabilization maneuver for the pediatric trauma victim. (From Emergency Cardiac Care Committee and Subcommittees, American Heart Association: Pediatric Basic Life Support, part 5. *JAMA* 1992;268:2251.)

sounds, chest rise, and instantaneous analysis of exhaled carbon dioxide (CO_2) by a colorimetric device placed within the respiratory tubing near the endotracheal tube (ETT). Confirmation of ETT position by exhaled CO_2 is most reliable with a perfusing rhythm. A chest x-ray then confirms the position. A simple formula for selecting the appropriate size ETT is as follows:

$$\text{Uncuffed ETT size (in mm)} = \left(\frac{\textit{age in years}}{4}\right) + 4$$

Optimal respiratory rates, based on the age of the patient, are indicated in Table 66-4.

In the field, competent bag-mask ventilation may be preferable to repeated attempts at endotracheal intubation by inadequately experienced personnel. The airway in children differs from that of the adult because it is smaller, more anteriorly placed, more difficult to visualize, and more prone to mucosal injuries, leading to subglottic stenosis.

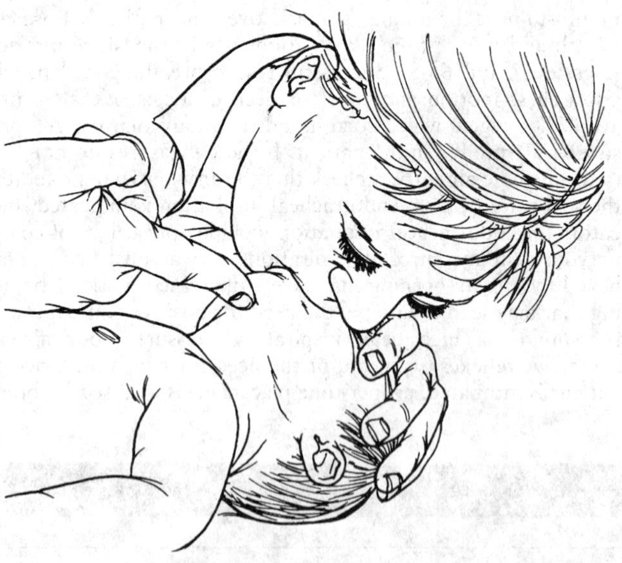

Figure 66-7. Rescue breathing in an infant. The rescuer's mouth covers the infant's nose and mouth, creating a seal. One hand performs the head-tilt while the other hand lifts the infant's jaw. Avoid head-tilt if the infant has sustained head or neck trauma. (From Emergency Cardiac Care Committee and Subcommittees, American Heart Association: Pediatric Basic Life Support, part 5. *JAMA* 1992;268:2251.)

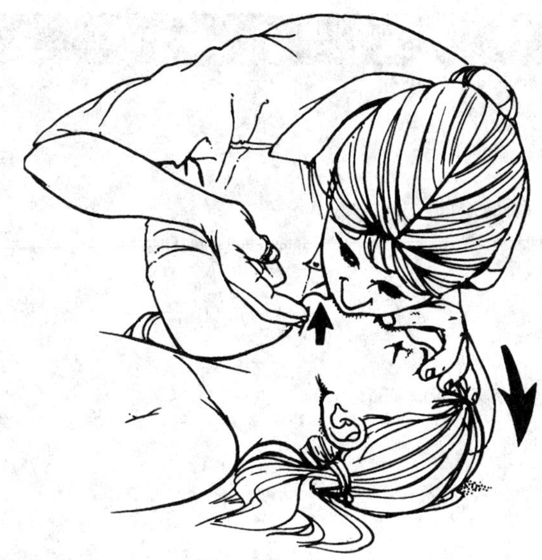

Figure 66-8. Rescue breathing in a child. The rescuer's mouth covers the child's mouth, creating a mouth-to-mouth seal. One hand maintains the head-tilt; the thumb and forefinger of the same hand are used to pinch the child's nose. (From Emergency Cardiac Care Committee and Subcommittees, American Heart Association: Pediatric Basic Life Support, part 5. *JAMA* 1992;268:2251.)

Foreign body aspiration should be suspected if respiratory distress has had a sudden onset (see Chapter 384) or if the chest does not rise when ventilation is first attempted in an unconscious, apneic infant or child. A conscious child suspected of a foreign body partial obstruction should be permitted to cough spontaneously until coughing is not effective (or aphonic), respiratory distress and stridor increase, or the child becomes unconscious. The airway is then opened with the head-tilt/chin-lift maneuver, and ventilation is attempted. If unsuccessful, the airway is repositioned and ventilation attempted again. If there is still no chest rise, attempts to remove a foreign body are indicated. In the infant younger than 1 yr, a combination of 5 back blows and 5 chest thrusts is administered (Fig. 66-9). The foreign body is removed if it is seen. If no foreign body is visualized, ventilation is again attempted. If this is unsuccessful, the head is repositioned and ventilation attempted again. If there is no chest rise, the series of back blows and chest thrusts is repeated.

A conscious child older than 1 yr is administered a series of 5 abdominal thrusts (Heimlich maneuver) with the child standing or sitting (Fig. 66-10). If the child is unconscious, this is done with the child lying down (Fig. 66-11). After the abdominal thrusts, the airway is examined for a foreign body, which should be removed if visualized. If no foreign body is seen, the head is repositioned and ventilation attempted. If it is unsuccessful, the head is repositioned and ventilation is attempted again. If these efforts are unsuccessful, the Heimlich sequence is repeated.

CARDIOVASCULAR SUPPORT. As resuscitation proceeds and ventilation is accomplished, support of the circulation should be provided to sustain adequate blood flow to deliver oxygen to the tissues (Figs. 66-12 to 66-14). Circulation is assessed by lay rescuers without checking for a pulse, whereas health care workers or trained parents should check for a pulse (see Table 66-4). If there is no pulse or if the pulse is <60 beats/min with poor perfusion, chest compressions must be given. Chest compressions are given without interrupting ventilations. The effectiveness of chest compressions is determined by the presence of a palpable pulse. The rate of chest compressions varies with age and size (see Table 66-4). Chest compressions in small infants and newborns may be performed by placing 2 thumbs on the midsternum with the

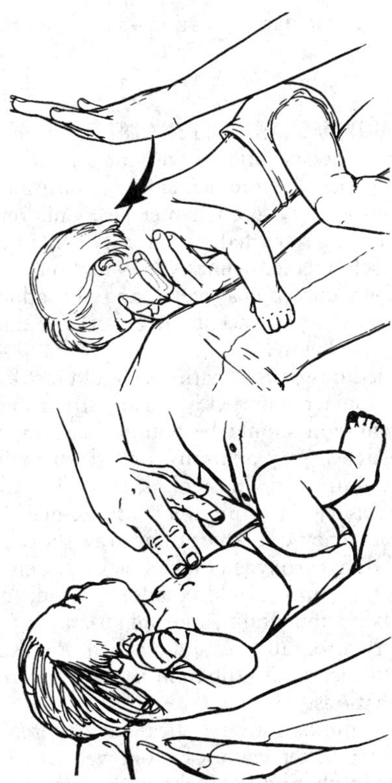

Figure 66-9. Back blows *(top)* and chest thrusts *(bottom)* to relieve foreign body airway obstruction in the infant. (From Emergency Cardiac Care Committee and Subcommittees, American Heart Association. Pediatric Basic Life Support, part 5. *JAMA* 1992;268:2251.)

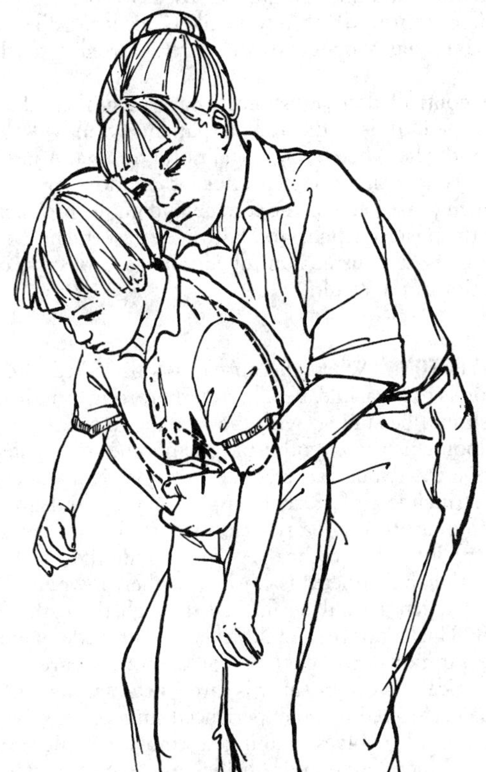

Figure 66-10. Abdominal thrusts with the victim standing or sitting (conscious). (From Emergency Cardiac Care Committee and Subcommittees, American Heart Association: Pediatric Basic Life Support, part 5. *JAMA* 1992;268:2251.)

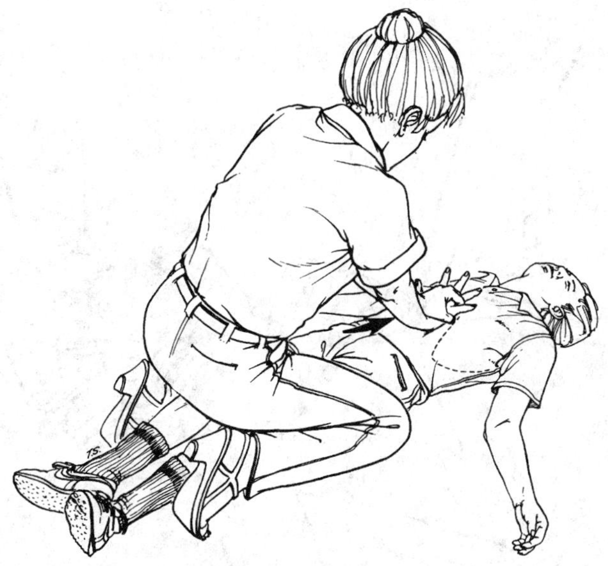

Figure 66-11. Abdominal thrusts with victim lying (conscious or unconscious). (From Emergency Cardiac Care Committee and Subcommittees, American Heart Association: Pediatric Basic Life Support, part 5. *JAMA* 1992;268:2251.)

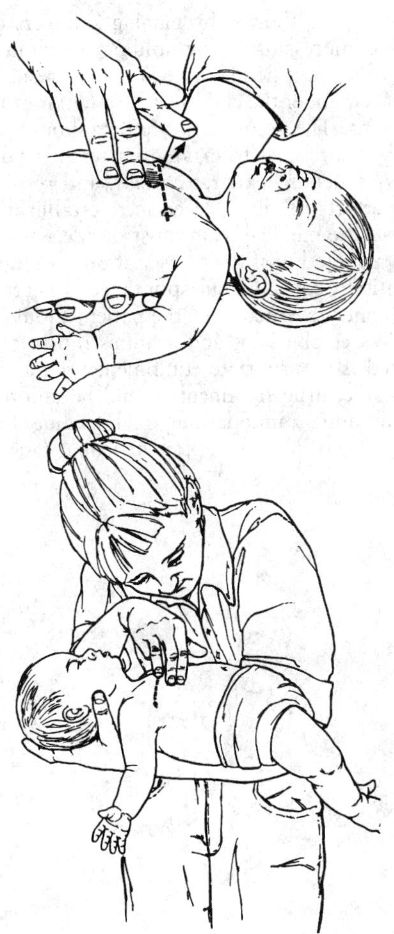

Figure 66-12. Cardiac compressions. *Top,* The infant is supine on the palm of the rescuer's hand. *Bottom,* Performing CPR while carrying an infant or small child. Note that the head is kept level with the torso. (From Emergency Cardiac Care Committee and Subcommittees, American Heart Association: Pediatric Basic Life Support, part 5. *JAMA* 1992;268:2251.)

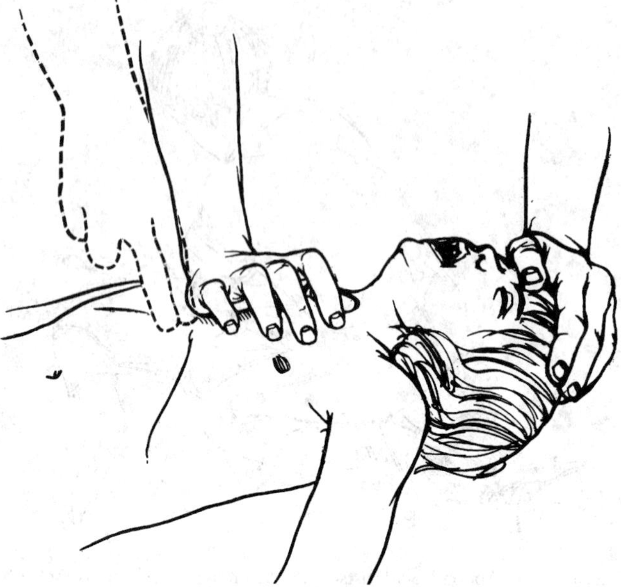

Figure 66-13. Locating the hand position for chest compression in a child. Note that the rescuer's other hand is used to maintain the head position to facilitate ventilation. (From Emergency Cardiac Care Committee and Subcommittees, American Heart Association: Pediatric Basic Life Support, part 5. *JAMA* 1992;268:2251.)

hands encircling the thorax, by placing 2 fingers over the midsternum and compressing, or by holding the child in the supine posture on one's lap. When feasible, a cardiac resuscitation board should be placed under the child's back to maximize the efficiency of compressions. The resuscitation effort should pause periodically to allow the rescuer to make an assessment of the possible return of spontaneous heart rate, pulse, and respirations. If the resuscitative efforts do not succeed in re-establishing respiration and heartbeat, the medical team must decide whether continued efforts are warranted or if the resuscitation should be stopped. If resuscitation is to continue but spontaneous heart rate and respirations have not returned, then the patient should be intubated, vascular access established, and administration of resuscitative drugs initiated. If appropriate equipment for monitoring of the ECG is available, drug treatment should be tailored to the particular dysrhythmia (amiodarone or lidocaine for ventricular tachycardia, adenosine for supraventricular tachycardias, cardioversion for ventricular fibrillation—usually used in older children only).

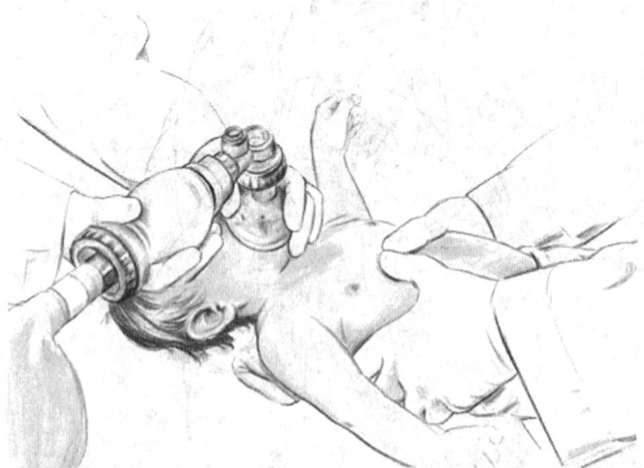

Figure 66-14. Two thumb-encircling hands used to perform chest compression in an infant (2 rescuers). (From Emergency Cardiac Care Committee and Subcommittees, American Heart Association: Pediatric Basic Life Support, part 9. *Circulation* 2000;102:1–253.)

INTUBATION AND MECHANICAL VENTILATION. Although it is possible to intubate awake infants without sedation, analgesia, or paralysis, analgesia is recommended to reduce metabolic stress, discomfort, and anxiety (see Chapter 76). Children 1 mo of age or older should be pretreated with a sedative, an analgesic, and possibly a muscle relaxant unless the situation is an emergency (apnea, asystole, unresponsiveness) and the administration of drugs would cause an unacceptable delay. The intubation technique is shown in Figure 66-15.

In a controlled intubation, patients should fast for at least 4 hr or have their stomach emptied by nasogastric tube. History and physical examination should be obtained for any allergies, evidence of unusual airway anatomy, or risk of malignant hyperthermia, and informed consent should be obtained. The equipment necessary for intubation and bag-mask ventilation as well as an emergency cricothyrotomy tray should be available. After a period of hyperoxygenation, a benzodiazepine (diazepam, midazolam, lorazepam) should be administered, followed by an opiate (fentanyl, remifentanil, morphine) and a paralytic agent (vecuronium, rocuronium). A sodium pentothal/succinylcholine combination to facilitate intubation is used most often in rapid sequence intubations.

Because many intubations in critically ill children are emergent, the foregoing steps often cannot be followed, and procedures for **rapid sequence intubation** (RSI) should be initiated (Table 66-7). The goals of RSI are to induce anesthesia and paralysis and complete intubation rapidly. This minimizes elevations of intracranial and blood pressure that may accompany intubation in awake or lightly sedated patients. Because the stomach generally cannot be emptied before RSI, the **Sellick maneuver** (compression of the cricoid cartilage backward, compressing the esophagus against the vertebral column) should be used to prevent aspiration of gastric contents, which is very likely to occur due to reflexes when the laryngoscope and ETT are inserted into the upper airway.

Under controlled circumstances, nasotracheal intubation may be performed. It is indicated in patients who will be lightly sedated and when there is significant oral trauma. A nasotracheal tube causes less noxious sensations than does an orotracheal tube, which passes across the tongue and gums, producing a gag reflex in the posterior pharynx. However, nasotracheal tubes may obstruct sinus and eustachian tube drainage, and sinus or middle ear infections may result.

CRICOTHYROTOMY. When the airway is obstructed and tracheal intubation is not feasible, needle cricothyrotomy is indicated. The patient should be supine, with the face looking directly upward. The midpoint of the cricothyroid membrane is palpated, and a 14-gauge intravenous catheter with a stylet is advanced slowly through it, inclined inferiorly at approximately 45 degrees. Quick aspiration of air through a syringe connected to the catheter indicates entry into the trachea. At this point, the metal stylet is removed and the catheter is pushed farther downward into the trachea. Oxygen should be flushed through the catheter at 10–15 L/min. This supports a child, even 1 with little or no spontaneous respirations, while plans for a more secure airway are made. Surgical cricothyrotomy is rarely necessary in children and should be performed by an experienced surgeon, except in severe emergencies. It involves making a transverse incision in the cricothyroid membrane and advancing a large catheter through the incision downward into the lower trachea. Although similar in principle to a needle cricothyrotomy, the risk of bleeding, upper airway obstruction, and pneumothorax are significantly greater.

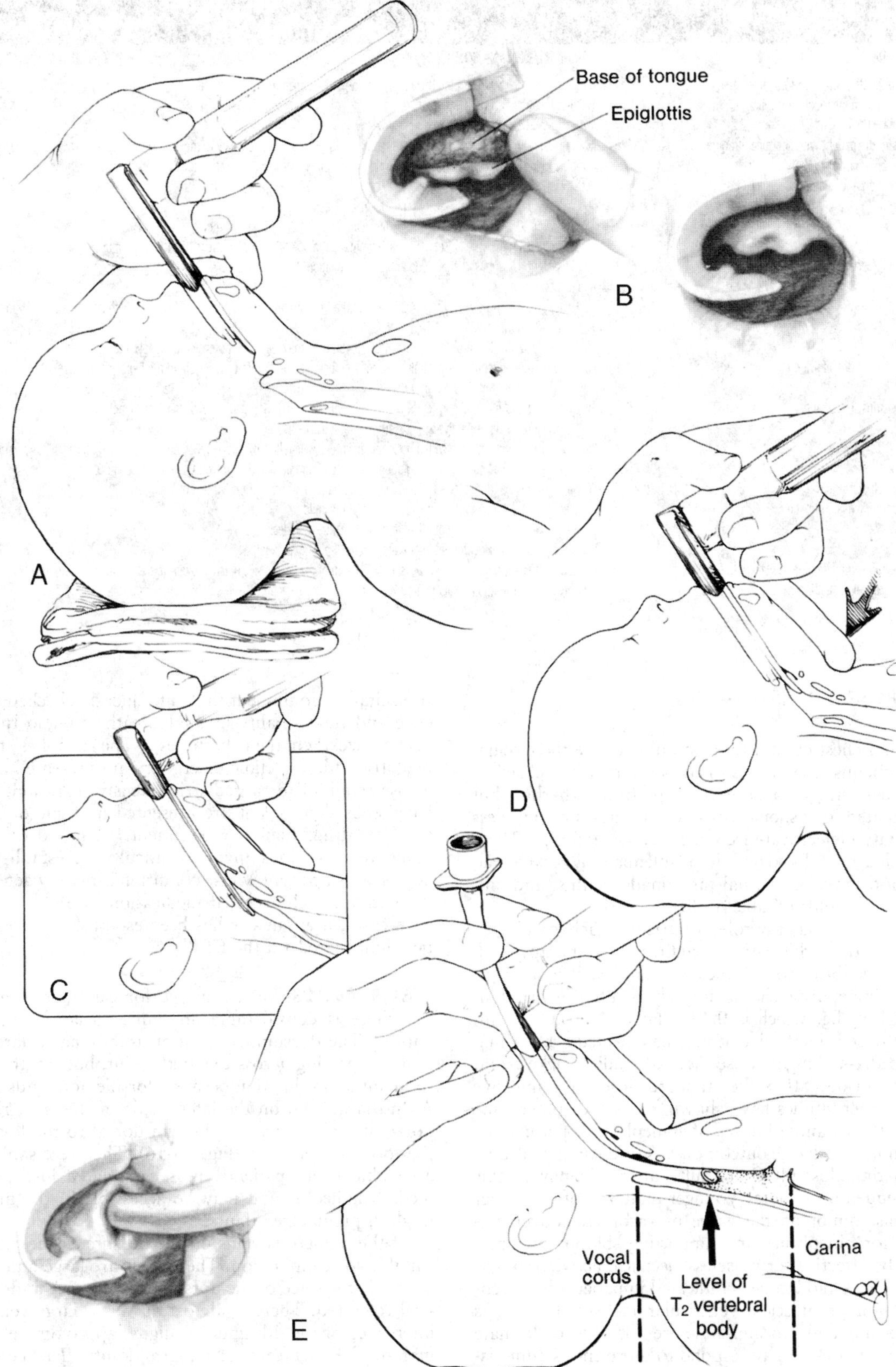

Figure 66-15. Intubation technique. (From Fleisher G, Ludwig S: *Textbook of Pediatric Emergency Medicine*. Baltimore, Williams & Wilkins, 1983, p 1250.)

TABLE 66-7. Rapid Sequence Intubation

STEP	PROCEDURE	COMMENT/EXPLANATION
1	Obtain a brief history and perform an assessment	Rule out drug allergies; examine the airway anatomy (e.g., micrognathia, cleft palate).
2	Assemble equipment, medications, etc.	See lists below.
3	Preoxygenate the patient	With bag/mask, nasal cannula, hood or "blow-by."
4	Premedicate the patient with lidocaine, atropine	Lidocaine minimizes the ICP rise with intubation and can be applied topically to the airway mucosa for local anesthesia. Atropine helps blunt the bradycardia associated with upper airway manipulation and reduces airway secretions.
5	Induce sedation and analgesia	Sedatives: *Thiopental* (2–5 mg/kg)—very rapid onset; can cause hypotension. *Diazepam* (0.1 mg/kg)—onset 2–5 min; elimination in 30–60 min or more. *Ketamine* (2 mg/kg)—onset 1–2 min, elimination in 30–40 min. May cause hallucinations if used alone; causes higher ICP, mucous secretions, increased vital signs, and bronchodilation. Analgesics: *Fentanyl:* 3–10 μg/kg, may repeat 3–4×. Rapid administration risks "tight chest" response, with no effective ventilation. Effects wear off in 20–30 min. *Morphine:* 0.05–0.1 mg/kg dose; may last 30–60 min, may lead to hypotension in hypovolemic patients.
6	Pretreat with nondepolarizing paralytic agent	Small dose of a nondepolarizing paralytic agent (see below), with intent of diminishing the depolarizing effect of succinylcholine, which is administered next.
7	Administer muscle relaxants	Succinylcholine dose is 1–2 mg/kg; causes initial contraction of muscles, then relaxation. This depolarization can, however, raise ICP and blood pressure. Onset of paralysis in 30–40 sec; duration 5–10 min. Increased use of pretreatment with a nondepolarizing muscle relaxant, especially rocuronium (1 mg/kg), which has a very rapid onset and short duration. Other nondepolarizing agents include vecuronium and pancuronium, both dosed at 0.1 mg/kg.
8	Perform a Sellick maneuver	Pressure on the cricoid cartilage, to occlude the esophagus and prevent regurgitation or aspiration.
9	Perform endotracheal intubation	ET: select the proper size for the age and weight of the child. Laryngoscope blades: a variety of Miller and the Macintosh blades. Patient supine: the neck extended moderately to the "sniffing" position.
10	Secure the tube and verify the position with a roentgenogram	ET tube secured with tape to the cheeks and upper lip or to an adhesive patch applied to the skin near the mouth.
11	Begin mechanical ventilation	Verify tube placement before ventilating with positive pressure; if an ET is in one bronchus, barotraumas may occur.

ET, endotracheal tube; ICP, intracranial pressure.

DRUG THERAPY AND DEFIBRILLATION

If ventilation and chest compressions do not restore the circulation and spontaneous respirations, medication may be needed. If there is ECG evidence of a potentially perfusing rhythm, but no pulse is palpated, one should consider the causes of **pulseless electrical activity** (electrical-mechanical dissociation). These include hypothermia, hypoxia, hypovolemia, hyperkalemia, tension pneumothorax, pericardial tamponade, toxins, and pulmonary thromboembolism (Table 66-8).

If there is bradycardia, asystole, ventricular tachycardia, or ventricular fibrillation, the patient requires drug therapy and, when indicated, defibrillation (Tables 66-9 and 66-10; see Figs. 66-1 to 66-4). Epinephrine should initially be used in the standard dose (0.01 mg/kg, which is 0.1 mL/kg of 1 : 10,000 solution). If the 1st dose is ineffective, it may be repeated every 3 min or increased to 0.1–0.2 mg/kg dose. Several studies suggest that high-dose epinephrine (≥10 × the standard dose) may improve outcomes, but other studies have shown high-dose epinephrine to be no better than standard doses of epinephrine, or it may be associated with more adverse outcomes. Vasopressin may also be effective as a 1-time dose (40 U in adults) after epinephrine; this is not recommended for children younger than 8 yr of age; other studies have cast doubt on the value of vasopressin over epinephrine or norepinephrine in supporting blood pressure. Atropine may be effective for pulseless electrical activity, bradycardia, or asystole. Amiodarone is indicated in patients with ventricular fibrillation or pulseless ventricular tachycardia that is refractory; lidocaine and procainamide are 2nd-choice alternate drugs. Torsades de pointes may respond to intravenous administration of 25 mg/kg of magnesium sulfate.

Intravenous or intraosseous fluids should be normal saline or lactated Ringer without glucose to support the circulation and avoid hyperglycemia, which is a poor prognostic factor during an arrest.

EQUIPMENT AND DRUGS FOR RESUSCITATION. An emergency department or intensive care unit should have a full supply of resuscitation equipment that is frequently checked for both presence and functionality (available catheters and tubes in appropriate sizes, charged batteries). The supplies needed for a pediatric office or clinic emergency are presented in Chapter 62. Those required for a pediatric intensive care unit (PICU) or an emergency department are presented in Table 66-11. See Table 66-9 for drugs that may be urgently required for resuscitation. Some resuscitations involve difficulty in establishing vascular access, and a patient whose condition is rapidly deteriorating may die without such access if medications are not administered. In such cases, if an airway has been established, certain drugs may be administered via the ETT.

VENOUS ACCESS. Veins suitable for cannulation are numerous, but there is considerable anatomic variation from patient to patient. The dorsum of the foot usually has a large vein in the midline, passing across the ankle joint, but a catheter is difficult to maintain in this vein because dorsiflexion tends to dislodge it. A 2nd large vein on the lateral side of the foot, running in the horizontal plane, usually 1–2 cm dorsal to the lower margin of the foot, is preferable (Fig. 66-16). The great saphenous vein is accessible in all patients. It is cannulated just anterior to the medial malleolus and may be accessible in the medial leg and thigh in premature infants.

Of the numerous veins on the dorsum of the hand, many are suitable for cannulation. The vessels are large and often secured on the flat surface of the dorsum of the hand, and cannulation is well tolerated. There is almost always a large vein lying in the interspace of the 4th and 5th digits, approximately 1 cm proximal to the metacarpophalangeal joints. The cephalic vein is usually cannulated at the wrist, along the forearm, or at the elbow (Fig. 66-17). The median vein of the forearm is also suitable because it lies along a flat surface of the forearm. The basilic vein is prone to sliding around when attempts are made to cannulate it.

Samples of blood may be obtained from the external and internal jugular veins or, in neonates, from various scalp veins. The 2 jugular veins are also potential sites for indwelling catheters (Fig.

TABLE 66-8. Potentially Treatable Conditions Associated with Cardiac Arrest

CONDITION	COMMON CLINICAL SETTINGS	CORRECTIVE ACTIONS
Acidosis	Pre-existing acidosis, diabetes, diarrhea, drugs and toxins, prolonged resuscitation, renal disease, and shock	Reassess the adequacy of cardiopulmonary resuscitation, oxygenation, and ventilation; reconfirm endotracheal tube placement Hyperventilate Consider intravenous bicarbonate if pH <7.20 after above actions have been taken
Cardiac tamponade	Hemorrhagic diathesis, cancer, pericarditis, trauma, after cardiac surgery, and after myocardial infarction	Administer fluids; obtain bedside echocardiogram, if available Perform pericardiocentesis; immediate surgical intervention is appropriate if pericardiocentesis is unhelpful but cardiac tamponade is known or highly suspected
Hypothermia	Alcohol abuse, burns, central nervous system disease, debilitated patient, drowning, drugs and toxins, endocrine disease, history of exposure, homelessness, extensive skin disease, spinal cord disease, and trauma	If hypothermia is severe (temperature <30° C), limit initial shocks for ventricular fibrillation or pulseless ventricular tachycardia to 3; initiate active internal rewarming and cardiopulmonary support; hold further resuscitation medications or shocks until core temperature is >30°C. If hypothermia is moderate (temperature 30–34° C), proceed with resuscitation (space medications at intervals greater than usual), passively rewarm, and actively rewarm truncal body areas
Hypovolemia, hemorrhage, anemia	Major burns, diabetes, gastrointestinal losses, hemorrhage, hemorrhagic diathesis, cancer, pregnancy, shock, and trauma	Administer fluids Transfuse packed red cells if hemorrhage or profound anemia is present Thoracotomy is appropriate when a patient has cardiac arrest from penetrating trauma and a cardiac rhythm and the duration of cardiopulmonary resuscitation before thoracotomy is <10 min
Hypoxia	Consider in all patients with cardiac arrest	Reassess the technical quality of cardiopulmonary resuscitation, oxygenation, and ventilation, reconfirm endotracheal tube placement
Hypomagnesemia	Alcohol abuse, burns, diabetic ketoacidosis, severe diarrhea, diuretics, and drugs (e.g., cisplatin, cyclosporine, pentamidine)	Administer 1–2 g magnesium sulfate IV over 2 min
Poisoning	Alcohol abuse, bizarre or puzzling behavioral or metabolic presentation, classic toxicologic syndrome, occupational or industrial exposure, and psychiatric disease	Consult a toxicologist for emergency advice on resuscitation and definitive care, including an appropriate antidote Prolonged resuscitation efforts may be appropriate; immediate cardiopulmonary bypass should be considered, if available
Hyperkalemia	Metabolic acidosis, excessive administration of potassium, drugs and toxins, vigorous exercise, hemolysis, renal disease, rhabdomyolysis, tumor lysis syndrome, and clinically significant tissue injury	If hyperkalemia is identified or strongly suspected, treat* with all of the following: 10% calcium chloride (5–10 mL by slow IV push; do not use if hyperkalemia is secondary to digitalis poisoning), glucose and insulin (50 mL of 50% dextrose in water and 10 units of regular insulin IV), sodium bicarbonate (50 mmol IV; most effective if concomitant metabolic acidosis is present), and albuterol (15–20 mg nebulized or 0.5 mg by IV infusion)
Hypokalemia	Alcohol abuse, diabetes, use of diuretics, drugs and toxins, profound gastrointestinal losses, hypomagnesemia	If profound hypokalemia (<2–2.5 mmol of potassium V) is accompanied by cardiac arrest, initiate urgent IV replacement (2 mmol/min IV for 10–15 mmol)*; then reassess
Pulmonary embolism	Hospitalized patient, recent surgical procedure, peripartum, known risk factors for venous thromboembolism, history of venous thromboembolism, or pre-arrest presentation consistent with a diagnosis of acute pulmonary embolism	Administer fluids; augment with vasopressors as necessary Confirm the diagnosis, if possible; consider immediate cardiopulmonary bypass to maintain patient's viability Consider definitive care (e.g., thrombolytic therapy, embolectomy by interventional radiology or surgery)
Tension pneumothorax	Placement of a central catheter, mechanical ventilation, pulmonary disease (including asthma, chronic obstructive pulmonary disease, and necrotizing pneumonia), thoracentesis, and trauma	Needle decompression, followed by chest tube insertion

*Adult dose. Adjust for size of child. See Table 66-9.
From Eisenbery MS, Mengert TJ: Cardiac resuscitation. *N Engl J Med* 2001; 344:1304–1313.

TABLE 66-9. Medications for Pediatric Resuscitation and Arrhythmias

MEDICATION	DOSE	REMARKS
Adenosine	0.1 mg/kg (maximum 6 mg) Repeat: 0.2 mg/kg (maximum 12 mg)	Monitor ECG Rapid IV/IO bolus
Amiodarone	5 mg/kg IV/IO; repeat up to 15 mg/kg Maximum: 300 mg	Monitor ECG and blood pressure Adjust administration rate to urgency (give more slowly when perfusing rhythm is present) Use caution when administering with other drugs that prolong Q-T (consider expert consultation)
Atropine	0.02 mg/kg IV/IO 0.03 mg/kg ET* Repeat once if needed Minimum dose: 0.1 mg Minimum single dose: Child, 0.5 mg Adolescent, 1 mg	Higher doses may be used with organophosphate poisoning
Calcium chloride (10%)	20 mg/kg IV/IO (0.2 mL/kg)	Slowly Adult dose: 5–10 mL
Epinephrine	0.01 mg/kg (0.1 mL/kg 1 : 10,000) IV/IO 0.1 mg/kg (0.1 mL/kg 1 : 1,000) ET* Maximum dose: 1 mg IV/IO; 10 mg ET	May repeat q3–5 min
Glucose	0.5–1 g/kg IV/IO	D10W: 5–10 mL/kg D25W: 2–4 mL/kg D50W: 1–2 mL/kg
Lidocaine	Bolus: 1 mg/kg IV/IO Maximum dose: 100 mg Infusion: 20–50 µg/kg/min ET*: 2–3 mg	
Magnesium sulfate	25–50 mg/kg IV/IO over 10–20 min; faster in torsades Maximum dose: 2 g	
Naloxone	<5 yr or ≤20 kg: 0.1 mg/kg IV/IO/ET* ≥5 yr or >20 kg: 2 mg IV/IO/ET*	Use lower doses to reverse respiratory depression associated with therapeutic opioid use (1–15 µg/kg)
Procainamide	15 mg/kg IV/IO over 30–60 min Adult dose: 20 mg/min IV infusion up to total maximum dose of 17 mg/kg	Monitor EGG and blood pressure Use caution when administering with other drugs that prolong QT (consider expert consultation)
Sodium bicarbonate	1 mEq/kg/dose IV/IO slowly	After adequate ventilation

*Flush with 5 mL of normal saline and follow with 5 ventilations.
From American Heart Association Guidelines for Cardiopulmonary Resuscitation and Emergency Cardiovascular Care. *Circulation* 2005; 112:IV-167–IV-187.
ECG, electro cardiogram; ET, endotracheal tube; IO, intraosseous; IV, intravenous.

TABLE 66-10. Medications to Maintain Cardiac Output and for Postresuscitation Stabilization*

MEDICATION	DOSE RANGE	COMMENT
Inamrinone	0.75–1 mg/kg IV/IO over 5 min; may repeat 2×; then: 2–20 μg/kg/min	Inodilator
Dobutamine	2–20 μg/kg/min IV/IO	Inotrope; vasodilator
Dopamine	2–20 μg/kg/min IV/IO in low doses; pressor in higher doses	Inotrope; chronotrope; renal and splanchnic vasodilator
Epinephrine	0.1–1 μg/kg/min IV/IO	Inotrope; chronotrope; vasodilator in low doses; pressor in higher doses
Milrinone	50–75 μg/kg IV/IO over 10–60 min then 0.5–0.75 μg/kg/min	Inodilator
Norepinephrine	0.1–2 μg/kg/min	Inotrope; vasopressor
Sodium nitroprusside	1–8 μg/kg/min	Vasodilator; prepare only in D5W

*Alternative formula for calculating an infusion: Infusion rate (mL/hr) = [weight (kg) × dose (μg/kg/min) × 60 (min/hr)]/concentration μg/mL)
From American Heart Association Guidelines for Cardiopulmonary Resuscitation and Emergency Cardiovascular Care. *Circulation* 2005; 112:IV-167–IV-187.
IO, intraosseous; IV, intravenous.

66-18). The most notable scalp veins are the superficial temporal (just anterior to the ear) and posterior auricular (just behind the ear).

Deeper and larger veins are very valuable because they provide reliable access for medication, nutritive solutions, and blood sampling. They may be reached by percutaneous cannulation or surgical exposure. To cannulate the femoral vein, after the skin is cleaned, a needle is inserted approximately 0.5 cm medial to the pulsing femoral artery (or, if there is no pulse, ≈⅔ of the way from the anterior-superior spine to the pubic tubercle (Fig. 66-19). Slight backward pressure on the plunger of a connected syringe is maintained so that blood flows easily into the syringe once the vessel is punctured. After the vessel is located, a small wire is advanced through the needle into the lumen of the vessel. The needle and syringe are then removed, and the catheter is threaded over the wire into the vessel (**Seldinger technique**). In small infants, the vein is only approximately 0.5–1 cm below the surface, so the needle puncture should be at a shallow angle. In large adolescents or very obese patients, the needle may need to be nearly perpendicular to the skin. In either case, once the vein is entered, the needle should be flattened out before it is advanced farther into the vein. Similar, but distinctive, cannulation techniques are used in providing access to the subclavian vein and the internal jugular vein. They involve the risk of pneumothorax in addition to bleeding. Because of its proximity to the

TABLE 66-11. Supplies Needed for Pediatric Intensive Care/Emergency Department

Storage cart for equipment/materials
Defibrillator/portable ECG monitor
Oxygen cylinder
Airway equipment:
Laryngoscope handle with batteries
Assortment of blades—Miller 0, 1, 2, 3 and MacIntosh 2, 3
Large assortment of endotracheal tubes, cuffed and uncuffed, with stylets
Nasal and oral airways
Self-inflating resuscitation bags
Anesthesia bags with oxygen adapter
Suction equipment, including tongue blades, Yankauer suction tip, several catheters
Various nasogastric tubes
Tapes, sponges, IV adapters, T connectors, stopcocks
Masks for bag-mask ventilation, many sizes
Mapleson system with varied bag sizes
Cardiac equipment:
Cardiac arrest board for compressions
IVs, butterflies, intraosseous needles
Blood pressure measuring equipment
Several unit doses of epinephrine, bicarbonate, calcium chloride, lidocaine, naloxone D25W
IV fluids and medications:
Various crystalloid and colloid fluids
Fully equipped IV tray—catheters, alcohol, needles, tape, tourniquets, arm boards
Cutdown tray
Umbilical catheter tray
Tracheostomy tray
Chest tube tray
Pleurovac pump
Cardiac surgery open chest tray (if unit cares for postoperative hearts)
ICP monitor tray
General minor surgical procedure tray
Military antishock trousers kit
Warm packs, sandbags, and so on
Monitoring equipment: pulse oximetry ECG, end-tidal CO_2, blood pressure

ECG, electrocardiogram; ICP, intracranial pressure; IV, intravenous.

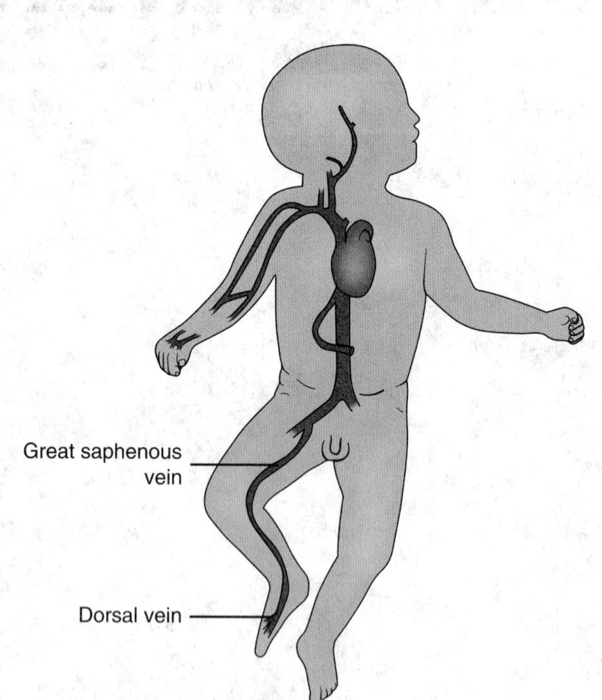

Figure 66-16. Veins of the lower extremity. (From Roberts JR, Hedges JR (editors): *Clinical Procedures in Emergency Medicine,* 4th ed. Philadelphia, Saunders, 2004.)

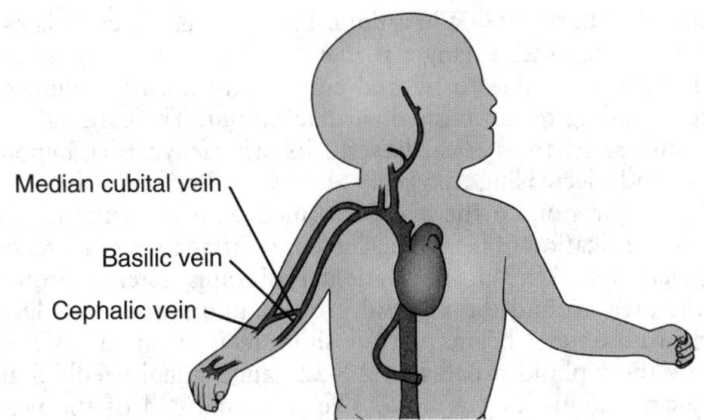

Figure 66-17. Veins of the upper extremity. (From Roberts JR, Hedges JR (editors): *Clinical Procedures in Emergency Medicine,* 4th ed. Philadelphia, Saunders, 2004.)

median nerve, the brachial vein is not often recommended for cannulation.

A **portable ultrasonic device** may be a great help in locating and cannulating veins, especially those of the neck and groin. This device provides a visual image of the vessel being cannulated, and even allows direct visual confirmation of the location of the target vein and entry of the needle into it. Skilled use of this device can improve the efficiency of placing catheters and minimizes stress and discomfort for the patient.

INTRAOSSEOUS VASCULAR ACCESS. Intraosseous needles are special rigid, large-bore needles that resemble those used for marrow aspiration. Current recommendations urge the use of intraosseous cannulation in patients for whom intravenous access proves difficult or unattainable, even in older children. If venous access is not available in an arrest situation within 1 min, an intraosseous line [IO] should be placed in the anterior tibia (with care taken to avoid traversing the epiphyseal plate). The needle should penetrate the anterior layer of compact bone, and its tip advanced into the spongy interior of the bone. Most medications, blood products, and fluids may be administered through this route, including most involved in emergency resuscitations. Once the patient has received initial drug and fluid therapy through the IO line, every effort should be made to obtain more conventional central venous access and remove the IO line as soon as possible, to minimize risk to the bone. Because such needles are often inserted in haste, consideration should be given to empirical antibiotic coverage after the needle is placed and the patient stabilized.

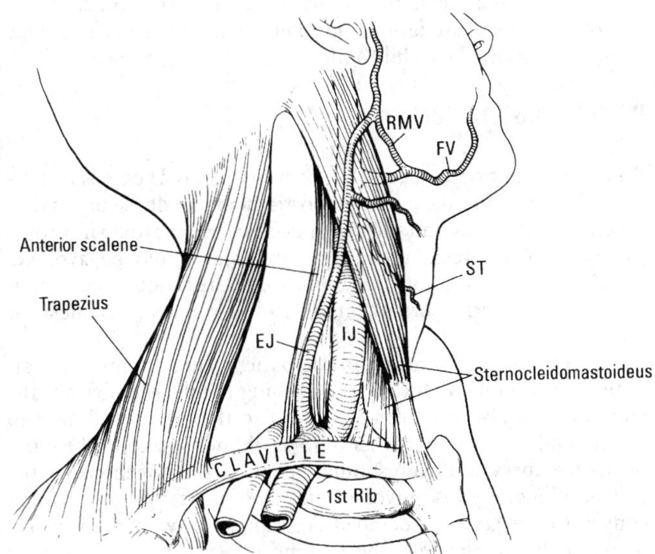

Figure 66-18. Internal and external jugular veins. EJ, external jugular vein; FV, facial vein; IJ, internal jugular vein; RMV, retromandibular vein; ST, superior thyroid vein. The 2 heads of the sternocleidomastoideus are indicated by the *lines*. (From Mathers LW, Smith DW, Frankel L: Anatomic considerations in placement of central venous catheters. *Clin Anat* 1992;5:89. Reprinted by permission of Wiley-Liss.)

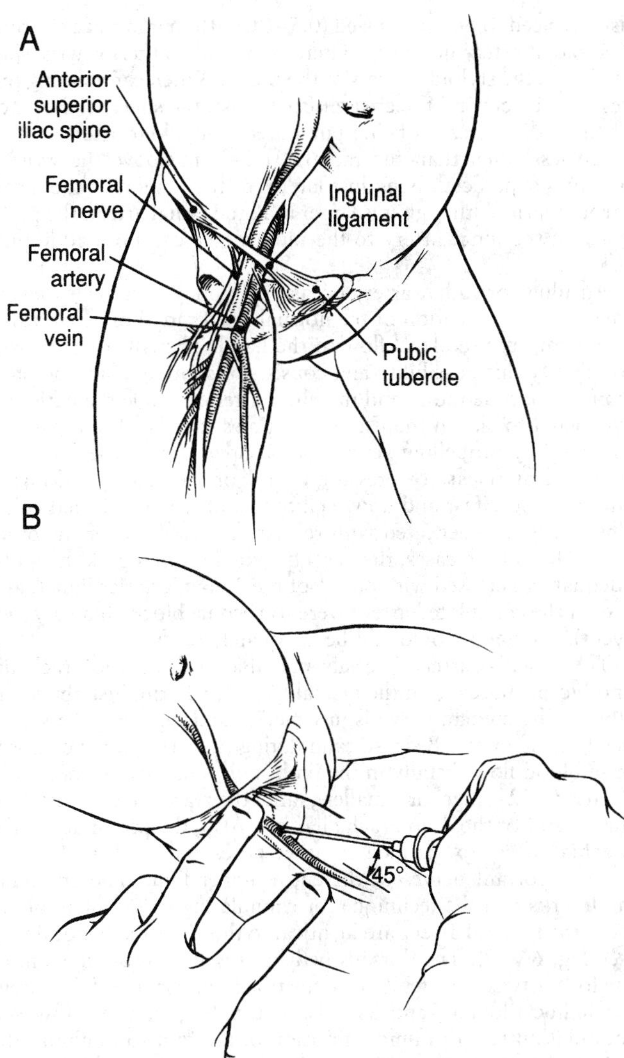

Figure 66-19. Femoral vein anatomy *(A)* and cannulation technique *(B)*. (From American Heart Association: Pediatric Advanced Life Support Student CD. © 2006, American Heart Association, Inc. Reproduced with permission.)

ENDOTRACHEAL TUBE DRUG ADMINISTRATION. Administration of certain drugs is also possible through the ETT. Drugs that are effective through this route include lidocaine, atropine, naloxone, and epinephrine. When given through an ETT, epinephrine should be given at 10 times the intravenous dose.

ARTERIAL ACCESS. Arterial catheters require special care for insertion and subsequent management because the blood flow to tissue can be compromised and considerable hemorrhage can occur if a catheter is dislodged. In most instances, the child should be in the PICU. The adequacy of perfusion distal to the catheter must be monitored (warmth, capillary filling, edema). Catheters usually need to be heparinized (0.5–1 U/mL) to minimize clotting. The radial artery lies on the lateral side of the anterior wrist, just medial to the styloid process of the radius. When cannulating this vessel at or beyond the crease of the wrist, the superficial branch of the radial artery is being punctured. The ulnar artery is used much less often than the radial. At 2–3 cm above the wrist it becomes superficial, lying just lateral to the tendon of the flexor carpi ulnaris. Although it is larger than the radial artery, the proximity of the ulnar artery to the ulnar nerve can pose additional risk.

An ulnar or radial artery occasionally may be absent or very small, and cannulation of the normal-sized radial or ulnar vessel may compromise blood flow to the hand. The **Allen test** is used to identify this possibility and consists of simultaneous compression of both the radial and the ulnar arteries, while the patient is instructed to clench the fist several times (to blanch the palm of the hand by propelling venous blood upward into the forearm), followed by release of pressure over 1 of the vessels and observation of how fast and how well the hand regains normal color. The test is then repeated with release of pressure over the other vessel. If, in both cases, the hand quickly becomes pink, it can be adequately perfused with only 1 of the 2 main arteries intact, and even if the cannulated artery were to become blocked (a very rare event), the hand would still be adequately perfused.

The brachial artery is easily palpable between the brachialis and biceps muscles, on the medial side of the arm, just above the elbow. The median nerve is just medial and may even lie superficial to the artery. Because cannulating this artery may compromise blood flow distally in the limb, only small catheters should be used (22-gauge or smaller), and they are placed distal to the takeoff of the deep brachial artery. Also, the proximity of the brachial artery to the median nerve poses extra risk to 1 of the most important nerves of the entire upper limb. The anatomic landmarks and the technique for cannulating or sampling blood from the femoral artery are identical to those for the femoral vein (see Fig. 66-19). The dorsalis pedis artery lies on the dorsum of the foot between the tendons of the tibialis anterior and the extensor hallucis longus, and its pulse is usually palpable. However, cannulation requires immobilization of the foot to minimize the risk of dislodging the catheter with flexion and extension of the ankle. Cannulation of the posterior tibial artery as it passes posterior to the medial malleolus is another useful alternative, particularly in neonates and infants.

THORACENTESIS AND CHEST TUBE PLACEMENT. See Chapters 71 and 409. Thoracentesis is the placement of a needle or catheter (chest tube) into the pleural space to evacuate fluid, blood, or air. Most insertions are performed in one of the intercostal spaces between the 4th and 9th ribs, along the midclavicular line in the anterior chest wall (in adolescents and adults), or in the plane of the midaxillary line. After appropriate systemic and local anesthesia/sedation, a skin incision is made and dissection through the chest wall is accomplished in layers, using blunt dissection techniques. The needle (and later, the chest tube) that enters the pleural space should penetrate the intercostal space by passing over the superior edge of the lower rib, because there are larger vessels along the inferior edge of the rib. Ideally, the chest tube should lie anterior in the pleural space for air and posterior for fluid accumulation. Final penetration of the intercostal membranes, to enter the pleural space, often takes considerable force, and the instrument (usually a hemostat) inserted into the pleural cavity should be grasped in such a way that there is no risk of uncontrolled deep penetration into the mediastinum, with possible contusion of the lung or heart. After the chest tube is inserted, it should be secured firmly to the chest wall and connected to a source of suction (a water-column suction chamber attached to wall suction) at a pressure of 15–20 cm H_2O. A radiograph should be obtained to verify chest tube placement and evacuation of the pleural space.

PERICARDIOCENTESIS. When fluid, blood, or gas accumulates in the pericardial sac, a danger is that the heart will be compressed and will not be able to fill and empty with normal volumes of blood, leading to diminished cardiac output. The cardinal signs of such a restrictive pericardial effusion are tachycardia, hypotension, and decreasing oxygen saturation. Pericardiocentesis is needle aspiration of the sac performed with or without ultrasound verification of needle placement or attachment of a recording electrode. After proper patient positioning, sterile cleansing of the area around the xiphoid process, and sedation/analgesia, pericardiocentesis begins with a short incision in the skin just below the xiphoid process. A 20–22-gauge spinal needle that is 6.25 cm (2.5 in) long is used. The proximal end of the needle is attached to a stopcock and a collection syringe. The needle is inserted through the incision and then positioned so that it points toward the space between the left nipple and the medial end of the clavicle. Once the needle is through the skin, its angle should be flattened considerably with respect to the chest wall so that penetration is not too deep (in larger children or adults, the angle must be steeper). During insertion, the syringe attached to the needle is continuously aspirated with gentle pressure so that, when the needle enters the pericardial space, there will be a rush of gas or fluid. Once the procedure is concluded, a sterile dressing should be placed over the skin incision and a chest radiograph obtained to rule out complications.

THE FAMILY AND PEDIATRIC RESUSCITATIONS

Some family members wish to be present throughout a resuscitation and do not respond well to any attempt to exclude them. The critically ill patient certainly is the highest priority, but for many parents and family members, their presence at a resuscitation, even if it is destined to fail, is a matter of deep importance to them. No universal guidelines have been developed for this situation, although most centers allow for some family presence. The fear that family members may lose their composure and require support, taking attention away from the patient, can be met if there is a member of the treatment team who can explain events as they are happening and answer questions. Although this remains a controversial area of policy and practice, it has been our experience that the family members' presence at a resuscitation, if requested, helps the family in the long run to accept the outcome of the resuscitation and to understand what efforts were made to support their child's life.

POST-RESUSCITATION CARE

When resuscitation is successful, continuous PICU care is usually needed to attend to the potential postischemic multiple organ dysfunction syndromes and the continued need for cardiac inotropic support. **Hyperglycemia** and **hyperthermia** should be avoided. Continuous observation for immediate neurologic deterioration and long-term permanent neurodevelopmental sequelae is imperative.

When resuscitation fails and the patient dies, attention is naturally focused on comforting the grieving family. Members of the medical team also need time to adjust to the events and need to understand how and why their efforts did not succeed. The more senior members of a team should recognize and acknowledge the contributions of those involved in the resuscitation and should convey to the family a detailed description of what took place. Increasingly, families may be present at resuscitations and may need a special kind of "debriefing" to help them accept what they witnessed. When appropriate, families should be reassured that any further data that become available shortly after a death (e.g., autopsy results) can be shared with them, if they wish. Finally, someone on the team must be mindful of the legal and procedural duties involved in a death, such as notification of the coroner, contact with the organ/tissue transplant bank, completion of the death certificate, and arrangements for disposition of the remains of the deceased, depending on local regulations, family wishes, and customs.

American Heart Association: 2005 American Heart Association (AHA) guidelines for cardiopulmonary resuscitation (CPR) and emergency cardiovascular care (ECC) of pediatric and neonatal patients: pediatric advanced life support. *Pediatrics* 2006;117:e1005-e1004–1028.

American Heart Association: 2005 American Heart Association (AHA) guidelines for cardiopulmonary resuscitation (CPR) and emergency cardiovascular care (ECC) of pediatric and neonatal patients: pediatric basic life support. *Pediatrics* 2006;117:e989–e1004.

Burns JP, Rushton CH: End-of-life care in the pediatric intensive care unit: Research review and recommendations. *Crit Care Clin* 2004;20:467–485.

Cummins RO, Hazinski MF: The most important changes in the international EED and CPR Guidelines 2000. *Circulation* 2000;102:1371–1376.

Eisenberg MS, Mengert TJ: Cardiac resuscitation. *N Engl J Med* 2001;344:1304–1313.

Hallstrom A, Cobb L, Johnson E, et al: Cardiopulmonary resuscitation by chest compression alone or with mouth-to-mouth ventilation. *N Engl J Med* 2000;342:1546–1553.

Janakiraman L: Pediatric Advanced Life Support (PALS): The current guidelines. *Indian J Pediatr* 2003;70(Suppl 1):S34–S38.

Kern K, Halperin HR, Field J: New guidelines for cardiopulmonary resuscitation and emergency cardiac care. *JAMA* 2001;285:1267–1269.

Kochanek MK, Clark RS, Ruppel RA, et al: Cerebral resuscitation after traumatic brain injury and cardiopulmonary arrest in infants and children in the new millennium. *Pediatr Clin North Am* 2001;48:661–681.

Lockey AS, Nolan JP: Cardiopulmonary resuscitation in adults. *BMJ* 2001;323:819–820.

Masutani S, Senzaki H, Ishido H, et al: Vasopressin in the treatment of vasodilatory shock in children. *Pediatr Int* 2005;47:132–136.

Nadkarni VM, Larkin GL, Peberdy MA, et al: First documented rhythm and clinical outcome from in-hospital cardiac arrest among children and adults. *JAMA* 2006;295:50–57.

Parfitt A: Resuscitation guidelines. *Lancet* 2006;367:282–284.

Perondi MB, Reis AG, Paiva EF, et al: A comparison of high-dose and standard-dose epinephrine in children with cardiac arrest. *N Engl J Med* 2004;350:1708–1709.

Reis AG, Nadkarni V, Perondi MB, et al: A prospective investigation into the epidemiology of in hospital pediatric cardiopulmonary resuscitation using internations Utstein reporting style. *Pediatrics* 2002;109:200–209.

Samson RA, Nadkarni VM, Meaney PA, et al: Outcomes of in-hospital ventricular fibrillation in children. *N Engl J Med* 2006;354:2328–2339.

Sorrentino A: Update on pediatric resuscitation drugs: High dose, low dose, or no dose at all. *Curr Opin Pediatr* 2005;17:223–226.

Tsai E: Should family members be present during cardiopulmonary resuscitation? *N Engl J Med* 2002;346:1019–1021.

Chapter 67 ■ Neurologic Emergencies and Stabilization

Lorry R. Frankel

Acute neurologic deterioration may be a life-threatening event, with numerous causes and a few typical clinical presentations (coma, seizures, weakness, altered mental status). The clinician must act quickly to stabilize the child with an evolving neurologic illness to reverse the process and avoid further permanent neurologic injury. The initial event produces the **primary injury** to the brain that gives rise to the typical signs and symptoms. If the primary events are not recognized, the child may be at significant risk for further injury, referred to as **secondary injury.** This involves systemic hypotension, respiratory failure, and hypoxia, as well as progressive cerebral or brainstem herniation resulting from the development of cerebral edema or intracranial bleeding, which if unrecognized and untreated, can worsen the outcome for the child.

Preservation of global neurologic function, prevention of secondary cerebral edema, and optimizing regeneration are goals for the stabilization and ongoing care of the child. Several disease states can profoundly affect neurologic function, either temporarily or permanently. The physician must recognize states that have the potential for permanent dysfunction and support the child in ways that optimize the return toward normal. The most common causes of acute global neurologic dysfunction in children are head trauma, hypoxia-ischemia, central nervous system (CNS) infection, and encephalopathies from endogenous metabolites or exogenous toxins. Idiopathic status epilepticus can also cause moderate or severe encephalopathy. Global neurologic dysfunction, coupled with focal signs, may be a late presentation of a CNS tumor or abscess.

The manifestations of an acute or evolving neurologic process can produce generalized or focal findings. Coma, stupor, and lethargy are more general findings suggestive of an advancing process that has global cerebral implications. Focal findings may reflect a more well-defined process localized to 1 part of the brain. **Coma** refers to a state in which the patient is unable to arouse or respond to noxious stimuli and is completely unaware of self and surroundings. **Stupor** may be confused with normal sleep, but the patient can be aroused with painful stimuli. **Lethargy** is more subjective and is used to indicate drowsiness or decreased wakefulness. These patients may be confused, but are able to communicate. Because these terms are often used by different physicians with different meanings, it is best to record the physical findings and use a quantitative score, such as the Glasgow Coma Scale (GCS). This score may be adjusted for age (see Table 66-5).

HEAD TRAUMA. Traumatic brain injury (TBI) is the primary injury that is caused by the direct mechanical disruption of brain tissue and the subsequent secondary injuries that result from the various cerebral and systemic processes worsened by events in the post-traumatic period. TBI in children is different than in adults because of the unique pathophysiology of children and the epidemiologic characteristics of pediatric injury. The causes of TBI in children may be separated into injuries associated with child abuse, contact injuries, and inertial injuries.

Nonaccidental trauma (NAT), or **child abuse,** has been thought to produce primary brain injury from repetitive acceleration-deceleration forces, which accompany shaking (therefore, the term *shaken baby;* see Chapter 36). The injuries sustained may be compatible with hypoxic injury secondary to brainstem and spinal cord injury or the direct effects of the traumatic force. Victims of child abuse may not have signs of external trauma (bruises, fractures). Instead, they may have mental status changes (lethargy, irritability), poor feeding, apnea, or seizures. If NAT is suspected, the clinician must obtain a head CT scan to evaluate for acute and subacute injuries, such as subdural and epidural hematomas or effusions, punctate intracerebral hemorrhages, skull fractures, cerebral edema, atrophy, and/or hydrocephalus (Figs. 67-1 to 67-4).

Contact injuries occur when an object strikes the head. The force generated by the impact may result in a skull fracture (depressed or linear), cerebral contusion (both coup and contrecoup), or intracranial bleeding (epidural hematoma, subdural hematoma, subarachnoid hemorrhage, or deep intracerebral hematoma). In severe forms of contact injuries, all of these findings may exist. Those with severe intraparenchymal and intraventricular hemorrhages have a poorer prognosis. In addition, diffuse cerebral edema may develop; this is not always evident on presentation and is not always related to the severity of the trauma (Figs. 67-5 to 67-7).

Inertial injuries usually occur from rapid acceleration-deceleration forces. This mechanism of injury results from the move-

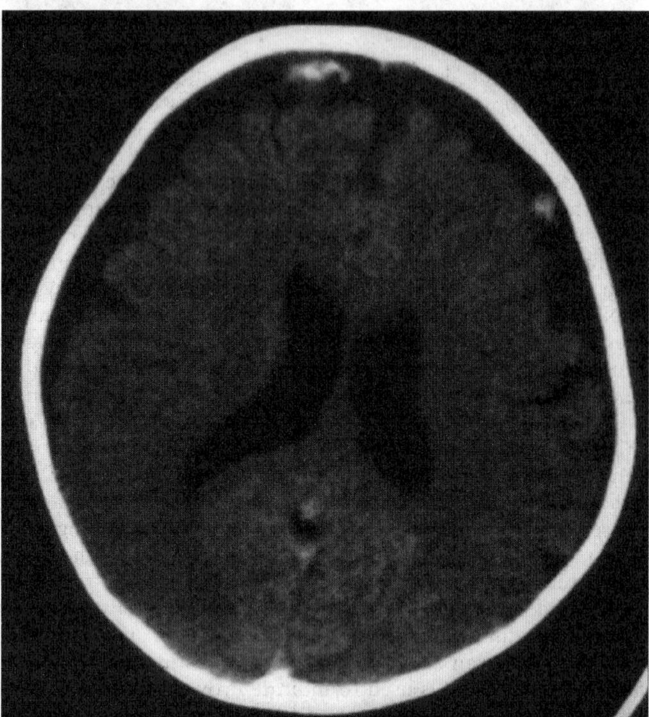

Figure 67-1. Nonaccidental trauma in an infant. Note the subdural fluid collections, dilated ventricles, and blood.

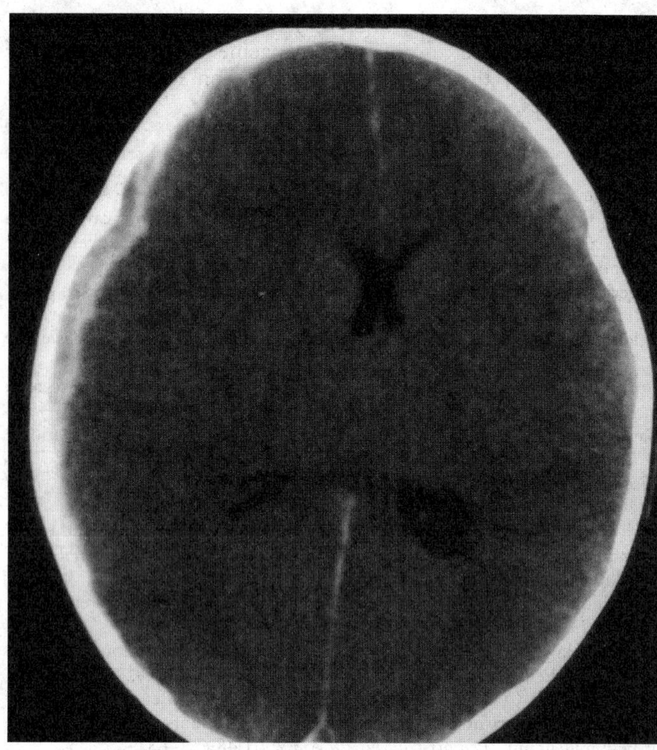

Figure 67-2. Nonaccidental trauma with a subdural collection of fluid and a midline shift.

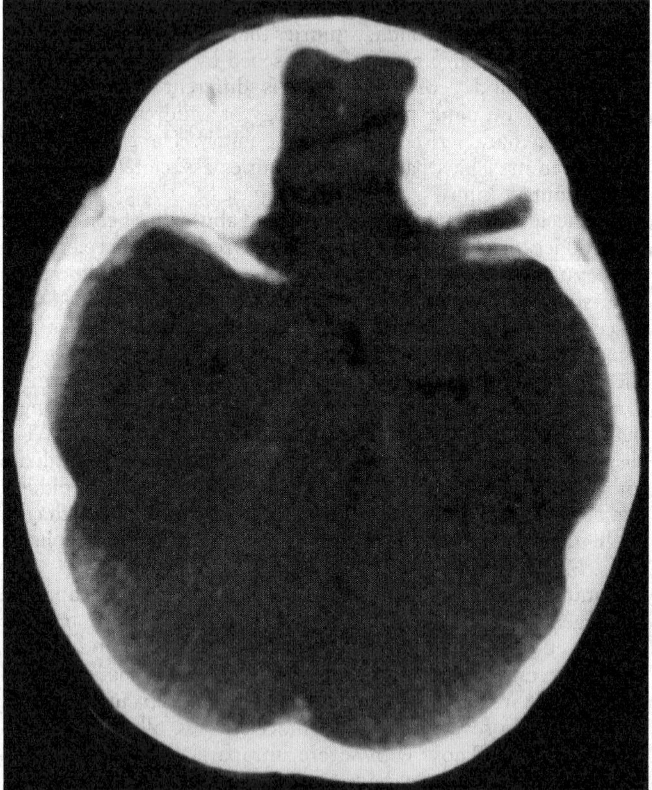

Figure 67-3. Nonaccidental trauma with massive cerebral edema, with loss of gray-white differentiation, loss of the ventricular system, and probable herniation of the brainstem.

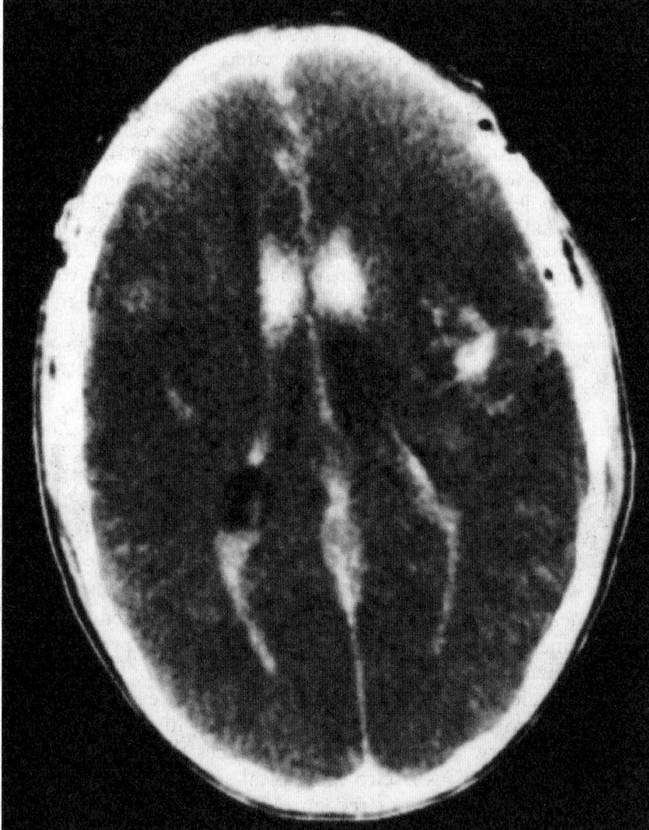

Figure 67-4. Nonaccidental trauma with significant intraventricular, intracerebral, and subdural hematomas, with loss of gray-white differentiation, suggestive of massive cerebral edema.

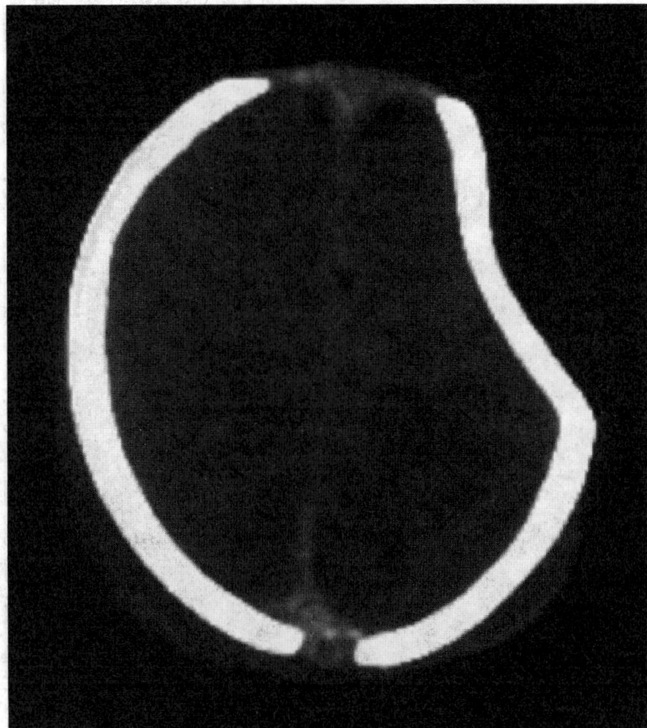

Figure 67-5. Contact head injury: a depressed skull fracture as a result of traumatic delivery with forceps. Brain swelling is seen.

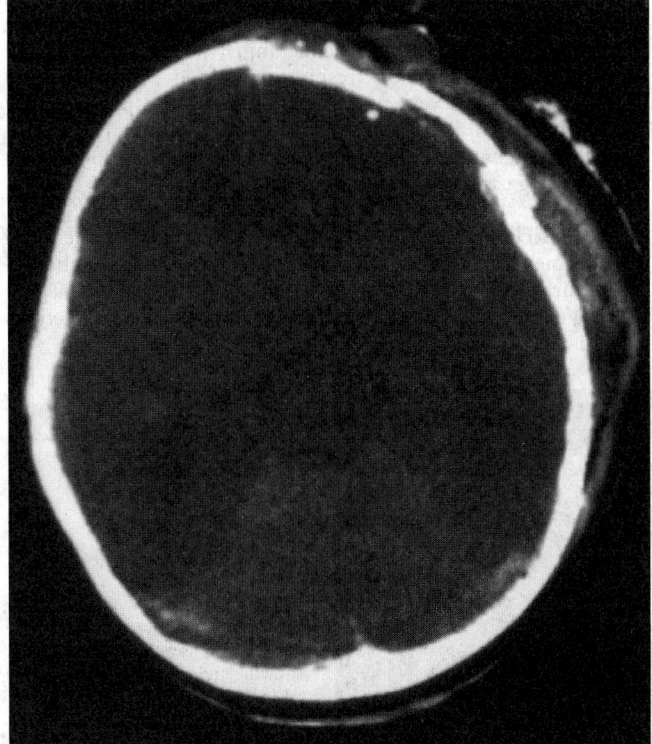

Figure 67-6. Contact head injury with malignant brain edema (hyperemia), a common pattern in severe head injury that is associated with significant secondary brain injury and a very high mortality rate. Cisterns are absent on CT scan. This type of injury is associated with hypoxia and hypotension. The reported mortality rates varies, with Bruce et al. reporting a rate of 12% in a 1981 article in the *Journal of Neurosurgery,* and Aldrich et al. reporting a rate of 53% in a 1992 article in the same publication.

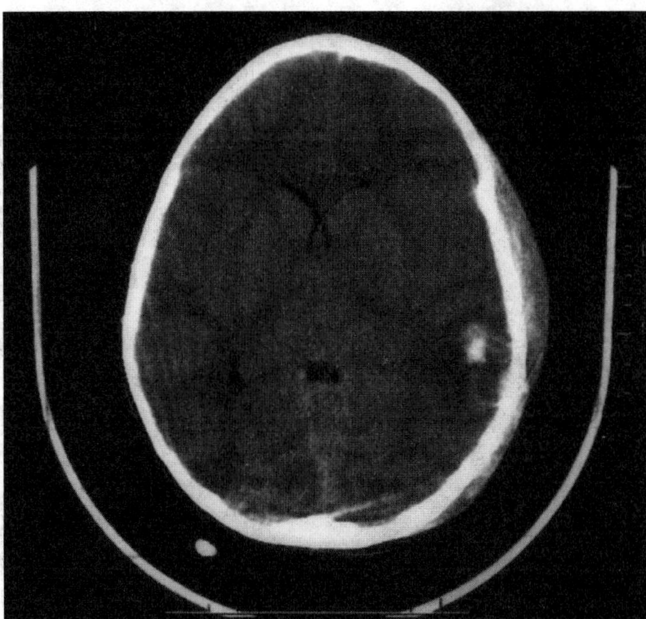

Figure 67-7. Significant closed head injury with subgaleal hematoma, intracerebral hemorrhage, and loss of gray-white differentiation.

ment of the intracranial structures within the cranial vault. This may produce severe forms of microscopic injury to the axons, resulting in **diffuse axonal injury (DAI).** Inertial injuries may occur in isolation or in association with contact injuries. The clinical significance of DAI is dependent on the extent and location with the brain. DAI of the brainstem may have more serious consequences than DAI in other parts of the brain (Figs. 67-8 to 67-10).

Secondary brain injuries associated with trauma may occur in the immediate post-traumatic period or develop over the next several days. Secondary injury is associated with systemic hypotension, hypoxia, intracranial hemorrhages, or increased metabolic needs. **Cerebral edema** is a significant secondary injury that may lead to further neuronal damage, cerebral herniation, and death. TBI may also produce events that may lead to neuronal death via the release of a variety of mediators, such as excitatory amino acids. This occurs after a generalized depolarization of neurons after the primary brain injury. When this happens, there appears to be cerebrovascular dysfunction (loss of autoregulation), cerebral edema alterations in the blood-brain barrier, release of free radicals, damage to the mitochondria, apoptosis, and neuronal death.

Patients with acute head injury and a GCS score of <8 should be admitted to a pediatric intensive care unit that is capable of caring for the acutely injured child. This includes capabilities for mechanical ventilation, neurosurgical intervention, and skilled nursing that can manage intracranial pressure (ICP) monitoring equipment as well advanced hemodynamic monitoring. Children with traumatic head injury may take a long time to recover, but often regain significant function during rehabilitation.

HYPOXIA-ISCHEMIA. Encephalopathy from poor or absent cerebral perfusion (both hypoxia and ischemia) often heralds a poorer outcome than that from trauma; the physician has little to offer to improve the outcome. Often there is diffuse, global brain injury. These children may have experienced a period of asystole and may have required CPR, such as after near-drowning episodes, acute life-threatening events, smoke inhalation, upper or lower airway obstruction, shock, or electrical injury. The lack of oxygen and perfusion produces primary neuronal damage. Secondary injury occurs from the response of the acti-

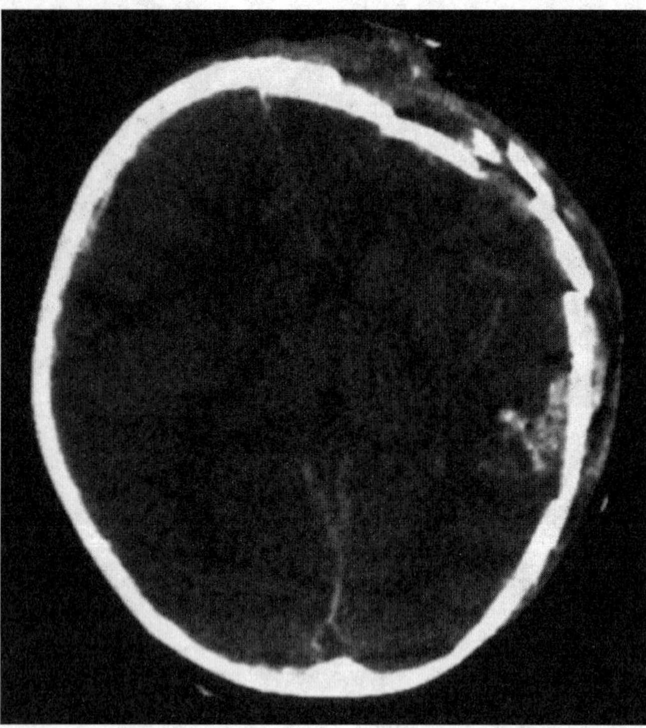

Figure 67-8. Significant head injury with multiple depressed skull fractures and intraparenchymal hemorrhage.

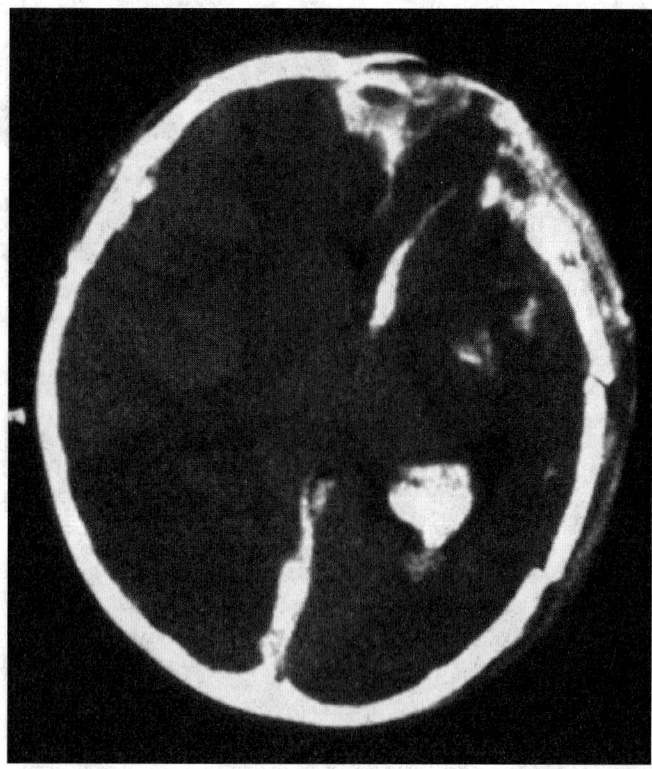

Figure 67-9. Significant head injury with multiple depressed skull fractures and intraparenchymal hemorrhage.

vation of mediators, which initiate a cascade of events that result in cerebral edema and apoptosis.

Imaging studies may be helpful in evaluating the structural damage seen with hypoxic-ischemic encephalopathy. These changes may not be immediately apparent; they provide an insight into the extent of the cerebral injury. Rapid diffusion weighted imaging (MRI) demonstrates lesions faster than any other imaging modality. There is often preservation of brainstem function. Other organ systems may reflect hypoxic-ischemic injury, such as the liver, kidneys, intestines, lung, and heart. A poor prognosis is associated with a low GCS score (<5), hypotension, cerebral edema, persistent apnea, CPR for >25 min, persistent loss of cranial nerve reflexes (gag, corneal), or a coma for >24 hr. Patients who have required significant support for these other organ systems have very poor outcomes. Children who have sustained serious hypoxic-ischemic injury but have preserved other vital organ function (respiration, blood pressure, pulse) may survive with severe neurologic function and possibly in a persistent vegetative state. These survivors may require technology when discharged from the intensive care unit, including tracheostomy, gastrostomy, and/or fundoplication.

CENTRAL NERVOUS SYSTEM INFECTION. Infections of the CNS include meningitis, meningoencephalitis, encephalitis, subdural or epidural empyema, and brain abscess (see Chapters 602 and 603). Viruses and bacteria cause meningitis; fungal infections

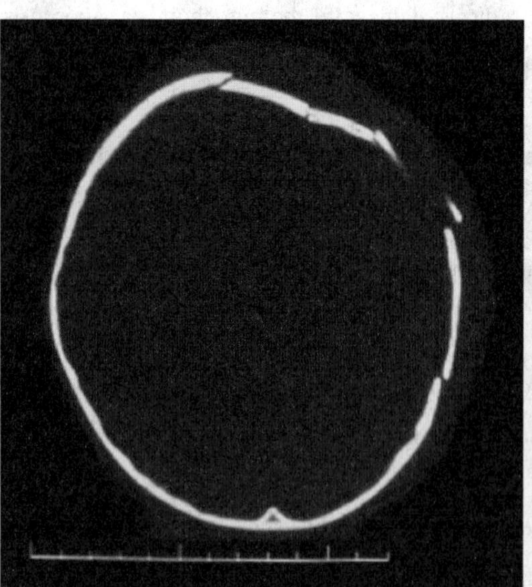

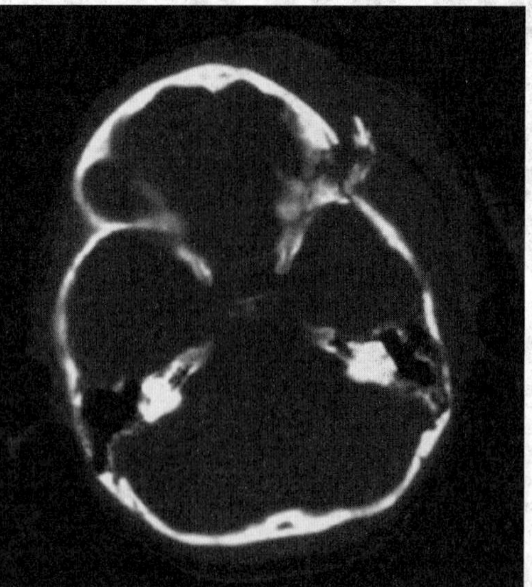

Figure 67-10. Bone widows associated with severe head injury, showing multiple skull fractures and edema.

may be noted in immunosuppressed patients. Important treatable causes of stupor and coma include bacterial meningitis, herpes simplex encephalitis, bacterial abscess, cerebral toxoplasmosis, and tuberculosis meningitis. An infectious cause must be considered in any patient with acute neurologic deterioration associated with fever or in those without a history of trauma. Signs of meningeal irritation, such as nuchal rigidity or the Kernig or Brudzinski sign, may be present. Infants may not always have a bulging fontanel. Patients with CNS infection may also have global encephalopathy, such as coma or status epilepticus. Patients who have had certain infections, such as acute demyelinating encephalomyelitis, may also have altered mental status, seizures, and focal neurologic deficits (see Chapter 600).

Early diagnosis and treatment with appropriate antibiotics or antiviral drugs are important. If the patient demonstrates any manifestations of systemic complications (hypotension, apnea) the clinician must address them immediately to prevent secondary neuronal injury and other organ dysfunction. This includes airway management, mechanical ventilation, and cardiovascular support. Complications from acute neurologic infections include cerebrovascular infarction, cerebritis, cranial nerve compression, and the development of hydrocephalus, subdural effusions, cerebral edema, and cerebral herniation. These findings are detected with imaging studies, which should be performed if the patient is not improving within 24–48 hr. In addition, patients whose condition continues to deteriorate, with the development of focal findings, should be evaluated for signs of ICP, such as hypertension, bradycardia, irregular respirations, or signs of compression of cranial nerves III or VI. Neurosurgical consultation may be indicated.

ENCEPHALOPATHIES FROM ENDOGENOUS METABOLITES OR EXOGENOUS TOXINS. Profound encephalopathy may result from metabolic defects (inborn errors of metabolism producing hypoglycemia, hyperammonemia, or lactic or organic acidosis); fulminant hepatic failure (hyperammonemia plus other unmeasured neurotoxins); or the ingestion of certain drugs and substances (ethanol, anticonvulsant drugs). Accidental ingestions are very common in toddlers and young children. Older children may experiment with various chemical substances or ingest wild mushrooms, which may produce acute cerebral signs. A **drug toxicology screen** is indicated in any patient who has an altered level of consciousness without a clear explanation.

Other laboratory tests may be helpful in the assessment of the child who presents with obtundation. These tests include routine electrolyte measurements to evaluate for an increased **anion gap** (acidosis from endogenous acids or exogenous acids, such as salicylates); **serum osmolarity** to detect differences between calculated and measured osmolarity (alcohol, ethylene glycol ingestion); and arterial blood gas analysis to determine if there is a respiratory alkalosis (early salicylate poisoning or hyperammonemia), a respiratory acidosis (opiate or barbiturate ingestion producing respiratory depression), or a metabolic acidosis (late salicylate ingestion or endogenous lactic or organic acidosis).

One must always determine if there are alterations in glucose homeostasis because diabetic ketoacidosis may produce altered levels of consciousness. In addition, hypoglycemia also produces obtundation, stupor, and coma. Hypoglycemia occurs frequently as a result of various metabolic and endocrine disorders and with intoxication with alcohol. Young infants and children are especially prone to episodes of hypoglycemia because they have limited glycogen stores and can become seriously hypoglycemic as a result of prolonged fasting, inborn errors of metabolism, hyperinsulinism, liver failure, or ingestions. Hypoglycemia is easily reversible and should be aggressively pursued in every comatose child (see Chapter 92).

DIABETES MELLITUS. Cerebral edema may occur during the treatment of diabetic ketoacidosis (DKA; see Chapter 590). This is likely due to the action of *idiogenic osmoles,* osmotically active particles formed within the cerebral cells during the acute phase to counteract the effects of hyperglycemia. If serum osmolality declines too quickly, these osmolar particles can act to attract water into the cell. Cerebral edema in DKA may be associated with significant morbidity and mortality. Coma may also occur in severe DKA or when it is associated with severe **hyperosmolar states** before treatment. Stress-induced hyperglycemia and a lactic acidosis (without ketonuria) are common during the hypoxic-ischemic encephalopathy and have a poor prognosis.

STATUS EPILEPTICUS. Severe status epilepticus results in stupor or coma and has the potential for permanent cellular damage if the seizures are prolonged or are associated with hypoxia, hypercarbia, and hypotension (see Chapter 593). Seizures lasting >10 min must be treated aggressively. Intensive therapies are aimed at halting epileptic activity and reducing neurologic cell metabolism to limit the extent of the primary neuronal injury. **Electrical status** produces coma and may severely affect the brain in the absence of clinically evident seizures; an electroencephalogram will confirm the diagnosis. Because patients may become apneic with the administration of anticonvulsants, the treating physician must be prepared to control the airway.

INTRACRANIAL HYPERTENSION. Acute intracranial hypertension often initially presents with headache and confusion, but may advance at various rates to combativeness, somnolence, and coma. It may be seen as a complication of global or focal encephalopathies or mass lesions. An increase in the volume of cerebral contents within the rigid cranial cavity (blood, edema, masses, cerebral [ventricular] spinal fluid) produces an increase in ICP. This may result from trauma from hemorrhage or hyperemia; hydrocephalus with cerebrospinal fluid accumulation; tumors or abscesses; severe CNS infections; and metabolic aberrations, including hypoxia-ischemia. As ICP increases, the effective cerebral perfusion pressure (CPP) decreases. CPP is equal to mean arterial pressure minus ICP. Autoregulation of the cerebral vasculature provides the initial protection to maintain cerebral perfusion. However, as ICP increases, autoregulation may be lost. CPP may be reduced by increased ICP, hypotension, or both. Additional manifestations of increased ICP include papilledema, Cushing triad (bradycardia, hypertension, irregular respirations), bulging fontanel, and signs of compression of cranial nerve III (ptosis, anisocoria) or VI (lateral rectus weakness). Increased ICP produces confusion, which may mimic global encephalopathy; increasing confusion and combativeness may progress to coma and brainstem compression. These are late signs of increased ICP and indicate that herniation of brain structures is occurring; this situation is life-threatening and requires immediate intervention.

HERNIATION. Coma may precede herniation of the intracranial contents. Brainstem herniation proceeds from higher to lower brain centers. Coma is followed by decorticate rigidity, small pupils, and Cheyne-Stokes breathing. As the midbrain and pons become involved, posturing changes to decerebrate, pupils become mid-position and nonreactive, and the breathing pattern is hyperpneic. As the medulla is compromised, blood pressure and heart rate fluctuate greatly, the patient becomes flaccid, and breathing is irregular and then absent. **Unilateral uncal lobe herniation** may be heralded by ipsilateral anisocoria, loss of papillary reflexes, and ptosis caused by compression of the cranial nerve III.

INFRATENTORIAL LESIONS. Lesions in the infratentorial region can cause coma, cranial nerve palsy, and respiratory abnormalities at an earlier stage in the disease than supratentorial lesions. Obstructive hydrocephalus may result from compression of the circulatory or cerebrospinal fluid pathways. Such compression is seen with posterior fossa tumors. These may produce brainstem compression without the depth or severity of encephalopathy seen in more global cortical disease. The hallmark of infratentorial herniation is early respiratory and autonomic impairment, whereas papillary responses may be preserved. Neck pain may be present as well as vocal cord paralysis.

PRINCIPLES OF SUPPORT FOR GLOBAL NEUROLOGIC DYSFUNCTION

NORMALIZE THE CIRCULATION AND RESPIRATION. The basics of neurologic stabilization include the ABCs of resuscitation (airway, breathing, and circulation; see Chapter 66) and maintenance of adequate oxygenation and perfusion. The decision to intubate the trachea and institute mechanical ventilation is determined by the need to control the airway: Is the patient able to protect the airway (intact cough and gag reflexes) from aspiration? In some patients with stupor, the respiratory drive may be intact but the gag reflex may be absent or upper airway muscle tone is lax. In the case of Guillain-Barré syndrome, one should not wait for respirations to be shallow. If the patient is unable to protect the airway, intubation is indicated. The work of breathing must be maintained to ensure adequate gas exchange and avoid hypercarbia and hypoxemia (Fig. 67-11). Intubation may be needed to hyperventilate the patient to produce mild hypocarbia, thus helping to reduce ICP. Intubation requires a degree of sophistication as well as the availability of the appropriate equipment, medication, and personnel to facilitate intubation in as rapid and atraumatic a manner as possible. The medication and procedure should not further raise ICP. A form of rapid sequence intubation is used, with appropriate positioning of the patient to support the neck (see Chapter 76). Once the airway is secured and the patient's oxygenation and ventilation have been stabilized, the clinician can focus on maintaining adequate cardiac output to ensure appropriate tissue perfusion.

Circulation should be normalized in an effort to optimize organ perfusion to vital organs. If evidence of poor perfusion still exists after appropriate fluid resuscitation, the use of inotropic agents to enhance cardiac output should be considered. In addition, ongoing fluid or blood loss is a concern. Once the patient has stable cardiac output, modest fluid restriction is beneficial and may help to avoid hypervolemia. Little benefit has been demonstrated from severe fluid restriction. However, serum electrolytes and urine output must be monitored. Fluid restriction may be used if the patient becomes hyponatremic from the syndrome of inappropriate antidiuretic hormone secretion (SIADH).

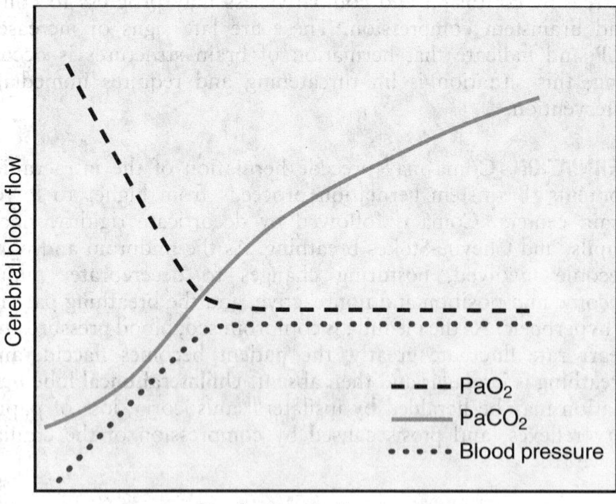

Figure 67-11. Changes in cerebral blood flow (CBF) in relation to Pa_{O_2}, Pa_{CO_2} and blood pressure. Note that CBF is fairly constant over a wide blood pressure range.

Fluid Management in the Presence of SIADH or Diabetes Insipidus. Inappropriate secretion of antidiuretic hormone is a frequent accompaniment of CNS injury or infection and can occur with many types of brain injury as well as with pulmonary disease (see Chapters 52 and 560). The diagnosis of SIADH is suggested by analyzing the osmolality of both urine (higher than expected) and serum (lower than expected) of hyponatremic patients. Urine osmolality is often higher than serum osmolality. The effects of SIADH can be reduced by fluid restriction. SIADH is usually self-limited, although it may persist while the patient is on mechanical ventilation. Patients with SIADH are normotensive and not edematous, in contrast to patients with hyponatremia and heart or hepatic failure (dilutional hyponatremia) or adrenal or renal insufficiency (salt-losing states).

Diabetes insipidus heralds a very poor outcome in the child with significant brain injury (see Chapter 559). A damaged pituitary or hypothalamus can induce massive unregulated urine output, dehydration, and a rapidly rising serum sodium concentration. The sodium level can rise as much as 30 mEq/L in a few hours. Diabetes insipidus can be managed with vigorous intravenous fluid intake, but is better controlled with vasopressin or desmopressin.

REDUCE INTRACRANIAL HYPERTENSION. The goal of therapy is to maintain CPP in the appropriate range for the patient's age: for infants and toddlers, >40 mm Hg; for young children, >50 mm Hg; and for adolescents, >60–70 mm Hg.

Intubation, Ventilation, and Positioning. The initial and most rapid therapeutic intervention for reducing intracranial hypertension requires endotracheal intubation and monitoring of blood gases to ensure appropriate oxygenation and ventilation and to keep Pa_{CO_2} at 30–35 mm Hg. Mild hyperventilation is helpful because it acutely reduces cerebral blood flow through cerebral vasoconstriction; significant hyperventilation (Pa_{CO_2} <25 mm Hg) may cause cerebral ischemia. Having the patient's head midline and elevated 30 degrees allows optimal venous drainage and may be helpful in reducing ICP. Deep sedation may be helpful to minimize patient movement; muscle relaxants may be helpful (intermittent or continuous infusion of benzodiazepines, narcotics, and vecuronium).

Ventricular Drainage, Diuretics, Steroids, and Other Therapies. Reduction in the cerebrospinal fluid volume may be helpful in managing increased ICP. If a ventriculostomy has been placed, periodic fluid removal will reduce ICP and hence improve CPP. Diuretics in the forms of mannitol and furosemide further reduce the circulating blood volume and have been used. Mannitol (0.25–0.5 g/kg/dose) is useful in the acute treatment of intracranial hypertension. It is an osmotic diuretic and promotes a shift of fluid from the intracellular to the vascular compartment. Mannitol is less beneficial with severe disruption of the blood-brain barrier because it may enter the CNS and draw fluid into the brain. Mannitol can produce renal failure and hemolysis because of the very hyperosmolar state it creates. Furosemide is a safer but less effective alternative. Usually, the combination of both agents is prescribed. Hypertonic saline infusions may be beneficial. The use of intravenous steroids is not indicated if there is diffuse cerebral injury. However, steroids may be of benefit when the edema is localized around an intracranial mass (abscess, tumor). Surgical decompression and evacuation of extravascular blood under pressure is essential. The use of barbiturate coma with continuous electroencephalographic monitoring is used with variable success to reduce the cerebral metabolic demands and ICP. Barbiturate coma may have many side effects, such as a reduction in cardiac output, producing systemic hypotension.

SEIZURES

BENZODIAZEPINES VS OTHER ANTIEPILEPTICS. Both benzodiazepines and other anticonvulsant drugs reduce cerebral metabolism and are effective in suppressing seizure activity. Seizures that last >10 min must be treated aggressively. Patients are considered to be in status if seizures last >20–30 min. A state of refractory seizures has evolved if seizures persist >60 min, despite anticonvulsant therapy. Benzodiazepines are very effective as a 1st-line agent for treating seizures in patients with hypoxic-ischemic encephalopathy and other causes of status. Both lorazepam and diazepam are very effective, with a rapid onset of action (3–5 min). Because benzodiazepines have a relatively short half-life, longer-acting agents are then needed. Phenytoin or phenobarbital is usually used next. Phenobarbital has a very long half-life, and at high serum levels, it may affect the neurologic examination. Phenytoin should not cause sedation, nor should it affect the neurologic examination. Fosphenytoin is often substituted for phenytoin. Other agents commonly used include midazolam and valproic acid. Seizures that are refractory require repeated dosing of phenobarbital to achieve levels of 50–100 mg/dL. Propofol has been used with some success in the treatment of refractory seizures.

BARBITURATE-INDUCED COMA. If seizures are refractory to barbiturates and phenytoin drugs, a barbiturate-induced coma may be necessary. Therapy may be titrated to a burst suppression pattern when using a barbiturate coma. This requires 24-hr electroencephalogram (EEG) monitoring with a portable bedside EEG. Complications of barbiturate-induced coma include cardiovascular depression with decreased cardiac output that may require inotropic support.

HYPOTHERMIA. Mild hypothermia (32–34°C) in non-neonates results in a decrease in cerebral metabolism and a reduction in ICP, but has the added potential risks of superinfection and dysrhythmias. Hypothermia has not been shown to reliably improve outcome in severe CNS illness in older children. Moderate hypothermia may be of benefit in patients with a GCS score of 5–7 when used for 24 hr. Those with a GCS score of <4 may not benefit from hypothermia treatment. Patients with nonpenetrating trauma who are younger than 30 yr of age, have CPP of >50, and are kept hypothermic (<35°C) on admission tend to have a better response to induced hypothermia. Hypothermia has been successful in neonates with hypoxic-ischemia injury after birth (see Chapter 99).

Beaumont A, Marmarou A: Treatment of raised intracranial pressure following traumatic brain injury. *Crit Rev Neurosurg* 1999;28:207–216.

Bernard SA, Gray TW, Buist MD, et al: Treatment of comatose survivors of out-of-hospital arrests with induced hypothermia. *N Engl J Med* 2002; 346:557–563.

Bishop NB: Traumatic brain injury: a primer for primary care physicians. *Curr Probl Pediatr Adolesc Health Care* 2006;36:313–340.

Clark RS, Lai Y, Hickey RW, et al: Hypoxic-ischemic encephalopathy: Pathobiology and therapy of the postresuscitation syndrome in children. In Fuhrman BP, Zimmerman J (editors): *Pediatric Critical Care,* 3rd ed. St. Louis, Mosby/Elsevier, 2006, pp 904–928.

Dias MS: Traumatic brain and spinal cord injury. *Pediatr Clin North Am* 2004;51:271–303.

Dunning J, Daly JP, Lomas JP, et al: Derivation of the children's head injury algorithm for the prediction of important clinical events decision rule for head injury children. *Arch Dis Child* 2006;91:885–891.

Guidelines for the acute medical management of severe traumatic brain injury in infants, children, and adolescents. *J Trauma* 2003;54:S235–S310.

Hypothermia after Cardiac Arrest Study Group: Mild therapeutic hypothermia to improve the neurologic outcome after cardiac arrest. *N Engl J Med* 2003;346:549–556.

Meyer PG, Ducrocq S, Carli P: Pediatric neurologic emergencies. *Curr Opin Crit Care* 2001;7:81–87.

Morris CG, McCoy W, Lavery GG: Spinal immobilization for unconscious patients with multiple injuries. *BMJ* 2004;329:495–499.

Rekate HL: Head injuries: Management of primary injuries and prevention of secondary damage. A consensus conference on pediatric neurosurgery. *Childs Nerv Syst* 2001;17:632–634.

Roppolo LP, Walters K: Airway management in neurological emergencies. *Neurocrit Care* 2004;1:405–414.

Servadei F: Coma scales. *Lancet* 2006;376:548–549.

Stevenson KL, Adelson PD: Neurointensive care of non-accidentally injured child. *Neurosurg Clin North Am* 2002;13:213–226.

67.1 • Brain Death • Lawrence H. Mathers and Lorry R. Frankel

Brain death is a clinical diagnosis which, when confirmed, can be the foundation for many significant decisions, including the discontinuation of further medical support or the decision to continue support while the family ponders the opportunity to donate organs. In most states, brain death is now recognized as legal death, meaning that cessation of heartbeat and interruption of the circulation of blood need not be part of a legal declaration of death.

EPIDEMIOLOGY. Brain death can result from a wide variety of insults, including immersion injuries, blunt force trauma, smoke inhalation, intracranial hemorrhage, hypoxic-ischemic insult, profound hypotension, and severe hypoglycemia. Trauma is the most common preceding event. In all of these situations, CNS neurons, which are almost completely dependent on adequate blood flow to ensure oxygen and glucose supply, will sustain serious injury after only a few minutes of insufficient perfusion and inadequate oxygen and glucose supply. Unlike other body tissues, the neurons of the human CNS have virtually no capacity to regenerate and replace themselves after significant injury. It is widely believed that the neurons of newborns and young infants may tolerate these CNS insults better than those of older children and adults. This may result from the fact that neurons in the very young are still developing and may possess some plasticity, making possible some tissue repair in response to significant injury.

DEFINING BRAIN DEATH. Brain death requires that **all** functions of the CNS (cortex and brainstem) be inactive; some reflex functions involving the spinal cord and the musculature of the trunk and limbs may persist in the presence of a diagnosis of brain death. The following features must be present in brain death: (1) irreversible unconsciousness; (2) irreversible absence of brainstem reflexes; and (3) absence of any factors that might impair CNS function. These factors include drugs that depress CNS function and hypothermia, which can also depress CNS function.

Laws often require documentation of multiple physical examinations, possibly coupled with confirmatory tests. It is not uncommon to require that **2 physicians** must examine and evaluate the patient and enter separate notes in the patient's chart confirming the finding of brain death. Criteria for appropriate declaration of brain death are not the same for patients of all ages. Most authorities, in the case of a child younger than 1 yr of age, require at least 2 assessments of brain injury, separated by 12–24 hr, before a declaration of brain death can be made.

TABLE 67-1. Age-specific Criteria for Brain Death*

Children 1 wk–2 mo of age: fulfillment of the criteria listed in **Table 67-2** in 2 separate examinations at least 48 hr apart, or 1 clinical examination followed by an isoelectric EEG at least 48 hr later

Children 2 mo–1 yr: fulfillment of the clinical criteria described in **Table 67-2** in 2 separate examinations, at least 24 hr apart, or 1 clinical examination followed by an isoelectric EEG or negative results of a cerebral blood flow study at least 24 hr later

Children >1 yr: fulfillment of the clinical criteria described in **Table 67-2** in 2 separate examinations at 12 hr apart

*Criteria for brain death in infants younger than 1 wk of age have not been delineated but should be at least as stringent as for those 1 wk–2 mo of age. It is often very difficult to diagnose brain death in premature infants; the wait period should be at least 72 hr. The standard wait period for adults is 6 hr. Some believe the wait period may be shortened if confirmatory testing is used. Once brain death is determined, that is the medical time of death.

EEG, electroencephalogram.

This level of caution is necessary because there is limited knowledge of the mechanisms and time course of the development of such severe injuries to the nervous systems of these very young children. Declaring brain death in infants younger than 1 wk of age and in premature infants requires serial neurologic examinations over 72 hr or more. Table 67-1 describes the criteria required for a diagnosis of brain death in children of different ages.

In addition to the clinical findings observed on neurologic examination, various confirmatory tests may be used, even though they are not required to support a diagnosis of brain death. These include EEG, cerebral perfusion study, and ICP monitoring. Complete brain death can be inferred from an isoelectric EEG, the absence of blood flow into the cranium, or measured IPC that is high enough to prevent arterial blood flow from the carotid and vertebral arterial systems into the intracranial compartment.

A number of tests for brain death have gained acceptance among those caring for acutely brain-injured children. Their overall intent is to provoke the brainstem into responding to external stimuli; if such stimuli provoke a response, even though faint, then brain death does not exist. If all provocative stimuli fail to evoke a response, then the patient's condition may be said to be consistent with brain death. Table 67-2 lists several widely used tests to confirm brain death. Individual tests are designed to test the integrity of the visual system, the auditory system, the vestibular system, proprioception in the upper neck and spinal muscles, or the regulation of eye position. If the child has no response to any of these stimuli, it may be inferred that there is serious injury involving **all** of the brainstem, from the lower medulla to the upper mesencephalon, and that 1 of the criteria for a declaration of brain death has been met.

The Apnea Test. Of particular importance is the **apnea test**, because it is by design more quantitative and reproducible. The goal of this test is to provide a strong physiologic stimulus to the brainstem, to elicit breathing. If the patient **does** breathe in the course of an apnea test, it is evidence that the brainstem, containing centers for monitoring of blood CO_2 levels and for production of coordinated muscle contractions leading to breathing, is not fully dysfunctional. To perform the apnea test, the patient's ventilator is set to deliver 100% O_2, the ventilator rate is adjusted to produce an arterial blood PCO_2 level normal for that patient, and a low level of positive end-expiratory pressure (PEEP) is set. After several minutes with these settings, an arterial blood gas sample is drawn to confirm that the patient's pH is in the normal range, the PCO_2 is in the range of 35–45 mm Hg, and the PO_2 is 100 mm Hg or greater. The ventilator rate is then set to zero; however, the ventilator delivers an inspired gas with an FIO_2 of 1.0. The patient is carefully observed for the next 5–30 min. Arte-

TABLE 67-2. Diagnosis of Brain Death

BRAIN DEATH CRITERIA	EVALUATED BY
PREREQUISITES	
1. A recognized cause of coma, sufficient to explain the irreversible cessation of all brain function	History, clinical examination, laboratory, technical investigations
2. Potentially reversible causes of coma must be excluded:	
a. Sedatives and neuromuscular blocking drugs	
b. Hypothermia	
c. Metabolic and endocrine disturbances:	
• Severe electrolyte disturbances	
• Severe hypo- or hyperglycemia	
d. Uncontrolled hypotension	
e. Surgically remediable intracranial conditions	
f. Any other sign that suggests a potentially reversible cause of coma	
CLINICAL EVALUATION	
1. Absence of higher brain function	Lack of consciousness, voluntary movement or responsiveness except for spinal reflexes (stimuli applied to any body region may not elicit a motor response within the cranial nerve distribution); preferably test in a cranial (trigeminal) dermatome rather than a spinal dermatome; no decorticate or decerebrate posturing, no convulsions
2. Absence of brainstem function	
a. Absence of sympathetic and parasympathetic regulation of the pupils	Pupils in midposition or dilated, showing neither direct nor indirect reaction to light
b. Disruption of the pathways controlling eye movement in the brainstem	Absence of spontaneous eye movement, absence of reaction to injection of iced water into the ear (vestibulo-ocular reflex), absence of doll's eye phenomenon (oculocephalic reflexes)
c. Disruption of the afferent trigeminal and efferent facial nerve pathways	Absence of blink response to (careful) corneal stimulation
d. Disruption of afferent and efferent pathways of cranial nerves IX and X in the medulla oblongata	Absence of gag response to stimulation of the posterior pharynx, absence of cough on suctioning of the trachea
e. Absence of vagal efferent activity	No significant increase of heart rate on administration of intravenous atropine or on pressure applied to the eyeballs (oculocardiac reflex)
f. Disruption of the respiratory control centers of the medulla oblongata	No respiratory movement (as assessed by observation ± capnography) at a $PaCO_2$ above a set limit during standardized apnea testing
"CONFIRMATORY" TESTS	
1. Confirmation of absence of higher brain function	Electrocerebral silence on EEG during at least 30 min
2. Confirmation of complete infarction of the brain and brainstem by confirmation of absence of blood flow	Four-vessel contrast angiography or radionuclide imaging
OBSERVATION	
Confirmation of irreversibility	Observation during a set time, ± repeat formal physical examination and confirmatory tests

From Lutz-Dettinger N, de Jaeger A, Kerremans I: Care of the potential pediatric organ donor. *Pediatr Clin North Am* 2001;48:715–749.

EEG, electroencephalogram; $PaCO_2$, partial pressure of carbon dioxide in arterial blood.

rial blood gas samples are periodically drawn, and the patient is monitored for any respiratory effort. If the patient breathes at all over the next 10 min, the patient is not apneic, the test is terminated, and the criteria for brain death have not been met. However, if the Pco_2 rises to >80 mm Hg and the patient has no spontaneous respirations, then the diagnosis of brain death can be made. The patient is usually placed back on the ventilator and a series of discussions then follows to help guide the family. The apnea test proves that the presence of high levels of CO_2 in the blood, normally a powerful stimulus to breathing, does not provoke breathing, supporting the diagnosis of brain death.

Confirming the Diagnosis. Great care must be taken to confirm the diagnosis of brain death and to exclude other conditions that may involve major impairment of nervous system function. The **persistent vegetative state** involves permanent unconsciousness, but some responses to external stimuli persist, even though they may be purposeless. A certain diagnosis of persistent vegetative state requires that significant time (≈6 mo) pass with no improvement in neurologic status. An especially frightening possibility is **locked-in syndrome,** in which outward signs of responsiveness are lacking, due to muscular dysfunction, but consciousness persists. It usually involves injuries to the lower brainstem.

WORKING WITH THE FAMILY DURING THE WITHDRAWAL OF SUPPORTIVE CARE AND ALLOWING A NATURAL DEATH. Once a firm diagnosis of brain death has been established, attention should turn to informing the family about the meaning of brain death and the steps to be taken next. For many families, it takes time to comprehend the finality of the injuries the child has suffered. The treating staff should not attempt to force the family into early decisions about further care and the withdrawal of support. The medical staff should reassure the family that the brain-dead child is not feeling any discomfort or pain and is, in fact, in a profound and irreversible coma. The total dependence of the patient on mechanical ventilation and other technologic devices should be strongly and repeatedly emphasized. The family may need time for relatives and friends to come to the hospital to say good-bye to the child and support the family. Every effort should be made to accommodate these requests. Many families who initially seem unable to face the prospect of withdrawing support will, in a relatively short time, accept the fact that further physiologic support of their brain-dead child is futile. Once the family is prepared, supportive care may be withdrawn so that the child will experience a natural death. It is not uncommon for families to hold the child during this process. It is helpful to have a special room set aside where the family and friends can be with the parents for support.

ORGAN DONATION. In many states, it is mandatory that the subject of organ donation be discussed with the family when the diagnosis of brain death has been made. This is usually the correct time to refer the family to an organ procurement program. The organ procurement service, if appropriate and medically indicated, will approach the family. These professionals are uniquely qualified to counsel families during this most distressing time and have an excellent rate of organ donation from these families.

If a decision is made to pursue possible organ donation, the organ procurement service will assume responsibility for the care of the patient in preparation for organ retrieval and placement. To provide optimal support of the organs to be transplanted, changes in the strategy of caring for the patient may occur to maintain acceptable organ perfusion, such as increasing the rate of intravenous fluid infusion, providing nutritional support, minimizing the use of vasopressors, and treating the patient with antibiotics. In addition, the organ procurement organization assumes full financial responsibility for the organ placement process.

Although acceptance and social approval for organ donation is growing, 3 in 4 opportunities to transplant such organs into needy potential recipients are still lost, and continued public education about the importance of organ donation is needed.

AAP Policy Statement: Pediatric organ donation and transplantation. *Pediatrics* 2002;109:982–984.

Banasiak KJ, Lister G: Brain death in children. *Curr Opin Pediatr* 2003;15:288–293.

Bernat JL: Chronic disorders of consciousness. *Lancet* 2006;367:1181–1192.

Goh AY-T, Mok Q: Clinical course and determination of brainstem death in a children's hospital. *Acta Paediatr* 2004;93:47–52.

Morenski JD, Oro JJ, Tobias JD, et al: Determination of death by neurological criteria. *J Intensive Care Med* 2003;18:211–221.

Oropello JM: Determination of brain death: Theme, variations, and preventable errors. *Crit Care Med* 2004;32:1417–1418.

Servadei F: Coma scales. *Lancet* 2006;367:548–549.

Tsai E, Shemie SD, Cox PN, et al: Organ donation in children: Role of the pediatric intensive care unit. *Pediatr Crit Care Med* 2000;1:156–160.

Wang MY, Wallace P, Gruen JP: Brain death documentation: Analysis and issues. *Neurosurgery* 2002;51:731–735; discussion 735–736.

Chapter 68 ■ Shock

Lorry R. Frankel and Saraswati Kache

Shock is an acute, dramatic syndrome, characterized by inadequate circulatory provision of oxygen, so that the metabolic demands of vital organs and tissues are not met. Insufficient oxygen is available to support aerobic cellular metabolism. There is a shift to less efficient anaerobic metabolism, which leads to lactic acidosis (see Chapter 52.7). The brain has no capacity for anaerobic metabolism and can be severely affected during periods of poor oxygen supply. If inadequate tissue perfusion continues, various adverse endocrine, vascular, inflammatory, metabolic, cellular, and systemic responses occur, and the patient becomes more physiologically unstable (see Chapter 176). Shock is a progressive process because of the continued presence of the initiating factor plus exaggerated and potentially harmful neurohumoral, inflammatory, and cellular responses. Initially, shock may be compensated, but may progress to an uncompensated condition, which requires greater interventions to respond to therapy. Untreated shock will lead to irreversible tissue injury (irreversible shock) and death. The specific pattern of response and the related pathophysiology, clinical manifestations, and treatments vary with the etiology of shock.

EPIDEMIOLOGY. Shock occurs in approximately 2% of all hospitalized children and adults in the United States (≈400,000 cases/yr). The mortality rate varies from 20–50%. Most patients do not die in the acute hypotensive phase of shock, but rather as a result of 1 or more associated complications. **Multiple organ dysfunction syndrome** increases the probability of death (1 organ system involved, 25%; 2 organ systems, 60%; 3 or more organ systems, >85%). The mortality rate in infected patients increases if the patient progresses from sepsis to septic shock to refractory sepsis. The mortality rate for shock in pediatric patients has decreased as a consequence of educational efforts (pediatric advanced life support), which emphasize early recognition and intervention and rapid transfer of critically ill patients to a pediatric intensive care unit via a transport service.

DEFINITION. There are 5 major types of shock: hypovolemic, septic, cardiogenic, distributive, and obstructive (Table 68-1). Hypovolemic (diarrhea-dehydration, hemorrhage) and septic

TABLE 68-1. Types of Shock

HYPOVOLEMIC	CARDIOGENIC	DISTRIBUTIVE	SEPTIC	OTHER
Decreased preload secondary to internal or external losses	Cardiac pump failure secondary to poor myocardial function	Abnormalities of vasomotor tone Loss of venous capcitance decreases preload Loss of arterial capcitance decreases afterload or systemic blood pressure	Includes multiple forms of shock Hypovolemic: third spacing Distributive: early shock with decreased afterload Cardiogenic: depression of myocardial function by endotoxins	Obstructive: significant direct obstruction to right or left heart function, or restriction of all cardiac chambers Heat stroke: hypovolemia due to salt and water losses, and decreased peripheral vascular resistance
SAMPLE CAUSES				
Loss of components of intravascular volume Blood: hemorrhage Plasma: burns, nephrotic syndrome Water and electrolytes: diarrhea, vomiting, diabetes	Congenital heart disease Cardiomyopathies: infectious or acquired, dilated or restrictive Ischemia Dysrhythmias	Anaphylaxis Neurologic: loss of sympathetic vascular tone secondary to spinal cord or brainstem injury Drugs	Bacterial Viral Fungal (immunocompromised patients are at increased risk)	Obstructive: large pulmonary embolism leading to right-sided heart failure, critical coarctation of aorta leading to left-sided heart failure Pericardial tamponade Tension pneumothorax Pericardial tamponade

TABLE 68-2. Definitions of Systemic Inflammatory Response Syndrome Infection, Sepsis, Severe Sepsis, and Septic Shock*

SYSTEMIC INFLAMMATORY RESPONSE SYNDROME†

The presence of at least 2 of the following 4 criteria, 1 of which must be abnormal temperature or leukocyte count:

- Core-temperature of >38.5℃ or <36℃
- Tachycardia, defined as a mean heart rate >2 SD above normal for age in the absence of external stimulus, long-term drug use or painful stimuli; or otherwise unexplained persistent elevation over a 0.5- to 4-hr period **OR for children <1 yr old: bradycardia, defined as a mean heart rate <10th percentile for age in the absence of external vagal stimulus, β-blocker drugs, or congenital heart disease; or otherwise unexplained persistent depression over a 0.5-hr period**
- Mean respiratory rate >2 SD above normal for age or mechanical ventilation for an acute process not related to underlying neuromuscular disease or the receipt of general anesthesia
- Leukocyte count elevated or depressed for age (not secondary to chemotherapy-induced leukopenia) or >10% immature neutrophils.

INFECTION

Suspected or proven (by positive culture, tissue stain, or polymerase chain reaction test) infection caused by any pathogen OR a clinical syndrome associated with a high probability of infection. Evidence of infection includes positive findings on clinical exam, imaging, or laboratory tests (e.g., white blood cells in a normally sterile body fluid, perforated viscus, chest radiograph consistent with pneumonia, petechial or purpuric rash, or purpura fulminans)

SEPSIS

Systemic inflammatory response syndrome in the presence of suspected or proven infection

SEVERE SEPSIS

Sepsis plus 1 of the following: cardiovascular organ dysfunction OR acute respiratory distress syndrome OR 2 or more other organ dysfunctions (defined in Table 68-4)

SEPTIC SHOCK

Sepsis and cardiovascular organ dysfunction as defined in Table 68-4

*Modifications from the adult definitions are shown in boldface.
†See Table 68-3 for age-specific ranges for physiologic and laboratory variables.
Core temperature must be measured by rectal, bladder, oral, or central catheter probe.
SD, standard deviation.
From Goldstein B, Giroir B, Randolph A, et al: International pediatric sepsis consensus conference: Definitions for sepsis and organ dysfunction in pediatrics. *Pediatr Crit Care Med* 2005;6:2–8.

TABLE 68-3. Age-specific Vital Signs and Laboratory Variables (Lower Values for Heart Rate, Leukocyte Count, and Systolic Blood Pressure are for the 5th and Upper Values for Heart Rate, Respiration Rate, or Leukocyte Count for the 95th Percentile)

	HEART RATE (BEATS/MIN)		RESPIRATORY RATE (BREATHS/MIN)	LEUKOCYTE COUNT (LEUKOCYTES ×10³/MM)	SYSTOLIC BLOOD PRESSURE (MM HG)
AGE GROUP	TACHYCARDIA	BRADYCARDIA			
0 day–1 wk	>180	<100	>50	>34	<65
1 wk–1 mo	>180	<100	>40	>19.5 or <5	<75
1 mo–1 yr	>180	<90	>34	>17.5 or <5	<100
2–5 yr	>140	NA	>22	>15.5 or <6	<94
6–12 yr	>130	NA	>18	>13.5 or <4.5	<105
13–18 yr	>110	NA	>14	>11 or <4.5	<117

From Goldstein B, Giroir B, Randolph A, et al: International pediatric sepsis consensus conference: Definitions for sepsis and organ dysfunction in pediatrics. *Pediatr Crit Care Med* 2005;6:2–8.
NA, not applicable.

shock are the most common causes of shock in children. Cardiogenic shock is seen in patients with congenital heart disease, immediately after cardiac surgery to repair a congenital heart defect, in patients with cardiomyopathy or myocarditis (viral, Kawasaki disease), or in those experiencing organ rejection after heart transplant.

Sepsis is defined as a systemic inflammatory response syndrome (SIRS) associated with an infection (see Chapter 176). Sepsis is the most common cause of mortality in children worldwide. In the United States, infants are at the greatest risk for sepsis. An international consensus conference defined SIRS, infection, sepsis, severe sepsis, and septic shock for the pediatric population (Table 68-2) and identified age-specific vital signs for SIRS (Table 68-3) and the criteria for multiorgan dysfunction (Table 68-4).

PATHOPHYSIOLOGY. An initial insult triggers shock, thus disrupting blood flow to end-organs, leading to inadequate tissue perfusion. The body's compensatory mechanisms are initiated to

TABLE 68-4. Criteria for Organ Dysfunction

CARDIOVASCULAR DYSFUNCTION

Despite administration of isotonic intravenous fluid bolus ≥40 mL/kg in 1 hr

Decrease in BP (hypotension) <5th percentile for age or systolic BP <2 SD below normal for age (see Table 68-3)

OR

Need for vasoactive drug to maintain BP in normal range (dopamine >5 μg/kg/min or dobutamine, epinephrine, or norepinephrine at any dose)

OR

Two of the following:
Unexplained metabolic acidosis: base deficit >5.0 mEq/L
Increased arterial lactate >2 × upper limit of normal
Oliguria: urine output <0.5 mL/kg/hr
Prolonged capillary refill: >5 sec
Core to peripheral temperature gap >3° C

RESPIRATORY*

PaO_2/FIO_2 <300 in absence of cyanotic heart disease or pre-existing lung disease

OR

$PaCO_2$ >65 torr or 20 mm Hg over baseline $PaCO_2$

OR

Proven need[†] or >50% FIO_2 to maintain saturation ≥92%

OR

Need for nonelective invasive or noninvasive mechanical ventilation[‡]

NEUROLOGIC

Glasgow Coma score ≤11

OR

Acute change in mental status with a decrease in Glasgow Coma score ≥3 points from abnormal baseline

HEMATOLOGIC

Platelet count <80,000/mm³ or a decline of 50% in the platelet count from the highest value recorded over the last 3 days (for patients with chronic hematologic or oncologic disorders)

OR

International normalized ratio >2

RENAL

Serum creatinine ≥2 × upper limit of normal for age or 2-fold increase in baseline creatinine

HEPATIC

Total bilirubin ≥4 mg/dL (not applicable for newborn)
Alanine transaminase level 2 × upper limit of normal for age

*Acute respiratory distress syndrome must include a PaO_2/FIO_2 ratio ≤200 mm Hg, bilateral infiltrates, acute onset, and no evidence of left-sided heart failure. Acute lung injury is defined identically except the PaO_2/FIO_2 ratio must be ≤300 mm Hg.
†Proven need assumes that the oxygen requirement was tested by decreasing flow, with a subsequent increase in flow if required.
‡In postoperative patients, this requirement can be met if the patient has an acute inflammatory or infectious process in the lungs that prevents him or her from being extubated.
From Goldstein B, Giroir B, Randolph A, et al: International pediatric sepsis consensus conference: Definitions for sepsis and organ dysfunction in pediatrics. *Pediatr Crit Care Med* 2005;6:2–8.
BP, blood pressure; FIO_2, fractional inspired oxygen; $PaCO_2$, partial pressure of carbon dioxide in arterial blood; PaO_2, partial pressure of oxygen in arterial blood.

maintain perfusion to vital organs, leading to **compensated shock.** If treatment is not introduced during this period of compensated shock, **decompensated shock** develops, causing tissue damage that leads to multisystem organ dysfunction and death (Fig. 68-1).

In the early phases of shock, multiple compensatory physiologic mechanisms act to maintain blood pressure (BP) and preserve tissue perfusion. These responses include increases in heart rate, stroke volume, and vascular smooth muscle tone, regulated through neurohormonal changes in sympathetic nervous system activation and other hormonal responses, to help preserve blood flow to vital organs, such as the brain, heart, and kidneys. The respiratory rate is increased to promote the excretion of CO_2 to compensate for increased CO_2 production and the metabolic acidosis that occurs due to poor tissue perfusion. Increased renal excretion of hydrogen ions and retention of bicarbonate occurs in an effort to maintain normal pH (see Chapter 52.7). Maintenance of vascular volume is facilitated by the renin-angiotensin-aldosterone and atrial natriuretic factor axes (through regulation of sodium), cortisol and catecholamine synthesis and release, and

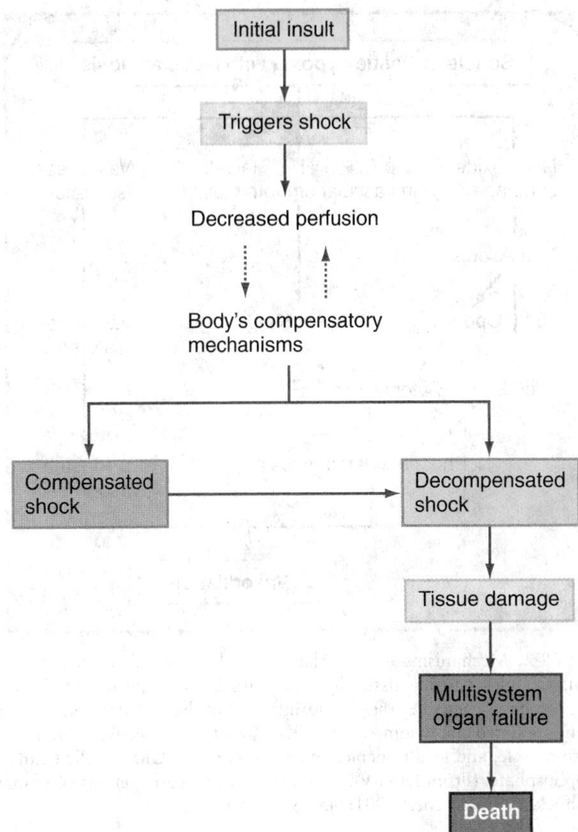

Figure 68-1. Algorithm for decompensated shock.

secretion of antidiuretic hormone. Despite these compensatory mechanisms, intravascular fluid leaks into the interstitial extracellular space because of vascular endothelial cell injury and loss of tight junctions.

All forms of shock affect heart rate—preload, afterload, or myocardial contractility—or a combination of all 3 components, leading to poor tissue perfusion (Table 68-5). More than 1 of these processes may occur simultaneously. Fluid loss commonly accompanies vomiting and diarrhea, hemorrhagic trauma, or severe burns, and can result in an initial increase in vascular resistance as the body attempts to maintain BP and restore circulating intravascular volume. Subsequently, hypotension develops and produces tissue ischemia. Significant electrolyte alterations

TABLE 68-5. Pathophysiology of Shock

EXTRACORPOREAL FLUID LOSS

Hypovolemic shock may be due to direct blood loss through hemorrhage or abnormal loss of body fluids (diarrhea, vomiting, burns, diabetes mellitus or insipidus, nephrosis)

LOWERING PLASMA ONCOTIC FORCES

Hypovolemic shock may also result from hypoproteinemia (liver injury, or as a progressive complication of increased capillary permeability)

ABNORMAL VASODILATION

Distributive shock (neurogenic, anaphylaxis, or septic shock) occurs when there is loss of vascular tone—venous, arterial, or both (sympathetic blockade, local substances affecting permeability, acidosis, drug effects, spinal cord transection)

INCREASED VASCULAR PERMEABILITY

Sepsis may change the capillary permeability in the absence of any change in capillary hydrostatic pressure (endotoxins from sepsis, excess histamine release in anaphylaxis)

CARDIAC DYSFUNCTION

Peripheral hypoperfusion may result from any condition that affects the heart's ability to pump blood efficiently (ischemia, acidosis, drugs, constrictive pericarditis, pancreatitis, sepsis)

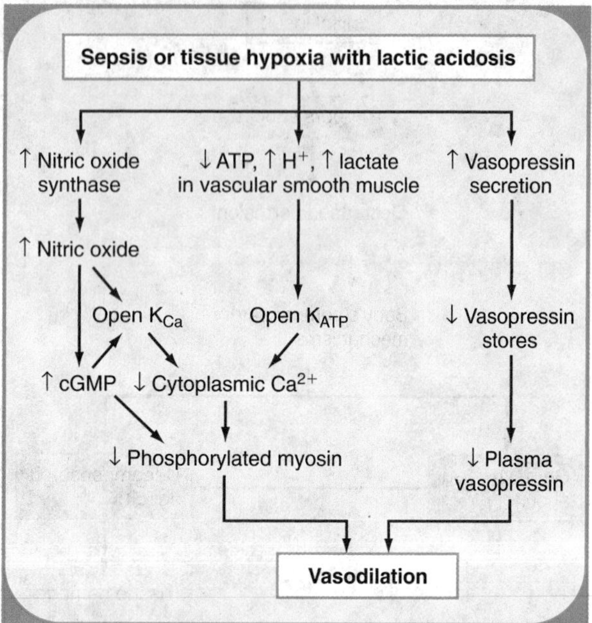

Figure 68-2. Mechanisms of vasodilatory shock. Septic shock and states of prolonged shock causing tissue hypoxia with lactic acidosis increase nitric oxide synthesis, activate the adenosine triphosphate (ATP)-sensitive and calcium-regulated potassium channel (K_{ATP} and K_{Ca}, respectively) in vascular smooth muscle, and lead to depletion of vasopressin. cGMP, cyclic guanosine monophosphate. (From Landry DW, Oliver JA: The pathogenesis of vasodilatory shock. *N Engl J Med* 2001;345:588–595.)

may accompany the fluid loss. When there is a pre-existing low plasma oncotic pressure (nephrotic syndrome, malnutrition, hepatic dysfunction, acute severe burns), there may be even greater capillary leaking; this results in decreased intravascular volume, which exacerbates shock, produces more edema, and potentially worsens the respiratory status. Abnormal vasodilation results in vasodilatory shock and is usually caused by sepsis, hypoxia, poisonings (carbon monoxide, cyanide, metformin), anaphylaxis, neurogenic events, or mitochondrial dysfunction (Fig. 68-2). The lower systemic vascular resistance (SVR) is usually accompanied by an increase in cardiac output and a redistribution of blood flow away from vital organs to nonvital organs; hence, the term **distributive shock.** Prolonged states of intense vasoconstriction due to hemorrhagic or cardiogenic shock may lead to vascular collapse, which then may result in terminal vasodilatory shock. Increased vascular permeability is most common with sepsis or anaphylaxis, but is also seen in hemorrhagic shock. Bacterial products (endotoxin) and inflammatory mediators (tumor necrosis factor, interleukins) are implicated and result in significant transcapillary depletion of intravascular volume. Cardiogenic shock, although rare in children, may be associated with cardiomyopathy, severe congenital heart disease, significant dysrhythmias, or the period immediately after surgery for congenital heart disease (see Chapter 434). Sepsis, pancreatitis, and SIRS can produce direct myocardial depressant effects, adding a cardiogenic component to patients with septic shock.

A significant misconception is that shock occurs only with low BP (hypotension). Through various compensatory mechanisms, hypotension is often a late finding. Tachycardia, with or without tachypnea, may be the 1st or only sign of early compensated shock. Hypotension is an advanced state of decompensated shock and has a high mortality rate. Shock may be present with normal BP if other factors do not permit the patient to maintain adequate tissue oxygen delivery. Anemia and hypoxia result in reduced oxygen delivery at any given cardiac output. Fever and trauma may increase tissue oxygen and metabolic requirements. Progression of any of the mechanisms that lead to shock results in hypoxia and lactic acidosis. Conversely, if blood pressure is low, but tissue perfusion is adequate to meet the metabolic demands of the body, shock may not be present. The clinical circumstances should be determined, including vital signs, physical examination findings, laboratory studies, and presence or absence of acidosis, to determine if the pediatric patient is in shock.

TABLE 68-6. Inflammatory Mediators

PROINFLAMMATORY MEDIATORS	ANTI-INFLAMMATORY MEDIATORS
Tumor necrosis factor	Interleukin-4
Interleukin-1	Interleukin-10
Interleukin-6	Soluble receptor and receptor antagonists
Interleukin-8	
Interleukin-γ	
HMGB-1	

From Balk RA, Ely EW, Goyette RE: *Sepsis Handbook,* 2nd ed. Society of Critical Care Medicine, 2006.
HMGB-1, high mobility group box chromosomal protein 1.

Mediators of tissue damage may cause progression from compensated shock to decompensated shock. The vascular endothelium is both a target of tissue injury and a source of mediators that lead to further tissue injury. Other significant systemic factors include the complement pathway, the coagulation system, activation of white blood cells, platelet-activating factor, nitric oxide, and oxygen free radical production from reperfusion injury. Bacterial sources of tissue injury include circulating endotoxin or exotoxin, as well as translocation of gut flora or endotoxin, if the intestinal mucosa is compromised. Exotoxins and endotoxins induce the production of various inflammatory molecules, such as the interleukins, and amplify the systemic factors that maintain shock. Both proinflammatory and anti-inflammatory mediators have been identified (Table 68-6). The balance between proinflammatory and anti-inflammatory mediators, along with individual gene polymorphisms of mediators and their receptors, have an important effect on the patient's ability to survive.

CLINICAL MANIFESTATIONS. A classification of shock is shown in Table 68-1. There is significant overlap in these categories, especially between septic and distributive shock. The clinical presentation of shock depends, in part, on the cause; if shock is unrecognized and untreated, a very similar untoward progression of clinical signs and pathophysiologic changes occurs and leads to a common final path (Table 68-7). The clinical features of shock also relate to the stage (duration vs progression) of the process (early vs late).

Hypovolemic shock usually presents as changes in mental status, tachypnea, tachycardia, hypotension, poor peripheral pulses, cool extremities, and oliguria (see Chapters 53–55). Table 68-7 outlines the clinical signs of a progressive decrease in perfusion. Supine hypotension and tachycardia are hallmarks of hypovolemia. Neonates and infants may also have poor urine output. Dry mucous membranes, dry axillae, and poor skin turgor are variably present. Hypovolemic shock may initially present with normal or only slightly cool distal extremities. **Septic shock,** in particular, has 2 phases: **Early, or warm, shock** is diagnosed by low SVR, and **late, or cold, shock** is diagnosed by high SVR. Septic shock may present initially with warm extremities (from peripheral vasodilation secondary to low SVR), bounding pulses (from high stroke volume and widened pulse pressure), tachycardia, tachypnea, adequate urination, and mild metabolic acidosis (see Chapter 176). **Cardiogenic shock** presents with cool extremities, delayed (>2–3 sec) capillary filling time, hypotension, poor peripheral or central pulses, tachypnea, increasing obtundation, and decreased urination (all caused by peripheral vasoconstriction and decreased cardiac output; see Chapter 434).

TABLE 68-7. Signs of Decreased Perfusion

ORGAN SYSTEM	↓PERFUSION	↓↓PERFUSION	↓↓↓PERFUSION
Central nervous system	—	Restless, apathetic, anxious	Agitated/confused, stuporous, coma
Respiration	—	↑Ventilation	↑↑Ventilation
Metabolism	—	Compensated metabolic acidemia	Uncompensated metabolic acidemia
Gut	—	↓Motility	Ileus
Kidney	↓Urine volume ↑Urinary specific gravity	Oliguria (<0.5 mL/kg/hr)	Oliguria/anuria
Skin	Delayed capillary refill	Cool extremities	Mottled, cyanotic, cold extremities
Cardiovascular system	↑Heart rate	↑↑Heart rate ↓Peripheral pulses	↑↑Heart rate, ↓blood pressure, central pulses only

Adapted from Lister G, Apkon M, Fabry JT: Shock. In Emmanouilides GC, Riemenschneider TA, Allen HD, et al (editors): *Moss & Adam's Heart Disease in Infants, Children and Adolescents: Including the Fetus and Young Adult,* 5th ed. Baltimore, Williams & Wilkins, 1994, pp 1725–1746.
↑, increased; ↓, decreased.

Uncompensated shock (high vascular resistance, decreased cardiac output, obtundation, oliguria) occurs late in the progression of shock, regardless of its etiology. Hemodynamic findings in various shock states are noted in Table 68-8.

The transition from compensated to decompensated shock is not always easy to identify. An increase in lactic acid production and very low **mixed venous oxygen saturation,** indicating inadequate oxygen delivery, are hallmarks of uncompensated shock. Measurement of the oxygen saturation of central mixed venous blood (Mvo_2) from the pulmonary artery, right ventricle, right atrium, superior vena cava, or inferior vena cava can determine if overall peripheral oxygen delivery (the true standard for such measurements is the pulmonary artery) is adequate. The Mvo_2 should be 20–25% < the arterial oxygen saturation (normally, Mvo_2 is 75–80%). A low Mvo_2, as measured by co-oximetry, suggests poor perfusion, requiring increased oxygen extraction by the end-organs and, in turn, decreasing the Mvo_2. This can guide caregivers in the use of fluid support and inotropic agents to improve cardiac output in the treatment of shock.

An unusual form of shock is **hemorrhagic shock encephalopathy syndrome.** This syndrome initially looks similar to heatstroke. It is usually seen in children younger than 3 yr of age and is characterized by encephalopathy, fever, shock, watery diarrhea, severe disseminated intravascular coagulation, and renal and hepatic dysfunction. In addition to the hemodynamic changes associated with poor perfusion and hypotension, affected patients may have seizures and other severe neurologic findings as a result of cerebral edema. These children have an associated rapid onset of abnormal liver function studies and coagulation tests. These abnormalities persist for 3–4 days. Therapy is directed at fluid resuscitation, maintaining adequate cardiac output, supporting the renal and hepatic failure, and ameliorating acute neurologic abnormalities. Other complications may include myoglobinuria due to rhabdomyolysis. These children have a very high mortality rate, and survivors have a high incidence of neurologic problems.

TABLE 68-8. Hemodynamic Variables in Different Shock States

	CO	SVR	MAP	WEDGE	CENTRAL VENOUS PRESSURE
Hypovolemic	↓	↑	↔ or ↓	↓↓↓	↓↓↓
Cardiogenic*					
Systolic	↓↓	↑↑↑	↔ or ↓	↑↑	↑↑
Diastolic	↔	↑↑	↔	↑↑	↑
Obstructive	↓	↑	↔ or ↓	↑↑†	↑↑†
Distributive	↑↑	↓↓↓	↔ or ↓	↔ or ↓	↔ or ↓
Septic					
Early	↑↑↑	↓↓↓	↔ or ↓‡	↓	↓
Late	↓↓	↓↓	↓↓	↑	↑ or ↔

*Systolic or diastolic dysfunction.
†Wedge pressure, central venous pressure, and pulmonary artery diastolic pressures are equal.
‡Wide pulse pressure.
From McConnell MS, Perkin RM: Shock states. In Fuhrman BP, Zimmerman JJ (editors): *Pediatric Critical Care,* 2nd ed. Philadelphia, CV Mosby, 1998.
MAP, mean arterial pressure; SVR, systemic vascular resistance.

TREATMENT

Improved outcomes are noted if shock is reversed early.

INITIAL MANAGEMENT. The ABCs of resuscitation (**airway, breathing,** and **circulation**) must be evaluated and stabilized for all patients in shock (see Chapter 66). Neonates and infants in particular may also have profound hypoglycemia associated with shock; it maybe helpful to recognize the ABCDs, with the D standing for **dextrose** in the pediatric population. Once the patient's airway, breathing, circulatory access, and dextrose are stabilized, treatment specific to shock can be initiated.

In most patients with early shock, an initial fluid bolus of 20 mL/kg of normal saline or lactated Ringer solution should be given rapidly (5–10 min). If it is not possible to insert an intravenous catheter into a peripheral vein within 90 sec or within 3 attempts, an intraosseous needle should be inserted to administer fluids (see Chapters 62 and 66). If cardiogenic shock is a concern, the fluid bolus should be held or a smaller volume given over a longer period to avoid exacerbating heart failure. After this infusion, the patient is reassessed to determine if more fluid is required or if other forms of therapy should be initiated (antibiotics, vasoactive agents, colloids). If the patient is decompensating during the fluid bolus, other interventions should be initiated concomitantly. Children in severe hypovolemic, septic, or anaphylactic shock may require additional fluid boluses (60–80 mL/kg within the 1st 1–2 hr of presentation). Fluid therapy should be titrated until improvements are noted in heart rate, blood pressure, urine output, level of consciousness, and capillary refill time (Fig. 68-3). After initial stabilization, ongoing losses (continued diarrhea, vomiting, burns) should be replaced with appropriate fluids, and the deficit and maintenance fluid requirements should be addressed. If the patient has a central venous catheter in place, the clinician may titrate fluid administration to restore central venous pressure to within the normal range (4–8 cm H_2O). The risk of fluid overload must also be continually reassessed. If the child's hypovolemia is from loss of blood or protein-rich fluid, replacement with whole blood or packed red blood cells or with fresh frozen plasma or albumin, respectively, may be appropriate. The use of dextrans (hydroxyethyl starch) or gelatins may be indicated if there is a need to increase plasma oncotic pressure but blood component therapy cannot be administered or is ineffective. There is a debate about the relative risks and benefits of choosing crystalloid solutions (normal saline, lactated Ringer solution) vs colloid (albumin, hetastarch) for fluid resuscitation. The concern with colloid solutions

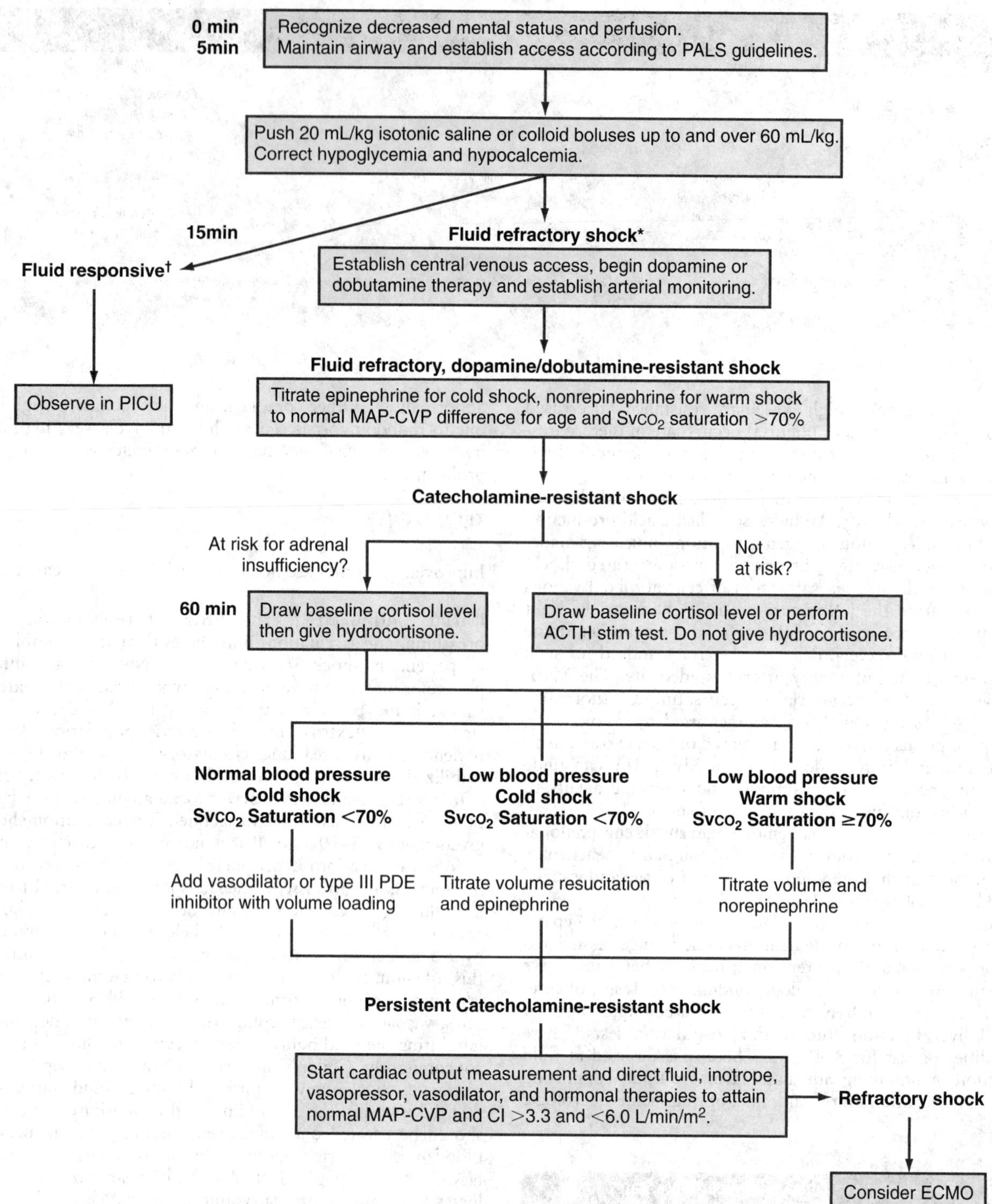

Figure 68-3. Resuscitation of pediatric septic shock. *Normalization of blood pressure and tissue perfusion. †Hypotension, abnormal capillary refill, or extremity coolness. ACTH, adrenocorticotropic hormone; CI, cardiac index; ECMO, extracorporeal membrane oxygenation; MAP-CVP, mean arterial pressure-central venous pressure-perfusion pressure; PALS, pediatric advanced life support; PDE, phosphodiesterase; PICU, pediatric intensive care unit. (From Dellinger RP, Carlet JM, Masur H: Surviving sepsis campaign guidelines for management of severe sepsis and septic shock. *Crit Care Med* 2004;32:858–873.)

for patients with vascular endothelial injury and leaky capillaries is that albumin may leak into the interstitial space and may be difficult to reabsorb. The organs of particular concern are the lungs and the gut; leaked albumin may decrease pulmonary compliance, increasing difficulty in oxygenation and ventilation. Nonetheless, for most patients, isotonic crystalloid solutions are appropriate. In refractory cases, hypertonic saline (3%) may be beneficial.

If, after appropriate fluid resuscitation, the patient continues to show poor perfusion and shock, vasoactive agents are needed (see Fig. 68-3). Restoration of normal oxygen delivery to vital tissues can be accomplished by improving oxygen-carrying capacity (maintaining normal hematocrit at 35–40%), improving oxygen saturation (95–99%) and Pa_{O_2} (if severely anemic), and enhancing depressed cardiac output. Cardiac output is influenced by heart rate, preload (fluid status), afterload (systemic vascular

TABLE 68-9. Cardiovascular Drug Treatment of Shock

DRUG	EFFECT(S)	DOSE RANGE	COMMENTS
Dopamine	Strengthens contractions (throughout dose range) Increases renal blood flow (low/intermediate doses) Vasoconstriction (high doses)	Intermediate dose = 5–15 μg/kg/min High dose = 15–25 μg/kg/min	Increasing risk of dysrhythmias at high dose Should be administered in a central vein
Epinephrine	Increases heart rate and strength of contractions Potent vasoconstrictor	0.05–3.0 μg/kg/min	May lessen renal perfusion Causes high O_2 consumption in the heart High risk of dysrhythmia
Dobutamine	Increases strength of heart contraction Little effect on heart rate Peripheral vasodilator, especially in vessels to viscera	1–20 μg/kg/min	Very weak vasoconstriction (high dose) Good for cardiogenic shock; strengthens heart contraction and produces afterload reduction
Norepinephrine	Strong vasoconstrictor Weak effect on strength of heart contraction	0.05–1.5 μg/kg/min	Produces short-term rise in blood pressure (high systemic vascular resistance) Causes increase in O_2 consumption, tendency for dysrhythmias
Phenylephrine	Strong vasoconstrictor Can be used to slow tachycardia through reflex cardiac slowing	0.5–2.0 μg/kg/min	Can cause sudden hypertension Causes increase in O_2 consumption
Milrinone	Potent inotrope Potent chronotrope Peripheral vasodilator	Load 50 μg/kg over 15 min 0.5–1 μg/kg/min	Phosphodiesterase inhibitor—slows cyclic adenosine monophosphate breakdown

resistance), and the state of myocardial contractility. Oxygen delivery should not exceed (supranormal) normal expectations because the *supply-dependency* oxygen relationship is not believed to be a critical factor in managing shock. When achieved, supranormal oxygen delivery does not improve outcome and may increase complications. When oxygen requirements are excessively high (seizures, burns, fever), along with providing adequate metabolite delivery, it is important to reduce metabolic stress (anticonvulsants, antipyretic agents).

For patients with obstructive shock, the primary insult must be addressed. A pulmonary embolus needs to be removed or undergo clot lysis, or a critical coarctation of the aorta needs to be repaired for the patient to improve. Patients with symptomatic pericardial effusions or a pneumothorax need immediate removal of fluid or air, respectively. Before pericardiocentesis, a rapid bolus of normal saline may improve cardiac output. Nonetheless, the patient will not improve until the obstructive lesion is corrected.

CARDIOVASCULAR MANAGEMENT. Also see Chapters 434 and 442. Septic, cardiogenic, distributive, and rarely, hypovolemic shock may require various drugs to stimulate heart rate (chronotropic) and cardiac contractility (inotropic) and enhance peripheral vascular resistance (blood pressure; see Fig. 68-3). These agents should be administered continuously through a central venous catheter. The rate of administration is titrated by careful monitoring of BP with an indwelling intra-arterial catheter. The type of shock guides the specific vasoactive agents used. Patients may be started on several agents concomitantly or sequentially, as the individual clinical course dictates. It is important to recognize that all cardiovascular drugs increase myocardial oxygen consumption and the risk of dysrhythmias (Table 68-9).

For patients in hypovolemic shock, adequate fluid resuscitation must be provided before the initiation of vasoactive agents. The fluids replaced should be the fluids lost; patients with traumatic injury can be transfused with whole blood to provide both packed red blood cells and coagulation factors. These patients may occasionally have poor cardiac output, despite appropriate preload, if the myocardium was ischemic or stunned. In such situations, dopamine infusion may be required until myocardial function improves and the metabolic abnormalities are corrected.

The initial treatment in pediatric shock is to stabilize the ABCDs and provide appropriate fluid resuscitation (see Table 68-3). If the patient continues in a state of shock, inotropic support should be initiated. Dopamine is the 1st-line agent and should be quickly optimized before the initiation of other agents. If the patient is in "warm shock," as recognized by hyperdynamic cardiac output, bounding pulses, and widened pulse pressure, then norepinephrine may be initiated. In adults, norepinephrine is considered the 1st-line drug for patients in septic shock. Patients in "cold shock," as diagnosed by signs of poor peripheral perfusion (prolonged capillary refill), should be started on epinephrine instead because their SVR is already presumably high. There is also a rationale for using intravenous vasopressin to treat **catecholamine-resistant shock.** Intravenous hydrocortisone in stress doses should be considered in some patients with septic shock (purpura fulminans) and in all patients receiving or recently weaned from steroids. A significant number of patients with septic shock have secondary adrenal insufficiency; a spot serum cortisol level will confirm the diagnosis, but empirical therapy may need to be started before the laboratory result is known. Hypoproteinemia may cause false low total cortisol levels; free cortisol levels are more accurate. Adequate infection therapy should also be provided for patients with septic shock; abscesses should be drained and appropriate bacteriocidal antibiotic therapy (usually 2 antibiotics) should be started.

Patients in cardiogenic shock require both systolic and diastolic myocardial support to improve the poor cardiac output associated with an elevated SVR. The ideal agents optimize cardiac output while decreasing SVR. Dobutamine improves systolic function and decreases SVR without a significant increase in heart rate. Milrinone offers the same advantages, with the added benefit of providing diastolic relaxation and improving ventricular preload. Dopamine can be considered as a 1st-line agent for patients in cardiogenic shock, particularly those with significant hypotension. For patients with profound hypotension, epinephrine is used to improve blood pressure, despite the significant increase in myocardial oxygen consumption.

A high SVR, as diagnosed by poor peripheral perfusion and acidosis, despite adequate cardiac output with the support of inotropic agents, may persist. This is often seen in patients with septic and

TABLE 68-10. Vasodilators/Afterload Reducers

Nitroprusside	Vasodilator (mainly arterial)	0.5–4.0 μg/kg/min	Rapid effect Prolonged use (>48 hr risks cyanide toxicity)
Nitroglycerin	Vasodilator (mainly venous)	1.0–20 μg/kg/min	Rapid effect Risk of high intracranial pressure
Prostaglandin E_1	Vasodilator Maintains an open ductus arteriosus in the newborn with ductal-dependent congenital heart disease	0.01–0.2 μg/kg/min	Can lead to hypotension Risk of apnea when given continuously

TABLE 68-11. Goal-directed Therapy of Organ System Dysfunction in Shock

SYSTEM	DISORDERS	GOALS	THERAPIES
Respiratory	Acute respiratory distress syndrome Respiratory muscle fatigue Central apnea	Prevent/treat: hypoxia and respiratory acidosis Prevent barotrauma Decrease work of breathing	Oxygen Early endotracheal intubation and mechanical ventilation PEEP Permissive hypercapnia High-frequency ventilation ECMO
Renal	Prerenal failure Renal failure	Prevent/treat: hypovolemia, hypervolemia, hyperkalemia, metabolic acidosis, hyper-/hyponatremia, and hypertension Establish normal urine output and blood pressure for age	Judicious fluid resuscitation Monitoring of serum electrolytes Low-dose dopamine Furosemide (Lasix) Dialysis, ultrafiltration, hemofiltration
Hematologic	Coagulopathy (DIC)	Prevent/treat: bleeding	Vitamin K Fresh frozen plasma Platelets
	Thrombosis	Prevent/treat: abnormal clotting	Heparinization Activated protein C
Gastrointestinal	Stress ulcers	Prevent/treat: gastric bleeding Avoid aspiration, abdominal distention	H_2-blocking agents or proton pump inhibitors Nasogastric tube
	Ileus Bacterial translocation	Avoid mucosal atrophy	Early enteral feedings
Endocrine	Adrenal insufficiency primary or secondary to chronic steroid therapy	Prevent/treat: adrenal crisis	Stress dose steroids in patients previously given steroids Physiologic dose for presumed primary insufficiency in sepsis
Metabolic	Metabolic acidosis	Correct etiology Normalize pH	Treatment of hypovolemia (fluids), poor cardiac function (fluids, inotropic agents) Improvement of renal acid excretion Low-dose (0.5–2 mEq/kg) sodium bicarbonate if the patient is not responding and pH < 7.1 and ventilation (CO_2 elimination) is adequate

DIC, disseminated intravascular coagulation; ECMO, extracorporeal membrane oxygenation; H_2, histamine$_2$ receptor; PEEP, positive end-expiratory pressure.

cardiogenic shock. Continuous infusion of a vasodilatory agent that can be easily titrated should be initiated (Table 68-10).

Distributive shock can be easily managed because these patients often have adequate cardiac output, but poor vascular tone. Initiating an agent that will provide vasoconstriction only, pure alpha support, may be the ideal. Phenylephrine and vasopressin are the 2 agents that fall into this category and may be considered in the treatment for patients with spinal cord injury. Epinephrine is the **treatment of choice** for patients with anaphylaxis because the release of various inflammatory mediators will also cause myocardial depression (see Chapter 148).

OTHER MODES OF SUPPORT IN SHOCK. Goal-directed therapy for complications of shock is noted in Table 68-11. Coagulation disorders are frequently found in severe shock and should be corrected, particularly if the patient is experiencing active bleeding (see Chapter 483). Correction of severe acidosis and hypercarbia is important because myocardial contractility and the efficacy of inotropic agents are decreased (see Chapter 52.7). Calcium can act as a direct myocardial stimulant, particularly in the neonate; therefore, hypocalcemia should be aggressively corrected (see Chapter 572).

Rarely, other invasive techniques may be needed to support children in shock who are not responding to fluid, pharmacologic support, or other modes of treatment, when the cause of shock is considered treatable and reversible. **Extracorporeal membrane oxygenation (ECMO)** or ventricular assist devices may be effective in treating young children with septic shock or severe cardiogenic shock, as a bridge to recovery (for those who recently underwent cardiac surgery and cannot be weaned from bypass) or cardiac transplant. Systemic anticoagulation is required while patients are receiving circulatory assistance. Given the precarious position of the large ECMO cannulas, the standard of care is to maintain patients in a state of deep sedation with minimal movement. Complications that are of greatest concern are intracranial hemorrhage due to anticoagulation and infection secondary to large invasive intravascular cannulas. Left ventricular or biventricular assist devices have also been used in older adolescent patients to manage severe cardiomyopathy and cardiogenic shock, as a bridge to transplantation. Although 2 different types exist, for long-term support, a pneumatic paracorporeal device may be more useful in patients of all sizes. Ventricular assist devices have the advantage of requiring a lower level of anticoagulation, and patients can be more mobile with these devices. Unlike ECMO, these devices do not provide respiratory support. A patient with poor pulmonary function may require significant ventilatory assistance (see Chapters 69 and 70) and may not be a candidate for an assist device. Renal replacement therapy (dialysis, hemofiltration) can be used to manage fluid overload or pulmonary edema and remove inflammatory mediators (see Chapter 535.1).

Barron ME, Wilkes MM, Navickis RJ: A systematic review of the comparative safety of colloids. *Arch Surg* 2004;139:552–563.

Beale RJ, Hollenberg SM, Vincent JL, et al: Vasopressor and inotropic support in septic shock: An evidence-based review. *Crit Care Med* 2004 32(11 Suppl):S445–S465.

Branco RG, Russell RR: Should steroids be used in children with meningococcal shock? *Arch Dis Child* 2005;90:1195–1196.

Cabrales P, Intaglietta M, Tsai AG: Increase plasma viscosity sustains microcirculation after resuscitation from hemorrhagic shock and continuous bleeding. *Shock* 2005;23:549–555.

Carcillo JA: Pediatric septic shock and multiple organ failure. *Crit Care Clin* 2003;19:413–440, viii.

Carcillo JA, Fields AI: Clinical practice parameters for hemodynamic support of pediatric and neonatal patients in septic shock. *Crit Care Med* 2002;30:1–30.

Carlotti AP, Troster EJ, Fernandes JC, et al: A critical appraisal of the guidelines for the management of pediatric and neonatal patients with septic shock. *Crit Care Med* 2005;33:1182.

Cooper MS, Stewart PM: Corticosteroid insufficiency in acutely ill patients. *N Engl J Med* 2003;348:727–734.
Dellinger RP, Carlet JM, Masur H, et al: Surviving sepsis campaign guidelines for management of severe sepsis and septic shock. *Crit Care Med* 2004;32:858–873.
Duke T, Molyneux EM: Intravenous fluids for seriously ill children: Time to reconsider. *Lancet* 2003;362:1320–1323.
Goldstein B, Giroir B, Randolph A: International pediatric sepsis consensus conference: Definitions for sepsis and organ dysfunction in pediatrics. *Pediatr Crit Care Med* 2005;6:2–8.
Hamrahian AH, Oseni TS, Arafah BM: Measurements of serum free cortisol in critically ill patients. *N Engl J Med* 2004;350:1629–1638.
Otieno H, Were E, Ahmed I: Are bedside features of shock reproducible between different observers? *Arch Dis Child* 2004;89:977–979.
Pope PE: Shock in polytrauma. *BMJ* 2003;327:1119–1120.
Safe Study Investigators: A comparison of albumin and saline for fluid resuscitation in the intensive care unit. *N Engl J Med* 2004;350:2247–2256.
Schortgen F, Lacherade JC, Bruneel F, et al: Effects of hydroxyethylstarch and gelatin on renal function in severe sepsis: A multicentre randomized study. *Lancet* 2001;357:911–916.
Sparrow A, Hedderley T, Nadel S: Choice of fluid for resuscitation of septic shock. *Emerg Med J* 2002;19:114–116.
Vincent JL: Resuscitation using albumin in critically ill patients. *BMJ* 2006;333:1029–1030.
Vincent JL, Gerlach H: Fluid resuscitation in severe sepsis and septic shock: An evidence-based review. *Crit Care Med* 2004;32(11Suppl):S451–S454.
Wills BA, Dung NM, Loan HT, et al: Comparison of three fluid solutions for resuscitation in dengue shock syndrome. *N Engl J Med* 2005;353:877–888.
Yunge M, Petros A: Angiotensin for septic shock unresponsive to noradrenaline. *Arch Dis Child* 2000;82:388–389.

Chapter 69 ■ Respiratory Distress and Failure

Lorry R. Frankel

Respiratory distress or failure is the primary diagnosis in nearly 50% of children admitted to the pediatric intensive care unit (PICU) and is a common cause of cardiopulmonary arrest in children. There is substantial variability in the etiology and severity of illness. Respiratory failure arises from derangements in pulmonary gas exchange. The 4 principal derangements are hypoventilation, diffusion impairment, intrapulmonary shunting, and ventilation-perfusion ($\dot{V}/\dot{Q}$) mismatch. The causes may be classified by age, anatomic lesions, or abnormalities involving lung and chest wall mechanics, neuromuscular systems, and central nervous system (CNS) control or respiratory drive. The presenting clinical findings usually help to determine the type of problem. Increased respiratory rate and effort (tachypnea and dyspnea) suggest mechanical problems with the lung or chest wall. Neuromuscular disease may result in progressively weaker respiratory effort and eventually fatigue. CNS pathology may present as other neurologic features (coma, areflexia, weakness) and a variety of respiratory patterns, including bradypnea, apnea, and Cheyne-Stokes respirations (Fig. 69-1). The heterogeneous group of pediatric diseases that can cause respiratory distress and failure requiring mechanical ventilation are shown in Table 69-1.

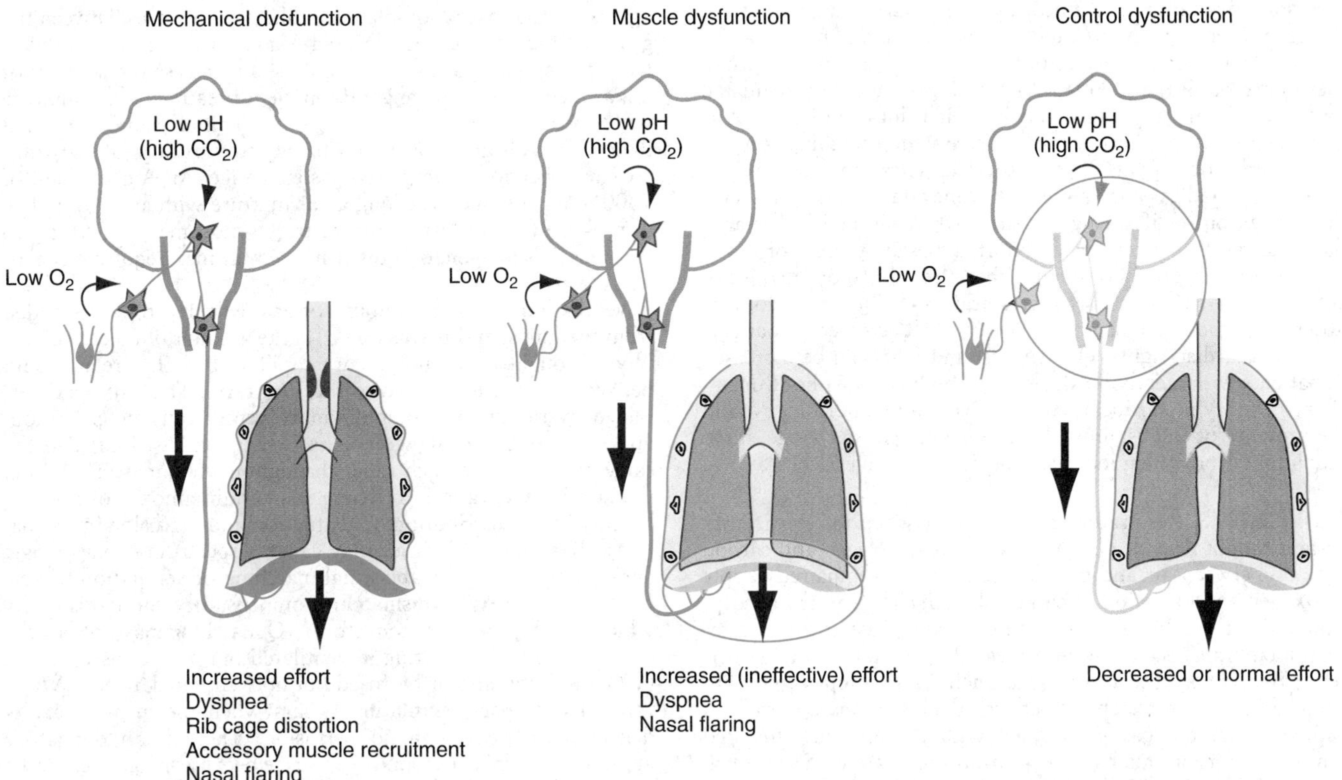

Figure 69-1. Presentation profiles of respiratory failure in childhood. When a mechanical dysfunction is present (by far, the most common circumstance), arterial hypoxemia and hypercapnia (and hence pH) are sensed by peripheral (carotid bodies) and central (medullary) chemoreceptors. After being integrated with other sensory information from the lungs and chest wall, chemoreceptor activation triggers an increase in the neural output to the respiratory muscles *(vertical arrows)*, which results in the physical signs that characterize respiratory distress. When the problem resides with the respiratory muscles (or their innervation), the same increase in neural output occurs *(arrow)*, but the respiratory muscles cannot increase their effort as demanded; therefore, the physical signs of distress are more subtle. Finally, when the control of breathing is itself affected by disease, the neural response to hypoxemia and hypercapnia is absent or blunted and the gas exchange abnormalities are not accompanied by respiratory distress.

TABLE 69-1. Anatomic Classification of Respiratory Failure

LUNG	RESPIRATORY PUMP
CENTRAL AIRWAY OBSTRUCTION	***CHEST WALL DEFORMITY***
Tracheomalacia	Kyphoscoliosis
Subglottic stenosis	Diaphragmatic hernia
Epiglottitis	Flail chest
Croup	Eventration of diaphragm
Vocal cord paralysis	Prune-belly syndrome
Foreign body aspiration	Asphyxiating thoracic dystrophy
Vascular ring	Pulmonary hypoplasia
Adenotonsillar hypertrophy	***BRAINSTEM***
Near-strangulation	Sleep apnea
PERIPHERAL AIRWAY OBSTRUCTION	Central hypoventilation
Bronchiolitis	Poisoning
Asthma	Trauma
Aspiration	Central nervous system infection
Cystic fibrosis	***SPINAL CORD***
Bronchomalacia	Trauma
DIFFUSE ALVEOLAR DAMAGE (acute respiratory distress syndrome)	Poliomyelitis
	Werdnig-Hoffmann disease
Sepsis	***NEUROMUSCULAR***
Pneumonia	Postoperative phrenic nerve injury
Pulmonary edema	Birth trauma
Near-drowning	Infant botulism
Pulmonary embolism	Guillain-Barré syndrome
Lung contusion	Muscular dystrophy
Shock	
Systemic inflammatory response syndrome	

Adapted from Helfaer M, Nichols D, Rogers M: Developmental physiology of the respiratory system. In Rogers MC (editor): *Textbook of Pediatric Intensive Care*, 2nd ed. Baltimore, Williams & Wilkins, 1992, pp 104–133.

Respiratory failure is defined, in general terms, as inability of the respiratory system to fulfill the gas exchange needs of the patient. Traditionally, respiratory failure is defined by abnormalities in arterial PO_2 and PCO_2. PO_2 and PCO_2 are tightly regulated by the CNS, and any alterations in their values can be taken as an indication that either the regulatory system (breathing control) or its effector organs (respiratory muscles and lungs) are impaired. Blood gas analysis requires time and should never delay the institution of lifesaving measures when the physical examination suggests that blood gas abnormalities are present or imminent. Moreover, an alteration in either arterial PO_2 or PCO_2 is not sufficient for the diagnosis of respiratory failure, nor does its absence exclude this diagnosis. PO_2 can be decreased in patients with intracardiac right-to-left shunts, and PCO_2 can be increased in patients with metabolic alkalosis, in both cases without intrinsic respiratory impairment. Arterial PO_2 may be normal, even in the presence of a substantial derangement in gas exchange, if the individual is breathing increased inspired oxygen concentrations.

PATHOGENESIS. Respiratory failure occurs when the respiratory system cannot provide adequate exchange of oxygen and carbon dioxide between air and blood, resulting in an impaired supply of oxygen and excretion of carbon dioxide. The oxygen absorption and carbon dioxide excretion that take place at the respiratory membrane occur because these 2 gases move along their respective concentration gradients, achieving complete equilibrium of pressure for each gas between the blood phase in the end capillary and the gas phase (air) with the alveolus. Inspired atmospheric room air has a PO_2 of approximately 159 mm Hg, and gas inside the alveoli, the **alveolar air**, normally has a PO_2 of 104 mm Hg. Alveolar air has this lower PO_2 because of humidification and because the oxygen in the alveoli is constantly being absorbed into the pulmonary blood. If the atmospheric air is supplemented with a higher concentration of oxygen, then alveolar PO_2 (PAO_2) will be higher, and the increased oxygen gradient between alveolar air and pulmonary blood results in increased absorption of oxygen. Carbon dioxide diffuses through the respiratory membrane so quickly that the mixed venous and alveolar PCO_2 are nearly the same. Atmospheric air has a PCO_2 of approximately zero, and a healthy person's alveolar and venous PCO_2 is approximately 40 mm Hg.

These relationships are described by the **alveolar gas equation:**

$$PAO_2 = [FIO_2(Pb - PH_2O)] - (PaCO_2/R)$$

where FIO_2 is the fraction of inspired oxygen (e.g., breathing oxygen at room air with a concentration of 21%—an FIO_2 of 0.21), Pb is barometric pressure (assumed to be 760 mm Hg at sea level), and PH_2O is water vapor pressure (which dilutes the dry oxygen content of the atmosphere, ≈47 mm Hg). R represents respiratory quotient, assumed to be 0.8, which can be calculated as follows:

$$R = CO_2\ \text{produced}/O_2\ \text{consumed}$$

Thus, the PAO_2 of a patient who breathes room air and has a $PaCO_2$ of 40 mm Hg would be predicted as:

$$PAO_2 = [0.21(760 - 47)] - (40/0.8) = 100\ \text{mm Hg}$$

If a patient were breathing a gas mixture with an FIO_2 of 0.5, then the PAO_2 would be 306 mm Hg.

$$PAO_2 = [0.5(760 - 47)] - (40/0.8) = 306\ \text{mm Hg}$$

The **alveolar-arterial oxygen gradient** (**A-a gradient**) is the difference between the predicted PAO_2 and the measured arterial PO_2 (PaO_2). The normal A-a gradient of healthy young subjects breathing air at sea level is <10 mm Hg because no lung pathology exists to prevent complete equilibration of gases between the gas and blood phases. An elevated A-a gradient represents underlying pulmonary pathology and is used to assess the severity of impairment of gas exchange. If a patient breathing a gas mixture with an FIO_2 of 0.5 has a PaO_2 of 100 mm Hg and a normal $PaCO_2$, the A-a gradient would be elevated to 206 (306 – 100), a clear indication of impaired gas exchange. An A-a gradient of >300 mm Hg while breathing a gas mixture with an FIO_2 of 1.0, a marker of acute respiratory distress syndrome (ARDS), signifies a serious oxygenation disturbance that may require mechanical ventilation.

Ventilation ($\dot{V}$) is the amount of gas delivered to and exhaled from the lungs, and **perfusion** ($\dot{Q}$) is the amount of mixed venous blood brought to the pulmonary capillary bed. The relationship between these 2 is referred to the **$\dot{V}/\dot{Q}$ ratio.** This ratio is determined by the amount of pulmonary ventilation and perfusion, and optimal gas exchange occurs if they are distributed in the same proportion to each other throughout the lungs. Therefore, the normal $\dot{V}/\dot{Q}$ ratio is 1. There is a certain amount of nonuniformity in the distribution of ventilation and perfusion in normal lungs. Respiratory diseases may cause a spectrum of pathologic derangement from the abnormal matching of ventilation to perfusion, termed **$\dot{V}/\dot{Q}$ mismatch.** Compensatory mechanisms by which the lungs attempt to restore $\dot{V}/\dot{Q}$ matching may not be adequate, potentially resulting in ventilated but nonperfused alveoli ($\dot{V}/\dot{Q}$ = infinity) and/or perfused but nonventilated alveoli ($\dot{V}/\dot{Q}$ = zero). **Dead space ventilation** occurs when the inspired gas is delivered to areas with no perfusion. There is an obligatory amount of normal anatomic dead space because inspired gas must traverse the nose, nasopharynx, trachea, and larger conducting airways. Pathologic alveolar (pulmonary) dead space occurs when alveoli are ventilated but not perfused. This results from a pathophysiologic process that impedes blood flow through the pulmonary capillary bed, such as pulmonary embolism, pulmonary hypotension or hypertension, or obstructive lung disease.

The volume of gas entering and leaving the mouth or nose per breath is the tidal volume. Alveolar ventilation, the volume of air entering and leaving the alveoli per min, is defined by the equation. Alveolar ventilation determines the rate of carbon dioxide excretion. Diseases that cause increased dead space result in decreased alveolar ventilation, and, unless the tidal volume or the frequency of respiration increases enough to compensate, the $PaCO_2$ will rise.

An **intrapulmonary shunt** occurs when the alveoli are perfused but not ventilated, with mixed venous blood being shunted to the systemic arterial circulation without coming into contact with any inspired oxygen. This blood does not participate in gas exchange. The resultant increase in carbon dioxide content of arterial blood is usually rapidly buffered, so the effect on $PaCO_2$ is negligible, but the dilution of oxygen content significantly lowers PaO_2. Therefore, diseases that cause increased intrapulmonary shunt cause hypoxemia. The hypoxemia associated with shunt can be severe and is often an indication for mechanical ventilation. Examples of diseases increasing intrapulmonary shunting are ARDS, pneumonia, pulmonary hemorrhage, atelectasis, and pulmonary edema. Supplemental oxygen does not always enhance PaO_2 in patients with shunting because the oxygen never reaches the alveolar capillary membrane.

Respiratory failure may also be classified as due to either lung disease or respiratory pump dysfunction (see Table 69-1). Common causes of respiratory failure in children include asthma, croup, respiratory syncytial virus infection, acute chest syndrome in sickle cell anemia, and pneumonia, whereas chronic respiratory failure is seen in bronchopulmonary dysplasia, cystic fibrosis, and progressive neuromuscular disorders. Lung diseases involve the airways, alveoli, or pulmonary circulation, alone or in combination, and result in hypoxemia. When lung disease leads to respiratory failure, patients have dyspnea, increased respiratory drive, and increased alveolar ventilation, which causes respiratory alkalosis unless the patient has fatigue leading to failure of the respiratory pump as well. The coordinated activities of the CNS and the respiratory muscles act like a respiratory pump; respiratory failure can result from CNS, neuromuscular, or muscular dysfunction. Failure of the respiratory pump causes hypoventilation, a decrease in alveolar ventilation, and hypercarbia. Hypoxemia may also occur when the respiratory pump fails; it is treated with supplemental oxygen or positive pressure ventilation.

CLINICAL MANIFESTATIONS. The limited ability of the developing respiratory system to compensate for disease-induced mechanical abnormalities makes early recognition of respiratory failure critical. Respiratory failure should be anticipated rather than recognized so that alterations in gas exchange can be prevented.

Children with impending respiratory failure due to lung disease have respiratory distress characterized by rapid breathing, or **tachypnea,** and exaggerated use of accessory muscles, as reflected by intercostal, supraclavicular, and subcostal **retractions,** which may be much more striking in a child than in an adult because of the increased compliance of the chest wall. Impending respiratory failure caused by respiratory pump dysfunction (CNS or neuromuscular disease) may be more difficult to recognize because these children may not have any signs of respiratory distress. A patient with a neuromuscular disease, such as muscular dystrophy or Werdnig-Hoffman disease, may be weak, and the degree of retractions may not be obvious. Other causes of respiratory pump failure, such as narcotic ingestion or brain tumor, cause decreased ventilatory drive and hypoventilation. An abnormally low respiratory rate, bradypnea, or shallow breathing may identify these children.

During physical examination, the clinician should avoid interfering with the patient's own mechanisms of compensation. An awake child with upper airway obstruction caused by croup or epiglottitis may be more stable in a parent's arms because the increased gas flow and the increased forces generated during crying worsen the obstruction and can precipitate failure. Similarly, most patients with severe restrictive and obstructive disease tolerate the supine position poorly because it promotes gravity-dependent perfusion of poorly ventilated areas and the weight of the abdominal organs imposes an additional burden on the diaphragm.

In a child suspected of respiratory failure, evaluation should always start with a rapid assessment of the adequacy of ventilation, including the presence and vigor of respiratory movements, the breathing rate, the presence of cyanosis, and the presence of signs of upper airway obstruction. A child with grossly inadequate respiratory effort or complete airway obstruction will die unless ventilation of the lungs is restored immediately. Special attention must be paid to the patient's state of consciousness. Hypoxemia and hypercarbia frequently cause lethargy and confusion, sometimes alternating with agitation. Whether resulting from these or concurrent mechanisms, CNS depression requires immediate attention because it further limits the ability of the respiratory system to deal with mechanical loads and leaves the airway unprotected against obstruction and aspiration of foreign materials.

Acute hypoxemia and hypercapnia result in dilation of the cerebral blood vessels and increased blood flow, often accompanied by severe headache. The sudden increased work of the accessory muscles of breathing may result in lower back pain. Although moderate to severe hypercapnia can cause peripheral vasodilation, mild to moderate hypoxemia can cause peripheral vasoconstriction and the patient may have cold extremities, a finding that may divert attention toward a circulatory dysfunction when the main problem is respiratory. Other symptoms of hypoxia include restlessness, dizziness, and impaired thought.

DIAGNOSIS. Respiratory distress is a clinical diagnosis made by the bedside clinician; respiratory failure is confirmed by diagnostic studies. Respiratory distress in children is usually diagnosed by history and physical examination; severe distress may need immediate treatment before diagnostic procedures or tests are performed. Some patients may not tolerate procedures such as an arterial puncture for a blood gas determination or a radiologic study; a change into an uncomfortable position may make it more difficult to breathe. It may be best to leave the patient in the position of greatest comfort, provide supplemental oxygen by face mask, and use aerosolized treatments and noninvasive pulse oximetry. If these measures are not tolerated and do not result in improvement, then endotracheal intubation is required to secure the airway.

LABORATORY FINDINGS. Although the clinical presentation may require immediate intubation and mechanical ventilation, for the majority of children, it is possible and helpful to first obtain an arterial blood sample to analyze blood gas tensions (PaO_2, $PaCO_2$, and pH) and initiate continuous noninvasive monitoring by pulse oximetry. *Hypoxemic respiratory failure* is defined as a PaO_2 of <60 mm Hg with an FIO_2 of >0.6 (in the absence of cyanotic heart disease); *acute hypercarbic respiratory failure* is defined as an acute $PaCO_2$ of >50 mm Hg. In addition to analysis of blood gases, the decision to initiate mechanical ventilation should consider the cause of respiratory failure, the possibility of reversing the cause of the failure via other interventions, and the overall trend in a patient's clinical status. A patient with respiratory pump failure from narcotic overdose may have an acute $PaCO_2$ of >50 mm Hg, but should respond quickly to administration of a narcotic antagonist and may not require ventilatory support. Conversely, a patient whose lung disease results in hypoxemia and dyspnea that seem adequately treated with supplemental oxygen may have a $PaCO_2$ that is initially lower than normal (respiratory alkalosis). However, if this patient tires, an acute increase in the $PaCO_2$ may indicate impending respiratory failure, even if the $PaCO_2$ is still <50 mm Hg.

TABLE 69-2. Noninvasive Modes of Respiratory Support

Oxygen only	Nasal cannula	Deliver up to 4 L O_2
	Simple face mask	Deliver up to 10 L O_2
	Non-rebreather face mask	Deliver up to 15 L O_2
Oxygen + noninvasive pressure support	Nasal CPAP: effective in neonates and patients < 8 kg	Can provide continuous positive airway pressure with a backup rate
	BiPAP: in older children or patients > 8 kg	Can provide 2 levels of support with inspiratory positive airway pressure and expiratory positive airway pressure

BiPAP, bilevel positive airway pressure; CPAP, continuous positive airway pressure.

TREATMENT. If the patient is not in impending respiratory failure, noninvasive methods of ventilatory support should be attempted before the initiation of mechanical ventilation (Table 69-2). Some of the advantages of noninvasive ventilation include decreased risk of pneumonia, no risk of the development of ventilator-induced lung injury, and the need for less overall sedation.

The goal of treatment is the restoration of adequate gas exchange with a minimum of complications. This is achieved by eliminating the initiating factors as quickly as possible. Thus, respiratory failure caused by cardiogenic pulmonary edema is treated with inotropic medications and diuretics. The child with asthma should be managed with bronchodilators and anti-inflammatory medications. Unfortunately, even in acute illnesses such as these, the response to treatment is not immediate, and frequently the entire function of the respiratory system must be artificially supported.

Hypoxemia is more dangerous than hypercarbia. Administration of supplemental oxygen is a safe and wise precaution in all patients who are at risk for acute respiratory failure or an exacerbation of chronic respiratory insufficiency, even if there is no initial evidence of hypoxemia (see Table 69-2).

The indication for ventilatory support in a child with respiratory failure is usually based on the persistence or worsening of gas exchange (see Chapter 70). Mechanical ventilation is necessary in a child with pneumonia in whom severe hypoxemia and hypercarbia develop because even the most effective antibiotic therapy requires time (at least 24 hr). On occasion, ventilatory support must be instituted in the absence of alterations in arterial P_{CO_2} when dysfunction of other systems places gas exchange in jeopardy by limiting the compensatory ability of the respiratory system; cardiovascular shock is a typical example. In shock, decreased blood flow and substrate delivery to the respiratory muscles may reduce the force that these muscles can develop and can precipitate secondary respiratory failure, even in the absence of substantial mechanical abnormalities of the respiratory system.

Ventilatory support often requires intubation of the trachea with an endotracheal tube or, less often, a tracheostomy cannula (see Chapter 70). Regardless of the type of ventilator, the objective of mechanical ventilation is not to normalize arterial blood gas tensions, but rather to provide "adequate" gas exchange. The definition of *adequate* includes some degree of hypercarbia and hypoxemia to minimize oxygen- and stretch-induced lung injury. Moderate hypercarbia (arterial P_{CO_2}, 60–80 mm Hg) has no detectable negative consequences because its effects on arterial pH are eventually minimized through renal retention of bicarbonate. Moderate hypoxemia (oxygen saturation, 85–90%) is similarly well tolerated in otherwise stable patients, particularly if the hemoglobin concentration and cardiac output are maintained at physiologic values and conditions such as fever and agitation, which increase tissue oxygen demands, are avoided. Artificial mechanical ventilation is usually initiated with conventional volume-driven ventilators; oscillator ventilators are often used as rescue therapy if conventional ventilators do not improve oxygenation, but their efficacy is not proven in many circumstances (see Chapter 70).

Extracorporeal membrane oxygenation (ECMO) is used in the treatment of newborns and small infants with life-threatening, refractory respiratory failure that is unresponsive to mechanical ventilation and is expected to resolve in a short time (see Chapter 101). Because of its risks (from vascular cannulation and anticoagulation) and the fact that its benefits over conventional management in non-neonatal patients have not been unequivocally demonstrated, indications for ECMO require considerable experience, caution, and judgment. Inhaled nitric oxide may acutely improve oxygenation by reducing increased pulmonary vascular resistance, ant this treatment and has replaced the use of ECMO in many intensive care situations. Inhaled helium is beneficial in patients with respiratory failure from abnormal airways, such as croup. Exogenous surfactant delivered into the trachea has improved oxygenation and survival in pediatric patients with ARDS.

DeBruin W, Notterman DA, Magid M, et al: Acute hypoxemic respiratory failure in infants and children: Clinical and pathologic characteristics. *Crit Care Med* 1992;20:1223–1234.

Guillemin K, Krasnow MA: The hypoxic response: Huffing and HIFing. *Cell* 1997;89:9–12.

The National Heart, Lung, and Blood Institute Acute Respiratory Distress Syndrome (ARDS) Clinical Trials Network: Comparison of two fluid-management strategies in acute lung injury. *N Engl J Med* 2006;354:2564–2574.

The National Heart, Lung, and Blood Institute Acute Respiratory Distress Syndrome (ARDS) Clinical Trials Network: Efficacy and safety of corticosteroids for persistent acute respiratory distress syndrome. *N Engl J Med* 2006;354:1671–1684.

Taylor RW, Zimmerman JL, Dellinger RP, et al: Low-dose inhaled nitric oxide in patients with acute lung injury A randomized controlled trial. *JAMA* 2004;291:1603–1609.

Wilson DF, Thomas NJ, Markovitz BP, et al: Effect of exogenous surfactant (calfactant) in pediatric acute lung injury. *JAMA* 2005;293:470–476.

Chapter 70 ■ Mechanical Ventilation

Lorry R. Frankel and Saraswati Kache

UNDERLYING CONCEPTS AND TERMINOLOGY

See also Chapter 370. Natural spontaneous ventilation occurs when the respiratory muscles (diaphragm, intercostal muscles) create negative inspiratory pressure, in part by expanding the rib cage, leading to lung inflation, which pulls air into the alveoli and allows gas exchange to occur. Intubated ventilated patients have compressed gas delivered to the lungs by positive pressure ventilation. This difference affects cardiopulmonary dynamics as well as the integrity of lung tissue. Positive pressure ventilators are the mainstay of mechanical ventilation in the adult, pediatric, and neonatal intensive care unit (ICU). During positive pressure mechanical ventilation, the flow of gas during inspiration and exhalation is driven by the airway pressure gradient between the airway opening and the alveoli. In a pediatric ICU, ventilator support is most frequently provided by intubation of the trachea, with placement of an endotracheal tube (ETT) and, on occasion, with a tracheostomy cannula. The ETT adapter, which attaches to the ventilator tubing, is considered the airway opening. During inspiration, airway opening pressure is greater than alveolar pressure, thereby driving gas into the lungs and inflating them. Exhalation is usually passive and occurs because, at the end of inspiration, alveolar pressure becomes greater than airway pressure. Important terms required to understand mechanical ventilation are shown in Table 70-1.

TABLE 70-1. Ventilator Parameters

ABBREVIATION	TERM	DEFINITION
PIP	Peak inspiratory pressure	Point of maximal airway pressure
PEEP	Positive end-expiratory pressure	Pressure maintained in airways at the end of exhalation
DP	Delta pressure	Difference between PIP and PEEP
V_T	Tidal volume	Volume of gas entering the patient's lung during inspiration
I_T	Inspiratory time	Duration of time in inspiration
E_T	Expiratory time	Duration of time in expiration
MAP	Mean airway pressure	Average of the pressure that the airway is experiencing throughout the respiratory cycle
R	Rate	Respiratory rate as set on the ventilator

Peak inspiratory pressure (PIP) occurs during maximal inspiration. **Positive end-expiratory pressure (PEEP)** maintains end-expiratory resting lung volume. The maximum pressure gradient is the difference between PIP and PEEP. **Mean airway pressure** is a measure of the average pressure to which the lungs are exposed during the respiratory cycle. Mean airway pressure can be increased by increasing PEEP, PIP, the ratio of inspiratory time to expiratory time (I : E ratio), or inspiratory flow (Fig. 70-1). Adjusting the ventilator to increase mean airway pressure is the therapy for hypoxemia that is not responding to an increasing FIO_2. This probably improves oxygenation by decreasing the number of collapsed alveoli or redistributing lung fluid.

COMPONENTS OF THE VENTILATOR BREATH

Each complete ventilator breath has an allotted time for inspiration **(I-time)** before the ventilator must cycle into exhalation time **(E-time).** The sum of the I-time and E-time equals the allotted time per breath. The ventilator delivers a set number of breaths per min, or **ventilator frequency.** The frequency determines the length of each breath. A frequency of 20 would result in 3 sec/breath. Most ventilators allow setting either the I-time or the **I : E ratio.** If an I-time of 1 sec is ordered and the breath is

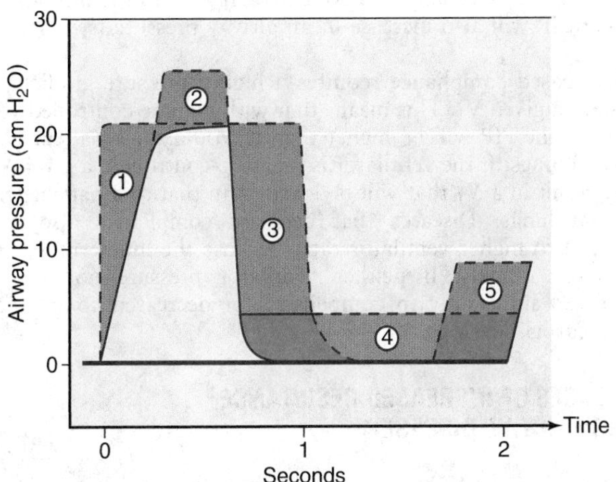

Figure 70-1. Five different ways to increase mean airway pressure: (1) Increase the respiratory flow rate, producing a square-wave inspiratory pattern; (2) increase peak inspiratory pressure; (3) reverse the inspiratory-expiratory ratio or prolong the inspiratory time without changing the rate; (4) increase positive end-expiratory pressure; and (5) increase the ventilatory rate by reducing the expiratory time without changing the inspiratory time. (From Harris TR, Wood BR: Physiologic principles. In Goldsmith JP, Karotkin EH [editors]: *Assisted Ventilation of the Neonate,* 3rd ed. Philadelphia, WB Saunders, 1996.)

TABLE 70-2. Comparison of Pressure-Controlled and Volume-Controlled Ventilation

COMPARING PRESSURE VS VOLUME VENTILATION	PRESSURE VENTILATION	VOLUME VENTILATION
Parameters set by the operator	PIP, PEEP, rate, FIO_2, I-time	V_T, PEEP, rate, FIO_2, I-time
Parameters determined by the ventilator	V_T, E-time	PIP, E-time
Advantages	Higher MAP provided with the same PIP; lung protective for noncompliant lungs	Guaranteed minute ventilation
Disadvantages	Does not accommodate for rapid changes in pulmonary compliance	Not optimal for patients with an endotracheal tube with large leaks
	Minute ventilation not guaranteed	May reach dangerous levels of PIP if compliance is worsening

E-time, expiratory time; FIO_2, fractional inspired oxygen; I-time, inspiratory time; MAP, mean airway pressure; PEEP, positive end-expiratory pressure; PIP, peak inspiratory pressure; V_T, tidal volume.

3 sec, the I : E ratio will be 1 : 2. If an I : E ratio of 1 : 3 is ordered, then the I-time would be 0.75 sec and the E-time would be 2.25 sec.

The change in lung volume during the inspiratory period is defined as the **tidal volume (V_T).** It is the volume above the **functional residual capacity (FRC),** that is, the volume above the end-expiratory lung volume. Gas flow is expressed in units of liters per min and I-time is expressed in sec; in pediatrics, V_T is usually expressed in milliliters rather than as fractions of a liter. Pulmonary compliance is the change in volume divided by the change in pressure (Compliance = $\Delta V/\Delta P$). This formula provides the basis for understanding pulmonary and ventilator interactions; it allows the physician to monitor patient progression or recovery from the pulmonary process by tracking ventilator parameters (see Chapter 69).

PRESSURE-CONTROLLED VS VOLUME-CONTROLLED VENTILATION

These are the 2 primary methods for positive pressure ventilation (Table 70-2).

Pressure-controlled ventilators allow a clinician to set the PIP and PEEP. The increase in airway pressure occurs swiftly at the initiation of inspiration to achieve the set PIP. This PIP is then maintained throughout the I-time. In pressure-controlled ventilation, lung volume rises until it reaches its capacity at that PIP or until the ventilator cycles into exhalation. Thus, V_T is not set, but rather is determined by both the pressure gradient of the ventilator and the patient's pulmonary compliance. In volume-controlled ventilation, V_T is preset as a product of setting flow and I-time. Airway pressure rises throughout inspiration and reaches its peak when the entire V_T is delivered. PIP is not set, but rather is determined by both V_T and the patient's pulmonary compliance.

VENTILATOR-PATIENT INTERACTIONS

When children are not attempting to breathe spontaneously, the ventilator completely controls the respiratory pattern. For children who can attempt to breathe, the degree to which a ventilator is able to synchronize with the patient's own respiratory efforts may have significant clinical effects. Patients whose lung disease is improving and who thus are receiving less sedation in an attempt to wean them from ventilator support may find that when they need to, they are unable to draw a breath, thereby experiencing dyspnea. Patients also may experience anxiety as gas is pushed into their airway while they are trying to exhale. This dyssynchrony often necessitates pharmacologic interventions with sedation or paralytic agents, which may result in prolonged intubation and ventilation. Patient-ventilator dyssynchrony may also cause barotrauma (pressure injury) to the lungs. Advances in mechanical ventilation have attempted to improve patient-ventilator synchronization.

MODES OF VENTILATION

ASSIST CONTROL. The **assist control mode** provides maximal support for the patient. Every breath, whether mechanical or spontaneous, is fully supported, with each breath having the same PIP or V_T and the same I-time. This mode can be either a volume or a pressure mode. Pressure support is unnecessary in this mode.

SYNCHRONIZED INTERMITTENT MANDATORY VENTILATION. Synchronized intermittent mandatory ventilation (SIMV) allows better response by the ventilator to the patient. During SIMV, the ventilator allows the child to trigger a breath by spontaneously attempting to inspire (Fig. 70-2). If the patient takes too long to initiate a spontaneous breath, then inspiration is time-triggered by the ventilator: **a mandatory breath.** Ventilator frequency determines the total time allotted per breath, and some percentage of that time is the window allowed for the patient to initiate inspiration. If the patient does not spontaneously try to breathe during this window of time, then the ventilator initiates inspiration. SIMV may be either volume-controlled or pressure-controlled. A patient may also breathe spontaneously more often than the set frequency of SIMV, inspiring fresh gas from the circuit at the set PEEP. These spontaneous breaths are assisted by the set **pressure support,** and the patient controls the I-time of these respirations.

PRESSURE SUPPORT. The **pressure support mode** allows for spontaneous breathing by patients. The ventilator assists every breath a child initiates by applying a predetermined amount of airway pressure above the set PEEP. A child can control the rate of breathing and the duration of inspiration, so the breathing pattern may truly be called spontaneous. Many ventilators allow both pressure support and SIMV. Pressure support breaths can occur whenever a child attempts to inspire, unless the patient is breathing within that window of time that results in an SIMV breath.

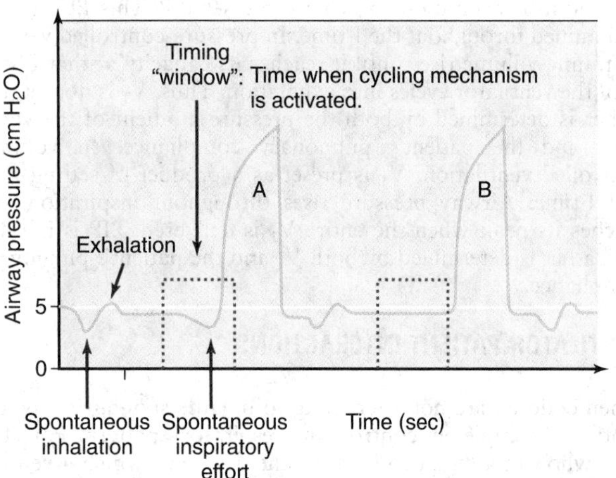

Figure 70-2. Synchronized intermittent mandatory ventilation. At set intervals, the ventilator's timing circuit becomes activated and a timing "window" appears *(shaded area)*. If the patient initiates a breath in the timing window, then the ventilator delivers a mandatory breath. If no spontaneous effort occurs, then the ventilator delivers a mandatory breath at a fixed time after the timing window. (From Banner MJ, Gallagher TJ: Respiratory failure in the adult: Ventilatory support. In Kirby RR, Smith RA, Desautels DA [editors]: *Mechanical Ventilation*. New York, Churchill Livingstone, 1985.)

MONITORING AND ALARMS

What is not controllable is monitored. In pressure-controlled ventilation, V_T is monitored. In volume-controlled ventilation, airway pressure is monitored; safety precautions include popoff limits to the peak airway pressure. An oxygen analyzer allows monitoring of FIO_2.

Alarms can be set for a wide array of events. The common alarms are for high or low airway pressure, absence of flow (apnea), loss of electrical power, high or low exhaled V_T, and high or low minute volume. When alarms occur, they must be evaluated to determine if there is a malfunction of the ventilator or a change in the patient. The importance of frequent physical examination cannot be overemphasized; it is the fastest means of diagnosing a variety of ventilator problems, such as patient-ventilator dyssynchrony, ETT obstruction, pneumothorax, and inadvertent extubation.

APPROACH TO MECHANICAL VENTILATION. The pressure gradient that inflates the lungs must overcome the pulmonary mechanics of the patient's respiratory system. See Chapter 370 for a discussion of the compliance, resistance, and time constant of the respiratory system. Respiratory diseases result in decreased lung compliance, increased airway resistance, or both. Ventilator strategies are designed to ameliorate physiologic derangements resulting in ventilation-perfusion mismatch.

DISEASES OF DECREASED COMPLIANCE (RESTRICTIVE DISEASE)

Compliance is decreased in various diseases that affect the lung parenchyma, such as acute respiratory distress syndrome, atelectasis, pneumonia, pulmonary edema, and pulmonary hemorrhage. In all of these diseases, FRC is reduced as terminal airways become fluid-filled or collapse. These smaller alveoli are more difficult to inflate. Intrapulmonary shunt is increased when blood flows to poorly ventilated lung units, worsening hypoxemia. One goal of mechanical ventilation when lung compliance is decreased is to decrease shunting by improving ventilation to the perfused lung units. The ventilator approach to decreased FRC is to increase mean airway pressure to recruit atelectatic areas of lung; this increase is usually achieved by a higher PEEP, although a higher PIP will also increase mean airway pressure (see Fig. 70-1).

Decreased compliance requires a higher pressure gradient to achieve a given V_T. This means that with volume-controlled ventilation, the PIP will be higher than it would for a patient with normal lungs. If the ventilator is pressure-controlled, a given PIP may result in a V_T that will be lower than that of a patient with normal lungs. Diseases that decrease compliance also may respond to higher ventilator rates because the lungs empty and fill more quickly. If neither ventilator pressure nor rate is increased sufficiently to compensate for decreased compliance, hypercarbia develops.

DISEASES OF INCREASED RESISTANCE (OBSTRUCTIVE DISEASE)

Resistance is increased in various diseases that decrease the caliber of the airway lumen by edema, spasm, or obstructing material. Because airways decrease in caliber during exhalation, increased resistance affects expiratory flow more than inspiratory flow. Diseases in which airway resistance is increased include asthma, bronchiolitis, bronchopulmonary dysplasia, smoke inhalation, and cystic fibrosis.

Diseases of increased resistance are often accompanied by both increased intrapulmonary shunt and dead space ventilation.

TABLE 70-3. Guidelines for Initiating Mechanical Ventilation

	NORMAL LUNGS	DECREASED COMPLIANCE	INCREASED RESISTANCE
Tidal volume (V_T)	8–12 mL/kg (set of volume-controlled and derived if pressure-controlled ventilation)	10–12 mL/kg (may need to use less if the inflating pressures are too high, i.e., risk for volutrauma)	10–12 mL/kg (may need to use less volume if the inflating pressures required are too high; i.e., barotrauma)
Rate (breaths/min)	Physiologic norm for age or lower, depending on the V_T used (e.g., infant rate = 30, toddler rate = 20, adolescent rate = 16)	May require higher rates to maintain adequate minute ventilation	Often requires lower rates to allow adequate emptying time
Peak inspiratory pressure (PIP) [cm H_2O]	Initial PIP = 20–25 cm H_2O; monitor for adequate chest expansion and V_T	May require higher PIP to obtain an acceptable V_T	May require higher PIP to obtain acceptable V_T
Positive end-expiratory pressure (PEEP)	2–4 cm H_2O to prevent atelectasis	Frequently requires higher PEEP to achieve oxygenation and improved compliance (e.g., 6–10 cm H_2O); anticipate decreased venous return and cardiac output	May need to maintain low PEEP to avoid exacerbation of gas trapping and overinflation
Oxygen concentration (FIO_2)	May not need supplemental oxygen; however, one usually begins with FIO_2 of 1.0 and may then quickly wean to an FIO_2 of ≤0.5	Begin with an FIO_2 of 1.0; attempt to wean to ≤0.6 by adjusting mean airway pressure/PEEP	Begin with an FIO_2 of 1.0; wean to maintain adequate oxygenation and avoid oxygen toxicity
Inspiratory time (I-time)	Normal for age I : E = 1 : 2, 1 : 3	Allow a generous I-time to allow recruitment of collapsed lung segments (e.g., 1 : 1.2)	Ensure adequate I-time and E-time, especially E-time, to avoid gas trapping (e.g., I : E of 1 : 3 or 1 : 4)

E-time, expiratory time.

Shunt occurs if the increased resistance greatly impedes gas flow, decreasing ventilation to alveoli that remain perfused. Dead space ventilation occurs if the increased resistance leads to gas trapping in areas of the lung that contain hyperinflated alveoli. These areas of hyperinflated lung units exert pressure on the surrounding structures, resulting in a reduction of pulmonary capillary blood flow. The increases in both shunt and dead space mean that these diseases produce both significant hypoxemia and hypercarbia. Increased resistance requires that a higher pressure must occur for the flow of gas to reach the terminal air sacs. Therefore, if volume-controlled ventilation is used, an increase in PIP is required to deliver a given V_T. If pressure-controlled ventilation is used, V_T is lower than in a normal lung at the same pressure.

Increased resistance may result in significant increases in time constant (see Chapter 370), unless there is a proportional decrease in compliance, which rarely happens in diseases of increased resistance. A longer time constant (time necessary for gas to fill or empty the alveoli) necessitates long inspiratory and expiratory times. Therefore, patients with these lung diseases may be adversely affected if the ventilator frequency is too high and expiratory and inspiratory times are too short. This results in a phenomenon known as **gas trapping** as the ventilator cycles back into inspiration before the lung has had sufficient time to empty. The ventilator breaths stack on each other as more and more gas is trapped, resulting in an increase in FRC. This eventually leads to lung hyperinflation, a predisposition to pneumothorax and barotrauma, and reduction in compliance.

INITIAL VENTILATOR SETTINGS

Mechanical ventilation is initiated to provide support for lungs that function normally or for diseases of decreased compliance or increased resistance (Table 70-3). **For supporting normal lungs,** ventilator frequency may be slightly lower than the normal respiratory rate for age because ventilator V_T is usually set higher than a healthy person's V_T of 5–7 mL/kg. The customary range for ventilator V_T has been lowered to 8–10 mL/kg from 10–15 mL/kg. For pressure-controlled ventilation, an initial PIP of 20–25 H_2O is usually sufficient to move an adequate V_T, but this must be immediately assessed by observation of chest expansion and measurement of V_T. To initiate **support for diseases of decreased compliance,** mean airway pressures must be higher and a higher PEEP is often used to achieve this goal. PEEP is titrated upward to re-recruit atelectatic areas and to provide adequate oxygenation at an FIO_2 of <0.6. Despite the mode of ventilation used, efforts should be made to maintain V_T of 6–8 mL/kg and to limit PIP to 30–35 cm H_2O. These lung-protective strategies recruit atelectatic areas while preventing overdistention of normal lung **parenchyma** (Fig. 70-3). Significant hypoxemia results from these diseases, and it is customary to start with an FIO_2 of 100% and then to reduce it to 60% or lower to avoid oxygen toxicity. The ventilator frequency may be set higher than normal because a decreased time constant permits a faster rate. A common inspiratory time is 0.8–1 sec.

Diseases of increased resistance often have very high time constants. Ventilator frequency may need to be set as low as 12–16 breaths/min in severe status asthmaticus to allow adequate inspiratory and expiratory times.

COMPLICATIONS

There are many pulmonary and systemic complications of mechanical ventilation (Table 70-4 and Fig. 70-4). Lung injury may result from positive pressure (**barotrauma**), **oxygen toxicity,** or excessive volume changes in the lung, or **volutrauma.** Volutrauma may be manifested acutely as pulmonary air leak, such as pneumothorax, pneumomediastinum, pulmonary interstitial emphysema, and bronchopleural fistula. Volutrauma may also be a cause of chronic repetitive lung injury, exacerbating the primary disease. This may result from subjecting alveolar units to repeated overdistention, such as with excessive V_T, or to cyclic collapse and re-expansion, such as with insufficient PEEP to stabilize the resting lung volume. In diseases of decreased compliance, more compliant lung units may receive more of the V_T than less compliant units, leading to volutrauma of the healthier segments of lung. This mechanism may contribute to the chronic lung injury that can develop in acute respiratory distress syndrome or any heterogenous pulmonary process. In diseases of increased resistance, the lung units with higher resistance need more time to fill and empty. This leads to overfilling of the lung units with lower resistance and time constants and to gas trapping and overdistention of the alveoli in the units with high time constants and severely obstructed airways.

Positive pressure ventilation also may affect the cardiovascular system. Some portion of the mean airway pressure is transmitted through the lungs and raises intrathoracic pressure. This may impede venous return and decrease right ventricular filling. Elevated intrathoracic pressure also may compress the pulmonary circulation and increase the afterload on the right ventricle, which may cause the interventricular septum to shift toward the left ventricle, resulting in a decrease in volume of the left ventricle and a reduction in left ventricular stroke volume. Cardiac output may thus be impeded. Alternatively, elevations in intrathoracic pressure may cause an afterload reduction for the left ventricle. The net result of these many cardiovascular effects may be beneficial or detrimental, depending on the overall cardiovascular status of

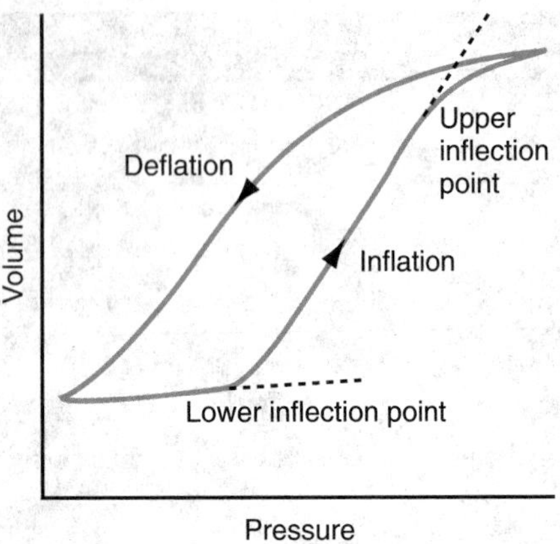

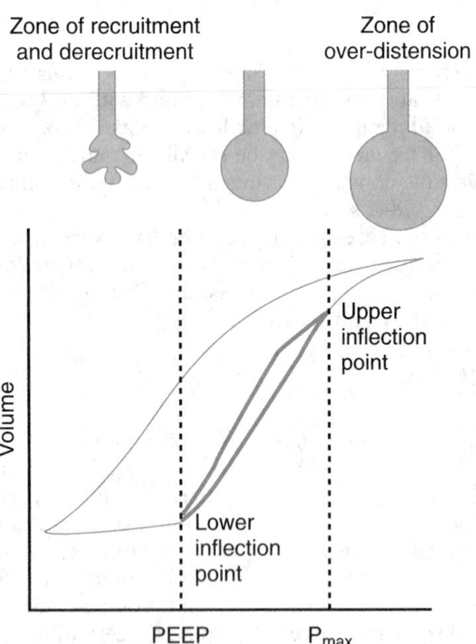

Figure 70-3. Pulmonary pressure-volume relationship of a patient with acute lung injury. *Top,* The lower inflection point is typically 12–18 cm H_2O, and the upper inflection point is 26–32 cm H_2O. *Bottom,* Specific protective ventilation strategies require that the positive end-expiratory pressure (PEEP) is set just above the lower inflection point and that the pressure limit (P_{max}) is just below the upper inflection point. Hence, the lung is ventilated in the safe zone between the zone of recruitment and derecruitment and the zone of overdistention, and both high- and low-volume injury is avoided. (From Pinhu L, Whitehead T, Evans T, et al: Ventilator-associated lung injury. *Lancet* 2003;361:332–340.)

the child. In general, high mean airway pressures require close observation for possible hemodynamic compromise and may necessitate support with fluids and inotropic drugs (see Chapter 68).

An ETT may become obstructed because of mucus, purulent material, or blood from trauma to the airway, or from the child biting on the tube. These are immediately life-threatening complications. An ETT also may cause injury to the tracheal mucosa, resulting in subglottic stenosis, which is usually not symptomatic until the tube is removed. Subglottic stenosis may resolve with time or may ultimately require surgical intervention.

Prolonged intubation and mechanical ventilation may predispose the child to nosocomial infections, often by bacteria resistant to numerous antibiotics. Nosocomial infection, sepsis, and

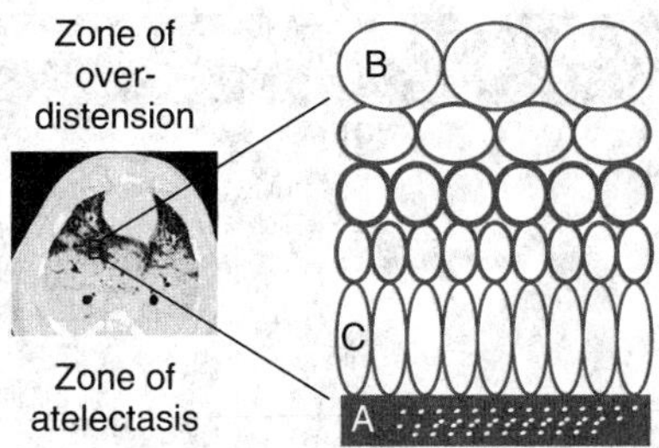

Figure 70-4. Atelectotrauma. The interface between collapsed and consolidated lung *(A)* and overdistended lung units *(B)* is heterogeneous and unstable. Depending on ambient conditions, this region is prone to cyclic recruitment and derecruitment and localized asymmetric stretch of lung units *(C)* immediately apposed to regions of collapsed lung. (From Pinhu L, Whitehead T, Evans T, et al: Ventilator-associated lung injury. *Lancet* 2003;361:332–240.)

TABLE 70-4. Components of Ventilator-Associated Lung Injury

VOLUTRAUMA
Damage caused by overdistention; sometimes called high-volume or high end-inspiratory volume injury
ATELECTOTRAUMA
Lung injury associated with repeated recruitment and collapse, theoretically prevented by using a level of positive end-expiratory pressure greater than the lower inflection point of the pressure-volume curve; sometimes called low-volume or low end-expiratory volume injury
BIOTRAUMA
Pulmonary and systemic inflammation caused by the release of mediators from lungs subjected to injurious mechanical ventilation
OXYGEN TOXIC EFFECTS
Damage caused by a high concentration of inspired oxygen; the oxygen concentration-toxic effect relationship for a damaged lung is not known
BAROTRAUMA
High-pressure–induced lung damage

From Pinhu L, Whitehead T, Evans T, et al: Ventilator-associated lung injury. *Lancet* 2003;361:332–340.

other organ system failures are the leading cause of death in patients with respiratory failure.

Other approaches to the care of the critically ill child with acute respiratory failure include high-frequency modes of ventilation, the application of permissive hypercapnia or hypoxia, and the use of natural surfactants or inhaled nitric oxide. High-frequency modes of ventilation can be divided into 3 distinct groups: oscillatory, jet, and flow interruption. All 3 modes use a very small V_T (<1 mL/kg), very rapid rates (150–1,000 breaths/min), and lower mean airway pressures to provide a gentler form of mechanical ventilation. **Permissive hypercapnia** allows the patient's $Pa{CO_2}$ to rise to 60–70 mm Hg; the patient is able to tolerate the degree of acidosis. To prevent oxygen toxicity, a permissive hypoxia strategy can be considered by accepting $Pa{O_2}$ of >50 mm Hg or saturation of >85%, ensuring that adequate end-organ oxygen delivery is being maintained. This is used to limit the amount of barotrauma and volutrauma to the patient. Positioning the patient in the prone position improves oxygenation and reduces ventilator-induced lung injury in patients with severe lung injury, but the outcome may not be improved.

Arnold JH, Anas NG, Luckett P, et al: High-frequency oscillatory ventilation in pediatric respiratory failure: A multicenter experience. *Crit Care Med* 2000;28:3941–3942.

Matthews BD, Noviski N: Management of oxygenation in pediatric acute hypoxemic respiratory failure. *Pediatr Pulmonol* 2001;32:459–470.

Mehta NM, Arnold, JH: Mechanical ventilation in children with acute respiratory failure. *Curr Opin Crit Care* 2004;10:7–12.

National Heart, Lung, and Blood Institute ARDS Clinical Trials Network: Higher versus lower positive end-expiratory pressures in patients with the acute respiratory distress syndrome. *N Engl J Med* 2004;351:327–336.

Nuckton TJ, Alonso JA, Kallet RH, et al: Pulmonary dead-space fraction as a risk factor for death in the acute respiratory distress syndrome. *N Engl J Med* 2002;346:1281–1286.
Pinhu L, Whitehead T, Evans T, et al: Ventilator-associated lung injury. *Lancet* 2003;361:332–340.
Priestley MA, Helfaer MA: Approaches in the management of acute respiratory failure in children. *Curr Opin Pediatr* 2004;16:293–298.
Squadrone V, Coha M, Cerutti E, et al: Continuous positive airway pressure for treatment of postoperative hypoxemia. *JAMA* 2005;293:589–595.
Steinbrook R: How best to ventilate? Trial design and patient safety in studies of the acute respiratory distress syndrome. *N Engl J Med* 2003;348:1393–1401.
Taylor RW, Zimmerman JL, Dellinger RP, et al: Low-dose inhaled nitric oxide in patients with acute lung injury. *JAMA* 2004;291:1603–1609.
Willson DF, Thomas NJ, Markovitz BP, et al: Effect of exogenous surfactant (calfactant) in pediatric acute lung injury. *JAMA* 2005;293:470–476.

70.1 • Long-Term Mechanical Ventilation •

Lorry R. Frankel and Saraswati Kache

Improvements in treating acute respiratory failure and advancements in invasive and noninvasive ventilation have led to an increased number of pediatric patients receiving long-term mechanical ventilation. Children younger than 10 yr of age with life-shortening or life-threatening medical conditions commonly require long-term ventilator assistance. Patients are often maintained on long-term ventilation until they recover from the initial pulmonary insult, or indefinitely, for progressive neuromuscular disease. The location of patient management varies from high-skilled nursing facilities to complete home care, depending on the technologic dependence of the child and the level of comfort of the caretakers.

DEFINITION. Chronic respiratory failure is pulmonary insufficiency for a protracted period, usually 28 days. This time limit is an approximation and varies with the specific clinical situation (Tables 70-5 and 70-6).

PATHOPHYSIOLOGY. The pathophysiology of chronic respiratory failure is divided into 3 major etiologies (see Table 70-6). The **1st group** is patients who have an acute pulmonary insult that has improved after aggressive ICU treatment, but will require prolonged rehabilitation to return to spontaneous unsupported breathing. The normal supply of respiratory muscle strength cannot meet the increased requirements of a pulmonary disease process. The **2nd group** is patients who have progressive neuromuscular disease in which respiratory failure develops slowly, over the course of mo to yr, and who require long-term ventilation. The decreased effort of respiratory muscles does not meet the normal demands of the lungs. The **3rd group** is patients who lack the appropriate neuronal input required to maintain respiration. Although both the lungs and the respiratory muscles are normal, lack of central nervous system stimulation prevents appropriate respiratory drive. All groups may have components of obstructive and restrictive disease over the course of time.

TABLE 70-5. Chronic Respiratory Failure

Patient symptoms: dyspnea, orthopnea, poor sleep, daytime fatigue and somnolence, morning headaches
ABG while the patient is awake with a $Pa\text{CO}_2$ of ≥45 mm Hg
Pulse oximetry during a sleep study with saturations of ≤88% for 5 consecutive min or longer
Forced vital capacity <50% of predicted

ABG, arterial blood gus; $Pa\text{CO}_2$, partial pressure of carbon dioxide in arterial blood.

TABLE 70-6. Disease Requiring Chronic Mechanical Ventilation

PARENCHYMAL INJURY WITH INCREASED WORK OF BREATHING
Bronchopulmonary dysplasia
Congenital anamolies
Tracheoesophgeal fistula
Airway anomalies
Congenital diaphragmatic hernia
Ventral wall anamolies
RESPIRATORY MUSCLE INSUFFICIENCY
Diaphragmatic paralysis
Infant botulism
Duchenne and other types of muscular dystrophy
Anterior horn cell disorders
Other neuromuscular disease
CENTRAL NERVOUS SYSTEM ABNORMALITIES PRODUCING HYPOVENTILATION
Central hypoventilation syndrome
Postinfectious
Brain tumor
Arnold-Chiari type I malformation
Spinal cord injury

Adapted from Pilmer S: Prolonged mechanical ventilation in children. *Pediatr Clin North Am* 1994;41(3):473–512.

INDICATIONS. Patients in an ICU in whom extubation is unsuccessful because of muscle weakness are candidates for long-term support. These patients may require more than 4–6 wk for the acute pulmonary process to completely resolve and to regain respiratory muscle strength; they also need some rehabilitation. Patients who have progressive neuromuscular disease and signs and symptoms of muscle fatigue should be considered for this treatment. Patients who have any central nervous system insult and cannot appropriately protect their airway should be considered for a tracheostomy, but may also need mechanical ventilation due to hypoventilation or apnea.

MODES OF VENTILATORY SUPPORT

NONINVASIVE VENTILATORY SUPPORT. Negative pressure ventilator jackets are not widely used for patients who need long-term ventilatory support. These jackets may be comfortable, depending on the specific model, and do not require an artificial airway. The disadvantage is that negative pressure ventilation is not as effective as positive pressure ventilation in providing adequate respiratory support.

Positive pressure systems are the preferred method for long-term ventilation. To provide positive pressure ventilation, an interface is required to provide the support from the mechanical system to the patient's pulmonary system. The possibilities include nasal, oronasal, and oral airways. The various devices available are nasal prongs for infants younger than 1 yr of age and nasal and face masks for older children and adolescents. These devices should be comfortable for the patient, should provide a tight seal to prevent significant loss of airflow, and should not elicit a gag or cough response. Chafing of the skin, particularly over the nasal bridge, with loss of skin integrity, is the most frequent problem with nasal and face masks. Long-term use of face masks may affect facial growth and cause midface hypoplasia. One strategy to prevent abnormal facial development is to alternate between the nasal and face mask. Another potential side effect of long-term use is orthodontic deformities.

Any ventilator used for intubated patients can be used to provide noninvasive positive pressure support. The settings usually include inspiratory positive airway pressure, expiratory positive airway pressure, a backup rate, and an inspiratory time (I-time). Inspiratory positive airway pressure is usually set at 15–20 cm H_2O, but the correct pressure required should be

TABLE 70-7. Appropriate Size Tracheostomy Tubes for Pediatric Patients

PATIENT AGE	PATIENT WEIGHT	UNCUFFED TUBE	CUFFED TUBE
Neonate–1 yr	6.4 kg	3.5 mm	3.0 mm
1–2 yr	10.5 kg	4.0 mm	3.5 mm
2–4 yr	13.7 kg	4.5 mm	4.0 mm
4–6 yr	17.1 kg	5.0 mm	4.5 mm
6–8 yr	24.5 kg	5.5 mm	5.0 mm
8–10 yr	27 kg	6.0 mm	5.5 mm
10–12 yr	37.1 kg	6.5 mm	6.0 mm
12–14 yr	42.3 kg	7.0 mm	6.5 mm
14–16 yr	54.3 kg	7.5 mm	7.0 mm

Adapted from Weiss M, Dullenkopf A, Gysin C, et al: Shortcomings of cuffed paediatric tracheal tubes. *Br J Anaesth* 2004;92:78–88.

From Weiss M, Gerber AC, Dullenkopf A: Appropriate placement of intubation depth marks new cuffed paediatric tracheal tube. *Br J Anaesth* 2005;94:80–87.

determined by the patient's chest rise. Expiratory positive airway pressure can be set at physiologic levels of 2–4 cm H_2O for patients at home or in long-term care facilities. During periods of acute illness, for example, if pneumonia develops in a patient with spinal muscular atrophy, expiratory positive airway pressure can be increased to as high as 8–10 cm H_2O to be used as a recruitment maneuver to prevent intubation. The rate can be set higher or lower than the patient's spontaneous respirations, depending on the amount of support the patient requires. Usually, the respiratory rate is set at 25–30 breaths/min for infants, 15–20 breaths/min for children, and 10–12 breaths/min for adolescents. Any volume mode on the ventilator should not be used for noninvasive ventilation because the leak in the system is usually large and the amount of support delivered is unpredictable.

INVASIVE VENTILATORY SUPPORT

Tracheostomy. Patients who cannot be maintained on noninvasive ventilation require invasive mechanical ventilation. A tracheotomy is performed and a tracheostomy tube secured in place to allow for long-term invasive mechanical support. Appropriate tracheostomy tube sizes based on age are listed in Table 70-7. The narrowest portion of the pediatric airway is below the glottis, at the level of the vocal cords in adults. Uncuffed tracheostomy tubes are preferred to cuffed tubes to prevent subglottic stenosis.

Ventilators. Pneumatically and electronically powered ventilators are available. The ideal **home ventilator** should be compact, reliable, and user-friendly. In addition, it should be comfortable and have appropriate alarms. Home ventilators can also be set to either the volume or the pressure mode, similar to ventilators in the ICU. In the pressure mode, the operator sets the desired PIP and PEEP; the ventilator determines the delivered volume, based on the patient's pulmonary compliance. This is usually the ideal mode for use in younger patients with uncuffed tracheostomy tubes because there is usually a large leak in the system, making the volume mode inappropriate. If the volume mode is used in older patients with cuffed tracheostomy tubes, the operator sets the desired V_T and the ventilator determines the required PIP, depending on pulmonary compliance. In either mode, with a home ventilator, the final decision on the appropriate pressure or V_T should be determined by the observed chest rise on physical examination. The respiratory rate should also be set by the physician, as required, to provide adequate ventilatory support.

INITIATION AND MANAGEMENT OF LONG-TERM MECHANICAL VENTILATION

Long-term ventilatory support should ideally be initiated in an inpatient setting. Once all of the appropriate equipment is acquired (face mask, ventilator), the ventilator settings should be adjusted to optimize patient oxygenation and ventilation. The patient should be monitored for adequate oxygenation with continuous pulse oximetry and intermittent blood gas sampling. Ventilation should be monitored with either a transcutaneous CO_2 monitor or an end-tidal CO_2 monitor for patients with tracheostomy tubes; these should be correlated with arterial blood gas measurements. The patient must be monitored during sleep to ensure that hypoxia or hypoventilation is not developing. Before discharge, the family should be appropriately educated and feel comfortable handling the equipment. They should also be given appropriate resources and contacts should questions or emergencies arise.

The duration of mechanical ventilation should be considered. This is usually determined by the patient's underlying disease process. A patient who is being transitioned to long-term mechanical ventilation after multisystem organ failure should initially be given 24-hr support and may eventually transition to ventilatory support at night, as the lungs and respiratory muscles recover. This type of patient may eventually be weaned from ventilation support. A patient who requires long-term home ventilation for Duchenne muscular dystrophy may initially require nighttime support, but may progress to 24-hr support as muscular strength worsens.

Multiple locations are available for patients who require long-term ventilation, and the appropriate facility should be determined based on the individual patient's needs. Possible locations include long-term rehabilitation hospitals, skilled nursing facilities, and the patient's home. During transfer, the referring facility should ensure that full information is given to the accepting facility regarding the patient's history and current ventilatory and medical management. If the patient is being discharged home, appropriate home health nursing should be arranged not only to provide medical care, but also to ensure a smooth transition to the home environment.

Nutrition is another important aspect of long-term mechanical ventilation. The metabolic requirements of these patients are usually high, and adequate caloric intake should be provided to prevent malnutrition and failure to thrive. A significant secondary effect of poor nutritional support can be decreased respiratory muscle mass and strength and slowed progress to recovery. A diet high in carbohydrates can increase CO_2 production and make weaning from ventilatory support difficult. Therefore, many practitioners provide up to 50% of calories in fats. Overfeeding is a problem in patients with neuromuscular disease and poor respiratory effort; caloric intake should be limited to prevent obesity and further interfere with respiratory function.

Infections (tracheitis, bronchitis, pneumonia) are common and may be due to community-acquired viruses (adenovirus, influenza, respiratory syncytial virus, parainfluenza) or community- and hospital-acquired bacteria; many of the latter organisms are gram-negative, highly antimicrobial-resistant pathogens that cause further deterioration in pulmonary function. Bacterial infection is most likely in the presence of fever, deteriorating lung function (hypoxia, hypercarbia, tachypnea, retractions), leukocytosis, and mucopurulent sputum, or in patients with secretions with leukocytes and organisms seen on Gram stain, as well as new infiltrates seen on x-ray. This must be distinguished from tracheal colonization, which is asymptomatic and associated with normal amounts of clear tracheal secretions. If infection is suspected, it must be treated with intravenous antibiotics, based on the culture and sensitivities of organisms recovered from the tracheal aspirate. Inhaled tobramycin, started early, may avert more serious infection, whereas inhaled deoxyribonuclease may help clear thick secretions. Infections should be **prevented** by appropriate immunizations (influenza, pneumococcus, *Haemophilus influenzae* type b), passive immunity (respiratory syncytial virus), and good tracheostomy care. Antibiotics should be used judiciously to prevent further colonization with drug-resistant organisms.

Ambrosino N, Clini E: Long-term mechanical ventilation and nutrition. *Respir Med* 2003:98:413–420.
Bach JR, Niranjan V: Noninvasive ventilation in children. In Bach JR (editor): *Noninvasive Mechanical Ventilation.* Philadelphia, Hanley & Belfus, 2002, pp 203–222.
Kacmarek RM, Steven D, Mack CW: *Home Respiratory Care and Mechanical Ventilation: The Essentials of Respiratory Care.* St. Louis, Elsevier Mosby, 2005, pp 569–589.
MacDuff A, Grant IS: Critical care management of neuromuscular disease, including long-term ventilation. *Curr Opin Crit Care* 2003;9:106–112.
Simonds AK: Home ventilation. *Eur Respir J* 2003;22(Suppl 47):38S–46S.
Slutsky AS, Hudson LD: PEEP or no PEEP-lung recruitment may be the solution. *N Engl J Med* 2006;354:1839–1841.
Weiss M, Dullenkopf A, Gysin C, et al: Shortcomings of cuffed paediatric tracheal tubes. *Br J Anaesth* 2004;92:78–88.
Weiss M, Gerber AC, Dullenkopf A: Appropriate placement of intubation depth marks new cuffed paediatric tracheal tube. *Br J Anaesth* 2005:94:80–87.

TABLE 71-1. Children Requiring Pediatric Trauma Center Care

Patients with serious injury to >1 organ or system
Patients with 1-system injury who require critical care or monitoring in an intensive care unit
Patients with signs of shock who require >1 transfusion
Patients with fracture complicated by suspected neurovascular or compartment injury
Patients with fracture of the axial skeleton
Patients with ≥2 long-bone fractures
Patients with potential replantation of an extremity
Patients with suspected or actual spinal cord or column injury
Patients with head injury with any 1 of the following:
Orbital or facial bone fracture
Cerebrospinal fluid leak
Altered state of consciousness
Changing neurologic signs
Open-head injury
Depressed skull fracture
Requiring intracranial pressure monitoring
Patients suspected of requiring ventilator support

From Krug SE: The acutely ill or injured child. In Behrman RE, Kliegman RM (editors): *Nelson Essentials of Pediatrics,* 4th ed. Philadelphia, WB Saunders, 2002, p 96.

Chapter 71 ■ Acute Care of the Victim of Multiple Trauma

Peter S. Dayan and Bruce L. Klein

EPIDEMIOLOGY. Injury is the leading cause of death for children aged 1–17 yr in industrialized nations (see Chapter 61). According to a 2001 UNICEF report, traffic accidents, intentional injuries, drownings, falls, fires, poisonings, and other traumatic events result in >20,000 childhood deaths annually in the world's wealthiest countries. Traffic accidents alone cause 41% of injury-related deaths.

Deaths represent only a small fraction of the total trauma burden. In the Netherlands, for every child who dies of injury, there are another 160 hospital admissions and 2,000 emergency department (ED) visits. Many survivors have permanent or temporary functional limitations.

Trauma is usually classified by the number of significantly injured body parts (1 or more), the severity of injury (mild, moderate, or severe), and the mechanism of injury (blunt, penetrating). In childhood, blunt trauma predominates, accounting for >90% of admissions. In adolescence, penetrating trauma increases in frequency and has a higher mortality rate.

REGIONALIZATION AND TRAUMA TEAMS. Mortality and morbidity rates have decreased in geographic regions with comprehensive, coordinated trauma systems. Designated trauma centers, in particular, have been associated with decreased mortality. At the scene, paramedics should administer necessary advanced life support and perform triage (Table 71-1). It is usually preferable to bypass local hospitals and rapidly transport a seriously injured child directly to a pediatric trauma center (or a trauma center with pediatric commitment).

When the receiving ED is notified before the child's arrival, the trauma team should be mobilized. Each member has defined tasks. A senior surgeon or, sometimes, an emergency physician leads the team. Designating an identifiable leader improves patient outcome. Team compositions vary somewhat from hospital to hospital; the model used at Children's National Medical Center (Washington, DC) is shown in Figure 71-1. Consultants,

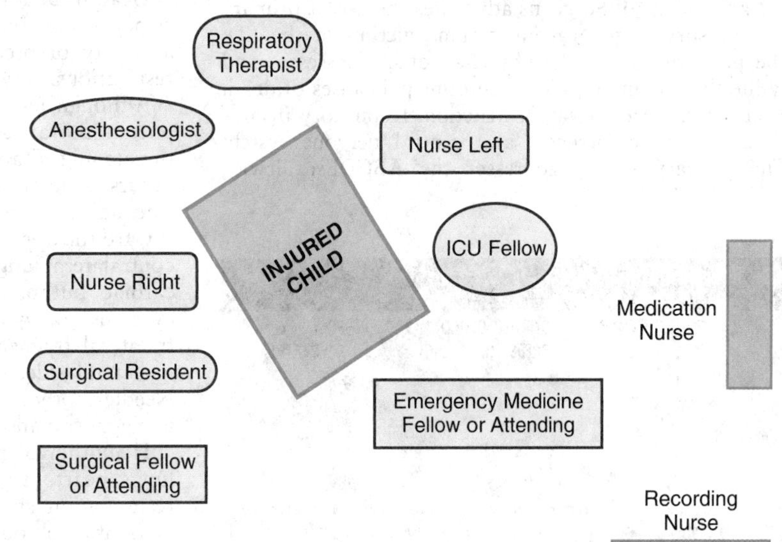

Figure 71-1. Members of the inner core of the trauma team at Children's National Medical Center (Washington, DC). Members of the outer core include a nursing administrator, a social worker, a radiology technician, a transport technician, and a security officer. ICU, intensive care unit.

TABLE 71-2. Injury Evaluation Scoring Systems*

I. INJURY SEVERITY SCORE (ISS)

A. ABBREVIATED INJURY SCALE (AIS) [USED TO CALCULATE ISS]†

AIS CODE	DESCRIPTION
1	Minor
2	Moderate
3	Serious
4	Severe
5	Critical
6	Maximum

B. ISS

The sum of the squares of the highest AIS in each of the ISS body regions:

1. Head and neck
2. Face
3. Chest
4. Abdomen and pelvic contents
5. Extremities and pelvic ring
6. External

PEDIATRIC TRAUMA SCORE‡

COMPONENT	CATEGORY		
	+2	+1	−1
Size	>20 kg	10–20 kg	<10 kg
Airway	Normal	Maintainable	Unmaintainable
Systolic BP	>90 mm Hg	90–50 mm Hg	<50 mm Hg
CNS	Awake	Obtunded/LOC	Coma/decerebrate
Open wound	None	Minor	Major/penetrating
Skeletal	None	Closed fracture	Open/multiple fractures

*Both the ISS and the Pediatric Trauma Score scoring systems correlate with survival outcome in children.

†Each organ or body structure injured has a specific code modified by the adjacent number corresponding to the severity of injury to that structure.

‡Sum of grades for each of 6 categories. This is a physiologically based scoring system.

From O'Neill JA Jr: *Principles of Pediatric Surgery*, 2nd ed. St. Louis, CV Mosby, 2003, p 148.

BP, blood pressure; CNS, central nervous system; LOC, loss of consciousness.

especially neurosurgeons and orthopedic surgeons, must be immediately available; the operating room staff should be alerted.

Physiologic status, anatomic locations, and/or mechanism of injury are used to determine whether to activate the trauma team. More importance should be placed on physiologic compromise and less on mechanism of injury. Scoring scales using similar parameters have been developed to predict patient outcome (see Chapter 61; Tables 71-2 and 71-3).

PRIMARY SURVEY

The American College of Surgeons advocates the use of primary and secondary surveys to evaluate trauma victims in the ED. During the primary survey, the physician quickly assesses and treats any life-threatening injuries. The principal causes of death shortly after trauma are airway obstruction, respiratory insufficiency, shock from hemorrhage, and central nervous system injury. The primary survey addresses the ABCDEs: airway, breathing, circulation, neurologic deficit, and exposure of the patient and control of the environment.

TABLE 71-3. Revised Trauma Score*

REVISED TRAUMA SCORE	GLASGOW COMA SCALE SCORE	SYSTOLIC BLOOD PRESSURE (MM HG)	RESPIRATORY RATE (BREATHS/MIN)
4	13–15	>89	10–20
3	9–12	76–89	>29
2	6–8	50–75	6–9
1	4–5	1–49	1–5
0	3	0	0

*A score of 0–4 is given for each variable, then added (range, 1–12). A score ≤11 indicates potentially important trauma.

From Fitzmaurice LS: Approach to multiple trauma. In Barkin RM (editor): *Pediatric Emergency Medicine*, 2nd ed. St. Louis, CV Mosby, 1997, p 224.

AIRWAY/CERVICAL SPINE. Optimizing oxygenation and ventilation while protecting the cervical spine from potential further injury is of paramount importance. Initially, any child sustaining multiple, blunt trauma must be suspected of having a cervical spine injury. Children are at risk for such injuries because of their relatively large heads, which augment flexion-extension forces, and weak neck muscles, which predispose them to ligament injuries. Unnecessary movement of the cervical spine can lead to paralysis. The cervical (and thoracic and lumbar spine) should be immobilized in the neutral position with a stiff collar, head blocks, and tape or cloth placed across the forehead, torso, and thighs to restrain the child to a rigid backboard.

Airway obstruction presents as snoring, gurgling, hoarseness, stridor, and/or diminished breath sounds, despite good respiratory effort. Children are more likely than adults to have airway obstruction because of their smaller oral cavities, proportionately larger tongues and greater amounts of tonsillar and adenoidal tissue, higher and more anterior glottic openings, and narrower tracheas. Obstruction is common in patients with severe head injuries for several reasons, including decreased muscle tone that allows the tongue to fall posteriorly, occluding the airway. With trauma, obstruction also can result from fractures of the mandible or facial bones, crush injuries of the larynx or trachea, secretions such as blood or vomitus, or foreign body aspiration.

If it is necessary to open the airway, a jaw-thrust **without head-tilt** is recommended (see Chapter 66). This procedure minimizes cervical spine motion. In an unconscious child, an oropharyngeal airway can be inserted to prevent posterior displacement of the mandibular tissues. A semiconscious child will gag with an oropharyngeal airway, but may tolerate a nasopharyngeal airway. If these maneuvers plus suctioning do not clear the airway, oral endotracheal intubation is indicated. Emergent cricothyrotomy is needed in <1% of victims.

BREATHING. Breathing is assessed by counting the respiratory rate; visualizing chest wall motion for symmetry, depth, and accessory muscle use; and auscultating breath sounds in both axillae. In addition to looking for cyanosis, pulse oximetry is standard. If breathing is inadequate, bag-valve-mask ventilation with 100% oxygen must be initiated immediately, followed by endotracheal intubation. End-expiratory CO_2 detectors help to verify accurate tube placement and are recommended by the pediatric advanced life support course.

Head trauma is the most common cause of respiratory insufficiency. An unconscious child with a severe head injury may have a variety of breathing abnormalities, including Cheyne-Stokes respirations, slow irregular breaths, or apnea.

Although less common than a pulmonary contusion, tension pneumothorax and massive hemothorax are immediately life-threatening (Tables 71-4 and 71-5). **Tension pneumothorax** occurs when air accumulates under pressure in the pleural space. The adjacent lung is compacted, the mediastinum is pushed toward the opposite hemithorax, and the heart, great vessels, and contralateral lung are compressed or kinked. Both ventilation and cardiac output are impaired. Characteristic findings include cyanosis, tachypnea, retractions, asymmetric chest rise, contralateral tracheal deviation, diminished breath sounds on the ipsilateral side, subcutaneous emphysema, and signs of shock. Needle thoracentesis, followed by thoracostomy tube insertion, is diagnostic and lifesaving.

Hemothorax results from injury to the intercostal vessels, lungs, heart, or great vessels. When ventilation is adequate, fluid resuscitation should begin before evacuation, because a large amount of blood may drain through the chest tube, resulting in shock.

TABLE 71-4. Life-Threatening Chest Injuries

TENSION PNEUMOTHORAX
One-way valve leak from the lung parenchyma
Complete collapse with mediastinal and tracheal shift to the side opposite the leak
Compromises venous return and decreases ventilation of the other lung
Clinically, manifests as respiratory distress, unilateral absent breath sounds, tracheal deviation, distended neck veins, tympany to percussion of the Involved side, and cyanosis
Relieve first with needle aspiration, then with chest tube drainage

OPEN PNEUMOTHORAX (SUCKING CHEST WOUND)
Effect on ventilation depends on size

MAJOR FLAIL CHEST
Usually caused by blunt injury resulting in multiple rib fractures
Loss of bone stability of the thoracic cage
Major disruption of synchronous chest wall motion
Mechanical ventilation and positive end-expiratory pressure required

MASSIVE HEMOTHORAX
Must be drained with a large-bore tube
Initiate drainage only with concurrent vascular volume replacement

CARDIAC TAMPONADE
Beck triad:
1. Decreased or muffled heart sounds
2. Distended neck veins from increased venous pressure
3. Hypotension with pulsus paradoxus (decreased pulse pressure during inspiration)

Must be drained

From Krug SE: The acutely ill or injured child. In Behrman RE, Kliegman RM (editors): *Nelson Essentials of Pediatrics,* 4th ed. Philadelphia, WB Saunders, 2002, p 97.

CIRCULATION. The most common type of shock in trauma is hypovolemic shock due to hemorrhage (see Chapter 68). Signs of shock include tachycardia; weak pulse; delayed capillary refill; cool, mottled, pale skin; and altered mental status. Early in shock, blood pressure remains normal because of compensatory increases in heart rate and peripheral vascular resistance. An individual can lose up to 25% of blood volume before blood pressure declines. It is important to note that 25% of blood volume equals 20 mL/kg, which is only 200 mL in a 10-kg child. With losses of >25%, hypotension ensues. Losses of >50% cause severe hypotension that, if prolonged, may become irreversible.

Direct pressure should be applied to control external hemorrhage. Blind clamping of bleeding vessels is not advisable because of the risk of damage to adjacent structures.

Cannulating a larger vein, such as an antecubital vein, is usually the quickest way to achieve intravenous access. A short, large-bore catheter offers less resistance to flow, allowing for more rapid administration. Ideally, a 2nd catheter should be placed within the 1st few minutes of resuscitation in a severely injured child. If intravenous access proves difficult, an intraosseous catheter can be inserted; all medications and fluids can be administered intraosseously (see Chapter 66). Other alternatives include central venous access using the Seldinger technique (femoral vein) or surgical cutdown (saphenous vein). Ultrasound can facilitate central venous catheter placement.

Aggressive, intravenous fluid resuscitation is essential early in shock to prevent further deterioration. Isotonic crystalloid solution, such as lactated Ringer or normal saline (20 mL/kg), should be infused rapidly. No consensus exists supporting the routine use of colloid or hypertonic (3%) saline solution. When necessary, repeated crystalloid boluses should be given. Most children stabilize with administration of crystalloid solution alone. However, if the patient remains in shock after boluses totaling 40–60 mL/kg of crystalloid, then 10–15 mL/kg of cross-matched, packed red blood cells should be transfused. Although less desirable, type-specific or O-negative cells can be substituted pending availability of cross-matched blood. When shock persists despite these measures, surgery to stop internal hemorrhage is usually indicated.

TABLE 71-5. Differential Diagnosis of Immediately Life-Threatening Cardiopulmonary Injuries

	TENSION PNEUMOTHORAX	MASSIVE HEMOTHORAX	CARDIAC TAMPONADE
Breath sounds	Ipsilaterally decreased	Ipsilaterally decreased	Normal
Percussion note	Hyper-resonant	Dull	Normal
Tracheal location	Contralaterally shifted	Midline or shifted	Midline
Neck veins	Distended	Flat	Distended
Heart tones	Normal	Normal	Muffled

From Cooper A, Foltin GL: Thoracic trauma. In Barkin RM (editor): *Pediatric Emergency Medicine,* 2nd ed. St. Louis, CV Mosby, 1997, p 325.

NEUROLOGIC DEFICIT. In the primary survey, neurologic status is briefly assessed by evaluating the level of consciousness and determining pupil size and reactivity. The level of consciousness can be classified using the **mnemonic AVPU:** **a**lert, responsive to **v**erbal commands, responsive to **p**ainful stimuli, or **u**nresponsive.

Head injuries account for approximately 70% of pediatric blunt trauma deaths. Primary direct cerebral injury occurs within seconds of the event and is irreversible. Secondary injury is caused by subsequent anoxia or ischemia. The goal is to minimize secondary injury by ensuring adequate oxygenation, ventilation, and perfusion, and maintaining normal intracranial pressure (ICP). A child with severe neurologic impairment, such as a Glasgow Coma Scale (GCS; see Table 66-5) score of 8 or less, should be intubated (see Chapter 66).

Signs of increased ICP, including progressive neurologic deterioration or evidence of transtentorial herniation, must be treated immediately (see Chapter 67). Hyperventilation lowers $Paco_2$, resulting in cerebral vasoconstriction, reduced cerebral blood flow, and decreased ICP. Vigorous, prolonged hyperventilation is not recommended because the consequent vasoconstriction may excessively decrease cerebral oxygenation or perfusion. Brief hyperventilation remains an immediate option for patients with acute increases in ICP. Mannitol lowers ICP and may improve survival. Because mannitol acts via osmotic diuresis, it can exacerbate hypovolemia and must be used cautiously. Hypertonic saline may be a useful agent to control ICP in patients with severe head injury. Neurosurgical consultation is mandatory. If signs of increased ICP persist, the neurosurgeon must decide whether to operate emergently.

EXPOSURE AND ENVIRONMENTAL CONTROL. All clothing should be cut away to reveal any injuries. Cutting is quickest and minimizes unnecessary patient movement.

Children often arrive mildly hypothermic because of their higher body surface area-to-mass ratios. They can be warmed using radiant heat as well as heated blankets and intravenous fluids.

SECONDARY SURVEY

During the secondary survey, the physician completes a detailed, head-to-toe physical examination.

HEAD TRAUMA. A GCS or Pediatric GCS score (see Table 66-5) should be assigned to every child with significant head trauma (see Chapter 67). This scale assesses eye opening and motor and verbal responses. In the Pediatric GCS, the verbal score is modified for age. The GCS further categorizes neurologic disability, and serial measurements identify improvement or deterioration over time. Patients with low scores 6–24 hr after injury have poorer prognoses.

Head CT scan without contrast has become standard to determine the type of injury. In severely injured children, diffuse cerebral injury with edema is a common and serious finding on CT scan. Focal evacuable hemorrhagic lesions (epidural hematoma)

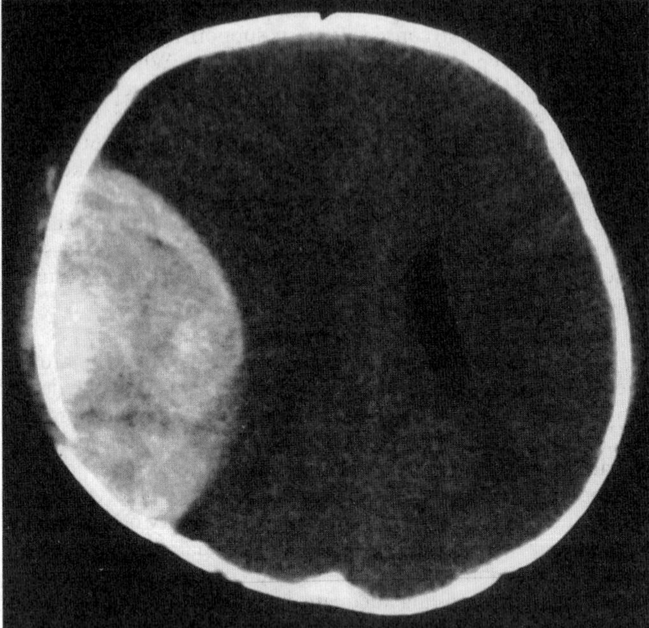

Figure 71-2. According to the history provided, this 7-mo-old girl did not wake up for her nightly feeding and began vomiting in the morning. The mother's boyfriend reported that the infant fell from a chair the previous day. CT scan shows a large epidural hematoma associated with the right parietal brain and marked shift of the midline from right to left. The right lateral ventricle is compressed as a result of the mass effect, and the left lateral ventricle is slightly prominent. The infant was taken emergently to the operating room for evacuation of the epidural hematoma and recovered uneventfully. (From O'Neill JA Jr: *Principles of Pediatric Surgery,* 2nd ed. St. Louis, Mosby, 2003, p 191.)

occur less commonly, but may require immediate neurosurgical intervention (Fig. 71-2).

Monitoring of ICP is frequently, although variably, used for children with severe brain injury (GCS score of 8 or less with abnormal CT scan findings). An advantage of an intraventricular catheter, in contrast to an intraparenchymal device, is that cerebrospinal fluid can be drained to treat acute increases in ICP. Hypotension, hypercarbia, hypoxia, and hyperthermia must be aggressively managed to prevent secondary brain injury. Cerebral perfusion pressure must be maintained at 40 mm Hg. Induced hypothermia to treat traumatic brain injury remains an experimental and unproven therapy.

A child with a severe brain injury must be treated aggressively in the ED because it is very difficult to accurately predict long-term neurologic outcome. Compared with adults with similar injuries, children have better functional outcomes.

CERVICAL SPINE TRAUMA. Cervical spine injuries occur in <2% of children with multisystem trauma, but are associated with significant mortality and morbidity. Bony injuries occur mainly from C1–C4 in children younger than 8 yr of age. In older children, they occur equally in the upper and lower cervical spine. The mortality rate, however, is significantly higher in patients with upper cervical spine injuries. Cervical spinal cord injury without radiographic (bone) abnormalities on plain films (SCIWORA) occurs in approximately 20% of children with cervical spine injuries. Patients with SCIWORA have persistent neurologic symptoms and obvious spinal cord abnormalities noted on MRI scan. Approximately 30% of all patients with cervical spine injuries have permanent neurologic deficits.

Evaluation begins with a detailed history and neurologic examination. Identifying the mechanism of injury helps in estimating the likelihood of a cervical spine injury. Both the patient and the

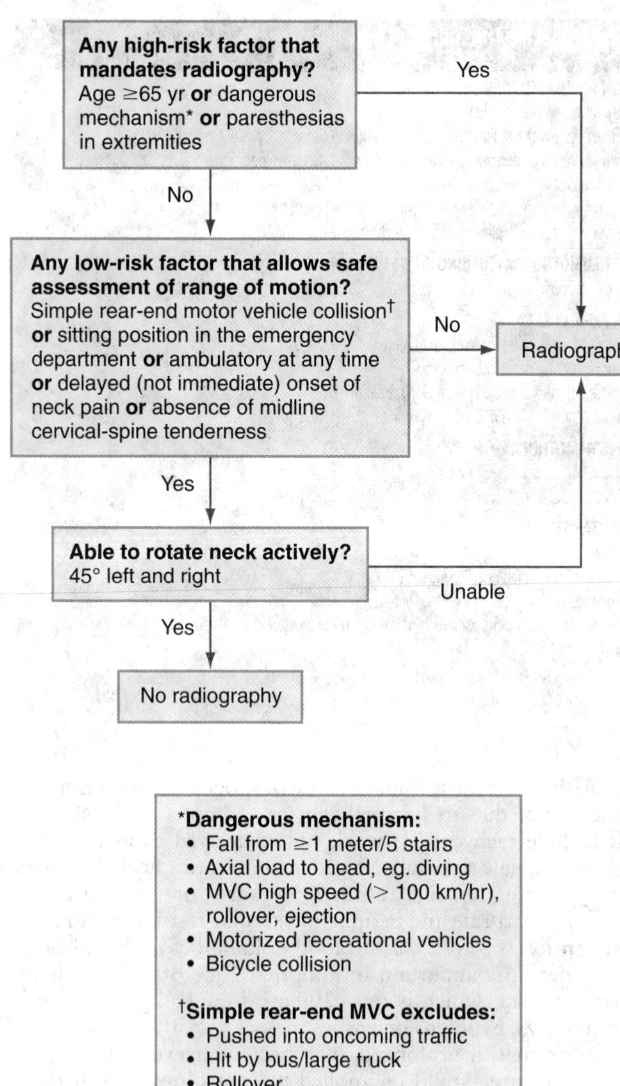

Figure 71-3. The Canadian C-spine rule. For adult patients with trauma who are alert (as indicated by a score of 15 on the Glasgow Coma Scale) and in stable condition and in whom cervical spine injury is a concern, the determination of risk factors guides the use of cervical spine radiography. A dangerous mechanism is considered to be a fall from an elevation of 3 ft or 5 stairs; an axial load to the head (e.g., diving); a motor vehicle collision at high speed (>100 km/hr, or ≈62 miles/hr) or with rollover or ejection; a collision involving a motorized recreational vehicle; or a bicycle collision. A simple rear-end motor vehicle collision excludes being pushed into oncoming traffic, being hit by a bus or a large truck, a rollover, and being hit by a high-speed vehicle. (From Stiell IG, Clement CM, McKnight RD, et al: The Canadian C-spine rule versus the NEXUS low-risk criteria in patients with trauma. *N Engl J Med* 2003;349:26:2510–2518.)

paramedic should be asked whether there were any neurologic symptoms or signs, such as weakness or abnormal sensation, that resolved before arrival. In a child with transient neurologic symptoms and normal plain x-ray films, SCIWORA still must be considered.

Whenever the history, physical examination, or mechanism of injury suggests a cervical spine injury, radiographs (including lateral, anteroposterior, and odontoid views) should be obtained after initial resuscitation. In adults, the Canadian C-spine rule helps to identify low-risk patients who may not require x-rays (Fig. 71-3). Cervical spine CT scan can be a valuable adjunct to plain films; some centers use CT as the primary diagnostic tool.

TABLE 71-6. Indications for Operation in Thoracic Trauma

THORACOTOMY IMMEDIATELY OR SHORTLY AFTER INJURY
Massive continuing pneumothorax
Cardiac tamponade
Open pneumothorax
Esophageal injury
Massive air leak from tracheobronchial injury
Aortic or other vascular injury
Acute rupture of the diaphragm
DELAYED THORACOTOMY
Chronic rupture of the diaphragm
Clotted hemothorax
Persistent chylothorax
Traumatic intracardiac defects
Evacuation of large foreign bodies
Chronic atelectasis from traumatic bronchial stenosis

From O'Neill JA Jr: *Principles of Pediatric Surgery,* 2nd ed, St. Louis, CV Mosby, 2003, p 157.

CT is helpful if an odontoid fracture is suspected because young children typically do not cooperate enough to obtain an "open-mouth" (odontoid) plain x-ray view. MRI is indicated in a child with suspected SCIWORA.

Rapid diagnosis of spinal cord injury is essential. Initiating high-dose intravenous methylprednisolone within 8 hr of spinal cord injury may improve motor outcome and has become standard therapy.

THORACIC TRAUMA. Pulmonary contusions occur frequently in young children with blunt chest trauma. A child's chest wall is relatively pliable; therefore, less force is absorbed by the rib cage and more is transmitted to the lungs. Respiratory distress may be noted in the ED or may develop during the 1st 24 hr of hospitalization.

Rib fractures result from significant external force. They are noted in patients with more severe injuries and are associated with a higher mortality rate. Flail chest, which is caused by multiple rib fractures, is rare in children. Indications for operative management are noted in Table 71-6.

ABDOMINAL TRAUMA. Liver and spleen contusions, hematomas, and lacerations account for the majority of intra-abdominal injuries due to blunt trauma. The kidneys, pancreas, and duodenum are relatively spared because of their retroperitoneal location. Pancreatic and duodenal injuries are more common after a bicycle handlebar impact or a direct blow to the abdomen (Table 71-7).

Although a thorough examination for intra-abdominal injuries is essential, this often proves difficult. Misleading findings can result from gastric distention from crying or an uncooperative toddler. Calm reassurance, distraction, and gentle, persistent palpation help with the examination. Important findings include distention, bruises, and tenderness. The usefulness of a rectal examination to evaluate for intra-abdominal and genitourinary trauma has been challenged, especially in young children. Specific symptoms and signs give insight into the mechanism of injury and the potential for particular injuries. Pain in the left shoulder may signify splenic trauma. A lap belt mark across the abdomen suggests a bowel or mesentery injury.

An abdominal CT scan with intravenous contrast medium enhancement rapidly identifies structural and functional abnormalities and is the preferred study in a stable child. It has excellent sensitivity and specificity for splenic (Fig. 71-4), hepatic (Fig. 71-5), and renal injuries, but should not be the sole test used to exclude intestinal, diaphragmatic, or pancreatic injuries. Administering oral contrast adds little information about most injuries and is not routinely recommended. The use of oral contrast in children with possible bowel perforation is controversial, because false-negative scans are common. Focused abdominal sonography in trauma helps to detect hemoperitoneum; the variably low

TABLE 71-7. Frequency of Abdominal Organ Injured by Injury Mechanism

BLUNT		PENETRATING	
ORGAN	**%**	**ORGAN**	**%**
Spleen	30	Gastrointestinal tract	70
Liver	28	Liver	27
Kidneys	28	Blood vessels	19
Gastrointestinal tract	14	Kidneys	10
Bladder/urethra/ureters	4	Spleen	9
Pancreas	3	Bladder/urethra/ureters	8
Blood vessels	3	Pancreas	6

From O'Neill JA Jr: *Principles of Pediatric Surgery,* 2nd ed. St. Louis, CV Mosby, 2003, p 159.

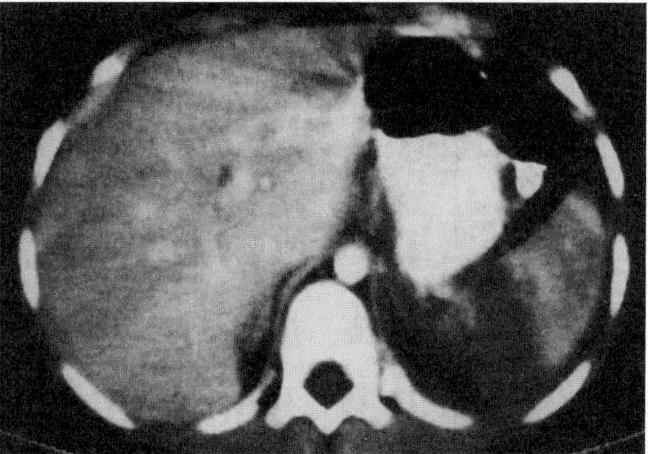

Figure 71-4. CT scan with intravenous contrast material and gastrointestinal contrast enhancement shows isolated splenic rupture that resulted from blunt trauma. This patient responded to nonoperative management, as do most patients with splenic injuries. (From O'Neill JA Jr: *Principles of Pediatric Surgery,* 2nd ed. St. Louis, Mosby, 2003, p 166.)

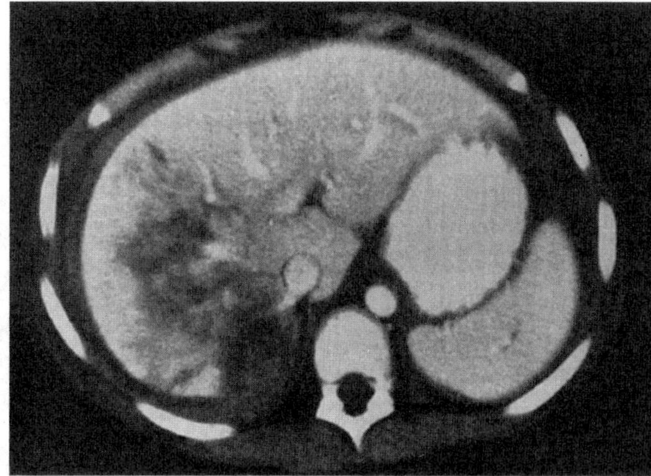

Figure 71-5. CT scan performed after severe blunt injury of the abdomen shows a bursting injury of the liver. The patient was stable and no operative intervention was required, although most patients with injuries this severe who are seen immediately after injury probably would be operated on. (From O'Neill JA Jr: *Principles of Pediatric Surgery,* 2nd ed. St. Louis, Mosby, 2003, p 168.)

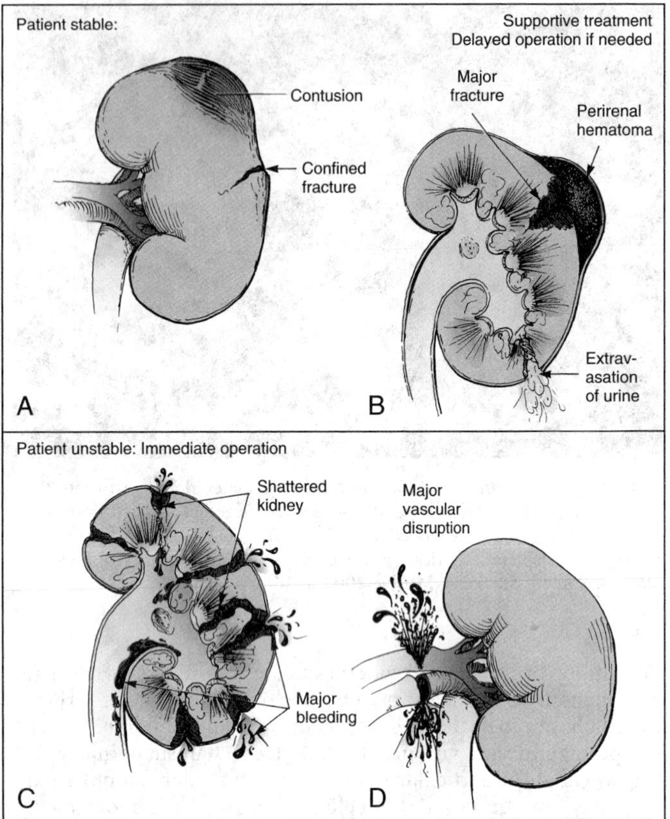

Figure 71-6. Types of blunt renal trauma. Types *A* and *B* often respond to nonoperative treatment. Types *C* and *D* usually require operative treatment. Although type *C* injuries often may be operated on in a delayed fashion, unless vascular disruptive injuries are recognized immediately and treated promptly, loss of the kidney usually occurs, and successful repair is rare. (From O'Neill JA Jr: *Principles of Pediatric Surgery,* 2nd ed. St. Louis, Mosby, 2003, p 173.)

sensitivity of this test in children suggests that it should not be used to exclude intra-abdominal injury.

Nonoperative treatment has become standard for hemodynamically stable children with splenic, hepatic, and renal (Fig. 71-6) injuries from blunt trauma. The majority of such children can be treated nonsurgically. In addition to avoiding perioperative complications, nonoperative treatment decreases the need for blood transfusions and shortens hospital stay. Indications for laparotomy are noted in Table 71-8. Splenic repair, if possible, is preferable to splenectomy.

TABLE 71-8. Indications for Laparotomy: Abdominal Injury

BLUNT INJURIES
Continued hemodynamic instability despite resuscitation
Signs of continuing hemorrhage
Need for blood replacement in excess of 1/2 of blood volume
Pneumoperitoneum
Physical signs of peritoneal irritation
Signs of significant injury to the intestine, pancreas, bladder, ureter, renal vasculature, or rectum
PENETRATING INJURIES
Most gunshot wounds
Selective operation for stab wounds with:
Hypotension
Unexplained blood loss
Evisceration
Physical signs of peritoneal irritation
Signs of significant amounts of blood or intestinal contents on peritoneal lavage or CT

From O'Neill JA Jr: *Principles of Pediatric Surgery,* 2nd ed. St. Louis, CV Mosby, 2003, p 163.

LOWER GENITOURINARY TRAUMA. The perineum should be inspected and the stability of the bones of the pelvis assessed. Urethral injuries are more common in males. Findings suggestive of urethral injury include scrotal or labial ecchymoses, blood at the urethral meatus, gross hematuria, and a superiorly positioned prostate on rectal examination (in an adolescent male). A pelvic fracture is also a risk factor for potential genitourinary injury. Any of these findings is a contraindication to urethral catheter insertion and warrants consultation with a urologist. Retrograde urethrocystogram and CT scan of the pelvis and abdomen are used to determine the extent of injury.

EXTREMITY TRAUMA. Thorough examination of the extremities is essential because extremity fractures are among the most frequently missed injuries in children with multiple trauma (see Chapter 682). All limbs should be inspected for deformity, swelling, and bruises; palpated for tenderness; and assessed for active and passive range of motion, sensory function, and perfusion. Extremity fractures may initially be missed in a severely injured patient as clinicians attend to more life-threatening injuries.

Before x-ray films are obtained, suspected fractures and dislocations should be immobilized and an analgesic administered. Splinting a femur fracture helps alleviate pain and may decrease blood loss. An orthopedic surgeon must be consulted immediately to evaluate a child with a compartment syndrome, another cause of neurovascular compromise, or an open fracture (see Chapter 682).

RADIOLOGIC AND LABORATORY EVALUATION. To avoid misdiagnoses, some authorities recommend routinely obtaining multiple studies in the ED. These include lateral cervical spine, anteroposterior chest, and anteroposterior pelvis x-ray films; arterial blood gas analysis; complete blood cell count; electrolytes; blood glucose; blood urea nitrogen; creatinine; amylase; liver function tests; prothrombin and partial thromboplastin times; type and cross match; and urinalysis. One benefit of standardizing the evaluation of patients with major trauma is that fewer decisions need to be made on an individual basis, which sometimes expedites ED management.

There are some advantages and limitations of these laboratory and radiologic studies. The lateral cervical spine x-ray film can miss significant injuries. When it is necessary to assess oxygenation, ventilation, and acid-base status, an arterial blood gas sample is useful. A large base deficit is associated with a higher mortality rate. Hemoglobin and hematocrit levels provide baseline values in the ED, but may not have equilibrated after a hemorrhage at the time of measurement. Abnormal liver function test results or an elevated serum amylase level may be noted in patients with significant abdominal trauma, but most patients with significant trauma to the abdomen have clinical indications for CT scanning or surgery. The majority of previously healthy children have normal coagulation profiles; these may become abnormal after major head trauma. Although routine urinalysis or dipstick testing for blood has been recommended for children, data from large adult studies suggest that this may be unnecessary in patients without gross hematuria or hypotension.

CARDIOPULMONARY ARREST. Preventing physiologic deterioration is crucial. Children who sustain multiple injuries from blunt trauma have a 0–2% survival rate once pulseless cardiac arrest occurs. Unfortunately, those few who survive resuscitation after pulseless arrest are likely to have severe neurologic impairment.

PSYCHOLOGIC AND SOCIAL SUPPORT. Serious multisystem trauma may result in significant long-term psychologic and social difficulties for the child and family, particularly when there is a major head injury. Like adults, children are at risk for depressive symptoms and post-traumatic stress disorder. Caregivers face persistent stress and have been noted to have more psychologic symptoms. Psychologic and social support, therefore, is extremely important.

Adelson PD, Bratton SL, Carney NA, et al: Guidelines for the acute medical management of severe traumatic brain injury in infants, children, and adolescents. *Pediatr Crit Care Med* 2003;4:S1–75.
American College of Surgeons: *Advanced Trauma Life Support for Doctors: Student Course Manual.* Chicago, American College of Surgeons, 2004.
Carli P, Orliaguet G: Severe traumatic brain injury in children. *Lancet* 2004;363:584–585.
CRASH Trial Collaborators: Effect of intravenous corticosteroids on death within 14 days in 10008 adults with clinically significant head injury (MRC CRASH trial): Randomized placebo-controlled trial. *Lancet* 2004;364:1321–1338.
Davis DH, Localio AR, Stafford PW, et al: Trends in operative management of pediatric splenic injury in a regional trauma system. *Pediatrics* 2005;115:89–94.
Dowd MD, McAneney C, Lacher M, et al: Maximizing the sensitivity and specificity of pediatric trauma team activation criteria. *Acad Emerg Med* 2000;7:1119–1125.
Feliz A, Shultz B, McKenna C, Gaines A: Diagnostic and therapeutic laparoscopy in pediatric abdominal trauma. *J Pediatr Surg* 2006;41:72–77.
McIntyre LA, Fergusson DA, Hebert PC, et al: Prolonged therapeutic hypothermia after traumatic brain injury in adults. *JAMA* 2003;289: 2992–2998.
Morris CG, McCoy W, Lavery GG: Spinal immobilization for unconscious patients with multiple injuries. *BMJ* 2004;329:495–499.
Osler TM, Vane DW, Tepas JJ, et al: Do pediatric trauma centers have better survival rates than adult trauma centers? An examination of the National Pediatric Trauma Registry. *J Trauma* 2001;50:95–101.
Sever MS, Vanholder R, Lameire N: Management of crush-related injuries after disasters. *N Engl J Med* 2006;354:1052–1063.
Shann F: Hypothermia for traumatic brain injury: How soon, how cold, and how long? *Lancet* 2003;362:1950–1951.
Stiell IG, Clement CM, McKnight RD, et al: The Canadian C-spine rule versus the NEXUS low-risk criteria in patients with trauma. *N Engl J Med* 2003;349:26:2510–2518.
UNICEF Innocenti Research Centre: A league table of child deaths by injury in rich nations. Innocenti Report Card No. 2, February 2001. *(www.unicef-icdc. org/publications/pdf/repcard2e.pdf).*

Chapter 72 ■ Nutritional Stabilization

Joseph V. DiCarlo

Critically ill children (surgery, trauma, infection, starvation) need nutritional support to ameliorate the negative nitrogen balance resulting from excess catabolism (Table 72-1). A child in the intensive care unit (ICU) is just as likely to be overfed as underfed, with food composition, especially high-carbohydrate intake, responsible for a respiratory quotient of >1.0. Daily energy requirements are most often estimated using weight, age, findings on physical examination, biochemical parameters, predictive equations, and correction factors. Predictive equations inaccurately predict energy expenditure in ventilated, critically ill children in the acute phase of illness (Table 72-2). In a minority of PICUs, energy expenditure is regularly measured by indirect calorimetry, a method that remains the gold standard. Most children have good long-term outcome in terms of nutritional status after discharge.

OVERFEEDING. Excessive intake of carbohydrates manifested as hyperglycemia may result in hyperosmolarity, osmotic diuresis, and dehydration. Subsequently, increased carbon dioxide production and an increase in the respiratory quotient may tax an already compromised respiratory system. Excessive administration of lipids can produce hypertriglyceridemia and fatty liver and may increase the risk of infection. Children who are supported with long-term mechanical ventilation may have lower energy expenditure than healthy children of the same age. This can be attributed to their lower activity levels and reduced muscle mass. Although weight gain in these children is similar to that in healthy children, it is disproportionately higher in fat.

TABLE 72-1. Caloric and Protein Requirements in the Critically Ill Child

Critical illness	25–30 kcal/kg/24 hr
Mechanical ventilation	20–25 kcal/kg/24 hr
Receiving growth hormone	15–20 kcal/kg/24 hr as carbohydrate
Bur or trauma	40–45 kcal/kg/24 hr
Protein (maintenance)	1.5–2.5 g/kg/24 hr
Protein (burn > 20%)	2.0–3.0 g/kg/24 hr

COMPONENTS OF FEEDING. Carbohydrate (glucose infusion of 3–5 mg/kg/min) is given to inhibit catabolism of endogenous protein. Generally, 70% of calories should be derived from carbohydrates and 30% from lipids. It is often difficult to deliver adequate calories to critically ill children because of enteral intolerance or restrictions in fluid volume, but the caloric goals should be attainable within the 1st week of hospitalization.

Amino acids should be provided in reasonable amounts, in any form (1.5 g/kg in older children, 2.0 g/kg in infants). Adequate amounts of glutamine, alanine, and the essential amino acids should be included, but branched-chain amino acids (leucine, cysteine, valine, lysine) may not confer any special benefit.

Vitamins, particularly water-soluble B complex and C, are best administered enterally. Vitamin deficiencies can develop even in children receiving parenteral nutrition (thiamine deficiency leading to Wernicke encephalopathy or riboflavin deficiency). Essential minerals and trace elements, including zinc, magnesium, and selenium, should also be provided.

HYPERGLYCEMIA AND GLUCOSE CONTROL. Endocrinopathy during sepsis can manifest as hyperglycemia and insulin resistance. The prevalence of hyperglycemia is quite high in pediatric critical care units, with the relative risk of dying increased when the maximum glucose level is >150 mg/dL in the first 24 hr of admission. Normoglycemia can be safely reached and maintained during intensive care by using insulin titration guidelines. In adults, intensive insulin therapy (maintaining blood glucose levels at 80–110 mg/dL) reduces morbidity and mortality rates in a surgical ICU. Preventing even moderate hyperglycemia with insulin

TABLE 72-2. Relative Effects of Starvation and Hypermetabolism

EVENT	STARVATION	HYPERMETABOLISM
Energy expenditure	↓	++
Respiratory quotient	0.7	0.8–0.85
Energy source	Glucose/fat	Mixed
Mediator activation	+	+++
Gluconeogenesis	+	+++
Catabolism	+	+++
Protein synthesis relative to catabolism	↓	↓↓
Amino acid oxidation	±	+++
Ureagenesis	±	++
Ketonemia	+++	±
Rate of malnutrition	+	+++

From Wesley JR: Nutrient metabolism in relation to systemic stress response. In Furhman BR Zimmerman JJ (editors): *Pediatric Critical Care.* St. Louis, CV Mosby, 1998. Adapted from Barton R, Cerra FB: *Chest* 1989:96:1153.
+, Increase; ↓, decrease; ±, minimal change.

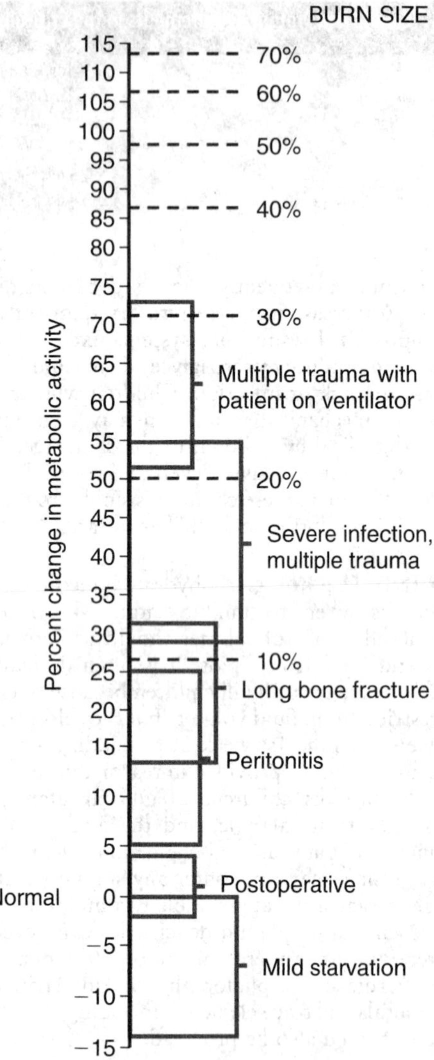

Figure 72-1. Index of per cent change in metabolic activity caused by various types of stress. (From Wesley JR, Khalidi N, Faubion WC, et al: *The University of Michigan Hospitals Parenteral and Enteral Nutrition Manual*, 6th ed. Chicago, Abbott Laboratories Hospital Products Division, 1990.)

during intensive care may protect the central and peripheral nervous systems. Ongoing studies will address these issues in children.

ENTERAL FEEDING. Early enteral feeding in critically ill children, particularly those with sepsis, may avert ulcerative complications, preserve the indigenous intestinal flora, avoid overgrowth by pathogens, and prevent atrophy of the mucosa. Normal flora also may be restored, in part, by the administration of probiotic agents. Enteral feeding improves the intestinal mucosal barriers, thus preventing bacterial or endotoxin translocation into the systemic circulation. If the stomach is relatively atonic, early feeding may be accomplished through a weighted tube passed through the pylorus into the jejunum; fluoroscopic guidance or placement via endoscopy may be necessary. Continuous and intermittent gastric feeding regimens are tolerated similarly with respect to the number of stools per day and the prevalence of diarrhea and vomiting. Children with sepsis often have ileus that precludes enteral nutrition. Enteral feeding is not necessarily prescribed in the child receiving vasoactive infusions if an ileus is absent or clinically resolving. Enteral feeding has been shown to be feasible in neonates supported with extracorporeal membrane oxygenation. Enteral feeding tolerance has not been studied in older patients receiving this therapy.

PARENTERAL NUTRITION. If the gastrointestinal tract cannot be used, parenteral nutrition is necessary. Conversion of maintenance intravenous fluids to parenteral nutrition is often indicated by the 2nd or 3rd day of hospitalization. There is no need to administer amino acids gradually, although protein restriction may be indicated for renal failure. Children undergoing hemofiltration lose large amounts of amino acids and should be supplemented.

IMMUNOMODULATION THROUGH DIET. Unfed patients in the PICU, in general, have the highest complication rate. Attempts to enhance immune function through dietary supplementation with glutamine, arginine, omega-3 fatty acids, and nucleotides have not shown benefit.

Calder PC: Immunonutrition. *BMJ* 2003;327:117–118.

Faustino EV, Apkon M: Persistent hyperglycemia in critically ill children. *J Pediatr* 2005;146:30–34.

Horn D, Chaboyer W: Gastric feeding in critically ill children: A randomized controlled trial. *Am J Crit Care* 2003;12:461–468.

Hulst JM, vanGoudoever TB, Zimmerman LJ, et al: Adequate feeding and the usefulness of the respiratory quotient in critically ill children. *Nutrition* 2005; 21:192–198.

King W, Petrillo T, Pettignano R: Enteral nutrition and cardiovascular medications in the pediatric intensive care unit. *J Parenter Enteral Nutr* 2004;28:334–338.

Rogers EJ, Gilbertson HR, Heine RG, et al: Barriers to adequate nutrition in critically ill children. *Nutrition* 2003;19:865–868.

Vazquez Martinez JL, Martinez-Romillo PD, Diez Sebastian J, et al: Predicted versus measured energy expenditure by continuous, online indirect calorimetry in ventilated, critically ill children during the early post injury period. *Pediatr Crit Care Med* 2004;5:19–27.

Chapter 73 ■ Drowning and Submersion Injury

Harry J. Kallas

Childhood drowning is a common cause of injury and fatality. After submersion in a liquid medium, suffocation and asphyxia may occur, with or without pulmonary aspiration. Within a few minutes, hypoxia and ischemia can lead to irreversible multisystem injury and death. Treatment initiated in the prehospital setting by bystanders performing CPR, followed by the rapid response of experienced emergency medical personnel and continued aggressive care in the emergency department (ED) and pediatric intensive care unit (PICU), reduces the mortality from the cardiorespiratory consequences of submersion. Neurologic injury from hypoxemia and ischemia continues to be the primary cause of mortality and long-term morbidity.

The definition of drowning adopted by the 2002 World Congress on Drowning and the World Health Organization (WHO) should be widely used: "drowning is the process of experiencing respiratory impairment from submersion or immersion in liquid." Drowning outcomes are classified as death, survival with morbidity, and survival without morbidity.

EPIDEMIOLOGY

The WHO estimates that 450,000 persons died from drowning in 2000 (≈1 person every min), a fatality rate of 6.8/100,000 population. The actual incidence is unknown, but is likely higher because many drowning deaths are not reported. Ninety-seven percent of unintentional drowning deaths occur in low- and middle-income countries. China and India have particularly high drowning mortality rates (10.2/100,000 and 8.5/100,000, respectively) and together constitute 43% of all drowning deaths worldwide. Another ⅓ of all drowning deaths occur in the Western Pacific region. The highest regional drowning rate is in Africa (14.2/100,000), and the lowest rates are in the Americas (3/100,000) and Europe (4.3/100,000), although there is wide variability within these regions associated with economic status. Drowning is 2nd only to traffic injuries as a leading cause of death from unintentional injury.

Drowning is a major cause of death from injury in children. More than ½ of all global drowning deaths occur in children younger than 14 yr old. In 2000, the drowning rate was 18.9/100,000 for children 0–4 yr old and 9.5/100,000 for children 5–14 yr old. Among global leading causes of death, drowning ranks 3rd for children 5–14 yr old (1st among boys and 5th among girls) and 11th for children younger than 5 yr old. In China, drowning is the leading cause of death from injury in children 1–14 yr old. In Bangladesh, 20% of all deaths in children 1–4 yr old are due to drowning (> respiratory infection or diarrheal illness).

In the USA, drowning is the 2nd leading cause of death from unintentional injury in children 1–14 yr old. Children younger than 5 yr old account for nearly 40% of all USA drowning fatalities. The U.S. National Center for Injury Prevention and Control reported 1,239 drowning deaths in children younger than 19 yr old in 2002 (crude mortality rate, 1.53/100,000). Between 1999 and 2002, the highest childhood age-adjusted drowning rates occurred predominantly in the southern USA (Mississippi, Florida, Louisiana, Arkansas, and Alabama) and the lowest rates were seen mostly in the northeastern states; there is up to a 6-fold difference in drowning rates between various states.

Fatality statistics convey only part of the problem because many submersion victims are resuscitated and survive with morbidity (predominantly neurologic sequelae). According to the WHO Global Burden of Disease Project in 2000, nonfatal submersion injuries continue to constitute a leading cause of burden of disease. For children younger than 15 yr old, drowning annually accounts for the loss of 8.3 million disability-adjusted life-years. These estimates are surely low because morbidity rates for nonfatal drowning are often unreliable from low- and middle-income countries.

In the USA, there are an estimated 500,000 significant submersion events each year; approximately 50,000 of those affected require some type of assessment or treatment. Many also require higher levels of hospital-based care. In the USA, between 2001 and 2003, there were 15,012 patients with nonfatal drowning injuries who were treated in the ED. Eighty-three percent of these ED visits were for persons younger than 20 yr old and 57% were for children 0–4 yr old. Fifty-five percent of the children required hospitalization or transfer to another facility. During this same period, there were >2,500 pediatric drowning deaths; almost ½ of those who die of drowning are declared dead at the scene and never present to medical facilities for care.

Compared with other injuries, drowning is particularly lethal. In the USA, among children younger than 15 yr old, there are approximately 6 nonfatal ED visits for drowning for each fatality. This nonfatal injury-to-fatality ratio is much higher than that seen in other major categories of injury, including falls (19,000 : 1), motor vehicle collisions (150 : 1), and suffocations (14 : 1). Morbidity among survivors of drowning is also much higher compared with other types of injury, primarily due to neurologic sequelae. In the USA and Australia, in 2000, the age-specific drowning morbidity rates for children 0–4 yr old were 26.5/100,000 and 24.1/100,000, respectively.

RISK FACTORS

Risk factors for drowning include age, sex, and race. Drowning fatality rates are highest in children younger than 5 yr old and 2nd highest in 15–19 yr olds (predominantly adolescent males). In almost every country, male drowning victims predominate at all ages. In the USA, males account for 75% of drowning deaths; the male-to-female ratio increases dramatically from 2 : 1 in toddlers to >10 : 1 in teenagers. Ethnic minority groups generally have higher drowning rates, possibly due to different environmental exposures and fewer opportunities to learn to swim. In the USA, black children have almost double the overall drowning rate of white children.

The proportion of drowning events at various sites is greatly influenced by the accessibility to various bodies of water, socioeconomic status, and geographic area. Any body of water can pose a hazard to a child (young children have drowned in a few centimeters of water). In the USA, 32% of all childhood drowning occurs in artificial pools, 9% at domestic sites (mostly bathtubs), 47% in natural freshwater (rivers, lakes), and only 4% in saltwater. Almost 40% of drowning deaths happen during swimming.

The most common site of drowning varies depending on age. In the USA, of children younger than 1 yr old who drowned, most did so in domestic sites (78%), predominantly in the bathtub, but also in artificial pools, buckets, and toilets. In victims 1–4 yr old, 55% drowned in artificial pools (mostly residential swimming pools) and 26% died at natural freshwater sites. In most industrialized countries, the swimming pool is the most common drowning site for young children. For children 5–9 yr old, 54% died in freshwater and 31% in artificial pools. In young adolescents (10–14 yr old), 61% died in freshwater and 21% died in artificial pools. Older teenagers (15–19 yr old) drown predominantly in freshwater sites (69%) and less commonly in artificial pools (12%) or saltwater (10%). The distribution of drowning locations varies significantly in different countries.

In warmer climates in the USA, Australia, and South Africa, 50–90% of drowning deaths occur in residential swimming pools. The U.S. Consumer Product Safety Commission estimated that 3,000 children younger than 5 yr old are seen annually in the ED after submersion in residential pools; up to 80% of these children are hospitalized for at least 1 day. Most pool submersion events occur at the child's own home, and nearly ½ occur within the 1st 6 mo of initial pool exposure. Brief lapses (<5 min) in supervision are associated with most submersion events.

Rural and farm settings have special considerations. In an Australian farm injury study, 58% of deaths in children younger than 5 yr old were due to drowning; 78% of the deaths were associated with access to farm dams and irrigation canals. In rural settings in the USA and Canada, drowning is a leading cause of pediatric farm injury death, accounting for 1 in 6 farm fatalities during 1995–2000.

In the USA, >½ of unintentional infant drowning deaths occur in the bathtub. After the 1st year of life, bathtub drowning becomes progressively less common (<10%). Often, these infants have inadequate supervision and parents who overestimate the child's abilities or coordination. Almost ½ of bathtub fatalities occur during brief lapses in adult supervision and while the tub is being shared by a slightly older "supervising" sibling. In Japan, where bathtubs are commonly left filled with water, ½ of all drownings occur in the bathtub; this is the most common drowning site for children younger than 4 yr old.

Hot tubs and spas pose special hazards, because many have suction devices that can entrap hair, clothing, or body parts, preventing children from surfacing. Brief lapses in supervision are noted in most circumstances; drowning from entrapment may occur even when parents are present and directly supervising the child. Children younger than 2 yr old are the most frequent victims.

Children may also drown in buckets, toilets, washing machines, sinks, and other common household objects containing water. Bucket drowning is common, constituting up to 24% of all toddler drownings in some regions. Young children fall headfirst into these water containers and may not be able to extricate themselves because they have a relatively cephalad center of gravity and/or have insufficient body mass to tip the bucket over. The mortality rate is high, in part because of cleaning fluids and other caustic substances that buckets may contain.

In older children and teenagers, as many as 70% of drowning deaths occur in open bodies of water, such as lakes, ponds, streams, ocean beaches, or irrigation ditches, usually where little or no adult supervision exists. At locations where a lifeguard is present, the risk of drowning is dramatically reduced.

The risk of drowning is significantly increased by the use of alcohol or illicit drugs. Alcohol clouds judgment, increasing the likelihood of injudicious risk-taking behavior, and retards motor coordination. Intoxicated adults are also incapable of providing adequate supervision for younger children near water. In a U.S. survey, 70% of males and 66% of females reported using alcohol while participating in aquatic activities; the largest group of positive respondents was 16–20 yr old. Positive blood alcohol levels are found in 10–50% of adolescent drowning victims.

One fifth of open-water drowning events involve boats or other watercraft, and almost 50% are associated with alcohol or drug use. In 2002, the U.S. Coast Guard received reports of 5,705 boating incidents that resulted in 4,062 injuries and 750 deaths. The majority of the deaths (70%) were caused by drowning.

Concomitant medical conditions may also increase the likelihood of drowning. Children with epilepsy have a 4–13-fold increased risk of drowning compared with nonepileptic children. Indeed, drowning is the most likely cause of death from unintentional injury in this population. Epilepsy-associated drowning occurs predominantly in bathtubs or swimming pools (86%); the majority of cases are in children older than age 5 yr. In nonepileptic children, other mental or motor disabilities (cerebral palsy) may also increase drowning risk.

Child abuse or homicide by submersion does occur, and its detection requires a careful history, a high index of suspicion, and an understanding of normal childhood developmental capabilities (see Chapter 36). Child abuse or neglect may be a factor in 5–19% of submersions in children 1–4 yr of age and in 10–67% of bathtub-related events. Approximately 1 in 30 child homicides are by intentional drowning, mostly in the bathtub. Eighty-five per cent of intentional bathtub drowning occurs in children 15–30 mo old, an age at which bathtub drowning should be unlikely due to age-dependent developmental capabilities. Compared with unintentional injuries, victims of abuse are less likely to have resuscitation attempted by bystanders and are more likely to die.

PATHOPHYSIOLOGY

Most pediatric victims drown silently and do not signal distress or call for help. Young children can struggle for only 10–20 sec before a final submersion event occurs. A drowning victim's splashing or efforts to breathe may be misconstrued by nearby persons as merely "playing" in the water.

Once submersion occurs, all organs and tissues are at risk for hypoxia. In minutes, hypoxia can lead to cardiac arrest, adding ischemia to the succession of events. This global hypoxic-ischemic injury is a common mechanism associated with drowning, with the severity of injury primarily dependent on its duration. Pulmonary aspiration can further exacerbate hypoxia and subsequent respiratory failure. With restoration of perfusion, resuscitated victims of severe drowning events have initiation of a myriad of biochemical and physiologic responses. The brain is particularly susceptible to the damaging effects of this hypoxic-ischemic and reperfusion injury.

ANOXIC-ISCHEMIC INJURY. After experimental submersion, a conscious animal will initially panic, trying to surface. During this stage, small amounts of water enter the hypopharynx, triggering laryngospasm. Most animals struggle violently and swallow copious amounts of water. There is a progressive decrease in arterial blood oxygen saturation (Sa_{O_2}), and the animal soon loses consciousness from hypoxia. Vomiting may ensue, accompanied by involuntary gastric fluid aspiration. In approximately 10% of animals, the initial laryngospasm persists until death without significant aspiration into the lungs (aspiration is absent or very scant in 10–15% of drowning fatalities). Profound hypoxia and medullary depression lead to terminal apnea. Superimposed on these events, cardiovascular changes include initial tachycardia followed by severe hypertension with reflex bradycardia, presumably from intense catecholamine release; arrhythmias may be seen. Cardiac output and oxygen delivery progressively decrease. By 3–4 min, the circulation abruptly fails as myocardial hypoxia supervenes. The heart may continue to have ineffective contractions with electrical activity for a short time, but there is no effective perfusion (pulseless electrical activity). Some drowning victims have a primary cardiac arrest secondary to 1 of the variants of the inherited prolonged Q-T syndromes (see Chapters 435 and 436). Successful resuscitation quickly becomes impossible because hypoxia-ischemia causes rapid, progressive, and irreversible global injury.

The diving reflex may potentially enhance cerebral and myocardial blood flow when the face is submerged in very cold water (<20°C) and is believed by some to contribute to cerebral protection during submersion. Although this reflex is prominent in many sea mammals, it is relatively weak in humans. The extent of neurologic protection afforded humans by the diving reflex is controversial, but is probably small.

With modern intensive care, the cardiorespiratory consequences of resuscitated drowning victims are usually manageable and are less often the cause of mortality than irreversible hypoxic-ischemic central nervous system (CNS) injury. CNS injury is the most frequent cause of mortality and long-term morbidity. Although the duration of anoxia before irreversible CNS injury begins is uncertain, it is probably on the order of 3–5 min.

Central Nervous System Injury. Myriad pathophysiologic events occur in the CNS as a result of hypoxemia and ischemia (see Chapter 67). The brain has minimal energy stores and requires constant delivery of oxygen and nutrients. After approximately 2 min of anoxia, adenosine triphosphate is critically depleted. Adenosine triphosphate is necessary to maintain neuronal metabolic functions and ionic gradients; its depletion is a likely trigger for a number of pathogenic cascades.

Cerebral blood flow aberrations and impaired autoregulation may persist after resuscitation. The uncoupling of cerebral blood flow autoregulation and CNS metabolic demands increases the potential for further injury as cerebral oxygen usage increases after the ischemic period while cerebral blood flow remains low.

Secondary CNS injury during reperfusion may be exacerbated by the release of glutamate and other "excitatory" amino acids (EAAs). Glutamate is the predominant excitatory neurotransmitter of the brain, and it acts through specific receptors. Activation of these EAA receptors on neural cell membranes leads to an influx of calcium and sodium. Glutamate also acts on metabotropic receptors, triggering secondary messenger systems that lead to the release of calcium from intracellular stores. Increased intracellular calcium after hypoxia-ischemia is likely a final pathway toward irreversible cellular injury and death.

After cardiopulmonary arrest, **cerebral edema** may occur. The mechanisms causing cerebral edema are not completely elucidated, but are likely mostly due to swelling in astrocyte foot processes and, to a lesser degree, vasogenic edema from disruption of the blood-brain barrier. Astrocyte-mediated uptake of EAAs from the extracellular space appears to be coupled to intracellular sodium and water accumulation. Acidosis, potassium, and arachidonic acid also mediate astrocyte swelling. The traditional concept of "cytotoxic" cerebral edema due to cellular energy failure (the pump-leak model) is deficient, although the inability to maintain ionic gradients may still play some role in the production of cerebral edema. Severe cerebral edema can elevate **intracranial pressure (ICP)**, contributing to further ischemia; intracranial hypertension is an ominous sign of profound CNS damage.

After drowning, children with initial serum glucose concentrations >250 mg/dL are more likely to die or survive in a persistent vegetative state compared with normoglycemic victims. **Hyperglycemia** after hypoxia-ischemia may exacerbate CNS injury through multiple physiologic pathways. Correction of hyperglycemia with insulin improves CNS injury in animals to a level equivalent to that in normoglycemic animals; insulin-induced hypoglycemia after hypoxia-ischemia leads to increased mortality, seizures, and a greater extent of neurologic injury. Control of hyperglycemia with insulin after drowning cannot be recommended in humans until clinical trials are performed. Currently, it seems prudent to correct hypoglycemia aggressively and avoid iatrogenic hyperglycemia.

Injury to Other Organs and Tissues. All other organs and tissues may be injured by hypoxia-ischemia. In the lung, damage to the pulmonary vascular endothelium, increasing vascular permeability and inflammation, can lead to acute respiratory distress syndrome (ARDS; see Chapter 69). Aspiration may also compound pulmonary injury (see Chapter 394). Myocardial dysfunction, arterial hypotension, decreased cardiac output, arrhythmias, and cardiac infarction may also occur (see Chapters 66 and 68). Acute tubular necrosis, cortical necrosis, and renal failure are common complications of major hypoxic-ischemic events (see Chapters 535 and 536). Vascular endothelial injury can initiate disseminated intravascular coagulation, hemolysis, and thrombocytopenia (see Chapter 483). Many factors contribute to gastrointestinal damage, including hypoxia-ischemia, hypothermia, catecholamine infusions, and perhaps the diving reflex; bloody diarrhea with mucosal sloughing may be seen after severe hypoxic-ischemic events and often portends a fatal injury. Levels of hepatic transaminases and serum pancreatic enzymes are often acutely elevated. Violation of normal mucosal protective barriers predisposes the victim to bacteremia and sepsis (see Chapter 176).

ASPIRATION AND PULMONARY INJURY. Pulmonary aspiration (see Chapter 394) occurs in a majority of drowning victims, but the amount aspirated is usually small. Nonaspirating victims may acutely succumb from laryngospasm and the consequences of hypoxia. The amount and composition of aspirated material can affect the patient's clinical course: Gastric contents, water salinity, pathogenic organisms, toxic chemicals, and other foreign matter can injure the lung or cause airway obstruction. A few children may have massive aspiration, increasing the likelihood of severe pulmonary dysfunction.

Clinical management is not significantly different in seawater or freshwater aspiration. Seawater is hypertonic (approximately 3% normal saline), establishing an osmotic gradient that draws interstitial and intravascular fluid into the alveoli; furthermore, seawater inactivates surfactant, increasing alveolar surface tension, making the alveolus unstable and prone to atelectasis. Hypotonic freshwater aspiration washes out surfactant, also causing alveolar instability and collapse. In either case, hypoxemia and pulmonary insufficiency result from ventilation-perfusion mismatch, increased intrapulmonary shunting, decreased lung compliance, and increased small airway resistance. In humans, aspiration of 1–3 mL/kg can lead to marked hypoxemia and a 10–40% reduction in lung compliance.

Noncardiogenic pulmonary edema may develop from aspiration of liquid or foreign material, hypoxia-ischemia, or marked hypothermia. When the PaO_2 to FiO_2 ratio is <200, with diffuse bilateral pulmonary infiltrates, ARDS is a common etiology (see Chapters 69 and 393). In some cases, pulmonary edema may be cardiogenic (due to severely impaired myocardial function) or, uncommonly, neurogenic. Pneumonia may result from aspirated contaminated material. Gastric acid or caustic agent aspiration can directly injure the lung without infection being present. Ventilator-associated lung injury (see Chapter 70) can also occur with excessive tidal volumes or pressures or with prolonged exposure to high concentrations of oxygen.

FLUID AND ELECTROLYTE ALTERATIONS (SEE CHAPTER 52). The majority of submersion victims do not aspirate large enough volumes of fluid to result in significant electrolyte disturbances. Many do swallow copious amounts of fluid, but even this does not appear to lead to a significant incidence of clinically relevant fluid or electrolyte aberrations. Children who survive long enough to be seen in the ED rarely have electrolyte aberrations requiring specific therapy.

Uncommonly, massive ingestion or aspiration of seawater can lead to hypernatremia and fluid shifts because of its high sodium concentration and osmolarity. Because fluid is osmotically drawn into the lungs or gastrointestinal tract, hemoconcentration may be observed. Hypernatremia and hemoconcentration in drowning victims may also be due to hyposmolar diuresis from brain injury–associated diabetes insipidus (see Chapter 559), usually a sign of profound CNS injury after hypoxic-ischemic events.

Water intoxication rarely occurs with massive freshwater aspiration or ingestion, causing hyponatremia and hemodilution. Sudden hypo-osmolarity can result in red blood cell swelling and hemolysis, hypothetically leading to hyperkalemia or hemoglobinuria with renal tubular damage. Plasma-free hemoglobin levels in human drowning are typically <500 mg/dL, usually insufficient to cause renal dysfunction from this mechanism alone. Alternatively, free water overload may be seen with excess antidiuretic hormone (SIADH), which can accompany pulmonary or brain injury (see Chapter 52). Excess free water may also increase cerebral edema and ICP.

HYPOTHERMIA (SEE CHAPTER 75). Hypothermia is common after submersion. It is often categorized, based on core body temperature measurement, as mild (34–36°C), moderate (30–34°C), or severe (<30°C).

Heat loss through conduction and convection is very efficient in water and, if the water is sufficiently cold, cannot be matched by the body's thermogenic mechanisms (shivering and nonshivering thermogenesis, vasoconstriction, active movements). Children are at increased risk for hypothermia because they have a relatively high ratio of body surface area to mass, decreased subcutaneous fat, and limited thermogenic capacity. Hypothermia can develop as a result of prolonged surface contact with cold water while the head is above water (immersion) or after submersion involving the potential additional impact of swallowing or aspirating large quantities of very cold fluid.

The minority of all drownings are **immersion** incidents in which the victim remains afloat, keeping the head above water without respiratory impairment. Surface heat loss can lead to significant core temperature decreases, depending on water and air temperature, insulation, body surface area, thermogenic capacity, and physical condition. Data from the early days of cardiopulmonary bypass indicate that surface cooling of anesthetized infants with ice packs and ice water decreases rectal temperature by as little as 2.5°C in the 1st 10 min; it takes a further 32 min for the temperature to fall to 24–26°C. As core temperature drops to <35°C, cognition, coordination, and muscle strength become progressively impaired. The likelihood of self-rescue becomes less likely at this point. With progressive hypothermia, there may be loss of consciousness, water aspiration, decreased heart rate and cardiac output, ineffective breathing, and cardiac arrest.

Submersion is a more common mechanism. Surface heat loss mechanisms are likely similar to those of immersion, but additionally, victims may swallow or aspirate significant quantities of cold fluid that contribute additively to hypothermia. In human adults, immersion in icy water results in intense involuntary reflex hyperventilation and decreased breath-holding ability to <10 sec. Victims of ice-water submersions may be more likely to have involuntary respiration and fluid aspiration, contributing to more rapid and deep hypothermia. It may theoretically be possible for the brain to rapidly cool to a neuroprotective level, if the water is cold enough and cardiac output lasts long enough for sufficient heat exchange to occur. Once submersion-associated hypoxia, apnea, and cardiovascular compromise decrease blood circulation, the rate of temperature drop is mitigated.

After the child is removed from the water, further drops in body temperature may occur as a result of cold air, wet clothes, hypoxia, and hospital transport. **Hypothermia** in pediatric drowning victims is observed even after drowning in relatively warm water and in warm climates. Unrecognized progressive hypothermia can lead to further patient decompensation. In hypothermic victims, compensatory mechanisms will usually attempt to restore normothermia at body temperatures >32°C; at lower temperatures, thermoregulation may fail and spontaneous rewarming will not occur. Moderate hypothermia increases oxygen consumption through shivering thermogenesis and increased sympathetic tone. As shivering ceases, as in patients with severe hypothermia or those receiving neuromuscular blockade, the metabolic rate decreases approximately 7%/°C.

With moderate to severe hypothermia, progressive bradycardia, impaired myocardial contractility, and loss of vasomotor tone contribute to inadequate perfusion, hypotension, and possible shock. Below 28°C, extreme bradycardia is usually present and the propensity for spontaneous ventricular fibrillation (VF) or asystole is high. Central respiratory center depression with moderate to severe hypothermia results in hypoventilation and eventual apnea. A deep coma, with fixed and dilated pupils and absent reflexes at very low body temperatures (<25–29°C), may give the false appearance of death.

Depending on the duration and severity of the temperature aberration, other systemic adverse consequences of hypothermia may occur acutely and persist even after rewarming. ARDS secondary to hypothermia can be seen in the absence of submersion or aspiration. Depressed hepatorenal metabolism and perfusion reduce drug clearance. Either hypoglycemia from glycogen store exhaustion or hyperglycemia due to catecholamines, altered pancreatic insulin release, and depressed peripheral glucose metabolism may be observed. Thrombocytopenia, platelet dysfunction, and disseminated intravascular coagulation may also occur. Although hypothermia slows bacterial replication, it also renders the host more susceptible to bacterial and fungal invasion and sepsis by impairing neutrophil and reticuloendothelial function.

During initial rewarming efforts, core body temperature may initially decline. This "**afterdrop**" may occur secondary to the return of colder blood from the extremities to the relatively warmer central core or through the conduction of heat from the warmer core to cooler surface layers. In patients with severe hypothermia, afterdrop may induce arrhythmias or further compromise cardiac, respiratory, or neurologic function. Afterdrop in moderate to severe hypothermia may be mitigated if rewarming measures are not applied to the extremities, focusing efforts instead on core rewarming.

"**Rewarming shock**" may be observed after rescue. When subjected to the additional metabolic requirements of increasing body temperature and the vasodilation accompanying surface rewarming, victims with borderline myocardial function may not be able to meet the increased physiologic demands. Hypotension, metabolic acidosis, tissue ischemia, and other consequences of shock (see Chapter 68) may therefore be exacerbated during rewarming.

HYPOTHERMIA AND NEUROPROTECTION. The theoretical benefits, implications, and consequences of hypothermia in drowning victims are areas of controversy. There are known adverse effects associated with hypothermia, and these must be balanced against the potential benefits observed in experimental data. One should clearly differentiate among: (1) controlled hypothermia, such as that used in the operating room before the onset of hypoxia or ischemia; (2) accidental hypothermia, such as in drowning, which is uncontrolled and variable, with onset during or shortly after hypoxia-ischemia; and (3) therapeutic hypothermia, involving the purposeful and controlled lowering and maintenance of body (or brain) temperature at some time after a hypoxic-ischemic event.

In drowning victims with uncontrolled accidental hypothermia associated with icy water submersion, there are a few case reports of good neurologic recovery after prolonged (10–150 min) cardiopulmonary arrest. These rare survivors have been in freezing water (<5°C) and have core body temperatures <30°C (often much lower). Presumably, these fortunate survivors must have had very rapid and sufficiently deep hypothermia develop before irreversible hypoxic-ischemic injury occurred. Under what circumstances such accidental neuroprotective hypothermia occurs in drowning is unknown, but it is rare.

Most often, in human drowning series, hypothermia is a poor prognostic sign and a neuroprotective effect has not been demonstrated. In King County, Washington, where the water is cold but rarely icy, 92% of survivors with good neurologic outcomes had initial temperatures >34°C, whereas 61% of those who died or had severe neurologic injury had temperatures <34°C. In another study of comatose drowning patients admitted to the PICU, 65% of hypothermic patients (<35°C) died compared with a 27% observed mortality rate in nonhypothermic victims. Similarly, in Finland (where the median water temperature was 16°C), a beneficial effect of hypothermia was not seen in pediatric submersion victims; submersion duration <10 min was most related to good outcome.

Human trials using therapeutic hypothermia in perinatal hypoxic-ischemic encephalopathy and in adults with out-of-hospital cardiac arrest have shown some benefit, but in traumatic brain injury results have been mixed or equivocal. The optimal temperature management and the conditions in which therapeutic hypothermia can be applied in human drowning victims have not been determined.

CLINICAL MANIFESTATIONS AND TREATMENT

The clinical course and outcome for a submersion victim are primarily determined by the circumstances of the incident, the duration of submersion, the speed of the rescue, and the effectiveness of resuscitative efforts (Table 73-1). Two groups may be identified, based on responsiveness at the scene. Children who require minimal resuscitation at the scene commonly have good outcomes and experience a low incidence of complications. These victims quickly regain spontaneous respiration and typically regain consciousness rapidly. They should be transported to the ED for further evaluation.

Victims in cardiac arrest require aggressive or prolonged resuscitation and have a high risk of multiorgan system complications, major neurologic morbidity, or death. Initial management requires coordinated and experienced prehospital care following the ABCs of emergency resuscitation (see Chapter 66). These children often remain comatose and lack brainstem reflexes despite the restoration of oxygenation and circulation. Subsequent ED and PICU care often involves advanced life support strategies and management of multiorgan dysfunction.

INITIAL EVALUATION AND RESUSCITATION (SEE CHAPTER 66). *Once a submersion has occurred, immediate institution of cardiopulmonary resuscitative efforts at the scene is imperative.* Every minute that passes without the re-establishment of adequate breathing and circulation dramatically decreases the possibility

TABLE 73-1. Essential Factors Concerning Submersion Incidents

FACTOR	IMPLICATIONS
Submersion duration	Submersion duration <5 min associated with favorable outcome. Submersion duration >10 min highly associated with poor outcome.
Resuscitation duration	Resuscitation duration <10 min for return of spontaneous circulation associated with favorable outcome. Resuscitation duration >25 min highly associated with poor outcome.
Scene CPR	Children with good outcome more likely to have received immediate bystander CPR. Delays in the institution of CPR associated with worse outcomes.
Core body temperature	Hypothermia very common in pediatric submersion and can affect vital signs, mental status, and resuscitative efforts.
Cardiac rhythm at scene	Patients with normal sinus rhythm at scene likely to have good outcome.
Neurologic responsiveness at scene	Patients with neurologic responsiveness and reactive pupils at scene likely to have good outcomes.
Circumstances of incident	Consider cervical trauma in shallow water and diving incidents. In boating accidents, consider trauma and carbon monoxide intoxication.
Gastric aspiration	Emesis and subsequent aspiration of gastric contents common during resuscitative efforts.
Nature of fluid medium	Consider possibility of caustic or toxic substance aspiration, such as in bucket drowning. Also, consider possible infectious pathogens that may pose a higher risk in some mediums, such as hot tubs, lakes, and rivers.
Temperature of fluid medium	Patients drowning in icy water (<5°C) may have potential for neuroprotective effects from rapid cooling of core body temperature.
Concomitant medical conditions	Consider factors that may contribute to submersion events, such as alcohol or drug intoxication, trauma, epilepsy, airway foreign body, and prolonged QT syndrome.
Child abuse	High index of suspicion and careful evaluation needed. Most abusive events involving submersion occur in bathtubs in older toddlers (>15 mo).

of a good outcome. When safe for the victim and the rescuer, institution of in-water resuscitation for nonbreathing victims by trained personnel may improve the likelihood of survival. Victims usually need to be extricated from the drowning medium as quickly as possible so that advanced lifesaving measures can be applied.

Bystander CPR is administered in only 40–60% of drownings. Children with good outcomes are almost 5 times as likely to have had immediate resuscitation at the scene compared with children with poor outcomes, although this is not demonstrated in all series. In drowning victims who receive bystander CPR, 50–80% survive to hospital discharge; these patients often do not have complete cardiac arrest and most respond quickly to resuscitative efforts with return of normal vital signs by ED arrival. In victims with full cardiac arrest who receive prehospital CPR, only 0–21% have neurologically intact survival. Waiting for paramedics to arrive takes too long in these circumstances, and bystander resuscitative efforts should not be delayed (even in a model prehospital system, paramedics took >10 min to arrive in 91% of submersion cases).

Initial resuscitation must focus on rapidly restoring oxygenation, ventilation, and adequate circulation. The airway should be clear of vomitus or foreign material, which may cause obstruction or aspiration. Abdominal thrusts should not be used for lung fluid removal because their effectiveness is not established; because many victims have a distended abdomen from swallowed water, abdominal thrusts may increase the risk of regurgitation and aspiration. In cases of suspected airway foreign body, chest compressions or back blows are preferable maneuvers.

The cervical spine should be protected in anyone with potential traumatic neck injury (see Chapters 67 and 71). Only approximately 0.5% of submersion victims have cervical spine injuries. Victims with spine injuries generally have a history of diving, a motorized vehicle crash, a fall from height, a water sport accident, child abuse, or drowning in open bodies of water with other clinical signs of serious injury. In such cases, the neck should be in a neutral position and protected with a well-fitting cervical collar. Patients rescued from unknown circumstances may also warrant cervical spine precautions. In low-impact submersions, spinal injuries are exceedingly rare and routine spinal immobilization is not warranted.

If the victim has ineffective respiration or apnea, ventilatory support must be initiated immediately (see Chapter 66). Mouth-to-mouth or mouth-to-nose breathing by trained bystanders often restores spontaneous ventilation. As soon as it is available, supplemental oxygen should be administered to all victims. Positive pressure bag-mask ventilation with 100% inspired oxygen fraction (FIO_2) should be instituted in patients with respiratory insufficiency.

Gastric distention is often exacerbated by mouth-to-mouth or bag-mask ventilation. Vomiting with possible aspiration is seen in 25–75% of victims during resuscitation. Cricoid pressure (the Sellick maneuver) during positive pressure breathing and early nasogastric decompression may decrease the risk of vomiting and aspiration (see Chapter 66).

If apnea, cyanosis, hypoventilation, or labored respiration persists, trained personnel should perform endotracheal tube (ETT) intubation as soon as possible. Intubation is also indicated to protect the airway in patients with depressed mental status or hemodynamic instability. Hypoxia must be corrected rapidly to optimize the chance of recovery. Oxygen alone may not correct hypoxia in patients with significant pulmonary edema or aspiration; in such cases, the application of positive end-expiratory pressure (PEEP) is often necessary. The routine use of PEEP in drowning has made early death from pulmonary insufficiency uncommon. Initial PEEP should be approximately 5 cm H_2O; it can be increased incrementally up to 10–15 cm H_2O if SaO_2 is not >90%. During bag-ETT ventilation, PEEP can be maintained by using an adjustable PEEP valve on the expiratory limb. Tidal volume and breath frequency should initially attempt to achieve normal ventilation (goal $PaCO_2$ 35–40 torr) without contributing to lung injury. Attempts to hyperventilate victims acutely or aggressively may be harmful.

Concurrent with securing airway control, oxygenation, and ventilation, the child's cardiovascular status must be evaluated. Heart rate and rhythm, blood pressure, temperature, and end-organ perfusion require urgent assessment. CPR should be instituted immediately in pulseless, bradycardic, or severely hypotensive victims (see Chapter 66). Continuously monitoring the electrocardiogram (ECG) greatly assists with the diagnosis and treatment of arrhythmias. Slow capillary refill, cool extremities, and altered mental status are potential indicators of shock (see Chapter 68). Core temperature must be evaluated, especially in children, because moderate to severe hypothermia can depress myocardial function and cause arrhythmias.

Often, intravenous fluids and cardioactive medications are required to improve circulation and perfusion (see Chapter 66). Venous access should be established as quickly as possible for the administration of fluids or pressors. Intraosseous catheter placement is a potentially lifesaving vascular access technique that avoids the delay usually associated with multiple attempts to establish intravenous access in critically ill children (see Chapter 66). Epinephrine is usually the initial drug of choice in victims with cardiopulmonary arrest (IV dose is 0.01 mg/kg of 1 : 10,000 solution given Q3–5 min as needed). Epinephrine can be given intratracheally (ETT dose is 0.1–0.2 mg/kg of 1 : 1,000 solution) if no intravenous access is available. Bolus intravascular administration of lactated Ringer solution or 0.9% normal saline (10–20 mL/kg) is often used to augment preload; repeated doses may be necessary. Hypotonic or glucose-containing solutions should not be used for intravascular volume administration.

In children with cardiac arrest after submersion, the 1st recorded rhythm is asystole in 55%, ventricular tachycardia (VT) or VF in 29%, and bradycardia in 16%. Electrical defibrillation (initially 2 J/kg, then 4 J/kg) is immediately necessary for children with VF or pulseless VT (see Chapter 66); these rhythms may be relatively refractory in drowning patients. Other cardioactive medications may be necessary to restore a perfusing rhythm (see Chapter 66). Post-resuscitation cardioactive medication infusions may be required to augment myocardial function and support blood pressure: Epinephrine infusion is usually the drug of choice (0.05–1 μg/kg/min IV) and should be titrated to blood pressure and perfusion (see Chapters 66 and 68).

HOSPITAL-BASED EVALUATION AND TREATMENT. ED and hospital management of the submersion victim includes and extends the aforementioned resuscitative efforts. Patient acuity determines the extent of further interventions. Some children present to the ED alert and with minimal symptoms. More ill children require hospitalization for ongoing evaluation and monitoring. Critically ill victims must be stabilized and transferred to a PICU (see Chapter 63).

All pediatric submersion victims probably should be hospitalized or observed for at least 6–12 hr, even if they are asymptomatic on presentation to the ED. At a minimum, serial monitoring of vital signs (respiratory rate, heart rate, blood pressure, and temperature), repeated careful pulmonary examination and neurologic assessment, chest radiography, and assessment of oxygenation by arterial blood gas or pulse oximetry should be performed on all submersion victims. Other studies may also be warranted, depending on the specific circumstances (possible traumatic injuries or suspected intoxication). Among asymptomatic or minimally symptomatic children (those who do not require advanced life support in the prehospital setting or during the 1st 4 hr in the ED and who have an initial ED Glasgow Coma Scale [GCS] score of 13 or greater), almost ½ may have respiratory deterioration or hypoxemia, usually during the 1st 4–8 hr post-submersion. Mild to rarely severe delayed respiratory symptoms and pulmonary edema can occur, even in children with initially normal findings on chest examination and radiography. Conversely, most children with minor early respiratory symptoms become asymptomatic by 18 hr post-submersion. Usually, these children have the return of normal room air Sa_{O_2} and pulmonary examination by 4–6 hr and are unlikely to have subsequent delayed respiratory deterioration. Select low-risk patients who are alert and asymptomatic with normal physical examination and oxygenation may be considered for discharge after 6–12 hr of observation, as long as appropriate follow-up can be assured.

For patients with persistent cardiopulmonary arrest on arrival in the ED after non-icy water drowning, there are no absolute clinically relevant parameters regarding withholding or stopping resuscitative efforts. In a representative study of 89 patients receiving ongoing CPR in the ED, 41 patients (46%) survived (8/41 intact and 33/41 with persistent vegetative state). Overall, 0–24% of victims requiring ongoing CPR in the ED have good functional recovery. Death or severe neurologic sequelae are quite likely in patients with submersion durations >10 min, deep coma and apnea in the ED, or arterial pH <7.0. In another comprehensive case series, 100% of children with resuscitation durations >25 min either died or had severe neurologic morbidity, and all victims with submersion duration >25 min died. On the other hand, extreme parameters, including submersion duration of 66 min, central body temperature of 13.7°C, pH of 6.29, or base excess of −36.5, have been rarely reported in survivors with good outcome. Given the level of prognostic uncertainty in the ED, almost all drowning victims should be treated aggressively, stabilized as much as possible, and admitted with close monitoring for at least 24–48 hr. However, for children who do not readily respond to aggressive resuscitative efforts, prolonged ongoing CPR after non-icy water submersion almost invariably predicts death or persistent vegetative state. Consequently, in most cases, discontinuation of CPR in the ED is probably warranted for victims of non-icy water submersion who do not respond to aggressive advanced life support within 25–30 min. Final decisions regarding if and when to discontinue resuscitative efforts must be individualized, with the understanding that protracted resuscitation efforts generally will not result in survivors with a possibility of good outcome.

MANAGEMENT OF BODY TEMPERATURE. Attention to core body temperature in the field, during transport, and in the hospital is very important. Core temperature is best measured at the tympanic membrane, which correlates most closely to brain temperature; rectal temperature determinations are often inadequate, owing to insufficient depth of thermometer insertion; oral and axillary temperature readings are unreliable. A low-recording thermometer is necessary to diagnose and monitor severe hypothermia. Continuous monitoring of core body (or brain) temperature is mandatory in the ED and PICU and should also be done to the extent possible in the prehospital setting.

Rewarming measures are generally categorized as passive, active external, or active internal. Passive rewarming measures can be applied in the prehospital or hospital setting and include the provision of dry blankets, a warm environment, and protection from further heat loss. All victims should have damp clothes removed and the skin dried. Passive rewarming relies on the patient's thermogenic ability, which is less in young children, and alone is not sufficient for moderate or severe hypothermia.

Active external rewarming (warm blankets, radiant warmers) restores temperature more rapidly (0.8 ± 0.4°C/hr), but decreased surface circulation makes this method less effective. In poorly perfused hypothermic victims, the application of warm packs and other cutaneous rewarming devices may cause significant burns. Moderate sources of external heat (forced-air blanket at ≈100 W) may result in skin rewarming and inhibition of shivering, but offer little rewarming advantage compared with shivering itself. Placing the subject in a forced warm air box (400 W) produces rates of rewarming double that of shivering (6.1 vs 3°C/hr).

Active core rewarming more rapidly improves body temperature and is necessary for moderate to severe hypothermia or for victims with impaired shivering thermogenesis. Simple active core rewarming measures include administration of warmed intravenous fluids (36–40°C) and heated humidified inspired oxygen (40–44°C), although the efficacy of these measures is not established. Gastric, bladder, or peritoneal lavage with warmed saline may be instituted relatively easily. Esophageal warming tubes also achieve good rewarming rates. More aggressive methods include hemodialysis, extracorporeal rewarming (venovenous or arteriovenous), or cardiopulmonary bypass (CPB). Rewarming rates for extracorporeal rewarming (2.1 ± 0.7°C/hr) are significantly higher than those for external active rewarming methods. For profound hypothermia, especially with circulatory collapse, CPB may be required and has a very rapid rewarming rate (6.9 ± 1.9°C/hr). Indications for CPB after drowning are not well established; this complex decision requires physician anticipation and rapid transfer to a tertiary care center.

Temperature Management in Hypothermic Victims Without Cardiopulmonary Arrest. Hypothermic drowning victims without cardiac arrest should have rewarming measures instituted as soon as possible (see Chapter 75). Passive and active external rewarming measures are necessary for victims with mild to moderate hypothermia. For victims with core temperatures <34°C, external rewarming measures should be applied only to truncal areas, attempting to avoid afterdrop. Patients with severe hypothermia (core temperature <30°C) also require active internal warming measures as soon as possible. Repeated frequent temperature measurements are important to assess the efficacy of rewarming efforts.

The cardiorespiratory management of patients with deep hypothermia (temperature <28°C) but without cardiopulmonary arrest is controversial. Ventricular arrhythmias have been temporally associated with ETT intubation or chest compressions in occasional reports of severely hypothermic patients. Therefore, to avoid precipitating VF, some authors advocate withholding intubation or chest compressions if any respiratory activity or perfusing rhythm is present. However, in a prospective case series of severely hypothermic victims, ventricular arrhythmia associated with ETT intubation was not observed. Therefore, gentle ETT placement should be performed in deeply hypothermic children with hypoxia or insufficient respiration.

No prospective studies are available to guide the clinician regarding chest compressions in severely hypothermic victims who are not in full cardiac arrest. Some authors would withhold chest compressions if core temperature is <28°C and the ECG shows a perfusing rhythm with a pulse, almost regardless of heart rate or hypotension. These recommendations in patients with deep hypothermia are based on observations that effective perfusion often returns with rewarming; rewarming is more effective when any circulation is present; VF or asystole slows rewarming efforts; chest compressions may precipitate VF; and CPR is less effective during severe hypothermia. However, given the lack of relevant data, other practitioners would initiate CPR and rewarming efforts in an effort to thwart life-threatening compromises of cardiac output (see Chapter 75).

Temperature Management in Hypothermic Victims with Cardiopulmonary Arrest. Full CPR with chest compressions is indicated for hypothermic victims if no pulse can be found or if narrow-complex QRS activity is absent on ECG (see Chapters 66 and 75). When core body temperature is >30°C, resuscitative efforts should proceed according to the current American Heart Association and American Academy of Pediatrics (AAP) guidelines for CPR, but intravenous medications may be given at a lower frequency in moderate hypothermia due to decreased drug clearance. When VF is present in severely hypothermic victims (<30°C), up to 3 defibrillation attempts should initially be delivered, but further defibrillation attempts should be held until the core temperature is >30°C, at which time successful defibrillation may be more likely.

There is significant controversy regarding the discontinuation of prolonged resuscitative efforts in hypothermic drowning victims. Victims with profound hypothermia may appear clinically dead, but full neurologic recovery is possible, although rare. Attempts at lifesaving resuscitation should not be withheld based on initial clinical presentation unless the victim is obviously dead (dependent lividity or rigor mortis). Body temperature should be taken into account before resuscitative efforts are terminated. Rewarming efforts should usually be continued until the temperature is 32–34°C; if the victim continues to have no effective cardiac rhythm and remains unresponsive to aggressive CPR, then resuscitative efforts may be discontinued.

Complete rewarming is not indicated for all arrest victims before resuscitative efforts are abandoned. In most situations, discontinuing resuscitation in victims of non-icy water submersion who remain asystolic despite 30–45 min of aggressive advanced CPR is probably warranted. Physicians must use their individual clinical judgment when deciding to stop resuscitative efforts, taking into account the unique circumstances of each incident.

Temperature Management After Cardiopulmonary Resuscitation. Once a drowning victim has had successful cardiopulmonary resuscitation after a cardiac arrest, temperature management should be carefully considered and body temperature should be continuously monitored. In victims who have had brief resuscitation durations and are awake soon after resuscitation, attempts to restore and maintain normothermia are warranted. Careful monitoring is necessary to prevent unrecognized worsening hypothermia that can lead to untoward consequences.

Victims who have had longer resuscitation durations are more likely to remain comatose; temperature management in these individuals is an active area of controversy. *There is general consensus that fever or hyperthermia (core body temperature >37.5°C) in comatose drowning victims resuscitated from cardiac arrest should be prevented at all times in the acute recovery period (at least the 1st 24–48 hr).* Based on experimental evidence and limited clinical evaluations, hyperthermia after drowning or other types of brain injury may increase the risk of mortality and exacerbate hypoxic-ischemic CNS damage.

For drowning victims who remain comatose after successful cardiopulmonary resuscitation, more contentious issues include: (1) rewarming of hypothermic victims, and (2) controlled application of therapeutic hypothermia. There are no human trials indicating that hypothermia improves the outcome of drowning patients.

Although there is no consensus of opinion, many investigators now cautiously recommend that hypothermic drowning victims who remain unresponsive due to hypoxic-ischemic encephalopathy after restoration of adequate spontaneous circulation **should not be actively rewarmed** to normal body temperatures. Active rewarming should be limited to such victims with core body temperatures <32°C, but temperatures 32–37.5°C should be allowed without further rewarming efforts.

More controversial is the induction of therapeutic hypothermia in drowning victims who remain comatose due to hypoxic-ischemic encephalopathy after cardiopulmonary resuscitation for cardiac arrest. The 2002 World Congress on Drowning recommended that hypothermia (32–34°C) should be instituted as soon as possible after resuscitation and sustained for 12–24 hr. These patients should be intubated, mechanically ventilated, and treated with sedatives and/or analgesics (with or without neuromuscular blocking agents) as necessary to prevent shivering and maintain hypothermia. Rewarming after this period should be very gradual.

A specific recommendation for therapeutic hypothermia, especially in children, is not yet generally accepted. The Advanced Life Support Task Force of the International Liaison Committee on Resuscitation (2002) did not recommend therapeutic hypothermia in children resuscitated after cardiopulmonary arrest, citing insufficient evidence and older studies demonstrating a potential deleterious effect in pediatric drowning victims. Until additional pediatric data become available, they suggest that clinicians should tailor temperature management for individual patients based on an assessment of available risk and benefit information, taking into account emerging laboratory and clinical reports.

BLOOD GLUCOSE MANAGEMENT. Both hyperglycemia and hypoglycemia are considered detrimental to the injured brain. Assessment of blood glucose should be obtained in the field and monitored frequently thereafter to maintain normoglycemia.

There is no conclusive data as to how hyperglycemia should be corrected in drowning victims and whether such correction influences outcome. *It would seem prudent to avoid iatrogenic hyperglycemia by not providing dextrose-containing fluids to victims who are already hyperglycemic.* In most victims, especially those with hyperglycemia, non–dextrose-containing solutions (normal saline) should be administered initially, with repeated blood sugar assessments to avoid unrecognized subsequent hypoglycemia. Although some preliminary data suggest that correction of hyperglycemia with insulin may improve outcome, its use after pediatric hypoxic-ischemic events cannot yet be recommended. Once the serum glucose concentration has returned to a normal value, appropriate dextrose-containing maintenance fluids may be started as a continuous infusion, with a goal of maintaining normoglycemia.

If a child is found to be hypoglycemic, 0.5–1 g/kg intravenous dextrose should be administered as either 10% or 25% solution (maximum, 25 g/dose), and continuous infusion of appropriate dextrose-containing fluids started or adjusted to maintain normoglycemia.

RESPIRATORY MANAGEMENT. The level of respiratory support should be appropriate to the patient's condition and is a continuation of prehospital management. One must frequently ensure that adequate oxygenation, ventilation, and airway control are maintained. Supplemental oxygen should be provided to all victims initially. High FIO_2 alone may not resolve hypoxia, and ETT intubation (see Chapter 66) and PEEP are often needed. PEEP increases functional residual capacity, decreases intrapulmonary shunting, improves ventilation-perfusion matching, and may improve pulmonary compliance. *The level of PEEP and FIO_2 should restore oxygenation, usually to a goal SaO_2 of >90%* (see Chapter 70). Excessive PEEP can impair venous blood return and depress cardiac output. Prolonged use of high FIO_2 (>70%) may contribute to pulmonary oxygen toxicity. An arterial catheter is often required for reliable and frequent arterial blood gas assessment and continuous blood pressure monitoring in critically ill patients.

Unintubated alert children with mild to moderate hypoxemia despite supplemental oxygen who can protect their airway may be candidates for mask continuous positive airway pressure or bilevel positive airway pressure. These noninvasive measures can improve oxygenation and possibly avert the need for ETT intubation. A nasogastric tube may be necessary to prevent gaseous gastric distention. Persistent hypoxemia, impaired ventilation, labored respiration, depressed mental status, or patient intolerance usually requires ETT intubation to secure the airway and breathing (see Chapters 66 and 70).

Hypercapnia should generally be avoided in potentially brain-injured children. Patients with actual or potential hypoventilation or markedly elevated work of breathing should have assisted or controlled mechanical ventilation to avoid hypercapnia and decrease the energy expenditures of labored respiration. The usual initial ventilatory goal is a $PaCO_2$ of 35–40 mm Hg. *Excessive hyperventilation is contraindicated;* even moderate acute hyperventilation may potentially contribute to cerebral vasoconstriction and hypoperfusion.

Children with **bronchospasm** after drowning may benefit from β_2-agonist therapy (see Chapter 388); however, pulmonary edema or an airway foreign body may also cause wheezing and should be considered. Bronchoscopy is indicated if a foreign body is suspected (see Chapter 384). The routine use of diuretics or corticosteroids for pulmonary edema or lung injury is not recommended. Prophylactic antibiotics are not generally helpful, except in cases where the aspirate is likely to be grossly contaminated.

A serious complication in some submersion victims is **ARDS** (see Chapters 69 and 70). ARDS can have detrimental effects on oxygenation and pulmonary compliance. Patients administered high airway pressures or tidal volumes during mechanical ventilation are at increased risk for ventilator-induced lung injury. The application of peak airway pressures >30–35 cm H_2O may lead to alveolar overdistention and damage, exacerbating lung injury, and promoting pulmonary and systemic inflammatory responses. The use of lower tidal volumes and pressures is associated with decreased ARDS-related mortality. Patients with ARDS and brain injury pose a difficult challenge because permissive hypercapnia—a strategy commonly used in ARDS—is normally contraindicated in patients with brain injury or intracranial hypertension. Sedation and, less often, neuromuscular blockade may be necessary to improve thoracic compliance, patient-ventilator synchrony, and gas exchange; however, these medications may also obscure neurologic evaluation, making prognostication and decision-making more difficult.

Various modes of high-frequency ventilation have been successfully used in drowning victims in whom conventional mechanical ventilation has failed (see Chapter 70). In a few cases, inhaled nitric oxide may help improve ventilation-perfusion matching and decrease pulmonary hypertension (see Chapter 70). Exogenous surfactant use after drowning has been reported, but indications and guidelines for effective delivery in this population do not exist. Extracorporeal life support in drowning has been reported; however, its general application in drowning victims is very controversial and should be limited until better selection criteria and more accurate predictors of neurologic outcome exist.

CARDIOVASCULAR MANAGEMENT. Cardiovascular stabilization is a continuation of measures instituted in the prehospital setting. Causes contributing to myocardial insufficiency include hypoxic-ischemic injury, ongoing hypoxia, hypothermia, acidosis, high airway pressures during mechanical ventilation, alterations of intravascular volume, and electrolyte disorders. Heart failure, shock, arrhythmias, or cardiac arrest may occur. Continuous ECG monitoring is mandatory to recognize and treat arrhythmias (see Chapter 435). Arterial catheterization facilitates continuous blood pressure and laboratory monitoring. Echocardiography, central venous pressure monitoring, or pulmonary artery catheter placement may aid in the assessment of intravascular volume status and myocardial function in select patients (see Chapter 64).

The provision of adequate oxygenation and ventilation is a prerequisite to improving myocardial function. Fluid resuscitation and inotropic agents are often necessary to improve heart function and restore tissue perfusion (see Chapter 66). Increasing preload with intravenous fluids may be beneficial by improving stroke volume and cardiac output. Overzealous fluid administration, especially in the presence of poor myocardial function, can worsen pulmonary edema. Epinephrine (dose range, 0.05–1 µg/kg/min IV) is usually the drug of choice for patients with cardiac dysfunction or hypotension after hypoxic-ischemic events. Others suggest that dobutamine (dose range, 2–20 µg/kg/min IV) may more effectively improve cardiac output in normotensive patients. Some patients may require other cardioactive medications, depending on individual cardiovascular dysfunction (see Chapters 66 and 68). Electrolyte abnormalities, particularly hypocalcemia, and body temperature should be corrected to optimize myocardial performance. Calcium gluconate (50–100 mg/kg IV) or calcium chloride (10–30 mg/kg IV) may be administered to treat hypocalcemia; care must be taken to avoid extravasation injury and these medications should preferably be administered through a central venous catheter.

Exertion, voluntary apnea, cold water exposure, and face immersion are gene-specific *(KVLQT1)* arrhythmogenic triggers for long Q-T syndrome (see Chapter 435). This uncommon diagnosis should be considered in cases of unexplained drowning during swimming.

NEUROLOGIC MANAGEMENT. Drowning victims who present to the hospital awake and alert usually have normal neurologic outcomes. In comatose victims, the possibility of irreversible CNS injury is a major concern. Current therapy emphasizes reducing both the duration of the primary insult (prompt resuscitation) and the potential secondary CNS injury. The most critical and effective neurologic intensive care measures after drowning are rapid restoration and maintenance of adequate oxygenation, ventilation, and perfusion. As previously discussed, core body temperature and glucose management may also be important modulators of neurologic injury after hypoxia-ischemia.

Head CT scans are not generally helpful unless there is a suspicion of associated traumatic injury or to rule out other possible causes of coma. The great majority of comatose drowning victims initially have normal scans. An acutely abnormal CT scan is most frequently associated with death. After 24 hr, poor gray-white differentiation and cerebral edema may be seen in most (but not all) children with severe hypoxic-ischemic injuries. Head CT scans cannot adequately distinguish patients with good outcomes from those with poor ones. MRI scans may detect changes associated with hypoxic-ischemic injury earlier than head CT scans, but these scans are rarely clinically indicated. There is no advantage of head CT scans or MRI scans over neurologic examination for prognostication or management of nontraumatic drowning.

Comatose drowning patients are at risk for **intracranial hypertension.** Although ICP monitoring and therapy to reduce intracranial hypertension would seem likely to preserve cerebral perfusion and prevent herniation, in fact, there is little evidence that they improve the outcome of drowning victims. Patients with elevated ICP usually have poor outcomes—either death or persistent vegetative state—regardless of ICP management. Children with normal ICP can also have poor outcomes, although less frequently. Conventional neurologic intensive care therapies, such as osmotic agents, diuretics, fluid restriction, muscle relaxants, hyperventilation, barbiturates, and steroids (measures often used in victims with elevated ICP from different causes), so far have not been shown to benefit the drowning victim, either individually or in combination. Indeed, there is some evidence that these therapies may decrease overall mortality, but only by increasing the number of survivors with severe neurologic morbidity. They do not seem to increase the number of neurologically intact survivors or reduce the severity of neurologic morbidity.

Electroencephalographic monitoring has only limited value and is generally not recommended, except to detect seizures (see Chapter 594) or as an adjunct in the clinical evaluation of brain death (see Chapter 67.1). *Seizures should be treated if possible,* although they tend to be very refractory. There is no evidence that treatment of seizures after drowning improves outcome. Fosphenytoin or phenytoin (loading dose of 10–20 mg of phenytoin equivalents [PE]/kg, followed by maintenance dosing of 5–8 mg of PE/kg/day in 2–3 divided doses; levels should be monitored) may be considered as an anticonvulsant; it may have some neuroprotective effects and may mitigate neurogenic pulmonary edema. Benzodiazepines, barbiturates, and other anticonvulsants may also have some role in seizure therapy in these patients (see Chapter 594).

With optimal management, many initially comatose children can have impressive neurologic improvement, usually within the 1st 24–72 hr. Unfortunately, almost ½ of deeply comatose children admitted to the PICU die of their brain injury or survive with severe neurologic damage. Many children become brain dead (see Chapter 67.1); submersion injury is the 2nd leading cause of brain death in the PICU. Deeply comatose drowning victims who do not substantially improve on neurologic examination after 24–72 hr of aggressive cardiorespiratory support and whose coma cannot be otherwise explained should be seriously considered for limitation or withdrawal of support (see Chapter 67).

OTHER MANAGEMENT ISSUES. A few submersion victims may have traumatic injury (see Chapter 71), especially if they were participating in water sports, such as boating, diving, or surfing. A high index of suspicion is required. Spinal precautions should be maintained in victims with altered mental status and suspected traumatic injury. Significant anemia suggests trauma and internal hemorrhage.

Hypoxic-ischemic injury can have multiple systemic effects, although protracted organ dysfunction is uncommon in the absence of severe CNS injury. Even after initially severe pulmonary injury, with careful supportive management, lung function returns to normal in most drowning victims. Acute renal failure (see Chapter 536) after hypoxic-ischemic injury from acute tubular or cortical injury can result in proteinuria, glucosuria, hemoglobinuria, oliguria, or anuria. Diuretics, fluid restriction, and dialysis are occasionally needed to treat fluid overload or electrolyte disturbances; renal function usually normalizes in survivors. Rhabdomyolysis after drowning has been reported. Profuse bloody diarrhea and mucosal sloughing usually portend a grim prognosis; conservative management includes bowel rest, nasogastric suction, and gastric pH neutralization. Nutritional support for most drowning victims is usually not difficult, because the majority of children either die or recover quickly and resume a normal diet within a few days; enteral tube feeding or parenteral nutrition is occasionally indicated in children who do not recover quickly.

Almost half of drowning victims have a fever during the 1st 48 hr after submersion. Aggressive control of fever in comatose patients is warranted because hyperthermia may exacerbate brain injury after hypoxia-ischemia. Hyperthermia is usually not due to infection and resolves without antibiotics in approximately 80% of patients. Generally, prophylactic antibiotics are not recommended.

Occasionally, infection may occur after drowning and antimicrobial therapy should be considered in victims with persistent fever, worsening pulmonary or general clinical status, or other evidence of infection. Cultures should be obtained from the respiratory system and blood and, occasionally, the stomach, early in the hospital course. Different pathogens are associated with drowning in freshwater, seawater, and other contaminated water sources, and they vary geographically. Also, aspiration can lead to infection with organisms from the victim's own respiratory and gastrointestinal tracts. Therapeutic hypothermia may increase the risk of infectious complications. Patients are also at risk for nosocomial infection during hospitalization.

Aerobic gram-negative bacterial infection (see Chapters 201 and 202), especially with *Pseudomonas* and similar species, such as *Aeromonas* and *Burkholderia pseudomallei* (endemic to Southeast Asia), has been reported after drowning. These and other virulent gram-negative organisms may cause severe pneumonia or sepsis (see Chapter 176). Aerobic gram-positive bacteria, such as *Streptococcus pneumoniae* and *Staphylococcus aureus,* are seldom cultured from water at a drowning site, but may be part of a victim's endogenous flora and may be aspirated, leading to infection (see Chapters 180 and 181). Many species of fungi inhabit polluted water, but only a few have been reported as pathogens after drowning. *Pseudallescheria boydii* is the most commonly reported fungus, with incubation times reported from 1 wk to 6 mo. Generalized infection rarely causes late neurologic deterioration. This fungus is often resistant to treatment with amphotericin B, and miconazole is advised when invasive disease is diagnosed (see Chapter 230). In victims at risk for atypical pathogens, a consultation with an infectious disease specialist should be considered.

Severe permanent encephalopathy is seen in 10–30% of PICU survivors after drowning. Chronic neurologic sequelae (see Chapter 38) include lowered mentation, cerebral dysfunction, spastic quadriplegia, extrapyramidal syndromes, optic and cerebral atrophy, cortical blindness, peripheral neuromuscular damage, and persistent vegetative state.

Psychiatric and psychosocial sequelae are common (see Chapters 19 and 20). Grief, guilt, and anger are frequent. Divorce rates of up to 80% are reported within a few years of severe injury to children, and parents often report difficulties with employment or substance abuse. Friends and family may blame the parents for the event. Professional counseling, pastoral care, or social work referral should be considered for drowning victims and their families.

PROGNOSIS

Of hospitalized pediatric drowning victims, 15% die and as many as 20% survive with severe permanent neurologic damage. In children requiring PICU admission, only approximately ½ survive neurologically intact, 13–35% die, and 7–27% survive with severe brain damage. The outcomes for drowning victims are remarkably bimodal: The great majority of victims either have a good outcome (intact or mild neurologic injury) or a bad outcome (persistent vegetative state or death), with very few exhibiting intermediate neurologic injury.

Prehospital predictors of non-icy water immersion outcomes in King County, Washington, have been comprehensively evaluated.

Intact survival or mild neurologic impairment occurred in 91% of children with submersion duration <5 min and in 87% with resuscitation duration <10 min. Children with normal sinus rhythm, reactive pupils, or neurologic responsiveness at the scene virtually always had good outcomes (99%). In cases requiring advanced CPR, death or severe neurologic morbidity occurred in 93% of patients with submersion duration >10 min and in 100% of victims requiring resuscitation for >25 min. All victims with submersion duration of >25 min died in this study. However, there are rare case reports of intact recovery in non-icy water drowning after longer submersion or resuscitation duration, highlighting the difficulty in assigning absolute prognostic classifications based on prehospital and ED variables alone.

The GCS (see Chapter 66) has some limited utility in predicting recovery. Children with a score of 6 or more on hospital admission generally have a good outcome, whereas those with a score of 5 or less have a much higher probability of poor neurologic outcome. However, occasionally, children with a GCS score of 3 or 4 in the ED have complete recovery. Upward trends in the GCS score during the 1st several hours of hospitalization may indicate a better prognosis. Overall, early GCS assessments fail to adequately distinguish children who will survive intact from those with major neurologic injury.

Neurologic examination and progression during the 1st 24–72 hr are currently the best prognosticators of long-term CNS outcome. Children who regain consciousness within 48–72 hr, even after prolonged resuscitation, are unlikely to have serious neurologic sequelae. In a small series of comatose victims of non-icy water submersion, all survivors with a good outcome had spontaneous purposeful movements and normal brainstem function within 24 hr; good recovery did not occur in any child with abnormal brainstem function or absence of purposeful movements at 24 hr. In another small series of drowning victims who remained unconscious >24 hr and survived for at least 1 yr, 73% remained in a persistent vegetative state and the rest had severe neurologic impairment. These victims continued to have many complications and a high mortality rate: 45% died during the study's 1-year follow-up period.

The prognostic value of neurologic responsiveness during the 1st 48–72 hr of hospitalization was also observed in a larger retrospective series of 274 pediatric drowning victims. Of the victims who had an initial GCS score of 3 in the ED, only 14% survived intact. Overall, 67.5% were intact survivors. Of these, 95% demonstrated purposeful neurologic function within 48 hr. Patients with a documented 1st purposeful neurologic response within 6 hr all survived intact. Conversely, only 5.6% of children with poor outcomes (persistent vegetative state or death) had "purposeful" movement documented in the 1st 48 hr. Laboratory and technologic methods to improve prognostication have not yet proved superior to neurologic examination.

Early prognostic certainty in drowning can be elusive in many cases. Serial neurologic evaluation after cardiopulmonary resuscitation should be performed over the ensuing 48–72 hr, with consideration given to limitation or withdrawal of support in patients who do not have significant neurologic recovery, even though this may occur before absolute prognostic certainty is achieved.

PREVENTION

The best hope for a "cure" for drowning and its serious consequences lies in prevention (rather than rescue or resuscitation). The vast majority of drownings can be prevented (Table 73-2). The circumstances and events associated with drowning differ across situations, cultures, regions, and countries.

Physicians should be part of legislative and educational efforts toward change. Unfortunately, too few physicians are an adequate resource. Although drowning is a leading cause of injury and death in children, only ½ of pediatricians give any anticipatory guidance to their patients' parents and only ⅓ give any guidance to teenagers. Part of the problem is that only 17.9% of pediatricians noted having received formal drowning prevention education during their residency training.

TABLE 73-2. Strategies for Drowning Prevention in Recreational Water Settings

MULTIPLE LAYERS OF PROTECTION ARE NECESSARY TO EFFECTIVELY DECREASE RISK OF DROWNING.

Control of Environment:

Preventive measures for residential swimming pools:

- Isolation fencing should completely isolate the pool from the home.
  - Fence should be ≥5-ft-tall ornamental iron fence with vertical bars 3.25 in apart, horizontal crossbars at least 45 in apart, and no decorative cutouts.
  - Gates should be self-closing and self-latching, with latches mounted near top and inside of fenced area.
  - Minimize availability of chairs, boxes, and other implements that a child can use to climb the fence or reach the gate latch.
- Constant supervision by responsible sober adults is imperative whenever children are in or around water. Individual responsible for supervision should be clearly identified, and that person should not leave the site or be distracted by any other activities.
- Remove toys from pool area after swim time.
- Avoid soft pool covers. Pool covers should be American Society for Testing Materials approved.
- Door alarms, pool alarms, or automatic door locks may be helpful when used in conjunction with fencing and other preventative measures.

Additional preventive measures at recreational natural bodies of water:

- Environmental design of aquatic facilities is effective at reducing drowning risk, including buoys and markers delimiting swim areas, availability of life-saving devices, and prominent signs.
- Swim only at sites where a trained lifeguard is present.
- U.S. Coast Guard-approved personal flotation devices should be worn by adults and children at all times during boating activities.
- Know the local weather conditions and forecast before boating or swimming.

Education:

- Patients and parents should receive anticipatory guidance regarding drowning prevention during physician visits.
- Swimming lessons should be provided for all children >4 yr old.
- Teach children never to swim alone or in unsupervised areas.
- Parents and teenagers should receive CPR instruction.
- Teenagers should receive education regarding increased risk of drowning in conjunction with alcohol and drug use.
- Pediatricians should receive formal drowning prevention education during their residency training.

Legislation:

- Physicians should take an active role in legislative efforts to reduce drowning risk.

Multiple layers of protection are necessary to minimize the risk of pediatric drowning. Preventive efforts should include hazard assessment and removal, creation of barriers, and protection of those at risk. Unfortunately, most prevention research deals with drowning in recreational settings (swimming pools), but drowning in low- and middle-income countries occurs primarily in locations associated with everyday activities (canals, wells, dams). Prevention strategies must take into account specifics regarding the setting and situation.

Environmental design changes can reduce the risk of drowning. The U.S. Army Corps of Engineers found that environmental design changes at aquatic facilities, such as inland lakes, played a role in reducing recreation-related drownings by 73% between 1981 and 1995, even though public use of these facilities increased by 66%. Changes included buoys and markers to delimit swimming areas, availability of lifesaving devices, and prominent signs. In Bangladesh, environmental design changes aimed at changing flood control embankments had the unintended consequence of reducing accidental drowning deaths in children younger than 5 yr old. Environmental and equipment design is a primary means for drowning prevention recommended by the WHO.

Whenever possible, removal of the hazard by eliminating or draining unnecessary accumulations of water (baths, buckets, ponds) should be undertaken. Barriers are an effective method of drowning prevention. Flood control embankments should be created in flood-prone areas. Fencing should be used in various situations, such as around swimming pools, rural fishponds, irrigation canals, and construction ditches that can fill with rainwater. For rural homes or farmhouses in proximity to water, fencing around the home can be an effective barrier to contain children. Wells should be fitted with locked protective grills.

The residential swimming pool is an important focus of preventive efforts because of the high drowning rate at this site. In 1 study of pools where children drowned, 75% of pools were inadequately fenced. Brief lapses in supervision were involved in the great majority of drownings. Only 18% of submersions were witnessed, even though a supervising adult could be identified 84% of the time. Fewer than ½ of households had any member who knew basic CPR, and ½ of the children who died did not receive CPR until paramedics arrived.

Appropriate pool fencing could prevent up to 80% of drownings in young children. Fences should completely isolate the pool from the house and yard (isolation fencing). Isolation fencing is greatly superior to perimeter fencing (a 3-sided fence that encloses the property and pool) because perimeter fencing allows pool access through the home. Studies indicate that isolation fencing dramatically reduces the risk of drowning by nearly ½ compared with 3-sided fencing. Proper gates are also important and should be self-closing and self-latching, with latches mounted inside and near the top of the fence.

Not all fences are equally effective. In 1 study, the commonly used 4-ft-tall, large chain link (2.5-in mesh) fence could be scaled by 75% of 2 yr olds in an average time of 25.6 sec and by 100% of 4 yr olds in an average time of 11.5 sec. Obviously, no commonly used barrier is universally insurmountable to young children. However, in this study, the only barrier insurmountable to children 4 yr of age and younger was a 5-ft-tall ornamental iron fence (vertical bars 3.25 in apart, horizontal crossbars 45 in apart, and no decorative cutouts). Clever children may still be able to climb any fence using aids such as chairs or boxes, again emphasizing the need for multiple layers of preventive strategies.

Parents need to closely supervise children at every moment during swimming. Toys should be removed from the pool area at the end of swim time. Pool covers should be approved by the American Society for Testing Materials. However, because pool covers are often cumbersome, they are unlikely to be replaced immediately after swim time and therefore are not likely to be an effective barrier. The use of lightweight covers should be discouraged, because they do not prevent the child from entering the pool and may obscure visualization of the submerged child. Door alarms and automatically closing and locking doors are untested in efficacy. Swimming pool alarms alone cannot be recommended at this time; in all alarms tested, a significant number of false alarms and failure to alarm were noted.

Parents must be made aware that any body of water, no matter how innocuous, poses a drowning risk, especially to children 4 yr of age and younger. Educating parents about the risks of common household implements, such as bathtubs, buckets, toilets, and washing machines, should be every pediatrician's task. Community education should also be increased. Parents must be taught to remain with children throughout the entire bath time and should be warned not to trust supervisory responsibilities to other children. Buckets containing water should never be left unattended. Toilet covers and bathroom doors should be closed at all times. Children with epilepsy can enjoy swimming as long as close supervision is maintained; these children should be encouraged to shower in a glass-free cubicle rather than in a bathtub.

All persons should learn how to swim. Swimming instruction for school-aged children emphasizing swimming and water safety skills, especially in low- and middle-income countries, is associated with significant reductions in drowning fatalities. In the Australian state of Victoria, reduction of drowning deaths by >50% was observed in association with the introduction of widespread and well-documented school-based swimming and water safety training for children 5–14 yr old. Nonetheless, even children who know how to swim should be prevented from swimming in unsupervised circumstances. Infant and toddler swimming programs are popular throughout the USA, but children are not developmentally ready for swimming lessons until they are at least 4 yr old (AAP recommendations). Aquatic programs for infants and toddlers have not been shown to decrease the risk of drowning, and parents should not feel secure that their child is safe in water or safe from drowning as a result of such programs.

Supervision by lifeguards is a positive factor in reducing the likelihood of drowning. The U.S. Lifeguards Association (USLA) estimates that approximately 100,000 persons are saved annually by lifeguards; the chance that a person will drown while attending a beach protected by a USLA-affiliated lifeguard is calculated to be only 1 in 18 million. According to USLA data during 1988–1997, >¾ of drowning deaths at USLA sites occurred at times when beaches were unguarded. In Brazil, an extensive lifeguard system is also credited with significant contributions to drowning prevention and rescue. Basic resuscitation skills must be learned by all volunteer and professional rescuers as well as laypersons who frequent aquatic areas or supervise others in water environments. The immediate institution of optimal CPR techniques is the most important factor for survival after drowning has occurred.

A National Transportation Safety Board review found that only 15% of boaters who drowned wore a personal flotation device (PFD). In a study of boaters in the northwest USA, only 25% wore a PFD. Use was highest in children younger than age 5 yr (91%) and lowest in those older than age 14 yr (13%). If no adult on a boat wore a PFD, then only 65% of children wore a PFD; if at least 1 adult wore a PFD, then 95% of children wore a PFD as well. Intensive community boating education efforts have been shown to substantially increase PFD use. Water safety education for children, teenagers, and parents that encourages PFD use and emphasizes the importance of never swimming alone should be reinforced in the school, community, and physician's office. Teenagers should learn CPR and receive counseling about alcohol and drug use (see Chapter 113), which significantly contributes to submersion and drowning.

American Heart Association: 2005 American Heart Association Guidelines for cardiopulmonary resuscitation and emergency cardiovascular care. *Circulation* 2005;112(Suppl):IV-133–IV-138.

Bierens JJ, Knape JT, et al: Drowning. *Curr Opin Crit Care* 2002;8:578–586.

Brenner RA: Prevention of drowning in infants, children, and adolescents. *Pediatrics* 2003;112:440–445.

Centers for Disease Control and Prevention: Nonfatal and fatal drownings in recreational water settings—United States, 2001–2002. *MMWR* 2004: 53:447–452.

Christensen DW, Jansen P, Perkin RM: Outcome and acute care hospital costs after warm water near-drowning in children. *Pediatrics* 1997;99:715–721.

Harries M: Near drowning. *BMJ* 2003;327:1336–1338.

Jacinto SJ, Gieron-Korthals M, et al: Predicting outcome in hypoxic-ischemic brain injury. *Pediatr Clin North Am* 2001;48:647–660.

Quan L, Cummings P: Characteristics of drowning by different age groups. *Inj Prev* 2003;9:163–168.

Thompson DC, Rivara FP: Pool fencing for preventing drowning in children. *Cochrane Database Syst Rev* 2000;2:CD001047.

Zuckerman GB, Gregory PM, Santos-Damiani SM: Predictors of death and neurologic impairment in pediatric submersion injuries. *Arch Pediatr Adolesc Med* 1998;152:134–140.

Chapter 74 ■ Burn Injuries

Alia Y. Antoon and Mary K. Donovan

Burns are a leading cause of unintentional death in children, 2nd only to motor vehicle crashes. There has been a decline in the incidence of burn injury requiring medical care over the last decade. This has coincided with an increased focus on burn treatment and prevention, increased fire and burn prevention education, greater availability of regional treatment centers, widespread use of smoke detectors, greater regulation of consumer products and occupational safety, and societal changes such as reduced smoking and alcohol abuse.

EPIDEMIOLOGY. Approximately 1.2 million people in the United States require medical care for burn injuries each year, with 51,000 requiring hospitalization. Approximately 30–40% of these patients are younger than 15 yr of age, with an average age of 32 mo. Fires are a major cause of mortality in children, accounting for up to 34% of fatal injuries in those younger than 16 yr. Scald burns account for 85% of total injuries and are most prevalent in children younger than 4 yr of age. Although the incidence of hot water scalding has been reduced by legislation requiring new water heaters to be preset at 120°F, scald injury remains the leading cause of hospitalization for burns. Steam inhalation used as a home remedy to treat respiratory infections is another potential cause for burns. Flame burns account for 13%; the remaining are electrical and chemical burns. Clothing ignition has declined since passage of the Federal Flammable Fabric Act, requiring sleepwear to be flame-retardant; however, the Consumer Product Safety Commission voted to relax the existing children's sleepwear flammability standard. Approximately 18% of burns are the result of child abuse (usually scalds), making it important to assess the pattern and site of injury and their consistency with the patient history (see Chapter 36). Friction burns from treadmills are also a problem. Hands are the most commonly injured sites, with deep 2nd-degree friction injury sometimes associated with fractures of the fingers. Anoxia, not the actual burn, is a major cause of morbidity and mortality in house fires.

Review of the history usually shows a common pattern: scald burns to the side of the face, neck, and arm if liquid is pulled from a table or stove; burns in the pant leg area if clothing ignites; burns in a splash pattern from cooking; and burns on the palm of the hand from contact with a hot stove. However, "glove or stocking" burns of the hands and feet; single-area deep burns on the trunk, buttocks, or back; and small, full-thickness burns (cigarette burns) in young children should raise the suspicion of child abuse (see Chapter 36).

Burn care involves a range of activities: prevention, acute care and resuscitation, wound management, pain relief, reconstruction, rehabilitation, and psychosocial adjustment. Children with massive burns require early and appropriate psychologic and social support as well as resuscitation. Surgical débridement, wound closure, and rehabilitative efforts should be instituted concurrently to promote optimal rehabilitation. Aggressive surgical removal of devitalized tissue, infection control, and judicious use of antibiotics, as well as early nutrition and cautious use of intubation and mechanical ventilation, are necessary to maximize survival. Children who have sustained burn injuries differ in appearance from their peers, necessitating supportive efforts for re-entry to school and social and sporting activities.

PREVENTION. The aim is a continuing reduction in the number of serious burn injuries (Table 74-1). Effective first aid and triage can decrease both the extent (area) and the severity (depth) of injuries. The use of flame-retardant clothing and smoke detectors, control of hot water temperature (thermostat settings) within buildings, and prohibition of cigarette smoking have been partially successful in reducing the incidence of burn injuries. Treatment of children with significant burn injuries in dedicated burn centers facilitates medically effective care, improves survival, and leads to greater cost efficiency. Survival of at least 80% of patients with burns of 90% of the body surface area (BSA) is possible; the overall survival rate of children with burns of all sizes is 99%. Death is more likely in children with irreversible anoxic brain injury sustained at the time of the burn.

Pediatricians can play a major role in preventing the most common burns by educating parents and health care providers. The growing number of treadmill injuries indicates the need for consumer education to reduce and prevent these injuries. These efforts must be geared to the various stages of child development. Simple, effective, efficient, and cost-effective preventive measures include the use of appropriate clothing, smoke detectors, and planned routes for emergency exit from the home. Child neglect and abuse must be seriously considered when the history of the injury and the distribution of the burn do not match.

TABLE 74-1. Burn Prophylaxis

PREVENT FIRES
Install and use smoke detectors
Control the hot water thermostat;—in public buildings, the maximum water temperature should be 120°F
Keep fire, matches, and lighters out of the reach of children
Avoid cigarette smoking, especially in bed
Do not leave lit candles unattended
Use flame retardant–treated clothing
Use caution when cooking, especially with oil
Keep cloth items off heaters
PREVENT INJURY
Roll, but do not run, if clothing catches fire; wrap in a blanket
Practice escape procedures
Crawl beneath smoke if a fire occurs indoors
Use educational materials*

*National Fire Protection Association pamphlets and videos.

ACUTE CARE, RESUSCITATION, AND ASSESSMENT

INDICATIONS FOR ADMISSION. Burns covering >10–15% of total BSA, burns associated with smoke inhalation, burns resulting from high-tension (voltage) electrical injuries, and burns associated with suspected child abuse or neglect should be treated as emergencies and the child hospitalized (Table 74-2). Small 1st- and 2nd-degree burns of the hands, feet, face, perineum, and joint surfaces also require admission if close follow-up care is difficult to provide. Children who have been in enclosed-space fires and those who have face and neck burns should be hospitalized for at least 24 hr for observation for signs of central nervous system (CNS) effects of anoxia from carbon monoxide poisoning or pulmonary effects from smoke inhalation.

FIRST AID MEASURES. Acute care should include the following:

TABLE 74-2. Indications for Hospitalization for Burns

Burns affecting >15% of body surface area
Electrical burns caused by high-tension wires
Inhalation injury, regardless of the amount of body surface area burned
Inadequate home situation
Suspected child abuse or neglect
Burns to the hands, feet, or genitals

1. Extinguish flames by rolling on the ground; cover the child with a blanket, coat, or carpet.
2. After determining that the airway is patent, remove smoldering clothing or clothing saturated with hot liquid. Jewelry, particularly rings and bracelets, should be removed or cut away to prevent constriction and vascular compromise during the edema phase in the 1st 24–72 hr after burn injury.
3. In cases of chemical injury, brush off any remaining chemical, if powdered or solid; then use copious irrigation or wash the affected area with water. Call Poison Control for the neutralizing agent to treat a chemical ingestion.
4. Cover the burned area with clean, dry sheeting and apply cold (not iced) wet compresses to small injuries. Significant large burn injury (>15–20% of BSA) decreases body temperature control and contraindicates the use of cold compress dressings.
5. If the burn is caused by hot tar, use mineral oil to remove the tar.
6. Administer analgesic medications.

TABLE 74-3. Acute Treatment of Burns
First aid
Fluid resuscitation
Provision of energy requirements
Control of pain
Prevention of infection—early excision and grafting
Prevention of excessive metabolic expenditures
Control of bacterial wound flora
Use of biologic and synthetic dressings to close the wound

EMERGENCY CARE. Life support measures should include the following (Table 74-3):

1. Rapidly review the cardiovascular and pulmonary status and document pre-existing or physiologic lesions (asthma, congenital heart disease, renal or hepatic disease).
2. Ensure and maintain an adequate airway and provide humidified oxygen by mask or endotracheal intubation (Fig. 74-1). The latter may be needed in children who have facial burns or a burn sustained in an enclosed space, before facial or laryngeal edema becomes evident. If hypoxia or carbon monoxide poisoning is suspected, 100% oxygen should be used (see Chapters 62 and 69).
3. Children with burns of >15% of BSA require intravenous fluid resuscitation to maintain adequate perfusion. All inhalation injuries, regardless of the extent of BSA burn, require venous access to control fluid intake. All high-tension and electrical injuries require venous access to ensure forced alkaline diuresis in case of muscle injury to avoid myoglobinuric renal damage. Lactated Ringer solution, 10–20 mL/kg/hr (normal saline may be used if lactated Ringer is not available), is initially infused until proper fluid replacement can be calculated. Consultation with a specialized burn unit should be made to coordinate fluid therapy, the type of fluid, the preferred formula for calculation, and preferences for the use of colloid agents, particularly if transfer to a burn center is anticipated.
4. Evaluate the child for associated injuries, which are common in patients with a history of high-tension electrical burn, especially if there has been a fall from a height. Injuries to the spine, bones, and thoracic or intra-abdominal organs may occur (see Chapter 71). The child should be placed on cervical spine precaution until this injury is ruled out. There is a very high risk of cardiac abnormalities, including ventricular tachycardia or ventricular fibrillation, resulting from conductivity of the high electric voltage. Cardiopulmonary resuscitation should be instituted promptly at the scene, and the patient should be placed on a cardiac monitor on arrival at the emergency department (see Chapter 62).

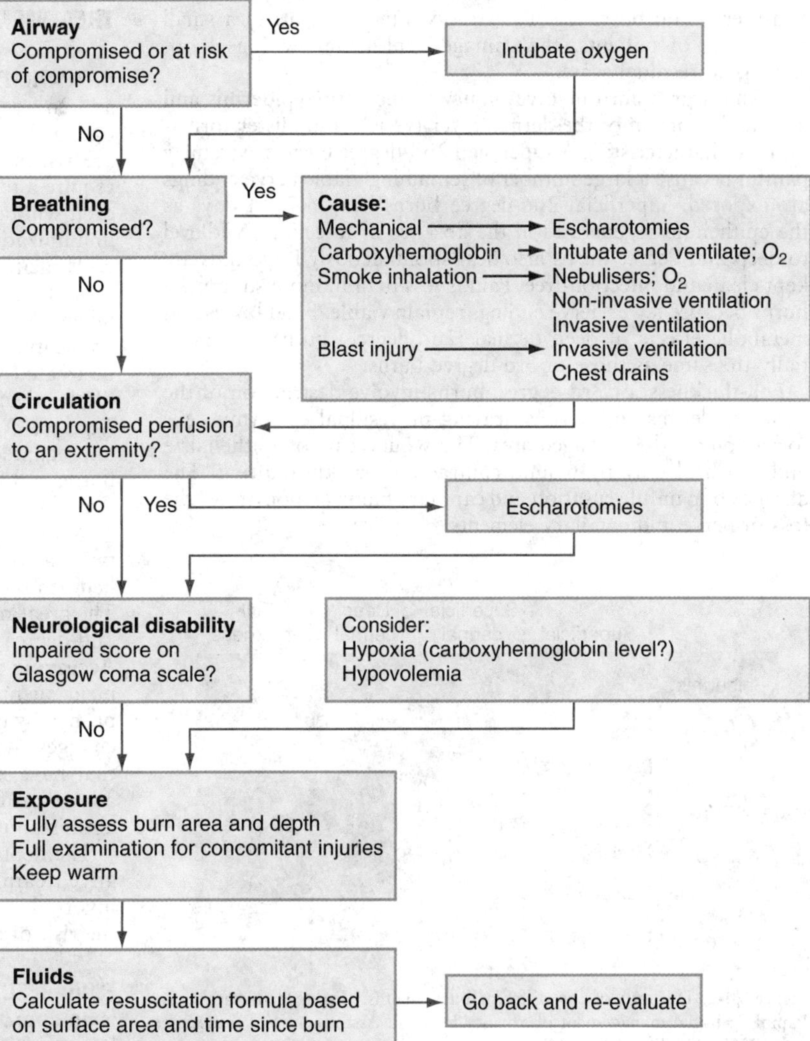

Figure 74-1. Algorithm for the primary survey of a major burn injury. O_2, oxygen. (From Hettiaratchy S, Papini R: Initial management of a major burn: I. Overview. *BMJ* 2004;328:1555–1557.)

TABLE 74-4. Categories of Burn Depth

	1ST-DEGREE BURN	2ND-DEGREE, OR PARTIAL-THICKNESS BURN	3RD-DEGREE, OR FULL-THICKNESS BURN
Surface appearance	Dry, no blisters. Minimal or no edema. Erythematous. Blanches, bleeds.	Moist blebs, blisters. Underlying tissue is mottled pink and white, with fair capillary refill. Bleeds.	Dry, leathery eschar. Mixed white, waxy, khaki, mahogany, soot-stained. No blanching or bleeding.
Pain	Very painful	Very painful	Insensate
Histologic depth	Epidermal layers only	Epidermis, papillary, and reticular layers of dermis. May include domes of subcutaneous layers.	Down to and may include fat, subcutaneous tissue, fascia, muscle, and bone
Healing time	2–5 days with no scarring	Superficial: 5–21 days with no grafting. Deep partial: 21–35 days with no infection. If infected, converts to full-thickness burn.	Large areas require grafting, but small areas may heal from the edges after wks.

5. **Children with burns of >15% of BSA should not receive oral fluids (initially), because gastric distention may develop. These children require insertion of a nasogastric tube in the emergency department to prevent aspiration.**
6. **A Foley catheter should be inserted to monitor urine output in all children who require intravenous fluid resuscitation.**
7. **All wounds should be wrapped with sterile towels until a decision is made about whether to treat the patient on an outpatient basis or refer the patient to an appropriate facility for treatment.**
8. **A carbon monoxide level (carboxy hemoglobin) should be obtained for fire victims and 100% oxygen administered until the result is known.**

CLASSIFICATION OF BURNS. Proper triage and treatment of burn injury require assessment of the extent and depth of the injury (Table 74-4 and Fig. 74-2). **First-degree burns** involve only the epidermis and are characterized by swelling, erythema, and pain (similar to a mild sunburn). Tissue damage is usually minimal, and there is no blistering. Pain resolves in 48–72 hr; in a small percentage of patients, the damaged epithelium will peel off, leaving no residual scars.

A **2nd-degree burn** involves injury to the entire epidermis and a variable portion of the dermal layer (vesicle and blister formation are characteristic). A **superficial** 2nd-degree burn is extremely painful because a large number of remaining viable nerve endings are exposed. Superficial 2nd-degree burns heal in 7–14 days as the epithelium regenerates in the absence of infection. Midlevel to deep 2nd-degree burns also heal spontaneously if wounds are kept clean and infection-free. Pain is less than in more superficial burns because fewer nerve endings remain viable. Fluid losses and metabolic effects of deep dermal (2nd-degree) burns are essentially the same as those of 3rd-degree burns.

Full-thickness, or 3rd-degree, burns involve destruction of the entire epidermis and dermis, leaving no residual epidermis cells to repopulate the damaged area. The wound cannot epithelialize and can heal only by wound contraction or skin grafting. The absence of painful sensation and capillary filling demonstrates the loss of nerve and capillary elements.

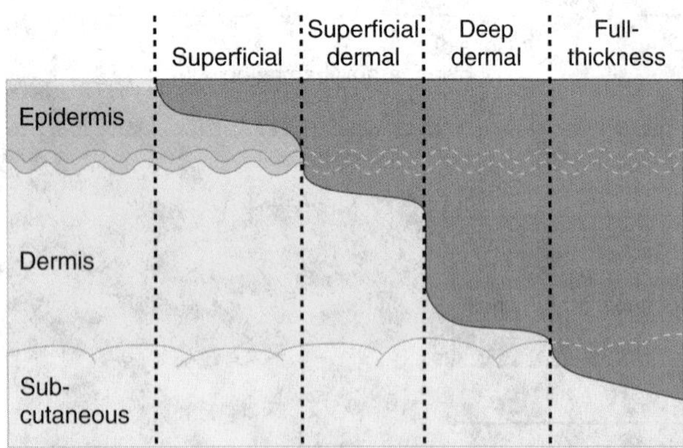

Figure 74-2. Diagram of the different burn depths. (From Hettiaratchy S, Papini R: Initial management of a major burn: II. Assessment and resuscitation. *BMJ* 2004;329:101–103.)

ESTIMATION OF BODY SURFACE AREA FOR A BURN. Appropriate burn charts for different childhood age groups should be used to accurately estimate the extent of BSA burned. The volume of fluid needed in resuscitation is calculated from the estimation of the extent and depth of burn surface. Mortality and morbidity also depend on the extent and depth of the burn. The variable growth rate of the head and extremities throughout childhood makes it necessary to use BSA charts, such as that modified by Lund and Brower or the chart used at the Shriners Hospital in Boston (Fig. 74-3). The **rule of nines** used in adults may be used only in children older than age 14 yr or as a very rough estimate to institute therapy before transfer to a burn center. In small burns of <10% of BSA, the **rule of palm** may be used, especially in outpatient settings. The area from the wrist crease to the finger crease (the palm) in the child equals 1% of the child's BSA.

TREATMENT

OUTPATIENT MANAGEMENT OF MINOR BURNS. A patient with 1st- and 2nd-degree burns of <10% of BSA may be treated on an outpatient basis unless there is inadequate family support or there are issues of child neglect or abuse. These outpatients do not require a tetanus booster or prophylactic penicillin therapy. Children who are not current with immunizations should have their immunizations updated. Blisters should be left intact and dressed with bacitracin or silver sulfadiazine cream (Silvadene). Dressings should be changed once daily, after the wound is washed with lukewarm water to remove any cream left from the previous application. Very small wounds, especially those on the face, may be treated with bacitracin ointment and left open. Débridement of the devitalized skin is indicated when the blisters rupture. Aquacel Ag^+ dressing (ConvaTec) is a soft felt-like material impregnated with silver ion that may be applied to 2nd-degree burns and wrapped with a dry sterile dressing. When this dressing is applied, silver ion is directly in contact with the wound. This kind of dressing should be kept on for 10 days, but checked twice a week. Burns to the palm with large blisters usually heal beneath the blisters, with close follow-up on an outpatient basis. The great majority of superficial burns heal in 10–20 days. Deep 2nd-degree burns take longer to heal and may benefit from Accuzyme ointment (HealthPoint), which is an enzyme débridement agent to be applied daily. Pain control should be accomplished by using acetaminophen with codeine 1 hr before dressing changes. Wounds that appear deeper than at initial assessment or that have not healed by 21 days may require a short hospital admission for grafting. Pruritus during healing is managed with antihistamines.

The depth of scald injuries is difficult to assess early; conservative treatment is appropriate initially, with the depth of the area involved determined before grafting is attempted. This obviates the risk of anesthesia and unnecessary grafting.

FLUID RESUSCITATION. For most children, the Parkland formula is an appropriate starting guideline for fluid resuscitation (4 mL lactated Ringer/kg/% BSA burned). Half of the fluid is given over

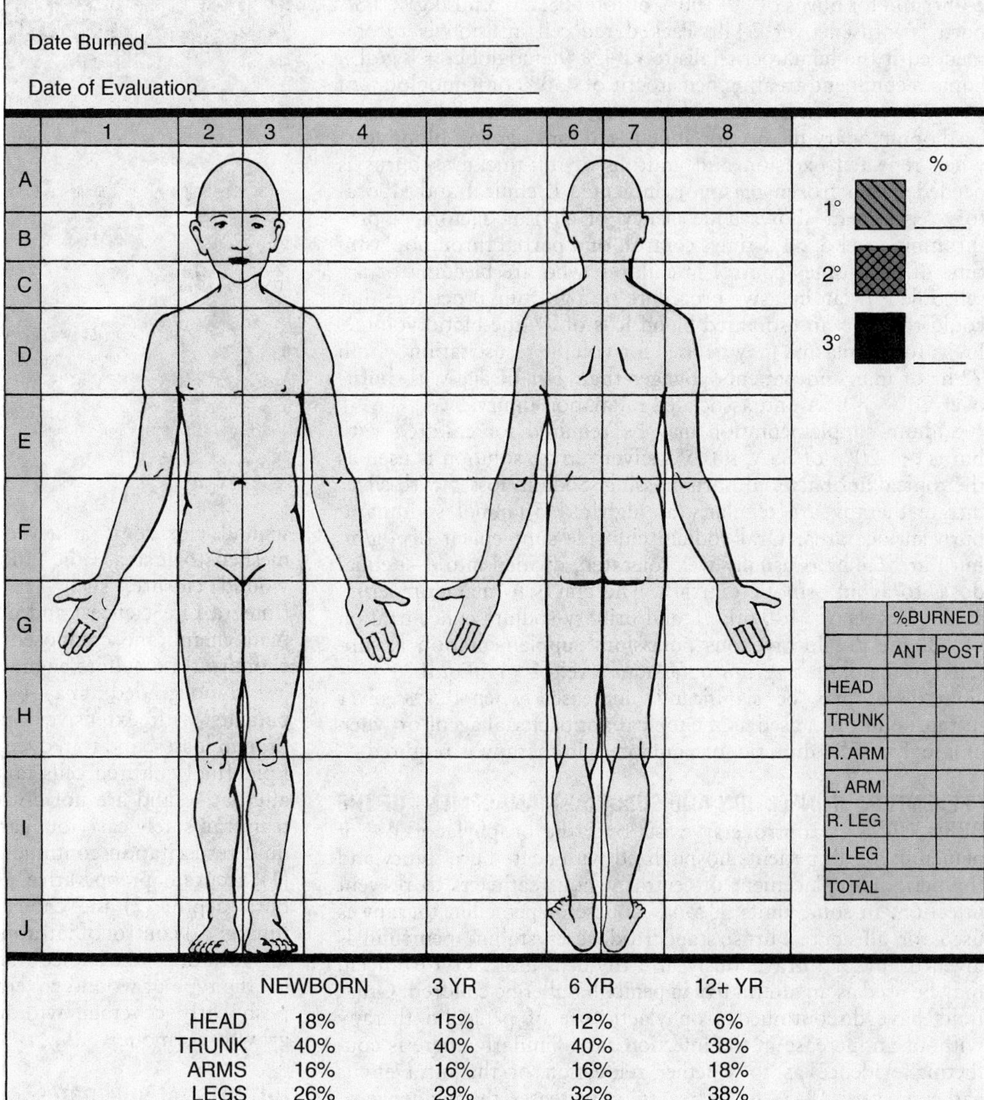

Figure 74-3. Chart to determine the developmentally related percentage of body surface area affected by a burn injury. ANT, anterior; POST, posterior; R., right; L., left. (Courtesy of Shriners Hospital for Crippled Children, Burn Institute, Boston Unit.)

the 1st 8 hr, calculated from the time of onset of injury. The remaining ½ is given at an even rate over the next 16 hr. The rate of infusion is adjusted according to the patient's response to therapy. Pulse and blood pressure should return to normal, and an adequate urine output (>1 mL/kg/hr in children; 0.5–10 mL/kg/hr in adolescents) should be accomplished by varying the intravenous infusion rate. Vital signs, acid-base balance, and mental status reflect the adequacy of resuscitation. Because of interstitial edema and sequestration of fluid in muscle cells, patients may gain up to 20% over baseline pre-burn body weight. Patients with burns of 30% of BSA require a large venous access (central venous line) to deliver the fluid required over the critical 1st 24 hr. Patients with burns of >60% of BSA may require a multilumen central venous catheter; these patients are best cared for in a specialized burn unit. In addition to fluid resuscitation, children should receive standard maintenance fluids (see Chapter 53).

During the 2nd 24 hr after the burn, patients begin to reabsorb edema fluid and to diurese. Half of the 1st day's fluid requirement is infused as lactated Ringer solution in 5% dextrose. Children younger than age 5 yr may require the addition of 5% dextrose in the 1st 24 hr of resuscitation. Controversy exists as to whether colloid should be provided in the early period of burn resuscitation. One preference is to use colloid replacement concurrently if the burn is >85% of total BSA. Colloid is usually instituted 8–24 hr after the burn injury. In children younger than 12 mo of age, sodium tolerance is limited; the volume and sodium concentration of the resuscitation solution should be decreased if urinary sodium is rising. The adequacy of resuscitation should be constantly assessed using vital signs, urine output, blood gases, hematocrit, and protein levels. Some patients require arterial and central venous lines, particularly those undergoing multiple excision and grafting procedures, as needed, for monitoring and replacement purposes. Central venous pressure monitoring may be indicated to assess circulation in patients with hemodynamic or cardiopulmonary instability. Femoral vein cannulation is a safe access for fluid resuscitation, especially in infants and children. Burn patients who require frequent blood gas monitoring benefit from radial or femoral arterial catheterization.

Oral supplementation may start as early as 48 hr postburn. Milk formula, artificial feedings, homogenized milk, or soy-based products can be given by bolus or constant infusion through a nasogastric or small bowel feeding tube. As oral fluids are tolerated, intravenous fluids are decreased proportionately in an effort to keep the total fluid intake constant, particularly if pulmonary dysfunction is present.

A 5% albumin infusion may be used to maintain the serum albumin levels at a desired 2 g/dL. The following rates are effective: For burns of 30–50% of total BSA, 0.3 mL of 5% albumin/kg/% BSA burn is infused over a 24-hr period; for burns of 50–70% of total BSA, 0.4 mL/kg/% BSA burn is infused over

24 hr; and for burns of 70–100% of total BSA, 0.5 mL/kg/% BSA burn is infused over 24 hr. Packed red cell infusion is recommended if the hematocrit falls to <24% (hemoglobin = 8 g/dL). Some recommend treating hematocrit of <30% or hemoglobin of <10 g/dL in patients with systemic infection, hemoglobinopathy, cardiopulmonary disease, or anticipated (or ongoing) blood loss, when repeated excision and grafting of full-thickness burns is needed. Fresh frozen plasma is indicated if clinical and laboratory assessment shows a deficiency of clotting factors, a prothrombin level of >1.5 times control, or a partial thromboplastin time of >1.2 times control in children who are bleeding or are scheduled for an invasive procedure or a grafting procedure that could result in an estimated blood loss of >½ the blood volume. Fresh frozen plasma may be used for volume resuscitation within 72 hr of injury in patients younger than 2 yr of age with burns over 20% of BSA and associated inhalation injury.

Sodium supplementation may be required for children with burns of >20% of BSA, if 0.5% silver nitrate solution is used as the topical antibacterial burn dressing. Sodium losses with silver nitrate therapy are regularly as high as 350 mmol sodium/m^2 burn surface area. Oral sodium chloride supplement of 4 g/m^2 burn area/24 hr is usually well tolerated, divided into 4–6 equal doses to avoid osmotic diarrhea. The aim is to maintain serum sodium levels of >130 mEq/L and urinary sodium concentration of >30 mEq/L. Intravenous potassium supplementation is supplied to maintain a serum potassium level of >3 mEq/dL. Potassium losses may be significantly increased when 0.5% silver nitrate solution is used as the topical antibacterial agent or when aminoglycoside, diuretic, or amphotericin therapy is required.

PREVENTION OF INFECTION AND SURGICAL MANAGEMENT OF THE BURN WOUND. Controversy exists over the prophylactic use of penicillin for all patients hospitalized with acute burn injury and the periodic replacement of central venous catheters to prevent infection. In some units, a 5-day course of penicillin therapy is used for all acute burns; standard-dose crystalline penicillin is given orally or intravenously in 4 divided doses. Erythromycin may be used as an alternative in penicillin-allergic children. Other units have discontinued prophylactic use of penicillin therapy without an increase in the infection rate. Similarly, there is conflicting evidence as to whether relocation of the intravenous catheter every 48–72 hr decreases or increases the incidence of catheter-related sepsis. Some recommend that the central venous catheter be replaced and relocated every 5–7 days, even if the site is not inflamed and there is no suspicion of catheter-related sepsis.

Mortality related to burn injury is associated not with the toxic effect of thermally injured skin, but with the metabolic and bacterial consequences of a large open wound, reduction of the patient's host resistance, and malnutrition. These abnormalities set the stage for life-threatening bacterial infection originating from the burn wound. Wound treatment and prevention of wound infection also promote early healing and improve aesthetic and functional outcomes. Topical treatment of the burn wound with 0.5% silver nitrate solution, silver sulfadiazine cream, or mafenide acetate (Sulfamylon) cream or topical solution aims at prevention of infection (Table 74-5). These 3 agents have tissue-penetrating capacity. Regardless of the choice of topical antimicrobial agent, it is essential that all 3rd-degree burn tissue be fully excised before bacterial colonization occurs and that the area be grafted as early as possible to prevent deep wound sepsis. Children with a burn of >30% of BSA should be housed in a bacteria-controlled nursing unit to prevent cross-contamination and to provide a temperature- and humidity-controlled environment to minimize hypermetabolism.

Deep 2nd-degree burns of >10% of BSA benefit from early excision and grafting. To improve outcome, sequential excision and grafting of 3rd-degree and deep 2nd-degree burns is required in children with large burns. Prompt excision with immediate wound closure is achieved with autografts, which are often meshed to increase the efficiency of coverings. Alternatives for wound closure, such as allografts, xenografts, and Integra (Integra LifeSciences) and other synthetic skin coverings (bilaminate membrane composed of a porous lattice of cross-linked chondroitin-6-sulfate engineered to induce neovascularization as it is biodegraded), may be important for wound coverage in patients with extensive injury to limit fluid, electrolyte, and protein losses, and to reduce pain and minimize temperature loss. Epidermal cultured cells (autologous keratinocytes) are a costly alternative and are not always successful. An experienced burn team can safely carry out early-stage or total excision while burn fluid resuscitation continues. Important keys to success include: (1) accurate preoperative and intraoperative determination of burn depth; (2) the choice of excision area and appropriate timing; (3) control of intraoperative blood loss; (4) specific instrumentation; (5) the choice and use of perioperative antibiotics; and (6) the type of wound coverage chosen. This process can accomplish early coverage without the use of recombinant human growth hormone.

TABLE 74-5. Topical Agents Used for Burns

AGENT	EFFECTIVENESS	EASE OF USE
Silver sulfadiazine Silvadene cream	Broad spectrum Good penetration	Closed dressings Changed twice daily Residue *must* be washed off with each dressing change
Mafenide acetate	Broad spectrum, including *Pseudomonas* Rapid and deep wound penetration	Closed dressings Changed twice daily Residue *must* be washed off with each dressing changed
0.5% silver nitrate solution	Bacteriostatic	Closed bulky dressing soaked every 2 hr and changed once daily
Aquacel Ag[+]	• Broad spectrum, including some fungi Superficial penetration Dressing impregnated with silver	Applied directly to 2nd-degree burn; occlusive dressing kept for 10 days
Accuzyme ointment	Topical enzymatic débridement	Applied daily

NUTRITIONAL SUPPORT. Supporting the increased energy requirements of a patient with a burn is a high priority. The burn injury produces a hypermetabolic response characterized by both protein and fat catabolism. Depending on the time since the burn, children with a burn of 40% of total BSA require approximately 50–100% > predicted basal energy expenditure (oxygen consumption) for their age. Early excision and grafting can decrease the energy requirement. Pain, anxiety, and immobilization increase the physiologic demands. Additional energy expenditure is caused by cold stress if environmental humidity and temperature are not controlled; this is especially true in young infants, in whom the large surface area-mass ratio allows proportionately > heat loss than in adolescents and adults. Providing environmental temperatures of 28–33°C, adequate covering during transport, and liberal use of analgesics and anxiolytics can decrease calorie demands. Special units to control ambient temperature and humidity may be necessary for children with large surface area burns. Appropriate sleep intervals are necessary and should be part of the regimen. Sepsis increases metabolic rates, and early enteral nutrition initially with high-carbohydrate, high-protein caloric support (1,800 cal/m^2/24 hr maintenance plus 2,200 cal/m^2 of burn/24 hr) reduces metabolic stress.

The objective of caloric supplementation programs is to maintain body weight and minimize weight loss by meeting metabolic demands. This reduces the loss of lean body mass. Calories are provided at approximately 1½ times the basal metabolic rate, with 3–4 g/kg of protein/day. The focus of nutritional therapy is to support and compensate for the metabolic needs. Multivitamins, particularly the B vitamin group, vitamin C, vitamin A, and zinc, are also necessary.

Alimentation should be started as soon as is practical, both enterally and parenterally, to meet all of the caloric needs and keep the gastrointestinal tract active and intact after the resuscitative phase. Patients with burns of >40% of total BSA need a flexible nasogastric or small bowel feeding tube to facilitate continuous delivery of calories without the risk of aspiration. To decrease the risk of infectious complications, parenteral nutrition is discontinued as soon as is practical, after delivery of sufficient enteral calories is established. Continuous gastrointestinal feeding is essential, even if feeding is interrupted, causing frequent visits to the operating room until full grafting takes place. The use of anabolic agents (growth hormone, oxandrolone, low-dose insulin) or anticatabolic agents (propranolol) remains controversial, although β-blocking may reduce metabolic stress.

TOPICAL THERAPY. Topical therapy is widely used and is effective against most burn pathogens (see Table 74-5). A number of topical agents are used: 0.5% silver nitrate solution, sulfacetamide acetate cream or solution, silver sulfadiazine cream, and Accuzyme ointment or Aquacel Ag^+. Accuzyme is an enzymatic débridement agent and may cause a stinging feeling for 15 min after application. Preferences vary among burn units. Each topical agent has advantages and disadvantages in application, comfort, and bacteriostatic spectrum. Sulfacetamide acetate is a very effective broad-spectrum agent with the ability to diffuse through the burn eschar; thus, it is the treatment of choice in injury to cartilaginous surfaces, such as the ears. The carbonic anhydrase inhibition activity of sulfacetamide may cause acid-base imbalance if large surface areas are treated, and adverse reactions to the sulfur-containing agents may produce transient leukopenia. This latter reaction is mostly noted with the use of silver sulfadiazine cream when applied over large surface areas in children younger than 5 yr. This phenomenon is transient, self-limiting, and reversible. No sulfa-containing agent should be used if the child has a history of sulfa allergies.

INHALATIONAL INJURY. Inhalational injury is serious in the infant and child, particularly if pre-existing pulmonary conditions are present (see Chapter 69). Mortality estimates vary, depending on the criteria for diagnosis, but are 45–60% in adults; exact figures are not available in children. Evaluation aims at early identification of inhalation airway injuries. These may occur from (1) direct heat (greater problems with steam burns); (2) acute asphyxia; (3) carbon monoxide poisoning; and (4) toxic fumes, including cyanides from combustible plastics. Sulfur and nitrogen oxides and alkalis formed during the combustion of synthetic fabrics produce corrosive chemicals that may erode mucosa and cause significant tissue sloughing. Exposure to smoke may cause degradation of surfactant and decrease its production, resulting in atelectasis. Inhalation injury and burn injury are synergistic, and the combined effect can increase morbidity and mortality.

The pulmonary complications of burns and inhalation can be divided into 3 syndromes that have distinct clinical manifestations and temporal patterns:

1. **Early carbon monoxide poisoning, airway obstruction, and pulmonary edema are major concerns.**
2. **The acute respiratory distress syndrome usually becomes clinically evident later, at 24–48 hr, although it can occur even later (see Chapter 69).**
3. **Late complications (days to weeks) include pneumonia and pulmonary emboli.**

Inhalation injury should be assessed by the evidence of obvious injury (swelling or carbonaceous material in the nasal passages), wheezing, crackles or poor air entry, and laboratory determination of carboxyhemoglobin (HbCO) and arterial blood gases.

Treatment is initially focused on establishing and maintaining a patent airway through prompt and early nasotracheal or orotracheal intubation and adequate ventilation and oxygenation. Wheezing is common, and β-agonist aerosols or inhaled corticosteroids are useful. Aggressive pulmonary toilet and chest physiotherapy are necessary in those with prolonged nasotracheal intubation or in the rare patient with a tracheotomy. The availability of less irritating endotracheal tube materials, as well as improved tube and cuff design, has allowed progressively longer periods of translaryngeal intubation. An endotracheal tube can be maintained for months without the need for tracheostomy. If tracheotomy has to be performed, it should be delayed until burns at and near the site have healed, and then it should be performed electively, with the child under anesthesia and using optimal tracheal positioning and hemostasis. In children with inhalation injury or burns of the face and neck, upper airway obstruction can develop rapidly; endotracheal intubation becomes a lifesaving intervention. Extubation should be delayed until the patient meets the accepted criteria for maintaining the airway.

Signs of CNS injury from hypoxemia due to asphyxia or carbon monoxide poisoning vary from irritability to depression. Carbon monoxide poisoning may be mild (<20% HbCO), with slight dyspnea, headache, nausea, and decreased visual acuity and higher cerebral functions; moderate (20–40% HbCO), with irritability, agitation, nausea, dimness of vision, impaired judgment, and rapid fatigue; or severe (40–60% HbCO), producing confusion, hallucination, ataxia, collapse, acidosis, and coma. Measurement of HbCO is important for diagnosis and treatment. Pa_{O_2} may be normal and the oxyhemoglobin saturation values misleading because HbCO is not detected by the usual tests of oxygen saturation. Carbon monoxide poisoning is assumed until the tests are performed, and it is treated with 100% oxygen. Significant carbon monoxide poisoning requires hyperbaric oxygen therapy (see Chapter 58).

Patients with severe inhalation injury or with other causes of respiratory deterioration that lead to acute respiratory distress syndrome who do not improve with conventional pressure-controlled ventilation (progressive oxygenation failure, as manifested by oxygen saturation of <90% while on F_{IO_2} of 0.9–1.0 and positive end-expiratory pressure of at least 12.5 cm H_2O) may benefit from high-frequency ventilation or nitric oxide inhalation treatment. Nitric oxide usually is administered through the ventilator at 5 parts per million (ppm) and increased to 30 ppm. This method of therapy reduces the need for extracorporeal membrane oxygenation.

PAIN RELIEF AND PSYCHOLOGIC ADJUSTMENT. See Chapter 66. It is important to provide adequate analgesia, anxiolytics, and psychologic support to reduce early metabolic stress, decrease the potential for post-traumatic stress syndrome, and allow future stabilization and physical and psychologic rehabilitation. Patients and family members require team support to work through the grieving process and accept long-term changes in appearance.

Children with burn injury show frequent and wide fluctuations in pain intensity. Appreciation of pain depends on the depth of the burn; the stage of healing; the patient's age and stage of emotional development and cognition; the experience and efficiency of the treating team; the use of analgesics and other drugs; the patient's pain threshold; and interpersonal and cultural factors. From the onset of treatment, **preemptive pain control** during dressing changes is of paramount importance. The use of a variety of nonpharmacologic interventions as well as pharmacologic agents needs to be reviewed throughout the treatment period. Opiate analgesia, prescribed in an adequate dose and timed to cover dressing changes, is essential to comfort management. A supportive person who is consistently present and "knows" the patient profile can integrate and encourage patient participation in burn care. The problem of undermedication is most prevalent in adolescents, in whom fear of drug dependence may inappropriately influence treatment. A related problem is that the child's specific pain experience may be misinterpreted; for anxious patients, those who are confused and alone, or those with preexisting emotional disorders, even small wounds may illicit intense pain. Anxiolytic medication added to the analgesic is usually helpful and has more than a synergistic effect. Equal attention is necessary to decrease stress in the intubated patient. Other modalities of pain and anxiety relief (relaxation techniques) can decrease the physiologic stress response. Oral morphine sulfate (immediate-release) is recommended on a consistent schedule at a dose of 0.3–0.6 mg/kg every 4–6 hr initially and until wound cover is accomplished. Morphine sulfate intravenous bolus at a dose of 0.05–0.1 mg/kg every 2 hr is administered in older patients using a patient-controlled analgesia protocol. Morphine sulfate rectal suppositories may be useful at an added dose of 0.3–0.6 mg/kg every 4 hr. For anxiety, lorazepam is given on a consistent schedule, 0.05–0.1 mg/kg/dose every 8 hr. To control pain during a procedure (dressing changes or débridement), oral morphine at a dose of 0.3–0.6 mg/kg is given 1–2 hr before the procedure, and this is supplemented by a morphine intravenous bolus at a dose of 0.05–0.1 mg/kg given immediately before the procedure. Lorazepam at a dose of 0.04 mg/kg is given orally, or intravenously if necessary, for anxiety before the procedure. Midazolam (Versed) is also very useful for conscious sedation, given at a dose of 0.05–0.1 mg/kg/hr as an infusion or a bolus; it may be repeated in 10 min, with a maximum dose of 0.2 mg/kg. During the process of weaning from analgesics, the dose of oral opiates is reduced by 25% over 1–3 days, sometimes with the addition of acetaminophen as opiates are tapered. Antianxiety medications are tapered by reducing the dose of benzodiazepines at 25–50%/dose daily over 1–3 days.

For ventilated patients, pain control is accomplished by using morphine sulfate intermittently as an intravenous bolus at a dose of 0.05–0.1 mg/kg every 2 hr. Doses may need to be increased gradually, and some children may need continuous infusion; a starting dose of 0.05 mg/kg/hr given as an infusion is increased gradually as the need of the child changes. Naloxone is rarely needed, but should be immediately available to reverse the effect of morphine, if necessary; if needed for an airway crisis, it should be given in a dose of 0.1 mg/kg up to a total of 2 mg, either intramuscularly or intravenously. For patients on assisted respiration who require treatment of anxiety, midazolam is used as an intermittent intravenous bolus (0.04 mg/kg given by slow push every 4–6 hr) or as a continuous infusion. Intubated patients do not require opiates to be discontinued during the process of weaning from the ventilator. Benzodiazepine should be reduced to approximately ½ the dose over 24–72 hr before extubation; too-rapid weaning from a benzodiazepine can lead to seizures.

RECONSTRUCTION AND REHABILITATION. To ensure maximum cosmetic and functional outcome, occupational and physical therapy must begin on the day of admission, continue throughout hospitalization, and for some patients, continue after discharge. Physical rehabilitation involves body and limb positioning, splinting, exercises (active and passive movement), assistance with activities of daily living, and gradual ambulation. These measures maintain adequate joint and muscle activity with as normal a range of movement as possible after healing or reconstruction. Pressure therapy is necessary to reduce hypertrophic scar formation; a variety of prefabricated and custom-made garments are available for use in different body areas for prevention of hypertrophic scarring. These custom-made garments deliver consistent pressure on scarred areas; they shorten the time of scar maturation and decrease the thickness of the scar as well as the redness and associated itching. Continued adjustments to scarred areas (scar release, grafting, rearrangement) and multiple minor cosmetic surgical procedures are necessary to optimize long-term function and improve appearance. Replacement of areas of alopecia and scarring has been achieved using tissue expander techniques.

SCHOOL RE-ENTRY AND LONG-TERM OUTCOME. It is best for the child to return to school immediately after discharge. Occasionally, a child may need to attend a few half-days (because of rehabilitation needs). However, it is important for the child to return to his or her normal routine of attending school and being with peers. Planning for a return to home and school often requires a *school re-entry program* that is individualized to each child's needs. For a school-aged child, planning for the return to school occurs simultaneously with planning for discharge. The hospital schoolteacher contacts the local school and plans the program with the school faculty, nurses, social workers, recreational/child life therapists, and rehabilitation therapists. This team should work with students and staff to ease anxiety, answer questions, and provide information. Burns and scars evoke fears in those who are not familiar with this type of injury and can result in a tendency to withdraw from or reject the burned child. A school re-entry program should be appropriate to a child's development and changing educational needs.

Major advances have made it possible to save the lives of children with massive burns; whereas some children have had lingering physical difficulties, most have a satisfactory quality of life. The comprehensive burn care that includes experienced multidisciplinary aftercare plays an important role in recovery. Long-term complications of burns are noted in Table 74-6.

TABLE 74-6. Common Long-Term Disabilities in Patients with Burn Injuries

DISABILITIES AFFECTING THE SKIN AND SOFT TISSUE
Hypertrophic scars
Susceptibility to minor trauma, chemicals, or cold
Dry skin
Contractures
Itching and neuropathic pain
Alopecia
Chronic open wounds
Skin cancers
ORTHOPEDIC DISABILITIES
Amputations
Contractures
Heterotopic ossification
Osteoporosis
METABOLIC DISABILITIES
Heat exhaustion
Obesity
PSYCHIATRIC AND NEUROLOGIC DISABILITIES
Sleep disorders
Adjustment disorders
Post-traumatic stress syndrome
Depression
Neuropathy and neuropathic pain
Long-term neurologic effects of carbon monoxide poisoning
Anoxic brain injury
LONG-TERM COMPLICATIONS OF CRITICAL CARE
Deep-vein thrombosis, venous insufficiency, or varicose veins
Tracheal stenosis, vocal cord disorders, or swallowing disorders
Renal or adrenal dysfunction
Hepatobiliary or pancreatic disease
Cardiovascular disease
Reactive airway disease or bronchial polyposis
PRE-EXISTING DISABILITIES THAT CONTRIBUTED TO THE INJURIES
Substance abuse
Risk-taking behavior
Untreated or poorly treated psychiatric disorder

Modified from Sheridan RL, Schultz JT, Ryan CM, et al: Case 6-2004: A 35-year-old woman with extensive, deep burns from a nightclub fire. *N Engl J Med* 2004;350:810–821.

SPECIAL SITUATIONS

ELECTRICAL BURNS. There are 3 types of electrical burns. Minor electrical burns usually occur as a result of biting on an extension cord. These injuries produce localized burns to the mouth, which usually involve the portions of the upper and lower lips that come in contact with the extension cord. The injury may involve or spare the corners of the mouth. Because these are nonconductive injuries (do not extend beyond the site of injury), hospital admission is not necessary and care is focused on the area of the injury visible in the mouth. Treatment with topical antibiotic creams is sufficient until the patient is seen in a burn unit outpatient department or by a plastic surgeon.

A more serious category of electrical burn is the high-tension electrical wire burn, for which children need to be admitted for observation, regardless of the extent of the surface area burn. Deep muscle injury is typical and cannot be readily assessed initially. These injuries result from high voltage (>1,000 V) and occur particularly at high-voltage installations, such as electric power stations or railroads; children climb an electric pole and touch an electric box out of curiosity or accidentally touch a high-tension electric wire. Such injuries have a mortality rate of 3–15% for children who arrive at the hospital for treatment. Survivors have a high rate of morbidity, including major limb amputations. Points of entry of current through the skin and the exit site show characteristic features consistent with current density and heat. The majority of entrance wounds involve the upper extremity, with small exit wounds in the lower extremity. The electrical path, from entrance to exit, takes the shortest distance between the 2 points and may produce injury in any organ or tissue in the path of the current. Multiple exit wounds in some patients attest to the possibility of several electrical pathways in the body, placing virtually any structure in the body at risk (Table 74-7). Damage to the abdominal viscera, thoracic structures, and the nervous system in areas remote from obvious extremity injury occurs and must be sought, particularly in injuries with multiple current pathways or those in which the victim falls from a high pole. Sometimes **arcing** occurs and results in concurrent flame burn and clothing fire. Cardiac abnormalities manifested by ventricular fibrillation or cardiac arrest are common; patients with high-tension electrical injury need cardiac monitoring until they are stable and have been fully assessed. Higher-risk patients have an abnormal electrocardiogram and a history of loss of consciousness. Renal damage from deep muscle necrosis and subsequent myoglobinuria is another complication; such patients need forced alkaline diuresis to minimize renal damage. Aggressive removal of all dead and devitalized tissue, even with the risk of functional loss, remains the key to effective management of the electrically damaged extremity. Early débridement facilitates early closure of the wound. Damaged major vessels must be isolated and buried in a viable muscle to prevent exposure. Survival depends on immediate intensive care, whereas a functional result depends on long-term care and delayed reconstructive surgery.

Lightning burns occur when a high-voltage current directly strikes a person (most dangerous) or when the current strikes the ground or an adjacent (in-contact) object. A step voltage burn is observed when lightning strikes the ground and travels up 1 leg and down the other leg (the path of least resistance). Lightning burns are dependent on the current path, the type of clothing worn, the presence of metal, and cutaneous moisture. Entry, exit, and path lesions are possible; the prognosis is poorest for lesions of the head or legs. Internal organ injury along the path is common and does not relate to the severity of the cutaneous burn. Linear burns, usually 1st- or 2nd-degree, are in the locations where sweat is present. Feathering or an arborescent pattern is characteristic of lightning injury. Lightning may ignite clothing or produce serious cutaneous burns from heated metal in the clothing. Internal complications of lightning burns include cardiac arrest caused by asystole, transient hypertension, premature ventricular contractions, ventricular fibrillation, and myocardial ischemia. Most severe cardiac complications resolve if the patient is supported with cardiopulmonary resuscitation (see Chapter 66). CNS complications include cerebral edema, hemorrhage, seizures, mood changes, depression, and paralysis of the lower extremities. Rhabdomyolysis and myoglobinuria (with possible renal failure) also occur.

TABLE 74-7. Electrical Injury: Clinical Considerations

	CLINICAL MANIFESTATIONS	MANAGEMENT
General		Extricate the patient; perform ABCs of resuscitation; immobilize the spine History: voltage, type of current CBC with platelets, electrolytes, BUN, creatinine, glucose
Cardiac	Dysrhythmias: asystole, ventricular fibrillation, sinus tachycardia, sinus bradycardia, PVC, PAC, conduction defects, atrial fibrillation, ST-T wave changes	Treat dysrhythmias Cardiac monitor, ECG, and chest x-ray film with suspected thoracic injury CPK with isoenzymes if indicated
Pulmonary	Respiratory arrest, acute respiratory distress, aspiration syndrome	Protect and maintain the airway Mechanical ventilation if indicated, chest x-ray film, ABG level
Renal	Acute renal failure, myoglobinuria	Provide aggressive fluid management unless a CNS injury is present Maintain adequate urine output >1 mL/kg/hr Consider CVP or pulmonary artery pressure monitoring Measure urine myoglobin; perform urinalysis; measure BUN, creatinine
Neurologic	**Immediate:** loss of consciousness, motor paralysis, visual disturbances, amnesia, agitation; intracranial hematoma **Secondary:** pain, paraplegia, brachial plexus injury, SIADH, autonomic disturbances, cerebral edema **Delayed:** paralysis, seizures, headache, peripheral neuropathy	Treat seizures Provide fluid restriction if indicated Consider spine x-ray films, especially cervical CT scan of the brain if indicated
Cutaneous/oral	Oral commissure burns, tongue and dental injuries; skin burns resulting from ignition of clothes, entrance and exit burns, and arc burns	Search for the entrance/exit wound Treat cutaneous burns; determine the tetanus status Obtain a plastic surgery of ENT consult if needed
Abdominal	Viscus perforation and solid organ damage; ileus; abdominal injury rare without visible abdominal burns	Place an NG tube if the patient has airway compromise or ileus Obtain SGOT, SGPT, amylase, BUN, and creatinine measurements and, CT radiographs as indicated
Musculoskeletal	Compartment syndrome from subcutaneous necrosis limb edema and deep burns Long bone fractures, spine injuries	Follow the patient for compartment syndrome Obtain x-ray films and orthopedic/general surgery consultations as indicated
Ocular	Visual changes, optic neuritis, cataracts, extraocular muscle paresis	Obtain an ophthalmology consultation as indicated

From Hall ML, Sills RM: Electrical and lightning injuries. In Barkin RM (editor): *Pediatric Emergency Medicine.* St. Louis, CV Mosby, 1997, p 484.

ABC, airway, breathing, circulation; ABG, arterial blood gas; BUN, blood urea nitrogen; CBC, complete blood cell count; CNS, central nervous system; CPK, creatinine phosphokinase; CVP, central venous pressure; ECG, electrocardiogram; ENT, ear, nose, and throat; NG, nasogastric; PAC, premature atrial contractions; PVC, premature ventricular contractions; SIADH, syndrome of inappropriate secretion of antidiuretic hormone; SGOT, serum glutamate oxaloacetate transaminase (aspartate aminotransferase); SGPT, serum glutamate pyruvate transaminase (alanine aminotransferase).

RENAL FAILURE IN BURN INJURY. See Chapter 535. Renal failure in burn injury is best classified in relation to the time of onset after the burn injury. Most cases present as nonoliguric renal failure; careful monitoring of fluids and electrolytes is critical. Special considerations concerning renal failure in a child with burn injury include the initial phase of capillary leak, making resuscitation difficult; severe catabolic stress, with increased risk of hyperkalemia; and rapid development of azotemia. Such children require high caloric and protein intake to prevent catabolic stress and promote wound healing.

Renal failure may occur early or late, after 1–3 wk. Early renal failure may occur immediately after the burn injury if late resuscitation with subsequent hypovolemia occurs (acute tubular necrosis) or if severe pigment nephropathy (hemoglobinuria with burn injury in an enclosed space or myoglobinuria secondary to deep muscle injury or after escharotomy) develops. This is associated with early maximal catabolic stress, and frequently, dialysis is necessary to sustain the circulation in the presence of marked capillary leak and to provide sufficient calories and protein to minimize catabolic stress. Late renal failure may result from sepsis or drug toxicity. At this time, there is less catabolic stress, and standard indications for dialysis apply.

Ali SN, O'Toole G, Tyler M: Milk bottle burns. *J Burn Care Rehabil* 2004;25:461–462.
Arnoldo B, Purdue GF, Kowalske K, et al: Electrical injuries: A 20-year review. *J Burn Care Rehabil* 2004;25:479–484.
Benson A, Dickson WA, Boyce DE: Burns. *BMJ* 2006;332:649–652.
Collier ML, Ward RS, Saffle JR, et al: Home treadmill friction injuries: A five-year review. *J Burn Care Rehabil* 2004;25:441–444.
Faustino EV, Apkon M: Persistent hyperglycemia in critically ill children. *J Pediatr* 2005;146:30–34.
Garrel D: Burn scars: A new cause of vitamin D deficiency. *Lancet* 2004;363:259–260.
Gosain A, Gamelli RL: Role of the gastrointestinal tract in burn sepsis. *J Burn Care Rehabil* 2005;26:85–91.
Herndon DN, Hart DW, Wolf SE, et al: Reversal of catabolism by beta-blockade after severe burns. *N Engl J Med* 2001;345:1223–1229.
Herndon DN, Tompkins RG: Support of the metabolic response to burn injury. *Lancet* 2004;363:1895–1902.
Hettiaratchy S, Dziewulski P: Pathophysiology and types of burns. *BMJ* 2004;328:1427–1429.
Hettiaratchy S, Papini R: Initial management of a major burn: I. Overview. *BMJ* 2004;328:1555–1557.
Hettiaratchy S, Papini R: Initial management of a major burn: II. Overview. *BMJ* 2004;329:101–103.
Hohlfeld J, de Buys Roessingh A, Hiti-Burri N, et al: Tissue engineered fetal skin constructs for paediatric burns. *Lancet* 2006;366:840–842.
Hudspith J, Rayatt S: First aid and treatment of minor burns. *BMJ* 2004;328:1487–1489.
Istre GR, McCoy MA, Osborn L, et al: Deaths and injuries from house fires. *N Engl J Med* 2001;344:1911–1916.
Juurlink DN, Buckley NA, Stanbrook MB, et al: Hyperbaric oxygen for carbon monoxide poisoning. *Cochrane Database Syst Rev* 2005;1:CD002041.
Milner S, Hodgetts T, Rylah L: The burns calculator: A simple proposed guide for fluid resuscitation. *Lancet* 1993;342:1089–1091.
Moore P, Blackeney P, Broemeling L, et al: Psychologic adjustment after childhood burn injuries as predicted by personality traits. *J Burn Care Rehabil* 1993;14:80–82.
Musgrave MA, Fingland R, Gomez M, et al: The use of inhaled nitric oxide as adjuvant therapy in patients with burn injuries and respiratory failure. *J Burn Care Rehabil* 2000;21:551–557.
Remensnyder JP: Acute electrical injuries. In Martyn JAJ (editor): *Acute Management of the Burned Patient.* Philadelphia, WB Saunders, 1990, pp 66–86.
Sheridan RL, Hinson M, Liang MH, et al: Long-term outcomes of children surviving massive burns. *JAMA* 2000;283:69–73.
Sheridan RL, Schultz JT, Ryan CM, et al: Case 6–2004: A 35-year-old woman with extensive, deep burns from a nightclub fire. *N Engl J Med* 2004;350:810–821.
Wiechman SA, Patterson DR: Psychosocial aspects of burn injuries. *BMJ* 2004;329:391–393.
Wright JB, Lam K, Burrell RE: Wound management in an era of increasing bacterial antibiotic resistance: A role for topical silver treatment. *Am J Infect Control* 1998;26:572–577.
Volinsky J, Hanson J, Lustig J: Lightning burns. *Arch Pediatr Adolesc Med* 1994;148:529–530.
Walker A: Emergency department management of house fire burns and carbon monoxide poisoning in children. *Curr Opin Pediatr* 1996;8:239–242.
Zaritsky A, Nadkarni VM, Hickey RW, et al: PALS Provider Manual. American Academy of Pediatrics, 2002.

Chapter 75 ■ Cold Injuries

Alia Y. Antoon and Mary K. Donovan

The involvement of children and youth in snowmobiling, mountain climbing, winter hiking, and skiing places them at risk for cold injury. Cold injury may produce either local tissue damage, with the injury pattern depending on exposure to damp cold (frostnip, immersion foot, or trench foot), dry cold (which leads to local frostbite), or generalized systemic effects (hypothermia).

PATHOPHYSIOLOGY. Ice crystals may form between or within cells, interfering with the sodium pump, and lead to rupture of cell membranes. Further damage may result from clumping of red blood cells or platelets, causing microembolism or thrombosis. Blood may be shunted away from an affected area by secondary neurovascular responses to the cold injury; this shunting often further damages an injured part while improving perfusion of other tissues. The spectrum of injury ranges from mild to severe and reflects the result of structural and functional disturbance in small blood vessels, nerves, and skin.

ETIOLOGY. In general, body heat may be lost by conduction (wet clothing, contact with metal or other solid conducting objects), convection (wind chill), evaporation, and radiation. Susceptibility to cold injury may be increased by dehydration, alcohol or drug use, substance abuse, impaired consciousness, exhaustion, hunger, anemia, impaired circulation due to cardiovascular disease, and sepsis, as well as in very young or aged persons.

Hypothermia occurs when the body can no longer sustain normal core temperature by physiologic mechanisms, such as vasoconstriction, shivering, muscle contraction, and nonshivering thermogenesis. When shivering ceases, the body is unable to maintain its core temperature; when the body core temperature falls to <35°C, the syndrome of hypothermia occurs. Wind chill, wet or inadequate clothing, and other factors increase local injury and may cause dangerous hypothermia, even in the presence of an ambient temperature that is not <17–20°C (50–60°F).

CLINICAL MANIFESTATIONS

FROSTNIP. Frostnip results in the presence of firm, cold, white areas on the face, ears, or extremities. Blistering and peeling may occur over the next 24–72 hr, occasionally leaving mild increased hypersensitivity to cold for some days or weeks. Treatment consists of warming the area with an unaffected hand or a warm object before the lesion reaches a stage of stinging or aching and before numbness supervenes.

IMMERSION FOOT (TRENCH FOOT). Immersion foot occurs in cold weather when the feet remain in damp or wet, poorly ventilated boots. The feet become cold, numb, pale, edematous, and clammy. Tissue maceration and infection are likely, and prolonged autonomic disturbance is common. This autonomic disturbance leads to increased sweating, pain, and hypersensitivity to temperature changes, which may persist for years. The treatment is largely prophylactic and consists of using well-fitting, insulated, waterproof, nonconstricting footwear. Once damage has occurred, patients must choose clothing and footwear that are more appropriate, dry, and well-fitting. The disturbance in skin integrity is managed by keeping the affected area dry and well ventilated and preventing or treating infection. Only supportive measures are possible for control of autonomic symptoms.

FROSTBITE. With frostbite, initial stinging or aching of the skin progresses to cold, hard, white anesthetic and numb areas. On rewarming, the area becomes blotchy, itchy, and often red, swollen, and painful. The injury spectrum ranges from complete normality to extensive tissue damage, even gangrene, if early relief is not obtained.

Treatment consists of warming the damaged area. It is important not to cause further damage by attempting to rub the area with ice or snow; initial warming, as in frostnip, may be tried. The area may be warmed against an unaffected hand, the abdomen, or an axilla while in transfer to a facility where more rapid warming with a water bath is possible. If the skin becomes painful and swelling occurs, anti-inflammatory agents are helpful and an analgesic agent is necessary. Freeze and re-thaw cycles are most likely to cause permanent tissue injury, and it may be necessary to delay definitive warming and apply only mild measures if the patient is required to walk on the damaged feet en route to definitive treatment. In the hospital, the affected area should be immersed in warm water (approximately 42°C), being careful not to burn the anesthetized skin. Vasodilating agents, such as prazosin or phenoxybenzamine, may be helpful. Anticoagulants (heparin, dextran) have provided equivocal results; results of chemical and surgical sympathectomy have also been equivocal. Oxygen is of help only at high altitudes. Meticulous local care, prevention of infection, and keeping the rewarmed area dry, open, and sterile provide optimal results. Recovery can be complete, and prolonged observation with conservative therapy is justified before any excision or amputation of tissue is considered. Analgesia and maintenance of good nutrition are necessary throughout the prolonged waiting period.

HYPOTHERMIA. Hypothermia may occur in winter sports when injury, equipment failure, or exhaustion decreases the degree of exertion, particularly if sufficient attention is not paid to wind chill. Immersion in frozen bodies of water and wet wind chill rapidly produce hypothermia. As the core temperature of the body falls, insidious onset of extreme lethargy, fatigue, incoordination, and apathy occurs, followed by mental confusion, clumsiness, irritability, hallucinations, and finally, bradycardia. A number of medical conditions, such as cardiac disease, diabetes mellitus, hypoglycemia, sepsis, β-blocking agent overdose, and substance abuse, may need to be considered in a differential diagnosis. The decrease in rectal temperature to <34°C (93°F) is the most helpful diagnostic feature. Hypothermia associated with drowning is discussed in Chapter 73.

Prevention is a high priority. Of extreme importance for those who participate in winter sports is wearing layers of warm clothing, gloves, socks within insulated boots that do not impede circulation, and a warm head covering, as well as applying adequate waterproofing and protecting against the wind. Thirty per cent of heat loss occurs from the head. Ample food and fluid need to be provided during exercise. Those who participate in sports should be alert to the presence of cold or numbing of body parts, particularly the nose, ears, and extremities, and they should review methods to produce local warming and know to seek shelter if they detect symptoms of local cold injury. Application of petrolatum (Vaseline) to the nose and ears gives certain protection against frostbite.

Treatment at the scene aims at prevention of further heat loss and early transport to adequate shelter. Dry clothing should be provided as soon as practical, and transport should be undertaken if the victim has a pulse. If no pulse is detected at the initial review, cardiopulmonary resuscitation is indicated (see Chapters 61 and 66; Fig. 75-1). During transfer, jarring and sudden motion should be avoided because these may cause ventricular arrhythmia. It is often difficult to attain a normal sinus rhythm during hypothermia.

If the patient is conscious, mild muscle activity should be encouraged and a warm drink offered. If the patient is unconscious, external warming should be initially undertaken using blankets and a sleeping bag, often with snuggling with a warm companion to increase the efficiency of warming. On arrival at a treatment center, while a warming bath of 45–48°C (113–118°F) is prepared, the patient should be warmed through inhalation of warm, moist air or oxygen or with heating pads or thermal blankets. Monitoring of serum chemistry values and an electrocardiogram are necessary until the core temperature rises to >35°C and can be stabilized. Control of fluid, pH, blood pressure, and oxygen is necessary in the early phases of the warming period and resuscitation. In severe hypothermia, there may be a combined respiratory and metabolic acidosis. Hypothermia may falsely elevate pH; nonetheless, most recommend warming the arterial blood gas specimen to 37°C before analysis and considering the result as in a normothermic patient. In patients with marked abnormalities, warming measures, such as gastric or colonic irrigation with warm saline or peritoneal dialysis, may be considered, but the effectiveness of these measures in treating hypothermia is unknown. In accidental deep hypothermia (core temperature, 28°C) with circulatory arrest, rewarming with cardiopulmonary bypass may be lifesaving for previously healthy young individuals.

CHILBLAIN (PERNIO). Chilblain (pernio) is a form of cold injury in which erythematous, vesicular, or ulcerative lesions occur. The lesions are presumed to be of vascular or vasoconstrictive origin. They are often itchy and may be painful and result in swelling and scabbing. The lesions are most often found on the ears, the tips of the fingers and toes, and on exposed areas of the legs. The lesions last for 1–2 wk, but may persist for longer. Treatment consists of prophylaxis: avoiding prolonged chilling and protecting potentially susceptible areas with a cap, gloves, and stockings. Prazosin and phenoxybenzamine may be helpful in improving circulation if this is a recurrent problem. For significant itching, local corticosteroid preparations may be helpful.

COLD-INDUCED FAT NECROSIS (PANNICULITIS). This common, usually benign injury occurs on exposure to cold air, snow, or ice and is manifested in exposed (or, less often, covered) surfaces as red (or, less often, purple to blue) macular, papular, or nodular lesions. Treatment is with nonsteroidal anti-inflammatory agents. The lesions may last 10 days to 3 wk (see Chapter 659).

Britt LD, Dascombe WH, Rodriguez A: New horizons in management of hypothermia and frostbite injury. *Surg Clin North Am* 1991;71:345–370.

Cold injury. Berkow R (editor): *The Merck Manual of Diagnosis and Therapy 16th edition.* Rahway, NJ, Merck, Sharp, & Dohme, 1992.

Shephard RJ: Metabolic adaptations to exercise in the cold: An update. *Sports Med* 1993;16:266–289.

Walpoth BH, Walpoth-Aslan BN, Mattle HP, et al: Outcome of survivors of accidental deep hypothermia and circulatory arrest treated with extracorporeal blood warming. *N Engl J Med* 1997;337:1500–1505.

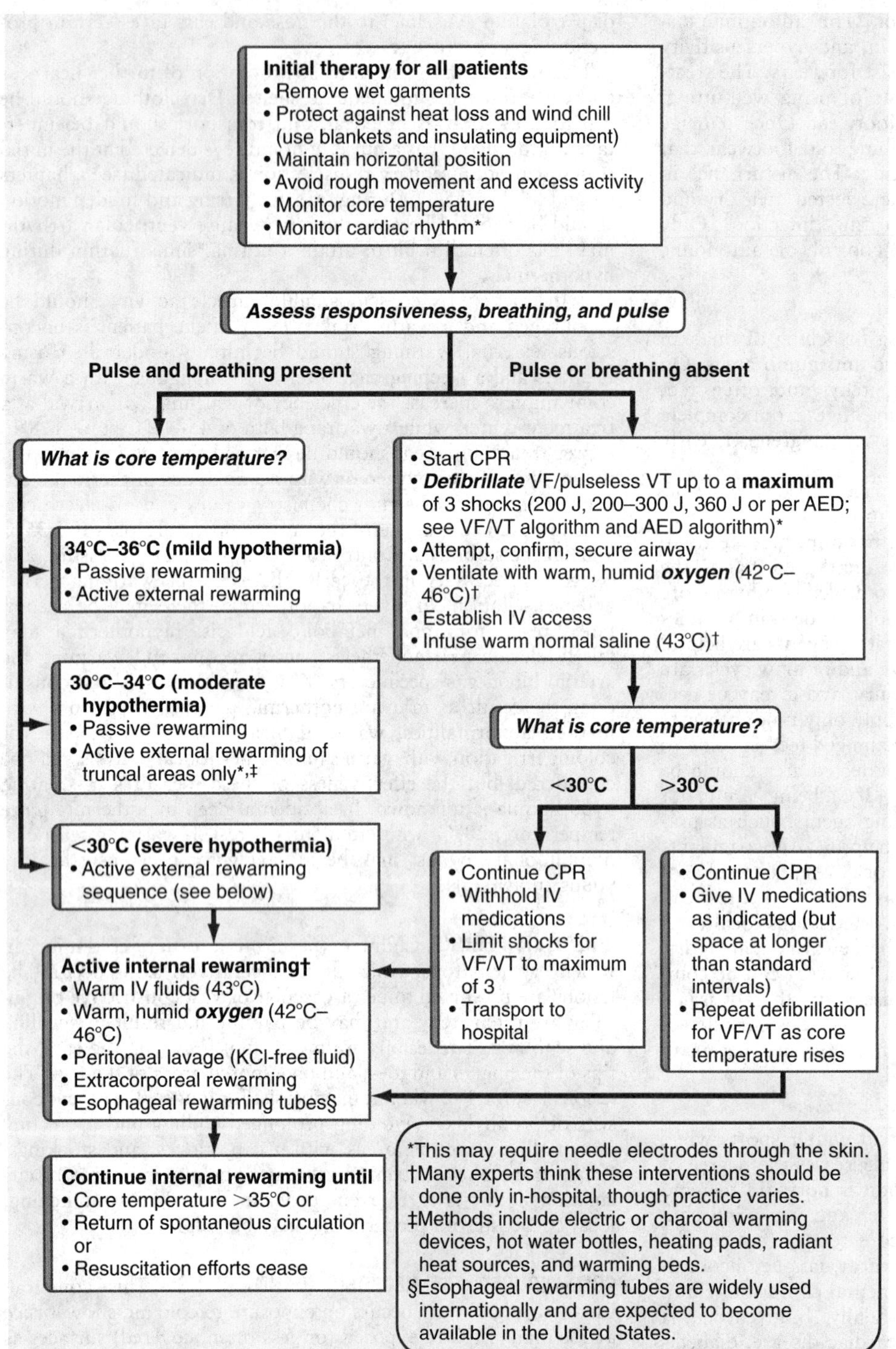

Figure 75-1. Hypothermia treatment algorithm for adult-size children and adolescents. AED, automated external defibrillator; VF, ventricular fibrillation; VT, ventricular tachycardia. *Fig. 66-3. (From American Heart Association: ECC guidelines. Part 8: Advanced challenges in resuscitation. Section 3: Special challenges in ECC. *Circulation* 2002;102: 1229.)

Chapter 76 ■ Anesthesia and Perioperative Care Randall C. Wetzel

The perioperative period is a high-risk time for infants and children. Potent drugs are used to blunt physiologic responses to what would be otherwise life-threatening trauma (surgery). Anesthesia is necessary on humane grounds. In addition, the appropriate application of anesthetic principles decreases the rate of mortality from surgery and painful procedures and enhances the child's ability to survive the surgical experience. Intraoperatively, the anesthesiologist is responsible for providing analgesia as well as physiologic and metabolic stability (Table 76-1). This is facilitated by obtaining a good preanesthesia history (Table 76-2). The increased risk of morbidity and mortality in the perioperative period demands the utmost vigilance. The risk is increased in certain disease states (Table 76-3). The primary purpose of general anesthesia is to suppress the conscious perception of, and physiologic response to, noxious stimuli and to render the patient unconscious.

TABLE 76-1. Goals of Anesthesia

Analgesia
Amnesia and a decreased level of consciousness
Akinesia
Physiologic support and homeostatic management throughout the perioperative process
Vigilance

GENERAL ANESTHESIA

ANALGESIA. Providing analgesia for procedures both in and out of the operating room is a major responsibility and functions within a spectrum of care (Table 76-4). Techniques exist to provide profound pain relief during operative procedures for all patients, including the most critically ill infants. Blunting the physiologic responses to painful stimuli inhibits the stress response and its multiple deleterious physiologic and metabolic consequences. The response to painful and stressful stimuli is a potent stimulus of the **systemic inflammatory response syndrome (SIRS)**, which leads to increased catabolism, physiologic instability, and increased mortality. Appropriate use of medication, such as fentanyl anesthesia in neonates, reduces the incidence of postoperative bradycardia, hypotension, acidosis, and hypoglycemia.

HYPNOSIS AND AMNESIA. The blunting of both consciousness (**hypnosis**) and conscious recall (**amnesia**) is a crucial feature of pediatric anesthesia care. Awareness of painful, anxiety-provoking, and stressful conditions for children is just as deleterious, physically and psychologically, as the painful procedures themselves. Management is aimed at blunting the fear and emotional response during surgery, painful procedures (bone marrow aspiration, lumbar punctures), or nonpainful but anxiety-provoking procedures (MRI, CT). Many drugs provide anxiolysis, blunting of recall, and amnesia for such events (Table 76-5). Obtundation of consciousness may accompany the provision of analgesia. Hypnotic and sedative agents can induce altered consciousness without producing any analgesia; *analgesia* and *obtunded consciousness* are not synonymous. It is also possible to provide analgesia (local, spinal, or epidural analgesia) without obtunding consciousness.

Sedation describes a medically induced state that is on a continuum between the awakened state and general anesthesia (see Table 76-4). General anesthesia obtunds or ablates critical physiologic reflexes; the most important are **airway-protective reflexes:** coughing, gagging, and swallowing. Cardiorespiratory reflexes are also obtunded with general anesthesia; respiratory depression and hemodynamic compromise may occur. As sedation deepens toward general anesthesia, loss of airway patency, loss of airway-protective reflexes, and loss of cardiovascular stability occur. Light (minimal) sedation is anxiolysis without loss of these reflexes and airway patency. Deep sedation occurs when these reflexes are obtunded or lost (see Table 76-4). Adequate sedation in children may be accompanied by the actual or potential loss of vital reflexes. It is mandatory that those providing sedation for children be able to detect the transition into deep sedation and general anesthesia and be prepared to manage the child's airway and provide CPR if required.

AKINESIA (IMMOBILITY OR MUSCULAR RELAXATION). *Akinesia* is the absence of movement and is necessary to ensure safe and adequate operative conditions and to provide ideal conditions for advanced and meticulous surgery. Akinesia is produced with muscle relaxants (see Table 76-5). These agents facilitate respiratory management in the perioperative period and in critically ill patients. The absence of movement is neither the absence of pain nor the presence of amnesia. Whenever neuromuscular

TABLE 76-2. The Preanesthetic History

CHILD'S PREVIOUS ANESTHETIC AND SURGICAL PROCEDURES
Review the anesthetic record for information about the mask and endotracheal tube size, the type and size of laryngoscope used, difficulties with mask ventilation or intubation, and a history of **hyperthermia** or **acidosis**

PERINATAL PROBLEMS (ESPECIALLY FOR INFANTS)
Need for prolonged hospitalization
Need for supplemental oxygen or intubation
History of apnea and bradycardia

OTHER MAJOR ILLNESSES AND HOSPITALIZATIONS

FAMILY HISTORY OF ANESTHETIC COMPLICATIONS, MALIGNANT HYPERTHERMIA, OR PSEUDOCHOLINESTERASE DEFICIENCY

RESPIRATORY PROBLEMS
Chronic exposure to environmental tobacco smoke
Obstructive apnea, breathing irregularities, or cyanosis (especially in infants younger than age 6 mo)
History of snoring or an obstructive breathing pattern
Recent upper respiratory tract infection
Recurrent respiratory infections
Previous laryngotracheitis (croup)
Asthma or wheezing during respiratory infections

CARDIAC PROBLEMS
Murmur
Dysrhythmia
Exercise intolerance
Syncope
Cyanosis

GASTROINTESTINAL PROBLEMS
Reflux and vomiting
Feeding difficulties
Failure to thrive
Liver disease

EXPOSURE TO EXANTHEMS OR POTENTIALLY INFECTIOUS PATHOGENS

NEUROLOGIC PROBLEMS
Seizures
Developmental delay
Neuromuscular diseases
Increased intracranial pressure

HEMATOLOGIC PROBLEMS
Anemia
Bleeding diathesis
Tumor
Immunocompromise
Prior blood transfusions and reactions

RENAL PROBLEMS
Renal insufficiency, oliguria, anuria
Fluid and electrolyte abnormalities

PSYCHOSOCIAL CONSIDERATIONS
Post-traumatic stress
Drug abuse, use of cigarettes or alcohol
Physical or sexual abuse
Family dysfunction
Previous traumatic medical or surgical experience
Psychosis, anxiety, depression

GYNECOLOGIC CONSIDERATIONS
Sexual history (sexually transmitted infections)
Possibility of pregnancy

CURRENT MEDICATIONS
Prior administration of corticosteroids

ALLERGIES
Drugs
Iodine
Latex products
Surgical tape
Food allergies (especially soya and egg albumin)

DENTAL CONDITION (LOOSE OR CRACKED TEETH)

WHEN AND WHAT THE CHILD LAST ATE (ESPECIALLY IN EMERGENCY PROCEDURES)

TABLE 76-3. Specific Pediatric Diseases and Their Anesthetic Implications

DISEASE	IMPLICATIONS
RESPIRATORY SYSTEM	
Asthma	Intraoperative bronchospasm that may be severe
	Pneumothorax or atelectasis
	Optimal preoperative medical management is essential; may require preoperative steroids
Difficult airway	May require special equipment and personnel
	Should be anticipated in children with dysmorphic features or acute airway obstruction, as in epiglottitis or laryngotracheobronchitis or with an airway foreign body
	Patients with Down syndrome may require evaluation of the atlanto-occipital joint
	Patients with storage diseases may be at high risk
Bronchopulmonary dysplasia	Barotrauma with positive pressure ventilation
	Oxygen toxicity, pneumothorax a risk
Cystic fibrosis	Airway reactivity, bronchorrhea
	Risk of pneumothorax, pulmonary hemorrhage
	Atelectasis
	Assess for cor pulmonale
Sleep apnea	Must exclude pulmonary hypertension and cor pulmonale
	Requires careful postoperative observation for obstruction
CARDIAC	
	Need for antibiotic prophylaxis for bacterial endocarditis
	Use of air filters; careful purging of air from the intravenous equipment
	Need to understand the effects of various anesthetics on the hemodynamics of specific lesions
	Preload optimization and avoidance of hyperviscous states in cyanotic patients
	Possible need for preoperative evaluation of myocardial function and pulmonary vascular resistance
	Provide information about pacemaker function and ventricular device function
HEMATOLOGIC	
Sickle cell disease	Possible need for simple or exchange transfusion based on preoperative hemoglobin and percent hemoglobin S
	Importance of avoiding acidosis, hypoxemia, hypothermia, dehydration, and hyperviscosity states
Oncology	Pulmonary evaluation of patients who have received bleomycin, *bis*-chloroethyl-nitrosourea, chloroethyl-cyclohexyl-nitrosourea, methotrexate, or radiation to the chest
	Avoidance of high oxygen concentration
	Cardiac evaluation of patients who have received anthracyclines; risk of severe myocardial depression with volatile agents
	Potential for coagulopathy
RHEUMATOLOGIC	
	Limited mobility of the temporomandibular joint, cervical spine, arytenoid cartilages
	Requires careful preoperative evaluation
	Possible difficult airway
GASTROINTESTINAL	
Esophageal, gastric	Potential for reflux and aspiration
Liver	High overall morbidity and mortality in patients with hepatic dysfunction
	Altered metabolism of some drugs
	Potential for coagulopathy
RENAL	
	Altered electrolyte and acid-base status
	Altered clearance of some drugs
	Need for preoperative dialysis in selected cases
	Succinylcholine to be used with extreme caution and only when the serum potassium level was recently shown to be normal
NEUROLOGIC	
Seizure disorder	Avoid anesthetics that may lower the threshold
	Ensure optimal control preoperatively
	Preoperative anticonvulsant levels
Increased intracranial pressure	Avoid agents that increase cerebral blood flow
	Avoid hypercarbia
Neuromuscular disease	Avoid depolarizing relaxants; at risk for hyperkalemia
	May be at risk for malignant hyperthermia
Developmental delay	May be uncooperative at induction
Psychiatric	Monoamine oxidase inhibitor (or cocaine) may interact with meperidine, resulting in hyperthermia and seizures
	Selective serotonin reuptake inhibitors may induce or inhibit various hepatic enzymes that may alter anesthetic drug clearance
	Illicit drugs may have adverse effects on cardiorespiratory homeostasis and may potentiate the action of anesthetics
ENDOCRINE	
Diabetes	Greatest risk is unrecognized intraoperative hypoglycemia; if insulin is administered, monitor blood glucose level intraoperatively; must provide glucose and insulin with adjustment for fasting condition and surgical stress
SKIN	
Burns	Difficult airway
	Risk of rhabdomyolysis and hyperkalemia from succinylcholine
	Fluid shifts
	Bleeding
	Coagulopathy
IMMUNOLOGIC	
	Retroviral drugs may inhibit benzodiazepine clearance
	Immunodeficiency requires careful infection control practices
	May require cytomegalovirus-negative blood products, irradiation, or leukofiltration
METABOLIC	
	Careful assessment of glucose homeostasis in infants

TABLE 76-4. Definitions of Anesthesia Care

Monitored anesthesia care: A specific anesthesia service in which an anesthesiologist has been requested to participate in the care of a patient undergoing a diagnostic or therapeutic procedure.
Monitored anesthesia care includes all aspects of anesthesia care: a preprocedure visit, intraprocedure care, and postprocedure anesthesia management.
During monitored anesthesia care, the anesthesiologist or a member of the anesthesia care team provides a number of specific services, which may include some or all of, but are not limited to, the following:

- Monitoring of vital signs, maintenance of the patient's airway, and continual evaluation of vital functions
- Diagnosis and treatment of clinical problems that occur during the procedure
- Administration of sedatives, analgesics, hypnotics, anesthetic agents, or other medications as necessary to ensure patient safety and comfort
- Provision of other medical services as needed to accomplish the safe completion of the procedure
- Anesthesia care often includes the administration of medications for which the loss of normal protective reflexes or loss of consciousness is likely.

Monitored anesthesia care refers to those clinical situations in which the patient remains able to protect the airway for the majority of the procedure.
If the patient is rendered unconscious and/or loses normal protective reflexes for an extended period, this will be considered a general anesthetic.
Light sedation: Administration of anxiolysis and/or analgesia that obtunds consciousness, but does not obtund normal protective reflexes (cough, gag, swallow, hemodynamic reflexes).
Deep sedation: Sedation that obtunds consciousness and normal protective reflexes or possesses a significant risk of blunting normal protective reflexes (cough, gag, swallow, hemodynamic reflexes).
General anesthesia: Administration of hypnosis, sedation, and analgesia that results in the loss of normal protective reflexes.
Regional anesthesia: Induction of neural blockade (either central, neuraxial, epidural, or spinal; or peripheral nerve block, e.g., digital nerve block, brachial plexus block), which provides analgesia and is associated with regional motor blockade. Consciousness is not obtunded. Special expertise is required. Frequently, in children, anxiolysis and sedation are also necessary for this technique to be successful. Regional anesthesia (e.g., caudal epidural blockade) is used to supplement general anesthesia and provide postoperative analgesia.
Local anesthesia: Provision of analgesia by local infiltration of an appropriate anesthetic agent. Does not require the presence or involvement of an anesthesiologist, although an anesthesiologist may provide local anesthesia services.
No anesthesiologist: An anesthesiologist will not be involved in the care of the child in any way.

blocking agents are used, analgesia and sedation must be provided.

PHYSIOLOGIC SUPPORT. The need for anesthesia increases the need to monitor and support physiologic integrity and homeostasis. Sedation and anesthesia have significant and potentially life-threatening physiologic consequences (see Tables 76-4 and 76-5). Maintenance of adequate cardiorespiratory function, fluid management, electrolyte control, thermoregulation, and concern for all aspects of the child's health are critical during anesthesia.

VIGILANCE. Constant, critical attention by physicians who understand the demands of the surgical procedure as well as the changes in physiologic status and their implications is mandatory to provide safe perioperative care for all children. Careful attention to the child's preoperative condition is mandatory for minimizing the risk in perioperative care (see Tables 76-3 and 76-4).

INDUCTION OF GENERAL ANESTHESIA

The goal of induction of general anesthesia is to rapidly achieve surgical anesthesia by using intravenous or, more commonly in children, inhalational induction agents. In children who are too young to tolerate the establishment of vascular access before the induction of anesthesia, it is routine to induce anesthesia by mask inhalation of volatile anesthetics. In the operating room, a child is often accompanied by the parents and placed on the operating room table. Before the induction of anesthesia, monitors are usually placed on the child. These include a pulse oximeter, electrocardiogram (ECG) electrodes, and frequently a blood pressure cuff. The child is then cautiously introduced to the face mask, which contains a high gas flow (5–7 L/min of oxygen), frequently mixed with nitrous oxide (N_2O). Inhalation of nitrous oxide and oxygen for 60–90 sec induces a state of euphoria. The airway responses to inhalational anesthetics are now blunted, and sevoflurane or halothane can be introduced into the inhaled gas mixture. This leads to unconsciousness within 30–60 sec while the child continues to breathe spontaneously.

The child is now "asleep," and the parents can be asked to leave. An intravenous line is then started and comprehensive intraoperative monitoring initiated. Surgical anesthesia can be maintained by spontaneous ventilation with a mask; this is safe only when the airway is secure and patent, the stomach is empty, and the child is older than 6 mo of age. Procedures longer than 1 hr are not usually performed with mask inhalational anesthesia. If these conditions are not met, if the surgeon needs to approach the airway, or if muscular paralysis is required, then the airway must be secured with endotracheal intubation. Although endotracheal intubation can be performed under deep inhalational anesthesia with respiratory depression and obtunded cough and gag reflexes, the depth of anesthesia required to ablate airway reflexes is very close to that which induces hemodynamic instability. After anesthetic induction, intravenous access is secured and anesthesia is deepened with intravenous agents. Muscle relaxation with intravenous, nondepolarizing muscle relaxants is induced to facilitate endotracheal intubation. Succinylcholine is rarely used. After paralysis is induced, direct laryngoscopy and airway intubation can be performed. Correct endotracheal tube placement is confirmed by direct laryngoscopy, end-tidal CO_2 measurement, endotracheal tube fogging, fiberoptic bronchoscopy, the finding of bilateral equal breath sounds during positive pressure ventilation, and chest radiograph, if necessary.

After endotracheal intubation, spontaneous ventilation may be permitted, if muscle relaxants are not used or have worn off; however, it is routine to provide controlled mechanical ventilation. When the child is completely anesthetized, positioned for surgery, and hemodynamically stable, and maintenance anesthesia is achieved, the surgery can begin.

INHALATIONAL ANESTHETICS. General anesthesia may be induced and maintained by either inhalation or the intravenous route. Inhalational anesthetics include halothane, enflurane, isoflurane, sevoflurane, and desflurane. Halothane is the prototypical pediatric inhalational anesthetic agent; its use has decreased since the availability of isoflurane and sevoflurane. Enflurane is rarely used in children.

The minimal alveolar concentration (MAC) of an inhalational anesthetic is the alveolar concentration that provides sufficient depth of anesthesia for surgery in 50% of patients. For potent inhalational agents, the alveolar concentration of anesthetic reflects the arterial concentration of anesthetic in the blood perfusing the brain. Thus, the MAC level is an indication of anesthetic potency and is analogous to the ED_{50} of a drug. MAC is age-dependent, is lower in premature infants than in full-term infants, and decreases from term through infancy to preadolescence. In adolescence, MAC again increases, falling thereafter. Inhalational anesthetic agents are poorly soluble in blood, but rapidly equilibrate between alveolar gas and blood. The less soluble an anesthetic agent is in blood (low blood gas partition coefficient), the more rapid are both the induction and the emergence from inhalational anesthesia. Sevoflurane (0.69) and desflurane (0.42) have lower blood gas partition coefficients (ratio of the anesthetic concentration in the blood to the alveolar gas at equilibrium) than halothane (2.4).

RESPIRATORY EFFECTS. The advantages of inhalational anesthesia are rapid onset, rapid offset, convenient route of delivery and excretion (respiratory), and the ability to provide profound analgesia and amnesia. Inhalational anesthetics are all airway irritants and, in low doses, can cause laryngospasm. All inhalational anesthetics depress ventilation in a dose-dependent manner: 1 MAC of inhalation anesthesia decreases minute ventilation by approx-

TABLE 76-5. Selected Drugs Used in Anesthesia

DRUG	USES AND IMPLICATIONS
MUSCLE RELAXANTS	
Succinylcholine	Used to facilitate endotracheal intubation and maintain muscle relaxation A depolarizing neuromuscular blocking agnent with rapid onset and offset properties Associated with the development of malignant hyperthermia in susceptible patients Degraded by plasma cholinesterase, which may be deficient in some individuals and result in prolonged effect Fasciculations may be associated with immediate increases in intracranial and intraocular pressure as well as postoperative muscle pain
Pancuronium, vecuronium, *cis*-atracurium, D-tubocurarine (curare)	Nondepolarizing neuromuscular blockers Less rapid onset than succinylcholine, but longer-acting Pancuronium is vagolytic, which may be of benefit in newborns, who have high levels of vagal tone Vecuronium and rocuronium are metabolized by the liver and excreted in bile *Cis*-atracurium is metabolized by plasma cholinesterase and therefore may be of benefit in patients with hepatic or renal disease; curare releases histamine and is long-acting
HYPNOTICS	
Thiopental	Used to induce a state of unconsciousness Rapidly acting hypnotic, but not an analgesic Offset is by redistribution, not by metabolism May cause hypotension because of its myocardial depressant effects and by vasodilation Causes respiratory depression Releases histamine and may be associated with bronchospasm in susceptible individuals Increases the seizure threshold
Ketamine	Hypnotic analgesic and amnestic Causes sialorrhea and should be co-administered with an antisalogogue, such as atropine or glycopyrrolate May be associated with laryngospasm Causes endogenous catecholamine release, tachycardia, and bronchodilation Increases intracranial and intraocular pressure Decreases the seizure threshold
Etomidate	Cardiovascular stability on induction with no increase in intracranial pressure May inhibit corticosteroid synthesis Associated with myoclonus, potential difficulty with assisted ventilation, and pain on injection
Propofol	Rapidly acting hypnotic; amnestic, but not analgesic Like pentothal, may cause hypotension Causes respiratory depression May increase the seizure threshold Great utility in titrated doses for sedation and with local anesthetic and short-acting opioid for outpatient procedures May suppress nausea
SEDATIVE-ANXIOLYTICS	
Benzodiazepines	May produce sedation, anxiolysis, or hypnosis, depending on the dose May produce antegrade but not retrograde amnesia All raise the seizure threshold, are metabolized by the liver, and depress respiration, especially when administered with opioids Frequently administered as premedicants Diazepam may be painful on injection and has active metabolites Midazolam can be administered by various routes and has a short half-life Lorazepam has no active metabolites Sedation effected by all benzodiazepines may be reversed by flumazenil, but respiratory depression may not be reliably reversed
ANALGESIC-SEDATIVES	
Opioids	Gold standard for providing analgesia May cause respiratory depression Morphine and, to a lesser extent, hydromophone may cause histamine release The synthetic opioids fentanyl, sufentanil, and short-acting alfentanil may have a greater propensity to cause chest wall rigidity when administered rapidly or in high doses and are also associated with the rapid development of tolerance; these 3 drugs have particular utility in cardiac surgery because of the hemodynamic stability associated with their use Remifentanil is an ultra–short-acting synthetic opioid that is metabolized by plasma cholinesterase; it may have particular utility when deep sedation and analgesia are required along with the ability to assess neurologic status intermittently
INHALATIONAL AGENTS	
Nitrous oxide	Causes amnesia and mild analgesia at low concentrations Danger of hypoxic mixture if the oxygen concentration is not monitored and preventive safety mechanisms are not in place
Potent vapors	"Complete anesthetics"—they induce a state of hypnosis, analgesia, and amnesia All are myocardial depressants, and some are vasodilators May trigger malignant hyperthermia in susceptible individuals Isoflurane and enflurane are fluorinated ethers and isomers Enflurane may lower the seizure threshold Halothane has been the gold standard for performing inhalation induction of anesthesia in children, but sevoflurane, a newer drug, is also well tolerated and has more rapid kinetics (onset and offset) because of its low solubility in blood Sevoflurane is the most commonly used for inhalational induction All are bronchodilators at equipotent concentrations Isoflurane, enflurane, and especially desflurane are associated with a higher incidence of laryngospasm, when used for anesthetic induction, than either halothane or sevoflurane Halothane may be associated with acute fulminant hepatitis, although this is extremely rare in children

imately 25%, resulting in smaller tidal volumes and decreased respiratory rates. Thus, expired CO_2 and $Paco_2$ increase. In addition, 1 MAC of anesthesia also decreases end-expiratory lung volume to approximately 30% < functional residual capacity. Small lung volumes result in decreased lung compliance, increased total pulmonary resistance, increased work of breathing, increased intrapulmonary arteriovenous shunting, and a restrictive lung defect. Inhalational anesthetics also shift the CO_2 response curve to the right, thus decreasing, but not ablating, the increase in minute ventilation with increasing $Paco_2$.

Inhalational anesthetics may induce apnea and hypoxia in premature infants and newborns and are less frequently used in premature infants and children. In neonates and young infants, general anesthesia always necessitates endotracheal intubation and controlled mechanical ventilation. In older children, spontaneous breathing through a mask, or a laryngeal mask airway, without controlled ventilation, is possible for shorter operations. The decreased end-expiratory lung volume and increased work of breathing always necessitate increased inspired oxygen tension.

CARDIOVASCULAR EFFECTS. Cardiovascular effects include depressed cardiac output and peripheral vasodilation; hypotension is frequent. This is accentuated in hypovolemic patients. This hypotensive effect is more pronounced in neonates than in older children and adults. Inhalational anesthetics also decrease baroreceptor and heart rate responses. At 1 MAC of halothane, cardiac output and ejection fraction are depressed by approximately 25%. At MAC doses of halothane, the heart rate is frequently increased; at higher concentrations, bradycardia may result, whereas profound bradycardia during anesthesia may indicate an overdose. Halothane sensitizes the heart to catecholamines and may produce arrhythmias. Inhalational anesthesia also blunts the hypoxic pulmonary vasomotor response in the pulmonary circulation, which may contribute to hypoxemia during inhalational anesthesia.

The net effect of inhalational anesthesia is decreased oxygen delivery. Perioperatively, catabolism is enhanced and oxygen demands are increased; there may be a profound imbalance between oxygen demand and oxygen delivery. Development of a metabolic acidosis may reflect this imbalance. Because the cardiovascular depressant effects of inhalational anesthesia are greater in premature and newborn infants, they are of limited use in these patients. However, they are widely used for the induction and maintenance of anesthesia in older children.

All inhalational anesthetic agents cause cerebrovasodilation. Halothane is a more potent cerebrovasodilator than sevoflurane or isoflurane. Thus, in children with elevated intracranial pressure, impaired cerebral perfusion, or head trauma, and in premature neonates at risk for intraventricular hemorrhage, halothane and other inhalational agents should be used with extreme caution. Although inhalational anesthetic agents decrease cerebral oxygen consumption, they may disproportionately decrease blood flow, thus worsening oxygen delivery.

SPECIFIC ANESTHETICS.

Halothane. Agents that are more pleasant to breathe and induce anesthesia more rapidly have replaced halothane. Halothane hepatitis is a well-recognized sequela of halothane and is most likely an idiosyncratic, allergic response. Hepatitis, which may be mild, leading to elevated levels of liver enzymes and jaundice, or severe, leading to acute hepatic necrosis, occurs in between 1 : 6,000 and 1 : 35,000 cases in adults. This appears to be rare in children, occurring in between 1 : 80,000 and 1 : 200,000 exposures in children. There is no reason to particularly avoid halothane in children with liver disease.

Isoflurane. Isoflurane maintains cardiac output and cerebral perfusion more effectively than halothane. The therapeutic ratio for inducing anesthesia without hemodynamic instability is greater for isoflurane. It is also less of a respiratory depressant than halothane. Isoflurane is pungent and a significant airway irritant, with an unacceptably high incidence of complications, such as laryngospasm. Emergence from anesthesia with isoflurane is quite smooth and faster than with halothane. Cerebral blood flow is only minimally affected, and cerebral oxygen delivery is maintained. Because isoflurane is not a suitable induction agent, induction with halothane or sevoflurane and maintenance with isoflurane is common pediatric anesthesia practice.

Sevoflurane. Sevoflurane has a low blood gas partition coefficient, predicting rapid alveolar equilibration and a faster rate of induction. Sevoflurane is not a significant airway irritant and leads to smoother induction than isoflurane and quicker induction than halothane. Sevoflurane appears to have fewer hemodynamic effects than halothane; the profile of respiratory effects at 1 MAC appears similar. Emergence from sevoflurane is quite rapid; however, there is a significant amount of emergence delirium, especially if pain has been inadequately controlled. This can be blunted with pretreatment with midazolam and adequate use of opioids; these delay recovery from anesthesia.

The major use of sevoflurane is for induction of inhalational anesthesia in children. Because isoflurane is less expensive than sevoflurane and has a similar physiologic profile, anesthesia is maintained with isoflurane. Metabolism of sevoflurane yields free fluoride, which may cause renal damage; therefore, the U.S. Food and Drug Administration has restricted the use of sevoflurane to <2 MAC hours, preferably with fresh gas flow rates >2 L/min.

Desflurane. Desflurane has the lowest blood gas solubility coefficient (0.42) of commonly used anesthetics. It would be predicted that desflurane would provide rapid induction and emergence from anesthesia. Unfortunately, it is a potent airway irritant and causes coughing, breath-holding, and laryngospasm during induction and therefore is unsuitable for induction.

Nitrous Oxide. Nitrous oxide is a tasteless, colorless, odorless gas with potent analgesic properties. It induces a state of euphoria (laughing gas). The MAC of nitrous oxide is >1; therefore, it is not suitable as a sole agent to maintain anesthesia. Nevertheless, nitrous oxide has few complications and produces little or no hemodynamic or respiratory depression. Commonly, during maintenance of anesthesia, the inhalational gas mixture is 70% nitrous oxide and 30% oxygen, with the addition of an inhalational anesthetic or potentiation of analgesia with an opioid or a hypnotic agent. It has a remarkably low blood gas partition (0.47), so it rapidly reaches alveolar equilibrium. Induction with and emergence from nitrous oxide–induced anesthesia is quite rapid. The deleterious effects of nitrous oxide are a suspicion of increased postoperative emesis and, in long-term use (days), bone marrow suppression. There is no evidence of harmful sequelae of the use of nitrous oxide for routine pediatric anesthesia. Nitrous oxide is a potent analgesic that is safely used in a mixture of 50% nitrous oxide and oxygen (Entonox) in obstetrics and emergency departments to provide analgesia. Although this combination appears to be quite safe, it potentiates the respiratory depressive effects of opioids, and its use, in combination with any other sedative, hypnotic, or opioid agent, requires very close monitoring because it may produce general anesthesia.

INTRAVENOUS ANESTHETIC AGENTS. Anesthesia can be both induced and maintained with either intermittent boluses or continuous infusions of intravenous anesthetic agents. Intravenous anesthetics include barbiturates, opioids, benzodiazepines, and miscellaneous drugs, such as ketamine. Intravenous anesthetic agents can induce anesthesia more rapidly than inhalational anesthetics, with fewer complications. An intravenous line needs to be placed and, unless intravenous access has already been obtained, inhalation induction may remain the preferred route. For children arriving in the operating room with intravascular access, intravenous induction should be routine, because it rapidly takes the child from the awake state to the anesthetized state with less hemodynamic and cardiorespiratory compromise than occurs with inhalational induction. All intravenous agents affect cardiorespiratory function. The one exception to this may be ketamine, which, in lower doses, releases catecholamines, which maintain cardiac function and blood pressure.

Barbiturates. The most commonly used barbiturate for intravenous induction is sodium thiopental, although propofol has nearly completely replaced it. Thiopental depresses respiration, induces apnea, and can cause hypotension in the hypovolemic patient. It generally has little effect on myocardial function, and in the euvolemic well child, it is a useful anesthetic induction agent. Induction with 3–5 mg/kg of thiopental usually produces 5–10 min of unconsciousness within seconds. Although loss of consciousness can rapidly be induced, barbiturates do not provide analgesia. After intravenous induction with sodium thiopental, maintenance anesthesia can be established using benzodiazepines, intravenous opioids, or inhalational anesthetics.

Pentobarbital is commonly used for sedation in children. Pentobarbital is an intravenous drug that induces loss of consciousness. It is also a potent respiratory depressant, particularly in conjunction with opioids and benzodiazepines. It has a very prolonged effect. It is not an analgesic agent, and painful procedures cannot be performed with pentobarbital sedation without supplemental analgesia. Pentobarbital sedation that is deep enough for anxiolysis and nonpainful procedures generally results in prolonged sleep. Its potency and long duration of action make it difficult to titrate. It is not an ideal drug for sedation for short or painful procedures. It is rarely, if ever, used by anesthesiologists for outpatient procedures.

Sodium methohexitone (Brevital) is another intravenous induction agent. It is similar to sodium thiopental and has a similar spectrum of respiratory depression.

Propofol. Propofol is the most commonly used intravenous induction agent in pediatric anesthesiology and has a rapid onset. In doses of 2–3 mg/kg, propofol induces less respiratory depression than thiopental, but does produce hypotension. Propofol can sometimes burn and itch on injection; this frequently leads the child to withdraw or otherwise respond after a propofol bolus. After induction of anesthesia, propofol is also a useful agent for maintaining hypnosis and amnesia and can be used as a sole anesthetic agent for nonpainful procedures, such as radiation therapy, MRI, and CT. Combined with opioids, it provides excellent, brief anesthesia for painful procedures, such as lumbar puncture and bone marrow aspiration. Propofol is a general anesthetic agent and obtunds airway reflexes, respiration, and hemodynamic function and should not be considered a "sedation agent." Although hemodynamic stability, and even spontaneous respirations, can be maintained with propofol sedation, its use for prolonged sedation over several hours to days in children younger than age 12 yr is associated with hemodynamic collapse, metabolic acidosis, cardiac failure, profound shock, and death. Its use for prolonged sedation (>12 hr) in the critical care setting in children is **contraindicated.**

Ketamine. Ketamine rapidly induces general anesthesia that lasts for 15–30 min when given at 2 mg/kg IV. It has few side effects and can maintain adequate blood pressure and cardiac output. Ketamine is also effective given either intramuscularly, subcutaneously, or orally; the dose must be increased for these alternative routes. Ketamine is not only a hypnotic agent, providing obtundation and loss of consciousness, but also an analgesic agent, and can act as a sole intravenous agent for the provision of general anesthesia. In low doses, airway reflexes and spontaneous ventilation may be maintained; in higher doses, loss of airway reflexes, apnea, and respiratory depression occur. It is unwise to rely on ketamine to prevent aspiration of gastric contents during deep sedation. Intravenous ketamine is a useful general anesthetic agent for short procedures.

Ketamine produces disturbing postanesthetic dreams and hallucinations. These can occur at the time of emergence from anesthesia and for up to weeks later. In adults, the incidence is 30–50%. In prepubertal children, it may be 5–10%. Premedication with a benzodiazepine, such as midazolam, greatly reduces these sequelae; a benzodiazepine is routinely added in children receiving ketamine anesthesia. The other side effect of ketamine is that it is a potent secretagogue, enhancing bronchial secretions. A drying agent, such as atropine or glycopyrrolate, is administered before the administration of ketamine.

Ketamine is a bronchial smooth muscle relaxant (bronchodilator) and is a useful agent for sedating asthmatic patients and others in the intensive care unit (ICU). Ketamine has been reported to increase intracranial pressure and therefore is not indicated in patients at risk for elevated intracranial pressure. Ketamine can increase myocardial oxygen demand and should be used cautiously in patients with impaired myocardial oxygen delivery or cardiac outflow tract obstruction.

Opioids. Opioids are superb analgesic agents, providing analgesia for painful procedures and postprocedural pain (see Chapter 77). Large doses of morphine, combined with nitrous oxide, provide adequate analgesia for painful procedures and surgery. Opioids suppress the CO_2 response, can induce apnea, and are respiratory depressants. Morphine is often associated with hypotension and bronchospasm from histamine release; it is used with caution in children with asthma. Morphine is a long-acting agent, and an equivalent dose per kilogram gives much higher blood levels in neonates than in older children, with plasma concentrations approximating 3 times those in adults. This is caused by a prolonged elimination half-life (14 hr) compared with adults (2 hr). Because of the prolonged activity and hemodynamic instability induced by morphine, the fentanyl class of synthetic opioids has largely replaced morphine.

Fentanyl is an effective agent to provide pain relief, analgesia, and sedation for painful procedures, with a shorter duration of action and a more stable hemodynamic profile than morphine. In equal analgesic doses, all opioids are equally potent respiratory depressants. Other anesthetic agents potentiate this respiratory depression, whether they are inhalational anesthetics or intravenous barbiturates or benzodiazepines.

Fentanyl use at 30–50 μg/kg causes absence of abnormal hemodynamic response to surgery and provides stable operative conditions. Effective analgesia and anesthesia can be provided with intravenous fentanyl in a 2–3 μg/kg bolus followed by a 1–3 μg/kg/hr continuous infusion. Hemodynamic effects can be blunted and recall totally obtunded using a nitrous-narcotic anesthetic technique, although muscle tone may remain high and spontaneous movements can occur. Nitrous-narcotic anesthetics usually contain a nondepolarizing muscle relaxant during maintenance anesthesia. If the patient will be extubated and resume spontaneous ventilation, reversal of the muscle relaxant is necessary.

Other synthetic opioids (sufentanil, alfentanil, remifentanil) have gained some use; fentanyl is the most commonly used. The indications and use for these other synthetic opioids are guided by their different potencies and altered pharmacokinetics. Both sufentanil and alfentanil have been used for cardiac anesthesia; they have a different potency than fentanyl. Alfentanil appears to cause an increased incidence of muscle rigidity, convulsions, and prolonged respiratory depression compared with fentanyl, and is not used in children.

Remifentanil has very rapid onset and offset of action. In doses of 0.25 μg/kg/min, surgical anesthesia can be maintained. Its short half-life and rapid offset are advantageous for rapid emergence. Unfortunately, its rapid offset of action also leads to postprocedural and postoperative pain and requires analgesic supplementation, frequently with an opioid, which removes the advantage of anesthesia with a short-acting opioid. Remifentanil may have a role in providing rapidly deepening anesthesia for particularly painful events or rapidly inducing analgesia. It is a potent respiratory depressant and provides no postprocedural analgesia, which limits its use.

Benzodiazepines. Benzodiazepines induce hypnosis, anxiolysis, sedation, and amnesia, and have anticonvulsant activity. In larger doses, they cause respiratory depression and apnea; they are synergistic with opioids and barbiturates in their respiratory depressant effects. Benzodiazepines inhibit neurally mediated γ-aminobutyric acid receptors to induce sedation.

The most commonly used benzodiazepine in pediatric anesthesia is midazolam. It is short-acting and water-soluble, and can be injected intravenously without pain. It is a potent hypnotic-anxiolytic-anticonvulsant and is approximately 4 times more potent than diazepam. In anxiolytic doses, midazolam (0.15 mg/kg) has no effect on respiratory rate, heart rate, or blood pressure and provides excellent preoperative sedation, frequently accompanied by amnesia. It can be administered orally, nasally, rectally, intravenously, or intramuscularly. Use of oral midazolam at a dose of 0.5–1.0 mg/kg, mixed in sweet flavored syrup, induces anxiolysis in approximately 90% of children. Although there are no hemodynamic, oxygenation, or respiratory depressant effects at this dose level, when midazolam is used as a sole agent, children may frequently lose their balance and head control, may have blurred vision, and rarely may become dysphoric. A child sedated with midazolam should not be left unattended and is not safe walking. Most children rapidly accept an inhalational anesthetic mask after oral midazolam premedication.

COMPLICATIONS DURING INDUCTION OF ANESTHESIA. The period between full wakefulness, with the child in control of airway reflexes, and general anesthesia, with total loss of control, is fraught with difficulty. During induction, laryngospasm, bronchospasm, vomiting, aspiration of the gastric contents, and subsequent aspiration pneumonitis pose a constant threat, but rarely occur. Concern about vomiting and aspiration dictates the use of preanesthetic fasting (NPO) guidelines and the indication for rapid sequence anesthetic induction.

Laryngospasm is the most common complication. During induction of anesthesia, especially with inhalational anesthetics, a period of excitement may occur. This period is associated with heightened airway reflexes, which can lead to coughing, gagging, laryngospasm, and bronchospasm. Laryngospasm is reflex closure of the larynx, which makes it impossible for the child to breathe or for ventilation to be used. The child may be making violent respiratory efforts against a closed glottis, generating significantly negative intrathoracic pressure, with an effect on cardiovascular function and an increased risk of postobstructive pulmonary edema. Laryngospasm can be prolonged, and hypoxia may ensue. Laryngospasm occurs in up to 2% of all anesthetic inductions in children younger than age 9 yr and is half as common in older patients. Laryngospasm occurs twice as frequently in children with active or recent upper respiratory tract infection (URI). A history of passive smoking from environmental (parental) tobacco smoke increases the likelihood of laryngospasm by 10-fold, and even more if the smoker is the child's mother.

Laryngospasm can be relieved during induction of anesthesia by deepening the anesthetic, either intravenously or by inhalational anesthesia (although with the glottis closed, further administration of inhalational anesthesia is not possible). Muscle relaxation will relieve laryngospasm, and in an acute situation, this may be an indication for succinylcholine. Constant positive airway pressure by someone skilled in airway management to ensure patency of the soft tissues of the oropharynx may be beneficial in alleviating the laryngospasm. Laryngospasm may also occur during emergence because a state of excitement is again traversed between deep anesthesia and wakefulness.

Bronchospasm can occur during induction, either in response to histamine release as a result of many of the anesthetic agents or as part of a hyperexcitable stage. Endotracheal intubation may also induce bronchospasm during induction. Bronchospasm during induction is particularly common in children with asthma. Bronchospasm secondary to intubation in a patient with reactive airway disease can be severe, may be associated with life-threatening hypoxemia, and may make it impossible to ventilate the child. The use of histamine-releasing anesthetic agents has been associated with total airway obstruction, respiratory failure, and cardiac arrest. Environmental tobacco smoke is a risk factor.

Other pulmonary problems with induction of anesthesia include massive atelectasis with hypoxemia, impaired ventilation and perfusion, blunted hypoxic pulmonary vasoconstriction, and increased airway secretions with decreased bronchociliary function. **Hypersecretion** is prevented by the routine use of antisialagogues, such as atropine. The newer inhalation agents are less potent secretagogues, and the use of atropine premedication is less common, but is probably indicated if ketamine is used.

Hemodynamic complications on induction include **hypotension**, which can be profound in hypovolemic patients; decreased myocardial function, which can be severe in patients with compromised cardiac function; and tachycardia and cardiac dysrhythmias. Some inhalational anesthetics, such as halothane, sensitize the myocardium to circulating catecholamines, and induction and excitement are associated with a hypercatecholaminergic state.

PARENTAL PRESENCE DURING INDUCTION OF ANESTHESIA. Parents may expect to be with their child during the induction of anesthesia, known as parental presence during induction of anesthesia (PPI). Removing a terrified child from the comforting arms of a parent is stressful for the child, the parent, and the caregivers. If this parental separation cannot be achieved comfortably with preoperative psychoprophylaxis and behavioral modification, including education and desensitization to the operative environment, or with pharmacologic aids, such as preoperative medications including benzodiazepine and barbiturates, then there may be a need to defer parent-child separation until general anesthesia has been induced. Preoperative oral benzodiazepine premedication more frequently provides calm, smooth induction conditions than parental presence without pharmacologic preparation. Although PPI in the hands of a confident, competent anesthesia practitioner can replace the need for preoperative medication, it does not reliably predict smooth induction. PPI appears to decrease neither emergence phenomena nor the incidence of postoperative behavioral changes, and it does not appear to add an advantage for the child over that provided by preoperative sedative medication, such as oral midazolam.

MAINTENANCE OF ANESTHESIA

Maintenance of anesthesia is the period between induction and emergence. The child should be asleep, unaware of pain, unresponsive with either motion or hemodynamic responses to painful stimuli, and homeostatically supported. The child is comatose, without airway-protective reflexes and with suppressed or absent respiration, and has received drugs that suppress hemodynamic adaptive responses. The child is also exposed to surgical trauma, and there may be blood loss and significant fluid shifts (3rd spacing), decreased intravascular volume, and hypothermia.

Anesthesia is usually maintained with nitrous oxide, an inhalational anesthetic such as isoflurane or sevoflurane, and an opioid for intraoperative analgesia, potentiation and deepening of anesthesia, and postoperative analgesia. A benzodiazepine is added either during premedication or intraoperatively to supplement hypnosis and amnesia. A nondepolarizing muscle relaxant (vecuronium or rocuronium) completes the pharmacologic maintenance of anesthesia. Agents can be given by continuous inhalational anesthesia or by continuous or bolus intravenous infusion.

During maintenance, the child may breathe spontaneously through an anesthetic mask or endotracheal tube or may be mechanically ventilated. All general anesthetic agents leads to decreased end-expiratory lung volume, which is generally lower than functional residual capacity, with an increase in pulmonary closing capacity and increased intrapulmonary shunt. Hypoxia would occur without supplemental oxygenation. These effects are compounded by respiratory depressant effects and the depressed CO_2 response curve. Therefore, it is generally considered that anesthetics that last for >1 hr require endotracheal intubation and positive pressure ventilation. For long procedures, spontaneous breathing through a mask is possible; however, in smaller children, in whom the surgical field and the airway may be close together, the need to maintain a patent airway necessitates endotracheal intubation.

Muscle relaxation to facilitate endotracheal intubation was once accomplished with succinylcholine. Succinylcholine has a high risk profile and is associated with postoperative pain (muscle spasms); hyperkalemia; elevated intracranial, intraocular, and intragastric pressures; malignant hyperthermia; and myoglobinuria and renal damage. Succinylcholine is rarely used, except to provide rapid relief of laryngospasm. Intubation of the airway is facilitated with a nondepolarizing muscle relaxant of short-acting duration; for procedures that last >40 min, vecuronium and alcuronium are adequate. After intubation of the airway, the decision must be made whether to maintain muscle relaxation to facilitate surgery or to allow the child to resume spontaneous respiration. Prolonged use of a nondepolarizing muscle relaxant is common practice, but may contribute to postoperative respiratory compromise if it is not fully reversed with appropriate agents.

Thermoregulation is critical during anesthesia. The absence of movement and the inhibition of shivering lead to difficulty in thermogenesis. All factors of heat loss—convection, radiation, evaporation, and conduction—occur during anesthesia. Humidification and warming of inspired air are required. Additional warming devices are commonly used, such as the BAIR© hugger. General anesthetic agents increase the interthreshold range (the minimal temperature change that will lead to sympathetic response, generally 0.3°C). Although temperature sensing may remain normal, an autonomic response to hypothermia is not triggered. Anesthetic agents cause vasoparesis, and this further impairs thermoregulation and causes increased heat loss. In newborns, inhalational anesthetics inhibit nonshivering thermogenesis from brown fat, placing them at higher risk for hypothermia.

INTRAOPERATIVE MONITORING. Routine monitoring includes electrocardiography, with common chest and limb leads to monitor rate, rhythm, and ST segment depression. Pulse oximetry and monitoring of end-tidal CO_2 are mandatory. The fraction of inspired oxygen is continuously measured. The fraction of anesthetic vapor in the inspiratory (and expired) gas mixture can be continuously monitored, and the mixture of oxygen, air, and nitrous oxide is continuously visualized, either through the use of rotameters or through direct measurement of the inspiratory gas mixture and digital display. Respiratory rate, tidal volume, and respiratory mechanics may be monitored intraoperatively (compliance and resistance). Blood pressure monitoring, with systolic, diastolic, and mean pressures is also routine. This can be done by Doppler ultrasonic or pneumatic techniques.

FLUID MAINTENANCE DURING SURGERY AND ANESTHESIA. Fluid maintenance differs from the normal resting state because of the effects of anesthesia and surgery. Patients who are unconscious and immobile have lost venous pump mechanisms and have venous pooling in the periphery. Anesthetic agents cause vasodilation, and patients have relative hypovolemia. Intravascular volume expansion is frequently required after the induction of anesthesia to maintain adequate perfusion, tissue oxygenation, urine output, and blood pressure. This volume expansion can be an isotonic salt-containing solution (normal saline, lactated Ringer). Surgery may lead to increased autonomic responses as part of the surgical stress response, with vasoconstriction and intravascular volume contraction, diuresis, and intravascular volume loss from hemorrhage and from 3rd-space (interstitial space) fluid losses caused by the inflammatory response to stress. Abnormalities in the distribution of renal blood flow and secretion of antidiuretic hormone further complicate the regulation of intravascular volume.

Hypoglycemia due to preoperative fasting was a concern and supported the recommendations that infants and small children receive isotonic solutions with 5% glucose. The occurrence of hyperglycemia and potential neurologic injury during cardiopulmonary bypass, or during neurosurgery and other situations in which central nervous system injury can occur, and with the recognition that hypoglycemia is rare in non-neonates, has called into question the routine use of glucose-containing solutions. In neonates, glucose monitoring during and after anesthesia is indicated. In older children with normal nutritional status, isotonic salt solutions without additional glucose are adequate. In children who are receiving parenteral alimentation with a solution containing a high glucose concentration (>10%), continuation of these glucose concentrations should be ensured to avoid hypoglycemia when these high-glucose solutions are stopped.

Intraoperative fluid maintenance includes: (1) current maintenance fluids and replacement of usual deficits while NPO; (2) replacement of 3rd-space losses; and (3) replacement of extraordinary losses (hemorrhage). Infants should receive glucose-containing isotonic fluids, such as D5W with 0.25 normal saline or isotonic crystalloid solutions. A guideline for determining fluid deficits and maintenance requirements in the operating room is shown in Table 76-6. Replacements of the fluid deficits should be done over the first 2 or 3 hr of intraoperative management. Deficits are generally calculated as the number of hr that a child was NPO times the hourly maintenance rate for the child. Half of this is replaced during the 1st hr and ½ during each of the subsequent 2 hr. If hypotension or tachycardia occurs or persists in the early stages of anesthesia, more rapid replacement of the deficit is indicated. The deficit is replaced with isotonic crystalloid solutions.

Third-space losses are replaced with isotonic salt solutions. For large operations, such as abdominal or thoracic procedures, where there may be a large amount of evaporative loss as well as a significant amount of 3rd-space losses, 8–10 mL/kg/hr of surgery is generally given as intravenous fluid replacement. For smaller operations, such as herniorrhaphy, pyloromyotomy, and minor procedures, 3–5 mL/kg/hr of fluid replacement for 3rd-space losses is indicated. Even when surgery involves the extremities and 3rd-space losses are minor, it is wise to give an additional 1–2 mL/kg/hr to replace these losses.

Crystalloid is indicated for blood loss at 3 mL of crystalloid/mL of blood loss. This formula could be reduced somewhat if blood is replaced on a milliliter per milliliter basis with packed red blood cells or whole blood equivalent. The use of albumin or other suitable colloid, such as fresh frozen plasma in neonatal surgery, also decreases the amount of crystalloid replacement needed for blood loss. During maintenance anesthesia, if large-volume transfusions are required, warming the blood and crystalloid solutions avoids hypothermia.

With major surgery and the resultant systemic inflammatory response, capillary integrity is lost and losses of interstitial fluid are common. Failure to replace this 3rd-space loss and restore

TABLE 76-6. Intraoperative Pediatric Fluid Replacement

4 mL/kg/hr	1–10 kg
2 mL/kg/hr	10–20 kg
1 mL/kg/hr	per kg >20 kg

Example: 22 kg child requires: (4 × 10) + (2 × 10) + (1 × 2) = 62 mL/hr intravascular volume leads to hypotension, shock, acidemia, and renal failure, and further stimulates the systemic inflammatory response and worsens physiologic impairment.

RECOVERY FROM ANESTHESIA

Recovery from anesthesia includes emergence and postoperative recovery from surgery and anesthetics. **Emergence** describes the time and the physiologic response to decreasing depth of anesthesia during return to consciousness. During emergence, patients experience decreased anesthetic effect, increased stress responses, physiologic and psychologic responses to painful stimuli, excitement, and anxiety. Conscious realization of pain may lead to physiologic responses during emergence. The resumption of normal physiologic functions, such as spontaneous ventilation and improved hemodynamic function, occurs. For routine elective procedures, before leaving the operating room, the child should be fully conscious, with intact airway reflexes, the ability to follow simple commands, the effects of muscle relaxants reversed, and airway patency maintained. If the child is going to the ICU, or if for surgical reasons the decision is made to leave the child intubated, then analgesia and sedation should be maintained, along with mechanical ventilation, in the postoperative period. Ideally, emergence should be as brief as possible, with maintenance of analgesia and anxiolysis and restoration of cardiorespiratory function. Inhalational anesthetic agents leave the system rapidly during ventilation, and muscle relaxants can be reversed; however, the effects of opioids, benzodiazepines, and intravenous hypnotic agents may be prolonged.

During emergence, the decision must be made whether to reverse the effects of muscle relaxants. The effects of long-acting, nondepolarizing muscle relaxants (vecuronium and pancuronium) can be reversed using neostigmine, an acetylcholinesterase inhibitor. Atropine, or glycopyrrolate, is frequently administered along with the anticholinesterase drug to prevent bradycardia, to which children are particularly sensitive. If the child appears to be weak or to have respiratory depression in the postoperative phase, then consideration of prolonged neuromuscular blockade is indicated.

TABLE 76-7. Recovery Scores

ALDRETE RECOVERY SCORE	>9 REQUIRED FOR DISCHARGE
ACTIVITY—VOLUNTARILY OR ON COMMAND	
Moves 4 extremities	2
Moves 2 extremities	1
No motion	0
BREATHING	
Deep breath, cough, cry	2
Dyspnea or shallow breathing	1
Apnea	0
BLOOD PRESSURE	
Within 20% of preanesthetic value	2
Within 20%–50% of preanesthetic value	1
>50% outside preanesthetic value	0
COLOR	
Pink	2
Pale, blotchy, dusky	1
Cyanotic	0
CONSCIOUSNESS	
Fully aware, responds	2
Arouses to stimulus	1
Unresponsive	0
STEWARD RECOVERY SCORE	**6 REQUIRED FOR DISCHARGE**
ACTIVITY	
Moves limbs purposefully	2
Nonpurposeful movement	1
Still	0
CONSCIOUSNESS	
Awake	2
Responsive	1
Unresponsive	0
AIRWAY	
Coughing on command or crying	2
Maintaining patent airway	1
Requires airway maintenance	0

POSTANESTHETIC CARE UNIT

In the postanesthetic care unit (PACU), the child is observed until there is adequate recovery from anesthesia. Parents should be permitted to comfort their children in the PACU. Achievement of spontaneous breathing, adequate arterial saturation >95%, and hemodynamic stability are key recovery end-points. The child should be arousable, responsive, and oriented before discharge from the PACU. The amount of time spent in the PACU will depend on whether the child is being discharged to an inpatient nursing unit, to an ICU, to a postrecovery area, or directly home. Discharge from the PACU depends on the child's overall functional status, not merely the physiologic end-points, but also the behavioral end-points as well as the adequate provision of analgesia and control of postoperative nausea and vomiting. There are several scoring systems (Table 76-7) for determining whether a child is ready to be discharged from the PACU.

COMPLICATIONS IN THE PACU.

Respiratory Depression. Prolonged emergence from anesthesia and respiratory depression can be caused by opioids or inadequate antagonism of neuromuscular blocking agents. Pain can cause significant hypoventilation, especially after thoracic or abdominal surgery. Delayed emergence from anesthesia can occur as a result of retention of inhaled anesthetic agents worsened by hypoventilation. Hypothermia, especially in neonates, delays metabolism and excretion of anesthetics and also aggravates neuromuscular blockade. If respiratory depression is profound, then maintenance of the airway may require an oral airway. If the depression is severe, endotracheal intubation and mechanical ventilation are indicated.

Only in rare cases, where **opioid suppression** is suspected, is reversal of the effects of opioid with naloxone indicated. The reversal of the effects of opioids with naloxone is not only reversal of respiratory depression, but also reversal of analgesia. A somnolent child with respiratory depression may become excited, agitated in severe pain, uncontrollable, and/or hypertensive after naloxone. Opioid reversal necessitates bedside attention by the physician to monitor the child's behavioral, hemodynamic, and respiratory status. Naloxone is shorter-acting than most opioid analgesics.

Atelectasis is another respiratory complication occurring in the first 48 hr after anesthesia. Although atelectasis suggests an inhaled foreign body, it is most likely caused by secretions and decreased respiratory effort secondary to pain. Microatelectasis may lead to postoperative infections. Aspiration pneumonia is another postoperative complication.

Postoperative stridor occurs in up to 2% of all pediatric patients. The use of uncuffed, atraumatic, nonirritant endotracheal tubes has decreased the incidence of airway trauma. The use of appropriately sized endotracheal tubes and assurance of an air leak <30 cm H_2O pressure further decreases the risk of airway trauma. A history of stridor increases the likelihood of postoperative complications. Stridor may be severe enough after extubation to require re-intubation. Retractions and respiratory distress in the postoperative period should suggest this complication, and stridor or wheezing should confirm the diagnosis. Racemic epinephrine aerosols are effective therapy; their use requires prolonged observation because of the potential for recurrence of the airway obstruction. Stridor in infants suggests the need for overnight observation.

Hemodynamic instability is much less common in the PACU. Volume expansion may be required to maintain adequate blood pressure, peripheral perfusion, and urine output. Excessive volume replacement (>30 mL/kg) that is required to maintain blood pressure, perfusion, and urine output in the postoperative period is an indication of shock and occult bleeding, and it requires surgical consultation.

Emergence delirium is noted in <3% of children and is more common in those 3–9 yr old. In the immediate hr after surgery, the child may become extremely restless, combative, and disoriented, and may be screaming, crying, or poorly communicative. These children pose a danger to themselves. This phenomenon is more common when barbiturates are used as part of premedication or induction and inhalational anesthetics or ketamine forms part of the maintenance anesthetic. Although disorientation is common in the postanesthetic stage, erratic, delirious behavior requires attention, with gentle restraint, a quiet environment, and comforting. Potential postoperative complications, such as hypoglycemia and hypoxemia, should be ruled out. Occasionally, it is necessary to sedate the child with benzodiazepines, although these prolong postanesthesia recovery time, and when they wear off, emergence delirium may occur.

Awareness Under Anesthesia. One of the primary goals of anesthesiology is obtunding consciousness to ablate both awareness during procedures and recall afterward. In adults, certain anesthetic techniques are associated with an unacceptably high incidence of recall during anesthesia. Awareness and recall of events during a surgical procedure can be unpleasant and terrifying; the long-term sequelae of such recall in children are unknown. Continuous monitoring of cerebral electroencephalographic function by monitoring the bispectral index (BIS) has been recommended. Unfortunately, data in children do not confirm the efficacy of BIS monitoring as a means of determining anesthetic depth, and this, combined with the absence of meaningful data on intraoperative awareness and recall in infants and children does not currently support the routine use of BIS monitoring.

Postoperative Nausea and Vomiting. After general anesthesia, as many as 40–50% of children may experience nausea and vomiting. More than 80% of all high-risk children receiving inhalational anesthesia experience postoperative nausea and vomiting (PONV). This may occur in the immediate postoperative period, within the first 1–2 hr, or several hours after surgery and anesthesia. The etiology may be related to the stress and trauma of surgery, combined with the emetic effects of anesthetic agents. Pain is an important cause of nausea and vomiting. Opioid analgesics also induce nausea and vomiting. Preoperative fasting does not decrease the incidence of nausea and vomiting. Indeed, hydration and glucose supplementation appear to be important factors in decreasing PONV. The use of analgesic agents other than opioids (acetaminophen, ketorolac) and regional or local anesthesia is associated with decreased PONV.

This complication prolongs recovery room times, requires significant nursing attention, and increases the use of potent antiemetic agents (ondansetron, other serotonin antagonists). Droperidol is beneficial prophylactically and for established vomiting; metoclopramide is useful prophylactically. Droperidol must be used with caution, due to the rare occurrence of a prolonged Q-T interval and ventricular arrhythmias. Ondansetron is very efficacious as a prophylactic and in the treatment of PONV. Ondansetron and other serotonin antagonists are recommended for high-risk patients (strabismus surgery) or for actual treatment of PONV. They are contraindicated in children taking serotonin reuptake inhibitors for migraine headaches.

Thermoregulation and Malignant Hyperthermia. In the PACU, thermoregulation remains abnormal for several hours. Shivering is common in the postoperative state, and a feeling of extreme cold is common. Warm blankets are very comforting and seem to decrease shivering. **Hypothermia,** especially in neonates, leads to hypotension, bradycardia, acidosis, apnea, and prolongation of the effect of opioids and neuromuscular blocking agents. Although there are deleterious effects of hypothermia, rewarming must be done cautiously to avoid burning and cutaneous hyperthermia. **Hyperthermia,** with temperatures in excess of 39°C, is of concern in the postoperative period. If this occurs within hours of the use of an inhalational anesthetic, especially if succinylcholine was used, malignant hyperthermia must be suspected.

Malignant hyperthermia is an acute hypermetabolic syndrome that is triggered by inhalational anesthetic agents and succinylcholine. It resembles neuroleptic malignant syndrome. The onset of malignant hyperthermia may be acute, and its course may be fulminant and rapidly fatal. This condition, albeit rare (approximately 1 : 60,000 pediatric patients given anesthesia) is a constant concern. The disease is familial, and hence a family history of death or a febrile reaction during anesthesia should alert the anesthesiologist to its potential. Its clinical course is characterized by rapid onset of fever, acidosis, hypercarbia, and increased expired CO_2. High fever (38.5–46.0°C, rising 1°C every 5 min), muscle rigidity, metabolic acidosis, and hemodynamic collapse can occur. Death ensues from shock and cardiac dysrhythmias with unresponsive ventricular fibrillation. The mortality rate for malignant hyperthermia was once >70%. Aggressive therapy, including discontinuation of all inhalational anesthetic administration, correction of the metabolic acidosis, and treatment with the muscle relaxant sodium dantrolene, has reduced the mortality rate to <5%. Dantrolene and a kit containing supplies necessary to treat malignant hyperthermia should be present at every site where pediatric anesthesia is provided.

Malignant hyperthermia is probably genetically heterogeneous, with >10 genes contributing to susceptibility. Genetic mutations in the ryanodine receptor (the calcium channel of the sarcoplasmic reticulum) have been reported in 20–40% of humans with malignant hyperthermia.

Malignant hyperthermia appears to occur from a massive triggering of excitation-contraction coupling, sarcolemmal calcium release, and propagation of contraction by a complex biochemical process. The prolonged ischemic contraction leads to myolysis, with release of myoglobin, very high serum creatine phosphokinase (CPK) levels, and renal failure secondary to myoglobinuria. Malignant hyperthermia generally occurs within the 1st 2 hr of anesthesia, but rarely can occur up to 24 hr later.

Certain phenomena are clues to the risk of malignant hyperthermia. The occurrence of masseter spasm during induction, with rigid clenching of the masseter muscles and an inability to open the mouth, may presage full-blown disease. Acute myoglobinuria associated with a malignant hyperthermia–triggering agent is another clue. The child may not be hypermetabolic or febrile, but may have dark urine and high serum CPK levels, with the risk of myoglobin-induced renal tubular damage. The finding of dark urine after an anesthetic requires investigation for malignant hyperthermia. An elevated CPK value and heme-positive urine in the absence of red blood cells in the urine indicates a need for renal protection with mannitol and alkaline diuresis.

Certain myopathies are associated with the risk of malignant hyperthermia; these include Duchenne muscular dystrophy, Noonan phenotype, and, in children with a history of ptosis, squint, scoliosis, and muscle cramping. It is wise to avoid the use of succinylcholine in children with myopathies.

Rapid therapy is essential. All known triggering agents must be stopped. Intravenous administration of dantrolene sodium (2.5 mg/kg IV) as an initial dose is given as soon as possible. The need for repeated doses is indicated by the persistence of muscle rigidity, acidosis, and tachycardia, up to a maximum dose of 10 mg/kg. After control of the symptoms, the patient should be observed for at least 24 hr after the laboratory values have returned to normal because relapse can occur.

Prevention of malignant hyperthermia in susceptible patients requires the avoidance of triggering agents, which include inhalational anesthetics. Most anesthesiology departments are capable of delivering general anesthetics using anesthesia machines from which all traces of anesthetic vapors have been removed. Intravenous anesthesia and a nitrous-opioid technique are safe. Dantrolene prophylaxis is not recommended because the disease is rapidly treatable and because the drug causes respiratory depression and muscle weakness. If a child is suspected of having malignant hyperthermia, the malignant hyperthermia hotline, 1-800-MHHYPER, should be notified. This hotline will register susceptible patients and provides diagnostic and therapeutic information. Preanesthesia susceptibility testing includes genetic analysis of the ryanodine receptor gene, muscle biopsies, in vitro contraction studies, and possibly measuring muscle CO_2 production in response to intramuscular caffeine.

Postoperative Apnea. Apnea within the first 24–48 hr after surgery and anesthesia in premature infants is common; both central and obstructive apnea (mixed apnea) may occur. The use of respiratory depressants may impair respiratory control in neonates. Apnea is also a recognized stress response in neonates, and inadequate anesthesia is associated with increased apnea and respiratory complications.

The risk of postoperative apnea in premature neonates is inversely proportional to postconceptual age at the time of surgery. This risk is minimal by the time premature infants have reached the postconceptual age of 60 wk. Apnea is most common within the first 12 hr after surgery; postanesthetic apnea has been reported in premature infants up to 48 hr later. The incidence of apnea in full-term infants is debatable and not clearly demonstrated. It is generally agreed that general anesthesia should be avoided, except for emergent surgery, in full-term children younger than 44 wk postconceptual age. If surgery is required within the 1st mo of life, overnight observation and monitoring is indicated. Theophyllines decrease the incidence of postoperative apnea; they do not ablate it and therefore are not routinely used. The safest course is to monitor premature infants younger than 60 wk postconceptual age and full-term infants younger than 1 mo old for at least 24 hr after anesthesia.

PREANESTHETIC EVALUATION

Most previously healthy children require minimal preoperative assessment. The American Society of Anesthesiologists (ASA) classification system for anesthetic care is the ASA Physical Status (PS) classification (Table 76-8).

For ASA PS-1 patients, a brief history, notation of medical allergies, and a physical examination, focusing on the airway, lungs, and cardiac function, are sufficient. All children who are being assessed for anesthesia risk should have a family history obtained for reactions to anesthetics, for drug allergies, and for sudden death intraoperatively or hyperthermia after surgery, which may indicate a risk of malignant hyperthermia. In children who have had a previous anesthetic, questions should be asked regarding intraoperative anesthetic complications. The history should focus on determining whether the child is at risk for anesthetic or surgical stress as well as cardiorespiratory disease and airway compromise.

Recent URIs should be noted. A URI is an upper respiratory illness associated with fever, mucopurulent green or yellow nasal discharge, productive cough, injected sclerae, and increased mucous secretions. Clear rhinorrhea is generally not a concern. URIs can increase airway reactivity for up to 6 wk in both normal children and children with a history of reactive airway disease. URIs can also increase the risk of laryngospasm and bronchospasm, cause decreased mucociliary clearance, and increase the risk of intraoperative atelectasis and hypoxemia. It is generally recommended to avoid general anesthesia for elective procedures for 4–6 wk after a URI. In patients with chronic sinusitis and nasal polyps, infection should be thoroughly treated before elective anesthesia.

Acute, fatal bronchospasm can occur during induction of anesthesia and endotracheal intubation for routine, minor surgery in children with asthma. Those children at particular risk for anesthetic complications with asthma are those who have been (1) admitted to the hospital within the previous yr for their asthma, (2) seen in an emergency department in the last 6 mo, (3) admitted to an ICU, or (4) treated with parenteral systemic steroids. The child should be free of wheezing for at least several days before surgery, even if this necessitates an increase in β-agonists and the addition of steroids. Preoperative steroids are indicated for all children with asthma who have received or are receiving asthma therapy within the last yr. Prednisone, 1 mg/kg given 24 and 12 hr before surgery, significantly decreases airway reactivity perioperatively. Active wheezing is an indication for canceling elective surgery. If wheezing cannot be controlled on an outpatient basis with β-agonists, steroids, and other asthma therapy, then admission for more aggressive therapy before surgery is indicated.

Bronchopulmonary dysplasia also provides significant intraoperative risks. The same applies to children with cystic fibrosis and other chronic lung diseases. Every effort should be made to ensure that these children achieve the best possible respiratory status before surgery. Infections should be treated and reactive airways optimally treated without evidence of wheezing.

AIRWAY EVALUATION. Because the induction of anesthesia is associated with loss of spontaneous ventilation and airway reflexes, predicting the inability to bag-and-mask ventilate or endotracheally intubate a child before anesthesia is critical. The anesthesiologist must be made aware of children who have congenital anomalies that affect the airway (Table 76-9). They include

TABLE 76-8. American Society of Anesthesiology Physical Status Classification

Class 1: Healthy patient, no systemic disease
Class 2: Mild systemic disease with no functional limitations (mild chronic renal failure, iron deficiency anemia, mild asthma)
Class 3: Severe systemic disease with functional limitations (hypertension, poorly controlled asthma or diabetes, congenital heart disease, cystic fibrosis)
Class 4: Severe systemic disease that is a constant threat to life (critically and/or acutely ill patients with major systemic disease)
Class 5: Moribund patients not expected to survive 24 hr, with or without surgery
Additional classification: "E"—emergency surgery

TABLE 76-9. Syndromes Causing Difficult Airways

Choanal atresia
Beckwith-Wiedemann
Mucopolysaccharidosis
Pierre Robin
Treacher-Collins
Goldenhar's
DiGeorge
Apert
Achondroplasia
Turner
Cornelia de Lange
Smith-Lemli-Opitz
Juvenile rheumatoid arthritis
Fractured mandible
Airway tumors, hemangiomas
Cystic hygroma/teratoma
Trisomy 21

micrognathia syndromes, macroglossia syndromes, and some thoracic anomalies. Congenital anomalies associated with airway compromise should be diagnosed preoperatively. Conditions that impair mouth opening (temporomandibular joint disease) should be noted. A history of wheezing or stridor may indicate postoperative airway complications and difficult intraoperative airway management.

MEDIASTINAL MASSES. Children with anterior mediastinal masses, such as lymphomas and primary mediastinal tumors, are at serious risk for airway compromise, cardiac tamponade, and vascular obstruction. Induction of general anesthesia and even mild sedation can rapidly lead to total loss of the airway, with inability to ventilate the child and cardiovascular collapse. These patients often present in a semi-emergent fashion, with the need for both a tissue diagnosis before treatment is initiated and a surgically placed central line.

Significant compression of vital structures can occur with seemingly mild symptoms. Tachypnea, orthopnea, wheezing, and sleep disturbances or avoidance of prone or supine positions are significant indications of serious risk. Pericardial tamponade or superior vena cava syndromes are more concerning findings. A CT scan showing >50% compression of the airway at the carina is an indication to prohibit general anesthesia and provide only mild sedation. Echocardiographic or CT evidence of pericardial tamponade, right ventricular compression, or compression of the pulmonary artery suggests severe risk. Biopsy under local anesthesia may be indicated. If anesthesia is required, cardiopulmonary bypass should be considered in the event that it becomes impossible to ventilate the child. In high-risk children, consideration should be given to initiating treatment with steroids, radiation therapy, and chemotherapy before obtaining a tissue diagnosis.

DOWN SYNDROME. Children with Down syndrome are occasionally behaviorally difficult and are especially fearful of medical caregivers. Their cardiac anomalies, macroglossia, and upper airway obstruction can be challenging. Children with Down syndrome have atlantoaxial instability caused by odontoid hypoplasia and joint laxity. In younger children, extension of the neck, routinely used to maintain and intubate the airway, may lead to cervical dislocation and spinal cord trauma. Some anesthesiologists recommend extension and flexion lateral neck films to detect instability before anesthesia. In these children, it is wise to exercise caution in stabilizing the cervical spine and also to avoid flexion and extension.

CARDIOVASCULAR SYSTEM. Because of the depressant effects of anesthetics and the increased metabolic demands of surgery, any compromise of myocardial function should be clearly delineated preoperatively. A preoperative ECG, an echocardiogram, and a cardiology consultation are indicated for children with a history of heart disease. An intracardiac shunt will affect oxygenation status intraoperatively. Because of the significant effect on the oxygen supply and demand relationship caused by general anesthesia and surgical stress, obstructive lesions, such as a valvular stenosis, must also be clearly defined. A history of cardiac dysrhythmias should be clearly understood, because inhalational anesthetics are dysrhythmogenic.

In neonates, ductus arteriosus, myocardial compromise, pulmonary edema, or congenital heart disease can significantly complicate oxygen delivery during anesthesia. Accurate diagnosis of cardiac murmurs in neonates is essential. Any cardiovascular compromise preoperatively will be worsened intraoperatively and can catastrophically complicate the perioperative course.

Anemia should be diagnosed and corrected preoperatively if possible. A hematocrit >30% is generally acceptable for routine elective anesthesia. If there are reasons to expect significant blood loss or prolonged convalescence, anemia should be corrected preoperatively. In the emergent setting, transfusion may be required. Although lower hematocrits can be tolerated in unstressed children, the significant threat to oxygen delivery posed by anesthesia and surgery, especially if blood loss is expected, requires maintenance of an adequate hemoglobin concentration perioperatively.

Evidence of coagulopathy should be sought. Easy bruising, the use of aspirin, or familial bleeding disorders should be discussed. Intraoperative hemorrhagic bleeding can be difficult to control; massive perioperative blood transfusions have significant risk of morbidity and mortality. Preoperative correction of coagulopathic disorders is indicated. In neonates, assurance of vitamin K prophylaxis and adequate coagulation status is critical before any significant surgery. In neonates and critically ill children, adequate platelet count and, where indicated, coagulation factors, prothrombin time, and partial thromboplastin time should be assured.

NEUROBEHAVIORAL CONSIDERATIONS. The child's level of interaction and understanding form a backdrop for providing safe and comfortable anesthesia. Seizures, significant neurologic impairment, altered level of consciousness, respiratory airway compromise secondary to neurologic disease, and neuromuscular disease should be sought and evaluated. Anticonvulsant drug metabolism is often altered perioperatively, and this may alter anticonvulsant drug levels. Anticonvulsants may also complicate anesthetic management. Maintenance of appropriate anticonvulsant therapy postoperatively is important to avoid new seizures. Cerebrospinal fluid secretion is increased during surgery and general anesthesia. This is significant in patients suspected of having elevated intracranial pressure or in children with ventriculoperitoneal shunts. In infants or older children with ventriculoperitoneal shunts, shunt patency and function should be assured before surgery.

Illness and the need for surgery or painful medical procedures are psychologically traumatic events for children and their families. Children are also remarkably adept at sensing stressful signals from their parents and caregivers. Many children who require anesthesia may have significant levels of fear and anxiety. Most children undergoing surgery have new-onset negative behavioral changes in the postoperative period, such as maladaptive behavioral responses that include generalized anxiety, enuresis, enhanced separation anxiety, temper tantrums, nighttime crying, and fear of strangers, doctors, and hospitals. Approximately 20% show these negative behavioral adaptations for 6 mo after surgery. Sleep quality is also altered postoperatively, resulting in further behavioral compromise.

The risk factors for postoperative behavioral changes include preoperative or induction anxiety and behaviors indicating extreme stress, as well as emergence excitation. The type of surgery may be important, with tonsillectomy and genitourinary surgery having a high incidence of postoperative behavioral changes, whereas simple procedures (tympanostomy tubes) seem to be associated with fewer changes. Another risk factor is recurrent procedures, such as anesthesia for laser surgery, strabismus surgery, or repeated eye examinations, which lead to difficult behavioral changes and have a significant effect on family dynamics.

Preoperative psychologic preparation programs decrease the incidence of postoperative behavioral changes, which last for up to 1 mo. PPI does not improve postoperative behavior. Oral midazolam (0.5 mg/kg) may decrease negative behavioral changes after surgery. Midazolam has the benefit of providing not only rapid-onset anxiolysis in 10–20 min, but also very effective and rapid (10 min) amnesia.

PREOPERATIVE PREPARATION. The child should be in the best possible nutritional state, and nutritional supplementation,

TABLE 76-10. Guidelines for Preoperative Fasting* (2-4-6-8 Rule)

TIME BEFORE SURGERY (HR)	ORAL INTAKE
2	Clear, sweet liquids
4	Breast milk
6	Infant formula, fruit juices, gelatin
8	Solid food

*These are general guidelines and may differ among hospitals.

even hyperalimentation in chronically ill children, may be worthwhile.

Preoperative Fasting. Aspiration of gastric contents is a perioperative disaster, and if superimposed on lung disease, may be rapidly fatal. Aspiration may lead to laryngospasm and bronchospasm, with hypoxemia and hypoxic ischemic encephalopathy. It may also produce intraoperative atelectasis and postoperative pneumonia. It is vital to ensure that the stomach is as empty as possible before the induction of anesthesia. Acid aspiration is less likely with an empty stomach. Preoperative fasting (NPO) guidelines are noted in Table 76-10.

Clear, sweet liquids (Pedialyte, D5W) facilitate gastric emptying, help avoid hypoglycemia, and can be given up to 2 hr before anesthesia in any child. For older infants and children, a fasting period of 4 hr for liquids provides optimal safety and minimal discomfort. Solids must be avoided for at least 8 hr before surgery. Because surgery is frequently scheduled in the morning, and for ease and clarity of understanding, the general guideline is NPO for solids after midnight. Many conditions delay gastric emptying, and prolonged periods of fasting may be required in the presence of stress, anxiety, illness, trauma, gross obesity, or biliary atresia, or in children with delayed gastric emptying for other reasons.

The Full Stomach. Because of the serious complications of aspiration of gastric contents, it is desirable to secure the airway as rapidly as possible after obtundation in patients at risk for having a full stomach. Gastric emptying may be delayed for up to 96 hr after an acute episode of trauma or surgical illness. Under these circumstances, induction of general anesthesia and endotracheal intubation are performed in a rapid sequence (**rapid sequence induction**).

Preparation is of utmost importance. All airway equipment should be available: a selection of laryngoscope blades, 2 laryngoscope handles (in case 1 fails), and appropriately sized endotracheal tubes, with 1 size above and 1 size below the appropriately sized endotracheal tube for age. Two sources of suction with 2 large-volume suction catheters (Yankauer suction catheters, or "tonsil suckers") should be available, because vomiting can be copious. The goal is to place an endotracheal tube through the vocal cords as rapidly as possible after the loss of airway reflexes. Because muscle relaxation with succinylcholine can take 30–45 sec and nondepolarizing muscle relaxants can take 45–90 sec, concurrent administration of sedation and muscle relaxation is indicated.

The risks of rapid sequence induction include the possibility that if the airway cannot be intubated, the child is paralyzed without a protected airway and ventilation may be hazardous or impossible. Rapid sequence induction should be performed by those who can definitely achieve rapid endotracheal intubation. It should be avoided in patients with a history of failed oral endotracheal intubation, or with 1 of many syndromes (micrognathia) associated with difficult intubation. Under these circumstances, bronchoscopic awake intubation may be indicated.

Before rapid sequence induction, the child should be preoxygenated by breathing 100% oxygen for 2 min to give an extra margin of safety should intubation be difficult. The child should not be assist-ventilated either before or after the administration of drugs because this may lead to increased gastric air and actually increase the likelihood of vomiting, regurgitation, and aspiration.

A standard regimen for rapid sequence induction includes the administration of 3–6 mg/kg of sodium thiopental or 1.5–3 mg/kg of propofol concurrently with either 0.9–1.2 mg/kg of rocuronium or 1.5 mg/kg of vecuronium. Immediately after the administration of sedation and muscle relaxants, the Sellick maneuver (cricoid pressure) should be performed by applying firm pressure in a posterior direction against the cricoid cartilage. This displaces the cricoid cartilage into the esophagus, forming an artificial sphincter to prevent reflux of the gastroesophageal contents. Cricoid pressure should be maintained until correct placement of the endotracheal tube is verified by direct visualization, fogging of the tube, and in all circumstances, positive end-tidal CO_2.

POSTOPERATIVE PAIN MANAGEMENT

Continuation of analgesia and anxiolysis should follow surgery or painful procedures (see Chapter 77). Incision and operative pain will persist for hours to days, depending on the type and location of the surgery. Complete freedom from pain is not possible. To indicate that a hospital perioperative service or a physician can provide a "pain-free" environment is misrepresentation and will disappoint children, families, and caregivers. Preoperative education about the surgery and a pain management plan, development of skills designed to decrease anticipatory anxiety, and active participation in treatment planning can be helpful for some children and families. Adjunctive therapy, such as visual reality, hypnosis, pet therapy, and play therapy, also can decrease the need for potent analgesics postoperatively.

The combination of opioid and nonopioid analgesic agents and an understanding of the benefits and risks provide the foundation of pain management. A judicious combination of nonsteroidal anti-inflammatory drugs, cyclo-oxygenase-2 (COX-2) inhibitors, opioids, and regional analgesia has a role in postoperative pain management. Repeated evaluation is as important as the modality of pain management. Continuous and repetitive small doses of analgesia around the clock are more effective at reducing pain than occasional prn dosing intervals.

Patient-controlled analgesia (PCA), nurse-controlled analgesia, and parent-controlled analgesia are all used postoperatively (see Chapter 77). PCA provides continuous pain treatment and self-medication (vs intermittent or prn pain control) as well as control and comfort in an otherwise personally uncontrolled circumstance. PCA provides both a background low-dose infusion rate of a continuous opioid and the opportunity to supplement analgesia with bolus doses as needed. The practitioner can determine the continuous infusion rate, the bolus dose, the lockout interval, and the number of boluses per unit time that the patient may receive. PCA relies on the theory that patients cannot or will not overdose themselves because somnolence will decrease repeated self-administration. In young children, the use of the *pain button* (for pain relief) may be more difficult to ensure; children as young as 5 yr have been able to use PCA successfully. In older children and adolescents, PCA should be a standard modality of postoperative pain management.

The concern with nurse-controlled analgesia or parent-controlled analgesia is that an overdose is possible. However, with careful observation and monitoring, as well as intelligent design of the continuous infusion rate, lockout periods, frequency of dosing, and bolus dose, this is a safe modality of therapy.

REGIONAL ANESTHESIA. Regional anesthesia is the use of anesthetics to block the conduction of afferent neural impulses to the CNS. These can be local analgesic techniques, peripheral nerve blocks, nerve-plexus blocks, or epidural and subarachnoid (spinal) nerve blocks. They may be administered either by a single injection (single shot) or by continuous infusion, as is common with epidural and occasionally subarachnoid blocks. They may be used for intraoperative anesthesia and postoperative analgesia, and they have the potential to decrease intraoperative analgesia and anesthetic use as well as provide postoperative pain management.

Analgesia at the site of need, without central cardiorespiratory depressant effects, can be valuable. Local anesthesia, with injection of lidocaine or bupivacaine into the affected area, can provide procedural analgesia that lasts for several hours. Infiltration of the wound site and the edges of an incision decreases postoperative pain in the initial hours after surgery. This can be injected by the surgeon at the conclusion of surgery and may supplement postoperative analgesia.

Epidural analgesia is common in pediatric practice. The epidural space lies between the dura and the pia and arachnoid membranes, an area through which all nerve roots pass. Bathing these nerve roots in local anesthetics inhibits conduction of pain impulses centrally. A single dose of epidural anesthetic may provide hours of pain relief, and a continuous infusion may provide effective pain relief for hours to days. The epidural injection of opioids can provide analgesia for 12–24 hr and is a potential supplement to postoperative analgesia.

A lumbar epidural is placed in the lumbar area to provide analgesia for labor and surgery below the thorax. Caudal epidural analgesia is placed through the sacral hiatus, inferior to the distal end of the spinal cord. This is the site most commonly used for regional anesthesia and analgesia in children and is efficacious for the provision of pelvic and lower limb anesthetic as well as beneficial in orthopedic and urologic surgery. A continuous infusion of bupivacaine is the most common means of providing postoperative epidural pain relief; this may be mixed with an opioid (fentanyl or preservative-free morphine). It is also possible to provide epidural PCA with a continuous infusion pump and the ability for the patient to self-medicate with bolus prn dosing. Epidural analgesia can also provide pain relief in patients with chronic pain or pain caused by advanced malignant conditions.

The most serious complications of neuraxial anesthesia include cephalad spread of blockade with respiratory depression, paralysis of respiratory muscles, and in extreme cases, brainstem analgesia and depression. The most common complications of neuraxial analgesia include mild discomfort; a paresthesia-like feeling of numbness and tingling; pruritus, which, if opioids are used, can be quite distressing; and occasional nausea and vomiting. Infection and epidural hematoma are extremely rare. Neuraxial opioids, especially administered intrathecally, can cause respiratory depression; their use requires postoperative monitoring. The use of neuraxial opioids often requires treatment with antipruritic as well as antiemetic drugs.

SEDATION AND PROCEDURAL PAIN. The same drugs that induce general anesthesia are often used to provide sedation (see Table 76-5). Sedation is on the continuum between wakefulness and general anesthesia (see Table 76-4). The term **conscious sedation** refers to a condition in which a patient is sleepy, comfortable, and cooperative, but maintains airway-protective and ventilatory reflexes. Unfortunately, for most children, this level of sedation provides little or no analgesia, and both psychologic and physiologic responses to painful stimuli persist. Sedation that is sufficient to obtund painful responses is most likely deep sedation. **Deep sedation** is a state of unarousability to voice and is accompanied by suppression of reflex responses. Management of sedated children requires vigilance and knowledge to ensure their safety and is governed by the same guidelines as anesthesia care (Table 76-11). A dose of sedative medication that causes minimal sedation in 1 subject may produce complete unconsciousness and apnea in another. Careful attention to guidelines for appropriate monitoring and management of sedation in children is imperative. For threatening and nonpainful procedures, anxiolysis or light sedation is frequently sufficient. For painful procedures (e.g., bone marrow aspiration, insertion of percutaneous intravenous catheter lines, lumbar punctures), the combination of sedation with analgesia that is required in children produces deep sedation.

TABLE 76-11. Systematic Approach to Sedation in Children

Thorough medical history, anticipating underlying medical problems predisposing the patient to sedation problems
Careful physical examination focused on the cardiorespiratory system and airway
Appropriate fasting
Informed consent
Pediatric drug dosing (milligrams per kilogram)
Appropriate-sized equipment
A separate, dedicated observer to monitor sedated patients who may have airway compromise (induced or pre-existing)
Documentation of vital signs and condition on a time-based record
Emergency backup system, code team, and crash cart
Fully equipped and staffed recovery area
Discharge criteria documenting recovery from sedation

Sedation with chloral hydrate, pentobarbital, or benzodiazepines is often adequate for nonpainful procedures. Nevertheless, there can be a high failure rate as well as complications, such as prolonged sedation (hours to overnight), ataxia, nausea and vomiting, desaturation, and the occasional need for rapid intervention. The temptation to add opioids and deepen sedation increases the risk of complications. The most rapid way to ensure safely reversible sedation is with potent anesthetic agents. The ultra–short-acting anesthetics (methohexital, remifentanil, propofol, thiopental) provide effective procedural sedation, but there is a higher likelihood of inadvertent oversedation and induction of general anesthesia. These anesthetics offer efficient and rapidly reversible procedural sedation. However, their use requires the presence of an anesthesiologist and/or specially trained, experienced, and qualified physicians.

American Academy of Pediatrics, Committee on Drugs, Section on Anesthesiology: Guidelines for monitoring and management of pediatric patients during and after sedation for diagnostic and therapeutic procedures. *Pediatrics* 1992;89:1110–1115.

Betz E: Incidence of PONV not influenced by choice of air or nitrous oxide. *Anesthesiology* 2002;28:2–4.

Bouwmeester NJ, Anand KJ, van Dijk M, et al: Hormonal and metabolic stress responses after major surgery in children aged 0–3 years: A double-blind, randomized trial comparing the effects of continuous versus intermittent morphine. *Br J Anaesth* 2001;87:390–399.

Campagna JA, Miller KW, Forman SA: Mechanisms of actions of inhaled anesthetics. *N Engl J Med* 2003;348:2110–2124.

Cook-Sather SD, Harris KA, Chiavacci R, et al: A liberalized fasting guideline for formula-fed infants does not increase average gastric fluid volume before elective surgery. *Anesth Analg* 2003;96:965–969.

Cote CJ, Notterman DA, Karl HW, et al: Adverse sedation events in pediatrics: A critical incident analysis of contributing factors. *Pediatrics* 2000;105: 805–814.

Cravero JP, Blike GT: Review of pediatric sedation. *Anesth Analg* 2004;99:1355–1364.

Crawford MW, Rohan D, MacGowan CK, et al: Effect of propofol anesthesia and continuous positive airway pressure on upper airway size and configuration in infants. *Anesthesiology* 2006;105:45–50.

Golianu B, Krane EJ, Galloway KS, et al: Pediatric acute pain management. *Pediatr Clin North Am* 2000;47:559–587.

Hall SC: General pediatric emergencies: Malignant hyperthermia syndrome. *Anesthesiol Clin North Am* 2001;19:367–382.

Hoffmann GM, Nowakowski R, Troshynski TJ, et al: Risk reduction in pediatric procedural sedation by application of an American Academy of Pediatrics/American Society of Anesthesiologists process model. *Pediatrics* 2002;109:236–243.

Jayabose S, Levendoglu-Tugal O, Giamelli J, et al: Intravenous anesthesia with propofol for painful procedures in children with cancer. *J Pediatr Hematol Oncol* 2001;23:290–293.

Kain ZN: Postoperative behavioral changes in children. *ASA Newsl* 2002;66:14–16.
Krauss B, Green SM: Sedation and analgesia for procedures in children. *N Engl J Med* 2000;342:938–945.
Markakis DA: Regional anesthesia in pediatrics. *Anesthesiol Clin North Am* 2000;18:355–381.
Maxwell LG, Yaster M: Perioperative management issues in pediatric patients. *Anesthesiol Clin North Am* 2000;18:601–632.
Melzer W, Dietze B: Malignant hyperthermia and excitation-contraction coupling. *Acta Physiol Scand* 2001;171:367–378.
Monitto CL, Greenberg RS, Kost-Byerly S, et al: The safety and efficacy of parent/nurse-controlled analgesia in patients less than six years of age. *Anesth Analg* 2000;91:573–579.
Practice guidelines for sedation and analgesia by non-anesthesiologists: A report by the American Society of Anesthesiologists Task Force on Sedation and Analgesia by Non-anesthesiologists. *Anesthesiology* 1996;84:459–471.
Tobias JD: Therapeutic applications of regional anesthesia in paediatric-aged patients. *Paediatr Anaesth* 2002;12:272–277.
Urwyler A, Deufel T, McCarthy T, et al: Guidelines for molecular genetic detection of susceptibility to malignant hyperthermia. *Br J Anaesth* 2001; 86:283–287.
Welborn LG, Greenspun JC: Anesthesia and apnea: Perioperative considerations in the former preterm infant. *Pediatr Clin North Am* 1994;41: 181–198.
Yaster M: The dose response of fentanyl in neonatal anesthesia. *Anesthesiology* 1987;66:433–435.

Chapter 77 ■ Pediatric Pain Management

Lonnie K. Zeltzer and Heather Krell

DEVELOPMENT OF PAIN PERCEPTION AND EFFECTS OF PAIN ON THE NEWBORN

The neural progression of pain transmission begins with the development of skin and mouth sensory neurons by the end of the first 2 wk of gestation (Table 77-1). There is a progression in the growth of the neural apparatus involved in pain transmission throughout fetal development until the appearance of the beginning of the pain inhibitory apparatus, starting at approximately 32 wk of gestation and continuing into the newborn period. There are a number of sources of pain in the newborn period. These include acute pain (diagnostic and therapeutic procedures, minor surgery, monitoring), continuous pain (pain from thermal/chemical burns, postsurgical and inflammatory pain), and chronic or disease-related pain (repeated heelsticks, indwelling catheters, necrotizing enterocolitis, nerve injury, chronic conditions, thrombophlebitis). The most common sources of pain in healthy infants are acute procedures, including heel lances, surgeries, and, in males, circumcisions. In 2004, there were 1.2 million infant circumcisions and 1.4 million operative procedures performed on newborns in the United States. In premature infants in the neonatal intensive care unit (NICU), there are more procedures. In the 1st wk of life, approximately 94% of preterm infants <28 wk of gestational age are ventilated. There are many procedures performed in preterm infants, with most being heelsticks; only a few are preceded by any type of analgesia. In the NICU, procedures such as airway suctioning are common; the majority of these procedures are not preceded by any analgesia. Repeated handling and acute pain episodes sensitize the neonate to increased reactivity and stress responses to subsequent procedures as neonates or children.

TABLE 77-1. Fetal Development of Pain Systems

FETAL AGE (WK)	NEURAL DEVELOPMENT
7	Skin receptors and sensory nerves around the mouth
8–10	Cortex begins to form
13	Maturation of neurons in the dorsal horn of the spinal cord
15	Subplate zone of the cortex formed (signaling station)
16	Nonthalamic fibers reach the cortex; appearance of hormonal and circulatory stress responses
18	Thalamic fibers enter the cortex
19	First EEG signals recorded
20	Skin receptors and sensory nerves present throughout the fetus; amygdala, hippocampus, and other subcortical areas developed and functional; thalamic fibers completely penetrate the cortex; responses to light, sound, touch, and taste recorded
32	Appearance of inhibitory mechanisms

EEG, electroencephalogram.

Responses to pain depend on the development of the stress response system, which varies with development. Typical responses include increased heart rate, respiratory rate, blood pressure, and intracranial pressure. Cardiac vagal tone, transcutaneous oxygen saturation, carbon dioxide levels, and peripheral blood flow are decreased. Autonomic signs include changes in skin color, vomiting, gagging, hiccupping, diaphoresis, dilated pupils, and palmar and forehead sweating. To assess pain in the newborn, it is critical to observe the infant for facial expression, body movements, cry, and any other atypical functional behaviors. The observer needs to consider the context in which the behavior is experienced. The infant's state (agitated, alert, asleep) and gestational and post-gestational age also affect behavioral stress responses.

There are serious short-term and longer-term consequences of untreated pain in the newborn. There is a shift in most NICUs to more liberal use of opioids. Nonetheless, morphine, the traditional "gold standard" of analgesia for acute pain, may not be very effective and may have adverse long-term consequences. No differences have been found in the incidence of severe intraventricular hemorrhage or in the mortality rate when infants receiving morphine are compared with the placebo group, and there are no changes in assessed pain from tracheal suctioning in ventilated infants receiving morphine compared with those receiving a placebo infusion. Morphine may not alleviate acute pain in *ventilated preterm* neonates, although there are few data on the effects of morphine and fentanyl in nonventilated newborns. The lack of opioid effects for acute pain in neonates may be due to an immaturity of opioid receptors; acute pain may cause the uncoupling of m-opioid receptors in the forebrain. Repetitive acute pain may create central neural changes in the newborn that may have long-term consequence for later pain vulnerability, cognitive effects, and opioid tolerance.

Most neonatologists use opioids in painful situations. Sucrose and pacifiers are also being used in the NICU. The effects of sucrose (sweet taste) are believed to be opioid-mediated because they are reversed with naloxone; stress and pain relief are integrated through the endogenous opioid system. Taste is functioning in the fetus by 12 wk and is well formed by 20 wk of gestational age. Sucrose, with or without a pacifier, may be effective for acute pain and stress control. Other nonpharmacologic strategies for stress and pain control include infant care by an individual primary nurse, tactile-kinesthetic stimuli (massage), "kangaroo care," and soothing sensorial saturation.

CLINICAL ASSESSMENT OF PAIN

Pain is both a sensory and an emotional experience. Whenever feasible, pain is best assessed by directly asking children about the character, location, quality, duration, frequency, and intensity of their pain. Some children may not report pain because of fears, such as talking to doctors, disappointing or bothering others, receiving an injection of medication, finding out they are sick, or returning to the hospital. For infants and nonverbal children, parents, pediatricians, nurses, and other caregivers are constantly challenged to interpret whether the distressed behaviors of the children represent pain, fear, hunger, or a range of other perceptions or emotions. Therapeutic trials of comfort measures (cuddling, feeding) and analgesic medications may be helpful in clarifying the situation.

Behavior and physiologic signs are useful, but can be misleading. A toddler may scream and grimace during an ear examination because of fear rather than from pain. Conversely, children with inadequately relieved persistent pain from cancer, sickle cell disease, trauma, or surgery may withdraw from their surroundings and appear very quiet, leading observers to conclude falsely that they are comfortable or sedated. In these situations, increased dosing of analgesics may make the child become more, not less, interactive and alert. Similarly, neonates and young infants may close their eyes, furrow their brows, and clench their fists in response to pain. Adequate analgesia is often associated with eye opening and increased involvement in the surroundings. A child who is experiencing significant chronic pain may play "normally" as a way to distract attention from pain. This coping behavior is sometimes misinterpreted as evidence of the child "faking" pain at other times.

Investigators have devised a range of behavioral distress scales for infants and young children, mostly emphasizing the patient's facial expressions, crying, and body movement. Facial expression measures appear most useful and specific in neonates. Autonomic signs can indicate pain, but are nonspecific and may reflect other processes, including fever, hypoxemia, and cardiac or renal dysfunction.

Children 3–7 yr old become increasingly articulate in describing the intensity, location, and quality of pain. Pain is occasionally referred to adjacent areas; referral of hip pain to the leg or knee is not rare in this age range. There are self-report measures for children this age, using drawings, pictures of faces, or graded color intensity (Table 77-2). Children age 8 yr and older can usually use verbal or visual analog pain scales accurately (Fig. 77-1). Verbal ratings may be as in Figure 77-1 or using a scale of 0–10 where 0 is no pain and 10 is the most (worst) pain possible. In the United States, regularly documented pain assessments are now required for children who are hospitalized and for those attending outpatient hospital clinics and emergency departments.

The measurement of pain in cognitively impaired children remains a challenge, and methods are being studied to determine ways of assessing pain in this group. Understanding pain expression and experience in this population is important because behaviors may be misinterpreted as indicating that cognitively impaired children are more insensitive to pain. Children with Down syndrome may express pain less precisely and more slowly than the general population. Pain in individuals with autism spectrum disorders may be difficult to assess because they may be both hyposensitive and hypersensitive to many different types of sensory stimuli and may have limited communication abilities.

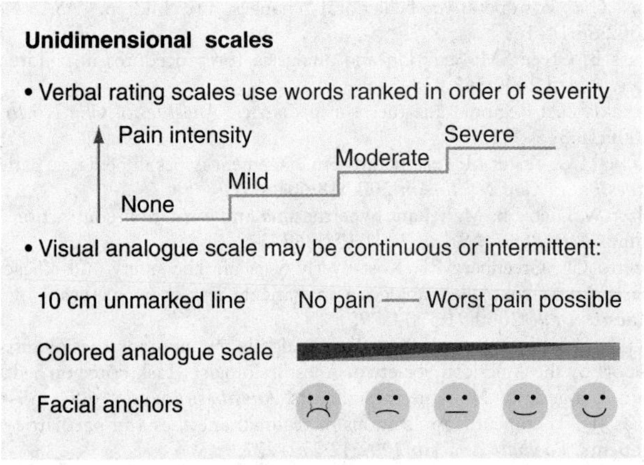

Unidimensional scales

• Verbal rating scales use words ranked in order of severity

Pain intensity: None — Mild — Moderate — Severe

• Visual analogue scale may be continuous or intermittent:

10 cm unmarked line — No pain —— Worst pain possible

Colored analogue scale

Facial anchors

Figure 77-1. Subjective measures of pain based on word descriptors. (From Holdcroft A, Power I: Management of pain. *BMJ* 2003;326:635–639.)

NONPHARMACOLOGIC APPROACHES TO PAIN MANAGEMENT

Numerous nonpharmacologic methods can be used to relieve pain, fear, and anxiety. These approaches have excellent safety profiles and increasing evidence of effectiveness. Studies of childhood chronic headaches provide robust evidence of the greater effectiveness of **cognitive-behavioral treatments** compared with that of many pharmacologic treatments. Many of these methods are also useful because children can generalize them to new situations and benefit from an increased sense of mastery by managing their symptoms. A child who has cancer and who learns self-hypnosis to reduce distress from lumbar punctures may successfully apply this skill to other stressful situations. Clinical attention to the environment, optimal positioning, physical comfort, and choice/control should be provided to every patient and family. Nonpharmacologic techniques alone may not work for some children and should not be used as an excuse for withholding appropriate analgesics.

Information should be given to children (and family members) in a developmentally and situationally appropriate manner as to

TABLE 77-2. Pain Measurement Tools

NAME	FEATURES	AGE RANGE	ADVANTAGES	LIMITATIONS
Visual Analog Scale (VAS)	Vertical 10-cm line; subject marks a spot on the line between "no pain" (or neutral face) and "worst pain imaginable" (or sad face)	8 yr and older	Good psychometric properties; gold standard	Cannot be used in younger children or those with cognitive limitations
Faces Scale (e.g., Wong-Baker, Oucher, Bieri, McGrath scales)	Subjects compare their pain with line drawings of faces or photos of children	4 yr and older	Can use at younger ages than VAS	Choice of "no pain" face affects responses (neutral vs smiling)
Color and other analog scales	Horizontal or vertical ruler, on which increasing intensity of red signifies more pain; pain ladder; pain thermometer; blocks	4 yr and older	Can use at younger ages than VAS; converges to VAS at older ages	Cannot be used in toddlers or those with cognitive limitations
Behavioral or combined behavioral-physiologic scales (e.g., CHEOPS, OPS, FACS, NIPS)	Scoring of observed behaviors (e.g., facial expression, limb movement) ± heart rate and blood pressure	Some work for any ages; some are specific age groups, including preterm infants	Can be used even for infants and nonverbal children	Nonspecific; over-rates feat in toddlers and preschool children; under-rates persistent pain; some measures are convenient, others require videotaping and complex processing; changes can occur unrelated to pain
Autonomic measures (e.g., heart rate, blood pressure, heart rate spectral analyses)	Scores changes in heart rate, blood pressure, or measures of heart rate variability (e.g., "vagal tone")	All ages	Can be used at all ages Useful for patients receiving mechanical ventilation	Nonspecific; changes can occur unrelated to pain
Hormonal-metabolic measures	Plasma or salivary sampling of hormones (e.g., cortisol, epinephrine)	All ages	Can be used at all ages	Nonspecific; changes can occur unrelated to pain; inconvenient; cannot provide "real-time" information

what to expect, given the child's medical condition, procedures, and treatments. Clinicians should include patients and their families in decision-making for pain control to ensure that the option chosen is the most appropriate for the situation and to optimize adherence to treatment protocols.

Relaxation techniques promote muscle relaxation and the reduction of anxiety, which often accompanies and increases pain. Controlled breathing and progressive muscle relaxation are commonly used relaxation techniques for preschool-aged and older children.

Distraction helps a child of any age shift attention away from pain and onto other activities. Common attention-sustainers in the environment include bubbles, music, video games, television, the telephone, conversation, school, and play.

Hypnotherapy involves helping a child to focus on an imaginative experience that is comforting, safe, fun, or intriguing. Hypnotherapy acts to capture the child's attention, alter sensory experiences, reduce distress, reframe pain experiences, create time distortions, help the child dissociate from the pain, and enhance feelings of mastery and self-control. This intervention is best for children of school age or older.

Biofeedback involves controlled breathing, relaxation, or hypnotic techniques with a mechanical device that provides visual or auditory "feedback" to the child when the desired action is approximated. Common targets of change include muscle tension, peripheral skin temperature through peripheral vasodilation, and anal control through rectal muscle contraction and relaxation. Biofeedback also enhances the child's sense of mastery and control and is especially useful for the child who needs more "proof" of change than that generated through hypnotherapy alone.

Iyengar yoga is a specific type of yoga developed to achieve balance in mind, body, and spirit. This form of therapeutic yoga is especially effective for chronic pain and also for improving mood, energy, and sleep, and reducing anxiety. Iyengar yoga involves a series of *asanas* (body poses) that are oriented for the specific medical condition or symptoms. It involves the use of props, such as blankets, bolsters, blocks, and belts to support the body and allow the patient to assume more healing poses. Yoga promotes a sense of energy, relaxation, strength, balance, and flexibility, and over time, enhances a sense of mastery and control. In more advanced yoga, certain types of breathing *(pranayama)* may be learned for added benefit.

Massage therapy can be very useful for children with chronic pain. Reductions in pain in children with juvenile rheumatoid arthritis and cancer and in adolescents with fibromyalgia have been noted using deep tissue massage. In addition to pain reduction and increased function, children in several studies were found to have short-term reductions in cortisol levels and improved sleep and mood. Massage is especially helpful in patients with myofascial pain. There are several types of massage, including craniosacral therapy.

Individual psychotherapy can be used to address the cognitive, behavioral, and psychologic contributors to pain and pain behaviors. Assessing and treating maladaptive coping, anxiety, depression, learning disorders, social problem-solving deficits, communication problems, relationship issues, unresolved grief or trauma, school avoidance, or other identified problems can reduce acute distress and chronic stress load on the central nervous system, thereby reducing excessive arousal and pain.

Family education and/or psychotherapy may be used to help family members understand the mechanisms and appropriate treatment of pain; alter family patterns that may inadvertently exacerbate pain; help parents cope with their own and their child's distress; and develop a plan for the child's optimal self-management of symptoms and independent functioning. Cognitive-behavioral family approaches have been shown to be effective for pediatric chronic pain.

Physical therapy can be very useful, especially for children with chronic musculoskeletal pain and/or those who have become deconditioned from inactivity. Exercise appears to have both specific benefits related to muscle functioning and posture and more generalized benefits related to improved body image, body mechanics, sleep, and mood.

Acupuncture is an important and popular part of a pain management plan for children with chronic pain and is feasible and very helpful for many children. Studies have shown its usefulness in chronic nausea, fatigue, and many chronic pain states, including migraines, chronic daily headaches, abdominal pain, and myofascial pain. Adult studies have also shown its efficacy in myofascial pain, primary dysmenorrhea, sickle cell crisis pain, and sore throat pain.

Transcutaneous electrical nerve stimulation (TENS) is quite safe and can be tried for many forms of localized pain. Children often find TENS helpful and effective; there are no randomized clinical trials of TENS for pain in children.

Music, art, dance, and aromatherapy have also been used and may be successful with some children.

The most successful way to treat chronic pain is to develop a communication plan among the different therapists, typically with the pediatrician as the case manager, so that each type of therapy is building on the other and all of the therapists are giving the same messages to the child and parent (integrative team approach).

DEVELOPMENTAL PHARMACOLOGY

Because the pharmacokinetics and pharmacodynamics of analgesics vary with age, drug response in infants and young children differs from that in older children and adults. The elimination half-life of most analgesics is prolonged in neonates and young infants because of their immature hepatic enzyme systems. Clearance of analgesics also may be variable in young infants and children. Renal blood flow, glomerular filtration, and tubular secretion increase dramatically in the 1st few wk and approach adult values by 3–5 mo of age. Renal clearance of analgesics is often greater in toddlers and preschool-aged children than in adults, whereas premature infants tend to have reduced renal clearance of analgesics. There also are age-related differences in body composition and protein binding. Total body water as a fraction of body weight is greater in neonates. Tissues with greater perfusion, such as the brain and heart, account for a larger proportion of body mass in neonates than do other tissues, such as muscle and fat. Because of decreased serum concentrations of albumin and α_1-acid glycoprotein, neonates have reduced protein binding of some drugs, resulting in higher amounts of free, unbound drug. Drug dosing in infants and younger children is often extrapolated from studies in adults and older children using weight-based scaling.

ACETAMINOPHEN, ASPIRIN, AND NONSTEROIDAL ANTI-INFLAMMATORY MEDICATIONS. Acetaminophen and nonsteroidal anti-inflammatory drugs (NSAIDs) have replaced aspirin as the most commonly used antipyretics and oral nonopioid analgesics (Table 77-3).

Acetaminophen is generally a safe nonopioid analgesic and antipyretic that has the advantage of rectal and oral routes of administration. In addition, acetaminophen is not associated with the gastrointestinal or antiplatelet effects of aspirin and NSAIDs, making it a particularly useful drug in patients with cancer. Unlike aspirin and NSAIDs, acetaminophen has little anti-inflammatory action. Toxicity from acetaminophen can occur from either large single doses or excessive cumulative dosing over days (see Chapter 710.2). Acetaminophen overdoses have been associated with fulminant hepatic failure in infants and children. Fever, alcohol, and dehydration may be risk factors for hepatic injury.

Aspirin is indicated for certain rheumatologic conditions and for inhibition of platelet adhesiveness, as in the treatment of

TABLE 77-3. Commonly Used Nonopioid Medications

Acetaminophen	10–15 mg/kg PO q4h 20–30 mg/kg/PR q4h 35 mg/kg/PR q6–8h *Maximum daily dosing:* 90 mg/kg/24 hr (children) 60 mg/kg/24 hr (infants) 30–45 mg/kg/24 hr (neonates)	No anti-inflammatory action; no antiplatelet or gastric effects; toxic dosing can produce hepatic failure
Aspirin	10–15 mg/kg PO q4h *Maximum daily dosing:* 120 mg/kg/24 hr (children)	Anti-inflammatory effects; prolonged antiplatelet effects; can cause gastritis; risk of Reye syndrome
Ibuprofen	8–10 mg/kg PO q6h	Anti-inflammatory effects; reversible antiplatelet effects; can cause gastritis; extensive pediatric safety experience
Naprosyn	5–7 mg/kg PO q8–12h	Anti-inflammatory effects; reversible antiplatelet effects; can cause gastritis; more prolonged duration than that of ibuprofen
Ketorolac	Loading dose 0.5 mg/kg then 0.25–0.5 mg/kg IV q6h to a maximum of 5 days; maximum dose 30 mg loading with maximum dosing of 15 mg q6h after that	Anti-inflammatory effects; reversible antiplatelet effects; can cause gastritis; useful for short-term situations when oral dosing is not feasible
Choline magnesium salicylate	10–20 mg/kg PO q8–12h	Weak anti-inflammatory effects; lower risk of bleeding and gastritis than with conventional NSAIDs
Nortriptyline, amitriptyline	Amitriptyline 0.2–0.5 mg/kg PO qhs, typically with maximum dose at 10–20 mg hs Nortriptyline is typically used at twice the doses described above	Useful for neuropathic pain; facilitates sleep; can enhance opioid effect; can be useful in sickle cell pain; rare risk of dysrhythmia; should screen for rhythm disturbances, check for normal QTc before beginning; side effects include dry mouth, sedation, constipation, urinary retention, orthostatic hypotension, palpitations
Gabapentin (Neurontin)	Start with 100 mg bid or tid and then increase; can use up to 3600 mg/24 h, but no good studies in children to indicate minimum or maximum dosing	Anticonvulsant used for neuropathic pain; can be associated with sedation or headache
Quetiapine, risperidone, thorazine, haloperidol	Quetiapine. Begin with 6.25 or 12.5 mg PO qd (hs) and can use q 6 hr prn, acute agitation with pain. Escalate dose to 25 mg/dose; risperidone can be especially useful for children with PDD spectrum or tic disorder and chronic pain; dose is 0.25–1 mg (in 0.25-mg increments) qd or bid; see PDR for other dosing.	Useful when arousal is clearly amplifying pain signaling; often used when first starting SSRI and then weaned off after on therapeutic doses of SSRI for at least 2 wk; check for normal QTc before beginning; side effects include extrapyramidal reactions and sedation; in high doses, can lower the seizure threshold in children with a seizure disorder; diphenhydramine (Benadryl) can be used to treat or prevent dystonic reactions
SSRIs (e.g., fluoxetine)	SSRI dosing per psychiatrist recommendation; fluoxetine can be used in very low doses (e.g., 1 mg) for children with chronic pain and PDD spectrum disorders	Useful for children with anxiety disorders in which arousal amplifies sensory signaling; useful in PDD spectrum disorders in very low doses; best to use in conjunction with psychiatric evaluation
Sucrose solution via pacifier or gloved finger	*Preterm infants (gestational age):* <28 wk: 0.2 mL swabbed into mouth; 28–32 wk: 0.2–2 mL, depending on suck/swallow; >32 wk: 2 mL *Term infants:* 1.5–2 mL PO over 2 min	Wait 2 min before starting procedure; analgesia may last up to 8 min; the dose may be repeated once

NSAIDs, nonsteriodal anti-inflammatory drugs; PDD, pervasive developmental disorder; PDR, Physicians' Desk Reference; QTc, correted QT interval on an electrocardiogram; SSRI, selective serotonin reuptake inhibitor.

Kawasaki disease. Concerns about Reye hepatic encephalopathy have resulted in a substantial decline in pediatric aspirin use during the last 20 yr (see Chapter 358).

The **NSAIDs** are used widely for the treatment of pain and fever in children. In children with juvenile rheumatoid arthritis, ibuprofen and aspirin are equally effective, but ibuprofen is associated with fewer side effects and better compliance. NSAIDs used adjunctively in surgical patients reduce opioid requirements (and opioid side effects) by as much as 35–40%. Although NSAIDs can be useful postoperatively, they should not be used as an excuse to withhold opioids from patients with unrelieved pain. Ketorolac is useful in treating moderate to severe acute pain when patients are unable to swallow oral medications. Adverse effects of NSAIDs are rare, but include gastrointestinal bleeding, renal dysfunction, and impaired platelet function. Although the overall incidence of bleeding is very low, NSAIDs should be avoided in children at risk for bleeding or when surgical hemostasis is a prominent concern. Renal injury from short-term use of ibuprofen in euvolemic children is quite rare; the risk is increased by hypovolemia or cardiac dysfunction. The safety of both ibuprofen and acetaminophen for short-term use is well established (see Table 77-3). NSAIDs and aspirin act by inhibition of cyclo-oxygenase (COX), which is an enzyme that catalyzes the production of prostanoids to form arachidonic acid. COX has 2 predominant isoenzymes: a constitutively synthesized form, COX-1, found in platelets, the gastric mucosa, liver, and kidneys; and an inducible form, COX-2, found in monocytes, peripheral nerves, and spinal cord, and induced by injury and inflammation. Inhibition of COX-1 produces side effects, and inhibition of COX-2 produces analgesia. It was once thought that COX-2 inhibitors were safer NSAIDs. Although these agents are associated with fewer gastric side effects, most have been withdrawn from the market because of serious cardiac side effects in adults.

OPIOIDS. Opioids are administered for moderate and severe pain, such as acute postoperative pain, sickle cell crisis pain, and cancer pain. Opioids can be administered by the oral, rectal, oral transmucosal, transdermal, intranasal, intravenous, epidural, intrathecal, subcutaneous, or intramuscular route. Infants and young children are often underdosed with opioids for fear of significant respiratory side effects. With proper understanding of the pharmacokinetics and pharmacodynamics of opioids, children can receive effective relief of pain and suffering with a good margin of safety (Tables 77-4 and 77-5).

Opioids act by mimicking the actions of endogenous opioid peptides in binding to receptors in the brain, brainstem, spinal cord, and peripheral nervous system. Opioids have dose-dependent respiratory depressant effects and blunt ventilatory responses to hypoxia and hypercarbia. The respiratory depressant effects of opioids can be increased with co-administration of other sedating drugs, such as benzodiazepines or barbiturates. Other common side effects include constipation, nausea, vomiting, urinary retention, and pruritus. Optimal use of opioids requires proactive and anticipatory management of these side effects. The most common easily treatable side effect is constipation. Stool softeners and stimulant laxatives should be administered to most patients receiving opioids for more than a few days. Constipation often continues to be a problem with long-term opioid administration. Specific bowel opiate receptor antagonists may prevent this complication. Nausea sometimes subsides with

TABLE 77-4. Practical Aspects of Prescribing Opioids

Morphine is typically regarded as 1st choice for severe pain.
The right dose is the dose that relieves pain with a good margin of safety.
Dosing should be titrated and individualized. There is no "right" dose for everyone.
Dosing should be more cautious with younger infants, in patients with coexisting diseases that increase risk or impair drug clearance, and with concomitant administration of sedatives.
Anticipate and treat peripheral side effects, including constipation, nausea, and itching.
Give doses at sufficient frequency to prevent the return of severe pain before the next dose.
With opioid dosing for more than 1 wk, taper gradually to avoid withdrawal symptoms.
When converting between parenteral and oral opioid doses, use appropriate potency ratios.
Tolerance refers to decreasing effect on continued administration of a drug or the need for increased dosing to achieve the same effect; patients receiving opioids continually may need increasing doses to achieve analgesia; tolerance to respiratory depression develops parallel with tolerance to analgesic action; thus, with higher doses, patients do not have respiratory depression.
Dependence refers to the need for continued opioid dosing to prevent withdrawal symptoms (irritability, agitation, autonomic arousal, nasal congestion, piloerection, diarrhea and/or jitteriness; and in neonates, yawning); produced by regular or high-dose opioids for ≥ 7 days, especially if the opioid is abruptly stopped; slow tapering may be needed.
Addiction refers to psychological craving with compulsive drug-seeking behavior. Opioid underdosing does not prevent addiction and may increase drug-seeking behavior for relief of pain; good pain relief takes the focus off opioids.

long-term dosing, but often requires treatment with antiemetics, such as phenothiazine, butyrophenones, antihistamines, and the new serotonin receptor antagonists. The combination of morphine and gabapentin may be more effective than either agent alone for relief of chronic pain. It is important for pediatricians to understand the phenomena of tolerance, dependence, withdrawal, and addiction (see Table 77-4).

Continuous intravenous infusion of opioids is a safe and effective option that permits more constant plasma concentrations and clinical effects than intermittent intravenous bolus dosing. One approach is to permit patients to titrate their own dosing using a **patient-controlled analgesia (PCA)** device (see Chapter 76). A basal continuous infusion is often also delivered. Children as young as 5–6 yr can effectively use PCA; parents or nurses can assist younger patients. Compared with children given intermittent intramuscular morphine, children using PCA reported better pain scores and satisfaction. PCA has the advantage of adjusting dosing to account for individual pharmacokinetic and pharmacodynamic variation, as well as changing pain intensity during the day. It also has the psychologic advantage of promoting patient control and active coping. There may be lower overall opioid consumption and fewer side effects with the use of PCA. Overdoses have been reported when well-meaning, inadequately instructed parents pushed the PCA button in medically complicated situations.

LOCAL ANESTHETICS. Local anesthetics are widely used in children for topical application, cutaneous infiltration, peripheral nerve block, epidural injection, and intraspinal punctures (see Chapter 76). Local anesthetics can be used with excellent safety and effectiveness. Excessive systemic concentrations can cause seizures, central nervous system depression, arrhythmia, or cardiac depression. Unlike opioids, there is a strict maximum dosing schedule for local anesthetics. Pediatricians should be aware of the need to calculate these doses and adhere to the guidelines.

Topical local anesthetic preparations have diverse uses in reducing pain, such as for suturing lacerations, intravenous catheter placements, lumbar punctures, and accessing indwelling central ports. The application of tetracaine, epinephrine (Adrenalin), and cocaine results in good anesthesia for suturing wounds. It should not be used on mucous membranes. Cocaine is not essential; combinations of tetracaine with phenylephrine or lidocaine-epinephrine-tetracaine are equally effective. **EMLA** is a topical eutectic mixture of lidocaine and prilocaine that is used to anesthetize intact skin and is commonly applied for venipuncture, lumbar puncture, and other needle procedures. EMLA is safe for use in neonates. It is more effective than placebo, but probably is less effective than ring block of the penis in providing analgesia for circumcision. EMLA should be used with caution for circumcision, because there was a report of redness and blistering on the penis in a study comparing dorsal penile block with EMLA. A small area should be tested for hypersensitivity before EMLA is applied more widely.

Lidocaine is the most commonly used local anesthetic for cutaneous infiltration. Maximum safe doses of lidocaine are 5 mg/kg without epinephrine and 6 mg/kg with epinephrine. Concentrated solutions (2%) should be avoided, because solutions as dilute as 0.3% are equally effective as 1–2% solutions; dilute solutions permit larger volumes. A lidocaine topical patch (Lidoderm) has been used as topical anesthetic for longer-term pain (complex regional pain syndrome).

REGIONAL ANESTHESIA. Regional anesthesia is widely used for postoperative pain relief in children after many types of surgery, such as abdominal, orthopedic, and thoracic procedures. It also can reduce the need for systemic opioids in patients with severe lung disease. Epidural analgesia and peripheral nerve blocks provide excellent analgesia and are safe, even in term and preterm infants. Spinal anesthesia can be used to avoid the need for general anesthesia as well as in intubated infants with moderate and severe lung disease who are undergoing herniorrhaphy or lower-extremity procedures (see Chapter 76).

PSYCHOTROPIC MEDICATIONS IN PEDIATRIC PAIN

It has been demonstrated that children and adolescents with chronic pain with no identified cause, as well as those with identified medical causes of pain, have significantly more psychiatric disorders than healthy children. The psychiatric illnesses that are most commonly seen in youths with chronic pain include depressive disorders, sleep disorders, and anxiety disorders, including generalized anxiety disorder, separation anxiety, post-traumatic stress disorder, and panic disorder. Pervasive developmental disorders are also common among the population with chronic pain. This increase in comorbid psychiatric disorders may be explained by the disruption of the serotonergic and noradrenergic systems that are the common pathways in both pain disorders and psychiatric disorders. Even without diagnosable psychiatric comorbidity, psychologic factors can affect a youth's ability to cope with a pain disorder, with a conditioned response of pain leading to a feeling of being out of control, and then to increased anxiety, which then increases the pain. Alternatively, the feeling of helplessness can prime the pain, leading the child to perseverate on the pain, think catastrophically, and feel hopeless, which then can lead to an increase in the subjective experience of pain as well as the development of a depressive disorder.

Most of the currently used pharmacologic strategies are extrapolated from adult trials without evidence of their efficacy in children and adolescents. Although several of the psychotropic medications have been approved by the U.S. Food and Drug Administration (FDA) for alternate uses, few of these medications have been specifically approved for use in youth with chronic pain. Thus, these medications should be used with caution, with a focus on minimization of pain to allow the child to participate effectively in therapies and return to normal activity as soon as possible. The use of psychotropic medications in this population should be guided by the same principles applied to pharmacologic treatment of any symptom or disease. Target symptoms should be identified and monitored, as should side effects. Dosing regimens should consider the child's weight and the effect of the particular medical condition and the other medications the child may be taking on the metabolism of the psychotropic medication. Side effects should be specifically addressed with both parent and

TABLE 77-5. Initial Dosage Guidelines for Analgesics

	EQUIANALGESIC DOSES		USUAL STARTING IV OR SC DOSES AND INTERVALS			USUAL STARTING ORAL DOSES AND INTERVALS		
DRUG	PARENTERAL	ORAL	CHILD < 50 KG	CHILD > 50 KG	PARENTERAL/ ORAL DOSE RATIO	CHILD < 50 KG	CHILD > 50 KG	COMMENTS
Codeine	N/A	200 mg	N/A	N/A	1 : 2	0.5–1 mg/kg q3–4h	30–60 mg q3–4h	Weak opioid; typically given with acetaminophen; not good for severe pain; some children are not codeine responders.
Morphine	10 mg	30 mg	*Bolus:* 0.1 mg/kg q2–4h	*Bolus:* 5–8 mg q2–4h	1 : 3	*Immediate release:* 0.3 mg/kg q3–4h	*Immediate release:* 15–20 mg q3–4h	Potent opioid for moderate/severe pain; can cause histamine release and wheezing in children with asthma; least expensive opioid.
			infusion: 0.01 mg/kg/hr in younger infants to 0.3 mg/kg/hr in older infants and children	*Infusion:* 1–1.5 mg/hr		*Sustained release:* 20–35 kg: 10–15 mg q8–12h 35–50 kg: 15–30 mg q8–12h	*Sustained release:* 30–45 mg q8–12h	Sustained-release form must be swallowed whole; cannot be crushed or it becomes immediate-acting.
Oxycodone	N/A	30 mg	N/A	N/A	N/A	0.1–0.2 mg q3–4h; available in liquid (1 mg/mL)	5–10 mg q3–4h; available in tablet (5 mg); also comes in long-acting form (q12h) in varying strengths	Weak opioid, but more potent than codeine, with fewer gastrointestinal side effects; more potent and preferable to hydrocodone, which is always combined with acetaminophen (e.g., Vicodin); available alone without acetaminophen (Percocet is combined form). Underutilized.
Methadone	10 mg	20 mg	0.1 mg/kg q4–8h	5–8 mg q4–8h	1 : 2	0.2 mg/kg q4–8h PO; available in liquid or tablet	10 mg q4–8h	12–24-hr duration; useful in certain types of chronic pain; requires additional vigilance, because it can accumulate and produce delayed sedation. If sedation occurs, doses should be withheld until sedation resolves, then substantially reduced and/or the dosing interval should be extended to 8–12 hr. When patients who are tolerant to morphine or hydromorphone are switched to methadone, they sometimes show incomplete cross tolerance and improved efficacy.
Fentanyl	100 μg (0.1 mg)	N/A	*Bolus:* 0.5–1 μg/kg q1–2h *Infusion:* 0.5–1.5 μg/kg/hr	*Bolus:* 25–50 μg q1–2h *Infusion:* 25–75 μg/hr	N/A	Transdermal patch 12.5-μg/hr dose if on morphine ≥30 mg/day	Transdermal patches available; patch reaches steady state at 24 hr and should be changed q72h	Potent analgesic 70–100 times as potent as morphine; rapid onset and shorter duration. With high doses and rapid administration, can cause chest wall rigidity (which can be reversed with naloxone or neuromuscular blockade). Useful for short procedures; low gastrointestinal side effect and pruritus profile. Transmucosal form is fast-acting, good for break-through pain.
Hydromorphone	1.5–2 mg	6–8 mg	*Bolus:* 0.02 mg q2–4h *Infusion:* 0.006 mg/kg/hr	*Bolus:* 1 mg q2–4h *Infusion:* 0.3 mg/hr	1 : 4	0.04–0.08 mg/kg q3–4h	2–4 mg q3–4h	Similar to morphine except 5 times as potent; less histamine release than with morphine.
Meperidine	75 mg	300 mg	*Bolus:* 0.8–1 mg/kg q2–3h	*Bolus:* 50–75 mg q2–3h	1 : 4	2–3 mg/kg q3–4h	100–150 mg q3–4h	Avoid if other opioids are available (especially for chronic use) because its metabolite, normeperidine, can cause dysphoria, agitation, and seizures. Primary use in low doses is for treatment of rigors and shivering with amphotericin or blood products.

N/A, not applicable.

child in detail, with specific instructions given on how to respond if adverse events occur. Directly addressing concerns about issues of addiction, dependence, and tolerance may be necessary to decrease treatment-related anxiety and increase adherence.

ANTIDEPRESSANT MEDICATIONS. Antidepressant medications have been demonstrated as useful in adults with chronic pain, including neuropathic pain, headaches, and rheumatoid arthritis, independent of their effects on depressive disorders. In children, clinical trials have been limited, and the practitioner should be cautious in the use of antidepressants, particularly serotonin reuptake inhibitors, whether for the treatment of chronic pain or for associated depressive or anxiety symptoms. The U.S. FDA issued an advisory informing the public of a small but significant increase in suicidal thoughts and attempts, although not completed suicides, found in a meta-analysis of studies involving children and adolescents. This issue in particular should be considered, and contingency plans developed with regard to this specific finding.

TRICYCLIC ANTIDEPRESSANTS. Tricyclic antidepressants (TCAs) have been most studied with relation to chronic pain in children and have been found effective in pain relief for symptoms including neuropathic pain, functional abdominal pain, and migraine prophylaxis. This may be based on inhibition of the neurochemical pathways involved in norepinephrine and serotonin reuptake and their interference with other neurochemicals involved in the perception of pain. These medications are also effective in the treatment of sleep disorders, which frequently accompany pediatric pain syndromes. Because biotransformation of TCAs is extensive in healthy children, the child should be started on a bedtime dose, which should then be titrated to a daily divided dose, with the larger dose remaining at bedtime. It is important to note that pain symptoms frequently remit at lower doses than those recommended for the treatment of depression in children. Typically, most children and adolescents do not require >10 mg of amitriptyline once a day at bedtime. Attention should be paid to hepatic microsomal enzyme metabolism because CYP2D6 inhibitors, such as cimetidine and quinidine, can increase the levels of TCAs. Anticholinergic side effects may occur and often remit over time. Issues of constipation, orthostatic hypotension, and dental caries as a result of dry mouth should be addressed, with the importance of hydration and diet emphasized. Other side effects include mild bone marrow suppression and liver dysfunction; thus, the results of complete blood count (CBC) and liver function tests (LFTs) should be monitored. Blood levels of TCAs can be obtained as well, but monitoring generally should occur on an individual basis, particularly with issues of adherence, overdose, or sudden changes in mental status. In the early 1990s, sudden cardiac death occurred in several children taking TCAs, leading to concerns about cardiotoxicity. A careful history regarding cardiac arrhythmias, heart disease, syncope, and family history should be obtained before the initiation of treatment. If there is any positive family history, then a baseline electrocardiogram (ECG) should be obtained, with care taken to ensure that the QTc is <445 msec. If the dose is increased >20 mg of amitriptyline at bedtime, then another ECG should be repeated with each dosing change. The patient should be referred to a cardiologist with any positive findings. Although there is no addiction problem with TCAs, there is a known **discontinuation syndrome,** including agitation, sleep disturbances, appetite changes, and gastrointestinal symptoms. These medications should be tapered slowly to assist in distinguishing among rebound, withdrawal, and symptoms indicating the need for medication continuation.

SEROTONIN REUPTAKE INHIBITORS. Serotonin reuptake inhibitors (SSRIs) have demonstrated modest improvement in the treatment of a variety of pain syndromes in adults, leading to a supposition that noradrenergic pathways are more significant in the treatment of pain than serotonergic pathways. SSRIs are indicated when symptoms of depressive or anxiety disorders are prominent. Although many SSRIs are used in practice with children, only fluoxetine has been approved by the U.S. FDA for use in children and adolescents. These medications have a less severe side effect profile than TCAs, with common side effects largely transient. These include gastrointestinal symptoms, headaches, agitation, sexual dysfunction, and anxiety. Rarely, hyponatremia, or syndrome of inappropriate antidiuretic hormone, may occur, so a baseline and regular chemistry panels should be followed. A baseline ECG should also be obtained because tachycardia may occur. There may be interactions with other medications with serotonergic effects (tramadol, trazodone, tryptophan). When these medications are used in combination, there is increased likelihood of the occurrence of a life-threatening **serotonergic syndrome,** with associated symptoms of myoclonus, hyperreflexia, autonomic instability, muscle rigidity, and delirium. There is also a **discontinuation syndrome** associated with shorter-acting SSRIs (paroxetine), which includes dizziness, lethargy, paresthesias, irritability, and vivid dreams. These medications should be tapered slowly over the course of several wk.

ATYPICAL ANTIDEPRESSANTS. Antidepressants such as duloxetine and venlafaxine have demonstrated efficacy with chronic pain syndromes because they inhibit both serotonin and norepinephrine reuptake and may directly block associated pain receptors. These medications have fewer anticholinergic properties than TCAs, and adherence to these medications is better than that of TCAs in psychiatric populations. Side effects of both medications include gastrointestinal symptoms, hyperhydrosis, dizziness, and agitation, but they generally improve over time. Hypertension and orthostatic hypotension may occur; in addition, the patient's blood pressure should be closely followed and appropriate hydration should be stressed.

ANTICONVULSANTS. Traditional anticonvulsants, such as **carbamazepine** and **valproic acid,** are believed to relieve chronic pain by blocking calcium channels at the cellular level and suppressing the hypersensitive sensory fibers without affecting normal nerve conduction. These medications are particularly useful in patients with mood disorders and neuropathic pain. In adults, valproic acid has been approved by the U.S. FDA for migraine prophylaxis, and carbamazepine has been approved for trigeminal neuralgia. Anticonvulsant medications generally have gastrointestinal side effects in addition to sedation, anemia, ataxia, rash, and hepatotoxicity, with an increased incidence of potentially fatal Stevens-Johnson syndrome associated with carbamazepine and oxcarbamazine. Baseline LFTs and CBC should be obtained and monitored. These medications have narrow therapeutic windows and may have extreme variability in medication levels with drug interactions, liver disease, and renal impairment, so drug levels should be obtained with each dose increase, and regularly thereafter. Carbamazepine, in particular, auto-induces hepatic microsomal enzyme, which can further complicate obtaining a therapeutic medication level. Frequent pregnancy tests are useful with menstruating female adolescents taking valproic acid, because severe neural tube defects are associated with this medication.

Gabapentin has demonstrated efficacy in the treatment of children with chronic pain, particularly neuropathic pain. Smaller studies of chronic headaches, reflex sympathetic dystrophy, and chronic regional pain syndrome have also shown great promise. The exact mechanism of action of this medication is unclear. It is theorized that it increases gabaminergic transmission and decreases glutaminergic transmission while binding to the voltage-dependent calcium channels, producing antineuralgic effects. Gabapentin has a relatively benign side effect profile and few drug interactions. Side effects include somnolence, dizziness, and ataxia, with rare incidences of new-onset oppositional behavior at high doses.

Topiramate has demonstrated greater success than traditional anticonvulsants in the treatment of trigeminal neuralgia in adults and the prevention of migraines. The increased efficacy is likely related to its multiple mechanisms of action. Although rare, topiramate may cause cognitive dulling, which may be problematic with school-aged children, and dosing of the medication should consider school hours. It should be noted, particularly with female adolescents, that significant weight gain is associated with all anticonvulsants other then topiramate, which is associated with weight loss.

BENZODIAZEPINES. Benzodiazepines are anxiolytic medications that have anticonvulsant and muscle relaxant effects. **Clonazepam,** a long-acting benzodiazepine, has demonstrated efficacy in neuropathic pain in blinded studies. These medications are most appropriate in acute situations because dependence, tolerance, and withdrawal may occur with prolonged use. These medications may also cause behavioral disinhibition, respiratory depression, and psychosis, further limiting their utility. However, studies have demonstrated the utility of benzodiazepines in children with severe anxiety and anticipatory anxiety, for example, with planned painful procedures. When dosing these medications, the practitioner should consider that many of the benzodiazepines are metabolized by the P450 microsomal enzyme system before conjugation, decreasing their duration of action. These differences may be less significant in benzodiazepines such as lorazepam and oxazepam, which undergo first-pass conjugation. Side effects common to benzodiazepines include sedation, ataxia, anemia, increased bronchial secretions, and depressed mood. Baseline CBC and LFTs should be obtained and monitored. These medications should be slowly tapered over several wk because withdrawal is potentially lethal and includes autonomic instability, delirium, and seizures, if abruptly discontinued.

ANTIPSYCHOTICS. Low doses of antipsychotic medications are often used to address the severe anxiety and agitation frequently associated with chronic pain in youth. The use of these medications is controversial, however, because the adverse events associated may be severe. Typical antipsychotics, including thioridazine (Mellaril), haloperidol, and chlorpromazine, are associated with a decrease in seizure threshold, agranulocytosis, weight gain, cardiac conduction disturbances, tardive dyskinesia, orthostatic hypotension, hepatic dysfunction, and life-threatening laryngeal dystonia. These side effects are generally less severe with atypical antipsychotics; however, they may still occur, and baseline ECG, LFTs, and CBC are essential and should be followed. With typical antipsychotics, an inventory of movement disturbances, such as the AIMS test (abnormal voluntary movement scale), should also be done at baseline and at every follow-up visit because these symptoms can be irreversible and may in fact worsen with abrupt withdrawal of medications. Atypical antipsychotics are generally associated with less severe side effect profiles, particularly with regard to dyskinesias and dystonias. With olanzapine, which may be particularly helpful with insomnia, blood glucose, cholesterol, and triglyceride levels should be assessed and monitored because diabetes and hypercholesterolemia may be side effects of this medication or the significant weight gain associated with its use. The anticholinergic side effects associated with quetiapine warrant frequent monitoring of blood pressure. Risperidone at doses >6 mg may cause side effects similar to those of typical antipsychotics. Clozapine has an increased incidence of life-threatening agranulocytosis, and should generally be avoided as a treatment for children and adolescents with chronic pain. All antipsychotics are associated with the rare, but potentially lethal neuroleptic malignant syndrome, which includes severe autonomic instability, muscular rigidity, catatonia, and altered mental status.

The utility of psychotropic medications in the treatment of children with chronic pain is becoming increasingly apparent. These medications, when used judiciously, have proven successful, even when common psychiatric comorbidities, such as depression and anxiety, are not apparent. Gabapentin and duloxetine are among the most promising of these medications, based not only on efficacy, but also on their mild side effect profiles and limited medication interactions; however, further testing should be pursued. Low-dose quetiapine also appears similarly useful for children with symptoms of agitation or severe anxiety. Most important when working with these medications is the team approach. A relationship with a consulting child and adolescent psychiatrist is essential, in light of the complexities in working with these medications. The psychiatrist or a team psychologist should also be consulted to elucidate common psychiatric comorbidities or isolated symptoms, such as feelings of helplessness and hopelessness, which may complicate the medical picture and decrease the patient's level of functioning.

SPECIFIC TYPES OF PAIN

Pharmacologic and nonpharmacologic approaches to pain management should be considered for all pain treatment plans, regardless of the type of pain. Many simple interventions designed to promote relaxation and patient control can be expected to work synergistically with pain medications for optimal relief of pain and related distress. More than 1 type of pain may be present in the same patient.

BRIEF PROCEDURAL PAIN. There is no 1 way to manage pain and distress for all procedures. The specific approach might vary according to the expected intensity and duration of the pain, the context and meaning of the procedure for the child and family, the coping styles and temperaments of the child and parents, the type of procedure, and the child's pain history (especially during procedures). Interventions that reduce distress for parents and children have been associated with reductions in children's report of pain and observations of their pain behavior. Therefore, optimal preparation might include education about the procedure, management of procedure-related expectations, development of skills designed to increase active participation and improved coping during the procedure, rehearsal of the procedure to increase mastery, and positive reinforcement for successful coping after the procedure is complete. Imagery, relaxation, and self-regulation and complementary approaches, such as massage or the application of cold or heat, may be especially beneficial. Depending on the situation, it may be helpful to have the parents present, if they are prepared with specific ways to comfort and distract the child. All pain management strategies will be most effective in a quiet environment (other than entertaining auditory distractors), with calm adults, and with clear and confident instructions.

During some procedures, analgesia may be required to make the procedure more comfortable, anxiolysis may be needed to make the procedure less terrifying, and/or sedation may be needed to permit the child to lie motionless. Local anesthetics, along with interventions to soothe the child and minimize distress, should be considered, even for simple procedures, such as venipuncture. Newborn circumcisions cause significant distress during the procedure and are associated with irritability and feeding disturbances for several days. For predictably severe procedural pain, such as bone marrow aspirations, local measures are often insufficient; systemic agents are then required. The use of anxiolytics alone does not provide analgesia and can make a child less able to communicate pain and distress (see Chapter 76 and Table 77-6).

OPERATIVE PAIN AND CONSCIOUS SEDATION

TRAUMA PAIN. See Chapter 76.The management of trauma pain and distress may be given minimal attention because of the emphasis on life-supporting, critical care interventions. Pain may be caused by the original trauma, surgical procedures, restricted movement, or underlying disease as well as by the presence of lines, tubes, and drains. It may be significantly exacerbated by biologic and psychologic post-traumatic stress responses. The selection of analgesics, including dosage, timing, and route of administration, should be tailored to the individual patient, given the overall context of what is best for the patient and desired by the family. Frequent communication with the family can also optimize appropriate expectations in family members, allowing

TABLE 77-6. Drugs Used for Conscious Sedation in Children*

DRUG	SUGGESTED STARTING DOSE(S)	COMMENTS
Midazolam	0.05-mg/kg incremental doses IV q 5–10 min up to 3–5 doses (to a maximum incremental dose of 1 mg) 0.1–0.2 mg/kg IM (maximum dose, 10 mg) 0.3–0.6 mg/kg PO (maximum dose, 20 mg)	Good anxiolytic Flumazenil is a reversal agent Dose more cautiously when combined with opioids
Fentanyl	0.5-μg/kg increments q 5 min up to 3–5 doses	Rapid infusion of large doses can produce chest wall rigidity Respiratory depression is amplified by co-administration of sedatives
Pentobarbital	1-mg/kg increments IV q 10 min up to 3 doses 2–4 mg/kg IM 4–6 mg/kg PO	Good sedative No analgesia Used often for radiologic procedures Can produce prolonged sedation
Chloral hydrate	25–100 mg/kg PO or PR 30–40 min before the procedure	High incidence of failed sedation with 25–50 mg/kg
Ketamine	0.2–0.5-mg/kg increments q 10 min × 3 1–2 mg/kg IM	Co-administration of midazolam or other benzodiazepines can reduce the risk of dysphoria or bad dreams Use should be restricted to cases managed by physicians with deep sedation qualifications
Propofol	Dosing per anesthesiologist	IV anesthetic often referred to as "milk of amnesia" Should be administered by an anesthesiologist

*To ensure that patients receive optimal, safe care, it is now required in the United States that hospitals develop conscious sedation guidelines, such as those established by the American Academy of Pediatrics. These guidelines should include recommendations for withholding feeding before procedures, drug dosages, strategies to achieve patient comfort, necessary monitoring, required resuscitation equipment, and a quality improvement program for tracking outcomes and ensuring efficacy and safety. The guidelines also should specify which subgroups of patients are at increased risk and should have sedation performed by pediatric anesthesiologists.

them to better attend to the needs of the child. When pain is prolonged, dosages should be adjusted to compensate for physical tolerance, and weaning strategies should be used to minimize withdrawal symptoms. Attention should be paid to the child's sleep-wake cycles (because sufficient sleep will enable the child to cope better when awake) and to the child's and family's psychologic response to the trauma. Parents can benefit from psychoeducation and/or consultation with a mental health provider to help them monitor the child for signs and symptoms of psychologic trauma and respond to these symptoms in a therapeutically helpful manner.

CANCER PAIN. The World Health Organization (WHO) proposed a model for analgesic therapy for cancer pain known as the *analgesic ladder* (Table 77-7). This consists of a hierarchy of oral pharmacologic interventions designed to treat pain of increasing magnitude. It presents a framework for the rational use of oral medication before the application of other techniques of drug administration, because of the simplicity and demonstrated efficacy of oral medication. Opioid therapy is the preferred approach for moderate or severe pain. Nonopioid analgesics are used for mild pain, a weak opioid is added for moderate pain, and strong opioids are administered for more severe pain. Adjuvant analgesics can be added, and side effects and comorbid symptoms are actively managed.

TABLE 77-7. World Health Organization Analgesic Ladder for Cancer Pain

STEP 1

Patients who present with mild to moderate pain should be treated with a nonopioid.

STEP 2

Patients who present with moderate to severe pain or who fail the 1st-step regimen should be treated with an oral opioid for moderate pain combined with a nonopioid analgesic.

STEP 3

Patients who present with very severe pain or who fail the 2nd-step regimen should be treated with an opioid used for severe pain, with or without a nonopioid analgesic.

Medications for persistent cancer-related pain should be administered on an around-the-clock basis, with additional "as-needed" doses, because regularly scheduled dosing maintians a constant level of drug in the body and helps to prevent a recurrence of pain.

Adjuvant medications can be used to treat opioid side effects and comorbid conditions.

Adjuvant analgesics represent a diverse group of drug classes that have other indications, but are analgesic in specific circumstances. Adjuvant medications should be used when indications exist at any step.

Some of the commonly used adjuvant analgesics include anticonvulsants, antidepressants, local anesthetics, corticosteroids, antihistaminics, muscle relaxants, neuroleptics, anticholinergics (for visceral pain caused by bowel obstruction), and psychostimulants (to decrease the sedation caused by opioid analgesia).

Although the oral route of opioid administration should be encouraged, some children are unable to take oral opioids. Intravenous infusions with a PCA are used next. Small, portable infusion pumps are convenient for home use. If venous access is limited, a useful alternative is to administer opioids (especially morphine or hydromorphone, not methadone or meperidine) through continuous subcutaneous infusion, with or without a bolus option. A small (e.g., 22-gauge) cannula is placed under the skin and secured on the thorax, abdomen, or thigh. Sites may be changed every 3–7 days, as needed. Alternative routes for opioids include the transdermal and oral transmucosal routes. These latter routes are preferred over IV or SQ drug delivery when at home.

PAIN ASSOCIATED WITH ADVANCED DISEASE. Patients with advanced disease, including cancer, AIDS, neurodegenerative disorders, and cystic fibrosis, need approaches to palliative care that focus on optimal quality of life. Nonpharmacologic and pharmacologic management of pain and other distressing symptoms is a key component of palliative care. Differences among these conditions related to the progression of underlying illness, associated distressing symptoms, and common emotional responses should shape individual treatment plans (see Chapter 40).

More than 90% of children and adolescents dying of cancer can be made comfortable by standard escalation of opioids according to the WHO protocol. A small subgroup (5%) will have enormous opioid dose escalation to >100 times the standard morphine or other opiate infusion rate. In most of these cases, there is spread of solid tumors to the spinal cord, roots, or plexus, and signs of neuropathic pain are evident.

The type of pain experienced by the patient (neuropathic, myofascial) should determine the need for adjunctive agents. Complementary measures, such as massage, hypnotherapy, or spiritual care, should also be considered in palliative care.

CHRONIC AND RECURRENT NONMALIGNANT PAIN. A large proportion of otherwise healthy children experience recurrent episodes or continuous nonspecific headache, chest pain, abdominal pain, or limb pain. These children, who often simply have a neurosensory pain signaling problem, may appear to be growing as expected and may show no signs suggestive of serious disease (see Chapter 167).

A thorough biopsychosocial history, review of systems, and physical examination comprise the cornerstone of diagnosis. It is also important to understand how the pain affects the child's social functioning and school functioning and attendance, as well as parental behaviors toward the child. Laboratory testing and diagnostic procedures should be minimal and guided by clinical indication. Gastrointestinal barium roentgenographic studies in children with recurrent abdominal pain that appears "benign", based on the history and physical findings, have a low yield. Recurrent abdominal pain may be one of a variety of functional abdominal symptoms, such as nausea, vomiting, bloating, diarrhea, or constipation, with mechanisms related to neuroenteric dysregulation rather than gastrointestinal structural or inflammatory problems. The absence of findings on radiographic or endoscopic procedures does not indicate that "the problem is fake or is psychologic."

Overall, management of chronic pain should emphasize nonpharmacologic approaches, rather than excessive reliance on medications in isolation. When it is concluded that a patient's pain is not disease related it is very important for the pediatrician to: (1) avoid overmedication because this can exacerbate the pain and associated disability; (2) maintain an open mind in terms of reassessing the diagnosis if the clinical presentation changes; and (3) understand and communicate to the family that the pain has a biologic basis (likely related to neural signaling and neurotransmitter dysregulation) and is naturally distressing to the child and family. All patients and families should receive a simple explanation of pain physiology that helps them to understand the importance of functional rehabilitation to normalize pain signaling, the low risk of causing further injury with systematic increases in normal functioning, and the risks associated with treating the pain as if it were acute. It is counterintuitive for most people to move a part of the body that hurts, and many patients with chronic pain have atrophy or contractures of a painful extremity because of disuse. Additionally, associated increases in worry and anxiety may exacerbate pain and leave the body even more vulnerable to further illness, injury, and disability.

For a small subgroup of children with chronic pain, school absenteeism is a significant problem. An especially detailed assessment of possible family, cognitive, learning, peer, and anxiety or other emotional problems is indicated to ensure that a successful plan for school re-entry can be developed and implemented. Home schooling for these patients has been shown to predict poor outcome and therefore is not recommended as a long-term solution.

NEUROPATHIC PAIN. Neuropathic pain is caused by abnormal excitability in the peripheral or central nervous system that may persist after an injury heals or inflammation subsides. The pain, which can be acute or chronic, is often described as *burning* or *stabbing* and may be associated with cutaneous hypersensitivity (**allodynia**). Neuropathic pain conditions may be responsible for >35% of referrals to chronic pain clinics and commonly include post-traumatic and postsurgical peripheral nerve injuries, phantom pain after amputation, pain after spinal cord injury, and pain due to metabolic neuropathies. Neuropathic pain frequently responds poorly to opioids. In adults, evidence suggests the efficacy of TCAs (nortriptyline, amitriptyline) and anticonvulsants (carbamazepine, gabapentin) for treatment of neuropathic pain. **Complex regional pain syndrome** type I (formerly known as *reflex sympathetic dystrophy*) is the term applied to an affected body part that has become sensitized without any specific nerve injury. Hyperalgesia can occur anywhere in the body, often in no particular neural distribution, including internal organs (stomach or esophagus). Treatment emphasizes targeted physical therapy and facilitation of functioning.

Akporehwe NA, Wilkinson PR, Quibell R, Akporehwe KA: Ketamine: a misunderstood analgesic? *BMJ* 2006;332:1466.

American Academy of Pediatrics, Committee on Fetus and Newborn, Committee on Drugs, Section on Anesthesiology, Section on Surgery: Prevention and management of pain and stress in the neonate. *Pediatrics* 2000;105:545–561.

American Academy of Pediatrics, Committee on Psychosocial Aspects of Child and Family Health: The assessment and management of acute pain in infants, children, and adolescents. *Pediatrics* 2001;108:793–797.

American Academy of Pediatrics, Subcommittee on Chronic Abdominal Pain: Chronic abdominal pain in children. *Pediatrics* 2005:115:812–815.

American Pain Society: *Guideline for the Management of Cancer Pain in Adults and Children,* Glenview, IL 2005.

American Pain Society: *Guideline for the Management of Fibromyalgia Pain in Adults and Children,* Glenview, IL 2005.

American Pain Society: Pediatric chronic pain: A position statement from the American Pain Society. *Am Pain Soc Bull* 2001;1.

Anand KJS, Hall RW, Desai N, et al: Effects of morphine analgesia in ventilated preterm neonates: Primary outcomes from the NEOPAIN randomized trial. *Lancet* 2004;363:1673–1682.

Berde CB, Sethna NF: Analgesia for the treatment of pain in childhood. *N Engl J Med* 2002;347:1094–1103.

Colvin L, Forbes K, Fallon M: Difficult pain. *BMJ* 2006;332:1081–1083.

Gilron I, Bailey JM, Tu D, et al: Morphine, gabapentin, or their combination for neuropathic pain. *N Engl J Med* 2005;352:1324–1334.

Holdcroft A, Power I: Management of pain. *BMJ* 2003;326:635–639.

Howard RF: Current status of pain management in children. *JAMA* 2003;290:2464–2469.

Marco CA, Plewa MC, Buderer N, et al: Self-reported pain sores in the emergency department: lack of association with vital signs. *Acad Emerg Med* 2006;13:974–979.

Quigley C: The role of opioids in cancer pain. *BMJ* 2005;331:825–829.

The Medical Letter: Acupuncture. *Med Lett* 2006;48:38–39.

Zeltzer LK, Schlank CB: *Conquering Your Child's Chronic Pain: A Pediatrician's Guide for Reclaiming a Normal Childhood.* New York, HarperCollins, 2005.

Zempsky WT, Cravero JP, Committee on Pediatric Emergency Medicine, and Section on Anesthesiology and Pain Medicine: Relief of pain and anxiety in pediatric patients in emergency medical systems. *Pediatrics* 2004:114: 1348–1356.

Part IX ▪ Human Genetics

Chapter 78 ▪ The Genetic Approach in Pediatric Medicine

Bruce R. Korf

With the completion of the human genome sequence and the haplotype map, investigative and diagnostic tools are available to determine the genetic contributions to both uncommon and common disorders. Information about the genetic aspects of all pediatric diseases has grown tremendously and is readily available on multiple websites and in other locations (Table 78-1).

THE BURDEN OF GENETIC DISORDERS IN CHILDHOOD. Although genetic disorders can present at any age, some of the most obvious and severe diseases begin in childhood. A single gene or multifactorial genetic condition was a major contributor to pediatric hospital admissions (in 1978) in approximately 25% of patients. The majority of chronic diseases in children has an obvious genetic component or is influenced by genetic susceptibility. Thirty-four percent of deaths of hospitalized children are associated with an underlying genetic disorder. Major categories of genetic disorders in children include single gene, chromosomal, and multifactorial conditions.

Individually, **single-gene disorders** are rare, but collectively they represent an important contribution to childhood disease. They include disorders such as sickle cell anemia and cystic fibrosis, as well as a myriad of extremely rare conditions that have been seen in only a few families. Single-gene disorders tend to occur when mutations have a profound effect on function of the gene product. Such effects include product (structural protein, enzyme, metabolite) deficiency as well as loss or gain of function. The phenotypes associated with single-gene disorders can be variable and modified by the action of other genes or the environment. The hallmark of a single-gene disorder is that the phenotype is overwhelmingly determined by mutation in an individual gene. Single-gene disorders may occur sporadically, owing to new mutations (mainly true for dominant disorders), but many are seen with increased frequency in specific populations. In some cases this is due to the **founder effect,** in which a mutation achieves relatively high frequency in a population derived from a small number of founders that remains closed to interbreeding with those outside the population. This is the case for Tay-Sachs disease in Ashkenazi Jews and French Canadians. Other mutations may be subject to positive selection in the heterozygous carrier state, such as hemoglobin mutations that confer relative resistance to malaria.

Chromosomal disorders such as Down syndrome are associated with the presence of an extra copy (**trisomy**) of chromosome 21. Only a few trisomies are compatible with live birth (chromosomes 13, 18, and 21, as well the X and Y chromosomes); most lead to early miscarriage as a result of severe genetic imbalance. Subtle changes of individual chromosome structure (**microdeletions**) have also been identified. Many of these are associated with distinctive phenotypes that can be recognized clinically; some produce nondescript phenotypes of developmental impairment with variable effects on intellect as well as growth and physical appearance.

Multifactorial inheritance occurs when multiple genes or gene-environmental effects cause a disorder. Multifactorial inheritance in pediatrics is seen with certain congenital anomalies, such as spina bifida or cleft lip/palate. These traits may cluster in families but usually do not segregate in accordance with mendelian dominant or recessive inheritance. The responsible genes are unknown, and genetic counseling is based on empirical data. The concept of multifactorial inheritance extends to common disorders, such as asthma and diabetes mellitus.

THE CHANGING PARADIGM OF GENETICS IN MEDICINE. Relatively few genetic disorders were amenable to treatment in the past; management was focused largely on prevention and management of chronic illnesses. Inborn errors of metabolism were the first genetic disorders to be recognized; many are amenable to treatment by dietary manipulation (see Chapter 84). These conditions result from genetically determined deficiency of specific enzymes, leading to the buildup of toxic substrates and/or deficiency of critical end products. The expansion of newborn genetic and metabolic screening includes a much larger array of screened disorders, made possible by the use of tandem mass spectrometry, permitting detection of a wide variety of metabolites in a single, inexpensive assay. Expanded newborn screening will dramatically increase the number of metabolic disorders in children that are amenable to treatment (see Chapters 84 and 94).

In addition to available screening programs, more therapies are in development for the treatment of many lysosomal storage disorders that were lethal or associated with intractable chronic illness. The basis for treatment in this case is **enzyme replacement,** using specially modified enzymes that are administered by intravenous infusion and are then taken up by cells and incorporated into lysosomes. Conditions such as Gaucher disease and Fabry disease are routinely treated; treatments for others such as Pompe disease and mucopolysaccharidosis are in development. This places an added responsibility on the pediatrician to establish an early diagnosis, which is a challenge given the rarity of these disorders and relatively nonspecific nature of early symptoms.

Therapeutic advances are extending to other nonmetabolic genetic disorders as well. Improvements in surgical treatment of congenital anomalies such as heart defects are extending the survival of children with birth defects or conditions such as Down syndrome. The life expectancy of those with cystic fibrosis has steadily increased, largely owing to improvements in antibiotic therapy as well as the management of both chronic pulmonary disease and malabsorption. A major consequence of these advances is that affected individuals survive into adulthood, creating a need to transition care from pediatric to adult providers. Gene replacement therapies have long been anticipated, though there have been major challenges in development of safe and effective approaches for the insertion of genes into diseased tissues and achievement of physiologically meaningful levels of gene expression. The advent of therapeutics based on use of stem cells also offers the possibility of treatment for previously intractable disorders.

Longstanding and highly successful carrier screening programs have existed for disorders such as Tay-Sachs disease and many other rare, single-gene disorders that are prevalent in specific populations. Couples are commonly offered screening for a variety of conditions, in part based on ancestry (Tay-Sachs disease, hemoglobinopathies, cystic fibrosis). Couples found to be at risk can be offered prepregnancy or prenatal testing, which is based on genetic tests aimed at detection of specific mutations. Pre-

TABLE 78-1. Useful Internet Genetic Reference Sites

WEB ADDRESS	DATA BASE
http://www.ncbi.nlm.nih.gov	General reference maintained by National Library of Medicine
http://www.ncbi.nlm.nih.gov/Omim	Online Mendelian Inheritance in Man (extremely useful for clinicians—over 10,000 entries of genetic traits indexed by gene name, symptoms, and so forth)
http://www.ncbi.nlm.nih.gov/genemap	General reference to current efforts to map the human genome
http://www.ncbi.nlm.nih.gov/Web/Genbank	Searchable repository of all DNA sequence data
http://www.ncbi.nlm.nih.gov/ncicgap	Cancer Genome Anatomy Project (National Cancer Institute)
http://www.nhgri.nih.gov	National Human Genome Research Institute Web Site (useful information about human genetics and ethical issues)
http://www.uwcm.ac.uk/uwcm/mg/hgmd0.html	Human Gene Mutation Database (searchable index of all described mutations in human genes with phenotypes and references)
http://www.genetests.org	Directory of clinics and labs for testing of genetic disorders
	Testing and counseling data
http://www.geneletter.com	Health, clinical, legal, social, and ethical issues
http://www.ashg.org	American Society of Human Genetics site
http://www.aap.org/VISIT/cmte18.htm	Committee on Genetics of the American Academy of Pediatrics site. Educational Genetics Compoundium. Health supervision guidelines for common genetic disorders.

natal testing is also offered for chromosomal disorders such as Down syndrome, with an increasing number of affected pregnancies being recognized by noninvasive screening tests such as maternal serum marker screening and fetal ultrasound. Prenatal diagnosis can be confirmed by amniocentesis at 16–18 weeks or chorionic villus sampling at 10–12 weeks. **Preimplantation genetic diagnosis (PGD)** of early embryos by analysis of single blastomeres can select only unaffected embryos for implantation. Approaches to noninvasive prenatal diagnosis by sampling of fetal cells or fetal DNA in maternal blood are also being developed in specialized laboratories.

Genetic testing is increasingly available for a wide variety of both rare and relatively common genetic disorders. Testing can resolve uncertainty regarding diagnosis, provide a basis for genetic counseling, and, in some instances, serve as a prelude for specific treatment. Genetic testing will play an increasingly central role in all aspects of pediatric practice. Genetic variations in enzymes involved in drug metabolism underlie differences in therapeutic effect and toxicity, and should be taken into account in the determination of drug dosage. Based on their genome, different individuals will respond differently to specific drugs. Tailoring treatment to individual variations in drug metabolism, responsiveness, and susceptibility to toxicity will lead to personalization of medical treatment. Genetic tests will come to underlie a high proportion of all medical decisions and will be seamlessly incorporated into routine medical care. Genetic tests will also be used in predictive testing for predisposition to disease to the extent that such testing can lead to strategies to prevent disease or improve outcome (see Chapter 83).

GENETICS AND PEDIATRIC PRACTICE. Genetics professionals (Table 78-2) include physicians who complete residencies in genetics and are certified by the American Board of Medical Genetics, recognized by the American Board of Medical Specialties. Genetic counselors receive a master's degree in genetic counseling and are certified by the American Board of Genetic Counseling. There are also nurse-geneticists who receive advanced training in genetics following completion of nursing education.

For rare single-gene disorders, the pediatrician will work closely with specialists in many disciplines (Table 78-3). Management will focus on achieving a correct diagnosis, counseling the family regarding natural history and management of the disorder as well as recurrence risk, and implementation of a management and treatment plan. As the scope of genetic testing increases, the pediatrician will be increasingly challenged to recognize relatively rare disorders that are amenable to treatment or to identify children who are at risk on the basis of family history who may not yet display symptoms of disease. Testing panels may be developed for common, complex problems, such as developmental delay. Some disorders for which early treatment is critical may be added to newborn or early childhood screening panels; others will be the subject of clinical practice guidelines. **Family history** will be an increasingly valuable tool to recognize children at risk, who can be tested and then offered personalized approaches to prevention or management. Genetic tests will increasingly underlie day-to-day treatment decisions for common disorders not traditionally viewed as genetic.

ETHICAL ISSUES. Genetic testing, diagnosis, and treatment must be performed with a high degree of confidentiality, avoiding any stigma for the patient. Genetic discrimination should be illegal because subtle or not so subtle effects of having a personal or family genetic diagnosis may occasionally affect employment or the ability to obtain health or life insurance. Nothing is so personal as one's genetic material. The decision to undergo genetic testing is complicated. The decision about whether to perform a

TABLE 78-2. Types of Genetics Professionals

PROFESSIONAL	TRAINING	CERTIFICATION	ROLE
Medical geneticist	MD and residency in medical genetics	American Board of Medical Genetics	Diagnosis and management of patients with genetic disorders
Genetic counselor	MS	American Board of Genetic Counseling	Genetic counseling and coordination of care
Laboratory geneticist	PhD or MD and 2-yr fellowship	American Board of Medical Genetics	Supervision of laboratory testing in cytogenetics, biochemical genetics, and molecular genetics
Nurse-geneticist	Advanced Practice Nurse in Genetics (master's) or Genetics Clinical Nurse (baccalaureate)	Genetic Nursing Credentialing Commission	Nursing care of patients with genetic disorders

TABLE 78-3. Role of Pediatrician, Specialist, and Geneticist in Care of Children with Rare and Common Disorders

TYPE OF DISORDER	PEDIATRICIAN	SPECIALIST	MEDICAL GENETICIST
Rare single-gene or chromosomal disorder	Recognize signs and symptoms; make referral; support family; manage longitudinal care	Manage specialty-specific problems	Perform diagnosis, counseling, and longitudinal care; advise on interpretation of test results; discuss genetic-based therapy
Common multifactorial disorder	Use genetic tests to guide treatment	Use genetic tests to guide treatment	Design and interpret tests; manage complex cases; perform family counseling; discuss genetic-based therapy

genetic test on a child is even more difficult, because the child cannot always participate in discussions about the testing. The ultimate decision hinges on how the results of the test will help or harm the child. The interest of the child is always foremost; thus, open discussion of the pros and cons of testing should always center on the child's interests. Molecular diagnostic tests are often used to diagnose malformation syndromes, mental retardation, or other disabilities wherein there is a clear benefit to the child. In other cases, the decision whether to test a child is more difficult.

Policies regarding genetic testing of children have been issued jointly by the American Society of Human Genetics and American College of Medical Genetics (*Amer J Hum Genet* 1995;57: 1233–1241) and by the American Academy of Pediatrics (*Pediatr* 2001;107:1451–1455). The AAP recommendations include the following:

1. **Established newborn screening tests should be reviewed and evaluated periodically to permit modification of the program or elimination of ineffective components. The introduction of new newborn screening tests should be conducted through carefully monitored research protocols.**
2. **Genetic tests, like most diagnostic or therapeutic endeavors for children, require a process of informed parental consent and the older child's assent. Newborn screening programs are encouraged to evaluate protocols in which informed consent from parents is obtained. The frequency of informed refusals should be monitored. Research to improve the efficiency and effectiveness of informed consent for newborn screening is warranted.**
3. **The AAP does not support the broad use of carrier testing or screening in children or adolescents. Additional research needs to be conducted on carrier screening in children and adolescents. The risks and benefits of carrier screening in the pediatric population should be evaluated in carefully monitored clinical trials before it is offered on a broad scale. Carrier screening for pregnant adolescents or for some adolescents considering pregnancy may be appropriate.**
4. **Genetic testing for adult-onset conditions generally should be deferred until adulthood or until an adolescent interested in testing has developed mature decision-making capacities. The AAP believes that genetic testing of children and adolescents to predict late-onset disorders is inappropriate when the genetic information has not been shown to reduce morbidity and mortality through interventions initiated in childhood.**
5. **Because genetic screening and testing may not be well understood, pediatricians need to provide parents the necessary information and counseling about the limits of genetic knowledge and treatment capabilities, the potential harm that may be done by gaining certain genetic information, including the possibilities for psychological harm, stigmatization, and discrimination, and medical conditions and disability and potential treatments and services for children with genetic conditions. Pediatricians can be assisted in managing many of the complex issues involved in genetic testing by collaboration with geneticists, genetic counselors, and prenatal care providers.**
6. **The AAP supports the expansion of educational opportunities in human genetics for medical students, residents, and practicing physicians and the expansion of training programs for genetic professionals.**

Boright AP, Kere J, Scherer SW: The genetics of childhood disease and development: A series of review articles. *Pediatr Res* 2003;53:4–9.

Braude P: Preimplantation diagnosis for genetic susceptibility. *N Engl J Med* 2006;355:541–543.

Burton PR, Tobin MD, Hopper JL: Key concepts in genetic epidemiology. *Lancet* 2005;366:941–950.

Greely HT: Banning genetic discrimination. *N Engl J Med* 2005;353:865–867.

Guttmacher AE, Collins FS: Genomic medicine—A primer. *N Engl J Med* 2002;347:1512–1520.

Hall JG, Powers EK, McLlvaine RT, et al: The frequency and financial burden of genetic disease in a pediatric hospital. *Am J Med Genet* 1978;1:417.

McCandless SE, Brunger JW, Cassidy SB: The burden of genetic disease on inpatient care in a children's hospital. *Am J Hum Genet* 2004;74:121–127.

Stevenson DA, Carey JC: Contribution of malformations and genetic disorders to mortality in a children's hospital. *Am J Med Genet A* 2004;126:393–337.

Chapter 79 ■ The Human Genome

Bruce R. Korf

Knowledge of the structure and function of DNA ushered in the era of molecular biology, with an increasingly rich understanding of the processes of DNA replication, transcription, translation, and protein processing. Many genetic disorders are understood at the molecular level, resulting in specific diagnostic tests and appropriate treatments. The Human Genome Project, culminating in the sequencing of the human genome, made it possible to study virtually any human gene and to explore the roles of genes in both rare and common disorders. It has also become apparent that the genome includes far more than a coded store of information to produce proteins.

The human genome has approximately 25,000 genes, which are the individual units of heredity of all traits. Reproductive or germline cells contain one copy (N) of this genetic complement and are **haploid,** whereas somatic (non-germline) cells contain two complete copies (2N) and are **diploid.** The genes are organized into long segments of DNA, which, during cell division, are compacted into intricate structures with proteins to form chromosomes. Each somatic cell has 46 chromosomes (22 pairs of autosomes, or non–sex chromosomes, and 1 pair of sex chromosomes [XY in a male, XX in a female]). Germ cells (eggs, sperm) contain 22 autosomes and 1 sex chromosome, for a total of 23. At fertilization, the full diploid chromosome complement of 46 is again realized in the embryo.

Most of the genetic material is contained in the cell's nucleus. The mitochondria (the cell's energy-producing organelles) contain their own unique genome. The **mitochondrial chromosome** consists of a double-stranded circular piece of DNA, which contains 16,568 base pairs (bp) of DNA and is completely sequenced. The proteins that comprise the mitochondria may either be produced in the mitochondria (from information contained in the mitochondrial genome) or produced from information contained in the nuclear genome and transported into the organelle. All mitochondria are maternally derived (because sperm do not usually carry mitochondria into fertilized eggs); different mitochondria within a single cell with a variety of genomes reflect the maternal lines from which they descended.

FUNDAMENTALS OF MOLECULAR GENETICS. The central tenet of molecular genetics is that information encoded in DNA predominantly located in the cell nucleus is transcribed into messenger RNA (mRNA), which is then transported to the cytoplasm, where it is translated into protein. A gene is a unit that includes a regulatory region and a coding region that stores information corresponding to the sequence of amino acids in a specific protein.

DNA consists of a pair of chains of a sugar-phosphate backbone linked by pyrimidine and purine bases to form a **double helix** (Fig. 79-1). The sugar in DNA is deoxyribose. The pyrimidines are cytosine (C) and thymine (T); the purines are guanine (G) and adenine (A). The bases are linked by hydrogen bonds such that A always pairs with T and G with C. Each strand of the double helix has polarity, with a free phosphate at one end (5′) and an unbonded hydroxyl on the sugar at the other end (3′). The two strands are oriented in opposite polarity in the double helix.

The replication of DNA follows the paring of bases in the parent DNA strand. The original two strands unwind by breaking the hydrogen bonds between base pairs. Free nucleotides, consisting of a base attached to a sugar-phosphate, form new hydrogen bonds with their complementary bases on the parent strand; new phosphodiester bonds are created by the enzyme **DNA polymerase.** Replication of chromosomes begins simulta-

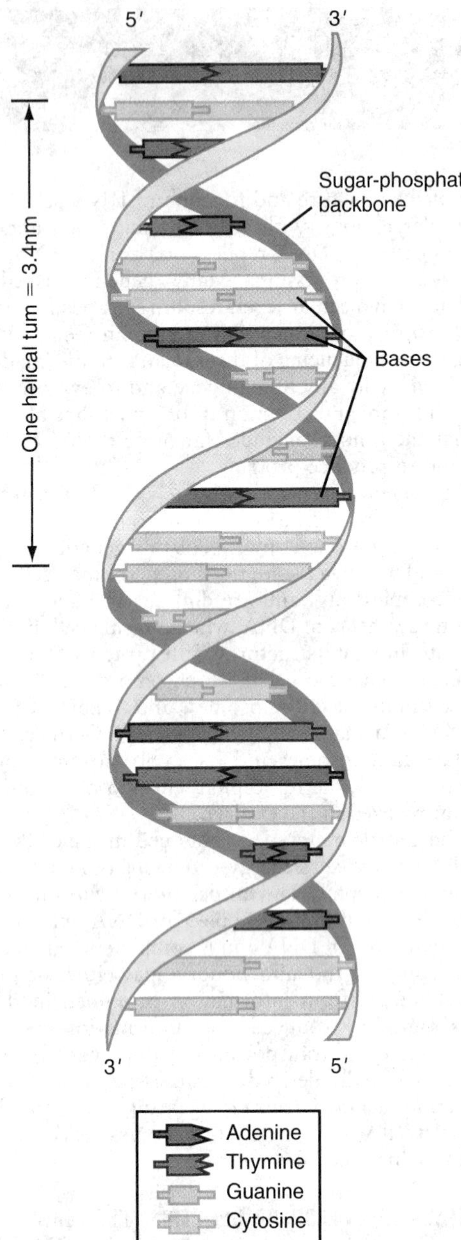

Figure 79-1. DNA double helix, with sugar-phosphate backbone and nitrogenous bases. (From Jorde LB, Carey JC, Bamshad MJ, et al [editors]: *Medical Genetics,* 2nd ed. St. Louis, Mosby, 1999, p 8.)

neously at multiple sites, forming replication bubbles that expand bidirectionally until the entire DNA molecule (chromosome) is replicated. Errors in DNA replication, or mutations induced by environmental mutagens such as irradiation or chemicals, are detected and potentially corrected by DNA repair systems.

A prototypical gene consists of a regulatory region, segments called **exons** that encode the amino acid sequence of a protein, and intervening segments called **introns** (Fig. 79-2). **Transcription** starts at the promoter region and continues through the entire length of the gene to form mRNA. The introns are then removed and the exons spliced together to form a mature message, which is then exported to the cytoplasm. There the mRNA is bound to ribosomes and translated into protein.

Transcription is initiated by attachment of RNA polymerase to the promoter site upstream of the beginning of the coding sequence. Specific proteins bind to the region to either repress or derepress transcription by opening up the chromatin, which is a complex of DNA and histone proteins. It is the production of these regulatory proteins (**transcription factors**) that determines when a gene is turned on or off. Some genes on specific chromosomes in defined areas are turned off more or less permanently by **epigenetic** methylation of cytosine bases that are adjacent to guanines (CpG bases). Gene regulation is flexible and responsive, with genes being turned on or off during development or in response to environmental stimuli.

Transcription proceeds through the full length of the gene, synthesizing mRNA in a 5′ to 3′ direction. RNA, like DNA, is a sugar-phosphate chain with pyrimidines and purines. The sugar in this case is ribose; uracil replaces thymine in RNA. The RNA reads off one strand of DNA to copy a complementary RNA sequence. A "cap" consisting of 7-methylguanosine is added to the 5′ end of the RNA in a 5′-5′ bond and, for most transcripts several hundred adenine bases are enzymatically added to the 3′ end after transcription. mRNA **processing** occurs in the nucleus and consists of excision of the introns and splicing together of the exons. Specific sequences at the start and end of introns mark the sites where the splicing machinery will act on the transcript. In some cases, there may be tissue-specific patterns to splicing, so that the same primary transcript can produce multiple distinct proteins.

The processed transcript is next exported to the cytoplasm, where it binds to ribosomes, which are protein-RNA complexes. The genetic code is then read in triplets of bases, each triplet corresponding with a specific amino acid or providing a signal that terminates **translation.** The triplet codons are recognized by transfer RNAs (tRNAs) that include complementary "anticodons" and bind the corresponding amino acid, delivering it to the growing peptide. A new amino acid is enzymatically attached to the peptide; each time an amino acid is added, the ribosome moves one triplet codon "step" along the mRNA. Eventually a stop codon is reached, at which point translation ends and the peptide is released. In some proteins, there may be **post-translational modifications** such as attachment of sugars (glycosylation); the protein is then delivered to its destination within or outside the cell by trafficking mechanisms that recognize portions of the peptide.

GENETIC VARIATION. The process of production of protein from a gene is subject to disruption at multiple levels owing to alterations in the coding sequence (Fig. 79-3). Changes in the promoter region can lead to altered gene regulation, including increased or decreased rates of transcription, failure of gene activation, or activation of the gene at inappropriate times or in inappropriate cells. Changes in the coding sequence can lead to **substitution** of one amino acid for another **(missense mutation)** or creation of a stop codon in the place of an amino acid codon. Some single-base changes do not affect the amino acid, since there may be several codons that correspond with a single amino acid (silent mutation). Amino acid substitutions may have a profound effect on protein function if the chemical properties of the substituted amino acid are markedly different from the usual one; substitutions may have a subtle or no effect on protein function if the substituted amino acid is chemically similar to the original one.

Genetic changes may also include **insertions** or **deletions.** Insertions or deletions of a non-integral multiple of three bases into the coding sequence leads to a **frameshift,** altering the grouping of bases into triplets. This leads to translation of an incorrect amino acid sequence and usually the eventual production of a stop codon. Insertion or deletion of an integral multiple of three bases into the coding sequence will insert or delete a corresponding number of amino acids from the protein. Larger scale insertions or deletions can disrupt a coding sequence or result in complete deletion of an entire gene or group of genes.

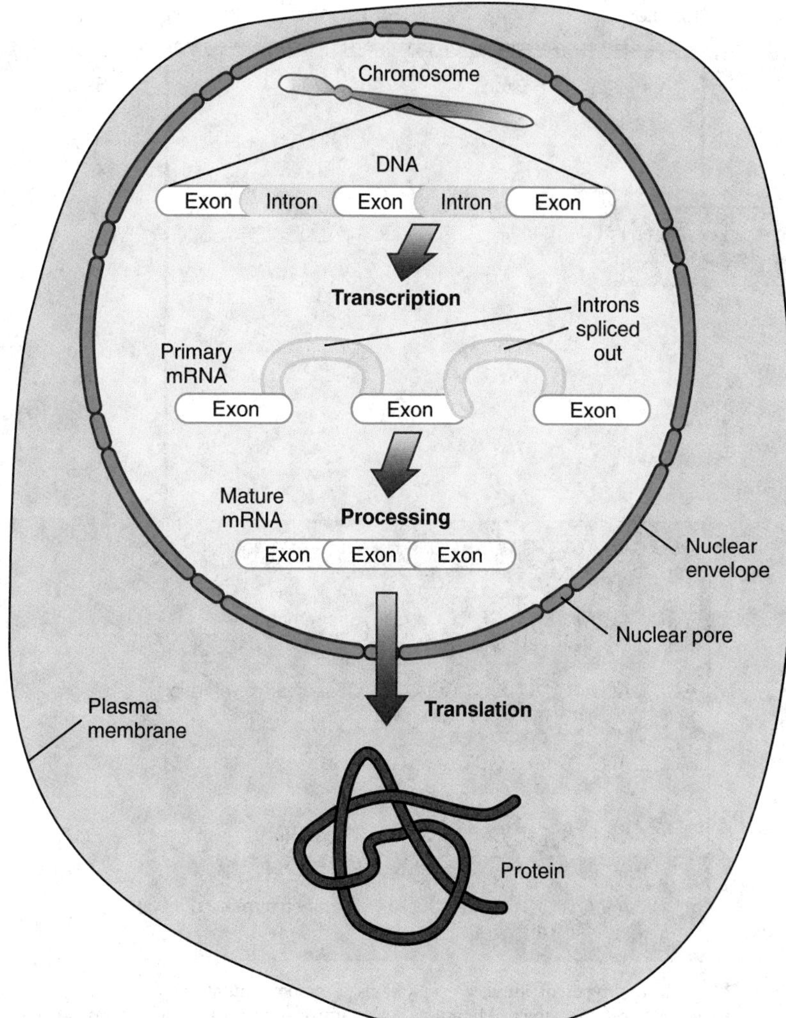

Figure 79-2. Summary of the steps leading from DNA to proteins. Replication and transcription occur in the cell nucleus. The mRNA is then transported to the cytoplasm, where translation of the mRNA into amino acid sequences composing a protein occurs. (From Jorde LB, Carey JC, Bamshad MJ, et al [editors]: *Medical Genetics,* 2nd ed. St. Louis, Mosby, 1999, p 12.)

Mutations usually can be classified as causing gain of function or loss of function. A **gain-of-function mutation** can result in an increase in the ability of a protein molecule to perform one or more normal functions, or, more commonly, it can result in overexpression or inappropriate expression of a gene product. Gain-of-function mutations most frequently produce autosomal dominant disorders (see Chapter 80). **Charcot-Marie-Tooth disease, type 1A,** or peroneal muscular atrophy, the most common form of chronic peripheral neuropathy of childhood, results from duplication of the gene for peripheral myelin protein 22, resulting in overexpression of the gene product. The gain-of-function mutation in **achondroplasia,** the most common of the short-limbed skeletal dysplasias, exemplifies the enhanced function of a normal protein. Achondroplasia results from a mutation in fibroblast growth receptor 3 (FGFR3), which leads to activation of the receptor, even in the absence of fibroblast growth factor (FGF). **Loss-of-function mutations** are frequently observed in autosomal recessive disorders in which loss of 50% enzyme activity in the heterozygote continues to allow for normal function. Alternatively, loss-of-function mutations can result in conditions in which 50% of the gene product is insufficient for normal function (**haploinsufficiency**). Loss-of-function mutations can have a dominant negative effect when the abnormal protein product actively interferes with the function of the normal protein product.

Another category of mutations may confer a novel property on the protein synthesized, without altering the protein's normal functions. In **sickle cell disease,** an amino acid is substituted into the hemoglobin molecule that has no effect on the ability of the protein to transport oxygen. However, unlike normal hemoglobin, under conditions of deoxygenation, sickle hemoglobin chains aggregate, forming fibers that deform the red cells. A final category of mutations results in abnormal expression of a gene over space and time. Many cancer-causing genes (**oncogenes**) are normal regulators of cellular proliferation during development; when expressed in adult life, and in cells in which they usually are not expressed, they may result in neoplasia.

Deletions can vary in their extent and, even when not visible at the cytogenetic level, can involve several genes; these are often termed **microdeletions.** By a variety of rearrangements, conditions referred to as **contiguous gene syndromes** may be generated. The clinician may be alerted to this possibility by an unusually diverse array of clinical features in any individual or the presence of additional features to a known condition. For example, owing to the close physical proximity of a series of genes, different deletions involving the short arm of the X chromosome can produce individuals with various combinations of the following features: ichthyosis, Kallmann syndrome, ocular albinism, mental retardation, chondrodysplasia punctata, and short stature. The individ-

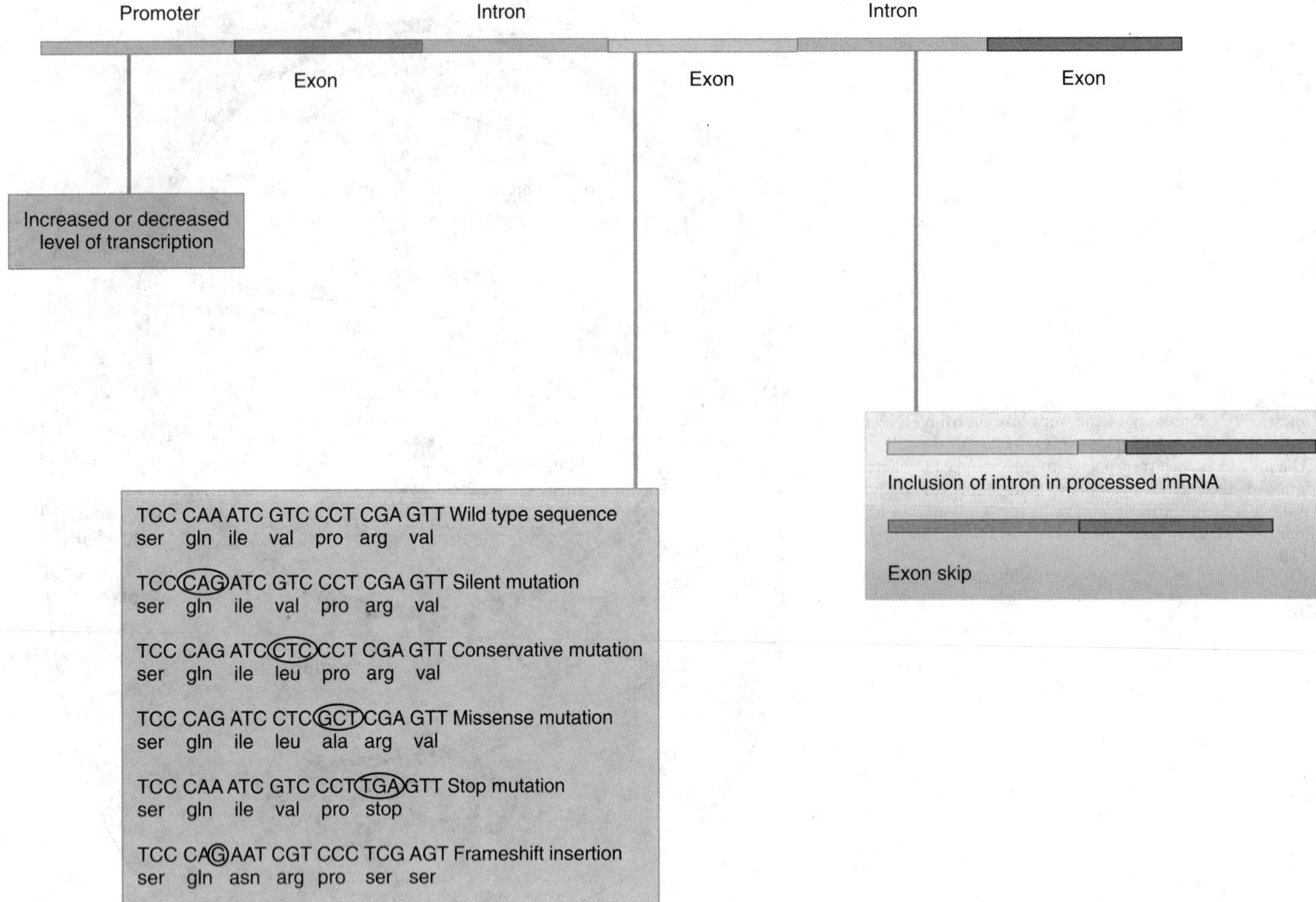

Figure 79-3. Various types of intragenic mutations. Promoter mutations alter rate of transcription or disrupt gene regulation. Base changes within exons can have various effects, as shown. Mutations within introns can lead to inclusion of some intronic sequence in the final processed mRNA, or can lead to exon skipping.

ual features in each case depend on the involvement of these genes and the loss of DNA sequences in the underlying rearrangement. Many other chromosome deletion syndromes have been described in humans, including Smith-Magenis, Rubinstein-Taybi, DiGeorge, William, and Prader-Willi syndromes.

Rearrangements such as **translocations** also take place in somatic cells. The best understood are the rearrangements that occur in lymphoid cells. Some rearrangements are required for the formation of functional immunoglobulin in B cells and antigen-recognizing receptors on the T cell. Large segments of DNA, which code for the variable and the constant regions of either immunoglobulin or the T-cell receptor, are physically joined at a specific stage in the development of an immunocompetent lymphocyte. The rearrangements take place during development of the lymphoid cell lineage in humans and result in the extensive diversity of immunoglobulin and T-cell receptor molecules. It is as a result of this post-germline DNA rearrangement that no two individuals, not even identical twins, are really identical, because mature lymphocytes from each will have undergone random DNA rearrangements at these loci.

Studies of the human genome sequence reveal that any two individuals differ in about one base in a thousand. Some of these differences are silent; some result in changes that explain phenotypic differences (hair or eye color, physical appearance); some have medical significance, causing single gene disorders such as sickle cell anemia or explaining susceptibility to common disorders such as asthma. Genetic variants within the same gene occur commonly in the population and are referred to as **polymorphisms.** These may be silent or subtle or have significant phenotypic effects.

GENOTYPE-PHENOTYPE CORRELATIONS IN GENETIC DISEASE. **Genotype** is the genetic constitution of an individual and refers to which particular alternative version (**allele**) of a gene is present at a specific location (**locus**) on a chromosome. **Phenotype** is the observed structural, biochemical, and physiologic characteristics of an individual, determined by the genotype, and refers to the observed structural and functional effects of a mutant allele at a specific locus. Many mutations result in predictable phenotypes. Therefore, identification of a specific mutation in an individual often can be used to predict clinical outcomes and plan appropriate treatment strategies.

The **long QT syndrome** exemplifies a disorder with predictable genotype-phenotype correlations (see Chapter 435.5). Long QT syndrome (phenotype) can be caused by mutations in several genes (genotypes), which are designated *LQT1*, *LQT2*, and *LQT3*, all encoding cardiac ion channels. The risk for cardiac events (syncope, aborted cardiac arrest, or sudden death) is higher with mutations at the *LQT1* locus (63%) or the *LQT2* locus (46%) than among subjects with mutations at the *LQT3* locus (18%). In addition, those with *LQT1* mutations experience most of their episodes during exercise and rarely during rest or sleep; those with *LQT2* and *LQT3* mutations are more likely to have episodes during sleep or rest, and rarely during exercise.

Mutations in the fibrillin-1 gene associated with **Marfan syndrome** represent another example of predictable genotype-phenotype correlations (see Chapter 700). Marfan syndrome is characterized by the combination of skeletal, ocular, and aortic manifestations, with the most devastating outcome being aortic root dissection and sudden death. Sixty-five exons make up the fibrillin-1 gene, and mutations have been found in almost all of these exons. The location of the mutation within the gene (genotype) may play a significant role in determining the severity of the condition (phenotype). Neonatal Marfan syndrome is caused by mutations in exons 24–27 and 31–32, whereas milder forms are caused by mutations in exons 59–65 and in exons 37 and 41.

Genotype-phenotype correlations have occasionally been observed in **cystic fibrosis** (CF) [see Chapter 400]. CF is a chronic lung disease caused by mutations in the CF transmembrane conductance regulator (CFTR) gene. More than 1,000 different mutations have been identified; the most common is the ΔF508 mutation, which accounts for 70% of all mutations and is associated with severe disease. Several mutations associated with mild disease have been identified, including 3272-26A→G, 3849+10 kb C→T, IVS8-5T, and 2789+5G→A. Patients with at least one 3272-26A→G allele and a second mutated allele (**compound heterozygote**) associated with severe disease are more likely to be diagnosed later and have better lung function, a lower incidence of *Pseudomonas aeruginosa* colonization, and normal pancreatic function. Homozygotes for this mutation are not observed and may not have clinical disease. Conversely, those with 2183AA→G mutations, either homozygous or heterozygous with another CF mutation, are more likely to have early-onset, severe disease. Those with this mutation tended to have severe pancreatic involvement, failure to thrive, variable lung involvement, and relatively early death.

With any given mutation, **modifier genes** for a different gene product may attenuate the mutated gene's phenotype. When sickle cell anemia is co-inherited with the gene for hereditary persistence of fetal hemoglobin, the sickle cell phenotypic expression is less severe. Modifier genes in CF may influence the development of congenital meconium ileus, or colonization with *P. aeruginosa.* Modifier genes may also affect the manifestations of Hirschsprung disease, neurofibromatosis type 2, craniosynostosis, and congenital adrenal hyperplasia. The combination of genetic mutations producing glucose-6-phosphate dehydrogenase deficiency and Gilbert disease (promoter of glucuronyl transferase) exacerbates neonatal physiologic hyperbilirubinemia.

HUMAN GENOME PROJECT. Gene mapping is performed by genetic linkage analysis, which is based on the principle that alleles at two genetic loci that are located near one another will segregate together in a family unless they are separated by genetic **recombination.** The frequency of recombination between the loci is a measure of physical distance. A set of polymorphic genetic loci is identified and is closely spaced along the entire human genome and could be used to map any genetic trait.

Physical mapping of the genome involves isolation of segments of the human genome with lengths from hundreds or thousands to a few million base pairs and placing them in microorganisms such as bacteria or yeast. Automated sequencing systems permit the base sequence of these segments to be determined. The segments could then be pieced together by examining the sequence of overlap regions and by relating the sequenced segments to polymorphic markers on the gene map. An alternative strategy involves breaking the entire genome into random fragments, sequencing the fragments, and then using a computer to order the fragments based on overlapping segments.

Analysis of the human genome has produced some surprising results as well. The number of genes is still not known precisely but appears to be around 25,000. This is fewer than had been expected and is in the same range as many simpler organisms. The number of proteins encoded, however, is far greater because of alternative promoter regions in some genes, alternative splicing, and post-translational modifications.

It is also apparent that most of the genome does not encode protein (less than 5% is transcribed and translated). Many transcribed sequences are not translated but represent genes that encode RNAs that serve a regulatory role. A high proportion of the genome consists of repeated sequences that are interspersed among the genes. Some of these are transposable genetic elements that have the ability to move from place to place in the genome. Others are static elements that were expanded and dispersed in the past during human evolution. Other repeated sequences may play a structural role. There are also regions of duplication of genomic regions. Such duplications are substrate for evolution, allowing genetic motifs to be copied and modified to serve new roles in the cell. Duplications may also form the basis for chromosomal rearrangement, permitting nonhomologous chromosome segments to pair during meiosis and exchange material. This is another source of evolutionary change, and also serves as a potential source of chromosomal instability leading to congenital anomalies or cancer.

Availability of the genome sequence permits the study of large groups of genes, looking for patterns of gene expression or genome alteration. Microarrays have been developed that permit tens or hundreds of thousands of genes to be analyzed on a small glass chip. Patterns of gene expression provide signatures for particular disease states, such as cancer, or in response to therapy (Fig. 79-4).

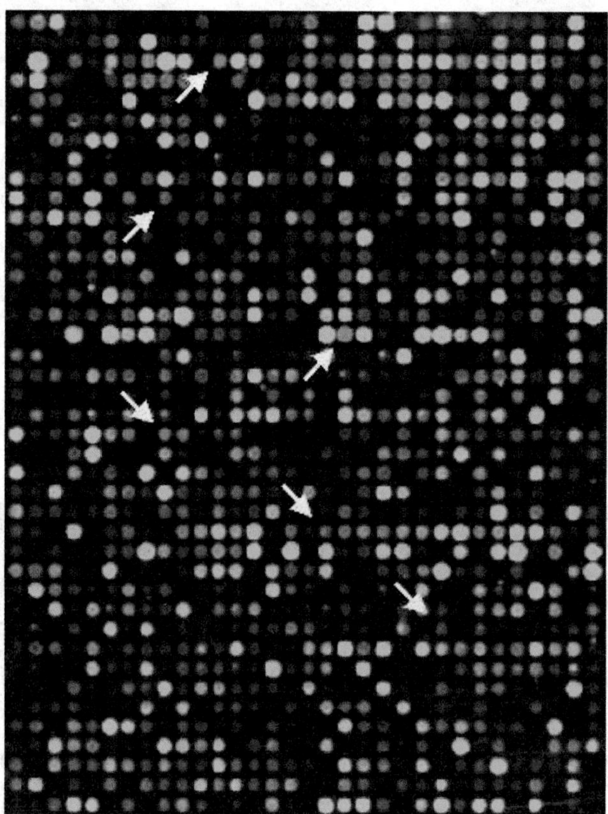

Figure 79-4. Microarray containing 36,000 oligonucleotides. The microarray was exposed to RNA from normal fibroblasts (labeled red; see arrows) and fibroblasts from a patient with Niemann-Pick disease, type C (labeled green). *Arrows* point to regions in which there was a strong hybridization signal with either normal or disease RNA. This microarray was used to search for genes that are highly expressed in the fibroblasts of patients. (From Jorde LB, Carey JC, Bamshad MJ, et al [editors]: *Medical Genetics,* 3rd ed. St. Louis, Mosby, 2006, p 116.)

Christensen K, Murray JC: What genome-wide association studies can do for medicine. *N Engl J Med* 2007;356:1094–1097.
Cordell HJ, Clayton DG: Genetic association studies. *Lancet* 2005;366:1121–1130.
Hattersley AT, McCarthy MI: What makes a good genetic association study? *Lancet* 2005;366:1315–1323.
Jarvis JN, Centola M: Gene-expression profiling: Time for clinical application? *Lancet* 2005;365:199–200.
Lander ES, Linton LM, Birren B, et al: Initial sequencing and analysis of the human genome. *Nature* 2001;409(6822):860–921.
McGhee SA, McCabe ERB: Genome-wide testing: genomic medicine. *Pediatr Res* 2006;60:243–244.
Teare MD, Barrett JH: Genetic linkage studies. *Lancet* 2005;366:1036–1044.
Venter JC, Adams MD, Myers EW, et al: The sequence of the human genome. *Science* 2001;291(5507):1304.

Chapter 80 ■ Patterns of Genetic Transmission

Nathaniel H. Robin

FAMILY HISTORY AND PEDIGREE NOTATION. The family history remains the most important screening tool for pediatricians in identifying a patient's risk for developing a wide range of diseases, including multifactorial conditions, like diabetes and attention deficit disorder, to single-gene disorders such as osteogenesis imperfecta and cystic fibrosis. Through a detailed family history the physician can ascertain the mode of genetic transmission and the risks to family members. Because not all familial clustering of disease is due to genetic factors, a family history can also identify common environmental and behavioral factors that influence the occurrence of disease. The main goal of the family history is to identify genetic susceptibility, and the cornerstone of the family history is a systematic and standardized pedigree.

A **pedigree** provides a graphic depiction of a family's structure and medical history. The person providing the information is termed the **proband,** and is typically designated by an arrow. It is important when taking a pedigree to be systematic and use standard symbols and configurations (Fig. 80-1) so that anyone can read and understand the information. A three-generation pedigree should be obtained as an initial screen for every new patient to identify possible genetic disorders segregating within the family, the inheritance pattern, and the risk to the patient. The closer the relationship of the proband to the person in the family with the genetic disorder, the greater is the shared genetic complement. **First-degree** relatives, such as a parent, full sibling, or child, share ½ their genetic information on average; 1st cousins share ⅛. Sometimes a disease in a more distant relative may create a greater risk; for that reason, a more extended pedigree may be needed to identify risk for certain disorders. A history of a distant maternally related cousin with mental retardation due to fragile X syndrome may have little significance for the male infant you are examining, or it may mean that this child is at elevated risk for fragile X syndrome.

MENDELIAN INHERITANCE

There are three classic forms of genetic inheritance: **autosomal dominant, autosomal recessive,** and **X-linked.** These are referred to as mendelian inheritance forms, after Gregor Mendel, the 19th century monk whose experiments led to the laws of **segregation of characteristics, dominance,** and **independent assortment.** These remain the foundation of single-gene inheritance. With mendelian inheritance, a single gene's effect is *necessary* and *sufficient* to cause a particular phenotype. This is in contrast to other forms

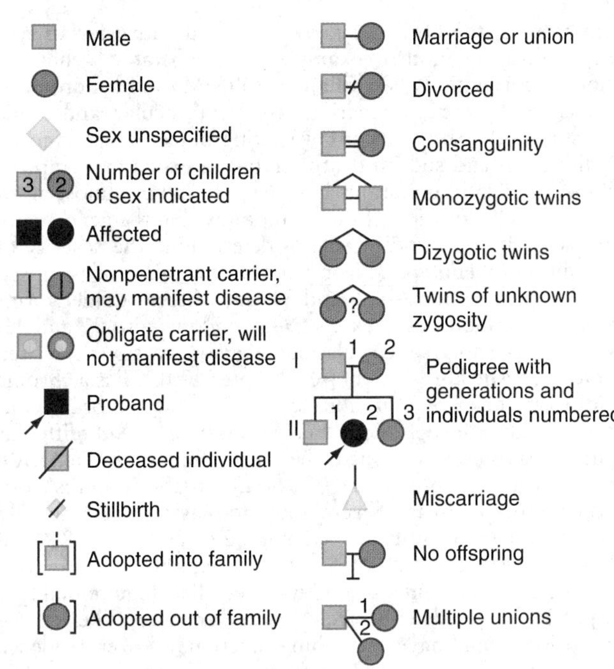

Figure 80-1. Pedigree notation. Symbols commonly used in pedigree charts. Although there is no uniform system of pedigree notation, the symbols shown here are according to recent recommendations made by professionals in the field of genetic counseling. (From Bennett RL, Steinhaus KA, Uhrich SB, et al: Recommendations for standardized pedigree nomenclature. *J Genet Counsel* 1995;4:267–279.)

of genetically determined traits, such as imprinting conditions, triplet repeat disorders, and multifactorial traits, in which other factors influence whether the disease will be present in someone who carries the genetic change.

Autosomal Dominant Inheritance. Autosomal dominant inheritance is determined by the presence of one abnormal gene on one of the autosomes (chromosomes 1–22). The genes on these chromosomes exist in pairs, with each parent contributing one copy. With an autosomal dominant trait, one of the paired genes has an effect on the phenotype that dominates the effect of the other of the pair. Phenotype refers not only to physical manifestations but also to behavioral characteristics or to differences detectable only through laboratory tests, such as biochemical abnormalities.

The pedigree for an autosomal dominant disorder (Fig. 80-2) demonstrates certain characteristics. (1) The disorder is transmitted in a vertical (parent to child) pattern, appearing in multiple generations. This is illustrated by individual I.1 (see Fig 80-2) passing on the changed gene to II.2 and II.5. (2) An affected individual has a 50% (1 in 2) chance of passing on the deleterious genes for *each* pregnancy, and therefore of having a child affected by the disorder. This is referred to as the **recurrence risk** for the disorder. (3) Unaffected individuals (family members who do not manifest the trait) do not pass the disorder to their children. (4) Males and females are equally affected. Although not a characteristic per se, (5) the finding of male-to-male transmission essentially confirms autosomal dominant inheritance. Vertical transmission can also be seen with X-linked traits. However, since a father passes on his Y chromosome to a son, male-to-male transmission cannot be seen with an X-linked trait. Therefore, male-to-male transmission eliminates X-linked inheritance as a possible explanation. While male-to-male transmission can occur with Y-linked genes as well, there are very few Y-linked disorders compared with thousands having the autosomal dominant inheritance pattern.

Although parent to child transmission is a characteristic of autosomal dominant inheritance, for many patients with an autosomal dominant disorder there is no history of an affected family member. There are several possible reasons: first, the patient may represent a **new mutation;** second, many autosomal dominant conditions demonstrate **incomplete penetrance,** meaning that not all individuals who carry the mutation have phenotypic manifestations. In a pedigree this may appear as a **skipped generation,** in which an unaffected individual links two affected persons (Fig. 80-3). There are many potential reasons that a disorder may exhibit incomplete penetrance, including the effect of modifier genes, environmental factors, gender, and age. Third, individuals with the same autosomal dominant mutation will manifest the disorder to different degrees. This is termed **variable expression** and is a characteristic of many autosomal dominant disorders. Fourth, some spontaneous genetic mutations occur not in the egg or sperm that forms a child but rather in a cell in the developing embryo. Such events are referred to as **somatic mutations.** The resulting phenotype caused by a somatic mutation can be varied, but it is usually milder than if all cells contain the mutation. In **germline mosaicism,** the mutation occurs in cells that populate the germline that produce eggs or sperm. A germline mosaic will have no manifestations of the disorder but will produce multiple eggs or sperm that carry the mutation.

Autosomal Recessive Inheritance. Autosomal recessive inheritance involves mutations in both copies of a gene. Examples of autosomal recessive diseases are cystic fibrosis and sickle cell disease. Characteristics of autosomal recessive traits (Fig. 80-4) include (1) **horizontal transmission,** the observation of multiple affected members of a kindred in the same generation, but no affected family members in other generations; (2) recurrence risk of 25% for parents with a previous affected child; (3) males and females being equally affected, though some traits exhibit different expression in males and females (ovarian cancer, hypospadias); (4) increased frequency of consanguinity, particularly for rare traits.

The chance that any two parents carry an identical mutant allele is increased if the couple is consanguineous. **Consanguinity** is relationship by descent from a common ancestor. Consanguinity between parents of a child with a suspected genetic disorder implies (but does not prove) autosomal recessive inheritance. Although consanguineous unions are uncommon in Western society, in other parts of the world (southern India, Japan, the Middle East) they are common. The risk of a genetic disorder for the offspring of a first-cousin marriage (6–8%) is about double the risk in the general population (3–4%). There are some genetic isolates (small populations separated by geography, religion, culture, or language) in which rare recessive disorders are more common than in the general population. Even though consanguinity may not be increased in these populations, because of limited mate choice, the chance of a couple from an isolated genetic region having a child with an autosomal recessive condition may be as high as that observed in first-cousin marriages. Screening programs have been developed in such groups to de-

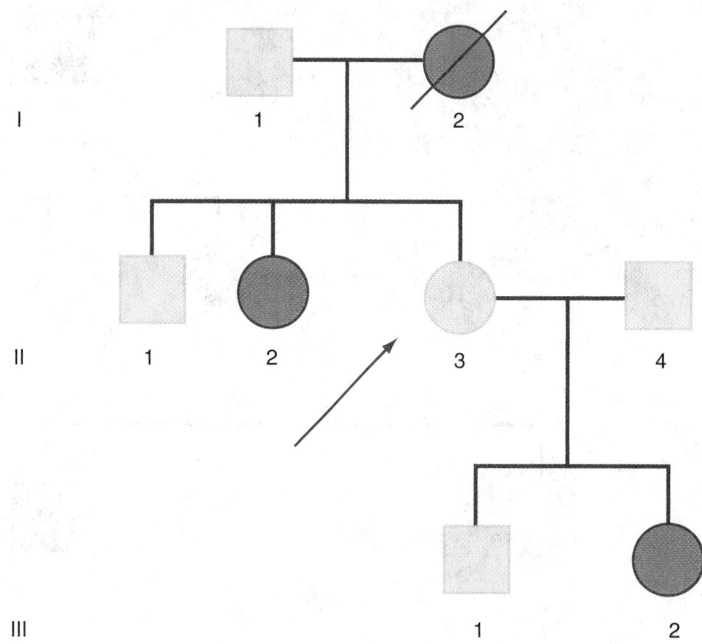

Figure 80-3. Incomplete penetrance. This family segregates a familial cancer syndrome, familial adenomatous polyposis. Individual II.3 is an obligate carrier, but there are no findings to suggest the disorder. She is termed nonpenetrant.

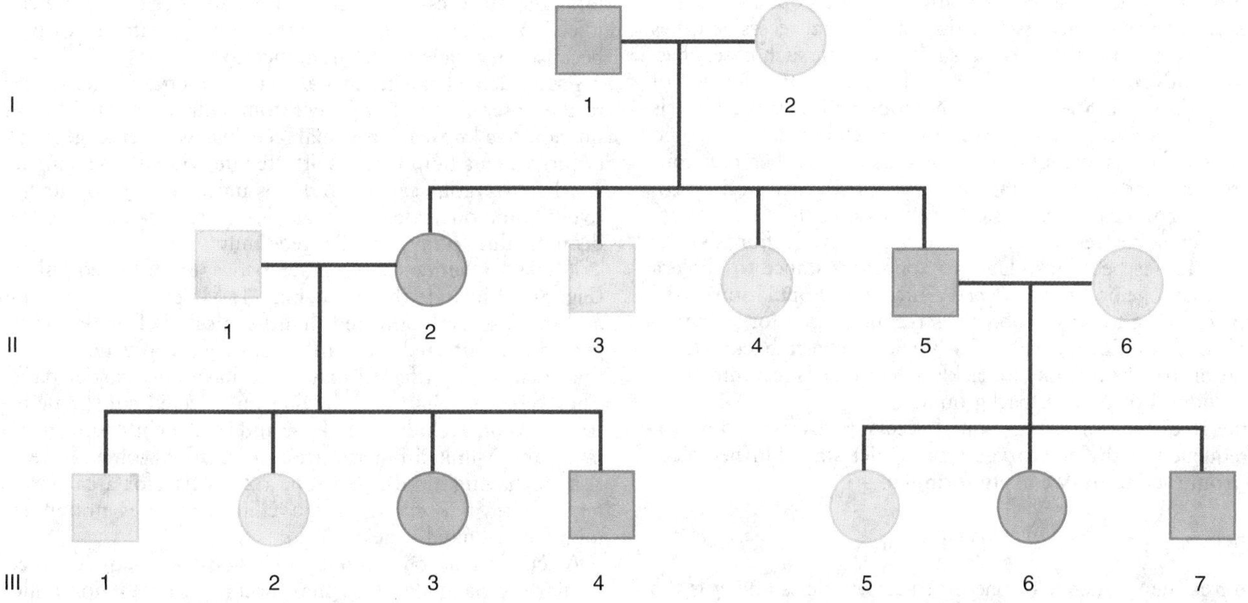

Figure 80-2. Autosomal dominant pedigree. Pedigree showing typical inheritance of a form of sensorineural deafness *(DFNA8)* inherited as an autosomal dominant trait. Blue, affected patients.

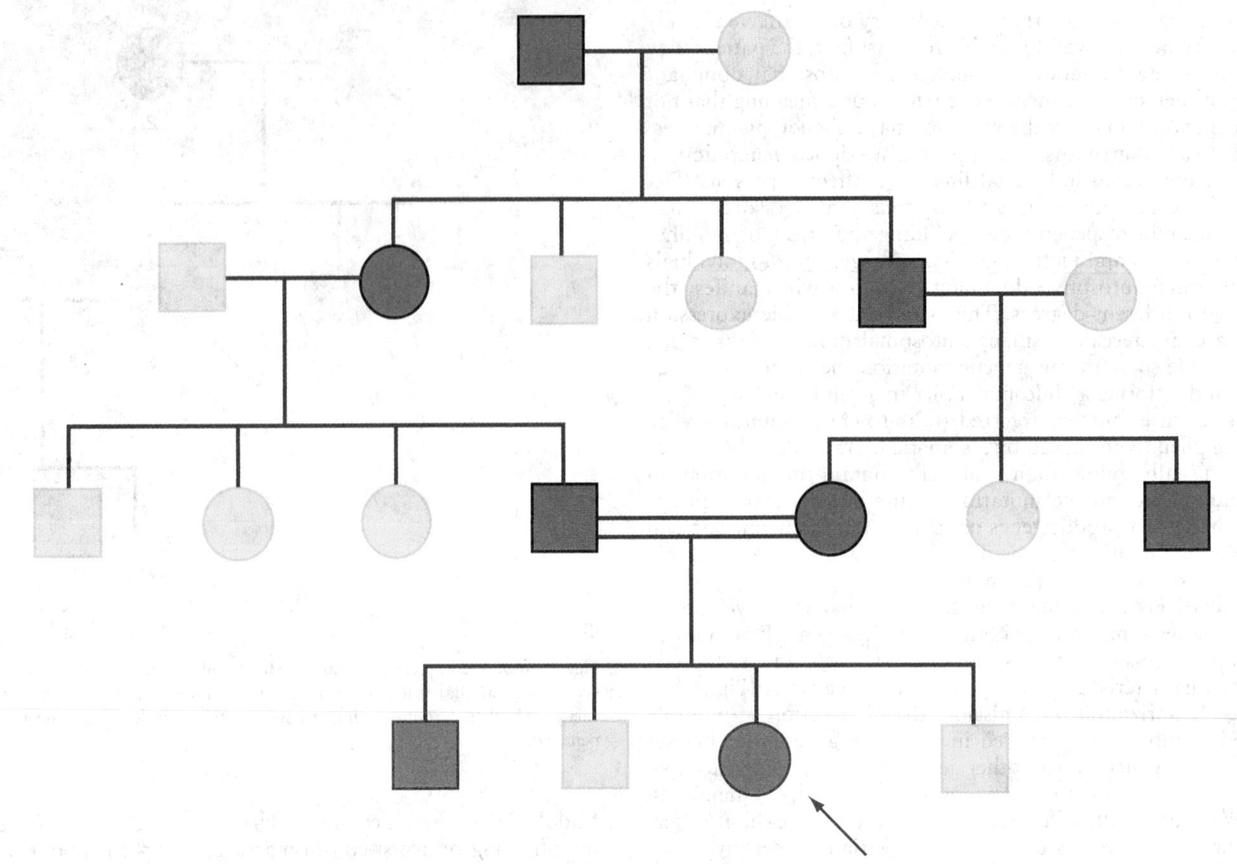

Figure 80-4. Autosomal recessive pedigree with parental consanguinity. Purple, carriers; Red, affected patients.

tect heterozygotes at risk for having affected children. A variety of autosomal recessive conditions are more common among Ashkenazi Jews than in the general population. National practice guidelines recommend screening asymptomatic Ashkenazi Jews for the neurodegenerative disorder Tay-Sachs disease, and Canavan disease carrier screening for other disorders (Fanconi anemia, Gaucher disease, cystic fibrosis, familial dysautonomia, nesidioblastosis) is under consideration for this population.

The prevalence of carriers of certain autosomal recessive genes in some larger populations is unusually high. In such cases, heterozygote advantage is postulated. The carrier frequencies of sickle cell disease in the African population and of cystic fibrosis in the northern European population are much higher than would be expected from new mutations. It is possible that heterozygous carriers have had an advantage in terms of survival and reproduction over noncarriers. In sickle cell disease, the carrier state may confer some resistance to malaria; in cystic fibrosis, the carrier state has been postulated to confer resistance to cholera or enteropathogenic *Escherichia coli* infections. Population-based carrier screening for cystic fibrosis is recommended for individuals of northern European and Ashkenazi Jewish background; population-based screening for sickle cell disease is recommended for individuals of African background.

If the frequency of an autosomal recessive disease is known, the frequency of the heterozygote or carrier state can be calculated from the **Hardy-Weinberg formula:**

$$p^2 + 2pq + q^2 = 1$$

where p is the frequency of one of a pair of alleles and q is the frequency of the other. For example, if the frequency of cystic fibrosis among white Americans is 1 in 2,500 (p^2), then the frequency of the heterozygote (2pq) can be calculated: if $p^2 = 1/_{2,500}$, then $p = 1/_{50}$ and $q = 49/_{50}$; $2pq = 2 \times 1/_{50} \times 49/_{50}$, or approximately $1/_{25}$ (or 3.92%).

Every human probably has several rare, harmful, recessive genes. Because these mutant genes are frequently not identifiable by laboratory tests, the heterozygous adult usually learns about these harmful recessive genes after the birth of a homozygous (and therefore affected) child. Related parents are much more likely to be heterozygous for the same harmful recessive genes because they have a common ancestor.

Pseudodominant Inheritance. Pseudodominant inheritance refers to the observation of apparent dominant (parent to child) transmission of a known autosomal recessive disorder (Fig. 80-5). This occurs when a homozygous affected individual has a partner who is a heterozygous carrier, and it is most likely to occur for relatively common traits, such as sickle cell anemia or congenital deafness due to *connexin26* gene mutation.

X-linked Inheritance. Characteristics of X-linked inheritance (Fig. 80-6) include the following: (1) Males are more commonly and more severely affected than females. (2) Female carriers are generally unaffected, or if affected, they are affected more mildly than males. (3) Affected males will have only carrier daughters. They have no chance of having an affected son (male-to-male transmission excludes X-linkage and is seen with autosomal dominant and Y-linked inheritance). (4) Carrier women have a 25% risk for having an affected son, a 25% risk for a carrier daughter, and a 50% chance for a child that does not inherit the mutated X-linked gene.

A female may occasionally exhibit signs of an X-linked trait similarly to a male. This may occur owing to nonrandom X-inactivation, homozygosity for an X-linked trait, or presence of a sex chromosome abnormality (45,X or 46,XY female).

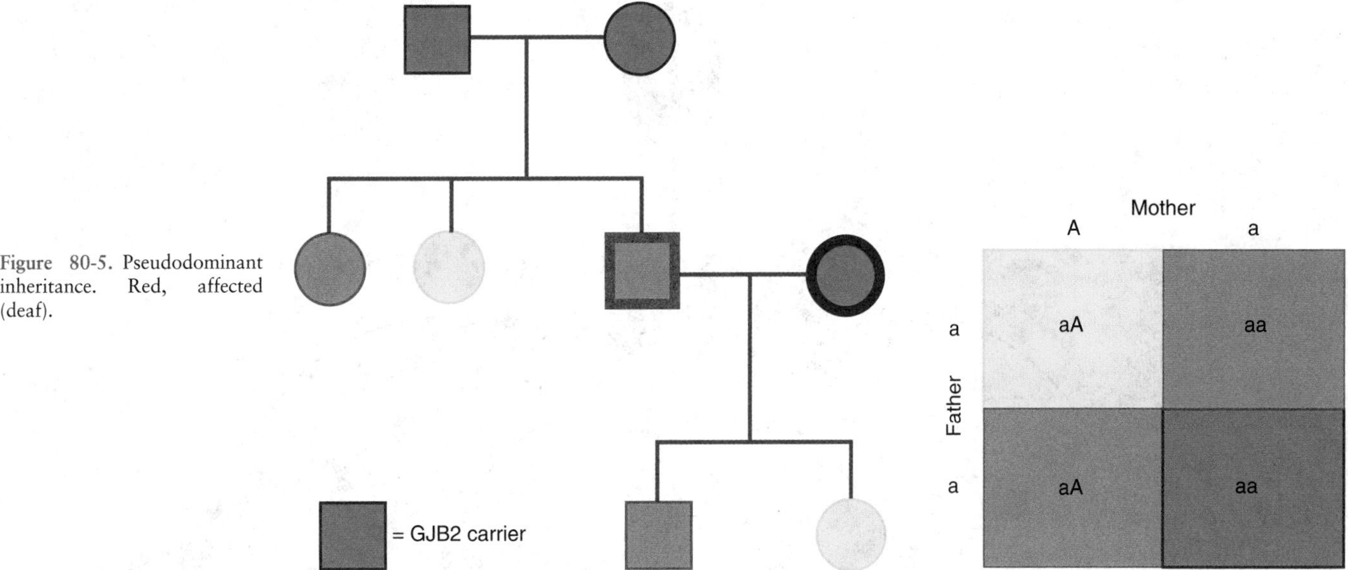

Figure 80-5. Pseudodominant inheritance. Red, affected (deaf).

X chromosome inactivation occurs early in development and involves random and irreversible inactivation of most genes on one X chromosome by each cell (Fig. 80-7). In some cases, a preponderance of cells may inactivate the same X chromosome, resulting in phenotypic expression of an X-linked mutation if it resides on the active chromosome. This may occur owing to chance or to selection against cells that have inactivated a normal X if the other X carries a structural rearrangement.

There are some X-linked disorders, called **X-linked dominant,** in which female carriers typically manifest abnormal findings. An affected man will have only affected daughters and unaffected sons, and half of the offspring of an affected woman will be affected (Fig. 80-8). Some X-linked dominant conditions are lethal in males. An example is incontinentia pigmenti (see Chapter 651). The pedigree shows only affected females, and an overall ratio of 2 : 1 females to males with an increased number of miscarriages (Fig. 80-9).

Y-LINKED INHERITANCE. There are few Y-linked traits. These demonstrate *only* male-to-male transmission, and only males are affected (Fig. 80-10). Most Y-linked genes are related to male sex determination and reproduction, and are associated with infertility. Therefore, it is rare to see familial transmission of a Y-linked disorder. Advances in assisted reproductive technologies may make possible familial transmission of male infertility.

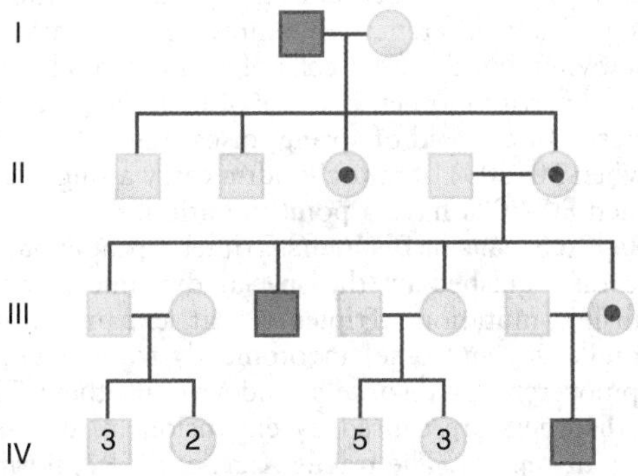

Figure 80-6. Pedigree demonstrating X-linked recessive inheritance. (From Nussbaum RL, McInnes RR, Willard HF: *Thompson & Thompson Genetics in Medicine,* 6th ed. Philadelphia, WB Saunders, 2001.)

Of special note is the pseudoautosomal region on the Y chromosome, the small region of homology that is shared by both Xp and Yp. Very few genes reside in this region. One of the few is *SHOX*. Heterozygous *SHOX* mutations cause **Leri-Weil dyschondrosteosis,** a rare skeletal dysplasia that involves bilateral bowing of the forearms with dislocations of the ulna at the wrist and generalized short stature. Homozygous mutations cause the much more severe **Langer mesomelic dwarfism.**

DIGENIC INHERITANCE. Digenic inheritance explains the occurrence of **retinitis pigmentosa** (RP) in children of parents who each carry a different RP-associated gene. Both parents have normal vision, as would be expected, but the offspring who were **double heterozygotes** developed RP. Digenic pedigrees (Fig. 80-11) exhibit characteristics of both autosomal dominant (vertical transmission) and autosomal recessive inheritance (1 in 4 recurrence risk). A couple in which the two partners are carriers for two different genes may have affected children. Any child, however, might transmit both mutations to an offspring, as in dominant inheritance.

PSEUDOGENETIC INHERITANCE AND FAMILIAL CLUSTERING. There are nongenetic reasons for the occurrence of a disease in multiple family members; these can mimic genetic transmission. Possible explanations include environmental factors, teratogen exposure, and as yet undetermined and undefined factors. Multiple siblings may have asthma due to exposure to cigarette smoke from their parents. A woman may have multiple children with small size, developmental delay, and unusual facial appearance owing to her use of alcohol during pregnancy. Alternatively, the disease may be very common in the general population. Breast cancer will affect 11% of all women; it is possible that several women in a family will develop breast cancer because of yet undetermined factors. It is usually possible to differentiate families with genetically determined high-risk cancer syndromes, such as that associated with a *BRCA1* mutation, by their earlier age of onset of breast cancer in multiple family members.

NONTRADITIONAL INHERITANCE

Some genetic disorders are inherited in a manner that does not follow classical mendelian patterns. This nontraditional inheritance pattern includes mitochondrial disorders, triplet repeat expansion diseases, and imprinting defects.

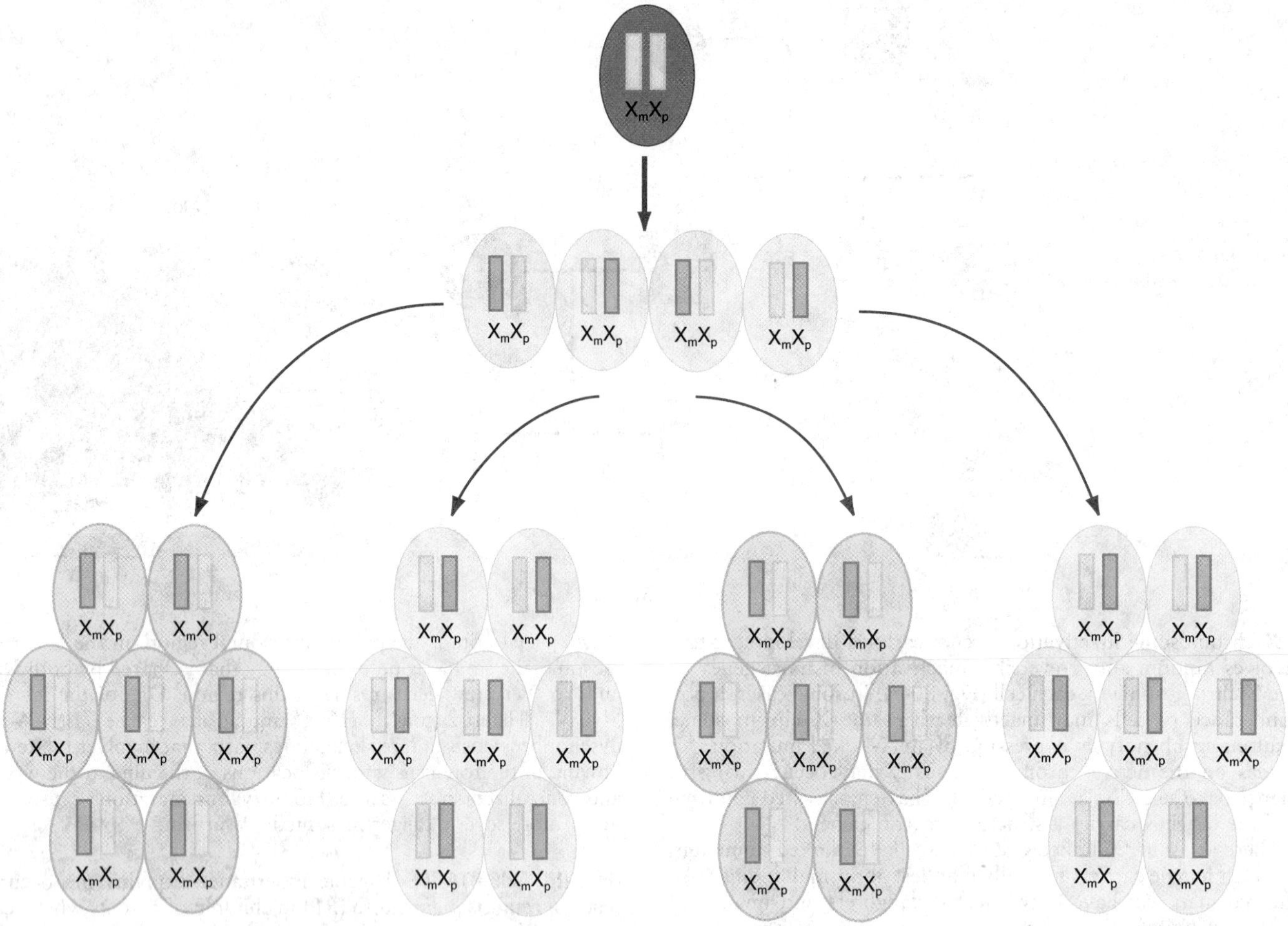

Figure 80-7. X-inactivation.

Mitochondrial Inheritance. An individual's mitochondrial genome is entirely derived from the mother (Fig. 80-12). Sperm contain few mitochondria, most of which are shed upon fertilization. Mitochondrial disorders exhibit maternal inheritance; a woman with a mitochondrial genetic disorder will have only affected offspring of either sex, while an affected father will have no affected offspring (Fig. 80-13). Although such an inheritance pattern can be explained by autosomal dominant or X-linked inheritance, it suggests a mitochondrial basis (Table 80-1).

The mitochondria are the cell's suppliers of energy, so that the organs that are most affected by the presence of abnormal mitochondria are those that have the greatest energy requirements, such as the brain, muscle, heart, and liver (see Chapters 87.4, 358, and 598). Common manifestations include developmental delay, seizures, cardiac dysfunction, decreased strength and tone, as well as hearing and vision problems. Examples include **MELAS** (*m*yopathy, *e*ncephalopathy, *l*actic *a*cidosis, and *s*trokelike episodes), **MERRF** (*m*yoclonic *e*pilepsy associated with *r*agged *r*ed *f*ibers), and **Kearns-Sayre syndrome** (ophthalmoplegia, pigmentary retinopathy, and cardiomyopathy) [see Chapter 598]. Mitochondrial diseases can be highly variable in clinical manifestations. Cells may contain a mixture of mutant and normal mitochondria, referred to as **heteroplasmy.** Unequal segregation of mutant and normal mitochondria (replicative advantage) can result in significant differences in expression of a mitochondrial trait in the ovum and different cells of an individual or different offspring of a carrier mother. Because of this, the mother may be asymptomatic. In affected offspring, disease manifestations tend to occur when 50–60% of mitochondria carry a single large deletion or when 80–90% have a point mutation.

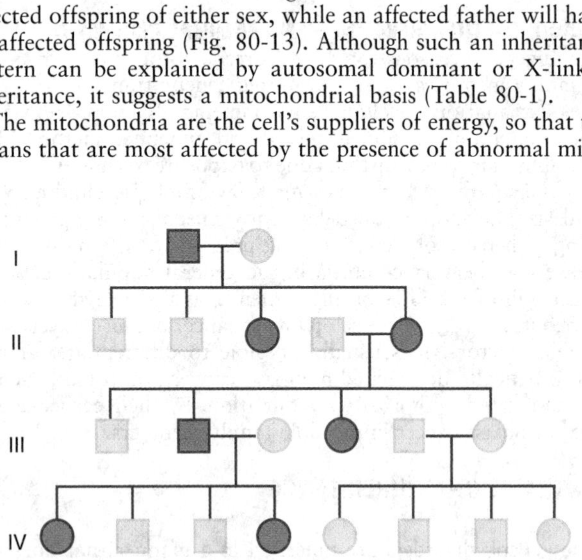

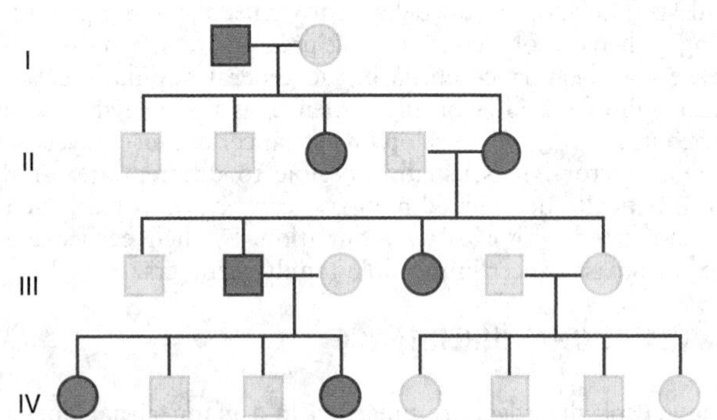

Figure 80-8. Pedigree pattern demonstrating X-linked dominant inheritance. (From Nussbaum RL, McInnes RR, Willard HF: *Thompson & Thompson Genetics in Medicine,* 6th ed. Philadelphia, WB Saunders, 2001.)

Triplet Repeat Expansion Disorders. Triplet repeat expansion disorders are distinguished by the special dynamic nature of the disease-causing mutation. Triplet repeat expansion disorders include fragile X syndrome, myotonic dystrophy, Huntington disease, spinocerebellar disorders, and several others (Table 80-2). These disorders are caused by expansion in the number of three-base-pair repeats. The **fragile X gene,** *FMR1,* normally has between 5 and 50 CGG triplets. An error in replication can result in expansion of that number, referred to as **premutation.** For fragile X, premutation comprises 50–200 repeats. Individuals

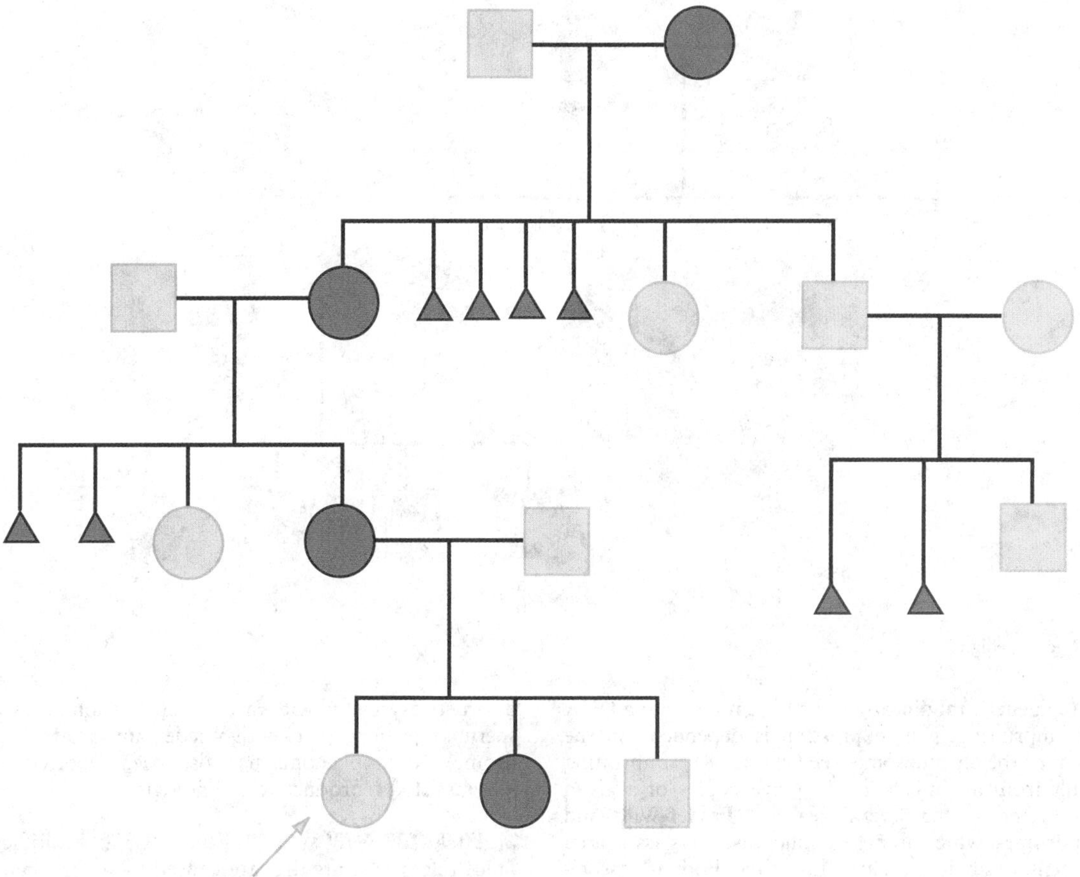

Figure 80-9. Pedigree of an X-linked dominant disorder with male lethality, such as incontinentia pigmenti.

with a premutation are at risk for having the gene expand further in subsequent meiosis, crossing into the range of full mutation. In fragile X, that boundary is above 200 repeats. With this number of repeats, the *FMR1* gene becomes hypermethylated, and protein production is lost. Some male carriers of the premutation develop a syndrome as adults characterized by ataxia, tremor, and cognitive decline.

The effect of the expansion is different in other genes. In **Huntington disease,** the expansion causes the gene product to have a new, toxic effect on the neurons of the basal ganglia. For most triplet repeat disorders, there is a clinical correlation to the size of the expansion, with a greater expansion causing more severe and/or earlier age of onset for the disease. The observation of increasing severity of disease and early age of onset in subsequent generations is termed **genetic anticipation** and is a defining characteristic of triplet repeat expansion disorders (Fig. 80-14).

Genetic Imprinting. The two copies of most genes are functionally equivalent. In a small number, only one of the pair is transcribed. The active gene will be that inherited from a specific parent, and the other copy is silenced associated with methyla-

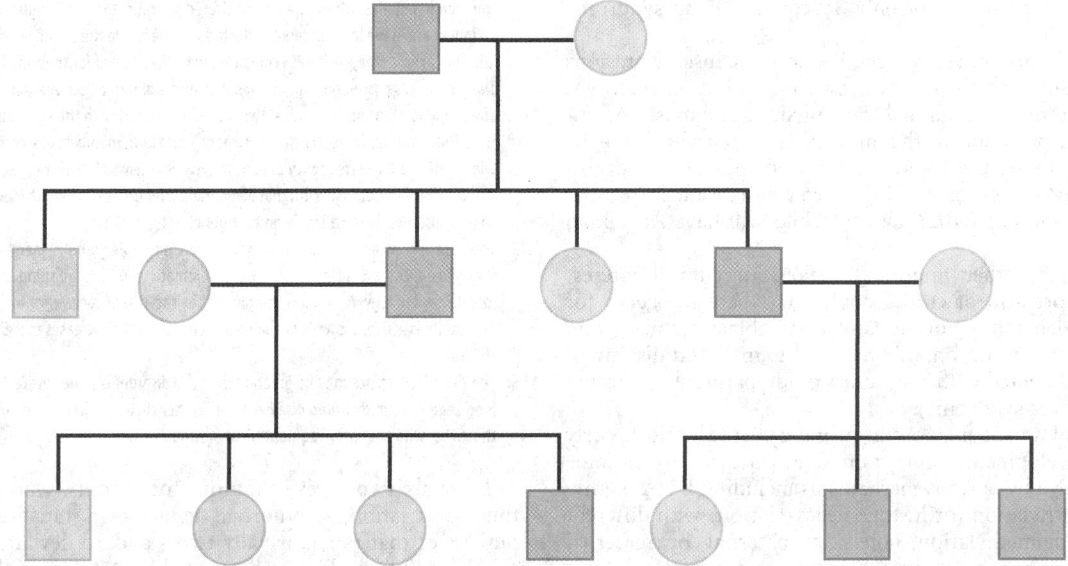

Figure 80-10. Y-linked inheritance. Blue, affected patient.

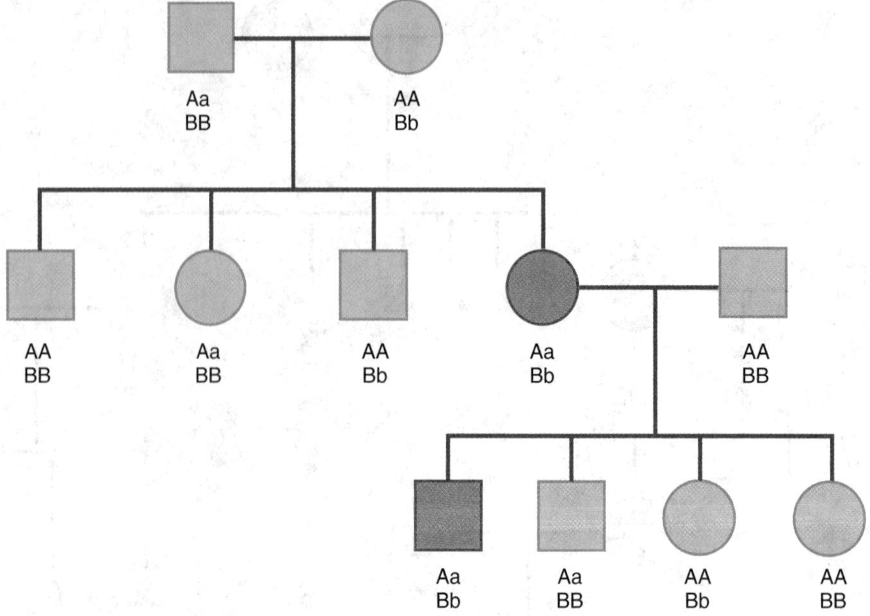

Figure 80-11. Digenic pedigree.

tion of DNA (**epigenetic modification** of a gene not due to a DNA mutation). In imprinting, gene expression is dependent on the parent of origin of the chromosome (see Chapter 81). Imprinting disorders result from an imbalance of active copies of a given gene, which can occur for several reasons. **Prader-Willi** and **Angelman syndromes,** which are two distinct disorders associated with developmental impairment, are illustrative. Both are associated with microdeletions of chromosome 15q11–12. The microdeletion in Prader-Willi syndrome is always on the paternally derived chromosome 15, whereas in Angelman syndrome it is on the maternal copy. *UBE3* is the specific gene for Angelman syndrome, and as expected, the paternal copy of *UBE3* is transcriptionally silenced in the brain.

Uniparental disomy (UPD), the rare occurrence of a child inheriting both copies of a chromosome from the same parent, is another genetic mechanism that can cause Prader-Willi and Angelman syndromes. Inheriting both chromosomes 15 from the mother is functionally the same as deletion of the paternal 15q12 and will result in Prader-Willi syndrome. About 30% of cases of Prader-Willi syndrome is caused by paternal UPD15, whereas maternal UPD15 accounts for only 3% of Angelman syndrome (see Chapter 81).

A mutation in an imprinted gene is another cause. Mutations in *UBE3* account for almost 30% of patients with Angelman syndrome and also result in familial transmission. The most uncommon cause is a mutation in the imprinting center, which results in an inability to set the imprint. In a woman, the inability to reset the father's chromosome 15 imprint will result in passing on no active copies of *UBE3*, and the child will have Angelman syndrome.

Besides 15q12, other imprinted regions of clinical interest include the short arm of chromosome 11 (where the genes for Beckwith-Wiedemann syndrome and nesidioblastosis map) and the long arm of chromosome 7 (maternal uniparental disomy of 7q has been associated with some cases of idiopathic short stature and Russell-Silver syndrome).

Imprinting of a gene may occur during gametogenesis or early embryonic development (reprogramming). Genes may become inactive or active by various mechanisms including DNA methylation or demethylation (or histone deacytylation) with different patterns of (de)methylation noted on paternal or maternal imprintable chromosome regions. Some genes demonstrate tissue specific imprinting. There is an increased incidence of imprinting disorders associated with in vitro fertilization or intracytoplasmic sperm injection (Beckwith-Wiedemann and Angelman syndrome). Retinoblastoma has also been reported in association with assisted reproductive technologies.

MULTIFACTORIAL/POLYGENIC INHERITANCE. Multifactorial inheritance refers to traits that are caused by a combination of inherited, environmental, and stochastic factors (Fig. 80-15). Multifactorial traits differ from polygenic inheritance, which refers to traits that result from the additive effects of multiple genes. Multifactorial traits segregate within families but do not exhibit a consistent or recognizable inheritance pattern. Characteristics include the following:

1. There is a similar rate of recurrence (typically 3–5%) among all 1st-degree relatives (parents, siblings, offspring of the affected child). It is unusual to find a substantial increase in risk for relatives related more distantly than 2nd degree to the index case.
2. The risk of recurrence is related to the incidence of the disease.
3. Some disorders have a sex predilection, as indicated by an unequal male : female incidence. Pyloric stenosis is more common in males, whereas congenital dislocation of the hips is more common in females. Where there is an altered sex ratio, the risk is higher for the relatives of an index case in the less commonly affected sex. The risk to the son of an affected female with infantile pyloric stenosis is 18% compared with the 5% risk for the son of an affected male. The female has passed on a greater genetic susceptibility to her offspring.
4. The likelihood that both identical twins will be affected with the same malformation is less than 100% but much greater than the chance that both members of a nonidentical twin pair will be affected. The frequency of concordance for identical twins ranges from 21% to 63%. This distribution contrasts with that of mendelian inheritance, in which identical twins always share a disorder due to a single mutant gene.
5. The risk of recurrence is increased when multiple family members are affected; these instances are often the most problematic for distinguishing multifactorial from mendelian etiology. A simple example is that the risk of recurrence for unilateral cleft lip and palate is 4% for a couple with one affected child and increases to 9% with two affected children.
6. The risk of recurrence may be greater when the disorder is more severe. The infant who has long-segment Hirschsprung disease has a greater chance of having an affected sibling than the infant who has short-segment Hirschsprung disease.

There are two types of multifactorial traits. One exhibits continuous variation, with normal defined by a statistical range, and outliers of that range, usually two standard deviations, are considered "abnormal" (intelligence, blood pressure, height, head circumference). Offspring represent a modified average of their

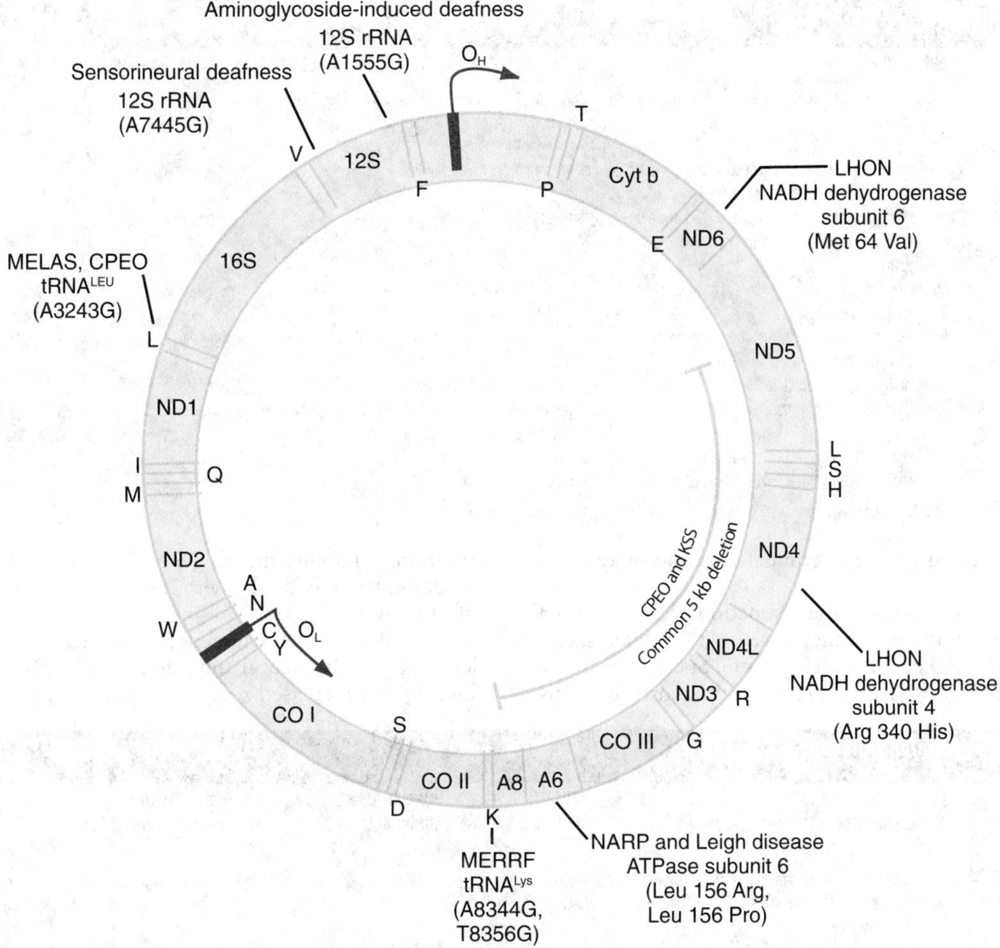

Figure 80-12. The human mitochondrial DNA molecule, showing the location of genes encoding 22 tRNAs, two rRNAs, and 13 proteins of the oxidative phosphorylation (OXPHOA) complex. Some of the most common disease-causing substitutions and deletions in the mtDNA genome are also illustrated. OH and OL are the origins of replication of the two DNA strands, respectively; 12S, 12S ribosomal RNA; 16S, 16S ribosomal RNA. The tRNAs are indicated by the single letter code for their corresponding amino acids (e.g., L for leucine, K for lysine). The 13 OXPHOS polypeptides encoded by mtDNA include components of complex I: NADH dehydrogenase (ND1, ND2, ND3, ND4, ND4L, ND5, and ND6); complex III: cytochrome *b* (Cyt *b*); complex IV: cytochrome *c* oxidase I, or Cyt *c* (COI, COII, COIII); and complex V: ATPase 6 (ATP-6, ATP-8). See Table 80-1 for representative diseases. (Adapted from Shoffner JM, Wallace DC: Oxidative phosphorylation disease. In Scriver CR, Beaudet AL, Sly WS, et al [editors]: *The Metabolic and Molecular Basis of Inherited Disease,* 7th ed. New York, McGraw-Hill, 1995; and Johns DR: Mitochondrial DNA and disease. *N Engl J Med* 1995;333:638–644. From Nussbaum RL, McInnes RR, Willard HF: *Thompson & Thompson Genetics in Medicine,* 6th ed. Philadelphia, WB Saunders, 2001.)

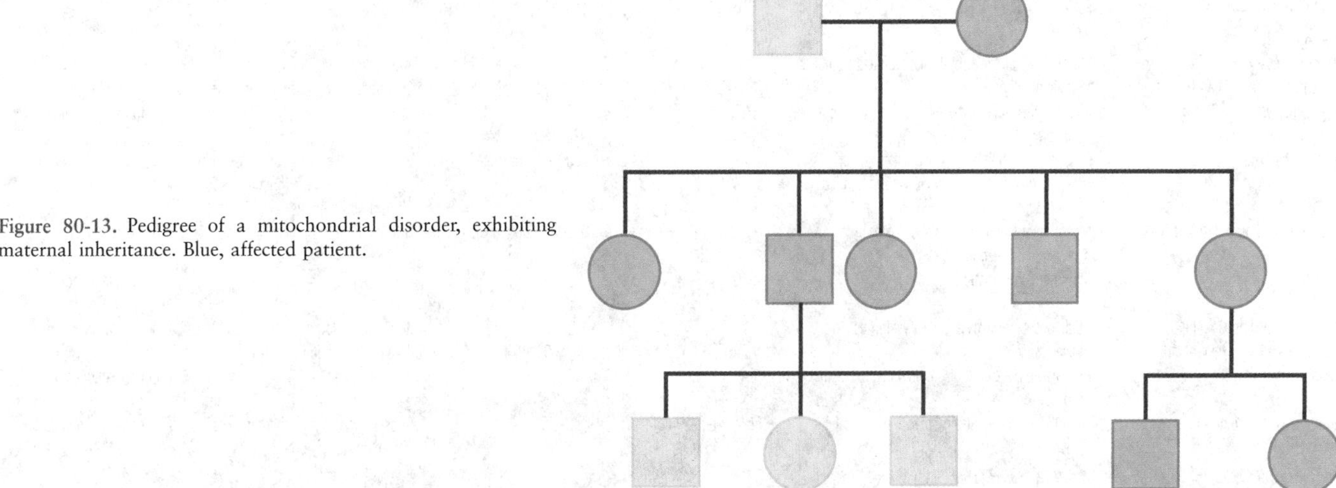

Figure 80-13. Pedigree of a mitochondrial disorder, exhibiting maternal inheritance. Blue, affected patient.

TABLE 80-1. Representative Examples of Disorders Due to Mutations in Mitochondrial DNA and Their Inheritance

DISEASE	PHENOTYPE	MOST FREQUENT MUTATION IN MTDNA MOLECULE	HOMOPLASMY VS HETEROPLASMY	INHERITANCE
Leber's hereditary optic neuropathy	Rapid optic nerve death, leading to blindness in young adult life	Substitution Arg340His in *ND1* gene of complex I of electron transport chain; other complex I missense mutations	Homoplasmic (usually)	Maternal
NARP, Leigh disease	*N*europathy, *a*taxia, *r*etinitis *p*igmentosa, developmental delay, mental retardation, lactic acidemia	Point mutations in ATPase subunit 6 gene	Heteroplasmic	Maternal
MELAS	*M*itochondrial *e*ncephalomyopathy, *l*actic *a*cidosis, and *s*trokelike episodes; may manifest only as diabetes mellitus	Point mutation in $tRNA^{Leu}$	Heteroplasmic	Maternal
MERRF	*M*yoclonic *e*pilepsy, *r*agged *r*ed *f*ibers in muscle, ataxia, sensorineural deafness	Point mutation in $tRNA^{Lys}$	Heteroplasmic	Maternal
Deafness	Progressive sensorineural deafness, often induced by aminoglycoside antibiotics	A1555G mutation in 12S rRNA	Homoplasmic	Maternal
	Nonsyndromic sensorineural deafness	A7445G mutation in 12S rRNA	Homoplasmic	Maternal
Chronic progressive external ophthalmoplegia (CPEO)	Progressive weakness of extraocular muscles	The common MELAS point mutation in $tRNA^{Lys}$; large deletions similar to KSS	Heteroplasmic	Maternal if point mutations
Pearson syndrome	Pancreatic insufficiency, pancytopenia, lactic acidosis	Large deletions	Heteroplasmic	Sporadic, somatic mutations
Kearns-Sayre syndrome (KSS)	PEO of early onset with heart block, retinal pigmentation	The 5 kb large deletion	Heteroplasmic	Sporadic, somatic mutations

From Nussbaum RL, McInnes RR, Willard HF (editors): *Thompson and Thompson Genetics in Medicine*, 6th ed. Philadelphia, WB Saunders, 2001, p. 246

parents, with nutritional and environmental factors playing an important role.

With other multifactorial traits, the distinction between normal and abnormal is clearer (pyloric stenosis, neural tube defects, congenital heart defects, and cleft lip, cleft palate). Such traits follow a threshold model (Fig. 80-16). There is postulated to be a distribution of liability due to genetic and nongenetic factors in the population. Individuals who exceed a threshold liability are affected by the trait.

The balance between genetic and environmental factors is demonstrated by **neural tube defects.** Genetic factors are implicated by the increased recurrence risk for parents of an affected

TABLE 80-2. Diseases Associated with Repeat Expansions

DISEASE	DESCRIPTION	REPEAT SEQUENCE	NORMAL RANGE, ABNORMAL RANGE	PARENT IN WHOM EXPANSION USUALLY OCCURS	LOCATION OF EXPANSION
Category 1					
Huntington disease	Loss of motor control, dementia, affective disorder	CAG	6–34; 36–100 or more	More often through father	Exon
Spinal and bulbar muscular atrophy	Adult-onset motor-neuron disease associated with androgen insensitivity	CAG	11–34; 40–62	More often through father	Exon
Spinocerebellar ataxia type 1	Progressive ataxia, dysarthria, dysmetria	CAG	6–39; 41–81	More often through father	Exon
Spinocerebellar ataxia type 2	Progressive ataxia, dysarthria	CAG	15–29; 35–59	—	Exon
Spinocerebellar ataxia type 3 (Machado-Joseph disease)	Dystonia, distal muscular atrophy, ataxia, external ophthalmoplegia	CAG	13–36; 68–79	More often through father	Exon
Spinocerebellar ataxia type 6	Progressive ataxia, dysarthria, nystagmus	CAG	4–16; 21–27	—	Exon
Spinocerebellar ataxia type 7	Progressive ataxia, dysarthria, retinal degeneration	CAG	7–35; 38–200	More often through father	—
Spinocerebellar ataxia type 17	Progressive ataxia, dementia, bradykinesia, dysmetria	CAG	29–42; 47–55	—	Exon
Dentatorubral-pallidoluysian atrophy/Haw River syndrome	Cerebellar atrophy, ataxia, myoclonic epilepsy, choreoathetosis, dementia	CAG	7–25; 49–88	More often through father	Exon
Category 2					
Pseudoachondroplasia/multiple epiphyseal dysplasia	Short stature, joint laxity, degenerative joint disease	GAC	5; 6–7	—	Exon
Oculopharyngeal muscular dystrophy	Proximal limb weakness, dysphagia, ptosis	GCG	6; 7–13	—	Exon
Cleidocranial dysplasia	Short stature, open skull sutures with bulging calvaria, clavicular hypoplasia, shortened fingers, dental anomalies	GCG, GCT, GCA	17; 27 (expansion observed in one family)	—	Exon
Synpolydactyly	Polydactyly and syndactyly	GCG, GCT, GCA	15; 22–25	—	Exon
Category 3					
Myotonic dystrophy (DMI; chromosome 19)	Muscle loss, cardiac arrhythmia, cataracts, frontal balding	CTG	5–37; 100 to several thousand	Either parent, but expansion to congenital form through mother	3′ untranslated region
Myotonic dystrophy (DM2; chromosome 3)	Muscle loss, cardiac arrhythmia, cataracts, frontal balding	CCTG	<75; 75–11,000	—	3′ untranslated region
Friedreich ataxia	Progressive limb ataxia, dysarthria, hypertrophic cardiomyopathy, pyramidal weakness in legs	GAA	7–2; 200–900 or more	Autosomal recessive inheritance, so disease alleles are inherited from both parents	Intron
Fragile X syndrome (FRAXA)	Mental retardation, large ears and jaws, macroorchidism in males	CGG	6–52; 200–2,000 or more	Exclusively through mother	5′ untranslated region
Fragile site (FRAXE)	Mild mental retardation	GCC	6–35; >200	More often through mother	5′ untranslated region
Spinocerebellar ataxia type 8	Adult-onset ataxia, dysarthria, nystagmus	CTG	16–37; 107–127	More often through mother	3′ untranslated region
Spinocerebellar ataxia type 10	Ataxia and seizures	ATTCT	12–16; 800–4,500	More often through father	Intron
Spinocerebellar ataxia type 12	Ataxia, eye movement disorders; variable age at onset	CAG	7–28; 66–78	—	5′ untranslated region
Progressive myoclonic epilepsy type 1	Juvenile-onset convulsions, myoclonus, dementia	12-bp repeat motif	2–3; 30–75	Autosomal recessive inheritance, so transmitted by both parents	5′ untranslated region

From Jorde LB, Carey JC, Bamshad MJ, White RL: *Medical Genetics*, 3rd ed. St. Louis, Mosby, 2006, p. 82

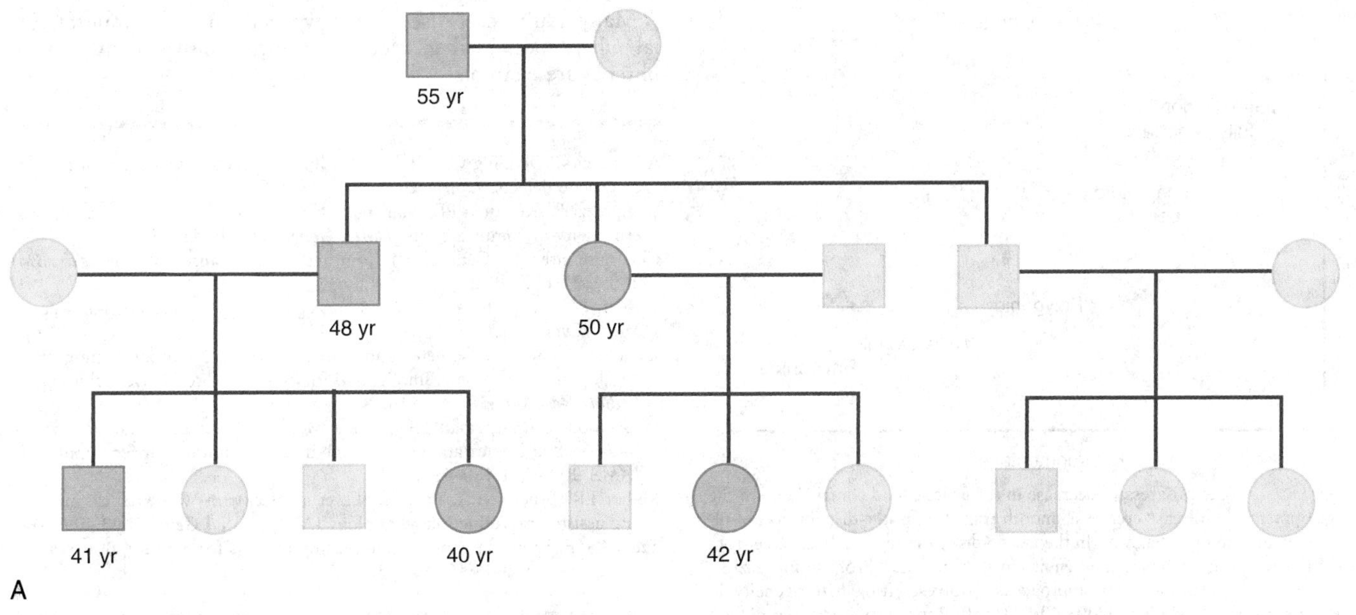

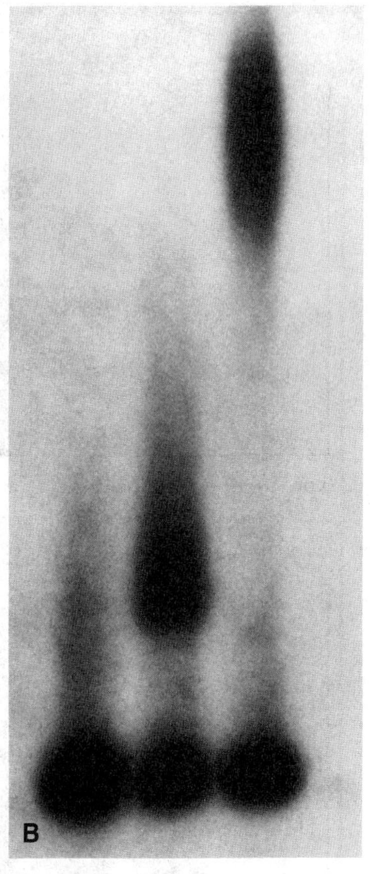

Figure 80-14. *A*, Myotonic dystrophy pedigree illustrating anticipation. In this case, the age of onset for family members affected with an autosomal dominant disease is lower in more recent generations. Blue, affected patients. *B*, An autoradiogram from a Southern blot analysis of the myotonic dystrophy gene in three individuals. Individual A is homozygous for a 4- to 5-repeat allele of 175 repeats; this individual has myotonic dystrophy. Individual C is also affected with myotonic dystrophy and has one normal allele and a disease-causing allele of approximately 900 repeats. (*B*, Courtesy of Drs. Kenneth and Elaine Lyon, University of Utah Health Sciences Center. From Jorde LB, Carey JC, Bamshad MJ, et al: *Medical Genetics*, 3rd ed. St. Louis, Mosby, 2006, p 81.)

child compared to the general population. This risk is 3%, less than what would be expected if the trait was caused by a single gene. Further emphasizing the role of nongenetic environmental factors is that the recurrence risk can be lowered by up to 70% if the mother-to-be takes folic acid at 4 mg/day starting 3 mo prior to conception. Another example is that a sequence variation in the interferon regulatory factor 6 gene is associated with an increased risk for cleft lip and palate.

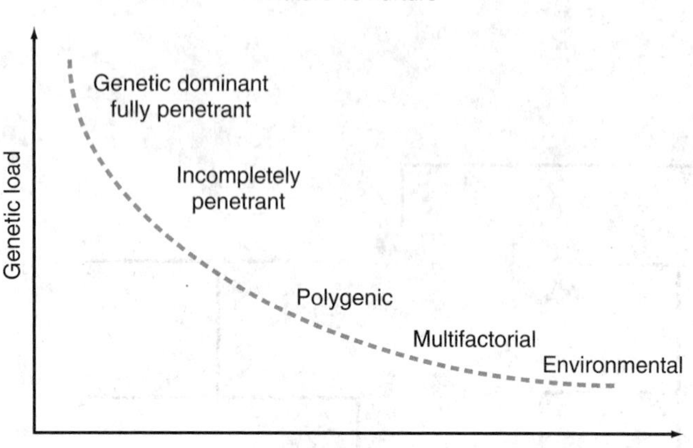

Figure 80-15. The progressive decrease in the genetic load contributing to the development of a disease creates a smooth transition in the distribution of illnesses on an etiologic diagram. In theory, no diseases are completely free from the influence of both genetic and environmental factors. (From Bomprezzi R, Kovanen PE, Martin R: New approaches to investigating heterogeneity in complex traits. *J Med Genet* 2003;40:553–559. Reproduced with permission from the BMJ Publishing Group.)

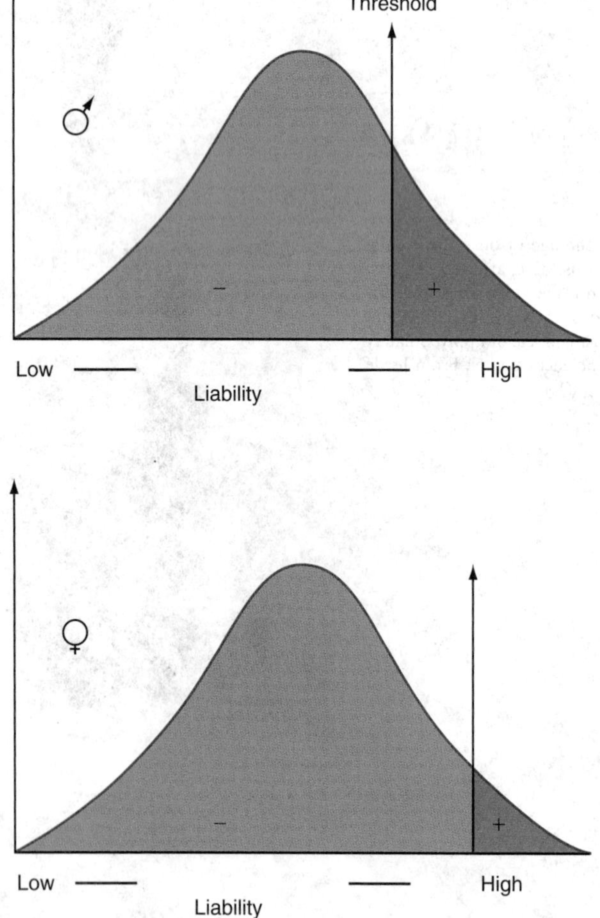

Figure 80-16. Typical linear erythema and blistering in a female infant with incontinentia pigmenti. As the child grows older, the skin lesions will become flattened, pigmented streaks. (Photograph courtesy of Virginia Sybert, University of Washington, Seattle. From Nussbaum RL, McInnes RR, Willard HF: *Thompson & Thompson Genetics in Medicine,* 6th ed. Philadelphia, WB Saunders, 2001.)

Many adult-onset diseases behave as if caused by multifactorial inheritance. Diabetes, coronary artery disease, and schizophrenia are examples.

Allegrucci C, Denning C, Priddle H, et al: Stem-cell consequences of embryo epigenetic defects. *Lancet* 2004;364:206–208.

Bomprezzi R, Kovanen PE, Martin R: New approaches to investigating heterogeneity in complex traits. *J Med Genet* 2003;40:553–559.

Clayton-Smith J: Genomic imprinting as a cause of disease. *BMJ* 2003;327:1121–1122.

Gosden RG, Feinberg AP: Genetics and epigenetics—nature's pen-and-pencil set. *N Engl J Med* 2007;356:731–733.

Jacob S, Moley KH: Gametes and embryo epigenetic reprogramming affect developmental outcome: Implication for assisted reproductive technologies. *Pediatr Res* 2005;58:437–446.

Jacquemont S, Hagerman RJ, Leehey MA, et al: Penetrance of the fragile X-associated tremor/ataxia syndrome in a permutation carrier population. *JAMA* 2004:291:460–468.

Maher ER, Brueton LA, Bowdin SC, et al: Beckwith-Wiedemann syndrome and assisted reproduction technology (ART). *J Med Genet* 2003;40:62–64.

Teebi AS, El-Shanti H: Consanguinity: Implications for practice, research and policy. *Lancet* 2006;367:970–971.

Chapter 81 ■ Cytogenetics

Maria Descartes and Andrew J. Carroll

Clinical cytogenetics is the study of chromosomes: their structure, inheritance, and abnormalities. Chromosome abnormalities occur in approximately 1% of live births and are responsible for a large proportion of early fetal losses, multiple congenital malformations, and cases of mental retardation. They have a significant role in the development of neoplasias.

Chromosome analysis is indicated in the child with multiple congenital anomalies and/or dysmorphic features. It is indicated for the pregnant woman with advanced maternal age (>35 yr). It is also warranted in patients with (1) two major malformations and/or three minor malformations; (2) problems in early growth and development, including ambiguous genitalia or mental retardation; (3) fertility problems or recurrent miscarriage (≥3), stillbirth, and neonatal death; (4) a first-degree relative with a known or suspected structural chromosome abnormality.

METHODS OF CHROMOSOME ANALYSIS. Cytogenetic studies are usually performed on peripheral blood lymphocytes; cultured fibroblasts may also be used. Prenatal chromosome studies are performed with cells obtained from the amniotic fluid, chorionic villus tissue, and fetal blood, or in preimplantation diagnosis, by analysis of a blastomere. Cytogenetic studies of bone marrow have an important role in tumor surveillance, particularly among patients with leukemia.

Chromosome anomalies include abnormalities of number and structure and are the result of errors in cell division. There are two types of cell division: mitosis, which occurs in most somatic cells, and meiosis, which is limited to the production of germ cells.

In **mitosis,** two genetically identical daughter cells are produced from a single parent cell. DNA duplication has already occurred during interphase, so at the beginning of mitosis the chromosomes consist of two DNA strands joined together at the centromere. Mitosis has four stages: prophase, metaphase, anaphase, and telophase. Prophase is characterized by condensation of the DNA. Also during prophase, the nuclear membrane and the nucleolus disappear and the mitotic spindle forms. In metaphase, the chromosomes are maximally compacted and are clearly

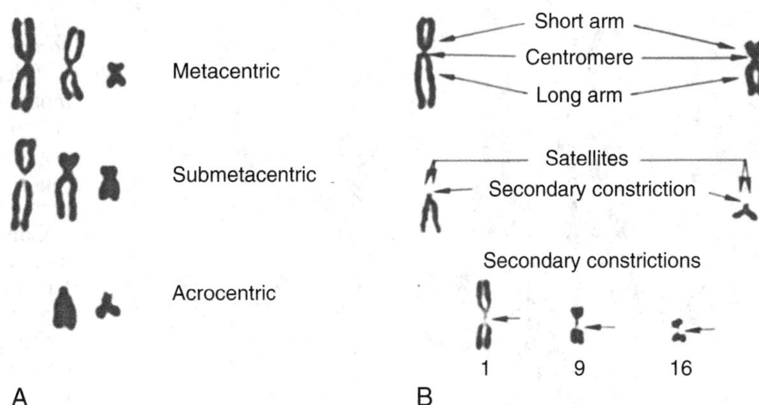

Figure 81-1. *A,* Centromere position determining the three types of chromosome seen in the normal human karyotype—metacentric, submetacentric, and acrocentric. *B,* Morphologic landmarks useful in chromosome identification.

visible as distinct structures. The chromosomes align at the center of the cell and spindle fibers connect to the centromere of each chromosome and extend to centrioles at the two poles of the mitotic figure (Fig. 81-1). In anaphase, the chromosomes divide along their longitudinal axes to form two daughter chromatids, which then migrate to opposite poles of the cell. Telophase is characterized by formation of two new nuclear membranes and nucleoli, duplication of the centrioles, and cytoplasmic cleavage to form the two daughter cells.

Meiosis begins in the female oocyte during fetal life and is completed years to decades later. In males, it begins in a particular spermatogonial cell sometime between adolescence and adult life and is completed in a few days. Meiosis is preceded by DNA replication so that at the outset each of the 46 chromosomes consists of two chromatids. In meiosis, a **diploid cell** (2n = 46 chromosomes) divides to form **haploid cells** (n = 23 chromosomes). Meiosis consists of two major rounds of cell division. In meiosis I, each of the homologous chromosomes pair precisely so that **genetic recombination,** involving exchange between two DNA strands **(crossing over),** may occur. This results in a reshuffling of alleles on the recombined chromosomes. Each daughter cell then receives one of each of the 23 homologous chromosomes. In oogenesis, one of the daughter cells receives most of the cytoplasm and becomes the egg, whereas the other smaller cell becomes the first polar body. Meiosis II is similar to a mitotic division but without a preceding round of DNA duplication (replication). Each of the 23 chromosomes divides longitudinally, and the homologous chromatids migrate to opposite poles of the cell. This produces four spermatogonia, or an egg cell and a second polar body, each with a haploid (n = 23 chromosomes) set. Consequently, meiosis fulfills two crucial roles: It reduces the chromosome number from diploid (46) to haploid (23) so that upon fertilization a diploid number is restored, and it allows for genetic recombination.

Two errors of cell division commonly occur during meiosis or mitosis, and both can result in an abnormal number of chromosomes. The first is **nondisjunction,** in which two chromosomes fail to separate and thus migrate together into one of the new cells, producing one cell with two copies of the chromosome and another with no copy. The second is **anaphase lag,** in which a chromatid or chromosome is lost because it fails to move quickly enough during anaphase to become incorporated into one of the new daughter cells (Fig. 81-2).

For chromosome analysis, cells are cultured (for varying periods depending on cell type), arrested in mitosis during metaphase (or prophase), exposed to a hypotonic solution, fixed, and then stained. The most frequently used staining method is trypsin-Giemsa which produces G- or GTG-banding, a unique combination of dark (G-positive) and light (G-negative) bands. Many other banding techniques and special stains including quinacrine (Q-banding), reverse (R-banding), and centromere (C-banding) are available for use in certain circumstances. Metaphase chromosome spreads are first evaluated microscopically, then their images are captured by a video camera and stored on a computer. Homologous chromosomes from a metaphase spread can be paired and arranged systematically into a karyotype. The chromosomes are arranged by size in pairs, the largest autosome being designated chromosome 1 and the smallest chromosome 22. The sex chromosomes (X and Y) make up the 23rd pair. A description of the karyotype includes two or three parts: (1) the number of chromosomes, (2) the sex chromosome constitution, and (3) any abnormalities noted. A normal karyotype is 46,XX for females and 46,XY for males (Fig. 81-3). If present, abnormalities are noted after the sex chromosome complement.

While the internationally accepted system for human chromosome classification relies largely on the length and banding

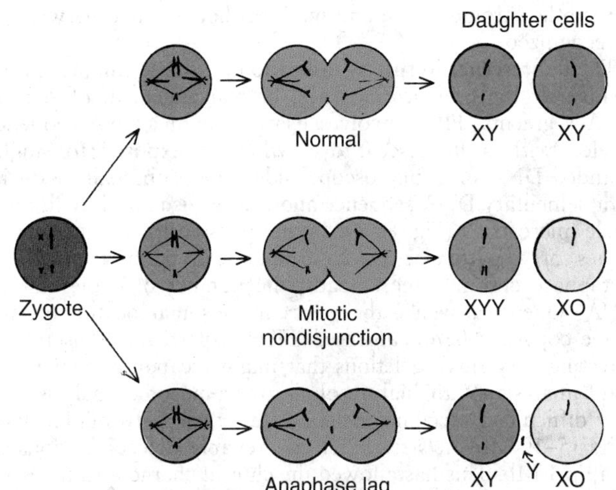

Figure 81-2. Formation of mosaicism. The X and Y chromosomes are used to illustrate two common errors leading to chromosomally abnormal cell populations. In normal mitosis *(top),* duplicated chromosomes separate and become incorporated into daughter cells. If one replicated chromosome fails to separate, mitotic nondisjunction occurs *(middle).* Occasionally, normal separation occurs, but one member fails to migrate. This is known as anaphase lag *(bottom).* (Used, with permission, from Wisniewski LP, Hirschhorn K: *A Guide to Human Chromosome Defects,* 2nd ed. White Plains, NY, March of Dimes Birth Defects Foundation, Birth Defects: Original Article Series, vol 16, sec 6, 1980.)

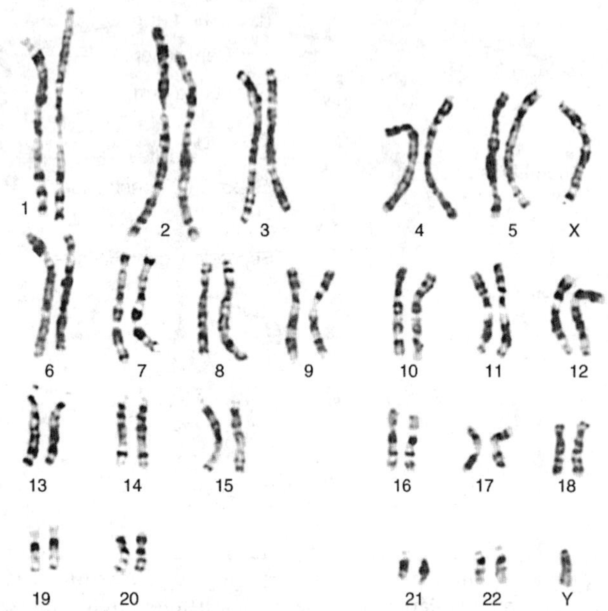

Figure 81-3. Karyotype of normal male with chromosomes in late prophase. The chromosomes are longer, and a greater number of bands are seen than when chromosomes are photographed at metaphase.

pattern of each chromosome, the position of the centromere relative to the ends of the chromosome also is a useful distinguishing feature (see Fig. 81-1). The centromere divides the chromosome in two, with the short arm designated as the p arm and the long arm designated as the q arm. A plus or minus sign before the number of a chromosome indicates that there is an extra or missing chromosome, respectively. Table 81-1 shows some of the abbreviations used for the description of chromosomes and their abnormalities. A metaphase chromosome spread will usually show 350–500 bands. Prophase and prometaphase chromosomes are longer, are less condensed, and often show 500–850 bands. High-resolution analysis is useful for detecting subtle chromosome abnormalities that might otherwise go unrecognized.

The **fluorescence in situ hybridization** (FISH) technique is used to identify the presence, absence, or rearrangement of specific DNA segments. FISH involves using a unique DNA sequence labeled with a fluorescent dye, which is exposed to single-stranded DNA on a microscope slide. The probe pairs with its complementary DNA sequence and can be visualized by fluorescence microscopy (Fig. 81-4). In interphase cells, the number of copies of a particular DNA segment can be determined. In metaphase chromosome spreads, the number of copies of the DNA sequence as well as the exact chromosomal location of each probe copy can be documented. FISH is particularly useful for detecting very small deletions that might escape notice with G-band analysis. With high-resolution chromosome analysis it is very difficult to recognize deletions less than 5–10 million base pairs (5–10 Mb) in size; FISH can reliably detect deletions as small a 1 Mb. This has allowed the clinical characterization of a number of microdeletion syndromes. In addition to gene- or locus-specific probes, complex mixtures of DNA from one part of a chromosome arm, an entire chromosome arm, or an entire chromosome are available for fluorescence staining of large chromosome sections or entire chromosomes. The probe mixtures are referred to as chromosome paints (Fig. 81-5).

Spectral karyotyping (SKY) and **multicolor FISH** (M-FISH) are similar molecular cytogenetic techniques that use 24 different chromosome painting probes and 5 fluorochromes to simultaneously visualize every chromosome in a metaphase spread. Each of the 24 different chromosome paints is labeled with a different combination of the 5 fluorescent dyes (which emit at different wavelengths). Each of the 22 autosomes and the X and Y chromosomes have their own unique spectra of wavelengths of fluorescence. Special filters, cameras, and image processing software are required to identify each chromosome. SKY and M-FISH are especially useful for identifying the complex chromosome rearrangements found in many tumors.

Comparative genomic hybridization (CGH) is a FISH-based method that can be used as a genome-wide screen to measure differences in copy number of a particular DNA sequence or chromosomal segment between two different DNA samples. The technique involves differentially labeling patient DNA with a fluorescent dye (green) and normal reference DNA with another fluorescent dye (red). Equal amounts of the two-label DNA samples are mixed and then used as a painting probe for FISH with normal metaphase chromosomes. The ratio of green-to-red fluorescence is measured along each chromosome. Regions of amplification of patient DNA would display an excess of green fluorescence, while regions of loss of patient DNA would show excess red fluorescence. If patient and control DNA are equally represented, the green-to-red ratio would be 1 : 1 and the chromosomes would appear yellow.

High-resolution CGH-based microarrays (array CGH) have the probe preparation that is the same as traditional CGH, but rather than hybridizing the probe to metaphase chromosome spreads, large-insert clones (such as bacterial artificial chromosomes; BACs) spotted on microarrays serve as the target. The resolution of array CGH is limited only by the size of the insert and the distance between clones, whereas chromosome CGH has a resolution of only 5–10 Mb. Targeted array-based CGH is an

TABLE 81-1. Some Abbreviations Used for Description of Chromosomes and Their Abnormalities

ABBREVIATION	MEANING	EXAMPLE	CONDITION
XX	Female	46,XX	Normal female karyotype
XY	Male	46,XY	Normal male karyotype
[##]	Number (#) of cells		Number of cells in each clone
cen	Centromere		
del	Deletion	46,XY,del(5p)	Male with deletion of part of chromosome 5 short arm
der	Derivative		A structurally rearranged chromosome
dup	Duplication		
ins	Insertion		
inv	Inversion	46,XY,inv(2)(p21q31)	Male with pericentric inversion of chromosome 2 with breakpoints at bands p21 and q31
ish	Metaphase FISH		Refers to *in situ* hybridization
nuc ish	Interphase FISH		Refers to *in situ* hybridization
mar	Marker	47,XY,+mar	Male with extra, unidentified chromosome material
mos	Mosaic	mos 45,X[14]/46,XX[16]	Turner syndrome mosaicism (analysis of 30 cells showed that 14 cells were 45,X and 16 cells were 46,XX)
p	Short arm		
q	Long arm		
r	Ring chromosome	46,X,r(X)(p21q27)	Female with one normal X chromosome and a ring X chromosome
t	Translocation	t(2;8)(q33;q24.1)	The interchange of material between chromosomes 2 and 8 with breakpoints at bands 2q33 and 8q24.1
ter	Termininal		
/	Slash	45,X,-Y/46,XY	Separate lines or clones
+	Gain of	47,XX,+21	Female with trisomy 21
–	Loss of	45,XY,–21	Male with monosomy 21

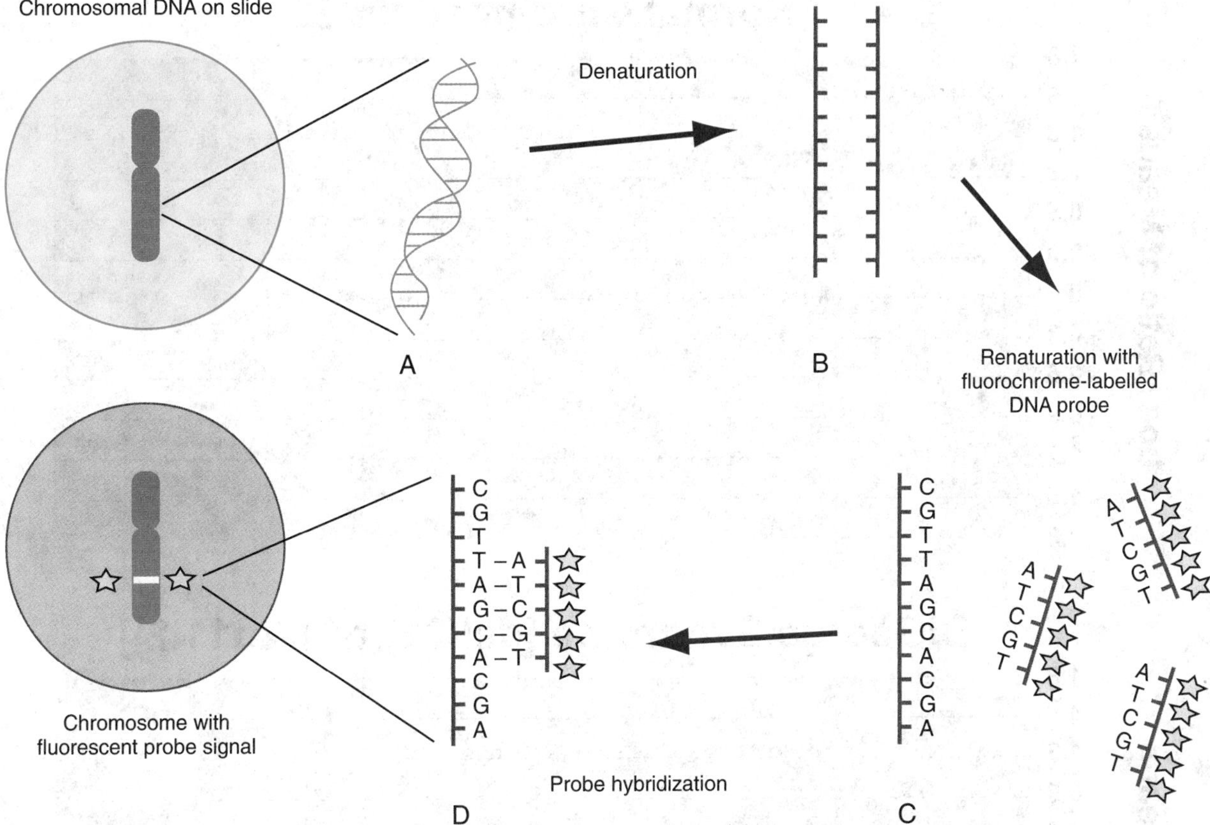

Figure 81-4. Fluorescence in situ hybridization (FISH) involves denaturation of double-stranded DNA as present in metaphase chromosomes or interphase nuclei on cytogenetic slide preparations *(A)* into single-stranded DNA *(B)*. The slide-bound (in situ) DNA is then renatured or reannealed in the presence of excess copies of a single-stranded, fluorochrome-labeled DNA base-pair sequence or probe *(C)*. The probe anneals or "hybridizes" to sites of complementary DNA sequence *(D)* within the chromosomal genome. Probe signal is visualized and imaged on the chromosome by fluorescent microscopy. (From Lin RL, Cherry AM, Bangs CD, et al: FISHing for answers: The use of molecular cytogenetic techniques in adolescent medicine practice. In Hyme HE, Greydanus D [editors]: *Genetic Disorders in Adolescents.* State of the Art Reviews. Adolescent Medicine. Philadelphia, Hanley and Belfus, 2002, pp 305–313.)

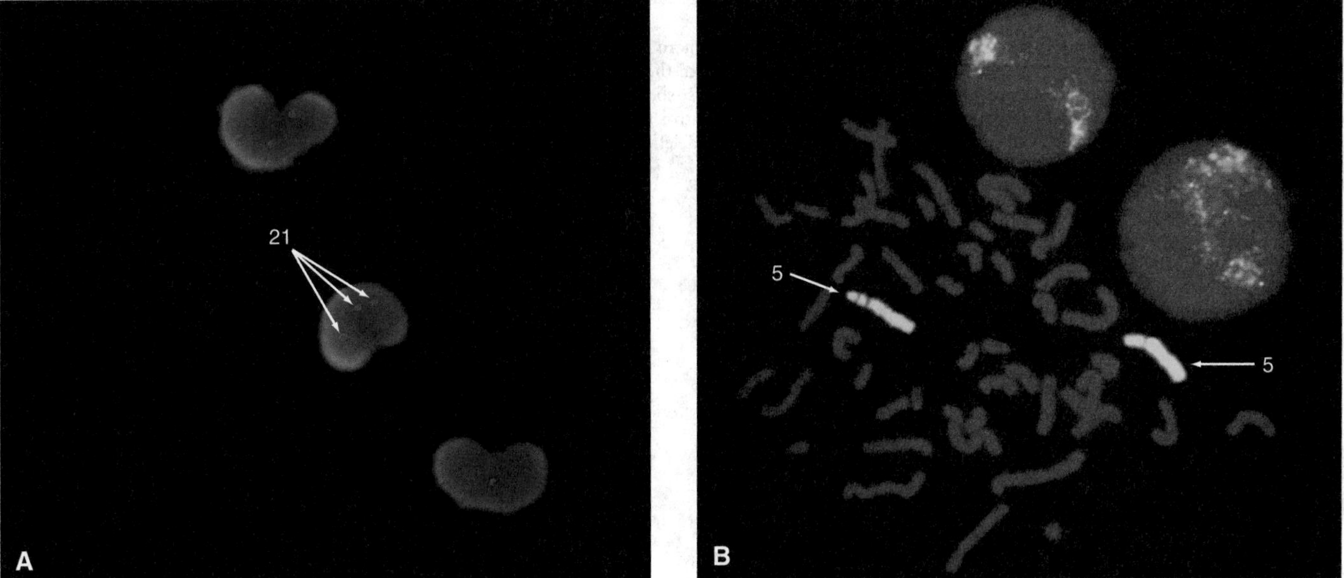

Figure 81-5. *A,* Fluorescence in situ hybridization (FISH) analysis of interphase peripheral blood cells from a patient with Down syndrome using a chromosome 21–specific probe. The 3 red signals mark the presence of 3 chromosomes 21. *B,* FISH analysis of a metaphase chromosome spread from a clinically normal individual using a whole-chromosome paint specific for chromosome 5. Both chromosomes 5 are completely labeled (yellow) along their entire length.

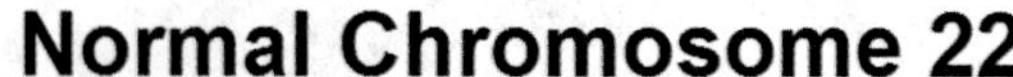

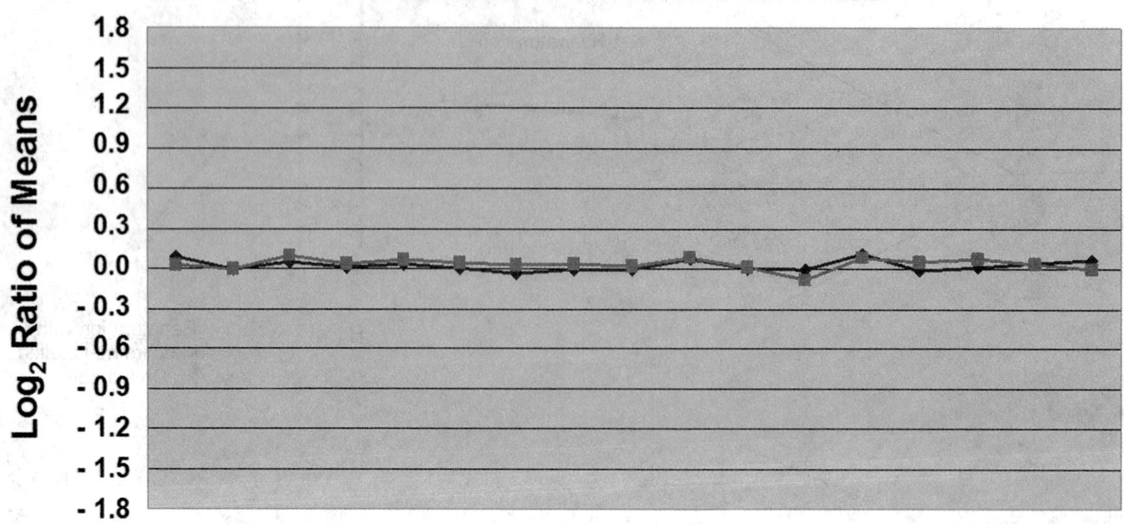

DiGeorge Syndrome [del(22)(q11.2q11.2)]

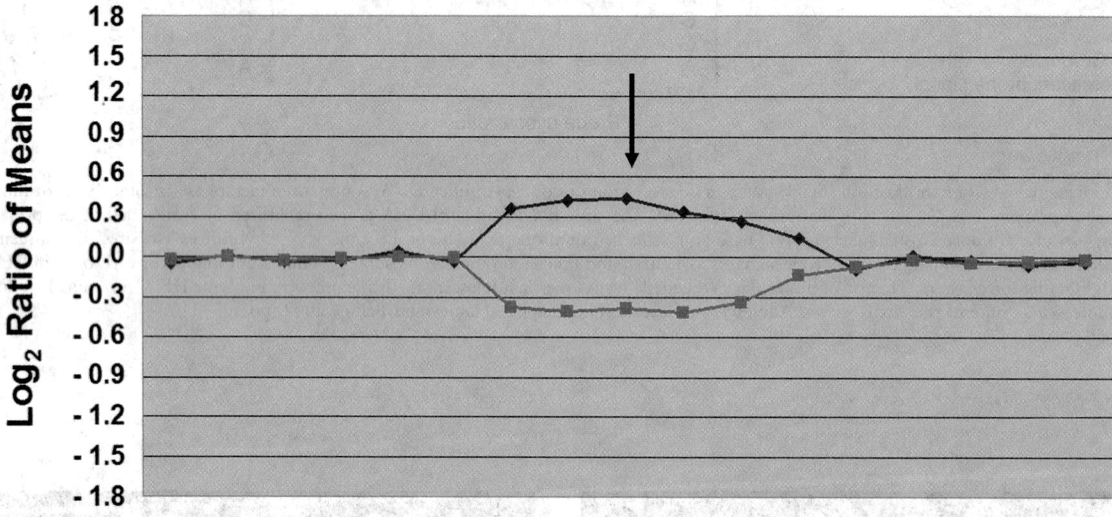

Figure 81-6. Representative array CGH plots from a normal control and from an individual with the 22q11.2 deletion seen in DiGeorge syndrome. Each clone is arranged along the *x*-axis according to its location on the chromosome with the most distal/telomeric p-arm clones on the left and the most distal/telomeric q-arm clones on the right. The blue line plots represent the ratios from the first slide (control Cy5/patient Cy3), and the pink plots represent the ratios obtained from the second slide in which the dyes have been reversed (patient Cy5/control Cy3). The top panel is a normal plot for chromosome 22. The lower plot is from an individual with DiGeorge syndrome in whom clones in the critical deletion region are deleted *(arrow)*. (Plots courtesy of BA Bejjani and LG Shaffer, Signature Genomic Laboratories, LLC.)

effective and efficient technique for detecting cryptic chromosomal aberrations, which may be an important adjunct to FISH and conventional chromosome analysis (Fig. 81-6).

ABNORMALITIES OF CHROMOSOME NUMBER

Aneuploidy and Polyploidy. Human cells contain a multiple of 23 chromosomes ($n = 23$). A haploid cell (n) has 23 chromosomes (ova or sperm). If a cell's chromosomes are an exact multiple of 23 (46, 69, 92 in humans), the cell is referred to as euploid. **Polyploid** or heteroploid cells are euploid cells with more than the normal **diploid** number of 46 (2n) chromosomes. While polyploid conceptions are usually not viable, the presence of mosaicism with a karyotypically normal line may allow for survival. Abnormal cells that do not contain a multiple of 23 chromosomes are termed **aneuploid** cells. Aneuploidy is the most common and clinically significant type of human chromosome abnormality, occurring in at least 3–4% of all clinically recognized pregnancies.

Triploid cells, those with three sets of chromosomes (3n), are viable in a mosaic form. Triploid infants can be liveborn but do not survive long. Triploidy is frequently the result of fertilization by two sperm (dispermy). Failure of one of the meiotic divisions, resulting in a diploid egg or sperm, can also result in triploidy. The phenotype of a triploid conception depends on the origin of the extra chromosome set. If the extra set is of **paternal origin,** it will result in a **hydatidiform mole.** Those that have an extra set of maternal chromosomes are spontaneously aborted.

Aneuploidies usually consist of monosomy and trisomy. **Monosomy,** which may be complete or partial, occurs when only one instead of the normal two chromosomes is present in an otherwise diploid cell. In humans, all complete autosomal monosomies appear to be lethal early in development; survival is possible in **mosaic forms.** An exception is monosomy for the X chromosome (karyotype 45,X), seen in the Turner syndrome.

The most common cause of aneuploidy is **nondisjunction,** the failure of chromosomes to disjoin normally during meiosis (see Fig. 81-2). Nondisjunction can occur during meiosis I or II or during mitosis. After meiotic nondisjunction, the resulting gamete either lacks a chromosome or has 2 copies, resulting in a monosomic or trisomic zygote, respectively.

Trisomy, characterized by the presence of 3 instead of the normal 2 of any particular chromosome, is the most common form of aneuploidy. Trisomy can be complete and present in all cells or it may be in mosaic form. Most individuals with trisomy exhibit a consistent and specific phenotype depending on the chromosome involved. FISH is commonly used in the prenatal detection of fetal aneuploidy and in the rapid diagnosis of newborns suspected to have a trisomy.

The major numerical disorders of chromosomes are 3 autosomal trisomies (trisomy 21, trisomy 18, trisomy 13), and 4 types of sex chromosomal aneuploidies: Turner syndrome (usually 45,X); Klinefelter syndrome (47,XXY); 47,XXX; and 47,XYY. By far the most common type of trisomy in liveborn infants is trisomy 21 (karyotype 47,XX,+21 or 47,XY,+21) or Down syndrome. Trisomy 18 and trisomy 13 are also relatively common and are associated with a characteristic set of congenital anomalies and mental retardation (Table 81-2).

Down syndrome is associated with cognitive impairment and characteristic facial and other dysmorphic features (Figs. 81-7 to 81-9). Affected individuals are more prone to congenital heart defects (atrioventricular septal defects, ventricular septal defects, isolated secundum atrial septal defects, PDA, tetralogy of Fallot),

TABLE 81-2. Chromosomal Trisomies and Their Clinical Findings

SYNDROME	INCIDENCE	CLINICAL MANIFESTATIONS
Trisomy 13, Patau syndrome	1/10,000 births	Cleft lip often midline; flexed fingers with polydactyly; ocular hypotelorism, bulbous nose; low-set malformed ears; small abnormal skull; cerebral malformation, especially holoprosencephaly; microphthalmia, cardiac malformations; scalp defects; hypoplastic or absent ribs; visceral and genital anomalies
Trisomy 18, Edwards syndrome	1/6,000 births	Low birthweight, closed fists with index finger overlapping the 3rd digit and the 5th digit overlapping the 4th, narrow hips with limited abduction, short sternum, rocker-bottom feet, microcephaly, prominent occiput, micrognathia, cardiac and renal malformations, and mental retardation; 95% of cases are lethal in the 1st yr
Trisomy 21, Down syndrome	1/600–800 births	Hypotonia, flat face, upward and slanted palpebral fissures and epicanthic folds, speckled irises (Brushfield sports); varying degrees of mental and growth retardation; dysplasia of the pelvis, cardiac malformations, and simian crease; short, broad hands, hypoplasia of middle phalanx of 5th finger, duodenal atresia, and high arched palate; 5% of patients with Down syndrome are the result of a translocation—t(14q21q), t(15q21q), and t(13q21q)—in which the phenotype is the same as trisomy 21 Down syndrome
Trisomy 8, mosaicism	1/20,000 births	Long face, high prominent forehead, wide upturned nose, thick everted lower lip, microretrognathia, low-set ears, high arched, sometimes cleft palate; osteoarticular anomalies common; moderate mental retardation

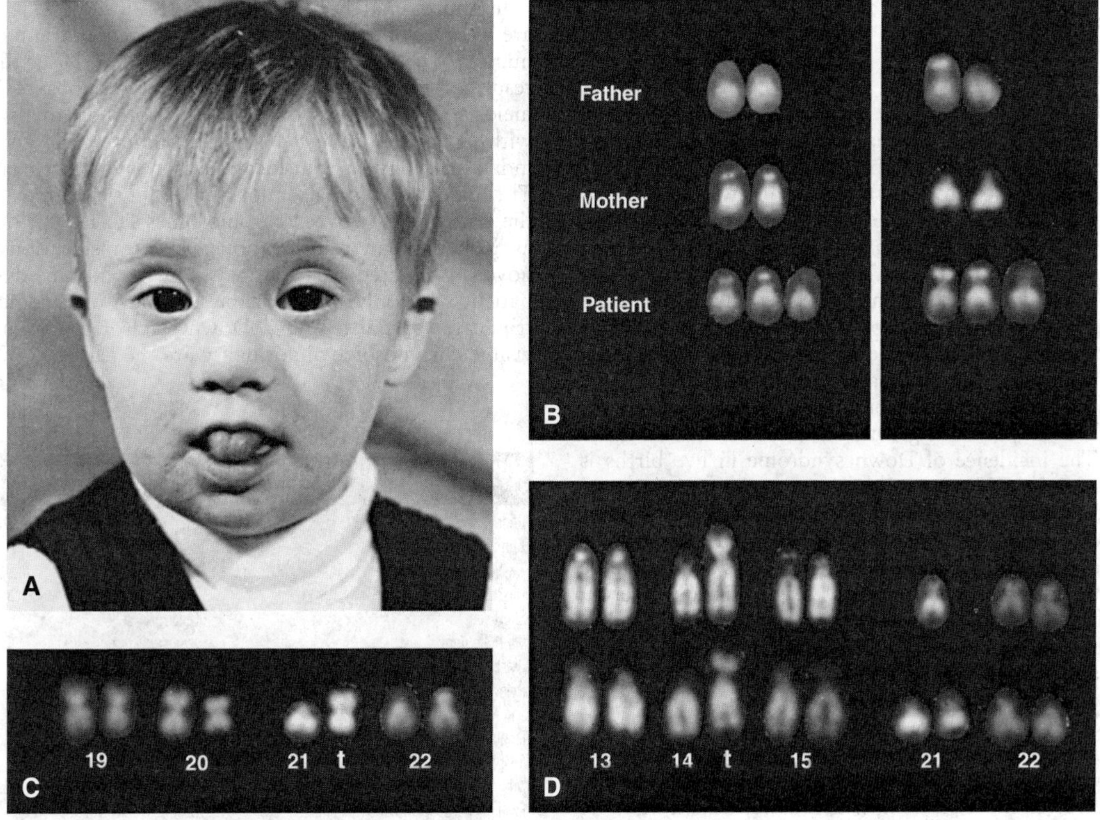

Figure 81-7. Partial karyotypes from patients with Down syndrome. *A,* Patient with trisomy 21. *B,* Chromosome 21 from 2 patients and their parents. *Left,* 2 of a patient's chromosomes with brightly fluorescent satellites were transmitted by the mother. *Right,* Another patient's 2 chromosomes with bright satellites resulted from paternal nondisjunction at second meiotic division. *C,* 21q21q translocation. *D,* 14q21q translocation in a mother *(above)* and her affected child *(below).*

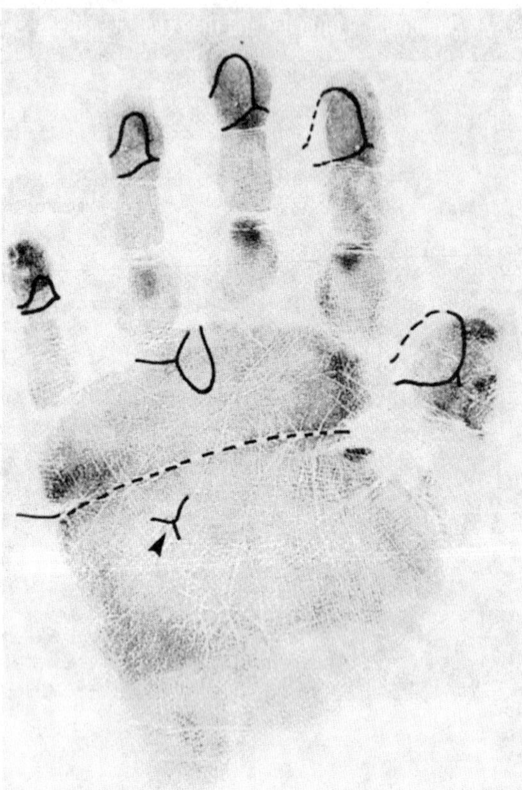

Figure 81-8. Characteristic dermal patterns of the palm of a child with Down syndrome: a single flexion crease (simian crease), axial triradius *(arrow)* in distal position, a pattern area on the palm between the third and fourth digits, and ulnar loops on all 10 digits. (From Nussbaum RL, McInnes RR, Willard HF: *Thompson & Thompson Genetics in Medicine,* 6th ed. Philadelphia, WB Saunders, 2004, p 160.)

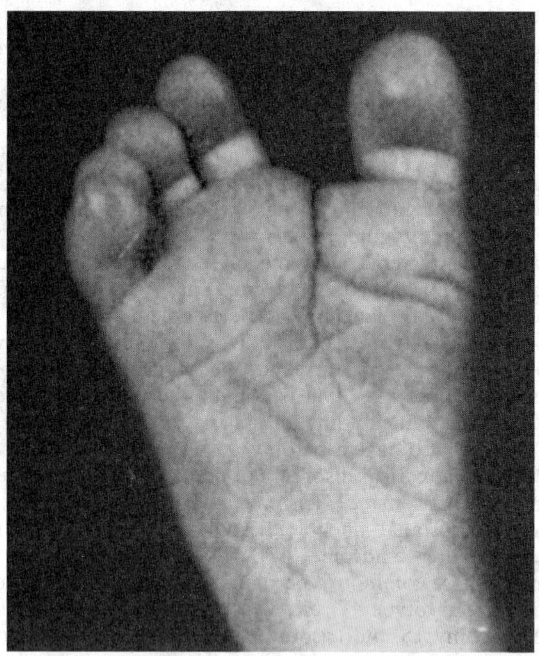

Figure 81-9. Prehensile foot in a 1-mo-old child. (From Wiedemann HR, Kunze J, Dibbern H: *Atlas of Clinical Syndromes: A Visual Guide to Diagnosis,* 3rd ed. St. Louis, Mosby, 1989.)

gastrointestinal anomalies, leukemia, Alzheimer disease, immune dysfunction, hypothyroidism, diabetes mellitus, and problems with hearing and vision (Table 81-3). Most males with Down syndrome are sterile; some females have been able to reproduce. Individuals with Down syndrome often benefit from programs aimed at stimulation, development, and education. They also benefit from anticipatory guidance, which establishes the protocol for screening, evaluation, and care for patients with genetic syndromes and chronic disorders. The life expectancy for children with Down syndrome is approximately 50 yr.

Down syndrome is the most common chromosome disorder and the single most common genetic cause of moderate mental retardation. The incidence of Down syndrome in live births is approximately 1 in 750; the incidence at conception is more than twice that rate. The occurrence of trisomy 21 as well as other autosomal trisomies increases with advanced maternal age (≥35 yr). Due to this increased risk, women at this age should be offered genetic counseling and prenatal diagnostic tools (serum screening, ultrasonography, amniocentesis, and chorionic villus sampling) [see Chapter 96].

Even though younger women have a lower risk, they represent half of all mothers with babies with Down syndrome because of their higher overall birth rate. All women should be offered screening for Down syndrome in their second trimester by means of 3 maternal serum tests (free β-hCG, unconjugated estriol, and α-fetoprotein). Even more efficient, with a detection rate of 95%, is a method of screening using maternal age and fetal nuchal translucency (NT) thickness along with maternal serum β-hCG, PAPP-A (pregnancy-associated plasma protein-A), unconjugated estriol, and α-fetoprotein. Increased levels of maternal serum α-fetoprotein (MSAFP) are also linked to other abnormal fetal conditions, including open neural tube defects and defects of the gastrointestinal system and genitourinary system.

In approximately 95% of the cases of Down syndrome there are 3 copies of chromosome 21. The parental origin of the supernumerary chromosome 21 is maternal in 97% of the cases as a result of errors in meiosis. The majority occurs in maternal meiosis I (78%). Approximately 1% of individuals are mosaics with some cells having 46 chromosomes, while another 4% of individuals have a **translocation** that involves chromosome 21. The majority of translocations in Down syndrome are fusions at the centromere between chromosomes 13, 14, 15, or 21, known as Robertsonian translocations. The translocations can be de novo or inherited. Very rarely is Down syndrome diagnosed in a patient with only a part of the long arm of chromosome 21 in triplicate (**partial trisomy**). Down syndrome patients without a visible chromosome abnormality are the least common.

TABLE 81-3. Additional Disorders in Children with Down Syndrome

	Increased Risk for Development of
Duodenal atresia	Leukemia: AML, ALL
Annular pancreas	Myelodysplasia
Tracheoesophageal fistula	Transient lymphoproliferative syndrome
Hirschsprung disease	Celiac disease
Short stature	Hypothyroidism
Short sternum	Diabetes mellitus
Brachycephaly	Obesity
Delayed fontanel closure	Refractive errors
Three fontanels	Strabismus
Frontal sinus hypoplasia	Mitral valve prolapse
Peripheral joint laxity	Conductive and/or sensorineural hearing loss
Atlantoaxial instability (C1–C2 subluxation)	Obstructive sleep apnea
Exaggerated space between 1st and 2nd toes	Epilepsy
Mottled skin in infancy	Alzheimer disease
Dry coarse skin in adolescence	Conduct oppositional disorders
	ADHD

TABLE 81-4. Other Rare Aneuploidies and Partial Autosomal Aneuploidies

DISORDER	KARYOTYPE	CLINICAL MANIFESTATIONS
Trisomy 8	47,XX/XY,+8	Growth and mental deficiency are variable. The majority of patients are mosaics. The presence of deep palmar and plantar furrows is characteristic.
Trisomy 9	47,XX/XY,+9	The majority of patients are mosaics. Clinical features include craniofacial (high forehead, microphthalmia, low-set malformed ears, bulbous nose) and skeletal (joint contractures) malformations and heart defects (60%).
Trisomy 16	47,XX/XY,+16	The most frequently observed autosomal aneuploidy in spontaneous abortions. The recurrence risk is negligible.
Tetrasomy	47,XX/XY,+i(12p)	Known as Pallister-Killian syndrome. Sparse anterior scalp hair, eyebrows, and eyelashes, prominent forehead, chubby cheeks, long philtrum with thin upper lip and cupid-bow configuration Polydactyly and streaks of hyper/hypopigmentation have been reported.

It is not possible to distinguish the phenotypes of individuals with full trisomy 21 and those with a translocation. Patients who are mosaic tend to have a milder phenotype.

Chromosome analysis is indicated in individuals suspected of having Down syndrome. If a translocation is identified, parental chromosome studies must be performed to determine whether one of the parents is a translocation carrier, which carries a high recurrence risk for having another affected child. That parent may also have other family members at risk. Translocation (21;21) carriers have a 100% recurrence risk for a chromosomally abnormal child. Genomic dosage imbalance contributes through direct and indirect pathways to the Down syndrome phenotype and its phenotypic variation.

Tables 81-4 and 81-5 provide more information on other aneuploidies and partial autosomal aneuploidies (Figs. 81-10 to 81-13).

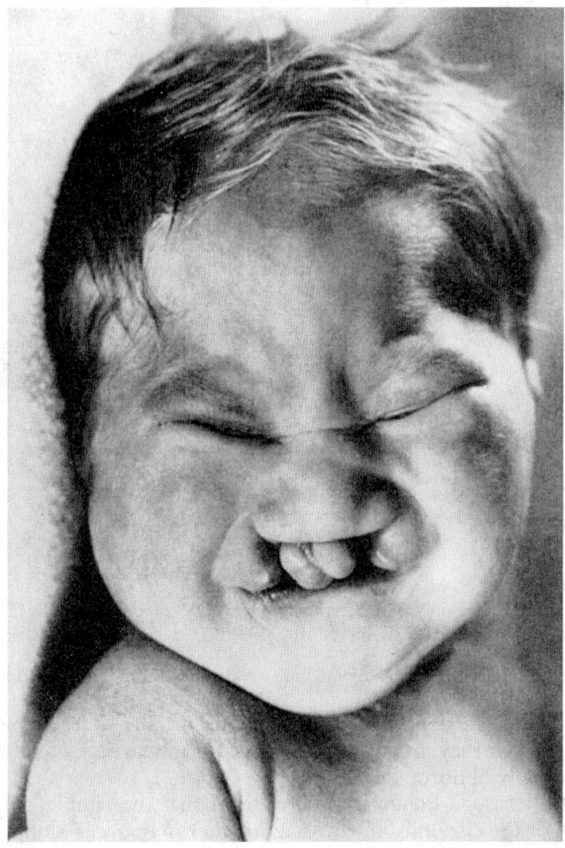

Figure 81-10. Facial appearance of a child with trisomy 13. (From Wiedemann HR, Kunze J, Dibbern H: *Atlas of Clinical Syndromes: A Visual Guide to Diagnosis,* 3rd ed. St. Louis, Mosby, 1989.)

ABNORMALITIES OF CHROMOSOME STRUCTURE

Translocations. Translocations, which involve the transfer of material from one chromosome to another, occur with a frequency of 1 in 500 liveborn human infants. They may be inherited from a carrier parent or appear de novo, with no other affected family member. Translocations may be either reciprocal or robertsonian (Fig. 81-14).

Reciprocal translocations are the result of breaks in nonhomologous chromosomes with reciprocal exchange of the broken segments. Carriers of a reciprocal translocation are usually phenotypically normal but are at an increased risk both for miscarriage due to unbalanced reciprocal translocation and for bearing chromosomally abnormal offspring. Unbalanced translocations are the result of abnormalities in the segregation/crossover of the translocation carrier chromosomes in the germ cells.

Robertsonian translocations involve two acrocentric chromosomes (chromosomes 13, 14, 15, 21, and 22) that fuse near the centromeric region with a subsequent loss of the short arms. Because the short arms of all 5 pairs of acrocentric chromosomes have multiple copies of genes for ribosomal RNA, loss of the short arm of 2 acrocentric chromosomes has no deleterious effect. The resulting karyotype has only 45 chromosomes, including the translocated chromosome that is made up of the long arm of the two fused chromosomes. Carriers of Robertsonian translocations are usually phenotypically normal. However, they are at increased risk for miscarriage and unbalanced abnormal offspring.

Inversions. An inversion requires that a single chromosome break at two points; the broken piece is then inverted and joined into the same chromosome. Inversions occur in 1 in 100 live births. There are two types of inversions: pericentric and paracentric. In **pericentric inversions,** the breaks are in the two opposite arms of the chromosome and include the centromere. They are usually discovered because they change the position of the centromere. The breaks in **paracentric inversions** occur in only

TABLE 81-5. Findings That May Be Present in Trisomy 13 and Trisomy 18

	TRISOMY 13	TRISOMY 18
Head and face	Scalp defects (e.g., cutis aplasia) Microphthalmia, corneal abnormalities Cleft lip and palate in 60%–80% of cases Microcephaly Microphthalmia Sloping forehead Holoprosencephaly (arhinencephaly) Capillary hemangiomas Deafness	Small and premature appearance Tight palpebral fissures Narrow nose and hypoplastic nasal alae Narrow bifrontal diameter Prominent occiput Micrognathia Cleft lip or palate Microcephaly
Chest	Congenital heart disease (e.g., VSD, PDA, and ASD) in 80% of cases Thin posterior ribs (missing ribs)	Congenital heart disease (e.g., VSD, PDA, and ASD) Short sternum, small nipples
Extremities	Overlapping of fingers and toes (clinodactyly) Polydactyly Hypoplastic nails, hyperconvex nails	Limited hip abduction Clinodactyly and overlapping fingers; index over 3rd, 5th over 4th; closed fist Rocker-bottom feet Hypoplastic nails
General	Severe developmental delays and prenatal and postnatal growth retardation Renal abnormalities Nuclear projections in neutrophils Only 5% live longer than 6 mo	Severe developmental delays and prenatal and postnatal growth retardation Premature birth, polyhydramnios Inguinal or abdominal hernias Only 5% live longer than 1 year

From Behrman RE, Kliegman RM: *Nelson Essentials of Pediatrics,* 4th ed. Philadelphia, WB Saunders, 2002, p 142. ASD, atrial septal defect; PDA, patent ductus arteriosus; VSD, ventricular septal defect.

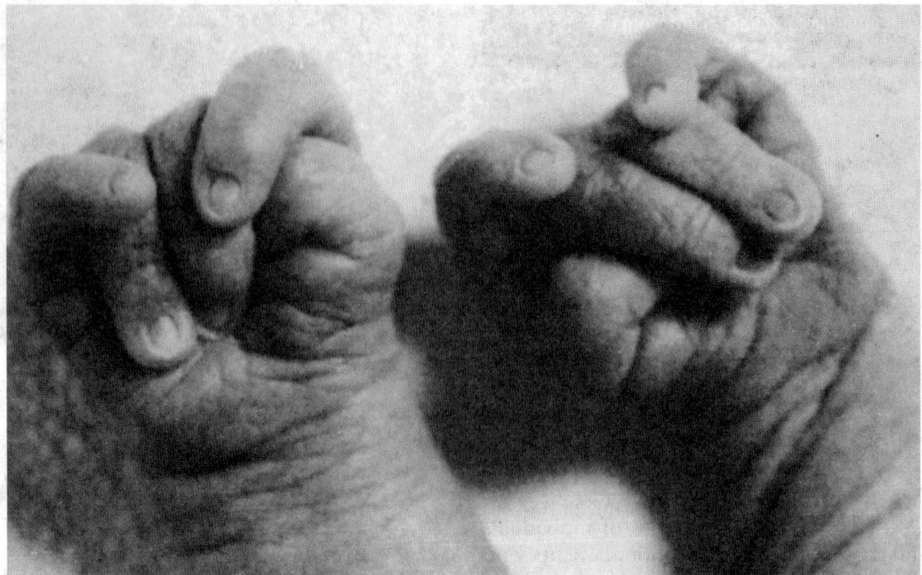

Figure 81-11. Trisomy 18: overlapping fingers and hypoplastic nails. (From Wiedemann HR, Kunze J, Dibbern H: *Atlas of Clinical Syndromes: A Visual Guide to Diagnosis,* 3rd ed. St. Louis, Mosby, 1989.)

one arm. Carriers of inversions are usually phenotypically normal, but they are at increased risk for miscarriages and chromosomally abnormal offspring.

Deletions and Duplications. Deletions may be simple, with a piece of the chromosome missing, or they may occur along with a duplication of another chromosome segment, resulting in an unbalanced reciprocal chromosomal translocation. The latter is usually due to abnormal crossover or segregation in a translocation or inversion carrier.

Deletions may be located at the end of the chromosome or in interstitial segments. A carrier of a deletion is monosomic for the genetic information of the missing segment. Deletions are usually associated with mental retardation and malformations. The most commonly observed deletions in routine chromosome preparations include 1p-, 4p-, 5p-, 9p-, 11p-, 13q-, 18p-, 18q-, and 21q- (Table 81-6 and Fig. 81-15). Deletions may be observed in routine chromosome preparations, with deletions and translocations larger than 5–10 Mb usually visible microscopically.

High-resolution banding techniques, FISH, and DNA studies can reveal deletions that are too small to be seen in ordinary or routine chromosome spreads. **Microdeletions** are small chromosome deletions, the largest of which are detectable only with prophase chromosome studies and/or DNA probes. For submicroscopic deletions, the missing piece can only be detected using FISH or DNA/molecular studies.

The presence of extra genetic material from the same chromosome is referred to as **duplication.** Duplications or partial (segmental) trisomies are less frequent than whole trisomies. Duplications may be sporadic or result from abnormal segregation in translocation or inversion carriers.

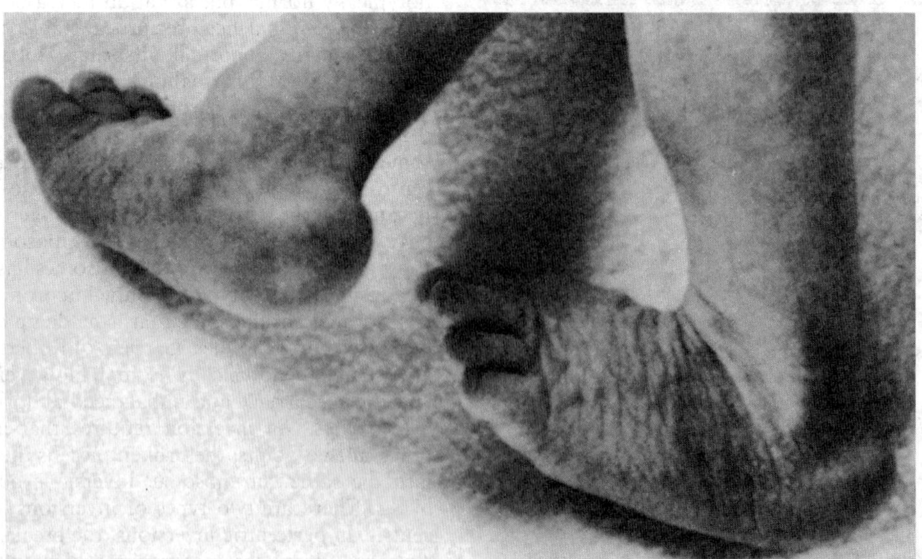

Figure 81-12. Trisomy 18: rocker-bottom feet (protruding calcanei). (From Wiedemann HR, Kunze J, Dibbern H: *Atlas of Clinical Syndromes: A Visual Guide to Diagnosis,* 3rd ed. St. Louis, Mosby, 1989.)

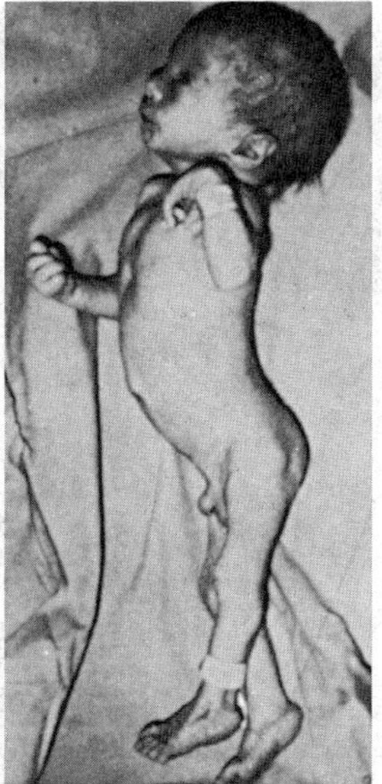

Figure 81-13. Male infant with trisomy 18 at age 4 days. Note prominent occiput, micrognathia, low-set ears, short sternum, narrow pelvis, prominent calcaneus, and flexion abnormalities of the fingers.

TABLE 81-6. Common Deletions and Their Clinical Manifestations

DELETION	CLINICAL ABNORMALITIES
4p-	Wolf-Hirschhorn syndrome. The main features are a typical "Greek helmet" facies with ocular hypertelorism, prominent glabella, and frontal bossing; microcephaly, dolichocephaly, hypoplasia of the eye socket, ptosis, strabismus, nystagmus, bilateral epicanthic folds, cleft lip and palate, beaked nose with prominent bridge, hypospadias, cardiac malformations, and mental retardation.
5p-	Cri-du-chat syndrome. The main features are hypotonia, short stature, characteristic cry, microcephaly with protruding metopic suture, moonlike face, hypertelorism, bilateral epicanthic folds, high arched palate, wide and flat nasal bridge, and mental retardation.
9p-	The main features are craniofacial dysmorphology with trigonocephaly, slanted palpebral fissures, discrete exophthalmos, arched eyebrows, flat and wide nasal bridge, short neck with pterygium colli, genital anomalies, long fingers and toes, cardiac malformations, and mental retardation.
13q-	The main features are low birthweight, failure to thrive, and severe mental retardation. Facial features include microcephaly, flat wide nasal bridge, hypertelorism, ptosis, micrognathia. Ocular malformations are common. The hands have hypoplastic or absent thumbs and syndactyly.
18p-	A few patients (15%) are severely affected and have cephalic and ocular malformations, cleft lip and palate, and varying degrees of mental retardation. Most (80%) have only minor malformations and mild mental retardation.
18q-	The main features are hypotonia with "froglike" position with the legs flexed, externally rotated, and in hyperabduction. The face is characteristic with depressed midface and apparent protrusion of the mandible, deep-set eyes, short upper lip, everted lower lip ("carplike" mouth); antihelix of the ears is very prominent; varying degrees of mental retardation and belligerent personality.
21q-	The main features are hypertonia, microcephaly, downward-slanting palpebral fissures, high palate, prominent nasal bridge, large low-set ears, micrognathia, and varying degrees of mental retardation. They may have skeletal malformations.

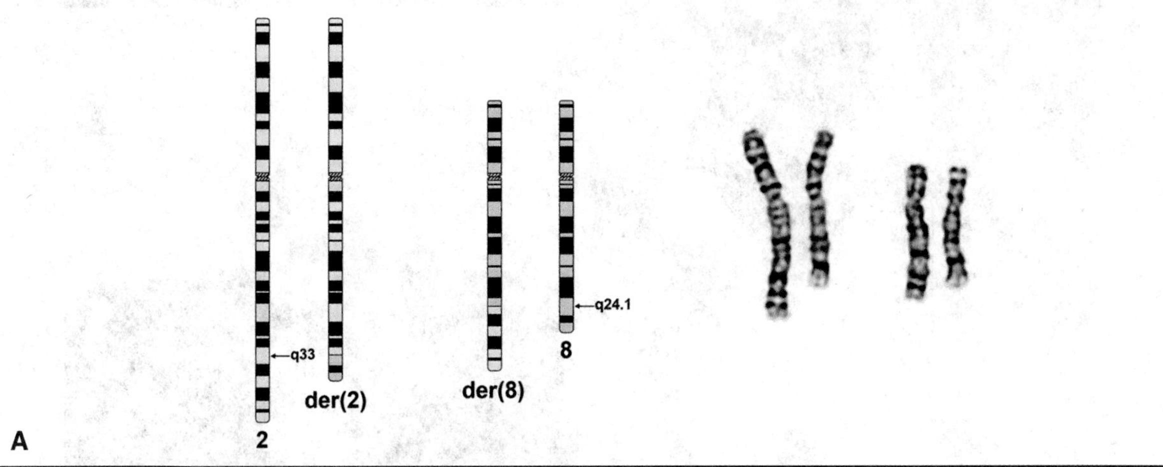

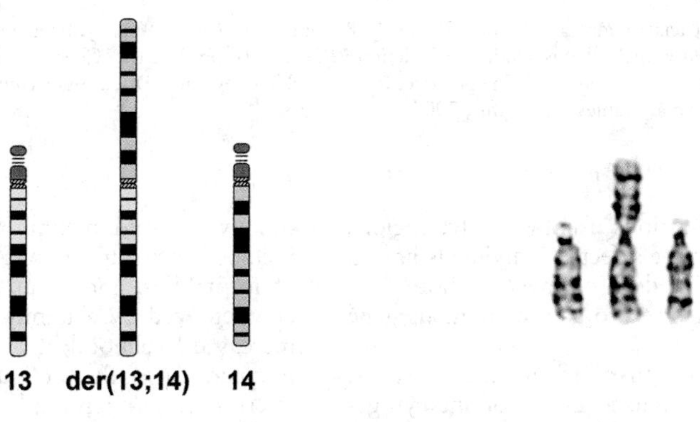

Figure 81-14. *A,* Schematic diagram *(left)* and partial G-banded karyotype *(right)* of a reciprocal translocation between chromosome 2 (blue) and chromosome 8 (pink). The breakpoints are on the long (q) arm of both chromosomes at bands 2q33 and 8q24.1 with the reciprocal exchange of material between the derivative (der) chromosomes 2 and 8. This translocation is balanced, with no net gain or loss of material. The nomenclature for this exchange is t(2;8)(q33:q24.1). *B,* Schematic diagram *(left)* and partial G-banded karyotype *(right)* of a Robertsonian translocation between chromosomes 13 (blue) and 14 (pink). The breakpoints are at the centromere (band q10) of both chromosomes with fusion of the long arms into a single derivative chromosome and loss of the short (p) arm material. The nomenclature for this exchange is der(13;14)(q10;q10).

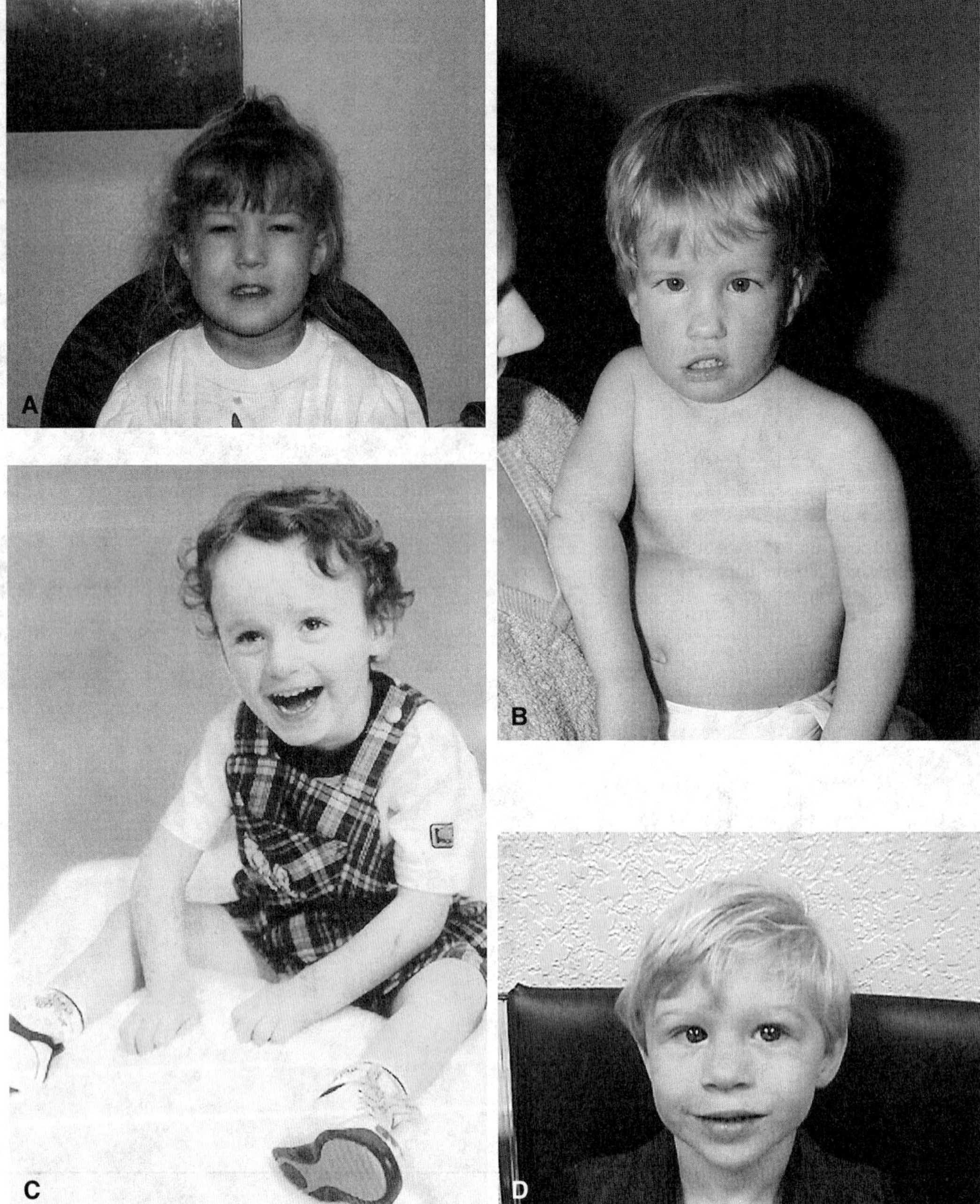

Figure 81-15. A, Child with velocardiofacial syndrome (deletion 22q11.2). B, Child with Prader-Willi syndrome (deletion 15q11–13). C, Child with Angelman syndrome (deletion 15q11–13). D, Child with Williams syndrome (deletion 7q11.23). (From Lin RL, Cherry AM, Bangs CD, et al: FISHing for answers: The use of molecular cytogenetic techniques in adolescent medicine practice. In Hyme HE, Greydanus D [editors]: *Genetic Disorders in Adolescents*. State of the Art Reviews. Adolescent Medicine. Philadelphia, Hanley and Belfus, 2002, pp 305–313.)

Microdeletions and microduplications usually involve regions that include several genes, so that the affected individuals have a distinctive phenotype. When such a deletion involves more than a single gene, the condition is referred to as a **contiguous gene syndrome** (Table 81-7).

Subtelomeric regions are often involved in chromosomal rearrangements that cannot be visualized using routine cytogenetics. Telomeres, which are the distal ends of the chromosomes, are gene-rich regions. Small subtelomeric deletions/duplications or rearrangements (translocations, inversions) may be relatively common in nonspecific mental retardation with minor anomalies. Subtelomeric rearrangements have been found in 3–7% of children with moderate to mild mental retardation and 0.5% of children with mild mental retardation. Clinical features (>30%) include short stature, microcephaly, hypertelorism, nasal and ear abnormalities, and cryptorchidism in males. This group is also characterized by a family history of mental retardation and an increased likelihood of retarded growth beginning in the prenatal period. Both the subtelomeric rearrangements and the microdeletion/microduplication syndromes are diagnosed by FISH or other molecular means.

Insertions. Insertions occur when a piece of a chromosome broken at two points is incorporated into a break in another part of a chromosome. A total of three breakpoints are then required, and they may occur between two or within one chromosome. A form of nonreciprocal translocation, insertions are rare. Insertion carriers are at risk of having offspring with deletions or duplications of the inserted segment.

Isochromosomes. Isochromosomes consist of two copies of the same chromosome arm joined through a single centromere and forming mirror images of one another. The most frequently reported autosomal isochromosomes tend to involve chromosomes with small arms. Some of the more common chromosome arms involved in this formation include 5p, 8p, 9p, 12p, 18p, and 18q. Individuals with 46 chromosomes one of which is an isochromosome are monosomic for genes in the lost arm and trisomic for the genes present in the isochromosome.

MARKER AND RING CHROMOSOMES. Marker chromosomes are rare and are usually chromosome fragments that are too small to be identified by banded cytogenetics; they usually occur in addition to the normal 46 chromosomes. Most are sporadic (70%); mosaicism is often (50%) noted because of the mitotic instability of the marker chromosome. The incidence in newborn infants is 1 in 3,300, and the incidence in individuals with mental retardation is 1 in 300. Their phenotype ranges from normal to severely abnormal.

Ring chromosomes, which are found for all human chromosomes, are rare. A ring chromosome is formed when both ends of a chromosome are deleted and the ends are then joined to form a ring. Depending on the amount of chromosome material that is lacking or in excess (if the ring is in addition to the normal chromosomes), a patient with a ring chromosome can appear normal or nearly normal or may have mental retardation and multiple congenital anomalies.

SEX CHROMOSOME ANEUPLOIDY. About 1 in 400 males and 1 in 650 females have some form of sex chromosome abnormality. Considered together, sex chromosome abnormalities are the most common chromosome abnormalities seen in liveborn infants, children, and adults. Sex chromosome abnormalities can be either structural or numerical and can be present in all cells or in a mosaic form. Those affected with these abnormalities may have few or no physical or developmental problems (Table 81-8).

TABLE 81-8. Sex Chromosome Abnormalities

DISORDER	KARYOTYPE	APPROXIMATE INCIDENCE
Klinefelter syndrome	47,XXY	1/575–1/1,000 Males
	48,XXXY	1/50,000–1/80,000 Male births
	Other (48,XXYY; 49,XXXYY; mosaics)	
XYY syndrome	47,XYY	1/800–1,000 Males
Other X or Y chromosome abnormalities		1/1,500 Males
XX males	46,XX	1/20,000 Males
Turner syndrome	45,X	1/2,500–1/5,000 Females
	Variants and mosaics	
Trisomy X	47,XXX	1/1,000 Females
	48,XXXX and 49,XXXXX	Rare
Other X chromosome abnormalities		1/3,000 Females
XY females	46,XY	1/20,000 Females

Turner Syndrome. Turner syndrome, a condition characterized by the complete or partial absence of the second sex chromosome, is defined by a combination of phenotypic features (Table 81-9). Half of the patients with Turner syndrome have a 45,X chromosome complement. The other half exhibits mosaicism and varied structural abnormalities of the X or Y chromosome. Parental age is not a factor in the 45,X abnormality; its variants occur in approximately 1 in 5,000 female live births. In 75% of patients, the lost chromosome is of paternal origin. 45,X is one of the chromosome abnormalities most frequently associated with spontaneous abortion. It has been estimated that 95–99% of 45,X conceptions are miscarried.

The phenotype in the newborn can include short stature, prominent ears, webbing of the neck, and edema of the hands

TABLE 81-7. Microdeletion/Contiguous Gene Syndromes and Their Clinical Manifestations

DELETION	SYNDROME	CLINICAL MANIFESTATIONS
1p36	1p deletion	Growth retardation, dysmorphic features with flat nasal bridge, abnormal ears, deep-set eyes, hearing loss, seizures, mental retardation
5q35	Sotos (50%)	Overgrowth, macrocephaly, large hands and feet, distinctive facial features, mental disabilities
6p25	Axenfeld-Rieger	Axenfeld-Rieger malformation, hearing loss, congenital heart defects, dental anomalies, developmental delays, facial dysmorphism
7q11.23	Williams	Round face with full cheeks and lips, stellate pattern in iris, strabismus, supravalvular aortic stenosis and other cardiac malformations, varying degrees of mental retardation, friendly personality
8p11	8p11	Kallman syndrome 2, spherocytosis, multiple congenital anomalies, mental retardation
8p23.1		Microcephaly, developmental delays, ASD, VSD, pulmonic stenosis, congenital behavioral abnormalities
8q24.1-q24.13	Langer-Giedion or tricho-rhino-phalangeal, type II	Sparse hair, multiple cone-shaped epiphyses, multiple cartilaginous exostoses, bulbous nasal tip, thickened alar cartilage, upturned nares, prominent philtrum, large protruding ears, mild mental retardation
9q22	Gorlin	Multiple basal cell carcinomas, odontogenic keratocysts, palmoplantar pits, calcification falx cerebri
9q34	9q34 deletion	Distinct face with synophrys, anteverted nares, tented upper lip, protruding tongue, midface hypoplasia, conotruncal heart defects, mental retardation
10p12-p13	DiGeorge 2	Many of the DiGeorge 1 and velocardiofacial 1 features
11p11.2-p14	Potocki-Shaffer	Multiple exostoses, enlarged parietal foramina, craniosynostosis, facial dysmorphism, mental handicap
11p13	WAGR	Hypernephroma (Wilms tumor), aniridia, male genital hypoplasia of varying degrees, gonadoblastoma, long face, upward slanting palpebral fissures, ptosis, beaked nose, low-set poorly formed auricles, mental retardation
11q24.1-11qter	Jacobsen	Mental and growth retardation, cardiac and digit anomalies, thrombocytopenia
15q11-q13 (pat)	Prader-Willi	Severe hypotonia at birth, obesity, short stature (responsive to growth hormone), small hands and feet, hypogonadism, mental retardation
15q11-q13 (mat)	Angelman	Hypotonia, fair hair, midface hypoplasia, prognathism, seizures, jerky ataxic movements, uncontrollable bouts of laughter, severe mental retardation
15q21	15q21 deletion	Growth retardation, beaked nose, thin upper lip, small hands and feet, mental retardation
16p13.3	Rubinstein-Taybi	Microcephaly, ptosis, beaked nose with low-lying philtrum, broad thumbs and large toes, mental retardation
17p11.2	Smith-Magenis	Brachycephaly, midfacial hypoplasia, prognathism, myopia, cleft palate, short stature, behavioral problems, mental retardation
17p13.3	Miller-Dieker	Microcephaly, lissencephaly, pachygyria, narrow forehead, hypoplastic male external genitals, growth retardation, seizures, profound mental retardation
20p12	Alagille syndrome	Bile duct paucity with cholestasis; heart defects, particularly pulmonary artery stenosis; ocular abnormalities (posterior embryo toxin); skeletal defects such as butterfly vertebrae; long nose with broad mid-nose
22q11.2	Velocardiofacial-DiGeorge syndrome	Hypoplasia or agenesis of the thymus and parathyroid glands, hypoplasia of auricle and external auditory canal, conotruncal cardiac anomalies, cleft palate, short stature, behavioral problems
22q13.3 deletion		Hypotonia, developmental delay, normal or accelerated growth, ptosis, dysplastic toenails, abnormal ears, pointed chin
Xp21.2-p21.3		Duchenne muscular dystrophy, retinitis pigmentosa, adrenal hypoplasia, mental retardation, glycerol kinase deficiency
Xp22.2-p22.3		Ichthyosis, Kallman syndrome, mental retardation, chondrodysplasia punctata
Xp22.3	Microphthalmia with linear defects (MLS)	Microphthalmia, linear skin defects, poikiloderma, congenital heart defects, seizures, mental retardation

TABLE 81-9. Disorders Associated with Turner Syndrome

Short stature
Congenital lymphedema
Horseshoe kidney
Patella dislocation
Increased carrying angle of elbow
Madelung deformity (chondrodysplasia of distal radial epiphysis)
Congenital hip dislocation
Scoliosis
Widespread nipples
Shield chest
Redundant nuchal skin (in utero cystic hygroma)
Low posterior hairline
Coarctation of aorta
Bicuspid aortic valve
Cardiac conduction abnormalities
Hypoplastic left heart syndrome?
Gonadal dysgenesis (infertility, primary amenorrhea)
Gonadoblastoma (if Y chromosome material present)
Learning disabilities (nonverbal perceptual motor and visuospatial skills) [in 70%]
Developmental delay (in 10%)
Social awkwardness
Hypothyroidism (acquired in 15–30%)
Type 2 diabetes mellitus (insulin resistance)
Strabismus
Cataract
Red-green colorblindness (as in males)
Recurrent otitis media
Sensorineural hearing loss
Inflammatory bowel disease
Celiac disease?

and feet, but many newborns are phenotypically normal (Fig. 81-16). Older children and adults have short stature and exhibit variable dysmorphic features. Congenital heart defects (40%) and structural renal anomalies (60%) are common. The most common heart defects are bicuspid aortic valves, coarctation of the aorta, aortic stenosis, and mitral valve prolapse. The gonads are generally streaks of fibrous tissue (**gonadal dysgenesis**). There is primary amenorrhea and lack of secondary sexual characteristics. These children should receive regular endocrinologic testing (see Chapter 587). Patients tend to be of normal intelligence but are at increased risk for behavioral problems and deficiencies in spatial and motor perception. Guidelines for health supervision for children with Turner syndrome are published by the AAP.

TABLE 81-10. Disorders Associated with Noonan Syndrome

Short stature	Short webbed neck
Failure to thrive	Shield chest
Epicanthal folds	Pectus excavatum or carinatum
Ptosis	Scoliosis
Hypertelorism	Cubitus valgus
Low nasal bridge	Pulmonary valve stenosis
Downward slanting palpebral fissures	Hypertrophic cardiomyopathy
Myopia	Atrial septal defect (ASD)
Nystagmus	Tetralogy of Fallot
Low-set auricles	Cryptorchidism
Dental malocclusion	Small penis
Low posterior hairline	Bleeding disorders, including thrombocytopenia

Approximately 10% of patients with **45,X/46,XY mosaicism** have external genitalia that are either ambiguous or female. The remaining 90% will have normal appearing external male genitalia. This variant is estimated to represent approximately 6% of patients with mosaic Turner syndrome. Some of the patients with Turner syndrome phenotype and a Y cell line will exhibit masculinization. Phenotypic females with 45,X/46,XY mosaicism have a 15–30% risk of developing **gonadoblastoma.** The risk for the patients with a male phenotype and external testes is not so high, but tumor surveillance is nevertheless recommended. The AAP has recommended the use of FISH analysis to look for Y-chromosome mosaicism in all 45,X patients. If Y chromosome material is identified, laparoscopic gonadectomy is recommended.

Noonan syndrome is an autosomal dominant disorder due in some patients (60%) to a mutation in *PTPN1,* which encodes a nonreceptor tyrosine kinase (SHP-2) on chromosome 12q24.1. Features common to Noonan syndrome include short stature, low posterior hairline, shield chest, congenital heart disease, and a short or webbed neck (Table 81-10). In contrast to Turner syndrome, Noonan syndrome affects both sexes and has a different pattern of congenital heart disease.

Klinefelter Syndrome. Eighty-percent of children with Klinefelter syndrome have a male karyotype with an extra chromosome X—47,XXY; the remaining 20% have a higher grade of sex chromosome aneuploidy (48,XXXY; 48,XXYY; 49,XXXXY), mosaicism (46,XY/47,XXY), or structurally abnormal X chromosomes. The greater the aneuploidy, the more severe the sexual and mental impairment and dysmorphism. Individuals with

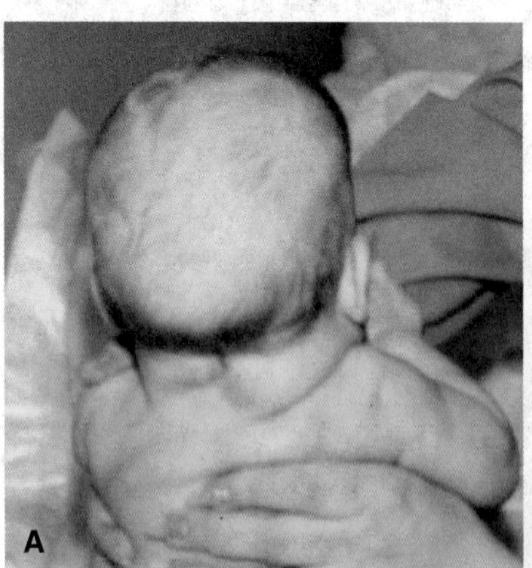

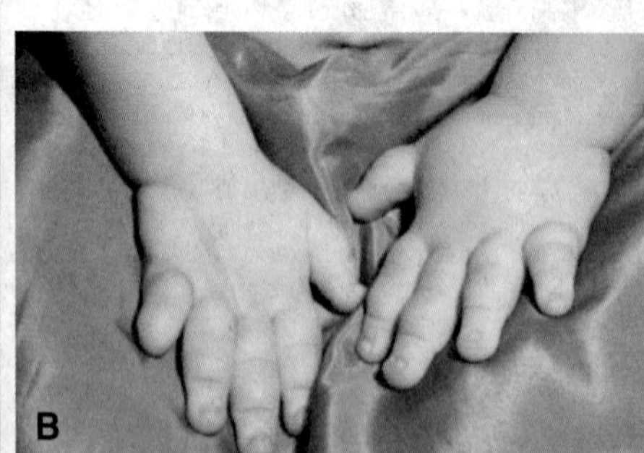

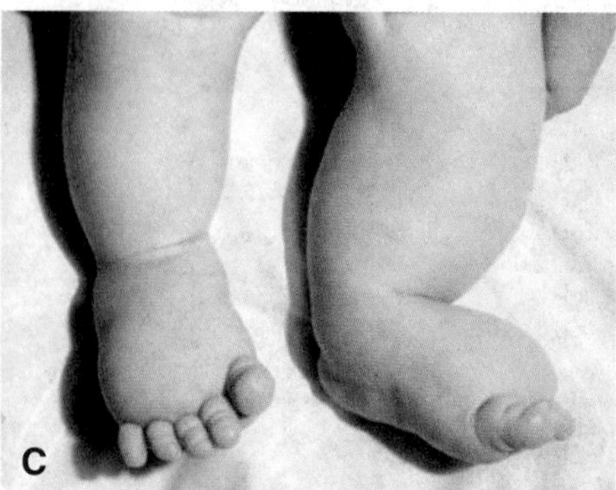

Figure 81-16. Redundant nuchal skin *(A)* and puffiness of the hands *(B)* and feet *(C)* in Turner's syndrome. (From Sybert VP, McCauley E: Turner's syndrome. *N Engl J Med* 2004;351:1227–1238. Copyright © 2004 Massachusetts Medical Society. All rights reserved.)

Klinefelter are male; this syndrome is the most common cause of hypogonadism and infertility in males and the most common sex chromosome aneuploidy in humans (see Chapter 584). The incidence is approximately 1 in 575 liveborn males. Errors in paternal nondisjunction in meiosis I (MI) account for half of the cases.

Puberty occurs at the normal age, but the testes remain small. Patients develop secondary sexual characteristics late; 50% will develop gynecomastia. Because many patients with Klinefelter syndrome are phenotypically normal until puberty, they often go undiagnosed until adulthood, when their infertility aids in clinical identification. Individuals with 46,XY/47,XXY have a better prognosis for testicular function. Although individuals with Klinefelter do not have a reduced intellect, they show deficits in language and executive functions.

47,XYY. The incidence of 47,XYY is approximately 1 in 800 to 1,000 males, with many cases remaining undiagnosed, since most affected individuals have a normal appearance and normal fertility. The extra Y is the result of nondisjunction at paternal meiosis II (MII). Those with this abnormality are of normal intelligence but are at risk for learning disabilities and hyperactive behavior.

FRAGILE SITES. Fragile sites are regions of chromosomes that show a tendency for separation, breakage, or attenuation under particular growth conditions. They appear as a gap in the staining. At least 120 chromosomal loci, many of them heritable, have been identified as fragile sites in the human genome (see Table 80-1). One fragile site that has clinical significance is that on the distal long arm of chromosome Xq27.3 associated with the **fragile X syndrome.** Fragile X accounts for 3% of the cases of males with mental retardation. There is another fragile site on the X chromosome (FRAXE on Xq28) that has also been implicated with mild mental retardation. The FRA11B (11q23.3) breakpoints are associated with Jacobsen syndrome. Fragile sites may also play a role in tumorigenesis.

The main **clinical manifestations** of fragile X syndrome in affected males are mental retardation, autistic behavior, macroorchidism, large size, and characteristic facial features. The macroorchidism may not be evident until puberty. The facial features, which include a long face and prominent jaw, become more obvious with age. Females affected with fragile X show varying degrees of mental retardation and/or learning disabilities. Diagnosis of fragile X is possible by its molecular characterization and by the observation that it is associated with an expanded DNA segment. The expansion involves an area of the gene that contains a variable number of trinucleotide (CGG) repeats.

MOSAICISM. Mosaicism describes an individual with 2 or more different cell lines derived from a single zygote and is usually the result of mitotic nondisjunction (see Fig. 81-2). Study of placental tissue from chorionic villus samples collected at or before the 10th wk of gestation has shown that 2% or more of all conceptions are mosaic for a chromosome abnormality. With the exception of chromosomes 13, 18, and 21, complete autosomal trisomies are usually nonviable; the presence of a normal cell line may allow these other trisomic conceptions to survive to term. Depending on the point at which the new cell line arises during early embryogenesis, mosaicism may be present in some tissues but not in others. Germline mosaicism, which refers to the presence of mosaicism in the germ cells of the gonad, is associated with an increased risk for recurrence of an affected child.

Pallister-Killian Syndrome. This disorder is characterized by coarse facies, pigmentary skin anomalies, localized alopecia, diaphragmatic hernias, cardiovascular anomalies, supernumerary nipples, and profound mental retardation. The syndrome is due to mosaicism for isochromosome 12p. The presence of the isochromosome 12p in cells gives four copies of 12p in the affected cells. The isochromosome 12p is preferentially cultured from fibroblasts and is seldom present in lymphocytes. The abnormalities seen in affected individuals probably reflect the presence of abnormal cells during early embryogenesis.

Hypomelanosis of Ito. This entity is characterized by unilateral or bilateral macular hypopigmented whorls, streaks, and patches (see Chapter 652). Abnormalities of the eyes, musculoskeletal system, and central nervous system may also be present. Patients with hypomelanosis of Ito have two genetically distinct cell lines. The mosaic chromosome anomalies that have been observed involve both autosomes and sex chromosomes and have been demonstrated in about 50% of patients. The mosaicism may not be visible in lymphocyte-derived chromosome studies; it is more likely to be found when chromosomes are analyzed from skin fibroblasts. The distinct cell lines may not always be due to observable chromosomal anomalies but to single gene mutations or other mechanisms.

CHROMOSOME INSTABILITY SYNDROMES. Chromosome instability syndromes, formerly known as chromosome breakage syndromes, are characterized by an increased risk of malignancy and specific phenotypes. They display autosomal recessive inheritance and have an increased frequency of chromosome breakage and/or rearrangement, whether spontaneous or induced. They result from specific defects in DNA repair, cell cycle control, and apoptosis. The resulting chromosomal instability leads to the increased risk of developing neoplasms. The classic chromosome instability syndromes are Fanconi anemia, ataxia telangiectasia, Nijmegen syndrome, ICF (immunodeficiency, centromere instability, and facial anomalies) syndrome, Roberts syndrome, Werner syndrome, and Bloom syndrome.

UNIPARENTAL DISOMY. Uniparental disomy (UPD) occurs when both chromosomes of a pair of chromosomes in a person with a normal number of chromosomes have been inherited from only one parent. **Uniparental isodisomy** means that the two chromosomes are identical, whereas **uniparental heterodisomy** means that the two chromosomes are different members of a pair, both of which were inherited from one parent. The phenotypical result of UPD varies according to the chromosome involved, the parent who contributed the chromosomes, and whether it is isodisomy or heterodisomy. Three types of phenotypic effects are seen in UPD: (1) those related to imprinted genes, that is, the absence of a gene that is expressed only when inherited from a parent of a specific gender, (2) those related to autosomal recessive disorders, and (3) those related to a vestigial aneuploid producing mosaicism (see Chapter 80).

In uniparental isodisomy, both chromosomes (and thus the genes) in the pair are identical. This is particularly important when the parent is a carrier of an autosomal recessive disorder. If the offspring of a carrier parent has uniparental disomy with isodisomy for a chromosome that carries an abnormal gene, the abnormal gene will be present in two copies and the phenotype will be that of the autosomal recessive disorder; the child has an autosomal recessive disorder even though one parent is a carrier of that recessive disorder. It is estimated that all human beings carry 5 to 8 abnormal autosomal recessive genes. The autosomal recessive disorders spinal muscular atrophy, cystic fibrosis, cartilage-hair hypoplasia, α- and β-thalassemias, and Bloom syndrome have occurred because of uniparental disomy. The possibility of uniparental isodisomy should also be considered when an individual is affected with more than one recessive disorder because the abnormal genes for both disorders could be carried on the same isodisomic chromosome. Uniparental isodisomy is a *rare* cause of recessively inherited disorders.

Maternal uniparental disomy involving chromosomes 2, 7, 14, and 15 and **paternal uniparental disomy** involving chromosomes 6, 11, 15, and 20 are associated with phenotypic abnormalities of growth and behavior. UPD maternal 7 is associated with a phe-

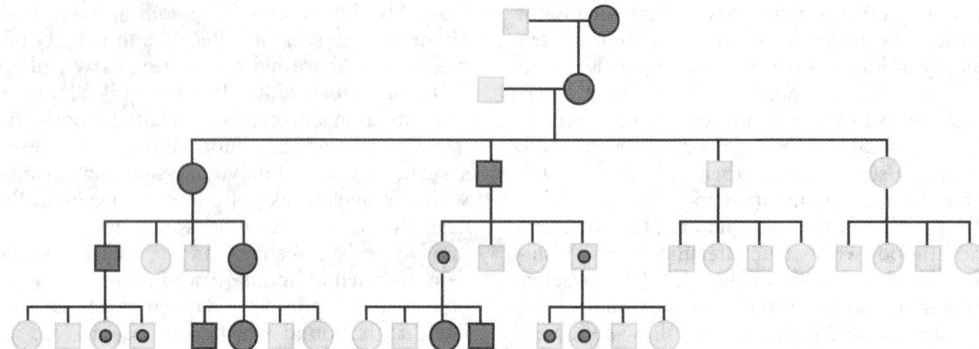

Figure 81-17. In pedigrees suggestive of paternal imprinting, phenotypic effects occur only when the gene is transmitted from the mother but not when transmitted from the father. Equal numbers of males and females are affected and not affected phenotypically in each generation. A non-manifesting transmitter gives a clue to the sex of the parent who passes the expressed genetic information; in other words, in paternal imprinting, there are "skipped" non-manifesting females.

notype similar to Russell-Silver syndrome with intrauterine growth restriction. These phenotypic effects may be related to imprinting (see Imprinting, below).

UPD for chromosome 15 is seen in some cases of Prader-Willi syndrome and Angelman syndrome. In Prader-Willi syndrome, about 60% of cases have maternal UPD (missing the paternal chromosome 15). In about 5% of individuals with Angelman syndrome, paternal UPD of chromosome 15 is observed (missing the maternal chromosome 15). The phenotype for both Prader-Willi syndrome and Angelman syndrome in cases of UPD is thought to be due to the lack of the functional contribution from a particular parent of their chromosome 15. These findings suggest there are differences in function of certain regions of chromosome 15, depending on whether it is inherited from the mother or from the father.

Uniparental disomy most likely arises when a pregnancy starts off as a **trisomy.** Most trisomies are lethal, and the fetus survives only if a cell line loses one of the extra chromosomes to become disomic. One third of the time, the disomic cell line is uniparental. Usually, the viable cell line outgrows the trisomic cell line. When mosaic trisomy is found at prenatal diagnosis, care should be taken to determine whether uniparental disomy has resulted and whether the chromosome involved is one of the disomies known to be associated with phenotypic abnormalities. There must always be concern that some residual cells that are trisomic will be present in some tissues, leading to malformations or dysfunction. The presence of aggregates of trisomic cells may account for the spectrum of abnormalities seen in individuals with UPD.

IMPRINTING. Genomic imprinting occurs when the phenotypic expression depends on the parent of origin for certain genes and chromosome segments. Whether the genetic material is expressed depends on the gender of the parent from whom it was derived. Genomic imprinting is suspected on the basis of a pedigree (Figs. 81-17 and 81-18) with unusual transmission. Imprinting probably occurs in many different parts of the human genome but is thought to be particularly important in gene expression related to development, growth, cancer, and behavior.

Imprinting in humans is noted by phenotypic differences seen in Prader-Willi and Angelman syndromes, which are associated with deletion and uniparental disomy of the same region of chromosome 15. Thus, in uniparental maternal disomy, there is also lack of the paternal segment of chromosome 15, resulting in Prader-Willi syndrome as well. In Prader-Willi syndrome, the deletion, when it occurs, is always of the paternally derived chromosome 15, suggesting that the phenotype of Prader-Willi is due to a lack of paternally derived genetic information carried on that segment of chromosome 15. In contrast, when there is a deleted chromosome 15 in Angelman syndrome, the deleted chromosome is always maternal in origin, and the UPD is always paternal, that is, there is lack of maternal information. There are likely to be many other disorders with this type of parent of origin effect.

ACQUIRED CYTOGENETIC ABNORMALITIES. Acquired (clonal) cytogenetic changes can be found in most tumor cells. Chromosome analysis is an important tool for the classification of many hematologic disorders. Most leukemias display numerical chromosome

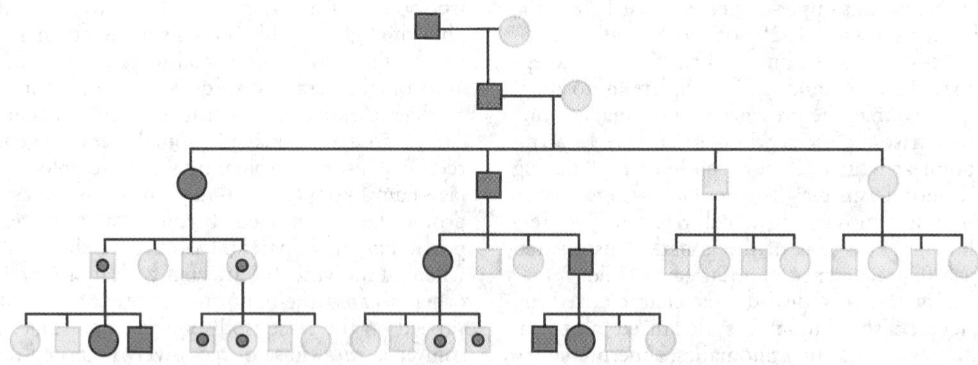

Figure 81-18. In pedigrees suggestive of maternal imprinting, phenotypic effects occur only when the gene is transmitted from the father but not when transmitted from the mother. Equal numbers of males and females are affected and not affected phenotypically in each generation. A non-manifesting transmitter gives a clue to the sex of the parent who passes the expressed genetic information; in other words, in maternal imprinting, there are "skipped" non-manifesting males.

abnormalities, structural rearrangements (mainly translocations), or both (see Chapter 495). Many of the chromosomal abnormalities are nonrandom and have been shown to be useful in diagnosing the leukemia subtype and predicting treatment outcome. This has been especially true in the case of acute lymphoblastic leukemia (ALL).

PRENATAL DIAGNOSIS. Prenatal diagnosis is indicated when there is a familial, maternal, or fetal condition that represents an increased risk for malformation, chromosome abnormality, or genetic disorder. Advanced maternal age (≥35), which is associated with an increased risk for aneuploidies, is the most common reason for prenatal diagnosis. Chromosome analysis and genetic counseling are also warranted in the event of (1) an abnormal screening result; (2) a chromosome abnormality in a previous offspring, parent, or close relative; (3) a previous offspring with multiple congenital anomalies on whom no chromosome study was obtained; (4) the need for fetal sex determination in pregnancies at risk for serious X-linked disorders for which specific prenatal diagnostic tests are not available (see Chapter 83).

Prenatal diagnosis using cell or tissue samples for chromosomal, biochemical, or molecular genetic studies may be performed using a number of techniques, including transabdominal amniocentesis, chorionic villus sampling (CVS), fetal blood sampling, and preimplantation genetic diagnosis (PGD). In addition, fetal cells and free fetal DNA have been detected in the mother's circulation and can aid in the prenatal diagnosis of fetal conditions (see Chapter 96).

Alfirevic Z, Neilson JP: Antenatal screening for Down's syndrome. *BMJ* 2004;329:811–812.

Antonarakis SE, Lyle R, Dermitzakis ET, et al: Chromosome 21 and Down syndrome: From genomics to pathophysiology. *Nat Rev Genet* 2004;5:725–738.

Bandyopadhyay R, Heller A, Knox-DuBois C, et al: Parental origin and timing of de novo Robertsonian translocation formation. *Am J Hum Genet* 2002;71:1456–1462.

Bejjani BA, Saleki R, Ballif BC, et al: Use of targeted array-based CGH for the clinical diagnosis of chromosomal imbalance: Is less more? *Am J Med Genet* 2005;134A:259–267.

Bondy CA, Van PL, Bakalov VK, et al: Prolongation of the cardiac QTc interval in Turner syndrome. *Medicine* 2006;85:75–81.

Caine A, Maltby AE, Parkin CA, et al: Prenatal detection of Down's syndrome by rapid aneuploidy testing for chromosomes 13, 18, and 21 by FISH or PCR without a full karyotype: A cytogenetic risk assessment. *Lancet* 2005;366:123–128.

Carrel AL, Moerchen V, Myers SE, et al: Growth hormone improves mobility and body composition in infants and toddlers with Prader-Willi syndrome. *J Pediatr* 2004;145:744–749.

Cicero S, Bindra R, Rembouskos G, et al: Integrated ultrasound and biochemical screening for trisomy 21 using fetal nuchal translucency, absent fetal nasal bone, free β-hCG and PAPP-A at 11 to 14 weeks. *Prenat Diagn* 2003;23:306–310.

Crolla JA, Youings SA, Ennis S, et al: Supernumerary marker chromosomes in man: Parental origin, mosaicism and maternal age revisited. *Eur J Hum Genet* 2005;13:154–160.

Cunniff C; American Academy of Pediatricians Committee on Genetics: Prenatal screening and diagnosis for pediatricians. *Pediatrics* 2004;114:889–894.

De Vries BBA, Lees M, Knight SJ, et al: Clinical studies of submicroscopic subtelomeric rearrangements: A checklist. *J Med Genet* 2001;38:145–150.

Douglas SD: Down syndrome: Immunologic and epidemiologic associations—Enigmas remain. *J Pediatr* 2005;147:723–725.

Dyken ME, Lin-Dyken DC, Poulton S, et al: Prospective polysomnographic analysis of obstructive sleep apnea in Down syndrome. *Arch Pediatr Adolesc Med* 2003;157:655–660.

Garrison MM, Jeffries H, Christakis DA: Risk of death for children with Down syndrome and sepsis. *J Pediatr* 2005;147:748–752.

Gibson PA, Newton RW, Selby K, et al: Longitudinal study of thyroid function in Down's syndrome in the first two decades. *Arch Dis Child* 2005;90:574–578.

Gicquel C, Rossignol S, Cabrol S, et al: Epimutation of the telomeric imprinting center region on chromosome 11p15 in Silver-Russell syndrome. *Nat Genet* 2005;37:1003–1007.

Heffner LJ: Advanced maternal age—How old is too old? *N Engl J Med* 2004;351:1927–1929.

Jacquemont S, Hagerman RJ, Hagerman PJ, Leehey MA: Fragile-X syndrome and fragile X associated tremor/ataxia syndrome: two faces of FMRI. *Lancet Neurol* 2007;6:45–55.

Kleefstra T, Yntema HG, Nillesen WM, et al: *MECP2* analysis in mentally retarded patients: Implications for routine DNA diagnostics. *Eur J Hum Genet* 2004;12:24–28.

Lanfranco F, Kamischke A, Zitzmann M, et al: Klinefelter's syndrome. *Lancet* 2004;364:273–283.

Malone FD, Canick JA, Ball RH, et al: First-trimester or second-trimester screening, or both, for Down's syndrome. *N Engl J Med* 2005;353:2001–2010.

Massa G, Verlinde F, De Schepper J, et al: Trends in age at diagnosis of Turner syndrome. *Arch Dis Child* 2005;90:267–268.

Mazzanti L, Cicognani A, Baldazzi L, et al: Gonadoblastoma in Turner syndrome and Y-chromosome-derived material. *Am J Med Genet* 2005;135A:150–154.

Neilson JP: Optimising prenatal diagnosis of Down's syndrome. *BMJ* 2006;332:433–434.

Rappold GA, Shanske A, Saenger P: All shook up by SHOX deficiency. *J Pediatr* 2005;147:422–424.

Rio M, Molinari F, Heuertz S, et al: Automated fluorescent genotyping detects 10% of cryptic subtelomeric rearrangements in idiopathic syndromic mental retardation. *J Med Genet* 2002;39:266–270.

Robin NH, Shprintzen RJ: Defining the clinical spectrum of deletion 22q11.2. *J Pediatr* 2005;147:90–96.

Roizen NJ, Patterson D: Down's syndrome. *Lancet* 2003;361:1281–1288.

Schubbert S, Zenker M, Rowe SL, et al: Germline *KRAS* mutations cause Noonan syndrome. *Nat Genet* 2006;38:331–336.

Schwartz S, Graf MD: Microdeletion syndromes: Characteristics and diagnosis. *Methods Mol Biol* 2002;204:275–290.

Sybert VP, McCauley E: Turner's syndrome. *N Engl J Med* 2004;351:1227–1238.

Tartaglia M, Pennacchio LA, Zhao C, et al: Gain-of-function SOSI mutations cause a distinctive form of Noonan syndrome. *Nat Genetics* 2007;39:75–79.

Vissers LELM, van Ravenswaaji CMA, Admiraal R, et al: Mutations in a new member of the chromodomain gene family cause CHARGE syndrome. *Nat Genet* 2004;36:955–957.

Walter S, Sandig K, Hinkel GK, et al: Subtelomere FISH in 50 children with mental retardation and minor anomalies, identified by a checklist, selects 10 rearrangements including a de novo balanced translocation of chromosomes 17p13.3 and 20q13.33. *Am J Med Genet* 2004;128A:364–373.

Wapner R, Thom E, Simpson JL, et al: First-trimester screening for trisomies 21 and 18. *N Engl J Med* 2003;349:1405–1412.

Warburton D, Dallaire L, Thangavelu M, et al: Trisomy recurrence: A reconsideration based on North American data. *Am J Hum Genet* 2004;75:376–385.

Yagi H, Furutani Y, Hamada H, et al: Role of *TBX1* in human del22q11.2 syndrome. *Lancet* 2003;362:1366–1373.

Youings S, Ellis K, Ennis S, et al: A study of reciprocal translocations and inversions detected by light microscopy with special reference to origin, segregation, and recurrent abnormalities. *Am J Med Genet* 2004;126A:46–60.

Zenker M, Gernot Buheitel G, Rauch R, et al: Genotype-phenotype correlations in Noonan syndrome. *J Pediatr* 2004;144:368–374.

Chapter 82 ■ Genetics of Common Disorders

Helen N. Lyon and Bruce R. Korf

Genetic studies are useful in diagnosing and treating rare pediatric conditions, often alleviating suffering, extending life, and in the case of neonatal metabolic screening, preventing injury before symptoms develop. Genetic studies may also identify the causes of more common diseases such as asthma and obesity. An understanding of the complex and potentially multiple pathways leading to disease is crucial to the development of appropriate prevention strategies (including screening of presymptomatic parents), as well as effective and specific therapies.

Common pediatric diseases are often multifactorial, with the combination of many genes and environmental factors triggering a complex sequence of events leading to disease. Each individual has variations in his or her set of genes; the interactions of the individual's gene variants with each other and with the environment determine susceptibility to disease. The complexity in the combination of factors increases the challenge of finding genetic variants that cause disease. Genetic tools include the completed human genome sequence, public databases of genetic variants, and the human haplotype map. The incorporation of these tools into large well-designed population studies is the field of **genetic epidemiology.**

82.1 • Major Genetic Approaches to the Study of Common Pediatric Disorders

A model for the genetic contribution to health is shown in Figure 82-1. Genetic liability is present from conception in all persons. Sometimes this liability is predominant and results in a single-gene disorder such as cystic fibrosis or sickle cell anemia. In most the liability is latent at birth but over time contributes to the emergence of specific medical conditions, particularly upon exposure to environmental factors. The goal in medical genetics is to identify the genetic factors in the hope of preventing the occurrence of disease, either by avoiding inciting environmental factors or by instituting treatments that reduce risk. For individuals who cross the threshold of disease, the goal is to better understand the pathogenesis in the hope that this will suggest better approaches to treatment.

A starting point in the genetic analysis of a complex trait is to obtain evidence in support of a genetic contribution and to estimate the relative strength of genetic and environmental factors (Fig. 82-2). This is done by determining whether a trait clusters in families and is seen among related individuals more often than in the general population. Possible inheritance models are delineated by such **segregation analyses.** The relative strength of genetic and nongenetic risk factors can be estimated by variance components analysis, and the amount of variability of a trait that is due to inherited factors is termed the **heritability** of a trait. Chromosomal regions with genes that may contribute to disease susceptibility can be located with **linkage mapping,** which locates regions of DNA that are inherited in families with the specific disease. Genetic **association studies** seek to determine relative risk of disease in individuals with specific genetic variants. Detection of the modest effect of each variant and interactions with environmental factors requires well-powered studies.

Both linkage mapping and association studies require markers along the DNA that can be ascertained, or **genotyped,** with large-scale laboratory techniques. Markers that are typically used are in the form of microsatellites and **single-nucleotide polymorphisms** (SNPs) [Fig. 82-3]. While humans all have the same genetic material, every person's genome is slightly different. A comparison of any two copies of the same region of genome will reveal that about one in every 1,200 bases will be different, usually in the form of a SNP. Most SNPs identified by comparing two chromosomes are common and are essentially the equivalent of genetic dialect, or random differences in coding with no significance or functional consequence. A few of these polymorphisms will alter the biologic function of a gene, either by affecting the structure of the protein or by altering the location, amount, or time at which the protein is made. Some of these functional alterations may affect susceptibility to disease.

Outcomes in genetic studies are clinical **phenotypes** and can be a clinical diagnosis of a disease or a discrete measurement or trait related to disease. A phenotype can be measured by the presence or absence of a disease as a qualitative trait, or by using a marker of disease, such as pulmonary function tests in asthma or body mass index in obesity, as a quantitative trait. A homogeneous phenotype is ideal to avoid conflicting results from the study of a trait that has two or more etiologies. **Genetic heterogeneity** refers to a trait resulting from more than one genetic mechanism. The development of a trait or disease from a different mechanism results in a **phenocopy,** the occurrence of which would diminish the detectibility of the responsible gene. A particular gene variant may not cause the same outcome, and this **pleiotropic effect** of each variant depends on other genetic effects and environmental exposures.

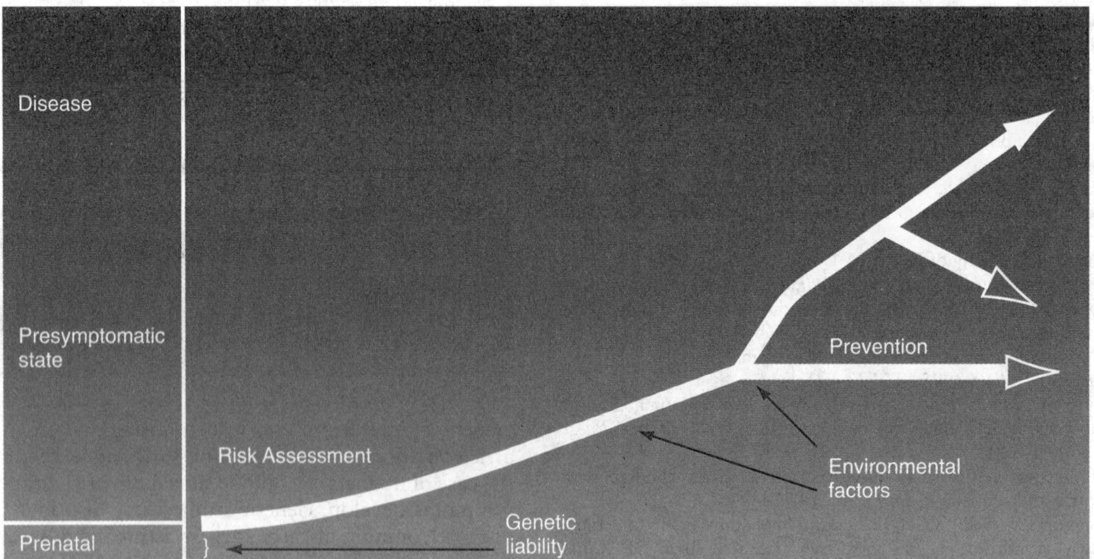

Figure 82-1. Model for the influence of genetics on health. Everyone inherits some genetic liability for disease risk, but for multifactorial disorders this is insufficient to produce disease on its own. Over time, exposure to environmental factors leads from a presymptomatic to a disease state. Identification of the genes responsible for risk can lead to prevention strategies or treatments.

$$V_P = \underbrace{V_A + V_D}_{\text{Genetic variance}} + \underbrace{V_E + V_I}_{\text{Environmental variance}} + COV_{GE} + \underbrace{V_M}_{\text{Measurement variance}}$$

V_A=Additive genetic variance
V_D=Deviation due to dominance and epistasis
V_E=Environmental variance
V_I=Interaction variance
CoV_{GE}=Covariance of genetics and environment

Relationship	Heritability
Monozygotic twins	$h^2=r$
Sib-sib or Dizygotic twins	$h^2=2r$
One parent–One offspring	$h^2=2r$
Midparent–Offspring	$h^2=r/\sqrt{0.5}=r/0.7071$
First cousins	$h^2=8r$
Uncle–Nephew	$h2=4r$

Figure 82-2. Heritability concept. Phenotypic variance can be partitioned into genetic variance, environmental variance, the covariance between the two, and measurement variance. Genetic variance can be further partitioned into additive affects and gene-gene interactions (epistasis); environmental variance can likewise be partitioned into additive and interactive effects. Heritability is defined as the proportion of phenotypic variance accounted for by genetic variance. One can estimate heritability in the narrow sense from correlation of a quantitative trait between relatives, as shown in the table.

There are many factors that may complicate segregation and heritability studies. Many diseases that are found to track in families may appear to skip a generation; a person could inherit an **allele** (inherited unit, DNA segment, or chromosome) and not show any sign of the disease, a phenomenon called **incomplete penetrance.** Some diseases manifest signs only later in life, while others become less obvious as the child grows older; study participants could be misclassified as unaffected who actually have the disease-producing gene. Many common diseases manifest with varying severity in families, and this **variable expressivity** is another factor that could cause misclassification of people.

To maximize the ability to detect a gene with disease association, environmental exposures need to be measured and accounted for in a population. The interaction between genes and the environment is called **epistasis.** Epistatic effects could affect the expressivity of a trait as well as the penetrance. An example of this is G6PD deficiency. An individual could carry the altered gene and be deficient in the enzyme, yet would never have a hemolytic crisis unless exposed to an oxidative stress. People with inherited propensity for malignant melanoma who live in darker geographic regions or limit their sun exposure may never express the phenotype of cancer. Asthma in some susceptible people may develop only after exposure to certain antigens or pollutants.

Linkage Mapping. Linkage studies were used in the past to isolate genes that cause rare genetic syndromes; modified methods have been used to identify chromosomal regions linked to more common diseases. Linkage studies involve tagging segments of a person's genome with markers that allow identification of seg-

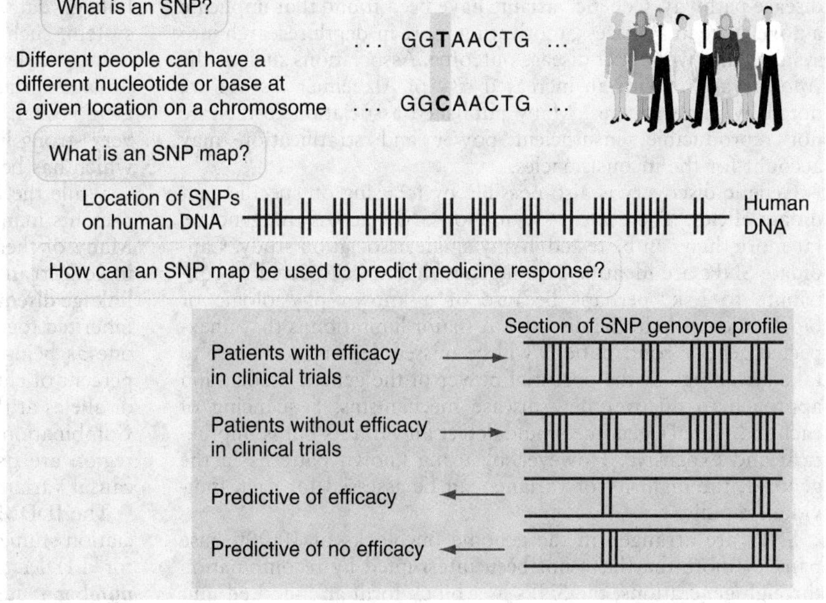

Figure 82-3. Different combinations of single nucleotide polymorphisms (SNPs) are found in different individuals. The locations of these SNPs can be pinpointed on maps of human genes. Subsequently, they can be used to create profiles that are associated with difference in response to a drug, such as efficacy and nonefficacy. (Adapted from Roses A: Pharmacogenetics and the practice of medicine. *Nature* 2000;405:857–865. Copyright 2000. Reprinted by permission for Macmillan Publishers Ltd.)

ments that have been inherited through the family along with disease. The markers are typically **microsatellites** or **SNPs** that define which type of an allele any person carries. The type of an allele is referred to as a **genotype.** Linkage analyses of common diseases have shown inconsistent results. Factors such as heterogeneity, pleiotropy, variable expressivity, and reduced penetrance in addition to variability in environmental exposures weaken the power of linkage studies in complex traits.

Genetic Association. For multifactorial common diseases, association analyses may be better suited to detect small effects than linkage studies. Genetic association studies are similar to traditional disease association studies, with a person's genotype being used as a predictor of a disease or trait. The goal is to identify the actual alleles at a locus that confer the risk for a disease. Three basic designs are used: (1) a case-control design, with a comparison of the frequency of an allele in affected people compared with unaffected people, (2) a population-based study, in which an increase in a quantitative trait or continuous measurement is correlated with genotype, and (3) a family-based test, in which transmission of alleles to affected and unaffected offspring is tested. This last type of analysis, known as a **transmission disequilibrium test** (TDT), looks for an allele that is transmitted to an affected person more often than the other allele. If there is no association between an allele and disease, the transmission of each allele should be equal, with each having a 50/50 ratio. If an allele confers risk of disease, the transmission ratio will be distorted, with one allele showing higher transmission to affected children.The success of all 3 types of association analysis depends on the design of a well-powered study, with enough subjects, and an accurately measured trait to avoid misclassification due to variable expressivity or reduced penetrance and to minimize the effect of genetic heterogeneity and pleiotropy. In large population-based studies, confounding by ethnicity or population stratification could distort results. Some genetic variants are more frequently found in people from a particular ethnic group, which could cause an apparent association of a variant with a disease, when the disease rate happens to be higher in that group. This association would not be a true association between an allele and a disease, as the association would be confounded by ethnicity, which is often referred to as **population stratification**. The family-based tests using the TDT are immune to population stratification because the association is not with a specific allele, but with a distortion of transmission in affected people within a family.

Association studies should be a powerful tool to find genetic variation that confers risk to an individual; the effect of any one genetic variant will be a very small contribution to the complex disease pathway. Genetic variants have been found that implicate a novel gene in a process, motivating more in-depth research into systems that will affect disease outcome. Associations such as the *ApoE4* variant with an increased risk of Alzheimer disease are noted by many studies. Many published association results are not reproducible; insufficient power and stratification may account for the inconsistencies.

Genetic discovery is also possible by focusing on specific **candidate alleles.** There are 5–10 million SNPs across the genome, far more than can be tested in any single association study. Candidate SNPs are identified from genes that are suspected to contribute to risk, perhaps because of a known physiologic or biochemical role in the disorder. A major limitation is that unexpected genetic contributions will be missed, leading to failure to take advantage of the potential power of the genetic association approach to uncover new disease mechanisms. Sequencing of each individual's genome would detect all variants but is impractical and expensive. However, by using known patterns in the genome, the majority of variants can be assessed for each individual rapidly.

SNPs are arranged in the genome on blocks of 10,000 base pairs or more that have not been interrupted by recombination through generations; the SNPs in a block form an inherited unit called a haplotype. The **HapMap project** has defined these blocks in four populations around the world, providing measurements of the relationship between SNPs in the blocks. This allows for the selection of SNPs that are proxies or "tags" for a haplotype block. Genotyping this smaller subset of SNPs captures most of the common variation in a region with far fewer genotypes. Current estimates show that 500,000 SNPs are sufficient to represent about 90% of variation in the human genome. The HapMap is available as a public database, a valuable resource for the design of association studies that can be tailored to specific populations.

82.2 • Current Understanding of Genetics of Common Disorders in Children

The impact of genetic studies of common pediatric disease is being realized. Prevention and intervention may soon be possible using valid genetic association results to identify children at risk. Three examples of diseases under intense scrutiny for genetic risk factors are type I diabetes mellitus, asthma, and obesity.

TYPE 1 DIABETES MELLITUS

Type 1 diabetes mellitus (T1DM) is the best characterized of the polygenic, multifactorial pediatric illnesses (see Chapter 590). It is a common disease with a well-defined phenotype and evidence of environmental and genetic components. Linkage studies in families with an affected child yield many loci that appear to be consistently linked to increased risk for T1DM. A few gene variants have been found that confer risk for disease, and some environmental factors have been identified including viral infections triggering the autoimmune process. While there are rare syndromic forms, such as **Wolfram syndrome,** resulting from known monogenic mutations, most children diagnosed with T1DM have a currently unidentified etiology.

Heritability estimates for T1DM are estimated between 66% and 72%, with twin concordance of 30% to 50%. Although these studies may be confounded by shared environment, it is evident that, at least in part, there is an inherited component to T1DM risk. The relative risk to a child in the general population is 0.4%, whereas for the sibling of a child with diabetes it is 15 times higher at 6%. The **Type 1 Diabetes Consortium** *(www.t1dgc.org)* has undertaken a meta-analysis of all of the linkage data. They have also devised a uniform nomenclature system, such that promising linkage regions have been assigned numbers, designated IDDM 1–18. Many early studies detected linkage at the MHC locus on chromosome 6p21 within the HLA gene region. A meta-analysis of these linkage studies showed a very strong linkage signal with a LOD score of 65 at this locus, which has been designated IDDM1.

While the HLA/IDDM1 locus has been studied extensively, it presents many challenges in detecting causal genetic alterations. Many of the genes in the region have similar functions and act in concert in the Th2 immune system. The region also has high **linkage disequilibrium** (LD); many of the proposed risk alleles are inherited together, making it difficult to isolate a signal from any one as being directly responsible for the increased risk. Thirty percent of children diagnosed with T1DM have the combination of alleles at this locus that code for HLA-DQ2/DQ8 (genotype). Combinations of alleles (haplotypes) at two loci in the HLA region are risk alleles; none of these has pinpointed distinctive causal variants.

The IDDM2 locus encompasses the insulin *(INS)* gene. Association studies identified variants in this gene that conferred risk for T1DM. A repeat region (known as a **VNTR,** or **variable number tandem repeat**) near the *INS* gene has been associated with diabetes risk, with a longer repeat correlated with increased risk for T1DM. The mechanism of gene dysfunction due to the repeat is unknown, and it is very likely that it is in LD with another variant that does alter function or interaction to predispose an individual to diabetes.

A variant of the *CTLA4* gene is found in the coding region of this gene, suggesting that a functional change in the protein could cause susceptibility. Additional studies found a variant in the 3′ untranslated region in LD with the coding SNP to be an even better predictor of risk. This SNP was in the promoter region of the gene, which could also suggest a functional role in transcription regulation. The mechanism by which alterations in this gene increases susceptibility to T1DM requires a thorough search for regulatory genes that may interact with the promoter region.

OBESITY

Childhood obesity in the United States is increasing at an alarming rate (see Chapter 44). Obesity is a multifactorial disease, with many of the contributing factors still unknown. It is likely a heterogeneous phenotype resulting from dysfunction in many different pathways. Contributing factors may include a modern environment of plentiful calories and low physical activity, which combined with inherited risk genes results in obesity.

Previously, childhood obesity was rare enough that a severely obese child warranted consideration of rare syndromes such as POMC (proopiomelanocortin) deficiency, Prader-Willi syndrome, and Bardet-Biedl syndrome. A few studies have suggested that childhood obesity is due to rare genes that act as a recessive trait and can explain a larger fraction of the variation in body mass. Melanocortin 4 receptor (*MC4R*) is an example of a gene with recessive mutations that are found in 3% of children with severe early-onset obesity. Polymorphisms in *MC4R* have not been found to be associated with more common polygenic obesity observed in the general population.

Common forms of obesity show a complex pattern of family segregation. Family studies and twin studies yield estimates of heritability ranging from 30% to 70%, with the typical estimate at 50%, meaning that about half of the variation in body mass within a population is due to inherited factors.

Body mass index (BMI) is a phenotype obtained in many cohort collections. Whole genome linkage studies have shown evidence of linkage regions on every chromosome, but a number of regions have been detected in several studies that hold promise for genes associated with common obesity. Linkage studies in children have resulted in the discovery of rare mutations in genes such as leptin and melanocortin that account for some of the severe early-onset obesity; these genes have not been consistently found to contribute to common obesity.

Studies have also focused on candidate genes thought to be involved in obesity-related pathways, such as insulin signaling, fatty acid oxidation, and appetite regulation. More than 100 genetic associations with obesity have been reported in positional and functional candidate genes, yet very few of these findings are reproducible; none have led to a novel prevention or therapy for common obesity. Haplotypes in the **ghrelin receptor,** ***ENPP1*****,** **leptin,** and **insulin signaling protein 2** are reported to be associated with common obesity, yet only the *INSIG2* finding has been replicated.

ASTHMA

Asthma is a common childhood condition; it is increasing at an epidemic rate (see Chapter 143). In the United States, asthma is more prevalent in Hispanic and African-American children. Atopy and asthma are heritable. Asthma is a heterogeneous diagnosis and is defined as reversible airway narrowing with obstruction associated with small airway bronchospasm and inflammation. It may result from dysregulation of the Th2 inflammatory cells with higher serum levels of IgE. Children with two parents affected with asthma have a 60% increased risk of atopy. The odds of asthma diagnosis in children aged 3 to 6 yr increase by 2-fold in children with two rather than one affected parent. Twin studies in Sweden and Finland have found asthma heritability estimates of 80%, with much higher concordance in monozygotic twins than in dizygotic twins. Children of asthmatic mothers have a higher risk than those with asthmatic fathers, suggesting the possibility of in utero mechanisms influencing risk of developing disease.

In utero exposure to tobacco and maternal asthma are associated with increased IgE levels in infants and a higher rate of asthma. Early pulmonary infections with respiratory syncytial virus (RSV), rhinovirus, and *Chlamydia* pneumonia have also been implicated in the development of asthma. Associations have been demonstrated with environmental exposures such as endotoxin, cockroach and dust mite antigens, and diesel particles. The lack of exposure to a different set of pathogens has been shown to increase immune deregulation and asthma, as proposed in the **hygiene hypothesis.** Exposure to parasites in early childhood has been correlated with protection against asthma and atopy.

Asthma has quantifiable markers such as pulmonary function tests. Linkage studies of asthma and its markers have demonstrated some overlap of DNA regions on chromosomes 5q, 6p, 12q, and 13q. Linkage to 20p13 has motivated association studies in the gene *ADAM33* (a member of the a disintegrin and metalloprotease domain family); this finding has not been reproducible. Interleukins 4 and 13 are associated with increased IgE levels, while IL-4 and -10 are associated with airway resistance as measured by FEV_1. Increased TNFα levels in bronchial secretions led to a study of polymorphisms in that gene with levels and asthma severity.

In childhood asthma there is great variability in response to medications. Large cohort studies in children (such as the Childhood Asthma Management Program and the Tucson Children's Respiratory Study) have provided evidence of subgroups of children with asthma that differ in the natural history of the disease as well as in drug response. Children vary greatly in response to leukotriene inhibitors and corticosteroids, another heterogeneous aspect of the asthma phenotype. Variation in the β_2-receptor has been shown to influence response to β-agonist therapy with one particular genotype in the receptor causing resistance to the stabilizing and dilating effects of the drug.

SUMMARY. It is clear that there is much yet to be discovered about the common diseases affecting most children. Successful therapies and prevention strategies will depend on the dissection of complex pathways in which many small changes and environmental interactions can act in order for a person to encounter a threshold for disease development. Gene therapy techniques could be applied as treatment focused on modifying the actual genetic risk factor, but will require identification of specific targets in disease pathways. Efforts in the past to supply a gene to take the place of a mutated gene had some success, but were limited by host rejection of the vectors. New discoveries promise more precise modulation of gene products using techniques such as RNAi (RNA interference) with synthetic RNA molecules targetted for specific genes.

The new tools available to researchers have allowed detection of a number of novel genes and pathways for common diseases, and the advent of whole genome association studies promises an acceleration of these results. Interactions between verifiable risk alleles and environmental factors as well as epistatic interactions will be increasingly possible. Whole genome association studies will provide vast amounts of data, requiring new analytic tools to dissect the true effects and interactions. Whole genome association testing promises to highlight many genetic variants that, in relation to each other and environmental factors will elucidate the pathways leading to common disease, leading to treatment and ultimately prevention of disease.

Altshuler D, et al: A haplotype map of the human genome. *Nature* 2005;437:1299–1320.

Balicki D, Beutler E: Gene therapy of human disease. *Medicine* 2002;81:69–86.

Bracken MB, Belanger K, Cookson WO, et al: Genetic and perinatal risk factors for asthma onset and severity: A review and theoretical analysis. *Epidemiol Rev* 2002;24,176–189.

Carroll W: Asthma genetics: Pitfalls and triumphs. *Paediatr Respir Rev* 2005;6:68–74.

Cavazzana-Calvo M, Fischer A: Efficacy of gene therapy for SCID is being confirmed. *Lancet* 2004;364:2155–2156.

Escolar DM, Scacheri CG: Pharmacologic and genetic therapy for childhood muscular dystrophies. *Curr Neurol Neurosci Rep* 2001;1:168–174.

Ferry N, Heard JM: Liver-directed gene transfer vectors. *Hum Gene Ther* 1998;9:1975–1981.

Fischer A: Gene therapy of lymphoid primary immunodeficiencies. *Curr Opin Pediatr* 2000;12:557–562.

Grimm D, Kay MA: Therapeutic short hairpin RNA expression in the liver: viral targets and vectors. *Gene Therapy* 2006;13(6):563–575.

High KA: Gene transfer as an approach to treating hemophilia. *Circ Res* 2001;88:137–144.

Hirschhorn JN: Genetic epidemiology of type 1 diabetes. *Pediatr Diabetes* 2003;4:87–100.

Kaiser J: Seeking the cause of induced leukemias in X-SCID trial. *Science* 2003;299:495.

Kozarsky KF: Gene therapy for cardiovascular disease. *Curr Opin Pharmacol* 2001;1:197–202.

Kwon HL, Belanger K, Bracken MB: Effect of pregnancy and stage of pregnancy on asthma severity: A systematic review. *Am J Obstet Gynecol* 2004;190:1201–1210.

Lyon HN, Hirschhorn JN: Genetics of common forms of obesity: A brief overview. *Am J Clin Nutr* 2005;82:215S–217S.

Liu F, Huang L: Development of non-viral vectors for systemic gene delivery. *J Control Release* 2002;18:259–266.

McCormick F: Cancer gene therapy: Fringe or cutting edge? *Nat Rev Cancer* 2001;1:130–141.

Onengut-Gumuscu S, Concannon P: The genetics of type 1 diabetes: Lessons learned and future challenges. *J Autoimmun* 2005;25:S34–S39.

Richardson PD, Kren BT, Steer CJ: Gene repair in the new age of gene therapy. *Hepatology* 2002;35:512–518.

Schmidt-Wolf GD, Schmidt-Wolf IG: Immunomodulatory gene therapy for haematological malignancies. *Br J Haematol* 2002;117:23–32.

Thomas CE, Ehrhardt A, Kay MA: Progress and problems with the use of viral vectors for gene therapy. *Nature Review Genetics* 2003;4(5):346–358.

Weiss ST, Raby BA: Asthma genetics 2003. *Hum Mol Genet* 2004;13(Spec No 1):R83–R89.

Yoon JW, Jun HS: Recent advances in insulin gene therapy for type 1 diabetes. *Trends Mol Med* 2002;8:62–68.

Chapter 83 ■ Integration of Genetics into Pediatric Practice

Bruce R. Korf

GENETIC TESTING. Genetic testing involves analysis of genetic material to obtain information related to an individual's health status using either chromosomal analysis (see Chapter 81) or DNA-based testing.

DIAGNOSTIC TESTING. Diagnostic genetic testing helps explain a set of signs and/or symptoms of a disease. The list of disorders for which specific genetic tests is available is extensive. The website *www.genetests.org* provides a database of available tests.

Single-gene disorders can be tested by two approaches: linkage analysis and direct mutation analysis. The former is used if the responsible gene is mapped but not yet identified, or if it is impractical to find specific mutations, usually because of the large size and larger number of different mutations in some genes. Direct mutation analysis is preferred and is facilitated as the human genome sequence is further elucidated and technologies for mutation analysis improve.

Linkage testing involves tracking a genetic trait through a family using closely linked polymorphic markers as a surrogate for the trait (Fig. 83-1). It requires testing an extended family and is vulnerable to several pitfalls, such as genetic recombination, genetic heterogeneity, and incorrect diagnosis in the proband. **Genetic recombination** occurs between any pair of loci, the frequency being proportional to the distance between them. This problem can be ameliorated by the use of very closely linked markers, and, if possible, using markers that flank the specific gene. **Genetic heterogeneity** can be problematic for a linkage-based test if there are multiple distinct loci that can cause the same phenotype, resulting in risk that the locus tested is not the one responsible for disease in the family. **Incorrect proband diagnosis** also leads to tracking the wrong gene. Linkage testing remains useful for several genetic conditions. It is critically important that genetic counseling be provided to the family to explain the complexities of interpretation of test results.

Direct mutation testing avoids the pitfalls of linkage testing by detection of the specific gene mutation. The specific approach used is customized to the biology of the gene being tested. In some disorders one or a few distinct mutations occur in all affected individuals. This is the case in sickle cell anemia, in which the same single base substitution occurs in everyone with the disorder. In other conditions, there may be many possible mutations that account for the disorder in different individuals. Cystic fibrosis is an example: over a thousand distinct mutations have been found in the *CFTR* gene. Mutation analysis will be challenging because no single technique will detect all possible mutations.

Direct mutation tests are interpreted in light of 3 factors: analytical validity, clinical validity, and clinical utility. **Analytical validity** is test accuracy—does the test correctly detect the presence or absence of mutation? Most genetic tests have a very high analytical validity, assuming that human error such as sample mix-up has not occurred. Such errors are possible, and unlike

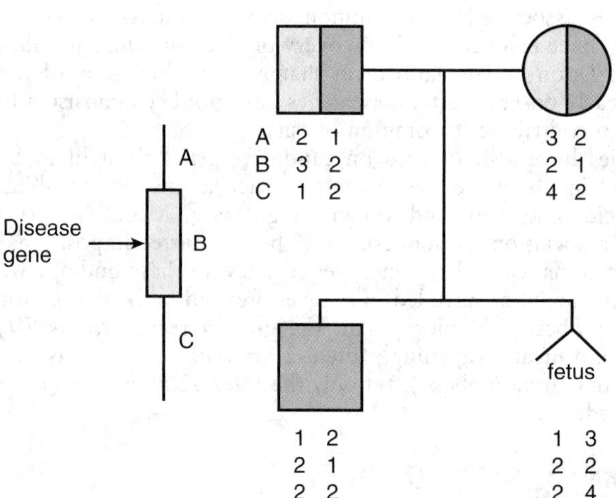

Figure 83-1. Use of linkage analysis in prenatal diagnosis of an autosomal recessive disorder. Both parents are carriers, and they have one affected son. The numbers below the symbols indicate alleles at 3 polymorphic loci: A, B, and C. Locus B resides within the disease gene. The affected son inherited the 1-2-2 chromosome from his father and the 2-1-2 chromosome from his mother. The fetus has inherited the same chromosome from the father, but the 3-2-4 chromosome from the mother, and therefore is most likely to be a carrier.

most medical tests, a genetic test is unlikely to be repeated, since it is assumed that the result will not change over time. Therefore, human errors may go undetected for long periods.

Clinical validity is the degree to which the test correctly predicts presence or absence of disease. Both false-positive and false-negative tests results may occur. **False-positive results** are more likely for predictive tests than for diagnostic tests. An important contributing factor is **non-penetrance;** an individual with an at-risk genotype may not express the condition. Another factor is the finding of a genetic variant of unknown significance. Detection of a base sequence variation in an affected individual does not prove that it is the cause of the individual's disorder. Various lines of evidence are used to establish pathogenicity. These include: finding the variant only in affected individuals; inferring that the variant alters the function of the gene product; determining whether the amino acid altered by the mutation is conserved in evolution; and determining whether the mutation segregates with disease in the family. In some cases, it may not be possible to be sure whether the variant is pathogenic or incidental.

False-negative results reflect an inability to detect a mutation in an affected individual. This occurs principally in disorders where genetic heterogeneity (allelic or gene locus heterogeneity) is the rule. It is difficult to detect all possible mutations within a gene, since mutations can be varied both in location within the gene and type of mutation. Direct sequencing will miss gene deletions or rearrangements, and mutations may be found within noncoding sequences such as introns or the promoter; a negative DNA test does not necessarily exclude a diagnosis.

Clinical utility is the degree to which the results of a test guide clinical management. For genetic testing, clinical utility includes establishing a diagnosis that obviates the need for additional workup or guiding surveillance or treatment. Test results may also be used as a basis for genetic counseling. There are some disorders for which genetic testing is possible but in which the test results do not add to the clinical assessment. If the diagnosis and genetic implications are already clear, it may not be necessary to pursue genetic testing.

PREDICTIVE TESTING. Predictive genetic testing involves performance of a test in an individual who is at risk of developing a genetic disorder (**presymptomatic**), usually on the basis of family history, yet does not manifest signs or symptoms. This is usually done for disorders that display age-dependent penetrance; the likelihood of manifesting signs and symptoms increases with age, as in cancer or Huntington disease.

A major caution with predictive testing is that presence of a gene mutation does not necessarily mean that the disease will develop. Many of the disorders with age-dependent penetrance display incomplete penetrance. An individual who inherits a mutation may never develop signs of the disorder. There is concern that a positive DNA test may result in stigmatization of an individual and may not as yet provide information that will guide medical management. Stigmatization might include psychological stress, but could also include discrimination, including denial of health, life, or disability insurance or employment (see Chapter 78). It is generally agreed that predictive genetic tests should be performed for children if the results of the test will benefit the medical management of the child. Otherwise, the test should be deferred until the child has grown up to the point of understanding the risks and benefits of testing and can provide informed consent. Individual states offer varying degrees of protection from discrimination on the basis of genetic testing; federal legislation has not yet passed through the U.S. Congress.

PREDISPOSITIONAL TESTING. It is expected that genetic tests may become available that will predict risk of disease. Common disorders are multifactorial in etiology; there may be many different genes that contribute to risk of any specific condition (see Chapter 82). Most of the genetic variants that have been found to correlate with risk of a common disease add small increments of relative risk, probably in most cases too little to guide management. It is possible, however, that further discovery of genes that contribute to common disorders will reveal examples of variants that convey more significant levels of risk. It is also possible that testing several genes together will provide more information about risk than any individual gene variant would confer. The rationale for predispositional testing is that the results would lead to strategies aimed at risk reduction. This might include avoidance of environmental exposures that would increase risk of disease, medical surveillance, or, in some cases, pharmacological treatment. The value of predispositional testing will need to be critically appraised through outcomes studies as these tests are developed.

PHARMACOGENETIC TESTING. Polymorphisms in drug metabolism genes may result in distinctive patterns of drug absorption, metabolism, excretion, or effectiveness (see Chapters 56 and 82). Knowledge of individual genotypes will guide pharmacological therapy, allowing customization of choice of drug and dosage to avoid toxicity and provide a therapeutic response.

83.1 • Genetic Counseling

Genetic counseling is a communication process in which the genetic contribution to health is explained, along with specific risks of transmission of a trait, and options to manage the condition and its inheritance (Table 83-1). The counselor is expected to present information in a neutral, non-directive manner and to provide support to the individual/family to cope with decisions that are made.

Genetic counseling has evolved from a model of care that was developed in the context of prenatal diagnosis and pediatrics (see Table 83-1). For prenatal diagnosis, the task is to assess risk to a couple of having a child with a genetic condition and advise the couple about options to manage that risk, including reproductive options such as artificial insemination and prenatal or preimplantation genetic diagnosis. In pediatrics, the task is to establish a diagnosis in a child, provide longitudinal care for the child, and advise the parents about risk of recurrence as well as options to deal with that risk.

The genetic counseling role has expanded, particularly with advances in understanding the genetics of adult-onset or common disorders. Genetic counseling has a major role in risk assessment for cancer, especially breast and ovarian cancer or colon cancer, for which well-defined genetic tests are available to assess risk to an individual.

TALKING TO FAMILIES. The type of information provided to a family depends on the urgency of the situation, the need to make decisions, and the need to collect additional information. There are 3 situations in which genetic counseling is particularly important.

The first is the **prenatal diagnosis** of a congenital anomaly or genetic disease. The need for information is urgent because a family must often decide whether to continue or to terminate a pregnancy. Risks to the mother must also be considered. The second type of situation occurs when a child is born with a life-threatening congenital anomaly or genetic disease. Decisions must be made immediately with regard to how much support should be provided for the child and whether certain types of therapy should be attempted. The third situation arises later in life when (1) a diagnosis with a genetic implication is made; (2) a couple is planning a family and there is a family history of a

TABLE 83-1. Indications for Genetic Counseling

Advanced parental age
Maternal age ≥35 yr
Paternal age ≥50 yr
Previous child with or family history of
Congenital abnormality
Dysmorphology
Mental retardation
Isolated birth defect
Metabolic disorder
Chromosome abnormality
Single-gene disorder
Adult-onset genetic disease (presymptomatic testing)
Cancer
Huntington disease
Consanguinity
Teratogen exposure (occupational, abuse)
Repeated pregnancy loss or infertility
Pregnancy screening abnormality
Maternal serum α-fetoprotein
Maternal triple screen or variant of this test
Fetal ultrasonography
Fetal karyotype
Heterozygote screening based on ethnic risk
Sickle cell anemia
Tay-Sachs, Canavan, Gaucher diseases
Thalassemias
Follow-up to abnormal neonatal genetic testing

genetic problem, including whether one member of a couple carries a translocation or is a carrier of an abnormal gene for an autosomal recessive or X-linked disorder; (3) an adolescent or young adult has a family history of an adult-onset genetic disorder (Huntington disease, breast cancer); (4) unusual features are present and a diagnosis is wanting or not possible; and (5) there is suspected exposure to a toxic substance or teratogen. It is often necessary to have several meetings with a family in this third category. Urgency is not as much of an issue as being sure that they have as much information and as many options as are available.

GENETIC COUNSELING. Providing accurate information to families requires (1) taking a careful family history and constructing a pedigree that lists the patient's relatives (including abortions, stillbirths, deceased individuals) with their sex, age, and state of health, up to and including third-degree relatives; (2) gathering information from hospital records about the affected individual (in some cases, about other family members); (3) documenting prenatal, pregnancy, and delivery histories; (4) reviewing the latest available medical, laboratory, and genetic information concerning the disorder; (5) careful physical examination of the affected individual (photographs, measurements) and of apparently unaffected individuals in the family; (6) establishing or confirming the diagnosis by the diagnostic tests available; (7) giving the family information about support groups; (8) providing new information to the family as it becomes available (a mechanism for updating needs to be established).

Counseling sessions must include the following information:

The Specific Condition or Conditions. If a specific diagnosis is made and confirmed, that should be discussed with the family and information provided in writing. However, often the disorder fits into a spectrum (1 of many types of arthrogryposis) or the diagnosis is clinical rather than laboratory based. In those situations, the family needs to understand the limits of present knowledge and that additional research will probably lead to better information in the future.

Knowledge of the Diagnosis of the Particular Condition. Although it is not always possible to make an exact diagnosis, having as accurate a diagnosis as possible is important. Estimates of recurrence risk for various family members depend on an accurate diagnosis. When a specific diagnosis cannot be made (as in many cases of multiple congenital anomalies), the various differential diagnoses should be discussed with the family and empirical information provided. If specific diagnostic tests are available, they should be discussed.

Natural History of the Condition. It is very important to discuss the natural history of the specific genetic disorder in the family. Affected individuals and their families will have questions regarding the prognosis and potential therapy that can be answered only with knowledge of the natural history. If there are other possible differential diagnoses, their natural history may also be discussed. If the disorder is associated with a spectrum of clinical outcomes or complications, the worst and best scenarios, as well as treatment and referral to the appropriate specialist, should be addressed.

Genetic Aspects of the Condition and Recurrence Risk. This information is important for the family because all family members need to be aware of their reproductive choices. The genetics of the disorder can be explained with visual aids (figures of chromosomes). It is important to provide accurate occurrence and recurrence risks for various members of the family, including unaffected individuals. If a definite diagnosis cannot be made, it is necessary to use empirical recurrence risks. Counseling should give the individuals the necessary information to understand the various options and let the patients make their own informed decisions regarding pregnancy, adoption, artificial insemination, prenatal diagnosis, screening, carrier detection, and termination of pregnancy. It may be necessary to have more than one counseling session.

Prenatal Diagnosis and Prevention. Many different methods of prenatal diagnosis are available, depending on the specific genetic disorder (see Chapter 96). The use of ultrasonography allows prenatal diagnosis of anatomic abnormalities such as congenital heart defects. Amniocentesis and chorionic villus sampling are used to obtain fetal tissue for analysis of chromosomal abnormalities, biochemical disorders, and DNA studies. Maternal blood or serum sampling is used for some types of screening. Fetal cells can be retrieved from the umbilical cord or from maternal blood for testing, although mothers may harbor cells from all previous pregnancies.

Therapies and Referral. A number of genetic disorders require the care of a specialist. Individuals with Turner syndrome usually need to be evaluated by an endocrinologist. Prevention of known complications is a priority. The psychologic adjustment of the family may require specific intervention.

Support Groups. A large number of community lay support groups have been formed to provide information and to fund research on specific genetic and nongenetic conditions. An important part of genetic counseling is to give information about these groups to individuals and to suggest a contact person for the families. Many groups have established websites with very helpful information.

Follow-up. Families should be encouraged to continue to ask questions and keep up with new information about the specific disorder. New developments often influence the diagnosis and therapy of specific genetic disorders. Lay support groups are a good source of new information.

Nondirective Counseling. Genetic counseling is usually nondirective; choices about reproduction are left to the family to decide what is right for them. The role of the counselor (physician, genetic counselor, nurse, medical geneticist) is to provide information in understandable terms and outline the range of options available.

83.2 • Management and Treatment of Genetic Disorders

Genetic conditions are often chronic disorders; few are amenable to curative therapies. Nevertheless, there are many management options available. All individuals/families should be provided information about the disorder, genetic counseling, anticipatory guidance, and appropriate medical surveillance. Surgical management is available for many conditions that are associated with congenital anomalies or predisposition to tumors. Resources available with patient information include the National Organization of Rare Disorders *(www.rarediseases.org)*, the Genetic Alliance *(www.geneticalliance.org)*, the National Library of Medicine *(www.nlm.nih.gov/medlineplus/geneticdisorders.html#specificconditions)*, and a large number of disease-specific sites. Specific medical therapies for genetic disorders can be classified into physiologic, pharmacologic, and replacement therapies.

PHYSIOLOGIC THERAPIES. Physiologic therapies attempt to ameliorate the phenotype of a genetic disorder by modification of the physiology of the affected individual. The underlying defect itself is not altered by treatment. Physiologic therapies are used in the treatment of **inborn errors of metabolism.** These include dietary manipulations, such as avoidance of phenylalanine for individuals with phenylketonuria; coenzyme supplementation for some patients with methylmalonicacidemia; provision of substrates to excrete ammonia for those with urea cycle disorders; bisphosphonate treatment for those with osteogenesis imperfecta to reduce bone fractures; and avoidance of cigarette smoking for individuals with α_1-antitrypsin deficiency. Physiologic treatments can be highly effective, but usually need to be maintained for a lifetime, given that they do not affect the underlying genetic disorder. Many of these treatments are most effective when begun early in life before irreversible damage has occurred, which is the rationale for newborn screening for inborn errors of metabolism.

PHARMACOLOGIC THERAPIES. Many physiologic therapies use pharmaceuticals (e.g., to remove ammonia in those with urea cycle disorders). Pharmacologic treatments directly target a defective cellular pathway that is altered by an abnormal or a missing gene product. There are relatively few such therapies. One example is the development of imatinib to treat chronic myelogenous leukemia (CML). CML is usually associated with a chromosome 9;22 translocation (the Philadelphia chromosome) that creates a fusion protein of BCR and the *Abl* oncogene. Imatinib is a small molecule that blocks ATP binding in the fusion protein; it is highly effective in treatment of CML and several other malignancies.

REPLACEMENT THERAPIES. Replacement therapies include replacement of a missing metabolite, an enzyme, an organ, or even a specific gene. **Enzyme replacement** is a component of the treatment of cystic fibrosis to manage intestinal malabsorption. Pancreatic enzymes are easily administered orally, since they must be delivered to the gastrointestinal tract. Enzyme replacement strategies are effective for some lysosomal storage disorders. Enzymes are targeted for the lysosome by modification with mannose-6-phosphate, which binds to a specific receptor. This receptor is also present on the cell surface, so lysosomal enzymes with exposed mannose-6-phosphate residues can be infused into the blood and are taken into cells and transported to lysosomes. Enzyme replacement therapies are available for Gaucher and Fabry diseases, some mucopolysaccharidoses, and Pompe disease.

Organ transplantation is a potentially effective approach to replacement of a defective gene. Aside from transplantation to replace damaged tissues, transplantation of liver or bone marrow is also used for several diseases, mainly inborn errors of metabolism, and hematologic or immunologic disorders. A successful transplant is essentially curative, though there may be significant risks and side effects (see Chapter 134).

Replacement of a defective gene (gene therapy) may offer a less invasive means of achieving a cure of a genetic disorder (see Chapter 82).

Alliance of Genetic Support Groups: *Directory of National Genetic Voluntary Organizations,* 35 Wisconsin Circle, Suite 440, Chevy Chase, MD 20815–7015.

Bartels DM, LeRoy BS, McCarthy P, et al: Nondirectiveness in genetic counseling: A survey of practitioners. *Am J Med Genet* 1997;72:172–179.

Bowles-Biesecker B, Marteau TM: The future of genetic counseling: An international perspective. *Nat Genet* 1999;22:133–137.

Burke W: Genetic testing. *N Engl J Med* 2002;347:1867–1876.

Farrell MH, Certain LK, Farrell PM: Genetic counseling and risk communication services of newborn screening programs. *Arch Pediatr Adolesc Med* 2001;155:120–126.

Fryer AE: Clinical genetic services: Activity, outcome, effectiveness and quality. Summary of a report of the Clinical Genetics Committee of the Royal College of Physicians. *J Roy Coll Physicians Lond* 1997;31:624–627.

Geneclinics: geneclinics@geneclinics.org.

Hayflick SJ, Eiff, MP, Carpenter L, et al: Primary care physicians' utilization and perceptions of genetics services. *Genet Med* 1998;1:13–21.

Holtzman NA, Watson MS: Promoting safe and effective genetic testing in the United States: Final report of the task force on genetic testing, Bethesda, MD, Human Genome Research Institute, 1997.

Hubbard R, Lewontin RC: Pitfalls of genetic testing. *N Engl J Med* 1996;334:1192–1194.

Preimplantation genetic diagnosis—For or against humanity? *Lancet* 2004;364:1729–1730.

Press N, Browner CH: Characteristics of women who refuse an offer of prenatal diagnosis: Data from the California maternal serum alpha fetoprotein blood test experience. *Am J Med Genet* 1998;78:433–445.

Sermon K, Van Steirteghem A, Liebaers I: Preimplantation genetic diagnosis. *Lancet* 2004;363:1633–1640.

Verlinsky Y, Rechitsky S, Sharapova T, et al: Preimplantation HLA testing. *JAMA* 2004;291:2079–2085.

Verlinsky Y, Rechitsky S, Verlinsky O, et al: Preimplantation diagnosis for sonic hedgehog mutation causing familial holoprosencephaly. *N Engl J Med* 2003;348:1449–1454.

Part X ▪ Metabolic Diseases

Chapter 84 ▪ An Approach to Inborn Errors of Metabolism

Iraj Rezvani

Many childhood conditions are caused by gene mutations that encode specific proteins. These mutations can result in the alteration of primary protein structure or the amount of protein synthesized. The functional ability of protein, whether it is an enzyme, receptor, transport vehicle, membrane, or structural element, may be relatively or seriously compromised. These hereditary biochemical disorders are collectively termed **inborn errors of metabolism.**

Most mutations are clinically inconsequential and represent polymorphic differences that set individuals apart *(genetic polymorphism)*. Some mutations produce disease states that range from very mild to lethal. Severe forms of inborn errors of metabolism usually present in the newborn period or shortly thereafter.

It is both technologically and economically possible to screen for a large number of metabolic conditions in the 1st few days of life, before any clinical manifestations of the disease become apparent (Tables 84-1 and 84-2). Institution of early treatment often prevents the deleterious effects of these conditions, especially on the central nervous system. Mass screening also identifies mild forms of inborn errors of metabolism, some of which may never cause clinical disease in the lifetime of the individual. Potential psychosocial implications of such findings can be devastating and deserves serious considerations. Intrauterine diagnosis of most genetic conditions is now feasible and has been used routinely to detect affected fetuses in the population at risk (see Chapter 96).

Children with inborn errors of metabolism may present with one or more of a large variety of signs and symptoms. These may include metabolic acidosis, persistent vomiting, failure to thrive, developmental delay, hypoglycemia, elevated blood or urinary levels of a particular metabolite (an amino acid, organic acid, ammonia), a peculiar odor (Table 84-3), or physical changes such as hepatomegaly. Considering those presenting in the neonatal period separately from children presenting later in life facilitates diagnosis.

NEONATAL PERIOD. Inborn errors of metabolism causing *clinical manifestations* in the neonatal period are usually severe and are often lethal if proper therapy is not initiated promptly. Clinical findings are usually nonspecific and similar to those seen in infants with sepsis. An inborn error of metabolism should be considered in the differential diagnosis of a severely ill neonatal infant, and special studies should be undertaken if the index of suspicion is high (Fig. 84-1).

Infants with metabolic disorders are usually normal at birth; signs and symptoms such as lethargy, poor feeding, convulsions, and vomiting may develop as early as a few hours after birth. A history of clinical deterioration in a previously normal neonate should suggest an inborn error of metabolism. Occasionally, vomiting may be severe enough to suggest the diagnosis of pyloric stenosis, which is usually not present, although it may simultaneously occur in such infants. Lethargy, poor feeding, convulsions, and coma may also be seen in infants with hypoglycemia (see Chapters 92 and 107) or hypocalcemia (see Chapters 48 and 572). Measurements of blood concentrations of glucose and calcium and response to intravenous injection of glucose or calcium usually establish these diagnoses. Because most inborn errors of metabolism are inherited as autosomal recessive traits, a history of consanguinity and/or death in the neonatal period should increase suspicion of this diagnosis. Some of these disorders have a high incidence in specific population groups. Tyrosinemia type 1 is more common among French-Canadians of Quebec than in the general population. Therefore, knowledge of the ethnic background of the patient may be helpful in diagnosis. *Physical examination* usually reveals nonspecific findings, with most signs related to the central nervous system. Hepatomegaly is a common finding in a variety of inborn errors of metabolism. Occasionally, a peculiar odor may offer an invaluable aid to the diagnosis (see Table 84-3). A physician caring for a sick infant should smell the patient and his or her excretions; for example, patients with maple syrup urine disease have the unmistakable odor of maple syrup in their urine and on their bodies.

Diagnosis usually requires a variety of specific *laboratory studies*. Measurements of serum concentrations of ammonia, bicarbonate, and pH are often very helpful initially in differentiating major causes of metabolic disorders (see Fig. 84-1). Elevation of blood ammonia is usually caused by defects of urea cycle enzymes. Infants with elevated blood ammonia levels from urea cycle defects commonly have normal serum pH and bicarbonate values; without measurement of blood ammonia, they may remain undiagnosed and succumb to their disease. Elevation of serum ammonia is also observed in some infants with certain organic acidemias. These infants are severely acidotic because of accumulation of organic acids in body fluids.

When blood ammonia, pH, and bicarbonate values are normal, other aminoacidopathies (such as hyperglycinemia) or galactosemia should be considered; galactosemic infants may also manifest cataracts, hepatomegaly, ascites, and jaundice.

Most inborn errors of metabolism presenting in the neonatal period are lethal if specific *treatment* is not initiated immediately. Specific diagnosis, even in an infant in whom death seems inevitable, is of great importance for genetic counseling of the family (see Chapter 83). Every effort should be made to determine the diagnosis while the infant is alive; postmortem examination is not always helpful. A specific diagnosis may be established by measurement of abnormal metabolites in body fluids, by assay of the specific enzyme activity, or by identification of the mutant gene.

CHILDREN AFTER THE NEONATAL PERIOD. Most inborn errors of metabolism that cause symptoms in the 1st few days of life exhibit milder variant forms that have a more insidious onset. These forms may escape detection during the neonatal period, and the diagnosis may be delayed for months or even years. Early clinical manifestations in children with these forms are commonly nonspecific and may be attributed to perinatal insults.

Clinical manifestations, such as mental retardation, motor deficits, developmental regression, convulsions, myopathy, recurrent emesis, and cardiomyopathy are the common findings in older children. There may be an episodic or intermittent pattern, with episodes of acute clinical manifestations separated by periods of seemingly disease-free states. The episodes are usually triggered by stress or a nonspecific catabolic insult such as an infection. The child may die during one of these acute attacks. An inborn error of metabolism should be considered in any child

TABLE 84-1. Disorders Recommended by the ACMG Task Force for Inclusion in Newborn Screening*

DISORDERS OF ORGANIC-ACID METABOLISM	DISORDERS OF AMINO-ACID METABOLISM
Isovaleric acidemia	Phenylketonuria
Glutaric aciduria type I	Maple syrup urine disease
3-Hydroxy-3-methylglutaric aciduria	Homocystinuria
Multiple carboxylase deficiency	Citrullinemia
Methylmalonic acidemia, mutase deficiency form	Argininosuccinic acidemia
3-Methylcrotonyl-CoA carboxylase deficiency	Tyrosinemia type I
Methylmalonic acidemia, Cbl A and Cbl B forms	**HEMOGLOBINOPATHIES**
Propionic acidemia	Sickle cell anemia
Beta-ketothiolase deficiency	Hemoglobin S-β-thalassemia
DISORDERS OF FATTY ACID METABOLISM	Hemoglobin SC disease
Medium-chain acyl-CoA dehydrogenase deficiency	**OTHER DISORDERS**
Very long-chain acyl-CoA dehydrogenase deficiency	Congenital hypothyroidism
Long-chain L-3-hydroxy acyl-CoA dehydrogenase deficiency	Biotinidase deficiency
Trifunctional protein deficiency	Congenital adrenal hyperplasia
Carnitine uptake defect	Galactosemia
	Hearing deficiency
	Cystic fibrosis

*The American College of Medical Genetics task force also recommended reporting an additional 25 disorders ("secondary targets") that can be detected through screening but that do not meet the criteria for primary disorders. At this time, there is state-to-state variation in newborn screening; a list of the disorders that are screened for by each state is available at http://genes-r-us.uthscsa.edu.

Cbl A, cobalamin A; Cbl B, cobalamin B; CoA, coenzyme A.

From Natowicz M: Newborn screening—Setting evidence-based policy for protection. *N Engl J Med* 2005;353:867–870.

TABLE 84-2. SECONDARY ("REPORT ONLY") CONDITIONS RECOMMENDED BY ACMG

ORGANIC ACID METABOLISM DISORDERS
Methylmalonic acidemia, Cbl C and Cbl D forms
2-Methyl 3-hydroxy butyric aciduria
Isobutyryl-CoA dehydrogenase deficiency
2-Methybutyryl-CoA dehydrogenase deficiency
3-Methylglutaconic aciduria
Malonic acidemia
FATTY ACID OXIDATION DISODERS
Medium/short chain L-3-OH acyl-CoA dehydrogenase deficiency
Short chain acyl-CoA dehydrogenase deficiency
Medium-chain ketoacyl-CoA thiolase deficiency
Glutaric acidemia type 2
Carnitine palmitoyltranferase I deficiency
Carnitine palmitoyltransferase II deficiency
Carnitine acylcarmitine translocase deficiency
Dienoyl-CoA reductase deficiency
AMINO ACID METABOLISM DISORDERS
Hyperphenylalaninemia, benign (not PKU)
Tyrosinemia Type 2
Tyrosinemia Type 3
Defects of biopterin cofactor biosynthesis
Defects of biopterin cofactor regeneration
Argininemia
Hypermethioninemia
Citrullinermia Type 2
HEMOGLOBINOPATHICS
Hemoglobin variants (including Hemoglobin E)
OTHERS
Galactose epimerase deficiency
Galactokinase deficiency

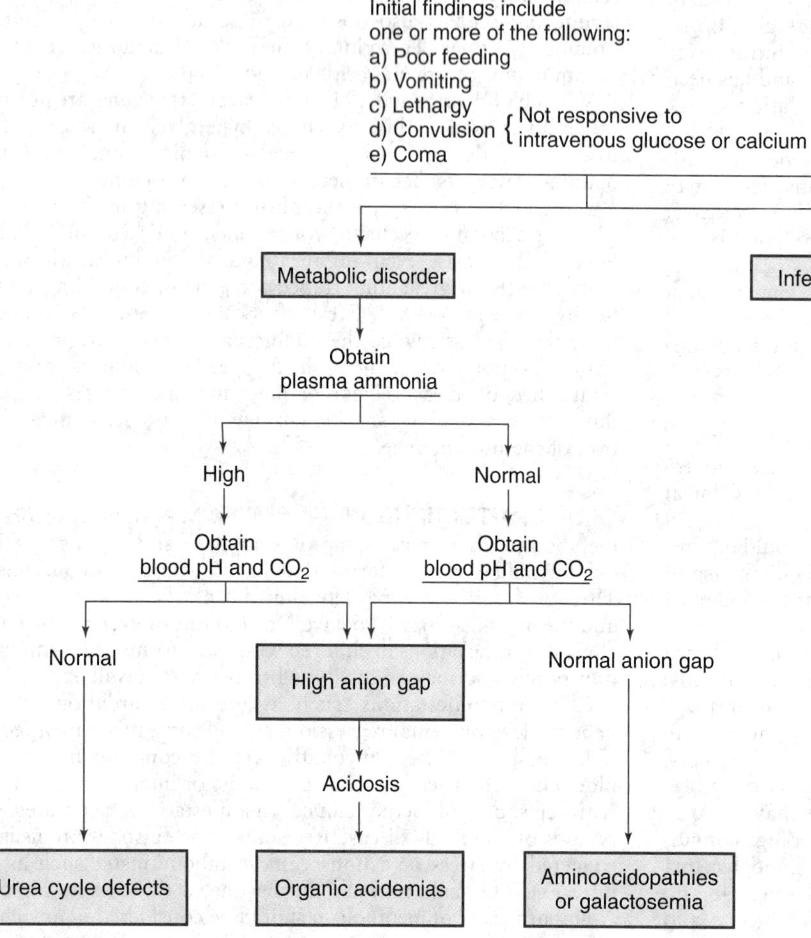

Figure 84-1. Clinical approach to a newborn infant with a suspected metabolic disorder. This schema is a guide to the elucidation of some of the metabolic disorders in newborn infants. Although some exceptions to this schema exist, it is appropriate for most cases.

TABLE 84-3. Inborn Errors of Amino Acid Metabolism Associated with Peculiar Odor

INBORN ERROR OF METABOLISM	URINE ODOR
Glutaric acidemia (type II)	Sweaty feet, acrid
Hawkinsinuria	Swimming pool
Isovaleric acidemia	Sweaty feet, acrid
Maple syrup urine disease	Maple syrup
Hypermethioninemia	Boiled cabbage
Multiple carboxylase deficiency	Tomcat urine
Oasthouse urine disease	Hops-like
Phenylketonuria	Mousey or musty
Trimethylaminuria	Rotting fish
Tyrosinemia	Boiled cabbage, rancid butter

with one or more of the following manifestations: unexplained mental retardation, developmental delay or regression, or motor deficit or convulsions; unusual odor, particularly during an acute illness; intermittent episodes of unexplained vomiting, acidosis, mental deterioration, or coma; hepatomegaly; renal stones; or muscle weakness or cardiomyopathy.

Grosse SD, Dezateux C: Newborn screening for inherited metabolic disease. *Lancet* 2007;369:5–6.

Marsden D, Larson C, Levy HL: Newborn Screening for metabolic disorders. *J Pediatr* 2006;148:577–584.

McBryde KD, Kershaw DB, Bunchman TE, et al: Renal replacement therapy in the treatment of confirmed or suspected in born errors of metabolism. *J Pediatr* 2006;148:770–778.

Waisbren SE: Newborn Screening for metabolid disorders. *JAMA* 2006;296:993–994.

Chapter 85 ■ Defects in Metabolism of Amino Acids

85.1 • Phenylalanine • Iraj Rezvani

Phenylalanine is an essential amino acid. Dietary phenylalanine not utilized for protein synthesis is normally degraded by way of the tyrosine pathway (Fig. 85-1). Deficiency of the enzyme phenylalanine hydroxylase or of its cofactor tetrahydrobiopterin causes accumulation of phenylalanine in body fluids and the central nervous system (CNS). The severity of hyperphenylalaninemia depends on the degree of enzyme deficiency and may vary from very high plasma concentrations (>20 mg/dL or >1,200 µmole/L, **classic phenylketonuria [PKU]**) to mildly elevated levels (2–6 mg/dL or 120–360 µmole/L). In affected infants with plasma concentrations >20 mg/dL, excess phenylalanine is metabolized to phenylketones (phenylpyruvate and phenylacetate; see Fig. 85-1) that are excreted in the urine, giving rise to the term *phenylketonuria* (PKU). These metabolites have no role in pathogenesis of CNS damage in patients with PKU; their presence in the body fluids simply signifies the severity of the condition. The brain is the main organ affected by hyperphenylalaninemia. The CNS damage in affected patients is caused by the elevated concentration of phenylalanine in brain tissue, which interferes with the cerebral transport of other large neutral amino acids (tyrosine, tryptophan). There are a few adults with classic PKU and normal intelligence who have never been treated with a phenylalanine-restricted diet. Phenylalanine content of the brain in these individuals was found to be close to that of normal subjects when studied by magnetic resonance spectroscopy (MRS) and imaging (MRI) techniques.

CLASSIC PHENYLKETONURIA (PKU). Severe hyperphenylalaninemia (plasma phenylalanine levels >20 mg/dL), if untreated, invariably results in the development of signs and symptoms of classic PKU, except in rare unpredictable occasions

Clinical Manifestations. The affected infant is normal at birth. Mental retardation may develop gradually and may not be evident for the 1st few months. It is usually severe, and most patients require institutional care if the condition remains untreated. Vomiting, sometimes severe enough to be misdiagnosed as pyloric stenosis, may be an early symptom. Older untreated children become hyperactive, with purposeless movements, rhythmic rocking, and athetosis.

On physical examination, these infants are lighter in their complexion than unaffected siblings. Some may have a seborrheic or eczematoid rash, which is usually mild and disappears as the child grows older. These children have an unpleasant odor of phenylacetic acid, which has been described as musty or mousey. There are no consistent findings on neurologic examination. Most infants are hypertonic with hyperactive deep tendon reflexes. About 25% of children have seizures, and more than 50% have electroencephalographic abnormalities. Microcephaly, prominent maxilla with widely spaced teeth, enamel hypoplasia, and growth retardation are other common findings in untreated children. The clinical manifestations of classic PKU are rarely seen in those countries in which neonatal screening programs for the detection of PKU are in effect.

MILDER FORMS OF HYPERPHENYLALANINEMIA, NON-PKU HYPERPHENYLALANINEMIAS. In any screening program for PKU, a group of infants are identified in whom initial plasma concentrations of phenylalanine are above normal (2 mg/dL, 120 µmole/L) but <20 mg/dL (1,200 µmole/L). These infants do not excrete phenylketones. Clinically, these infants may remain asymptomatic, but progressive brain damage may occur gradually with age. These patients have milder deficiencies of phenylalanine hydroxylase or its cofactor tetrahydrobiopterin (BH_4) than those with classic PKU. Attempts have been made to classify these patients in different subgroups depending on the degree of hyperphenylalaninemia, but such a practice has little clinical or therapeutic advantage. As with classic PKU, deficiency of BH_4 should be investigated in all infants with milder forms of hyperphenylalaninemia (see later).

Diagnosis. Because of gradual development of clinical manifestations of hyperphenylalaninemia, early diagnosis can only be achieved by mass screening of all newborn infants (see later). In infants with positive results from the screen for hyperphenylalaninemia, diagnosis should be confirmed by quantitative measurement of plasma phenylalanine. Identification and measurement of phenylketones in the urine has no place in any screening program. In countries and places where such programs are not in effect, however, identification of phenylketones in the urine by ferric chloride may offer a simple test for diagnosis of infants with developmental and neurologic abnormalities. Once the diagnosis of hyperphenylalaninemia is established, deficiency of cofactor (BH_4) should be ruled out in all affected infants with proper studies (see later).

Neonatal Screening for Hyperphenylalaninemia. Effective and relatively inexpensive methods for mass screening of newborn infants have been developed and are used in the United States and several other countries. The bacterial inhibition assay of Guthrie, which was the 1st method for the purpose, has been replaced by more precise and quantitative methods (fluorometric and tandem mass spectrometry). All these methods require a few drops of blood, which are placed on a filter paper and mailed to a central laboratory for assay. Blood phenylalanine in affected infants with PKU may rise to diagnostic levels as early as 4 hr after birth even

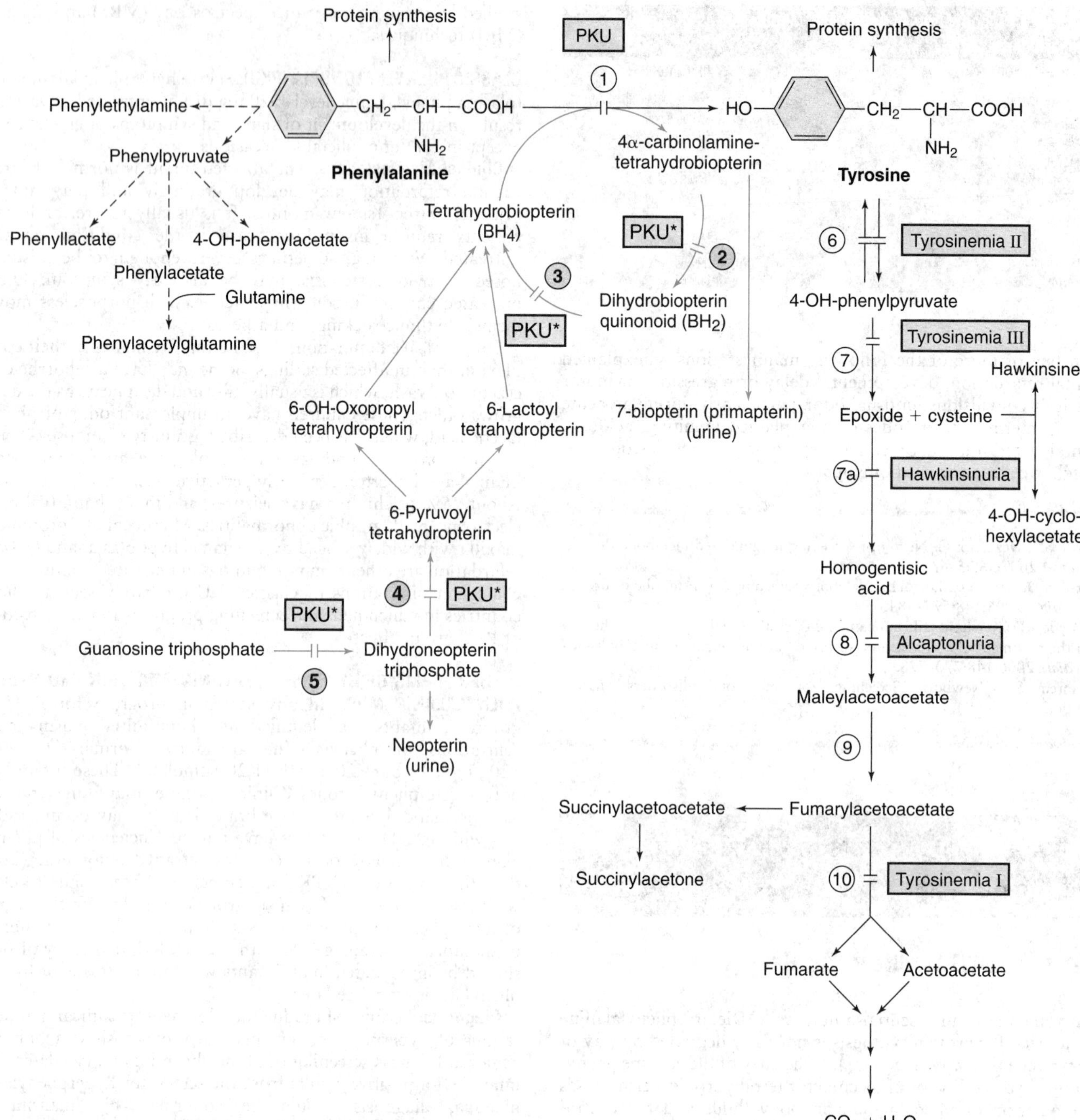

Figure 85-1. Pathways of phenylalanine and tyrosine metabolism. Inborn errors are depicted as bars crossing the reaction *arrow(s)*. Pathways for synthesis of cofactor BH_4 are shown in *purple*. PKU* refers to defects of BH_4 metabolism that affect the phenylalanine, tyrosine, and tryptophan hydroxylases (see Figs. 85-2 and 85-5). **Enzymes:** (1) phenylalanine hydroxylase, (2) carbinolamine dehydratase, (3) dihydrobiopterin reductase, (4) 6-pyruvoyltetrahydropterin synthase, (5) guanosine triphosphate (GTP) cyclohydrolase, (6) tyrosine aminotransferase, (7a) intramolecular rearrangement, (7+7a) 4-hydroxyphenylpyruvate dioxygenase, (8) homogentisic acid dioxygenase, (9) maleylacetoacetate isomerase, (10) fumarylacetoacetate hydroxylase.

in the absence of protein feeding. It is recommended, however, that the blood for screening be obtained in the 1st 24–48 hr of life after feeding protein to reduce the possibility of false negative results, especially in the milder forms of the condition.

Treatment. The goal of therapy is to reduce phenylalanine in the body; formulas low in or free of this amino acid are available commercially. The diet should be started as soon as diagnosis is established. It is generally accepted that infants with persistent plasma levels of phenylalanine >6 mg/dL (360 µmole/L) should be treated with a phenylalanine-restricted diet similar to that for classic PKU. No dietary restriction is currently recommended for infants whose phenylalanine levels are between 2 and 6 mg/dL. Plasma concentrations of phenylalanine in treated patients should be maintained as close to normal as possible. Because phenylalanine is not synthesized by the body, **overtreatment** may lead to phenylalanine deficiency manifested by lethargy, failure to thrive, anorexia, anemia, rashes, diarrhea, and death; moreover, tyrosine becomes an essential amino acid in this disorder and its adequate intake must be ensured. Controversies exist regarding the "allowable" degree of residual hyperphenylalaninemia in treated patients. It is generally believed that plasma phenylalanine levels should be maintained between 2 and 6 mg/dL (120–360 µmole/L) at least in the 1st 12 yr of life. The duration of diet therapy is also controversial. Discontinuation of therapy, even in adulthood, may cause deterioration of IQ and cognitive performance. The current recommendation is that all patients be kept on a phenylalanine-restricted diet for life.

Oral administration of the **cofactor tetrahydrobiopterin** (BH_4) to patients with milder forms of hyperphenylalaninemia due to phenylalanine hydroxylase deficiency may reduce plasma levels of phenylalanine without the need to remain on a low phenylalanine diet. Significant reduction in plasma phenylalanine levels (>30%) also has been observed in some patients with classic PKU following administration of a single dose of oral BH_4 (10 mg/kg). The response to BH_4 cannot be predicted consistently on the basis of genotype, especially in compound heterozygous patients. Dietary management of hyperphenylalaninemia requires close monitoring of blood levels of phenylalanine, expert nutritional input, and well-designed educational materials for the patient and the family. Proper management of these patients is best achieved through a regional treatment center.

Pregnancy in Women with Hyperphenylalaninemia (Maternal PKU). Pregnant women with hyperphenylalaninemia who are not receiving a phenylalanine-restricted diet have a very high risk of having offspring with mental retardation, microcephaly, and congenital heart disease. These complications are related to high levels of maternal plasma phenylalanine during pregnancy and not to the genetic defect of PKU in the fetus. Prospective mothers who have been treated for hyperphenylalaninemia should be maintained on a phenylalanine-restricted diet before and during pregnancy; every effort should be made to keep blood phenylalanine levels below 6 mg/dL (360 μmole/L) throughout the pregnancy. All women with hyperphenylalaninemia who are of childbearing age should be counseled properly as to the risk of the just described congenital anomalies in their offspring.

HYPERPHENYLALANINEMIA FROM DEFICIENCY OF THE COFACTOR BH_4. In 1–2% of infants with hyperphenylalaninemia, the defect resides in one of the enzymes necessary for production or recycling of the cofactor BH_4 (Fig. 85-2). These infants are diagnosed as having PKU, but they deteriorate neurologically despite adequate control of plasma phenylalanine. BH_4 is the cofactor for phenylalanine, tyrosine, and tryptophan hydroxylases. The latter two hydroxylases are essential for biosynthesis of the neurotransmitters dopamine (see Fig. 85-2) and serotonin (see Fig. 85-5). BH_4 is also a cofactor for nitric oxide synthase, which catalyzes the generation of nitric oxide from arginine. Patients with BH_4 deficiency are diagnosed very early in life because all patients with PKU and hyperphenylalaninemia are tested for the possibility of this cofactor deficiency.

BH_4 is synthesized from guanosine triphosphate through several enzymatic reactions (see Fig. 85-1). Four enzyme deficiencies leading to defective BH_4 formation have been described. More than half of the reported patients have had a deficiency of 6-pyruvoyltetrahydropterin synthase (PTPS).

Clinical Manifestations. Infants with cofactor deficiency are identified during screening programs for PKU because of evidence of hyperphenylalaninemia. Plasma phenylalanine levels may be as high as those in classic PKU or in the range of milder forms of hyperphenylalaninemia. Neurologic manifestations, such as loss of head control, truncal hypotonia (floppy baby), drooling, swallowing difficulties, and myoclonic seizures, develop after 3 mo of age despite adequate dietary therapy.

Diagnosis. BH_4 deficiency and the responsible enzyme defect may be diagnosed by the following tests: measurement of neopterin (oxidative product of dihydroneopterin triphosphate) and biopterin (oxidative product of dihydrobiopterin and tetrahydrobiopterin) in body fluids, especially urine (see Fig. 85-1). In patients with guanosine triphosphate (GTP) cyclohydrolase deficiency, urinary excretion of both neopterin and biopterin is very low. In patients with 6-pyruvoyltetrahydropterin synthase deficiency, there is a marked elevation of neopterin excretion and a concomitant decrease in biopterin excretion. In patients with dihydropteridine reductase deficiency, neopterin is normal, but biopterin is very high. Excretion of biopterin increases in this enzyme deficiency because the quinonoid dihydrobiopterin cannot be recycled into BH_4. Patients with carbinolamine dehydratase deficiency excrete 7-biopterin (an unusual isomer of biopterin) in their urine.

BH_4 LOADING TEST. An oral dose of BH_4 (20 mg/kg) normalizes plasma phenylalanine in patients with BH_4 deficiency within 4 to 8 hr. The blood phenylalanine should be elevated (>400 μmole/L) to enable interpretation of the results. This may be achieved by discontinuing diet therapy for 2 days before the test or by administering a loading dose of phenylalanine (100 mg/kg) 3 hr before the test.

ENZYME ASSAY. The activity of dihydropteridine reductase can be measured in the dry blood spots on the filter paper used

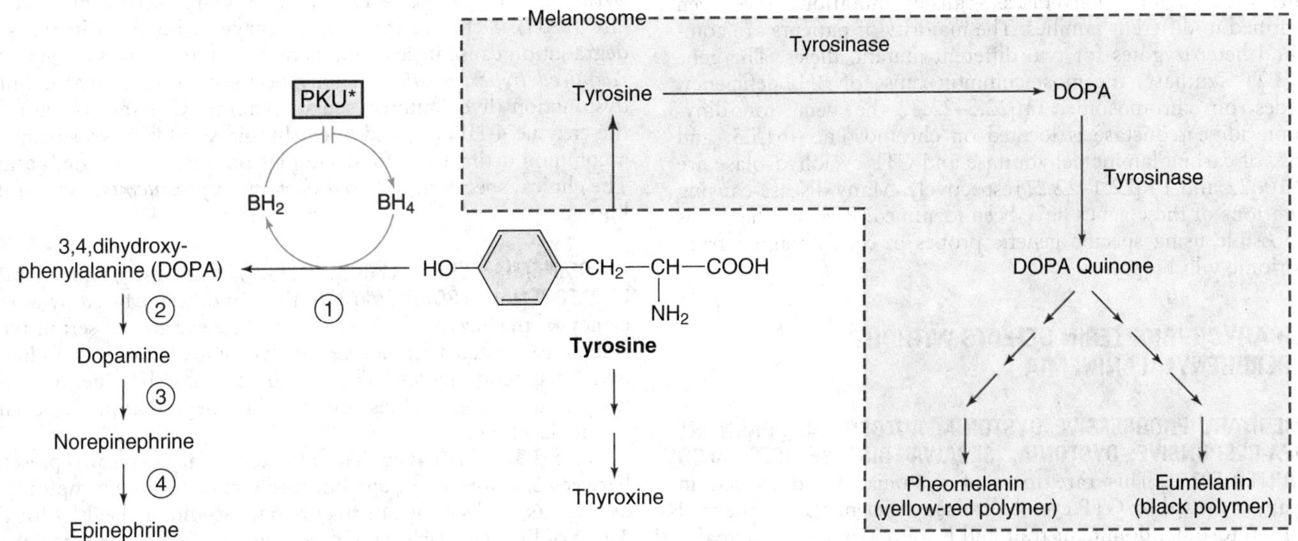

Figure 85-2. Other pathways involving tyrosine metabolism. PKU* indicates hyperphenylalanemia due to tetrahydrobiopterin (BH_4) deficiency (see Fig. 85-1). **Enzymes:** (1) tyrosine hydroxylase, (2) aromatic L-amino acid decarboxylase (AADC), (3) dopamine hydroxylase, (4) phenylethanolamine-N-methyltransferase (PNMT).

for screening purposes. 6-Pyruvoyltetrahydropterin synthase activity can be measured in the liver, kidneys, and erythrocytes. Carbinolamine dehydratase activity can be measured in the liver and kidneys. GTP cyclohydrolase activity can be measured in the liver and in cytokine (interferon-γ) stimulated mononuclear cells or fibroblasts (the enzyme activity is normally very low in unstimulated cells).

Treatment. The goals of therapy are to correct hyperphenylalaninemia and to restore neurotransmitter deficiencies in the CNS.

The control of hyperphenylalaninemia is important in patients with cofactor deficiency, because high levels of phenylalanine interfere with the transport of neurotransmitter precursors (tyrosine, tryptophan) into the brain. Plasma phenylalanine should be maintained as close to normal as possible (<6 mg/dL). This can be achieved by a combination of a low phenylalanine diet and oral supplementation of BH_4. Infants with GTP cyclohydrolase or PTPS deficiencies respond more readily to BH_4 therapy (5–10 mg/kg/day) than those with dihydropteridine reductase deficiency. In the latter patients, doses as high as 20 mg/kg/day may be required. BH_4 for replacement therapy is commercially available, although it is expensive.

Administration of deficient neurotransmitters (L-dopa and 5-hydroxytryptophan) is recommended even when treatment with BH_4 normalizes plasma levels of phenylalanine. BH_4 does not readily enter the brain to restore neurotransmitter production. Supplementation with folinic acid is also recommended in patients with dihydropteridine reductase deficiency.

Hyperprolactinemia occurs in patients with BH_4 deficiency and may be due to dopamine deficiency (which is the major prolactin inhibiting factor) in the hypothalamic region. Measurement of serum prolactin levels may be a convenient method for monitoring adequacy of neurotransmitter replacement in affected patients.

Some drugs such as trimetoprin sulfamethoxazole, methotrexate, and other antileukemic agents are known to inhibit dihydropteridine reductase enzyme activity and should be used with great caution in patients with BH_4 deficiency.

Genetics and Prevalence. All defects causing hyperphenylalaninemia are inherited as autosomal recessive traits. The prevalence of PKU in the United States is estimated at 1/14,000 to 1/20,000 live births. The prevalence of non-PKU hyperphenylalaninemia is estimated at 1/50,000. The condition is more common in whites and Native Americans and less prevalent in blacks, Hispanics, and Asians.

The gene for phenylalanine hydroxylase is located on chromosome 12q24.1 and many disease-causing mutations have been identified in different families. The majority of patients are compound heterozygotes for two different mutant alleles. The gene for PTP synthase, the most common cause of BH_4 deficiency, resides on chromosome 11q22.3–23.3, the gene for dihydropteridine reductase is located on chromosome 4p15.3, and those of carbinolamine dehydratase and GTP cyclohydrolase are on 10q22 and 14q22.1–22.2, respectively. Many disease-causing mutations of these genes have been identified. Prenatal diagnosis is possible using specific genetic probes in cells obtained from chorionic villi biopsy.

TETRAHYDROBIOPTERIN DEFECTS WITHOUT HYPERPHENYLALANINEMIA

HEREDITARY PROGRESSIVE DYSTONIA, AUTOSOMAL DOMINANT DOPA-RESPONSIVE DYSTONIA, SEGAWA DISEASE (SEE ALSO CHAPTER 597.3). This rare form of dystonia, 1st described in Japan, is caused by GTP cyclohydrolase deficiency. It is inherited as an autosomal dominant trait and is more common in females than males (4:1)

Clinical manifestations usually occur around 5–6 yr of age and are heralded by dystonia of the lower limbs, which may spread to all extremities within a few years. Torticollis, dystonia of the arms, and poor coordination may precede dystonia of the lower limbs in some patients. Early development is generally normal. The symptoms usually have an impressive diurnal variation, becoming worse by the end of the day and improving with sleep. Parkinsonian signs may also be present or develop subsequently with advancing age. Patients may be misdiagnosed as having cerebral palsy. Late presentation in adult life has also been reported.

Laboratory findings show no hyperphenylalaninemia, but reduced levels of BH_4 and neopterin are found in the spinal fluid. Dopamine and its metabolites (homovanillic acid) may also be reduced in the spinal fluid. It is believed that the enzyme deficiency in this condition is less severe than that of the autosomal recessive form of GTP cyclohydrolase deficiency, which is associated with hyperphenylalaninemia (see earlier). The existence of asymptomatic carriers indicates that other factors or genes may play a role in pathogenesis of the phenotype. The asymptomatic carrier may be identified by measuring the ratio of plasma phenylalanine to tyrosine after an oral dose of phenylalanine (100 mg/kg); the ratio increases significantly (≈3 times above normal value at 2 hr) in the asymptomatic carrier.

Diagnosis may be confirmed by reduced levels of BH_4 and neopterin in the spinal fluid, by measurement of the enzyme activity, and by identification of the gene defect (see earlier). Clinically, the condition should be differentiated from other causes of dystonias and childhood Parkinsonism, especially tyrosine hydroxylase (see Chapter 85.2) and aromatic amino acid decarboxylase deficiencies. The striking diurnal pattern of dystonia is an important clinical finding in favor of GTP cyclohydrolase deficiency.

Treatment with L-dopa in conjunction with a peripheral dopa decarboxylase inhibitor usually produces dramatic improvement.

85.2 • TYROSINE • Grant A. Mitchell and Iraj Rezvani

Tyrosine, obtained from ingested proteins and synthesized endogenously from phenylalanine, is used for protein synthesis and is a precursor of dopamine, norepinephrine, epinephrine, melanin, and thyroxine. Excess tyrosine is metabolized to carbon dioxide and water (see Fig. 85-1). Hypertyrosinemia is observed with deficiencies of tyrosine aminotransferase, 4-hydroxyphenpyruvate dioxygenase (4-HPPD), or fumarylacetoacetate hydrolase (FAH). Deficiencies of other enzymes involved in tyrosine degradation cause little or no increase in blood levels of tyrosine. *Acquired hypertyrosinemia* may occur in severe hepatocellular dysfunction (liver failure), scurvy (vitamin C is the cofactor for the enzyme 4-HPPD), and hyperthyroidism; hypertyrosinemia is a common artifact in blood samples obtained soon after eating, The clinical spectrum of *hereditary hypertyrosinemias* is not fully known.

TYROSINEMIA TYPE I (TYROSINOSIS, HEREDITARY TYROSINEMIA, HEPATORENAL TYROSINEMIA). In this condition, caused by a deficiency of the enzyme FAH, a moderate elevation of serum tyrosine is associated with severe involvement of the liver, kidneys, and peripheral nerves. These findings may be due to accumulation of metabolites of tyrosine degradation, especially succinylacetone.

Clinical Manifestations. The affected infant typically presents between 2 and 6 mo of age but rarely may become symptomatic as early as 2 wks of age or may remain seemingly healthy for the 1st yr of life. The earlier the presentation, the poorer is the prognosis. The 1 yr mortality, which is about 60% in infants who develop symptoms before 2 mo of age, decreases to 4% in infants who become symptomatic after 6 mo of age.

The major organs affected are the liver, peripheral nerves, and kidneys. An acute **hepatic crisis** commonly heralds the onset of the disease and is usually precipitated by an intercurrent illness that produces a catabolic state. Fever, irritability, vomiting, hemorrhage, hepatomegaly, jaundice, elevated levels of serum transaminases, and hypoglycemia are common. An odor resembling boiled cabbage may be present, due to increased methionine metabolites. Most hepatic crises resolve spontaneously, but may progress to liver failure and death. Between the crises, varying degrees of failure to thrive, hepatomegaly, and clotting abnormalities often persist. Cirrhosis of the liver and, eventually, hepatocellular carcinoma occur with increasing age; carcinoma is unusual before 2 yr of age.

Episodes of acute **peripheral neuropathy** resembling acute porphyria occur in ≈40% of affected children. These crises, often triggered by a minor infection, are characterized by severe pain, often in the legs, associated with hypertonic posturing of the head and trunk, vomiting, paralytic ileus, and, occasionally, self-induced injuries of the tongue or buccal mucosa. Marked weakness and paralysis occur in ≈30% of the episodes, which may lead to respiratory failure requiring mechanical ventilation. Crises typically last 1 to 7 days.

Renal involvement is manifested as a Fanconi-like syndrome with normal anion gap metabolic acidosis, hyperphosphaturia, hypophosphatemia, and vitamin D–resistant rickets. Nephromegaly and some degree of nephrocalcinosis are often found by ultrasound examination.

Hypertrophic cardiomyopathy is occasionally seen in these infants.

Laboratory Findings. In untreated patients, liver function tests are perturbed in a characteristic fashion. α-Fetoprotein level is increased, often markedly, and liver-synthesized coagulation factors are decreased in most patients; serum levels of transaminases are increased, particularly during acute hepatic episodes. Serum concentration of bilirubin is increased with liver failure. Increased levels of α-fetoprotein are present in the cord blood of affected infants, indicating intrauterine liver damage. Plasma tyrosine level is dependent on diet; tyrosine level has less diagnostic value than that of succinylacetone (see later). Elevations in serum concentrations of methionine and other amino acids, characteristic of liver failure, may also be present. Hyperphosphaturia and hypophosphatemia are common. Generalized aminoaciduria may occur. The urinary level of 5-aminolevulinic acid is elevated (due to inhibition of 5-aminolevulinic hydratase by succinylacetone). The presence of elevated levels of succinylacetone in serum and urine is diagnostic (see Fig. 85-1).

Diagnosis is usually established by demonstration of elevated levels of succinylacetone in urine or blood. Neonatal screening methods detect hypertyrosinemia; only a minority of patients with tyrosinemia type I are identified by these methods. Succinylacetone, which is not detected by the current screening methods, is the preferable initial metabolite tested. Tyrosinemia type I should be differentiated from other causes of hepatitis and hepatic failure in infants, including galactosemia, hereditary fructose intolerance, neonatal iron storage disease, giant cell hepatitis, and citrullinemia type II (see Chapter 85.11).

Treatment and Outcome. A diet low in phenylalanine and tyrosine can slow down but not halt the progression of the condition. The **treatment of choice** is nitisinone (NTBC, 2-(nitro-4-trifluoromethylbenzoyl)-1,3-cyclohexanedione), which inhibits tyrosine degradation at 4-HPPD (see Fig. 85-1). This treatment prevents acute hepatic and neurologic crises. Patients treated with nitisinone are also prescribed a diet low in phenylalanine and tyrosine. Although nitisinone stops or greatly slows progression of the disease, much pretreatment liver damage is not reversible. Therefore, patients must be followed for development of **hepatocellular carcinoma.** On imaging, the presence of a liver nodule usually indicates generalized cirrhosis. Accurate distinction between benign nodules and malignant ones is difficult to obtain through imaging. Liver transplantation is an effective therapy and alleviates the risk of hepatocellular carcinoma. The impact of nitisinone treatment on the need for liver transplantation is still under study but depends on the stage of the disease at which therapy begins.

Genetics and Prevalence. Tyrosinemia type I is an autosomal recessive trait. The gene for FAH has been mapped to chromosome 15q; numerous mutations have been identified. DNA analysis is useful for molecular prenatal diagnosis and for testing in groups at risk for specific mutations such as French-Canadians from the Saguenay-Lac Saint-Jean region of Quebec. Tyroninemia type I is panethnic; lack of French-Canadian or Scandinavian ancestry does not exclude the diagnosis. The prevalence of the condition is estimated to be 1/1,846 live births in the Saguenay-Lac Saint-Jean region. The worldwide prevalence is estimated to be 1/100,000 to 1/120,000. Prenatal diagnosis has been achieved by measurement of succinylacetone in amniotic fluid, by the enzyme assay in amniocytes or chorionic villi biopsy, and by DNA analysis.

TYROSINEMIA TYPE II (RICHNER-HANHART SYNDROME, OCULOCUTANEOUS TYROSINEMIA). This rare autosomal recessive disorder is caused by deficiency of tyrosine aminotransferase enzyme, which results in palmar and plantar hyperkeratosis, herpetiform corneal ulcers, and mental retardation (see Fig. 85-1). **Ocular manifestations** of excessive tearing, redness, pain, and photophobia often occur before skin lesions. Corneal lesions are presumed to be due to tyrosine deposition. In contrast to herpetic ulcers, corneal lesions in tyrosinemia type II stain poorly with fluorescin and often are bilateral. **Skin lesions,** which may develop later in life, include painful, nonpruritic hyperkeratotic plaques on the soles, palms, and fingertips. Mental retardation, which occurs in <50% of patients, is usually mild to moderate.

Abnormal **laboratory findings** are limited to significant hypertyrosinemia (20–50 mg/dL; 110–2,750 µmole/L) and tyroiluria. Surprisingly, 4-hydroxyphenypyruvic acid and its metabolites are also elevated in urine despite being downstream from the metabolic block (see Fig. 85-1). This is presumed to be due to shunting of tyrosine via other transaminases in the presence of high tyrosine concentrations. The condition is due to the deficiency of the cytosolic fraction of hepatic tyrosine aminotransferase. In contrast to tyrosinemia type I, liver and kidney function, as well as serum concentrations of other amino acids, are normal.

Diagnosis is established by assay of plasma tyrosine concentration. Sustained hypertyrosinemia on a nonrestricted diet is also seen in liver failure; the level of plasma tyrosine is higher in tyrosinemia type II and oculocutaneous manifestations are absent in liver failure. Diagnosis of type II tyrosinemia may be confirmed by assay of tyrosine aminotransferase activity in liver or by DNA analysis of the mutant gene.

Treatment with a diet low in tyrosine and phenylalanine improves the biochemical abnormalities and may result in dramatic healing of the skin and eye lesions. Some observations support the reasonable claim that mental retardation may be prevented by early dietary restriction of tyrosine. The gene for tyrosine aminotransferase is mapped to chromosome 16q and several disease-causing mutations have been identified. About half the reported cases are of Italian descent.

TYROSINEMIA TYPE III (PRIMARY DEFICIENCY OF 4-HPPD). Only a few cases have been reported; most were detected by amino acid determinations performed for various neurologic findings. There is doubt as to whether this enzyme deficiency causes any clinical abnormalities. Age of onset has been from 1 to 17 mo. Developmental delay, seizures, intermittent ataxia, and self-destructive behavior are reported. No liver or renal abnormalities are present. Asymptomatic infants have been identified in neonatal screening programs.

The diagnosis is suspected in children with sustained moderate increases in plasma levels of tyrosine (350–700 µmole/L) and the presence of 4-hydroxyphenylpyruvic acid and its metabolites (4-hydroxyphenyllactic and 4-hydroxyphenylacetic acids) in urine. Diagnosis may be confirmed by demonstration of low activity of 4-HPPD enzyme in liver biopsy or presence of mutations in the 4-HPPD gene.

Given the possible association with neurologic abnormalities, dietary reduction of plasma tyrosine levels is reasonable. It is also logical to attempt a trial of vitamin C, the cofactor for 4-HPPD. The condition is inherited as an autosomal recessive trait. The gene for 4-HPPD is mapped to chromosome 12q24-qter.

TRANSIENT TYROSINEMIA OF THE NEWBORN. In a small number of newborns, plasma tyrosine may rise to as high as 60 mg/dL (3,300 µmole/L) during the 1st 2 wk of life. Most affected infants are premature and are receiving high-protein diets. The condition is presumably due to delayed maturation of 4-HPPD enzyme (see Fig. 85-1). Lethargy, poor feeding, and decreased motor activity are noted in some patients; most are asymptomatic and come to medical attention because of a high blood phenylalanine level, rendering the screening test for PKU positive. **Laboratory findings** include marked elevation of plasma tyrosine with a moderate increase in plasma phenylalanine. The presence of marked hypertyrosinemia differentiates this condition from phenylketonuria. 4-Hydroxyphenylpyruvic acid and its metabolites (4-hydroxyphenyllactic and 4-hydroxyphenylacetic acids) are also present in the urine. Hypertyrosinemia usually resolves spontaneously in the 1st mo of life. The condition is often corrected promptly by reducing the amount of protein in the diet (to 2 g/kg/24 hr) and by administering vitamin C (200–400 mg/24 hr). Mild intellectual deficits have been reported in some full-term infants with this disorder, but the causal relationship to hypertyrosinemia is not conclusively established.

HAWKINSINURIA. This rare condition (named after the 1st affected family) is caused by a mutant 4-HPPD enzyme that catalyzes a partial reaction and releases an intermediate compound used for diagnosis (see Fig. 85-1). This intermediate is either reduced to form 4-hydroxycyclohexylacetic acid (4-HCAA) or reacts with glutathione to form the unusual organic acid hawkinsin (2-L-cysteine-S-yl-1-4-dihydroxycyclohex-5-en-1-yl-acetic acid); secondary glutathione deficiency may occur.

Individuals with this disorder become symptomatic only during infancy. The symptoms usually appear after weaning from breast-feeding with the introduction of a high-protein diet. Severe metabolic acidosis, ketosis, failure to thrive, mild hepatomegaly, and an unusual odor (of a swimming pool) are described. Mental development is usually normal.

Affected children and adults excrete the organic acids 4-HCAA, 4-hydroxyphenylpyruvic acid and its metabolites (4-hydroxyphenyllactic and 4-hydroxyphenylacetic acids), 5-oxoproline (owing to secondary glutathione deficiency), and hawkinsin in their urine. Plasma tyrosine level is usually normal.

Treatment consists of a low-protein diet (breast milk) or a diet low in phenylalanine and tyrosine. A trial with large doses of vitamin C (up to 1,000 mg/24 hr) is also recommended. No therapy is needed after 1 yr of age. The same mutation, a substitution of threonine for the normal alanine codon at position 33 of the 4-HPPD gene, has been identified in unrelated patients with hawkinsinuria.

ALCAPTONURIA. This rare (incidence ≈1/250,000) autosomal recessive disorder is due to a deficiency of homogentisic acid oxidase, which causes large amounts of homogentisic acid to accumulate in the body and then to be excreted in the urine (see Fig. 85-1).

Clinical manifestations of alcaptonuria consist of ochronosis and arthritis, which occur in adulthood. The only sign of the disorder in children is a blackening of the urine on standing. This is caused by oxidation and polymerization of the homogentisic acid. Urine with acid pH may not darken even after many hours. This sign may never be noted, delaying the diagnosis until adulthood. *Ochronosis,* seen clinically as dark spots on the sclera or ear cartilage, results from the accumulation of the black polymer of homogentisic acid. *Arthritis* can be disabling and occurs in almost all affected subjects with advancing age. It involves the large joints (spine, hip, and knee) and is usually more severe in males. Like rheumatoid arthritis, the arthritis has acute exacerbations, but the radiologic findings are typical of osteoarthritis, with characteristic narrowing of the joint spaces and calcification of the intervertebral discs. High incidences of heart disease (mitral and aortic valvulitis, calcification of the heart valves, and myocardial infarction) have been noted.

The **diagnosis** is confirmed by finding massive excretion of homogentisic acid in urine. The enzyme is expressed only in the liver and kidneys. The gene for alcaptonuria maps to chromosome 3q and several diseases-causing mutations have been identified. Alcaptonuria is most common in the Dominican Republic and Slovakia.

There is no effective **treatment** for this disorder. Nitisinone (see treatment of tyrosinemia type I) inhibits homogentisic production; its administration to patients with alcaptonuria before pigment deposition may be useful in prevention of arthritis.

TYROSINE HYDROXYLASE DEFICIENCY (INFANTILE PARKINSONISM, AUTOSOMAL RECESSIVE DOPA-RESPONSIVE DYSTONIA) [SEE CHAPTER 597.3]. Tyrosine hydroxylase catalyzes the formation of L-dopa from tyrosine (see Fig. 85-2). Deficiency of this enzyme has been reported in a few children with dystonia and parkinsonism. The clinical picture resembles the autosomal dominant dystonia due to GTP cyclohydrolase deficiency (see Chapter 85.1). The spectrum of the condition is not fully appreciated.

Clinical manifestations such as jerky movements of the limbs leading to spasticity and muscle rigidity, expressionless face, ptosis, drooling, oculogyric crises, and parkinsonism may start in early infancy. Psychomotor retardation has been seen in some patients. No diurnal variation of the symptoms has been noted.

Laboratory findings include reduced levels of dopamine and its metabolite homovanillic acid (HVA) and normal concentrations of tetrahydrobiopterin and neopterin in the spinal fluid. Serum prolactin levels are usually elevated.

Diagnosis should be considered in any patients with dystonia and parkinsonism. GTP cyclohydroxylase deficiency should be ruled out by proper studies (see earlier). Diagnosis is established by the laboratory findings (see earlier) and gene study.

Treatment with L-dopa results in a dramatic improvement. Patients unresponsive to L-dopa have recently been reported, however. The condition is inherited as an autosomal recessive trait. The gene for tyrosine hydroxylase is mapped to chromosome 11p.

ALBINISM. Albinism is due to defects in the biosynthesis and distribution of melanin (Table 85-1). Melanin is synthesized by melanocytes from tyrosine in a membrane-bound intracellular organelle, the melanosome. Melanocytes originate from the embryonic neural crest and migrate to the skin, eyes (choroid and iris), and hair follicles. The melanin in the eye is not secreted into the adjacent tissues, whereas the pigment in skin and hair follicles is secreted into the epidermis and the hair shaft. The rate of melanogenesis is very low in the eye and very high in the skin and hair. The biosynthetic pathway for melanin synthesis is not completely elucidated (see Fig. 85-2). The end products are two pigments: *pheomelanin,* which is a yellow-red pigment; and *eumelanin,* a brown-black pigment.

Clinical manifestations common in generalized albinism are hypopigmentation of the skin and hair. Patients with involvement

TABLE 85-1. Classification of Albinism

TYPE	GENE	CHROMOSOME
OCULOCUTANEOUS ALBINISM (OCA)		
OCA_1 (tyrosinase deficient)	*TYR*	11q
OCA_1A (severe deficiency)	*TYR*	11q
OCA_1B (mild deficiency)*	*TYR*	11q
OCA_2 (tyrosinase positive)†	P (pink-eyed dilution)	15q
Prader-Willi and Angelman syndromes	P	15q
OCA_3 (Rufous, red OCA)	*TYRP1***	9p
Hermansky-Pudlak syndrome	*HPS1*	10q
Chédiak-Higashi syndrome	*CHS1*	1q
OCULAR ALBINISM		
OA_1 (Nettleship-Falls type)	OA	XP
LOCALIZED ALBINISM		
Piebaldism	*KIT*	4q
Waardenburg syndrome I & III	*PAX3*	2q
Waardenburg syndrome II	*MITF*	3p

*This includes Amish, minimal pigment, yellow albinism, and platinum and temperature-sensitive variants.
**Tyrosinase related protein 1.
†Includes brown OCA.

of the eyes may have strabismus, photophobia, decreased visual acuity, and the presence of red reflex. Irides are translucent and pink in infancy and change to light blue or brown with age. Biocular (stereoscopic) vision is absent because of an abnormal decussation and misrouting of the optic fibers at the chiasm. About 90% of optic nerve fibers from one eye cross to the other side at the chiasma in patients with albinism. This defect also causes asymmetric visual evoked potentials. Blindness and skin cancer are major late sequelae of albinism in its severe forms. Melanin is also present in the cochlea. Albino individuals may be more susceptible to ototoxic agents such as gentamicin.

Many clinical forms of albinism have been identified. Some of the seemingly distinct clinical forms are caused by different mutations of the same gene. Several genes located on different chromosomes are shown to be involved in melanogenesis (see Table 85-1). Attempts to differentiate types of albinism based on the mode of inheritance, tyrosinase activity, or the extent of hypopigmentation have failed to yield a comprehensive classification. The following classification is based on the distribution of albinism in the body and the type of mutated gene. Not all conditions associated with albinism are discussed. Interested readers are referred to more comprehensive sources (see references).

Oculocutaneous (Generalized) Albinism (OCA). Lack of pigment is generalized, affecting skin, hair, and eyes. Three genetically distinct forms exist: OCA_1, OCA_2, and OCA_3. The lack of pigment is usually more severe in patients with OCA_1; these types may not be distinguishable clinically, however, because of a great degree of overlap. All are inherited as autosomal recessive traits.

OCA_1 (TYROSINASE-DEFICIENT ALBINISM). The defect in these patients resides in the tyrosinase gene, which is located on chromosome 11q. Many mutant alleles have been identified. Most affected individuals are compound heterozygote for two different mutant alleles. The condition can be subdivided to OCA_1 A and OCA_1 B based on enzyme activity and, to a lesser extent, clinical manifestations.

OCA_1 A (Tyrosinase-Negative OCA). A number of mutations in the tyrosinase gene render the enzyme completely inactive. Individuals with this form usually have the most severe case of generalized albinism. Clinically, lack of pigment in the skin (milky white), hair (white hair), and eyes (red gray irides) is evident at birth and remains unchanged throughout life. They do not tan and do not develop pigmented nevi or freckles.

OCA_1 B. These mutations in the tyrosinase gene result in enzymes with some residual activities. Clinically these individuals, although completely depigmented at birth, are capable of developing some pigment with age and become light blond with light blue or hazel eyes. They develop pigmented nevi and freckles and they may tan. These patients, depending on the degree of pigmentation, were once subdivided into different groups and were thought to be genetically different. One interesting form is the temperature-sensitive albinism in which the tyrosinase becomes more active in cooler parts of the body such as limbs. These individuals have no pigment in the scalp and trunk but develop some pigment in arms and legs.

OCA_2 (TYROSINASE-POSITIVE OCA). This is the most common form of generalized albinism. It is particularly common in African blacks. Clinically, these individuals demonstrate some pigmentation of the skin and eyes at birth and continue to collect pigment throughout their lives. The hair is yellow at birth and may become darker with age. They have pigmented nevi and freckles but do not tan. They may be clinically indistinguishable from OCA_1 B. These individuals have normal tyrosinase activity. The defect is in the p (pink-eyed dilution) gene, which is located on chromosome 15q. This gene produces the P protein, a melanosome membrane protein, the function of which is not completely understood. Patients with Prader-Willi and Angelman syndromes who have deletion of chromosome 15 lack one copy of the OCA_2 gene and have mild pigmentary dilution (see Chapter 80).

OCA_3 (RUFOUS ALBINISM). This form has been identified only in Africans, African-Americans, and natives of New Guinea. Patients have reddish hair with reddish brown skin as an adult. The color of the skin is peculiar to this form. In the young, the manifestation may be confused with that of OCA_2. Patients with OCA_3 can make pheomelanine but not eumelanine. The mutation is in the tyrosinase related protein 1 (TYRP1) gene, the function of which is not understood.

HERMANSKY-PUDLAK SYNDROME. This is a group of disorders, each caused by mutation of one of the seven genes *HPS1* to *HPS7*. These genes are necessary for normal structure and function of lysosome-derived organelles including melanosomes and platelet dense bodies. In most forms, a tyrosinase-positive OCA of highly variable severity is associated with platelet dysfunction (owing to the absence of platelet dense bodies) and an accumulation of a ceroid-like material in tissues. The condition is transmitted as an autosomal recessive trait and is most prevalent in Puerto Rico (types 1 and 3, frequency about 1:2,000). Bleeding tendencies, often manifested as epistaxis and a prolonged bleeding time, are common. The ceroid-like material is histochemically similar to that found in neuronal ceroid lipofuscinosis. The accumulation of this material in tissues results in restrictive lung disease, inflammatory bowel disease, kidney failure, and cardiomyopathy in the 3rd or 4th decade of life. The majority of patients have mutations in *HPS1,* which is located on chromosome 10q.

CHÉDIAK-HIGASHI SYNDROME. Patients with this rare autosomal recessive condition have partial albinism and susceptibility to infection with the presence of giant peroxidase-positive lysosomal granules in granulocytes (see Chapter 129). These patients have a reduced number of melanosomes, which are abnormally large (macromelanosomes). Patients who survive early childhood may develop a lymphofollicular malignancy. Mutations in *CHS1* gene (located on the long arm of chromosome 1) have been identified in these patients.

Ocular Albinism (OA). Albinism is limited to the eyes. All the eye findings of albinism (see earlier) are present. The X-linked recessive form (OA_1) has been segregated as a separate entity. Most cases of autosomal recessive ocular albinism are felt to be mild variants of OCA_2.

OCULAR ALBINISM 1 (OA_1 NETTLESHIP-FALLS TYPE). Only the hemizygote male has the complete manifestation while some abnormal retinal pigmentation may be present in heterozygote female carriers. The gene for this condition is located on the short arm of the X chromosome. An X-linked ocular albinism with late-onset sensorineural deafness has also been reported.

Localized Albinism. This disorder is characterized by localized areas of hypopigmentation of skin and hair, which may be present at birth or develop with time.

PIEBALDISM. In this autosomal dominant inherited condition, the individual is usually born with a white forelock. The underlying skin is depigmented. In addition, there are usually white macules on the face, trunk, and extremities. The white hair lock and the depigmented underlying skin are devoid of melanocytes. Mutations in the *KIT* gene have been shown in affected patients.

WAARDENBURG SYNDROME. In this syndrome, lateral displacement of inner canthi, broad nasal bridge, heterochromia of irides and sensorineural deafness are associated with a white forelock. This condition is inherited as an autosomal dominant trait. Four types of this syndrome have been identified. Patients with type I have displacement of inner canthi. The condition is caused by mutations in the *PAX3* gene. Type II patients have normal inner canthi, and mutations in the *MITF* gene have been shown in some patients. Patients with type III have all the findings seen in individuals with type I, plus hypoplasia and contractures of the upper limbs. The gene abnormality is in the *PAX3*. Type IV is associated with Hirschsprung disease, is heterogeneous, and mutations in different genes (*EDN3, EDNRB*, or *SOX10*) have been identified in different patients.

85.3 • METHIONINE • Iraj Rezvani and David S. Rosenblatt

The normal pathway for catabolism of methionine, an essential amino acid, produces S-adenosylmethionine, which serves as a methyl group donor for methylation of a variety of compounds in the body, and cysteine, which is formed through a series of reactions called trans-sulfuration (Fig. 85-3).

HOMOCYSTINURIA (HOMOCYSTINEMIA). Most homocysteine, an intermediate compound of methionine degradation, is normally remethylated to methionine. This methionine-sparing reaction is catalyzed by the enzyme methionine synthase, which requires a metabolite of folic acid (5-methyltetrahydrofolate) as a methyl donor and a metabolite of vitamin B_{12} (methylcobalamin) as a cofactor (see Fig. 85-3). Only 20–30% of total homocysteine (and its dimer homocystine) is in free form in the plasma of normal individuals. The rest is bound to proteins as mixed disulfides. Three major forms of homocystinemia and homocystinuria have been identified.

Homocystinuria Due to Cystathionine β-Synthase (CBS) Deficiency (Classic Homocystinuria). This is the most common inborn error of methionine metabolism. About 40% of affected patients respond to high doses of vitamin B_6 and usually have milder clinical manifestations than those who are unresponsive to vitamin B_6 therapy. These patients possess some residual enzyme activity.

Infants with this disorder are normal at birth. **Clinical manifestations** during infancy are nonspecific and may include failure to thrive and developmental delay. The diagnosis is usually made after 3 yr of age, when subluxation of the ocular lens (**ectopia lentis**) occurs. This causes severe myopia and iridodonesis (quivering of the iris). Astigmatism, glaucoma, staphyloma, cataracts, retinal detachment, and optic atrophy may develop later in life. Progressive **mental retardation** is common. Normal intelligence, however, has been reported. In an international survey of >600 patients, IQ scores ranged from 10 to 135. The higher IQ scores were noted in vitamin B_6 responsive patients. **Psychiatric and behavioral disorders** have been observed in >50% of affected patients. Convulsions occur in ≈20% of patients. Affected individuals with homocystinuria manifest *skeletal abnormalities* resembling those of Marfan syndrome (see Chapter 700); they are usually tall and thin, with elongated limbs and arachnodactyly. Scoliosis, pectus excavatum or carinum, genu valgum, pes cavus, high arched palate, and crowding of the teeth are commonly seen. These children usually have fair complexions, blue eyes, and a peculiar malar flush. Generalized osteoporosis, especially of the spine, is the main roentgenographic finding. **Thromboembolic episodes** involving both large and small vessels, especially those of the brain, are common and may occur at any age. Optic atrophy, paralysis, cor pulmonale, and severe hypertension (due to renal infarcts) are among the serious consequences of thromboembolism, which is caused by changes in the vascular walls and increased platelet adhesiveness secondary to elevated homocystine levels. The risk of thromboembolism increases after surgical procedures. Spontaneous pneumothorax and acute pancreatitis are rare complications.

Elevations of both methionine and homocystine (or homocysteine) in body fluids are the diagnostic **laboratory findings.** Freshly voided urine should be tested for homocystine, since this compound is unstable and may disappear as the urine is stored. Cystine is low or absent in plasma. The **diagnosis** may be established by assay of the enzyme in liver biopsy specimens, cultured fibroblasts, or phytohemagglutinin-stimulated lymphocytes or by DNA analysis.

Treatment with high doses of vitamin B_6 (200–1,000 mg/24 hr) causes dramatic improvement in most patients who are responsive to this therapy. The degree of response to vitamin B_6 treatment may be different in different families. Some patients may not respond because of folate depletion; a patient should not be considered unresponsive to vitamin B_6 until folic acid (1–5 mg/24 hr) has been added to the treatment regimen. Restriction of methionine intake in conjunction with cysteine supplementation is recommended for patients who are unresponsive to vitamin B_6. The need for dietary restriction and its extent remains controversial in patients with vitamin B_6 responsive form. In some patients with this form, addition of betaine may obviate the need for any dietary restriction. Betaine (trimethylglycine, 6–9 g/24 hr for adults or 200–250 mg/kg/day for children) lowers homocysteine levels in body fluids by remethylating homocysteine to methionine (see Fig. 85-3); this may result in further elevation of plasma methionine levels. This treatment has produced clinical improvement (preventing vascular events) in patients who are unresponsive to vitamin B_6 therapy. Cerebral edema has occurred in a patient with vitamin B_6 nonresponsive homocystinuria and dietary noncompliance during betaine therapy. Administration of large doses of vitamin C (1 g/day) has improved the endothelial function; long-term clinical efficacy is not known.

More than 100 pregnancies in women with the classic form of homocystinuria have been reported with favorable outcomes for both mothers and infants. The majority of infants were full term and normal. Postpartum thromboembolic events occurred in a few mothers. All but one of the 38 affected male patients has had normal offspring.

The screening of newborn infants for classic homocystinuria has been performed worldwide and a prevalence of 1/200,000 to 1/350,000 has been estimated. The condition seems more common in New South Wales, Australia (1/60,000) and Ireland. Early treatment of patients identified by the screening process has produced favorable results. The mean IQ of 16 patients with vitamin B_6 unresponsive form treated in early infancy was 94 ± 4. Dislocation of the lens seemed to be prevented in some patients.

Homocystinuria is inherited as an autosomal recessive trait. The gene for cystathionine β-synthase is located on chromosome 21q22.3. Prenatal diagnosis is feasible by performing an enzyme assay of cultured amniotic cells or chorionic villi or by DNA analysis. Many disease-causing mutations have been identified in different families. The majority of affected patients are compound

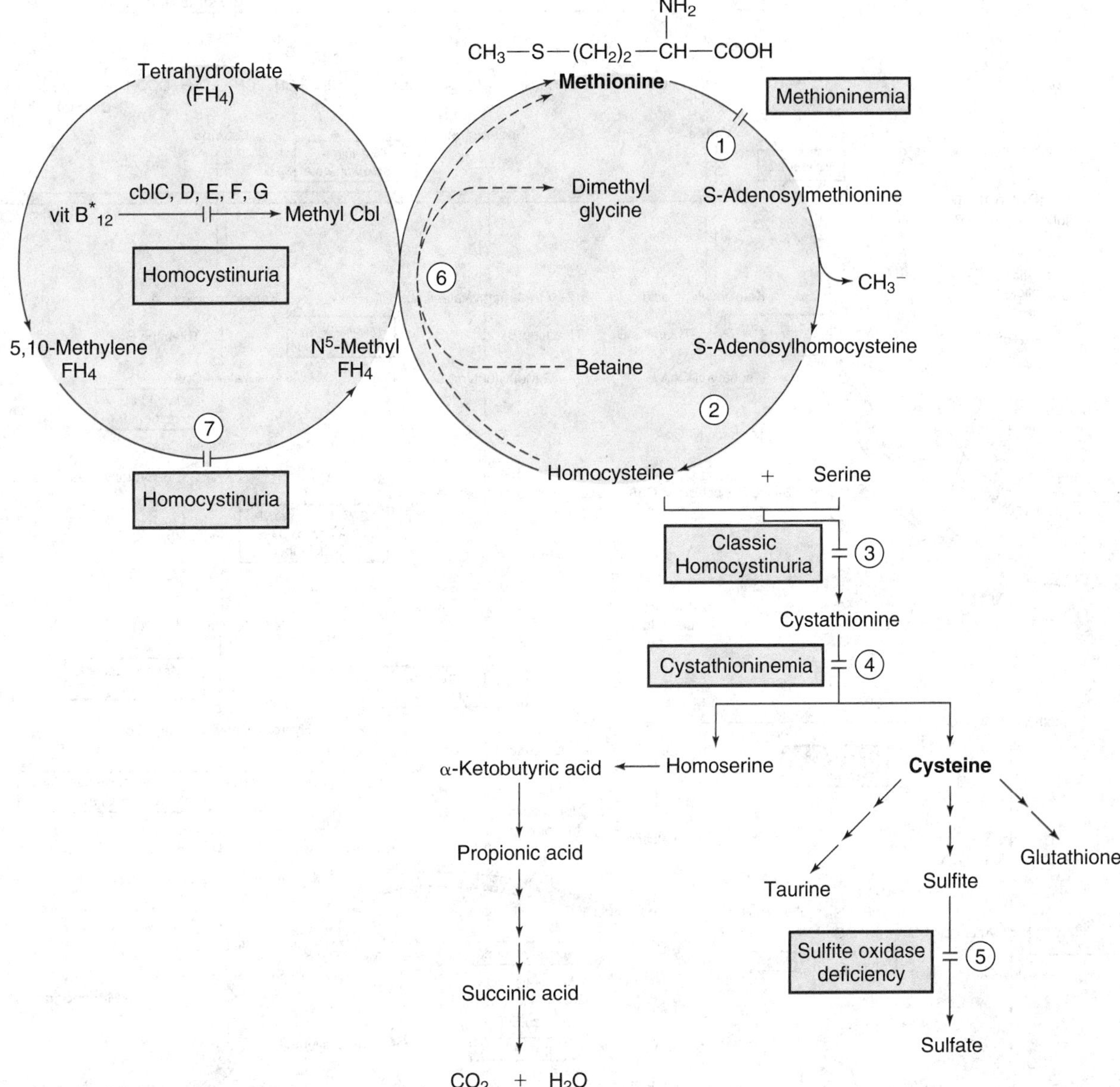

Figure 85-3. Pathways in the metabolism of sulfur-containing amino acids. **Enzymes:** (1) methionine adenosyltransferase, (2) adenosylhomocysteine hydrolase, (3) cystathion synthase, (4) cystathionase, (5) sulfite oxidase, (6) betaine homocysteine methyltransferase, (7) methylene tetrahydrofolate reductase.

heterozygotes for two different alleles. Heterozygous carriers are usually asymptomatic; thromboembolic events and coronary heart disease are more common in these individuals than in the normal population.

Homocystinuria Due to Defects in Methylcobalamin Formation. Methylcobalamin is the cofactor for the enzyme methionine synthase, which catalyzes remethylation of homocysteine to methionine. There are at least five distinct defects in the intracellular metabolism of cobalamin that may interfere with the formation of methylcobalamin. To better understand the metabolism of cobalamin, see methylmalonic acidemia (see Chapter 85.6 and Figs. 85-3 and 85-4). The five defects are designated as *cbl*C, *cbl*D, *cbl*E *(methionine synthase reductase)*, *cbl*G *(methionine synthase)*, and *cbl*F. Patients with *cbl*C, *cbl*D, and *cbl*F defects have methylmalonic acidemia in addition to homocystinuria because formation of both adenosylcobalamin and methylcobalamin is impaired (see Chapter 85.6).

Patients with *cbl*E and *cbl*G defects are unable to form methylcobalamin and develop homocystinuria without methylmalonic acidemia (see Fig. 85-4); fewer than 40 patients are known with each of these diseases.

The **clinical manifestations** are similar in patients with all of these defects. Vomiting, poor feeding, lethargy, hypotonia, and developmental delay may occur in the 1st few months of life. One patient with the *cbl*G defect was not symptomatic (except for mild developmental delay) until she was 21 yr old, however, when she developed difficulty in walking and numbness of the hands. **Laboratory findings** include megaloblastic anemia, homocystinuria, and hypomethioninemia. The presence of megaloblastic anemia differentiates these defects from homocystinuria due to methylenetetrahydrofolate reductase deficiency (see later). The presence of hypomethioninemia differentiates both of these conditions from cystathionine β-synthase deficiency (see earlier).

Diagnosis is established by complementation studies performed in cultured fibroblasts. Prenatal diagnosis has been accomplished by studies in amniotic cell cultures. The gene for *cbl*E (*MTRR*) is mapped to chromosome 5p15.3–p15.2 and that for *cbl*G (*MTR*) is mapped to chromosome 1q43; several disease-causing

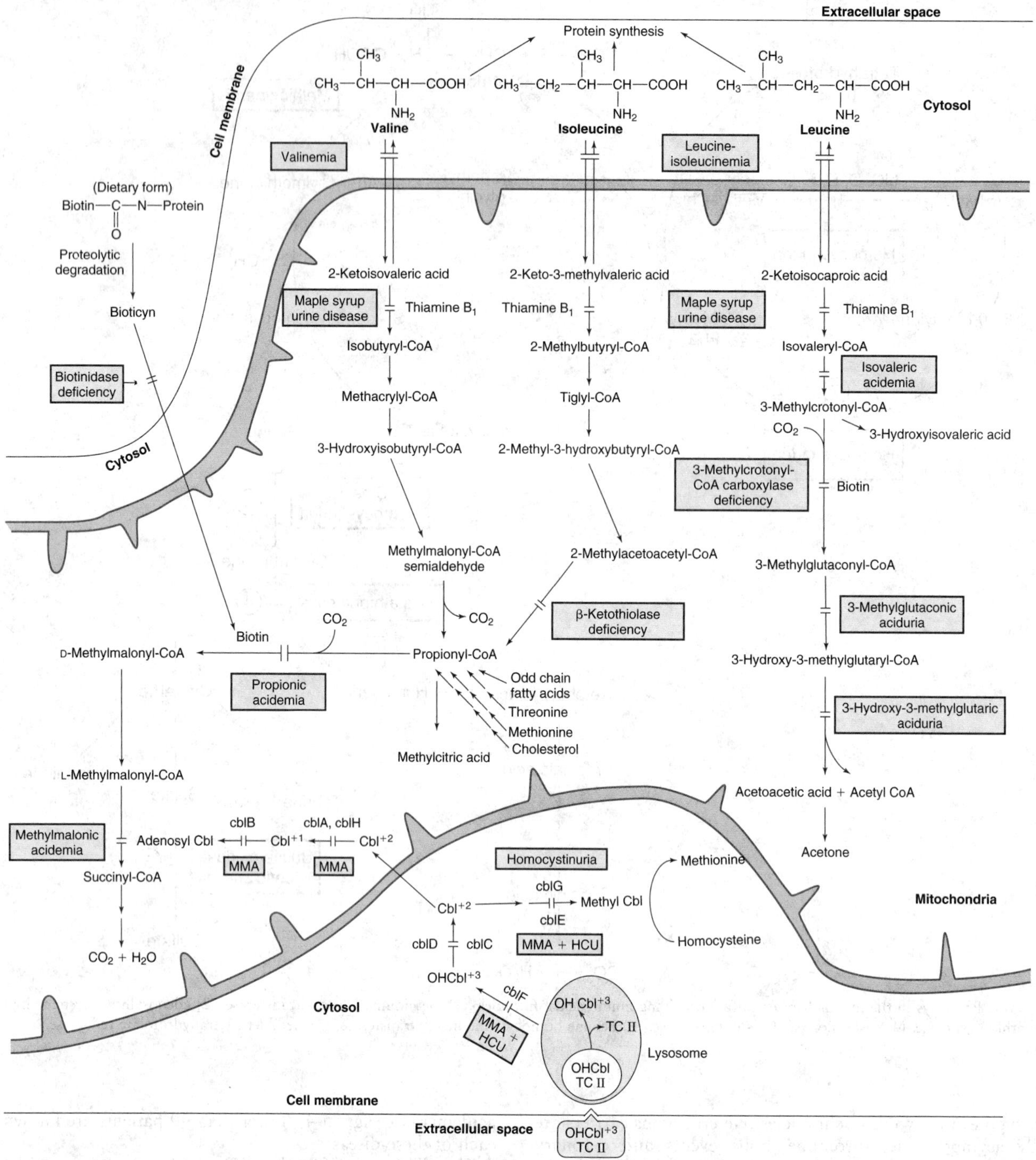

Figure 85-4. Pathways in the metabolism of the branched-chain amino acids, biotin, and vitamin B_{12} (cobalamin). MMA, methylmalonic acidemia; HCU, homocystinuria; Cbl, cobalamin; OHCbl, hydroxycobalamin; cbl, defect in metabolism of cobalamin; TC, transcobalamine.

mutations, including a common missense mutation (P1173L) in the *MTR* gene, have been described.

Treatment with vitamin B_{12} in the form of hydroxycobalamin (1–2 mg/24 hr) is used to correct the clinical and biochemical findings. Results vary among both diseases and sibships.

Homocystinuria Due to Deficiency of Methylenetetrahydrofolate Reductase (MTHFR). This enzyme reduces 5–10 methylenetetrahydrofolate to form 5-methyltetrahydrofolate, which provides the methyl group needed for remethylation of homocysteine to methionine (see Fig. 85-3).

The severity of the enzyme defect and of the clinical manifestations varies considerably in different families. **Clinical findings** vary from apnea, seizure, microcephaly, coma, and death to developmental delay, ataxia, and motor abnormalities or even psychiatric manifestations. Premature vascular disease or peripheral neuropathy has been reported as the only manifestation of this enzyme deficiency in some patients. Adults with severe enzyme deficiency may even be completely asymptomatic. Exposure to the anesthetic nitrous oxide (which inhibits methionine synthase) in patients with MTHFR deficiency may result in neurologic deterioration and death.

Laboratory findings include moderate homocystinemia and homocystinuria. The methionine concentration is low or low normal. This finding differentiates this condition from classic homocystinuria caused by cystathionine synthase deficiency. Absence of megaloblastic anemia distinguishes this condition from homocystinuria caused by methylcobalamin formation (see earlier). Thromboembolism of vessels has also been observed in these patients. **Diagnosis** may be confirmed by the enzyme assay in cultured fibroblasts or leukocytes or by finding causal mutation in the *MTHR* gene.

A number of polymorphisms have been described in the *MTHR* gene. Two of these (677C > T and 1298A > C) may affect levels of plasma total homocysteine and have been studied as possible risk factors for a wide variety of medical conditions, ranging from birth defects to vascular disease and even risk for cancer, prognosis for survival in leukemia, and risk for Alzheimer disease. To date, the best data support a role for 677C > T polymorphism as a risk factor for neural tube defects. Although a clinical test for polymorphism is widely available, its predictive value in any given individual has yet to be determined.

Treatment of severe MTHFR deficiency with a combination of folic acid, vitamin B_6, vitamin B_{12}, methionine supplementation, and betaine has been tried. Of these, early treatment with betaine seems to have the most beneficial effect.

The condition is inherited as an autosomal recessive trait; the gene for the enzyme has been located on chromosome 1p36.3 and many disease-causing mutations have been reported. Prenatal diagnosis can be offered by measuring MTHFR enzyme activity in cultured chorionic villi cells or amniocytes, by linkage analysis in informative families, or by DNA analysis of the mutation.

HYPERMETHIONINEMIA. **Secondary hypermethioninemia** occurs in liver disease, tyrosinemia type I, and classic homocystinuria. Hypermethioninemia has also been found in premature and some full-term infants receiving high-protein diets, in whom it may represent delayed maturation of the enzyme methionine adenosyltransferase. Lowering the protein intake usually resolves the abnormality. **Primary hypermethioninemia** caused by the deficiency of hepatic methionine adenosyltransferase (see Fig. 85-3) has been reported in a few patients. The majority of these patients have been diagnosed in the neonatal period through screening for homocystinuria. Affected individuals with residual enzyme activity remain asymptomatic throughout life despite persistent hypermethioninemia. Some complain of unusual odor to their breath (boiled cabbage). A few patients with complete enzyme deficiency have had neurologic abnormalities related to demyelination (mental retardation, dystonia, dyspraxia). The gene for methionine adenosyltransferase is on chromosome 10q22 and several disease-causing mutations have been identified. A novel defect, glycine N-methyltransferase deficiency, also causes isolated hypermethioninemia.

CYSTATHIONINEMIA (CYSTATHIONINURIA). Secondary cystathioninuria occurs in patients with vitamin B_6 or B_{12} deficiency, liver disease (particularly damage caused by galactosemia), thyrotoxicosis, hepatoblastoma, neuroblastoma, ganglioblastoma, or defects in remethylation of homocysteine.

Cystathionase deficiency results in massive cystathioninuria and mild to moderate cystathioninemia; cystathionine is not normally detectable in blood. Deficiency of this enzyme is inherited as an autosomal recessive trait and its prevalence is estimated to be about 1/14,000 live births. Affected subjects with a wide variety of clinical manifestations have been reported. Lack of a consistent clinical picture and the presence of cystathioninuria in a number of normal persons suggest that cystathionase deficiency may be of no clinical significance. A majority of reported cases are responsive to oral administration of large doses of vitamin B_6 (≥100 mg/24 hr). When cystathioninuria is discovered in a patient, vitamin B_6 treatment seems indicated, but its beneficial effect has not been established. The gene encoding for cystathionase is located on chromosome 16.

85.4 • Cysteine/Cystine • Iraj Rezvani

Cysteine is a sulfur-containing nonessential amino acid that is synthesized from methionine (see Fig. 85-3). In the presence of oxygen, two molecules of cysteine are oxidized to form cystine. The most common disorders of cysteine/cystine metabolism, cystinuria (see Chapter 547) and cystinosis (see Chapter 529.3), are discussed elsewhere.

SULFITE OXIDASE DEFICIENCY (MOLYBDENUM COFACTOR DEFICIENCY). At the last step in cysteine metabolism, sulfite is oxidized to sulfate by sulfite oxidase, and the sulfate is excreted in the urine (see Fig. 85-3). This enzyme requires a molybdenum-pterin complex named molybdenum cofactor. This cofactor is also necessary for the function of two other enzymes in humans: xanthine dehydrogenase (which oxidizes xanthine and hypoxanthine to uric acid) and aldehyde oxidase. Three enzymes, encoded by three different genes, are involved in the synthesis of the cofactor. The genes are mapped to chromosomes 14q24, 6p21.3, and 5q11. Deficiency of any of the three enzymes causes cofactor deficiency with identical phenotype. Most patients who were originally diagnosed as having sulfite oxidase deficiency have been proven to have molybdenum cofactor deficiency. Both conditions are inherited as autosomal recessive traits.

The enzyme and the cofactor deficiencies produce identical **clinical manifestations.** Refusal to feed, vomiting, severe intractable seizures (tonic, clonic, myoclonic), and severe developmental delay may develop within a few weeks after birth. Bilateral dislocation of ocular lenses is a common finding in patients who survive the neonatal period.

These children excrete large amounts of sulfite, thiosulfate, S-sulfocysteine, xanthine, and hypoxanthine in their urine. Urinary and serum levels of uric acid and urinary concentration of sulfate are diminished. Fresh urine should be used for screening purposes and for quantitative measurements of sulfite, because oxidation at room temperature may produce false-negative results.

Diagnosis is confirmed by measurement of sulfite oxidase and molybdenum cofactor in fibroblasts and liver biopsies, respectively. Prenatal diagnosis is possible by performing an assay of sulfite oxidase activity in cultured amniotic cells or in samples of chorionic villi.

No effective **treatment** is available, and most children die in the 1st 2 yr of life. The prevalence of neither of the deficiencies is known.

85.5 • Tryptophan • Iraj Rezvani

Tryptophan is an essential amino acid and a precursor for nicotinic acid and serotonin (Fig. 85-5). Presumed deficiencies of a variety of different enzymes involved in tryptophan catabolism have been reported, but no distinct clinical entity has yet emerged. Hartnup disorder causes disturbance in tryptophan absorption.

HARTNUP DISORDER. In this autosomal recessive disorder, named after the 1st reported family, there is a defect in the transport of monoamino-monocarboxylic amino acids (neutral amino acids) by the intestinal mucosa and renal tubules. Most children with Hartnup defect remain asymptomatic. The major **clinical manifestation** in the rare symptomatic patient is cutaneous photosensitivity. The skin becomes rough and red after moderate exposure to the sun, and with greater exposure, a pellagra-like rash may develop. The rash may be pruritic, and a chronic eczema may appear. The skin changes have been reported in affected infants as young as 10 days of age. Some patients may have intermittent ataxia manifested as an unsteady, wide-based gait. The ataxia may last a few days and usually recovers spontaneously. Mental

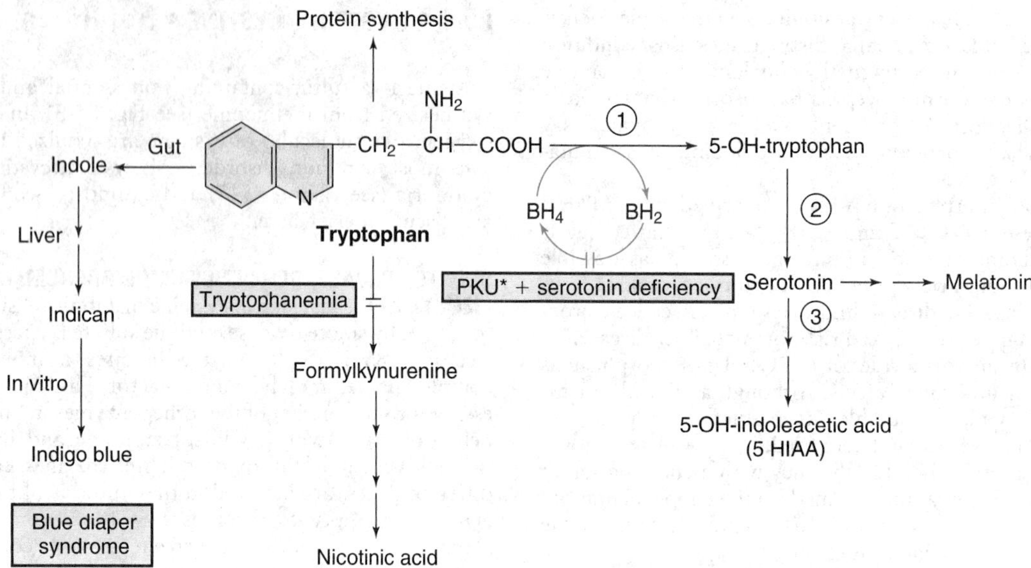

Figure 85-5. Pathways in the metabolism of tryptophan. PKU* indicates hyperphenylalanemia due to tetrahydrobiopterin deficiency (see Fig. 85-1). **Enzymes:** (1) tryptophan hydroxylase, (2) aromatic L-amino acid decarboxylase (AADC), (3) monoamine oxidase (MAO).

development is usually normal. Two individuals in the original kindred were mentally retarded, however. Episodic psychologic changes, such as irritability, emotional instability, depression, and suicidal tendencies, have been observed; these changes are usually associated with bouts of ataxia. Short stature and atrophic glossitis are seen in some patients.

Most children diagnosed with Hartnup disorder by neonatal screening have remained asymptomatic. This indicates that other factors are also involved in pathogenesis of the clinical condition.

The main **laboratory finding** is aminoaciduria, which is restricted to neutral amino acids (alanine, serine, threonine, valine, leucine, isoleucine, phenylalanine, tyrosine, tryptophan, histidine). Urinary excretion of proline, hydroxyproline, and arginine remains normal. This finding differentiates Hartnup disorder from other causes of generalized aminoaciduria, such as Fanconi syndrome. Plasma concentrations of neutral amino acids are usually normal. This seemingly unexpected finding is because these amino acids are absorbed as dipeptides and the transport system for small peptides is intact in Hartnup disorder. The indole derivatives (especially indican) may be found in large amounts in some patients, owing to bacterial breakdown of unabsorbed tryptophan in the intestines.

Diagnosis is established by the striking intermittent nature of symptoms and the just described urinary findings.

Treatment with nicotinic acid or nicotinamide (50–300 mg/24 hr) and a high-protein diet results in a favorable response in symptomatic patients. Because of the intermittent nature of the clinical manifestations, the efficacy of these treatments is difficult to evaluate. The prevalence of the disorder is estimated to be 1/30,000. Normal outcome both for mother and fetus is reported in affected pregnant women. The gene for this condition has not yet been identified.

85.6 • Valine, Leucine, Isoleucine, and Related Organic Acidemias • Iraj Rezvani and David S. Rosenblatt*

The early steps in the degradation of these three essential amino acids, the *branched-chain amino acids,* are similar (see Fig. 85-4). The intermediate metabolites are all organic acids, and deficiency of any of the degradative enzymes, except for the transaminases, causes acidosis; in such instances, the organic acids before the enzymatic block accumulate in body fluids and are excreted in the urine. These disorders commonly cause metabolic acidosis, which usually occurs in the 1st few days of life. Although most of the clinical findings are nonspecific, some manifestations may provide important clues to the nature of the enzyme deficiency. An approach to infants suspected of having an organic acidemia is presented in Figure 85-6. Definitive diagnosis is usually established by identifying and measuring specific organic acids in body fluids (blood, urine), by the enzyme assay, and by identification of the mutant gene.

Organic acidemias are not limited to defects in the catabolic pathways of branched-chain amino acids. Disorders causing accumulation of other organic acids include those derived from lysine (see Chapter 85.13), those associated with lactic acid (see Chapter 87), and dicarboxylic acidemias associated with defective fatty acid degradation (see Chapter 86.1).

*David S. Rosenblatt contributed to the section on methylmalonic acidemia.

MAPLE SYRUP URINE DISEASE (MSUD). Decarboxylation of leucine, isoleucine, and valine is accomplished by a complex enzyme system (branched-chain α-ketoacid dehydrogenase) using thiamine pyrophosphate (vitamin B_1) as a coenzyme. This mitochondrial enzyme consists of four subunits: $E_{1\alpha}$, $E_{1\beta}$, E_2, and E_3. The E_3 subunit is shared with two other dehydrogenases in the body, namely pyruvate dehydrogenase and α-ketoglutarate dehydrogenase. Deficiency of this enzyme system causes MSUD (see Fig. 85-4), named after the sweet odor of maple syrup found in body fluids, especially urine. Based on clinical findings and response to thiamine administration, five phenotypes of MSUD have been identified.

Classic MSUD. This form has the most severe **clinical manifestations.** Affected infants who are normal at birth develop poor feeding and vomiting in the 1st wk of life; lethargy and coma may ensue within a few days. Physical examination reveals hypertonicity and muscular rigidity with severe opisthotonos. Periods of hypertonicity may alternate with bouts of flaccidity. Neurologic findings are often mistaken for generalized sepsis and meningitis. Cerebral edema may be present; convulsions occur in most infants, and hypoglycemia is common. In contrast to most hypoglycemic states, correction of the blood glucose concentration does not improve the clinical condition. Routine **laboratory**

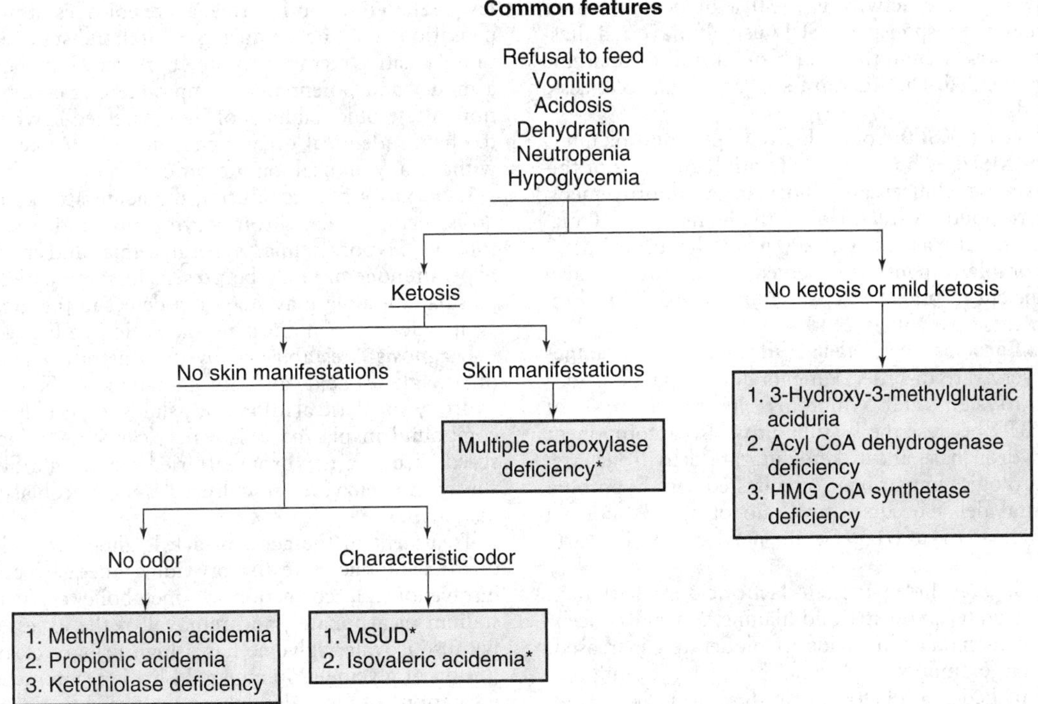

Figure 85-6. Clinical approach to infants with organic acidemia. *Asterisks* indicate disorders in which patients have a characteristic odor (see text and Table 84-2). MSUD, maple syrup urine disease.

findings are usually unremarkable, except for metabolic acidosis. Death usually occurs in untreated patients in the 1st few weeks or months of life.

Diagnosis is often suspected because of the peculiar odor of maple syrup found in urine, sweat, and cerumen (see Fig. 85-6). It is usually confirmed by amino acid analysis showing marked elevations in plasma levels of leucine, isoleucine, valine, and alloisoleucine (a stereoisomer of isoleucine not normally found in blood) and depression of alanine. Leucine levels are usually higher than those of the other three amino acids. Urine contains high levels of leucine, isoleucine, and valine and their respective ketoacids. These ketoacids may be detected qualitatively by adding a few drops of 2,4-dinitrophenylhydrazine reagent (0.1% in 0.1 N HCl) to the urine; a yellow precipitate of 2,4-dinitrophenylhydrazone is formed in a positive test. Neuroimaging during the acute state may show cerebral edema, which is most prominent in the cerebellum, dorsal brainstem, cerebral peduncle, and internal capsule. After recovery from the acute state and with advancing age, hypomyelination and cerebral atrophy may be seen in neuroimaging of the brain. The enzyme activity can be measured in leukocytes and cultured fibroblasts.

Treatment of the acute state is aimed at hydration and quick removal of the branched-chain amino acids and their metabolites from the tissues and body fluids. Because renal clearance of these compounds is poor, hydration alone may not produce a rapid improvement. Peritoneal dialysis or hemodialysis is the most effective mode of therapy in critically ill infants and should be instituted promptly; significant decreases in plasma levels of leucine, isoleucine, and valine are usually seen within 24 hr of institution of treatment. Providing sufficient calories and nutrients intravenously or orally should reverse the patient's catabolic state. Cerebral edema may need to be treated with mannitol, lasix, or hypertonic saline.

Treatment after recovery from the acute state requires a diet low in branched-chain amino acids. Synthetic formulas devoid of leucine, isoleucine, and valine are available commercially. Because these amino acids cannot be synthesized endogenously, small amounts of them should be added to the diet; the amount should be titrated carefully by performing frequent analyses of the plasma amino acids. A clinical condition resembling **acrodermatitis enteropathica** occurs in affected infants whose plasma isoleucine concentration becomes very low; addition of isoleucine to the diet causes a rapid and complete recovery. Patients with MSUD should remain on the diet for the rest of their lives. Liver transplantation has been performed in a small number of patients with classic MSUD with promising results. These children have been able to tolerate a normal diet.

The long-term **prognosis** of affected children remains guarded. Severe ketoacidosis, cerebral edema, and death may occur during any stressful situation such as infection or surgery, especially in mid-childhood. Mental and neurologic deficits are common sequelae.

Intermittent MSUD. In this form of MSUD, seemingly normal children develop vomiting, odor of maple syrup, ataxia, lethargy, and coma during any stress or catabolic state such as infection or surgery. During these attacks, laboratory findings are indistinguishable from those of the classic form, and death may occur. **Treatment** of the acute attack of intermittent MSUD is similar to that of the classic form. After recovery, although a normal diet is tolerated, a diet low in branched-chain amino acids is recommended. Activity of dehydrogenase in patients with the intermittent form is higher than in the classic form and may reach 5–20% of the normal activity.

Mild (Intermediate) MSUD. In this form, affected children develop milder disease after the neonatal period. **Clinical manifestations** are insidious and limited to the central nervous system. Patients have mild to moderate mental retardation (usually after 5 mo of age) with or without seizures. They have the odor of maple syrup and excrete moderate amounts of the branched-chain amino acids and their ketoacid derivatives in the urine. Plasma concentrations of leucine, isoleucine, and valine are moderately increased whereas those of lactate and pyruvate are normal. These children are commonly diagnosed during an intercurrent illness when signs and symptoms of classic MSUD may occur. The dehydrogenase activity is 3–30% of normal. Since patients with thiamine-responsive MSUD usually have manifestations similar to those seen in the mild form, a trial of thiamine therapy is recommended. Diet therapy, similar to that of classic MSUD, is needed.

Thiamine-Responsive MSUD. Some children with mild or intermediate forms of MSUD who are treated with high doses of thiamine have dramatic clinical and biochemical improvement. Although some respond to treatment with thiamine at 10 mg/24 hr, others may require as much as 200 mg/24 hr for at least 3 wk before a favorable response is observed. These patients also require diets deficient in branched-chain amino acids. The enzymatic activity in these patients is 2–40% of normal.

MSUD Due to a Deficiency of E_3 Subunit (Dihydrolipoyl Dehydrogenase). This is a very rare disorder. Patients develop lactic acidosis in addition to signs and symptoms similar to those of intermediate MSUD because the E_3 subunit is also a component of pyruvate dehydrogenase and α-ketoglutarate dehydrogenase. Progressive neurologic impairment manifested by hypotonia and developmental delay occurs after 2 mo of age. Abnormal movements progress to ataxia. Death may occur in early childhood.

Laboratory findings include persistent lactic acidosis with high levels of plasma lactate, pyruvate, and alanine. Plasma concentrations of branched-chain amino acids are moderately increased. Patients excrete large amounts of lactate, pyruvate, α-glutarate, and the three branched-chain ketoacids in their urine.

No effective **treatment** is available. Dietary restriction of branched-chain amino acids and treatment with high doses of thiamine, biotin, and lipoic acid has been ineffective.

Genetics and Prevalence of MSUD. All forms of MSUD are inherited as an autosomal recessive trait. The gene for each subunit resides on different chromosomes. The $E_{1\alpha}$ gene is on chromosome 19q13.1-q13.2; $E_{1\beta}$ is on chromosome 6p22-p21; E_2 is on chromosome 1p31; and E_3 is on chromosome 7q31-q32. Many different disease-causing mutations have been identified in patients with different forms of MSUD. A given phenotype is caused by a variety of genotypes; patients from different pedigrees with the classic form of MSUD have been shown to have mutations in genes for $E_{1\alpha}$, $E_{1\beta}$, or E_2. Most patients are compound heterozygotes inheriting two different mutant alleles.

The prevalence is estimated at 1/185,000. The classic form of MSUD is more prevalent in the Old Order of Mennonites in the United States, with estimated prevalence of 1/358. Affected patients in this population are homozygous for a specific mutation (Y394N) in the $E_{1\alpha}$ subunit gene.

Early detection of MSUD is feasible by mass screening of newborn infants. Prenatal diagnosis has been accomplished by enzyme assay of the cultured amniocytes, cultured chorionic villi tissue, or direct assay of the chorionic villi samples and by identification of the mutant gene.

Several successful pregnancies have occurred in women with different forms of MSUD. No ill effects have been observed in the offspring of these patients. Episodes of metabolic decompensations have occurred in the mothers during pregnancy and the postpartum period.

ISOVALERIC ACIDEMIA. This rare condition is due to the deficiency of isovaleryl coenzyme A (CoA) dehydrogenase (see Fig. 85-5).

Clinical manifestations in the *acute form* include vomiting and severe acidosis in the 1st few days of life. Lethargy, convulsions, and coma may ensue, and death may occur if proper therapy is not initiated. The vomiting may be severe enough to suggest pyloric stenosis. The characteristic odor of "sweaty feet" may be present (see Fig. 85-6). Infants who survive this acute episode will go on to have the chronic intermittent form later on in life. A milder form of the disease *(chronic intermittent form)* also exists; in this, the 1st clinical manifestation (vomiting, lethargy, acidosis or coma) may not appear until the child is a few months or a few years old. In both forms, acute episodes of metabolic decompensations may occur during a catabolic state such as an infection. Sensitive methods for newborn screening have identified yet a milder and potentially asymptomatic phenotype of the condition; a few older siblings of these affected newborns were found to have identical genotype and biochemical abnormalities without any clinical manifestations.

Laboratory findings during the acute attacks include ketoacidosis, neutropenia, thrombocytopenia, and occasionally pancytopenia. Hypocalcemia, hyperglycemia, and moderate to severe hyperammonemia may be present in some patients. Increases in plasma ammonia may suggest a defect in the urea cycle. In urea cycle defects the infant is not acidotic (see Fig. 85-6).

Diagnosis is established by demonstrating marked elevations of isovaleric acid and its metabolites (isovalerylglycine, 3-hydroxyisovaleric acid) in body fluids, especially urine. The main compound in plasma is isovalerylcarnitine, which can be measured even in a few drops of dried blood on a filter paper. Measuring the enzyme in cultured skin fibroblasts confirms the diagnosis.

Treatment of the acute attack is aimed at hydration, reversal of the catabolic state (by providing adequate calories orally or intravenously), correction of metabolic acidosis (by infusing sodium bicarbonate), and removal of the excess isovaleric acid. Because isovalerylglycine has a high urinary clearance, administration of glycine (250 mg/kg/24 hr) is recommended to enhance formation of isovalerylglycine. L-carnitine (100 mg/kg/24 hr orally) also increases removal of isovaleric acid by forming isovalerylcarnitine, which is excreted in the urine. In patients with significant hyperammonemia (blood ammonia > 200 μM), measures that reduce blood ammonia should be employed (see Chapter 85.11). Exchange transfusion and peritoneal dialysis may be needed if the just described measures fail to induce significant clinical and biochemical improvement. After recovery from the acute attack, the patient should receive a low-protein diet (1.0–1.5 g/kg/24 hr) and should be given glycine and carnitine supplements. Pancreatitis (acute or recurrent forms) has been reported in survivors. Normal development can be achieved with early and proper treatment.

Prenatal diagnosis may be accomplished by measuring isovalerylglycine in amniotic fluid, by enzyme assay in cultured amniocytes, or by identification of the mutant gene. Successful pregnancy with favorable outcomes both for the mother and the infant has been reported. Mass screening of newborn infants is in use in the United States and other countries. Isovaleric acidemia is inherited as an autosomal recessive trait. The gene has been mapped to chromosome 15q14–15q15 and many disease-causing mutations have been identified. The prevalence of the condition is estimated from 1/62,500 (in parts of Germany) to 1/250,000 (in the United States).

MULTIPLE CARBOXYLASE DEFICIENCIES (DEFECTS IN UTILIZATION OF BIOTIN). Biotin is a water-soluble vitamin that is a cofactor for all four carboxylase enzymes in humans: pyruvate carboxylase, acetyl CoA carboxylase, propionyl CoA carboxylase, and 3-methylcrotonyl CoA carboxylase. The latter two are involved in the metabolic pathways of leucine, isoleucine, and valine (see Fig. 85-4).

Dietary biotin is bound to proteins; free biotin is generated in the intestine by the action of digestive enzymes, by intestinal bacteria, and perhaps by biotinidase. The latter enzyme, which is found in serum and most tissues in the body, is also essential for the recycling of biotin in the body by releasing it from the apoenzymes (carboxylases, see Fig. 85-4). Free biotin must form a covalent peptide bond with the apoprotein of the four carboxylases to activate them (holocarboxylase). This binding is catalyzed by holocarboxylase synthetase. Deficiencies in this enzyme or in biotinidase result in malfunction of all the carboxylases and in organic acidemia.

Holocarboxylase Synthetase Deficiency (Multiple Carboxylase Deficiency—Infantile or Early Form). Infants with this rare autosomal recessive disorder become symptomatic in the 1st few weeks of life. Symptoms may appear as early as a few hours after birth to 21 mo of age. **Clinically**, the affected infants who seem normal at birth develop breathing difficulties (tachypnea and apnea) shortly after birth. Feeding problems, vomiting, and hypotonia are also commonly present. If the condition remains untreated, generalized erythematous rash with exfoliation and alopecia (partial or total), failure to thrive, irritability, seizures, lethargy, and even coma may occur. Developmental delay is common. Immune deficiency manifests with susceptibility to infection. The urine may have a peculiar odor, which has been described as similar to tomcat urine. The rash, when present, differentiates this condition from other organic acidemias (see Fig. 85-6).

Laboratory findings include metabolic acidosis, ketosis, hyperammonemia, and the presence of a variety of organic acids, which include lactic acid, propionic acid, 3-methylcrotonic acid, 3-methylcrotonylglycine, tiglylgycine, methylcitrate, and 3-hydroxyisovaleric acid in body fluids. **Diagnosis** is confirmed by the enzyme assay in lymphocytes or cultured fibroblasts. The mutant enzyme usually has an increased K_m value for biotin; the enzyme activity may be restored by the administration of large doses of biotin.

Treatment with biotin (10 mg/day orally) usually results in an improvement in clinical manifestations and may normalize the biochemical abnormalities. Early diagnosis and treatment are critical to prevent irreversible neurologic damage. In some patients, however, complete resolution may not be achieved even with large doses (up to 80 mg/day) of biotin.

The gene for holocarboxylase synthetase is located on chromosome 21q22.1 and many disease-causing mutations have been identified in different families. Prenatal diagnosis has been accomplished by assaying enzyme activity in cultured amniotic cells and by measurement of intermediate metabolites (3-hydroxyisovalerate and methylcitrate) in amniotic fluid. Pregnant mothers who had previous offspring with holocarboxylase synthetase deficiency have been treated with biotin late in pregnancy. Affected infants were normal at birth, but the efficacy of the treatment as related to the outcome remains unclear.

Biotinidase Deficiency (Multiple Carboxylase Deficiency—Juvenile or Late Form). The absence of biotinidase results in biotin deficiency. Infants with this deficiency may develop **clinical manifestations** similar to those seen in infants with holocarboxylase synthetase deficiency, but, unlike the latter, symptoms may appear later, when the child is several months or several years old; symptoms may develop as early as 1 wk of age. Therefore, the term "late form" does not apply to all cases and can be misleading. The delay is presumably because of the presence of sufficient free biotin derived from the mother or the diet. Atopic or seborrheic dermatitis, alopecia, ataxia, myoclonic seizures, hypotonia, developmental delay, sensorineural hearing loss, and immunodeficiency (from T-cell abnormalities) may occur. A small number of children with intractable seborrheic dermatitis and partial (15–30% activity) deficiency of the enzyme for whom the dermatitis resolved with biotin therapy has been reported; these children were otherwise asymptomatic. Asymptomatic children and adults with this enzyme deficiency have been identified in screening programs. Most of these individuals have shown to have partial deficiency of the enzyme activity.

Laboratory findings and the pattern of organic acids in body fluids resemble those associated with holocarboxylase synthetase deficiency (see earlier). **Diagnosis** can be established by measurement of the enzyme activity in the serum. A simplified method for mass screening of newborn infants is now available and is in use in the United States and around the world.

Treatment with free biotin (5–20 mg/24 hr) results in a dramatic clinical and biochemical response. Treatment with biotin is also suggested for individuals with partial biotinidase deficiency.

The prevalence of this autosomal recessive trait is estimated at 1/60,000. The gene for biotinidase is located on chromosome 3p25 and many disease-causing mutations have been identified in different families. Prenatal diagnosis is possible by the measurement of the enzyme activity in the amniotic cells or by identification of the mutant gene.

Multiple Carboxylase Deficiency Due to Dietary Biotin Deficiency. Acquired deficiency of biotin may occur in infants receiving total parenteral nutrition without added biotin, in patients receiving prolonged anticonvulsant drugs (phenytoin, primidone, carbamazepine) or in children with short bowel syndrome or chronic diarrhea who are receiving formulas low in biotin. Excessive ingestion of raw eggs may also cause biotin deficiency because the protein avidin in egg white binds biotin and makes it unavailable for absorption. Infants with biotin deficiency develop dermatitis, alopecia, and candidal skin infections.

ISOLATED 3-METHYLCROTONYL COA CARBOXYLASE DEFICIENCY. This enzyme is one of four carboxylase enzymes in the body that require biotin as a cofactor (see Fig. 85-4). An isolated deficiency of this enzyme must be differentiated from disorders of biotin metabolism (multiple carboxylase deficiency), which cause diminished activity of all four carboxylases. 3-Methylerotonyl CoA carboxylase is a heteromeric enzyme consisting of α (biotin containing) and β subunits.

Clinical manifestations are highly variable, ranging from fatal neonatal onset with acidosis, severe hypotonia, and seizures to asymptomatic adults. In the severe form of the condition, the affected infant who has been seemingly normal develops an acute episode of vomiting, hypotonia, lethargy, and convulsions after a minor infection. Death may occur during the acute episode.

Laboratory findings during acute episodes include mild to moderate acidosis, ketosis, severe hypoglycemia, hyperammonemia, and elevated serum levels of liver transaminases. Large amounts of 3-hydroxyisovaleric acid and 3-methylcrotonylglycine are found in the urine. Urinary excretion of 3-methylcrotonic acid is not usually increased in this condition because the accumulated 3-methylcrotonyl CoA is converted to 3-hydroxyisovaleric acid. Severe secondary carnitine deficiency is common. The condition should be differentiated biochemically from multiple carboxylase deficiency (see earlier) in which lactic acid and metabolites of propionic acid are present in body fluids in addition to 3-hydroxyisovaleric acid. **Diagnosis** may be confirmed by measurement of the enzyme activity in cultured fibroblasts. Documentation of normal activities of other carboxylases is necessary for definitive diagnosis.

Aggressive **treatment** of acute episodes with hydration, intravenous infusion of glucose, and alkali is recommended. These patients are unresponsive to biotin therapy. Patients who in earlier reports were found to be biotin responsive were most probably suffering from multiple carboxylase deficiency due to biotinidase deficiency (see earlier). Long-term treatment includes a diet restricted in leucine in conjunction with the oral administration of L-carnitine (75–100 mg/kg/24 hr) and the prevention of catabolic states. Normal growth and development are expected in these patients.

The condition is inherited as an autosomal recessive trait. The gene for α subunit (*MCC1*) is located on chromosome 3q25–27 and that for the β subunit (*MCC2*) is mapped to chromosome 5q12–13. Mutation in either of these genes may result in the deficiency of the enzyme activity. Similar phenotype may be caused by different genotype. Several disease-causing mutations in either gene have been identified in different families. Newborn screening programs using tandem mass spectrometry have identified an unexpectedly high number of infants with 3-methylcrotonyl CoA carboxylase deficiency (1:50,000), suggesting that this condition may be one of the most common organic acidemias in certain populations.

3-METHYLGLUTACONIC ACIDURIA. At least three inherited conditions are known to be associated with excessive excretion of 3-methylglutaconic acid in the urine. Deficiency of the enzyme 3-methylglutaconyl CoA hydratase (see Fig. 85-4) has been documented in only one condition (type I). In the other two conditions, the enzyme activity is normal despite a modest 3-methylglutaconic aciduria.

3-Methylglutaconic Aciduria Type I (3-Methylglutaconyl CoA Hydratase Deficiency) [see Fig. 85-4]. This rare autosomal recessive condition is manifested by speech retardation, choreoathetoid movements, optic atrophy, mild psychomotor delay, and the development of metabolic acidosis during a catabolic state. Asymptomatic affected adults have also been reported. Patients excrete large amounts of 3-methylglutaconic acid and moderate amounts of 3-hydroxyisovaleric and 3-methylglutaric acids. Deficiency of 3-methylglutaconyl CoA hydratase has been shown in cultured fibroblasts and lymphoblasts. **Treatment** with a low-protein diet has been suggested. Beneficial effects of this therapy on the clinical course of the disease remain doubtful. Administration of L-carnitine has resulted in clinical improvement in one patient. The gene for the enzyme (*AUH*) is mapped to chromosome 9.

3-Methylglutaconic Aciduria Type II (X-Linked Cardiomyopathy, Neutropenia, Growth Retardation, and 3-Methylglutaconic Aciduria with Normal 3-Methylglutaconyl CoA Hydratase, Barth syndrome). **Clinical manifestations** of this condition, which usually occur shortly after birth, include dilated **cardiomyopathy** (manifested as respiratory distress and heart failure), hypotonia, growth retardation, and moderate to severe neutropenia. Mild lactic aciduria and/or hypoglycemia have been reported in some patients. If patients survive infancy, relative improvement may occur with advancing age. Cognitive development is usually normal despite delayed motor function.

Laboratory findings include mild to moderate increases in urinary excretion of 3-methylglutaconic, 3-methylglutaric, and 2-ethylhydracrylic acids. Neutropenia is a common finding. Lactic acidosis, hypoglycemia, and abnormal mitochondrial ultrastructure have been shown in some patients. Unlike 3-methylglutaconic aciduria type I, urinary excretion of 3-hydroxyoisovaleric acid is not elevated. Total cardiolipin and subclasses of cardiolipin are very low in skin fibroblast cultures from these patients. This finding may be useful for establishing the diagnosis.

The condition is inherited as an X-linked recessive trait. The gene has been mapped to chromosome Xq28 and several disease-causing mutations have been identified. The activity of the enzyme 3-methylglutaconyl CoA hydratase is normal. The reason for the increased excretion of the herein described organic acids is not yet understood. No effective **treatment** is available.

3-Methylglutaconic Aciduria Type III (Costeff Optic Atrophy Syndrome). **Clinical manifestations** in these patients include early onset optic atrophy and later development of choreoathetoid movements, spasticity, ataxia, dysarthria, and mild developmental delay. All reported patients except one were Iraqi Jews living in Israel. These patients excrete moderate amounts of 3-methylglutaconic and 3-methylglutaric acids. As in 3-methyglutaconic aciduria type II, the reason for the increased excretion of these organic acids has not been elucidated. Activity of the enzyme 3-methylglutaconyl CoA hydratase has been normal. The condition is inherited as an autosomal recessive trait. The gene for this condition (*OPA3*) is mapped to chromosome 19q13.2–13.3. No effective **treatment** is available.

β-KETOTHIOLASE DEFICIENCY (MITOCHONDRIAL ACETOACETYL COA THIOLASE DEFICIENCY). This reversible mitochondrial enzyme cleaves 2-methylacetoacetyl CoA (see Fig. 85-4) or acetoacetyl CoA in one direction and synthesizes these compounds in a reverse action (Fig. 85-7).

Clinical manifestations are quite variable, ranging from an asymptomatic course in an adult to severe episodes of acidosis starting in the 1st yr of life. These children have intermittent episodes of unexplained ketosis and acidosis. These episodes usually occur after an intercurrent infection and respond quickly to intravenous fluids and bicarbonate therapy. Mild to moderate hyperammonemia may also be present during attacks. Both hypoglycemia and hyperglycemia have been reported in isolated cases. The child may be completely asymptomatic between episodes and may tolerate a normal protein diet well. Mental development is normal in most children. The episodes may be misdiagnosed as salicylate poisoning because of the similarity of clinical findings and the interference of elevated blood levels of acetoacetate with the colorimetric assay for salicylate.

Laboratory findings during the acute attack include acidosis, ketosis, and hyperammonemia. The urine contains large amounts of 2-methylacetoacetate and its decarboxylation product butanone, 2-methyl-3-hydroxybutyrate, and tiglylglycine. Lower concentrations of these urinary metabolites persist during the seemingly well periods. Mild hyperglycinemia may also be present. The clinical and biochemical findings should be differentiated from those seen with propionic and methylmalonic acidemias (see later). **Diagnosis** may be established by assay of the enzyme in cultured fibroblasts or identification of the mutant gene.

Treatment of acute episodes includes hydration and infusion of bicarbonate to correct the acidosis; a 10% glucose solution with the appropriate electrolytes and intravenous lipids may be used to minimize the catabolic state. Restriction of protein intake (1–2 g/kg/24 hr) is recommended for long-term therapy. Oral L-carnitine (50–100 mg/kg/24 hr) is also recommended to prevent possible secondary carnitine deficiency. Long-term prognosis for achieving normal life seems very favorable. Three patients graduated from high school and one has attended college. All patients continued to have abnormal metabolites in body fluids. Successful pregnancy with normal outcomes for both mother and infant has been reported.

The pathogenesis of ketosis in this condition is not adequately explained because, in this enzyme deficiency, one expects impaired ketone formation (see Fig. 85-7). It is postulated that excess acetoacetyl CoA produced from other sources is used as a substrate for 3-hydroxy 3-methylglutaryl (HMG) CoA synthesis in the liver.

This condition is inherited as an autosomal recessive trait and may be more prevalent than has been appreciated. It is most prevalent in Tunisia. The gene (*ACAT1*) for this enzyme (T_2) is located on chromosome 11q22.3–23.1.

CYTOSOLIC ACETOACETYL COA THIOLASE DEFICIENCY. This enzyme catalyzes the cytosolic production of acetoacetyl CoA from two moles of acetyl CoA (see Fig. 85-7). Cytosolic acetoacetyl CoA is the precursor of hepatic cholesterol synthesis. Cytosolic acetoacetyl CoA thiolase is a completely different enzyme from that of mitochondrial thiolase (see earlier and Fig. 85-4). **Clinical manifestations** in patients with this rare enzyme deficiency are similar to those in patients with mevalonic acidemia (see later). Severe progressive developmental delay, hypotonia, and choreoathetoid movements develop in the 1st few months of life. **Laboratory findings** are nonspecific; elevated levels of lactate, pyruvate, acetoacetate, and 3-hydroxybutyrate may be found in blood and urine. One patient had normal levels of acetoacetate and 3-hydroxybutyrate. **Diagnosis** can be established by demonstrating a deficiency in cytosolic thiolase activity in liver biopsy or in cultured fibroblasts or by DNA analysis. No effective **treatment** is available. The gene for this condition is mapped to chromosome 6q25.3-q26.

Mitochondrial 3-Hydroxy 3-Methylglutaryl (HMG) CoA Synthase Deficiency. This enzyme catalyzes synthesis of HMG-CoA from acetoacetyl CoA in the mitochondria. This is a critical step in ketone body synthesis in the liver (see Fig. 85-7). Only a few

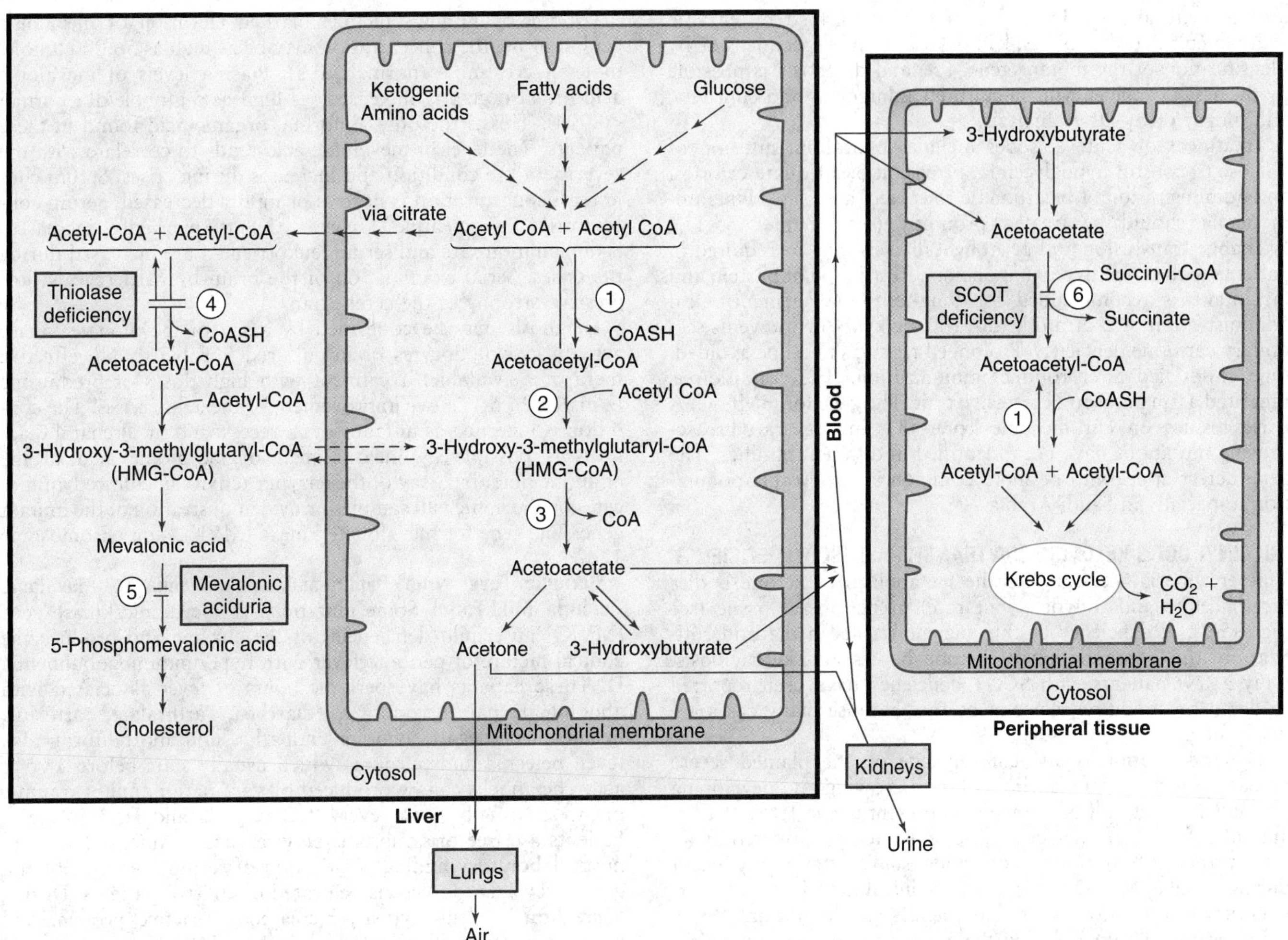

Figure 85-7. Formation (liver) and metabolism (peripheral tissues) of ketone bodies and cholesterol synthesis. **Enzymes:** (1) mitochondrial acetoacetyl CoA thiolase, (2) HMG-CoA synthase, (3) HMG-CoA lyase, (4) cytosolic acetoacetyl CoA thiolase, (5) mevalonic kinase, (6) succinyl CoA:3-ketoacid CoA transferase (SCOT).

patients with deficiency of this enzyme have been reported. All patients have had similar presentations and outcomes. Signs and symptoms of acute hypoglycemia have occurred after an acute illness (gastroenteritis). Age at presentation has ranged from 18 mo to 6 yr. All children were asymptomatic before the episodes and remained normal after the recovery (except for mild hepatomegaly with fatty infiltration). None of the patients has had a second episode, perhaps as a result of preventive measures to avoid prolonged fasting during ensuing intercurrent illnesses. Hepatomegaly was a consistent **physical finding** in all patients. **Laboratory findings** included hypoglycemia, acidosis with mild or no ketosis, elevation of liver function tests, and massive dicarboxylic aciduria. The clinical and laboratory findings may be confused with those of patients with defects in fatty acid metabolism (see Chapter 86.1). In contrast to the latter, blood concentrations of acylcarnitine conjugates are normal in patients with HMG-CoA synthase deficiency. Fasting of these patients has produced the here mentioned clinical and biochemical abnormalities.

Treatment consisted of provision of adequate calories and avoidance of prolonged periods of fasting. No dietary protein restriction was needed.

The condition is inherited as an autosomal recessive trait. The gene for this condition is located on chromosome 1p13-p12 and several disease-causing mutations have been identified. The condition should be considered in any child with fasting hypoglycemia and is perhaps more common than appreciated.

3-HYDROXY-3-METHYLGLUTARIC ACIDURIA. This condition is due to a deficiency of HMG-CoA lyase (see Fig. 85-4). This enzyme catalyzes the conversion of HMG-CoA to acetoacetate and is a rate-limiting enzyme for ketogenesis (see Fig. 85-7). **Clinically,** >60% of patients become symptomatic between 3 and 11 mo of age, whereas about 30% develop symptoms in the 1st few days of life. One child remained asymptomatic until 15 yr of age. Episodes of vomiting, severe hypoglycemia, hypotonia, acidosis with mild or no ketosis, and dehydration may rapidly lead to lethargy, ataxia, and coma. These episodes often occur during a catabolic state such as fasting or an intercurrent infection. Hepatomegaly is common. These manifestations may be mistaken for Reye syndrome or medium-chain acyl CoA dehydrogenase (MCAD) deficiency. Patients are usually clinically asymptomatic between the attacks; one patient died of acute cardiomyopathy at age 7 mo during a febrile illness. Development is usually normal, but mental retardation and seizure with abnormalities of white matter (shown by MRI) have been observed in patients with prolonged episodes of hypoglycemia.

Laboratory findings include hypoglycemia, moderate to severe hyperammonemia, and acidosis. There is mild or no ketosis (see Fig. 85-7). Urinary excretion of 3-hydroxy-3-methylglutaric acid and other proximal intermediate metabolites of leucine catabolism (3-methylglutaconic acid and 3-hydroxyisovaleric acid) is markedly increased. These organic acids are excreted in the urine as carnitine conjugates, resulting in secondary carnitine deficiency. Glutaric and adipic acids may also be increased in urine during acute attacks. **Diagnosis** may be confirmed by enzyme assay in cultured fibroblasts, leukocytes, or liver specimens or by identification of the mutant gene. Prenatal diagnosis is possible by the assay of the enzyme in cultured amniocytes or a chorionic villi biopsy or by DNA analysis.

Treatment of acute episodes includes hydration, infusion of glucose to control hypoglycemia, provision of adequate calories, and administration of bicarbonate to correct acidosis. Hyperammonemia should be treated promptly (see Chapter 85.11). Exchange transfusion and peritoneal dialysis may be required in patients with severe hyperammonemia. Restriction of protein and fat intake is recommended for long-term management. Oral administration of L-carnitine (50–100 mg/kg/24 hr) prevents secondary carnitine deficiency. Prolonged fasting should be avoided. One child died after routine immunization. The condition is inherited as an autosomal recessive trait. The gene for HMG-CoA lyase resides on chromosome 1pter-p33 and several disease-causing mutations have been identified in different families. The gene defect appears to be more common in the Arabic population, especially in Saudi Arabia.

SUCCINYL COA:3-KETOACID COA TRANSFERASE (SCOT) DEFICIENCY. This enzyme is necessary for the metabolism of ketone bodies (acetoacetate and 3-hydroxybutyrate) in peripheral tissue (see Fig. 85-7). A deficiency of this enzyme results in the underutilization and accumulation of ketone bodies and ketoacidosis. Only a few patients with SCOT deficiency have been reported to date; the condition may not be rare because many cases are undiagnosed.

The presentation is an acute episode of unexplained severe ketoacidosis in an infant who had been growing and developing normally. About half of the patients present in the 1st wk of life and all before 2 yr. The acute episode is often precipitated by an intercurrent infection or a catabolic state. Death may occur during these episodes. A chronic subclinical ketosis usually persists between the attacks. Development is usually normal.

Laboratory findings during the acute episode are nonspecific and include metabolic acidosis and ketonuria with high levels of acetoacetate and 3-hydroxybutyrate in blood and urine. No other organic acids are found in the blood or in the urine. Blood glucose levels are usually normal, but hypoglycemia has been reported in two newborn infants with severe ketoacidosis. Plasma amino acids are usually normal. **Diagnosis** can be established by demonstrating a deficiency of enzyme activity in cultured fibroblasts or by DNA analysis.

Treatment of acute episodes consists of hydration, correction of acidosis, and the provision of a diet adequate in calories. Long-term treatment with a high-carbohydrate diet and avoidance of catabolic states is recommended. *This condition should be considered in any infant with unexplained bouts of ketoacidosis.* The condition is inherited as an autosomal recessive trait. The gene for this enzyme is located on chromosome 5p13, and several disease-causing mutations have been found in different families.

MEVALONIC ACIDURIA. Mevalonic acid, an intermediate metabolite of cholesterol synthesis, is converted to 5-phosphomevalonic acid by the action of the enzyme mevalonate kinase (see Fig. 85-7). Based on clinical manifestations, two forms of this condition have been recognized.

Mevalonic Aciduria, Severe Form. **Clinical manifestations** include mental retardation, failure to thrive, growth retardation, hypotonia, ataxia, hepatosplenomegaly, cataracts, and facial dysmorphism (dolichocephaly, frontal bossing, low-set ears, downward slanting of the eyes, and long eyelashes). Recurrent crises, characterized by fever, vomiting, diarrhea, arthralgia, edema, lymphadenopathy, further enlargement of liver and spleen, and morbilliform rash have been observed in all patients. These episodes last 4–5 days and recur up to 25 times/yr. Death may occur during these crises.

Laboratory findings include marked elevation of mevalonic acid in urine; the concentration may be as high as 56,000 μmole/mole of creatinine (normal <0.3). Plasma levels of mevalonic acid are also greatly increased (as high as 54 μmole/dL; normal <0.004). This is the only abnormal organic acid found in these patients. The level of mevalonic acid tends to correlate with the severity of the condition and increases during crises. Serum cholesterol concentration is normal or mildly decreased. Serum concentration of creatine kinase (CK) is markedly increased. Sedimentation rate and serum leukotriene-4 are increased during the crises. Serial examination of the brain by MRI reveals progressive atrophy of the cerebellum.

Diagnosis may be confirmed by assay of mevalonate kinase activity in lymphocytes or in cultured fibroblasts. No effective therapy is available. **Treatment** with high doses of prednisone (2 mg/kg/24 hr) causes improvement of the acute crises. The condition is inherited as an autosomal recessive trait. Prenatal diagnosis is possible by measurement of mevalonic acid in the amniotic fluid, by assay of the enzyme activity in cultured amniocytes or chorionic villi samples or by demonstration of the mutant gene. The gene for mevalonate kinase (MVK) is on chromosome 12q24.

Periodic Fever with Hyperimmunoglobulinemia D (Mevalonic Aciduria, Mild Form). Some mutations of mevalonic kinase gene (MVK) cause mild deficiencies of the enzyme and produce the **clinical picture** of periodic fever with hyperimmunogobulinemia D. These patients have periodic bouts of fever associated with abdominal pain, vomiting, diarrhea, arthralgia, arthritis, hepatosplenomegaly, lymphadenopathy, and morbiliform rash (even petechia and purpura) which usually start before 1 yr of age. The attacks can be produced by vaccination, minor trauma, or stress; usually occur every 1–2 months and last 2–7 days. Patients are free of symptoms between acute attacks. The diagnostic **laboratory finding** is elevation of serum immunoglobulin gamma D (IgD); IgA is also elevated in 80% of patients. During acute attacks, leukocytosis, increased C-reactive protein, and mild mevalonic aciduria may be present. High concentration of serum IgD differentiates this condition from familial Mediterranean fever.

Treatment of acute attacks remains symptomatic. The condition is inherited as an autosomal recessive trait; most patients are white and are from western European countries (60% are either Dutch or French). The enzyme activity is usually about 5–15% of normal. The pathogenesis of the condition remains unclear. Several disease-causing mutations of the gene (located on chromosome 12q24) have been identified, but one mutation (V377I) is present in 80% of patients. Long-term prognosis is usually good, but amyloidosis has occurred in a few patients.

PROPIONIC ACIDEMIA (PROPIONYL COA CARBOXYLASE DEFICIENCY). Propionic acid is an intermediate metabolite of isoleucine, valine, threonine, methionine, odd-chain fatty acids, and cholesterol catabolism. It is normally carboxylated to methylmalonic acid by the mitochondrial enzyme propionyl CoA carboxylase, which requires biotin as a cofactor (see Fig. 85-4). The enzyme is composed of two nonidentical subunits, α and β. Biotin is bound to the α subunit.

Clinical findings are nonspecific. In the severe form of the condition, patients develop symptoms in the 1st few days or weeks of life. Poor feeding, vomiting, hypotonia, lethargy, dehydration, and clinical signs of severe ketoacidosis progress rapidly to coma and death. Seizures occur in ≈30% of affected infants. If an infant survives the 1st attack, similar episodes may occur during an intercurrent infection or constipation or after ingestion of a high-protein diet. Moderate to severe mental retardation and neurologic abnormalities such as dystonia, choreoathetosis, tremor, and pyramidal signs are common sequelae in the older survivors. In the milder forms, the older infant may have mental retardation without acute attacks of ketosis. Some affected children may have episodes of unexplained severe ketoacidosis separated by periods of seemingly normal health. Mass screening of newborns has identified milder forms of the condition; a few of theses infants were completely asymptomatic at diagnosis. The severity of clinical manifestations may also be variable within a family; in one kindred, a brother was diagnosed at 5 yr of age whereas his 13 yr old sister, with the same level of enzyme deficiency, was asymptomatic.

Laboratory findings during the acute attack include severe metabolic acidosis with a large anion gap, ketosis, neutropenia, thrombocytopenia, and hypoglycemia. Moderate to severe hyperammonemia is common; plasma ammonia concentrations usually correlate with the severity of the disease. Measurement of plasma ammonia is especially helpful in planning therapeutic strategy during episodes of exacerbation in a patient whose diagnosis has been established. Pathogenesis of hyperammonemia is not well understood. Hyperglycinemia is a common finding. Elevations in plasma and urinary levels of glycine have also been observed in patients with methylmalonic acidemia. These disorders were collectively referred to as *ketotic hyperglycinemia* before the specific enzyme deficiencies were elucidated. Concentrations of propionic acid and methylcitric acid (presumably made by the condensation of propionyl CoA with oxaloacetic acid) are markedly elevated in the plasma and urine of infants with propionic acidemia. 3-Hydroxypropionic acid, propionylglycine, and other intermediate metabolites of isoleucine catabolism, such as tiglic acid, tiglyglycine, and 2-methyloacetoacetic acid, are also found in urine. Moderate elevations in blood levels of ammonia, glycine, and previously mentioned organic acids usually persist between the acute attacks. CT scan and MRI of the brain may reveal evidence of cerebral atrophy, demyelination, and abnormalities in globus pallidus and basal ganglia. These findings represent past infarctions caused by a cerebral vascular accident, which may occur during an acute episode of metabolic decompensation. This complication (**metabolic stroke**) may also occur in patients with other organic acidemias and is a major cause of neurologic sequelae.

The **diagnosis** of propionic acidemia should be differentiated from multiple carboxylase deficiencies (see earlier and Fig. 85-6). Infants with the latter condition may have skin manifestations and excrete large amounts of lactic acid, 3-methylcrotonic acid, and 3-hydroxyisovaleric acid in addition to propionic acid. The presence of hyperammonemia may suggest a genetic defect in the urea cycle enzymes. Infants with defects in the urea cycle are usually not acidotic (see Fig. 84-1). Definitive diagnosis of propionic acidemia can be established by measuring the enzyme activity in leukocytes or cultured fibroblasts.

Treatment of acute attacks includes hydration, correction of acidosis, and amelioration of the catabolic state by provision of adequate calories through parenteral hyperalimentation. Minimal amounts of protein (0.25 g/kg/24 hr), preferably a protein deficient in propionate precursors, should be provided in the hyperalimentation fluid very early in the course of treatment. To curtail the possible production of propionic acid by intestinal bacteria, sterilization of the intestinal tract flora by antibiotics (oral neomycin, or metronidazole) should be promptly initiated. Constipation should also be treated. Patients with propionic acidemia may develop carnitine deficiency, presumably as a result of urinary loss of propionylcarnitine formed from the accumulated organic acid. Administration of L-carnitine (50–100 mg/kg/24 hr orally or 10 mg/kg/24 hr intravenously) normalizes fatty acid oxidation and improves acidosis. In patients with concomitant hyperammonemia, measures to reduce blood ammonia should be employed (see Chapter 85.11). Very ill patients with severe acidosis and hyperammonemia require peritoneal dialysis or hemodialysis to remove ammonia and other toxic compounds efficiently. Although infants with true propionic acidemia are rarely responsive to biotin, this compound should be administered (10 mg/24 hr orally) to all infants during the 1st attack and until the diagnosis is established.

Long-term treatment consists of a low-protein diet (1.0–1.5 g/kg/24 hr) and administration of L-carnitine (50–100 mg/kg/24 hr orally). Synthetic proteins deficient in propionate precursors (isoleucine, valine, methionine, and threonine) may be used to increase the amount of dietary protein (to 1.5–2.0 g/kg/24 hr) while causing minimal change in propionate production. Excessive supplementation with these proteins may cause a deficiency of the essential amino acids. To avoid this problem, natural proteins should comprise most of the dietary protein (50–75%). Some patients may require chronic alkaline therapy to correct chronic acidosis. The concentration of ammonia in the blood usually normalizes between attacks, and chronic treatment of hyperammonemia is not usually needed. Catabolic states that may trigger acute attacks (infections, constipation) should be treated promptly and aggressively. Close monitoring of blood pH, amino acids, urinary content of propionate and its metabolites, and growth parameters is necessary to ensure the proper balance of the diet and the success of therapy.

Long-term prognosis is guarded. Death may occur during an acute attack. Normal psychomotor development is possible, especially in the mild forms identified through screening programs; most children identified clinically manifest some degree of permanent neurodevelopmental deficit such as dystonia, chorea, and pyramidal signs despite adequate therapy. These neurologic findings may be sequelae of a **metabolic stroke** occurring during an acute decompensation (see earlier).

Prenatal diagnosis is achieved by measuring the enzyme activity in cultured amniotic cells or in samples of uncultured chorionic villi, by measurement of methylnitrate in amniotic fluid, or by identification of the mutant gene.

The condition is inherited as an autosomal recessive trait and can be identified by mass screening of newborns. It is more prevalent in Saudi Arabia (1 : 2,000 to 1 : 5,000). The gene for the α subunit (*PCCA* gene) is located on chromosome 13q32 and that of the β subunit (*PCCB* gene) is mapped to the chromosome 3q21-q22. Many mutations in either gene have been identified in different patients. Pregnancy with normal outcome has been reported in affected females.

METHYLMALONIC ACIDEMIA. Methylmalonic acid, a structural isomer of succinic acid, is normally derived from propionic acid as part of the catabolic pathways of isoleucine, valine, threonine, methionine, cholesterol, and odd-chain fatty acids. Two enzymes are involved in the conversion of D-methylmalonic acid to succinic acid: methylmalonyl CoA racemase, which forms the L-isomer; and methylmalonyl CoA mutase, which converts the L-methylmalonic acid to succinic acid (see Fig. 85-4). The latter enzyme requires adenosylcobalamin, a metabolite of vitamin B_{12}, as a coenzyme. Deficiency of either the mutase or its coenzyme causes the accumulation of methylmalonic acid and its precursors in body fluids. A deficiency of the racemase has not been confirmed.

At least two forms of mutase apoenzyme deficiencies have been identified. These are designated *mut*^{0}, meaning no detectable enzyme activity, and *mut*$^-$, indicating residual, although abnormal, mutase activity. The majority of reported patients with methylmalonic acidemia have a deficiency of the mutase apoenzyme (*mut*^{0} or *mut*$^-$). These patients are not responsive to vitamin B_{12} therapy. In the remaining patients with methylmalonic acidemia, the defect resides in the formation of adenosylcobalamin.

Defects in Metabolism of Vitamin B_{12} (Cobalamin). Dietary vitamin B_{12} requires intrinsic factor, a glycoprotein secreted by the gastric parietal cells, for absorption in the terminal ileum. It is transported in the blood by haptocorrin (TCI) and transcobalamin II (TCII). The complex of transcobalamin II-cobalamin (TCII-Cbl) is recognized by a specific receptor on the cell membrane and enters the cell by endocytosis. The TCII-Cbl complex is hydrolyzed in the lysosome, and free cobalamin is released into the cytosol (see Fig. 85-4). The cobalt of the molecule is reduced in the cytosol from three valences (cob[III]alamin) to two (cob[II]alamin) before it enters the mitochondria, where further reduction to cob(I)alamin occurs. The latter compound reacts with adenosine to form adenosylcobalamin (coenzyme for methylmalonyl CoA mutase). The free cobalamin in the cytosol may also undergo a series of poorly understood enzymatic steps to form methylcobalamin (coenzyme for methionine synthase, see Fig. 85-3).

At least eight different defects in the intracellular metabolism of cobalamin have been identified. These are designated *cbl*A through H (*cbl* stands for a defect in any step of cobalamin metabolism). *cbl*A, *cbl*H, and *cbl*B cause methylmalonic acidemia only; *cbl*B is caused by a deficiency of adenosylcobalamin transferase. In patients with *cbl*C, *cbl*D, and *cbl*F defects, synthesis of both adenosylcobalamin and methylcobalamin is impaired, causing homocystinuria in addition to methylmalonic acidemia. The *cbl*E defect and the *cbl*G defect involve only the synthesis of methylcobalamin, resulting in homocystinuria without methylmalonic aciduria but usually with megaloblastic anemia.

Clinical manifestations of patients with methylmalonic acidemia due to *mut*^{0}, *mut*$^-$, *cbl*A, *cbl*B, and *cbl*H are similar. There are wide variations in clinical presentation, ranging from very sick newborn infants to asymptomatic adults, regardless of the nature of the enzymatic defect or the biochemical abnormalities. In severe forms, lethargy, feeding problems, vomiting, tachypnea (due to acidosis), and hypotonia may develop in the 1st few days of life and may progress to coma and death if untreated. Infants who survive the 1st attack may go on to develop similar acute metabolic episodes during a catabolic state (such as infection) or after ingestion of a high-protein diet. Between the acute attacks, the patient commonly continues to exhibit hypotonia and feeding problems with failure to thrive. In milder forms, patients may present later in life with hypotonia, failure to thrive, and developmental delay. Asymptomatic patients with typical biochemical abnormalities of methylmalonic acidemia are also reported. It is important to note that mental development and IQ of patients with methylmalonic acidemia may remain within the normal range despite repeated acute attacks and regardless of the nature of the enzyme deficiency. In one study of patients with different forms of the condition, developmental retardation was noted in only 47%. One adolescent girl with a *mut*$^-$ deficiency had an IQ of 129.

The episodic nature of the condition and its biochemical abnormalities may be confused with those of ethylene glycol (antifreeze) ingestion. The peak of propionate in the assay has been mistaken as that of ethylene glycol.

Laboratory findings include ketosis, acidosis, anemia, neutropenia, thrombocytopenia, hyperglycinemia, hyperammonemia, hypoglycemia, and the presence of large quantities of methylmalonic acid in body fluids (see Fig. 85-6). Propionic acid and its metabolites 3-hydroxypropionate and methylitcrate are also found in the urine. Hyperammonemia may suggest the presence of genetic defects in the urea cycle enzymes; patients with defects in urea cycle enzymes are not acidotic (see Fig. 84-1). The reason for hyperammonemia is not well understood.

Diagnosis can be confirmed by measuring propionate incorporation or mutase activity, by performing complementation studies in cultured fibroblasts, or by identifying the mutant gene.

Treatment of acute attacks is similar to that of attacks in patients with propionic acidemia (see earlier), except that large doses (1 mg/24 hr) of vitamin B_{12} are used instead of biotin. Long-term treatment consists of administration of a low-protein diet (1.0–1.5 g/kg/24 hr), L-carnitine (50–100 mg/kg/24 hr orally), and vitamin B_{12} (1 mg/24 hr for patients with defects in vitamin B_{12} metabolism; the dose can be decreased depending on the clinical response). The protein composition of the diet is similar to that prescribed for patients with propionic acidemia. Chronic alkaline therapy is usually required to correct chronic acidosis, especially during infancy and early childhood. Blood levels of ammonia usually normalize between the attacks, and chronic treatment of hyperammonemia is rarely needed. Constipation and stressful situations that may trigger acute attacks (such as infection) should be prevented or treated promptly.

Inadequate oral intake secondary to poor appetite is a common and bothersome complication in long-term management of these patients. Consequently, enteral feeding (through a nasogastric tube or gastrostomy) should be considered early in the course of the treatment. Close monitoring of blood pH, amino acid levels, blood and urinary concentrations of methylmalonate, and growth parameters is necessary to ensure proper balance in the diet and the success of therapy. Glutathione deficiency, responsive to high doses of ascorbate, has been described in one patient. Liver and combined liver and kidney transplantations have been attempted with variable success.

Prognosis depends on the severity of symptoms and the occurrence of complications (see later). In general, patients with mutase apoenzyme deficiency (*mut*^{0}, *mut*$^-$) have a less favorable prognosis and those with *cbl*A defect have a better outcome than those with *cbl*B.

A few **complications** have been noted in the survivors. Infarcts of the brain, especially those of the basal ganglia (globus pallidus) and internal capsule, have been reported in a few patients during an acute episode of metabolic decompensation (**metabolic stroke**). These patients have survived with major extrapyramidal (tremor, dystonia) and pyramidal (paraplegia) sequelae. The pathogenesis of this complication also remains unclear.

Chronic renal failure necessitating renal transplant has been reported in a number of older patients with the condition. This complication has been observed in all genetic forms of the condition. **Tubulointerstitial nephritis** has been documented in some of these patients and is thought to be the major cause of renal failure. The pathogenesis remains unclear.

Acute and recurrent pancreatitis has been reported in the affected patients as young as 13 months of age. This complication may account for a fair number of hospitalizations of these children.

The prevalence of the condition is estimated at 1/48,000. All defects causing methylmalonic acidemia are inherited as autosomal recessive traits. Successful mass screening of newborns has been achieved by the tandem mass spectrometry method. The gene for the mutase has been mapped to the short arm of chromosome 6, and at least 160 different mutations have been identified in the *mut* gene including a number of ethnic-specific mutations. Neonates with methylmalonic acidemia and severe diabetes due to the absence of β cells who have paternal uniparental isodisory of chromosome 6 have been reported. Mutations in the gene for *cbl*A (*MMAA,* located on chromosome 4q31-q31.2) and in the gene for *cbl*B (*MMAB,* mapped to chromosome 12q24) have been identified in a number of affected patients. The gene for *cbl*H has not yet been found.

Successful pregnancy with normal outcomes for both the mother and the baby has been reported.

COMBINED METHYLMALONIC ACIDURIA AND HOMOCYSTINURIA (*cbl*C, *cbl*D, AND *cbl*F DEFECTS). Almost 200 patients with methylmalonic acidemia and homocystinuria due to *cbl*C, *cbl*D, and *cbl*F defects (see Figs. 85-3 and 85-4) are reported. The majority of the patients had the *cbl*C defect; five patients with *cbl*D and nine with *cbl*F defects have been identified. The *cbl*C defect is now subdivided into two variants, one with dysfunction of only methionine synthase and one with dysfunction of methylmanolyl CoA mutase.

Neurologic findings are prominent in patients with *cbl*C and *cbl*D defects. Most patients with the *cbl*C defect present in the 1st few months of life because of failure to thrive, lethargy, poor feeding, mental retardation, and seizures. Late-onset defects with sudden development of dementia and myelopathy have been reported. Megaloblastic anemia was a common finding in patients with *cbl*C defect. Mild to moderate increases in concentrations of methylmalonic acid and homocysteine were found in body fluids. Unlike patients with classic homocystinuria, plasma levels of methionine are low to normal in these defects. Neither hyperammonemia nor hyperglycinemia is present in these patients. The 1st two patients with *cbl*F defect were females in whom poor feeding, growth and developmental delay, and persistent stomatitis manifested in the 1st 3 wk of life. The 1st patient did not have megaloblastic anemia and homocystinuria, but these signs were present in the 2nd infant. Moderate methylmalonic acidemia was present in both infants. One patient was not diagnosed until age 10 yr and had findings suggestive of rheumatoid arthritis, a pigmented skin abnormality, and encephalopathy. Vitamin B_{12} malabsorption has been noted in patients with *cbl*F defect.

Experience with **treatment** of patients with *cbl*C, *cbl*D, and *cbl*F defects is limited. Large doses of hydroxycobalamin (1–2 mg/24 hr) in conjunction with betaine (6–9 g/24 hr) seem to produce biochemical improvement with little clinical effect. Unexplained severe hemolytic anemia, hydrocephalus, and congestive heart failure have been major complications in patients with *cbl*C defect. The gene for *cblC* is mapped to chromosme 1.

Patients with *cbl*E and *cbl*G defects do not have methylmalonic acidemia (see Chapter 85.3).

85.7 • Glycine • Iraj Rezvani

Glycine is a nonessential amino acid synthesized mainly from serine and threonine. The main catabolic pathway requires the complex glycine cleavage enzyme to cleave the 1st carbon of glycine and convert it to carbon dioxide (Fig. 85-8). The glycine cleavage protein, a mitochondrial multienzyme, is composed of four proteins: P protein, H protein, T protein, and L protein, which are encoded by four different genes.

HYPERGLYCINEMIA. Elevated levels of glycine in body fluids occur in propionic acidemia and methylmalonic acidemia that are collectively referred to as **ketotic hyperglycinemia** because episodes of severe acidosis and ketosis occur. The pathogenesis of hyperglycinemia in these disorders is not fully understood, but inhibition of the glycine cleavage enzyme system by the various organic acids has been shown to occur in some of the patients. The term **nonketotic hyperglycinemia** is reserved for the clinical condition caused by the genetic deficiency of the glycine cleavage enzyme system (see Fig. 85-8). In this condition, hyperglycinemia is present without ketosis.

NONKETOTIC HYPERGLYCINEMIA (NKH), GLYCINE ENCEPHALOPATHY. Four forms of this condition have been identified: neonatal, infantile, late onset, and transient.

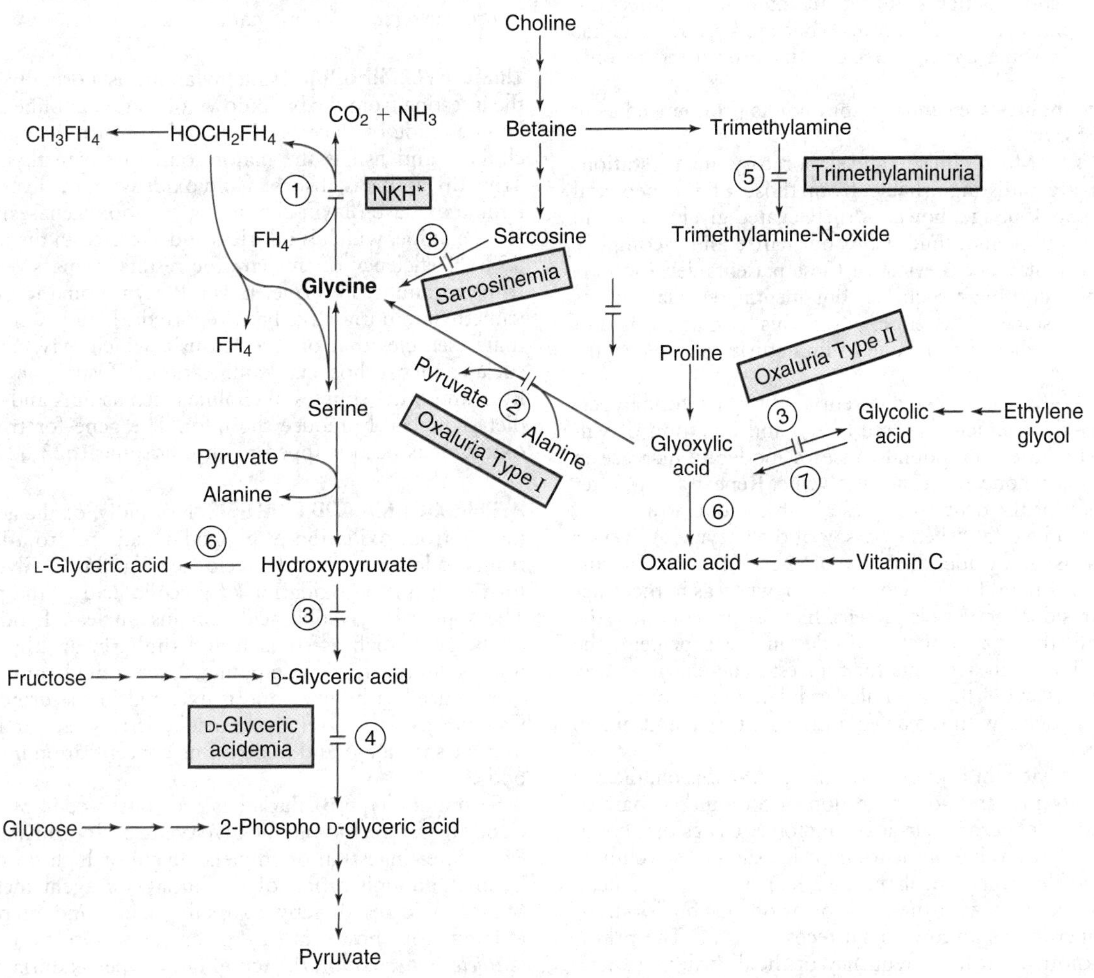

Figure 85-8. Pathways in the metabolism of glycine and gloxylic acid. **Enzymes:** (1) glycine cleavage enzyme, (2) alanine:glyoxylate aminotransferase, (3) D-glyceric acid dehydrogenase, (4) glycerate kinase, (5) trimethylamine oxidase, (6) lactate dehydrogenase, (7) glycolate oxidase, (8) sarcosine dehydrogenase. FH_4, tetrahydrofolate; NkH*, nonketotic hyperglycinemia.

Neonatal Hyperglycemia. This is the most common form of NKH. **Clinical manifestations** develop in the 1st few days of life (between 6 hr and 8 days after birth). Poor feeding, failure to suck, lethargy, and profound hypotonia may progress rapidly to a deep coma, apnea, and death. Convulsions, especially myoclonic seizures and hiccups, are common.

Laboratory findings reveal moderate to severe hyperglycinemia (as high as eight times normal) and hyperglycinuria. The unequivocal elevation of glycine concentration in the spinal fluid (15 to 30 times normal) and the high ratio of glycine concentration in spinal fluid to that in plasma (a value >0.08) are diagnostic of NKH. Serum pH is normal; plasma serine levels are usually low.

About 30% of affected infants die despite supportive therapy. Those who survive develop profound psychomotor retardation and intractable seizure disorders (myoclonic and/or grand mal seizures). **Hydrocephalus**, requiring shunting, and **pulmonary hypertension** have been noted in some survivors.

Infantile NKH. These previously normal infants develop **signs and symptoms** of neonatal NKH (see earlier) after 6 mo of age. Seizures are the common presenting signs. This condition appears to be a milder form, infants usually survive, and mental retardation is not as profound as in the neonatal form.

Laboratory findings in these patients are identical to the neonatal form.

Late-Onset NKH, Mild Episodic Form. Progressive spastic diplegia, optic atrophy, and choreoathetotic movements are the main **clinical manifestations.** Age of onset has been between 2 and 33 yr. Symptoms of delirium, chorea, and vertical gaze palsy may occur episodically in some patients during an intercurrent infection. Mental development is usually normal, but mild retardation has been reported in some patients. Seizures have occurred in only one patient.

Laboratory findings are similar to but not as pronounced as in the neonatal form.

Transient NKH. Most clinical and laboratory manifestations of this form are indistinguishable from those of the neonatal form. By 2 to 8 wk of age, however, the elevated glycine levels in plasma and cerebrospinal fluid (CSF) normalize and a complete clinical recovery may occur. Most of these patients develop normally with no neurologic sequelae, but mental retardation has been noted in some. The etiology of this condition is not known, but it is believed to be due to immaturity of the enzyme system.

All forms of NKH should be differentiated from ketotic hyperglycinemia, D-glyceric aciduria (see later), and ingestion of valproic acid. The latter compound causes a moderate increase in blood and urinary concentrations of glycine. Repeat assays after discontinuation of the drug should establish the diagnosis.

Diagnosis can be established by assay of the enzyme in liver or brain specimens or by identification of the mutation. Enzyme activity in the neonatal form is close to zero, whereas in the other forms, some residual activity is present. In most patients with the neonatal form, the enzyme defect resides in the P protein; the defect in the T protein accounts for the rest. The enzyme assay in three patients with the infantile and late-onset forms has revealed two patients with the defect in the T protein and one in the H protein.

No effective **treatment** is known. Exchange transfusion, dietary restriction of glycine, and administration of sodium benzoate or folate have not altered the neurologic outcome. Drugs that counteract the effect of glycine on neuronal cells, such as strychnine, diazepam, and dextromethorphan, have shown some beneficial effects only in patients with the mild forms of the condition.

NKH is inherited as an autosomal recessive trait. The prevalence is not known, but high frequency of the disorder has been noted in northern Finland (1/12,000). The gene for P protein is located on chromosome 9p22. The gene for H protein is mapped to chromosome 16p24 and that for T protein is mapped to chromosome 3p21-p21.1. Several disease-causing mutations have been identified. Prenatal diagnosis has been accomplished by performing an assay of the enzyme activity in chorionic villi biopsy specimens or by identification of the mutant gene.

SARCOSINEMIA. Increased concentrations of sarcosine (N-methylglycine) are observed in both blood and urine, but no consistent clinical picture has been attributed to this metabolic defect. This is a recessively inherited inborn error involving sarcosine dehydrogenase, the enzyme that converts sarcosine to glycine (see Fig. 85-8). The gene for this enzyme is located on chromosome 9q33-q34.

D-GLYCERIC ACIDURIA. D-glyceric acid is an intermediate metabolite of serine and fructose metabolism (see Fig. 85-8). At least two forms of this rare condition have been identified. In one form, clinical manifestations of severe encephalopathy (hypotonia, seizures, and mental and motor deficits) and the laboratory findings of hyperglycinemia and hyperglycinuria were suggestive of nonketotic hyperglycinemia. These patients excreted large quantities of D-glyceric acid (this compound is not normally detectable in urine). Enzyme studies indicated a deficiency of glycerate kinase in one patient and decreased activity of D-glyceric dehydrogenase in another.

In the other form, the major findings are persistent metabolic acidosis and developmental delay. This infant excreted large amounts of D-glyceric acid without hyperglycinemia. The enzyme defect in this patient is not known.

No effective therapy is available. Restriction of fructose improved seizures in one patient.

TRIMETHYLAMINURIA. Trimethylamine is normally produced in the intestine from the breakdown of dietary choline and trimethylamine oxide by bacteria. Eggs and liver are the main sources of choline, and fish is the major source of trimethylamine oxide. Trimethylamine is absorbed and oxidized in the liver by trimethylamine oxidase (flavin-containing monooxygenases) to trimethylamine oxide, which is odorless and excreted in the urine (see Fig. 85-8). Deficiency of this enzyme results in massive excretion of trimethylamine in urine. Several asymptomatic patients with trimethylaminuria have been reported; there is a foul body odor that resembles that of a rotten fish, which may have significant social and psychosocial ramifications. Restriction of fish, eggs, liver, and other sources of choline (such as nuts and grains) in the diet significantly reduce the odor. The gene for trimethylamine oxidase has been mapped to chromosome 1q23-q25.

HYPEROXALURIA AND OXALOSIS. Normally, oxalic acid is derived mostly from oxidation of glyoxylic acid and, to a lesser degree, from oxidation of ascorbic acid (see Fig. 85-8). Glyoxylic acid is formed from the oxidation of glycolic acid in the preoxisomes. The source of glycolic acid remains unclear. Foods containing oxalic acid, such as spinach and rhubarb, are the main exogenous sources of this compound. Oxalic acid cannot be further metabolized in humans and is excreted in the urine as oxalates. Calcium oxalate is relatively insoluble in water and precipitates in tissues (kidneys and joints) if its concentration increases in the body.

Secondary hyperoxaluria has been observed in pyridoxine deficiency (cofactor for alanine-glyoxylate aminotransferase, see Fig. 85-8) after ingestion of ethylene glycol or high doses of vitamin C, after administration of the anesthetic agent methoxyflurane (which oxidizes directly to oxalic acid), and in patients with inflammatory bowel disease or extensive resection of the bowel *(enteric hyperoxaluria)*. Acute, fatal hyperoxaluria may develop after ingestion of plants with a high oxalic acid content such as sorrel. Precipitation of calcium oxalate in tissues causes hypocalcemia, liver necrosis, renal failure, cardiac arrhythmia, and death.

The lethal dose of oxalic acid is estimated to be between 5 and 30 g.

Primary hyperoxaluria is a rare genetic disorder in which large amounts of oxalates accumulate in the body. Two types of primary hyperoxaluria have been identified. The term **oxalosis** refers to deposition of calcium oxalate in parenchymal tissue.

Primary Hyperoxaluria Type I. This rare condition is the most common form of primary hyperoxaluria. It is due to a deficiency of the peroxisomal enzyme alanine-glyoxylate aminotransferase, which is expressed only in the liver peroxisomes and requires pyridoxine (vitamin B_6) as its cofactor. In the absence of this enzyme, glyoxylic acid, which cannot be converted to glycine, is transferred to the cytosol, where it is oxidized to oxalic acid in peroxisomes (see Fig. 85-8).

There is a wide variation in the age of presentation. The majority of patients become symptomatic before 5 yr of age. In ≈10% of cases, symptoms develop before 1 yr of age (neonatal oxaluria). The initial **clinical manifestations** are related to renal stones and nephrocalcinosis. Renal colic and asymptomatic hematuria lead to a gradual deterioration of renal function, manifested by growth retardation and uremia. Most patients die before 20 yr of age from renal failure if the disorder is untreated. Acute arthritis is a rare manifestation and may be misdiagnosed as gout because uric acid is usually elevated in patients with type I hyperoxaluria. Late forms of the disease presenting during adulthood have also been reported. Crystalline retinopathy and optic neuropathy causing visual loss have occurred in a few patients.

A marked increase in urinary excretion of oxalate (normal excretion 10–50 mg/24 hr) is the most important **laboratory finding**. The presence of oxalate crystals in urinary sediment is rarely helpful for diagnosis because such crystals are often seen in normal individuals. Urinary excretion of glycolic acid and glyoxylic acid is increased. **Diagnosis** can be confirmed by performing an assay of the enzyme in liver specimens or by identification of the mutant gene.

Medical treatment has been largely unsuccessful. In some patients, administration of large doses of pyridoxine reduces urinary excretion of oxalate. Renal transplantation in patients with renal failure has not improved the outcome in most cases, because oxalosis has recurred in the transplanted kidney. Combined liver and kidney transplants have resulted in a significant decrease in plasma and urinary oxalate in a few patients, and this may be the most effective treatment of this disorder.

The condition is inherited as an autosomal recessive trait. The gene for this enzyme is mapped to chromosome 2q36-q37. Several mutations of the gene have been described in patients with this condition. The most common mutation results in the mistargeting of the enzyme to the mitochondria instead of the peroxisomes. The in vitro enzyme activity in these patients may reach the level found in obligate heterozygotes. In vivo function remains defective, however. About 30% of patients with hyperoxaluria type 1 are estimated to have this defect.

Prenatal diagnosis has been achieved by the measurement of fetal hepatic enzyme activity obtained by needle biopsy or by DNA analysis of chorionic villi samples.

Primary Hyperoxaluria Type II (L-Glyceric Aciduria). This rare condition is due to a deficiency of D-glycerate dehydrogenase (hydroxypyruvate reductase)/glyoxylate reductase enzyme complex (see Fig. 85-8). A deficiency in the activity of this enzyme results in an accumulation of two intermediate metabolites, hydroxypyruvate (the ketoacid of serine) and glyoxylic acid. Both these compounds are further metabolized by lactate dehydrogenase (LDH) to L-glyceric acid and oxalic acid, respectively. About 30% of reported patients are from the Saulteaux-Ojibway Indians of Manitoba.

Clinically, these patients are indistinguishable from those with hyperoxaluria type I. Renal stones presenting with renal colic and hematuria may develop before age 2 yr. Renal failure is less common in this condition than in hyperoxaluria type I; the urine contains large amounts of L-glyceric acid in addition to high levels of oxalate (L-glyceric acid is not normally present in urine). Urinary excretion of glycolic acid and glyoxylic acid is not increased. The presence of L-glyceric acid without increased levels of glycolic and glyoxylic acids in urine differentiates this type from type I hyperoxaluria. The gene is mapped to chromosome 9cen.

No effective **therapy** is available.

CREATINE DEFICIENCY. Creatine is synthesized in the liver, pancreas, and kidneys from arginine and glycine (Fig. 85-9) and is transported to muscles and the brain, in which there is high creatine kinase activity. Phosphorylation and dephosphorylation of creatine by this enzyme in conjunction with adenosine diphosphate and triphosphate (ADP/ATP) provide high-energy phosphate reactions in these organs. Creatine is nonenzymatically metabolized to creatinine at a constant daily rate and is excreted in the urine. Three genetic conditions are known to cause creatine deficiency in tissues. Two are due to deficiency of the enzymes involved in the biosynthesis of creatine. The enzymes are arginine-glycine aminotransferase (AGAT) and quanidinoacetate methyltransferase (GAMT) (see Fig. 85-9). Both conditions respond well to creatine supplementation. The third condition is caused by the defect in the creatinine transporter (CRTR) and is not responsive to creatinine administration.

Clinical manifestations of the three defects are similar, relate to the brain and muscles, and may appear in the 1st few weeks or months of life. Developmental delay, mental retardation, speech delay, and seizures are common. Dystonic hyperkinetic movements are seen in severe GAMT deficiency.

Laboratory findings include decreased creatine and creatinine in blood and urine in patients with AGAT and GAMT defects. Marked elevations of guanidinoacetate in blood, urine, and especially in CSF are diagnostic of GAMT defects. Low levels of guanidinoacetate are found with the AGAT defect. Absence of creatine and creatine phosphate (in all three defects) and high levels of guanidinoacetate (with GAMT defects) can be demonstrated in the brain by MRS. MRI shows signal hyperintensity of the globus pallidus. **Diagnosis** of AGAT or GAMT defects may be confirmed by measurement of the enzyme in the liver, cultured fibroblasts, or stimulated lymphoblasts or by DNA analysis of the gene. Diagnosis of CRTR is confirmed by genetic analysis or creatine uptake by fibroblasts.

Treatment with creatine monohydrate (350 mg–2 g/kg/day) orally has resulted in a dramatic improvement in muscle tone and overall mental development and has normalized MRI and electroencephalographic findings in patients with AGAT and GAMT defects. It is believed that early treatment may assure normal development. No therapy is available for the CRTR defect.

AGAT and GAMT defects are inherited as autosomal recessive traits. CRTR is an X-linked trait. The prevalence of the enzyme deficiency is not known; four patients with GAMT defects (three from one family) were identified among 180 institutionalized patients with severe mental handicap. This condition must be considered in any patient with brain and muscle disorders, since treatment can produce a dramatic response.

85.8 • Serine • Iraj Rezvani

Serine is a nonessential amino acid synthesized from glucose and glycine (see Fig. 85-9).

3-PHOSPHOGLYCERATE DEHYDROGENASE DEFICIENCY. Deficiency of this enzyme causes deficiencies of serine and glycine in the body. **Clinical manifestations**, which are developed in the 1st few months of life, include microcephaly, severe psychomotor retar-

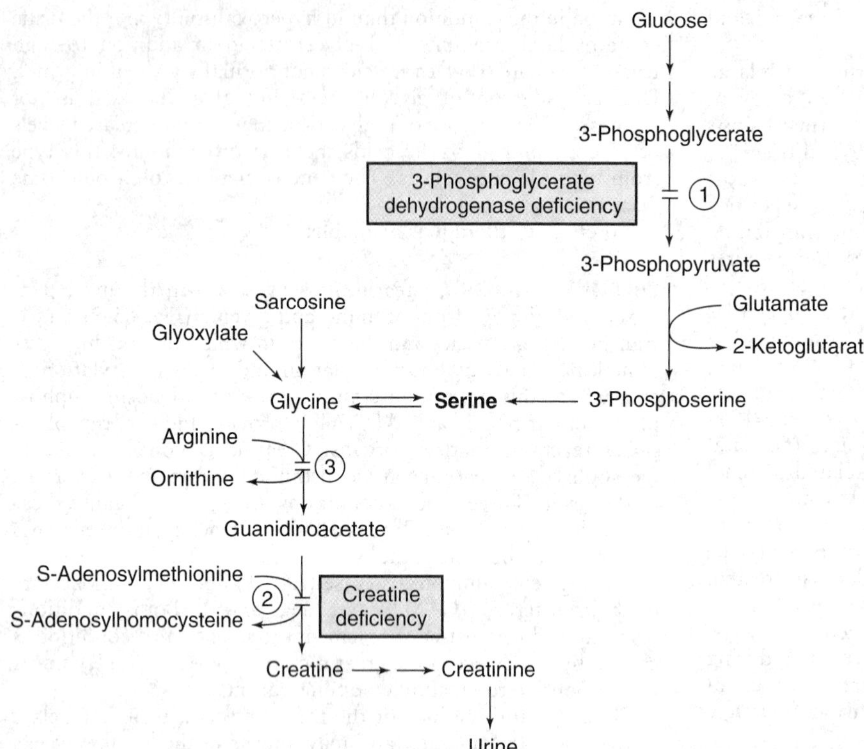

Figure 85-9. Pathways for the synthesis of serine and creatine. **Enzymes:** (1) 3-phosphoglycerate dehydrogenase, (2) guanidinoacetate methyltransferase (GAMT). (3) arginine:glycine aminotransferase (AGAT).

dation, and intractable seizures. Other findings such as failure to thrive, spastic tetraplegia, nystagmus, cataracts, hypogonadism, and megaloblastic anemia may also be present.

Laboratory findings include low levels of serine and glycine in plasma and very low levels of serine and glycine in CSF. No abnormal organic acid is found in the urine. Magnetic resonance imaging of the brain shows significant attenuation of white matter and incomplete myelination.

Diagnosis can be confirmed by measurement of the enzyme activity in cultured fibroblasts and by DNA analysis.

Treatment with serine (200–600 mg/kg/24 hr, orally) alone or in conjunction with glycine (200–300 mg/kg/24 hr) normalizes the serine levels in the blood and CSF. This treatment produces significant improvement in all clinical findings except for the psychomotor retardation; seizure activity subsides within a few days of therapy and may be halted completely. Microcephaly improves in young affected infants. There is evidence to indicate that psychomotor retardation may be prevented if the treatment starts in the 1st few days of life.

The condition is inherited as an autosomal recessive trait. The gene for 3-phosphoglycerate dehydrogenase enzyme has been mapped to chromosome 1q12 and a few disease-producing mutations have been identified in different families. Prenatal diagnosis has been achieved by DNA analysis in a family with previously affected offspring; administration of serine to the mother corrected microcephaly in the affected fetus as evidenced by ultrasound imaging. The favorable response of this condition to a simple treatment makes this diagnosis an important consideration in any child with microcephaly and neurologic defects such as psychomotor delay or a seizure disorder.

85.9 • Proline • Iraj Rezvani

Proline and hydroxyproline are found in high concentrations in collagen. Neither of these amino acids is normally found in urine in the free form except in early infancy. Excretion of "bound" hydroxyproline (dipeptides and tripeptides containing hydroxyproline) reflects collagen turnover and is increased in disorders of accelerated collagen turnover, such as rickets or hyperparathyroidism.

HYPERPROLINEMIA. Two types of this rare autosomal recessive condition have been described. *Type I hyperprolinemia* is due to a deficiency of proline dehydrogenase, and *type II* is due to a defect in Δ′-pyrroline-5-carboxylic acid dehydrogenase enzyme (Fig. 85-10). Neither type causes any specific clinical manifestation attributable to hyperprolinemia. Increased blood concentrations of proline (more pronounced in type II) and prolinuria are found in both types. Hydroxyproline and glycine are also excreted in abnormal amounts in the urine because of the saturation of the common tubular reabsorption mechanism by the massive prolinuria. The presence of Δ′-pyrroline-5-carboxylic acid in plasma and urine differentiates type II from type I. No treatment is recommended for the affected individuals.

The gene for proline dehydrogenase is mapped to chromosome 22q11.2 and several disease-causing mutations have been identified; some mutations have been associated with an increased risk of **schizophrenia.** Microdeletion of chromosome 22q11.2 causes velocardiofacial (**DiGeorge,** Shpritzen) syndrome. In a study, eight out of 15 patients with this syndrome also had type I hyperprolinemia. It has been suggested that patients with hyperprolinemia be screened (by FISH analysis) for presence of microdeletion of chromosome 22q11.2. The gene for Δ′-pyrroline-5-carboxylic acid dehydrogenase is mapped to chromosome 1p36.

PROLIDASE DEFICIENCY. During collagen degradation, imidodipeptides (such as glycylproline) are released and are normally cleaved by tissue prolidase. This enzyme requires manganese for its proper activity. Deficiency of prolidase, which is inherited as an autosomal recessive trait, results in the accumulation of imidodipeptides in body fluids.

The **clinical manifestations** of this rare condition and the age at onset are quite variable (19 mo to 19 yr) and include recur-

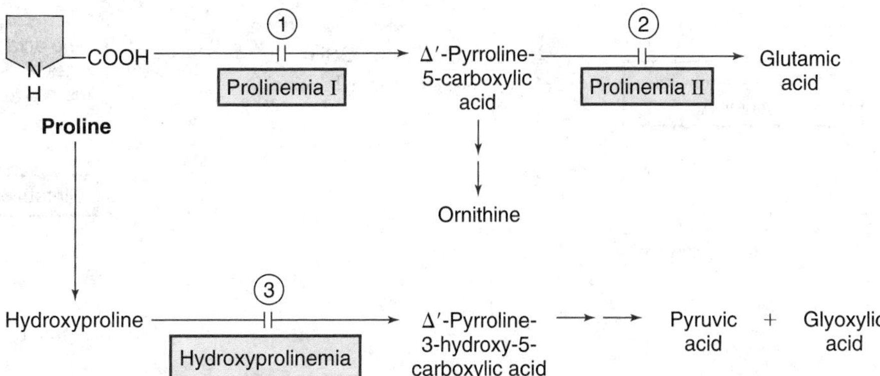

Figure 85-10. Pathways in the metabolism of proline. **Enzymes:** (1) proline oxidase, (2) Δ′-pyrroline-5-carboxylic acid dehydrogenase, (3) hydroxyproline oxidase.

rent, painful skin ulcers, which are typically on hands and legs. Other skin lesions that may precede ulcers by several years may include scaly erythematous maculopapular rash, purpura, and telangiectasia. Most ulcers become infected. Healing of the ulcers may take 4 to 7 mo. Mild to severe mental and motor deficits and susceptibility to infections are also present in most patients (recurrent otitis media, sinusitis, respiratory infection, splenomegaly). Infection is the cause of death. Some patients may have some craniofacial abnormalities such as ptosis, ocular proptosis, and prominent cranial sutures. Asymptomatic cases have also been reported. Development of systemic lupus erythematosus (SLE) has been noted in affected children of one family; young patients with SLE should be screened for prolidase deficiency. High levels of urinary excretion of imidodipeptides are diagnostic. Enzyme assay may be performed in erythrocytes or cultured skin fibroblasts.

Oral supplementation with proline, ascorbic acid, and manganese and the topical use of proline and glycine result in an improvement in leg ulcers. These treatments have not been found consistently effective in all patients.

The gene for prolidase enzyme has been mapped to chromosome 19cen-q13.11 and several disease-causing mutations have been identified in different families.

85.10 • Glutamic Acid • Iraj Rezvani

Glutathione (γ-glutamylcysteinylglycine) is the major product of glutamic acid in the body. This ubiquitous tripeptide is synthesized and degraded through a complex cycle called the γ-glutamyl cycle (Fig. 85-11). Because of its free sulfhydryl (-SH) group and its abundance in the cell, glutathione protects other sulfhydryl-containing compounds (such as enzymes and coenzyme A) from oxidation. It is also involved in the detoxification of peroxides, including hydrogen peroxide, and in keeping the cell content in a reduced state. The common consequence of glutathione deficiency is hemolytic anemia. Glutathione also participates in amino acid transport across the cell membrane through the γ-glutamyl cycle.

GLUTATHIONE SYNTHETASE DEFICIENCY (FIG. 85-11). Three forms of this condition have been reported. In the **severe form**, which is due to generalized deficiency of the enzyme, severe acidosis and massive 5-oxoprolinuria are the rule. In the **mild form**, in which the enzyme deficiency causes glutathione deficiency only in erythrocytes, neither 5-oxoprolinuria nor acidosis has been observed. A **moderate form** has also been observed in which the hemolytic anemia is associated with variable degrees of acidosis and 5-oxoprolinuria. In all forms, patients have hemolytic anemia secondary to glutathione deficiency. All forms are rare (a total of 65 patients have been reported).

Glutathione Synthetase Deficiency, Severe Form (Pyroglutamic Acidemia, Severe 5-Oxoprolinuria) and Moderate Form. **Clinical manifestations** of this rare condition occur in the 1st few days of life and include metabolic acidosis, jaundice, and mild to moderate hemolytic anemia. Chronic acidosis continues after recovery. Similar episodes of life-threatening acidosis may occur during gastroenteritis or an infection or after a surgical procedure. Progressive neurologic damage manifested by mental retardation, spastic tetraparesis, ataxia, tremor, dysarthria, and seizures develops with age. Susceptibility to infection, presumably due to granulocyte dysfunction, is observed in some patients. Patients with the moderate form have milder acidosis and less 5-oxoprolinuria than with the severe form; neurologic manifestations are also absent.

Laboratory findings include metabolic acidosis, mild to moderate degrees of hemolytic anemia, and 5-oxoprolinuria. High concentrations of 5-oxoproline are also found in blood. The glutathione content of erythrocytes is markedly decreased. Increased synthesis of 5-oxoproline in this disorder is believed to be due to the conversion of γ-glutamylcysteine to 5-oxoproline by the enzyme γ-glutamyl cyclotransferase (see Fig. 85-11). γ-Glutamylcysteine production increases greatly because the normal inhibitory effect of glutathione on the γ-glutamylcysteine synthetase enzyme is removed. A deficiency of glutathione synthetase has been demonstrated in a variety of cells including erythrocytes.

Treatment of acute attack includes hydration, correction of acidosis (by infusion of sodium bicarbonate), and measures to correct anemia and hyperbilirubinemia. Chronic administration of alkali is usually needed indefinitely. Administration of large doses of vitamins C and E has been recommended. Drugs and oxidants that are known to cause hemolysis and stressful catabolic states should be avoided. Oral administration of glutathione analogs has been tried with variable success.

Prenatal diagnosis can be achieved by the measurement of 5-oxoproline in amniotic fluid, by enzyme analysis in cultured amniocytes or chronic villi samples, or by DNA analysis of the gene. Successful pregnancy in an affected female (moderate form) with favorable outcomes for both mother and infant has been reported.

Glutathione Synthetase Deficiency, Mild Form. This form has been reported in only a few patients. Mild to moderate hemolytic anemia has been the only **clinical finding** in these patients. Splenomegaly has been reported in some patients. Mental development is normal; metabolic acidosis and increased concentrations of 5-oxoproline do not occur. This condition is due to mutations in the gene that encodes for glutathione synthetase enzyme. These mutations, however, presumably render the enzyme unstable but with normal catalytic function. The expedited rate of enzyme turnover caused by these mutations is of no consequence for all tissues with normal protein synthesis except for erythrocytes in which the absence of protein synthesis results

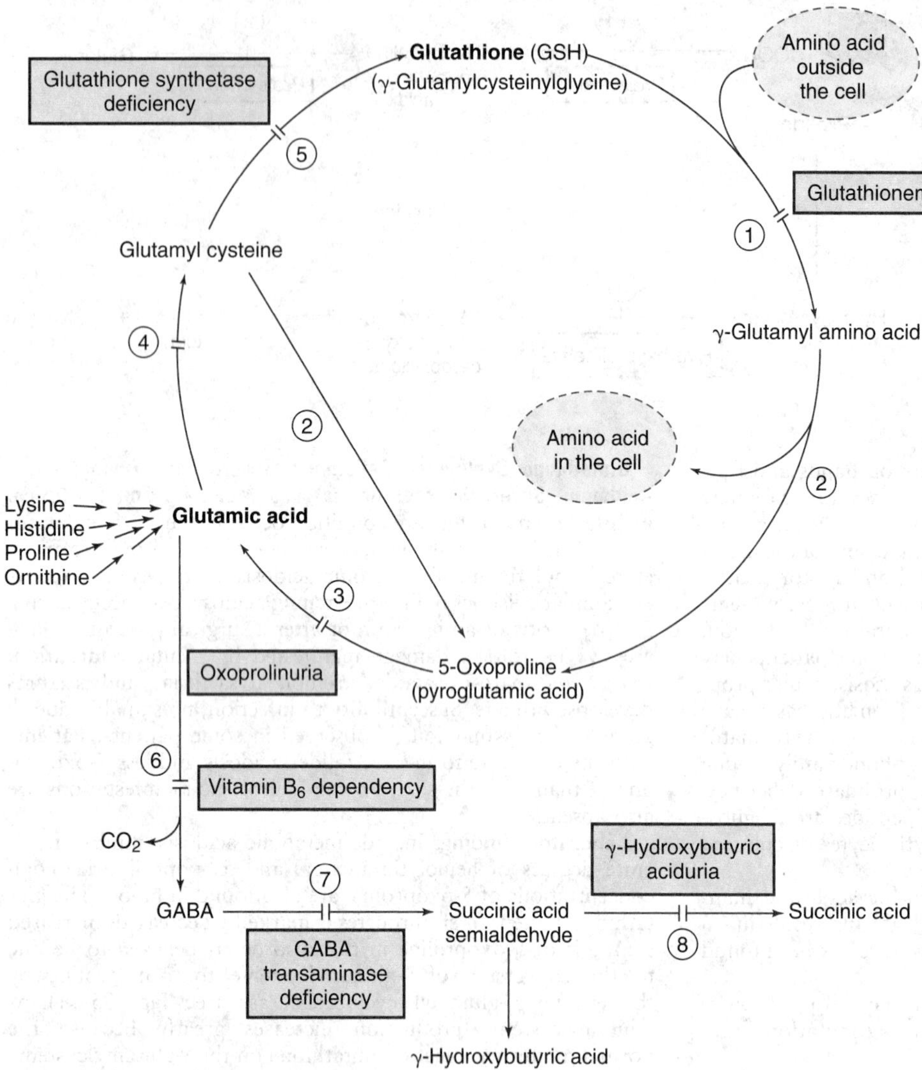

Figure 85-11. The γ-glutamyl cycle. Defects of the glutathione synthesis and degradation are noted. **Enzymes:** (1) γ-glutamyl transpeptidase, (2) γ-glutamyl cyclotransferase, (3) 5-oxoprolinase, (4) γ-glutamylcysteine synthetase, (5) glutathione synthetase, (6) glutamic acid decarboxylase, (7) GABA transaminase, (8) succinic semialdehyde dehydrogenase.

in a serious deficiency of glutathione. **Treatment** is that of hemolytic anemia and avoidance of drugs and oxidants that can trigger the hemolytic process.

All forms of the condition are inherited as an autosomal recessive trait. The gene for this enzyme is located on chromosome 20q11.2. Several disease-causing mutations have been identified in different families

5-Oxoprolinase Deficiency (5-Oxoprolinuria). The main cause of massive 5-oxoprolinuria is glutathione synthetase deficiency (see earlier). Moderate 5-oxoprolinuria has been found in a variety of metabolic and acquired conditions, such as in patients with severe burns, Stevens-Johnson syndrome, homocystinuria, urea cycle defects, and tyrosinemia type I.

A few individuals with moderate 5-oxoprolinuria (4–10 g/day) due to 5-oxoprolinase deficiency have been identified. No specific clinical picture has yet emerged. Moderate to severe mental retardation has been reported in two patients. Asymptomatic individuals with the enzyme deficiency have also been identified, however. It is, therefore, not clear whether 5-oxoprolinase deficiency is of any clinical consequence. No treatment has been recommended.

γ-Glutamylcysteine Synthase Deficiency. Only a few patients with this enzyme deficiency have been reported. The most consistent **clinical manifestation** has been mild chronic hemolytic anemia. Acute attacks of hemolysis have occurred after exposure to sulfonamides. Peripheral neuropathy and progressive spinocerebellar degeneration have been noted in two siblings in adulthood. **Laboratory findings** of chronic hemolytic anemia were present in all patients. Generalized aminoaciduria is also present because the γ-glutamyl cycle is involved in amino acid transport in cells (see Fig. 85-11). **Treatment** is that of hemolytic anemia and avoidance of drugs and oxidants that may trigger the hemolytic process. The condition is inherited as an autosomal recessive trait.

GLUTATHIONEMIA (γ-GLUTAMYL TRANSPEPTIDASE [GGT] DEFICIENCY). This enzyme is present in any cell that has secretory or absorptive functions. It is especially abundant in the kidneys, pancreas, intestines, and liver. The enzyme is also present in the bile. Measurement of this enzyme in the blood is commonly performed to evaluate liver and bile duct diseases.

Deficiency of this enzyme causes elevation in glutathione concentrations in body fluids, but the cellular levels remain normal. Only a few patients with enzyme deficiency have been reported; therefore, the scope of **clinical manifestations** has not yet been defined. Mild to moderate mental retardation and severe behavioral problems were observed in three patients. One of the two sisters with this condition had normal intelligence as an adult, however, and the other had Prader-Willi syndrome.

Laboratory findings include marked elevations in urinary concentrations of glutathione (up to 1 g/day), γ-glutamylcysteine, and cysteine. None of the reported patients has had generalized aminoaciduria, a finding that would have been expected to occur in this enzyme deficiency (see Fig. 85-11).

Diagnosis can be confirmed by measurement of the enzyme activity in leukocytes or cultured skin fibroblasts. No effective **treatment** is available.

The condition is inherited as an autosomal recessive trait. The enzyme GGT is a complex protein and is encoded by at least seven genes.

INBORN ERRORS OF METABOLISM OF γ-AMINOBUTYRIC ACID (GABA). Decarboxylation of glutamic acid by glutamic acid decarboxylase (GAD) is the main biosynthetic pathway for GABA production in the brain and other organs, especially the kidneys and the β cells of the pancreas. This enzyme requires pyridoxine (vitamin B_6) as a cofactor (see Fig. 85-11). Two GAD enzymes (GAD_{65} and GAD_{67}) have been identified. GAD_{67} is the main enzyme in the brain and GAD_{65} is the major one in the β cells. Antibodies against GAD_{65} and GAD_{67} are the major markers for type I diabetes and stiff man syndrome, respectively. The gene for GAD_{65} is mapped to chromosome 10p11.23 and that for GAD_{67} to chromosome 2q31. Knockout of the gene for GAD_{67} in mice causes cleft palate; the association of mutations in GAD_{67} gene with cleft lip in human has been shown in one study.

Pyridoxine (Vitamin B_6) Dependency with Seizures. This autosomal recessive condition is due to GABA deficiency in the brain, which is presumably caused by decreased activity of GAD. The main **clinical manifestation** of this condition is seizures, which usually occur in the 1st few hours of life and are unresponsive to conventional anticonvulsant therapy. Administration of vitamin B_6 in large doses (10–100 mg/kg) usually results in a dramatic improvement of both seizures and electoencephalographic abnormalities. Late onset forms of the condition (as late as 5 yr of age) have been reported. A trial with vitamin B_6 therapy has, therefore, been recommended in any infant with intractable seizures. The dependency is usually lifelong. Other neurologic findings such as delayed speech have been noted in some patients.

Laboratory studies have revealed increased glutamate and decreased GABA levels in the brain and in the spinal fluid.

The pathogenesis of this condition remains unclear. Although an increase in the Km of the GAD enzyme for its cofactor (vitamin B_6) in the brain seems a logical explanation, no abnormality in the GAD activity in the brain has been documented. DNA studies of the gene for GAD_{65} and GAD_{67} have likewise revealed no mutations. Linkage studies have mapped the condition to the long arm of chromosome 5q31.2, a locus completely different from loci of GAD genes.

Treatment with high daily doses of vitamin B_6 is necessary indefinitely.

GABA Transaminase Deficiency. This is a very rare autosomal recessive condition that has been reported in three infants from two different families. **Clinical manifestations** include severe psychomotor retardation, hypotonia, hyperreflexia, lethargy, and refractory seizures. Increased linear growth was present in the original report of two siblings but not in the third patient. Increased concentrations of GABA and β-alanine are found in the spinal fluid. Evidence of leukodystrophy was noted in the postmortem examination of the brain. GABA transaminase deficiency is demonstrated in the brain and lymphocytes. No effective treatment is available. Treatment with vitamin B_6 has been ineffective. The gene for this enzyme is located on chromosome 16p13.3.

γ-Hydroxybutyric Aciduria (Succinic Semialdehyde Dehydrogenase Deficiency). More than 150 patients with this enzyme deficiency (see Fig. 85-11) have been reported. **Clinical manifestations**, which usually begin in early infancy, include mild to moderate mental retardation, delayed speech, marked hypotonia, ataxia, and seizures. Other associated findings are oculomotor apraxia, choreoathetosis, autistic features, and aggressive behavior. Ataxia may improve with advancement of age.

Laboratory studies reveal marked elevations in γ-hydroxybutyric acid concentrations in the blood (up to 200-fold), spinal fluid (up to 1,200-fold), and urine (up to 800-fold). There is no acidosis. Urinary excretion of γ-hydroxybutyric acid decreases with age. Increased concentrations of glycine may also be present in plasma, urine, and spinal fluid.

Diagnosis can be confirmed by measurement of the enzyme activity in lymphocytes. Prenatal diagnosis has been achieved by measurement of γ-hydroxybutyric acid in the amniotic fluid and assay of the enzyme activity in the amniocytes or in biopsy specimens of chorionic villi.

Treatment has been largely ineffective; vigabatrine has produced some improvement in ataxia and mental status in some patients.

The condition is inherited as an autosomal recessive trait. The gene for succinic semialdehyde dehydrogenase has been mapped to chromosome 6p22; several disease-causing mutations have been identified in different families.

The role of γ-hydroxybutyric acid in the pathogenesis of this condition remains unclear and somewhat confusing because administration of this compound to humans and animals has produced some opposite effects. γ-Hydroxy-butyrate (GHB) has been used illicitly as a recreational drug with anesthetic effect and is one of the date-rape drugs (see also Chapter 113).

Congenital Glutamine Deficiency. This uncommon disorder is due to a deficiency of glutamine synthase. Glutamine is absent in plasma, urine, and CSF but plasma levels of glutamate remain normal. Manifestations include cerebral malformations (abnormal gyration, white matter lesions), multiorgan failure including respiratory failure, and neonatal death. It may be inherited as an autosomal trait; the gene is mapped to chromosome 1q31.

85.11 • Urea Cycle and Hyperammonemia (Arginine, Citrulline, Ornithine) • Iraj Rezvani

Catabolism of amino acids results in the production of free ammonia, which is highly toxic to the central nervous system. Ammonia is detoxified to urea through a series of reactions known as the Krebs-Henseleit or urea cycle (Fig. 85-12). Five enzymes are required for the synthesis of urea: carbamyl phosphate synthetase (CPS), ornithine transcarbamylase (OTC), argininosuccinate synthetase (AS), argininosuccinate lyase (AL), and arginase. A sixth enzyme, *N*-acetylglutamate synthetase, is also required for synthesis of *N*-acetylglutamate, which is an activator of the CPS enzyme. Individual deficiencies of these enzymes have been observed and, with an overall estimated prevalence of 1/30,000 live births, they are the most common genetic causes of hyperammonemia in infants.

GENETIC CAUSES OF HYPERAMMONEMIA. In addition to genetic defects of the urea cycle enzymes, a marked increase in plasma level of ammonia is observed in other inborn errors of metabolism (Table 85-2).

CLINICAL MANIFESTATIONS OF HYPERAMMONEMIA. In the **neonatal period**, symptoms and signs are mostly related to brain dysfunction and are similar regardless of the cause of the hyperammonemia. The affected infant is normal at birth but becomes symptomatic within a few days of protein feeding. Refusal to eat, vomiting, tachypnea, and lethargy quickly progress to a deep coma. Convulsions are common. Physical examination may reveal hepatomegaly in addition to the neurologic signs of deep coma. In **infants and older children** acute hyperammonemia is manifested by vomiting and neurologic abnormalities such as ataxia, mental confusion, agitation, irritability, and combativeness. These manifestations may alternate

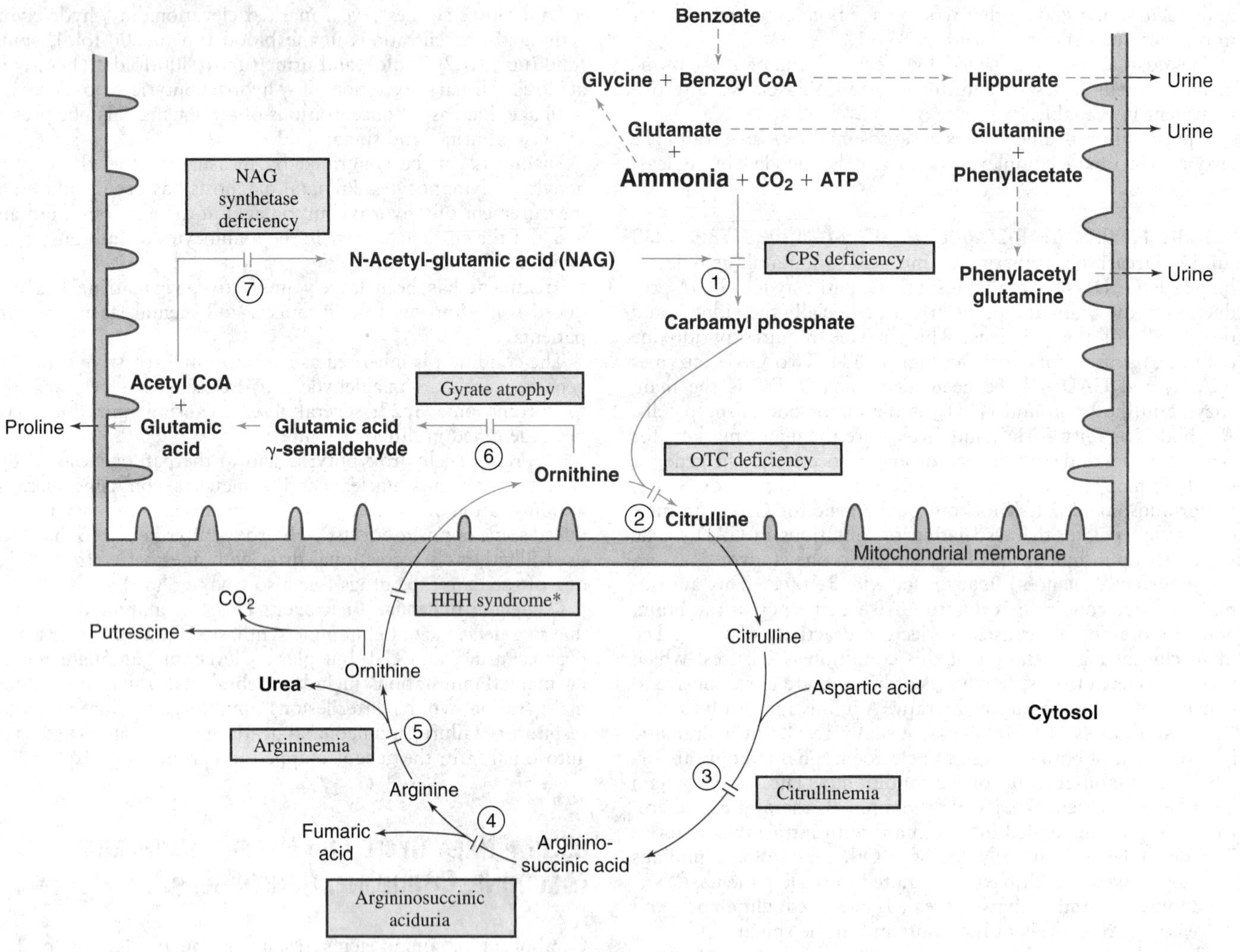

Figure 85-12. Urea cycle: pathways for ammonia disposal and ornithine metabolism. Reactions occurring in the mitochondria are depicted in *purple*. Reactions shown with *interrupted arrows* are the alternate pathways for the disposal of ammonia. **Enzymes:** (1) carbamyl phosphate synthetase (CPS), (2) ornithine transcarbamylase (OTC), (3) argininosuccinic acid synthetase (AS), (4) argininosuccinic acid lyase (AL), (5) arginase, (6) ornithine 5-aminotransferase, (7) *N*-acetylglutamate (NAG) synthetase.* HHH syndrome, hyperammonemia-hyperornithinemia-homocitrullinemia.

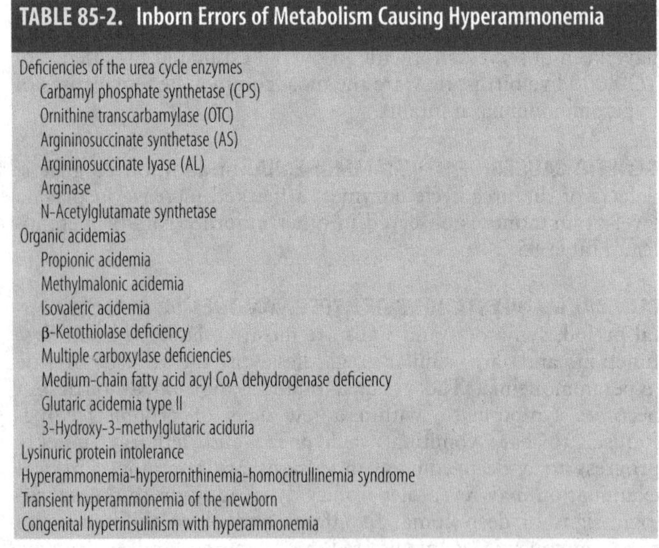

TABLE 85-2. Inborn Errors of Metabolism Causing Hyperammonemia

Deficiencies of the urea cycle enzymes
Carbamyl phosphate synthetase (CPS)
Ornithine transcarbamylase (OTC)
Argininosuccinate synthetase (AS)
Argininosuccinate lyase (AL)
Arginase
N-Acetylglutamate synthetase
Organic acidemias
Propionic acidemia
Methylmalonic acidemia
Isovaleric acidemia
β-Ketothiolase deficiency
Multiple carboxylase deficiencies
Medium-chain fatty acid acyl CoA dehydrogenase deficiency
Glutaric acidemia type II
3-Hydroxy-3-methylglutaric aciduria
Lysinuric protein intolerance
Hyperammonemia-hyperornithinemia-homocitrullinemia syndrome
Transient hyperammonemia of the newborn
Congenital hyperinsulinism with hyperammonemia

with periods of lethargy and somnolence that may progress to coma.

Routine **laboratory studies** show no specific findings when hyperammonemia is due to defects of the urea cycle enzymes. Blood urea nitrogen is usually low. Serum pH is usually normal or mildly elevated. In infants with organic acidemias, hyperammonemia is commonly associated with severe acidosis. Newborn infants with hyperammonemia are often misdiagnosed as having sepsis; they may succumb without a correct diagnosis. CT may reveal cerebral edema (Fig. 85-13). Autopsy is usually unremarkable. It is imperative to measure plasma ammonia levels in any ill infant whose clinical manifestations cannot be explained by an obvious infection.

DIAGNOSIS. The main criterion for diagnosis is hyperammonemia. The plasma ammonia concentration in the ill infant is usually >200 µmole/L (normal values <35 µmole/L). An approach to the differential diagnosis of hyperammonemia in the newborn infant is illustrated in Figure 85-14. Patients with a deficiency of CPS or OTC have no specific abnormalities of plasma amino acids except for increased levels of glutamine, aspartic acid, and alanine secondary to hyperammonemia. A marked increase in urinary orotic acid in patients with OTC deficiency

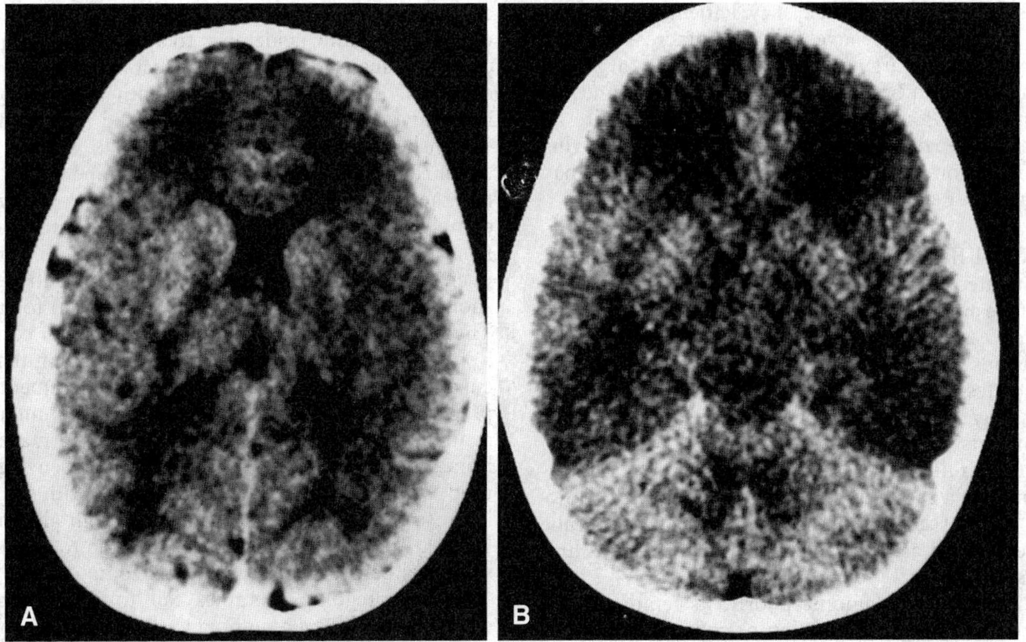

Figure 85-13. Computer axial tomographic scans of the head of hyperammonemic encephalopathy in the composite case of ornithine transcarbamylase deficiency. *A*, Image done on admission to the community hospital. *B*, Image done 24 hours later demonstrates bilateral hemispheric edema with effacement of cerebrospinal fluid spaces. (From Brusiloe SW: Hyperammonemic encephalopathy. *Medicine* 2002;81:240.)

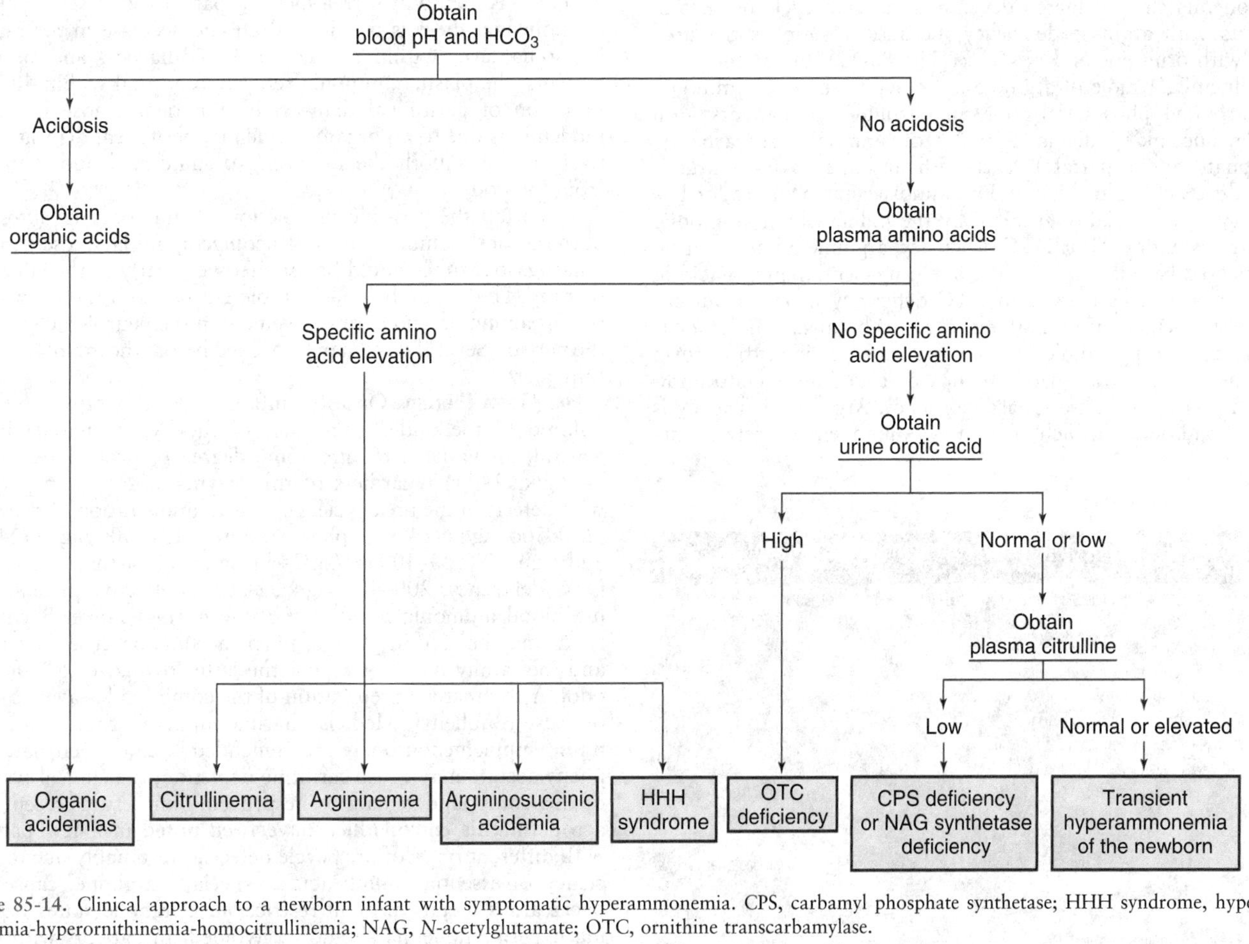

Obtain blood pH and HCO_3

Acidosis

Obtain organic acids

No acidosis

Obtain plasma amino acids

Specific amino acid elevation

No specific amino acid elevation

Obtain urine orotic acid

High

Normal or low

Obtain plasma citrulline

Low

Normal or elevated

Organic acidemias

Citrullinemia

Argininemia

Argininosuccinic acidemia

HHH syndrome

OTC deficiency

CPS deficiency or NAG synthetase deficiency

Transient hyperammonemia of the newborn

Figure 85-14. Clinical approach to a newborn infant with symptomatic hyperammonemia. CPS, carbamyl phosphate synthetase; HHH syndrome, hyperammonemia-hyperornithinemia-homocitrullinemia; NAG, *N*-acetylglutamate; OTC, ornithine transcarbamylase.

differentiates this defect from CPS deficiency. Patients with a deficiency of AS, AL, or arginase have a marked increase in the plasma level of citrulline, argininosuccinic acid, or arginine, respectively. Differentiation between the CPS deficiency and the *N*-acetylglutamate (NAG) synthetase deficiency may require an assay of the respective enzymes. Clinical improvement occurring after oral administration of carbamylglutamate, however, may suggest NAG synthetase deficiency.

TREATMENT OF ACUTE HYPERAMMONEMIA. Acute hyperammonemia should be treated promptly and vigorously. The goal of therapy is to remove ammonia from the body and to provide adequate calories and essential amino acids to halt further breakdown of endogenous proteins (Table 85-3). Adequate calories, fluid, and electrolytes should be provided intravenously. Intravenous lipids (1 g/kg/24 hr) provide an effective source of calories. Minimal amounts of protein (0.25 g/kg/24 hr), preferably in the form of essential amino acids, should be added to the intravenous fluid to prevent a catabolic state. Oral feeding with a low-protein formula (0.5–1.0 g/kg/24 hr) through a nasogastric tube should be started as soon as sufficient improvement in the clinical condition is seen.

Because the kidneys clear ammonia poorly, its removal from the body must be expedited by formation of compounds with a high renal clearance. Sodium benzoate forms hippuric acid with endogenous glycine (see Fig. 85-12). Each mole of benzoate removes 1 mole of ammonia as glycine. Phenylacetate conjugates with glutamine to form phenylacetylglutamine, which is readily excreted in the urine. One mole of phenylacetate removes 2 moles of ammonia as glutamine from the body (see Fig. 85-12).

Arginine administration is effective in the treatment of hyperammonemia that is due to defects of the urea cycle (except in patients with arginase deficiency) because it supplies the urea cycle with ornithine and NAG (see Fig. 85-12). In patients with citrullinemia, 1 mole of arginine reacts with 1 mole of ammonia (as carbamyl phosphate) to form citrulline. In patients with argininosuccinic acidemia, 2 moles of ammonia (as carbamyl phosphate and aspartate) react with arginine to form argininosuccinic acid. Citrulline and argininosuccinic acid are far less toxic and more readily excreted by the kidneys than ammonia. In patients with CPS or OTC deficiency, arginine administration is indicated because arginine becomes an essential amino acid in these disorders. Patients with OTC deficiency benefit from citrulline supplementation (200 mg/kg/24 hr) because 1 mole of citrulline can accept 1 mole of ammonia (as aspartic acid) to form arginine. Administration of arginine or citrulline is **contraindicated** in patients with arginase deficiency. Arginase deficiency is a rare condition in which acute hyperammonemia rarely occurs as a presenting sign. In patients whose hyperammonemia is secondary to organic acidemias, treatment with arginine is not indicated because no beneficial effect from such therapy can be expected. In a newborn infant with a 1st attack of hyperammonemia, arginine should be used until the diagnosis is established.

TABLE 85-3. Treatment of Acute Hyperammonemia in an Infant

1. Provide adequate calories, fluid, and electrolytes intravenously (10% glucose and intravenous lipids 1 g/kg/24 hr). Add minimal amounts of protein preferably as a mixture of essential amino acids (0.25 g/kg/24 hr) during the 1st 24 hr of therapy.
2. Give priming doses of the following compounds:
   To be added to 20 mL/kg of 10% glucose and infused within 1–2 hr
   Sodium benzoate 250 mg/kg (5.5 g/nm^2)*
   Sodium phenylacetate 250 mg/kg (5.5 g/nm^2)*
   Arginine hydrochloride 200–600 mg/kg (4.0–12.0 g/nm^2) as a 10% solution
3. Continue infusion of sodium benzoate* (250–500 mg/kg/24 hr), sodium phenylacetate* (250–500 mg/kg/24 hr), and arginine (200–600 mg/kg/24 hr†) following the above priming doses. These compounds should be added to the daily intravenous fluid.
4. Initiate peritoneal dialysis or hemodialysis if above treatment fails to produce an appreciable decrease in plasma ammonia.

*These compounds are usually prepared as a 1–2% solution for intravenous use. Sodium from these drugs should be included as part of the daily sodium requirement.

†The higher dose is recommended in the treatment of patients with citrullinemia and argininosuccinic aciduria. Arginine is not recommended in patients with arginase deficiency and in those whose hyperammonemia is secondary to organic acidemia.

Benzoate, phenylacetate, and arginine may be administered together for maximal therapeutic effect. A priming dose of these compounds is followed by continuous infusion until recovery from the acute state occurs (see Table 85-3). Both benzoate and phenylacetate are usually supplied as concentrated solutions and should be properly diluted (1–2% solution) for intravenous use. The recommended therapeutic doses of both compounds deliver a substantial amount of sodium to the patient that should be calculated as part of the daily sodium requirement. A commercial preparation of sodium benzoate plus sodium phenylacetate is available for intravenous use (Medicis Pharmaceutical Corporation, www.medicis.com). Benzoate and phenylacetate should be used with caution in newborn infants with hyperbilirubinemia because they may displace bilirubin from albumin (see Chapter 102.4). In infants at risk, it is advisable to reduce bilirubin to a safe level before administering benzoate or phenylacetate.

If the foregoing therapies fail to produce any appreciable change in the blood ammonia level within a few hours, hemodialysis or peritoneal dialysis should be used. Exchange transfusion has little effect on reducing total body ammonia. It should be used only if dialysis cannot be employed promptly or when the patient is a newborn infant with hyperbilirubinemia (see earlier). Hemodialysis, although the most effective measure for removal of ammonia, is technically difficult to perform and may not be readily available. Peritoneal dialysis is the most practical and expeditious method for treatment of patients with severe hyperammonemia; there is usually a dramatic decrease in the plasma ammonia level within a few hours of dialysis, and in most patients, the plasma ammonia returns to normal within 48 hr of initiation of peritoneal dialysis. In a patient whose hyperammonemia is due to an organic acidemia, peritoneal dialysis effectively removes both the offending organic acid and ammonia from the body.

To curtail the possible production of ammonia by intestinal bacteria, oral administration of neomycin and lactulose through a nasogastric tube should be initiated very early in the course of therapy. There may be considerable lag between the normalization of ammonia and an improvement in the neurologic status of the patient. Several days may be needed before the infant becomes fully alert.

Long-Term Therapy. Once the infant is alert, therapy should be tailored to the underlying cause of the hyperammonemia. In general, all patients require some degree of protein restriction (1–2 g/kg/24 hr) regardless of the enzymatic defect. In patients with defects in the urea cycle, chronic administration of benzoate (250–500 mg/kg/24 hr), phenylacetate (250–500 mg/kg/24 hr), and arginine (200–400 mg/kg/24 hr) or citrulline (in patients with OTC deficiency, 200–400 mg/kg/24 hr) is effective in maintaining blood ammonia levels within the normal range. Phenylbutyrate may be used in place of phenylacetate, because the patient and the family may not accept the latter owing to its offensive odor. A commercial preparation of the compound is available for oral use (Buphenyl, Medicis Pharmaceutical Corporation). Carnitine supplementation is recommended because benzoate and phenylacetate may cause carnitine depletion; the clinical benefits of this compound remain to be proved. Skin lesions resembling **acrodermatitis entropathica** have been noted in a few patients with different types of urea cycle defects, presumably due to deficiency of essential amino acids, especially arginine, caused by overzealous dietary protein restriction. Catabolic states triggering hyperammonemia should be avoided. In patients with CPS, OTC, and AS deficiencies, acute hyperammonemic attacks may be precipitated by valporate administration.

CARBAMYL PHOSPHATE SYNTHETASE (CPS) AND *N*-ACETYLGLUTAMATE (NAG) SYNTHETASE DEFICIENCIES (SEE FIG. 85-12). Deficiencies of these two enzymes produce similar **clinical and biochemical manifestations.** There is a wide variation in severity of symptoms and in the age of presentation. Most commonly, the affected infant becomes symptomatic during the 1st few days of life with signs and symptoms of hyperammonemia (refusal to eat, vomiting, lethargy, convulsion, and coma). Late forms (as late as 32 yr of age) may present as an acute bout of hyperammonemia in a seemingly normal individual. Coma and death may occur during these episodes (a previously asymptomatic 26 yr old female died from hyperammonemia during childbirth). Intermediate forms with mental retardation and chronic subclinical hyperammonemia interspersed with bouts of acute hyperammonemia have also been observed.

Laboratory findings include hyperammonemia without an increase in any specific amino acids in plasma; marked elevations in plasma concentrations of glutamine and alanine seen in these patients are secondary to hyperammonemia. Urinary orotic acid is usually low or may be absent (see Fig. 85-14).

Treatment of acute hyperammonemic attacks and the long-term therapy of the condition is outlined earlier (see Table 85-3). Patients with NAG synthetase deficiency benefit from oral administration of carbamylglutamate. It is therefore important to differentiate between CPS and NAG synthetase deficiencies by assay of the enzyme activities in biopsy specimens obtained from the liver. Deficiency of NAG synthetase is rare in North America.

CPS deficiency is inherited as an autosomal recessive trait; the enzyme is normally present in the liver and intestine. The gene is mapped to chromosome 2q35. Several disease-causing mutations have been found in different families. The prevalence of the condition is not known.

ORNITHINE TRANSCARBAMYLASE (OTC) DEFICIENCY (SEE FIG. 85-12). In this X-linked partially dominant disorder, the hemizygote males are more severely affected than heterozygote females. The heterozygous females may have a mild form of the disease, but the majority (≈75%) are asymptomatic. This is the most common form of all the urea cycle disorders.

Clinical manifestations in a male newborn infant are usually those of severe hyperammonemia (see earlier) occurring in the 1st few days of life. Milder forms of the condition are commonly seen in heterozygous females and in some affected males. **Mild** forms characteristically have episodic manifestations, which may occur at any age (usually after infancy). Episodes of hyperammonemia (manifested by vomiting and neurologic abnormalities such as ataxia, mental confusion, agitation, and combativeness) are separated by periods of wellness. These episodes usually occur after ingestion of a high-protein diet or as a result of a catabolic state such as infection. Hyperammonemic coma, cerebral edema (see Fig. 85-13), and death may occur during one of these attacks. Mental development may proceed normally. Mild to moderate mental retardation is common. Gallstones have been seen in the survivors; the mechanism remains unclear.

The major **laboratory finding** during the acute attack is hyperammonemia without an increase in any specific amino acid in the blood. Elevation of the plasma concentrations of glutamine and alanine are secondary to hyperammonemia. A marked increase in the urinary excretion of orotic acid differentiates this condition from CPS deficiency (see Fig. 85-14). Orotates may precipitate in urine as gravel or stones. In the mild form, these laboratory abnormalities may revert to normal between attacks. This form should be differentiated from all the episodic conditions of childhood. In particular, lysinuric protein intolerance (see Chapter 85.13) mimics the clinical and biochemical characteristics of OTC deficiency. Increased urinary excretions of lysine, ornithine, and arginine and elevated blood concentrations of citrulline, which are salient features of lysinuric protein intolerance, are not seen in patients with OTC deficiency.

The **diagnosis** may be confirmed by performing an assay of enzyme activity that is normally present only in the liver or by identification of the mutant gene. Prenatal diagnosis has been achieved by means of fetal liver biopsy or by DNA studies of chorionic villi samples. An oral protein load, which increases plasma ammonia and urinary orotic acid levels, may identify asymptomatic heterozygous female carriers. A marked increase in urinary excretion of orotidine after an allopurinol loading test also detects obligate female carriers. Mild cerebral dysfunction may be present in asymptomatic female carriers.

Treatment of acute hyperammonemic attacks and the long-term therapy of the condition is outlined in earlier pages of this chapter. Citrulline is used in place of arginine in patients with OTC deficiency. Liver transplantation is a successful and definite treatment for patients with OTC deficiency who have been well controlled and have avoided multiple hyperammonemic crises.

The gene for ornithine transcarboxylase has been mapped to X chromosome (Xp21.1). Many disease-causing mutations (>200) have been identified in different patients. The degree of enzyme deficiency and the genotype dictate the severity of the phenotype in most cases. Mothers of affected infants are expected to be carriers of the mutant gene. A mother who gave birth to two affected male offspring was found to have normal genotype, suggesting gonadal mosaicism in the mother.

ARGININOSUCCINATE SYNTHETASE (AS) DEFICIENCY (CITRULLINEMIA) [SEE FIG. 85-12]. Two clinically and genetically distinct forms of citrullinemia have been identified. The classic form (type I) is due to the deficiency of the AS enzyme. The adult form (type II) is due to deficiency of a mitochondrial transport protein named citrin.

Citrullinemia Type I (Classic Citrullinemia, CTLN 1). This condition is caused by the deficiency of AS (see Fig. 85-12) and has variable clinical manifestation depending on the degree of the enzyme deficiency. Two major forms of the condition have been identified. The **severe or neonatal form**, which is the most common form of the condition, appears in the 1st few days of life with sign and symptoms of hyperammonemia (see earlier). In the **subacute or mild form**, clinical findings such as failure to thrive, frequent vomiting, developmental delay, and dry, brittle hair appear gradually after 1 yr of age. Acute hyperammonemia, triggered by an intercurrent catabolic state, may bring the diagnosis to light.

Laboratory findings are similar to those found in patients with OTC deficiency except that the plasma citrulline concentration is markedly elevated (50–100 times normal) in patients with citrullinemia type I (see Fig. 85-14). Urinary excretion of orotic acid is moderately increased; crystalluria due to precipitation of orotates may also occur. The **diagnosis** is confirmed by performing an assay of the enzyme activity in cultured fibroblasts or by DNA analysis. Prenatal diagnosis is accomplished by the assay of the enzyme activity in cultured amniotic cells or by DNA analysis of cells obtained from chorionic villi biopsy.

Treatment of acute hyperammonemic attacks and the long-term therapy of the condition are outlined in the earlier pages of this chapter. Plasma concentration of citrulline remains elevated at all times and may increase further after administration of arginine. Although prognosis is poor for symptomatic neonates, patients with the mild disease usually do well on a protein-restricted diet in conjunction with sodium benzoate and arginine therapy. Mild to moderate mental deficiency is a common sequela, even in a well-treated patient.

Citrullinemia is inherited as an autosomal recessive trait. The gene is located on chromosome 9q34. Several disease-causing mutations have been identified in different families. The majority of patients are compound heterozygotes for two different alleles. The prevalence of the condition is not known.

Citrurullinemia Due to Citrin Deficiency (Citrullinemia Type II, CTLN 2). Citrin is a mitochondrial transport protein encoded by a gene (*SLC25A13*) located on chromosome 7q21.3. One of the functions of this protein is to transport aspartate from mitochondria to cytoplasm; aspartate is required for converting citrulline to argininosuccinic acid (see Fig. 85-12). Citrin deficiency causes disruption of the urea cycle. AS activity is deficient in the liver of these patients, but no mutation in the gene for AS has been found. It is postulated that citrin deficiency or its mutated gene interferes with translation of mRNA for AS enzyme in the liver. Mutation in the gene for citrin produces two distinct clinical entities. The condition is reported almost exclusively in Japan.

Neonatal Intrahepatic Cholestasis (Citrullinemia Type II–Neonatal Form). **Clinical and laboratory manifestations**, which usually starts at 3 mo of age, include cholestatic jaundice with mild to moderate direct (conjugated) hyperbilirubinemia, marked hypoproteinemia, clotting dysfunction (increased prothrombin time and partial thromboplastin times), and increased serum γ-glutamyltranspeptidase (GGTP) and alkaline phosphatase activities; liver transaminases are usually normal. Plasma concentrations of ammonia and citrulline are usually normal, but moderate elevations are reported. There may be also increases in plasma concentrations of methionine, tyrosine, alanine, and threonine. Elevation in serum galactose levels has been found in some patients; all enzymes involved in galactose metabolism are normal. The reason for hypergalactosemia is not known. Marked elevation in serum level of α-fetoprotein is also present. These findings resemble those of tyrosinemia type I, but unlike the latter condition, urinary excretion of succinylacetone is not elevated (see Chapter 85.2). Liver biopsy shows fatty infiltration, cholestasis with dilated canaliculi, and a moderate degree of fibrosis. The condition is usually self-limiting and the majority of infants recover spontaneously by 1 yr of age with only supportive and symptomatic treatment. Hyperammonemia and hypercitrullinemia, if present, should be treated with low-protein diet and other appropriate measures (see earlier). Hepatic failure requiring liver transplantation has occurred in a few cases. Although the condition is almost exclusively seen in Japan, the diagnosis should be considered in any neonatal hepatitis syndrome with cholestasis. Data on the long-term prognosis and the natural history of the condition are limited; development into the adult form of the condition (see later) after several years of seemingly asymptomatic hiatus has been observed.

Citrullinemia Type II, Adult Form (Adult-Onset Citrullinemia, Citrullinemia Type II–Mild Form). This form starts suddenly in a previously normal individual and manifests with neuropsychiatric symptoms such as disorientation, delirium, delusion, aberrant behavior, tremors, and frank psychosis. Moderate degrees of hyperammonemia and hypercitrullinemia are present. The age of onset is usually between 20 and 40 yr (range 11 to 79 yr). Patients who recover from the 1st episode will have recurrent attacks and most will die within a few years of diagnosis mainly from cerebral edema. Pancreatitis, hyperlipidemia, and hepatoma are major complications among the survivors. Medical **treatment** has been mostly ineffective for prevention of future attacks. Liver transplantation is the most effective therapy.

Several disease-causing mutations of the gene have been identified in affected families in Japan. The pathogenesis of citrullinemia type II (neonatal and adult forms) remains enigmatic. Although the frequency of abnormal gene is quite high in Japan (1;20,000 homozygosity), the clinical condition has a frequency of only 1:100,000. This indicates that a substantial number of homozygous individuals remain asymptomatic. Only a few non-Japanese patients have been identified.

ARGININOSUCCINATE LYASE (AL) DEFICIENCY (ARGININOSUCCINIC ACIDURIA) [SEE FIG. 85-12]. The severity of the **clinical and biochemical manifestations** varies considerably. In the **neonatal form**, signs and symptoms of severe hyperammonemia (see earlier) develop in the 1st few days of life and mortality is usually high. Infants who survive the 1st acute episode follow the clinical course of the subacute form. In the **subacute or late form**, the major finding is mental retardation, which is associated with failure to thrive and hepatomegaly. Abnormalities of the hair characterized by dryness and brittleness are of special diagnostic value. Gallstones have been seen in some of the survivors. Acute attacks of severe hyperammonemia commonly occur during a catabolic state.

Laboratory findings include hyperammonemia, moderate elevations in liver enzymes, nonspecific increases in plasma levels of glutamine and alanine, moderate increase in plasma levels of citrulline (less than that seen in citrullinemia), and marked increase in plasma levels of argininosuccinic acid (see Fig. 85-14). In most amino acid analyzers, argininosuccinic acid appears within the isoleucine or methionine region, which may cause confusion in the diagnosis. Argininosuccinic acid can also be found in large amounts in urine and spinal fluid. The levels in the spinal fluid are usually higher than those in plasma. The enzyme is normally present in erythrocytes, the liver, and cultured fibroblasts. Prenatal diagnosis is possible by measurement of the enzyme activity in cultured amniotic cells or by identification of the mutant gene. Argininosuccinic acid is also elevated in the amniotic fluid of affected fetuses.

Treatment of acute hyperammonemic attacks and the long-term therapy of the condition are outlined in the earlier pages of this chapter. Mental retardation, persistent hepatomegaly with mild increases in liver enzymes, and bleeding tendencies due to abnormal clotting factors are common sequelae of the disease. This deficiency is inherited as an autosomal recessive trait with a prevalence of ≈1/70,000 live births. The gene is located on chromosome 7cen-q11.2

ARGINASE DEFICIENCY (HYPERARGININEMIA) [SEE FIG. 85-12]. This defect is inherited as an autosomal recessive trait. There are two genetically distinct arginases in humans. One is cytosolic (A1) and is expressed in the liver and erythrocytes, and the other (A2) is found in the renal and brain mitochondria. The gene for cytosolic enzyme, which is the one deficient in patients with arginase deficiency, is mapped to chromosome 6q23. The role of the mitochondrial enzyme is not well understood; its activity increases in patients with argininemia but has no protective effect. Several disease-causing mutations have been identified in different families.

The **clinical manifestations** of this rare condition are quite different from those of other urea cycle enzyme defects. The onset is insidious; the infant usually remains asymptomatic in the 1st few months or, sometimes, years of life. A **progressive spastic diplegia** with scissoring of the lower extremities, choreoathetotic movements, and loss of developmental milestones in a previously normal infant may suggest a degenerative disease of the central nervous system. Two children were treated for several years as cerebral palsy before the diagnosis of arginase deficiency was confirmed. Mental retardation is progressive; seizures are common, but episodes of severe hyperammonemia are not usually seen in this disorder. Hepatomegaly may be present. The acute neonatal form with intractable seizures, cerebral edema, and death has also been reported.

Laboratory findings include marked elevations of arginine in plasma and CSF (see Fig. 85-14). Urinary orotic acid is moderately increased. Plasma ammonia levels may be normal or mildly elevated. Urinary excretions of arginine, lysine, cystine, and ornithine are usually increased, but normal levels have also been noted. Therefore, determination of amino acids in plasma is a critical step in the diagnosis of argininemia. The guanidino compounds (α-keto-guanidinovaleric acid, argininic acid) are markedly increased in urine. The **diagnosis** is confirmed by assaying arginase activity in erythrocytes.

Treatment consists of a low-protein diet devoid of arginine. Administration of a synthetic protein made of essential amino acids usually results in a dramatic decrease in plasma arginine concentration and an improvement in neurologic abnormalities.

The composition of the diet and the daily intake of protein should be monitored by frequent plasma amino acid determinations. Sodium benzoate (250–375 mg/kg/24 hr) is also effective in controlling hyperammonemia, when present; lowering of plasma arginine levels has been noted with this treatment. Mental retardation is a common sequela of the condition. One patient developed type 1 diabetes at age 9 yr while his argininemia was under good control.

TRANSIENT HYPERAMMONEMIA OF THE NEWBORN. Although plasma levels of ammonia in normal full-term infants are within normal limits, very low birthweight infants may have a **mild transient hyperammonemia** (40–50 µmole/L), which lasts for about 6–8 wk. These infants are asymptomatic, and follow-up studies up to 18 mo of age have not revealed any significant neurologic deficits.

Severe transient hyperammonemia has been observed in newborn infants. The majority of affected infants are premature and have mild respiratory distress syndrome. Hyperammonemic coma may develop within 2–3 days of life, and the infant may succumb to the disease if treatment is not started immediately. Laboratory studies reveal marked hyperammonemia (plasma ammonia as high as 4,000 µmole/L) with moderate increases in plasma levels of glutamine and alanine. Plasma concentrations of urea cycle intermediate amino acids are usually normal except for citrulline, which may be moderately elevated. The cause of the disorder is unknown. Urea cycle enzyme activities are normal. **Treatment** of hyperammonemia should be initiated promptly and continued vigorously (see earlier). Recovery without sequelae is common, and hyperammonemia does not recur even with a normal protein diet.

ORNITHINE. Ornithine is one of the intermediate metabolites of the urea cycle that is not incorporated into natural proteins. Rather, it is generated in the cytosol from arginine and must be transported into the mitochondria where it is used as a substrate for the enzyme OTC to form citrulline. Excess ornithine is catabolized by two enzymes, ornithine 5-aminotransferase, which is a mitochondrial enzyme and converts ornithine to a proline precursor, and ornithine decarboxylase, which resides in the cytosol and converts ornithine to putrescine (see Fig. 85-12). Two genetic disorders result in hyperornithinemia: gyrate atrophy of the retina and hyperammonemia-hyperornithinemia-homocitrullinemia syndrome.

Gyrate Atrophy of the Retina and Choroid. This is a rare autosomal recessively inherited disorder caused by the deficiency of the enzyme ornithine 5-aminotransferase (see Fig. 85-12). About 30% of the reported cases are from Finland. **Clinical manifestations** are limited to the eyes and include night blindness, myopia, loss of peripheral vision, and posterior subcapsular cataracts. These eye changes start between 5 and 10 yr of age and progress to complete blindness by the 4th decade of life. Atrophic lesions in the retina resemble cerebral gyri. These patients usually have normal intelligence. There is a 10- to 20-fold increase in plasma levels of ornithine (400–1,400 µmole/L). There is no occurrence of hyperammonemia and no increases in any other amino acids; plasma levels of glutamate, glutamine, lysine, creatine, and creatinine are moderately decreased. Some patients respond partially to high doses of pyridoxine (500–1,000 mg/24 hr). Arginine-restricted diet in conjunction with supplemental lysine, proline, and creatine has been successful in reducing plasma ornithine concentration and has produced some clinical improvements. The gene for ornithine 5-aminotransferase is mapped to chromosome 10q26. Many (at least 60) disease- causing mutations have been identified in different families.

HYPERAMMONEMIA-HYPERORNITHINEMIA-HOMOCITRULLINEMIA (HHH) SYNDROME. In this rare autosomal recessively inherited disorder, the defect is in the transport system of ornithine from the cytosol into the mitochondria, which causes an accumulation of ornithine in the cytosol and a deficiency of ornithine inside the mitochondria. The former causes hyperornithinemia and the latter results in disruption of the urea cycle and hyperammonemia (see Fig. 85-12). Homocitrulline is presumably formed from the reaction of mitochondrial carbamyl phosphate with lysine, which occurs because of the intramitochondrial deficiency of ornithine. **Clinical manifestations** of hyperammonemia may develop shortly after birth or may be delayed until adulthood. Acute episodes of hyperammonemia manifest as refusal to feed, vomiting, and lethargy; coma may occur during infancy. Progressive neurologic signs, such as lower limb weakness, increased deep tendon reflexes, spasticity, clonus, seizures, and varying degrees of psychomotor retardation may develop if the condition remains undiagnosed. No clinical ocular findings have been observed in these patients.

Laboratory findings reveal marked increases in plasma levels of ornithine and homocitrulline in addition to hyperammonemia. Restriction of protein intake improves hyperammonemia. Ornithine supplementation may produce clinical improvement in some patients. The gene for this disorder (*SLC25A15*) is located on chromosome 13q14.

85.12 • Histidine • Iraj Rezvani

Histidine is an essential amino acid only during infancy. Its biosynthetic pathway in older children and adults is poorly understood. Histidine is degraded through the urocanic acid pathway to glutamic acid. Several genetic conditions involving the degradative pathway of histidine have been reported, but none has any clinical consequence.

85.13 • Lysine • Iraj Rezvani

The major pathway in the catabolism of lysine involves its condensation with α-ketoglutaric acid to form saccharopine. Saccharopine is then degraded to α-aminoadipic acid semialdehyde and glutaric acid. These 1st two steps are catalyzed by α-aminoadipic semialdehyde synthase, which has two activities; lysine-ketoglutarate reductase; and saccharopine dehydrogenase (Fig. 85-15). In a minor pathway for lysine degradation, lysine is transaminated first and then condensed to the cyclic form, pipecolic acid. This is the major pathway for D-lysine in the body and for the L-lysine in the brain (see Fig. 85-15).

Hyperlysinemia, α-aminoadipic acidemia and *α-ketoadipic acidemia* are three conditions that are due to inborn errors of metabolism of lysine. Individuals with these conditions are usually asymptomatic.

GLUTARIC ACIDURIA TYPE I. Glutaric acid is an intermediate in the degradation of lysine (see Fig. 85-15), hydroxylysine, and tryptophan. Glutaric aciduria type I, a disorder caused by a deficiency of glutaryl CoA dehydrogenase, should be differentiated from glutaric aciduria type II, a distinct clinical and biochemical disorder caused by defects in the electron transport system (see Chapter 86.1).

Clinical Manifestations. Affected infants with glutaric aciduria type I may develop normally up to 2 yr of life; **macrocephaly** is a common finding in these infants. Symptoms of hypotonia, loss of head control, choreoathetosis, seizures, generalized rigidity, opisthotonos, and dystonia may occur suddenly in a seemingly normal infant after a minor infection. Recovery from the 1st attack usually occurs slowly, but some residual neurologic abnormalities, especially dystonia and extrapyramidal movements, may

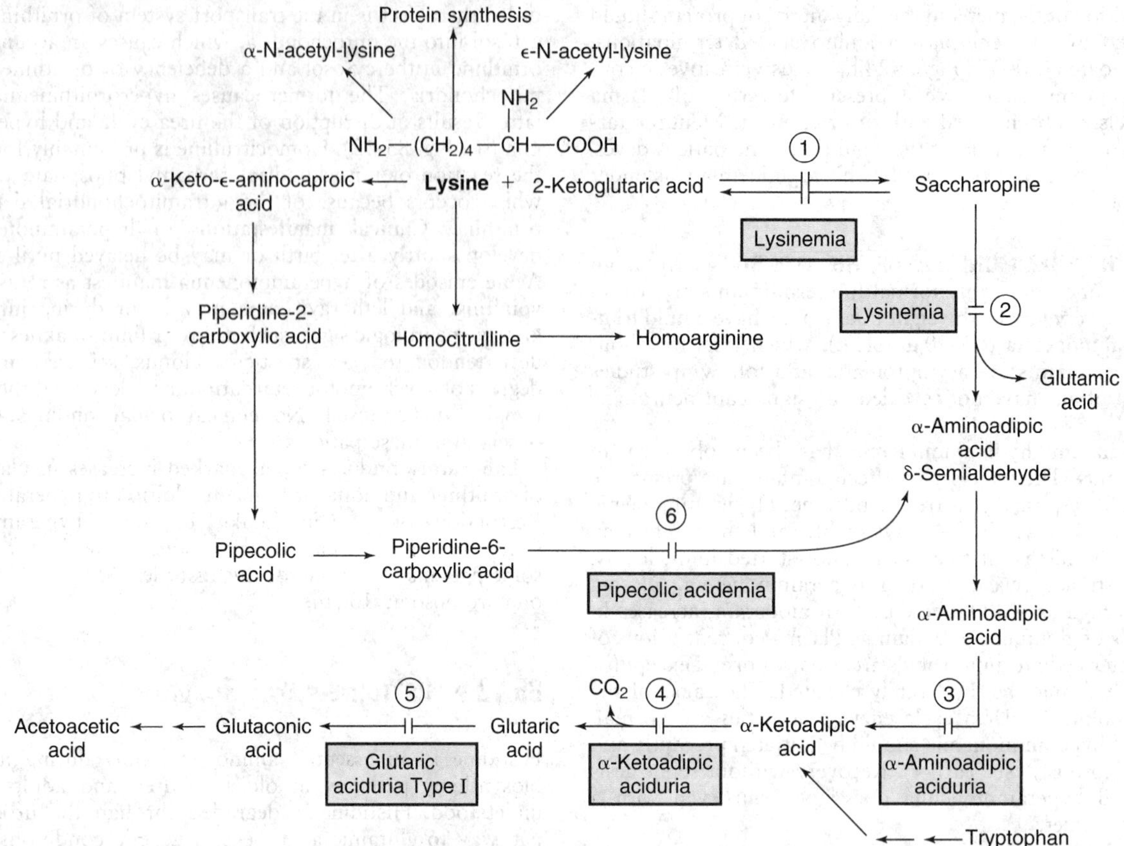

Figure 85-15. Pathways in the metabolism of lysine. **Enzymes:** (1) lysine ketoglutarate reductase, (2) saccharopine dehydrogenase, (3) α-aminoadipic acid transferase, (4) α-ketoadipic acid dehydrogenase, (5) glutaryl CoA dehydrogenase, (6) α-aminoadipic semialdehyde oxidase.

persist. Additional acute episodes resembling the 1st one usually occur during an intercurrent infection. In other patients, these signs and symptoms may develop gradually in the 1st few years of life and hypotonia and choreoathetosis may gradually progress into rigidity and dystonia. Acute episodes of metabolic decompensation with vomiting, ketosis, seizures, and coma also commonly occur in these patients after infection or other catabolic states. Death usually occurs in the 1st decade of life during one of these episodes. The intellectual abilities usually remain relatively normal in most patients.

Laboratory Findings. During acute episodes, mild to moderate metabolic acidosis and ketosis may occur. Hypoglycemia, hyperammonemia, and elevations of serum transaminases are seen in some patients. High concentrations of glutaric acid are usually found in urine, blood, and CSF. 3-Hydroxyglutaric acid may also be present in the urine. This finding differentiates glutaric aciduria type I from type II. In glutaric aciduria type II, 2-hydroxyglutaric rather than 3-hydroxyglutaric acid is elevated. Plasma amino acid concentrations are usually within normal limits. Laboratory findings may be unremarkable between attacks. Severely affected children without glutaric aciduria have also been reported. In some of these patients, the glutaric acid is elevated only in the spinal fluid. In any child with progressive dystonia and dyskinesia, activity of the enzyme glutaryl CoA dehydrogenase should be measured in leukocytes or cultured fibroblasts. CT and MRI of the brain reveal macrocephaly, dilated lateral ventricles, cortical atrophy, fibrosis, and atrophy of striatum (putamen and caudate).

Treatment. A low-protein diet (especially a diet restricted in lysine and tryptophan) and high doses (200–300 mg/24 hr) of riboflavin (the coenzyme for glutaryl CoA dehydrogenase) and L-carnitine (50–100 mg/kg/24 hr orally) produce a dramatic decrease in the levels of glutaric acid in body fluids, but the clinical effect has been variable. The addition of a GABA analog (baclofen) and valproic acid to the therapeutic regimen produces improvement in some affected children.

The condition is inherited as an autosomal recessive trait. The prevalence is not known. The condition is more prevalent in Sweden and among the Old Order Amish population in the United States. The gene is located on chromosome 19p13.2 and many disease-causing mutations have been reported in different families. A single mutation (*A421V*) accounts for all the patients from Lancaster County Old Order Amish.

Prenatal diagnosis may be accomplished by demonstrating increased concentrations of glutaric acid in amniotic fluid, by the assay of the enzyme activity in amniocytes or chorionic villi samples, or by identification of the mutant gene.

LYSINURIC PROTEIN INTOLERANCE (FAMILIAL PROTEIN INTOLERANCE). This rare autosomal recessive disorder is due to a defect in the transport of the cationic amino acids lysine, ornithine, and arginine in both kidneys and intestine. Unlike patients with cystinuria, urinary excretion of cystine is not increased in these patients. About half of the reported cases have been from Finland, where the prevalence has been estimated to be 1/60,000.

Clinical manifestations consist of refusal to feed, nausea, aversion to protein, vomiting, and mild diarrhea, which may result in failure to thrive, wasting, and hypotonia. Breast-fed infants usually remain asymptomatic until shortly after weaning. This may be due to the low protein content of breast milk. Episodes of hyperammonemia may occur after ingestion of a high-protein diet. Mild to moderate hepatosplenomegaly, osteoporosis, sparse brittle hair, thin extremities with moderate centripetal adiposity, and growth retardation are common physical findings in patients whose condition has remained undiagnosed. Mental development is usually normal, but moderate mental retardation has been observed in 20% of patients. **Interstitial pneumonitis** manifesting with fever, fatigue, cough, and dyspnea occur as an acute episode or as a chronic progressive process. Some patients have remained undiagnosed until the appearance of pulmonary manifestations. Radiographic evidence of pulmonary fibrosis has been observed in up to 65% of patients without clinical manifestations of pulmonary involvement. Acute pulmonary proteinosis with renal involvement resembling glomerulonephritis has occurred in older patients and may cause death.

Laboratory findings may reveal hyperammonemia and an elevated concentration of urinary orotic acid, which develop only after protein feeding. Fasting blood ammonia and urinary orotic acid excretion are usually normal. Plasma concentrations of lysine, arginine, and ornithine are usually mildly decreased, but urinary levels of these amino acids, especially lysine, are greatly increased. The mechanism producing hyperammonemia is not clear. All enzymes of the urea cycle are normal. Hyperammonemia may be related to a disturbance of the urea cycle secondary to a deficiency of arginine and ornithine. In patients with cystinuria who also have defects in the transport of lysine, arginine, and ornithine in both intestine and kidneys hyperammonemia is not observed. Plasma concentrations of alanine, glutamine, serine, glycine, proline, and citrulline are usually increased. These abnormalities may be secondary to hyperammonemia and are not specific to this disorder.

Mild anemia and increased serum levels of ferritin, lactic dehydrogenase (LDH), and thyroxine-binding globulin have also been observed in these patients. This condition should be differentiated from hyperammonemia due to urea cycle defects (see Chapter 85.11), especially in heterozygous females with OTC deficiency. Increased urinary excretion of lysine, ornithine, and arginine and elevated blood levels of citrulline are not seen in patients with OTC deficiency.

The transport defect in this condition resides in the basolateral (antiluminal) membrane of enterocytes and renal tubular epithelia. This explains the observation that cationic amino acids are unable to cross these cells even when administered as dipeptides. Lysine in the form of dipeptide crosses the luminal membrane of the enterocytes but hydrolyzes to free lysine molecules in the cytoplasm. Free lysine, unable to cross the basolateral membrane of the cells, is diffused back into the lumen.

Treatment with a low-protein diet (1.0–1.5 g/kg/24 hr) supplemented with citrulline (3–8 g/day) has produced biochemical and clinical improvements. Episodes of hyperammonemia should be treated promptly (see Chapter 85.11). Supplementation with lysine is not useful because it is poorly absorbed and tends to produce diarrhea and abdominal pain. Treatment with high doses of prednisone and bronchoalveolar lavage has been effective in the management of acute pulmonary complications.

The gene for lysinuric protein intolerance (*SLC7A7*) is mapped to chromosome 14q11.2 and several disease-causing mutations have been identified in different families. Pregnancies in affected mothers have been complicated by anemia, thrombocytopenia, toxemia, and bleeding, but offspring have been normal.

85.14 • Aspartic Acid (Canavan Disease) • Reuben K. Matalon

N-acetylaspartic acid, a derivative of aspartic acid, is synthesized in the brain and is found in a high concentration, similar to that of glutamic acid. Its function is unknown, but excessive amounts of *N*-acetylaspartic acid in urine and deficiency of the enzyme aspartoacylase that cleaves the *N*-acetyl group from *N*-acetylaspartic acid are associated with Canavan disease.

CANAVAN DISEASE. Canavan disease, an autosomal recessive disorder characterized by spongy degeneration of the white matter of the brain, leads to a severe form of leukodystrophy. It is more prevalent in individuals of Ashkenazi Jewish descent than in other ethnic groups.

Etiology and Pathology. The deficiency of the enzyme aspartoacylase leads to the accumulation of *N*-acetylaspartic acid in the brain, especially in white matter, and massive urinary excretion of this compound. Excessive amounts of *N*-acetylaspartic acid are also present in the blood and CSF. There is striking vacuolization and astrocytic swelling in white matter. Electron microscopy reveals distorted mitochondria. As the disease progresses, the ventricles enlarge, owing to cerebral atrophy.

Clinical Manifestations. The severity of Canavan disease covers a wide spectrum. Infants usually appear normal at birth and may not manifest symptoms of the disease until 3–6 mo of age, when they develop progressive macrocephaly, severe hypotonia, and persistent head lag. As the infant grows older, delayed milestones become evident. These children become hyperreflexic and hypertonic; joint stiffness may be encountered. As they grow older, seizures and optic atrophy develop. Feeding difficulties, poor weight gain, and gastroesophageal reflux may occur in the 1st yr of life; swallowing deteriorates in the 2nd and 3rd yr of life, and nasogastric feeding or permanent gastrostomy may be required. Most patients die in the 1st decade of life; with improved nursing care, they may survive through the 2nd decade.

Atypical Canavan Disease. Some patients with Canavan disease may have a mild allele (Y288C), a substitution of tyrosine with cysteine or (R71H) substitution, or arginine with histidine. Such patients have very mild delays and are not suspected of having Canavan disease. The excretion of *N*-acetylaspartic acid is increased moderately in urine, which raises the question of Canavan disease and the MRI of the brain shows a different image, not global white matter disease, but increased signal intensities with the basal ganglia, which may be confused with mitochondrial disease.

Diagnosis. CT scans and MRI reveal diffuse white matter degeneration, primarily in the cerebral hemispheres, with less involvement in the cerebellum and brainstem (Fig. 85-16). Repeated evaluations may be required. MRS performed at the time MRI is done can show the high peak of *N*-acetylaspartic acid, suggesting Canavan disease. The differential diagnosis of Canavan disease should include Alexander disease, which is another leukodystrophy with macrocephaly. Progression is usually slow in Alexander disease; hypotonia is not as pronounced as it is in Canavan disease. Brain biopsy shows spongy degeneration of the myelin fivers, astrocytic swelling, and elongated mitochondria. Definitive diagnosis can be established by finding elevated amounts of *N*-acetylaspartic acid in the urine or blood. A deficiency of aspartoacyclase can be found in cultured skin fibroblasts. The biochemical method is the preferred choice for diagnosis. Levels of *N*-acetylaspartic acid in normal urine are only trace amounts (24 ± 16 µmol/mmol creatinine), whereas in patients with Canavan disease they are in the range of 1,440 ± 873 µmol/mmol creatinine. High levels of *N*-acetylaspartic acid in plasma, CSF, and brain tissue can also be detected. The activity of aspartoacylase in the fibroblasts of obligate carriers is about half or less of the activity found in normal individuals.

The gene for aspartoacylase is cloned, and mutations leading to Canavan disease are identified. There are two mutations predominant in the Ashkenazi Jewish population. The 1st is an amino acid substitution (E285A) in which glutamic acid is substituted to alanine. This mutation is the most frequent and encompasses 83% of 100 mutant alleles examined in Ashkenazi Jewish patients. The second common mutation is a change from tyrosine to a nonsense mutation, leading to a stop in the coding sequence (Y231X). This mutation accounts for 13% of the 100 mutant alleles. In the non-Jewish population, more diverse mutations have been observed; the two mutations common in Jewish

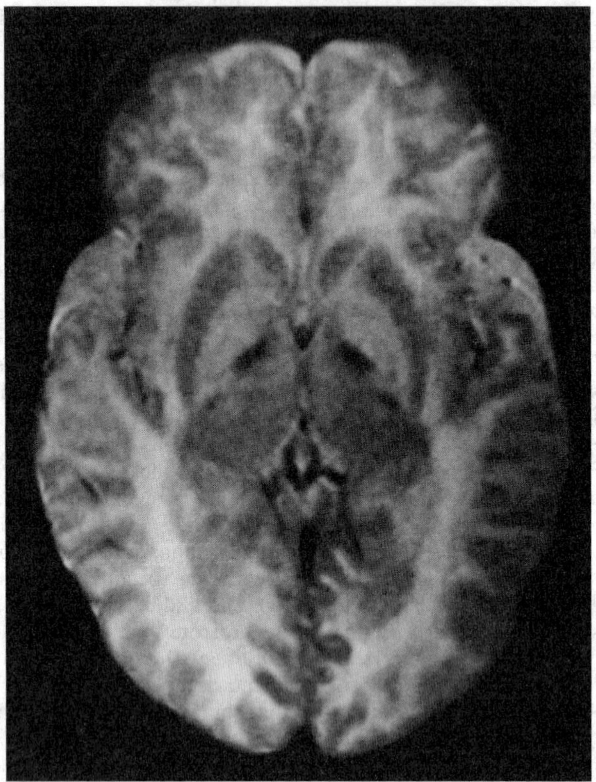

Figure 85-16. Axial T weighted MRI of a 2 yr old patient with Canavan disease. Extensive thickening of the white matter is seen.

people are rare. A different mutation (A305E), substitution of alanine for glutamic acid, accounts for 40% of 62 mutant alleles in non-Jewish patients. With the diagnosis of Canavan disease, it is important to obtain a molecular diagnosis because this will lead to accurate counseling and prenatal for the family. If the mutations are not known, prenatal diagnosis relies on the level of *N*-acetylaspartic acid in the amniotic fluid. In Ashkenazi Jewish patients, the carrier frequency can be as high as 1:36, which is close to that of Tay-Sachs disease. Ashkenazi Jewish individuals may need to be screened for Canavan disease.

Treatment and Prevention. No specific treatment is available. Feeding problems and seizures should be treated on an individual basis. Genetic counseling, carrier testing, and prenatal diagnosis are the only methods of prevention. Injection of liposomes with the human aspartoacyclase gene was introduced to the ventricles of two children with Canavan disease. The results of this gene therapy have not been encouraging.

General

Crombez E, Koch R, Cederbaum S: Pitfalls in newborn screening. *J Pediatr* 2005;147:119–120.

Holtzman NA: Expanding newborn screening. *JAMA* 2003;290:2606–2608.

McKusick VA: Online Mendelian Inheritance in Man (OMIM). Available at www.ncbi.nlm.nih. gov/entrez/query.fcgi?db-omim

Morioka D, Kasahara M, Takada Y, et al: Living donor liver transplantation for pediatric patients with inheritable metabolic disorders. *Am J Transplant* 2005;11:2754–2763.

Natowicz M: Newborn screening—Setting evidence-based policy for protection. *N Engl J Med* 2005;353:867–870.

Schulz A, Lindner M, Kohlmuller D, et al: Expanded newborn screening for inborn errors of metabolism by electrospray ionization-tandem mass spectrometry: Results, outcome, and implications. *Pediatrics* 2003;11: 1399–1406.

Scriver CR, Beaudet AL, Valle D, et al (eds): *The Metabolic and Molecular Basis of Inherited Disease,* 8th ed. New York, McGraw-Hill, 2001.

Waisbren SE, Albers S, Amato S, et al: Effect of expanded newborn screening for biomedical genetic disorders on child outcomes and parental stress. *JAMA* 2003;290:2564–2572.

Phenylalanine

Blau N, Koch R, Matalon R, et al: New development in phenylketonuria and tetrahydrobiopterin research. *Mol Genet Metab (Suppl 1)* 2005;86: 1–156.

Blau N, Seriver Cr: New approaches to treat PKU: How far are we? *Mol Genet Metab* 2004;81:1–2.

Crone Mr, van Spronsen FJ, Oudshoom K, et al: Behavioural factors related to metabolic control in patients with phenylketonuria. *J Inherit Metab Dis* 2005;28:627–637.

Desviat Lr, Perez B, Belanger-Quintana A, et al: Tetrahydrobiopterin responsiveness: Results of the BH4 loading test in 31 Spanish PKU patients and correlation with their genotype. *Mol Genet Metab* 2004;83:157–162.

Gassio R, Fuste E, Lopez-Sala A, et al: School performance in early and continuously treated phenylketonuria. *Pediatr Neurol* 2005;33:267–271.

Koch R: Maternal phenylketonuria: The importance of early control during pregnancy. *Arch Dis Child* 2005;90:114–115.

Koch R, de la Cruz F, Azen CG, et al: The maternal phenylketonuria collaborative study: New developments and the need for new strategies. *Pediatrics* 2003;112(Suppl):1513–1584.

Levy HL, Guldberg P, Guttler F, et al: Congenital heart disease in maternal phenylketonuria: Report from the maternal PKU collaborative study. *Pediatr Res* 2001;49:636–642.

Matalon R, Koch R, Michals-Matalon K, et al: Biopterin responsive phenylalanine hydroxylase deficiency. *Genet Med* 2004;6:27–32.

Muntau AC, Röschinger W, Habich M, et al: Tetrahydrobiopterin as an alternative treatment for mild phenylketonuria. *N Engl J Med* 2002;347:2122–2132.

Segawa M, Nomura Y, Nishiyama N: Autosomal dominant guanosine triphosphate cyclohydrolase I deficiency (Segawa disease). *Ann Neurol* 2003;54:S32–S45.

Waisbren SE, Hanley W, Levy HL, et al: Outcome at age 4 years in offspring of women with maternal phenylketonuria: The maternal PKU collaborative study. *JAMA* 2000;283:756–762.

Walter JH, White FJ, Hall SK, et al: How practical are recommendations for dietary control in phenylketonuria? *Lancet* 2002;360:55–57.

Tyrosine

Cerone R, Fantasia AR, Castellano E, et al: Pregnancy and tyrosinaemia type II. *J Inherit Metab Dis* 2002;25:317–318.

Crone J, Moslinger D, Bodamer OA, et al: Reversibility of cirrhotic regenerative liver nodules upon NTBC treatment in a child with tyrosinaemia type I. *Acta Paediatr* 2003;92:625–628.

Dionisi-Vivi C, Hoffmann GF, Leuzzi V, et al: Tyrosine hydroxylase deficiency with severe clinical course: Clinical and biochemical investigations and optimization of therapy. *J Pediatr* 2000;136:560–562.

Ellaway CJ, Holme E, Standing S, et al: Outcome of tyrosinaemia type III. *J Inherit Metab Dis* 2001;24:824–832.

Furukawa Y: Update on dopa-responsive dystonia: Locus heterogeneity and biochemical features. *Adv Neurol* 2004;94:127–138.

Held PK: Disorders of tyrosine catabolism *J Mol Genet Metab* 2006;88:103–106.

Magera MJ, Gunawardena ND, Hahn SH, et al: Quantitative determination of succinylaction in dried blood spots for newborn screening of tyrosinemia type I. *J Mol Genet Metab* 2006;88:16–21.

Macsai MS, Schwartz TL, Hinkle D, et al: Tyrosinemia type II: Nine cases of ocular signs and symptoms. *Am J Ophthalmol* 2001;132:522–527.

Madan V, Gupta U: Tyrosinaemia type II with diffuse plantar keratoderma and self-mutilation. *Clin Exp Dermatol* 2006;31:54–56.

Moller LB, Romstad A, Paulsen M, et al: Pre- and postnatal diagnosis of tyrosine hydroxylase deficiency. *Prenat Diagn* 2005;25:671–675.

Phornphutkul C, Introne WJ, Perry MB, et al: Natural history of alkaptonuria. *N Engl J Med* 2002;347:2111–2121.

Russell-Eggitt I: Albinism. *Ophthalmol Clin North Am* 2001;14:533–546.

Schiller A, Wevers RA, Steenbergen GC, et al: Long-term course of L-dopa responsive dystonia caused by tyrosine hydroxylase deficiency. *Neurology* 2004;63:1524–1526.

Techakittiroj C, Cunningham A, Hooper PF, et al: High protein diet mimics hypertyrosinemia in newborn infants. *J Pediatr* 2005;146:281–282.

Tomita Y, Suzuki T: Genetics of pigmentary disorders. *Am J Med Genet C Semin Med Genet* 2004;131C:75–81.

Van Spronsen FJ, Bijleveld CM, van Maldegem BT, Wijburg FA: Hepatocellular carcinoma in hereditary tyrosinemia type I despite 2-(2 nitro-4–3 trifluoro-methylbenzoyl)-1,3-cyclohexanedione treatment. *J Pediatr Gastroenterol Nutr* 2005;40:90–93.

Methionine

Carmel R, Green R, Roesnblatt DS, Watkins D: Update on cobalamin, folate, and homocysteine. Genetic diseases and polymorphisms. *Hematology Am Soc Hematol Educ Program* 2003;62–81.

Lawson-Yuen A, Levy HL: The use of betaine in the treatment of elevated homocysteine. *J Mol Genet Metab* 2006;88:201–207.

Lee SJ, Lee DH, Yoo HW, et al: Identification and functional analysis of cystathionine beta-synthase gene mutations in patients with homocystinuria. *J Hum Genet* 2005;50:648–654.

Lerner-Ellis JP, Tirone JC, Pawelek PD, et al: Identification of the gene responsible for methylmalonic aciduria and homocystinuria, *cbl*C type. *Nat Genet* 2006;38:93–100.

Morel CF, Scott, P, Christenson E, et al: Prenatal diagnosis for severe methylenetetrahydrofolate reductase deficiency by linkage analysis and enzymatic assay. *Mol Genet Metab* 2005;85:115–120.

Selzer RR, Rosenblatt DS, Laxova R, Hogan K: Adverse effect of nitrous oxide in a child with 5,10-methylenetertahydrofolate reductase deficiency. *N Engl J Med* 2003;349:45–50.

Sibani S, Leclerc D, Weisberg IS, et al: Characterization of mutations in severe methylenetetrahydrofolate reductase deficiency reveals an FAD-responsive mutation. *Hum Mut* 2003;21:509–520.

Topaloglu AK, Sansaricq C, Snyderman SE: Influence of metabolic control on growth in homocystinuria due to cystathionine β-synthase deficiency. *Pediatr Res* 2001;49:796–798.

Ueland PM, Holm, PI, Hustad S: Betaine: A key modulator of one-carbon metabolism and homocysteine status. *Clin Chem Lab Med* 2005;43: 1069–1075.

Vilaseca MA, Cuartero ML, Martinez de Salinas M, et al: Two successful pregnancies in pyridoxine-nonresponsive homocystinuria. *J Inherit Metab Dis* 2004;27:775–777.

Yaghmai R, Kashani AH, Greaghty MT, et al: Progressive cerebral edema associated with high methionine levels and betaine therapy in a patient with cystathionine beta-synthase (CBS) deficiency. *Am J Med Genet* 2002;108: 57–63.

Yap S, Rushe H, Howard PM, et al: The intellectual abilities of early treated individuals with pyridoxine-nonresponsive homocystinuria due to cystathionine beta-synthase deficiency. *J Inherit Metab Dis* 2001;24:437–447.

Cysteine/Cystine, Tryptophan

Karakas E, Wilson HL, Graf TN, et al: Structural insights into sulfite oxidase deficiency. *J Biol Chem* 2005;280:33506–33515.

Kleta R, Bernardini I, Arcos-Burgos M, et al: Molecular basis of the Hartnup disorder. *Mol Genet Metab* 2005;84:226.

Leimkuhler S, Charcosset M, Latour P, et al: Ten novel mutations in the molybdenum cofactor genes *MOCS1* and *MOCS2* and in vitro characterization of a *MOCS2* mutation that abolishes the binding ability of molybdopterin synthase. *Hum Genet* 2005;117:565–570.

Tan WH, Eichler FS, Hoda S, et al: Isolated sulfite oxidase deficiency: A case report with a novel mutation and review of the literature. *Pediatrics* 2005;116:757–766.

Valine, Leucine, Isoleucine, and Related Organic Acidemias

Acquaviva C, Benoist JF, Callebaut I, et al: N219Y, a new frequent mutation among *mut*^{0} forms of methylmalonic acidemia in Caucasian patients. *Eur J Hum Genet* 2001;9:577–582.

Anikster Y, Kleta R, Shaag A, et al: Type III 3-methylglutaconic aciduria (optic atrophy plus syndrome, or Costeff optic atrophy syndrome): Identification of the *OPA3* gene and its founder mutation in Iraqi Jews. *Am J Hum Genet* 2001;69:1218–1224.

Barshop BA, Khanna A: Domino hepatic transplantation in maple syrup urine disease. *N Engl J Med* 2005;353:2410–2411.

Barth PG, Valianpour F, Bowen VM, et al: X-linked cardioskeletal myopathy and neutropenia (Barth syndrome): An update. *Am J Med Genet* 2004;126A:349–354.

Baumgatner MR: Molecular mechanism of dominant expression in 3-methylcrotonyl CoA carboxylase deficiency. *J Inherit Metab Dis* 2005; 28:301–309.

Bodner-Leidecker A, Wendel U, Saudubray JM, et al: Branched-chain L-amino acid metabolism in classical maple syrup urine disease after orthotopic liver transplantation. *J Inherit Metab Dis* 2000;23:805–818.

Chakrapani A, Sivakumar P, McKiernan PJ, et al: Metabolic stroke in methylmalonic acidemia five years after liver transplantation. *J Pediatr* 2002;140:261–263.

Dantas MF, Suormala T, Randolph A, et al: 3-Methylcrotonyl-CoA carboxylase deficiency: Mutation analysis in 28 probands, 9 symptomatic and 19 detected by newborn screening. *Hum Mutat* 2005;26:164.

Desviat LR, Perez B, Perez-Cerda C, et al: Propionic acidemia: Mutation update and functional and structural effects of the variant alleles. *Mol Genet Metab* 2004;83:28–37.

D'Osualdo A, Picco P, Caroli F, et al: MVK mutations and associated clinical features in Italian patients affected with autoinflammatory disorders and recurrent fever. *Eur J Hum Genet* 2005;13:314–320.

Ensenauer R, Vockley J, Willard J, et al: A common mutation is associated with a mild, potentially asymptomatic phenotype in patients with isovaleric acidemia diagnosed by newborn screening. *Am J Hum Genet* 2004;75:1136–1142.

Fukao T, Scriver CR, Kondo N, et al: The clinical phenotype and outcome of mitochondrial acetoacetyl-CoA thiolase deficiency (beta-ketothiolase or T2 deficiency) in 26 enzymatically proved and mutation-defined patients. *Mol Genet Metab* 2001;72:109–114.

Harding CO, Pillers DA, Steiner RD, et al: Potential for misdiagnosis due to lack of combined methylmalonic aciduria/hyperhomocysteinemia (*cblC*) in the neonate. *J Perinatol* 2003;23:384–386.

Hoffmann B, Helbling C, Schadewaldt P, Wendel U: Impact of longitudinal plasma leucine levels on the intellectual outcome in patients with classic MSUD. *Pediatr Res* 2006;59:17–20.

Houten SM, Frenkel J, Rijkers GT, et al: Temperature dependence of mutant mevalonate kinase activity as a pathogenic factor in hyper-IgD and periodic fever syndrome. *Hum Mol Genet* 2002;22:3115–3124.

Hymes J, Stanley CM, Wolf B: Mutation in BTD causing biotinidase deficiency. *Hum Mutat* 2001;18:375–381.

Kayser M: Disorders of ketone production and utilization. *J Mol Genet Metab* 2006;87:281–283.

Koeberl DD, Millington DS, Smith WE, et al: Evaluation of 3-methylcrotonyl-CoA carboxylase deficiency detected by tandem mass spectrometry newborn screening. *J Inherit Metab Dis* 2003;26:25–35.

Lerner-Ellis JP, Gradinger AB, Watkins D, et al: Mutation and biochemical analysis of patients belonging to the *cbl* B complementation class of vitamin B_{12}–dependent methylmalonic aciduria. *Mol Genet Metab* 2006;87: 219–225.

Longo N, Fukao T, Singh R, et al: Succinyl-CoA:3-ketoacid transferase (SCOT) deficiency in a new patient homozygous for an R217X mutation. *J Inherit Metab Dis* 2004;27:691–692.

Mardach R, Verity MA, Cederbaum SD: Clinical, pathological, and biochemical studies in a patient with propionic acidemia and fatal cardiomyopathy. *Mol Genet Metab* 2005;85:286–290.

Morel CF, Scott P, Christensen E, et al: Prenatal diagnosis for severe methylenetetrahydrofolate reductase deficiency by linkage analysis and enzymatic assay. *Mol Genet Metab* 2005;85:115–120.

Morel CF, Watkins D, Scott P, et al: Prenatal diagnosis for methylmalonic acidemia and inborn errors of vitamin B_{12} metabolism and transport. *Mol Genet Metab* 2005;86:160–171.

Morrone A, Malyagia S, Donati MA, et al: Clinical findings and biochemical and molecular analysis of four patients with holocarboxylase synthetase deficiency. *Am J Med Genet* 2002;111:10–18.

Morton DH, Strauss KA, Robinson DL, et al: Diagnosis and treatment of maple syrup disease: A study of 36 patients. *Pediatrics* 2002;109:999–1008.

Moslinger D, Muhl A, Suormala T, et al: Molecular characterization and neuropsychological outcome of 21 patients with profound biotinidase deficiency detected by newborn screening and family studies. *Eur J Pediatr* 2003;162:S46–S49.

Nellis MM, Kasinski A, Carlson M, et al: Relationship of causative genetic mutations in maple syrup urine disease with their clinical expression. *Mol Genet Metab* 2003;80:189–195.

Prasad C, Nurko S, Borovoy J, Korson MS: The importance of gut motility in the metabolic control of propionic acidemia. *J Pediatr* 2004;144:532–535.

Prietsch V, Mayateper E, Krastel H, et al: Mevalonate kinase deficiency: Enlarging the clinical and biochemical spectrum. *Pediatrics* 2003;111: 258–261.

Sass JO, Hofmann M, Skladal D, et al: Propionic acidemia revisited: A workshop report. *Clin Pediatr (Phila)* 2004;43:837–843.

Valianpour F, Waners RJA, Overmars H, et al: Cardiolipin deficiency in X-linked cardioskeletal myopathy and neutropenia (Barth syndrome,

MIM 302060): A study in cultured skin fibroblasts. *J Pediatr* 2002;141: 729–733.

Varvogli L, Repetto GM, Waisbren SE, et al: High cognitive outcome in an adolescent with *mut*-methylmalonic acidemia. *Am J Med Genet* 2000; 96:192–195.

Wolf NI, Rahman S, Clayton PT, Zschocke J: Mitochondrial HMG-CoA synthase deficiency: Identification of two further patients carrying two novel mutations. *Eur J Pediatr* 2003;162:279–280.

Worgan LC, Niles K, Tirone JC, et al: The spectrum of mutations in *mut* methylmalonic acidemia and identification of a common Hispanic mutation and haplotype. *Hum Mutat* 2006;27:31–43.

Yorifuji T, Muroi J, Uematsu A, et al: Living related liver transplantation for neonatal-propionic acidemia. *J Pediatr* 2000;137:572–574.

Glycine

Almeida LS, Verhoeven NM, Roos B, et al: Creatine and guanidinoacetate: Diagnostic markers for inborn errors in creatine biosynthesis and transport. *Mol Genet Metab* 2004;82:214–219.

Caldeira Araujo H, Smit W, Verhoeven NM, et al: Guanidinoacetate methyltransferase deficiency identified in adults and a child with mental retardation. *Am J Med Genet A* 2005;133:122–127.

Cochat P, Nogeeria PCK, Mahmoud MA, et al: Primary hyperoxaluria in infants: Medicoethical and economic issues. *J Pediatr* 1999;135:746–750.

Dampure CJ: Molecular etiology of primary hyperoxaluria type 1: New directions for treatment. *Am J Nephrol* 2005;25:303–310.

Dinopoulos A, Matsubara Y, Kure S: Atypical variants of nonketotic hyperglycinemia. *Mol Genet Metab* 2005;86:61–69.

Hoover-Fong JE, Shah S, Van Hove JL, et al: Natural history of nonketotic hyperglycinemia in 65 patients. *Neurology* 2004;63:1847–1853.

Jamieson NV, European PHI Transplantation Study Group: A 20-year experience of combined liver/kidney transplantation for primary hyperoxaluria (PH1): The European PH1 transplant registry experience 1984–2004. *Am J Nephrol* 2005;25:282–289.

Milliner DS: The primary hyperoxalurias: An algorithm for diagnosis. *Am J Nephrol* 2005;25:154–160.

Rosenberg EH, Almeida LS, Kleefstra T, et al: High prevalence of SLC6A8 deficiency in X-linked mental retardation. *Am J Hum Genet* 2004;75:97–105.

Sellner L, Edkins E, Greed L, Lewis B: Detection of mutations in the glycine decarboxylase gene in patients with nonketotic hyperglycinaemia. *Mol Genet Metab* 2005;84:167–171.

Stromberger C, Bodamer OA, Stockler-Ipsiroglu S: Clinical characteristics and diagnostic clues in inborn errors of creatine metabolism. *J Inherit Metab Dis* 2003;26:299–308.

Verhoven NM, Salomons GS, Jakobs C: Laboratory diagnosis of defects of creatine biosynthesis and transport. *Clin Chim Acta* 2005;361:1–9.

Serine

de Koning TJ, Klomp LW: Serine-deficiency syndromes. *Curr Opin Neurol* 2004;17:197–204.

de Koning TJ, Klomp LW, van Oppen AC, et al: Prenatal and early postnatal treatment in 3-phosphoglycerate-dehydrogenase deficiency. *Lancet* 2004;364:2221–2222.

Pollitt RJ, Sharrard MJ: Treating rare inborn errors of metabolism. *Lancet* 2004;364:2158–2160.

Proline

Forlino A, Lupi A, Vaghi P, et al: Mutation analysis of five new patients affected by prolidase deficiency: The lack of enzyme activity causes necrosis-like cell death in cultured fibroblasts. *Hum Genet* 2002;111: 314–322.

Lupi A, DeRiso A, Torre SD, et al: Characterization of new PEPD allele causing prolidase deficiency in two unrelated patients: Natural-occurrent mutations as a tool to investigate structure-function relationship. *J Hum Genet* 2004;49:500–506.

Glutamic Acid

Gordon N: Succinic semialdehyde dehydrogenase deficiency (SSADH) (4-hydroxybutyric aciduria, gamma-hydroxybutyric aciduria). *Eur J Paediatr Neurol* 2004;8:261–265.

Haberle J, Gorg B, Rutsch F, et al: Congenital glutamine deficiency with glutamine synthetase mutations. *N Engl J Med* 2005;353:1926–1933.

Medina-Kauwe LK, Tobin AJ, DeMeirleir L, et al: 4-Aminobutyrate aminotransferase (GABA transaminase) deficiency. *J Inherit Metab Dis* 1999;22:414–427.

Njalsson R: Glutathione synthetase deficiency. *Cell Mol Life Sci* 2005;62: 1939–1945.

Njalsson R, Ristoff E, Carlsson K, et al: Genotype, enzyme activity, glutathione level, and clinical phenotype in patients with glutathione synthetase deficiency. *Hum Genet* 2005;116:384–389.

Pearl PL, Gibson KM: Clinical aspects of the disorders of GABA metabolism in children. *Curr Opin Neurol* 2004;17:107–113.

Pearl PL, Gibson KM, Acosta MT, et al: Clinical spectrum of succinic semialdehyde dehydrogenase deficiency. *Neurology* 2003;60:1413–1417.

Ristoff E, Larsson A: Oxidative stress in inborn errors of metabolism: Lessons from glutathione deficiency. *J Inherit Metab Dis* 2002;25:223–226.

Wong CG, Bottiglieri T, Snead OC III: GABA, gamma-hydroxybutyric acid, and neurological disease. *Ann Neurol* 2003;54:S3–S12.

Urea Cycle

Anadiotis G, Ierardi-Curto L, Kaplan PB, et al: Ornithine transcarbamylase deficiency and pancreatitis. *J Pediatr* 2001;138:123–124.

Arvio P, Arvio M: Progressive nature of aspartylglucosaminuria. *Acta Paediatr* 2002;91:255–257.

Brusilow SW: Hyperammonemic encephalopathy. *Medicine (Baltimore)* 2002;81:240–249.

Crombez EA, Cederbaum SD: Hyperargininemia due to liver arginase deficiency. *Mol Genet Metab* 2005;84:243–251.

Ensenauer R, Tuchman M, El-Youssef M, et al: Management and outcome of neonatal-onset ornithine transcarbamylase deficiency following liver transplantation at 60 days of life. *Mol Genet Metab* 2005;84:363–366.

Gropman AL, Batshaw ML: Cognitive outcome in urea cycle disorders. *Mol Genet Metab* 2004;81:S58–S62.

Haberle J, Koch HG: Genetic approach to prenatal diagnosis in urea cycle defects. *Prenat Diagn* 2004;24:378–383.

Horslen SP, McCowan TC, Goertzen TC, et al: Isolated hepatocyte transplantation in an infant with a severe urea cycle disorder. *Pediatrics* 2003;111:1262–1267.

Kaiser-Kupfer MI, Caruso RC, Valle D: Gyrate atrophy of the choroid and retina: Further experience with long-term reduction of ornithine levels in children. *Arch Ophthalmol* 2002;120:146–153.

Kaiser-Kupfer MI, Caruso RC, Valle D, Reed GF: Use of an arginine-restricted diet to slow progression of visual loss in patients with gyrate atrophy. *Arch Ophthalmol* 2004;122;982–984.

Kleijer WJ, Garrisen VH, Linnebank M, et al: Clinical, enzymatic, and molecular genetic characterization of a biochemical variant type of argininosuccinic aciduria: Prenatal and postnatal diagnosis in five unrelated families. *J Inherit Metab Dis* 2002;25:499–410.

Korman SH, Kanazawa N, Abu-Libdeh B, et al: Hyperornithinemia, hyperammonemia, and homocitrullinuria syndrome with evidence of mitochondrial dysfunction due to a novel SLC25A15 (*ORNT1*) gene mutation in a Palestinian family. *J Neurol Sci* 2004;218:53–58.

Linnebank M, Tschiedel E, Haberle J, et al: Argininosuccinate lyase (ASL) deficiency: Mutation analysis in 27 patients and a completed structure of the human ASL gene. *Hum Genet* 2002;111:350–359.

McBride KL, Miller G, Carter S, et al: Developmental outcomes with early orthotopic liver transplantation for infants with neonatal-onset urea cycle defects and a female patient with late-onset ornithine transcarbamylase deficiency. *Pediatrics* 2004;114:e523–e526.

Morioka D, Kasahara M, Takada Y, et al: Current role of liver transplantation for the treatment of urea cycle disorders: A review of the worldwide English literature and 13 cases at Kyoto University. *Liver Transpl* 2005;11:1332–1342.

Nagasaka H, Komatsu H, Ohura T, et al: Nitric oxide synthesis in ornithine transcarbamylase deficiency: Possible involvement of low no synthesis in clinical manifestations of urea cycle defect. *J Pediatr* 2004;145:259–262.

Nicolaides P, Liebsch D, Dale N, et al: Neurological outcome of patients with ornithine carbamoyltransferase deficiency. *Arch Dis Child* 2002;86:54–56.

Picker JD, Puga AC, Levy HL, et al: Arginase deficiency with lethal neonatal expression: Evidence for the glutamine hypothesis of cerebral edema. *J Pediatr* 2003;142:349–352.

Robininath T, Costello DJ, Lynch T, et al: Fatal presentation of ornithine transcarbamylase deficiency in a 62-year-old man and family studies. *J Inherit Metab Dis* 2004;27:285–288.

Saheki T, Kobayashi K, Iijima M, et al: Metabolic derangements in deficiency of citrin, a liver-type mitochondrial aspartate-glutamate carrier. *Hepatol Res* 2005;33:181–184.

Saheki T, Kobayashi K, Iijima M, et al: Adult-onset type II citrullinemia and idiopathic neonatal hepatitis caused by citrin deficiency: Involvement of the aspartate glutamate carrier for urea synthesis and maintenance of the urea cycle. *Mol Genet Metab* 2004;81:S20–S26.

Santinelli R, Costagliola C, Tolone C, et al: Low-protein diet and progression of retinal degeneration in gyrate atrophy of the choroid and retina: A 26-year follow-up. *J Inherit Metab Dis* 2004;27:187–196.

Scaglia F, O'Brien WE, Henry J, et al: An integrated approach to the diagnosis and prospective management of partial ornithine transcarbamylase deficiency. *Pediatrics* 2002;109:150–152.

Summar M, Tuchman M: Proceedings of a consensus conference for the management of patients with urea cycle disorders. *J Pediatr* 2001;138:S6–S10.

Tazawa Y, Kobayashi K, Abukawa D, et al: Clinical heterogeneity of neonatal intrahepatic cholestasis caused by citrin deficiency: Case reports from 16 patients. *Mol Genet Metab* 2004;83:213–219.

Wilcken B: Problems in the management of urea cycle disorders. *Mol Genet Metab* 2004;81:S86–S91.

Zammarchi E, Ciani F, Pasquini E, et al: Neonatal onset of hyperornithinemia, hyperammonemia, homocitrullinemia syndrome with favorable outcome. *J Pediatr* 1997;131:440–443.

Lysine

Bjugstad KB, Goodman SI, Freed CR: Age at symptom onset predicts severity of motor impairment and clinical outcome of glutaric aciduria type I. *J Pediatr* 2000;137:681–686.

Kolker S, Ramaekers VT, Zschocke J, et al: Acute encephalopathy despite early therapy in a patient with homozygosity for E365K in the glutamyl coenzyme A dehydrogenase gene. *J Pediatr* 2001;138:277–279.

Palacin M, Bertran J, Chillaron J, et al: Lysinuric protein intolerance: Mechanisms of pathophysiology. *Mol Genet Metab* 2004;81:S27–S37.

Sperandeo MP, Annunziata P, Ammendola V, et al: Lysinuric protein intolerance: Identification and functional analysis of mutations of the *SLC7A7* gene. *Hum Mutat* 2005;25:410.

Strauss KA: Glutaric aciduria type 1: A clinician's view of progress. *Brain* 2005;128:697–699.

Strauss KA, Puffenberger EG, Robinson DL, Morton DH: Type I glutaric aciduria, part 1: Natural history of 77 patients. *Am J Med Genet C Semin Med Genet* 2003;121:38–51.

Aspartic Acid

Leone P, Janson CG, Bilianuk L, et al: Aspartoacylase gene transfer to the mammalian central nervous system with therapeutic implications for Canavan disease. *Ann Neurol* 2000;48:27–38.

Matalon R, Michals K: Molecular basis of Canavan disease. *Eur J Paediatr Neurol* 1998;2:69–76.

Matalon R, Michals-Matalon K: Spongy degeneration of the brain, Canavan disease: Biochemical and molecular findings. *Front Biosci* 2000;5:307–311.

Surendran S, Bamforth FJ, Chan A, et al: Mild elevation of *N*-acetylaspartic acid and macrocephaly: Diagnostic problem. *J Child Neurol* 2003;18:809–812.

Tacke U, Olbrich H, Sass JO, et al: Possible geneotype-phenotype correlations in children with mild clinical course of Canavan disease. *Neuropediatrics* 2005;36:252–255.

Topcu M, Erdem G, Saatsi I, et al: Clinical and magnetic resonance imaging features of L-2-hydroxyglutaric aciduria: Report of three cases in comparison with Canavan disease. *J Child Neurol* 1996;11:373–377.

Yalcinkaya C, Benbir G, Salomons GS, et al: Atypical MRI findings in Canavan disease: A patient with a mild course. *Neuropediatrics* 2005;36:336–339.

Chapter 86 ■ Defects in Metabolism of Lipids

86.1 • Disorders of Mitochondrial Fatty Acid β–Oxidation • Charles A. Stanley and Michael J. Bennett

Mitochondrial β-oxidation of fatty acids is an essential energy-producing pathway. It is a particularly important pathway during prolonged periods of starvation, and during periods of reduced caloric intake due to gastrointestinal illness or increased energy expenditure during febrile illness. Under these conditions, the body switches from using predominantly carbohydrate to predominantly fat as its major fuel. Fatty acids are also important fuels for exercising skeletal muscle and are the preferred substrate for the heart. In these tissues, fatty acids are completely oxidized to carbon dioxide and water. The end products of hepatic fatty acid oxidation are the ketone bodies β-hydroxybutyrate and acetoacetate. These cannot be oxidized by the liver but serve as important fuels in peripheral tissues, particularly the brain.

Genetic defects have been identified in nearly all of the known steps in the fatty acid oxidation pathway; all are recessively inherited (Table 86-1).

Clinical manifestations characteristically involve the tissues with a high β-oxidation flux including liver, skeletal, and cardiac muscle. The most common presentation is an acute episode of life-threatening coma and hypoglycemia induced by a period of fasting due to defective hepatic ketogenesis. Other manifestations include chronic cardiomyopathy and muscle weakness or exercise-induced acute rhabdomyolysis. The fatty acid oxidation defects can be asymptomatic during periods when there is no fasting stress. Acutely presenting disease may be misdiagnosed as Reye syndrome or, if fatal, as sudden unexpected infant death. Fatty acid oxidation disorders are easily overlooked because the only specific clue to the diagnosis may be the finding of inappropriately low concentrations of urinary ketones in an infant who has hypoglycemia. Genetic defects in ketone body utilization may be overlooked because ketosis is an expected finding with fasting hypoglycemia. In some circumstances, clinical manifestations appear to arise from toxic effects of fatty acid metabolites rather than simply inadequate energy production. These include disorders (LCHAD, CPT-IA, SCAD, TFP; see later) in which the presence of an affected fetus (homozygous) increases the risk of a life-threatening illness in the heterozygote mother, resulting in acute fatty liver of pregnancy or preeclampsia with HELLP (hemolysis, elevated liver enzymes, low platelets) syndrome. Malformations of the brain and kidneys have been described in severe electron transfer flavoprotein (ETF), ETF dehydrogenase (ETF-DH), and carnitine palmitoyltransferase-2 (CPT-II) deficiencies that might reflect in utero toxicity of fatty acid metabolites. Progressive retinal degeneration and chronic progressive liver disease have been identified in LCHAD deficiency. Newborn screening programs using tandem mass spectrometry (MS/MS) detect characteristic acylcarnitines seen in many of these disorders and permit presymptomatic diagnosis. Screening programs have provided evidence that all the fatty acid oxidation disorders combined are among the most common inborn errors of metabolism.

Figures 86-1 and 86-2 outline the steps involved in the oxidation of a typical long-chain fatty acid. In the *carnitine cycle,* fatty acids are transported across the barrier of the inner mitochondrial membrane as acylcarnitine esters. Within the mitochondria, successive turns of the four-step β-oxidation cycle convert the coenzyme A (CoA)–activated fatty acid to acetyl CoA units. Two to three different chain-length specific isoenzymes are needed for each of these β-oxidation steps to accommodate the different-sized fatty acyl CoA species. The electron transfer pathway carries electrons generated in the 1st β-oxidation step (acyl CoA dehydrogenase) to the *electron transport chain* for adenosine triphosphate (ATP) production, while electrons generated from the third step (3-hydroxyacyl CoA dehydrogenase) enter the *respiratory chain* at the level of complex 1. Most of the acetyl CoA generated from hepatic β-oxidation flows through the *pathway of ketogenesis* to form β-hydroxybutyrate and acetoacetate.

TABLE 86-1. Mitochondrial Fatty Acid Oxidation Disorders—Clinical and Biochemical Features

ENZYME DEFICIENCY	GENE	CLINICAL PHENOTYPE	LABORATORY FINDINGS
Carnitine transporter	*OCTN2*	Cardiomyopathy, skeletal myopathy, liver disease, sudden death, endocardial fibroelastosis, prenatal and NB screening diagnosis reported	↓ Total and free carnitine, normal acylcarnitines, acylglycine, and organic acids
Long-chain fatty acid transporter	*FATP1-6*	Rare, acute liver failure in childhood requiring liver transplantation	Reduced intracellular C_{14}–C_{18} fatty acids, reduced fatty acid oxidation
Carnitine palmitoyl transferase-I	*CPT-I*	Liver failure, skeletal myopathy, renal tubulopathy, and sudden death. Prenatal and NB screening diagnosis reported, maternal preeclampsia, HELLP syndrome association described in a few patients.	Normal or ↑ free carnitine, normal acylcarnitines, acylglycine, and organic acids
Carnitine translocase	*CACT*	Chronic progressive liver failure, persistent ↑ NH_3, hypertrophic cardiomyopathy	Normal or ↓ free carnitine, abnormal acylcarnitine profile
Carnitine palmitoyl transferase-II	*CPT-II*	Early and late onset types. Liver failure, encephalopathy, cardiomyopathy, renal cystic changes, NB screening diagnosis reported.	Normal or ↓ free carnitine, abnormal acylcarnitine profile
Short-chain acyl CoA dehydrogenase	*SCAD*	Benign to a severe presentation, to include encephalopathic disease to progressive myopathy. NB screening diagnosis possible, maternal preeclampsia, HELLP syndrome association described in few patients.	Normal or ↓ free carnitine, elevated urine ethylmalonic acid, inconsistently abnormal acylcarnitine profile
Medium-chain acyl CoA dehydrogenase	*MCAD*	Hypoglycemia, hepatic encephalopathy, sudden death. NB screening diagnosis possible, maternal preeclampsia, HELLP syndrome association described rarely.	Normal or ↓ free carnitine, ↑ plasma acylglycine, plasma C_6–C_{10} free fatty acids, ↑ C_8–C_{10} acyl-carnitine
Very long chain acyl CoA dehydrogenase	*VLCAD*	Dilated cardiomyopathy, arrhythmias, hypoglycemia, and hepatic steatosis. Late-onset, stress-induced rhabdomyolysis, episodic myopathy. Prenatal and NB screening diagnosis possible	Normal or ↓ free carnitine, ↑ plasma $C_{14:1}$, C_{14} acylcarnitine, ↑ plasma C_{10}–C_{16} free fatty acids
ETF dehydrogenase*	*ETF-DH*	Nonketotic fasting hypoglycemia, congenital anomalies, milder forms of liver disease, cardiomyopathy, and skeletal myopathy	Normal or ↓ free carnitine, increased ratio of acyl to free carnitine, ↑ acyl-carnitine, urine organic acid and acylglycines
Electron transport flavoprotein-α*	*α-ETF*	Nonketotic fasting hypoglycemia, congenital anomalies, liver disease, cardiomyopathy, and skeletal myopathy also described	Normal or ↓ free carnitine, increased ratio of acyl to free carnitine, ↑ acyl-carnitine, urine organic acid and acylglycines
Electron transport flavoprotein-β*	*β-ETF*	Fasting hypoglycemia, congenital anomalies, liver disease, cardiomyopathy, and skeletal myopathy also described	Normal or ↓ free carnitine, increased ratio of acyl to free carnitine, ↑ acyl-carnitine, urine organic acid and acylglycines
Short-chain L-3-hydroxyacyl CoA dehydrogenase	*SCHAD*	Hypoglycemia, hyperinsulinemia, cardiomyopathy, myopathy. NB screening diagnosis possible.	Normal or ↓ free carnitine, elevated free fatty acids, inconsistently abnormal urine organic acid and plasma acylcarnitines
Long-chain L-3-hydroxyacyl CoA dehydrogenase	*LCHAD*	NB screening diagnosis possible, maternal preeclampsia, HELLP syndrome, and AFLP association described frequently	Normal or ↓ free carnitine, increased ratio of acyl to free carnitine, ↑ free fatty acids, ↑ C_{16}-OH and C_{18}-OH carnitines
Mitochondrial trifunctional protein	*MTP*	Severe cardiac and skeletal myopathy, hypoglycemia, acidosis, hyper NH_3, sudden death, elevated liver enzymes, retinopathy. Maternal preeclampsia, HELLP syndrome, and AFLP association described frequently.	Normal or ↓ free carnitine, increased ratio of acyl to free carnitine, ↑ free fatty acids, ↑ C_{16}-OH and C_{18}-OH carnitines
Long-chain 3-ketoacyl-CoA thiolase	*LKAT*	Severe neonatal presentation, hypoglycemia, acidosis, ↑ creatine kinase, cardiomyopathy, neuropathy, and early death. Late onset presents with myopathy. Maternal preeclampsia, HELLP syndrome association frequent.	Normal or ↓ free carnitine, increased ratio of acyl to free carnitine, ↑ free fatty acids, ↑ 2-trans, 4-cis decadienoylcarnitine
2,4-Dienoyl-CoA reductase	*DECR1*	Only one patient described, hypotonia in the newborn, mainly severe skeletal myopathy, and respiratory failure. Hypoglycemia rare.	Normal or ↓ free carnitine, ↑ acyl to free carnitine ratio, normal urine organic acids and acylglycines
HMG CoA synthetase	*HMGCS2*	Hypoketosis and hypoglycemia, rarely myopathy	Elevated total plasma fatty acids, enzymes studies in fibroblasts may be diagnostic
HMG CoA lyase	*HMGCL*	Hypoketosis and hypoglycemia, rarely myopathy	Normal free carnitine, ↑ C_5-OH, and methylglutaryl-carnitine, enzymes studies in fibroblasts may be diagnostic

*Also known as glutaric acidemia type II.
HELLP, hemolysis, elevated liver enzymes, low platelets; NB, newborn.
From Shekhawat PS, Matern D, Strauss AW: Fetal fatty oxidation disorders, their effect on maternal health and neonatal outcome: Impact of expanded newborn screening on their diagnosis and management. *Pediatr Res* 2005;57:78R–84R.

DEFECTS IN THE β-OXIDATION CYCLE

MEDIUM-CHAIN ACYL COA DEHYDROGENASE (MCAD) DEFICIENCY. MCAD deficiency is the most common of the fatty acid oxidation disorders. The disorder shows a strong founder effect; most patients have a northwestern European ancestry, and the majority of patients are homozygous for a single common missense mutation, an A–G transition at cDNA position 985 that changes a lysine to glutamic acid at residue 329 (K329E).

Clinical Manifestations. Affected patients usually present in the 1st 3 mo–3 yr of life with episodes of acute illness triggered by prolonged fasting lasting longer than 12–16 hr. Signs and symptoms include vomiting and lethargy, which rapidly progress to coma or seizures and cardiorespiratory collapse. Sudden unexpected infant death may occur. The liver may be slightly enlarged with fat deposition. Attacks are rare until the infant is beyond the 1st few months of life, presumably due to more frequent feedings at a younger age. Affected older infants are at higher risk of illness as they begin to fast through the night or are exposed to fasting stress during an intercurrent childhood illness. Presentation in the 1st days of life has been reported in newborns that were fasted inadvertently before successful breast-feeding. Diagnosis of MCAD has occasionally been documented in previously healthy teenage and adult individuals, indicating that even patients who have been asymptomatic in infancy are still at risk for metabolic decompensation if exposed to sufficient periods of fasting.

Laboratory Findings. During acute episodes, hypoglycemia is usually present. Plasma and urinary ketone concentrations are inappropriately low (**hypoketotic hypoglycemia**). Because of the relative hypoketonemia, there is little or no metabolic acidemia. Tests of liver function are abnormal, with elevations of liver enzymes (ALT, AST), elevated blood ammonia, and prolonged prothrombin (PT) and partial thromboplastin times (PTT). Liver biopsy at times of acute illness shows microvesicular or macrovesicular steatosis due to triglyceride accumulation. During fasting stress or at times of acute illness, urinary organic acid profiles by gas chromatography/mass spectrometry show inappropriately low concentrations of ketones and elevated levels of medium-chain dicarboxylic acids (adipic, suberic, and sebacic acids) that derive from microsomal and peroxisomal omega oxidation of fatty acids. Plasma and tissue concentrations of total carnitine are reduced to 25–50% of normal, and the fraction of total esterified carnitine is increased. This pattern of **secondary carnitine deficiency** is seen in almost all the fatty acid oxidation defects and reflects competition between increased acylcarnitine levels and free carnitine transport at the plasma membrane. Significant exceptions to this rule are the plasma membrane carnitine transporter CPT-IA and β-hydroxy-β-methylglutaryl CoA (HMG CoA) synthase deficiencies.

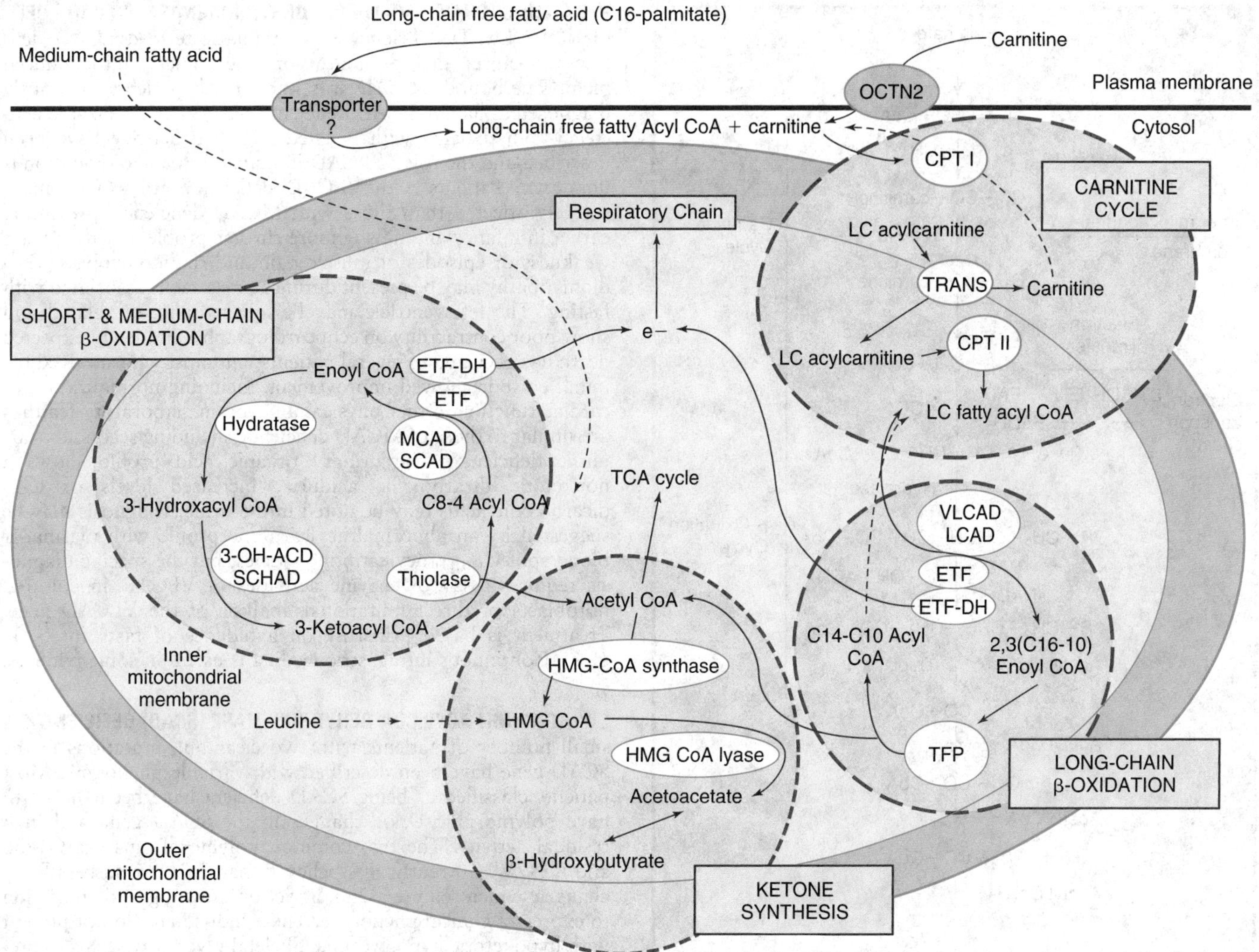

Figure 86-1. Mitochondrial fatty acid oxidation. Carnitine enters the cell through the action of the organic cation/carnitine transporter (OCTN2). Palmitate, a typical 16-carbon long-chain fatty acid, is transported across the plasma membrane and can be activated to form a long-chain (LC) fatty acyl coenzyme A (CoA). It then enters into the carnitine cycle, where it is transesterified by carnitine palmitoyltransferase-I (CPT-I), translocated across the inner mitochondrial membrane by carnitine/acylcarnitine translocase (TRANS), and then reconverted into a long-chain fatty acyl CoA by carnitine palmitoyltransferase-II (CPT-II) to undergo β-oxidation. Very long chain acyl CoA dehydrogenase (VLCAD/LCAD) leads to the production of (C16–10) 2,3 enoyl CoA. Trifunctional protein (TFP) contains the activities of enoyl CoA hydratase (hydratase), 3-OH-hydroxyacyl CoA dehydrogenase (3-OH-ACD), and β-ketothiolase (thiolase). Acetyl CoA, FADH, and NADH are produced. Medium- and short-chain fatty acids (C8–4) can enter the mitochondrial matrix independent of the carnitine cycle. Medium-chain acyl CoA dehydrogenase (MCAD), short-chain acyl CoA dehydrogenase (SCAD), and short-chain hydroxy acyl CoA dehydrogenase (SCHAD) are required. Acetyl CoA can then enter the Krebs (TCA) cycle. Electrons are transported from FADH to the respiratory chain via the electron transfer flavoprotein (ETF) and the electron transfer flavoprotein dehydrogenase (ETF-DH). NADH enters the electron transport chain through complex I. Acetyl CoA can be converted into hydroxymethylglutaryl (HMG) CoA by β-hydroxy-β-methylglutaryl CoA synthase (HMG CoA synthase) and then the ketone body acetoacetate by the action of β-hydroxy-β-methylglutaryl CoA lyase (HMG CoA lyase).

Diagnostic markers include increased plasma $C_{8:0}$, $C_{10:0}$, and $C_{10:1}$ acylcarnitine species and increased urinary acylglycines including hexanoyl-, suberyl- and 3-phenylpropionyl glycines. Newborn screening programs using tandem mass spectrometry can diagnose presymptomatic infants based on the detection of the abnormal acylcarnitines in filter paper blood spots. In many cases, the diagnosis can be confirmed by finding the common A985G mutation. A second common mutation, T199C, has been detected in infants with characteristic acylcarnitines in newborn screening tests. Interestingly, this allele has not been seen to date in symptomatic MCAD patients; it may represent a mild mutation.

Treatment. Acute illnesses should be promptly treated with intravenous fluids containing 10% dextrose to treat or prevent hypoglycemia and to suppress lipolysis as rapidly as possible (see Chapter 92). Chronic therapy consists of avoiding fasting. This usually requires simply adjusting the diet to ensure that overnight fasting periods are limited to <10–12 hr. Restricting dietary fat or treatment with carnitine is controversial. The necessity for active therapeutic intervention for individuals with the T199C mutation has not yet been established.

Prognosis. Up to 25% of unrecognized patients may die during their 1st attack of illness. There is frequently a history of a previous sibling death due to unrecognized MCAD deficiency. Some patients may develop permanent brain injury during an attack of profound hypoglycemia. The prognosis for survivors without brain damage is excellent because muscle weakness or cardiomyopathy does not occur in MCAD deficiency. Fasting tolerance improves with age and the risks of illness decreases. As many as 50% of affected patients have never had an episode; therefore, testing of siblings of affected patients is important to detect asymptomatic family members.

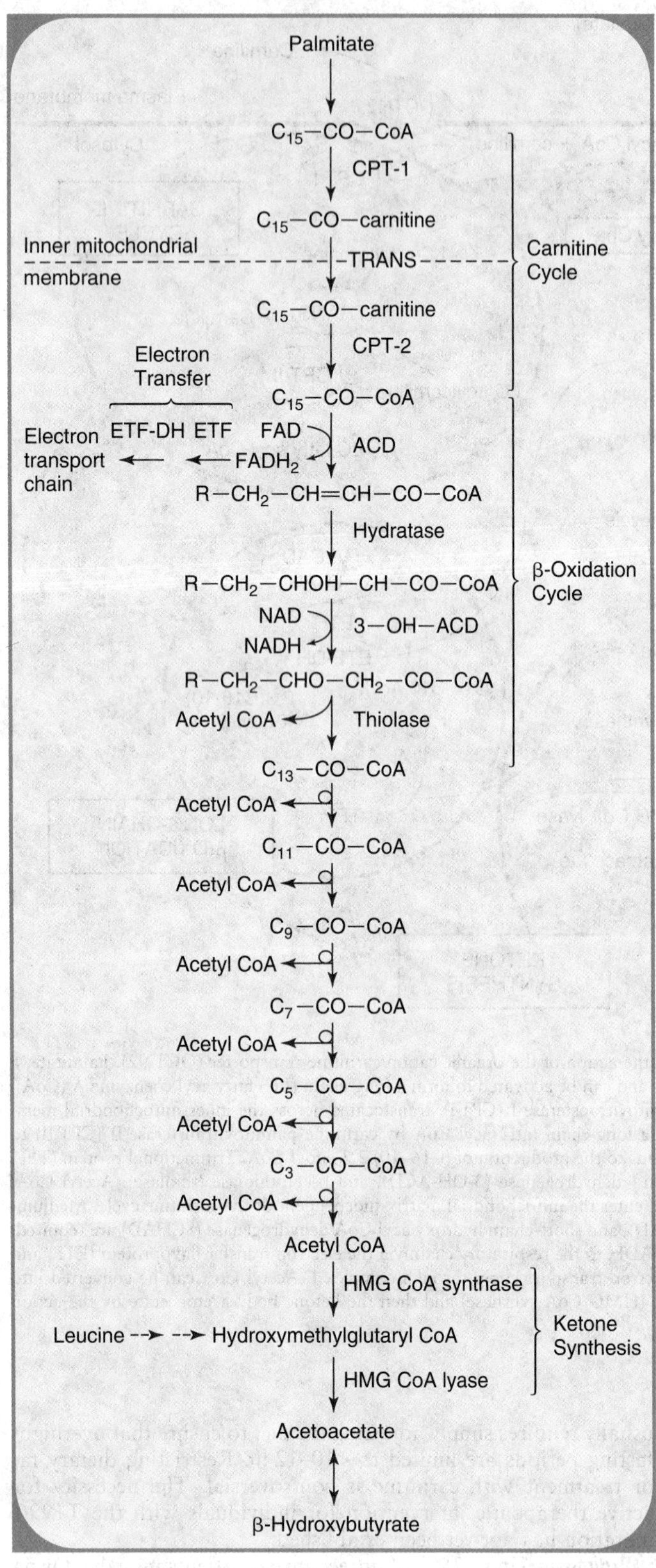

Figure 86-2. Pathway of mitochondrial oxidation of palmitate, a typical 16-carbon long-chain fatty acid. Enzyme steps include carnitine palmitoyltransferase (CPT) 1 and 2, carnitine/acylcarnitine translocase (TRANS), electron transfer flavoprotein (ETF), ETF dehydrogenase (ETF-DH), acyl CoA dehydrogenase (ACD), enoyl CoA hydratase (hydratase), 3-hydroxy-acyl CoA dehydrogenase (3-OH-ACD), β-ketothiolase (thiolase), β-hydroxy-B-methylglutaryl CoA (HMG CoA) synthase, and lyase.

VERY LONG CHAIN ACYL COA DEHYDROGENASE (VLCAD) DEFICIENCY. VLCAD deficiency was originally termed LCAD deficiency before the existence of the inner mitochondrial membrane-bound VLCAD was known. All patients previously diagnosed as having LCAD deficiency have VLCAD enzyme deficiency. No patients with isolated LCAD deficiency have been described and the role of LCAD in human fatty acid oxidation is unknown. Patients with VLCAD deficiency are usually more severely affected than those with MCAD deficiency, presenting earlier in infancy and having more chronic problems with muscle weakness or episodes of muscle pain and rhabdomyolysis. Cardiomyopathy may be present during acute attacks associated with fasting. The left ventricle may be hypertrophic or dilated and show poor contractility on echocardiography. Sudden unexpected death has occurred in several patients, but most who survived the initial episode showed improvement, including normalization of cardiac function. Other physical and routine laboratory features are similar to those of MCAD deficiency, including secondary carnitine deficiency. The urinary organic acid profile shows a nonketotic dicarboxylic aciduria. Increased levels of C_{6-12} dicarboxylic acids may be noted in the urine. Diagnosis may be suggested by an abnormal acylcarnitine profile with plasma or blood spot $C_{14:1,14:0}$ acylcarnitine species, but the specific diagnosis requires assay of enzyme activities of VLCAD in cultured fibroblasts or direct mutational analysis of the VLCAD gene. Treatment is based primarily on avoidance of fasts for >10–12 hr. Continuous intragastric feeding is useful in some patients.

SHORT–CHAIN ACYL COA DEHYDROGENASE (SCAD) DEFICIENCY. A small number of patients with two clear null mutations in the SCAD gene have been described with variable phenotype. Most patients classified as being SCAD deficient have been shown to have polymorphic DNA changes in the SCAD gene and high residual activity. The two common polymorphisms are G185S and R147W. Currently, it is believed that these are susceptibility changes, which require a 2nd, as yet unknown, genetic mutation to express a clinical phenotype. These individuals do not present with hypoketotic hypoglycemia. Skeletal myopathy seems to predominate, but a consistent clinical phenotype has not been identified. Some patients have severe metabolic acidosis. Neurologic signs are present in most patients, although mildly affected individuals may be asymptomatic. Diagnosis is indicated by elevated levels of butyrylcarnitine on blood spots or plasma and increased excretion of urinary ethylmalonic acid and butyrylglycine. These metabolic abnormalities are most pronounced in patients with null mutations and variably present in patients who are homozygous for the polymorphisms. Confirmation of diagnosis requires mutation analysis. Some of the clinical features suggest a toxicity syndrome, perhaps owing to accumulation of short-chain fatty acid metabolites. One reported patient had normal ketogenesis, implying that there is no impairment of longer chain fatty acid oxidation.

Treatment is limitation of fasting stress and dietary fat.

LONG–CHAIN 3–HYDROXYACYL COA DEHYDROGENASE (LCHAD)/MITOCHONDRIAL TRIFUNCTIONAL PROTEIN (TFP) DEFICIENCY. LCHAD deficiency is the second most common of the fatty acid oxidation disorders. The LCHAD enzyme is part of a mitochondrial trifunctional protein (TFP), which also contains two other steps in β-oxidation, long-chain enoyl CoA hydratase and long-chain β-ketothiolase. It is a hetero-octameric protein composed of 4α and 4β chains that derive from distinct contiguous genes with a common promoter region. In some patients, only the LCHAD activity of the TFP is affected (LCHAD deficiency), whereas others have deficiencies of all three activities (TFP deficiency). **Clinical manifestations** include attacks of acute hypoketotic hypoglycemia similar to MCAD deficiency; patients often show evidence of more severe disease, including cardiomyopathy, muscle cramps and weakness, and abnormal liver function (cholestasis). Toxic effects of fatty acid metabolites may produce pigmented retinopathy, progressive liver failure, peripheral neuropathy, and rhabdomyolysis. Life-threatening obstetric complications; acute fatty liver of pregnancy; and hemolysis, elevated liver enzymes, low platelets (HELLP) syndrome are observed in heterozygous mothers carrying homozygotic fetuses affected with LCHAD/TFP deficiency. Sudden unexpected infant death may occur. **Diagnosis** is indicated by elevated levels of blood spot or plasma 3-hydroxy acylcarnitines of chain lengths C_{16}–C_{18}. Urinary organic acid profile in patients may show increases in levels of 3-hydroxydicarboxylic acids of chain lengths C_6–C_{14}. Secondary carnitine deficiency is common. A common mutation in the α subunit, E474Q, is seen in >60% of LCHAD deficient patients. This mutation in the fetus is significantly associated with the obstetric complications, but other mutations in either subunit may also be associated with maternal illness.

Treatment is similar to that for MCAD or LCAD/VLCAD deficiency, that is, avoiding fasting stress. Some investigators have suggested that dietary supplements with medium-chain triglyceride oil and docosahexaenoic acid (DHA) may be useful. Liver transplantation does not ameliorate the metabolic abnormalities.

SHORT-CHAIN 3-HYDROXYACYL-COA DEHYDROGENASE (SCHAD) DEFICIENCY. Very few patients with this inborn error have been described. Only five patients with proven mutations of SCHAD have been reported. Four cases in three families with recessive mutations of SCHAD presented with episodes of hypoketotic hypoglycemia that was shown to be due to hyperinsulinism. In contrast to patients with other forms of fatty acid oxidation disorders, these cases required specific therapy for hyperinsulinism to avoid recurrent hypoglycemia. A 5th child presented with fulminant hepatic failure at age 10 mo and was compound heterozygous for two different SCHAD mutations. Other reports include a child with attacks of fasting hypoglycemia and myoglobinuria associated with deficiency of SCHAD in muscle but not in cultured fibroblasts, three children with fatal liver disease, and an infant who died suddenly and unexpectedly. This variable phenotype may be due to genetic heterogeneity. Specific metabolic markers for SCHAD deficiency have not yet been identified, making this a particularly difficult diagnosis to establish.

DEFECTS IN THE CARNITINE CYCLE

PLASMA MEMBRANE CARNITINE TRANSPORT DEFECT (PRIMARY CARNITINE DEFICIENCY). Primary carnitine deficiency is the only genetic defect in which carnitine deficiency is the cause, rather than the consequence, of impaired fatty acid oxidation. The most common presentation is progressive cardiomyopathy with or without skeletal muscle weakness beginning at 1–4 yr of age. A smaller number of patients may present with fasting hypoketotic hypoglycemia in the 1st yr of life before the cardiomyopathy becomes symptomatic. The underlying defect involves the plasma membrane sodium gradient–dependent carnitine transporter that is present in heart, muscle, and kidney. This transporter is responsible both for maintaining intracellular carnitine concentrations 20- to 50-fold higher than plasma concentrations and for renal conservation of carnitine.

Diagnosis of the carnitine transporter defect is aided by the fact that patients have extremely reduced carnitine levels in plasma and muscle (1–2% of normal). Heterozygote parents have plasma carnitine levels ≈50% of normal. Fasting ketogenesis may be normal because liver carnitine transport is normal, but it may be impaired if dietary carnitine intake is interrupted. The fasting urinary organic acid profile may show a hypoketotic dicarboxylicaciduria pattern if hepatic fatty acid oxidation is impaired, but it is otherwise unremarkable. The defect in carnitine transport can be demonstrated clinically by severe reduction in renal carnitine threshold or in vitro by assay of carnitine uptake using cultured fibroblasts or lymphoblasts. Mutations in the organic cation/carnitine transporter (*OCTN2*) underlie this disorder. **Treatment** of this disorder with pharmacologic doses of oral carnitine (100–200 mg/kg/day) is highly effective in correcting the cardiomyopathy and muscle weakness as well as any impairment in fasting ketogenesis. Muscle total carnitine concentrations remain <5% of normal on treatment.

CARNITINE PALMITOYLTRANSFERASE-IA (CPT-IA) DEFICIENCY. Several dozen infants and children have been described with a deficiency of the liver and kidney isozyme of CPT-IA. **Clinical manifestations** include fasting hypoketotic hypoglycemia, occasionally with markedly abnormal liver function tests and, rarely, with renal tubular acidosis. The heart and skeletal muscle are not involved because the muscle isozyme is unaffected. Fasting urinary organic acid profile shows a hypoketotic C_6–C_{12} dicarboxylicaciduria but may be normal. Plasma acylcarnitine analysis demonstrates mostly free carnitine with very little acylated carnitine. This observation has been used to establish CPT-IA diagnosis on newborn screening by tandem mass spectrometry. CPT-IA deficiency is the only fatty acid oxidation disorder in which plasma total carnitine levels are elevated to 150–200% of normal. This may be explained by the fact that the inhibitory effects of long-chain acylcarnitines on the renal tubular carnitine transporter are absent in CPT-IA deficiency. The enzyme defect can be demonstrated in cultured fibroblasts or lymphoblasts. CPT-IA deficiency in the fetus has been associated with acute fatty liver of pregnancy in the mother in a single case report. **Treatment** is similar to that for MCAD deficiency with avoidance of situations where fasting ketogenesis is necessary.

CARNITINE-ACYLCARNITINE TRANSLOCASE (CACT) DEFICIENCY. This defect of the inner mitochondrial membrane carrier protein for fatty acylcarnitines blocks the entry of long-chain fatty acids into the mitochondria for oxidation. The clinical phenotype of this disorder is characterized by a severe and generalized impairment of fatty acid oxidation. Most newborn patients present with attacks of fasting-induced hypoglycemia, hyperammonemia, and cardiorespiratory collapse. All symptomatic newborns have had evidence of cardiomyopathy and muscle weakness. Several patients with a partial translocase deficiency and milder disease without cardiac involvement have also been identified. No distinctive urinary or plasma organic acids are noted, although increased levels of plasma long-chain acylcarnitines are reported. **Diagnosis** can be made using cultured fibroblasts or lymphoblasts. The human gene has been cloned, and mutations have been identified in affected patients. **Treatment** is similar to that of other fatty acid oxidation disorders.

CARNITINE PALMITOYLTRANSFERASE-II (CPT-II) DEFICIENCY. Three forms of CPT-II deficiency have been described. The antenatal presentation of this disorder is associated with a profound enzyme deficiency, and neonatal death has been reported in several newborns with dysplastic kidneys, cerebral malformations, and mild facial anomalies. A severe deficiency of enzyme activity is associated with an infantile-onset form. This form shares all the clinical and laboratory features of CACT deficiency. A milder defect is associated with an adult presentation of episodic rhabdomyolysis. The 1st episode usually does not occur until late childhood or early adulthood. Attacks may be precipitated by prolonged exercise. There is aching muscle pain and myoglobinuria that may be severe enough to cause renal failure. Serum levels of creatine kinase are elevated to 5,000–100,000 U/L. Fasting hypoglycemia has not been described, but fasting may contribute to attacks of myoglobinuria. Muscle biopsy shows increased deposition of neutral fat. The myopathic presentation of CPT-II deficiency is associated with a common mutation S113L. An intermediate form of CPT-II deficiency presents in infancy/early childhood with fasting-induced hepatic failure, cardiomyopathy, and skeletal myopathy with hypoketotic hypoglycemia but does not have the severe developmental changes seen in the neonatal presentation. This pattern is more like that seen in VLCAD deficiency and management is identical. Patients are generally heterozygous for one of the severe mutations and one of the milder mutations.

Diagnosis of all forms of CPT-II deficiency can be made by demonstrating deficient enzyme activity in muscle or other tissues and in cultured fibroblasts. Mutation analysis is available.

DEFECTS IN ELECTRON TRANSFER PATHWAY

ELECTRON TRANSFER FLAVOPROTEIN (ETF) AND ELECTRON TRANSFER FLAVOPROTEIN DEHYDROGENASE (ETF–DH) DEFICIENCIES (GLUTARIC ACIDURIA TYPE 2, MULTIPLE ACYL COA DEHYDROGENATION DEFICIENCIES). ETF and ETF-DH function to transfer electrons into the mitochondrial electron transport chain from dehydrogenation reactions catalyzed by VLCAD, MCAD, and SCAD, as well as glutaryl CoA dehydrogenase and at least four enzymes involved in branch-chain amino acid oxidation. Deficiencies of ETF or ETF-DH produce illness that combines the features of impaired fatty acid oxidation and impaired oxidation of several amino acids. Complete deficiencies of either protein are associated with severe illness in the newborn period, characterized by acidosis, hypoglycemia, coma, hypotonia, cardiomyopathy, and an unusual odor of sweaty feet due to isovaleryl CoA dehydrogenase inhibition. Some affected neonates have had facial dysmorphia and polycystic kidneys similar to that seen in severe CPT-II deficiency, which suggests that toxic effects of accumulated metabolites may occur in utero.

Diagnosis can be made from the urinary organic acid profile, which shows abnormalities corresponding to blocks in oxidation of fatty acids (ethylmalonate and C_6–C_{10} dicarboxylic acids), lysine (glutarate), and branched-chain amino acids (isovaleryl-, isobutyryl-, and α-methylbutyryl-glycine). Most severely affected infants do not survive the neonatal period.

Partial deficiencies of ETF and ETF-DH produce a disorder that may mimic MCAD deficiency or other milder fatty acid oxidation defects. These patients have attacks of fasting hypoketotic coma. The urinary organic acid profile reveals primarily elevations of dicarboxylic acids and ethylmalonate, derived from short-chain fatty acid intermediates. Secondary carnitine deficiency is present. Some patients with mild forms of ETF/ETF-DH deficiency benefit from treatment with high doses of riboflavin, which is a cofactor for the pathway of electron transfer.

DEFECTS IN KETONE SYNTHESIS PATHWAY

β-HYDROXY-β-METHYLGLUTARYL COA (HMG COA) SYNTHASE DEFICIENCY. HMG CoA synthase is the rate-limiting step in the conversion of acetyl CoA derived from fatty acid β-oxidation in the liver to ketones. Several patients with this defect have recently been identified. The presentation is one of fasting hypoketotic hypoglycemia without evidence of impaired cardiac or skeletal muscle function. Urinary organic acid profile showed only a hypoketotic dicarboxylic aciduria. Plasma and tissue carnitine levels are normal, in contrast to all the other disorders of fatty acid oxidation. A separate synthase enzyme, present in cytosol for cholesterol biosynthesis, is not affected. The HMG CoA synthase defect is expressed only in the liver and cannot be demonstrated in cultured fibroblasts. The gene has been cloned, and mutations in the affected patients have been characterized. Avoiding fasting is usually a successful treatment.

β-HYDROXY-β-METHYLGLUTARYL COA LYASE DEFICIENCY. See Chapter 85.6.

DEFECTS IN KETONE UTILIZATION

The ketones β-hydroxybutyrate and acetoacetate are the end products of hepatic fatty acid oxidation and are important as metabolic fuels for the brain during fasting. Two defects in utilization of ketones in brain and other peripheral tissues present as episodes of "hyperketotic" coma, with or without hypoglycemia.

SUCCINYL-COA:3-KETOACID COA TRANSFERASE (SCOT) DEFICIENCY. Several patients with SCOT deficiency have been reported. Characteristic presentation is an infant with recurrent episodes of severe ketoacidosis induced by fasting. Plasma acylcarnitine and urine organic acid abnormalities do not distinguish from other causes of ketoacidosis. **Treatment** of episodes requires infusion of glucose and large amounts of bicarbonate until metabolically stable. All patients exhibit inappropriate hyperketonemia even between catabolic episodes. SCOT is responsible for activating acetoacetate in peripheral tissues using succinyl CoA as a donor to form acetoacetyl CoA. Deficient activity can be demonstrated in brain, muscle, and fibroblasts from affected patients. The gene has been cloned, and numerous mutations have been characterized.

β-KETOTHIOLASE DEFICIENCY. See Chapter 85.6.

Andresen BS, Dobrowolski SF, O'Reilly L, et al: Medium-chain acyl-CoA dehydrogenase (MCAD) mutations identified by MS/MS-based prospective screening of newborns differ from those observed in patients with clinical symptoms: Identification and characterization of a new, prevalent mutation that results in mild MCAD deficiency. *Am J Hum Genet* 2001;68:1408–1418.

Bonnefont JP, Djouadi F, Prip-Buus C, et al: Carnitine palmitoyltransferases 1 and 2: Biochemical, molecular and medical aspects. *Mol Aspects Med* 2004;25:495–520.

Clayton PT, Eaton S, Aynsley-Green A, et al: Hyperinsulinism in short-chain L-3-hydroxyacyl-CoA dehydrogenase deficiency reveals the importance of beta-oxidation in insulin secretion. *J Clin Invest* 2001;108:457–465.

Den Boer MEJ, Dionisi-Vici C, Chakrapani A, et al: Mitochondrial trifunctional protein deficiency: A severe fatty acid oxidation disorder with cardiac and neurologic involvement. *J Pediatr* 2003;142:s684–s688.

Den Boer MEJ, Wanders RJA, Morris AAM, et al: Long-chain 3-hydroxyacyl-CoA dehydrogenase deficiency: Clinical presentation and follow-up of 50 patients. *Pediatrics* 2002;109:99–104.

Elpeleg ON, Hammerman C, Saada A, et al: Antenatal presentation of carnitine palmitoyltransferase II deficiency. *Am J Med Genet* 2001;102:183–187.

Fukao T, Mitchell GA, Song XQ, et al: Succinyl-CoA:3-ketoacid CoA transferase (SCOT): Cloning of the human SCOT gene, tertiary structural modeling of the human SCOT monomer, and characterization of three pathogenic mutations. *Genomics* 2000;68:144–151.

Gregersen N, Andresen BS, Corydon MJ, et al: Mutation analysis in mitochondrial fatty acid oxidation defects: Exemplified by acyl-CoA dehydrogenase deficiencies, with special focus on genotype-phenotype relationship. *Hum Mutat* 2001;18:169–189.

Klose DA, Kolker S, Heinrich B, et al: Incidence and short-term outcome of children with symptomatic presentation of organic acid and fatty acid oxidation disorders in Germany. *Pediatrics* 2002;110:1204–1210.

Mathur A, Sims HF, Gopalakrishnan D, et al: Molecular heterogeneity in very-long-chain acyl-CoA dehydrogenase deficiency causing pediatric cardiomyopathy and sudden death. *Circulation* 1999;99:1337–1343.

Shekhawat PS, Matern D, Strauss AW: Fetal fatty acid oxidation disorders, their effect on maternal health and neonatal outcome: Impact of expanded newborn screening on their diagnosis and management. *Pediatr Res* 2005;57:78R–86R.

Stanley CA, Bennett MJ, Mayatepek E: Disorders of mitochondrial fatty acid oxidation and related metabolic pathways. *In:* Fernandes J, Saudubray J-M, Van den Bergh G, Walter JH (eds). Inborn Metabolic Diseases: Diagnosis and Treatment 4th edition: Heidelberg: Springer-Verlag, 2006 pp. 175–188.

Wilcken B, Haas M, Joy P, et al: Outcome of neonatal screening for medium-chain acyl-CoA dehydrogenase deficiency in Australia: a cohort study. *Lancet* 2007;369:37–42.

Yang Z, Yamada J, Zhao Y, et al: Prospective screening for pediatric mitochondrial protein defects in pregnancies complicated by liver disease. *JAMA* 2002;288:2163–2166.

86.2 • Disorders of Very Long Chain Fatty Acids • Hugo W. Moser

PEROXISOMAL DISORDERS

The peroxisomal diseases are genetically determined disorders caused either by the failure to form or maintain the peroxisome or by a defect in the function of a single enzyme that is normally located in this organelle. These disorders cause serious disability in childhood and occur more frequently and present a wider range of phenotype than has been recognized in the past.

ETIOLOGY. Peroxisomal disorders are subdivided into two major categories (Table 86-2).

In category A, the **peroxisomal biogenesis disorders (PBD)**, the basic defect is the failure to import one or more proteins into the organelle. In category B, **defects affect a single peroxisomal protein.** The peroxisome is present in all cells except mature erythrocytes and is a subcellular organelle surrounded by a single membrane; >50 peroxisomal enzymes are identified. Some enzymes are involved in the production and decomposition of hydrogen peroxide; others are concerned with lipid and amino acid metabolism. Most peroxisomal enzymes are 1st synthesized in their mature form on free polyribosomes and enter the cytoplasm. Proteins that are destined for the peroxisome contain specific peroxisome targeting sequences (PTS). Most peroxisomal matrix proteins contain PTS1, a 3-amino acid sequence at the carboxyl terminus. PTS2 is an amino-terminal sequence that is critical for the import of enzymes involved in plasmalogen and branched-chain fatty acid metabolism. Import of proteins involves a complex series of reactions that involves at least 23 distinct proteins. These proteins are referred to as peroxins encoded by *PEX* genes. Table 86-3 summarizes the *PEX* genes that are defective in human disease states.

TABLE 86-2. Classification of Peroxisomal Disorders

A: DISORDERS OF PEROXISOME IMPORT
A1: Zellweger syndrome
A2: Neonatal adrenoleukodystrophy
A3: Infantile Refsum disease
A4: Rhizomelic chondrodysplasia punctata
B: DEFECTS OF SINGLE PEROXISOMAL ENZYME
B1: X-linked adrenoleukodystrophy
B2: Acyl CoA oxidase deficiency
B3: Bifunctional enzyme deficiency
B4: Peroxisomal thiolase deficiency
B5: Classic Refsum disease
B6: 2-Methylacyl CoA racemase deficiency
B7: DHAP acyltransferase deficiency
B8: Alkyl-DHAP synthase deficiency
B9: Mevalonic aciduria
B10: Glutaric aciduria type III
B11: Hyperoxaluria type I
B12: Acatalasemia

EPIDEMIOLOGY. Except for X-linked adrenoleukodystrophy (X-ALD), all the peroxisomal disorders in Table 86-2 are autosomal recessive traits. X-ALD is the most common peroxisomal disorder, with an estimated incidence of 1/17,000. The combined incidence of the other peroxisomal disorders is estimated to be 1/50,000.

PATHOLOGY. Absence or reduction in the number of peroxisomes is pathognomonic for disorders of peroxisome biogenesis. In most disorders, there are membranous sacs that contain peroxisomal integral membrane proteins, which lack the normal complement of matrix proteins; these are peroxisome "ghosts." Pathologic changes are observed in many organs and include profound and characteristic defects in neuronal migration; micronodular cir-

TABLE 86-3. Peroxisome Biogenesis Factors (PEX) and Their Alterations in Human Peroxisomal Biogenesis Disorders (PBD)

		COMPLEMENTATION GROUP			NO. PATIENTS STUDIED AT KKI		
PEROXIN#	CHARACTERISTIC	KKI	JAPAN	AMS	KKI	PHENOTYPE	CHROMOSOME
1	143-kd AAA ATPase	1	E	2	99	ZS, NALD, IRD	7q21-22
2	C_3HC_4 zinc binding integral peroxisomal membrane protein 35–52 kd	10	F	5	2	ZS	
3	51–52 kd Integral peroxisomal membrane protein						
4	21–24 kd Peroxisomal associated ubiquitin-conjugating enzyme						
5	PTS 1 receptor	2		4	2	ZS, NALD	12p13.3
6	12–127 kd AAA ATPase	4	C	3	16	ZS, NALD	6p21.1
7	PTS 2 receptor	11		1	43	RCDP	6q22-24
8	71–81 kd Peroxisomal associated protein						
9	42-kd Integral peroxisomal membrane protein						
10	C_3HC_4 zine-binding integral peroxisomal membrane protein	7	B		5	ZS, NALSD	8q21.1
11	27–32 kd Peroxisomal membrane protein involved in peroxisomal proliferation						
12	48-kd C_3HC_4 zinc binding integral peroxisomal membrane protein	3			6	ZS, NALSD, IRD	
13	SH-3 containing 40–43 kd peroxisomal integral peroxisomal membrane protein		H		2	ZS, NALSD	
14	41-kd Integral membrane protein						
15	48-kd Cytosolic protein						
16	39-kd Peripheral peroxisomal membrane protein	9	D		1	ZS	
17	27–30 kd Peroxisomal? intrinsic membrane protein						
18	35–39 kd Peroxisomal membrane protein zinc finger motif						
19	Peroxisomal membrane protein, prenylated		J			ZS	
		8	A		7	ZS, NALSD, IRD	
			G			ZS	
26	? Docking factor for Pex1p and Pex6p						

Ams, Amsterdam; KKI, Kennedy Krieger Institute.
From Moser HW: Genotype-phenotype correlations in disorders of peroxisome biogenesis. *Mol Genet Metab* 1999;68:316.

TABLE 86-4. Abnormal Laboratory Findings Common to Disorders of Peroxisome Biogenesis

Peroxisomes absent to reduced in number
Catalase in cytosol
Deficient synthesis and reduced tissue levels of plasmalogens
Defective oxidation and abnormal accumulation of very long chain fatty acids
Deficient oxidation and age-dependent accumulation of phytanic acid
Defects in certain steps of bile acid formation and accumulation of bile acid intermediates
Defects in oxidation and accumulation of L-pipecolic acid
Increased urinary excretion of dicarboxylic acids

rhosis of the liver; renal cysts; chondrodysplasia punctata; corneal clouding, congenital cataracts, glaucoma, and retinopathy; congenital heart disease; and dysmorphic features.

PATHOGENESIS. It is likely that all pathologic changes are secondary to the peroxisome defect. Multiple peroxisomal enzymes fail to function in the PBD (Table 86-4). The enzymes that are diminished or absent are synthesized but are degraded abnormally fast because they may be unprotected outside of the peroxisome. It is not clear how defective peroxisome functions lead to the widespread pathologic manifestations.

The PBD are associated with genetically determined import defects. The PBD have been subdivided into 12 complementation groups. The molecular defects have been defined in 10 of these groups (see Table 86-3). The pattern and severity of pathologic features vary with the nature of the import defects and the degree to which import is impaired. These gene defects lead to disorders that were named before their relationship to the peroxisome was recognized, namely, Zellweger syndrome (ZS), neonatal adrenoleukodystrophy (NALD), infantile Refsum disease (IRD), and rhizomelic chondrodysplasia punctata (RCDP). The 1st three disorders are now considered to form a clinical continuum, with ZS the most severe, IRD the least severe, and NALD intermediate. They can be caused by 11 different gene defects, which involve mainly the import of proteins that contain the PTS1 targeting signal; the gene defects cannot be distinguished on the basis of clinical features. The clinical severity varies with the degree to which protein import is impaired. Mutations that abolish import completely are often associated with the ZS phenotype, whereas a missense mutation, in which some degree of import function is retained, leads to the somewhat milder phenotypes. A defect in *PEX7*, which involves the import of proteins that utilize PTS2, is associated with RCDP. *PEX7* defects that leave import partially intact are associated with milder phenotypes, some of which resemble classic Refsum disease.

The genetic disorders that involve single peroxisomal enzymes usually have clinical manifestations that are more restricted and present subsequent to the neonatal period and not infrequently in adolescents or adults. The clinical manifestations may be related to the biochemical defect. The primary adrenal insufficiency of X-ALD is caused by accumulation of very long chain fatty acids (VLCFA) in the adrenal cortex, and the peripheral neuropathy in Refsum disease is caused by the accumulation of phytanic acid in Schwann cells and myelin.

PBD with Milder or Atypical Phenotypes. Newborn infants with **Zellweger syndrome** show striking and consistent, recognizable abnormalities. Of central diagnostic importance are the typical facial appearance (high forehead, unslanting palpebral fissures, hypoplastic supraorbital ridges, and epicanthal folds; Fig. 86-3), severe weakness and hypotonia, neonatal seizures, and eye abnormalities (cataracts, glaucoma, corneal clouding, Brushfield spots, pigmentary retinopathy, and nerve dysplasia). Because of the hypotonia and "mongoloid" appearance, Down syndrome may be suspected. Infants with Zellweger syndrome rarely live more than a few months. More than 90% show postnatal growth failure. Table 86-5 lists the main clinical abnormalities.

Patients with **neonatal ALD** show fewer and, occasionally, no dysmorphic features. Neonatal seizures occur frequently. Some degree of psychomotor development is present; function remains in the severely or profoundly retarded range, and development may regress after 3–5 yr of age, probably from a progressive leukodystrophy. Several patients are now in a stable, albeit disabled, state in their 3rd or 4th decade. Hepatomegaly, impaired liver function, pigmentary degeneration of the retina, and severely impaired hearing are invariably present. Adrenocortical function is usually impaired, but overt Addison disease is rare. Chondrodysplasia punctata and renal cysts are absent.

Patients with **infantile Refsum disease** have survived to the 2nd decade or longer. They are able to walk, although gait may be ataxic and broad based. Cognitive function is in the severely retarded range. All have sensorineural hearing loss and pigmentary degeneration of the retina. They have moderately dysmorphic features that may include epicanthal folds, a flat bridge of the nose, and low-set ears. Early hypotonia and hepatomegaly with impaired function are common. Levels of plasma cholesterol and high- and low-density lipoprotein are often moderately reduced. Chondrodysplasia punctata and renal cortical cysts are absent. Postmortem study in infantile Refsum disease reveals micronodular liver cirrhosis and small hypoplastic adrenals. The brain shows no malformations, except for severe hypoplasia of the cerebellar granule layer and ectopic locations of the Purkinje cells in the molecular layer. The mode of inheritance is autosomal recessive.

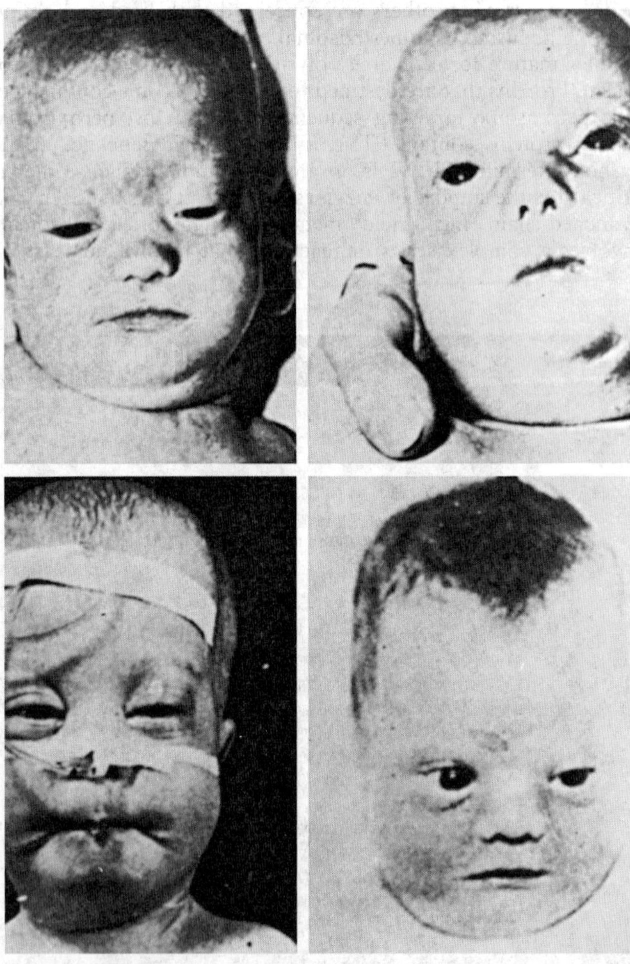

Figure 86-3. Four patients with Zellweger cerebrohepatorenal syndrome. Note the high forehead, epicanthal folds, and hypoplasia of supraorbital ridges and midface. (Courtesy of Hans Zellweger, MD)

TABLE 86-5. Main Clinical Abnormalities in Zellweger Syndrome

	CASE IN WHICH INFORMATION ABOUT THE FEATURE WAS AVAILABLE		CASES IN WHICH THE FEATURE WAS PRESENT	
ABNORMAL FEATURE	NO.	%	NO.	%
High forehead	60	53	58	97
Flat occiput	16	14	13	81
Large fontanelle(s), wide sutures	57	50	55	96
Shallow orbital ridges	33	29	33	100
Low/broad nasal bridge	23	20	23	100
Epicanthus	36	32	33	92
High arched palate	37	32	35	95
External ear deformity	40	35	39	97
Micrognathia	18	16	18	100
Redundant skinfold of neck	13	11	13	100
Brushfield spots	6	5	5	83
Cataract/cloudy cornea	35	31	30	86
Glaucoma	12	11	7	58
Abnormal retinal pigmentation	15	13	6	40
Optic disc pallor	23	20	17	74
Severe hypotonia	95	83	94	99
Abnormal Moro response	26	23	26	100
Hyporeflexia or areflexia	57	50	56	98
Poor sucking	77	68	74	96
Gavage feeding	26	23	26	100
Epileptic seizures	61	54	56	92
Psychomotor retardation	45	39	45	100
Impaired hearing	21	18	9	40
Nystagmus	37	32	30	81

From Heymans HAS: Cerebro-hepato-renal (Zellweger) syndrome: Clinical and biochemical consequences of peroxisomal dysfunctions. Thesis, University of Amsterdam, 1984.

Some patients with PBD disorders have milder and atypical phenotypes. They may present with peripheral neuropathy or with retinopathy, impaired vision, or cataracts in childhood, adolescence, or adulthood and have been diagnosed to have Charcot-Marie-Tooth disease or Usher syndrome. Some patients have survived to the 5th decade. Defects in *PEX7,* which most commonly lead to the RCDP phenotype, may also lead to a milder phenotype with clinical manifestations similar to those of classical Refsum disease (phytanoyl CoA hydroxylase deficiency).

Rhizomelic Chondrodysplasia Punctata (RCDP). This disorder is characterized by the presence of stippled foci of calcification within the hyaline cartilage and is associated with dwarfing, cataracts (72%), and multiple malformations due to contractures. Vertebral bodies have a coronal cleft filled by cartilage that is a result of an embryonic arrest. Disproportionate short stature affects the proximal parts of the extremities (Fig. 86-4*A*). Radiologic abnormalities consist of shortening of the proximal limb bones, metaphyseal cupping, and disturbed ossification (Fig. 86-4*B*). Height, weight, and head circumference are less than the 3rd percentile, and these children are severely retarded mentally. Skin changes such as those observed in ichthyosiform erythroderma are present in ≈25% of patients.

Isolated Defects of Peroxisomal Fatty Acid Oxidation. The disorders labeled B1 through B3 (see Table 86-2) each involve one of three enzymes involved in peroxisomal fatty acid oxidation. Their clinical manifestations resemble those of the Zellweger syndrome/neonatal ALD/infantile Refsum disease continuum; they can be distinguished from disorders of peroxisome biogenesis by laboratory tests. Defects of bifunctional enzyme are common and are found in ≈15% of patients with the Zellweger syndrome/neonatal ALD/infantile Refsum disease phenotype. Patients with isolated acyl CoA oxidase deficiency have a somewhat milder phenotype that resembles that of neonatal ALD.

Isolated Defects of Plasmalogen Synthesis. Plasmalogens are lipids in which the 1st carbon of glycerol is linked to an alcohol rather than a fatty acid. They are synthesized through a complex series of reactions, the 1st two steps of which are catalyzed by the peroxisomal enzymes dihydroxyacetone phosphate alkyl transferase and synthase. Deficiency of either of these enzymes (B4 and B5 in Table 86-2) leads to a phenotype that is clinically indistinguishable from the peroxisomal import disorder RCDP. This latter disorder is caused by a defect in *PEX7,* the receptor for peroxisome targeting sequence 2. It shares the severe deficiency of plasmalogens with disorders B4 and B5 but, in addi-

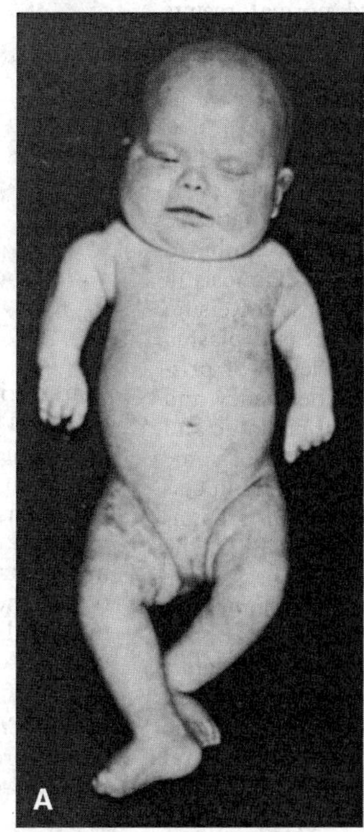

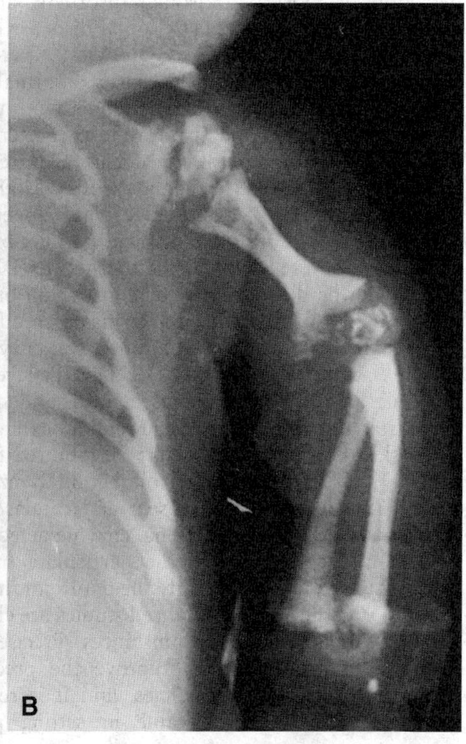

Figure 86-4. *A,* Newborn infant with rhizomelic chondrodysplasia punctata (RCDP). Note the severe shortening of the proximal limbs, the depressed bridge of the nose, hyperlorism, and widespread scaling skin lesions. *B,* Note the marked shortening of the humerus and epiphyseal stippling at the shoulder and elbow joints. (Courtesy of John P. Dorst, MD)

tion, has defects of phytanic oxidation. The fact that disorders B4 and B5 are associated with the full phenotype of RCDP suggests that a deficiency of plasmalogens is sufficient to produce it.

Classic Refsum Disease. The defective enzyme (phytanoyl CoA oxidase) is localized to the peroxisome. The manifestation of classic Refsum disease includes impaired vision from retinitis pigmentosa, ichthyosis, peripheral neuropathy, ataxia, and, occasionally, cardiac arrhythmias. In contrast to infantile Refsum disease, cognitive function is normal and there are no congenital malformations. Classic Refsum disease often does not manifest until young adulthood, but visual disturbances such as night blindness, ichthyosis, and peripheral neuropathy may already be present in childhood and adolescence. Early diagnosis is important because institution of a phytanic acid–restricted diet can reverse the peripheral neuropathy and prevent the progression of the visual and central nervous system manifestations. The classical Refsum disease phenotype may also be caused by defects in *PEX7*.

2-Methylacyl CoA Racemase Deficiency. This disorder is caused by an enzyme defect that leads to the accumulation of the branched-chain fatty acids (phytanic and pristanic acid) and bile acids. Patients present with adult-type peripheral neuropathy and may also have pigmentary degeneration of the retina.

LABORATORY FINDINGS. Laboratory tests for peroxisomal disorders can be viewed at three levels of complexity.

Level 1: Does the Patient Have a Peroxisomal Disorder? This can be resolved by noninvasive tests that are generally available (Table 86-6). Measurement of plasma VLCFA is the most commonly used assay. Whereas plasma VLCFA levels are elevated in many patients with peroxisomal disorders, this is not always the case. The most important exceptions are RCDP, in which VLCFA levels are normal, but plasma phytanic acid levels are increased and red blood cell plasmalogen levels are reduced. In some other peroxisomal disorders, the biochemical abnormalities are still more restricted. Therefore, a panel of tests is recommended and includes plasma levels of VLCFA and of phytanic, pristanic, and pipecolic acids and levels of plasmalogens in red blood cells. Tandem mass spectrometry techniques also permit convenient quantitation of bile acids in plasma and urine. This panel of tests can be performed on 2 mL samples of venous blood and permits detection of most peroxisomal disorders, and normal results make the presence of a peroxisomal disorder unlikely.

Level 2: What Is the Precise Nature of the Peroxisomal Disorder? Table 86-6 lists the main biochemical abnormalities in the various peroxisomal disorders. When combined with the clinical presentation, the just mentioned panel of tests is often sufficient to identify the precise nature of the defect. Elevated plasma VLCFA levels permit the precise diagnosis of X-ALD in male patients. Marked reduction of erythrocyte plasmalogen levels combined with elevated plasma phytanic acid permits precise diagnosis in a patient with the clinical features of RCDP. Classic Refsum disease can be diagnosed by demonstration of increased plasma phytanic acid combined with normal or reduced levels of pristanic acid levels, while in D-bifunctional enzyme deficiency and 2-methylacyl CoA racemase deficiency, the levels of pristanic and phytanic acid are both increased. Precise identification of some peroxisomal disorders may require more extensive studies in cultured skin fibroblasts. This may be required for the differentiation of PBD from defects in bifunctional enzyme. In PBD, the patient's peroxisomes are absent and catalase is in the soluble fraction, whereas in bifunctional enzyme defect, peroxisomes are present and catalase is in the particulate fraction. Fibroblast studies are required to identify the nature of the molecular defect in PBD. Whether such specialized studies are clinically warranted depends on individual circumstances. Precise definition of the defect in a proband may improve the precision of prenatal diagnosis in at-risk pregnancies, and it is required for carrier detection. It is also of value in setting prognosis. Precise characterization is of prognostic value in patients with *PEX1* defects. This defect is present in ≈60% of PBD patients, and about half of the *PEX1* defects have the G843D allele, which is associated with a significantly milder phenotype than is found in other mutations.

TABLE 86-6. Peroxisomal Disorders That Involve Fatty Acid Oxidation: Diagnostic Assays

DISEASE	ASSAY		FINDING
Zellweger syndrome	Plasma	VLCFA	Increased
Neonatal adrenoleukodystrophy		Phytanic acid	Age-dependent increase
Infantile Refsum disease		Pristanic acid	Age-dependent increase
		Pipecolic acid	Increased
		Bile acid	Increased, abnormal pattern
	RBCs,	Plasmalogen levels	Variably decreased
	Fibroblasts	VLCFA levels	Increased
		VLCFA oxidation	Decreased
		Plasmalogen synthesis	Decreased
		Phytanic, pristanic oxidation	Decreased
		Catalase localization	Cytosolic
		Immunocytochemistry	Peroxisomes absent
		Complementation	See Table 86-1
		DNA	See Table 86-1
Rhizomelic chondrodysplasia punctata	Plasma	Phytanic acid	Increased
		VLCFA	Normal
	RBCs	Plasmalogen levels	Decreased
	Fibroblasts	Plasmalogen synthesis	Decreased
		Phytanic acid oxidation	Decreased
		DNA	*PEX7* defect
X-linked ALD hemizygote	Plasma	VLCFA	Increased
	Fibroblasts	VLCFA levels	Increased
		VLCFA oxidation	Decreased
		ALDP immunoreactivity	Absent 70%
		DNA	*ABCD1* mutation
X-linked ALD heterozygote	Plasma	VLCFA	Variable increase in 85%
	Fibroblasts	VLCFA levels	Variable increase in 90%
		ALDP immunoreactivity	Variable decrease
		DNA	*ABCD1* mutation
Bifunctional enzyme defect	Plasma	VLCFA	Increased
		Phytanic acid	Increased
		Pristanic acid	Increased
		Bile acids	Increased, abnormal pattern
	Fibroblasts	VLCFA levels	Increased
		Pristanic acid oxidation	Decreased
		Catalase localization	Peroxisomal
		Enzyme	D-bifunctional protein deficiency
Acyl CoA oxidase deficiency	Plasma	VLCFA	Increased
	Fibroblasts	VLCFA levels	Increased
		VLCFA oxidation	Decreased
		Enzyme	Acyl CoA oxidase defect
2-Methyl acyl CoA racemase deficiency	Plasma	Pristanic acid	Increased
		Bile acids	Increased, abnormal pattern
	Fibroblasts	Pristanic acid oxidation	Decreased
		Enzyme	2-Methyl acyl CoA oxidase defect
Classic Refsum disease	Plasma	Phytanic acid	Increased
		Pristanic acid	Decreased
	Fibroblasts	Enzyme	Phytanoyl CoA deficiency

ALD, adrenoleukodystrophy; VLCFA, very long chain fatty acids.

Level 3: What Is the Molecular Defect? Table 86-3 shows that the molecular defects in most of the PBD have been defined. Definition of the molecular defect in the proband, which is now offered in several laboratories, is essential for carrier detection and speeds prenatal diagnosis.

DIAGNOSIS. There are several noninvasive laboratory tests that permit precise and early diagnosis of peroxisomal disorders (see Table 86-6). The challenge in PBD is to differentiate them from the large variety of other conditions that can cause hypotonia, seizures, failure to thrive, or dysmorphic features. Experienced clinicians can readily recognize classic Zellweger syndrome by its clinical manifestations. PBD patients often do not show the full clinical spectrum of disease and may be identifiable only by laboratory assays. Clinical features that may serve as indications for these diagnostic assays include severe psychomotor retardation; weakness and hypotonia; dysmorphic features; neonatal seizures; retinopathy, glaucoma, or cataracts; hearing deficits; enlarged liver and impaired liver function; and chondrodysplasia punctata. The presence of one or more of these abnormalities increases the likelihood of this diagnosis. Atypical milder forms presenting as peripheral neuropathy have also been described.

Some patients with the isolated defects of peroxisomal fatty acid oxidation (group B) resemble those with group A disorders and can be detected by the demonstration of abnormally high levels of VLCFA.

Patients with RCDP must be distinguished from patients with other causes of chondrodysplasia punctata. In addition to warfarin embryopathy and Zellweger syndrome, these disorders include the milder autosomal dominant form of chondrodysplasia punctata (Conradi-Hunermann syndrome), which is characterized by longer survival, absence of severe limb shortening, and usually intact intellect; an X-linked dominant form; and an X-linked recessive form associated with a deletion of the terminal portion of the short arm of the X chromosome. RCDP is suspected clinically because of the shortness of limbs, psychomotor retardation, and ichthyosis. The most decisive laboratory test is the demonstration of abnormally low plasmalogen levels in red blood cells and an impaired capacity to synthesize plasmalogens in cultured skin fibroblasts. These biochemical defects are not present in other types of chondrodysplasia punctata. Chondrodysplasia punctata may also be associated with a defect of 3β-hydroxysteroid-Δ^8,Δ^7-isomerase, an enzyme involved in biosynthesis of cholesterol.

COMPLICATIONS. Patients with Zellweger cerebrohepatorenal syndrome have multiple disabilities involving muscle tone, swallowing, cardiac abnormalities, liver disease, and seizures. These conditions are treated symptomatically, but the prognosis is poor, and most patients succumb in the 1st few months of life. Patients with RCDP may develop quadriparesis owing to compression at the base of the brain.

PREVENTION. See Chapters 83 and 84.

TREATMENT. The most effective therapy is the dietary treatment of classic Refsum disease with a phytanic acid–restricted diet.

For patients with the somewhat milder variants of the peroxisome import disorders, considerable success has been achieved with multidisciplinary early intervention, including physical and occupational therapy, hearing aids, alternative communication, nutrition, and support for the parents. Although most patients continue to function in the profoundly or severely retarded range, some make significant gains in self-help skills, and several are in stable condition in their teens or even early 20s.

Studies to mitigate some of the secondary biochemical abnormalities include the oral administration of docosahexaenoic acid in a dosage of 50–100 mg/24 hr either as the ethyl ester or in the form of a triglyceride in which one of the fatty acids has been replaced by docosahexaenoic acid. This therapy normalizes the plasma and erythrocyte levels of this substance, which has important physiologic functions in retina and brain, but the levels of which are reduced greatly in patients with disorders of peroxisome biogenesis because the last step of its synthesis takes place in the peroxisome. There are anecdotal reports of clinical improvement. The oral administration of cholic acid and chenodeoxycholic acid in a dosage of 100–250 mg/24 hr, with the aim of reducing the levels of presumably toxic bile acid intermediates, may be effective.

GENETIC COUNSELING. All the peroxisomal disorders, except hyperoxaluria type 1, can be diagnosed prenatally in the 1st or 2nd trimester. The tests are similar to those described for postnatal diagnosis (see Table 86-6) and use chorionic villus sampling or amniocytes. More than 300 pregnancies have been monitored, and more than 60 affected fetuses have been identified without diagnostic error. Because of the 25% recurrence risk, couples with an affected child must be advised about the availability of prenatal diagnosis. Heterozygotes can be identified in X-ALD and in those disorders in which the molecular defect has been identified (see Table 86-3).

ADRENOLEUKODYSTROPHY (X-LINKED)

X-ALD is a genetically determined disorder associated with the accumulation of saturated VLCFA and a progressive dysfunction of the adrenal cortex and central and peripheral nervous system white matter.

ETIOLOGY. The key biochemical abnormality is the tissue accumulation of unbranched saturated VLCFA, with a carbon chain length of 24 or more. Excess hexacosanoic acid (C26:0) is the most striking and characteristic feature. This accumulation of fatty acids is caused by genetically deficient peroxisomal degradation of fatty acid. The key biochemical defect involves the impaired function of peroxisomal lignoceroyl CoA ligase, the enzyme that catalyzes the formation of the CoA derivative of VLCFA. The gene that is defective (*ABCD1*) codes for a peroxisomal membrane (ALDP). More than 400 distinct mutations have been identified, and most families have a mutation that is "private" (unique to that kindred) and are updated on the website http://www.x-ald.nl. The gene has been mapped to chromosome Xq28. The mechanism by which the ALDP defect leads to VLCFA accumulation and the pathology of X-ALD is unknown.

EPIDEMIOLOGY. The minimum incidence of X-ALD in males is 1/21,000, and the combined incidence of X-ALD males and heterozygous females in the general population is estimated to be 1/17,000. All races are affected. The various phenotypes often occur in members of the same kindred.

PATHOLOGY. Characteristic lamellar cytoplasmic inclusions can be demonstrated with the electron microscope in adrenocortical cells, testicular Leydig cells, and nervous system macrophages. These inclusions probably consist of cholesterol esterified with VLCFA. They are most prominent in cells of the zona fasciculata of the adrenal cortex, which at 1st are distended with lipid and later atrophy.

The nervous system can display two types of lesions. In the severe childhood cerebral form and in the rapidly progressive adult forms, demyelination is associated with an inflammatory response manifested by the accumulation of perivascular lymphocytes that is most intense in the parieto-occipital region. In the slowly progressive adult form, adrenomyeloneuropathy (AMN), the main finding is a distal axonopathy that affects the long tracts in the spinal cord. The inflammatory response is mild or absent.

PATHOGENESIS. The adrenal dysfunction is probably a direct consequence of the accumulation of VLCFA. The cells in the zona fasciculata are distended with abnormal lipids. Cholesterol esterified with VLCFA is relatively resistant to adrenocorticotropic hormone (ACTH)–stimulated cholesterol ester hydrolases, and this limits the capacity to convert cholesterol to active steroids. In addition, C26:0 excess increases the viscosity of the plasma membrane and this may interfere with receptor and other cellular functions.

There is no correlation between the neurologic phenotype and the nature of the mutation or the severity of the biochemical defect as assessed by plasma levels of VLCFA or between the degree of adrenal involvement and nervous system involvement. The severity of the illness and rate of progression correlate with the intensity of the inflammatory response. The inflammatory response may be cytokine mediated and may involve an autoimmune response triggered in an unknown way by the excess of VLCFA. A CD1 lipid antigen has been implicated. Mitochondrial damage and oxidative stress also contribute. Approximately half of the patients do not experience the inflammatory response. A modifier gene that sets the "thermostat" for the inflammatory response is postulated.

CLINICAL MANIFESTATIONS. There are five relatively distinct phenotypes, three of which present in childhood with symptoms and signs. In all the phenotypes, development is usually normal in the 1st 3–4 yr.

In the **childhood cerebral form** of ALD, symptoms are 1st noted most commonly between the ages of 4 and 8 yr (21 months is the earliest onset reported). The most common initial manifestations are hyperactivity, which is often mistaken for an attention deficit disorder, and worsening school performance in a child who had previously been a good student. **Auditory discrimination** is often impaired, although tone perception is preserved. This may be evidenced by difficulty in using the telephone and greatly impaired performance on intelligence tests in items that are presented verbally. Spatial orientation is often impaired. Other initial symptoms are disturbances of vision, ataxia, poor handwriting, seizures, and strabismus. Visual disturbances are often due to involvement of the cerebral cortex, which leads to variable and seemingly inconsistent visual capacity. **Seizures** occur in nearly all patients and may represent the 1st manifestation of the disease. Some patients present with increased intracranial pressure or with unilateral mass lesions. Impaired cortisol response to ACTH stimulation is present in 85% of patients, and mild hyperpigmentation is noted. In most patients with this phenotype, however, adrenal dysfunction is recognized only after the condition is diagnosed because of the cerebral symptoms. Cerebral childhood ALD tends to progress rapidly with increasing spasticity and paralysis, visual and hearing loss, and loss of ability to speak or swallow. The mean interval between the 1st neurologic symptom and an apparently vegetative state is 1.9 yr. Patients may continue in this apparently vegetative state for 10 yr or more.

Adolescent ALD designates patients who experience neurologic symptoms between the ages of 10 and 21 yr. The manifestations resemble those of childhood cerebral ALD except that progression is slower.

About 10% of patients present acutely with status epilepticus, adrenal crisis, acute encephalopathy, or coma.

Adrenomyeloneuropathy 1st manifests in late adolescence or adulthood as a progressive paraparesis caused by long tract degeneration in the spinal cord. Approximately half of the patients also have involvement of the cerebral white matter.

The **"Addison only"** phenotype is an important and underdiagnosed condition. Of male patients with Addison disease, 25% may have the biochemical defect of ALD. Many of these patients have intact neurologic systems, whereas others have subtle neurologic signs. Many acquire adrenomyeloneuropathy in adulthood.

The term "asymptomatic ALD" is applied to persons who have the biochemical defect of ALD but are free of neurologic or endocrine disturbances. Nearly all persons with the gene defect eventually become neurologically symptomatic. A few have remained asymptomatic even in the 6th or 7th decade.

Approximately 50% of female heterozygotes acquire a syndrome that resembles adrenomyeloneuropathy but is milder and of later onset. Adrenal insufficiency is rare.

LABORATORY AND RADIOGRAPHIC FINDINGS. The most specific and important laboratory finding is the demonstration of abnormally high levels of VLCFA in plasma, red blood cells, or cultured skin fibroblasts. The test should be performed in a laboratory that has experience with this specialized procedure. Positive results are obtained in all male patients with X-ALD and in ≈85% of female carriers of X-ALD. Mutation analysis is the most reliable method for the identification of carriers.

CT and MRI. Patients with childhood cerebral or adolescent ALD show cerebral white matter lesions that are characteristic with respect to location and attenuation patterns on MRI. In 80% of patients, the lesions are symmetric and involve the periventricular white matter in the posterior parietal and occipital lobes. About 50% show location of a garland of accumulated contrast material adjacent and anterior to the posterior hypodense lesions (Fig. 86-5*A*). This zone corresponds to the zones of

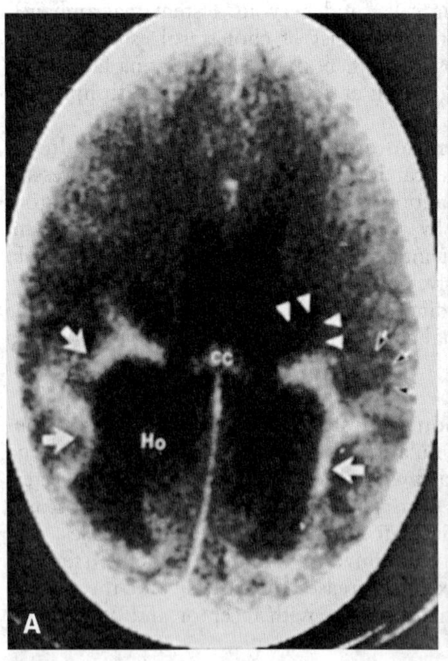

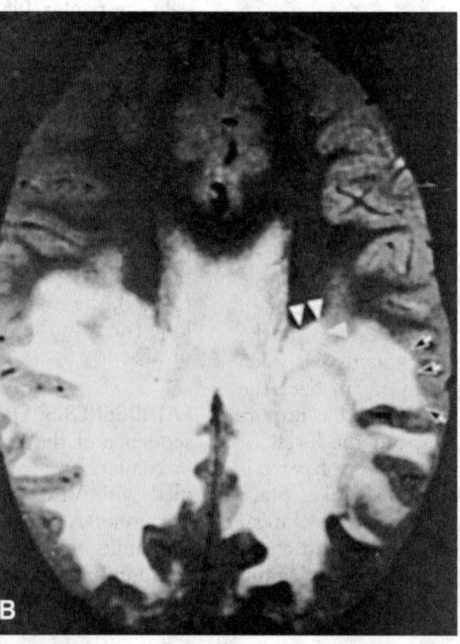

Figure 86-5. *A,* Contrast enhanced CT abnormalities in adrenoleukodystrophy (ALD) with typical parieto-occipital location, showing symmetric bilateral hypodense inactive zones (HO). The enhancing active periphery zone of hypodensity is demarcated by *arrows.* Compare the anterior zone of hypodensity *(arrowheads)* with that on the MRI in *B.* CC, corpus callosum. *B,* MRI of the same pattern and area shown by CT. MRI T2 weighted image shows a high-intensity signal of the abnormally bright parieto-occipital white matter. Subcortical involvement is better identified on MRI. Separation of active zones may be better appreciated by CT, because both inactive and active zones are seen at high-signal areas on MRI. It is assumed, however, that such major distinctions afforded by CT will also be demonstrable when IV enhancement (paramagnetic enhancement) becomes readily available. Note the hypodense involvement of CT (*arrowheads* and *arrows* in *A*) compared with the well-resolved lesions on MRI in *B.* (From Kumar AJ, Rosenbaum WE, Naidu S, et al: Adrenoleukodystrophy: Corresponding MR imaging with CT. *Radiology* 1987;165:497–504.)

intense perivascular lymphocytic infiltration where the blood-brain barrier breaks down. In 12% of patients, the initial lesions are frontal. Unilateral lesions that produce a mass effect suggestive of a brain tumor may occur. MRI provides a clearer delineation of normal and abnormal white matter than does CT and may demonstrate abnormalities missed by CT (Fig. 86-5*B*).

Impaired Adrenal Function. More than 85% of patients with the childhood form of ALD have elevated levels of ACTH in plasma and a subnormal rise of cortisol levels in plasma following intravenous injection of 250 μg of ACTH (Cortrosyn).

DIAGNOSIS AND DIFFERENTIAL DIAGNOSIS. The earliest manifestations of childhood cerebral ALD are difficult to distinguish from the more common attention deficit disorders or learning disabilities. Rapid progression, signs of dementia, or difficulty in auditory discrimination suggest ALD. Even in early stages, CT or MRI may show strikingly abnormal changes. Other leukodystrophies (see Chapters 599 and 612.10) or multiple sclerosis (see Chapter 600.1) may mimic these radiographic findings. Definitive diagnosis depends on demonstration of VLCFA excess, which occurs only in X-ALD and the other peroxisomal disorders. The latter may be distinguished from X-ALD by their clinical presentation during the neonatal period.

Cerebral forms of ALD may present as increased intracranial pressure and unilateral mass lesions. These have been misdiagnosed as gliomas, even after brain biopsy, and several patients have received radiotherapy before the correct diagnosis was made. Measurement of VLCFA in plasma or brain biopsy specimens is the most reliable differentiating test.

Adolescent or adult cerebral ALD can be confused with psychiatric disorders, dementing disorders, or epilepsy. The 1st clue to the diagnosis of ALD may be the demonstration of white matter lesions by CT or MRI; assays of VLCFA are confirmatory.

ALD cannot be distinguished clinically from other forms of Addison disease; it is recommended that assays of VLCFA levels be performed in all male patients with Addison disease. ALD patients do not usually have antibodies to adrenal tissue in their plasma.

COMPLICATIONS. An avoidable complication is the occurrence of adrenal insufficiency. The most difficult neurologic problems are those related to bed rest, contracture, coma, and swallowing disturbances. Other complications involve behavioral disturbances and injuries associated with defects of spatial orientation, impaired vision and hearing, and seizures.

TREATMENT. Corticosteroid replacement for adrenal insufficiency or adrenocortical hypofunction is effective (see Chapter 576). It may be lifesaving and increase general strength and well-being, but it does not alter the course of the neurologic disability.

Bone Marrow Transplantation. Bone marrow transplantation (BMT) benefits patients who show early evidence of the inflammatory demyelination that is characteristic of the rapidly progressive neurologic disability in boys and adolescents with the cerebral X-ALD phenotype. BMT is a high-risk procedure, and patients must be selected with great care. The mechanism of the beneficial effect is incompletely understood. Bone marrow–derived cells do express ALDP, the protein that is deficient in X-ALD; ≈50% of brain microglial cells are bone marrow derived. It is possible that replacement of affected cells by cells that contain the normal gene changes the brain milieu sufficiently to correct the brain metabolic disturbance. The favorable effect may also be caused by modification of the brain inflammatory response. Five to 10 yr follow-up of boys and adolescents who had early cerebral involvement has shown stabilization and, in some instances, improvement. On the other hand, BMT has not shown favorable effects in patients who had already severe brain involvement and may accelerate disease progression under these circumstances. The nonverbal IQ has been found to be of predictive value, and transplant is not recommended in patients with nonverbal IQ significantly below 80. Unfortunately, in more than half the patients who are diagnosed because of neurologic symptoms, the illness is so advanced that they are not candidates for transplant.

Consideration of BMT is most relevant in neurologically asymptomatic or mildly involved patients. Screening at-risk relatives of symptomatic patients identifies these patients most frequently. Screening by measurement of plasma VLCFA levels in patients with Addison disease may also identify candidates for BMT. Because of its risk (10–20% mortality) and the fact that up to 50% of untreated patients with X-ALD do not develop inflammatory brain demyelination, transplant is not recommended in patients who are free of demonstrable brain involvement. The MRI is also of key importance for the crucial decision of whether transplant should be performed. MRI abnormalities precede clinically evident neurologic or neuropsychologic abnormalities. The brain MRI should be monitored at 6 mo to 1 yr intervals in neurologically asymptomatic boys and adolescents between the ages of 3 and 15 yr. If the MRI is normal, BMT is not indicated. If brain MRI abnormalities develop, the patient should be evaluated at 3 mo intervals to determine if the abnormality is progressive, in combination with careful neurologic and neuropsychologic evaluation; and if early progressive involvement is confirmed, transplant should be considered. Magnetic resonance spectroscopy improves the capacity to determine whether the brain involvement is progressive. It is not known whether BMT has a favorable effect on the noninflammatory spinal cord involvement in adults with the adrenomyeloneuropathy phenotype.

Lorenzo's Oil Therapy. The administration of Lorenzo's oil to asymptomatic boys reduces the risk of developing the childhood cerebral phenotype by a factor of two or more. Lorenzo's oil (4:1 mixture of glyceryl trioleate and glyceryl trierucate) combined with a dietary regimen is recommended for neurologically asymptomatic boys who have a normal brain MRI and are younger than 8 yr old, but must be supervised carefully. Adrenal function and brain MRI must be monitored. Patients who develop progressive MRI abnormalities are evaluated for hematopoietic stem cell transplant when changes are still in an early phase. Lorenzo's oil has not been shown to alter disease progression in patients who already have cerebral involvement.

Other Therapies. Interferon-β and immunosuppressive therapies have not been found to be effective. Therapies with lovastatin and with 4-phenylbutyrate have been proposed and are being tested in clinical trials. Gene therapy has shown promise in cultured cells and the mouse model of X-ALD but is not yet available for human trial.

Supportive Therapy. The progressive behavioral and neurologic disturbances associated with the childhood form of ALD are extremely difficult for the family. ALD patients require the establishment of a comprehensive management program and partnership among the family, physician, visiting nursing staff, school authorities, and counselors. In addition, parent support groups are often helpful (United Leukodystrophy Foundation, 2304 Highland Drive, Sycamore, IL 60178). Communication with school authorities is important because under the provisions of Public Law 94–142, children with ALD qualify for special services as "other health impaired" or "multihandicapped." Depending on the rate of progression of the disease, special needs might range from relatively low-level resource services within a regular school program to home- and hospital-based teaching programs for children who are not mobile.

Management challenges vary with the stage of the illness. The early stages are characterized by subtle changes in affect, behavior, and attention span. Counseling and communication with school authorities are of prime importance. Changes in the sleep-wake cycle can be benefited by the judicious use at night of sedatives such as chloral hydrate (10–50 mg/kg), pentobarbital (5 mg/kg), or diphenhydramine (2–3 mg/kg).

As the leukodystrophy progresses, the modulation of muscle tone and support of bulbar muscular function are major concerns. Baclofen in gradually increasing doses (5 mg bid to 25 mg qd) is the most effective pharmacologic agent for the treatment of acute episodic painful muscle spasms. Other agents may also be used, with care being taken to monitor the occurrence of side effects and drug interactions. As the leukodystrophy progresses, bulbar muscular control is lost. Although initially this can be managed by changing the diet to soft and pureed foods, most patients eventually require a nasogastric tube or a gastrostomy. At least one third of patients have focal or generalized seizures that usually readily respond to standard anticonvulsant medications.

GENETIC COUNSELING AND PREVENTION. Genetic counseling and primary and secondary prevention of X-ALD are of crucial importance. Extended family screening should be offered to all at-risk relatives of symptomatic patients; one program led to the identification of more than 250 asymptomatic affected males and 1,200 women heterozygous for X-ALD. The plasma assay permits reliable identification of affected males in whom plasma VLCFA levels are increased already on the day of birth. Identification of asymptomatic males permits institution of steroid replacement therapy when appropriate and prevents the occurrence of adrenal crisis, which may be fatal. Monitoring of brain MRI also permits identification of patients who are candidates for BMT at a stage when this procedure has the greatest chance of success. Plasma VLCFA assay is recommended in all male patients with Addison disease. X-ALD has been shown to be the cause of adrenal insufficiency in >25% of boys with Addison disease of unknown cause. Identification of women heterozygous for X-ALD is more difficult than that of affected males. Plasma VLCFA levels are normal in 15–20% of heterozygous women, and failure to note this has led to serious errors in genetic counseling. If VLCFA levels are normal both in plasma and cultured skin fibroblasts, the risk of false-negative results is reduced but not eliminated. DNA analysis permits accurate identification of carriers, provided that the mutation has been defined in a family member, and is the procedure recommended for the identification of heterozygous women. Mutation analysis is available on a service basis.

Prenatal diagnosis of affected male fetuses can be achieved by measurement of VLCFA levels in cultured amniocytes or chorionic villus cells and by mutation analysis. Whenever a new patient with X-ALD is identified, a detailed pedigree should be constructed and efforts should be made to identify all at-risk female carriers and affected males. These investigations should be accompanied by careful and sympathetic attention to social, emotional, and ethical issues during counseling.

Peroxisomal Disorders

Baumgartner MR, Poll-The BT, Verhoeven NM, et al: Clinical approach to inherited peroxisomal disorders: A series of 27 patients. *Ann Neurol* 1998;44:720–730.

Ferdinandusse S, Ylianttila MS, Gloerich J, et al: Mutational spectrum of D-bifunctional protein deficiency and structure-based genotype-phenotype analysis. *Am J Hum Genet* 2006;78:112–124.

Martinez M, Pineda M, Vidal R, et al: Docosahexaenoic acid—A new therapeutic approach to peroxisomal-disorder patients: Experience with two cases. *Neurology* 1993;43:1389–1397.

Moser HW: Genotype-phenotype correlations in disorders of peroxisome biogenesis. *Mol Genet Metab* 1999;68:316–327.

Motley AM, Brites P, Gerez L, et al: Mutational spectrum in the *PEX7* gene and functional analysis of mutant alleles in 78 patients with rhizomelic chondrodysplasia punctata type 1. *Am J Hum Genet* 2002;70:612–624.

Preuss N, Brosius U, Biermanns M, et al: *PEX1* mutations in complementation group 1 of Zellweger spectrum patients correlate with severity of disease. *Pediatr Res* 2002;51:706–714.

Steinberg S, Chen L, Wei L, Moser A, et al: The *PEX* gene screen: Molecular diagnosis of peroxisome biogenesis disorders in the Zellweger syndrome spectrum. *Mol Genet Metab* 2004;83:252–263.

Walter C, Gootjes J, Mooijer PA: Disorders of peroxisome biogenesis due to mutations in *PEX1*: Phenotypes and *PEX1* protein levels. *Am J Hum Genet* 2001;69:35–48.

Wanders RJ, Jansen GA, Skjeldal OH: Refsum disease, peroxisomes and phytanic acid oxidation: A review. *J Neuropathol Exp Neurol* 2001;60:1021–1031.

Adrenoleukodystrophy (X-Linked)

Bezman L, Moser AB, Raymond GV, et al: Adrenoleukodystrophy: Incidence, new mutation rate, and results of extended family screening. *Ann Neurol* 2001;49:512–517.

Boehm CD, Cutting GR, Lachtermacher MB, et al: Accurate DNA-based diagnostic and carrier testing for X-linked adrenoleukodystrophy. *Mol Genet Metab* 1999;66:128–136.

Kemp S, Pujol A, Waterham HR, et al: X-linked adrenoleukodystrophy mutation database: Role in diagnosis and clinical correlations. *Hum Mutat* 2001;18:499–515.

Moser AB, Kreiter N, Bezman L, et al: Plasma very long chain fatty acids in 3,000 peroxisome disease patients and 29,000 controls. *Ann Neurol* 1999;45:100–110.

Moser HW, Loes DJ, Melhem ER, et al: X-linked adrenoleukodystrophy: Overview and prognosis as a function of age and brain magnetic resonance imaging abnormality: A study involving 372 patients. *Neuropediatrics* 2000;31:227–239.

Moser HW, Raymond GV, Dubey P: Adrenoleukodystrophy: New approaches to a neurodegenerative disease. *JAMA* 2005;294:3131–3134.

Moser HW, Raymond GV, Lu SE, et al: Follow-up of 89 Lorenzo's Oil treated asymptomatic adrenoleukodystrophy patients. *Arch Neurol* 2005;62:1073–1080.

Peters C, Charnas LR, Tan Y, et al: Cerebral X-linked adrenoleukodystrophy: The international hematopoietic cell transplantation experience from 1982 to 1999. *Blood* 2004;104:881–888.

Stephenson DJ, Bezman L, Raymond GV: Acute presentation of childhood adrenoleukodystrophy. *Neuropediatrics* 2000;31:293–297.

Van Geel BM, Assies J, Haverkort EB, et al: Progression of abnormalities in adrenomyeloneuropathy and neurologically asymptomatic X-linked adrenoleukodystrophy despite treatment with "Lorenzo's oil." *J Neurol Neurosurg Psychiatry* 1999;67:290–299.

86.3 • Disorders of Lipoprotein Metabolism and Transport • William A. Neal

EPIDEMIOLOGY OF BLOOD LIPIDS AND CARDIOVASCULAR DISEASE

The relationship between dietary fat consumption and plasma cholesterol was demonstrated nearly a century ago. Well-fed Americans had higher rates of coronary heart disease (CHD) than postwar Europeans who subsisted on limited rations. The Seven Countries Study of geographic, social class, and ethnic differences in CHD around the world found strong associations between average intake of saturated fats, plasma cholesterol, and mortality from CHD. In 1960, the mean total blood cholesterol level among Americans was 220 mg/dL. By 1991, the level declined to a mean of 205 mg/dL.

In 1977, the Cooperative Lipoprotein Phenotyping Study showed that there is an inverse relationship between HDL and CHD. Clinical trials of dietary and drug interventions directed toward modulation of cholesterol levels were begun during the 1970s, ultimately providing the basis for screening and treatment standards as promulgated by the National Cholesterol

Education Program (NCEP). Further refinement of the molecular basis of lipoprotein metabolism has better characterized phenotypic abnormalities and more directed interventional strategies.

Of all common chronic diseases, none is so clearly influenced by both environmental and genetic factors as CHD. This multifactorial disorder is strongly associated with increasing age and male gender, though it is increasingly apparent that heart disease is under recognized in women. Tobacco use confers a twofold higher lifetime risk. Sedentary activity and high intake of saturated fats, leading to adiposity, increase risk through differences in the plasma levels of lipoproteins that are atherogenic. Family history is a reflection of the combined influence of lifestyle and genetic predisposition to early heart disease. Risk of premature heart disease associated with positive family history is 1.7 times higher than in families with no such history.

The pathogenesis of atherosclerosis begins during childhood. Korean and Vietnam war casualties were noted to have surprisingly advanced fatty streak and plaque formation in the coronary arteries and aorta. The Johns Hopkins Precursors Study demonstrated that white male medical students with blood cholesterol levels in the lowest quartile showed only a 10% incidence of CHD three decades later, whereas those in the highest quartile had a 40% incidence. The Pathobiological Determinants of Atherosclerosis in Youth (PDAY) Study demonstrated a significant relationship between the weight of the abdominal fat pad and the extent of atherosclerosis found at autopsy on subjects 15–34 yr of age. The Bogalusa Heart Study of >3,000 black and white children and adolescents has provided the most comprehensive longitudinal data relating the presence and severity of CHD risk factors with semiquantifiable severity of atherosclerosis.

The "fetal origins hypothesis" is based on the observation that babies born with low birthweight have a higher incidence of heart disease as adults. Epidemiologic studies support the idea that prenatal and early postnatal conditions may affect adult health status. Children who are large for gestational age at birth and exposed to an intrauterine environment of either diabetes or maternal obesity are at increased risk of eventually developing the "metabolic syndrome" (insulin resistance, type II diabetes, obesity, CHD). Breast-feeding preterm infants confers a long-term cardioprotective benefit 13–16 yr later. Those adolescents who were breast-fed as infants had lower C-reactive protein concentrations and a 14% lower LDL to HDL ratio compared to those fed infant formulas.

Poverty is also associated with numerous negative health outcomes. The Young Hearts Project in Northern Ireland has shown that behavioral risk factors are influenced by socioeconomic status, and they are well established by adolescence, even though no biologic differences are apparent.

BLOOD LIPIDS AND ATHEROGENESIS

Numerous epidemiologic studies have demonstrated the association of hypercholesterolemia, referring to elevated total blood cholesterol, with atherosclerotic disease. Advances in clinical laboratory techniques for measurement of other selected lipoprotein particles have increased our understanding of the role of blood lipids in relation to heart disease. The ability to measure subcomponents within classes of lipid particles, as well as markers of inflammation, have further elucidated the process of atherogenesis and plaque rupture leading to acute coronary syndromes. Atherosclerosis affects primarily the coronary arteries but also often involves the aorta, arteries of the lower extremities, and carotid arteries.

The early stage of development of atherosclerosis is thought to begin with vascular endothelial dysfunction and intima media thickness, which has been shown to occur in preadolescent children with risk factors such as obesity or familial hypercholesterolemia. The complex process of penetration of the intimal lining of the vessel may be due to a variety of insults, including the presence of highly toxic oxidized LDL particles. Lymphocytes and monocytes penetrate the damaged endothelial lining, where they become macrophages laden with LDL lipids and then become foam cells. Such accumulation is counterbalanced by HDL particles capable of removing lipid deposits from the vessel wall. Fundamental to plaque formation is an inflammatory process (elevated C-reactive protein) involving macrophages and the arterial wall. The deposition of lipid within the subendothelial lining of the arterial wall appears macroscopically as fatty streaks, which may to some degree be reversible. A later stage of plaque development involves disruption of arterial smooth muscle cells stimulated by the release of tissue cytokines and growth factors. The atheroma is composed of a core of fatty substance separated from the lumen by collagen and smooth muscle (Fig. 86-6). Growth of the atherosclerotic plaque may result in ischemia of the tissue supplied by the artery. Chronic inflammation within the atheroma, perhaps caused by infectious agents such as *Chlamydia pneumoniae*, results in plaque instability and subsequent rupture. Platelet adherence leads to clot formation at the site of rupture, resulting in myocardial infarction or a cerebrovascular event.

PLASMA LIPOPROTEIN METABOLISM AND TRANSPORT

Abnormalities of lipoprotein metabolism are associated with diabetes mellitus and premature atherosclerosis. Lipoproteins are soluble complexes of lipids and proteins that effect transport of fat absorbed from the diet, or synthesis by the liver and adipose

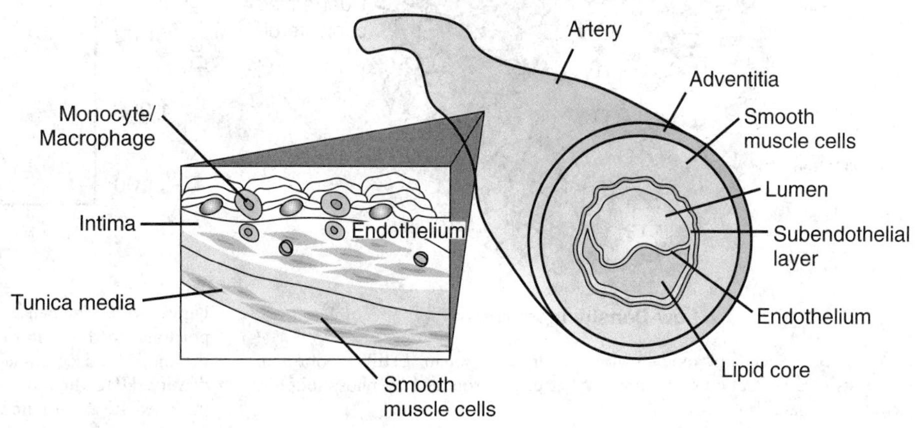

Figure 86-6. The early stage of development of atherosclerosis begins with penetration of the intimal lining of the vessel by inflammatory cells. Deposition of lipid within the subendothelial lining of the arterial wall eventually leads to disruption of smooth muscle cells to form an atheromatous lipid core that impinges on the lumen. Chronic inflammation leads to plaque instability, setting the stage for plaque rupture and complete occlusion of the vessel lumen by clot formation.

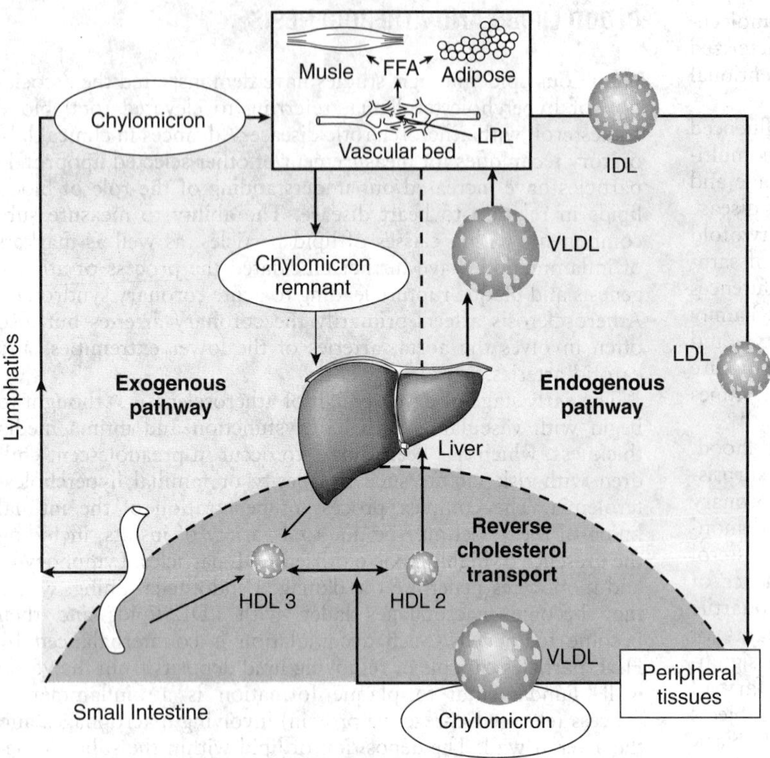

Figure 86-7. The exogenous, endogenous, and reverse cholesterol pathways. The exogenous pathway transports dietary fat from the small intestine as chylomicrons to the periphery and the liver. The endogenous pathway denotes the secretion of very low density lipoprotein (VLDL) from the liver and its catabolism to intermediate density lipoprotein (IDL) and low-density lipoprotein (LDL). Triglycerides are hydrolyzed from the VLDL particle by the action of lipoprotein lipase (LPL) in the vascular bed, yielding free fatty acids (FFAs) for utilization and storage in muscle and adipose tissue. High-density lipoprotein (HDL) metabolism is responsible for the transport of excess cholesterol from the peripheral tissues back to the liver for excretion in the bile. Nascent HDL-3 particles derived from the liver and small intestine are esterified to more mature HDL-2 particles by enzyme-mediated movement of chylomicron and VLDL into the HDL core, which is removed from the circulation by endocytosis.

tissues, for utilization and storage. Dietary fat is transported from the small intestine as chylomicrons. Lipids synthesized by the liver as very low density lipoproteins (VLDL) are catabolized to intermediate density lipoproteins (IDL) and low-density lipoproteins (LDL). High-density lipoproteins (HDL) are fundamentally involved in VLDL and chylomicron metabolism and cholesterol transport. Nonesterified free fatty acids (FFAs) are metabolically active lipids derived from lipolysis of triglycerides stored in adipose tissue bound to albumin for circulation in the plasma (Fig. 86-7).

Lipoproteins consist of a central core of triglycerides and cholesteryl esters (CE) surrounded by phospholipids, cholesterol, and proteins (Fig. 86-8). The density of the several classes of lipoproteins is inversely proportional to the ratio of lipid to protein (Fig. 86-9).

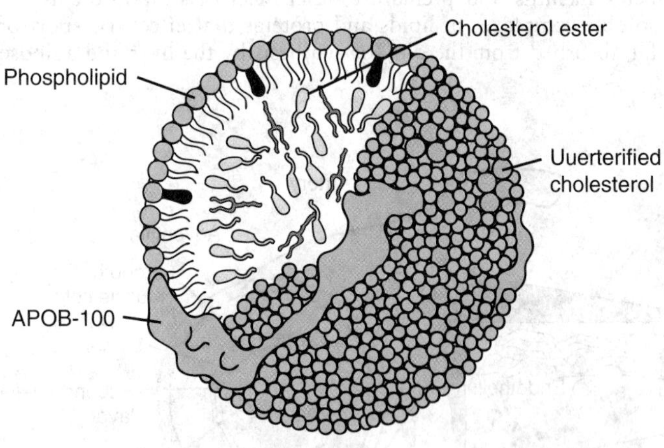

Figure 86-8. Schematic model of low-density lipoprotein (LDL). Lipoprotein consists of a central core of cholesteryl esters, surrounded by phospholipids, cholesterol, and protein.

Constituent proteins are known as apolipoproteins (Table 86-7). They are responsible for a variety of metabolic functions in addition to their structural role, including cofactors or inhibitors of enzymatic pathways, and mediators of lipoprotein binding to cell surface receptors. ApoA is the major apoliprotein of HDL. ApoB is present in LDL, VLDL, IDL, and chylomicrons. ApoB-100 is derived from the liver, whereas apoB-48 comes from the small intestine. ApoC-I, C-II, and C-III are small peptides important in triglyceride metabolism. Likewise, apoE, which is present in VLDL, HDL, chylomicrons, and chylomicron remnants, plays an important role in the clearance of triglycerides.

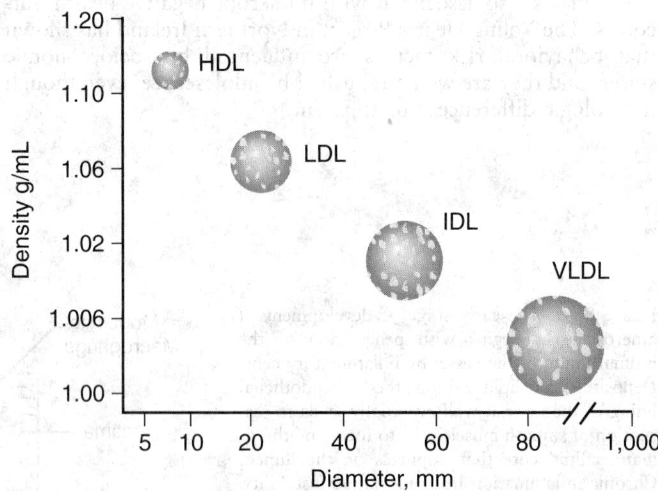

Figure 86-9. The density of the several classes of lipoprotein is inversely proportional to the ratio of lipid to protein. As lipid is less dense than protein, the more lipid contained in the particle increases its size and decreases its density. HDL, high-density lipoprotein; LDL, low-density lipoprotein; IDL, intermediate density lipoprotein; VLDL, very low density lipoprotein.

TABLE 86-7. Characteristics of the Major Lipoproteins

LIPOPROTEIN*	SOURCE	SIZE (nm)	DENSITY (g/mL)	COMPOSITION % PROTEIN	COMPOSITION % LIPID	APOLIPOPROTEINS*
Chylomicrons	Intestine	80–1,200	<0.95	1–2	98–99	C-I, C-II, C-III, E, A-I, A-II, A-IV, B-48
Chylomicron remnants	Chylomicrons	40–150	<1.0006	6–8	92–94	B-48, E
VLDL	Liver, intestine	30–80	0.95–1.006	7–10	90–93	B-100, C-I, C-II, C-III
IDL	VLDL	25–35	1.006–1.019	11	89	B-100, E
LDL	VLDL	18–25	1.019–1.063	21	79	B-100
HDL	Liver, intestine VLDL, Chylomicrons	5–20	1.125–1.210	32–57	43–68	A-I, A-II, A-IV C-I, C-II, C-III D, E

*Lipoproteins consist of a central core of triglycerides and cholestenyl esters surrounded by phospholipids, cholesterol, and proteins. Constituent proteins are known as apolipoproteins.
HDL, high-density lipoprotein; IDL, intermediate density lipoprotein; LDL, low-density lipoprotein; VLDL, very low density lipoprotein.

TRANSPORT OF EXOGENOUS (DIETARY) LIPIDS. All dietary fat with the exception of medium-chain triglycerides is efficiently carried into the circulation by way of lymphatic drainage from the intestinal mucosa. Triglyceride (TG) and CE combine with apoA and apoB-48 in the intestinal mucosa to form chylomicrons, which are carried into the peripheral circulation via the lymphatic system. HDL particles contribute apoC-II to the chylomicrons, required for the activation of lipoprotein lipase (LPL) within the capillary endothelium of adipose, heart, and skeletal muscle tissue. Free fatty acids are oxidized, resterified for storage as triglycerides, or released into the circulation bound to albumin for transport to the liver. After hydrolysis of the TG core from the chylomicron, apoC particles are recirculated back to HDL. The subsequent contribution of apoE from HDL to the remnant chylomicron facilitates binding of the particle to hepatic LDL receptors (LDL-R). Within the hepatocyte, the chylomicron remnant may be incorporated into membranes, resecreted as lipoprotein back into the circulation, or secreted as bile acids. Normally, all dietary fat is disposed of within 8 hrs after the last meal, an exception being individuals with a disorder of chylomicron metabolism. Postprandial hyperlipidemia is a risk factor for atherosclerosis. Abnormal transport of chylomicrons and their remnants may result in their absorption into the blood vessel wall as foam cells, caused by the ingestion of CE by macrophages, the earliest stage in the development of fatty streaks.

TRANSPORT OF ENDOGENOUS LIPIDS FROM THE LIVER. The formation and secretion of VLDL from the liver and its catabolism to IDL and LDL particles describe the endogenous lipoprotein pathway. Fatty acids used in the hepatic formation of VLDL are derived primarily by uptake from the circulation. VLDL appears to be transported from the liver as rapidly as it is synthesized, and it consists of triglycerides, cholesteryl esters, phospholipids, and apoB-100. Nascent particles of VLDL secreted into the circulation combine with apoliproteins C's and E. The size of the VLDL particle is determined by the amount of triglyceride present, progressively shrinking in size as TG is hydrolyzed by the action of LPL, yielding free fatty acids for utilization or storage in muscle and adipose tissue. Hydrolysis of ≈80% of the TG present in VLDL particles produces IDL particles containing an equal amount of cholesterol and TG. The remaining remnant IDL is converted to LDL for delivery to peripheral tissues or to the liver. ApoE is attached to the remnant IDL particle to allow binding to the cell and subsequent incorporation into the lysosome. Individuals with deficiency of either apoE2 or hepatic triglyceride lipase (HTGL) accumulate IDL in the plasma.

LDL particles account for ≈70% of the plasma cholesterol in normal individuals. LDL receptors are present on the surfaces of nearly all cells. Most LDL is taken up by the liver, and the rest is transported to peripheral tissues such as the adrenal glands and gonads for steroid synthesis. Dyslipidemia is greatly influenced by LDL-R activity. The efficiency with which VLDL is converted into LDL is also important in lipid homeostasis.

HDL AND REVERSE CHOLESTEROL TRANSPORT. As hepatic secretion of lipid particles into the bile is the only mechanism by which cholesterol can be removed from the body, transport of excess cholesterol from the peripheral cells is a vitally important function of HDL. HDL is heavily laden with apoA-I containing lipoproteins, which is nonatherogenic in contrast to B lipoproteins. Cholesterol-poor nascent HDL particles secreted by the liver and small intestine are esterified to more mature HDL-2 particles by the action of the enzyme lecithin-cholesterol acyltransferase (LCAT), which facilitates movement of chylomicrons and VLDL into the HDL core. HDL-2 may transfer cholesteryl esters back to apoB lipoproteins mediated by cholesteryl ester transfer protein (CETP), or the cholesterol-rich particle may be removed from the plasma by endocytosis, completing reverse cholesterol transport. Low HDL may be genetic (deficiency of apoA-I) or secondary to increased plasma TG.

HYPERLIPOPROTEINEMIAS

HYPERCHOLESTEROLEMIA (TABLE 86-8)

Familial Hypercholesterolemia (FH). FH is a monogenic autosomal co-dominant disorder caused by mutations affecting the LDL

TABLE 86-8. Hyperlipoproteinemias

DISORDER	LIPOPROTEINS ELEVATED	CLINICAL FINDINGS	GENETICS	ESTIMATED INCIDENCE
Familial hypercholesterolemia	LDL	Tendon xanthomas, CHD	AD	1/500
Familial defective ApoB-100	LDL	Tendon xanthomas, CHD	AD	1/1,000
Autosomal recessive hypercholesterolemia	LDL	Tendon xanthomas, CHD	AR	<1/1,000,000
Sitosterolemia	LDL	Tendon xanthomas, CHD	AR	<1/1,000,000
Polygenic hypercholesterolemia	LDL	CHD		1/30?
Familial combined hyperlipidemia (FCHL)	LDL, TG	CHD	AD	1/200
Familial dysbetalipoproteinemia	LDL, TG	Tubereruptive xanthomas, peripheral vascular disease	AD	1/10,000
Familial chylomicronemia (Frederickson type I)	TG↑↑	Eruptive xanthomas, hepatosplenomegaly, pancreatitis	AR	1/1,000,000
Familial hypertriglyceridemia (Frederickson type IV)	TG↑	±CHD	AD	1/500
Familial hypertriglyceridemia (Frederickson type V)	TG↑↑	Xanthomas ±CHD	AD	
Familial hepatic lipase deficiency	VLDL	CHD	AR	<1/1,000,000

AD, autosomal dominant; AR, autosomal recessive; CHD, coronary heart disease; LDL, low-density lipoproteins, TG, triglycerides; VLDL, very low density lipoproteins.

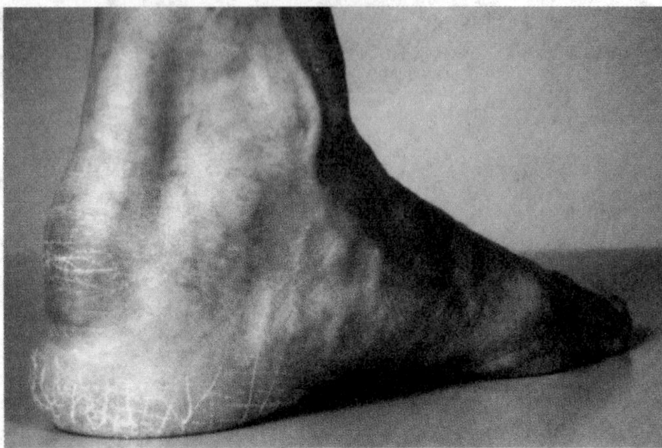

Figure 86-10. Achilles tendon xanthoma (heterozygous familial hypercholesterolemia). (From Durrington P: Dyslipidaemia. *Lancet* 2003;362:717–731.)

receptor. It is characterized by strikingly elevated LDL cholesterol, premature cardiovascular disease, and tendon xanthomas. Molecular studies have identified five classes of mutations affecting the ability of LDL cholesterol to bind with the LDL receptor. Of the nearly 800 mutations described, some result in failure of synthesis of the LDL receptor (receptor negative) and others cause defective binding or release at the lipoprotein-receptor interface. Receptor negative mutations result in more severe phenotypes than receptor defective mutations.

Homozygous FH. FH homozygotes inherit two abnormal LDL receptor genes, resulting in markedly elevated plasma cholesterol levels ranging between 500 and 1,200 mg/dL. Triglyceride levels are normal to mildly elevated, and HDL levels may be slightly decreased. The condition occurs in 1/1,000,000 persons. Receptor negative patients have <2% normal LDL receptor activity, whereas those who are receptor defective may have as much 25% normal activity and a better prognosis.

The prognosis is poor regardless of the specific LDL receptor aberration. Severe atherosclerosis involving the aortic root and coronary arteries is present by early to mid-childhood. These children usually present with xanthomas, which may cause thickening of the Achilles tendon or extensor tendons of the hands, or cutaneous lesions on the hands, elbows, knees, or buttocks (Figs. 86-10, 86-11, and 86-12). Corneal arcus may be present. Family

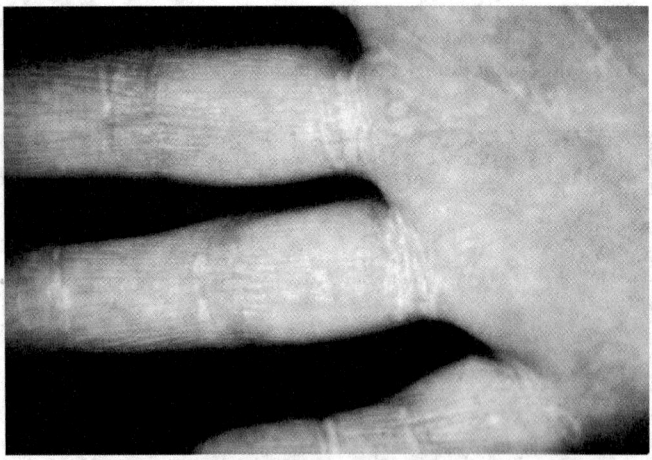

Figure 86-11. Striate palmar xanthomata. (From Durrington P: Dyslipidaemia. *Lancet* 2003;362:717–731.)

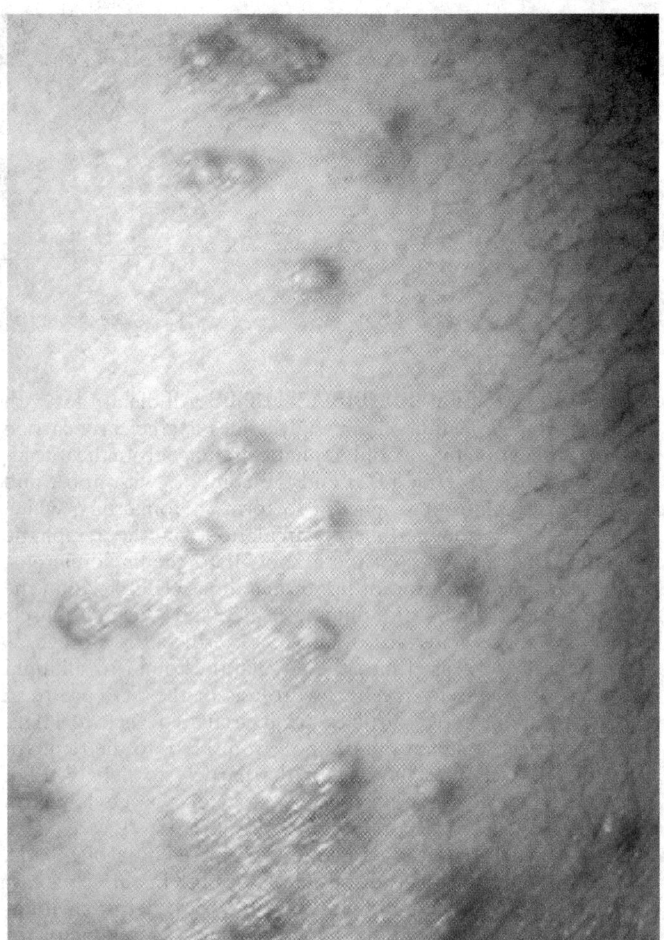

Figure 86-12. Eruptive xanthomata on extensor surface of forearm. (From Durrington P: Dyslipidaemia. *Lancet* 2003;362:717–731.)

history is informative because premature heart disease is strongly prevalent among relatives of both parents. The diagnosis may be confirmed by measuring LDL receptor activity in cultured skin fibroblasts. Phenotypic expression of the disease may also be assessed by measuring receptor activity on the surface of lymphocytes by using cell sorting techniques.

Untreated homozygous patients rarely survive to adulthood. Symptoms of coronary insufficiency may occur; sudden death is common. LDL apheresis to selectively remove LDL particles from the circulation is recommended for many children and has been shown to slow the progression of atherosclerosis. Liver transplantation has also been successful in decreasing LDL cholesterol levels, but complications related to immunosuppression are common. HMG CoA reductase inhibitors are often effective depending on the specific class of LDL receptor defect present. Combination therapy with ezetimibe, selectively blocking cholesterol adsorption in the gut, usually results in further modest decline in LDL levels; it has largely replaced the use of bile acid sequestrants.

Heterozygous FH. Heterozygous FH is one of the most common single gene mutations associated with acute coronary syndromes and atherosclerotic CHD in adults. Its prevalence is ≈1/500 individuals worldwide, but the frequency may be as high as 1/250 in selected populations such as French-Canadians, Afrikaners, and Christian Lebanese due to the founder effect of unique new mutations.

Heart disease accounts for more than half of all deaths in Western society. The pathogenesis of CHD is both environmental and genetic, and the complex interrelationship between the two determines the phenotypic expression of disease. Chinese people with heterozygous FH living in China have a mean LDL cholesterol of 168 mg/dL, whereas immigrant Chinese with the disease living in Canada average 288 mg/dL. This dramatic disparity in lipoprotein levels between geographic locations is expected to narrow as dietary and physical activity practices in China approximate those of the industrialized West.

Since heterozygous FH is a co-dominant condition with nearly full penetrance 50% of first-degree relatives of affected individuals will have the disease, as will 25% of second-degree relatives. An estimated 10 million people have FH worldwide. Symptoms of CHD usually occur at the mean age of 45–48 yr in males, and a decade later in females.

The World Health Organization (WHO) has targeted FH for individualized intervention strategies because of its large effect on morbidity and mortality. A relatively small percentage of the population accounts for a disproportionately high share of the burden of cardiovascular disease. The clinical expression of the disease is straightforward and treatment is effective.

One cannot overemphasize the importance of family history for suspecting the possibility of FH. Indeed, the whole basis for deciding which children should have blood cholesterol testing is determined by a family history of premature CHD and/or parental hypercholesterolemia.

Plasma levels of LDL cholesterol do not allow unequivocal diagnosis of FH heterozygotes, but values are generally twice normal for age because of one absent or dysfunctional allele. The U.S. MED-PED ("make early diagnosis–prevent early death") Program based in Utah has formulated diagnostic criteria. Similar criteria with minor variation exist in the United Kingdom and Holland. The diagnosis within well-defined FH families is predictable according to LDL cut points. More stringent criteria are required to establish the diagnosis in previously undiagnosed families, requiring strong evidence of an autosomal inheritance pattern and higher LDL cut points. At a total cholesterol level of 310 mg/dL, only 4% of persons in the general population would have FH, whereas 95% of persons who were first-degree relatives of known cases would have the disease. The mathematical probability of FH, verified by molecular genetics, is derived from a U.S. population cohort and may not be applicable to other countries.

Very high cholesterol levels in children should prompt extensive screening of adult first- and second-degree relatives ("reverse" cholesterol screening). A child younger than 18 yr with total plasma cholesterol of 270 mg/dL and/or LDL-C of 200 mg/dL has an 88% chance of having FH. If there is a first-degree relative with proven FH, the diagnosis in the child is virtually certain (Table 86-9). Conversely, criteria for diagnosing probable FH in a child whose first-degree relative has known FH require only modest elevation of total cholesterol to 220 mg/dL (LDL-C 155 mg/dL).

Treatment of children with FH should begin with a rather rigorous low-fat diet (see later). Diet alone is rarely sufficient for decreasing blood cholesterol levels to acceptable levels (LDL-C <130 mg/dL). The Expert Panel on Blood Cholesterol Levels in Children and Adolescents (National Cholesterol Education Program) has promulgated guidelines for the consideration of cholesterol lowering medication in children at least 10 years of age. Such consideration should be given if the LDL-C is >160 mg/dL in the presence of a strong history of premature heart disease in the family; or >190 mg/dL even in the absence of a positive family history, for example, if the child is adopted and family history is not available.

Today, bile acid sequestrants are rarely used because of poor patient compliance and they have only modest benefit. Their safety is well established. Ezetimibe blocks cholesterol adsorption in the gastrointestinal tract and has a low risk of side effects. Preliminary data suggest that ezetimibe will lower total cholesterol by 20–30 mg/dL. This medication has not been evaluated by controlled clinical trials in children. HMG CoA reductase inhibitors have become the drug of choice for treatment of FH because of their remarkable effectiveness and acceptable risk profile. There is sufficient clinical experience with this class of drugs in children to document that they are as effective in children as adults, and the risks of elevated hepatic enzymes and myositis are no greater than in adults (see below).

TABLE 86-9. Percentage of Youths Under Age 18 Expected to Have FH According to Cholesterol Levels and Closest Relative with FH

TOTAL CHOL. (MG/DL)	LDL CHOL. (MG/DL)	PERCENTAGE WITH FH AT THAT LEVEL			
		DEGREE OF RELATIVE			
		FIRST	SECOND	THIRD	GENERAL POPULATION
180	122	7.2	2.4	0.9	0.01
190	130	13.5	5.0	2.2	0.03
200	138	26.4	10.7	4.9	0.07
210	147	48.1	23.6	11.7	0.19
220	155	73.1	47.5	27.9	0.54
230	164	90.0	75.0	56.2	1.8
240	172	97.1	93.7	82.8	6.3
250	181	99.3	97.6	95.3	22.2
260	190	99.9	99.5	99.0	57.6
270	200	100.0	99.9	99.8	88.0
280	210	100.0	100.0	100.0	97.8
290	220	100.0	100.0	100.0	99.6
300	230	100.0	100.0	100.0	99.9
310	210	100.0	100.0	100.0	100.0

Chol., cholesterol; FH, familial hypercholesterolemia; LDL, low-density lipoprotein.

From Williams RR, Hunt SC, Schumacher MC, et al: Diagnosing heterozygous familial hypercholesterolemia using new practical criteria validated by molecular genetics. *Am J Cardiol* 1993;72:171–176.

Familial Defective ApoB-100 (FDB). FDB is an autosomal dominant condition that is indistinguishable from heterozygous FH. LDL cholesterol levels are increased, triglycerides are normal, adults often develop tendon xanthomas, and premature CHD occurs. FDB is caused by mutation in the receptor binding region of apoB-100, the ligand of the LDL receptor, with an estimated frequency of 1/700 people in Western cultures. It is usually caused by substitution of glutamine for arginine in position 3500 in apoB-100, which results in reduced ability of the LDL receptor to bind LDL cholesterol, thus impairing its removal from the circulation. Specialized laboratory testing can distinguish FDB from FH, but this is not necessary, except in research settings, since treatment is the same.

Autosomal Recessive Hypercholesterolemia (ARH). This rare condition, caused by a defect in LDL receptor mediated endocytosis in the liver, clinically presents with severe hypercholesterolemia at levels intermediate between those found in homozygous and heterozygous FH. It is disproportionately present among Sardinians, and is modestly responsive to treatment with HMG CoA reductase inhibitors.

Sitosterolemia. A rare autosomal recessive condition characterized by excessive intestinal adsorption of plant sterols, sitosterolemia is caused by mutations in the ATP-binding cassette transporter system which is responsible for limiting adsorption of plant sterols in the small intestine and promotes biliary excretion of the small amounts adsorbed. Plasma cholesterol levels may be severely elevated, resulting in tendon xanthomas and premature atherosclerosis. Diagnosis can be confirmed by measuring elevated plasma sitosterol levels. Treatment with HMG CoA reductase inhibitors is not effective, but cholesterol adsorption inhibitors such as ezetimibe and bile acid sequestrants are effective.

Polygenic Hypercholesterolemia. Primary elevation in LDL cholesterol among children and adults is most often polygenic; the small effects of many genes are impacted by environmental influences (diet). Plasma cholesterol levels are modestly elevated; triglyceride levels are normal. Polygenic hypercholesterolemia aggregates in families sharing a common lifestyle but does not follow predictable hereditary patterns found in single gene lipoprotein defects. Treatment of children with polygenic hypercholesterolemia is directed toward adoption of a healthy lifestyle: reduced total and saturated fat consumption and at least 1 hr of physical activity daily. Cholesterol lowering medication is rarely necessary.

HYPERCHOLESTEROLEMIA WITH HYPERTRIGLYCERIDEMIA

Familial Combined Hyperlipidemia (FCHL). This is an autosomal dominant condition characterized by moderate elevation in plasma LDL cholesterol and triglycerides, and reduced plasma HDL cholesterol. It is the most common primary lipid disorder, occurring in ≈1/200 people. No single metabolic aberration has been identified linking FCHL with atherogenesis, but it is well documented that ≈20% of individuals who develop CHD by 60 yr of age have FCHL. Family history of premature heart disease is typically positive; the formal diagnosis requires that at least two first-degree relatives have evidence of one of three variants of dyslipidemia: (1) >90th percentile plasma LDL cholesterol; (2) >90th percentile LDL cholesterol and triglycerides; and (3) >90th percentile triglycerides. Individuals switch from one phenotype to another. Xanthomas are not a feature of FCHL. Elevated plasma apoB levels with increased small dense LDL particles support the diagnosis.

Children and adults with FCHL have co-existing adiposity, hypertension, and hyperinsulinemia, suggesting the presence of the *metabolic syndrome.* Formal diagnosis of this multiplex syndrome as defined by the NCEP's Adult Treatment Panel III (ATP III) identifies six major components: abdominal obesity, atherogenic dyslipidemia, hypertension, insulin resistance with or without impaired glucose tolerance, evidence of vascular inflammation, and hypercoaguability. It is estimated that 30% of overweight adults fulfill criteria for the diagnosis of metabolic syndrome, including two thirds of those with FCHL. Hispanics and South Asians from the Indian subcontinent are especially susceptible.

The mechanisms associating visceral adiposity with the metabolic syndrome and type II diabetes are not fully understood. A plausible unifying principal is that obesity causes endoplasmic reticulum stress, leading to suppression of insulin receptor signaling and thus insulin resistance and heightened inflammatory response. How this relates to atherogenesis is unclear. It is assumed that hypercholesterolemia and, with less certainty, hypertriglyceridemia confer risk for cardiovascular disease in patients with FCHL. When features of the metabolic syndrome are included in logistic models shared etiologic features such as increased visceral adiposity become apparent. Visceral adiposity increases with age and its importance in children as a risk factor for heart disease and diabetes is limited by the relative paucity of data. Though longitudinal measurement of waist circumference and the presence of intra-abdominal fat as determined by MRI is being conducted in the research setting, body mass index (BMI) remains the surrogate for adiposity in the pediatric clinical setting.

The metabolic syndrome is a dramatic illustration of the interaction of genetics and the environment. Genetic susceptibility is essential as an explanation for premature heart disease in individuals with FCHL. Unhealthy lifestyle, poor diet, and physical inactivity contribute to obesity and attendant features of the metabolic syndrome.

The cornerstone of management is lifestyle modification. This includes a diet low in saturated fats, trans fats, and cholesterol, as well as reduced consumption of simple sugars. Increased dietary intake of fruits and vegetables is important, as is 1 hr of moderate physical activity daily. Compliance among children and their parents is often a problem, but small incremental steps are more likely to succeed than aggressive weight-loss strategies. It is very important that the child's caregivers participate in the process. Plasma triglyceride levels are usually quite responsive to dietary restriction, especially reduction in the amount of sweetened drinks consumed. Blood cholesterol levels may decrease by 10–15%, but if LDL cholesterol remains >160 mg/dL, drug therapy should be considered.

Familial Dysbetalipoproteinemia (FDBL, Type III Hyperlipoproteinemia). FDBL is caused by mutations in the gene for apolipoprotein E (apoE), which when exposed to environmental influences such as high fat, high caloric diet, or excessive alcohol intake, results in a mixed type of hyperlipidemia. Patients tend to have elevated plasma cholesterol and triglycerides to a relatively similar degree. HDL cholesterol is typically normal in contrast to other causes of hypertriglyceridemia associated with low HDL. This rare disorder affects ≈1/10,000 persons. ApoE mediates removal of chylomicron and VLDL remnants from the circulation by binding to hepatic surface receptors. The polymorphic *apoE* gene expresses in three isoforms: *apoE3, apoE2,* and *apoE4. E4* is the "normal" allele present in the majority of the population. The *apoE2* isoform has lower affinity for the LDL receptor and its frequency is ≈7%. About 1% of the population is homozygous for *apoE2/E2,* the most common mutation associated with FDBL, but only a minority express the disease. Expression requires precipitating illnesses such as diabetes, obesity, renal disease, or hypothyroidism. Individuals homozygous for *apoE4/E4* are at risk for late-onset Alzheimer disease.

Most patients with FDBL present in adulthood with distinctive xanthomas. Tuberoeruptive xanthomas resemble small grapelike clusters on the knees, buttocks, and elbows. Prominent orange-yellow discoloration of the creases of the hands (palmar xanthomas) is also typically present. Atherosclerosis, often presenting with peripheral vascular disease, usually occurs in the 4th or 5th decade. Children may present with a less distinctive rash and generally have precipitating illnesses.

The diagnosis of FDBL is established by lipoprotein electrophoresis, which demonstrates a broad beta band containing remnant lipoproteins. Direct measurement of VLDL by ultracentrifugation can be performed in specialized lipid laboratories. A VLDL/total triglyceride ratio >0.30 supports the diagnosis. *ApoE* genotyping for *apoE2* homozygosity can be performed, confirming the diagnosis in the presence of the distinctive physical findings. A negative result does not necessarily rule out the disease as other mutations in *apoE* may cause even more serious manifestations.

Pharmacologic treatment of FDBL is necessary to decrease the likelihood of symptomatic atherosclerosis in adults. HMG CoA reductase inhibitors, nicotinic acid, and fibrates are all effective. FDBL is quite responsive to recommended dietary restriction.

HYPERTRIGLYCERIDEMIAS

The familial disorders of triglyceride-rich lipoproteins include both common and rare variants of the Frederickson classification system. These include chylomicronemia (type I), familial hypertriglyceridemia (type IV), and the more severe combined hypertriglyceridemia and chylomicronemia (type V). Hepatic lipase (HL) deficiency also results in a similar combined hyperlipidemia.

Familial Chylomicronemia (Type I Hyperlipidemia). This rare single gene defect, like familial hypercholesterolemia, is due to mutations affecting clearance of apoB-containing lipoproteins. Deficiency or absence of lipoprotein lipase (LPL) or its cofactor apoC-II, which facilitates lipolysis by LPL, causes severe elevation of triglyceride rich plasma chylomicrons. HDL cholesterol levels are decreased. As clearance of these particles is markedly delayed, the plasma is noted to have a turbid appearance even after prolonged fasting (Fig. 86-13). Chylomicronemia caused by LPL deficiency is associated with modest elevation in triglycerides, whereas this is not the case when the cause is deficient or

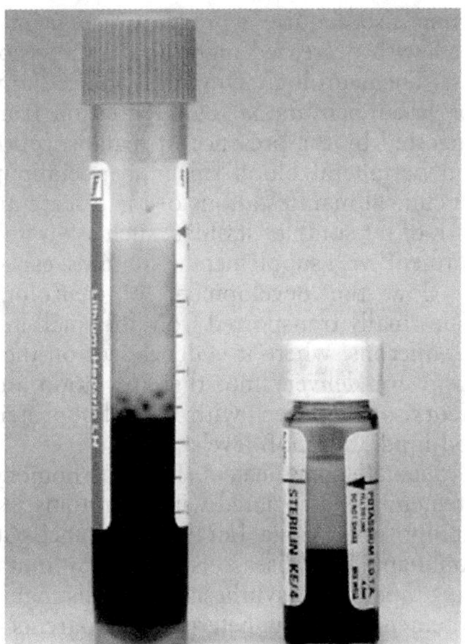

Figure 86-13. Milky plasma from patient with acute abdominal pain. (From Durrington P: Dyslipidaemia. *Lancet* 2003;362:717–731.)

absent apoC-II. Both are autosomal recessive conditions with a frequency of ≈1/1,000,000. The disease usually presents during childhood with acute pancreatitis. Eruptive xanthomas on the arms, knees, and buttocks may be present, and there may be hepatosplenomegaly. The diagnosis is established by assaying triglyceride lipolytic activity. Treatment of chylomicronemia is by vigorous dietary fat restriction supplemented by fat-soluble vitamins. Medium-chain triglycerides that are adsorbed into the portal venous system may augment total fat intake, and administration of fish oils may also be beneficial.

Familial Hypertriglyceridemia (FHTG, Type IV Hyperlipidemia). FHTG is an autosomal dominant disorder of unknown etiology, which occurs in ≈1/500 individuals. It is characterized by elevation of plasma triglycerides >90th percentile (250–1,000 mg/dL range), often accompanied by slight elevation in plasma cholesterol and low HDL. FHTG does not usually manifest until adulthood, though it is expressed in ≈20% of affected children. In contrast to FCHL, FHTG is not thought to be highly atherogenic. It is most likely caused by defective breakdown of VLDL, or less often by overproduction of this class of lipoproteins.

The diagnosis should include the presence of at least one first-degree relative with hypertriglyceridemia. FHTG should be distinguished from FCHL and FDBL, as the latter require more vigorous treatment to prevent coronary or peripheral vascular disease. The differentiation is usually possible on clinical grounds, in that lower LDL cholesterol levels accompany FHTG, but measurement of normal apoB levels in FHTG may be helpful in ambiguous situations.

A more severe hypertriglyceridemia characterized by increased levels of chylomicrons as well as VLDL particles (Frederickson type V) may occasionally be encountered. Triglyceride levels are often >1,000 mg/dL. The disease is rarely seen in children. In contrast to chylomicronemia (Frederickson type I), LPL or apoC-II deficiency is not present. These patients often develop eruptive xanthomas in adulthood, whereas type IV hypertriglyceridemia individuals do not. Acute pancreatitis may be the presenting illness. As with other hypertriglyceridemias, excessive alcohol consumption and estrogen therapy can exacerbate the disease.

Secondary causes of transient hypertriglyceridemia should be ruled out before making a diagnosis of FHTG. A diet high in simple sugars and carbohydrates, or excessive alcohol consumption as well as estrogen therapy may exacerbate hypertriglyceridemia. Adolescents and adults should be questioned about excessive consumption of soda and other sweetened drinks, as it is common to encounter people who drink supersized drinks or multiple 12 oz cans of sweetened drinks daily. Cessation of this practice often results in dramatic fall in triglyceride levels as well as weight among those who are obese. HDL cholesterol levels will tend to rise as BMI stabilizes.

Pediatric diseases associated with hyperlipidemia include hypothyroidism, nephrotic syndrome, biliary atresia, glycogen storage disease, Niemann-Pick disease, Tay-Sachs disease, systemic lupus erythematosus, hepatitis, and anorexia nervosa (Table 86-10).

Certain medications exacerbate hyperlipidemia, including isotretinoin (Accutane), thiazide diuretics, oral contraceptives, steroids, β blockers, immunosuppressants, and protease inhibitors used in the treatment of HIV.

Treatment of hypertriglyceridemia in children rarely requires medication unless levels >1,000 mg/dL persist after dietary restriction of fats, sugars, and carbohydrates, accompanied by increased physical activity. In such cases, the aim is to prevent episodes of pancreatitis. The common use of fibrates and niacin in adults with hypertriglyceridemia is not recommended in children. HMG CoA reductase inhibitors are reasonably effective in lowering triglyceride levels, and there is considerably more experience documenting the safety and efficacy of this class of lipid lowering medications in children.

Hepatic Lipase Deficiency. Hepatic lipase deficiency is a very rare autosomal recessive condition causing elevation in both plasma cholesterol and triglycerides. Hepatic lipase (HL) hydrolyzes triglycerides and phospholipids in VLDL remnants and IDL, preventing their conversion to LDL. HDL cholesterol levels tend to be increased rather than decreased, suggesting the diagnosis. Laboratory confirmation is established by measuring HL activity in heparinized plasma.

DISORDERS OF HDL METABOLISM

Primary Hypoalphaliproteinemia. Isolated low HDL cholesterol is a familial condition that often follows a pattern suggestive of autosomal dominant inheritance but may occur independent of family history. It is the most common disorder of HDL metabolism. It is defined as HDL cholesterol <10th percentile for gender

TABLE 86-10. Secondary Causes of Hyperlipidemia

HYPERCHOLESTEROLEMIA
Hypothyrodism
Nephrotic syndrome
Cholestasis
Anorexia nervosa
Drugs: progesterone, thiazides, tegretol, cyclosporine
HYPERTRIGLYCERIDEMIA
Obesity
Type II diabetes
Alcohol
Renal failure
Sepsis
Stress
Cushing syndrome
Pregnancy
Hepatitis
AIDS, protease inhibitions
Drugs: anabolic steroids, β blockers, estrogen, thiazides
REDUCED HDL
Smoking
Obesity
Type II diabetes
Malnutrition
Drugs: β Blockers, anabolic steroids

HDL, high-density lipoprotein.

and age with normal plasma triglycerides and LDL cholesterol. Whether it is associated with more rapid atherosclerosis is uncertain. It appears to be related to a reduction in apoA-I synthesis and increased catabolism of HDL. Secondary causes of low HDL cholesterol, such as the metabolic syndrome, and rare diseases such as LCAT deficiency and Tangier disease must be ruled out.

Familial Hyperalphalipoproteinemia. This is an unusual condition conferring deceased risk for CHD among family members. Plasma levels of HDL cholesterol exceed 80 mg/dL.

Familial ApoA–I Deficiency. Mutations in the *apoA-I* gene may result in complete absence of plasma HDL. Nascent HDL is produced in the liver and small intestine. Free cholesterol from peripheral cells is esterified by LCAT, enabling formation of mature HDL particles. ApoA-I is required for normal enzymatic functioning of LCAT. The resultant accumulation of free cholesterol in the circulation eventually leads to corneal opacities, planar xanthomas, and premature atherosclerosis. Some patients, however, may have mutations of *apoA-I* that result in very rapid catabolism of the protein not associated with atherogenesis, despite HDL cholesterol levels in the 15–30 mg/dL range.

Tangier Disease. This is an autosomal co-dominant disease associated with levels of HDL cholesterol <5 mg/dL. It is caused by mutations in ABCA1, a protein that facilitates the binding of cellular cholesterol to apoA-I. This results in free cholesterol accumulation in the reticuloendothelial system manifested by tonsillar hypertrophy of a distinctive orange color and hepatosplenomegaly. Intermittent peripheral neuropathy may occur from cholesterol accumulation in Schwann cells. Diagnosis should be suspected in children with enlarged orange tonsils and extremely low HDL cholesterol levels.

Familial Lecithin–Cholesterol Acyltransferase (LCAT) Deficiency. Mutations affecting LCAT interfere with the esterification of cholesterol, thereby preventing formation of mature HDL particles. This is associated with rapid catabolism of apoA-I. Free circulating cholesterol in the plasma is greatly increased, which leads to corneal opacities and HDL cholesterol levels <10 mg/dL. Partial LCAT deficiency is known as "fish-eye" disease. Complete deficiency causes hemolytic anemia and progressive renal insufficiency early in adulthood. This rare disease is not thought to cause premature atherosclerosis. Laboratory confirmation is based on demonstration of decreased cholesterol esterification in the plasma.

Cholesteryl Ester Transfer Protein (CETP) Deficiency. Mutations involving the CETP gene are localized to chromosome 16y21. CETP facilitates the transfer of lipoproteins from mature HDL to and from VLDL and chylomicron particles, thus ultimately regulating the rate of cholesterol transport to the liver for excretion in the bile. About half of mature HDL2 particles are directly removed from the circulation by HDL receptors on the surface of the liver. The other half of cholesteryl esters in the core of HDL exchange with triglycerides in the core of apoB lipoproteins (VLDL, IDL, LDL) for transport to the liver. Homozygous deficiency of CETP has been observed in subsets of the Japanese population with extremely high HDL cholesterol levels (>150 mg/dL).

CONDITIONS ASSOCIATED WITH LOW CHOLESTEROL. Disorders of apoB-containing lipoproteins and intracellular cholesterol metabolism are associated with low plasma cholesterol.

Abetalipoproteinemia. This rare autosomal recessive disease is caused by mutations in the gene encoding microsomal triglyceride transfer protein necessary for the transfer of lipids to nascent chylomicrons in the small intestine and VLDL in the liver. This results in absence of chylomicrons, VLDL, LDL, and apoB, and very low levels of plasma cholesterol and triglycerides. Fat malabsorption, diarrhea, and failure to thrive present in early childhood. Spinocerebellar degeneration, secondary to vitamin E deficiency, manifests in loss of deep tendon reflexes progressing to ataxia and lower extremity spasticity by adulthood. Patients with abetalipoproteinemia also acquire a progressive pigmented retinopathy associated with decreased night and color vision and eventual blindness. The neurologic symptoms and retinopathy may be mistaken for Friedreich ataxia. Differentiation from Friedreich ataxia is suggested by the presence of malabsorption and acanthocytosis on peripheral blood smear in abetalipoproteinemia. Many of the clinical manifestations of the disease are a result of malabsorption of fat-soluble vitamins, such as vitamins E, A, and K. Early treatment with supplemental vitamins, especially E, may significantly slow the development of neurologic sequelae. Vitamin E is normally transported from the small intestine to the liver by chylomicrons, where it is dependent on the endogenous VLDL pathway for delivery into the circulation and peripheral tissues. Parents of children with abetalipoproteinemia have normal blood lipid and apoB levels.

Familial Hypobetalipoproteinemia. Familial homozygous hypobetalipoproteinemia is associated with symptoms very similar to those of abetalipoproteinemia, but the inheritance pattern is autosomal co-dominant. The disease is caused by mutations in the gene encoding apoB-100 synthesis. It is distinguishable from abetalipoproteinemia in that heterozygous parents of probands have plasma LDL cholesterol and apoB levels less than half normal. There are no symptoms or sequelae associated with the heterozygous condition.

The selective inability to secrete apoB-48 from the small intestine results in a condition resembling abetalipoproteinemia or homozygous hypobetalipoproteinemia. Sometimes referred to as Anderson disease, the failure of chylomicron absorption causes steatorrhea and fat-soluble vitamin deficiency. The blood level of apoB-100, derived from normal hepatocyte secretion, is normal in this condition.

Smith–Lemli–Opitz Syndrome (SLOS). Patients with SLOS often have multiple congenital anomalies and developmental delay caused by low plasma cholesterol and accumulated precursors (Tables 86-11 and 86-12). Family pedigree analysis has revealed its autosomal recessive inheritance pattern. Mutations in the *DHCR7* (7 dehydrocholesterol-Δ^7 reductase) gene result in deficiency of the microsomal enzyme DHCR7, which is necessary to compete the final step in cholesterol synthesis. It is not known why defects in cholesterol synthesis result in congenital malformations, but as cholesterol is a major component of myelin, neu-

TABLE 86-11. Major Clinical Characteristics of Smith-Lemli-Opitz Syndrome: Frequent Anomalies (>50% of Patients)

CRANIOFACIAL
Microcephaly
Blepharoptosis
Anteverted nares
Retromicrognathia
Low-set, posteriorly rotated ears
Midline cleft palate
Broad maxillary alveolar ridges
Cataracts (<50%)
SKELETAL ANOMALIES
Syndactyly of toes II/III
Postaxial polydactyly (<50%)
Equinovarus deformity (<50%)
GENITAL ANOMALIES
Hypospadias
Cryptorchidism
Sexual ambiguity (<50%)
DEVELOPMENT
Pre- and postnatal growth retardation
Feeding problems
Mental retardation
Behavioral abnormalities

From Haas D, Kelley RI, Hoffmann GF: Inherited disorders of cholesterol biosynthesis. *Neuropediatrics* 2001;32:113–122.

TABLE 86-12. Characteristic Malformations of Internal Organs in Severely Affected Smith-Lemli-Opitz Patients

CENTRAL NERVOUS SYSTEM
- Frontal lobe hypoplasia
- Enlarged ventricles
- Agenesis of corpus callosum
- Cerebellar hypoplasia
- Holoprosencephaly

CARDIOVASCULAR
- Atrioventricular canal
- Secundum atrial septal defect
- Patent ductus arteriosus
- Membranous ventricular septal defect

URINARY TRACT
- Renal hypoplasia or aplasia
- Renal cortical cysts
- Hydronephrosis
- Ureteral duplication

GASTROINTESTINAL
- Hirschsprung disease
- Pyloric stenosis
- Refractory dysmotility
- Cholestatic and noncholestatic progressive liver disease

PULMONARY
- Pulmonary hypoplasia
- Abnormal lobation

ENDOCRINE
- Adrenal insufficiency

From Haas D, Kelley RI, Hoffmann GF: Inherited disorders of cholesterol biosynthesis. *Neuropediatrics* 2001;32:113–122.

rodevelopment is severely impaired. The incidence of SLOS is estimated to be 1/20,000–60,000 births among whites, with a somewhat higher frequency in Hispanics and lower incidence in individuals of African descent.

Spontaneous abortion of SLOS fetuses may occur. Type II SLOS often leads to death by the end of the neonatal period. Survival is unlikely when the plasma cholesterol level is <20 mg/dL. Laboratory measurement should be performed by gas chromatography, as standard techniques for lipoprotein assay include measurement of cholesterol precursors, which may yield a false positive result. Milder cases may not present until late childhood. Phenotypic variance ranges from microcephaly, cardiac and brain malformation, and multiple organ-system failure to only subtle dysmorphic features and mild developmental delay. Treatment includes supplemental dietary cholesterol (egg yolk) and possibly HMG CoA reductase inhibition to prevent the synthesis of toxic precursors proximal to the enzymatic block.

DISORDERS OF INTRACELLULAR CHOLESTEROL METABOLISM

Cerebrotendinous Xanthomatosis. This autosomal recessive disorder presents clinically in late adolescence with tendon xanthomas, cataracts, and progressive neurodegeneration. It is caused by tissue accumulation of bile acid intermediates shunted into cholestanol resulting from mutations in the gene for sterol 27-hydroxylase. This enzyme is necessary for normal mitochondrial synthesis of bile acids in the liver. Early treatment with chenodeoxycholic acid reduces cholesterol levels and prevents the development of symptoms.

Wolman Disease and Cholesterol Ester Storage Disease (CESD). These autosomal recessive disorders are caused by lack of lysosomal acid lipase. After LDL cholesterol is incorporated into the cell by endocytosis, it is delivered to lysosomes where it is hydrolyzed by lysosomal lipase. Failure of hydrolysis because of complete absence of the enzyme causes accumulation of cholesteryl esters within the cells. Hepatosplenomegaly, steatorrhea, and failure to thrive occur during early infancy, leading to death by the age of 1 yr. In CESD, a less severe form than Wolman disease, there is low but detectable acid lipase activity.

Niemann–Pick Disease Type C. This is a disorder of intracellular cholesterol transport characterized by accumulation of cholesterol and sphingomyelin in the central nervous and reticuloendothelial systems. Death from this autosomal recessive neurologic disease usually occurs by adolescence.

LIPOPROTEIN PATTERNS IN CHILDREN AND ADOLESCENTS. Table 86-13, derived primarily from the Lipid Research Clinics Population Studies, shows the distribution of lipoprotein levels in American youth at various ages. Total plasma cholesterol rises rapidly from a mean of 68 mg/dL at birth to a level approximately twice that by the end of the neonatal period. A very gradual rise in total cholesterol level occurs until puberty, at which time the mean level reaches 160 mg/dL. Total cholesterol falls transiently during puberty, in males due to a small decrease in HDL cholesterol, and in females secondary to a slight fall in LDL cholesterol. Blood cholesterol levels track reasonably well as individuals age. High blood cholesterol tends to aggregate in families, a reflection of genetic and environmental influences.

An acceptable total cholesterol among children and adolescents is <170 mg/dL; borderline is 170–199 mg/dL; and high >200 mg/dL. An acceptable LDL cholesterol is <110 mg/dL; bor-

TABLE 86-13 Plasma Cholesterol and Triglyceride Levels in Childhood and Adolescence: Means and Percentiles

	TOTAL TRIGLYCERIDE (MG/DL)					TOTAL CHOLESTEROL (MG/DL)					LOW-DENSITY LIPOPROTEIN CHOLESTEROL (MG/DL)					HIGH-DENSITY LIPOPROTEIN CHOLESTEROL (MG/DL)*				
	5TH	MEAN	75TH	90TH	95TH	5TH	MEAN	75TH	90TH	95TH	5TH	MEAN	75TH	90TH	95TH	5TH	10TH	25TH	MEAN	95TH
Cord	14	34	—	—	84	42	68	—	—	103	17	29	—	—	50	13	—	—	35	60
1–4 yr																				
Male	29	56	68	85	99	114	155	170	190	203	—	—	—	—	—	—	—	—	—	—
Female	34	64	74	95	112	112	156	173	188	200	—	—	—	—	—	—	—	—	—	—
5–9 yr																				
Male	28	52	58	70	85	125	155	168	183	189	63	93	103	117	129	38	42	49	56	74
Female	32	64	74	103	126	131	164	176	190	197	68	100	115	125	140	36	38	47	53	73
10–14 yr																				
Male	33	63	74	94	111	124	160	173	188	202	64	97	109	122	132	37	40	46	55	74
Female	39	72	85	104	120	125	160	171	191	205	68	97	110	126	136	37	40	45	52	70
15–19 yr																				
Male	38	78	88	125	143	118	153	168	183	191	62	94	109	123	130	30	34	39	46	63
Female	36	73	85	112	126	118	159	176	198	207	59	96	111	29	137	35	38	43	52	74

*Note that different percentiles are listed for HDL cholesterol.

Data for cord blood from Strong W: Atherosclerosis: Its pediatric roots. In Kaplan N, Stamler J (eds): *Prevention of Coronary Heart Disease.* Philadelphia, WB Saunders, 1983. Data for children 1–4 yr from Tables 6, 7, 20 and 21, and all other data from Tables 24, 25, 32, 33, 36, and 37 in *Lipid Research Clinics Population Studies Data Book, Vol. 1, The Prevalence Study.* NIH publication No. 80-1527. Washington, DC, National Institutes of Health, 1980.

derline 110–129 mg/dL; and high >130 mg/dL. HDL cholesterol should be >40 mg/dL.

BLOOD CHOLESTEROL SCREENING. NCEP's Expert Panel on Blood Cholesterol Levels in Children and Adolescents established guidelines for cholesterol measurement that were published in 1991. The panel recommended a *selective* approach to screening based on the following criteria:

Screen children and adolescents whose parents or grandparents have documented coronary artery disease before the age of 55 yr.

Screen the offspring of a parent who has been found to have a blood cholesterol level of >240 mg/dL.

Screen children and adolescents for whom family history is unobtainable, particularly those with other risk factors.

The American Academy of Pediatrics and the American Heart Association (AHA) have endorsed these criteria. Application of these criteria will result in the screening of 25% of American youth, representing those most likely to have a familial basis for their hypercholesterolemia. A predicted 59% of children with elevated levels of blood cholesterol will avoid detection because of the lack of universal screening, and therein lies the source of considerable controversy and confusion. Reliance on family history of premature heart disease or known parental cholesterol >240 mg/dL is considered by some to be too insensitive and difficult to apply.

The rationale is basically sound, though admittedly the guidelines are fraught with problems of compliance. If family history of widespread premature atherosclerotic heart disease is obtained, offspring are indeed at significantly greater risk of dyslipidemia than children without such family history. The converse applies to children who do not fulfill criteria for screening; they are not likely to have a strong genetic predisposition to heart disease. The 59% of children with hypercholesterolemia not detected by clinicians following the guidelines are likely to have only modest elevation of cholesterol due to environmental influences such as diet and sedentary lifestyle. Primary prevention strategies applicable to the population as a whole include daily physical activity and a diet low in saturated fats. Children and adolescents for whom there may be consideration of using cholesterol lowering medication will nearly always be correctly identified by following current guidelines.

Early diagnosis and treatment of individuals who are at risk of premature CHD because of genetic susceptibility is an important public health strategy. It is estimated that no more than 20% of people with heterozygous familial hypercholesterolemia are diagnosed, and <10% are being adequately treated. A detailed study from the United Kingdom has established the cost-effectiveness of "cascade screening," which means tracking and testing family members of FH probands. It is even more cost-effective to screen younger people because of more life years gained after preventive treatment.

It is well documented that many parents are unaware of their own cholesterol levels, making the use of that criterion problematic. The evidence that cholesterol screening of children may cause psychological harm to the child is less than compelling, as is the concern that universal screening might lead to overuse of cholesterol lowering medication. The worrisome epidemic of childhood obesity, approaching 50% in some disadvantaged high-risk populations, supports broader screening to identify those with the metabolic syndrome. A fasting lipid profile rather than nonfasting total blood cholesterol measurement is indicated if screening is being conducted because of obesity as a risk factor for heart disease and type 2 diabetes in order to detect hypertriglyceridemia and/or low HDL cholesterol. NCEP guidelines do not specify the age at which at-risk children should be tested. Five years of age is a reasonable age to screen since dietary interventions for those children with hypercholesterolemia can be safely applied at this stage of neurodevelopment.

RISK ASSESSMENT AND TREATMENT OF HYPERLIPIDEMIA. NCEP recommends risk assessment based on LDL cholesterol levels (Fig. 86-14). The follow-up interval and modification of diet is determined by the severity of dyslipidemia. Borderline hypercholesterolemia (LDL 110–129 mg/dL) should prompt initiation of the child on the AHA Step I diet:

Calories consumed as fat should not exceed 30% of total calories consumed per day.

Calories consumed as saturated fat should not exceed 10% of total calories per day.

Total cholesterol intake should be limited to <300 mg/dL per day.

Instruction regarding avoidance of other risk factors for heart disease such as tobacco use should be provided, and the child should be reevaluated in 1 yr.

Persistence of elevated LDL cholesterol >130 mg/dL indicates the need for more comprehensive evaluation and lifestyle modification. History and physical examination and additional laboratory tests aimed at ruling out secondary causes of hyperlipidemia (see Table 86-10) should be performed. Other family members should have blood cholesterol screening. If the LDL cholesterol level does not achieve the minimal goal of <130 mg/dL, the AHA Step II diet should be recommended. This diet allows the same average fat consumption of no more than 30% of total calories, but restricts saturated fats to <7–8% of total calories and cholesterol intake to <200 mg/day. Follow-up lab tests, measurement of height and weight for the calculation of body mass index (BMI), and dietary history should be scheduled at 3–6 mo intervals.

The 2004 revision of the NCEP ATP III raised the minimal acceptable level of HDL cholesterol from 35 mg/dL to 40 mg/dL. If low HDL cholesterol is present, counseling directed toward weight management, tobacco avoidance, and daily physical activity should be provided.

No restriction of fat or cholesterol is recommended for infants <2 yr of age because of rapid growth and development, especially involving the central nervous system and the possibility of developing failure to thrive. Overfeeding should be discouraged, however, as, increasingly, infants and toddlers are exceeding weight for height standards published by the U.S. Centers for Disease Control and Prevention. The myth that "a bigger baby is a healthier baby" persists.

The safety of a heart healthy diet among children 3–19 yr has been established by the National Health and Nutrition Examination Survey (NHANES III). Despite a decrease in the average level of fat intake from the second survey, there was no evidence of poor growth or compromised nutritional status. The prospective, well-controlled Dietary Intervention Study in Children (DISC) compared children consuming a low-fat Step I diet with subjects consuming the "usual" diet, containing 33–34% of calories as fat and 13% as saturated fat. No differences between groups with regard to height, weight, micronutrients, or psychologic well-being were observed. Children on the low-fat diet had lower LDL cholesterol levels.

The Committee on Nutrition of the American Academy of Pediatrics suggests that as children >2 yr consume fewer calories from fat, they should eat more grain products, fruits, vegetables, low-fat milk products, beans, lean meats, poultry, fish, and other protein-rich foods. Low-carbohydrate, high-fat diets have become popular in the last decade as a means to achieve weight reduction. Unlimited fat intake is strongly discouraged, as is unrestricted sugar and carbohydrate consumption. Carbohydrates should comprise ≈55% of calories, achieved by consuming complex carbohydrates such as pasta, certain vegetables, potatoes, legumes, and whole grain cereals and bread.

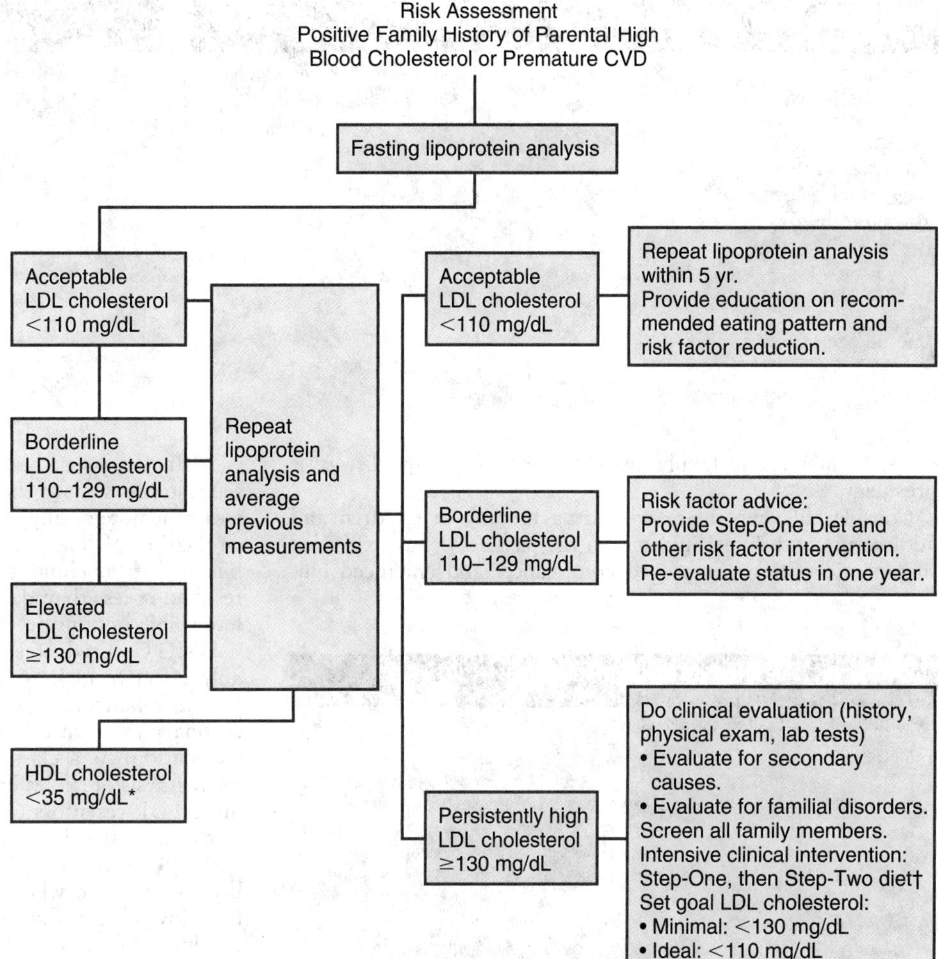

Figure 86-14. Flow chart of classification, education, and follow-up of children based on low-density lipoprotein (LDL) cholesterol levels. CVD, cardiovascular disease; HDL, high-density lipoprotein. (From Williams CL, Hagman LL, Daniels SR, et al: Cardiovascular health in childhood. *Circulation* 2002;106:143–160.)

Protein should provide ≈15–20% of calories, and should contain all of the essential fatty acids. The exclusion of meat or fish from the diet necessitates a healthy mixture of plant proteins in order to achieve appropriate nutrient balance. Thus, foods high in fiber, such as fruits, vegetables, and whole grains, are recommended because of their excellent nutrient content as components of an eating pattern low in saturated fats. Children should eat five or more fruits and vegetables daily. Canned and frozen vegetables and soups should be selected for low sodium content.

These dietary recommendations, if followed, provide adequate calories for optimal growth and development without promoting obesity. Compliance on the part of children and their caregivers is challenging in today's society. Children learn eating habits from their parents. Successful adoption of a healthier diet is far more likely to occur if meals and snacks in the home are applicable to the entire family rather than an individual child. A regular time for meals together as a family is desirable. Grandparents and other nonparental caregivers sometimes need to be reminded not to indulge the child who is on a restricted diet. The rise in obesity is prompting some school districts to restrict sweetened drink availability and offer more nutritious cafeteria selections.

The rise in sedentary activity among our youth is contributing to the nationwide increase in obesity, which, in turn, is increasing the prevalence of other risk factors such as dyslipidemia and hypertension. The National Association for Sport and Physical Education (NASPE) recommends that children should accumulate at least 60 minutes of age-appropriate physical activity on most days of the week. Extended periods (>2 hr) of daytime inactivity are discouraged, as is >2 hr of television and other forms of screen time.

Drug Therapy (Tables 86-14 and 86-15). The NCEP Expert Panel for Children and Adolescents recommends that consideration be given to pharmacologic treatment of hyperlipidemia if the child is at least 10 yr of age and an adequate period of dietary restriction, at least 6 mo, has not achieved therapeutic goals. Drug therapy should be considered when:

- **LDL cholesterol remains >190 mg/dL**
- **LDL cholesterol remains >160 mg/dL and there is a positive family history of premature cardiovascular disease (CVD) before 55 yr of age or two or more other risk factors for CVD are present after vigorous attempts at lifestyle modification.**

These arbitrary but sensible guidelines are based on the statistical probability of the child having an inherited form of dyslipidemia such as familial hypercholesterolemia (FH). Ten years of age was selected because that is the age at which fatty streak formation in the coronary arteries and aorta has been observed. The guidelines further specify that, in rare cases, an individual may begin therapy earlier when extremely high levels of cholesterol

TABLE 86-14. Drugs Used for the Treatment of Hyperlipidemia

DRUG	MECHANISM OF ACTION	INDICATION	STARTING DOSE
HMG CoA reductase inhibitors (statins)	↓ Cholesterol and VLDL synthesis ↑ Hepatic LDL receptors	Elevated LDL	5–80 mg qhs
Bile acid sequestrants:	↑ Bile and excretion	Elevated LDL	
Cholestyramine			4–32 g daily
Colestipol			5–40 g daily
Nicotinic acid	↓ Hepatic VLDL synthesis	Elevated LDL Elevated TG	100–2,000 mg tid
Fibric acid derivitives: Gemfibrozil	↑ LPL ↓ VLDL	Elevated TG	600 mg bid
Fish oils	↓ VLDL production	Elevated TG	3–10 g daily
Cholesterol absorption inhibitors: Ezetamibe	↓ Intestinal absorption cholesterol	Elevated LDL	10 mg daily

LDL, low-density lipoprotein; LPL, lipoprotein lipase; TG, triglyceride; VLDL, very low density lipoprotein.

are encountered and family history of early coronary disease is prevalent.

Considerable experience with drug therapy in children and adolescents with hyperlipidemia in the past 15 yr has expanded therapeutic options, improved compliance, and enhanced efficacy. In the past, the mainstay of drug therapy was bile acid sequestrants such as cholestyramine and cholestipol because they were not systemically absorbed. Interruption of the enterohepatic circulation of bile acids promotes synthesis in the liver of new bile acids from cholesterol. Gastrointestinal side effects and taste resulted in less than desirable compliance, even when there were few viable options.

TABLE 86-15. Side Effects of Lipid-Lowering Drugs

DRUG AND SITE OR TYPE OF EFFECT	EFFECT
STATINS	
Skin	Rash
Nervous system	Loss of concentration, sleep disturbance, headache, peripheral neuropathy
Liver	Hepatitis, loss of appetite, weight loss, and increases in serum aminotransferases to two to three times the upper limit of the normal range
Gastrointestinal tract	Abdominal pain, nausea, diarrhea
Muscles	Muscle pain or weakness, myositis (usually with serum creatine kinase > 1,000 U/L), rhabdomyolysis with renal failure
Immune system	Lupus-like syndrome (lovastatin, simvastatin, or fluvastatin)
Protein binding	Diminished binding of warfarin (lovastatin, simvastatin, fluvastatin)
BILE ACID-BINDING RESINS	
Gastrointestinal tract	Abdominal fullness, nausea, gas, constipation, hemorrhoids, anal fissure, activation of diverticulitis, diminished absorption of vitamin D in children
Liver	Mild serum aminotransferase elevations, which can be exacerbated by concomitant treatment with a statin
Metabolic system	Increases in serum triglycerides of ≈10% (greater increases in patients with hypetriglyceridemia)
Electrolytes	Hyperchloremic acidosis in children and patients with renal failure (cholestyramine)
Drug interactions	Binding of warfarin, digoxin, thiazide diuretics, thyroxine, statins
NICOTINIC ACID	
Skin	Flushing, dry skin, pruritus, ichthyosis, acanthosis nigricans
Eyes	Conjunctivitis, cystoid macular edema, retinal detachment
Respiratory tract	Nasal stuffiness
Heart	Supraventricular arrhythmias
Gastrointestinal tract	Heartburn, loose bowel movements or diarrhea
Liver	Mild increase in serum aminotransferases, hepatitis with nausea and fatigue
Muscles	Myositis
Metabolic system	Hyperglycemia (incidence, ≈5% higher in patients with diabetes), increase of 10% in serum uric acid
FIBRATES	
Skin	Rash
Gastrointestinal tract	Stomach upset, abdominal pain (mainly gemfibrozil), cholesterol-saturated bile, increase of 1–2% in gallstone incidence
Genitourinary tract	Erectile dysfunction (mainly clofibrate)
Muscles	Myositis with impaired renal function
Plasma proteins	Interference with binding of warfarin, requiring reduction in the dose of warfarin by ≈30%
Liver	Increased serum aminotransferases

From Knopp RH: Drug treatment of lipid disorders. *N Engl J Med* 1999;341:498–512.

HMG CoA reductase inhibitors, known as statins, are remarkably effective in lowering LDL cholesterol levels and reducing plaque inflammation, thereby reducing the likelihood of a sudden coronary event in an at-risk adult within weeks of starting the medication. As a class, they work by blocking the intrahepatic biosynthesis of cholesterol, thereby stimulating the production of more LDL receptors on the cell surface. The NCEP ATP advocates aggressive lowering of LDL to <70 mg/dL in individuals with known coronary heart disease. This information is relevant because children who fulfill criteria for consideration of cholesterol lowering medication will almost always have inherited the condition from one parent. Not infrequently, when providing care for the child, questions come up about screening and treatment of parents or grandparents. Statins are equally effective in children, capable of lowering LDL cholesterol levels by half when necessary. They also effect modest reduction in triglycerides and inconsistent increase in HDL cholesterol. Statins have been shown to improve intima-media thickness in carotid arteries in affected children 8–18 yr old. Their side-effect profile, mainly liver dysfunction and rarely rhabdomyolysis with secondary renal failure, should be taken into consideration before prescribing the drug. There has been no evidence to date, however, that complications are any more frequent in children than in adults, and skeletal muscle discomfort seems to be somewhat less of a problem. Statins are contraindicated in patients with active liver disease and during pregnancy and lactation. Children should have liver enzymes monitored regularly, and creatine phosphokinase (CPK) measured if muscle ache or weakness occurs. Liver enzymes can be allowed to rise threefold before discontinuing the drug. It should be reemphasized that children with modest elevations in cholesterol, such as that seen in polygenic hypercholesterolemia, are not candidates for statins as a rule because of their side-effect profile.

Other cholesterol lowering medications such as nicotinic acid and fibrates have been used far less often in children than bile acid sequestrants and statins. Nicotinic acid has been used selectively in children with marked hypertriglyceridemia at risk for acute pancreatitis, though dietary restriction of complex sugars and carbohydrates usually results in significant lowering of triglyceride levels.

Ezetimibe is useful in the pediatric population because of its efficacy and low side-effect profile. Ezetimibe reduces plasma LDL cholesterol by blocking sterol absorption in enterocytes. The drug is marketed as an adjunct to statins when adult subjects are not achieving sufficient blood lipid lowering with statins alone.

Large clinical trials of ezetimibe used as monotherapy in children have not been conducted. Nevertheless there are sufficient reports in the literature documenting the impressive effectiveness of this medication without worrisome side effects that the clinician can feel on relatively safe grounds recommending it instead of a statin when moderate hypercholesterolemia is encountered. The dose is 10 mg taken once daily. Parents concerned about the possibility of lifelong use of statins as a treatment are generally much more receptive to the use of ezetimibe. Regardless of which drug is selected for a given child or adolescent in need of pharmacologic treatment, the goal is to decrease the LDL cholesterol to <130 mg/dL or, more ideally, <110 mg/dL. There is no reason to push LDL levels lower as is recommended for high-risk adults.

Austin MA, Hutter CH, Zimmern RL, et al: Familial hypercholesterolemia and coronary heart disease: A huge association review. *Am J Epidemiol* 2004;160:421–429.

De Jongh S, Ose L, Szamosi T, et al: Efficacy and safety of statin therapy in children with familial hypercholesterolemia. *Circulation* 2002;106:2231–2237.

Demerath E, Muratova V, Spangler E, et al: School-based obesity screening in rural Appalachia. *Prev Med* 2003;37:553–560.

Durrington P: Dyslipidaemia. *Lancet* 2003;362:717–731.

Goldberg AC, Aditi S, Ji L, et al: Efficacy and safety of ezetimibe coadministered with simvastatin in patients with primary hypercholesterolemia: A randomized, double-blind, placebo-controlled trial. *Mayo Clin Proc* 2004;79:620–629.

Grundy SM, Hansen B, Smith SC, et al: Clinical management of metabolic syndrome: Report of the American Heart Association/National Heart, Lung, Blood Institute/American Diabetes Association Conference on Scientific Issues Related to Management. *Circulation* 2004;109:551–556.

Hopkins PN, Heiss G, Ellison C, et al: Coronary artery disease risk in familial combined hyperlipidemia and familial hypertriglyceridemia: A case-control comparison from the National Heart, Lung, and Blood Institute Family Heart Study. *Circulation* 2003;108:519–523.

Leren T: Cascade genetic screening for familial hypercholesterolemia. *Clin Genet* 2004;66:483–487.

Merkens LS, Connor WE, Linck LM, et al: Effects of dietary cholesterol on plasma lipoproteins in Smith-Lemli-Opitz syndrome. *Pediatr Res* 2004;56:726–732.

Raitakari OT: Arterial abnormalities in children with familial hypercholesteremia. *Lancet* 2004;363:342–343.

Singhal A, Cole TJ, Fewtrell M, et al: Breast milk feeding and lipoprotein profile in adolescents born preterm: Follow-up of a prospective randomized study. *Lancet* 2004;363:1571–1578.

Wiegman A, Hutten BA, de Groot E, et al: Efficacy and safety of statin therapy in children with familial hypercholesterolemia. *JAMA* 2004;292:331–337.

86.4 • Lipidoses • Margaret M. McGovern and Robert J. Desnick

The lysosomal lipid storage diseases are diverse disorders each due to an inherited deficiency of a lysosomal hydrolase leading to the lysosomal accumulation of the enzyme's particular substrate (Table 86-16). With the exception of Wolman disease and cholesterol ester storage disease, the lipid substrates share a common structure that includes a ceramide backbone (2-N-acyl-sphingosine) from which the various sphingolipids are derived by substitution of hexoses, phosphorylcholine, or one or more sialic acid residues on the terminal hydroxyl group of the ceramide molecule. The pathway of sphingolipid metabolism in nervous tissue (Fig. 86-15) and in visceral organs (Fig. 86-16) is known; each catabolic step has a genetically determined metabolic defect. Because sphingolipids are essential components of all cell membranes, the inability to degrade these substances and their subsequent accumulation results in the physiologic and morphologic alterations and characteristic clinical manifestations of the lipid storage disorders (see Table 86-16). Progressive lysosomal accumulation of glycosphingolipids in the central nervous system leads to neurodegeneration, whereas storage in visceral cells can lead to organomegaly, skeletal abnormalities, pulmonary infiltration, and other manifestations. The storage of a substrate in a specific tissue is dependent on its normal distribution in the body.

Diagnostic assays for the identification of affected individuals rely on the measurement of the specific enzymatic activity in isolated leukocytes or cultured fibroblasts. For most disorders, carrier identification and prenatal diagnosis are available; a specific diagnosis is essential to permit genetic counseling. The characterization of the genes that encode the specific enzymes required for sphingolipid metabolism permit the development of therapeutic options, such as recombinant enzyme replacement therapy, as well as the potential of gene therapy. Identification of specific disease-causing mutations improves diagnosis, prenatal detection, and carrier identification. For some disorders (Gaucher disease), it has been possible to make genotype-phenotype correlations that predict disease severity and allow more precise genetic counseling. Inheritance is autosomal recessive except for X-linked Fabry disease.

GM_1 GANGLIOSIDOSIS. GM_1 gangliosidosis most frequently presents in early infancy (type 1 disease) but has been described in patients with a juvenile onset (type 2). Both are autosomal recessive traits; each results from the deficient activity of β-galactosidase, a lysosomal enzyme encoded by a gene on chromosome 3 (3p21.33). Although the disorder is characterized by pathologic accumulation of GM_1 gangliosides in the lysosomes of both neural and visceral cells, GM_1 ganglioside accumulation is most marked in the brain. In addition, keratan sulfate, a mucopolysaccharide, accumulates in liver and is excreted in the urine of patients with GM_1 gangliosidosis. The β-galactosidase gene has been isolated and sequenced; mutations causing either type 1 or type 2 disease have been identified.

The **clinical manifestations** of the infantile form of GM_1 gangliosidosis (type 1 disease) may be evident in the newborn as hepatosplenomegaly, edema, and skin eruptions (**angiokeratomata**). It most frequently presents in the 1st 6 mo of life with developmental delay followed by progressive psychomotor retardation and the onset of tonic-clonic seizures. A typical facies is characterized by low-set ears, frontal bossing, a depressed nasal bridge, and abnormally long philtrum. Up to 50% of patients have a **macular cherry red spot**. Hepatosplenomegaly and skeletal abnormalities similar to those of the mucopolysaccharidoses, including anterior beaking of the vertebrae, enlargement of the sella turcica, and thickening of the calvarium, are present. By the end of the 1st yr of life, most patients are blind and deaf, with severe neurologic impairment characterized by decerebrate rigidity. Death usually occurs by 3–4 yr of age. The juvenile-onset form of GM_1 gangliosidosis (type 2) is clinically distinct, with a variable age at onset. Affected patients present primarily with neurologic symptoms including ataxia, dysarthria, mental retardation, and spasticity. Deterioration is slow; patients may survive through the 4th decade of life. These patients lack the visceral involvement, facial abnormalities, and skeletal features seen in type 1 disease. There is no specific treatment for either form of GM_1 gangliosidosis.

The **diagnosis** of GM_1 gangliosidosis should be suspected in infants with typical clinical features and is confirmed by the demonstration of the deficiency of β-galactosidase activity in peripheral leukocytes or cultured skin fibroblasts. Other disorders that share some of the features of the GM_1 gangliosidoses include Hurler disease (mucopolysaccharidosis type I), I-cell disease, and Niemann-Pick disease (NPD) type A, which can each be distinguished by the demonstration of their specific enzymatic deficiencies. Carriers of the disorder are detected by the measurement of the enzymatic activity in white blood cells or cul-

TABLE 86-16. Differential Findings in Lipidoses Lysosomal Storage Diseases

NOMENCLATURE	ENZYME DEFECT	HYDROPS FETALIS	COARSE FACIAL FEATURES DYSOSTOSIS MULTIPLEX	HEPATOSPLENOMEGALY	CARDIAC INVOLVEMENT CARDIAC FAILURE	MENTAL DETERIORATION	MYOCLONUS	SPASTICITY	PERIPHERAL NEUROPATHY	CHERRY-RED SPOT	CORNEAL CLOUDING	ANGIOKERATOMATA	VACUOLATED LYMPHOCYTES	↑ GAG (URINE)	↑ PATHOLOGIC OLIGOSACCHARIDES
MUCOLIPIDOSES															
Mucolipidoses II, I-cell disease	*N*-Acetylglucosaminylphosphotransferase	(+)	++	+	++	++	–	–	–	–	(+)	–	+	–	–
Mucolipidosis III, Pseudo-Hurler	*N*-Acetylglucosaminylphosphotransferase	–	+	(+)	–	(+)	–	–	–	–	+	–	+	–	–
Mucolipidosis IV	Unknown	–	–	+	–	(+)	–	–	–	–	–	–	–	–	–
SPHINGOLIPIDOSES															
Fabry disease	α-Galactosidase	–	–	–	+	–	–	–	–	–	+	++	–	–	–
Farber disease	Ceramidase	–	–	(+)	++	+	–	–	+	(+)	–	–	–	–	–
Galactosialidosis	β-Galactosidase and sialidase	(+)	++	++	+	++	(+)	+	–	+	+	+	+	–	+
G_{M1}gangliosidosis	β-Galactosidase	(+)	++	+	(+)	++	–	(+)	–	++	+	+	–	–	+
G_{M2}gangliosidosis (Tay-Sachs disease, Sandhoff disease)	β-Hexosaminidases A and B	–	–	(+)	–	++	+	+	–	++	–	–	–	–	+
Gaucher type I	Glucocerebrosidase	–	–	+	–	–	–	–	–	–	–	–	–	–	+
Gaucher type II	Glucocerebrosidase	(+)	–	+	–	++	+	+	–	–	–	–	–	–	+
Gaucher type III	Glucocerebrosidase	(+)	–	+	–	+	(+)	(+)	–	–	–	–	–	–	+
Niemann-Pick type I (= A & B)	Sphingomyelinase	(+)	–	++	–	+	(+)	–	(+)	(+)	(+)	–	+	–	–
Metachromatic leukodystrophy	Arylsulfatase A	–	–	–	–	++	–	+	++	(+)	–	–	–	–	–
Krabbe disease	β-Galactocerebrosidase	–	–	–	–	++	–	+	++	(+)	–	–	–	–	–
LIPID STORAGE DISORDERS															
Niemann-Pick type II (= C & D)	Intracellular cholesterol transport	–	–	(+)	–	+	–	–	–	(+)	–	–	+	–	–
Wolman disease	Acid lipase	(+)	–	+	(+)	–	–	–	–	(+)	–	–	+	–	–
Ceroid lipofuscinosis, infantile (Santavuori-Hantia)	Palmitoyl-proteinthioesterase (CLN1)	–	–	–	–	+	+	+	–	–	–	–	+	–	–
Ceroid lipofuscinosis, late infantile (Jansky-Bielschowsky)	Pepstatin-insensitive peptididase (CLN2). Variants in Finland (CLN5), Turkey (CLN7), and Italy (CLN6)	–	–	–	–	+	+	+	–	–	–	–	+	–	–
Ceroid lipofuscinosis, juvenile (Spielmeyer-Vogt)	CLN3, membrane protein	–	–	–	–	+	–	(+)	–	–	–	–	(+)	–	–
Ceroid lipofuscinosis, adult (Kufs, Parry)	CLN4, probably heterogeneous	(+)	–	–	–	+	–	–	–	–	–	–	(+)	–	–
OLIGOSACCHARIDOSES															
Aspartylglucosaminuria	Aspartylglucosaminase	–	+	(+)	(+)	+	–	–	–	–	(+)	(+)	+	–	+
Fucosidosis	α-Fucosidase	–	++	(+)	+	++	+	+	–	–	–	(+)	+	–	+
α-Mannosidosis	α-Mannosidase	–	++	+	–	++	–	(+)	–	–	++	(+)	+	–	+
β-Mannosidosis	β-Mannosidase	–	+	(+)	–	+	–	+	+	–	–	(+)	–	–	+
Schindler disease	α-*N*-Acetylgalactosaminidase	–	–	–	–	+	+	+	–	–	–	–	–	–	+
Sialidosis I	Sialidase	(+)	–	–	–	–	++	+	+	++	(+)	–	+	–	+
Sialidosis II	Sialidase	(+)	++	+	+	++	(+)	–	–	++	–	+	+	–	+

++, prominent; +, often present, (+), inconstant or occuring later in the disease course; –, not present.
GAG, glycosaminoglycans.
Modified from Hoffmann GF, Nyhan WL, Zschoke J, et al: *Storage Disorders in Inherited Metabolic Diseases.* Philadelphia, Lippincott, Williams & Wilkins, 2002, pp 346–351.

tured skin fibroblasts; prenatal diagnosis is accomplished by determination of the enzymatic activity in cultured aminocytes or chorionic villi.

THE GM_2 GANGLIOSIDOSES. The GM_2 gangliosidoses include **Tay-Sachs disease** and **Sandhoff disease**; each results from the deficiency of β-hexosaminidase activity and the lysosomal accumulation of GM_2 gangliosides, particularly in the central nervous system. Both disorders have been classified into infantile-, juvenile-, and adult-onset forms based on the age at onset and clinical features. β-Hexosaminidase occurs as two isozymes: β-hexosaminidase A, which is composed of one α and one β subunit, and β-hexosaminidase B, which has two β subunits. β-Hexosaminidase deficiency results from mutations in the α subunit and causes Tay-Sachs disease, whereas mutations in the β-subunit gene result in the deficiency of both β-hexosaminidases A and B and cause Sandhoff disease. Both are autosomal recessive traits, with Tay-Sachs disease having a predilection in the Ashkenazi Jewish population, where the carrier frequency is about 1/25.

More than 50 mutations have been identified; most are associated with the infantile forms of disease. Three mutations account for >98% of mutant alleles among Ashkenazi Jewish carriers of Tay-Sachs disease, including one allele associated with the adult-onset form. Mutations that cause the subacute or chronic forms result in enzyme proteins with residual enzymatic activities, the levels of which correlate with the severity of the disease.

Patients with the infantile form of Tay-Sachs disease have **clinical manifestations** in infancy of loss of motor skills, increased startle reaction, and macular pallor and **retinal cherry red spots** (see Table 86-16). Affected infants usually develop normally until 4–5 mo of age when decreased eye contact and an exaggerated startle response to noise (**hyperacusis**) are noted. **Macrocephaly,** not associated with hydrocephalus, may develop. In the 2nd yr of life, seizures requiring anticonvulsant therapy develop. Neurodegeneration is relentless, with death occurring by the age of 4

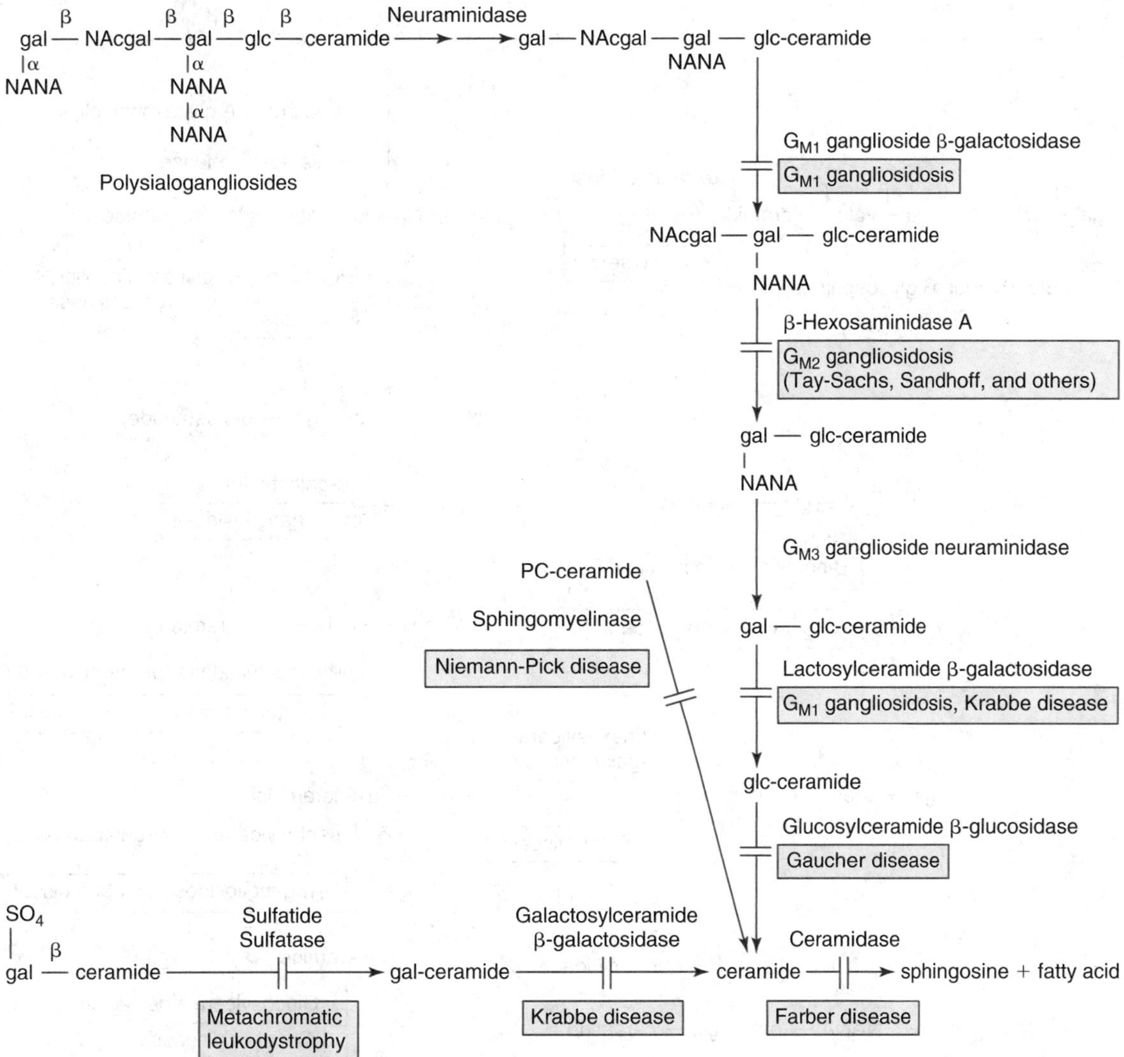

Figure 86-15. Pathways in the metabolism of sphingolipids found in nervous tissues. The name of the enzyme catalyzing each reaction is given with the name of the substrate acted on. Inborn errors are depicted as *bars* crossing the reactions *arrows,* and the name of the associated defect or defects is given in the nearest *box*. The gangliosides are named according to the nomenclature of Svennerholm. Anomeric configurations are given only at the largest starting a compound. Gal, galactose; glc, glucose; NAcgal, N-acetylgalactosamine; NANA, N-acetylneuraminic acid; PC, phosphorylcholine.

or 5 yr. The juvenile-onset form initially presents with ataxia and dysarthria and may not be associated with a macular cherry red spot.

The **clinical manifestations** of Sandhoff disease are similar to those for Tay-Sachs disease. Infants with Sandhoff disease, however, have hepatosplenomegaly, cardiac involvement, and mild bony abnormalities. The juvenile form of this disorder presents as ataxia, dysarthria, and mental deterioration, but without visceral enlargement or a macular cherry red spot. There is no treatment available for Tay-Sachs disease or Sandhoff disease.

The **diagnosis** of infantile Tay-Sachs disease and Sandhoff disease is usually suspected in an infant with neurologic features and a cherry red spot. Definitive diagnosis is by determination of the level of β-hexosaminidases A and B in isolated blood leukocytes. The two disorders are distinguished by the enzymatic assay, because in Tay-Sachs disease only the β-hexosaminidase A isozyme is deficient, whereas in Sandhoff disease both the β-hexosaminidase A and B isozymes are deficient. Future at-risk pregnancies for both disorders can be monitored by prenatal diagnosis by amniocentesis or chorionic villus sampling. Identification of carriers in families is also possible by β-hexosaminidases A and B determination. Indeed, for Tay-Sachs disease, carrier screening of all couples in which at least one member is of Ashkenazi Jewish descent is recommended before the initiation of pregnancy to identify couples at risk. These studies can be conducted by the determination of the level of β-hexosaminidase A activity in peripheral leukocytes or plasma. Molecular studies to identify the exact molecular defect in enzymatically identified carriers should also be performed to permit more specific identification of carriers in the family and to allow prenatal diagnosis in at-risk couples by both enzymatic and genotype determinations. The incidence of Tay-Sachs disease has been markedly reduced since the introduction of carrier screening programs in the Ashkenazi Jewish population. Newborn screening may be possible by measuring specific glycosphingolipid markers.

GAUCHER DISEASE. This disease is a multisystemic lipidosis characterized by hematologic problems, organomegaly, and skeletal involvement, the latter usually manifesting as bone pain and pathologic fractures (see Table 86-16). It is the most common lysosomal storage disease and the most prevalent genetic defect among Ashkenazi Jews. There are three clinical subtypes delineated by the absence or presence and progression of neurologic manifestations: Type 1 or the adult, non-neuronopathic form; type 2, the infantile or acute neuronopathic form; and type 3, the

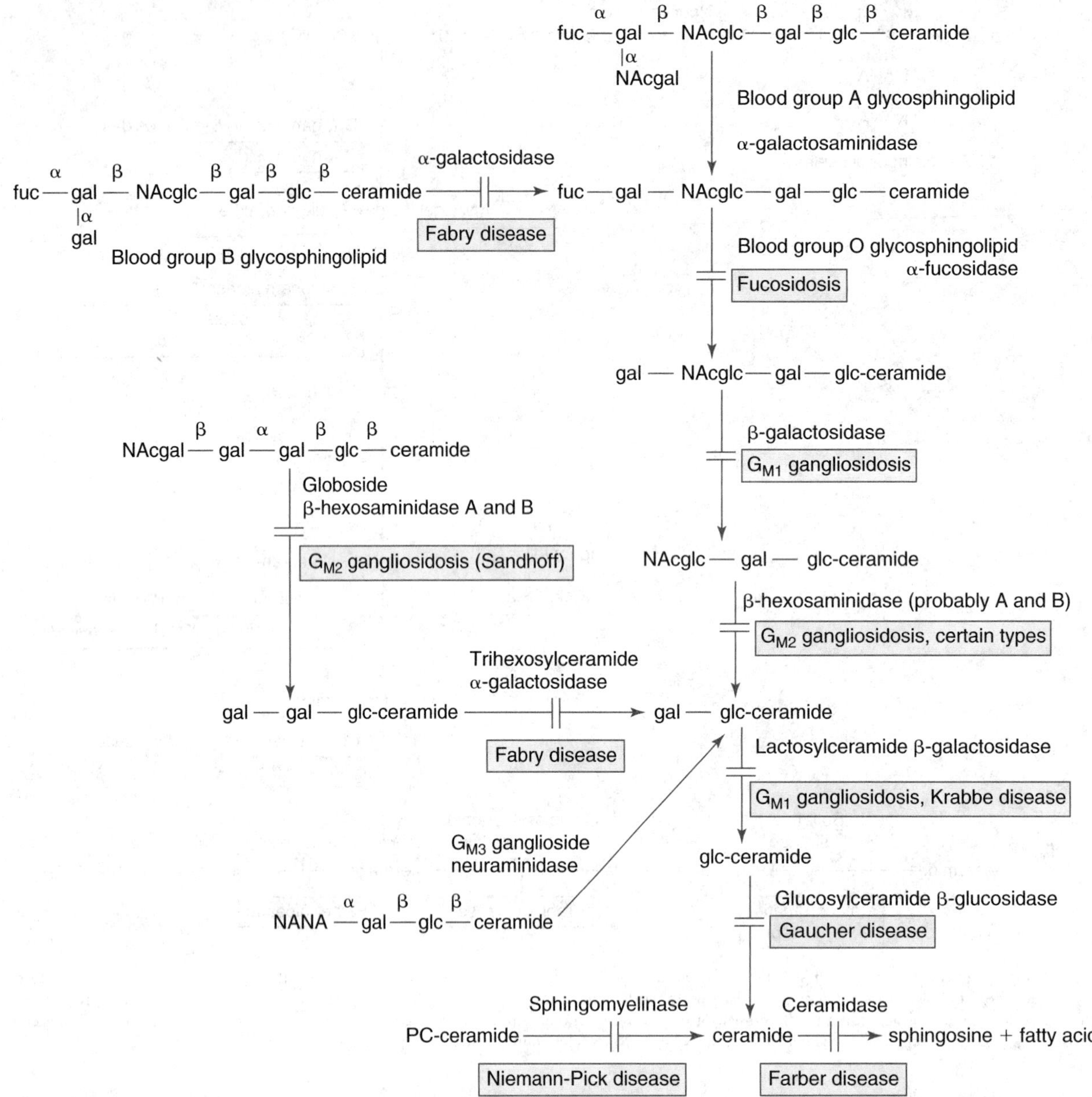

Figure 86-16. Pathways in the degradation of sphingolipids found in visceral organs and red or white blood cells. See also the legend for Figure 86-15. Fuc, fucose; NAcglc, N-acetylglucosamine.

juvenile or Norrbottnian form. All are autosomal recessive traits. Type 1, which accounts for 99% of cases, has a striking predilection for Ashkenazi Jews, with an incidence of about 1/1,000 and a carrier frequency of 1/18.

Gaucher disease results from the deficient activity of the lysosomal hydrolase, acid β-glucosidase, which is encoded by a gene located on chromosome 1q21-q31. The enzymatic defect results in the accumulation of undegraded glycolipid substrates, particularly glucosylceramide, in cells of the reticuloendothelial system. This progressive deposition results in infiltration of the bone marrow, progressive hepatosplenomegaly, and skeletal complications. Four mutations—N370S, L444P, 84insG, and IVS2—account for ≈95% of mutant alleles among Ashkenazi Jewish patients, permitting screening for this disorder in this population. Genotype-phenotype correlations have been noted, providing the molecular basis for the clinical heterogeneity seen in Gaucher disease type 1, which has a wide range of severity and age at onset. Patients who are homozygous for the N370S mutation tend to have later onset, with a more indolent course than patients with one copy of N370S and another common allele.

Clinical manifestations of type 1 Gaucher disease have a variable age at onset, from early childhood to late adulthood, with most symptomatic patients presenting by adolescence. At presentation, patients may have bruising from thrombocytopenia, chronic fatigue secondary to anemia, hepatomegaly with or without elevated liver function test results, splenomegaly, and bone pain. Occasional patients have pulmonary involvement at the time of presentation. Patients presenting in the 1st decade frequently are not Jewish and have growth retardation and a more malignant course. Other patients may be discovered fortuitously during evaluation for other conditions or as part of routine examinations; these patients may have a milder or even a benign course. In symptomatic patients, splenomegaly is progressive and can become massive. Most patients develop radiologic evidence of skeletal involvement, including an Erlenmeyer flask deformity of the distal femur. Clinically apparent bony involvement, which

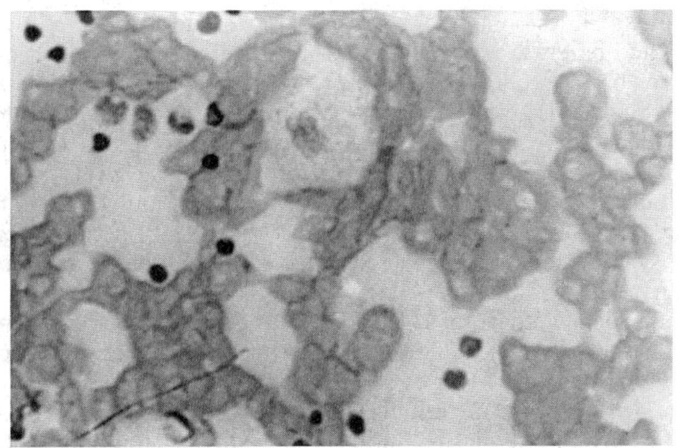

Figure 86-17. Cells from the spleen of a patient with Gaucher disease. A characteristic spleen cell is shown engorged with glucocerebroside.

occurs in >20% of patients, can present as bone pain or pathologic fractures. Lytic lesions can develop in the long bones, including the femur, ribs, and pelvis; osteosclerosis may be evident at an early age. Bone crises with severe pain and swelling can occur. Bleeding secondary to thrombocytopenia may manifest as epistaxis or bruising and is frequently overlooked until other symptoms become apparent. With the exception of the severely growth-retarded child, who may experience developmental delay secondary to the effects of chronic disease, development and intelligence are normal.

The pathologic hallmark of Gaucher disease is the Gaucher cell in the reticuloendothelial system, particularly in the bone marrow (Fig. 86-17). These cells, which are 20–100 µm in diameter, have a characteristic wrinkled paper appearance resulting from the presence of intracytoplasmic substrate inclusions. The cytoplasm of the Gaucher cell reacts strongly positively with the periodic acid–Schiff stain. The presence of this cell in bone marrow and tissue specimens is highly suggestive of Gaucher disease, although it also may be found in patients with granulocytic leukemia and myeloma.

Gaucher disease type 2 is much less common and does not have an ethnic predilection. It is characterized by a rapid neurodegenerative course with extensive visceral involvement and death within the 1st 2 yr of life. It presents in infancy with increased tone, strabismus, and organomegaly. Failure to thrive and stridor caused by laryngospasm are typical. After a several-year period of psychomotor regression, death occurs secondary to respiratory compromise. **Gaucher disease type 3** presents as clinical manifestations that are intermediate to those seen in types 1 and 2, with presentation in childhood and death by age 10–15 yr. It has a predilection for the Swedish Norrbottnian population, among which the incidence is 1/50,000. Neurologic involvement is present but occurs later and with decreased severity compared with type 2 disease. Type 3 disease is further classified as types 3a and 3b based on the extent of neurologic involvement and whether there is progressive myotonia and dementia (type 3a) or isolated supranuclear gaze palsy (type 3b).

Gaucher disease should be considered in the differential diagnosis of patients with unexplained organomegaly, who bruise easily, have bone pain, or have a combination of these conditions. Bone marrow examination usually reveals the presence of Gaucher cells. All suspected diagnoses should be confirmed by determination of the acid β-glucosidase activity in isolated leukocytes or cultured fibroblasts. The identification of carriers can be achieved by enzymatic assay, with confirmation of results by molecular testing in most Jewish families. Testing should be offered to all family members, keeping in mind that heterogeneity, even among members of the same kindred, can be so great that nonsymptomatic affected individuals may be diagnosed. Prenatal diagnosis is available by determination of enzyme activity in chorionic villi or cultured amniotic fluid cells.

Treatment of patients with Gaucher disease type 1 includes enzyme replacement therapy, with recombinant acid β-glucosidase (imiglucerase). Most extraskeletal symptoms (organomegaly, hematologic indices) are reversed by an initial debulking dose of enzyme (60 IU/kg) administered by intravenous infusion every other week. Monthly maintenance enzyme replacement improves bone structure, decreases bone pain, and induces compensatory growth in affected children. A small number of patients have undergone bone marrow transplantation, which is curative but results in significant morbidity and mortality from the procedure, making the selection of appropriate candidates limited. Although enzyme replacement does not alter the neurologic progression of patients with Gaucher disease types 2 and 3, it has been used in selected patients as a palliative measure, particularly in type 3 patients with severe visceral involvement. Alternative treatments, including the use of agents designed to decrease the synthesis of glucosylceramide by chemical inhibition of glucoslceramide synthase, are being evaluated and efforts are also under way to develop gene therapy for type 1 disease.

NEIMANN–PICK DISEASE (NPD). The original description of NPD was what is now known as type A NPD, a fatal disorder of infancy characterized by failure to thrive, hepatosplenomegaly, and a rapidly progressive neurodegenerative course that leads to death by 2–3 yr of age. Type B is a non-neuronopathic form observed in children and adults. Type C is a neuronopathic form that results from defective cholesterol transport. All the subtypes are inherited as autosomal recessive traits and display variable clinical features (see Table 86-16).

NPD types A and B result from the deficient activity of acid sphingomyelinase, a lysosomal enzyme encoded by a gene on chromosome 11 (11p15.1-p15.4). The enzymatic defect results in the pathologic accumulation of sphingomyelin, a ceramide phospholipid, and other lipids in the monocyte-macrophage system, the primary pathologic site. The progressive deposition of sphingomyelin in the central nervous system results in the neurodegenerative course seen in type A, and in non-neural tissue in the systemic disease manifestations of type B, including progressive lung disease in some patients. The acid sphingomyelinase gene is sequenced, and a variety of mutations that cause types A and B NPD are known.

The **clinical manifestations** and course of type A NPD is uniform and is characterized by a normal appearance at birth (although the newborn period is sometimes complicated by prolonged jaundice). Hepatosplenomegaly, moderate lymphadenopathy, and psychomotor retardation are evident by 6 mo of age, followed by neurodevelopmental regression and death by 3 yr. With advancing age, the loss of motor function and the deterioration of intellectual capabilities are progressively debilitating; and in later stages, spasticity and rigidity are evident. Affected infants lose contact with their environment. In contrast to the stereotyped type A phenotype, the clinical presentation and course of patients with type B disease are more variable. Most are diagnosed in infancy or childhood when enlargement of the liver or spleen, or both, is detected during a routine physical examination. At diagnosis, type B NPD patients usually have evidence of mild pulmonary involvement, usually detected as a diffuse reticular or finely nodular infiltration on the chest radiograph. **Pulmonary symptoms** usually present in adults. In most patients, hepatosplenomegaly is particularly prominent in childhood, but with increasing linear growth, the abdominal protuberance decreases and becomes less conspicuous. In mildly affected patients, the splenomegaly may not be noted until adulthood, and there may be minimal disease manifestations.

In some type B patients, decreased pulmonary diffusion caused by alveolar infiltration becomes evident in late childhood or early adulthood and progresses with age. Severely affected individuals may experience significant pulmonary compromise by 15–20 yr of age. Such patients have low PO_2 values and dyspnea on exertion. Life-threatening bronchopneumonias may occur, and cor pulmonale has been described. Severely affected patients may have liver involvement leading to life-threatening cirrhosis, portal hypertension, and ascites. Clinically significant pancytopenia due to secondary **hypersplenism** may require partial or complete splenectomy; this should be avoided if possible because splenectomy frequently causes progression of pulmonary disease, which can be life-threatening. In general, type B patients do not have neurologic involvement and have a normal IQ. Some patients with type B disease have cherry red maculae or haloes and subtle neurologic symptoms (peripheral neuropathy).

Type C NPD patients often present with prolonged neonatal jaundice, appear normal for 1–2 yr, and then experience a slowly progressive and variable neurodegenerative course. Their hepatosplenomegaly is less severe than that of patients with types A or B NPD, and they may survive into adulthood. The underlying biochemical defect in type C patients is an abnormality in cholesterol transport, leading to the accumulation of sphingomyelin and cholesterol in their lysosomes and a secondary partial reduction in acid sphingomyelinase activity (see Chapter 86.3).

In type B NPD patients, splenomegaly is usually the 1st manifestation detected. The splenic enlargement is noted in early childhood; however, in very mild disease, the enlargement may be subtle and detection may be delayed until adolescence or adulthood. The presence of the characteristic NPD cells in the bone marrow aspirates supports the diagnosis of type B NPD. Patients with type C NPD, however, also have extensive infiltration of NPD cells in the bone marrow and, thus, all suspected cases should be evaluated enzymatically to confirm the clinical diagnosis by measuring the acid sphingomyelinase activity level in peripheral leukocytes, cultured fibroblasts, or lymphoblasts, or a combination of these cells. Patients with types A and B NPD have markedly decreased levels (1–10%), whereas patients with type C NPD have somewhat decreased acid sphingomyelinase activities. The enzymatic identification of NPD carriers is problematic. In families in which the specific molecular lesion has been identified, however, family members can be accurately tested for heterozygote status by DNA analysis. Prenatal diagnosis of types A and B NPD can be made reliably by the measurement of acid sphingomyelinase activity in cultured amniocytes or chorionic villi; molecular analysis of fetal cells can provide the specific diagnosis or serve as a confirmatory test. The clinical diagnosis of type C NPD can be supported by the demonstration of filipin stain positivity in cultured fibroblasts and/or by identifying a specific mutation in the *NPC* gene.

There is no specific **treatment** for NPD. Orthotopic liver transplantation in an infant with type A disease and amniotic cell transplantation in several type B NPD patients have been attempted with little or no success. Bone marrow transplantation in a small number of type B NPD patients has been shown to be successful in reducing the spleen and liver volumes, the sphingomyelin content of the liver, the number of Niemann-Pick cells in the marrow, and radiologically detected infiltration of the lungs. In one patient, however, liver biopsies taken up to 33 mo post transplantation showed only a moderate reduction in stored sphingomyelin. To date, lung transplantation has not been performed in any severely compromised patient with type B disease, although two patients who underwent whole lung lavages with variable results have been reported.

Future prospects for treatment of type B disease include enzyme replacement and gene therapy. Treatment of types A and C disease is presently precluded by the severe neurologic involvement.

FABRY DISEASE. This condition is an inborn error of glycosphingolipid metabolism characterized by angiokeratomas (telangiectatic skin lesions), hypohidrosis, corneal and lenticular opacities, acroparesthesias, and vascular disease of the kidney, heart, and/or brain (see Table 86-16). The disease is an X-linked recessive trait that is manifested in affected males and has an estimated prevalence of ≈1/40,000 males. Later-onset affected males with residual α-galactosidase A activity may present with cardiac and/or renal disease including hypertrophic cardiomyopathy and renal failure. Heterozygous females for the classic phenotype can be asymptomatic or as severely affected as the males, the variability due to random X-inactivation. The disease results from the deficient activity of α-galactosidase A, a lysosomal enzyme encoded by a gene located on the long arm of the X chromosome (Xq22). The enzymatic defect leads to the systemic accumulation of neutral glycosphingolipids, primarily globotriaosylceramide, particularly in the plasma and lysosomes of vascular endothelial and smooth muscle cells. The progressive vascular glycosphingolipid deposition in affected males results in ischemia and infarction, leading to the major disease manifestations. The cDNA and genomic sequences encoding α-galactosidase A have identified more than 200 different mutations in the α-galactosidase A gene that are responsible for this lysosomal storage disease, including amino acid substitutions, gene rearrangements, and mRNA splicing defects.

Affected males with the classic phenotype have the skin lesions, acroparesthesias, hypohidrosis, and ocular changes, whereas males with the later onset phenotypes lack these findings and present with cardiac and/or renal disease in adulthood. The classic **angiokeratomas** usually occur in childhood and may lead to early diagnosis. They increase in size and number with age and range from barely visible to several mm in diameter. The lesions are punctate, dark red to blue-black, and flat or slightly raised. They do not blanch with pressure, and the larger ones may show slight hyperkeratosis. Characteristically, the lesions are most dense between the umbilicus and knees, in the "bathing trunk area," but may occur anywhere, including the oral mucosa. The hips, thighs, buttocks, umbilicus, lower abdomen, scrotum, and glans penis are common sites, and there is a tendency toward symmetry. Variants without skin lesions have been described. Sweating is usually decreased or absent. Corneal opacities and characteristic lenticular lesions, observed under slit-lamp examination, are present in affected males as well as in ≈70% of asymptomatic heterozygotes. Conjunctival and retinal vascular tortuosity is common and results from the systemic vascular involvement.

Pain is the most debilitating symptom in childhood and adolescence. **Fabry crises**, lasting from minutes to several days, consist of agonizing, burning pain in the hands, feet, and proximal extremities and are usually associated with exercise, fatigue, fever, or a combination of these factors. These painful acroparesthesias usually become less frequent in the 3rd and 4th decades of life, although in some men, they may become more frequent and severe. Attacks of abdominal or flank pain may simulate appendicitis or renal colic.

The major morbid symptoms result from the progressive involvement of the vascular system. Early in the course of the disease, casts, red cells, and lipid inclusions with characteristic birefringent "Maltese crosses" appear in the urinary sediment. Proteinuria, isosthenuria, and gradual deterioration of renal function and development of azotemia occur in the 2nd through 4th decades. Cardiovascular findings may include hypertension, left ventricular hypertrophy, anginal chest pain, myocardial ischemia or infarction, and heart failure. Mitral insufficiency is the most common valvular lesion. Abnormal electrocardiographic and echocardiographic findings are common. Cerebrovascular manifestations result from multifocal small vessel involvement. Other features may include chronic bronchitis and dyspnea, lymphedema of the legs without hypoproteinemia, episodic diarrhea, osteoporosis, retarded growth, and delayed puberty. Death most often results from uremia or vascular disease of the heart or brain.

Before hemodialysis or renal transplantation, the mean age at death for affected men was 41 yr. Later onset cardiac variants with residual α-galactosidase A activity have cardiac disease and may have mild proteinuria but usually have normal renal function for age. The cardiac manifestations include hypertrophy of the left ventricular wall and interventricular septum, and electrocardiographic abnormalities consistent with cardiomyopathy. Others have had hypertrophic cardiomyopathy or myocardial infarction, or both.

The **diagnosis** in classically affected males is most readily made from the history of painful acroparesthesias, hypohidrosis, the presence of characteristic skin lesions, and the observation of the characteristic corneal opacities and lenticular lesions. The disorder is often misdiagnosed as rheumatic fever, erythromelalgia, or neurosis. The skin lesions must be differentiated from the benign angiokeratomas of the scrotum (Fordyce disease) or from angiokeratoma circumscriptum. **Angiokeratomas** identical to those of Fabry disease have been reported in fucosidosis, aspartylglycosaminuria, late-onset GM_1 gangliosidosis, galactosialidosis, α-N-acetylgalactosaminidase deficiency, and sialidosis. Later onset variants have been identified among chronic hemodialysis patients. Like the cardiac variants, these renal variants lack the early classic manifestations such as the angiokeratomas, acroparesthesias, hypohidrosis, and corneal opacities. The diagnosis of classic and variant patients is confirmed biochemically by the demonstration of markedly decreased α-galactosidase A activity in plasma, isolated leukocytes, or cultured fibroblasts or lymphoblasts.

Heterozygous females may have corneal opacities, isolated skin lesions, and intermediate activities of α-galactosidase A in plasma or cells. Rare female heterozygotes may have manifestations as severe as those in affected males. Asymptomatic at-risk females in families affected by Fabry disease, however, should be optimally diagnosed by the direct analysis of their family's specific mutation. Prenatal detection of affected males can be accomplished by the demonstration of deficient α-galactosidase A activity or the family's specific gene mutation in chorionic villi obtained in the 1st trimester or in cultured amniocytes obtained by amniocentesis in the 2nd trimester of pregnancy. Fabry disease can potentially be detected by newborn screening.

Treatment for Fabry disease was once nonspecific and limited to supportive care, which included the use of phenytoin and/or carbamazepine to decrease the frequency and severity of the chronic acroparesthesias and the periodic crises of excruciating pain. Renal transplantation and long-term hemodialysis are lifesaving procedures for patients with renal failure. Recombinant α-galactosidase (Fabrazyme, Genzyme Corporation, Cambridge, MA; Replagal, TKT Corporation, Cambridge, MA) is a safe and effective enzyme replacement therapy for Fabry disease at a dose of 1mg/kg every other week.

FUCOSIDOSIS. This is a rare autosomal recessive disorder caused by the deficient activity of α-fucosidase and the accumulation of fucose-containing glycosphingolipids, glycoproteins, and oligosaccharides in the lysosomes of the liver, brain, and other organs (see Table 86-16). The α-fucosidase gene is on chromosome 1 (1p24), and specific mutations are known. Although the disorder is panethnic, most affected patients are from Italy and the United States. There is wide variability in the clinical phenotype, with the most severely affected patients presenting in the 1st yr of life with developmental delay and somatic features similar to those of the mucopolysaccharidoses. These features include frontal bossing, hepatosplenomegaly, coarse facial features, and macroglossia. The central nervous system storage results in a relentless neurodegenerative course, with death in childhood. Patients with milder disease have angiokeratomas and longer survival. No specific therapy exists for the disorder, which can be diagnosed by the demonstration of deficient α-fucosidase activity in peripheral leukocytes or cultured fibroblasts. Carrier identification studies and prenatal diagnosis are possible by determination of the enzymatic activity.

SCHINDLER DISEASE. This is an autosomal recessive neurodegenerative disorder that results from the deficient activity of α-N-acetylgalactosaminidase and the accumulation of sialylated and asialoglycopeptides and oligosaccharides (see Table 86-16). The gene for the enzyme is mapped to chromosome 22 (22q13.1–13.2). The disease is clinically heterogeneous, and two major phenotypes have been identified. Type I disease is an infantile-onset neuroaxonal dystrophy. Affected infants have normal development for the 1st 9–15 mo of life followed by a rapid neurodegenerative course that results in severe psychomotor retardation, cortical blindness, and frequent myoclonic seizures. Type II disease is characterized by a variable age at onset, mild retardation, and angiokeratomas. There is no specific therapy for either form of the disorder. The diagnosis is by demonstration of the enzymatic deficiency in leukocytes or cultured skin fibroblasts.

METACHROMATIC LEUKODYSTROPHY (MLD). This is an autosomal recessive white matter disease caused by a deficiency of arylsulfatase A (ASA), which is required for the hydrolysis of sulfated glycosphingolipids. Another form of MLD is caused by a deficiency of a sphingolipid activator protein (SAP1), which is required for the formation of the substrate-enzyme complex. The deficiency of this enzymatic activity results in the white matter storage of sulfated glycosphingolipids, which leads to **demyelination** and a **neurodegenerative** course. The ASA gene is on chromosome 22 (22q13.31qter); specific mutations are known to fall into two groups that correlate with disease severity.

The **clinical manifestations** of the late **infantile** form of MLD, which is most common, usually presents between 12 and 18 mo of age as irritability, inability to walk, and hyperextension of the knee, causing genu recurvatum. Deep tendon reflexes are diminished or absent. Gradual muscle wasting, weakness, and hypotonia become evident and lead to a debilitated state. As the disease progresses, nystagmus, myoclonic seizures, optic atrophy, and quadriparesis appear, with death in the 1st decade of life (see Table 86-16). The **juvenile** form of the disorder has a more indolent course with onset that may occur as late as 20 yr of age. This form of the disease presents as gait disturbances, mental deterioration, urinary incontinence, and emotional difficulties. The **adult** form, which presents after the 2nd decade, is similar to the juvenile form in its clinical manifestations, although emotional difficulties and psychosis are more prominent features. Dementia, seizures, diminished reflexes, and optic atrophy also occur in both the juvenile and adult forms. The pathologic hallmark of MLD is the deposition of metachromatic bodies, which stain strongly positive with periodic acid–Schiff and alcian blue, in the white matter of the brain. Neuronal inclusions may be seen in the midbrain, pons, medulla, retina, and spinal cord; demyelination occurs in the peripheral nervous system. Bone marrow transplantation has resulted in normal enzymatic levels in peripheral blood but no clear evidence for clinical efficacy in terms of the neurologic course; supportive care remains the primary intervention.

The **diagnosis** of MLD should be suspected in patients with the clinical features of leukodystrophy. Decreased nerve conduction velocities, increased cerebrospinal fluid protein, metachromatic deposits in sampled segments of sural nerve, and metachromatic granules in urinary sediment are all suggestive of MLD. Confirmation of the diagnosis is based on the demonstration of the reduced activity of ASA in leukocytes or cultured skin fibroblasts. Sphingolipid activator protein deficiency is diagnosed by measuring the concentration of SAP1 in cultured fibroblasts using a specific antibody to the protein. Carrier detection and prenatal diagnosis is available for all forms of the disorder.

MULTIPLE SULFATASE DEFICIENCY. This is an autosomal recessive disorder that results from the deficiency of three enzymatic activities: arylsulfatases A, B, and C. Sulfatides, mucopolysaccharides, steroid sulfates, and gangliosides accumulate in the cerebral cortex and visceral tissues, resulting in a clinical phenotype with features of **leukodystrophy** as well as those of the **mucopolysaccharidoses.** Severe **ichthyosis** may also occur. Carrier testing and prenatal diagnosis by measurement of the enzymatic activities can be performed. There is no specific treatment for multiple sulfatase deficiency other than supportive care.

KRABBE DISEASE. This condition, also called globoid cell leukodystrophy, is an autosomal recessive fatal disorder of infancy. It results from the deficiency of the enzymatic activity of galactocerebrosidase and the white matter accumulation of galactosylceramide, which is normally found almost exclusively in the myelin sheath. The galactocerebrosidase gene is on chromosome 14 (14q31), and specific disease-causing mutations are known. The **infantile** form of Krabbe disease is rapidly progressive and patients present in early infancy with irritability, seizures, and hypertonia (see Table 86-16). Optic atrophy is evident in the 1st yr of life, and mental development is severely impaired. As the disease progresses, optic atrophy and severe developmental delay become apparent; affected children exhibit opisthotonos and die before 3 yr of age. A second, **late infantile** form of Krabbe disease also exists and patients present after the age of 2 yr. Affected individuals have a disease course similar to that of the early infantile form. Bone marrow transplantation has been attempted in several patients with later onset disease but without significant results. Umbilical cord blood transplantation of presymptomatic patients in the 1st 2 mo of life results in engraftment and normal blood galactocerebrosidase levels. Developmental milestones, cerebral myelination, and cognitive function up to 3 yr of age have been near age-appropriate expectations. Nonetheless, some patients demonstrate mild to moderate language delays and mild to severe gross motor delays. The diagnosis of Krabbe disease relies on the demonstration of the specific enzymatic deficiency in white blood cells or cultured skin fibroblasts. Carrier identification and prenatal diagnosis are available.

FARBER DISEASE. This is an autosomal recessive disorder that results from the deficiency of the lysosomal enzyme ceramidase and the accumulation of ceramide in various tissues, especially the joints. Symptoms can begin as early as the 1st yr of life with painful joint swelling and nodule formation (Fig. 86-18), which is sometimes diagnosed as rheumatoid arthritis. As the disease progresses, nodule or granulomatous formation on the vocal cords can lead to hoarseness and breathing difficulties; failure to thrive is common. In some patients, moderate central nervous system dysfunction is present (see Table 86-16). Patients may die of recurrent pneumonias in their teens; there is currently no specific therapy. The diagnosis of this disorder should be suspected in patients who have nodule formation over the joints but no other findings of rheumatoid arthritis. In such patients, ceramidase activity should be determined in cultured skin fibroblasts or white blood cells. Carrier detection and prenatal diagnosis are available.

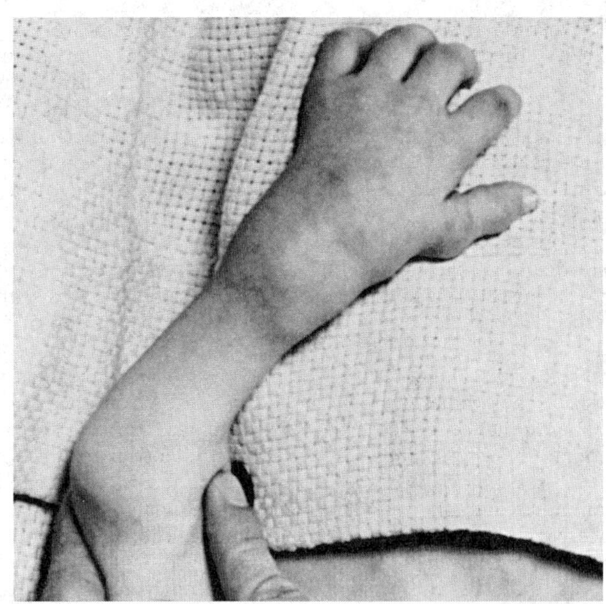

Figure 86-18. Forearm of an 18 mo old girl with Farber disease. Note the painful joint swelling and the nodule formation. The infant was suspected of having rheumatoid arthritis.

WOLMAN DISEASE AND CHOLESTEROL ESTER STORAGE DISEASE (CESD). These are autosomal recessive lysosomal storage diseases that result from the deficiency of acid lipase and the accumulation of cholesterol esters and triglycerides in histiocytic foam cells of most visceral organs. The gene for lysosomal acid lipase is on chromosome 10 (10q24-q25). Wolman disease is the more severe clinical phenotype and is a fatal disorder of infancy. The clinical features of the disease become apparent in the 1st wk of life and include failure to thrive, relentless vomiting, abdominal distention, steatorrhea, and hepatosplenomegaly (see Table 86-16). There usually is hyperlipidemia. Hepatic dysfunction and fibrosis may occur. **Calcification of the adrenal glands** is pathognomonic for the disorder. Death usually occurs within 6 mo.

Cholesterol ester storage disease is a less severe disorder that may not be diagnosed until adulthood. Hepatomegaly can be the only detectable abnormality, but affected individuals are at significant risk for premature atherosclerosis. Adrenal calcification is not a feature.

Diagnosis and carrier identification are based on measuring acid lipase activity in leukocytes or cultured skin fibroblasts. Prenatal diagnosis depends on measuring decreased enzyme levels in cultured chorionic villi or amniocytes. There is no specific therapy available for either disorder, although pharmacologic agents to suppress cholesterol synthesis, in combination with cholestyramine and diet modification, have been used in patients with cholesterol ester storage disease (see Chapter 86.3).

Charrow J, Anderson HC, Kaplan P, et al: Enzyme replacement therapy and monitoring for children with type 1 Gaucher disease: Consensus recommendations. *J Pediatr* 2004;144:112–120.

Clark JTR: Narrative review: Fabry disease. *Ann Intern Med* 2007;146: 425–433.

Desnick RJ, Brady R, Barranger J, et al: Fabry disease, an under-recognized multi-systemic disorder: Expert recommendations for diagnosis, management, and enzyme replacement therapy. *Ann Intern Med* 2003;138: 338–346.

Elstein D, Abrahamov A, Hadas-Halpern I, et al: Gaucher's disease. *Lancet* 2001;358:324–337.

Escolar ML, Poe MD, Provenzale JM, et al: Transplantation of umbilical-cord blood in babies with infantile Krabbe's disease. *N Engl J Med* 2005;20:2069–2080.

Johnson WG: The clinical spectrum of hexosaminidase deficiency diseases. *Neurology* 1981;31:1453–1456.

Kaplan P, Anderson HC, Kacena KA, Yee JD: the clinical and demographic characteristics of nonneuronpathic Gaucher disease in 887 children at diagnosis. *Arch Pediatr Adolesc Med* 2006;160:603–608.

Meikle PJ, Ranieri E, Simonsen H, et al: Newborn screening for lysosomal storage disorders: Clinical evaluation of a two-tier strategy. *Pediatrics* 2004;114:909–916.

Mistry PK, Abrahamov A: A practical approach to diagnosis and management of Gaucher's disease. *Baillieres Clin Haematol* 1997;10:817–838.

Schuchman EH, Desnick RJ: Types A and B Niemann Pick disease. In Scriver CR, Beaudet AL, Sly WS, et al (eds): *The Metabolic and Molecular Bases of Inherited Disease,* 8th ed. New York, McGraw-Hill, 2001.

Wilcox WR, Banikazemi M, Guffon N, et al: Long-term safety and efficacy of enzyme replacement therapy for Fabry disease. *Am J Hum Genet* 2004;75:65–74.

86.5 • Mucolipidoses • Margaret M. McGovern and Robert J. Desnick

I-cell disease (mucolipidosis II [ML-II]) and **pseudo-Hurler polydystrophy (mucolipidosis III [ML-III])** are biochemically related, rare autosomal recessive disorders that share some clinical features with Hurler syndrome. These diseases result from the abnormal transport of newly synthesized lysosomal enzymes that are normally targeted to the lysosome by the presence of mannose-6-phosphate residues and are recognized by specific lysosomal membrane receptors. These mannose-6-phosphate recognition markers are synthesized in a two-step reaction that occurs in the Golgi apparatus and is mediated by two enzymatic activities. The enzyme that catalyzes the 1st step, the UDP-N-acetylglucosamine : lysosomal enzyme *N*-acetylglucosamine-1-phosphotransferase, is defective in both ML-II and ML-III. This enzyme deficiency results in abnormal targeting of the lysosomal enzymes that are then secreted into the extracellular matrix. Because the lysosomal enzymes require the acidic medium of the lysosome to function, patients with this defect accumulate a variety of different substrates due to the cellular deficiency of all lysosomal enzymes. The diagnosis of ML-II and ML-III can be made by the determination of the serum lysosomal enzymatic activities, which are elevated, or by the demonstration of reduced enzymatic levels in cultured skin fibroblasts. Direct measurement of the phosphotransferase activity is possible. Prenatal diagnosis and carrier identification studies are available for both disorders by measurement of lysosomal enzymatic activities in cultured cells. Neonatal screening by tandem mass spectroscopy may detect I-cell disease.

I-CELL DISEASE. This disorder shares many of the clinical manifestations of Hurler syndrome, although there is no mucopolysacchariduria and the presentation is earlier (see Table 86-16). Some patients have clinical features evident at birth, including coarse facial features, craniofacial abnormalities, restricted joint movement, and hypotonia. Nonimmune hydrops may be present in the fetus. The remainder of patients present in the 1st yr with severe psychomotor retardation, coarse facial features, and skeletal manifestations that include kyphoscoliosis and a lumbar gibbus. Patients may also have congenital dislocation of the hips, inguinal hernias, and gingival hypertrophy. Progressive, severe psychomotor retardation leads to death in early childhood. No treatment is available.

PSEUDO-HURLER POLYDYSTROPHY. Pseudo-Hurler polydystrophy is a less severe disorder than I-cell disease, with later onset and survival to adulthood reported. Affected children may present around the age of 4 or 5 yr with joint stiffness and short stature. Progressive destruction of the hip joints and moderate dysostosis multiplex are evident. Radiographic evidence of low iliac wings, flattening of the proximal femoral epiphyses with valgus deformity of the femoral head, and hypoplasia of the anterior third of the lumbar vertebrae are characteristic findings. Ophthalmic findings include corneal clouding, retinopathy, and astigmatism; visual complaints are uncommon (see Table 86-16). Some patients have learning disabilities or mental retardation. Treatment, which should include orthopedic care, is symptomatic.

Chapter 87 ■ Defects in Metabolism of Carbohydrates Priya S. Kishnani and Yuan-Tsong Chen

Carbohydrate synthesis and degradation provide the energy required for most metabolic processes. The important carbohydrates include three monosaccharides—glucose, galactose, and fructose—and a polysaccharide, glycogen. The relevant biochemical pathways of these carbohydrates are shown in Figure 87-1. Glucose is the principal substrate of energy metabolism. A continuous source of glucose from dietary intake, gluconeogenesis, and glycogenolysis of glycogen maintains normal blood glucose levels. Metabolism of glucose generates adenosine triphosphate (ATP) via glycolysis (conversion of glucose or glycogen to pyruvate), mitochondrial oxidative phosphorylation (conversion of pyruvate to carbon dioxide and water), or both. Dietary sources of glucose come from ingesting polysaccharides, primarily starch and disaccharides, including lactose, maltose, and sucrose. Oral intake of glucose is intermittent and unreliable. Glucose made de novo from amino acids, primarily alanine (gluconeogenesis) contributes to maintaining the euglycemic state, but this process requires time to be active. The breakdown of hepatic glycogen provides the rapid release of glucose, which maintains a constant blood glucose concentration. Glycogen is also the primary stored energy source in muscle, providing glucose for muscle activity during exercise. Galactose and fructose are monosaccharides that provide fuel for cellular metabolism; their role is less significant than that of glucose. Galactose is derived from lactose (galactose + glucose), which is found in milk and milk products. Galactose is an important energy source in infants, but it is 1st metabolized to glucose. Galactose (exogenous or endogenously synthesized from glucose) is also an important component for certain glycolipids, glycoproteins, and glycosaminoglycans. The dietary sources of fructose are sucrose (fructose + glucose, sorbitol) and fructose itself, which is found in fruits, vegetables, and honey.

Defects in glycogen metabolism typically cause an accumulation of glycogen in the tissues, hence the name *glycogen storage disease* (Table 87-1). Defects in gluconeogenesis or the glycolytic pathway, including galactose and fructose metabolism, do not result in an accumulation of glycogen (see Table 87-1). The defects in pyruvate metabolism in the pathway of the conversion of pyruvate to carbon dioxide and water via mitochondrial oxidative phosphorylation are more often associated with lactic acidosis and some tissue glycogen accumulation.

87.1 • Glycogen Storage Diseases • Priya S. Kishnani and Yuan-Tsong Chen

The disorders of glycogen metabolism, the glycogen storage diseases (GSDs), result from deficiencies of various enzymes or transport proteins in the pathways of glycogen metabolism (see Fig. 87-1). The glycogen found in these disorders is abnormal in quantity, quality, or both. GSDs are categorized by numeric type in accordance with the chronologic order in which these enzymatic defects were identified. This numeric classification is still widely used, at least up to number VII. The glycogen storage diseases can also be classified by organ involvement and clinical manifestations into liver and muscle glycogenoses (see Table 87-1).

There are more than 12 forms of glycogenoses. Glucose-6-phosphatase deficiency (type I), lysosomal acid α-glucosidase deficiency (type II), debrancher deficiency (type III), and liver

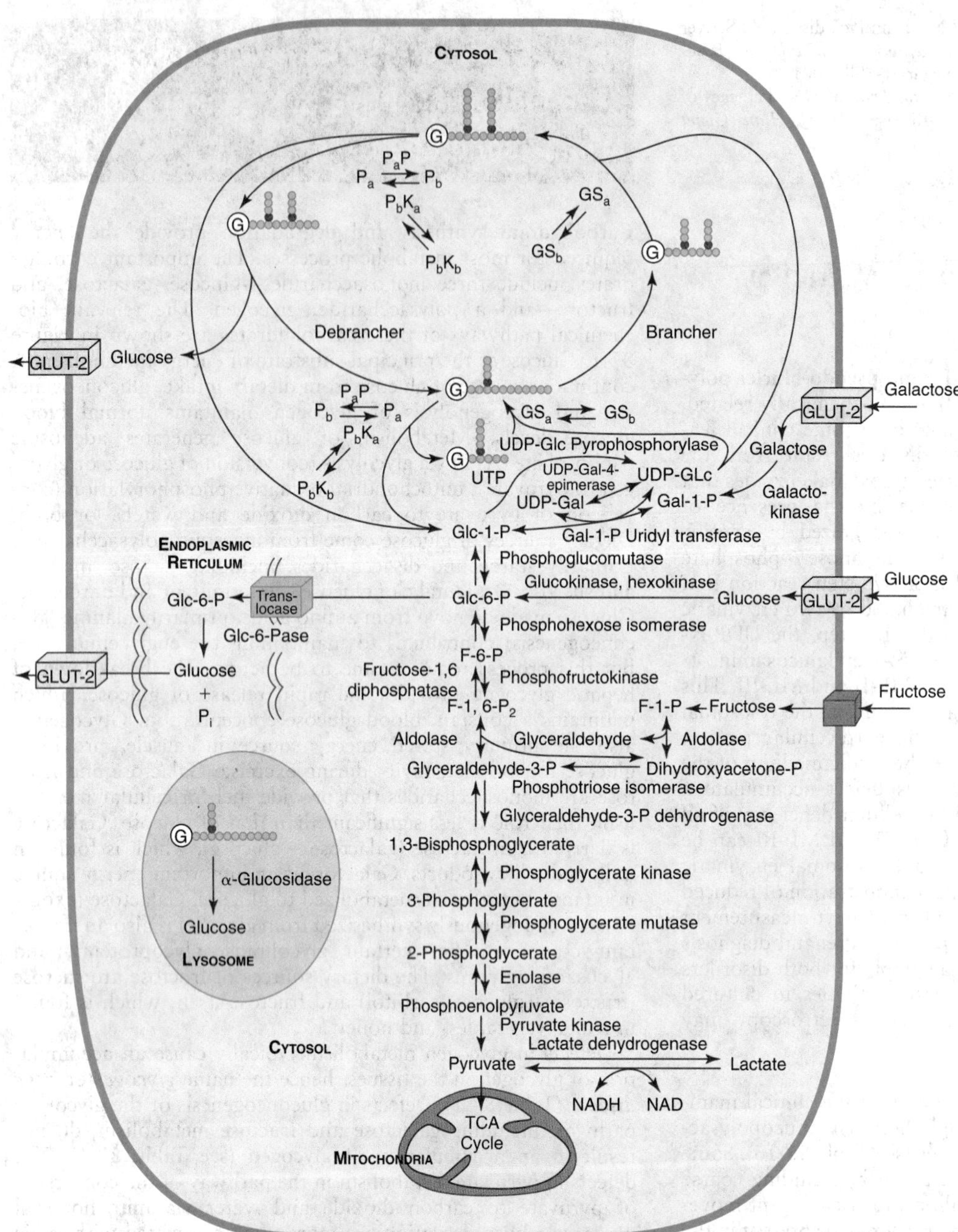

Figure 87-1. Pathway related to glycogen storage diseases and galactose and fructose disorders. GSa, active glycogen synthetase; GSb, inactive glycogen synthetase; Pa, active phosphorylase; Pb, inactive phosphorylase; PaP, phosphorylase a phosphatase; PbKa, active phosphorylase b kinase; PbKb, inactive phosphorylase b kinase; G, glycogen, the primer for glycogen synthesis; UDP, uridine diphosphate; GLUT-2, glucose transporter 2; NAD/NADH, nicotinamide-adenine dinucleotide. (Modified from Beaudet AR: Glycogen storage disease. In Isselbacher KJ, et al [eds]: *Harrison's Principles of Internal Medicine,* 13th ed. New York, McGraw-Hill, 1994. Reproduced with permission of The McGraw-Hill Companies.)

phosphorylase kinase deficiency (type IX) are the most common that typically present in early childhood; myophosphorylase deficiency (type V, McArdle disease) is the most common in adolescents and adults. The frequency of all forms of GSD is ≈1/20,000 live births.

LIVER GLYCOGENOSES

The GSDs that principally affect the liver include glucose-6-phosphatase deficiency (type I), debranching enzyme deficiency (type III), branching enzyme deficiency (type IV), liver phosphorylase deficiency (type VI), phosphorylase kinase deficiency (type IX, formerly termed GSD VIa), glycogen synthetase deficiency (type 0), and glucose transporter-2 defect. Because hepatic carbohydrate metabolism is responsible for plasma glucose homeostasis, this group of disorders typically causes fasting hypoglycemia and hepatomegaly. Some (type III, type IV, type IX) can be associated with cirrhosis. Other organs can also be involved and may manifest as renal dysfunction in type I and myopathy (skeletal and/or cardiomyopathy) in types III and IV, as well as in some rare forms of phosphorylase kinase deficiency.

TYPE I GLYCOGEN STORAGE DISEASE (GLUCOSE-6-PHOSPHATASE OR TRANSLOCASE DEFICIENCY, VON GIERKE DISEASE). Type I GSD is caused by the absence or deficiency of glucose-6-phosphatase activity in the liver, kidney, and intestinal mucosa. It can be divided into two subtypes: type Ia, in which the glucose-6-phosphatase enzyme is defective; and type Ib, in which a translocase that transports glucose-6-phosphate across the microsomal membrane is defective. The defects in both type Ia and type Ib lead to inadequate hepatic conversion of glucose-6-phosphate to glucose through normal glycogenolysis and gluconeogenesis and make affected individuals susceptible to fasting hypoglycemia.

Type I GSD is an autosomal recessive disorder. The structural gene for glucose-6-phosphatase is located on chromosome 17q21; the gene for translocase is on chromosome 11q23. Common mutations responsible for the disease are known. Carrier detec-

TABLE 87-1. Features of the Disorders of Carbohydrate Metabolism

DISORDERS	BASIC DEFECTS	CLINICAL PRESENTATION	COMMENTS
LIVER GLYCOGENOSES			
Type/Common Name			
Ia/Von Gierke	Glucose-6-phosphatase	Growth retardation, hepatomegaly, hypoglycemia; elevated blood lactate, cholesterol, triglyceride, and uric acid levels	Common, severe hypoglycemia
Ib	Glucose-6-phosphate translocase	Same as type Ia, with additional findings of neutropenia and impaired neutrophil function	10% of type Ia
IIIa/Cori or Forbes	Liver and muscle debrancher deficiency (amylo, 1, 6 glucosidase)	Childhood: hepatomegaly, growth retardation, muscle weakness, hypoglycemia, hyperlipidemia, elevated transaminase levels; liver symptoms improve with age	Common, intermediate severity of hypoglycemia
IIIb	Liver debrancher deficiency; normal muscle enzyme activity	Liver symptoms same as in type IIIa; no muscle symptoms	15% of type III
IV/Andersen	Branching enzyme	Failure to thrive, hypotonia, hepatomegaly, splenomegaly, progressive cirrhosis (death usually before 5th yr), elevated transaminase levels	Rare neuromuscular variants exist
VI/Hers	Liver phosphorylase	Hepatomegaly, mild hypoglycemia, hyperlipidemia, and ketosis	Rare, benign glycogenosis
Phosphorylase kinase deficiency	Phosphorylase kinase	Hepatomegaly, mild hypoglycemia, hyperlipidemia, and ketosis	Common, benign glycogenosis
Glycogen synthetase deficiency	Glycogen synthetase	Early morning drowsiness and fatigue, fasting hypoglycemia, and ketosis	Decreased liver glycogen store
Fanconi-Bickel syndrome	Glucose transporter 2 (GLUT-2)	Failure to thrive, rickets, hepatorenomegaly, proximal renal tubular dysfunction, impaired glucose and galactose utilization	GLUT-2 expressed in liver, kidney, pancreas, and intestine
MUSCLE GLYCOGENOSES			
Type/Common Name			
II/Pompe Infantile	Acid α-glucosidase (acid maltase)	Cardiomegaly, hypotonia, hepatomegaly; onset: birth–6 mo	Common, cardiorespiratory failure leading to death by age 2 yr
Juvenile	Acid α-glucosidase (acid maltase)	Myopathy, variable cardiomyopathy; onset: childhood	Residual enzyme activity
Adult	Acid α-glucosidase (acid maltase)	Myopathy, respiratory insufficiency; onset: adulthood	Residual enzyme activity
Danon disease	Lysosome-associated membrane protein 2 (LAMP2)	Hypertrophic cardiomyopathy	Rare, X-linked
PRKAG2 deficiency	AMP-activated protein kinase γ	Hypertrophic cardiomyopathy	Autosomal dominant
V/McArdle	Myophosphorylase	Exercise intolerance, muscle cramps, increased fatigability	Common, male predominance
VII/Tarui	Phosphofructokinase	Exercise intolerance, muscle cramps, hemolytic anemia, myoglobinuria	Prevalent in Japanese and Ashkenazi Jews
Phosphoglycerate kinase deficiency	Phosphoglycerate kinase	As with type V	Rare, X-linked
Phosphoglycerate mutase deficiency	M subunite of phosphoglycerate mutase	As with type V	Rare, majority of patients are African-American
Lactate dehydrogenase deficiency	M subunit of lactate dehydrogenase	As with type V	Rare
GALACTOSE DISORDERS			
Galactosemia with transferase deficiency	Galactose-1-phosphate uridyltransferase	Vomiting, hepatomegaly, cataracts, aminoaciduria, failure to thrive	African-American patients tend to have milder symptoms
Galactokinase deficiency	Galactokinase	Cataracts	Benign
Generalized uridine diphosphate galactose-4-epimerase deficiency	Uridine diphosphate galactose-4-epimerase	Similar to transferase deficiency with additional findings of hypotonia and nerve deafness	A benign variant also exists
FRUCTOSE DISORDERS			
Essential fructosuria	Fructokinase	Urine reducing substance	Benign
Hereditary fructose intolerance	Fructose-1-phosphate aldolase	Acute: vomiting, sweating, lethargy Chronic: failure to thrive, hepatic failure	Prognosis good with fructose restriction
DISORDERS OF GLUCONEOGENESIS			
Fructose-1, 6-diphosphatase deficiency	Fructose-1, 6-diphosphatase	Episodic hypoglycemia, apnea, acidosis	Good prognosis, avoid fasting
Phosphoenolpyruvate carboxykinase deficiency	Phosphoenolpyruvate carboxykinase	Hypoglycemia, hepatomegaly, hypotonia, failure to thrive	Rare
DISORDERS OF PYRUVATE METABOLISM			
Pyruvate dehydrogenase complex defect	Pyruvate dehydrogenase	Severe fatal neonatal to mild late onset, lactic acidosis, psychomotor retardation, and failure to thrive	Most commonly due to E1 α subunit, defect X-linked
Pyruvate carboxylase deficiency	Pyruvate carboxylase	Same as above	Rare, autosomal recessive
Respiratory chain defects (oxidative phosphorylation disease)	Complex I to V, many mitochondrial DNA mutations	Heterogeneous with multisystem involvement	Mitochondrial inheritance
DISORDERS IN PENTOSE METABOLISM			
Pentosuria	L-xylulose reductase	Urine reducing substance	Benign
Transaldolase deficiency	Transaldolase	Liver cirrhosis and failure, cardiomyopathy	Autosomal recessive
Ribose-5-phosphate isomerase deficiency	Ribose-5-phosphate isomerase	Progressive leukoencephalopathy and peripheral neuropathy	

tion and prenatal diagnosis are possible with the DNA-based diagnosis.

Clinical Manifestations. Patients with type I GSD may present in the neonatal period with hypoglycemia and lactic acidosis; they more commonly present at 3–4 mo of age with hepatomegaly, hypoglycemic seizures, or both. These children often have **doll-like faces** with fat cheeks, relatively thin extremities, short stature, and a protuberant abdomen that is due to massive hepatomegaly; the kidneys are also enlarged, whereas the spleen and heart are normal.

The biochemical hallmarks of the disease are hypoglycemia, lactic acidosis, hyperuricemia, and hyperlipidemia. Hypoglycemia and lactic acidosis can develop after a short fast. Hyperuricemia is present in young children; gout rarely develops before puberty. Despite marked hepatomegaly, the liver transaminase levels are usually normal or only slightly elevated. Intermittent diarrhea may occur (the mechanism is unknown). Easy bruising and epistaxis are common and are associated with a prolonged bleeding time as a result of impaired platelet aggregation and adhesion.

The plasma may be "milky" in appearance as a result of a striking elevation of triglyceride levels. Cholesterol and phospholipids are also elevated, but less prominently. The lipid abnormality resembles type IV hyperlipidemia and is characterized by increased levels of very low density lipoprotein, low-density lipoprotein, and a unique apolipoprotein profile consisting of increased levels of apo B, C, and E, with relatively normal or reduced levels of apo A and D. The histologic appearance of the liver is characterized by a universal distention of hepatocytes by glycogen and fat. The lipid vacuoles are particularly large and prominent. There is little associated fibrosis.

All these findings apply to both type Ia and type Ib GSD, but **type Ib** has additional features of recurrent bacterial infections from **neutropenia** and impaired neutrophil function. Oral and intestinal mucosal ulceration and **inflammatory bowel disease** are common. Exceptional cases of type Ib without neutropenia and type Ia with neutropenia have been reported.

Although type I GSD affects mainly the liver, multiple organ systems are involved. Puberty is often delayed. Virtually all females have ultrasound findings consistent with **polycystic ovaries;** other features of polycystic ovary syndrome (acne, hirsuitism) are not seen. It is uncertain whether this affects long-term ovulation and fertility. There have been multiple reports of successful pregnancy in adult women with GSD I. Symptoms of gout usually start around puberty from long-term hyperuricemia. Secondary to the lipid abnormalities, there is an increased risk of **pancreatitis.** The dyslipidemia, together with elevated erythrocyte aggregation, predisposes these patients to atherosclerosis. Premature atherosclerosis has not yet been clearly documented except for rare cases. Impaired platelet aggregation and increased antioxidative defense to prevent lipid peroxidation may function as a protective mechanism to help reduce the risk of atherosclerosis. Frequent fractures and radiographic evidence of **osteopenia** are common; bone mineral content is reduced even in prepubertal patients.

By the 2nd or 3rd decade of life, most patients with type I GSD exhibit **hepatic adenomas** that can hemorrhage and, in some cases, become malignant. **Pulmonary hypertension** has been seen in some long-term survivors of the disease.

Renal disease is another complication, and most patients with type I GSD who are >20 yr of age have proteinuria. Many also have hypertension, renal stones, nephrocalcinosis, and altered creatinine clearance. Glomerular hyperfiltration, increased renal plasma flow, and microalbuminuria are often found in the early stages of renal dysfunction and can occur before the onset of proteinuria. In younger patients, hyperfiltration and hyperperfusion may be the only signs of renal abnormalities. With the advancement of renal disease, focal segmental glomerulosclerosis and interstitial fibrosis become evident. In some patients, renal function has deteriorated and progressed to failure, requiring dialysis and transplantation. Other renal abnormalities include amyloidosis, a Fanconi-like syndrome, hypocitraturia, hypercalciuria, and a distal renal tubular acidification defect.

Diagnosis. The diagnosis of type I GSD is suspected on the basis of clinical presentation and the laboratory findings of hypoglycemia, lactic acidosis, hyperuricemia, and hyperlipidemia. Neutropenia is noted in GSD Ib patients, typically after the 1st 2–3 yr of life. Administration of glucagon or epinephrine results in little or no rise in blood glucose level, but the lactate level rises significantly. Before the glucose-6-phosphatase and glucose-6-phosphate translocase genes were cloned, a definitive diagnosis required a liver biopsy. Gene-based mutation analysis now provides a noninvasive way of diagnosis for most patients with types Ia and Ib disease.

Treatment. Treatment is designed to maintain normal blood glucose levels and is achieved by continuous nasogastric infusion of glucose or oral administration of uncooked cornstarch. Nasogastric drip feeding can be introduced in early infancy from the time of diagnosis. It can consist of an elemental enteral formula or contain only glucose or a glucose polymer to provide sufficient glucose to maintain normoglycemia during the night. Frequent feedings with high-carbohydrate content are given during the day.

Uncooked cornstarch acts as a slow-release form of glucose and can be introduced at a dose of 1.6 g/kg every 4 hr for infants <2 yr of age. The response of young infants is variable. As the child grows older, the cornstarch regimen can be changed to every 6 hr at a dose of 1.75–2.5 g/kg of body weight. Because fructose and galactose cannot be converted directly to glucose in GSD type I, these sugars are restricted in the diet. Sucrose (table sugar, cane sugar, other ingredients), fructose (fruit, juice, high fructose corn syrup), lactose (dairy foods), and sorbitol should be avoided or limited. Due to these dietary restrictions, vitamins and minerals such as calcium and vitamin D may be deficient and supplementation is required to prevent nutritional deficiencies. Dietary therapy improves hyperuricemia, hyperlipidemia, and renal function, slowing the development of renal failure. This therapy fails, however, to normalize blood uric acid and lipids levels completely in some individuals, despite good metabolic control, especially after puberty. The control of hyperuricemia can be further augmented by the use of allopurinol, a xanthine oxidase inhibitor. The hyperlipidemia can be reduced with lipid-lowering drugs such as HMG-CoA reductase inhibitors and fibrate (see Chapter 86). Microalbuminuria, an early indicator of renal dysfunction in type I disease, is treated with angiotensin-converting enzyme (ACE) inhibitors. Citrate supplements can be beneficial for patients with hypocitraturia by preventing or ameliorating nephrocalcinosis and development of urinary calculi.

In patients with type Ib GSD, granulocyte and granulocyte-macrophage colony–stimulating factors are successful in correcting the neutropenia, decreasing the number and severity of bacterial infections, and improving the chronic inflammatory bowel disease.

Orthotopic liver transplantation is a potential cure of type I GSD, but the inherent short- and long-term complications leave this as a treatment of last resort, usually for patients with liver malignancy, multiple liver adenomas, metabolic derangements refractory to medical management, and/or liver failure. Large adenomas (>2 cm) that are rapidly increasing in size and/or number may require partial hepatic resection. Smaller adenomas (<2 cm) can be treated with percutaneous ethanol injection or transcatheter arterial embolization.

Before any surgical procedure, the bleeding status must be evaluated and good metabolic control established. Prolonged bleeding times can be normalized by the use of intensive intravenous glucose infusion for 24–48 hr before surgery. Use of 1-deamino-8-D-arginine vasopressin (DDAVP) can reduce bleeding complications. Lactated ringer solution should be avoided because it contains lactate and no glucose. Glucose levels should be maintained in the normal range throughout surgery with the use of 10% dextrose.

Prognosis. Previously, many patients with type I GSD died at a young age, and the prognosis was guarded for those who survived. The long-term complications occur mostly in adults whose disease was not adequately treated during childhood. Early diagnosis and effective treatment have improved the outcome; renal disease and formation of hepatic adenomas with potential risk for malignant transformation remain serious complications.

TYPE III GLYCOGEN STORAGE DISEASE (DEBRANCHER DEFICIENCY, LIMIT DEXTRINOSIS). Type III GSD is caused by a deficiency of glycogen debranching enzyme activity. Debranching enzyme, together with phosphorylase, is responsible for complete degradation of glycogen. When debranching enzyme is defective, glycogen breakdown is incomplete and an abnormal glycogen with short outer branch chains and resembling limit dextrin accumulates. Deficiency of glycogen debranching enzyme causes hepatomegaly, hypoglycemia, short stature, variable skeletal myopathy, and variable cardiomyopathy. The disorder usually involves both liver and muscle and is termed type IIIa GSD. In ≈15% of patients, the disease appears to involve only liver and is classified as type IIIb.

Type III glycogenosis is an autosomal recessive disease that has been reported in many different ethnic groups; the frequency is relatively high in non-Ashkenazi Jews from North Africa (Sephardic). The gene for debranching enzyme is located on chromosome 1p21. More than 30 different mutations are identified; two exon 3 mutations (17delAG and Q6X) are specifically associated with glycogenosis IIIb. Carrier detection and prenatal diagnosis are possible using DNA-based linkage or mutation analysis.

Clinical Manifestations. During infancy and childhood, the disease may be indistinguishable from type I GSD, because hepatomegaly, hypoglycemia, hyperlipidemia, and growth retardation are common (Fig. 87-2). Splenomegaly may be present, but the kidneys are not enlarged. Remarkably, hepatomegaly and hepatic symptoms in most patients with type III GSD improve with age and usually resolve after puberty. Progressive liver cirrhosis and failure can occur. **Hepatocellular carcinoma** has also been reported, more typically in patients with progressive liver cirrhosis. The frequency of adenomas in individuals with GSD III is far less, compared to GSD I. Furthermore, the relationship of hepatic adenomas and malignancy in GSD III is unclear. A single case of malignant transformation at the site of adenomas has been noted. In patients with muscular involvement (type IIIa), muscle weakness is usually minimal during childhood but can become severe after the 3rd or 4th decade of life, as evidenced by slowly progressive weakness and wasting. Myopathy does not follow any particular pattern of involvement; both proximal and distal muscles are involved. Electromyography reveals a widespread myopathy; nerve conduction studies may be abnormal. Ventricular hypertrophy is a frequent finding, but overt cardiac dysfunction is rare. Hepatic symptoms in some patients may be so mild that the diagnosis is not made until adulthood, when the patients show symptoms and signs of neuromuscular disease. The initial diagnosis has been confused with Charcot-Marie-Tooth disease. Polycystic ovaries are common; fertility, however, is not reduced.

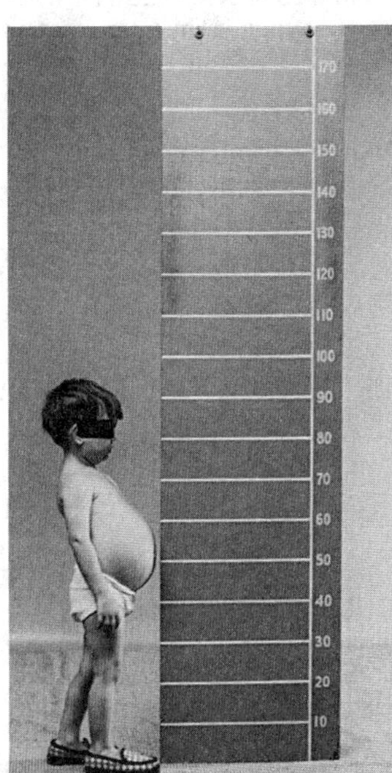

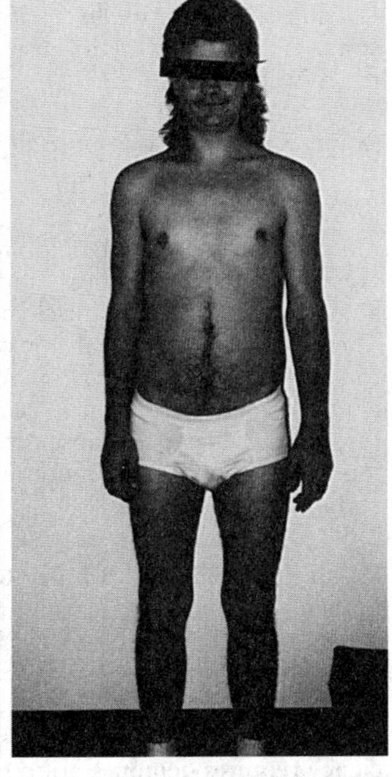

Figure 87-2. Growth and development in a patient with type IIIb glycogen storage disease. The patient has debrancher deficiency in liver but normal activity in muscle. As a child, he had hepatomegaly, hypoglycemia, and growth retardation. After puberty, he no longer had hepatomegaly or hypoglycemia, and his final adult height is normal. He had no muscle weakness or atrophy; this is in contrast to type IIIa patients, in whom a progressive myopathy is seen in adulthood.

Hypoglycemia and hyperlipidemia are common. In contrast to type I GSD, elevation of liver transaminase levels and fasting ketosis are prominent, but blood lactate and uric acid concentrations are usually normal. Serum creatine kinase levels can be useful to identify patients with muscle involvement; normal levels do not rule out muscle enzyme deficiency. The administration of glucagon 2 hr after a carbohydrate meal provokes a normal increase in blood glucose; after an overnight fast, glucagon may provoke no change in blood glucose level.

Diagnosis. The histologic appearance of the liver is characterized by a universal distention of hepatocytes by glycogen and the presence of fibrous septa. The fibrosis and the paucity of fat distinguish type III glycogenosis from type I. The fibrosis, which ranges from minimal periportal fibrosis to micronodular cirrhosis, appears in most cases to be nonprogressive. Overt cirrhosis has been seen in some patients with GSD III.

Patients with myopathy and liver symptoms have a generalized enzyme defect (type IIIa). The deficient enzyme activity can be demonstrated not only in liver and muscle, but also in other tissues such as heart, erythrocytes, and cultured fibroblasts. Patients with hepatic symptoms without clinical or laboratory evidence of myopathy have debranching enzyme deficiency only in the liver, with enzyme activity retained in the muscle (type IIIb). Definite diagnosis requires enzyme assay in liver, muscle, or both. Mutation analysis can provide a noninvasive method for diagnosis and subtype assignment in the majority of patients.

Treatment. Dietary management is less demanding than in type I GSD. Patients do not need to restrict dietary intake of fructose and galactose. If hypoglycemia is present, frequent meals high in carbohydrates with cornstarch supplements or nocturnal gastric drip feedings are usually effective. A high-protein diet during the daytime plus overnight protein enteral infusion can also be effective in preventing hypoglycemia and preventing endogenous protein breakdown because protein can be used as a substrate for gluconeogenesis, a pathway that is intact in type III GSD. There is no satisfactory treatment for the progressive myopathy other than recommending a high-protein diet and an exercise program. Liver transplantation has been performed in patients with end-stage cirrhosis and/or hepatic carcinoma.

TYPE IV GLYCOGEN STORAGE DISEASE (BRANCHING ENZYME DEFICIENCY, AMYLOPECTINOSIS, OR ANDERSEN DISEASE). Deficiency of branching enzyme activity results in accumulation of an abnormal glycogen with poor solubility. The disease is referred to as type IV GSD or amylopectinosis because the abnormal glycogen has fewer branch points, more α 1–4 linked glucose units, and longer outer chains, resulting in a structure resembling amylopectin.

Type IV GSD is an autosomal recessive disorder. The glycogen branching enzyme gene is located on chromosome 3p21. Mutations responsible for type IV GSD have been identified, and their characterization in individual patients can be useful in predicting the clinical outcome. Some mutations are associated with a good prognosis and lack of progression of liver disease.

Clinical Manifestations. This disorder is clinically variable. The most common and classic form is characterized by progressive cirrhosis of the liver and is manifested in the 1st 18 mo of life as hepatosplenomegaly and failure to thrive. The cirrhosis progresses to portal hypertension, ascites, esophageal varices, and liver failure that usually leads to death by 5 yr of age. Rare patients survive without progression of liver disease.

A **neuromuscular** form of the disease has been reported. Patients may present at birth with severe hypotonia, muscle atrophy, and neuronal involvement with death in the neonatal period; others may present in late childhood with myopathy or cardiomyopathy; or present as adults with diffuse central and peripheral nervous system dysfunction accompanied by accumulation of polyglucosan body disease in the nervous system (so-called adult polyglucosan body disease). For adult polyglucosan disease, leukocyte or nerve biopsy is needed to establish the diagnosis because the branching enzyme deficiency is limited to those tissues.

Diagnosis. Tissue depostion of amylopectin-like materials can be demonstrated in liver, heart, muscle, skin, intestine, brain, spinal cord, and peripheral nerve. The hepatic histologic findings are characterized by micronodular cirrhosis and faintly stained basophilic inclusions in the hepatocytes. The inclusions consist of coarsely clumped, stored material that is periodic acid–Schiff positive and partially resistant to diastase digestion. Electron microscopy shows, in addition to the conventional α and β glycogen particles, accumulation of the fibrillar aggregations that are typical of amylopectin. The distinct staining properties of the cytoplasmic inclusions, as well as electron microscopic findings, could be diagnostic. However, polysaccharidoses with histologic features reminiscent of type IV disease, but without enzymatic correlation, have been observed. The definitive diagnosis rests on the demonstration of the deficient branching enzyme activity in liver, muscle, cultured skin fibroblasts, or leukocytes. Prenatal diagnosis is possible by measuring the enzyme activity in cultured amniocytes or chorionic villi.

Treatment. There is no specific treatment for type IV GSD. Liver transplantation has been performed for patients with progressive hepatic failure, but because it is a multisystem disorder involving many organ systems, the long-term success of liver transplantation is unknown.

TYPE VI GLYCOGEN STORAGE DISEASE (LIVER PHOSPHORYLASE DEFICIENCY, HERS DISEASE). There are few patients with documented liver phosphorylase deficiency. Such patients have a benign course and present with hepatomegaly and growth retardation in early childhood. Hypoglycemia, hyperlipidemia, and hyperketosis are usually mild if present. Lactic acid and uric acid levels are normal. The heart and skeletal muscles are not involved. The hepatomegaly and growth retardation improve with age and usually disappear around puberty. Treatment is symptomatic. A high-carbohydrate diet and frequent feeding are effective in preventing hypoglycemia; most patients require no specific treatment. GSD VI is an autosomal recessive disease. Diagnosis rests on enzyme analysis of the liver biopsy. The liver phosphorylase gene (PYGL) is on chromosome 14q21–22 and has 20 exons. Many mutations are known in this gene, a splice site mutation in intron 13 has been identified in the Mennonite population.

TYPE IX GLYCOGEN STORAGE DISEASE (PHOSPHORYLASE KINASE DEFICIENCY). This disorder represents a heterogeneous group of glycogenoses. Phosphorylase, the rate-limiting enzyme of glycogenolysis, is activated by a cascade of enzymatic reactions involving adenylate cyclase, cyclic adenosine monophosphate–dependent protein kinase (protein kinase A), and phosphorylase kinase. The latter enzyme has four subunits (α, β, γ, δ), each encoded by different genes on different chromosomes and differentially expressed in various tissues. This cascade of reactions is stimulated primarily by glucagon. This glycogenosis could be the result of any enzyme deficiency along this pathway; the most common is the deficiency of phosphorylase kinase.

The numeric classification of phosphorylase kinase deficiency is confusing, ranging from type VIa to VIII to IX. It is advisable to refrain from such a designation and to classify the various disorders according to organ involvement and mode of inheritance.

X-LINKED LIVER PHOSPHORYLASE KINASE DEFICIENCY. X-linked liver phosphorylase kinase deficiency is the most common form of liver glycogenoses. In addition to liver, enzyme activity can also be deficient in erythrocytes and leukocytes; it is normal in muscle. Typically, a 1–5 yr old presents with growth retardation and an incidental finding of hepatomegaly. Cholesterol, triglycerides, and liver enzymes are mildly elevated. Ketosis may occur after fasting. Lactate and uric acid levels are normal. Hypoglycemia is mild, if present. The response in blood glucose to glucagon is normal. Hepatomegaly and abnormal blood chemistries gradually become normal with age. Most adults achieve a normal final height and are usually asymptomatic despite a persistent phosphorylase kinase deficiency. Liver histologic appearance shows glycogen-distended hepatocytes. The accumulated glycogen (β particles, rosette form) has a frayed or burst appearance and is less compact than the glycogen seen in type I or type III GSD. Fibrous septal formation and low-grade inflammatory changes may be present.

The structural gene for the common liver isoform of the phosphorylase kinase subunit, liver α subunit is on the X chromosome (αL at Xp22.2). Mutations of this gene are known.

AUTOSOMAL LIVER AND MUSCLE PHOSPHORYLASE KINASE DEFICIENCY. Several patients have been reported with phosphorylase kinase deficiency in liver and blood cells and an autosomal mode of inheritance. As with the X-linked form, hepatomegaly and growth retardation apparent in early childhood are the predominant symptoms. Some patients also exhibit muscle hypotonia. When measured in a few cases, reduced activity of the enzyme has been demonstrated in muscle. Mutations causing autosomally transmitted liver and muscle phosphorylase kinase deficiency are found in the autosomal β subunit gene of the PK gene (chromosome 16q12-q13).

AUTOSOMAL LIVER PHOSPHORYLASE KINASE DEFICIENCY. This form of phosphorylase kinase deficiency is due to mutations in the testis/liver isoform of the γ subunit of the gene (TL, PHKG2). In contrast to the benign course of X-linked phosphorylase kinase deficiency, patients with mutations in the PHKG2 gene have more severe phenotypes with recurrent hypoglycemia and often develop a progressive liver cirrhosis. PHKG2 maps to chromosome 16p12.1 and many disease-causing mutations are known for this gene

MUSCLE-SPECIFIC PHOSPHORYLASE KINASE DEFICIENCY. A few cases of phosphorylase kinase deficiency restricted to muscle are known. Patients, both male and female, present either with muscle cramps and myoglobinuria with exercise or with progressive muscle weakness and atrophy. Phosphorylase kinase activity is decreased in muscle but normal in liver and blood cells. There is no hepatomegaly or cardiomegaly. The structural gene for muscle specific form α subunit (αM) is located at Xq12. Mutations of this gene have been found in male patients with this disorder. The gene for muscle γ subunit (γM, PHKG1) is on chromosome 7p12 (29). No mutations in this gene have been reported so far.

PHOSPHORYLASE KINASE DEFICIENCY LIMITED TO HEART. These patients present with cardiomyopathy in infancy and rapidly progress to heart failure and death. Phosphorylase kinase deficiency is demonstrated in the heart with normal enzyme activity in skeletal muscle and liver.

Diagnosis. Definitive diagnosis of phosphorylase kinase deficiency requires demonstration of the enzymatic defect in affected tissues. Phosphorylase kinase can be measured in leukocytes and erythrocytes, but because the enzyme has many isozymes, the diagnosis can be missed without studies of liver, muscle, or heart in certain instances.

Treatment. The treatment for liver phosphorylase kinase deficiency includes a high-carbohydrate diet and frequent feedings to prevent hypoglycemia; most patients require no specific treatment. Prognosis for the X-linked and certain autosomal forms is good. Patients with mutations in the γ subunit typically have a more severe clinical course with progressive liver disease. There is no treatment for the fatal form of isolated cardiac phosphorylase kinase deficiency other than heart transplantation.

GLYCOGEN SYNTHETASE DEFICIENCY (GSD 0). Deficiency of hepatic glycogen synthetase leads to a marked decrease of glycogen stored in the liver. The patients present in infancy with early-morning (before eating breakfast) drowsiness, pallor, emesis, and fatigue and sometimes convulsions associated with hypoglycemia and hyperketonemia. Blood lactate and alanine levels are low, and there is no hyperlipidemia or hepatomegaly. Prolonged hyperglycemia, glycosuria, and elevation of lactate with normal insulin levels after administration of glucose or a meal suggest a possible diagnosis of deficiency of glycogen synthetase. Definitive diagnosis requires a liver biopsy to measure the enzyme activity or identification of mutations in the liver glycogen synthetase gene, located on chromosome 12p12.2. Treatment consists of frequent meals, rich in protein, and nighttime supplementation with uncooked cornstarch.

HEPATIC GLYCOGENOSIS WITH RENAL FANCONI SYNDROME (FANCONI-BICKEL SYNDROME). This rare autosomal recessive disorder is caused by defects in the facilitative glucose transporter 2 (GLUT-2), which transports glucose in and out of hepatocytes, pancreatic β cells, and the basolateral membranes of intestinal and renal epithelial cells. The disease is characterized by proximal renal tubular dysfunction, impaired glucose and galactose utilization, and accumulation of glycogen in liver and kidney.

The affected child typically presents in the 1st yr of life with failure to thrive, rickets, and a protuberant abdomen from hepatomegaly and nephromegaly. Laboratory findings include glucosuria, phosphaturia, generalized aminoaciduria, bicarbonate wasting, hypophosphatemia, increased serum alkaline phosphatase levels, and radiologic findings of rickets. Mild fasting hypoglycemia and hyperlipidemia may be present. Liver transaminase, plasma lactate, and uric acid levels are usually normal. Oral galactose or glucose tolerance tests show intolerance, which could be explained by the functional loss of GLUT-2 preventing liver uptake of these sugars.

Tissue biopsy results show marked accumulation of glycogen in hepatocytes and proximal renal tubular cells, presumably owing to the altered glucose transport out of these organs.

There is no specific treatment. Growth retardation persists through adulthood. Symptomatic replacement of water, electrolytes, and vitamin D; restriction of galactose intake; and a diet similar to that used for diabetes mellitus presented in frequent and small meals with an adequate caloric intake may improve growth.

MUSCLE GLYCOGENOSES

The role of glycogen in muscle is to provide substrates for the generation of ATP for muscle contraction. The muscle GSDs are broadly divided into 2 groups. The 1st group is characterized by hypertrophic cardiomyopathy, progressive skeletal muscle weakness and atrophy, or both, and is represented by a lysosomal glycogen degrading enzyme deficiency of acid α-glucosidase (type II GSD) and deficiencies of lysosomal-associated membrane protein 2 (LAMP2) and AMP-activated protein kinase γ2 (PRKAG2). The 2nd group comprises muscle energy disorder characterized by muscle pain, exercise intolerance, myoglobinuria, and susceptibility to fatigue. This group includes myophosphorylase deficiency (McArdle disease, type V) and deficiencies of phosphofructokinase (type VII), phosphoglycerate kinase, phosphoglycerate mutase, and lactate dehydrogenase. Some of these latter enzyme deficiencies can also be associated with a compensated hemolysis, suggesting a more generalized defect in glucose metabolism.

TYPE II GLYCOGEN STORAGE DISEASE (LYSOSOMAL ACID α 1,4-GLUCOSIDASE DEFICIENCY, POMPE DISEASE). Pompe disease, also referred to as GSD type II or acid maltase deficiency, is caused by a deficiency of acid α-1,4-glucosidase (acid maltase), an enzyme responsible for the degradation of glycogen in lysosomes. This enzyme defect results in lysosomal glycogen accumulation in multiple tissues and cell types, with cardiac, skeletal, and smooth muscle cells being the most seriously affected. The disease is characterized by accumulation of glycogen in lysosomes, as opposed to its accumulation in cytoplasm in the other glycogenoses.

Pompe disease is an autosomal recessive disorder with an incidence of ≈1/40,000 live births. The gene for acid α-glucosidase is on chromosome 17q25.2. Multiple pathogenic mutations have been identified that could be helpful in delineating the phenotypes. An example is a splice site mutation (IVS1–13T→G), commonly seen in late-onset patients of caucasian descent.

Clinical Manifestations. The disorder encompasses a range of phenotypes, each including myopathy but differing in age at onset, organ involvement, and clinical severity. **Infantile-onset Pompe disease** is thought to be uniformly lethal without specific therapy. Affected infants present in the 1st few months of life with hypotonia, a generalized muscle weakness with a "floppy infant appearance," feeding difficulties, macroglossia, hepatomegaly, and a hypertrophic cardiomyopathy followed by death from cardiorespiratory failure or respiratory infection usually by 1 yr of age. **Juvenile and adult-onset disease** (late-onset forms) is characterized by a lack or absence of severe cardiac involvement and a less severe short-term prognosis. Symptoms can start at any age and are related to progressive dysfunction of skeletal muscles. The clinical picture is dominated by slowly progressive proximal muscle weakness with truncal involvement and greater involvement of the lower limbs than the upper limbs. The pelvic girdle, paraspinal muscles, and diaphragm are the muscle groups most seriously affected. With disease progression, patients become confined to wheelchairs and require artificial ventilation. The initial symptoms in some patients may be respiratory insufficiency manifested by somnolence, morning headache, orthopnea, and exertional dyspnea, which eventually lead to sleep-disordered breathing and respiratory failure. Respiratory failure is the cause of significant morbidity and mortality in this form of the disease. The age of death varies from early childhood to late adulthood, depending on the rate of disease progression and the extent of respiratory muscle involvement.

Laboratory Findings. These include elevated levels of serum creatine kinase, aspartate aminotransferase, and lactate dehydrogenase. In the infantile form a chest x-ray showing massive cardiomegaly is frequently the 1st symptom detected. Electrocardiographic findings include a high-voltage QRS complex and a shortened PR interval. Echocardiography reveals thickening of both ventricles and/or the intraventricular septum and/or left ventricular outflow tract obstruction. Muscle biopsy shows the presence of vacuoles that stain positively for glycogen; acid phosphatase is increased, presumably from a compensatory increase of lysosomal enzymes. Electron microscopy reveals glycogen accumulation within the membranous sac and in the cytoplasm. Electromyography reveals myopathic features with excessive electrical irritability of muscle fibers and pseudomyotonic discharges. Serum creatine kinase is not always elevated in adult patients. Depending on the muscle sampled or tested, the muscle histologic appearance on electromyography may not be abnormal. It is prudent to examine the affected muscle.

Diagnosis. The confirmatory step for a diagnosis of Pompe disease is enzyme assay demonstrating deficient acid α-glucosidase. This assay is usually done in muscle, cultured skin fibroblasts, dried blood spots, leukocytes, or blood mononuclear cells using maltose, glycogen, or 4-methylumbelliferyl-α-D-glucopyranoside (4MUG) as a substrate. Deficiency is usually more severe in the infantile form than in the juvenile and adult forms. The skin fibroblast assay is usually preferred to muscle biopsy because it is a less invasive procedure with the advantage of maintaining a cell line for future use and providing information on residual enzyme activity. Blood-based assays have the advantage of a rapid turn-around time. A muscle biopsy can yield faster results and provide additional information about glycogen content and site of glycogen storage within and outside the lysosomes of muscle cells. A major limitation of a muscle biopsy in late-onset patients is the variable pathology and glycogen accumulation in different muscles and within muscle fibers; muscle histology and glycogen content can vary depending on the site of muscle biopsy. There is also a risk from anesthesia. Prenatal diagnosis using amniocytes or chorionic villi is available in the fatal infantile form.

Treatment. Treatment options were once limited to supportive or palliative care. Clinical trials of enzyme replacement therapy (ERT) have been promising and ERT with myozyme is available for treatment of Pompe disease. Recombinant acid α-glucosidase is capable of improving cardiac and skeletal muscle functions (Fig. 87-3). For patients with the late-onset form of the disease, a high-protein diet may be beneficial. Nocturnal ventilatory support, when indicated, should be used. It has been shown to improve the quality of life and is particularly beneficial during a period of respiratory decompensation.

GLYCOGEN STORAGE DISEASES MIMICKING HYPERTROPHIC CARDIOMYOPATHY. Deficiencies of lysosomal-associated membrane protein 2 (LAMP2, also called Danon disease) and AMP-activated protein kinase γ2 (PRKAG2) result in accumulation of glycogen in the heart and skeletal muscle. These patients present primarily as a hypertrophic cardiomyopathy, but can be distinguished from the usual causes of hypertrophic cardiomyopathy due to defects in sarcomere protein genes by their electrophysiologic abnormalities, particularly ventricular pre-excitation and conduction defects. The onset of cardiac symptoms, including chest pain, palpitation, syncope, and cardiac arrest, can occur between the ages of 8 and 15 yr for LAMP2 deficiency, younger than the average age for patients with PRKAG2 deficiency, which is 33 yr. The prognosis for LAMP2 deficiency is poor with progressive end-stage heart failure early in adulthood. Cardiomyopathy due to PRKAG mutations is compatible with long-term survival, although some patients may necessitate the implantation of a pacemaker and aggressive control of arrhythmias.

TYPE V GLYCOGEN STORAGE DISEASE (MUSCLE PHOSPHORYLASE DEFICIENCY, MCARDLE DISEASE). This is caused by the deficiency of muscle phosphorylase activity. Lack of this enzyme limits muscle ATP generation by glycogenolysis, results in glycogen accumulation, and is the prototype of muscle energy disorders. A deficiency of myophosphorylase impairs the cleavage of glucosyl molecules from the straight chain of glycogen.

Clinical Manifestations. Symptoms usually 1st develop in late childhood or as an adult and are characterized by exercise intolerance with muscle cramps/pain. Two types of activity tend to cause symptoms: brief exercise of great intensity, such as sprinting or carrying heavy loads; and less intense but sustained activity, such as climbing stairs or walking uphill. Moderate exercise, such as walking on level ground, can be performed by most patients for long periods. Many patients experience a characteristic "second wind" phenomenon. If they slow down or pause briefly at the 1st appearance of muscle pain, they can resume exercise with more ease. Due to the underlying myopathy, these patients may be at risk for statin-induced myositis and rhabdomyolysis.

About half report burgundy-colored urine after exercise, which is the consequence of exercise-induced **myoglobinuria** secondary to **rhabdomyolysis.** Intense myoglobinuria after vigorous exercise may cause acute renal failure. In rare cases, electromyographic findings may suggest an inflammatory myopathy and the diagnosis can be confused with polymyositis.

The level of serum creatine kinase is usually elevated at rest and increases more after exercise. Exercise also increases the levels of blood ammonia, inosine, hypoxanthine, and uric acid. The latter abnormalities are attributed to accelerated recycling of muscle purine nucleotides owing to insufficient ATP production.

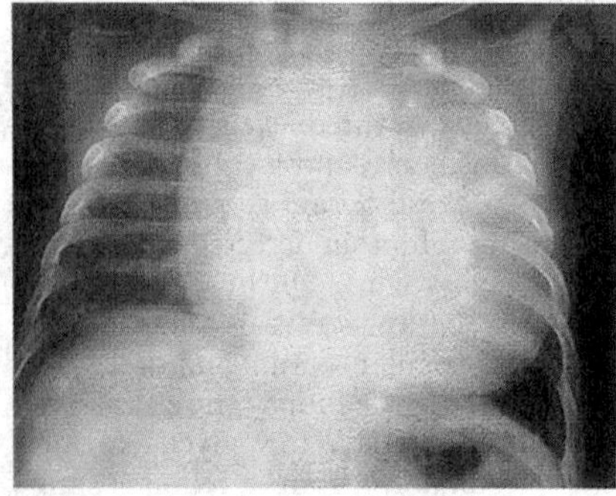

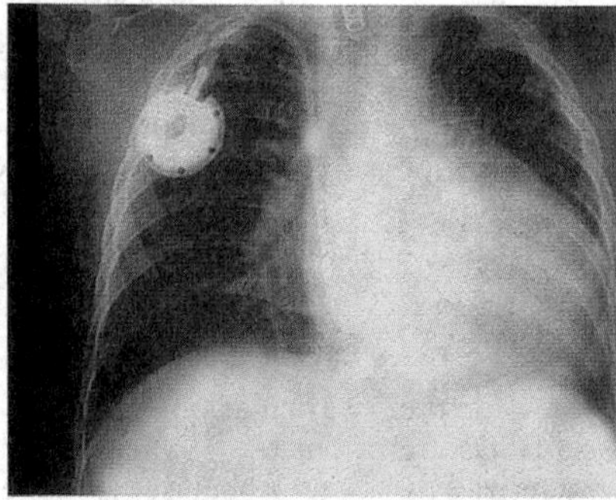

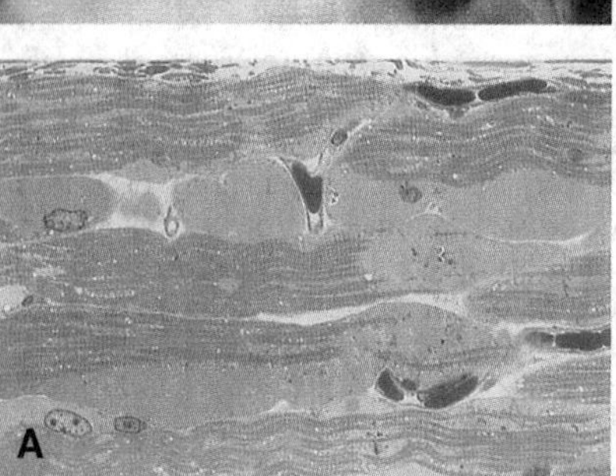

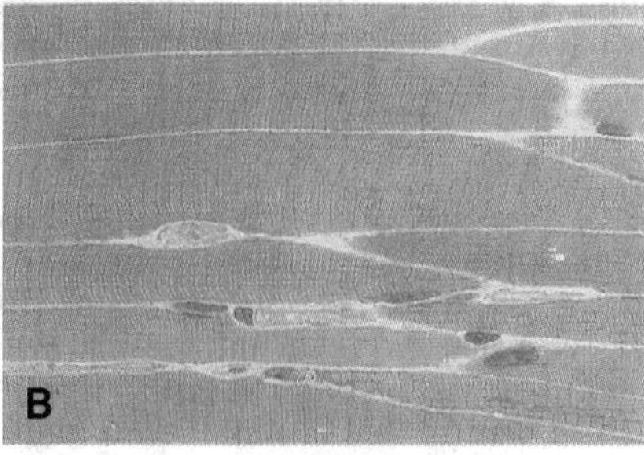

Figure 87-3. Chest x-ray and muscle histology findings of an infantile-onset Pompe disease patient before *(A)* and after *(B)* enzyme replacement therapy. Note the decrease in heart size and muscle glycogen with the therapy. (Modified from Amalfitano A, Bengur AR, Morse RP, et al: Recombinant human acid alpha-glucosidase enzyme therapy for infantile glycogen storage disease type II: Results of a phase I/II clinical trial, *Genet Med* 2001;3:132–138.)

Type V GSD is an autosomal recessive disorder. The gene for muscle phosphorylase (PYGM) has been mapped to chromosome 11q13.

Clinical heterogeneity is uncommon in type V GSD, but late-onset disease with no symptoms as late as the 8th decade and an early-onset, fatal form with hypotonia, generalized muscle weakness, and progressive respiratory insufficiency have been described.

Diagnosis. An ischemic exercise test offers a rapid diagnostic screening for patients with a metabolic myopathy. Lack of an increase in blood lactate levels and exaggerated blood ammonia elevations indicate muscle glycogenosis and suggest a defect in the conversion of muscle glycogen or glucose to lactate. The abnormal ischemic exercise response is not limited to type V GSD. Other muscle defects in glycogenolysis or glycolysis produce similar results (deficiencies of muscle phosphofructokinase, phosphoglycerate kinase, phosphoglycerate mutase, or lactate dehydrogenase).

Phosphorus magnetic resonance imaging (^{31}P MRI) allows for the noninvasive evaluation of muscle metabolism. Patients with type V GSD have no decrease in intracellular pH and have excessive reduction in phosphocreatine in response to exercise. The diagnosis should be confirmed by enzymatic evaluation of muscle. A common nonsense mutation R49X in exon 1 is found in 90% of white patients, and a deletion of a single codon in exon 17 is found in 61% of Japanese patients. Other common mutations in whites (G204S in exon 5 and K542T in exon 14) make DNA-based diagnosis and carrier testing for McArdle disease possible for the 2 populations.

Treatment. Avoidance of strenuous exercise prevents the symptoms; however, regular and moderate exercise is recommended to improve exercise capacity. **Sucrose** given before exercise can markedly improve tolerance in these patients. A high-protein diet may increase muscle endurance and creatine supplement has been shown to improve muscle function in some patients. Longevity is not generally affected.

TYPE VII GLYCOGEN STORAGE DISEASE (MUSCLE PHOSPHOFRUCTOKINASE DEFICIENCY, TARUI DISEASE). Type VII GSD is caused by a deficiency of muscle phosphofructokinase, which catalyzes the ATP-dependent conversion of fructose-6-phosphate to fructose-1,6-diphosphate and is a key regulatory enzyme of glycolysis. Phosphofructokinase is composed of 3 isoenzyme subunits (M [muscle], L [liver], and P [platelet]) that are encoded by different genes and differentially expressed in tissues. Skeletal muscle contains only the M subunit, and red blood cells contain a hybrid of L and M forms. Type VII disease is due to a defective M isoenzyme, which causes a complete enzyme defect in muscle and a partial defect in red blood cells.

Type VII GSD is an autosomal recessive disorder and is prevalent among Japanese people and Ashkenazi Jews. The gene for muscle phosphofructokinase is located on chromosome 1cen-1q32. A splicing defect and a nucleotide deletion in the muscle phosphofructokinase gene accounts for 95% of mutant alleles in Ashkenazi Jews. Diagnosis based on molecular testing is thus possible in this population.

Clinical Manifestations. Six features of type VII are distinctive: (1) Exercise intolerance, usually evident in childhood, is more severe than in type V disease and may be associated with nausea, vomiting, and severe muscle pain; vigorous exercise causes severe muscle cramps and myoglobinuria. (2) A compensated hemolysis occurs as evidenced by an increased level of serum bilirubin and an elevated reticulocyte count. (3) Hyperuricemia is common and exaggerated by muscle exercise to a more severe degree than that observed in type V or III GSD. (4) An abnormal glycogen resembling amylopectin is present in muscle fibers; it is periodic acid–Schiff positive but resistant to diastase digestion. (5) Exercise intolerance is particularly acute after meals that are rich in carbohydrates because glucose cannot be utilized in muscle and because glucose inhibits lipolysis and thus deprives muscle of fatty acid and ketone substrates. In contrast, patients with type V disease can metabolize blood-borne glucose derived from either liver glycogenolysis or exogenous glucose; indeed, glucose infusion improves exercise tolerance in type V patients. (6) There is no spontaneous second-wind phenomenon because of the inability to metabolize blood glucose.

Two rare type VII variants occur. One variant presents in infancy with hypotonia and limb weakness and proceeds to a rapidly progressive myopathy that leads to death by 4 yr of age. The other variant presents in adults and is characterized by a slowly progressive, fixed muscle weakness rather than cramps and myoglobinuria.

Diagnosis. To establish a diagnosis, a biochemical or histochemical demonstration of the enzymatic defect in the muscle is required. The absence of the M isoenzyme of phosphofructokinase can also be demonstrated in blood cells and fibroblasts.

Treatment. There is no specific treatment. Avoidance of strenuous exercise is advisable to prevent acute attacks of muscle cramps and myoglobinuria.

OTHER MUSCLE GLYCOGENOSES WITH MUSCLE ENERGY IMPAIRMENT. Six additional defects in enzymes—phosphoglycerate kinase, phosphoglycerate mutase, lactate dehydrogenase, fructose-1,6-biphosphate aldolase A, muscle pyruvate kinase, and β-enolase in the pathway of the terminal glycolysis—cause symptoms and signs of muscle energy impairment similar to those of types V and VII GSD. The failure of blood lactate to increase in response to exercise is a useful diagnostic test and can be used to differentiate muscle glycogenoses from disorders of lipid metabolism, such as carnitine palmitoyl transferase II deficiency and very long chain acyl-CoA dehydrogenase deficiency, which also cause muscle cramps and myoglobinuria. Muscle glycogen levels can be normal in the disorders affecting terminal glycolysis and assaying the muscle enzyme activity is needed to make a definite diagnosis. There is no specific treatment. Avoidance of strenuous exercise prevents acute attacks of muscle cramps and myoglobinuria. Avoidance of drugs such as statins, and malignant hyperthermia precautions for patients undergoing anesthesia should be followed.

87.2 • Defects in Galactose Metabolism •

Priya S. Kishnani and Yuan-Tsong Chen

Milk and dairy products contain lactose, the major dietary source of galactose. The metabolism of galactose produces fuel for cellular metabolism through its conversion to glucose-1-phosphate (see Table 87-1). Galactose also plays an important role in the formation of galactosides, which include glycoproteins, glycolipids, and glycosaminoglycans. Galactosemia denotes the elevated level of galactose in the blood and is found in 3 distinct inborn errors of galactose metabolism defective in 1 of the following enzymes: galactose-1-phosphate uridyl transferase, galactokinase, and uridine diphosphate galactose-4-epimerase. The term *galactosemia,* although adequate for the deficiencies in any of these disorders, generally designates the transferase deficiency.

GALACTOSE-1-PHOSPHATE URIDYL TRANSFERASE DEFICIENCY GALACTOSEMIA. Two forms of the deficiency exist: Infants with complete or near complete deficiency of the enzyme (classic galactosemia) and those with partial transferase deficiency. **Classic galactosemia** is a serious disease with onset of symptoms typically by the 2nd half of the 1st wk of life. The incidence is 1/60,000. The newborn infant receives high amounts of lactose (up to 40% in breast milk and certain formulas), which consists of equal parts of glucose and galactose. Without the transferase enzyme, the infant is unable to metabolize galactose-1-phosphate, the accumulation of which results in injury to kidney, liver, and brain. This injury may begin prenatally in the affected fetus by transplacental galactose derived from the diet of the heterozygous mother or by endogenous production of galactose in the fetus.

Clinical Manifestations. The diagnosis of uridyl transferase deficiency should be considered in newborn or young infants with any of the following features: jaundice, hepatomegaly, vomiting, hypoglycemia, convulsions, lethargy, irritability, feeding difficulties, poor weight gain or failure to regain birth weight, aminoaciduria, nuclear cataracts, vitreous hemorrhage, hepatic failure, liver cirrhosis, ascites, splenomegaly, or mental retardation. Symptoms are milder and improve when milk is temporarily withdrawn and replaced by intravenous or lactose-free nutrition. Patients with galactosemia are at increased risk for *Escherichia coli* neonatal sepsis; the onset of sepsis often precedes the diagnosis of galactosemia. Death from liver and kidney failure and sepsis may follow within days. When the diagnosis is not made at birth, damage to the liver (cirrhosis) and brain (mental retardation) becomes increasingly severe and irreversible.

Partial transferase deficiency is generally asymptomatic. It is more frequent than classic galactosemia and is diagnosed in newborn screening because of moderately elevated blood galactose and/or low transferase activity. Galactosemia should be considered for the newborn or young infant who is not thriving or who has any of the preceding findings. Light and electron microscopy of hepatic tissue reveals fatty infiltration, the formation of pseudoacini, and eventual macronodular cirrhosis. These changes are consistent with a metabolic disease but do not indicate the precise enzymatic defect.

Diagnosis. The preliminary diagnosis of galactosemia is made by demonstrating a reducing substance in several urine specimens collected while the patient is receiving human milk, cow's milk, or any other formula containing lactose. The reducing substance found in urine by Clinitest (glucose, galactose, others) can be identified by chromatography or by an enzymatic test specific for galactose. Galactosuria is present, provided the last milk feed does not date back more than a few hours and the child is not vomiting excessively. Clinistix urine test results are negative because the test materials rely on the action of glucose oxidase, which is specific for glucose and is nonreactive with galactose. Owing to a proximal renal tubular syndrome, however, the acutely ill baby may also excrete glucose together with amino acids. Because galactose is injurious to persons with galactosemia, diagnostic challenge tests dependent on administering galactose orally or intravenously should not be used. Direct enzyme assay using erythrocytes establishes the diagnosis. One needs to confirm that the patient did not receive a blood transfusion before the collection of the blood sample, as a diagnosis could be missed. Deficient activity of galactose-1-phosphate uridyl transferase is demonstrable in hemolysates of erythrocytes, which also exhibit increased concentrations of galactose-1-phosphate.

Genetics. Transferase deficiency galactosemia is an autosomal recessive disorder. There are several enzymatic variants of galactosemia. The Duarte variant, a single amino acid substitution (N314D), has diminished red cell enzyme activity but usually no clinical significance. Some African-American patients have milder symptoms despite the absence of measurable transferase activity in erythrocytes; these patients retain 10% enzyme activity in liver and intestinal mucosa, whereas most white patients have no detectable activity in any of these tissues. In African-Americans, 62% of alleles are represented by the S135L mutation, a mutation that is responsible for a milder disease course. In the white population, 70% of alleles are represented by the Q188R and K285N missense mutations and are associated with severe disease. Carrier testing and prenatal diagnosis can be performed by direct enzyme analysis of amniocytes or chorionic villi; testing can also be DNA based.

Treatment and Prognosis. Because of newborn screening for galactosemia, patients are being identified and treated early. Various milk substitutes are available (casein hydrolysates, soybean-based formula). Elimination of galactose from the diet reverses growth failure and renal and hepatic dysfunction. Cataracts regress, and most patients have no impairment of eyesight. Early diagnosis and treatment have improved the prognosis of galactosemia; however, on long-term follow-up, patients still manifest ovarian failure with primary or secondary amenorrhea, decreased bone mineral density, developmental delay, and learning disabilities that increase in severity with age. Most manifest speech disorders, whereas a smaller number demonstrate poor growth and impaired motor function and balance (with or without overt ataxia). The relative control of galactose-1-phosphate levels does not always correlate with long-term outcome, leading to the belief that other factors, such as elevated galactitol, decreased uridine diphosphate galactose (UDP-galactose, a donor for galactolipids and proteins), and endogenous galactose production may be responsible.

GALACTOKINASE DEFICIENCY. The deficient enzyme is galactokinase, which normally catalyzes the phosphorylation of galactose. The principal metabolites accumulated are galactose and galactitol. Two genes have been reported to encode galactokinase: GK1 chromosome 17q24 and GK2 on chromosome 15. Cataracts are usually the sole manifestation of galactokinase deficiency; pseudotumor cerebri is a rare complication. The affected infant is otherwise asymptomatic. Heterozygote carriers may be at risk for presenile cataracts. Affected patients have an increased concentration of blood galactose levels, provided they have been fed a lactose-containing formula. The diagnosis is made by demonstrating an absence of galactokinase activity in erythrocytes or fibroblasts. Transferase activity is normal. Treatment is dietary restriction of galactose.

URIDINE DIPHOSPHATE GALACTOSE-4-EPIMERASE DEFICIENCY. The abnormally accumulated metabolites are similar to those in transferase deficiency; however, there is also an increase in cellular UDP-galactose. There are 2 distinct forms of epimerase deficiency. The 1st is benign form discovered incidentally through neonatal screening programs. Affected persons are healthy and without problems; the enzyme deficiency is limited to leukocytes and erythrocytes. No treatment is required. The 2nd form of epimerase deficiency is severe, and clinical manifestations resemble transferase deficiency, with the additional symptoms of hypotonia and nerve deafness. The enzyme deficiency is generalized, and clinical symptoms respond to restriction of dietary galactose. Although this form of galactosemia is rare, it must be considered in a symptomatic patient with measurable galactose-1-phosphate who has normal transferase activity. Diagnosis is confirmed by the assay of epimerase in erythrocytes.

Patients with the severe form of epimerase deficiency cannot synthesize galactose from glucose and are galactose dependent. Because galactose is an essential component of many nervous system structural proteins, patients are placed on a galactose-restricted diet rather than a galactose-free diet.

Infants with the mild form of epimerase deficiency have not required treatment. It is advisable to follow urine specimens for reducing substances and exclude aminoaciduria within a few weeks of diagnosis while the infant is still on lactose-containing formula.

The gene for UDP-galactose-4-epimerase is located on chromosome 1 at 1p36. Carrier detection is possible by measurement of epimerase activity in the erythrocytes. Prenatal diagnosis for the severe form of epimerase deficiency, using an enzyme assay of cultured amniotic fluid cells, is possible.

87.3 • Defects in Fructose Metabolism •

Priya S. Kishnani and Yuan-Tsong Chen

Two inborn errors are known in the specialized pathway of fructose metabolism: benign or essential fructosuria and hereditary fructose intolerance (HFI). Fructose-1,6-bisphosphatase deficiency, although strictly speaking not a defect of the specialized fructose pathway, is discussed in Chapter 87.4

DEFICIENCY OF FRUCTOKINASE (ESSENTIAL OR BENIGN FRUCTOSURIA). Deficiency of fructokinase is not associated with any clinical manifestations. It is an accidental finding usually made because the asymptomatic patient's urine contains a reducing substance. No treatment is necessary and the prognosis is excellent. Inheritance is autosomal recessive with an incidence of 1/120,000. The gene encoding fructokinase is located on chromosome 2p23.3.

Fructokinase catalyzes the 1st step of metabolism of dietary fructose: conversion of fructose to fructose-1-phosphate (see Fig. 87-1). Without this enzyme, ingested fructose is not metabolized. Its level is increased in the blood, and it is excreted in urine because there is practically no renal threshold for fructose. Clinitest results reveal the urinary-reducing substance, which can be identified as fructose by chromatography.

DEFICIENCY OF FRUCTOSE-1,6-BISPHOSPHATE ALDOLASE (ALDOLASE B, HEREDITARY FRUCTOSE INTOLERANCE). Deficiency of fructose-1,6-bisphosphate aldolase is a severe condition of infants that appears with the ingestion of fructose-containing food and is caused by a deficiency of fructose aldolase B activity in the liver, kidney, and intestine. The enzyme catalyzes the hydrolysis of fructose-1,6-bisphosphate into triose phosphate and glyceraldehyde phosphate. The same enzyme also hydrolyzes fructose-1-phosphate. Deficiency of this enzyme activity causes a rapid accumulation of fructose-1-phosphate and initiates severe toxic symptoms when exposed to fructose.

Epidemiology and Genetics. The true incidence of hereditary fructose intolerance (HFI) is unknown but may be as high as 1/26,000. The gene for aldolase B is on chromosome 9q22.3. Several mutations causing hereditary fructose intolerance are known. A single missense mutation, a G→C transversion in exon 5 resulting in the normal alanine at position 149 being replaced by a proline, is the most common mutation identified in northern Europeans. This mutation, plus 2 other point mutations, account for 80–85% of hereditary fructose intolerance in Europe and the United States. Diagnosis of hereditary fructose intolerance can be made by direct DNA analysis.

Clinical Manifestations. Patients with HFI are perfectly healthy and asymptomatic until fructose or sucrose (table sugar) is ingested (usually from fruit, fruit juice, or sweetened cereal). Symptoms may occur early in life, soon after birth if foods or formulas containing these sugars are introduced into the diet. Certain patients are very sensitive to fructose, whereas others can tolerate moderate intakes (up to 250 mg/kg/day). The average intake of fructose in Western societies is 1–2 g/kg/day. Early clinical manifestations resemble galactosemia and include jaundice, hepatomegaly, vomiting, lethargy, irritability, and convulsions. Laboratory findings include a prolonged clotting time, hypoalbuminemia, elevation of bilirubin and transaminase levels, and proximal tubular dysfunction. Acute fructose ingestion produces symptomatic hypoglycemia; the higher the intake, the more severe is the clinical picture. Chronic ingestion results in failure to thrive and hepatic disease. If the intake of the fructose persists, hypoglycemic episodes recur, and liver and kidney failure progress, eventually leading to death.

Diagnosis. Suspicion of the enzyme deficiency is fostered by the presence of a reducing substance in the urine during an episode. An intravenous fructose tolerance test, administered with great caution, is 1 step in facilitating diagnosis. The fructose challenge will cause a rapid fall, 1st of serum phosphate and then of blood glucose, and a subsequent increase in uric acid and magnesium. An oral tolerance test should not be performed because patients can become acutely ill. Definitive diagnosis is made by assay of fructaldolase B activity in the liver. Gene-based diagnosis is available for most patients with this disease; a common mutation (substitution of *Pro* for *Ala* at position 149) accounts for 53% of HFI alleles worldwide.

Treatment. Treatment consists of the complete elimination of all sources of sucrose, fructose, and sorbitol from the diet. It may be difficult because these sugars are widely used additives, found even in most medicinal preparations. With treatment, liver and kidney dysfunction improves, and catch-up in growth is common. Intellectual development is usually unimpaired. As the patient matures, symptoms become milder even after fructose ingestion; the long-term prognosis is good. Because of voluntary dietary avoidance of sucrose, affected patients have few dental caries.

87.4 • Defects in Intermediary Carbohydrate Metabolism Associated with Lactic Acidosis •

Priya S. Kishnani and Yuan-Tsong Chen

Lactic acidosis occurs with defects of carbohydrate metabolism that interfere with the conversion of pyruvate to glucose via the pathway of gluconeogenesis or to carbon dioxide and water via the mitochondrial enzymes of the citric acid cycle. Figure 87-4 depicts the relevant metabolic pathways. Type I GSD, fructose-1,6-diphosphatase deficiency, and phosphoenolpyruvate carboxylase deficiency are disorders of gluconeogenesis associated with lactic acidosis. Pyruvate dehydrogenase complex deficiency, respiratory chain defects, and pyruvate carboxylase deficiency are disorders in the pathway of pyruvate metabolism causing lactic acidosis. Lactic acidosis can also occur in defects of fatty acid oxidation, organic acidurias (see Chapters 85.6, 85.10, and 86.1), or biotin utilization diseases. These disorders are easily distinguishable by the presence of abnormal acylcarnitine profiles and amino acids in the blood and unusual organic acids in the urine. Blood lactate, pyruvate, and acylcarnitine profiles and the presence of these unusual urine organic acids should be determined in infants and children with unexplained acidosis, especially if there is an increase of anion gap (see Chapter 55).

Lactic acidosis unrelated to an enzymatic defect occurs in hypoxemia. In this case, as well as in defects in the respiratory chain, the serum pyruvate concentration may remain normal (<1.0 mg/dL with an increased lactate : pyruvate ratio), whereas pyruvate is usually increased when lactic acidosis results from an enzymatic defect in gluconeogenesis or pyruvate dehydrogenase complex (both lactate and pyruvate are increased and the ratio is normal). Lactate and pyruvate should be measured in the same blood specimen and on multiple blood specimens obtained when the patient is symptomatic because lactic acidosis can be intermittent. An algorithm for the differential diagnosis of lactic acidosis is shown in Figure 87-5.

DISORDERS OF GLUCONEOGENESIS

DEFICIENCY OF GLUCOSE-6-PHOSPHATASE (TYPE I GLYCOGEN STORAGE DISEASE). Type I GSD is the only glycogenosis associated with significant lactic acidosis. The chronic metabolic acidosis predisposes these patients to osteopenia; after prolonged fasting, the acidosis associated with hypoglycemia is a life-threatening condition (see Chapter 87.1).

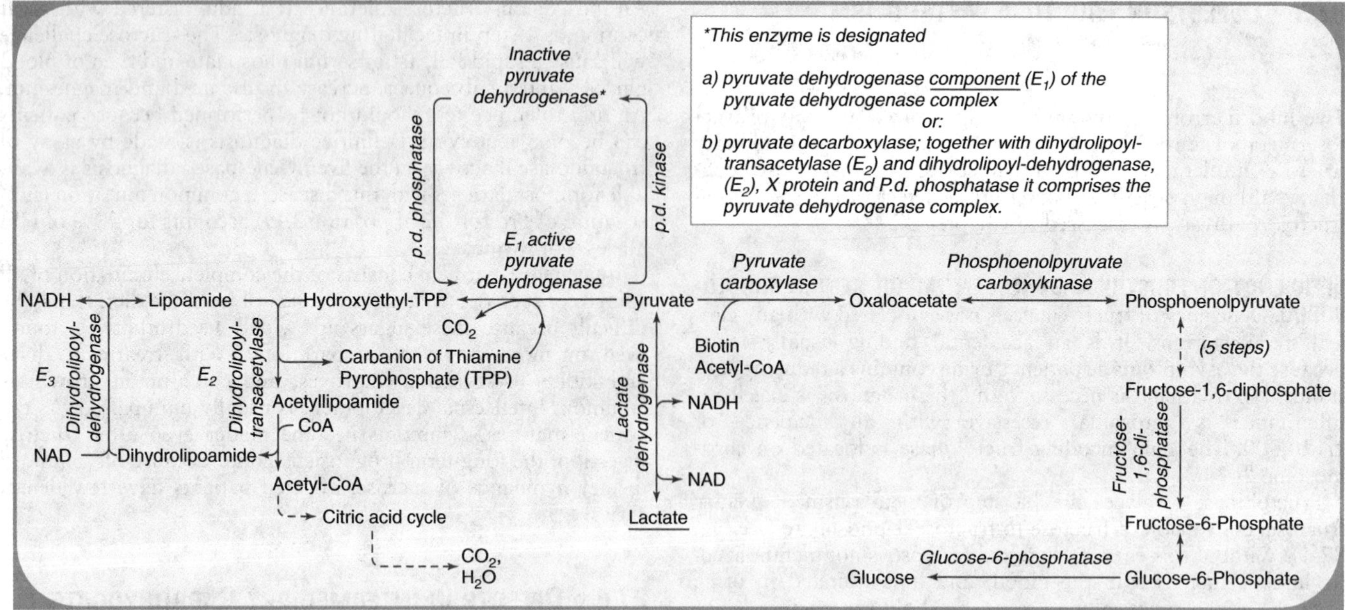

Figure 87-4. Enzymatic reactions of carbohydrate metabolism, deficiencies of which can give rise to lactic acidosis, pyruvate elevations, or hypoglycemia. The pyruvate dehydrogenase complex comprises, in addition to E_1, E_2, and E_3, an extra lipoate-containing protein (not shown), called protein X, and pyruvate dehydrogenase phosphatase.

FRUCTOSE-1,6-DIPHOSPHATASE DEFICIENCY. Fructose-1,6-diphosphatase deficiency impairs the formation of glucose from all gluconeogenic precursors, including dietary fructose. Hypoglycemia occurs when glycogen reserves are limited or exhausted. The **clinical manifestations** are characterized by life-threatening episodes of acidosis, hypoglycemia, hyperventilation, convulsions, and coma. In about ½ of the cases, the deficiency presents in the 1st wk of life. In infants and small children, episodes are triggered by febrile infections and gastroenteritis if oral food intake decreases. The frequency of the attacks decreases with age. Laboratory findings include low blood glucose, high lactate and uric acid levels, and metabolic acidosis. In contrast to hereditary fructose intolerance, there is usually no aversion to sweets; renal tubular and liver functions are normal.

The diagnosis is established by demonstrating an enzyme deficiency in either liver or intestinal biopsy. The enzyme defect can also be demonstrated in leukocytes in some cases. The gene coding for fructose-1,6-diphosphatase is located on chromosome 9q22; mutations are characterized making carrier detection and prenatal diagnosis possible. Treatment of acute attacks consists of correction of hypoglycemia and acidosis by intravenous glucose infusion; the response is usually rapid. Avoidance of fasting, aggressive management of infections and restriction of fructose and sucrose from the diet can prevent further episodes. For long-term prevention of hypoglycemia, a slowly released carbohydrate such as cornstarch is useful. Patients who survive childhood develop normally.

PHOSPHOENOLPYRUVATE CARBOXYKINASE (PEPCK) DEFICIENCY. PEPCK is a key enzyme in gluconeogenesis. It catalyzes the conversion of oxaloacetate to phosphoenolpyruvate (see Fig. 87-4). PEPCK deficiency is both a mitochondrial enzyme deficiency and a cytosolic enzyme deficiency, encoded by 2 distinct genes.

The disease has been reported in only a few cases. The clinical features are heterogeneous, with hypoglycemia, lactic acidemia, hepatomegaly, hypotonia, developmental delay, and failure to thrive as the major manifestations. There may be multisystem involvement, with neuromuscular deficits, hepatocellular damage, renal dysfunction, and cardiomyopathy. The diagnosis is based on the reduced activity of PEPCK in liver, fibroblasts, or lymphocytes. Fibroblasts and lymphocytes are not suitable for diagnosing the cytosolic form of PEPCK deficiency because these tissues possess only mitochondrial PEPCK. To avoid hypoglycemia, patients should be treated with slow-release carbohydrates such as cornstarch and fasting should be avoided.

DISORDERS OF PYRUVATE METABOLISM

Pyruvate is formed from glucose and other monosaccharides, from lactate, and from alanine. It is metabolized through 4 main enzyme systems: lactate dehydrogenase, alanine aminotransferase, pyruvate carboxylase, and pyruvate dehydrogenase complex. Deficiency of the M subunit of lactate dehydrogenase causes exercise intolerance and myoglobinuria (see Chapter 87.1). Genetic deficiency of alanine aminotransferase has not been reported in humans.

PYRUVATE DEHYDROGENASE COMPLEX DEFICIENCY. After entering the mitochondria, pyruvate is converted into acetyl coenzyme A (acetyl CoA) by the pyruvate dehydrogenase complex (PDHC), which catalyzes the oxidation of pyruvate to acetyl CoA, which then enters the tricarboxylic acid cycle for ATP production. The complex comprises 5 components: E_1, an α-keto acid decarboxylase; E_2, a dihydrolipoyl transacylase; E_3, a dihydrolipoyl dehydrogenase; protein X, an extra lipoate-containing protein; and pyruvate dehydrogenase phosphatase. The most common is a defect in the E_1 (see Fig. 87-4).

Deficiency of the pyruvate dehydrogenase complex is the most common of the disorders leading to lactic acidemia and central nervous system dysfunction. The central nervous system dysfunction is because the brain obtains its energy primarily from oxidation of glucose. Brain acetyl CoA is synthesized nearly exclusively from pyruvate.

The E_1 defects are caused by mutations in the gene coding for E_1 α subunit, which is X-linked. Although X-linked, its deficiency is a problem in both males and females, even though only 1 E_1 α allele in females carries a mutation.

Clinical Manifestations. The disease has a wide spectrum of presentations from the most severe neonatal presentation to a mild

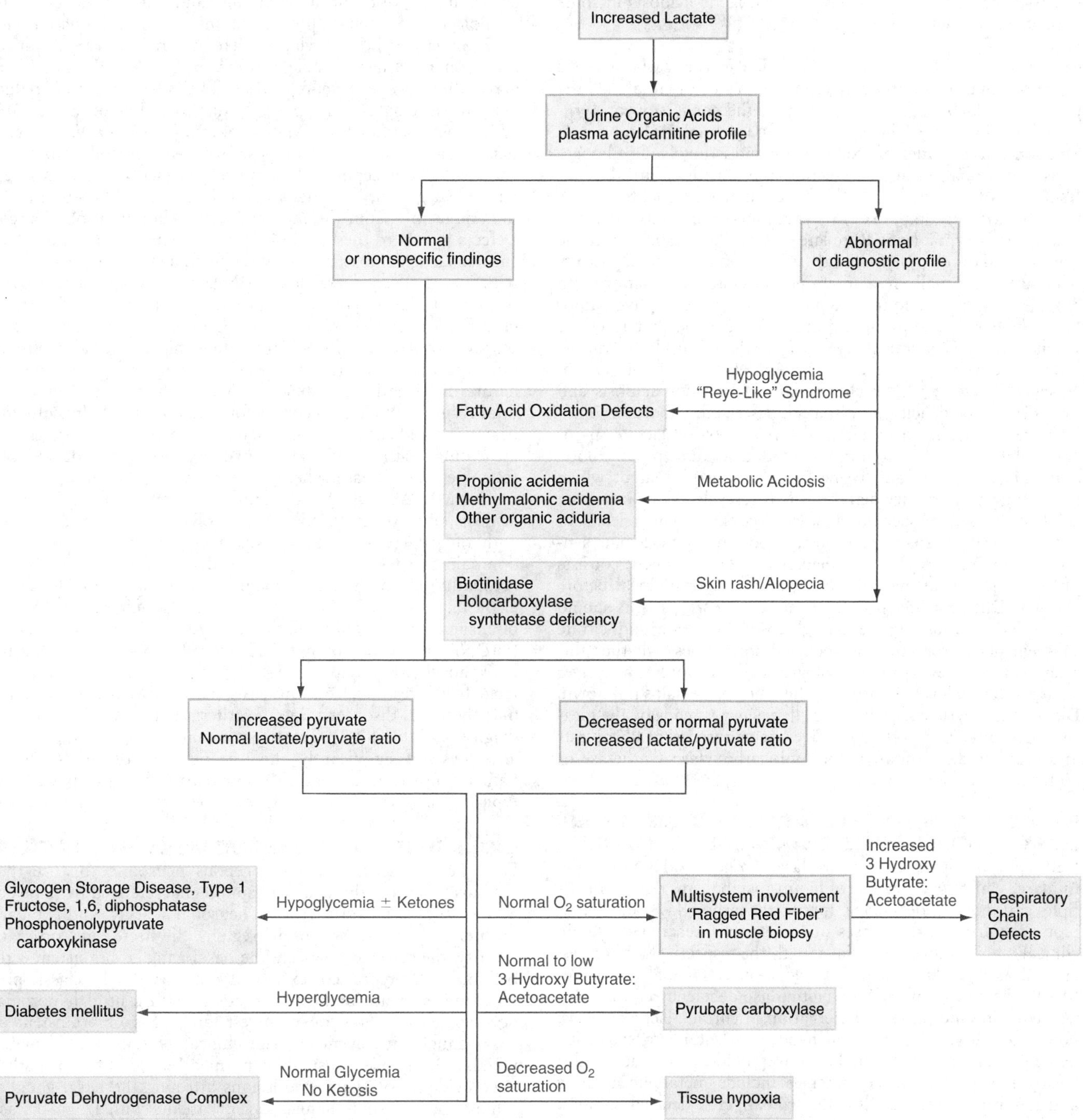

Figure 87-5. Algorithm of the differential diagnosis of lactic acidosis.

late-onset form. The neonatal onset is associated with lethal lactic acidosis, white matter cystic lesions, **agenesis of the corpus callosum,** and the most severe enzyme deficiency. Infantile onset can be lethal or associated with psychomotor retardation and chronic lactic acidosis, cystic lesions in the brainstem and basal ganglia, and pathologic features resembling **Leigh disease.** Older children, usually boys, may have less acidosis, have greater enzyme activity, and manifest ataxia with high-carbohydrate diets. Intelligence may be normal. Patients of all ages may have **facial dysmorphology,** features similar to those of fetal alcohol syndrome.

The E_2 and protein X-lipoate defects are rare and result in severe psychomotor retardation. The E_3 lipoamide dehydrogenase defect leads to deficient activity not only in the pyruvate dehydrogenase complex, but also in the α-keto glutarate and branched-chain keto acid dehydrogenase complexes. Pyruvate dehydrogenase phosphatase deficiency has also been reported. These other PDHC defects have clinical manifestations within the variable spectrum associated with PDHC deficiency due to E_1 deficiency.

Treatment. The general prognosis is poor except in rare cases in which mutation is associated with altered affinity for thiamine pyrophosphate, which may respond to thiamine supplementation. Because carbohydrates can aggravate lactic acidosis, a ketogenic diet is recommended. The diet has been found to lower the blood lactate level, but limited or no long-term benefit is seen. A potential treatment strategy is to maintain any residual PDHC in its active form by **dichloroacetate,** an inhibitor of E_1 kinase. Beneficial effects in controlling postprandial lactic acidosis in some patients have been shown.

DEFICIENCY OF PYRUVATE CARBOXYLASE. Pyruvate carboxylase is a mitochondrial, biotin-containing enzyme essential in the process of gluconeogenesis; it catalyzes the conversion of pyruvate to oxaloacetate. The enzyme is also essential for Krebs cycle function as a provider of oxaloacetate and is involved in lipogenesis and formation of nonessential amino acids. **Clinical manifestations** of this deficiency have varied from neonatal severe lactic acidosis accompanied by hyperammonemia, citrullinemia, and hyperlysinemia (**type B**) to late-onset mild to moderate lactic acidosis and developmental delay (**type A**). In both types, patients who survived usually had severe psychomotor retardation with seizures, spasticity, and microcephaly. Some patients have pathologic changes in the brainstem and basal ganglia that resemble **Leigh disease.** The clinical severity appears to correlate with the level of the residual enzyme activity. A "benign" form of PC deficiency characterized by recurrent attacks of lactic acidosis and mild neurologic deficits has also been described. Laboratory findings are characterized by elevated levels of blood lactate, pyruvate, alanine, and ketonuria. In the case of type B, blood ammonia, citrulline, and lysine levels are also elevated, which might suggest a primary defect of the urea cycle. The mechanism is likely caused by depletion of oxaloacetate, which leads to reduced levels of aspartate, a substrate for argininosuccinate synthetase in the urea cycle (see Chapter 85.11). **Treatment** consists of avoidance of fasting, and eating a carbohydrate meal before bedtime. During acute episodes of lactic acidosis, patients should receive continuous intravenous glucose. Aspartate and citrate supplements restore the metabolic abnormalities; whether this treatment can prevent the neurologic deficits is not known. Liver transplantation has been attempted; its benefit remains unknown. Diagnosis of pyruvate carboxylase deficiency is made by the measurement of enzyme activity in liver or cultured skin fibroblasts and must be differentiated from holocarboxylase synthetase or biotinidase deficiency.

DEFICIENCY OF PYRUVATE CARBOXYLASE SECONDARY TO DEFICIENCY OF HOLOCARBOXYLASE SYNTHETASE OR BIOTINIDASE. Deficiency of either holocarboxylase synthetase (HCS) or biotinidase, which are enzymes of biotin metabolism, result in multiple carboxylase deficiency (pyruvate carboxylase and other biotin-requiring carboxylases and metabolic reactions) and in clinical manifestations associated with the respective deficiencies, as well as rash, lactic acidosis, and alopecia (see also Chapter 85.6). The course of HCS or biotinidase deficiency can be protracted, with intermittent exacerbation of chronic lactic acidosis, failure to thrive, seizures, and hypotonia leading to spasticity, lethargy, coma, and death. Late-onset milder forms have also been reported. Laboratory findings include metabolic acidosis and abnormal organic acids in the urine. In HCS deficiency, biotin concentrations in plasma and urine are normal. **Diagnosis** can be made in skin fibroblasts or lymphocytes by assay for HCS activity, and in the case of biotinidase, in the serum by a screening blood spot. **Treatment** consists of biotin supplementation, 5–20 mg/day, and is generally effective if treatment is started before the development of brain damage. Patients identified through newborn screening and treated with biotin have remained asymptomatic.

Both enzyme deficiencies are autosomal recessive traits. HCS and biotinidase are located on chromosome 21q22 and 3p25, respectively. Ethnic-specific mutations in the HCS gene have been identified. Two common mutations (del7/ins3 and R538C) in the biotinidase gene account for 52% of all mutant alleles in symptomatic patients with biotinidase deficiency.

MITOCHONDRIAL RESPIRATORY CHAIN DEFECTS (OXIDATIVE PHOSPHORYLATION DISEASE). The mitochondrial respiratory chain catalyzes the oxidation of fuel molecules and transfers the electrons to molecular oxygen with concomitant energy transduction into ATP (oxidative phosphorylation). The respiratory chain produces ATP from nicotinamide-adenine dinucleotide (NADH) or $FADH_2$ and includes 5 specific complexes (I: NADH–coenzyme Q reductase; II: succinate–coenzyme Q reductase; III: coenzyme QH_2 cytochrome C reductase; IV: cytochrome C oxidase; V: ATP synthase). Each complex is composed of 4–35 individual proteins and, with the exception of complex II (which is encoded solely by nuclear genes), is encoded by nuclear or mitochondrial DNA (inherited only from the mother by mitochondrial inheritance). Defects in any of these complexes or assembly systems produce chronic lactic acidosis presumably due to a change of redox state with increased concentrations of NADH. In contrast to PDHC or pyruvate carboxylase deficiency, skeletal muscle and heart are usually involved in the respiratory chain disorders; and in muscle biopsy, "ragged red fibers" (indicating mitochondrial proliferation) are often seen (see Fig. 87-5). Because of the ubiquitous nature of oxidative phosphorylation, a defect of the mitochondrial respiratory chain accounts for a vast array of clinical manifestations and should be considered in patients in all age groups presenting with multisystem involvement. Some deficiencies resemble **Leigh disease,** whereas others cause infantile myopathies such as **MELAS** (mitochondrial myopathy, encephalopathy, lactic acidosis, and strokelike episodes), **MERRF** (myoclonus epilepsy, with ragged red fibers), and **Kearns-Sayre syndrome** (external ophthalmoplegia, acidosis, retinal degeneration, heart block, myopathy, and high cerebrospinal fluid protein) [Table 87-2; see also Chapters 598.2 and 610.4]. Diagnosis requires measurement of enzyme activities in tissues or analysis of mitochondrial DNA (mtDNA) mutation, or both (Fig. 87-6). Analysis of oxidative phosphorylation complexes I–IV from intact mitochondria isolated from fresh skeletal muscle is the most sensitive assay for mitochondrial disorders. Specific criteria may assist in making a diagnosis (Table 87-3). **Treatment** remains largely symptomatic and does not significantly alter the outcome of disease. Some patients, however, appear to respond to cofactor supplements, typically coenzyme Q10 plus L-carnitine at pharmacologic doses.

LEIGH DISEASE (SUBACUTE NECROTIZING ENCEPHALOMYELOPATHY). Leigh disease is a heterogenous neurologic disease that remains a neuropathologic description characterized by demyelination, gliosis, necrosis, relative neuronal sparing, and capillary proliferation in specific brain regions. In decreasing order of severity, the affected areas are the basal ganglia, brainstem cerebellum, and cerebral cortex (see Chapter 598). The classic presentation is of an infant who presents with central hypotonia, developmental regression or arrest, and signs of brainstem or basal ganglia involvement. The clinical presentation is highly variable. Diagnosis is usually confirmed by radiologic or pathologic evidence of symmetric lesions affecting the basal ganglia, brainstem, and subthalamic nuclei. Patients with Leigh disease have defects in several enzyme complexes. Dysfunction in cytochrome C oxidase (complex IV) is the most commonly reported defect, followed by NADH–coenzyme Q reductase (complex I), PDHC, and pyruvate carboxylase. Mutations in the nuclear SURF1 gene, which encodes a factor involved in the biogenesis of cytochrome C oxidase and mitochondrial DNA mutations in the ATPase 6 coding region, are common molecular findings in patients with Leigh disease.

87.5 • Defects in Pentose Metabolism •

Priya S. Kishnani and Yuan-Tsong Chen

About 90% of glucose metabolism in the body is via the glycolytic pathway, with the remaining 10% via the hexose

TABLE 87-2. Clinical and Genetic Heterogeneity of Disorders Related to Mutations in Mitochondrial DNA (mtDNA)*

	GIANT DELETIONS IN mtDNA			MUTATION IN TRANSFER RNA		MUTATION IN RIBOSOMAL RNA	MUTATION IN MESSENGER RNA		
SYMPTOMS, SIGNS, AND FINGDINGS	KSS	PEO	PS	MERRF	MELAS	AID	NARP	MILS	LHON
CENTRAL NERVOUS SYSTEM									
Seizures	−	−	−	[+]	+	−	−	+	−
Ataxia	+	−	−	[+]	+	−	[+]	±	−
Myoclonus	−	−	−	[+]	±	−	−	−	−
Psychomotor retardation	−	−	−	−	−	−	−	+	−
Psychomotor regression	+	−	−	±	+	−	−	−	−
Hemiparesis and hemianopia	−	−	−	−	[+]	−	−	−	−
Cortical blindness	−	−	−	−	[+]	−	−	−	−
Migraine-like headaches	−	−	−	−	[+]	−	−	−	−
Dystonia	−	−	−	−	+	−	−	+	±
PERIPHERAL NERVOUS SYSTEM									
Peripheral neuropathy	±	−	−	±	±	−	[+]	−	−
MUSCLE									
Weakness and exercise intolerance	+	[+]	−	+	+	−	+	+	−
Ophthalmoplegia	+	[+]	±	−	−	−	−	−	−
Ptosis	[+]	[+]	−	−	−	−	−	−	−
EYE									
Pigmentary retinopathy	[+]	−	−	−	−	−	[+]	±	−
Optic atrophy	−	−	−	−	−	−	±	±	[+]
BLOOD									
Sideroblastic anemia	±	−	[+]	−	−	−	−	−	−
ENDOCRINE SYSTEM									
Diabetes mellitus	±	−	−	−	±	−	−	−	−
Short stature	+	−	−	+	+	−	−	−	−
Hypoparathyroidism	±	−	−	−	−	−	−	−	−
HEART									
Conduction disorder	[+]	[−]	−	−	±	−	−	−	±
Cardiomyopathy	±	−	−	−	±	[+]	−	±	−
GASTROINTESTINAL SYSTEM									
Exocrine pancreatic dysfunction	±	−	[+]	−	−	−	−	−	−
Intestinal pseudo-obstruction	−	−	−	−	+	−	−	−	−
EAR, NOSE, AND THROAT									
Sensorineural hearing losss	±	−	−	+	+	[+]	±	−	−
KIDNEY									
Fanconi's syndrome	±	−	±	−	±	−	−	−	−
LABORATORY FINDINGS									
Lactic acidosis	+	±	+	+	+	−	−	±	−
Ragged-red fibers on muscle biopsy	+	+	±	+	+	−	−	−	−
MODE OF INHERITANCE									
Maternal	−	−	−	+	+	−	+	+	+
Sporadic	+	+	+	−	−	−	−	−	−

*Characteristic constellations of symptoms and signs are boxed.

+, presence of a symptom, sign, or finding; −, absence of a symptom, sign, or finding; ±, possible presence of a symptom, sign, or finding; AID, aminoglycoside-induce deafness; KSS, Kearns-Sayre syndrome; LHON, Leber's hereditary optic neuropathy. MELAS, mitochondrial encephalomyopathy, lactic acidosis, and strokelike episodes; MERRE, myoclonic epilepsy with ragged-red fibers; MILS, maternally inherited Leigh syndrome; NARP, neuropathy, ataxia, and retinitis pigmentosa; PEO, progressive external ophthalmoplegia; PS, Pearson syndrom.

From DiMauro S, Schon EA: Mitochondrial respiratory-chain diseases. *N Engl J Med* 2003;348:2656–2628.

TABLE 87-3. Modified Walker Criteria Applied to Children Referred for Evaluation of Mitochondrial Disease

	MAJOR CRITERIA	MINOR CRITERIA
Clinical	Clinically complete RC encephalomyopathy[†] or a mitochondrial cytopathy defined as fulfilling all 3 of the following[‡]	Symptoms compatible with an RC defect[§]
Histology	>2% ragged red fibers (RRF) in skeletal muscle	Smaller numbers of RRF, SSAM, or widespread electron microscopy abnormalities of mitochondria
Enzymology	Cytochrome c oxidase negative fibers or residual activity of an RC complex <20% in a tissue; <30% in a cell line, or <30% in 2 or more tissues	Antibody-based demonstration of an RC defect or residual activity of an RC complex 20–30% in a tissue, 30–40% in a cell line, or 30–40% in 2 or more tissues
Functional	Fibroblast ATP synthesis rates >3 SD below mean	Fibroblast ATP synthesis rates 2–3 SD below mean, or fibroblasts unable to grow in galactose media
Molecular	Nuclear or mtDNA mutation of undisputed pathogenicity	Nuclear or mtDNA mutation of probable pathogenicity
Metabolic		One or more metabolic indicators of impaired metabolic function

ATP, indicates adenosine triphosphate; RC, respiratory chain; SSAM, subsarcolemmal accumulation of mitochondria.

[†]Leigh disease, Alpers disease, LIMD, Pearson syndrome, Kearns-Sayre syndrome, MELAS, MERRF, NARP, MNGIE, and LHON.

[‡]1) Unexplained combination of multisystemic symptoms that is essentially pathognomic for an RC disorder, 2) a progressive clinical course with episodes of exacerbation or a family history strongly indicative of an mtDNA mutation, 3) other possible metabolic or nonmetabolic disorders have been excluded by appropriate testing.

[§]Added pediatric features: stillbirth associated with a paucity of intrauterine movement, neonatal death or collapse, movement disorder, severe failure to thrive, neonatal hypotonia, and neonatal hypertonia as minor clinical criteria.

From Scaglia F, Towbin JA, Craigen WJ, et al: Clinical spectrum, morbidity and mortality in 113 pediatric patients with mitochondrial disease. *Pediatrics* 2004;114:925–931.

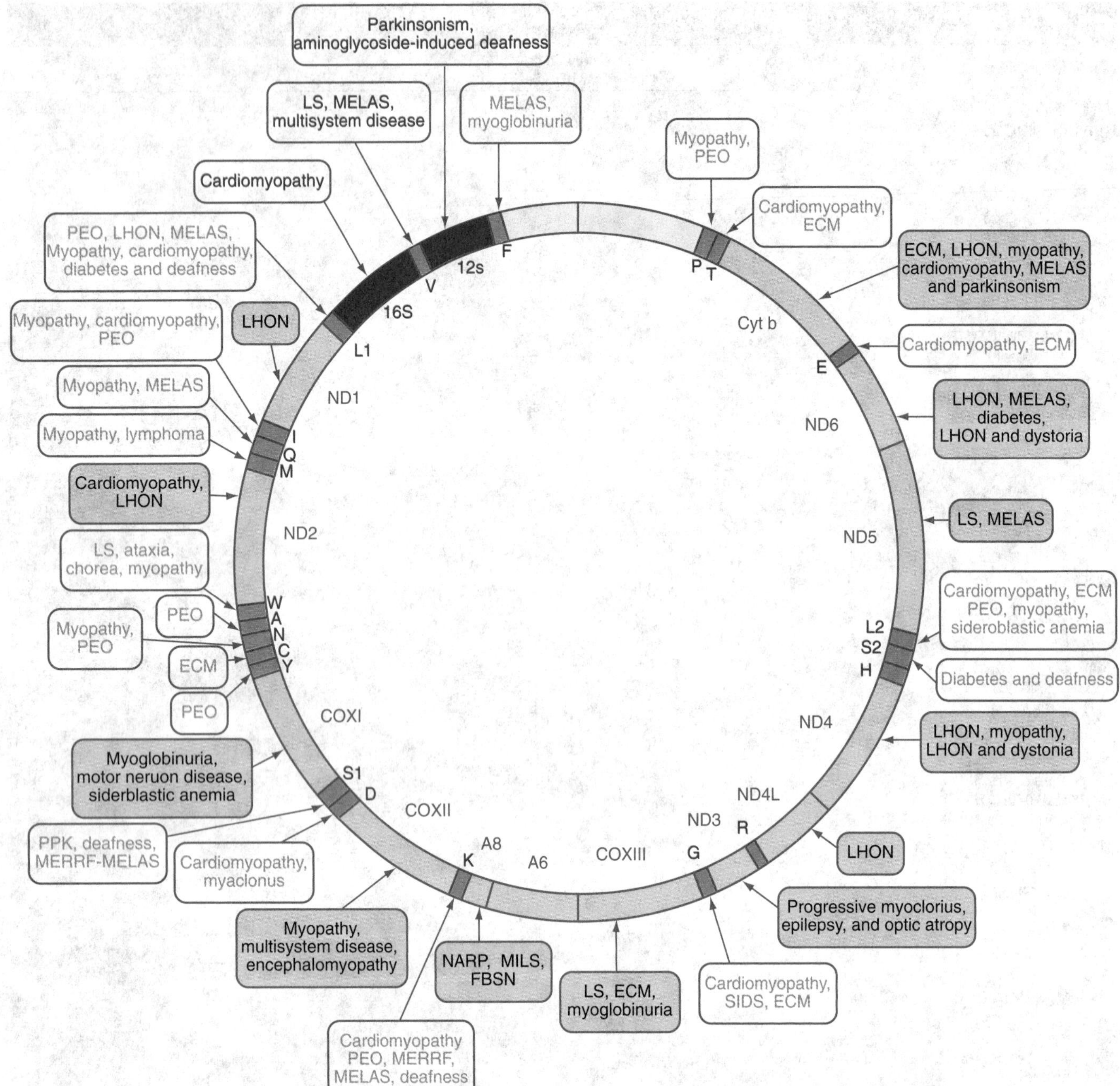

Figure 87-6. Mutations in the human mitochondrial genome that are known to cause disease. Disorders that are frequently or prominently associated with mutations in a particular gene are shown in *bold*. Diseases due to mutations that impair mitochondrial protein synthesis are shown in *blue*. Diseases due to mutations in protein-coding genes are shown in *red*. ECM, encephalomyopathy; FBSN, familial bilateral striatal necrosis; LHON, Leber hereditary optic neuropathy; LS, Leigh syndrome; MELAS, mitochondrial encephalomyopathy, lactic acidosis, and strokelike episodes; MERRF, myoclonic epilepsy with ragged-red fibers; MILS, maternally inherited Leigh syndrome; NARP, neuropathy, ataxia, and retinitis pigmentosa; PEO, progressive external ophthalmoplegia; PPK, palmoplantar keratoderma; and SIDS, sudden infant death syndrome. (From DiMauro S, Schon EA: Mitochondrial respiratory-chain diseases. *N Engl J Med* 2003;348:2656–2668. Copyright © 2003 Massachusetts Medical Society. All rights reserved.)

monophosphate pathway. The hexose monophosphate shunt leads to formation of pentoses, as well as providing NADH. One of the metabolites is ribose-5-phosphate, which is used in the biosynthesis of ribonucleotides and deoxyribonucleotides. Through the transketolase and transaldolase reactions, the pentose phosphates can be converted back to fructose-6-phosphate and glucose-6-phosphate.

ESSENTIAL PENTOSURIA. Essential pentosuria is a benign disorder encountered principally in Ashkenazi Jews and is an autosomal trait. The urine contains L-xylulose, which is excreted in increased amounts because of a block in the conversion of L-xylulose to xylitol due to xylitol dehydrogenase deficiency. The condition is usually discovered accidentally in a urine test for reducing substances; no treatment is required.

TRANSALDOLASE DEFICIENCY. To date, only 2 patients are reported; 1 presented with liver cirrhosis and hepatosplenomegaly in early infancy and the other presented with severe neonatal hepatopathy and cardiomyopathy. Biochemical abnormalities revealed elevated levels of arabitol, ribitol, and eythritol in the urine. Enzyme assay in the lymphoblasts/fibroblasts demonstrated low transaldolase activity, which was confirmed by mutations in the transaldolase gene.

RIBOSE-5-PHOSPHATE ISOMERASE DEFICIENCY. Only 1 case has been reported. The affected male had psychomotor retardation from early in life and developed epilepsy at 4 yr of age. Thereafter, a slow neurologic regression developed, with prominent cerebellar ataxia, some spasticity, optic atrophy, and a mild sensorimotor neuropathy. MRI of the brain at ages 11 yr and 14 yr showed extensive abnormalities of the cerebral white matter. Proton magnetic resonance spectroscopy (MRS) of the brain revealed elevated levels of ribitol and D-arabitol. These pentitols were also increased in urine and plasma similar to the patient found in transaldolase deficiency. Enzyme assays in cultured fibroblasts showed deficient ribose-5-phosphate isomerase activity, which was confirmed by a molecular study.

Amalfitano A, Bengur AR, Morse RP, et al: Recombinant human acid alpha-glucosidase enzyme therapy for infantile glycogen storage disease type II: Results of a phase I/II clinical trial. *Genet Med* 2001;3:132–138.

Arad M, Maron BJ, Gorham JM, et al: Glycogen storage disease presenting as hypertrophic cardiomyopathy. *N Engl J Med* 2005;352:362–372.

Bachrach BE, Weinstein DA, Orbo-Melander M, et al: Glycogen synthase deficiency (glycogen storage disease type O) presenting with hyperglycemia and glucosuria: Report of three new mutations. *J Pediatr* 2002;140:781–783.

Bosch AM, Grootenhuis MA, Bakker HD, et al: Living with classical galactosemia: Health-related quality of life consequences. *Pediatrics* 2004;113:e423–e428.

Chamoles NA, Niizawa G, Blanco M, et al: Glycogen storage disease type II: Enzymatic screening in dried blood spots on filter paper. *Clin Chim Acta* 200;347:97–s102.

Chen YT: Glycogen storage diseases. In Scriver CR, Beaudet AL, Sly WS, Valle D (eds): *The Metabolic and Molecular Bases of Inherited Disease,* 8th ed. New York, McGraw-Hill, 2001, pp 1521–1551.

Crimi M, Papadimitrious A, Galbiati S, et al: A new mitochondrial DNA mutation in ND3 gene causing severe Leigh syndrome with early lethality. *Pediatr Res* 2004;55:842–846.

De Meirleir L: Defects of pyruvate metabolism and the Krebs cycle. *J Child Neruol* 2002;17(Suppl 3):3S26–3S34.

Den Boer MEJ, Dionisi-Vici C, Chakrapani A, et al: Mitochondrial trifunctional protein deficiency: A severe fatty acid oxidation disorder with cardiac and neurologic involvement. *J Pediatr* 2003;142:684–689.

DiMauro S, Schon EA: Mitochondrial respiratory-chain diseases. *N Engl J Med* 2003;348:2656–2668.

Elpeleg O: Inherited mitochondrial DNA depletion. *Pediatr Res* 2003;54:153–159.

Franco LM, Krishnamurthy V, Bali D, et al: Hepatocellular carcinoma in glycogen storage disease type Ia: A case series. *J Inherit Metab Dis* 2005;28:153–162.

Garcoa-Cazorla A, De Lonlay P, Nassogne MC, et al: Long-term follow-up of neonatal mitochondrial cytopathies: A study of 57 patients. *Pediatrics* 2005;116:1170–1177.

Haller RG, Vissing J: No spontaneous second wind in muscle phosphofructokinase deficiency. *Neurology* 2004;62:82–86.

Holton JB, Walter JH, Tyfield IA, et al: Galactosemia. In Scriver CM, Beaudet AL, Sly WS, Valle D (eds): *The Metabolic and Molecular Bases of Inherited Disease,* 8th ed. New York, McGraw-Hill, 2001, pp 1553–1587.

Huck JH, Verhoeven NM, Struys EA, et al: Ribose-5-phosphate isomerase deficiency: New inborn error in the pentose phosphate pathway associated with a slowly progressive leukoencephalopathy. *Am J Hum Genet* 2004;74:745–751.

Huntsman RJ, Sinclair DB, Bhargava R, Chan A: Atypical presentations of Leigh syndrome: A case series and review. *Pediatr Neurol* 2005;32:334–340.

Kishnani PS, Howell RR: Pompe disease in infants and children. *J Pediatr* 2004;144:S35–S43.

Livingstone C, Al Riyami S, Wilkins P, Ferns GA: McArdle's disease diagnosed following statin-induced myositis. *Ann Clin Biochem* 2004;41:338–340.

Scaglia F, Towbin JA, Craigen WJ, et al: Clinical spectrum, morbidity, and mortality in 113 pediatric patients with mitochondrial disease. *Pediatrics* 2004;114:925–931.

Scheers I, Bachy V, Stephenne X, Sokal EM: Risk of hepatocellular carcinoma in liver mitochondrial respiratory chain disorders. *J Pediatr* 2005;146: 414–417.

Shen JJ, Chen YT: Molecular characterization of glycogen storage disease type III. *Curr Mol Med* 2002;2:167–175.

Shoffner JM: Oxidative phosphorylation diseases. In Scriver CR, Beaudet AL, Sly WS, Valle D (eds): *The Metabolic and Molecular Bases of Inherited Disease,* 8th ed. New York, McGraw-Hill, 2001, pp 2367–2423.

Stacpoole PW, Kerr DS, Barnes C, et al: Controlled Clinical trial of dichloroacetate for treatment of congenital lactic acidosis in children. Pediatrics 2006;117:1519–1531.

Uusimaa J, Finnila S, Remes AM, et al: Molecular epidemiology of childhood mitochondrial encephalomyopathies in a Finnish population: Sequence analysis of entire mtDNA of 17 children reveals heteroplasmic mutations in tRNA Arg, tRNAGlu, and tRNA Leu(UUR) genes. *Pediatrics* 2004;114: 443–450.

Van den Hout JMP, Kamphoven JHJ, Winkel LPF, et al: Long-term intravenous treatment of pompe disease with recombinant human α-glucosidase from milk. *Pediatrics* 2004;113:e448–e457.

Verhoeven NM, Wallot M, Huck JH, et al: A newborn with severe liver failure, cardiomyopathy and transalodase deficiency. *J Inherit Metab Dis* 2005;28:169–179.

Vissing J, Haller RG: The effect of oral sucrose on exercise tolerance in patients with McArdle's disease. *N Engl J Med* 2003;349:2503–2509.

Webb AL, Singh RH, Kennedy MJ, Elsas LJ: Verbal dyspraxia and galactosemia. *Pediatr Res* 2003;53:396–402.

Weber P, Scholl S, Baumgartner ER: Outcome in patients with profound biotinidase deficiency: Relevance of newborn screening. *Dev Med Child Neurol* 2004;46:481–484.

Winkel LP, Van den Hout JM, Kamphoven JH, et al: Enzyme replacement therapy in late-onset Pompe's disease: A three-year follow-up. *Ann Neurol* 2004;55:495–502.

Zeviani M, Di Donato S: Mitochondrial disorders. *Brain* 2004;127: 2153–2172.

87.6 • Disorders of Glycoprotein Degradation and Structure • Margaret M. McGovern and Robert J. Desnick

The disorders of glycoprotein degradation and structure include several lysosomal storage diseases that result from defects in glycoprotein degradation, and the congenital disorders of glycoprotein (CDGs), which are pathophysiologically unrelated. Glycoproteins are macromolecules that are composed of oligosaccharide chains linked to a peptide backbone. They are synthesized by 2 pathways: the glycosyltransferase pathway, which synthesizes oligosaccharides linked O-glycosidically to serine or threonine residues; and the dolichol, lipid-linked pathway, which synthesizes oligosaccharides linked N-glycosidically to asparagine.

The glycoprotein lysosomal storage diseases result from the deficiency of the enzymes that normally participate in the degradation of oligosaccharides and include sialidosis, galactosialidosis, aspartylglucosaminuria, and α-mannosidosis. In some instances, the underlying abnormality that leads to glycoprotein accumulation also results in abnormal degradation of other classes of macromolecules that contain similar oligosaccharide linkages, such as certain glycolipids and proteoglycans. In these instances, the underlying enzymatic deficiency results in the accumulation of both glycoproteins and glycolipids. The classification of these types of disorders as lipidoses or glycoproteinoses is dependent on the nature of the predominantly stored substance. In general, the glycoprotein disorders are characterized by autosomal recessive inheritance and a progressive disease course with clinical features that resemble those seen in the mucopolysaccharidoses.

SIALIDOSIS AND GALACTOSIALIDOSIS. Sialidosis is an autosomal recessive disorder that results from the primary deficiency of neuraminidase due to mutations in the gene that encodes this protein, which is located on chromosome 10. In contrast, galactosialidosis is due to the deficiency of 2 lysosomal enzymes, neuraminidase and β-galactosidase. The loss of these enzymatic activities results from mutations in a gene located on chromosome 20 that encodes protective protein/cathepsin A (PPCA), which functions to stabilize these enzymatic activities. Neuraminidase normally cleaves terminal sialyl linkages of several oligosaccharides and glycoproteins. Its deficiency results in the accumulation of oligosaccharides, and the urinary excretion of sialic acid terminal oligosaccharides and sialylglycopeptides. Examination of tissues from affected individuals reveals pathologic storage of substrate in many tissues including liver, bone marrow, and brain.

The **clinical phenotype** associated with **neuraminidase deficiency** is variable and includes type I sialidosis which usually presents in the 2nd decade of life with myoclonus and the presence of a cherry red spot. These patients typically come to attention secondary to gait disturbances, myoclonus, or visual complaints. In contrast, **type II sialidosis** occurs as congenital, infantile, and juvenile forms. The congenital and infantile forms result from isolated neuraminidase deficiency, whereas the juvenile form results from both neuraminidase and β-galactosidase deficiency. The **congenital type II disease** is characterized by hydrops fetalis, neonatal ascites, hepatosplenomegaly, stippling of the epiphyses, periosteal cloaking, and stillbirth or death in infancy. The **type II infantile form** presents in the 1st yr of life with dysostosis multiplex, moderate mental retardation, visceromegaly, corneal clouding, cherry red spot, and seizures. The **juvenile type II** form of sialidosis, which is sometimes designated *galactosialidosis,* has a variable age of onset ranging from infancy to adulthood. In infancy, the phenotype is similar to that of GM_1 gangliosidosis, with edema, ascites, skeletal dysplasia, and cherry red spot. Patients with later-onset disease have dysostosis multiplex, visceromegaly, mental retardation, dysmorphism, corneal clouding, progressive neurologic deterioration, and bilateral cherry red spots. No specific therapy exists for any form of the disease, although studies in animal models have demonstrated improvement in the phenotype after bone marrow transplantation. The diagnosis of sialidosis and galactosialidosis is achieved by the demonstration of the specific enzymatic deficiency. Prenatal diagnosis using cultured amniotic cells is also possible.

ASPARTYLGLUCOSAMINURIA (AGU). This is a rare autosomal recessive lysosomal storage disorder, except in Finland, where the carrier frequency is estimated at 1/36. The disorder results from the deficient activity of aspartylglucosaminidase and the subsequent accumulation of aspartylglucosamine, particularly in the liver, spleen, and thyroid. The gene for the enzyme has been localized to the long arm of chromosome 4 and the cDNA has been cloned and sequenced. In the Finnish population, a single mutation in the gene (C163S) accounts for most mutant alleles, whereas outside of Finland, a large number of private mutations have been described. Affected individuals with AGU typically present in the 1st yr of life with recurrent infections, diarrhea, and hernias. Coarsening of the facies and short stature usually develop later. Other features include joint laxity, macroglossia, hoarse voice, crystal-like lens opacities, hypotonia, and spasticity. Psychomotor development is usually near normal until the age of 5 when a decline is noted. Behavioral abnormalities are typical and IQ values in affected adults are usually <40. Survival to adulthood is common, with most early deaths attributable to pneumonia or other pulmonary causes. Definitive diagnosis requires measurement of the enzyme in peripheral blood leukocytes. Molecular diagnosis by analysis of DNA for the C163S mutation is possible for Finnish patients. Several patients have undergone allogeneic bone marrow transplants, but this approach has not been proven effective and no specific treatment is available. Prenatal diagnosis by the determination of the level of aspartylglucosaminidase in cultured amniocytes or chorionic villi has been reported.

αS-MANNOSIDOSIS. This autosomal recessive disorder results from the deficient activity of α-mannosidase and the accumulation of mannose-rich compounds. The gene encoding the enzyme has been localized to chromosome 19p13.2-q12, although the cDNA has not been cloned. Affected patients with this disorder display clinical heterogeneity. There is a severe infantile form, or type I disease, and a milder juvenile variant, type II disease. All patients have psychomotor retardation, facial coarsening, and dysostosis multiplex. The infantile form of the disorder, however, is characterized by more rapid mental deterioration, with death occurring between the ages of 3 and 10 yr. Patients with the infantile form also have more severe skeletal involvement and hepatosplenomegaly. The juvenile disorder is characterized by onset of symptoms in early childhood or adolescence with milder somatic features and survival to adulthood. Hearing loss, destructive synovitis, pancytopenia, and spastic paraplegia have been reported in type II patients. No specific therapy exists for the disorder. The diagnosis is made by the demonstration of the deficiency of α-mannosidase activity in white blood cells or cultured fibroblasts, and prenatal diagnosis has also been achieved.

CONGENITAL DISORDERS OF GLYCOSYLATION (CDGS). These are a heterogenous group of autosomal recessive disorders that result from defects in the processing and synthesis of the carbohydrate moiety of glycoproteins.

There are at least 22 identifiable disorders; type Ia is the most common (Table 87-4). One main group includes those with defects in biosynthesis or transfer of sugar chains from a lipid-linked oligosaccharide precursor to a new protein in the endoplasmic reticulum (group Ia to IL). Group II (IIa to IIf) is characterized by defects in N-linked sugar chain Golgi processing. Undefined disorders are temporarily assigned to group X.

A distinctive biochemical marker of the disorder is the presence of carbohydrate-deficient transferrin in serum and cerebrospinal fluid. The most consistent clinical features of the disorder include psychomotor retardation, which varies in severity, and facial dysmorphic features that include a prominent jaw and ears and inverted nipples. Frequent neurologic findings in infancy include cerebellar atrophy (Fig. 87-7), hypotonia, weakness, hyperreflexia, and strokelike episodes.

In childhood, ataxia, muscle atrophy, decreased deep tendon reflexes, toe walking, and continued strokelike episodes are observed. The latter events may be related to coagulopathies characterized by reduced factor XI, protein C, and antithrombin III. Strabismus is a consistent finding and retinitis pigmentosa is common. Growth failure, liver dysfunction, retinal degeneration, and skeletal abnormalities have also been described. The skeletal features can include contractures, kyphoscoliosis, and pectus carinatum, all of which may be secondary to the neurologic effects of the disorder. Pericardial effusion in older patients and hypertrophic obstructive cardiomyopathy in the infant also occur.

Transferrin studies have also revealed that infantile **olivopontinecerebellar atrophy** is a severe form of CDG. Lipodystrophy with prominent fat pads on the buttocks is a distinctive feature. The disorder should be considered in patients with mental retardation, cerebellar hypoplasia, hepatic dysfunction, and episodic strokelike episodes, and in patients with various combinations of the features detailed in the previous paragraph. The diagnosis can be confirmed by analysis of the transferrin pattern by isoelectric focusing. Although prenatal diagnosis by analysis of transferrin has been attempted, it has not proven reliable. Treatment of these disorders is symptomatic, except for CDGIb, which responds to oral mannose (100–150 mg/kg/day every 4–6 hr), and possible CDGIIc, which may respond to oral fucose (25 mg/kg/day tid).

TABLE 87-4. Characteristics of Representative Congenital Disorders of Glycosylation (CDG)

NAME	DEFECT	DYSMORPHOLOGY	NEUROLOGIC SIGNS	GASTROINTESTINAL SIGNS	OTHER SIGNS
CDGIa	Phosphomannomutase 2 M6P ⟶ M1P Incidence 1/80,000	Fat maldistribution: narrow waist, fat in axilla, groin, buttock High nasal bridge Prominant jaw Large ears Inverted nipples	Hypotonia Hyporeflexia Strabismus Ataxia: olivopontocerebellar atrophy or hypoplasia Mental retardation (IQ 40–60) Strokelike episodes Hemorrhagic cerebral infarcts Polyneuropathy Muscle wasting Scoliosis Spinal stenosis Kyphosis Pigmentary retinal degeneration Contractures Seizures	Poor feeding Failure to thrive Carnitine deficiency Diarrhea Liver failure	Cardiomyopathy Pericardial effusions Nephrotic syndrome Renal tubulopathy Severe infections Hypogonadism Absent puberty TBG deficiency ↓ Levels of: antithrombin III, α_1 acid glycoprotein, α_1-antitrypsin, ferritin, ceruloplasmin, proteins C + S, factor XI, complement-C1, C3a, C4a
CDGIb	Phosphomannose isomerase F6P ⟶ M6P	None	Normal development	Protein-losing enteropathy Failure to thrive Chronic intractable diarrhea Hepatic fibrosis Hyperinsulinemic hypoglycemia Vomiting	Coagulopathy ↓ proteins C, S, antithrombin III
CDGIc	Glucosyltransferase: prevents glucose addition to endoplasmic reticulum lumen	None	Similar to CDGIa but milder Mild cerebellar hypoplasia No neuropathy Pigmentary retinal degeneration Seizures	Failure to thrive	Recurrent eyelid edema Frequent infections Coagulopathy
CDGId	Mannosyltransferase: prevents mannose addition to endoplasmic reticulum lumen	High arched palate Microcephaly	Developmental delay Seizures (severe) CNS atrophy	Failure to thrive	Coagulopathy
CDGIe	Dolichol-phosphate-mannose synthetase: DPM donates mannose	High arched palate Microcephaly Down slanting palpebral fissures Hemangiomas Short arms Small hands Dysplastic nails	Developmental delay Hypotonia Seizures (severe) Cortical blindness Hyperreflexia Delayed myelination	Failure to thrive	↑ CPK
CDGIIa	*N*-acetyl-glucosaminyl-transferase II	Facial dysmorphology	Stereotypic hand movements Seizures Developmental delay No neuropathy or cerebellar hypoplasia	Failure to thrive	Coagulopathy
CDGIIb	Glucosidase I	Facial dysmorphology	Hypotonia Retardation Seizures	Hepatomegaly	Coagulopathy
CDGIIc	GDP-fucose transporter I	Facial dysmorphology	Developmental delay Hypotonia	Failure to thrive	Recurrent infections with leukocytosis
CDGx or CDGIx	Unknown Unclassified	Like CDGIa Microcephaly	Hypotonia Seizures Cerebellar hypoplasia Developmental delay	Intractable diarrhea Failure to thrive	Nonimmune hydrops Cataracts Thrombocytopenia Renal tubulopathy Distal bone demineralization
CDG-Ih	h*ALG8* gene*	Facial dysmorphology	Seizures Hypotonia Developmental delay	Chronic diarrhea Protein-losing enteropathy Chronic liver disease	Coagulopathy Renal microcysts Nephrotic syndrome
CDG-X variant	Unknown	None	None	Asymptomatic cryptogenic Chronic liver disease	Coagulopathy
CDGIIX	Unknown	None	Developmental delay Hypotonia Cerebral atrophy	Chronic diarrhea Liver cirrhosis	Recurrent infections

*enzyme, dolichyl-phosphate glucose; mannose 9-N acetylglucosamine 2-PP-Dol-α-1,3-glucosyl transferase.
CNS, central nervous system; DPM, dolichol-phosphate-mannose; FGP, fructose-6-phosphate; M6P, mannose-6-phosphate; MIP, mannose-1-phosphate; TBG, thyroid-binding globulin.

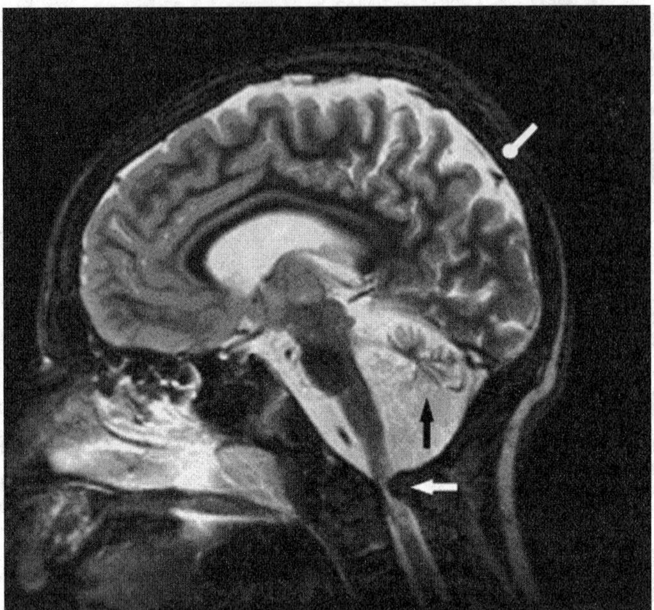

Figure 87-7. Sagital T2-weighted MR image shows severe spinal cord compression with myelopathy *(white arrow)*, together with cerebellar atrophy *(black arrow)*, and cortical atrophy of the parietal lobe *(blunt arrow)*. (From Schade van Westrum SM, Nederkoorn PJ, Schuurman PR, et al: Skeletal dysplasia and myelopathy in congenital disorder of glycosylation type 1A. *J Pediatr* 2006;145:115–117.)

Collins AE, Ferriero DM: The expanding spectrum of congenital disorders of glycosylation. *J Pediatr* 2005;147:728–730.

Denecke J, Kranz C, Von Kleist-Retzow JCh, et al: Congenital disorder of glycosylation type 1d: clinical phenotype, molecular analysis, prenatal diagnosis, and glycosylation of fetal proteins. *Pediatr Res* 2005;58:248–253.

Dinopoulos A, Mohamed I, Jones B, et al: Radiologic and neurophysiologic aspects of stroke-like episodes in children with congenital disorder of glycosylation Type 1a. *Pediatrics* 2007;119:e768–e772.

Eklund EA, Sun L, Westphal V, et al: Congenital disorder of glycosylation (CDG)-Ih patient with a severe hepato-intestinal phenotype and evolving central nervous system pathology. *J Pediatr* 2005;147:847–880.

Leroy JG: Congenital disorders of N-glycosylation including diseases associated with O- as well as N-glycosylation defects. *Pediatr Res* 2006;60: 643–656.

Mandato C, Brive L, Miura Y, et al: Cryptogenic liver disease in four children: A novel congenital disorder of glycosylation. *Pediatr Res* 2006;59:293–298.

Miura Y, Tay SK, Aw MM, et al: Clinical and biochemical characterization of a patient with congenital disorder of glycosylation (CDG) IIx. *J Pediatr* 2005;147:851–853.

Schade van Westrum SM, Nederkoorn PJ, Schuurman PR, et al: Skeletal dysplasia and myelopathy in congenital disorder of glycosylation type 1A. *J Pediatr* 2006;148;115–117.

Chapter 88 ■ Mucopolysaccharidoses

Jürgen Spranger

Mucopolysaccharidoses are hereditary, progressive diseases caused by mutations of genes coding for lysosomal enzymes needed to degrade glycosaminoglycans (acid mucopolysaccharides). Glycosaminoglycan (GAG) is a long-chain complex carbohydrate composed of uronic acids, amino sugars, and neutral sugars. The major glycosaminoglycans are chondroitin-4-sulfate, chondroitin-6-sulfate, heparan sulfate, dermatan sulfate, keratan sulfate, and hyaluronan. These substances are synthesized and, with the exception of hyaluronan, linked to proteins to form proteoglycans, major constituents of the ground substance of connective tissue, as well as nuclear and cell membranes. Degradation of proteoglycans starts with the proteolytic removal of the protein core followed by the stepwise degradation of the glycosaminoglycan moiety. Failure of this degradation due to absent or grossly reduced activity of mutated lysosomal enzymes results in the intralysosomal accumulation of GAG fragments (Fig. 88-1). Distended lysosomes accumulate in the cell, interfere with cell function, and lead to a characteristic pattern of clinical, radiologic, and biochemical abnormalities (Table 88-1, Fig. 88-2). Within this pattern, specific diseases can be recognized that evolve from the intracellular accumulation of different degradation products (Table 88-2). As a general rule, the impaired degradation of heparan sulfate is more closely associated with mental deficiency and the impaired degradation of dermatan sulfate, chondroitin sulfates, and keratan sulfate with mesenchymal abnormalities. Variable expression within a given entity results from allelic mutations and varying residual activity of mutated enzymes. Allelic mutations of the gene encoding L-iduronidase may result in severe Hurler disease with early death or in mild Scheie disease manifesting only with limited joint mobility, mild skeletal abnormalities, and corneal opacities. Mucopolysaccharidoses are autosomal recessive disorders, with the exception of Hunter disease, which is X-linked recessive. Their overall frequency is between 3.5/100,000 and 4.5/100,000. The most common subtype is MPS-III, followed by MPS-I and MPS-II.

CLINICAL ENTITIES

MUCOPOLYSACCHARIDOSIS I. MPS I is caused by mutations of the *IUA* gene on chromosome 4p16.3 encoding α-L-iduronidase. Mutation analysis reveals 2 major alleles, W402X and Q70X, that account for more than ½ the MPS-I alleles in the white population. The mutations introduce stop codons with ensuing absence of functional enzyme (null alleles); homozygosity or compound heterozygosity gives rise to Hurler disease. Other mutations occur in only 1 or a few individuals.

Deficiency of α-L-iduronidase results in a broad clinical spectrum, from severe **Hurler** disease to mild **Scheie** diseases. Homozygous nonsense mutations result in severe forms of MPS I, whereas missense mutations are more likely to preserve some residual enzyme activity associated with a milder form of the disease.

TABLE 88-1. Recognition Pattern of Mucopolysaccharidoses

	MUCOPOLYSACCHARIDOSIS TYPE						
MANIFESTATIONS	I-H	I-S	II	III	IV	VI	VII
Mental deficiency	+	−	±	+	−	−	±
Coarse facial features	+	(+)	+	+	−	+	±
Corneal clouding	+	+	−	−	(+)	+	±
Visceromegaly	+	(+)	+	(+)	−	+	+
Short stature	+	(+)	+	−	+	+	+
Joint contractures	+	+	+	−	−	+	+
Dysostosis multiplex	+	(+)	+	(+)	+	+	+
Leucocyte inclusions	+	(+)	+	+	−	+	+
Mucopolysaccharidurla	+	+	+	+	+	+	+

I-H, Hurler disease; I-S, Scheie disease; II, Hunter disease; III, Sanfilipppo disease; IV, Morquio disease; VI, Maroteaux-Lamy disease; VII, Sly disease.

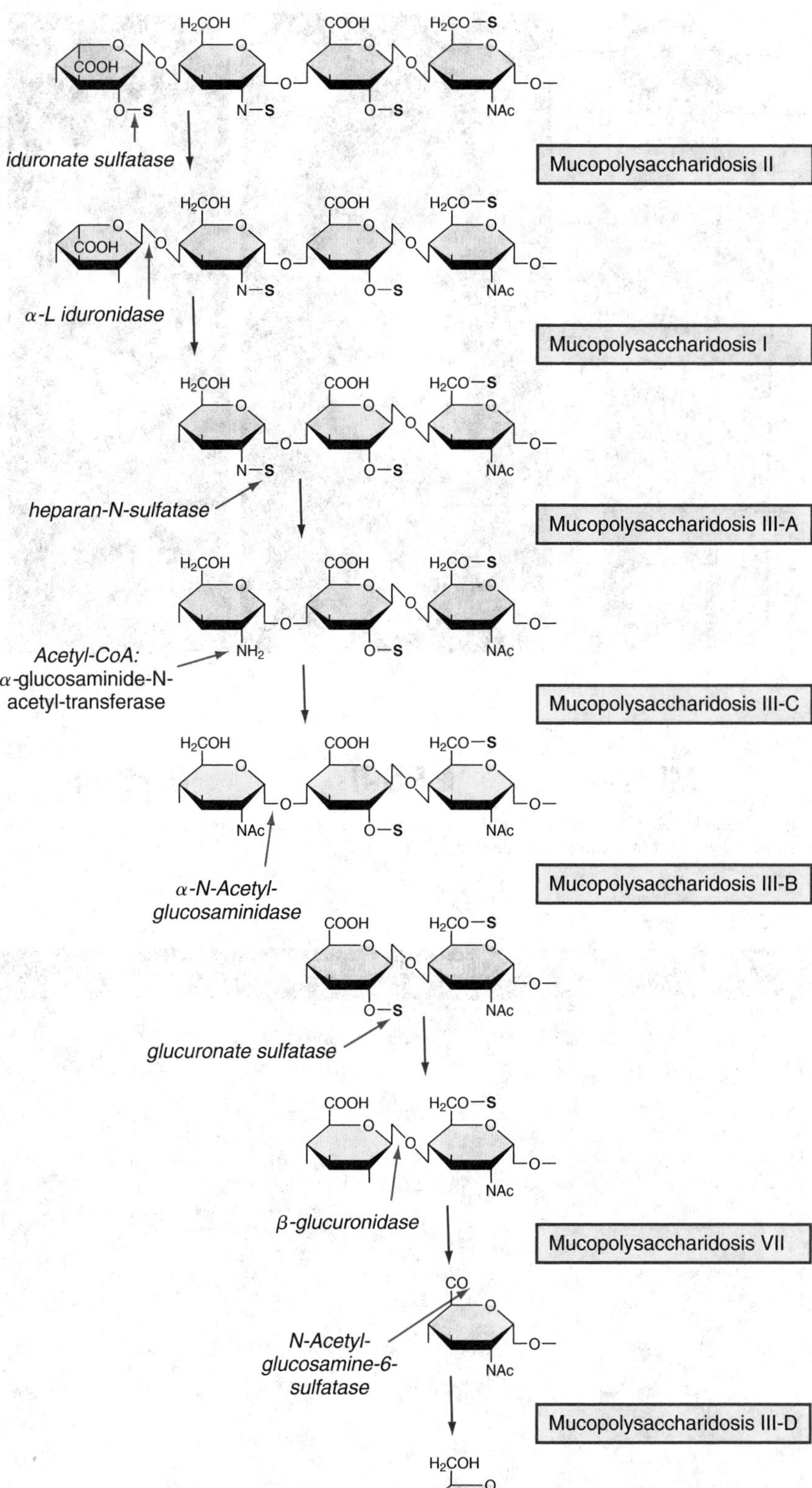

Figure 88-1. Degradation of heparan sulfate and mucopolysaccharidoses resulting from the deficiency of individual enzymes. Some of the enzymes are also involved in the degradation of other glycosaminoglycans (not shown).

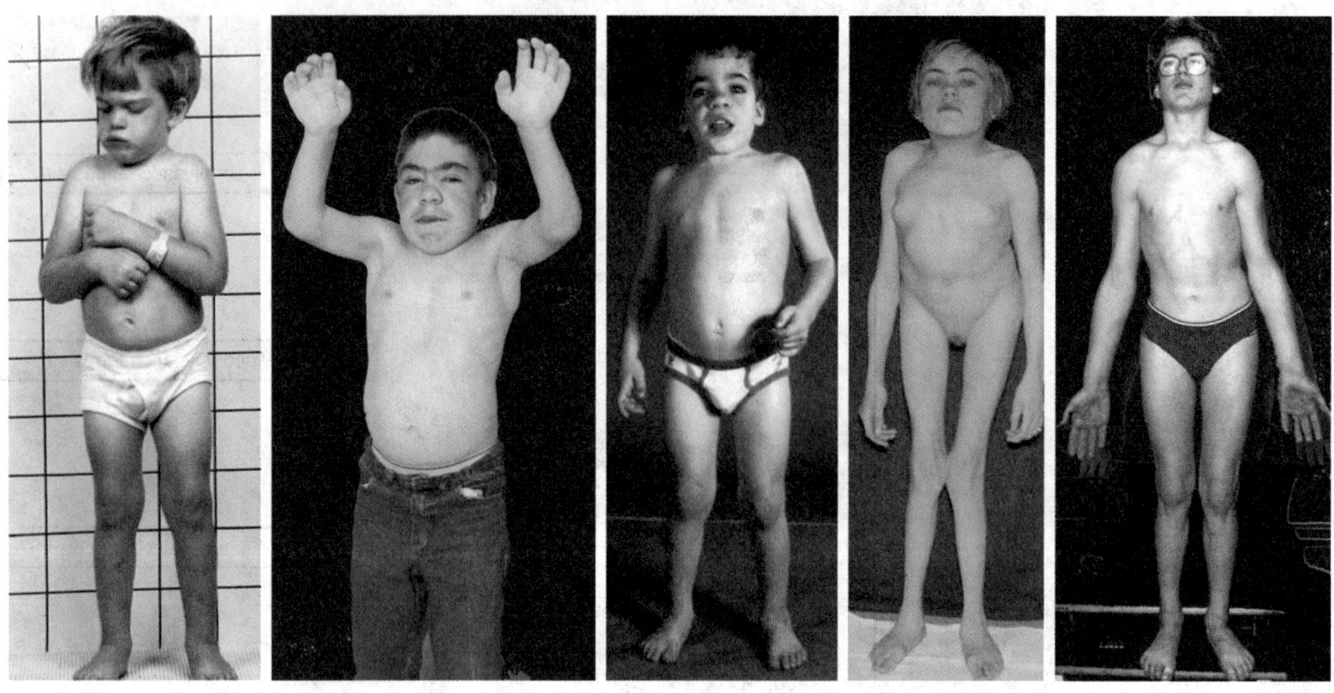

MPS-I MPS-II MPS-III MPS-IV MPS-VI

Figure 88-2. Patients with various types of mucopolysaccharidoses. I: Hurler disease, 3 yr; II: Hunter disease, 12 yr; III: Sanfilippo disease, 4 yr; IV: Morquio disease, 10 yr; VI: Maroteaux-Lamy disease, 15 yr.

TABLE 88-2. Mucopolysaccharidoses: Clinical, Molecular, and Biochemical Aspects

MPS TYPE	EPONYM	INHERITANCE	GENE CHROMOSOME	MAIN CLINICAL FEATURES	DEFECTIVE ENZYME	*ASSAY*	*MIM NUMBER*
I-H	Pfaundler-Hurler	AR	*IDA* 4p16.3	Severe Hurler phenotype, mental deficiency, corneal clouding, death usually before age 14 years	α-L-iduronidase	L,F,Ac,C V	252 800 607 014
I-S	Scheie	AR	*IDA* 4p16.4	Stiff joints, corneal clouding, aortic valve disease, normal intelligence, survive to adulthood	α-L-iduronidase	L,F,Ac,C V	607 016
I-HS	Hurler-Scheie	AR	*IDA* 4p16.4	Phenotype intermediate between I-H and I-S	α-L-iduronidase	L,F,Ac,Cv	607 015
II	Hunter	XLR	*IDS* Xq27.3-28	Severe course similar to I-H but clear corneas. Mild course: less pronounced features, later manifestation, survival to adulthood with mild or no mental deficiency	Iduronate sulfate sulfatase	S,F, Af, Ac, Cv	309 900
III-A	Sanfilippo A	AR	*HSS* 17q25.3	Behavioral problems, sleeping disorder, aggression, progressive dementia, mild dysmorphism, coarse hair, clear corneas, survival to adulthood possible	Heparan-S-sulfamidase	L,F,Ac,Cv	252 900 605 270
II-IB	Sanfilippo B	AR	*NAGLU* 17q21		N-ac-α-glucosaminidase	S,F,Ac,Cv	252 920
III-C	Sanfilippo C	AR	*HGSNAT 8p11-q13*		Ac-CoA-glucosaminide-N-acetyltransferase	F,Ac	252 930
III-D	Sanfilippo D	AR	*GNS* 12q14		N-ac-glucosaminine-6-sulfate sulfatase	F,Ac	252 940 607 664
IV-A	Morquio A	AR	*GALNS* 16q24.3	Short-trunk dwarfism, fine corneal opacities, characteristic bone dysplasia; final height <125 cm	N-ac-galactosamine-6-sulfate sulfatase	L,F,Ac	253 000
IV-B	Morquio B	AR	*GLB1* 3p21.33	Same as IV-A, but milder; adult height >120 cm	β-Galactosidase	L,F,Ac,Cv	253 010 230 500
VI	Maroteaux-Lamy	AR	*ARSB* 5q11-q13	Hurler phenotype with marked corneal clouding but normal intelligence; mild, moderate, and severe expression in different families	N-ac-galactos-amine-α-4-sulfate sulfatase (arylsulfatase B)	L,F,Ac	253 200
VII	Sly	AR	*GUSB* 7q21.11	Varying from fetal hydrops to mild dysmorphism; dense inclusions in granulocytes	β-glucuronidase	S,F,Ac,Cv	253 220
IX	Hyaluronidase deficiency	AR	*HYAL1* 3p21.3	Periarticular masses, no Hurler phenotype	Hyaluronidase 1	S	601 492

Ac, cultured amniotic cells; Af, amniotic fluid; Cv, chorionic villi; F, cultured fibroblasts; L, leukocytes; MIM, Mendelian Inheritance in Man Catalog; S, serum.

Hurler Disease. This form of MPS I (MPS I-H) is a severe, progressive disorder with multiple organ and tissue involvement that results in premature death, usually by 10 yr of age. An infant with Hurler syndrome appears normal at birth, but inguinal hernias are often present. **Diagnosis** is usually made between 6 and 24 mo of age with evidence of hepatosplenomegaly, coarse facial features, corneal clouding, large tongue, prominent forehead, joint stiffness, short stature, and skeletal dysplasia (see Fig. 88-2). Acute cardiomyopathy has been found in some infants <1 yr of age. Most patients have recurrent upper respiratory tract and ear infections, noisy breathing, and persistent copious nasal discharge. Valvular heart disease with incompetence, notably of the mitral and aortic valves, regularly develops, as does coronary artery narrowing. Obstructive airway disease, notably during sleep, may necessitate tracheotomy. Obstructive airway disease, respiratory infection, and cardiac complications are the common causes of death.

Most children with Hurler syndrome acquire only limited language skills because of developmental delay, combined conductive and neurosensory hearing loss, and an enlarged tongue. Progressive ventricular enlargement with increased intracranial pressure caused by communicating hydrocephalus also occurs. Corneal clouding, glaucoma, and retinal degeneration are common. Radiographs show a characteristic skeletal dysplasia known as **dysostosis multiplex** (Figs. 88-3 and 88-4). The earliest radiographic signs are thick ribs and ovoid vertebral bodies. Skeletal abnormalities in addition to those shown in the figures include enlarged, coarsely trabeculated diaphyses of the long bones with irregular metaphyses and epiphyses. With progression of the disease, macrocephaly develops, with thickened calvarium, premature closure of lambdoid and sagittal sutures, shallow orbits, enlarged J-shaped sella, and abnormal spacing of teeth with dentigerous cysts.

Hurler-Scheie Disease. The clinical phenotype of MPS I-H/S is intermediate between Hurler and Scheie diseases and is characterized by progressive somatic involvement, including dysostosis multiplex with little or no intellectual dysfunction. The onset of symptoms is usually observed between 3 and 8 yr of age; survival to adulthood is common. Cardiac involvement and upper airway obstruction contribute to clinical morbidity. Some patients have spondylolisthesis, which may cause cord compression.

Scheie Disease. MPS I-S is a comparatively mild disorder characterized by joint stiffness, aortic valve disease, corneal clouding, and mild dysostosis multiplex. Onset of significant symptoms is usually after the age of 5 yr, with diagnosis made between 10 and 20 yr of age. Patients with Scheie disease have normal intelligence and stature but have significant joint and ocular involvement. A carpal tunnel syndrome often develops. Ophthalmic features include corneal clouding, glaucoma, and retinal degeneration. Obstructive airway disease, causing sleep apnea, develops in some patients, necessitating tracheotomy. Aortic valve disease is common and has required valve replacement in some patients.

MUCOPOLYSACCHARIDOSIS II. Hunter disease (MPS II) is an X-linked disorder caused by the deficiency of iduronate 2-sulfatase (IDS). The gene encoding IDS is mapped to Xq28. Point mutations of the *IDS* gene have been detected in about 80% of patients with MPS II. Major deletions or rearrangements of the *IDS* gene have been found in the rest; these are usually associated with a more severe clinical phenotype (see Fig. 88-2). Hunter disease manifests almost exclusively in males; it has been observed in a few females and this is explained by skewed inactivation of the X chromosome carrying the normal gene.

Marked molecular heterogeneity explains the wide clinical spectrum of Hunter disease. Patients with severe MPS II have fea-

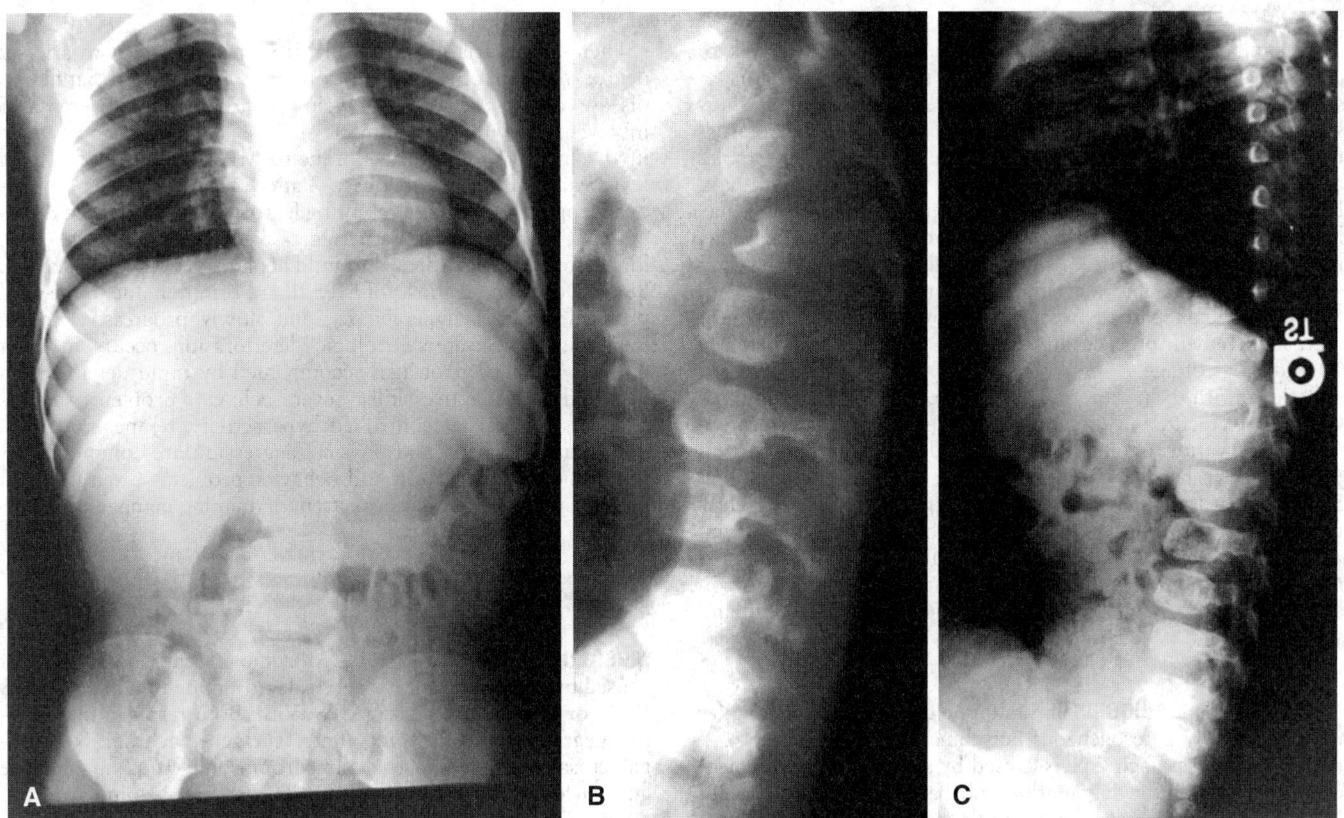

Figure 88-3. Dysostosis multiplex. *A,* Sanfilippo disease, 4 yr: The ribs are wide. *B,* Sanfilippo disease, 4 yr: immature, ovoid configuration of the vertebral bodies. *C,* Hurler disease, 18 mo: anterior-superior hypoplasia of L-1 resulting in hook-shaped appearance.

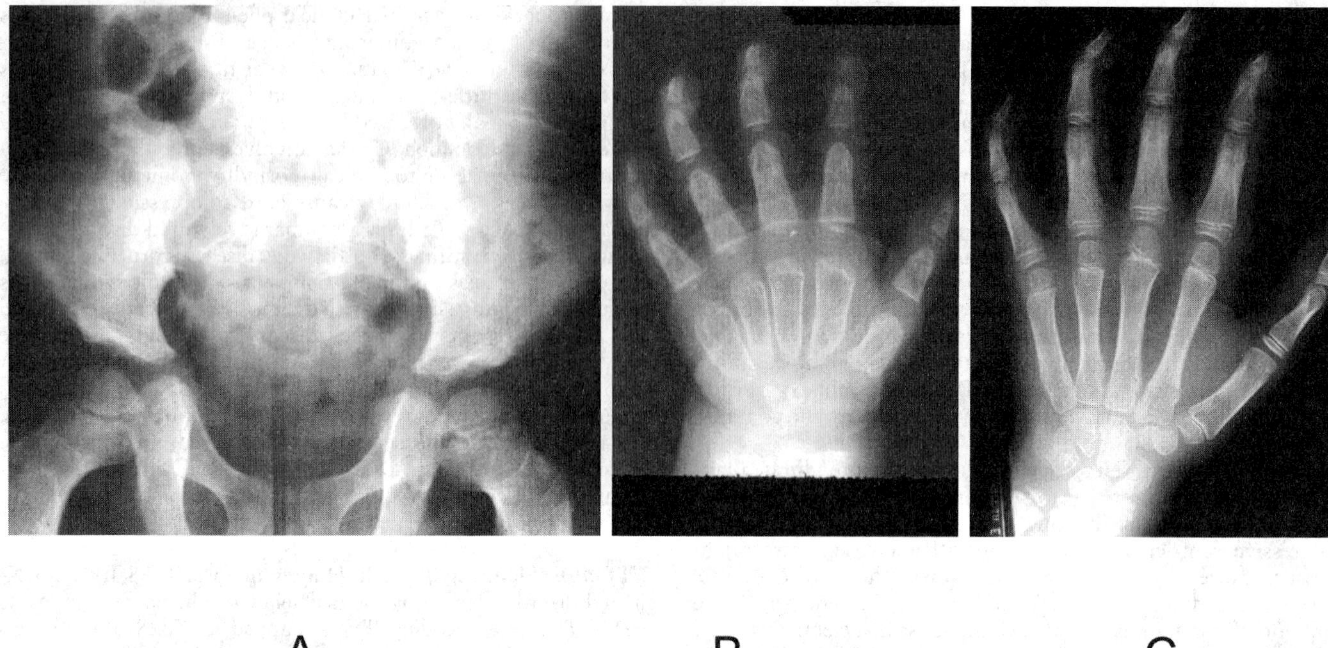

Figure 88-4. Dysostosis multiplex. *A,* Mucopolysaccharidosis (MPS) I-H, 10 yr. The inferior portions of the ilia are hypoplastic with resulting iliac flare and shallow acetabular fossae. The femoral necks are in valgus position. *B,* MPS I-H, 4 yr. Metacarpals and phalanges are abnormally short, wide, and deformed with proximal pointing of the metacarpals and bullet-shaped phalanges. Bone trabeculation is coarse and the cortices are thin. *C,* MPS I-S, 13 yr. The carpal bones are small leading to a V-shaped configuration of the digits. The short tubular bones are well modeled. Flexion of the middle and distal phalanges II–V is caused by joint contractures.

tures similar to those of Hurler disease except for the lack of corneal clouding and the somewhat slower progression of somatic and CNS deterioration. Coarse facial features, short stature, dysostosis multiplex, joint stiffness, and mental retardation manifest between 2 and 4 yr of age. Grouped skin papules are present in some patients. Extensive Mongolian spots have been observed in African and Asian patients since birth and may be an early marker of the disease. Gastrointestinal storage may produce chronic diarrhea. Communicating hydrocephalus and spastic paraplegia may develop due to thickened meninges. In severely affected patients, extensive, slowly progressive neurologic involvement precedes death, which usually occurs between 10 and 15 yr of age.

Patients with the mild form have a prolonged life span, minimal CNS involvement, and slow progression of somatic deterioration with preservation of intelligence in adult life. Survival to ages 65 and 87 yr has been reported; some patients had children. Somatic features are Hurler-like but milder with a greatly reduced rate of progression. Adult height may exceed 150 cm. Airway involvement, valvular cardiac disease, hearing impairment, carpal tunnel syndrome, and joint stiffness are common and can result in significant loss of function in both the mild and severe forms.

MUCOPOLYSACCHARIDOSIS III. Sanfilippo disease (MPS III) makes up a genetically heterogeneous but clinically similar group of 4 recognized types. Each type is caused by a different enzyme deficiency involved in the degradation of heparan sulfate (see Fig. 88-1). Mutations have been found in all the MPS III disorders for which the genes have been isolated.

Phenotypic variation exists in MPS III patients but to a lesser degree than in other MPS disorders. Patients with Sanfilippo disease are characterized by slowly progressive, severe CNS involvement with mild somatic disease. Such disproportionate involvement of the CNS is unique to MPS III. Onset of clinical features usually occurs between 2 and 6 yr in a child who previously appeared normal. Presenting features include delayed development, hyperactivity with aggressive behavior, coarse hair, hirsutism, sleep disorders, and mild hepatosplenomegaly (see Fig. 88-2). Delays in diagnosis of MPS III are common due to the mild physical features, hyperactivity, and slowly progressive neurologic disease. Severe neurologic deterioration occurs in most patients by 6–10 yr of age, accompanied by rapid deterioration of social and adaptive skills. Severe behavior problems such as sleep disturbance, uncontrolled hyperactivity, temper tantrums, destructive behavior, and physical aggression are common. Profound mental retardation and behavior problems often occur in patients with normal physical strength, making management particularly difficult.

MUCOPOLYSACCHARIDOSIS IV. Morquio disease (MPS IV) is caused by a deficiency of N-acetylgalactosamine-6-sulfatase (MPS IV-A) or of β-galactosidase (MPS IV-B). Both result in the defective degradation of keratan sulfate. The gene encoding N-acetylgalactosamine-6-sulfatase is on chromosome 16q24.3 and the gene encoding β-galactosidase, *GLB1,* on chromosome 3p21.33. β-galactosidase catalyzes G_{M1} ganglioside in addition to keratan sulfate, and most mutations of *GLB1* result in generalized gangliosidosis, a spectrum of neurodegenerative disorders associated with dysostosis multiplex. A W273L mutation of the *GLB1* gene, either in the homozygous state or as part of compound heterozygosity, commonly results in Morquio B disease.

Both types of Morquio disease are characterized by short-trunk dwarfism, fine corneal deposits, a skeletal dysplasia that is distinct from other mucopolysaccharidoses, and preservation of intelligence. MPS IV-A is usually more severe than MPS IV-B, with adult heights of <125 cm in the former and >150 cm in the latter. There is considerable variability of expression in both subtypes, however. The appearance of genua valga, kyphosis, growth retardation with short trunk and neck, and waddling gait with a tendency to fall are early symptoms of MPS IV (see Fig. 88-2). Extra skeletal manifestations include mild corneal clouding, small teeth with abnormally thin enamel, frequent caries formation, and, occasionally, hepatomegaly and cardiac valvular lesions. Instability of the odontoid process and ligamentous laxity are regularly present and can result in life-threatening atlantoaxial instability and dislocation. Surgery to stabilize the upper cervical spine, usually by posterior spinal fusion before the development of cervical myelopathy, can be lifesaving.

MUCOPOLYSACCHARIDOSIS VI. **Maroteaux-Lamy** disease (MPS VI) is caused by mutations of the *ARSB* gene on chromosome 5q11–13 encoding N-acetylgalactosamine-4-sulfatase (arylsulfatase B). It is characterized by severe to mild somatic involvement, as seen in MPS I, but with preservation of intelligence. The somatic involvement of the severe form of MPS VI is characterized by corneal clouding, coarse facial features, joint stiffness, valvular heart disease, communicating hydrocephalus, and dysostosis multiplex (see Fig. 88-2). In the severe form, growth can be normal for the 1st few years of life but seems virtually to stop after age 6–8 yr. The mild to intermediate forms of Maroteaux-Lamy disease can be easily confused with Scheie syndrome. Spinal cord compression from thickening of the dura in the upper cervical canal with resultant myelopathy is a frequent occurrence in patients with MPS VI.

MUCOPOLYSACCHARIDOSIS VII. **Sly syndrome** (MPS VII) is caused by mutations of the *GUSB* gene located on chromosome 7q21.11. Mutations result in a deficiency of β-glucuronidase, intracellular storage of glycosaminoglycan fragments and a very wide range of clinical involvement. The most severe form presents as lethal nonimmune fetal hydrops and may be detected in utero by ultrasound. Some severely affected newborns survive for some months and have, or develop, signs of lysosomal storage including thick skin, visceromegaly, and dysostosis multiplex. Less severe forms of MPS VII present in the 1st years of life with features of MPS-I but slower progression. Corneal clouding varies. Patients with manifestation after 4 yr of life have skeletal abnormalities of dysostosis multiplex but normal intelligence and usually clear corneae. They may be found incidentally on the basis of a blood smear that shows coarse granulocytic inclusions.

MUCOPOLYSACCHARIDOSIS IX. The disorder is caused by a mutation in the *HYAL1* gene on chromosome 3p21.2–21.2 encoding 1 of 3 hyaluronidases. Clinical findings in the only known patient, a 14 yr old girl, were bilateral nodular soft tissue periarticular masses, lysosomal storage of GAGs in histiocytes, mildly dysmorphic craniofacial features, short stature, normal joint movement, and normal intelligence. Small erosions in both acetabulae were the only radiographic findings.

DIAGNOSIS AND DIFFERENTIAL DIAGNOSIS

Radiographs of chest, spine, pelvis, and hands are useful to detect early signs of dysostosis multiplex (see Figs. 88-3 and 88-4). Semiquantitative spot tests for increased urinary GAG excretion are quick, inexpensive, and useful for initial evaluation but are subject to both false-positive and false-negative results. Chemical quantification of uronic acid–containing substances is required to assess the total urinary excretion of GAG. Quantitative analysis of single GAG by various methods, or of oligosaccharides by tandem mass spectrometry, reveals type-specific profiles. Morquio disease is often missed in urinary assays but can reliably be diagnosed in serum using monoclonal antibodies to keratan sulfate. Any individual who is suspected of an MPS disorder based on clinical features, radiographic results, or urinary GAG screening tests should have a definitive diagnosis established by enzyme assay. Serum, leukocytes, or cultured fibroblasts are used as the tissue source for measuring lysosomal enzymes (see Table 88-2). Prenatal diagnosis is available for all mucopolysaccharidoses and is carried out on cultured cells from amniotic fluid or chorionic villus biopsy. Measurement of GAGs in amniotic fluid is unreliable. Carrier testing in Hunter syndrome, an X-linked disorder, requires analysis of *IDS* gene once the specific mutation or chromosome arrangement in the family under consideration is known. Molecular analysis in patients with other mucopolysaccharidoses or in known carriers requires a specific rationale. Attempts are being made to develop methods for routine newborn screening.

Mucolipidoses and oligosaccharidoses manifest with the same clinical and radiographic features as mucopolysaccharidoses (see Chapters 86.4 and 86.5). In these conditions, the urinary excretion of glycosaminoglycans is not elevated. Hurler-like facial features, joint contractures, dysostosis multiplex, and elevated urinary GAG excretion differentiate the mucopolysaccharidoses from other neurodegenerative and dwarfing conditions.

TREATMENT

Bone marrow transplantation from related or unrelated donors or **cord blood transplantation** results in significant clinical improvement of somatic disease in MPS I, II, and VI. Clinical effects include increased life expectancy, resolution or improvement of growth failure, hepatosplenomegaly, joint stiffness, facial appearance, pebbly skin changes in MPS II, obstructive sleep apnea, heart disease, communicating hydrocephalus, and hearing loss. Enzyme activity in serum and urinary GAG excretion normalize. Transplantation does not significantly improve the neuropsychologic outcome of MPS patients if there is impaired mentation at the time of transplantation. This is true for MPS I-H, II, and III. Patients with MPS I who have undergone transplantation before 24 mo of age and with a baseline mental development index >70 have improved long-term outcome. Early transplantation in MPS II may have the same effect. Transplantation in MPS VI stabilizes or improves cardiac manifestations, posture, and joint mobility. Stem cell transplantation does not correct skeletal and ocular anomalies; they have to be treated with appropriate orthopedic and ophthalmologic procedures. Cord blood transplantation is the therapy of choice in children with MPS I-H, and possibly MPS II, before the age of 2 yr, but transplantation-related death or primary graft failure, which occurs in ≈30% of the patients, must be weighed against other therapeutic options.

Enzyme replacement using recombinant enzymes is approved for patients with MPS I, MPS II, and MPS VI. It reduces organomegaly, ameliorates rate of growth and joint mobility, and reduces the number of episodes of sleep apnea and urinary GAG excretion. The enzymes do not cross the blood-brain barrier and do not prevent deterioration of neurocognitive involvement. Consequently, this therapy is the domain for patients with mild central nervous involvement. To stabilize extraneural manifestations, it is also recommended in young patients before stem cell transplantation. The combination of enzyme replacement therapy and stem cell transplantation may offer the best treatment. Recombinant iduronate-2-sulfatase ameliorates the non-neurologic manifestations of Hunter disease, and recombinant N-Ac-gal4-sulfatase has been successfully tested in patients with MPS VI.

Primary prevention through genetic counseling and tertiary prevention to avoid or treat complications remains the mainstay of supportive pediatric care. Multidisciplinary attention to respiratory and cardiovascular complications, hearing loss, carpal tunnel syndrome, spinal cord compression, hydrocephalus, and other problems can greatly improve the quality of life for patients and their families (Table 88-3). The progressive nature of clinical involvement in MPS patients dictates the need for specialized and coordinated evaluation.

TABLE 88-3. Management of Mucopolysaccharidoses

PROBLEM	PREDOMINANTLY IN	MANAGEMENT
NEUROLOGIC		
Hydrocephalus	MPS I, II, VI, VII	Fundoscopy, CT scan, ventriculoperitoneal shunting
Chronic headaches	All	See behavioral disturbances
Behavioral disturbance	MPS III	Behavioral or medication therapy, sometimes CT scan, ventriculoperitoneal shunting
Disturbed sleep/wake circle	MPS III	Melatonin
Seizures	MPS I, II, III	EEG, anticonvulsants
Odontoid hypoplasia	MPS IV	Cervical MRI, upper cervical fusion
Spinal cord compression	All	Laminectomy, dural excision
OPHTHALMOLOGIC		
Corneal opacity	MPS I, VI, VII	Corneal transplant
Glaucoma	MPS I, VI, VII	Medication, surgery
Retinal degeneration	MPS I, II	Night light
EARS, AIRWAYS		
Recurrent otitis media	MPS I, II, VI, VII	Ventilating tubes
Impaired hearing	All except MPS IV	Audiometry, hearing aids
Obstruction	All except MPS III	Adenotomy, tonsillectomy, bronchodilator therapy, CPAP at night, laser excision of tracheal lesions, tracheotomy
CARDIAC		
Cardiac valve disease	MPS I, II, VI, VII	Endocarditis prevention, valve replacement
Coronary insufficiency	MPS I, II, VI, VII	Medical therapy
Arrhythmias	MPS I, II, VI, VII	Antiarrhythmic medication, pacemaker
ORAL, GASTROINTESTINAL		
Hypertrophic gums, poor teeth	MPS I, II, VI, VII	Dental care
Chronic diarrhea	MPS II	Diet modification, loperamide
MUSCULOSKELETAL		
Joint stiffness	All except MPS IV	Physical therapy
Weakness	All	Physical therapy, wheelchair
Gross long bone malalignment	All	Corrective osteotomies
Carpal tunnel syndrome	MPS I, II, VI, VII	Electromyography, surgical decompression
ANESTHESIA	All except III	Avoid atlantoaxial dislocation, use angulated videointubation laryngoscope and small endotracheal tubes

CPAP, continuous positive air pressure.

Allen JL: Treatment of respiratory system (not just lung) abnormalities in mucopolysaccharidosis I. *J Pediatr* 2004;144:561–562.

Beesley CE, Meaney CA, Greenland G, et al: Mutational analysis of 85 mucopolysaccharidosis type I families: Frequency of known mutations, identification of 17 novel mutations and in vitro expression of missense mutations. *Hum Genet* 2001;109:503–511.

Broadhead DM, Kirk JM, Burt A, et al: Full expression of Hunter's disease in a female with an X-chromosome deletion leading to non-random inactivation. *Clin Genet* 1986;30:392–398.

Cheng Y, Verp MS, Knutel T, Hibbard JU: Mucopolysaccharidosis type VII as a cause of recurrent non-immune hydrops fetalis. *J Perinat Med* 2003;31:535–537.

Fuller M, Rozaklis T, Ramsay SL, et al: Disease-specific markers for the mucopolysaccharidoses. *Pediatr Res* 2004;56:733–738.

Grewal SS, Wynn R, Abdenur JE, et al: Safety and efficacy of enzyme replacement therapy in combination with hematopoietic stem cell transplantation in Hurler syndrome. *Genet Med* 2005;7:143–146.

Harmatz P, Gingliani R, Schwartz I, et al: Enzyme replacement therapy for mucopolysaccharidosis VI: A phase 3, randomized, double-blind, placebo-controlled, multinational study of recombinant human N-acetylgalactosamine 4-sulfatase (recombinant human arylsulfatase Bor RHASB) and follow-on, open-label extension study. *J Pediatr* 2006;148: 533–539.

Harmatz P, Whitley CV, Waber L, et al: Enzyme replacement therapy in mucopolysaccharidosis VI (Maroteaux-Lamy syndrome). *J Pediatr* 2004;144:574–580.

Hershkovitz E, Young E, Cooper A, et al: Bone marrow transplantation for Maroteaux-Lamy syndrome. *J Inherit Metab Dis* 1999;22:50–62.

Ito K, Ochiai T, Suzuki H, et al: The effect of haematopoietic stem cell transplant on papules with 'pebbly' appearance in Hunter's syndrome. *Br J Dermatol* 2004;151:207–211.

Meikle PJ, Ranieri E, Skimonsen H, et al: Newborn screening for lysosomal storage disorders: Clinical evaluation of a two-tier strategy. *Pediatrics* 2004;114:909–914.

Muenzer J: The mucopolysaccharidoses: A heterogeneous group of disorders with variable pediatric presentations. *J Pediat* 2004;44:S27–S33.

Nelson J, Crowhurst J, Carey B, Greed L: Incidence of the mucopolysaccharidoses in Western Australia. *Am J Med Genet A* 2003;123A:310–313.

Ochiai T, Ito K, Okada T, et al: Significance of extensive Mongolian spots in Hunter's syndrome. *Br J Dermatol* 2003;148:1173–1178.

Robertson SP, Klug GL, Rogers JG: Cerebrospinal fluid shunts in the management of behavioural problems in Sanfilippo syndrome (MPS III). *J Pediatr* 1998;157:653–655.

Souillet G, Guffon N, Maire I, et al: Outcome of 27 patients with Hurler's syndrome transplanted from either related or unrelated haematopoietic stem cell sources. *Bone Marrow Transplant* 2003;31:1105–1117.

Staba SL, Escolar ML, Poe M, et al: Cord-blood transplants from unrelated donors in patients with Hurler's syndrome. *New Engl J Med* 2004;350: 1960–1969.

Tomatsu S, Okamura K, Taketani T, et al: Development and testing of new screening method for keratan sulfate in mucopolysaccharidosis IVA. *Pediatr Res* 2004;55:592–597.

Triggs-Raine B, Salo TJ, Zhang H, et al: Mutations in HYAL1, a member of a tandemly distributed multigene family encoding disparate hyaluronidase activities, cause a newly described lysosomal disorder, mucopolysaccharidosis IX. *Proc Nat Acad Sci U S A* 1999;96:6296–6300.

Vellodi A, Young E, Cooper A, et al: Long-term follow-up following bone marrow transplantation for Hunter disease. *J Inherit Metab Dis* 1999;22:638–648.

Wilcox WR: Lysosomal storage disorders: The need for better pediatric recognition and comprehensive care. *J Pediatr* 2004;144: S3–S14.

Wraith JE, Clarke LA, Beck M: Enzyme replacement therapy for mucopolysaccharidosis I: A randomized, double-blinded, placebo-controlled multinational study of recombinant human α-iduronidase (Laronidase). *J Pediatr* 2004;144:581–588.

Chapter 89 ■ Disorders of Purine and Pyrimidine Metabolism James. C. Harris

The inherited disorders of purine and pyrimidine metabolism cover a broad spectrum of illnesses with various presentations. These include hyperuricemia, acute renal failure, renal stones, gout, unexplained neurologic deficits (seizures, muscle weakness, choreoathetoid and dystonic movements), developmental disability, intellectual disability, compulsive self-injury and aggression, autistic-like behavior, unexplained anemia, failure to thrive, susceptibility to recurrent infection (immune deficiency), and deafness. When identified, all family members should be screened.

Purines are involved in all biologic processes; all cells require a balanced supply of purines for growth and survival. They provide the primary source of cellular energy through adenosine triphosphate (ATP) and, together with pyrimidines, provide the source for the RNA and DNA that stores, transcribes, and translates genetic information. Purines provide the basic coenzymes (NAD, NADH) for metabolic regulation and play a major role in signal transduction (GTP, cAMP, cGMP). Metabolically active nucleotides are formed from heterocyclic nitrogen-containing purine bases (guanine and adenine) and pyrimidine bases (cytosine, uridine, and thymine). The early steps in the biosynthesis of the purine ring are shown in Figure 89-1. Purines are primarily produced from endogenous sources and, in usual circumstances, dietary purines have a small role. The end product of purine metabolism in humans is uric acid (2,6,8-trioxypurine).

Uric acid is not a specific disease marker, so the cause of its elevation must be determined. The level of uric acid present at any time depends on the size of the purine nucleotide pool, which is derived from de novo purine synthesis, catabolism of tissue nucleic acids, and increased turnover of preformed purines. Uric acid is poorly soluble and must be excreted continuously to avoid toxic accumulations in the body. Its renal excretion involves the following components: (1) glomerular filtration, (2) reabsorption in the proximal convoluted tubule, (3) secretion near the terminus of the proximal tubule, and (4) limited reabsorption near these secretory sites. Thus, renal loss of uric acid is a result of renal tube excretion and is a function of serum uric acid concentration and a homeostatic mechanism to avoid hyperuricemia. Because renal tubule excretion is greater in children than in adults, serum uric acid levels are a less reliable indicator of uric acid production in children than in adults, and consequently, measurement of the level in urine may be required to determine excessive production. Clearance of a smaller portion of uric acid is via the gastrointestinal tract (biliary and intestinal secretion). Owing to poor solubility of uric acid under normal circumstances, uric acid is near the maximal tolerable limits, and small alterations in production or solubility or changes in secretion may result in high serum levels. In renal insufficiency, urate excretion is increased by residual nephrons and by the gastrointestinal tract. **Increased production of uric acid** is found in malignancy; Reye syndrome; Down syndrome; psoriasis; sickle cell anemia; cyanotic congenital heart disease; pancreatic enzyme replacement; glycogen storage disease types I, III, IV, and V; hereditary fructose intolerance; acyl coenzyme A dehydrogenase deficiency; and gout.

The **metabolism** of both purines and pyrimidines can be divided into two biosynthetic pathways and a catabolic pathway. The 1st, the de novo pathway, involves a multistep biosynthesis of phosphorylated ring structures from precursors such as CO_2, glycine, and glutamine. Purine and pyrimidine nucleotides are produced from ribose-5-phosphate or carbamyl phosphate, respectively. The second, a single-step salvage pathway, recovers purine and pyrimidine bases derived from either dietary intake or the catabolic pathway (see Figs. 89-1, 89-2, and 89-3). In the de novo pathway, the nucleosides guanosine, adenosine, cytidine, uridine, and thymidine are formed by the addition of riose-1-phosphate to the purine bases guanine or adenine, and to the pyrimidine bases cytosine, uracil, and thymine. The phosphorylation of these nucleosides produces monophosphate, diphosphate, and triphosphate nucleotides. Under usual circumstances, the salvage pathway predominates over the biosynthetic pathway. Synthesis is most active in tissues with high rates of cellular turnover, such as gut epithelium, skin, and bone marrow. The

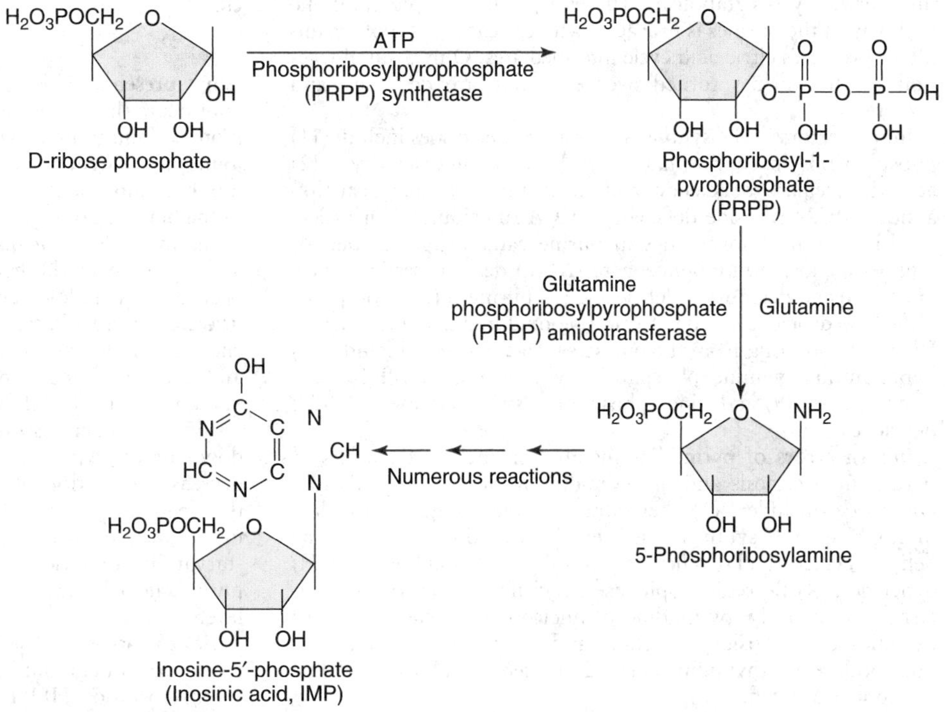

Figure 89-1. Early steps in the biosynthesis of the purine ring.

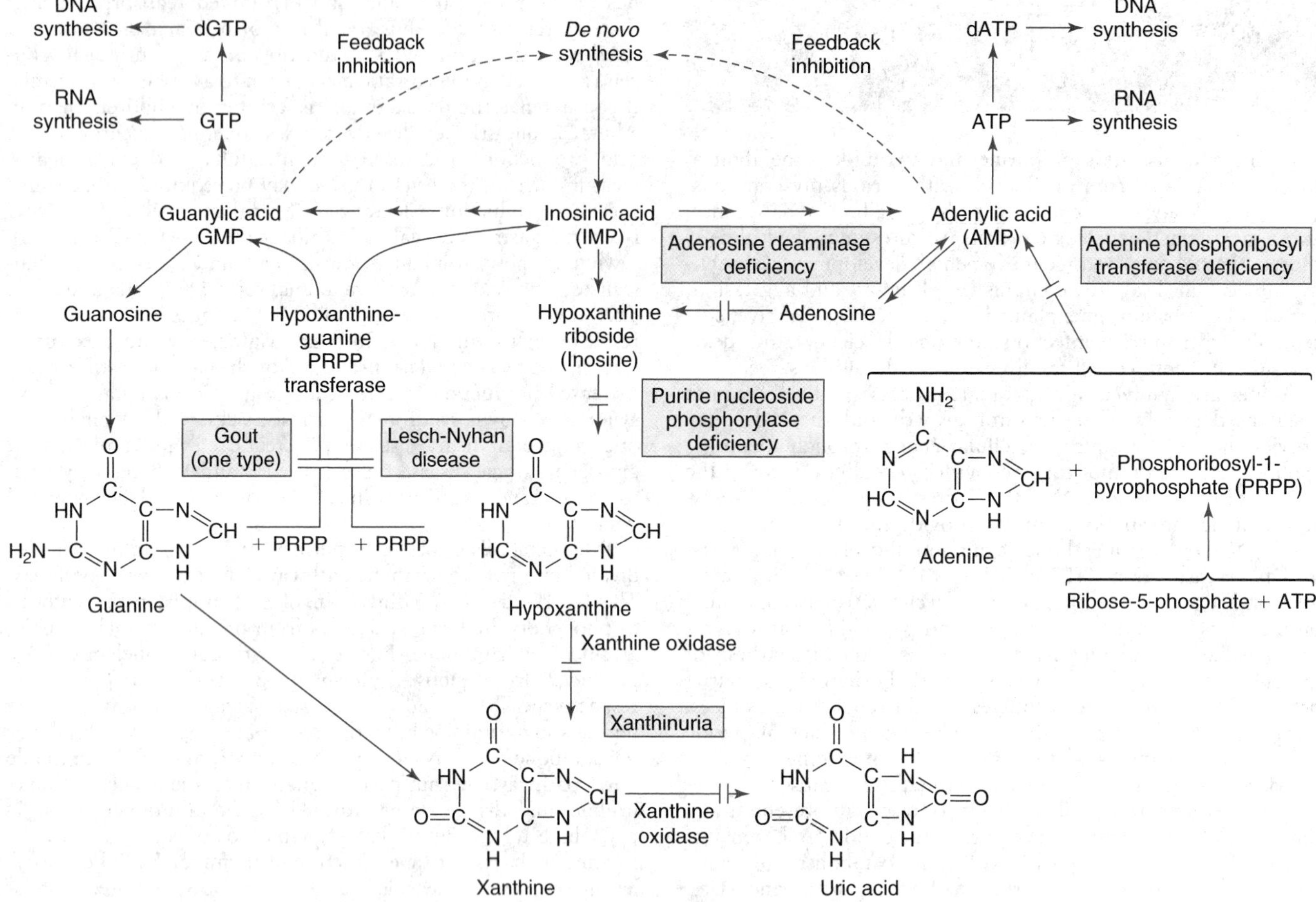

Figure 89-2. Pathways in purine metabolism and salvage.

third pathway is catabolism. The end product of the catabolic pathway of the purines is uric acid, whereas catabolism of pyrimidines produces citric acid cycle intermediates. Only a small fraction of the purines turned over each day are degraded and excreted.

Inborn errors in the **synthesis** of purine nucleotides include: (1) phosphoribosylpyrophosphate synthetase superactivity, (2) adenylosuccinase deficiency, and (3) 5-amino-4-imizolecarboxamide (AICA) riboside deficiency (AICA-ribosiduria). Disorders resulting from abnormalities in purine **catabolism** include: (4) muscle adenosine monophosphate (AMP) deaminase deficiency, (5) adenosine deaminase deficiency, (6) purine nucleoside phosphorylase deficiency, and (7) xanthine oxidoreductase deficiency. Disorders resulting from the purine **salvage** pathway include: (8) hypoxanthine-guanine phosphoribosyltransferase (HPRT) deficiency, and (9) adenine phosphoribosyltransferase (APRT) deficiency.

Inborn errors of pyrimidine metabolism include disorders of pyrimidine synthesis and of pyrimidine nucleotide degradation. Disorders include: (1) hereditary orotic aciduria (uridine monophosphate synthase deficiency), (2) dihydropyrimidine dehydrogenase (DPD) deficiency, (3) dihydropyrimidinase (DPH) deficiency, (4) β-ureidopropionase deficiency, (5) UMPH-1 deficiency (previously pyrimidine 5′-nucleotidase deficiency), (6) pyrimidine nucleoside depletion and overactive cytosolic 5′-nucleotidase, (7) thymidine kinase 2 deficiency, and (8) thymidine phosphorylase deficiency.

GOUT

Gout presents with hyperuricemia, uric acid nephrolithiasis, and acute inflammatory arthritis. Gouty arthritis is due to monosodium urate crystal deposits that result in inflammation in joints and surrounding tissues. The presentation is most commonly monoarticular, typically in the metatarsophalangeal joint of the big toe. Tophi, deposits of monosodium urate crystals, may occur over points of insertion of tendons at the elbows, knees, and feet or over the helix of the ears. **Primary gout**, ordinarily occurring in middle-aged men, results from overproduction of uric acid, decreased renal excretion of uric acid, or both. The biochemical etiology of gout is unknown for most of those affected, and it is considered to be a polygenic trait. When hyperuricemia and gout occur in childhood, it is most often **secondary gout**, the result of another disorder in which there is rapid tissue breakdown or cellular turnover leading to increased production or decreased excretion of uric acid. Gout occurs in any condition that leads to reduced clearance of uric acid: during therapy for malignancy or with dehydration, lactic acidosis, ketoacidosis, starvation, diuretic therapy, and renal shutdown. Excessive purine, alcohol, or carbohydrate ingestion may increase uric acid levels.

Gout is associated with hereditary disorders in three different enzyme disorders that result in hyperuricemia. These include the severe form of HPRT deficiency (Lesch-Nyhan disease) and

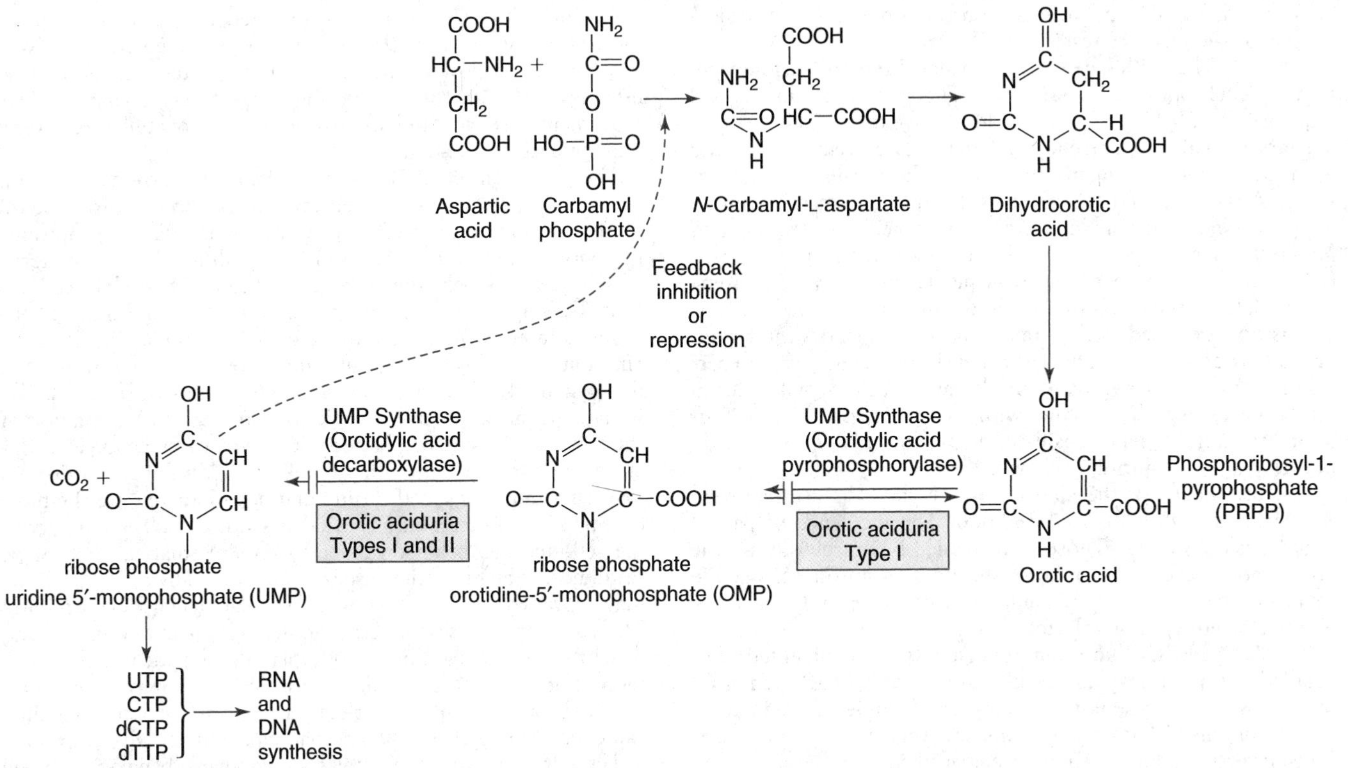

Figure 89-3. Pathways in pyrimidine biosynthesis.

partial HPRT deficiency, superactivity of PP-ribose-P synthetase, and glycogen storage disease type I (glucose-6-phosphatase deficiency) [see Chapter 87.1]. In the 1st two, the basis of hyperuricemia is purine nucleotide and uric acid overproduction, whereas in the third, it is both excessive uric acid production and diminished renal excretion of urate. Glycogen storage disease types III, V, and VII are associated with exercise-induced hyperuricemia, the consequence of rapid ATP utilization and failure to regenerate it effectively during exercise (see Chapter 87.1). Autosomal dominant juvenile hyperuricemia, gouty arthritis, medullary cysts, and progressive renal insufficiency are features associated with **familial juvenile hyperuricemic nephropathy (FJHN)**, medullary cystic kidney disease type 1 (MCKD1) and type 2 (MCKD2). MCKD1 has been mapped to chromosome 1q21. FJHN and MCKD2 have been mapped to chromosome 16p11.2. FJHN and MCKD2 are proposed to be allelic and can result from uromodulin (UMOD) mutations; the term *uromodulin-associated kidney disease* (UAKD) has been proposed. Unlike the three inherited purine disorders that are X-linked and the recessively inherited glycogen storage disease, these are autosomal dominant conditions. **Familial juvenile gout** or familial juvenile hyperuricemic nephropathy is associated with severe renal hypoexcretion of uric acid. Although it most commonly presents from puberty up to the 3rd decade, it has been reported in infancy. It is characterized by early onset, hyperuricemia, gout, familial renal disease, and low urate clearance relative to glomerular filtration rate. It occurs in both males and females and is frequently associated with a rapid decline in renal function that may lead to death unless diagnosed and treated early. Once FJHN is recognized, presymptomatic detection is of critical importance to identify asymptomatic family members with hyperuricemia and to begin treatment, when indicated, to prevent nephropathy.

Treatment of hyperuricemia involves the combination of allopurinal (a xanthine oxidase inhibitor) to decrease uric acid production, probenecid to increase uric acid clearance in those with normal renal function, alkalinization of the urine to increase the solubility of uric acid, and increased fluid intake to reduce the concentration of uric acid. A low-purine diet, weight reduction, and reduced alcohol intake are recommended.

ABNORMALITIES IN PURINE SALVAGE

LESCH-NYHAN DISEASE (LND). This is a rare X-linked disorder of purine metabolism that results from HPRT deficiency. This enzyme is normally present in each cell in the body, but its highest concentration is in the brain, especially in the basal ganglia. **Clinical manifestations** include hyperuricemia, intellectual disability, dystonic movement disorder that may be accompanied by choreoathetosis and spasticity, dysarthric speech, and compulsive self-biting, usually beginning with the eruption of teeth.

There are several clinical presentations of HPRT deficiency. HPRT levels are related to the extent of motor symptoms, to the presence or absence of self-injury, and possibly to the level of cognitive function. The majority of individuals with classic LND have low or undetectable levels of the HPRT enzyme. Partial deficiency in HPRT (**Kelley-Seegmiller syndrome**) with >1.5–2.0% enzyme is associated with hyperuricemia and variable neurologic dysfunction (neurologic HPRT deficiency). HPRT deficiency with levels >8% leads to a severe form of gout, with apparently normal cerebral functioning (**HPRT-related hyperuricemia**) although cognitive deficits may occur. Qualitatively similar cognitive deficit profiles have been reported in both LND and variant cases. Variants produced scores that are intermediate between those of patients with LND and normal controls on nearly every neuropsychologic measure tested.

Genetics. The *HPRT* gene has been localized to the long arm of the X chromosome (q26-q27). The complete amino acid sequence for *HPRT* is known (≈44 kb; 9 exons). The disorder appears in males; occurrence in females is extremely rare and ascribed to nonrandom inactivation of the normal X chromosome. Absence of *HPRT* prevents the normal metabolism of hypoxanthine resulting in excessive uric acid production and manifestations of gout, necessitating specific drug treatment (allopurinol). Because of the enzyme deficiency, hypoxanthine accumulates in the cerebrospinal fluid, but uric acid does not; uric acid is not produced in the brain and does not cross the blood-brain barrier. The behavior disorder is not caused by hyperuricemia or excess hypoxanthine because patients with partial HPRT deficiency, the variants with hyperuricemia, do not self-injure and infants having isolated hyperuricemia from birth do not develop self-injurious behavior.

The prevalence of the classic Lesch-Nyhan disease has been estimated at 1/100,000 to 1/380,000. The incidence of partial variants is not known. Those with classic LND rarely survive the 3rd decade because of renal or respiratory compromise. The life span may be normal for patients with partial HPRT deficiency without severe renal involvement.

Pathology. No specific brain abnormality is documented after detailed histopathology and electron microscopy of affected brain regions. Magnetic resonance imaging has documented reductions in the volume of basal ganglia nuclei. Abnormalities in neurotransmitter metabolism have been identified in three autopsied cases. All three patients had very low HPRT levels (<1% in striatal tissue and 1–2% of control in thalamus and cortex). There was a functional loss of 65–90% of the nigrostriatal and mesolimbic dopamine terminals, although the cells of origin in the substantia nigra did not show dopamine reduction. The brain regions primarily involved were the caudate nucleus, putamen, and nucleus accumbens. It is proposed that the neurochemical changes may be linked to functional abnormalities, possibly resulting from a diminution of arborization or branching of dendrites rather than cell loss. A neurotransmitter abnormality is demonstrated by changes in cerebral spinal fluid neurotransmitters and their metabolites, and confirmed by positron emission tomography scans of dopamine function. Reductions in vivo in the presynaptic dopamine transporter have been documented in the caudate and putamen of six individuals.

The mechanism whereby HPRT leads to the neurologic and behavioral symptoms is unknown. Both hypoxanthine and guanine metabolism is affected; guanosine triphosphate (GTP) and adenosine have substantial effects on neural tissues. There is a functional link between purine nucleotides and the dopamine system that involves guanine, the precursor of GTP. Dopamine binding to its receptor results in either an activation (D_1 receptor) or an inhibition (D_2 receptor) of adenylcyclase. Both receptor effects are mediated by G proteins (GTP-binding proteins) dependent on guanosine diphosphate (GDP) in the GDP/GTP exchange for cellular activation. Dopamine and adenosine systems are also linked through the role of adenosine as a neuroprotective agent in preventing neurotoxicity. Adenosine agonists mimic the biochemical and behavioral actions of dopamine antagonists, whereas adenosine receptor antagonists act as functional dopamine agonists. Dopamine reduction in brain is documented in HPRT-deficient strains of mutant mice.

Clinical Manifestations. At birth, infants with LND have no apparent neurologic dysfunction. After several months, developmental delay, intellectual disability, and neurologic signs become apparent. Before the age of 4 mo, hypotonia, recurrent vomiting, and difficulty with secretions may be noted. By ≈8–12 mo, extrapyramidal signs appear, primarily dystonic movements. In some cases, spasticity may become apparent at this time or, in some instances, later in life.

Cognitive function is usually reported to be in the mild-to-moderate range of intellectual disability, although some individuals test in the low normal range. Because test scores may be influenced by difficulty in testing the subjects owing to their movement disorder and dysarthric speech, overall intelligence may be underestimated.

The age of onset of self-injury may be as early as 1 yr and, occasionally, as late as the teens. Self-injury occurs, although all sensory modalities, including pain, are intact. The self-injurious behavior usually begins with self-biting, although other patterns of self-injurious behavior emerge with time. Most characteristically, the fingers, mouth, and buccal mucosa are mutilated. Self-biting is intense and causes tissue damage and may result in the amputation of fingers and substantial loss of tissue around the lips (Fig. 89-4). Extraction of primary teeth may be required. The biting pattern can be asymmetric, with preferential mutilation of the left or right side of the body. The type of behavior is different from that seen in other intellectual disability syndromes involving self-injury; self-hitting and head banging are the most common initial presentations in other syndromes. The intensity of the self-injurious behavior generally requires that the patient be restrained. When restraints are removed, the individual with LND may appear terrified, and stereotypically place a finger in the mouth. The patient may ask for restraints to prevent elbow movement; when the restraints are placed or replaced, the patient may appear relaxed and better humored. Dysarthric speech may cause interpersonal communication problems; the higher-functioning children can express themselves fully and participate in verbal therapy.

The self-mutilation presents as a compulsive behavior that the child tries to control but frequently is unable to resist. Older individuals may enlist the help of others and notify them when they are comfortable enough to have restraints removed. In some instances, the behavior may lead to deliberate self-harm. Individuals with LND may also show compulsive aggression and inflict injury to others through pinching, grabbing, or hitting or by using verbal forms of aggression. Afterwards they may apologize, stating that their behavior was out of their control. Other maladaptive behaviors include head or limb banging, eye poking, and psychogenic vomiting.

Diagnosis. The presence of dystonia along with self-mutilation of the mouth and fingers suggests Lesch-Nyhan disease. With partial HPRT deficiency, recognition is linked to either hyperuricemia alone or hyperuricemia and a dystonic movement disorder. Serum levels of uric acid >4–5 mg uric acid/dL and a urine uric acid:creatinine ratio of 3:4 or more are highly suggestive of HPRT deficiency, particularly when associated with neurologic symptoms. The definitive diagnosis requires an analysis of the HPRT enzyme. This is assayed in an erythrocyte lysate. Individuals with classic LND have near 0% enzyme activity and those with partial variants show values between 1.5% and 60%. The intact cell HPRT assay in skin fibroblasts offers a good correlation between enzyme activity and the severity of the disease. Molecular techniques are used for gene sequencing and the identification of carriers.

Differential diagnosis includes other causes of infantile hypotonia and dystonia. Children with LND are often initially incorrectly diagnosed as having athetoid cerebral palsy. When a diagnosis of cerebral palsy is suspected in an infant with a normal prenatal, perinatal, and postnatal course, LND should be considered. Partial HPRT deficiency may be associated with acute renal failure in infancy; therefore, clinical awareness of partial HPRT deficiency is of particular importance.

An understanding of the molecular disorder has led to effective drug treatment for uric acid accumulation and arthritic tophi, renal stones, and neuropathy. Reduction in uric acid alone does not influence the neurologic and behavioral aspects of LND. Despite treatment from birth for uric acid elevation, behavioral and neurologic symptoms are unaffected. The most significant complications of LND are renal failure and self-mutilation.

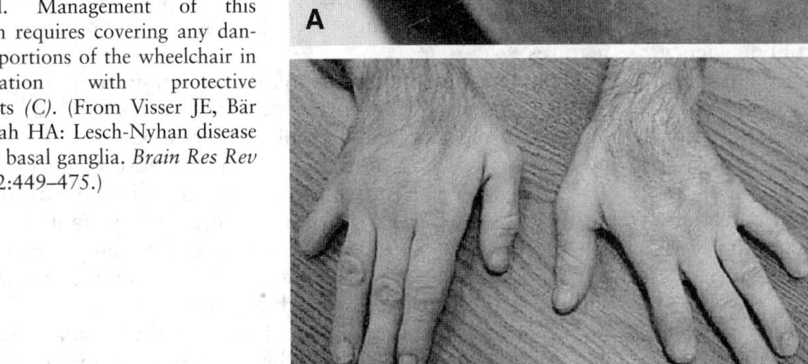

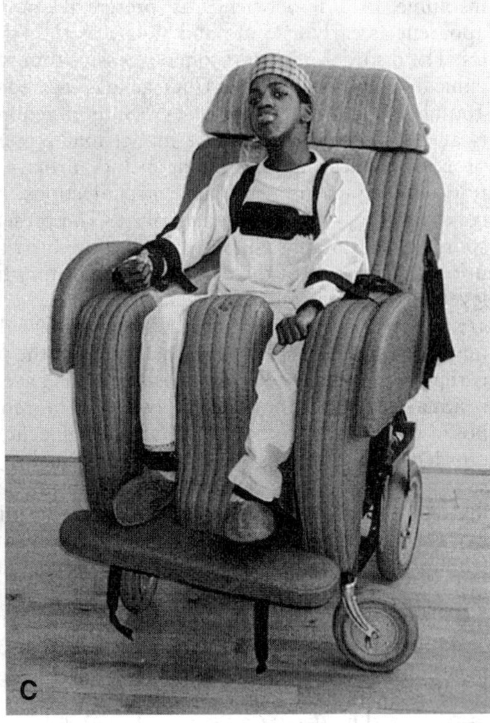

Figure 89-4. Self-injury in Lesch-Nyhan disease. Tissue damage to the lip *(A)* and fingers *(B)* was self-inflicted. Management of this problem requires covering any dangerous portions of the wheelchair in combination with protective restraints *(C)*. (From Visser JE, Bär PR, Jinah HA: Lesch-Nyhan disease and the basal ganglia. *Brain Res Rev* 2000;32:449–475.)

Treatment. Medical management of this disorder focuses on the prevention of renal failure by pharmacologic treatment of hyperuricemia with high fluid intake along with alkali and allopurinol. Allopurinol treatment must be monitored because urinary oxypurine excretion is sensitive to allopurinol, resulting in an increased concentration of xanthine, which is extremely insoluble. Self-mutilation is reduced through behavior management and the use of restraints, removal of teeth, or both. Injection of botulism toxin into the masseter muscles was useful in one patient. Pharmacologic approaches to decrease anxiety and spasticity with medication have mixed results. Drug therapy focuses on symptomatic management of anticipatory anxiety, mood stabilization, and reduction of self-injurious behavior. Diazepam may be helpful for anxiety symptoms, and carbamazepine or gabapentin for mood stabilization. Each of these medications may reduce self-injurious behavior by helping to reduce anxiety and stabilize mood.

Bone marrow transplantation (BMT) has been carried out in several patients, based on the possibility that the CNS damage is produced by a circulating metabolic toxin. Several infant patients have died of complications of BMT. In one adult case in which the transplantation was successful, there was no change in neurologic symptoms or in behavior. In this case, dopamine receptors measured by positron emission tomography before and after BMT showed no changes in receptor density after the transplantation. To date, there is no evidence that BMT is a beneficial treatment approach; it remains an experimental and potentially dangerous therapy.

Two patients received partial exchange transfusions every 2 mo for 3 to 4 yr. Erythrocyte HPRT activity was 10–70% of normal during this period, but no reduction of neurologic or behavioral symptoms was apparent. Successful *preimplantation genetic diagnosis* and in vitro fertilization for LND has been reported with the birth of an unaffected male infant.

Both the motivation for self-injury and its biologic basis must be addressed in treatment programs. Yet behavioral techniques alone, using operant conditioning approaches, have not proved to be an adequate general treatment. Although behavioral procedures have had some selective success in reducing self-injury, generalization outside the experimental setting limits this approach and patients under stress may revert to their previous self-injurious behavior. Behavioral approaches may also focus on reducing the self-injurious behavior through the treatment of phobic anxiety associated with being unrestrained. The most common techniques are systematic desensitization, extinction, and differential reinforcement of other (competing) behavior. Stress management has been recommended to assist patients to develop more effective coping mechanisms. Individuals with LND do not respond to contingent electric shock or similar aversive behavioral measures. An increase in self-injury may be observed when aversive methods are utilized.

Restraint (day and night) and dental procedures are common means to prevent self-injury. The time in restraints is linked to the age of onset of self-injury. Children with LND can participate in making decisions regarding restraints and the type of restraints. The time in restraints may potentially be reduced with systematic behavior treatment programs. Many patients have teeth extracted to prevent self-injury. Others use a protective mouth guard designed by a dentist. Most parents suggest that stress reduction and awareness of the patient's needs are the most effective in reducing self-injury. Positive behavioral techniques of reinforcing appropriate behavior are rated effective by almost half of the families.

ADENINE PHOSPHORIBOSYLTRANSFERASE (APRT) DEFICIENCY. APRT, a purine salvage enzyme, catalyzes the synthesis of AMP from adenine and 5-phosphoribosyl-1-pyrophosphate (PP-ribose-P). The absence of this enzyme results in the inability to utilize adenine and accumulated adenine being oxidized by xanthine dehydrogenase to 2,8-dihydroxyadenine, which is extremely insoluble. APRT deficiency is present from birth, becoming apparent as early as 5 mo and as late as the 7th decade. **Genetics:** The disorder is an autosomal recessive trait with considerable clinical heterogeneity. The *APRT* gene is located on chromosome 16q (16q24.3) and encompasses 2.8 kb of genomic DNA. There is an APRT knockout mouse model that replicates the disease process. **Clinical manifestations** include urinary calculus formation with crystalluria, urinary tract infections, hematuria, renal colic, dysuria, and acute renal failure. The presence of brownish spots on the infant's diaper or of yellow-brown crystals in the urine is suggestive of the diagnosis. **Laboratory findings:** Urinary levels of adenine, 8-hydroxyadenine, and 2,8-dihydroxyadenine are elevated, whereas plasma uric acid is normal. The deficiency may be complete (type I) or partial (type II); the partial deficiency is reported in Japan. The diagnosis is made based on the level of residual enzyme in erythrocyte lysates. The renal calculi, composed of 2,8-dihydroxyadenine, are radiolucent, soft, and easily crushed. These stones are not distinguishable from uric acid stones by routine tests but require high-pressure liquid chromatography (HPLC), ultraviolet or infrared radiation detection, mass spectroscopy (MS), x-ray crystallography, or capillary electrophoresis for diagnosis, particularly to distinguish from stones in HPRT deficiency.

Treatment includes high fluid intake, dietary purine restriction, and allopurinol, which inhibits the conversion of adenine to its metabolites, further 2,8-dihydroxyadenine excretion, and further stone formation. Alkalinization of the urine is to be avoided, because, unlike that of uric acid, the solubility of 2,8-dihydroxyadenine does not increase up to a pH of 9. Shock-wave lithotripsy has been reported to be successful. The prognosis depends on renal function at the time of diagnosis. Early treatment is critical in the prevention of stones because severe renal insufficiency may accompany late recognition.

DISORDERS LINKED TO PURINE NUCLEOTIDE SYNTHESIS

PHOSPHORIBOSYLPYROPHOSPHATE (PRPP) SYNTHETASE SUPERACTIVITY. PRPP is a substrate involved in the synthesis of essentially all nucleotides and important in the regulation of the de novo pathways of purine and pyrimidine nucleotide synthesis. This enzyme produces PRPP from ribose-5-phosphate and ATP, as shown in Figures 89-1 and 89-2. PRPP is the 1st intermediary compound in the de novo synthesis of purine nucleotides that lead to the formation of inosine monophosphate. Superactivity of the enzyme results in an increased generation of PRPP. Because PRPP amidotransferase, the 1st enzyme of the de novo pathway, is not physiologically saturated by PRPP, the synthesis of purine nucleotides increases, and, consequently, the production of uric acid is increased. PRPP synthetase superactivity is one of the few hereditary disorders in which there is enhancement of the activity of an enzyme.

Genetics: Phosphoribosylpyrophosphate synthetase (PRS) superactivity is inherited as an X-linked trait and presents with two clinical phenotypes with varying degrees of severity. Three distinct PRS cDNAs have been cloned and sequenced. Two forms are X linked to Xq22-q24 and Xp22.2-p.22.3 (escapes X inactivation), respectively, and are widely expressed; the third maps to human chromosome 7 and appears to be transcribed only in the testes. Even though the defect is X linked it should be considered in a child or young adult of either sex with hyperuricemia and/or hyperuricosuria and normal HPRT activity in lysed red cells. **Clinical manifestations** in the more severe type in affected hemizygous males include signs of uric acid overproduction that are apparent in infancy or early childhood, neurodevelopmental retardation, and, in some cases, sensorineural deafness. Hypotonia, delays in motor milestones, ataxia, and autistic-like behavior have been described. Heterozygous female carriers may also develop gout and hearing impairment. The late juvenile to early adult onset type is found in males who show gout or uric acid urolithiasis but no neurologic signs. A mechanism for the neurologic symptoms is unknown. **Laboratory findings:** Blood uric acid may be two to three times normal values, and the urinary excretion of uric acid is increased. The *diagnosis* requires enzyme analysis of erythrocytes and cultured fibroblasts. This disorder must be differentiated from partial HPRT deficiency involving the salvage pathway, which also results in neurologic HPRT deficiency or hyperuricemia without neurologic features.

Treatment is with allopurinol, which inhibits xanthine oxidase, the last enzyme of the purine catabolic pathway. Uric acid production is reduced and is replaced by hypoxanthine, which is more soluble, than xanthine. The initial dose of allopurinol is 10–20 mg/kg/24 hr in children and is adjusted to maintain normal uric acid levels in plasma. Occasionally, xanthine calculi may form. Consequently, a low-purine diet (one free of organ meats, dried beans, and sardines), high fluid intake, and alkalinization of the urine to establish a urinary pH of 6.0–6.5 is necessary. These measures control the hyperuricemia and urate neuropathy but do not affect the neurologic symptoms. There is no known treatment for the neurologic complications.

ADENYLOSUCCINATE LYASE (ADSL) DEFICIENCY. This is an inherited deficiency of de novo purine synthesis in humans. Adenylosuccinase lyase is an enzyme that catalyzes two pathways in de novo synthesis and purine nucleotide recycling. These are the conversion of succinylaminoimidazole carboxamide ribotide (SAICAR) into aminoimidazole carboxamide ribotide (AICAR) in the de novo synthesis of purine nucleotides, and the conversion of adenylosuccinate (S-AMP) into adenosine monophosphate (AMP); the latter is the 2nd step in the conversion of inosine monophosphate (IMP) into AMP in the purine nucleotide cycle. ADSL deficiency results in the accumulation in urine, cerebrospinal fluid, and, to a smaller extent, in plasma, of SAICA riboside (SAICAr) and succinyladenosine (S-Ado), dephosphorylated derivatives of SAICAR and S-AMP, respectively. **Genetics:** This is an autosomal recessive disorder; the gene has been mapped to chromosome 22q13.1-q13.2 and ≈20 gene mutations have been identified. **Laboratory** investigations show the presence in urine and cerebrospinal fluid of succinylpurines, which are normally undetectable.

Clinical manifestations include varying degrees of psychomotor retardation, generally accompanied by a seizure disorder and/or autistic-like behaviors (poor eye contact and repetitive behaviors). Neonatal seizures and a severe infantile epileptic encephalopathy are often the 1st manifestations of this disorder. Others demonstrate moderate to severe intellectual disability sometimes associated with growth retardation and muscle hypotonia. One reported case, a girl, tested in the mild range of intellectual disability. The form with profound intellectual disability has been designated type I, the variant case with mild intellectual disability as type II. Other patients have an intermediate clinical symptom pattern with moderately delayed psychomotor development, seizures, stereotypies, and agitation. **Pathology:** CT and MRI of the brain may show hypotrophy or **hypoplasia of the cerebellum,** particularly the vermis. It is proposed that rather than being caused by purine nucleotide deficiency, the symptoms are due to the neurotoxic effects of accumulating succinyl purines. The ratio of S-Ado/SAICAr has been linked to phenotype severity suggesting that SAICAr is the more toxic compound and that S-Ado might be neuroprotective. The **laboratory diagnosis** is based on the presence in urine and cerebrospinal fluid of SAICAr and S-Ado; both are usually undetectable. No successful **treatment** has been demonstrated for this disorder. Prenatal diagnosis has been reported. Systematic screening with the Bratton-Marshall test is suggested in infants and children with unexplained psychomotor retardation and/or seizure disorders.

5-AMINO-4-IMIDAZOLECARBOXAMIDE (AICA) RIBOSIDE DEFICIENCY (AICA-RIBOSIDURIA). AICA riboside is the dephosphorylated product of AICAR, also termed ZMP. It, along with its diphosphates and triphosphates, accumulates in red blood cells and fibrocytes in AICA riboside deficiency. The enzyme defect is in the conversion of AICAR to FAICAR (formyl-AICAR), catalyzed by the bifunctional enzyme AICAR transformylase/IMP cyclohydrolase (ATIC). The transformylase is deficient in fibroblasts in this disorder. **Genetics:** This is an inborn error of purine biosynthesis caused by a mutation of *ATIC* gene effecting AICAR transformylase activity. In a reported case, AICAR transformylase was profoundly deficient, whereas the IMP cyclohydrolase level was 40% of normal. **Clinical features:** The disorder is described in a female infant with profound intellectual disability, epilepsy, dysmorphic features (prominent forehead and metopic suture, brachycephaly, wide mouth with thin upper lip, low-set ears, and prominent clitoris due to fused labia minora), and congenital blindness. **Laboratory findings:** Urinary screening with the Bratton-Marshall test resulted in the identification of this disorder. No successful treatment is described.

DISORDERS RESULTING FROM ABNORMALITIES IN PURINE CATABOLISM

MYOADENYLATE DEAMINASE DEFICIENCY (MUSCLE ADENOSINE MONOPHOSPHATE DEAMINASE DEFICIENCY). Myoadenylate deaminase is a muscle-specific isoenzyme of AMP deaminase that is active in skeletal muscle. During exercise, the deamination of AMP leads to increased levels of IMP and ammonia in proportion to the work performed by the muscle. Two forms of myoadenylate deaminase deficiency are known: an inherited (primary) form that may be asymptomatic or associated with cramps or myalgia with exercise, and a secondary form that may be associated with other neuromuscular or rheumatologic disorders. **Clinical manifestations** are, most commonly, isolated muscle weakness, fatigue, myalgias after moderate-to-vigorous exercise, or cramps. Myalgias may be associated with an increased serum creatine kinase level and detectable electromyelographic abnormalities. Muscle wasting or histologic changes on biopsy are absent. The age of onset may be as early as 8 mo of life with ≈25% of cases recognized between 2 and 12 years of age. The enzyme defect has been identified in asymptomatic family members. Secondary forms of muscle AMP deaminase deficiency have been identified in Werdnig-Hoffmann disease, Kugelberg-Welander syndrome, polyneuropathies, and amyotrophic lateral sclerosis (see Chapter 611). The metabolic disorder involves the purine nucleotide cycle. The enzymes involved in this cycle are AMP deaminase, adenylosuccinate synthetase, and adenylosuccinase (see Fig. 89-2). It is proposed that muscle dysfunction in AMP deaminase deficiency results from impaired energy production during muscle contraction. It is unclear how individuals may carry the deficit and be asymptomatic. In addition to muscle dysfunction, a mutation of liver AMP deaminase has been proposed as a cause of primary gout, leading to overproduction of uric acid.

The inherited form of the disorder is an autosomal recessive trait. *AMP-D1*, the gene responsible for encoding muscle AMP deaminase, is located on the short arm of chromosome 1 (1p13–21). Population studies reveal that this mutant allele is found at high frequency in Caucasian populations. The disorder may be screened for by performing the forearm ischemic exercise test. The normal elevation of venous plasma ammonia after exercise that is seen in normal subjects is absent in AMP deaminase deficiency. The final diagnosis is made by histochemical or biochemical assays of a muscle biopsy. The primary form is distinguished by the finding of enzyme levels <2% with little or no immunoprecipitable enzyme. Affected individuals are advised to exercise with caution to prevent rhabdomyolysis and myoglobinuria. Although there are no documented fully effective treatments, it has been proposed that enhancing the rate of replenishment of the ATP pool might be beneficial. Using this rationale, **treatment** with ribose (2–60 g/24 hr orally, in divided doses) or xylitol, which is converted to ribose, has been reported to improve endurance and muscle strength in some cases but is ineffective in others. Genetic approaches may be feasible in the future for inherited cases, whereas treatment of the underlying condition is essential in secondary cases.

ADENOSINE DEAMINASE DEFICIENCY. See Chapter 125.1.

PURINE NUCLEOSIDE PHOSPHORYLASE DEFICIENCY. See Chapter 125.2.

XANTHINE OXIDOREDUCTASE DEFICIENCY, HEREDITARY XANTHINURIA/MOLYBDENUM COFACTOR DEFICIENCY. Xanthine oxidoreductase (XOR) is the catalylic enzyme in the final step of the purine catabolic pathway and oxides hypoxanthine to xanthine and xanthine to uric acid. Because XOR exists in two forms, xanthine dehydrogenase and xanthine oxidase, the deficiency is also referred to as xanthine dehydrogenase/xanthine oxidase (XDH/XO) deficiency. Xanthine, the immediate precursor of uric acid, is less soluble than uric acid in urine and deficiency of the enzyme results in xanthinuria. Xanthine oxidoreductase deficiency may occur in an isolated form (xanthinuria type I), in a combined form involving xanthine oxidoreductase deficiency and aldehyde oxidase deficiency (xanthinuria type II), or in a combined form with deficiency of xanthine oxidoreductase, aldehyde oxidase, and sulfite oxidase (molybdenum cofactor deficiency). The isolated form results in an almost total replacement of uric acid by hypoxanthine and xanthine. Patients can oxidize allopurinol to oxypurinal via aldehyde oxidase. Patients with the isolated form are usually asymptomatic or have mild symptoms; however, renal stones, often not visible on radiography, are a risk for renal damage and may appear at any age. Crystalline xanthine deposits in muscle may result in muscle pain following exertion. Rarely, xanthine stones have been reported as a result of allopurinol administration. In type II, the clinical presentation is similar to type I. Type II patients are deficient in both oxidases and cannot metabolize allopurinol. Molybdenum cofactor deficiency (failure to synthesize the molybdenum cofactor) involves all three molybdoenzymes and, like isolated sulfite oxidase deficiency, results in neonatal feeding problems, neonatal seizures, increased or decreased muscle tone, ocular lens dislocation, severe intellectual disability, and death in early childhood.

The inheritance of types I and II is autosomal recessive; the human XOR gene is located on chromosome 2p22. In both forms of the deficiency, the **diagnosis** is made by measuring plasma concentrations of uric acid; plasma uric acid is low (<1 mg/dL) and xanthine is elevated in plasma and urine. Urinary uric acid is reduced, being replaced by xanthine and hypoxanthine. In molybdenum cofactor deficiency, there is, in addition, an excessive excretion of sulfite and other sulfur-containing metabolites. Enzyme diagnostic measurement requires jejunal or liver biopsy because these are the only human tissues that contain appreciable amounts of xanthine oxidoreductase. Sulfite oxidase and the molybdenum cofactor can be measured in liver and fibroblasts. Although the isolated deficiency is generally benign, **treatment** with a low-purine diet and increased fluid intake are recommended. Allopurinol has been recommended for those with residual xanthine oxidoreductase activity. It completely blocks the conversion of hypoxanthine into the far less soluble xanthine. The prognosis for molybdenum cofactor deficiency is very poor, and drug trials to date have been unsuccessful. This disorder may be a candidate for somatic gene therapy in the future.

DISORDERS OF PYRIMIDINE METABOLISM

The pyrimidines are the building blocks of DNA and RNA and involved in the formation of coenzymes, as active intermediates in carbohydrate and phospholipid metabolism, glucuronidation in detoxification processes, and glycocylation of proteins and lipids. Pyrimidine synthesis differs from that of purines in that the single pyrimidine ring is 1st assembled and then linked to ribose phosphate to form uridine 5′-monophosphate (UMP). The pyrimidines uracil and thymine are degraded in four steps, as shown in Figure 89-3. Eight disorders of pyrimidine metabolism are reviewed. Purine metabolism has an easily measurable end point in uric acid; however, there is no equivalent compound in pyrimidine metabolism. The 1st defect, hereditary orotic aciduria, is in the de novo synthetic pathway, whereas the other disorders involve overactivity (in one syndrome) or defects in the pyrimidine degradation pathway. Degradation disorders may present as anemia, neurologic disorders, or multisystem mitochondrial disorders. The 1st three steps of the degradation pathways for thymine and uracil make use of the same enzymes (DPD, DPH, and UP). These three steps result in the conversion into β-alanine from uracil. There is increasing evidence that pyrimidines play an important role in the regulation of the nervous system. Reduced production of the neurotransmitter function of β-alanine is hypothesized to produce clinical symptoms. Clinically, these rare disorders may be overlooked because symptoms are not highly specific; however, they should be considered as possible causes of anemia and neurologic disease and are a contraindication for treatment of cancer patients with certain pyrimidine analogs.

HEREDITARY OROTIC ACIDURIA (URIDINE MONOPHOSPHATE SYNTHASE TYPE 1 DEFICIENCY). This is a disorder of pyrimidine synthesis associated with deficient activity of the last two enzymes of the de novo pyrimidine synthetic pathway, orotate phosphoribosyltransferase (OPRT) and orotidine-5′-monophosphate decarboxylase (ODC). The activities of these two enzymes reside in separate domains to a single polypeptide coded by a single gene. This bifunctional protein, uridine 5′-monophosphate (UMP) synthase, catalyzes the two-step conversion of orotic acid to UMP, via orotidine monophosphate (OMP). Hereditary orotic aciduria results in the excessive accumulation of orotic acid. **Genetics:** This disorder is autosomal recessive. Two functional domains are encoded on a single gene. The gene for UMP synthase is located on the long arm of chromosome 3 (3q13). Genetic metabolic defects that involve four of the six enzymes associated with the urea cycle may result in orotic aciduria secondary to PP-ribose-P depletion resulting from a substantial increased flux through the de novo pathway. **Clinically,** patients with hereditary orotic aciduria (UMP synthase type 1 deficiency) have a macrocytic hypochromic megablastic anemia that is unresponsive to the usual forms of therapy (iron, folic acid, and B_{12}) and may have leukopenia. Onset is usually in the 1st months of life. Untreated, this disorder can lead to developmental disability, intellectual disability, failure to thrive, cardiac disease, strabismus, crystalluria, and occasional ureteric obstruction. Renal function is generally normal. Heterozygotes may have mild orotic aciduria but are not otherwise affected. The clinical features may be related to pyrimidine nucleotide depletion. Metabolities derived from several pharmacologic agents (5-azauridine, allopurinol) produce secondary orotic aciduria and orotidinuria by specifically inhibiting ODC. Orotic aciduria may also occur in association with parenteral nutrition, essential amino acid deficiency, and Reye syndrome. The enzymatic defect may be demonstrated in liver, lymphoblasts, erythrocytes, leukocytes, and cultured skin fibroblasts. A carrier detection test is available, as is prenatal diagnosis. In ODC deficiency (UMP synthase type 2 deficiency), the **clinical** symptoms show neurologic abnormalities without megaloblastic anemia. In reported cases, both orotidinuria and orotic aciduria were found.

The administration of uridine in doses of 50–300 mg/kg/day has been an effective **treatment** in most cases and led to clinical improvement and reduction in orotic acid excretion. Lifelong treatment is required. Uracil is ineffective because, unlike purines, pyrimidine salvage occurs at the nucleoside (uridine) level. The long-term **prognosis** in uncomplicated cases is good; however, congenital malformations and other associated features may adversely affect outcome.

DIHYDROPYRIMIDINE DEHYDROGENASE (DPD) DEFICIENCY. DPD catalyzes the initial and rate-limiting step in the degradation of the pyrimidine bases uracil and thiamine. DPD has been identified in most tissues, with the highest activity being in lymphocytes. **Genetics:** DPD deficiency is an autosomal recessive disorder mapping to chromosome 1p22 with at least 32 polymorphisms detected. It is estimated that the frequency of the heterozygote may be as high as 3%. The **clinical manifestations** in children may include seizure disorder, intellectual disability, and motor delay. Less frequent are growth retardation, microcephaly, and autistic-like behavior and ocular anomalies. Others do not show developmental abnormalities but may have milder neurologic symptoms and language disorder. In most cases, there is an initial period of normal psychomotor development, followed by subsequent developmental delays. Symptoms may be linked to altered uracil, thymine, and β-alanine homeostasis. DPD is the initial and rate-limiting enzyme in the catabolism of the neoplastic drug 5-fluorouracil (5-FU), being responsible for 80% of its catabolism. Patients with a partial deficiency of this enzyme are at risk for developing a severe 5-FU-associated toxicity. In adult patients, neurotoxicity (headache, somnolence, visual illusions, and memory impairment) linked to pyrimidinemia after 5-FU treatment for cancer is reported in previously healthy individuals.

Prenatal **diagnosis** has been reported. **Laboratory findings:** DPD deficiency is characterized by a variable phenotype and diagnosed by the accumulation of thiamine and uracil in urine, plasma, and cerebrospinal fluid and no activity in fibroblasts. Diagnostic tests use high-pressure liquid chromatography (HPLC) or gas chromatography–mass spectroscopy (GC-MS). Alternatively, DPD deficiency may be confirmed by measuring the enzyme in cultured fibroblasts and leukoblasts. Uric acid levels have been reported to be normal. Because β-alanine is a structural analog of γ-aminobutyric acid (GABA) and glycine, it has been proposed that it may affect inhibitory neurotransmission. There is no established **treatment** for this disorder; patients with seizures do respond to anticonvulsant medications. Patients with DPD deficiency should not be given 5-FU, and this deficiency should be suspected when neurologic symptoms emerge after cancer treatment with 5-FU.

DIHYDROPYRIMIDINASE (DPH) DEFICIENCY (DIHYDROPYRIMIDINURIA). DPH is the second enzyme in the three-step degradation pathway of uracil and thiamine leading to increased urinary excretion. DPH deficiency is characterized by increased urinary secretion of dihydrouracil and dihydrothymine as well as uracil and thymine. There is a variable clinical phenotype. **Genetics:** There is an autosomal recessive form of inheritance with the gene mapped to chromosome 8q22. In one study, there was no significant difference in residual activity between mutations observed in symptomatic and asymptomatic individuals. Population prevalence in a Japanese sample is 0.1% **Clinical manifestations** in three unrelated affected cases include seizures with dysmorphic features and developmental delay in two of these cases. Three unrelated infant and two adult asymptomatic cases were identified, however, in a screening program for pyrimidine-degradation disorders in Japan and were asymptomatic despite the accumulation of pyrimidine degradation products in body fluids. **Laboratory findings:** Organic acid screening by GC-MS may identify increased amounts of these compounds in urine. Oral loading tests with uracil, dihydrouracil, thymine, and dihydrothymine have been used to differentiate this disorder from DPD deficiency. In symptomatic cases, **treatment** with β-alanine has been attempted with equivocal results. Although it has not been reported, increased sensitivity to fluorouracil is expected because of its role in pyrimidine metabolism.

N-CARBAMYL-β-AMINO ACIDURIA (DEFICIENCY OF β-UREIDOPROPIONASE). The pyrimidine bases uracil and thymine are degraded via the consecutive action of three enzymes to β-alanine and β-aminoisobutyric acid, respectively. The third enzyme in the pathway is β-ureidopropionase (UP) and its deficiency leads to N-carbamyl-β-amino aciduria. Urinary analysis in a reported case showed elevated levels of N-carbamyl-β-alanine and N-carbamyl-β-aminoisobutyric acid. The enzyme is expressed only in the liver and no activity of β-ureidopropionase is detected in a liver biopsy. **Genetics:** Fluorescence in situ hybridization localized the human β-ureidopropionase gene to 22q11.2 **Clinical manifestations** in a reported case included muscular hypotonia, dystonic movements, and severe developmental delay. **Laboratory findings:** Neuropathology involves both gray and white matter. UP deficiency leads to pathologic accumulation of 3-UPA in body fluids. 3-UPA acts as an endogenous neurotoxin via inhibition of mitochondrial energy metabolism, resulting in the initiation of secondary, energy-dependent excitotoxic mechanisms. There is no known **treatment** for UP deficiency.

URIDINE MONOPHOSPHATE HYDROLASE 1 DEFICIENCY (PYRIMIDINE 5′-NUCLEOTIDASE DEFICIENCY). Erythrocyte maturation is accompanied by RNA degradation and the release of mononucleotides. Pyrimidine 5′-nucleotidase is the 1st degradative enzyme of the pyrimidine salvage cycle and catalyzes the hydrolysis of pyrimidine 5′-nucleotides to the corresponding nucleosides. Enzyme deficiency results in the accumulation of high levels of cytidine and uridine nucleotides in the erythrocytes of those affected, which results, in turn, in hemolysis. Deficiency of pyrimidine 5′-nucleotidase is at least in part compensated in vivo by other nucleosidases or perhaps other nucleotide metabolic pathways. **Genetics:** This is an autosomal recessive disorder involving a gene on chromosome 7 (7p15). In pyrimidine 5′-nucleotidase deficiency, patients, who are homozygotes, **clinically** present with a defect restricted to erythrocytes that is characterized by nonspherocytic hemolytic anemia with basophilic stippling. Other characteristic features include splenomegaly, increased indirect bilirubin, and hemoglobinuria. Lead is a powerful inhibitor of pyrimidine 5′-nucleotidase and assessment of lead levels should be included whenever the hemolytic anemia, pyrimidine 5′-nucleotidase deficiency, and basophilic stippling are found together. Diagnosis requires demonstration of a complete deficiency of the major isoenzyme uridine monophosphate hydrolase-1. The enzyme defect should be suspected in patients with nonspherocytic hemolytic anemia with basophilic stippling. The anemia is usually moderate, and transfusions are rarely necessary. There is no specific **treatment**. Splenectomy has not proved to be an effective treatment. Lead-induced acquired pyrimidine 5′-nucleotidase deficiency is treatable, unlike the congenital deficiency.

PYRIMIDINE NUCLEOSIDE DEPLETION AND OVERACTIVE CYTOSOLIC 5′-NUCLEOTIDASE. Pyrimidine nucleoside depletion and overactive cytosolic 5′-nucleotidase may lead to a neurodevelopmental disorder. Four unrelated patients showed sixfold to 10-fold elevation in the activity of pyrimidine 5′-nucleotidase in fibroblasts with both purine and pyrimidine substrates. Investigation in cultured fibroblasts derived from these patients showed normal incorporation of purine bases into nucleotides but decreased incorporation of uridine and orotic acid. **Clinical manifestations** include developmental delay, seizures, ataxia, recurrent infections, severe language deficit, hyperactivity, short attention span, and aggressive behavior appearing in the 1st few yr of life. Affected patients show electroencephalogram (EEG) abnormalities. Metabolic testing is normal except for persistent hypouricosuria. It is proposed that increased catabolic activity and decreased pyrimidine salvage cause a deficiency of pyrimidine nucleotides. **Treatment** is with oral uridine, based on its effects on reversing increased nucleotide catabolism. All reported patients treated with uridine show improved speech and behavior, decreased seizure activity with discontinuation of seizure medications, and decreased frequency of infections.

THYMIDINE PHOSPHORYLASE DEFICIENCY. Thymidine phosphorylase catalyzes the conversion of thymidine to thymine. This enzyme is also known as **platelet-derived endothelial cell growth factor** due to its angiogenic or "gliostatin" properties, indicating its inhibitory effects on glial cell proliferation. It has been implicated in mitochondrial nucleoside metabolism. Plasma thymidine level is increased >20-fold in patients compared to controls. Loss of function of thymidine phosphorylase causes mitochondrial neurogastrointestinal encephalomyopathy (MNGIE), an autosomal recessive disorder with mitochondrial DNA alterations. **Genetics:** It is an autosomal recessive disorder, and the gene encoding thymidine phosphorylase has been identified as the MNGIE gene and mapped to chromosome 22q13.32-qter. **Clinical manifestations of MNGIE** include ptosis, progressive external ophthalmoparesis, gastrointestinal dysmotility and malabsorption, cachexia, peripheral neuropathy, skeletal muscle myopathy, and leukoencephalopathy. **Laboratory findings:** Muscle biopsies typically reveal mitochondrial abnormalities. The **diagnosis** is made by assay of thymidine phosphorylase activity in peripheral leukocytes. Increased thymidine may cause mitochondrial nucleotide pool imbalance resulting in mitochondrial DNA alterations through a mitochondria-specific thymidine salvage pathway. Supportive **treatment** is indicated.

THYMIDINE KINASE 2 (TK2) DEFICIENCY. Thymidine kinase 2 (TK2) is a key enzyme in mitochondrial DNA (mtDNA) precursor synthesis. TK deficiencies cause tissue-specific depletion of mtDNA.

TK2 normally phosphorylates deoxythymidine, deoxycytidine, and deoxyuridine. **Genetics:** The gene is located on chromosome 16q22. **Clinically**, in TK2 deficiency, affected individuals have severe myopathy and depletion of muscular mitochondrial DNA in infancy. No specific treatment is available. Supportive **treatment** is indicated.

Augoustides-Savvopoulou P, Papachristou F, Fairbanks LD, et al: Partial hypoxanthine-guanine phosphoribosyltransferase deficiency as the unsuspected cause of renal disease spanning three generations: A cautionary tale. *Pediatrics* 2002;109:E17.

Cameron JS, Moro F, Simmonds HA: Gout, uric acid and purine metabolism in paediatric nephrology. *Pediatr Nephrol* 1993;7:105–118.

Cameron JS, Simmonds HA: Hereditary hyperuricemia and renal disease. *Semin Nephrol* 2005;25:9–18.

Dabrowski E, Smathers SA, Ralstrom CS, et al: Botulinum toxin as a novel treatment for self-mutilation in Lesch-Nyman Syndrome. *Dev Med Child Neurol* 2005;47:636–639.

Jinnah HA, De Gregorio L, Harris JC, et al: The spectrum of inherited mutations causing HPRT deficiency: 75 new cases and a review of 196 previously reported cases. *Mutat Res* 2000;463:309–326.

Loffler M, Fairbanks LD, Zameitat E, et al: Pyrimidine pathways in health and disease. *Mol Med* 2005;11:430–437.

Marinaki AM, Escuredo E, Duley JA, et al: Genetic basis of hemolytic anemia caused by pyrimidine 5' nucleotidase deficiency. *Blood* 2001;97:3327–3332.

Nishino I, Spinazzola A, Hirano M: MNGIE: From nuclear DNA to mitochondrial DNA. *Neuromuscul Disord* 2001;11:7–10.

Nyhan WL: Disorders of purine and pyrimidine metabolism. *Mol Genet Metab* 2005;86:25–33.

Nyhan WL, Vuong LU, Broock R: Prenatal diagnosis of Lesch-Nyhan disease. *Prenat Diagn* 2003;23:807–809.

Race V, Marie S, Vincent MF, et al: Clinical, biochemical and molecular genetic correlations in adenylosuccinate lyase deficiency. *Hum Mol Genet* 2000;9:2159–2165.

Schretlen DJ, Harris JC, Park K, et al: Neurocognitive functioning in Lesch-Nyhan disease and partial hypoxanthine-guanine phosphoribosyltransferase deficiency. *J Int Neuropsychol Soc* 2001;7:805–812.

Schretlen DJ, Ward J, Meyer SM, et al: Behavioral aspects of Lesch-Nyhan disease and its variants. *Dev Med Child Neurol* 2005;47:673–677.

Scriver CR, Beaudet AL, Sly WS, et al (eds): *The Metabolic and Molecular Basis of Inherited Disease,* Vol. 2, 8th ed. New York, McGraw-Hill, 2001, pp 2513–2702.

Simmonds HA, Duley JA, Fairbanks LD, et al: When to investigate for purine and pyrimidine disorders: Introduction and review of clinical and laboratory indications. *J Inherit Metab Dis* 1997;20:214–226.

van Gennip AH, van Kuilenburg AB: Defects of pyrimidine degradation: Clinical, molecular, and diagnostic aspects. *Adv Exp Med Biol* 2000;486:233–241.

Wong DF, Harris JC, Naidu S, et al: Dopamine transporters are markedly reduced in Lesch-Nyhan disease in vivo. *Proc Natl Acad Sci U S A* 1996;93:5539–5543.

Chapter 90 ■ Progeria

W. Ted Brown

Progeria's most striking feature resembles accelerated aging. This rare syndrome, also referred to as the Hutchinson-Gilford progeria syndrome (HGPS), has an incidence of ≈1/8,000,000. Affected children do not become sexually mature or reproduce as a result of severe failure to thrive; parent-to-child transmission has not been observed. The clinical diagnosis of HGPS is based on recognition of common clinical features and exclusion of other syndromes that have overlapping features. Mutations in *LMNA*, the gene encoding lamin A/C, are the only mutations known to be associated with HGPS. Approximately 90% of individuals with HGPS have had an identifiable *LMNA* mutation.

CLINICAL MANIFESTATIONS. Children with progeria usually appear normal in early infancy, but manifestations such as midfacial cyanosis, "sculpted nose," and "sclerodema" may suggest the existence of the syndrome at birth. Profound growth failure occurs in the 1st yr of life. The characteristic facies, alopecia, loss of subcutaneous fat, abnormal posture, stiffness of joints, and bone and skin changes usually become apparent in the 2nd yr of life (Fig. 90-1). Motor and mental development is normal. The dominant clinical manifestations include short stature; weight distinctly low for height; diminished subcutaneous fat; head disproportionately large for face; micrognathia; prominent scalp veins; generalized alopecia; prominent eyes; delayed and abnormal dentition; pyriform thorax; short, dystrophic clavicles; "horse-riding" stance; wide-based shuffling gait; coxa valga, thin limbs, and prominent, stiff joints; and failure to complete sexual maturation.

Features frequently present are skin that is thin, taut, dry, wrinkled, and brown-spotted in various areas; sclerodermatous skin over the lower abdomen, proximal thighs, and buttocks; prominent superficial veins; loss of eyebrows and eyelashes; persistently patent anterior fontanel; sculpted, beaked nasal tip; faint nasolabial cyanosis; thin lips; protruding ears; absence of ear lobules; thin, high-pitched voice; dystrophic nails; and progressive radiolucency of the terminal phalanges and distal clavicles (acro-osteolysis). Differential diagnosis includes mandibular-acral dysplasia, Cockayne syndrome, Hallermann-Streiff syndrome, and neonatal progeroid syndrome (Wiedemann-Rautenstrauch). **Werner syndrome** is another disease of premature aging due predominantly to mutations in the DNA helicase gene (Table 90-1).

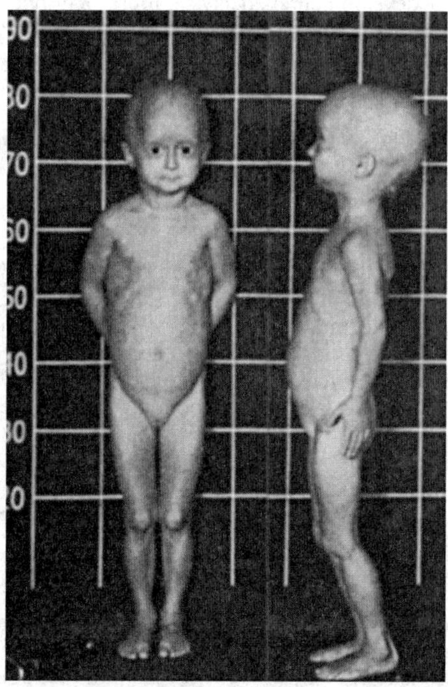

Figure 90-1. A 4.5 yr old girl with height of 1.75 yr and bone age of 4 yr. (From Wilkins L: *Diagnosis and Treatment of Endocrine Disorders in Childhood and Adolescence,* 3rd ed. Springfield, IL, Charles C Thomas, 1965.)

TABLE 90-1. Features of Werner and Hutchinson-Gilford Syndromes

FEATURE	WERNER SYNDROME	HUTCHINSON-GILFORD SYNDROME
MIM number	277700	176670
Causative gene(s)	*WRN, LMNA*	*LMNA*
Genetics	Autosomal recessive	Sporadic, autosomal dominant
Onset	Young adulthood	Childhood
Hair graying	+	+
Hair loss	Male pattern	Total
Skin thinning	+	+
Subcutaneous tissue loss	+	+
Skin calcification	+	–
Ankle ulceration	+	–
Hyperkeratosis	+	–
Cataracts	+	–
Short stature	+	+
Coxa valga	–	+
Mandibular hypoplasia	–	+
Atherosclerosis	+	+
Osteopenia/osteoporosis	+	+
Laryngeal atrophy (high voice)	+	+
Thymic atrophy	+	–
Diabetes	Variable	–
Hypogonadism	+	+
Cancer susceptibility	+	–

MIM, Mendelian Inheritance in Man; +, present; –, absent.
Modified from Hegele RA: Drawing the line in progeria syndromes. *Lancet* 2003;362:416–417.

LABORATORY FINDINGS. Variable degrees of insulin resistance (occasionally, insulin-dependent diabetes mellitus), abnormalities of collagen, increased metabolic rate, and inconsistent abnormalities of serum cholesterol and other lipids are found, but there are no demonstrable abnormalities of thyroid, parathyroid, pituitary, or adrenal function.

MOLECULAR PATHOGENESIS. The nuclear lamina, a protein-containing layer attached to the inner nuclear membrane, is composed of a family of polypeptides, with the major components being the lamins A, B1, B2, and C. Lamins A and C are formed by alternative splicing of the *LMNA* gene transcript. Separate genes encode lamin B1 and B2. Lamin A is normally synthesized as a precursor molecule (prelamin A). Alternative splicing within exon 10 gives rise to two different mRNAs that code for prelamin A and lamin C. Prelamin A, with 664 amino acids, has 98 unique carboxy-terminal amino acids. Lamin C has six unique carboxy-terminal amino acids. Because prelamin A contains a CAAX (cysteine-aliphatic-aliphatic-any amino acid) box at its carboxyl terminus, it is modified by farnesylation, whereas lamin C is not. After **farnesylation**, cleavage of the last three amino acids, and methylation of the C-terminus, an internal proteolytic cleavage occurs, removing the last 15 coding amino acids, to generate mature lamin A with 646 amino acids. The **most common HGPS** mutation is a G608G (GGC > GGT) mutation in exon 11. This mutation results in an activation of a cryptic splice site within exon 11, resulting in production of a transcript that deletes 50 amino acids near the C-terminus. The HGPS G608G mutation and consequent abnormal splicing produces a prelamin A that retains the CAAX box but is missing the site for endoproteolytic cleavage. This HGPS mutation acts as a **dominant negative mutation.**

A growing list of other diseases is associated with different mutations in *LMNA*, which have come to be known as laminopathies. These include Emery-Dreifuss muscular dystrophy type 2, familial dilated cardiomyopathy and conduction system defects, Dunnigan-type familial partial lipodystrophy, limb girdle muscular dystrophy 1B, Charcot-Marie-Tooth disease 2B1, mandibuloacral dysplasia, and atypical Werner syndrome (see Table 90-1).

PROGNOSIS. Children with progeria usually have severe atherosclerosis, and death occurs as a result of complications of cardiac or cerebrovascular disease, generally between age 5 and 20 yr, with a median life span of ≈13 yr. Cataracts and tumors have infrequently been noted, but many changes associated with normal aging in adults, such as presbycusis, presbyopia, arcus senilis, osteoarthritis, senile personality changes, or Alzheimer disease, are not found.

TREATMENT. No specific treatment for this condition exists. There is a progeria foundation (www.progeriaresearch.org), which maintains a Progeria Registry to help with diagnosis and to define more clearly the incidence and molecular basis of the disorder.

Brown WT, Gordon LB, Collis FS: Hutchinson-Gilford progeria syndrome. In Gene Reviews at Gene Tests: Medical Genetics Information Rescurce [database online]. Available at http://www.genetests.org/(updated August 2006).

Capell BC, Erdos MR, Madigan JP, et al: Inhibiting farnesylation of progerin prevents the characteristic nuclear blebbing of Hutchinson-Gilford progeria syndrome. *Proc Natl Acad Sci U S A* 2005;102:12879–12884.

Chen L, Lee L, Kudlow A, et al: *LMNA* mutations in atypical Werner's syndrome. *Lancet* 2003;363:440–445.

Eriksson M, Brown WT, Gordon LB, et al: Recurrent de novo point mutations in lamin A cause Hutchinson-Gilford progeria syndrome. *Nature* 2003;423:293–298.

Hegele RA: Drawing the line in progeria syndromes. *Lancet* 2003;362: 416–417.

Chapter 91 ■ The Porphyrias

Karl E. Anderson, Chul Lee, and Robert J. Desnick

Porphyrias are metabolic diseases resulting from deficiencies of specific enzymes of the heme biosynthetic pathway. These enzymes are most active in bone marrow and liver. When these diseases are manifest, accumulation of 1 or more intermediates occurs initially in 1 of these tissues. Erythropoietic porphyrias, in which overproduction of heme pathway intermediates occurs primarily in bone marrow erythroid cells, usually present at birth or in early childhood with cutaneous photosensitivity, or in the case of congenital erythropoietic porphyria, even in utero as nonimmune hydrops. Most porphyrias are hepatic, with overproduction and initial accumulation of porphyrin precursors or porphyrins occurring 1st in the liver. Regulatory mechanisms for heme biosynthesis in liver are distinct from those in the bone marrow and appear to account for activation of hepatic porphyrias during adult life rather than childhood. Homozygous forms of the hepatic porphyrias may manifest clinically prior to puberty, and asymptomatic heterozygous children may present with nonspecific and unrelated symptoms. Parents often request advice about long-term prognosis and information about management of these disorders and drugs that can be taken safely to treat other common conditions.

The DNA sequences and chromosomal locations are established for the human genes of the enzymes in this pathway, and multiple disease-related mutations have been found for each porphyria. All but 3 of the inherited porphyrias display autosomal dominant inheritance. Although initial diagnosis of porphyria by biochemical methods remains essential, it is especially important in children to confirm the diagnosis by demonstrating a specific gene mutation(s).

THE HEME BIOSYNTHETIC PATHWAY

Heme is required for a variety of hemoproteins such as hemoglobin, myoglobin, respiratory cytochromes, and cytochrome P450 enzymes (CYPs). It is believed that the 8 enzymes in the pathway for heme biosynthesis are active in all tissues. Hemoglobin synthesis in erythroid precursor cells accounts for ≈85% of daily heme synthesis in humans. Hepatocytes account for most of the rest, primarily for synthesis of CYPs, which are especially abundant in the liver endoplasmic reticulum (ER), and turn over more rapidly than many other hemoproteins, such as the mitochondrial respiratory cytochromes. As shown in Figure 91-1, pathway intermediates are the porphyrin precursors δ-aminolevulinic acid (ALA, also known as 5-aminolevulinic acid) and porphobilinogen (PBG), and porphyrins (mostly in their reduced forms, known as porphyrinogens). At least in humans, these intermediates do not accumulate in significant amounts under normal conditions or have important physiologic functions.

A deficiency of each enzyme in the pathway, with the exception of the 1st, is associated with a different porphyria (Table 91-1). The 1st enzyme, ALA synthase (ALAS), occurs in 2 forms. An erythroid specific form, termed ALAS2, is deficient in X-linked sideroblastic anemia, due to mutations of the *ALAS2* gene on chromosome Xp11.2. The ubiquitous form of this enzyme, termed ALAS1, is found in all tissues including liver, and its gene is located on chromosome 3p21.1. Disease-related mutations of ALAS1 have not been described.

Regulation of heme synthesis differs in the 2 major heme-forming tissues. Liver heme biosynthesis is primary controlled by ALAS1. Synthesis of ALAS1 in liver is regulated by a "free" heme pool (see Fig. 91-1), which can be augmented by newly synthesized heme or by existing heme released from hemoproteins and destined for breakdown to biliverdin by heme oxygenase.

In the erythron, novel regulatory mechanisms allow for the production of the very large amounts of heme needed for hemoglobin synthesis. The response to stimuli for hemoglobin synthesis occurs during cell differentiation, leading to an increase in cell number. Also, unlike the liver, heme has a stimulatory role in hemoglobin formation, and the stimulation of heme synthesis in erythroid cells is accompanied by increases not only in ALAS2, but also by sequential induction of other heme biosynthetic enzymes. Separate erythroid-specific and nonerythroid or "housekeeping" transcripts are known for the 1st 4 enzymes in the pathway. The separate forms of ALAS are encoded by genes on different chromosomes, but for each of the other 3, erythroid and nonerythroid transcripts are transcribed by alternative promoters in the same gene. Heme also regulates the rate of its synthesis in erythroid cells by controlling the transport of iron into reticulocytes.

Intermediates of the heme biosynthetic pathway are efficiently converted to heme and, normally, only small amounts of the intermediates are excreted. Some may undergo chemical modifications before excretion. Whereas the porphyrin precursors ALA and PBG are colorless, nonfluorescent, and largely excreted unchanged in urine, PBG may degrade to colored products such as the brownish pigment called porphobilin or spontaneously polymerize to uroporphyrins. Porphyrins are red in color and display bright red fluorescence when exposed to long wavelength ultraviolet light. Porphyrinogens, which are colorless and nonfluorescent, are the reduced form of porphyrins, and when they accumulate, are readily autoxidized to the corresponding porphyrins outside the cell. Only the type III isomers of uroporphyrinogen and coproporphyrinogen are converted to heme (see Fig. 91-1).

ALA and PBG are excreted in urine. Excretion of porphyrins and porphyrinogens in urine or bile is determined by the number of carboxyl groups. Those with many carboxyl groups, such as uroporphyrin (octacarboxyl porphyrin) and heptacarboxyl porphyrin), are water soluble and readily excreted in urine. Those with fewer carboxyl groups, such as protoporphyrin (dicarboxyl porphyrin), are not water soluble and are excreted in bile and feces. Coproporphyrin (tetracarboxyl porphyrin) is excreted

TABLE 91-1. The Human Porphyrias, the Causative Heterozygous or Homozygous Mutations of Specific Enzymes of the Heme Biosynthetic Pathway, the Usual Time of Presentation, and Classifications for Each Disease Based on the Major Tissue Sites of Overproduction of Heme Pathway Intermediates (Hepatic vs Erythropoietic) or the Type of Major Symptoms (Acute Neurovisceral vs Cutaneous)

				CLASSIFICATIONS			
DISEASE (ABBREVIATION)	ENZYME (ABBREVIATION)	MUTATIONS OF THIS ENZYME	PRESENTATION	HEPATIC	ERYTHROPOIETIC	ACUTE/NEUROLOGIC	CUTANEOUS
δ-Aminolevulinic acid dehydratase porphyria (ADP)	*δ-Aminolevulinic acid dehydratase (ALAD)*	Homozygous	Mostly post puberty	X	X*	X	
Acute intermittent porphyria (AIP)	*Porphobilinogen deaminase (PBGD)*	Heterozygous	Post puberty	X		X	
Homozygous AIP		Homozygous	Childhood	X	X	X	
Congenital erythropoietic porphyria (CEP)	*Uroporphyrinogen III synthase (UROS)*	Homozygous	In utero or infancy		X		X
Porphyria cutanea tarda (PCT) type 1	*Uroporphyrinogen decarboxylase (UROD)*	None	Adults	X			X
PCT type 2¶		Heterozygous	Adults	X			
PCT type 3		None	Adults	X			
Hepatoerythropoietic porphyria (HEP)		Homozygous	Childhood	X	X*		X
Hereditary coproporphyria (HCP)	*Coproporphyrinogen oxidase (CPO)*	Heterozygous	Post puberty	X		X	X
Homozygous HCP		Homozygous	Childhood	X	X	X	X
Variegate porphyria (VP)	*Protoporphyrinogen oxidase (PPO)*	Heterozygous	Post puberty	X		X	X
Homozygous VP		Homozygous	Childhood	X	X	X	X
Erythropoietic protoporphyria (EPP)	*Ferrochelatase (FECH)*	Heterozygous (heteroallelic with low expression normal allele) or homozygous	Childhood		X		X

*ADP and HEP are considered primarily hepatic porphyrias, but substantial increases in erythrocyte zinc protoporphyrin suggest an erythropoietic component.

¶PCT is due to inhibition of hepatic UROD. Autosomal dominant inheritance of a partial deficiency of UROD is a predisposing factor in cases defined as familial (type 2) PCT.

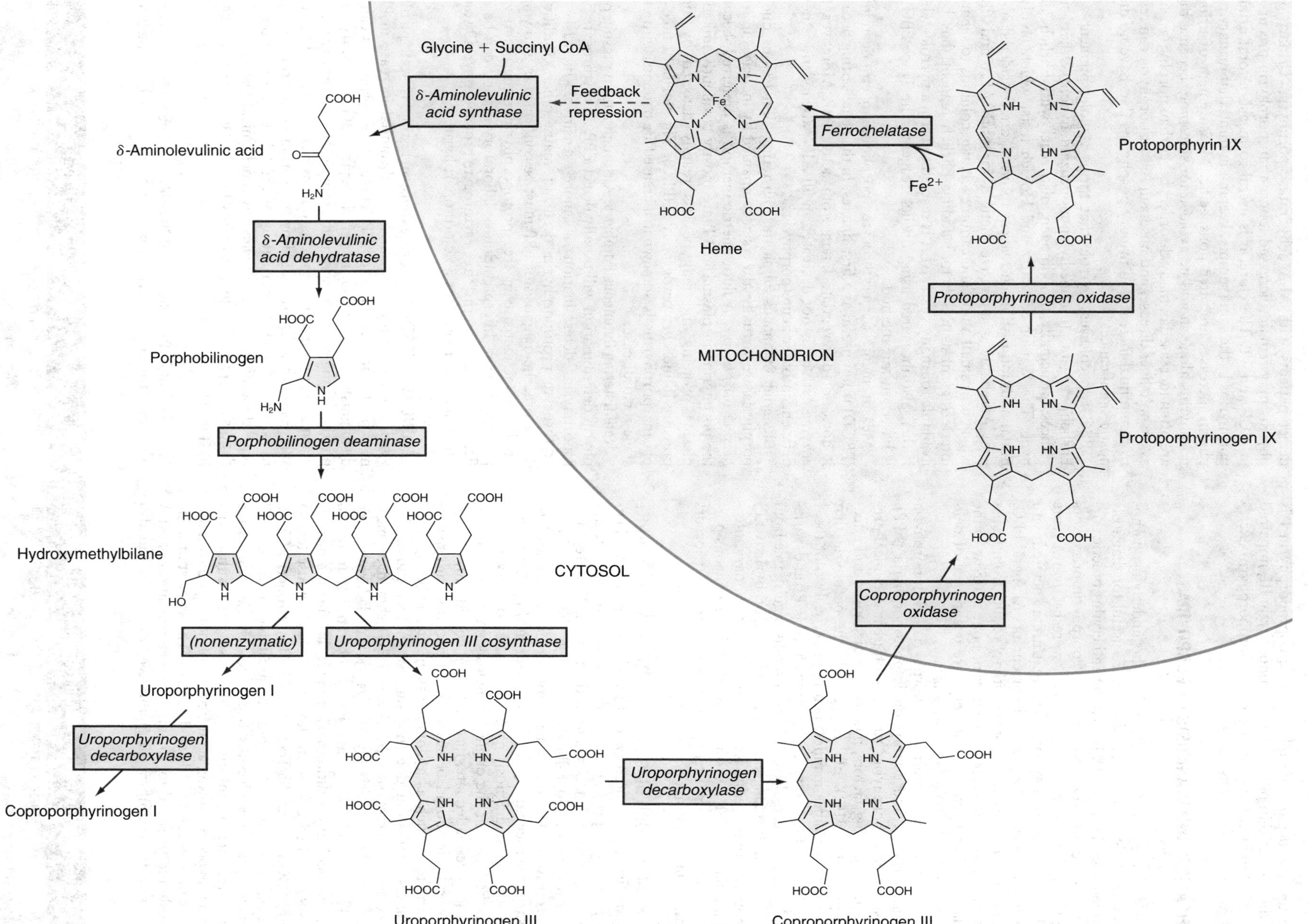

Figure 91-1. Enzymes and intermediates of the heme biosynthetic pathway. The pathway is regulated in the liver by the end product, heme, mainly by feedback repression *(dashed arrow)*.

partly in urine and partly in bile. Because coproporphyrin I is more readily excreted in bile than is coproporphyrin III, impaired hepatobiliary function may increase total coproporphyrin excretion and the ratio of these isomers.

CLASSIFICATION AND DIAGNOSIS OF PORPHYRIAS

Two classification schemes reflect either the underlying pathophysiology or clinical features, and both are useful for diagnosis and treatment (see Table 91-1). In **hepatic** and **erythropoietic** porphyrias, the source of excess production of porphyrin precursors and porphyrins is the liver and bone marrow, respectively. **Acute porphyrias** cause neurologic symptoms that are associated with increases of 1 or both of the porphyrin precursors ALA and PBG. In the **cutaneous porphyrias,** photosensitivity results from transport of porphyrins in blood from the liver or bone marrow to the skin. **Dual porphyria** refers to the very rare occurrence of deficiencies of 2 different heme pathway enzymes.

It is notable that acute intermittent porphyria (AIP), porphyria cutanea tarda (PCT), and erythropoietic protoporphyria (EPP), the 3 most common porphyrias, are very different in clinical presentation, precipitating factors, methods of diagnosis, and effective therapy (Table 91-2). EPP is probably the porphyria that most commonly becomes manifest before puberty. Two of the 4 acute porphyrias, hereditary coproporphyria (HCP) and variegate porphyria (VP), can also cause lesions indistinguishable from PCT (see Table 91-1). Congenital erythropoietic porphyria (CEP) causes more severe blistering lesions, often with secondary infection and mutilation. EPP is distinct from the other cutaneous porphyrias in causing nonblistering photosensitivity that occurs acutely after sun exposure.

FIRST-LINE LABORATORY DIAGNOSTIC TESTING. A few sensitive and specific first-line laboratory tests should be relied on whenever symptoms or signs suggest the diagnosis of porphyria. If a first-line or screening test is significantly abnormal, more comprehensive testing should follow to establish the type of porphyria. Overuse of laboratory tests for screening can lead to unnecessary expense and even delay in diagnosis. In patients who present with a past diagnosis of porphyria, laboratory reports that were the basis for the original diagnosis must be reviewed, and if these were inadequate, further testing considered.

Acute porphyria should be suspected in patients with neurovisceral symptoms such as abdominal pain after puberty, when initial clinical evaluation does not suggest another cause, and *urinary porphyrin precursors (ALA and PBG)* should be measured. Urinary PBG is virtually always increased during acute attacks of AIP, HCP, and VP, and is not substantially increased in any other medical conditions. Therefore, this measurement is both sensitive and specific. A method for rapid, in-house testing for urinary PBG, such as the Trace PBG kit (Trace America/Trace Diagnostics, Louisville, CO), should be available in-house at all major medical facilities. Results from **spot (single void)** urine specimens are highly informative because very substantial increases are expected during acute attacks of porphyria. A 24 hr collection can unnecessarily delay diagnosis. The same spot urine specimen should be saved for quantitative determination of ALA and PBG, in order to confirm the qualitative PBG result, and also detect patients with ALA dehydratase porphyria. Urinary porphyrins may remain increased longer than porphyrin precursors in HCP and VP. Therefore, it is useful to measure total urinary porphyrins in the same sample, keeping in mind that urinary porphyrin increases are often nonspecific. Measurement of urinary porphyrins alone should be avoided for screening, because these are often increased in many disorders other than porphyrias, such as chronic liver disease, and misdiagnoses of porphyria can result from minimal increases in urinary porphyrins that have no diagnostic significance.

PBG is a colorless pyrrole that forms a violet pigment with Ehrlich reagent (*p*-dimethylaminobenzaldehyde). Other substances, principally urobilinogen, also react with Ehrlich aldehyde. The Watson-Schwartz and Hoesch tests, which involved initial addition of Ehrlich reagent to urine, are considered obsolete. A reliable quantitative method for both ALA and PBG, which uses small anion and cation exchange columns to separate interfering substances before adding Ehrlich reagent, has been available for many years. ALA is reacted to form a pyrrole, which is then also measured using Ehrlich reagent. The Trace PBG kit is based on this method.

Measurement of erythrocyte porphobilinogen deaminase (PBGD) is not useful as a first-line test in the acute setting because it does not differentiate latent from active AIP. Moreover, the enzyme activity is not decreased in all AIP patients and is never deficient in other acute porphyrias.

Blistering Cutaneous Porphyrias. Blistering skin lesions due to porphyria are virtually always accompanied by increases in *total plasma porphyrins*. A fluorometric method is preferred, because the porphyrins in plasma in VP are mostly covalently linked to plasma proteins and may be less readily detected by high-pressure liquid chromatography (HPLC). The normal range for plasma porphyrins is somewhat increased in patients with end-stage renal disease.

Nonblistering Cutaneous Porphyria. Although a total plasma porphyrin determination will usually detect EPP, an erythrocyte protoporphyrin determination is more sensitive. Increases in erythrocyte protoporphyrin occur in many other conditions. Therefore, the diagnosis of EPP must be confirmed by showing a predominant increase in free protoporphyrin rather than zinc protoporphyrin. Interpretation of laboratory reports can be difficult, because the term "free erythrocyte protoporphyrin" sometimes actually represents zinc protoporphyrin.

SECOND-LINE TESTING. More extensive testing is well justified when a first-line test is positive. A substantial increase in PBG may be due to AIP, HCP, or VP. These acute porphyrias can be distinguished by measuring erythrocyte PBGD, urinary porphyrins (using the same spot urine sample), fecal porphyrins, and plasma porphyrins. The various porphyrias that cause blistering skin lesions are differentiated by measuring porphyrins in urine, feces, and plasma. Confirmation at the DNA level is important once the diagnosis is established by biochemical testing. Further details are provided in the following sections on each type of porphyria.

TESTING FOR SUBCLINICAL PORPHYRIA. It is often difficult to diagnose or "rule out" porphyria in patients who had suggestive

TABLE 91-2. The Three Most Common Human Porphyrias and Their Major Features

	PRESENTING SYMPTOMS	EXACERBATING FACTORS	MOST IMPORTANT SCREENING TESTS	TREATMENT
Acute intermittent porphyria	Neurologic	Drugs (mostly P450-inducers), progesterone, dietary restriction	Urinary porphobilinogen	Hemin, glucose
Porphyria cutanea tarda	Skin blistering and fragility (chronic)	Iron, alcohol, smoking, estrogens, hepatitis C, HIV, halogenated hydrocarbons	Plasma (or urine) porphyrins	Phlebotomy, low-dose hydroxychloroquine or chloroquine
Erythropoietic protoporphyria	Skin pain and swelling (mostly acute)		Erythrocyte (or plasma) porphyrins	β-Carotene

symptoms months or years in the past, and in relatives of patients with acute porphyrias, because porphyrin precursors and porphyrins may be normal. More extensive testing and consultation with a specialist laboratory and physician may be needed. Before evaluating relatives, the diagnosis of porphyria should be firmly established in an index case, and the laboratory results reviewed to guide the choice of tests for the family members. The index case or another family member with confirmed porphyria should be retested if necessary. Identification of a disease-causing mutation in an index case greatly facilitates detection of additional gene carriers.

δ-AMINOLEVULINIC ACID DEHYDRATASE PORPHYRIA (ADP)

This is the most recently described human porphyria and is sometimes termed *Doss porphyria* after the investigator who described the 1st 2 cases. The term *plumboporphyria* emphasizes the similarity of this condition to lead poisoning, but incorrectly implies that it is due to lead exposure.

ETIOLOGY. This porphyria results from a deficiency of δ-aminolevulinic acid dehydratase (ALAD), which is inherited as an autosomal recessive trait. Only 6 cases have been confirmed by mutation analysis. The prevalence of heterozygous ALAD deficiency was estimated to be <1% in Germany and ≈2% in Sweden.

PATHOLOGY AND PATHOGENESIS. ALAD catalyzes the condensation of two molecules of ALA to form the pyrrole PBG (see Fig. 91-1). The enzyme is subject to inhibition by a number of exogenous and endogenous chemicals. ALAD is the principal lead-binding protein in erythrocytes, and lead can displace the zinc atoms of the enzyme. Erythrocyte ALAD activity is also a sensitive index of lead exposure.

All ADP cases inherited a different ALAD mutation from each parent. Eleven ALAD mutations, mostly point mutations, have been identified, some expressing partial activity, such that heme synthesis is partially preserved. The amount of residual enzyme activity may predict the phenotypic severity of this disease. Immunochemical studies in 3 cases demonstrated nonfunctional enzyme protein that cross reacted with anti-ALAD antibodies. Late-onset cases associated with a myeloproliferative disorder may be heterozygous or have a somatic mutation, with expansion of an affected clone of erythroid cells.

ADP is often classified as a hepatic porphyria, although the site of overproduction of ALA is not established. A patient with severe, early-onset disease underwent liver transplantation, without significant clinical or biochemical improvement, which might suggest that the excess intermediates did not originate in the liver. Excess urinary coproporphyrin III in ADP might originate from metabolism of ALA to porphyrinogens in a tissue other than the site of ALA overproduction. Administration of large doses of ALA to normal subjects also leads to substantial coproporphyrinuria. Increased erythrocyte protoporphyrin may, as in all other homozygous porphyrias, be explained by accumulation of earlier pathway intermediates in bone marrow erythroid cells during hemoglobin synthesis, followed by their transformation to protoporphyrin after hemoglobin synthesis is complete. As in other acute porphyrias, the pathogenesis of the neurologic symptoms is poorly understood (see section on AIP).

CLINICAL MANIFESTATIONS. In most cases, symptoms resemble other acute porphyrias, including acute attacks of abdominal pain and neuropathy. Precipitating factors, such as exposure to harmful drugs, have not been evident in most cases. Four of the 6 reported cases were adolescent males. A Swedish infant had more severe disease, with neurologic impairment and failure to thrive. A 63 yr old man in Belgium developed an acute motor polyneuropathy concurrently with a myeloproliferative disorder.

LABORATORY FINDINGS. Urinary ALA, coproporphyrin III, and erythrocyte zinc protoporphyrin are substantially increased. Urinary PBG is normal or slightly increased. Erythrocyte ALAD activity is markedly reduced, and both parents should have approximately half-normal activity of this enzyme and normal urinary ALA.

DIAGNOSIS AND DIFFERENTIAL DIAGNOSIS. The 3 other acute porphyrias are characterized by substantial increases in both ALA and PBG. In contrast, ALA but not PBG is substantially increased in ADP. A marked deficiency of erythrocyte ALAD and half-normal activity in the parents support the diagnosis. Other causes of ALAD deficiency, such as **lead poisoning,** must be excluded. Succinylacetone accumulates in hereditary tyrosinemia type 1 and is structurally similar to ALA, inhibits ALAD, and can cause increased urinary excretion of ALA and clinical manifestations that resemble acute porphyria. Idiopathic acquired ALAD deficiency has been reported. Unlike lead poisoning, the deficient ALAD activity is not restored by the in vitro addition of sulfhydryl reagents such as dithiothreitol. Even if no other cause of ALAD deficiency is found, it is essential to confirm the diagnosis of ADP by molecular studies.

TREATMENT. Treatment experience is limited but is similar to other acute porphyrias. Glucose seems not very effective but may be tried for mild symptoms. Hemin therapy was apparently effective for acute attacks in adolescent male cases, and weekly infusions prevented attacks in 1 of these cases. Hemin was not effective either biochemically or clinically in the Swedish child with severe disease, and produced a biochemical response but no clinical improvement in the Belgian man with a late-onset form, who had a peripheral neuropathy but no acute attacks. Hemin is also effective in treating porphyria-like symptoms associated with hereditary tyrosinemia, and can significantly reduce urinary ALA and coproporphyrin in lead poisoning. Avoidance of drugs that are harmful in other acute porphyrias is advisable. Liver transplantation was not effective in the child with severe disease.

PROGNOSIS. The outlook is generally good in typical cases, although recurrent attacks may occur. The course was unfavorable in the Swedish child with more severe disease, and is uncertain in adults with late-onset disease associated with myeloproliferative disorders.

PREVENTION AND GENETIC COUNSELING. Heterozygous parents should be aware that subsequent children are at risk for the disease, as in any autosomal recessive disorder. Diagnosis in utero is possible, but has not been reported.

ACUTE INTERMITTENT PORPHYRIA (AIP)

This disorder has also been termed *pyrroloporphyria, Swedish porphyria,* and *intermittent acute porphyria* and is the most common type of acute porphyria in most countries.

ETIOLOGY. AIP results from the deficient activity of the housekeeping form of PBG deaminase (PBGD). This enzyme is also known as hydroxymethylbilane (HMB) synthase; the prior term uroporphyrinogen I synthase is obsolete. PBGD catalyzes the deamination and head-to-tail condensation of 4 PBG molecules to form the linear tetrapyrrole, HMB (also known as preuroporphyrinogen; see Fig. 91-1). A unique dipyrromethane cofactor binds the pyrrole intermediates at the catalytic site until 6 pyrroles (including the dipyrrole cofactor) are assembled in a linear fashion, after which the tetrapyrrole HMB is released. The apo-deaminase generates the dipyrrole cofactor to form the holo-deaminase, and this occurs more readily from HMB than from PBG. Indeed, high concentrations of PBG may inhibit formation of the holo-deaminase. The product HMB can cyclize nonenzymatically to form nonphysiological uroporphyrinogen I, but in the presence of the next enzyme in the pathway is more rapidly cyclized to form uroporphyrinogen III.

Erythroid and housekeeping forms of the enzyme are encoded by a single gene on human chromosome 11 (11q24.1–>q24.2), which contains 15 exons. The 2 isoenzymes are both monomeric proteins and differ only slightly in molecular weight (≈40 and 42 kd, respectively), and result from alternative splicing of exons 1 and 2. The erythroid-specific isoenzyme, therefore, is encoded by exons 2 through 15, and the erythroid promoter, which functions only in erythroid cells, is located immediately upstream from exon 2. The housekeeping isozyme is encoded by exons 1 and 3 through 15, and its promoter is immediately upstream from exon 1. Cis-acting sequences bind the erythroid-specific DNA-binding factors NF-E1 and NF-E2, leading to expression of the erythroid promoter. The housekeeping promoter functions in all cell types, including erythroid cells.

The pattern of inheritance of AIP is autosomal dominant, with very rare homozygous cases that present in childhood. More than 200 *PBGD* mutations, including missense, nonsense, and splicing mutations and insertions and deletions have been identified in AIP, and in many population groups, including blacks. Most mutations are found in only 1 or a few families. But due to founder effects, some are more common in certain geographic areas such as northern Sweden (W198X), Holland (R116W), Argentina (G116R), Nova Scotia (R173W), and Switzerland (W283X). De novo mutations may be found in ≈3% of cases. *Chester porphyria* was initially described as a variant form of acute porphyria in a large English family, but was found to be due to a *PBGD* mutation. The nature of the *PBGD* mutation does not account for the severity of the clinical presentation, which varies markedly within families.

Most mutations lead to approximately half-normal activity of the housekeeping and erythroid isozymes and half-normal amounts of their respective enzyme proteins in all tissues of heterozygotes. In ≈5% of unrelated AIP patients, the housekeeping isozyme is deficient, but the erythroid-specific isozyme is normal. Mutations causing this variant are usually found within exon 1 or its 5′ splice donor site or initiation of translation codon. Immunochemical methods can distinguish mutations that are CRIM-positive (i.e., having excess cross-reactive immunologic material [CRIM] relative to the mutant enzyme activity), whereas CRIM-negative mutations either do not synthesize a mutant enzyme protein, or the protein is not stable and not immunologically detectable using anti-PBGD antibodies. A child with homozygous AIP was found to have inherited a different CRIM-positive mutation from each parent.

PATHOLOGY AND PATHOGENESIS. Induction of the rate-limiting hepatic enzyme ALAS1 is thought to underlie acute exacerbations of this and the other acute porphyrias. AIP remains latent (or asymptomatic) in the great majority of those who are heterozygous carriers of *PBGD* mutations, and this is almost always the case before puberty. In those with no history of acute symptoms, porphyrin precursor excretion is usually normal, suggesting that half-normal hepatic PBGD activity is sufficient and hepatic ALAS1 activity is not increased. Many nongenetic factors that lead to clinical expression of AIP, including certain drugs and steroid hormones, have the capacity to induce hepatic ALAS1 and CYPs. Under conditions in which heme synthesis is increased in the liver, half-normal PBGD activity may become limiting and ALA, PBG, and other heme pathway intermediates may accumulate. In addition, heme synthesis becomes impaired and heme-mediated repression of hepatic ALAS1 is less effective.

It is not proven, however, that hepatic PBGD remains constant at ≈50% of normal activity during exacerbations and remission of AIP, as in erythrocytes. An early report suggested that the enzyme activity is considerably less than half-normal in the liver during an acute attack. Hepatic PBGD activity might be reduced further once AIP becomes activated if, as recently suggested, excess PBG interferes with assembly of the dipyrromethane cofactor for this enzyme. It also seems likely that currently unknown genetic factors play a contributing role in, for example, patients who continue to have attacks even when known precipitants are avoided.

The fact that AIP is almost always latent before puberty suggests that **endocrine factors,** adult levels of steroid hormones, are important for clinical expression. Symptoms are more common in women, which suggests a role for female hormones. Premenstrual attacks are probably due to endogenous progesterone. Acute porphyrias are sometimes exacerbated by exogenous steroids, including oral contraceptive preparations containing progestins. Surprisingly, pregnancy is usually well tolerated, suggesting that beneficial metabolic changes may ameliorate the effects of high levels of progesterone.

Drugs that are unsafe in acute porphyrias (Table 91-3) include those having the capacity to induce hepatic ALAS1, which is closely associated with induction of CYPs. Griseofulvin is an example of a chemical that can increase heme turnover by promoting the destruction of specific CYPs to form an inhibitor of ferrochelatase (FECH, the final enzyme in the pathway), such as N-methyl protoporphyrin. Sulfonamide antibiotics are harmful but apparently not inducers of hepatic heme synthesis. Ethanol and other alcohols are inducers of ALA synthase and some CYPs.

Nutritional factors, principally reduced intake of calories and carbohydrates, as may occur with illness or attempts to lose

TABLE 91-3. Drugs Regarded as Unsafe and Safe in Acute Porphyrias

UNSAFE	SAFE
Barbiturates*	Narcotic analgesics
Sulfonamide antibiotics*	Aspirin
Meprobamate* (also mebutamate,* tybutamate*)	Acetaminophen
Carisoprodol*	Phenothiazines
Glutethimide*	Penicillin and derivatives
Methyprylon	Streptomycin
Ethchlorvynol*	Glucocorticoids
Mephenytoin	Bromides
Phenytoin*	Insulin
Succinimides	Atropine
Carbamazepine*	Cimetidine
Clonazepam	Ranitidine†
Primidone*	Acetaminophen (paracetamol)
Valproic acid*	Acetazolamide
Pyrazolones (aminopyrine, antipyrine)	Allopurinol
Griseofulvin*	Amiloride
Ergots	Bethanidine
Metoclopramide*	Bumetanide
Rifampin*	Cimetidine
Pyrazinamide*	Coumarins
Diclofenac*	Fluoxetine
Progesterone and synthetic progestins*	Gabapentin
Danazol*	Gentamicin
Alcohol	Guanethidine
ACE inhibitors (especially enalapril)	Ofloxacin
Calcium channel blockers (especially nifedipine)	Propranolol
Ketoconazole	Succinylcholine
Rifampin	Tetracycline

This partial listing does not include all available information about drug safety in acute porphyrias. Other sources should be consulted for drugs not listed here.

* Porphyria is listed as a contraindication, warning, precaution, or adverse effect in U.S. labeling for these drugs. Estrogens are also listed as harmful in porphyria, but have been implicated as harmful in acute porphyrias mostly based only on experience with estrogen-progestin combinations. While estrogens can exacerbate PCT, there is little evidence they are harmful in the acute porphyrias.

† Porphyria is listed as a precaution in U.S. labeling for this drug. However, this drug is regarded as safe by other sources.

weight, can increase porphyrin precursor excretion and induce attacks of porphyria. Increased carbohydrate intake may ameliorate attacks. Recent findings indicate that hepatic ALAS1 is regulated by the peroxisome proliferator-activated receptor γ coactivator 1α (PGC-1α), which may represent an important link between nutritional status and acute porphyrias.

Other factors have been implicated. Chemicals in cigarette smoke, such as polycyclic aromatic hydrocarbons, can induce hepatic CYPs and heme synthesis. A survey of AIP patients found an association between smoking and repeated porphyric attacks. Attacks may result from metabolic stress and impaired nutrition associated with major illness, infection, or surgery.

The additive effect of multiple predisposing factors, including drugs, endogenous hormones, nutritional factors, and smoking, is suggested by clinical observations. Exposure to drugs and other precipitating factors is less likely to cause an attack in patients who have had no recent symptoms than in those with recent and frequent porphyric symptoms.

Neurologic Mechanisms. The mechanism of neural damage in acute porphyrias is poorly understood. Convincing evidence for the hypothesis that heme formation is decreased in the nervous system is lacking. Vasospasm resulting from decreased nitrous oxide production by nitrous oxide synthase (a hemoprotein) has been suggested, however, to cause cerebral manifestations in AIP. The most favored hypothesis at present is that one or more heme precursors, or perhaps a derivative, are neurotoxic. Increased ALA in AIP, HCP, VP, ADP, plumbism, and hereditary tyrosinemia type 1, which have similar neurologic manifestations, suggests that this substance or a derivative may be neuropathic. Porphyrins derived from ALA after its uptake into cells may have toxic potential. ALA can also interact with γ-aminobutyric acid (GABA) receptors. A single report of a woman with severe AIP who improved markedly after allogeneic liver transplant supports the hypothesis that heme precursors from the liver cause the neurologic manifestations.

EPIDEMIOLOGY. AIP occurs in all races and is the most common acute porphyria, with a prevalence in most countries of ≈5/100,000. In Sweden, prevalence was estimated to be 7.7/100,000, including latent cases with normal porphyrin precursors. A much higher prevalence of 60–100/100,000 in northern Sweden is due to a common mutation and a founder effect. The combined prevalence of AIP and VP in Finland is ≈3.4/100,000. A survey of chronic psychiatric patients in the United States using an erythrocyte PBGD determination found a high prevalence (210/100,000) of PBGD deficiency, but a study in Mexico found a similar prevalence in psychiatric patients and controls. Population screening by erythrocyte PBGD activity or DNA analysis revealed a prevalence of ≈200 heterozygotes per 100,000 in Finland, and 1 in about 1,675 (60/100,000) in France. Therefore, carriers of PBGD mutations that can cause AIP may be common. The suggestion that AIP accounts for the vampire legends is also unfounded and portrays the disease unfavorably. Proposals that patients with poorly understood conditions such as multiple chemical sensitivity syndrome actually have acute porphyria are also poorly founded and based on inadequate diagnostic criteria.

CLINICAL MANIFESTATIONS. Neurovisceral manifestations of acute porphyrias may appear any time after puberty, but rarely before. Very rare cases of homozygous AIP develop severe neurologic manifestations early in childhood, and acute attacks do not occur.

In affected heterozygotes, acute attacks are characterized by a constellation of nonspecific symptoms, which may become severe and life-threatening. Abdominal pain occurs in 85–95% of cases, is usually severe, steady, and poorly localized, but sometimes cramping, and accompanied by signs of ileus, including abdominal distention and decreased bowel sounds. Nausea, vomiting, and constipation are common, and increased bowel sounds and diarrhea may occur. Bladder dysfunction may cause hesitancy and dysuria. **Tachycardia,** the most common physical sign, occurs in up to 80% of attacks. This is often accompanied by hypertension, restlessness, course or fine tremors, and excess sweating, which are attributed to sympathetic overactivity and increased catecholamines. Other common manifestations include mental symptoms; pain in the extremities, head, neck, or chest; muscle weakness; and sensory loss. Because all these manifestations are neurologic rather than inflammatory, there is little or no abdominal tenderness, fever, or leukocytosis.

Porphyric neuropathy is primarily motor and appears to result from axonal degeneration rather than demyelinization. Sensory involvement is indicated by pain in the extremities, which may be described as muscle or bone pain, and by numbness, paresthesias, and dysesthesias. Paresis may occur early in an attack, but is more often a late manifestation in an attack that is not recognized and adequately treated. Rarely, severe neuropathy develops when there is little or no abdominal pain. Motor weakness most commonly begins in the proximal muscles of the upper extremities and then progresses to the lower extremities and the periphery. It is usually symmetric, but occasionally asymmetric or focal. Initially, tendon reflexes may be little affected or hyperactive and become decreased or absent. Cranial nerves, most commonly the 10th and 7th, may be affected, and blindness from involvement of the optic nerves or occipital lobes has been reported. More common central nervous system manifestations include seizures, anxiety, insomnia, depression, disorientation, hallucinations, and paranoia. Seizures may result from hyponatremia, porphyria itself, or an unrelated cause. Chronic depression and other mental symptoms occur in some patients, but attribution to porphyria is often difficult.

Hyponatremia is common during acute attacks. Inappropriate antidiuretic hormone (ADH) secretion is often the most likely mechanism, but it is difficult to document and other mechanisms must be considered in individual cases. Salt depletion from excess renal sodium loss, gastrointestinal loss, and poor intake have been suggested as causes of hyponatremia in AIP. In some patients, unexplained reductions in total blood and red blood cell volumes were found and increased ADH secretion might then be an appropriate physiologic response. Other electrolyte abnormalities may include hypomagnesemia and hypercalcemia.

The attack usually resolves quite rapidly, unless treatment is delayed. Abdominal pain may resolve within a few hours and paresis within a few days. Even severe motor neuropathy can improve over months or several years, but may leave some residual weakness. Progression of neuropathy to respiratory and bulbar paralysis and death is uncommon with appropriate treatment and removal of harmful drugs. Sudden death may result from cardiac arrhythmia.

LABORATORY FINDINGS. Levels of ALA and PBG are substantially increased during acute attacks and these may decrease after an attack but usually remain increased unless the disease becomes asymptomatic for a prolonged period. A population-based study in Sweden indicated that symptoms suggestive of porphyria may occur in heterozygotes during childhood, in contrast to adults, even when urinary porphyria precursors are not elevated. This study lacked, however, a comparison with the frequency of such nonspecific symptoms in a control group of children.

Porphyrins are also markedly increased, which accounts for reddish urine in AIP. These are predominantly uroporphyrins, which can form nonenzymatically from PBG. But because the increased urinary porphyrins in AIP are predominantly isomer III, their formation is likely to be largely enzymatic, which might occur if excess ALA produced in liver enters cells in other tissues and is then converted to porphyrins via the heme biosynthetic pathway. Porphobilin, a degradation product of PBG, and dipyrrylmethenes appear to account for brownish urinary discoloration. Total fecal porphyrins and plasma porphyrins are normal or slightly increased in AIP. Erythrocyte protoporphyrin may be somewhat increased in patients with manifest AIP.

Erythrocyte PBGD activity is approximately half-normal in most patients (70–80%) with AIP. The normal range is wide, however, and overlaps with the range for AIP heterozygotes. As noted, some PBGD gene mutations cause the enzyme to be deficient only in nonerythroid tissues. Also, PBGD is highly dependent on erythrocyte age, and an increase in erythropoiesis due to concurrent illness in an AIP patient may raise the activity into the normal range.

DIAGNOSIS AND DIFFERENTIAL DIAGNOSIS. An increased urinary PBG establishes that a patient has 1 of the 3 most common acute porphyrias (see Table 91-2). Measuring PBG in serum is preferred when there is coexistent severe renal disease, but is less sensitive when renal function is normal. Measurement of urinary ALA is less sensitive than PBG and also less specific, but will detect ADP, the fourth type of acute porphyria. Erythrocyte PBGD activity is decreased in most AIP patients, and helps confirm the diagnosis in a patient with high PBG. A normal enzyme activity in erythrocytes does not exclude AIP, however, for reasons discussed earlier. Measuring erythrocyte PBGD is quite useful for screening family members of a patient with AIP known to have low enzyme activity in erythrocytes. However, 5–15% of individuals can be misclassified using the enzymatic assay. This is not useful in infants <4 mo of age, when the enzyme can be physiologically increased in erythrocytes. Erythrocyte PBGD activity may be falsely low if processing, storage, or transport of the sample is compromised. Simultaneous measurement of multiple heme biosynthetic pathway enzymes, as offered by some commercial laboratories, is less reliable than assays that utilize specific substrates. A report of low activities of both erythrocyte ALAD and PBGD suggests an unreliable result.

Knowledge of the PBGD mutation in a family enables reliable identification of other gene carriers. PBGD deficiency can be documented in a fetus by measuring the enzyme activity in amniotic fluid cells, or more reliably by finding a PBGD mutation in these cells.

COMPLICATIONS. AIP and other acute porphyrias are commonly associated with mild abnormalities in liver function. The risk of more advanced liver disease and hepatocellular carcinoma is also increased during adult life, perhaps 60- to 70-fold, even in asymptomatic individuals who have increased porphyrins or porphyrin precursors. Few patients who developed this neoplasm had increases in serum α-fetoprotein. Therefore, current recommendations are that patients with acute porphyrias, especially >50 yr old, be screened at least yearly by ultrasound or an alternative imaging method.

The risk of chronic hypertension and impaired renal function appears to be increased in AIP. Hypertension or a possible nephrotoxic effect of ALA may explain impaired renal function in AIP, which may progress to severe renal failure and require renal transplantation.

Increased serum thyroxin levels due to increased thyroxin-binding globulin occur in some AIP patients. Hypercholesterolemia and elevated low-density lipoprotein cholesterol appear to be less common in this disorder than previously thought.

TREATMENT

Hemin. Intravenous hemin, combined with symptomatic and supportive measures, is the treatment of choice for most acute attacks of porphyria. There is a favorable biochemical and clinical response to early treatment with hemin, and less response if treatment is delayed. It is no longer recommended that therapy with hemin for a severe attack be started only after an unsuccessful trial of intravenous glucose for several days. Mild attacks, without severe manifestations such as paresis and hyponatremia, may be treated initially with intravenous glucose. After intravenous administration, hemin binds to hemopexin and albumin in plasma and is taken up primarily in hepatocytes. Hemin then enters and augments the regulatory heme pool in hepatocytes, represses the synthesis of hepatic ALAS1, and dramatically reduces porphyrin precursor overproduction.

Hemin* is available for intravenous administration in the United States as a lyophilized hematin preparation (Panhematin, Ovation). Degradation products begin to form as soon as the lyophilized product is reconstituted with sterile water, and these are responsible for phlebitis at the site of infusion and a transient anticoagulant effect. Loss of venous access due to phlebitis is common after repeated administration. Stabilization of lyophilized hematin by reconstitution with 30% human albumin can prevent these adverse effects, and is recommended, especially if a peripheral vein is used for the infusion. Uncommon side effects of hemin include fever, aching, malaise, hemolysis, anaphylaxis, and circulatory collapse. Heme arginate, a more stable hemin preparation, is available in Europe and South Africa.

Hemin treatment should be instituted only after a diagnosis of acute porphyria has been initially confirmed by a marked increase in urinary PBG (determined most rapidly using a kit, as described earlier). When prior documentation of the diagnosis is available for review, it is not essential to confirm an increase in PBG with every recurrent attack, if other causes of the symptoms are excluded clinically. The standard regimen of hemin for treatment of acute porphyric attacks is 3–4 mg/kg daily for 4 days. Lower doses have less effect on porphyrin precursor excretion and probably less clinical benefit. An investigational approach is to combine heme therapy with an inhibitor of heme breakdown, such as tin protoporphyrin or tin mesoporphyrin, to prolong the efficacy of the administered heme.

General and Supportive Measures. Drugs that may exacerbate porphyrias (see Table 91-3) should be discontinued whenever possible, and other precipitating factors identified. Hospitalization is warranted, except for mild attacks, for treatment of severe pain, nausea, and vomiting; for administration of hemin and fluids; and for monitoring vital capacity, nutritional status, neurologic function, and electrolytes. Pain usually requires a narcotic analgesic; there is low risk for addiction after recovery from the acute attack. A phenothiazine such as chlorpromazine is needed for nausea, vomiting, anxiety, and restlessness. Chloral hydrate or low doses of short-acting benzodiazepines can be given for restlessness or insomnia. β-Adrenergic blocking agents may be useful during acute attacks to control tachycardia and hypertension, but may be hazardous in patients with hypovolemia and incipient cardiac failure, because increased catecholamine secretion may in this situation be an important compensatory mechanism.

Carbohydrate Loading. The effects of carbohydrates on repressing hepatic ALAS1 and reducing porphyrin precursor excretion are weak compared to those of hemin. Therefore, only mild attacks (mild pain, no paresis or hyponatremia) are treated with carbohydrate loading. Glucose polymer solutions by mouth are sometimes tolerated. At least 300 g of intravenous glucose, usually given as a 10% solution, has been recommended for adults hospitalized with attacks of porphyria. Amounts up to 500 g daily may be more effective, but large volumes may favor development of hyponatremia.

*Hemin is the generic name for all heme preparations used for intravenous administration. *Hemin* is also a chemical term that refers to the oxidized (ferric) form of *heme* (iron protoporphyrin IX), and is usually isolated as hemin chloride. In alkaline solution, the chloride is replaced by the hydroxyl ion, forming hydroxyheme, or *hematin.*

Enzyme Replacement. Treatment with recombinant human erythrocyte PBGD is currently being studied. When administered intravenously to asymptomatic patients, the drug markedly decreases circulating levels of PBG without adverse effects. Studies of its efficacy for treating acute attacks are in progress. Early studies of gene therapy using fibroblasts from patients and mice with PBGD deficiency, and whole mice with adenoviral or nonviral delivery of plasmids encoding the normal enzyme, have provided evidence for correction of the metabolic defect.

Other Therapies. Liver transplantation was effective in 1 patient with severe AIP. Further evidence of efficacy is needed, however, before this can be recommended. Cimetidine, a well-known inhibitor of hepatic CYPs, can prevent experimental forms of porphyria induced by chemical agents that undergo activation by these enzymes, but these models are not highly relevant to human AIP. The drug's use is based on uncontrolled observations.

Seizures and Other Complications. Seizures due to hyponatremia or other electrolyte imbalances may not require prolonged treatment with anticonvulsant drugs, most of which have at least some potential for exacerbating acute porphyrias. Bromides, gabapentin, and probably vigabatrin are safe. Clonazepam may be less harmful than phenytoin or barbiturates. Control of hypertension may help prevent chronic renal impairment, which can progress and require renal transplantation.

Safe and Unsafe Drugs. Patients often do well with avoidance of harmful drugs. Some drugs known or strongly suspected to be harmful or safe in the acute porphyrias are listed in Table 91-6. Updated and more extensive listings are available on an interactive website of the European Porphyria Initiative (www.porphyria-europe.com) and from the American Porphyria Foundation (www.porphyriafoundation.com). Information regarding safety is lacking for many drugs, especially for those recently introduced, and sometimes opinions are conflicting.

Exogenous progestins, usually in combination with estrogens, can induce attacks of porphyria. Estrogens are seldom reported to be harmful when given alone or in animal and hepatocyte culture systems. Synthetic steroids with an ethynyl substituent can cause a mechanism-based destruction of hepatic CYPs and should probably be avoided in patients with acute porphyria. Danazol is especially contraindicated.

Other Conditions. Major surgery can be carried out safely in patients with acute porphyria, especially if barbiturates are avoided. Halothane has been recommended as an inhalation agent and propofol and midazolam as intravenous induction agents.

Pregnancy is usually well tolerated, which is surprising, because levels of progesterone, a potent inducer of hepatic ALAS1, are considerably increased during pregnancy. Some women do experience continuing attacks during pregnancy, however. These sometimes result from reduced caloric intake or metoclopramide, a contraindicated drug sometimes used to treat hyperemesis gravidarum.

Diabetes mellitus and other endocrine conditions are not known to precipitate attacks of porphyria. In fact, the onset of diabetes mellitus and resulting high circulating glucose levels may decrease the frequency of attacks and lower porphyrin precursor levels in AIP.

PROGNOSIS. The outlook for patients with acute porphyrias has improved markedly in the past several decades. In Finland, for example, 74% of patients with AIP or VP reported that they led normal lives, and less than ⅓ had recurrent attacks during several years of follow-up. In those presenting with acute symptoms, recurrent attacks were most likely within the next 1–3 yr. Moreover, only 6% of gene carriers who had never had attacks developed symptoms. The improved outlook may result from earlier detection, better treatment of acute attacks, and replacement of harmful drugs such as barbiturates and sulfonamides with safer drugs. A smaller number of patients, however, continue to have recurrent attacks, chronic pain, and other symptoms even after avoiding known exacerbating factors.

PREVENTION. For prevention of attacks, it is important to identify multiple inciting factors and remove as many as possible. Drugs for concurrent medical conditions should be reviewed. Because dietary factors are often inapparent, consultation with a dietitian may be useful. A well-balanced diet that is somewhat high in carbohydrate (60–70% of total calories) and sufficient to maintain weight is recommended. There is little evidence that additional dietary carbohydrate helps further in preventing attacks, and it may lead to weight gain. Patients who wish to lose excess weight should do so gradually and when they are clinically stable. Iron deficiency, which can be detected by a low serum ferritin, should be corrected.

GnRH analogs, which reversibly suppress ovulation, can be dramatically effective for preventing frequently recurring luteal phase attacks, but baseline and continuing gynecologic evaluation and bone density measurements are important, and transdermal estrogen or a biphosphonate may be added to prevent bone loss. Hemin administered once or twice weekly can prevent frequent, noncyclic attacks of porphyria in some patients.

GENETIC COUNSELING. Children with a family history of porphyria are often seen by pediatricians for evaluation and counseling. Information and laboratory results from a relative with proven porphyria must be reviewed in order to guide testing of the child, which is different depending on the type of acute porphyria. A mutation identified in the index case can be sought in the child. If the child is found to have inherited the mutation, counseling to avoid potentially harmful drugs is appropriate. Counseling should also emphasize that the great majority of those who inherit a PBGD mutation never develop symptoms, and the prognosis of those who do is favorable. Therefore, a normal, healthy life is expected, especially with avoidance of harmful drugs and other factors and prompt recognition and treatment of symptoms should they occur. Given the favorable outlook for most mutation carriers, even during pregnancy, having children is not precluded, and prenatal diagnosis of acute porphyrias is less important than it is for many other inherited diseases. Inheritance of a PBGD mutation should be regarded as confidential information and not interfere with employment or insurance eligibility.

CONGENITAL ERYTHROPOIETIC PORPHYRIA (CEP)

Also termed *Günther disease,* this rare disease usually presents with photosensitivity shortly after birth, or in utero as nonimmune hydrops.

ETIOLOGY. CEP is an autosomal recessive disease due to a marked deficiency of uroporphyrinogen III synthase (UROS). Many UROS mutations have been identified among CEP families. Later-onset disease in adults is likely to be associated with myeloproliferative disorders and expansion of a clone of erythroblasts that carry a UROS mutation.

PATHOLOGY AND PATHOGENESIS. UROS, which is markedly deficient in CEP, catalyzes inversion of pyrrole ring D of HMB (the pyrrole ring shown on the right end of the molecule in Figure 91-1) and rapid cyclization of the linear tetrapyrrole to form uroporphyrinogen III. This enzyme is also termed uroporphyrinogen cosynthase. The human enzyme is a monomer. The gene for the enzyme is found on chromosome 10q25.3–>q26.3, and contains 10 exons. Erythroid and housekeeping transcripts are generated by alternative promoters but encode the same enzyme. The housekeeping transcript contains exon 1 (untranslated) spliced to exons

2B through 10, while the erythroid transcript contains exon 2A (untranslated) also spliced to exons 2B through 10. The housekeeping promoter is upstream of exon 1, whereas the erythroid-specific proximal promoter is upstream of exon 2A and contains erythroid transcription factor binding sites including GATA1 and NF-E2. Thus, there is erythroid-specific regulation, but the enzyme product is the same in all tissues.

In CEP, large amounts of HMB accumulate in erythroid cells during hemoglobin synthesis and cyclize nonenzymatically to form uroporphyrinogen I, which is auto-oxidized to uroporphyrin I. Some of the uroporphyrinogen I that accumulates is metabolized to coproporphyrinogen I, which accumulates because it is not a substrate for coproporphyrinogen oxidase. Thus, both uroporphyrin I and coproporphyrin I accumulate in the bone marrow and are then found in circulating erythrocytes, plasma, urine, and feces.

A variety of UROS mutations have been identified in CEP, including missense and nonsense mutations, large and small deletions and insertions, splicing defects, and intronic branch point mutations. At least 4 mutations have been identified in the erythroid-specific promoter. Many patients inherited a different mutation from each parent, and most mutations have been detected in only 1 or a few families. An exception is a common mutation, C73R, which is at a mutational hotspot and was found in ≈33% of alleles.

Genotype-phenotype correlations have been based on the in vitro expression of various CEP mutations and the severity of associated phenotypic manifestations. The C73R allele, which is associated with a severe phenotype in homozygotes or in patients heteroallelic for C73R and another mutation expressing little residual activity, resulted in < 1% of normal enzyme activity. Patients with the C73R allele and heteroallelic for other mutations expressing more residual activity have milder disease.

Hemolysis is a common feature of CEP. Excess porphyrins in circulating erythrocytes cause cell damage, perhaps by a phototoxic mechanism, leading to both intravascular hemolysis and increased splenic clearance of erythrocytes. Also important is ineffective erythropoiesis, with intramedullary destruction of porphyrin-laden erythroid cells and breakdown of heme. Expansion of the bone marrow due to erythroid hyperplasia may contribute to **bone loss.** Nutrient deficiencies sometimes cause erythroid hypoplasia. Despite the marked deficiency of UROS, heme production in the bone marrow is increased, due to hemolysis and a compensatory increase in hemoglobin production. This occurs, however, at the expense of marked accumulation of HMB, which is converted to porphyrinogens and porphyrins.

CLINICAL MANIFESTATIONS. In severe cases, CEP can cause fetal loss, or be recognized in utero as intrauterine hemolytic anemia and **nonimmune hydrops fetalis.** CEP may be associated with neonatal hyperbilirubinemia, and **phototherapy may unintentionally induce severe photosensitivity.**

The most characteristic presentation is reddish urine or pink staining of diapers by urine or meconium shortly after birth (Fig. 91-2). With sun exposure, severe blistering lesions appear on exposed areas of skin on the face and hands, and have been termed *hydroa aestivale* because they are more severe with greater sunlight exposure during summer (Fig. 91-3). Vesicles and bullae, as well as friability, hypertrichosis, scarring, thickening, and areas of hypo- and hyperpigmentation are very similar to those seen in PCT, but usually much more severe. Infection and scarring sometimes cause loss of facial features and fingers and damage to the cornea, ears, and nails. Porphyrins are deposited in dentine and bone in utero. Reddish-brown teeth in normal light, an appearance termed **erythrodontia,** display reddish fluorescence under long-wave ultraviolet light (Fig. 91-4). Hemolysis and splenomegaly are features of many cases. Bone marrow compensation may be adequate, especially in milder cases. Patients with severe phenotypes, however, are often transfusion-dependent.

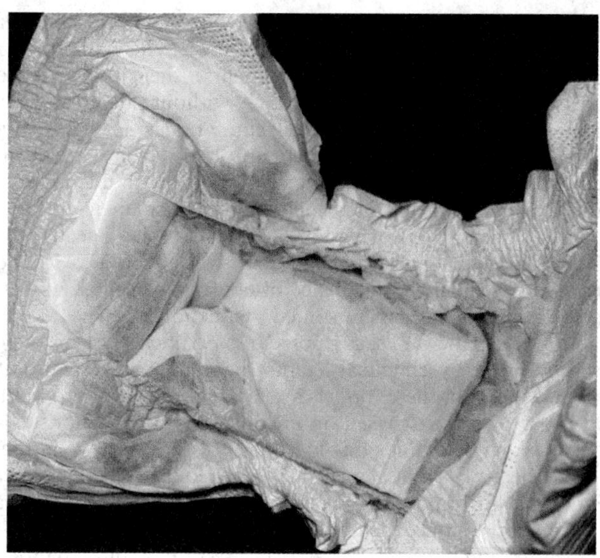

Figure 91-2. Congenital erythropoietic porphyria. The diaper of an affected baby demonstrates the red color of urine. (From Paller AS, Macini AJ: *Hurwitz Clinical Pediatric Dermatology,* 3rd ed. Philadelphia, Elsevier Saunders, 2006, p 517.)

Splenomegaly may contribute to the anemia and cause leukopenia and thrombocytopenia, which may be complicated by significant bleeding. Neuropathic symptoms are absent, and there is no sensitivity to drugs, hormones, and carbohydrate restriction. The liver may be damaged by iron overload or hepatitis acquired from blood transfusions.

Milder cases of CEP with onset of symptoms in adult life and without erythrodontia may more closely mimic PCT. These late-onset cases are likely to be associated with myeloproliferative disorders, and expansion of a clone of cells carrying a UROS somatic mutation.

LABORATORY FINDINGS. Urinary porphyrin excretion and circulating porphyrin levels in CEP are much higher than in almost all other porphyrias. Urinary porphyrin excretion can be as high as 50–100 mg daily, and consists mostly of uroporphyrin I and coproporphyrin I. ALA and PBG are normal. Fecal porphyrins are markedly increased, with a predominance of coproporphyrin I.

Marked increases in erythrocyte porphyrins in CEP consist mostly of uroporphyrin I and coproporphyrin I. These porphyrins are also increased in bone marrow, spleen, plasma, and, to a lesser extent, liver. The porphyrin pattern in erythrocytes is influenced by rates of erythropoiesis and erythroid maturation. A predominance of protoporphyrin has been noted in some CEP

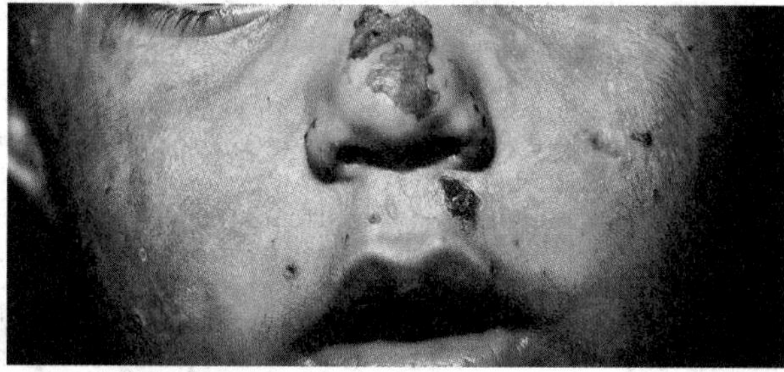

Figure 91-3. Congenital erythropoietic porphyria. Vesicles, bullae, and crusts on sun-exposed areas. (From Paller AS, Macini AJ: *Hurwitz Clinical Pediatric Dermatology,* 3rd ed. Philadelphia, Elsevier Saunders, 2006, p 517.)

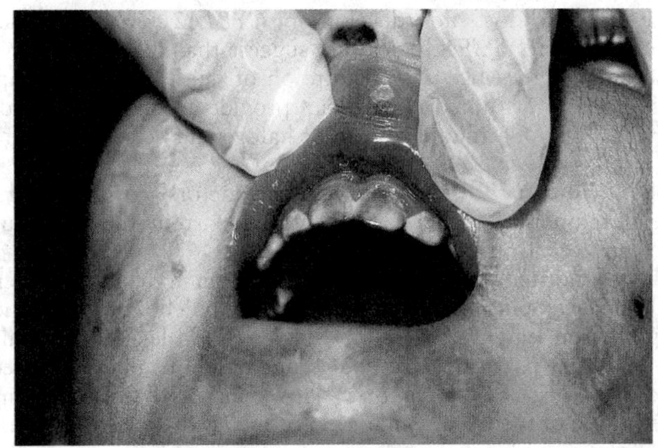

Figure 91-4. Congenital erythropoietic porphyria. Brownish teeth that fluoresce under Wood lamp examination. (From Paller AS, Macini AJ: *Hurwitz Clinical Pediatric Dermatology,* 3rd ed. Philadelphia, Elsevier Saunders, 2006, p 517.)

patients, and in 1 such patient, uroporphyrin and coproporphyrin increased when erythropoiesis was stimulated by blood removal.

DIAGNOSIS AND DIFFERENTIAL DIAGNOSIS. The diagnosis of CEP should be documented by full characterization of porphyrin patterns and identification of the underlying mutations. In later onset cases, an underlying myeloproliferative disorder and a UROS somatic mutation should be suspected and studied in detail.

The clinical picture in hepatoerythropoietic porphyria (HEP) may be very similar, but the porphyrin patterns in urine and feces in HEP resemble PCT. A predominant increase in erythrocyte protoporphyin is unusual in CEP, but is characteristic of EPP, HEP, and rare homozygous cases of AIP, HCP, and VP. EPP is also distinguished by normal urinary porphyrins and by increases in erythrocyte free protoporphyrin, whereas the increased protoporphyrin in other conditions is complexed with zinc.

CEP should be suspected as a cause of nonimmune hydrops or hemolytic anemia in utero. With recognition of the disease at this stage, intrauterine transfusion can be considered, and severe, scarring photosensitivity from photodynamic therapy for hyperbilirubinemia avoided. Prenatal diagnosis is feasible by finding red-brown discoloration and increased porphyrins in amniotic fluid, measuring porphyrins in fetal erythrocytes and plasma and UROS activity in cultured amniotic fluid cells, or identifying UROS gene mutations in chorionic villi or cultured amniotic cells.

TREATMENT. Protection from sunlight exposure, minimizing skin trauma, and prompt treatment of any cutaneous infections are highly important in managing CEP (see Table 91-4). Sunscreen lotions and beta-carotene are sometimes beneficial. Transfusions to achieve a level of hemoglobin sufficient to suppress erythropoiesis significantly can be quite effective in reducing porphyrin levels and photosensitivity. Concurrent deferoxamine to reduce iron overload, and hydroxyurea to suppress erythropoiesis further may provide additional benefit. Splenectomy reduces hemolysis and transfusion requirements in some patients. Oral charcoal may increase fecal loss of porphyrins, but may contribute little in more severe cases. Intravenous hemin may be somewhat effective, but has not been extensively studied and seems unlikely to provide long-term benefit. Chloroquine has not been beneficial.

Bone marrow or stem cell transplantation, which has markedly reduced porphyrin levels and photosensitivity and increased long-term survival, should be considered, especially for severe disease. Gene therapy may be accomplished in the future. To date, human UROS cDNA has been subcloned into retroviral vectors, which have been used to transduce fibroblasts and lymphoblasts from patients with CEP, resulting in significant levels of enzyme expression. Transduction of hematopoietic progenitor cells and early erythroid cells was also achieved.

PROGNOSIS. The outlook is favorable in milder cases and in patients with more severe disease treated by transfusions sufficient to suppress erythropoiesis and bone marrow porphyrin production at least partially. Successful bone marrow or stem cell transplantation has proven effective.

PREVENTION AND GENETIC COUNSELING. Genetic counseling is important for affected families, because CEP can be recognized before birth and a severe phenotype can often be predicted by identifying the nature of the UROS mutations.

PORPHYRIA CUTANEA TARDA (PCT)

This is the most common and readily treated human porphyria (see Table 91-2). It occurs in mid or late adult life, and is rare in children. Previous terms include *symptomatic porphyria, PCT symptomatica,* and *idiosyncratic porphyria.* The underlying cause is a liver-specific, acquired deficiency of uroporphyrinogen decarboxylase (UROD) with contributions by several types of genetic factors. UROD mutations are found in familial PCT. The homozygous form of familial PCT is HEP, which has a more severe presentation, usually in childhood.

ETIOLOGY. PCT is due to a marked deficiency of hepatic UROD. This enzyme deficiency must be substantial (≈20% of normal activity or less) for PCT to become manifest, and its development is attributed to generation of a UROD inhibitor specifically in the liver. This inhibitor, which has not been characterized, is derived from a heme pathway intermediate such as uroporphyrinogen, and CYPs such as CYP1A2, as well as iron, are involved in its formation (Fig. 91-5). Even with substantial inhibition of hepatic UROD activity, the amount of enzyme protein measured immunochemically remains at its genetically determined level.

UROD catalyzes the decarboxylation of the 4 acetic acid side chains of uroporphyrinogen (an octacarboxyl porphyrinogen) to form coproporphyrinogen (a tetracarboxyl porphyrinogen) (see

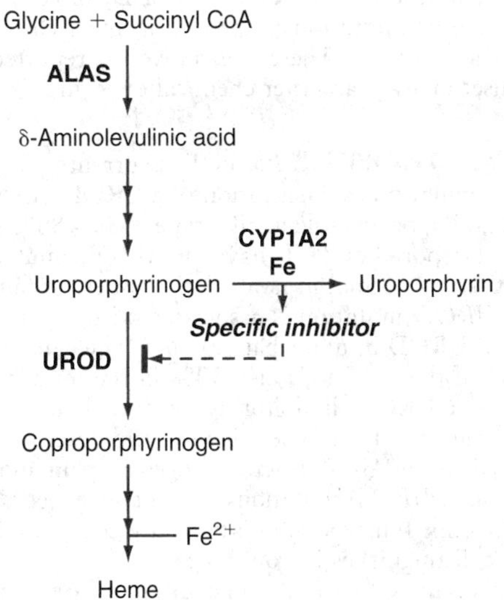

Figure 91-5. Formation of a specific inhibitor of uroporphyrinogen decarboxylase in the liver in porphyria cutanea tarda. ALAS, δ-aminolevulinic acid synthase; CYP1A2, cytochrome P450 1A2; UROD, uroporphyrinogen decarboxylase.

Fig. 91-1). The enzyme reaction occurs in a sequential, clockwise fashion, with the intermediate formation of hepta-, hexa-, and pentacarboxyl porphyrinogens. Uroporphyrinogen III, as compared with other uroporphyrinogen isomers, is the preferred substrate. Human UROD is a dimer with the 2 active site clefts juxtaposed. The UROD gene is on chromosome 1p34 and contains 10 exons, with only 1 promoter. Therefore, the gene is transcribed as a single mRNA in all tissues.

The majority of PCT patients (≈80%) have no *UROD* mutations and are said to have sporadic (type 1) disease. Some are heterozygous for *UROD* mutations and are said to have familial (type 2) PCT. Described mutations include missense, nonsense, and splice site mutations, several small and large deletions, and small insertions, with only a few identified in more than 1 family. A few of these mutations may be located near the active site cleft, but most appear to involve regions with important structural roles. Being heterozygous for a *UROD* mutation is insufficient to cause PCT unless a UROD inhibitor is also generated. Because penetrance of the genetic trait is low, many patients with familial PCT have no family history of the disease.

Induction of hepatic ALAS1 is not a prominent feature in PCT, although alcohol may increase this enzyme slightly. Iron and estrogens are also not potent inducers of ALAS1 and drugs that are potent inducers of ALAS1 and CYPs are much less commonly implicated in PCT than in acute porphyrias.

Blistering skin lesions result from porphyrins that are released from the liver. Sunlight exposure leads to generation of reactive oxygen species in the skin, complement activation, and lysosomal damage.

EPIDEMIOLOGY. Different prevalences probably relate to geographic variations in susceptibility factors such as hepatitis C and ethanol use. The yearly incidence in the United Kingdom was estimated at 2–5/ 1,000,000, and the prevalence in the United States and Czechoslovakia was estimated at ≈1/25,000 and 1/5,000, respectively. The disease was reported to be prevalent in the Bantus of South Africa in association with iron overload. PCT is more common in males, possible due to greater alcohol intake, and in women it is commonly associated with estrogen use.

A massive outbreak of PCT occurred in eastern Turkey in the 1950s. Wheat intended for planting and treated with hexachlorobenzene as a fungicide was consumed by many at a time of food shortage. Cases and small outbreaks of PCT after exposure to other chemicals including di- and trichlorophenols and 2,3,7,8-tetrachlorodibenzo-*p*-dioxin (TCDD, dioxin) have been reported. The manifestations improved in most cases when the exposure was stopped. There are, however, reported cases of delayed onset many years after chemical exposure.

PATHOLOGY AND PATHOGENESIS. PCT is currently classified into 3 clinically similar types. Generation of a UROD inhibitor in the liver plays an important role in all 3 types. The ≈80% of patients with type 1 (sporadic) PCT have no UROD mutations, and UROD activity is normal in nonhepatic tissues. In familial (type 2) PCT, a *UROD* mutation is associated with a partial (≈50%) deficiency of UROD in nonhepatic tissues. The genetically determined level of the enzyme is also 50% in the liver, but is much lower when a UROD inhibitor is generated and the disease becomes clinically active. Type 3 is rare, and describes PCT with normal erythrocyte UROD activity occurring in more than 1 family member. *UROD* mutations or another genetic basis have not been identified in type 3, and familial occurrence is the only feature that distinguishes it from type 1.

CYPs, especially CYPY1A2, can catalyze the oxidation of uroporphyrinogen to uroporphyrin. This uroporphyrinogen oxidase (URO-OX) activity is enhanced by iron, and leads to formation of a UROD inhibitor (see Fig. 91-5). CYP1A2 seems essential for development of uroporphyria in rodents, because experimental uroporphyria does not develop in *CYP1A2* knockout mice. Studies with *CYP2E1* knockouts suggest that this enzyme may also contribute. Mice with disruption of one *UROD* allele and either 1 or 2 disrupted *HFE* alleles provide an important model for PCT without administration of halogenated chemicals.

SUSCEPTIBILITY FACTORS. The following factors are implicated in the development of PCT, and these coexist in the individual patient.

Iron. A normal or increased amount of iron in the liver is essential for developing PCT, and treatment by phlebotomy to reduce hepatic iron leads to remission. Serum ferritin levels are usually in the upper part of the normal range or moderately increased, and liver histology commonly shows increased iron staining. Prevalence of the C282Y mutation of the *HFE* gene, which is the major cause of hemochromatosis in white people, is increased in both type 1 and type 2 PCT, and ≈10% of patients are C282Y homozygotes. In southern Europe, where the C282Y is less prevalent, the H63D mutation is more commonly associated. PCT may occur with secondary iron overload.

Hepatitis C. This viral infection is highly prevalent in PCT in most geographic locations; in the United States, for example, it is present in 56–74% of cases, which is similar to the rate cited in earlier reports from southern Europe. Prevalence of hepatitis C in PCT is lower in northern Europe (<20%). Steatosis and oxidative stress in hepatitis C may favor iron-mediated generation of reactive oxygen species and a UROD inhibitor.

HIV. Many reports suggest HIV infection can contribute to the development of PCT, although less commonly than does hepatitis C. The mechanism is not known.

Ethanol. The long-recognized association between alcohol and PCT may be explained by the generation of active oxygen species, which may cause oxidative damage, mitochondrial injury, depletion of reduced glutathione and other antioxidant defenses, increased production of endotoxin, and activation of Kupffer cells.

Smoking and Cytochrome P450 Enzymes. Smoking has not been extensively studied as a susceptibility factor, but is commonly associated with alcohol use in PCT. It may act to induce hepatic CYPs and oxidative stress. Hepatic CYPs are thought to be important in oxidizing uroporphyrinogen and generating a UROD inhibitor (see Fig. 91-5). Genetic polymorphisms of CYP1A2 and 1A1 have been implicated in human PCT. The frequency of an inducible genotype was more common in PCT patients than in controls in 2 studies.

Antioxidant Status. Ascorbic acid deficiency has been implicated in contributing to uroporphyria in laboratory models and human PCT. In 1 series, plasma ascorbate levels were substantially reduced in 84% of patients with PCT. Low levels of serum carotenoids were also described, further suggesting that oxidant stress in hepatocytes is important in PCT.

Estrogens. Use of estrogen-containing oral contraceptives or postmenopausal estrogen replacement is very commonly associated with PCT (type 1 or 2) in women. PCT sometimes occurs during pregnancy, although it is not clear whether the risk is increased.

CLINICAL MANIFESTATIONS

Cutaneous Manifestations. PCT is readily recognized by blistering and crusted skin lesions on the backs of the hands, which are the most sun-exposed areas of the body, and somewhat less commonly on the forearms, face, ears, neck, legs, and feet. The fluid-filled vesicles commonly rupture and become crusted or denuded areas, heal slowly, and are subject to infection. The skin on the backs of the hands is characteristically friable, and minor trauma may cause blisters or denudation of skin. Small white plaques, termed *milia,* may precede or follow vesicle formation. Facial hypertrichosis and hyperpigmentation are also common. Severe scarring and thickening of sun-exposed skin may resemble scleroderma. Skin biopsy findings include subepidermal blistering and deposition of PAS-positive material around blood vessels and fine fibrillar material at the dermoepithelial junction, which may relate to excessive skin fragility. IgG, other immunoglobulins, and complement are also deposited at the dermoepithelial junction and around dermal blood vessels. The skin lesions and histologic changes are not specific for PCT. The same findings occur in VP and HCP, and resemble those of CEP and HEP but are usually less severe. Onset of the disease in childhood is rare, and is more common in type 2 disease.

Liver Abnormalities. PCT is almost always associated with nonspecific liver abnormalities, especially increased transaminases and γ-glutamyltranspeptidase, even in the absence of heavy alcohol intake or hepatitis C. Most histologic findings, such as necrosis, inflammation, increased iron, and increased fat, are nonspecific. More specific findings are red fluorescence of liver tissue, and fluorescent, birefringent, needlelike inclusions presumably consisting of porphyrins. Electron microscopy shows these inclusions are in lysosomes, and paracrystalline inclusions are found in mitochondria. Distorted lobular architecture and cirrhosis are more common with long-standing disease.

The risk of developing hepatocellular carcinoma is increased, with reported incidences ranging from 4 to 47% in PCT. These tumors seldom contain large amounts of porphyrins.

Other Findings and Associations. Mild or moderate erythrocytosis in some adult patients is not well understood, but chronic lung disease due to smoking may contribute. An earlier onset of symptoms may be noted in patients with genetic predisposing factors, such as an inherited partial deficiency of UROD or the C282Y/C282Y *HFE* genotype. Iron overload secondary to conditions such as myelofibrosis and end-stage renal disease may be associated with PCT. The disease can be especially severe in patients with end-stage renal disease, because the lack of urinary excretion leads to much higher concentrations of porphyrins in plasma, and the excess porphyrins are poorly dialyzable. PCT occurs more frequently in patients with systemic lupus erythematosis and other immunologic disorders than would have been expected by chance, but the basis of this association is not known.

LABORATORY FINDINGS. Porphyrin accumulates in the liver mostly as the oxidized porphyrins rather than porphyrinogens in PCT, as indicated by the immediate red fluorescence observed in liver tissue. This develops in weeks or months, and then porphyrins appear in plasma and are transported to the skin, causing photosensitivity. Only a very small increase in synthesis of heme pathway intermediates and little or no increase in hepatic ALAS1 are required to account for the excess porphyrins excreted.

Hepatic UROD deficiency leads to a complex pattern of excess porphyrins, which initially accumulate as porphyrinogens, and then undergo nonenzymatic oxidation to the corresponding porphyrins (uro-, hepta-, hexa-, and pentacarboxyl porphyrins, and isocoproporphyrins). Uroporphyrin and heptacarboxyl porphyrin predominate in urine, with lesser amounts of coproporphyrin and penta- and hexacarboxyl porphyrin. A normally minor pathway is accentuated by UROD deficiency, whereby pentacarboxyl porphyrinogen is oxidized by coproporphyrinogen oxidase (CPO; the next enzyme in the pathway), forming isocoproporphyrinogen, an atypical tetracarboxyl porphyrinogen. Relative to normal values, urinary porphyrins are increased to a greater extent than fecal porphyrins. The total amount of porphyrins excreted in feces in PCT exceeds that in urine, however, and total excretion of type III isomers (including isocoproporphyrins, which are mostly derived from the type III series) exceeds that of type I isomers. Perhaps because uroporphyrinogen III is the preferred substrate for UROD, excess uroporphyrin in PCT is predominantly isomer I. Hepta- and hexacarboxyl porphyrin are mostly isomer III; and pentacarboxyl porphyrin and coproporphyrin are approximately equal mixtures of isomers I and III.

DIAGNOSIS AND DIFFERENTIAL DIAGNOSIS. Plasma porphyrins are always increased in clinically manifest PCT, and a total plasma porphyrin determination is most useful for screening. A normal value rules out PCT and other porphyrias that produce blistering skin lesions. If increased, it is useful to determine the plasma fluorescence emission maximum at neutral pH, because a maximum near 619 nm is characteristic of PCT (as well as CEP and HCP) and, most important, excludes VP, which has a distinctly different fluorescence maximum. Increased urinary porphyrins, with a predominance of uroporphyrin and heptacarboxyl porphyrin, is confirmatory. Urine porphyrins are less useful for initial screening because nonspecific increases, especially of coproporphyrin, occur in liver disease and other medical conditions. Urinary ALA may be increased slightly, and PBG is normal.

Familial (type 2) and sporadic (type 1) PCT can be distinguished by finding decreased erythrocyte UROD activity (in type 2), or more reliably by finding a disease-related *UROD* mutation. Type 3 is distinguished from type 1 only by occurrence of PCT in a relative. Biochemical findings in HEP are similar to those in PCT, but with an additional marked increase in erythrocyte zinc protoporphyrin.

Pseudoporphyria (also known as pseudo-PCT) presents with skin lesions that closely resemble PCT, but without significant increases in plasma porphyrins. A photosensitizing drug such as a nonsteroidal anti-inflammatory agent is sometimes implicated. Both PCT and pseudoporphyria may occur in patients with end-stage renal disease.

COMPLICATIONS. Cutaneous blisters may rupture and become infected, sometimes leading to cellulitis. In more severe disease in patients with end-stage renal disease, repeated infections can be mutilating, as in CEP. Pseudoscleroderma, with scarring, contraction, and calcification of skin and subcutaneous tissue, is a rare complication. Other complications, such as advanced liver disease and hepatocellular carcinoma, were already discussed.

TREATMENT. Management of PCT includes choice of 2 specific and effective forms of treatment, phlebotomy or low-dose hydroxychloroquine, and removal of susceptibility factors when possible. The diagnosis of PCT must be firmly established, and conditions that produce identical cutaneous lesions excluded, because these do not respond to treatments used in PCT. Treatment can usually be started after demonstrating an increase in plasma total porphyrins and excluding VP by analysis of the fluorescence spectrum at neutral pH, while urine and fecal studies are still pending. Patients should be evaluated for use of alcohol, estrogens (in women), and smoking, which should be stopped, and tested for hepatitis C, HIV, and *HFE* mutations. Some susceptibility factors influence the choice of treatment.

Phlebotomy is considered standard therapy, and is effective both in children and adults with PCT because it reduces hepatic iron content. Treatment is guided by plasma (or serum) ferritin and porphyrin levels. Hemoglobin or hematocrit levels should be followed to prevent symptomatic anemia. For adults, a unit of blood (≈450 mL) is removed at ≈2 wk intervals until a target serum ferritin near the lower limit of normal (≈15 ng/mL) is achieved. A total of 6 to 8 phlebotomies is often sufficient. After this, plasma porphyrin concentrations continue to fall from pretreatment levels (generally 10–25 μg/dL) to below the upper limit of normal (≈1 μg/dL), usually after several more weeks. This is followed by gradual clearing of skin lesions, sometimes including pseudoscleroderma. Liver function abnormalities may improve, and hepatic siderosis, needle-like inclusions, and red fluorescence of liver tissue will disappear. Although remission usually persists even if ferritin levels later return to normal, it is advisable to follow porphyrin levels and reinstitute phlebotomies if these begin to rise. Infusions of deferoxamine, an iron chelator, may be used when phlebotomy is contraindicated.

An alternative when phlebotomy is contraindicated or poorly tolerated is a low-dose regimen of chloroquine or hydroxychloroquine. Normal doses of these 4-aminoquinoline antimalarials increase plasma and urinary porphyrin levels and increase photosensitivity in PCT, reflecting an outpouring of porphyrins from the liver. This is accompanied by acute hepatocellular damage, with fever, malaise, nausea, and increased serum transaminases, but is followed by complete remission of the porphyria. These adverse consequences of normal doses are largely avoided by a low-dose regimen (chloroquine 125 mg or hydroxychloroquine 100 mg, ½ of a normal tablet, twice weekly), which can be continued until plasma or urine porphyrins are normalized. There is at least some risk of retinopathy, which may be lower with hydroxychloroquine. Prospective treatment trials comparing this treatment with phlebotomy are lacking. Low-dose chloroquine may not be effective in patients homozygous for the *C282Y* mutation in the *HFE* gene. Therefore, the degree of excess hepatic iron may influence response to this treatment. The mechanism of action of 4-aminoquinolines in PCT is not known, but is quite specific, since these drugs are not useful in other porphyrias.

In patients with PCT and hepatitis C, PCT should be treated 1st because this condition is more symptomatic and can be treated more quickly and effectively. Treatment of PCT by phlebotomy may not be possible once interferon-ribavirin treatment is complicated by anemia. Moreover, treatment of hepatitis C may be more effective after iron reduction. Resistance of hepatitis C to treatment with interferon-α or pegylated interferon and ribavirin has been reported in patients previously treated for PCT, but prospective studies are lacking (see Chapter 355).

PCT in patients with end-stage renal disease is often more severe and difficult to treat. Although phlebotomy is often contraindicated initially, erythropoietin administration can correct anemia, mobilize iron, and support phlebotomy in many cases. Response may also occur after renal transplantation, due in part to resumption of endogenous erythropoietic production.

Liver imaging and a serum α-fetoprotein determination may be advisable in all PCT patients, perhaps at 6–12 mo intervals for early detection of hepatocellular carcinoma. Finding low erythrocyte UROD activity or a *UROD* mutation identifies those with an underlying genetic predisposition, which does not alter treatment but is useful for genetic counseling (see later).

PROGNOSIS. PCT is the most readily treated form of porphyria, and complete remission is expected with treatment either by phlebotomy or low-dose hydroxychloroquine. There is little information on rates of recurrence and long-term outlook. Risk for hepatocellular carcinoma is increased, and some susceptibility factors such as hepatitis C can lead to complications even after PCT is in remission.

PREVENTION AND GENETIC COUNSELING. Patients with PCT may have concerns about risk to other family members. A heritable *UROD* mutation can usually be detected or excluded by measuring erythrocyte UROD activity, although DNA studies are more sensitive. Relatives of patients with *UROD* mutations have an increased risk for developing PCT, and may have increased motivation to avoid adverse behaviors such as ethanol and tobacco use and exposures to hepatitis C and HIV. Such counseling would be given to anyone, however. The finding of *HFE* mutations, and especially *C282Y,* should prompt screening of relatives, some of whom may be C282Y homozygotes and warrant lifelong monitoring of serum ferritin.

HEPATOERYTHROPOIETIC PORPHYRIA

Hepatoerythropoietic porphyria (HEP), which is the homozygous form of familial (type 2) PCT, resembles CEP clinically. Excess porphyrins originate mostly from liver, with a pattern consistent with severe UROD deficiency. This rare disorder has no particular racial predominance.

ETIOLOGY. HEP is an autosomal recessive disorder, although most patients have inherited a different mutation from unrelated parents. In contrast to most mutations in familial (type 2) PCT, most causing HEP are associated with expression of some residual enzyme activity. At least 1 genotype is associated with the predominant excretion of pentacarboxyl porphyrin.

PATHOLOGY AND PATHOGENESIS. Excess porphyrins originate primarily from the liver in HEP, although the substantial increase in erythrocyte zinc protoporphyrin indicates that the heme biosynthetic pathway is also impaired in bone marrow erythroid cells. Apparently, porphyrinogens accumulate in the marrow while hemoglobin synthesis is most active, and are metabolized to protoporphyrin after hemoglobin synthesis is complete. The cutaneous lesions are due to photoactivation of porphyrins in skin, as in other cutaneous porphyrias.

CLINICAL MANIFESTATIONS. Like CEP, this disease usually presents with blistering skin lesions, hypertrichosis, scarring, and red urine in infancy or childhood. Sclerodermoid skin changes are sometimes prominent. Unusually mild cases have been described. Concurrent conditions that affect liver function can alter disease severity. For example, hepatitis A caused the disease to become manifest in a 2 year old child, and then improved with recovery of liver function.

LABORATORY FINDINGS. Biochemical findings resemble those in PCT with accumulation and excretion of uroporphyrin, heptacarboxyl porphyrin and isocoproporphyrin. But in addition, erythrocyte zinc protoporphyrin is substantially increased.

DIAGNOSIS AND DIFFERENTIAL DIAGNOSIS. HEP is distinguished from CEP by increases in both uroporphyrin and heptacarboxyl porphyrin, and isocoproporphyrins. In CEP the excess erythrocyte porphyrins are predominantly uroporphyrin and coproporphyrin rather than protoporphyrin. Blistering skin lesions are unusual in EPP, the excess erythrocyte protoporphyrin in that disease is free and not complexed with zinc, and urinary porphyrins are normal.

TREATMENT AND PROGNOSIS. Avoiding sunlight exposure is most important in managing this disease, as in CEP. Oral charcoal was helpful in a severe case associated with dyserythropoiesis. Phlebotomy has shown little or no benefit. The outlook depends on the severity of the enzyme deficiency and may be favorable if sunlight can be avoided. Retrovirus-mediated gene transfer corrected porphyria in transduced lymphoblastoid cells from HEP patients, suggesting that gene therapy may eventually be developed.

PREVENTION AND GENETIC COUNSELING. As part of genetic counseling in affected families, it is feasible to diagnose HEP in utero, either by analysis of porphyrins in amniotic fluid or DNA studies.

HEREDITARY COPROPORPHYRIA (HCP)

This autosomal dominant hepatic porphyria is due to a deficiency of coproporphyrinogen oxidase (CPO). The disease presents with acute attacks, as in AIP. Cutaneous photosensitivity may occur, but much less commonly than in VP. Rare homozygous cases present in childhood.

ETIOLOGY. A partial (≈50%) deficiency in CPO activity has been found in all cells studied from patients with HCP. A much more profound deficiency is found in homozygous cases. Human CPO is a homodimer composed of ≈39 kd subunits, and contains no metals or prosthetic groups. The enzyme requires molecular oxygen, and is localized in the mitochondrial intermembrane space. A single active site on the enzyme catalyzes the oxidative decarboxylation of 2 of the 4 proprionic acid groups of coproporphyrinogen III to form the 2 vinyl groups at positions 2 and 4, on rings A and B, respectively, of protoporphyrinogen IX (see Fig. 91-1). Most of the intermediate tricarboxyl porphyrinogen, termed *harderoporphyrinogen,* is not released before undergoing the second decarboxylation to protoporphyrinogen IX. Coproporphyrinogen I is not a substrate for this enzyme.

The human CPO gene contains 7 exons and is located on chromosome 3q12.1. A single promoter contains elements for both housekeeping and erythroid-specific expression. A variety of CPO gene mutations have been described in HCP, with a predominance of missense mutations and no genotype-phenotype correlations. Harderoporphria, a biochemical variant form of HCP, is due to CPO mutations that impair substrate binding, leading to premature release of harderoporphyrinogen.

EPIDEMIOLOGY. HCP is less common than AIP and VP, but its prevalence has not been carefully estimated. There is no obvious racial predominance. Homozygous HCP is rare and presents during childhood. Harderoporphyria, a biochemically distinguishable variant of HCP, has been recognized in heterozygous and homozygous forms.

PATHOLOGY AND PATHOGENESIS. Increased ALA and PBG during acute attacks of HCP may be explained by induction of ALAS1 and by the normally relatively low activity of PBGD in the liver. Hepatic ALAS1 is increased during acute attacks, but is normal when the disease is latent and porphyrin precursor excretion is normal. Because coproporphyrinogen III concentration in the liver is probably less than the Km for CPO, the reaction rate is likely to be determined in part by substrate concentration. The substrate coproporphyrinogen appears to be lost more readily from the liver cell than, for example, uroporphyrinogen, especially when heme synthesis is stimulated. Coproporphyrin and coproporphyrinogen are both transported into bile and excreted in urine, and do not appear to accumulate in the liver in HCP.

CLINICAL MANIFESTATIONS. Symptoms are identical to those of AIP except that attacks are generally milder, and cutaneous lesions that resemble those in PCT develop occasionally. Severe motor neuropathy and respiratory paralysis can occur. Like other acute porphyrias, HCP is almost always latent before puberty, and symptoms are most common in adult women. Attacks are precipitated by the same factors that cause attacks in AIP, including fasting, oral contraceptive steroids, and hormone increases during the luteal phase of the menstrual cycle. Concomittant liver diseases may increase porphyrin retention and photosensitivity. The risk of hepatocellular carcinoma is increased, as in other acute porphyrias.

The clinical features of homozygous HCP, which begin in early childhood, may include jaundice, hemolytic anemia, hepatosplenomegaly, and skin photosensitivity. These symptoms are generally quite distinct from those seen in heterozygotes.

LABORATORY FINDINGS. The porphyrin precursors ALA and PBG are increased during acute attacks, but may decrease more rapidly than in AIP. Marked increases in coproporphyrin III in urine and feces are more persistent. In homozygous cases, porphyrin excretion may be more markedly increased and are accompanied by substantial increases in erythrocyte zinc protoporphyrin. Harderoporphyria is characterized by a marked increase in fecal excretion of harderoporphyrin (tricarboxyl porphyrin) as well as coproporphyrin. Plasma porphyrins are usually normal or only slightly increased.

DIAGNOSIS AND DIFFERENTIAL DIAGNOSIS. The diagnosis of HCP is readily established in patients with clinically manifest disease, although urinary ALA, PBG, and uroporphyrin may revert to normal more quickly than in AIP. Urinary coproporphyrin III is increased. Urinary porphyrins, especially coproporphyrin, can be increased in many medical conditions, however, such as liver disease, and small increases may not be clinically significant and lead to an incorrect diagnosis of HCP. Fecal porphyrins are mostly coproporphyrin (isomer III) in HCP, whereas in VP, coproporphyrin III and protoporphyrin are often increased approximately equally. Plasma porphyrins are usually normal in HCP and increased in VP.

The ratio of fecal coproporphyrin III to coproporphyrin I is especially sensitive for detecting latent heterozygotes (especially adults). Assays for CPO, a mitochondrial enzyme, require cells such as lymphocytes and are not widely available. Identification of a CPO mutation in an index case greatly facilitates screening family members.

TREATMENT AND PROGNOSIS. Acute attacks of HCP are treated as in AIP, which includes intravenous hemin and identifying and avoiding precipitating factors. Cholestyramine may be of some value for photosensitivity occurring with liver dysfunction. Phlebotomy and chloroquine are not effective. GnRH analogues can be effective for prevention of cyclic attacks. The prognosis is generally better than in AIP.

PREVENTION AND GENETIC COUNSELING. These are the same as in other acute porphyrias.

VARIEGATE PORPHYRIA (VP)

This hepatic porphyria is due to a deficiency of protoporphyrinogen oxidase (PPO), which is inherited as an autosomal dominant trait. The disorder is termed *variegate* because it can present with neurologic or cutaneous manifestions. Other terms have included *porphyria variegata, protocoproporphyria,* and *South African genetic porphyria.* Rare cases of homozygous VP are symptomatic in childhood.

ETIOLOGY. PPO is approximately half normal in all cells studied in patients with VP. The enzyme is more markedly deficient in rare cases of homozygous VP, with approximately half-normal enzyme activity in parents.

Human PPO is a homodimer that contains FAD and is localized to the cytosolic side of the inner mitochondrial membrane. Membrane-binding domains may be docked onto human FECH, the next enzyme in the pathway, which is embedded in the opposite side of the membrane. PPO catalyzes the oxidation of protoporphyrinogen IX to protoporphyrin IX by the removal of 6 hydrogen atoms (see Fig. 91-1). The enzyme requires molecular oxygen. The substrate is readily oxidized nonenzymatically to protoporphyrin under aerobic conditions, or if exported into the cytosol. PPO is highly specific for protoporphyrinogen IX, and is inhibited by tetrapyrroles such as heme, biliverdin, and bilirubin and by certain herbicides that cause protoporphyrin to accumulate and induce phototoxicity in plants. Inhibition by bilirubin may account for decreased PPO activity in Gilbert disease.

The human PPO gene on chromosome 1q22–q23 consists of 1 noncoding and 12 coding exons. A single PPO transcript is produced in a variety of tissues, but putative transcriptional element binding sequences may allow for erythroid-specific expression. Many PPO mutations have been reported in VP families. A missense mutation, R59W, is prevalent in South Africa. No convincing genotype-phenotype correlations have been identified. Mutations in homozygous cases of VP are more likely to encode enzyme proteins with residual activity.

EPIDEMIOLOGY. VP is less common than AIP in most countries. The R59W mutation is highly prevalent in South African whites (≈3/1,000). This example of genetic drift or "founder effect" has been traced to a man or his wife who emigrated from Holland to South Africa in 1688. In Finland, the prevalence is ≈1.3/100,000 and is about as common as AIP.

PATHOLOGY AND PATHOGENESIS. Acute attacks develop in a minority (≈25%) of heterozygotes for PPO deficiency, and are often attributable to drugs, steroids, and nutritional factors that play a role in other acute porphyrias. Protoporphyrinogen IX accumulates and undergoes auto-oxidation to protoporphyrin IX. Coproporphyrinogen III may accumulate due to a close functional association between PPO in the inner mitochondrial membrane and CPO in the intermembrane space. Liver porphyrin content is not increased. The increased porphyrin content in plasma consists of porphyrin-peptide conjugates, which may be formed from protoporphyrinogen. Increased ALA and PBG during acute attacks may be explained, as in HCP, by induction of ALAS1 by exacerbating factors, and by the normally relatively low activity of PBGD in liver. Furthermore, PBGD is inhibited by protoporphyrinogen, the substrate for PPO.

CLINICAL MANIFESTATIONS. Symptoms develop in some heterozygotes after puberty. Neurovisceral symptoms occurring as acute attacks are identical to AIP, but are generally milder and less often fatal. Drugs, steroids, and nutritional alterations such as fasting, which are harmful in AIP, can also induce attacks of VP. Attacks occur equally in males and females, at least in South Africa. Cutaneous fragility, vesicles, bullae, hyperpigmentation, and hypertrichosis of sun-exposed areas are much more common than in HCP. They are likely to occur apart from and be more long lasting than the neurovisceral symptoms. Oral contraceptives can precipitate cutaneous manifestations. Acute attacks have become less common, and skin manifestations are more frequently the initial presentation; this may be due to earlier diagnosis and counseling. The risk of hepatocellular carcinoma is increased in VP, as in other acute porphyrias.

Symptoms of homozygous VP begin in infancy or childhood. These children generally have severe photosensitivity, neurologic symptoms, convulsions, developmental disturbances, and sometimes growth retardation, but do not have acute attacks.

LABORATORY FINDINGS. Urinary ALA, PBG, and uroporphyrin are increased during acute attacks but often less so than in AIP, and these may be normal or only slightly increased during remission. Plasma porphyrins, urinary and fecal coproporphyrin III, and fecal coproporphyrin III and protoporphyrin are more persistently increased between attacks. Erythrocyte zinc protoporphyrin levels are markedly increased in homozygous VP, and may be modestly increased in heterozygous cases.

DIAGNOSIS AND DIFFERENTIAL DIAGNOSIS. VP is readily distinguished from AIP and HCP, which also present with acute attacks and increases in PBG. Plasma porphyrin analysis is especially useful, because the plasma porphyrins in VP are tightly protein bound, resulting in a characteristic fluorescence emission spectrum at neutral pH. Fecal porphyrins are increased, with approximately equal amounts of coproporphyrin III and protoporphyrin. Fluorometric detection of plasma porphyrins is more sensitive than stool porphyrin analysis in asymptomatic VP. PPO assays using cells that contain mitochondria, such as lymphocytes, are sensitive for identifying asymptomatic carriers but are not widely available.

TREATMENT. Acute attacks are treated as in AIP. Hemin is beneficial for acute attacks but not for cutaneous symptoms. Light protection is important in patients with skin manifestations, using long-sleeved clothing, gloves, a broad-brimmed hat, and opaque sunscreen preparations. Exposure to short-wavelength ultraviolet light, which does not excite porphyrins, may increase skin pigmentation and provide some protection. Phlebotomy and chloroquine are not effective. Surprisingly, oral activated charcoal was reported to increase porphyrin levels and worsen skin manifestations.

PROGNOSIS AND PREVENTION. The outlook of patients with VP has improved, which may be attributed to improved treatment, earlier diagnosis, and detection of latent cases. Cyclic acute attacks in women can be prevented with a GnRH analog, as in AIP. A diagnosis of VP or any other acute porphyria should not lead to difficulty obtaining insurance, because the prognosis is usually good once the diagnosis is established.

GENETIC COUNSELING. These are the same as in other acute porphyrias.

ERYTHROPOIETIC PROTOPORPHYRIA (EPP)

In this autosomal dominant disorder, protoporphyrin accumulates due to a partial deficiency of FECH, the last enzyme in the heme biosynthetic pathway. EPP is sometimes termed *protoporphyria* or *erythrohepatic protoporphyria,* although the liver does not contribute substantially to production of excess protoporphyrin in uncomplicated cases.

ETIOLOGY. FECH, the enzyme that is deficient in EPP, catalyzes the final step in heme synthesis, which is insertion of ferrous iron (Fe^{2+}) into protoporphyrin IX (see Fig. 91-1). The enzyme is also termed *heme synthetase* or *protoheme ferrolyase.* The human enzyme is a dimer, and each homodimer contains a [2Fe-2S] cluster, which may have a role in bridging homodimers. FECH is found in the mitochondrial inner membrane where its active site faces the mitochondrial matrix. It may be associated with complex I of the mitochondrial electron transport chain, and the ferrous iron substrate may be produced upon nicotinamide-adenine dinucleotide (NADH) oxidation. FECH is specific for the reduced form of iron, but can utilize other metals such as Zn^{2+} and Co^{2+} and other dicarboxyl porphyrins. Accumulation of free protoporphyrin rather than zinc protoporphyrin in EPP indicates that formation of the latter is dependent on FECH activity in vivo.

The human FECH gene is located on chromosome 18q21.3, has a single promoter sequence, and contains 11 exons. Two mRNAs of ≈1.6 and ≈2.5 kb were described, which may be explained by the use of 2 alternative polyadenylation signals. The larger transcript is more abundant in murine erythroid cells, suggesting erythroid-specific regulation of FECH. A variety of FECH mutations have been reported in EPP, including missense, nonsense, and splicing mutations, small and large deletions, and an insertion.

The inheritance of 2 alleles associated with reduced FECH activity is required for disease expression. This is consistent with FECH activities as low as 15–25% of normal in EPP patients. In most patients, a disabling mutation on one FECH allele is combined with a common polymorphism affecting the other allele, which produces less than normal amounts of enzyme. This intronic single nucleotide polymorphism, IVS3-48T/C, results in the expression of an aberrantly spliced mRNA that is degraded by a nonsense-mediated RNA decay mechanism, which decreases the steady-state level of FECH mRNA. Inheritance of EPP in most affected families is correctly termed autosomal dominant because the IVS3-48T/C polymorphism by itself does not cause disease, even when homozygous. In a few families, however, 2 FECH mutations and a pattern of autosomal recessive inheritance have been found, and EPP with autosomal recessive inheritance occurs naturally in cattle and in mouse models. Another potential and less common mechanism is that a defective subunit might interact with a normal subunit in a "dominant-negative" fashion to render the dimer nonfunctional, such that only the 25% of dimers with 2 normal subunits would have enzyme activity.

In variant cases of EPP, FECH activity is normal, and both free and zinc protoporphyrin are increased. In these cases, a genetic defect in iron delivery to normal FECH is postulated.

EPP is sometimes associated with myelodysplastic syndromes and expansion of a clone of hematopoietic cells with deletion of one *FECH* allele. In such cases, there is late onset of the disease.

EPIDEMIOLOGY. EPP is the 3rd most common porphyria, although its prevalence is not precisely known (see Table 91-2). It is described mostly in white people, but occurs in other races as well, including blacks. The IVS3-48T/C polymorphism is common in whites and East Asians but rare in Africans, which would be predictive of a lower disease prevalence in populations of African origin.

PATHOLOGY AND PATHOGENESIS. FECH is deficient in all tissues in EPP, but bone marrow reticulocytes are thought to be the primary source of the excess protoporphyrin, some of which enters plasma and circulates to the skin. Accumulated protoporphyrin in circulating erythrocytes, which are no longer synthesizing heme and hemoglobin, also contributes. The liver functions as an excretory organ for excess protoporphyrin rather than a source. FECH deficiency in tissues other than bone marrow may be important, as tissue transplantation studies in mice suggest that skin photosensitivity and liver damage occur only when FECH is deficient in these tissues.

Patients with EPP are maximally sensitive to light in the 400 nm range, which corresponds to the so-called Soret band (the narrow peak absorption maximum that is characteristic for protoporphyrin and other porphyrins). Having absorbed light, porphyrins enter an excited energy state and release energy as fluorescence, singlet oxygen, and other reactive oxygen species. Tissue damage is accompanied by lipid peroxidation, oxidation of amino acids, cross linking of proteins in cell membranes, and damage to capillary endothelial cells. Such damage may be mediated by photoactivation of the complement system and release of histamine, kinins, and chemotactic factors. Repeated acute damage leads to thickening of the vessel walls and perivascular deposits from accumulation of serum components. Deposition of amorphous material containing immunoglobulin, complement components, glycoproteins, acid glycosaminoglycans, and lipids around blood vessels occurs in the upper dermis.

There is little evidence for impaired erythropoiesis or hemolysis in EPP. Iron accumulation in erythroblasts and ring sideroblasts has been noted in the bone marrow of some patients, however, suggesting that FECH deficiency sometimes impairs erythroid heme synthesis.

Liver damage that develops in a small proportion of EPP patients is attributed to excess protoporphyrin, which is insoluble in water and is excreted only by hepatic uptake and biliary excretion. Some may be reabsorbed by the intestine and undergo enterohepatic circulation. Excess protoporphyrin can decrease hepatic bile formation and flow, form crystalline structures in hepatocytes, and impair mitochondrial function.

CLINICAL MANIFESTATIONS. Symptoms of cutaneous photosensitivity begin in childhood, and consist of pain, redness, and itching occurring within minutes of sunlight exposure. Swelling may resemble angioneurotic edema. These are referred to as solar urticaria and are usually worse in the spring and summer. Petechiae and purpuric lesions may be seen, but blisters are usually absent. Chronic changes may include lichenification, leathery pseudovesicles, labial grooving, and nail changes, but changes in pigmentation and pronounced scarring are unusual. Neuropathy develops only in some patients with severe hepatic decompensation.

Unless hepatic or other complications develop, protoporphyrin levels and symptoms of photosensitivity remain remarkably stable for many years in most patients. Factors that exacerbate hepatic porphyrias play little or no role in EPP. Anemia is seldom prominent. Mild anemia with hypochromia and microcytosis is sometimes noted, and depletion of iron stores may be relatively common even in the absence of anemia. Mild, unexplained hypertriglyceridemia and somewhat lower levels of erythrocyte protoporphyrin and increased sunlight tolerance during pregnancy have been described.

LABORATORY FINDINGS. Protoporphyrin is substantially increased in circulating erythrocytes in EPP, and consists almost entirely of free protoporphyrin. In a variant form of EPP without FECH deficiency, zinc protoporphyrin as well as free protoporphyrin is increased, although the latter still predominates. Protoporphyrin is also increased in bone marrow, plasma, bile, and feces. Other porphyrins and porphyrin precursors are normal in uncomplicated EPP.

DIAGNOSIS AND DIFFERENTIAL DIAGNOSIS. A diagnosis of EPP is confirmed primarily by finding a substantially elevated concentration of erythrocyte protoporphyrin, which is predominantly free and not complexed with zinc. Erythrocyte zinc protoporphyrin concentration is increased in some homozygous porphyrias, iron deficiency, lead poisoning, anemia of chronic disease, hemolytic conditions, and many other erythrocytic disorders. Because many assays for erythrocyte protoporphyrin or "free erythrocyte protoporphyrin" measure both zinc and free protoporphyrin, and specific assays for metal-free protoporphyrin are less widely available, reports of increased erythrocyte protoporphyrin must be interpreted with care.

The increase in plasma total porphyrin concentration in EPP is often less than in other cutaneous porphyrias. Great care must be taken to avoid light exposure during sample processing, because plasma porphyrins in EPP are particularly subject to photodegradation. Other findings include normal levels of urinary porphyrin precursors and porphyrins.

Measurement of FECH activity requires cells containing mitochondria and is not widely available. Demonstration of normal FECH activity and a greater than expected proportion of zinc protopoporphyrin in erythrocytes is important in identifying variant EPP. DNA studies are increasingly important for confirming the mode of inheritance and for genetic counseling.

The development of life-threatening hepatic complications of EPP is accompanied by abnormal liver function tests, increasing erythrocyte and plasma protoporphyrin levels, and increased photosensitivity. Increases in urinary porphyrins, especially coproporphyrin, are attributable to liver dysfunction.

COMPLICATIONS. Biliary stones containing protoporphyrin are sometimes symptomatic and require cholecystectomy. Liver disease occurs in 1–2% of EPP patients, including children, and may be chronic or progress rapidly to death from liver failure. Liver disease is sometimes the major presenting feature of EPP. Upper abdominal pain may suggest biliary obstruction, and unnecessary laparotomy to exclude this possibility can be detrimental. Concurrent conditions that impair liver function, such as viral hepatitis, alcohol intake, iron deficiency, fasting, or oral contraceptive steroids, may contribute. Liver histology shows marked deposition of protoporphyrin in liver cells and bile canaliculi. Patients with protoporphyric liver failure, which represents a severe phenotype, most often have "null mutations" and the IVS3–48T/C polymorphism in the nonmutant allele, but some may have 2 mutant alleles and autosomal recessive inheritance. The bone marrow is probably the major source of protoporphyrin, even in EPP patients with hepatic failure.

TREATMENT. Exposure to sunlight should be avoided whenever possible, which is aided by wearing closely woven clothing. Oral beta-carotene leads to clinical improvement and greater tolerance to light in some patients, usually 1 to 3 mo after starting treatment. In most adults, doses of 120–180 mg daily will maintain serum carotene levels in the recommended range of 600–800 mg/dL, but doses up to 300 mg daily may be needed. Mild skin discoloration due to carotenemia is expected. The recommended product is Solatene (Tishcon), which was developed as a drug specifically for treating this disease, rather than nutritional products that are less standardized. Beta-carotene may quench singlet oxygen or free radicals, but does not substantially alter circulating porphyrin levels. Better tolerance of sunlight may result in tanning, which provides additional protection. Oral cysteine may also quench excited oxygen species and was found more recently to increase tolerance to sunlight in EPP.

Other measures to darken the skin may also be helpful. This may be accomplished by narrow-band UV-B phototherapy or with topical products such as dihydroxyacetone and lawsone (naphthoquinone). Caloric restriction and drugs or hormone preparations that impair hepatic excretory function should be avoided, and iron deficiency should be corrected if present.

Treatment of protoporphyric liver disease must be individualized and results are unpredictable. Ursodeoxycholic acid may be of some value in early stages. Cholestyramine or activated charcoal may interrupt the enterohepatic circulation of protoporphyrin, promote its fecal excretion, and reduce liver protoporphyrin content. Splenectomy may be beneficial when EPP is complicated by hemolysis and splenomegaly. Spontaneous resolution may occur, especially if another reversible cause of liver dysfunction, such as viral hepatitis or alcohol abuse, is contributing. Otherwise, exchange transfusion, plasma exchange, and intravenous hemin to suppress erythroid and hepatic protoporphyrin production may be beneficial.

Motor neuropathy resembling that seen in acute porphyrias sometimes develops in EPP patients with liver disease after transfusion or liver transplantation and is sometimes reversible. Artificial lights, such as operating room lights during liver transplantation or other surgery, may cause severe photosensitivity, with extensive burns of the skin and peritoneum and photodamage of circulating erythrocytes in patients with protoporphyric liver disease.

With continued progression of liver disease, liver transplantation may be considered. But because liver disease may recur in the transplanted liver due to continued bone marrow production of excess protoporphyrin, bone marrow transplantation (BMT) should also be considered if a suitable donor is available. BMT did ameliorate liver disease in a murine model of protoporphyria, and led to remission of protoporphyria in a patient who underwent BMT for acute myelogenous leukemia. Gene therapy strategies are under study in murine models. For example, a dual gene therapy approach allowed selection of hematopoietic stem cells with erythroid-specific expression of the therapeutic FECH gene, leading to a progressive increase of normal erythrocytes and correction of photosensitivity.

PROGNOSIS. Typical EPP patients have lifelong photosensitivity, but can otherwise expect normal longevity. Protoporphyric liver disease is often life-threatening; however, the incidence is low.

PREVENTION. Symptoms can be prevented by avoiding sunlight. Avoiding agents that may cause liver damage may help prevent liver complications.

GENETIC COUNSELING. DNA studies are increasingly important for genetic counseling, especially in families in which a child or adult has developed protoporphyric hepatopathy. This will usually identify a disabling FECH mutation and the IVS3–48T/C polymorphism. In some EPP families, however, 2 disease-associated mutations are found, with a pattern of autosomal recessive inheritance. EPP may improve during pregnancy.

DUAL PORPHYRIA

Dual porphyria refers to patients with porphyria who have deficiencies of more than 1 enzyme of the heme biosynthetic pathway. Molecular documentation is important in such cases. For example, an unusual pattern of porphyrin precursors and porphyrins in a patient presenting with an acute attack was explained by heterozygous mutations in both the *CPO* and *ALAD* genes. Kindreds with individuals having both PCT and either AIP, HCP, or VP have been described, with individuals developing either neurovisceral or cutaneous symptoms. One patient with symptoms of AIP and PCT was documented to have both *PBGD* and *UROD* mutations. An infant with severe porphyria was found, based on enzyme measurements, to have inherited CPO deficiency from 1 parent and UROS deficiency from both parents. Coexistence of UROS and UROD deficiencies were described in a patient with an erythropoietic porphyria. A family with deficiencies of both PBGD and CPO has also been described.

PORPHYRIA DUE TO TUMORS

Very rarely, hepatocellular tumors contain and presumably produce excess porphyrins, but such cases have not been studied carefully. Hepatocellular carcinomas complicating PCT and acute hepatic porphyrias usually are not described as containing large amounts of porphyrins. Erythropoietic porphyrias can develop late in life due to clonal expansion of erythroid cells containing a specific enzyme deficiency in patients who have developed myelodysplastic or myeloproliferative syndromes.

General

Anderson KE, Sassa S, Bishop DF, Desnick RJ: Disorders of heme biosynthesis: X-linked sideroblastic anemias and the porphyrias. In Scriver CR, Beaudet AL, Sly WS, et al (eds): *The Metabolic and Molecular Basis of Inherited Disease,* vol II, 8th ed. New York, McGraw-Hill, 2001, pp 2991–3062.

Hift RJ, Meissner PN: An analysis of 112 acute porphyric attacks in Cape Town, South Africa. *Medicine* 2005;84:48–60.

Kauppinen R: Porphyrias. *Lancet* 2005;365:241–252.

Congenital Erythropoietic Porphyria

Dupuis-Girod S, Akkari V, Ged C, et al: Successful match-unrelated donor bone marrow transplantation for congenital erythropoietic porphyria (Gunther disease). *Eur J Pediatr* 2005;164:104–107.

Piomelli S, Poh-Fitzpatrick MB, Seaman C, et al: Complete suppression of the symptoms of congenital erythropoietic porphyria by long-term treatment with high-level transfusions. *N Engl J Med* 1986;314:1029–1031.

Solis C, Aizencang GI, Astrin KH, et al: Uroporphyrinogen III synthase erythroid promoter mutations in adjacent GATA1 and CP2 elements cause congenital erythropoietic porphyria. *J Clin Invest* 2001;107:753–762.

Verstraeten L, Van Regemorter N, Pardou A, et al: Biochemical diagnosis of a fatal case of Gunther's disease in a newborn with hydrops-fetalis. *Eur J Clin Chem Clin Biochem* 1993;31:121–128.

Acute Intermittent Porphyria

Andant C, Puy H, Bogard C, et al: Hepatocellular carcinoma in patients with acute hepatic porphyria: Frequency of occurrence and related factors. *J Hepatol* 2000;32:933–939.

Anderson KE, Bloomer JR, Bonkovsky HL, et al: Recommendations for the diagnosis and treatment of the acute porphyrias. *Ann Intern Med* 2005;142:439–450.

Meyer UA, Schuurmans MM, Lindberg RLP: Acute porphyrias: Pathogenesis of neurological manifestations. *Semin Liver Dis* 1998;18:43–52.

Solis C, Martinez-Bermejo A, Naidich TP, et al: Acute intermittent porphyria: Studies of the severe homozygous dominant disease provide insights into the neurologic attacks in acute porphyrias. *Arch Neurol* 2004;61:1764–1770.

Soonawalla ZF, Orug T, Badminton MN, et al: Liver transplantation as a cure for acute intermittent porphyria. *Lancet* 2004;363:705–706.

Winkler M, Anderson KE: Vampires, porphyria and the media: The medicalization of a myth. *Perspect Biol Med* 1990;33:598–611.

Hereditary Coproporphyria and Variegate Porphyria

Hift RJ, Meissner PN: An analysis of 112 acute porphyric attacks in Cape Town, South Africa: Evidence that acute intermittent porphyria and variegate porphyria differ in susceptibility and severity. *Medicine (Baltimore)* 2005;84:48–60.

Long C, Smyth SJ, Woolf J, et al: Detection of latent variegate porphyria by fluorescence emission spectroscopy of plasma. *Br J Dermatol* 1993;129:9–13.

Martasek P: Hereditary coproporphyria. *Semin Liver Dis* 1998;18:25–32.

Porphyria Cutanea Tarda

Egger NG, Goeger DE, Payne DA, et al: Porphyria cutanea tarda: Multiplicity of risk factors including HFE mutations, hepatitis C, and inherited uroporphyrinogen decarboxylase deficiency. *Dig Dis Sci* 2002;47:419–426.

Elder GH: Porphyria cutanea tarda and related disorders. In Kadish KM, Smith K, Guilard R (eds): *Porphyrin Handbook,* part II, vol 14. San Diego, Academic Press, 2003, pp 67–92.

Erythropoietic Protoporphyria

Cox TM: Protoporphyria. In Kadish KM, Smith K, Guilard R (eds): *Porphyrin Handbook,* part II, vol 14. San Diego, Academic Press, 2003, pp 121–149.

Goodwin RG, Kell WJ, Laidler P, et al: Photosensitivity and acute liver injury in myeloproliferative disorder secondary to late-onset protoporphyria caused by deletion of a ferrochelatase gene in hematopoietic cells. *Blood* 2006;107:60–62.

Magnus IA, Jarrett A, Prankert TAJ, Rimington C: Erythropoietic protoporphyria: A new porphyria syndrome with solar urticaria due to protoporphyrinaemia. *Lancet* 1961;2:448–451.

McGuire BM, Bonkovsky HL, Carithers RL Jr, et al: Liver transplantation for erythropoietic protoporphyria liver disease. *Liver Transpl* 2005; 11:1590–1596.

Chapter 92 ■ Hypoglycemia

Mark A. Sperling

Glucose has a central role in fuel economy and is a source of energy storage in the form of glycogen, fat, and protein (see Chapter 87). Glucose, an immediate source of energy, provides 38 mol of adenosine triphosphate (ATP) per mol of glucose oxidized. It is essential for cerebral energy metabolism because it is usually the preferred substrate and its utilization accounts for nearly all the oxygen consumption in the brain. Cerebral glucose uptake occurs through a glucose transporter molecule or molecules that are not regulated by insulin. Cerebral transport of glucose is a carrier-mediated, facilitated diffusion process that is dependent on blood glucose concentration. Deficiency of brain glucose transporters can result in seizures because of low cerebral and cerebrospinal fluid (CSF) glucose concentrations (hypoglycorrhachia) despite normal blood glucose levels. To maintain the blood glucose concentration and prevent it from falling precipitously to levels that impair brain function, an elaborate regulatory system has evolved.

The defense against hypoglycemia is integrated by the autonomic nervous system and by hormones that act in concert to enhance glucose production through enzymatic modulation of glycogenolysis and gluconeogenesis while simultaneously limiting peripheral glucose utilization. Hypoglycemia represents a defect in one or several of the complex interactions that normally integrate glucose homeostasis during feeding and fasting. This process is particularly important for neonates, in whom there is an abrupt transition from intrauterine life, characterized by dependence on transplacental glucose supply, to extrauterine life, characterized ultimately by the autonomous ability to maintain euglycemia. Because prematurity or placental insufficiency may limit tissue nutrient deposits, and genetic abnormalities in enzymes or hormones may become evident in the neonate, hypoglycemia is common in the neonatal period.

DEFINITION

In neonates, there is not always an obvious correlation between blood glucose concentration and the classic clinical manifestations of hypoglycemia. The absence of symptoms does not indicate that glucose concentration is normal and has not fallen to less than some optimal level for maintaining brain metabolism. There is evidence that hypoxemia and ischemia may potentiate the role of hypoglycemia in causing permanent brain damage. Consequently, the lower limit of accepted normality of the blood glucose level in newborn infants with associated illness that already impairs cerebral metabolism has not been determined (see Chapter 107). Out of concern for possible neurologic, intellectual, or psychologic sequelae in later life, many authorities recommend that any value of blood glucose <50 mg/dL in neonates be viewed with suspicion and vigorously treated. This is particularly applicable after the initial 2–3 hr of life, when glucose normally has reached its nadir; subsequently, blood glucose levels begin to rise and achieve values of 50 mg/dL or higher after 12–24 hr. In older infants and children, a whole blood glucose concentration of <50 mg/dL (10–15% higher for serum or plasma) represents hypoglycemia.

SIGNIFICANCE AND SEQUELAE

Metabolism by the adult brain accounts for the majority of total basal glucose turnover. Most of the endogenous hepatic glucose production in infants and young children can be accounted for by brain metabolism. Furthermore, there is a correlation between glucose production and estimated brain weight at all ages.

Because the brain grows most rapidly in the 1st yr of life and because the larger proportion of glucose turnover is used for brain metabolism, sustained or repetitive hypoglycemia in infants and children can retard brain development and function. Transient isolated hypoglycemia of short duration does not appear to be associated with these severe sequelae. In the rapidly growing brain, glucose may also be a source of membrane lipids and, together with protein synthesis, it can provide structural proteins and myelination that are important for normal brain maturation. Under conditions of severe and sustained hypoglycemia, these cerebral structural substrates may become degraded to energy-usable intermediates such as lactate, pyruvate, amino acids, and ketoacids, which can support brain metabolism at the expense of brain growth. The capacity of the newborn brain to take up and oxidize ketone bodies is about fivefold greater than that of the adult brain. The capacity of the liver to produce ketone bodies, however, may be limited in the newborn period, especially in the presence of hyperinsulinemia, which acutely inhibits hepatic glucose output, lipolysis, and ketogenesis, thereby depriving the brain of any alternate fuel sources. Although the brain may metabolize ketones, these alternate fuels cannot completely replace glucose as an essential central nervous system (CNS) fuel. The deprivation of the brain's major energy source during hypoglycemia and the limited availability of alternate fuel sources during hyperinsulinemia have predictable adverse consequences on brain metabolism and growth: decreased brain oxygen consumption and increased breakdown of endogenous structural components with destruction of functional membrane integrity. Hypoglycemia may thus lead to permanent impairment of brain growth and function. The potentiating effects of hypoxia may exacerbate brain damage or indeed be responsible for it when blood glucose values are not in the classic hypoglycemic range.

The major long-term sequelae of severe, prolonged hypoglycemia are mental retardation, recurrent seizure activity, or both. Subtle effects on personality are also possible but have not been clearly defined. Permanent neurologic sequelae are present in 25–50% of patients with severe recurrent symptomatic hypoglycemia who are younger than 6 mo of age. These sequelae may be reflected in pathologic changes characterized by atrophic gyri, reduced myelination in cerebral white matter, and atrophy in the cerebral cortex. Infarcts are absent if hypoxia-ischemia did not contribute to cerebral manifestations; the cerebellum is spared if hypoglycemia is the sole insult. These sequelae are more likely when alternative fuel sources are limited, as occurs with hyperinsulinemia, when the episodes of hypoglycemia are repetitive or prolonged, or when they are compounded by hypoxia. There is no precise knowledge relating the duration or severity of hypoglycemia to subsequent neurologic development of children in a predictable manner. Although less common, hypoglycemia in older children may also produce long-term neurologic defects through neuronal death mediated, in part, by cerebral excitotoxins released during hypoglycemia.

SUBSTRATE, ENZYME, AND HORMONAL INTEGRATION OF GLUCOSE HOMEOSTASIS

IN THE NEWBORN (SEE CHAPTER 107). Under nonstressed conditions, fetal glucose is derived entirely from the mother through placental transfer. Therefore, fetal glucose concentration usually reflects but is slightly lower than maternal glucose levels. Catecholamine release, which occurs with fetal stress such as hypoxia, mobilizes fetal glucose and free fatty acids (FFAs) through β-adrenergic mechanisms, reflecting β-adrenergic activity in fetal liver and adipose tissue. Catecholamines may also inhibit fetal insulin and stimulate glucagon release.

The acute interruption of maternal glucose transfer to the fetus at delivery imposes an immediate need to mobilize endogenous glucose. Three related events facilitate this transition: changes in hormones, changes in their receptors, and changes in key enzyme activity. There is a three- to fivefold abrupt increase in glucagon concentration within minutes to hours of birth. The level of insulin usually falls initially and remains in the basal range for several days without demonstrating the usual brisk response to physiologic stimuli such as glucose. A dramatic surge in spontaneous catecholamine secretion is also characteristic. Epinephrine can also augment growth hormone secretion by α-adrenergic mechanisms; growth hormone levels are elevated at birth. Acting in unison, these hormonal changes at birth mobilize glucose via glycogenolysis and gluconeogenesis, activate lipolysis, and promote ketogenesis. As a result of these processes, plasma glucose concentration stabilizes after a transient decrease immediately after birth, liver glycogen stores become rapidly depleted within hours of birth, and gluconeogenesis from alanine, a major gluconeogenic amino acid, can account for ≈10% of glucose turnover in the human newborn infant by several hours of age. FFA concentrations also increase sharply in concert with the surges in glucagon and epinephrine and are followed by rises in ketone bodies. Glucose is thus partially spared for brain utilization while FFAs and ketones provide alternative fuel sources for muscle as well as essential gluconeogenic factors such as acetyl coenzyme A (CoA) and the reduced form of nicotinamide-adenine dinucleotide (NADH) from hepatic fatty acid oxidation, which is required to drive gluconeogenesis.

In the early postnatal period, responses of the endocrine pancreas favor glucagon secretion so that blood glucose concentration can be maintained. These adaptive changes in hormone secretion are paralleled by similarly striking adaptive changes in hormone receptors. Key enzymes involved in glucose production also change dramatically in the perinatal period. Thus, there is a rapid fall in glycogen synthase activity and a sharp rise in phosphorylase after delivery. Similarly, the amount of rate-limiting enzyme for gluconeogenesis, phosphoenolpyruvate carboxykinase, rises dramatically after birth, activated in part by the surge in glucagon and the fall in insulin. This framework can explain several causes of neonatal hypoglycemia based on inappropriate changes in hormone secretion and unavailability of adequate reserves of substrates in the form of hepatic glycogen, muscle as a source of amino acids for gluconeogenesis, and lipid stores for the release of fatty acids. In addition, appropriate activities of key enzymes governing glucose homeostasis are required (see Fig. 87-1).

IN OLDER INFANTS AND CHILDREN. Hypoglycemia in older infants and children is analogous to that of adults, in whom glucose homeostasis is maintained by glycogenolysis in the immediate postfeeding period and by gluconeogenesis several hours after meals. The liver of a 10 kg child contains ≈20–25 g of glycogen, which is sufficient to meet normal glucose requirements of 4–6 mg/kg/min for only 6–12 hr. Beyond this period, hepatic gluconeogenesis must be activated. Both glycogenolysis and gluconeogenesis depend on the metabolic pathway summarized in Figure 87-1. Defects in glycogenolysis or gluconeogenesis may not be manifested in infants until the frequent feeding at 3–4 hr intervals ceases and infants sleep through the night, a situation usually present by 3–6 mo of age. The source of gluconeogenic precursors is derived primarily from muscle protein. The muscle bulk of infants and small children is substantially smaller relative to body mass than that of adults, whereas glucose requirements/unit of body mass are greater in children, so the ability to compensate for glucose deprivation by gluconeogenesis is more limited in infants and young children, as is the ability to withstand fasting for prolonged periods. The ability of muscle to generate alanine, the principal gluconeogenic amino acid, may also be limited. Thus, in normal young children, the blood glucose level falls after 24 hr of fasting, insulin concentrations fall appropriately to levels of <5–10 μU/mL, lipolysis and ketogenesis are activated, and ketones may appear in the urine.

The switch from glycogen synthesis during and immediately after meals to glycogen breakdown and later gluconeogenesis is governed by hormones, of which insulin is of central importance. Plasma insulin concentrations increase to peak levels of 50–100 μU/mL after meals, which serve to lower the blood glucose concentration through the activation of glycogen synthesis, enhancement of peripheral glucose uptake, and inhibition of glucose production. In addition, lipogenesis is stimulated, whereas lipolysis and ketogenesis are curtailed. During fasting, plasma insulin concentrations fall to ≤5–10 μU/mL, and together with other hormonal changes, this fall results in activation of gluconeogenic pathways (see Fig. 87-1). Fasting glucose concentrations are maintained through the activation of glycogenolysis and gluconeogenesis, inhibition of glycogen synthesis, and activation of lipolysis and ketogenesis. It should be emphasized that a plasma insulin concentration of >5 μU/mL, in association with a blood glucose concentration of ≤40 mg/dL (2.2 mM), is abnormal, indicating a **hyperinsulinemic state** and failure of the mechanisms that normally result in suppression of insulin secretion during fasting or hypoglycemia.

The hypoglycemic effects of insulin are opposed by the actions of several hormones whose concentration in plasma increases as blood glucose falls. These **counter-regulatory hormones,** glucagon, growth hormone, cortisol, and epinephrine, act in concert by increasing blood glucose concentrations via activating glycogenolytic enzymes (glucagon, epinephrine); inducing gluconeogenic enzymes (glucagon, cortisol); inhibiting glucose uptake by muscle (epinephrine, growth hormone, cortisol); mobilizing amino acids from muscle for gluconeogenesis (cortisol); activating lipolysis and thereby providing glycerol for gluconeogenesis and fatty acids for ketogenesis (epinephrine, cortisol, growth hormone, glucagon); and inhibiting insulin release and promoting growth hormone and glucagon secretion (epinephrine).

Congenital or acquired deficiency of any one of these hormones is uncommon but will result in hypoglycemia, which occurs when endogenous glucose production cannot be mobilized to meet energy needs in the postabsorptive state, that is, 8–12 hr after meals or during fasting. Concurrent deficiency of several hormones (**hypopituitarism**) may result in hypoglycemia that is more severe or appears earlier during fasting than that seen with isolated hormone deficiencies. Most of the causes of hypoglycemia in infancy and childhood reflect inappropriate adaptation to fasting.

CLINICAL MANIFESTATIONS (SEE CHAPTER 107)

Clinical features generally fall into two categories. The 1st includes symptoms associated with the activation of the autonomic nervous system and epinephrine release, usually seen with a rapid decline in blood glucose concentration (Table 92-1). The 2nd category includes symptoms due to decreased cerebral glucose utilization, usually associated with a slow decline in blood glucose level or prolonged hypoglycemia (see Table 92-1). Although these classic symptoms occur in older children, the symptoms of hypoglycemia in infants may be subtler and include

TABLE 92-1. Manifestations of Hypoglycemia in Childhood

FEATURES ASSOCIATED WITH ACTIVATION OF AUTONOMIC NERVOUS SYSTEM AND EPINEPHRINE RELEASE*
Anxiety[†]
Perspiration[†]
Palpitation (tachycardia)[†]
Pallor
Tremulousness
Weakness
Hunger
Nausea
Emesis
Angina (with normal coronary arteries)
FEATURES ASSOCIATED WITH CEREBRAL GLUCOPENIA
Headache[†]
Mental confusion[†]
Visual disturbances (↓ acuity, diplopia)[†]
Organic personality changes[†]
Inability to concentrate[†]
Dysarthria
Staring
Paresthesias
Dizziness
Amnesia
Ataxia, incoordination
Somnolence, lethargy
Seizures
Coma
Stroke, hemiplegia, aphasia
Decerebrate or decorticate posture

*Some of these features will be attenuated if the patient is receiving β-adrenergic blocking agents.
[†]Common.

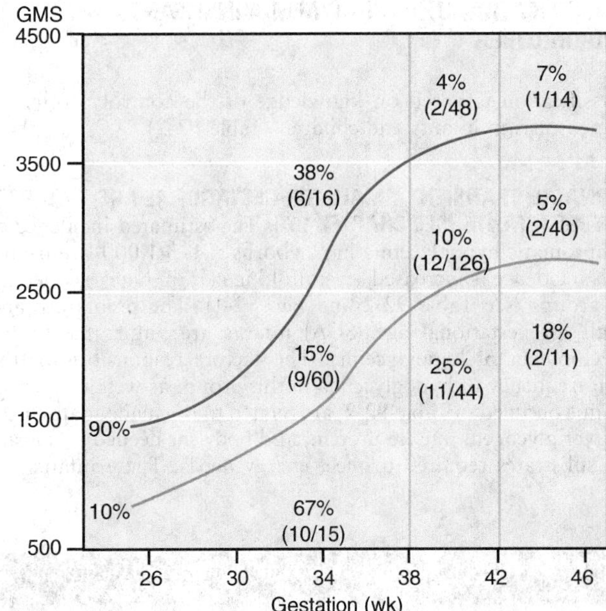

Figure 92-1. Incidence of hypoglycemia by birthweight, gestational age, and intrauterine growth. (From Lubchenco LO, Bard H: Incidence of hypoglycemia in newborn infants classified by birthweight and gestational age. *Pediatrics* 1971;47:831–838.)

cyanosis, apnea, hypothermia, hypotonia, poor feeding, lethargy, and seizures. Some of these symptoms may be so mild that they are missed. Occasionally, hypoglycemia may be asymptomatic in the immediate newborn period. Newborns with hyperinsulinemia are often large for gestational age; older infants with hyperinsulinemia may eat excessively because of chronic hypoglycemia and become obese. In childhood, hypoglycemia may present as behavior problems, inattention, ravenous appetite, or seizures. It may be misdiagnosed as epilepsy, inebriation, personality disorders, hysteria, and retardation. A blood glucose determination should always be performed in sick neonates, who should be vigorously treated if concentrations are <50 mg/dL. At any age level, hypoglycemia should be considered a cause of an initial episode of convulsions or a sudden deterioration in psychobehavioral functioning.

Many neonates have asymptomatic (chemical) hypoglycemia. In contrast to the frequency of chemical hypoglycemia, the incidence of symptomatic hypoglycemia is highest in small for gestational age infants (Fig. 92-1). The exact incidence of symptomatic hypoglycemia has been difficult to establish because many of the symptoms in neonates occur **together** with other conditions such as infections, especially sepsis and meningitis; central nervous system anomalies, hemorrhage, or edema; hypocalcemia and hypomagnesemia; asphyxia; drug withdrawal; apnea of prematurity; congenital heart disease; or polycythemia.

The onset of symptoms in neonates varies from a few hours to a week after birth. In approximate order of frequency, symptoms include jitteriness or tremors, apathy, episodes of cyanosis, convulsions, intermittent apneic spells or tachypnea, weak or high-pitched cry, limpness or lethargy, difficulty feeding, and eye rolling. Episodes of sweating, sudden pallor, hypothermia, and cardiac arrest and failure also occur. Frequently, a clustering of episodic symptoms may be noted. Because these clinical manifestations may result from various causes, it is critical to measure serum glucose levels and determine whether they disappear with the administration of sufficient glucose to raise the blood sugar to normal levels; if they do not, other diagnoses must be considered.

CLASSIFICATION OF HYPOGLYCEMIA IN INFANTS AND CHILDREN

Classification is based on knowledge of the control of glucose homeostasis in infants and children (Table 92-2).

NEONATAL, TRANSIENT, SMALL FOR GESTATIONAL AGE, AND PREMATURE INFANTS (SEE CHAPTER 107). The estimated incidence of symptomatic hypoglycemia in newborns is 1–3/1,000 live births. This incidence is increased severalfold in certain high-risk neonatal groups (see Table 92-2 and Fig. 92-1). The premature and small for gestational age (SGA) infants are vulnerable to the development of hypoglycemia. The factors responsible for the high frequency of hypoglycemia in this group, as well as in other groups outlined in Table 92-2, are related to the inadequate stores of liver glycogen, muscle protein, and body fat needed to sustain the substrates required to meet energy needs. These infants are small by virtue of prematurity or impaired placental transfer of nutrients. Their enzyme systems for gluconeogenesis may not be fully developed. Transient hyperinsulinism responsive to diazoxide has also been reported as contributing to hypoglycemia in asphyxiated, SGA, and premature newborn infants. In most cases, the condition resolves quickly, but it may persist to 7 mo of life.

In contrast to deficiency of substrates or enzymes, the hormonal system appears to be functioning normally at birth in most low-risk neonates. Despite hypoglycemia, plasma concentrations of alanine, lactate, and pyruvate are higher, implying their diminished rate of utilization as substrates for gluconeogenesis. Infusion of alanine elicits further glucagon secretion but causes no significant rise in glucose. During the initial 24 hr of life, plasma concentrations of acetoacetate and β-hydroxybutyrate are lower in SGA infants than in full-term infants, implying diminished lipid stores, diminished fatty acid mobilization, impaired ketogenesis, or a combination of these conditions. Diminished lipid stores are most likely because fat (triglyceride) feeding of newborns results

TABLE 92-2. Classification of Hypoglycemia in Infants and Children

NEONATAL TRANSIENT HYPOGLYCEMIA

Associated with inadequate substrate or immature enzyme function in otherwise normal neonates
Prematurity
Small for gestational age
Normal newborn

Transient neonatal hyperinsulinism also present in:
Infant of diabetic mother
Small for gestational age
Discordant twin
Birth asphyxia
Infant of toxemic mother

NEONATAL, INFANTILE, OR CHILDHOOD PERSISTENT HYPOGLYCEMIAS

Hormonal disorders
Hyperinsulinism
- Recessive K_{ATP} channel HI
- Focal K_{ATP} channel HI
- Dominant K_{ATP} channel HI
- Dominant glucokinase HI
- Dominant glutamate dehydrogenase HI (hyperinsulinism/hyperammonemia syndrome)
- Acquired islet adenoma
- Beckwith-Wiedemann syndrome
- Insulin administration (Munchausen syndrome by proxy)
- Oral sulfonylurea drugs
- Congenital disorders of glycosylation

Counter-regulatory hormone deficiency
Panhypopituitarism
Isolated growth hormone deficiency
Adrenocorticotropic hormone deficiency
Addison disease
Epinephrine deficiency

Glycogenolysis and gluconeogenesis disorders
Glucose-6-phosphatase deficiency (GSD 1a)
Glucose-6-phosphate translocase deficiency (GSD 1b)
Amylo-1,6-glucosidase (debranching enzyme) deficiency (GSD 3)
Liver phosphorylase deficiency (GSD 6)
Phosphorylase kinase deficiency (GSD 9)
Glycogen synthetase deficiency (GSD 0)
Fructose-1,6-diphosphatase deficiency
Pyruvate carboxylase deficiency
Galactosemia
Hereditary fructose intolerance

Lipolysis disorders

Fatty acid oxidation disorders
Carnitine transporter deficiency (primary carnitine deficiency)
Carnitine palmitoyltransferase-1 deficiency
Carnitine translocase deficiency
Carnitine palmitoyltransferase-2 deficiency
Secondary carnitine deficiencies
Very long, long-, medium-, short-chain acyl CoA dehydrogenase deficiency

OTHER ETIOLOGIES

Substrate-limited
Ketotic hypoglycemia
Poisoning—drugs
Salicylates
Alcohol
Oral hypoglycemic agents
Insulin
Propranolol
Pentamidine
Quinine
Disopyramide
Ackee fruit (unripe)—hypoglycin
Vacor (rate poison)
Trimethoprim-sulfamethoxazole (with renal failure)

Liver disease
Reye syndrome
Hepatitis
Cirrhosis
Hepatoma

Amino acid and organic acid disorders
Maple syrup urine disease
Propionic acidemia
Methylmalonic acidemia
Tyrosinosis
Glutaric aciduria
3-Hydroxy-3-methylglutaric aciduria

Systemic disorders
Sepsis
Carcinoma/sarcoma (secreting—insulin-like growth factor II)
Heart failure
Malnutrition
Malabsorption
Anti-insulin receptor antibodies
Anti-insulin antibodies
Neonatal hyperviscosity
Renal failure
Diarrhea
Burns
Shock
Postsurgical
Pseudohypoglycemia (leukocytosis, polycythemia)
Excessive insulin therapy of insulin-dependent diabetes mellitus
Factitious
Nissen fundoplication (dumping syndrome)
Falciparum malaria

GSD, glycogen storage disease; HI, hyperinsulinemia; K_{ATP}, regulated potassium channel.

in a rise in the plasma levels of glucose, FFAs, and ketones. Some infants with perinatal asphyxia and some SGA newborns may have transient hyperinsulinemia, which promotes hypoglycemia and diminishes the supply of FFAs.

The role of FFAs and their oxidation in stimulating neonatal gluconeogenesis is essential. The provision of FFAs as triglyceride feedings from formula or human milk together with gluconeogenic precursors may prevent the hypoglycemia that usually ensues after neonatal fasting. For these and other reasons, milk feedings are introduced early (at birth or within 2–4 hr) after delivery. In the hospital setting, when feeding is precluded by virtue of respiratory distress or when feedings alone cannot maintain blood glucose concentrations at levels >50 mg/dL, intravenous glucose at a rate that supplies 4–8 mg/kg/min should be started. Infants with transient neonatal hypoglycemia can usually maintain the blood glucose level spontaneously after 2–3 days of life, but some require longer periods of support. In these latter infants, insulin values >5 uU/ml at the time of hypoglycemia should be treated with diazoxide.

INFANTS BORN TO DIABETIC MOTHERS (SEE CHAPTER 107). Of the transient hyperinsulinemic states, infants born to diabetic mothers are the most common. Gestational diabetes affects some 2% of pregnant women, and ≈1/1,000 pregnant women have insulin-dependent diabetes. At birth, infants born to these mothers may be large and plethoric, and their body stores of glycogen, protein, and fat are replete.

Hypoglycemia in infants of diabetic mothers is mostly related to hyperinsulinemia and partly related to diminished glucagon secretion. Hypertrophy and hyperplasia of the islets is present, as is a brisk, biphasic, and typically mature insulin response to glucose; this insulin response is absent in normal infants. Infants born to diabetic mothers also have a subnormal surge in plasma glucagon immediately after birth, subnormal glucagon secretion in response to stimuli, and, initially, excessive sympathetic activity that may lead to adrenomedullary exhaustion as reflected by decreased urinary excretion of epinephrine. The normal plasma hormonal pattern of low insulin, high glucagon, and high catecholamines is reversed to a pattern of high insulin, low glucagon, and low epinephrine. As a consequence of this abnormal hormonal profile, the endogenous glucose production is significantly inhibited compared with that in normal infants, thus predisposing them to hypoglycemia.

Mothers whose diabetes has been well controlled during pregnancy, labor, and delivery generally have infants near normal size who are less likely to acquire neonatal hypoglycemia and other complications formerly considered typical of such infants (see Chapter 107). In supplying glucose to hypoglycemic infants, it is important to avoid hyperglycemia that evokes a prompt exuberant insulin release, which may result in rebound hypoglycemia. When needed, glucose should be provided at continuous infusion rates of 4–8 mg/kg/min, but the appropriate dose for each patient should be individually adjusted. During labor and delivery, maternal hyperglycemia should be avoided because it results in fetal hyperglycemia, which predisposes to hypoglycemia when the glucose supply is interrupted at birth. Hypoglycemia persisting or occurring after 1 wk of life requires an evaluation for the causes listed in Table 92-2.

Infants born with **erythroblastosis fetalis** may also have hyperinsulinemia and share many physical features, such as large body size, with infants born to diabetic mothers. The cause of the hyperinsulinemia in infants with erythroblastosis is not clear.

PERSISTENT OR RECURRENT HYPOGLYCEMIA IN INFANTS AND CHILDREN

HYPERINSULINISM. Most children with hyperinsulinism that causes hypoglycemia present in the neonatal period or later in infancy; hyperinsulinism is the most common cause of persistent hypoglycemia in early infancy. Hyperinsulinemic infants may be macrosomic at birth, reflecting the anabolic effects of insulin in utero. There is no history or biochemical evidence of maternal diabetes. The onset is from birth to 18 mo of age, but occasionally it is 1st evident in older children. Insulin concentrations are inappropriately elevated at the time of documented hypoglycemia; with non-hyperinsulinemic hypoglycemia, plasma insulin concentrations should be <5 μU/mL and no higher than 10 μU/mL. In affected infants, plasma insulin concentrations at the time of hypoglycemia are commonly >5–10 μU/mL. Some authorities set more stringent criteria, arguing that any value of insulin >2 μU/mL with hypoglycemia is abnormal. The insulin (μU/mL):glucose (mg/dL) ratio is commonly >0.4; plasma insulin-like growth factor binding protein-1 (IGFBP-1), ketones, and FFA levels are low. Macrosomic infants may present with hypoglycemia from the 1st days of life. Infants with lesser degrees of hyperinsulinemia, however, may manifest hypoglycemia after the 1st few weeks to months, when the frequency of feedings has been decreased to permit the infant to sleep through the night and hyperinsulinism prevents the mobilization of endogenous glucose. Increasing appetite and demands for feeding, wilting spells, jitteriness, and frank seizures are the most common presenting features. Additional clues include the rapid development of fasting hypoglycemia within 4–8 hr of food deprivation compared with other causes of hypoglycemia (Tables 92-3 and 92-4); the need for high rates of exogenous glucose infusion to prevent hypoglycemia, often at rates >10–15 mg/kg/min; the absence of ketonemia or acidosis; and elevated C-peptide or proinsulin levels at the time of hypoglycemia. The latter insulin-related products are also absent in **factitious hypoglycemia** from exogenous administration of insulin as a form of child abuse (Munchausen by proxy syndrome). [See Chapter 36.2.] Provocative tests with tolbutamide or leucine are not necessary in infants; hypoglycemia is invariably provoked by withholding feedings for several hours, permitting simultaneous measurement of glucose, insulin, ketones, and FFAs in the same sample at the time of clinically manifested hypoglycemia. This is termed the "critical sample." The glycemic response to glucagon at the time of hypoglycemia reveals a brisk rise in glucose of at least 40 mg/dL, which implies that glucose mobilization has been restrained by insulin but that glycogenolytic mechanisms are intact (Tables 92-5, 92-6, and 92-7).

The measurement of serum IGFBP-1 concentration may help diagnose hyperinsulinemia. The secretion of IGFBP-1 is acutely inhibited by insulin; IGFBP-1 concentrations are low during hyperinsulinism-induced hypoglycemia. In patients with spontaneous or fasting-induced hypoglycemia with a low insulin level (ketotic hypoglycemia, normal fasting), IGFBP-1 concentrations are significantly higher.

The differential diagnosis of endogenous hyperinsulinism includes **diffuse β-cell hyperplasia or focal β-cell microadenoma.** The distinction between these two major entities is important because the former, if unresponsive to medical therapy, requires

TABLE 92-3. Hypoglycemia in Infants and Children: Clinical and Laboratory Features

GROUP	AGE AT DIAGNOSIS (MO)	GLUCOSE (MG/DL)	INSULIN (μU/ML)	FASTING TIME TO HYPOGLYCEMIA (HR)
HYPERINSULINEMIA (*N* = 12)				
Mean	7.4	23.1	22.4	2.1
SEM	2.0	2.7	3.2	0.6
NONHYPERINSULINEMIA (*N* = 16)				
Mean	41.8	36.1	5.8	18.2
SEM	7.3	2.4	0.9	2.9

Adapted from Antunes JD, Geffner ME, Lippe BM, et al: Childhood hypoglycemia: Differentiating hyperinsulinemic from nonhyperinsulinemic causes. *J Pediatr* 1990;116:105–108.

TABLE 92-4. Correlation of Clinical Features with Molecular Defects in Persistent Hyperinsulinemic Hypoglycemia in Infancy

TYPE	MACROSOMIA	HYPOGLYCEMIA/ HYPERINSULINEMIA	FAMILY HISTORY	MOLECULAR DEFECTS	ASSOCIATED CLINICAL, BIOCHEMICAL, OR MOLECULAR FEATURES	RESPONSE TO MEDICAL MANAGEMENT	RECOMMENDED SURGICAL APPROACH	PROGNOSIS
Sporadic	Present at birth	Moderate/severe in 1st days to weeks of life	Negative	? *SUR1*/K_{IR}6.2 Mutations not always identified in diffuse hyperplasia	Loss of heterozygosity in microadenomatous tissue	Generally poor; may respond better to somatostatin than to diazoxide	Partial pancreatectomy if frozen section shows β-cell crowding with small nuclei—microadenoma	Excellent
							Subtotal >95%	Guarded; diabetes mellitus develops in 50% of patients; hypoglycemia persists in 33% pancreatectomy if frozen section shows giant nuclei in β-cells —diffuse hyperplasia
Autosomal recessive	Present at birth	Severe in 1st days to weeks of life	Positive	*SUR*/K_{IR}6.2	Consanguinity a feature in some populations	Poor	Subtotal pancreatectomy	Guarded
Autosomal dominant	Unusual	Moderate onset usually post 6 mo of age	Positive	Glucokinase (activating) Some cases gene unknown	None	Very good to excellent	Surgery usually not required Partial pancreatectomy only if medical management fails	Excellent
Autosomal dominant	Unusual	Moderate onset usually post 6 mo of age	Positive	Glutamate Dehydrogenase (activating)	Modest hyperammonemia	Very good to excellent	Surgery usually not required	Excellent
Beckwith-Wiedemann syndrome	Present at birth	Moderate, spontaneously resolves post □ 6 mo of age	Negative	Duplicating/imprinting in chromosome 11p15.1	Macroglossia, omphalocele, hemihypertrophy	Good	Not recommended	Excellent for hypoglycemia; associated with embryonal tumors (Wilms hepatoblastoma)
Congenital disorders of glycosylation	Not usual	Moderate/onset post 3 mo of age	Negative	Phosphomannose isomerase deficiency	Hepatomegaly, vomiting, intractable diarrhea	Good with mannose supplement	Not recommended	Fair

near total pancreatectomy, despite which hypoglycemia may persist or diabetes mellitus may ensue at some later time. By contrast, focal adenomas diagnosed preoperatively or intraoperatively permit localized curative resection with subsequent normal glucose metabolism. About 50% of the autosomal recessive or sporadic forms of neonatal/infantile hyperinsulinism are due to focal microadenomas, which may be distinguished from the diffuse form by the pattern of insulin response to selective insulin secretagogues infused into an artery supplying the pancreas with sampling via the hepatic vein. Positron emission tomography (PET scanning) using 18 fluoro-L-dopa can distinguish the diffuse form (uniform fluorescence throughout the pancreas) from the focal form (focal uptake of 18 fluoro-L-dopa and localized fluorescence) [See Fig. 92-3.].

TABLE 92-5. Analysis of Critical Blood Sample During Hypoglycemia and 30 Minutes After Glucagon*

SUBSTRATES
- Glucose
- Free fatty acids
- Ketones
- Lactate
- Uric acid
- Ammonia

HORMONES
- Insulin
- Cortisol
- Growth hormone
- Thyroxine, thyroid-stimulating hormone
- IGFBP-1[†]

*Glucagon 50 μg/kg with maximum of 1 mg IV or IM.

[†]Measure once only before or after glucagon administration. Rise in glucose of ≥40 mg/dL after glucagon given at the time of hypoglycemia strongly suggests a hyperinsulinemic state with adequate hepatic glycogen stores and intact glycogenolytic enzymes. If ammonia is elevated to 100–200 μM, consider activating mutation of glutamate dehydrogenase.

IGFBP-1, insulin-like growth factor binding protein–1.

Insulin-secreting macroadenomas are rare in childhood and may be diagnosed preoperatively via CT or MRI. The plasma levels of insulin alone, however, cannot distinguish the aforementioned entities. The diffuse or microadenomatous forms of islet cell hyperplasia represent a variety of genetic defects responsible for abnormalities in the endocrine pancreas characterized by autonomous insulin secretion that is not appropriately reduced when blood glucose declines spontaneously or in response to provocative maneuvers such as fasting (see Tables 92-7 and 92-8). Clinical, biochemical, and molecular genetic approaches now permit classification of congenital hyperinsulinism, formerly termed **nesidioblastosis,** into distinct entities. **Persistent hyperinsulinemic hypoglycemia of infancy (PHHI)** may be inherited or sporadic, is severe, and is caused by mutations in the regulation of the potassium channel intimately involved in insulin secretion by the pancreatic β cell (Fig. 92-2). Normally, glucose entry into the β cell is enabled by the non–insulin-responsive glucose transporter GLUT-2. On entry, glucose is phosphorylated to glucose-6-phosphate by the enzyme glucokinase, enabling glucose

TABLE 92-6. Criteria for Diagnosing Hyperinsulinism Based on "Critical" Samples (Drawn at a Time of Fasting Hypoglycemia: Plasma Glucose <50 mg/dL)

1. Hyperinsulinemia (plasma insulin >2 μU/mL)*
2. Hypofattyacidemia (plasma free fatty acids <1.5 mmol/L)
3. Hypoketonemia (plasma β-hydroxybutyrate: <2.0 mmol/L)
4. Inappropriate glycemic response to glucagon, 1 mg IV (delta glucose >40 mg/dL)

*Depends on sensitivity of insulin assay.

From Stanley CA, Thomson PS, Finegold DN, et al: Hypoglycemia in Infants and Neonates. In Sperling MA (editor): *Pediatric Endocrinology,* 2nd ed., Philadelphia, WB Saunders, 2002, pp 135–159.

TABLE 92-7. Diagnosis of Acute Hypoglycemia in Infants and Children

ACUTE SYMPTOMS PRESENT

1. Obtain blood sample before and 30 min after glucagon administration.
2. Obtain urine as soon as possible. Examine for ketones; if not present and hypoglycemia confirmed, suspect hyperinsulinemia or fatty acid oxidation defect; if present, suspect ketotic, hormone deficiency, inborn error of glycogen metabolism, or defective gluconeogenesis.
3. Measure glucose in the original blood sample. If hypoglycemia is confirmed, proceed with substrate-hormone measurement as in Table 92-5.
4. If glycemic increment after glucagon exceeds 40 mg/dL above basal, suspect hyperinsulinemia.
5. If insulin level at time of confirmed hypoglycemia is >5 μU/mL, suspect endogenous hyperinsulinemia; if >100 μU/mL, suspect factitious hyperinsulinemia (exogenous insulin injection). Admit to hospital for supervised fast.
6. If cortisol is <10 μg/dL or growth hormone is <5 ng/mL, or both, suspect adrenal insufficiency or pituitary disease, or both. Admit to hospital for hormonal testing and neuroimaging.

HISTORY SUGGESTIVE: ACUTE SYMPTOMS NOT PRESENT

1. Careful history for relation of symptoms to time and type of food intake, bearing in mind age of patient. Exclude possibility of alcohol or drug ingestion. Assess possibility of insulin injection, salt craving, growth velocity, intracranial pathology.
2. Careful examination for hepatomegaly (glycogen storage disease; defect in gluconeogenesis); pigmentation (adrenal failure); stature and neurologic status (pituitary disease)
3. Admit to hospital for provocative testing:
   a. 24 hr fast under careful observation; when symptoms provoked, proceed with steps 1–4 as when acute symptoms present
   b. Pituitary-adrenal function using arginine-insulin stimulation test if indicated
4. Liver biopsy for histologic and enzyme determinations if indicated
5. Oral glucose tolerance test (1.75 g/kg; max 75 g) if reactive hypoglycemia suspected (dumping syndrome, etc.)

metabolism to generate ATP. The rise in the molar ratio of ATP relative to adenosine diphosphate (ADP) closes the ATP-sensitive potassium channel in the cell membrane (K_{ATP} channel). This channel is composed of two subunits, the K_{IR} 6.2 channel, part of the family of inward-rectifier potassium channels, and a regulatory component in intimate association with K_{IR} 6.2 known as the sulfonylurea receptor (SUR). Together, K_{IR} 6.2 and SUR constitute the potassium-sensitive ATP channel K_{ATP}. Normally, the K_{ATP} is open, but with the rise in ATP and closure of the channel, potassium accumulates intracellularly, causing depolarization of the membrane, opening of voltage-gated calcium channels, influx of calcium into the cytoplasm, and secretion of insulin via exocytosis. The genes for both SUR and K_{IR} 6.2 are located close together on the short arm of chromosome 11, the site of the insulin gene. Inactivating mutations in the gene for SUR or, less often, K_{IR} 6.2 prevent the potassium channel from opening. It remains essentially closed with constant depolarization and, therefore, constant inward flux of calcium; hence, insulin secretion is continuous. A milder autosomal dominant form of these defects is also reported. Likewise, an activating **mutation in glucokinase** or **glutamate dehydrogenase** results in closure of the potassium channel through overproduction of ATP and hyperinsulinism. Inactivating mutations of the glucokinase gene are responsible for inadequate insulin secretion and form the basis of maturity-onset diabetes of youth (see Chapter 590).

The familial forms of PHHI are more common in certain populations, notably Arabic and Ashkenazi Jewish communities, where it may reach an incidence of about 1/2,500, compared with the sporadic rates in the general population of ≈1/50,000. These **autosomal recessive forms** of PHHI typically present in the

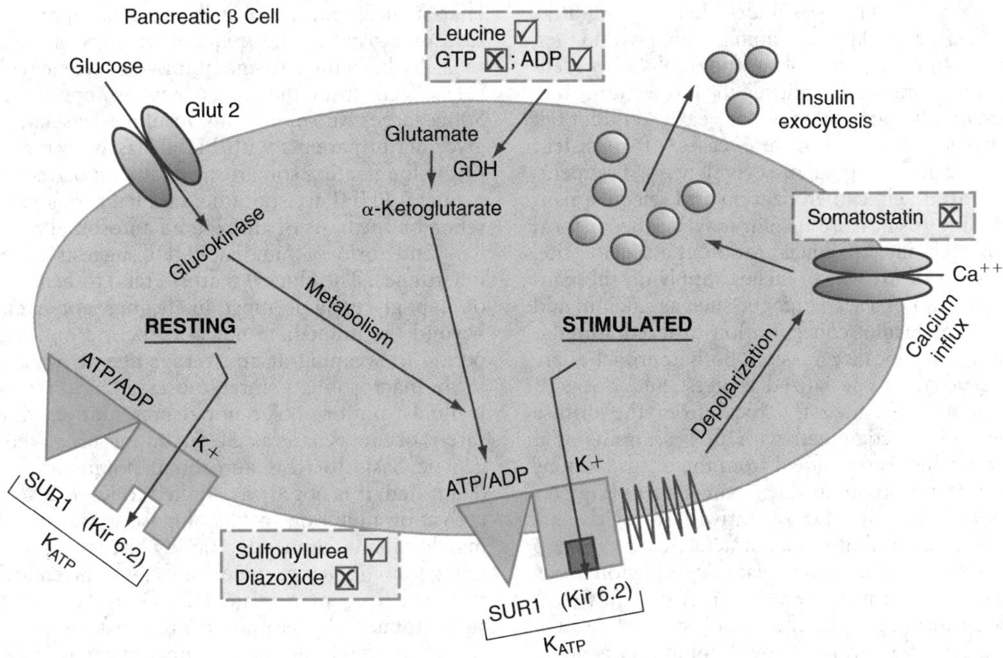

Figure 92-2. Schematic representation of the pancreatic cell with some important steps in insulin secretion. The membrane-spanning, adenosine triphosphate (ATP)–sensitive potassium (K^+) channel (K_{ATP}) consists of two subunits: the sulfonylurea receptor (SUR) and the inward rectifying K channel (K_{IR} 6.2). In the resting state, the ratio of ATP to adenosine diphosphate (ADP) maintains K_{ATP} in an open state, permitting efflux of intracellular K^+. When blood glucose concentration rises, its entry into the β cell is facilitated by the GLUT-2 glucose transporter, a process not regulated by insulin. Within the β cell, glucose is converted to glucose-6-phosphate by the enzyme glucokinase and then undergoes metabolism to generate energy. The resultant increase in ATP relative to ADP closes K_{ATP}, preventing efflux of K^+, and the rise of intracellular K^+ depolarizes the cell membrane and opens a calcium (Ca^{2+}) channel. The intracellular rise in Ca^{2+} triggers insulin secretion via exocytosis. Sulfonylureas trigger insulin secretion by reacting with their receptor (SUR) to close K_{ATP}; diazoxide inhibits this process, whereas somatostatin, or its analog octreotide, inhibits insulin secretion by interfering with calcium influx. Genetic mutations in *SUR* or K_{IR} 6.2 that prevent K_{ATP} from being open are responsible for autosomal recessive forms of persistent hyperinsulinemic hypoglycemia of infancy (PHHI). One form of autosomal dominant PHHI is due to an activating mutation in glucokinase. The amino acid leucine also triggers insulin secretion by closure of K_{ATP}. Metabolism of leucine is facilitated by the enzyme glutamate dehydrogenase (GDH), and overactivity of this enzyme in the pancreas leads to hyperinsulinemia with hypoglycemia, associated with hyperammonemia from overactivity of GDH in the liver. √, stimulation; GTP, guanosine triphosphate; X, inhibition.

TABLE 92-8. Clinical Manifestations and Differential Diagnosis in Childhood Hypoglycemia

CONDITION	HYPOGLYCEMIA	URINARY KETONES OR REDUCING SUGARS	HEPATOMEGALY
Normal	0	0	0
Hyperinsulinemia	Recurrent severe	0	0
Ketotic hypoglycemia	Severe with missed meals	Ketonuria +++	0
Fatty acid oxidation disorder	Severe with missed meals	Absent	0 to + Abnormal liver function test results
Hypopituitarism	Moderate with missed meals	Ketonuria ++	0
Adrenal insufficiency	Severe with missed meals	Ketonuria ++	0
Enzyme deficiencies	Severe-constant	Ketonuria +++	+++
Glucose-6-phosphatase debrancher	Moderate with fasting	Ketonuria ++	++
Phosphorylase	Mild-moderate	Ketonuria ++	+
Fructose-1, 6-diphosphatase	Severe with fasting	Ketonuria +++	+++
Galactosemia	After milk or milk products	0 Ketones;(s) +	+++
Fructose intolerance	After fructose	0 Ketones;(s) +	+++

Details of each condition are discussed in the text. 0, absence; ↑ or ↓ indicates respectively small increase or decrease; ↑↑ or ↓↓ indicates respectively large increase or decrease.

immediate newborn period as macrosomic newborns with a weight >4.0 kg and severe recurrent or persistent hypoglycemia manifesting in the initial hours or days of life. Glucose infusions as high as 15–20 mg/kg/min and frequent feedings fail to maintain euglycemia. Diazoxide, which acts by opening K_{ATP} channels (see Fig. 92-2), fails to control hypoglycemia adequately. Somatostatin, which also opens K_{ATP} and inhibits calcium flux, may be partially effective in ≈50% of patients (see Fig. 92-2). Calcium channel blocking agents have had inconsistent effects. When affected patients are unresponsive to these measures, pancreatectomy is strongly recommended to avoid the long-term neurologic sequelae of hypoglycemia. If surgery is undertaken, preoperative CT or MRI rarely reveals an isolated adenoma, which would then permit local resection. Intraoperative ultrasonography may identify a small impalpable adenoma, permitting local resection. Adenomas often present in late infancy or early childhood. Distinguishing between **focal** and **diffuse** cases of **persistent hyperinsulinism** has been attempted in several ways. Preoperatively, transhepatic portal vein catheterization and selective pancreatic venous sampling to measure insulin may localize a focal lesion from the step-up in insulin concentration at a specific site. Selective catheterization of arterial branches supplying the pancreas, followed by infusion of a secretagogue such as calcium and portal vein sampling for insulin concentration (arterial stimulation-venous sampling) may localize a lesion. Both approaches are highly invasive, restricted to specialized centers, and not uniformly successful in distinguishing the focal from the diffuse forms. 18F-labeled L-dopa combined with PET scanning is a promising means to distinguish the focal from the diffuse lesions of hyperinsulinism unresponsive to medical management (Fig. 92-3). The "gold standard" remains intraoperative histologic characterization. Diffuse hyperinsulinism is characterized by large β cells with abnormally large nuclei, whereas focal adenomatous lesions display small and normal β cell nuclei. Although *SUR1* mutations are present in both types, the focal lesions arise by a random loss of a maternally imprinted growth-inhibitory gene on maternal chromosome 11p in association with paternal transmission of a mutated *SUR1* or K_{IR} 6.2 paternal chromosome 11p. Thus the focal form represents a double hit-loss of maternal repressor and transmission of a paternal mutation. Local excision of focal adenomatous islet cell hyperplasia results in a cure with little or no recurrence. For the diffuse form, near-total resection of 85–90% of the pancreas is recommended. The near-total pancreatectomy required for the diffuse hyperplastic lesions is, however, often associated with persistent hypoglycemia with the later development of hyperglycemia or frank, insulin-requiring diabetes mellitus.

Further resection of the remaining pancreas may occasionally be necessary if hypoglycemia recurs and cannot be controlled by medical measures, such as the use of somatostatin or diazoxide.

Experienced pediatric surgeons in medical centers equipped to provide the necessary preoperative and postoperative care, diagnostic evaluation, and management should perform surgery. In some patients who have been managed medically, hyperinsulinemia and hypoglycemia regress over months. This is similar to what occurs in children with the hyperinsulinemic hypoglycemia seen in **Beckwith-Wiedemann syndrome.**

If hypoglycemia 1st manifests between 3 and 6 mo of age or later, a therapeutic trial using medical approaches with diazoxide, somatostatin, and frequent feedings can be attempted for up to 2–4 wk. Failure to maintain euglycemia without undesirable side effects from the drugs may prompt the need for surgery. Some success in suppressing insulin release and correcting hypoglycemia in patients with PHHI has been reported with the use of the long-acting somatostatin analog octreotide. Most cases of neonatal PHHI are sporadic; familial forms permit genetic counseling on the basis of anticipated autosomal recessive inheritance.

A 2nd form of familial PHHI suggests **autosomal dominant inheritance.** The clinical features tend to be less severe, and onset of hypoglycemia is most likely, but not exclusively, to occur beyond the immediate newborn period and usually beyond the period of weaning at an average age at onset of about 1 yr. At birth, macrosomia is rarely observed, and response to diazoxide is almost uniform. The initial presentation may be delayed and rarely occur as late as 30 yr, unless provoked by fasting. The genetic basis for this autosomal dominant form has not been delineated; it is not always linked to K_{IR} 6.2/*SUR1*. However, the activating mutation in glucokinase is transmitted in an autosomal dominant manner. If a family history is present, genetic counseling for a 50% recurrence rate can be given for future offspring.

A 3rd form of persistent PHHI is associated with **mild and asymptomatic hyperammonemia,** usually as a sporadic occurrence, although dominant inheritance occurs. Presentation is more like the autosomal dominant form than the autosomal recessive form. Diet and diazoxide control symptoms, but pancreatectomy may be necessary in some cases. The association of hyperinsulinism and hyperammonemia is caused by an inherited or de novo gain-of-function mutation in the enzyme glutamate dehydrogenase. The resulting increase in glutamate oxidation in the pancreatic β cell raises the ATP concentration and, hence, the ratio of ATP:ADP, which closes K_{ATP}, leading to membrane depolarization, calcium influx, and insulin secretion (see Fig. 92-2). In the liver, the excessive oxidation of glutamate to β-ketoglutarate may generate ammonia and divert glutamate from being

SERUM		EFFECT OF 24–36 HR FAST ON PLASMA					GLYCEMIC RESPONSE TO GLUCAGON		GLYCEMIC RESPONSE TO INFUSION OF	
LIPIDS	URIC ACID	GLUCOSE	INSULIN	KETONES	ALANINE	LACTATE	FED	FASTED	ALANINE	GLYCEROL
Normal	Normal	↓	↓	↑	↓	Normal	↑	↓	Not indicated	
Normal or ↑	Normal	↓↓	↑↑	↓↓	Normal	Normal	↑	↑	Not indicated	
Normal	Normal	↓↓	↓	↑↑	↓↓	Normal	↑	↓↓	Not indicated	
Abnormal	↑		Contraindicated				↑	↓	Not indicated	
Normal	Normal	↓↓	↓	↑↑	↓↓	Normal	↑	↓↓	↑	↑
Normal	Normal	↓↓	↓	↑↑	↓↓	Normal	↑	↓↓	↑	↑
↑↑	↑↑	↓↓	↓	↑↑	↑↑	↑↑	0	0–↓↓	0	0
Normal	Normal	↓↓	↓	↑↑	↓↓	Normal	↑	0–↓↓	↑	↑
Normal	Normal	↓	↓	↑↑	↓↓	Normal	0–↑	0–↓↓	↑	↑
↑↑	↑↑	↓↓	↓	↑↑	↑↑	↑↑	↑	0–↓↓	↓	↓
Normal	Normal	↓	↓	↑	↓	Normal	↑	0–↓↓	↑	↑
Normal	Normal	↓	↓	↑	↓	Normal	↑	0–↓↓	↑	↑

processed to *N*-acetylglutamate, an essential cofactor for removal of ammonia through the urea cycle via activation of the enzyme carbamoyl phosphate synthetase. The hyperammonemia is mild, with concentrations of 100–200 μM/L, and produces no CNS symptoms or consequences, as seen in other hyperammonemic states. Leucine, a potent amino acid for stimulating insulin secretion and implicated in leucine-sensitive hypoglycemia, acts by allosterically stimulating glutamate dehydrogenase. Thus, **leucine-sensitive hypoglycemia** may be a form of the hyperinsulinemia-hyperammonemia syndrome or a potentiation of mild disorders of the K_{ATP} channel.

Hypoglycemia associated with hyperinsulinemia is also seen in ≈50% of patients with the **Beckwith-Wiedemann syndrome.** This syndrome is characterized by omphalocele, gigantism, macroglossia, microcephaly, and visceromegaly. Distinctive lateral earlobe fissures and facial nevus flammeus are present; hemihypertrophy occurs in many of these infants. Diffuse islet cell hyperplasia occurs in infants with hypoglycemia. The diagnostic and therapeutic approaches are the same as those discussed previously, although microcephaly and retarded brain development may occur independently of hypoglycemia. Patients with the Beckwith-Wiedemann syndrome may acquire tumors, including Wilms tumor, hepatoblastoma, adrenal carcinoma, gonadoblastoma, and rhabdomyosarcoma. This overgrowth syndrome is caused by mutations in the chromosome 11p15.5 region close to the genes for insulin, SUR, K_{IR} 6.2, and IGF-2. Duplications in this region and genetic imprinting from a defective or absent copy of the maternally derived gene are involved in the variable features and patterns of transmission. Hypoglycemia may resolve in weeks to months of medical therapy. Pancreatic resection may also be needed.

Hyperinsulinemic hypoglycemia in infancy is reported as a manifestation of one form of congenital disorder of glycosylation. Disorders of protein glycosylation usually present with neurologic symptoms but may also include liver dysfunction with hepatomegaly, intractable diarrhea, protein-losing enteropathy,

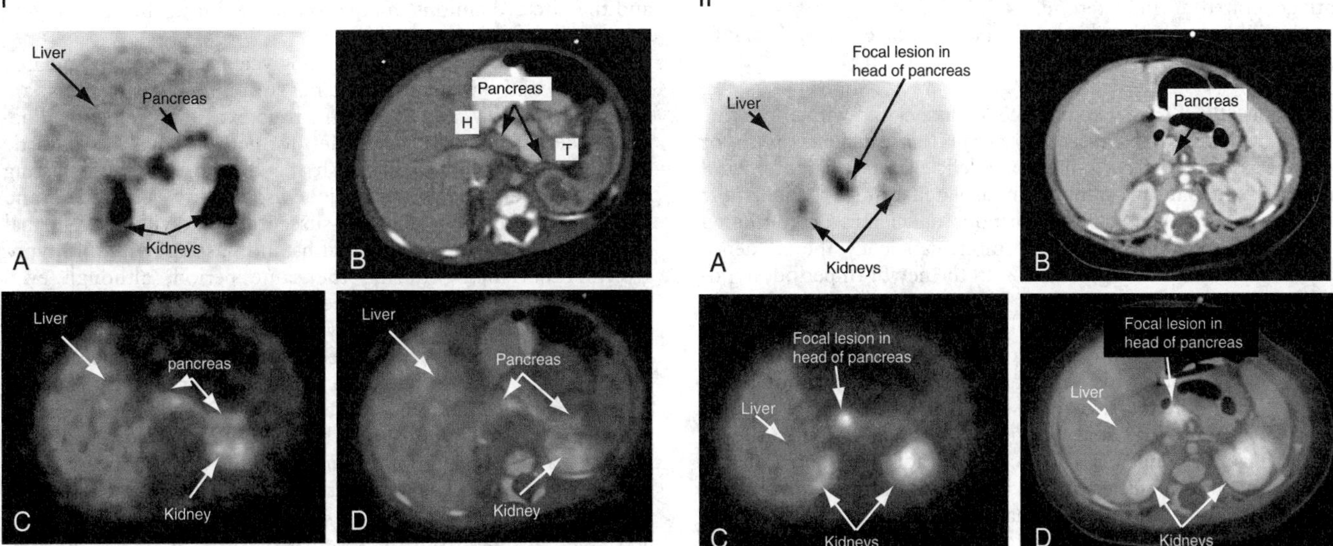

Figure 92-3. Congenital hyperinsulinism. I panels (Diffuse): [18F]-DOPA PET of patient with diffuse form of congenital hyperinsulinism. *A,* Diffuse uptake of [18F]-DOPA is visualized throughout the pancreas. Transverse views show *B,* normal pancreatic tissue on abdominal CT; *C,* diffuse uptake of [18F]-DOPA in pancreas; and *D,* confirmation of pancreatic uptake of [18F]-DOPA with coregistration. H, head of pancreas; T, tail of pancreas. **II** panels (Focal): [18F]-DOPA PET of patient with focal form of congenital hyperinsulinism. *A,* Discrete area of increased [18F]-DOPA uptake is visualized in the head of the pancreas. The intensity of this area is greater than that observed in the liver and neighboring normal pancreatic tissue. Transverse views show *B,* normal pancreatic tissue on abdominal CT; C, focal uptake of [18F]-DOPA in pancreatic head; and *D,* confirmation of [18F]-DOPA uptake in the pancreatic head with coregistration. (Courtesy of Dr Olga Hardy, Children's Hospital of Philadelphia).

and hypoglycemia (see Chapter 87.6). These disorders are often underdiagnosed. One entity associated with hyperinsulinemic hypoglycemia is caused by phosphomannose isomerase deficiency, and clinical improvement followed supplemental treatment with oral mannose at a dose of 0.17 g/kg six times per day.

After the 1st 12 mo of life, hyperinsulinemic states are uncommon until islet cell adenomas reappear as a cause after the patient is several years of age. Hyperinsulinemia due to **islet cell adenoma** should be considered in any child 5 yr or older presenting with hypoglycemia. The diagnostic approach is outlined in Tables 92-7 and 92-8. Fasting for up to 24–36 hr usually provokes hypoglycemia; coexisting hyperinsulinemia confirms the diagnosis, provided that factitious administration of insulin by the parents, a form of **Munchausen syndrome by proxy,** is excluded. Occasionally, provocative tests may be required. Exogenously administered insulin can be distinguished from endogenous insulin by simultaneous measurement of C-peptide concentration. If C-peptide levels are elevated, endogenous insulin secretion is responsible for the hypoglycemia; if C-peptide levels are low but insulin values are high, exogenous insulin has been administered, perhaps as a form of child abuse. Islet cell adenomas at this age are treated by surgical excision; familial multiple endocrine adenomatosis type I (Wermer syndrome) should be considered. Antibodies to insulin or the insulin receptor (insulin mimetic action) are also rarely associated with hypoglycemia. Some tumors produce insulin-like growth factors, thereby provoking hypoglycemia by interacting with the insulin receptor. The astute clinician must also consider the possibility of deliberate or accidental ingestion of drugs such as a sulfonylurea or related compound that stimulates insulin secretion. In such cases, insulin and C-peptide concentrations in blood will be elevated. Inadvertent substitution of an insulin secretagogue by a dispensing error should be considered in those taking medications who suddenly develop documented hypoglycemia.

A rare form of hyperinsulinemic hypoglycemia has been reported after exercise. Whereas glucose and insulin remain unchanged in most people after moderate, short-term exercise, rare patients manifest severe hypoglycemia with hyperinsulinemia 15–50 min after the same standardized exercise. This form of exercise-induced hyperinsulinism may be caused by an abnormal responsiveness of β-cell insulin release in response to pyruvate generated during exercise.

Nesidioblastosis has also rarely been reported after bariatric surgery for obesity.

ENDOCRINE DEFICIENCY. Hypoglycemia associated with endocrine deficiency is usually caused by adrenal insufficiency with or without associated growth hormone deficiency (see Chapters 558 and 576). In panhypopituitarism, isolated adrenocorticotropic hormone (ACTH) or growth hormone deficiency, or combined ACTH deficiency plus growth hormone deficiency, the incidence of hypoglycemia is as high as 20%. In the newborn period, hypoglycemia may be the presenting feature of hypopituitarism; in males, a microphallus may provide a clue to a coexistent deficiency of gonadotropin. Newborns with hypopituitarism often have a form of "hepatitis" and the syndrome of **septo-optic dysplasia.** When adrenal disease is severe, as in congenital adrenal hyperplasia caused by cortisol synthetic enzyme defects, adrenal hemorrhage, or congenital absence of the adrenal glands, disturbances in serum electrolytes with hyponatremia and hyperkalemia or ambiguous genitals may provide diagnostic clues (see Chapter 577). In older children, failure of growth should suggest growth hormone deficiency. Hyperpigmentation may provide the clue to Addison disease with increased ACTH levels or adrenal unresponsiveness to ACTH owing to a defect in the adrenal receptor for ACTH. The frequent association of Addison disease in childhood with hypoparathyroidism (hypocalcemia), chronic mucocutaneous candidiasis, and other endocrinopathies should be considered. Adrenoleukodystrophy should also be considered in the differential diagnosis of primary Addison disease in older children (see Chapter 86.2).

Hypoglycemia in cortisol–growth hormone deficiency may be caused by decreased gluconeogenic enzymes with cortisol deficiency, increased glucose utilization due to a lack of the antagonistic effects of growth hormone on insulin action, or failure to supply endogenous gluconeogenic substrate in the form of alanine and lactate with compensatory breakdown of fat and generation of ketones. Deficiency of these hormones results in reduced gluconeogenic substrate, which resembles the syndrome of ketotic hypoglycemia. Investigation of a child with hypoglycemia, therefore, requires exclusion of ACTH-cortisol or growth hormone deficiency and, if diagnosed, its appropriate replacement with cortisol or growth hormone.

Epinephrine deficiency could theoretically be responsible for hypoglycemia. Urinary excretion of epinephrine has been diminished in some patients with spontaneous or insulin-induced hypoglycemia in whom absence of pallor and tachycardia was also noted, suggesting that failure of catecholamine release, due to a defect anywhere along the hypothalamic-autonomic-adrenomedullary axis, might be responsible for the hypoglycemia. This possibility has been challenged, owing to the rarity of hypoglycemia in patients with bilateral adrenalectomy, provided that they receive adequate glucocorticoid replacement, and because diminished epinephrine excretion is found in normal patients with repeated insulin-induced hypoglycemia. Many of the patients described as having hypoglycemia with failure of epinephrine excretion fit the criteria for ketotic hypoglycemia.

Glucagon deficiency in infants or children may rarely be associated with hypoglycemia.

SUBSTRATE LIMITED

Ketotic Hypoglycemia. This is the **most common** form of childhood hypoglycemia. This condition usually presents between the ages of 18 mo and 5 yr and remits spontaneously by the age of 8–9 yr. Hypoglycemic episodes typically occur during periods of intercurrent illness when food intake is limited. The classic history is of a child who eats poorly or completely avoids the evening meal, is difficult to arouse from sleep the following morning, and may have a seizure or be comatose by midmorning. Another common presentation occurs when parents sleep late and the affected child is unable to eat breakfast, thus prolonging the overnight fast.

At the time of documented hypoglycemia, there is associated ketonuria and ketonemia; plasma insulin concentrations are appropriately low, ≤5–10 μU/mL, thus excluding hyperinsulinemia. A ketogenic provocative diet, formerly used as a diagnostic test, is not essential to establish the diagnosis because fasting alone provokes a hypoglycemic episode with ketonemia and ketonuria within 12–18 hr in susceptible individuals. Normal children of similar age can withstand fasting without hypoglycemia developing during the same period, although even normal children may acquire these features by 36 hr of fasting.

Children with ketotic hypoglycemia have plasma alanine concentrations that are markedly reduced in the basal state after an overnight fast and decline even further with prolonged fasting. Alanine, produced in muscle, is a major gluconeogenic precursor. Alanine is the only amino acid that is significantly lower in these children, and infusions of alanine (250 mg/kg) produce a rapid rise in plasma glucose without causing significant changes in blood lactate or pyruvate levels, indicating that the entire gluconeogenic pathway from the level of pyruvate is intact, but that there is a deficiency of substrate. Glycogenolytic pathways are also intact because glucagon induces a normal glycemic response in affected children in the fed state. The levels of hormones that counter hypoglycemia are appropriately elevated, and insulin is appropriately low.

The etiology of ketotic hypoglycemia may be a defect in any of the complex steps involved in protein catabolism, oxidative deamination of amino acids, transamination, alanine synthesis, or alanine efflux from muscle. Children with ketotic hypoglycemia are frequently smaller than age-matched controls and often have a history of transient neonatal hypoglycemia. Any decrease in muscle mass may compromise the supply of gluconeogenic substrate at a time when glucose demands per unit of body weight are already relatively high, thus predisposing the patient to the rapid development of hypoglycemia, with ketosis representing the attempt to switch to an alternative fuel supply. Children with ketotic hypoglycemia may represent the low end of the spectrum of children's capacity to tolerate fasting. Similar relative intolerance to fasting is present in normal children, who cannot maintain blood glucose after 30–36 hr of fasting, compared with the adult's capacity for prolonged fasting. Although the defect may be present at birth, it may not be evident until the child is stressed by more prolonged periods of calorie restriction. Moreover, the spontaneous remission observed in children at age 8–9 yr might be explained by the increase in muscle bulk with its resultant increase in supply of endogenous substrate and the relative decrease in glucose requirement per unit of body mass with increasing age. There is also some evidence to support the contention that impaired epinephrine secretion from immaturity of autonomic innervation contributes to ketotic hypoglycemia. Rarely, inborn errors of fatty acid metabolism present as ketotic hypoglycemia, although, typically, fatty acid oxidation defects produce hypoketotic hypoglycemia.

In anticipation of spontaneous resolution of this syndrome, **treatment** of ketotic hypoglycemia consists of frequent feedings of a high-protein, high-carbohydrate diet. During intercurrent illnesses, parents should test the child's urine for the presence of ketones, the appearance of which precedes hypoglycemia by several hours. In the presence of ketonuria, liquids of high carbohydrate content should be offered to the child. If these cannot be tolerated, the child should be admitted to the hospital for intravenous glucose administration.

Branched-Chain Ketonuria (Maple Syrup Urine Disease) [See Chapter 85.6]. The hypoglycemic episodes were once attributed to high levels of leucine, but evidence indicates that interference with the production of alanine and its availability as a gluconeogenic substrate during calorie deprivation is responsible for hypoglycemia.

GLYCOGEN STORAGE DISEASE. See Chapter 87.1.

Glucose-6-Phosphatase Deficiency (Type I Glycogen Storage Disease). Affected children usually display a remarkable tolerance to their chronic hypoglycemia; blood glucose values in the range of 20–50 mg/dL are not associated with the classic symptoms of hypoglycemia, possibly reflecting the adaptation of the CNS to ketone bodies as an alternative fuel.

Affected untreated children manifest growth failure, mental retardation, and a shortened life span unless they are treated. Continuous intragastric feeding improves the metabolic and clinical findings by reducing the frequency and severity of hypoglycemia, thereby avoiding the secondary hormonal changes that appear to be responsible for the metabolic derangements. Continuous intragastric feeding at night, combined with frequent daytime feedings, produces equally effective amelioration of the biochemical disturbances and avoids the inconvenience of 24 hr continuous gastric feeding. The daytime feedings are given every 3–4 hr: 60–70% of the calories as carbohydrate low in fructose and galactose, 12–15% of the calories as protein, and 15–25% of the calories as fat. At night, a small nasogastric tube is passed by the patient (or a parent for younger children), and approximately one third of the daily caloric requirements is continuously infused over 8–12 hr using a small continuous infusion pump. One commercially available formula for nocturnal infusion contains 89% of the calories as glucose and glucose oligosaccharides, 1.8% as safflower oil, and 9.2% as crystalline amino acids (Vivonex, Novartis Nutrition, St. Louis Park MN 55416). Nocturnal cornstarch therapy is also beneficial. Transient nocturnal hypoglycemia is not completely prevented, and renal glomerular dysfunction plus formation of hepatic adenoma remain serious complications. Liver transplantation offers promise of long-term cure.

Amylo-1,6-Glucosidase Deficiency (Debrancher Enzyme Deficiency; Type III Glycogen Storage Disease). See Chapter 87.

Liver Phosphorylase Deficiency (Type VI Glycogen Storage Disease) [See Chapter 87]. Low hepatic phosphorylase activity may result from a defect in any of the steps of activation; a variety of defects have been described. Hepatomegaly, excessive deposition of glycogen in liver, growth retardation, and occasional symptomatic hypoglycemia occur. A diet high in protein and reduced in carbohydrate usually prevents hypoglycemia.

Glycogen Synthetase Deficiency (See Chapter 87). The inability to synthesize glycogen is rare. There is hypoglycemia and hyperketonemia after fasting because glycogen reserves are markedly diminished or absent. After feeding, however, hyperglycemia with glucosuria may occur because of the inability to assimilate some of the glucose load into glycogen. During fasting hypoglycemia, levels of the counter-regulatory hormones, including catecholamines, are appropriately elevated or normal, and insulin levels are appropriately low. The liver is not enlarged. Protein-rich feedings at frequent intervals result in dramatic clinical improvement, including growth velocity. This condition mimics the syndrome of ketotic hypoglycemia and should be considered in the differential diagnosis of that syndrome.

DISORDERS OF GLUCONEOGENESIS

Fructose-1,6-Diphosphatase Deficiency (See Chapter 87.3). A deficiency of this enzyme results in a block of gluconeogenesis from all possible precursors below the level of fructose-1,6-diphosphate. Infusion of these gluconeogenic precursors results in lactic acidosis without a rise in glucose; acute hypoglycemia may be provoked by inhibition of glycogenolysis. Glycogenolysis remains intact, and glucagon elicits a normal glycemic response in the fed, but not in the fasted, state. Accordingly, affected individuals have hypoglycemia only during caloric deprivation, as in fasting, or during intercurrent illness. As long as glycogen stores remain normal, hypoglycemia does not develop. In affected families, there may be a history of siblings with known hepatomegaly who died in infancy with unexplained metabolic acidosis.

Clinical features simulate those of type I glycogen storage disease. Hepatomegaly in individuals with fructose-1,6-diphosphatase deficiency is due to lipid storage rather than glycogen storage. Lactic acidosis, ketosis, hyperlipidemia, and hyperuricemia occur; their pathogenesis is related to the severity and duration of hypoglycemia and the resultant low levels of insulin and high levels of counter-regulatory hormones. Therapy for these infants, consisting of a diet high in carbohydrates (56%, excluding fructose, which cannot be utilized), low in protein (12%), and normal in fat composition (32%), has permitted normal growth and development. Continuous nocturnal provision of calories through the intragastric infusion system described earlier for type I glycogen storage disease is also applicable to children with fructose-1,6-diphosphatase deficiency. During intercurrent illnesses with vomiting, intravenous glucose infusion is necessary to prevent severe hypoglycemia.

Defects in Fatty Acid Oxidation (See Chapter 86). The important role of fatty acid oxidation in maintaining gluconeogenesis is underscored by examples of congenital or drug-induced defects in fatty acid metabolism that may be associated with fasting hypoglycemia.

Various congenital enzymatic deficiencies causing defective carnitine or fatty acid metabolism occur. A severe and relatively common form of fasting hypoglycemia with hepatomegaly, cardiomyopathy, and hypotonia occurs with long- and medium-chain fatty acid coenzyme-A dehydrogenase deficiency (LCAD and MCAD). Plasma carnitine levels are low, ketones are not present in urine, but dicarboxylic aciduria is present. Clinically, patients with **acyl CoA dehydrogenase deficiency** present with a Reye-like syndrome (see Chapter 358), recurrent episodes of severe fasting hypoglycemic coma, and cardiorespiratory arrest (sudden infant death syndrome–like events). Severe hypoglycemia and metabolic acidosis without ketosis also occur in patients with multiple acyl CoA dehydrogenase disorders. Hypotonia, seizures, and acrid odor are other clinical clues. Survival depends on whether the defects are severe or mild; diagnosis is established from studies of enzyme activity in liver biopsy tissue or in cultured fibroblasts from affected patients. Tandem mass spectrometry can be employed for blood samples, even those on filter paper, for screening of congenital inborn errors. The frequency of this disorder is at least 1/10,000–15,000 births. Avoidance of fasting and supplementation with carnitine may be lifesaving in these patients who generally present in infancy.

Interference with fatty acid metabolism also underlies the fasting hypoglycemia associated with Jamaican vomiting sickness, with atractyloside, and with the drug valproate. In **Jamaican vomiting sickness,** the unripe ackee fruit contains a water-soluble toxin, hypoglycin, which produces vomiting, CNS depression, and severe hypoglycemia. The hypoglycemic activity of hypoglycin derives from its inhibition of gluconeogenesis secondary to its interference with the acyl CoA and carnitine metabolism essential for the oxidation of long-chain fatty acids. The disease is almost totally confined to Jamaica, where ackee forms a staple of the diet for the poor. The ripe ackee fruit no longer contains this toxin. *Atractyloside* is a reagent that inhibits oxidative phosphorylation in mitochondria by preventing the translocation of adenine nucleotides, such as ATP, across the mitochondrial membrane. Atractyloside is a perhydrophenanthrenic glycoside derived from *Atractylis gummifera.* This plant is found in the Mediterranean basin; ingestion of this "thistle" is associated with hypoglycemia and a syndrome similar to Jamaican vomiting sickness. The anticonvulsant drug **valproate** is associated with side effects, predominantly in young infants, which include a Reye-like syndrome, low serum carnitine levels, and the potential for fasting hypoglycemia. In all these conditions, hypoglycemia *is not associated with ketonuria.*

Acute Alcohol Intoxication. The liver metabolizes alcohol as a preferred fuel, and generation of reducing equivalents during the oxidation of ethanol alters the NADH:NAD ratio, which is essential for certain gluconeogenic steps. As a result, gluconeogenesis is impaired and hypoglycemia may ensue if glycogen stores are depleted by starvation or by pre-existing abnormalities in glycogen metabolism. In toddlers who have been unfed for some time, even the consumption of small quantities of alcohol can precipitate these events. The hypoglycemia promptly responds to intravenous glucose, which should always be considered in a child who presents initially with coma or seizure, after taking a blood sample to determine glucose concentration. The possibility of the child's ingesting alcoholic drinks must also be considered if there was a preceding adult evening party. A careful history allows the diagnosis to be made and may avoid needless and expensive hospitalization and investigation.

Salicylate Intoxication (See Chapter 58). Both hyperglycemia and hypoglycemia occur in children with salicylate intoxication. Accelerated utilization of glucose, resulting from augmentation of insulin secretion by salicylates, and possible interference with gluconeogenesis may contribute to hypoglycemia. Infants are more susceptible than are older children. Monitoring of blood glucose levels with appropriate glucose infusion in the event of hypoglycemia should form part of the therapeutic approach to salicylate intoxication in childhood. Ketosis may occur.

Phosphoenol Pyruvate Carboxykinase Deficiency. Deficiency of this rate-limiting gluconeogenic enzyme is associated with severe fasting hypoglycemia and variable onset after birth. Hypoglycemia may occur within 24 hr after birth, and defective gluconeogenesis from alanine can be documented in vivo. Liver, kidney, and myocardium demonstrate fatty infiltration, and atrophy of the optic nerve and visual cortex may occur. Hypoglycemia may be profound. Lactate and pyruvate levels in plasma have been normal, but a mild metabolic acidosis may be present. The fatty infiltration of various organs is caused by increased formation of acetyl CoA, which becomes available for fatty acid synthesis. Diagnosis of this rare entity can be made with certainty only through appropriate enzymatic determinations in liver biopsy material. Avoidance of periods of fasting through frequent feedings rich in carbohydrate should be helpful because glycogen synthesis and breakdown are intact.

Pyruvate Carboxylase Deficiency (See Chapter 87). This is predominantly a disease of the CNS characterized by a subacute necrotizing encephalomyelopathy and high levels of blood lactate and pyruvate. Hypoglycemia is not a prominent feature of this syndrome, presumably because gluconeogenesis from precursors other than alanine remains intact, and these precursors bypass the pyruvate carboxylase step. The utilization of alanine as well as lactate through pyruvate cannot proceed, however, so these substrates accumulate in blood, and modest hypoglycemia may result during fasting. Affected patients usually die of progressive CNS disease.

OTHER ENZYME DEFECTS

Galactosemia (Galactose-1-Phosphate Uridyl Transferase Deficiency). See Chapter 87.

Fructose Intolerance (Fructose-1-Phosphate Aldolase Deficiency) [See Chapter 87]. Acute hypoglycemia is due to the inhibition by fructose-1-phosphate of glycogenolysis via the phosphorylase system and of gluconeogenesis at the level of fructose-1,6-diphosphate aldolase. Affected individuals usually learn spontaneously to eliminate fructose from their diet.

DEFECTS IN GLUCOSE TRANSPORTERS

GLUT-1 Deficiency. Two infants with a seizure disorder were found to have low cerebrospinal fluid (CSF) glucose concentrations despite normal plasma glucose. Lactate concentrations in CSF were also low, suggesting decreased glycolysis rather than bacterial infection, which causes low CSF glucose with high lactate. The erythrocyte glucose transporter was defective, suggesting a similar defect in the brain glucose transporter responsible for the clinical features. A ketogenic diet reduced the severity of seizures by supplying an alternate source of brain fuel that bypassed the defect in glucose transport.

GLUT-2 Deficiency. Children with hepatomegaly, galactose intolerance, and renal tubular dysfunction (**Fanconi-Bickel syndrome**) have been shown to have a deficiency of the GLUT-2 glucose transporter of plasma membranes. In addition to liver and kidney tubules, GLUT-2 is also expressed in pancreatic β cells. Hence, the clinical manifestations reflect impaired glucose release from liver and defective tubular reabsorption of glucose plus phosphaturia and aminoaciduria.

SYSTEMIC DISORDERS. Several systemic disorders are associated with hypoglycemia in infants and children. Neonatal sepsis is often associated with hypoglycemia, possibly as a result of diminished caloric intake with impaired gluconeogenesis. Similar mechanisms may apply to the hypoglycemia found in severely malnourished infants or those with severe malabsorption. Hyperviscosity with a central hematocrit of >65% is associated with hypoglycemia in at least 10–15% of affected infants. **Falciparum malaria** has been associated with hyperinsulinemia and hypoglycemia. Heart and renal failure have also been associated with hypoglycemia, but the mechanism is obscure. Infants and children with **Nissen fundoplication,** a relatively common procedure used to ameliorate gastroesophageal reflux, frequently have an associated "dumping" syndrome with hypoglycemia. Characteristic features include significant hyperglycemia of up to

500 mg/dL 30 minutes postprandially and severe hypoglycemia (average 32 mg/dL in one series) 1.5–3.0 hr later. The early hyperglycemia phase is associated with brisk and excessive insulin release that causes the rebound hypoglycemia. Glucagon responses have been inappropriately low in some. Although the physiologic mechanisms are not always clearly apparent, and attempted treatments not always effective, **acarbose,** an inhibitor of glucose absorption, has been reported to be successful in one small series.

DIAGNOSIS AND DIFFERENTIAL DIAGNOSIS

Table 92-8 lists the pertinent clinical and biochemical findings in the common childhood disorders associated with hypoglycemia. A careful and detailed history is essential in every suspected or documented case of hypoglycemia (see Table 92-7). Specific points to be noted include age at onset, temporal relation to meals or caloric deprivation, and a family history of prior infants known to have had hypoglycemia or of unexplained infant deaths. In the 1st wk of life, the majority of infants have the transient form of neonatal hypoglycemia either as a result of prematurity/intrauterine growth retardation or by virtue of being born to diabetic mothers. The absence of a history of maternal diabetes, but the presence of macrosomia and the characteristic large plethoric appearance of an "infant of a diabetic mother" should arouse suspicion of hyperinsulinemic hypoglycemia of infancy probably due to a K_{ATP} channel defect that is familial (autosomal recessive) or sporadic; plasma insulin concentrations >10 μU/mL in the presence of documented hypoglycemia confirm this diagnosis. The presence of hepatomegaly should arouse suspicion of an enzyme deficiency; if non–glucose-reducing sugar is present in the urine, galactosemia is most likely. In males, the presence of a microphallus suggests the possibility of hypopituitarism, which also may be associated with jaundice in both sexes.

Past the newborn period, clues to the cause of persistent or recurrent hypoglycemia can be obtained through a careful history, physical examination, and initial laboratory findings. The temporal relation of the hypoglycemia to food intake may suggest that the defect is one of gluconeogenesis, if symptoms occur 6 hr or more after meals. If hypoglycemia occurs shortly after meals, galactosemia or fructose intolerance is most likely, and the presence of reducing substances in the urine rapidly distinguishes these possibilities. The autosomal dominant forms of hyperinsulinemic hypoglycemia need to be considered, with measurement of glucose, insulin, and ammonia, and careful history for other affected family members of any age. Measurement of IGFBP-1 may be useful; it is low in hyperinsulinemia states and high in other forms of hypoglycemia. The presence of hepatomegaly suggests one of the enzyme deficiencies in glycogen breakdown or in gluconeogenesis, as outlined in Table 92-8. The absence of ketonemia or ketonuria at the time of initial presentation strongly suggests hyperinsulinemia or a defect in fatty acid oxidation. In most other causes of hypoglycemia, with the exception of galactosemia and fructose intolerance, ketonemia and ketonuria are present at the time of fasting hypoglycemia. At the time of the hypoglycemia, serum should be obtained for determination of hormones and substrates, followed by repeated measurement after an intramuscular or intravenous injection of glucagon, as outlined in Table 92-7. Interpretation of the findings is summarized in Table 92-8. Hypoglycemia with ketonuria in children between ages 18 mo and 5 yr is most likely to be ketotic hypoglycemia, especially if hepatomegaly is absent. The ingestion of a toxin, including alcohol or salicylate, can usually be excluded rapidly by the history. Inadvertent or deliberate drug ingestion and errors in dispensing medicines should also be considered.

When the history is suggestive, but acute symptoms are not present, a 24–36 hr supervised fast can usually provoke hypoglycemia and resolve the question of hyperinsulinemia or other conditions (see Table 92-8). Such a fast is contraindicated if a fatty acid oxidation defect is suspected; other approaches such as mass tandem spectrometry or molecular diagnosis, or both, should be considered. Because adrenal insufficiency may mimic ketotic hypoglycemia, plasma cortisol levels should be determined at the time of documented hypoglycemia; increased buccal or skin pigmentation may provide the clue to primary adrenal insufficiency with elevated ACTH (melanocyte-stimulating hormone) activity. Short stature or a decrease in the growth rate may provide the clue to pituitary insufficiency involving growth hormone as well as ACTH. Definitive tests of pituitary-adrenal function such as the arginine-insulin stimulation test for growth hormone IGF-1, IGFBP-1, and cortisol release may be necessary.

In the presence of hepatomegaly and hypoglycemia, a presumptive diagnosis of the enzyme defect can often be made through the clinical manifestations, presence of hyperlipidemia, acidosis, hyperuricemia, response to glucagon in the fed and fasted states, and response to infusion of various appropriate precursors (see Tables 92-7 and 92-8). These clinical findings and investigative approaches are summarized in Table 92-8. Definitive diagnosis of the glycogen storage disease may require an open liver biopsy (see Chapter 87). Occasional patients with all the manifestations of glycogen storage disease are found to have normal enzyme activity. These definitive studies require special expertise available only in certain institutions.

TREATMENT

The prevention of hypoglycemia and its resultant effects on CNS development are important in the newborn period. For neonates with hyperinsulinemia not associated with maternal diabetes, subtotal or focal pancreatectomy may be needed, unless hypoglycemia can be readily controlled with long-term diazoxide or somatostatin analogs.

Treatment of **acute symptomatic neonatal** or infant hypoglycemia includes intravenous administration of 2 mL/kg of D_{10} W, followed by a continuous infusion of glucose at 6–8 mg/kg/min, adjusting the rate to maintain blood glucose levels in the normal range. If hypoglycemic seizures are present, some recommend a 4 mL/kg bolus of D_{10} W.

The management of **persistent** neonatal or infantile hypoglycemia includes increasing the rate of intravenous glucose infusion to 10–15 mg/kg/min or more, if needed. This may require a central venous or umbilical venous catheter to administer a hypertonic 15–25% glucose solution. If hyperinsulinemia is present, it should be medically managed initially with diazoxide and then somatostatin analogs or calcium channel blockers. If hypoglycemia is unresponsive to intravenous glucose plus diazoxide (maximal doses up to 25 mg/kg/day) and somastostatin analogs, surgery via partial or near-total pancreatectomy should be considered.

Oral diazoxide, 10–25 mg/kg/24 hr given in divided doses every 6 hr, may reverse hyperinsulinemic hypoglycemia but may also produce hirsutism, edema, nausea, hyperuricemia, electrolyte disturbances, advanced bone age, IgG deficiency, and, rarely, hypotension with prolonged use. A long-acting somatostatin analog (octreotide, formerly SMS 201–995) is sometimes effective in controlling hyperinsulinemic hypoglycemia in patients with islet cell disorders not caused by genetic mutations in K_{ATP} channel and islet cell adenoma. Octreotide is administered subcutaneously every 6–12 hr in doses of 20–50 μg in neonates and young infants. Potential but unusual complications include poor growth due to inhibition of growth hormone release, pain at the injection site, vomiting, diarrhea, and hepatic dysfunction (hepatitis, cholelithiasis). Octreotide is usually employed as a temporizing agent for various periods before subtotal pancreatectomy for K_{ATP} channel disorders. It may be particularly useful for the treatment of refractory hypoglycemia despite subtotal pancreatectomy. Total pancreatectomy is not optimal therapy, owing to the risks of surgery, permanent diabetes mellitus, and exocrine pancreatic insufficiency. Continued prolonged medical therapy without pancreatic resection if hypoglycemia is controllable is worthwhile because some children have a spontaneous resolution of the hyperinsulinemic hypoglycemia. This should be balanced against the risk of hypoglycemia-induced CNS injury and the toxicity of drugs.

PROGNOSIS

The prognosis is good in asymptomatic neonates with hypoglycemia of short duration. Hypoglycemia recurs in 10–15% of infants after adequate treatment. Recurrence is more common if intravenous fluids are extravasated or discontinued too rapidly before oral feedings are well tolerated. Children in whom ketotic hypoglycemia later develops have an increased incidence of neonatal hypoglycemia.

The prognosis for normal intellectual function must be guarded because prolonged, recurrent, and severe symptomatic hypoglycemia is associated with neurologic sequelae. Symptomatic infants with hypoglycemia, particularly low-birthweight infants, those with persistent hyperinsulinemic hypoglycemia, and infants of diabetic mothers, have a poorer prognosis for subsequent normal intellectual development than asymptomatic infants do.

Ahmad A, Kahler SG, Kishnani PS, et al: Treatment of pyruvate carboxylase deficiency with high doses of citrate and aspartate. *Am J Med Genet* 1999;87:331–338.

Bachrach BE, Weinstein DA, Orbo-Melander M, et al: Glycogen synthase deficiency (glycogen storage disease type 0) presenting with hyperglycemia and glucosuria: Report of three new mutations. *J Pediatr* 2002;140: 781–783.

Dacou-Voutetakis C, Psychou F, Maniati-Christidis M: Persistent hyperinsulinemic hypoglycemia of infancy: Long term results. *J Pediatr Endocrinol Metab* 1998;11:131–141.

Dalgic N, Ergenekon E, Soysal S, et al: Transient neonatal hypoglycemia—Long-term effects on neurodevelopmental outcome. *J Pediatr Endocrinol Metab* 2002;15:319–324.

DeBaun MR, King AA, White N: Hypoglycemia in Beckwith-Wiedemann syndrome. *Semin Perinatol* 2000;24:164–171.

de Lonlay P, Benelli C, Fouque F, et al: Hyperinsulinism and hyperammonemia syndrome: Report of 12 unrelated patients. *Pediatr Res* 2001;50:353–357.

de Lonlay P, Cuer M, Vuillaumier-Barrot S, et al: Hyperinsulinemic hypoglycemia as a presenting sign in phosphomannose isomerase deficiency: A new manifestation of carbohydrate-deficient glycoprotein syndrome treatable with mannose. *J Pediatr* 1999;135:379–383.

de Lonlay P, Giurgea I, Touati G, et al: Neonatal hypoglycaemia: Aetiologies. *Semin Neonatol* 2004;9:49–58.

de Lonlay-Debeney P, Poggi-Travert F, Fournet J-C, et al: Clinical features of 52 neonates with hyperinsulinism. *N Engl J Med* 1999;340:1169–1175.

DeVivo DC, Trifiletti RR, Jacobson RI, et al: Defective glucose transport across the blood-brain barrier as a cause of persistent hypoglycorrhachia, seizures, and developmental delay. *N Engl J Med* 1991;325:703–709.

Dunne MJ, Kane C, Shepherd RM, et al: Familial persistent hyperinsulinemic hypoglycemia of infancy and mutations in the sulfonylurea receptor. *N Engl J Med* 1997;336:703–706.

Freckmann ML, Thorburn DR, Kirby DM, et al: Mitochondrial electron transport chain defect presenting as hypoglycemia. *J Pediatr* 1997;130: 431–436.

Giurgea I, Laborde K, Touati G, et al: Acute insulin responses to calcium and tolbutamide do not differentiate focal from diffuse congenital hyperinsulinism. *J Clin Endocrinol Metab* 2004;89:925–929.

Glaser B, Kesavan P, Heyman M, et al: Familial hyperinsulinism caused by an activating glucokinase mutation. *N Engl J Med* 1998;338:226–230.

Hardy OT, Hernandez-Pampaloni M, Saffer JR, et al: Diagnosis and localization of focal congenital hyperinsulinism by 18f-fluorodopa PET scan. *J Pediatr* 2007;150:140–145.

Huopio H, Reimann F, Ashfield R, et al: Dominantly inherited hyperinsulinism caused by a mutation in the sulfonylurea receptor type 1. *J Clin Invest* 2000;106:897–906.

Katz LE, Ferry RJ Jr, Stanley CA, et al: Suppression of insulin over-secretion by subcutaneous recombinant human insulin-like growth factor 1 in children with congenital hyperinsulinism due to defective beta-cell sulfonylurea receptor. *J Clin Endocrinol Metab* 1999;84:3117–3124.

Kelly A, Ng D, Ferry RJ Jr, et al: Acute insulin responses to leucine in children with the hyperinsulinism/hyperammonemia syndrome. *J Clin Endocrinol Metab* 2001;86:3724–3728.

Kinnala A, Rikalainen H, Lapinleimu H, et al: Cerebral magnetic resonance imaging and ultrasonography findings after neonatal hypoglycemia. *Pediatrics* 1999;103:724–729.

Lucas A, Morley R, Cole TJ: Adverse neurodevelopmental outcome of moderate neonatal hypoglycemia. *Br Med J* 1988;297:1304–1308.

Magge SN, Shyng SL, MacMullen C, et al: Familial leucine-sensitive hypoglycemia of infancy due to a dominant mutation of the beta-cell sulfonylurea receptor. *J Clin Endocrinol Metab* 2004;89:4450–4456.

Mayefsky JH, Sarnaik AP, Postellon DC: Factitious hypoglycemia. *Pediatrics* 1982;69:804–805.

Meissner T, Wendel U, Burgard P, et al: Long-term follow-up of 114 patients with congenital hyperinsulinism. *Eur J Endocrinol* 2003;149:43–51.

Melis D, Parenti G, Della CR, et al: Brain damage in glycogen storage disease type I. *J Pediatr* 2004;144:637–642.

Menni F, deLonlay P, Sevin C, et al: Neurologic outcomes of 90 neonates and infants with persistent hyperinsulinemic hypoglycemia. *Pediatrics* 2001;107:476–479.

Molven A, Rishaung U, Matre GE, et al: Hunting for a hypoglycemia gene: Severe neonatal hypoglycemia in a consanguineous family. *Am J Med Genet* 2002;113:40–46.

Ng DD, Ferry RJ Jr, Kelly A, et al: Acarbose treatment of postprandial hypoglycemia in children after Nissen fundoplication. *J Pediatr* 2001;139: 877–879.

Njuguna P, Newton C: Management of severe falciparum malaria. *J Postgrad Med* 2004;50:45–50.

Osier FH, Berkley JA, Ross A, et al: Abnormal blood glucose concentrations on admission to a rural Kenyan district hospital: Prevalence and outcome. *Arch Dis Child* 2003;88:621–625.

Otonkoski T, Nanto-Salonen K, Seppanen M, et al: Noninvasive diagnosis of focal hyperinsulinism of infancy with [18F]-DOPA positron emission tomography. *Diabetes* 2006;55:13–18.

Otonkoski T, Kaminen N, Ustinov J, et al: Physical exercise-induced hyperinsulinemic hypoglycemia is an autosomal-dominant trait characterized by abnormal pyruvate-induced insulin release. *Diabetes* 2003;52:199–204.

Raizen DM, Brooks-Kayal A, Steinkrauss L, et al: Central nervous system hyperexcitability associated with glutamate dehydrogenase gain of function mutations. *J Pediatr* 2005;146:388–394.

Ribeiro MJ, de Lonlay P, Delzescaux T, et al: Characterization of hyperinsulinism in infancy assessed with PET and 18F-Fluoro-L-DOPA. *J Nucl Med* 2005;46:560–566.

Spar JA, Lewine JD, Orrison WW Jr: Neonatal hypoglycemia: CT and MR findings. *Am J Neuroradiol* 1994;15:1477–1478.

Sperling MA, Menon RK: Differential diagnosis and management of neonatal hypoglycemia. *Pediatr Clin North Am* 2004;51:703–723.

Stanley CA: Advances in diagnosis and treatment of hyperinsulinism in infants and children. *J Clin Endocrinol Metab* 2002;87:4857–4859.

Stanley CA, Thornton PS, Ganguly A, et al: Preoperative evaluation of infants with focal or diffuse congenital hyperinsulinism by intravenous acute insulin response tests and selective pancreatic arterial calcium stimulation. *J Clin Endocrinol Metab* 2004;89:288–296.

Steinkrauss L, Lipman TH, Hendell CD, et al: Effects of hypoglycemia on developmental outcome in children with congenital hyperinsulinism. *J Pediatr Nurs* 2005;20:109–118.

Sun L, Eklund EA, Chung WK, et al: Congenital disorder of glycosylation is presenting with hyperinsulinemic hypoglycemia and islet cell hyperplasia. *J Clin Endocrinol Metab* 2005;90:4371–4375.

Taylor SI, Barbetti F, Accili D, et al: Syndromes of autoimmunity and hypoglycemia: Autoantibodies directed against insulin and its receptor. *Endocrinol Metab Clin North Am* 1989;18:123–143.

Thornton PS, Satin-Smith MS, Herold K, et al: Familial hyperinsulinism with apparent autosomal dominant inheritance: Clinical and genetic differences from the autosomal recessive variant. *J Pediatr* 1998;132:9–14.

Traill Z, Squier M, Anslow P: Brain imaging in neonatal hypoglycaemia. *Arch Dis Child Fetal Neonatal Ed* 1998;79:F145–F147.

Vannucci RC, Vannucci SJ: Hypoglycemic brain injury. *Semin Neonatal* 2001;6:147–155.

Wang ML, Dorer DJ, Fleming MP, et al: Clinical outcomes of near-term infants. *Pediatrics* 2004;114:372–376.

Weber TA, Antognetti MR, Stacpoole PW, et al: Caveats when considering ketogenic diets for the treatment of pyruvate dehydrogenase complex deficiency. *J Pediatr* 2001;138:390–395.

Wolfsdorf JI, Crigler JF Jr: Effect of continuous glucose therapy begun in infancy on the long-term clinical course of patients with type I glycogen storage disease. *J Pediatr Gastroenterol Nutr* 1999;29:136–143.

Wiesli P, Brandle M, Schmid C, et al: Selective arterial calcium stimulation and hepatic venous sampling in the evaluation of hyperinsulinemic hypoglycemia: Potential and limitations. *J Vasc Interv Radiol* 2004;15: 1251–1256.

Part XI ▪ The Fetus and the Neonatal Infant

Chapter 93 ▪ Overview of Mortality and Morbidity

Barbara J. Stoll

Fetal and extrauterine life forms a continuum during which human growth and development are influenced by genetic, environmental, and social factors. The perinatal period is most often defined as the period from the 28th wk of gestation through the 7th day after birth (additional definitions include the 20th wk of gestation to the 7th day and the 20th wk of gestation to the 28th day). The neonatal period is defined as less than 28 days of life and may be further subdivided into the very early (birth to less than 24 hr), early (birth to less than 7 days), and late neonatal periods (7 days to less than 28 days).

Perinatal mortality is influenced by prenatal, maternal, and fetal conditions and by circumstances surrounding delivery. Perinatal deaths are associated with intrauterine growth restriction (IUGR); conditions that predispose the fetus to asphyxia, such as placental insufficiency; severe congenital malformations; and overwhelming early-onset neonatal infections (Table 93-1). Major causes of neonatal mortality are diseases associated with preterm birth and low birthweight (LBW) and lethal congenital anomalies. Neonatal mortality is highest during the 1st 24 hr of life and accounts for 65% of all infant deaths (deaths before 1 yr of age). Between 1980 and 2004, neonatal mortality rates in the United States declined by almost 50% to 4.7 per 1,000 live births (Fig. 93-1). Factors related to the decline include improved obstetric and neonatal management with a significant reduction in birthweight-specific neonatal mortality (Fig. 93-2). Further reduction in neonatal mortality will depend on prevention of preterm delivery and LBW, prenatal diagnosis and early management of congenital anomalies and infections, and timely effective diagnosis and treatment of diseases that result from adverse factors during pregnancy, labor, and/or delivery (see Table 93-1).

In the United States each year, approximately 6 million pregnancies, 4 million live births, 18,000 neonatal deaths, and 28,000 infant deaths occur. Eleven per cent of births are to teenage women between the ages of 15 and 19 yr; 34% are to unmarried women. Births among teenagers (especially 1st births) declined 31% between 1991 and 2002 (Fig. 93-3). Births to girls 10–14 years, very young mothers at great social and medical risk, declined substantially over this period. Births to unmarried women remain stable.

Infant mortality rates (deaths occurring from birth to 12 mo of age per 1,000 live births) vary by country; in 2002, rates were lowest in Singapore (2.4/1,000 births), moderate in the United States (7.0/1,000), and highest in developing countries (30–150/1,000). Medical, socioeconomic, and cultural factors influence perinatal and neonatal mortality. Preventive variables such as health education, prenatal care, nutrition, social support, risk identification, and obstetric care can effectively reduce perinatal and neonatal mortality. In the United States, 50% of infant deaths in 2002 were due to four causes (classified according to the International Classification of Diseases, 10th edition): congenital malformations, disorders relating to prematurity and unspecified LBW, sudden infant death syndrome (SIDS), and newborns affected by maternal complications of pregnancy. LBW (as a result of preterm delivery and/or IUGR) is a major determinant of both neonatal and infant mortality rates and, together with congenital anomalies (cardiac, central nervous system, respiratory), contributes significantly to childhood morbidity. The LBW rate is directly related to the variance of infant mortality rates among different countries. In the United States, increases in preterm births, especially of the most immature infants (under 750 g BW), may result in increases in both neonatal and infant mortality rates. In developing countries, malnutrition as well as respiratory and gastrointestinal infections are major causes of infant deaths.

The **LBW rate** (infants weighing 2,500 g or less at birth each year) in the United States increased from 6.6% to 8.1% between 1981 and 2004, whereas the very low birthweight (VLBW) rate (infants weighing 1,500 g or less at birth) increased from 1.1% to 1.47% of all births. In the past decade, LBW has increased among white infants, mainly because of an increase in multiple births (often associated with assisted reproduction), whereas among blacks, LBW has decreased (Fig. 93-4). Nonetheless, LBW and VLBW rates remain highest among black infants. Reasons for the racial disparity in LBW remain unclear. Despite advances in prenatal and obstetric care, racial disparity in birthweight persists, thus suggesting the need for novel prevention programs. Furthermore, although preterm LBW survival is better among black neonates (see Fig. 93-2), overall neonatal and infant mortality rates remain highest among blacks (Fig. 93-5), even those born to extremely low-risk mothers (married, aged 20–34 yr, ≥13 yr of education, adequate prenatal care, no medical risk factors, no alcohol or tobacco use during pregnancy). A reduction in the racial disparity in mortality is an important public health issue reflected in the U.S. National Health Objectives for the Year 2010.

LBW is caused by preterm birth, IUGR, or both factors. The predominant cause of LBW in the United States is preterm birth, whereas in developing countries, the cause is more often IUGR. Although IUGR does not appear to further increase the risk of mortality in preterm infants, both morbidity and mortality are increased in term growth-restricted infants. VLBW infants are most often premature (<37 wk of gestation), although IUGR may also complicate their early delivery. Even though VLBW occurs in only 1–2% of all infants in the United States, these births represent a large proportion of the neonatal and infant mortality and infants with both short- and long-term complications, including neurodevelopmental handicaps. The etiology of preterm birth is complex, multifactorial, and not completely understood. Causes include maternal diseases such as severe preeclampsia requiring elective delivery, premature rupture of membranes, uterine abnormalities, placental bleeding (abruptio, previa), multifetus gestation, drug misuse, maternal chronic illnesses, fetal distress, and infection. A complex interaction can be noted between infection, inflammation, and both preterm premature rupture of membranes and preterm birth. Infectious antecedents include maternal urinary tract infection, chorioamnionitis, bacterial vaginosis, and upper and lower genitourinary tract infection with a variety of agents (*Chlamydia trachomatis, Ureaplasma urealyticum, Mycoplasma hominis, Gardnerella vaginalis,* and group B streptococcus). In many cases, the cause of preterm delivery is unknown.

Although 99% of births occur in hospitals, only 83% of pregnant women receive the ideal of prenatal care in the 1st trimester. Many women who receive inadequate prenatal care are at risk for perinatal complications. Barriers to prenatal care include absent or insufficient money or insurance to pay for care; poor

TABLE 93-1. Major Causes of Perinatal and Neonatal Mortality

FETAL	PRETERM	FULL TERM
Placental insufficiency	Severe immaturity	Congenital anomalies
Intrauterine infection	Respiratory distress syndrome	Birth asphyxia, trauma
Severe congenital malformations (anomalies)	Intraventricular hemorrhage	Infection
Umbilical cord accident	Congenital anomalies	Meconium aspiration pneumonia
Abruptio placentae	Infection	Persistent pulmonary hypertension (PPHN)
Hydrops fetalis	Necrotizing enterocolitis	
	Bronchopulmonary dysplasia (BPD)	

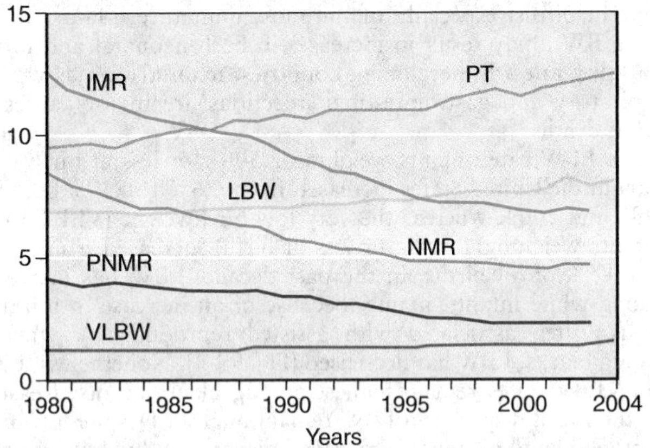

Figure 93-1. Infant, neonatal, and postneonatal mortality, low birthweight (LBW) and very low birthweight (VLBW), and preterm delivery: United States, 1980–2004. IMR indicates infant deaths per 1,000 live births; NMR, neonatal deaths per 1,000 live births; PNMR, postneonatal deaths per 1,000 live births; LBW, per cent LBW (<2,500 g); VLBW, per cent VLBW (<1,500 g); PT, per cent preterm (<37 weeks of gestation). (From Hoyert DL, Mathews TJ, Menacker F, et al: Annual summary of vital statistics: 2004. *Pediatrics* 2006;117:168–183).

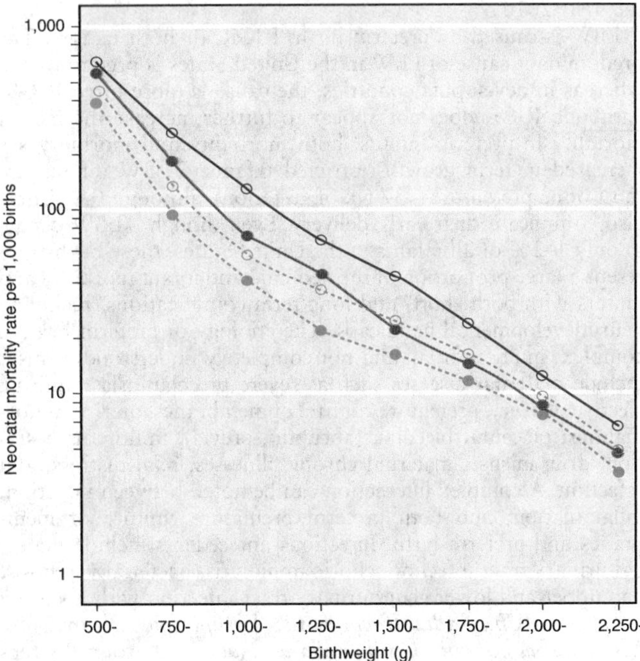

Figure 93-2. Neonatal mortality, by birthweight categories, for black *(filled circles)* and for white *(open circles)* infants in the United States. *Solid lines* denote data for 1989; *dashed lines* are for 1997. Data shown are for births of newborn infants weighing <2,250 g only. (From Demissie K, Rhoads GG, Ananth CV, et al: Trends in preterm birth and neonatal mortality among blacks and whites in the United States from 1989 to 1997. *Am J Epidemiol* 2001;154:307–315.)

coordination of services, including language and cultural issues; and inadequate effective education about the importance of prenatal care. Successful and adequate provision of high-quality prenatal care requires competent health care professionals and coordination of services among physicians' offices, clinics, community hospitals, special regionalized programs for high-risk mothers and infants, and tertiary care centers. Regional perinatal programs should provide continuing education and consultation in both the community and the referral center and transportation for pregnant women and newborn infants to appropriate hospitals; they should also include a regional hospital with facilities, equipment, and personnel for obstetric and neonatal intensive care (Table 93-2).

Fetal deaths slightly exceed neonatal deaths in their contribution to perinatal mortality. Obstetricians have a central role in reducing perinatal mortality and morbidity. Intrapartum fetal deaths have declined more than antepartum fetal deaths, reflecting improvements in care during labor and delivery. It is important to emphasize the need to be able to predict the maturity and functional reserve of a fetus both before and during labor so that fetuses and infants at greatest risk can be identified as early as possible. The obstetrician and pediatrician must effectively interact to anticipate perinatal problems and take prompt preventive and therapeutic measures.

Postneonatal mortality refers to deaths between 28 days and 1 yr of life. Historically, these infant deaths were due to causes outside the neonatal period, such as SIDS, infections (respiratory, enteric), and trauma. With the advent of modern neonatal care, many VLBW infants who would have died in the 1st mo of life now survive the neonatal period only to succumb to the seque-

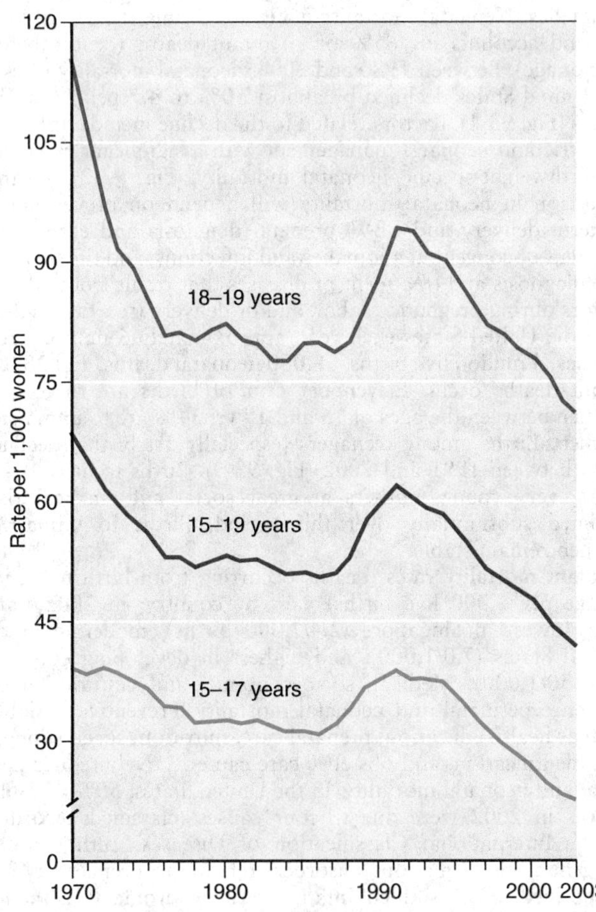

Figure 93-3. Birthrates for teenagers by age: United States, 1970–2003. (From Hamilton BE, Martin JA, Sutton PD: Births: Preliminary data for 2003. *Natl Vital Stat Rep* 2004;53:1–17.)

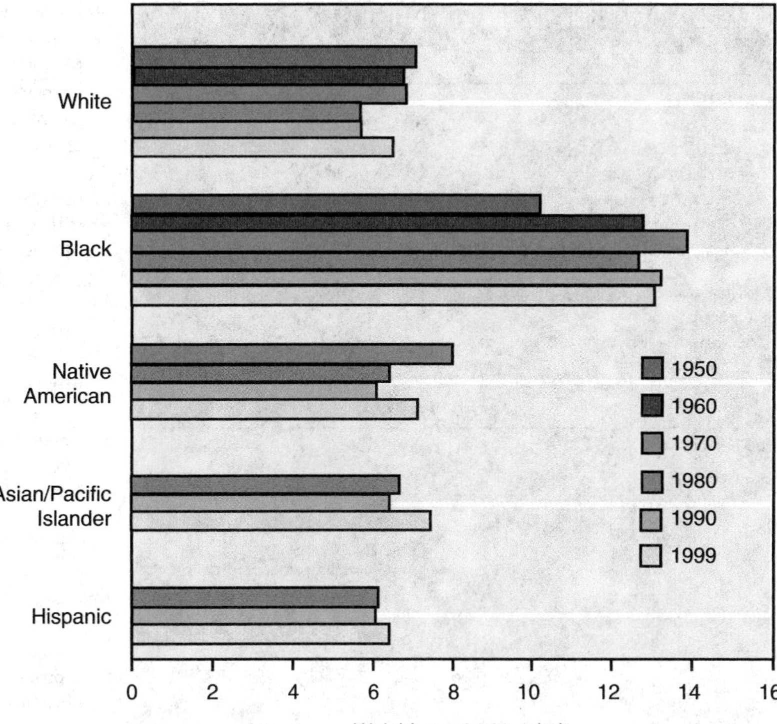

Figure 93-4. Per cent low birthweight by race and ethnicity, selected years: United States, 1950–1999. (From Guyer B, Freedman MA, Strobino DM, et al: Annual summary of vital statistics: Trends in the health of Americans during the 20th century. *Pediatrics* 2000;106:1307–1317.)

lae noted in Table 93-3. This delayed neonatal mortality is an important contributor to postneonatal mortality.

For the most immature infants at the limit of viability (22–25 wk gestation), decision-making regarding care is a complex process that involves the physician and other health professionals, and the family. The challenge for all premature infants is not only to improve survival, but also to reduce short-term complications and improve long-term neurodevelopmental outcome.

Adverse neurodevelopmental sequelae include cerebral palsy, seizures, and hydrocephalus requiring a shunt, blindness, deafness, and cognitive impairment. The risk of an adverse outcome

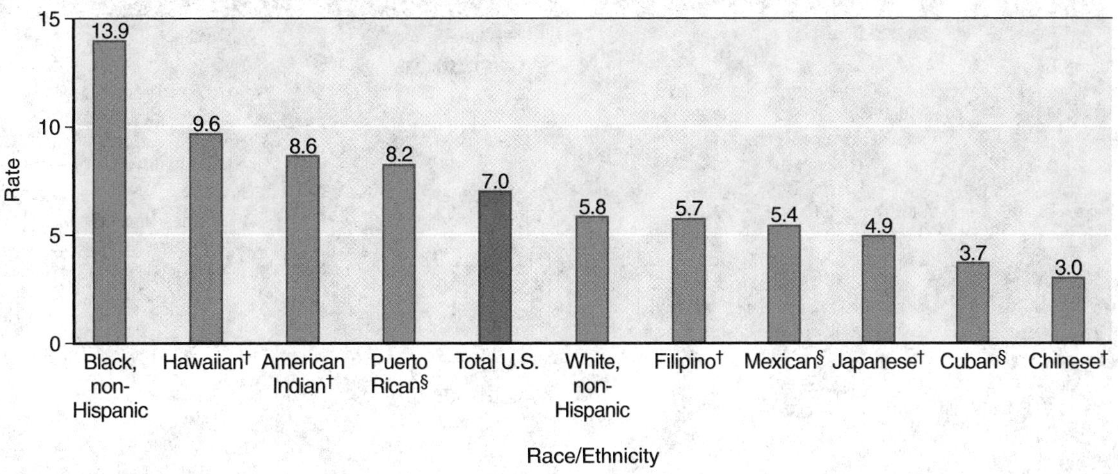

Figure 93-5. Infant mortality rates* by race and ethnicity, 2002. In 2002, the infant mortality rate was highest for infants of non-Hispanic black mothers. Infants of Hawaiian, Native American, and Puerto Rican mothers also had high rates. The lowest rates were observed for infants of Cuban and Chinese mothers. Additional birth data are available at http://www.cdc.gov/nchs/births.htm. (From Mathews TJ, Menacker F, MacDorman MF: Infant mortality statistics from the 2002 period linked birth/infant death data set. Available at http://www.cdc.gov/nchs/data/nvsr/nvsr53/nvsr53_10.pdf.)

*Per 1,000 live births.

†Can include persons of Hispanic and non-Hispanic origin.

‡Persons of Hispanic origin might be of any race.

TABLE 93-2. Levels of In-Hospital Perinatal Care

MATERNAL	NEONATE
BASIC	
Monitor and care for low-risk patients	Resuscitation Stabilization
Triage for high risk for transfer	Well neonatal care
Detection and care of unanticipated labor problems	Nursery care
Emergency cesarean delivery within 30 min	Visitation General pediatrician staff (capable of neonatal resuscitation)
Blood bank, anesthesia, radiology, ultrasound, and laboratory support	
Care of postpartum problems	
Obstetrician, nurse, midwife staff	
SPECIAL CARE	
Basic services plus	*Basic services plus*
Care of high-risk pregnancies	Care of high-risk neonate with short-term problems
Triage, transfer of high-risk pregnancies (<32 wk, IUGR, preeclampsia, severe maternal medical illness)	Stabilization before transfer (<1,500 g, <32 wk, critically ill)
	Accept convalescing back (reverse) transfers
SUBSPECIALTY CARE	
Basic plus specialty care plus	*Basic plus specialty care plus*
Experienced perinatologist (24-hr coverage)	Experienced neonatologist (24-hr coverage)
Evaluation of high-risk therapies	Inborn plus transferred patients
Care for severe maternal medical or obstetric illnesses	Evaluation of high-risk therapies All pediatric medical, radiologic, and surgical subspecialties
High-risk fetal care (Rh disease, nonimmune hydrops, life-threatening anomalies)	NICU with operating room capabilities High-risk follow-up
Outcomes research	Outcomes research
Community education	Community education

IUGR, intrauterine growth retardation; NICU, neonatal intensive care unit.

From American Academy of Pediatrics, American College of Obstetricians and Gynecologists: *Guidelines for Perinatal Care,* 5th ed. Elk Grove Village, IL, American Academy of Pediatrics, 2002.

increases with decreasing gestational age at birth. Early morbidity and prognostic variables that contribute to adverse neurodevelopmental outcomes include grades 3–4 intraventricular hemorrhage, periventricular leukomalacia, necrotizing enterocolitis requiring extensive bowel resection, neonatal infections, bronchopulmonary dysplasia, and postnatal steroid therapy. The association of postnatal steroid use with adverse neurodevelopmental outcome highlights the importance of high-risk infant follow-up after hospital discharge to assess the long-term impact of new and/or frequently used therapies. Many studies have documented the impact of social and family risk factors on outcome. At school age, VLBW infants have poorer physical growth, cognitive function, and school performance. All VLBW infants must be monitored after discharge to detect neurodevelopmental impairment as early as possible and to ensure that children and families receive any interventions available and adequate support to optimize long-term outcome. Although disadvantages may persist into adulthood, recent data suggest that there may be cognitive improvement throughout childhood.

Baker LC, Afendulis CC, Chandra A, et al: Differences in neonatal mortality among whites and Asian American subgroups. *Arch Pediatr Adolesc Med* 2007;161:69–76.

Barrington KJ: Postnatal steroids and neurodevelopmental outcomes: A problem in the making. *Pediatrics* 2001;107:1425–1426.

Bhandari V, Bizzarro MJ, Shetty A, et al: Familial and genetic susceptibility to major neonatal morbidities in preterm twins. *Pediatrics* 2006;117:1901–1906.

Craig ED, Thompson JMD, Mitchell EA: Socioeconomic status and preterm birth: New Zealand trends, 1980 to 1999. *Arch Dis Child Fetal Neonatal Ed* 2002;86:F142–F146.

Department of Health and Human Services Centers for Disease Control and Prevention: Racial/ethnic disparities in neonatal mortality—United States, 1995–2002. *MMWR* 2004;54:553–556.

Goldenberg RL, Hauth JC, Andrews WW: Mechanisms of disease: Intrauterine infection and preterm delivery. *N Engl J Med* 2000;342:1500–1507.

TABLE 93-3. Morbidities and Sequelae of Perinatal and Neonatal Illness

MORBIDITIES	EXAMPLES
CENTRAL NERVOUS SYSTEM	
Spastic diplegic-quadriplegic cerebral palsy	Hypoxic-ischemic encephalopathy, periventricular leukomalacia, undetermined antenatal factors
Choreoathetotic cerebral palsy	Bilirubin encephalopathy (kernicterus)
Microcephaly	Hypoxic-ischemic encephalopathy, intrauterine infection (rubella, CMV)
Communicating hydrocephalus	Intraventricular hemorrhage, meningitis
Seizures	Hypoxic-ischemic encephalopathy, hypoglycemia
Encephalopathy	Congenital infections (rubella, CMV, human immunodeficiency virus, toxoplasmosis)
Educational failure and/or mental retardation	Immaturity, hypoxia, hypoglycemia, cerebral palsy, intraventricular hemorrhage low socioeconomic status
SENSATION—PERIPHERAL NERVES	
Reduced visual acuity (blindness)	Retinopathy of prematurity (ROP)
Strabismus	Undetermined, prematurity
Hearing impairment (deafness) encephalopathy, hypoxia ± hyperventilation	Drug toxicity (furosemide, aminoglycosides), bilirubin
Poor speech	Immaturity, chronic illness, hypoxia, prolonged endotracheal intubation, hearing deficit
Paralysis-paresis	Birth trauma—brachial plexus, phrenic nerve, spinal cord
RESPIRATORY	
Bronchopulmonary dysplasia (BPD)	Oxygen toxicity, barotrauma
Subglottic stenosis	Endotracheal tube injury
Sudden infant death syndrome	Prematurity, BPD, infant of illicit drug user
Choanal stenosis, nasal septum destruction	Nasotracheal intubation
	Growth failure
CARDIOVASCULAR	
Cyanosis	Precorrective palliative care of congenital cyanotic heart disease, cor pulmonale from BPD, reactive airway
Heart failure	Precorrective palliative care of complex congenital heart disease, BPD, ventricular septal defect
GASTROINTESTINAL	
Short-gut syndrome	Necrotizing enterocolitis, gastroschisis, malrotation-volvulus, cystic fibrosis, intestinal atresia
Cholestatic liver disease (cirrhosis, hepatic failure)	Hyperalimentation toxicity, sepsis, short-gut syndrome
Failure to thrive	Short-gut syndrome, cholestasis, BPD, cerebral palsy, severe congenital heart disease
Inguinal hernia	Unknown
MISCELLANEOUS	
Cutaneous scars	Chest tube or IV placement, hyperalimentation, subcutaneous infiltration, fetal puncture, intrauterine varicella, cutis aplasia
Absent radial artery pulse	Frequent arterial puncture
Hypertension	Renal thrombi, repair of coarctation of aorta

BPD, bronchopulmonary dysplasia; CMV, cytomegalovirus; ROP, retinopathy of prematurity.

Goodman DC, Fisher ES, Little GA, et al: The relation between the availability of neonatal intensive care and neonatal mortality. *N Engl J Med* 2002;346:1538–1544.

Gross SJ, Mettelman BB, Dye TD, et al: Impact of family structure and stability on academic outcome in preterm children at 10 years of age. *J Pediatr* 2001;138:169–175.

Hack M, Flannery DJ, Schluchter M, et al: Outcomes in young adulthood for very-low-birth-weight infants. *N Engl J Med* 2002;346:149–157.

Hamilton BE, Martin JA, Sutton PD, Centers for Disease Control and Prevention, National Center for Health Statistics: Births: Preliminary data for 2003. *Natl Vital Stat Rep* 2004;53:1–17.

Healthy People 2010, 2nd ed. Washington, DC, US Government Printing Office (Conference ed in 2 vol) (GPO stock No. 017-001-00547-9).

Hessol NA, Fuentes-Afflick E: Ethnic differences in neonatal and postneonatal mortality. *Pediatrics* 2005;115:e44–e51.

Horbar JD, Badger GJ, Carpenter JH, et al: Trends in mortality and morbidity for very low birth weight infants, 1991–1999. *Pediatrics* 2002; 110:143–151.

Hoyert DL, Mathews TJ, Menacker F, et al: Annual summary of vital statistics: 2004. *Pediatrics* 2006;117:168–183.

Lawn JE, Cousens S, Bhutta ZA, et al: Why are 4 million newborn babies dying each year? *Lancet* 2004;364:399–401.

Lawn JE, Cousens S, Zupan J, et al: 4 million neonatal deaths: When? Where? Why? *Lancet* 2004;365:891–908.

MacDorman MF, Martin JA, Mathews TJ, et al: Explaining the 2001–02 infant mortality increase: Data from the linked birth/infant death data set. *Natl Vital Stat Rep* 2005;53:1–22.

Martin JA, Kochanek KD, Strobino DM, et al: Annual summary of vital statistics—2003. *Pediatrics* 2005;115:619–634.

Menacker F, Martin JA, MacDorman MF, et al: Births to 10–14 year old mothers, 1990–2002: Trends and health outcomes. *Natl Vital Stat Rep* 2004;53:1–18.

Ment LR, Vohr B, Allan W, et al: Change in cognitive function over time in very low-birth-weight infants. *JAMA* 2003;289:705–711.

Chapter 94 ■ The Newborn Infant (see also Chapter 7) Barbara J. Stoll

The neonatal period is a highly vulnerable time for an infant, who is completing many of the physiologic adjustments required for extrauterine existence. The high neonatal morbidity and mortality rates attest to the fragility of life during this period; in the United States, of all deaths occurring in the 1st yr, two thirds are in the neonatal period. The annual rate of deaths during the 1st yr is unequaled until the 7th decade.

An infant's transition from intrauterine to extrauterine life requires many biochemical and physiologic changes. No longer dependent on maternal circulation via the placenta, the newborn's respiratory system must function for exchange of oxygen and carbon dioxide. Newborn infants are also dependent on gastrointestinal tract function for absorbing food, renal function for excreting waste and maintaining chemical homeostasis, hepatic function for neutralizing and excreting toxic substances, and function of the immunologic system for protecting against infection. The neonatal cardiovascular and endocrine systems also adapt for self-sufficient functioning. Many of a newborn infant's special problems are related to poor adaptation because of asphyxia, premature birth, life-threatening congenital anomalies, or the adverse effects of delivery.

94.1 • History in Neonatal Pediatrics

The neonatal history should (1) identify disabling diseases that are amenable to prompt preventive action or treatment (respiratory distress syndrome), (2) anticipate conditions that may be of later importance (gonococcal conjunctivitis), and (3) uncover possible causative factors that may explain pathologic conditions regardless of their immediate or future significance (screening for inborn errors of metabolism). The perinatal history should include demographic and social data (socioeconomic status, age, race); past medical illnesses in the mother and family, including previous siblings (cardiopulmonary disorders, infectious diseases, genetic disorders, anemia, jaundice, diabetes mellitus); previous maternal reproductive problems (stillbirth, prematurity, blood group sensitization); events occurring in the present pregnancy (vaginal bleeding, medications, acute illness, duration of rupture of membranes); and a description of the labor (duration, fetal presentation, fetal distress, fever) and delivery (cesarean section, anesthesia or sedation, use of forceps, Apgar score, need for resuscitation).

94.2 • Physical Examination of the Newborn Infant

Many physical and behavioral characteristics of a normal newborn infant are described in Chapters 7 and 591.

The **initial examination** of a newborn infant should be performed as soon as possible after delivery to detect abnormalities and to establish a baseline for subsequent examination. Infants should have temperature, pulse, respiratory rate, color, type of respiration, tone, activity, and level of consciousness monitored every 30 min after birth for 2 hr or until stabilized. For high-risk deliveries, this examination should take place in the delivery room and focus on congenital anomalies and pathophysiologic problems that may interfere with normal cardiopulmonary and metabolic adaptation to extrauterine life. Congenital anomalies may be present in 3–5% of infants. After a stable delivery room course, a 2nd and more detailed examination should be performed within 24 hr of birth. If an infant remains in the hospital longer than 48 hr, a **discharge examination** should be performed within 24 hr of discharge. With a healthy infant, the mother should be present during this examination; even minor, seemingly insignificant anatomic variations may worry a family and should be explained. The explanation must be careful and skillful so that otherwise unworried families are not unduly alarmed. No infant should be discharged from the hospital without a final examination because certain abnormalities, particularly heart murmurs, often appear or disappear in the immediate neonatal period; in addition, evidence of disease that has just been acquired may be noted. The pulse (normal, 120–160 beats/min), respiratory rate (normal, 30–60 breaths/min), temperature, weight, length, head circumference, and dimensions of any visible or palpable structural abnormality should be recorded. Blood pressure is determined if a neonate appears ill or has a heart murmur.

Examining a newborn requires patience, gentleness, and procedural flexibility. Thus, if the infant is quiet and relaxed at the beginning of the examination, palpation of the abdomen or auscultation of the heart should be performed 1st before other, more disturbing manipulations are attempted.

GENERAL APPEARANCE. Physical activity may be absent during the relaxation of normal sleep, or it may be decreased by the effects of illness or drugs; an infant may be either lying with the extremities motionless, to conserve energy for the effort of difficult breathing, or be vigorously crying with accompanying activity of the arms and legs. Both active and passive muscle tone and any unusual posture should be recorded. Coarse, tremulous movements with ankle or jaw **myoclonus** are more common and less significant in newborn infants than at any other age. Such movements tend to occur when an infant is active, whereas convulsive twitching usually occurs in a quiet state. **Edema** may produce a superficial appearance of good nutrition. Pitting after applied pressure may or may not be noted, but the skin of the fingers and toes lacks the normal fine wrinkles when filled with fluid. Edema of the eyelids commonly results from irritation caused by the administration of silver nitrate. Generalized edema may occur with prematurity, hypoproteinemia secondary to severe erythroblastosis fetalis, nonimmune hydrops, congenital nephrosis, Hurler syndrome, or unknown cause. Localized edema suggests a congenital malformation of the lymphatic system; when confined to one or more extremities of a female infant, it may be the initial sign of Turner syndrome (Chapters 81 and 587.1).

SKIN. Vasomotor instability and peripheral circulatory sluggishness are revealed by deep redness or purple lividity in a crying infant, whose color may darken profoundly with closure of the glottis preceding a vigorous cry, and by harmless cyanosis (**acrocyanosis**) of the hands and feet, especially when they are cool. Mottling, another example of general circulatory instability, may be associated with serious illness or related to a transient fluctuation in skin temperature. An extraordinary division of the body from the forehead to the pubis into red and pale halves is known as **harlequin color change**, a transient and harmless condition. Significant **cyanosis** may be masked by the pallor of circulatory failure or anemia; alternatively, the relatively high hemoglobin content of the 1st few days and the thin skin may combine to produce an appearance of cyanosis at a higher Pao_2 than in older children. Localized cyanosis is differentiated from ecchymosis by the momentary blanching pallor (with cyanosis) that occurs after pressure. The same maneuver also helps in demonstrating icterus, possibly significant but unnoticed if the skin is suffused with blood. **Pallor** may represent asphyxia, anemia, shock, or edema. Early recognition of anemia may lead to a diagnosis of erythroblastosis fetalis, subcapsular hematoma of the liver or spleen, subdural hemorrhage, or fetal-maternal or twin-twin transfusion. Without being anemic, postmature infants tend to have paler and thicker skin than term or premature infants do. The ruddy red appearance of plethora is seen with polycythemia.

The vernix and common transitory macular capillary hemangiomas of the eyelids and neck are described in Chapter 646. Cavernous hemangiomas are deeper, blue masses that if large, may trap platelets and produce disseminated intravascular coagulation or interfere with local organ function. Scattered petechiae may be seen on the presenting part (usually the scalp or face) after a difficult delivery. Slate-blue, well-demarcated areas of pigmentation are seen over the buttocks, back, and sometimes other parts of the body in more than 50% of black, Native American, or Asian infants and occasionally in white ones. These patches have no known anthropologic significance despite their name, **mongolian spots**; they tend to disappear within the 1st year. The vernix, skin, and especially the cord may be stained brownish yellow if the amniotic fluid has been colored by the passage of meconium during or before birth.

The skin of premature infants is thin and delicate and tends to be deep red; in extremely premature infants, the skin appears almost gelatinous and bleeds and bruises easily. Fine, soft, immature hair, **lanugo**, frequently covers the scalp and brow and may also cover the face of premature infants. Lanugo has usually been lost or replaced by vellus hair in term infants. **Tufts of hair** over the lumbosacral spine suggest an underlying abnormality such as occult spina bifida, a sinus tract, or a tumor. The nails are rudimentary in very premature infants, but they may protrude beyond the fingertips in infants born past term. Post-term infants may have a peeling, parchment-like skin (Fig. 94-1), a severe degree of which suggests ichthyosis congenita (Chapter 657).

In many neonates, small, white, occasionally vesiculopustular papules on an erythematous base develop 1–3 days after birth.

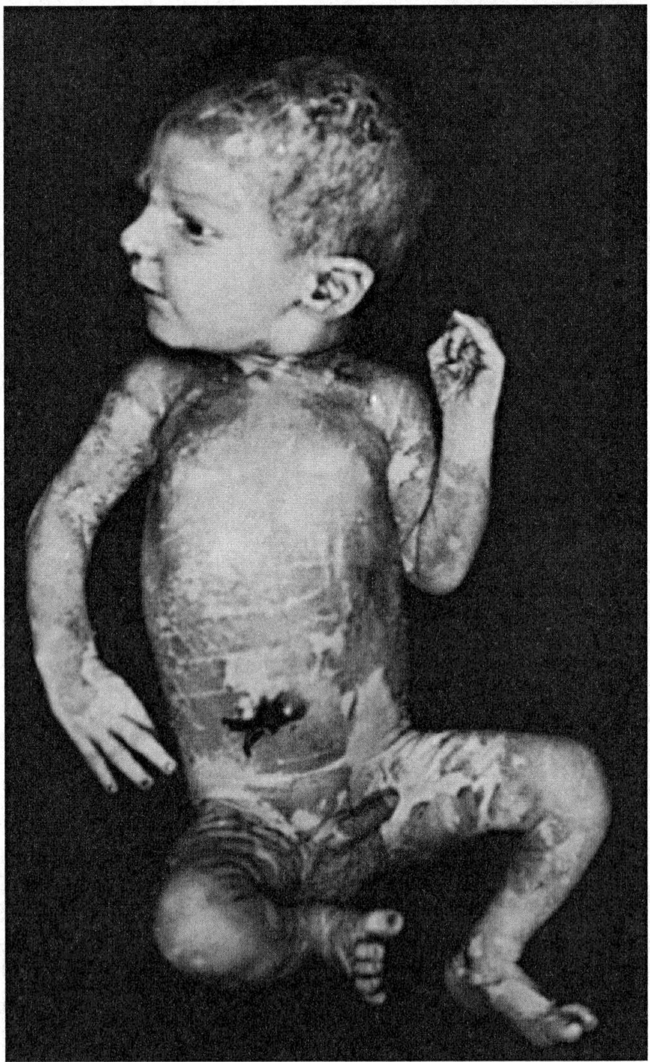

Figure 94-1. Infant with intrauterine growth retardation as a result of placental insufficiency. Note the long, thin appearance with peeling, parchment-like dry skin, alert expression, meconium staining of the skin, and long nails. (From Clifford S: *Advances in Pediatrics*, vol 9. Chicago, Year Book, 1962.)

This benign rash, **erythema toxicum**, persists for as long as 1 wk, contains eosinophils, and is usually distributed on the face, trunk, and extremities (Chapter 646). **Pustular melanosis**, a benign lesion seen predominantly in black neonates, contains neutrophils and is present at birth as a vesiculopustular eruption around the chin, neck, back, extremities, and palms or soles; it lasts 2–3 days. Both lesions need to be distinguished from more dangerous vesicular eruptions such as herpes simplex (Chapter 249) and staphylococcal disease of the skin (Chapter 180.1).

Amniotic bands may disrupt the skin, extremities (amputation, ring constriction, syndactyly), face (clefts), or trunk (abdominal or thoracic wall defects). Their cause is uncertain but may be related to amniotic membrane rupture or vascular compromise with fibrous band formation. Excessive skin fragility and extensibility with joint hypermobility suggest Ehlers-Danlos syndrome, Marfan syndrome, congenital contractural arachnodactyly, or other disorders of collagen synthesis.

SKULL. All infants should have their head circumference charted. The skull may be molded, particularly if the infant is the first-born and if the head has been engaged for a considerable time. The parietal bones tend to override the occipital and frontal

TABLE 94-1. Disorders Associated with a Large Anterior Fontanel

Achondroplasia	Intrauterine growth retardation
Apert syndrome	Kenny syndrome
Athyrotic hypothyroidism	Osteogenesis imperfecta
Cleidocranial dysostosis	Prematurity
Congenital rubella syndrome	Pyknodysostosis
Hallermann-Streiff syndrome	Russell-Silver syndrome
Hydrocephaly	13-, 18-, 21-trisomies
Hypophosphatasia	Vitamin D deficiency rickets

bones. The head of an infant born by cesarean section or from a breech presentation is characterized by its roundness. The suture lines and the size and fullness of the anterior and posterior fontanels should be determined digitally by palpation. Premature fusion of sutures (**cranial synostosis**) is identified by a hard nonmovable ridge over the suture and an abnormally shaped skull. Great variation in the size of the **fontanels** exists at birth; if small, the anterior fontanel usually tends to enlarge during the 1st few months of life. The persistence of excessively large anterior (normal, 20 ± 10 mm) and posterior fontanels has been associated with several disorders (Table 94-1). Persistently small fontanels suggest microcephaly, craniosynostosis, congenital hyperthyroidism, or wormian bones; a 3rd fontanel suggests trisomy 21 but is seen in preterm infants. Soft areas (**craniotabes**) are occasionally found in the parietal bones at the vertex near the sagittal suture; they are more common in premature infants and in infants who have been exposed to uterine compression. Though usually insignificant, their possible pathologic cause should be investigated if they persist. Soft areas in the occipital region suggest the irregular calcification and wormian bone formation associated with osteogenesis imperfecta, cleidocranial dysostosis, lacunar skull, cretinism, and, occasionally, Down syndrome. Transillumination of an abnormal skull in a dark room followed by ultrasound or computed tomography will rule out hydranencephaly or hydrocephaly (Chapter 592). An excessively large head (megalencephaly) suggests hydrocephaly, storage disease, achondroplasia, cerebral gigantism, neurocutaneous syndromes, or inborn errors of metabolism, or it may be familial. The skull of a premature infant may suggest hydrocephaly because of the relatively larger brain growth in comparison to that of other organs. Depression of the skull (indentation, fracture, ping-pong ball deformity) is usually of prenatal onset from prolonged focal pressure by the bony pelvis. Atrophic or alopecic scalp areas may represent aplasia cutis congenita, which may be sporadic or autosomal dominant or be associated with trisomy 13, chromosome 4 deletion, or Johanson-Blizzard syndrome. Deformational plagiocephaly may be due to in utero positioning forces on the skull and is manifested as an asymmetric skull and face with ear malalignment. It is associated with torticollis and vertex positioning. Any significant and persistent abnormality in shape or size of the skull should be evaluated by cranial CT.

FACE. The general appearance should be noted with regard to dysmorphic features, such as epicanthal folds, widely or narrowly spaced eyes, microphthalmos, asymmetry, long philtrum, and low-set ears, which are often associated with congenital syndromes. The face may be asymmetric as a result of a 7th nerve palsy, hypoplasia of the depressor muscle at the angle of the mouth, or an abnormal fetal posture (Chapter 108); when the jaw has been held against a shoulder or an extremity during the intrauterine period, the mandible may deviate strikingly from the midline. Symmetric facial palsy suggests absence or hypoplasia of the 7th nerve nucleus (**Möbius syndrome**).

Eyes. The eyes often open spontaneously if the infant is held up and tipped gently forward and backward. This maneuver, a result of labyrinthine and neck reflexes, is more successful for inspecting the eyes than is forcing the lids apart. Conjunctival and retinal hemorrhages are usually benign. Retinal hemorrhages are more common with vacuum-assisted deliveries (75%) than after cesarean section (7%). They resolve in most infants by 2 wk (85%) and in all infants by 4 wk of age. **Pupillary reflexes** are present after 28–30 wk of gestation. The iris should be inspected for colobomas and heterochromia. A cornea larger than 1 cm in diameter in a term infant (with photophobia and tearing) suggests congenital glaucoma and requires prompt ophthalmologic consultation. The presence of bilateral red reflexes suggests the absence of cataracts and intraocular pathology (Chapters 618, 626–632). **Leukokoria** (white pupillary reflex) suggests cataracts, tumor, chorioretinitis, retinopathy of prematurity, or a persistent hyperplastic primary vitreous and warrants an immediate ophthalmologic consultation.

Ears. Deformities of the pinnae are occasionally seen. Unilateral or bilateral preauricular skin tags occur frequently; if pedunculated, they can be tightly ligated at the base, and dry gangrene and sloughing result. The tympanic membrane, easily seen otoscopically through the short, straight external auditory canal, normally appears dull gray.

Nose. The nose may be slightly obstructed by mucus accumulated in the narrow nostrils. The nares should be symmetric and patent. Dislocation of the nasal cartilage from the vomerian groove results in asymmetric nares. Anatomic obstruction of the nasal passages secondary to unilateral or bilateral choanal atresia results in respiratory distress.

Mouth. A normal mouth may rarely have precocious dentition, with natal (present at birth) or neonatal (eruption after birth) teeth in the lower incisor position or aberrantly placed; these teeth are shed before the deciduous ones erupt (Chapter 304). Alternatively, such teeth occur in Ellis-van Creveld, Hallermann-Streiff, and other syndromes. Extraction is not usually indicated. Premature eruption of deciduous teeth is even more unusual. The soft and hard palate should be inspected and palpated for a complete or submucosal cleft and the contour noted if the arch is excessively high or the uvula is bifid. On the hard palate on either side of the raphe may be temporary accumulations of epithelial cells called Epstein pearls. Retention cysts of similar appearance may also be seen on the gums. Both disappear spontaneously, usually within a few weeks of birth. Clusters of small white or yellow follicles or ulcers on an erythematous base may be found on the anterior tonsillar pillars, most frequently on the 2nd–3rd day of life. Of unknown cause, they clear without treatment in 2–4 days.

Neonates do not have active salivation. The tongue appears relatively large; the frenulum may be short, but rarely is shortness (**tongue-tied** or **ankyloglossia**) a reason for cutting it. If there are problems with feedings (breast or bottle) and the frenulum is short, frenulotomy may be indicated. The sublingual mucous membrane occasionally forms a prominent fold. The cheeks have a fullness on both the buccal and the external aspects as a result of the accumulation of fat making up the sucking pads. These pads, as well as the labial tubercle on the upper lip (**sucking callus**), disappear when suckling ceases. A marble-sized buccal mass is usually due to benign idiopathic fat necrosis.

The throat of a newborn infant is hard to see because of the low arch of the palate; it should be clearly viewed because it is easy to miss posterior palatal or uvular clefts. The tonsils are small.

NECK. The neck appears relatively short. Abnormalities are not common but include goiter, cystic hygroma, branchial cleft rests, teratoma, hemangioma, and lesions of the sternocleidomastoid muscle that are presumably traumatic or due to a fixed positioning in utero that produces either a hematoma or fibrosis, respectively. Congenital torticollis causes the head to turn toward and the face to turn away from the affected side. Plagiocephaly, facial asymmetry, and hemihypoplasia may develop if it is untreated

(Chapter 679.1). Redundant skin or webbing in a female infant suggests intrauterine lymphedema and Turner syndrome (Chapter 587.1). Both clavicles should be palpated for fractures.

CHEST. Breast hypertrophy is common, and milk may be present (but should not be expressed). Asymmetry, erythema, induration, and tenderness should suggest mastitis or a breast abscess. Look for supernumerary nipples, inverted nipples, or widely spaced nipples with a shield-shaped chest; the latter suggests Turner syndrome.

LUNGS. Much can be learned by observing breathing. Variations in rate and rhythm are characteristic and fluctuate according to the infant's physical activity, state of wakefulness, or the presence of crying. Because fluctuations are rapid, the respiratory rate should be counted for a full minute with the infant in the resting state, preferably asleep. Under these circumstances, the usual rate for normal term infants is 30–40/min; in premature infants the rate is higher and fluctuates more widely. A rate consistently over 60/min during periods of regular breathing usually indicates pulmonary, cardiac, or metabolic disease (acidosis). Premature infants may breathe with a Cheyne-Stokes rhythm, known as periodic respiration, or with complete irregularity. Irregular gasping, sometimes accompanied by spasmodic movements of the mouth and chin, strongly indicates serious impairment of the respiratory centers.

The breathing of newborn infants is almost entirely diaphragmatic, so during inspiration the soft front of the thorax is usually drawn inward while the abdomen protrudes. If the baby is quiet, relaxed, and of good color, this "paradoxical movement" does not necessarily signify insufficient ventilation. On the other hand, labored respiration with retractions is important evidence of respiratory distress syndrome, pneumonia, anomalies, or mechanical disturbance of the lungs. A weak persistent or intermittent groaning, whining cry or **grunting** during expiration signifies potentially serious cardiopulmonary disease or sepsis and warrants immediate attention. When benign, the grunting resolves between 30 and 60 min after birth. Flaring of the alae nasi and retraction of the intercostal muscles and sternum are common signs of pulmonary pathology.

Normally, the breath sounds are bronchovesicular. Suspicion of pulmonary pathology because of diminished breath sounds, rales, retractions, or cyanosis should always be verified with a chest radiograph.

HEART. Normal variation in the size and shape of the chest makes it difficult to estimate the size of the heart. The location of the heart should be determined to detect dextrocardia. Transitory murmurs usually represent a closing ductus arteriosus. Although congenital heart disease may not initially produce the murmur that will appear later, a substantial portion of infants with murmurs detected during routine neonatal examination have an underlying malformation. Evaluation of the heart by echocardiography and electrocardiography is essential when the possibility of a significant lesion exists. The pulse may vary normally from 90/min in relaxed sleep to 180/min during activity. The still higher rate of supraventricular tachycardia (>220) may be determined better on a cardiac monitor or electrocardiogram than by ear. Premature infants, whose resting heart rate is usually 140–150/min, may have a sudden onset of sinus bradycardia. Pulses should be palpated in the upper and lower extremities to detect coarctation of the aorta on both admission and discharge from the nursery.

Blood pressure measurements may be a valuable diagnostic aid in ill infants (Chapter 425). The oscillometric method is the easiest and most accurate noninvasive method available. Continuous or intermittent direct measurement of blood pressure with an umbilical artery catheter may be indicated in special circumstances for infants who are under close observation in an intensive care unit (Fig. 94-2).

ABDOMEN. The liver is usually palpable, sometimes as much as 2 cm below the rib margin. Less commonly, the tip of the spleen may be felt. The approximate size and location of each kidney can usually be determined on deep palpation. At no other period of life does the amount of air in the gastrointestinal tract vary so much, nor is it usually so great under normal circumstances. Gas should normally be present in the rectum on roentgenogram by 24 hr of age. The abdominal wall is normally weak (especially in premature infants), and diastasis recti and umbilical hernias are common, particularly among black infants.

Unusual masses should be investigated immediately by ultrasonography. Renal pathology is the cause of most neonatal abdominal masses. **Cystic abdominal masses** include

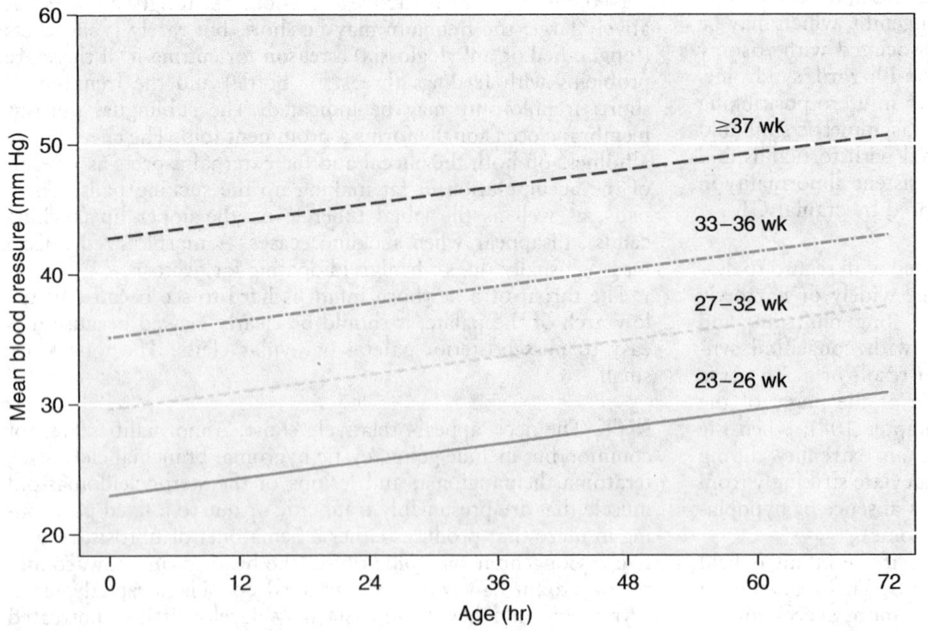

Figure 94-2. Nomogram for mean blood pressure (BP) in neonates with gestational ages of 23–43 wk derived from continuous arterial BP measurements obtained from 103 infants admitted to the neonatal intensive care unit. The graph shows the predicted mean BP of neonates of different gestational age during the 1st 72 hours of life. Each line represents the lower limit of the 80% confidence interval (two-tail) of the mean BP for each gestational age group; 90% of infants for each gestational age group will be expected to have a mean BP value equal to or above the value indicated by the corresponding line, the lower limit of the confidence interval. (From Nuntnarumit P, Yang W, Bada-Ellzey SB: Blood pressure measurements in the newborn. *Clin Perinatol* 1999;26:981–996.)

hydronephrosis, multicystic-dysplastic kidneys, adrenal hemorrhage, hydrometrocolpos, intestinal duplication, and choledochal, ovarian, omental, or pancreatic cysts. **Solid masses** include neuroblastoma, congenital mesoblastic nephroma, hepatoblastoma, and teratoma. A solid flank mass may be caused by **renal vein thrombosis**, which becomes clinically apparent with hematuria, hypertension, and thrombocytopenia. Renal vein thrombosis in infants is associated with polycythemia, dehydration, diabetic mothers, asphyxia, sepsis, nephrosis, and hypercoagulable states such as antithrombin III or protein C deficiency.

Abdominal distention at birth or shortly afterward suggests either obstruction or perforation of the gastrointestinal tract, often as a result of meconium ileus; later distention suggests lower bowel obstruction, sepsis, or peritonitis. A scaphoid abdomen in a newborn suggests diaphragmatic hernia. Abdominal wall defects produce an omphalocele (Chapter 105) when they occur through the umbilicus and gastroschisis when they occur lateral to the midline. Omphaloceles are associated with other anomalies and syndromes such as Beckwith-Wiedemann, conjoined twins, trisomy 18, meningomyelocele, and imperforate anus. **Omphalitis** is an acute local inflammation of the periumbilical tissue that may extend to the abdominal wall, the peritoneum, the umbilical vein or portal vessels, or the liver and may result in later portal hypertension. The umbilical cord should have two arteries and one vein. A single umbilical artery suggests an occult renal anomaly.

GENITALS. The genitals and mammary glands normally respond to transplacentally acquired maternal hormones to produce enlargement and secretion of the breasts in both sexes and prominence of the female genitals, often with considerable nonpurulent discharge. These transitory manifestations require observation but no intervention.

An imperforate hymen may result in **hydrometrocolpos** and a lower abdominal mass. A normal scrotum at term is relatively large; its size may be increased by the trauma of breech delivery or by a transitory hydrocele, which is distinguished from a hernia by palpation and transillumination. The testes should be in the scrotum or palpable in the canals in term infants. Black male infants usually have dark pigmentation of the scrotum before the rest of the skin assumes its permanent color.

The prepuce of a newborn infant is normally tight and adherent. Severe hypospadias or epispadias should always lead one to suspect either that abnormal sex chromosomes are present (Chapter 81) or that the infant is actually a masculinized female with an enlarged clitoris because this finding may be the 1st evidence of adrenogenital syndrome (Chapter 577). Erection of the penis is common and has no significance. Urine is usually passed during or immediately after birth; a period without voiding may normally follow. Most void by 12 hr, and about 95% of preterm and term infants void within 24 hr.

ANUS. Some passage of meconium usually occurs within the 1st 12 hr after birth; 99% of term infants and 95% of premature infants pass meconium within 48 hr of birth. Imperforate anus is not always visible and may require evidence obtained by gentle insertion of the little finger or a rectal tube. Roentgenographic study is required. Passage of meconium does not rule out an imperforate anus if a rectal-vaginal fistula is present. The dimple or irregularity in skinfold often normally present in the sacrococcygeal midline may be mistaken for an actual or potential neurocutaneous sinus.

EXTREMITIES. In examining the extremities, the effects of fetal posture (Chapter 671) should be noted so that their cause and usual transitory nature can be explained to the mother. Such explanations are particularly important after breech presentations. Observing the extremities in spontaneous or stimulated activity more commonly than by any other means arouses the suspicion of a fracture or nerve injury associated with delivery. The hands and feet should be examined for polydactyly, syndactyly, and abnormal dermatoglyphic patterns such as a simian crease.

The hips of all infants should be examined with specific maneuvers to rule out congenital dislocation (Chapter 677.1).

NEUROLOGIC EXAMINATION (See Chapters 7 and 591). In utero neuromuscular diseases associated with limited fetal motion produce a constellation of signs and symptoms that are independent of the specific disease. Severe positional deformation and contractures produce arthrogryposis. Other manifestations of fetal neuromuscular disease include breech presentation, polyhydramnios, failure to breathe at birth, pulmonary hypoplasia, dislocated hips, undescended testes, thin ribs, and clubfoot.

94.3 • Routine Delivery Room Care

Low-risk infants may initially be placed head downward after delivery to clear the mouth, pharynx, and nose of fluid, mucus, blood, and amniotic debris by gravity; gentle suction with a bulb syringe or soft rubber catheter may also be helpful if there is a significant amount of fluid. Wiping the palate and pharynx with gauze may lead to abrasions and the development of thrush, pterygoid ulcers (Bednar aphthae), or rarely, tooth bud infection with maxillary osteomyelitis and retrobulbar abscess formation. The stomachs of infants delivered by cesarean section may contain more fluid than those of infants delivered vaginally. Their stomachs may need to be emptied by gastric tube if a significant amount of fluid is suspected to prevent aspiration of gastric contents. Naso or orogastric tube placement is a potentially noxious stimulus that may predispose to future poor experiences with pain. If not necessary, tube placement should be avoided. Most healthy infants who appear to be in satisfactory condition may be given directly to their mothers for immediate bonding and nursing without undergoing oropharyngeal or gastric suctioning. If respiratory distress is a concern, infants should be placed under a warmer with the head dependent.

The **Apgar score** is a practical method of systematically assessing newborn infants immediately after birth to help identify those requiring resuscitation and to predict survival in the neonatal period (Table 94-2). The 1-min Apgar score may signal the need for immediate resuscitation, and the 5-, 10-, 15-, and 20-min scores may indicate the probability of successfully resuscitating an infant. A low score may be due to a number of factors, including drugs given to the mother during labor and immaturity (Table 94-3). The Apgar score was not designed to predict neurologic outcome. Indeed, the score is normal in most patients in whom cerebral palsy subsequently develops, and the incidence of cerebral palsy is low in infants with Apgar scores of 0–3 at 5 min (but higher than in infants with Apgar scores of 7–10). The Apgar score and umbilical artery blood pH both predict neonatal death.

TABLE 94-2. Apgar Evaluation of Newborn Infants

SIGN	0	1	2
Heart rate	Absent	Below 100	Over 100
Respiratory effort	Absent	Slow, irregular	Good, crying
Muscle tone	Limp	Some flexion of extremities	Active motion
Response to catheter in nostril (tested after oropharynx is clear)	No response	Grimace	Cough or sneeze
Color	Blue, pale	Body pink, extremities blue	Completely pink

Sixty sec after complete birth of the infant (disregarding the cord and placenta), the five objective signs above are evaluated, and each is given a score of 0, 1, or 2. A total score of 10 indicates an infant in the best possible condition. An infant with a score of 0–3 requires immediate resuscitation. Modified from Apgar V: *Res Anesth Analg* 1953;32:260.

TABLE 94-3. Factors Affecting the Apgar Score

FALSE-POSITIVE (NO FETAL ACIDOSIS OR HYPOXIA; LOW APGAR)	FALSE-NEGATIVE (ACIDOSIS; NORMAL APGAR)
Immaturity	Maternal acidosis
Analgesics, narcotics, sedatives	High fetal catecholamine levels
Magnesium sulfate	Some full-term infants
Acute cerebral trauma	
Precipitous delivery	
Congenital myopathy	
Congenital neuropathy	
Spinal cord trauma	
Central nervous system anomaly	
Lung anomaly (diaphragmatic hernia)	
Airway obstruction (choanal atresia)	
Congenital pneumonia and sepsis	
Previous episodes of fetal asphyxia (recovered)	
Hemorrhage-hypovolemia	

Regardless of the etiology, a low Apgar score because of fetal asphyxia, immaturity, central nervous system depression, or airway obstruction identifies an infant needing immediate resuscitation.

An Apgar score of 0–3 at 5 min is uncommon but is a better predictor of neonatal death (in both term and preterm infants) than an umbilical artery pH of 7.0 or less; the presence of both variables increases the relative risk of neonatal mortality in term and preterm infants (Table 94-4).

Infants who fail to initiate respiration should receive prompt resuscitation and close observation (Chapter 100).

MAINTENANCE OF BODY HEAT. Relative to body weight, the body surface area of a newborn infant is approximately three times that of an adult, and in low birthweight infants, the insulating layer of subcutaneous fat is thinner. The estimated rate of heat loss in a newborn is approximately four times that of an adult. Under the usual delivery room conditions (20–25°C), an infant's skin temperature falls approximately 0.3°C/min and deep body temperature decreases approximately 0.1°C/min during the period immediately after delivery; these rates generally result in a cumulative loss of 2–3°C in deep body temperature (corresponding to a heat loss of approximately 200 kcal/kg). The heat loss occurs by convection of heat energy to the cooler surrounding air, by conduction of heat to the colder materials on which the infant is resting, by heat radiation from the infant to other nearby cooler solid objects, and by evaporation from moist skin and lungs (a function of alveolar ventilation).

Metabolic acidosis, hypoxemia, hypoglycemia, and increased renal excretion of water and solutes may develop in term infants exposed to cold after birth because of their effort to compensate for heat loss. Heat production is augmented by increasing the metabolic rate and oxygen consumption in part by releasing norepinephrine, which results in nonshivering thermogenesis through oxidation of fat, particularly brown fat. In addition, muscular activity may increase. Hypoglycemic or hypoxic infants cannot increase their oxygen consumption when exposed to a cold environment, and their central temperature decreases. After labor and vaginal delivery, many newborn infants have mild to moderate metabolic acidosis, for which they may compensate by hyperventilating, a response that is more difficult for infants with CNS depression (asphyxia, drugs) and infants exposed to cold stress in the delivery room. Therefore, to reduce heat loss, it is desirable to ensure that infants are dried and either wrapped in blankets or placed under a warmer. **Skin-to-skin contact** with the mother is the optimal method to maintain temperature in the stable newborn. Because carrying out resuscitative measures on a covered infant or one enclosed in an incubator is difficult, a radiant heat source should be used to warm the baby during resuscitation.

TABLE 94-4. Incidence of Neonatal Death in 132,228 Singleton Infants Born at Term (37th wk of Gestation or Later) in Relation to Apgar Scores at 5 min of Age*

5-MIN APGAR SCORE	NO. OF LIVE BIRTHS	NO. NEONATAL DEATHS (RATE PER 1,000 BIRTHS)	RELATIVE RISK (95% CI)
0–3	86	21 (244)	1,460 (835–2,555)
4–6	561	5 (9)	53 (20–140)
7–10	131,581	22 (0.2)	1

*Infants with 5-min Apgar scores of 7–10 served as the reference group.
CI, confidence interval.
From Casey BM, McIntire DD, Leveno KJ: The continuing value of the Apgar score for the assessment of newborn infants. *N Engl J Med* 2001;344:467–471.

ANTISEPTIC SKIN AND CORD CARE. Careful removal of blood from the skin shortly after birth may reduce the risk of infection with blood-borne agents. Once a healthy infant's temperature has stabilized, the entire skin and cord should be cleansed with warm water or a mild nonmedicated soap solution and rinsed with water to reduce the incidence of skin and periumbilical colonization with pathogenic bacteria and subsequent infectious complications. To avoid heat loss, infants are then dried and wrapped in sterile blankets. To reduce colonization with *Staphylococcus aureus* and other pathogenic bacteria, the umbilical cord may be treated daily with bactericidal or antimicrobial agents such as triple dye or bacitracin. One application of triple dye followed by twice-daily alcohol swabbing (until the cord falls off) reduces colonization, exudates, and foul odor of the umbilicus when compared to dry care (soap and water when soiled). Alternatively, chlorhexidine washing or, on rare occasion during *S. aureus* epidemics, a single hexachlorophene bath may be used. Routine or repeated total body exposure to hexachlorophene may be neurotoxic, particularly in low-birthweight infants, and is thus contraindicated. Nursery personnel should use chlorhexidine or iodophor-containing antiseptic soaps for routine handwashing before caring for each infant. Rigidly enforcing hand-to-elbow washing for 2 min in the initial wash and 15–30 sec in the 2nd wash is essential for staff and visitors entering the nursery. Equally thorough washes between handling infants are also required.

OTHER MEASURES. The eyes of all infants must be protected against gonococcal infection by instilling 1% silver nitrate drops, the best-proven therapy; erythromycin (0.5%) and tetracycline (1.0%) sterile ophthalmic ointments are alternative measures that add coverage against chlamydia. Povidone-iodine (2.5% solution) may also be effective as a one-time prophylactic agent. This procedure may be delayed during the initial short-alert period after birth to promote bonding, but once applied, drops should not be rinsed out. Also see Chapters 191 and 223.3.

Although hemorrhage in newborn infants can be due to factors other than vitamin K deficiency, an intramuscular injection of 1 mg of water-soluble vitamin K_1 (phytonadione) is recommended for all infants immediately after birth to prevent hemorrhagic disease of the newborn (see Chapter 103.4). Higher dose, repeated administration of oral vitamin K may also be useful, but this treatment is not yet established. Larger intravenous doses predispose to the development of hyperbilirubinemia and kernicterus and should be avoided. Administration of vitamin K to the mother during labor is not recommended because of unpredictable placental transfer.

Neonatal screening is available for various genetic, metabolic, hematologic, and endocrine diseases. All states have neonatal screening programs, although the specific tests required vary (Chapter 84). Laboratory tests performed on infant heel puncture blood samples include those for hypothyroidism, phenylketonuria, galactosemia, maple syrup urine disease, homocystinuria, biotinidase deficiency, adrenal hyperplasia, hemoglobinopathy, cystic fibrosis, tyrosinemia, and other organic acid defects or aminoacidopathies. To be effective in the timely identification and prompt management of treatable diseases, screening programs must include not only high-quality laboratory tests but also follow-up of infants with abnormal test results; education, counseling, and psychologic support for families; and prompt referral of the neonate for accurate diagnosis and therapy. Routine screening of the hematocrit or blood glucose is not necessary in the absence of risk factors. Hearing impairment, a serious morbidity that affects speech and language development, may be severe in 2/1,000 and overall affects 5/1,000 births. Universal screening of infants is recommended to ensure early detection of hearing loss and appropriate, timely intervention.

94.4 • Nursery Care

Non–high-risk healthy infants may be taken to the "regular" newborn nursery or be placed in the mother's room if the hospital has rooming-in.

The bassinet, preferably of clear plastic to allow for easy visibility and care, should be cleaned frequently. All professional care should be given in the bassinet, including the physical examination, clothing changes, temperature taking, skin cleansing, and other procedures that if performed elsewhere, would establish a common contact point and possibly provide a channel for cross infection. The clothing and bedding should be minimal, only that needed for an infant's comfort; the nursery temperature should be kept at approximately 24°C (75°F). The infant's temperature should be taken by axillary measurement. Although the interval between temperature taking depends on many circumstances, it need not be shorter than 4 hr during the 1st 2–3 days and 8 hr thereafter. Axillary temperatures of 36.4–37.0°C (97.0–98.5°F) are within normal limits. Weighing at birth and daily thereafter is sufficient. Healthy infants should be placed supine to reduce the risk of sudden infant death syndrome.

Vernix is spontaneously shed within 2–3 days, much of it adhering to the clothing, which should be completely changed daily. The diaper should be checked before and after feeding and when the baby cries; it should be changed when wet or soiled. Meconium or feces should be cleansed from the buttocks with sterile cotton moistened with sterile water. The foreskin of a male infant should not be retracted. Circumcision is an elective procedure.

Early discharge (<48 hr) or very early discharge (<24 hr) may increase the risk of rehospitalization for hyperbilirubinemia, sepsis, failure to thrive, dehydration, and missed congenital anomalies. Early discharge requires careful ambulatory follow-up at home (visiting nurse) or in the office within 48 hr. Additional criteria for the early discharge of term neonates have been developed by the American Academy of Pediatrics and American College of Obstetrics and Gynecology (Table 94-5).

TABLE 94-5. Recommendations for Early Discharge from the Normal Newborn Nursery*

- Uncomplicated antepartum, intrapartum, postpartum courses
- Vaginal delivery
- Singleton at 38–42 wk: appropriate for gestational age
- Normal vital signs including respiratory rate < 60 breaths/min; axillary temperature 36.1–37°C (97.0–98.6°F) in open crib
- Physical examination reveals no abnormalities requiring immediate attention
- Urination; stool × 1
- At least two uneventful, successful feedings
- No excessive bleeding after (2 hr) circumcision
- No jaundice within 24 hr of birth
- Evidence of parental knowledge, ability, and confidence to care for the baby at home
  - Feeding
  - Cord, skin, genital care
  - Recognition of illness (jaundice, poor feeding, lethargy, fever, etc.)
  - Infant safety (car seat, supine sleep position, etc.)
- Availability of family and physician support (physician follow-up)
- Laboratory evaluation
  - Venereal Disease Research Laboratories (VDRL)
  - Hepatitis B surface antigen and vaccination or appointment for vaccination
  - State screening (e.g., phenylketonuria, thyroid, galactosemia, sickle cell)
  - Coombs' test
- No social risks
  - Substance abuse
  - History of child abuse
  - Domestic violence
  - Mental illness
  - Teen mother
  - Homeless

*It is not likely that all these criteria will be met before 48 hr of age.
Adapted from American Academy of Pediatrics, American College of Obstetricians and Gynecologists: *Guidelines for Perinatal Care*, 5th ed. Elk Grove Village, IL, American Academy of Pediatrics, 2002.

94.5 • Parent-Infant Bonding (see also Chapter 7)

Normal infant development depends partly on a series of affectionate responses exchanged between a mother and her newborn infant that binds them together psychologically and physiologically. This bonding is facilitated and reinforced by the emotional support of a loving family. The attachment process may be important in enabling some mothers to provide loving care during the neonatal period and subsequently during childhood. It is initiated before birth with the planning and confirmation of the pregnancy and with the growing acceptance of the fetus as an individual. After delivery and during the ensuing weeks, sensory (visual, auditory, olfactory) and physical contact between the mother and baby triggers various mutually rewarding and pleasurable interactions such as the mother touching the infant's extremities and face with her fingertips and encompassing and gently massaging the infant's trunk with her hands. Touching an infant's cheek elicits responsive turning toward the mother's face or toward the breast with nuzzling and licking of the nipple, a powerful stimulus for prolactin secretion. An infant's initial quiet alert state provides the opportunity for eye-to-eye contact, which is particularly important in stimulating the loving and possessive feelings of many parents for their babies. An infant's crying elicits the maternal response of touching the infant and speaking in a soft, soothing, higher-toned voice. Initial contact between the mother and infant should take place in the delivery room, and opportunities for extended intimate contact should be provided within the 1st hours after birth. Delayed or abnormal maternal-infant bonding, as occurs because of prematurity, infant or maternal illness, birth defects, or family stress, may harm infant development and maternal caretaking ability. Hospital routines should be designed to encourage parent-infant contact.

NURSERIES AND BREAST-FEEDING. See Chapter 42 for full discussions of breast-feeding and formula feeding. Many hospital practices contribute to difficulties in breast-feeding by enforcing 4-hr feeding schedules, limiting nursing time, using only one breast at a feeding, washing nipples with substances other than water, delaying the 1st feeding, providing formula supplements, and using heavy intrapartum sedation. The Baby-Friendly Hospital Initiative is a global effort (sponsored by the World Health Organization and the United Nations Children's Fund) to promote breast-feeding, which recommends 10 steps to successful breast-feeding (Table 94-6).

Hospital practices that encourage successful breast-feeding include immediate postpartum mother-infant contact with suckling, rooming-in, demand feeding, inclusion of fathers in prena-

TABLE 94-6. Ten Steps to Successful Breast-Feeding

Every facility providing maternity services and care for newborn infants should accomplish the following:

1. Have a written breast-feeding policy that is routinely communicated to all health care staff.
2. Train all health care staff in the skills necessary to implement this policy.
3. Inform all pregnant women about the benefits and management of breast-feeding.
4. Help mothers initiate breast-feeding within a half hour of birth.
5. Show mothers how to breast-feed and how to maintain lactation even if they should be separated from their infants.
6. Give newborn infants no food or drink other than breast milk unless *medically* indicated.
7. Practice rooming-in (allow mothers and infants to remain together) 24 hr a day.
8. Encourage breast-feeding on demand.
9. Give no artificial teats or pacifiers (also called *dummies* or *soothers*) to breast-feeding infants.
10. Foster the establishment of breast-feeding support groups and refer mothers to them on discharge from the hospital or clinic.

From *Protecting, Promoting and Supporting Breastfeeding: The Special Role of Maternity Services.* A Joint WHO/UNICEF Statement Published by the World Health Organization, 1211 Geneva 27, Switzerland, 1989.

tal breast-feeding education, and support from experienced women. Nursing at least 5 min at each breast is reasonable and allows a baby to obtain most of the available breast contents and provides effective stimulation for increasing the milk supply. Nursing episodes should then be extended according to the comfort and desire of the mother and infant. A confident and relaxed mother, supported by an encouraging home and hospital environment, is likely to nurse well.

DRUGS AND BREAST-FEEDING. Maternal medications may affect the production and safety of breast milk (Table 94-7). Although most commonly used medications are safe, the safety of any drug to be used while a woman is breast-feeding must be confirmed before a new drug is initiated and/or breast-feeding is continued. Maternal sedatives may result in sedation of the infant. Maternal drugs that are weak acids, composed of large molecules, plasma bound, or poorly absorbed from the maternal or neonatal intestine are less likely to affect a neonate. When fresh breast milk is fed by tube or bottle, bacteriologic evaluation of stored milk should be performed within 24 hr.

Medical contraindications to breast-feeding in the United States include infection with HIV, human T-cell leukemia virus types 1 and 2, cytomegalovirus (preterm infants), active tuberculosis (until appropriately treated ≥2 wk and not considered contagious), and hepatitis B virus (until an infant receives hepatitis B immune globulin and vaccine) (Table 94-8).

TABLE 94-7. Drugs and Breast-Feeding

CONTRAINDICATED	AVOID OR GIVE WITH CAUTION	PROBABLY SAFE
Amphetamines	Alcohol	Acetaminophen
Antineoplastic agents	Amiodarone	Acyclovir
Bromocriptine	Anthroquinones (laxatives)	Aldomet
Chloramphenicol	Aspirin (salicylates)	Anesthetics
Clozapine	Atropine	Antibiotics (not chloramphenicol)
Cocaine	β-adrenergic blocking agents	Antiepileptics
Cyclophosphamide	Birth control pills	Antihistamines*
Diethylstilbestrol	Bromides	Antithyroid (not methimazole)
Doxorubicin	Calciferol	Bishydroxycoumarin
Ergots	Cascara	Chlorpromazine*
Gold salts	Ciprofloxacin	Codeine*
Heroin	Danthron	Cyclosporine
Immunosuppressants	Dihydrotachysterol	Depo-Provera
Iodides	Domperidone	Digoxin
Lithium	Estrogens	Dilantin (phenytoin)
Methimazole	Metoclopramide	Diuretics
Methylamphetamine	Metronidazole	Fluoxetine
Phencyclidine (PCP)	Meperidine	Furosemide
Radiopharmaceuticals	Phenobarbital*	Haloperidol*
Thiouracil	Primidone	Hydralazine
	Psychotropic drugs	Indomethacin, other nonsteroidal anti-inflammatory drugs
	Reserpine	
	Salicylazosulfapyridine (sulfasalazine)	Low molecular weight heparius
		Metformin
		Methadone*
		Morphine
		Muscle relaxants
		Paroxetine
		Prednisone
		Propranolol
		Propylthiouracil
		Sedatives*
		Sertraline
		Theophylline
		Vitamins
		Warfarin

*Watch for sedation.

Ainsworth SB, Wyllie JP, Wren C: Prevalence and clinical significance of cardiac murmurs in neonates. *Arch Dis Child Fetal Neonatal Ed* 1999; 43F–45F.

American Academy of Pediatrics Committee on Drugs: The transfer of drugs and other chemicals into human milk. *Pediatrics* 2001;108:776–789.

American Academy of Pediatrics Committee on Fetus and Newborn: The APGAR score. *Pediatrics* 2006;117:1444–1447.

American Academy of Pediatrics Section on Breastfeeding: Breastfeeding and the use of human milk. *Pediatrics* 2005;115:496–506.

Casey BM, McIntire DD, Leveno KJ: The continuing value of the Apgar score for the assessment of newborn infants. *N Engl J Med* 2001;344:467–471.

Dore S, Buchan D, Coulas S, et al: Alcohol versus natural drying for newborn cord care. *JOGNN* 1998;27:621–627.

Elliman DAC, Dezateux C, Bedford HE: Newborn and childhood screening programmes: Criteria, evidence, and current policy. *Arch Dis Child* 2002; 87:6–9.

Emerson MV, Pieramici DJ, Stoessel KM, et al: Incidence and rate of disappearance of retinal hemorrhage in newborns. *Ophthalmology* 2001;108: 36–39.

Friedman MA, Spitzer AR: Discharge criteria for the term newborn. *Pediatr Clin N Am* 2004;51:599–618.

Hall DMB, Renfrew MJ: Tongue tie. *Arch Dis Child* 2005;90:1211–1215.

Hampton T: FDA warns against breast milk drug. *JAMA* 2004;292:322.

Howard L: Safety of antipsychotic drugs for pregnant and breastfeeding women with non-affective psychosis. *Br Med J* 2004;329:933–934.

Janssen PA, Selwood BL, Dobson SR, et al: To dye or not to dye: A randomized, clinical trial of a triple dye/alcohol regime versus dry cord care. *Pediatrics* 2003;111:15–20.

Kennell JH, Klaus MH: Bonding: Recent observations that alter perinatal care. *Pediatr Rev* 1998;19:4–12.

Kerschner JE: Neonatal hearing screening: To do or not to do. *Pediatr Clin N Am* 2004;51:725–736.

Lawrence RM, Lawrence RA: Breast milk and infection. *Clin Perinatol* 2004;31:501–528.

Lindford AJ, Hettiaratchy S, Schonauer F: Postpartum splinting of ear deformities. *BMJ* 2007;334:366–368.

Liu LL, Clemens CJ, Shay DK, et al: The safety of newborn early discharge. *JAMA* 1997;278:293–298.

Mehl AL, Thomson V: The Colorado newborn hearing screening project, 1992–1999: On the threshold of effective population-based universal newborn hearing screening. *Pediatrics* 2002;109(1):E7.

Moster D, Lie RT, Irgens LM, et al: The association of Apgar score with subsequent death and cerebral palsy: A population-based study in term infants. *J Pediatr* 2001;138:798–803.

Nicoll A, Williams A: Breast feeding. *Arch Dis Child* 2002;87:91–92.

Nuntnarumit P, Yang W, Bada-Ellzey SB: Blood pressure measurements in the newborn. *Clin Perinatol* 1999;26:981–996.

Ostrea EM Jr, Mantaring JB, Silvestre MA: Drugs that affect the fetus and newborn infant via the placenta or breast milk. *Pediatr Clin N Am* 2004; 51:539–579.

Philipp BL, Merewood A: The baby-friendly way: The best breastfeeding start. *Pediatr Clin N Am* 2004;51:761–783.

Puckett RM, Offringa M: Prophylactic vitamin K for vitamin K deficiency bleeding in neonates. *Cochrane Database Syst* 2000;4:CD002776.

Radford A, Southall DP: Successful application of the baby-friendly hospital initiative contains lessons that must be applied to the control of formula feeding in hospitals in industrialized countries. *Pediatrics* 2001;108: 766–768.

TABLE 94-8. Summary of Infectious Agents Detected in Milk and Newborn Disease

INFECTIOUS AGENT	DETECTED IN BREAST MILK?	BREAST MILK REPORTED CAUSE OF NEWBORN DISEASE?	MATERNAL INFECTION CONTRAINDICATION TO BREAST-FEEDING?
Bacteria			
Mastitis/*Staphylococcus aureus*	Yes	No	No, unless breast abscess present
Mycobacterium tuberculosis			
Active disease	Yes	No	Yes, because of aerosol spread, or TB mastitis
PPD+/CXR–	No	No	No
Escherichia coli, other GNR	Yes, stored	Yes, stored	—
Group B streptococci	Yes	Yes	No*
Listeria monocytogenes	Yes	Yes	No*
Coxiella burnetii	Yes	Yes	No*
Syphilis	No	No	No[3]
Viruses			
HIV	Yes	Yes	Yes, developed countries
Cytomegalovirus			
Term infant	Yes	Yes	No
Preterm infant	Yes	Yes	Evaluate on an individual basis
Hepatitis B virus	Yes, surface antigen	No	No, developed countries[1]
Hepatitis C virus	Yes	No	No[†]
Hepatitis E virus	Yes	No	No
HTLV-1	Yes	Yes	Yes, developed countries
HTLV-2	Yes	?	Yes, developed countries
Herpes simplex virus	Yes	No/?yes	No, unless breast vesicles present
Rubella			
Wild type	Yes	Yes, rare	No
Vaccine	Yes	No	No
Varicella-zoster virus	Yes	No	No, cover active lesions[2]
Epstein-Barr virus	Yes	No	No
HHV-6	No	No	No
HHV-7	Yes	No	No
West Nile virus	Possible	Possible	Unknown
Parasites			
Toxoplesma gondii	Yes	Yes, one case	No

*Provided that the mother and child are taking appropriate antibiotics.
[†]Provided that the mother is HIV-seronegative. Mothers should be counseled that breast milk transmission of hepatitis C virus has not been documented, but is theoretically possible.
[1]Immunize and immune globulin at birth.
[2]Provide appropriate antivaricella therapy or prophylaxis to newborn.
[3]Treat mother and child if active disease.
CXR, chest x-ray; GNR, gram-negative rods; HHV, human herpesvirus; HTLV, human T-cell leukemia virus; *PPD*, purified protein derivative.
From Jones CA: Maternal transmission of infectious pathogens in breast milk. *J Paediatr Child Health* 2001;37:576–82.

Rein AJJT, Omokhodion SI, Nir A: Significance of a cardiac murmur as the sole clinical sign in the newborn. *Clin Pediatr* 2000;39:511–520.
Rhead WJ, Irons M: The call from the newborn screening laboratory: Frustration in the afternoon. *Pediatr Clin N Am* 2004;51:803–818.
Shoup AG, Owen KE, Jackson G, et al: The Parkland Memorial Hospital experience in ensuring compliance with universal newborn hearing screening follow-up. *J Pediatr* 2005;146:66–72.
Srinivasan R, Arora RS: Do well infants born with an isolated single umbilical artery need investigation? *Arch Dis Child* 2004;90:100–101.
Wolke D, Dave S, Hayes J, et al: Routine examination of the newborn and maternal satisfaction: A randomized controlled trial. *Arch Dis Child* 2002;86: F155–F160.
Yost GC, Young PC, Buchi KF: Significance of grunting respirations in infants admitted to a well-baby nursery. *Arch Pediatr Adolesc* 2001;155:372–375.

Chapter 95 ■ High-Risk Pregnancies

Barbara J. Stoll

High-risk pregnancies are those that increase the likelihood of abortion, fetal death, premature delivery, intrauterine growth restriction, poor cardiopulmonary or metabolic transitioning at birth, fetal or neonatal disease, congenital malformations, mental retardation, or other handicaps (Table 95-1; see also Chapter 96). Some factors, such as ingestion of a teratogenic drug in the 1st trimester, are causally related to the risk; others, such as hydramnios, are associations that alert a physician to determine the etiology and avoid the inherent risks associated with excessive amniotic fluid. Based on their history, 10–20% of pregnant women can be identified as high risk; nearly half of all perinatal mortality and morbidity is associated with these pregnancies. Although assessing antepartum risk is important in reducing perinatal mortality and morbidity, some women become high risk only during labor and delivery; therefore, careful monitoring is critical throughout the intrapartum course.

Identifying high-risk pregnancies is important not only because it is the 1st step toward prevention but also because therapeutic steps may often be taken to reduce the risks to the fetus or neonate if the physician knows of the potential for difficulty.

GENETIC FACTORS. The occurrence of chromosomal abnormalities, congenital anomalies, inborn errors of metabolism, mental retardation, or any familial disease in blood relatives increases the risk of the same condition in the infant. Because many parents recognize only obvious clinical manifestations of genetically determined diseases, specific inquiry should be made about any disease affecting one or more blood relatives.

MATERNAL FACTORS. The lowest neonatal mortality rate occurs in infants of mothers who receive adequate prenatal care and who are 20–30 yr of age. Both teenage pregnancies and those in women older than 40 yr, particularly primiparous women, are at

TABLE 95-1. Factors Associated with High-Risk Pregnancy

ECONOMIC	Prolonged gestation
Poverty	Prolonged labor
Unemployment	Previous infant with cerebral palsy, mental retardation, birth trauma, congenital anomalies
Uninsured, underinsured health insurance	Abnormal lie (breech)
Poor access to prenatal care	Multiple gestations
CULTURAL-BEHAVIORAL	Premature rupture of membranes
Low educational status	Infections (systemic, amniotic, extra-amniotic, cervical)
Poor health care attitudes	Preeclampsia or eclampsia
No care or inadequate prenatal care	Uterine bleeding (abruptio placentae, placenta previa)
Cigarette, alcohol, illicit drug use	Parity (0 or more than 5)
Age less than 20 or over 35 yr	Uterine or cervical anomalies
Unmarried	Fetal disease
Short interpregnancy interval	Abnormal fetal growth
Lack of support group (husband, family, religion)	Idiopathic premature labor
Stress (physical, psychologic)	Iatrogenic prematurity
Black race	High or low levels of maternal serum α-fetoprotein
BIOLOGIC-GENETIC	**MEDICAL**
Previous low birthweight or preterm infant	Diabetes mellitus
Low weight for height	Hypertension
Poor weight gain during pregnancy	Congenital heart disease
Short stature	Autoimmune disease
Poor nutrition	Sickle cell anemia
Inbreeding (autosomal recessive?)	TORCH infection
Intergenerational effects	Intercurrent surgery or trauma
Low maternal birthweight	Sexually transmitted disease
Hereditary diseases (inborn error of metabolism)	Maternal hypercoagulable states
REPRODUCTIVE	Exposure to prescription medications
Previous cesarean section	
Previous infertility	
Conception by reproductive technology	

TORCH, toxoplasmosis, other agents, rubella, cytomegalovirus, herpes simplex.

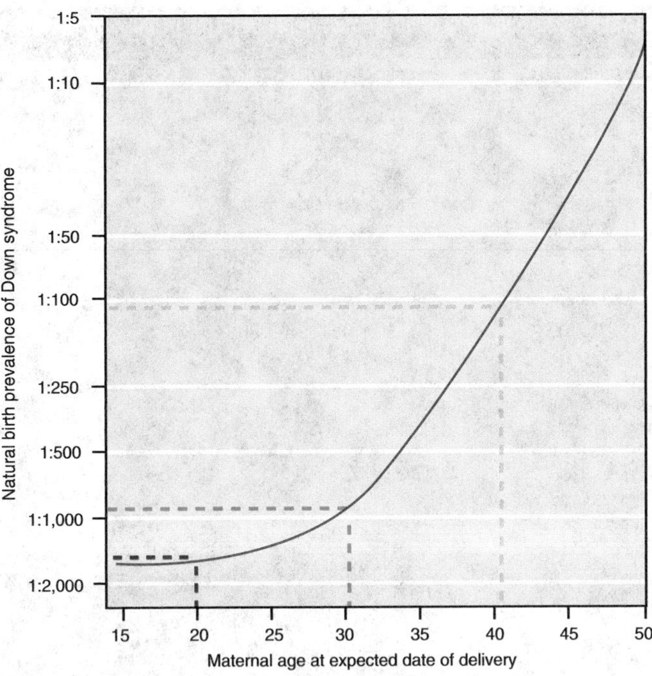

Figure 95-1. Natural birth prevalence of Down syndrome according to maternal age. (From Wald NJ, Leck I: *Antenatal and Neonatal Screening,* 2nd ed. Oxford, Oxford University Press, 2000.)

increased risk for intrauterine growth restriction, fetal distress, and intrauterine death. Advanced maternal age increases the risk of both chromosomal and non-chromosomal fetal malformations (Fig. 95-1).

Maternal illness (Table 95-2), multiple pregnancies, particularly those involving monochorionic twinning, infections (Table 95-3), and certain drugs (Chapter 96) increase the risk for the fetus. The use of assisted reproductive technology (in vitro fertilization, intracytoplasmic sperm injection) increases the risk of low birthweight and very low birthweight, as well as major birth defects and multiple-fetus pregnancies. Low birthweight, prematurity, and twinning in these infants also increases the risk of cerebral palsy.

Preterm birth is common in high-risk pregnancies (Chapter 97). Factors associated with prematurity are noted in Table 95-1 and

TABLE 95-2. Maternal Conditions Affecting the Fetus or Neonate

DISORDER	EFFECTS	MECHANISM
Autoantibody against folate receptors	Neural tube defects	Block cellular uptake of folate
Cervical neoplasia	Preterm premature rupture of membranes	Associated with loop electrosurgical excision procedure or laser cone therapy
Cholestasis	Preterm delivery	Unknown, possibly hepatitis E
Cyanotic heart disease	Intrauterine growth restriction	Low fetal oxygen delivery
Diabetes mellitus		
Mild	Large for gestational age, hypoglycemia	Fetal hyperglycemia—produces hyperinsulinemia; insulin promotes growth
Severe	Growth restriction	Vascular disease, placental insufficiency
Drug addiction	Intrauterine growth restriction, neonatal withdrawal	Direct drug effect plus poor diet
Endemic goiter	Hypothyroidism	Iodine deficiency
Graves disease	Transient neonatal thyrotoxicosis	Placental immunoglobin passage of thyroid-stimulating antibody
Herpes gestationalis (noninfectious)	Bullous rash	Unknown
Hyperparathyroidism	Neonatal hypocalcemia	Maternal calcium crosses to fetus and suppresses fetal parathyroid gland
Hypertension	Intrauterine growth restriction, intrauterine fetal demise	Placental insufficiency, fetal hypoxia
Idiopathic thrombocytopenic purpura	Thrombocytopenia	Nonspecific maternal platelet antibodies cross placenta
Isoimmune neutropenia or thrombocytopenia	Neutropenia or thrombocytopenia	Specific antifetal neutrophil or platelet antibody crosses placenta after sensitization of mother
Malignant melanoma	Placental or fetal tumor	Metastasis
Myasthenia gravis	Transient neonatal myasthenia	Immunoglobin to acetylcholine receptor crosses placenta
Myotonic dystrophy	Neonatal myotonic dystrophy, congenital contractures, respiratory insufficiency	Genetic anticipation
Obesity	Macrosomia, hypoglycemia	Unknown
Phenylketonuria	Microcephaly, retardation	Elevated fetal phenylalanine levels
Poor nutrition	Intrauterine growth restriction, adult insulin resistance, schizophrenia (?)	Reduced fetal nutrients, nutritional programming
Preeclampsia, eclampsia	Intrauterine growth restriction, thrombocytopenia, neutropenia, fetal demise	Uteroplacental insufficiency, fetal hypoxia, vasoconstriction
Renal transplant	Intrauterine growth restriction	Uteroplacental insufficiency
Rhesus or other blood group sensitization	Fetal anemia, hypoalbuminemia, hydrops, neonatal jaundice	Antibody crosses placenta directed to fetal cells with antigen
Sickle cell anemia	Preterm birth, intrauterine growth restriction	Maternal sickling producing fetal hypoxia
Systemic lupus erythematosus	Congenital heart block, rash, anemia, thrombocytopenia, neutropenia	Antibody directed to fetal heart, red and white blood cells, and platelets

?, possible.

TABLE 95-3. Maternal Infections Affecting the Fetus or Newborn

INFECTION	MODE OF TRANSMISSION	OUTCOME
Bacteria		
Group B streptococcus	Ascending cervical	Sepsis, pneumonia
Escherichia coli	Ascending cervical	Sepsis, pneumonia
Listeria monocytogenes	Transplacental	Sepsis, pneumonia
Ureaplasma urealyticum	Ascending cervical	Pneumonia, meningitis
Mycoplasma hominis	Ascending cervical	Pneumonia
Chlamydia trachomatis	Vaginal passage	Conjunctivitis, pneumonia
Syphilis	Transplacental, vaginal passage	Congenital syphilis
Borrelia burgdorferi	Transplacental	Prematurity, fetal demise
Neisseria gonorrhoeae	Vaginal passage	Ophthalmia (conjunctivitis), sepsis, meningitis
Mycobacterium tuberculosis	Transplacental	Prematurity, fetal demise, congenital tuberculosis
Granulocytic ehrlichiosis	Transplacental	Sepsis
Virus		
Rubella	Transplacental	Congenital rubella
Cytomegalovirus	Transplacental, breast milk (rare)	Congenital cytomegalovirus or asymptomatic
Human immunodeficiency virus	Transplacental, vaginal passage, breast milk	Congenital acquired immunodeficiency syndrome
Hepatitis B	Vaginal passage, transplacental, breast milk	Neonatal hepatitis, chronic HBsAg carrier
Hepatitis C	Transplacental	Uncommon but neonatal hepatitis, chronic carrier possible
Lymphocytic choriomeningitis	Transplacental	Fetal, neonatal death; hydrocephalus, chorioretinitis
Herpes simplex type 2 or 1	Transplacental	Congenital herpes simplex virus
	Vaginal passage, ascending	Neonatal encephalitis, disseminated viremia
Varicella-zoster	Transplacental, early	Congenital anomalies
	Transplacental, late	Neonatal varicella
Parvovirus	Transplacental	Fetal anemia, hydrops
Coxsackie B	Fecal-oral	Myocarditis, meningitis, hepatitis
Poliomyelitis	Transplacental	Congenital poliomyelitis
Epstein-Barr	Transplacental	Anomalies (?)
Rubeola	Transplacental	Abortion, fetal measles
West Nile	Transplacental	Chorioretinitis, focal cerebral necrosis
Parasites		
Toxoplasmosis	Transplacental	Congenital toxoplasmosis or asymptomatic
Malaria	Transplacental	Abortion, prematurty, intrauterine growth restriction
Trypanosomiasis	Transplacental	Congenital Chagas disease
Hookworm	None	Maternal anemia, LBW
Fungi		
Candida	Ascending, cervical	Sepsis, pneumonia, rash
Prion		
Creutzfeld-Jakob disease	Transplacental, colostrum	Hypothetical route, no long-term data

HBsAg, hepatitis B surface antigen; LBW, low birthweight.

include biologic markers such as cervical shortening, genital infection, fetal fibronectin in cervicovaginal secretions, and preterm premature rupture of membranes (PROM). The latter occurs in 1% of pregnancies but is noted in 30–40% of preterm deliveries, and it is a leading identifiable cause of prematurity. Premature delivery is often difficult to predict. Although women with preterm delivery have more spontaneous uterine contractions before the start of labor, this finding plus the length of the cervix and the presence of fetal fibronectin in cervical secretions has low sensitivity and poor positive predictive value for premature births.

Polyhydramnios and **oligohydramnios** indicate high-risk pregnancies. Although the turnover rate is rapid, during normal pregnancy the amniotic fluid volume gradually increases at a rate of <10 mL/day until about the 34th wk of pregnancy, after which it slowly diminishes. Volumes vary widely in normal pregnancy; term volume may be 500–2,000 mL. A volume estimated at greater than 2,000 mL in the 3rd trimester constitutes polyhydramnios, and a volume estimated at <500 mL indicates oligohydramnios. Polyhydramnios complicates 1–3% and oligohydramnios complicates 1–5% of pregnancies. The ultrasonographic criteria for these diagnoses are based on the amniotic fluid index, which is determined by measuring the vertical diameter of amniotic fluid pockets in four quadrants; an index >24 cm suggests polyhydramnios, whereas one <5 cm suggests oligohydramnios.

Acute polyhydramnios is rare and is usually associated with premature labor and delivery before 28 wk. **Chronic polyhydramnios** is diagnosed in the 3rd trimester by the discrepancy between uterine size and gestational age; it is occasionally not diagnosed until the patient has dysfunctional labor or an abnormally large amount of amniotic fluid is noted during delivery. Polyhydramnios is associated with premature labor, abruptio placentae, multiple congenital anomalies, and fetal neuromuscular dysfunction or obstruction of the gastrointestinal tract that interferes with reabsorption of the amniotic fluid swallowed by the fetus (Table 95-4). Increased fetal urination or edema formation is also associated with excessive amniotic fluid volume. Ultrasound demonstrates the increased amniotic fluid surrounding the fetus and detects associated fetal anomalies, hydrops, pleural effusions, and ascites. In 60% of patients, no cause is identified. Polyhydramnios may be managed by serial amniocentesis or by short-course maternal indomethacin if it is due to excessive fetal urination. **Treatment** is indicated for acute maternal respiratory distress and threatened preterm labor or to provide time for the administration of corticosteroids to enhance fetal lung maturity.

Oligohydramnios is associated with congenital anomalies; intrauterine growth restriction; severe renal, bladder, or urethral anomalies; and drugs that interfere with fetal urination (see Table 95-4). Oligohydramnios becomes most evident after 20 wk of gestation, when fetal urination is the major source of amniotic fluid. Rupture of the membranes must be ruled out when oligo-

TABLE 95-4. Conditions Associated with Disorders of Amniotic Fluid Volume

OLIGOHYDRAMNIOS	POLYHYDRAMNIOS
Intrauterine growth restriction Fetal anomalies Twin-twin transfusion (donor) Amniotic fluid leak Renal agenesis (Potter syndrome) Urethral atresia Prune-belly syndrome Pulmonary hypoplasia Amnion nodosum Indomethacin Angiotensin-converting enzyme inhibitors Intestinal pseudo-obstruction	*Congenital anomalies*: Anencephaly, hydrocephaly, tracheoesophageal fistula, duodenal atresia, spina bifida, cleft lip or palate, cystic adenomatoid lung malformation, diaphragmatic hernia *Syndromes*: Achondroplasia, Klippel-Feil, trisomy 18, trisomy 21, TORCH, hydrops fetalis, multiple congenital anomalad *Other*: Diabetes mellitus, twin-twin transfusion (recipient), fetal anemia, fetal heart failure, polyuric renal disease, neuromuscular diseases, nonimmune hydrops, chylothorax, teratoma *Idiopathic*

TORCH, toxoplasmosis, other agents, rubella, cytomegalovirus, herpes simplex.

hydramnios is suspected, especially if a normal-sized bladder is seen on fetal ultrasonography. Oligohydramnios causes fetal compression abnormalities such as clubfoot, spadelike hands, and a flattened nasal bridge. The most serious complication of chronic oligohydramnios is **pulmonary hypoplasia**. The risk of umbilical cord compression during labor and delivery is increased in pregnancies complicated by oligohydramnios and may be alleviated by saline amnio-infusion. Ultrasonography may reveal small (1–2 cm) pockets of fluid in addition to the associated growth restriction or anomalies. Oligohydramnios in combination with an elevated α-fetoprotein level, uterine bleeding, or intrauterine growth restriction has an increased risk of intrauterine fetal demise.

Antenatal screening can be used to detect a number of disorders, including Down syndrome and other chromosomal abnormalities, neural tube defects and other structural anomalies, Tay-Sachs disease and other metabolic genetic diseases, hemoglobinopathies and other blood disorders, and cystic fibrosis. Screening methods include maternal blood tests, fetal ultrasound, and diagnostic tests on cells or fluid obtained by amniocentesis or chorionic villus sampling and by fetal blood or tissue sampling.

Second-trimester screening (15–18 wk) of maternal serum α-fetoprotein (MSAFP) levels is used to screen for open neural tube defects. About 90% of affected pregnancies can be detected by an elevated MSAFP level. Gastroschisis, omphalocele, congenital nephrosis, twins, and other abnormal conditions can also be identified. Low MSAFP is associated with incorrect gestational age estimates, trisomy 18 or 21, and intrauterine growth restriction.

Several effective screening strategies can be used to detect Down syndrome (Fig. 95-2), including a combination of maternal age, nuchal translucency on ultrasound, and a number of serum markers: α-fetoprotein, unconjugated estriol, total human chorionic gonadotropin (HCG), the free β subunit of HCG, inhibin A, and pregnancy-associated plasma protein A. The most effective strategy, the integrated test, combines 1st- and 2nd-trimester screening and can identify 94% of affected pregnancies with a 5% false-positive rate or 85% with a 1% false-positive rate. Absence of the fetal nasal bone is also noted in trisomy 21. Chromosomal analysis of cells obtained by amniocentesis or chorionic villus biopsy makes the diagnosis.

A pregnancy should be considered high risk when the uterus is inappropriately large or small. A uterus large for the estimated stage of gestation suggests the presence of multiple fetuses, hydramnios, or an excessively large infant; an inappropriately small one suggests oligohydramnios or poor intrauterine growth. **PROM** earlier than 24 hr before delivery carries a risk of fetal infection; it also increases the risk of premature birth. PROM at term usually results in the onset of labor within 48 hr but poses a risk of chorioamnionitis and umbilical cord compression. PROM before 37 wk has a longer latency until labor starts and has the added risks of cord prolapse, oligohydramnios, abruptio placentae, fetal malposition, and if present for more than 7 days in a fetus between 20 and 30 wk gestation, pulmonary hypoplasia, uterine-induced deformations, and extremity contractures.

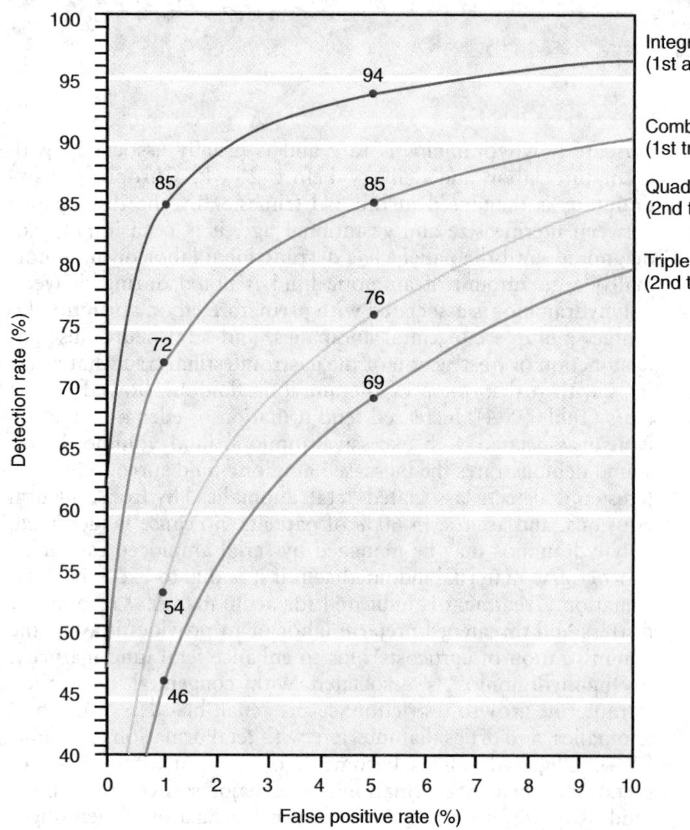

Figure 95-2. Rates of detection of Down syndrome and false-positive rates for various screening tests. The triple test includes measurements of serum α-fetoprotein, unconjugated estriol, human chorionic gonadotropin in the second trimester. The quadruple test includes the measurements of the triple test plus inhibin A in the 2nd trimester. The combined test includes measurements of serum pregnancy-associated plasma protein A, free β subunit of human gonadotropin, and nuchal translucency in the 1st trimester. The integrated test includes measurements of serum, α-fetoprotein, unconjugated estriol, human chorionic gonadotropin, and inhibin A in the 2nd trimester. (From Wald NJ, Watt HC, Hackshaw AK: Integrated screen for Down syndrome based on tests performed during the first and second trimester. *N Engl J Med* 1999; 341:461–467.)

Prolonged and difficult labor increases the risk for mechanical and hypoxic damage. A tumultuous short labor with a precipitous delivery increases the risk of birth asphyxia and intracranial hemorrhage. **Placental separation** at any time before delivery and abnormal implantation or compression of the cord increase the possibility of brain damage from fetal hypoxia; brown or muddy amniotic fluid suggests that meconium has been passed, possibly during an episode of fetal hypoxia.

Although the safety of any type of delivery depends on the skill of the obstetrician, additional hazards accompany particular methods and result from the circumstances that dictated them. The risk of **intracranial hemorrhage** is greater in infants delivered by vacuum extraction, or forceps than in those with unassisted spontaneous vaginal deliveries. Neonatal deaths after deliveries by mid and high forceps, breech extraction, and version are likely to be related to traumatic intracranial injury.

Infants born by **cesarean section** present problems possibly related to the unfavorable obstetric circumstance that necessitated the operation or to prolonged maternal anesthesia. In normal term pregnancies without any indication of fetal distress, surgical delivery through the abdomen carries a greater risk than delivery through the birth canal. Controversy exists regarding the safest type of delivery for a non-distressed, viable immature fetus, especially in a breech presentation; cesarean section may involve less risk than the "stress" of labor and the potentially hypoxic effects of uterine contractions during vaginal delivery. Term breech positions (≈3–4% of term births) that do not become vertex after external cephalic version will also benefit from cesarean section. A small percentage of mature infants delivered by cesarean section have some degree of respiratory difficulty for 1–2 days. Although transient tachypnea is the most frequently associated problem, hyaline membrane disease may develop, particularly in infants born to women not in labor, those with uncertain dates or pulmonary maturity, and those born to diabetic mothers or after asphyxia. A trial of labor after a previous cesarean section is associated with increased risk to both mother and fetus, including uterine rupture and hypoxic-ischemic encephalopathy.

Anesthesia and analgesia affect the fetus as well as the mother; mild maternal hypoxemia secondary to hypoventilation or hypotension resulting from epidural anesthesia may result in severe fetal hypoxia and shock. Skilled use of medication avoids severe fetal narcosis while securing the benefits of gentle and unhurried delivery. Even skilled administration may result in a mildly depressed infant whose crying and breathing may be delayed 1–2 min and who may be somewhat inactive for several hours. When anesthesia and analgesia are carelessly used or when their milder effects are added to already unfavorable fetal circumstances such as prematurity, hypoxia, or trauma, the result may be catastrophic.

ACOG Practice Bulletin. Assessment of risk factors for preterm birth. Clinical management guidelines for obstetrician-gynecologists. *Obstet Gynecol* 2001;98:709–716.

Chitty LS, Kagan KO, Molina FS, et al: Fetal nuchal translucency scan and early prenatal diagnosis of chromosomal abnormalities by rapid aneuploidy screenining: observational study. *BMJ* 2006;332:452–454.

Christian P, Khatry SK, West KP Jr: Antenatal anthelmintic treatment, birthweight, and infant survival in rural Nepal. *Lancet* 2004;364:981–983.

Cunniff C: Prenatal screening and diagnosis for pediatricians. *Pediatrics* 2004;114:889–894.

Ecker JL, Frigoletto Jr. FD: Cesarean delivery and the risk–benefit calculus. *N Engl J Med* 2007;356:885–888.

Epstein FH, Parry S, Strauss JF III: Premature rupture of the fetal membranes. *N Engl J Med* 1998;338:663–670.

Goldenberg RL, Iams JD, Mercer BM, et al: The preterm prediction study: Toward a multiple-marker test for spontaneous preterm birth. *Am J Obstet Gynecol* 2001;185:643.

Guise JM, McDonagh MS, Osterweil P, et al: Systematic review of the incidence and consequences of uterine rupture in women with previous caesarean section. *Br Med J* 2004;329:19–22.

Hansen M, Kurinczuk JJ, Bower C, et al: The risk of major birth defects after intracytoplasmic sperm injection and in vitro fertilization. *N Engl J Med* 2002;346:725–730.

Hollier LM, Leveno KJ, Kelly MA, et al: Maternal age and malformations in singleton births. *Obstet Gynecol* 2000;96:701–706.

Holmes W, Toole M: Micronutrient supplements in pregnant Nepalese women. *Lancet* 2005;365:916–917.

James D: Caesarean section for fetal distress. *Br Med J* 2001;322:1316–1317.

MMWR: Intrauterine West Nile Virus infection—New York, 2002. *MMWR* 2002;51:1135–1136.

Landon MB, Hauth JC, Leveno KJ, et al: Maternal and perinatal outcomes associated with a trial of labor after prior cesarean delivery. *N Eng J Med* 2004;351:2581–2589.

Neugebauer R: Accumulating evidence for prenatal nutritional origins of mental disorders. *JAMA* 2005;294:621–623.

O'Leary DR, Kuhn S, Kniss KL, et al: Birth outcomes following West Nile virus infection of pregnant women in the United States: 2003–2004. *Pediatrics* 2006;117:e537–e545.

Petrou S, Mugford M: Should prenatal diagnostic testing be offered to all pregnant women on economic grounds? *Lancet* 2004;363:258–259.

Pinborg A, Loft A, Schmidt L, et al: Neurological sequelae in twins born after assisted conception: Controlled national cohort study. *Br Med J* 2004;329:311–314.

Rothenberg SP, da Costa MP, Sequeria JM, et al: Autoantibodies against folate receptors in women with a pregnancy complicated by neural-tube defect. *N Engl J Med* 2004;350:134–142.

Sadler L, Saftlas A, Wang W, et al: Treatment for cervical intraepithelial neoplasia and risk of preterm delivery. *JAMA* 2004;291:2100–2106.

Schieve LA, Meikle SF, Ferre C, et al: Low and very low birth weight in infants conceived with use of assisted reproductive technology. *N Engl J Med* 2002;346:731–736.

Shennan A, Bewley S: How to manage term breech deliveries. *Br Med J* 2001;323:244–245.

Stromberg B, Dahlquist G, Ericson A, et al: Neurological sequelae in children born after in vitro fertilization: A population-based study. *Lancet* 2002;359:461–465.

Whitby EH, Griffiths PD, Rutter S, et al: Frequency and natural history of subdural haemorrhages in babies and relation to obstetric factors. *Lancet* 2004;362:846–850.

Chapter 96 ■ The Fetus

Barbara J. Stoll and Ira Adams-Chapman

The major emphasis in fetal medicine involves (1) assessment of fetal growth and maturity, (2) evaluation of fetal well-being or distress, (3) assessment of the effects of maternal disease on the fetus, (4) evaluation of the effects of drugs administered to the mother on the fetus, and (5) identification and treatment of fetal disease or anomalies. Increasing knowledge of fetal physiology has paved the way for effective fetal therapy, intervention during fetal distress, and improved adaptation of a newborn infant to extrauterine life, particularly a premature infant. Some aspects of human fetal growth and development are summarized in Chapter 6.

96.1 • Fetal Growth and Maturity

Ultrasonography of the fetus, a common obstetric procedure, is both safe and accurate. Indications for antenatal ultrasonography include estimation of gestational age (unknown dates, discrepancy between uterine size and dates or suspected growth restriction), assessment of amniotic fluid volume, estimation of fetal weight, determination of the location of the placenta and the number and position of fetuses, and identification of congenital anomalies.

Fetal growth can be assessed by ultrasonography as early as 6–8 wk. The most accurate assessment of gestational age is by 1st-trimester ultrasound measurement of crown-rump length. The biparietal diameter is used to assess gestational age beginning in the 2nd trimester. Through 34 wk the biparietal diameter accurately estimates gestation to within ±10 days. Later in gestation, accuracy falls to ±3 wk. Methods used to assess gestational age at term include measurement of abdominal circumference and femoral length. If a single ultrasound examination is performed, the most information can be obtained with a scan at 18–20 wk, when both gestational age and fetal anatomy can be evaluated. Serial scans may be useful in assessing fetal growth. Two patterns of fetal growth restriction have been identified: continuous fetal growth 2 SD below the mean for gestational age or a normal fetal growth curve that abruptly slows or flattens later in gestation (Fig. 96-1).

Fetal maturity is usually assessed by accurate ultrasonographic dating of gestational age, but it may also be estimated by determining the surfactant content of amniotic fluid (Chapter 101.4). Determination of the extent of calcification by ultrasound (placental maturity index), detection of the 1st audible fetal heart tones (16–18 wk), and observation of the initial fetal movements (18–20 wk) may also aid in evaluating the maturity of a fetus. An estimate of gestational age by dating of the last menstrual period should also be obtained.

96.2 • Fetal Distress

Fetal compromise may occur during the antepartum or intrapartum periods; it may be asymptomatic in the antenatal period. Antepartum fetal surveillance is warranted for women at increased risk for fetal distress, including those with a history of stillbirth, intrauterine growth restriction (IUGR), oligohydramnios or polyhydramnios, multiple gestation, rhesus sensitization, hypertensive disorders, diabetes mellitus or other chronic maternal disease, decreased fetal movement, and post-term pregnancy. The predominant cause of antepartum fetal distress is uteroplacental insufficiency. Fetal distress may be manifested clinically as IUGR, fetal hypoxia, increased vascular resistance in fetal blood vessels (Figs. 96-2 and 96-3), and when severe, mixed respiratory and metabolic (lactic) acidosis. The goals of antepartum fetal surveillance are to prevent intrauterine fetal demise, prevent hypoxic brain injury, and prolong gestation in women at risk for preterm delivery when such prolongation is safe or deliver a fetus when it is in jeopardy. The most commonly used noninvasive tests are the nonstress test (NST), the contraction stress test (CST), and the biophysical profile (BPP). Methods for assessing fetal well-being are listed in Table 96-1.

The **NST** monitors the presence of fetal heart rate accelerations that follow fetal movement. A reactive (normal) NST result demonstrates two fetal heart rate accelerations of at least 15 beats/min lasting 15 sec. A nonreactive NST result suggests fetal compromise and requires further assessment with a CST or the BPP. A **CST** observes the fetal heart rate response to spontaneous, nipple-, or oxytocin-stimulated uterine contractions. Fetal compromise is suggested when three contractions in 10 min are followed by late decelerations. A CST is contraindicated in women with preterm premature rupture of membranes or a previous uterine scar from a classic cesarean section and in those with multiple gestations, an incompetent cervix, or placenta previa. The goals of fetal monitoring are to prevent intrauterine fetal demise and hypoxic brain injury. Although the CST and NST have low false-negative rates, both have high false-positive rates. The **BPP** assesses fetal breathing, body movement, tone, heart rate, and amniotic fluid volume, and it is used to improve the accurate and safe identification of fetal compromise (Table 96-2). A score of 2

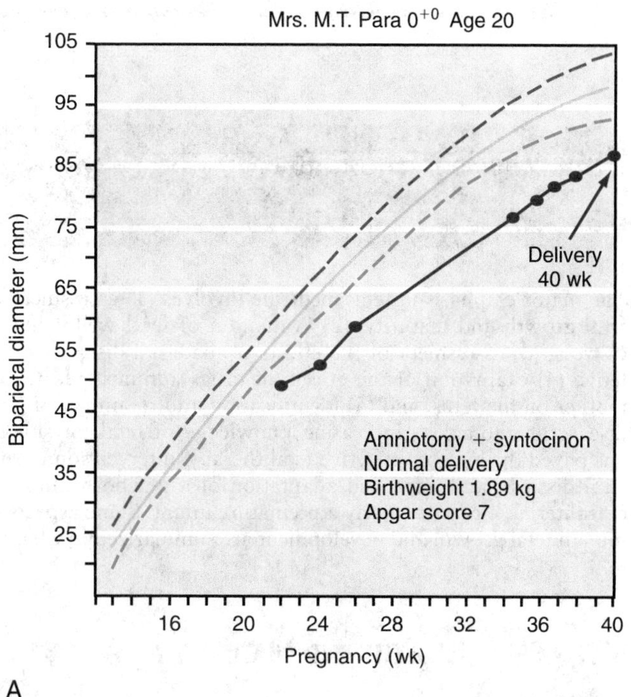

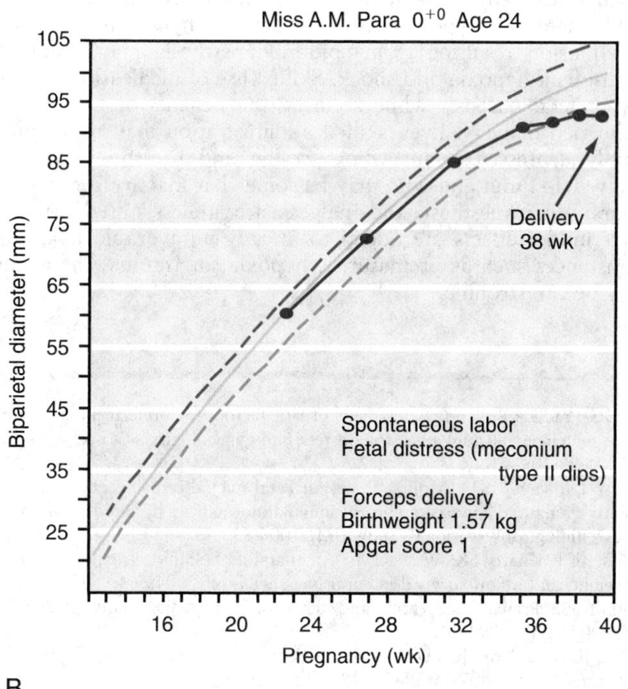

Figure 96-1. *A*, Example of a "low-profile" growth retardation pattern in an uneventful pregnancy and labor. The baby cried at 1 min and hypoglycemia did not develop. Birthweight was below the 5th percentile for gestational age. *B*, Example of a "late-flattening" growth retardation pattern. The mother had a typical history of preeclampsia, and the infant had intrapartum fetal distress, a low Apgar score, and postnatal hypoglycemia. Birthweight was below the 5th percentile for gestational age. (From Campbell S: *Clin Obstet Gynecol* 1974;1:41.)

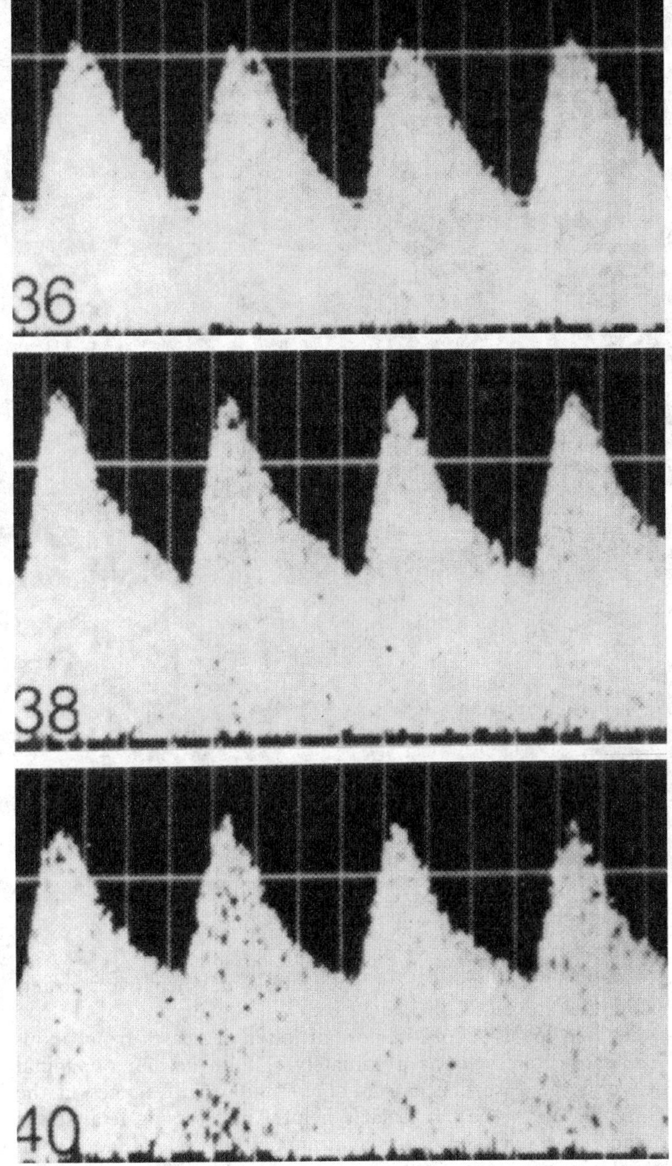

Figure 96-2. Normal Doppler velocity in sequential studies of fetal umbilical artery flow velocity waveforms from one normal pregnancy. Note the systolic peak flow with lower but constant heart flow during diastole. The systolic : diastolic ratio can be determined and, in normal pregnancies, is less than 3 after the 30th wk of gestation. The numbers indicate the week of gestation. (From Trudinger B: Doppler ultrasound assessment of blood flow. In Creasy RK, Resnik R [eds]: *Maternal-Fetal Medicine: Principles and Practice,* 3rd ed. Philadelphia, WB Saunders, 1994.)

is given for each observation present. A total score of 8–10 is reassuring; a score of 6 is equivocal, and retesting should be done in 12–24 hr; and a score of 4 or less warrants immediate evaluation and possible delivery. The BPP has good negative predictive value. Signs of compromise seen on Doppler ultrasonography include a reduced, absent, or reversed diastolic waveform velocity in the fetal aorta or umbilical artery (see Fig. 96-3 and Table 96-1). High-risk fetuses often have combinations of abnormalities, such as oligohydramnios, reversed diastolic Doppler umbilical artery blood flow velocity, and a low BPP.

Fetal distress during labor may be detected by monitoring the fetal heart rate, uterine pressure, and fetal scalp blood pH (Fig. 96-4).

Continuous fetal heart rate monitoring detects abnormal cardiac patterns by instruments that compute the beat-to-beat fetal heart rate from a fetal electrocardiographic signal. Signals are derived from an electrode attached to the fetal presenting part, from an ultrasonic transducer placed on the maternal abdominal wall to detect continuous ultrasonic waves reflected from the contractions of the heart, or from a phonotransducer placed on the mother's abdomen. Uterine contractions are simultaneously recorded from an amniotic fluid catheter and pressure transducer or from a tocotransducer applied to the maternal abdominal wall overlying the uterus.

Fetal heart rate patterns show various characteristics, some of which suggest fetal distress. The baseline fetal heart rate is the average rate between uterine contractions, which gradually decreases from about 155 beats/min in early pregnancy to about 135 beats/min at term; the normal range at term is 120–160 beats/min. **Tachycardia** (>160 beats/min) is associated with early fetal hypoxia, maternal fever, maternal hyperthyroidism, maternal β-sympathomimetic or atropine therapy, fetal anemia, infection, and some fetal arrhythmias. The latter do not generally occur with congenital heart disease and may resolve spontaneously at birth. **Fetal bradycardia** (<120 beats/min) occurs with fetal hypoxia, placental transfer of local anesthetic agents and β-adrenergic blocking agents, and, occasionally, heart block with or without congenital heart disease.

Normally, the baseline fetal heart rate is variable, with long-term changes of 3–6 cycles/min as well as short-term beat-to-beat variation. This variability may be decreased or lost with fetal hypoxemia or the placental transfer of drugs such as atropine, diazepam, promethazine, magnesium sulfate, and most sedative and narcotic agents. Prematurity, the sleep state, and fetal tachycardia may also diminish beat-to-beat variability.

Periodic accelerations or decelerations of the fetal heart rate in response to uterine contractions may also be monitored (see Fig. 96-4). **Early deceleration (type I)**, associated with head compression, is a repetitive pattern of slowing that is synchronous with and proportional to the amplitude of the uterine contraction. **Variable deceleration** (associated with cord compression) is characterized by variable shape, abrupt onset and occurrence with consecutive contractions, and return to baseline at or after the conclusion of the contraction. **Late deceleration (type II)**, associated with fetal hypoxemia, occurs repetitively after a uterine contraction is well established, is proportional to its amplitude, and persists into the interval following contractions. The late deceleration pattern is usually associated with maternal hypotension or excessive uterine activity, but it may be a response to any maternal, placental, umbilical cord, or fetal factor that limits effective oxygenation of the fetus. Reflex late decelerations with normal beat-to-beat variability are associated with chronic compensated fetal hypoxia, and they occur during uterine contrac-

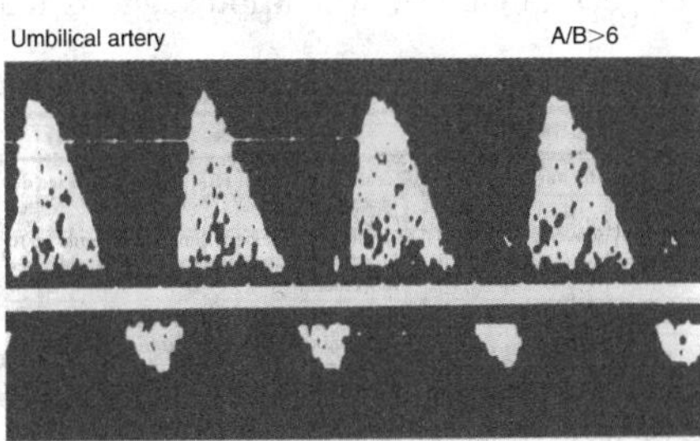

Figure 96-3. Abnormal Doppler velocimetry. On an umbilical artery Doppler flow velocity waveform, the umbilical placental impedance is so high that the diastolic component shows flow in a reverse direction. This finding is an indication of severe intrauterine hypoxia and intrauterine growth restriction. (From Trudinger B: Doppler ultrasound assessment of blood flow. In Creasy RK, Resnik R [eds]: *Maternal-Fetal Medicine: Principles and Practice,* 3rd ed. Philadelphia, WB Saunders, 1994.)

TABLE 96-1. Fetal Diagnosis and Assessment

METHOD	COMMENT AND INDICATIONS
IMAGING	
Ultrasound (real-time)	Biometry (growth), anomaly (morphology) detection. Biophysical profile. Amniotic fluid volume, hydrops. Determine gestational age and IUGR
Ultrasound (Doppler)	Velocimetry (blood flow velocity). Detection of increased vascular resistance secondary to fetal hypoxia, IUGR
Embryoscopy	Early diagnosis of limb anomaly
Fetoscopy	Detection of facial, limb, cutaneous anomalies
MRI	Best to define lesions before fetal surgery
FLUID ANALYSIS	
Amniocentesis	Fetal maturity (L:S ratio), karyotype (cytogenetics), biochemical enzyme analysis, molecular genetic DNA diagnosis, bilirubin, or α-fetoprotein determination. Bacterial culture, pathogen antigen, or genome detection
Fetal urine	Prognosis of obstructive uropathy?
CORDOCENTESIS (PERCUTANEOUS UMBILICAL BLOOD SAMPLING)	Detection of blood type, anemia, hemoglobinopathies, thrombocytopenia, acidosis, hypoxia, polycythemia, IgM antibody response to infection. Rapid karyotyping and molecular DNA genetic diagnosis. Fetal therapy (see Table 96-5)
FETAL TISSUE ANALYSIS	
Chorionic villus biopsy	Karyotype, molecular DNA genetic analysis, enzyme assays
Skin biopsy	Hereditary skin disease*
Liver biopsy	Enzyme assay*
Circulating fetal cells or DNA in maternal blood or plasma	Molecular DNA genetic analysis
MATERNAL SERUM α-FETOPROTEIN	
Elevated	Twins, neural tube defects (anencephaly, spina bifida), intestinal atresia, hepatitis, nephrosis, fetal demise, incorrect gestational age
Reduced	Trisomies, aneuploidy
MATERNAL CERVIX	
Fetal fibronectin	Indicates risk of preterm birth
Bacterial culture	Identifies risk of fetal infection (group B streptococcus, *Neisseria gonorrhoeae*)
Fluid	Determination of premature rupture of membranes
ANTEPARTUM BIOPHYSICAL MONITORING	
Nonstress test	Fetal distress; hypoxia
Contraction stress test	Fetal distress; hypoxia
Biophysical profile	Fetal distress; hypoxia
INTRAPARTUM FETAL HEART RATE MONITORING	See Fig. 96-4

*DNA genetic analysis on chorionic villus samples, amniocytes from amniocentesis, or fetal cells recovered from the maternal circulation may obviate the need for direct fetal tissue biopsy if the gene or genetic marker is available (e.g., the gene for Duchenne muscular dystrophy).
IUGR, intrauterine growth restriction; L:S, lecithin : sphingomyelin ratio.

tions that temporarily impede oxygen transport to the heart. Nonreflex late decelerations are more ominous and indicate severe hypoxic depression of myocardial function. The latter, together with decreased beat-to-beat variability or spontaneous decelerations in the absence of uterine contractions, either warrants further assessment by fetal blood sampling or is an indication for delivery.

Fetal scalp blood sampling during labor through a slightly dilated cervix may aid in confirming fetal distress suspected on the basis of variations in fetal heart rate or the presence of meconium in amniotic fluid. The proper use of this technique may result in earlier delivery of depressed infants, who thus have a better chance of successful resuscitation, increased survival, and less morbidity. Alternatively, when continuous fetal heart rate monitoring or general clinical evaluation suggests that a fetus is at risk, a normal fetal scalp blood sample may help avert obstetric intervention.

Fetal scalp blood pH in normal labor decreases from about 7.33 early in labor to approximately 7.25 at the time of vaginal delivery; the base deficit is about 4–6 mEq/L. Changes in the buffer base may be particularly helpful in assessing fetal status because they correspond to the accumulation of fetal lactic acid. A pH <7.25 suggests fetal distress, and a pH <7.20 is an indication for further assessment and intervention. Determination of the lactate concentration in fetal scalp blood is another tool for monitoring the condition of the fetus.

Complications of fetal scalp sampling and internal monitoring devices are relatively uncommon but include bleeding (usually because of an underlying coagulation defect), puncture of the fontanel, and scalp abscesses with or without adjacent

TABLE 96-2. Biophysical Profile Scoring: Technique and Interpretation

BIOPHYSICAL VARIABLE	NORMAL SCORE (2)	ABNORMAL SCORE (0)
Fetal breathing movements	At least 1 episode of FBM of at least 30 sec duration in 30 min observation	Absent FBM or no episode of ≥30 sec in 30 min
Gross body movement	At least 3 discrete body/limb movements in 30 min (episodes of active continuous movement considered a single movement)	2 or fewer episodes of body/limb movements in 30 min
Fetal tone	At least 1 episode of active extension with return to flexion of fetal limb(s) or trunk. Opening and closing of hand considered normal tone	Either slow extension with return to partial flexion or movement of limb in full extension or absent fetal movement with fetal hand held in complete or partial deflection
Reactive FHR	At least 2 episodes of FHR acceleration of ≥15 beats/min and at least 15 sec duration associated with fetal movement in 30 min	Less than 2 episodes of acceleration of FHR or acceleration of <15 beats/min in 30 min
Qualitative AFV*	At least 1 pocket of AF that measures at least 2 cm in 2 perpendicular planes	Either no AF pockets or a pocket <2 cm in 2 perpendicular planes

*Modification of the criteria for reduced amniotic fluid from less than 1 cm to less than 2 cm would seem reasonable. Ultrasound is used for biophysical assessment of the fetus.
AF, amniotic fluid; AFV, amniotic fluid volume; FBM, fetal breathing movement; FHR, fetal heart rate.
From Creasy RK, Resnik R (eds): *Maternal-Fetal Medicine: Principles and Practice*, 3rd ed. Philadelphia, WB Saunders, 1994.

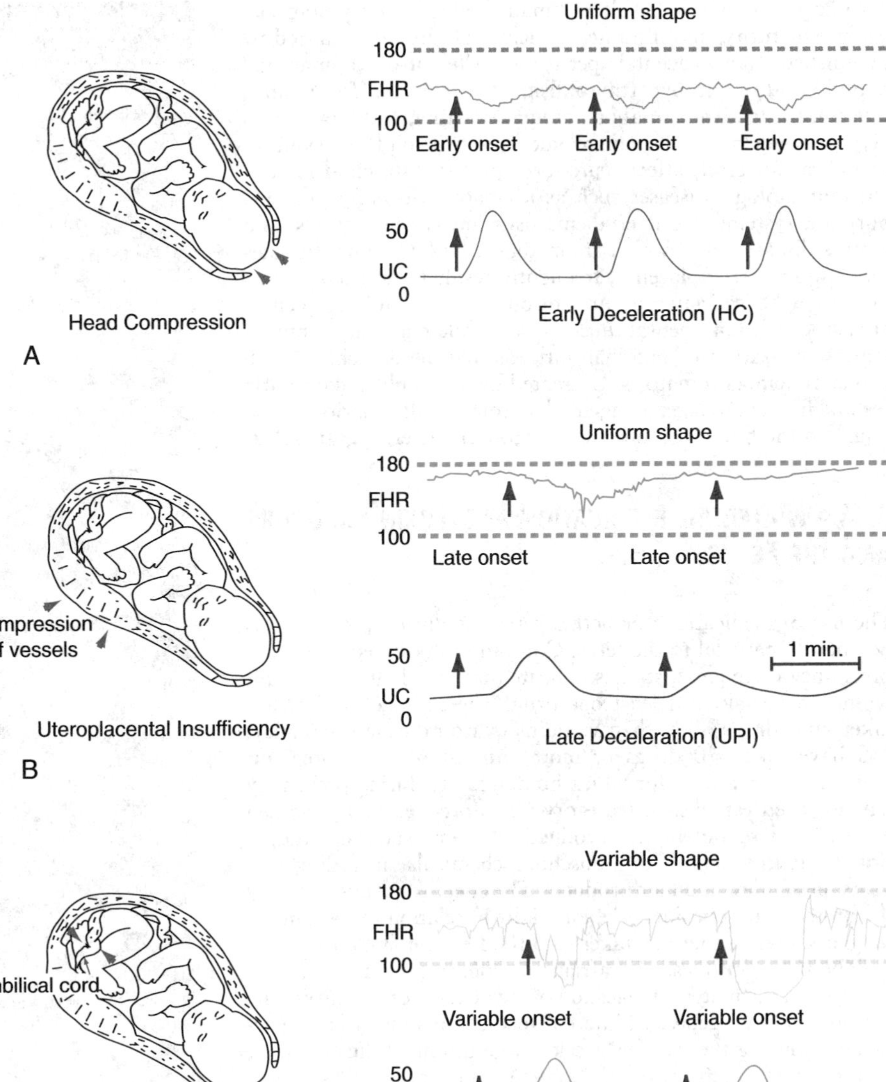

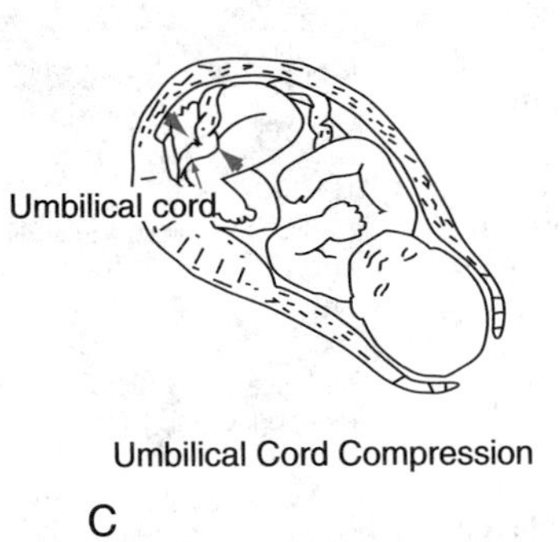

Figure 96-4. Patterns of periodic fetal heart rate (FHR) deceleration. The tracing in *A* shows early deceleration occurring during the peak of uterine contractions as a result of pressure on the fetal head. *B,* Late deceleration caused by uteroplacental insufficiency. *C,* Variable deceleration as a result of umbilical cold compression. *Arrows* denote the time relationship between the onset of FHR changes and uterine contractions. (From Hon EH: *An Atlas of Fetal Heart Rate Patterns.* New Haven, CT, Harty Press, 1968.)

osteomyelitis. Abscesses may be due to *Staphylococcus aureus* or gram-negative rods; more often they are sterile.

Umbilical cord blood samples obtained at the time of delivery are useful to document fetal acid-base status. Although the exact cord blood pH value that defines significant fetal acidemia is unknown, an umbilical artery pH <7.0 has been associated with greater need for resuscitation and a higher incidence of respiratory, gastrointestinal, cardiovascular, and neurologic complications. Nonetheless, when a low pH is detected, many newborn infants will be neurologically normal.

Intrapartum fetal pulse oximetry provides more accurate assessment of fetal oxygenation in labor and may be utilized to assess fetal well-being. It appears that oximetry decreases the cesarean section rate for nonreassuring fetal heart rate status detected by cardiotocography without adversely affecting fetal/neonatal outcome. Further studies are warranted.

96.3 • Maternal Disease and the Fetus

INFECTIOUS DISEASES (SEE TABLE 95-2). Almost any maternal infection with severe systemic manifestations may result in miscarriage, stillbirth, or premature labor. Whether these results are due to infection of the fetus or are secondary to stress is not always clear. Maternal hyperthermia during infections may be associated with an increased incidence of congenital anomalies. Regardless of the severity of the maternal infection, certain agents frequently infect a fetus and result in serious sequelae. Such fetuses are often small for gestational age. Some infections, such as rubella, may also produce congenital malformations if they occur during the period of organogenesis. Intrauterine infection/chorioamnionitis may be an important risk factor for cerebral white matter injury and subsequent cerebral palsy. Infections that affect maternal nutrition (hookworm) may also result in low birthweight (LBW) babies.

NONINFECTIOUS DISEASES (SEE TABLE 95-1). Maternal diabetes may result in organomegaly, hypertrophy and hyperplasia of the β cells of the fetal pancreas, and metabolic derangements in the neonate (see Chapter 107.1). A high incidence of intrauterine death occurs after the 36th wk of gestation in unmonitored and poorly controlled diabetic mothers. Moreover, maternal diabetes is a risk factor for cardiovascular and other malformations. **Eclampsia-preeclampsia** of pregnancy, chronic hypertension, and chronic renal disease result in small fetal size for gestational age, prematurity, and intrauterine death, all probably caused by diminished uteroplacental perfusion. Uncontrolled maternal hypothyroidism or hyperthyroidism is responsible for relative infertility, a tendency to abort, premature labor, and fetal death. Hypothyroidism in pregnant women (even if mild or asymptomatic) can adversely affect neurodevelopment of the child. Maternal immunologic diseases such as idiopathic thrombocytopenic purpura, systemic lupus erythematosus, myasthenia gravis, and Graves disease, all of which are mediated by IgG autoantibodies that can cross the placenta, frequently result in transient illness in the newborn. Maternal autoantibodies to the folate receptor are associated with neural tube defects, while maternal immunologic sensitization to paternal antigens may be associated with neonatal hemochromatosis. Untreated maternal phenylketonuria results in miscarriage, congenital cardiac malformations, and injury to the brain of a nonphenylketonuric heterozygotic fetus.

96.4 • Maternal Medication and Toxin Exposure and the Fetus

The use of medications or herbal remedies during pregnancy is potentially harmful to the fetus. Consumption of medications in pregnancy is frequent; studies indicate that over half of pregnant women have taken at least one drug. The average mother has taken four drugs other than vitamins or iron during pregnancy; 4% have taken 10 drugs or more. Almost 40% of pregnant women receive a drug for which human safety during pregnancy has not been established (category C). Moreover, many women are exposed to potential reproductive toxins, such as occupational, environmental, or household chemicals, including solvents, pesticides, and hair products. The effects of drugs taken by the mother vary considerably, especially in relation to the time in pregnancy when they are taken and the fetal genotype for drug-metabolizing enzymes. Miscarriage or congenital malformations result from the maternal ingestion of teratogenic drugs during the period of organogenesis. Maternal medications taken later, particularly during the last few weeks of gestation or during labor, tend to affect the function of specific organs or enzyme systems, and they adversely affect the neonate rather than the fetus (Table 96-3 and Table 96-4).

The effects of drugs may be evident immediately in the delivery room or later in the neonatal period, or they may be delayed even longer. The administration of diethylstilbestrol during pregnancy has resulted in vaginal adenosis and vaginal adenocarcinoma in females in the 2nd or 3rd decade. In addition to in utero carcinogenesis, various reproductive problems have been reported in these women, including cervical anomalies and premature births, ectopic pregnancies, and spontaneous pregnancy loss.

Evidence has confirmed an interaction between genetic factors and susceptibility to certain drugs or environmental toxins. Phenytoin teratogenesis may be mediated by genetic differences in the enzymatic production of epoxide metabolites; specific genes may influence the adverse effects of benzene exposure during pregnancy. Polymorphisms of genes encoding enzymes that metabolize the polycyclic aromatic hydrocarbons in cigarette smoke influence the growth-restricting effects of smoking on the fetus.

Often the risk of controlling maternal disease must be balanced with the risk of possible complications in the fetus. The majority of women with epilepsy have normal fetuses. Nonetheless, several commonly used antiepileptic drugs (AEDs) are associated with congenital malformations. Infants exposed to valproic acid may have multiple anomalies including neural tube defects, hypospadius, facial anomalies, cardiac anomalies, and limb defects. In addition, they have lower developmental index scores compared to those unexposed infants or those exposed to other commonly used AEDs.

TABLE 96-3. Agents Acting on Pregnant Women That May Adversely Affect the Structure or Function of the Fetus and Newborn

DRUG	EFFECT ON FETUS
Accutane (isotretinoin)	Facial-ear anomalies, heart disease, CNS anomalies
Alcohol	Congenital cardiac, CNS, limb anomalies; IUGR; developmental delay; attention deficits; autism
Aminopterin	Abortion, malformations
Amphetamines	Congenital heart disease, IUGR, withdrawal
Azathioprine	Abortion
Busulfan (Myleran)	Stunted growth; corneal opacities; cleft palate; hypoplasia of ovaries, thyroid, and parathyroids
Carbamazepine	Spina bifida, possible neurodevelopmental delay
Carbimazole	Scalp defects, choanal atresia, esophageal atresia, developmental delay
Carbon monoxide	Cerebral atrophy, microcephaly, seizures
Chloroquine	Deafness
Chorionic villus sampling	Probably no effect, possibly limb reduction
Cigarette smoking	Low birthweight for gestational age
Cocaine/crack	Microcephaly, LBW, IUGR, behavioral disturbances
Cyclophosphamide	Multiple malformations
Danazol	Virilization
17α-Ethinyl testosterone (Progestoral)	Masculinizaition of female fetus
Hyperthermia	Spina bifida
Lithium	Ebstein anomaly, macrosomia
6-Mercaptopurine	Abortion
Methyl mercury	Minamata disease, microcephaly, deafness, blindness, mental retardation
Methyltestosterone	Masculinization of female fetus
Misoprostol	Arthrogryposis, cranial neuropathies (Möbius syndrome), equinovarus
Norethindrone	Masculinization of female fetus
Penicillamine	Cutis laxa syndrome
Phenytoin	Congenital anomalies, IUGR, neuroblastoma, bleeding (vitamin K deficiency)
Polychlorinated biphenyls	Skin discoloration—thickening, desquamation, LBW, acne, developmental delay
Prednisone	Oral clefts
Progesterone	Masculinization of female fetus
Quinine	Abortion, thrombocytopenia, deafness
Statins	IUGR, limb deficiencies, VACTERAL
Stilbestrol (diethylstilbestrol [DES])	Vaginal adenocarcinoma in adolescence
Streptomycin	Deafness
Tetracycline	Retarded skeletal growth, pigmentation of teeth, hypoplasia of enamel, cataract, limb malformations
Thalidomide	Phocomelia, deafness, other malformations
Toluene (solvent abuse)	Craniofacial abnormalities, prematurity, withdrawal symptoms, hypertonia
Trimethadione and paramethadione	Abortion, multiple malformations, mental retardation
Valproate	CNS, facial and cardiac anomalies, limb defects, impaired neurologic function
Vitamin D	Supravalvular aortic stenosis, hypercalcemia
Warfarin (Coumadin)	Fetal bleeding and death, hypoplastic nasal structures

CNS, central nervous system; IUGR, intrauterine growth restriction; LBW, low birthweight; VACTERAL, vertebral, anal, cardiac, tracheoesophageal fistula, renal, arterial, limb.

Methotrexate is used for medical termination of pregnancy; surviving exposed infants may be at higher risk for congenital anomalies, IUGR, hypotonia, and developmental delay.

In view of the limits of current knowledge on the fetal effects of maternal medication, no drugs or herbal agent should be prescribed during pregnancy without weighing maternal need against the risk of fetal damage. All women should be specifically counseled to abstain from the use of alcohol, tobacco, and illicit drugs during pregnancy.

96.5 • Teratogens

When an infant or child has a congenital malformation or is developmentally delayed, the parents often wrongly blame themselves and attribute the child's problems to events that occurred

TABLE 96-4. Agents Acting on Pregnant Women That May Adversely Affect the Newborn Infant

Acebutolol—IUGR, hypotension, bradycardia	Intravenous fluids during labor (e.g., salt-free solutions)—electrolyte disturbances, hyponatremia, hypoglycemia
Acetazolamide—metabolic acidosis	Iodide (radioactive)—goiter
Amiodarone—bradycardia, hypothyroidism	Iodides—goiter
Anesthetic agents (volatile)—CNS depression	Lead—reduced intellectual function
Adrenal corticosteroids—adrenocortical failure (rare)	Magnesium sulfate—respiratory depression, meconium plug, hypotonia
Ammonium chloride—acidosis (clinically inapparent)	Methimazole—goiter, hypothyroidism
Aspirin—neonatal bleeding, prolonged gestation	Morphine and its derivatives (addiction)—withdrawal symptoms (poor feeding, vomiting, diarrhea, restlessness, yawning and stretching, dyspnea and cyanosis, fever and sweating, pallor, tremors, convulsions)
Atenolol—IUGR, hypoglycemia	Naphthalene—hemolytic anemia (in G6PD-deficient infants)
Baclofen—withdrawal	Nitrofurantoin—hemolytic anemia (in G6PD-deficient infants)
Blue cohosh herbal tea—neonatal heart failure	Oxytocin—hyperbilirubinemia, hyponatremia
Bromides—rash, CNS depression, IUGR	Phenobarbital—bleeding diathesis (vitamin K deficiency), possible long-term reduction in IQ, sedation
Captopril, enalapril—transient anuric renal failure, oligohydramnios	Primaquine—hemolytic anemia (in G6PD-deficient infants)
Caudal-paracervical anesthesia with mepivacaine (accidental introduction of anesthetic into scalp of baby)—bradypnea, apnea, bradycardia, convulsions	Propranolol—hypoglycemia, bradycardia, apnea
Cholinergic agents (edrophonium, pyridostigmine)—transient muscle weakness	Propylthiouracil—goiter, hypothyroidism
CNS depressants (narcotics, barbiturates, benzodiazepines) during labor—CNS depression, hypotonia	Pyridoxine—seizures
Cephalothin—positive direct Coombs test reaction	Reserpine—drowsiness, nasal congestion, poor temperature stability
Dexamethasone—periventricular leukomalacia	Sulfonamides—interfere with protein binding of bilirubin; kernicterus at low levels of serum bilirubin, hemolysis with G6PD deficiency
Fluoxetine and other SSRIs—transient neonatal withdrawal, hypertonicity, minor anomalies	Sulfonylurea agents—refractory hypoglycemia
Haloperidol—withdrawal	Sympathomimetic (tocolytic β-agonist) agents—tachycardia
Hexamethonium bromide—paralytic ileus	Thiazides—neonatal thrombocytopenia (rare)
Ibuprofen—oligohydramnios, pulmonary hypertension	
Imipramine—withdrawal	
Indomethacin—oliguria, oligohydramnios, intestinal perforation, pulmonary hypertension	

CNS, central nervous system; G6PD, glucose-6-phosphate dehydrogenase; IUGR, intrauterine growth restriction; SSRI, selective serotonin reuptake inhibitor.

during pregnancy. Because benign infections occur and several nonteratogenic drugs are often taken during many pregnancies, the pediatrician must evaluate the presumed viral infections and the drugs ingested to help parents understand their child's birth defect. The causes of approximately 40% of congenital malformations are unknown. Although only a relatively few agents are recognized to be teratogenic in humans (see Tables 96-1–96-4), new agents continue to be identified. Overall, only 10% of anomalies are due to recognizable teratogens. The time of exposure is usually at less than 60 days' gestation during organogenesis. Specific agents produce predictable lesions. Some agents have a dose or threshold effect; below the threshold, no alterations in growth, function, or structure occur. Genetic variables such as the presence of specific enzymes may metabolize a benign agent into a more toxic-teratogenic form (phenytoin conversion to its epoxide). In many circumstances, the same agent and dose may not consistently produce the lesion.

Reduced enzyme activity of the folate methylation pathway, particularly the formation of 5-methyltetrahydrofolate, may be responsible for neural tube or other birth defects. The common thermolabile mutation of 5,10-methylene tetrahydrofolate reductase may be one of the enzymes responsible. Folate supplementation for all pregnant women (by direct fortification of cereal grains, mandatory in the United States) during organogenesis may overcome this genetic enzyme defect, thus reducing the incidence of neural tube and perhaps other birth defects.

The Food and Drug Administration classifies drugs into five pregnancy risk categories. **Category A** suggests no risk based on evidence from controlled human trials. **Category B** suggests either no risk shown in animal studies but no adequate studies in humans or some risk in animal studies that are not confirmed by human studies. **Category C** is either definite risk shown in animal studies but no adequate human studies or no available data for animals or humans. **Category D** includes drugs with some risk but with a benefit that may exceed that risk for the treated life-threatening condition, such as streptomycin for tuberculosis. **Category X** is for drugs that are contraindicated in pregnancy on the basis of animal and human evidence and whose risk exceeds the benefits.

The specific mechanism of action is known or postulated for very few teratogens. Warfarin, an anticoagulant because it is a vitamin K antagonist, prevents the carboxylation of γ-carboxyglutamic acid, which is a component of osteocalcin and other vitamin K–dependent bone proteins. The teratogenic effect on developing cartilage, especially nasal cartilage, appears to be avoided if the pregnant woman's anticoagulation treatment between weeks 6 and 12 of gestation is switched from warfarin to heparin. Hypothyroidism in the fetus may be caused by the maternal ingestion of an excessive amount of iodides or propylthiouracil; each interferes with the conversion of inorganic to organic iodides. Phenytoin may be teratogenic because of the accumulation of a metabolite as a result of deficiency of epoxide hydrolase.

Recognition of teratogens offers the opportunity for prevention of related birth defects. If a pregnant woman is informed of the potentially harmful effects of alcohol on her unborn infant, she may be motivated to control this problem during pregnancy. A woman with insulin-dependent diabetes mellitus may significantly decrease her risk for having a child with birth defects by achieving good control of her disease before conception.

96.6 • Radiation (See also Chapter 706)

Accidental exposure of pregnant women to radiation is a common cause for anxiety about whether the fetus will have birth defects or genetic abnormalities. It is unlikely that exposure to diagnostic radiation will cause gene mutations; no increase in genetic abnormalities has been identified in the offspring exposed as unborn fetuses to the atomic bomb explosions in Japan in 1945.

A more realistic concern is whether the exposed human fetus will show birth defects or a higher incidence of malignancy. The recommended occupational limit of maternal exposure to radiation from all sources is 500 mrad for the entire 40 wk of a pregnancy. See Chapter 706 for a discussion of gonadal exposure in the mother and whole body exposure of the fetus. The limited data on human fetuses show that large doses of radiation (20,000–50,000 mrad) are harmful to the central nervous system, as evidenced by microcephaly, mental retardation, and IUGR. Leukemia is another risk.

Therapeutic abortion is often recommended when exposure exceeds 10,000 mrad. It is more likely that a human fetus will be exposed to 1,000–3,000 mrad, an amount not shown to cause malformations. Whether this level of fetal exposure is associated with an increased risk for childhood cancer or leukemia is controversial.

96.7 • Intrauterine Diagnosis of Fetal Disease (see Table 96-1)

See section 96.2 for a discussion of fetal distress.

Diagnostic procedures are used to identify fetal diseases when abortion is being considered, when direct fetal treatment is possible, or when a decision is made to deliver a viable but premature infant to avoid intrauterine fetal demise. Fetal assessment is also indicated in a broader context when the family, medical, or reproductive history of the mother suggests the presence of a high-risk pregnancy or a high-risk fetus (see Chapters 95 and 96.3).

Various methods are used for identifying fetal disease (see Table 96-1). Fetal ultrasonographic imaging may detect fetal growth abnormalities (by biometric measurements of biparietal diameter, femoral length, or head or abdominal circumference) or fetal malformations (Fig. 96-5). Although 95% of fetuses whose biparietal diameter is 9.5 cm or more are at least 37 wk of gestation, the lungs of these fetuses may not be mature. Serial determination of growth velocity and the head-to-abdominal circumference ratio enhances the ability to detect IUGR. Real-time ultrasonography may identify placental abnormalities (abruptio placentae, placenta previa) and fetal anomalies such as hydrocephalus, neural tube defects, duodenal atresia, diaphragmatic hernia, renal agenesis, bladder outlet obstruction, congenital heart disease, limb abnormalities, sacrococcygeal teratoma, cystic hygroma, omphalocele, gastroschisis, and hydrops (Table 96-5).

Real-time ultrasonography also facilitates performance of cordocentesis and the BPP by imaging fetal breathing, body movements, tone, and amniotic fluid volume (see Table 96-2). Doppler velocimetry assesses fetal arterial blood flow (vascular resistance) (see Figs. 96-2 and 96-3). Roentgenographic examination of the fetus has been replaced by real-time ultrasonography, MRI, and fetoscopy.

Amniocentesis, the transabdominal withdrawal of amniotic fluid during pregnancy for diagnostic purposes (see Table 96-1), is frequently performed to determine the timing of the delivery of fetuses with erythroblastosis fetalis or the need for fetal transfusion. It is also done for genetic indications, usually between the 15th and 16th wk of gestation, with results available within 1–2 wk. The most common indication for genetic amniocentesis is advanced maternal age (the risk for chromosome abnormality at age 21 is 1:526 vs 1:8 at age 49). The amniotic fluid may be directly analyzed for amino acids, enzymes, hormones, and abnormal metabolic products, and amniotic fluid cells may be cultivated to permit detailed cytologic analysis for prenatal detection of chromosomal abnormalities and DNA-gene or enzymatic

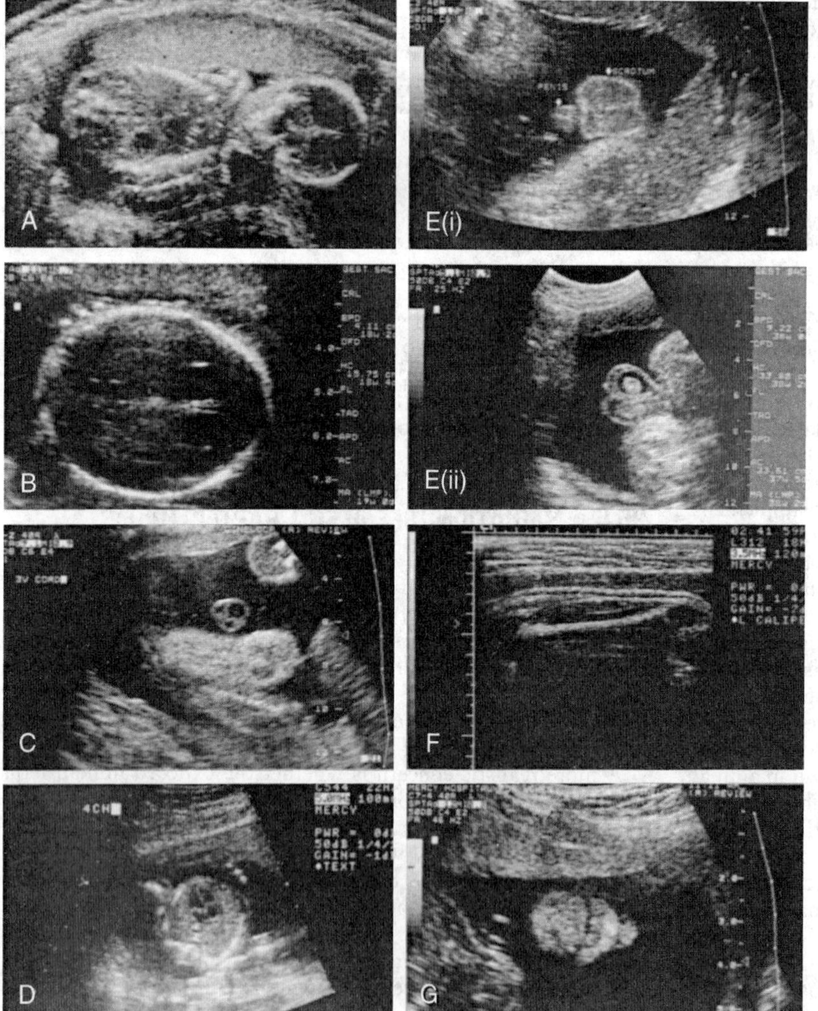

Figure 96-5. Assessment of fetal anatomy. *A,* Overall view of the uterus at 24 wk showing a longitudinal section of the fetus and an anterior placenta. *B,* Transverse section at the level of the lateral ventricle at 18 wk showing (*right*) prominent anterior horns of the lateral ventricles on either side of the midline echo of the falx. *C,* Cross section of the umbilical cord showing that the lumen of the umbilical vein is much wider than that of the two umbilical arteries. *D,* Four-chambered view of the heart at 18 wk with equal-sized atria. *E,* (*i*) normal male genitals near term; (*ii*) hydrocele outlining a testicle within the scrotum projecting into a normal-sized pocket of amniotic fluid at 38 wk. Approximately 2% of male infants after birth have clinical evidence of a hydrocele that is often bilateral, not to be confused with subcutaneous edema occurring during vaginal breech birth. *F,* Section of a thigh near term showing thick subcutaneous tissue (4.6 mm between markers) above the femur of a fetus with macrosomia. *G,* Fetal face viewed from below showing (*from right to left*) the nose, alveolar margin, and chin at 20 wk. (From Special investigative procedures. In Beischer NA, Mackay EV, Colditz PB [eds]: *Obstetrics and the Newborn,* 3rd ed. Philadelphia, WB Saunders, 1997.)

TABLE 96-5. Significance of Fetal Ultrasonographic Anatomic Findings

PRENATAL OBSERVATION	DEFINITION	DIFFERENTIAL DIAGNOSIS	SIGNIFICANCE	POSTNATAL EVALUATION
Dilated cerebral ventricles	Ventriculomegaly ≥ 10 mm	Hydrocephalus Hydrancephalus Dandy-Walker cyst Agenesis of corpus callosum	Transient isolated ventriculomegaly common and usually benign. Persistent or progressive more worrisome. Identify associated cranial and extracranial anomalies. Bilateral increases risk of developmental delay. Unilateral may be normal variant	Serial head US or CT. Evaluate for extracranial anomalies
Choroid plexus cysts	1–3% incidence Size ~10 mm: unilateral or bilateral	Abnormal karyotype (trisomy 18, 21) Aneuploidy risk 1 : 100 if isolated. ↑ Risk (1 : 3) with other anomalies. Risk ↑ if large, complex, or bilateral cysts or advanced maternal age	Often isolated, benign; resolves by 24–28 wk. Examine for other organ anomalies, then amniocentesis for karyotype	Head US or CT. Examine for extracranial anomalies; karyotype if indicated
Nuchal pad thickening	≥6 mm at 15–20 wk; cystic hygroma	Trisomy 21, 18 Turner syndrome (XO) Nonchromosomal syndromes Normal (~25%)	~50% have chromosome abnormalities Amniocentesis for karyotype	Evaluate for multiple organ malformations; karyotype if indicated
Dilated renal pelvis	Pyelectasis ≥ 5 to 10 mm 0.6–1% incidence	UPJ obstruction Vesicoureteral reflux Posterior ureteral valves Etopic ureterocele Large-volume nonobstruction	Often "physiologic" and transient Reflux is common If >10 mm or with caliectasis, consider pathologic cause. If large bladder, consider posterior urethral valves, megacystic syndrome	Repeat US day 5 and 1 mo; VCUG, prophylactic antibiotics
Echogenic bowel	0.6% incidence	CF, meconium peritonitis, trisomy 21 or 18, other chromosomal abnormalities CMV, toxoplasmosis, GI obstruction	Often normal (65%) 10% have CF 1.5% have aneuploidy	Sweat chloride and DNA testing Karyotype Surgery for obstruction TORCH evaluation
Stomach appearance	Small or absent or double bubble	Upper GI obstruction (esophageal atresia) Double bubble signifies duodenal atresia Abnormal karyotype Polyhydramnios Stomach in chest signifies diaphragmatic hernia	Must also consider neurologic disorders that reduce swallowing. Over 30% with double bubble have trisomy 21	Chromosomes, KUB if indicated, upper GI series, neurologic evaluation

CF, cystic fibrosis; CMV, cytomegalovirus; GI, gastrointestinal; KUB, kidney, ureter, and bladder; TORCH, toxoplasmosis, other agents, rubella, CMV, herpes simplex; UPJ, ureteropelvic junction; US, ultrasonography; VCUG, voiding cystourethrogram.

analysis for the detection of inborn metabolic errors. Analysis of amniotic fluid may also help in identifying neural tube defects (elevation of α-fetoprotein), adrenogenital syndrome (elevation of 17-ketosteroids and pregnanetriol), and thyroid dysfunction. Chorionic villus biopsy (transvaginal or transabdominal) performed in the 1st trimester also provides fetal cells but may pose a slightly increased risk for fetal loss or limb reduction defects. Fetal cells circulating in maternal blood and fetal DNA in maternal plasma are potential noninvasive sources of material for prenatal diagnosis. This technology may eliminate the need for amniocentesis or chorionic villus sampling.

The best available chemical indices of fetal maturity are provided by determination of amniotic fluid creatinine and lecithin, which reflect the maturity of the fetal kidneys and lungs, respectively. Lecithin is produced in the lungs by type II alveolar cells and eventually reaches the amniotic fluid via the effluent from the trachea. Until the middle of the 3rd trimester, its concentration nearly equals that of sphingomyelin; thereafter, sphingomyelin remains constant in amniotic fluid while lecithin increases. By 35 wk, the lecithin:sphingomyelin (L:S) ratio averages about 2:1, indicative of lung maturity.

Earlier lung maturation may occur in the presence of severe premature separation of the placenta, premature rupture of the fetal membranes, narcotic addiction, or maternal hypertensive and renal vascular disease. A delay in pulmonary maturation may be associated with hydrops fetalis or maternal diabetes without vascular disease. The likelihood of hyaline membrane disease is greatly reduced with L:S ratios of 2:1 or more, although hypoxia, acidosis, and hypothermia may increase the risk despite this "mature" L:S ratio. Maternal and fetal blood have an L:S ratio of about 1:4; thus, contamination will not alter the significance of a ratio of 2:1 or more. Meconium contamination, storage, and centrifugation all may reduce the reliability of the L : S ratio.

Saturated phosphatidylcholine or phosphatidylglycerol concentrations in amniotic fluid may be more specific and sensitive predictors of pulmonary maturity, especially in high-risk pregnancies such as those occurring in women with diabetes (see Chapters 101 and 107.1).

Although amniocentesis can be carried out with little discomfort to the mother, even in experienced hands the procedure entails some small risk, such as direct damage to the fetus, placental puncture and bleeding with secondary damage to the fetus, stimulation of uterine contraction and premature labor, amnionitis, and maternal sensitization to fetal blood. The earlier in gestation that amniotic puncture is done, the greater the risk to the fetus. Using ultrasound for placental and fetal localization can reduce the risk of complications. The procedure should be limited to cases in which the potential benefits of the findings will outweigh the risk.

Cordocentesis, or percutaneous umbilical blood sampling, is used to diagnose fetal hematologic abnormalities, genetic disorders, infections, and fetal acidosis (see Table 96-1). Under direct ultrasonographic visualization, a long needle is passed into the umbilical vein at its entrance to the placenta or fetal abdominal wall. Blood may be withdrawn to determine fetal hemoglobin, platelet concentration, lymphocyte DNA, the presence of infection, or Pao_2, pH, Pco_2, and lactate levels.

Transfusion or administration of drugs can be given through the umbilical vein (Table 96-6). Serum screening is offered to pregnant women at midgestation to evaluate the risk for Down syndrome (trisomy 21) and congenital malformations known to cause elevations of various markers, including abdominal wall and neural tube defects. A combination of these biochemical markers (including α-fetoprotein, inhibin A, estriol, pregnancy-associated plasma protein A, and β-HCG [human chorionic gonadotropin]) and ultrasound increases the positive predictive value of these screening tests. Additionally, families with a known genetic syndrome may be offered prenatal genetic testing from amniotic fluid or amniocytes obtained via amniocentesis or chorionic villus sampling.

TABLE 96-6. FETAL Therapy

DISORDER	POSSIBLE TREATMENT
Hematology	
Anemia with hydrops (erythroblastosis fetalis)	Umbilical vein packed red blood cell transfusion
Thalassemia	Fetal stem cell transplantation
Thrombocytopenia	
Isoimmune	Umbilical vein platelet transfusion, maternal IVIG
Autoimmune (ITP)	Maternal steroids and IVIG
Chronic granulomatous disease	Fetal stem cell transplantation
Metabolic-Endocrine	
Maternal phenylketonuria (PKU)	Phenylalanine restriction
Fetal galactosemia	Galactose-free diet (?)
Multiple carboxylase deficiency	Biotin if responsive
Methylmalonic acidemia	Vitamin B_{12} if responsive
21-Hydroxylase deficiency	Dexamethasone
Maternal diabetes mellitus	Tight insulin control during pregnancy, labor, and delivery
Fetal goiter	Maternal hyperthyroidism—maternal propylthiouracil Fetal hypothyroidism—intra-amniotic thyroxine
Bartter syndrome	Maternal indomethacin may prevent nephrocalcinosis and postnatal sodium losses
Fetal Distress	
Hypoxia	Maternal oxygen, position
Intrauterine growth restriction	Maternal oxygen, position, improve macro- and micronutrients if deficient
Oligohydramnios, premature rupture of membranes with variable deceleration	Amnioinfusion (antepartum and intrapartum)
Polyhydramnios	Amnioreduction (serial), indomethacin (if due to ↑ urine output) if indicated
Supraventricular tachycardia	Maternal digoxin,* flecainide, procainamide, amiodarone, quinidine
Lupus anticoagulant	Maternal aspirin, prednisone
Meconium-stained fluid	Amnioinfusion
Congenital heart block	Dexamethasone, pacemaker (with hydrops)
Premature labor	Sympathomimetics, magnesium sulfate, antibiotics
Respiratory	
Pulmonary immaturity	Betamethasone
Bilateral chylothorax—pleural effusions	Thoracentesis, pleuroamniotic shunt
Congenital Abnormalities†	
Neural tube defects	Folate, vitamins (prevention); fetal surgery‡
Obstructive uropathy (with oligohydramnios but without renal dysplasia)	>24 wk <32 wk, vesicoamniotic shunt plus amnioinfusion
Cystic adenomatoid malformation (with hydrops)	Pleuroamniotic shunt or resection‡
Fetal neck masses	Secure an airway with EXIT procedure‡
Infectious Disease	
Group B streptococcus	Ampicillin, penicillin (prevention)
Chorioamnionitis	Antibiotics
Toxoplasmosis	Spiramycin, pyrimethamine, sulfadiazin, and folic acid
Syphilis	Penicillin
Tuberculosis	Antituberculosis drugs
Lyme disease	Penicillin, ceftriaxone
Parvovirus	Intrauterine red blood cell transfusion for hydrops, severe anemia
Chlamydia trachomatis	Erythromycin
HIV-AIDS	Zidovudine (AZT) plus protease inhibitors
Cytomegalovirus	Ganciclovir by umbilical vein
Other	
Nonimmune hydrops (anemia)	Umbilical vein packed red blood cell transfusion
Narcotic abstinence (withdrawal)	Maternal low-dose methadone
Severe combined immunodeficiency disease	Fetal stem cell transplantation
Sacrococcygeal teratoma (with hydrops)	In utero resection or vessel obliteration
Twin-twin transfusion syndrome	Repeated amniocentesis, YAG laser photocoagulation of shared vessels
Twin reversed arterial perfusion (TRAP) syndrome	Digoxin, indomethacin, cord occlusion
Multifetal gestation	Selective reduction
Neonatal hemochromatosis	Maternal IVIG

(?) Denotes possible but not proved efficacy.
*Drug of choice (may require percutaneous umbilical cord sampling and umbilical vein administration if hydrops is present). Most drug therapy is given to the mother, with subsequent placental passage to the fetus.
†Detailed fetal ultrasonography is needed to detect other anomalies; karyotype is also indicated.
‡Ex utero intrapartum treatment permits surgery and other procedures.
IVIG, intravenous immunoglobulin.

96.8 • Treatment and Prevention of Fetal Disease

Management of fetal diseases depends on coordinated advances in diagnostic accuracy and knowledge of the disease's natural history; an understanding of fetal nutrition, pharmacology, immunology, and pathophysiology; the availability of antimicrobial and antiviral drugs; and therapeutic procedures. Progress in providing specific treatments for accurately diagnosed diseases has improved with the advent of real-time ultrasonography and cordocentesis (see Tables 96-1 and 96-6).

The incidence of sensitization of Rh-negative women by Rh-positive fetuses has been reduced by prophylactic administration of Rh(D) immunoglobulin to mothers early in pregnancy and after each delivery or abortion, thus reducing the frequency of hemolytic disease in their subsequent offspring. Fetal erythroblastosis (see Chapter 103.2) may be accurately diagnosed by amniotic fluid analysis and treated with intrauterine intraperitoneal or, more often, intraumbilical vein transfusions of packed Rh-negative blood cells to maintain the fetus until it is mature enough to have a reasonable chance of survival.

Fetal hypoxia or distress may now be diagnosed with moderate success. Treatment, however, remains limited to supplying the mother with high concentrations of oxygen, positioning the uterus to avoid vascular compression, and initiating operative delivery before severe fetal injury occurs.

Pharmacologic approaches to fetal immaturity (administration of steroids to the mother to accelerate fetal lung maturation and to decrease the incidence of respiratory distress syndrome [see Chapter 101.4] in prematurely delivered infants) are successful. Inhibiting labor with β-sympathomimetic tocolytic agents is unfortunately not successful in most patients with premature labor. Management of definitively diagnosed fetal genetic disease or congenital anomalies consists of parental counseling or abortion; rarely, high-dose vitamin therapy for a responsive inborn error of metabolism (biotin-dependent disorders) or fetal transfusion (with red blood cells or platelets) may be indicated. Fetal surgery (see Table 96-6) remains an experimental approach to therapy and is available only in a few highly specialized perinatal centers. The nature of the defect and its consequences, as well as ethical implications for the fetus and the parents, must be considered.

Folic acid supplementation decreases the incidence and recurrence of neural tube defects (NTD). Because the neural tube closes within the 1st 28 days of conception, periconceptional supplementation is needed for prevention. It is recommended that women without a prior history of a NTD, ingest 400 µg/day throughout their reproductive years. Women with a history of a prior pregnancy complicated by a NTD or a 1st-degree relative with a NTD should have preconceptual counseling and they should ingest 4 mg/day of supplemental folic acid at least 1 mo before conception. Fortification of cereal grain flour with folic acid is established policy in the United States and some other countries. The optimal concentration of folic acid in enriched grains is somewhat controversial. The incidence of NTD in the United States and other countries has decreased significantly since these public health initiatives were implemented. Use of some antiepileptic drugs (valproate, carbamazepine) during pregnancy is associated with an increased risk of NTD. Women taking these medications should ingest 1–5 mg of folic acid/day in the preconception period.

Andrade SE, Gurwitz JH, Davis RL, et al: Prescription drug use in pregnancy. *Am J Obstet Gynecol* 2004;191:398–407.

Benn PA, Kaminsky LM, Ying J, et al: Combined second trimester biochemical and ultrasound screening for Down's syndrome. *Obstet Gynecol* 2002;100:1168–1176.

Bianchi DW, Lo YM: Fetomaternal cellular and plasma DNA trafficking: The yin and the yang. *Ann N Y Acad Sci* 2001;945:119–131.

Boyle RJ: Effects of certain prenatal drugs on the fetus and newborn. *Pediatr Rev* 2002;23:17–23.

Castilla EE, Lopez-Camelo JS, Campana H, et al: Epidemiological methods to assess the correlation between industrial contaminants and rates of congenital anomalies. *Mutat Res* 2001;489:123–145.

Czeizel AE. The primary prevention of birth defects: Multivitamins or folic acid? *Int J Med Sci* 2004;1:50–61.

Coles CD: Fetal alcohol exposure and attention: Moving beyond ADHD. *Alcohol Res Health* 2001;25:199–203.

DeMarini DM, Preston RJ: Smoking while pregnant: Transplacental mutagenesis of the fetus by tobacco smoke. *JAMA* 2005;293:1264–1265.

East CE, Chan FY, Colditz PB: Fetal pulse oximetry for fetal assessment in labour. *Cochrane Database Syst Rev* 2004;4:CD004075.

Edison RJ, Muenke M: Mechanistic and epidemiologic considerations in the evaluation of adverse birth outcomes following gestational exposure to statins. *Am J Med Gen* 2004;131A:287–298.

[no authors listed] Fetal therapy—ethical considerations. American Academy of Pediatrics. Committee on Bioethics. *Pediatrics* 1999;103:1061–1063.

Flake AW, Zanjani ED: In utero hematopoietic stem cell transplantation. *JAMA* 1997;278:932–937.

Foulds N, Walpole I, Elmslie F, et al: Carbimazole embryopathy: An emerging phenotype. *Am J Med Gen* 2005;132A:130–135.

Gonzalez C, Marquez-Dias M, Kim C, et al: Congenital abnormalities in Brazilian children associated with misoprostol misuse in the first trimester of pregnancy. *Lancet* 1998;351:1624–1627.

Graham JM Jr, Edwards MJ, Edwards MJ: Teratogen update: Gestational effects of maternal hyperthermia due to febrile illnesses and resultant patterns of defects in humans. *Teratology* 1998;58:209–221.

Grimes DA: When to deliver a stunted fetus. *Lancet* 2004;364:483–484.

Haddow JE, Palomaki GE, Allan WC, et al: Maternal thyroid deficiency during pregnancy and subsequent neuropsychological development of the child. *N Engl J Med* 1999;341:549–555.

Holmes N, Harrison MR, Baskin LS: Fetal surgery for posterior urethral valves: Long-term postnatal outcomes. *Pediatrics* 2001;108:E7.

Honein MA, Paulozzi LJ, Mathews TJ, et al: Impact of folic acid fortification of the US food supply on the occurrence of neural tube defects. *JAMA* 2001;285:2981–2986.

Ismaili K, Avni FE, Wissing M, et al: Long-term clinical outcome of infants with mild and moderate fetal pyelectasis: Validation of neonatal ultrasound as a screening tool to detect significant nephrouropathies. *J Pediatr* 2004; 144:759–765.

Johnson MP, Sutton LN, Rintoul N, et al: Fetal myelomeningocele repair: Short-term clinical outcomes. *Am J Obstet Gynecol* 2003;189:582–587.

Jones KJ, Lacro RV, Johnson KA, et al: Pattern of malformations in the children of women treated with carbamazepine during pregnancy. *N Engl J Med* 1989;320:1661–1666.

Kaufman RH, Adam E, Hatch EE, et al: Continued follow-up of pregnancy outcomes in diethylstilbestrol-exposed offspring. *Obstet Gynecol* 2000; 96:483–489.

Khattak S, K-Moghtader G, McMartin K, et al: Pregnancy outcome following gestational exposure to organic solvents: A prospective controlled study. *JAMA* 1999;281:1106–1109.

Kiss H, Petricevic L, Husslein P: Prospective randomized controlled trial of an infection screening programme to reduce the rate of preterm delivery. *Br Med J* 2004;329:371–374.

Klauser CK, Christensen EE, Chauhan SP, et al: Use of fetal pulse oximetry among high-risk women in labor: A randomized clinical trial. *Am J Obstet Gynecol* 2005;192:1810–1819.

Koren G, Pastuszak A, Ito S: Drugs in pregnancy. *N Engl J Med* 1998; 338:1128–1137.

Kulin NA, Pastuszak A, Sage SR, et al: Pregnancy outcome following maternal use of the new selective serotonin reuptake inhibitors. *JAMA* 1998; 279:609–610.

Lammer EJ, Chen CT, Hoar RM, et al: Retinoic acid embryopathy. *N Engl J Med* 1985;313:837–841.

Leviton A, Paneth N, Reuss ML, et al: Maternal infection, fetal inflammatory response, and brain damage in very low birth weight infants. *Pediatr Res* 1999;46:566–575.

Li Y, DiNiro E, Vitucci A, et al: Detection of paternally inherited fetal point mutations for β-thalassemia using size-fractionated cell-free DNA in maternal plasma. *JAMA* 2005;293:843–849.

Loffredo CA, Wilson PD, Ferencz C: Maternal diabetes: An independent risk factor for major cardiovascular malformations with increased mortality of affected infants. *Teratology* 2001;64:98–106.

Lumley J, Watson L, Watson M, et al: Periconceptional supplementation with folate and/or multivitamins for preventing neural tube defects. *Cochrane Database Syst Rev* 2005:3.

Mann K, Donaghue C, Fox SP, et al: Strategies for the rapid prenatal diagnosis of chromosomal aneuploidy. *Eur J Hum Genet* 2004;12:907–915.

Manning FA, Snijders R, Harman CR, et al: Fetal biophysical profile score. VI. Correlation with antepartum umbilical venous fetal pH. *Am J Obstet Gynecol* 1993;169:755–763.

McDonald SD, Ferguson S, Tam L, et al: The prevention of congenital anomalies with periconceptional folic acid supplementation. *J Obstet Gynaecol Can* 2003:25:115–121.

Mercer BM, Miodovnik M, Thurnau GR, et al: Antibiotic therapy for reduction of infant morbidity after preterm premature rupture of the membranes. *JAMA* 1997;278:989–995.

Mitchell AA: Systematic identification of drugs that cause birth defects—a new opportunity. *N Engl J Med* 2003;26:2556–2559.

Molloy AM, Daly S, Mills JL, et al: Thermolabile variant of 5,10-methylenetetrahydrofolate reductase associated with low red cell folates: Implications for folate intake recommendations. *Lancet* 1997;349:1591–1593.

Moran LR, Almeida PG, Worden S, et al: Intrauterine baclofen exposure: A multidisciplinary approach. *Pediatrics* 2004;114:e267–e269.

Osrin D, Vaidya A, Shrestha Y, et al: Effects of antenatal multiple micronutrient supplementation on birthweight and gestational duration in Nepal: Double-blind, randomized controlled trial. *Lancet* 2005;365:955–962.

Ott WJ: Intrauterine growth restriction and Doppler ultrasonography. *J Ultrasound Med* 2000;19:661.

Park-Wyllie L, Mazzotta P, Pastuszak A, et al: Birth defects after maternal exposure to corticosteroids: Prospective cohort study and meta-analysis of epidemiological studies. *Teratology* 2000;62:385–392.

Pauli RM, Lian JB, Mosher DF, et al: Association of congenital deficiency of multiple vitamin K–dependent coagulation factors and the phenotype of the warfarin embryopathy: Clues to the mechanism of teratogenicity of coumadin derivatives. *Am J Hum Genet* 1987;41:566–583.

Prontera W, Jaeggi ET, Pfizenmaier M, et al: Ex utero intrapartum treatment (EXIT) of severe fetal hydrothorax. *Arch Dis Child* 2002;86:F58–F60.

Senat MV, Deprest J, Boulvain M, et al: Endoscopic laser surgery versus serial amnioreduction for severe twin-to-twin transfusion syndrome. *N Engl J Med* 2004;351:136–144.

Stenhouse EJ, Crossley JA, Aitken DA, et al: First trimester combined ultrasound and biochemical screening for Down syndrome in routine clinical practice. *Prenat Diagn* 2004:24:774–780.

Strickler SM, Dansky LV, Miller MA, et al: Genetic predisposition to phenytoin-induced birth defects. *Lancet* 1985;2:746–749.

Sutton L, Sun P, Adzick N: Fetal neurosurgery. *Neurosurgery* 2001;48:124–142.

Thacker SB, Stroup D, Chang M: Continuous electronic heart rate monitoring for fetal assessment during labor. *Cochrane Database Syst Rev* 2001;2:CD000063.

Tomson T, Battino D: Teratogenicity of antiepileptic drugs: State of the art. *Curr Opin Neurol* 2005;18:135–140.

Toriello HV: Folic acid and neural tube defects. *Genet Med* 2005;7:283–284.

Wachtel SS, Shulman LP, Sammons D: Fetal cells in maternal blood. *Clin Genet* 2001;59:74–79.

Wang X, Chen D, Niu T, et al: Genetic susceptibility to benzene and shortened gestation: Evidence of gene-environment interaction. *Am J Epidemiol* 2000;152:693–700.

Wang X, Zuckerman B, Pearson C, et al: Maternal cigarette smoking, metabolic gene polymorphism, and infant birth weight. *JAMA* 2002;287:195–202.

Whitington PF, Hibbard JU: High-dose immunoglobulin during pregnancy for recurrent neonatal haemochromatosis. *Lancet* 2004;364:1690–1698.

Wu YW, Colford JM Jr: Chorioamnionitis as a risk factor for cerebral palsy. *JAMA* 2000;284:1417–1424.

Wyldes M, Watkinson M: Isolated mild fetal ventriculomegaly. *Arch Dis Child Fetal Neonatal Ed* 2004;89:F9–F13.

Chapter 97 ■ The High-Risk Infant

Barbara J. Stoll and Ira Adams-Chapman

Neonates at risk should be identified as early as possible to decrease neonatal morbidity and mortality (see also Chapter 93). The term high-risk infant designates an infant who should be under close observation by experienced physicians and nurses. Infants in the high-risk category are listed in Table 97-1. Approximately 9% of all births require special or neonatal intensive care. Usually needed for only a few days, such observation may last from a few hours to several months. Some institutions find it advantageous to provide a special or transitional care nursery for high-risk infants, often within the labor and delivery suite. This facility should be equipped and staffed similar to a neonatal intensive care area.

Examination of fresh placenta, cord, and membranes may alert the physician to newborn infants at high risk and may help confirm a diagnosis in a sick infant. **Fetal blood loss** may be indicated by placental pallor, retroplacental hematoma, and tears in the velamentous cords or chorionic blood vessels supplying the succenturiate lobes. Placental edema and secondary possible immunoglobulin G deficiency in newborns may be associated with fetofetal transfusion syndrome, hydrops fetalis, congenital nephrosis, or hepatic disease. **Amnion nodosum** (granules on the amnion) and **oligohydramnios** are associated with pulmonary hypoplasia and renal agenesis, whereas small whitish nodules on the cord suggest a candidal infection. Short cords and noncoiled

TABLE 97-1. High-Risk Infants

Demographic Social Factors
Maternal age <16 or >40 yr
Illicit drug, alcohol, cigarette use
Poverty
Unmarried
Emotional or physical stress
Past Medical History
Genetic disorders
Diabetes mellitus
Hypertension
Asymptomatic bacteriuria
Rheumatologic illness (SLE)
Long-term medication (see Tables 96-3 and 96-4)
Previous Pregnancy
Intrauterine fetal demise
Neonatal death
Prematurity
Intrauterine growth restriction
Congenital malformation
Incompetent cervix
Blood group sensitization, neonatal jaundice
Neonatal thrombocytopenia
Hydrops
Inborn errors of metabolism
Present Pregnancy
Vaginal bleeding (abruptio placentae, placenta previa)
Sexually transmitted infections (colonization: herpes simplex, group B streptococcus), chlamydia, syphilis, hepatitis B, HIV
Multiple gestation
Preeclampsia
Premature rupture of membranes
Short interpregnancy time
Poly/oligohydramnios
Acute medical or surgical illness
Inadequate prenatal care
Familial or acquired hypercoagulable states
Abnormal fetal ultrasonography
Treatment of infertility
Labor and Delivery
Premature labor (<37 wk)
Postdates (>42 wk)
Fetal distress
Immature L : S ratio; absent phosphatidylglycerol
Breech presentation
Meconium-stained fluid
Nuchal cord
Cesarean section
Forceps delivery
Apgar score <4 at 1 min
Neonate
Birthweight <2,500 or >4,000 g
Birth before 37 or after 42 wk of gestation
SGA, LGA growth status
Tachypnea, cyanosis
Congenital malformation
Pallor, plethora, petechiae

L : S, lecithin : sphingomyelin ratio; LGA, large for gestational age; SGA, small for gestational age; SLE, systemic lupus erythematosus.

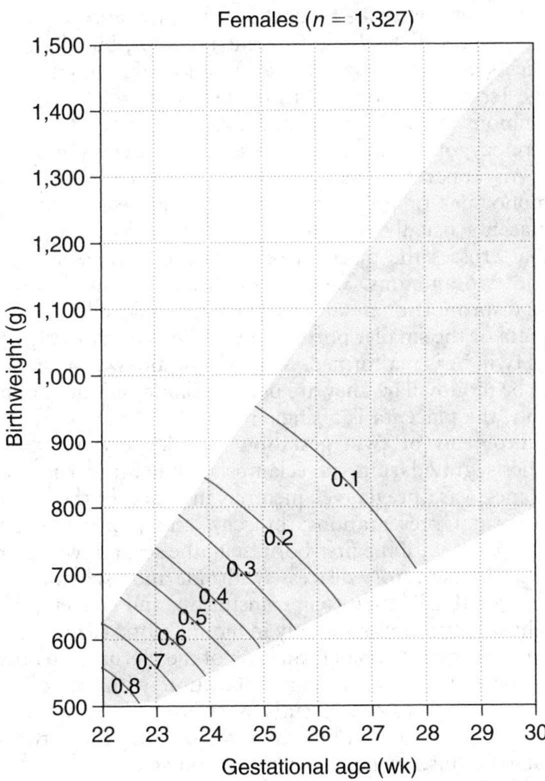

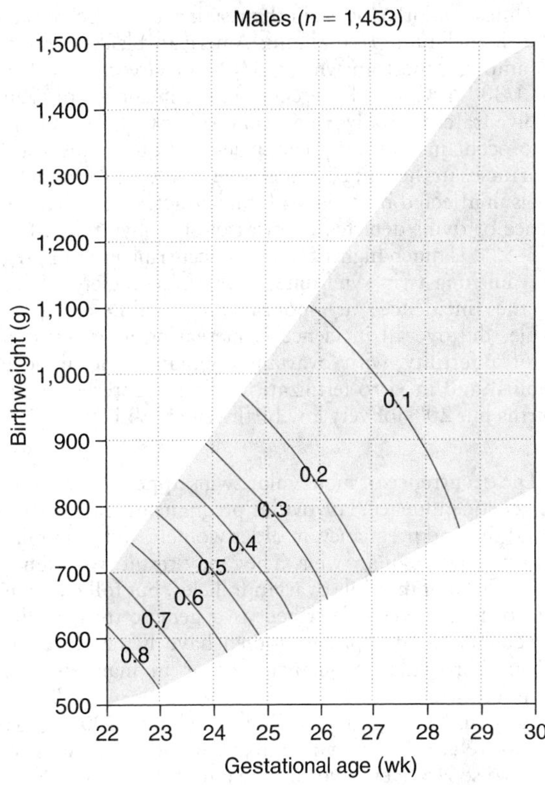

Figure 97-1. Estimated mortality risk by birthweight and gestational age based on singleton infants in NICHD Neonatal Research Network centers between January 1, 1995, and December 31, 1996. (From Lemons JA, Bauers CR, Oh W, et al: Very low birthweight outcomes of the National Institute of Child Health and Human Development Neonatal Research Network, January 1995 through December 1996. *Pediatrics* 2001;107 [available at http://www.pediatrics.org.cgi/content/full/107/1/el].)

cords occur with chromosome abnormalities and omphalocele. True umbilical cord knots are seen in approximately 1% of births and are associated with a long cord, small fetal size, polyhydramnios, monoamniotic twinning, fetal demise, and low Apgar scores.

Chorioangiomas are associated with prematurity, abruptio, polyhydramnios, and intrauterine growth restriction (IUGR). **Meconium staining** suggests in utero stress and opacity of the fetal placental surface suggests infection. Single umbilical arteries are associated with an increased incidence of congenital renal abnormalities and syndromes.

Many infants who are born prematurely, are small for gestational age (SGA), have significant perinatal asphyxia, are breech, or are born with life-threatening congenital anomalies do not have previously identified risk factors. For any given duration of gestation, the lower the birthweight, the higher the neonatal mortality; for any given weight, the shorter the gestational duration, the higher the neonatal mortality (Fig. 97-1). The highest risk of neonatal mortality occurs in infants who weigh <1,000 g at birth and whose gestation was <28 wk. The lowest risk of neonatal mortality occurs in infants with a birthweight of 3,000–4,000 g and a gestational age of 38–42 wk. As birthweight increases from 500 to 3,000 g, a logarithmic decrease in neonatal mortality occurs; for every week of increase in gestational age from the 25th to the 37th wk, the neonatal mortality rate decreases by approximately half. Nevertheless, approximately 40% of all perinatal deaths occur after 37 wk of gestation in infants weighing 2,500 g or more; many of these deaths take place in the period immediately before birth and are more readily preventable than those of smaller and more immature infants. Neonatal mortality rates rise sharply for infants weighing over 4,000 g at birth and for those whose gestational period is 42 wk or longer. Because neonatal mortality largely depends on birthweight and gestational age, Figure 97-1 can be used to help identify high-risk infants quickly. This analysis is based on total live births and therefore describes the mortality risk only at birth. Because most neonatal mortality occurs within the 1st hours and days after birth, the outlook improves dramatically with increasing postnatal survival.

Airas U, Heinonen S: Clinical significance of true umbilical knots: A population-based analysis. *Am J Perinatol* 2002;19:127–132.

Amini SB, Catalano PM, Hirsch V, et al: An analysis of birth weight by gestational age using a computerized perinatal data base, 1975–1992. *Obstet Gynecol* 1994;83:342–352.

Grether JK, Eaton A, Redline R, et al: Reliability of placental histology using archived specimens. *Paediatr Perinat Epidemiol* 1999;13:489–495.

Hansen AR, Collins MH, Genest D, et al: Very low birthweight infant's placenta and its relation to pregnancy and fetal characteristics. *Pediatr Dev Pathol* 2000;3:419–430.

Lemons JA, Bauer CR, Oh W, et al: Very low birth weight outcomes of the National Institute of Child Health and Human Development Neonatal Research Network, January 1995 through December 1996. *Pediatrics* 2001;107 (available at http://www.pediatrics.org/cgi/content/full/107/1/e1).

Seri I: Low superior vena cava flow during the first postnatal day and neurodevelopment in preterm neonate. *J Pediatr* 2004;145:573–575.

Vogler C, Petterchak J, Sotelo-Avila C, et al: Placental pathology for the surgical pathologist. *Adv Anat Pathol* 2000;7:214–229.

97.1 • Multiple Gestation Pregnancies

INCIDENCE. The reported incidence of spontaneous twinning is highest among blacks and East Indians, followed by northern

European whites, and it is lowest in the Asian races. Specific rates include 1/56 in Belgium, 1/70 among American blacks, 1/86 in Italy, 1/88 among American whites, 1/130 in Greece, 1/150 in Japan, and 1/300 in China. Differences in the incidence of twins mainly involve fraternal (polyovular) dizygotic twins. Triplets are estimated to occur in 1 in 86^2 pregnancies and quadruplets in 1 in 86^3 pregnancies in the United States. The incidence of monozygotic twins is unaffected by racial or familial factors (3–5/1,000). The incidence of twins detected by ultrasonography at 12 wk of gestation (3–5%) is much higher than that occurring later in pregnancy; the **vanishing twin syndrome** results in a singleton fetus. Although the incidence of spontaneous multifetal gestation is stable, the overall incidence is increasing as a result of treatment of infertility with ovarian stimulants (clomiphene, gonadotropins) and in vitro fertilization. Twins represent about 2.5% of births but 20% of very low birthweight (VLBW) infants.

ETIOLOGY. The occurrence of monovular twins appears to be independent of genetic influence. Polyovular pregnancies are more frequent beyond the 2nd pregnancy, in older women, and in families with a history of polyovular twins. They may result from simultaneous maturation of multiple ovarian follicles, but follicles containing two ova have been described as a genetic trait leading to twin pregnancies. Twin-prone women have higher levels of gonadotropin. Polyovular pregnancies occur in many women treated for infertility.

Conjoined twins (Siamese twins—incidence, 1/50,000) probably result from relatively late monovular separation, as does the presence of two separate embryos in one amniotic sac. The latter condition has a high fatality rate that is due to obstruction of the circulation secondary to intertwining of the umbilical cords. The prognosis for conjoined twins depends on the possibility of surgical separation, which in turn depends on the degree that vital organs are shared. The site of connections varies: thoraco-omphalopagus (28% of conjoined twins), thoracopagus (18%), omphalopagus (10%), craniopagus (6%), and incomplete duplication (10%). Difficult to separate conjoined twins have occasionally survived to adulthood. Most conjoined twins are female.

Superfecundation, or fertilization of an ovum by an insemination that takes place after one ovum has already been fertilized, and **superfetation,** or fertilization and subsequent development of an ovum when a fetus is already present in the uterus, have been proposed as uncommon explanations for differences in size and appearance of certain twins at birth.

A prenatal diagnosis of pregnancy with twins is suggested by a uterine size that is greater than that expected for gestational age, auscultation of two fetal hearts, and elevated maternal serum α-fetoprotein or human chorionic gonadotropin levels, and it is confirmed by ultrasound. Ninety per cent of twins are detected before delivery.

MONOZYGOTIC VS DIZYGOTIC TWINS. Identifying twins as monozygotic or dizygotic (monovular or polyovular) is important because studying monozygotic twins is useful in determining the relative influence of heredity and environment on human development and disease. Twins of widely discrepant size are usually monochorionic. Twins not of the same sex are dizygotic. In twins of the same sex, zygosity should be determined and recorded at birth through careful examination of the placenta or detailed blood typing, gene analysis, or tissue (HLA) typing. Monozygotic twins may have physical and cognitive differences because their in utero environment may be different; differences may exist in the mitochondrial genome, in post-translational gene product modification, and in the expression of nuclear genes in response to environmental factors (nutrition). Indeed differential epigenetic modification of identical genes may be a common postnatal factor responsible for discordant phenotypes among monozygotic twins.

Examination of the Placenta. If the placentas are separate, they are always dichorionic (present in 75%), but the twins are not necessarily dizygotic because initiation of monovular twinning at the 1st cell division or during the morula stage may result in two amnions, two chorions, and even two placentas. One third of monozygotic twins are dichorionic and diamnionic.

An apparently single placenta may be present with either monovular or polyovular twins; yet inspection of a polyovular placenta usually reveals that each twin has a separate chorion that crosses the placenta between the attachments of the cords and two amnions. Separate or fused dichorionic placentas may be disproportionate in size. The fetus attached to the smaller placenta or the smaller portion of the placenta is usually smaller than its twin or is malformed. **Monochorionic twins** may be presumed to be monovular. They are usually diamnionic and, almost invariably, the placenta is a single mass.

Problems of twin gestation include polyhydramnios, hyperemesis gravidarum, preeclampsia, premature rupture of membranes, vasa previa, velamentous insertion of the umbilical cord, abnormal presentations (breech), and premature labor. When compared with the first-born twin, the second twin is at increased risk for respiratory distress syndrome and asphyxia. Twins are at risk for IUGR, twin-twin transfusion, and congenital anomalies, which occur predominantly in monozygotic twins. Anomalies are due to compression deformation of the uterus from crowding (hip dislocation), vascular communication with embolization (ileal atresia, porencephaly, cutis aplasia) or without embolization (acardiac twin), and unknown factors that cause twinning (conjoined twins, anencephaly, meningomyelocele).

Placental vascular anastomoses occur with high frequency only in monochorionic twins. In monochorionic placentas, the fetal vasculature is usually joined, sometimes in a very complex manner. The vascular anastomoses in monochorionic placentas may be artery to artery, vein to vein, or artery to vein. They are usually balanced so that neither twin suffers. Artery-to-artery communications cross over placental veins, and when anastomoses are present, blood can readily be stroked from one fetal vascular bed to the other. Vein-to-vein communications are similarly recognized but are less common. A combination of artery-to-artery and vein-to-vein anastomoses is associated with the condition of lethal **acardiac fetus.** This rare lethal anomaly (1/35,000) is secondary to the **TRAP sequence**—twin reversed arterial perfusion. Nd : YAG laser ablation of the anastomosis or cord occlusion in utero can be used to treat heart failure in the surviving twin. In rare cases, one umbilical cord may arise from the other after leaving the placenta. In such cases, the twin attached to the secondary cord is usually malformed or dies in utero.

In the **fetal transfusion syndrome,** an artery from one twin acutely or chronically delivers blood that is drained into the vein of the other. The latter becomes plethoric and large, and the former is anemic and small. Generally, with chronicity, a 5 g/dL hemoglobin and 20% body weight difference can be noted in this syndrome. Maternal hydramnios in a twin pregnancy suggests fetal transfusion syndrome. Anticipating this possibility by preparing to transfuse the donor twin or bleed the recipient twin may be lifesaving. Death of the donor twin in utero may result in generalized fibrin thrombi in the smaller arterioles of the recipient twin, possibly as the result of transfusion of thromboplastin-rich blood from the macerating donor fetus. Disseminated intravascular coagulation may develop in the surviving twin. Table 97-2 lists the more frequent changes associated with a large uncompensated arteriovenous shunt from the placenta of one twin to that of the other. Treatment of this highly lethal problem includes maternal digoxin, aggressive amnioreduction for polyhydramnios, selective twin termination, or Nd : YAG laser or fetoscopic ablation of the anastomosis.

Postnatal Identification. The following physical criteria can be used to determine whether twins are monovular: (1) both must

TABLE 97-2. Characteristic Changes in Monochorionic Twins with Uncompensated Placental Arteriovenous Shunts

TWIN ON	
ARTERIAL SIDE—DONOR	VENOUS SIDE—RECIPIENT
Prematurity	Prematurity
Oligohydramnios	Polyhydramnios
Small premature	Hydrops
Malnourished	Large premature
Pale	Well nourished
Anemic	Plethoric
Hypovolemia	Polycythemic
Hypoglycemia	Hypervolemic
Microcardia	Cardiac hypertrophy
Glomeruli small or normal	Myocardial dysfunction
Arterioles thin walled	Tricuspid valve regurgitation
	Right ventricular outflow obstruction
	Glomeruli large
	Arterioles thick walled

be of the same sex; (2) their features, including ears and teeth, must be obviously alike (but they need not resemble each other more than the lateral halves of one individual); (3) their hair must be identical in color, texture, natural curl, and distribution; (4) their eyes must be of the same color and shade; (5) their skin must be of the same texture and color (nevi may be differently apportioned and distributed); (6) their hands and feet must be of the same conformation and of similar size; and (7) their anthropometric values must show close agreement.

PROGNOSIS. Most twins are born prematurely, and maternal complications of pregnancy are more common than with single pregnancies. Although monochorionic twins have a significant increase in perinatal mortality, there is no significant difference between the neonatal mortality rates of twin and single births in comparable weight and gestational age groups (Fig. 97-2). Because most twins are premature by weight, their overall mortality is higher than that of single births. The perinatal mortality of twins is about four times that of singletons. Monoamnionic twins have an increased likelihood of entangling their cords,

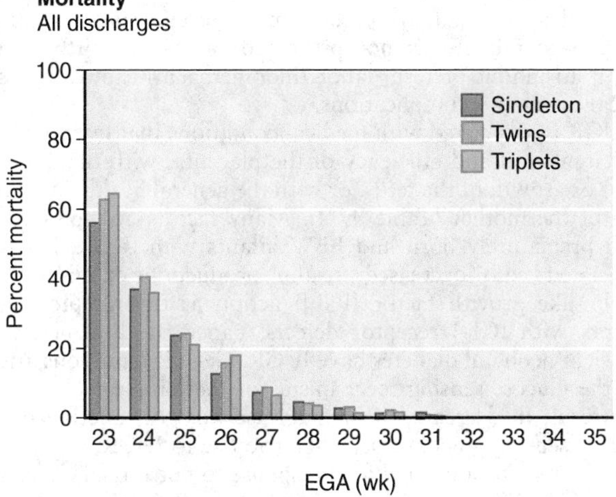

Figure 97-2. Mortality. All Discharges. The neonatal mortality rate for all babies who died during the original hospitalization at each week of gestational age is given. The *bars on the left* represent singletons; the *middle bars* represent twins, and the *bars on the right* represent triplets. There are no differences seen among singleton births, twin births, or triplet births. EGA, estimated gestational age. (From Garite TJ, Clark RH, Elliott JP, et al: Twins and triplets: The effect of plurality and growth on neonatal outcome compared with singleton infants. *Am J Obstet Gynecol* 2004;191:700–707.)

which may lead to asphyxia. Theoretically, the 2nd twin is more subject to anoxia than the 1st because the placenta may separate after birth of the 1st twin and before birth of the 2nd. In addition, delivery of the 2nd twin may be difficult because it may be in an abnormal presentation (breech, entangled), uterine tone may be decreased, or the cervix may begin to close after the 1st twin's birth. A growth-retarded twin is at high risk for hypoglycemia. Any notable difference in the size of monovular twins at birth usually disappears by the time the infants are 6 mo of age. The mortality for multiple gestations with four or more fetuses is excessively high for each fetus. Because of this poor prognosis, selective fetal reduction (with transabdominal intrathoracic fetal injection of KCl) to two to three fetuses has been offered as a treatment option. Monozygotic twins have an increased risk of one twin dying in utero. The surviving twin has a greater risk for cerebral palsy and other neurodevelopmental sequelae.

TREATMENT. Prenatal diagnosis enables the obstetrician and pediatrician to anticipate the birth of infants who are at high risk because of twinning. Close observation is indicated during labor and in the immediate neonatal period so that prompt treatment of asphyxia or fetal transfusion syndrome can be initiated. The decision to perform an immediate blood transfusion in a severely anemic "donor twin" or to perform a partial exchange transfusion of a "recipient twin" must be based on clinical judgment.

Cohen J: Associated multiple gestation-ART. *Clin Obstet Gynecol* 2003;46:363–374.

Dechaud H, Picot MC, Hedon B, et al: First-trimester multifetal pregnancy reduction: Evaluation of technical aspects and risks from 2,756 cases in the literature. *Fetal Diagn Ther* 1998;13:261–265.

Donovan EF, Ehrenkranz RA, Shankaran S, et al: Outcomes of very low birth weight twins cared for in the National Institute of Child Health and Human Development Neonatal Research Network's intensive care units. *Am J Obstet Gynecol* 1998;179:742–749.

Fauser BCJM, Devroey P, Macklon NS: Multiple birth resulting from ovarian stimulation for subfertility treatment. *Lancet* 2005;365:1807–1816.

Fraga MF, Ballestar E, Paz MF, et al: Epigenetic differences arise during the lifetime of monozygotic twins. *PNAS* 2005;102:10606–10609.

Garite TJ, Clark RH, Elliott JP, et al: Twins and triplets: the effect of plurality and growth on neonatal outcome compared with singleton infants. *Am J Obstet Gynecol* 2004;191:700–707.

Hartley RS, Emanuel I, Hitti J: Perinatal mortality and neonatal morbidity rates among twin pairs at different gestational ages: Optimal delivery timing at 37 to 38 weeks' gestation. *Am J Obstet Gynecol* 2001;184:451–458.

Mari G, Roberts A, Detti L, et al: Perinatal morbidity and mortality rates in severe twin-twin transfusion syndrome: Results of the International Amnioreduction Registry. *Am J Obstet Gynecol* 2001;185:708–715.

Norwitz ER, Hoyte LPJ, Jenkins KJ, et al: Brief report: Separation of conjoined twins with the twin reversed-arterial-perfusion sequence after prenatal planning with three-dimensional modeling. *N Engl J Med* 2000;343:399–402.

Pearn J: Bioethical issues in caring for conjoined twins and their parents. *Lancet* 2001;357:1968.

Pharoah PO: Twins and cerebral palsy. *Acta Paediatr Suppl* 2001;436:6–10.

Steer P: Perinatal death in twins. *BMJ* 2007;334:545–546.

97.2 • Prematurity and Intrauterine Growth Retardation

DEFINITIONS. Liveborn infants delivered before 37 wk from the 1st day of the last menstrual period are termed premature by the World Health Organization. Low birthweight (LBW; birthweight of 2,500 g or less) is due to prematurity, poor intrauterine growth (IUGR, also referred to as SGA), or both. Prematurity and IUGR are associated with increased neonatal morbidity and mortality. Ideally, definitions of LBW for individual populations should be based on data that are as genetically and environmentally homogeneous as possible. Figure 97-1 presents variations in neonatal mortality based on birthweight, gestational age, and gender.

INCIDENCE. There is an increasing percentage of deaths in children less than 5 yr of age that occur in the neonatal period. Approximately 38% of deaths in this age group occur within the 1st mo of life, of which 28% are attributable to premature birth. In 2003, 7.9% of liveborn neonates in the United States weighed <2,500 g; the rate for blacks was almost twice that for whites. Over the past 2 decades, the LBW rate has increased primarily because of an increased number of preterm births. Women whose 1st births are delivered before term are at increased risk for recurrent preterm delivery. Approximately 30% of LBW infants in the United States have IUGR and are born after 37 wk. At LBW rates greater than 10%, the contribution of IUGR increases and that of prematurity decreases. In developing countries, approximately 70% of LBW infants have IUGR. Infants with IUGR have greater morbidity and mortality than do appropriately grown, gestational age–matched infants (see Fig. 97-1). Although U.S. infant mortality rates have fallen since 1971, the ethnic disparity between blacks and white or Hispanic infants remains unchanged. Black infants have higher neonatal mortality rates and comprise a larger percentage of low birthweight births in the United States.

VERY LOW BIRTHWEIGHT INFANTS. VLBW infants weigh <1,500 g and are predominantly premature. In the United States in 2003, the VLBW rate was approximately 1.4%, 3.1% among blacks and 1.2% among whites. The VLBW rate is an accurate predictor of the infant mortality rate. VLBW infants account for over 50% of neonatal deaths and 50% of handicapped infants; their survival is directly related to birthweight, with approximately 20% of those between 500 and 600 g and over 90% of those between 1,250 and 1,500 g surviving. The VLBW rate has remained unchanged for black Americans but has increased among whites, perhaps because of a rise in multiple births among whites. Perinatal care has improved the rate of survival of VLBW infants. When compared with term infants, VLBW neonates have a higher incidence of rehospitalization during the 1st yr of life for sequelae of prematurity, infections, neurologic complications, and psychosocial disorders.

FACTORS RELATED TO PREMATURE BIRTH AND LOW BIRTHWEIGHT. It is difficult to separate completely the factors associated with prematurity from those associated with IUGR (see also Chapters 94 and 95). A strong positive correlation exists between both preterm birth and IUGR and low socioeconomic status. Families of low socioeconomic status have higher rates of maternal undernutrition, anemia, and illness; inadequate prenatal care; drug misuse; obstetric complications; and maternal histories of reproductive inefficiency (abortions, stillbirths, premature or LBW infants). Other associated factors such as single-parent families, teenage pregnancies, short interpregnancy interval, and mothers who have borne more than four previous children are also encountered more frequently. Systematic differences in fetal growth have also been described in association with maternal size, birth order, sibling weight, social class, maternal smoking, and other factors. The degree to which the variance in birthweight among various populations is due to environmental (extrafetal) rather than genetic differences in growth potential is difficult to determine.

The etiology of preterm birth is multifactorial and involves a complex interaction between fetal, placental, uterine, and maternal factors (Table 97-3).

TABLE 97-3. Identifiable Causes of Preterm Birth

Fetal
Fetal distress
Multiple gestation
Erythroblastosis
Nonimmune hydrops
Placental
Placental dysfunction
Placenta previa
Abruptio placentae
Uterine
Bicornuate uterus
Incompetent cervix (premature dilatation)
Maternal
Preeclampsia
Chronic medical illness (cyanotic heart disease, renal disease)
Infection (*Listeria monocytogenes*, group B streptococcus, urinary tract infection, bacterial vaginosis, chorioamnionitis)
Drug abuse (cocaine)
Other
Premature rupture of membranes
Polyhydramnios
Iatrogenic
Trauma

Premature birth of infants whose LBW is appropriate for their preterm gestational age is associated with medical conditions characterized by an inability of the uterus to retain the fetus, interference with the course of the pregnancy, premature rupture of the amniotic membranes or premature separation of the placenta, multifetal gestation, or an undetermined stimulus to effective uterine contractions before term.

Overt or asymptomatic bacterial infection (group B streptococci, *Listeria monocytogenes, Ureaplasma urealyticum, Mycoplasma hominis, Chlamydia, Trichomonas vaginalis, Gardnerella vaginalis, Bacteroides* spp.) of the amniotic fluid and membranes (chorioamnionitis) may initiate preterm labor. Bacterial products may stimulate the production of local inflammatory mediators (interleukin 6, prostaglandins), which may induce premature uterine contractions or a local inflammatory response with focal amniotic membrane rupture. Appropriate antibiotic therapy reduces the risk of fetal infection and may prolong gestation. The use of β-sympathomimetic receptor agonists (ritodrine, terbutaline) has not prevented premature birth. Other agents to inhibit preterm labor (indomethacin) can lead to significant neonatal complications.

IUGR is associated with medical conditions that interfere with the circulation and efficiency of the placenta, with the development or growth of the fetus, or with the general health and nutrition of the mother (Table 97-4). Many factors are common to both prematurely born and LBW infants with IUGR. IUGR is associated with decreased insulin production or insulin (or insulin-like growth factor [IGF]) action at the receptor level. Infants with IGF-I receptor defects, pancreatic hypoplasia, or transient neonatal diabetes have IUGR. Genetic mutations affecting the glucose-sensing mechanisms of the pancreatic islet cells that result in decreased insulin release (loss of function of the glucose-sensing glucokinase gene) give rise to IUGR.

IUGR may be a normal fetal response to nutritional or oxygen deprivation. Therefore, the issue is not the IUGR but rather the ongoing risk of malnutrition or hypoxia. Similarly, some preterm births signify a need for early delivery from a potentially disadvantageous intrauterine environment. IUGR is often classified as reduced growth that is symmetric (head circumference, length, and weight equally affected) or asymmetric (with relative sparing of head growth) (see Fig. 96-1). **Symmetric IUGR** often has an earlier onset and is associated with diseases that seriously affect

TABLE 97-4. Factors Often Associated with Intrauterine Growth Restriction

Fetal
Chromosomal disorders (autosomal trisomies)
Chronic fetal infections (cytomegalic inclusion disease, congenital rubella, syphilis)
Congenital anomalies—syndrome complexes
Irradiation
Multiple gestation
Pancreatic hypoplasia
Insulin deficiency
Insulin-like growth factor type I deficiency

Placental
Decreased placental weight or cellularity, or both
Decrease in surface area
Villous placentitis (bacterial, viral, parasitic)
Infarction
Tumor (chorioangioma, hydatidiform mole)
Placental separation
Twin transfusion syndrome

Maternal
Toxemia
Hypertension or renal disease, or both
Hypoxemia (high altitude, cyanotic cardiac or pulmonary disease)
Malnutrition (micro- or macronutrient deficiencies)
Chronic illness
Sickle cell anemia
Drugs (narcotics, alcohol, cigarettes, cocaine, antimetabolites)

fetal cell number, such as conditions with chromosomal, genetic, malformation, teratogenic, infectious, or severe maternal hypertensive etiologies. **Asymmetric IUGR** is often of late onset, demonstrates preservation of Doppler waveform velocity to the carotid vessels, and is associated with poor maternal nutrition or with late onset or exacerbation of maternal vascular disease (preeclampsia, chronic hypertension). Problems of infants with IUGR are noted in Table 97-5.

TABLE 97-5. Problems of IUGR (SGA) Infants

PROBLEM	PATHOGENESIS
Intrauterine fetal demise	Hypoxia, acidosis, infection, lethal anomaly
Perinatal asphyxia	↓ Uteroplacental perfusion during labor ± chronic fetal hypoxia-acidosis; meconium aspiration syndrome
Hypoglycemia	↓ Tissue glycogen stores, ↓ gluconeogenesis, hyperinsulinism, ↑ glucose needs of hypoxia, hypothermia, large brain
Polycythemia-hyperviscosity	Fetal hypoxia with ↑ erythropoietin production
Reduced oxygen consumption/ hypothermia	Hypoxia, hypoglycemia, starvation effect, poor subcutaneous fat stores
Dysmorphology	Syndrome anomalads, chromosomal-genetic disorders, oligohydramnios-induced deformation, TORCH infection

Other problems include pulmonary hemorrhage and those common to the gestational age–related risks of prematurity if born at less than 37 wk.
IUGR, intrauterine growth restriction; SGA, small for gestational age; TORCH, toxoplasmosis, other agents, rubella, cytomegalovirus, herpes simplex.

ASSESSMENT OF GESTATIONAL AGE AT BIRTH. When compared with a premature infant of appropriate weight, an infant with IUGR has a reduced birthweight and may appear to have a disproportionately larger head relative to body size; infants in both groups lack subcutaneous fat. Neurologic maturity (nerve conduction velocity), in the absence of asphyxia, correlates with gestational age despite reduced fetal weight. Physical signs may be useful in estimating gestational age at birth. Commonly used, the Ballard scoring system is accurate to ±2 wk (Figs. 97-3–97-5). An infant should be presumed to be at high risk for mortality or morbidity if a discrepancy exists between the estimation of gestational age by physical examination, the mother's estimated date of her last menstrual period, and fetal ultrasonic evaluation.

SPECTRUM OF DISEASE IN LOW-BIRTHWEIGHT INFANTS. Immaturity increases the severity but reduces the distinctiveness of the clinical manifestations of most neonatal diseases. Immature organ function, complications of therapy, and the specific disorders that caused the premature onset of labor contribute to neonatal mor-

Physical maturity	−1	0	1	2	3	4	5
Skin	Sticky, friable, transparent	Gelatinous, red, translucent	Smooth, pink, visible veins	Superficial peeling and/or rash, few veins	Cracking, pale areas, rare veins	Parchment, deep cracking, no vessels	Leathery, cracked, wrinkled
Lanugo	None	Sparse	Abundant	Thinning	Bald areas	Mostly bald	
Plantar surface	Heel–toe 40–50 mm: −1 <40 mm: −2	<50 mm, no crease	Faint red marks	Anterior transverse crease only	Creases on ant. 2/3	Creases over entire sole	
Breast	Impercep-tible	Barely perceptible	Flat areola–no bud	Stripped areola, 1–2 mm bud	Raised areola, 3–4 mm bud	Full areola, 5–10 mm bud	
Eye/ear	Lids fused loosely (−1), tightly (−2)	Lids open, pinna flat, stays folded	Slightly curved pinna; soft; slow recoil	Well-curved pinna, soft but ready recoil	Formed and firm, instant recoil	Thick cartilage, ear stiff	
Genitals, male	Scrotum flat, smooth	Scrotum empty, faint rugae	Testes in upper canal, rare rugae	Testes descending, few rugae	Testes down, good rugae	Testes pendulous, deep rugae	
Genitals, female	Clitoris prominent, labia flat	Prominent clitoris, small labia minora	Prominent clitoris, enlarging minora	Majora and minora equally prominent	Majora large, minora small	Majora cover clitoris and minora	

Figure 97-3. Physical criteria for maturity. The expanded New Ballard Score includes extremely premature infants and has been refined to improve accuracy in more mature infants. (From Ballard JL, Khoury JC, Wedig K, et al: New Ballard Score, expanded to include extremely premature infants. *J Pediatr* 1991;119:417–423.)

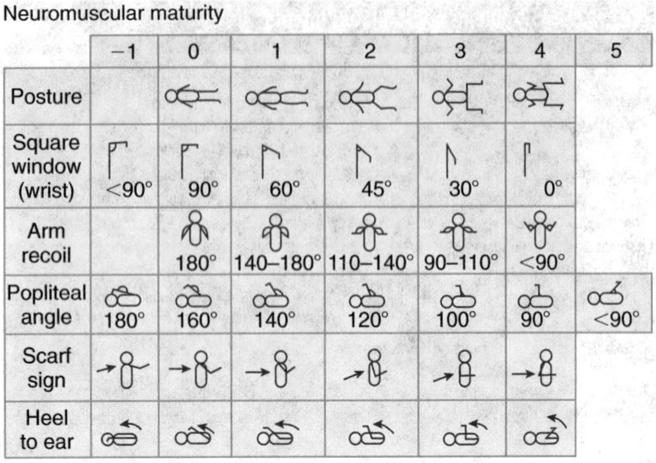

Neuromuscular maturity

	−1	0	1	2	3	4	5
Posture							
Square window (wrist)	<90°	90°	60°	45°	30°	0°	
Arm recoil		180°	140–180°	110–140°	90–110°	<90°	
Popliteal angle	180°	160°	140°	120°	100°	90°	<90°
Scarf sign							
Heel to ear							

Figure 97-4. Neuromuscular criteria for maturity. The expanded New Ballard Score includes extremely premature infants and has been refined to improve accuracy in more mature infants. (From Ballard JL, Khoury JC, Wedig K, et al: New Ballard Score, expanded to include extremely premature infants. *J Pediatr* 1991;119:417–423.)

bidity and mortality associated with premature, LBW infants (Table 97-6). Among VLBW infants, morbidity is inversely related to birthweight. Respiratory distress syndrome is noted in approximately 80% of infants 501–750 g; in 65% of those 751–1,000 g; in 45% between 1,001 and 1,250 g; and in 25% between 1,251 and 1,500 g. Severe intraventricular hemorrhage (IVH) is noted in approximately 25% of infants 501–750 g; in 12% between 751 and 1,000 g; in 8% between 1,001 and 1,250 g; and in 3% between 1,251 and 1,500 g. Overall, the risk of late sepsis (24%), bronchopulmonary dysplasia (23%), severe IVH (11%), necrotizing enterocolitis (7%), and prolonged hospitalization (45–125 days) is high in VLBW infants. Problems

Maturity Rating

Score	Weeks
−10	20
−5	22
0	24
5	26
10	28
15	30
20	32
25	34
30	36
35	38
40	40
45	42
50	44

Figure 97-5. Maturity rating. The physical and neurologic scores are added to calculate gestational age. (From Ballard JL, Khoury JC, Wedig K, et al: New Ballard Score, expanded to include extremely premature infants. *J Pediatr* 1991;119:417–423.)

associated with IUGR LBW infants are noted in Table 97-5; these added problems are often superimposed on those noted in Table 97-6 if an infant with IUGR is also premature. Poor postnatal growth is an important problem for both preterm and IUGR infants.

NURSERY CARE. At birth, the measures needed to clear the airway, initiate breathing, care for the umbilical cord and eyes, and administer vitamin K are the same for immature infants as for those of normal weight and maturity (Chapter 94). Special care is required to maintain a patent airway and avoid potential aspiration of gastric contents. Additional considerations are the need for (1) thermal control and monitoring of the heart rate and respiration, (2) oxygen therapy, and (3) special attention to the details of feeding. Safeguards against infection can never be relaxed. Routine procedures that disturb these infants may result in hypoxia. The need for regular and active participation by the parents in the infant's care in the nursery, the need to instruct the mother in at-home care of her infant, and the question of prognosis for later growth and development require special consideration.

Thermal Control. The survival rate of LBW and sick infants is higher when they are cared for at or near their **neutral thermal environment.** This environment is a set of thermal conditions, including air and radiating surface temperatures, relative humidity, and airflow, at which heat production (measured experimentally as oxygen consumption) is minimal and the infant's core temperature is within the normal range. It is a function of the size and postnatal age of an infant; larger, older infants require lower environmental temperatures than smaller, younger infants do. Isolettes (incubators) or radiant warmers can be used to maintain body temperature. Body heat is conserved through provision of a warm environment and standard conditions of humidity. The optimal environmental temperature for minimal heat loss and oxygen consumption for an unclothed infant is one that maintains the infant's core temperature at 36.5–37.0°C. It depends on an infant's size and maturity; the smaller and more immature the infant, the higher the environmental temperature required. An additional Plexiglas heat shield or head cap and body clothing may be required to keep an extremely LBW (ELBW) preterm infant warm. Infant warmth can be maintained by heating the air to a desired temperature or by servo-controlling the infant's body temperature at a desired set point. Continuous monitoring of the infant's temperature is required so that the environmental temperature can be adjusted to maintain optimal body temperature. Kangaroo mother care with direct skin to skin contact and a hat and blanket covering the infant is a safe alternative, with careful monitoring to avoid the risk of serious hypothermia when incubators are unavailable or when the infant is stable and the parents desire close contact with their infant.

Maintaining a relative humidity of 40–60% aids in stabilizing body temperature by reducing heat loss at lower environmental temperatures; by preventing drying and irritation of the lining of respiratory passages, especially during the administration of oxygen and after or during endotracheal intubation (usually 100% humidity); and by thinning viscid secretions and reducing insensible water loss from the lungs. An infant should be weaned and then removed from the isolette or radiant warmer only when the gradual change to the atmosphere of the nursery does not result in a significant change in the infant's temperature, color, activity, or vital signs.

Administering oxygen to reduce the risk of injury from hypoxia and circulatory insufficiency must be balanced against the risk of hyperoxia to the eyes (retinopathy of prematurity) and oxygen injury to the lungs. Oxygen should be administered via a head hood, nasal cannula, continuous positive airway pressure apparatus, or endotracheal tube to maintain stable and safe inspired oxygen concentrations. Although cyanosis must be treated immediately, oxygen is a drug and its use must be carefully regulated

TABLE 97-6. Neonatal Problems Associated with Premature Infants

Respiratory
Respiratory distress syndrome (hyaline membrane disease)*
Bronchopulmonary dysplasia
Pneumothorax, pneumomediastinum; interstitial emphysema
Congenital pneumonia
Pulmonary hypoplasia
Pulmonary hemorrhage
Apnea*
Cardiovascular
Patent ductus arteriosus*
Hypotension
Hypertension
Bradycardia (with apnea)*
Congenital malformations
Hematologic
Anemia (early or late onset)
Subcutaneous, organ (liver, cranial, adrenal) hemorrhage*
Disseminated intravascular coagulopathy
Vitamin K deficiency
Hydrops—immune or nonimmune
Gastrointestinal
Poor gastrointestinal function—poor motility*
Necrotizing enterocolitis
Hyperbilirubinemia—direct and indirect*
Congenital anomalies producing polyhydramnios
Spontaneous gastrointestinal isolated perforation
Metabolic-Endocrine
Hypocalcemia*
Hypoglycemia*
Hyperglycemia*
Late metabolic acidosis
Hypothermia*
Euthyroid but low-thyroxine status
Central Nervous System
Intraventricular hemorrhage*
Periventricular leukomalacia
Hypoxic-ischemic encephalopathy
Seizures
Retinopathy of prematurity
Deafness
Hypotonia*
Congenital malformations
Kernicterus (bilirubin encephalopathy)
Drug (narcotic) withdrawal
Renal
Hyponatremia*
Hypernatremia*
Hyperkalemia*
Renal tubular acidosis
Renal glycosuria
Edema
Other
Infections* (congenital, perinatal, nosocomial: bacterial, viral, fungal, protozoal)

*Common.

to maximize benefit and minimize potential harm. The concentration of inspired oxygen must be adjusted in accordance with the oxygen tension of arterial blood (Pa_{O_2}) or noninvasive methods such as continuous pulse oximetry or transcutaneous oxygen measurements. Capillary blood gases are inadequate for estimating arterial oxygen levels.

Fluid Requirements. Fluid needs vary according to gestational age, environmental conditions, and disease states. Assuming minimal water loss in the stool of infants not receiving oral fluids, their water needs are equal to their insensible water loss, excretion of renal solutes, growth, and any unusual ongoing losses. Insensible water loss is indirectly related to gestational age; very immature preterm infants (<1,000 g) may lose as much as 2–3 mL/kg/hr, partly because of immature skin, lack of subcutaneous tissue, and a large exposed surface area. Insensible water loss is increased under radiant warmers, during phototherapy, and in febrile infants. It is diminished when infants are clothed, are covered by a Plexiglas inner heat shield, breathe humidified air, or are of advanced postnatal age. Larger premature infants (2,000–2,500 g) nursed in an incubator may have an insensible water loss of approximately 0.6–0.7 mL/kg/hr.

Adequate fluid intake is essential for excretion of the urinary solute load (urea, electrolytes, phosphate). The amount varies with dietary intake and the anabolic or catabolic state of nutrition. Formulas with a high solute load, high protein intake, and catabolism increase the end products that require urinary excretion and thus increase the requirement for water. **Renal solute loads** may vary between 7.5 and 30 mOsm/kg. Newborn infants, especially those with VLBW, are also less able to concentrate urine; their fluid intake required to excrete solutes increases.

Water intake in term infants is usually begun at 60–70 mL/kg on day 1 and increased to 100–120 mL/kg by days 2–3. Smaller, more premature infants may need to start with 70–80 mL/kg on day 1 and advance gradually to 150 mL/kg/day. Fluid volumes should be titrated individually, although it is unusual to exceed 150 mL/kg/24 hr. Infants weighing <750 g in the 1st wk of life have immature skin and a large surface area, characteristics that lead to a high rate of transepidermal fluid loss, at times requiring higher rates of intravenous fluids. Daily weights, urine, and serum urea nitrogen and sodium levels should be monitored carefully to determine water balance and fluid needs. Clinical observation and physical examination are poor indicators of the state of hydration of premature infants. Conditions that increase fluid loss, such as glycosuria, the polyuric phase of acute tubular necrosis, and diarrhea, may place additional strain on kidneys that have not yet acquired their maximal capacity to conserve water and electrolytes, the results of which may be severe dehydration. Alternatively, fluid overload may lead to edema, heart failure, patent ductus arteriosus, and bronchopulmonary dysplasia.

Total Parenteral Nutrition. Before complete enteral feeding has been established or when enteral feeding is impossible for prolonged periods, total intravenous alimentation may provide sufficient fluid, calories, amino acids, electrolytes, and vitamins to sustain the growth of LBW infants. This technique has been lifesaving for VLBW infants and those who have had intractable diarrheal syndromes or extensive bowel resection. Infusions may be administered through a percutaneously or less often surgically placed indwelling central venous catheter or through a peripheral vein. The umbilical vein may also be used for a short time.

The goal of parenteral alimentation is to deliver sufficient calories from glucose, protein, and lipids to promote optimal growth. The infusate should contain 2.5–3 g/dL of synthetic amino acids and glucose usually in the range of 10–15 g/dL, in addition to appropriate quantities of electrolytes, trace minerals, and vitamins. If a peripheral vein is used, it is advisable to keep the glucose concentration below 12.5 g/dL. If a central vein is used, glucose concentrations as high as 25 g/dL may be used (rarely). Intravenous fat emulsions such as 20% Intralipid (2.2 kcal/mL) may be administered to provide calories without an appreciable osmotic load, thereby decreasing the need for infusion of the higher concentrations of glucose by central or peripheral vein while preventing the development of essential fatty acid deficiency. Intralipid may be initiated at 0.5 g/kg/24 hr and advanced to 3 g/kg/24 hr, if triglyceride levels remain normal; 0.5 g/kg/24 hr is sufficient to prevent essential fatty acid deficiency. Electrolytes, trace minerals, and vitamin additives are included in amounts approximating established intravenous maintenance requirements. The content of each day's infusate should be determined after carefully assessing the infant's clinical and biochemical status. Slow and continuous infusion is advisable. A well-trained pharmacist should mix all solutions under a laminar flow hood.

After a caloric intake of >100 kcal/kg/24 hr is established by total parenteral intravenous nutrition, LBW infants can be expected to gain about 15 g/kg/24 hr, with a positive nitrogen balance of 150–200 mg/kg/24 hr, in the absence of episodes of sepsis, surgical procedures, or other severe stress. This goal can usually be achieved (and the catabolic tendency during the 1st wk of life reversed with subsequent weight gain) by peripheral vein infusion of 2.5–3.5 g/kg/24 hr of an amino acid mixture, 10 g/dL of glucose, and 2–3 g/kg/24 hr of Intralipid.

Complications of intravenous alimentation are related to both the catheter and metabolism of the infusate. Sepsis is the most important problem of central vein infusions and can be minimized only by meticulous catheter care and aseptic preparation of the infusate; a vancomycin-heparin solution also reduces the risk of line sepsis. Coagulase-negative staphylococcus is the most common infecting organism. Treatment includes appropriate antibiotics. If an infection persists (repeatedly positive blood cultures while receiving appropriate antibiotics), the line must be removed. Thrombosis, extravasation of fluid, and accidental dislodgment of catheters have also occurred. Although sepsis is less often attributable to peripheral vein infusion, phlebitis, cutaneous sloughing, and superficial infection may occur. Metabolic complications of parenteral nutrition include hyperglycemia from the high glucose concentration of the infusate, which may lead to osmotic diuresis and dehydration; azotemia; a possible increased risk of nephrocalcinosis; hypoglycemia from sudden accidental cessation of the infusate; hyperlipidemia and possibly hypoxemia from intravenous lipid infusions; and hyperammonemia, which may be due to high levels of certain amino acids. Metabolic bone disease and/or cholestatic jaundice and liver disease may develop in infants who require long-term parenteral nutrition and receive no enteral nutrition. Biochemical and physiologic monitoring of infants receiving intravenous alimentation is indicated because of the frequency and seriousness of complications.

Feeding. The method of feeding each LBW infant should be individualized. It is important to avoid fatigue and aspiration of food by regurgitation or by the feeding process. No feeding method averts these problems unless the person feeding the infant has been well trained in the method. Oral feeding (nipple) should not be initiated or should be discontinued in infants with respiratory distress, hypoxia, circulatory insufficiency, excessive secretions, gagging, sepsis, central nervous system depression, severe immaturity, or signs of serious illness. These high-risk infants require parenteral nutrition or gavage feeding to supply calories, fluid, and electrolytes. The process of oral alimentation requires, in addition to a strong sucking effort, coordination of swallowing, epiglottal and uvular closure of the larynx and nasal passages, and normal esophageal motility, a synchronized process that is usually absent before 34 wk of gestation.

Preterm infants at 34 wk of gestation or more can often be fed by bottle or at the breast. Because the effort of sucking is usually the limiting factor, breast-feeding is less likely to succeed until the infant matures. Bottle-feeding of expressed breast milk may be a temporary alternative. In bottle-feeding, effort may be reduced by use of special small, soft nipples with large holes. Smaller or less vigorous infants should be fed by gavage: A soft plastic tube with No. 5 French external and approximately 0.05 cm internal diameters and with a rounded atraumatic tip and two holes on alternate sides is preferable. The tube is passed through the nose until approximately 2.5 cm (1 inch) of the lower end is in the stomach. The free end of the tube has an adapter into which the tip of a syringe is fitted, and a measured amount of fluid is given by pump or by gravity. Such tubes may be left in place for 3–7 days before being replaced by a similar tube through the alternate nostril. Infants occasionally have enough local irritation from an indwelling tube that they may gag or troublesome secretions may gather around it in the nasopharynx. In such cases, a catheter may be passed through the mouth by a skilled person and removed at the end of each feeding.

The LBW infant may be fed with intermittent bolus feedings or continuous feeding. In the occasional infant with feeding intolerance, nasojejunal feeding may be successful. Intestinal perforation is a risk with nasojejunal feeding. A change to breast- or bottle-feeding may be instituted gradually as soon as an infant displays general vigor adequate for oral feeding without fatigue.

Gastrostomy feeding is not usually indicated in premature infants except as an adjunct to surgical management of specific gastrointestinal conditions or in permanently neurologically injured patients unable to suck and swallow normally.

Initiation of Feeding. The optimal time to introduce enteral feeding to a sick LBW infant is controversial. **Trophic feeding** is the practice of feeding very small amounts of enteral nourishment to VLBW preterm infants to stimulate development of the immature gastrointestinal tract. The benefits of trophic feeding include enhanced gut motility, improved growth, decreased need for parenteral nutrition, fewer episodes of sepsis, and shortened hospital stays. Once the infant is stable, small-volume feedings are given in addition to intravenous fluids/nutrition. Feeding is gradually advanced and parenteral nutrition decreased. This approach may reduce the incidence of necrotizing enterocolitis. The main principle in feeding premature infants is to proceed cautiously and gradually. Careful early feeding of breast milk or formula tends to reduce the risk of hypoglycemia, dehydration, and hyperbilirubinemia without the additional risk of aspiration, provided that the presence of respiratory distress or other disorders does not present an indication for withholding oral feedings and administering electrolytes, fluids, and calories intravenously.

If an infant is well, is making sucking movements, and is in no distress, oral feeding may be attempted, although most infants weighing <1,500 g require tube feeding because they are unable to coordinate breathing, sucking, and swallowing. Intestinal tract readiness for feeding may be determined by active bowel sounds, passage of meconium, and the absence of abdominal distention, bilious gastric aspirates, or emesis. For infants under 1,000 g, the initial feedings are either half- or full-strength breast milk or preterm formula at 10 mL/kg/24 hr as a continuous nasogastric tube drip (or given by intermittent gavage every 2–3 hr). If the initial feeding is tolerated, the volume is increased by 10–15 mL/kg/24 hr. The daily milk volume increment should not exceed 20–30 mL/kg/24 hr. Once a volume of 150 mL/kg/24 hr has been achieved, the caloric content may be increased to 24 or 27 kcal/oz. With high caloric density, infants are at risk for dehydration, edema, lactose intolerance, diarrhea, flatus, and delayed gastric emptying with emesis. Intravenous fluids are needed until feedings provide approximately 120 mL/kg/24 hr. The feeding protocol for premature infants weighing over 1,500 g is initiated at a volume of 20–25 mL/kg/24 hr of full-strength breast milk or preterm formula given as a bolus every 3 hr. Thereafter, increments in total daily formula volume should not exceed 20 mL/kg/24 hr. The expected weight increments for premature infants of various birthweights are projected from Figure 97-6. Infants with IUGR may not demonstrate the initial weight loss noted in premature infants.

Regurgitation, vomiting, abdominal distention, or gastric residuals from previous feedings should arouse suspicion of sepsis, necrotizing enterocolitis, or intestinal obstruction; these conditions are indications to drop back in the schedule and increase subsequent feedings slowly or to change to intravenous alimentation and evaluate for more serious problems (Chapter 102.2). Weight gain may not be achieved for 10–12 days, and a daily intake of 130–150 mL/kg or more may be necessary for some infants. Alternatively, in vigorous infants whose feeding schedule is advanced successfully in calories or volume, weight gain may appear within a few days.

When tube feeding is used, the contents of the stomach should be aspirated before each feeding. If only air or small amounts of mucus are obtained, the feeding is given as planned. If all or a substantial part of the previous feeding is aspirated, it is advis-

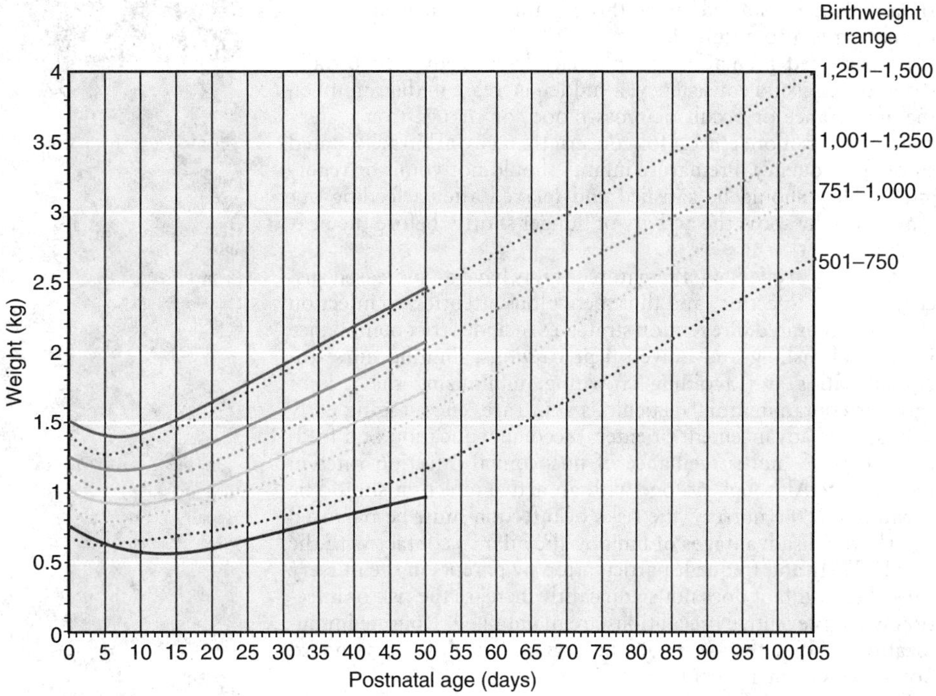

Figure 97-6. Average daily weight (kg) vs postnatal age (days) for infants with birthweight ranges of 501–750 g, 751–1,000 g, 1,001–1,250 g, and 1,251–1,500 g *(dotted lines),* plotted with the curves of Dancis and colleagues for infants with birthweights of 750 g, 1,000 g, 1,250 g, and 1,500 g *(solid lines).* (From Wright K, Dawson JP, Fallis D, et al: New postnatal growth grids for very low birth weight infants. *Pediatrics* 1993; 91:922–926.)

able to reduce the amount of the feeding and proceed more gradually with subsequent increases.

The digestive enzyme systems of infants older than 28 wk gestation are mature enough to permit adequate digestion and absorption of protein and carbohydrate. Fat is less well absorbed, primarily because of inadequate amounts of bile salt; unsaturated fats and the fat of human milk are absorbed better than those of cow's milk. The weight gain of infants weighing under 2,000 g at birth should be adequate when human milk or "humanized" milk premature formula (40% casein and 60% whey) with a protein intake of 2.25–2.75 g/kg/24 hr is fed. These two alternatives should provide all amino acids essential for premature infants, including tyrosine, cystine, and histidine. Higher protein intake may be well tolerated and is generally safe, especially in older, rapidly growing infants. Protein intake as high as 4–5 g/kg/24 hr may be hazardous. Although linear growth may be promoted, high-protein formulas may cause abnormal plasma aminograms; elevations in blood urea nitrogen, ammonia, and sodium concentrations; metabolic acidosis (cow's milk formulas); and untoward effects on neurologic development. Furthermore, the high protein and mineral contents of balanced cow's milk formulas with a high caloric content constitute a large solute load for the kidneys, a fact important in maintaining water balance, especially in infants with diarrhea or fever.

Breast milk from the infant's mother is the preferred milk for all infants, including VLBW infants. In addition to nutritional advantages, the benefits of breast milk include protection against a wide range of infections (through both specific and nonspecific anti-infective factors in breast milk and beneficial effects on intestinal flora), a decreased risk of necrotizing enterocolitis in preterm infants, a lower risk of sudden infant death syndrome, and possible long-term effects, including a lower risk of childhood/adolescent obesity and improved neurodevelopmental outcome. Once a premature infant takes 120 mL/kg/ 24 hr, **breast milk fortifiers** are added to supplement breast milk with protein, calcium, and phosphorus. If breast milk is unavailable, special preterm formulas should be used. At approximately 34–36 wk gestation, infants who are not receiving breast milk should be switched to a term formula (unless metabolic bone disease is present—see Chapter 106) because hypercalcemia may develop as a result of the preterm formula's higher calcium and vitamin D levels.

Although formula in amounts necessary for adequate growth probably contains adequate quantities of all vitamins, the volume of milk sufficient to satisfy these requirements may not be ingested for several weeks. Therefore, LBW infants should be given supplemental vitamins. Because requirements for these infants have not been precisely established, the recommended daily allowances for term infants should be given (see Chapter 41). Furthermore, these infants may have a special need for certain vitamins. Intermediary metabolism of phenylalanine and tyrosine depends, in part, on vitamin C. Decreased fat absorption with increased fecal fat loss may be associated with decreased absorption of vitamin D, other fat-soluble vitamins, and calcium in premature infants. VLBW infants are particularly prone to the development of osteopenia, but their total intake of vitamin D should not exceed 1,500 IU/24 hr. Folic acid is essential for the formation of DNA and production of new cells; serum and erythrocyte levels decrease in preterm infants during the 1st few wk of life and remain low for 2–3 mo. Therefore, folic acid supplementation is recommended, although it does not result in improved growth or an increased hemoglobin concentration. Deficiency of vitamin E is uncommon but is associated with increased hemolysis and, if severe, with anemia and edema in premature infants. Vitamin E functions as an antioxidant to prevent the peroxidation of excessive polyunsaturated fatty acids in red blood cell membranes; its need may increase because of the increased membrane content of these fatty acids when formulas with high polyunsaturated fatty acids are used. Vitamin A supplementation has been shown to reduce bronchopulmonary dysplasia in VLBW infants. Vitamin K deficiency is discussed in Chapter 103.4.

In LBW infants, **physiologic anemia** as a result of postnatal suppression of erythropoiesis is exacerbated by smaller fetal iron stores and greater expansion of blood volume from the more rapid growth than that of term infants; therefore, the anemia develops earlier and reaches a lower ultimate level. Fetal or neonatal blood loss accentuates this problem. Iron stores, even in VLBW neonates, are usually adequate until an infant's birthweight has doubled; iron supplementation (2 mg/kg/24 hr) should then be started. If erythropoietin is used, iron supplementation is also required.

Properly fed premature infants may have from 1 to 6 daily stools of semisolid consistency; a sudden increase in their number, the appearance of occult or gross blood, or change to a watery consistency is more reason for concern than any arbitrarily stated stooling frequency. Premature infants should not vomit or regurgitate. They should be satisfied and relaxed after a feeding but may normally show the activity of hunger shortly before the next feeding.

Prevention of Infection. Premature infants have an increased susceptibility to infection, and thus meticulous attention to infection control is required. Prevention strategies include strict compliance with handwashing and universal precautions, limiting nurse-to-patient ratios and avoiding crowding, minimizing the risk of catheter contamination, meticulous skin care, encouraging early appropriate advancement of enteral feeding, education and feedback to staff, and surveillance of nosocomial infection rates in the nursery. Although no one with an active infection should be permitted in the nursery, the risks of infection must be balanced against the disadvantages of limiting the infant's contact with the family. Early and frequent participation by parents in the nursery care of their infant does not significantly increase the risk of infection when preventive precautions are maintained. Routine immunizations should be given on the regular schedule at standard doses (see Chapter 170).

Preventing transmission of infection from infant to infant is difficult because often neither term nor premature newborn infants have clear clinical evidence of an infection early in its course. When epidemics occur within a nursery, cohort nursing and isolation rooms should be used. Universal precautions require gloves to be worn with all patient contact.

TABLE 97-7. Potential Adverse Reactions to Drugs Administered to Premature Infants

DRUG	REACTION
Oxygen	Retinopathy of prematurity, bronchopulmonary dysplasia
Sulfisoxazole	Kernicterus
Chloramphenicol	Gray baby syndrome—shock, bone marrow suppression
Vitamin K analogs	Jaundice
Novobiocin	Jaundice
Hexachlorophene	Encephalopathy
Benzyl alcohol	Acidosis, collapse, intraventricular bleeding
Intravenous vitamin E	Ascites, shock
Phenolic detergents	Jaundice
$NaHCO_3$	Intraventricular hemorrhage
Amphotericin	Anuric renal failure, hypokalemia, hypomagnesemia
Reserpine	Nasal stuffiness
Indomethacin	Oliguria, hyponatremia, intestinal perforation
Cisapride	Prolonged Q-Tc interval
Tetracycline	Enamel hypoplasia
Tolazoline	Hypotension, gastrointestinal bleeding
Calcium salts	Subcutaneous necrosis
Aminoglycosides	Deafness, renal toxicity
Enteric gentamicin	Resistant bacteria
Prostaglandins	Seizures, diarrhea, apnea, hyperostosis, pyloric stenosis
Phenobarbital	Altered state, drowsiness
Morphine	Hypotension, urine retention, withdrawal
Pancuronium	Edema, hypovolemia, hypotension, tachycardia, vecuronium contractions, prolonged hypotonia
Iodine antiseptics	Hypothyroidism, goiter
Fentanyl	Seizures, chest wall rigidity, withdrawal
Dexamethasone	Gastrointestinal bleeding, hypertension, infection, hyperglycemia, cardiomyopathy, reduced growth
Furosemide	Deafness, hyponatremia, hypokalemia, hypochloremia, nephrocalcinosis, biliary stones
Heparin (not low-dose prophylactic use)	Bleeding, intraventricular hemorrhage, thrombocytopenia
Erythromycin	Pyloric stenosis

IMMATURITY OF DRUG METABOLISM. Renal clearance of almost all substances excreted in the urine is diminished in newborn infants, but more so in premature ones. The glomerular filtration rate increases with increasing gestational age; therefore drug dosing recommendations vary with age. Intervals between doses may therefore need to be extended when administering drugs excreted chiefly by the kidneys. Longer intervals are required for many drugs administered to preterm infants. Drugs detoxified in the liver or requiring chemical conjugation before renal excretion should also be given with caution and in doses smaller than usual.

When possible, blood levels should be determined for potentially toxic drugs, especially if renal or hepatic dysfunction is present. Decisions about the choice and dose of antibacterial agents and the route of administration should be made on an individual basis rather than routinely because of the dangers of (1) development of infections with organisms resistant to antibacterial agents, (2) inhibition of intestinal bacteria that manufacture significant amounts of essential vitamins (vitamin K and thiamine), and (3) harmful interference in important metabolic processes.

Many drugs apparently safe for adults on the basis of toxicity studies may be harmful to newborn infants, especially premature ones. Oxygen and a number of drugs have proved toxic to premature infants in amounts not harmful to term infants (Table 97-7). Thus, administering any drug, particularly in high doses, without pharmacologic testing in premature infants should be undertaken carefully after weighing risks against benefits.

PROGNOSIS. Infants born weighing 1,501–2,500 g have a 95% or greater chance of survival, but those weighing less still have significantly higher mortality (see Fig. 97-1). Intensive care has extended the period during which a VLBW infant is at increased risk of dying of complications of prematurity, such as bronchopulmonary dysplasia, necrotizing enterocolitis, or nosocomial infection (Table 97-8). The postdischarge mortality rate of LBW infants is higher than that of term infants during the 1st 2 yr of life. Because many of these deaths are attributable to infection (respiratory syncytial virus [RSV]), they are at least theoretically preventable. In addition, premature infants have an increased incidence of failure to thrive, sudden infant death syndrome, child abuse, and inadequate maternal-infant bonding. The biologic risk associated with poor cardiorespiratory regulation because of immaturity or complications of underlying perinatal disease and the social risk associated with poverty also contribute to the high mortality and morbidity of these infants. Congenital anomalies are present in approximately 3–7% of LBW infants.

In the absence of congenital abnormalities, central nervous system injury, VLBW, or marked IUGR, the physical growth of LBW infants tends to approximate that of term infants by the

TABLE 97-8. Sequelae of Low Birthweight

IMMEDIATE	LATE
Hypoxia, ischemia	Mental retardation, spastic diplegia, microcephaly, seizures, poor school performance
Intraventricular hemorrhage	Mental retardation, spasticity, seizures, hydrocephalus
Sensorineural injury	Hearing, visual impairment, retinopathy of prematurity, strabismus, myopia
Respiratory failure	Bronchopulmonary dysplasia, cor pulmonale, bronchospasm, malnutrition, subglottic stenosis, iatrogenic cleft palate, recurrent pneumonia
Necrotizing enterocolitis	Short-bowel syndrome, malabsorption, malnutrition, infectious diarrhea
Cholestatic liver disease	Cirrhosis, hepatic failure, hepatic carcinoma, malnutrition
Nutrient deficiency	Osteopenia, fractures, anemia, vitamin E, growth failure
Social stress	Child abuse or neglect, failure to thrive, divorce
Other	Sudden infant death syndrome, infections, inguinal hernia, cutaneous scars (chest tube, patent ductus arteriosus ligation, intravenous infiltration), gastroesophageal reflux, hypertension, craniosynostosis, cholelithiasis, nephrocalcinosis, cutaneous hemangiomas

2nd yr; it occurs earlier in premature infants with larger birth size. VLBW infants may not catch up, especially if they have severe chronic sequelae, insufficient nutritional intake, or an inadequate caretaking environment (see Table 97-8). Infants with IUGR (SGA) who grow poorly and don't demonstrate catch-up growth (which most do) may benefit from recombinant human growth hormone therapy beginning at age 4 yr. Premature birth in itself may prejudice later development. The greater the immaturity and the lower the birthweight, the greater the likelihood of intellectual and neurologic deficit; as many as 50% of 500–750 g infants have a significant neurodevelopmental impairment (blindness, deafness, mental retardation, cerebral palsy). Small head circumference at birth may be similarly related to a poor neurobehavioral prognosis. Many surviving LBW infants have hypotonia before 8 mo corrected age, which improves by the time they are 8 mo–1 yr old. This transient hypotonia is not a poor prognostic sign. Thirty to 50% of VLBW children have poor school performance at 7 yr of age (repeat grades, special classes, learning disorders, poor speech and language), despite a normal IQ. Factors posing a risk for poor academic performance include birthweight below 750 g, severe IVH, periventricular leukomalacia, bronchopulmonary dysplasia, cerebral atrophy, posthemorrhagic hydrocephalus, IUGR, low socioeconomic status, and, possibly, low thyroxine levels. Adolescents who were VLBW report satisfactory health; 94% are integrated in regular classes despite neurosensory disabilities (hearing, vision, cerebral palsy, cognition) in 24%.

Both premature and IUGR infants are at risk for significant metabolic conditions (obesity, type II diabetes) and cardiovascular disorders (ischemic heart disease, hypertension) as adults. This **fetal origins** hypothesis of adult morbidities may be due to insulin resistance, which may be evident in early childhood.

PREDICTING NEONATAL MORTALITY. Birthweight and gestational age have traditionally been used as strong indicators for the risk of neonatal death. Indeed, survival at 22 wk of gestation is poor, particularly in those infants requiring aggressive resuscitation in the delivery room. With increasing gestational age, survival rates increase to approximately 15% at 23 wk, 56% at 24 wk, and 79% at 25 wk. The survival of infants <24 wk gestation, weighing <750 g with a 1-min Apgar score <3 is 30%. These infants are also at risk for poor neurodevelopmental outcome. Birthweight-specific neonatal diseases such as grade IV IVH, severe group B streptococcal pneumonia, and pulmonary hypoplasia also contribute to a poor outcome. **Scoring systems** that have been developed take into consideration physiologic abnormalities (hypotension-hypertension, acidosis, hypoxia, hypercapnia, anemia, neutropenia), as in the **Score for Neonatal Acute Physiology (SNAP),** or clinical parameters (gestational age, birthweight, anomalies, acidosis, $F{IO_2}$), as in the **Clinical Risk Index for Babies (CRIB).** CRIB includes six parameters collected in the 1st 12 hr after birth, and SNAP has 26 variables collected in the 1st 24 hr. Although these risk scoring systems may provide prognostic information for mortality, they may not be useful for predicting morbidity in survivors. Furthermore, when compared with the clinical judgment of experienced neonatologists (based on birthweight, illness severity, low Apgar score, BPD, IUGR, therapeutic requirements), objective risk scores provide similar predictability. Combining a physician's judgment and an objective score may produce a more accurate assessment of the risk of mortality.

DISCHARGE FROM THE HOSPITAL. Before discharge, a premature infant should be taking all nutrition by nipple, either bottle or breast (Table 97-9). Some medically fragile infants may be discharged home on gavage feedings after the parents have received appropriate training and education. Growth should be occurring at steady increments of approximately 10–30 g/24 hr. Temperature should be stabilized in an open crib. Infants should have had no recent episodes of apnea or bradycardia, and parenteral drug administration should have been discontinued or converted to oral dosing. Stable infants recovering from bronchopulmonary dysplasia may be discharged on a regimen of oxygen given by nasal cannula as long as careful follow-up is arranged with frequent pulse oximetry monitoring and outpatient visits. All infants with a birthweight under 1,500 g and those between 1,500 and 2,000 g with an unstable clinical course requiring oxygen should have an eye examination to screen for retinopathy of prematurity. All LBW infants should have a hearing test prior to discharge. Those who had indwelling umbilical arterial catheters should have their blood pressure measured to check for renal vascular hypertension. The hemoglobin level or hematocrit should be determined to evaluate for possible anemia. If all major medical problems have resolved and the home setting is adequate, premature infants may then be discharged when their weight approaches 1,800–2,100 g; close follow-up plus easy access to health care providers is essential for early discharge protocols. Alternatively, if the medical or social environment is not ideal, high-risk neonates who have been transported to neonatal intensive care units and whose major illness has resolved may be returned to their hospital of birth for an additional period of hospitalization. Standard vaccinations with full doses should commence after discharge or, if in the hospital, with vaccines that do not contain live viruses. For RSV prophylaxis, see Chapter 257.

TABLE 97-9. Recommendations for the Discharge of High-Risk Low-Birthweight Infants

- Resolution of acute life-threatening illnesses
- Ongoing follow-up for chronic but stable problems
    - Bronchopulmonary dysplasia
    - Intraventricular hemorrhage
    - Necrotizing enterocolitis
    - Ventricular septal defect, other cardiac lesions
    - Anemia
    - Retinopathy of prematurity
    - Hearing
    - Apnea
    - Cholestasis
- Stable temperature regulation
- Gaining weight on oral feedings
    - Breast-feeding
    - Bottle-feeding
    - Gastric tube
- Free of significant apnea; home monitoring for apnea if needed
- Appropriate immunizations and planning for respiratory syncytial virus prophylaxis if indicated
- Hearing screenings
- Ophthalmologic examination if <27 wk or <1,250 g at birth
- Mother's knowledge, skill, confidence documented in
    - Administration of medications (diuretics, methylxanthines, aerosols, etc.)
    - Use of oxygen, apnea monitors, oximeters
    - Nutritional support
        - Timing
        - Volume
        - Mixing concentrated formulas
    - Recognition of illness and deterioration
    - Basic cardiopulmonary resuscitation
    - Infant safety (see Table 97-1)
- Scheduling of referrals
    - Primary care provider
    - Neonatal follow-up clinic
    - Occupational therapy/physical therapy
    - Imaging (head ultrasound)
- Assessment of and solution to social risks (Table 97-1)

Adapted from American Academy of Pediatrics, American College of Obstetrcians: *Guidelines for Perinatal Care,* 5th ed. Elk Grove Village, IL, American Academy of Pediatrics, 2002.

HOME CARE. While the infant is in the hospital, the mother should receive instruction on how to care for the baby after discharge.

Ideally, this program should include at least one visit to her home by someone capable of evaluating domestic arrangements and advising about any needed improvements.

97.3 • Post-Term Infants

Post-term infants are those born after 42 wk of gestation, as calculated from the mother's last menstrual period, regardless of weight at birth. This designation is often used synonymously with the term "postmature" for infants whose gestation exceeds the normal 280 days by 7 or more days. Approximately 25% of all pregnancies end on or after the 287th day of gestation, 12% on or after the 294th day, and 5% on or after the 301st day. The cause of post-term birth or postmaturity is unknown. Large size of the infant correlates poorly with late delivery but does correlate with large size of either parent, multigravidity, or a prediabetic or diabetic state in the mother.

CLINICAL MANIFESTATIONS. Post-term infants may be clinically indistinguishable from term infants, but some have received the designation postmature because their appearance and behavior suggest those of an infant 1–3 wk of age. These post-term, postmature infants often have increased birthweight and are characterized by the absence of lanugo, decreased or absent vernix caseosa, long nails, abundant scalp hair, white parchment-like or desquamating skin, and increased alertness. If placental insufficiency occurs, the amniotic fluid and fetus may be meconium stained, and abnormal fetal heart rates may be observed; the infant may have growth retardation. Although this syndrome is frequently confused with postmaturity, only about 20% of infants with placental insufficiency syndrome are post-term. The majority of those affected are term and preterm infants, particularly those SGA who are infants of toxemic mothers, older primigravidas, and women with chronic hypertension. The placentas are often small or poorly attached. This syndrome has been postulated to result from degenerative changes in the placenta that progressively reduce oxygen and nourishment to the fetus.

Infants born post-term in association with presumed placental insufficiency may have various physical signs. Desquamation, long nails, abundant hair, pale skin, alert faces, and loose skin, especially around the thighs and buttocks, give them the appearance of having recently lost weight; meconium-stained nails, skin, vernix, umbilical cord, and placental membranes may also be noted (see Fig. 94-1).

PROGNOSIS. When delivery is delayed 3 wk or more beyond term, mortality is significantly increased and, in some series, has been approximately three times that of a control group of infants born at term. Mortality has been lowered markedly through improved obstetric management.

MANAGEMENT. Careful obstetric monitoring, including nonstress testing, biophysical profile, or Doppler velocimetry, usually provides a rational basis for choosing a course of nonintervention, induction of labor, or cesarean section. Induction of labor or cesarean section may be indicated in older primigravidas who go more than 2–4 wk beyond term, particularly if evidence of fetal distress is present. Medical problems in the newborn are treated if they arise.

97.4 • Large for Gestational Age

See also Chapter 107.1.

Neonatal mortality rates decrease with increasing birthweight until approximately 4,000 g, after which mortality increases. These oversized infants are usually born at term, but preterm infants with weights high for gestational age also have a significantly higher mortality than do infants of the same size born at term; maternal diabetes and obesity are predisposing factors. Infants who are very large, regardless of their gestational age, have a higher incidence of birth injuries such as cervical and brachial plexus injuries, phrenic nerve damage with paralysis of the diaphragm, fractured clavicles, cephalohematomas, subdural hematomas, and ecchymoses of the head and face.

The incidence of congenital anomalies, particularly congenital heart disease, is also higher than in term infants of normal weight. Intellectual and developmental retardation is statistically more common in high birthweight term and preterm infants than in babies of appropriate weight for gestational age.

97.5 • Infant Transport

With the advent of regionalized care of high-risk neonates, increasing numbers of sick infants are being transported to neonatal intensive care units in hospitals at which they were not born. Ideally, high-risk mothers should be transported to and their babies delivered at centers where these specialized units are located. Neonatal transport should include consultation about the infant's problem and care before transport, ease of access to the transport team, and transport and stabilization by the team before moving the infant. Securing an airway, providing oxygen, assisting with infant ventilation, providing antimicrobial therapy, maintaining the circulation, providing a warmed environment, and placing intravenous or arterial lines or chest tubes should all be initiated, if indicated, before transport. Infant and maternal records, laboratory reports, and a tube of clotted maternal blood should also be provided. Before departing, the mother should be briefly reassured and allowed to see her stabilized infant, if practical; the father should follow the transport vehicle to the unit. The transport officer or nurse should also call ahead to inform the receiving unit about the nature of the patient's illness.

The transport vehicle should be equipped with appropriate medicines, fluids, oxygen tanks, catheters, chest tubes, endotracheal tubes, laryngoscopes, and an infant warming device. It should be well illuminated and have ample room for emergency procedures and monitoring equipment. With efficient transport and appropriately educated nursing and medical staff at the referring hospitals, the mortality of "outborn" neonates should be no higher than that of those born within the tertiary care center.

Alberry M, Soothill P: Management of fetal growth restriction. *Arch Dis Child Fetal Neonatal Ed* 2007;92:F62–F67.

Alexander GR, Kogan M, Bader D, et al: US birth weight/gestational age-specific neonatal mortality: 1995-1997 rates for whites, Hispanics, and blacks. Pediatrics 2003;111:e61–e66.

American Academy of Pediatrics: Hospital discharge of the high-risk neonate—proposed guidelines. *Pediatrics* 1998;22:411–417.

Bonhoeffer J, Siegrist CA, Heath PT: Immunisation of premature infants. *Arch Dis Child* 2006;91:929–935.

Caple J, Armentrout D, Huseby V, et al: Randomized, controlled trial of slow versus rapid feeding volume advancement in preterm infants. *Pediatrics* 2004:114:1597–1600.

Clandinin MT, van Aerde JE, Merkel KL, et al: Growth and development of preterm infants fed infant formulas containing docosahexaenoic acid and arachidonic acid. *J Pediatr* 2005:146:461–468.

DeFelice C, Tassi R, De Capua B, et al: A new phenotypical variant of intrauterine growth restriction? *Pediatrics* 2007;119:e983–e990.

Eriksson JG: The fetal origins hypothesis—10 years on. *Br Med J* 2005;330:1096–1097.

Fawzi WW, Msamanga GI, Urassa W, et al: Vitamins and perinatal outcomes among HIV-negative women in Tanzania. *N Engl J Med* 2007;356:1423–2431.

Gardner F, Johnson A, Yudkin P, et al: Behavioral and emotional adjustment of teenagers in mainstream school who were born before 29 weeks' gestation. *Pediatrics* 2004;114:676–682.

Garite TJ, Clark R, Thorp JA: Intrauterine growth restriction increases morbidity and mortality among premature neonates. *Am J Obstet Gynecol* 2004;191:481–487.

Gilbert WM, Danielsen B: Pregnancy outcomes associated with intrauterine growth restriction. *Am J Obstet Gynecol* 2003;188:1596–1601.

Gupta P, Ray M, Dua T, et al: Multimicronutrient supplementation for undernourished pregnant women and the birth size of their offspring. *Arch Pediatr Adolesc Med* 2007;161:58–64.

Hack M, Taylor HG, Drotar D, et al: Chronic conditions, functional limitations, and special health care needs of school-aged children born with extremely low birth weight in the 1990s. *JAMA* 2005;294:318–325.

Hack M, Wilson Costello D: Decrease in frequency of cerebral palsy in preterm infants. *Lancet* 2007;369:7–8.

Hessol NA, Fuentes-Afflick E: Ethnic differences in neonatal and postneonatal mortality. *Pediatrics* 2005;115:e44–e51.

Hofman PL, Regan F, Jackson WE, et al: Premature birth and later insulin resistance. *N Engl J Med* 2004;351:2179–2188.

Hollo O, Rautava P, Korhonen T, et al: Academic achievement of small for gestational age children at age 10 years. *Arch Pediatr Adolesc Med* 2002;156:179–187.

Johnston LB, Savage MO: Should recombinant human growth hormone therapy be used in short small for gestational age children? *Arch Dis Child* 2004;89:740–744.

Lawn JE, Cousens S, Zupan J, et al: 4 million neonatal deaths: When? Where? Why? *Lancet* 2005;365:891–900.

Lee SK, Zupancic JAF, Pendray M, et al: Transport risk index of physiologic stability: A practical system for assessing infant transport care. *J Pediatr* 2001;139:220–226.

Lorenz JM, Paneth N, Jetton JR, et al: Comparison of management strategies for extreme prematurity in New Jersey and the Netherlands: Outcomes and resource expenditure. *Pediatrics* 2001;108:1269–1274.

Marlow N, Wolke D, Bracewell MA, et al: Neurologic and developmental disability at six years of age after extremely preterm birth. *N Eng J Med* 2005;352:9–19.

McCormick MC, Behrman RE: The quiet epidemic of premature birth: commentary on a recent institute of medicine report. *Ambul Pediatr* 2007;7:8–9.

McGuire W, Henderson G, Fowlie PW: Feeding the preterm infant. *Br Med J* 2004;329:1227–1230.

McGuire W, McEwan P, Fowlie PW: Care in the early newborn period. *Br Med J* 2004;329:1087–1089.

Modi N: Management of fluid balance in the very immature neonate. *Arch Dis Child* 2004;89:F108–F111.

Platt MJ, Cans C, Johnson A, et al: Trends in cerebral palsy among infants of very low birthweight (<1500 g) or born prematurely (<32 weeks) in 16 European centres: a database study. *Lancet* 2007;369:43–50.

Ruiz-Pelaez JG, Charpak N, Cuervo LG: Kangaroo mother care, an example to follow from developing countries. *Br Med J* 2004;329:1179–1181.

Schanler RH, Shulman RJ and Lau C: Feeding strategies for premature infants: Beneficial outcomes of feeding fortified human milk versus preterm formula. *Pediatrics* 1999;103:1150–1157.

Sedin G: To avoid heat loss in very preterm infants. *J Pediatr* 2004;145:720–722.

Shankaran S, Johnson Y, Langer JC, et al: Outcome of extremely low birth weight infants at highest risk: Gestational age <24 weeks, birth weight <750 g, and 1 minute Apgar <3. *Am J Obstet Gynecol* 2004;191:1084–1091.

Strömberg B, Dahiquist G, Ericson A, et al: Neurological sequelae in children born after in-vitro fertilisation: A population-based study. *Lancet* 2002;359:461.

Tommiska V, Ostberg M, Fellman V: Parental stress in families of 2 year old extremely low birthweight infants. *Arch Dis Child Fetal Neonatal Ed* 2002;86:F161–F164.

Tucker J, McGuire W: Epidemiology of preterm birth. *Br Med J* 2004;329:675–678.

Walsh MC, Morris BH, Wrage LA, et al: Extremely low birthweight neonates with protracted ventilation mortality and 18-month neurodevelopmental outcomes. *J Pediatr* 2005;146:798–804.

Wilson-Costello D, Friedman H, Minich N, et al: Improved survival rates with increased neurodevelopmental disability for extremely low birth weight in infants in the 1990s. *Pediatrics* 2005;115:997–1003.

Chapter 98 ■ Clinical Manifestations of Diseases in the Newborn Period

Barbara J. Stoll

The wide variety of disorders that affect the newborn originate in utero, during birth, or in the immediate postnatal period. These disorders may represent genetic mutations, chromosomal aberrations, or acquired diseases and injuries. Recognizing disease in newborn infants depends on knowledge of the disorder and evaluation of a limited number of relatively nonspecific clinical signs and symptoms.

Central cyanosis has respiratory, cardiac, central nervous system (CNS), hematologic, and metabolic causes (Table 98-1).

TABLE 98-1. Differential Diagnosis of Cyanosis in the Newborn

Central or peripheral nervous system hypoventilation
Birth asphyxia
Intracranial hypertension, hemorrhage
Oversedation (direct or through maternal route)
Diaphragm palsy
Neuromuscular diseases
Seizures
Respiratory disease
Upper airway
Choanal atresia/stenosis
Pierre Robin syndrome
Intrinsic airway obstruction (laryngeal/bronchial/tracheal stenosis)
Extrinsic airway obstruction (bronchogenic cyst, duplication cyst, vascular compression)
Lower airway
Respiratory distress syndrome
Transient tachypnea
Meconium aspiration
Pneumonia (sepsis)
Pneumothorax
Congenital diaphragmatic hernia
Pulmonary hypoplasia
Cardiac right-to-left shunt
Abnormal connections (pulmonary blood flow normal or increased)
Transposition of great vessels
Total anomalous pulmonary venous return
Truncus arteriosus
Hypoplastic left heart syndrome
Single ventricle or tricuspid atresia with large ventricular septal defect but without pulmonic stenosis
Obstructed pulmonary blood flow (pulmonary blood flow decreased)
Pulmonic atresia with intact ventricular septum
Tetralogy of Fallot
Critical pulmonic stenosis with patent foramen ovale or atrial septal defect
Tricuspid atresia
Single ventricle with pulmonic stenosis
Ebstein malformation of the tricuspid valve
Persistent fetal circulation (persistent pulmonary hypertension of newborn)
Methemoglobinemia
Congenital (hemoglobin M, methemoglobin reductase deficiency)
Acquired (nitrates, nitrites)
Inadequate ambient O_2 or less O_2 delivered than expected (rare)
Disconnection of O_2 supply to nasal cannula, head hood
Connection of air, rather than O_2, to a mechanical ventilator
Spurious/artifactual
Oximeter artifact (poor contact between probe and skin, poor pulse searching)
Arterial blood gas artifact (contamination with venous blood)
Other
Hypoglycemia
Adrenogenital syndrome
Polycythemia
Blood loss

From Smith F: Cyanosis. In Kliegman: *Practical Strategies in Pediatric Diagnosis and Therapy*. Philadelphia, WB Saunders, 1996.

Respiratory insufficiency may be due to pulmonary conditions or may be secondary to CNS depression as a result of drugs, intracranial hemorrhage, or anoxia. If caused by the former, respirations tend to be rapid and may be accompanied by retraction of the thoracic cage. If it is due to the latter, respirations tend to be irregular and weak and are often slow. Cyanosis unaccompanied by obvious signs of respiratory difficulty suggests cyanotic congenital heart disease or methemoglobinemia. Cyanosis resulting from congenital heart disease may, however, be difficult to distinguish clinically from cyanosis caused by respiratory disease. Episodes of cyanosis may also be the initial sign of hypoglycemia, bacteremia, meningitis, shock, or pulmonary hypertension. Peripheral acrocyanosis is common and does not usually warrant concern.

Pallor, in addition to anemia or acute hemorrhage, should suggest hypoxia, asphyxia, hypoglycemia, sepsis, shock, or adrenal failure.

Hypotension in term infants suggests shock from hypovolemia (hemorrhage, dehydration), the systemic inflammatory response syndrome (bacterial sepsis, intrauterine infection), cardiac dysfunction (left heart obstructive lesions—hypoplastic left heart syndrome, myocarditis, asphyxia-induced myocardial stunning, anomalous coronary artery), pneumothorax, pneumopericardium, pericardial effusion, or metabolic disorders (hypoglycemia, adrenal insufficiency–salt-losing adrenogenital syndrome). Hypotension is a common problem in sick preterm infants and may be due to any of the problems noted in a term infant. It may develop in preterm infants with severe respiratory distress syndrome. Strategies used to support blood pressure include volume expansion (normal saline is equally as effective as 5% albumin), pressors (dopamine, dobutamine, epinephrine), and corticosteroids. Some infants weighing <1,000 g do not respond to fluids or inotropic agents but may respond to therapy with intravenous hydrocortisone. Sudden onset of hypotension in a very low birthweight infant suggests pneumothorax, intraventricular hemorrhage, or subcapsular hepatic hematoma.

Convulsions (see Chapter 593.7) usually point to a disorder of the CNS and suggest hypoxic-ischemic encephalopathy, intracranial hemorrhage, cerebral anomaly, subdural effusion, meningitis, hypocalcemia, hypoglycemia, cerebral infarction, benign familial seizures, and, rarely, pyridoxine dependence, hyponatremia, hypernatremia, inborn errors of metabolism, or drug withdrawal. Seizures beginning in the delivery room or shortly thereafter may be due to the unintentional injection of maternal local anesthetic into the fetus. Convulsions may also result from hyponatremia and water intoxication in the infant after the administration of large amounts of hypotonic fluid to the mother shortly before and during delivery.

Convulsions should be distinguished from the jitteriness that may be present in normal newborns, in infants of diabetic mothers, in those who experienced birth asphyxia or drug withdrawal, and in polycythemic neonates. Jitteriness resembling simple tremors may be stopped by holding the infant's extremity; it often depends on sensory stimuli and occurs when the infant is active, and it is not associated with abnormal eye movements. Tremors are often more rapid with a smaller amplitude than are tonic clonic seizures. Seizures in premature infants are often subtle and associated with abnormal eye (fluttering, deviation, stare) or facial (chewing, tongue thrusting) movements; the motor component is often that of tonic extension of the limbs, neck, and trunk. Term infants may have focal or multifocal, clonic or myoclonic movements, but they may also have more subtle seizure activity. Apnea may be the 1st manifestation of seizure activity, particularly in a premature infant. Seizures may adversely affect the subsequent neurodevelopmental outcome and even predispose to non-neonatal seizures. Seizures should be treated aggressively.

After severe birth asphyxia, infants may have **motor automatisms** characterized by oral-buccal-lingual movements, rotary limb activities (rowing, pedaling, swimming), tonic posturing, or myoclonus. These motor activities are not usually accompanied by time-synchronized electroencephalographic discharges, may not signify cortical epileptic activity, respond poorly to anticonvulsant therapy, and are associated with a poor prognosis. Such automatisms may represent cortical depression that produces a brainstem release phenomenon or subcortical seizures.

Lethargy may be a manifestation of infection, asphyxia, hypoglycemia, hypercapnia, sedation from maternal analgesia or anesthesia, a cerebral defect, and, indeed, almost any severe disease, including inborn errors of metabolism. Lethargy appearing after the 2nd day should, in particular, suggest infection. Lethargy with emesis suggests increased intracranial pressure or an inborn error of metabolism.

Irritability may be a sign of discomfort accompanying intra-abdominal conditions, meningeal irritation, drug withdrawal, infections, congenital glaucoma, or any condition producing pain. As in later infancy, the eardrums should always be examined as a possible source of pain. Hyperactivity, especially in a premature infant, may be a sign of hypoxia, pneumothorax, emphysema, hypoglycemia, hypocalcemia, CNS damage, drug withdrawal, neonatal thyrotoxicosis, bronchospasm, esophageal reflux, or discomfort from a cold environment.

Failure to feed well is seen in most sick newborn infants and should always occasion a careful search for infection, a central or peripheral nervous system disorder, intestinal obstruction, and other abnormal conditions.

Fever may be the result of too high an environmental temperature because of weather, overheated nurseries or isolettes/radiant warmers, or too many clothes. It is also noted in "dehydration fever" of newborn infants. If these causes of fever can be eliminated, serious infection (pneumonia, bacteremia, meningitis, and viral infections, particularly herpes simplex or enteroviruses) must be considered, although such infections often occur without provoking a febrile response in newborn infants (see Chapters 174 and 175). An unexplained fall in body temperature may accompany infection or other serious disturbances of the circulation or CNS. A sudden servo-controlled increase in isolette ambient temperature to maintain body temperature is a sign of temperature instability and may be associated with sepsis.

Periods of **apnea**, particularly in premature infants, may be associated with various disturbances (see Chapter 101.2). When apnea recurs or when the intervals are longer than 20 sec or are associated with cyanosis or bradycardia, an immediate diagnostic evaluation is needed.

Jaundice during the 1st 24 hr of life warrants diagnostic evaluation and should be considered to be due to hemolysis until proved otherwise. Septicemia and intrauterine infections such as syphilis, cytomegalovirus, and toxoplasmosis should also be considered, especially in infants with an increase in plasma direct-reacting bilirubin.

Jaundice after the 1st 24 hr may be "physiologic" or may be due to septicemia, hemolytic anemia, galactosemia, hepatitis, congenital atresia of the bile ducts, inspissated bile syndrome after erythroblastosis fetalis, syphilis, herpes simplex, or other congenital infections (see Chapter 102.3).

Vomiting during the 1st day of life suggests obstruction in the upper digestive tract or increased intracranial pressure. Roentgenographic studies are indicated when obstruction is suspected. Vomiting may also be a nonspecific symptom of an illness such as septicemia. It is a common manifestation of overfeeding or inexperienced feeding technique, pyloric stenosis, milk allergy, duodenal ulcer, stress ulcer, inborn errors of metabolism (hyperammonemia, metabolic acidosis), or adrenal insufficiency. Vomitus containing dark blood is usually a sign of a serious illness; the benign possibility of swallowed maternal blood should also be considered. Bile-stained vomitus strongly suggests obstruction below the ampulla of Vater and warrants contrast radiography.

Diarrhea may be a symptom of overfeeding (especially high–caloric density formula), acute gastroenteritis, or malabsorption, or it may be a nonspecific symptom of infection. Diarrhea may occur in conditions accompanied by compromised circulation of part of the intestinal or genital tract, such as mesenteric thrombosis, necrotizing enterocolitis, strangulated hernia, intussusception, and torsion of the ovary or testis.

Abdominal distention, usually a sign of intestinal obstruction or an intra-abdominal mass, may also be seen in infants with enteritis, necrotizing enterocolitis, isolated intestinal perforation, ileus accompanying sepsis, respiratory distress, ascites, or hypokalemia.

Failure to move an extremity (**pseudoparalysis**) suggests fracture, dislocation, or nerve injury. It is also seen in osteomyelitis and other infections that cause pain on movement of the affected part.

Pain in neonates may be unrecognized and/or undertreated. The intensive care of neonates may involve a number of painful procedures, including blood sampling, (heel stick, venous or arterial puncture), endotracheal intubation and suctioning, mechanical ventilation, and insertion of chest tubes and intravascular catheters. Pain in neonates results in obvious distress and acute physiologic stress responses, which may have developmental implications for pain in later life. Moreover, the knowledge that infants may experience pain contributes to the stress of parents of sick newborns.

Pain and discomfort are potentially avoidable problems during the treatment of sick infants. Preemptive relief from painful stimuli should be provided before pain or anxiety develops. The most frequently used drugs are intermittent or continuous doses of opioids (morphine, fentanyl) or benzodiazepines (midazolam, lorazepam). Although the long-term effects of opioids and sedatives are not well established, the 1st concern should be the treatment and/or prevention of acute pain. Continuous opiate infusions should be used with caution. Some minor but painful procedures on well neonates have also been managed with oral sucrose solutions, although the optimal dose is undetermined (Table 98-2).

CONGENITAL ANOMALIES

Congenital anomalies are a major cause of stillbirths and neonatal deaths, but they are perhaps even more important as causes of acute illness and long-term morbidity. Anomalies are discussed in general in Chapters 81 and 108 and specifically in the chapters on the various systems of the body. Early recognition of anomalies is important for planning care; with some, such as tracheoesophageal fistula, diaphragmatic hernia, choanal atresia, and intestinal obstruction, immediate medical and surgical therapy is essential for survival (Table 98-3). Parents are likely to feel anxious and guilty on learning of the existence of a congenital anomaly and require sensitive counseling.

TABLE 98-2. Pain in the Neonate: General Considerations

- Pain in newborns is often unrecognized and/or undertreated.
- If a procedure is painful in adults, it should be considered painful in newborns.
- Health care institutions should develop and implement patient care policies to assess, prevent, and manage pain in neonates.
- Pharmacologic agents with known pharmacokinetic and pharmacodynamic properties and demonstrated efficacy in neonates should be used. Agents known to compromise cardiorespiratory function should be administered only by persons experienced in neonatal airway management and in settings with the capacity for continuous monitoring.
- Educational programs to increase the skills of health care professionals in the assessment and management of stress and pain in neonates should be provided.
- Further research is needed to develop and validate neonatal pain assessment tools that are useful in the clinical setting; to determine optimal behavioral and pharmacologic interventions; and to study long-term effects of pain and pain management

Adapted from Anonymous: Prevention and management of pain and stress in the neonate. *Pediatrics* 2000;105:454–461; and Anand KJS, International Evidence-Based Group for Neonatal Pain: Consensus statement for the prevention and management of pain in the newborn. *Arch Pediatr Adolesc Med* 2001;155:173–180.

TABLE 98-3. Common Life-Threatening Congenital Anomalies

NAME	MANIFESTATIONS
Choanal atresia	Respiratory distress in delivery room, apnea, unable to pass nasogastric tube through nares. Suspect CHARGE syndrome
Pierre Robin syndrome	Micrognathia, cleft palate, airway obstruction
Diaphragmatic hernia	Scaphoid abdomen, bowel sounds present in chest, respiratory distress
Tracheoesophageal fistula	Polyhydramnios, aspiration pneumonia, excessive salivation, unable to place nasogastric tube in stomach. Suspect VATER syndrome
Intestinal obstruction: volvulus, duodenal atresia, ileal atresia	Polyhydramnios, bile-stained emesis, abdominal distention. Suspect trisomy 21, cystic fibrosis, cocaine
Gastroschisis, omphalocele	Polyhydramnios, intestinal obstruction
Renal agenesis, Potter syndrome	Oligohydramnios, anuria, pulmonary hypoplasia, pneumothorax
Neural tube defects: anencephalus, meningomyelocele	Polyhydramnios, elevated α-fetoprotein, decreased fetal activity
Ductal-dependent congenital heart disease	Cyanosis, hypotension, murmur

CHARGE, coloboma of the eye, heart anomaly, choanal atresia, retardation, and genital and ear anomalies; VATER, vertebral defects, imperforate anus, tracheoesophageal fistula, and radial and renal dysplasia.

American Academy of Pediatrics Committee on Fetus and Newborn and Section on Surgery, Canadian Paediatric Society Fetus and Newborn Committee: Prevention and management of pain in the neonate: an update. *Pediatrics* 2006;223:2231–2241.

Anand KJS, International Evidence-Based Group for Neonatal Pain: Consensus statement for the prevention and management of pain in the newborn. *Arch Pediatr Adolesc Med* 2001;155:173–180.

Brady-Fryer B, Wiebe N, Lander JA: Pain relief for neonatal circumcision. *Cochrane Database Syst Rev* 2005;2:1.

Brunquell PJ, Glennon CM, DiMario FJ, et al: Prediction of outcome based on clinical seizure type in newborn infants. *J Pediatr* 2002;140:707–712.

Derbyshire SWG: Can fetuses feel pain? *BMJ* 2006;332:909–912.

Franck LS, Allen A, Cox S, Winter I: Parents' view about infant pain in neonatal intensive care. *Clin J Pain* 2005;21:133–139.

Levene M: The clinical conundrum of neonatal seizures. *Arch Child Dis Fetal Neonatal Ed* 2002;86:F75–F77.

Ng PC, Lee CH, Lam CWK, et al: Transient adrenocortical insufficiency of prematurity and systemic hypotension in very low birthweight infants. *Arch Dis Child* 2004;89:F119–126.

Pignotti MS, Indolfi G, Ciuti R, Donzelli G: Perinatal asphyxia and inadvertent neonatal intoxication from local anesthetics given to the mother during labour. *Br Med J* 2005;330:34–35.

Seri I, Evans J: Controversies in the diagnosis and management of hypotension in the newborn infant. *Curr Opin Pediatr* 2001;13:116–123.

Simons SHP, van Dijk M, van Longen RA, et al: Routine morphine infusion in preterm newborns who received ventilatory support. *JAMA* 2003; 290:2419–2427.

Stevens B, Yamada J, Ohlsson A: Sucrose for analgesia in newborn infants undergoing painful procedures. *Cochrane Database Syst Rev* 2005;2:1.

Taddio A, Lee C, Yip A, et al: Intravenous morphine and topical tetracaine for treatment of pain in preterm neonates undergoing central line placement. *JAMA* 2006;295:793–800.

Chapter 99 ■ Nervous System Disorders

Ira Adams-Chapman and Barbara J. Stoll

Central nervous system (CNS) disorders are important causes of neonatal mortality and both short- and long-term morbidity. The

CNS can be damaged as a result of hypoxia, asphyxia, hemorrhage, trauma, hypoglycemia, or direct cytotoxicity. The etiology of CNS damage is often multifactorial and includes acute perinatal complications, postnatal hemodynamic instability and developmental abnormalities that may be genetic and/or environmental. Predisposing factors for brain injury include chronic and acute maternal illness resulting in uteroplacental dysfunction, intrauterine infection, macrosomia/dystocia, malpresentation, prematurity, and intrauterine growth restriction. Acute and often unavoidable emergencies during the delivery process frequently result in mechanical and/or hypoxic ischemic brain injury.

99.1 • The Cranium

Erythema, abrasions, ecchymoses, and subcutaneous fat necrosis of facial or scalp soft tissues may be noted after forceps or vacuum-assisted deliveries. Their location depends on the area of application of the forceps. Ecchymoses may be seen after manipulative deliveries and occasionally in premature infants for no discernible reason. Traumatic hemorrhage may involve any layer of the scalp, as well as intracranial contents (Fig. 99-1).

Subconjunctival and **retinal hemorrhages** are frequent; petechiae of the skin of the head and neck are also common. All are probably secondary to a sudden increase in intrathoracic pressure during passage of the chest through the birth canal. Parents should be assured that these hemorrhages are temporary and the result of normal events of delivery. They resolve rapidly within the 1st 2 wk of life.

Caput succedaneum is a diffuse, sometimes ecchymotic, edematous swelling of the soft tissues of the scalp involving the area presenting during vertex delivery (see Fig. 99-1). It may extend across the midline and across suture lines. The edema disappears within the 1st few days of life. Molding of the head and overriding of the parietal bones are frequently associated with caput succedaneum and become more evident after the caput has receded; they disappear during the 1st weeks of life. Rarely, a hemorrhagic caput may result in shock and require blood transfusion. Analogous swelling, discoloration, and distortion of the face are seen in face presentations. No specific treatment is needed, but if extensive ecchymoses are present, hyperbilirubinemia may develop.

Cephalohematoma (Fig. 99-2) is a subperiosteal hemorrhage, hence always limited to the surface of one cranial bone. Cephalohematomas occur in 1–2% of live births. No discoloration of the overlying scalp occurs, and swelling is not usually visible for several hours after birth because subperiosteal bleeding is a slow process. The lesion becomes a firm tense mass with a palpable rim localized over 1 area of the skull. Most cephalohematomas are resorbed within 2 wk–3 mo, depending on their size. They may begin to calcify by the end of the 2nd week. A few remain for years as bony protuberances and are detectable by x-ray as widening of the diploic space; cystlike defects may persist for months or years. An underlying skull fracture, usually linear and not depressed, may be associated with 10–25% of cases. A sensation of central depression suggesting but not indicative of an underlying fracture or bony defect is usually encountered on palpation of the organized rim of a cephalohematoma. Cephalohematomas require no treatment, although phototherapy may be necessary to treat hyperbilirubinemia.

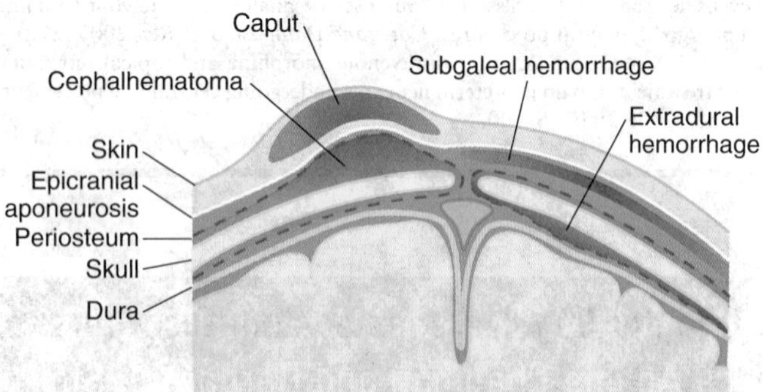

Figure 99-1. Sites of extracranial (and extradural) hemorrhages in the newborn. Schematic diagram of important tissue planes from skin to dura. From Volpe JJ: *Neurology of the Newborn,* 4th ed. Philadelphia, WB Saunders, 2001.)

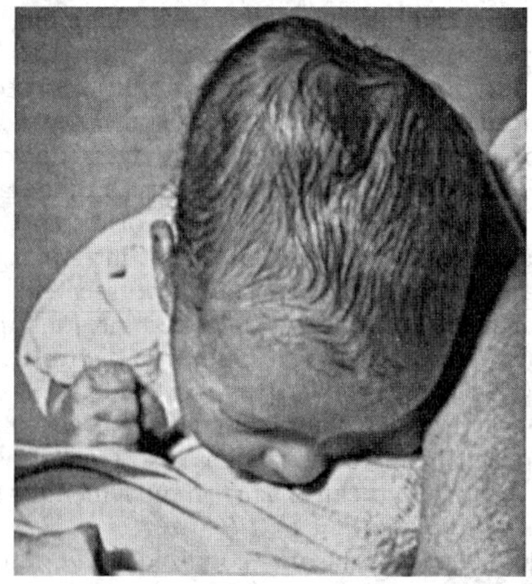

Figure 99-2. Cephalohematoma of the right parietal bone.

A **subgaleal hemorrhage** is a collection of blood beneath the aponeurosis that covers the scalp the entire length of the occipital-frontalis muscle. Bleeding can be very extensive into this large potential space and even dissect into the subcutaneous tissues of the neck. There is often an association with vacuum-assisted delivery. The mechanism of injury is most likely secondary to a linear skull fracture, suture diastasis or fragmentation of the superior margin of the parietal bone, and/or rupture of the emissary vein. Extensive subgaleal bleeding is occasionally secondary to a hereditary coagulopathy (hemophilia). A subgaleal hemorrhage presents as a firm fluctuant mass, which increases in size after birth. Many patients develop a consumptive coagulopathy due to massive blood loss. Patients should be monitored for hypotension and the development of hyperbilirubinemia. These lesions typically resolve over a 2–3 week period.

Fractures of the skull may occur as a result of pressure from forceps or from the maternal symphysis pubis, sacral promontory, or ischial spines. Linear fractures, the most common, cause no symptoms and require no treatment. Depressed fractures are usually indentations of the calvaria similar to a dent in a ping-pong ball; they are generally a complication of forceps delivery or fetal compression. Affected infants may be asymptomatic unless they have associated intracranial injury; it is advisable to elevate severe depressions to prevent cortical injury from sustained pressure. Fracture of the occipital bone with separation of the basal and squamous portions almost invariably causes fatal hemorrhage because of disruption of the underlying vascular sinuses. Such fractures may result during breech deliveries from traction on the hyperextended spine of the infant with the head fixed in the maternal pelvis.

99.2 • Traumatic, Epidural, Subdural, and Subarachnoid Hemorrhage

Traumatic epidural, subdural, or subarachnoid hemorrhage is especially likely when the fetal head is large in proportion to the size of the mother's pelvic outlet, with prolonged labor, in breech or precipitous deliveries, or as a result of mechanical assistance with delivery. Massive subdural hemorrhage, often associated with tears in the tentorium cerebelli or, less frequently, in the falx cerebri, is rare but is encountered more often in full-term than in premature infants. Patients with massive hemorrhage caused by tears of the tentorium or falx cerebri rapidly deteriorate and may die after birth. The majority of subdural and epidural hemorrhages resolve without intervention; consultation with a neurosurgeon is recommended. The diagnosis of subdural hemorrhage may be delayed until the chronic subdural fluid volume expands and produces megalocephaly, frontal bossing, a bulging fontanel, anemia, and sometimes seizures. CT scan and MRI are useful imaging techniques to confirm these diagnoses. Symptomatic subdural hemorrhage in large term infants should be treated by removing the subdural fluid collection with a spinal needle placed through the lateral margin of the anterior fontanelle. In addition to birth trauma, child abuse must be suspected in all infants with subdural effusion outside of the immediate neonatal period.

Subarachnoid hemorrhage (SAH) is rare and typically clinically silent. The anastomoses between the penetrating leptomeningeal arteries or the bridging veins are the most likely source of the bleeding. The majority of affected infants have no clinical symptoms, but the SAH may be detected due to an elevated number of red blood cells on a lumbar puncture sample. Some infants develop benign seizures, which tend to occur on the 2nd day of life. Rarely, an infant has a life-threatening catastrophic hemorrhage and dies. There are usually no neurologic abnormalities during the acute episode or on follow-up. Significant neurologic findings should suggest an arteriovenous malformation. This lesion can easily be detected by CT or MRI; ultrasonography is a less sensitive tool.

99.3 • Intracranial-Intraventricular Hemorrhage and Periventricular Leukomalacia

ETIOLOGY. Intracranial hemorrhage may result from trauma or asphyxia and, rarely, from a primary hemorrhagic disturbance or congenital vascular anomaly. Primary hemorrhagic disturbances and vascular malformations are rare and usually give rise to subarachnoid or intracerebral hemorrhage. In utero hemorrhage associated with maternal idiopathic or, more often, fetal alloimmune thrombocytopenia may occur as severe cerebral hemorrhage or a porencephalic cyst after resolution of a fetal cortical hemorrhage. Intracranial bleeding may be associated with disseminated intravascular coagulopathy, isoimmune thrombocytopenia, and neonatal vitamin K deficiency, especially in infants born to mothers receiving phenobarbital or phenytoin. Intracranial hemorrhage often involves the ventricles (intraventricular hemorrhage [IVH]) of premature infants delivered spontaneously without apparent trauma.

EPIDEMIOLOGY. The overall incidence of IVH has decreased over the past decade secondary to improved perinatal care and increased use of antenatal corticosteroids; however, it continues to be a significant cause of morbidity in preterm infants. Approximately 30% of premature infants <1,500 g will have an IVH. The risk is inversely related to gestational age and birthweight, with the smallest and most immature infants being at the highest risk. In LBW infants, 5% of infants 1,250–1,500 g will have a severe IVH (grade III or IV) compared to 11.4% of infants <1,000 g. Sixty to 70% of infants 500–750 g will develop an IVH. The overall incidence for severe cranial ultrasound abnormalities (IVH, periventricular leukomalacia [PVL]) among preterm infants <1,000 g is 22%; the incidence of PVL has increased from 2% to 7% over a 15 yr period.

PATHOGENESIS. The major neuropathologic lesions associated with VLBW infants are IVH and PVL. IVH in premature infants occurs in the gelatinous subependymal germinal matrix. This periventricular area is the site of orgin for embryonal neurons and fetal glial cells, which migrate outwardly to the cortex. Immature blood vessels in this highly vascular region of the brain combined with poor tissue vascular support predispose premature infants to hemorrhage. The germinal matrix involutes as the infant approaches full term gestation and the tissue's vascular integrity improves, therefore IVH is much less common in the term infant. **Periventricular hemorrhagic infarction** (grade IV hemorrhage) often develops after a severe IVH due to venous congestion. Predisposing factors for IVH include prematurity, respiratory distress syndrome, hypoxic-ischemic or hypotensive injury, reperfusion injury of damaged vessels, increased or decreased cerebral blood flow, reduced vascular integrity, increased venous pressure, pneumothorax, hypervolemia, and hypertension.

Understanding of the pathogenesis of PVL is evolving and it appears to involve both intrauterine and postnatal events. A complex interaction exists between the development of the cerebral vasculature and regulation of cerebral blood flow (both gestational-age dependent), disturbances in the oligodendrocyte precursors required for myelination, and maternal/fetal infection and/or inflammation. Similar factors (hypoxia-ischemia), venous obstruction from an IVH, or undetected fetal stress may result in decreased perfusion to the brain leading, in turn, to periventricular hemorrhage and necrosis. PVL is characterized by focal necrotic lesions in the periventricular white matter and/or more diffuse white matter damage. The risk for PVL increases in infants with severe IVH and/or ventriculomegaly. The corticospinal tracts descend through the periventricular white matter, hence the association between cerebral white matter injury/PVL and motor abnormalities, including cerebral palsy. The possible interaction of various factors in the pathogenesis of white matter damage is shown in Figure 99-3.

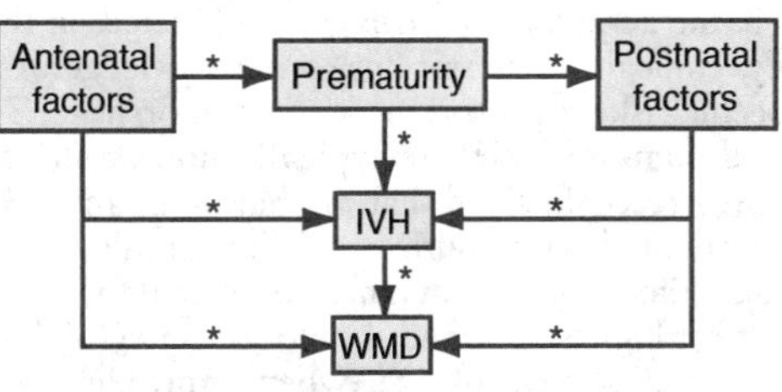

The * represents places in this scheme where factors may diminish or promote the likelihood of developing WMD.

Possible Promoters of WMD Occurrence
Fetal growth restriction
Hypothyroxinemia
Hypocarbia/hypercarbia
Fetal vasculitis
Maternal/placental infection
Other cytokine-promoting factors

Possible Protectors Against WMD Occurrence
Antenatal corticosteroids
Prostaglandin inhibitors
Toxemia/magnesium

Figure 99-3. Schematic of possible associations linking prematurity, intraventricular hemorrhage (IVH), and white matter disorder (WMD). Antenatal factors may represent factors that both lead to prematurity and act as an independent marker of risk for IVH and WMD. Factors that occur as a result of or in association with prematurity may, in turn, modify the likelihood of having IVH or WMD. IVH in its own right may contribute to WMD. (From Kuban K, Sanochka U, Leviton A, et al: White matter disorders of prematurity: Association with intraventricular hemorrhage and ventriculomegaly. The Developmental Epidemiology Network. *J Pediatr* 1999:134:539–546.)

CLINICAL MANIFESTATIONS. The majority of patients with IVH have no clinical symptoms, including some with moderate to severe hemorrhages. Some premature infants who develop a severe IVH may have an acute deterioration on the 2nd or 3rd day of life. Periods of apnea, pallor, or cyanosis; poor suck; abnormal eye signs; a high-pitched, shrill cry; muscular twitching, convulsions, or decreased muscle tone; metabolic acidosis; shock; and a decreased hematocrit or failure of the hematocrit to increase after transfusion may be the 1st clinical indications. IVH is rarely present at birth; 50% occur within the 1st day of life and up to 75% within the 1st 3 days of life. A small percentage of infants will have a late hemorrhage between days 14 and 30. The more immature infants tend to hemorrhage earlier in the course as compared to larger, more mature preterm infants. IVH is rare after the 1st month of life as a primary event.

PVL is usually clinically asymptomatic until the neurologic sequelae of white matter damage become apparent in later infancy as spastic motor deficits. PVL may be present at birth but usually occurs later as an early echodense phase (3–10 days of life), followed by the typical echolucent (cystic) phase (14–20 days of life).

The severity of hemorrhage may be defined by the location and degree of ventricular dilatation from CT scans. **Grade I** hemorrhage represents bleeding isolated to the subependymal area. **Grade II** hemorrhage represents bleeding within the ventricle but without evidence of ventricular dilatation. **Grade III** hemorrhage represents intraventricular hemorrhage with ventricular dilatation. **Grade IV** hemorrhage represents intraventricular and parenchymal hemorrhage. Another grading system describes 3 levels of increasing severity of IVH detected by ultrasound: **Grade I** is bleeding confined to the germinal matrix–subependymal region or to <10% of the ventricle (≈35% of IVH cases), **grade II** is intraventricular bleeding with 10–50% filling of the ventricle (≈40% of IVH cases), and **grade III** is more than 50% involvement with dilated ventricles (Fig. 99-4). **Ventriculomegaly** is defined as mild (0.5–1 cm), moderate (1.0–1.5 cm), or severe (>1.5 cm).

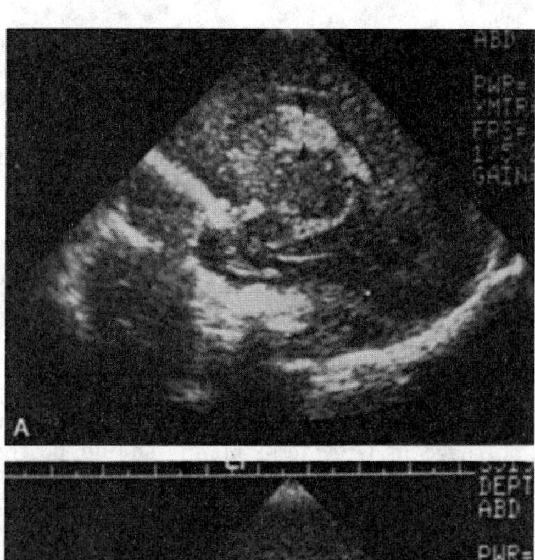

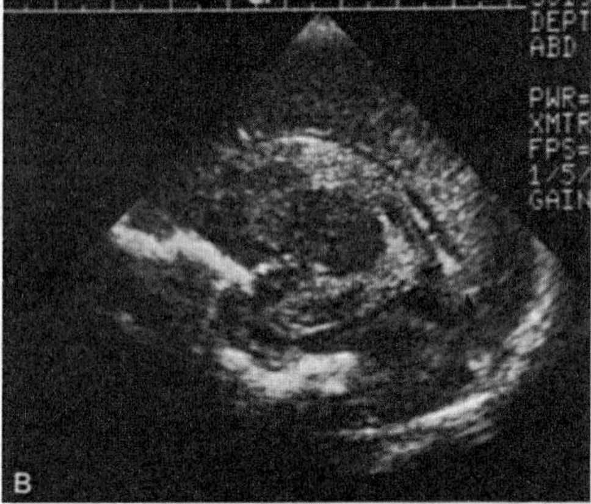

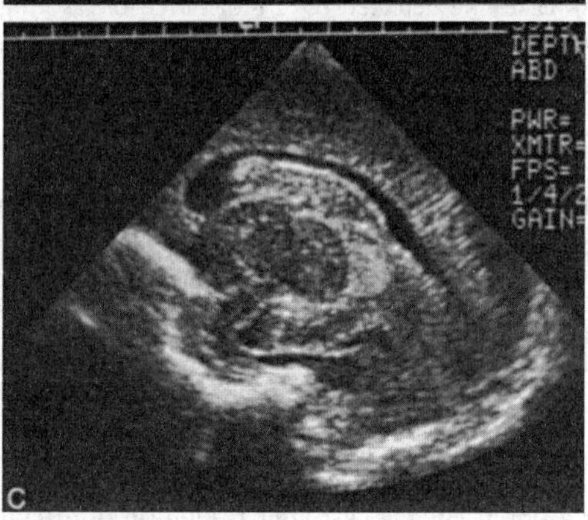

Figure 99-4. Grading the severity of germinal matrix intraventricular hemorrhage with parasagittal ultrasound scans. *A,* Grade I. Note the echogenic blood in the germinal matrix *(arrowheads)* just anterior to the anterior tip of the choroid plexus, which (normally) is also echogenic. *B,* Grade II. Note the echogenic blood *(arrowheads)* filling <50% of the ventricular area. *C,* Grade III. Note the large blood clot nearly completely filling and distending the entire lateral ventrical. (From Intracranial hemorrhage: Germinal matrix-intraventricular hemorrhage of the premature infant. In Volpe JJ: *Neurology of the Newborn,* 4th ed. Philadelphia, WB Saunders, 2001.)

DIAGNOSIS. Intracranial hemorrhage is suspected on the basis of the history, clinical manifestations, and knowledge of the birth-weight-specific risks for intraventricular hemorrhage. The associated clinical signs of IVH are typically nonspecific or absent; therefore, it is recommended that premature infants <34 wk gestation be evaluated with routine real-time cranial ultrasonography through the anterior fontanel to screen for IVH. Infants <1,000 g are at highest risk and should have a cranial ultrasound within the 1st 3–5 days of age, when approximately 75% of lesions will be detectable. Ultrasound is the preferred imaging technique for screening because it is noninvasive, portable, reproducible and sensitive and specific for detection of IVH. Infants weighing 1,001–1,500 g should be examined within the 1st 7–14 days of life. All at-risk infants should have a follow-up ultrasound performed at 36–40 wk postmenstrual age to evaluate adequately for PVL, because cystic changes related to perinatal injury may not be visible for at least 2-4 wk. Twenty-nine per cent of LBW infants who later developed cerebral palsy did not have radiographic evidence of PVL until after 28 days. Ultrasound examination also detects the precystic and cystic symmetric lesions of PVL and the asymmetric intraparenchymal echogenic lesions of cortical hemorrhagic infarction. Furthermore, the delayed development of cortical atrophy, porencephaly, and the severity, progression, or regression of posthemorrhagic hydrocephalus can be determined by serial ultrasonography.

Approximately 3–5% of VLBW infants will develop posthemorrhagic hydrocephalus and require ventriculoperitoneal shunt insertion; if the initial scan is abnormal, additional interval ultrasonographic studies are indicated to monitor for the development of hydrocephalus.

IVH represents only one facet of brain injury in the term or preterm infant. MRI is a more sensitive tool for evaluation of extensive periventricular injury and may be more predictive for adverse long-term outcome. CT or diffusion-weighted MRI is indicated for term infants in whom brain injury is suspected because ultrasound may not reveal edema or intraparenchymal hemorrhage and infarction.

PROGNOSIS. The majority of infants with grade I or II IVH have normal neurodevelopmental outcome; however, up to 30% of infants with birth weight <1,000 g with normal cranial ultrasounds have CP or low cognitive performance at 18 mo adjusted age. Severe IVH (grade III or IV), progressive hydrocephalus requiring ventricular-peritoneal shunting, intraparenchymal hem-

TABLE 99-1. Developmental Outcome at 18–22 Months Adjusted Age in VLBW Infants with Posthemorrhagic Hydrocephalus Requiring Shunt Insertion

	MDI SCORE		PDI SCORE	
GROUP	MEAN ± S.E.	MEDIAN	MEAN ± S.E.	MEDIAN
No IVH/no shunt	80.7 ± 0.3	82	84.9 ± 0.3	87
IVH 3-4/no shunt	74.1 ± 0.6	75	76.3 ± 0.7	81
IVH 3-4/shunt	63.3 ± 1.2	55	59.8 ± 1.1	49

Adams-Chapman, et al. *NICHD Neonatal Research Network*.

orrhage, and extensive PVL are each independently associated with a poor prognosis (cerebral palsy and abnormal psychomotor, or cognitive outcome). IVH with intraparenchymal echodensities larger than 1 cm are associated with high mortality and a high incidence of motor and cognitive deficits. Severe IVH (grade III or IV) and PVL occur in approximately 18% of infants <1,000 g and are associated with cerebral palsy and adverse neurodevelopmental and functional outcomes. The highest risk group (<24 wk gestation, <750 g, and 1-min Apgar <3) has a 32% incidence of severe IVH and 9% incidence of PVL. These infants are at the highest risk for death or cerebral palsy. Infants with parenchymal lesions or ventricular enlargement have a high risk of mental retardation at 6 yr follow-up.

Most infants with IVH and acute ventricular distention do not develop **posthemorrhagic hydrocephalus (PHH)**. Ten to 15% of LBW neonates with IVH develop hydrocephalus, which may initially be present without clinical signs such as an enlarging head circumference, apnea, bradycardia, lethargy, a bulging fontanel, or widely split sutures. In infants in whom symptomatic hydrocephalus develops, clinical signs may be delayed 2–4 wk despite progressive ventricular distention with compression and thinning of the cerebral cortex. The majority of infants with PHH have spontaneous regression; 3–5% of VLBW infants with PHH will require shunt insertion. Infants <1,000 g with PHH requiring shunt insertion have lower cognitive and psychomotor performance at 18–22 mo (Table 99-1).

PREVENTION. Improved perinatal care is imperative to minimize traumatic brain injury and decrease the risk of preterm delivery. The incidence of traumatic intracranial hemorrhage may be reduced by judicious management of cephalopelvic disproportion and operative (forceps, vacuum) delivery. Fetal or neonatal hemorrhage caused by maternal idiopathic thrombocytopenic purpura or alloimmune thrombocytopenia may be reduced by maternal treatment with steroids, intravenous immunoglobulin, or fetal platelet transfusion and cesarean section. Intravenous vitamin K should be given before delivery to all women receiving phenobarbital or phenytoin during the pregnancy. Tenacious care of the LBW infants' respiratory status and fluid and electrolyte management including avoiding acidosis, hypocarbia, hypoxia, hypotension, wide fluctuations in neonatal blood pressure, and pneumothorax are important factors that may impact the risk for development of IVH and PVL.

A single course of antenatal corticosteroids is recommended in pregnancies 24–34 wk gestation at risk for preterm delivery. Antenatal steroids decrease the risk of death, grade III and IV IVH (betamethasone and dexamethasone), and PVL (betamethasone only). The safety plus efficacy of multiple courses of antenatal steroids is unknown.

The prophylactic administration of low-dose indomethacin (0.1 mg/kg/day for 3 days) to VLBW preterm infants reduces the incidence of severe IVH but does not improve the overall long-term developmental outcome. Indomethacin can transiently decrease cerebral blood flow and potentially put the infant at higher risk for cerebral ischemia. The frequency of indomethacin use in the LBW population varies throughout the country.

TREATMENT. Although no treatment is available for IVH, it may be associated with other complications that require therapy. Seizures are aggressively treated with anticonvulsant drugs. Anemia and coagulopathy require transfusion with packed red blood cells or fresh frozen plasma. Shock and acidosis is treated by the judicious and slow administration of sodium bicarbonate and fluid resuscitation.

Insertion of a VP shunt is the preferred method to treat progressive and symptomatic posthemorrhagic hydrocephalus; some infants require a temporary cerebrospinal fluid diversion before a permanent shunt can be safety inserted. Diuretics and acetazolamide are not effective. Serial lumbar punctures, ventricular taps, reservoirs, and externalized ventricular drains are potential temporizing interventions; they have an associated risk of infection and of "puncture porencephaly" due to injury to the surrounding parenchyma. A ventriculosubgaleal shunt inserted from the ventricle into a surgically created subgaleal pocket provides a closed system for constant ventricular decompression without these additional risk factors. Decompression is regulated by the pressure gradient between the ventricle and the subgaleal pocket.

99.4 • Brain Injury from Inflammation, Infection, and Medications

Severe IVH and PVL are the most commonly associated risk factors for adverse outcome in the VLBW infant. Other factors are also involved in the etiology of perinatal brain injury. Cytokines and pre- or postnatal infections or inflammation may contribute to brain injury. A systemic inflammatory response syndrome in the mother, fetus, or infant may induce the production of various inflammatory mediators that are directly cytotoxic or cause decreased CNS perfusion (Fig. 99-5). Preterm infants with evidence (often subclinical) of intrauterine or postnatal infection or maternal chorioamnionitis are more likely than uninfected infants to have adverse neurodevelopmental outcome, cerebral palsy, and delayed growth.

In utero infections may involve the developing central nervous system and directly impair cell growth or produce cell neurosis, resulting in microcephaly, developmental delay, mental retardation, or cerebral palsy. These specific congenital or perinatal acquired infections include those due to cytomegalovirus (Chapter 252), toxoplasmosis (Chapter 287), herpes simplex

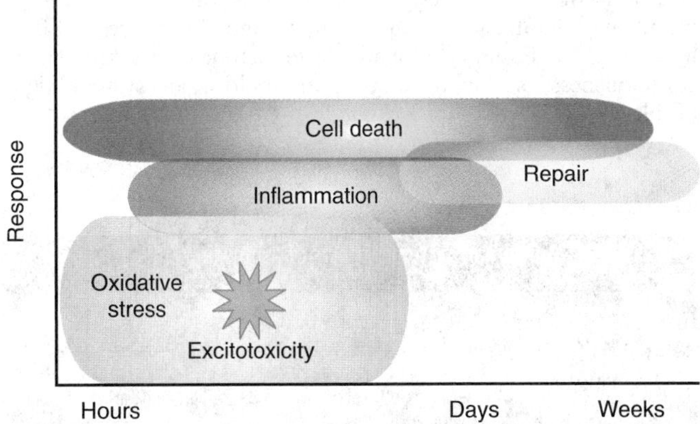

Figure 99-5. Mechanisms of brain injury in the term neonate. Oxidative stress and excitotoxicity, through downstream intracellular signaling, produce both inflammation and repair. Cell death begins immediately and continues during a period of days to weeks. The cell-death phenotype changes from an early necrotic morphology to a pathology resembling apoptosis. This evolution is called the necrosis–apoptosis continuum. (From Ferriero DM: Neonatal brain injury. *N Engl J Med* 2004;351:1985–1995. Copyright © 2004 Massachusetts Medical Society. All rights reserved.)

(Chapter 249), syphilis (Chapter 215), rubella (Chapter 244), and human immunodeficiency virus (Chapter 273). Postnatal acquired bacterial meningitis in the 1st year, but even more so in the 1st month of life, is another major risk factor for CNS injury and associated adverse neurodevelopmental outcome (Chapters 109.5, 602).

Long-term adverse neurodevelopmental outcomes are also associated with postnatal corticosteroid use in VLBW infants. Early postnatal exposure to dexamethasone within the 1st wk of life is associated with metabolic derangements, poor growth, increased risk for sepsis, and an increased risk of spontaneous bowel perforation. Infants exposed to postnatal steroids after the 1st wk of life have an increased risk of cerebral palsy and developmental delay. The risk may be increased with prolonged steroid use (>6 wk). At 8 yrs of age, dexamethasone-treated children are smaller, have smaller head circumferences, poorer motor skills and coordination, more difficulty with visual motor integration, and lower full scale verbal IQ and performance IQ scores. The AAP recommends that postnatal corticosteroid use in VLBW infants should be limited to exceptional clinical circumstances and the parents should be informed of the potential adverse side effects, including increased risk for developmental delay, cerebral palsy, and impaired growth.

Necrotizing enterocolitis (NEC) affects approximately 9–14% of LBW infants and is associated with significant morbidity and mortality (Chapter 102.2). Patients with NEC requiring surgery are more likely to have MDI <70, PDI <70, and evidence of overall neurodevelopmental impairment. Infants with severe NEC are reported to have a higher incidence of PVL, postnatal infections, and poor growth.

99.5 • Hypoxia-Ischemia

Anoxia is a term used to indicate the consequences of complete lack of oxygen as a result of a number of primary causes. **Hypoxia** refers to decreased arterial concentration of oxygen. **Ischemia** refers to blood flow to cells or organs that is insufficient to maintain their normal function. Hypoxic-ischemic encephalopathy is an important cause of permanent damage to CNS tissues that may result in neonatal death or manifest later as cerebral palsy or developmental delay. Fifteen to 20% of infants with hypoxic-ischemic encephalopathy (HIE) die in the neonatal period, and 25–30% of survivors are left with permanent neurodevelopmental abnormalities (cerebral palsy, mental retardation). The greatest risk of adverse outcome is seen in infants with fetal acidosis (pH <7.0), a 5-min Apgar score of 0–3, hypoxic-ischemic encephalopathy (altered tone, depressed level of consciousness, seizures), and other multiorgan system signs (Table 99-2).

TABLE 99-2. Multiorgan Systemic Effects of Asphyxia

SYSTEM	EFFECT
Central nervous system	Hypoxic-ischemic encephalopathy, infarction, intracranial hemorrhage, seizures, cerebral edema, hypotonia, hypertonia
Cardiovascular	Myocardial ischemia, poor contractility, cardiac stun, tricuspid insufficiency, hypotension
Pulmonary	Pulmonary hypertension, pulmonary hemorrhage, respiratory distress syndrome
Renal	Acute tubular or cortical necrosis
Adrenal	Adrenal hemorrhage
Gastrointestinal	Perforation, ulceration with hemorrhage, necrosis
Metabolic	Inappropriate secretion of antidiuretic hormone, hyponatremia, hypoglycemia, hypocalcemia, myoglobinuria
Integument	Subcutaneous fat necrosis
Hematology	Disseminated intravascular coagulation

ETIOLOGY. Most neonatal encephalopathic or seizure disorders, in the absence of major congenital malformations or syndromes, appear to be due to perinatal events rather than prenatal events. Brain MRI or autopsy findings of full-term neonates with encephalopathy demonstrated that 80% have acute injuries, <1% have prenatal injuries, and 3% have non-hypoxic ischemic diagnoses. Fetal hypoxia may be caused by various disorders in the mother, including (1) inadequate oxygenation of maternal blood from hypoventilation during anesthesia, cyanotic heart disease, respiratory failure, or carbon monoxide poisoning; (2) low maternal blood pressure from acute blood loss, spinal anesthesia, or compression of the vena cava and aorta by the gravid uterus; (3) inadequate relaxation of the uterus to permit placental filling as a result of uterine tetany caused by the administration of excessive oxytocin; (4) premature separation of the placenta; (5) impedance to the circulation of blood through the umbilical cord as a result of compression or knotting of the cord; and (6) placental insufficiency from toxemia or postmaturity.

Placental insufficiency often remains undetected on clinical assessment. Intrauterine growth restriction may develop in chronically hypoxic fetuses without the traditional signs of fetal distress. Doppler umbilical waveform velocimetry (demonstrating increased fetal vascular resistance) and cordocentesis (demonstrating fetal hypoxia and lactic acidosis) identify a chronically hypoxic infant (Chapter 96). Uterine contractions may further reduce umbilical oxygenation and depress the fetal cardiovascular system and CNS and result in low Apgar scores and postnatal hypoxia in the delivery room.

After birth, hypoxia may be caused by (1) failure of oxygenation as a result of severe forms of cyanotic congenital heart disease or severe pulmonary disease; (2) anemia severe enough to lower the oxygen content of the blood (severe hemorrhage, hemolytic disease); (3) shock severe enough to interfere with the transport of oxygen to vital organs from overwhelming sepsis, massive blood loss, and intracranial or adrenal hemorrhage.

PATHOPHYSIOLOGY AND PATHOLOGY. Animal studies suggest that hypoxia will not cause lethal brain injury without ischemia. The topography of injury typically correlates to areas of decreased cerebral blood flow. After an episode of hypoxia and ischemia, anaerobic metabolism occurs, which generates increased amounts of lactate and inorganic phosphates. Excitatory and toxic amino acids, particularly glutamate, accumulate in the damaged tissue. Increased amounts of intracellular sodium and calcium may result in tissue swelling and cerebral edema. There is also increased production of free radicals and nitric oxide in these tissues. The initial circulatory response of the fetus is increased shunting through the ductvs venosus, ductus arteriosus, and foramen ovale, with transient maintenance of perfusion of the brain, heart, and adrenals in preference to the lungs, liver, kidneys, and intestine.

The pathology of hypoxia-ischemia is dependent on the affected organ and the severity of the injury. Early congestion, fluid leak from increased capillary permeability, and endothelial cell swelling may then lead to signs of coagulation necrosis and cell death. Congestion and petechiae are seen in the pericardium, pleura, thymus, heart, adrenals, and meninges. Prolonged intrauterine hypoxia may result in inadequate perfusion of the periventricular white matter, resulting, in turn, in PVL. Pulmonary arteriole smooth muscle hyperplasia may develop, which predisposes the infant to pulmonary hypertension (Chapter 101.8). If fetal distress produces gasping, the amniotic fluid contents (meconium, squames, lanugo) are aspirated into the trachea or lungs.

The combination of chronic fetal hypoxia and acute hypoxic-ischemic injury after birth results in gestational age-specific neuropathology (Table 99-3). Term infants demonstrate neuronal necrosis of the cortex (later, cortical atrophy) and parasagittal ischemic injury. Preterm infants demonstrate PVL (later, spastic

TABLE 99-3. Topography of Brain Injury in Term Infants with Hypoxic-Ischemic Encephalopathy and Clinical Correlates

AREA OF INJURY	LOCATION OF INJURY	CLINICAL CORRELATE	LONG-TERM SEQUELAE
Selective neuronal necrosis	Entire neuroaxis, deep cortical area, brainstem and pentocubicular	Stupor or coma Seizures Hypotonia Oculomotor abnormalities Suck/swallow abnormalities	Cognitive delay Cerebral palsy Dystonia Seizure disorder Ataxia Bulbar and pseudobulbar palsy
Parasagittal injury	Cortex and subcortical white matter Parasagittal regions, esp. posterior	Proximal limb weakness Upper extremities affected greater than lower extremities	Spastic quadriparesis Cognitive delay Visual and auditory processing Difficulty
Focal ischemic necrosis	Cortex and subcortical white matter Vascular injury (usually MCA distribution)	Unilateral findings Seizures common and typically focal	Hemiparesis Seizures Cognitive delays
Periventricular injury	Injury to motor tracts, especially lower extremity	Bilateral and symmetric weakness in lower extremity More common in preterm infants	Spastic diplegia

MCA, middle cerebral artery.
Modified from Volpe JJ: *Neurology of the Newborn*, 4th ed. Philadelphia, WB Saunders, 2001.

diplegia), status marmoratus of the basal ganglia, and IVH. Term more often than preterm infants have focal or multifocal cortical infarcts that clinically manifest as focal seizures and hemiplegia.

CLINICAL MANIFESTATIONS. Intrauterine growth restriction with increased vascular resistance may be the 1st indication of fetal hypoxia. During labor, the fetal heart rate slows, and beat-to-beat variability declines. Continuous heart rate recording may reveal a variable or late (type II) deceleration pattern (see Fig. 96-4), and fetal scalp blood analysis may show a pH <7.20 (Chapter 96). The acidosis usually has both metabolic and respiratory components. Particularly in infants near term, these signs should lead to the administration of high concentrations of oxygen to the mother and immediate delivery to avoid fetal death or CNS damage.

At delivery, the presence of yellow, meconium-stained amniotic fluid is evidence that fetal distress has occurred. At birth, these infants are frequently depressed and fail to breathe spontaneously. During the ensuing hours, they may remain hypotonic or change from hypotonic to hypertonic, or their tone may appear normal (Table 99-4). Pallor, cyanosis, apnea, a slow heart rate, and unresponsiveness to stimulation are also signs of hypoxic-ischemic encephalopathy. Cerebral edema may develop during the next 24 hr and result in profound brainstem depression. During this time, seizure activity may occur; it may be severe and refractory to the usual doses of anticonvulsants. Phenobarbital, the drug of choice, is given with an intravenous loading dose (20 mg/kg); additional doses of 5–10 mg/kg (up to 40–50 mg/kg total) may be needed. Phenytoin (20 mg/kg loading dose) or lorazepam (0.1 mg/kg) may be needed for refractory seizures. Phenobarbital levels should be monitored 24 hr after the loading dose and maintenance therapy (5 mg/kg/24 hr) are begun. Therapeutic phenobarbital levels are 20–40 μg/mL. Though most often a result of the hypoxic-ischemic encephalopathy, seizures in asphyxiated newborns may also be due to hypocalcemia, hypoglycemia, or infection.

In addition to CNS dysfunction, heart failure and cardiogenic shock, persistent pulmonary hypertension, respiratory distress syndrome, gastrointestinal perforation, hematuria, and acute tubular necrosis are associated with perinatal asphyxia secondary to inadequate perfusion (see Table 99-2).

After delivery, hypoxia is due to respiratory failure and circulatory insufficiency. The severity of neonatal encephalopathy depends on the duration and timing of injury. Symptoms develop over a series of days, making it important to perform serial neurological examinations (see Table 99-4). During the initial hours after an insult, infants have a depressed level of consciousness. Periodic breathing with apnea or bradycardia is present, but cranial nerve functions are often spared with intact pupillary responses and spontaneous eye movement. Seizures are common with extensive injury. Hypotonia is also common as an early manifestation.

TABLE 99-4. Hypoxic-Ischemic Encephalopathy in Term Infants

SIGNS	STAGE 1	STAGE 2	STAGE 3
Level of consciousness	Hyperalert	Lethargic	Stuporous, coma
Muscle tone	Normal	Hypotonic	Flaccid
Posture	Normal	Flexion	Decerebrate
Tendon reflexes/clonus	Hyperactive	Hyperactive	Absent
Myoclonus	Present	Present	Absent
Moro reflex	Strong	Weak	Absent
Pupils	Mydriasis	Miosis	Unequal, poor light reflex
Seizures	None	Common	Decerebration
Electroencephalographic	Normal	Low voltage changing to seizure activity	Burst suppression to isoelectric
Duration	<24 hr if progresses; otherwise, may remain normal	24 hr to 14 days	Days to weeks
Outcome	Good	Variable	Death, severe deficits

Modified from Sarnat HB, Sarnat MS: Neonatal encephalopathy following fetal distress: A clinical and electroencephalographic study. *Arch Neurol* 1976;33:696–705. Copyright 1976, American Medical Association.

DIAGNOSIS. Ultrasound has limited utility in evaluation of hypoxic injury in the term infant; it is the preferred modality in evaluation of the preterm infant. CT scans are helpful in identification of focal hemorrhagic lesions, diffuse cortical injury, and damage to the basal ganglia; CT has limited ability to identify cortical injury within the 1st few days of life. Diffusion-weighed MRI is the preferred imaging modality because of its increased sensitivity and specificity early in the process and its ability to outline the topography of the lesion.

Amplitude integrated EEG (aEEG) is a promising modality to determine which infants are at highest risk for significant brain injury. A single channel tracing is generated from 2 electrodes placed in the biparietal area. A filter is used to filter and attenuate the signal between 2 Hz and 15 Hz. This technique is simple to perform and correlates with standard EEG. It has good reliability and positive predictive value of 85% and negative predictive value of 91–96% for infants who will have adverse neurodevelopmental outcome. It provides information quickly within the window where intervention is most likely to be useful. aEEG is also able to detect seizure activity, which is common in patients with HIE. Continuous aEEG monitoring detects subclinical seizure activity during the subacute phase.

TREATMENT. Systemic or selective cerebral hypothermia for the acute management of HIE is promising because it may decrease the rate of apoptosis and suppresses production of mediators known to be neurotoxic, including extracellular glutamate, free radicals, NO, and lactate. The neuroprotective effects are thought to be secondary to downregulating the secondary mediators of injury resulting from cerebral edema, accumulation of cytokines, and seizures. Animal data suggest that the intervention is most effective when implemented within 6 hr of the event.

Several trials demonstrated that either isolated cerebral cooling or whole body hypothermia are safe and well tolerated by term or near-term infants with HIE. Systemic hypothermia may result in more uniform cooling of the brain and deeper CNS structures. Infants treated with systemic hypothermia have a lower incidence of cortical neuronal injury on MRI. Early small clinical trials demonstrated no significant adverse short-term effects and a trend toward improved neurodevelopmental outcome at 18 mo among infants with moderate to severe encephalopathy. Selective head cooling is not effective in infants with the most severe aEEG findings, but is effective in those with less severe aEEG changes.

Additional therapy for infants with HIE includes supportive care directed at management of organ system dysfunction. Careful attention to ventilatory status and adequate oxygenation, blood pressure, hemodynamic status, acid-base balance, and possible infection is important. Secondary hypoxia or hypotension due to complications of HIE must be prevented. Aggressive treatment of seizures is critical and may necessitate continuous electroencephalographic monitoring.

PROGNOSIS. The outcome of HIE correlates to the timing and severity of the insult and ranges from complete recovery to death. The prognosis varies depending on whether the metabolic and cardiopulmonary complications (hypoxia, hypoglycemia, shock) are treated, the infant's gestational age (outcome is poorest if the infant is preterm), and the severity of the encephalopathy. Severe encephalopathy (see Table 99-4), characterized by flaccid coma, apnea, absent oculocephalic reflexes, and refractory seizures, is associated with a poor prognosis. A low Apgar score at 20 min, absence of spontaneous respirations at 20 min of age, and persistence of abnormal neurologic signs at 2 wk of age also predict death or severe cognitive and motor deficits. The combined use of an early electroencephalogram (EEG) and MRI is useful in predicting outcome in term infants with HIE. Normal MRI and EEG findings are associated with a good recovery, whereas severe MRI and EEG abnormalities predict a poor outcome. Infants with stage 2 and 3 encephalopathy are at the highest risk for adverse outcome. Microcephaly and poor head growth during the 1st year of life also correlate with injury to the basal ganglia and white matter and adverse developmental outcome at 12 mo. All survivors of moderate to severe encephalopathy require comprehensive high-risk medical and developmental follow-up. Early identification of neurodevelopmental problems allows prompt referral for developmental, rehabilitative, neurologic care, and early intervention services so that the best possible outcome can be achieved.

Brain death after neonatal HIE is diagnosed by the clinical findings of coma unresponsive to pain, auditory, or visual stimulation; apnea with P_{CO_2} rising from 40 to over 60 mm Hg without ventilatory support; and absent brainstem reflexes (pupil, oculocephalic, oculovestibular, corneal, gag, sucking). These findings must occur in the absence of hypothermia, hypotension, and elevated levels of depressant drugs (phenobarbital). An absence of cerebral blood flow on radionuclide scans and no electrical activity on EEG (electrocerebral silence) is inconsistently observed in clinically brain-dead neonatal infants. Persistence of the clinical criteria for 2 days in term and 3 days in preterm infants predicts brain death in most asphyxiated newborns. Nonetheless, no universal agreement has been reached regarding the definition of neonatal brain death. Consideration of withdrawal of life support should include discussions with the family, the health care team, and, if there is disagreement, an ethics committee. The best interest of the infant involves judgments about the benefits and harm of continuing therapy or avoiding ongoing futile therapy.

99.6 • Spine and Spinal Cord

Injury to the spine/spinal cord is rare, but can be devastating. Strong traction exerted when the spine is hyperextended or when the direction of pull is lateral, or forceful longitudinal traction on the trunk while the head is still firmly engaged in the pelvis, especially when combined with flexion and torsion of the vertical axis, may produce fracture and separation of the vertebrae. Such injuries are most likely to occur when difficulty is encountered in delivering the shoulders in cephalic presentations and the head in breech presentations. The injury occurs most commonly at the level of the 4th cervical vertebra with cephalic presentations and the lower cervical–upper thoracic vertebrae with breech presentations. Transection of the cord may occur with or without vertebral fractures; hemorrhage and edema may produce neurologic signs that are indistinguishable from those of transection except that they may not be permanent. Areflexia, loss of sensation, and complete paralysis of voluntary motion occur below the level of injury, although the persistence of a withdrawal reflex mediated through spinal centers distal to the area of injury is frequently misinterpreted as representing voluntary motion. If the injury is severe, the infant, who from birth may be in poor condition because of respiratory depression, shock, or hypothermia, may deteriorate rapidly to death within several hours before any neurologic signs are obvious. Alternatively, the course may be protracted, with symptoms and signs appearing at birth or later in the 1st wk; immobility, flaccidity, and associated brachial plexus injuries may not be recognized for several days. Constipation may also be present. Some infants survive for prolonged periods, their initial flaccidity, immobility, and areflexia being replaced after several weeks or months by rigid flexion of the extremities, increased muscle tone, and spasms. Apnea on day 1 and poor motor recovery by 3 mo are poor prognostic signs.

The **differential diagnosis** includes amyotonia congenita and myelodysplasia associated with spina bifida occulta. Ultrasonography or, more often, MRI confirms the diagnosis. **Treatment** of the survivors is supportive, including home ventilation; patients often remain permanently disabled. When a fracture or dislocation is causing compression, the prognosis is related to the time elapsed before the compression is relieved.

99.7 • Peripheral Nerve Injuries

BRACHIAL PALSY. Brachial plexus injury is a common problem, with an incidence of 0.6–4.6 per 1,000 live births. Injury to the brachial plexus may cause paralysis of the upper part of the arm with or without paralysis of the forearm or hand or, more commonly, paralysis of the entire arm. These injuries occur in macrosomic infants and when lateral traction is exerted on the head and neck during delivery of the shoulder in a vertex presentation, when the arms are extended over the head in a breech presentation, or when excessive traction is placed on the shoulders. Approximately 45% of brachial plexus injuries are associated with shoulder dystocia. In **Erb-Duchenne paralysis**, the injury is limited to the 5th and 6th cervical nerves. The infant loses the power to abduct the arm from the shoulder, rotate the arm exter-

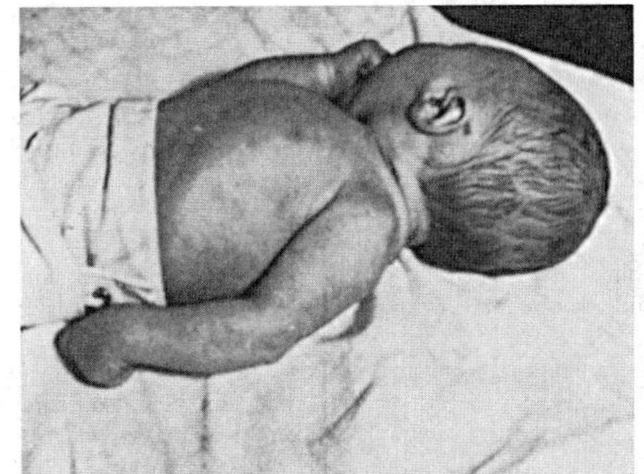
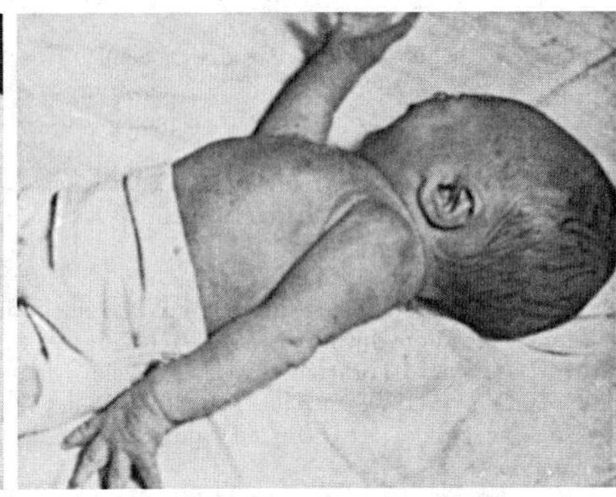

Figure 99-6. Brachial palsy of the left arm (asymmetric Moro reflex).

nally, and supinate the forearm. The characteristic position consists of adduction and internal rotation of the arm with pronation of the forearm. Power to extend the forearm is retained, but the biceps reflex is absent; the Moro reflex is absent on the affected side (Fig. 99-6). The outer aspect of the arm may have some sensory impairment. Power in the forearm and hand grasp are preserved unless the lower part of the plexus is also injured; the presence of hand grasp is a favorable prognostic sign. When the injury includes the phrenic nerve, alteration in diaphragmatic excursion may be observed fluoroscopically. **Klumpke paralysis** is a rare form of brachial palsy; injury to the 7th and 8th cervical nerves and the 1st thoracic nerve produces a paralyzed hand and ipsilateral ptosis and miosis (**Horner syndrome**) if the sympathetic fibers of the 1st thoracic root are also injured. Mild cases may not be detected immediately after birth. Differentiation must be made from cerebral injury; from fracture, dislocation, or epiphyseal separation of the humerus; and from fracture of the clavicle. MRI demonstrates nerve root rupture or avulsion.

Full recovery occurs in most patients, the prognosis depending on whether the nerve was merely injured or was lacerated. If the paralysis was due to edema and hemorrhage about the nerve fibers, function should return within a few months; if due to laceration, permanent damage may result. Involvement of the deltoid is usually the most serious problem and may result in shoulder drop secondary to muscle atrophy. In general, paralysis of the upper part of the arm has a better prognosis than paralysis of the lower part.

Treatment consists of partial immobilization and appropriate positioning to prevent the development of contractures. In upper arm paralysis, the arm should be abducted 90 degrees with external rotation at the shoulder, full supination of the forearm, and slight extension at the wrist with the palm turned toward the face. This position may be achieved with a brace or splint during the 1st 1–2 wk. Immobilization should be intermittent through the day while the infant is asleep and between feedings. In lower arm or hand paralysis, the wrist should be splinted in a neutral position and padding placed in the fist. When the entire arm is paralyzed, the same treatment principles should be followed. Gentle massage and range-of-motion exercises may be started by 7–10 days of age. Infants should be closely monitored with active and passive corrective exercises. If the paralysis persists without improvement for 3–6 mo, neuroplasty, neurolysis, end-to-end anastomosis, and nerve grafting offer hope for partial recovery.

The type of treatment and the prognosis depend on the mechanism of injury and the number of nerve roots involved. The mildest injury to a peripheral nerve (neurapraxia) is due to edema and heals spontaneously within a few weeks. Axonotmesis is more severe and is due to nerve fiber disruption with an intact myelin sheath; function usually returns in a few months. Total disruption of nerves (neurotmesis) or root avulsion is the most severe, especially if it involves C5–T1; microsurgical repair may be indicated. Fortunately, most (75%) injuries are at the root level C5–C6, involve neurapraxia and axonotmesis, and should heal spontaneously. Botulism toxin may be used to treat biceps-triceps co-contractions.

PHRENIC NERVE PARALYSIS. Phrenic nerve injury (3rd, 4th, 5th cervical nerves) with diaphragmatic paralysis must be considered when cyanosis and irregular and labored respirations develop. Such injuries, usually unilateral, are associated with ipsilateral upper brachial palsy. Because breathing is thoracic in type, the abdomen does not bulge with inspiration. Breath sounds are diminished on the affected side. The thrust of the diaphragm, which may often be felt just under the costal margin on the normal side, is absent on the affected side. The diagnosis is established by ultrasonography or fluoroscopic examination, which reveals elevation of the diaphragm on the paralyzed side and seesaw movements of the 2 sides of the diaphragm during respiration.

No specific treatment is available; infants should be placed on the involved side and given oxygen if necessary. Initially, intravenous feedings may be needed; later, progressive gavage or oral feeding may be started, depending on the infant's condition. Pulmonary infections are a serious complication. Recovery usually occurs spontaneously by 1–3 mo; rarely, surgical plication of the diaphragm may be indicated.

FACIAL NERVE PALSY. Facial palsy is usually a peripheral paralysis that results from pressure over the facial nerve in utero, from efforts during labor, or from forceps use during delivery. Rarely, it may result from nuclear agenesis of the facial nerve. Peripheral paralysis is flaccid and, when complete, involves the entire side of the face, including the forehead. When the infant cries, movement occurs only on the nonparalyzed side of the face, and the mouth is drawn to that side. On the affected side the forehead is smooth, the eye cannot be closed, the nasolabial fold is absent, and the corner of the mouth droops. The forehead wrinkles on the affected side with central paralysis because only the lower $^{2}/_{3}$ of the face is involved. The infant also usually has other manifestations of intracranial injury, most commonly a 6th nerve palsy. The prognosis depends on whether the nerve was injured by pressure or whether the nerve fibers were torn. Improvement occurs within a few weeks in the former instance. Care of the exposed eye is essential. Neuroplasty may be indicated when the paralysis is persistent. Facial palsy may be confused with absence of the depressor muscles of the mouth, which is a benign problem.

Other peripheral nerves are seldom injured in utero or at birth except when they are involved in fractures or hemorrhage.

AAP Committee of the Fetus and Newborn: Postnatal corticosteroids to treat or prevent chronic lung disease in preterm infants. *Pediatrics* 2002;109:330–338.

Accardo J, Kammann H, Hoon AH Jr: Neuroimaging in cerebral palsy. *J Pediatr* 2004;145:S19–S27.

Ambalavonan N, Carlo WA, Shankaran S, et al: Predicting outcomes of neonates diagnosed with hypoxic-ischemic encephalopathy. *Pediatrics* 2006;118:2084–2093.

Bager B: Perinatally acquired brachial plexus palsy—a persisting challenge. *Acta Paediatr* 1997;86:1214–1219.

Baud O, Foix-L'Helias L, Kaminski M, et al: Antenatal glucocorticoid treatment and cystic periventricular leukomalacia in very premature infants. *N Engl J Med* 1999;341:1190–1196.

Biagioni E, Mercuri E, Rutherford M, et al: Combined use of electroencephalogram and magnetic resonance imaging in full-term neonates with acute encephalopathy. *Pediatrics* 2001;107:461–468.

Brown T, Cupido C, Scarfone H, et al: Developmental apraxia arising from neonatal brachial plexus palsy. *Neurology* 2000;55:24–30.

Cooke R: Head cooling in neonatal hypoxic-ischaemic encephalopathy. *Lancet* 2005;365:632–634.

Crowley P: Prophylactic corticosteroids for preterm birth. *Cochrane Database Syst Rev* 2002;2:CD000065.

De Felice C, Toti P, Laurini RN, et al: Early neonatal brain injury in histologic chorioamnionitis. *J Pediatr* 2001;138:101–104.

De Vries LS, Hellstrom-Westas: Role of cerebral function monitoring in the newborn. *Arch Dis Child Fetal Neonatal Ed* 2005;90:F201–F207.

De Vries LS, Van Haastert IC, Rademaker KJ, et al: Ultrasound abnormalities preceding cerebral palsy in high risk preterm infants. *J Pediatr* 2004; 144:815–820.

Ekert P, Perlman M, Steinlin M, et al: Predicting the outcome of postasphyxial hypoxic-ischemic encephalopathy within 4 hours of birth. *J Pediatr* 1997;131:613–617.

Evans D, Levene M: Neonatal seizures. *Arch Dis Child* 1998;78:F70–F75.

Ferriero DM: Neonatal brain injury. *N Engl J Med* 2004;351:1985–1995.

Gluckman PD, Wyatt JS, Azzopardi D, et al: Selective head cooling and mild systemic hypothermia after neonatal encephalopathy: Multicenter randomized trial. *Lancet* 2005;365:663–670.

Gressens P, Rogido M, Paindaveine B, et al: The impact of frequent neonatal intensive care practices on the developing brain. *J Pediatr* 2002;140: 646–653.

Hall RT, Hall FK, Daily DK: High-dose phenobarbital therapy in term newborn infants with severe perinatal asphyxia: A randomized, prospective study with three-year follow-up. *J Pediatr* 1998;132:345–348.

Hamrick SE, Ferriero DM: The injury response in the term newborn brain: Can we neuroprotect? *Curr Opin Neurol* 2003:15:147–154.

Hellstrom-Westas L, Rosen I, Svenningsen NW: Predictive value of early continuous amplitude integrated EEG recordings on outcome after severe birth asphyxia in full term infants. *Arch Dis Child Fetal Neonatal Ed* 1995;72:34F–38F.

Heuchan AM, Evans N, Henderson DJ, et al: Perinatal risk factors for major intraventricular haemorrhage in the Australian and New Zealand neonatal network, 1995–1997. *Arch Dis Child* 2002;86:F86–F90.

Hintz SR, Kendrick DE, Stoll BJ: Neurodevelopmental and growth outcomes of extremely low birth weight infants after necrotizing enterocolitis. *Pediatrics* 2005;115:696–703.

Hoeksma AF, Wolf H, Oei SL: Obstetrical brachial plexus injuries: Incidence, natural course and shoulder contracture. *Clin Rehabil* 2000;14:523–526.

Inder T, Huppi PS, Zientara GP, et al: Early detection of periventricular leukomalacia by diffusion-weighted magnetic resonance imaging techniques. *J Pediatr* 1999;134:631–634.

Inder TE, Hunt RW, Morley CJ, et al: Randomized trial of systemic hypothermia selectively protects the cortex on MRI in term hypoxic-ischemic Encephalopathy. *J Pediatr* 2004;145:835–837.

Kennedy CR, Ayers S, Campbell MJ, et al: Randomized, controlled trial of acetazolamide and furosemide in posthemorrhagic ventricular dilation in infancy: Follow-up at 1 year. *Pediatrics* 2001;108:597–607.

Klinger G, Beyene J, Shah P, et al: Do hyperoxaemia and hypocapnia add to the risk of brain injury after intrapartum asphyxia? *Arch Dis Child* 2005;90:F49–F52.

Laptook AR, O'Shea TM, Shankaran S, et al: Adverse neurodevelopmental outcomes among extremely low birth weight infants with a normal head ultrasound: Prevalence and antecedents. *Pediatrics* 2005;115:673–680.

MacKinnon JA, Perlman M, Kirpalani H, et al: Spinal cord injury at birth: Diagnostic and prognostic data in 22 patients. *J Pediatr* 1993;122:431–437.

Maunu J, Ekholm E, Parkkola R, et al: Antenatal doppler measurements and early brain injury in very low birthweight infants. *J Pediatr* 2007;150: 51–56.

Mercuri E, Ricci D, Cowan FM, et al: Head growth in infants with hypoxic-ischemic encephalopathy: Correlation with neonatal magnetic resonance imaging. *Pediatrics* 2000;106:235–243.

Miller SP, Ramaswamy V, Michelson D, et al: Patterns of brain injury in term neonatal encephalopathy. *J Pediatr* 2005;146:453–460.

Mills JF, Dargaville PA, Coleman LT, et al: Upper cervical spinal cord injury in neonates: The use of magnetic resonance imaging. *J Pediatr* 2001;138: 105–108.

Munro MJ, Walker AM, Barfield CP: Hypotensive extremely low birth weight infants have reduced cerebral blood flow. *Pediatrics* 2004;114:1591–1596.

Narayan P, Mapstone TB: Shunting techniques: Ventriculosubgaleal shunting: Techniques in Neurosurgery. 2002;7:212–215.

Noetzel MJ, Wolpaw JR: Emerging concepts in the pathophysiology of recovery from neonatal brachial plexus injury. *Neurology* 2000;55:5–6.

Paneth N: Cerebral palsy in term infants—birth or before birth? *J Pediatr* 2001;138:791–792.

Pierrat V, Duquennoy C, van Haastert IC, et al: Ultrasound diagnosis and neurodevelopmental outcome of localized and extensive cystic periventricular leukomalacia. *Arch Dis Child* 2002;84:F151–F156.

Pierrat V, Haiuari N, Liska A, et al: Prevalence, causes, and outcome at 2 years of age of newborn encephalopathy: Population based study. *Arch Dis Child* 2005;90:F257–F261.

Rickards AL, Kelly EA, Doyle LW, et al: Cognition, academic progress, behavior and self-concept at 14 years of very low birth weight children. *J Dev Behav Pediatr* 2001;22:11–18.

Rollnik JD, Hierner R, Schubert M, et al: Botulinum toxin treatment of co-contractions after birth-related brachial plexus lesions. *Neurology* 2000;55:112–114.

Saigal S, Stoskopf BL, Streiner DL, et al: Physical growth and current health status of infants who were of extremely low birth weight and controls at adolescence. *Pediatrics* 2001;108:407–415.

Salhab WA, Perlman JM, Silver L, et al: Necrotizing enterocolitis and neurodevelopmental outcome in extremely low birth weight infants <1000 g. *J Perinatol* 2004;24:534–540.

Schmidt B, Davis P, Moddemann PD, et al: Long-term effects of indomethacin prophylaxis in extremely-low-birth-weight infants. *N Engl J Med* 2001;344:1966–1972.

Shankaran S, Johnson Y, Langer J, et al: Outcome of extremely-low-birth-weight infants at highest risk: Gestational age ≤24 weeks, birthweight ≤750 g, and 1-minute Apgar ≤3. *Am J Obstet Gynecol* 2004;191:1084–1091.

Soul JS, Eichenwald E, Walter G, et al: CSF removal in infantile posthemorrhagic hydrocephalus results in significant improvements in cerebral hemodynamics. *Pediatr Res* 2004;55:872–876.

Stark AR, Carlo WA, Tyson JE, et al: Adverse effects of early dexamethasone treatment in extremely low birth weight infants. *N Engl J Med* 2001;344:95–101.

Stoll BJ, Hansen NI, Adams-Chapman I, et al: Neurodevelopmental and growth impairment among extremely low-birth-weight infants with neonatal infections. *JAMA* 2004;292:2357–2365.

Strombeck C, Krumlinde-Sundholm L, Forrsberg H: Functional outcome at 5 years in children with obstetrical brachial plexus palsy with and without microsurgical reconstruction. *Dev Med Child Neurol* 2000;42: 148–157.

Toet MC, Hellstrom-Westas L, Broenendaal F, et al: Amplitude integrated EEG 3 and 6 hours after birth in full term neonates with hypoxic-ischaemic encephalopathy. *Arch Dis Child Fetal Neonatal Ed* 1999;81:19F–23F.

Vergani P, Locatelli A, Doria V, et al: Intraventricular hemorrhage and periventricular leukomalacia in preterm infants. *Obstet Gynecol* 2004;104: 225–231.

Vincer MJ, Allen AC, Joseph KS, et al: Increasing prevalence of cerebral palsy among very preterm infants: a population-based study. *Pediatrics* 2006; 118:e1621–e1626.

Whitelaw A: Repeated lumbar or ventricular punctures in newborns with intraventricular hemorrhage. *Cochrane Database Syst Rev* 2002;1: CD000216.

Whitelaw A, Thoresen, Pople I: Posthaemorrhagic ventricular dilatation. *Arch Dis Child* 2002;86:F72–F74.

Wood NS, Costeloe K, Gibson AT, et al: The EPICure Study: Associations and antecedents of neurological and developmental disability at 30 months of age following extremely preterm birth. *Arch Dis Child Fetal Neonatal Ed* 2005;90:F134–F140.

Wu YW, Colford JM Jr: Chorioamnionitis as a risk factor for cerebral palsy: A meta-analysis. *JAMA* 2000;284:1417–1424.

Yang SH, Choi SJ, Roh CR, et al: Multiple courses of antenatal corticosteroid therapy in patients with preterm premature rupture of membranes. *J Perinat Med* 2004;32:42–48.

Yeh TF, Lin YJ, Hung C, et al. Outcomes at school age after postnatal dexamethasone therapy for lung disease of prematurity. *N Eng J Med* 2004;350:1304–1313.

Chapter 100 ■ Delivery Room Emergencies

Barbara J. Stoll and Ira Adams-Chapman

Most infants complete the transition to extrauterine life without difficulty; however, a small percentage will require resuscitation after birth. The most common delivery room emergency for neonates is secondary to failure to initiate and maintain effective respirations. Less frequently, but of major importance are shock (Chapter 98), severe anemia (Chapter 103.1), plethora (Chapter 103.2), convulsions (Chapter 593.7), and management of life-threatening congenital malformations (Chapter 98). Improved perinatal care and prenatal diagnosis of fetal anomalies allows for appropriate maternal transports for high-risk deliveries.

RESPIRATORY DISTRESS AND FAILURE. Disorders of respiration in newborn infants can be categorized as either central nervous system (CNS) failure representing depression or failure of the respiratory center, or peripheral respiratory difficulty indicating interference with the alveolar exchange of oxygen and carbon dioxide. Cyanosis occurs in both groups (see Table 98-1). Respiratory problems encountered in the delivery room are most frequently those of airway obstruction and depression of the CNS (maternal medications, asphyxia) with an absence of adequate respiratory effort.

Respiratory distress in the presence of good respiratory effort should lead to an immediate consideration of the underlying cause and is an indication for x-ray examination of the chest.

If respiratory movements are made with the mouth closed but the infant fails to move air in and out of the lungs, bilateral **choanal atresia** (Chapter 373) or other obstruction of the upper respiratory tract should be suspected. The mouth should be opened and the mouth and posterior of the pharynx cleared of secretions by gentle suction. An oropharyngeal airway should be inserted and the source of the obstruction sought immediately. If effective respiratory flow is not produced by opening the infant's mouth and clearing the airway, laryngoscopy is indicated. With obstructive malformations of the mandible, epiglottis, larynx, or trachea, an endotracheal tube should be inserted; prolonged endotracheal intubation or tracheostomy may be required. Respiratory failure caused by CNS depression or injury may require continuous mechanical ventilation.

Hypoplasia of the mandible (Pierre Robin, DiGeorge, and other syndromes; see Chapters 305, 308) with posterior displacement of the tongue may result in symptoms similar to those of choanal atresia and may be temporarily relieved by pulling the tongue or mandible forward. A scaphoid abdomen suggests a **diaphragmatic hernia** or **eventration**, as does asymmetry in contour or movement of the chest or a shift of the apical impulse of the heart; these latter manifestations are also compatible with **tension pneumothorax.** A pneumothorax on the 1st day of life suggests pulmonary hypoplasia, renal malformations, or both.

Pulmonary causes of respiratory difficulty are discussed in Chapter 101.

FAILURE TO INITIATE OR SUSTAIN RESPIRATION. Failure to initiate or sustain respiratory effort usually originates in the CNS as a result of asphyxia or peripherally due to neuromuscular disorders. Prematurity alone is seldom a causative factor except in infants weighing <1,000 g. Intrapulmonary problems, such as the pulmonary hypoplasia associated with oligohydramnios as in Potter syndrome or neuromuscular diseases, bilateral pleural effusions (hydrops fetalis), and severe intrauterine pneumonia, may at times result in poorly sustained ventilation. The lungs in these infants may be noncompliant, and standard efforts to begin respirations may be inadequate to initiate sufficient ventilation.

Narcosis results from administration of morphine, meperidine, fentanyl, barbiturates, or tranquilizers to the mother shortly before delivery or from maternal anesthesia given during the 2nd stage of labor. This should be avoided by using appropriate analgesic and anesthetic practices. **Treatment** includes initial physical stimulation and securing of a patent airway. If effective ventilation is not initiated, artificial breathing with a mask and bag must be instituted. At the same time, if the respiratory depression is due to morphine or its derivatives, naloxone hydrochloride (Narcan), 0.1 mg/kg, should be given by the intravenous, subcutaneous, intratracheal, or intramuscular routes and repeated 2 to 3 times if needed. Narcan is contraindicated in infants born to mothers with opiate addiction because it precipitates acute neonatal withdrawal with severe seizures. Ventilation is essential before and during administration of this antidote. If depression is due to other anesthetics or analgesics, artificial respiration should be continued until the infant is able to sustain ventilation. CNS stimulant drugs should not be used because they are ineffective and may be harmful.

Prenatal or perinatal hypoxia of whatever cause, if sufficiently severe, produces brainstem depression and secondary apnea that is unresponsive to sensory stimulation. Death from apnea may be prevented by resuscitation, provided that the basic cause of the hypoxia can be eliminated within a reasonable time while artificial respiration continues. External cardiac massage, correction of acidosis, and circulatory support with drugs may be important adjuncts to ventilation in the severely asphyxiated infant.

NEONATAL RESUSCITATION. While the majority of babies undergo a smooth physiologic transition and breathe effectively after delivery, 5–10% require active intervention to establish normal cardiorespiratory function. The goals of neonatal resuscitation are to prevent the morbidity and mortality associated with hypoxic-ischemic tissue (brain, heart, kidney) injury and to reestablish adequate spontaneous respiration and cardiac output. High-risk situations should be anticipated by the history of the pregnancy, labor, and delivery and identification of signs of fetal distress. Although the Apgar score is helpful in evaluating patients in need of attention, infants who are born limp, cyanotic, apneic, or pulseless require immediate resuscitation before assignment of the 1-min Apgar score. Rapid and appropriate resuscitative efforts improve the likelihood of preventing brain damage and achieving a successful outcome.

Guidelines for neonatal resuscitation propose an "integrated" assessment/response approach for the initial evaluation of an infant with simultaneous assessment of infant color, general appearance, and risk factors. The fundamental principles include evaluation of the airway, establishing effective respiration and adequate circulation; the guidelines also highlight the assessment and response to the neonatal heart rate and the management of infants with meconium-stained fluid.

Immediately after birth, an infant in need of resuscitation should be placed under a radiant heater and dried (to avoid hypothermia), positioned head down and slightly extended, the airway cleared by suctioning, and gentle tactile stimulation provided (slapping the foot, rubbing the back). Simultaneously, the infant's color, heart rate, and respiratory effort should be assessed (Fig. 100-1).

The steps in neonatal resuscitation follow the ABCs: **A**, anticipate and establish a patent airway by suctioning and, if necessary, performing endotracheal intubation; **B**, initiate breathing by using tactile stimulation or positive-pressure ventilation with a bag and mask or through an endotracheal tube; **C**, maintain the circulation with chest compression and medications, if needed. Steps to follow for immediate neonatal evaluation and resuscitation are outlined in Figure 100-1 (also see Chapter 66).

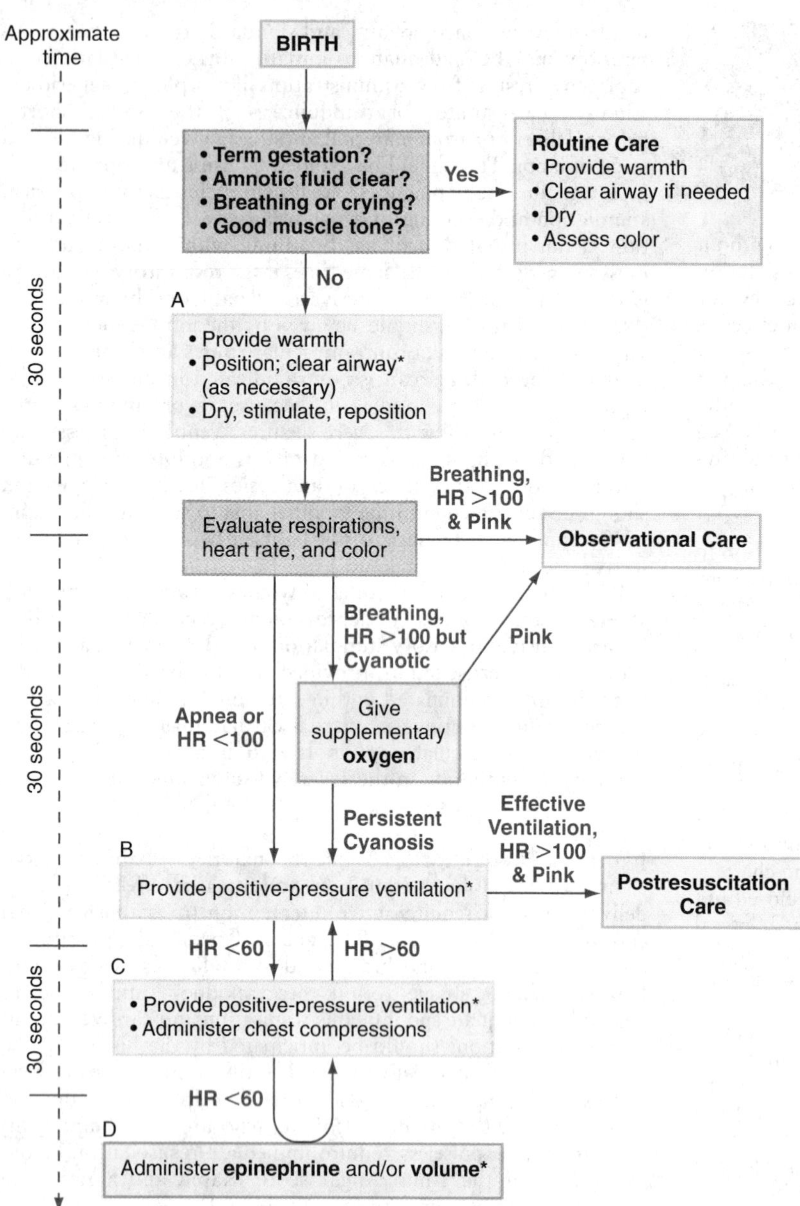

Figure 100-1. Neonatal flow algorithm. HR, heart rate. (From Part 13: Neonatal Resuscitation Guidelines. *Circulation* 2005;112:IV188–IV195.)

If no respirations are noted or if the heart rate is below 100/min, positive pressure ventilation is given through a tightly fitted face mask and bag for 15–30 sec. In infants with severe respiratory depression who do not respond to positive pressure ventilation via bag and mask, endotracheal intubation should be performed. Many recommend early intubation for extremely low birthweight preterm infants. Guidelines for endotracheal tube size and depth of insertion in infants with different birthweights are shown in Table 100-1. If the heart rate does not improve after 30 sec with bag and mask (or endotracheal) ventilation and remains below 100/min, ventilation is continued and chest compression should be initiated over the lower third of the sternum at a rate of 120/min. The ratio of compressions to ventilation is 3:1. If the heart rate remains <60 despite effective compressions and ventilation, administration of epinephrine should be considered. Persistent bradycardia in neonates is usually due to hypoxia resulting from respiratory arrest and often responds rapidly to effective ventilation alone. Persistent bradycardia despite what appears to be adequate resuscitation suggests more severe cardiac compromise or inadequate ventilation technique. Poor response to ventilation may be due to a loosely fitted mask, poor positioning of the endotracheal tube, intraesophageal intubation, airway obstruction, insufficient pressure, pleural effusions, pneumothorax, excessive air in the stomach, asystole, hypovolemia, diaphragmatic hernia, or prolonged intrauterine asphyxia.

TABLE 100-1. Guidelines for Tracheal Tube Size and Depth of Insertion

TUBE SIZE (mm ID)	DEPTH OF INSERTION FROM UPPER LIP (cm)	WEIGHT (g)	GESTATION (wk)
2.5	6.5–7	<1,000	<28
3	7–8	1,000–2,000	28–34
3/3.5	8–9	2,000–3,000	34–38
3.5/4.0	≥9	>3,000	>38

ID, internal diameter.
From Kattwinkel J, Niermeyer S, Nadkarni, et al: Resuscitation of the newly born infant: An advisory statement from the Pediatric Working Group of the International Liaison Committee on Resuscitation. *Circulation* 1999;99:1927–1938. By permission of the American Heart Association, Inc.

Traditionally, the inspired gas for neonatal resuscitation has been 100% oxygen. Resuscitation with room air is equally effective and may reduce the risk of hyperoxia, with decreased cerebral blood flow, and generation of oxygen free radicals. Currently 100% O_2 is recommended. Room air may become the preferred initial gas for neonatal resuscitation in the future; if the neonate does not achieve normal oxygen saturations within 90 sec, increasing concentrations of oxygen should be blended in (up to 100% oxygen) until normal oxygen saturations are achieved. If pulmonary hypertension is suspected (meconium aspiration, diaphragmatic hernia) one may consider 100% oxygen as the initial gas for resuscitation. Particular attention is required during the resuscitation of VLBW neonates, to monitor oxygen saturation to minimize the risk of hyperoxia.

Although the 1st breath normally requires pressures as low as 15–20 cm H_2O, pressures as high as 30–40 cm H_2O may be needed. Subsequent breaths are given at a rate of 40–60/min with a pressure of 15–20 cm H_2O. Noncompliant stiff lungs secondary to respiratory distress syndrome, congenital pneumonia, pulmonary hypoplasia, or meconium aspiration may require higher pressures. Successful ventilation is determined by adequate chest rise, symmetric breath sounds, improved pink color, heart rate >100/min, spontaneous respirations, presence of end-tidal CO_2, and improved tone. Various devices to detect exhaled CO_2 and to confirm accurate placement of an endotracheal tube are commercially available. A laryngeal mask airway may be an effective tool to establish an airway, especially if bag mask ventilation is ineffective or intubation is unsuccessful.

If the infant has respiratory depression and the mother has a history of analgesic narcotic drug administration within 4 hr prior to delivery, naloxone hydrochloride (0.1 mg/kg) is given while adequate ventilation is maintained. Breathing in the depressed infant should be maintained until a response to naloxone is noted. Continuous observation of the infant is important because repeated doses of naloxone may be needed even after the infant has been transferred to the nursery due to the short half-life of the drug.

Medications are rarely required but should be administered when the heart rate is < 60/min after 30 sec of combined ventilation and chest compressions or during asystole. The umbilical vein can generally be readily cannulated and used for immediate administration of medications during neonatal resuscitation (Fig. 100-2). The endotracheal tube may be used for the administration of epinephrine if intravenous access is not available and/or for naloxone hydrochloride. Epinephrine (0.1–0.3 mL/kg of a 1 : 10,000 solution, intravenously or intratracheally) is given for asystole or for failure to respond to 30 sec of combined resuscitation. The dose may be repeated every 3–5 min. Data in neonates are insufficient to recommend higher doses in infants who are unresponsive to the standard dose. Emergency volume expansion is accomplished with 10–20 mL/kg of an isotonic crystalloid solution or O-negative red blood cells (in acute hemorrhage). Volume infusions should be used cautiously during the resuscitation of a VLBW infant. Sodium bicarbonate (2 mEq/kg, 0.5 mEq/mL of a 4.2% solution) should be given slowly (1 mEq/kg/min) if metabolic acidosis has been documented and the resuscitation is prolonged. Sodium bicarbonate should be given only after effective ventilation has been established because such therapy may increase blood CO_2 and produce respiratory acidosis complicating an existing metabolic acidosis. Restoration of oxygenation and tissue perfusion is the main treatment of metabolic acidosis associated with asphyxia.

Severe asphyxia may also depress myocardial function and cause cardiogenic shock despite the recovery of heart and respiratory rates. Dopamine or dobutamine administered as a continuous infusion (5–20 μg/kg/min) and fluids should be started after the initial resuscitation effort to improve cardiac output in an infant with poor peripheral perfusion, weak pulses, hypotension, tachycardia, and poor urine output. Epinephrine (0.1–1.0 μg/kg/min) may be indicated for infants in severe shock who do not respond to dopamine or dobutamine (Chapter 66).

Less severe degrees of asphyxia can usually be managed by brief periods of bag and mask ventilation. Chest compression and medications are not needed for most neonates who have mild to moderate birth depression. Regardless of the severity of asphyxia or the response to resuscitation, asphyxiated infants should be monitored closely for signs of multiorgan hypoxic-ischemic tissue injury (see Table 99-1).

MECONIUM. Meconium staining of the amniotic fluid may be an indication of fetal stress; therefore, personnel skilled at endotracheal intubation and resuscitation should be present at the delivery. Previously the decision to intubate a neonate was based on the presence and thickness/consistency of the meconium-stained

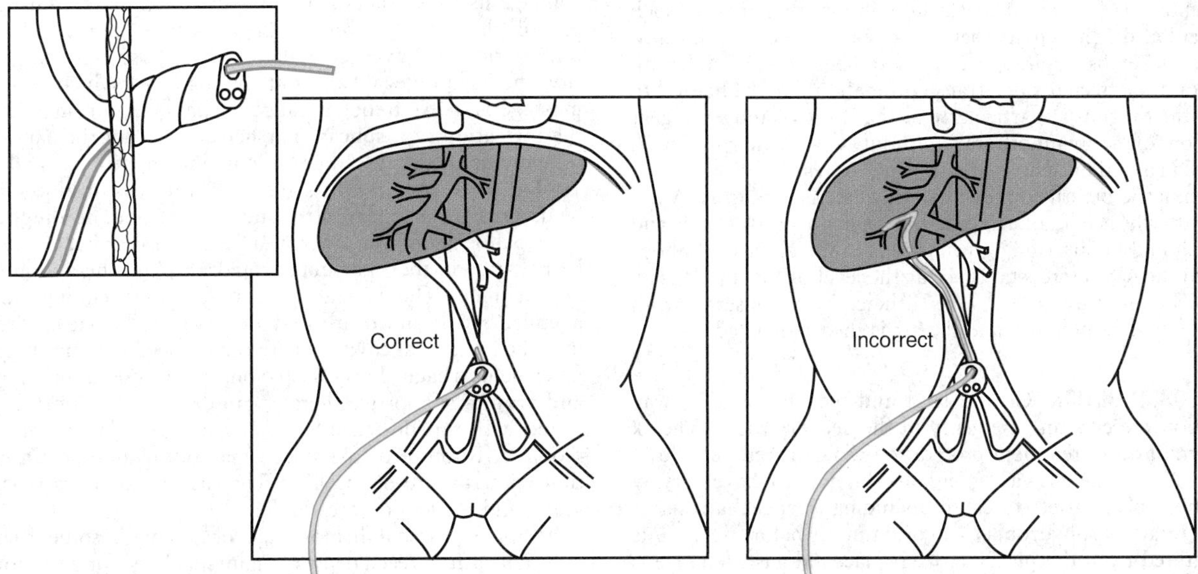

Figure 100-2. Use of the umbilical vein for administration of medications during neonatal resuscitation. (From Kattwinkel J, Bloom RS [eds]: *Neonatal Resuscitation Textbook*, 5th ed. Elk Grove, IL, American Academy of Pediatrics, American Heart Association, 2006, with permission.)

fluid; current evidence no longer supports this practice. If any meconium staining is present in the amniotic fluid, the obstetrician should suction the mouth, nose, and hypopharynx immediately after delivery of the head but before delivery of the shoulders. If the infant is vigorous with good respiratory effort and a heart rate >100/min, tracheal intubation to aspirate meconium should not be attempted and the mouth and nose should be suctioned with a bulb or suction catheter. If the infant is depressed with poor muscle tone and/or a heart rate < 100/min, tracheal intubation and suctioning should be performed. The endotracheal tube should be attached to a suction device and free flow oxygen should be provided throughout the procedure.

SHOCK. Circulatory insufficiency may be present at birth as a result of severe asphyxia or hemorrhage during gestation, labor, or delivery. Causes of bleeding include hemolysis; placental abruption, previa, or tear; traumatic injury to the umbilical cord or internal organs; and intracranial bleeding. Clinical manifestations include signs of respiratory distress, cyanosis, pallor, flaccidity, cold mottled skin, tachycardia or bradycardia, hepatosplenomegaly, and, rarely, convulsions. Edema and hepatosplenomegaly suggest hydrops fetalis or heart failure without shock. Shock from overwhelming infection may also be present after birth.

Supportive treatment with type O Rh-negative blood or normal saline is indicated for hemorrhage or hypovolemia, respectively. Oxygen should be administered and the metabolic acidosis corrected with sodium bicarbonate. Sympathomimetic agents such as dopamine or dobutamine may be needed to support cardiac output and blood pressure. The diagnosis and treatment of erythroblastosis fetalis are discussed in Chapter 103.2. If infection is present, appropriate antibiotics must be started as soon as possible.

After supportive measures have stabilized the infant's condition, a specific diagnosis should be established and appropriate continuing treatment instituted.

PNEUMOTHORAX. Infants may develop a pneumothorax in the delivery room resulting in respiratory distress and hypoxia. Approximately 1–2 % of infants develop a pneumothorax after birth; only 0.05–0.07% have symptoms (Chapter 101.13). The risk is higher in infants requiring positive pressure ventilation or those with meconium-stained amniotic fluid. Rarely, an infant has a congenital malformation that results in lung hypoplasia, such as congenital diaphragmatic hernia or renal agenesis. Clinically, the infant develops respiratory distress and has diminished breath sounds on the affected side. Transillumination may be helpful to confirm the diagnosis, particularly in the LBW infant. Emergent evacuation of a pneumothorax without x-ray confirmation is indicated in an infant who is unresponsive to resuscitation efforts, has asymmetric breath sounds, bradycardia, and cyanosis. A 23-gauge butterfly needle or Angiocath attached to a stopcock and syringe should be inserted perpendicular to the chest wall above the rib in the 4th intercostal space at the level of the nipple (Fig. 100-3). The air is evacuated. The catheter is then inserted with constant negative pressure and the air is then evacuated.

AIRWAY OBSTRUCTION. Critical fetal and then neonatal airway obstruction presents an emergency in the delivery room. The ex utero intrapartum treatment procedure (**EXIT procedure**) allows time to secure the airway in infants known to have airway obstruction for a variety of causes including laryngeal atresia or stenosis, teratomas, hydromas, and oral tumors before the infants are separated from the placenta. Uteroplacental gas exchange is maintained throughout the procedure. High risk perinatal care has led to more frequent prenatal diagnosis of many disorders known to cause critical airway obstruction (Fig. 100-4).

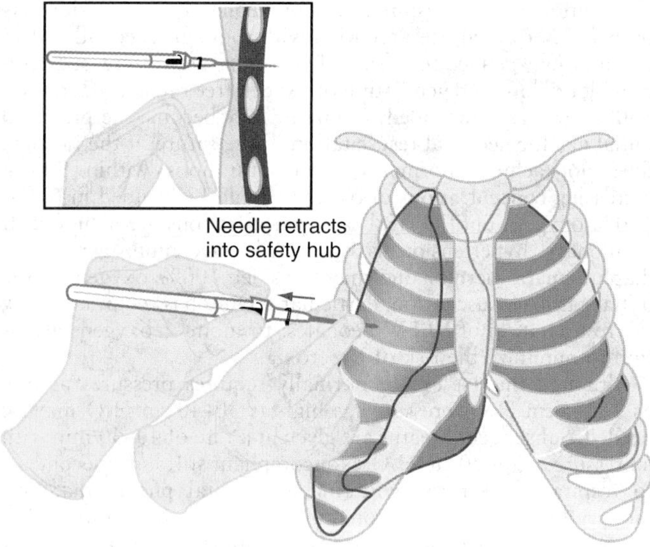

Figure 100-3. Decompression of a pneumothorax. (From Kattwinkel J, Bloom RS [eds]: *Neonatal Resuscitation Textbook*, 5th ed. Elk Grove, IL, American Academy of Pediatrics, American Heart Association, 2006.)

ABDOMINAL WALL DEFECTS. Appropriate management of patients with abdominal wall defects (omphalocele, gastroschisis) in the delivery room prevents excessive fluid loss and minimizes the risk for injury to the exposed viscera. Gastroschisis is the more common defect and typically is not covered by a membrane. The exposed intestines should be gently placed in a sterile clear plastic bag after delivery. A membrane often covers an omphalocele and care should be taken to prevent rupture. Infants should be transferred to a tertiary referral center for surgical consultation and evaluation for other associated anomalies (see Chapter 105).

INJURY DURING DELIVERY

CENTRAL NERVOUS SYSTEM. See Chapter 99.

VISCERA. The **liver** is the only internal organ other than the brain that is injured with any frequency during the delivery process. Damage usually results from pressure on the liver during delivery of the head in breech presentations. Large infant size, intrauterine asphyxia, coagulation disorders, extreme prematurity, and hepatomegaly are contributing factors. Incorrect cardiac massage is a less frequent cause. Hepatic rupture may result in the formation of a **subcapsular hematoma,** but the capsule may tamponade further bleeding. Infants may appear normal for the 1st 1–3 days. Nonspecific signs related to loss of blood into the hematoma may appear early and include poor feeding, listlessness, pallor, jaundice, tachypnea, and tachycardia. A mass may be palpable in the right upper quadrant, and the abdomen may appear blue. The hematoma may be large enough to cause anemia. Shock and death may occur if the hematoma ruptures into the peritoneal cavity, where the reduced pressure may allow fresh hemorrhage. Early suspicion, ultrasonographic diagnosis, and prompt supportive therapy can decrease the mortality associated with this disorder. Surgical repair of a laceration may be required. Rupture of the spleen may occur alone or in connection with rupture of the liver. The causes, complications, treatment, and prevention are similar.

Although adrenal hemorrhage occurs with some frequency, especially after breech delivery, in infants large for gestational age or infants of diabetic mothers, its cause is often undetermined; it may be due to trauma, anoxia, or severe stress, as in overwhelming infection. Ninety per cent are unilateral; 75% are right-

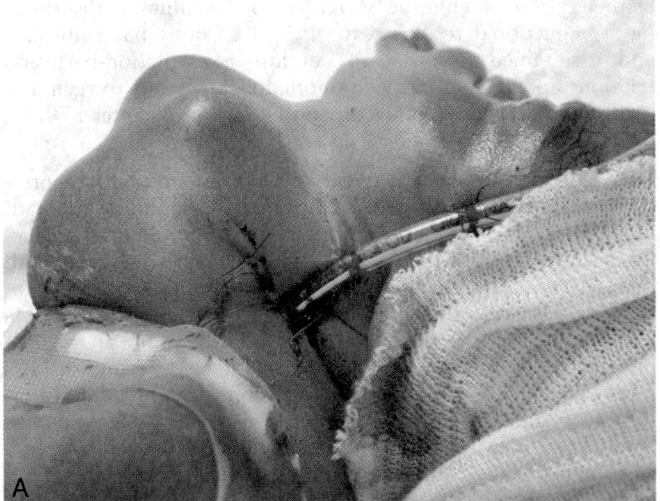

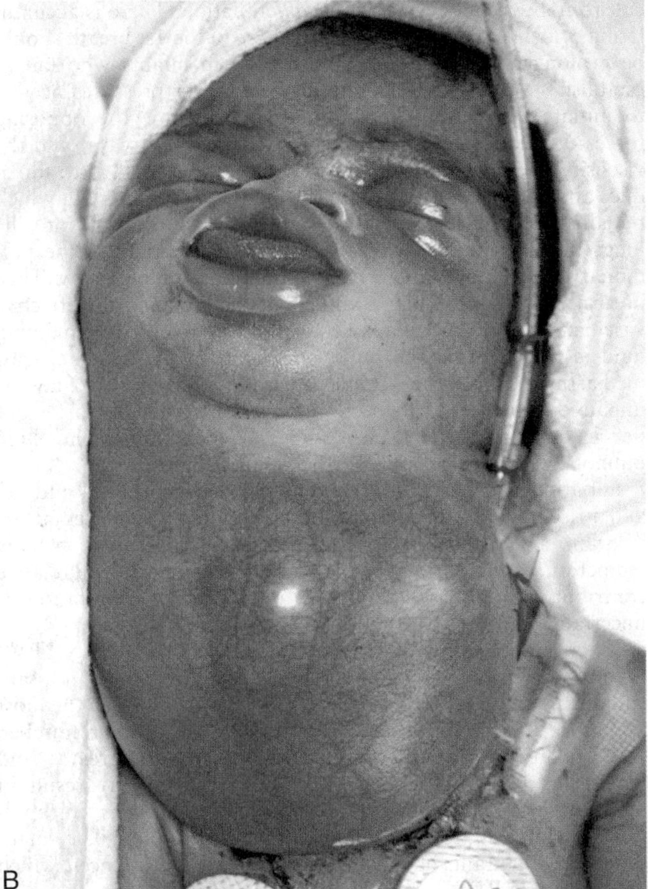

Figure 100-4. EXIT procedure. Baby with teratoma and critical airway obstruction. Trachea displaced to the lateral neck. (Photograph compliments of Dr. Mark Wulkan, pediatric surgeon at Emory University.)

sided. Calcified central hematomas of the adrenal, identified by x-ray or autopsy in older infants and children, suggest that not all adrenal hemorrhages are immediately fatal. In severe cases, the diagnosis is usually made at postmortem examination. The symptoms are profound shock and cyanosis. A mass may be present in the flank along with overlying skin discoloration; jaundice may also develop. If adrenal hemorrhage is suspected, abdominal ultrasonography may be helpful, and treatment of acute adrenal failure may be indicated (Chapter 576).

FRACTURES

Clavicle. The clavicle is fractured during labor and delivery more frequently than any other bone; it is particularly vulnerable with difficult delivery of the shoulder in vertex presentations and the extended arms in breech deliveries. The infant characteristically does not move the arm freely on the affected side; crepitus and bony irregularity may be palpated, and discoloration is occasionally visible over the fracture site. The Moro reflex is absent on the affected side, and spasm of the sternocleidomastoid muscle with obliteration of the supraclavicular depression at the site of the fracture can be noted. Infants with greenstick fractures may not have any limitation of movement, and the Moro reflex may be present. The prognosis is excellent. **Treatment,** if any, consists of immobilization of the arm and shoulder on the affected side. A remarkable degree of palpable callus develops at the site within a week and may be the initial evidence of the fracture. Fracture of the humerus or brachial palsy may also be responsible for limitation of movement of an arm and absence of a Moro reflex on the affected side.

Extremities. In fractures of the long bones, spontaneous movement of the extremity is usually absent (pseudoparalysis). The Moro reflex is often absent from the involved extremity. Associated nerve involvement may occur. Satisfactory results of treatment of a fractured humerus are obtained with 2–4 wk of immobilization during which the arm is strapped to the chest, a triangular splint and a Velpeau bandage are applied, or a cast is applied. For fracture of the femur, good results are achieved with traction-suspension of both lower extremities, even if the fracture is unilateral; the legs are immobilized in a spica cast. Splints are effective for treatment of fractures of the forearm or leg. Healing is usually accompanied by excess callus formation. The prognosis is excellent for fractures of the extremities. Fractures in VLBW infants may be related to osteopenia (Chapter 106).

Dislocations and epiphyseal separations rarely result from birth trauma. The upper femoral epiphysis may be separated by forcible manipulation of the infant's leg as, for example, in breech extraction or after version. The affected leg shows swelling, slight shortening, limitation of active motion, painful passive motion, and external rotation. The diagnosis is established roentgenographically. The prognosis is good for milder injuries, but coxa vara frequently results from extensive displacement.

Nose. The most prevalent injury to the nose is dislocation of the cartilaginous portion of the septum from the vomerine groove and the columella. The infant may have difficulty nursing and some impairment of nasal respiration. On physical examination, the nares appear asymmetric and the nose flattened. An oral airway is rarely needed, and surgical consultation should be obtained for definitive treatment.

American Heart Association, American Academy of Pediatrics: 2005 American Heart Association (AHA) guidelines for cardiopulmonary resuscitation (CPR) and emergency cardiovascular care (ECC) of pediatric and neonatal patients: neonatal resuscitation guidelines. *Pediatrics* 2006;117:e1029–e1038.

Carrasco M, Martell M, Estol PC: Oronasopharyngeal suction at birth: Effects on arterial oxygen saturation. *J Pediatr* 1997;130:832–834.

Davis PG, Tan A, O'Donnell CPF, Schulze A: Resuscitation of newborn infants with 100% oxygen or air: A systematic review and meta-analysis. *Lancet* 2004;364:1329–1333.

DeBacker A, Madern GC, Van de Ven CP, et al: Strategy for management of newborns with cervical teratoma. *J Perinat Med* 2004;32:500–508.

Gunn AJ, Bennet L: Is temperature important in delivery room resuscitation? *Semin Neonatol* 2001;6:241–249.

Hansmann G: Neonatal resuscitation on air: Is it time to turn down the oxygen tanks? *Lancet* 2004;364:1293–1294.

Hirose S, Farmer DL, Lee H, et al: The ex utero intrapartum treatment procedure: Looking back at the EXIT. *J Pediatr Surg* 2004;39:375–380.

Lindner W, Vofsbeck S, Hummler H, et al: Delivery room management of extremely low birth weight infants: Spontaneous breathing or intubation? *Pediatrics* 1999;103:961–967.

Niermeyer S, Kattwinkel J, Van Reempts P, et al: International guidelines for neonatal resuscitation: An excerpt from the Guidelines 2000 for Cardiopulmonary Resuscitation and Emergency Cardiovascular Care: International Consensus on Science. *Pediatrics* 2000;106:E29.
Paneth N: The evidence mounts against use of pure oxygen in newborn resuscitation. *J Pediatr* 2005;147:4–6.
Shih JC, Hsu WC, Chou HC, et al: Prenatal three-dimensional ultrasound and magnetic resonance imaging evaluation of a fetal oral tumor in preparation for the ex-utero intrapartum treatment (EXIT) procedure. *Ultrasound Obstet Gynecol* 2005;25:76–79.
Wolkoff LI, Davis JM: Delivery room resuscitation of the newborn. *Clin Perinatol* 1999;26:641–658.

Chapter 101 ■ Respiratory Tract Disorders

Golde G. Dudell and Barbara J. Stoll

Respiratory disorders are the most frequent cause of admission for neonatal intensive care in both term and preterm infants. Signs and symptoms include cyanosis, grunting, nasal flaring, retractions, tachypnea, decreased breath sounds with rales and/or rhonchi, pallor, and apnea. A wide variety of pathologic lesions may be responsible for respiratory disturbances (see Tables 98-1 and 98-2), including hyaline membrane disease (HMD; respiratory distress syndrome [RDS]), aspiration (meconium or amniotic fluid) syndrome, pneumonia, sepsis, congenital heart disease, heart failure, pulmonary hypertension, choanal atresia, hypoglycemia, hypoplasia of the mandible with posterior displacement of the tongue, macroglossia, malformation of the epiglottis, malformation or injury of the larynx, cysts or neoplasms of the larynx or chest, pneumothorax, lobar emphysema, pulmonary sequestration, cystic adenomatoid malformations, pulmonary agenesis or hypoplasia, congenital pulmonary lymphangiectasis, tracheoesophageal fistula, avulsion of the phrenic nerve, hernia or eventration of the diaphragm, intracranial lesions, neuromuscular disorders, and metabolic disturbances.

It is occasionally difficult to distinguish respiratory from cardiovascular causes or sepsis on the basis of clinical signs alone. Any sign of postnatal respiratory distress is an indication for immediate examination and diagnostic evaluation, including a blood gas or pulse oximetry determination and x-ray of the chest. Timely and appropriate therapy is essential to prevent ongoing injury and improve outcome. As a result of important advances in understanding the pathophysiology of respiratory disease, neonatal and infant deaths from early respiratory disease have declined markedly. The challenge is not only to continue to improve survival, but also to reduce short- and long-term complications related to early lung disease.

101.1 • Transition to Pulmonary Respiration

Successful establishment of adequate lung function at birth is dependent on airway patency, functional lung development, and maturity of respiratory control. Fetal lung fluid must be removed and replaced with gas. This process begins before birth as active sodium transport across the pulmonary epithelium drives liquid from the lung lumen into the interstitium with subsequent absorption into the vasculature. Increased levels of circulating catecholamines, vasopressin, prolactin, and glucocorticoids enhance lung fluid adsorption and trigger the change in lung epithelia from a chloride secretory to a sodium reabsorptive mode. Functional residual capacity (FRC) must be established and maintained in order to develop a ventilation-perfusion relationship that will provide optimal exchange of oxygen and carbon dioxide between alveoli and blood (see Chapter 370).

THE 1ST BREATH. During vaginal delivery, intermittent compression of the thorax facilitates removal of lung fluid. Surfactant lining the alveoli enhances the aeration of gas-free lungs by reducing surface tension, thereby lowering the pressure required to open alveoli. Although spontaneously breathing infants do not need to generate an opening pressure to create airflow, infants requiring positive pressure ventilation at birth require an opening pressure of 13–32 cm H_20 and are more likely to establish FRC if they generate a spontaneous, negative pressure breath. Expiratory esophageal pressures associated with the 1st few spontaneous breaths in term newborns range from 45 to 90 cm H_2O. This high pressure, due to expiration against a partially closed glottis, may aid in the establishment of FRC but would be difficult to mimic safely using artificial ventilation. There is accumulating evidence that the inspiratory phase of the 1st breath should be prolonged in order to establish FRC in infants who fail to establish spontaneous respirations. The higher pressures needed to initiate respiration are required to overcome the opposing forces of surface tension (particularly in small airways) and the viscosity of liquid remaining in the airways, as well as to introduce about 50 mL/kg of air into the lungs, 20–30 mL/kg of which remains after the 1st breath to establish FRC. Air entry into the lungs displaces fluid, decreases hydrostatic pressure in the pulmonary vasculature, and increases pulmonary blood flow. This, in turn, increases the blood volume of the lung and the effective vascular surface area available for fluid uptake. The remaining fluid is removed via the pulmonary lymphatics, upper airway, mediastinum, and the pleural space. Fluid removal may be impaired after cesarean section or as a result of surfactant deficiency, endothelial cell damage, hypoalbuminemia, high pulmonary venous pressure, or neonatal sedation.

Initiation of the 1st breath is due to a decline in $Pa{O_2}$ and pH and a rise in $Pa{CO_2}$ as a result of interruption of the placental circulation, a redistribution of cardiac output, a decrease in body temperature, and various tactile and sensory inputs. The relative contribution of these stimuli to the onset of respiration is uncertain.

When compared with term infants, low birthweight (LBW) infants who have a very compliant chest wall may be at a disadvantage in drawing the 1st breath. The FRC is lowest in the most immature infants because of the decrease in alveolar number. Abnormalities in ventilation-perfusion ratio are greater and persist for longer periods in LBW infants and may result in hypoxemia and hypercarbia as a result of atelectasis, intrapulmonary shunting, hypoventilation, and gas trapping. The smallest immature infants have the most profound disturbances, which may resemble RDS.

BREATHING PATTERNS IN NEWBORNS. During sleep in the 1st months of life, normal full-term infants may have infrequent episodes when regular breathing is interrupted by short pauses. This **periodic breathing** pattern, which shifts from a regular rhythmicity to cyclic brief episodes of intermittent apnea, is more common in premature infants, who may have apneic pauses of 5–10 sec followed by a burst of rapid respirations at a rate of 50–60/min for 10–15 sec. They rarely have an associated change in color or heart rate, and it often stops without apparent reason. Intermittent periodic breathing persists beyond 36 wks postconceptional age (PCA; gestational age at birth plus postnatal age) in the premature infant. The duration of periodic breathing, however, decreases between 33 and 35 wk PCA. If an infant is hypoxic, an increase in inspired oxygen concentration often converts periodic to regular breathing. Periodic breathing, a normal characteristic of neonatal respiration, has no prognostic significance.

Boon AW, Milner AD, Hopkin IE: Lung expansion, tidal exchange and formation of the functional residual capacity during resuscitation of asphyxiated neonates. *J Pediatr* 1979;95:1031–1036.
Jain L: Alveolar fluid clearance in developing lungs and its role in neonatal transition. *Clin Perinatol* 1999;26:585–599.
Saugstad OD: Oxygen saturations immediately after birth. *J Pediatr* 2006;148:569–570.
Saunders RA, Milner AD: Pulmonary pressure/volume relationships during the last phase of delivery and the first postnatal breaths in human subjects. *J Pediatr* 1979;93:667–673.
Venkatesh VC, Katzberg HD: Glucocorticoid regulation of epithelial sodium channel genes in human fetal lung. *Am J Physiol* 1997;273:L227–L233.
Vyas H, Field D, Milner AD, et al: Determinants of the first inspiratory volume and functional residual capacity at birth. *Pediatr Pulmonol* 1986;2:189–193.
Walker AM, Alcorn DG, Cannata JC, et al: Effect of ventilation on pulmonary blood volume of the fetal lamb. *J Appl Physiol* 1975;39:969–975.

101.2 • Apnea

Apnea is a common problem in preterm infants that may be due to prematurity or an associated illness. In term infants, apnea is always worrisome and demands immediate diagnostic evaluation. Periodic breathing must be distinguished from prolonged apneic pauses because the latter may be associated with serious illnesses. Apnea is a feature of many primary diseases that affect neonates (Table 101-1). These disorders produce apnea by direct depression of the central nervous system's control of respiration (hypoglycemia, meningitis, drugs, hemorrhage, seizures), disturbances in oxygen delivery (shock, sepsis, anemia), or ventilation defects (pneumonia, RDS, persistent pulmonary hypertension of the newborn [PPHN], muscle weakness).

Idiopathic apnea of prematurity occurs in the absence of identifiable predisposing diseases. Apnea is a disorder of respiratory control and may be obstructive, central, or mixed. **Obstructive apnea** (pharyngeal instability, neck flexion, nasal occlusion) is characterized by absent airflow but persistent chest wall motion. Pharyngeal collapse may follow the negative airway pressures generated during inspiration, or it may result from incoordination of the tongue and other upper airway muscles involved in maintaining airway patency. In **central apnea,** which is caused by decreased central nervous system (CNS) stimuli to respiratory muscles, airflow and chest wall motion are absent. Gestational age is the most important determinant of respiratory control, with the frequency of apnea being inversely related to gestational age. The immaturity of the brainstem respiratory centers is manifested by an attenuated response to carbon dioxide and a paradoxical response to hypoxia that results in apnea rather than hyperventilation. The most common pattern of idiopathic apnea in preterm neonates has a mixed etiology (50–75%), with obstructive apnea preceding (usually) or following central apnea. Short episodes of apnea are usually central, whereas prolonged ones are often mixed.

Apnea is sleep state dependent; the frequency increases during active (rapid eye movement) sleep. Paradoxical chest wall movement (inspiratory abdominal expansion and inward chest wall movement) is common during active sleep and may cause a fall in $Pa{O_2}$ because of ventilation-perfusion defects. Furthermore, increased negative pressure during paradoxical breathing and inhibition of pharyngeal muscle tone during active sleep may contribute to upper airway collapse and obstructive apnea.

TABLE 101-1. Potential Causes of Neonatal Apnea and Bradycardia

Central nervous system	Intraventricular hemorrhage, drugs, seizures, hypoxic injury, herniation, neuromuscular disorders, Leigh syndrome, brainstem infarction or anomalies (e.g., olivopontocerebellar atrophy), after general anesthesia
Respiratory	Pneumonia, obstructive airway lesions, upper airway collapse, atelectasis, extreme prematurity (<1,000 g), laryngeal reflex, phrenic nerve paralysis, severe hyaline membrane disease, pneumothorax, hypoxia
Infectious	Sepsis, necrotizing enterocolitis, meningitis (bacterial, fungal, viral), respiratory syncytial virus, pertussis
Gastrointestinal	Oral feeding, bowel movement, esophagitis, intestinal perforation
Metabolic	↓ Glucose, ↓ calcium, ↓/↑ sodium, ↑ ammonia, ↑ organic acids, ↑ ambient temperature, hypothermia
Cardiovascular	Hypotension, hypertension, heart failure, anemia, hypovolemia, vagal tone
Other	Immaturity of respiratory center, sleep state

CLINICAL MANIFESTATIONS. The incidence of idiopathic apnea of prematurity varies inversely with gestational age. In preterm infants, it is rare on the 1st day of life; apnea immediately after birth signifies another illness. The onset of idiopathic apnea occurs on the 2nd–7th day of life. In preterm infants, **serious apnea** is defined as cessation of breathing for longer than 20 sec, or any duration if accompanied by cyanosis and bradycardia. The incidence of associated bradycardia increases with the length of the preceding apnea and correlates with the severity of hypoxia. Short apnea episodes (10 sec) are rarely associated with bradycardia, whereas longer ones (>20 sec) have a higher incidence of bradycardia. Bradycardia follows the apnea by 1–2 sec in more than 95% of cases and is most often sinus, but on occasion can be nodal. Vagal responses and, rarely, heart block are causes of bradycardia without apnea.

TREATMENT. Infants at risk for apnea should be placed on cardiorespiratory monitors. Gentle tactile stimulation is often adequate therapy for mild and intermittent episodes. Infants with recurrent and prolonged apnea may require suctioning, repositioning, and bag and mask ventilation. Oxygen should be administered judiciously to treat hypoxia. The onset of apnea in a previously well premature neonate after the 2nd wk of life or in a term infant at any time is a critical event that warrants immediate investigation. Recurrent apnea of prematurity may be treated with theophylline or caffeine. Methylxanthines increase central respiratory drive by lowering the threshold of response to hypercarbia, as well as enhancing contractility of the diaphragm and preventing diaphragmatic fatigue. The specific effects appear to vary to some degree between theophylline and caffeine. Evidence suggests that **caffeine** is a more potent centrally acting respiratory agent with fewer side effects than theophylline. Loading doses of 5–7 mg/kg of theophylline (orally) or aminophylline (intravenously) should be followed by doses of 1–2 mg/kg given every 6–12 hr by the oral or intravenous routes. Loading doses of 20 mg/kg of **caffeine citrate** are followed 24 hr later by maintenance doses of 5 mg/kg/24 hr qd orally or intravenously. These doses should be monitored by observation of vital signs, clinical response, and serum drug levels (therapeutic levels: theophylline, 6–10 µg/mL; caffeine, 8–20 µg/mL). Caffeine may reduce the risk of BPD. Doxapram, known to be a potent respiratory stimulant, acts predominantly on peripheral chemoreceptors and has been used in neonates with apnea of prematurity, but has a limited therapeutic role due to side effects. Transfusion of packed red blood cells to reduce the incidence of idiopathic apnea is reserved for severely anemic infants. Gastroesophageal reflux may also occur in infants with apnea of prematurity. Data do not support a causal relationship between gastroesophageal reflux and apneic events or the use of antireflux medications to reduce the frequency of apnea in preterm infants.

Nasal continuous positive airway pressure (CPAP, 2–5 cm H_2O) and high-flow humidified nasal cannula (1–2.5 L/min) are effective therapies for mixed or obstructive apnea. The efficacy of CPAP is related to its ability to splint the upper airway and prevent airway obstruction.

PROGNOSIS. Unless severe, recurrent, and refractory to therapy, apnea of prematurity does not alter an infant's prognosis. Associated problems of intraventricular hemorrhage (IVH), bronchopulmonary dysplasia (BPD), and retinopathy of prematurity are critical in determining the prognosis for apneic infants. Apnea of prematurity usually resolves by 36 wk PCA and does not predict future episodes of sudden infant death syndrome. Some infants with persistent apnea are discharged as long as cardiorespiratory monitoring can be performed at home. In the absence of significant events, home monitoring can be safely discontinued after 43 wk PCA.

Arad-Cohen N, Cohen A, Tirosh E: The relationship between gastroesophageal reflux and apnea in infants. *J Pediatr* 2000;137:321–326.

Darnall RA, Kattwinkel J, Nattie C, et al: Margin of safety for discharge after apnea in preterm infants. *Pediatrics* 1997;100:795–801.

Eichenwald EC, Aina A, Stark AR: Apnea frequently persists beyond term gestation in infants delivered at 24 to 28 weeks. *Pediatrics* 1997;100: 354–359.

Eichenwald EC, Blackwell M, Lloyd JS, et al: Inter-neonatal intensive care unit variation in discharge timing: Influence of apnea and feeding management. *Pediatrics* 2001;108:928–933.

Finer NN, Barrington KJ: Doxapram and neurodevelopmental outcome. *J Pediatr* 2002;141:296.

Kimball AL, Carlton DP: Gastroesophageal reflux medications in the treatment of apnea in premature infants. *J Pediatr* 2001;138:355–360.

Peter CS, Sprodowski N, Bohnhorst B, et al: Gastroesophageal reflux and apnea prematurity: No temporal relationship. *Pediatrics* 2002;109:8–11.

Ramanathan R, Corwin MJ, Hunt CE, et al: Cardiorespiratory events recorded on home monitors: Comparison of healthy infants with those at increased risk for SIDS. *JAMA* 2001;285:2199–2207.

Schmidt B, Roberts RS, Davis P, et al: Caffeine therapy for apnea of prematurity. *N Engl J Med* 2006;354:2112–2120.

Sreenan C, Lemke RP, Hudson-Mason A, et al: High-flow nasal cannulae in the management of apnea of prematurity: A comparison with conventional nasal continuous positive airway pressure. *Pediatrics* 2001;107:1081–1083.

Sychowski SP, Dodd E, Thomas P, et al: Home apnea monitor use in preterm infants discharged from newborn intensive care units. *J Pediatr* 2001; 139:245–248.

Tauman R, Sivan Y: Duration of home monitoring for infants discharged with apnea of prematurity. *Biol Neonate* 2000;78:168–173.

101.3 • Congenital Central Hypoventilation Syndrome (Ondine Curse) • Gabriel G. Haddad

The typical presentation of children with congenital central hypoventilation syndrome (CCHS, or Ondine curse) occurs in the neonatal period. The initial symptoms include periods of cyanosis when the newborn falls asleep, with diminished chest excursions and prolonged periods of respiratory pauses, with symptoms disappearing when the infant is awakened. CCHS can mimic many diseases; hence, other diagnoses must be entertained before the diagnosis of CCHS is made. There are usually no detectable gross anatomic abnormalities, although brainstem tumors and arteriovenous malformations have been described and other neurologic diseases must be considered. The primary defect is in the CNS, but there may be abnormalities in other elements of the respiratory control system (carotid bodies, peripheral chemosensitivity).

PATHOGENESIS AND PATHOPHYSIOLOGY. The cause and pathogenesis of CCHS are unknown. There are a number of reports of familial cases. Segregation analysis among families of 50 patients with CCHS demonstrates that CCHS is familial. There is one case of transmission of mother to child. In spite of these studies, the specific mode of inheritance is still unknown. A rare association of Hirschsprung disease with Ondine curse (Haddad syndrome) was first described in 1978. It is because of this association with aganglionosis of the bowel that a number of candidate genes have been considered. In one such case, a missense mutation in exon 12 of the RET proto-oncogene has been reported. Endothelin signaling pathway mutations (endothelin receptor and endothelin 3 gene) are noted in a small proportion of patients with Hirschsprung disease. A mutation has also been identified in a glial-derived neurotrophic factor in a patient with CCHS and growth hormone deficiency. Analysis of PHOX2b gene reveals that more than 97% of probands are heterozygous for exon 3–polyalanine expansion mutation of PHOX2b and that the length of the expansion is associated with the severity of the CCHS disease. Case control family studies have also shown that CCHS patients, their parents, and relatives were more likely to be affected than controls and controls' parents in terms of an imbalance in the autonomic nervous system (ANS). The best-fitting genetic model of CCHS is that of a mendelian inheritance of a major gene disturbing the ANS.

Pathologic studies have also supported the idea that CCHS is a disease involving the autonomic nervous system. One patient had neuronal loss in reticular nuclei and the nucleus ambiguus, hypoglossal, and dorsal motoneurons of the vagus nerve. Small carotid bodies have also been seen in some patients with CCHS. Some physiologic studies have lent support for ANS involvement and have shown that the heart rate in these infants is rather fixed with little, if any, heart rate variability.

Patients with CCHS or CCHS with Hirschsprung disease have no carbon dioxide sensitivity and no ventilatory response to carbon dioxide during sleep. During wakefulness, the carbon dioxide set point is much lower, and they respond to it, unless the condition is severe enough for hypoventilation to occur even in the awake state. These children also have been shown to have no sensitivity to hypoxia. This lack of sensitivity to carbon dioxide and the respiratory failure do not improve with time, and the oldest patients with CCHS still show the same failures. Older children with CCHS show an increase in ventilation when they are exercised at various work rates, and the increase in ventilation they exhibit may not be related to anaerobic stimuli (lactate or pH), but rather to neural reflexes (limb movements) or hormonal cues.

In CCHS, the condition expresses itself best during sleep, at which time sensory feedback plays a relatively minor role. The defect may be in the automatic control system, which resides mostly in the brainstem. Although physiologic evidence indicates that the respiratory failure in these children is mostly based on defects in central mechanisms, rather than on peripheral (carotid) mechanisms, the interactions between peripheral and central mechanisms also may be important. It is also important that premotor neurons, which communicate with phrenic or intercostal motor neurons, can be excited enough to drive the respiratory musculature in certain instances (wakefulness).

On postmortem examination of some CCHS patients, absence of the arcuate nucleus has been seen, but the relation of this anomaly to the disease is not clear. Gliosis in brainstem structures has also been noted, but this could be part of a more generalized response of the CNS to hypoxia and ischemia resulting from long-term and intermittent respiratory failure.

CLINICAL MANIFESTATIONS. Patients with CCHS usually present in the 1st few hours after delivery. Most children are the products of uneventful pregnancies and are term infants with appropriate weight for gestational age; Apgar scores have been variable. Symptoms of respiratory failure, with slow and irregular respiratory efforts, long respiratory pauses (lasting up to 40 sec), and cyanosis, appear in the 1st day of life. Cardiac, respiratory, infectious, and metabolic diseases, including intrauterine drug exposure, should be ruled out. One hallmark of this condition is that patients fail to respire adequately during sleep, not during wakefulness, although children with the most severe respiratory failure may hypoventilate in the waking state as well. In most neonates with CCHS, the $Paco_2$ accumulates during sleep to very high levels, sometimes up to 80–90 mm Hg, and declines to normal levels soon after the infants awaken. CCHS infants have been shown to have long respiratory pauses, a relatively normal tidal volume, and a very low respiratory rate (declining to as low a level as 8–10 breaths/min during sleep) with interspersed respiratory pauses, starting in the 1st few days of life. Respiratory rates are generally normal during wakefulness, and the lowest respiratory rates have been found in non–rapid eye movement or quiet sleep. Often, the respiratory rate and the tidal volume are normal in REM sleep in these infants. In rare instances, older children have presented for the 1st time with CCHS. In these cases, one should consider the possibility that the case was rather mild and the diagnosis was missed in the nursery. Older children may manifest pulmonary hypertension, cyanosis, and digital clubbing. Alternatively, other diagnoses should be followed and potentially treated.

Because respiratory failure in these infants has a central cause, the hypoxemia that ensues is commensurate with hypoventilation with little or no abnormality in the arterial-alveolar (A-a) gradient. In some children, however, the hypoventilation may be severe enough to produce airway closure, microatelectasis, and an increase in the A-a gradient.

In a sizable subset of these infants, abdominal distention, constipation, or complete failure to pass meconium occurs. Rarely, a child with CCHS also has diagnosed Hirschsprung disease with variable aganglionosis of the colon and small intestine. Whether all patients with congenital CCHS have some degree of aganglionosis of the large bowel is unknown.

Patients with CCHS also have a faster heart rate than normal for their age and low heart rate variability, an almost fixed heart rate with little sinus arrhythmia. Other anomalies found on autopsy suggesting abnormalities in the autonomic regulation of vital functions include multiple ganglioneuroblastomas of the sympathetic chain and the adrenal medulla.

DIFFERENTIAL DIAGNOSIS. Other neurologic diseases or conditions have to be excluded before this diagnosis is made. Brainstem infarction, tumors, arteriovenous malformations, syringomyelia, Leigh necrotizing encephalomyelopathy, olivopontocerebellar degeneration, and Möbius syndrome should be considered. Fatty acid metabolic defects and carnitine deficiency are other diagnoses that can give similar symptoms and clinical presentation. Variables that can render the diagnosis difficult include asphyxia, infection, and trauma.

Detailed respiratory physiology and sleep recordings are a necessity when CCHS is in the differential diagnosis. O_2 saturation monitoring, ECG halter, chest x-ray, echocardiogram, fluoroscopy of the diaphragm, MRI of the brain and brainstem, serum and urinary carnitine, muscle biopsy, and a rectal biopsy are all indicated depending on the history, physical examination, clinical presentation, and hospital course.

TREATMENT. Management should include general and nutritional care, ventilatory support (prolonged support necessitating tracheostomy), and prevention of acidosis, cerebral hypoxia, and ischemia. Careful monitoring at all times, especially during sleep, is important to prevent hypoventilation and its consequences. Some of these infants can grow and gain developmental and neurologic milestones that are close to normal for age, although hypoventilation abnormalities can persist. These abnormalities may be a result of episodes of hypoxia or part of the spectrum of CCHS. Pharmacologic respiratory stimulation is unsuccessful. Cardiorespiratory monitoring is very important as ventilatory needs change with age and it is through this monitoring that appropriate needs are detected and therefore provided as these infants grow older.

Phrenic nerve pacing is used in patients after the age of 2 yr. Although there are complications related to pacing, including phrenic nerve fibrosis, infections, and multiple surgeries, a number of these patients have eventually become independent of mechanical ventilators.

Bolk S, Angrist M, Schwartz S, et al: Congenital central hypoventilation syndrome mutation analysis of the receptor tyrosine kinase RET. *Am J Med Genet* 1996;63:603–609.

Croaker GD, Shi E, Simpson E, et al: Congenital central hypoventilation syndrome and Hirschsprung's disease. *Arch Dis Child* 1998;78:316–322.

Haddad GG, Mazza NM, Defendini R, et al: Congenital failure of automatic control of ventilation, gastrointestinal motility and heart rate. *Medicine (Baltimore)* 1978;57:517–526.

Marazita ML, Maher BS, Cooper ME, et al: Genetic segregation analysis of autonomic nervous system dysfunction in families of probands with idiopathic congenital central hypoventilation syndrome. *Am J Med Genet* 2001;100:229–236.

Mellins RB, Balfour HH Jr, Turino GM, et al: Failure of automatic control of ventilation (Ondine's curse): Report of an infant born with this syndrome and review of the literature. *Medicine (Baltimore)* 1970;49:487–504.

Sakai T, Wakizaka A, Matsuda H, et al: Point mutation in exon 12 of the receptor tyrosine kinase proto-oncogene RET in Ondine-Hirschsprung syndrome. *Pediatrics* 1998;101:924–926.

Shahar E, Shinawi M: Neurocristopathies presenting with neurologic abnormalities associated with Hirschsprung's disease. *Pediatr Neurol* 2003;28:385–391.

Verloes A, Elmer C, Lacombe D, et al: Ondine-Hirschsprung syndrome (Haddad syndrome): Further delineation in two cases and review of the literature. *Eur J Pediatr* 1993;152:75–77.

Weese-Mayer DE, Berry-Kravis EM, Zhou L, et al: Idiopathic congenital central hypoventilation syndrome:Aanalysis of genes pertinent to early autonomic nervous system embryologic development and identification of mutations in PHOX2b. *Am J Med Genet* 2003;123:267–278.

Weese-Mayer DE, Bolk S, Silvestri JM, et al: Idiopathic congenital central hypoventilation syndrome: Evaluation of brain-derived neurotrophic factor genomic DNA sequence variation. *Am J Med Genet* 2002;107:306–310.

101.4 • Respiratory Distress Syndrome (Hyaline Membrane Disease)

INCIDENCE. RDS occurs primarily in premature infants; its incidence is inversely related to gestational age and birthweight. It occurs in 60–80% of infants less than 28 wk of gestational age, in 15–30% of those between 32 and 36 wk, in about 5% beyond 37 wk, and rarely at term. The risk of developing RDS increases with maternal diabetes, multiple births, cesarean section delivery, precipitous delivery, asphyxia, cold stress, and a history of previously affected infants. The incidence is highest in preterm male or white infants. The risk of RDS is reduced in pregnancies with chronic or pregnancy-associated hypertension, maternal heroin use, prolonged rupture of membranes, and antenatal corticosteroid prophylaxis.

ETIOLOGY AND PATHOPHYSIOLOGY. Surfactant deficiency (decreased production and secretion) is the primary cause of RDS. The failure to attain an adequate FRC and the tendency of affected lungs to become atelectatic correlate with high surface tension and the absence of pulmonary surfactant. The major

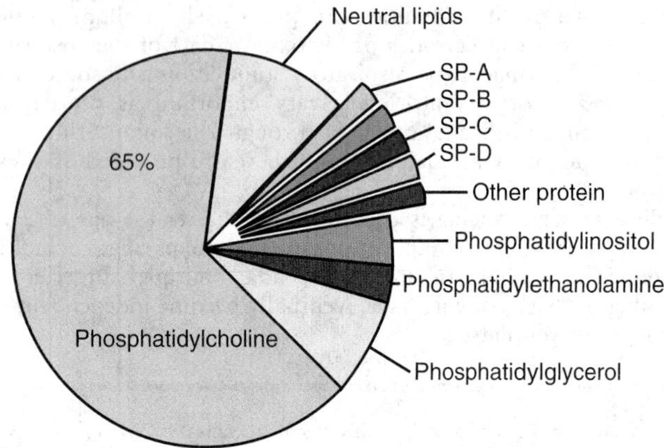

Figure 101-1. Composition of surfactant recovered by alveolar wash. The quantities of the different components are similar for surfactant from the mature lungs of mammals. (From Jobe AH: Fetal lung development, tests for maturation, induction of maturation, and treatment. In Creasy RK, Resnick R [eds]: *Maternal-Fetal Medicine: Principles and Practice,* 3rd ed. Philadelphia, WB Saunders, 1994.)

constituents of surfactant are dipalmitoyl phosphatidylcholine (lecithin), phosphatidylglycerol, apoproteins (surfactant proteins SP-A, -B, -C, -D), and cholesterol (Fig. 101-1). With advancing gestational age, increasing amounts of phospholipids are synthesized and stored in type II alveolar cells (Fig. 101-2). These surface-active agents are released into the alveoli, where they reduce surface tension and help maintain alveolar stability by preventing the collapse of small air spaces at end-expiration. The amounts produced or released may be insufficient to meet postnatal demands because of immaturity. Surfactant is present in high concentrations in fetal lung homogenates by 20 wk of gestation, but it does not reach the surface of the lungs until later. It appears in amniotic fluid between 28 and 32 wk. Mature levels of pulmonary surfactant are usually present after 35 wk. Though rare, genetic disorders may contribute to respiratory distress. Abnormalities in surfactant protein B and C genes as well as a gene responsible for transporting surfactant across membranes (ABC transporter 3 *[ABCA3]*) are associated with severe and often lethal familial respiratory disease. Other familial causes of respiratory distress (not RDS) include alveolar capillary dysplasia, acinar dysplasia, pulmonary lymphangiectasia, and mucopolysaccharidosis.

Synthesis of surfactant depends in part on normal pH, temperature, and perfusion. Asphyxia, hypoxemia, and pulmonary ischemia, particularly in association with hypovolemia, hypotension, and cold stress, may suppress surfactant synthesis. The epithelial lining of the lungs may also be injured by high oxygen concentrations and the effects of respirator management, thereby resulting in a further reduction in surfactant.

Alveolar atelectasis, hyaline membrane formation, and interstitial edema make the lungs less compliant, so greater pressure is required to expand the alveoli and small airways. In affected infants, the lower part of the chest wall is pulled in as the diaphragm descends, and intrathoracic pressure becomes negative, thus limiting the amount of intrathoracic pressure that can be produced; the result is the development of atelectasis. The highly compliant chest wall of preterm infants offers less resistance than that of mature infants to the natural tendency of the lungs to collapse. Thus, at end-expiration, the volume of the thorax and lungs tends to approach residual volume, and atelectasis may develop.

Deficient synthesis or release of surfactant, together with small respiratory units and a compliant chest wall, produces atelectasis and results in perfused but not ventilated alveoli, which causes **hypoxia.** Decreased lung compliance, small tidal volumes, increased physiologic dead space, increased work of breathing, and insufficient alveolar ventilation eventually result in **hypercapnia.** The combination of hypercapnia, hypoxia, and acidosis produces pulmonary arterial vasoconstriction with increased right-to-left shunting through the foramen ovale and ductus arteriosus and within the lung itself. Pulmonary blood flow is reduced, and ischemic injury to the cells producing surfactant and to the vascular bed results in an effusion of proteinaceous material into the alveolar spaces (Fig. 101-3).

PATHOLOGY. The lungs appear deep purplish red and are liverlike in consistency. Microscopically, extensive atelectasis with engorgement of the interalveolar capillaries and lymphatics can be observed. A number of the alveolar ducts, alveoli, and respiratory bronchioles are lined with acidophilic, homogeneous, or granular membranes. Amniotic debris, intra-alveolar hemorrhage, and interstitial emphysema are additional but inconstant findings; interstitial emphysema may be marked when an infant has been ventilated. The characteristic hyaline membranes are rarely seen in infants dying earlier than 6–8 hr after birth.

CLINICAL MANIFESTATIONS. Signs of RDS usually appear within minutes of birth, although they may not be recognized for several hours in larger premature infants until rapid, shallow respirations have increased to 60/min or greater. A late onset of tachypnea should suggest other conditions. Some patients require resuscitation at birth because of intrapartum asphyxia or initial severe

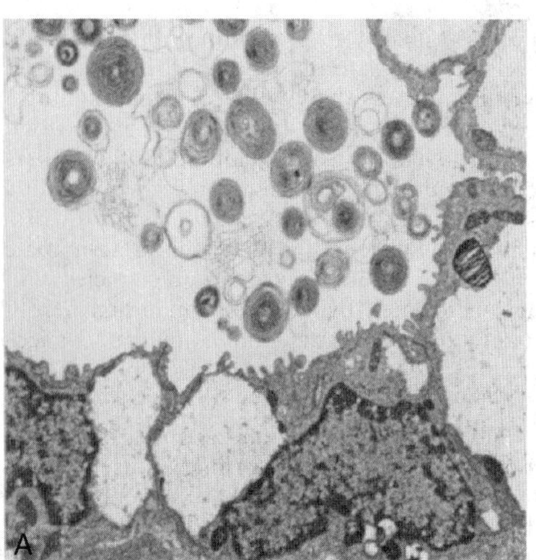

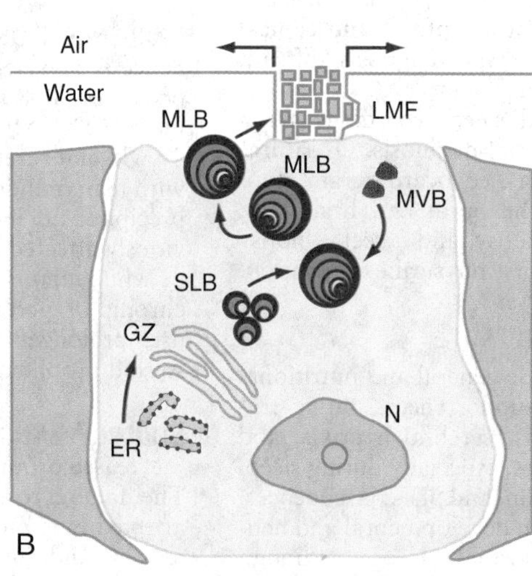

Figure 101-2. *A,* Fetal rat lung (low magnification), day 20 (term, day 22) showing developing type II cells, stored glycogen *(pale areas),* secreted lamellar bodies, and tubular myelin. (Courtesy of Mary Williams, MD, University of California, San Francisco.) *B,* Possible pathway for transport, secretion, and reuptake of surfactant. ER, endoplasmic reticulum; GZ, Golgi zone; LMF, lattic (tubular) myelin figure; MLB, mature lamellar body; MVB, multivesicular body; N, nucleus; SLB, small lamellar body. (From Hansen T, Corbet A: Lung development and function. In Taeusch HW, Ballard RA, Avery MA [eds]: *Schaffer and Avery's Diseases of the Newborn,* 6th ed. Philadelphia, WB Saunders, 1991.)

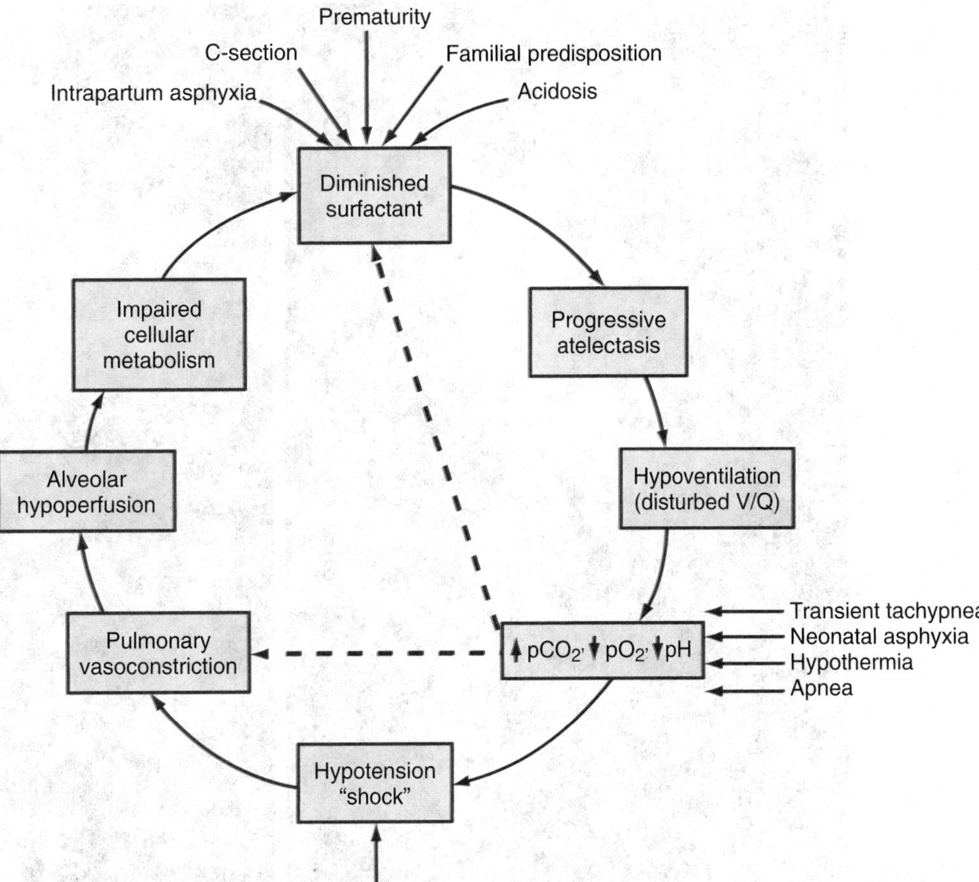

Figure 101-3. Contributing factors in the pathogenesis of hyaline membrane disease. The potential "vicious circle" perpetuated hypoxia and pulmonary insufficiency. (From Farrell P, Zachman R: In Quilligan EJ, Kretchmer N [eds]: *Fetal and Maternal Medicine.* New York, John Wiley, 1980. Reprinted by permission of John Wiley and Sons, Inc.)

respiratory distress (especially with a birthweight <1,000 g). Characteristically, tachypnea, prominent (often audible) grunting, intercostal and subcostal retractions, nasal flaring, and duskiness are noted. Cyanosis increases and is often relatively unresponsive to oxygen administration. Breath sounds may be normal or diminished with a harsh tubular quality and, on deep inspiration, fine rales may be heard, especially posteriorly over the lung bases. The natural course of untreated RDS is characterized by progressive worsening of cyanosis and dyspnea. If the condition is inadequately treated, blood pressure may fall; fatigue, cyanosis, and pallor increase, and grunting decreases or disappears as the condition worsens. Apnea and irregular respirations occur as infants tire and are ominous signs requiring immediate intervention. Patients may also have a mixed respiratory-metabolic acidosis, edema, ileus, and oliguria. Respiratory failure may occur in infants with rapid progression of the disease. In most cases, the symptoms and signs reach a peak within 3 days, after which improvement is gradual. Improvement is often heralded by spontaneous diuresis and the ability to oxygenate the infant at lower inspired oxygen levels or lower ventilator pressures. Death is rare on the 1st day of illness, usually occurs between days 2 and 7, and is associated with alveolar air leaks (interstitial emphysema, pneumothorax), pulmonary hemorrhage, or IVH. Mortality may be delayed weeks or months if BPD develops in mechanically ventilated infants with severe RDS.

DIAGNOSIS. The clinical course, x-ray of the chest, and blood gas and acid-base values help establish the clinical diagnosis. On x-ray, the lungs may have a characteristic, but not pathognomonic appearance that includes a fine reticular granularity of the parenchyma and air bronchograms, which are often more prominent early in the left lower lobe because of superimposition of the cardiac shadow (Fig. 101-4). The initial roentgenogram is occasionally normal, with the typical pattern developing at 6–12 hr. Considerable variation in films may be seen, depending on the phase of respiration and the use of CPAP or positive end-expiratory pressure (PEEP); this variation often results in poor correlation between roentgenograms and the clinical course. Laboratory findings are initially characterized by hypoxemia and later by progressive hypoxemia, hypercapnia, and variable metabolic acidosis.

In the **differential diagnosis,** early-onset sepsis may be indistinguishable from RDS. In pneumonia manifested at birth, the chest roentgenogram may be identical to that for RDS. Maternal group B streptococcal colonization, organisms on Gram stain of gastric or tracheal aspirates or a buffy coat smear, and/or the presence of marked neutropenia may suggest the diagnosis of early-onset sepsis. Cyanotic heart disease (total anomalous pulmonary venous return) can also mimic RDS both clinically and radiographically. Echocardiography with color flow imaging should be performed in infants who fail to respond to surfactant replacement to rule out cyanotic congenital heart disease as well as ascertain patency of the ductus arteriosus and assess pulmonary vascular resistance. Persistent pulmonary hypertension, aspiration (meconium, amniotic fluid) syndromes, spontaneous pneumothorax, pleural effusions, and congenital anomalies such as cystic adenomatoid malformation, pulmonary lymphangiectasia, diaphragmatic hernia, and lobar emphysema must be considered, but can generally be differentiated from RDS by roentgenographic evaluation. Transient tachypnea may be distinguished by its short and mild clinical course. Congenital alveolar proteinosis (congenital surfactant protein B deficiency) is a rare familial disease that manifests as severe and lethal RDS in predominantly term and near-term infants (see Chapter 404). In

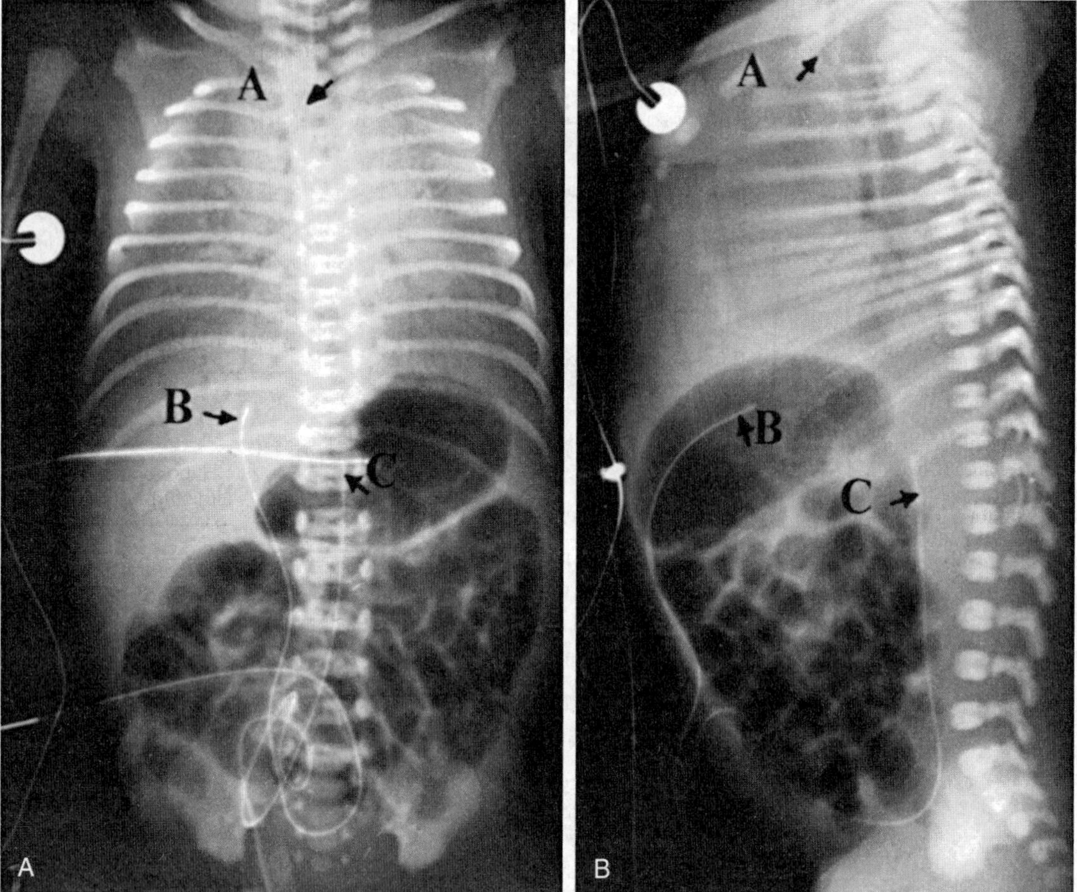

Figure 101-4. Infant with respiratory distress syndrome. Note the granular lungs, air bronchogram, and air-filled esophagus. Anteroposterior *(A)* and lateral *(B)* roentgenograms are needed to distinguish the umbilical artery from the vein catheter and to determine the appropriate level of insertion. The lateral view clearly shows that the catheter has been inserted into an umbilical vein and is lying in the portal system of the liver. *A* is the endotracheal tube; *B* is the umbilical venous catheter at the junction of the umbilical vein, ductus venosus, and portal vein; *C* is the umbilical artery catheter passed up the aorta to T12. (Courtesy of Walter E. Berdon, Babies Hospital, New York City.)

atypical cases of RDS, a lung profile (lecithin:sphingomyelin ratio and phosphatidylglycerol level) performed on a tracheal aspirate can be helpful in establishing a diagnosis of surfactant deficiency.

PREVENTION. Avoidance of unnecessary or poorly timed cesarean section, appropriate management of high-risk pregnancy and labor, and prediction and possible in utero acceleration of pulmonary immaturity (see Chapter 96) are important preventive strategies. In timing cesarean section or induction of labor, estimation of fetal head circumference by ultrasonography and determination of the lecithin concentration in amniotic fluid by the lecithin:sphingomyelin ratio (particularly useful with phosphatidylglycerol in diabetic pregnancies) decrease the likelihood of delivering a premature infant. Antenatal and intrapartum fetal monitoring may similarly decrease the risk of fetal asphyxia; asphyxia is associated with an increased incidence and severity of RDS.

Administration of betamethasone to women 48 hr before the delivery of fetuses between 24 and 34 wk of gestation significantly reduces the incidence, mortality, and morbidity of RDS. Corticosteroid administration is recommended for all women in preterm labor (24–34 wk gestation) who are likely to deliver a fetus within 1 wk. Repeated weekly doses of betamethasone until 32 wk may reduce neonatal morbidities and the duration of mechanical ventilation. Prenatal glucocorticoid therapy decreases the severity of RDS and reduces the incidence of other complications of prematurity, such as IVH, patent ductus arteriosus (PDA), pneumothorax, and necrotizing enterocolitis, without adversely affecting postnatal growth, lung mechanics or development, or the incidence of infection. Prenatal glucocorticoids may act synergistically with postnatal exogenous surfactant therapy. Prenatal dexamethasone may be associated with a higher incidence of periventricular leukomalacia than betamethasone. The relative risk of RDS, IVH and death is higher with antenatal dexamethasone treatment when compared with betamethasone.

Administration of a 1st dose of surfactant into the trachea of symptomatic premature infants immediately after birth (prophylactic) or during the 1st few hours of life (early rescue) reduces air leak and mortality from RDS, but does not alter the incidence of BPD.

TREATMENT. The basic defect requiring treatment is inadequate pulmonary exchange of oxygen and carbon dioxide; metabolic acidosis and circulatory insufficiency are secondary manifestations. Early supportive care of LBW infants, especially in the treatment of acidosis, hypoxia, hypotension (see Chapter 98), and hypothermia may lessen the severity of RDS. Therapy requires careful and frequent monitoring of heart and respiratory rates, oxygen saturation, PaO_2, $PaCO_2$, pH, bicarbonate, electrolytes, blood glucose, hematocrit, blood pressure, and temperature. Arterial catheterization is frequently necessary. Because most cases of RDS are self-limited, the goal of treatment is to minimize abnormal physiologic variations and superimposed iatrogenic problems. Treatment of these infants is best carried out in a specially staffed and equipped hospital unit, the neonatal intensive care unit (NICU).

The general principles for supportive care of any LBW infant should be adhered to, including developmental care and scheduled "touch times." To avoid hypothermia and minimize oxygen consumption, infants should be placed in an isolette or radiant warmer and core temperature maintained between 36.5 and 37°C (see Chapters 97 and 98). Use of an isolette is preferable in very low birthweight (VLBW) infants due to the high insensible water losses associated with radiant heat. Calories and fluids should initially be provided intravenously. For the 1st 24 hr, 10% glucose and water should be infused through a peripheral vein at a rate of 65–75 mL/kg/24 hr. Subsequently, electrolytes should be added and fluid volume increased gradually. Excessive fluids (>140 cc/kg/day) contribute to the development of PDA and BPD.

Warm humidified oxygen should be provided at a concentration initially sufficient to keep arterial levels between 50 and 70 mm Hg (85–95% saturation) to maintain normal tissue oxygenation while minimizing the risk of oxygen toxicity. If the PaO_2 cannot be maintained above 50 mm Hg at inspired oxygen concentrations of 60% or greater, applying CPAP at a pressure of 5–10 cm H_2O by nasal prongs is indicated and usually produces a sharp rise in PaO_2. Early use of CPAP for stabilization of at-risk VLBW infants beginning in the delivery room is also common. CPAP prevents collapse of surfactant-deficient alveoli, improves FRC, and improves ventilation-perfusion matching. Another approach is to intubate the VLBW infant, administer intratracheal surfactant, and then extubate to CPAP. The amount of CPAP required usually decreases abruptly at about 72 hr of age, and infants can be weaned from CPAP shortly thereafter. If an infant managed by CPAP cannot maintain an arterial oxygen tension above 50 mm Hg while breathing 70–100% oxygen, assisted ventilation is required.

Infants with severe RDS and those with complications that result in persistent apnea require assisted mechanical ventilation. Reasonable indications for its use are (1) arterial blood pH < 7.20, (2) arterial blood PCO_2 of 60 mm Hg or higher, (3) arterial blood PO_2 of 50 mm Hg or less at oxygen concentrations of 70–100% and CPAP of 6–10 cm H_2O, or (4) persistent apnea. Intermittent positive pressure ventilation delivered by time-cycled, pressure-limited, continuous flow ventilators is a common method of conventional ventilation for newborns. Other methods of conventional ventilation include synchronized intermittent mandatory ventilation (the set rate and pressure synchronized with the patient's own breaths), pressure support (the patient triggers each breath and a set pressure is delivered), and volume guarantee (a mode in which a specific tidal volume is set and the pressure delivered varies). Assisted ventilation for infants with RDS should always include PEEP (see Chapter 70). When using high ventilatory rates in a mode without inspiratory flow termination, care should be taken to avoid the administration of inadvertent PEEP.

The **goals of mechanical ventilation** are to improve oxygenation and elimination of carbon dioxide without causing pulmonary barotrauma or oxygen toxicity. Acceptable ranges of blood gas values, after balancing the risks of hypoxia and acidosis against those of mechanical ventilation, vary between institutions and range between a PaO_2 of 50–70 mm Hg, a $PaCO_2$ of 45–65 mm Hg, and a pH of 7.20–7.35. During mechanical ventilation, **oxygenation** is improved by increasing either the FIO_2 or the mean airway pressure. The latter can be increased by increasing the peak inspiratory pressure, gas flow, the inspiratory:expiratory ratio, or PEEP. Excessive PEEP may impede venous return, thereby reducing cardiac output and decreasing oxygen delivery despite improvement in PaO_2. PEEP levels of 4–6 cm H_2O are usually safe and effective. **Carbon dioxide elimination** is achieved by increasing the peak inspiratory pressure (tidal volume) or the rate of the ventilator. Many ventilated neonates receive sedation or pain relief with benzodiazepines or opiates (morphine, fentanyl), respectively. Midazolam is approved for use in neonates, and has demonstrated sedative effects. Adverse hemodynamic effects and myoclonus have been associated with its use in neonates. If used, a continuous infusion or administration of individual doses over at least 10 min is recommended to reduce these risks. Data are insufficient to assess the efficacy and safety of lorazepam. Diazepam is not recommended due to its long half-life, its long-acting metabolites, and concern about the benzyl alcohol content. Continuous infusion of morphine in VLBW neonates requiring mechanical ventilation does not improve mortality rates, severe intraventricular hemorrhage, or periventricular leukomalacia. The need for additional doses of morphine is associated with poor outcome.

High-frequency ventilation (HFV) was developed to reduce lung injury and/or improve gas exchange in patients with severe respiratory disease. HFV achieves desired minute ventilation by using smaller tidal volumes and high rates (300–1,200 breaths/min or 5–20 Hz). HFV may improve the elimination of carbon dioxide, decrease the mean airway pressure, and improve oxygenation in patients who do not respond to conventional ventilators and who have severe RDS, interstitial emphysema, recurrent pneumothoraces, or meconium aspiration pneumonia. High-frequency jet ventilation may cause necrotizing tracheal damage, especially in the presence of hypotension or poor humidification, and high-frequency oscillator therapy has been inconsistently associated with an increased risk of air leaks, IVH, and periventricular leukomalacia. Both methods can cause gas trapping. High-frequency oscillation strategies that promote lung recruitment, combined with surfactant therapy, may improve gas exchange, but have not been shown to reduce the risk for BPD. Elective use of high-frequency oscillation or jet ventilation, when compared with conventional ventilation, does not offer advantages if used as the initial ventilation strategy to treat VLBW infants with RDS. There may be a small reduction in the rate of BPD with high-frequency oscillation, but the evidence is weakened by the inconsistency of this effect across trials and this finding is not statistically significant. Of concern is the increase in acute brain injury in one trial, which used a low-volume strategy during jet ventilation.

Multidose endotracheal instillation of **exogenous surfactant** to VLBW infants requiring 30% oxygen and mechanical ventilation for the treatment (**rescue therapy**) of RDS dramatically improves survival and reduces the incidence of pulmonary air leaks, but it has not consistently reduced the incidence of BPD. Immediate effects include improved alveolar-arterial oxygen gradients, reduced ventilator mean airway pressure, increased pulmonary compliance, and improved appearance of the chest roentgenogram. A number of surfactant preparations are available, including synthetic surfactants and natural surfactants derived from animal sources. Exosurf is a synthetic surfactant. Natural surfactants include Survanta (bovine), Infasurf (calf), and Curosurf (porcine). Although both synthetic and natural surfactants are effective in the treatment and prevention of RDS, natural surfactants appear to be superior, perhaps because of their surfactant-associated protein content. Natural surfactants have a more rapid onset and are associated with a lower risk of pneumothorax and improved survival. Surfaxin, formerly known as KL4 surfactant, is a novel synthetic lung surfactant containing phospholipids and an engineered peptide, sinapultide, designed to mimic the actions of human surfactant protein B (SP-B). Surfaxin use for the prevention and treatment of respiratory distress syndrome (RDS) demonstrates a lower all-cause mortality compared to Exosurf and equivalency to the natural surfactants Survanta and Curosurf. Rapid testing of pulmonary maturity soon after birth by examining tracheal aspirate secretions may reduce the number of unaffected infants treated with surfactant and permit early rescue therapy within the 1st 1–2 hr of life.

Rescue treatment is initiated as soon as possible in the 1st 24 hr of life. Repeated dosing is given via the endotracheal tube every 6–12 hr for a total of 2 to 4 doses, depending on the preparation. Exogenous surfactant should be given by a physician who is qualified in neonatal resuscitation and respiratory management and who is able to care for the infant beyond the 1st hr of stabilization. Additional on-site staff support required includes nurses and respiratory therapists experienced in the ventilatory management of LBW infants. Appropriate monitoring equipment (radiology, blood gas laboratory, pulse oximetry) must also be available. Furthermore, each institution should have an approved protocol for the administration of surfactant. Complications of surfactant therapy include transient hypoxia, bradycardia and hypotension, blockage of the endotracheal tube, and pulmonary hemorrhage (see Chapter 101.9).

Premature infants requiring ventilator support after a week of age experience transient episodes of surfactant dysfunction associated with deficiency of SP-B and SP-C, which are temporally associated with episodes of infection and respiratory deterioration. Treatment with exogenous surfactant, SP-B, SP-C, or strategies to increase endogenous surfactant protein production may be beneficial in infants with respiratory failure and surfactant dysfunction. In one study of VLBW infants at 7–30 d with stable ventilatory requirements, a dose of surfactant produced a transient decrease in the concentration of supplemental oxygen. The associations between respiratory deteriorations and surfactant function and composition as well as the short- and long-term safety of surfactant treatment for these events in chronically ventilated infants need further investigation.

Inhaled nitric oxide (iNO) decreases the need for extracorporeal membrane oxygenation (ECMO) in term and near-term infants with hypoxic respiratory failure. The response to iNO is equivalent to that to HFOV in term or near-term infants with RDS. A positive response to combined therapy suggests that alveolar recruitment by HFOV may allow iNO gas to reach the pulmonary resistance vessels.

Low-dose iNO may decrease the incidence of BPD in critically ill premature infants. A reduction in the rate of death or BPD in infants <1,000 g treated with iNO was observed in one study. iNO treatment of RDS may also be associated with improved neurodevelopmental outcome.

Weaning strategies from ventilators vary widely and are influenced by lung mechanics as well as the availability of ventilatory modes (pressure support). Once extubated, many infants transition to nasal CPAP to avoid postextubation atelectasis and hypoxia. Synchronized nasal intermittent ventilation has been shown to decrease the need for reintubation in VLBW infants. High flow (1–2 L/min) or warmed, humidified high flow (2–8 LPM) nasal cannula oxygen is commonly used to support term and near-term infants following extubation and to wean premature infants off nasal CPAP. Preloading with caffeine may enhance the success of extubation.

Metabolic acidosis in RDS may be a result of perinatal asphyxia and hypotension and is often encountered when an infant has required resuscitation (see Chapter 100). Sodium bicarbonate, 1–2 mEq/kg, may be administered over a 15–20 min period through a peripheral or umbilical vein, with the acid-base determination repeated within 30 min, or it may be administered over a period of several hours. Often, sodium bicarbonate is administered on an emergency basis through an umbilical venous catheter. Alkali therapy may result in skin slough from infiltration, increased serum osmolarity, hypernatremia, hypocalcemia, hypokalemia, and liver injury when concentrated solutions are administered rapidly through an umbilical vein catheter wedged in the liver. Sodium bicarbonate may exacerbate a severe respiratory acidosis, especially if ventilation is ineffective.

Monitoring of aortic blood pressure through an umbilical or peripheral arterial catheter or by oscillometric technique is useful in managing the shocklike state that may occur during the 1st hr or so in VLBW infants who have been asphyxiated or have severe RDS (see Fig. 94-2). Hypotension and low flow in the superior vena cava (SVC) have been associated with increased CNS morbidity and increased mortality and should be treated with cautious administration of volume (crystalloid) and early use of vasopressors. Dopamine is more effective in raising blood pressure than dobutamine. Hypotension may be refractory to pressors, but glucocorticoid responsive, especially in neonates <1,000 g. This hypotension may be due to transient adrenal insufficiency in the ill VLBW infant. Treat with intravenous hydrocortisone (Solu-Cortef) at 1–2 mg/kg/dose Q 6–12 hr (see Chapter 98).

Periodic monitoring of $Pa{O_2}$, $Pa{CO_2}$, and pH is an important part of the management; if assisted ventilation is being used, such monitoring is essential. Blood should be obtained from the umbilical or peripheral artery. Tissue $P{O_2}$ may also be estimated continuously from transcutaneous electrodes or pulse oximetry (oxygen saturation). Capillary blood samples are of limited value for determining Po2, but may be useful for evaluating $Pa{CO_2}$ and pH. Radiopaque umbilical catheters should have their position checked roentgenographically after insertion (see Fig. 101-4). The tip of an umbilical artery catheter should lie just above the bifurcation of the aorta (L3–L5) or above the celiac axis (T6–T10). Preferred sites for peripheral catheters are the radial or posterior tibial arteries. Placement and supervision should be carried out by skilled and experienced personnel. Catheters should be removed as soon as patients no longer have any indication for their continued use—usually when the infant is stable and the $F{IO_2}$ is <40%.

Because of the difficulty of distinguishing **group B streptococcal** or other bacterial infections from RDS, empirical antibiotic therapy is indicated until the results of blood cultures are available. Penicillin or ampicillin with an aminoglycoside is suggested; however, the choice of antibiotics is based on the recent pattern of bacterial sensitivity in the hospital where the infant is being treated (see Chapter 109).

COMPLICATIONS OF RDS AND INTENSIVE CARE. The most serious complications of tracheal intubation are asphyxia from obstruction of the tube, cardiac arrest during intubation or suctioning, and the subsequent development of subglottic stenosis. Other complications include bleeding from trauma during intubation, posterior pharyngeal pseudodiverticula, need for tracheostomy, ulceration of the nares because of pressure from the tube, permanent narrowing of the nostril as a result of tissue damage and scarring from irritation or infection around the tube, erosion of the palate, avulsion of a vocal cord, laryngeal ulcer, papilloma of a vocal cord, and persistent hoarseness, stridor, or edema of the larynx.

Measures to reduce the incidence of these complications include skillful intubation, adequate securing of the tube, use of polyvinyl endotracheal tubes, use of the smallest size tube that will provide effective ventilation to reduce local pressure necrosis and ischemia, avoidance of frequent changes and motion of the tube in situ, avoidance of too frequent or vigorous suctioning, and prevention of infection through meticulous cleanliness and frequent sterilization of all apparatus attached to or passed through the tube. The personnel inserting and caring for the endotracheal tube should be experienced and skilled.

Risks associated with **umbilical arterial catheterization** include vascular embolization, thrombosis, spasm, and vascular perforation; ischemic or chemical necrosis of abdominal viscera; infection; accidental hemorrhage; and impaired circulation to a leg with subsequent gangrene. Although the reported incidence of thrombotic complications varies from 1% to 23% at necropsy, aortography has demonstrated that clots form in or about the tips of 95% of catheters placed in an umbilical artery. Aortic ultrasonography can also be used to investigate the presence of thrombosis. The risk of a serious clinical complication resulting from umbilical catheterization is probably between 2% and 5%.

Transient blanching of the leg may occur during catheterization of the umbilical artery. It is usually due to reflex arterial spasm, the incidence of which is lessened by using the smallest available catheter, particularly in very small infants. The catheter should be removed immediately; catheterization of the other artery may then be attempted. Persistent spasm after removal of the catheter may be relieved by topical nitroglycerin paste applied to the affected area or, rarely, by warming the opposite leg. Blood sampling from a radial artery may similarly result in spasm or thrombosis, and the same treatment is indicated. Intermittent severe spasm or unrelieved spasm may respond to the cautious use of topical nitroglycerin. Accidentally lodging the catheter in a smaller artery, either blocking it completely or causing unrecognized local vascular spasm, may result in gangrene of the organ or area supplied by the vessel. To prevent this complication, the catheter should be removed promptly if blood cannot be withdrawn from it.

Serious hemorrhage on removal of the catheter is rare. Thrombi may form in the artery or in the catheter, the incidence of which can be lowered by using a smooth-tipped catheter with a hole only at its end, by rinsing the catheter with a small amount of saline solution containing heparin, or by continuously infusing a solution containing 1–2 units/mL of heparin. The risk of thrombus formation with potential vascular occlusion can also be reduced by removing the catheter when early signs of thrombosis, such as narrowing of pulse pressure and disappearance of the dicrotic notch, are noted. Some prefer to use the umbilical artery for blood sampling only and leave the catheter filled with heparinized saline between samplings. **Renovascular hypertension** may occur days to weeks after umbilical arterial catheterization in a small number of neonates.

Umbilical vein catheterization is associated with many of the same risks as umbilical artery catheterization. An additional risk is cardiac perforation and pericardial tamponade if the catheter is incorrectly placed in the right atrium; portal hypertension can develop from portal vein thrombosis, especially in the presence of omphalitis.

Extrapulmonary extravasation of air is another complication of the management of RDS (see Chapter 101.3).

Some neonates with RDS may have clinically significant shunting through a **patent ductus arteriosus (PDA)**. Delayed closure of the PDA is associated with hypoxia, acidosis, increased pulmonary pressure secondary to vasoconstriction, systemic hypotension, immaturity, and local release of prostaglandins, which dilate the ductus. There is a relationship between early adrenal insufficiency, ductal patency, airway inflammation, and the development of BPD. Shunting through the PDA may initially be bidirectional or right to left. As RDS resolves, pulmonary vascular resistance decreases, and left-to-right shunting may occur and lead to left ventricular volume overload and pulmonary edema. Manifestations of PDA may include (1) apnea for unexplained reasons in an infant recovering from RDS; (2) a hyperdynamic precordium, bounding peripheral pulses, wide pulse pressure, and a continuous or systolic murmur with or without extension into diastole or an apical diastolic murmur, multiple clicks resembling the shaking of dice; (3) carbon dioxide retention; (4) increasing oxygen dependence; (5) x-ray evidence of cardiomegaly and increased pulmonary vascular markings; and (6) hepatomegaly. The **diagnosis** is confirmed by echocardiographic visualization of a PDA with Doppler flow demonstrating left-to-right or bidirectional shunting. VLBW infants with PDA are at increased risk of more prolonged and more severe RDS, bronchopulmonary dysplasia, and death. Prophylactic "closure," closure of the asymptomatic but clinically detected PDA, and closure of the symptomatic PDA are three strategies to manage a PDA. Interventions include fluid restriction, the use of diuretics, the use of cyclo-oxygenase inhibitors, and surgical closure. Short-term benefits have to be balanced against adverse effects such as transient renal dysfunction and a possible increase in the risk of intestinal perforation. There is no evidence available that any of the strategies examined result in long-term benefit, in particular, disability-free survival. Much uncertainty about "best practice" therefore remains. Many infants respond to general supportive measures, including diuretics and fluid restriction. Medical and/or surgical ductal closure is indicated in premature infants with PDA when there is a delay in clinical improvement or deterioration after initial clinical improvement of RDS. Pharmacologic or surgical closure of the PDA is often followed by a dramatic decrease in ventilatory and oxygen requirements. Indomethacin is **the drug of choice** for medical closure of the PDA. Intravenous indomethacin is given in three doses every 12–24 hr; treatment may be repeated 1 time. For infants <48 hr, the 1st dose is 0.2 mg/kg, while the 2nd and 3rd doses are 0.1 mg/kg. Between 2 and 7 days of life, all doses are 0.2 mg/kg. Over 7 days of life, the 1st dose is 0.2 mg/kg and subsequent doses are 0.25 mg/kg. Prophylactic low-dose indomethacin reduces the incidence of both IVH and PDA and improves the rate of permanent ductal closure, but it does not improve the long-term prognosis. **Contraindications** to indomethacin include thrombocytopenia ($<50{,}000/mm^3$), bleeding disorders, oliguria (<1 mL/kg/hr), necrotizing enterocolitis, isolated intestinal perforation, and an elevated plasma creatinine level (>1.8 mg/dL). Infants whose PDA fails to close with indomethacin or who have contraindications to indomethacin are candidates for surgical closure. Surgical mortality is very low even in the extremely low birthweight group. Complications of surgery include Horner syndrome, injury to the recurrent laryngeal nerve, chylothorax, transient hypertension, pneumothorax, and bleeding from the surgical site. Ligation rather than division can also result in recanalization, but this is rare. Inadvertent ligation of the left pulmonary artery or the transverse aortic arch has been reported.

Intravenous ibuprofen may be an alternative to indomethacin; it can be as effective in closing a PDA without reducing cerebral, mesenteric, or renal blood flow velocity. Compared to indomethacin, therapeutic ibuprofen reduces the risk of oliguria, but may increase the risk for BPD and pulmonary hypertension. Ibuprofen does not confer a net benefit over indomethacin.

Bronchopulmonary dysplasia (BPD) is a result of lung injury in infants requiring mechanical ventilation and supplemental oxygen. The clinical, radiographic, and lung histology of classic BPD described in 1967, in an era before the widespread use of antenatal steroids and postnatal surfactant, was a disease of more mature preterm infants with RDS treated with positive pressure ventilation and oxygen. BPD is a disease primarily of infants <1,000 g born at less than 28 wk gestation, many of whom have little or no lung disease at birth, but develop progressive respiratory failure over the 1st few weeks of life.

When compared with infants with classic BPD, most current infants with BPD do not have the prominent airway changes of squamous metaplasia and peribronchial fibrosis, severe alveolar septal fibrosis, or hypertensive vascular changes. Airway muscle thickening and derangements in elastic fiber architecture persist. The morphometric features currently found in BPD include alveolar hypoplasia, variable saccular wall fibrosis, and minimal airway disease. Some specimens also have decreased pulmonary microvasculature development. The histopathology of BPD indicates interference with normal lung anatomic maturation, which may prevent subsequent lung growth and development. The pathogenesis of BPD is multifactorial and affects both the lungs and the heart. RDS is a disease of progressive alveolar collapse. Alveolar collapse (atelectotrauma) as a result of insufficient PEEP, together with ventilator-induced phasic overdistention of the lung (volutrauma), promotes injury. Oxygen induces injury by producing free radicals that cannot be metabolized by the immature antioxidant systems of VLBW neonates. Mechanical ventilation and oxygen injure the lung by their effect on alveolar and vascular development. Moreover, inflammation (measured by circulating neutrophils, neutrophils and macrophages in alveolar fluid,

TABLE 101-2. Definition of Bronchopulmonary Dysplasia: Diagnostic Criteria

GESTATIONAL AGE	<32 WK	≥32 WK
Time point of assessment	36 wk PMA or discharge home, whichever comes first	>28 days' but <56 days' postnatal age or discharge home, whichever comes first.
	Treatment with >21% oxygen for at least 28 days **plus**	Treatment with >21% oxygen for at least 28 days **plus**
Mild BPD	Breathing room air at 36 wk PMA or discharge, whichever comes first	Breathing room air by 56 days' postnatal age or discharge, whichever comes first
Moderate BPD	Need* for <30% oxygen at 36 wk PMA or discharge, whichever comes first	Need* for <30% oxygen at 56 days' postnatal age or discharge, whichever comes first
Severe BPD	Need* for ≥30% oxygen and/or positive pressure (PPV or NCPAP) at 36 wk PMA or discharge, whichever comes first	Need* for ≥30% oxygen and/or positive pressure (PPV or NCPAP) at 56 days' postnatal age or discharge, whichever comes first

BPD usually develops in neonates being treated with oxygen and PPV for respiratory failure, most commonly respiratory distress syndrome. Persistence of the clinical features of respiratory disease (tachypnea, retractions, crackles) is considered common to the broad description of BPD and has not been included in the diagnostic criteria describing the severity of BPD. Infants treated with greater than 21% oxygen and/or positive pressure for nonrespiratory disease (e.g., central apnea or diaphragmatic paralysis) do not have BPD unless parenchymal lung disease also develops and they have clinical features of respiratory distress. A day of treatment with greater than 21% oxygen means that the infant received greater than 21% oxygen for more than 12 hr on that day. Treatment with greater than 21% oxygen and/or positive pressure at 36 wk PMA or at 56 days' postnatal age or discharge should not reflect an "acute" event, but should rather reflect the infant's usual daily therapy for several days preceding and after 36 wk PMA, 56 days' postnatal age, or discharge.

*A physiologic test confirming that the oxygen requirement at the assessment time point remains to be defined. This assessment may include a pulse oximetry saturation range.

BPD, bronchopulmonary dysplasia; NCPAP, nasal continuous positive airway pressure; PMA, postmenstrual age; PPV, positive pressure ventilation.

From Jobe AH, Bancalari E: Bronchopulmonary dysplasia. *Am J Respir Crit Care Med* 2001; 163:1723–1729.

and pro-inflammatory cytokines) contributes to the progression of lung injury. Several clinical factors, including immaturity, chorioamnionitis, or acquired infection potentially with genital mycoplasma species, symptomatic PDA, and malnutrition, contribute to the development of BPD.

BPD is usually defined as a need for supplemental oxygen at 36 wk after conception. Another definition of BPD is based on the severity of disease (Table 101-2). BPD can also be defined by standardized oxygen saturation monitoring at 36 wk PCA. Neonates on positive pressure support or receiving >30% supplemental oxygen are diagnosed with BPD. Those receiving 30% oxygen or less undergo a stepwise 2% reduction in supplemental oxygen to room air while under continuous observation and oxygen saturation monitoring. Outcomes are "no BPD" (saturations 88% or greater for 60 min) or "BPD" (saturation <88%). This test is highly reliable and correlated with discharge home in oxygen, length of hospital stay, and hospital readmissions in the 1st yr of life.

The occurrence of BPD is inversely related to gestational age. Instead of showing improvement on the 3rd–4th day, consistent with the natural course of RDS, some infants develop an increased need for oxygen and ventilatory support. Respiratory distress persists or worsens and is characterized by hypoxia, hypercapnia, oxygen dependence, and, in severe cases, the development of right-sided heart failure. The chest roentgenogram may reveal pulmonary interstitial emphysema, wandering atelectasis with concomitant hyperinflation, and cyst formation (Fig. 101-5). Four distinct pathologic stages of classic BPD have been identified, which are acute lung injury, exudative bronchiolitis, proliferative bronchiolitis, and obliterative fibroproliferative bronchiolitis. Histologic study at this stage (10–20 days) shows residual hyaline membrane formation, progressive alveolar coalescence with atelectasis of the surrounding alveoli, interstitial edema, coarse focal thickening of the basement membrane, and widespread bronchial and bronchiolar mucosal metaplasia and hyperplasia. These findings correspond to a severe maldistribution of ventilation. Pathologic examination of infants who die later in the course of BPD reveals cardiac enlargement and pulmonary changes consisting of focal areas of emphysema with hypertrophy of the peribronchial smooth muscle of the tributary bronchioles, perimucosal fibrosis, and widespread metaplasia of the bronchiolar mucosa, thickening of basement membranes, and separation of the capillaries from the alveolar epithelial cells.

Infants at risk for classic BPD usually have severe respiratory distress requiring prolonged periods of mechanical ventilation and oxygen therapy. Additional associations include the presence of interstitial emphysema, lower gestational age, male sex, low $Paco_2$ during the treatment of RDS, PDA, high peak inspiratory pressure, increased airway resistance in the 1st wk of life, increased pulmonary artery pressure, and possibly a family history of atopy or asthma. Genetic polymorphisms may increase the risk of developing BPD. In some VLBW infants without RDS who require mechanical ventilation for apnea or respiratory insufficiency, BPD that does not follow the classic pattern may develop. Overhydration during the 1st days of life may also contribute to the development of BPD. Vitamin A supplementation (5,000 IU intramuscularly 3×/wk for 4 wk) in VLBW infants reduces the risk of BPD (1 case prevented for every 14–15 treated). Early use of nasal CPAP and rapid extubation to nasal CPAP are associated with a decreased risk of BPD.

Severe BPD requires prolonged mechanical ventilation. Gradual weaning should be attempted despite elevations in $Paco_2$ since hypercarbia may be the result of air trapping rather than inadequate minute ventilation. Acceptable blood gas concentrations include a $Paco_2$ of 50–70 mm Hg (if pH >7.30) and a Pao_2 of 55–60 mm Hg with an oxygen saturation of 95% or higher. Lower levels of Pao_2 may exacerbate pulmonary hypertension with resultant cor pulmonale, and also inhibit growth. Airway obstruction in BPD may be due to mucus and edema production, bronchospasm, and airway collapse from acquired tracheobronchomalacia. These events may contribute to "blue spells." Alternatively, blue spells may be due to acute pulmonary vasospasm or right ventricular dysfunction.

Treatment of BPD includes nutritional support, fluid restriction, drug therapy, maintenance of adequate oxygenation, and prompt treatment of infection. Growth must be monitored because recovery is dependent on the growth of lung tissue and remodeling of the pulmonary vascular bed. Nutritional supplementation to provide added calories (24–30 calories/30 mL formula), protein (3–3.5 g/kg/24 hr) and fat (3 g/kg/24 hr) is needed for growth. Diuretic therapy results in a short-term improvement in lung mechanics and may result in decreased oxygen and ventilatory requirements. Furosemide (1 mg/kg/dose intravenously twice daily [bid] or 2 mg/kg/dose orally bid) given daily or every other day is the treatment of choice for fluid overload in infants with BPD. This loop diuretic has been demonstrated to decrease pulmonary interstitial emphysema (PIE) and pulmonary vascular resistance (VR), improve pulmonary function, and facilitate weaning from mechanical ventilation and oxygen. Adverse effects of long-term diuretic therapy are frequent and include hyponatremia, hypokalemia, alkalosis, azotemia, hypocalcemia, hypercalciuria, cholelithiasis, renal stones, nephrocalcinosis, and ototoxicity. Potassium chloride supplementation is often necessary. Hyponatremia should be treated with fluid restriction and a decrease in the dosage or frequency of furosemide. Sodium chloride supplementation should be avoided. Thiazide diuretics with inhibitors of aldosterone have been used in infants with BPD. Several trials of thiazide diuretics combined with spironolactone have shown increased urine output with or without improvement in pulmonary mechanics in infants with BPD. Adverse effects include electrolyte imbalance. Inhaled bronchodilators improve lung mechanics by decreasing airway resis-

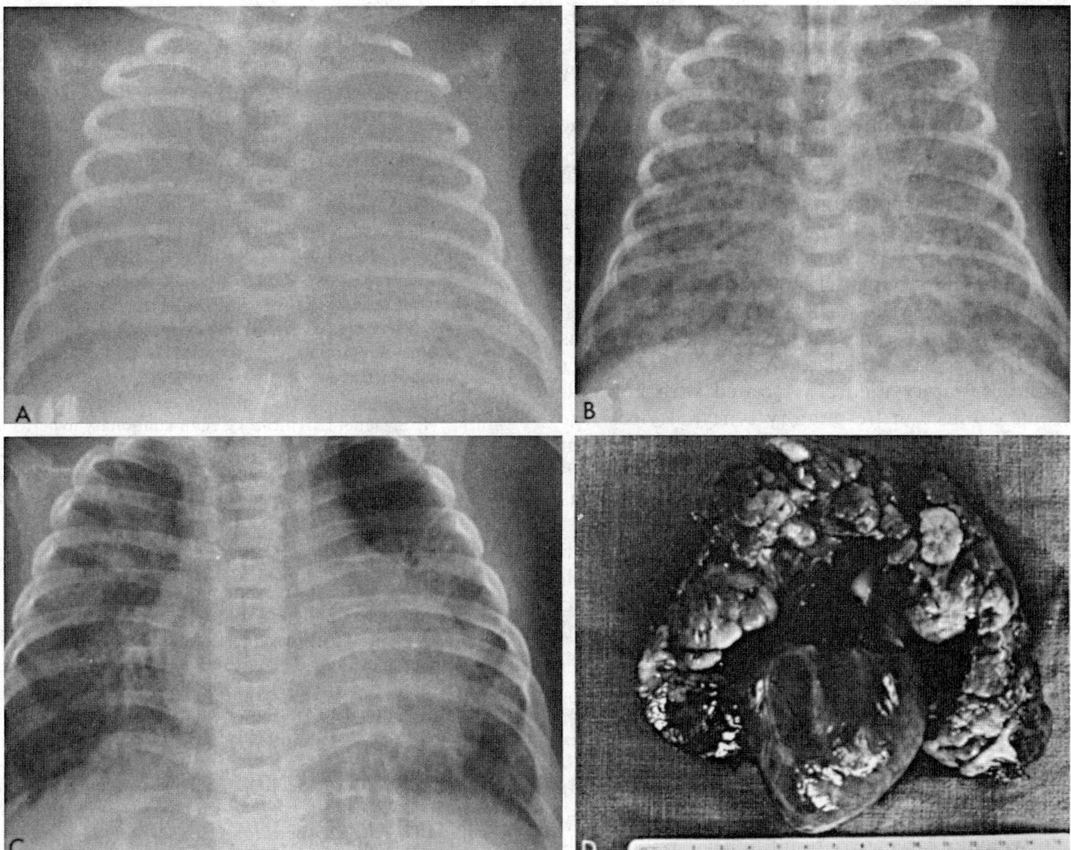

Figure 101-5. Pulmonary changes in infants treated with prolonged, intermittent positive pressure breathing with air containing 80–100% oxygen in the immediate postnatal period for the clinical syndrome of hyaline membrane disease. *A,* A 5-day-old infant with nearly complete opacification of the lungs. *B,* A 13-day-old infant with "bubbly lungs" simulating the roentgenographic appearance of the Wilson-Mikity syndrome. *C,* A 7-mo-old infant with irregular, dense strands in both lungs, hyperinflation, and cardiomegaly suggestive of chronic lung disease. *D,* Large right ventricle and a cobbly, irregular aerated lung of an infant who died at 11 mo of age. This infant also had a patent ductus arteriosus. (From Northway WH Jr, Rosan RC, Porter DY: Pulmonary disease following respirator therapy of hyaline-membrane disease. *N Engl J Med* 1967;276:357–368.)

tance. Albuterol is a specific β2-agonist used to treat bronchospasm in infants with BPD. Albuterol may improve lung compliance by decreasing airway resistance secondary to smooth muscle cell relaxation. Changes in pulmonary mechanics may last as long as 4–6 hr. Adverse effects include hypertension and tachycardia. Ipratropium bromide is a muscarinic antagonist related to atropine, but with more potent bronchodilator effects. Improvements in pulmonary mechanics have been demonstrated in BPD after ipratropium bromide inhalation. Combination therapy of albuterol and ipratropium bromide may be more effective than either agent alone. Few adverse effects have been noted. Cromolyn sodium inhibits release of inflammatory mediators from mast cells. Some studies have shown a decrease in inflammatory mediators in tracheobronchial aspirates of infants with BPD who were treated with this drug. With current aerosol administration strategies, exactly how much medication is delivered to the airways and lungs of infants with BPD, especially if they are ventilator dependent, is unclear. Because significant smooth muscle relaxation does not appear to occur within the 1st few weeks of life, aerosol therapy in the early stages of BPD is not indicated. Methylxanthines are used to increase respiratory drive, decrease apnea, and improve diaphragmatic contractility. These substances may also decrease pulmonary vascular resistance and increase lung compliance in infants with BPD, probably through direct smooth muscle relaxation. They also exhibit diuretic effects. All of the effects cited here may accelerate weaning from mechanical ventilation. Synergy between theophylline and diuretics has been demonstrated. Theophylline has a half-life of 30–40 hours, is metabolized primarily to caffeine in the liver, and may have adverse effects, such as tachycardia, gastroesophageal reflux, agitation, and seizures. Caffeine has a longer half-life than theophylline. Both are available in intravenous and enteral formulations. Caffeine has fewer adverse effects than theophylline.

Preventive therapy of BPD with postnatal dexamethasone may reduce the time to extubation and may decrease the risk of BPD, but is associated with substantial short- and long-term risks, including hypertension, hyperglycemia, gastrointestinal bleeding and perforation, hypertrophic cardiomyopathy, sepsis, and poor weight gain and head growth. Survival is not improved, and infants who have been treated with dexamethasone have an increased risk of neurodevelopmental delay and cerebral palsy. The use of dexamethasone for the prevention or treatment of BPD **is not recommended.** The routine use of dexamethasone in infants with established BPD is not currently recommended unless severe pulmonary disease exists. A rapid tapering course starting at 0.25 mg/kg/day and lasting for 5–7 days may be adequate. Inhaled beclomethasone does not prevent BPD, but decreases the need for systemic steroids. Inhaled corticosteroids facilitate earlier extubation of ventilated infants with BPD.

Physiologic abnormalities of the pulmonary circulation in BPD include elevated pulmonary vascular resistance (PVR) and abnormal vasoreactivity. Acute exposure to even modest levels of hypoxemia causes large elevations in pulmonary artery pressure in infants with BPD with pulmonary hypertension. Higher oxygen saturations are effective in lowering pulmonary artery pressure. The current recommendation for treatment of patients with BPD and pulmonary hypertension is to avoid oxygen saturations below 92%, and in those with established pulmonary hypertension to maintain levels of 94–96%.

Low-dose iNO has no acute effects on lung function, cardiac function, and oxygenation in evolving BPD. The use of low-dose iNO may improve oxygenation in some infants with severe BPD, allowing decreased FIO_2 and ventilator support (see RDS).

The **long-term prognosis** is good for infants who have been weaned from oxygen before discharge from the NICU. Prolonged ventilation, IVH, pulmonary hypertension, cor pulmonale, and oxygen dependence beyond 1 yr of life are poor prognostic signs. Mortality in infants with BPD ranges from 10% to 25% and is highest in infants who remain ventilator dependent for longer than 6 mo. Cardiorespiratory failure associated with cor pulmonale and acquired infection (respiratory syncytial virus) are common causes of death. Survivors with BPD often go home on a regimen of oxygen, diuretics, and bronchodilator therapy. Prevention of sleep-associated hypoxia and high caloric formulas improve growth and cardiorespiratory outcome.

Non-cardiorespiratory complications of BPD include growth failure, psychomotor retardation, and parental stress, as well as sequelae of therapy such as nephrolithiasis, osteopenia, and electrolyte imbalance. Airway problems such as tonsillar and adenoidal hypertrophy, vocal cord paralysis, subglottic stenosis, and tracheomalacia are common and may aggravate or cause pulmonary hypertension. Subglottic stenosis may require tracheotomy or an anterior cricoid–split procedure to relieve upper airway obstruction. Cardiac complications of BPD include pulmonary hypertension, cor pulmonale, systemic hypertension, left ventricular hypertrophy, and the development of aortopulmonary collateral vessels, which, if large, may result in heart failure. Pulmonary function slowly improves in most survivors due to continued lung and airway growth and healing. Rehospitalization for impaired pulmonary function is most common during the 1st 2 yr of life. There is a gradual decrease in symptom frequency in children aged 6–9 yr as compared to the 1st 2 yr of life. Persistence of respiratory symptoms and abnormal pulmonary function tests are present in children aged 7 and 10 yr. Airway obstruction and hyperactivity and hyperinflation are noted in some adolescent and adult survivors of BPD. High-resolution chest CT scanning or MRI studies in children and adults with a history of BPD reveal lung abnormalities that correlate directly with the degree of pulmonary function abnormality.

PROGNOSIS. Early provision of intensive observation and care of high-risk newborn infants can significantly reduce the morbidity and mortality associated with RDS and other acute neonatal illnesses. Antenatal steroids, postnatal surfactant use, improved modes of ventilation, and developmentally appropriate care have resulted in low mortality from RDS (≈10%). Mortality increases with decreasing gestational age. Optimal results depend on the availability of experienced and skilled personnel, specially designed and organized regional hospital units, proper equipment, and lack of complications such as severe asphyxia, intracranial hemorrhage, or irremediable congenital malformation. Surfactant therapy has reduced mortality from RDS approximately 40%; the incidence of BPD has not been measurably affected.

Although 85–90% of all infants surviving RDS after requiring ventilatory support with respirators are normal, the outlook is much better for those weighing more than 1,500 g. The long-term prognosis for normal pulmonary function in most infants surviving RDS is excellent. Survivors of severe neonatal respiratory failure may have significant pulmonary and neurodevelopmental impairment.

Anand KJS, Hall RW, Desai N, et al: Effects of morphine analgesia in ventilated preterm neonates: Primary outcomes from the NEOPAIN randomised trial. *Lancet* 2004;363:1673–1682.

Ballard RA, Truog WE, Cnaan A, et al: Inhaled nitric oxide in preterm infants undergoing mechanical ventilation. *N Engl J Med* 2006;355:343–352.

Brooks JM, Travadi JN, Patole SK, et al: Is surgical ligation of patent ductus arteriosus necessary? The western Australian experience of conservative management. *Arch Dis Child* 2005;90:F235–F239.

Clyman RI: Recommendations for the postnatal use of indomethacin: An analysis of four separate treatment strategies. *J Pediatr* 1996;128:601–607.

Clyman RI, Chome N: Patent ductus arteriosus: evidence for and against treatment. *J Pediatr* 2007;150:216–219.

Crowther CA, Haslam RR, Hiller JE, et al: Neonatal respiratory distress syndrome after repeat exposure to antenatal corticosteroids: a randomised controlled trial. *Lancet* 2006;367:1913–1919.

Flynn PA, Da Graca RL, Auld PAM, et al: The use of a bedside assay for plasma B-type natriuretic peptide as a biomarker in the management of patent ductus arteriosus in premature neonates. *J Pediatr* 2005;147:38–42.

Gournay V, Savagner C, Thiriez G, et al: Pulmonary hypertension after ibuprofen prophylaxis in very preterm infants. *Lancet* 2002;359:1486–1488.

Greenough A, Milner AD, Dimitriou G: Synchronized mechanical ventilation for respiratory support in newborn infants. *Cochrane Database Syst Rev* 2001;1:CD000456.

Hallman M: Lung surfactant, respiratory failure, and genes. *N Engl J Med* 2004;350:1278–1280.

Hammerman C, Kaplan M: Primum non nocere: Prophylactic versus curative ibuprofen. *Lancet* 2004;364:1920–1922.

Higgins RD, Bancalari E, Willinger M, Raju TNK: Executive summary of the workshop on oxygen in neonatal therapies: controversies and opportunities for research. *Pediatrics* 2007;119:790–796.

Kinsella JP, Cutter GR, Walsh WF, et al: Early inhaled nitric oxide therapy in premature newborns with respiratory failure. *N Engl J Med* 2006;355:354–364.

Kinsella JP, Greenough A, Abman SH: Bronchopulmonary dysplasia. *Lancet* 2006;367:1421–1430.

Konduri GG, Vohr B, Robertson C, et al: Early inhaled nitric oxide therapy for term and near-term newborn infants with hypoxic respiratory failure: neurodevelopmental follow-up. *J Pediatr* 2007;150:235–240.

Kotecha S, Allen J: Oxygen therapy for infants with chronic lung disease. *Arch Dis Child Fetal Neonatal Ed* 2002;87:F11–F14.

Lago P, Bettiol T, Salvadori S, et al: Safety and efficacy of ibuprofen versus indomethacin in preterm infants treated for patent ductus arteriosus: A randomized controlled trial. *Eur J Pediatr* 2002;161:202–207.

Laughon M, Bose C, Allred E, et al: Factors associated with treatment for hypotension in extremely low gestational age newborns during the first postnatal week. *Pediatrics* 2007;119:273–280.

LeFlore JL, Salhab WA, Broyles RS, et al: Association of antenatal and postnatal dexamethasone exposure with outcomes in extremely low birth weight neonates. *Pediatrics* 2002;110:275–279.

Lee BH, Stoll BJ, McDonald SA, et al: Adverse neonatal outcomes associated with antenatal dexamethasone versus antenatal betamethasone. *Pediatrics* 2006;117:1503–1510.

McIntosh N: High or low oxygen saturation for the preterm baby. *Arch Dis Child Fetal Neonatal Ed* 2001;84:F149–150.

Merrill JD, Ballard RA, Cnaan A, et al: Dysfunction of pulmonary surfactant in chronically ventilated premature infants. *Pediatr Res* 2004;56:918–926.

Mestan KKL, Marks JD, Hecox K, et al: Neurodevelopmental outcomes of premature infants treated with inhaled nitric oxide. *N Engl J Med* 2005;353:23–32.

Miller SP, Mayer EE, Clyman RI, et al: Prolonged indomethacin exposure is associated with decreased white matter injury detected with magnetic resonance imaging in premature newborns at 24 to 28 weeks' gestation at birth. *Pediatrics* 2006;117:1626–1631.

Montan S, Arul Kumaran S: Neonatal respiratory distress syndrome. *Lancet* 2006;367:1878–1879.

Moya FR, Sinha SS, Segal RS, et al: Comparison of incidences of all-cause mortality between the novel surfactant, Surfaxin (lucinactant) and the animal derived surfactants Survanta (beractant) and Curosurf (poractant alfa). *Pediatr Res* 2004;56:497.

Narayanan M, Cooper B, Weiss H, et al: Prophylactic indomethacin: Factors determining permanent ductus arteriosus closure. *J Pediatr* 2002;136:330–337.

Ng PC, Lee CH, Bnur FL, et al: A double-blind, randomized, controlled study of a "stress dose" of hydrocortisone for rescue treatment of refractory hypotension in preterm infants. *Pediatrics* 2006;117:367–375.

Northway WH Jr, Rosan RC, Porter DY: Pulmonary disease following respirator therapy of hyaline-membrane disease. Bronchopulmonary dysplasia. *N Engl J Med* 1976;276:357–368.

Osborn D, Evans N, Kluckow M: Randomized trial of dobutamine versus dopamine in preterm infants with low systemic blood flow. *J Pediatr* 2002;140:183–191.
Parikh NA, Lasky RE, Kennedy KA, et al: Postnatal dexamethasone therapy and cerebral tissue volumes in extremely low birth weight in infants. *Pediatrics* 2007;119:265–272.
Pillow JJ, Travadi JN: Bubble CPAP: Is the noise important? An invitro study. *Pediatr Res* 2005;57:826–830.
Sandri F, Ancora G, Lanzoni A, et al: Prophylactic nasal continuous positive airways pressure in newborns of 28–31 weeks gestation: Multicentre randomized controlled clinical trial. *Arch Dis Child* 2004;89:F394–F398.
Schmidt B, Davis P, Moddemann D, et al: Long-term effects of indomethacin prophylaxis in extremely low birth weight infants. *N Engl J Med* 2001;344:1966–1972.
Seri N: Hydrocortisone and vasopressor-resistant shock in preterm neonates. *Pediatrics* 2006;117:516–518.
Shah SS, Ohlsson A: Ibuprofen for the prevention of patent ductus arteriosus in preterm and/or low birth weight infants. *Cochrane Database Syst Rev* 2003;2:CD004213.
Shulenin S, Nogee LM, Annilo T, et al: ABCA3 gene mutations in newborns with fatal surfactant deficiency. *N Engl J Med* 2004;350:1296–1303.
Singer L, Yamashita T, Lilien L, et al: A longitudinal study of developmental outcome of infants with bronchopulmonary dysplasia and very low birth weight. *Pediatrics* 1997;100:987–993.
Smith VC, Zupanoc JAF, McCormick MC, et al: Trends in severe bronchopulmonary dysplasia rates between 1994–2002. *J Pediatr* 2005:146:469–473.
Soll RF, Blanco F: Natural surfactant extract versus synthetic surfactant for neonatal respiratory distress syndrome. *Cochrane Database Syst Rev* 2001;2:CD000144.
Stark AR: High-frequency oscillatory ventilation to prevent bronchopulmonary dysplasia—are we there yet? *N Engl J Med* 2002;347:682–684.
Stark AR, Carlo WA, Tyson JE, et al: Adverse effects of early dexamethasone treatment in extremely-low-birth-weight infants. *N Engl J Med* 2001; 344:95–101.
Steer P, Flenady V, Shearman A, et al: High dose caffeine citrate for extubation of preterm infants: A randomized controlled study. *Arch Dis Child* 2004;89:F499–F503.
Truog WE, Ballard PL, Norberg M, et al: Inflammatory markers and mediators in tracheal fluid of premature infants treated with inhaled nitric oxide. *Pediatrics* 2007;119:670–678.
Tyson JE: Does indomethacin prophylaxis benefit extremely low birth weight infants? Results of a placebo-controlled multicenter trial. *Pediatr Res* 2002;51:1.
Tyson JE, Wright LL, Oh W, et al: Vitamin A supplementation for extremely-low-birth-weight infants. *N Engl J Med* 1999;340:1962–1968.
Van Marter LJ: Strategies for preventing bronchopulmonary dysplasia. *Curr Opin Pediatr* 2005;17:174–180.
Van Meurs KP, Wright LL, Ehrenkranz RA, et al: Inhaled nitric oxide for premature infants with severe respiratory failure. *N Engl J Med* 2005; 353:13–22.
Van Overmeire B, Van de Broek H, Van Laer P, et al: Early versus late indomethacin treatment for patent ductus arteriosus in premature infants with respiratory distress syndrome. *J Pediatr* 2001;138:205–211.
Walsh MC, Yao Q, Gettner P, et al, for the National Institute of Child Health and Human Development Neonatal Research Network: Impact of a physiologic definition on bronchopulmonary dysplasia rates. *Pediatrics* 2004; 114:1305–1311.
Watkinson M: Hypertension in the newborn baby. *Arch Dis Child Fetal Neonatal Ed* 2002;86:F78–F81.
Watterberg KL, Gerdes JS, Cole CH, et al: Prophylaxis of early adrenal insufficiency to prevent bronchopulmonary dysplasia: A multicenter trial. *Pediatrics* 2004;114:1649–1657.
Yeh TF, Lin YJ, Lin HC, et al: Outcomes at school age after postnatal dexamethasone therapy for lung disease of prematurity. *N Engl J Med* 2004;350:1304–1312.

101.5 • Transient Tachypnea of the Newborn

Transient tachypnea usually follows uneventful normal preterm or term vaginal delivery or cesarean delivery. It may be characterized by the early onset of tachypnea, sometimes with retractions, or expiratory grunting and, occasionally, cyanosis that is relieved by minimal oxygen (<40%). Patients usually recover rapidly within 3 days. The lungs are generally clear without rales or rhonchi, and the chest x-ray shows prominent pulmonary vascular markings, fluid in the intralobar fissures, overaeration, flat diaphragms, and, rarely, pleural effusions. Hypercapnia and acidosis are uncommon. Distinguishing the disease from RDS may be difficult; the distinctive features of transient tachypnea are sudden recovery of the infant and the absence of x-ray findings of RDS (hypoaeration, diffuse reticulogranular pattern, air bronchograms). The syndrome is believed to be secondary to slow absorption of fetal lung fluid resulting in decreased pulmonary compliance and tidal volume and increased dead space. In severe cases, retained fetal fluid can interfere with the normal postnatal fall in pulmonary vascular resistance resulting in persistent pulmonary hypertension. Treatment is supportive. There is no evidence for the use of oral furosemide in this disorder.

Severe respiratory morbidity and mortality have been reported in infants born by elective cesarean section who initially present with signs and symptoms of transient tachypnea. These infants develop refractory hypoxemia due to pulmonary hypertension and require ECMO support. The term "malignant TTN" has been used to describe this condition.

Avery ME, Gatewood OB, Brumley G: Transient tachypnea of newborn. Possible delayed reabsorption of fluid at birth. *Am J Dis Child* 1966;111:380–385.
Gross TL, Sokol RJ, Kwong MS, et al: Transient tachypnea of the newborn: The relationship to preterm delivery and significant neonatal morbidity. *Am J Obstet Gynecol* 1983;146:236–241.
Heritage CK, Cunningham MD: Association of elective repeat cesarean delivery and persistent pulmonary hypertension of the newborn. *Am J Obstet Gynecol* 1985;152:627–629.
Keszler M, Carbone MT, Cox C, et al: Severe respiratory failure after elective repeat cesarean delivery: A potentially preventable condition leading to extracorporeal membrane oxygenation. *Pediatrics* 1992;89: 670–672.
Sundell H, Garrott J, Blankenship WJ, et al: Studies on infants with type II respiratory distress syndrome. *J Pediatr* 1971;78:754–764.
Wiswell TE, Rawlings JS, Smith FR: Effect of furosemide on the clinical course of transient tachypnea of the newborn. *Pediatrics* 1985;75:908–910.

101.6 • Aspiration of Foreign Material (Fetal Aspiration Syndrome, Aspiration Pneumonia)

During prolonged labor and difficult deliveries, infants often initiate vigorous respiratory movements in utero because of interference with the supply of oxygen through the placenta. Under such circumstances, the infant may aspirate amniotic fluid containing vernix caseosa, epithelial cells, meconium, blood, or material from the birth canal, which may block the smallest airways and interfere with alveolar exchange of oxygen and carbon dioxide. Pathogenic bacteria may accompany the aspirated material, and pneumonia may ensue, but even in noninfected cases, respiratory distress accompanied by roentgenographic evidence of aspiration is seen (Fig. 101-6).

Postnatal pulmonary aspiration may also occur in newborn infants as a result of tracheoesophageal fistula, esophageal and duodenal obstruction, gastroesophageal reflux, improper feeding practices, and administration of depressant medicines.

To avoid aspiration of gastric contents, the stomach should be aspirated using a soft catheter just before surgery or other major procedures that require anesthesia or conscious sedation. If aspiration is sudden and overwhelming, immediate laryngoscopy and suctioning under direct visualization may prevent the aspirated material from reaching the lungs. The treatment of aspiration pneumonia is symptomatic and may include respiratory support

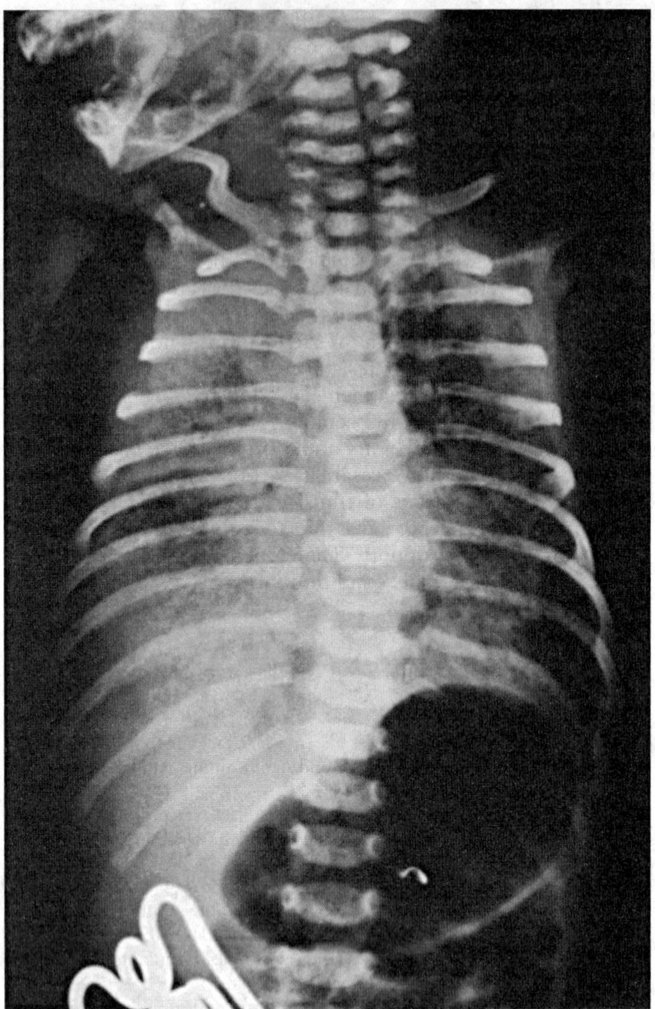

Figure 101-6. Fetal aspiration syndrome (aspiration pneumonia). Note the coarse granular pattern with irregular aeration typical of fetal distress from the aspiration of material contained in amniotic fluid, such as vernix caseosa, epithelial cells, and meconium. (From Goodwin SR, Grave SA, Haberkern CM: Aspiration in intubated premature infants. *Pediatrics* 1985;75:85–88.)

and systemic antibiotics (see Chapters 109.8 and 394). Gradual improvement generally occurs over 3–4 days.

Goodwin SR, Graves SA, Haberkern CM: Aspiration in intubated premature infants. *Pediatrics* 1985;75:85–88.

101.7 • Meconium Aspiration

Meconium-stained amniotic fluid is found in 10–15% of births and usually occurs in term or post-term infants. Meconium aspiration pneumonia develops in 5% of such infants; 30% of them require mechanical ventilation, and 3–5% expire. Usually, but not invariably, fetal distress and hypoxia occur before the passage of meconium into amniotic fluid. These infants are meconium stained and may be depressed and require resuscitation at birth. The pathophysiology is noted in Figure 101-7. Meconium inactivates surfactant.

CLINICAL MANIFESTATIONS. Either in utero or more often with the 1st breath, thick, particulate meconium is aspirated into the lungs. The resulting small airway obstruction may produce respiratory distress within the 1st hours, with tachypnea, retractions, grunting, and cyanosis observed in severely affected infants. Partial obstruction of some airways may lead to pneumothorax or pneumomediastinum, or both. Prompt treatment may delay the onset of respiratory distress, which may consist of only tachypnea without retractions. Overdistention of the chest may be prominent. The condition usually improves within 72 hr, but when its course requires assisted ventilation, it may be severe with a high risk for mortality. Tachypnea may persist for many days or even several weeks. The typical chest roentgenogram is characterized by patchy infiltrates, coarse streaking of both lung fields, increased anteroposterior diameter, and flattening of the diaphragm. A normal chest roentgenogram in an infant with severe hypoxia and no cardiac malformation suggests the diagnosis of pulmonary hypertension (see Chapter 101.8). Arterial Po_2 may be low in either disease and, if hypoxia has occurred, metabolic acidosis is usually present.

PREVENTION. The risk of meconium aspiration may be decreased by rapid identification of fetal distress and initiating prompt delivery in the presence of fetal acidosis, late decelerations, or poor beat-to-beat variability. Despite initial enthusiasm for amnioinfusion, it does not reduce the risk of meconium aspira-

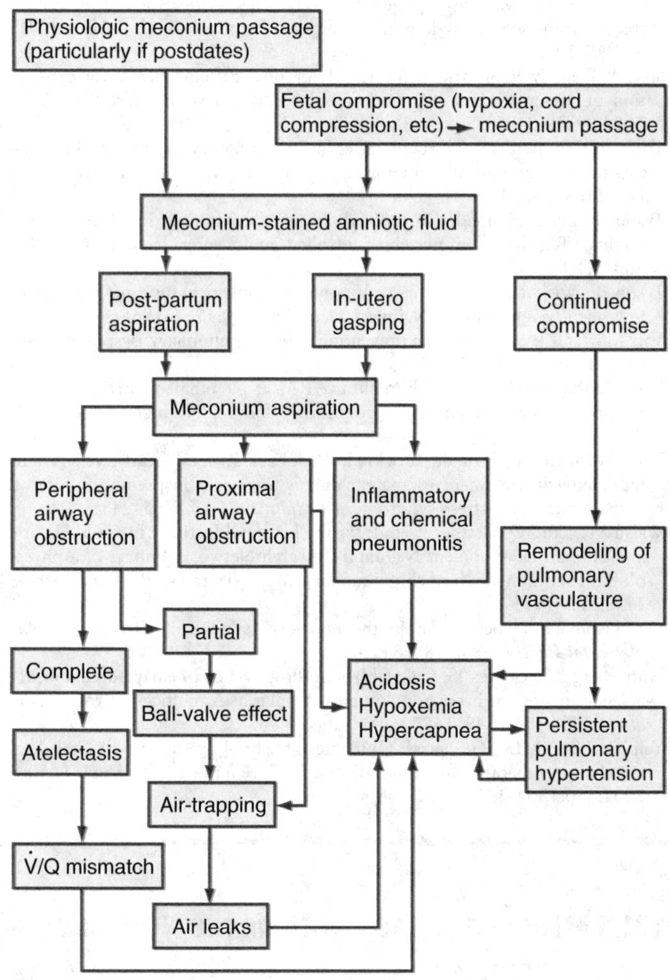

Figure 101-7. Pathophysiology of meconium passage and the meconium aspiration syndrome. V/Q, ventilation-perfusion ratio. (From Wiswell TE, Bent RC: Meconium staining and the meconium aspiration syndrome: Unresolved issues. *Pediatr Clin North Am* 1993;40:955–981.)

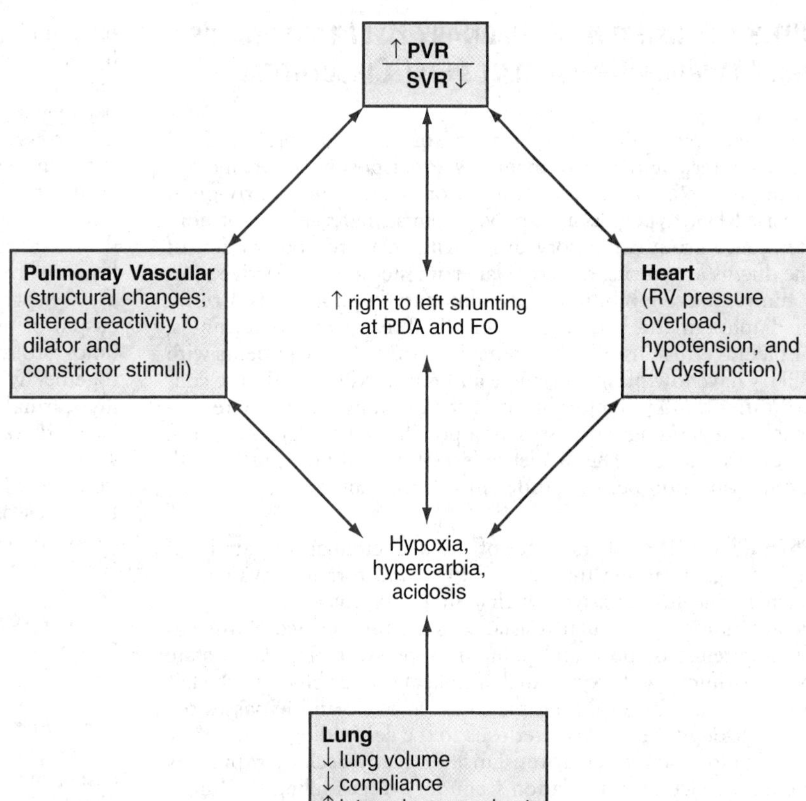

Figure 101-8. Cardiopulmonary interactions in persistent pulmonary hypertension of the newborn (PPHN). FO, foramen ovale; LV, left ventricular; PDA, patent ductus arteriosus; PVR, pulmonary vascular resistance; RV, right ventricular; SVR, systemic vascular resistance. (From Kinsella JP, Abman SH: Recent developments in the pathophysiology and treatment of persistent pulmonary hypertension of the newborn. *J Pediatr* 1995;126:853–864.)

tion syndrome, cesarean delivery, or other major indicators of maternal or neonatal morbidity. Nasopharyngeal suctioning of meconium-stained infants after delivery of the head was once considered a low-risk method of reducing the incidence of meconium aspiration syndrome (MAS). Routine intrapartum nasopharyngeal suctioning in pregnancies with meconium-stained amniotic fluid does not reduce the risk for MAS and, on rare occasions, may cause nasopharyngeal trauma or cause a cardiac arrhythmia.

TREATMENT. Routine intubation to aspirate the lungs of vigorous infants born through meconium-stained fluid is not recommended. Depressed infants (those with hypotonia, bradycardia, fetal acidosis, or apnea) should undergo endotracheal intubation, and suction should be applied directly to the endotracheal tube to remove meconium from the airway. The risk associated with laryngoscopy and endotracheal intubation (bradycardia, laryngospasm, hypoxia, posterior pharyngeal laceration with pseudodiverticulum formation) is less than the risk of MAS in these high-risk circumstances.

Treatment of meconium aspiration pneumonia includes supportive care and standard management for respiratory distress. The beneficial effect of mean airway pressure on oxygenation must be weighed against the risk of pneumothorax. Administration of exogenous surfactant to infants with MAS requiring mechanical ventilation decreases the need for ECMO support; the effect is greatest in those infants treated early. Severe meconium aspiration may be complicated by persistent pulmonary hypertension. Patients who are refractory to conventional mechanical ventilation may benefit from HFV, iNO, or ECMO (see Chapter 101.8).

PROGNOSIS. The mortality rate of meconium-stained infants is considerably higher than that of non-stained infants. A decline in neonatal deaths due to meconium aspiration syndrome is related to improvements in obstetric and neonatal care. Residual lung problems are rare, but include symptomatic cough, wheezing, and persistent hyperinflation for up to 5–10 yr. The ultimate prognosis depends on the extent of CNS injury from asphyxia and the presence of associated problems such as pulmonary hypertension.

American Academy of Pediatrics, American College of Obstetricians and Gynecologists: *Guidelines for Perinatal Care,* 5th ed. Washington DC, American Academy of Pediatrics/American College of Obstetricians and Gynecologists, 2002.

Cuttini M: Intrapartum prevention of meconium aspiration syndrome. *Lancet* 2004;364:560–561.

Dargaville PA, South M, McDougall PN: Surfactant and surfactant inhibitors in meconium aspiration syndrome. *J Pediatr* 2001;138:113–115.

Findlay RD, Taeusch HW, Walther FJ: Surfactant replacement therapy for meconium aspiration syndrome. *Pediatrics* 1996;97:48–52.

Fraser WD, Hofmeyr J, Lede R, et al: Amnioinfusion for prevention of the meconium aspiration syndrome. *N Engl J Med* 2005;353:909–916.

Gregory GA, Gooding CA, Phibbs RH, et al: Meconium aspiration in infants—a prospective study. *J Pediatr* 1974;85:848–852.

Halliday HL: Endotracheal intubation at birth for preventing morbidity and mortality in vigorous, meconium-stained infants born at term. *Cochrane Database Syst Rev* 2001;1:CD000500.

Ramin KD, Leveno KJ, Kelly MA, et al: Amniotic fluid meconium: A fetal environmental hazard. *Obstet Gynecol* 1996;87:181–184.

Vain NE, Szyld EG, Prudent LM: Oropharyngeal and nasopharayngeal suctioning of meconium-stained neonates before delivery of their shoulders: Multicentre, randomized controlled trial. *Lancet* 2004;364:597–602.

Wiswell TE, Gannon CM, Jacob J, et al: Delivery room management of the apparently vigorous meconium-stained neonate: Results of the multicenter, international collaborative trial. *Pediatrics* 2000;105:1–7.

Wiswell TE, Knight GR, Finer NN, et al: A multicenter, randomized, controlled trial comparing Surfaxin (lucinactant) lavage with standard care for treatment of meconium aspiration syndrome. *Pediatrics* 2002;109:1081–1087.

101.8 • Persistent Pulmonary Hypertension of the Newborn (Persistent Fetal Circulation)

Persistent pulmonary hypertension of the newborn (PPHN) occurs in term and post-term infants. Predisposing factors include birth asphyxia, meconium aspiration pneumonia, early-onset sepsis, RDS, hypoglycemia, polycythemia, maternal use of nonsteroidal anti-inflammatory drugs with in utero constriction of the ductus arteriosus, maternal late trimester use of selective serotonin reuptake inhibitors, and pulmonary hypoplasia as a result of diaphragmatic hernia, amniotic fluid leak, oligohydramnios, or pleural effusions. PPHN is often idiopathic. Some patients with PPHN have low plasma arginine and nitric oxide metabolite concentrations and polymorphisms of the carbamoyl phosphate synthase gene, findings suggestive of a possible subtle defect in nitric oxide production. The incidence is 1/500–1,500 live births with a wide variation between different clinical centers.

PATHOPHYSIOLOGY. Persistence of the fetal circulatory pattern of right-to-left shunting through the PDA and foramen ovale after birth is due to excessively high pulmonary vascular resistance. Fetal pulmonary vascular resistance is usually elevated relative to fetal systemic or postnatal pulmonary pressure. This fetal state permits shunting of oxygenated umbilical venous blood to the left atrium (and brain) through the foramen ovale and bypasses the lungs through the ductus arteriosus to the descending aorta. After birth, pulmonary vascular resistance normally declines rapidly as a consequence of vasodilation secondary to gas filling the lungs, a rise in postnatal Pao_2, a reduction in $Paco_2$, increased pH, and release of vasoactive substances. Increased neonatal pulmonary vascular resistance may (1) be maladaptive from an acute injury (not demonstrating normal vasodilation in response to increased oxygen and other changes after birth); (2) be the result of increased pulmonary artery medial muscle thickness and extension of smooth muscle layers into the usually nonmuscular, more peripheral pulmonary arterioles in response to chronic fetal hypoxia; (3) be due to pulmonary hypoplasia (diaphragmatic hernia, Potter syndrome); or (4) be obstructive as a result of polycythemia or total anomalous pulmonary venous return, or alveolar capillary dysplasia, which is a lethal autosomal recessive disorder characterized by thickened alveolar septa, increased muscularization of the pulmonary arterioles, a reduced number of capillaries, and misalignment of the intrapulmonary veins. Regardless of etiology, profound hypoxia from right-to-left shunting and normal or elevated $Paco_2$ are present (Fig. 101-8).

CLINICAL MANIFESTATIONS. Infants become ill in the delivery room or within the 1st 12 hr of life. PPHN related to polycythemia, idiopathic causes, hypoglycemia, or asphyxia may result in severe cyanosis with tachypnea, although, initially, signs of respiratory distress may be minimal. Infants who have PPHN associated with meconium aspiration, group B streptococcal pneumonia, diaphragmatic hernia, or pulmonary hypoplasia usually exhibit cyanosis, grunting, flaring, retractions, tachycardia, and shock. Multiorgan involvement may be present (see Table 99-1). Myocardial ischemia, papillary muscle dysfunction with mitral and tricuspid regurgitation, and biventricular dysfunction produce cardiogenic shock with decreased pulmonary blood flow, tissue perfusion, and oxygen delivery. The hypoxia is quite labile and often out of proportion to the findings on chest roentgenograms.

DIAGNOSIS. PPHN should be suspected in all term infants who have cyanosis with or without fetal distress, intrauterine growth restriction, meconium-stained amniotic fluid, hypoglycemia, polycythemia, diaphragmatic hernia, pleural effusions, and birth asphyxia. Hypoxia is universal and is unresponsive to 100% oxygen given by oxygen hood, but it may respond transiently to hyperoxic hyperventilation administered after endotracheal intubation or to the application of a bag and mask. A Pao_2 gradient between a preductal (right radial artery) and a postductal (umbilical artery) site of blood sampling >20 mm Hg suggests right-to-left shunting through the ductus arteriosus, as does a saturation gradient >5% between a preductal and postductal site by pulse oximetry. Real-time echocardiography combined with Doppler flow studies demonstrates right-to-left shunting across a patent foramen ovale and a ductus arteriosus. Deviation of the intra-atrial septum into the left atrium is seen in severe PPHN. Tricuspid or mitral insufficiency may be noted on auscultation as a holosystolic murmur and can be visualized echocardiographically together with poor contractility when PPHN is associated with myocardial ischemia. The degree of tricuspid regurgitation can be used to estimate pulmonary artery pressure. The 2nd heart sound is accentuated and not split. In asphyxia-associated and idiopathic PPHN, the chest roentgenogram is normal, whereas in PPHN associated with pneumonia and diaphragmatic hernia, it shows parenchymal opacification and bowel and/or liver in the chest, respectively. The **differential diagnosis** of PPHN includes cyanotic heart disease (especially obstructed total anomalous pulmonary venous return) and the associated etiologic entities that predispose to PPHN (hypoglycemia, polycythemia, sepsis).

TREATMENT. Therapy is directed toward correcting any predisposing disease (hypoglycemia, polycythemia) and improving poor tissue oxygenation. The response to therapy is often unpredictable, transient, and complicated by the adverse effects of drugs or mechanical ventilation. Initial management includes oxygen administration and correction of acidosis, hypotension, and hypercapnia. Persistent hypoxia should be managed with intubation and mechanical ventilation.

The optimal approach to mechanical ventilation is controversial. In the pre–nitric oxide era, one approach to the treatment of severe PPHN consisted of instituting mechanical ventilation without the use of muscle relaxants; ventilator settings were adjusted to achieve a Pao_2 of 50–70 mm Hg and a $Paco_2$ of 50–60 mm Hg. Tolazoline (1 mg/kg), a nonselective α-adrenergic antagonist, was sometimes used as an adjunct to non-selectively vasodilate the pulmonary arterial system, but it also resulted in systemic hypotension, which was treated with volume expansion and dopamine. Another approach incorporated hyperventilation to reduce pulmonary vasoconstriction by lowering the $Paco_2$ (≈25 mm Hg) and increasing the pH (7.50–7.55). This strategy required high peak inspiratory pressures and rapid respiratory rates, often necessitating the use of muscle relaxants for control of ventilation. Ventilator settings were adjusted to achieve a Pao_2 between 90 and 100 mm Hg. Alkalinization with sodium bicarbonate was also used to elevate serum pH.

Forced alkalosis using sodium bicarbonate and hyperventilation were popular therapies because of their ability to produce acute pulmonary vasodilation and rapid increases in Pao_2. Hypocarbia constricts the cerebral vasculature and reduces cerebral blood flow. Extreme alkalosis and hypocarbia are associated with later neurodevelopmental deficits, including cerebral palsy and neurosensory hearing loss. Other complications of hyperventilation included air trapping, reduced cardiac output due to decreased venous return, barotrauma, pneumothorax, increased fluid requirements, and edema. Sodium bicarbonate and THAM infusions, on the other hand, require careful monitoring of serum electrolytes and blood gases to assure that ventilation is adequate to allow carbon dioxide clearance. The use of alkali infusions is associated with an increased need for ECMO and an increased rate of BPD. Currently, infants with PPHN are managed without hyperventilation and/or alkalinization. In skilled hands, "gentle ventilation" with permissive hypercarbia results in excellent outcomes and a low incidence of BPD.

Because of their lability and ability to fight the ventilator, newborns with PPHN usually require sedation. Fentanyl may decrease sympathetic tone during stressful interventions and maintain a more relaxed pulmonary vascular bed. The use of paralytic agents is controversial and reserved for the newborn that cannot be treated with sedatives alone. Muscle relaxants may promote atelectasis of dependent lung regions and ventilation-perfusion mismatch. Paralysis may be associated with an increased risk of death. In survivors of congenital diaphragmatic hernia, prolonged administration of pancuronium during the neonatal period is associated with sensorineural hearing loss as well as acute myopathy.

Inotropic therapy is frequently needed to support blood pressure and perfusion. Whereas dopamine is frequently used as a 1st-line agent, other agents such as dobutamine, epinephrine, and milrinone are helpful when myocardial contractility is poor. Some of the sickest newborns with PPHN develop hypotension refractory to vasopressor administration. This results from desensitization of the cardiovascular system to catecholamines by overwhelming illness and relative adrenal insufficiency. Hydrocortisone rapidly upregulates cardiovascular adrenergic receptor expression and serves as a hormone substitute in cases of adrenal insufficiency.

Nitric oxide gas is an endothelial-derived signaling molecule that relaxes vascular smooth muscle and can be delivered to the lung by an inhalation device. Two large randomized controlled trials have shown that iNO reduces the need for ECMO support by approximately 40%. The optimal starting dose is 20 ppm. Higher doses have not been shown to be more effective and are associated with side effects including methemoglobinemia and increased levels of nitrogen dioxide, a pulmonary irritant. Most newborns require iNO for less than 5 days. Although nitric oxide has been used chronically in children and adults with primary pulmonary hypertension, prolonged dependency is rare in neonates and suggests the presence of lung hypoplasia, congenital heart disease, or alveolar capillary dysplasia. The maximal safe duration of iNO therapy is unknown. The dose can be weaned to 5 ppm after 6–24 hr of therapy. The dose can then be weaned slowly and discontinued when the FiO_2 is <0.6 and the iNO dose is 1 ppm. Abrupt discontinuation should be avoided as it may cause rebound pulmonary hypertension. iNO should only be used at institutions that offer ECMO support or have the capability of transport on iNO if a referral for ECMO is necessary. Some neonates with PPHN do not respond adequately to iNO. Therapy with continuous inhaled or intravenous prostacyclin (PGI_2) has improved oxygenation and outcome in infants with PPHN. Intravenous continuous PGI_2 is also effective in treating older children with primary pulmonary hypertension. Oral sildenafil (a type 5 phosphodiesterase inhibitor) improves exercise tolerance in adults with moderately severe pulmonary artery hypertension. The safety and efficacy of intravenous sildenafil is under investigation in newborns with PPHN.

Extracorporeal Membrane Oxygenation. In 5–10% of patients with PPHN (approximately 1/4,000 births), the response to 100% oxygen, mechanical ventilation, and drugs is poor. In such patients, the alveolar-arterial oxygen gradient (roughly at sea level, $[760 - 47] - PaCO_2 - PaO_2$) or the oxygenation index (OI) has been used to predict mortality rates >80%.

$$OI = (\text{Mean airway pressure} \times FiO_2 \times 100) \div \text{Postductal } PaO_2$$

Alveolar-arterial gradients >620 for 8–12 hr and an OI over 40 that is unresponsive to nitric oxide inhalation predict a high mortality rate and are indications for ECMO. ECMO is used to treat carefully selected, severely ill infants with hypoxemic respiratory failure caused by RDS, meconium aspiration pneumonia, congenital diaphragmatic hernia, PPHN, or sepsis.

ECMO is a form of cardiopulmonary bypass that augments systemic perfusion and provides gas exchange. Most experience has been with venoarterial bypass, which requires carotid artery ligation and the placement of large catheters in the right internal jugular vein and carotid artery. Venovenous bypass avoids carotid artery ligation and provides gas exchange, but it does not support cardiac output. Blood is initially pumped through the ECMO circuit at a rate that approximates 80% of the estimated cardiac output of 150–200 mL/kg/min. Venous return passes through a membrane oxygenator, is rewarmed, and returns to the aortic arch in venoarterial ECMO and to the right atrium in venovenous ECMO. Venous oxygen saturation values are used to monitor tissue oxygen delivery and subsequent extraction on venoarterial ECMO, whereas arterial oxygen saturation values are used to monitor oxygenation on venovenous ECMO. The rate of ECMO flow is adjusted to achieve satisfactory venous oxygen saturation (>65%) and cardiovascular stability on venoarterial ECMO and an arterial saturation of 85–95% on venovenous ECMO. When ECMO is started in an infant, the FiO_2 is weaned to room air and ventilatory settings are minimized to reduce the risk of oxygen toxicity and barotrauma, thus permitting time for the lungs to rest and heal.

Because ECMO requires complete heparinization to prevent clotting in the circuit, patients with or at high risk for IVH (weight <2 kg, age <34 wk gestation) are not candidates for this therapy. In addition, infants for whom ECMO is being considered should have reversible lung disease, no signs of systemic bleeding, an absence of severe asphyxia or lethal malformations, and they should have been ventilated for less than 10 days. Complications of ECMO include thromboembolism, air embolization, bleeding, stroke, seizures, atelectasis, cholestatic jaundice, thrombocytopenia, neutropenia, hemolysis, infectious complications of blood transfusions, edema formation, and systemic hypertension.

The number of neonatal respiratory ECMO cases has shown a progressive decline from a high of 1,500/year in 1992 to 750/year in 2004. The probable reasons for this are improved perinatal management and neonatal care, including the use of lung protective ventilation and iNO.

PROGNOSIS. Survival in patients with PPHN varies with the underlying diagnosis. The long-term outcome for infants with PPHN is related to the associated hypoxic-ischemic encephalopathy and the ability to reduce pulmonary vascular resistance. The long-term prognosis for infants who have PPHN and who survive after treatment with hyperventilation is comparable to that for infants who have underlying illnesses of equivalent severity (birth asphyxia, hypoglycemia, polycythemia). The outcome for infants who have PPHN treated with ECMO is also favorable; 70–80% survive, and 60–75% of survivors appear normal at 1–3.5 yr of age. Survival of infants born with congenital diaphragmatic hernia (CDH) has increased over the past 10 yr to 67%; benchmark institutions are reporting survival rates of >80%. Those infants with CDH who require ECMO continue to have a lower survival than the general neonatal ECMO population (52%).

Alano MA, Ngougmna E, Ostrea EM Jr, et al: Analysis of nonsteroidal anti-inflammatory drugs in meconium and its relation to persistent pulmonary hypertension of the newborn. *Pediatrics* 2001;107:519–523.

Baquero H, Soliz A, Neira F, et al: Oral sildenafil in infants with persistent pulmonary hypertension of the newborn: a pilot randomized blinded study. *Pediatrics* 2006;117:1077–1083.

Bennett CC, Johnson A, Field DJ, et al: UK collaborative randomized trial of neonatal extracorporeal membrane oxygenation: Follow-up to age 4 years. *Lancet* 2001;357:1094–1096.

Chambers CD, Hernandez-Díaz S, van Marter LJ, et al: Selective serotonin-reuptake inhibitors and risk of persistent pulmonary hypertension of the newborn. *N Engl J Med* 2006;354:579–587.

Finer NN, Sun JW, Rich W, et al: Randomized, prospective study of low-dose verus high-dose inhaled nitric oxide in the neonate with hypoxic respiratory failure. *Pediatrics* 2001;108:949–955.

Gill BS, Neville HL, Khan AM, et al: Delayed institution of extracorporeal membrane oxygenation is associated with increased mortality rate and prolonged hospital stay. *J Pediatr* Surg 2002;37:7–10.

Hoffman GM, Ross GA, Day SE, et al: Inhaled nitric oxide reduces the utilization of extracorporeal membrane oxygenation in persistent pulmonary hypertension of the newborn. *Crit Care Med* 1997;25:352–359.

Kelly LK, Porta NFM, Goodman DM, et al: Inhaled prostacyclin for term infants with persistent pulmonary hypertension refractory to inhaled nitric oxide. *J Pediatr* 2002;141:830–832.

Kinsella JP, Abman SH: Clinical approach to inhaled nitric oxide therapy in the newborn with hypoxemia. *J Pediatr* 2000;136:717–726.

Nakajima W, Ishida A, Arai H, et al: Methaemoglobinaemia after inhalation of nitric oxide in infants with pulmonary hypertension. *Lancet* 1997; 350:1002–1003.

Pearson DL, Dawling S, Walsh WF, et al: Neonatal pulmonary hypertension: Urea cycle intermediates, nitric oxide production, and carbamoyl-phosphate synthetase function. *N Engl J Med* 2001;344:1832–1838.

Roy BJ, Rycus P, Conrad SA, et al: The changing demographics of neonatal extracorporeal membrane oxygenation patients reported to the extracorporeal life support organization (ELSO) registry. *Pediatrics* 2000;106: 1334–1338.

Sen P, Thakur N, Stockton DW, et al: Expanding the phenotype of alveolar capillary dysplasia (ACD). *J Pediatr* 2004;145:646–651.

Walsh-Sukys MC, Tyson JE, Wright LL, et al: Persistent pulmonary hypertension of the newborn in the era before nitric oxide: Practice variation and outcomes. *Pediatrics* 2000;105:14–20.

101.9 • Diaphragmatic Hernia • Peter F. Ehrlich and Arnold G. Coran

A diaphragmatic hernia is defined as a communication between the abdominal and thoracic cavities with or without abdominal contents in the thorax (Fig. 101-9). The etiology may be congenital or traumatic. The symptoms and prognosis depend on the location of the defect and associated anomalies. The defect may be at the esophageal hiatus (hiatal), paraesophageal (adjacent to the hiatus), retrosternal (Morgagni), or at the posterolateral (Bochdalek) portion of the diaphragm. The term *congenital diaphragmatic hernia (CDH)* typically refers to the Bochdalek form. These lesions may cause significant respiratory distress at birth, can be associated with other congenital anomalies, and have a significant mortality and long-term morbidity. The overall survival from the CDH Study Group is 67%. The Bochdalek hernia accounts for up to 90% of the hernias seen in the newborn period, with 80–90% occurring on the left side. The Morgagni hernia accounts for 2–6% of congenital diaphragmatic defects. The size of the defect is highly variable, ranging from a small hole to complete agenesis of this area of the diaphragm. The management strategy for a child with a CDH has evolved from an emergent operation to deferred repair of the defect until pulmonary hypertension is resolved. Specific attention is focused on monitoring the systemic and pulmonary circulation, ventilation strategies that stabilize the infant and avoid barotraumas, and long-term management of pulmonary function.

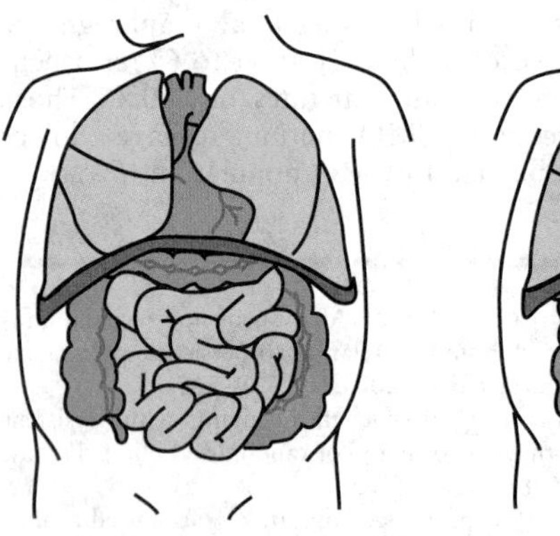

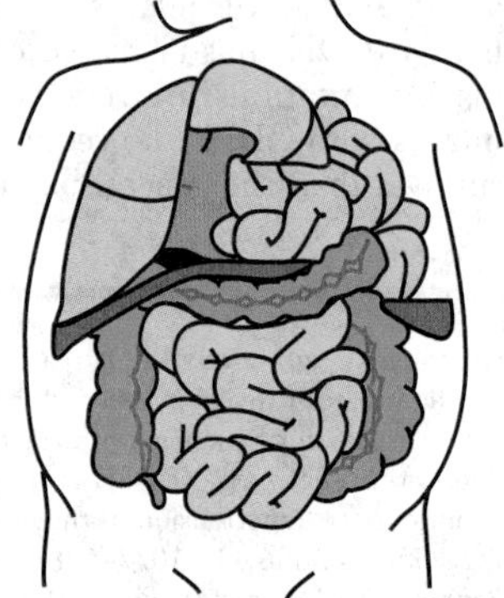

Figure 101-9. *A*, A normal diaphragm separating the abdominal and thoracic cavity. *B*, Diaphragmatic hernia with a small lung and abdominal contents in the thoracic cavity.

CONGENITAL DIAPHRAGMATIC HERNIA (BOCHDALEK)

EMBRYOLOGY, PATHOLOGY, AND ETIOLOGY. The diaphragm is a dome-shaped musculotendinous structure that is derived from four distinct fused structures. The septum transversum gives rise to the central tendon and separates the pericardial and peritoneal cavities. The central tendon constitutes 30% of the diaphragm and is the largest portion. The pleuroperitoneal membranes give rise to the dorsal lateral portions of the diaphragm; this separates the paired pleural cavities and the "fetal diaphragm" at approximately 8 wk gestation. The esophageal mesentery forms the dorsal crura and the intercostal muscle groups give rise to the muscular portion of the diaphragm. CDH may be due to defective formation of the pleuroperitoneal membrane. When the abdominal contents return to the abdomen from the umbilical sac at 10 wk gestation, herniation of the abdominal contents may occur.

Although CDH is characterized by a structural diaphragmatic defect, a major limiting factor for survival is the associated **pulmonary hypoplasia.** Fetal lung development is classified into 4 main stages. The *pseudoglandular* phase begins at the 5th wk with lung bud formation and ends at the 16–17th wk of gestation. During this stage, the major bronchi and terminal bronchi are formed. The next stage is the *canalicular* stage, characterized by the development of the respiratory bronchioles, alveolar ducts, and pulmonary vessels from wk 16 to 24–25. Initial alveolar or terminal sac development occurs during the *saccular* phase (24 wk term). Gas exchange is now possible. After delivery, alveoli continue to develop until approximately 8 yr of life. The stage is appropriately termed the *alveolar* stage. Lung hypoplasia was initially thought to be solely due to the compression of the lung from the herniated abdominal contents, which impaired lung growth. Pulmonary hypoplasia may occur, however, early in embryonic development, before the defect.

Pulmonary hypoplasia is characterized by a reduction in pulmonary mass and the number of bronchial divisions, respiratory bronchioles, and alveoli. The pathology of pulmonary hypoplasia and CDH includes abnormal septa in the terminal saccules, thickened alveoli, and thickened pulmonary arterioles. Biochemical abnormalities include relative surfactant deficiencies, increased glycogen in the alveoli with decreased levels of phosphatidylcholine, total DNA, and total lung protein. All these contribute to limited gas exchange.

EPIDEMIOLOGY. The incidence of CDH is between 1/2,000 and 1/5,000 live births, with females affected twice as often as males. Defects are more common on the left (85%) and are occasionally (<5%) bilateral. Pulmonary hypoplasia and malrotation of the intestine are part of the lesion, not associated anomalies. Most cases of CDH are sporadic, but familial cases have been reported. In one study, complete agenesis of the diaphragm had an autosomal recessive pattern of inheritance; in the majority of cases, genetic factors are multifactorial. Associated anomalies have been reported in up to 30% of cases; these include central nervous system lesions, esophageal atresia, omphalocele, and cardiovascular lesions. CDH is recognized as part of several chromosomal syndromes: trisomy 21, trisomy 13, trisomy 18, Fryn, Brachmann–de Lange, Pallister-Killian, and Turner.

DIAGNOSIS, CLINICAL PRESENTATION, AND TREATMENT. CDH can be diagnosed on prenatal ultrasound (between 16 and 24 wk) in over 50% of cases. High-speed magnetic resonance imaging can further define the lesion. Findings on ultrasound may include polyhydramnios, chest mass, mediastinal shift, gastric bubble or a liver in the thoracic cavity, and fetal hydrops. Certain imaging features may predict outcome; these include lung size to head size ratio (LHR). Nonetheless, there is no definitive characteristic that reliably predicts outcome. After delivery, a chest radiograph is needed to confirm the diagnosis (Fig. 101-10). In some instances with an echogenic chest mass, further imaging is required. The **differential diagnosis** may include a cystic lung lesion (pulmonary sequestration, cystic adenomatoid malformation) requiring an upper gastrointestinal series to confirm the diagnosis.

Arriving at the diagnosis early in pregnancy allows for prenatal counseling, possible fetal interventions, and planning for postnatal care. A referral to a center providing high-risk obstetrics, pediatric surgery, and tertiary care neonatology is advised. Careful evaluation for other anomalies should include echocardiography and amniocentesis. To avoid unnecessary termination and unrealistic expectations, an experienced multidisciplinary group must carefully counsel the parents of a child diagnosed with a diaphragmatic hernia.

Respiratory distress is a cardinal sign in babies with CDH. This may occur immediately or there may be a "honeymoon" period of up to 48 hr when the baby is relatively stable. Early respiratory distress within 6 hr of life is thought to be a poor prognostic sign. The clinical signs of respiratory distress are characterized by tachypnea, grunting, use of accessory muscles, and cyanosis.

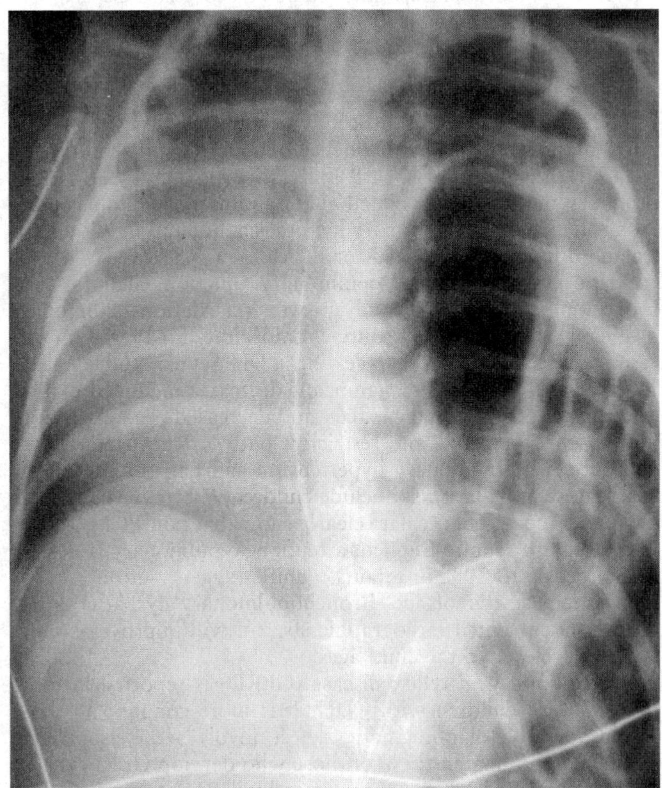

Figure 101-10. This chest radiograph shows a stomach, nasogastric tube, and small bowel contents in the thoracic cavity consistent with a congenital diaphragmatic hernia (CDH).

Children with CDH will also have a scaphoid abdomen and increased chest wall diameter. Bowel sounds may also be heard in the chest with decreased breath sounds bilaterally. The point of maximal cardiac impulse may be displaced away from the side of the hernia if mediastinal shift has occurred. A chest x-ray and nasal gastric tube is all that is usually required to confirm the diagnosis.

A small group will present beyond the neonatal period. Patients with a delayed presentation may experience vomiting as a result of intestinal obstruction or mild respiratory symptoms. Delayed presentation of a diaphragmatic hernia after a documented episode of group B streptococcal sepsis is well described. Occasionally, incarceration of the intestine will proceed to ischemia with sepsis and shock. Unrecognized diaphragmatic hernia is a rare cause of sudden death in infants and toddlers.

INITIAL MANAGEMENT. Aggressive respiratory support is often needed in children with CDH. This will include rapid endotracheal intubation, sedation, and possibly paralysis. Arterial (pre and postductal) and central venous (umbilical) lines are mandated, as are a urinary catheter and nasogastric tube. A preductal Sa_{O_2} of 85% or greater should be the minimum goal. Prolonged mask ventilation, which enlarges the stomach and small bowel thus making oxygenation more difficult, should be avoided. Barotrauma is a significant problem; therefore, peak inspiratory pressure (PIP) must be carefully monitored and kept below 25. Permissive hypercapnea with a Pa_{CO_2} of 45–60 is helpful as long the pH is above 7.3. Gentle ventilation with **permissive hypercapnea** reduces lung injury and mortality. Factors that contribute to pulmonary hypertension (hypoxia, acidosis, hypothermia) should be avoided. Echocardiography is a critically important imaging study that guides therapeutic decisions by measuring pulmonary and system vascular pressures and defining the presence of cardiac dysfunction. Routine use of inotropes is not supported in the absence of left ventricular dysfunction. Babies with CDH may be surfactant deficient. Although surfactant is commonly used, no study has proven that it is beneficial.

VENTILATION STRATEGIES. Conventional mechanical ventilation, high frequency oscillation ventilation (HFOV), and extracorporeal membrane oxygenation (ECMO) are the three main strategies to support respiratory failure in the newborn with CDH. The goals are to maintain oxygenation without inducing barotrauma. The first modality to be used is conventional ventilation. Pressure limited ventilation with the rate set between 30 and 60 and a PIP of 25cm H_2O or less reduces the risk of lung injury. Hyperventilation to induce alkalosis and decrease ductal shunting has not proven effective and should be avoided. Permissive hypercapnia has reduced lung injury and mortality in several studies. HFOV was initially used as a high pressure strategy to recruit alveolar units. This was unsuccessful resulting in increased barotrauma as the newborn with CDH has a nonrecruitable lung. The most logical approach to HFOV is to use it early, thus allowing ventilation at lower mean airway pressures.

Nitric oxide is a selective pulmonary vasodilator. Nitric oxide reduces ductal shunting and pulmonary pressures and results in improved oxygenation. Although helpful in persistent pulmonary hypertension of the newborn, randomized trials have not demonstrated improved survival or reduced need for ECMO when NO was used in newborns with CDH. Nonetheless, it is used in patients with CDH before starting ECMO (see Chapter 101.8)

ECMO. The availability of ECMO and the utility of preoperative stabilization have improved survival. ECMO combined with paralysis and nasogastric suction may produce a dramatic reduction of the volume of herniated viscera. ECMO is the therapeutic option in children who fail conventional ventilation or conventional ventilation and HFOV. ECMO is most commonly used before repair of the defect. Several objective criteria for ECMO have been developed (see Chapter 101.8).

Birthweight and the 5-min APGAR scores may be the best predictors of outcome in patients treated with ECMO. The lower limit of weight for ECMO is 2 kg. ECMO modes may be venoarterial (VA) or venovenous (VV), although VA is used most commonly (85%).

The duration of ECMO for neonates with diaphragmatic hernia is significantly longer (7–14 days) than for those with persistent fetal circulation or meconium aspiration, and may last up to 2–4 wk. Timing of repair of the diaphragm on ECMO is controversial; some centers prefer early repair to allow a greater duration of post repair on ECMO, whereas many centers defer repair until the infant has demonstrated the ability to tolerate weaning from ECMO. The recurrence of pulmonary hypertension has a high mortality, and weaning from ECMO support should be cautious. If the patient cannot be weaned from ECMO after repair, options include discontinuing support or, in rare cases, lung transplantation.

NOVEL STRATEGIES FOR INFANTS WITH CDH. There are no reliable prenatal prognosticators of outcomes in children with CDH. The most widely studied is fetal ultrasound (US). A prospective study using US at 24–26 wk compared fetal LHR. There were no survivors when the LHR was less than 1, and all babies survived with LHR greater then 1.4. A second important consideration was the presence of liver in the thoracic cavity, which is a poor prognostic feature. Human studies have shown no benefit for in utero repair of CDH.

Tracheal occlusion in utero is based on the observation that in utero fetal lung fluid plays a critical role in lung growth and maturity. A deficiency of lung fluid results in pulmonary hypoplasia. In experimental models, tracheal occlusion or ligation induces lung growth, reduces herniated viscera, and improves compliance and oxygenation. The technique has not been beneficial. Partial liquid ventilation (PLV) after birth is an experimental therapy under investigation in adults and children with severe respiratory failure. PLV increases functional residual capacity by recruiting collapsed alveoli, thereby improving ventilation perfusion mismatches and compliance. It also may reduce lung injury and increase surfactant production. A study is under way to evaluate the role of PLV in neonates with CDH.

SURGICAL REPAIR. The ideal time to repair the diaphragmatic defect is under debate. Most centers will wait at least 48 hr after stabilization and resolution of the pulmonary hypertension. A requirement for only conventional ventilation, a low PIP and FIO_2 below 50 are good relative indicators of stability. If the newborn was on HFOV, repair is delayed until the child can be back on a conventional ventilator. If the newborn was on ECMO, an ability to wean should be a consideration before surgical repair. In some centers, the repair is done with the cannulas in place; in other centers, the cannulas are removed. A subcostal approach is the most frequently used (Fig. 101-11). This allows for good visualization of the defect and, if the abdominal cavity cannot accommodate the herniated contents, a silastic patch can be placed. Both laparoscopic and thoracoscopic repairs have been reported, but these should be reserved only for the most stable infants.

The defect size and amount of native diaphragm present are variable. Whenever possible, a primary repair using native tissue is performed. If the defect is too large, a Gore-Tex patch is used.

There is a higher recurrence rate among children with patches (the patch does not grow as the child grows) compared to repairs with native tissue. A loosely fitted patch may reduce recurrence rates. Pulmonary hypertension must be monitored carefully and, in some instances, a postoperative course of ECMO is needed. Other recognized complications include bleeding, chylothorax, and bowel obstruction.

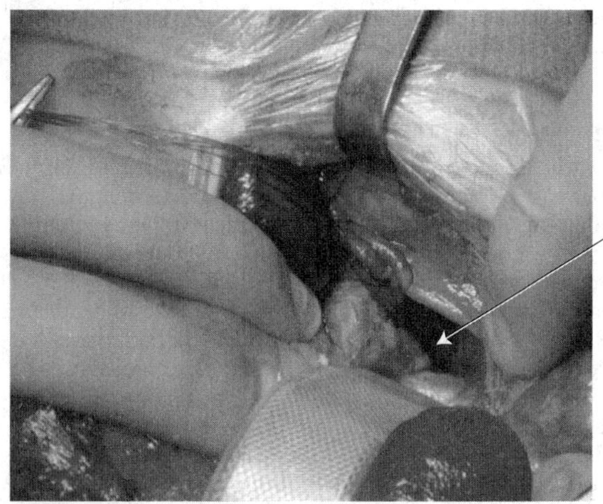

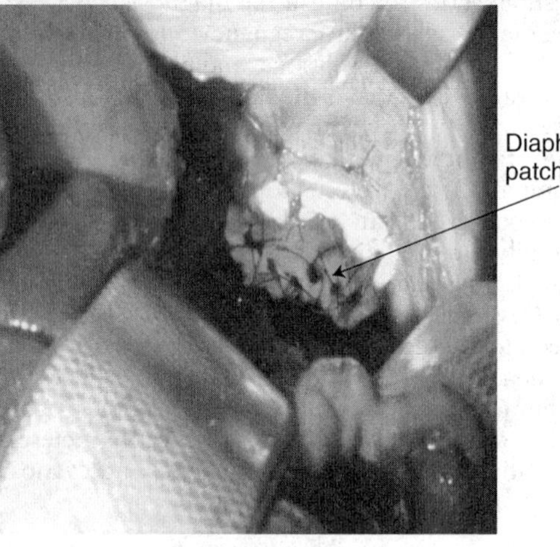

Figure 101-11. *A*, An intraoperative picture of a congenital diaphragmatic hernia (CDH) before repair. *B*, An intraoperative picture of a patch repair of a CDH.

OUTCOME AND LONG-TERM SURVIVAL. Overall survival of liveborn infants is 67%. The incidence of spontaneous fetal demise with CDH diagnosis is 7–10%. Relative predictors of a poor prognosis include an associated major anomaly, symptoms before 24 hr of age, severe pulmonary hypoplasia, herniation to the contralateral lung, and the need for ECMO.

Serious sequelae include pulmonary function changes, neurodevelopmental delays, and growth retardation. Pulmonary problems continue to be a source of morbidity for long-term survivors of CDH. Children receiving CDH repair studied at 6–11 yr of age demonstrate significant decreases in forced expiratory flow at 50% of vital capacity and decreased peak expiratory flow. Both obstructive and restrictive patterns can occur. Those without severe pulmonary hypertension and barotrauma do the best. Those at highest risk include children who required ECMO and patch repair, but the data clearly show that non-ECMO CDH survivors also require frequent attention to pulmonary issues. At discharge, up to 20% of infants require oxygen, but only 1–2% require it past 1 yr of age. **Bronchopulmonary dysplasia** is frequently documented radiographically, but will improve as more alveoli develop and the child ages.

Gastroesophageal reflux disease (GERD) is reported in more than 50% of children with CDH. It is more common in those children whose diaphragmatic defect involves the esophageal hiatus. Approximately 25% of those who develop GERD will be refractory to medical management and will require an antireflux procedure. Intestinal obstruction is reported in up to 20% of children. This could be due to a midgut volvulus, adhesions, or a recurrent hernia that incarcerated. Recurrent diaphragmatic hernia is reported in 5–20% in most series. Children with patch repairs are at highest risk.

Children with CDH typically have delayed growth in the 1st 2 yr of life. Contributing factors include poor intake, GERD, and a caloric requirement that may be higher because of the energy required to breathe. Many children will normalize and "catch up" by the time they are 2 yr old.

Neurocognitive defects are common and may be due to the disease or the interventions. The incidence of neurologic abnormalities is higher in those infants requiring ECMO (67% vs 24%). The abnormalities are similar to those seen in neonates treated with ECMO for other diagnoses and include transient and permanent developmental delay, abnormal hearing or vision, and seizures. Serious hearing loss may occur in up to 28% of children who were on ECMO. The majority of neurologic abnormalities are classified as mild to moderate.

Other long-term problems occurring in this population include pectus excavatum and scoliosis. Survivors of CDH repair, particularly those requiring ECMO support, have a variety of long-term abnormalities that appear to improve with time but require close monitoring and multidisciplinary support.

101.10 • Foramen of Morgagni Hernia • Peter F. Ehrlich and Arnold G. Coran

The anteromedial diaphragmatic defect through the foramen of Morgagni accounts for 2–6% of diaphragmatic hernias. Failure of the sternal and crural portions of the diaphragm to meet and fuse produces this defect. These defects are more commonly right-sided (90%) but may be bilateral (Fig. 101-12). The transverse colon or small intestine or liver is usually contained in the hernia sac. The majority of children with these defects are asymptomatic and are diagnosed beyond the neonatal period. The diagnosis is usually made on chest x-ray (CXR) when the children are evaluated for another reason. The CXR shows a structure behind the heart and a lateral film localizes the mass to the retrosternal area. A chest CT will confirm the diagnosis. When symptoms occur, they can be recurrent respiratory infections, cough, vomiting, or reflux; in rare instances, incarceration may occur. Repair is recommended for all patients and can be accomplished laparoscopically or by an open approach. Prosthetic material is rarely required.

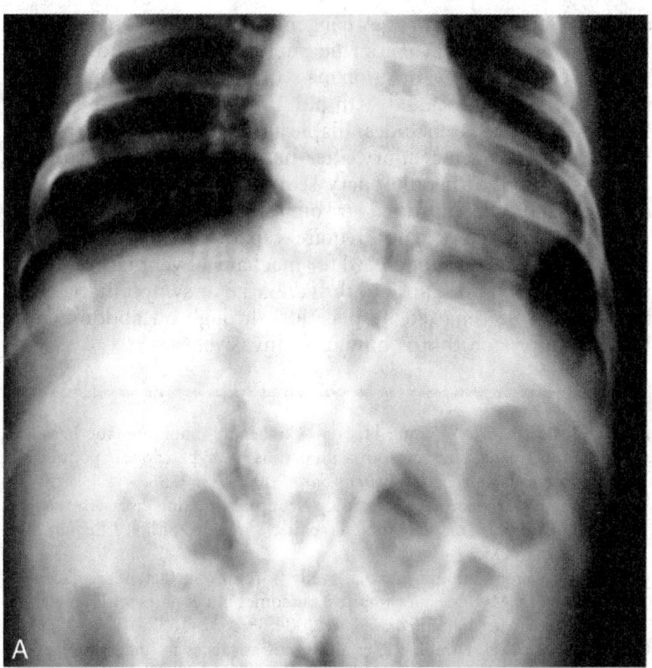

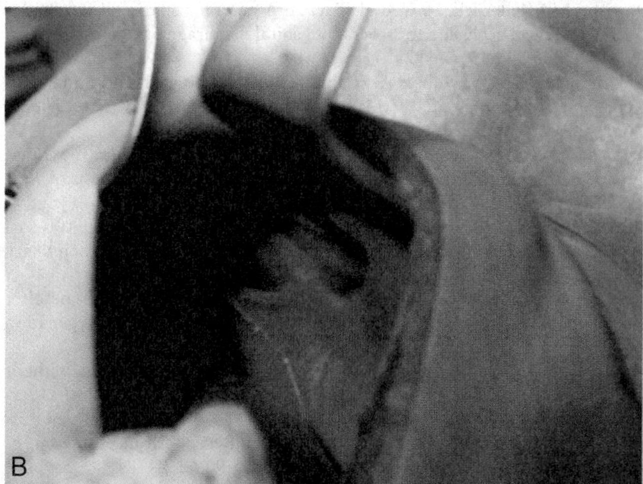

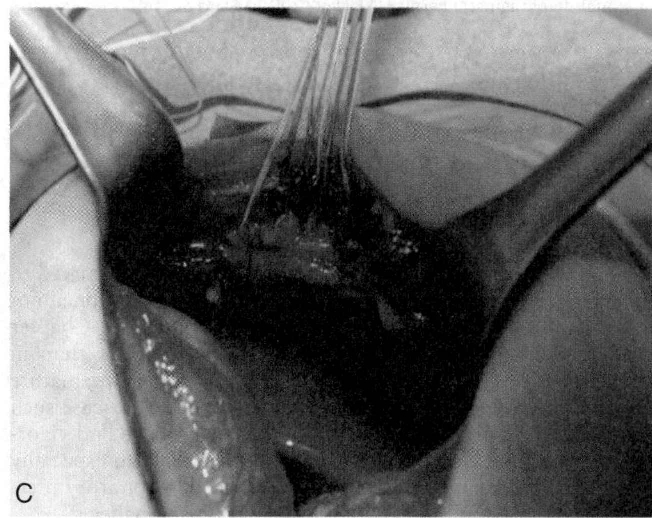

Figure 101-12. *A*, A chest radiograph demonstrating a Morgagni hernia. *B*, An intraoperative picture of a Morgagni hernia before repair. *C*, An intraoperative picture of a Morgagni hernia after closure.

101.11 • Paraesophageal Hernia • Peter F. Ehrlich and Arnold G. Coran

Paraesophageal hernia is differentiated from hiatal hernia in that the gastroesophageal junction is in the normal location. The herniation of the stomach alongside or adjacent to the gastroesophageal junction is prone to incarceration with strangulation and perforation. A previous Nissen fundoplication and other diaphragmatic surgeries are risk factors. This unusual diaphragmatic hernia should be repaired promptly after identification.

101.12 • Eventration • Peter F. Ehrlich and Arnold G. Coran

Eventration of the diaphragm is an abnormal elevation, consisting of a thinned diaphragmatic muscle producing elevation of the entire hemidiaphragm or, more commonly, the anterior aspect of the hemidiaphragm. This produces a paradoxical motion of the affected hemidiaphragm. Most eventrations are asymptomatic and do not require repair. A congenital form is the result of an incomplete development of the muscular portion or central tendon. Congenital eventration may affect lung development, but it has not been associated with pulmonary hypoplasia. The differential diagnosis includes diaphragmatic paralysis, traction injury, and iatrogenic injury after heart surgery. Eventration is also associated with pulmonary sequestration, congenital heart disease, and chromosomal trisomies. Most eventrations are asymptomatic and do not require repair. The indications for surgery include continued need for mechanical ventilation, recurrent infections, and failure to thrive. Large or symptomatic eventrations can be repaired by plication through an abdominal or thoracic approach that is minimally invasive.

Boloker J, Bateman DA, Wung JT, et al: Congenital diaphragmatic hernia in 120 infants treated consecutively with permissive hypercapnea/spontaneous respiration/elective repair. *J Pediatr Surg* 2002;37:357–366.

Congenital Diaphragmatic Hernia Study Group: Estimating disease severity of congenital diaphragmatic hernia in the first 5 minutes of life. *J Pediatr Surg* 2001;36:141–145.

Congenital Diaphragmatic Hernia Study Group: Surfactant replacement therapy on ECMO does not improve outcomes in neonates with congenital diaphragmatic hernia. *J Pediatr Surg* 2004;39:1632–1637.

Greer JJ, Allan DW, Babiuk RP, et al: Recent advances in understanding the pathogenesis of nitrogen-induced congenital diaphragmatic hernia. *Pediatr Pulmonol* 2000;29:394–399.

Harrison MR Keller RL, Hawgood SB, et al: A randomized trial of fetal endoscopic tracheal occlusion for severe congenital diaphragmatic hernia. *N Engl J Med* 2003;349:1916–1924.

Jaillard SM, Pierrat V, Dubois A, et al: Outcome at two years of infants with congenital diaphragmatic hernia: A population based study. *Ann Thorac Surg* 2003;75:250–256.

Jesudason EC: Challenging embryological theories on congenital diaphragmatic hernia: Future therapeutic implications for pediatric surgeons. *Ann R Coll Surg Engl* 2002;84:252–259.

Muratore CS, Kharasch V, Lund DP, et al: Pulmonary morbidity in 100 survivors of congenital diaphragmatic hernia monitored in a multidisciplinary clinic. *J Pediatr Surg* 2001;36:133–140.

Rasheed A, Tindall S, Cueny DL, et al: Neurodevelopmental outcome after congenital diaphragmatic hernia: Extracorporeal membrane oxygenation before and after surgery. *J Pediatr Surg* 2001;36:539–544.

Sbragia L, Paek BW, Filly RA, et al: Congenital diaphragmatic hernia without herniation of the liver: Does lung to head ratio predict survival? *J Ultrasound Med* 2000;19:845–848.

Smith NP, Jesudason EC, Featherstone NC, et al: Recent advances in congenital diaphragmatic hernia. *Arch Dis Child* 2005;90:426–428.

Van Meures K, Congenital Diaphragmatic Hernia Study Group: Is surfactant therapy beneficial in the treatment of the term newborn infant with congenital diaphragmatic hernia? *J Pediatr* 2004;145:312–316.

101.13 • Extrapulmonary Extravasation of Air (Pneumothorax, Pneumomediastinum, Pulmonary Interstitial Emphysema)

Asymptomatic pneumothorax, usually unilateral, is estimated to occur in 1–2% of all newborn infants; symptomatic pneumothorax and pneumomediastinum are less common (see Chapter 100). Pneumothorax occurs more frequently in males than in females and in term and post-term infants than in premature ones. The incidence is increased in infants with lung disease such as meconium aspiration and RDS; in those who have had vigorous resuscitation or are receiving assisted ventilation, especially if high inspiratory pressure and/or excessive end-expiratory pressure is used; and in infants with urinary tract anomalies.

ETIOLOGY AND PATHOPHYSIOLOGY. The most common cause of pneumothorax is overinflation resulting in alveolar rupture. It may be "spontaneous" or be due to underlying pulmonary disease such as lobar emphysema or rupture of a congenital lung cyst or pneumatocele, to trauma, or to a "ball-valve" type of bronchial or bronchiolar obstruction resulting from aspiration. Air leaks occur during the 1st 24–36 hr in infants with meconium aspiration pneumonia and in infants with RDS when lung compliance is reduced, and later during the recovery phase of RDS if inspiratory pressure and PEEP are not reduced simultaneously with improved respiratory function.

Pneumothorax associated with **pulmonary hypoplasia** is common, occurs on the 1st day of life, and is due to reduced alveolar surface area and poorly compliant lungs. It is associated with disorders of decreased amniotic fluid volume (Potter syndrome, renal agenesis, renal dysplasia, chronic amniotic fluid leak), decreased fetal breathing movement (oligohydramnios, neuromuscular disease), pulmonary space-occupying lesions (diaphragmatic hernia, pleural effusion, chylothorax), and thoracic abnormalities (asphyxiating thoracic dystrophies).

Air from a ruptured alveolus escapes into the interstitial spaces of the lung, where it may cause interstitial emphysema or dissect along the peribronchial and perivascular connective tissue sheaths to the hilum of the lung. If the volume of escaped air is great enough, it may collect in the mediastinal space (pneumomediastinum) or rupture into the pleural space (pneumothorax), subcutaneous tissue (subcutaneous emphysema), peritoneal cavity (pneumoperitoneum) and/or pericardial sac (pneumopericardium). Rarely, increased mediastinal pressure may compress the pulmonary veins at the hilum and thereby interfere with pulmonary venous return to the heart and cardiac output. On occasion, air may embolize into the circulation and produce cutaneous blanching, air in intravascular catheters, an air-filled heart on chest roentgenograms, and death.

Tension pneumothorax occurs if an accumulation of air within the pleural space is sufficient to elevate intrapleural pressure above atmospheric pressure. Unilateral tension pneumothorax results in impaired ventilation not only in the ipsilateral lung, but also in the contralateral lung due to a shift in the mediastinum toward the contralateral side. Compression of the vena cava and torsion of the great vessels may interfere with venous return.

CLINICAL MANIFESTATIONS. The physical findings of clinically asymptomatic pneumothorax are hyperresonance and diminished breath sounds over the involved side of the chest with or without tachypnea.

Symptomatic pneumothorax is characterized by respiratory distress, which varies from only an increased respiratory rate to severe dyspnea, tachypnea, and cyanosis. Irritability and restlessness or apnea may be the earliest signs. The onset is usually sudden but may be gradual; an infant may rapidly become critically ill. The chest may appear asymmetric with an increased anteroposterior diameter and bulging of the intercostal spaces on the affected side; other symptoms may be hyperresonance and diminished or absent breath sounds. The heart is displaced toward the unaffected side, resulting in displacement of the cardiac apex and point of maximal impulse (PMI) of the heart. The diaphragm is displaced downward, as is the liver with right-sided pneumothorax, and may result in abdominal distention. Because pneumothorax may be bilateral in approximately 10% of patients, symmetry of findings does not rule it out. In tension pneumothorax, signs of shock may be noted.

Pneumomediastinum occurs in at least 25% of patients with pneumothorax and is usually asymptomatic. The degree of respiratory distress depends on the amount of trapped air. If it is great, bulging of the midthoracic area is observed, the neck veins are distended, and blood pressure is low. The last two findings are a result of tamponade of the systemic and pulmonary veins. Although often asymptomatic, subcutaneous emphysema in newborn infants is almost pathognomonic of pneumomediastinum.

Pulmonary interstitial emphysema (PIE) may precede the development of a pneumothorax or may occur independently and result in increasing respiratory distress as a result of decreased compliance, hypercapnia, and hypoxia. The latter is due to an increased alveolar-arterial oxygen gradient and intrapulmonary shunting. Progressive enlargement of blebs of air may result in cystic dilatation and respiratory deterioration resembling pneumothorax. In severe cases, PIE precedes the development of BPD. Avoidance of high inspiratory or mean airway pressures may prevent the development of PIE. Treatment may include bronchoscopy in patients with evidence of mucous plugging, selective intubation and ventilation of the uninvolved bronchus, oxygen, general respiratory care, and HFV.

DIAGNOSIS. Pneumothorax and pneumomediastinum should be suspected in any newborn infant who shows signs of respiratory distress, is restless or irritable, or has a sudden change in condition. The diagnosis of pneumothorax is established by x-ray, with the edge of the collapsed lung standing out in relief against the pneumothorax (Fig. 101-13); pneumomediastinum is diagnosed by hyperlucency around the heart border and between the sternum and the heart border (Fig. 101-14). Transillumination of the thorax is often helpful in the emergency diagnosis of pneumothorax; the affected side transmits excessive light. Associated renal anomalies are identified by ultrasonography. **Pulmonary hypoplasia** is suggested by signs of uterine compression (extremity contractures), a small thorax on chest roentgenograms, severe hypoxia with hypercapnia, and signs of the primary disease (hypotonia, diaphragmatic hernia, Potter syndrome).

Pneumopericardium may be asymptomatic and require only general supportive treatment, but it usually manifests as sudden shock with tachycardia, muffled heart sounds, and poor pulses suggesting tamponade, which requires prompt evacuation of entrapped air. Pneumoperitoneum from air dissecting through the diaphragmatic apertures during mechanical ventilation may be confused with intestinal perforation. Paracentesis can be helpful in differentiating the two conditions. The presence of organisms on Gram stain or intestinal contents suggests the latter. Occasionally, pneumoperitoneum can result in an abdominal compartment syndrome requiring decompression.

TREATMENT. Without a continued air leak, asymptomatic and mildly symptomatic small pneumothoraces require only close observation. Frequent small feedings may prevent gastric dilatation and minimize crying, which can further compromise ventilation and worsen the pneumothorax. Breathing 100% oxygen accelerates the resorption of free pleural air into blood by reducing the nitrogen tension in blood and producing a resultant nitrogen pressure gradient from the trapped air in the blood, but the benefit must be weighed against the risks of oxygen toxicity. Nitrogen washout is not helpful in infants who develop a pneumothorax while in a high concentration of ambient oxygen. With severe respiratory or circulatory embarrassment, emergency needle aspiration is indicated. Either immediately or after needle

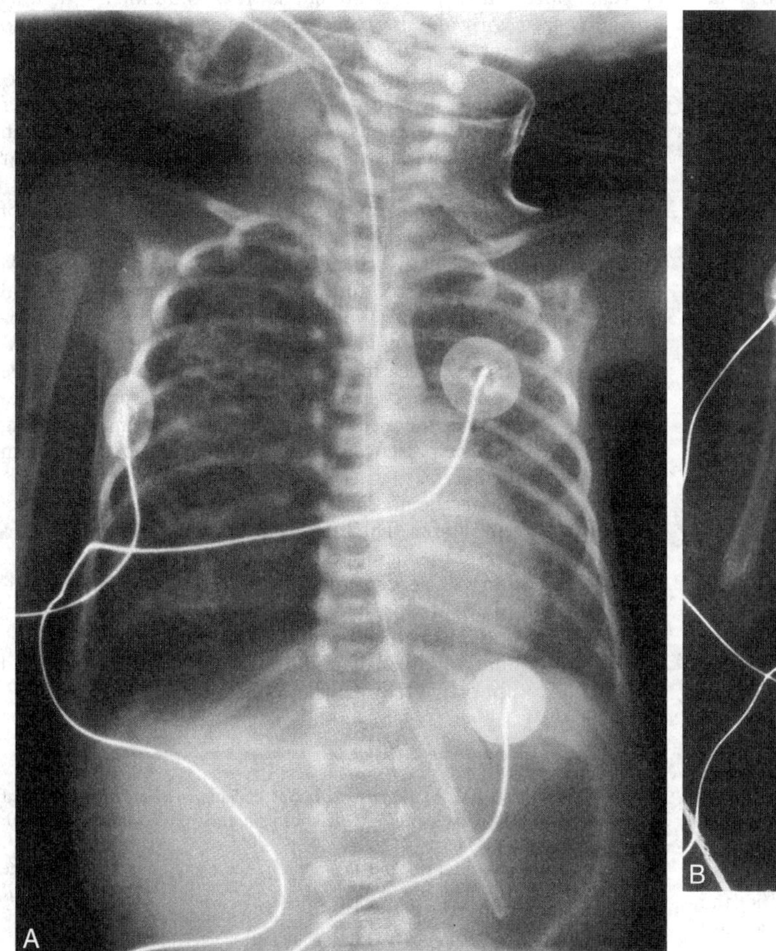

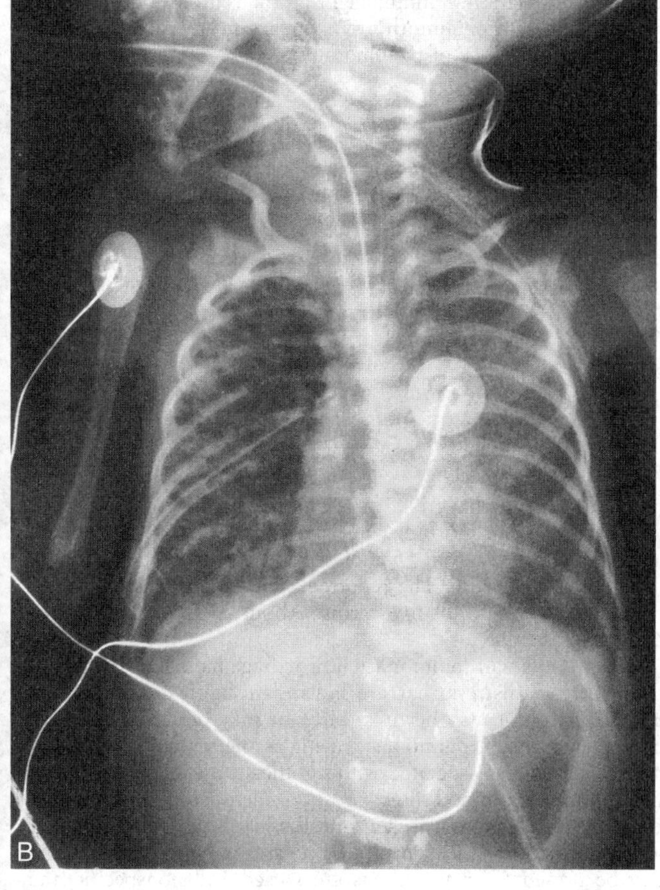

Figure 101-13. *A,* Right-sided tension pneumothorax and widespread right lung pulmonary interstitial emphysema in a preterm infant on intensive care. *B,* Resolution of pneumothorax with a chest tube in place. Pulmonary interstitial emphysema (PIE) persists. (From Meerstadt PWD, Gyll C: *Manual of Neonatal Emergency X-Ray Interpretation.* Philadelphia, WB Saunders, 1994: 73.)

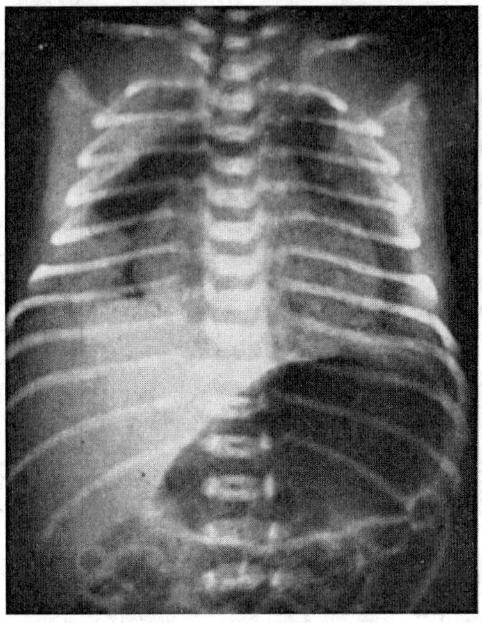

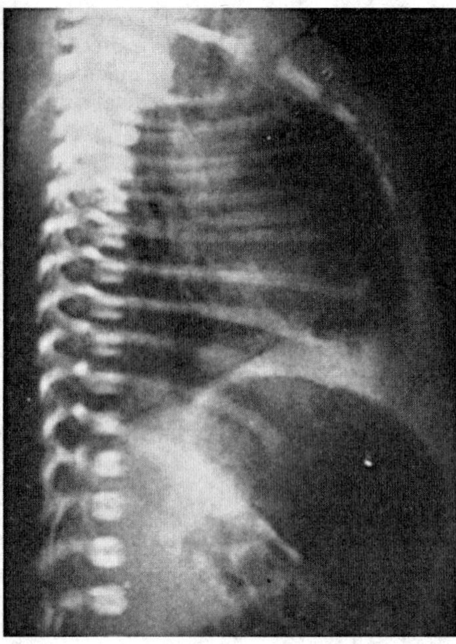

Figure 101-14. Pneumomediastinum in a newborn infant. The anteroposterior view demonstrates compression of the lungs, and the lateral view shows bulging of the sternum, each resulting from distention of the mediastinum by trapped air.

aspiration, a chest tube should be inserted and attached to underwater seal drainage (see Fig. 101-13). If the air leak is ongoing, continuous suction (–5 to –20 cm H_2O) may be needed to evacuate the pneumothorax completely. Severe localized interstitial emphysema may respond to selective bronchial intubation. Judicious use of sedation in infants fighting the ventilator may reduce the incidence of pneumothorax. Surfactant therapy for RDS reduces the incidence of pneumothorax.

Primhak RA: Factors associated with pulmonary air leak in premature infants receiving mechanical ventilation. *J Pediatr* 1983;102:764–768.

Ryan CA, Barrington KJ, Phillips HJ, et al: Contralateral pneumothoraces in the newborn: Incidence and predisposing factors. *Pediatrics* 1987; 79:417–421.

Watkinson M, Tiron I: Events before the diagnosis of a pneumothorax in ventilated neonates. *Arch Dis Child Fetal Neonatal Ed* 2001;85:F201–F203.

101.14 • Pulmonary Hemorrhage

Pulmonary hemorrhage is a rare, but catastrophic complication with a high risk of morbidity and mortality. Massive pulmonary hemorrhage is present in 15% of neonates who come to autopsy in the 1st 2 wk of life. The reported incidence at autopsy varies from 1 to 4 per 1,000 live births. About ¾ of patients weigh <2,500 g at birth.

Most infants with pulmonary hemorrhage have had symptoms of respiratory distress that are indistinguishable from those of HMD. The onset may occur at birth or may be delayed several days. Hemorrhagic pulmonary edema is the source of blood in many cases and is associated with significant ductal shunting and high pulmonary blood flow or severe left-sided heart failure resulting from hypoxia. In severe cases, cardiovascular collapse, poor lung compliance, profound cyanosis, and hypercapnia may be present. X-ray findings are varied and nonspecific and range from minor streaking or patchy infiltrates to massive consolidation.

The incidence of pulmonary hemorrhage is increased in association with acute pulmonary infection, severe asphyxia, HMD, assisted ventilation, PDA, congenital heart disease, erythroblastosis fetalis, hemorrhagic disease of the newborn, thrombocytopenia, inborn errors of ammonia metabolism, and cold injury. Pulmonary hemorrhage is the only severe complication associated with surfactant treatment; the relative risk for pulmonary hemorrhage after surfactant treatment is 1.47. Pulmonary hemorrhage is seen with all surfactants; incidence ranges from 1% to 5% of treated infants and is higher with natural surfactant. Bleeding is predominantly alveolar in about 65% of cases and interstitial in the rest. In severely ill neonates, bleeding into other organs is observed at autopsy, suggesting the possibility of an additional bleeding diathesis such as disseminated intravascular coagulation.

The little available information that describes the prognosis of infants who bleed through the mouth or nostrils suggests that it is extremely poor. Death occurs in the 1st 48 hr of life in 65% of infants who come to autopsy. **Treatment** includes blood replacement, PEEP, suctioning to clear the airway, intratracheal administration of epinephrine, and, in some cases, HFV. Although surfactant treatment has been associated with the development of pulmonary hemorrhage, administration of exogenous surfactant after the bleeding has occurred can improve lung compliance since the presence of intra-alveolar blood and protein can inactive surfactant.

Acute pulmonary hemorrhage may rarely occur in previously healthy full-term infants. The cause is unknown. Pulmonary hemorrhage may present as hemoptysis or blood in the nasopharynx or airway with no evidence of upper respiratory or gastrointestinal bleeding. Patients present with acute, severe respiratory failure requiring mechanical ventilation. Chest x-rays usually demonstrate bilateral alveolar infiltrates. Infants usually respond to intensive supportive treatment (see Chapter 406).

Berger TM, Allred EN, Van Marter LJ: Antecedents of clinically significant pulmonary hemorrhage among newborn infants. *J Perinatol* 2000;20: 295–300.

Centers for Disease Control and Prevention: Acute pulmonary hemorrhage among infants—Chicago, April 1992–November 1994. *MMWR* 1995;44:67,73–74.

Cole VA, Norman ICS, Reynolds EOR, et al: Pathogenesis of hemorrhagic pulmonary edema and massive pulmonary hemorrhage in the newborn. *Pediatrics* 1973;51:175–187.

Kluckow M, Evans N: Ductal shunting, high pulmonary blood flow, and pulmonary hemorrhage. *J Pediatr* 2000;137:68–72.

Pandit PB, Dunn MS, Colucci EA: Surfactant therapy in neonates with respiratory deterioration due to pulmonary hemorrhage. *Pediatrics* 1995;95: 32–36.
Pappin A, Shenker N, Hack M, et al: Extensive intra-alveolar pulmonary hemorrhage in infants dying after surfactant therapy. *J Pediatr* 1994;124: 621–626.

Chapter 102 ■ Digestive System Disorders

Anthony J. Piazza and Barbara J. Stoll

VOMITING. Vomiting or, more often, regurgitation is a relatively frequent symptom during the neonatal period. In the 1st few hours after birth, infants may vomit mucus, occasionally blood streaked. This vomiting rarely persists after the 1st few feedings; it may be due to irritation of the gastric mucosa by material swallowed during delivery. If vomiting is protracted, gastric lavage with physiologic saline solution may relieve it.

When vomiting occurs shortly after birth and is persistent, the possibilities of intestinal obstruction, metabolic disorders, and increased intracranial pressure must be considered. A history of maternal polyhydramnios suggests upper gastrointestinal (esophageal, duodenal, ileal) atresia. Bile-stained emesis suggests intestinal obstruction beyond the duodenum, but may also be idiopathic. Abdominal x-rays (kidney-ureter-bladder [KUB] and cross-table lateral views) should be performed in neonates with persistent emesis and in all infants with bile-stained emesis to detect air-fluid levels, distended bowel loops, characteristic patterns of obstruction (double bubble: duodenal atresia), and pneumoperitoneum (intestinal perforation). A contrast swallow roentgenogram with small bowel follow-through is indicated in the presence of bilious emesis.

Obstructive lesions of the digestive tract are the most frequent gastrointestinal anomalies (see Chapters 316, 326, 327, and 329). Vomiting from esophageal obstruction occurs with the 1st feeding. The diagnosis of esophageal atresia can be suspected if unusual drooling from the mouth is observed and if resistance is encountered during an attempt to pass a catheter into the stomach. The diagnosis should be made before the infant has trouble with oral feedings and develops aspiration pneumonia. Infantile achalasia (cardiospasm), a rare cause of vomiting in newborn infants, is demonstrable roentgenographically by obstruction at the cardiac end of the esophagus without organic stenosis. Regurgitation of feedings because of continuous relaxation of the esophageal-gastric sphincter, or chalasia, is a cause of vomiting. Keeping the infant in a semi-upright position, thickening the feeding, or administering prokinetic drugs can control it.

Vomiting because of obstruction of the small intestine usually begins on the 1st day of life and is frequent, persistent, usually non-projectile, copious, and, unless the obstruction is above the ampulla of Vater, bile stained; it is associated with abdominal distention, visible deep peristaltic waves, and reduced or absent bowel movements. Malrotation with obstruction from **midgut volvulus** is an acute emergency that not only must be considered but also urgently evaluated by an upper gastrointestinal contrast series. X-rays of the abdomen show the distribution of air in the intestine, which may point to the anatomic location of an obstruction; malrotation can be identified only by contrast studies. Normally, air can be demonstrated by x-ray in the jejunum by 15–60 min, in the ileum by 2–3 hr, and in the colon by 3 hr after birth. Absence of rectal gas at 24 hr is abnormal. Persistent vomiting may occur with congenital diaphragmatic hernia. The vomiting associated with pyloric stenosis may begin any time after birth but does not assume its characteristic pattern before the 2nd–3rd wk. Vomiting with obstipation is a common early sign of **Hirschsprung disease.** Vomiting may occur with many other disturbances that do not obstruct the digestive tract, such as milk allergy, adrenal hyperplasia of the salt-losing variety, galactosemia, hyperammonemias, organic acidemias, increased intracranial pressure, septicemia, meningitis, and urinary tract infection. In many infants, it is simply regurgitation from overfeeding or from failure to permit the infant to eructate swallowed air. (See Chapter 320 for a discussion of gastric emptying and gastroesophageal reflux.)

DIARRHEA. See Chapters 55.1, 55.2, 337, and 338.

CONSTIPATION. More than 90% of full-term newborn infants pass meconium within the 1st 24 hr. The possibility of intestinal obstruction should be considered in any infant who does not pass meconium by 24–36 hr. Intestinal atresia, stricture, or stenosis; Hirschsprung disease; milk bolus obstruction; meconium ileus; or meconium plugs may manifest as constipation or, more often, obstipation. About 20% of very low birthweight (VLBW) infants do not pass meconium within the 1st 24 hr. Constipation not present from birth but appearing during the 1st mo of life may be a sign of short-segment congenital aganglionic megacolon, hypothyroidism, strictures after necrotizing enterocolitis (NEC), or anal stenosis. It must be kept in mind that infrequent bowel movements do not necessarily mean constipation. A breast-fed infant usually has frequent bowel movements, whereas a formula-fed infant may have 1–2 movements a day or every other day.

MECONIUM PLUGS. Lower colonic or anorectal plugs (Fig. 102-1) with a lower than normal water content may cause intestinal obstruction. Rarely, a firm mass of meconium may form elsewhere in the intestine and cause intrauterine intestinal obstruction and meconium peritonitis unrelated to cystic fibrosis (CF). Anorectal plugs may also cause mucosal ulceration and intestinal perforation. **Meconium plugs** are associated with small left colon syndrome in infants of diabetic mothers and with CF, rectal aganglionosis, maternal opiate use, and magnesium sulfate therapy for preeclampsia. The plug may be evacuated by glycerin suppository

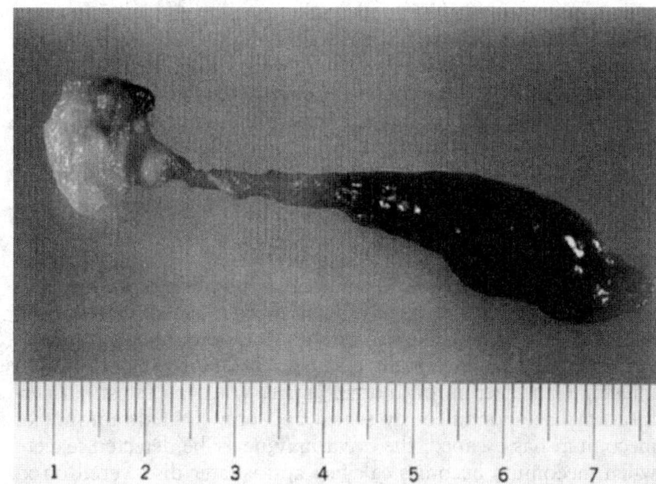

Figure 102-1. This plug of meconium and mucus (scale in cm) caused bowel obstruction in a premature infant. A radiograph showed marked gaseous distension and multiple fluid levels at 30 hr of age. Dramatic improvement occurred when the plug was passed after an enema. (From: The abnormal fetus. In Beischer NA, Mackay EV, Colditz PB [eds]: *Obstetrics and the Newborn*, 3rd ed. Philadelphia, WB Saunders, 1997.)

or rectal irrigation with isotonic saline. Enemas with the iodinated contrast medium Gastrografin usually induce passage of the plug, presumably because the high osmolarity (1,900 mOsm/L) of the solution draws fluid rapidly into the intestinal lumen and loosens inspissated material. Such rapid loss of fluid into the bowel may result in acute dehydration and shock, so it is advisable to dilute the contrast material with an equal amount of water, correct any existing dehydration, and provide intravenous fluids during and for several hours after the procedure. After removal of a meconium plug, the infant should be observed closely for the possible presence of congenital aganglionic megacolon.

102.1 • Meconium Ileus in Cystic Fibrosis

Impaction of meconium causes intestinal obstructions and may be associated with CF. The absence of fetal pancreatic enzymes in CF limits normal digestive activities in the intestine, and meconium becomes viscid and mucilaginous. It clings to the intestinal wall and moves with difficulty. The inspissated and impacted meconium fills the intestinal canal but is most concentrated in the lower part of the ileum. Clinically, the pattern is that of congenital intestinal obstruction with or without intestinal perforation. Abdominal distention is prominent, and vomiting becomes persistent. Infrequently, one or more inspissated meconium stools may be passed shortly after birth.

The **differential diagnosis** involves other causes of intestinal obstruction, including intestinal pseudo-obstruction and other causes of pancreatic insufficiency (see Chapter 346). A presumptive diagnosis can be made on the basis of a history of CF in a sibling, by palpation of doughy or cordlike masses of intestines through the abdominal wall, and by the x-ray appearance. In contrast to the generally evenly distended intestinal loops above an atresia, the loops may vary in width and are not as evenly filled with gas. At points of heaviest meconium concentration, the infiltrated gas may create a bubbly granular appearance (Figs. 102-2 and 102-3). It is technically difficult to do a sweat test in a neonate. Genetic testing confirms the diagnosis of CF.

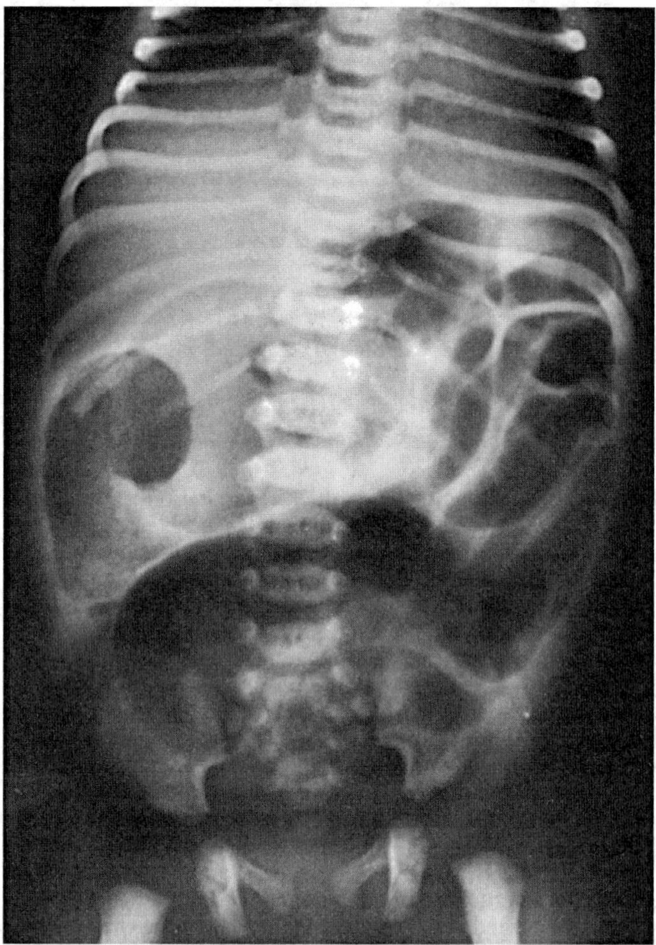

Figure 102-2. Meconium ileus. Impacted meconium with small amounts of air interspersed can be seen in loops of intestine on the right side of the abdomen. The intestinal loops above this impaction are greatly distended.

Treatment for meconium ileus is high Gastrografin enemas as described for meconium plug. If unsuccessful or perforation of the bowel wall is suspected, laparotomy is performed and the ileum opened at the point of greatest diameter of the impaction. Approximately 50% of these infants have associated intestinal atresia, stenosis, or volvulus that requires surgery. The inspissated meconium is removed by gentle and patient irrigation with warm isotonic sodium chloride or acetylcysteine (Mucomyst) solution through a catheter passed between the impaction and bowel wall. Most infants with meconium ileus survive the neonatal period. If associated with CF, the long-term prognosis depends on the severity of the underlying disease (see Chapter 400).

MECONIUM PERITONITIS. Perforation of the intestine may occur in utero or shortly after birth. Frequently, the intestinal perforation will seal naturally with relatively little meconium leakage into the peritoneal cavity. In some cases, with long-standing perforation, meconium peritonitis is more pronounced. Perforations occur most often as a complication of meconium ileus in infants with CF, but are occasionally due to a meconium plug or in utero intestinal obstruction of another cause. When an intestinal perforation has spontaneously sealed and only a small amount of meconium has escaped, the event may never be detected, except when meconium becomes calcified and is later discovered on x-rays of the abdomen. Alternatively, the clinical picture may be dominated by the signs of intestinal obstruction (as in meconium ileus) or chemical peritonitis. Characteristically noted are abdominal distention, vomiting, and absence of stools. Treatment consists primarily of elimination of the intestinal obstruction and drainage of the peritoneal cavity.

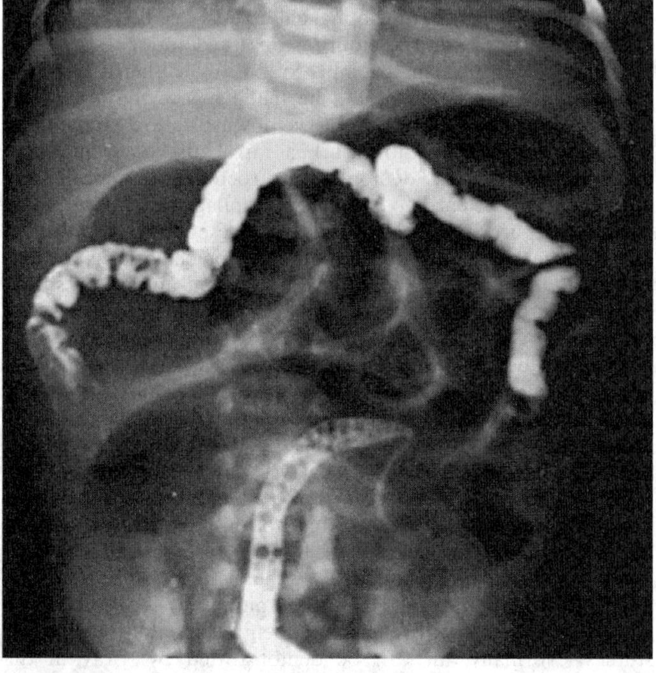

Figure 102-3. Meconium ileus. The colon, outlined by contrast material, is small because meconium has not reached it.

102.2 • Neonatal Necrotizing Enterocolitis (NEC)

NEC is the most common life-threatening emergency of the gastrointestinal tract in the newborn period. The disease is characterized by various degrees of mucosal or transmural necrosis of the intestine. The cause of NEC remains unclear but is most likely multifactorial. The incidence of NEC is 1–5% of infants in neonatal intensive care units. Both incidence and case fatality rates increase with decreasing birthweight and gestational age. Because very small, ill preterm infants are particularly susceptible to NEC, a rising incidence may reflect improved survival of this high-risk group of patients. Although rare, the disease does occur in term infants.

PATHOLOGY AND PATHOGENESIS. Many factors may contribute to the development of a necrotic segment of intestine, gas accumulation in the submucosa of the bowel wall (**pneumatosis intestinalis**), and progression of the necrosis to perforation, peritonitis, sepsis, and death. The distal part of the ileum and the proximal segment of colon are involved most frequently; in fatal cases, gangrene may extend from the stomach to the rectum. Although NEC is a multifactorial disease primarily associated with intestinal immaturity, the concept of "risk factors" for NEC is controversial. The triad of intestinal ischemia (injury), enteral nutrition (metabolic substrate), and pathogenic organisms has classically been linked to NEC. The greatest risk factor for NEC is prematurity. NEC probably results from an interaction between loss of mucosal integrity due to a variety of factors (ischemia, infection, inflammation) and the host's response to that injury (circulatory, immunologic, inflammatory) resulting in necrosis of the affected area. Coagulation necrosis is the characteristic histologic finding of intestinal specimens. Clustering of cases suggests a primary role for an infectious agent. Various bacterial and viral agents, including *Escherichia coli, Klebsiella, Clostridium perfringens, Staphylococcus epidermidis,* and rotavirus, have been recovered from cultures. Nonetheless, in most situations, no pathogen is identified. NEC rarely occurs before the initiation of enteral feeding and is much less common in infants fed human milk. Aggressive enteral feeding may predispose to the development of NEC.

CLINICAL MANIFESTATIONS. Infants with NEC have a variety of signs and symptoms and may have an insidious or sudden catastrophic onset (Table 102-1). The onset of NEC usually occurs in the 1st 2 wk of life but can be as late as 3 mo of age in VLBW infants. Age of onset is inversely related to gestational age. The 1st signs of impending disease may be nonspecific including lethargy and temperature instability or related to gastrointestinal pathology such as abdominal distention and gastric retention. Obvious bloody stools are seen in 25% of patients. Because of nonspecific signs, sepsis may be suspected before NEC. The spectrum of illness is broad and ranges from mild disease with only guaiac-positive stools to severe illness with bowel perforation, peritonitis, systemic inflammatory response syndrome, shock, and death. Progression may be rapid, but it is unusual for the disease to progress from mild to severe after 72 hr.

TABLE 102-1. Signs and Symptoms Associated with Necrotizing Enterocolitis

GASTROINTESTINAL	SYSTEMIC
Abdominal distention	Lethargy
Abdominal tenderness	Apnea/respiratory distress
Feeding intolerance	Temperature instability
Delayed gastric emptying	"Not right"
Vomiting	Acidosis (metabolic and/or respiratory)
Occult/gross blood in stool	Glucose instability
Change in stool pattern/diarrhea	Poor perfusion/shock
Abdominal mass	Disseminated intravascular coagulopathy
Erythema of abdominal wall	Positive results of blood cultures

From Kanto WP Jr, Hunter JE, Stoll BJ: Recognition and medical management of necrotizing enterocolitis. *Clin Perinatol* 1994;21:335–346.

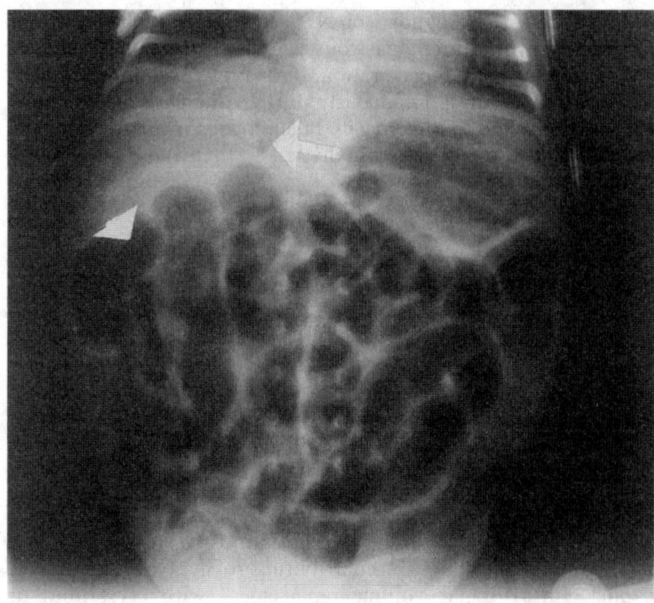

Figure 102-4. Necrotizing enterocolitis. A kidney-ureter-bladder film demonstrates abdominal distension, hepatic portal venous gas *(arrow)*, and a bubbly appearance of pneumatosis intestinalis (*arrowhead;* right lower quadrant). The latter two signs are thought to be pathognomonic for neonatal necrotizing enterocolitis.

DIAGNOSIS. A very high index of suspicion in treating preterm at-risk infants is crucial. Plain abdominal x-rays are essential to make a diagnosis of NEC. The finding of pneumatosis intestinalis (air in the bowel wall) confirms the clinical suspicion of NEC and is diagnostic; 50–75% of patients have pneumatosis when treatment is started (Fig. 102-4). Portal venous gas is a sign of severe disease, and pneumoperitoneum indicates a perforation (Figs. 102-4 and 102-5). Hepatic ultrasonography may detect portal venous gas despite normal abdominal roentgenograms.

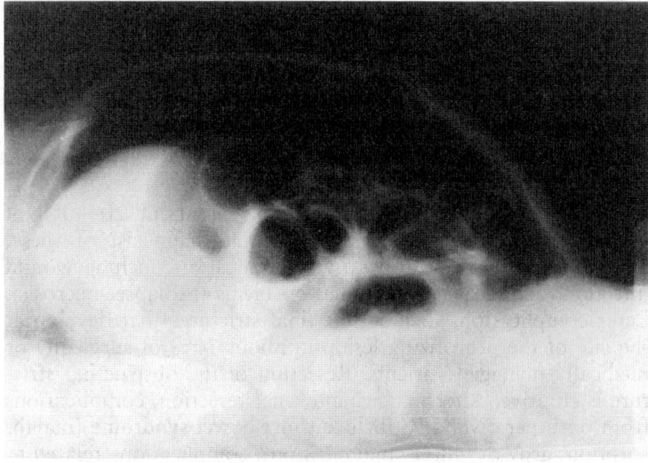

Figure 102-5. Intestinal perforation. A cross-table abdominal roentgenogram in a patient with a neonatal necrotizing enterocolitis demonstrates marked distention and massive pneumoperitoneum as evidenced by the free air below the anterior abdominal wall.

The **differential diagnosis** of NEC includes specific infections (systemic or intestinal), gastrointestinal obstruction, volvulus, and isolated intestinal perforation. Idiopathic focal intestinal perforation can occur spontaneously or after the early use of postnatal steroids and indomethacin. Pneumoperitoneum develops in such patients, but they are usually less ill than those with NEC.

TREATMENT. Rapid initiation of therapy is required for suspected as well as proven NEC cases. There is no definitive treatment for established NEC and, therefore, therapy is directed at supportive care and preventing further injury with cessation of feeding, nasogastric decompression, and administration of intravenous fluids. Careful attention to respiratory status, coagulation profile, and acid-base and electrolyte balance are important. Once blood has been drawn for culture, systemic antibiotics (with broad coverage based on the antibiotic sensitivity patterns of the gram-positive, gram-negative, and anaerobic organisms in the neonatal ICU) should be started immediately. If present, umbilical catheters should be removed while maintaining good intravenous access. Ventilation should be assisted in the presence of apnea or if abdominal distention is contributing to hypoxia and hypercapnia. Intravascular volume replacement with crystalloid or blood products, cardiovascular support with volume and/or inotropes, and correction of hematologic, metabolic, and electrolyte abnormalities are essential to stabilize the infant.

The patient's course should be monitored closely by performing frequent physical assessments; sequential anteroposterior and cross-table lateral or lateral decubitus abdominal x-rays to detect intestinal perforation; and serial determination of hematologic, electrolyte, and acid-base status. Gown and glove isolation and grouping infants at similar increased risks into cohorts separate from other infants should be instituted to contain an epidemic.

A surgeon should be consulted early in the course of treatment. **Indications for surgery** include evidence of perforation on abdominal roentgenograms (pneumoperitoneum) or positive abdominal paracentesis (stool or organism on Gram stain from peritoneal fluid). Failure of medical management, a single fixed bowel loop on roentgenograms, abdominal wall erythema, or a palpable mass are relative indications for exploratory laparotomy. Ideally, surgery should be performed after intestinal necrosis develops, but before perforation and peritonitis occurs. The role of **peritoneal drainage** in lieu of laparotomy in a patient with perforation secondary to NEC remains to be determined. Peritoneal drainage may be helpful for patients in extremis with peritonitis who are too unstable to undergo surgery. Peritoneal drainage tends to be more successful in patients with isolated intestinal perforation. In general, these patients tend to have a lower birth-weight, are less likely to be receiving oral feeding, and are prone to perforation at an earlier postnatal age than are patients with perforation related to NEC. In many patients with isolated intestinal perforation treated by drainage, no further surgical procedure is needed; a small subgroup may require later surgery to repair an intestinal stricture or fistula.

PROGNOSIS. Medical management fails in about 20–40% of patients with pneumatosis intestinalis at diagnosis; of these, 10–30% die. Early postoperative complications include wound infection, dehiscence, and stomal problems (prolapse, necrosis). Later complications include **intestinal strictures** that develop at the site of the necrotizing lesion in about 10% of surgically or medically managed patients. Resection of the obstructing stricture is curative. After massive intestinal resection, complications from postoperative NEC include **short-bowel syndrome** (malabsorption, growth failure, malnutrition), complications related to central venous catheters (sepsis, thrombosis), and cholestatic jaundice. Premature infants with NEC who require surgical intervention or who have concomitant bacteremia are at increased risk for adverse growth and neurodevelopmental outcome.

PREVENTION. Newborns exclusively breast-fed have a reduced risk of NEC. Whereas early initiation of aggressive feeding protocols may increase the risk of NEC in VLBW infants, a gut stimulation protocol of minimal enteral feeds followed by judicious volume advancement may decrease the risk. Probiotic preparations have also decreased the incidence of NEC.

Berseth CL, Bisquera JA, Paje VU: Prolonging small feeding volumes early in life decreases the incidence of necrotizing enterocolitis in very low birth weight infants. *Pediatrics* 2003;111:529–534.

Blakely ML, Tyson JE, Lally KP, et al: Laparotomy versus peritoneal drainage for necrotizing enterocolitis or isolated intestinal perforation in extremely low birth rate infants: Outcomes through 18 mo adjusted age. *Pediatrics* 2006;117:e680–e687.

Carroll D, Corfield A, Spicer R, et al: Faecal calprotectin concentrations and diagnosis of necrotizing enterocolitis. *Lancet* 2003;361:310–311.

Cass DL, Brandt ML, Patel DL, et al: Peritoneal drainage as definitive treatment for neonates with isolated intestinal perforation. *J Pediatr Surg* 2000;35:1531–1536.

Grosfeld JL, Molinari F, Chaet M, et al: Gastrointestinal perforation and peritonitis in infants and children: Experience with 179 cases over 10 years. *Surgery* 1996;120:650–655.

Hintz SR, Kendrick DE, Stoll, BJ et al: Neurodevelopment and growth outcomes of extremely low birth weight infants after necrotizing enterocolitis. *Pediatrics* 2005;115:1–8

Kliegman, RM: The relationship of neonatal feeding practices and the pathogenesis and prevention of necrotizing enterocolitis. *Pediatrics* 2003;111:671–672.

Kliegman RM, Willoughby RE: Prevention of necrotizing enterocolitis with probiotics. *Pediatrics* 2005;115:171–172.

Lin HC, Su BH, Chen AC, et al: Oral probiotics reduce the incidence and severity of necrotizing enterocolitis in very low birth weight infants. *Pediatrics* 2005;115:1–4.

Lin PW, Stoll BJ: Necrotizing enterocolitis. *Lancet* 2006;368:1271–1283.

Lucas A, Cole TJ: Breast milk and neonatal necrotizing enterocolitis. *Lancet* 1990;336:1519–1523.

Moss RL, Dimmitt RA, Barnhart DC, et al: Laparotomy versus peritoneal drainage for necrotizing enterocolitis and perforation. *N Engl J Med* 2006;354:2225–2234.

Moss RL, Dimmitt RA, Henry MC, et al: A meta-analysis of peritoneal drainage versus laparotomy for perforated necrotizing enterocolitis. *J Pediatr Surg* 2001;36:1210–1213.

Murdoch EM, Sinha AK, Shanmugalingam ST, et al: Doppler flow velocimetry in the superior mesenteric artery on the first day of life in preterm infants and the risk of neonatal necrotizing enterocolitis. *Pediatrics* 2006;118: 1999–2003.

Patole SK, de Klerk N: Impact of standardized feeding regimens on incidence of neonatal necrotizing enterocolitis: A systematic review and meta-analysis of observational studies. *Arch Dis Child* 2005;90:F147–F151.

Pietz J, Achanti B, Lilien L, et al: Prevention of necrotizing enterocolitis in preterm infants: a 20-year experience. *Pediatrics* 2007;119:e164–e170.

Reber KM, Nankervis CA: Necrotizing enterocolitis: preventative strategies. *Clin Perinatol* 2004;31:157–167.

Sharma R, Tepas III JJ, Hudak ML, et al: Portal venous gas and surgical outcome of neonatal necrotizing enterocolitis. *J Pediatr Surg* 2005;40:371–376.

Stoll BJ, Hansen NI, Adams-Chapman I, et al: Neurodevelopmental and growth impairment among extremely low-birth-weight infants with neonatal infection. *JAMA* 2004;292:2357–2365.

Williams H: Perforation: How to spot free intraperitoneal air on abdominal radiograph. *Arch Dis Child Educ Pract Ed* 2006;91:ep54–ep57.

102.3 • Jaundice and Hyperbilirubinemia in the Newborn

Hyperbilirubinemia is a common and, in most cases, benign problem in neonates. Jaundice is observed during the 1st wk of life in approximately 60% of term infants and 80% of preterm infants. The yellow color usually results from the accumulation of unconjugated, nonpolar, lipid-soluble bilirubin pigment in the skin. This unconjugated bilirubin (designated **indirect acting** by nature of the Van den Bergh reaction) is an end product of heme-protein catabolism from a series of enzymatic reactions by heme-oxygenase and biliverdin reductase and non-enzymatic reducing agents in the reticuloendothelial cells. It may also be due in part to deposition of pigment from conjugated bilirubin, the end product from indirect, unconjugated bilirubin that has undergone conjugation in the liver cell microsome by the enzyme uridine diphosphoglucuronic acid (UDP)–glucuronyl transferase to form the polar, water-soluble glucuronide of bilirubin (**direct reacting**). Although bilirubin may have a physiologic role as an antioxidant, elevated levels of indirect, unconjugated bilirubin are potentially neurotoxic. Even though the conjugated form is not neurotoxic, direct hyperbilirubinemia indicates potentially serious hepatic disorders or systemic illnesses.

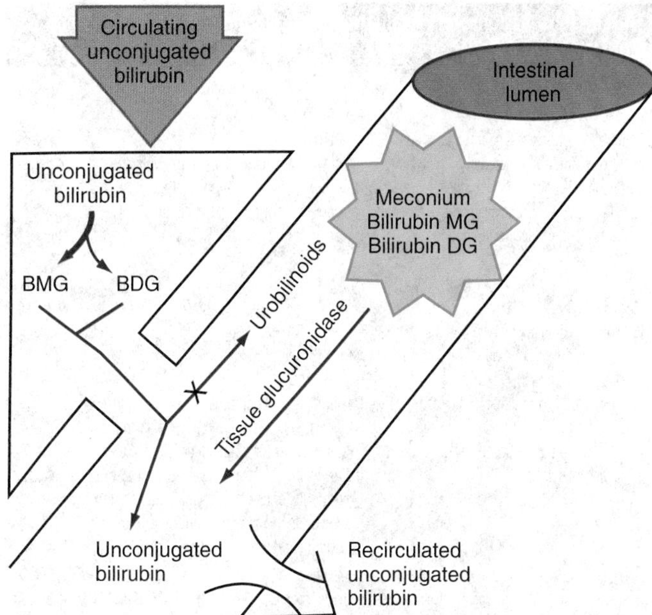

Figure 102-6. The neonatal production rate of bilirubin is 6–8 mg/kg/24 hr (in contrast to 3–4 mg/kg/24 hr in adults). Water-insoluble bilirubin is bound to albumin. At the plasma-hepatocyte interface, a liver membrane carrier (bilitranslocase) transports bilirubin to a cystolic binding protein (ligandin or Y protein, not known to be glutathione S-transferase), which prevents back-absorption to plasma. Bilirubin is converted to bilirubin monoglucuronide transferase (BMG). Neonates excrete more BMG than adults do. In the fetus, conjugated lipid-insoluble BMG and BDG must be deconjugated by tissue β-glucuronidases to facilitate placental transfer of lipid-soluble unconjugated bilirubin across the placental lipid membranes. After birth, intestinal or milk-containing glucuronidases contribute to the enterohepatic recirculation of bilirubin and possibly to the development of hyperbilirubinemia. BDG, bilirubin diglucoronide.

ETIOLOGY. During the neonatal period, metabolism of bilirubin is in transition from the fetal stage during which the placenta is the principal route of elimination of the lipid-soluble, unconjugated bilirubin to the adult stage, during which the water-soluble conjugated form is excreted from hepatic cells into the biliary system and gastrointestinal tract. Unconjugated hyperbilirubinemia may be caused or increased by any factor that (1) increases the load of bilirubin to be metabolized by the liver (hemolytic anemias, polycythemia, shortened red cell life as a result of immaturity or transfused cells, increased enterohepatic circulation, infection); (2) damages or reduces the activity of the transferase enzyme or other related enzymes (genetic deficiency, hypoxia, infection, thyroid deficiency); (3) competes for or blocks the transferase enzyme (drugs and other substances requiring glucuronic acid conjugation); or (4) leads to an absence or decreased amounts of the enzyme or to reduction of bilirubin uptake by liver cells (genetic defect, and prematurity). The toxic effects of elevated serum levels of unconjugated bilirubin are increased by factors that reduce the retention of bilirubin in the circulation (hypoproteinemia, displacement of bilirubin from its binding sites on albumin by competitive binding of drugs such as sulfisoxazole and moxalactam, Chuen-Lin herbal tea, acidosis, and increased free fatty acid concentration secondary to hypoglycemia, starvation, or hypothermia). Neurotoxic effects are directly related not only to the permeability of the blood-brain barrier and nerve cell membranes, but also to neuronal susceptibility to injury, all of which are adversely influenced by asphyxia, prematurity, hyperosmolality, and infection. Early and frequent feeding decreases whereas breast-feeding and dehydration increase serum levels of bilirubin. Delay in passage of meconium, which contains 1 mg bilirubin/dL, may contribute to jaundice by enterohepatic circulation after deconjugation by intestinal glucuronidase (Fig. 102-6). Drugs such as oxytocin and chemicals used in the nursery such as phenolic detergents may also produce unconjugated hyperbilirubinemia. Risk factors for unconjugated hyperbilirubinemia are noted in Table 102-2. Additional risk factors include polycythemia, infection, prematurity, and being an infant of a diabetic mother.

CLINICAL MANIFESTATIONS. Jaundice may be present at birth or may appear at any time during the neonatal period, depending on etiology. Jaundice usually becomes apparent in a cephalocaudal progression starting on the face and progressing to the abdomen and then feet, as serum levels increase. Dermal pressure may reveal the anatomic progression of jaundice (face, ≈ 5 mg/dL; mid-abdomen, ≈ 15 mg/dL; soles, ≈ 20 mg/dL), but clinical examination cannot be depended on to estimate serum levels. Jaundice to the mid-abdomen, signs or symptoms, high-risk factors that suggest nonphysiologic jaundice, or hemolysis must be evaluated further (Tables 102-2 and 102-3). Noninvasive techniques for transcutaneous measurement of bilirubin (TcB) that correlate with serum levels may be used to screen infants, but determina-

TABLE 102-2. Risk Factors for Development of Severe Hyperbilirubinemia in Infants of 35 or More Weeks' Gestation (in Approximate Order of Importance)

Major risk factors
- Predischarge TSB or TcB level in the high-risk zone (Fig 102-8)
- Jaundice observed in the first 24 hr
- Blood group incompatibility with positive direct antiglobulin test, other known hemolytic disease (G6PD deficiency), elevated $ETCO_c$
- Gestational age 35–36 wk
- Previous sibling received phototherapy
- Cephalohematoma or significant bruising
- Exclusive breastfeeding, particularly if nursing is not going well and weight loss is excessive
- East Asian race*

Minor risk factors
- Predischarge TSB or TcB level in the high intermediate-risk zone
- Gestational age 37–38 wk
- Jaundice observed before discharge
- Previous sibling with jaundice
- Macrosomic infant of a diabetic mother
- Maternal age ≥25 yr
- Male gender

Decreased risk (these factors are associated with decreased risk of significant jaundice, listed in order of decreasing importance)
- TSB or TcB level in the low-risk zone (Fig 102-8)
- Gestational age ≥41 wk
- Exclusive bottle feeding
- Black race
- Discharge from hospital after 72 hr

*Race as defined by mother's description.

ETCO, end tidal carbon monoxide; G6PD, glucose-6-phosphate dehydrogenase; TcB, transcutaneous bilirubin; TSB, total serum bilirubin.

From AAP Subcommittee on Hyperbilirubinemia: Management of hyperbilirubinemia in the newborn infant 35 or more weeks of gestation. *Pediatrics* 2004;114:297–316.

TABLE 102-3. Laboratory Evaluation of the Jaundiced Infant of 35 or More Weeks' Gestation

INDICATIONS	ASSESSMENTS
Jaundice in first 24 hr	Measure TcB and/or TSB
Jaundice appears excessive for infant's age	Measure TcB and/or TSB
Infant receiving phototherapy or TSB rising rapidly (i.e., crossing percentiles [Fig 102-8]) and unexplained by history and physical examination	Blood type and Coombs test, if not obtained with cord blood Complete blood count and smear Measure direct or conjugated bilirubin It is an option to perform reticulocyte count, G6PD, and $ETCO_c$, if available Repeat TSB in 4–24 hr depending on infant's age and TSB level
TSB concentration approaching exchange levels or not responding to phototherapy	Perform reticulocyte count, G6PD, albumin, $ETCO_c$, if available
Elevated direct (or conjugated) bilirubin level	Do urinalysis and urine culture. Evaluate for sepsis if indicated by history and physical examination
Jaundice present at or beyond age 3 wk, or sick infant	Total and direct (or conjugated) bilirubin level If direct bilirubin elevated, evaluate for causes of cholestasis Check results of newborn thyroid and galactosemia screen, and evaluate infant for signs or symptoms of hypothyroidism

$ETCO_c$, end tidal carbon monoxide; G6PD, glucose-6-phosphate dehydrogenase; TcB, transcutaneous bilirubin.
From AAP Subcommittee on Hyperbilirubinemia: Management of hyperbilirubinemia in the newborn infant 35 or more weeks of gestation. *Pediatrics* 2004;114:297–316.

tion of serum bilirubin level is indicated in patients with elevated age-specific transcutaneous measurement, progressing jaundice, or risk for either hemolysis or sepsis. Whereas jaundice from deposition of indirect bilirubin in the skin tends to appear bright yellow or orange, jaundice of the obstructive type (direct bilirubin) has a greenish or muddy yellow cast. Although signs of kernicterus rarely appear on the 1st day, affected infants may present with lethargy and poor feeding and, without treatment, can progress to acute bilirubin encephalopathy (Chapter 102.4).

DIFFERENTIAL DIAGNOSIS. Jaundice, consisting of either indirect or direct bilirubin, that is present at birth or appears within the 1st 24 hr of life requires immediate attention and may be due to erythroblastosis fetalis, concealed hemorrhage, sepsis, or congenital infections, including syphilis, cytomegalovirus, rubella, and toxoplasmosis. Hemolysis is suggested by a rapid rise in serum bilirubin (>0.5 mg/dL/hr), anemia, pallor, reticulocytosis, hepatosplenomegaly, and a positive family history. An unusually high proportion of direct-reacting bilirubin may characterize jaundice in infants who have received intrauterine transfusions for erythroblastosis fetalis. Jaundice that 1st appears on the 2nd or 3rd day is usually **physiologic** but may represent a more severe form. Familial non-hemolytic icterus (**Crigler-Najjar syndrome**) and early-onset breast-feeding jaundice are seen initially on the 2nd or 3rd day. Jaundice appearing after the 3rd day and within the 1st wk suggests bacterial sepsis or urinary tract infection; it may also be due to other infections, notably syphilis, toxoplasmosis, cytomegalovirus, or enterovirus. Jaundice secondary to extensive ecchymosis or blood extravasation may occur during the 1st day or later, especially in premature infants. Polycythemia may also lead to early jaundice.

There is a long differential diagnosis for jaundice 1st recognized after the 1st wk of life, including breast-milk jaundice, septicemia, congenital atresia or paucity of the bile ducts, hepatitis, galactosemia, hypothyroidism, CF, and congenital hemolytic anemia crises related to red cell morphology and enzyme deficiencies (Fig. 102-7). The differential diagnosis for persistent jaundice during the 1st mo of life includes hyperalimentation-associated cholestasis, hepatitis, cytomegalic inclusion disease, syphilis, toxoplasmosis, familial non-hemolytic icterus, congenital atresia of the bile ducts, galactosemia, or inspissated bile syndrome following hemolytic disease of the newborn. Rarely, physiologic jaundice may be prolonged for several wk, as in infants with hypothyroidism or pyloric stenosis.

Full-term, low-risk, asymptomatic infants may be evaluated by monitoring total serum bilirubin (TSB) levels. Regardless of gestation or time of appearance of jaundice, patients with significant hyperbilirubinemia and those with symptoms or signs require a complete diagnostic evaluation, which includes determination of direct and indirect bilirubin fractions, hemoglobin, reticulocyte count, blood type, Coombs test, and examination of a peripheral blood smear. Indirect hyperbilirubinemia, reticulocytosis, and a smear with evidence of red blood cell destruction suggest hemolysis (see Table 102-3). In the absence of blood group incompatibility, non–immunologically induced hemolysis should be considered. If direct hyperbilirubinemia is present, hepatitis, congenital bile duct disorders (atresia, paucity, Byler disease), cholestasis, inborn errors of metabolism, CF, and sepsis are diagnostic possibilities. If the reticulocyte count, Coombs test, and direct bilirubin are normal, physiologic or pathologic indirect hyperbilirubinemia may be present (see Fig. 102-7).

PHYSIOLOGIC JAUNDICE (ICTERUS NEONATORUM). Under normal circumstances, the level of indirect-reacting bilirubin in umbilical cord serum is 1–3 mg/dL and rises at a rate of <5 mg/dL/24 hr; thus, jaundice becomes visible on the 2nd–3rd day, usually peaking between the 2nd and 4th days at 5–6 mg/dL and decreasing to below 2 mg/dL between the 5th and 7th days of life. Jaundice associated with these changes is designated *physiologic* and is believed to be the result of increased bilirubin production from the breakdown of fetal red blood cells combined with transient limitation in the conjugation of bilirubin by the immature neonatal liver.

Overall, 6–7% of full-term infants have indirect bilirubin levels >12.9 mg/dL and less than 3% have levels >15 mg/dL. Risk factors for elevated indirect hyperbilirubinemia include maternal age, race (Chinese, Japanese, Korean, and Native American), maternal diabetes, prematurity, drugs (vitamin K_3, novobiocin), altitude, polycythemia, male sex, trisomy 21, cutaneous bruising, blood extravasation (cephalohematoma), oxytocin induction, breast-feeding, weight loss (dehydration or caloric deprivation), delayed bowel movement, and a family history/sibling who had physiologic jaundice (see Table 102-2). In infants without these variables, indirect bilirubin levels rarely rise above 12 mg/dL, whereas infants with several risk factors are more likely to have higher bilirubin levels. A combination of breast-feeding, variant UDP-glucuronosyl transferase activity (1A1) and alterations of the organic anion transporter 2 gene increases the risk in Asian children. Prediction of which neonates are at risk for exaggerated physiologic jaundice can be based on hour-specific bilirubin levels in the 1st 24–72 hr of life (Fig. 102-8). Indirect bilirubin levels in full-term infants decline to adult levels (1 mg/dL) by 10–14 days of life. Persistent indirect hyperbilirubinemia beyond 2 wk suggests hemolysis, hereditary glucuronyl transferase deficiency, breast-milk jaundice, hypothyroidism, or intestinal obstruction. Jaundice associated with pyloric stenosis may be due to caloric deprivation, deficiency of hepatic UDP-glucuronyl transferase, or an increase in the enterohepatic circulation of bilirubin from an ileus. In premature infants, the rise in serum bilirubin tends to be the same or somewhat slower but of longer duration than in term infants. Peak levels of 8–12 mg/dL are not usually reached until the 4th–7th day, and jaundice is infrequently observed after the 10th day, corresponding to the maturation of mechanisms for bilirubin metabolism and excretion.

The diagnosis of physiologic jaundice in term or preterm infants can be established only by precluding known causes of jaundice on the basis of the history, clinical findings, and laboratory data (Table 102-4). In general, a search to determine the cause of jaundice should be made if (1) it appears in the 1st 24–36 hr of life, (2) serum bilirubin is rising at a rate faster than 5 mg/dL/24 hr, (3) serum bilirubin is >12 mg/dL in full-term

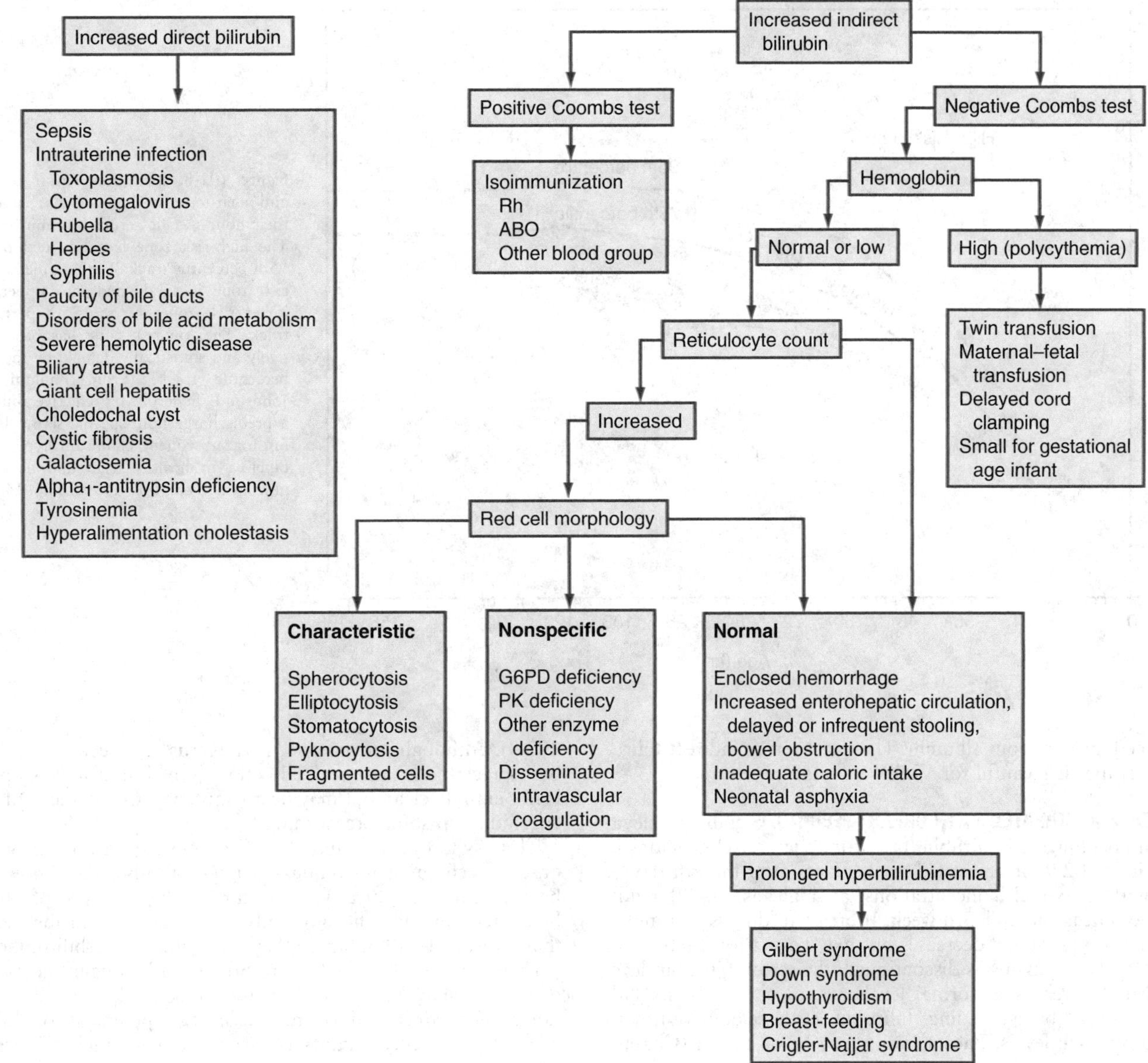

Figure 102-7. Schematic approach to the diagnosis of neonatal jaundice. G6PD, glucose-6-phosphate dehydrogenase; PK, pyruvate kinase. (From Oski FA: Differential diagnosis of jaundice. In Taeusch HW, Ballard RA, Avery MA [editors]: *Schaffer and Avery's Diseases of the Newborn*, 6th ed. Philadelphia, WB Saunders, 1991.)

infants (especially in the absence of risk factors) or 10–14 mg/dL in preterm infants, (4) jaundice persists after 10–14 days of life, or (5) direct-reacting bilirubin is >2 mg/dL at any time. Other factors suggesting a nonphysiologic cause of jaundice are family history of hemolytic disease, pallor, hepatomegaly, splenomegaly, failure of phototherapy to lower bilirubin, vomiting, lethargy, poor feeding, excessive weight loss, apnea, bradycardia, abnormal vital signs (including hypothermia), light-colored stools, dark urine positive for bilirubin, and signs of kernicterus (Chapter 102-4).

PATHOLOGIC HYPERBILIRUBINEMIA. Jaundice and its underlying hyperbilirubinemia are considered pathologic if the time of appearance, duration, or pattern varies significantly from that of physiologic jaundice or if the course is compatible with physiologic jaundice but other reasons exist to suspect that the infant is at special risk for neurotoxicity. It may not be possible to determine the precise cause of an abnormal elevation of unconjugated bilirubin, but many of these infants have associated risk factors such as Asian race, prematurity, breast-feeding, or weight loss. Frequently, the terms *exaggerated physiologic jaundice* and *hyperbilirubinemia of the newborn* are used for infants whose primary problem is probably a deficiency or inactivity of bilirubin glucuronyl transferase (Gilbert syndrome) rather than an excessive load of bilirubin for excretion (see Table 102-2). The combination of glucose-6-phosphate dehydrogenase (G6PD) deficiency and a mutation of the promoter region of UDP-glucuronyl transferase-1 produces indirect hyperbilirubinemia in the absence of signs of hemolysis. Nonphysiologic hyperbilirubinemia may also be caused by mutations in the gene for bilirubin UDP-glucuronyl transferase.

The greatest risk associated with indirect hyperbilirubinemia is the development of bilirubin-induced neurologic dysfunction, which typically occurs with high indirect bilirubin levels (Chapter 102.4). The development of kernicterus (bilirubin encephalopathy) is dependent on the level of indirect bilirubin, duration of exposure to elevated levels, the cause of jaundice, and the infant's well-being. Neurologic injury including kernicterus occurs at lower bilirubin levels in preterm infants and in the presence of asphyxia, intraventricular hemorrhage, hemolysis, or drugs that

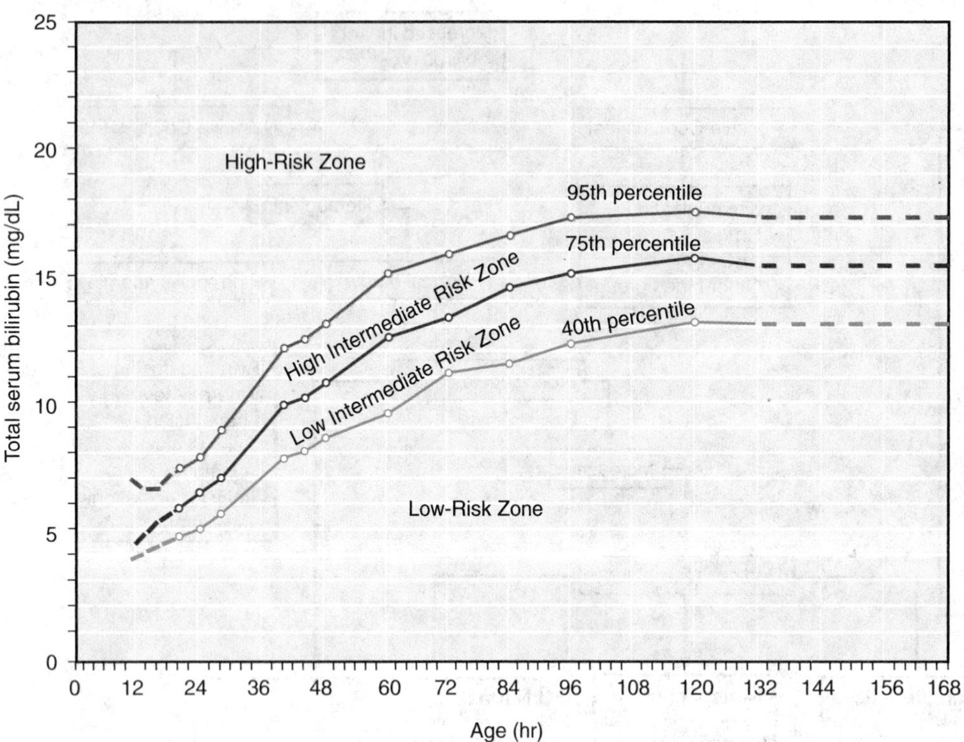

Figure 102-8. Risk designation of term and near-term well newborns based on their hour-specific serum bilirubin values. The high-risk zone is subdivided by the 95th percentile track. The intermediate at-risk zone is subdivided into upper and lower risk zones by the 75th percentile track. The low-risk zone has been electively and statistically defined by the 40th percentile track. (From Bhutani VK, Johnson L, Sivieri EM: Predictive ability of a predischarge hour-specific serum bilirubin for subsequent significant hyperbilirubinemia in healthy term and near-term newborns. *Pediatrics* 1999;103:6–14.)

displace bilirubin from albumin. The exact serum indirect bilirubin level that is harmful for VLBW infants is unclear.

JAUNDICE ASSOCIATED WITH BREAST-FEEDING. Significant elevation in unconjugated bilirubin (breast-milk jaundice) develops in an estimated 2% of breast-fed term infants after the 7th day of life, with maximal concentrations as high as 10–30 mg/dL reached during the 2nd–3rd week. If breast-feeding is continued, the bilirubin gradually decreases but may persist for 3–10 wk at lower levels. If nursing is discontinued, the serum bilirubin level falls rapidly, reaching normal levels within a few days. With resumption of breast-feeding, bilirubin levels seldom return to previously high levels. Phototherapy may be of benefit (Chapter 102.4). Although uncommon, kernicterus can occur in patients with breast-milk jaundice. The etiology of breast-milk jaundice is not entirely clear, but may be attributed to the presence of glucuronidase in some breast milk.

This syndrome should be distinguished from an early-onset, accentuated unconjugated hyperbilirubinemia known as breast-feeding jaundice which occurs in the 1st week of life, in breast-fed infants who normally have higher bilirubin levels than formula-fed infants (Fig. 102-9). Hyperbilirubinemia (>12 mg/dL) develops in 13% of breast-fed infants in the 1st wk of life and may be due to decreased milk intake with dehydration and/or reduced caloric intake. Giving supplements of glucose water to breast-fed infants is associated with higher bilirubin

TABLE 102-4. Diagnostic Features of the Various Types of Neonatal Jaundice

DIAGNOSIS	NATURE OF VAN DEN BERGH REACTION	JAUNDICE		PEAK BILIRUBIN CONCENTRATION		BILIRUBIN RATE OF ACCUMULATION (mg/dL/day)	REMARKS
		Appears	Disappears	mg/dL	Age in Days		
"Physiologic jaundice":							Usually relates to degree of maturity
Full-term	Indirect	2–3 days	4–5 days	10–12	2–3	<5	
Premature	Indirect	3–4 days	7–9 days	15	6–8	<5	
Hyperbilirubinemia due to metabolic factors							Metabolic factors: hypoxia, respiratory distress, lack of carbohydrate
Full-term	Indirect	2–3 days	Variable	>12	1st wk	<5	Hormonal influences: cretinism, hormones, Gilbert syndrome
Premature	Indirect	3–4 days	Variable	>15	1st wk	<5	Genetic factors: Crigler-Najjar syndrome, Gilbert syndrome Drugs: vitamin K, novobiocin
Hemolytic states and hematoma	Indirect	May appear in 1st 24 hr	Variable	Unlimited	Variable	Usually >5	Erythroblastosis: Rh, ABO, Kell Congenital hemolytic states: spherocytic, nonspherocytic Infantile pyknocytosis Drugs: vitamin K Enclosed hemorrhage—hematoma
Mixed hemolytic and hepatotoxic factors	Indirect and direct	May appear in 1st 24 hr	Variable	Unlimited	Variable	Usually >5	Infection: bacterial sepsis, pyelonephritis, hepatitis, toxoplasmosis, cytomegalic inclusion disease, rubella, syphilis Drugs: vitamin K
Hepatocellular damage	Indirect and direct	Usually 2–3 days, may appear by 2nd wk	Variable	Unlimited	Variable	Variable, can be >5	Biliary atresia; paucity of bile ducts, familial cholestasis, galactosemia; hepatitis and infection

From Brown AK: Neonatal jaundice. *Pediatr Clin North Am* 1962;9:575–603.

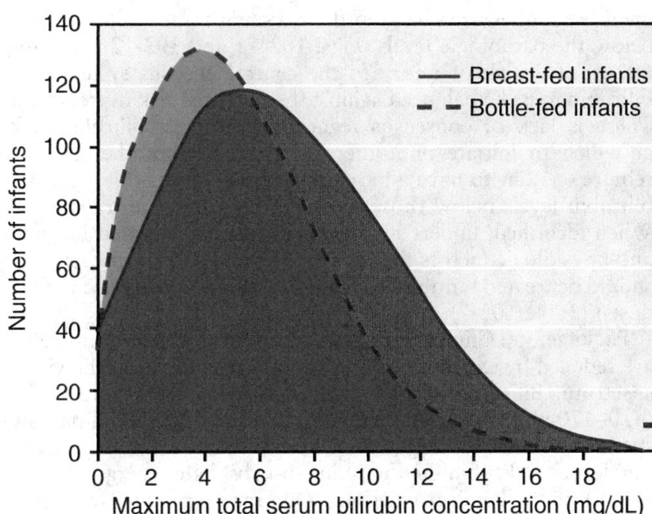

Figure 102-9. Distribution of maximal bilirubin levels during the 1st wk of life in breast-fed and formula-fed white infants weighing more than 2,500 g. (From Maisels MJ, Gifford K: Normal serum bilirubin levels in the newborn and the effect of breast-feeding. *Pediatrics* 1986;78:837–843.)

levels, in part because of reduced intake of the higher caloric density of breast milk. Frequent breast-feeding (>10/24 hr), rooming-in with night feeding, discouraging 5% dextrose or water supplementation, and ongoing lactation support may reduce the incidence of early breast-feeding jaundice.

NEONATAL HEPATITIS. See Chapter 353.1.

CONGENITAL ATRESIA OF THE BILE DUCTS. See Chapter 353.1. Jaundice persisting for more than 2 wk or associated with acholic stools and dark urine suggests biliary atresia. All such infants must have an immediate diagnostic evaluation, including determination of direct bilirubin.

INSPISSATED BILE SYNDROME. See Late Complications in Chapter 103.

102.4 • Kernicterus

Kernicterus, or bilirubin encephalopathy, is a neurologic syndrome resulting from the deposition of unconjugated (indirect) bilirubin in the basal ganglia and brainstem nuclei. The pathogenesis of kernicterus is multifactorial and involves an interaction between unconjugated bilirubin levels, albumin binding and unbound bilirubin levels, passage across the blood-brain barrier, and neuronal susceptibility to injury. Disruption of the blood-brain barrier by disease, asphyxia, and other factors and maturational changes in blood-brain barrier permeability affect risk.

The precise blood level above which indirect-reacting bilirubin or free bilirubin will be toxic for an individual infant is unpredictable, but kernicterus is rare in healthy term infants and in the absence of hemolysis if the serum level is <25 mg/dL. In previously healthy, predominantly breast-fed term infants, kernicterus has developed when bilirubin levels exceed 30 mg/dL, although the range is wide (21–50 mg/dL). Onset is usually in the 1st wk of life, but may be delayed to the 2nd–3rd wk. The risk in infants with hemolytic disease is directly related to serum bilirubin levels. The duration of exposure needed to produce toxic effects is unknown. Little evidence suggests that a level of indirect bilirubin <25 mg/dL affects the IQ of healthy term infants without hemolytic disease. Nonetheless, the more immature the infant is the greater the susceptibility to kernicterus. Factors that potentiate the movement of bilirubin across the blood-brain barrier and into brain cells are discussed in Chapter 102.3.

CLINICAL MANIFESTATIONS. Signs and symptoms of kernicterus usually appear 2–5 days after birth in term infants and as late as the 7th day in premature infants, but hyperbilirubinemia may lead to encephalopathy at any time during the neonatal period. The early signs may be subtle and indistinguishable from those of sepsis, asphyxia, hypoglycemia, intracranial hemorrhage, and other acute systemic illnesses in a neonate. Lethargy, poor feeding, and loss of the Moro reflex are common initial signs. Subsequently, the infant may appear gravely ill and prostrated, with diminished tendon reflexes and respiratory distress. Opisthotonos with a bulging fontanel, twitching of the face or limbs, and a shrill high-pitched cry may follow. In advanced cases, convulsions and spasm occur, with affected infants stiffly extending their arms in an inward rotation with the fists clenched (Table 102-5). Rigidity is rare at this late stage.

Many infants who progress to these severe neurologic signs die; the survivors are usually seriously damaged, but may appear to recover and for 2–3 mo show few abnormalities. Later in the 1st yr of life, opisthotonos, muscle rigidity, irregular movements, and convulsions tend to recur. In the 2nd yr, the opisthotonos and seizures abate, but irregular, involuntary movements, muscle rigidity, or, in some infants, hypotonia increase steadily. By 3 yr of age, the complete neurologic syndrome is often apparent and consists of bilateral choreoathetosis with involuntary muscle spasms, extrapyramidal signs, seizures, mental deficiency, dysarthric speech, high frequency hearing loss, squinting, and defective upward eye movements. Pyramidal signs, hypotonia, and ataxia occur in a few infants. In mildly affected infants, the syndrome may be characterized only by mild to moderate neuromuscular incoordination, partial deafness, or "minimal brain dysfunction," occurring singly or in combination; these problems may be inapparent until the child enters school (see Table 102-5).

PATHOLOGY. The surface of the affected brain is usually pale yellow. On pathologic section, certain regions are characteristically stained yellow by unconjugated bilirubin, particularly the corpus subthalamicum, hippocampus and adjacent olfactory areas, striate bodies, thalamus, globus pallidus, putamen, inferior clivus, cerebellar nuclei, and cranial nerve nuclei. Nonpigmented areas may also be damaged, characterized by neuronal loss, reactive gliosis, and atrophy of involved fiber systems in late disease. The pattern of injury has been related to the development of oxidative enzyme systems in various regions of the brain and overlaps with that found in hypoxic brain damage. Evidence favors the hypothesis that bilirubin interferes with oxygen utilization by cerebral tissue, possibly by injuring the cell membrane; antecedent hypoxic injury increases the susceptibility of brain cells to injury. Gross bilirubin staining without the specific microscopic changes of kernicterus may not be the same entity.

TABLE 102-5. Clinical Features of Kernicterus
ACUTE FORM
Phase 1 (1st 1–2 days): poor sucking, stupor, hypotonia, seizures
Phase 2 (middle of 1st wk): hypertonia of extensor muscles, opisthotonos, retrocollis, fever
Phase 3 (after the 1st wk): hypertonia
CHRONIC FORM
First year: hypotonia, active deep tendon reflexes, obligatory tonic neck reflexes, delayed motor skills
After 1st yr: movement disorders (choreoathetosis, ballismus, tremor), upward gaze, sensorineural hearing loss

From Dennery PA, Seidman DS, Stevenson DK: Neonatal hyperbilirubinemia. *N Engl J Med* 2001;344:581–590.

INCIDENCE AND PROGNOSIS. By pathologic criteria, kernicterus will develop in ⅓ of infants (all gestational ages) with untreated hemolytic disease and bilirubin levels >25–30 mg/dL. The incidence at autopsy in hyperbilirubinemic premature infants is 2–16% and is related to the risk factors discussed in Chapter 102.3. Reliable estimates of the frequency of the clinical syndrome are not available because of the wide spectrum of manifestations. Overt neurologic signs have a grave prognosis; more than 75% of such infants die, and 80% of affected survivors have bilateral choreoathetosis with involuntary muscle spasms. Mental retardation, deafness, and spastic quadriplegia are common.

PREVENTION. Although kernicterus has been thought to be a disease of the past, there are recent reports of neurotoxic effects of bilirubin in term and near-term infants discharged as healthy newborns. Some experts recommend universal screening for hyperbilirubinemia in the 1st 24–48 hr of life to detect infants at high risk for severe jaundice and bilirubin-induced neurologic dysfunction.

Effective prevention requires ongoing vigilance and a practical, system-based approach in order to distinguish infants with benign newborn jaundice from those whose course may be less predictable and potentially harmful. Protocols using the hour-specific bilirubin nomogram (see Fig. 102-8), physical examination and clinical risk factors have been successful in identifying patients at risk for hyperbilirubinemia and candidates for targeted management. The American Academy of Pediatrics (AAP) has identified potentially preventable causes of kernicterus: (1) early discharge (<48 hr) with no early follow-up (within 48 hr of discharge); this problem is particularly important in near-term infants (35–37 wk gestation); (2) failure to check the bilirubin level in an infant noted to be jaundiced in the 1st 24 hr; (3) failure to recognize the presence of risk factors for hyperbilirubinemia; (4) underestimation of the severity of jaundice by clinical (visual) assessment; (5) lack of concern regarding the presence of jaundice; (6) delay in measuring the serum bilirubin level despite marked jaundice or delay in initiating phototherapy in the presence of elevated bilirubin levels; and (7) failure to respond to parental concern regarding jaundice, poor feeding, or lethargy. The AAP subcommittee on hyperbilirubinemia provided an evidence-based management guideline for infants at least 35 wk (Fig. 102-10). They further recommend determining before discharge each infant's risk factors from established protocols (see Table 102-2). The following is further recommended: (1) any infant who is jaundiced before 24 hr requires measurement of the serum bilirubin level and, if it is elevated, the infant should be evaluated for possible hemolytic disease; and (2) follow-up should be provided within 2–3 days of discharge to all neonates discharged earlier than 48 hr after birth. Early follow-up is particularly important for infants younger than 38 weeks' gestation. The timing of follow-up depends on the age at discharge and the presence of risk factors. In some cases, follow-up within 24 hr is necessary. Post-discharge follow-up is essential for early recognition of problems related to hyperbilirubinemia and disease progression. Parental communication with regard to concerns about infant's skin color and behavioral activities should be addressed early and frequently, including education about potential risks and neurotoxicity. Ongoing lactation promotion, education, support, and follow-up services are essential throughout the neonatal period. Mothers should be advised to nurse their infant every 2–3 hr and avoid routine supplementation with water or glucose water in order to ensure adequate hydration and caloric intake.

TREATMENT OF HYPERBILIRUBINEMIA. Regardless of the cause, the goal of therapy is to prevent indirect-reacting bilirubin related neurotoxicity while not causing undo harm. Phototherapy and, if unsuccessful, exchange transfusion remain the primary treatment modalities used to keep the maximal total serum bilirubin below the pathologic levels (Figs. 102-11 and 102-12 and Table 102-6). The risk of injury to the central nervous system from bilirubin must be balanced against the potential risk of treatment. There is lack of consensus regarding the exact bilirubin level at which to initiate phototherapy. Because phototherapy may require 6–12 hr to have a measurable effect, it must be started at bilirubin levels below those indicated for exchange transfusion. When identified, underlying medical causes of elevated bilirubin and physiologic factors that contribute to neuronal susceptibility should be treated (antibiotics for septicemia and correction of acidosis) (Table 102-7).

Phototherapy. Clinical jaundice and indirect hyperbilirubinemia are reduced by exposure to a high intensity of light in the visible spectrum. Bilirubin absorbs light maximally in the blue range (420–470 nm). Broad-spectrum white, blue, and special narrow-spectrum (super) blue lights have been effective in reducing bilirubin levels. Bilirubin in the skin absorbs light energy, causing several photochemical reactions. One major product from phototherapy is a result of a reversible photo-isomerization reaction converting the toxic native unconjugated 4Z, 15Z-bilirubin into an unconjugated configurational isomer 4Z,15E-bilirubin, which can then be excreted in bile without conjugation. The other major product from phototherapy is lumirubin, which is an irreversible structural isomer converted from native bilirubin and can be excreted by the kidneys in the unconjugated state.

The therapeutic effect of phototherapy depends on the light energy emitted in the effective range of wavelengths, the distance between the lights and the infant, and the surface area of exposed skin, as well as the rate of hemolysis and in vivo metabolism and excretion of bilirubin. Available commercial phototherapy units vary considerably in spectral output and the intensity of radiance emitted; therefore, the wattage can be accurately measured only at the patient's skin surface. Dark skin does not reduce the efficacy of phototherapy. Maximal intensive phototherapy should be used when indirect bilirubin levels approach those noted in Figure 102-11 and Table 102-7. Such therapy includes "special blue" fluorescent tubes, placing the lamps within 15–20 cm of the infant, and placing a fiberoptic phototherapy blanket under the infant's back to increase the exposed surface area.

The use of phototherapy has decreased the need for exchange transfusion in term and preterm infants with hemolytic and nonhemolytic jaundice. When indications for exchange transfusion are present, phototherapy should not be used as a substitute; however, phototherapy may reduce the need for repeated exchange transfusions in infants with hemolysis. Conventional phototherapy is applied continuously, and the infant is turned frequently for maximal skin surface area exposure. It should be discontinued as soon as the indirect bilirubin concentration has reduced to levels considered safe with respect to the infant's age and condition. Serum bilirubin levels and hematocrit should be monitored every 4–8 hr in infants with hemolytic disease or those with bilirubin levels near toxic range for the individual infant. Others, particularly older infants, may be monitored less frequently. Serum bilirubin monitoring should continue for at least 24 hr after cessation of phototherapy in patients with hemolytic disease because unexpected rises in bilirubin may occur and require further treatment. Skin color cannot be relied on for evaluating the effectiveness of phototherapy; the skin of babies exposed to light may appear to be almost without jaundice in the presence of marked hyperbilirubinemia. Although not necessary for all affected infants, intravenous fluid supplementation added to oral feedings may be beneficial in dehydrated patients or those with high bilirubin levels nearing exchange transfusion.

Complications associated with phototherapy include loose stools, erythematous macular rash, purpuric rash associated with transient porphyrinemia, overheating, dehydration (increased insensible water loss, diarrhea), hypothermia from exposure, and a benign condition called *bronze baby syndrome*. Phototherapy

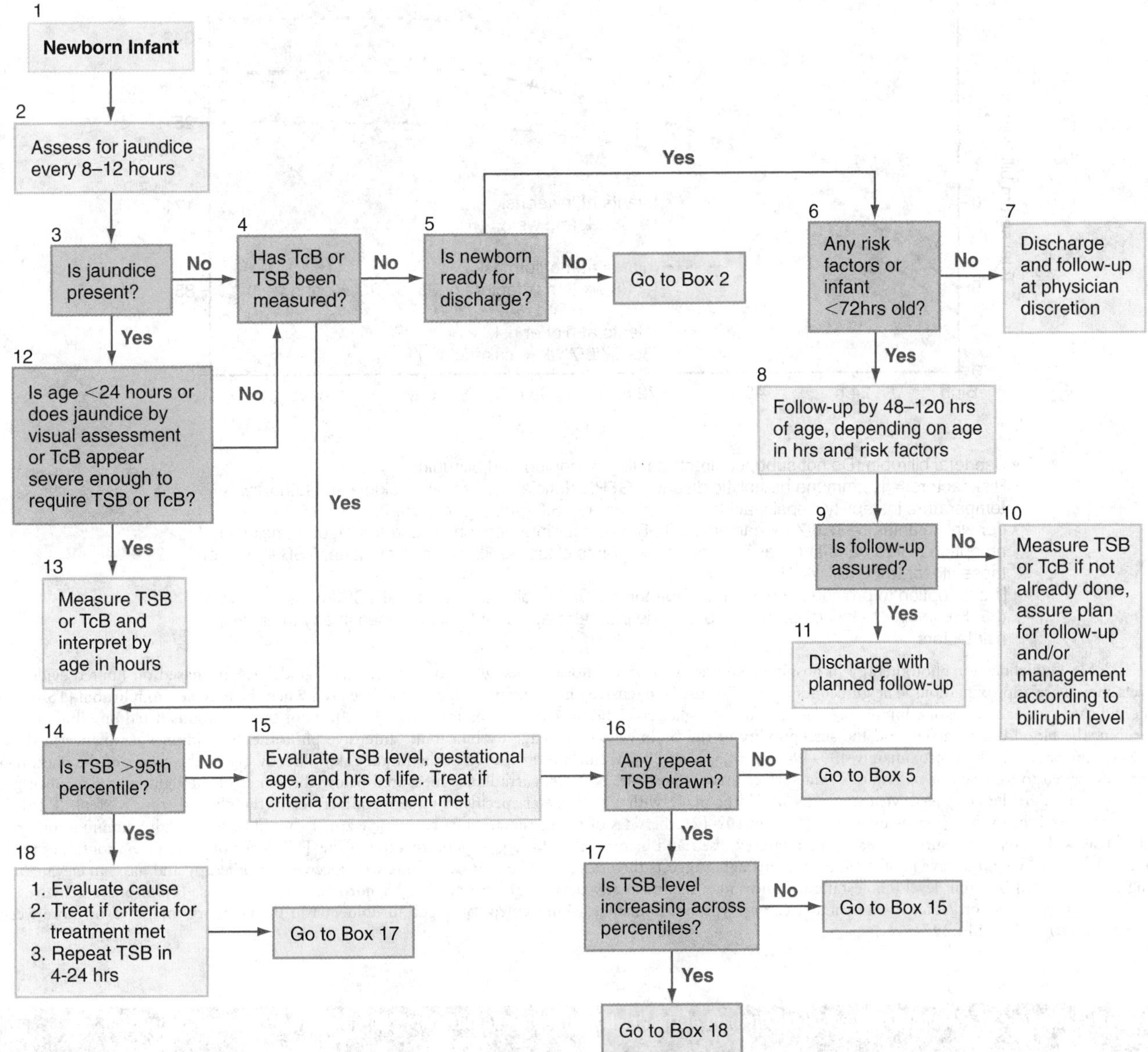

Figure 102-10. Algorithm for the management of jaundice in the newborn nursery. TcB, transcutaneous bilirubin; TSB, total serum bilirubin. (From American Academy of Pediatrics Subcommittee on Hyperbilirubinemia: Management of hyperbilirubinemia in the newborn infant 35 or more weeks of gestation. *Pediatrics* 2004;114:297–316.)

is contraindicated in the presence of porphyria. Before initiating phototherapy, the infant's eyes should be closed and adequately covered to prevent light exposure and corneal damage. Eye shields should be fitted properly to avoid pressure injury to the closed eyes, corneal excoriation if the eyes can be opened under the binding, and nasal occlusion. Body temperature should be monitored, and the infant should be shielded from bulb breakage. Irradiance should be measured directly and details of the exposure recorded (type and age of the bulbs, duration of exposure, distance from the light source to the infant). In infants with hemolytic disease, care must be taken to monitor for the development of anemia, which may require transfusion. Anemia may develop despite lowering of bilirubin levels. Clinical experience suggests that long-term adverse biologic effects of phototherapy are absent, minimal, or unrecognized.

The term **bronze baby syndrome** refers to a sometimes-noted dark, grayish-brown skin discoloration in infants undergoing phototherapy. Almost all infants observed with this syndrome have had significant elevation of direct-reacting bilirubin and other evidence of obstructive liver disease. The discoloration may be due to photo-induced modification of porphyrins, which are often present during cholestatic jaundice and may last for many months. Despite the bronze baby syndrome, phototherapy can continue if needed.

TABLE 102-6. Suggested Maximal Indirect Serum Bilirubin Concentrations (mg/dL) in Preterm Infants

BIRTHWEIGHT (g)	UNCOMPLICATED	COMPLICATED*
<1,000	12–13	10–12
1,000–1,250	12–14	10–12
1,251–1,499	14–16	12–14
1,500–1,999	16–20	15–17
2,000–2,500	20–22	18–20

Phototherapy is usually started at 50–70% of the maximal indirect level. If values greatly exceed this level, if phototherapy is unsuccessful in reducing the maximal bilirubin level, or if signs of kernicterus are evident, exchange transfusion is indicated.
*Complications include perinatal asphyxia, acidosis, hypoxia, hypothermia, hypoalbuminemia, meningitis, intraventricular hemorrhage, hemolysis, hypoglycemia, or signs of kernicterus.

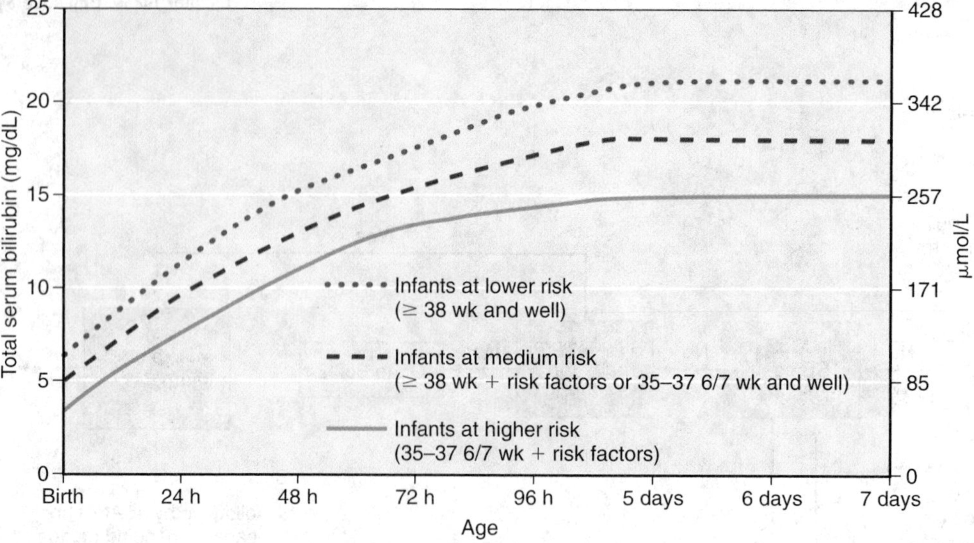

- Use total bilirubin. Do not subtract direct reacting or conjugated bilirubin.
- Risk factors = isoimmune hemolytic disease, G6PD deficiency, asphyxia, significant lethargy, temperature instability, sepsis, acidosis, or albumin < 3.0 g/dL (if measured).
- For well infants 35–37 6/7 wk can adjust TSB levels for intervention around the medium risk line. It is an option to intervene at lower TSB levels for infants closer to 35 wks and at higher TSB levels for those closer to 37 6/7 wk.
- It is an option to provide conventional phototherapy in hospital or at home at TSB levels 2–3 mg/dL (35–50mmol/L) below those shown but home phototherapy should not be used in any infant with risk factors.

Figure 102-11. Guidelines for phototherapy in hospitalized infants of 35 or more weeks' gestation. Note: These guidelines are based on limited evidence and the levels shown are approximations. The guidelines refer to the use of intensive phototherapy, which should be used when the total serum bilirubin (TSB) exceeds the line indicated for each category. Infants are designated as "higher risk" because of the potential negative effects of the conditions listed on albumin binding of bilirubin, the blood-brain barrier, and the susceptibility of the brain cells to damage by bilirubin. "Intensive phototherapy" implies irradiance in the blue-green spectrum (wavelengths approximately 430–490 nm) of at least 30 μW/cm²/nm (measured at the infant's skin directly below the center of the phototherapy unit) and delivered to as much of the infant's skin surface area as possible. Note that irradiance measured below the center of the light source is much greater than that measured at the periphery. Measurements should be made with a radiometer specified by the manufacturer of the phototherapy system. If TSB levels approach or exceed the exchange transfusion line (see Fig. 102-12), the sides of the bassinette, incubator, or warmer should be lined with aluminum foil or white material. This will increase the surface area of the infant exposed and increase the efficacy of phototherapy. If the TSB does not decrease or continues to rise in an infant who is receiving intensive phototherapy, this strongly suggests the presence of hemolysis. Infants who receive phototherapy and have an elevated direct-reacting or conjugated bilirubin level (cholestatic jaundice) may inconsistently develop the bronze-baby syndrome. G6PD, glucose-6-phosphate dehydrogenase. (From American Academy of Pediatrics Subcommittee on Hyperbilirubinemia: Management of hyperbilirubinemia in the newborn infant 35 or more weeks of gestation. *Pediatrics* 2004;114:297–316.)

TABLE 102-7. Example of a Clinical Pathway for Management of the Newborn Infant Readmitted for Phototherapy or Exchange Transfusion

Treatment
- Use intensive phototherapy and/or exchange transfusion as indicated in Figs. 102-11 and 102-12

Laboratory tests
- TSB and direct bilirubin levels
- Blood type (ABO, Rh)
- Direct antibody test (Coombs)
- Serum albumin
- Complete blood cell count with differential and smear for red cell morphology
- Reticulocyte count
- $ETCO_c$ (if available)
- G6PD if suggested by ethnic or geographic origin or if poor response to phototherapy
- Urine for reducing substances
- If history and/or presentation suggest sepsis, perform blood culture, urine culture, and cerebrospinal fluid for protein, glucose, cell count, and culture

Interventions
- If TSB ≥25 mg/dL (428 μmol/L) or ≥20 mg/dL (342 μmol/L) in a sick infant or infant <38 wk gestation, obtain a type and crossmatch, and request blood in case an exchange transfusion is necessary
- In infants with isoimmune hemolytic disease and TSB level rising in spite of intensive phototherapy or within 2–3 mg/dL (34–51 μmol/L) of exchange level (Fig. 102-12), administer intravenous immunoglobulin 0.5–1 g/kg over 2 hr and repeat in 12 hr if necessary
- If infant's weight loss from birth is >12% or there is clinical or biochemical evidence of dehydration, recommend formula or expressed breast milk. If oral intake is in question, give intravenous fluids.

For infants receiving intensive phototherapy
- Breastfeed or bottle-feed (formula or expressed breast mild) every 2–3 hr
- If TSB ≥25 mg/dL (428 μmol/L), repeat TSB within 2–3 hr
- If TSB 20–25 mg/dL (342–428 μmol/L), repeat within 3–4 hr. If TSB <20 mg/dL (342 μmol/L), repeat in 4–6 hr. If TSB continues to fall, repeat in 8–12 hr
- If TSB is not decreasing or is moving closer to level for exchange transfusion or the TSB/albumin ratio exceeds levels shown in Fig. 102-12, consider exchange transfusion (see Fig. 102-12 for exchange transfusion recommendations)
- When TSB is <13–14 mg/dL (239 μmol/L), discontinue phototherapy
- Depending on the cause of the hyperbilirubinemia, it is an option to measure TSB 24 hr after discharge to check for rebound

ETCO, end tidal carbon monoxide; G6PD, glucose-6-phosphate dehydrogenase; TSB, total serum bilirubin.

From AAP Subcommittee on Hyperbilirubinemia: Management of hyperbilirubinemia in the newborn infant 35 or more weeks of gestation. *Pediatrics* 2004;114:297–316.

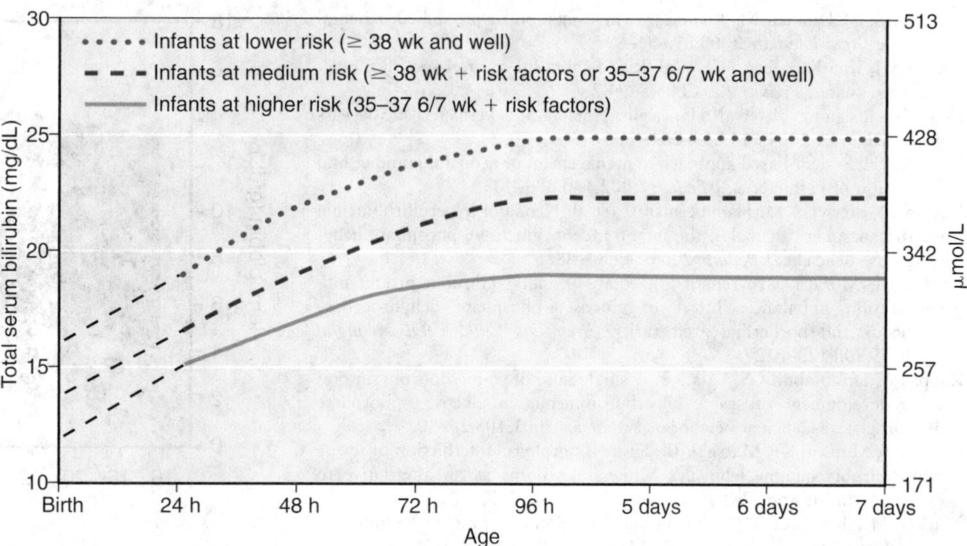
Infants at lower risk (≥ 38 wk and well)
Infants at medium risk (≥ 38 wk + risk factors or 35–37 6/7 wk and well)
Infants at higher risk (35–37 6/7 wk + risk factors)
Total serum bilirubin (mg/dL)
μmol/L
30
25
20
15
10
513
428
342
257
171
Birth
24 h
48 h
72 h
96 h
5 days
6 days
7 days
Age
• The dashed lines for the first 24 hours indicate uncertainty due to a wide range of clinical circumstances and a range of responses to phototherapy.
• Immediate exchange transfusion is recommended if infant shows signs of acute bilirubin encephalopathy (hypertonia, arching, retrocollis, opisthotonos, fever, high pitched cry) or if TSB is ≥ 5 mg/dL (85 μmol/L) above these lines.
• Risk factors = isoimmune hemolytic disease, G6PD deficiency, asphyxia, significant lethargy, temperature instability, sepsis, acidosis.
• Measure serum albumin and calculate B/A ratio (See legend).
• Use total bilirubin. Do not subtract direct reacting or conjugated bilirubin.
• If infant is well and 35–37 6/7 wk (median risk) can individualize TSB levels for exchange based on actual gestational age.

Figure 102-12. Guidelines for exchange transfusion in hospitalized infants of 35 or more weeks' gestation. Note: These suggested levels represent a consensus of most of the committee, but are based on limited evidence and the levels shown are approximations. During birth hospitalization, exchange transfusion is recommended if the total serum bilirubin (TSB) rises to these levels despite intensive phototherapy. For readmitted infants, if the TSB level is above the exchange level, repeat TSB measurement every 2–3 hr and consider exchange if the TSB remains above the levels indicated after intensive phototherapy for 6 hr. The following B : A ratios can be used together with but not in lieu of the TSB level as an additional factor in determining the need for exchange transfusion. G6PD, glucose-6-phosphate dehydrogenase. (From American Academy of Pediatrics Subcommittee on Hyperbilirubinemia: Management of hyperbilirubinemia in the newborn infant 35 or more weeks of gestation. *Pediatrics* 2004;114:297–316.)

Intravenous Immunoglobulin. The administration of intravenous immunoglobulin is an adjunctive treatment for hyperbilirubinemia due to isoimmune hemolytic disease. Its use is recommended when serum bilirubin is approaching exchange levels despite maximal interventions including phototherapy. Intravenous immunoglobulin (0.5–1.0 g/kg/dose; repeat in 12 hr) has been shown to reduce the need for exchange transfusion in both ABO and Rh hemolytic disease, presumably by reducing hemolysis.

Metalloporphyrins. A potentially important alternative therapy is the use of metalloporphyrins for hyperbilirubinemia. The metalloporphyrin Sn-mesoporphyrin (SnMP) offers promise as a drug candidate. The proposed mechanism of action is by competitive enzymatic inhibition of the rate limiting conversion of heme-protein to biliverdin (an intermediate metabolite to the production of unconjugated bilirubin) by heme-oxygenase. A single intramuscular dose on the 1st day of life may reduce the need for phototherapy. Such therapy may be beneficial when jaundice is anticipated, particularly in patients with ABO incompatibility or G6PD deficiency or when blood products are discouraged as with Jehovah's Witness patients. Complications from metalloporphyrins include transient erythema if the infant is receiving phototherapy. Administration of SnMP may reduce bilirubin levels and decrease both the need for phototherapy and length of hospital days; however, it remains unclear whether treatment with metalloporphyrins for unconjugated hyperbilirubinemia will alter risk of kernicterus or long-term neurodevelopment impairment. Data on efficacy, toxicity, and long-term benefit are currently being evaluated.

Exchange Transfusion. Double volume exchange transfusion is performed if intensive phototherapy has failed to reduce bilirubin levels to a safe range and if the risk of kernicterus exceeds the risk of the procedure. Potential complications from exchange transfusion are not trivial and include metabolic acidosis, electrolyte abnormalities, hypoglycemia, hypocalcemia, thrombocytopenia, volume overload, arrhythmias, NEC, infection, graft versus host disease, and death. This widely accepted treatment is repeated if necessary to keep indirect bilirubin levels in a safe range (see Fig. 102-12 and Table 102-7). See Exchange Transfusion in Chapter 103.

Various factors may affect the decision to perform a double volume exchange transfusion in an individual patient. The appearance of clinical signs suggesting kernicterus is an indication for exchange transfusion at any level of serum bilirubin. A healthy full-term infant with physiologic or breast-milk jaundice may tolerate a concentration slightly higher than 25 mg/dL with no apparent ill effect, whereas kernicterus may develop in a sick premature infant at a significantly lower level. A level approaching that considered critical for the individual infant may be an indication for exchange transfusion during the 1st or 2nd day of life when a further rise is anticipated, but not typically on the 4th day in term infants or on the 7th day in premature infants because an imminent fall may be anticipated as the hepatic conjugating mechanism becomes more effective.

American Academy of Pediatrics, Subcommittee on Hyperbilirubinemia: Clinical practice guideline: management of hyperbilirubinemia in the newborn infant 35 or more weeks of gestation. *Pediatrics* 2004;114:297–316.

Bhutani V, Johnson L, Sivier E: Predictive ability of a predischarge hour specific serum bilirubin for subsequent significant hyperbilirubinemia in healthy term and near-term newborns. *Pediatrics* 1999;103:6–14.

Bhutani VK, Johnson LH, Keren R: Diagnosis and management of hyperbilirubinemia in the term neonate: For a safer first week. *Pediatr Clin North Am* 2004;51:843–861.

Centers for Disease Control and Prevention: Kernicterus in full-term infants—United States, 1994–1998. *MMWR Morb Mortal Wkly Rep* 2001;50:491–494.

Chen SM, Chang MH, Du JC, et al: Screening for biliary atresia by infant stool color card in Taiwan. *Pediatrics* 2006;117:1147–1154.

Dennery PA, Seidman DS, Stevenson DK: Neonatal hyperbilirubinemia. *N Engl J Med* 2001;344:581.

Gottstein R, Cooke RWI: Systematic review of intravenous immunoglobulin in haemolytic disease of the newborn. *Arch Dis Child Fetal Neonatal Ed* 2003;88:F6–F10.

Hannam S, McDonnell M, Rennie JM: Investigation of prolonged neonatal jaundice. *Acta Paediatr* 2000;89:694–697.
Huang MJ, Kua KE, Teng HC, et al: Risk factors for severe hyperbilirubinemia in neonates. *Pediatr Res* 2004;56:682–689.
Ip S, Lau J, Chung M, et al: Hyperbilirubinemia and kernicterus: 50 years later. *Pediatrics* 2004;114:263–264.
Johnson LH: System-based approach to management of neonatal jaundice and prevention of kernicterus. *J Pediatr* 2002;140:396–403.
Kaplan M, Herschel M, Hammerman C, et al: Neonatal hyperbilirubinemia in African American males: the importance of glucose-6-phosphate dehydrogenase deficient. *J Pediatr* 2006;149:83–88.
Kaplan M, Muraca M, Vreman HJ, et al: Neonatal bilirubin production-conjugation imbalance: Effect of glucose-6-phosphate dehydrogenase deficiency and borderline prematurity. *Arch Dis Child Fetal Neonatal Ed* 2005;90:F123–F127.
Kappas A, Drummond GS, Valaes T: A single dose of sn-mesoporphyrin prevents development of severe hyperbilirubinemia in glucose-6-phosphate dehydrogenase–deficient newborns. *Pediatrics* 2001;108:25–30.
Kappas A, Munson DP, Marshall JR: Sn-mesoporphyrin interdiction of severe hyperbilirubinemia in Jehovah's Witness newborns as an alternative to exchange transfusion. *Pediatrics* 2001;108:1374–1377.
Maisels MJ, Kring E: The contribution of hemolysis to early jaundice in normal newborns. *Pediatrics* 2006;118:276–279.
Maisels MJ, Kring E: Rebound in serum bilirubin level following intensive phototherapy. *Arch Pediatr Adolesc Med* 2002;156:669–672.
Maisels MJ, Kring E: Transcutaneous bilirubin levels in the first 96 hours in a normal newborn population of ≥35 weeks' gestation. *Pediatrics* 2006;117:1169–1173.
Maisels MJ, Newman TB: Kernicterus in otherwise healthy, breast-fed term newborns. *Pediatrics* 1995;96:730–733.
Maruo Y, Nishizawa K, Sato H, et al: Association of neonatal hyperbilirubinemia with bilirubin UDP-glucuronosyltransferase polymorphism. *Pediatrics* 1999;103:1224–1227.
Mehta S, Kumar P, Narang A: A randomized controlled trial of fluid supplementation in term neonates with severe hyperbilirubinemia. *J Pediatr* 2005;147:781–785.
Monaghan G, Ryan M, Seddon R, et al: Genetic variation in bilirubin UDP-glucuronosyltransferase gene promoter and Gilbert's syndrome. *Lancet* 1996;347:578–581.
Newman TB, Liljestrand P, Jeremy RJ, et al; Outcomes among newborns with total serum bilirubin levels of 25 mg per deciliter or more. *N Engl J Med* 2006;354:1889–1900.
Oh W, Tyson JE, Fanaroff AA, et al: Association between peak serum bilirubin and neurodevelopmental outcomes in extremely low birth weight infants. *Pediatrics* 2003;112:773–779.
Patra K, Storfer-Isser A, Siner B, et al: Adverse events associated with neonatal exchange transfusion in the 1990s. *J Pediatr* 2004;144:626–631.
Rubaltelli FF, Da Riol R, D'Amore ESG, et al: The bronze baby syndrome: Evidence of increased tissue concentration of copper porphyrins. *Acta Paediatr* 1996;85:381–384.
Stevenson DK, Wong RJ, Vreman HJ, et al: NICHD conference on kernicterus: Research on prevention of bilirubin-induced brain injury and kernicterus: Bench-to-bedside—diagnostic methods and prevention and treatment strategies. *J Perinatol* 2004;24:521–525.
Suresh GK, Martin CL, Soll RF: Metalloporphyrins for treatment of unconjugated hyperbilirubinemia in neonates. Cochrane Database Syst Rev 2003;2:CD004207.
Wennberg RP, Ahlfors CE, Bhutani VD, et al: Toward understanding kernicterus: a challenge to improve the management of jaundiced newborns. *Pediatrics* 2006;117:474–485.

Chapter 103 ■ Blood Disorders

Barbara J. Stoll

103.1 • Anemia in the Newborn Infant

Hemoglobin increases with advancing gestational age: at term, cord blood hemoglobin is 16.8 g/dL (14–20 g/dL); hemoglobin

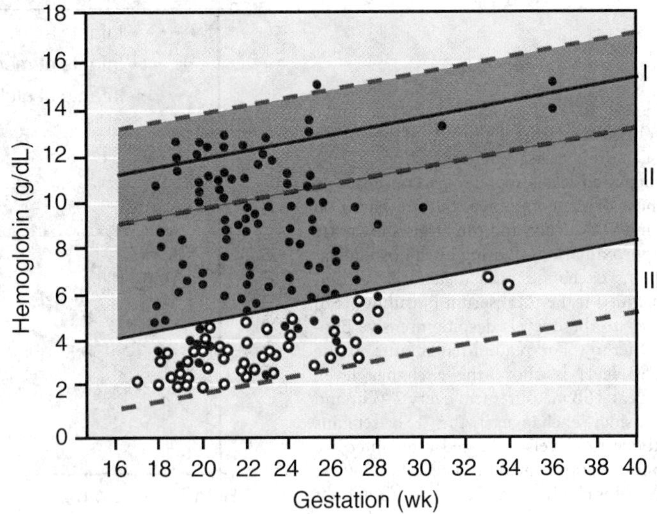

Figure 103-1. Range (mean and 95% confidence limits) of hemoglobin concentration from 10 to 40 wk of gestational age in normal (zone 1) fetuses obtained by cordocentesis (percutaneous umbilical blood sample). *Solid circles* depict maternal red blood cell isoimmunization; *open circles* indicate hemoglobin levels in fetuses with ultrasonographic evidence of hydrops (zone 3). (From Soothill PW: Cordocentesis: Role in assessment of fetal condition. *Clin Perinatol* 1989;16:755–770.)

levels in very low birthweight (VLBW) infants are 1–2 g/dL below those at term (Fig. 103-1). Less than the normal range of hemoglobin for birthweight and postnatal age is defined as anemia (Table 103-1). A "physiologic" decrease in hemoglobin content is noticed at 8–12 wk in term infants (hemoglobin, 11 g/dL) and at about 6 wk in premature infants (7–10 g/dL).

Infants born by cesarean section may have a lower hematocrit (Hct) than do those born vaginally. **Anemia at birth** is manifested as pallor, heart failure, or shock (Fig. 103-2). It may be due to acute or chronic fetal blood loss, hemolysis, or underproduction of erythrocytes. Specific causes include hemolytic disease of the newborn, tearing or cutting of the umbilical cord during delivery, abnormal cord insertion, communicating placental vessels, placenta previa or abruptio, nuchal cord, incision into the placenta, internal hemorrhage (liver, spleen, intracranial), α-thalassemia, congenital parvovirus infection or other hypoplastic anemias, and twin-twin transfusion in monozygotic twins with arteriovenous placental connections (see Chapter 97).

Transplacental hemorrhage with bleeding from the fetal into the maternal circulation has been reported in 5–15% of pregnancies, but, unless severe, it is not usually sufficient to cause clinically apparent anemia at birth. The cause of transplacental hemorrhage is not clear, but its occurrence has been proven by demonstrating significant amounts of fetal hemoglobin and red blood cells (RBCs) in maternal blood on the day of delivery by the **Kleihauer-Betke** test or by flow cytometry methods to detect fetal cells in maternal blood. If the infant has severe anemia with heart failure, emergency exchange transfusion to restore Hct and oxygen-carrying capacity may be needed.

Acute blood loss usually results in severe distress at birth, initially with a normal hemoglobin level, no hepatosplenomegaly, and early onset of shock. In contrast, chronic blood loss in utero produces marked pallor, less distress, a low hemoglobin level with microcytic indices, and, if severe, heart failure.

Anemia appearing in the first few days after birth is also most frequently a result of hemolytic disease of the newborn. Other causes are hemorrhagic disease of the newborn, bleeding from an improperly tied or clamped umbilical cord, large cephalohematoma, intracranial hemorrhage, or subcapsular bleeding from rupture of the liver, spleen, adrenals, or kidneys. Rapid decreases

TABLE 103-1. Normal Red Blood Cell Values from 18 Weeks' Gestation to 14 Weeks of Life

AGE	HEMOGLOBIN (g/dL)	HEMATOCRIT (%)	MCV (μ^3)	RETICULOCYTES (%)
Gestational (weeks)				
18–20*	11.5 ± 0.8	36 ± 3	134 ± 8.8	N/A
21–22*	12.3 ± 0.9	39 ± 3	130 ± 6.2	N/A
23–25*	12.4 ± 0.8	39 ± 2	126 ± 6.2	N/A
26–27	19.0 ± 2.5	62 ± 8	132 ± 14.4	9.6 ± 3.2
28–29	19.3 ± 1.8	60 ± 7	131 ± 13.5	7.5 ± 2.5
30–31	19.1 ± 2.2	60 ± 8	127 ± 12.7	5.8 ± 2.0
32–33	18.5 ± 2.0	60 ± 8	123 ± 15.7	5.0 ± 1.9
34–35	19.6 ± 2.1	61 ± 7	122 ± 10.0	3.9 ± 1.6
36–37	19.2 ± 1.7	64 ± 7	121 ± 12.5	4.2 ± 1.8
38–40	19.3 ± 2.2	61 ± 7	119 ± 9.4	3.2 ± 1.4
Postnatal (days)				
1	19.0 ± 2.2	61 ± 7	119 ± 9.4	3.2 ± 1.4
2	19.0 ± 1.9	60 ± 6	115 ± 7.0	3.2 ± 1.3
3	18.7 ± 3.4	62 ± 9	116 ± 5.3	2.8 ± 1.7
4	18.6 ± 2.1	57 ± 8	114 ± 7.5	1.8 ± 1.1
5	17.6 ± 1.1	57 ± 7	114 ± 8.9	1.2 ± 0.2
6	17.4 ± 2.2	54 ± 7	113 ± 10.0	0.6 ± 0.2
7	17.9 ± 2.5	56 ± 9	118 ± 11.2	0.5 ± 0.4
Postnatal (weeks)				
1–2	17.3 ± 2.3	54 ± 8	112 ± 19.0	0.5 ± 0.3
2–3	15.6 ± 2.6	46 ± 7	111 ± 8.2	0.8 ± 0.6
3–4	14.2 ± 2.1	43 ± 6	105 ± 7.5	0.6 ± 0.3
4–5	12.7 ± 1.6	36 ± 5	101 ± 8.1	0.9 ± 0.8
5–6	11.9 ± 1.5	36 ± 6	102 ± 10.2	1.0 ± 0.7
6–7	12.0 ± 1.5	36 ± 5	105 ± 12.0	1.2 ± 0.7
7–8	11.1 ± 1.1	33 ± 4	100 ± 13.0	1.5 ± 0.7
8–9	10.7 ± 0.9	31 ± 3	93 ± 12.0	1.8 ± 1.0
9–10	11.2 ± 0.9	32 ± 3	91 ± 9.3	1.2 ± 0.6
10–11	11.4 ± 0.9	34 ± 2	91 ± 7.7	1.2 ± 0.7
11–12	11.3 ± 0.9	33 ± 3	88 ± 7.9	0.7 ± 0.3
12–14	11.9	37	86.8	0.9

*Based on samples collected in utero. Results expressed as mean value ±1 standard deviation from the mean except for postnatal weeks 12–14 in which only the mean value is given.

From Bizzarro MJ, Colson E, Ehrenkranz RA: Differential diagnosis and management of anemia in the newborn. *Pediatr Clin North Am* 2004;51:1087–1107.

in hemoglobin or Hct values during the first few days of life may be the initial clue to these conditions.

Later in the neonatal period, delayed anemia may develop as a result of hemolytic disease of the newborn, with or without exchange transfusion or phototherapy. Congenital hemolytic anemia (spherocytosis) occasionally appears during the 1st mo of life, and hereditary nonspherocytic hemolytic anemia has been described during the neonatal period secondary to deficiency of glucose-6-phosphate dehydrogenase (G6PD) and pyruvate kinase. Bleeding from hemangiomas of the upper gastrointestinal tract or from ulcers caused by aberrant gastric mucosa in a Meckel diverticulum or duplication is a rare source of anemia in newborns. Repeated blood sampling of infants requiring frequent monitoring of blood gas and chemistry parameters is a common cause of anemia among hospitalized infants. Deficiency of minerals such as copper may cause anemia in infants maintained on total parenteral nutrition.

Anemia of prematurity occurs in low birthweight infants 1–3 mo after birth, is associated with hemoglobin levels below 7–10 g/dL, and is clinically manifested as pallor, poor weight gain, decreased activity, tachypnea, tachycardia, and feeding problems. Repeated phlebotomy for blood tests, shortened RBC survival, rapid growth, and the physiologic effects of the transition from fetal (low Pa_{O_2} and hemoglobin saturation) to neonatal life (high Pa_{O_2} and hemoglobin saturation) contribute to anemia of prematurity. The oxygen available to neonatal tissue is lower than that in adults, but a neonate's erythropoietin response is attenuated for the degree of anemia and, as a result, hemoglobin and reticulocyte levels are low. In VLBW infants, delayed clamping of the umbilical cord with the infant held below the level of the placenta may enhance placental-infant transfusion and reduce postnatal transfusion needs. This maneuver should not delay any needed resuscitation and may lead to hyperviscosity.

Treatment of neonatal anemia by blood transfusion depends on the severity of symptoms, the hemoglobin level, and the presence of co-morbid diseases (bronchopulmonary dysplasia, cyanotic congenital heart disease, respiratory distress syndrome) that interfere with oxygen delivery. The need for treatment with blood should be balanced against the risks of transfusion, including hemolytic transfusion reactions, exposure to blood product preservatives and other potential toxins, volume overload, possible increased risk of retinopathy of prematurity and necrotizing enterocolitis, graft vs host reaction, and transfusion-acquired infection (cytomegalovirus [CMV], HIV, parvovirus, hepatitis B and C) (see Chapter 474). The risk of CMV infection can be almost eliminated by the use of leukoreduced blood. In the infant under 1,500 g, CMV antibody-negative leukoreduced blood should be used. The risk of acquiring HIV and hepatitis B and C viruses is reduced but not eliminated by antibody screening of donated blood. Blood banking techniques that limit multiple donor exposure should be encouraged. Although transfusion guidelines for preterm infants have been proposed (Table 103-2), they have not been subjected to rigorous clinical study. Nonetheless, these guidelines have led to a decline in the number of unnecessary transfusions.

Asymptomatic full-term infants with a hemoglobin level of 10 g/dL may be monitored, whereas symptomatic neonates born after abruptio placentae or with severe hemolytic disease of the newborn warrant immediate transfusion. Preterm infants who

TABLE 103-2. Transfusion Protocol

Hct/Hgb	RESPIRATORY SUPPORT AND/OR SYMPTOMS	TRANSFUSION VOLUME
Hct ≤ 35/Hgb ≤ 11	Infants requiring moderate or significant mechanical ventilation (MAP > 8 cm H_2O and FI_{O_2} > 0.4)	15 mL/kg PRBCs* over period of 2–4 hr
Hct ≤ 30/Hgb ≤ 10	Infants requiring minimal respiratory support (any mechanical ventilation or endotracheal/nasal CPAP > 6 cm H_2O and FI_{O_2} ≤ 0.4)	15 mL/kg PRBCs over period of 2–4 hr
Hct ≤ 25/Hgb ≤ 8	Infants not requiring mechanical ventilation but who are receiving supplemental O_2 or CPAP with an FI_{O_2} ≤ 0.4 and in whom 1 or more of the following is present: • ≤24 hr of tachycardia (HR > 180) or tachypnea (RR > 80) • An increased oxygen requirement from the previous 48 hr, defined as a ≥4-fold increase in nasal canula flow (i.e., 0.25 to 1 L/min) or an increase in nasal CPAP ≥ 20% from the previous 48 hr (i.e., 5 to 6 cm H_2O) • Weight gain <10 g/kg/day over the previous 4 days while receiving ≥100 kcal/kg/day • An increase in episodes of apnea and bradycardia (>9 episodes in a 24-hr period or ≥2 episodes in 24 hr requiring bag and mask ventilation) while receiving therapeutic doses of methylxanthines • Undergoing surgery	20 mL/kg PRBCs over period of 2–4 hr (divide into 2–10 mL/kg volumes if fluid sensitive)
Hct ≤ 20/Hgb ≤ 7	Asymptomatic and an absolute reticulocyte count <100,000 cells/μL	20 mL/kg PRBCs over period of 2-4 hr (2–10 mL/kg volumes)

***RBC should be irradiated prior to transfusion.**

CPAP, continuous positive airway pressure; FI_{O_2}, fractional inspired oxygen; Hct, hematocrit; Hgb, hemoglobin; HR, heart rate; MAP, mean airway pressure; PRBC, packed red blood cells; RR, respiratory rate.

From Ohls RK, Ehrenkranz RA, Wright LL, et al: Effects of early erythropoietin therapy on the transfusion requirements of preterm infants below 1250 grams birth weight: A multicenter, randomized, controlled trial. *Pediatrics* 2001;108:934–942.

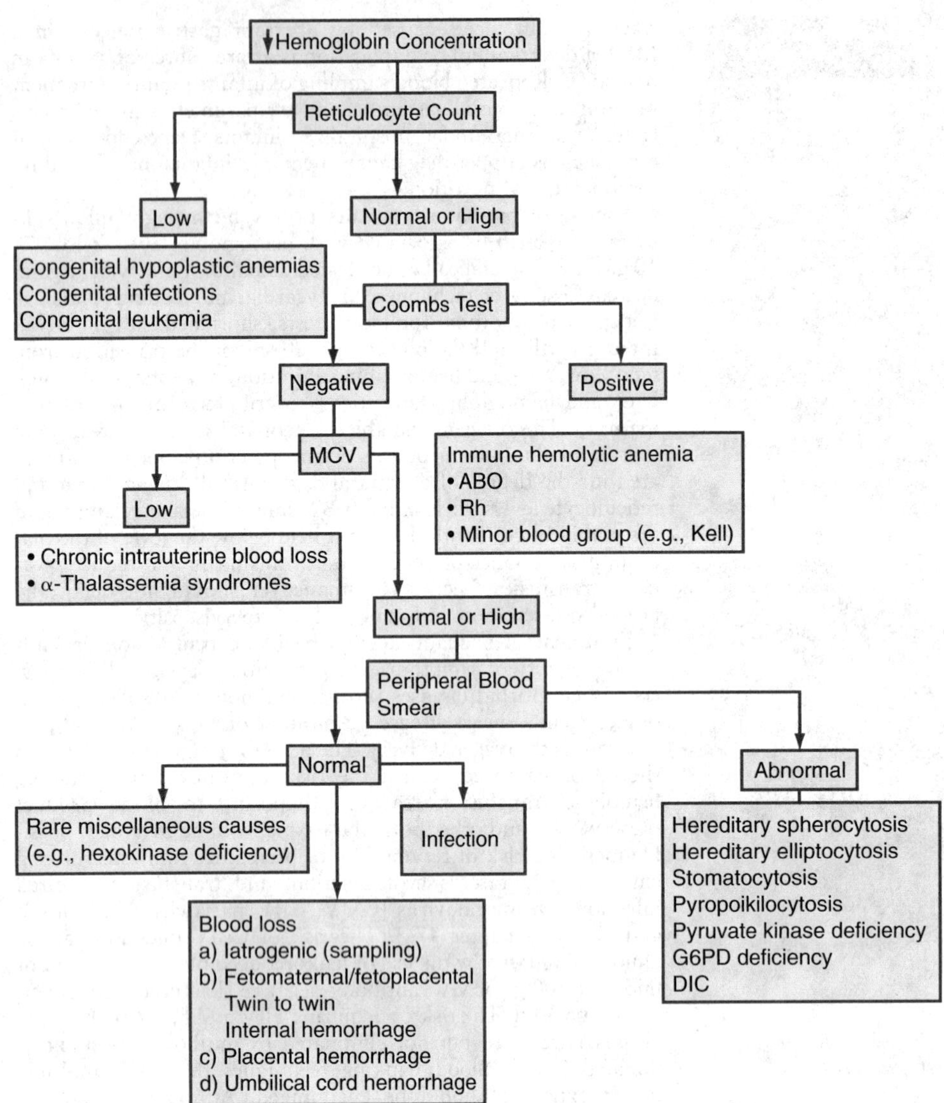

Figure 103-2. Diagnostic approach to anemia in newborn infants. DIC, disseminated intravascular coagulation; G6PD, glucose-6-phosphate dehydrogenase; MCV, mean corpuscular volume. (Modified from Blanchette VS, Zipursky A: Assessment of anemia in newborn infants. *Clin Perinatol* 1984;11: 489–510.)

have repeated episodes of apnea and bradycardia despite theophylline therapy and a hemoglobin level of 8 g/dL or lower may benefit from RBC transfusion. In addition, infants with respiratory distress syndrome or severe bronchopulmonary dysplasia may need hemoglobin levels of 12–14 g/dL to improve oxygen delivery. No transfusion is needed to replace blood removed for testing or for mild asymptomatic anemia. Asymptomatic neonates with reticulocytopenia and hemoglobin levels of 7 g/dL or lower may require transfusion; if a transfusion is not provided, close observation is essential. Packed RBC transfusion (10–20 mL/kg) is given at a rate of 2–3 mL/kg/hr to raise the hemoglobin concentration; 2 mL/kg raises the hemoglobin level 0.5–1 g/dL. Hemorrhage should be treated with whole blood if available; alternatively, fluid resuscitation is initiated and followed by packed RBC transfusion.

Recombinant human erythropoietin (r-HuEPO) has been used to prevent or treat chronic anemia associated with prematurity, bronchopulmonary dysplasia, and the hyporegenerative anemia of erythroblastosis fetalis. Anemia of prematurity is associated with abnormally low endogenous levels of serum erythropoietin but with r-HuEPO–responsive erythrocyte progenitor cells. Therapy with r-HuEPO must be supplemented with oral iron and possibly vitamin E. Doses and regimens vary. Treatment with erythropoietin and iron does not have a major impact on transfusion requirements and, therefore, routine use of erythropoietin in VLBW infants is not recommended.

103.2 • Hemolytic Disease of the Newborn (Erythroblastosis Fetalis)

Erythroblastosis fetalis is caused by the transplacental passage of maternal antibody active against paternal RBC antigens of the infant and is characterized by an increased rate of RBC destruction. It is an important cause of anemia and jaundice in newborn infants despite the development of a method of preventing maternal isoimmunization by Rh antigens. Although more than 60 different RBC antigens are capable of eliciting an antibody response, significant disease is associated primarily with the D antigen of the Rh group and with incompatibility of ABO factors. Rarely, hemolytic disease may be caused by C or E antigens or by other RBC antigens such as C^W, C^X, D^U, K (Kell), M, Duffy, S, P, MNS, Xg, Lutheran, Diego, and Kidd. Anti-Lewis antibodies do not cause disease.

HEMOLYTIC DISEASE OF THE NEWBORN CAUSED BY RH INCOMPATIBILITY

The Rh antigenic determinants are genetically transmitted from each parent, determine the Rh type, and direct the production of a number of blood group factors (C, c, D, d, E, and e). Each factor can elicit a specific antibody response under suitable conditions; 90% are due to D antigen and the remainder to C or E.

PATHOGENESIS. Isoimmune hemolytic disease from D antigen is approximately three times more frequent among white persons than among blacks. When Rh-positive blood is infused into an Rh-negative woman through error or when small quantities (usually more than 1 mL) of Rh-positive fetal blood containing D antigen inherited from an Rh-positive father enter the maternal circulation during pregnancy, with spontaneous or induced abortion, or at delivery, antibody formation against D antigen may be induced in the unsensitized Rh-negative recipient mother. Once sensitization has taken place, considerably smaller doses of antigen can stimulate an increase in antibody titer. Initially, a rise in IgM antibody occurs, which is later replaced by IgG antibody; the latter readily crosses the placenta and causes hemolytic manifestations.

Hemolytic disease rarely occurs during a first pregnancy because transfusion of Rh-positive fetal blood into an Rh-negative mother occurs near the time of delivery, too late for the mother to become sensitized and transmit antibody to her infant before delivery. The fact that 55% of Rh-positive fathers are heterozygous (D/d) and may have Rh-negative offspring and that fetal-to-maternal transfusion occurs in only 50% of pregnancies reduces the chance of sensitization, as does small family size, in which the opportunities for its reoccurrence are reduced. Finally, the capacity of Rh-negative women to form antibodies is variable, some producing low titers even after adequate antigenic challenge. Thus, the overall incidence of isoimmunization of Rh-negative mothers at risk is low, with antibody to D detected in less than 10% of those studied, even after five or more pregnancies; only about 5% ever have babies with hemolytic disease.

When the mother and fetus are also incompatible with respect to group A or B, the mother is partially protected against sensitization by the rapid removal of Rh-positive cells from her circulation by her preexisting anti-A or anti-B, which are IgM antibodies and do not cross the placenta. Once a mother has been sensitized, her infant is likely to have hemolytic disease. The severity of Rh illness worsens with successive pregnancies. The possibility that the first affected infant after sensitization may represent the end of the mother's childbearing potential for Rh-positive infants argues urgently for the prevention of sensitization. The injection of anti-D gamma globulin (RhoGAM) into the mother immediately after the delivery of each Rh-positive infant has been a successful strategy to reduce Rh hemolytic disease (see later).

CLINICAL MANIFESTATIONS. A wide spectrum of hemolytic disease occurs in affected infants born to sensitized mothers, depending on the nature of the individual immune response. The severity of the disease may range from only laboratory evidence of mild hemolysis (15% of cases) to severe anemia with compensatory hyperplasia of erythropoietic tissue leading to massive enlargement of the liver and spleen. When the compensatory capacity of the hematopoietic system is exceeded, profound anemia occurs and results in pallor, signs of cardiac decompensation (cardiomegaly, respiratory distress), massive anasarca, and circulatory collapse. This clinical picture of excessive abnormal fluid in two or more fetal compartments (skin, pleura, pericardium, placenta, peritoneum, amniotic fluid), termed **hydrops fetalis**, frequently results in death in utero or shortly after birth. With the use of RhoGAM to prevent Rh sensitization, nonimmune (nonhemolytic) conditions have become frequent causes of hydrops (Table 103-3). The severity of hydrops is related to the level of anemia and the degree of reduction in serum albumin (oncotic pressure), which is due in part to hepatic dysfunction. Alternatively, heart failure may increase right heart pressure, with the subsequent development of edema and ascites. Failure to initiate spontaneous effective ventilation because of pulmonary edema or bilateral pleural effusions results in birth asphyxia; after successful resuscitation, severe respiratory distress may develop. Petechiae, purpura, and thrombocytopenia may also be present in severe cases as a result of decreased platelet production or the presence of concurrent disseminated intravascular coagulation.

Jaundice may be absent at birth because of placental clearance of lipid-soluble unconjugated bilirubin, but in severe cases, bilirubin pigments stain the amniotic fluid, cord, and vernix caseosa yellow. Jaundice is generally evident on the 1st day of life because the infant's bilirubin-conjugating and excretory systems are unable to cope with the load resulting from massive hemolysis. Indirect-reacting bilirubin therefore accumulates postnatally and may rapidly reach extremely high levels and present a significant risk of bilirubin encephalopathy. The risk of kernicterus developing from hemolytic disease is greater than from comparable nonhemolytic hyperbilirubinemia, although the risk in an individual patient may be affected by other complications (anoxia, acidosis). Hypoglycemia occurs frequently in infants with severe isoimmune hemolytic disease and may be related to hyperinsulinism and hypertrophy of the pancreatic islet cells in these infants.

Infants born after intrauterine transfusion for prenatally diagnosed erythroblastosis may be severely affected because the indications for transfusion are evidence of already severe disease in utero (hydrops, fetal anemia). Such infants usually have very high (but extremely variable) cord levels of bilirubin, which reflects the severity of the hemolysis and its effects on hepatic function. Infants treated with intra-umbilical vein transfusions in utero may also have a benign postnatal course if the anemia and hydrops resolve before birth. Anemia from continuing hemolysis may be masked by the previous intrauterine transfusion, and the clinical manifestations of erythroblastosis may be superimposed on various degrees of immaturity resulting from spontaneous or induced premature delivery.

LABORATORY DATA. Before treatment, the direct Coombs test is usually positive, and anemia is generally present. The cord blood hemoglobin content varies and is usually proportional to the severity of the disease; with hydrops fetalis it may be as low as 3–4 g/dL. Alternatively, despite hemolysis, it may be within the normal range because of compensatory bone marrow and extramedullary hematopoiesis. The blood smear typically shows polychromasia and a marked increase in nucleated RBCs. The reticulocyte count is increased. The white blood cell count is usually normal but may be elevated; thrombocytopenia may develop in severe cases. Cord bilirubin is generally between 3 and 5 mg/dL; direct-reacting (conjugated) bilirubin may also be elevated, especially if there was an intrauterine transfusion. Indirect-reacting bilirubin rises rapidly to high levels in the 1st 6 hr of life.

After intrauterine transfusions, cord blood may show a normal hemoglobin concentration, negative direct Coombs test, predominantly type O Rh-negative adult RBCs, and a relatively normal smear.

DIAGNOSIS. Definitive diagnosis of erythroblastosis fetalis requires demonstration of blood group incompatibility and corresponding antibody bound to the infant's RBCs.

Antenatal Diagnosis. In Rh-negative women, a history of previous transfusions, abortion, or pregnancy should suggest the possibility of sensitization. Expectant parents' blood types should be tested for potential incompatibility, and the maternal titer of IgG antibodies to D antigen should be assayed at 12–16, 28–32, and 36 wk. Fetal Rh status may be determined by isolating fetal cells or fetal DNA (plasma) from the maternal circulation. The presence of elevated antibody titers at the beginning of pregnancy, a rapid rise in titer, or a titer of 1 : 64 or greater suggests significant hemolytic disease, although the exact titer correlates poorly with the severity of disease. If a mother is found to have anti-

TABLE 103-3. Etiology of Hydrops Fetalis*

CATEGORY	DISORDERS	CATEGORY	DISORDERS
Anemia	Immune (Rh, Kell) hemolysis	Teratomas	Choriocarcinoma
	α-Thalassemia		Sacrococcygeal teratoma
	Red blood cell enzyme deficiencies (G6PD)	Tumors and storage diseases	Neuroblastoma
	Fetomaternal hemorrhage		Hepatoblastoma
	Donor in twin-to-twin transfusion		Gaucher disease
Cardiac dysrhythmias	Supraventricular tachycardia		Niemann-Pick disease
	Atrial flutter		Mucolipidosis
	Congenital heart block		GM_1 gangliosidosis
Structural heart lesions	Premature closure of foramen ovale		Mucopolysaccharidosis
	Tricuspid insufficiency	Chromosome abnormalities	Trisomy 13, 15, 16, 18, 21
	Hypoplastic left heart		XX/XY, 45XO
	Endocardial cushion defect		Partial duplication of chromosome 11, 15, 17, 18
	Cardiomyopathy		Partial deletion of chromosome 13, 18
	Endocardial fibroelastosis		Triploidy
	Tuberous sclerosis with cardiac rhabdomyoma		Tetraploidy
	Pericardial teratoma	Bone diseases	Osteogenesis imperfecta
Vascular	Chorioangioma of placenta, chorionic vessels, or umbilical vessels		Asphyxiating thoracic dystrophy
	Umbilical artery aneurysm		Skeletal dysplasias
	Angiomyxoma of umbilical cord	Congenital infections	Cytomegalovirus
	True knot of umbilical cord		Parvovirus
	Hepatic hemangioma		Rubella
	Cerebral arteriovenous malformation (aneurysm of vein of Galen)		Toxoplasmosis
	Angiosteohypertrophy (Klippel-Trénaunay syndrome)		Syphilis
	Thrombosis of renal or umbilical vein or inferior vena cava		Leptospirosis
	Recipient in twin-to-twin transfusion		Chagas disease
Lymphatic	Lymphangiectasia	Others	Bowel obstruction with perforation and meconium peritonitis, volvulus
	Cystic hygroma		Hepatic fibrosis
	Chylothorax, chylous ascites		Beckwith-Wiedemann syndrome
	Noonan syndrome		Prune-belly syndrome
	Multiple pterygium syndrome		Congenital nephrosis
Central nervous system	Absent corpus callosum		Infant of a diabetic mother
	Encephalocele		Myotonic dystrophy
	Intracranial hemorrhage		Neu-Laxova syndrome
	Holoprosencephaly		Maternal therapy with indomethacin
Thoracic lesions	Cystic adenomatoid malformation of lung	Idiopathic	Multiple congenital anomaly syndromes
	Mediastinal teratoma		
	Diaphragmatic hernia		
	Sequestered lung		

*The incidence of nonimmune (nonhemolytic) hydrops fetalis is 1/2,000–1/3,500 births.
G6PD, glucose-6-phosphate dehydrogenase.
Modified from Phibbs R: In Polin N, Fox W (eds): Fetal and Neonatal Physiology, 2nd ed. Philadelphia, WB Saunders, 1998.

body against D antigen at a titer of 1 : 16 (15 IU/ml in Europe) or greater at any time during a subsequent pregnancy, the severity of fetal disease should be monitored by Doppler ultrasonography of the middle cerebral artery and then percutaneous umbilical blood sampling (PUBS) if indicated (see Chapter 96). If the mother has a history of a previously affected infant or a stillbirth, an Rh-positive infant is usually equally or more severely affected than the previous infant, and the severity of disease in the fetus should be monitored.

Assessment of the fetus may require information obtained from ultrasonography and PUBS. Real-time ultrasonography is used to detect the progression of disease, with hydrops defined as skin or scalp edema, pleural or pericardial effusions, and ascites. Early ultrasonographic signs of hydrops include organomegaly (liver, spleen, heart), the double–bowel wall sign (bowel edema), and placental thickening. Progression to polyhydramnios, ascites, pleural or pericardial effusions, and skin or scalp edema may then follow. If pleural effusions precede ascites and hydrops by a significant length of time, causes other than fetal anemia should be suspected (see Table 103-3). Extramedullary hematopoiesis and, less so, hepatic congestion compress the intrahepatic vessels and produce venous stasis with portal hypertension, hepatocellular dysfunction, and decreased albumin synthesis.

Hydrops is present when fetal hemoglobin is <5 g/dL, frequent when <7 g/dL, and variable between 7 and 9 g/dL. Real-time ultrasonography predicts fetal well-being by the biophysical profile (see Table 96-2), whereas Doppler ultrasonography assesses fetal distress by demonstrating increased vascular resistance in fetal arteries (middle cerebral). In pregnancies with ultrasonographic evidence of hemolysis (hepatosplenomegaly), early or late hydrops, or fetal distress, further and more direct assessment of fetal hemolysis should be performed.

Amniocentesis was classically used to assess fetal hemolysis. Hemolysis of fetal RBCs produces hyperbilirubinemia before the onset of severe anemia. Bilirubin is cleared by the placenta, but a significant proportion enters the amniotic fluid and can be measured by spectrophotometry. Ultrasonographically guided transabdominal aspiration of amniotic fluid may be performed as early as 18–20 wk of gestation. Spectrophotometric scanning of amniotic fluid wavelengths demonstrates a positive optical density (OD) deviation of absorption for bilirubin from normal at 450 nm. Amniocentesis and cordocentesis are invasive procedures with risks to both the fetus and mother, including fetal death, fetal bleeding, fetal bradycardia, worsening of alloimmunization, premature rupture of membranes, preterm labor, and chorioamnionitis. Noninvasive measurements to detect fetal anemia are desirable. In fetuses without hydrops, moderate to severe anemia can be detected noninvasively by demonstration of an increase in the peak velocity of systolic blood flow in the middle cerebral artery by Doppler ultrasound.

PUBS is the standard approach to assess the fetus if Doppler and real-time ultrasonography suggest an affected fetus. PUBS is performed to determine fetal hemoglobin levels and to transfuse packed RBCs in those with serious fetal anemia (Hct of 25–30%).

Postnatal Diagnosis. Immediately after the birth of any infant to an Rh-negative woman, blood from the umbilical cord or from the infant should be examined for ABO blood group, Rh type, Hct and hemoglobin, and reaction of the direct Coombs test. If the Coombs test is positive, a baseline serum bilirubin level should be measured, and a commercially available RBC panel should be used to identify RBC antibodies present in the mother's serum, both tests being performed not only to establish the diagnosis but also to ensure selection of the most compatible blood for exchange transfusion should it be necessary. The direct Coombs test is usually strongly positive in clinically affected infants and may remain so for a few days up to several months.

TREATMENT. The main goals of therapy are to (1) prevent intrauterine or extrauterine death from severe anemia and hypoxia, and (2) avoid neurotoxicity from hyperbilirubinemia.

Treatment of an Unborn Infant. Survival of severely affected fetuses has been improved by the use of fetal ultrasonography to identify the need for in utero transfusion. Intravascular (umbilical vein) transfusion of packed RBCs is the treatment of choice for fetal anemia, replacing intrauterine transfusion into the fetal peritoneal cavity. Hydrops or fetal anemia (Hct <30%) is an indication for umbilical vein transfusion in infants with pulmonary immaturity (see Fig. 103-1). **Intravascular fetal transfusion** is facilitated by maternal and hence fetal sedation with diazepam and by fetal paralysis with pancuronium. Packed RBCs are given by slow-push infusion after cross matching with the mother's serum. The cells should be obtained from a CMV-negative donor and irradiated to kill lymphocytes to avoid graft vs host disease. Of note, leukoreduction alone (without irradiation) does not prevent graft vs host disease. Transfusions should achieve a post-transfusion Hct of 45–55% and can be repeated every 3–5 wk. Indications for delivery include pulmonary maturity, fetal distress, complications of PUBS, or 35–37 wk of gestation. The survival rate for intrauterine transfusions is 89%; the complication rate is 3%. Complications include rupture of the membranes and preterm delivery, infection, fetal distress requiring emergency cesarean section, and perinatal death.

Treatment of a Liveborn Infant. The birth should be attended by a physician skilled in neonatal resuscitation. Fresh, low-titer, group O, leukoreduced, and irradiated Rh-negative blood cross matched against maternal serum should be immediately available. If clinical signs of severe hemolytic anemia (pallor, hepatosplenomegaly, edema, petechiae, ascites) are evident at birth, immediate resuscitation and supportive therapy, temperature stabilization, and monitoring before proceeding with exchange transfusion may save some severely affected infants. Such therapy should include correction of acidosis with 1–2 mEq/kg of sodium bicarbonate; a small transfusion of compatible packed RBCs to correct anemia; volume expansion for hypotension, especially in those with hydrops; and provision of assisted ventilation for respiratory failure.

Exchange Transfusion. When an infant's clinical condition at birth does not require an immediate full or partial exchange transfusion, the decision to perform one should be based on a judgment that the infant has a high risk of rapid development of a dangerous degree of anemia or hyperbilirubinemia. Cord hemoglobin of 10 g/dL or less and bilirubin of 5 mg/dL or more suggest severe hemolysis but inconsistently predict the need for exchange transfusion. Some physicians consider previous kernicterus or severe erythroblastosis in a sibling, reticulocyte counts >15%, and prematurity to be additional factors supporting a decision for early exchange transfusion (see Chapters 102.3 and 102.4). Intrauterine, intravascular transfusions have decreased the need for exchange transfusion.

The hemoglobin concentration, Hct, and serum bilirubin level should be measured at 4–6 hr intervals initially, with extension to longer intervals if and as the rate of change diminishes. The decision to perform an exchange transfusion is based on the likelihood that the trend of bilirubin levels plotted against hours of age indicates that serum bilirubin will reach the levels indicated in Figure 102-12 and Table 102-7. Term infants with levels of 20 mg/dL or higher have an increased risk of kernicterus. Ordinary transfusions of compatible Rh-negative, leukoreduced, and irradiated RBCs may be necessary to correct anemia at any stage of the disease up to 6–8 wk of age, when the infant's own blood-forming mechanism may be expected to take over. Weekly determinations of hemoglobin or Hct should be done until a spontaneous rise has been demonstrated.

Careful monitoring of the serum bilirubin level is essential until a falling trend has been demonstrated in the absence of phototherapy (see Chapter 102-3). Even then, an occasional infant, particularly if premature, may experience an unpredicted significant rise in serum bilirubin as late as the 7th day of life. Attempts to predict the attainment of dangerously high levels of serum bilirubin based on observed levels exceeding 6 mg/dL in the 1st 6 hr or 10 mg/dL in the 2nd 6 hr of life or on rates of rise exceeding 0.5–1.0 mg/dL/hr can be unreliable. Measurement of unbound bilirubin may be a more sensitive predictor of the risk associated with hyperbilirubinemia.

Blood for exchange transfusion should be as fresh as possible. Heparin or citrate-phosphate-dextrose-adenine solution may be used as an anticoagulant. If the blood is obtained before delivery, it should be taken from a type O, Rh-negative donor with a low titer of anti-A and anti-B antibodies and should be compatible with the mother's serum by the indirect Coombs test. After delivery, blood should be obtained from an Rh-negative donor whose cells are compatible with both the infant's and the mother's serum; when possible, type O donor cells are generally used, but cells of the infant's ABO blood type may be used when the mother has the same type. A complete cross match, including an indirect Coombs test, should be performed before the 2nd and subsequent transfusions. Blood should be gradually warmed and maintained at a temperature between 35 and 37°C throughout the exchange transfusion. It should be kept well mixed by gentle squeezing or agitation of the bag to avoid sedimentation; otherwise, the use of supernatant serum with a low RBC count at the end of the exchange will leave the infant anemic. Whole blood or packed leukoreduced and irradiated RBCs reconstituted with fresh frozen plasma to an Hct of 40% should be used. The infant's stomach should be emptied before transfusion to prevent aspiration, and body temperature should be maintained and vital signs monitored. A competent assistant should be present to help monitor, tally the volume of blood exchanged, and perform emergency procedures.

With strict aseptic technique, the umbilical vein is cannulated with a polyvinyl catheter to a distance no greater than 7 cm in a full-term infant. When free flow of blood is obtained, the catheter is usually in a large hepatic vein or the inferior vena cava. Alternatively, the exchange may be performed through peripheral arterial (drawn out) and venous (infused in) lines. The exchange should be carried out over a 45–60 min period, with aspiration of 20 mL of infant blood alternating with infusion of 20 mL of donor blood. Smaller aliquots (5–10 mL) may be indicated for sick and premature infants. The goal should be an isovolumetric exchange of approximately two blood volumes of the infant (2 × 85 mL/kg).

Infants with acidosis and hypoxia from respiratory distress, sepsis, or shock may be further compromised by the significant acute acid load contained in citrated blood, which usually has a pH between 7 and 7.2. The subsequent metabolism of citrate may result in metabolic alkalosis later if citrated blood is used. Fresh heparinized blood avoids this problem. During the exchange, blood pH and PaO_2 should be serially monitored because infants often become acidotic and hypoxic during exchange transfusions. Symptomatic hypoglycemia may occur before or during an exchange transfusion in moderately to severely affected infants; it may also occur 1–3 hr after exchange. Acute complications, noted in 5–10% of infants, include transient bradycardia with or without calcium infusion, cyanosis, transient vasospasm, thrombosis, apnea with bradycardia requiring resuscitation, and death. Infectious risks include CMV, HIV, and hepatitis. Necrotizing enterocolitis is a rare complication of exchange transfusion.

The risk of death from an exchange transfusion performed by an experienced physician is 0.3/100 procedures. With the decreasing use of this procedure because of the use of phototherapy and prevention of sensitization, the general level of physician competence is decreasing. Thus, it is best if this procedure is performed in experienced neonatal referral centers.

After exchange transfusion, the bilirubin level must be determined at frequent intervals (every 4–8 hr) because bilirubin may rebound 40–50% within hours. Repeated exchange transfusions should be carried out to keep the indirect fraction from exceeding the levels indicated in Table 102-7 for preterm infants and 20 mg/dL for term infants. Symptoms suggestive of kernicterus are mandatory indications for exchange transfusion at any time.

Late Complications. Infants who have hemolytic disease or who have had an exchange or an intrauterine transfusion must be observed carefully for the development of anemia and cholestasis. **Late anemia** may be hemolytic or hyporegenerative. Treatment with supplemental iron, erythropoietin, or blood transfusion may be indicated. A mild graft vs host reaction may be manifested as diarrhea, rash, hepatitis, or eosinophilia.

Inspissated bile syndrome refers to the rare occurrence of persistent icterus in association with significant elevations in direct and indirect bilirubin in infants with hemolytic disease. The cause is unclear, but the jaundice clears spontaneously within a few weeks or months.

Portal vein thrombosis and portal hypertension may occur in children who have been subjected to exchange transfusion as newborn infants. It is probably associated with prolonged, traumatic, or septic umbilical vein catheterization.

Prevention of Rh Sensitization. The risk of initial sensitization of Rh-negative mothers has been reduced to less than 1% by the intramuscular injection of 300 μg of human anti-D globulin (1 mL of RhoGAM) within 72 hr of delivery of an Rh-positive infant, ectopic pregnancy, abdominal trauma in pregnancy, amniocentesis, chorionic villus biopsy, or abortion. This quantity is sufficient to eliminate ≈ 10 mL of potentially antigenic fetal cells from the maternal circulation. Large fetal-to-maternal transfers of blood may require proportionately more RhoGAM. RhoGAM administered at 28–32 wk and again at birth (40 wk) is more effective than a single dose. The use of this technique, combined with improved methods of detecting maternal sensitization and measuring the extent of fetal-to-maternal transfusion, plus the use of fewer obstetric procedures that increase the risk of such fetal-to-maternal bleeding (version, manual separation of the placenta), should further reduce the incidence of erythroblastosis fetalis.

HEMOLYTIC DISEASE OF THE NEWBORN CAUSED BY BLOOD GROUP A AND B INCOMPATIBILITY

ABO incompatibility is the most common cause of hemolytic disease of the newborn. Approximately 15% of live births are at risk, but manifestations of disease develop in only 0.3–2.2%. Major blood group incompatibility between the mother and fetus generally results in milder disease than Rh incompatibility does. Maternal antibody may be formed against B cells if the mother is type A or against A cells if the mother is type B. Usually, the mother is type O and the infant is type A or B. Although ABO incompatibility occurs in 20–25% of pregnancies, hemolytic disease develops in only 10% of such offspring, and the infants are generally type A_1, which is more antigenic than A_2. Low antigenicity of the ABO factors in the fetus and newborn infant may account for the low incidence of severe ABO hemolytic disease relative to the incidence of incompatibility between the blood groups of the mother and child. Although antibodies against A and B factors occur without previous immunization ("natural" antibodies), they are usually IgM antibodies that do not cross the placenta. However, IgG antibodies to A antigen may be present and these do cross the placenta, so A-O isoimmune hemolytic disease may be found in first-born infants. Mothers who have become immunized against A or B factors from a previous incompatible pregnancy also exhibit IgG antibody. These "immune" antibodies are the primary mediators in ABO isoimmune disease.

CLINICAL MANIFESTATIONS. Most cases are mild, with jaundice being the only clinical manifestation. The infant is not generally affected at birth; pallor is not present, and hydrops fetalis is extremely rare. The liver and spleen are not greatly enlarged, if at all. Jaundice usually appears during the 1st 24 hr. Rarely, it may become severe, and symptoms and signs of kernicterus develop rapidly.

DIAGNOSIS. A presumptive diagnosis is based on the presence of ABO incompatibility, a weakly to moderately positive direct Coombs test result, and spherocytes in the blood smear, which may at times suggest the presence of hereditary spherocytosis. Hyperbilirubinemia is often the only other laboratory abnormality. The hemoglobin level is usually normal but may be as low as 10–12 g/dL. Reticulocytes may be increased to 10–15%, with extensive polychromasia and increased numbers of nucleated RBCs. In 10–20% of affected infants, the unconjugated serum bilirubin level may reach 20 mg/dL or more unless phototherapy is administered.

TREATMENT. Phototherapy may be effective in lowering serum bilirubin levels (see Chapter 102.4). In rare severe cases, treatment is directed at correcting dangerous degrees of anemia or hyperbilirubinemia by exchange transfusions with type O blood of the same Rh type as the infant. Indications for this procedure are similar to those previously described for hemolytic disease caused by Rh incompatibility. Some infants with ABO hemolytic disease may require transfusion of packed RBCs at several weeks of age because of slowly progressive anemia. Post-discharge monitoring of hemoglobin/Hct is essential in newborns with ABO hemolytic disease.

OTHER FORMS OF HEMOLYTIC DISEASE

Blood group incompatibilities other than Rh or ABO account for less than 5% of hemolytic disease of the newborn. The direct Coombs test is invariably positive, and exchange transfusion may be indicated for hyperbilirubinemia and anemia. Hemolytic disease, anemia, and hydrops fetalis as a result of anti-Kell antibodies are not predictable from the previous obstetric history, amniotic fluid bilirubin determinants, or the maternal antibody titer. Erythroid suppression may contribute to the anemia; PUBS is beneficial in actually measuring the fetal Hct.

Congenital infections such as cytomegalic inclusion disease, toxoplasmosis, rubella, and syphilis may be manifested as anemia, jaundice, hepatosplenomegaly, and thrombocytopenia, but the direct Coombs test result is negative and these conditions usually have other distinguishing clinical findings. Homozygous α-thalassemia may be associated with severe hemolytic anemia and a clinical picture resembling hydrops fetalis; it can be distinguished by a negative direct Coombs test result and characteristic clinical and laboratory findings (see Chapter 462.9). Anemia and jaundice may occur in infancy from hereditary spherocytosis (see Chapter 458) and other red cell membrane defects, and, if untreated, can result in kernicterus. Hemolytic anemia producing jaundice in the 1st wk of life may also be secondary to congenital deficiencies in RBC enzymes, such as pyruvate kinase or G6PD.

103.3 • Plethora in the Newborn Infant (Polycythemia) (See Chapter 467)

Plethora, a ruddy, deep red-purple appearance associated with a high Hct, is often due to polycythemia, defined as a central Hct of 65% or higher. Peripheral (heelstick) Hct values are higher than central values, whereas Coulter counter results are lower than Hct values determined by microcentrifugation. The incidence of neonatal polycythemia is increased at high altitudes (5% in Denver vs 1.6% in Texas); in postmature (3%) vs term (1–2%) infants; in small for gestational age (8%) vs large for gestational age (3%) vs average for gestational age (1–2%) infants; during the 1st day of life (peak, 2–3 hr); in the recipient infant of a twin-twin transfusion; after delayed clamping of the umbilical cord; in infants of diabetic mothers; in trisomy 13, 18, or 21; in adrenogenital syndrome; in neonatal Graves disease; in hypothyroidism; in infants of hypertensive mothers or those on propranolol; and in Beckwith-Wiedemann syndrome. Infants of diabetic or hypertensive mothers and those with growth restriction may have been exposed to chronic fetal hypoxia, which stimulates erythropoietin production and increases RBC production.

Clinical manifestations include irritability, lethargy, tachypnea, respiratory distress, cyanosis, feeding disturbances, hyperbilirubinemia, hypoglycemia, and thrombocytopenia. Severe complications include seizures, stroke, pulmonary hypertension, necrotizing enterocolitis, renal vein thrombosis, and renal failure. Many affected infants are asymptomatic. Hyperviscosity is present in most infants with central Hct values of 65% or higher and accounts for the symptoms of polycythemia. Hyperviscosity determined at constant shear rates (11.5 sec^{-1}) is present when whole blood viscosity is above 18 cycles/sec. Hyperviscosity is accentuated because neonatal RBCs have decreased deformability and filterability, which predisposes to stasis in the microcirculation.

Treatment of symptomatic polycythemic newborns is partial exchange transfusion (with normal saline). The Hct level (without measurement of viscosity) at which to perform a partial exchange transfusion in an **asymptomatic infant** is unclear but should not be considered if the Hct is ≤70–75%. Partial exchange will lower the Hct and viscosity and improve acute symptoms. The volume to be exchanged is calculated from the following formula:

Volume of exchange (mL) = Blood volume × (Observed − Desired hematocrit)/Observed hematocrit

The long-term prognosis of polycythemic infants is unclear. Reported adverse outcomes include speech deficits, abnormal fine motor control, reduced IQ, school problems, and other neurologic abnormalities. It is thought that the underlying etiology (chronic intrauterine hypoxia) and hyperviscosity contribute to adverse outcomes. It is unclear whether partial exchange transfusion improves the long-term outcome. Most asymptomatic infants develop normally.

103.4 • Hemorrhage in the Newborn Infant

HEMORRHAGIC DISEASE OF THE NEWBORN. A moderate decrease in factors II, VII, IX, and X normally occurs in all newborn infants by 48–72 hr after birth, with a gradual return to birth levels by 7–10 days of age. This transient deficiency of vitamin K–dependent factors is probably due to lack of free vitamin K from the mother and absence of the bacterial intestinal flora normally responsible for the synthesis of vitamin K. Rarely, in term infants and more frequently in premature infants, accentuation and prolongation of this deficiency between the 2nd and 7th days of life result in spontaneous and prolonged bleeding. Breast milk is a poor source of vitamin K, and hemorrhagic complications are more frequent in breast-fed than in formula-fed infants. This classic form of hemorrhagic disease of the newborn, which is responsive to and prevented by vitamin K therapy, must be distinguished from disseminated intravascular coagulopathy and from the more infrequent congenital deficiencies of one or more of the other factors that are unresponsive to vitamin K (see Chapter 482). Early-onset life-threatening vitamin K deficiency–induced bleeding (onset from birth to 24 hr) also occurs if the mother has been treated with drugs (phenobarbital, phenytoin) that interfere with vitamin K function. Late onset (>2 wk) is often associated with vitamin K malabsorption, as noted in neonatal hepatitis or biliary atresia (Table 103-4).

Hemorrhagic disease of the newborn resulting from severe transient deficiencies in vitamin K–dependent factors is characterized by bleeding that tends to be gastrointestinal, nasal, subgaleal, intracranial, or postcircumcision. Prodromal or warning signs (mild bleeding) may occur before serious intracranial hemorrhage. The prothrombin time (PT), blood coagulation time, and partial thromboplastin time are prolonged, and levels of prothrombin (II) and factors VII, IX, and X are significantly

TABLE 103-4. Hemorrhagic Disease of the Newborn

	EARLY ONSET	CLASSIC DISEASE	LATE ONSET
Age	0–24 hr	2–7 days	1–6 mo
Site of hemorrhage	Cephalohematoma Subgaleal Intracranial Gastrointestinal Umbilicus Intra-abdominal	Gastrointestinal Ear-nose-throat–mucosal Intracranial Circumcision Cutaneous Gastrointestinal Injection sites	Intracranial Gastrointestinal Cutaneous Ear-nose-throat–mucosal Injection sites Thoracic
Etiology/risks	Maternal drugs (phenobarbital, phenytoin, warfarin, rifampin, isoniazid) that interfere with vitamin K Inherited coagulopathy	Vitamin K deficiency Breast-feeding	Cholestasis—malabsorption of vitamin K (biliary atresia, cystic fibrosis, hepatitis) Abetalipoprotein deficiency Idiopathic in Asian breast-fed infants Warfarin ingestion
Prevention	Posible vitamin K at birth or to mother (20 mg) before birth Avoid high-risk medications	Prevented by parenteral vitamin K at birth. Oral vitamin K regimens require repeated dosing over time	Prevented by parenteral and high-dose oral vitamin K during periods of malabsorption or cholestasis
Incidence	Very rare	≈2% if not given vitamin K	Dependent on primary disease

decreased. Vitamin K facilitates post-transcriptional carboxylation of factors II, VII, IX, and X. In the absence of carboxylation, such factors form PIVKA (protein induced in vitamin K absence), which is a sensitive marker for vitamin K status. Bleeding time, fibrinogen, factors V and VIII, platelets, capillary fragility, and clot retraction are normal for maturity.

Intramuscular administration of 1 mg of vitamin K at the time of birth **prevents** the decrease in vitamin K–dependent factors in full-term infants, but it is not uniformly effective in the prophylaxis of hemorrhagic disease of the newborn in premature infants. The disease may be effectively **treated** with a slow intravenous infusion of 1–5 mg of vitamin K_1, with improvement in coagulation defects and cessation of bleeding noted within a few hours. Serious bleeding, particularly in premature infants or those with liver disease, may require a transfusion of **fresh frozen plasma** or whole blood. The mortality rate is low in treated patients.

A particularly severe form of deficiency of vitamin K–dependent coagulation factors has been reported in infants born to mothers receiving anticonvulsive medications (phenobarbital and phenytoin) during pregnancy. They may have severe bleeding, with onset within the 1st 24 hr of life; the bleeding is usually corrected by vitamin K_1, although in some the response is poor or delayed. A PT should be obtained on cord blood and the infant given 1–2 mg of vitamin K intravenously. If the PT is greatly prolonged and fails to improve, 10 mL/kg of fresh frozen plasma should be administered.

The routine use of intramuscular vitamin K for prophylaxis in the United States is safe and is not associated with an increased risk of childhood cancer or leukemia. Although oral vitamin K (birth, discharge, 3–4 wk: 1–2 mg) has been suggested as an alternative, the effectiveness of oral vitamin K has not been established and it cannot be recommended for routine therapy. The intramuscular route remains the method of choice.

Other forms of bleeding may be clinically indistinguishable from hemorrhagic disease of the newborn responsive to vitamin K, but they are neither prevented nor successfully treated with it. A clinical pattern identical to that of hemorrhagic disease of the newborn may also result from any of the congenital defects in blood coagulation (see Chapters 476 and 477). Hematomas, melena, and postcircumcision and umbilical cord bleeding may be present; only 5–35% of cases of factor VIII and IX deficiency become clinically apparent in the newborn period. Treatment of the rare congenital deficiencies of coagulation factors requires fresh frozen plasma or specific factor replacement.

Disseminated intravascular coagulopathy in newborn infants results in consumption of coagulation factors and bleeding. Affected infants are often premature; the clinical course is frequently characterized by asphyxia, hypoxia, acidosis, shock, hemangiomas, or infection. Treatment is directed at correcting the primary clinical problem, such as infection, and interrupting consumption and replacing clotting factors (see Chapter 483).

Infants with central nervous system or other bleeding posing an immediate threat to life should receive fresh frozen plasma, vitamin K, and blood if needed as soon as possible after blood has been drawn for coagulation studies, which should include a determination of the number of platelets.

The **swallowed blood syndrome,** in which blood or bloody stools are passed, usually on the 2nd or 3rd day of life, may be confused with hemorrhage from the gastrointestinal tract. The blood may be swallowed during delivery or from a fissure in the mother's nipple. Differentiation from gastrointestinal hemorrhage is based on the fact that the infant's blood contains mostly fetal hemoglobin, which is alkali-resistant, whereas swallowed blood from a maternal source contains adult hemoglobin, which is promptly changed to alkaline hematin after the addition of alkali. Apt devised the following test for this differentiation: (1) Rinse a blood-stained diaper or some grossly bloody (red) stool with a suitable amount of water to obtain a distinctly pink supernatant hemoglobin solution. (2) Centrifuge the mixture and decant the supernatant solution. (3) To five parts of the supernatant fluid add one part of 0.25 N (1%) sodium hydroxide. Within 1–2 min a color reaction takes place: A yellow-brown color indicates that the blood is maternal in origin; a persistent pink indicates that it is from the infant. A control test with known adult or infant blood, or both, is advisable.

Widespread subcutaneous ecchymoses in premature infants at or immediately after birth are apparently a result of fragile superficial blood vessels rather than a coagulation defect. Administering vitamin K_1 to the mother during labor has no effect on the incidence of ecchymoses. Occasionally, an infant is born with petechiae or a generalized bluish suffusion limited to the face, head, and neck, probably as a result of venous obstruction by a nuchal cord or sudden increases in intrathoracic pressure during delivery. It may take 2–3 wk for such suffusions to disappear.

NEONATAL THROMBOCYTOPENIC PURPURA. See Chapter 484.

Anderson C: Critical haemoglobin thresholds in premature infants. *Arch Dis Child Fetal Neonatal Ed* 2001;84:F146–F148.

Bednarek F, Weisberger S, Richardson DK, et al: Variations in blood transfusions among newborn intensive care units. *J Pediatr* 1998;133:601–607.

Bizzarro MJ, Colson E, Ehrenkranz RA: Differential diagnosis and management of anemia in the newborn. *Pediatr Clin North Am* 2004;51:1087–1107.

Davis BH, Olsen S, Bigelow NC, et al: Detection of fetal red cells in fetomaternal hemorrhage using a fetal hemoglobin monoclonal antibody by flow cytometry. *Transfusion* 1998;38:749–756.

Dempsey EM, Barrington K: Short and long term outcomes following partial exchange transfusion in the polycythaemic newborn: a systematic review. *Arch Dis Child Fetal Neonatal Ed* 2006;91:F2–F6.

Ferguson D, Hébert PC, Lee SK, et al: Clinical outcomes following institution of universal leukoreduction of blood transfusions for premature infants. *JAMA* 2003;289:1950–1956.

Franz AR, Pohlandt F: Red blood cell transfusions in very and extremely low birthweight infants under restrictive transfusion guidelines: Is exogenous erythropoietin necessary? *Arch Dis Child Fetal Neonatal Ed* 2001;84:F96–F100.

Greer FR: Are breast-fed infants vitamin K deficient? *Adv Exp Med Biol* 2001;501:391–395.

Hébert PC, Fergusson D, Blajchman MA, et al: Clinical outcomes following institution of the Canadian universal leukoreduction program for red blood cell transfusions. *JAMA* 2003;289:1941–1949.

Hermansen MC: Nucleated red blood cells in the fetus and newborn. *Arch Dis Child* 2001;84:F211–F215.

Janssens HM, de Haan MJJ, van Kamp IL, et al: Outcome for children treated with fetal intravascular transfusions because of severe blood group antagonism. *J Pediatr* 1997;131:373–380.

Klumper FJ, van Kamp IL, Vandenbussche FP, et al: Benefits and risks of fetal red-cell transfusion after 32 weeks gestation. *Eur J Obstet Gynecol Reprod Biol* 2000;92:91–96.

Kumar D, Greer FR, Super DM, et al: Vitamin K status of premature infants: Implications for current recommendations. *Pediatrics* 2001;108:1117–1122.

Kumar S, Regan: Management of pregnancies with RhD alloimmunization. *Br Med J* 2005;330:1255–1258.

Lo D, Hjelm N, Fidler C, et al: Prenatal diagnosis of fetal RhD status by molecular analysis of maternal plasma. *N Engl J Med* 1998;339:1734–1738.

Maier RF, Obladen M, Mueller-Hansen I, et al: Early treatment with erythropoietin β ameliorates anemia and reduces transfusion requirements in infants with birth weights below 1000 g. *J Pediatr* 2002;141:8–15.

Mari G, Deter RL, Carpenter RL, et al: Noninvasive diagnosis by Doppler ultrasonography of fetal anemia due to maternal red-cell alloimmunization. Collaborative Group for Doppler Assessment of the Blood Velocity in Anemic Fetuses. *N Engl J Med* 2000;342:9–14.

Moise Jr. KJ: Diagnosing hemolytic disease of the fetus—time to put the needles away. *N Engl J Med* 2006;355:192–194.

Naulaers G, Barten S, Vanhole C, et al: Management of severe neonatal anemia due to fetomaternal transfusion. *Am J Perinatol* 1999;16:193–196.

Nicaise C, Gire C, Casha P, et al: Erythropoietin as treatment for late hyporegenerative anemia in neonates with Rh hemolytic disease after in utero exchange transfusion. *Fetal Diagn Ther* 2002;17:22–24.

Pappas A, Delaney-Black V: Differential diagnosis and management of polycythemia. *Pediatr Clin North Am* 2004;51:1063–1086.
Patra K, Storfer-Isser A, Siner B, et al: Adverse events associated with neonatal exchange transfusion in the 1990s. *J Pediatr* 2004;144:626–631.
Puckett RM, Offringa M: Prophylactic vitamin K for vitamin K deficiency bleeding in neonates. *Cochrane Database Syst Rev* 2000;4:CD002776.
Rabe H, Wacker A, Hulskamp G, et al: A randomised controlled trial of delayed cord clamping in very low birth weight preterm infants. *Eur J Pediatr* 2000;159:775–777.
Rothenberg T: Partial plasma exchange transfusion in polycythemic neonates. *Arch Dis Child* 2002;86:60–62.
Schimmel MS, Bromiker R, Soll RF: Neonatal polycythemia: Is partial exchange transfusion justified? *Clin Perinatol* 2004;31:545–553.
Sekizawa A, Watanabe A, Kimura T, et al: Prenatal diagnosis of the fetal RhD blood type using a single fetal nucleated erythrocyte from maternal blood. *Obstet Gynecol* 1996;87:501–505.
Stephenson T, Zuccollo J, Mohajer M: Diagnosis and management of non-immune hydrops in the newborn. *Arch Dis Child Fetal Neonatal Ed* 1994;70:F151–F154.
van Kamp IL, Klumper FJ, Bakkum RS, et al: The severity of immune fetal hydrops is predictive of fetal outcome after intrauterine treatment. *Am J Obstet Gynecol* 2001;185:668–673.
van Kamp IL, Klumper FJ, Oepkes D, et al: Complications of intrauterine intravascular transfusion for fetal anemia due to maternal red-cell alloimmunization. *Am J Obstet Gynecol* 2005;192:171–177.
Vaughan JI, Manning M, Warwick RM, et al: Inhibition of erythroid progenitor cells by anti-Kell antibodies in fetal alloimmune anemia. *N Engl J Med* 1998;338:798–803.
Waldron P, de Alarcon P: ABO hemolytic disease of the newborn: A unique constellation of findings in siblings and review of protective mechanisms in the fetal-maternal system. *Am J Perinatol* 1999;16:391–398.
Wong W, Fok TF, Lee CH, et al: Randomized controlled trial: Comparison of colloid or crystalloid for partial exchange transfusion for treatment of neonatal polycythaemia. *Arch Dis Child* 1997;77:F115–F118.
Zipursky A: Prevention of vitamin K deficiency bleeding in newborns. *Br J Haematol* 1999;104:430–437.

Chapter 104 ■ Genitourinary System (see also Part XXIII) Barbara J. Stoll

Urinary tract anomalies (hydronephrosis, dysplasia, cystic or solitary kidney) are frequently identified by prenatal ultrasonography (see Table 96–5). After birth, the presence/extent of anomalies needs to be confirmed and followed by detailed evaluation and appropriate management. Follow-up of urinary anomalies diagnosed in utero requires renal ultrasonography after birth. For anomalies such as ureteropelvic junction obstruction and reflux, prenatal diagnosis provides the opportunity for early treatment to minimize functional deterioration and urinary tract infection.

One or both kidneys are often easily palpable in a newborn infant. When both are palpable and similar, infants usually do not have any particular diagnostic problems, but when only one kidney can be felt, a frequent impression is that it is larger than normal or is displaced by an intrinsic or extrinsic mass. Fetal lobulation may contribute to this impression. The problem usually resolves as the kidney becomes progressively less easily palpable during the early months of life. Because palpable enlargement or displacement of a kidney in a newborn may be due to hydronephrosis, neuroblastoma, mesoblastic nephroma, adrenal hemorrhage, or a cystic malformation, ultrasound examination is indicated.

THROMBOSIS OF THE RENAL VEIN. See Chapter 107.

CIRCUMCISION (SEE CHAPTER 544). Circumcision is the most common elective surgical procedure performed on newborn boys in the United States. The benefits relate to cultural or religious beliefs as well as medical benefits and include a reduced incidence of balanitis, penile cancer, sexually transmitted diseases (including HIV), and urinary tract infections. The risks are low (local infection, bleeding), but as with any surgical procedure, pain relief must be provided. Analgesia may include concentrated oral sucrose, a dorsal penile nerve block, or topical lidocaine-prilocaine cream.

Alanis MC, Lucidi RS: Neonatal circumcision: A review of the world's oldest and most controversial operation. *Obstet Gynecol Surv* 2004;59:379–395.
Brady-Fryer B, Wiebe N, Lander JA: Pain relief for neonatal circumcision. *Cochrane Database Syst Rev* 2004;4:CD004217.
Circumcision policy statement. American Academy of Pediatrics. Task Force on Circumcision. *Pediatrics* 1999;103:686–693.
Lannon CM, Bailey A, Fleischman A, et al: Circumcision debate. Task Force on Circumcision, 1999–2000. *Pediatrics* 2000;105:641–642.
Nelson CP, Dunn R, Wan J, et al: The increasing incidence of newborn circumcision: Data from the nationwide inpatient sample. *J Urol* 2005;173:978–981.
Schoen EJ, Colby CJ, Ray GT: Newborn circumcision decreases incidence and costs of urinary tract infections during the first year of life. *Pediatrics* 2000;105:789–793.
Schoen EJ, Wiswell TE, Moses S: New policy on circumcision—cause for concern. *Pediatrics* 2000;105:620–623.

Chapter 105 ■ The Umbilicus
Barbara J. Stoll

UMBILICAL CORD. The cord contains the two umbilical arteries, the vein, the rudimentary allantois, the remnant of the omphalomesenteric duct, and a gelatinous substance called Wharton jelly. The sheath of the umbilical cord is derived from the amnion. The muscular umbilical arteries contract readily, but the vein does not. The vein retains a fairly large lumen after birth. The normal cord at term is 55 cm long. Abnormally short cords are associated with antepartum abnormalities including fetal hypotonia, oligohydramnios, uterine constraint, and with increased risk for complications of labor and delivery for both mother and infant. Long cords (>70 cm) increase risk for true knots, wrapping around fetal parts (neck, arm) or prolapse, and straight untwisted cords are associated with fetal distress, anomalies, and intrauterine fetal demise.

When the cord sloughs after birth, portions of these structures remain in the base. The blood vessels are functionally closed, but anatomically patent for 10–20 days. The arteries become the lateral umbilical ligaments; the vein, the ligamentum teres; and the ductus venosus, the ligamentum venosum. During this interval, the umbilical vessels are potential portals of entry for infection. The umbilical cord usually sloughs within 2 wk. Delayed separation of the cord, after more than 1 mo, has been associated with neutrophil chemotactic defects and overwhelming bacterial infection (see Chapter 129.2).

A single umbilical artery is present in about 5–10/1,000 births; the frequency is about 35–70/1,000 in twin births. Approximately 30% of infants with a single umbilical artery have congenital abnormalities, usually more than one; many such infants are stillborn or die shortly after birth. Trisomy 18 is one of the more frequent abnormalities. Because abnormalities may not be apparent on physical examination, it is important that at every delivery the cut cord and the maternal and fetal surfaces of the placenta be inspected. The number of arteries present should be recorded as an aid to the early suspicion and identification of abnormalities in such infants. For infants with a single umbilical artery, many recommend renal ultrasonography.

Patency of the omphalomesenteric (vitelline) duct may be responsible for intestinal obstruction, intestinal fistula with fecal or bilious draining, prolapse of the bowel, a polyp (cyst), or a Meckel diverticulum (see Chapter 328.2). **Therapy** is surgical excision of the anomaly.

A persistent urachus (urachal cyst, sinus, patent urachus, or diverticulum) is due to failure of closure of the allantoic duct and is associated with bladder outlet obstruction. Patency should be suspected if a clear, light yellow, urine-like fluid is being discharged from the umbilicus. Symptoms include drainage, a mass or cyst, abdominal pain, local erythema, or infection. Urachal anomalies should be investigated by ultrasonography and a cystogram. **Therapy** is surgical excision of the anomaly and correction of any bladder outlet obstruction if present.

CONGENITAL OMPHALOCELE. An omphalocele is a herniation or protrusion of the abdominal contents into the base of the umbilical cord (Figs. 105-1 and 105-2). In contrast to the more common umbilical hernia, the sac is covered with peritoneum without overlying skin. The size of the sac that lies outside the abdominal cavity depends on its contents. Herniation of intestines into the cord occurs in about 1/5,000 births and herniation of liver and intestines in 1/10,000 births. The abdominal cavity is proportionately small because the impetus to grow and develop is deficient. Immediate surgical repair, before infection has taken place and before the tissues have been damaged by drying (saline-soaked sterile dressings should be applied immediately) or by rupture of the sac, is essential for survival. Mersilene mesh or similar synthetic material may be used to cover the viscera if the sac has ruptured or if excessive mobilization of the skin would be necessary to cover the mass and its intact sac.

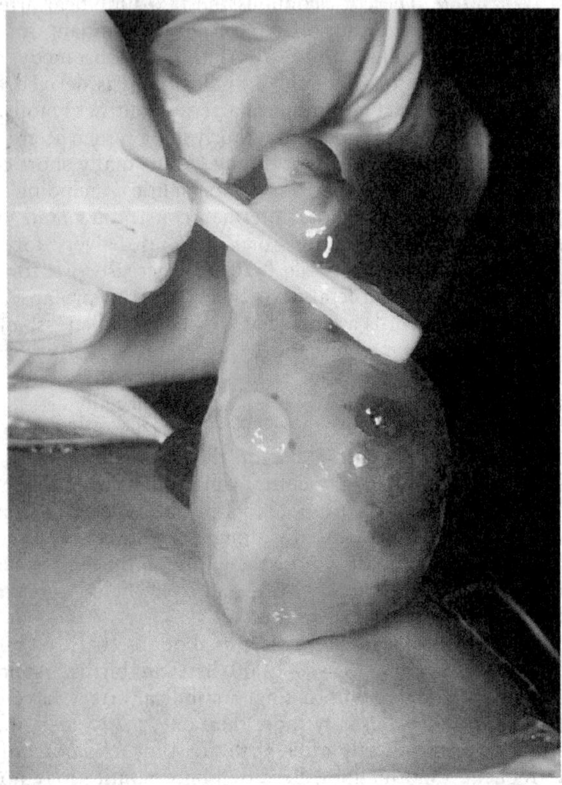

Figure 105-1. Small intact sac at the base of the umbilical cord. (From Clark DA, Thompson JE, Barnemeyer BM: *Atlas of Neonatology,* 7th ed. Philadelphia, WB Saunders, 2000.)

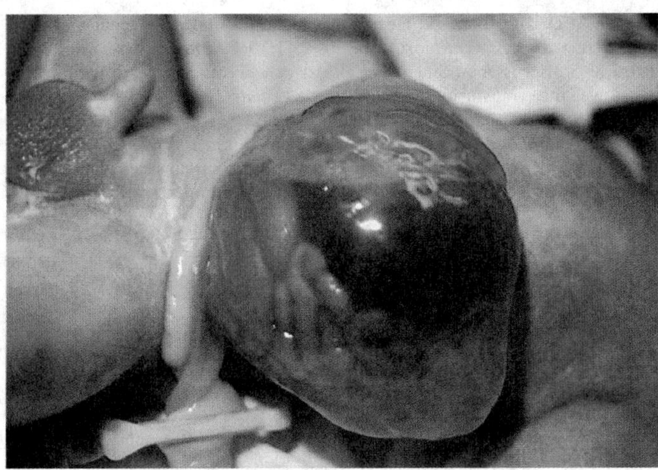

Figure 105-2. Intact sac with healthy organs visible. (From Clark DA, Thompson JE, Barnemeyer BM: *Atlas of Neonatology,* 7th ed. Philadelphia, WB Saunders, 2000.)

The risk of associated congenital anomalies/syndromes, including Beckwith-Wiedemann syndrome (omphalocele, macrosomia, hypoglycemia), trisomies 13 and 18, and cardiac anomalies, is increased in patients with omphalocele.

TUMORS. Tumors of the umbilicus are rare and include angioma, enteroteratoma, dermoid cyst, myxosarcoma, and cysts of urachal or omphalomesenteric duct remnants.

HEMORRHAGE. Hemorrhage from the umbilical cord may be due to trauma, inadequate ligation of the cord, or failure of normal thrombus formation. It may also indicate hemorrhagic disease of the newborn or other coagulopathies (especially factor XIII deficiency), septicemia, or local infection. The infant should be observed frequently during the first few days of life so that if hemorrhage does occur, it will be detected promptly.

GRANULOMA. The umbilical cord usually dries and separates within 6–8 days after birth. The raw surface becomes covered by a thin layer of skin; scar tissue forms, and the wound is usually healed within 12–15 days. The presence of saprophytic organisms delays separation of the cord and increases the possibility of invasion by pathogenic organisms. Mild infection or incomplete epithelialization may result in a moist granulating area at the base of the cord with a slight mucoid or mucopurulent discharge. Good results are usually obtained by cleansing with alcohol several times daily.

Persistence of granulation tissue at the base of the umbilicus is common. The tissue is soft, 3–10 mm in size, vascular and granular, and dull red or pink, and it may have a seropurulent secretion. **Treatment** is cauterization with silver nitrate, repeated at intervals of several days until the base is dry.

Umbilical granuloma must be differentiated from **umbilical polyp,** a rare anomaly resulting from persistence of all or part of the omphalomesenteric duct or the urachus. The tissue of the polyp is firm and resistant, is bright red, and has a mucoid secretion. If the polyp is communicating with the ileum or bladder, small amounts of fecal material or urine may be discharged intermittently. Histologically, the polyp consists of intestinal or urinary tract mucosa. **Treatment** is surgical excision of the entire omphalomesenteric or urachal remnant.

INFECTIONS. Although aseptic delivery and routine cord care (daily application of triple dye to the umbilical stump and surrounding skin) decrease the risk of umbilical infection, the necrotic tissue of the umbilical cord is an excellent medium for bacterial growth. **Omphalitis** may remain localized or may spread to the abdominal wall, the peritoneum, the umbilical or portal vessels, or the liver. Infants with abdominal wall cellulitis or those with **necrotizing fasciitis** have a high incidence of associated bacteremia. Portal vein phlebitis may develop and result in the later onset of **extrahepatic portal hypertension.** The general manifestations may be minimal (periumbilical erythema), even when septicemia or hepatitis has resulted. Treatment includes prompt antibiotic therapy (effective against *Staphylococcus aureus* and *Escherichia coli*) and, if abscess formation has occurred, surgical incision and drainage. Necrotizing fasciitis is often polymicrobial and has a high mortality. Changes in newborn bathing practices that replace antiseptics with nonantiseptic pH-balanced soap may be associated with increased risk of omphalitis.

UMBILICAL HERNIA. Often associated with diastasis recti, an umbilical hernia is due to imperfect closure or weakness of the umbilical ring. Predisposing factors include black race and low birthweight. The hernia appears as a soft swelling covered by skin that protrudes during crying, coughing, or straining and can be reduced easily through the fibrous ring at the umbilicus. The hernia consists of omentum or portions of the small intestine. The size of the defect varies from <1 cm in diameter to as much as 5 cm, but large ones are rare.

TREATMENT. Most umbilical hernias that appear before the age of 6 mo disappear spontaneously by 1 yr of age. Even large hernias (5–6 cm in all dimensions) have been known to disappear spontaneously by 5–6 yr of age. Strangulation is extremely rare. It is generally agreed that "strapping" is ineffective. Surgery is not advised unless the hernia persists to the age of 4–5 yr, causes symptoms, becomes strangulated, or becomes progressively larger after the age of 1–2 yr. Defects exceeding 2 cm are less likely to close spontaneously.

Ameh EA, Nmadu PT: Major complications of omphalitis in neonates and infants. *Pediatr Surg Int* 2002;18:413–416.

Holland AJ, Ford WD, Linke RJ, et al: Influence of antenatal ultrasound on the management of fetal exomphalos. *Fetal Diagn Ther* 1999;14:223–228.

Janssen PA, Selwood BL, Dobson SR, et al: To dye or not to dye: A randomized, clinical trial of a triple dye/alcohol regime versus dry cord care. *Pediatrics* 2003;111:15–20.

Krakowiak P, Smith EN, de Bruyn G, et al: Risk factors and outcomes associated with a short umbilical cord. *Obstet Gynecol* 2004;103:119–127.

Lurie S, Sherman D, Bukovsky I: Omphalocele delivery enigma: The best mode of delivery still remains dubious. *Eur J Obstet Gynecol Reprod Biol* 1999;82:19–22.

Pomeranz A: Anomalies, abnormalities, and care of the umbilicus. *Pediatr Clin North Am* 2004;51:819–827.

Weber DM, Freeman NV, Elhag KM: Periumbilical necrotizing fasciitis in the newborn. *Eur J Pediatr Surg* 2001;11:86–91.

Zupan J, Garner P, Omari AA: Topical umbilical cord care at birth. *Cochrane Database Syst Rev* 2004;3:CD001057.

Chapter 106 ■ Metabolic Disturbances

Barbara J. Stoll

HYPERTHERMIA IN THE NEWBORN (TRANSITORY FEVER OF THE NEWBORN, DEHYDRATION FEVER)

Elevations in temperature (38–39°C or 100–103°F) are occasionally noted on the 2nd–3rd day of life in infants whose clinical course has been otherwise satisfactory. This disturbance is especially likely to occur in breast-fed infants whose intake of fluid has been particularly low or in infants who are overdressed or are exposed to high environmental temperatures, either in an incubator, in a bassinette near a radiator, or in the sun.

The infant may lose weight. A consistent relationship may not be seen between the fever and the extent of weight loss or inadequacy of fluid intake. Urinary output and the frequency of voiding diminish. The fontanel may be depressed. The infant takes fluids avidly, but the apparent vigor of the infant contrasts with the usual appearance of "being sick" from an infection. The rise in temperature may be associated with an increase in serum levels of protein and sodium and with an increase in hematocrit. The possibility of local or systemic infection should be evaluated. Administering oral or parenteral fluids or lowering the environmental temperature leads to prompt reduction of the fever and alleviation of symptoms. Oral hydration should be with additional nursing or formula and not with pure water, due to the risk of hyponatremia.

A more severe form of neonatal hyperthermia occurs in both newborn and older infants when they are warmly dressed for outdoor low temperatures that do not exist in their immediate indoor environment. The diminished sweating capacity of newborn infants is a contributing factor. Warmly dressed infants left near stoves or radiators, traveling in well-heated automobiles, or left with bright sunlight shining directly on them through the windows of a closed room or automobile are likely to be victims. Excess clothing in hot weather, especially when the infant is left in the sun, is a less common cause. Body temperature may become as high as 41–44°C (106–111°F). The skin is hot and dry, and initially the infant usually appears flushed and apathetic. Tachypnea and irritability may be noted. This stage may be followed by stupor, grayish pallor, coma, and convulsions. Hypernatremia may contribute to the convulsions. Mortality and morbidity rates (brain damage) are high. Hyperthermia has been associated with sudden infant death and with hemorrhagic shock and encephalopathy syndrome (see Chapter 68). The condition is prevented by dressing infants in clothing suitable for the temperature of the immediate environment. In newborn infants, exposure of the body to usual room temperature or immersion in tepid water usually suffices to bring the temperature back to normal levels. Older infants may require cooling for a longer time by repeated immersion or by the use of a water-cooled mattress or other apparatus for induction of hypothermia. Attention to possible fluid and electrolyte disturbance is essential.

NEONATAL COLD INJURY

Neonatal cold injury usually occurs in abandoned infants or those in inadequately heated homes during damp cold spells when the outside temperature is in the freezing range (see Chapter 75). The initial features are apathy, refusal of food, oliguria, and coldness to touch. The body temperature is usually between 29.5 and 35°C (85–95°F), and immobility, edema, and redness of the extremities, especially the hands, feet, and face, are observed. Bradycardia and apnea may also occur. The facial erythema frequently gives a false impression of health and delays recognition that the infant is ill. Local hardening over areas of edema may lead to confusion with scleredema. Rhinitis is common, as are hypoglycemia and acidosis. Hemorrhagic manifestations are frequent; massive pulmonary hemorrhage is a common finding at autopsy. **Treatment** consists of warming and paying scrupulous attention to recognizing and correcting hypotension and metabolic imbalances, particularly hypoglycemia. Prevention consists of providing adequate environmental heat. The mortality rate is about 10%; about 10% of survivors have evidence of brain damage.

EDEMA

Generalized edema occurs in association with **hydrops fetalis** (see Chapter 103.2) and in the offspring of diabetic mothers. In premature infants, edema is often a consequence of a decreased ability to excrete water or sodium, although some have considerable edema without identifiable cause. Infants with respiratory distress syndrome may become edematous without heart failure. Edema of the face and scalp may be caused by pressure from the umbilical cord around the neck, and transient localized swelling of the hands or feet may similarly be due to intrauterine pressure. Edema may be associated with heart failure. A lag in renal excretion of electrolytes and water may result in edema after a sudden large increase in intake of electrolytes, particularly with feeding of concentrated cow's milk formulas. High-protein formulas may also cause edema as a result of the excessive renal solute load, particularly in premature infants. Rarely, idiopathic hypoproteinemia with edema lasting weeks or months is observed in term infants. The cause is unclear, and the disturbance is benign. Persistent edema of 1 or more extremities may represent congenital lymphedema (Milroy disease) or, in females, Turner syndrome. Generalized edema with hypoproteinemia may be seen in the neonatal period with congenital nephrosis and rarely with Hurler syndrome or after feeding hypoallergenic formulas to infants with cystic fibrosis of the pancreas. Sclerema is described in Chapter 646.

HYPOCALCEMIA (TETANY) (SEE CHAPTER 48)

METABOLIC BONE DISEASE. Metabolic bone disease is a common complication in very low birthweight preterm infants. The smallest sickest infants are at greatest risk. Progressive osteopenia with demineralized bones and occasionally pathologic fractures may develop. The major cause is inadequate intake of calcium to meet the requirements for growth. Poor intake of phosphorus and vitamin D are additional risk factors. Contributing factors include prolonged parenteral nutrition, vitamin D and calcium malabsorption, intake of unsupplemented human milk, immobilization, and urinary calcium losses from chronic diuretic use. The serum alkaline phosphatase level is used to monitor metabolic bone disease and can be over 1,000 U/L in severe cases. Fortified human milk and formulas designed for preterm infants provide improved intake of calcium, phosphorus, and vitamin D; promote bone mineralization; and may prevent metabolic bone disease. Many extremely low birthweight infants will require additional oral supplements of calcium, phosphorus, and vitamin D. Treatment of fractures requires immobilization and administration of calcium and, if needed, phosphorus (for hypophosphatemia) and vitamin D (not more than 1,000 IU/day unless severe cholestasis or vitamin D resistance is present). See also Chapters 48 and 571.

HYPOMAGNESEMIA

Rarely, hypomagnesemia of unknown cause may occur in newborn infants, usually in association with hypocalcemia. It may also be associated with insufficient stores of skeletal magnesium secondary to deficient placental transfer, decreased intestinal absorption, neonatal hypoparathyroidism, hyperphosphatemia, renal loss (primary or secondary to drugs, e.g., amphotericin B), a defect in magnesium and calcium homeostasis, or iatrogenic deficiency caused by loss incurred during exchange transfusion or insufficient replacement during total intravenous alimentation. Infants of diabetic mothers may have serum magnesium levels that are lower than normal. The clinical manifestations of hypomagnesemia are indistinguishable from those of hypocalcemia and tetany and may, in fact, contribute to the accompanying hypocalcemia.

Hypomagnesemia occurs when serum magnesium levels fall below 1.5 mg/dL (0.62 mmol/L), although clinical signs do not usually develop until serum magnesium levels fall below 1.2 mg/dL. During exchange transfusion with citrated blood, which is low in magnesium because of binding by citrate, serum magnesium decreases about 0.5 mg/dL (0.2 mmol/L); approximately 10 days are required for return to normal. In non-iatrogenic hypomagnesemia, the serum magnesium level may be <0.5 mg/dL. Serum calcium in either instance is usually at levels noted in hypocalcemic tetany, but the serum phosphorus value is normal or high. Because the hypocalcemia accompanying hypomagnesemia is inadequately corrected by administering calcium alone, hypomagnesemia should also be suspected in any patient with tetany not responding to calcium therapy.

Immediate **treatment** consists of intramuscular injection of magnesium sulfate. For newborn infants, 25–50 mg/kg/dose Q 8 hr for 3–4 doses usually suffices. The accompanying hypocalcemia usually corrects itself as the hypomagnesemia resolves. The same daily dose can be given for oral maintenance therapy. Four to 5 times higher doses may be required in malabsorptive states. In most cases, the metabolic defect is transient, and treatment can be discontinued after 1–2 wk. A few patients appear to have a permanent form of the disease that requires continuous oral supplementation with magnesium to prevent recurrence of hypomagnesemia. No residual damage to the central nervous system is evident after prompt treatment.

HYPERMAGNESEMIA

Hypermagnesemia may occur in newborn infants of mothers treated with magnesium sulfate during labor. At high serum levels, the central nervous system is depressed and infants have profound respiratory depression requiring mechanical ventilation. Lower levels may result in hypoventilation, lethargy, flaccidity, hyporeflexia, and poor sucking. Hypermagnesemia may be associated with failure to pass meconium (**meconium plug syndrome**). The upper limit of normal magnesium is 2.8 mg/dL (1.15 mmol/L), but serious symptoms rarely occur at levels below 5 mg/dL (2.1 mmol/L). In most cases, no specific therapy (beyond supportive care and maintenance of respiratory support) is required. Intravenous calcium and diuresis will reduce magnesium levels. In rare cases, exchange transfusion has been used for rapid removal of magnesium ion from the blood.

SUBSTANCE ABUSE AND NEONATAL ABSTINENCE (WITHDRAWAL)

Substance abuse during pregnancy is a serious problem for both the mother and her newborn. The mother may suffer adverse consequences of her addiction, including episodes of drug withdrawal during pregnancy and illnesses related to high-risk behavior. Effects on the fetus and newborn include chronic or intermittent drug exposure, acute withdrawal shortly after birth, poor maternal nutrition, and long-term effects on physical growth and neurodevelopment. Because infants with in utero drug exposure often have social and environmental risk factors and may have been exposed to multiple substances, it may be difficult to evaluate the effects of specific in utero drug exposure on long-term neurodevelopmental outcome.

Pregnancy in women who use illegal drugs or alcohol is, by definition, high risk. Prenatal care is usually inadequate, and these women have a higher incidence of sexually transmitted infections, including syphilis, HIV, and hepatitis. In addition, the risk of preterm labor, intrauterine growth restriction, premature rupture of membranes, and perinatal morbidity and mortality is higher. Physiologic addiction to narcotics occurs in most infants born to actively addicted mothers because opiates cross the placenta. Withdrawal may be manifested even before birth by increased activity of the fetus when the mother feels a need for the drug or withdrawal symptoms develop. Heroin and methadone are the drugs most frequently associated with withdrawal syndromes, but such syndromes may also occur with alcohol, nicotine, phenobarbital, pentazocine, codeine, propoxyphene, hydroxyzine, amphetamines, neuroleptics, antidepressants, and benzodiazepines.

Heroin addiction results in a 50% incidence of low birthweight infants, half of whom are small for gestational age. Chronic infections, maternal undernutrition, and a direct fetal growth-inhibiting effect are possible causes. The rate of stillbirths is increased, but not the incidence of congenital anomalies. Clinical manifestations of withdrawal occur in 50–75% of infants, usually beginning within the 1st 48 hr, depending on the daily maternal dose (<6 mg/24 hr is associated with no or mild symptoms), the duration of addiction (>1 yr has a >70% incidence of withdrawal), and the time of the last maternal dose (the incidence is higher if the last dose was taken within 24 hr of birth). Rarely, symptoms may appear as late as 4–6 wk of age. The incidence of respiratory distress syndrome and hyperbilirubinemia may be decreased in preterm infants of heroin users; accelerated production of pulmonary surfactant may explain the former, and enzyme induction of hepatic glucuronyl transferase the latter.

Tremors and hyperirritability are the most prominent symptoms. The tremors may be fine or jittery and indistinguishable from those of hypoglycemia, but they are more often coarse, "flapping," and bilateral; the limbs are frequently rigid, hyperreflexic, and resistant to flexion and extension. Irritability and hyperactivity are generally marked and may lead to skin abrasions. Other signs include wakefulness, hyperacusis, hypertonicity, tachypnea, diarrhea, vomiting, high-pitched cry, fist sucking, poor feeding with weight loss (disorganized sucking), and fever. Sneezing, yawning, hiccups, myoclonic jerks, convulsions, abnormal sleep cycles, nasal stuffiness, apnea, flushing alternating rapidly with pallor, and lacrimation are less common. The Neonatal Intensive Care Unit Neurobehavioral Scale (NNNS) is a useful way to evaluate opiate or other drug exposed neonates (Table 106-1). The risk of sudden infant death syndrome is increased. The diagnosis is generally established by the history and clinical findings. Examining the urine for opiates may reveal only low levels during withdrawal, but quinine, which is often mixed with heroin, may be present in higher concentrations. Meconium testing is more accurate than neonatal urine drug testing. Hypoglycemia and hypocalcemia should be excluded.

Methadone addiction is associated with severe withdrawal symptoms, the incidence varying from 20 to 90%. Mothers taking methadone usually have better prenatal care than those taking heroin; these mothers have a high incidence of polysubstance abuse, including alcohol, barbiturates, and tranquilizers, and they are often heavy smokers. The incidence of congenital anomalies is not increased. The average birthweight of infants of mothers taking methadone is higher than that of infants of heroin-addicted mothers; the clinical manifestations are similar except that the former group has a higher incidence of seizures (10–20%) and the late onset (2–6 wk of age) of withdrawal. Women who continue to abuse heroin, even if they enter a methadone program, are more likely to have preterm and/or low birthweight infants than those born to women who stop using heroin. They are also more likely to suffer withdrawal and have a higher risk of neonatal mortality.

Alcohol withdrawal is uncommon. Infants of women who have been drinking immediately before delivery may have alcohol on their breath for several hours because it rapidly crosses the placenta and blood levels in the infant are similar to those in the mother. Hypoglycemia and a metabolic acidosis may be present. Infants in whom withdrawal symptoms develop often become agitated and hyperactive, with marked tremors lasting 72 hr, followed by about 48 hr of lethargy before return to normal activity. Seizures may develop.

TABLE 106-1. Neurobehavioral Scale

DOMAIN	ITEMS
Physiological	Labored breathing
	Nasal flaring
Autonomic	Sweating
	Spit-up
	Hiccoughing
	Sneezing
	Nasal stuffiness
	Yawning
CNS	Abnormal sucking
	Choreiform movements
	Athetoid postures and movements
	Tremors
	Cogwheel movements
	Startles
	Hypertonia
	Back arching
	Fisting
	Cortical thumb
	Myoclonic jerks
	Generalized seizures
	Abnormal posture
Skin	Pallor
	Mottling
	Lividity
	Overall cyanosis
	Circumoral cyanosis
	Periocular cyanosis
Visual	Gaze aversion during orientation
	Pull-down during orientation
	Fuss/cry during orientation
	Obligatory following during orientation
	End point nystagmus during orientation
	Sustained spontaneous nystagmus
	Visual locking
	Hyperalertness
	Setting sun sign
	Roving eye movements
	Strabismus
	Tight blinking
	Other abnormal eye signs
Gastrointestinal	Gagging/choking
	Loose stools, watery stools
	Excessive gas, bowel sounds
State	High-pitch cry
	Monotone-pitch cry
	Weak cry
	No cry
	Extreme irritability
	Abrupt state changes
	Inability to achieve quiet awake state (state 4)

From Lester BM, Tronick EZ, Brazelton TB: The Neonatal Intensive Care Unit Network Neurobehavioral Scales procedures. *Pediatrics* 2004;113:641–667.

Phenobarbital withdrawal usually occurs in full-term, appropriate for gestational age infants of addicted mothers. Symptoms begin at a median age of 7 days (range, 2–14 days). Infants may have a brief acute stage consisting of irritability, constant crying, sleeplessness, hiccups, and mouthing movements, followed by a subacute stage consisting of voracious appetite, frequent regurgitation and gagging, episodic irritability, hyperacusis, sweating, and a disturbed sleep pattern, all of which may last 2–4 mo.

Cocaine abuse in pregnant women is common, but withdrawal in their infants is unusual; the pregnancy may be complicated by premature labor, abruptio placentae, and fetal asphyxia. Infants may have intrauterine growth restriction and neurobehavioral deficits characterized by impaired state regulation, impaired auditory information processing, developmental delay, and learning disabilities. At 24 mo of age, they score lower on the mental scale of the Bayley score and are twice as likely to have developmental delay. Family disorganization, polysubstance abuse, sexually transmitted infections, and child abuse and neglect may also be present. At 4 yr of age, infants exposed to cocaine prenatally demonstrate specific cognitive impairments (visual-spatial and math skills; general knowledge) and are less likely to have an IQ above the normative mean. A more enriching home environment is associated with IQ scores of cocaine-exposed children being similar to those of nonexposed children.

TREATMENT. Infants who are undergoing opiate withdrawal require care in a quiet environment with reduction of external stimuli and swaddling. Not all infants require drug therapy. Therapy is indicated for seizures, for diarrhea, or for such irritability that normal sleep and feeding patterns are disturbed and weight gain is poor. Treatment of heroin and methadone withdrawal has been successful with various combinations of narcotics, sedatives, and hypnotics. Methadone withdrawal may require larger amounts of medication for longer periods to control clinical manifestations than are needed for heroin withdrawal. Phenobarbital, 5–10 mg/kg/24 hr in 3 to 4 divided doses, can effectively reduce irritability and prevent seizures. Paregoric at a beginning dose of 0.05–0.1 mL/kg is given every 3–4 hr and increased by 0.05 mL every 4 hr if necessary, depending on the size and response of the infant. Paregoric abolishes most withdrawal symptoms, especially diarrhea. Tincture of opium (10 mg/mL) diluted 25-fold results in the same morphine equivalency as paregoric. The recommended dose of diluted tincture of opium is 0.1 mL/kg (≈2 drops/kg) with feedings every 4 hr. The dose may be increased by 2 drops every 4 hr if needed. The dose and duration of therapy may be adjusted according to the clinical response. A combination of an opiate plus phenobarbital may be the most effective approach to an opiate withdrawal. Parenteral administration of fluids may be necessary to prevent aspiration or dehydration until the symptoms are brought under control.

Mortality from withdrawal is under 5% and may be negligible with early recognition and treatment. The prognosis for normal development is affected by the adverse circumstances of high-risk pregnancy and delivery and by the environment to which the infant is returned after recovery, as well as by the effects of the particular drug on fetal and subsequent neonatal development.

106.1 • Maternal Selective Serotonin Reuptake Inhibitors and Neonatal Behavioral Syndromes

Women of childbearing age have a combined incidence of depression and anxiety of approximately 19%. Selective serotonin reuptake inhibitors (SSRIs; fluoxetine, paroxetine, sertraline, citalopram, fluvoxamine) and, less often, serotonin norepinephrine reuptake inhibitors (SNRI; venlafaxine, duloxetine) have been used to treat pregnant women with depression or anxiety disorders. Exposure to these agents during pregnancy does not produce major congenital malformations. Nonetheless, poor neonatal adaptation has been noted with the use of many of these agents but most often with paroxetine and fluoxetine.

It is unclear if poor neonatal adaptation is due to serotonin overstimulation (**serotonin syndrome**) or due to withdrawal (**serotonin discontinuation syndrome**). Indeed, both may occur with different agents. Paroxetine has a short half-life and few if any active metabolites, and is also a potent muscarinic blocking agent. Serum levels after birth decline rapidly. Neonatal adaptive symptoms after late pregnancy exposure to paroxetine may be withdrawal, with cholinergic overdrive. Symptoms may also be delayed. In contrast, fluoxetine and its active metabolite (nor-

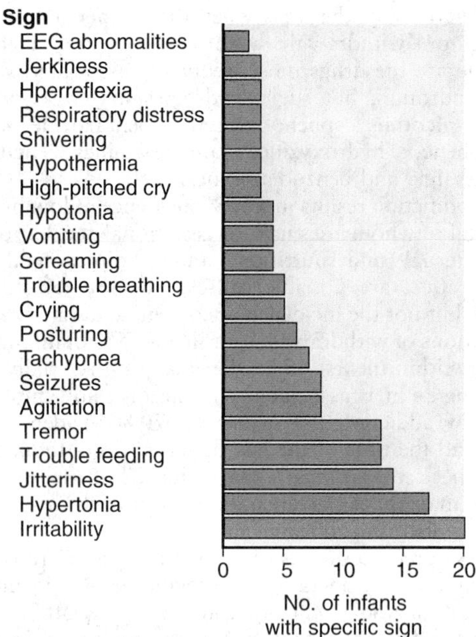

Figure 106-1. Neonatal signs after late in uteroexposure to serotonin reuptake inhibitors. Frequencies of specific signs reported to the FDA Adverse Events Reporting System. Ordered by frequency of occurrence ($n = 57$ infants). EEG, electroencephalographic; FDA, U.S. Food and Drug Administration. (From Moses-Kolko EL, Bogen D, Perel J, et al: Neonatal signs after late in utero exposure to serotonin reuptake inhibitors. *JAMA* 2005;293:2372–2383.)

fluoxetine) have long half-lives and may produce a serotonin syndrome of acute toxicity. Onset may be at birth or in the 1st 24 hr of life. Cord blood levels of fluoxetine are equal to that in the mother. All agents cross the placental and blood-brain barriers.

A neonatal behavorial syndrome that has features of both direct serotonin toxicity and withdrawal (cholinergic overdrive) is noted in Figure 106-1 and is characterized by central nervous system (irritability, excess or restless sleep), motor (agitation, tremor, hyperreflexia, rigidity, hypo- or hypertonia), respiratory (nasal congestion, respiratory distress, tachypnea), gastrointestinal (diarrhea, emesis, poor feeding) and systemic (hypo- or hyperthermia, hypoglycemia) manifestations. Most infants have only mild symptoms that resolve within 2 wks; a severe syndrome characterized by seizures, dehydration, weight loss, hyperpyrexia, and respiratory failure is present in <1%. No deaths have been reported.

Treatment is directed at the individual manifestations with supportive therapies. Prevention has been proposed by weaning the mother from the SSRI in the 3rd trimester of pregnancy. This must be weighed against the recurrence of material psychiatric symptoms during the last trimester and postpartum period.

106.2 • Fetal Alcohol Syndrome

High levels of alcohol ingestion during pregnancy can be damaging to embryonic and fetal development. A specific pattern of malformation identified as *fetal alcohol syndrome* has been documented, and major and minor components of the syndrome are expressed in 1–2 infants/1,000 live births (see Table 106–1). Both

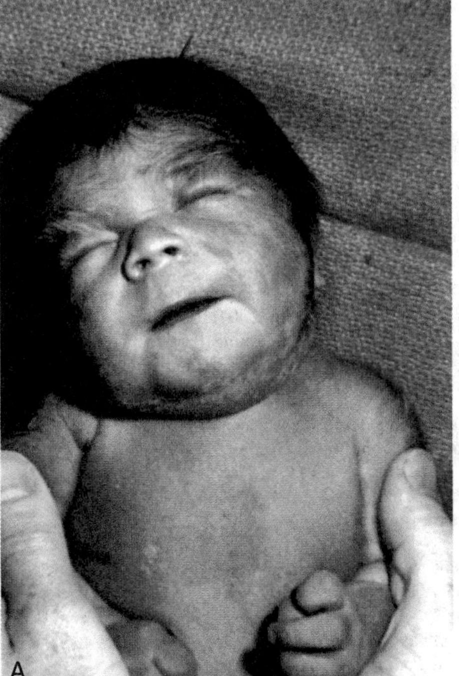

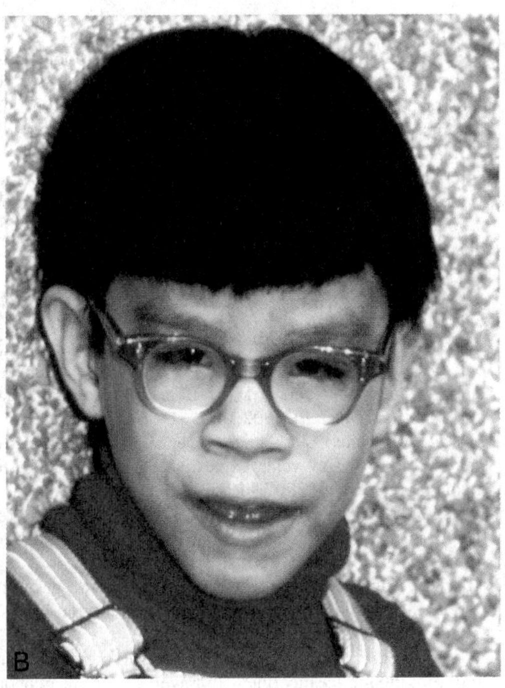

Figure 106-2. At birth *(A)* and at 4 yr of age *(B)*. Note the short palpebral fissures; long, smooth philtrum with vermillion border; and hirsutism in the newborn. (From Jones KL, Smith DW: Recognition of the fetal alcohol syndrome in early infancy. *Lancet* 1973;2:999–1001.)

moderate and high levels of alcohol intake during early pregnancy may result in alterations in growth and morphogenesis of the fetus; the greater the intake, the more severe the signs. Infants born to heavy drinkers have twice the risk of abnormality as those born to moderate drinkers; 32% of infants born to heavy drinkers had congenital anomalies as compared with 9% in the abstinent and 14% in the moderate group. Additional maternal risk factors associated with fetal alcohol syndrome are advanced maternal age, low socioeconomic status, poor psychologic indicators, and binge drinking.

Characteristics of fetal alcohol syndrome include (1) prenatal onset and persistence of growth deficiency for length, weight, and head circumference; (2) facial abnormalities, including short palpebral fissures, epicanthal folds, maxillary hypoplasia, micrognathia, smooth philtrum, and a thin, smooth upper lip (Fig. 106-2); (3) cardiac defects, primarily septal defects; (4) minor joint and limb abnormalities, including some restriction of movement and altered palmar crease patterns; and (5) delayed development and mental deficiency varying from borderline to severe (Table 106-2). Fetal alcohol syndrome is a common identifiable cause of mental retardation. The severity of dysmorphogenesis may range from severely affected infants with full manifestations of fetal alcohol syndrome to those mildly affected with only a few manifestations.

The detrimental effects may be due to the alcohol itself or to 1 of its breakdown products. Some evidence suggests that alcohol may impair placental transfer of essential amino acids and zinc, both necessary for protein synthesis, which may account for the intrauterine growth restriction.

Treatment of these infants is difficult because no specific therapy exists. These infants may remain hypotonic and tremulous despite sedation, and the prognosis is poor. Counseling with regard to recurrence is important. Prevention is achieved by eliminating alcohol intake after conception.

TABLE 106-2. Fetal Alcohol Syndrome Surveillance Network Case Definition Categories

	PHENOTYPE POSITIVE		
CASE DEFINITION CATEGORY	Face	Central Nervous System	Growth
Confirmed fetal alcohol syndrome (FAS) phenotype with or without maternal alcohol exposure*	Abnormal facial features consistent with FAS as reported by a physician *or* Two of the following: Short palpebral fissures, abnormal philtrum, thin upper lip	Frontal-occipital circumference ≤ 10th percentile at birth or any age *or* Standardized measure of intellectual function ≤1 SD below the mean *or* Standardized measure of developmental delay ≤1 SD below the mean *or* Developmental delay or mental retardation diagnosed by a qualified examiner (e.g., psychologist or physician) *or* Attention deficit disorder diagnosed by a qualified evaluator	Intrauterine weight or height corrected for gestational age ≤ 10th percentile *or* Postnatal weight or height ≤10th percentile for age *or* Postnatal weight for height ≤10th percentile
Probable FAS phenotype with or without maternal alcohol exposure*	Required; facial features same as above	Must meet either CNS or growth criteria as outlined above	

*Documentation in the records of some level of maternal alcohol use during the index pregnancy.
From Fetal alcohol syndrome—Alaska, Arizona, Colorado and New York, 1995–1997. *MMWR Morb Mortal Wkly Rep* 2002;51:433–435.

Backstrom MC, Kuusela AL, Maki R: Metabolic bone disease of prematurity. *Ann Med* 1996;28:275–282.
Bandstra ES, Morrow CE, Anthony JC, et al: Intrauterine growth of full-term infants: Impact of prenatal cocaine exposure. *Pediatrics* 2001;108: 1309–1319.
Centers for Disease Control and Prevention: Fetal alcohol syndrome—Alaska, Arizona, and New York, 1995–1997. *MMWR Morb Mortal Wkly Rep* 2002;51:433–435.
Cohen LS, Altshuler LL, Harlow BL, et al: Relapse of major depression during pregnancy in women who maintain or discontinue antidepressant treatment. *JAMA* 2006;295:499–507.
Coyle MG, Ferguson A, Lagasse L, et al: Neurobehavioral effects of treatment for opiate withdrawal. *Arch Dis Child Fetal Neonatal Ed* 2005;90:F73–F74.
Coyle MG, Ferguson A, Lagasse L, et al: Diluted tincture of opium (DTO) and phenobarbital versus DTO alone for neonatal opiate withdrawal in term infants. *J Pediatr* 2002;140:561–564.
Ferriera E, Carceller AM, Agogue C, et al: Effects of selective serotonin reuptake inhibitors and venlafaxine during pregnancy in term and preterm neonates. *Pediatrics* 2007;119:52–59.
Fewtrell MS, Cole TJ, Bishop NJ, et al: Neonatal factors predicting childhood height in preterm infants: Evidence for a persisting effect of early metabolic bone disease? *J Pediatr* 2000;137:668–673.
Frank DA, Augustyn M, Knight WG, et al: Growth, development, and behavior in early childhood following prenatal cocaine exposure: A systematic review. *JAMA* 2001;285:1613–1625.
Godding V, Bonnier C, Fiasse L, et al: Does in utero exposure to heavy maternal smoking induce nicotine withdrawal symptoms in neonates? *Pediatr Res* 2004;55:645–651.
Hulse GK, O'Neill G: Methadone and the pregnant user: A matter for careful clinical consideration. *Aust N Z J Obstet Gynaecol* 2001;41:329–332.
Iveli MF, Morales S, Rebolledo A, et al: Effects of light ethanol consumption during pregnancy: increased frequency of minor anomalies in the newborn and altered contractility of umbilical cord artery. *Pediatr Res* 2007;61: 456–461.
Jackson L, Ting A, Mckay S, et al: A randomized controlled trial of morphine versus phenobarbitone for neonatal abstinence syndrome. *Arch Dis Child Fetal Neonatal Ed* 2004; 89:F300–F304.
Jacobson SW, Carr LG, Croxford J, et al: Protective effects of the alcohol dehydrogenase-ASH1B allele in children exposed to alcohol during pregnancy. *J Pediatr* 2006;148:30–37.
Johnson K, Gerada C, Greenough A: Treatment of neonatal abstinence syndrome. *Arch Dis Child Fetal Neonatal Ed* 2003;88:F2–vF5.
Kable JA, Coles CD: The impact of prenatal alcohol exposure on neurophysiological encoding of environmental events at six months. *Alcohol Clin Exp Res* 2004;28:489–496.
Kallen B: Neonate characteristics after maternal use of antidepressants in late pregnancy. *Arch Pediatr Adolesc Med* 2004;158:312–316.
Koren G: Discontinuation syndrome following late pregnancy exposure to antidepressants. *Arch Pediatr Adolesc Med* 2004;158:307–308.
Laine K, Heikkinen T, Ekblad U, et al: Effects of exposure to selective serotonin reuptake inhibitors during pregnancy on serotonergic symptoms in newborns and cord blood monoamine and prolactin concentrations. *Arch Gen Psychiatry* 2003;60:720–726.
Lester BM, Tronick EZ, Brazelton TB: The neontal intensive care unit network neurobehavioral scale procedures. *Pediatrics* 2004;113:641–667.
Malisza KL, Allman AA, Shiloff D, et al: Evaluation of spatial working memory function in children and adults with fetal alcohol spectrum disorders: a functional magnetic resonance imaging study. *Pediatr Res* 2005;58: 1150–1157.
Mattson SN, Schoenfeld AM, Riley EP: Teratogenic effects of alcohol on brain and behavior. *Alcohol Res Health* 2001;25:185–191.
Moore ES, Ward RE, Jamison PL, et al: The subtle facial signs of prenatal exposure to alcohol: An anthropometric approach. *J Pediatr* 2001;139:215–219.
Moses-Kolko EL, Bogen D, Percel J, et al: Neonatal signs after late in utero exposure to serotonin reuptake inhibitors. *JAMA* 2005;293:2372–2383.
Ostrea EM Jr, Knapp DK, Tannenbaum L, et al: Estimates of illicit drug use during pregnancy by maternal interview, hair analysis, and meconium analysis. *J Pediatr* 2001;138:344–348.
Rauch F, Schoenau E: Skeletal development in premature infants: A review of bone physiology beyond nutritional aspects. *Arch Dis Child Fetal Neonatal Ed* 2002;86:F82–F85.
Ruchkin V, Martin A: SSRIs and the developing brain. *Lancet* 2005;365:451–453.
Ryan S: Nutritional aspects of metabolic bone disease in the newborn. *Arch Dis Child* 1996;74:F145–F148.
Sanz EJ, De-las-Cuevas C, Kiuru A, et al: Selective serotonin reuptake inhibitors in pregnant women and neonatal withdrawal syndrome: a database analysis. *Lancet* 2005;365:482–487.
Shankaran S, Das A, Bauer CR, et al: Association between patterns of maternal substance use and infant birth weight, length, and head circumference. *Pediatrics* 2004;114:e226–e234.
Singer LT, Minnes S, Short E, et al: Cognitive outcomes of preschool children with prenatal cocaine exposure. *JAMA* 2004;291:2448–2456,
Smith LM, La Gasse LL, Derauf C, et al: The infant development, environment, and lifestyle study: effects of prenatal methamphetamine exposure, polydrug exposure, and poverty or intrauterine growth. *Pediatrics* 2006;118:1149–1156.
Sood B, Delaney-Black V, Covington C, et al: Prenatal alcohol exposure and childhood behavior at age 6 to 7 years: I. Dose-response effect. *Pediatrics* 2001;108:e34.
Zeskind PS, Stephens LE: Maternal selective serotonin reuptake inhibitor use during pregnancy and newborn neurobehavior. *Pediatrics* 2004;113:368–375.
Zuckermann B, Frank DA, Mayes L: Cocaine-exposed infants and developmental outcomes. *JAMA* 2002;287:1990–1991.

Chapter 107 ■ The Endocrine System

Barbara J. Stoll

The endocrinopathies are discussed in detail in Part XXV.

Pituitary dwarfism is not usually apparent at birth, although panhypopituitary male infants may have neonatal hypoglycemia, hyperbilirubinemia, and micropenis. Conversely, constitutional dwarfs usually have length and weight consistent with prematurity when born after a normal gestational period; otherwise, their physical appearance is normal.

Primary hypothyroidism occurs in approximately 1/4,000 births. Because most of these infants are asymptomatic at birth, all states screen for this serious and treatable disease. Thyroid deficiency may also be apparent at birth in genetically determined cretinism or in infants of mothers treated with antithyroid medications or during a pregnancy complicated by maternal hyperthyroidism. Constipation, prolonged jaundice, goiter, lethargy, or poor peripheral circulation as shown by persistently mottled skin or cold extremities should suggest cretinism. Early diagnosis and treatment of congenital thyroid hormone deficiency improves intellectual outcome and is facilitated by screening all newborn infants for this deficiency. The optimal therapy for all infants with congenital hypothyroidism remains uncertain, however. **Transient hypothyroxinemia** of prematurity is most common in ill very low birthweight (VLBW) infants. These infants are probably chemically euthyroid, as suggested by normal levels of serum thyrotropin and other tests of the pituitary-hypothalamic axis. Because the relationship between low thyroid levels and neurodevelopmental outcome is unclear, it remains uncertain whether premature infants with this transient problem should be treated with thyroid hormone.

Transient hyperthyroidism may occur at birth in infants of mothers with hyperthyroidism or in infants whose mothers have been receiving thyroid medication.

Transient hypoparathyroidism may be manifested as tetany of the newborn (see Chapter 572).

The adrenal glands are subject to numerous disturbances, which may become apparent and require lifesaving treatment during the neonatal period. Acute **adrenal hemorrhage** and failure may occur after breech or other traumatic deliveries or in association with overwhelming infection. Congenital adrenal hyperplasia is suggested by vomiting, diarrhea, dehydration, hyperkalemia, hyponatremia, shock, ambiguous genitals, or clitoral enlargement. Some infants have ambiguous genitals and hypertension. Because the condition is genetically determined, newborn siblings of patients with the salt-losing variety of adrenocortical hyperplasia should be closely observed for manifestations of adrenal insufficiency. Newborn screening and early diagnosis and therapy for this disorder may prevent severe salt wasting and adverse outcomes. Congenitally hypoplastic adrenal glands may also give rise to adrenal insufficiency during the 1st few weeks of life.

Female infants with webbing of the neck, lymphangiectatic edema, hypoplasia of the nipples, cutis laxa, low hairline at the nape of the neck, low-set ears, high-arched palate, deformities of the nails, cubitus valgus, and other anomalies should be suspected of having gonadal dysgenesis.

Transient diabetes mellitus (see Chapter 590) is rare and is encountered only in newborns. It is usually manifested as dehydration, loss of weight, or acidosis in small for gestational age infants.

107.1 • Infants of Diabetic Mothers

Women with diabetes in pregnancy (Type 1, Type 2, and gestational) are all at increased risk for adverse pregnancy outcomes. Adequate glycemic control before and during pregnancy is crucial to improving outcome.

Diabetic mothers have a high incidence of polyhydramnios, preeclampsia, pyelonephritis, preterm labor, and chronic hypertension; their fetal mortality rate, which is high at all gestational ages, especially after 32 wk, is greater than that of nondiabetic mothers. Fetal loss throughout pregnancy is associated with poorly controlled maternal diabetes (especially ketoacidosis) and congenital anomalies. Most infants born to diabetic mothers are large for gestational age. If the diabetes is complicated by vascular disease, infants may be growth restricted, especially those born after 37 wk gestation. The neonatal mortality rate is over 5 times that of infants of nondiabetic mothers and is higher at all gestational ages and in every birthweight for gestational age category.

PATHOPHYSIOLOGY. The probable pathogenic sequence is that maternal hyperglycemia causes fetal hyperglycemia, and the fetal pancreatic response leads to fetal hyperinsulinemia; fetal hyperinsulinemia and hyperglycemia then cause increased hepatic glucose uptake and glycogen synthesis, accelerated lipogenesis, and augmented protein synthesis (Fig. 107-1). Related pathologic findings are hypertrophy and hyperplasia of the pancreatic islet β cells, increased weight of the placenta and infant organs except for the brain, myocardial hypertrophy, increased amount of cytoplasm in liver cells, and extramedullary hematopoiesis. Hyperinsulinism and hyperglycemia produce fetal acidosis, which may result in an increased rate of stillbirth. Separation of the placenta at birth suddenly interrupts glucose infusion into the neonate without a proportional effect on the hyperinsulinism, and hypoglycemia and attenuated lipolysis develop during the 1st hr after birth.

Hyperinsulinemia has been documented in infants of gestational diabetic mothers and in those of insulin-dependent diabetic mothers without insulin antibodies. The former group also has significantly higher fasting plasma insulin levels than normal newborns do despite similar glucose levels; they respond to glucose

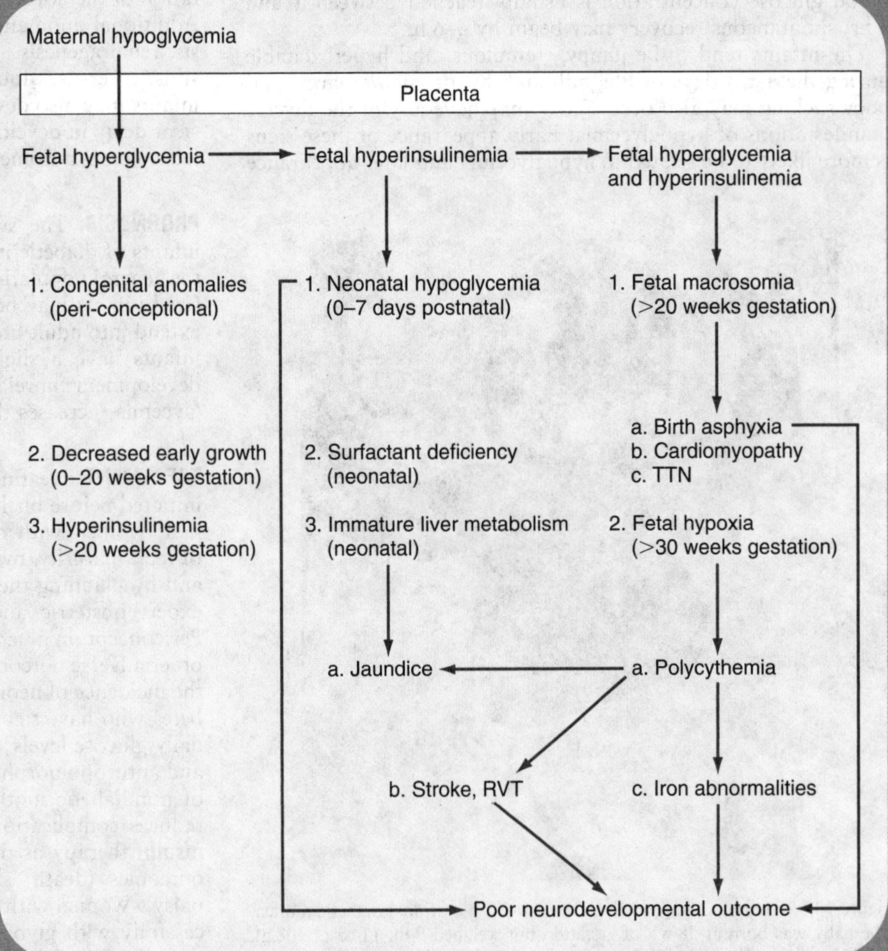

Figure 107-1. The fetal and neonatal events attributable to fetal hyperglycemia *(column 1)*, fetal hyperinsulinemia *(column 2)*, or both in synergy *(column 3)*. Time of risk is denoted in parentheses. RVT, renal vein thrombosis. (From Nold JL, Georgieff MK: Infants of diabetic mothers. *Pediatr Clin North Am* 2004;51: 619–637.)

with an abnormally prompt elevation in plasma insulin and assimilate a glucose load more rapidly. After arginine administration, they also have an enhanced insulin response and increased disappearance rates of glucose in comparison to normal infants. In contrast, fasting glucose production and utilization rates are diminished. The lower free fatty acid levels in infants of insulin-dependent diabetic mothers reflect their hyperinsulinemia. With good prenatal diabetic control, the incidence of macrosomia and hypoglycemia has decreased.

Although hyperinsulinism is probably the main cause of hypoglycemia, the diminished epinephrine and glucagon responses that occur may be contributing factors. Congenital anomalies correlate with poor metabolic control during the periconception and organogenesis periods and may be due to hyperglycemia-induced teratogenesis. Chronic fetal hypoxia, indicated by elevated amniotic fluid erythropoietin levels, is associated with increased fetal and neonatal morbidity.

CLINICAL MANIFESTATIONS. Infants of diabetic and gestational diabetic mothers often bear a surprising resemblance to each other (Fig. 107–2). They tend to be large and plump as a result of increased body fat and enlarged viscera, with puffy, plethoric facies resembling that of patients who have been receiving corticosteroids. These infants may also, however, be of normal or low birthweight, particularly if delivered before term or the mother has associated vascular disease.

Hypoglycemia develops in about 25–50% of infants of diabetic mothers and 15–25% of infants of mothers with gestational diabetes, but only a small percentage of these infants become symptomatic. The probability of hypoglycemia developing in the infant increases and glucose levels are likely to be lower at higher cord or maternal fasting blood glucose levels. The nadir in an infant's blood glucose concentration is usually reached between 1 and 3 hr; spontaneous recovery may begin by 4–6 hr.

The infants tend to be jumpy, tremulous, and hyperexcitable during the 1st 3 days of life, although hypotonia, lethargy, and poor sucking may also occur. They may have any of the diverse manifestations of hypoglycemia. Early appearance of these signs is more likely to be related to hypoglycemia and later appearance related to hypocalcemia; these abnormalities may also occur together. Perinatal asphyxia or hyperbilirubinemia may produce similar signs. Hypomagnesemia may be associated with the hypocalcemia. These manifestations may also occur in the absence of hypoglycemia, hypocalcemia, or asphyxia.

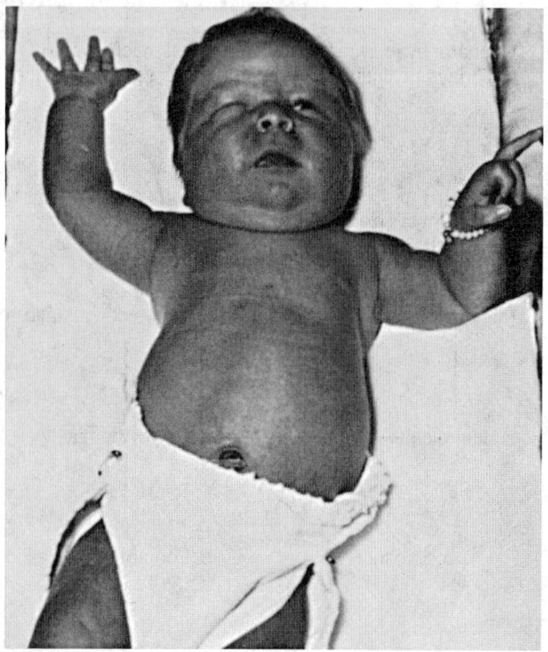

Figure 107-2. Large, plump, plethoric infant of a gestational diabetic mother. The baby was born at 38 wk of gestation but weighed 9 lb, 11 oz (4,408 g). Mild respiratory distress was the only symptom other than appearance.

Tachypnea develops in many infants of diabetic mothers during the 1st 2 days of life and may be a manifestation of hypoglycemia, hypothermia, polycythemia, cardiac failure, transient tachypnea, or cerebral edema from birth trauma or asphyxia. Infants of diabetic mothers have a higher incidence of **respiratory distress syndrome** than do infants of nondiabetic mothers born at comparable gestational age; the greater incidence is possibly related to an antagonistic effect of insulin on stimulation of surfactant synthesis by cortisol.

Cardiomegaly is common (30%), and heart failure occurs in 5–10% of infants of diabetic mothers. Asymmetric septal hypertrophy may occur and become manifested similar to transient idiopathic hypertrophic subaortic stenosis. Inotropic agents worsen the obstruction and are contraindicated. Congenital heart disease is more common in infants of diabetic mothers. Birth trauma is also a common sequela of fetal macrosomia.

Neurologic development and ossification centers tend to be immature and correlate with brain size (which is not increased) and gestational age rather than total body weight. In addition, these infants have an increased incidence of hyperbilirubinemia, polycythemia, and renal vein thrombosis; the latter should be suspected in infants with a flank mass, hematuria, and thrombocytopenia.

The incidence of **congenital anomalies** is increased threefold in infants of diabetic mothers; cardiac malformations (ventricular or atrial septal defect, transposition of the great vessels, truncus arteriosus, double-outlet right ventricle, tricuspid atresia, coarctation of the aorta) and lumbosacral agenesis are most common. Additional anomalies include neural tube defects, hydronephrosis, renal agenesis and dysplasia, duodenal or anorectal atresia, situs inversus, double ureter, and holoprosencephaly. These infants may also develop abdominal distention caused by a transient delay in development of the left side of the colon, the small left colon syndrome.

PROGNOSIS. The subsequent incidence of diabetes mellitus in infants of diabetic mothers is increased in comparison to that of the general population. Physical development is normal, but oversized infants may be predisposed to childhood obesity that may extend into adult life. Disagreement persists about whether these infants have a slightly increased risk of impaired intellectual development unrelated to hypoglycemia; symptomatic hypoglycemia increases the risk, as does maternal ketonuria.

TREATMENT. Treatment of infants of diabetic mothers should be initiated before birth by frequent prenatal evaluation of all pregnant women with overt or gestational diabetes, by evaluation of fetal maturity, by biophysical profile, by Doppler velocimetry, and by planning the delivery of these infants in hospitals where expert obstetric and pediatric care is continuously available. Periconception glucose control reduces the risk of anomalies and other adverse outcomes, and glucose control during labor reduces the incidence of neonatal hypoglycemia. Women with Type 1 diabetes who have tight glucose control during pregnancy (average daily glucose levels <95 mg/dL) deliver infants with birthweights and anthropomorphic features that are similar to those of infants of nondiabetic mothers. Treatment of gestational diabetes also reduces complications; dietary advice, glucose monitoring, and insulin therapy as needed decrease the rate of serious perinatal outcomes (death, shoulder dystocia, bone fracture, or nerve palsy). Women with gestational diabetes may also be treated successfully with glyburide, which may not cross the placenta. In these mothers, the incidence of macrosomia and neonatal hypoglycemia is similar to that in mothers with insulin-treated gestational diabetes. Regardless of size, all infants of diabetic mothers should initially receive intensive observation and care. Asymptomatic infants should have a blood glucose determination within 1 hr of birth and then every hour for the next 6–8 hr; if clinically well and normoglycemic, oral or gavage feeding with breast milk or formula should be started as soon as possible and continued at 3 hr intervals. If any question arises about an infant's ability to tolerate oral feeding, the feeding should be discontinued and glucose given by peripheral intravenous infusion at a rate of 4–8 mg/kg/min. Hypoglycemia should be treated, even in asymptomatic infants, by frequent feeding and/or intravenous infusion of glucose. Bolus injections of hypertonic glucose should be avoided because they may cause further hyperinsulinemia and potentially produce rebound hypoglycemia. Managing hypoglycemia in sick or symptomatic infants is discussed in the following section. For treatment of hypocalcemia and hypomagnesemia, see Chapter 106; for respiratory distress syndrome treatment, see Chapter 101.4; for treatment of polycythemia, see Chapter 103.3.

107.2 • Hypoglycemia (See Also Chapter 92)

The incidence of hypoglycemia varies with the category of fetal growth and the nursery feeding protocols (Fig. 107-3). Early feeding decreases the incidence, whereas prematurity, hypothermia, hypoxia, maternal diabetes, maternal glucose infusion in labor, and intrauterine growth restriction (IUGR) increase the incidence of hypoglycemia. Serum glucose levels decline after birth until 1–3 hr of age, when levels spontaneously increase in normal infants. In healthy term infants, serum glucose values are rarely <35 mg/dL between 1 and 3 hr of life, <40 mg/dL from 3 to 24 hr, and <45 mg/dL (2.5 mmol/L) after 24 hr. Both premature and full-term infants are at risk for serious neurodevelopmental deficits from equally low glucose levels. This risk is related to the depth and duration of the hypoglycemia.

CLINICAL MANIFESTATIONS. In contrast to the frequency of chemical hypoglycemia, the incidence of symptomatic hypoglycemia is highest in small for gestational age infants (see Fig. 107-3). The incidence of symptomatic hypoglycemia probably varies between 1 and 3 per 1,000 live births and affects about 5–15% of growth-restricted infants.

The onset of symptoms varies from a few hours to a week after birth. In approximate order of frequency, symptoms include jitteriness or tremors, apathy, episodes of cyanosis, convulsions, intermittent apneic spells or tachypnea, weak or high-pitched cry, limpness or lethargy, difficulty feeding, and eye rolling. Episodes of sweating, sudden pallor, hypothermia, and cardiac arrest and failure also occur. Frequently, a clustering of episodic symptoms may be noted. Because these clinical manifestations may result from various causes, it is critical to measure serum glucose levels and determine whether they disappear with the administration of sufficient glucose to raise the blood sugar to normal levels; if they do not, other diagnoses must be considered.

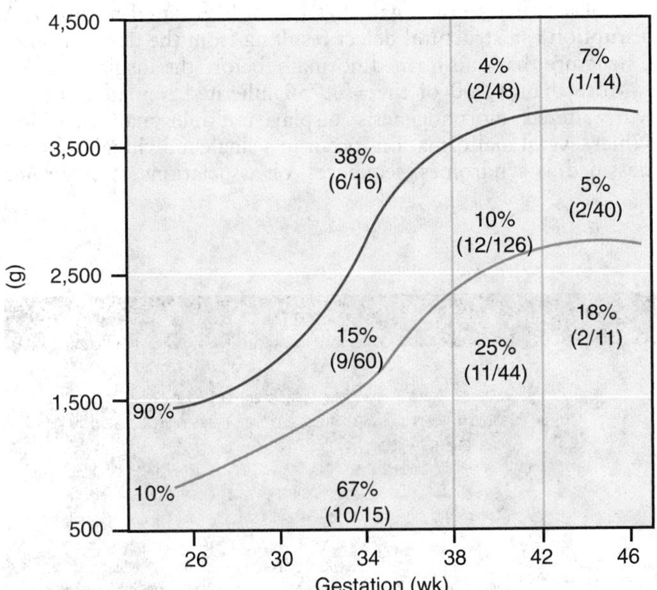

Figure 107-3. Incidence of hypoglycemia by birthweight, gestational age, and intrauterine growth. (From Lubchenco LO, Bard H: Incidence of hypoglycemia in newborn infants classified by birth weight and gestational age. *Pediatrics* 1971;47:831–838.)

TREATMENT. When symptoms other than seizures are present, an intravenous bolus of 200 mg/kg (2 mL/kg) of 10% glucose is effective in elevating the blood glucose concentration. In the presence of convulsions, 4 mL/kg of 10% glucose as a bolus injection is indicated.

After initial therapy, a glucose infusion should be given at 8 mg/kg/min. If hypoglycemia recurs, the infusion rate and concentration should be increased until 15–20% glucose is used. If intravenous infusions of 20% glucose are inadequate to eliminate symptoms and maintain constant normal serum glucose concentrations, hyperinsulinemia is probably present and diazoxide should be administered. If the diazoxide is unsuccessful, octreotide may be useful; infants with severe persistent hyperinsulinemic hypoglycemia may eventually need to undergo subtotal pancreatectomy (see Chapter 92). The serum glucose level should be measured every 2 hr after initiating therapy until several determinations are above 40 mg/dL. Subsequently, levels should be measured every 4–6 hr and the treatment gradually reduced and finally discontinued when the serum glucose value has been in the normal range and the baby asymptomatic for 24–48 hr. Treatment is usually necessary for a few days to a week, rarely for several weeks.

Infants at increased risk for hypoglycemia should have their serum glucose measured within 1 hr of birth, every 1–2 hr for the 1st 6–8 hr, and then every 4–6 hr until 24 hr of life. Normoglycemic high-risk infants should receive oral or gavage feeding with human milk or formula started at 1–3 hr of age and continued at 2–3 hr intervals for 24–48 hr. An intravenous infusion of glucose at 4 mg/kg/min should be provided if oral feedings are poorly tolerated or if asymptomatic transient neonatal hypoglycemia develops.

PROGNOSIS. The prognosis is good in asymptomatic patients with hypoglycemia of short duration. Hypoglycemia recurs in 10–15% of infants after adequate treatment. Recurrence is more common if intravenous fluids are extravasated or discontinued too rapidly before oral feedings are well tolerated. Children in whom ketotic hypoglycemia later develops have an increased incidence of neonatal hypoglycemia. The prognosis for normal intellectual function must be guarded because prolonged, recurrent, and severe symptomatic hypoglycemia is associated with neurologic sequelae. Symptomatic infants with hypoglycemia, particularly low birthweight infants, those with persistent hyperinsulinemic hypoglycemia, and infants of diabetic mothers, have a poorer prognosis for subsequent normal intellectual development than asymptomatic infants do.

Bongers-Schokking JJ, Koot HM, Wiersma D, et al: Influence of timing and dose of thyroid hormone replacement on development in infants with congenital hypothyroidism. *J Pediatr* 2000;136:292–297.

Briët JM, van Wassenaer AG, Dekker FW, et al: Neonatal thyroxine supplementation in very preterm children: Developmental outcome evaluated at early school age. *Pediatrics* 2001;107:712–718.
Clausen TD, Mathiesen E, Ekbom P, et al: Poor pregnancy outcome in women with type 2 diabetes. *Diabetes Care* 2005;28:323–328.
Cornblath M, Hawdon JM, Williams AF, et al: Controversies regarding definition of neonatal hypoglycemia: Suggested operational thresholds. *Pediatrics* 2000;105:1141–1145.
Crowther CA, Hiller JE, Moss JR, et al; Australian Carbohydrate Intolerance Study in Pregnant Women (ACHOIS) Trial Group: Effect of treatment of gestational diabetes mellitus on pregnancy outcomes. *N Engl J Med* 2005;352:2477–2486.
Duvanel CB, Fawer CL, Cotting J, et al: Long-term effects of neonatal hypoglycemia on brain growth and psychomotor development in small-for-gestational-age preterm infants. *J Pediatr* 1999;134:492–498.
Fisher DA: The importance of early management in optimizing IQ in infants with congenital hypothyroidism. *J Pediatr* 2000;136:273–274.
Hussain K, Aynsley-Green A: Hyperinsulinaemic hypoglycaemia in preterm neonates. *Arch Dis Child Fetal Neonatal Ed* 2004;89:F65–F67.
Jensen DM, Damm P, Moelsted-Pederson L, et al: Outcomes in type 1 diabetic pregnancies: A nationwide, population-based study. *Diabetes Care* 2004;27:2819–2823.
Langer O, Yogev Y, Most O, et al: Gestational diabetes: The consequences of not treating. *Am J Obstet Gynecol* 2005;192:989–997.
Langer O, Yogev Y, Xenakis E, et al: Insulin and glyburide therapy: Dosage, severity level of gestational diabetes, and pregnancy outcome. *Am J Obstet Gynecol* 2005;192:134–139.
Lilien L, Pildes R, Srinivasan G, et al: Treatment of neonatal hypoglycemia with minibolus and intravenous glucose infusion. *J Pediatr* 1980;97:295–298.
Menni F, de Lonlay P, Sevin C, et al: Neurologic outcomes of 90 neonates and infants with persistent hyperinsulinemic hypoglycemia. *Pediatrics* 2001;107:476–479.
Nold JL, Georgieff MK: Infants of diabetic mothers. *Pediatr Clin North Am* 2004;51:619–637.
Osborn DA: Thyroid hormones for preventing neurodevelopmental impairment in preterm infants. *Cochrane Database Syst Rev* 2001;4:CD001070.
Rapaport R, Rose SR, Freemark M: Hypothyroxinemia in the preterm infant: The benefits and risks of thyroxine treatment. *J Pediatr* 2001;139:182–188.
Rovet JF: In search of the optimal therapy for congenital hypothyroidism. *J Pediatr* 2004;144:698–700.
Stanley CA, Baker L: The causes of neonatal hypoglycemia. *N Engl J Med* 1999;340:1200–1201.
Teramo K, Kari MA, Eronen M, et al: High amniotic fluid erythropoietin levels are associated with an increased frequency of fetal and neonatal morbidity in type 1 diabetic pregnancies. *Diabetologia* 2004;47:1695–1703.
Vela-Huerta MM, Vargas-Origel A, Olvera-López A: Asymmetrical septal hypertrophy in newborn infants of diabetic mothers. *Am J Perinatol* 2000;17:89–94.
Wren C, Birrell G, Hawthorne G: Cardiovascular malformations in infants of diabetic mothers. *Heart* 2003;89:1217–1220.

Chapter 108 ■ Dysmorphology

Anthony Wynshaw-Boris and Leslie G. Biesecker

Dysmorphology is the study of abnormalities of human form and the mechanisms that cause these abnormalities. It is estimated that 1 in 40, or 2.5% of newborns, have a recognizable malformation or malformations at birth. In about half the cases, a single isolated malformation is found, while the other half display multiple malformations. It is estimated that 10% of pediatric hospital admissions have known genetic conditions, 18% have congenital defects of unknown etiology, and 40% of surgical admissions are patients with congenital malformations. Twenty to 30% of infant deaths and 30–50% of deaths after the neonatal period are due to congenital abnormalities (http://www.marchofdimes.com/peristats/). In 2001, birth defects accounted for 1 in 5 infant deaths in the United States, with a rate of 137.6 deaths per 100,000 live births, which is higher than other causes such as preterm/low birth weight (109.5/100,000), sudden infant death syndrome (55.5/100,000), maternal complications of pregnancy (37.3/100,000) and respiratory distress syndrome (25.3/100,000).

CLASSIFICATION OF BIRTH DEFECTS

Congenital birth defects are either isolated, single defects, or present as multiple anomalies in a single individual. Single primary defects can be classified by the nature of the presumed cause of the defect as a malformation, dysplasia, deformation, or disruption (Table 108-1). Malformations and dysplasias both affect intrinsic structure. A **malformation** is a primary structural defect arising from a localized error in morphogenesis, resulting in the abnormal formation of a tissue or organ. **Dysplasia** refers to an abnormal organization of cells into tissues. The distinction of a malformation from a dysplasia may be helpful, but there is much overlap. Deformations and disruptions are secondary effects that result from forces generated extrinsic to the affected tissue or organ. A **deformation** is an alteration in shape or structure of a structure or organ that has differentiated normally. A **disruption** is a structural defect resulting from the destruction of a structure that had formed normally before the insult.

More than 1,000 of the ≈ 1,750 inherited human disorders with altered morphogenesis display multiple malformations. When several malformations occur in a single individual, they are classified as syndromes, sequences, or associations. A **syndrome**

TABLE 108-1. Mechanisms, Terminology, and Definitions of Dysmorphology

TERMINOLOGY	DEFINITION	EXAMPLE
Malformation sequence	Single, local tissue morphogenesis abnormality that produces a chain of subsequent defects	DiGeorge sequence of primary fourth brachial arch and 3rd and 4th pharyngeal pouch defects that lead to aplasia or hypoplasia of the thymus and parathyroid glands, aortic arch anomalies, and micrognathia
Deformation sequence	Mechanical (uterine) forces that alter structure of intrinsically normal tissue	Oligohydramnios produces deformations by in utero compression of limbs (dislocated hips, equinovarus foot deformity), crumpled ears, dislocated nose, or small thorax
Disruption sequence	In utero tissue destruction after a period of normal morphogenesis	Amnionic membrane rupture sequence, leading to amputation of fingers/toes, tissue fibrosis, and destructive tissue bands
Dysplasia sequence	Poor organization of cells into tissues or organs	Neurocutaneous melanosis sequence with poor migration of melanocyte precursor cells from the neural crest to the periphery, manifesting as melanocytic hamartosis of skin, meninges, and so forth
Malformation syndrome	Appearance of multiple malformations in unrelated tissues without an understandable unifying cause; with enhanced genetic investigation, a single etiology may become identified	Trisomy 21 Teratogens

From Kliegman RM, Greenbaum LA, Lye PS: *Practical Strategies in Pediatric Diagnosis and Therapy*, 2nd ed. Philadelphia, Elsevier Saunders, 2004.

is defined as a pattern of multiple abnormalities that are related by pathophysiology and result from a common, defined etiology. **Sequences** consist of multiple malformations that are caused by a single event that can have many etiologies. An **association** refers to a nonrandom collection of malformations where there is an unclear relationship among the malformations such that they do not fit the criteria for a syndrome or sequence.

MALFORMATIONS AND/OR DYSPLASIAS. Human malformations and dysplasias are caused by the combined effects of genes and environmental factors (Table 108-2). Some malformations are caused by single gene defects or abnormalities of multiple genes acting in concert, while the environment causes others. In 1996, it was thought that malformations were due to monogenic defects in 7.5% of patients; in 6%, they were caused by chromosomal anomalies; in 20%, they were the result of multigenic defects; and in 6–7%, they resulted from known environmental factors such as maternal diseases, infections, and teratogens (Table 108-3). In the remaining 60–70% of patients, malformations were due to unknown etiologies. A decade later, the percentages are somewhat higher for all categories of known causes of malformations, which is due to improved methods of detection of small chromosomal abnormalities as well as techniques for mapping and cloning disease genes. We still do not know, however, the causes or even the diagnosis for 50% of children with birth defects.

Many developmental abnormalities are caused by mutations in a single gene and display characteristic mendelian patterns of inheritance. The molecular etiology for more than 100 single gene disorders is known. Affected genes are often part of evolutionarily conserved signal transduction pathways, transcription factors, or regulatory proteins required for key developmental events. Some examples are listed in Table 108-2, and include autosomal recessive spondylocostal dysostosis (SCD) syndrome, the autosomal recessive Smith-Lemli-Opitz syndrome (SLOS), the autosomal dominant Rubinstein-Taybi syndrome, and the X-linked lissencephaly ("smooth-brain") syndrome. The SCD syndrome is etiologically heterogeneous and is often caused by mutations in the gene coding for delta-like 3 (DLL3), a ligand of the Notch receptors. The Notch/delta pathway is conserved throughout evolution and regulates a number of developmental events. Patients with SCD display a characteristic pattern of abnormal vertebral segmentation associated with a number of other malformations such as neural tube defects. SLOS (Fig. 108-1) results from mutations in the sterol delta-7-reductase gene, an enzyme important in cholesterol biosynthesis. Patients with SLOS display syndactyly (fusion of the fingers and toes) often with polydactyly, upturned nose, ptosis, cryptorchidism, central nervous system hypoplasia, and holoprosencephaly. These mutations link cholesterol biosynthesis pathogenetically to the sonic hedgehog (SHH) pathway, since many of the features of the former disorder are related to defects in SHH, which is post-translationally modified by cholesterol (see Chapter 86). Rubinstein-Taybi syndrome (see Fig. 108-1) results from heterozygous loss-of-function mutations in the gene coding for a broadly acting transcriptional coactivator called CBP, or CREB-binding protein. The CBP coactivator regulates the transcription of a number of genes, which helps to explain why patients with mutations in CBP have a wide-ranging phenotype that includes mental retardation, broad thumbs and toes, and congenital heart disease. One of the transcription factors that binds to CBP is GLI3, a transcription factor that is

TABLE 108-2. Examples of Malformations with Distinct Causes, Clinical Features, and Pathogenesis

DISORDER	CAUSE/INHERITANCE	CLINICAL FEATURES	PATHOGENESIS
Spondylocostal dysostosis syndromes	Mendelian AR	Abnormal vertebral segmentation Neural tube defects	DLL3 mutation
Rubinstein-Taybi syndrome	Mendelian AR	Mental retardation Broad thumbs, toes Hypoplastic maxillae Prominent nose Congenital heart disease	CBP mutations
X-linked lissencephaly	Mendelian X-linked	Male Severe mental retardation Seizures Female Variable	DCX mutations
Aniridia	Autosomal semi-dominant	Reduced or absent iris	PAX6 mutations
Waardenburg syndrome	Autosomal semi-dominant	Deafness White forelock Wide-spaced eyes Pale eye pigment	PAX3 mutations MITF mutations
Holoprosencephaly	Loss of function or heterozygosity	Microcephaly Cyclopia Single central incisor	SHH mutations
Velocardiofacial syndrome	Microdeletion 22q 11.2	Conotruncal congenital heart disease Cleft palate T-cell defects Facial anomalies	TBX1 mutations
Down syndrome	Chromosomal	Mental retardation Characteristic dysmorphic features Congenital heart disease Increased risk of leukemia Alzheimer disease	50% increase of 250 genes of chromosome 21 Trisomy 21
Neural tube defects	Multifactorial	Meningomyelocele	Defects in folate sensitive enzymes or folic acid uptake
Fetal alcohol syndrome	Teratogenic	Microcephaly Developmental delay Facial abnormalities Behavioral abnormalities	Ethanol toxicity to developing brain
Retinoic acid embryopathy	Teratogenic	Microtia Congenital heart disease	Isotretinoin effects neural crest and branchial arch development

TABLE 108-3. Causes of Congenital Malformations

Monogenic (7.5% of Serious Anomalies)	***Environmental Agents (% Unknown)***
X-linked hydrocephalus	Polychlorinated biphenyls
Achondroplasia	Herbicides
Ectodermal dysplasia	Mercury
Apert disease	Alcohol
Treacher Collins syndrome	***Medications (% Unknown)***
Chromosomal (6% of Serious Anomalies)	Thalidomide
Trisomies 21, 18, 13	Diethylstilbestrol
XO, XXY	Phenytoin
Deletions 4p-, 5p, 7q-, 13q-, 18p-, 18q-, 22q-	Warfarin
Prader-Willi syndrome (50% have deletion of chromosome 15)	Cytotoxic drugs
	Paroxetine
Maternal Infection (2% of Serious Anomalies)	ACE inhibitors
Intrauterine infections (e.g., herpes simplex, CMV, varicella-zoster, rubella, and toxoplasmosis)	Isotretinoin (vitamin A)
	D-Penicillamine
Maternal Illness (3.5% of Serious Anomalies)	Valproic acid
Diabetes mellitus	***Unknown Etiologies***
Phenylketonuria	*Polygenetic*
Hyperthermia	Associated with infertility (spontaneous or with treatment)
Uterine Environment (% Unknown)	Anencephaly/spina bifida
Deformation	Cleft lip/palate
Uterine pressure, oligohydramnios: clubfoot, torticollis congenital hip dislocation, pulmonary hypoplasia, 7th nerve palsy	Pyloric stenosis
	Congenital heart disease
	Sporadic Syndrome Complexes (Anomalads)
Disruption	CHARGE syndrome
Amniotic bands, congenital amputations, gastroschisis, porencephaly, intestinal atresia	VATER syndrome
	Pierre Robin syndrome
Twinning	Prune-belly syndrome
Conjoined twins, intestinal atresia, porencephaly	***Nutritional***
	Low folic acid-neural tube defects

ACE, angiotensin-converting enzyme; CHARGE, coloboma, heart defects, atresia choanae, retarded growth, genital anomalies, ear anomalies (deafness); CMV, cytomegalovirus; VATER, vertebral defects, anal atresia, tracheoesophageal fistula with esophageal atresia, and radial and renal anomalies.
From Behrman RE, Kliegman RM (eds): *Nelson's Essentials of Pediatrics,* 4th ed. Philadelphia, WB Saunders, 2002.

part of the SHH pathway (see Fig. 108-1). X-linked lissencephaly, a severe neuronal migration defect in which males display a smooth brain with reduced or absent gyri and sulci, and females display a variable pattern of mental retardation and seizures, is caused by mutations in DCX, a protein that regulates the activity of dynein motors and moves the nucleus during neuronal migration.

Other malformation syndromes are caused by chromosomal imbalance, multifactorial inheritance, and teratogens (see Tables 108-2 and 108-3). Down syndrome results from an extra dose of part or all of chromosome 21, a small chromosome that contains ≈ 200 known or predicted genes. It is most commonly caused by trisomy 21, which means that individuals with Down syndrome have an increased dose of as many as 250 genes contained on this chromosome (see Chapter 81). Neural tube defects (NTDs) are an example of a disorder that displays multifactorial inheritance in the majority of cases. NTDs and a number of other congenital malformations such as cleft lip and palate recur in families, but several genes and environmental factors together contribute to the pathogenesis (see Table 108-2). Many of the genes involved in NTDs are unknown, so one cannot predict with certainty a mode of inheritance or a precise recurrence risk. Empiric risks can be provided based on population studies and the presence of single or multiple relatives with the same malformation. However, an important gene/environment interaction has been identified for NTDs (see Chapter 592.1). Folic acid status is associated with NTDs, and can result from a combination of dietary deficiencies and increased utilization during pregnancy, as well as a common variant in the gene for an enzyme in the folate recycling path-way, 5,10-methylene-tetrahydrofolate reductase that makes this enzyme less stable. These discoveries led to the recommendation that all women supplement their diets with 400–800 µg of folic acid per day 1 mo before pregnancy and during the 1st 2 mo of pregnancy. This supplementation has resulted in a reduction in the incidence of NTDs by 75%. Several teratogenic causes of birth defects have been described (see Tables 108-2 and 108-3). Ethanol causes a recognizable malformation syndrome called fetal alcohol syndrome (FAS) (see Chapter 106.2). Children with FAS display microcephaly, developmental delay, hyperactivity and facial dysmorphisms. Ethanol is toxic to the developing central nervous system, and causes cell death of developing neurons.

DEFORMATIONS. Most deformations involve the musculoskeletal system (Fig. 108-2). Fetal movement is required for the proper development of the normal musculoskeletal system, and anything that restricts fetal movement can cause a musculoskeletal deformation from intrauterine molding. It is important to recognize that deformations can be caused by problems either intrinsic or extrinsic to the developing fetus. Two major intrinsic causes of deformations are primary neuromuscular disorders and oligohydramnios, or decreased amniotic fluid, caused by renal defects. The major extrinsic causes of deformation are those that result in fetal crowding to restrict fetal movement, which is an important factor in development of the normal musculoskeletal system. Examples of such extrinsic causes are oligohydramnios from chronic leakage of amniotic fluid, breech presentation (Fig. 108-3), and abnormal shape of the amniotic cavity. When a fetus is in the breech position, the incidence of deformations is increased 10-fold. The shape of the amniotic cavity has a profound effect on the shape of the fetus and is influenced by many factors, including uterine shape; volume of amniotic fluid; size and shape of the fetus; presence of more than one fetus; site of placental implantation; presence of uterine tumors; shape of the abdominal cavity, which is influenced by the pelvis, sacral promontory, and neighboring abdominal organs; and tightness of the abdominal musculature.

It is important to determine if deformations result from intrinsic or extrinsic causes. Most children with deformations from extrinsic causes are otherwise completely normal, and their prognosis is usually excellent. Correction usually occurs spontaneously. Deformations caused by intrinsic factors, such as multiple joint contractures resulting from central nervous system defects, would have a different prognosis and a far greater significance to the child.

DISRUPTION. Disruption defects are caused by destruction of a previously normally formed part. At least two basic mechanisms are known to produce disruption. One involves entanglement followed by tearing apart or amputation of a normally developed structure, usually a digit, arm, or leg, by strands of amnion floating within amniotic fluid (**amniotic bands**) (Fig. 108-4). The second involves interruption of the blood supply to a developing part, which leads to infarction, necrosis, and/or resorption of structures distal to the insult. If interruption of the blood supply occurs early in gestation, the disruptive defect that is seen at term usually involves **atresia** or absence of a particular part. If the infarction occurs later, necrosis is more likely to be present. Examples of disruptive single primary defects for which infarction has been implicated include non-duodenal intestinal atresia, gastroschisis, porencephaly, and terminal transverse limb reduction defects. Genetic factors usually play a minor role in the pathogenesis of disruptions; most are sporadic events in otherwise normal families. The prognosis for a disruptive defect is determined entirely by the extent and location of the tissue loss.

MULTIPLE ANOMOLIES SYNDROME AND SEQUENCE. The pattern of multiple anomalies that occurs when a single primary defect in early morphogenesis produces multiple abnormalities through a cascading process of secondary and tertiary errors in morphogenesis is called a **sequence.** When evaluating a child with multiple anomalies, the physician must differentiate multiple

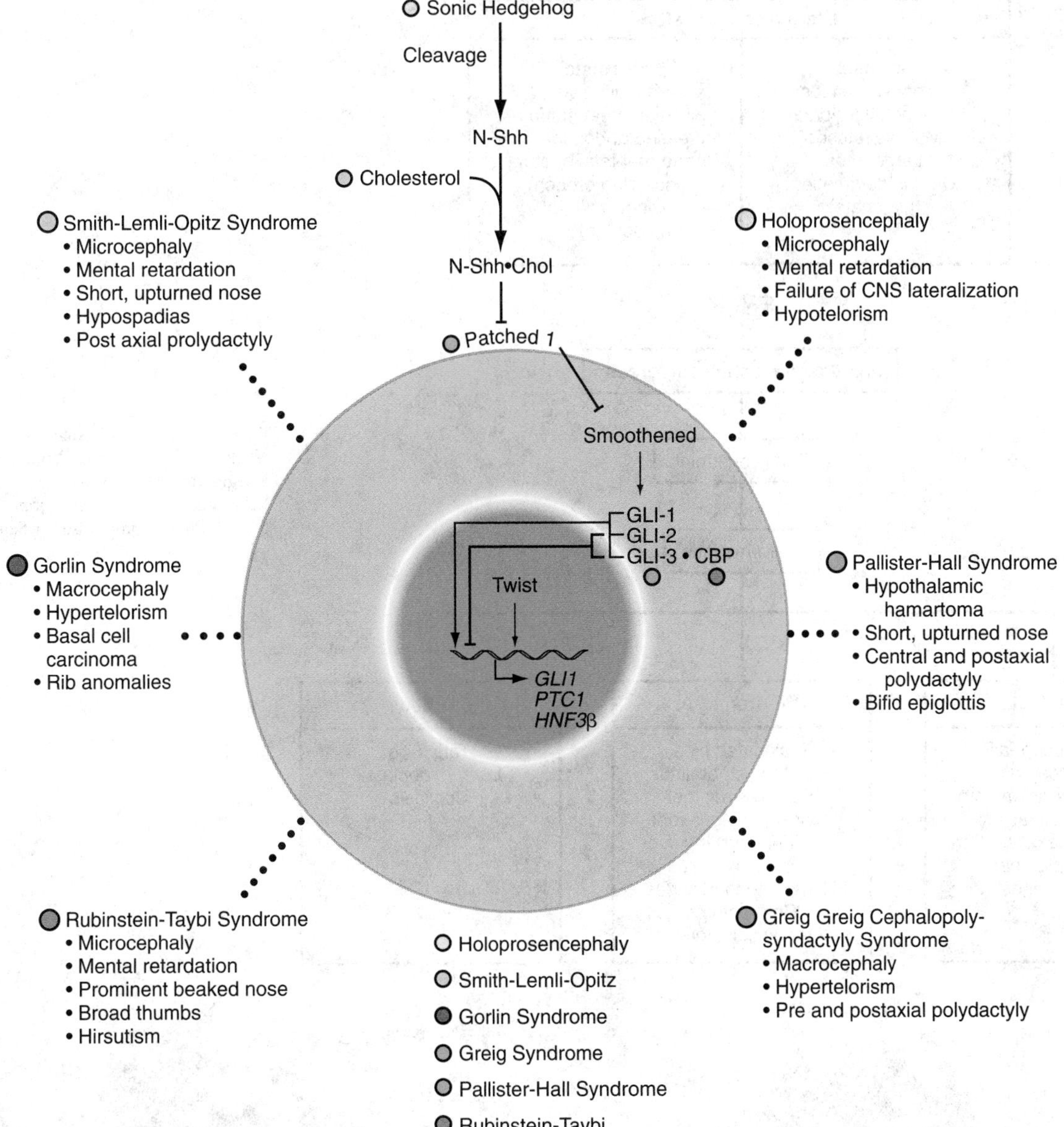

Figure 108-1. Mutations in genes that function together in a genetic developmental pathway commonly have overlapping clinical manifestations. Several components of the Sonic hegehog (SHH) pathway have been identified, and their relationships elucidated (see text for further details). Mutations in several members of this pathway result in phenotypes that have facial dysmorphisms, seen in holoprosencephaly, Smith-Lemli-Opitz syndrome, Gorlin syndrome, Greig cephalopolysyndactyly syndrome, Pallister-Hall syndrome, and Rubinstein-Taybi syndrome, which result from mutations in SHH, sterol delta-7-reductase, Patched 1, GLI3, GLI3, and CBP, respectively.

anomalies secondary to a single localized error in morphogenesis (a sequence) from a multiple malformation syndrome. In the former, recurrence risk counseling for the multiple anomalies depends entirely on the risk of recurrence for the single localized malformation. The Robin malformation sequence is a pattern of multiple anomalies produced by mandibular hypoplasia. Because the tongue is relatively large for the oral cavity, it drops back (glossoptosis), blocks closure of the posterior palatal shelves, and causes a U-shaped cleft palate. There are numerous causes of mandibular hypoplasia, all of which result in characteristic features of Robin sequence.

MOLECULAR MECHANISMS OF MALFORMATIONS: INBORN ERRORS OF DEVELOPMENT

The genes mutated in malformation syndromes (as well as genes whose expression is disrupted by environmental agents or teratogens) are part of evolutionarily conserved signal transduction pathways, transcription factors, or regulatory proteins required for key developmental events. We should consider malformations to be inborn errors of development. Consideration of malformations as alterations of important developmental pathways provides a molecular framework for understanding human birth defects.

SONIC HEDGEHOG (SHH) PATHWAY AS MODEL. The SHH pathway is developmentally important during embryogenesis to induce controlled proliferation in a tissue-specific manner; disruption of specific steps in this pathway results in a variety of related developmental disorders and malformations (see Fig. 108-1). Activation of this pathway in the adult leads to abnormal proliferation and cancer. The SHH pathway transduces an external signal in the form of a ligand into changes in gene transcription by binding of the ligand to specific cellular receptors. SHH is a ligand

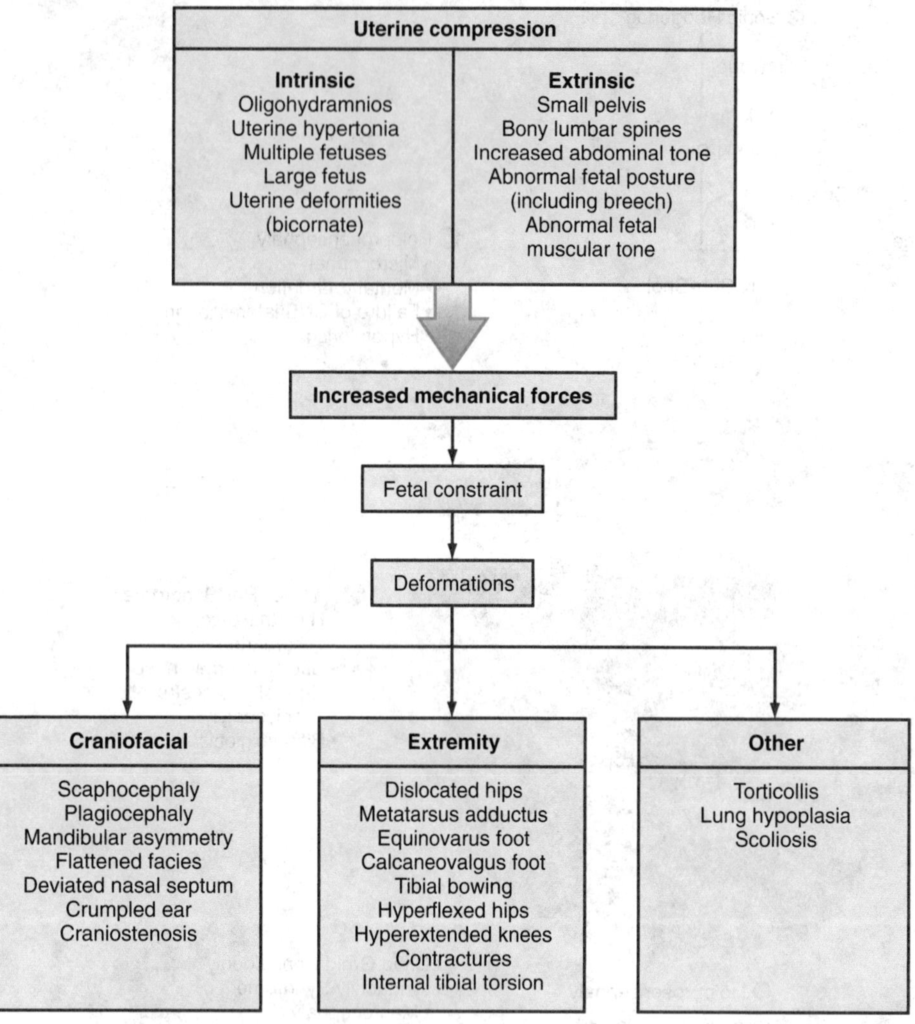

Figure 108-2. Deformation abnormalities resulting from uterine compression. (From Kliegman RM, Jenson HB, Marcdante KJ, Behrman RE: *Nelson Essentials of Pediatrics,* 5th ed. Philadelphia, Elsevier Saunders, 2005.)

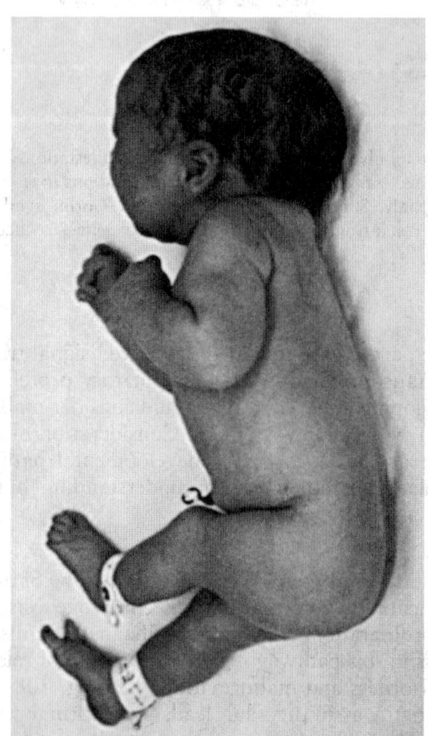

Figure 108-3. Breech deformation sequence.

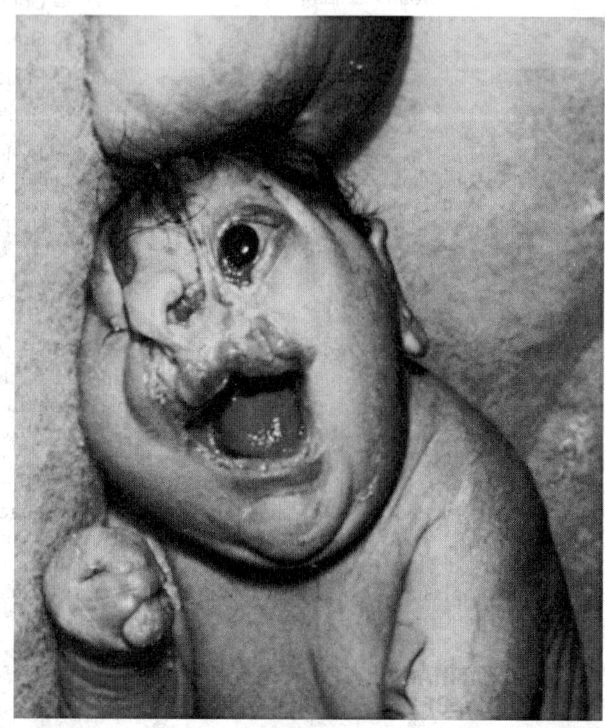

Figure 108-4. Amniotic band disruption sequence.

expressed in the embryo in a variety of areas important for development of the brain, face, limbs, and the gut. Sporadic and inherited mutations are found to cause **holoprosencephaly** (see Fig. 108-1), a variably severe midline defect with phenotypes ranging from a single maxillary incisor with hypotelorism to cyclopia. SHH is processed by proteolytic cleavage to an active N-terminal form, which is then further modified by the addition of cholesterol. Defects in cholesterol biosynthesis, in particular the sterol delta-7-reductase gene, result in **Smith-Lemli-Opitz syndrome** (SLOS; see Fig. 108-1). SLOS is also associated with holoprosencephaly. The modified and active form of SHH binds to its transmembrane receptor Patched (PTCH); there are two family members PTCH-1 and PTCH-2. SHH binding to PTCH inhibits the activity of the transmembrane protein Smoothened (SMOH). SMOH act to suppress downstream targets of the SHH pathway, the GLI family of transcription factors, so inhibition of SMOH by PTCH results in activation of GLI1, GLI2 and GLI3, resulting in alteration of transcription of GLI targets. Somatic inactivating mutations in PTCH-1 and PTCH-2 act as tumor suppressors, while activating mutations in SMOH function as oncogenes, particularly in basal cell carcinomas and medulloblastomas. Germline inactivating mutations in PTCH-1 result in **Gorlin syndrome** (see Fig. 108-1), an autosomal dominant disorder characterized by dysmorphic features (short metacarpals, rib defects, broad face, and dental abnormalities), basal cell nevi that undergo malignant transformation, and an increased risk of cancers such as rhabdomyosarcoma and medulloblastoma. GLI1 amplification has been found in several human tumors including glioblastoma, osteosarcoma, rhabdomyosarcoma, and B cell lymphomas, while mutations or alterations in GLI3 have been found in Greig cephalopolysyndactyly syndrome (GCPS), **Pallister-Hall syndrome** (PHS), and postaxial polydactyly type A (and A/B) and preaxial polydactyly type IV (see Fig. 108-1). GCPS consists of hypertelorism, syndactyly, preaxial polydactyly and broad thumbs, and great toes. PHS is an autosomal dominant disorder characterized by postaxial polydactyly, syndactyly, hypothalamic hamartomas, imperforate anus, and, occasionally, holoprosencephaly. GLI3 binds to CBP, the protein haploinsufficient in the **Rubinstein-Taybi syndrome** (RTS). Disorders that are caused by mutations in genes that function together in a genetic developmental pathway commonly have overlapping clinical manifestations. These overlapping manifestations result from the expression domains of SHH important for development of the brain, face, limbs, and gut in the embryo. Brain defects are found in holoprosencephaly, SLOS, and PHS. Facial abnormalities are found in holoprosencephaly, Gorlin syndrome, GCPS, and PHS. Limb defects are found in SLOS, Gorlin syndrome, GCPS, PHS, and the polydactyly syndromes. Overexpression or activating mutations of the SHH pathway results in cancer including basal cell carcinoma, medulloblastoma, glioblastoma, and rhabdomyosarcoma.

APPROACH TO THE DYSMORPHIC CHILD

A comprehensive and rational diagnostic approach to the dysmorphic child can be derived from the etiologic principles discussed. The history and physical examination considerations extend directly from the etiologic factors and couple the medical evaluation to human developmental biology. One approach to the dysmorphic child is the pattern recognition approach, which compares the manifestations of the patient against an enormous and memorized (or computerized) knowledge of human pleiotropic disorders. Although this approach is appropriate for the small number of experienced dysmorphologists, the systematic genetic-mechanism approach can be used by clinicians who are not experts in dysmorphology. By gathering and analyzing these clinical data, the general pediatrician can either diagnose the patient in straightforward cases or initiate a referral process to an appropriate expert.

HISTORY. The history for a child with birth defects includes a number of elements that are related to etiologic factors. The first is the pedigree or family history that is necessary to assess the **inheritance pattern,** or lack thereof, of the disorder. For disorders that have simple mendelian inheritance patterns, the recognition of that pattern can be critical to help narrow the differential diagnosis. A number of common birth defects have complex genetic contributions, such as isolated cleft palate and spina bifida. The recognition of a close relative (or the fetus of a close relative) affected with a birth defect that is similar to that of the proband can be quite useful. A three-generation pedigree is sufficient for this purpose (see Chapter 83).

The perinatal history is an essential component of the history (see Chapter 96). This includes the pregnancy history of the mother (useful for recognition of recurrent miscarriages that may be a sign of a familial chromosomal disorder), factors that may relate to deformations or disruptions (oligohydramnios), and maternal exposures to teratogenic drugs or chemicals (methyl mercury, isotretinoin, and ethanol are potential causes of microcephaly). Although recognition of known teratogens is an important part of the history, it is important to know that many more agents are impugned as teratogenic than are confirmed to be so. Physicians are encouraged to consult experts in teratology and expert information sources such as Teris (http://depts.washington.edu/~terisweb/teris/) to analyze specific potential teratogens.

One final component to the history that is often useful is the natural history of the phenotype. Malformation syndromes caused by chromosomal aneuploidy or aneusomy and single gene pleiotropic disorders are usually static. Although the patients can develop new complications over time, the phenotype is not progressive. In contrast, disorders that cause dysmorphic features by the mechanism of metabolic perturbations (Hunter syndrome, Sanfillipo syndrome) are either mild or inapparent at birth and progress relentlessly, causing deterioration of the patient over time.

EXAMINATION. The physical examination is essential to the diagnosis of a dysmorphic syndrome. The essential element of the evaluation is objective assessment of the structure of the child. The clinician needs to perform an organized and systematic cataloguing of the size and structure of various body structures. Familiarity with the nomenclature of dysmorphic signs is helpful (Table 108-4). The size and shape of the head is relevant, as many children with Down syndrome have mild microcephaly and brachycephaly (shortened anteroposterior dimension of the skull). Eye position and shape are useful signs for many disorders. There are a number of reference standards to which pediatric physical measurements (interpupillary distance) can be compared. It is also useful to categorize abnormalities as "major" or "minor" birth defects. The former are those that either cause dysfunction (absence of a digit) or require surgical correction (polydactyly) and the latter neither cause significant dysfunction nor require surgical correction (mild cutaneous syndactyly) (Table 108-5). By cataloguing every available physical parameter, the clinician can recognize the diagnosis, or at least have enough information for intelligent discussion of the patient with a consultant.

IMAGING STUDIES. Imaging studies can be critical in diagnosis of a dysmorphic disorder. If short stature or disproportionate stature (long trunk and short limbs) is noted, a full skeletal survey should be performed. The skeletal survey can yield numerous abnormal features that can be used to narrow the differential diagnosis. When there are abnormal neurologic signs or symptoms, central nervous system imaging is indicated. Some children with micro-

TABLE 108-4. Definitions of Common Clinical Signs

SIGN	DEFINITION
Brachycephaly	A condition in which head shape is shortened from front to back along the sagittal plane; the skull is rounder than normal
Brachydactyly	A condition of having short digits
Brushfield spots	Speckled white rings about two thirds of the distance to the periphery of the iris of the eye
Camptodactyly	Permanent flexion of one or more fingers associated with missing inner phalangeal creases indicating lack of finger movement from before 8 wk gestation
Clinodactyly	A medial or lateral curving of the fingers and usually refers to incurving of the 5th finger
Hypoplastic nail	An unusually small nail on a digit
Low-set ears	This designation is made when the helix meets the cranium at a level below a horizontal plane that is an extension of a line through both inner canthi
Melia	A suffix meaning "limb" (e.g., amelia—missing limb; brachymelia—short limb)
Ocular hypertelorism	Increased distance between the pupils of the two eyes
Plagiocephaly	A condition in which head shape is asymmetric in the sagittal or coronal planes; can result from asymmetry in suture closure or from asymmetry of brain growth
Posterior parietal hair whorl	A single whorl occurs to the right or left of midline and within 2 cm anterior to the posterior fontanel in 95% of cases. The whorl represents the focal point from which the posterior scalp skin was under growth tension during brain growth between the 10th and 16th wk of fetal development. Aberrant position of the whorl reflects an early defect in brain development
Postaxial polydactyly	Extra finger or toe present on the lateral side of the hand or foot
Preaxial polydactyly	Extra finger or toe present on the medial side of the hand or foot
Prominent lateral palatine ridges	Relative overgrowth of the lateral palatine ridges secondary to a deficit of tongue thrust into the hard palate
Scaphocephaly	A condition in which the head is elongated from front to back in the sagittal plane; most normal skulls are scaphocephalic
Shawl scrotum	The scrotal skin joins around the superior aspect of the penis and represents a mild deficit in full migration of the labial-scrotal folds
Short palpebral fissures	Decreased horizontal distance of the eye based on measurement from the inner to the outer canthus
Syndactyly	Incomplete separation of the fingers. It most commonly occurs between the 3rd and 4th fingers and between the 2nd and 3rd toes
Synophrys	Eyebrows that meet in the midline
Telecanthus	Lateral displacement of the inner canthi. The inner canthal distance is increased, but the inner pupillary distance is normal
Widow's peak	V-shaped midline, downward projection of the scalp hair in the frontal region. It represents an upper forehead intersection of the bilateral fields of periocular hair growth suppression. It usually occurs because the fields are widely spaced, as in ocular hypertelorism

cephaly will be recognized to have abnormal cortical migration (lissencephaly), which markedly narrows the differential diagnosis for microcephaly. Other studies such as echocardiography and renal ultrasonography can be useful to identify additional major or minor malformations.

LABORATORY. The laboratory evaluation of the dysmorphic child is helpful but complex. Cytogenetics with Giemsa-banded peripheral leukocyte karyotype (or chromosome analysis) is the gold standard and should be performed in most evaluations of the dysmorphic child (Table 108-6). A practical reason for ordering the karyotype early in the diagnostic process is that it typically takes 7–12 days for results. Due to many chromosome abnormalities including derangement of the termini (telomeres) of the chromosomes, assays should detect small (submicroscopic) duplications or deletions of the termini of the chromosomes. These tests are clinically available and may be considered if standard chromosome analysis is negative. Eventually, a whole genome assay by array comparative genomic hybridization (CGH) will be used to assess patients for chromosome imbalances.

TABLE 108-5. Minor Anomalies and Phenotype Variants

Craniofacial	**Hand**
Large fontanel	Simian creases
Flat or low nasal bridge	Bridged upper palmar creases
Saddle nose, upturned nose	Clinodactyly of fifth digit
Mild micrognathia	Hyperextensibility of thumbs
Cutis aplasia of scalp	Single flexion crease of fifth digit (hypoplasia of middle phalanx)
Eye	Partial cutaneous syndactyly
Inner epicanthal folds	Polydactyly
Telecanthus	Short, broad thumb
Slanting of palpebral fissures	Narrow, hyperconvex nails
Hypertelorism	Hypoplastic nails
Brushfield spots	Camptodactyly
Ear	Shortened fourth digit
Lack of helical fold	**Foot**
Posteriorly rotated pinna	Partial syndactyly of second and third toes
Preauricular with or without auricular skin tags	Asymmetric toe length
Small pinna	Clinodactyly of second toe
Auricular (preauricular) pit or sinus	Overlapping toes
Folding of helix	Nail hypoplasia
Darwinian tubercle	Wide gap between hallux and second toe
Crushed (crinkled) ear	Deep plantar crease between hallux and second toe
Asymmetric ear sizes	**Others**
Low-set ears	Mild calcaneovalgus
Skin	Hydrocele
Dimpling over bones	Shawl scrotum
Capillary hemangioma (face, posterior neck)	Hypospadias
Mongolian spots (African Americans, Asians)	Hypoplasia of labia majora
Sacral dimple	
Pigmented nevi	
Redundant skin	
Cutis marmorata	

Approximately 15% of newborns have one minor anomaly, 0.8% have two minor anomalies, and 0.5% have three. If two minor anomalies are present, the probability of an underlying syndrome or a major anomaly (congenital heart disease, renal, central nervous system, limbic) is fivefold that in the general population. If three minor anomalies are present, the probability that there is a major anomaly is 20–30%.

From Kliegman RM, Greenbaum LA, Lye PS: *Practical Strategies in Pediatric Diagnosis and Therapy*, 2nd ed. Philadelphia, Elsevier Saunders, 2004.

Molecular testing for mutations that cause pleiotropic developmental anomaly syndromes is available for many disorders. In most cases, however, such testing should not be performed as screening tests, but instead ordered thoughtfully after the differential diagnosis has been narrowed. It may eventually become feasible to implement high throughput genomic DNA sequencing as a diagnostic tool, but existing molecular diagnostics are not used for diagnostic screening purposes.

Historically, dysmorphic and metabolic disorders were considered distinct classes of disease. However, as in the case of the Smith-Lemli-Opitz syndrome, metabolic abnormalities of the fetus can cause malformations. A general metabolic screen should be performed unless the differential diagnosis leads the clinician to strongly suspect a nonmetabolic disease.

DIAGNOSIS. The examining physician should gather the following data: pedigree, perinatal, and pediatric (for older children) history and have an appreciation for the natural history of the disorder. At this point, the physician has examined the child and identified abnormal physical features, and obtained appropriate imaging studies and preliminary interpretations.

TABLE 108-6. Clinical Indications for Karyotype Analysis

At least one major and two minor malformations
At least two major malformations
Development OR growth retardation with two or more major or minor anomalies

Note: These are guidelines and prudence dictates the use of the chromosome analysis in cases that may not meet these general guidelines. These guidelines are for situations where such an analysis is strongly recommended.

The clinician now organizes the findings by their specificity into potential developmental pathophysiologic processes. The specificity assessment is the simplest. If a child has a patent ductus arteriosus (PDA), mild growth retardation, mild microcephaly, and holoprosencephaly (MRI finding of failure to lateralize the forebrain), micropenis, and ptosis, these findings can be prioritized. The PDA, ptosis, mild growth retardation, and mild microcephaly are nonspecific findings (present in many disorders or often as isolated features not part of a syndrome), whereas holoprosencephaly and micropenis are present in fewer syndromes and are never normal variants. By recognizing this, the clinician can search for disorders that include both holoprosencephaly and micropenis. This can be performed manually using the features index of a textbook such as *Smith's Recognizable Patterns of Human Malformation* (Jones, 2005) or a computerized database such as the Winter-Baraitser dysmorphology database (http://www.lmdatabases.com/about_lmd.html). Searching for disorders with both findings leads quickly to a modest list of only 21 disorders. One of these is SLOS. The identification of this possible diagnosis causes the physician to return to the bedside, realize that many of the nonspecific features in the child are common in SLOS, and make a tentative diagnosis of this disorder. Although holoprosencephaly is an uncommon manifestation of SLOS, this manifestation makes sense because of the known pathogenetic link between sonic hedgehog and cholesterol biosynthesis. Because this disorder is caused by mutations in the sterol delta-7-reductase gene and is associated with elevated 7-dehydrocholesterol, the pediatrician can initiate a consultation with the clinical geneticist for suspected SLOS. The consultant can then confirm the diagnosis and begin the process of identifying a laboratory to verify the diagnosis.

MANAGEMENT AND COUNSELING. Management of the affected patient and genetic counseling are essential aspects of the approach to the dysmorphic patient. Children with Down syndrome have a high incidence of hypothyroidism and children with achondroplasia have a high incidence of cervicomedullary junction constriction. Herein lies one of the many benefits of early and accurate diagnosis because anticipatory guidance and medical monitoring of patients for syndrome-specific medical risks can prolong and improve the quality of life. When a diagnosis is made, the treating physicians can refer to published information on the natural history and management of particular syndromes through articles, genetics reference texts, and, for more common disorders, general pediatric texts.

The second major benefit of an accurate diagnosis is that it provides data for appropriate recurrence risk estimates. Genetic disorders may only cause direct effects on one member of the family, but the diagnosis of the condition has implications for the entire family. One or both parents may be carriers; siblings may be carriers or may wish to know their at-risk status when they reach their reproductive years. Recurrence risk provision is one facet of genetic counseling, which should be a component of all evaluations for families affected with birth defects or other heritable disorders (Chapter 83).

Ang Jr. ESBC, Gluncic V, Duque A, et al: Prenatal exposure to ultrasound waves impacts neuronal migration in mice. *PNAS* 2006;103:12903–12910.

Berry RJ, Buehler JW, Strauss LT, et al: Birth weight–specific infant mortality due to congenital anomalies, 1960 and 1980. *Public Health Rep* 1987;102:171–181.

Boyle RJ: Effects of certain prenatal drugs on the fetus and newborn. *Pediatr Rev* 2002;23:17–24.

Breen DP, Davenport RJ: Teratogenicity of antiepileptic drugs. *BMJ* 2006; 333:615–616.

Cassidy SB, Allanson JE: *Management of Genetic Syndromes.* Hoboken, NJ, Wiley-Liss, 2005.

Cohen MM Jr: An introduction to sonic hedgehog signaling. In Epstein CJ, Erickson RP, Wynshaw-Boris A (eds): *Inborn Errors of Development: The Molecular Basis of Clinical Disorders of Morphogenesis.* New York, Oxford University Press, 2004.

Cooper WO, Hernandez-Diaz S, Arbogast PG, et al: Major congenital malformations after first-trimester exposure to ACE inhibitors. *N Engl J Med* 2006;354:2443–2451.

Epstein CJ: Human malformations and their genetic basis. In Epstein CJ, Erickson RP, Wynshaw-Boris A (eds): *Inborn Errors of Development: The Molecular Basis of Clinical Disorders of Morphogenesis.* New York, Oxford University Press, 2004.

Epstein CJ: The new dysmorphology: Application of insights from basic developmental biology to the understanding of human birth defects. Proc Natl Acad Sci U S A 1995;92:8566–8573.

Epstein CJ, Erickson RP, Wynshaw-Boris A (eds): *Inborn Errors of Development: The Molecular Basis of Clinical Disorders of Morphogenesis.* New York, Oxford University Press, 2004.

Gleeson JG: LIS1 and DCX and classical lissencephaly. In Epstein CJ, Erickson RP, Wynshaw-Boris A (eds): *Inborn Errors of Development: The Molecular Basis of Clinical Disorders of Morphogenesis.* New York, Oxford University Press, 2004.

Hall JG, Froster-Iskenius UG, Allanson JE: *Handbook of Normal Physical Measurements.* NewYork, Oxford Medical Publications, 1989.

Hassold TJ, Patterson D: *Down Syndrome: A Promising Future Together.* New York, Wiley-Liss, 1999.

Ho KS, Scott MP: Sonic hedgehog in the nervous system: Functions, modifications and mechanisms. *Curr Opin Neurobiol* 2002;12:57–63.

Hoekelman RA, Pless IB: Decline in mortality among young Americans during the 20th century: Prospects for reaching national mortality reduction goals for 1990. *Pediatrics* 1988;82:582–595.

Holmes LB: Inborn errors of morphogenesis. A review of localized hereditary malformations. *N Engl J Med* 1974;291:763–773.

Irons M: DHCR7 and the Smith-Lemli-Opitz (RSH) syndrome. In Epstein CJ, Erickson RP, Wynshaw-Boris A (eds): *Inborn Errors of Development: The Molecular Basis of Clinical Disorders of Morphogenesis.* New York, Oxford University Press, 2004.

Jones KL: *Smith's Recognizable Patterns of Human Malformation.* Philadelphia, WB Saunders, 2005.

Kingston HM: Genetic assessment and pedigree analysis. In Rimoin DL, Connor JM, Pyeritz RE, Korf BR (eds): *Emery and Rimoin's Principles and Practice of Medical Genetics,* 4th ed. New York, Churchill Livingstone, 2002.

Mitchell LE, Adzick NS, Melchionne J, et al: Spina bifida. *Lancet* 2004;364:1885–1895.

Miyamo A, Weinmaster G: Introduction to notch signaling. In Epstein CJ, Erickson RP, Wynshaw-Boris A (eds): *Inborn Errors of Development: The Molecular Basis of Clinical Disorders of Morphogenesis.* New York, Oxford University Press, 2004.

Mulliken JB: The craniofacial surgeon as amateur geneticist. *J Craniofac Surg* 2002;13:3–17.

Oskarsdottir S, Persson C, Eriksson BO, et al: Presenting phenotype in 100 children with 22q11 deletion syndrome. *Eur J Pediatr* 2005;164: 146–153.

Park SM, Mathur R, Smith GCS: Congenital anomalies after treatment for infertility. *BMJ* 2006;333:665–666.

Petrij F, Breuning MH, Hennekam RCM, et al: CBP and the Rubinstein-Taybi syndrome. In Epstein CJ, Erickson RP, Wynshaw-Boris A (eds): *Inborn Errors of Development: The Molecular Basis of Clinical Disorders of Morphogenesis.* New York, Oxford University Press, 2004.

Plunkett KS, Simpson JL: A general approach to genetic counseling. *Obstet Gynecol Clin North Am* 2002;29:265–276.

Rimoin DL, Connor JM, Pyeritz RE, Korf BR (eds): *Emery and Rimoin's Principles and Practice of Medical Genetics,* 4th ed. New York, Churchill Livingstone, 2002.

Salman M, Jhanwar SC, Ostrer H. 2004. Will the new cytogenetics replace the old cytogenetics? *Clin Genet* 66:265–275.

Turnpenny PD, Kusumi K: DLL3 and spondylocostal dysostosis. In Epstein CJ, Erickson RP, Wynshaw-Boris A (eds): *Inborn Errors of Development: The Molecular Basis of Clinical Disorders of Morphogenesis.* New York, Oxford University Press, 2004.

Villavicencio EH, Walterhouse DO, Iannaccone PM: The sonic hedgehog-patched-GLI pathway in human development and disease. *Am J Hum Genet* 2000;67:1047–1054.

Wilson GN. 1992. Genomics of human dysmorphogenesis. *Am J Med Genet* 42:187–196.

Yagi H, Furutani Y, Hamada H, et al: Role of TBX1 in human del22q11.2 syndrome. *Lancet* 2003;362:1366–1373.

Chapter 109 ■ Infections of the Neonatal Infant Barbara J. Stoll

109.1 • Pathogenesis and Epidemiology

Infections are a frequent and important cause of neonatal and infant morbidity and mortality. As many as 2% of fetuses are infected in utero, and up to 10% of infants have infections in the 1st mo of life. Neonatal infections are unique: (1) Infectious agents can be transmitted from the mother to the fetus or newborn infant by diverse modes. (2) Newborn infants are less capable of responding to infection because of 1 or more immunologic deficiencies. (3) Coexisting conditions often complicate the diagnosis and management of neonatal infections. (4) The clinical manifestations of newborn infections vary and include subclinical infection, mild to severe manifestations of focal or systemic infection, and, rarely, congenital syndromes resulting from in utero infection. The timing of exposure, inoculum size, immune status, and virulence of the etiologic agent influence the expression of disease. (5) Maternal infection that is the source of transplacental fetal infection is often undiagnosed during pregnancy because the mother was either asymptomatic or had nonspecific signs and symptoms at the time of acute infection. (6) A wide variety of etiologic agents infect the newborn, including bacteria, viruses, fungi, protozoa, and mycoplasmas. (7) Immature, very low birthweight (VLBW) newborns have improved survival but remain in the hospital for a long time in an environment that puts them at continuous risk for acquired infections.

109.2 • Modes of Transmission and Pathogenesis

PATHOGENESIS OF INTRAUTERINE INFECTION. Intrauterine infection is a result of clinical or subclinical maternal infection with a variety of agents (cytomegalovirus [CMV], *Treponema pallidum, Toxoplasma gondii,* rubella virus, varicella virus, parvovirus B19) by hematogenous transplacental transmission to the fetus. Transplacental infection may occur at any time during gestation, and signs and symptoms may be present at birth or be delayed for months or years (Fig. 109-1). Infection may result in early spontaneous abortion, congenital malformation, intrauterine growth restriction, premature birth, stillbirth, acute or delayed disease in the neonatal period, or asymptomatic persistent infection with sequelae later in life. In some cases, no apparent effects are seen in the newborn infant.

The timing of infection during gestation affects the outcome. First trimester infection may alter embryogenesis, with resulting congenital malformations (congenital rubella) (see Chapter 244). Third trimester infection often results in active infection at the time of delivery (toxoplasmosis, syphilis) (see Chapters 287 and 215). Infections that occur late in gestation may lead to a delay in clinical manifestations until some time after birth (syphilis).

Maternal infection is a necessary prerequisite for transplacental infection. For some etiologic agents (rubella), maternal immunity is effective and antibody is protective for the fetus. For other agents (CMV), maternal antibody may ameliorate the outcome of infection or have no effect (see Chapter 252). Even without maternal antibody, transplacental transmission of infection to a fetus is variable because the placenta may function as an effective barrier.

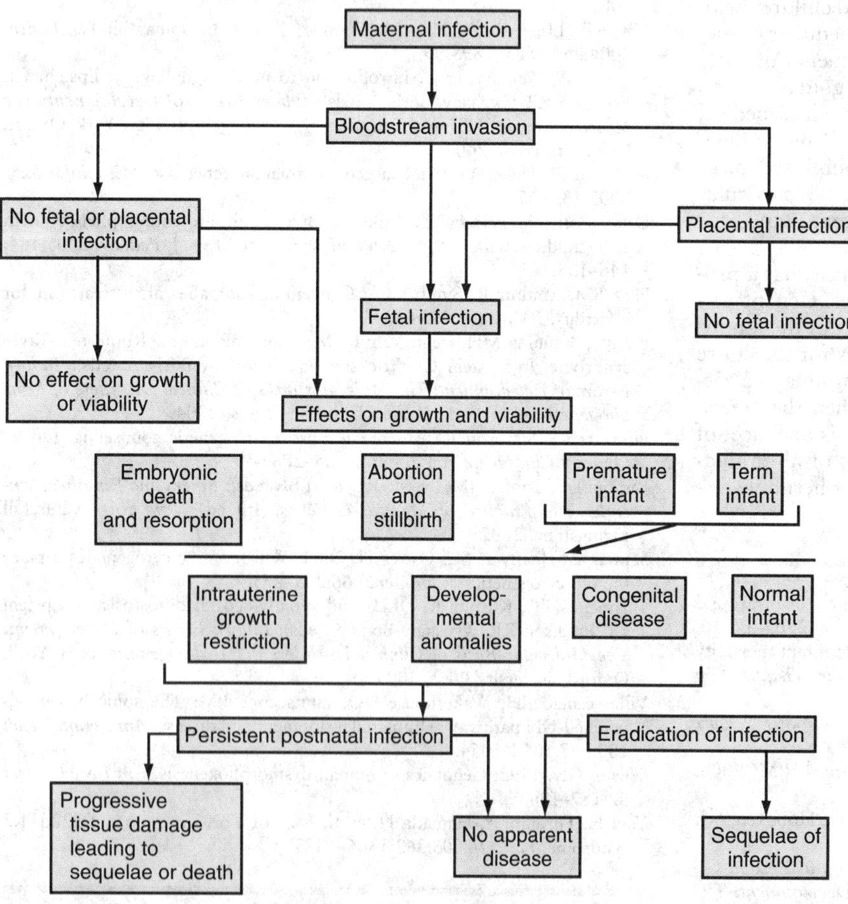

Figure 109-1. Pathogenesis of hematogenous transplacental infections. (From Klein JO, Remington JS: Current concepts of infections of the fetus and newborn infant. In Remington JS, Klein JO [eds]: *Infectious Diseases of the Fetus and Newborn Infant,* 5th ed. Philadelphia, WB Saunders, 2002.)

PATHOGENESIS OF ASCENDING BACTERIAL INFECTION. In most cases, the fetus or neonate is not exposed to potentially pathogenic bacteria until the membranes rupture and the infant passes through the birth canal and/or enters the extrauterine environment. The human birth canal is colonized with aerobic and anaerobic organisms that may result in ascending amniotic infection and/or colonization of the neonate at birth. Vertical transmission of bacterial agents that infect the amniotic fluid and/or vaginal canal may occur in utero or more commonly during labor and/or delivery (Fig. 109-2). **Chorioamnionitis** results from microbial invasion of amniotic fluid, often as a result of prolonged rupture of the chorioamniotic membrane. Amniotic infection may also occur with apparently intact membranes or with a relatively brief duration of membrane rupture. The term *chorioamnionitis* refers to the clinical syndrome of intrauterine infection, which includes maternal fever, with or without local or systemic signs of chorioamnionitis, (uterine tenderness, foul smelling vaginal discharge/amniotic fluid, maternal leukocytosis, maternal and/or fetal tachycardia). Chorioamnionitis may also be asymptomatic, only diagnosed by amniotic fluid analysis or pathologic examination of the placenta. Histologic chorioamnionitis is inversely related to gestational age at birth (Fig. 109-3) and directly related to duration of membrane rupture. Greater than 24 hr was once considered prolonged rupture of membranes because microscopic evidence of inflammation of the membranes is uniformly present when the duration of rupture exceeds 24 hr. At 18 hr of membrane rupture, however, the incidence of early-onset disease with group B streptococcus (GBS) increases significantly; longer than 18 hr is the appropriate cutoff for increased risk of neonatal infection. Difficult or traumatic delivery and premature delivery are also associated with an increased frequency of neonatal infection.

Bacterial colonization does not always result in disease. Factors influencing which colonized infant will develop disease are not well understood but include prematurity, underlying illness, invasive procedures, inoculum size, virulence of the infecting organism, the innate immune system and host response, and transplacental maternal antibodies (Fig. 109-4). Aspiration or ingestion of bacteria in amniotic fluid may lead to congenital pneumonia or systemic infection, with manifestations becoming apparent before delivery (fetal distress, tachycardia), at delivery (perinatal asphyxia), or after a latent period of a few hours (respiratory distress, shock). Aspiration or ingestion of bacteria during the birth process may lead to infection after an interval of 1–2 days.

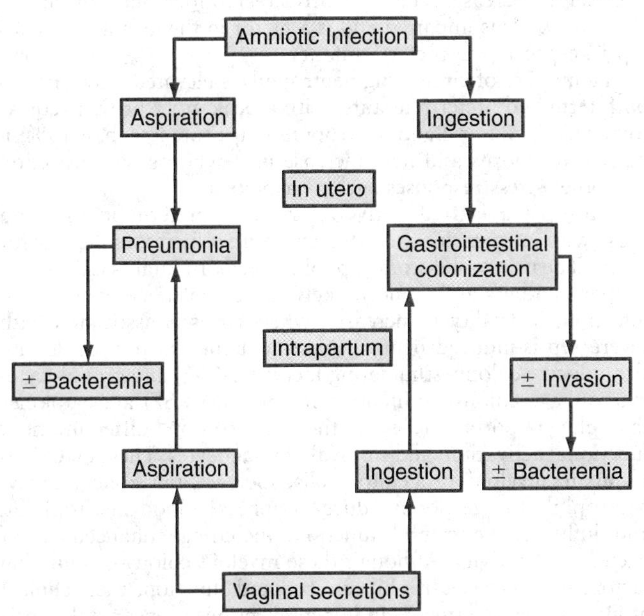

Figure 109-2. Pathways of ascending or intrapartum infection.

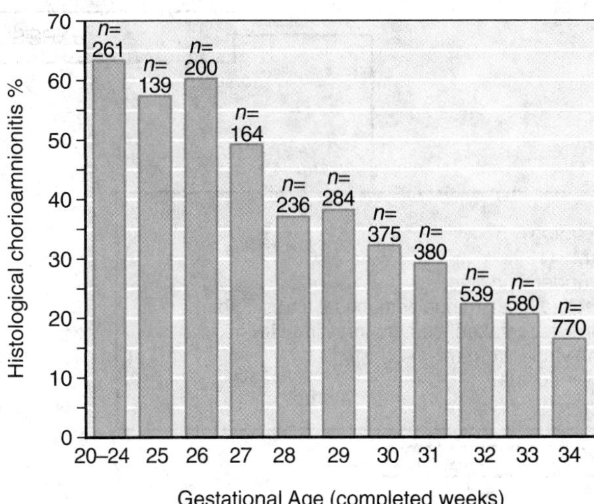

Figure 109-3. Histologic chorioamnionitis in liveborn preterm babies by gestational age (n = 3,928 babies). (From Lahra MM, Jeffery HE: A fetal response to chorioamnionitis is associated with early survival after preterm birth. *Am J Obstet Gynecol* 2004;190:147–151.)

Resuscitation at birth, particularly if it involves endotracheal intubation, insertion of an umbilical vessel catheter, or both, is associated with an increased risk of bacterial infection. Explanations include the presence of infection at the time of birth or acquisition of infection during the invasive procedures associated with resuscitation.

PATHOGENESIS OF LATE-ONSET POSTNATAL INFECTIONS. After birth, neonates are exposed to infectious agents in the nursery or in the community. Postnatal infections may be transmitted by direct contact with hospital personnel, the mother, or other family members; from breast milk (HIV, CMV); or from inanimate sources such as contaminated equipment. The most common source of postnatal infections in hospitalized newborns is hand contamination of health care personnel.

Most cases of meningitis result from hematogenous dissemination. Less often, meningitis results from contiguous spread as a result of contamination of open neural tube defects, congenital sinus tracts, or penetrating wounds from fetal scalp sampling or internal fetal electrocardiographic monitors. Abscess formation, ventriculitis, septic infarcts, hydrocephalus, and subdural effusions are complications of meningitis that occur more often in newborn infants than in older children.

109.3 • IMMUNITY

Decreased function of neutrophils, and other cells involved in the response to infection have been demonstrated in both term and preterm infants. Preterm infants may also have low concentrations of immunoglobulins. Both preterm and term infants have quantitative and qualitative defects of the complement system. Despite these alterations in immune function, the rate of systemic infection in newborns is low. All newborns enter an unsterile environment, but infection develops in only a few.

IMMUNOGLOBULINS. IgG is actively transported across the placenta, with concentrations in a full-term infant comparable to or higher than those in the mother. The specificity of IgG antibody in cord blood is dependent on the mother's previous antigenic

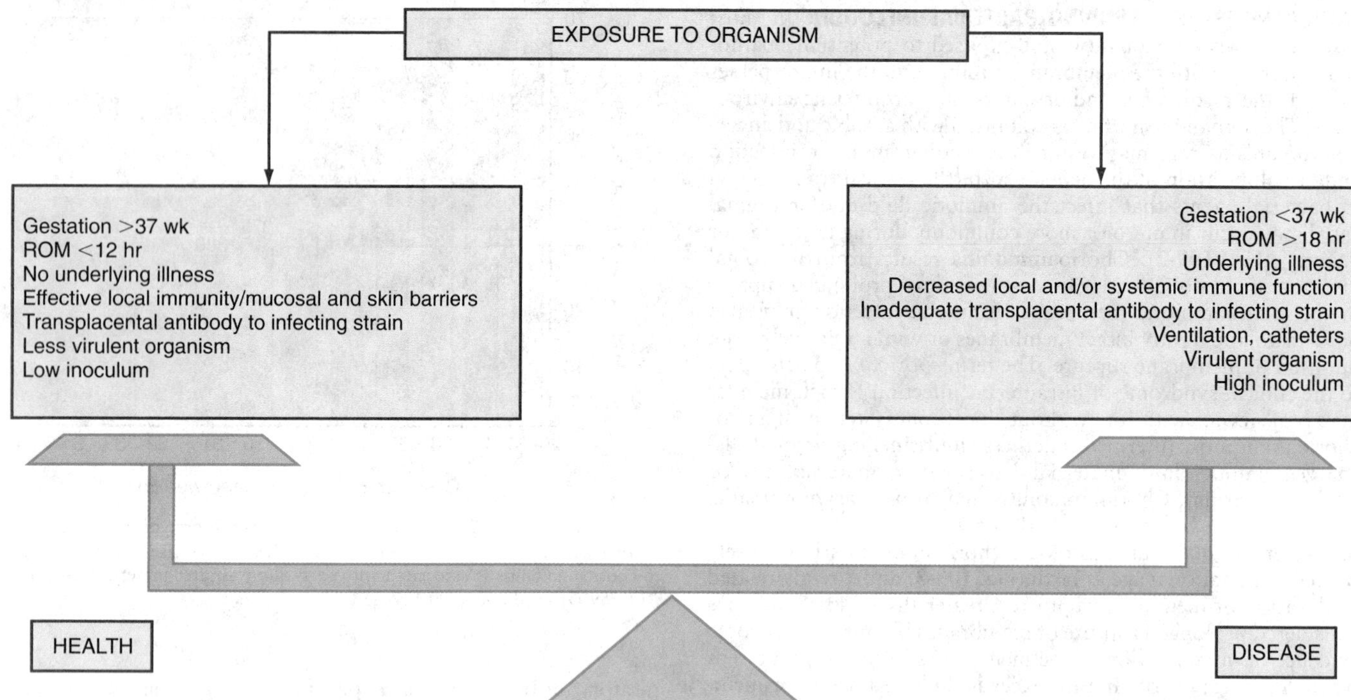

Figure 109-4. Factors influencing the balance between health and disease in neonates exposed to a potential pathogen. ROM, rupture of membranes. (Adapted from Baker CJ: Group B streptococcal infections. *Clin Perinatol* 1997;24:59–70.)

exposure and immunologic response. In premature infants, cord IgG levels are directly proportional to gestational age. Studies of type-specific IgG antibodies to GBS have shown that the ratio of cord to maternal serum concentrations is 1.0, 0.5, and 0.3 at term, 32 wk, and 28 wk of gestation, respectively. Levels of maternally derived IgG fall rapidly after birth. Infants with birthweights <1,500 g become significantly hypogammaglobulinemic, with mean plasma IgG concentrations in the range of 200–300 mg/dL in the 1st wk of life. Other classes of immunoglobulins are not transferred across the placenta, although a fetus can synthesize IgA and IgM in response to intrauterine infection.

The presence of passively transferred specific IgG antibody in adequate concentration provides neonates protection against infections to which protection is mediated by that antibody (tetanus, encapsulated bacteria such as GBS). Specific bactericidal and opsonic antibodies against enteric gram-negative bacteria are predominantly in the IgM class. Newborn infants usually lack antibody-mediated protection against *Escherichia coli* and other *Enterobacteriaceae*.

COMPLEMENT. The complement system mediates bactericidal activity against certain organisms such as *E. coli* and functions as an opsonin with antibody in the phagocytosis of bacteria such as GBS. No transplacental passage of complement from the maternal circulation takes place. A fetus begins to synthesize complement components as early as the 1st trimester. Full-term newborn infants have slightly diminished classical pathway complement activity and moderately diminished alternative pathway activity. Considerable variability, however, is seen in both the concentration and activity of complement components. Premature infants have lower levels of complement components and less complement activity than full-term newborns do. These deficiencies contribute to diminished complement-derived chemotactic activity and to a diminished ability to opsonize certain organisms in the absence of antibody. Opsonization of *Staphylococcus aureus* is normal in neonatal sera, but various degrees of impairment have been noted with GBS and *E. coli*.

NEUTROPHILS. Quantitative and qualitative deficiencies of the phagocyte system contribute to the newborns' susceptibility to infection. Neutrophil migration (chemotaxis) is abnormal at birth in both term and preterm infants. Neonatal neutrophils have decreased adhesion, aggregation, and deformability, all of which may delay the response to infection. Abnormal expression of cell membrane adhesion molecules (the β_2 integrins and selectins) and abnormalities in the neonatal neutrophil cytoskeleton contribute to abnormal chemotaxis. With adequate opsonization, phagocytosis and killing by neutrophils are comparable in newborn infants and adults. In the face of infectious or noninfectious stress (respiratory distress syndrome), however, the ability of neonatal neutrophils to phagocytose gram-negative (but not gram-positive) bacteria is decreased. The oxidative respiratory burst of neonatal neutrophils is impaired and is a factor in the increased risk of sepsis, especially in preterm infants.

The number of circulating neutrophils is elevated after birth in both term and preterm infants, with a peak at 12 hr that returns to normal by 22 hr. Band neutrophils constitute less than 15% in normal newborns and may increase in newborns with infection and other stress responses such as asphyxia.

Neutropenia is frequently observed in preterm infants and those with intrauterine growth restriction; it increases the risk for sepsis. The neutrophil storage pool in newborn infants is 20–30% of that in adults and is more likely to be depleted in the face of infection. Mortality is increased when sepsis is associated with severe sepsis-induced neutropenia and bone marrow depletion. Granulocyte colony–stimulating factor (G-CSF) and granulocyte-macrophage colony–stimulating factor (GM-CSF) are cytokines that play important roles in the proliferation, differentiation, functional activation, and survival of phagocytes. These cytokines stimulate myeloid progenitor cells, increase the bone marrow neutrophil storage pool, induce peripheral blood neutrophilia, and influence neutrophil function, including enhancement of bactericidal activity. Although these myeloid colony–stimulating factors influence neutrophil number and function, their clinical utility in the treatment and/or prevention of neonatal sepsis remains undetermined.

MONOCYTE-MACROPHAGE SYSTEM. The monocyte-macrophage system consists of circulating monocytes and tissue macrophages, particularly in the liver, spleen, and lung. Activated macrophages are involved in antigen presentation, phagocytosis, and immune modulation. The number of circulating monocytes in neonatal blood is normal, but the mass or function of macrophages in the reticuloendothelial system is diminished, particularly in preterm infants. In both term and preterm infants, chemotaxis of monocytes is impaired; this impairment affects the inflammatory response in tissues and the results of delayed hypersensitivity skin tests. Monocytes from neonates ingest and kill microorganisms as well as monocytes from adults.

NATURAL KILLER CELLS. Natural killer (NK) cells are a subgroup of lymphocytes that are cytolytic against cells infected with viruses. NK cells also lyse cells coated with antibody in a process called antibody-dependent cell-mediated cytotoxicity (ADCC). NK cells appear early in gestation and are present in cord blood in numbers equivalent to those in adults; neonatal NK cells have decreased cytotoxic activity and ADCC in comparison to adult cells. The diminished cytotoxicity against herpes simplex virus (HSV)–infected cells may predispose to disseminated HSV infection in newborns (see Chapter 249).

CYTOKINES/INFLAMMATORY MEDIATORS. The patient's response to infection and clinical outcome involves a balance between proinflammatory and anti-inflammatory cytokines. Several adverse neonatal outcomes, including brain injury, necrotizing enterocolitis, and bronchopulmonary dysplasia, may be mediated by the cytokine response to infection in the mother, fetus, or newborn. The mediators that have been studied in newborns include tumor necrosis factor-α (TNFα), interleukin 1 (IL-1), IL-4, IL-6, IL-8, IL-10, IL-12, platelet-activating factor, and the leukotrienes. The release of various inflammatory mediators in response to infection offers the potential opportunity to facilitate an early laboratory diagnosis of infection. Potential surrogate markers for bacterial sepsis, pneumonia, and necrotizing enterocolitis include TNFα, IL-6, and IL-8.

Innate immunity involves nonspecific cellular and humoral responses to an infectious agent without previous exposure. Recognition of pathogens is initiated by soluble components in plasma (including mannose binding lectin) and by recognition of receptors on monocytes and other cells. Toll-like receptors play an important role in pathogen recognition. Genetic polymorphisms (mutations) of various proteins involved in the immune response may increase the risk and severity of neonatal infections. The neutrophil is another important cellular component of innate immunity. Neutrophil granules contain many enzymes; 1 protein, bactericidal/permeability-increasing protein (BPI), binds to the endotoxin in the cell wall of gram-negative bacteria. It facilitates opsonization and prevents the inflammatory response to endotoxin. BPI activity may be decreased in neonates.

109.4 • Etiology of Fetal and Neonatal Infection

A number of agents may infect newborns in utero, intrapartum, or postpartum (Tables 109-1 and 109-2). Intrauterine transplacental infections of significance to the fetus and/or newborn include syphilis, rubella, CMV, toxoplasmosis, parvovirus B19, and varicella. Although HSV, HIV, hepatitis B virus (HBV), hepatitis C virus, and tuberculosis (TB) can each result in transplacental infection, the most common mode of transmission for these agents is intrapartum during labor and delivery with passage through an infected birth canal (HIV, HSV, HBV) or postnatal from contact with an infected mother or caretaker (TB).

TABLE 109-1. Bacterial Causes of Systemic Neonatal Infections

BACTERIA	EARLY ONSET	LATE ONSET, MATERNAL ORIGIN	LATE ONSET, NOSOCOMIAL	LATE ONSET, COMMUNITY
GRAM POSITIVE				
Clostridia	+		+	*
Enterococci	+		++	
Group B streptococcus	+++	+	+	+
Listeria monocytogenes	+	+		
Other streptococci	++			+
Staphylococcus aureus	+		++	+
Staphylococcus, coagulase negative	+		+++	
Streptococcus pneumoniae	+			++
Viridans streptococcus	+		++	
GRAM NEGATIVE				
Bacteroides	+		+	
Campylobacter	+			
Citrobacter			+	+
Enterobacter			+	
Escherichia coli	+++		+	++
Haemophilus influenzae	+			+
Klebsiella			+	
Neisseria gonorrhoeae	+			
Neisseria meningitidis	+		+	
Proteus			+	
Pseudomonas			+	
Salmonella		+		+
Serratia			+	
OTHERS				
Treponema pallidum	+	+		
Mycobacterium tuberculosis		+		

**Clostridium tetani* in some developing countries.
+, relative frequency.

Any microorganism inhabiting the genitourinary or lower gastrointestinal tract may cause intrapartum and postpartum infection. The most common bacteria are GBS, enteric organisms, gonococci, and chlamydiae. The more common viruses are CMV, HSV, and HIV.

Agents that commonly cause **nosocomial** infection are coagulase-negative staphylococci, gram-negative bacilli *(E. coli, Klebsiella pneumoniae, Salmonella, Enterobacter, Citrobacter, Pseudomonas aeruginosa, Serratia)*, enterococci, *S. aureus*, and *Candida*. Viruses contributing to nosocomial neonatal infection include enteroviruses, CMV, hepatitis A, adenoviruses, influenza, respiratory syncytial virus, rhinovirus, parainfluenza, HSV, and rotavirus. Community-acquired pathogens such as *Streptococcus pneumoniae* may also cause infection in newborn infants after discharge from the hospital.

Congenital pneumonia may be caused by CMV, rubella virus, and *T. pallidum* and, less commonly, by the other agents producing transplacental infection (Table 109-3). Microorganisms causing pneumonia acquired during labor and delivery include

TABLE 109-2. Nonbacterial Causes of Systemic Neonatal Infections

VIRUSES	MYCOPLASMA
Adenovirus	*M. hominis*
Cytomegalovirus	*Ureaplasma urealyticum*
Enteroviruses	**FUNGI**
Herpes simplex virus	*Candida* species
HIV	*Malassezia* species
Parvovirus	**PROTOZA**
Rubella virus	Plasmodia
Varicella-zoster virus	*Toxoplasma gondii*
	Trypanosoma cruzi

TABLE 109-3. Etiologic Agents of Neonatal Pneumonia According to Timing of Acquisition

TRANSPLACENTAL	PERINATAL	POSTNATAL
Cytomegalovirus	Anaerobic bacteria	Adenovirus
Herpes simplex virus	*Chlamydia*	*Candida* species*
Mycobacterium tuberculosis	Cytomegalovirus	Coagulase-negative staphylococci
Rubella virus	Enteric bacteria	Cytomegalovirus
Treponema pallidum	Group B streptococci	Echoviruses
Varicella-zoster virus	*Haemophilus influenzae*	Enteric bacteria*
	Herpes simplex virus	Influenza viruses A, B
	Listeria monocytogenes	Parainfluenza
	Mycoplasma	*Pseudomonas**
		Respiratory syncytial virus
		Staphylococcus aureus
		Mycobacterium tuberculosis

*More likely in infants undergoing mechanical ventilation, with indwelling catheters, or after abdominal surgery.

GBS, gram-negative enteric aerobes, *Listeria monocytogenes,* genital *Mycoplasma, Chlamydia trachomatis,* CMV, HSV, and *Candida* species.

The bacteria responsible for most cases of nosocomial pneumonia typically include staphylococcal species, gram-negative enteric aerobes, and occasionally, *Pseudomonas.* Fungi are responsible for an increasing number of systemic infections acquired during prolonged hospitalization of preterm neonates. Respiratory viruses cause isolated cases and outbreaks of nosocomial pneumonia. These viruses, usually endemic during the winter months and acquired from infected hospital staff or visitors to the nursery, include respiratory syncytial virus, parainfluenza virus, influenza viruses, and adenovirus. Respiratory viruses are the single most important cause of community-acquired pneumonia and are usually contracted from infected household contacts.

The most common bacterial causes of **neonatal meningitis** are GBS, *E. coli,* and *L. monocytogenes. S. pneumoniae,* other streptococci, non-typable *Haemophilus influenzae,* both coagulase-positive and coagulase-negative staphylococci, *Klebsiella, Enterobacter, Pseudomonas, T. pallidum,* and *Mycobacterium tuberculosis* may also produce meningitis.

109.5 • Epidemiology of Early- and Late-Onset Neonatal Infections

The terms *early-onset infection* and *late-onset infection* refer to the age at onset of infection in the neonatal period (Table 109-4). Originally divided arbitrarily as infections occurring before and after 1 wk of life, it is more useful to separate early- and late-onset infections according to peripartum pathogenesis. Early-onset infections are acquired before or during delivery. Late-onset infections are acquired after delivery in the normal newborn nursery, neonatal intensive care unit (NICU), or the community. The age at onset depends on the timing of vertical transmission and the virulence of the infecting organism. Pyogenic early infections such as GBS are usually clinically apparent within the 1st 24 hr of life. Late, late-onset infections (onset after 1 mo of life) occur, particularly in VLBW preterm infants or term infants requiring prolonged neonatal intensive care for other chronic problems.

The incidence of neonatal bacterial sepsis varies from 1 to 4 cases per 1,000 live births in developed countries, with considerable fluctuation over time and with geographic location. Term male infants have an approximately twofold higher incidence of sepsis than term females. This sex difference is less clear in preterm low-birthweight (LBW) infants. Attack rates of neonatal sepsis increase significantly in LBW infants in the presence of maternal chorioamnionitis, congenital immune defects, mutations of genes involved in the innate immune system, asplenia, galactosemia *(E. coli),* and malformations leading to high inocula of bacteria (obstructive uropathy).

Intrapartum antibiotics are used to reduce vertical transmission of GBS, as well as lessen neonatal morbidity after preterm rupture of membranes. After the introduction of selective intrapartum antibiotic prophylaxis to prevent perinatal transmission of GBS, rates of early-onset neonatal GBS infection in the United States declined from 1.7 cases per 1,000 live births to 0.6 per 1,000. Intrapartum chemoprophylaxis does not reduce the rates of late-onset GBS disease. Intrapartum antibiotics have little or no effect on the rates of non-GBS pathogens. Of concern is an increase in gram-negative infections (especially *E. coli*) in VLBW and possibly term infants in the face of a reduction in early GBS sepsis by intrapartum antibiotics.

The incidence of meningitis in newborn infants is 0.2–0.4 cases per 1,000 live births and is higher in preterm infants. Bacterial meningitis may be associated with sepsis or may occur as a local meningeal infection. Meningitis develops in fewer than 20% of newborn infants with early-onset invasive bacterial infections. One third of VLBW infants with late-onset meningitis have negative blood cultures. The discordance in blood and cerebrospinal fluid (CSF) cultures suggests that meningitis may be underdiagnosed among VLBW infants and emphasizes the need for culture of CSF in such infants when late-onset sepsis is suspected.

PREMATURITY. The most important neonatal factor predisposing to infection is prematurity or LBW. Preterm infants have a 3- to 10-fold higher incidence of infection than full-term normal birth-weight infants. Possible explanations include: (1) Maternal genital tract infection is considered to be an important cause of preterm labor, with an increased risk of vertical transmission to the newborn (Figs. 109-5 and 109-6). (2) The frequency of intra-amniotic infection is inversely related to gestational age (see Fig. 109-3). (3) Premature infants have documented immune dysfunction. (4) Premature infants often require prolonged intravenous access, endotracheal intubation, or other invasive procedures that provide a portal of entry or impair barrier and clearance mechanisms.

NOSOCOMIAL INFECTIONS. Nosocomial (hospital-acquired) infections are responsible for significant morbidity and late mortality in hospitalized newborns. Many define nosocomial infections as infections occurring after 3 days of life, which are not directly acquired from the mother's genital tract. The Centers for Disease Control and Prevention (CDC) defines a nosocomial infection as any infection occurring after admission to the NICU that was not transplacentally acquired. Rates of nosocomial infection in healthy term infants who are either rooming in with their mothers

TABLE 109-4. Neonatal Infection by Age of Onset

CHARACTERISTICS	EARLY ONSET	LATE ONSET	LATE, LATE (NOSOCOMIAL) ONSET
Age at onset	Birth to 7 days usually <72 hr	7 to 30 days	>30 days
Maternal obstetric complications	Common	Uncommon	Varies
Prematurity	Frequent	Varies	Usual
Organism source	Maternal genital tract	Maternal genital tract/environment	Environment/community
Manifestation	Multisystem	Multisystem or focal	Multisystem or focal
Site	Normal nursery, NICU, community	NICU, community	NICU, community

NICU, neonatal intensive care unit.

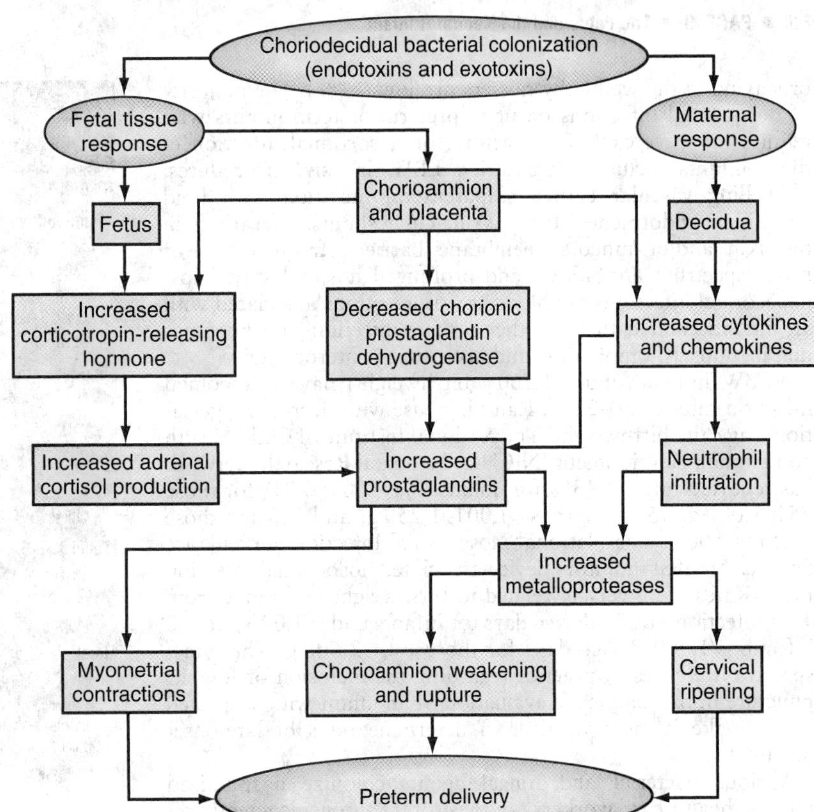

Figure 109-5. Potential pathways from choriodecidual bacterial colonization to preterm delivery. (From Goldenberg RL, Hauth JA, Andrews WW: Intrauterine infection and preterm delivery. *N Engl J Med* 2000;342:1500–1507. Copyright 2000, Massachusetts Medical Society.)

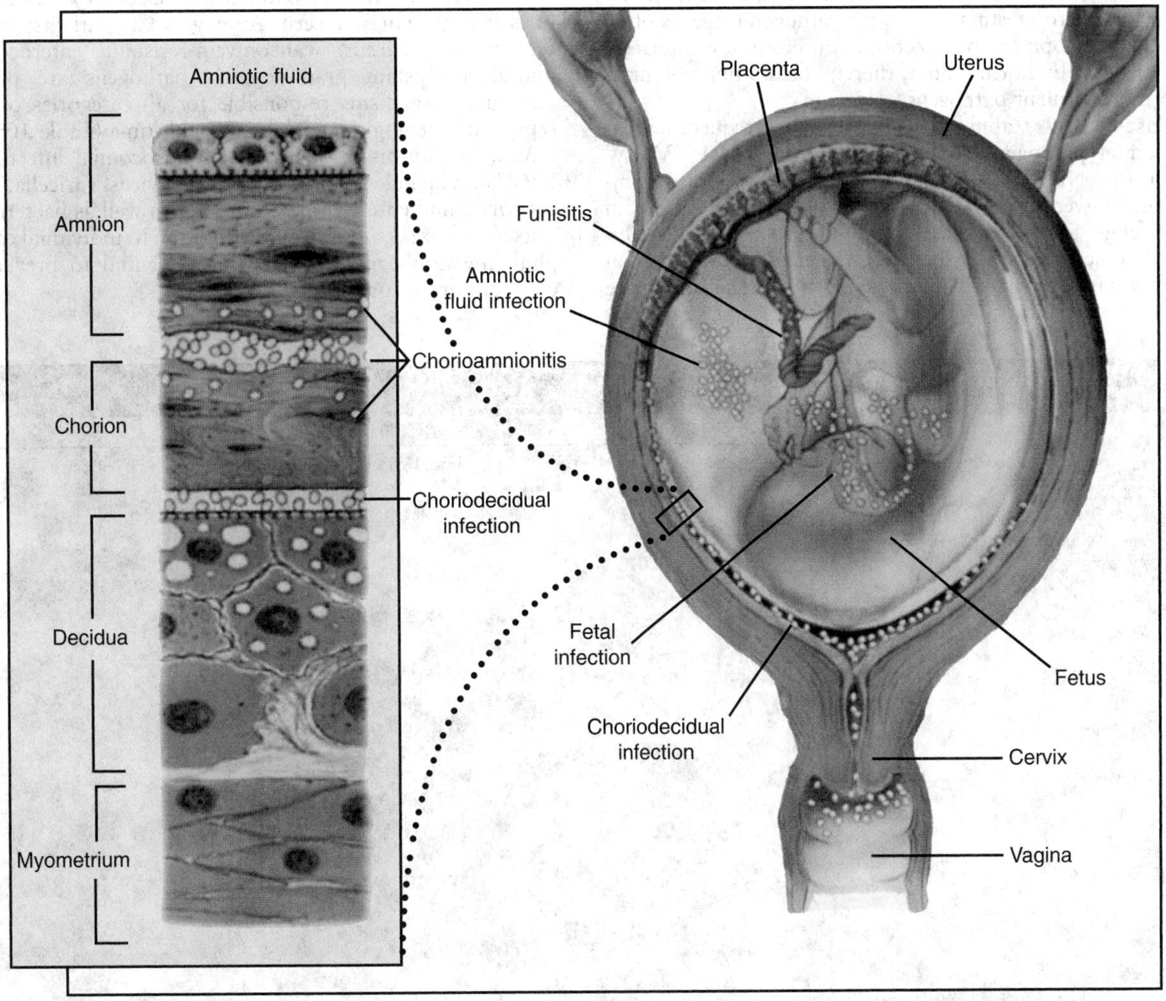

Figure 109-6. Potential sites of bacterial infection within the uterus. (From Goldenberg RL, Hauth JA, Andrews WW: Intrauterine infection and preterm delivery. *N Engl J Med* 2000;342:1500–1507. Copyright 2000, Massachusetts Medical Society.)

or staying in the well baby nursery are low (<1%). The majority of nosocomial infections occur in preterm or term infants who require intensive care. Risk factors for nosocomial infection in these infants include prematurity, LBW, invasive procedures, indwelling vascular catheters, parenteral nutrition with lipid emulsions, endotracheal tubes, ventricular shunts, alterations in the skin and/or mucous membrane barriers, frequent use of broad-spectrum antibiotics, and prolonged hospital stay. Most nosocomial infections are bloodstream infections associated with an intravascular catheter. Other serious infections are pneumonia, meningitis, omphalitis, and necrotizing enterocolitis.

VLBW infants (under 1,500 g birthweight) have nosocomial infection rates of 20–25%. Rates increase with decreasing gestational age and birthweight. The National Institute of Child Health and Human Development (NICHD) Neonatal Research Network has reported rates of 43% for infants 401–750 g; 28% for those 751–1,000 g; 15% for those 1,001–1,250 g; and 7% for those 1,251–1,500 g. The National Nosocomial Infection Surveillance System (NNISS) monitors device-associated nosocomial infection rates. Rates are inversely related to birthweight and range from 11.4 infections/1,000 device days for infants under 1,000 g to 3.8 infections/1,000 device days for those over 2,500 g. The widespread differences in practice regarding the inclusion of lumbar puncture in the diagnostic evaluation of an infant with suspected sepsis make it more difficult to determine rates of late-onset meningitis.

Various bacterial and fungal agents colonize hospitalized infants, health care workers, and visitors. Pathogenic agents can be transmitted by direct contact or indirectly via contaminated equipment, intravenous fluids, medications, blood products, or enteral feedings. Colonization of the infant's skin, umbilicus, and respiratory or gastrointestinal tract with pathogenic agents often precedes the development of infection. Antibiotic use interferes with colonization by normal flora, thereby facilitating colonization with more virulent pathogens.

Coagulase-negative staphylococci are the most frequent neonatal nosocomial pathogens. Among a cohort of 6,215 VLBW infants in the NICHD Neonatal Research Network, gram-positive agents were associated with 70%, gram-negative with 18%, and fungi with 12% of cases of late-onset sepsis (Table 109-5). Coagulase-negative staphylococcus, the single most common organism, was isolated in 48% of these infections. The emergence of nosocomial bacterial pathogens resistant to multiple antibiotics is a growing concern. Among NICU patients, methicillin-resistant *S. aureus,* vancomycin-resistant enterococci, and multidrug-resistant gram-negative pathogens are particularly alarming. Organisms responsible for all categories of neonatal sepsis and meningitis may change with time (Table 109-6).

Viral organisms may also cause nosocomial infection in the NICU and include respiratory syncytial virus, varicella, influenza, rotavirus, and enteroviruses. For viral as well as bacterial agents, nursery outbreaks may occur in addition to individual cases. Hospital infection control policies are essential to prevent and/or contain nursery outbreaks.

TABLE 109-5. Distribution of Pathogens Associated with the 1st Episode of Late-Onset Sepsis in VLBW Infants: NICHD Neonatal Research Network, September 1, 1998, Through August 31, 2000

ORGANISM*	N	%
Gram-positive organisms	**922**	**70.2**
Staphylococcus—coagulase negative	629	47.9
Staphylococcus aureus	103	7.8
Enterococcus spp.	43	3.3
Group B streptococci	30	2.3
Other	117	8.9
Gram-negative organisms	**231**	**17.6**
Escherichia coli	64	4.9
Klebsiella	52	4.0
Pseudomonas	35	2.7
Enterobacter	33	2.5
Serratia	29	2.2
Other	18	1.4
Fungi	**160**	**12.2**
Candida albicans	76	5.8
Candida parapsilosis	54	4.1
Other	30	2.3
Total	**1,313**	**100**

*Patients with dual infections and patients with presumed coagulase-negative staphylococci (CONS) contaminants excluded. According to the definitions in text, 276 (44%) CONS were definite infections and 353 (56%) were possible infections.

NICHD, National Institute of Child Health and Human Development; VLBW, very low birthweight.

From Stoll BJ, Hansen N, Fanaroff AA, et al: Late-onset sepsis in very low birthweight neonates: The experience of the NICHD neonatal research network. *Pediatrics* 2002;110:285–291.

TABLE 109-6. Neonatal Inborn Sepsis: 1928–2003

	% IN EACH STUDY*						
	1928–1932	1933–1943	1944–1957	1958–1965	1966–1978	1979–1988	1989–2003
Gram-positive aerobic bacteria							
S. aureus	28	9	13	3	5	3	8
Coagulase-negative staphylococcus				1	1	8	29
β-hemolytic streptococci							
Group B		5	6	1	32	37	12
Group D			2	10	4	8	9
Nongrouped and other	38	36	10				
Viridans streptococci		2		3	1	3	1
S. pneumoniae	5	11	5	3	1	1	
L. monocytogenes		2	2		1	1	<1
Gram-negative aerobic bacteria							
E. coli	26	25	37	45	32	20	11
Klebsiella-Enterobacter				11	12	3	11
Pseudomonas	3		21	15	2	3	3
Haemophilus				1	4	5	1
Salmonella			2		1	1	
Gram-negative anaerobic bacteria					1	3	
Fungi					2	1	8
Other		9	3	5	5	1	6
n	39	44	62	73	239	147	520

*Percentages do not always sum up to 100% as a result of rounding.

From Bizzarro MJ, Raskind C, Baltimore RS, et al: Seventy-five years of neonatal sepsis at Yale: 1928–2003. *Pediatrics* 2005;116:595–602.

The mean age at onset of the 1st episode of late-onset nosocomial sepsis is 2–3 wk, independent of the infecting pathogen. Nosocomial infections increase the risk of adverse outcomes, including prolonged hospitalization and mortality.

Active surveillance for nosocomial infection is essential in monitoring overall rates of infection, rates of infection with specific pathogens, and antibiotic susceptibility patterns and in identifying clusters of cases or true infectious outbreaks. Surveillance is based on the ongoing review of nursery infections and data from the microbiology laboratory; routine surveillance to detect colonization is not indicated. Culture results should indicate the bacterial isolate and the antimicrobial sensitivity pattern. Assessment of other microbial markers (biotype, serotype, DNA fingerprint) is helpful in epidemics. During epidemics, investigation of possible reservoirs of infection, modes of transmission, and risk factors is necessary. Identification of colonized infants and nursery personnel is also helpful.

Infections acquired after discharge from the nursery are usually community acquired. They have the same epidemiologic considerations as other community-acquired infections in infants and children, except for protection provided by maternal antibody.

109.6 • Clinical Manifestations of Transplacental Intrauterine Infections

Infection with agents that cross the placenta (CMV, *T. pallidum*, *T. gondii*, rubella, parvovirus B19) may be asymptomatic at birth or may cause a spectrum of disease ranging from relatively mild symptoms to multisystem involvement with severe and life-threatening complications. For some agents, disease is characterized by chronicity, recurrence, or both (in the mother and infant), and the agent may cause ongoing injury. Clinical signs and symptoms do not help make a specific etiologic diagnosis, but rather raise suspicion of an intrauterine infection and help distinguish these infections from acute bacterial infections that occur during labor and delivery. The following signs and symptoms are common to many of these agents (Table 109-7): intrauterine growth restriction, microcephaly or hydrocephalus, intracranial calcifications, chorioretinitis, cataracts, myocarditis, pneumonia, hepatosplenomegaly, direct hyperbilirubinemia, anemia, thrombocytopenia, hydrops fetalis, and skin manifestations, including petechiae, purpura, and vesicles. Many of these agents cause late sequelae, even if the infant is asymptomatic at birth. These adverse outcomes include sensorineural hearing loss, visual disturbances (including blindness), seizures, and neurodevelopmental abnormalities.

BACTERIAL SEPSIS

Neonates with bacterial sepsis may have either nonspecific signs and symptoms or focal signs of infection (Tables 109-8 and 109-9), including temperature instability, hypotension, poor perfusion with pallor and mottled skin, metabolic acidosis, tachycardia or bradycardia, apnea, respiratory distress, grunting, cyanosis, irritability, lethargy, seizures, feeding intolerance, abdominal distention, jaundice, petechiae, purpura, and bleeding. International criteria are noted in Table 109-10. The initial manifestation may involve only limited symptomatology and only 1 system, such as apnea alone or tachypnea with retractions or tachycardia, or it may be an acute catastrophic manifestation with multiorgan dysfunction. Infants should be reevaluated over time to determine whether the symptoms have progressed from mild to severe. Later complications of sepsis include respiratory failure, pulmonary hypertension, cardiac failure, shock, renal failure, liver dysfunction, cerebral edema or thrombosis, adrenal hemorrhage and/or insufficiency, bone marrow dysfunction (neutropenia, thrombo-

TABLE 109-7. Clinical Manifestations of Transplacental Infections

MANIFESTATION	PATHOGEN
Intrauterine Growth Restriction	*CMV, Plasmodium, rubella, toxoplasmosis, Treponema pallidum, Trypanosoma cruzi, VZV*
Congenital Anatomic Defects	
Cataracts	Rubella
Heart defects	Rubella
Hydrocephalus	HSV, lymphocytic choriomeningitis virus, rubella, toxoplasmosis
Intracranial calcification	CMV, HIV, toxoplasmosis, *T. cruzi*
Limb hypoplasia	VZV
Microcephaly	CMV, HSV, rubella, toxoplasmosis
Microphthalmos	CMV, rubella, toxoplasmosis
Neonatal Organ Involvement	
Anemia	CMV, parvovirus, *Plasmodium*, rubella, toxoplasmosis, *T. cruzi, T. pallidum*
Carditis	Coxsackieviruses, rubella, *T. cruzi*
Encephalitis	CMV, enteroviruses, HSV, rubella, toxoplasmosis, *T. cruzi, T. pallidum*
Hepatitis	CMV, enteroviruses, HSV
Hepatosplenomegaly	CMV, enteroviruses, HIV, HSV, *Plasmodium*, rubella, *T. cruzi, T. pallidum*
Hydrops	Parvovirus, *T. pallidum*, toxoplasmosis
Lymphadenopathy	CMV, HIV, rubella, toxoplasmosis, *T. pallidum*
Osteitis	Rubella, *T. pallidum*
Petechiae, purpura	CMV, enteroviruses, rubella, *T. cruzi*
Pneumonitis	CMV, enteroviruses, HSV, measles, rubella, toxoplasmosis, *T. pallidum*, VZV
Retinitis	CMV, HSV, lymphocytic choriomeningitis virus, rubella, toxoplasmosis, *T. pallidum*, West Nile virus
Rhinitis	Enteroviruses, *T. pallidum*
Skin lesions	Entroviruses, HSV, measles, rubella, *T. pallidum*, VZV
Thrombocytopenia	CMV, enteroviruses, HIV, HSV, rubella, toxoplasmosis, *T. pallidum*
Late Sequelae	
Convulsions	CMV, enteroviruses, rubella, toxoplasmosis
Deafness	CMV, rubella, toxoplasmosis
Dental/skeletal	Rubella, *T. pallidum*
Endocrinopathies	Rubella, toxoplasmosis
Eye pathology	HSV, rubella, toxoplasmosis, *T. cruzi, T. pallidum*. VZV
Hepatitis	Hepatitis B
Mental retardation	CMV, HIV, HSV, rubella, toxoplasmosis, *T. cruzi*, VZV
Nephrotic syndrome	*Plasmodium, T. pallidum*

CMV, cytomegalovirus; HSV, herpes simplex virus; VZV, varicella-zoster virus.

TABLE 109-8. Initial Signs and Symptoms of Infection in Newborn Infants

GENERAL	**CARDIOVASCULAR SYSTEM**
Fever, temperature instability	Pallor; mottling; cold, clammy skin
"Not doing well"	Tachycardia
Poor feeding	Hypotension
Edema	Bradycardia
GASTROINTESTINAL SYSTEM	**CENTRAL NERVOUS SYSTEM**
Abdominal distention	Irritability, lethargy
Vomiting	Tremors, seizures
Diarrhea	Hyporeflexia, hypotonia
Hepatomegaly	Abnormal Moro reflex
RESPIRATORY SYTEM	**IRREGULAR RESPIRATIONS**
Apnea, dyspnea	Full fontanel
Tachypnea, retractions	High-pitched cry
Flaring, grunting	**HEMATOLOGIC SYSTEM**
Cyanosis	Jaundice
RENAL SYSTEM	Splenomegaly
Oliguria	Pallor
	Petechiae, purpura
	Bleeding

TABLE 109-9. Manifestations of Neonatal Bacterial Infections

	TIME		OCCURRENCE	
	EARLY ONSET	LATE ONSET	COMMON	UNCOMMON
Abdomen				
Peritonitis	+	+	+	
Hepatitis	+	+		+
Adrenal abscess	+	+		+
Gallbladder hydrops	+	+		+
Brain				
Meningitis	+	+	+	
Abscess		+	+	
Subdural empyema		+	+	
Cerebritis	+	+	+	
Ventriculitis		+	+	
Cardiovascular				
Endovascular infection		+	+	
Endocarditis	+	+		+
Pericarditis	+	+		+
Myocarditis	+	+		+
Ocular				
Conjunctivitis	+	+	+	
Endophthalmitis	+	+		+
Chorioretinitis		+		+
Osteoarticular				
Arthritis	+	+		+
Osteomyelitis		+		+
Dactylitis		+		+
Respiratory Tract				
Pneumonia	+	+	+	
Ethmoiditis	+	+		+
Otitis media		+		+
Mastoiditis		+		+
Salivary glands		+		+
Retropharyngeal cellulitis		+		+
Empyema	+	+	+	
Skin, Soft Tissue				
Breast abscess	+	+	+	
Facial cellulitis	+	+		+
Adenitis		+		+
Fasciitis	+	+		+
Impetigo		+	+	
Purpura fulminans	+	+		+
Omphalitis		+		+
Scalp abscess	+	+		+
Abscess of cystic hygroma		+		+
Urinary tract infection	+	+	+	
No Focus				
Bacteremia	+	+	+	
Sepsis	+	+	+	

cytopenia, anemia), and disseminated intravascular coagulopathy (DIC).

A variety of noninfectious conditions can occur together with neonatal infection or can make the diagnosis of infection more difficult. Respiratory distress syndrome (RDS) secondary to surfactant deficiency can coexist with bacterial pneumonia. Because bacterial sepsis can be rapidly progressive, the physician must be alert to the signs and symptoms of possible infection and initiate diagnostic evaluation and empirical therapy in a timely manner. The **differential diagnosis** of many of the signs and symptoms that suggest infection is extensive; these noninfectious disorders must also be considered (Table 109-11).

SYSTEMIC INFLAMMATORY RESPONSE SYNDROME

The clinical manifestations of infection depend on the virulence of the infecting organism and the body's inflammatory response.

TABLE 109-10. Clinical Criteria for the Diagnosis of Sepsis

	IMCI CRITERIA FOR SEVERE BACTERIAL INFECTION*	WHO YOUNG INFANT STUDY GROUP†
Convulsions	X	X
Respiratory rate >60 breaths/min	X	X (divided by age group)
Severe chest indrawing	X	X
Nasal flaring	X	
Grunting	X	
Bulging fontanel	X	
Pus draining from the ear	X	
Redness around umbilicus extending to the skin	X	
Temperature > 37.7°C (or feels hot) or <35.5°C (or feels cold)	X	X
Lethargic or unconscious	X	X (not aroused by minimal stimulus)
Reduced movements	X	X (change in activity)
Not able to feed	X	X (not able to sustain such)
Not attaching to the breast	X	
No suckling at all	X	
Crepitations		X
Cyanosis		X
Reduced digital capillary refill time		

*Any of the signs listed implies high suspicion of serious bacterial infection.
†Each symptom or sign is associated with a score. The score indicates the probability of disease.
IMCI, Integrated Management of Childhood Illness.
From Vergnano S, Sharland M, Kazembe P, et al: Neonatal sepsis: An international perspective. *Arch Dis Child Fetal Neonatal Ed* 2005;90:F220–F224.

The term *systemic inflammatory response syndrome (SIRS)* is most frequently used to describe this unique process of infection and the subsequent systemic response (see Chapters 68 and 176). In addition to infection, SIRS may result from trauma, hemorrhagic shock, other causes of ischemia, and pancreatitis.

TABLE 109-11. Serious Systemic Illness in Newborns: Differential Diagnosis of Neonatal Sepsis

Cardiac
Congenital: Hypoplastic left heart syndrome, other structural disease, PPHN
Acquired: Myocarditis, hypovolemic or cardiogenic shock, PPHN

Gastrointestinal
Necrotizing enterocolitis
Spontaneous GI perforation
Structural abnormalities

Hematologic
Neonatal purpura fulminans
Immune-mediated thrombocytopenia
Immune-mediated neutropenia
Severe anemia
Malignancies (congenital leukemia)
Hereditary clotting disorders

Metabolic
Hypoglycemia
Adrenal disorders: Adrenal hemorrhage, adrenal insufficiency, congenital adrenal hyperplasia
Inborn errors of metabolism: Organic acidurias, lactic acidoses, urea cycle disorders, galactosemia

Neurologic
Intracranial hemorrhage: spontaneous, child abuse
Hypoxic-ischemic encephalopathy
Neonatal seizures
Infant botulism

Respiratory
Respiratory distress syndrome
Aspiration pneumonia: Amniotic fluid, meconium, or gastric contents
Lung hypoplasia
Tracheoesophageal fistula
Transient tachypnea of the newborn

PPHN, persistent pulmonary hypertension of the newborn.

TABLE 109-12. Definitions of SIRS and Sepsis: Pediatric Patients

SIRS: The systemic inflammatory response to a variety of clinical insults, manifested by 2 or more of the following conditions:
- Temperature instability <35°C or >38.5°C
- Respiratory dysfunction
  - Tachypnea > 2 SD above the mean for age
  - Hypoxemia (PaO_2 <70 mm Hg on room air)
- Cardiac dysfunction
  - Tachycardia > 2 SD above the mean for age
  - Delayed capillary refill >3 sec
  - Hypotension > 2 SD below the mean for age
- Perfusion abnormalities
  - Oliguria (urine output <0.5 mL/kg/hr)
  - Lactic acidosis (elevated plasma lactate and/or arterial pH <7.25)
  - Altered mental status

Sepsis: The systemic inflammatory response to an infectious process

From Adams-Chapman I, Stoll, BJ: Systemic inflammatory response syndrome. *Semin Pediatr Infect Dis* 2001; 12:5–16.

Patients with SIRS have a spectrum of clinical symptoms that represent progressive stages of the pathologic process. In adults, SIRS is defined by the presence of 2 or more of the following: (1) fever or hypothermia, (2) tachycardia, (3) tachypnea, and (4) abnormal WBC count or an increase in immature forms. In neonates and pediatric patients, SIRS is manifested as temperature instability, respiratory dysfunction (altered gas exchange, hypoxemia, acute respiratory distress syndrome [ARDS]), cardiac dysfunction (tachycardia, delayed capillary refill, hypotension), and perfusion abnormalities (oliguria, metabolic acidosis) (Table 109-12). Increased vascular permeability results in capillary leak into peripheral tissues and the lungs, with resultant pulmonary and peripheral edema. DIC results in the more severely affected cases. The cascade of escalating tissue injury may lead to multisystem organ failure and death.

FEVER. Only about 50% of infected newborn infants have a temperature higher than 37.8°C (axillary). Fever in newborn infants does not always signify infection; it may be caused by increased ambient temperature, isolette or radiant warmer malfunction, dehydration, central nervous system (CNS) disorders, hyperthyroidism, familial dysautonomia, or ectodermal dysplasia. A single temperature elevation is infrequently associated with infection; fever sustained over 1 hr is more likely to be due to infection. Most febrile infected infants have additional signs compatible with infection, although a focus of infection is not always apparent. Acute febrile illnesses occurring later in the neonatal period may be caused by urinary tract infection, meningitis, pneumonia, osteomyelitis, or gastroenteritis, in addition to sepsis, thus underscoring the importance of a diagnostic evaluation that includes blood culture, urine culture, lumbar puncture, and other studies as indicated (see later). Many agents may cause these late infections, including HSV, enteroviruses, respiratory syncytial virus, and bacterial pathogens. In premature infants, hypothermia or temperature instability requiring increasing ambient (isolette, warmer) temperatures is more likely to accompany infection.

RASH. Cutaneous manifestations of infection include impetigo, cellulitis, mastitis, omphalitis, and subcutaneous abscesses. **Ecthyma gangrenosum** is indicative of infection with *Pseudomonas* species. The presence of small salmon-pink papules suggests *L. monocytogenes* infection. A vesicular rash is consistent with herpesvirus infection. The mucocutaneous lesions of *Candida albicans* are discussed elsewhere (see Chapter 231.1). Petechiae and purpura may have an infectious cause. Purple papulonodular lesions are referred to as "blueberry-muffin" rash and represent dermal erythropoiesis. Causes include congenital viral infections (CMV, rubella, and parvovirus), congenital neoplastic disease, and Rh hemolytic disease.

OMPHALITIS. Omphalitis is a neonatal infection resulting from inadequate care of the umbilical cord, which continues to be a problem, particularly in developing countries. The umbilical stump is colonized by bacteria from the maternal genital tract and the environment (see Chapter 105). The necrotic tissue of the umbilical cord is an excellent medium for bacterial growth. Omphalitis may remain a localized infection or may spread to the abdominal wall, the peritoneum, the umbilical or portal vessels, or the liver. Abdominal wall cellulitis or necrotizing fasciitis with associated sepsis and a high mortality rate may develop in infants with omphalitis. Prompt diagnosis and treatment is necessary to avoid serious complications.

TETANUS (SEE CHAPTER 208). Neonatal tetanus is a serious neonatal infection in developing countries. It results from unclean delivery and unhygienic management of the umbilical cord in an infant born to a mother who has not been immunized against tetanus. The surveillance **case definition** of neonatal tetanus requires the ability of a newborn to suck at birth and for the 1st few days of life, followed by an inability to suck starting between 3 and 10 days of age, difficulty swallowing, spasms, stiffness, seizures, and death. Bronchopneumonia, presumably resulting from aspiration, is a common complication and cause of death. Neonatal tetanus is a preventable disease. It can be prevented by immunizing mothers before or during pregnancy and by ensuring a clean delivery, sterile cutting of the umbilical cord, and proper cord care after birth.

PNEUMONIA. Early signs and symptoms of pneumonia may be nonspecific, including poor feeding, lethargy, irritability, cyanosis, temperature instability, and the overall impression that the infant is not well. Respiratory symptoms include grunting, tachypnea, retractions, flaring of the alae nasi, cyanosis, apnea, and progressive respiratory failure. If the infant is premature, these signs of progressive respiratory distress may be superimposed upon RDS or bronchopulmonary dysplasia (BPD). If an infant is being ventilated at the time of infection, the most prominent change may be the need for an increase in ventilatory support.

Signs of pneumonia on physical examination, such as dullness to percussion, change in breath sounds, and the presence of rales or rhonchi, are very difficult to appreciate in a neonate. X-rays of the chest may reveal new infiltrates or an effusion, but if the neonate has underlying RDS or BPD, it is very difficult to determine whether the radiographic changes represent a new process or worsening of the underlying disease.

The progression of neonatal pneumonia can be variable. Fulminant infection is most commonly associated with pyogenic organisms such as GBS (see Chapter 183). Onset may be during the 1st hours or days of life, with the infant often manifesting rapidly progressive circulatory collapse and respiratory failure. With early-onset pneumonia, the clinical course and radiographs of the chest may be indistinguishable from severe RDS.

In contrast to the rapid progression of pneumonia when caused by pyogenic organisms, older infants with community-acquired infection often have an indolent course. The onset is usually preceded by upper respiratory tract symptoms or conjunctivitis. A nonproductive cough ensues, and the degree of respiratory compromise is variable. Fever is usually absent, and radiographic examination of the chest shows focal or diffuse interstitial pneumonitis. This infection has been called the **"afebrile pneumonia syndrome"** and is generally caused by *C. trachomatis,* CMV, *Ureaplasma urealyticum,* or one of the respiratory viruses. Although *Pneumocystis carinii* was implicated in the original description of this syndrome, its etiologic role is now in doubt, except in newborns infected with HIV.

109.7 • DIAGNOSIS

The maternal history may provide important information about maternal exposure to infection, maternal immunity (natural or acquired), maternal colonization, and obstetric risk factors (prematurity, prolonged ruptured membranes, maternal chorioamnionitis) (see Table 102-13).

Sexually transmitted infections (STIs) that infect a pregnant woman are of particular concern to the fetus and newborn because of the possibility for intrauterine or perinatal transmission. All pregnant women and their partners should be queried about a history of STIs. Women should also be counseled about the need for timely diagnosis and therapy for infections during pregnancy. The CDC recommends the following screening tests and appropriate treatment of infected mothers: (1) All pregnant women should be offered voluntary and confidential HIV testing at the 1st prenatal visit. For women at high risk of infection during pregnancy (multiple sexual partners or STIs during pregnancy, intravenous drug use), repeat testing in the 3rd trimester is recommended. (2) A serologic test for syphilis should be performed on all pregnant women at the 1st prenatal visit. Repeat screening early in the 3rd trimester and again at delivery is recommended for women who had positive serology in the 1st trimester and for those at high risk for infection during pregnancy. (3) A serologic test for hepatitis B surface antigen (HBsAg) should be performed at the 1st prenatal visit and repeated late in pregnancy in those who are initially negative but at high risk for infection. (4) A maternal genital culture for *C. trachomatis* should be performed at the 1st prenatal visit. Young women (under 25 yr) and those at increased risk for infection (new or multiple partners during pregnancy) should be retested during the 3rd trimester. (5) A maternal genital culture for *Neisseria gonorrhoeae* should be performed at the 1st prenatal visit for women at risk and for those who live in areas with a high prevalence of gonorrhea. Repeat testing in the 3rd trimester is recommended for those at continued risk. (6) Evaluation for bacterial vaginosis should be considered at the 1st prenatal visit for asymptomatic women at high risk for preterm labor. (7) The CDC has recommended universal screening for rectovaginal GBS colonization of all pregnant women at 35–37 wk gestation and a screening-based approach to selective intrapartum antibiotic prophylaxis against GBS (Fig. 109-7; see also Chapter 183).

SUSPECTED INTRAUTERINE INFECTION

The acronym *TORCH* refers to toxoplasmosis, other agents (syphilis, etc.), rubella, CMV, and HSV. Although the term may be helpful in remembering some of the etiologic agents of intrauterine infection, the TORCH battery of serologic tests has a poor diagnostic yield, and appropriate specific diagnostic studies should be selected for each etiologic agent under consideration. CMV and HSV require culture or polymerase chain reaction (PCR) methods, whereas syphilis, toxoplasmosis, and rubella are diagnosed by specific serologic methods (Table 109-13).

In most cases of suspected fetal infection, concern is not raised until the pregnant woman has been ill for several weeks or, in retrospect, after delivery. At this time, the maternal immune response to the suspected pathogen may no longer reflect an acute infection; that is, the specific IgM response is no longer detectable and the IgG response has already reached a plateau. Many of the pathogen-specific IgM serologic assays require considerable skill to perform and tend to be less reliable than the more common IgG assays. As a result, IgM assays can be either falsely negative or falsely positive.

Neonatal antibody titers are often difficult to interpret because IgG is acquired from the mother by transplacental passage and determination of neonatal IgM titers to specific pathogens is technically difficult to perform and not universally available. IgM titers to specific pathogens have high specificity but only moderate sensitivity; they should not be used to preclude infection. Paired maternal and fetal-neonatal IgG titers with higher newborn IgG levels or rising IgG titers during infancy may be used to diagnose some congenital infections (syphilis). Total cord blood IgM or IgA (neither are actively transported across the placenta to the fetus) and the presence of IgM-rheumatoid factor in neonatal serum are nonspecific tests for intrauterine infection.

If the likelihood of maternal infection with a known teratogenic agent is high, fetal ultrasound examination is recommended. If the examination demonstrates either a physical abnormality or delayed growth for gestational age, examination of a fetal blood sample may be warranted. **Cordocentesis** can provide a sufficient sample for both total and pathogen-specific IgM assays or for PCR or culture. The total IgM value is important because the normal fetal IgM level is <5 mg/dL. Any eleva-

TABLE 109-13. Evaluation of a Newborn for Infection or Sepsis

HISTORY (SPECIFIC RISK FACTORS)
Maternal infection during gestation or at parturition (type and duration of antimicrobial therapy)
Urinary tract infection
Chorioamnionitis
Maternal colonization with GBS, *Neisseria gonorrhoeae*, herpes simplex
Gestational age/birthweight
Multiple birth
Duration of membrane rupture
Complicated delivery
Fetal tachycardia (distress)
Age at onset (in utero, birth, early postnatal, late)
Location at onset (hospital, community)
Medical intervention
Vascular access
Endotracheal intubation
Parenteral nutrition
Surgery
EVIDENCE OF OTHER DISEASES*
Congenital malformations (heart disease, neural tube defect)
Respiratory tract disease (RDS, aspiration)
Necrotizing enterocolitis
Metabolic disease, e.g., galactosemia
EVIDENCE OF FOCAL OR SYSTEMIC DISEASE
General appearance, neurologic status
Abnormal vital signs
Organ system disease
Feeding, stools, urine output, extremity movement
LABORATORY STUDIES
Evidence of Infection
Culture from a normally sterile site (blood, CSF, other)
Demonstration of a microorganism in tissue or fluid
Antigen detection (urine, CSF)
Maternal or neonatal serology (syphilis, toxoplasmosis)
Autopsy
Evidence of Inflammation
Leukocytosis, increased immature/total neutrophil count ratio
Acute-phase reactants: CRP, ESR
Cytokines: interleukin 6
Pleocytosis in CSF or synovial or pleural fluid
Disseminated intravascular coagulation: fibrin split products
Evidence of Multiorgan System Disease
Metabolic acidosis: pH, P_{CO_2}
Pulmonary function: P_{O_2}, P_{CO_2}
Renal function: BUN, creatinine
Hepatic injury/function: bilirubin, ALT, AST ammonia, PT, PTT
Bone marrow function: neutropenia, anemia, thrombocytopenia

*Diseases that increase the risk of infection or may overlap with signs of sepsis.

ALT, alanine aminotransferase; AST, aspartate aminotransferase; BUN, blood urea nitrogen; CRP, C-reactive protein; CSF, cerebrospinal fluid; ESR, erythrocyte sedimentation rate; GBS, group B streptococci; P_{CO_2}, partial pressure of carbon dioxide; P_{O_2}, partial pressure of oxygen; PT, prothrombin time; PTT, partial thromboplastin time; RDS, respiratory distress syndrome.

Vaginal and rectal screening cultures at 35–37 wk gestation for ALL pregnant women (unless patient had GBS bacteriuria during the current pregnancy or a previous infant with invasive GBS disease)

Intrapartum prophylaxis indicated

Patients meeting any of the following criteria **SHOULD** receive intrapartum prophylaxis:

- Previous infant with invasive GBS disease, **OR**
- GBS bacteriuria during **current** pregnancy, **OR**
- Positive GBS screening culture during pregnancy (unless a planned cesarean delivery, in the absence of labor or amniotic membrane rupture, is performed), **OR**
- Unknown GBS status (culture not done, incomplete, or results unknown) **AND**
    - Delivery at <37 wk gestation,** **OR**
    - Amniotic membrane rupture ≥18 hours, **OR**
    - Intrapartum temperature ≥100.4°F (≥38.0°C)*

Intrapartum prophylaxis NOT indicated

If patient meets none of the stated criteria, intrapartum prophylaxis for GBS is **NOT** indicated. This includes the following circumstances:

- Previous pregnancy with a positive GBS screening culture (unless a culture was ALSO positive during the current pregnancy)
- Planned cesarean delivery performed in the absence of labor or membrane rupture (regardless of maternal GBS culture status)
- Negative vaginal and rectal GBS screening culture during the current pregnancy, regardless of intrapartum risk factors

*If amnionitis is suspected, broad-spectrum antibiotic therapy that includes an agent known to be active against GBS should replace GBS prophylaxis.
**If onset of labor or rupture of amniotic membranes occurs at <37 wk gestation AND there is a significant risk for preterm delivery (as assessed by the clinician), a suggested algorithm for GBS prophylaxis management is outlined below:

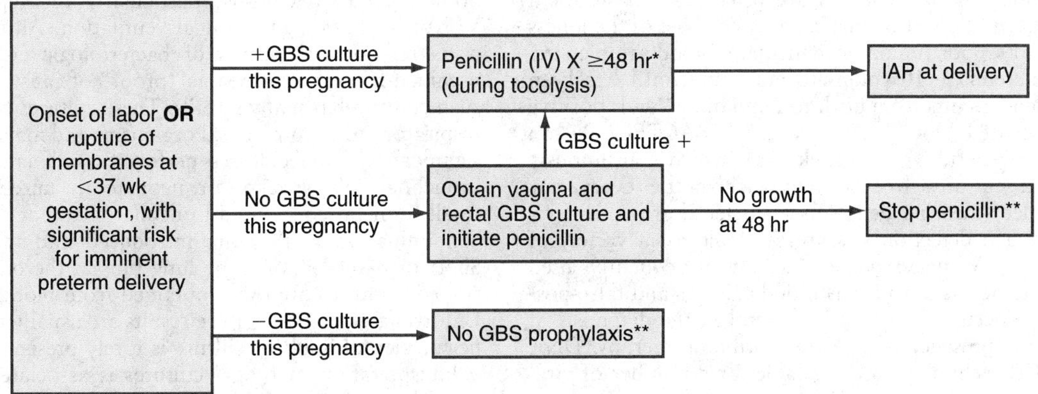

*Penicillin should be continued for a total of at least 48 hr, unless delivery occurs sooner. At the physician's discretion, antibiotic prophylaxis may be continued beyond 48 hr in a GBS culture-positive woman if delivery has not yet occurred. For women who are GBS culture positive, antibiotic

**If delivery has not occurred within 4 wk, a vaginal and rectal GBS screening culture should be repeated, and the patient should be managed as above, based on the result of the repeat culture.

Figure 109-7. Revised perinatal group B streptococcus (GBS) prevention guidelines. IAP, intrapartum antibiotic prophylaxis. (From Schrag S, Gorwitz R, Fultz-Butts K, et al: Prevention of perinatal group B streptococcal disease. Revised guidelines from CDC. *MMWR Recomm Rep* 2002;51:1–22.)

tion in total IgM may indicate an underlying fetal infection. Specific IgM antibody tests are available for CMV, *T. pallidum,* parvovirus B19, and toxoplasmosis. IgM tests are useful only when the results are strongly positive. A negative pathogen-specific IgM finding does not rule out that pathogen as a cause of fetopathy.

If maternal serologic studies point to a specific pathogen, it is sometimes possible to detect the organism in amniotic fluid or fetal blood (culture, PCR). Amniocentesis can be performed and the fluid sent for analysis. The presence of CMV, *Toxoplasma,* or parvovirus in amniotic fluid indicates that the fetus is infected and at high risk, but it does not always mean that the fetus will have severe sequelae. In contrast, HSV and varicella-zoster virus (VZV) are rarely isolated from amniotic fluid samples. CMV, *Toxoplasma,* and parvovirus can also be identified from cordocentesis sampling.

Parvovirus does not grow in the cell cultures commonly available in the virology laboratory. An IgM response is not always detectable in women with primary infection. When fetal parvovirus infection is suspected, testing of fetal blood or amniotic fluid by PCR is recommended in addition to testing for a specific IgM response in the fetus. PCR may also be used for the diagnosis of toxoplasmosis, CMV, HSV, rubella, and syphilis.

Neonatal infections with CMV, *Toxoplasma,* rubella, HSV, and syphilis present a diagnostic dilemma because: (1) their clinical features overlap and may initially be indistinguishable; (2) disease may be inapparent; (3) maternal infection is often asymptomatic; (4) special laboratory studies may be needed; and (5) appropriate treatment of toxoplasmosis, syphilis, and HSV, which may reduce significant long-term morbidity, is predicated on an accurate diagnosis. Common shared features that should suggest the diagnosis of an intrauterine infection include intrauterine growth restriction, hematologic involvement (anemia, neutropenia, thrombocytopenia, petechiae, purpura), ocular signs (chorioretinitis, cataracts, keratoconjunctivitis, glaucoma, microphthalmos), CNS signs (microcephaly, aseptic meningitis, hydrocephaly, intracranial calcifications), other organ system involvement (pneumonia, myocarditis, nephritis, hepatitis with hepatosplenomegaly, jaundice), and nonimmune hydrops. Diagnostic studies in newborns with suspected chronic intrauterine infection should specifically test for each diagnostic consideration. Systemic infections with CMV, HSV, and enteroviruses frequently involve the liver; if these infections are suspected, liver function tests should be performed. Neonatal HSV meningitis may be confirmed by isolation of the virus (or more often by PCR) from CSF or another site (skin, eye, mouth).

SUSPECTED BACTERIAL OR FUNGAL INFECTIONS

Bacterial or fungal infection is diagnosed by isolating the etiologic agent from a normally sterile body site (blood, CSF, urine, joint fluid). Obtaining 2 blood culture specimens by venipuncture from different sites avoids confusion caused by skin contamination and increases the likelihood of bacterial detection. Samples should be obtained from an umbilical catheter only at the time of initial insertion. A peripheral venous sample should also be obtained when blood is drawn for culture from central venous catheters. Although blood cultures are usually the basis for a diagnosis of bacterial infection, the bacteremic phase of the illness may be missed by poor timing or inadequate blood sample size. Low-level bacteremia (<10 colony-forming units/mL) has been observed in some infants from birth to 2 mo of age with positive cultures. Automated blood culture systems (BACTEC, Becton Dickinson; BacT/Alert, Organon Teknika), which continuously monitor blood cultures by checking each bottle every few minutes, have led to earlier detection of bacterial growth.

Bacterial antigen detection kits are available for a variety of organisms (GBS, *S. pneumoniae*) but are infrequently used because they are not as sensitive as blood cultures and false-positive results can occur. They may be helpful in the diagnosis of meningitis in the presence of previous antibiotic therapy. DNA probes and PCR technology are available for a number of viral and bacterial agents, but they are more often used in reference or research laboratories than in standard hospital microbiology laboratories.

Documentation of a positive blood culture is the first diagnostic criterion that must be met for sepsis (see Table 109-13). It is important to note, however, that some patients with bacterial infection may have negative blood cultures ("clinical infection"), and other approaches to identification of infection are needed. A variety of diagnostic markers of infection are being evaluated. Although the total WBC count and differential and the ratio of immature to total neutrophils have limitations in sensitivity and specificity, an immature-to-total neutrophil ratio of ≥0.2 suggests bacterial infection. Neutropenia is more common than neutrophilia in severe neonatal sepsis, but neutropenia also occurs in association with maternal hypertension, preeclampsia, and intrauterine growth restriction. Thrombocytopenia is a nonspecific indicator of infection. Tests to demonstrate an inflammatory response include C-reactive protein, procalcitonin, haptoglobin, fibrinogen, inflammatory cytokines (including IL-6, IL-8, and TNF-α), and cell surface markers. It is unclear which surrogate markers for infection are most helpful.

When the clinical findings suggest an acute infection and the site of infection is unclear, additional studies should be performed, including blood cultures, lumbar puncture, urine examination, and a chest x-ray. Urine should be collected by catheterization or suprapubic aspiration; urine culture for bacteria can be omitted in suspected early-onset infections because hematogenous spread to the urinary tract is rare at this point. Examination of the buffy coat with Gram or methylene blue stain may demonstrate intracellular pathogens. Demonstration of bacteria and inflammatory cells in Gram-stained gastric aspirates on the 1st day of life may reflect maternal amnionitis, which is a risk factor for early-onset infection. Stains of endotracheal secretions in infants with early-onset pneumonia may demonstrate intracellular bacteria, and cultures may reveal either pathogens or upper respiratory tract flora. Careful examination of the placenta can be helpful in the diagnosis of both chronic and acute intrauterine infections.

Diagnostic evaluation is indicated for asymptomatic infants born to mothers with chorioamnionitis. The probability of neonatal infection correlates with the degree of prematurity and bacterial contamination of the amniotic fluid. In an asymptomatic term infant whose mother has chorioamnionitis, 2 blood cultures should be performed and presumptive treatment initiated. There is controversy over whether a lumbar puncture is necessary for all term infants with suspected early-onset sepsis. If the blood culture result is positive or if the infant becomes symptomatic, lumbar puncture should definitely be performed. If the mother has been treated with antibiotics for chorioamnionitis, the newborn's blood culture result may be negative, and the clinician must rely on clinical observation and other laboratory tests.

The diagnosis of pneumonia in a neonate is usually presumptive; microbiologic proof of infection is generally lacking because lung tissue is not easily cultured. CDC definitions of pneumonia do not target newborns, particularly the high-risk group of VLBW infants on mechanical ventilation. Although some clinicians rely on the results of bacteriologic culture of material obtained from the trachea as "proof" of cause, interpretation of such cultures has many pitfalls. These cultures often reflect upper respiratory tract commensal organisms and may have no etiologic significance. Even cultures performed on material obtained by bronchoalveolar lavage in a neonate are unreliable because the small bronchoscopes used in neonates cannot be protected from contamination as they are introduced into the distal airways. Short of tissue obtained by lung biopsy, the only reliable bacteriologic cultures are those obtained from blood or pleural fluid. Unfortunately, blood culture results are usually negative, and sufficient pleural fluid for culture is rarely present.

Interpretation of fungal cultures is associated with the same problems as for bacterial cultures. Cultures of respiratory secretions for *U. urealyticum* and other genital *Mycoplasma* species are of little value because normal neonates are often colonized with these agents as a result of contamination with secretions from the maternal genital tract. Cultures for respiratory viruses and *C. trachomatis* may be valuable; they are never indigenous flora, and isolation of them therefore suggests an etiologic role.

Serologic tests may be helpful in evaluating neonates with suspected pneumonia. Although no serologic tests are useful for bacteria or fungi, reliable tests for respiratory viruses and *C. trachomatis* are available. Serologic tests for *U. urealyticum* are complicated, technically demanding, and therefore not clinically useful. Other tests of potential value in evaluating neonates with possible infectious pneumonitis are discussed under diagnosis of infections (see Chapter 169). The **differential diagnosis** of pneumonitis in neonates is broad and includes RDS, meconium aspiration syndrome, persistent pulmonary hypertension, diaphragmatic hernia, transient tachypnea of the newborn, congenital heart disease, and BPD.

The diagnosis of meningitis is confirmed by examination of CSF and identification of a bacterium, virus, or fungus by culture, antigen, or the use of PCR. The importance of the lumbar puncture (LP) as part of the diagnostic evaluation of the neonate with suspected sepsis has been the subject of debate; clinical practice varies. For term infants with suspected early-onset sepsis, many clinicians start with a blood culture and a complete blood count, because 70–85% of term neonates with bacterial meningitis have positive results on blood culture. Examination and culture of CSF are undertaken in term infants with symptoms and/or bacteremia. Many clinicians defer the LP in severely ill infants with suspected early-onset infection because of the fear of respiratory and/or cardiovascular compromise. In these situations, blood culture should be performed and treatment initiated for presumed meningitis until lumbar puncture can be safely performed.

Normal, uninfected infants from 0–4 wk of age may have elevated CSF protein levels of 84 ± 45 mg/dL, glucose of 46 ± 10 mg/dL, and elevated CSF leukocyte counts of 11 ± 10 with the 90th percentile being 22. The proportion of polymorphonuclear leukocytes is 2.2 ± 3.8%, with the 90th percentile being 6. Elevated CSF protein levels and leukocyte counts and hypoglycorrhachia may develop in preterm infants after intraventricular hemorrhage. Many nonpyogenic congenital infections (toxoplasmosis, CMV, HSV, syphilis producing an aseptic meningitis) can also produce alterations in CSF protein and leukocytes.

Gram stain of CSF yields a positive result in most patients with bacterial meningitis. The leukocyte count is usually elevated, with a predominance of neutrophils (>70–90%); the number is often >1,000 but may be <100 in infants with neutropenia or early in the disease. Microorganisms are recovered from most patients who have not been pretreated with antibiotics. Bacteria have also been isolated from CSF that did not have an abnormal number of cells (<25) or an abnormal protein level (<200 mg/dL), thus underscoring the importance of performing a culture and Gram stain on all CSF specimens. Contamination of CSF by bacteremia after traumatic lumbar puncture may occur rarely. Culture-negative meningitis may be seen with antibiotic pretreatment, a brain abscess, or infection with *Mycobacterium hominis, U. urealyticum, Bacteroides fragilis,* enterovirus, or HSV. Head ultrasonography or, more often, CT with contrast enhancement may be helpful in diagnosing ventriculitis and brain abscess.

109.8 • Treatment

Treatment of suspected bacterial infection is determined by the pattern of disease and the organisms that are common for the age of the infant and the flora of the nursery. Once appropriate cultures have been obtained, intravenous or, less often, intramuscular antibiotic therapy should be instituted immediately. Initial empirical treatment of early-onset bacterial infections should consist of ampicillin and an aminoglycoside (usually gentamicin). Nosocomial infections acquired in a NICU are more likely to be caused by staphylococci, various *Enterobacteriaceae, Pseudomonas* species, or *Candida* species. Thus, an antistaphylococcal drug (methicillin or nafcillin for *S. aureus* or, more often, vancomycin for coagulase-negative staphylococci or methicillin-resistant *S. aureus*) should be substituted for ampicillin. A history of recent antimicrobial therapy or the presence of antibiotic-resistant infections in the NICU suggests the need for a different aminoglycoside agent (amikacin). When the history or the presence of necrotic skin lesions suggests *Pseudomonas* infection, initial therapy should be piperacillin, ticarcillin, carbenicillin, or ceftazidime and an aminoglycoside. The use of antifungal therapy should be considered in VLBW infants who have had previous antibiotic therapy, may have mucosal colonization with *C. albicans,* and are at high risk for invasive disease (see Chapter 231.1). Doses of commonly used antibiotics are provided in Table 109-14. Peak and trough levels of gentamicin (peak, 5–10 µg/mL; trough, <2 µg/mL) and vancomycin (peak, 25–40 µg/mL; trough, < 10 µg/mL) are useful to ensure therapeutic levels and minimize toxicity if administered for more than 2–3 days.

Once the pathogen has been identified and antibiotic sensitivities determined, the most appropriate drug or drugs should be selected. For most gram-negative enteric bacteria, ampicillin and an aminoglycoside or a 3rd-generation cephalosporin (cefotaxime or ceftazidime) should be used. Enterococci should be treated with both a penicillin (ampicillin or piperacillin) and an aminoglycoside because the synergy of both drugs is needed. Ampicillin alone is adequate for *L. monocytogenes,* and penicillin suffices for GBS. Clindamycin or metronidazole is appropriate for anaerobic infections.

Third-generation cephalosporins such as cefotaxime are valuable additions for treating documented neonatal sepsis and meningitis because (1) the minimal inhibitory concentrations needed for treatment of gram-negative enteric bacilli are much lower than those for the aminoglycosides, (2) excellent penetration into CSF occurs, and (3) much higher doses can be given. The end result is much higher bactericidal titers in serum and CSF than achievable with ampicillin-aminoglycoside combinations. The routine use of 3rd-generation cephalosporins for suspected sepsis in NICU patients is inappropriate because of the potential for rapid emergence of resistant organisms and a possible link with candida sepsis.

The emergence of antibiotic resistance among pathogens that infect newborns is of great concern. Vancomycin-resistant enterococci and vancomycin-insensitive *S. aureus* are worrisome. Guidelines to limit the use of vancomycin must be followed. Although vancomycin use cannot be avoided in neonatal units where methicillin-resistant *S. aureus* is endemic, use can be reduced by limiting empirical therapy to patients with a high suspicion of severe infection with coagulase-negative staphylococci (severely ill neonate with an indwelling intravascular catheter) and discontinuing therapy after 2–3 days when blood cultures are negative. The rational use of antibiotics in neonates involves using narrow-spectrum drugs when possible, treating infection and not colonization, and limiting the duration of therapy.

Therapy for most bloodstream infections should be continued for a total of 7–10 days or for at least 5–7 days after a clinical response has occurred. A blood culture taken 24–48 hr after initiation of therapy should yield negative results. If the blood culture remains positive, the possibility of an infected indwelling catheter, endocarditis, an infected thrombus, an occult abscess, subtherapeutic antibiotic levels, or resistant organisms should be considered. A change in antibiotics, longer duration of therapy, or removal of the catheter may be indicated.

Treatment of newborn infants whose mothers received antibiotics during labor should be individualized. If early-onset sepsis is thought to be likely, treatment of the infant should be continued until it is shown that no infection has occurred (the infant remains asymptomatic for 24–72 hr) or clinical and laboratory evidence of recovery is apparent. Furthermore, in the context of intrapartum antibiotic use, it is important to consider that the organism causing infection may be resistant to the antibiotic given to the mother, which may influence choice of antibiotic use in the infant.

For pneumonia developing in the 1st 7–10 days of life, a combination of ampicillin and an aminoglycoside or cefotaxime is appropriate. Nosocomial pneumonia, generally manifested after this time, can be treated empirically with methicillin or vancomycin and an aminoglycoside or a 3rd-generation cephalosporin. *Pseudomonas* pneumonia should be treated with an aminoglycoside combined with ticarcillin or ceftazidime. Pneumonia caused by *C. trachomatis* is treated with either erythromycin or trimethoprim-sulfamethoxazole; *U. urealyticum* infection is treated with erythromycin.

Presumptive antimicrobial therapy for bacterial meningitis should include ampicillin in meningitic doses and cefotaxime or gentamicin unless staphylococci are likely, which is an indication for vancomycin. Susceptibility testing of gram-negative enteric organisms is important because resistance to cephalosporins and aminoglycosides is common. Most aminoglycosides administered by parenteral routes do not achieve sufficiently high antibiotic levels in the lumbar CSF or ventricles to inhibit the growth of gram-negative bacilli. Therefore, some experts recommend a combination of intravenous ampicillin and a 3rd-generation

TABLE 109-14. Suggested Dosage Schedules for Antibiotics Used in Newborns

		DOSAGE (MG/KG) AND INTERVAL OF ADMINISTRATION				
		Weight < 1,200 g*	Weight 1,200–2,000 g		Weight > 2,000 g	
ANTIBIOTIC	ROUTE	*Age 0–4 wk*	*Age 0–7 Days*	*Age > 7 Days*	*Age 0–7 Days*	*Age > 7 Days*
Amikacin[†] (SDD)	IV, IM	7.5 q12h	7.5 q12h	7.5 q8h	10 q12h	10 q8h
Amikacin[†] (ODD)	IV, IM	18 q48h	16 q36h	15 q24h	15 q24h	15 q24h
Ampicillin	IV, IM					
Meningitis		50 q12h	50 q12h	50 q8h	50 q8h	50 q6h
Other infections		25 q12h	25 q12h	25 q8h	25 q8h	25 q6h
Aztreonam	IV, IM	30 q12h	30 q12h	30 q8h	30 q8h	30 q6h
Cefazolin	IV, IM	20 q12h	20 q12h	20 q12h	20 q12h	20 q8h
Cefepime	IV, IM	50 q12h	50 q12h	50 q8h	50 q12h	50 q8h
Cefotaxime	IV, IM	50 q12h	50 q12h	50 q8h	50 q12h	50 q8h
Ceftazidime	IV, IM	50 q12h	50 q12h	50 q8h	50 q8h	50 q8h
Ceftriaxone	IV, IM	50 q24h	50 q24h	50 q24h	50 q24h	75 q24h
Cephalothin	IV	20 q12h	20 q12h	20 q8h	20 q8h	20 q6h
Chloramphenicol[‡]	IV, PO	25 q24h	25 q24h	25 q24h	25 q24h	25 q12h
Ciprofloxacin[§]	IV	—	—	10–20 q24h	—	20–30 q12h
Clindamycin	IV, IM, PO	5 q12h	5 q12h	5 q8h	5 q8h	5 q6h
Erythromycin	PO	10 q12h	10 q12h	10 q8h	10 q12h	10 q8h
Gentamicin[†] (SDD)	IV, IM	2.5 q18h	2.5 q12h	2.5 q8h	2.5 q12h	2.5 q8h
Gentamicin[†] (ODD)	IV, IM	5 q48h	4 q36h	4 q24h	4 q24h	4 q24h
Imipenem	IV, IM	—	20 q12h	20 q12h	20 q12h	20 q8h
Linezolid	IV	—	10 q12h	10 q8h	10 q12h	10 q8h
Methicillin	IV, IM					
Meningitis		50 q12h	50 q12h	50 q8h	50 q8h	50 q6h
Other infections		25 q12h	25 q12h	25 q8h	25 q8h	25 q6h
Metronidazole[‖]	IV, PO	7.5 q48h	7.5 q24h	7.5 q12h	7.5 q12h	15 q12h
Mezlocillin	IV, IM	75 q12h	75 q12h	75 q8h	75 q12h	75 q8h
Meropenem**	IV, IM	—	20 q12h	20 q12h	20 q12h	20 q8h
Nafcillin	IV	25 q12h	25 q12h	25 q8h	25 q8h	37.5 q6h
Netilmicin[†] (SDD)	IV, IM	2.5 q18h	2.5 q12h	2.5 q8h	2.5 q12h	2.5 q8h
Netilmicin (ODD)				Same as for gentamicin		
Oxacillin	IV, IM	25 q12h	25 q12h	25 q8h	25 q8h	37.5 q6h
Penicillin G (units)	IV					
Meningitis		50,000 q12h	50,000 q12h	50,000 q8h	50,000 q8h	50,000 q6h
Other infections		25,000 q12h	25,000 q12h	25,000 q8h	25,000 q8h	25,000 q6h
Penicillin benzathine (units)	IM	—	50,000 (one dose)	50,000 (one dose)	50,000 (one dose)	50,000 (one dose)
Penicillin procaine (units)	IM	—	50,000 q24h	50,000 q24h	50,000 q24h	50,000 q24h
Piperacillin	IV, IM	—	50–75 q12h	50–75 q8h	50–75 q8h	50–75 q6h
Peperacillin/tazobactam				Same as for piperacillin		
Rifampin	PO, IV	—	10 q24h	10 q24h	10 q24h	10 q24h
Ticarcillin	IV, IM	75 q12h	75 q12h	75 q8h	75 q8h	75 q6h
Ticarcillin-clavulanate				Same as for ticarcillin		
Tobramycin[†] (SDD)	IV, IM	2.5 q18h	2 q12h	2 q8h	2 q12h	2 q8h
Tobramycin (ODD)				Same as for gentamicin		
Vancomycin	IV	15 q24h	10 q12h	10 q12h	10 q8h	10 q8h

*Data from Prober CG, Stevenson DK, Benitz WE: The use of antibiotics in neonates weighing less than 1200 grams. *Pediatr Infect Dis J* 1990;9:111.
[†]Adjustments of further dosing intervals should be based on aminoglycoside half-lives calculated after serum peak and trough concentrations measurements.
[§]Doses suggested based on anecdotal clinical experience.
[‖]A loading intravenous dose of 15 mg/kg followed 24 hours later (term infants) and 48 hours later (preterm infants) by 7.5 mg/kg every 12 hours has been suggested by other investigators.
**Dosages of meropenem suggested are the same as those of imipenem.
IM, intramuscular; IV, intravenous; ODD, once-daily dosing; PO, oral; SDD, standard daily dosing.
Adapted from Sáez-Llorens X, McCraken GH, Jr: Clinical Pharmacology of Antibacterial Agents, In Remington JS, Klein JO, Wilson CB, Baker CJ (editors) *Infectious Diseases of the Fetus and Newborn Infant,* 6th edition. Philadelphia, Elsevier, 2005.

cephalosporin for the treatment of neonatal gram-negative meningitis. Cephalosporins should not be used as empirical monotherapy because *L. monocytogenes* and enterococcus are resistant to cephalosporins.

Meningitis caused by GBS usually responds within 24–48 hr and should be treated for 14–21 days. Gram-negative bacilli may continue to grow from repeated CSF samples for 72–96 hr after therapy despite the use of appropriate antibiotics. Treatment of gram-negative meningitis should be continued for 21 days or for at least 14 days after sterilization of the CSF, whichever is longer. *P. aeruginosa* meningitis should be treated with ceftazidime. Metronidazole is the treatment of choice for infection caused by *B. fragilis*. Prolonged antibiotic administration, with or without drainage for treatment and diagnosis, is indicated for neonatal cerebral abscesses. CT scans are recommended for patients with suspected ventriculitis, hydrocephalus, or cerebral abscess (initial and follow-up assessments) and for those with an unexpectedly complicated course (prolonged coma, focal neurologic deficits, persistent or recurrent fever). Neonatal herpes meningoencephalitis should be treated with acyclovir, and empirical therapy should be considered in symptomatic infants with a CSF mononuclear pleocytosis. Pleconaril was the treatment of choice for severe enteroviral infections such as meningoencephalitis, carditis, or hepatitis. Treatment of candidal meningitis is discussed in Chapter 231.

Treatment of sepsis and meningitis may be divided into antimicrobial therapy for the suspected or known pathogen and supportive care. Careful attention to respiratory and cardiovascular status is mandatory. Adequate oxygenation of tissues should be maintained; ventilatory support is frequently necessary for respiratory failure caused by sepsis, pneumonia, pulmonary hypertension, or ARDS. Refractory hypoxia and shock may require extracorporeal membrane oxygenation, which has reduced mortality rates in full-term infants with respiratory failure. Shock and metabolic acidosis should be identified and managed with fluid resuscitation and inotropic agents as needed. Corticosteroids should be administered only for adrenal insufficiency. Fluids, electrolytes, and glucose levels should be monitored carefully with correction of hypovolemia, hyponatremia, hypocalcemia, and hypoglycemia. Hyperbilirubinemia should be monitored and treated aggressively with phototherapy and/or exchange transfusion because the risk of kernicterus increases in the presence of sepsis and meningitis. Seizures should be treated with anticonvulsants. Parenteral nutrition is needed for any infant who cannot sustain enteral feeding.

DIC may complicate neonatal septicemia. Platelet counts, hemoglobin, and clotting studies should be monitored. DIC is treated by management of the underlying infection, but if bleeding occurs, DIC may require fresh frozen plasma, platelet transfusions, or whole blood.

Because neutrophil storage pool depletion has been associated with a poor prognosis, a number of clinical trials of granulocyte transfusion therapy have been conducted, with variable results. The use of G-CSF or GM-CSF abolishes sepsis-induced neutropenia, but the effect of these cytokines on sepsis-related mortality is unclear. Modern leukapheresis techniques and the use of G-CSF to mobilize polymorphonuclear cells in healthy donors for use in granulocyte transfusion is a promising approach that needs further study. The use of intravenous immunoglobulin (IVIG) has been shown to decrease mortality in patients with sepsis; a meta-analysis of several trials recommended administration of a single dose of 500–750 mg/kg as adjunctive therapy. Selected IVIG preparations containing specific monoclonal antibodies are being studied.

It is important to remember that nonbacterial infectious agents can produce the syndrome of neonatal sepsis. HSV infection requires immediate specific treatment, as does systemic *Candida* infection. Treatment and other aspects of various nonbacterial infections are discussed in detail in other sections: TB (Chapter 212), syphilis (Chapter 215), genital mycoplasmas (Chapter 221), *C. trachomatis* (Chapter 223), *Candida* (Chapter 231), rubella (Chapter 244), enteroviruses (Chapter 247); parvovirus B19 (Chapter 248); HSV (Chapter 249), VZV (Chapter 250), and CMV (Chapter 252).

109.9 • Complications and Prognosis

The sequelae of intrauterine infections with specific pathogens are described in their respective chapters. In general, complications of bacterial or fungal infections may be divided into those related to the inflammatory process per se and those that underlie neonatal problems such as respiratory distress and fluid and electrolyte abnormalities.

Complications of bacteremic infections include endocarditis, septic emboli, abscess formation, septic joints with residual disability, and osteomyelitis and bone destruction. Recurrent bacteremia is rare (<5% of patients). Candidemia may lead to vasculitis, endocarditis, and endophthalmitis, as well as abscesses in the kidneys, liver, lungs, and brain. Sequelae of sepsis may result from septic shock, DIC, or organ failure.

Mortality rates from the sepsis syndrome depend on the definition of sepsis. In adults, the mortality rate approaches 50%, and the rate in newborn infants is probably at least that high. Reported mortality rates in neonatal sepsis are as low as 10% because all bacteremic infections are included in the definition. Several studies have documented that the sepsis case fatality rate is highest for gram-negative and fungal infections (Table 109-15).

The case fatality rate for neonatal bacterial meningitis is between 20 and 25%. Many of these cases have associated sepsis.

TABLE 109-15. Infecting Pathogen vs Death Rate, Late-Onset Sepsis Review in VLBW Infants: NICHD Neonatal Research Network, September 1, 1998, through August 31, 2000

ORGANISM*	N	DEATH N[†]
All gram-positive organisms	**905**	**101 (11.2%)**
Staphylococcus—coagulase negative	606	55 (9.1%)
Staphylococcus aureus	99	17 (17.2%)
Group B streptococcus	32	7 (21.9%)
All other streptococci	65	7 (10.8%)
All gram-negative organisms	**257**	**93 (36.2%)**
Escherichia coli	53	18 (34.0%)
Klebsiella	62	14 (22.6%)
Pseudomonas	43	32 (74.4%)
Enterobacter	41	11 (26.8%)
Serratia	39	14 (35.9%)
All fungal organisms	**151**	**48 (31.8%)**
Candida albicans	82	36 (43.9%)
Candida parapsilosis	44	7 (15.9%)

*Organisms found on the last positive blood culture before death or discharge. Organism counts differ from those based on the 1st positive blood culture (Table 98-5) because of multiple sepsis episodes. Death rates are not shown for every organism found.

[†]The odds ratios for death, with control for gestational age, study center, race, and sex, were as follows: gram-positive vs other infections, 0.26 (0.19–0.35), $p < 0.001$; gram-negative vs other infections, 3.5 (2.5–4.9), $p < 0.001$; and fungi vs other infections, 2.0 (1.3–3.0), $p < 0.01$.

NICHD, National Institute of Child Health and Human Development; VLBW, very low birthweight.

From Stoll BJ, Hansen N, Fanaroff AA, et al: Late-onset sepsis in very low birthweight neonates: The experience of the NICHHD neonatal research network. *Pediatrics* 2002;110:285–291.

Risk factors for death or for moderate or severe disability include a duration of seizures for more than 72 hr, coma, necessity for the use of inotropic agents, and leukopenia. Immediate complications of meningitis include ventriculitis, cerebritis, and brain abscess. Late complications of meningitis occur in 40–50% of survivors and include hearing loss, abnormal behavior, developmental delay, cerebral palsy, focal motor disability, seizure disorders, and hydrocephalus. CT has demonstrated cerebritis, brain abscess, infarct, subdural effusions, cortical atrophy, and diffuse encephalomalacia in newborns surviving meningitis. A number of these sequelae may be encountered in infants with sepsis but without meningitis as a result of cerebritis or septic shock. Extremely low birthweight infants (<1,000 g) with sepsis are at increased risk for poor neurodevelopmental and growth outcomes in early childhood.

109.10 • Prevention

A number of intrauterine infections are preventable through maternal immunization, including hepatitis B, rubella, and VZV. CMV vaccines are under study. Toxoplasmosis is preventable with appropriate diet and avoidance of exposure to cat feces. Malaria during pregnancy can be minimized with chemoprophylaxis. Congenital syphilis is preventable by timely diagnosis and appropriate early treatment of infected pregnant women.

Neonatal tetanus can be prevented by maternal tetanus immunization and proper care of the umbilical cord. Aggressive management of suspected maternal chorioamnionitis with antibiotic therapy during labor, along with rapid delivery of the infant, reduces the risk of early-onset neonatal sepsis. Vertical transmission of GBS (see Chapter 183) is significantly reduced by selective intrapartum chemoprophylaxis. Neonatal infection with *Chlamydia* can be prevented by identification and treatment of infected pregnant women (see Chapter 223). Mother-to-child transmission of HIV is significantly reduced by maternal antiretroviral therapy during pregnancy, labor, and delivery, cesarean section delivery prior to rupture of membranes, and antiretroviral treatment of the infant after birth (see Chapter 273).

TABLE 109-16. Principles for the Prevention of Nosocomial Infection in the Neonatal Intensive Care Unit

Observe recommendations for universal precautions with all patient contact
Gloves
Gowns, mask, and isolation as indicated
Nursery design engineering
Appropriate nursing : patient ratio
Avoid overcrowding and excessive workload
Readily accessible sinks, antiseptic solutions, soap, and paper towels
Handwashing
Improve handwashing compliance
Wash hands before and after each patient encounter
Appropriate use of soap, alcohol-based preparations, or antiseptic solutions
Alcohol-based antiseptic solution at each patient bedside
Provide emollients for nursery staff
Education and feedback for nursery staff
Minimizing risk of CVC contamination
Maximal sterile barrier precautions during CVC insertion
Local antisepsis with chlorhexidine gluconate
Minimize repeated entry into the line for laboratory tests
Aseptic technique when entering the line
Minimize CVC days
Sterile preparation of all fluids to be administered via a CVC
Meticulous skin care
Encourage early and appropriate advancement of enteral feeding
Education and feedback for nursery personnel
Continuous monitoring and surveillance of nosocomial infection rates in the NICU

CVC, central venous catheter; NICU, neonatal intensive care unit.
From Adams-Chapman I, Stoll BJ: Prevention of nosocomial infections in the neonatal intensive care unit. *Curr Opin Pediatr* 2002; 14:157–164.

PREVENTION OF NOSOCOMIAL INFECTION

Principles for the prevention of nosocomial infection include adherence to universal precautions with all patient contact, avoiding nursery crowding and limiting nurse-to-patient ratios, strict compliance with handwashing, meticulous neonatal skin care, minimizing the risk of catheter contamination, decreasing the number of venipunctures and heelsticks, reducing the duration of catheter and mechanical ventilation days, encouraging appropriate advancement of enteral feedings, providing education and feedback to nursery personnel, and ongoing monitoring and surveillance of nosocomial infection rates in the NICU (Table 109-16).

Most nosocomial infections in the NICU are bloodstream infections associated with an intravascular catheter. Catheters used in neonates include peripheral intravenous catheters, umbilical catheters, peripherally inserted central catheters, and surgically placed central venous catheters (CVCs). Efforts to reduce catheter-related infections include proper antisepsis of the skin before insertion of the catheter, sterile precautions during catheter insertion, aseptic technique when entering the line, minimizing repeated entry into the line for blood sampling, sterile preparation of fluids to be used with a CVC, and, finally, minimizing the number of catheter days.

The skin is an important mechanical barrier to infection. VLBW infants are born with an ineffective epidermal barrier that results in increased transepidermal water loss and an increased risk for infection. Efforts to reduce traumatic injury to this immature skin are important, including a reduction in the number of heelsticks.

Handwashing remains the most important and effective means of reducing nosocomial infections. Several expert groups have established guidelines for effective handwashing. Antimicrobial soaps or alcohol-based preparations are recommended. Proper handwashing is essential before entering the NICU and before each patient contact. Barriers to compliance with handwashing include overcrowding, excessive patient-to-nurse ratios, poorly located sinks and inadequate supplies, lack of easy-to-use alcohol-based products at the bedside, concern about skin irritation, and inadequate knowledge, including the mistaken belief that the use of gloves obviates the need for handwashing.

Ongoing education of staff regarding practices that are likely to reduce nosocomial infections and active surveillance of infection rates are important components of nosocomial infection control.

Adams-Chapman I, Stoll BJ: Prevention of nosocomial infections in the neonatal intensive care unit. *Curr Opin Pediatr* 2002;14:157–164.

Adams-Chapman I, Stoll BJ: Systemic inflammatory response syndrome. *Semin Pediatr Infect Dis* 2001;12:5.

Ahmed A, Hickey SM, Ehrett S, et al: Cerebrospinal fluid values in the term neonate. *Pediatr Infect Dis J* 1996;15:298–303.

Ahrens P, Kattner E, Köhler B, et al: Mutations of genes involved in the innate immune system as predictors of sepsis in very low birth weight infants. *Pediatr Res* 2004;55:652–656.

Ameh EA, Nmadu PT: Major complications of omphalitis in neonates and infants. *Pediatr Surg Int* 2002;18:413–416.

Bang AT, Bang RA, Reddy MH, et al: Simple clinical criteria to identify sepsis or pneumonia in neonates in the community needing treatment or referral. *Pediatr Infect Dis J* 2005;24:325–341.

Bedford Russell AR, Emmerson AJB, Wilkinson N, et al: A trial of recombinant human granulocyte colony stimulating factor for the treatment of very low birthweight infants with presumed sepsis and neutropenia. *Arch Dis Child Fetal Neonatal Ed* 2001;84:F172–F176.

Benjamin DK Jr, Ross K, McKinney RE Jr, et al: When to suspect fungal infection in neonates: A clinical comparison of *Candida albicans* and *Candida parapsilosis* fungemia with coagulase-negative staphylococcal bacteremia. *Pediatrics* 2000;106:712–718.

Bernstein HM, Pollock BH, Calhoun DA, et al: Administration of recombinant granulocyte colony-stimulating factor to neonates with septicemia: A meta-analysis. *J Pediatr* 2001;138:917–920.

Bizzarro MJ, Raskind C, Baltimore RS, et al: Seventy-five years of neonatal sepsis at Yale: 1928–2003. *Pediatrics* 2005;116:595–602.

Buhimschi CS, Buhimschi IA, Abdel-Razeq S, et al: Proteomic biomarkers of intra-amniotic inflammation: relationship with funisitis and early-onset sepsis in the premature neonate. *Pediatr Res* 2007;61:318–324.

Buttery JP: Blood cultures in newborns and children: Optimizing an everyday test. *Arch Dis Child Fetal Neonatal Ed* 2002;87:F25–F28.

Centers for Disease Control and Prevention: Intrauterine West Nile virus infection—New York, 2002. *MMWR* 2002;51:1135–1136.

Centers for Disease Control and Prevention: Sexually transmitted diseases treatment guidelines 2002. *MMWR* 2002;51:1–78.

Cordero L, Ayers LW, Miller RR, et al: Surveillance of ventilator-associated pneumonia in very-low-birth-weight infants. *Am J Infect Control* 2002;30:32–39.

Daley AJ, Isaacs D, Australasian Study Group for Neonatal Infections: Ten-year study on the effect of intrapartum antibiotic prophylaxis on early onset group B streptococcal and *Escherichia coli* neonatal sepsis in Australasia. *Pediatr Infect Dis J* 2004;23:630–634.

Goldenberg RL, Hauth JC, Andrews WW: Mechanisms of disease: Intrauterine infection and preterm delivery. *N Engl J Med* 2000;342:1500–1507.

Gravett MG, Novy MJ, Rosenfeld RG, et al: Diagnosis of intra-amniotic infection by proteomic profiling and identification of novel biomarkers. *JAMA* 2004;292:462–469.

Hodge D, Puntis JWL: Diagnosis, prevention, and management of catheter related bloodstream infection during long-term parenteral nutrition. *Arch Dis Child Fetal Neonatal Ed* 2002;87:F21–F24.

Karlowicz MG, Buescher ES, Surka AE: Fulminant late-onset sepsis in a neonatal intensive care unit, 1988–1997, and the impact of avoiding empiric vancomycin therapy. *Pediatrics* 2000;106:1387–1390.

Kaufman D, Boyle R, Hazen KC, et al: Fluconazole prophylaxis against fungal colonization and infection in preterm infants. *N Engl J Med* 2002;345:1660–1666.

Klinger G, Chin CN, Beyene J, et al: Predicting the outcome of neonatal bacterial meningitis. *Pediatrics* 2000;106:477–482.

Kumar Y, Qunibi M, Neal TJ, et al: Time to positivity of neonatal blood cultures. *Arch Dis Child Fetal Neonatal Ed* 2001;85:F182–F186.

Lahra MM, Jeffery HE: A fetal response to chorioamnionitis is associated with early survival after preterm birth. *Am J Obstet Gynecol* 2004;190:147–151.

Levy O: Impaired innate immunity at birth: Deficiency of bactericidal/permeability-increasing protein (BPI) in the neutrophils of newborns. *Pediatr Res* 2002;51:667–669.

Levy O, Zarember KA, Roy RM, et al: Selective impairment of TLR-mediated innate immunity in human newborns: Neonatal blood plasma reduces monocyte TNF-alpha induction by bacterial lipopeptides, lipopolysaccharide, and imiquimod, but preserves the response to R-848. *J Immunol* 2004;173:4627–4634.

Lin F-YC, Philips JB III, Azimi PH, et al: Level of maternal antibody required to protect neonates against early-onset disease caused by group B streptococcus type Ia: A multicenter, seroepidemiology study. *J Infect Dis* 2001;184:1022–1028.

Miralles R, Hodge R, McParland PC, et al: Relationship between antenatal inflammation and antenatal infection identified by detection of microbial genes by polymerase chain reaction. *Pediatr Res* 2005;57:570–577.

Mylonakis E, Paliou M, Hohmann EL, et al: Listeriosis during pregnancy. *Medicine (Baltimore)* 2002;81:260–269.

Ng PC: Diagnostic markers of infection in neonates. *Arch Dis Child Fetal Neonatal Ed* 2004;89:F229.

Oddie S, Embleton ND: Risk factors for early onset neonatal group B streptococcal sepsis: Case-control study. *Br Med J* 2002;325:308.

Ronnestad A, Abrahamsen TG, Medbo S, et al: Late-onset septicemia in a Norwegian national cohort of extremely premature infants receiving very early full human milk feeding. *Pediatrics* 2005;115:e269–e276.

Ronnestad A, Abrahamsen TG, Medbo S, et al: Septicemia in the first week of life in a Norwegian national cohort of extremely premature infants. *Pediatrics* 2005;115:e262–e268.

Saiman L, Ludington E, Pfaller M, et al: Risk factors for candidemia in neonatal intensive care unit patients. *Pediatr Infect Dis J* 2000;19:319–324.

Schrag S, Gorwitz R, Fultz-Butts K, et al: Prevention of perinatal group B streptococcal disease. Revised guidelines from CDC. *MMWR Recomm Rep* 2002;51:1–22.

Schrag SJ, Zell ER, Lynfield R, et al: A population-based comparison of strategies to prevent early onset group B streptococcal disease in neonates. *N Engl J Med* 2002;347:233–239.

Stoll BJ, Hansen NI, Adams-Chapman I, et al: Neurodevelopmental and growth impairment among extremely low-birth-weight infants with neonatal infection. *JAMA* 2004;292:2357–2365.

Stoll BJ, Hansen N, Fanaroff AA, et al: To tap or not to tap: High likelihood of meningitis without sepsis among very low birth weight infants. *Pediatrics* 2004;113:1181–1186.

Stoll BJ, Hansen N, Fanaroff AA, et al: Changes in pathogens causing sepsis in very low birthweight infants. *N Engl J Med* 2002;347:240–247.

Stoll BJ, Hansen N, Fanaroff AA, et al: Late-onset sepsis in very low birthweight neonates: The experience of the NICHD Neonatal Research Network. *Pediatrics* 2002;110:285–291.

Stoll BJ, Hansen N, Higgins RD, et al: Very low birth weight preterm infants with early onset neonatal sepsis: The predominance of gram-negative infections continues in the NICHD Neonatal Research Network, 2002–2003. *Pediatr Infect Dis J* 2005, in press.

Vergnano S, Sharland M, Kasembe P, et al: Neonatal sepsis: An international perspective. *Arch Dis Child Fetal Neonatal Ed* 2005;90:F220–F224.

Yoon BH, Romero R, Moon JB, et al: Clinical significance of intra-amniotic inflammation in patients with preterm labor and intact membranes. *Am J Obstet Gynecol* 2001;185:1130–1136.

Part XII ■ Adolescent Medicine

Chapter 110 ■ The Epidemiology of Adolescent Health Problems

Renée R. Jenkins

Behavioral and psychosocial risks, including injuries, account for substantial causes of morbidity and mortality for U.S. youths. Adolescents make fewer visits to physicians for ambulatory office visits than does any other age group; yet school-aged children and adolescents are more likely than younger children to have unmet health needs and delayed medical care. Adolescents and young adults are less likely to be insured than all other age groups. Uninsured children and adolescents are less likely to receive preventive visits, have a regular source of care, and go without treatment of symptoms than the insured. Adolescents who receive preventive care may still be unlikely to discuss sexually transmitted diseases, HIV, or pregnancy prevention at those visits. Sexually experienced teens report the discussions more often than nonsexually experienced teens, but the frequency is still low at 64% for sexually experienced girls and 33.5% for sexually experienced boys.

In the general ambulatory setting, health supervision (10%) and acne led the lists of diagnoses for 10–14 yr olds and 15–19 yr olds, respectively, followed by acute upper respiratory infections and normal pregnancy. Children with disabilities, as a group, access health care services more frequently than do nondisabled children, and adolescents represent the largest proportion of children who are disabled, at 84.3 cases/1000 children ages 12–17 yr compared with 33.2 cases/1000 for children younger than 6 yr of age. Overall, impairments of speech, special senses, and intelligence (primarily mental retardation) as well as respiratory disease (primarily asthma) make up the largest categories of disability diagnoses.

TABLE 110-1. Percentage of Fatal Crashes by Characteristic, 2003

DRIVER AGE:	16	17–19	20–49
Driver error	77	73	57
Speeding	38	36	23
Single vehicle	50	45	39
3+ occupants	28	24	18
Drivers killed with 0.08+ BAC	13	27	42

BAC, blood alcohol concentration.
From Insurance Institute for Highway Safety, Beginning Teenage Drivers, available at: *www.iihs.org/safety/facts/teens/beginningdrivers.htm* (accessed October 3, 2005).

The leading causes of hospitalization in adolescents parallel the diagnoses of adolescents seen in the ambulatory setting, with the exception of mental disorders. Hospitalizations for mental disorders composed 21% of the top five discharge diagnoses in 2002 for 10–21 yr olds, with pregnancy and childbirth (49%), diseases of the digestive system (11%), injuries (9%), and respiratory tract diseases (5.5%) completing the list.

The health conditions having the greatest impact on the status of adolescent health are early unintended pregnancy, sexually transmitted infections, mental disorders, injuries, and substance use and abuse. Automobile and motorcycle accidents are the leading causes of adolescent morbidity and mortality. Alcohol is a factor in approximately one third of the fatal accidents involving adolescents. In addition, other factors such as driver error, less frequent use of seat belts, and the presence of other teen passengers increases the severity of crashes involving teen drivers (Table 110-1, Fig. 110-1). About 100 nonfatal injuries occur for

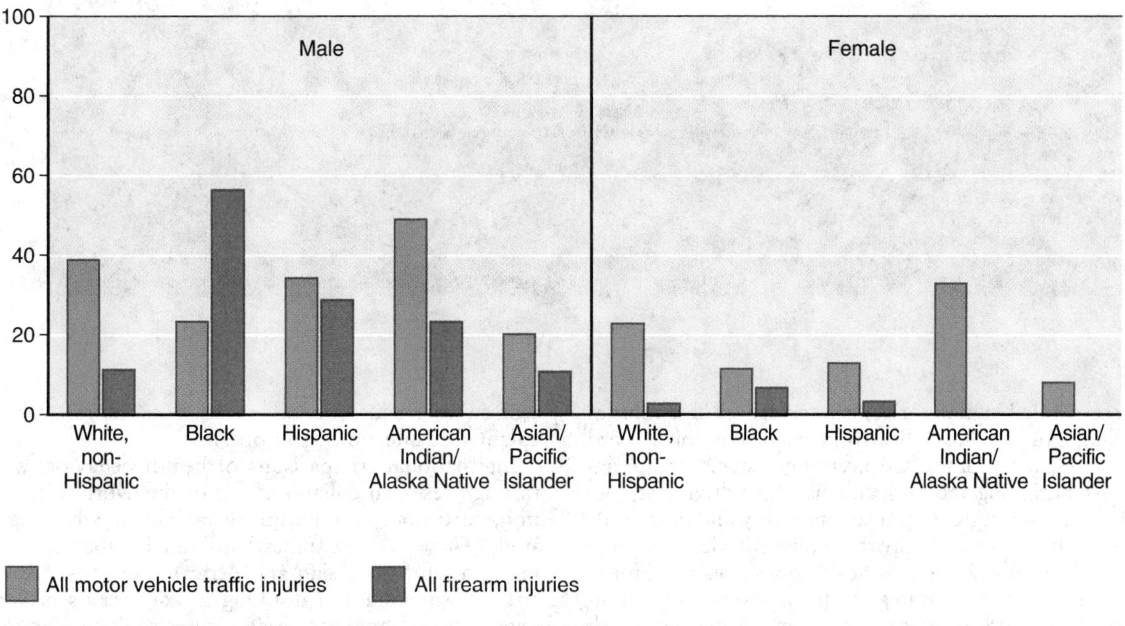

Figure 110-1. Injury death rates among adolescents ages 15–19 by gender, race, Hispanic origin, and type of injury, 2002. (Data from Centers for Disease Control and Prevention, National Center for Health Statistics, National Vital Statistics System; Figure from *America's Children: Key National Indicators of Well-Being 2005*.)

TABLE 110-2. Twenty-One Critical Health Objectives for Adolescents and Young Adults

OBJ. #	OBJECTIVE	BASELINE (YEAR)	2010 TARGET
16-03. (a,b,c)	*Reduce deaths of adolescents and young adults.*		(per 100,000)
	10 to 14 yr olds	21.5/100,000 (1998)	16.8
	15 to 19 yr olds	69.5/100,000 (1998)	39.8
	20 to 24 yr olds	92.7/100,000 (1998)	49.0
UNINTENTIONAL INJURY			
15-15. (a)	*Reduce deaths caused by motor vehicle crashes;* 15 to 24 yr olds	25.6/100,000 (1999)	*
26-01. (a)	*Reduce deaths and injuries caused by alcohol- and drug-related motor vehicle crashes;* 15 to 24 yr olds	13.5/100,000 (1998)	*
15-19.	Increase use of safety belts. 9th–12th grade students	84.0% (1999)	92.0%
26-06.	Reduce the proportion of adolescents who report that they rode, during the previous 30 days, with a driver who had been drinking alcohol; 9th–12th grade students	33.0% (1999)	30.0%
VIOLENCE			
18-01.	*Reduce the suicide rate.*		
	10 to 14 yr olds	1.2/100,000 (1999)	*
	15 to 19 yr olds	8.0/100,000 (1999)	*
18-02.	Reduce the rate of suicide attempts by adolescents who required medical attention; 9th–12th grade students	2.6% (1999)	1.0%
15-32.	*Reduce homicides.*		
	10 to 14 yr olds	1.2/100,000 (1999)	*
	15 to 19 yr olds	10.4/100,000 (1999)	*
15-38.	Reduce physical fighting among adolescents; 9th–12th grade students	36.0% (1999)	32.0%
15-39.	Reduce weapon carrying by adolescents on school property; 9th–12th grade students	6.9% (1999)	4.9%
SUBSTANCE ABUSE AND MENTAL HEALTH			
26-11. (d)	Reduce the proportion of persons engaging in binge drinking of alcoholic beverages; 12 to 17 yr olds	7.7% (1998)	2.0%
26-10. (b)	Reduce past-month use of illicit substances (marijuana); 12 to 17 yr olds	8.3% (1998)	0.7%
06-02.	Reduce the proportion of children and adolescents with disabilities who are reported to be sad, unhappy, or depressed; 4 to 17 yr olds	†	†
18-07.	Increase the proportion of children with mental health problems who receive treatment	59.0% (2001)	66.0%
REPRODUCTIVE HEALTH			
09-07.	*Reduce pregnancies among adolescent females;* 15 to 17 yr olds	68.0/1000 females (1996)	43.0/1000
13-05.	*Reduce the number of new cases of HIV/AIDS diagnosed among adolescents and adults;* 13 to 24 yr olds	16,479 (1998)‡	§
25-01. (a,b,c)	*Reduce the proportion of adolescents and young adults with Chlamydia trachomatis infections;* 15 to 24 yr olds		
	Females attending family-planning clinics	5.0% (1997)	3.0%
	Females attending sexually transmitted disease clinics	12.2% (1997)	3.0%
	Males attending sexually transmitted disease clinics	15.7% (1997)	3.0%
25-11. (a,b,c)	Increase the proportion of adolescents (9th–12th grade students) who:		
	Have never had sexual intercourse	50.0% (1999)	56.0%
	If sexually experienced, are not currently sexually active	27.0% (1999)	30.0%
	If currently sexually active, used a condom the last time they had sexual intercourse	58.0% (1999)	65.0%
CHRONIC DISEASES			
27-02. (a)	Reduce tobacco use by adolescents; 9th–12th grade students	40.0% (1999)	21.0%
19-03. (b)	*Reduce the proportion of children and adolescents who are overweight or obese,* 12 to 19 yr olds	11.0% (1988–1994)	5.0%
22-07.	Increase the proportion of adolescents who engage in vigorous physical activity that promotes cardiorespiratory fitness ≥3 days per week for ≥20 min per occasion; 9th–12th grade students	65.0% (1999)	85.0%

The 21 Critical Health Objectives represent the most serious health and safety issues facing adolescents and young adults (aged 10–24 yr): mortality, unintentional injury, violence, substance abuse and mental health, reproductive health, and the prevention of chronic diseases during adulthood.

Note: Critical health outcomes are italicized, and behaviors that substantially contribute to important health outcomes are in normal type.

*2010 target not provided for adolescent/young adult age group.

†Baseline and target inclusive of age groups outside of adolescent/young adult age parameters.

‡Proposed baseline is shown but has not yet been approved by the *Healthy People 2010* Steering Committee.

§Development objective: baseline and 2010 target to be provided by 2005.

From U.S. Department of Health and Human Services: *Healthy People 2010,* 1 and 2. Washington, DC, U.S. Government Printing Office, November 2000. This information can also be accessed at *http://wonder.cdc.gov/data2010/*.

every adolescent killed in a motor vehicle accident. These injuries are the leading cause of disability from head and spinal cord injuries for adolescents. Graduated licensing systems, more vigorously enforced drinking age laws, and nighttime driving restrictions are successful strategies to prevent mortality and morbidity.

The National Initiative to Improve Adolescent Health by the Year 2010 has identified 21 critical health objectives for adolescents and young adults as a strategy to focus state and community resources and health professionals on improving the health status of U.S. youths (Table 110-2). The progress to date includes significant improvement in incidence of teen pregnancy and tobacco use, small increments of improvement in some areas (i.e., physical fighting, weapon carrying, safety belt use), and worsening trends for others such as motor vehicle crashes, chlamydial infections, and obesity.

International comparisons of health behaviors are organized through research collaborations of the World Health Organization, particularly the Health Behaviour in School-aged Children study. These data are somewhat limited in that they do not reflect information from Asian and African countries. Health behavior data on smoking and drinking in adolescents between ages 11 and 15 years show the United States ranking 31st out of 35 for ever having smoked with 43% of girls and 55% of boys reporting ever smoking. Greenland, Lithuania, and the Ukraine lead the nations surveyed in reports of ever smoking, with more than 88% of 15 yr old boys with this behavior. Denmark and Wales led the

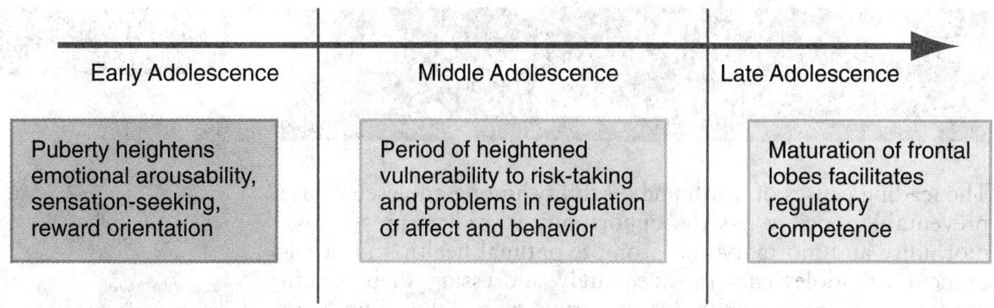
Early Adolescence
Middle Adolescence
Late Adolescence
Puberty heightens emotional arousability, sensation-seeking, reward orientation
Period of heightened vulnerability to risk-taking and problems in regulation of affect and behavior
Maturation of frontal lobes facilitates regulatory competence

Figure 110-2. It has been speculated that the impact of puberty on arousal and motivation occurs before the maturation of the frontal lobes is complete. This gap may create a period of heightened vulnerability to problems in the regulation of affect and behavior, which might help to explain the increased potential in adolescence for risk taking, recklessness, and the onset of emotional and behavioral problems. (From Steinberg L: Cognitive and affective development in adolescence. *Trends Cogn Sci* 2005;9:69–74.)

TABLE 110-3. Developmental Tasks of Adolescence

	BIOLOGIC	PSYCHOLOGIC	SOCIAL
Early adolescence	Early puberty (girls: breast bud and pubic hair development, start of growth spurt; boys: testicular enlargement, start of genital growth)	Concrete thinking but early moral concepts, progression of sexual identity development (sexual orientation), possible homosexual peer interest, reassessment of body image	Emotional separation from parents, start of strong peer identification, early exploratory behaviors (smoking, violence)
Mid-adolescence	Girls: mid-late puberty and end of growth spurt; menarche; development of female body shape with fat deposition; boys: mid-puberty, spermarche and nocturnal emissions; voice breaks; start of growth spurt	Abstract thinking but self still seen as "bullet proof," growing verbal abilities, identification of law with morality, start of fervent ideology (religious, political)	Emotional separation from parents, strong peer identification, increased health risk (smoking, alcohol, etc.), heterosexual peer interest, early vocational plans
Late adolescence	Boys: end of puberty, continued increase in muscle bulk and body hair	Complex abstract thinking, identification of difference between law and morality, increased impulse control, further development of personal identity, further development or rejection of religious and political ideology	Development of social autonomy, intimate relationships, development of vocational capability and financial independence

Adapted from McIntosh N, Helms P, Smyth R (editors): *Forfar and Arneil's Textbook of Paediatrics*, 6th ed. Edinburgh, Churchill Livingstone, 2003, pp 1757–1768 and Christie D, Viner R: Adolescent development. *Br Med J* 2005;350:301–304.

TABLE 110-4. Identified Risk and Protective Factors for Adolescent Health Behaviors

BEHAVIOR	RISK FACTORS	PROTECTIVE FACTORS
Smoking	Depression and other mental health problems, alcohol use, disconnectedness from school or family, difficulty talking with parents, minority ethnicity, low school achievement, peer smoking	Family connectedness, perceived healthiness, higher parental expectations, low prevalence of smoking in school
Alcohol and drug misuse	Depression and other mental health problems, low self-esteem, easy family access to alcohol, working outside school, difficulty talking with parents, risk factors for transition from occasional to regular substance misuse (smoking, availability of substances, peer use, other risk behaviors)	Connectedness with school and family, religious affiliation
Teenage pregnancy	Deprivation, city residence, low educational expectations, lack of access to sexual health services, drug and alcohol use	Connectedness with school and family, religious affiliation
Sexually transmitted infections	Mental health problems, substance misuse	Connectedness with school and family, religious affiliation

Adapted from McIntosh N, Helms P, Smyth R (editors): *Forfar and Arneil's Textbook of Paediatrics*, 6th ed. Edinburgh, Churchill Livingstone, 2003, pp 1757–1768 and Viner R, Macfarlane A: Health promotion. *Br Med J* 2005;330:527–529.

list of teenagers reporting drinking to the point of being drunk two or more times for 60% or more of 15 yr olds, whereas the United States reported about 22–30%. On health behaviors associated with risks for obesity, U.S. teens report more physical activity in comparison to other countries, but they also report eating breakfast less often than other teens and drinking soft drinks daily more often than most teens. Healthy behaviors such as daily fruit and vegetable consumption for U.S. teens are also below the average. Compiling and analyzing international data provide a sound basis for policy and intervention initiatives to improve adolescent health globally.

Adolescence is a time of immense biologic, psychologic, and social change (Table 110-3). Many of the psychologic changes have a biologic substrate in the development and eventual maturation of the central nervous system, particularly the frontal lobe areas responsible for executive functioning (Fig. 110-2). In addition to cognitive development, there are both risk and protective factors for adverse adolescent health behaviors that are dependent on the social environment as well as the mental health of an adolescent (Table 110-4).

American Medical Association: Guidelines for adolescent preventive services (GAPS). Available at: *www.ama-assn.org/ama/upload/mm/39/gapsmono.pdf* (accessed).

Christie D, Viner R: Adolescent development. *Br Med J* 2005;330:301–304.

Currie C, Roberts C, Morgan A, et al (editors): *Young People's Health in Context, Health Behaviour in School-aged Children (HBSC) Study: International Report from the 2001/2002 Survey.* Geneva, World Health Organization, Health Policy for Children and Adolescents (HEPCA), Series No. 4, 2004.

Dahl RE: Adolescent brain development: A period of vulnerabilities and opportunities. *Ann N Y Acad Sci* 2004;1021:1–22.

Eaton D, Kann L, Kinchen S, et al: Youth risk behavior surveillance—United States, 2005. *MMWR Surv Summ* 2006;55:1–108.

Federal Interagency Forum on Child and Family Statistics: *America's Children: Key National Indicators of Well-Being.* Washington, DC, Federal Interagency Forum on Child and Family Statistics, 2005.

Insurance Institute for Highway Safety, Beginning Teenage Drivers. Available at: *www.iihs.org/safety facts/teens/beginning drivers.htm* (accessed October 3, 2005).

Lancet: Who is responsible for adolescent health? *Lancet* 2004;363:2009.

Maternal and Child Health Bureau: *Child Health USA 2004.* Rockville, MD, U.S. Department of Health and Human Services, HRSA, MCHB, 2004.

McPherson A: Adolescents in primary care. *Br Med J* 2005;330:465–467.

Paus T: Mapping brain maturation and cognitive development during adolescence. *Trends Cogn Sci* 2005;9:60–68.

Steinberg L: Cognitive and affective development in adolescence. *Trends Cogn Sci* 2005;9:69–74.

Viner R, Booy R: Epidemiology of health and illness. *Br Med J* 2005;330:411–414.

Viner R, Macfarlane A: Health promotion. *Br Med J* 2005;330:527–529.

Chapter 111 ■ Delivery of Health Care to Adolescents

Renée R. Jenkins

The leading causes of death and disability among adolescents are preventable. Society has the opportunity to reduce preventable morbidity and mortality and promote optimal health and development of adolescents by adequately addressing their health needs. The World Health Organization in collaboration with United Nations International Children's Emergency Fund and United Nations Population Fund has developed a **common agenda** for action for healthy development in the 2nd decade of life by advocating for youths to have opportunities to "1) acquire accurate information about their health needs; 2) build the life skills needed to avoid risk-taking behavior, 3) obtain counseling, especially during crisis situation, 4) have access to health services (including reproductive health services) and 5) live in a safe and supportive environment."

The Society for Adolescent Medicine identified 10 program and policy characteristics to ensure comprehensive and high-quality care to adolescents. **Health insurance coverage** that is affordable, continuous, and not subject to exclusion for preexisting conditions should be available for all adolescents and young adults who have no access to private insurance. **Comprehensive, coordinated benefits** should meet the developmental needs of adolescents, particularly for reproductive, mental health, dental, and substance abuse services. **Safety net providers and programs** such as school-based health centers, community health centers, family planning, and sexually transmitted infections clinics that treat adolescents and young adults need to have assured funding for viability and sustainability. **Quality of care** data should be collected and analyzed by age so that the performance measures for age-appropriate health care needs of adolescents are monitored. Poor **affordability** is an obvious deterrent to access and should be removed as a barrier to preventive services. **Confidentiality** and access to care that requires consent by the adolescent should be available, while family involvement should be encouraged. Health plans and providers should be adequately **compensated** to support the range and intensity of services required to address the developmental and health service needs of adolescents. **Health care providers, trained and experienced,** to care for adolescents should be available in all communities. The creation and dissemination of provider education about adolescent preventive health guidelines have been demonstrated to improve the content of recommended care (Table 111-1). The ease of recognition or expectation that an adolescent needs can be addressed in a setting relates to the **visibility and flexibility** of sites and services. Staff at sites should be approachable, linguistically capable, and culturally competent. Health services should be **coordinated** to respond to goals for adolescent health at the local, state, and national levels. The coordination should address service financing and delivery in a manner that reduces disparities in care.

Adolescents have the lowest annual rate of visits to office-based physicians compared with all other age groups (Fig. 111-1). For all age groups, including adolescents, individuals without insurance receive less health care; insurance coverage is poorer for adolescents and young adults. In 2000, adolescents (12–17 yr olds) were more likely to be uninsured than children under 12 yr: 12.3% compared to 11.3%. Older adolescents and young adults (18–24 yr olds) were the least likely to have health insurance coverage, with 72.7% covered for some or all of 2000, more than double the rate of uninsured younger teenagers.

The complexity and interaction of physical, cognitive, and psychosocial developmental processes during adolescence require sensitivity and skill on the part of the health professional (see Chapter 110). Health education and promotion as well as disease prevention should be the focus of every visit. Clinicians who are trained in adolescent health guidelines and are provided charting tools for documentation improve the screening and counseling addressing high-risk behaviors at preventive care visits. Guidelines have been promulgated from several organizations. The U.S. Preventive Services Task Force use evidence-based criteria for recommendations, recognizing that evidence is insufficient in some instances. A comparative analysis of guidelines reveals more similarities than differences (Table 111-2). The American Medical Association's Guidelines for Adolescent Preventive Services (GAPS), having been designed exclusively for adolescents, are more specific in stating the criteria for intervention or referral. A companion document to the GAPS guidelines provides algorithms for each of the major preventive directives. Figure 111-2 provides a sample guideline using the algorithm for sexuality (see Chapter 116). A consistent element to the approach of each of the guidelines is the role of parents in support of the adolescent's health and development. Bright Futures goes even further in recommending the support and interaction of the community in the adolescent's life.

TABLE 111-1. Comparisons among Recommendations for Adolescent Preventive Services Developed by National Organizations*

	AAFP	AAP	AMA	BF	USPSTF
Immunizations					
ACIP recommendations	Yes	Yes	Yes	Yes	Yes
Health guidance for teens					
Normal development†‡	Yes	Yes	Yes	Yes	No
Injury prevention†§	Yes	Yes	Yes	Yes	Yes
Nutrition†	Yes	Yes	Yes	Yes	Yes
Physical activity†	Yes	Yes	Yes	Yes	Yes
Dental health†	Yes	Yes	No	Yes	Yes
Breast or testicular self-examination†	Yes	Yes	No	Yes	No
Skin protection†	Yes	Yes	Yes	Yes	Yes
Health guidance for parents†	No	Yes	Yes	Yes	No
Screening/counseling‖					
Obesity†	Yes	Yes	Yes	Yes	Yes
Contraception¶	Yes	Yes	Yes	Yes	Yes
Tobacco use†	Yes	Yes	Yes	Yes	Yes
Alcohol use†	Yes	Yes	Yes	Yes	Yes
Substance use†	Yes	Yes	Yes	Yes	Yes
Hypertension†	Yes	Yes	Yes	Yes	Yes
Depression/suicide†	No	Yes	Yes	Yes	No
Eating disorders†	No	Yes	Yes	Yes	No
School problems†	No	Yes	Yes	Yes	No
Abuse†	No	Yes	Yes	Yes	No#
Hearing†	Yes	Yes	No	Yes	No
Vision†	No	Yes	No	Yes	No
Tests					
Tuberculosis¶	Yes	Yes	Yes	Yes	Yes
Papanicolaou test¶	Yes	Yes	Yes	Yes	Yes
Human immunodeficiency virus infecion¶	Yes	Yes	Yes	Yes	Yes
Sexually transmitted diseases¶	Yes	Yes	Yes	Yes	Yes
Cholesterol¶	Yes	Yes	Yes	Yes	No
Urinalysis†	No	Yes	No	No	No
Hematocrit†	No	Yes	No	No	No
Periodicity of visits	Tailored	Annual	Annual	Annual	Tailored
Target age range, yr**	13–18	11–21	11–21	11–21	11–24

*AAFP indicates American Academy of Family Physicians (data from AAFP); AAP, American Academy of Pediatrics (data from AAP); AMA, American Medical Association (data from Elster and Kuznets); BF, Bright Futures (data from Green, ed.); and USPSTF, U.S. Preventive Services Task Force (data from USPSTF).

†Procedure is recommended for all adolescents/parents.

‡This includes providing adolescents with information on normal physical, psychosocial, and sexual development.

§This includes activities such as promoting the use of safety belts and safety helmets, placement of home fire alarms, and reducing the risk of injury from firearms and violence. Organizations differ in the activities they include for injury prevention.

‖The AAP recommends "developmental/behavioral assessment."

¶Procedure is recommended for selected adolescents who are at high risk of the medical problem.

#Child abuse is not addressed as a separate screening topic, but is included in the general screening for family violence.

**The AAP, AMA, and BF make a distinction among developmental stages of adolescence.

From *Adolescent Medicine: State of the Art Reviews*—Vol. 14, No. 2, June 2003. Philadelphia, Hanley & Belfus, an affiliate of Elsevier.

Table originally from: Elster AB: Comparison of recommendations for adolescent clinical preventive services developed by national organizations. *Arch Pediatr Adolesc Med* 1998;152:195.

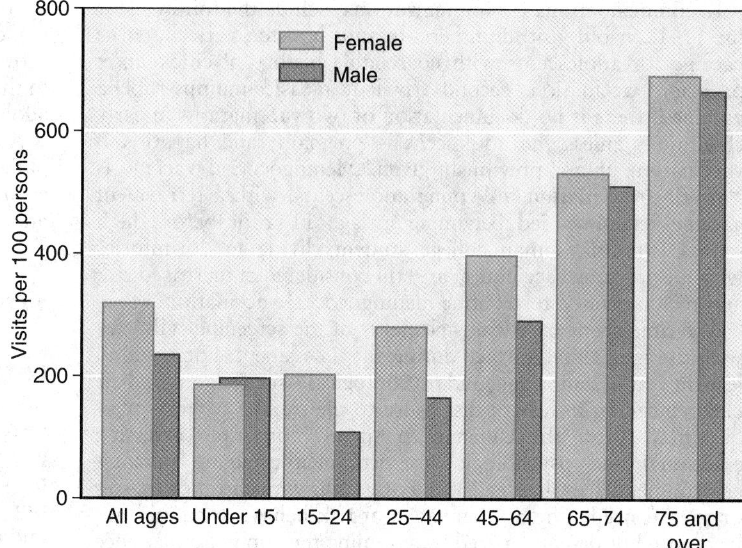

Figure 111-1. Annual rate of visits to office-based physicians by patient's age and sex: United States, 2002. (From National Center for Health Statistics, 2004.)

TABLE 111-2. Comparison of Supervision Guidelines

SOURCE *PERIODICITY*	AAP *ANNUALLY*	GAPS *ANNUALLY*	BRIGHT FUTURES *ANNUALLY*
ANTICIPATORY GUIDANCE			
Parenting	X	X	X
Adolescent development	X	X	X
Safety practices	X	X	X
Diet and fitness	X	X	X
Healthy lifestyles	X	X	X
Oral health	X		X
SCREENING HISTORY			
Tobacco use	X	X	X
Alcohol and drug use	X	X	X
Sexual behavior	X	X	X
School performance	X	X	X
Depression/suicide risk	X	X	X
Eating disorders	X	X	
Learning problems		X	X
Abuse	X	X	X
PHYSICAL ASSESSMENT WITH SPECIFIC RECOMMENDATIONS			
Hypertension	X*	X	
Obesity	X*	X	X
Breast cancer (self-examination)	X		X
Comprehensive examination	X	X	X
Scoliosis	X		X
TESTS			
Hyperlipidemia	X	X	X
Tuberculin	X†	X†	X‡
Vision	X		X
Anemia	X		X
GC, chlamydia, syphilis§	X	X	X
Genital warts (HPV)§		X	
HIV infection	X	X	X
Cervical cancer‖	X	X	X
IMMUNIZATIONS			
MMR	X	X	X
dT	X	X	X
Hepatitis B	X	X	X

*Recommends obtaining and plotting measures only.
†Under specific conditions.
‡At least one during adolescence (14–16 yr old).
§For adolescents who are sexually active.
‖For adolescent girls who are sexually active or ≥18 yr old.

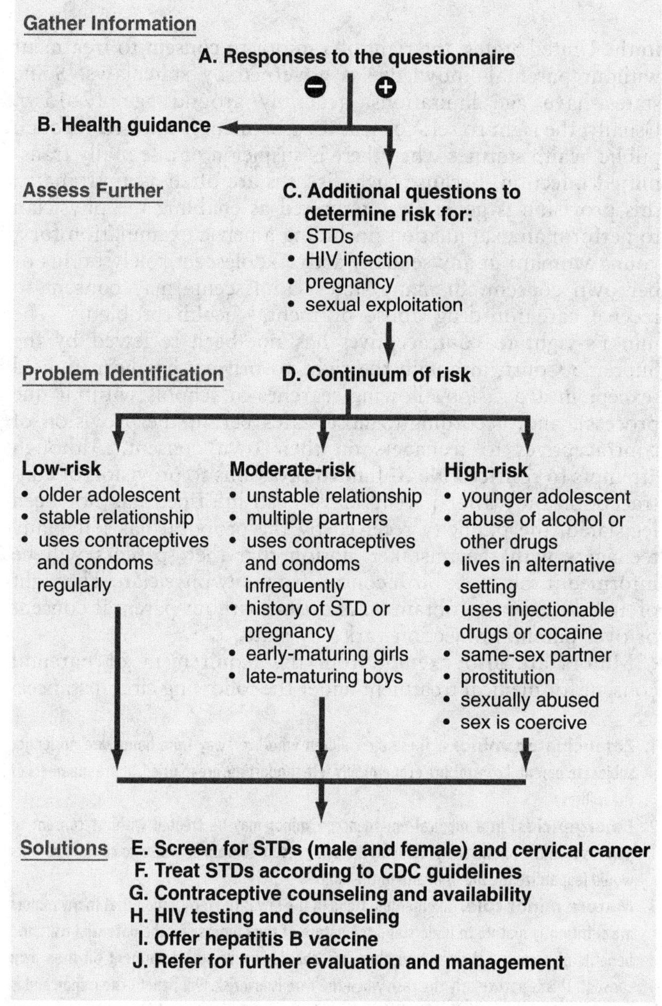

Figure 111-2. Sexuality algorithm. (From Levenberger PB, Elster AB: *Guidelines for Adolescent Preventive Services, Clinical Evaluation and Management Handbook*. Chicago, American Medical Association, 1995. © 1995 American Medical Association.)

Recommendations for immunizations include the following at the 11–12 yr old visit: diphtheria-tetanus booster; varicella virus vaccine for adolescents with no reliable history of chickenpox or prior vaccination; second trivalent measles-mumps-rubella vaccine if there is no documentation of two vaccinations in early childhood, unless the adolescent is pregnant; and hepatitis B vaccination, if not previously given. Meningococcal vaccine is a routine vaccination for young adolescents, with a tetravalent vaccine recommended beginning at age 11 yr or before high school entry. Freshman college students living in dormitories without previous vaccination are still considered at increased risk and recommended for routine meningococcal vaccination.

The time spent on various elements of the screening will vary with the issues that surface during the assessment. For gay and lesbian youths, emotional and psychological issues related to their experiences, from fear of disclosure to the trauma of homophobia, may direct the clinician to spend more time assessing emotional and psychologic supports in the young person's environment (see Chapter 13.2). For youths with chronic illnesses or special needs, the assessment of at-risk behaviors should not be omitted or de-emphasized by assuming they do not experience the "normal" adolescent vulnerabilities.

111.1 • Legal Issues

In the United States, the right of a minor to **consent** to treatment without parental knowledge is governed by state laws. Some states have age limitations, generally around age 12–15 yr. Usually, the right to self-consent for treatment is granted through public health statutes when there is suspicion of a sexually transmitted infection. Because such diseases are often asymptomatic, this provision is generally interpreted as enabling the physician to perform an examination (including a pelvic examination for a young woman) in any sexually active adolescent solely on his or her own consent. In many states, adolescents may consent to receive care for drug abuse or mental health problems. The minor's right to **contraceptives** has not been reviewed by the Supreme Court, although the right to privacy has been upheld (except in a decision allowing searches in schools without due process), and, accordingly, most states permit the provision of contraceptives to teenagers on their own consent. Although attempts to restrict Title X–funded programs to provision of contraception only after parents have been informed has not been legislated, the publicity received by the proposal has left many teenagers with the mistaken notion that their parents will be informed if they seek birth control from any physician. The right of an adolescent to obtain an **abortion** without parental consent or over parental objection varies by state.

Minors are also exempt from the requirement of parental consent for medical treatment under the following circumstances:

1. **Emancipated minors.** These are children who live away from home, are no longer subject to parental control, are economically self-supporting, are married, or are members of the military.
2. **Emergencies.** In a medical emergency, a minor may be treated without consent of parents if, in the physician's judgment, the delay resulting from attempts to contact parents would jeopardize the life or health of the minor.
3. **Mature minor rule.** An emerging trend in the law is the recognition that many minors are sufficiently mature to understand the nature of their illness and the potential risks and benefits of proposed therapy and, therefore, should receive such treatment on their own consent. This is particularly the case when the care is low risk, will benefit the minor, and is within established medical practice standards. In these cases, the physician should document that the adolescent has acted in a responsible manner.

Legal policies regarding the confidentiality of information are less consistent than those governing consent. In general, the right to self-consent for health care carries with it the right to confidentiality about that information. Exceptions exist when there are mandatory reporting requirements, as in abuse cases, some legal provision requiring parental disclosure, or a self-imposed danger to the minor. When exceptions exist, this should be divulged to the adolescent and an opportunity for assent or agreement provided.

A chaperone should be present whenever an adolescent female patient is examined by a male physician. The necessity for chaperones in the situation of a female physician examining a male adolescent patient has not yet become an issue.

111.2 • Screening Procedures

INTERVIEWING THE ADOLESCENT. The preparation for a successful interview with an adolescent patient varies based on the history of the relationship with the patient. Patients who are going from preadolescence to adolescence while seeing the same provider and their parents should be guided through the transition. Although the rules for confidentiality are the same for new and continuing patients, the change in the physician-patient relationship, allowing more privacy during the visit and more autonomy in the health process, may be threatening for the parent as well as the adolescent. For new patients, the initial phases of the interview are more challenging given the need to establish rapport rapidly with the patient in order to meet the goals of the encounter. Issues of confidentiality and privacy should be explicitly stated along with the conditions under which that confidentiality may need to be altered, that is, in life- or safety-threatening situations. For new patients, the parents should be interviewed with the adolescent or before the adolescent to ensure that the adolescent does not perceive a breach of confidentiality. The clinician who takes time to listen avoids judgmental statements and the use of street jargon and shows respect for the adolescent's emerging maturity will have an easier time communicating with him or her. The use of open-ended questions, rather than closed-ended questions, will further facilitate history taking (the closed-ended question "Do you get along with your father?" leading to the answer "Yes," compared with the question, "What would you like to change in your relationship with your father?," which may lead to an answer such as "I would like to stop him from always putting me down, especially in front of my friends").

The goals of the interview or clinical encounter are to establish an information base, identify problems and issues from the patient's perspective, and identify problems and issues from the perspective of the clinician based on knowledge of the health and other issues relevant to the adolescent age group. The adolescent should be given an opportunity to express concerns and the reasons for seeking medical attention. The adolescent as well as the parent should also be given an opportunity to express the strengths and successes of the adolescent, in addition to communicating problems.

Barriers to an effective interview occur when the interviewer is distracted by other events or individuals in the office, when there are extreme time limitations obvious to either party, or when there is expressible discomfort with either the patient or the interviewer. The need for an interpreter when a patient is hearing impaired or if the patient and interviewer are not language compatible provides a challenge but not necessarily a barrier under most circumstances (Chapter 4). Observations during the interview can be useful to the overall assessment of the patient's maturity, presence or absence of depression, and the parent-adolescent relationship. Given the key role of a successful interview in the screening process, adequate training and experience should be sought by clinicians wishing to give comprehensive care to adolescent patients.

PSYCHOSOCIAL ASSESSMENT. A few questions should be asked to detect the adolescent who is having difficulty with peer relation-

TABLE 111-3. HEADS/S F/FIRST

Home. Space, privacy, frequent geographic moves, neighborhood.
Education/School. Frequent school changes, repetition of a grade/in each subject, teachers' reports, vocational goals, after-school educational clubs (language, speech, math, etc.), learning disabilities.
Abuse. Physical, sexual, emotional, verbal abuse; parental discipline.
Drugs. Tobacco, alcohol, marijuana, inhalants, "club drugs," "rave" parties, others. Drug of choice, age at initiation, frequency, mode of intake, rituals, alone or with peers, quit methods, and number of attempts.
Safety. Seat belts, helmets, sports safety measures, hazardous activities, driving while intoxicated.
Sexuality/Sexual Identity. Reproductive health (use of contraceptives, presence of sexually transmitted diseases, feelings, pregnancy)
Family and Friends. Family: family constellation, genogram, single/married/separated/divorced/blended family, family occupations and shifts; history of addiction in 1st- and 2nd-degree relatives, parental attitude toward alcohol and drugs, parental rules; chronically ill physical or mentally challenged parent. **Friends:** peer cliques and configuration ("preppies," "jocks," "nerds," "computer geeks," cheerleaders), gang or cult affiliation.
Image. Height and weight perceptions, body musculature and physique, appearance (including dress, jewelry, tattoos, body piercing as fashion trends or other statement).
Recreation. Sleep, exercise, organized or unstructured sports, recreational activities (television, video games, computer games, Internet and chat rooms, church or community youth group activities [e.g., Boy/Girl Scouts; Big Brother/Sister groups, campus groups]). How many hours per day, days per week involved?
Spirituality and Connectedness. Use HOPE* or FICA† acronym; adherence, rituals, occult practices, community service or involvement.
Threats and Violence. Self-harm or harm to others, running away, cruelty to animals, guns, fights, arrests, stealing, fire setting, fights in school.

*HOPE: **h**ope or security for the future; **o**rganized religion; **p**ersonal spirituality and practices; **e**ffects on medical care and end of life issues.
†FICA: **f**aith beliefs; **i**mportance and influence of faith; **c**ommunity support.
From Dias PJ: Adolescent substance abuse. Assessment in the office. *Pediatr Clin North Am* 2002;49:269–300.

ships ("Do you have a best friend with whom you can share even the most personal secret?"), self-image ("Is there anything you would like to change about yourself?"), depression ("What do you see yourself doing 5 yr from now?"), school ("How are your grades this year compared with last year?"), personal decisions ("Are you feeling pressured to engage in any behavior for which you do not feel you are ready?"), and an eating disorder ("Do you ever feel that food controls you rather than vice versa?"). The GAPS and Bright Futures materials provide questions and patient encounter forms to structure the assessments that are available at their websites (*www.ama-assn.org; www.brightfutures.org*). The HEADS/SF/FIRST mnemonic, basic or expanded, can be useful in guiding the interview if encounter forms are not available (Table 111-3). Based on the assessments, appropriate counseling or referrals are recommended for more thorough probing or for in-depth interviewing.

PHYSICAL EXAMINATION

AUDIOMETRY. Highly amplified music of the kind enjoyed by many adolescents may result in hearing loss (see Chapter 636). Therefore, a hearing screening is recommended by the Bright Futures guidelines for adolescents who are exposed to loud noises regularly, have had recurring ear infections, or report problems.

VISION TESTING. The pubertal growth spurt may involve the optic globe, resulting in its elongation and myopia in genetically predisposed individuals. Vision testing should, therefore, be performed in order to detect this problem before it affects school performance.

BLOOD PRESSURE DETERMINATION. Criteria for a diagnosis of hypertension are based on age-specific norms that increase with pubertal maturation (see Chapter 445). An individual whose blood pressure exceeds the 95th percentile for his or her age is suspect for having hypertension, regardless of the absolute reading. Those adolescents with blood pressure between the 90th and 95th percentiles should receive appropriate counseling relative to weight and have a follow-up examination in 6 mo. Those with blood pressure above the 90th percentile should have their blood pressure measured on three separate occasions to determine the stability of the elevation before moving forward with an intervention strategy. The technique is important; false-positive results may be obtained if the cuff covers less than two thirds of the upper arm. The patient should be seated, and an average should be taken of the 2nd and 3rd consecutive readings, using the change rather than the disappearance as the diastolic pressure. Most adolescents with elevations of blood pressure have labile hypertension. If the blood pressure is below two standard deviations for age, anorexia nervosa and Addison disease should be considered.

SCOLIOSIS (SEE CHAPTER 678.1). Approximately 5% of male and 10–14% of female adolescents have a mild curvature of the spine. This is two to four times the rate in younger children. Scoliosis is typically manifested during the peak of the height velocity curve, at approximately 12 yr in females and 14 yr in males. Curves measuring greater than 10 degrees should be monitored by an orthopedist until growth is complete.

BREAST EXAMINATION (SEE CHAPTERS 114 AND 551). Examination of the female adolescent's breasts is performed to detect masses, evaluate progression of sexual maturation, provide reassurance about development, and teach the technique of self-examination with the hope that this practice will continue into the higher risk later years. Although self-examination is promoted in two of the three guidelines, there is disagreement on the justification for promoting this routinely, given the rare instances of malignant breast masses in this age group.

SCROTUM EXAMINATION. The peak incidence of germ cell tumors of the testes is in late adolescence and early adulthood. For that reason, palpation of the testes may have an immediate yield and should serve as a model for instruction of self-examination. Because varicoceles often appear during puberty, the examination also provides an opportunity to explain and reassure the patient about this entity (see Chapter 545).

PELVIC EXAMINATION. See Chapter 548.

LABORATORY TESTING. The increased incidence of iron-deficiency anemia after menarche mandates the performance of a hematocrit annually in young women with moderate to heavy menses. The reference standard for this test changes with progression of puberty, as estrogen suppresses erythropoietin (see Chapter 446). Populations with nutritional risk should also have the hematocrit monitored. Androgens have the opposite effect, causing the hematocrit to rise during male puberty; Sex Maturity Rating 1 males (see Chapter 12) have an average hematocrit of 39%, whereas those who have completed puberty (Sexual Maturation Rating 5: Chapter 12) have an average value of 43%. Tuberculosis testing on an annual basis is important in adolescents with risk factors, such as an adolescent with HIV, living in the household with someone with HIV, the incarcerated adolescent, or those with other risk factors, because puberty has been shown to activate this disease in those not previously treated. During adolescence, a screening urinalysis is indicated for the sexually active male and female. Polymorphonuclear leukocytes in the urinary sediment suggest the possibility of either cervicitis, vaginitis, or an asymptomatic infection of the urinary tract in adolescent females and urethritis in adolescent males.

Sexually active adolescents should undergo screening for sexually transmitted infections, regardless of symptoms (see Chapter 119). There are clear indications for chlamydia and gonorrhea screening of women younger than 25 yr old, but less sufficient evidence to support routine screening in young men. Screening young men is a clinical option and with newer noninvasive testing is being re-examined for benefit in reducing the spread of infection. HIV testing should be included for those at increased risk, those with a history of sexually transmitted infections, those with more than one sex partner in the past 6 mo, bisexual and homosexual males, sexual partners of at-risk individuals, and intravenous drug users, or those seen in high-risk or high-prevalence settings. Syphilis screening is recommended for pregnant adolescents and those at increased risk of infection. For sexually active females, the guidelines for Pap smears for cervical cancer screening suggest that screening can be delayed safely up to 3 yr after the onset of sexual activity or age 21 yr, whichever is earlier. Repeat screening can be performed every 2–3 yr contingent on past results and patient risk factors. Augmentation or replacement of the traditional Pap smear is occurring with techniques (Thin-Prep, AutoPap, Papnet, cervicography, human papillomavirus [HPV] DNA testing) that increase the sensitivity of the screen and add the ability to identify HPV, a potential cervical cancer risk.

Although not included in any of the guidelines, screening tests for genetic defect carrier states, such as sickle cell anemia, are commonly performed in affected populations. Age-appropriate counseling should be immediately available to ensure an opportunity to have questions answered and to have unspoken fears allayed.

111.3 • Health Enhancement

The health status of adolescents may be enhanced by application of principles of prevention and anticipatory guidance. Prevention of infectious disease should include immunization and counseling. Prevention of sexually transmitted infections and pregnancy is an important issue to be addressed in sexually active adolescents of both sexes. Prevention of the use of harmful illicit drugs and alcohol and the potential for related injuries should be reviewed. Prevention of automotive accidents and interpersonal conflicts ending violently, the leading killer of adolescents, and of smoking, the leading killer of adults, should also be discussed. Facilitating an optimal health outcome for the adolescent patient also includes supporting him or her in successfully negotiating adolescence through school, job, and personal and family relations.

Adolescent Medicine: State of the Art Reviews: The office visit. *Adolesc Med* 2003;14:263–272.

American Medical Association: *Guidelines for Adolescent Preventive Services, Recommendations Monograph,* 3rd ed. Chicago, American Medical Association, 1996.

Bilukha PP, Rosenstein N. Prevention and control of meningococcal disease. *MMWR* 2005;54(RR07);1–21.

Committee on Psychosocial Aspects of Child and Family Health 1995–1996: *Guidelines for Health Supervision III,* 3rd ed. Elk Grove Village, IL, American Academy of Pediatrics, 1997, updated 2002.

Elster AB: Comparison of recommendations for adolescent clinical preventive services developed by national organizations. *Arch Pediatr Adolesc Med* 1998;152:193–198.

Green M, Palfrey JS, Clark EM (editors): *Bright Futures: Guidelines for Health Supervision of Infants, Children, and Adolescents,* 2nd ed., update. Elk Grove Village, IL, American Academy of Pediatrics, 2002.

Larcher V: Consent, competence, and confidentiality. *Br Med J* 2005;350:353–356.

Loertscher L, Simmons P: Adolescents: Knowledge of and attitudes toward Minnesota laws concerning adolescent medical care. *J Pediat Adolesc Gynecol* 2006;19:205–207.

Society for Adolescent Medicine: Access to health care for adolescents and young adults: Position paper of the Society for Adolescent Medicine. *J Adolesc Health* 2004;35:342–344.

U.S. Preventive Services Task Force: Guide to Clinical Preventive Services, 2005. Recommendations of the U.S. Preventive Services Task Force (AHRQ publication no. 05-0570), available at: *www.ahrq.gov/clinic/pocketgd.htm* (accessed November 29, 2005).

Woodwell DA, Cherry DK: *National Ambulatory Medical Care Survey: 2002 Summary. Advance Data from Vital and Health Statistics* (publication no. 346). Hyattsville, MD, National Center for Health Statistics, 2004.

World Health Organization: Overview of Child and Adolescent Health and Development, available at: *www.who.int/child-adolescent-health/OVERVIEW/AHD/adh_over.htm* (accessed November 20, 2005).

Chapter 112 ■ Violent Behavior

Renée R. Jenkins

Interpersonal and community violence, physical abuse, and domestic violence lead to significant rates of injury and death for specific age, gender, and racial sectors of the population in the United States (also see Chapters 35 and 61). The World Health Organization (WHO) recognizes violence as a leading worldwide public health problem. WHO defines violence as "The intentional use of physical force or power, threatened or actual, against oneself, another person, or against a group or community that either results in or has a high likelihood of resulting in injury, death, psychologic harm, maldevelopment or deprivation." The Centers for Disease Control and Prevention (CDC) accept a definition of a violent injury as "a threatened or actual use of physical force against a person or group that either results or is likely to result in injury or death." Youths are perpetrators of violence, victims of violence, or observers of violence with varying severity of impact on the individual. Violent acts may result in, or are contributed to by, mental health problems or disorders. Pediatricians are challenged to screen for these disorders and counsel or refer adolescents with serious disorders to mental health professionals. The public health and educational communities have launched a spectrum of violence prevention interventions to increase youth prosocial behavior and reduce violence as a societal problem.

EPIDEMIOLOGY. In 2002, over 877,700 youths aged 10–24 yr old were injured from violent acts in the United States, with 1 in 13 requiring hospitalization. Firearm injuries present the most significant threat for injury and death, ranking second only to motor vehicles among causes of injury deaths. Although the rates of violent crime victimization have declined since the mid-1990s, rates in youths aged 12–24 yr are higher than in any other age group (Fig. 112-1). Worldwide, males are more likely to be homicide fatality victims than females (Table 112-1). Statistics Canada reported that the arrest rate of female youths for interpersonal offences increased twofold compared to their male counterparts between 1988 and 1998, while the same figures for adults increased only 6%. Homicide rates vary significantly from one region to another, from 36.4 per 100,000 in Latin America to 0.9 per 100,000 in high-income countries in Europe. Although the United States reported similar nonfatal violent behaviors in a cross-national study, the rate of violence-related mortality was considerably higher in the United States compared to those same countries, suggesting that the weapon of use, i.e., firearms, may play the explanatory role in the United States.

The Youth Risk Behavior Surveillance System reported a decrease in the proportion of youths carrying a weapon such as a gun, knife, or club in 2003 at 17.1% of students (26.9% male and 6.7% female) compared to 26.1% in 1991. Nationally, 33% of students in 2003 also reported being in a fight in the prior year; this too has declined from 42.5% in 1991. Adolescents also make up almost one fourth of the child abuse and neglect cases in the United States (see Chapter 36). Adolescents and children younger than 5 yr of age are the most likely victims of physical abuse that causes injury.

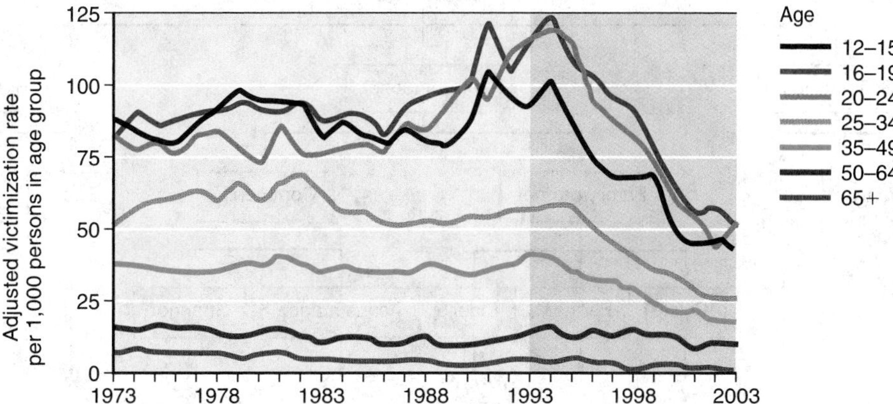

Figure 112-1. Violent crime rates by age of victim. Note: Violent crimes included are homicide, rape, robbery, and both simple and aggravated assault. The National Crime Victimization Survey redesign was implemented in 1993; the area with the lighter shading is before the redesign and the darker area after the redesign. The data before 1993 are adjusted to make them comparable to data collected since the redesign. The adjustment methods are described in *Criminal Victimization 1973–95*. Estimates for 1993 and beyond are based on collection year while earlier estimates are based on data year. For additional information about the methods used, see *Criminal Victimization 2003*. Additional information on this topic can be found in *Age Patterns of Victims of Serious Violent Crime*. For related data about homicide trends by age, see *Homicide Trends in the U.S.* Sources: Rape, robbery, and assault data are from the National Crime Victimization Survey (NCVS). Ongoing since 1972, this survey of households interviews about 75,000 persons age 12 and older in 42,000 households twice each year about their victimizations from crime. The homicide data are collected by the FBI's Uniform Crime Reports (UCR) from reports from law enforcement agencies. From *www.ojp.usdoj.gov/bjs/glance/vage.htm*.

ETIOLOGY. The WHO report places youth violence in a model within the context of three larger types of violence: self-inflicted, interpersonal, and collective (Fig. 112-2). Interpersonal violence is subdivided into violence largely between family members or partners and includes child abuse. Community violence occurs between individuals who are unrelated. Collective violence incorporates violence by people who are members of an identified group against another group of individuals with social, political, or economic motivation. The types of violence in this model have behavioral links, in that child abuse victims are more likely to experience violent and aggressive interpersonal behavior as adolescents and adults. Overlapping risk factors exist for the types of violence, such as firearm availability, alcohol abuse, and socioeconomic inequalities. The benefit to identifying common risk factors for the types of violence lies in the potential of intervening with prevention efforts and gaining positive outcomes for more than one type of violent behavior. The model further acknowledges four categories that explore the potential nature of violence as involving physical, sexual, or psychologic force, or deprivation.

Explanatory models of violence have emphasized intrapersonal and environmental influences. The development psychopathology model of Mofitt identifies two types of antisocial youths: one that is life course persistent and one that is life course limited.

TABLE 112-1. Estimated Global Homicide and Suicide Rates by Age Group, 2000

AGE GROUP (YR)	HOMICIDE RATE (PER 100,000 POPULATION)		SUICIDE RATE (PER 100,000 POPULATION)	
	MALES	FEMALES	MALES	FEMALES
0–4	5.8	4.8	0.0	0.0
5–14	2.1	2.0	1.7	2.0
15–29	19.4	4.4	15.6	12.2
30–44	18.7	4.3	21.5	12.4
45–59	14.8	4.5	28.4	12.6
≥60	13.0	4.5	44.9	22.1
Total*	13.6	4.0	18.9	10.6

*Age standardized.

From World Health Organization: *World Report on Violence and Health: Summary.* Geneva, World Health Organization, 2002 (Table 2, p 7).

Adolescent-limited offenders have no childhood aberrant behaviors and are more likely to commit status offenses such as vandalism, running away, and other behaviors symbolic of their struggle for autonomy from parents. **Life course–persistent offenders** exhibit aberrant behavior in childhood, such as problems with temperament, behavioral development, and cognition; as adolescents they participate in more victim-oriented crimes. The public health model emphasizes the environment and other external influences. A third theoretical model examines violent behaviors across the spectrum occurring within and outside the family and is referred to as the **cycle of violence.** This hypothesis proposes that precursors such as child abuse and neglect, a child witnessing violence, adolescent sexual and physical abuse, and adolescent exposure to violence and violent assaults predispose youths to outcomes of violent behavior, violent crime, delinquency, violent assaults, suicide, or premature death. An additional common paradigm for high-risk violence behavior poses a balance of risk and protective factors at the individual, family, and community levels. None of these theories successfully explains interpersonal or self-inflicted violent behavior. Although the media influence violence through a strong effect on aggressive behavior, many questions still remain about the causes of violent behavior.

CLINICAL MANIFESTATIONS. There are several clinical entities directly associated with violent behavior that require recognition and intervention. The most common behavioral diagnoses associated with aggressive behavior in adolescents are mental retardation (Chapter 38), learning disabilities (Chapter 32), moderately severe language disorders, and mental disorders such as attention-deficit/hyperactivity (Chapter 31), mood disturbance (Chapter 25), anxiety, and disruptive behavioral disorders (Chapter 28). Inability to master prosocial skills such as the establishment and maintenance of positive family and peer relations and the resolution of conflict may put adolescents with these disorders at higher risk of physical violence and other risky behaviors. **Conduct disorder** and **oppositional defiant disorder** are specific psychiatric diagnoses whose definitions are associated with violent behavior (Table 112-2). They occur co-morbidly with other disorders such as attention-deficit/hyperactivity disorder and increase an adolescent's vulnerability for juvenile delin-

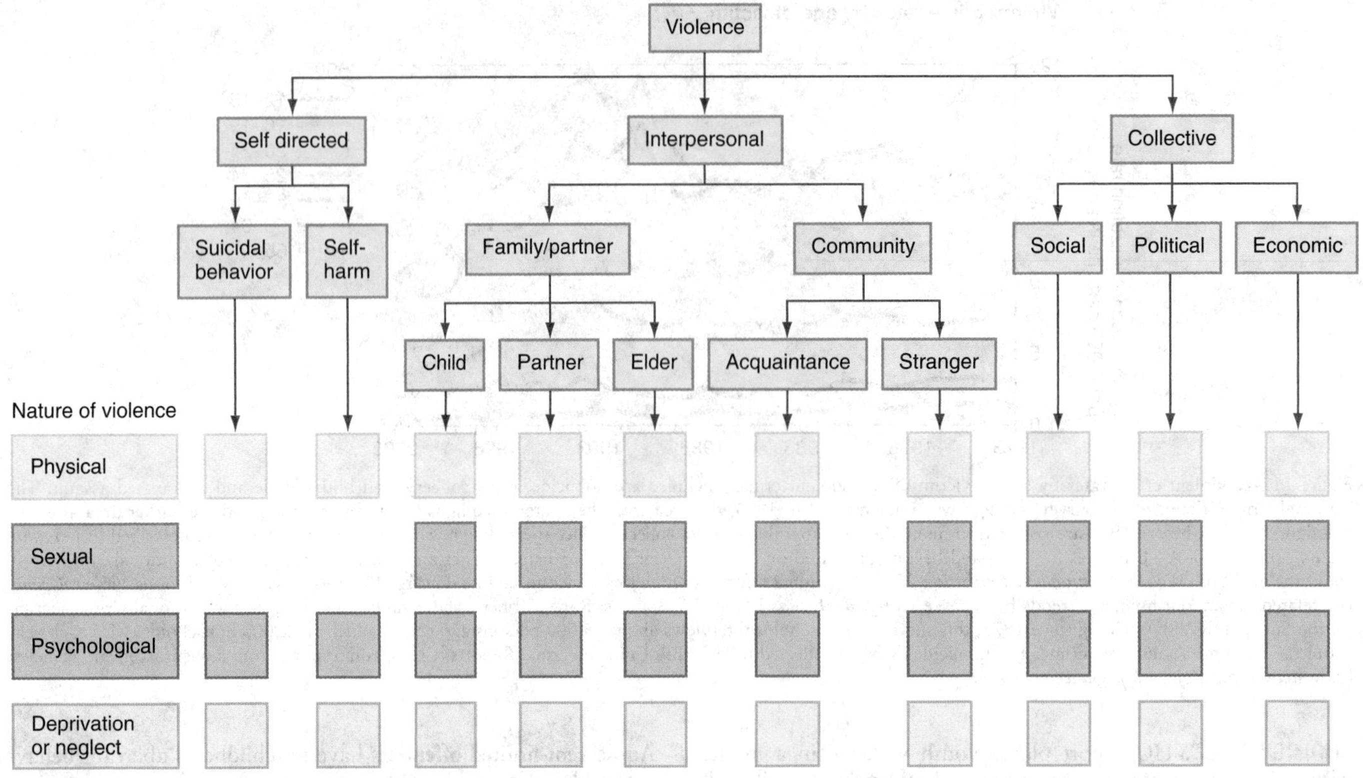

Figure 112-2. A typology of violence. (World Health Organization. *World Report on Violence and Health: Summary.* Geneva, World Health Organization, 2002, p 5.)

TABLE 112-2. Oppositional Defiant Disorder, Conduct Disorder, and Juvenile Delinquency

PSYCHIATRIC DISORDER LABELS		LEGAL LABEL JUVENILE DELINQUENCY
OPPOSITIONAL DEFIANT DISORDER	CONDUCT DISORDER	
Recurrent pattern of negativistic, defiant, disobedient, and hostile behavior toward authority figures that has a significant adverse effect on functioning (e.g., social, academic, occupational)	Repetitive and persistent pattern of behavior that violates the basic rights of others or major age-appropriate societal norms or rules	Offenses that are illegal because of age; illegal acts
Examples: losing temper; arguing with adults; defying or refusing to comply with request or rules of adults; annoying behavior; blaming others; and being irritable, spiteful, resentful	Examples: physical fighting, deceitfulness, stealing, destruction of property, threatening or causing physical harm to people or animals, driving without a license, prostitution, rape (even if not adjudicated in the legal system)	Examples: single or multiple instances of being arrested or adjudicated for any of the following: stealing, destruction of property, threatening or causing physical harm to people or animals, driving without a license, prostitution, rape
Diagnosed by a mental health clinician	Diagnosed by a mental health practitioner	Adjudicated in the legal system

From Greydanus DE, Pratt HD, Patel DR, Sloane MA: The rebellious adolescent. *Pediatr Clin North Am* 1997;44:1460.

quency, substance use or abuse, sexual promiscuity, adult criminal behavior, incarceration, and antisocial personality disorder.

In an emergency or urgent care setting, one is very likely to encounter victims of physical and/or sexual assault. Rather than treat the physical injury in isolation, the American Academy of Pediatrics has established a model protocol for physical assault victims and guidelines for caring for sexual assault victims. The guidelines recommend psychologic evaluation and support, social service evaluation of the circumstance surrounding the assault, and a treatment plan on discharge that is designed to protect the adolescent from subsequent injury episodes and minimize the development of psychologic disability. Victims as well as witnesses of violence are at risk of *post-traumatic stress disorder* (see Chapters 24 and 35).

DIAGNOSIS. The assessment of an adolescent at risk of, or with a history of, violent behavior or victimization should be a part of the health maintenance visit of all adolescents. The answers to questions about recent history of involvement in a physical fight, carrying a weapon, or firearms in the household, as well as concerns that the adolescent may have about his or her personal safety may suggest a problem requiring a more in-depth evaluation. The **FISTS mnemonic** provides guidance for structuring the assessment (Table 112-3). The additional factors of physical or sexual abuse, serious problems at school, poor school perfor-

TABLE 112-3. FISTS Mnemonic to Assess an Adolescent's Risk of Violence

F: Fighting (How many fights were you in last year? What was the last?)
I: Injuries (Have you ever been injured? Have you ever injured someone else?)
S: Sex (Has your partner hit you? Have you hit your partner? Have you ever been forced to have sex?)
T: Threats (Has someone with a weapon threatened you? What happened? Has any thing changed to make you feel safer?)
S: Self-defense (What do you do if someone tries to pick a fight? Have you carried a weapon in self-defense?)

From Knox L: *Connecting the Dots to Prevent Youth Violence: A Training and Outreach Guide for Physicians and Other Health Professionals.* Chicago, American Medical Association, 2002, p 24.

TABLE 112-4. Public Health Approach to Youth Violence Prevention Model with Examples

	VICTIM (HOST)	PERPETRATOR (VECTOR)	FIREARM (AGENT)	SOCIAL ENVIRONMENT	PHYSICAL ENVIRONMENT
Primary prevention	Conflict resolution Violence anticipatory guidance	Substance abuse treatment Home visiting programs for new and single parents	Handgun and assault weapons ban Firearm registration	Job opportunities Adult-supervised activities	Better lighting Zoning-enforced limits in liquor licenses
Secondary prevention	Medical services Psychologic services	Job training Psychosocial rehabilitation	Handgun locks Public education on risks of ownership	School incident debriefing Safe havens	Increased police presence Graffiti removal
Tertiary prevention	Physical rehabilitation Psychosocial services	Incarceration Educational-psychosocial rehabilitation	Firearm surveillance	Foster care Alternative schools	Urban planning, e.g., decrease population density in public housing and mixture of income levels

From Calhoun AD, Clark-Jones F: Theoretical frameworks: Developmental psychopathology, the public health approach to violence, and the cycle of violence. *Pediatr Clin North Am* 1998;45:287.

mance and attendance, multiple incidents of trauma, and symptoms associated with mental disorders are indications for evaluation by a mental health professional. In a situation of acute trauma, assault victims are not always forthcoming about the circumstances of their injuries for fear of retaliation or police involvement. Stabilization of the injury or the gathering of forensic evidence in sexual assault is the treatment priority; however, once this is achieved, addressing a more comprehensive set of issues surrounding the assault is appropriate.

TREATMENT. In the instance of acute injury secondary to violent assault, the treatment plan should follow standards established by the American Academy of Pediatrics model protocol, which includes, but is not limited to, the stabilization of the injury, evaluation and treatment of the injury, evaluation of the assault circumstance, psychologic evaluation of the functioning of the victim, rehabilitation of the injury, and outpatient follow-up of the behavioral and physical sequelae. See Chapter 118 for the management of sexual assault victims. Multiple treatment modalities are used simultaneously in managing adolescents with persistent violent and aggressive behavior and range from cognitive-behavioral therapy involving the individual and family to specific family interventions (parent management training, multisystemic treatment) and pharmacotherapy. Treatment of existing co-morbid conditions such as attention-deficit/hyperactivity disorder, depression appears to reduce aggressive behavior. Pharmacotherapy studies are underway examining the use of risperidone in patients with a conduct disorder diagnosis in whom aggressive behavior severely affects their functioning.

PREVENTION. The WHO report recognizes a multitiered approach to prevention: individual approaches, relationship approaches, community approaches, and societal approaches (Table 112-4). **Individual approaches** concentrate on changing attitudes and behaviors to avoid aggressive and violent behavior for all children as well as youths who have already displayed some violent tendencies. **Relationship approaches** focus more on victims, families, and peer relationships, especially those with the potential to trigger aggressive or violent responses. **Community-based approaches** raise public awareness in an effort to stimulate action by community members to reduce violence and protect vulnerable community members. **Societal approaches** include broader advocacy and legislative actions, as well as societal and cultural environmental changes. A specific prevention strategy can incorporate several approaches, such as the handgun/firearm prevention recommendations that include gun-lock safety, public education, and legislative advocacy. The CDC characterizes specific successful programs and summarizes program content on its website *(www.cdc.gov)*. For the clinician, three levels of competency are outlined for emergency medicine residency trainees that have broader clinician applicability: generalist level (I), specialist (II), and scholar/leader level (III). Table 112-5 describes the generalist competencies. Clinicians are encouraged to develop competencies consistent with the spectrum of approaches.

TABLE 112-5. Generalist Competencies for Youth Violence Prevention

Medical Knowledge

1. Recognize violence as a public health problem
2. Describe interconnection among different types of violence
3. Identify risk and protective factors for youth violence including the socioemotional competencies that research suggests are protective against violence
4. Understand violence is preventable

Practice-based Learning and Improvement

5. Recognize the value of research and evaluation on violence prevention
6. List interventions that have been found to be effective in the prevention of youth violence and know the characteristics common to effective interventions

Interpersonal and Communication Skills

7. Demonstrate skill in culturally appropriate and empowering communications with youths and their families around issues of violence
8. Engender "hope" in youths and families regarding violence prevention
9. Examine personal beliefs and experiences with violence and know their impact on professional practice and attitudes
10. Understand people do not want to live in a violent environment, nor do they want their families to live in a violent environment

Professionalism

11. Perceive youths, families, and communities as useful resources and partners/colleagues with health professional in reducing risk, increasing protection, and preventing violence

Systems-Based Practice

12. Know possible roles for all health professionals in youth violence prevention
13. Know legal requirements for health professionals as they relate to youth violence
14. Understand violence prevention is an appropriate and important role for health professionals and that this role occurs in the context of large multisector efforts to prevent violence
15. Demonstrate knowledge of role health professionals can play in social and political advocacy for the health of youths, families, and communities

Adapted from Denninghoff KR, Knox L, Cunningham R, Partain S: Emergency medicine: Competencies for youth violence prevention and control. *Acad Emerg Med* 2002;9:947–956.

American Academy of Pediatrics, Committee on Adolescence: Care of the adolescent sexual assault victim. *Pediatrics* 2001;107:1476–1479 *(www.aap.org)*.

American Academy of Pediatrics, Task Force on Adolescent Assault Victim Needs: Adolescent assault victim needs: A review of issues and a model protocol. *Pediatrics* 1996;98:991–1001 *(www.aap.org)*.

Brener N, Lowry R, Barrios L: Violence-related behaviors among high-school students—United States, 1991–2003. *MMWR* 2004;53:651–655.

Denninghoff KR, Knox L, Cunningham R, Partain S: Emergency medicine: Competencies for youth violence prevention and control. *Acad Emerg Med* 2002;9:947–956.

Duke N, Resnick MD, Borowsky IW: Adolescent firearm violence: Position paper of the Society for Adolescent Medicine. *J Adolesc Health* 2005;37:171–174.

Hennes HMA, Calhoun AD (editors): Violence among children and adolescents. *Pediatr Clin North Am* 1998;45:269–280.

Knox L: *Connecting the Dots to Prevent Youth Violence: A Training and Outreach Guide for Physicians and Other Health Professionals.* Chicago, IL, American Medical Association, 2002.

Krug EG, Dahlberg LL, Merch JA, et al: World Report on Violence and Health: Summary. Geneva, World Health Organization, 2002, available at: *www.who.int/violence_injury_prevention/violence/world_report/en/summary_en.pdf* (accessed August 11, 2005).

Rappaport N, Thomas C: Recent research findings on aggressive and violent behavior in youth: Implications for clinical assessment and intervention. *J Adolesc Health* 2004;35:260–277.

Rennison CM: Criminal Victimization 2000: Changes 1999–2000 with Trends 1993–2000. Bureau of Justice Statistics. National Crime Victimization Survey, June 2001, available at: *www.ojp.usdoj.gov/bjs/pub/pdf/cv00.pdf.*

Smith-Khuri, Iachan R, Scheidt PC, et al: A cross national study of violence-related behaviors in adolescents. *Arch Pediatr Adolesc Med* 2004; 158:539–544.

Zwi A, Grove N, Kelly P, et al: Child health in armed conflict: time to rethink. *Lancet* 2006;367:1886–1888.

Chapter 113 ■ Substance Abuse

Renée R. Jenkins and Hoover Adger

Cultural and societal attitudes frame acceptable behaviors for substance use. Adolescents are influenced by adult role models and environmental messages related to substances. In the context of the current decade, occasional or situational use of certain substances such as alcohol, marijuana, and cigarettes may be viewed as "normative" given the proportion of youths who report some experience with these substances. Others view the potential for adverse outcomes even with occasional use in immature adolescents, such as motor vehicle accidents and other injuries, sufficient justification to consider any drug use in younger adolescents a considerable risk.

Drug use in younger, less experienced adolescents can act as a substitute for developing age-appropriate coping strategies and enhance vulnerability to poor decision-making. The first use of the most commonly used drugs occurs before age 18 yr, with 88% of people reporting first alcohol use <21 yr old, the legal drinking age in the United States. When drug use begins to negatively alter functioning in older adolescents at school and in the family and risk-taking behavior is seen, intervention is warranted. Serious drug use is not an isolated phenomenon. It is a part of a complex set of family and individual issues that should be addressed in a comprehensive fashion. The challenge to the clinician is to determine which type of behavior one is observing and to take the necessary action. The challenge to the community and society is to create norms that decrease the likelihood of adverse health outcomes for adolescents and promote and facilitate opportunities for adolescents to choose healthier and safer options.

ETIOLOGY. Substance abuse is biopsychosocially determined. Biologic factors, including genetic predisposition, are established contributors. Behaviors such as rebelliousness, poor school performance, delinquency, criminal activity, and personality traits such as low self-esteem, anxiety, and lack of self-control are frequently associated with or predate the onset of drug use. The determinants of adolescent substance use and abuse are explained using a number of theoretical models, with factors at the individual level, the level of significant relationships with others, and the level of the setting or environment. Models include a balance of risk and protective or coping factors that tend to account for individual differences among adolescents with similar risk factors who escape adverse outcomes. Risk factors for adolescent drug use may differ from those associated with adolescent drug abuse. Adolescent **use** is more commonly related to social and peer factors, whereas **abuse** is more often a function of psychologic and biologic factors. The likelihood that an otherwise normal adolescent would experiment with drugs may be dependent on the availability of the drug to the adolescent, the perceived positive or otherwise functional value to the adolescent, and the presence or absence of restraints as determined by the adolescent's cultural or other important value systems. An abusing adolescent may have genetic or biologic factors coexisting with dependence on a particular drug for coping with day-to-day activities.

Specific historical questions can assist in determining the severity of the drug problem through a rating system (Table 113-1). The type of drug used (marijuana versus heroin), the circumstances of use (alone or in a group setting), the frequency and timing of use (daily before school versus rarely on a weekend), the premorbid personality (depressed versus happy), as well as the teenager's general functional status should all be considered in evaluating any youngster found to be abusing a drug. The stage of drug use/abuse should also be considered (Table 113-2). Certain protective factors play a part in buffering the risk factors as well as assisting in anticipating the long-term outcome of experimentation. Emotionally supportive parents with open communication styles, involvement in organized school activities, and recognition of the importance of academic achievement are examples of the important protective factors. Involvement in

TABLE 113-1. Assessing the Seriousness of Adolescent Drug Abuse

VARIABLE	0	+1	+2
Age (yr)	>15	<15	
Sex	Male	Female	
Family history of drug abuse		Yes	
Setting of drug use	In group		Alone
Affect before drug use	Happy	Always poor	Sad
School performance	Good, improving		Recently poor
Use before driving	None		Yes
History of accidents	None		Yes
Time of week	Weekend	Weekdays	
Time of day		After school	Before or during school
Type of drug	Marijuana, beer, wine	Hallucinogens, amphetamines	Whiskey, opiates, cocaine, barbiturates

Total score: 0–3 = less worrisome, 3–8 = serious, 8–18 = very serious.

TABLE 113-2. Stages of Adolescent Substance Abuse

STAGE	DESCRIPTION
1	Potential for abuse • Decreased impulse control • Need for immediate gratification • Available drugs, alcohol, inhalants • Need for peer acceptance
2	Experimentation: learning the euphoria • Use of inhalants, tobacco, marijuana, and alcohol with friends • Few, if any, consequences • Use may increase to weekends regularly • Little change in behavior
3	Regular use: seeking the euphoria • Use of other drugs, e.g., stimulants, LSD, sedatives • Behavioral changes and some consequences • Increased frequency of use; use alone • Buying or stealing drugs
4	Regular use: preoccupation with the "high" • Daily use of drugs • Loss of control • Multiple consequences and risk-taking • Estrangement from family and "straight" friends
5	Burnout: use of drugs to feel normal • Polysubstance use/cross-addiction • Guilt, withdrawal, shame, remorse, depression • Physical and mental deterioration • Increased risk-taking, self-destructive, suicidal

From Comerci GD: Recognizing the five stages of substance abuse. *Contemp Pediatr* 1985;2:57–68.

TABLE 113-3. Thirty-Day Prevalence (Recent) Use of Alcohol, Cigarettes, Marijuana, Inhalants, and Steroids (Anabolic-Androgenic) in 8th, 10th, and 12th Grades, 2001 and 2004

	8TH GRADE (%)	10TH GRADE (%)	12TH GRADE (%)
Alcohol			
2001	21.5	39.0	49.8
2004	18.6	35.2	48.0
Cigarettes			
2001	12.2	21.3	29.5
2004	9.2	16.0	25.0
Marijuana			
2001	9.2	19.8	22.4
2004	6.4	15.9	19.9
Inhalants			
2001	4.0	2.4	1.7
2004	4.5	2.4	1.5
Steroids (anabolic)			
2001	0.7	0.9	1.3
2004	0.5	0.8	1.6

From Johnston LD, O'Malley PM, Bachman JG, et al: National press release, Overall teen drug use continues gradual decline; but use of inhalants rises, December 21, 2004, University of Michigan News and Information Services, Ann Arbor, available at *www.monitoringthefuture.org/press.html* (accessed April 26, 2005).

organized sports activities is usually protective, but it may be a risk factor in regard to the use of anabolic steroids. Any use of a psychoactive drug in the context of the use of machinery or a motor vehicle or in a potentially volatile interpersonal interaction can add an increased health risk, regardless of the extent of any prior use.

EPIDEMIOLOGY. Surveys on adolescent substance use have a variety of limitations due to sampling and questionnaire differences. The National Survey on Drug Use and Health may reflect refusal to report use within a household, but has more diverse ethnic subgroup data. School-based surveys (Monitoring the Future study and Youth Risk Behavior Surveillance) do not capture school dropouts, school absenteeism, and high rates of refusal. The rates of drug use across surveys are not dramatically different and certain observations are consistent across surveys. In the United States, alcohol and cigarettes are the most prevalent drugs (Table 113-3). Marijuana is the most commonly reported illicit drug used. The prevalence of substance use varies by age, gender, geographic region, race, and other demographic and contextual factors. Younger teenagers tend to report less use of most drugs than do older teenagers, with the exception of inhalants (17.3% in 8th grade, 12.4% in 10th grade, 10.9% in 12th grade, 2004). Males strongly predominate in the lifetime prevalence reports for smokeless tobacco and anabolic steroids compared with females. Less urbanized areas report more binge drinking and daily cigarette use than urban ones. In school surveys, Hispanics report more experience with cocaine in 8th and 10th grades, whereas white students report high rates of smokeless tobacco and daily cigarette smoking in all grades. By 12th grade, blacks report less use of drugs across most categories. Methamphetamine and heroin use has become popular in rural poor whites and affluent suburban adolescents in the Midwest, respectively.

In examining trends in drug use, fewer students reported marijuana, alcohol, and cigarette use over the years since 2001 in 8th, 10th, and 12th grades (see Table 113-3). Inhalant use in 8th grade and anabolic steroid use in 12th grade have been increasing since 2001. Prescription drug abuse is increasing in prevalence among adolescents. Over 7% of high school seniors report nonmedical use of prescription sedatives. Abused medications include Vicodin, oxycodone, Percocet, and Ritalin. Younger adolescents may abuse over-the-counter medications (Benadryl) and have "skittle" parties ingesting "colored" pills for a high.

Since 1999, European nations have been surveying student drug use employing the same methods used in the United States. Among 15–16 yr old students, in the past 30 days, European students compared to U.S. students were more likely to have smoked tobacco (37% vs 26%) and to have consumed alcohol (61% vs 40%), while U.S. students were more likely to have used marijuana (41% vs 17%) and any other illicit drug (23% vs 6%). In Australia, 40% of students ages 12 to 17 yr report ever using marijuana, 9% hallucinogens, and 6% amphetamines.

Club drugs (rave dance parties) and date rape drugs are increasingly popular among older adolescents and young adults (Table 113-4).

PATHOGENESIS. The process of physical growth and development that characterizes puberty may be affected adversely by the use of drugs. One third of adolescent females who use heroin have secondary amenorrhea, even in the absence of weight loss. The higher incidence of menstrual abnormalities in the adolescent

TABLE 113-4. Common Names and Salient Features of New Club Drugs Used Recreationally

	MDMA	EPHEDRINE	γ-HYDROXYBUTYRATE	γ-BUTYROLACTONE	1,4-BUTANEDIOL	KETAMINE	FLUNITRAZEPAM	NITRITES
Common name	Ecstasy, XTC, E, X, adam, hug drug	Herbal Ecstasy, herbal fuel, zest	Liquid Ecstasy, goop soap, Georgia homeboy, grievous bodily harm	Blue nitro, longevity, revivarant, GH revitalizer, gamma G, nitro, insom-X, remforce, firewater, invigorate	Thunder nectar, serenity, pine needle extract, zen, enliven, revitalise plus, lemon drops	K, special K, vitamin K, ket, kat	Roofies, circles, rophies, rib, roche, roaches, forget pill, R2, Mexican valium, roopies ruffies	Poppers, ram, rock hard, thrust, TNT
Duration of action	4–6 hr	4–6 hr	1.5–3.5 hr	1.5–3.5 hr	1.5–3.5 hr	1–3 hr	6–12 hr	Minutes
Elimination half-life	8–9 hr	5–7 hr	27 min	ND	ND	2 hr	9–25 hr	ND
Peak plasma concentration	1–3 hr	2–3 hr	20–60 min*	15–45 min	15–45 min	20 min	1 hr	Seconds
Physical dependence	No	No	Yes	Yes	Yes	No	Yes	No
Antidote	No	No	No	No	No	No	Yes	No
DEA schedule	I	None	III	None	None	III	IV	None
Detection with routine drug screen	Yes†	Yes†	No	No	No	No‡	No‡	No
Best detection method (time frame)	GC/MS (4 hr–2 days)	GC/MS (4 hr–2 days)	GC/MS (1–12 hr)	GC/MS (1–12 hr)	GC/MS (1–12 hr)	GC/MS (1 day)	GC/MS (1–12 hr)	GC/MS (1–12 hr)

DEA, U.S. Drug Enforcement Agency, currently reviewing possibility of flunitrazepam being placed into schedule of the U.S. Controlled Substance Act; GC/MS, gas chromatography–mass spectroscopy. Duration, half-life, and peak plasma are probably different after high or sequential doses because of nonlinear kinetics; ND, not determined in human beings.

*Depends on dose.

†Concentrations that are sufficiently high can give positive results for amphetamine because of cross reactions.

‡Flunitrazepam can give positive results for benzodiazepines; ketamine can give positive results for phencyclidine.

From Ricaurte GA, McCann UD: Recognition and management of complication of new recreational drug use. *Lancet* 2005;365:2137–2145.

TABLE 113-5. The Most Common Toxic Syndromes

ANTICHOLINERGIC SYNDROMES	
Common signs	Delirium with numbling speech, tachycardia, dry, flushed skin, dilated pupils, myoclonus, slightly elevated temperature, urinary retention, and decreased bowel sounds. Seizures and dysrhythmias may occur in severe cases.
Common causes	Antihistamines, antiparkinsonian medication, atropine, scopolamine, amantadine, antipsychotic agents, antidepressant agents, antispasmodic agents, mydriatic agents, skeletal muscle relaxants, and many plants (notably jimson weed and *Amanita muscaria*).
SYMPATHOMIMETIC SYNDROMES	
Common signs	Delusions, paranoia, tachycardia (or bradycardia if the drug is a pure α-adrenergic agonist), hypertension, hyperpyrexia, diaphoresis, piloerection, mydriasis, and hyperreflexia. Seizures, hypotension, and dysrhythmias may occur in severe cases.
Common causes	Cocaine, amphetamine, methamphetamine (and its derivatives 3,4-methylenedioxyamphetamine, 3,4-methylenedioxymethamphetamine, 3,4-methylenedioxyethamphetamine, and 2,5-dimethoxy-4-bromoamphetamine), and over-the-counter decongestants (phenylpropanolamine, ephedrine, and pseudoephedrine). In caffeine and theophylline overdoses, similar findings, except for the organic psychiatric signs, result from catecholamine release.
OPIATE, SEDATIVE, OR ETHANOL INTOXICATION	
Common signs	Coma, respiratory depression, miosis, hypotension, bradycardia, hypothermia, pulmonary edema, decreased bowel sounds, hyporeflexia, and needle marks. Seizures may occur after overdoses of some narcotics, notably propoxyphene.
Common causes	Narcotics, barbiturates, benzodiazepines, ethchhlorvynol, glutethimide, methyprylon, methaqualone, meprobamate, ethanol, clonidine, and guanabenz.
CHOLINERGIC SYNDROMES	
Common signs	Confusion, central nervous system depression, weakness, salivation, lacrimation, urinary and fecal incontinence, gastrointestinal cramping, emesis, diaphoresis, muscle fasciculations, pulmonary edema, miosis, bradycardia or tachycardia, and seizures.
Common causes	Organophosphate and carbamate insecticides, physostigmine, edrophonium, and some mushrooms.

From Kulig K: Inital management of ingestions of toxic substances. *N Engl J Med* 1992;326:1678.

heroin user probably results from a greater vulnerability of the hypothalamic-pituitary-ovarian axis in the maturing individual. Experiments with naloxone, the opiate antagonist, suggest that endogenous opiates block the release of gonadotropin-releasing hormone. Amphetamines interfere with stage 4 sleep and may impair the relationship between sleep and augmentation of secretion of gonadotropin during early adolescence (also see Chapter 18). To derive calories mainly from ethanol during the peak of the pubertal growth spurt deprives the body of the protein necessary for normal muscle growth.

The metabolism of certain prescribed drugs may be affected by coincident abuse of illicit drugs or alcohol. Induction of hepatic enzymes by barbiturates or alcohol may accelerate the metabolism and enhance the excretion of substances requiring glucuronidation. Estrogen-containing oral contraceptives taken by an abuser of these substances may result in a vulnerability to pregnancy. The use of estrogens increases the risk of intoxication from alcohol as a result of decreased ethanol metabolism. The potentiating interaction of alcohol and barbiturates must also be considered when prescribing anticonvulsant medications. Abdominal pain and vomiting occur when metronidazole is ingested by an alcohol-abusing adolescent because of the antagonistic effect of alcohol on acetaldehyde.

CLINICAL MANIFESTATIONS. Although manifestations vary by the specific substance of use, adolescents who use drugs often present in an office setting with no obvious physical findings. Drug use is more frequently detected in adolescents who are victims of motor vehicle accidents or intentional injuries. Eliciting appropriate historical information regarding substance use, followed by blood alcohol and urine drug screens is recommended in emergency settings. An adolescent presenting to an emergency setting with an impaired sensorium as part of a toxic syndrome should be evaluated for substance use as a part of the differential diagnosis (Table 113-5). Certain psychiatric and behavioral diagnoses, including conduct disorders and personality disorders, are frequently associated with substance use and should be considered once such use is detected. Screening for substance use is recommended for patients with psychiatric and behavioral diagnoses. Other clinical manifestations of substance use are associated with the route of use; intravenous drug use is associated with venous "tracks" and needle marks, and nasal mucosal injuries are associated with nasal insufflation of drugs. Seizures can be a direct effect of drugs such as cocaine and amphetamines or an effect of drug withdrawal in the case of barbiturates or tranquilizers. Additional specific clinical manifestations are described in the following sections on each substance.

SCREENING FOR SUBSTANCE ABUSE DISORDERS. The annual health maintenance examination provides an opportunity for identifying adolescents with substance use or abuse issues (see Chapters 19 and 111). The direct questions as well as the assessment of school, family relations, and peer activities may necessitate a more in-depth interview if there are suggestions of difficulties in those areas. Several self-report screening questionnaires are available with varying degrees of standardization, length, and reliability. Mnemonics specifically designed for adolescents are in use (CRAFFT) (Table 113-6). The use of urine screening is recommended in select circumstances, most of which are constructed to provide for the confidentiality and informed choice of the adolescent. Involuntary screening with parental permission is strongly discouraged for older, competent adolescents. Lack of decision-making capacity or very strong medical indications may present a clinical situation in which consent may be waived. Indications for urine screening include (1) psychiatric symptoms to rule out co-morbidity or dual diagnoses, (2) significant changes in school performance or other daily behaviors, (3) frequently occurring accidents, (4) frequently occurring episodes of respiratory problems, (5) evaluation of serious motor vehicular of other injuries, and (6) as a monitoring procedure for a recovery program. Table 113-7 demonstrates the types of tests commonly used for detection by substance, along with the approximate retention time between the use and the identification of the substance in the urine. Most initial screening uses an immunoassay method such as the enzyme-multiplied immunoassay technique followed by a confirmatory test using highly sensitive, highly specific gas chromatography–mass spectrometry. The

TABLE 113-6. CRAFFT Mnemonic Tool

- Have you ever ridden in a **C**ar driven by someone (including yourself) who was high or had been using alcohol or drugs?
- Do you ever use alcohol or drugs to **R**elax, feel better about yourself or fit in?
- Do you ever use alcohol or drugs while you are by yourself (**A**lone)?
- Do you ever **F**orget things you did while using alcohol or drugs?
- Do your **F**amily or **F**riends ever tell you that you should cut down on your drinking or drug use?
- Have you ever gotten into **T**rouble while you were using alcohol or drugs?

Adapted from Anglin TM: Evaluation by interview and questionnaire. In Schydlower M (editor): *Substance Abuse: A Guide for Health Professionals*, 2nd ed. Elk Grove Village, IL, American Academy of Pediatrics, 2002, p 69.

TABLE 113-7. Urine Screening for Drugs Commonly Abused by Adolescents

DRUG	MAJOR METABOLITE	INITIAL	FIRST CONFIRMATION	SECOND CONFIRMATION	APPROXIMATE RETENTION TIME
Alcohol (blood)	Acetaldehyde	GC	IA		7–10 hr
Alcohol (urine)	Acetaldehyde	GC	IA		10–13 hr
Amphetamines		TLC	IA	GC, GC/MS	48 hr
Barbiturates		IA	TLC	GC, GC/MS	Short-acting (24 hr); long-acting (2–3 wk)
Benzodiazepines		IA	TLC	GC, GC/MS	3 days
Cannabinoids	Carboxy- and hydroxymetabolites	IA	TLC	GC/MS	3–10 days (occasional user); 1–2 mo (chronic user)
Cocaine	Benzoyl ecgonine	IA	TLC	GC/MS	2–4 days
Methaqualone	Hydroxylated metabolites	TLC	IA	GC/MS	2 wk
Opiates					
Heroin	Morphine Glucuronide	IA	TLC	GC, GC/MS	2 days
Morphine	Morphine Glucuronide	IA	TLC	GC, GC/MS	2 days
Codeine	Morphine Glucuronide	IA	TLC	GC, GC/MS	2 days
Phencyclidine		TLC	IA	GC, GC/MS	8 days

GC, gas chromatography; IA, immunoassay; MS, mass spectrometry; TLC, thin-layer chromatography.
Modified from Drugs of abuse—urine screening [Physician information sheet]. Los Angeles, Pacific Toxicology. From MacKenzie RG, Kipke MD: Substance use and abuse. In Friedman SB, Fisher M, Schonberg SK (editors): *Comprehensive Adolescent Health Care*. St. Louis, Quality Medical Publishing, 1992, p 783.

substances that can cause false-positive results should be considered, especially when there is a discrepancy between the physical findings and the urine drug screen result. Parental use of home drug-testing products is ill advised.

DIAGNOSIS. Substance abuse is characterized by a maladaptive pattern of use indicated by continued use despite consequences or recurrent use where such use may be physically hazardous. Chemical dependence can be defined as a chronic and progressive disease process characterized by loss of control over use, compulsion, and the establishment of an altered state where one requires continued administration of a psychoactive substance in order to feel good or to avoid feeling bad (see Table 113-2). Diagnosing substance abuse rests on the realization that all children and adolescents are at risk but that some are at substantially more risk than others. Making the diagnosis must be part of a comprehensive diagnostic approach. Sources of diagnostic information might include history and mental status examination, physical examination, self-report questionnaires, structured interview and standardized tests, and laboratory screening. Specific diagnostic codes are assigned to substance abuse (Table 113-8) and substance dependence. These criteria are used in adults and have limitations in use with adolescents due to differing patterns of use, developmental implications, and other age-related consequences; an additional adolescent-sensitive set of criteria specifically for diagnostic use has not been developed. Adolescents who meet diagnostic criteria should be referred to a specialist in or program for substance abuse treatment unless the primary care physician has additional training in addiction medicine.

TABLE 113-8. DSM-IV-TR Diagnostic Criteria for Substance Abuse and Substance Dependence

SUBSTANCE ABUSE: A maladaptive pattern of substance use leading to clinical significant impairment of distress as manifested by one or more of the following criteria:

- Recurrent substance use resulting in a failure to fulfill major role obligations at work, school, or home (e.g., substance-related absences or suspensions from school, being fired from a job)
- Recurrent substance use in circumstances that are physically hazardous (e.g., driving an automobile, skiing, swimming, rock climbing, riding a bicycle, scooter or skateboard, or operating machinery while impaired by a substance's effects)
- Recurrent substance-related legal problems (e.g., arrest for driving under the influence, disorderly conduct, or vandalism, while impaired by a substance's effects)
- Continued substance use despite persistent or recurrent social or interpersonal problems caused or exacerbated by the effects of the substance (e.g., physical fights or unpleasant argument, damaging furniture or punching holes in the wall, sexual behavior that is later regretted)

From American Psychiatric Association: *Diagnostic and Statistical Manual of Mental Disorders, Fourth Edition, Text Revision*. Washington, DC, American Psychiatric Association, 2000.

COMPLICATIONS. Substance use in adolescence has psychologic as well as physical risks. Youths may engage in robbery, burglary, drug dealing, or prostitution for the purpose of acquiring the money necessary to buy drugs or alcohol. Acts of delinquent behavior are more commonly associated with recent illicit drug use (Fig. 113-1). Regular use of any drug eventually diminishes judgment and is associated with unprotected sexual activity with its consequences of pregnancy (see Chapter 117) and sexually transmitted infections (see Chapter 119), including HIV as well as physical violence and trauma. Drug and alcohol use is closely associated with trauma in the adolescent population. Several studies of adolescent trauma victims have identified cannabinoids and cocaine in blood and urine samples in significant proportions, in addition to the more common identification of alcohol. Any use of injected substances involves the risk of hepatitis B and C viruses as well as HIV.

PREVENTION. The model of prevention relevant to the problem of adolescent drug or alcohol use is one that anticipates experimentation with some agent at some point in the normal development of the adolescent and that attempts to delay that event as long as possible, to make its use as limited in amount and setting as possible, and to prevent entirely any use while operating a motor vehicle or any other machinery. The Center for Substance Abuse Prevention created a National Registry of Effective Prevention Programs as a resource of science-based prevention programs, all theoretically driven and based on known risk and protective factors. See Table 113-9 for an example of the domains and the risk and protective factors within those domains. Programs on the registry were scored on 15 criteria that demonstrated strong implementation and evaluation characteristics. These programs are offered for dissemination and have program developers available to provide technical assistance.

TABLE 113-9. Domains of Risk and Protective Factors for Substance Abuse Interventions

RISK FACTORS	DOMAIN	PROTECTIVE FACTORS
Early aggressive behavior	Individual	Self-control
Lack of parental supervision	Family	Parental monitoring
Substance abuse	Peer	Academic competence
Drug availability	School	Anti–drug use policies
Poverty	Community	Strong neighborhood attachment

www.nida.nih.gov/Prevention/Prevopen.html.

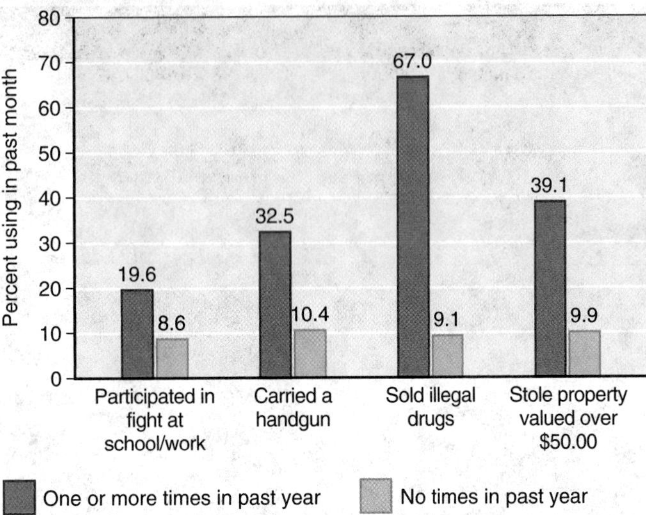

Figure 113-1. Past month illicit drug use among youths aged 12–17, by participation in delinquent behaviors: 2003. (From National Survey on Drug Use and Health Data, 2003. SAMHSA, Office of Applied Studies; available at: *www.oas.samhsa.gov* [accessed April 26, 2005]).

TREATMENT. Acute management is discussed in the following sections on specific agents. A variety of chronic treatment programs are available in inpatient and ambulatory settings. Brief interventions, including motivational interviewing, have been used in alcohol and tobacco users with some clinical effectiveness. These interventions are time limited and patient centered, with clear advice provided; they are useful in the primary care setting. Evidence-based practices for substance abuse disorder by hierarchy of evidence are provided in Table 113-10. Family, motivational, and cognitive-behavioral models have particular application for adolescents. Important features of successful long-term management of these adolescents include continuing medical evaluation after detoxification and the provision of developmentally appropriate psychosocial support systems.

PROGNOSIS. For adolescent substance abusers who have been referred to a drug treatment program, outcomes are directly related to regular attendance in post-treatment groups. For males with learning problems, these outcomes are poorer than those of their peers without learning problems. Peer use patterns and parental use have a major influence on outcome for males. For females, factors such as self-esteem and anxiety are more important influences on outcomes. The chronicity of a substance use disorder makes relapse an issue that must always be kept in mind when managing patients after treatment, and appropriate assistance from a health professional qualified in substance abuse management should be obtained.

113.1 • Alcohol

By 12th grade, close to 75% of adolescents in U.S. high schools report ever having an alcoholic drink, with over 25% having their first drink before age 13 yr. The initiation of alcohol use at an early age is associated with an increased risk of alcohol-related problems unless moderate use is deeply rooted in the adolescent's cultural tradition. The usual progression of alcohol use is from beer to wine to distilled spirits, although regional and national differences may alter this pattern. Four ounces of distilled spirits (86 proof) consumed on an empty stomach produces a plasma ethanol level of approximately 65 mg/dL in an adult male of average weight and 80 mg/dL in a premenstrual female of adult weight. The legal definition of intoxication in most statutes in the United States is a blood ethanol level of 80 or 100 mg/dL (0.08% or 0.10%).

Alcohol contributes to more deaths in young individuals than all the illicit drugs combined. Among studies of adolescent trauma victims, alcohol is reported to be present in 32–45% of hospital admissions. Motor vehicle crashes are the most frequent type of event associated with alcohol use, but the injuries spanned several types including self-inflicted wounds. Alcohol-positive adolescents are also more likely to report a history of injury. Pediatricians should not underestimate the need to recognize alcohol use and abuse and its short-term consequences in this age group.

PHARMACOLOGY AND PATHOPHYSIOLOGY. Alcohol (ethyl alcohol or ethanol) is rapidly absorbed in the stomach and is transported to the liver and metabolized by two pathways. The primary pathway involves removal of two hydrogen atoms to form acetaldehyde, a reaction catalyzed by alcohol dehydrogenase through reduction of a cofactor nicotinamide-adenine dinucleotide. The removed hydrogen atoms supply energy (7.1 kcal/g of alcohol) and contribute to the excess synthesis of triglycerides, a phenomenon that is responsible for producing a **fatty liver,** even in those who are well nourished. Engorgement of hepatocytes with fat causes necrosis, triggering an inflammatory process (**alcoholic hepatitis**), which is followed by fibrosis, the hallmark of **cirrhosis.** Early hepatic involvement may result in elevation in γ-glutamyl transpeptidase and serum glutamic-pyruvic transaminase. The second metabolic pathway, which is utilized at high serum alcohol levels, involves the microsomal enzyme system of the liver, in which the cofactor is reduced nicotinamide-adenine dinucleotide phosphate. The net effect of activation of this pathway is to decrease metabolism of drugs that share this system and to allow for their accumulation, enhanced effect, and possible toxicity (drinking alcohol and ingesting tranquilizers results in the potentiation of each).

CLINICAL MANIFESTATIONS. Alcohol acts primarily as a central nervous system (CNS) depressant. It produces euphoria, grogginess, talkativeness, impaired short-term memory, and an increased pain threshold. Alcohol's ability to produce vasodilation and hypothermia is also centrally mediated. At very high serum levels, respiratory depression occurs. Its inhibitory effect on pituitary antidiuretic hormone release is responsible for its diuretic effect. The gastrointestinal complications of alcohol use can occur from a single large ingestion. The most common is acute erosive **gastritis,** which is manifested by epigastric pain, anorexia, vomiting, and guaiac-positive stools. Less commonly, vomiting and midabdominal pain may be caused by acute alcoholic **pancreatitis;** diagnosis is confirmed by the finding of elevated serum amylase and lipase activities.

TABLE 113-10. Evidence-based Practices for Substance Abuse Disorders by Hierarchy of Evidence

PRACTICE	LEVEL OF EVIDENCE	PRACTICE	LEVEL OF EVIDENCE
Behavioral		Pharmacologic	
Brief intervention	2	Acamprosate	2
Brief strategic family	2	Buprenorphine	2
Cognitive-behavioral	2	Disulfiram	4
Drug counseling: individual and group	3	LAAM	2
		Methadone	2
		Naltrexone	2
Motivational enhancement therapy	2		
Multidimensional family therapy	2		
12-Step facilitation	3		

Level of evidence: 2 = systematic review of controlled trial; 3 = single randomized, controlled trial; 4 = systematic review of observational studies with outcomes.

From McGovern MP, Carroll KM: Evidence-based practices for substance use disorders. *Psychiatr Clin North Am* 2003;26:991–1010.

DIAGNOSIS. In addition to the general risk factors noted for substance use, a positive family history of alcohol abuse is significant. The genetic influences for the predisposition to alcoholism are supported by family, twin, and adoption studies. Children of alcoholic parents demonstrate a three- to fourfold increase in the risk of alcoholism. The **alcohol overdose syndrome** should be suspected in any teenager who appears disoriented, lethargic, or comatose. Although the distinctive aroma of alcohol may assist in diagnosis, confirmation by analysis of blood is recommended. There is a high correlation between results obtained by serum and breath analyses so that the latter method may be reliably used. At levels >200 mg/dL, the adolescent is at risk of death, and levels >500 mg/dL (median lethal dose) are usually associated with a fatal outcome. When the level of depression appears excessive for the reported blood level, head trauma or ingestion of other drugs should be considered as possible confounding factors.

Problem drinking during adolescence requiring a therapeutic intervention is not uncommon. Brief alcohol screening instruments (CRAFFT [see Table 113-6] or AUDIT [Alcohol Use Disorders Identification Test]) perform well in a clinical setting as techniques to identify DSM-IV–defined adolescents with alcohol use disorders.

TREATMENT. The usual mechanism of death from the alcohol overdose syndrome is respiratory depression, and artificial ventilatory support must be provided until the liver can eliminate sufficient amounts of alcohol from the body. In a patient without alcoholism, it generally takes 20 hr to reduce the blood level of alcohol from 400 mg/dL to zero. Dialysis should be considered when the blood level is >400 mg/dL. As a follow-up to acute treatment, referral for treatment of the alcohol use disorder is indicated. In emergency department settings, even brief interventions have shown some success in decreasing alcohol use and alcohol-related problems in adolescents.

113.2 • Tobacco

CIGARETTES. Compared to all other substances and firearms, tobacco kills more individuals in the United States each year than all these other causes combined. The average smoker in the United States starts at age 12 yr, and most are regular smokers by age 14 yr. More than 90% of adolescent smokers become adult smokers. Adolescent smokers may become nicotine dependent smoking fewer cigarettes a day than are necessary for adult smokers.

Additional exposure to second-hand smoke is also high with 70% of middle school and 57% of high school student smokers living in a home where someone else smokes. Nicotine absorbed from environmental tobacco smoke may predispose the child to subsequent cigarette use as adolescents. Worldwide, the Global Youth Tobacco Survey reports that 24% of youths surveyed began smoking before age 10, and younger women, aged 13–15 years are as likely to use tobacco products as young men. Tobacco use in Asia has been increasing over the past decade. Adolescents see the positive aspects of smoking as helping with boredom, dealing with stress, staying thin, and appearing more mature and ignore negative aspects such as making their teeth yellow, playing sports being harder, being harder to quit, and having bad breath.

PHARMACOLOGY. Human and animal studies confirm the addictive effect of nicotine, the primary active ingredient in cigarettes. It produces a syndrome of dependence as well as withdrawal. Nicotine is absorbed by multiple sites in the body, including the lungs, skin, gastrointestinal tract, and buccal and nasal mucosa. The average nicotine content of one cigarette is 10 mg and the average nicotine intake per cigarette ranges from 1.0 to 3 mg. Nicotine, as delivered in cigarette smoke, has a half-life of 10–20 min, with an elimination half-life of 2–3 hr. Nicotine's effect on the brain takes <20 sec. The action of nicotine is mediated through nicotinic acetylcholine receptors. These receptors are located on noncholinergic presynaptic and postsynaptic sites in the brain. **Cotinine** is the major metabolite of nicotine via C-oxidation. It has a biologic half-life of 19–24 hr and can be detected in urine, serum, and saliva.

CLINICAL MANIFESTATIONS. Adverse health effects of smoking may occur during adolescence. These adverse effects include an increased prevalence of chronic cough, sputum production, and wheezing. Smoking during pregnancy is associated with an average decrease in fetal weight of 200 g; this decrease, added to the already smaller size of infants born to teenagers, increases perinatal morbidity and mortality. Smoking in combination with the use of estrogen-containing oral contraceptives is associated with an increased risk of myocardial infarction. Tobacco smoke induces hepatic smooth endoplasmic reticulum enzymes and, as a result, may also influence metabolism of drugs and of endogenously produced hormones. Phenacetin, theophylline, and imipramine are examples of drugs affected in this manner.

TREATMENT. Adolescents counseled to quit smoking by health-care providers are highly influenced, with 60% agreeing to give up smoking. However, health supervision and supportive counseling are necessary components to smoking cessation management in adolescents since relapse is common.

The approach to smoking cessation in adolescents includes the **5 As (Ask, Advise, Assess, Assist, and Arrange)** and use of nicotine replacement therapy in addicted teens who are motivated to quit and are not using smokeless tobacco (SLT). Consensus panels recommend the 5 A's although evidence of efficacy in adolescents is limited. Nicotine patch studies to date in adolescents suggest a positive effect on reducing withdrawal symptoms and that pharmacotherapy should be combined with behavioral therapy to reach higher cessation and lower relapse rates. Medications such as bupropion are not approved for use under 18 yr old, however some pilot studies in adolescents report cessation efficacy. Caution in the use of antidepressant in teenagers is warranted (see Chapter 20.2). Additional options may be available through formal smoking cessation programs offered by community agencies. Clinical practice guidelines are available for practical office-based counseling strategies. Strong local and international policy efforts are directed at reducing tobacco use in adolescents through restricting youth access to tobacco products, increasing cigarette prices, and mass media counter-advertising. WHO sponsored a Framework Convention on Tobacco Control which produced a treaty containing tools to help countries build tobacco control policies to reduce the negative health and economic impacts of tobacco for all ages.

SMOKELESS TOBACCO. Surveys in the late 1980s and 1990s indicating the increased use of smokeless tobacco (SLT) prompted the National Cancer Institute to lead the U.S. federal government's effort to prevent SLT use, especially in adolescents. Surveys now indicate that from the early to mid-1990s to 2004, lifetime prevalence of SLT use continues to decline in 8th, 10th, and 12th graders. Regular users of SLT risk physical dependence on nicotine. Chewing tobacco may result in lesions, primarily in the mandibular mucobuccal fold. With chronic use, these lesions may become malignant.

113.3 • Marijuana

Lifetime use of marijuana among students 15 to 16 yr of age varies widely between nations, with >40% of youths from the United States, Canada, and Australia reporting use; 35% from

France; 4–5% in Asia; and 1% in Romania. In most countries, use begins at about age 14–15 yr. Marijuana may be a gateway drug that leads to the use of more dangerous and addictive drugs. In addition, marijuana use in vulnerable adolescents has been linked to the development of adult-onset psychosis.

Marijuana and alcohol share a number of psychopharmacologic qualities. Both decrease short-term memory and fine coordination, prolong reaction time, and produce "mental clouding." About 300 mg of cannabis is equivalent to 70 g of alcohol.

PHARMACOLOGY. Marijuana (THC, "pot," "weed," "hash," "grass") is derived from the *Cannabis sativa* plant, which flourishes in temperate and hot, dry climates. The tetrahydrocannabinol (THC) fraction of the resin is responsible for its hallucinogenic properties and has been synthesized (δ-9-THC). THC is absorbed rapidly by the nasal or oral routes, producing a peak of subjective effect at 10 min and 1 hr, respectively. Marijuana is generally smoked as a "reefer" or "joint," made by rolling the crushed plant material in paper. Although there is much variation in content, each cigarette contains 8–10% THC. Another popular form that is smoked, a "blunt," is a hollowed-out small cigar refilled with marijuana.

CLINICAL MANIFESTATIONS. In addition to the "desired" effects of elation and euphoria, marijuana may cause impairment of short-term memory, poor performance of tasks requiring divided attention (e.g., those involved in driving), loss of critical judgment, and distortion of time perception. Visual hallucinations and perceived body distortions occur rarely, but there may be "flashbacks" or recall of frightening hallucinations experienced under marijuana's influence that usually occur during stress or with fever.

Temperature may be lowered. Tachycardia is apparent within 20 min of smoking marijuana and is followed 1–2 hr later by transient systolic and diastolic hypertension, which disappears by 3 hr. Heavy users report pharyngitis, sinusitis, bronchitis, and asthma.

Smoking marijuana for a minimum of 4 days/wk for 6 mo appears to result in dose-related suppression of plasma testosterone levels and spermatogenesis, prompting concern about the potential deleterious effect of smoking marijuana before completion of pubertal growth and development. There is an antiemetic effect of oral THC or smoked marijuana, often followed by appetite stimulation, which is the basis of the drug's use in patients receiving cancer chemotherapy. Although the possibility of teratogenicity has been raised because of findings in animals, there is no evidence of such effects in humans. An **"amotivational" syndrome** has been described in long-term marijuana users who lose interest in age-appropriate behavior, yet proof of the causative relationship remains equivocal. The increased THC content of marijuana of almost five to 15 times in the 1990s as compared to the 1970s is related to the observation of a **withdrawal syndrome,** which had not occurred in the past, occurring 24 to 48 hr after discontinuing the drug. Heavy users experience malaise, irritability, agitation, insomnia, drug craving, shakiness, diaphoresis, night sweats, and gastrointestinal disturbance. The symptoms peak by the 4th day and resolve in 10–14 days. Certain drugs may interact with marijuana to potentiate sedation (alcohol, diazepam), potentiate stimulation (cocaine, amphetamines), or be antagonistic (propranolol, phenytoin). Long-term heavy cannabis users show memory and attention impairments that last beyond the period of intoxication and worsen with increasing years of regular use.

113.4 • Volatile Inhalants

The practice of inhalation of a variety of euphoriants is popular among younger adolescents. Young adolescents are attracted to these substances because of their rapid action, easy availability, and low cost. The most popular inhalants among adolescent are glue, gasoline, and volatile nitrites. **"Huffing,"** directly inhaling, or inhaling deeply from a paper bag containing a chemical-soaked cloth is the common method used by teens.

CLINICAL MANIFESTATIONS. The major effects of inhalants are psychoactive. Toluene, the main ingredient in airplane glue and some rubber cements, causes relaxation and pleasant hallucinations for up to 2 hr. Tolerance and physical dependence may occur. Gasoline, a popular substance among rural adolescents and Native American youths, contains a complex mixture of organic solvents. Euphoria is followed by violent excitement; coma may result from prolonged or rapid inhalation. Volatile nitrites, such as amyl nitrite, butyl nitrite, and related compounds marketed as room deodorizers, are used as euphoriants, enhancers of musical appreciation, and aphrodisiacs among older adolescents and young adults. They may result in headaches, syncope, and lightheadedness; profound hypotension and cutaneous flushing followed by vasoconstriction and tachycardia; transiently inverted T waves and depressed ST segments on electrocardiography; methemoglobinemia; increased bronchial irritation; and increased intraocular pressure (Table 113-11).

COMPLICATIONS. Airplane glue has been responsible for a wide range of complications, relating to chemical toxicity, to the method of administration (in plastic bags, with resultant suffocation), and to the often dangerous setting in which the inhalation occurs (inner-city roof tops). Gasoline toxicity is acute as well as chronic. Death in the acute phase may result from cerebral or pulmonary edema or myocardial involvement. Chronic use may cause pulmonary hypertension, restrictive lung defects or reduced diffusion capacity, peripheral neuropathy, acute rhabdomyolysis, hematuria, tubular acidosis, and possibly cerebral and cerebellar atrophy. Chronic inhalant abuse has long been linked to widespread brain damage and cognitive abnormalities that can range from mild impairment to severe dementia. MRI of inhalant abusers and long-term cocaine abusers show more frequent occurrence of abnormalities in the basal ganglia, cerebellum, pons, and thalamus for those who abused inhalants. These structures play a critical role in receiving sensory information from the peripheral nervous system and the spinal cord and relaying messages throughout the CNS that coordinate and control a variety of functions including voluntary and involuntary movements. Common pathologic changes reported in chronic inhalant abusers include difficulty coordinating movement, gait disorders, and spasticity, particularly in the legs.

TABLE 113-11. Hazards of Chemicals Found in Commonly Abused Inhalants

amyl nitrite, butyl nitrite *("poppers," "video head cleaner")* sudden sniffing death syndrome, suppressed immunologic function, injury to red blood cells (interfering with oxygen supply to vital tissues)

benzene *(found in gasoline)* bone marrow injury, impaired immunologic function, increased risk of leukemia, reproductive system toxicity

butane, propane *(found in lighter fluid, hair and paint sprays)* sudden sniffing death syndrome via cardiac effects, serious burn injuries (because of flammability)

freon *(used as a refrigerant and aerosol propellant)* sudden sniffing death syndrome, respiratory obstruction and death (from sudden cooling/cold injury to airways), liver damage

methylene chloride *(found in paint thinners and removers, degreasers)* reduction of oxygen-carrying of blood, changes to the heart muscle and heartbeat

nitrous oxide *("laughing gas")*, **hexane** death from lack of oxygen to the brain, altered perception and motor coordination, loss of sensation, limb spasms, blackouts caused by blood pressure changes, depression of heart muscle functioning

toluene *(found in gasoline, paint thinners and removers, correction fluid)* brain damage (loss of brain tissue mass, impaired cognition, gait disturbance, loss of coordination, loss of equilibrium, limb spasms, hearing and vision loss), liver and kidney damage

trichlorethylene *(found in spot removers, degreasers)* sudden sniffing death syndrome, cirrhosis of the liver, reproductive complications, hearing and vision damage

DIAGNOSIS. The brief effect of the inhalants makes it unlikely to diagnose unless there is a complication or death from use. Complete blood counts, coagulation studies, and hepatic and renal function studies may identify the complications. In extreme intoxication, a user may manifest symptoms of restlessness, general muscle weakness, dysarthria, nystagmus, disruptive behavior, and occasionally hallucinations, placing inhalant use in the differential diagnosis for acute intoxication of an adolescent. Toluene is excreted rapidly in the urine as hippuric acid, with the residual detectable in the serum by gas chromatography.

TREATMENT. Treatment is generally supportive and directed toward control of arrhythmia and stabilization of respirations and circulation. Withdrawal symptoms do not usually occur.

113.5 • Hallucinogens

Several naturally occurring and synthetic substances are used by adolescents for their hallucinogenic properties. Lysergic acid diethylamide (LSD) and methylenedioxymethamphetamine (MDMA) or Ecstasy are the most commonly reported hallucinogens in high school.

LYSERGIC ACID DIETHYLAMIDE. LSD (acid, big "d," blotters) is one of the constituents found in rye fungus. Morning glory seeds contain lysergic acid derivatives, although the commercially packaged varieties have often been treated with toxic chemicals such as insecticides and fungicides. Although the specific mechanisms of action of LSD are still under study, it is proposed to alter neurotransmitters mediated by serotonin. LSD is a very potent hallucinogen with doses as low as 20 μg causing effects in some individuals. Its high potency allows effective doses to be applied to objects as small as postage stamps and paper blotters. It is rapidly absorbed from the gastrointestinal tract.

The onset of action can be between 30 and 60 min, and it peaks between 2 and 4 hr. By 10–12 hr, an individual returns to the predrug state.

CLINICAL MANIFESTATIONS. The effects of LSD can be divided into three categories: somatic (physical effects), perceptual (altered changes in vision and hearing), and psychic effects (changes in sensorium). The common somatic symptoms are dizziness, dilated pupils, nausea, flushing, elevated temperature, and tachycardia. The sensation of synesthesia or "seeing" smells and "hearing" colors has been reported with LSD use. Delusional ideation, body distortion, and suspiciousness to the point of toxic psychosis are the more serious of the psychic symptoms.

TREATMENT. An individual is considered to have a "bad trip" when the setting causes the user to become terrified or panicked. These episodes should be treated by removing the individual from the aggravating situation or setting and attempting to re-establish contact with reality through calm verbal interaction. Any physical complications such as hyperthermia, seizure, or hypertension should be treated supportively. "Flashbacks" or LSD-induced states after the drug has worn off and tolerance to the effects of the drug are additional complications of its use.

METHYLENEDIOXYMETHAMPHETAMINE. MDMA ("X," Ecstasy), a phenylisopropylamine hallucinogen, is a synthetic compound similar to mescaline, commonly referred to as a "designer drug." Like other hallucinogens, this drug is proposed to interact with serotoninergic neurons in the CNS. It is the preferred drug at "raves," all night dance parties, and is also known as one of the "club drugs" along with γ-hydroxybutyrate (GHB) and ketamine (see Table 113-4).

CLINICAL MANIFESTATIONS. Euphoria, a heightened sensual awareness, and increased psychic and emotional energy are acute effects. Compared to other hallucinogens, MDMA is less likely to produce emotional lability, depersonalization, and disturbances of thought. Nausea, jaw clenching, teeth grinding, and blurred vision are somatic symptoms, whereas anxiety, panic attacks, and psychosis are the adverse psychic outcomes. A few deaths have been reported after ingestion of the drug. In high doses, MDMA can interfere with the body's ability to regulate temperature. The resultant hyperthermia in association with vigorous dancing at a "rave" has resulted in severe liver, kidney, and cardiovascular system failure and death. There are no specific treatment regimens recommended for acute toxicity. Research in humans suggests that chronic MDMA use can lead to changes in brain function, affecting cognitive tasks and memory. These symptoms may occur because of MDMA's effects on neurons that use serotonin as a neurotransmitter. The serotonin system plays an important role in regulating mood, aggression, sexual activity, sleep, and sensitivity to pain. Research in animals link MDMA exposure to long-term neurotoxicity and damage to serotonin containing neurons. A study in nonhuman primates showed that exposure to MDMA for only 4 days caused damage to serotonin nerve terminals that was evident 6–7 yr later.

PHENCYCLIDINE. PCP (sternyl, angel dust, "hog," "peace pill," "sheets") is an arylcyclohexalamine whose popularity is related, in part, to its ease of synthesis in home laboratories. One of the byproducts of home synthesis causes cramps, diarrhea, and hematemesis. The drug is thought to potentiate adrenergic effects by inhibiting neuronal reuptake of catecholamines. PCP is available as a tablet, liquid, or powder, which may be used alone or sprinkled on cigarettes ("joints"). The powders and tablets generally contain 2–6 mg of PCP, whereas joints average 1 mg for every 150 mg of tobacco leaves, or approximately 30–50 mg per joint.

CLINICAL MANIFESTATIONS. The clinical manifestations are dose related. Euphoria, nystagmus, ataxia, and emotional lability occur within 2–3 min after smoking 1–5 mg and last for hours. Hallucinations may involve bizarre distortions of body image that often precipitate panic reactions. With doses of 5–15 mg, a toxic psychosis may occur, with disorientation, hypersalivation, and abusive language lasting for >1 hr. Hypotension, generalized seizures, and cardiac arrhythmias commonly occur with plasma concentrations from 40–200 mg/dL. Death has been reported during psychotic delirium, from hypertension, hypotension, hypothermia, seizures, and trauma. The coma of PCP may be distinguished from that of the opiates by the absence of respiratory depression; the presence of muscle rigidity, hyperreflexia, and nystagmus; and lack of response to naloxone. PCP psychosis may be difficult to distinguish from schizophrenia. In the absence of a history of use, analysis of urine must be depended on for diagnosis.

TREATMENT. Management of the PCP-intoxicated patient includes placement in a darkened, quiet room on a floor pad, safe from injury. For recent oral ingestion, gastric absorption is poor and induction of emesis or gastric lavage is useful. Diazepam, in a dose of 5–10 mg orally or 2–5 mg intravenously, may be helpful if the patient is agitated and not comatose. Rapid excretion of the drug is promoted by acidification of the urine. Supportive therapy of the comatose patient is indicated with particular attention to hydration, which may be compromised by PCP-induced diuresis.

113.6 • Cocaine

Crack cocaine, the highly addictive smokable form of cocaine, has increased availability and severity of cocaine use in the face of a decrease in use in the overall population.

Cocaine, an alkaloid extracted from the leaves of the South American *Erythroxylon coca,* is supplied as the hydrochloride salt in crystalline form. It is rapidly absorbed from the nasal mucosa, detoxified by the liver, and excreted in the urine as benzoyl ecgonine. Its half-life is slightly more than 1 hr. The perceived effect of "snorting" cocaine may be influenced by some of the many diluents now being added to or actually substituted for the drug (heroin, amphetamines, PCP, or fillers such as mannitol or quinine). Smoking the cocaine alkaloid ("freebasing") in pipes or cigarettes, mixed with tobacco, marijuana, parsley, or as a paste has become a popular method of use. Accidental burns are potential complications of this practice. With crack cocaine, the smoker feels "high" in <10 sec. The risk of addiction with this method is higher and more rapidly progressive than from snorting cocaine. Tolerance develops and the user must increase the dose or change the route of administration, or both, to achieve the same effect. Drug dealers often place cocaine in plastic bags or condoms and swallow these containers during transport. Rupture of a container produces a sympathomimetic crisis (see Table 113-5).

CLINICAL MANIFESTATIONS. Cocaine produces euphoria, increased motor activity, decreased fatigability, and occasionally paranoid ideation. Its sympathomimetic properties are responsible for pupillary dilatation, tachycardia, hypertension, and hyperthermia. Binge patterns of use are common. Neurologic effects such as dizziness, paresthesias, and seizures can occur. Use in group settings has been associated with sexual promiscuity and increased risks of sexually transmitted infections. Lethal effects are possible, especially when cocaine is used in combination with other drugs, such as heroin, in an injectable form known as a "speedball." Pregnant adolescents who use cocaine place their fetus at risk of premature delivery, complications of low birthweight, and possibly developmental disorders.

TREATMENT. Intensive supportive therapy is directed at the clinical manifestations of acute intoxication.

113.7 • AMPHETAMINES

Stimulants, particularly amphetamines, are among the most frequently reported illicit drugs, other than marijuana used by high school seniors. Methamphetamine, commonly known as "ice," accounted for >25% of stimulant use. Methamphetamine is particularly popular among adolescents and young adults because of its potency and ease of absorption. It can be ingested by mouth, by snorting, by smoking, or absorbing across mucous membranes, such as vaginal mucosa. Amphetamines have multiple CNS effects, among them the release of neurotransmitters and an indirect catecholamine agonist effect. In high doses, they may also affect serotonergic receptors.

CLINICAL MANIFESTATIONS. The effects of amphetamines can be dose related. High doses produce slowing of cardiac conduction in the face of ventricular irritability. Hypertensive and hyperpyrexic episodes can occur as seizures (see Table 113-5). Binge effects result in the development of psychotic ideation with the potential for sudden violence. Cerebrovascular damage and psychosis can result from long-term use. There is a withdrawal syndrome associated with amphetamine use, with early, intermediate, and late phases. The early phase is characterized as a "crash" phase with depression, agitation, anergia, and desire for more of the drug. Loss of physical and mental energy, limited interest in the environment, and anhedonia mark the intermediate phase. In the final phase, drug craving returns, often triggered by particular situations or objects.

TREATMENT. Agitation and delusional behaviors can be treated with haloperidol or droperidol. Phenothiazines are contraindicated and may cause a rapid drop in blood pressure or seizure activity. Other supportive treatment consists of a cooling blanket for hyperthermia and treatment of the hypertension and arrhythmias, which may respond to sedation with lorazepam or diazepam.

113.8 • OPIATES

Heroin's popularity is growing in suburban middle class high school students. Heroin produces euphoria and analgesia. Heroin is hydrolyzed to morphine, which undergoes hepatic conjugation with glucuronic acid before excretion, usually within 24 hr of administration. It can be detected in urine by thin-layer chromatography up to 48 hr after administration. The route of administration influences the timing of the onset of action. When the drug is inhaled ("snorting"), it requires almost 30 min before the desired effect is achieved. Through smoking or by the subcutaneous route ("skin-popping"), the effect is achieved within minutes; when injected intravenously ("mainlining"), it has an immediate effect. Tolerance develops to the euphoric effect and only rarely to the inhibitory effect on smooth muscle, which causes both constipation and miosis.

Fentanyl, another opiate, is 50 to 100 times more potent than morphine. It has a rapid onset and short half life. It is often mixed with heroin to give an added high; street names include drop dead, flatline, and lethal injection. Fentanyl-laced drugs have been responsible for many deaths among street drug users.

CLINICAL MANIFESTATIONS. The clinical manifestations are determined by the pharmacologic effects of heroin or its adulterants, combined with the conditions and the route of administration. The cerebral effects include euphoria, diminution in pain, and pinpoint pupils (see Table 113-5). An effect on the hypothalamus is suggested by the lowering of body temperature. Vasodilation is a major cardiovascular manifestation related to the method of administration of the drug. Respiratory depression is mediated centrally and is characterized by alveolar underventilation. Pulmonary edema is common from the overdose syndrome, but it may also be seen as an incidental roentgenographic finding in an otherwise asymptomatic adolescent heroin abuser. The most common dermatologic lesions are the "tracks," the hypertrophic linear scars that follow the course of large veins. Smaller, discrete peripheral scars, resembling healed insect bites, may be easily overlooked. The adolescent who injects heroin subcutaneously may have fat necrosis, lipodystrophy, and atrophy over portions of the extremities. Attempts to conceal these stigmata may include amateur tattoos in unusual sites. Abscesses secondary to unsterile techniques of drug administration are commonly found. There is a loss of libido; the mechanism is unknown. The female heroin user may resort to prostitution to support the habit, thus increasing the risk of sexually transmitted disease (including HIV), pregnancy, and other hazards. Constipation results from decreased smooth muscle propulsive contractions and increased anal sphincter tone. The absence of sterile technique in injection may lead to cerebral microabscesses or endocarditis, usually caused by *Staphylococcus aureus.* Infection with HIV is another complication of needle use. Abnormal serologic reactions are also common, including false-positive Venereal Disease Research Laboratory and latex fixation tests.

WITHDRAWAL. After a period of ≥8 hr without heroin, the addicted individual undergoes, during a 24–36 hr period, a series of physiologic disturbances referred to collectively as "withdrawal" or the **abstinence syndrome.** The earliest sign is yawning, followed by lacrimation, mydriasis, insomnia, "goose flesh," cramping of the voluntary musculature, hyperactive bowel sounds and diarrhea, tachycardia, and systolic hypertension. While the administration of methadone has been the most common method of detoxification, the addition of buprenorphine, an opiate agonist-antagonist, is available for detoxification and maintenance treatment of heroin and other opiates. This medication has the advantage in that it offers less risk of addiction and can be dispensed in the privacy of a physician's office. Combined with behavioral interventions, it has a greater success rate of detoxification.

OVERDOSE SYNDROME. The overdose syndrome is an acute reaction after the administration of an opiate. It is the leading cause of death among drug users. The clinical signs include stupor or coma, seizures, miotic pupils (unless severe anoxia has occurred), respiratory depression, cyanosis, and pulmonary edema. The differential diagnosis includes CNS trauma, diabetic coma, hepatic (and other) encephalopathy, Reye syndrome, as well as overdose of alcohol, barbiturates, PCP, or methadone. Diagnosis of opiate toxicity is facilitated by intravenous administration of the opiate antagonist naloxone, 0.01 mg/kg (2 mg is a common initial dose for an adolescent), which causes dilation of pupils constricted by the opiate. Diagnosis is confirmed by the finding of morphine in the serum.

TREATMENT. This consists of maintaining adequate oxygenation and continued administration of naloxone every 5 min, when necessary, to improve and maintain adequate ventilation. Naloxone may have to be continued for 24 hr if methadone, rather than shorter acting heroin, has been taken. Naloxone kept in the home in the event of an overdose may hold potential to reduce heroin-related deaths.

113.9 • Anabolic Steroids

The quest for enhanced athletic performance has led to the abuse of anabolic steroids by competitive athletes of both sexes. As with other substances, prevalence data vary across surveys. Reports of anabolic steroids having ever been used range from 0.7% to 3.7%, usually with male use predominating. On the Youth Risk Behavior Surveillance, 9th grade girls reported ever using steroids more then twice as frequently as 12th grade girls (7.3% vs 3.3%). Use of anabolic steroids has been associated with a constellation of problem behaviors such as engaging in physical fights with injuries requiring medical attention, weapon carrying, binge drinking, and using other substances of abuse (Table 113-12). The evidence of increased muscle mass and strength are controversial but are supported by objective data. The effects appear to be related to the myotrophic action at androgen receptors as well as competitive antagonism at catabolism-mediating corticosteroid receptors. Erythropoietic and psychologic effects may also contribute to their enhancement effects. Anabolic steroids used for performance enhancement include nandrolone, stanozolol, methenolone, tibolone, oxandrolone, and testosterone preparations.

CLINICAL MANIFESTATIONS. Some of the adverse side effects of these drugs are reversible; others are not. The most immediate effect for all users is increasing acneform lesions. Other dermatologic manifestations include linear keloids, stria, oily hair, and hirsutism. These findings may be the first recognizable effects. Males can experience gynecomastia, breast pain, testicular atrophy, and azoospermia. Women experience more irreversible side effects such as breast atrophy, clitoral enlargement, and menstrual abnormalities. Serious psychologic effects also have been reported from the use of high doses of these agents (often 100 times the therapeutic doses), including uncontrollable rage,

TABLE 113-12. Summary of Performance-enhancing Supplements and Drugs

	BENEFITS	ADVERSE EFFECTS	CURRENT RECOMMENDATIONS AND LEGAL ISSUES
AAS	• DO increase muscle strength and mass at high doses • Do NOT increase endurance performance	• *Endocrine/reproductive*—testicular atrophy and irreversible gynecomastia in males and irreversible virilization in females • *Cardiovascular*—adverse changes in lipid profile and elevation of blood pressure • *Hepatic*—enzyme elevation, jaundice and possibly malignancy • *Musculoskeletal*—epiphyseal fusion and decreased tensile strength of tendons • *Psychiatric*—multiple effects including potential addiction and dependence	• ILLEGAL and punishable as a felony • Schedule III controlled substance • Banned by all major sports governing organizations • Condemned by both AAP and ACSM
Andro/DHEA	• *Andro*—Doses up to 100 mg do NOT increase testosterone production or strength • *Andro*—Higher doses might increase testosterone but at the cost of greatly increased estrogens • *DHEA*—Does NOT increase testosterone or enhance performance	• Adverse changes in lipid profile • Effects of increased estrogens • Possibly cause effects of increased androgens at higher doses • May promote growth of hormone sensitive malignancies	• Banned by IOC, NCAA, NFL, and recently NBA • Purchased OTC as dietary supplement • NOT recommended
Creatine	• DOES increase work capability over brief, repetitive, maximal exertion • Does NOT improve endurance or maximal exertion over 60 sec • Individual response varies with "responders" and "nonresponders" • No additional benefit for doses above 20 g/day × 4 day load or 2 g/day maintenance	• Appears relatively safe in small number of studies • No good information of long-term use, especially on heart and brain • No information in growing adolescents • Early weight gain from water retention • Anecdotal reports of cramping and hydration issues • Sporadic reports of reversible renal problems	• NOT banned by many sports governing organizations • Purchased OTC as dietary supplement • ACSM does NOT recommend for adolescent population • Use with caution in adults
Ephedra	• Does NOT improve endurance or weight loss when used alone • Seems to improve endurance when combined with caffeine • Seems to improve weight combined with caffeine in *obese* persons on *dietary restrictions* • No studies of weight loss when combined with caffeine in lean athletes	• Linked to serious adverse cardiovascular and CNS events such as hypertension, stroke, and sudden death • Effects potentiated by addition of caffeine • Combination of ephedrine and caffeine considered unsafe by FDA	• Systematic use banned by IOC and NCAA • Combinations of herbal forms of ephedra and caffeine found in OTC supplements NOT recommended

AAP, American Academy of Pediatrics; AAS, anabolic–androgenic steroids; ACSM, American College of Sports Medicine; Andro, androstenedione; CNS, central nervous system; DHEA, dehydroepiandrosterone; FDA, U.S. Food and Drug Administration; IOC, International Olympic Committee; NBA, National Basketball Association; NCAA, National Collegiate Athletic Association; NFL, National Football League; OTC, over the counter.
From Congeni J, Miller S: Supplements and drugs used to enhance athletic performance. *Pediatr Clin North Am* 2002;49:435–461.

depression, mania, mood fluctuations, and alterations in libido. Users choosing the injectable route increase the risk of HIV if injection equipment is shared with others.

Abnormalities of the liver can be acute, such as hepatitis and hepatomegaly, or more long term, such as the increased risk of hepatocellular carcinoma, particularly with the 17-α-alkylated forms. Fluid retention is a common side effect that prompts users to take diuretics. In addition to these effects, which occur in individuals of all ages, the early adolescent is at risk of growth retardation because of the possibility of accelerating epiphyseal closure.

DIAGNOSIS AND TREATMENT. The clinical signs noted, coupled with a complete history, provide a diagnosis in most instances. Patients should also be questioned about the use of other performance-enhancing substances. Although urine testing is available and performed at the Olympic and collegiate competitive levels, few laboratories perform these tests and they are very expensive. Therefore, the secondary school approach and the approach recommended for the clinician has focused on education and prevention, sharing factual information on the benefits and risks of using these substances. Treatment is supportive.

Arseneault L, Cannon M, Poulton R, et al: Cannabis use in adolescence and risk for adult psychosis: Longitudinal prospective study. *Br Med J* 2002;325:1212–1213.

Baca CT, Grant KJ: Take-home naloxone to reduce heroin death. *Addiction* 2005;100:1823–1831.

Becklake MR, Ghezzo H, Ernst P: Childhood predictors of smoking in adolescence: A follow-up study of Montreal schoolchildren. *CMAJ* 2005;173:377–379.

Boddiger D: Fentanyl-laced street drugs "kill hundreds." *Lancet* 2006;368: 569–570.

Bonomo Y, Proimos J: Substance misuse: Alcohol, tobacco, inhalants, and other drugs. *Br Med J* 2005;330:777–780.

Cami J, Farre M: Drug addiction. *N Engl J Med* 2003;349:975–986.

Centers for Disease Control and Prevention: Methamphetamine use and HIV risk behaviors among heterosexual men—preliminary results from five Northern California counties, December 2001–November 2003. *MMWR* 2006;55:273–278.

Congeni J, Miller S: Supplements and drug use to enhance athletic performance. *Pediatr Clin North Am* 2002;49:435–461.

Department of Health and Human Services Centers for Disease Control and Prevention: Atypical reactions associated with heroin use—five states, January–April 2005. *MMWR* 2005;54:793–796.

Farrelly MC, Davis KC, Haviland ML, et al: Evidence of a dose-response relationship between "truth" antismoking ads and youth smoking prevalence. *Am J Public Health* 2005;95:425–431.

Friedman RA: The changing face of teenage drug abuse—the trend toward prescription drugs. *N Engl J Med* 2006;354:1448–1450.

Global Youth Tobacco Survey Collaborating Group: Differences in worldwide tobacco use by gender: Findings from the Global Youth Tobacco Survey. *J School Health* 2003;73:207–215.

Global Youth Network. Drug Trends, 2005, available at: *www.unode.org/youthnet.*

Greydanus DE, Patel DR: The adolescent and substance abuse: Current concepts. *Curr Probl Pediatr Adolesc Health Care* 2005;35:73–104.

Hall W: Is cannabis use psychotogenic? *Lancet* 2006;367:193–194.

Johnston LD, O'Malley PM, Bachman JG, Schulenberg JE: *Monitoring the Future: National Results on Adolescent Drug Use: Overview of Key Findings, 2004* (NIH Publication no. 05-5726). Bethesda, MD, National Institute on Drug Abuse, 2005.

Kosten TR, O'Connor: Management of drug and alcohol withdrawal. *N Engl J Med* 2003;348:1786–1795.

Lynskey MT, Vink JM, Boomsma DI: Early onset cannabis use and progression to other drug use in a sample of Dutch twins. *Behav Genet* 2006;36:195–200.

Marsch LA, Bickel WK, Badger GJ, et al: Comparison of pharmacological treatments for opioid-dependent adolescents. *Arch Gen Psychiatry* 2005;62:1157–1164.

Medical Letter: Acute reactions to drugs of abuse. *Med Lett Drugs Ther* 2002;44:21–24.

Ogilvie D, Gruer L, Haw S: Young people's access to tobacco, alcohol, and other drugs. *Br Med J* 2005;331:393–396.

Poikolainen K: Ecstasy and the antecedents of illicit drug use. *BMJ* 2006;332: 803–804.

Ricaurte GA, McCann UD: Recognition and management of complications of new recreational drug use. *Lancet* 2005;365:2137–2145.

Rimsza ME, Moses KS: Substance abuse on the college campus. *Pediatr Clin North Am* 2005;52:307–319.

Schinke S, Brounstein P, Gardner S: *Science-Based Prevention Programs and Principles, 2002.* (DHHS Publication no. (SMA) 03-3764). Rockville, MD, Center for Substance Abuse Prevention, Substance Abuse and Mental Health Services Administration, 2002. *(www.modelprograms.samhsa.gov)*

Sindelar HA, Barnett NP, Spirito A: Adolescent alcohol use and injury: A summary and critical review of the literature. *Minerva Pediatr* 2004;56:291–309.

Snead III OC, Gibson KM: γ-Hydroxybutyric acid. *N Engl J Med* 2005;352:2721–2732.

Spoth RL, Clair S, Shin C, Redmond C: Long-term effects of universal preventive interventions on methamphetamine use among adolescents. *Arch Pediatr Adolesc Med* 2006;160:876–882.

Sunday SR, Folan P: Smoking in adolescence: What a clinician can do to help. *Med Clin North Am* 2004;88:1495–1515.

Tanski SE, Prokhorov AV, Klein JD: Youth and tobacco. *Minerva Pediatr* 2004;56:553–565.

Chapter 114 ■ The Breast

Renée R. Jenkins

Breast development is one of the first obvious signs of puberty. Whether the issue is normal progression, some variation in progression, or a definable disorder, it is often the focus of attention. Normal breast development during puberty is described using a Sex Maturity Rating scale of 1–5, as the breast becomes more mature (see Chapter 12).

NORMAL VARIANTS. Minor breast asymmetry is common in adult females and sexually mature adolescent females, but other rarely occurring conditions should be ruled out. **Poland syndrome** is marked by a hypoplastic breast nipple and areola with hypoplastic ipsilateral chest wall structures. **Accessory breast tissue (polymastia)** can also occur in males and females. This lesion can consist of a **supernumerary nipple (polythelia)** or breast tissue, or both, and usually occurs along both milk lines of the thorax and the abdomen. Accessory breast tissue beneath the umbilicus, though rare, can be associated with cardiovascular or genitourinary abnormalities. Unilateral or bilateral **juvenile (virginal) hypertrophy** occurs with specific histopathologic changes but without any known cause. The enlargement may be mild and cause back pain and postural problems or severe enough to be associated with tissue and skin necrosis. Embarrassment and possible psychologic problems should be addressed in the management of this condition. Reconstructive surgical repair is indicated in severe breast asymmetry or hypertrophy but is recommended after sex maturity rating 5 has been reached. A dramatic increase in adolescents desiring breast augmentation has occurred over the past decade. Breast augmentation in adolescents is discouraged due to associated psychologic and physical immaturity.

FEMALE DISORDERS (SEE CHAPTER 551)

MASSES. The most common adolescent breast disorder is a mass, the majority of which are benign **cysts** or **fibroadenomas.** The patient should be questioned about the variation in symptoms with the menstrual cycle, associated symptoms such as nipple discharge, recent trauma to the breast, family history of breast masses or cancer, and history of chest radiation or malignancy. Cysts vary in size over the course of a menstrual cycle, so a patient should be re-examined 2 wk after the initial examination. Persistence of the mass or its enlargement over three menstrual cycles is an indication for surgical consultation. Multiple fibroadenomas occur in 10–20% of patients. The **fibroadenoma** tends not to vary in size during the menstrual cycle, often distinguishing it from a cyst. **Cystosarcoma phylloides** is a rare variant of a fibroadenoma distinguished by having a more cellular stroma. It is typically larger than a fibroadenoma and rarely can be malignant. A contusion of the breast can result in a poorly defined tender mass or a hematoma presenting as a mass.

In a review of 15 retrospective surgical studies of women younger than age 22 yr, the most common lesion was the fibroadenoma (68.3%), followed by fibrocystic changes (18.5%). **Carcinoma** of the breast in the adolescent is rare. Adolescents with previous radiation to the chest, a family history of BRCA1 or 2, or with malignancies with the potential to metastasize to the breast should be monitored more closely for breast masses. The dense breast tissue of the adolescent obstructs the visualization of a palpable mass; thus, mammography is not advised for this age group. Ultrasonography is useful is distinguishing cystic from solid masses. Color Doppler ultrasound is useful in evaluating fibroadenomas and breast abscesses.

MASTALGIA. Physiologic swelling and tenderness occur on a cyclic basis, most commonly during the premenstrual phase, and are secondary to hormonal stimulation and resulting proliferative changes. Nodularity, poorly localized tenderness, and a soreness radiating to the axilla and arm are usual accompanying findings. The preferable term for these changes is *benign breast changes* rather than the classic "fibrocystic disease." Noncyclic mastalgia is less common in younger women compared to women in their 40s. Treatments recommended for this condition include firm support, heat, analgesics, hormonal therapy, diuretics, and evening primrose oil. Adult doses of evening primrose oil, two 500-mg capsules three times a day, has been associated with an overall response rate of 44%. A 3-mo trial is recommended with a follow-up treatment of 2 mo if the response is positive. A 3–6 mo course of topical nonsteroidal anti-inflammatory drugs has also been demonstrated to be effective. Clinical trials fail to support any benefit from the use of diuretics, vitamin B, B_6, or E.

NIPPLE DISCHARGE. Nipple discharge in adolescents is usually due to local stimulation, use of medications including oral contraceptives, and pregnancy. Rarely, it results from a pituitary or breast neoplasm or infection. Examination of the discharge assists in diagnosis: Benign conditions are associated with a milky, sticky, thick discharge; infection is associated with a purulent discharge; intraductal papilloma and cancer are associated with a serous, serosanguineous, or bloody discharge. Elevation of the serum prolactin level may occur in the **amenorrhea-galactorrhea syndromes,** associated with the use of certain antihypertensive medications, oral contraceptives, or tranquilizers, or secondary to a pituitary adenoma. The latter is associated with central nervous system signs and is evaluated with MRI of the head.

INFECTION. Infection in the non–breast-feeding adolescent is rare and may be secondary to a human bite or the initial symptom of diabetes mellitus. Shaving or plucking of areolar hair, trauma from sexual play, and nipple piercing can also be associated with infection. Erythema and increased warmth of skin may be the first signs of infection. Appropriate antibiotic therapy (usually directed against *Staphylococcus aureus*), with culture if any discharge is present, is indicated; surgical drainage is rarely necessary.

TABLE 114-1. Drugs That Can Cause Gynecomastia

DRUG	MECHANISM
Amiodarone	Unknown
Calcium channel blockers (diltiazem, verapamil, nifedipine)	Unknown
Central nervous system agents (amphetamines, diazepam, methyldopa, phenytoin, reserpine, tricyclic antipressants)	Unknown
Cimetidine	Androgen receptor antagonism
Cytotoxic agents (alkylating agents, vincristine, nitrosoureas, methotrexate	Primary hypogonadism due to Leydig cell damage
Flutamide	Androgen receptor antagonism
Highly active antiretroviral treatment (HAART)	Possible drug-mediated estrogen effects
Hormones	
Androgens	Aromatization to estrogens; other mechanisms?
Estrogens	Direct stimulation of the breast
Human chorionic gonadotropin	Stimulation of testicular Leydig cell estrogen secretion
Isoniazid	Possibly refeeding
Ketoconazole, metronidazole	Inhibition of testosterone synthesis
Marijuana	Androgen receptor antagonism
D-penicillamine	Unknown
Phenothiazines	Elevated serum prolactin
Spironolactone	Androgen receptor antagonism; at high doses, interference with testosterone biosynthesis
Theophylline	Unknown

Adapted from Bembo SA, Carlson HE: Gynecomastia: Its features, and when and how to treat it. *Clevel Clin J Med* 2004;71:514.

MALE DISORDERS. Gynecomastia (see Chapter 586) occurs in approximately one third of normal males during early to mid-puberty and often causes concern that may not be openly voiced. The response should be factual, with information and reassurance as to its usually transient nature. Rarely is it of such magnitude or persistence as to warrant surgery. Older adolescents and adult men with persistent gynecomastia have been treated for 3 mo with danazol (200 mg PO bid) or tamoxifen (10–20 mg PO bid) for nonsurgical management. Nonpubertal gynecomastia with hypogonadism is associated with Klinefelter syndrome and places a patient at a higher risk of breast cancer (see Chapter 584). Other conditions associated with nonpubertal gynecomastia are secondary to endocrine disorders, neoplasms, chronic disease, trauma, and medications as well as drugs of abuse (Table 114-1). Highly active antiretroviral therapy, particularly efavirenz, is also recognized as a cause.

Colak T, Ipek T, Kanik A, et al: Efficacy of topical nonsteroidal anti-inflammatory drugs in mastalgia treatment. *J Am Coll Surg* 2003;196:525–530.

Davis AJ, Kulig JW: Adolescent breast disorders. *Adolesc Health Update* 1996;9:1–8.

Khan HN, Blamey RW: Endocrine treatment of physiological gynaecomastia. *Br Med J* 2003;327:301–302.

Laufer MR, Goldstein DP: The breast: Examination and lesions. In Emans SJH, Laufer MR, Goldstein DP (editors): *Pediatric and Adolescent Gynecology,* 5th ed. Philadelphia, Lippincott Williams & Wilkins, 2005.

McGrath MH, Schooler WG: Elective plastic surgical procedures in adolescence. *Adolesc Med* 2004;15:487–502.

Rahim S, Ortiz O, Maslow M, Holzman R: A case-control study of gynecomastia in HIV-1-infected patients receiving HAART. *AIDS Read* 2004;14:23–4, 29–32, 35–40.

Chapter 115 ■ Menstrual Problems

Renée R. Jenkins

(See also Chapter 550.)

Some variety of menstrual dysfunction occurs at some time in about 50% of adolescent females. Although most of the problems are minor, severe dysmenorrhea or prolonged menstrual bleeding can be debilitating. Adolescents with mild dysfunction that does not require medical intervention should have their condition explained to them and should be reassured about their reproductive normalcy.

NORMAL MENSTRUATION

The age at the start of normal menarche varies according to the characteristics of the population. In a large office-based study in the United States, 35% of white girls and 62% of African-American girls had initiated menses between ages 12 and 13 yr. The age at menarche in Tanner's English series ranges from ages 9 to 16 yr, with a mean age of 13.46 yr. An international study surveying age at menarche in 67 countries calculated a mean age of menarche at 13.53 years with the variability reflecting differences in energy balance more so than nutritional status. In 2002 in the United States, the age at menarche was 12.52 yr for non-Hispanic whites, 12.06 yr for non-Hispanic blacks, and 12.09 yr for Mexican Americans. Overall, the age at menarche declined 2.3 mo between 1988 and 1994 and 1999 and 2002. The age at menarche is closely related to other parameters of pubertal maturation and correlated closely with bone age. The onset and continuation of normal menstrual cycling depend on the functional and anatomic integrity of (1) the hypothalamus together with higher centers, including possibly the pineal gland; (2) the anterior pituitary; (3) the ovary; and (4) the uterus. The percentage of body fat is also a factor in the onset of menarche, with a minimal fatness of 17% of body weight being necessary for the onset of menstrual cycles and a minimum of 22% fatness necessary to maintain regular ovulatory cycles (see Chapter 689). Menarche usually occurs about 2.3 yr after the initiation of puberty, with a range of 1–3 yr, and becomes regular after 2–2.5 yr. The length of the menstrual cycle from the first day of menses of one cycle to the first day of the next cycle can range from 21 to 45 days, although the average is about 28 days. Anovulatory cycles are generally longer. The average blood flow usually results in about 40 mL of blood loss, with a range of 25–70 mL. The later the age at which menarche occurs, the longer it is until the ovulatory cycles are established.

Menstrual cycle irregularities are described according to variation in frequency of menses, amount, and both frequency and amount (Table 115-1). A complete history for evaluating a patient with menstrual dysfunction should include questions specifically related to puberty and menstrual patterns, a family history of gynecologic problems and maternal onset of menarche, and a medical history noting hospitalizations, chronic illness, medication or substance use, and infections. The related associations of weight change, nutrition, exercise, and sports participation can be critically important in considering a differential diagnosis. Regardless of the age of the adolescent, an appropriate history of any type of sexual activity should be elicited, and the pediatrician should be cognizant of the need to rule out sexual abuse as an issue in young adolescents when other findings suggest sexual activity.

In addition to the basic growth parameters of weight, height, blood pressure, heart rate, and body mass index, signs of virilization should be assessed, such as hirsutism and clitoromegaly. A careful external and internal pelvic examination is necessary to eliminate anatomic defects and accumulating additional specimens for the evaluation. In the young adolescent, someone with expertise in this age group should perform the examination with the proper-sized equipment.

TABLE 115-1. Terms for Menstrual Cycle Irregularities

VARIATIONS IN FREQUENCY
Polymenorrhea: frequent regular or irregular bleeding at <21-day intervals
Oligomenorrhea: infrequent irregular bleeding at >45-day intervals
Primary amenorrhea: no menstrual flow by age 16 yr
Secondary amenorrhea: absence of vaginal bleeding for >3 mo
Irregular menses: bleeding at varying intervals, ≥21-day intervals but <45-day intervals

VARIATIONS IN AMOUNT
Hypomenorrhea: decreased menstrual flow at regular intervals
Hypermenorrhea: profuse menstrual flow of normal duration at regular intervals

VARIATIONS IN AMOUNT AND DURATION
Metrorrhagia: intermenstrual irregular bleeding between regular periods
Menorrhagia: excessive amount and increased duration of uterine bleeding occurring regularly
Menometrorrhagia: frequent irregular, excessive, and prolonged episodes of uterine bleeding
Dysfunctional uterine bleeding: prolonged excessive menstrual bleeding associated with irregular periods: usually due to immaturity of reproductive axis in adolescence if within first 2 yr of menarche

From Blythe MI: Common menstrual problems of adolescence. *Adolesc Med* 1997;8:87–109.

MENSTRUAL IRREGULARITIES

ETIOLOGY. The distinction among menstrual irregularities is somewhat artificial given that the causes of the entities are often similar; many of the problems of pubertal delay, such as Turner mosaic syndrome (see Chapter 587), may present as primary amenorrhea or secondary amenorrhea. Thyroid disorders also can be the source of secondary amenorrhea or abnormal vaginal bleeding. The common cause of all these disorders is a disturbance of the hypothalamic-pituitary-ovarian axis. The amenorrheic disorders are categorized on the basis of follicle-stimulating hormone (FSH) levels into **hypergonadotropic hypogonadism** (ovarian failure) and **hypogonadotropic hypogonadism** (hypothalamic or pituitary dysfunction). FSH-luteinizing hormone (LH) patterns in perimenarchal girls with anovulatory bleeding also suggest the prevalence of a maturational defect for normal negative feedback cyclicity. The rising levels of estrogen do not cause a fall in FSH and the subsequent suppression of estrogen secretion, and consequently the endometrium becomes thickened, promoting irregular and heavier blood flow with shedding.

Psychogenic factors have been implicated in amenorrhea. It is often difficult to separate psychologic from nutritional factors because weight loss is a common confounding variable in many of these situations, such as depression (see Chapter 25), anorexia nervosa (see Chapter 27), or stress.

CLINICAL MANIFESTATIONS. Amenorrhea, or absence of menses, may be primary or secondary. An adolescent has primary amenorrhea if by age 14 yr she has not menstruated and has no secondary sex characteristics or at age 16 yr has not menstruated but has secondary sex characteristics. The close concordance of the age of menarche between daughters and mothers and among siblings should suggest this diagnosis when the patient is more than 1 yr older than was the mother or sisters when their menarche occurred. The distinguishing characteristic of the clinical presentation of amenorrhea is the presence or absence of **virilization.** Clinical features such as clitoromegaly, hirsutism, or excessive acne are associated with adrenal or ovarian disease. Other clinical presentations such as slender or obese body habitus or short stature also are characteristic of syndromes associated with amenorrhea.

The first consideration in the adolescent who presents with secondary amenorrhea is **pregnancy.** This possibility also exists, albeit rarely, as a cause of primary amenorrhea, if fertilization of the first released ovum occurred before menses. A history of sexual intercourse, nausea, and breast tenderness and physical findings of increased pigmentation of nipples and linea alba, cyanosis and softening of the cervix, and an enlarged uterus form the classic picture.

In the clinical presentation of abnormal vaginal bleeding, mild to moderate bleeding may present without any specific clinical findings; severe bleeding is accompanied by the abnormal vital signs associated with hypovolemia (see Chapter 68). Very severe bleeding may progress to syncope and death, making this one of the few gynecologic emergencies of adolescence.

115.1 • Amenorrhea

DIFFERENTIAL DIAGNOSIS. In *primary amenorrhea,* chromosomal or congenital abnormalities, such as gonadal dysgenesis, the triple X syndrome, isochromosomal abnormalities, testicular feminization syndrome, and, rarely, true hermaphroditism, should be considered in addition to the conditions that cause secondary amenorrhea (Table 115-2). Elevated levels of FSH and LH suggest primary gonadal failure, and chromosome analysis elucidates its cause. When primary amenorrhea occurs with advanced pubertal development, a structural anomaly of the *müllerian duct system* (see Chapter 554) should be suspected. Imperforate hymen is most common and is associated with recurrent (monthly) abdominal pain and, after some time has passed, a midline, lower abdominal mass, the blood-filled vagina, or hematocolpos. Diagnosis is made by inspection of the introitus, revealing a bulging hymen with bluish discoloration. If the obstruction is at the level of the cervix, the blood-filled uterus (hematometrium) is apparent on bimanual examination or ultrasonography. Agenesis of the cervix or uterus is rare but occurs in association with sacral agenesis.

Primary or secondary amenorrhea may also be caused by chronic illness, particularly that associated with malnutrition or tissue hypoxia, such as diabetes mellitus, inflammatory bowel disease, cystic fibrosis, or cyanotic congenital heart disease. In most cases, the illness has been diagnosed previously, but, occasionally, the amenorrhea is its first manifestation. **Polycystic ovarian syndrome** (see Chapter 587.2) is one of the most common endocrine disorders affecting premenopausal women and presents with menstrual abnormalities from amenorrhea to dysfunctional uterine bleeding. The criterion for the diagnosis of PCOS is menstrual irregularity in the face of androgen excess with either hirsutism, acne, or increased serum androgens. When the androgen excess is coupled with insulin resistance and acanthosis nigricans, the term **HAIR-AN syndrome** is used. A central nervous system (CNS) tumor, most commonly a craniopharyngioma, may present with amenorrhea. **Prolactinomas,** although rare, are the most common pituitary tumor in adolescence. Abnormalities of the thyroid gland, typically hyperthyroidism, may first be suspected by delayed sexual maturation or amenorrhea, even in the absence of other signs and symptoms. Hypothyroidism may cause precocious puberty but may also be associated with delayed puberty or abnormal uterine bleeding. Anorexia nervosa, which may present with either primary or secondary amenorrhea, is occasionally confused with hyperthyroidism because of weight loss, hyperactivity, and personality changes seen in both entities. Amenorrhea is one of the components of the **female athlete triad** in association with disordered eating and osteoporosis (see Chapter 689). Ballerinas, gymnasts, and runners may be at disproportionate risk of this triad. Ingestion of drugs, both legal and illegal, may cause amenorrhea and, in the case of phenothiazines, even a false-positive urine pregnancy test. Some drugs, including phenothiazines and certain antihypertensive agents, may cause galactorrhea, further mimicking pregnancy. Amenorrhea can follow discontinuation of combined hormonal therapy (CHT). A thorough drug history is, therefore, necessary.

TABLE 115-2. Congenital Anatomic Causes of Primary Amenorrhea with Normal Breast Development*

DIAGNOSIS	MÜLLERIAN AGENESIS	ANDROGEN INSENSITIVITY (AI)	TRANSVERSE VAGINAL SEPTUM	IMPERFORATE HYMEN
Patients with primary amenorrhea†	15%	1%	3%	1%
Patients with primary amenorrhea and apparent obstruction or absence of vagina†	75%	5%	15%	5%
Chromosomes‡	46,XX	46,XY	46,XX	46,XX
Gonads	Ovaries	Testes	Ovaries	Ovaries
Serum testosterone‡	Normal female level	Normal male level (high)	Normal female level	Normal female level
Vagina	Absent or shallow	Absent or shallow	Obstructed by septum which may be thick or thin, high or low	Obstructed by thin membrane, which may look blue from hematocolpos
Axillary/pubic hair	+	Absent unless AI is incomplete	+	+
Cyclic pain	±	–	+	+
Uterus	Absent or rudimentary	–	+	+
Mass	–	–	+ Can present with acute urinary retention as hematocolpos mass obstructs urethra	+ Can present with acute urinary retention
Introitus bulges with Valsalva maneuver	–	–	–	+
Associated anomalies	Urinary tract and skeletal	Inguinal hernias; gonadal malignancy in adulthood	Major urinary tract abnormalities in 15%	Possibly some increase in urinary tract abnormalities
Treatment	Vaginal dilation or surgical neovagina	Gonadectomy after age 16–18 yr Vaginal dilation or surgical neovagina	Surgical approach depends on extent and location of septum; may be extensive; should be done as soon as possible	Excision of hymen as soon as possible; diagnostic needle aspiration contraindicated because of risk of infection
Fertility	Advanced reproductive technology required; in vitro fertilization surrogate with uterus to gestate pregnancy	Not fertile	Variable, low septa have a better prognosis than do high septa	Usually fertile

*Cervix not visible on pelvic examination. Short vagina; may be absent or obstructed.
†Data from Reindollar RH, Byrd JR, McDonough PG: Delayed sexual development: A study of 252 patients. *Am J Obstet Gynecol* 1981;140:371.
‡Sometimes useful in differentiating müllerian agenesis from androgen insensitivity.
+, present; –, absent; ±, may be present or absent.
From Kliegman RM, Greenbaum LA, Lye PS: *Practical Strategies in Pediatric Diagnosis and Therapy,* 2nd ed. Philadelphia, Elsevier, 2004, p 505.

LABORATORY FINDINGS. The approach to the clinical evaluation of amenorrhea suggests a stepwise progression initiated by the history and physical examination. The pregnancy test, preferably a qualitative serum ß subunit human chorionic gonadotropin, is the key laboratory test to perform in the evaluation of amenorrhea regardless of the history or sexual activity given by the patient or signs of virilization (Fig. 115-1). The next step for laboratory determinations follows the scheme in which gonadotropin levels and physical examination findings are central to the assessment. The direct correlation of bone age to menstrual age enhances the value of a radiograph before proceeding with an extensive work-up. The measurement of FSH is critical in determining whether chromosomal abnormalities (with FSH elevation >25 mIU/mL) or other endocrinopathies or CNS tumors (with normal or low FSH <5 mIU/mL) are present. Prolonged amenorrhea (>6 mo) and persistent oligomenorrhea without an explanation should prompt the measurement of thyroid-stimulating hormone, FSH, LH, and prolactin levels, even in the face of a normal progesterone challenge. Elevated LH and normal FSH levels require the measurement of androgen excess even in the absence of obvious virilization. An LH:FSH ratio >3 and elevated free testosterone and DHEAS (dihydroepiandrosterone sulfate) levels are common in adolescents with polycystic ovary syndrome (PCOS). Hyperinsulinemia is a characteristic feature of PCOS, and there is an increased risk of diabetes mellitus. An elevated prolactin level or other clinical features suggesting a CNS tumor should be followed up with cranial CT scan or, preferably, MRI.

Endometrial status can be assessed as part of the evaluation when other endocrinologic parameters are normal by a progesterone challenge in which 5 or 10 mg oral medroxyprogesterone acetate is given for 5–10 days. Withdrawal bleeding should occur 2–7 days thereafter when normal endometrium is present. If bleeding does not occur, one must consider insufficient estrogenic priming of the endometrium, an abnormal uterus, or an outflow tract obstruction.

TREATMENT. Determination of the cause of amenorrhea may permit the initiation of corrective intervention. When the disorder is not amenable to remediation, consideration should be given to establishing regular pseudomenses to allow the adolescent to feel like her peers (Table 115-3). Counseling the adolescent whose diagnosis renders her unable to conceive is especially challenging, and support and follow-up are important. If the result of a vaginal smear is positive for estrogen effect, regular cycling can be accomplished using medroxyprogesterone in a dose of 10 mg orally for 10–12 days at least every other month. Combination norgestimate- or drospirenone-containing oral contraceptives can also be used for this purpose in patients with PCOS. In a patient with gonadal dysgenesis, conjugated estrogens must be given first (Premarin in an oral dose of 0.3 mg and increased to 1.25 mg) for feminization to progress. This is followed by medroxyprogesterone, 10 mg orally on days 10–21 of the cycle. Lifestyle changes, particularly weight reduction and insulin sensitizers, specifically metformin, have been shown to re-establish menses and ovulation is some patients, but symptoms return when the medication is discontinued.

115.2 • Abnormal Uterine Bleeding

DIFFERENTIAL DIAGNOSIS. Most abnormal vaginal bleeding in adolescents results from anovulatory cycles, normally occurring in the 1st yr of menarche. This is called **dysfunctional uterine bleeding;** this term is used when no demonstrable organic lesion is identified to account for the abnormal bleeding. Organic lesions are found in about 9% of 10–20 yr old young women; the most common include ectopic pregnancy, threatened abortion, endometritis, and hormonal contraceptives (Fig. 115-2). Table 115-4 lists the extensive differential diagnosis; studies of severe cases that require hospitalization report coagulation disorders (idiopathic thrombocytopenic purpura, von Willebrand disease, Glanzmann disease, leukemia), hypothyroidism, thalassemia major, Fanconi syndrome, and rheumatoid arthritis as the more frequent diagnoses. Medications may cause abnormal uterine bleeding; these include estrogens, progestins, androgens, prolactin and drugs that cause prolactin release (estrogens, phenothiazines, tricyclic antidepressants, metoclopramide), and anticoagulants (heparin, warfarin, aspirin, and nonsteroidal anti-inflammatory drugs [NSAIDs]).

LABORATORY FINDINGS. The hemoglobin and hematocrit are the most important elements in the initial evaluation. They establish the **severity of the bleeding,** with levels less than a hemoglobin of 9 g/dL or a hematocrit of 27% considered severe, 9–11 g/dL and 27–33% considered moderate, and >11 g/dL and >33% considered mild. Hospitalization is generally recommended for adoles-

TABLE 115-3. Hormone Replacement Options for Amenorrheic Conditions*

	HORMONE REPLACEMENT	BENEFITS OF THERAPY	RISKS OF THERAPY
Chronic anovulation (estrogen present)	Progestin therapy with medroxyprogesterone acetate, 5–10 mg/day PO or 5 mg norethindrone acetate 12 days/mo every 1–3 mo	Diminishes risk of sudden menorrhagia and of endometrial hyperplasia/cancer later in life; creates predictable normal menses	Some premenstrual symptoms may occur while the patient is taking progestin; does not provide contraception or address cause of amenorrhea; does not suppress androgens to treat hirsutism
	Low-dose oral contraceptive pills (20–35 μg estrogen) or contraceptive patch	Same as for progestin therapy; provides contraception; improves hirsutism by suppressing ovarian androgens	Does not address cause of amenorrhea; some parents object to their daughters' taking oral contraceptives; side effects can include nausea, headache, and breakthrough bleeding
Hypogonadism (low-estrogen state)†	Oral medroxyprogesterone acetate 5–10 mg/day or 2.5–5 mg norethindrone acetate on days 1–12 of the month (by calendar) plus oral conjugated estrogens, 0.625 mg/day	Prevents osteoporosis,‡ heart disease, and atrophic vaginal changes; eliminates hot flashes if present	Does not address cause of amenorrhea; does not provide contraception (if ovulation is possible, given the diagnosis); premenstrual symptoms may occur while the patient is taking progestins; some adolescents prefer oral contraceptives to "medications"
	Low-dose oral contraceptive pills (20–35 μg estrogen)	Same as HRT; provides contraception in case of spontaneous ovulation (if that is a possibility); many adolescents prefer taking oral contraceptives to taking "medications"	Same as risks of oral contraceptives for chronic anovulation

*These options may need modification according to the individual's response.
†See Chapter 587 for treatment of pubertal delay.
‡Estrogen therapy may not prevent bone loss in girls with amenorrhea and low body weight.
HRT, hormone replacement therapy.
From Kliegman RM, Greenbaum LA, Lye PS: *Practical Strategies in Pediatric Diagnosis and Therapy,* 2nd ed. Philadelphia, Elsevier, 2004, p 508.

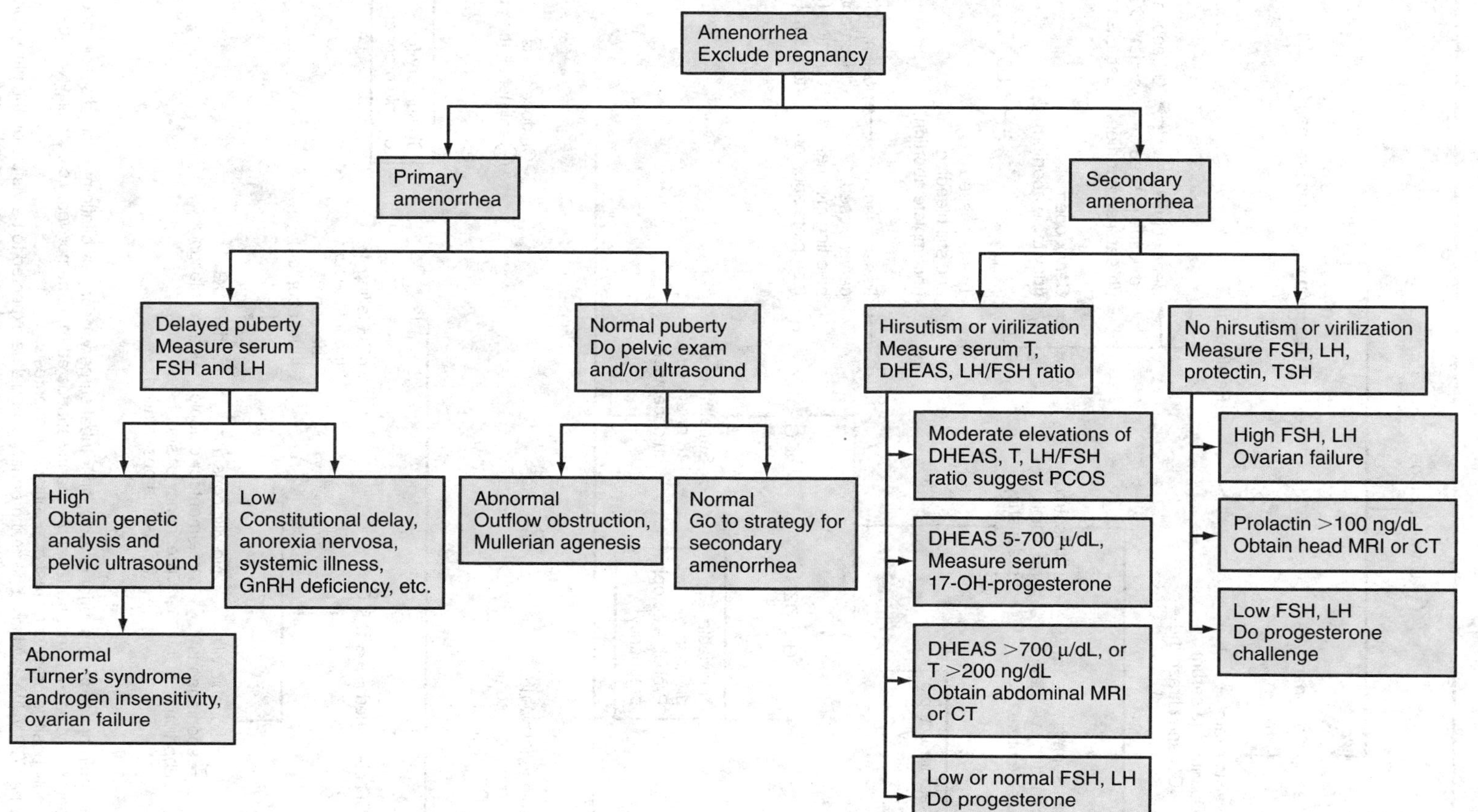

Figure 115-1. Approach to the adolescent with amenorrhea. DHEAS, dihydroepiandrotestosterone sulfate; FSH, follicle-stimulating hormone; GnRH, gonadotropin-releasing hormone; LH, luteinizing hormone; PCOS, polycystic ovary syndrome; T, testosterone. (From Slap GB: Menstrual disorders in adolescence. *Best Pract Res Clin Obstet Gynecol* 2003;17:75–92.)

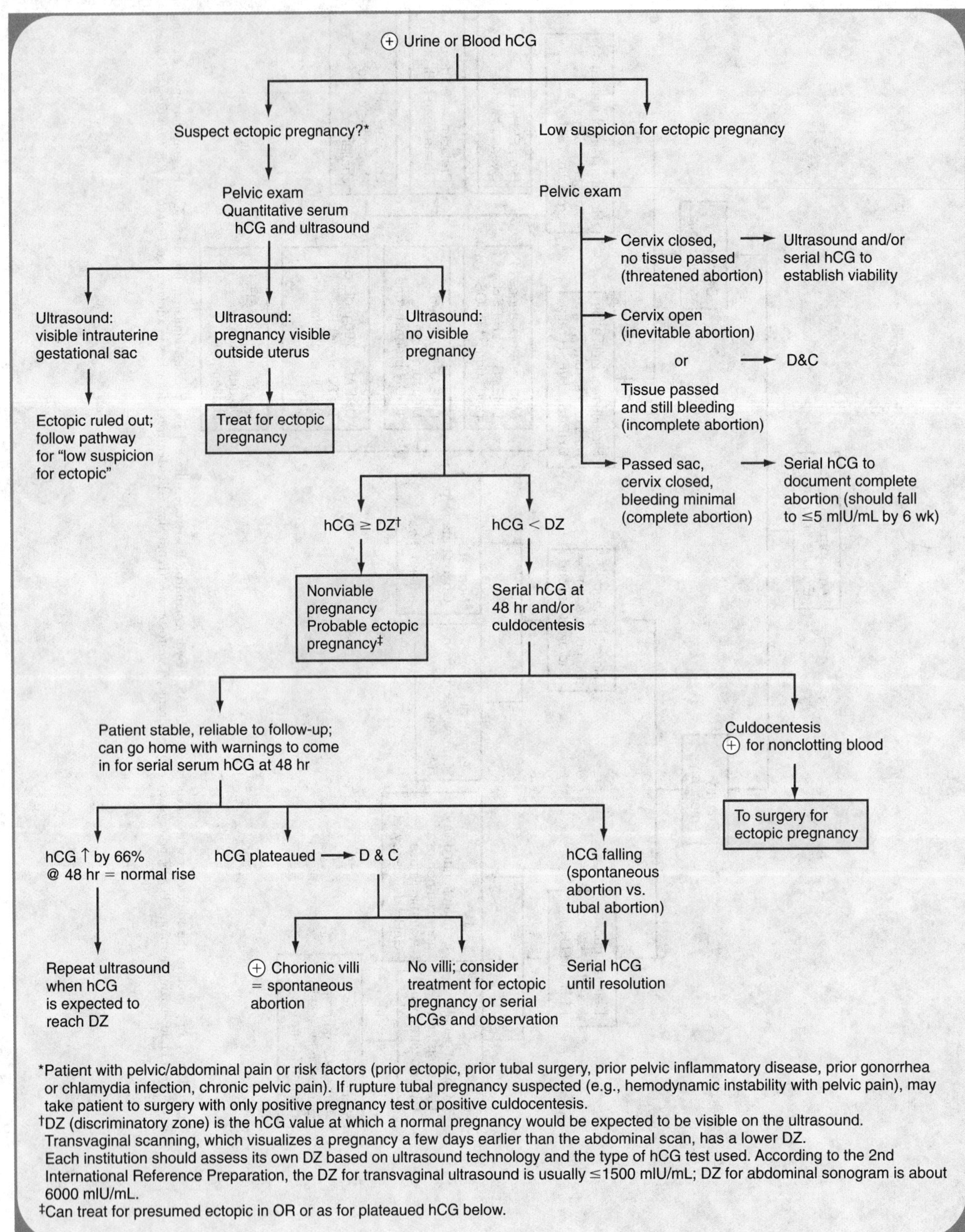

Figure 115-2. Evaluation of abnormal bleeding in pregnancy. D&C, dilation and curettage; DZ, discriminatory zone; hCG, human chorionic gonadotropin. (From Kliegman RM, Greenbaum LA, Lye PS: *Practical Strategies in Pediatric Diagnosis and Therapy,* 2nd ed. Philadelphia, Elsevier, 2005, p 503.)

TABLE 115-4. Differential Diagnosis of Abnormal Vaginal Bleeding in Adolescents

	BLEEDING PATTERN			EVALUATION	
	MR	*MMR*	*IB*	SUGGESTIVE FINDING; *DIAGNOSTIC FINDING*	TREATMENT
SOURCE: UTERUS				**COMMON CAUSES**	
Anovulation	+	+		No extrauterine source of bleeding seen on examination *Responds appropriately to treatment*	See text
Coagulopathy	+			More commonly found in cases of severe bleeding especially if onset at menarche; family history, ROS suggestive of clotting disorder; ecchymoses, petechiae may be seen on examination *Abnormal PT, PTT, platelet count, bleeding time, or test for von Willebrand disease*	Treat coagulopathy; oral contraceptives may help with menorrhagia; complete menstrual suppression sometimes required See also Chapters 476–484
Complication of pregnancy		+		History of late period; pregnancy symptoms (nausea, breast tenderness) *Positive urine or blood pregnancy test*	Fig. 115-2 and Chapter 117
SOURCE: VAGINA				**UNCOMMON CAUSES**	
Injury			+	History *Visible laceration*	Surgical or topical hemostasis; suture or allow to heal by secondary intention
Foreign body (e.g., retained tampon or contraceptive sponge)			+	History, foul discharge *Visible foreign body*	Removal
Cancer			+ +	Lesion seen, ± abnormal cytologic findings *Biopsy*	Referral to specialist; therapy chosen per type and stage of tumor
SOURCE: CERVIX				**LESS COMMON CAUSES**	
Neoplasia					
Dysplasia/carcinoma			+	Bleeding point on cervix; abnormal cytology *Colposcopy with directed biopsies*	LEEP, laser, cryotherapy, or cone biopsy
Cervical polyp			+	Polyp seen	Grasp with clamp or ring forceps and twirl off polyp in office; send specimen to pathologist
Hemangioma			+	Lesion seen	Conservative versus excision or ablation
Infection (cervicitis) (see Chapter 119)					
Herpes simplex			+	Cervical vesicles ± ulceration, ± pelvic pain, tenderness; Pap smear sometimes shows multinucleated giant cells *Culture positive for herpes*	If primary infection, consider oral famcyclovir, 250 mg b.i.d. × 7–10 days
Human papillomavirus (HPV)			+	Flat or raised warts seen on cervix *Pap smear + colposcopy necessary to differentiate from dysplasia; HPV typing may determine risk of cancer*	Laser, LEEP, cryotherapy, trichloroacetic acid or 5-fluorouracil cream after Pap smear and colposcopy; treat for dysplasia or symptoms
Trichomonas			+	Friable inflamed cervix; yellow-green vaginal discharge, pH 7–8 *Saline preparation: motile flagellates*	Metronidazole, 2 g orally once each for patient and sexual partners
SOURCE: UTERUS				**LESS COMMON CAUSES**	
Neoplasia					
Fibroid	±		±	± Enlarged uterus on examination; palpable fibroids *Abnormal findings on ultrasound and/or hysteroscopy*	NSAID sometimes helpful for menorrhagia; myomectomy via hysteroscope or laparoscope or laparotomy may be needed
Endometrial polyps			+	History of spotting superimposed on normal menstrual cycle *Hysteroscopy, saline sonogram, and/or D&C*	D&C or hysteroscopic excision
Malignant uterine tumor		±	±	Abnormal Pap smear, enlarged uterus, tissue at cervical os. *Biopsy*	Surgery determined by type of tumor and stage
Ovarian tumor producing estrogen (bleeding is uterine)		+		Adnexal mass on examination or ultrasonography *Surgical diagnosis and staging*	Surgery
Foreign body					
IUD	+		+	No other cause of bleeding (patient ovulatory, not pregnant, no PID) *IUD in uterus; responds to therapy*	NSAID sometimes useful for menorrhagia; removal if PID coexists or if necessary to control bleeding
Infection					
PID	+		+	Tender uterus and adnexae; purulent cervical discharge ± ↑ WBC count, ESR, or fever *Clinical diagnosis, tests often positive for gonorrhea, chlamydia*	CDC guidelines (see Chapter 119)
Postpartum or postabortal endometritis ± retained products of conception			+	± ↑ WBC count, ESR, fever *Recent pregnancy; tender uterus*	D&C if retained tissue seen on sonogram; broad-spectrum antibiotics, methergine
Congenital partially obstructed hemivagina or uterine horn			+	Foul, dark blood after menses *Abnormal pelvic examination and/or pelvic ultrasonography*	Refer for surgical treatment

CDC, Centers for Disease Control and Prevention; D&C, dilation and curettage; ESR, erythrocyte sedimentation rate; IB, intermenstrual bleeding; IUD, intrauterine device; LEEP, loop electroexcisional procedure; MMR, menometrorrhagia; MR, menorrhagia; NSAID, nonsteroidal anti-inflammatory drug; Pap, Papanicolaou; PID, pelvic inflammatory disease; PT, prothrombin time; PTT, partial thromboplastin time; ROS, review of systems; WBC, white blood cell.
From Kliegman RM, Greenbaum LA, Lye PS: *Practical Strategies in Pediatric Diagnosis and Therapy*, 2nd ed. Philadelphia, Elsevier, 2004, p 497–498.

cents with a hemoglobin <7 g/dL or a hemoglobin <10 g/dL with significant postural blood pressure changes or excessive heavy bleeding. For sexually active teenagers, tests for gonorrhea, chlamydia, and pregnancy are also performed. The secondary evaluation should include liver and thyroid function studies, prothrombin time, partial thromboplastin time, and bleeding time. If these studies are not performed at the first visit, they must be performed before any estrogen therapy is initiated that might interfere with interpreting the results.

TREATMENT. In **mild** cases, iron supplementation is recommended, and the patient should keep a menstrual calendar to follow the subsequent flow patterns. With **moderate** disturbances, cycling with oral contraceptives, barring any contraindications, should be considered along with monitoring the iron status and oral iron therapy. **Severe** bleeding, not requiring hospitalization, can usually be stopped with hormonal therapy, either medroxyprogesterone acetate (Provera) 10 mg/24 hr for 10–14 days or a combination oral contraceptive using two to four pills per day

TABLE 115-5. Differential Diagnosis of Dysmenorrhea

	DESCRIPTION OF PAIN	OCCURRENCE OF DYSMENORRHEA IN ANOVULATORY CYCLES	DIAGNOSIS	TREATMENT
Primary	Crampy lower abdominal/low back pain ± radiation to upper thighs ± nausea, vomiting, diarrhea, headache; begins at time of menstrual flow; lasts 1–3 days	No	Normal abdominal and pelvic examination; internal pelvic examination can be reserved for sexually active girls and older teenagers; rectoabdominal examination assesses pelvic pathology	NSAIDs and/or oral contraceptives; see Table 115-6
Secondary				
Congenital partial outflow obstruction (e.g., rudimentary uterine horn, obstructed hemivagina)	Pain begins at or shortly after menarche and occurs with bleeding	Yes	Pelvic examination ± ultrasonography ± laparoscopy; found in 8% of adolescents who underwent laparoscopy for pain	Surgical relief of obstruction
Endometriosis	Increasingly severe dysmenorrhea ± chronic pelvic pain exacerbated during menses	No	Found in 16–70% of adolescents who underwent laparoscopy for pelvic pain; pelvic examination finding may be normal or there may be tenderness of the uterosacral ligaments/cul-de-sac and/or ovarian masses; although congenital obstruction of menstrual outflow increases chance of endometriosis, most teenagers with endometriosis have normal anatomy; diagnosis is by laparoscopy	Surgical and/or hormonal therapy; post-treatment prophylaxis with oral contraceptives
Atypical secondary dysmenorrhea				
Pelvic inflammatory disease	Pain during or immediately after menses	Yes	Pelvic examination: tender uterus and adnexa, ± cervicitis, ± ↑ WBC count, ± ↑ ESR, ± fever	Follow CDC recommendations (see Chapter 119)
Pregnancy complication	Pain and bleeding may coincide and may be interpreted by the patient as a painful menstrual period	N/A	UCG, or serum hCG	See Figure 115-2

CDC, Centers for Disease Control and Prevention; ESR, erythrocyte sedimentation rate; hCG, human chorionic gonadotropin, N/A, not applicable; NSAIDs, nonsteroidal anti-inflammatory drugs; UCG, urinary chorionic gonadotropin; WBC, white blood cell.
From Kliegman RM, Greenbaum LA, Lye PS: *Practical Strategies in Pediatric Diagnosis and Therapy*, 2nd ed. Philadelphia, Elsevier, 2004, p 509.

until the bleeding stops, then one pill per day for the remainder of the cycle. Once a patient is hospitalized, Premarin 25 mg every 4 hr up to two to three doses given intravenously is required. At the same time, the combination oral contraceptive regimen or Depo-Provera (medroxyprogesterone acetate [DMPA]), 150 mg IM every 12 wk, required for maintenance, can be initiated. These estrogen doses are high, prompting some concern about the risk of thromboembolism, but no complications have been reported from short-term use. For severe cases, transfusion of packed red blood cells may be needed.

In the rare case of a patient whose bleeding cannot be controlled by one of these methods, an endometrial curettage may be indicated. Although this procedure is frequently undertaken in adult women with menometrorrhagia, the rarity of endometrial carcinoma and the usual efficacy of hormonal therapy in adolescence make this procedure unnecessarily invasive in this age group.

115.3 • DYSMENORRHEA

Painful menstrual cramps are experienced by nearly two thirds of postmenarchal teenagers in the United States. More than 10% of this group suffers sufficiently to miss school, making dysmenorrhea the leading cause of short-term school absenteeism in female adolescents. Dysmenorrhea may be primary or secondary. **Primary dysmenorrhea** is characterized by the absence of any specific pelvic pathologic condition and is the more commonly occurring form (Table 115-5). Prostaglandins F_2 and E_2, produced by the endometrium, stimulate local vasoconstriction and the myometrial contractions, producing pain. **Secondary dysmenorrhea** results from an underlying **structural abnormality** of the cervix or uterus, a **foreign body** such as an intrauterine device, **endometriosis,** or **endometritis.** Endometriosis, a condition in which implants of endometrial tissue are found at ectopic locations within the peritoneal cavity. Characteristically, there is severe pain at the time of menses; its specific location depends on the site of the implants.

A pelvic examination must be performed to exclude the causes of secondary dysmenorrhea, and if none is found, a diagnosis of primary dysmenorrhea should be considered. Adolescents suffering from dysmenorrhea have high levels of prostaglandins F_2 and E_2 and experience symptomatic relief when prostaglandin synthetase inhibitors are administered (Table 115-6). If given before a menstrual period (or shortly after it begins), administration of a rapidly absorbed prostaglandin synthetase inhibitor, such as naproxen sodium, is effective in destroying the prostaglandins

TABLE 115-6. Treatment of Primary Dysmenorrhea

	MEDICATION	REGIMEN	COMMENTS
NSAID	Ibuprofen, 200 mg	2 tablets PO q4-6h	Over-the-counter
	Naproxen sodium, 275 mg	2 tablets to start, then 1 PO q6h	
	Naproxen sodium, 550 mg	1 tablet PO q12h	12-hr regimen is appealing to patients
	Mefenamic acid, 250 mg	2 tablets to start, then 1 PO q6h	Suggested in some studies as most effective drug
Oral contraceptives or contraceptive patch	Any low-dose pill (≤35 μg of estrogen) or ortho Evra	Cyclic	Particularly useful if birth control method is needed; a few cycles may be needed to reach maximum effectiveness

*Aspirin has not been shown to be better than placebo in the treatment of primary dysmenorrhea. NSAID treatment is effective if started at the onset of cramping and bleeding.
NSAID, nonsteroidal antiinflammatory drug; PO, per os (orally).
From Kliegman RM, Greenbaum LA, Lye PS: *Practical Strategies in Pediatric Diagnosis and Therapy*, 2nd ed. Philadelphia, Elsevier, 2004, p 510.

before they produce pain (two tablets of 275 mg each taken with the onset of menses and one tablet taken every 6–8 hr after that for the 1st 24 hr). Medication is rarely needed beyond the 1st day. For the teenager with dysmenorrhea who requires contraception, combined hormonal therapy in the form of oral contraceptives, the contraceptive patch, or vaginal ring may be indicated. It is not certain whether the beneficial effect of such use derives from the ability of oral contraceptives to inhibit ovulation and thus eliminate progesterone production from the corpus luteum or from their ability to limit endometrial proliferation and therefore the production of prostaglandins.

In adolescent patients with **endometriosis,** danazol, an antigonadotropin, is rarely prescribed because of the unacceptable side effects of weight gain, irregular menses, edema, acne, oily skin, hirsutism, and a deep voice change. The use of gonadotropin-releasing hormone (GnRH) agonists such as nafarelin and leuprolide are more commonly used with the goal of the creation of an acyclic, low-estrogen environment. This prevents bleeding at the site of the implants and further seeding of the pelvis during retrograde menstruation. GnRH agonist can be given as a nasal spray or IM injection every 3 mo. Depot-leuprolide can be given at a dose of 11.25 mg every 3 mo. To reduce the risk of decreased bone density, a long-term side effect of GnRH analog therapy, prescriptions for courses of therapy lasting longer than 6 consecutive mo are not recommended. "Add back" hormonal therapy with norethindrone or conjugated estrogen has been shown to reduce bone and lipid metabolism side effects.

TABLE 115-7. Criteria for Premenstrual Dysphoric Disorder*

In most menstrual cycles during the past year, presence of ≥5 of the following symptoms for most of the last week of the luteal phase, with remission beginning within a few days after the onset of the follicular phase and absence of symptoms during the week after menses; inclusion of ≥1 of the first 4 symptoms:
- Markedly depressed mood, feelings of hopelessness, or self-deprecating thoughts
- Marked anxiety, tension, feelings of being "keyed up" or "on edge"
- Marked affective lability (e.g., feeling suddenly sad or tearful or having increased sensitivity to rejection)
- Persistent and marked anger or irritability or increased interpersonal conflicts
- Decreased interest in usual activities (e.g., work, school, friends, and hobbies)
- Subjective sense of difficulty in concentrating
- Lethargy, easy fatigability, or marked lack of energy
- Marked change in appetite, overeating, or specific food cravings
- Hypersomnia or insomnia
- Subjective sense of being overwhelmed or out of control
- Other physical symptoms, such as breast tenderness or swelling, headache, joint or muscle pain, a sensation of "bloating," weight gain

Marked interference with work or school or with usual social activities and relationships with others (e.g., avoidance of social activities or decreased productivity and efficiency at work or school)

Disturbance not a mere exacerbation of the symptoms of another disorder, such as major depressive disorder, panic disorder, dysthymic disorder, or a personality disorder (although possibly superimposed on any of these disorders)

Confirmation of three criteria above by prospective daily ratings during at least two consecutive symptomatic menstrual cycles (diagnosis may be made provisionally before such confirmation)

*The criteria are from the *Diagnostic and Statistical Manual of Mental Disorders, Fourth Edition, Text Revision.* In menstruating women, the luteal phase corresponds to the period between ovulation and the onset of menses, and the follicular phase begins with menses. In nonmenstruating women (e.g., women who have had a hysterectomy), determination of the timing of the luteal and follicular phases may require measurement of circulating reproductive hormones.

From Grady-Weliky TA: Premenstrual dysphoric disorder. *N Engl J Med* 2003;348:433–438.

115.4 • Premenstrual Syndrome

Premenstrual syndrome (PMS), or the late luteal phase syndrome, is a complex of physical signs and behavioral symptoms occurring during the 2nd half of the menstrual cycle, which may resolve with the onset of menses. **Clinical manifestations** may include breast fullness and tenderness; bloating; fatigue; headache; increased appetite, especially for sweets and salty foods; irritability and mood swings; and depression, inability to concentrate, tearfulness, and violent tendencies. About one third of women in the reproductive age group may have PMS, but the absence of objective findings makes this difficult to corroborate. It is not common among adolescents, and it does not relate to the presence of dysmenorrhea, which is much more common in this age group. For the diagnosis of PMS, documentation of symptoms using a special calendar for 2–3 mo should demonstrate the pattern of association with menses. NSAIDs, particularly mefenamic acid, diuretics, agnus castus fruit extract, and CHT have demonstrated some therapeutic efficacy in small trials. An open-label trial of an oral contraceptive containing drospirenone demonstrated effectiveness in reducing symptoms commonly associated with PMS. **Premenstrual dysphoric disorder** occurs less commonly in 3–8% of women of reproductive age, is a more severe form of premenstrual syndrome (Table 115-7), and requires more intensive therapy (Table 115-8).

TABLE 115-8. Recommended Treatment Strategies for Premenstrual Dysphoric Disorder*

MEDICATION	STARTING DOSE (MG)	THERAPEUTIC DOSE (MG)	COMMON SIDE EFFECTS
FIRST-LINE: SELECTIVE SEROTONIN REUPTAKE INHIBITORS			
Fluoxetine	10–20	20	Sexual dysfunction (anorgasmia and decreased libido), sleep alterations (insomnia, sedation, or hypersomnia), and gastrointestinal distress (nausea and diarrhea)
Sertraline	25–50	50–150	Same as fluoxetine
Paroxetine	10–20	20–30	Same as fluoxetine
Citalopram	10–20	20–30	Same as fluoxetine
SECOND-LINE			
Clomipramine	25	50–75	Dry mouth, fatigue, vertigo, sweating, headache, nausea
Alprazolam	0.50–0.75	1.25–2.25	Drowsiness, sedation
THIRD-LINE			
Leuprolide	3.75	3.75	Hot flashes, night sweats, headache, nausea

*For selective serotonin reuptake inhibitors and clomipramine, the starting and therapeutic doses are administered once daily and are the same with luteal-phase and continuous administration. For luteal-phase administration, the medication should be intiated at time of ovulation (usually approximately 2 wk before the expected onset of menses) and discontinued on the 1st day of menses. The therapeutic doses given for selective serotonin reuptake inhibitors are those that were reported in the randomized clinical trials. However, clinical experience has shown that a subgroup of patients with premenstrual dysphoric disorder may require slightly higher doses (up to 60 mg fluoxetine; up to 150 mg sertraline; up to 40 mg paroxetine; and up to 40 mg citalopram). If a patient is taking another selective serotonin reuptake inhibitor and tolerating it well but has a partial response at the doses listed, it would be appropriate to increase the dose of the specific selective serotonin reuptake inhibitor before switching to another agent. Alprazolam is administered three times a day; treatment should begin at 0.25 mg three times a day. Clinical trials of leuprolide used the depot form; leuprolide should be administered intramuscularly each month.

From Grady-Weliky TA: Premenstrual dysphoric disorder. *N Engl J Med* 2003;384:433–438.

Adams Hillard PJ, Deitch HR: Menstrual disorders in the college female. *Pediatr Clin North Am* 2005;52:179–197.
Anderson SE, Must A: Interpreting the continued decline in the average age at menarche: Results from two nationally representative surveys of U.S. girls studied 10 years apart. *J Pediatr* 2005;147:753–760.
Borenstein J, Yu H, Wade S, et al: Effect of an oral contraceptive containing ethinyl estradiol and drospirenone on premenstrual symptomatology and health-related quality of life. *J Reprod Med* 2003;48:79–85.
Grady-Weliky TA: Premenstrual dysphoric disorder. *N Engl J Med* 2003;348:433–438.
Lethaby A, Farquhar C: Treatments for heavy menstrual bleeding. *Br Med J* 2003;327:1243–1244.
Proctor M, Farquhar C: Diagnosis and management of dysmenorrhea. *BMJ* 2006;332:1134–1138.
Shin SY, Lee YY, Yang SY, et al: Characteristics of menstruation-related problems for adolescents and premarital women in Korea. *Eur J Obstet Gynecol Reprod Biol* 2005;121:236–242.
Slap GB: Menstrual disorders in adolescence. *Best Pract Res Clin Obstet Gynecol* 2003;17:75–92.

Chapter 116 ■ Contraception

Renée R. Jenkins

Adolescents bear a disproportionate risk of the adverse consequences of sexual activity, sexually transmitted infections (STIs) (see Chapter 119), and early, unintended pregnancy (see Chapter 117). An age-appropriate sexual history will identify adolescents at risk, and contraceptive counseling and management should be offered as part of a broad reproductive health intervention.

EPIDEMIOLOGY.

Sexual Activity. In the United States, the 2002 National Survey of Family Growth reported a decline in sexual activity from 1995 to 2002, with reports of ever having intercourse declining in young women and men aged 15–17 yr and in men aged 18–19 yr, but not significantly in 18–19 yr old women (Fig. 116-1). The Centers for Disease Control and Prevention's Youth Risk Behavior Survey supports this observation in high school students with "ever had intercourse" rates falling from 53.1% in 1995 to 46.7% in 2003, although the lowest rate for female students was reported in 2001 (42.9% in 2001 and 45.3% in 2003); 61.6% of high school seniors report ever having had intercourse, with 34.3% currently active sexually, defined as having had intercourse during the 3 mo preceding the survey. Males report sexual initiation at an earlier age, but by 12th grade there are no significant gender differences for ever or current sexual activity. The median age at first intercourse for women in Canada, Great Britain, Sweden, and the United States ranges from 17.1 to 17.5 yr, but is slightly higher (18.0 yr) in France. Among developing nations, there is greater diversity; 73% of Liberian women ages 15–19 have had intercourse, compared to 53% of Nigerian, 49% of Ugandan, and 32% of Botswanan women. Only 7% of Chinese university students report being sexually experienced (Fig. 116-2).

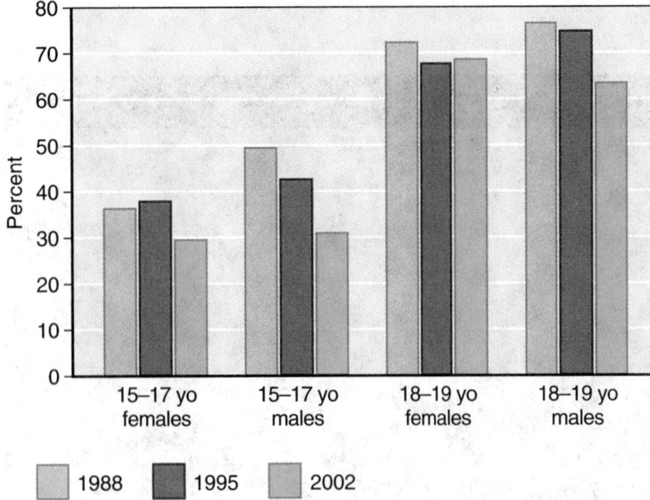

Figure 116-1. Percentage of never married females and males who ever had sexual intercourse: United States 1988–2002. (From Abma JC, Martinez GM, Mosher WD, et al: Teenagers in the United States: Sexual activity, contraceptive use, and childbearing, 2002. *Vital Health Stat 23* 2004;24:1–48.)

Factors associated with early sexual activity in nations worldwide include lower expectations for education, poor perception of life options, low school grades, and involvement in other high-risk behaviors. For those who have never had intercourse, being against their religion and morals, avoiding pregnancy or a sexually transmitted infection (STI), and waiting for the right person were the most frequent reasons adolescents report for abstaining.

Contraceptive Use. Recent use of any contraceptive method among currently sexually active adolescents aged 15–19 yr increased from 79.9% in 1988 to 83.2% in 2003 according to the National Survey of Family Growth. The frequency dipped slightly in 1995 to 70.7%. Condoms were the most frequently used method, with dramatic increases from 1995–2002 in non-Hispanic white females (40.8% to 60.8%) and non-Hispanic black males (71% to 86.1%). The type of hormonal method selected also varies by ethnicity, with non-Hispanic white women more likely to select pills (40.7%), and black women using pills as the first choice, but being more than twice as likely than whites to use an injectable method (Table 116-1). U.S. teens used medical methods at last intercourse less frequently compared to other teens; 52% in U.S. teens, 56% in Swedish 18–19 yr olds, 67% of French 15–19 yr olds, 72% of British 16–19 yr olds, and 73% of Canadian 15–19 yr olds. Sexually active adolescent women in the United States delay going to a clinic or a doctor for a medical contraceptive for an average of 6 mo after initiating intercourse. A higher likelihood of contraceptive use in women is associated with older age at sexual initiation, aspirations for higher academic achievement, acceptance of one's own sexuality, and a positive attitude toward contraception.

CONTRACEPTIVE COUNSELING. The health screening interview during the adolescent preventive visit offers the opportunity both to support the adolescent who is abstinent to continue to be so and to identify the sexually active adolescent who has unsafe sexual practices (see Chapter 111). Adolescents with chronic diseases are particularly vulnerable to having these issues omitted from the health maintenance visit. There may be particular cautions related to concurrent medication to be noted for these chronically ill teenagers; sexuality and contraceptive issues do need to be addressed. The goals of a counseling intervention with the adolescent are to understand the adolescent's perceptions and misperceptions about contraceptives, help him or her put the risk of unprotected intercourse in a personal perspective, and educate the adolescent regarding the real risk and contraindications for the various methods available.

The likelihood that an adolescent will use a contraceptive method depends on such factors as the developmental level of the adolescent, the reproductive history, the involvement in other high-risk behaviors, and the degree of readiness for using contraception. **Readiness to use contraception** progresses in stages, from (1) precontemplative, not thinking about using contracep-

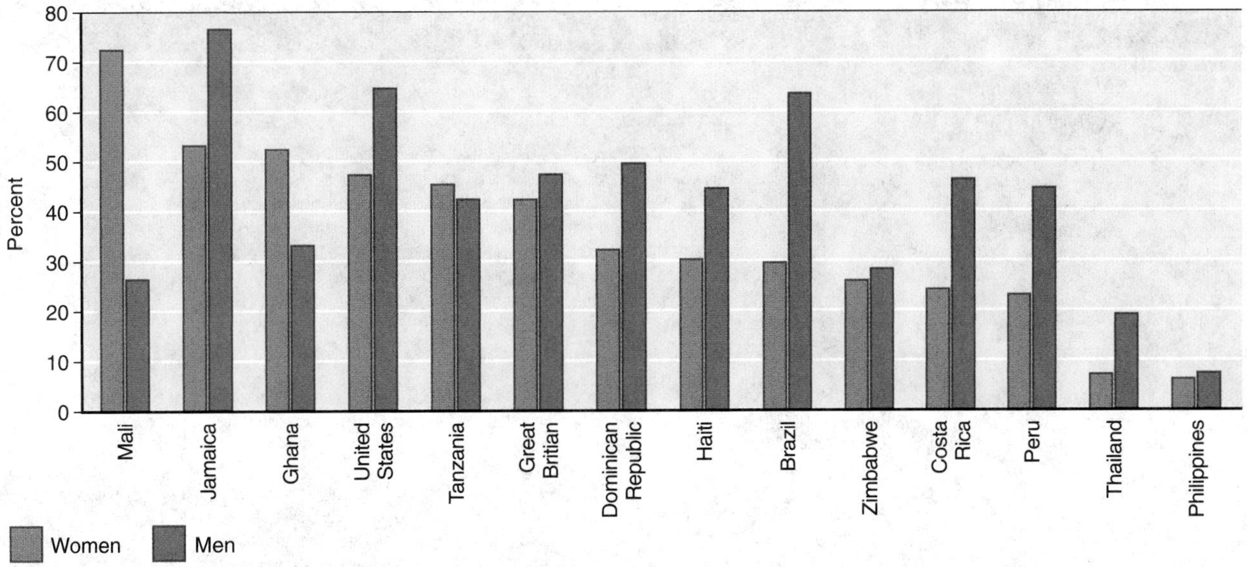

Figure 116-2. Range of 20–24 yr olds who were sexually active by 17 yr.

tion; (2) contemplative, giving it some thought, but having no immediate plans; (3) preparative, wanting to try a method in the near future; to (4) active, using contraception. The adolescent should also be made aware of the "perfect" use failure rates versus the "typical" failure rates based on the correct and consistent use of the method (Table 116-2). The pregnancy risk for withdrawal as a method is probably underestimated in adolescents, and its low efficacy rate should be specifically addressed with young adolescents. Once an adolescent chooses a method, recognition of the common side effects, with clear plans on management, communication with the provider about the realistic expectation for failure, and a contingency plan for that possibility between the adolescent and the provider give closure to the counseling session and provide strategies for close follow-up (see Table 116-2). The **pelvic examination** as a requirement to obtain medical contraception creates a barrier for some teenagers; consequently, clinicians have commonly delayed the examination for 3–6 mo for adolescents who might otherwise postpone the acceptance of a contraceptive device. Confidentiality and consent issues related to contraceptive management are discussed in Chapter 100).

TABLE 116-1. Percentage of Distribution of Non-Hispanic White and Non-Hispanic Black Contraceptive Users Aged 15–19 yr

	YEARS BY CURRENT METHOD, 1988–2002		
RACE/ETHNICITY AND METHOD	1988	1995	2002
NON-HISPANIC WHITE			
Pill	43	29.6	40.7
Other hormonal[†]	—	4.8	8.0
Male condom	31.3	40.8	60.8
All other methods[‡]	12	8.6	*
Dual methods (hormonal + condom)	*	10.0	22.5
No method	16.7	26.7	10.3
Any method	83.3	73.3	89.7
NON-HISPANIC BLACK			
Pill	48.3	15.3	27.8
Other hormonal[†]	—	15.6	18.6
Male condom	23.9	41.1	49.9
All other methods[‡]	*	*	—
Dual methods (hormonal + condom)	*	*	23.3
No method	32.3	26.7	25.2
Any method	67.7	73.3	74.8

*Figure does not meet standard of reliability or precision; quantity, zero.
[†]Includes Depo-Provera injectable, Lunelle injectable, Norplant implants, emergency contraception, and contraceptive patch in 2002; Depo-Provera and Norplant in 1995.
[‡]All other methods besides condom and hormonal methods.
—, data not available.
From Abma JC, Martinez GM, Mosher WD, et al: Teenagers in the United States: Sexual activity, contraceptive use, and childbearing, 2002. *Vital Health Stat 23* 2004;24:1–48.

116.1 • Barrier Methods

CONDOMS. This method prevents sperm from being deposited in the vagina. There are no major side effects associated with the use of a condom. The risk of AIDS may have increased the use of condoms among adolescents, with 46.2% of high school students in 1991 reporting using a condom at last sexual intercourse increasing to 63% in 2003. Condom use appears to be higher among sexually active youths in Great Britain and Canada. Condom use at first intercourse is higher in France compared to the United States. The main advantages of condoms are their low price, availability without prescription, little need for advance planning, and, most important for this age group, their effectiveness in preventing transmission of STIs, including HIV and HPV. Latex condoms are recommended as protection against STIs, to be used along with all nonbarrier medical methods for adolescents. A female condom is available over the counter in single size disposable units. It is a second choice over the male latex condom because of the complexity of properly using the device, its low typical efficacy rate, and the lack of studies in humans demonstrating its effectiveness against STDs. Most adolescents would require intensive education and hands-on practice to use it effectively.

DIAPHRAGM AND CERVICAL CAP. These methods have few side effects but are much less likely to be used by teenagers. Adolescents tend to object to the messiness of the jelly or to the fact that the insertion of a diaphragm may interrupt the spontaneity of sex, or they may express discomfort about touching their genitals.

TABLE 116-2. Contraceptive Methods

METHOD	FAILURE RATE (%) PERFECT USE	FAILURE RATE (%) TYPICAL USE	DOSING	MECHANISM OF ACTION	POTENTIAL SIDE EFFECTS	ADVANTAGES
HORMONAL CONTRACEPTIVES						
The patch	0.7	0.9	Weekly for 3 wk (off on 4th wk) 20 μg ethinyl estradiol 150 μg norelgestromin released daily	Combined hormonal method: thickens cervical mucus, inhibits ovulation, inhibits sperm's ability to fertilize egg, slows tubal mobility, disrupts ovum transport, induces endometrial atrophy	Breakthrough bleeding, nausea, headaches, breast tenderness, skin site reaction, less effective if patient >90 kg (198 lb)	Similar to OCPs but less frequent dosing
Oral contraceptive (the pill) combination	0.1	5	Daily Varies 20–50 μg estrogen Varies 0.15–1 μg progestogen	Combined hormonal method: (see above)	Breakthrough bleeding, nausea, headaches, breast tenderness	Decrease in: PID risk, ectopic pregnancy risk, menstrual blood loss, dysmenorrheal, acne
Progestin only	0.5	5	Daily (within 3-hr period) 0.35 mg norethindrone or 0.075 mg norgestrel	Progestin-only hormonal method: inhibits ovulation, thickens and decreases cervical mucus, atrophies endometrium	Irregular bleeding, breast tenderness, depression	No estrogen
Contraceptive injections progestin-only injection (Depo-Provera)	0.3	0.3	3 mo 150 mg depot medroxyprogesterone per injection	Progestin-only hormonal method: (see above)	Irregular bleeding or amenorrhea, weight gain, breast tenderness, acne, depression, possible decrease in bone density	No estrogen, decrease in: menstrual blood loss, dysmenorrhea, PID risk
Progestin-releasing IUD (Mirena)	0.1	0.1	5 yr Releases 20 μg/day levonorgestrel	Progestin-only hormonal effect and IUD effect of preventing sperm from fertilizing ovum	Breakthrough bleeding in first 3–6 mo, then hypo-, or amenorrhea	No estrogen, easy to use, long-acting Decrease in: menstrual blood loss, dysmenorrheal, (possible) PID risk
Vaginal ring (Nuva Ring)	0.65	N/A	Monthly (insert for 3 wk of each month) Serum levels of 15 μg ethinyl estradiol Releases 150 μg norelgestromin daily	Combined hormonal method: (see above)	Vaginal irritation, vaginal discharge, headache	Similar to OCs but less frequent dosing
NONHORMONAL CONTRACEPTIVES						
Male condom	3	14	Every act of intercourse	Barrier method: blocks passage of semen	Latex allergy	Recommended to be used in addition to another contraceptive; only method that decreased STD, HIV risk
Female condom	5	21	Every act of intercourse	Barrier method: lines the vagina fully and perineum partially	Vaginal discomfort, partner penile irritation	Provides some protection against STD, HIV
IUD Copper-containing (ParaGard)	0.6	0.8	10 yr 36 × 22 mm, copper wire wound around vertical stem of T	IUD: prevents sperm from fertilizing ova	Heavier menses	Easy to use, long-acting nonhormonal
Spermicides	18	29	Every act of intercourse nonoxynol-9 (in U.S.). Dose varies by formulation, e.g., gel, suppository, from 52.5 to 150 mg	Kills sperm by destroying sperm cell membrane	Allergy or sensitivity to ingredients, recurrent urinary tract infections	Recommended to be used in addition to another barrier contraceptive

IUD, intrauterine device; OCs, oral contraceptives; PID, pelvic inflammatory disease; STD, sexually transmitted disease.
From As-sanie S, Gantt A, Rosenthal MS: Pregnancy prevention in adolescents. *Am Fam Physician* 2004;70:1517–1524 and Hatcher RA, Trussell J, Stewart F, et al (editors): *Contraceptive Technology.* New York, Ardent Media, Inc., 2004.

116.2 • Spermicides

A variety of agents containing the spermicide nonoxynol-9 are available as foams, jellies, creams, films, or effervescent vaginal suppositories. They must be placed in the vaginal cavity shortly before intercourse and reinserted before each subsequent ejaculation in order to be effective. Rare side effects consist of contact vaginitis. There has been some concern regarding the vaginal and cervical mucosal damage observed with nonoxynol-9, and the overall impact on HIV transmission is unknown. The finding that nonoxynol-9 is gonococcicidal and spirocheticidal has not been substantiated in randomized clinical trials. Spermicides should be used in combination with condoms.

116.3 • Combination Methods

The conjoint use of the condom by the male and spermicidal foam by the female adolescent is extremely effective; the failure rate is 2% (perfect use), without any of the potential side effects and complications associated with the use of other forms of contraception having comparable efficacy. This combination also prevents STIs, including HIV and HPV.

116.4 • Hormonal Methods

Hormonal methods employ either an estrogenic substance in combination with a progestin or a progestin alone. The action of the estrogen-progestin combination is to prevent the surge of luteinizing hormone and, as a result, to inhibit ovulation. Progestin may prevent ovulation, but it is not reliable. Progestin does, however, affect fallopian tube transport and the composition of cervical mucus in such a way as to make fertilization or implantation less likely.

COMBINATION ORAL CONTRACEPTIVES. Oral contraceptives (OCs) are commonly referred to as "the pill" and currently contain 35, 30, or 20 μg of estrogenic substance, typically ethinyl estradiol, and a progestin. The pill is one of the most reliable contraceptive methods available. Typical-use failure rates in 15–19 yr old women have ranged up to 18.1%. Thrombophlebitis, hepatic adenomas, myocardial infarction, and carbohydrate intolerance are some of the more serious potential complications of exogenous estrogen use. These disorders are exceedingly rare in adolescents. Even though teenage smokers who use OCs have a relative risk of more than 2.0 for myocardial infarction, the likelihood of its occurrence is much smaller, and thus insignificant, than the risk of dying from pregnancy-related complications. Some long-range beneficial effects of estrogen use include decreased risks of benign breast disease, ovarian disease, and anemia.

The short-term adverse effects of OCs, such as nausea and weight gain, often interfere with compliance in adolescent patients. These effects are usually transient and may be overshadowed by the beneficial effects of a shortened menses and the relief of dysmenorrhea. The inhibition of ovulation or the suppressant effect of estrogens on prostaglandin production by the endometrium makes OCs effective in preventing dysmenorrhea (see Chapter 115). An initial thought for younger adolescents regarding the potentially unknown effect of estrogens on epiphyseal growth is no longer a concern. Acne may be worsened by some and improved by other OC preparations. The pills with nonandrogenic progestins are particularly effective in reducing acne and hirsutism. Drospirenone, a progestin with antimineralocorticoid activity, has been shown to reduce premenstrual symptomatology, but the potential for hyperkalemia as a side effect eliminates patients with renal, liver, or adrenal diseases and patients on certain medications. A beneficial cardiovascular effect occurs for adolescents taking estrogen-containing OCs; these young women have higher levels of cardioprotective high-density lipoproteins than controls. Although women <35 yr old who smoke are at less risk of cardiovascular complications, adolescents on OCs should be encouraged to stop smoking.

Extending cycling of OCs for adolescents has some anticipated benefits with increased ovarian activity suppression and improved contraceptive efficacy during treatment with drugs that reduce OC efficacy. Seasonale (0.15 mg levonorgestrel/30µg ethinyl estradiol) was approved by the U.S. Food and Drug Administration (FDA) in September 2003 for extended cycling with 84 active pills and seven placebo pills. The most common side effect is intermenstrual bleeding and/or spotting with the total days of bleeding over the first year of treatment being similar for Seasonale subjects and subjects on a 28-day cycle. The unscheduled bleeding pattern diminishes over time. Concerns have been noted over the lack of safety data on long-term effects, particularly on the return to reproductive function and fertility after discontinuing use.

Contraindications to the use of estrogen-containing OCs include hepatocellular disease, migraine headaches, breast disease, any condition in which hypercoagulability may be a problem (replaced cardiac valve, thrombophlebitis, sickle cell anemia) because of the increased levels of factor VIII and decreased production of antithrombin III, and known or suspected pregnancy (Table 116-3). The risks of pregnancy must be balanced against the benefits of reliable contraception in patients with chronic diseases such as diabetes, epilepsy, and sickle cell disease. The initial history taken before prescribing OCs should specifically address these risks. The World Health Organization ranks multiple medical eligibility criteria for safety with the use of hormonal contraception from 4, precluding use, to 1, conditions raising no concerns, and provides a thorough listing for reference purposes.

MISSED CONTRACEPTIVE PILLS. The effectiveness of OC is dependent on compliance, and unfortunately adolescent women may forget to take a pill each day. The risk of pregnancy may be higher if a 20-µg ethinyl estradiol pill is used compared to a 30–35 µg pill. A pill is considered missed if it is 12 hr late from the designated daily time. If three pills are missed, back up contraception is required and if intercourse has occurred, emergency contraception (EC) is indicated (Fig. 116-3). Rules for missed pills are noted in Table 116-4.

OTHER COMBINATION METHODS. The *transdermal patch* (Evra) releases 20 µg ethinyl estradiol and 150 µg norelgestromin daily and is applied to the lower abdomen, buttocks, or upper body. It is worn continuously for 1 wk and changed weekly for a total of 3 wk, then removed to allow menstrual bleeding (see Table 116-2). It should not be applied to the breast. Limited studies in adolescents suggest higher rates of partial or full detachment compared to adults, with high patient satisfaction and 50–83% continuation rates from 3–18 mo of use.

TABLE 116-3. Summary of Guidelines for the Use of Combination Estrogen-Progestin Oral Contraceptives in Women with Characteristics That Might Increase the Risk of Adverse Effect*

VARIABLE	ACOG GUIDELINES	WHO GUIDELINES
Smoker, >35 yr of age		
<15 cigarettes/day	Risk unacceptable	Risk usually outweighs benefit
≥15 cigarettes/day	Risk unacceptable	Risk unacceptable
Hypertension		
Blood pressure controlled	Risk acceptable; no definition of blood-pressure control	Risk usually outweighs benefit if systolic blood pressure is 140–159 mm Hg and diastolic blood pressure is 90–99 mm Hg
Blood pressure uncontrolled	Risk unacceptable; no definition of uncontrolled blood pressure	Risk unacceptable if systolic blood pressure is ≥160 mm Hg or diastolic blood pressure is ≥100 mm Hg
History of stroke, ischemic heart disease, or venous thromboembolism	Risk unacceptable	Risk unacceptable
Diabetes	Risk acceptable if no other cardiovascular risk factors and no end-organ damage	Benefit outweighs risk if no end-organ damage and diabetes is of ≤20 yr duration
Hypercholesterolemia	Risk acceptable if LDL cholesterol <160 mg/dL and no other cardiovascular risk factors	Benefit-risk ratio is dependent on the presence or absence of other cardiovascular risk factors
Multiple cardiovascular risk factors	Not addressed	Risk usually outweighs benefit or risk unacceptable, depending on risk factors
Migraine headache		
Age ≥35 yr	Risk usually outweighs benefit	Risk usually outweighs benefit
Focal symptoms	Risk unacceptable	Risk unacceptable
Breast cancer		
Current disease	Risk unacceptable	Risk unacceptable
Past disease, no active disease for 5 yr	Risk unacceptable	Risk usually outweighs benefit
Family history of breast or ovarian cancer	Risk acceptable	Risk acceptable

*The American College of Obstetricians and Gynecologists (ACOG) guidelines recommend the use of formulations containing <50 µg ethinyl estradiol with the "lowest progestin dose," without mention of the type of progestin. The World Health Organization (WHO) guidelines pertain explicitly to formulations containing ≤35 µg ethinyl estradiol and do not mention the dose or type of progestin. To convert values for low-density lipoprotein (LDL) cholesterol to millimoles per liter, multiply by 0.02586.

From Petitti DB: Combination estrogen-progestin oral contraceptives. *N Engl J Med* 2003;349:1443–1450. The full statement is available from the Faculty of Family Planning at www.ffprhc.org.uk.

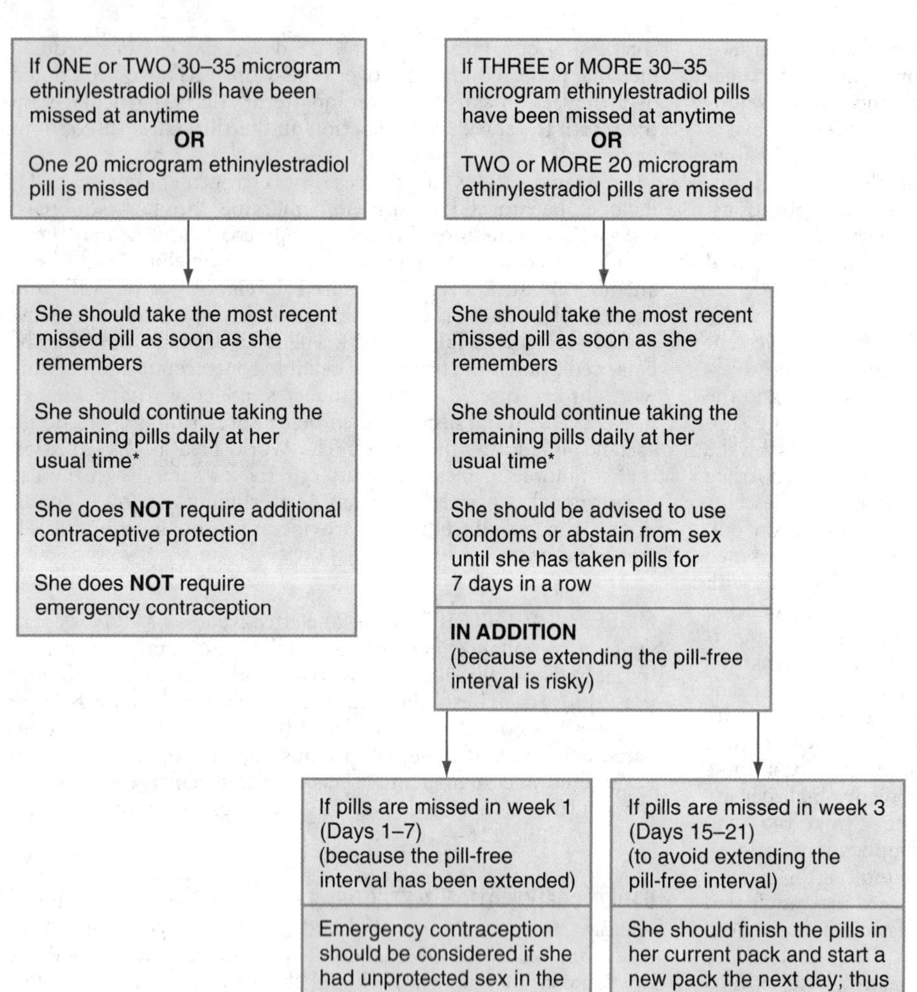

*Depending on when she remembers her missed pill she may take two pills on the same day (one at the moment of remembering and the other at the regular time) or even at the same time.

Figure 116-3. Advice for women missing combined oral contraceptives (30–35 µg and 20 µg ethinyl estradiol formulations). (From Faculty of Family Planning and Reproductive Health Care Effectiveness Unit. FFPRHC Guidance (July 2006) First Prescription of Combined Oral Contraception. The full statement is available at www.ffprhc.org.uk.)

The *vaginal contraceptive ring* (Nuva Ring) is a flexible, transparent, colorless vaginal ring that measures about 2.1 inches in diameter and is inserted into the vagina by the patient. It releases 15 µg ethinyl estradiol and 120 µg etonogestrel per day and remains in place for 3 wk, during which time these hormones are absorbed. If the ring is accidentally expelled, it should be reinserted; however, if it is out of place for more than 3 hr, a backup method of contraception should be used.

All these methods have contraindications similar to those to oral contraceptives (see Table 116-3).

ALL-PROGESTIN CONTRACEPTIVES. Progestin-only contraceptives are available for the adolescent in whom the use of estrogen is potentially deleterious: those with liver disease, replaced cardiac valves, or hypercoagulable states. These agents ("mini-pills") are less reliable in inhibiting ovulation and are associated with a 0.5%/yr pregnancy rate (perfect use). Acceptance by adolescents is limited by the necessity of taking the pill daily, the higher incidence of amenorrhea, and increased bleeding.

An *injectable progestin,* medroxyprogesterone (Depo-Provera, DMPA), is highly effective in birth control in a dose of 150 mg as a deep intramuscular injection, with failure rates typically at 0.3–0.4% (see Table 116-2). DMPA is particularly attractive for adolescents who have difficulty with compliance, mentally retarded teenagers, and teenagers with chronic illnesses who have a relative contraindication to estrogen use. Issues relative to transient of bone density loss while on DMPA are of particular concern during adolescence, the developmental period in which the accumulation of bone density is at its greatest. Depo-Provera carries a "black-box" warning noting significant risk for bone mineral density loss with unknown risk to adolescents of osteoporotic fracture in later life; increased duration of use appears to be associated with greater and possibly irreversible bone loss. DMPA should not be used by teens at risk of osteoporosis, such as those who have chronic renal disease, who are wheelchair bound, or who have eating disorders or chronic amenorrhea (see Chapter 705). It is not recommended for use for >2 yr unless other birth control methods are inadequate. Early studies suggest that estrogen supplementation may offer some protection from bone loss.

TABLE 116-4. Missed Pill Rules

- Whenever a woman realizes that she missed pills, the essential advice is "**just keep going**." She should take a pill as soon as possible and then resume her usual pill-taking schedule.
- **Also,** if the missed pills are in **wk 3**, she should **omit the pill-free interval**.
- **Also,** a back-up method (usually condoms) or abstinence should be used for 7 days if the following numbers of pills are missed:
  Two for 20 (if two or more 20 µg ethinylestradiol pills are missed)
  Three for 30 (if three or more 30–35 µg ethinylestradiol pills are missed)

From Faculty of Family Planning and Reproductive Health Care Clinical Effectiveness Unit: Missed pills: new recommendations, April 2005, available at: *www.ffprhc.org.uk/admin/uploads/MissedPillRules%20.pdf.*

The *long-acting progestational agent* levonorgestrel (Norplant) is not available in the United States. A 3-yr implant with a single rod containing etonogestrel releasing 60µg/day is available in nine European countries and is pending FDA approval in the United States.

116.5 • Emergency Contraception

Unprotected intercourse at mid-cycle carries a pregnancy risk of 20–30%. At any other time during the cycle, the risk drops to 2–4%. The risk may be reduced or eliminated by intervention as soon as possible after unprotected intercourse with a "window" up to 120 hr. Outside the United States, several agents are used for EC: oral high-dose estrogens, high-dose combination estrogen-progestins, high-dose progestins, danazol, mifepristone, and the postcoital insertion of a copper intrauterine device (IUD) (Table 116-5). Strategies are under way to promote more widespread use of EC to reduce unintended pregnancies. One controlled trial in adolescent women demonstrated more effective use of EC with advance provision and was not associated with more frequent unprotected intercourse or less condom or pill use. The **Yuzpe method** is commonly used in the United States, consisting of combination pills totaling 200 µg ethinyl estradiol and 2.0 mg norgestrel or 1.0 mg levonorgestrel. Pills that can be utilized for this method are shown in Table 116-6. The high-dose combination OCs disrupt the luteal phase hormone pattern, creating an unstable and unsuitable uterine lining for implantation. If used mid-cycle, when ovulation is about to occur, the high-dose estrogen and progestin blunt the luteinizing hormone surge and impair ovulation. This method is effective in reducing the risk of pregnancy by 75%. The most common side effect is nausea (50%) and vomiting (20%), prompting some clinicians to prescribe or recommend antiemetics along with the OCs. A urine pregnancy test is usually required prior to dispensing the pills to rule out an existing pregnancy. There is some controversy about the need to do this, since there is no evidence to suggest that OCs used in this manner affect early fetal development and the dose as prescribed would not disrupt a previously undetected pregnancy. The EC kit prepackaged for this method (Preven) was withdrawn from the market in 2004. A progestin-only EC kit was FDA approved in 1999 and contains two tablets, each with 0.75 mg levonorgestrel. Nausea and vomiting are uncommon side effects, and in a recent comparison, levonorgestrel proved more effective at preventing pregnancy. Mifepristone (RU-486) is a highly effective EC method with a nearly 0% failure rate; it functions as an abortifacient and its use is highly controversial. Teens can access EC information through a hotline at 1-888-NOT-2-LATE. A 2-wk follow-up appointment is recommended following any of the methods to determine the effectiveness of treatment and to diagnose a possible early pregnancy. The visit also provides an opportunity to counsel the adolescent, explore the situation leading up to the unprotected intercourse, test for STDs, and initiate continuing contraception when appropriate.

TABLE 116-5. Types of Emergency Contraception

CLASS	DOSE	BRANDS AVAILABLE IN THE UNITED STATES
Combined oral contraceptives	100 µg ethinyl estradiol and 0.5 mg levonorgestrel twice 12 hr apart	Preven (Gynétics) Ovral (Wyeth)*
Progestin-only oral contraceptives	1.5 mg levonorgestrel once or 0.75 mg twice 12 hr apart	Plan B (Women's Capital Corporation)
Copper T intrauterine device	—	ParaGard T 380A (Ortho-McNeil)
Antiprogestins	10 mg mifepristone	None at this dose

*Other hormonal contraceptives that are effective for emergency contraception, along with the doses and instructions for use, are listed at *www.not-2-late.com*.

From Westhoff C: Emergency contraception. *N Engl J Med* 2003;349:1830–1834.

TABLE 116-6. Twenty Oral Contraceptives That Can Be Used for Emergency Contraception in the United States

BRAND	COMPANY	PILLS PER DOSE†	ETHINYL ESTRADIOL PER DOSE (µg)	LEVONORGESTREL PER DOSE (mg)‡
Plan B*	Barr	1 white pill	0	0.75
Ogestrel	Watson	2 white pills	100	0.50
Ovral	Wyeth-Ayerst	2 white pills	100	0.50
Cryselle	Barr	4 white pills	120	0.60
Levora	Watson	4 white pills	120	0.60
Lo/Ovral	Wyeth-Ayerst	4 white pills	120	0.60
Low-Ogestrel	Watson	4 white pills	120	0.60
Levien	Berlex	4 light-orange pills	120	0.60
Nordette	Wyeth-Ayerst	4 light-orange pills	120	0.60
Portia	Barr	4 pink pills	120	0.60
Seasonale	Barr	4 pink pills	120	0.60
Trivora	Watson	4 pink pills	120	0.50
Tri-levlen	Berlex	4 yellow pills	120	0.50
Triphasil	Wyeth-Ayerst	4 yellow pills	120	0.50
Enpresse	Barr	4 orange pills	120	0.50
Alesse	Wyeth-Ayerst	5 pink pills	100	0.50
Lessina	Barr	5 pink pills	100	0.50
Levlite	Berlex	5 pink pills	100	0.50
Aviane	Barr	5 orange pills	100	0.50
Ovrette	Wyeth-Ayerst	20 yellow pills	0	0.75

*Plan B is the only dedicated product specifically marketed for emergency contraception. Alesse, Aviane, Cryselle, Enpresse, Lessina, Levlen, Levlite, Levora, Lo/Ovral, Low-Ogestrel, Nordette, Ogestrel, Ovral, Portia, Seasonale, Tri-levlen, Triphasil, and Trivora have been declared safe and effective for use as emergency contraceptive products by the U.S. Food and Drug Administration. Outside the United States, >20 emergency contraceptive products are specifically packaged, labeled, and marketed. For example, Gedeon Richter and HRA Pharma are marketing in many countries the levonorgestrel-only products Postinor-2 and Norlevo, respectively, each consisting of a two-pill strip with each pill containing 0.75 mg levonorgestrel. Norlevo became available over the counter without a prescription in Norway in October 2000 and in Sweden in late 2001.

†The treatment schedule is one dose within 120 hr after unprotected intercourse, and another dose ~12 hr later. However, recent research has found that both doses of Plan-B can be taken at the same time.

‡The progestin in Cryselle, Lo/Ovral, Low-Ogestrel, Ogestrel, Ovral, and Ovrette is norgestrel, which contains two isomers, only one of which (levonorgestrel) is bioactive; the amount of norgestrel in each tablet is twice the amount of levonorgestrel.

116.6 • Intrauterine Devices

IUDs are small, flexible, plastic objects introduced into the uterine cavity through the cervix. They differ in size, shape, and the presence or absence of pharmacologically active substances (copper or progesterone). The mechanism of action of IUDs is uncertain, although they render the endometrium unsuitable for implantation by inducing a local polymorphonuclear leukocyte response, production of prostaglandins E_2 and F_2, and stimulation of uterine contractility. They are effective in preventing pregnancy in 97–99% of women. Young patients and those with multiple sexual partners are at increased risk of infection, and the prescription of an IUD to teenagers who require passive contraception should be limited to the method of last resort.

Abma JC, Martinez GM, Mosher WD, et al: Teenagers in the United States: Sexual activity, contraceptive use, and childbearing. *Vital Health Stat 23* 2004;24:1–48.

American Academy of Pediatrics Committee on Adolescence: Emergency contraception. *Pediatrics* 2005;116:1026–1035.

Anderson J, Santelli J, Morrow B: Trends in adolescent contraceptive use, unprotected and poorly protected sex 1991–2003. *J Adol Health* 2006;38:734–739.

As-sanie S, Gantt A, Rosenthal MS: Pregnancy prevention in adolescents. *Am Fam Physician* 2004;70:1517–1524.

Bissell P, Anderson C: Enhanced access to emergency contraception. *Lancet* 2005;365:1668–1670.

Borenstein J, Yu H, Wade S, et al: Effect of an oral contraceptive containing ethinyl estradiol and drospirenone on premenstrual symptomatology and health-related quality of life. *J Reprod Med* 2003;48:79–85.

Cromer BA, Lazebnik R, Romer E, et al: Double-blinded randomized controlled trial of estrogen supplementation in adolescent girls who receive depot medroxyprogesterone acetate for contraception. *Am J Obstet Gynecol* 2005;92:42–47.

Darroch JE, Singh SS, Frost JJ, et al: Differences in teenage pregnancy rates among five developed countries: The roles of sexual activity and contraceptive use. *Fam Plann Perspect* 2001;33:244–250.

Department of Reproductive Health and Research (RHR), World Health Organization: What can a woman do if she missed combined oral contraceptives (COCs)?, available at: *www.who.int/reproductive-health/ publications/spr/spr_q17_missed_cocs.html.*

Faculty of Family Planning and Reproductive Health Care Clinical Effectiveness Unit: Missed pills: New recommendation, April 2005, available at: *www.ffprhc.org.uk/admin/uploads/MissedPillRules%20.pdf.*

FDA Talk Paper. Black box warning added concerning long-term use of Depo-Provera contraceptive injection, November 17, 2004, available at: *www.fda.gov/bbs/topics/ANSWERS/2004/ANS01325.html.*

Gold MA, Wolford JE, Smith KA, Parker AM: The effects of advance provision of emergency contraception on adolescent women's sexual and contraceptive behaviors. *J Pediatr Adolesc Gynecol* 2004;7:87–96.

Greydanus DE, Rimsza ME, Matytsina L: Contraception for college students. *Pediatr Clin North Am* 2005;52:135–161.

Grunbaum JA, Kann L, Kinchen S, et al: Youth risk behavior surveillance—United States 2003. *MMWR* 2004;53:1–13.

Mansour D, Fraser IS: Missed contraceptive pills and the critical pill-free interval. *Lancet* 2005;365:1670–1671.

Medical Letter. Emergency contraception OTC. *Med Lett Drugs Ther* 2004;46:10–11.

Peterson HB, Curtis KM: Long-acting methods of contraception. *N Engl J Med* 2005;353:2169–2175.

Petitti DB: Combination estrogen-progestin oral contraceptives. *N Engl J Med* 2003;349:1443–1450.

Scholes D, LaCroix AZ, Ichikawa LE, et al: Change in bone mineral density among adolescent women using and discontinuing depot medroxyprogesterone acetate contraception. *Arch Pediatr Adolesc* 2005;159:139–144.

Tripp J, Viner R: Sexual health, contraception, and teenage pregnancy. *Br Med J* 2005;330:590–593.

Wall LL, Brown D: Refusals by pharmacists to dispense emergency centraception: a critique. *Obstet Gynecol* 2006;107:1148–1151.

Westhoff C: Emergency contraception. *N Engl J Med* 2003;349:1830–1834.

Winer RL, Hughes JP, Feng Q, et al: Condom use and the risk of genital human papillomavirus infection in young women. *N Engl J Med* 2006; 354:2645–2654.

World Health Organization: Medical Eligibility for Contraceptive Use, third edition—2004, available at: *www.who.int/reproductive-health/publications/MEC_3/* (accessed April 23, 2005).

Chapter 117 ■ Adolescent Pregnancy

Dianne S. Elfenbein, Marianne E. Felice, and Renée R. Jenkins

EPIDEMIOLOGY. Annually approximately 13 million infants are born to adolescents worldwide. The annual number of live births per 1000 girls aged 15–19 yr is estimated at 50 per 1000 worldwide for the period 2000–2005, with the highest rate in Sub-Saharan Africa at 127 per 1000. It is 71 in Latin America and the Caribbean and 18 in East Asia and the Pacific.

The United States has the highest teen birth rate (41.2 births per 1000 teens in 2004) among all industrialized countries. U.S. teen birth rates are double the rate in Great Britain and Canada and nearly four times the rates in France and Sweden. Two thirds of teen births are to 18–19 yr old women who technically have reached the age of majority.

Adolescent birth rates in the United States have steadily decreased since the early 1990s for all ages, races, and ethnic groups (Table 117-1), but the decrease is most dramatic for African-American teens and for young women aged 15–17 yr. The 2004 birth rate for teens ages 15–19 yr is 33% lower than the 1991 rate of 61.8 and the birth rate for teens aged 15–17 yr at 22.4 is 42% lower than the 1991 rate. From 1991 to 2003, the birth rates for non-Hispanic black teens decreased 45%; for non-Hispanic white teens, 35%; and for Hispanic teens, 22%. Pregnancy rates, which include births, miscarriages, stillbirths, and induced abortions, have also decreased, indicating that the decline in birth rates is not due to an increase in pregnancy terminations.

The improvement in U.S. teen birth rates is attributed to three factors: more teens are delaying the onset of sexual intercourse, more teens are using some form of contraception when they do begin to have sexual intercourse, and there is increased use of the new, long-lasting hormonal contraceptives. In 2002, 46% of both adolescent males and females reported sexual experiences. In 2002, 75% of high school females and 82% of high school males indicated that they had used some form of contraception at the time of their most recent sexual experience.

ETIOLOGY. Adolescents who become pregnant are affected by multiple factors ranging from policy and environmental influences to family and individual factors. In industrialized countries with policies supporting access to protection against pregnancy and sexually transmitted infections (STIs), adolescents are more likely to use hormonal contraceptives and condoms, resulting in lower adolescent birth rates. Young teenagers are likely to be less deliberate and logical about their sexual decisions and their sexual activity is likely to be sporadic and coercive, factors contributing to inconsistent contraceptive use and a greater risk of pregnancy. Better hopes for employment as well as other lifestyle benefits are associated with lowered probability of childbearing. In nonindustrialized countries, laws permitting marriage of young and mid-adolescents, poverty, and limited female education are associated with increased adolescent pregnancy rates.

CLINICAL MANIFESTATIONS. Adolescents may experience the traditional symptoms of pregnancy: morning sickness (vomiting, nausea that may also occur any time of the day), swollen tender breasts, weight gain, and amenorrhea. Often the presentation is more vague. Headache, fatigue, abdominal pain, and scanty or irregular menses are common presenting symptoms.

Denial of sexual activity and menstrual irregularity should not preclude the diagnosis in face of other clinical or historical information. An unanticipated request for a complete check-up or a visit for contraception may uncover a suspected pregnancy. Pregnancy is still the most common diagnosis when an adolescent presents with **secondary amenorrhea.**

TABLE 117-1. Teen Birth Rates (Births per 1000 Females) in the U.S.A.

AGE	1940	1950	1960	1970	1980	1990	2000	2001	2002	2003	2004
15–19	54.1	81.6	89.1	68.3	53.0	59.9	47.7	45.9	43.0	41.7	41.2
15–17	—	—	43.9	38.8	32.5	37.5	26.9	25.3	23.2	22.4	22.1
18–19	—	—	166.7	114.7	82.1	88.6	78.1	75.8	72.8	70.8	70.8

Adapted from *Facts at a Glance*. Washington, DC, Child Trends, Inc., 2005.

TABLE 117-2. Diagnosis of Pregnancy Dated from First Day of Last Menstrual Cycle

CLASSIC SYMPTOMS
Missed menses, breast tenderness, nipple sensitivity, nausea, vomiting, fatigue, abdominal and back pain, weight gain, urinary frequency
Note: Teens may present with unrelated symptoms that enable them to visit the doctor and maintain confidentiality.
LABORATORY DIAGNOSIS
Tests for human chorionic gonadotropin in urine or blood may be positive 7–10 days after fertilization, depending on sensitivity.
Note: Irregular menses make ovulation/fertilization difficult to predict. Home pregnancy tests have a high error rate.
PHYSICAL CHANGES
2–3 wk after implantation: cervical softening and cyanosis
8 wk: uterus size of orange
12 wk: uterus size of grapefruit and palpable suprapubically
20 wk: uterus at umbilicus
Note: If physical findings are not consistent with dates, pelvic ultrasound will confirm.

DIAGNOSIS (TABLE 117-2). On physical examination, the findings of an enlarged uterus, cervical cyanosis (Chadwick sign), a soft uterus (Hegar sign), or a soft cervix (Goodell sign) are highly suggestive of an intrauterine pregnancy. A confirmatory pregnancy test is always recommended. The most commonly used method is a qualitative measurement of the ß subunit for human chorionic gonadotropin (hCG) by blood or urine. The results are positive in 98% of women within 7 days after implantation. The most sensitive test is a quantitative ß-hCG radioimmunoassay, in which results are reliable within 7 days after fertilization. This test is more expensive and less likely to be used under routine circumstances. Evaluations for a possible ectopic pregnancy, a retained placenta following an abortion, or a molar pregnancy are additional indications to measure ß-hCG levels. Urine pregnancy tests are the enzyme-linked immunosorbent assay type using highly specific monoclonal antibodies to ß-hCG. These tests may be positive as early as 3–4 days after implantation. One health department study reported 28% of adolescents requesting a pregnancy test had already performed home pregnancy tests prior to the visit. These tests are most often of lower sensitivity and specificity than tests used in the office and should be repeated with more reliable tests before proceeding with clinical management.

PREGNANCY COUNSELING. After the diagnosis of pregnancy is made, it is important to begin addressing the psychosocial aspects of the pregnancy. The patient's response to the pregnancy should be assessed and her emotional issues addressed. It should not be assumed that the pregnancy was unintended. Discussion of the patient's options should be initiated. These options may include releasing the child to an adoptive family, electively terminating the pregnancy, or raising the child herself with the help of family, father, friends, and other social resources. Options should be presented in a supportive, informative, nonjudgmental fashion; they may need to be discussed over several visits for some young women. Other issues that may need discussion are: informing and involving the patient's parents and the father of the infant; implementing strategies for insuring continuation of the young mother's education; discontinuation of tobacco, alcohol, and illicit drug use; starting folic acid, calcium, and iron supplements; proper nutrition; testing for STIs; discontinuance and avoidance of any medications that may be considered teratogenic. Especially in younger adolescents, the possibility of coercive sex should be considered and appropriate social/legal referrals made if abuse has occurred. Patients who are electing to continue their pregnancies should be referred as soon as possible to an adolescent-friendly obstetric provider.

CHARACTERISTICS OF TEEN PARENTS. Young women who become parents as teenagers tend to come from economically disadvantaged groups. Although the birth rates among black and Hispanic teens have decreased in the past decade, their rates are more than double those for non-Hispanic whites. Parenting teens frequently have poor school performance prior to becoming pregnant, and their families have low educational attainment. They frequently come from single-parent families where one or both parents became parents as teenagers. They may view pregnancy as having a positive social value and as not interfering with their long-term goals.

Teenaged men who become fathers as adolescents also have poorer educational achievement than their age-matched peers. They are more likely than peers to have been involved with illegal activities and with the use of illegal substances. Adult men who father the children of teen mothers are poorer and educationally less advanced than their age-matched peers and tend to be 2–3 yr older than the mother; any combination of age differences may exist. Younger teen mothers are more likely to have a greater age difference between themselves and the father of their child, raising the issue of coercive sex or statutory rape (see Chapter 118).

MEDICAL COMPLICATIONS OF MOTHERS AND BABIES. Although pregnant teens are at higher than average risk of complications of pregnancy, most teenagers have pregnancies that are without major medical complications, delivering healthy infants. In 2000, approximately 56% of teen pregnancies resulted in live births, about 28% were terminated as an induced abortion, and 15% ended in miscarriage or stillbirth. As expected, teen mothers have low rates of age-related chronic disease (diabetes) that might affect the outcomes of a pregnancy. They also have lower rates of twin pregnancies than older women. They tolerate childbirth well with few operative interventions. However, as compared with 20–39 yr old mothers, teens have higher incidences of very low birthweight infants, very preterm infants, neonatal deaths, and infant deaths within 1 yr after birth. The highest rate of poor outcomes occurs in the youngest mothers; in the United States from 2000–2002, the rates of preterm, low birthweight, and very low birthweight deliveries were twofold higher in mothers ages 10–14 yr as compared with all other mothers, and the rate of very preterm (<32 wk of gestation) infants was threefold higher for the youngest mothers. Teen mothers also have higher rates of anemia, pregnancy-associated hypertension, and eclampsia, with the youngest teens having rates of pregnancy-associated hypertension 40% higher than the rates of women in their 20s and 30s. Many, but especially the youngest, teens have poor weight gain (<16 lb per pregnancy). This correlates with a decrease in the birthweight of their children. Poor maternal weight gain also correlates strongly with teens' late entrance into prenatal care and with inadequate utilization of prenatal care. In addition, sexually active teens have higher rates of STIs than older sexually active women.

Teenage women have the highest rates of **violence** during pregnancy of any group. Violence is associated with injuries and death as well as preterm births, low birthweight, bleeding, substance abuse, and late entrance into prenatal care. An analysis of the Pregnancy Mortality Surveillance System indicates that from 1991 to 1999, homicide was the second leading cause of injury-related deaths in pregnant and postpartum women. Women ages 19 yr and younger had the highest pregnancy-related homicide rate (see Chapter 112).

Prematurity and low birthweight increase the perinatal morbidity and mortality for infants of teen mothers. These infants also have higher than average rates of sudden infant death syndrome, possibly because of less use of the supine sleep position, and are at higher risk of both intentional and unintentional injury (see Chapter 36). One study shows the risk of homicide to be 9 to 10 times higher if a child born to a teen mother is not the mother's firstborn as compared with the risk to a firstborn of a woman age 25 yr or older. The perpetrator is often a father, stepfather, or boyfriend of the mother.

After child birth, **depressive symptoms** may occur in 40–50% of teenaged mothers. Depression seems to be greater with additional social stressors and with decreased social supports. Support from the infant's father and the teen's mother seem to be especially important in preventing depression. Pediatricians who care for parenting teens should be sensitive to the possibility of depression as well as to inflicted injury to mother or child; appropriate diagnosis, treatment, and referral to mental health or social agencies should be offered.

PSYCHOSOCIAL OUTCOMES/RISKS FOR MOTHER AND CHILD

EDUCATIONAL. Teenage mothers often quit school prior to becoming pregnant or defer completion of their education for some time after the birth of their child. High school graduation or an equivalency degree is generally achieved eventually. Mothers who have given birth as teens generally remain 2 yr behind their age-matched peers in formal educational attainment at least through their 3rd decade. Lack of education limits the income of these young families (see Chapter 1).

SUBSTANCE USE. Most substance-abusing mothers appear to decrease their substance use while pregnant. However, use begins to increase again about 6 mo postpartum, complicating the parenting process and the mother's return to school.

REPEAT PREGNANCY. Approximately 30% of teen mothers become pregnant within 2 yr of their infant's birth, with about 50% of these pregnancies resulting in the birth of an infant. Prenatal care is begun even later with a second pregnancy, and the second infant is at increased risk of prematurity, early death, and homicide. Mothers at risk of repeat pregnancy include those who do not return to school within 6 mo of the index birth, those who are married or living with their infant's father, or those who receive so much child care assistance from the adolescent mother's mother that the teen is left with too little involvement in the child's care.

BEHAVIORAL, EDUCATIONAL, AND SOCIAL OUTCOMES OF INFANTS. Existing long-term follow-up studies involving infants of teen mothers suggest that many infants born to teen mothers have behavioral problems seen as early as the preschool period. Many drop out of school early (33%), become adolescent parents (25%), or, if male, are incarcerated (16%). Explanations for these poor outcomes include poverty, maternal and paternal learning difficulties, negative parenting styles in teen parents, maternal depression, parental immaturity, and conflicts with grandparents, especially grandmothers. Continued positive paternal involvement may be somewhat protective against negative outcomes. Comprehensive programs focused on supporting adolescent mothers and infants utilizing life skills training, medical care, and psychosocial support demonstrate higher employment rates, higher income, and less welfare dependency in adolescents exposed to the programs.

PREVENTION OF TEEN PREGNANCIES (TABLE 117-3). Adolescent pregnancy is a multifaceted problem that requires multifactorial solutions. The provision of contraception and education about fertility risk from the primary care physician is important, but insufficient to address the problem. Family and community involvement are also needed. Strategies for primary prevention (preventing first births) are different from the strategies needed for secondary prevention (preventing second or more births).

Since the late 1990s, there has been an emphasis on abstinence-only sexual education with large amounts of federal funding allocated to programs that teach youngsters to wait until marriage to initiate sexual activity and do not mention contraception. Abstinence education is sometimes coupled with "virginity pledges" in which teenagers pledge to remain abstinent until they marry. Other educational programs emphasize HIV and STI prevention and in the process prevent pregnancy, and others include both abstinence and contraception in their curricula. In many communities, programs that engage youths in community service and/or combine sex education and youth development are also successful in deterring pregnancy. Programs vary in their sites of service from schools, to social agencies, to health clinics, to youth organizations, to churches. Other countries have taken different approaches. In Sweden, family and sex education has been taught in schools since the 1950s and since 1975, abortion has been free on demand. Contraceptive counseling is free and readily available at family planning and youth health clinics along with STI screening.

Secondary prevention programs are fewer in number. In the United States, some communities have tried to "pay" young mothers to not become pregnant again, but these efforts have not been fruitful. Home visiting by nurses has been tried in several areas, and many communities have developed "Teen Tot" Clinics that provide a "one-stop shopping model" for health care for both the teen mother and the baby in the same site at the same time.

In the practice setting, the identification of the sexually active adolescent through a confidential clinical interview is a first step in pregnancy prevention. The primary care physician should provide the teenager with factual information in a nonjudgmental manner and then guide him or her in the decision-making process of choosing a contraceptive. In addition, the practice setting is an ideal setting to support the teenager who chooses to remain abstinent.

TABLE 117-3. Effective Strategies to Reduce Teen Pregnancy

1. There is no one prevention program that will work in all communities for all teenagers.
2. Little information is available on the impact of programs that stress abstinence as the only acceptable behavior for unmarried teens. However, adolescents who take virginity pledges may delay sexual activity for some time, but when they do engage in sexual activity, they are more likely to have unprotected intercourse than those who never pledged virginity.
3. Some sex and HIV education programs have produced credible evidence that they reduce sexual risk taking either by delaying the onset of sexual activity, reducing the frequency of sex, reducing the number of sexual partners, or by increasing the use of condoms or other forms of contraception. Such programs do not accelerate the onset or increase sexual activity.
4. School-based and school-linked clinics do not increase sexual activity, but it is not clear whether they increase condom or contraceptive use.
5. All successful secondary prevention programs find ways to maintain close relationships with the teen mother and her baby after the birth, and most programs emphasize contraception and school completion.

Alan Guttmacher Institute: Teen pregnancy: Trends and lessons learned. *Issues in Brief.* 2002; Series No. 1.

Chang J, Berg CJ, Saltzman LE, et al: Homicide: A leading cause of injury deaths among pregnant and postpartum women in the United States, 1991–1999. *Am J Public Health* 2005;95:471–477.

Child Trends: *Facts at a Glance 2003: Annual Newsletter on Teen Pregnancy.* Washington, DC, Child Trends, 2003.

Committee on Adolescence and Committee on Early Childhood, Adoption, and Dependent Care, American Academy of Pediatrics, 2000–2001: Care of Adolescent Parents and Their Children. *Pediatrics* 2001;107:429–434.

Edgardh K: Adolescent sexual health in Sweden. *Sex Transm Infect* 2002;78:352–356.

Elan-Evans LD, Strauss LT, Herndon J, et al: Abortion Surveillance U.S. 2000. *MMWR* 2003;52(SS12):1–32.

Elfenbein DS, Felice M: Adolescent Pregnancy. *Pediatr Clin North Am* 2003;50:781–800.

Klerman LV: Risk of poor pregnancy outcomes; is it higher among multiparous teenage mothers? *J Adol Health* 2006;38:761–764.

Menacker F, Martin JA, MacDorman MF, Ventura SJ: *Births to 10–14 Year Old Mothers, 1990–2002: Trends and Health Outcomes. National Vital Statistics Reports*, vol. 53, no. 7. Hyattsville, MD, National Center for Health Statistics, 2004.

National Campaign to Prevent Teen Pregnancy: Available at: *www.teenpregnancy.org*.

Nicoletti AM: Teen pregnancy. In Emans SJ, Laufer MR, Goldstein DP (editors): *Pediatric and Adolescent Gynecology*, 5th ed. Philadelphia, Lippincott Williams & Wilkins, 2005, pp 844–878.

Chapter 118 ■ Adolescent Rape

Christine Barron and Marianne Felice

Rape is coercive sexual intercourse involving physical force or psychologic manipulation of a female or a male. Rape is defined as penetration of any genital, oral, or anal orifice by a part of the assailant's body or any object. Rape is an act of violence, not an act of sex.

EPIDEMIOLOGY. Exact figures on the incidence of rape are unavailable because many rapes are not reported. In the United States, the annual rates of sexual victimization per 1000 persons were reported in 2004 by the U.S. Department of Justice, National Crime Victimization Survey to be 1.2 for ages 12–15 yr, 1.3 for ages 16–19 yr, and 1.7 for ages 20–24 yr. Rape occurs worldwide and is especially prevalent in war. An estimated one fourth to one half million adolescent and older women were raped during the 1994 conflict in Rwanda. During the Balkan conflict, with teenage girls particularly targeted, at least 20,000 girls and women were raped. In East Timor, 23% of adolescent and adult women reported being sexually assaulted during the 1999 armed conflict, declining to 10% during the postcrisis period.

Females exceed males as rape victims by nearly 10:1, but male rape may be more underreported than female rape. Female adolescents and young adults account for the highest rates of rape compared to any other age group. The normal developmental growth tasks of adolescence may contribute to this vulnerability in the following ways: (1) the emergence of independence from parents and the establishment of relationships outside the family may expose adolescents to environments with which they are unfamiliar and situations that they are unprepared to handle; (2) dating and becoming comfortable with one's sexuality may result in activities that are unwanted, but the adolescent is too inexperienced to stop the unwanted actions; and (3) young adolescents may be naïve and more trusting than they should be. Many teens are computer competent and very familiar with the World Wide Web. One of the most concerning negative features of the Internet is the ability of sexual perpetrators to have a communication conduit to unsuspecting vulnerable populations, such as teens, who were previously beyond their reach. Chat rooms represent a major risk for adolescents resulting in correspondence with individuals unknown to them or protective family members, while simultaneously providing a false sense of security due to remote electronic communications. A determined perpetrator can obtain specific information to identify the adolescent and arrange for a meeting that is primed for sexual victimization.

Some adolescents are at higher risk of being victims of rape than others (Table 118-1).

TABLE 118-1. Adolescents at High Risk of Rape Victimization

MALE AND FEMALE ADOLESCENTS
Drug and alcohol use
Runaways
Mental retardation or developmental delay
Street youths
Youths with a parental history of sexual abuse
PRIMARILY FEMALES
Survivors of prior sexual assault
Newcomers to a town or college
PRIMARILY MALES
Institutionalized settings (jail)
Young male homosexuals

TYPES OF RAPE

Acquaintance rape (by a person known to the victim) is the most common form of rape for victims between 16 and 24 yr of age. The acquaintance may be a neighbor, classmate, or friend of the family. The victim-assailant relationship may cause conflicting loyalties in families, and the teen's report may be received with disbelief and/or skepticism by her family. Adolescent acquaintance rape differs from adult acquaintance rape as weapons are less often used, and thus the victims are less likely to sustain physical injuries. Victims of acquaintance rape are also more likely to delay seeking medical care, may never report the crime (males greater than females), and are less likely to proceed with criminal prosecution even after reporting the incident(s).

Date rape (by a person dating the victim) is often drug facilitated and is prevalent in adolescent populations. Date rape drugs are pharmaceuticals administered in a clandestine manner to potential victims. Gamma-hydroxybutyric acid (GHB), flunitrazepam (Rohypnol), and ketamine hydrochloride are the leading agents used for these illegal purposes (see Chapter 113). The pharmacologic properties of these drugs make them suitable for this use as they have simple modes of administration, are easily concealed (colorless, odorless, tasteless), have rapid onsets of action with resulting induction of anterograde amnesia, and have rapid eliminations due to a short half-life. Detection of these drugs requires a high index of suspicion and medical evaluation within 8–12 hr, prompting specific testing because routine toxicology screening is insufficient.

Date rape victims are often new to a specific environment (college freshman, newcomer to a town) and lack strong social support. Victims may not be assertive in establishing boundaries or limits with their dates and may be intoxicated when the incident takes place. The date rape assailant may engage in more sexual activities than other men his age and often has a history of aggressive behavior toward women. He may interpret passivity as assent and deny the charge of coercion or force; he may also be intoxicated at the time of the assault.

A date rape victim often experiences long-term issues of trust, self-blame, and guilt. She may lose confidence in her judgment concerning men in the future. She is nearly always ashamed of the incident and is less likely to report the rape. She is reluctant to talk about the rape to family, friends, or a counselor and, hence, may never heal from the psychologic scars that ensue.

Male rape generally refers to same-sex rape of male teens by other males. Specific subgroups of young men are at high risk of being victims of rape (see Table 118-1). Male rape is most prevalent within institutional settings. Male rape outside institutions typically involves coercion of the male teen by someone considered an authority figure. Male rape victims often experience conflicted sexual identity whether or not they are homosexual. Issues of loss of control and powerlessness are particularly bothersome for male rape victims, and it is not uncommon for these young men to have symptoms of anxiety, depression, sleep disturbance, and suicidal ideation. Males are less likely than females to report rape and less likely to seek professional help.

Gang rape usually occurs when a group of young men rape a solitary female victim. This type of rape may be part of a ritualistic activity or rite of passage for some male group (gangs, college fraternity) or be displaced rage on the part of the assailants.

Female victims of gang rape may find it difficult to return to the environment in which the rape occurred for fear of confrontation with the assailants (college setting or place of employment) and may insist on moving away from the locale entirely.

Statutory rape refers to sexual activity between an adult and an adolescent under the age of legal consent, as defined by individual state law. Statutory rape laws are based on the premise that below a certain age, an individual is not legally capable of giving consent to engage in sexual intercourse. In some states in the United States, statutory rape laws apply to sexual contact or intercourse occurring between a minor and another individual with a specific age difference even when both are minors and both assert that the sexual act was voluntary (a 17 yr old male who has sexual intercourse with a 13 yr old female). The intent of such laws is to protect youths from being victimized, but they may inadvertently lead some teenagers to withhold pertinent sexual information from a clinician for fear that their sexual partner will be reported to the law. Clinicians must be familiar with the laws of the nation and/or state/province.

Stranger rape occurs less frequently within the adolescent population and is most similar to adult rape. Such rapes frequently occur with an abduction, use of weapons, and increased risk of physical injuries. These rapes are more likely to be reported and prosecuted.

CLINICAL MANIFESTATIONS. The adolescent's acute presentation following a rape may vary considerably, from histrionics to near-mute withdrawal. Even if they do not seem to be afraid, most victims are extremely fearful and very anxious about the rape examination, the rape report, and the entire process. Since adolescents are between the developmental lines of childhood and adulthood their responses to rape may have elements of both child and adult behaviors. Many teens, particularly young adolescents, may experience some level of cognitive disorganization.

Adolescents may be reluctant to report rape for a variety of reasons, including self-blame, fear, embarrassment, or in the circumstances of drug-facilitated rape, uncertainty of event details. Adolescent victims, unlike child victims who elicit sympathy and support, are often faced with intense scrutiny regarding their credibility and inappropriately misplaced societal blame for the assault. This view is baseless and should not be used during an evaluation of any teenage victim, including acquaintance rape.

When adolescents do not report a rape, they may present at a future date with symptoms of post-traumatic stress disorder, such as sleep disturbances, nightmares, mood swings, and flashbacks. Other teens may present with psychosomatic complaints or difficulties with schoolwork; all adolescents should be screened for the possibility of sexual abuse at nearly all health examination visits.

INTERVIEW AND PHYSICAL EXAMINATION. Although many teens delay seeking medical care, others present to a medical facility within 72 hr of the rape at which time forensic evidence collection should be completed. Experienced clinicians with training and knowledge of forensic evidence collection and medical-legal procedures should complete the rape evaluation or supervise the evaluation when possible.

The clinician's responsibilities are to provide support, to obtain the history in a nonjudgmental manner, to conduct a complete examination without re-traumatizing the victim, and to collect forensic evidence. The clinician must complete laboratory testing, administer prophylaxis treatment for STIs and emergency contraception, arrange for counseling services, and file a report to appropriate authorities. It is not the clinician's responsibility to decide whether a rape has occurred; the legal system will do so.

After obtaining a concise history including details of the physical contact that occurred between the victim and the assailant, the clinician should conduct a thorough and complete physical examination and document all injuries. Clinicians should provide sensitive, nonjudgmental support during the entire evaluation, as the adolescent victim has experienced a major trauma and is susceptible to retraumatization during this process. Each component of the evaluation should be explained in detail to the victim, allowing the adolescent as much control as possible, including refusal to complete any part or all of the forensic evidence collection process. It is often useful to permit a trusted supportive person, such as a family member, friend or rape crisis advocate, to be present during the evaluation if that is the adolescent's wish.

The examining clinician should be familiar with the **forensic evidence collection** kit (which is state specific) prior to initiating the examination. In the United States, each state's forensic evidence kit is different, but most include some or all of the following components: forensic evidence of semen deposits detected by a fluorescent lamp with a wavelength near 490 nm (many Woods lamps are inadequate), swabs of bite mark impressions to collect genetic markers (DNA, ABO group), and documentation of acute cutaneous injuries utilizing body diagram charts and/or photographs with visible standard measurements. Areas of restraint should be carefully inspected for injuries; these areas include extremities, neck, and the inner aspect of the oral mucosa where a dentition impression may be seen.

The genital examination of a female rape victim should be undertaken with the patient in the lithotomy position. The genital examination of a male rape victim should be undertaken with the patient in supine position. The clinician's examination should include careful inspection of the entire pelvic, genital, and perianal areas. The clinician should document any acute injuries such as edema, erythema, petechiae, hemorrhage, or tearing. Aqueous solution of toluidine blue (1%), which adheres to nucleated cells, may be used during the acute examination to improve visualization of microtrauma in the perianal area. Additionally, a colposcope may be used to provide photodocumentation of injuries.

LABORATORY DATA. The forensic evidence kit should be completed when clinically indicated and if the patient is evaluated within 72 hr of sexual assault. Additional laboratory studies required during initial evaluation are noted in Table 118-2. Follow-up evaluations should be scheduled to repeat these laboratory studies.

TREATMENT. Medical treatment includes prophylaxis treatment for STIs (see Chapter 119) and emergency contraception. The Centers for Disease Control and Prevention estimates that the risk for acquiring STIs following a sexual assault in adults is 6–12% for *Neisseria gonorrhoeae*, 4–17% for *Chlamydia trachomatis*,

TABLE 118-2. Laboratory Data for Evaluation of Rape Victims

WITHIN 8–12 HR
Urine and blood for date rape drugs (GHB, Rohypnol, and ketamine)
WITHIN 72 HR
Forensic evidence kit
Urinalysis
Pregnancy test
Hepatitis B screen
Syphilis (RPR, VDRL)
Herpes simplex virus titers (I & II)
HIV
Wet mount for the detection of spermatozoa, *Trichomonas vaginalis*, and bacterial vaginosis
Cultures obtained based on history of physical contact for
Oropharynx: *Neisseria gonorrhea*
Rectal: *N. gonorrhea* and *Chlamydia*
Urethral (male): *N. gonorrhea* and *Chlamydia*
Endocervical (female): *N. gonorrhea* and *Chlamydia*

GHB, gamma-hydroxybutyric acid; RPR, rapid plasma reagin; VDRL, Venereal Disease Research Laboratory.

TABLE 118-3. Prophylaxis Treatment for Rape Victims

Neisseria gonorrhoeae	Ciprofloxacin 500 mg PO × 1 dose or Ceftriaxone 125 mg IM × 1 dose
Chlamydia trachomatis	Azithromycin 1 g PO × 1 dose
Trichomonas vaginalis and bacterial vaginosis	Metronidazole 2 g PO × 1 dose
*HIV**	Combivir 1 tab PO bid × 28 days
Emergency contraception[†]	Ovral 2 tabs (0.05 mg ethinyl estradiol, 0.50 mg norgestrel) and second dose in 12 hr Plan B 1 tab (0.75 mg levonorgestrel) and second dose in 12 hr

*HIV postexposure Prophylaxis is provided for patients with penetration and the assailant is known to be HIV positive or at high risk due to a history of incarceration, intravenous drug use, or multiple sexual partners. If provided, follow-up must be arranged.

[†]Provided for patients with negative urine pregnancy screen. In addition, provide antiemetic (Compazine, Zofran) for patients receiving emergency contraception medication other than Plan B.

and 0.5–3.0% for syphilis. Antimicrobial prophylaxis is recommended for adolescent rape victims due to the risk of acquiring an STI and the risk of pelvic inflammatory disease (Table 118-3).

At the time of presentation, the clinician should address the need for follow-up care including psychologic counseling. Adolescent victims are at increased risk of post-traumatic stress disorder, depression, self-abusive behaviors, suicidal ideation, delinquency, substance abuse, eating disorders, and sexual revictimization. It is important for the adolescent victim and parents to understand the value of timely counseling services to decrease these potential long-term sequelae. Counseling services should be arranged during the initial evaluation, with follow-up arranged with the primary care physician to improve compliance. Counseling services for family members of the victim may improve their ability to provide appropriate support to the adolescent victim. Caution parents not to use the assault as a validation of their parental guidance, as it will only serve to place blame inappropriately on the adolescent victim.

PREVENTION. **Primary prevention** may be accomplished through education of preadolescents and adolescents on the issues of rape, healthy relationships, Internet dangers, and drug-facilitated rape. Prevention messages should be targeted to both males and females. High-risk situations that may increase the likelihood of a sexual assault (use of drugs or alcohol) should be discouraged. **Secondary prevention** includes informing adolescents of the benefits of timely medical evaluations when rape has occurred. Individual clinicians should ask adolescents about past experiences of forced and unwanted sexual behaviors and offer help in dealing with those experiences. The importance of prevention cannot be overstated since adolescents are disproportionately affected by rape and they are particularly vulnerable to long-term consequences.

Blythe MJ, Fortenberry JD, Temkit M, et al: Incidence and correlates of unwanted sex in relationships of middle and late adolescent women. *Arch Pediatr Adolesc Med* 2006;160:591–595.

Buzi RS, Tortolero SR, Ross MW, et al: The impact of a history of sexual abuse on high-risk sexual behaviors among females attending alternative schools. *Adolescence* 2003;38:595–605.

Catalano SM: Criminal Victimization 2003. Washington, DC, Bureau of Justice Statistics, 2004, available at: */www.ojp.usdoj.gov/bjs/abstract/cv03.htm*.

Coker AL, McKeown RE, Sanderson M, Davis KE: Severe dating violence and quality of life among South Carolina high school students. *Am J Prev Med* 2000;19:220–227.

Foshee VA, Bauman KE, Greene WF, et al: The Safe Dates Program: 1-Year follow-up results. *Am J Public Health* 2000;90:1619–1622.

Kaplan DW, Feinstein RA, Fisher MM, et al: Committee on Adolescence, Care of the Adolescent Sexual Assault Victim. *Pediatrics* 2001;107:1476–1479.

Nofzigen S, Stein RE: To tell or not to tell: lifestyle impects on whether adolescents tell about violent victimization. *Violence Vict* 2006;21:371–382.

Raj A, Silverman JG, Amaro H: The relationship between sexual abuse and sexual risk among high school students: Findings from the 1997 Massachusetts Youth Risk Behavior Survey. *Matern Child Health J* 2000;4:125–134.

Silverman JG, Raj A, Clements K: Dating violence and associated sexual risk and pregnancy among adolescent girls in the United States. *Pediatrics* 2004;114:e220–e225.

Silverman JG, Raj A, Mucci LA, Hathaway JE: Dating violence against adolescent girls and associated substance use, unhealthy weight control, sexual risk behavior, pregnancy, and suicidality. *JAMA* 2001;286:572–579.

Taylor CA, Sorenson SB: Injunctive social norms of adults regarding teen dating violence. *J Adolesc Health* 2004;34:468–479.

Chapter 119 ■ Sexually Transmitted Infections Renée R. Jenkins

The behavioral and physiologic characteristics of adolescence predispose sexually active adolescents to the increased acquisition and adverse consequences of sexually transmitted infections (STIs). When controlled for sexual activity, age-specific rates of many STIs are highest among sexually experienced adolescents. For STI pathogens, intimate sexual contact is the common mode of transmission; however, the clinical expression can be listed according to STI syndromes based on a constellation of clinical signs and symptoms. Different microorganisms are responsible for similar symptoms. Almost all STI pathogens can also infect an adolescent without manifesting any clinical symptoms. The approach to prevention and control of these infections lies in education, screening, and early diagnosis and treatment. (See chapters discussing specific microorganisms in Part XVI.)

ETIOLOGY. The risk of contracting an STI exists in any adolescent who has had sexual intercourse. The younger the adolescent is at the time of initiation of sexual activity, the higher the risk of infection. Physical, behavioral, and social factors contribute to the adolescent's higher risk (Table 119-1). Oral sex places the patient at risk of herpes simplex virus type 1 (HSV-1) infection as well as gonorrhea, syphilis, HIV, and papillomavirus infections. Drug and alcohol use add to the vulnerability of adolescents in con-

TABLE 119-1. Circumstances Contributing to Adolescents' Susceptibility to Sexually Transmitted Infections

PHYSICAL
Younger age at puberty
Cervical ectopy
Smaller introitus leading to traumatic sex
Asymptomatic nature of sexually transmitted infection
Uncircumcised penis
BEHAVIOR LIMITED BY COGNITIVE STAGE OF DEVELOPMENT
Early adolescence: have not developed ability to think abstractly
Middle adolescence: develop belief of uniqueness and invulnerability
SOCIAL FACTORS
Poverty
Limited access to "adolescent friendly" health care services
Adolescent health-seeking behaviors (forgoing care because of confidentiality concerns or denial of health problem)
Sexual abuse and violence
Homelessness
Young adolescent females with older male partners

From Shafii T, Burstein G. An overview of sexually transmitted infections among adolescents. *Adolesc Med Clin* 2004;15:207.

tracting an infection. Exposure to uncommon sexual pathogens is increased with anal sex. Young adolescents who inaccurately perceive oral sex as having no risk of infection increase their risk by failing to use barrier protection and require counseling. Educational interventions may have some impact in reducing the risky behaviors of adolescents who have sex with more than one partner in 6 mo and who fail to use condoms consistently. Adolescents who are victims of sexual abuse or rape may not consider themselves "sexually active," given the context of the encounter, and need reassurance, protection, and appropriate intervention when these circumstances are uncovered. Depot medroxyprogesterone acetate contraception may increase the risk of chlamydial infections.

EPIDEMIOLOGY. Adolescents and young adults younger than 25 yr of age have the highest reported prevalence of gonorrheal (see Chapter 191) and chlamydial (see Chapter 223) infection; rates of these infections in the United States are highest in women at ages 15–19 yr and in men ages 20–24 yr. Reported rates from 2000 to 2003 in women 15–19 yr have increased about 14% to 2687/100,000, while in young men of the same age, the increase is about 35% to 690/100,000. These rates reflect increased screening, more sensitive test methods, and improved reporting. After peaking in 1990, the rates for primary and secondary syphilis (see Chapter 215) are declining for women, but increasing from men over age 20 yr. Pelvic inflammatory disease (PID) rates are highest in females aged 15–25 yr when compared to older women. AIDS, but not HIV, is reportable in the United States, giving a somewhat skewed perception of a lower rate of infection in adolescents. In 2003, 2050 young people aged 13–24 yr were diagnosed with AIDS, whereas 3847 young people with HIV were reported from the 33 areas that conduct name-based confidential HIV infection surveillance. Epidemiologists using the best evidence available from screening programs and Centers for Disease Control and Prevention reports in 2000 estimate that human papillomavirus (HPV) is the most prevalent infection in 15–24 yr olds compared to other common STIs (Fig. 119-1). (See Chapter 263.)

Rates vary considerably between nations. Among 15–19 yr olds from 16 developed nations, syphilis rates range from 0/100,000 in Norway, 0.2/100,000 in England and Wales to 211.4/100,000 in the Russian Federation; gonorrhea rates range from 0.6/100,000 in Belgium to 596.5/100,000 in the Russian Federation; and chlamydia rates range from 12.2/100,000 in Belgium to 1131.8/100,000 in the United States. Rates generally have been decreasing except in the Russian Federation where substantial increases were witnessed during the 1990s. STIs are a significant problem among adolescents in many African nations.

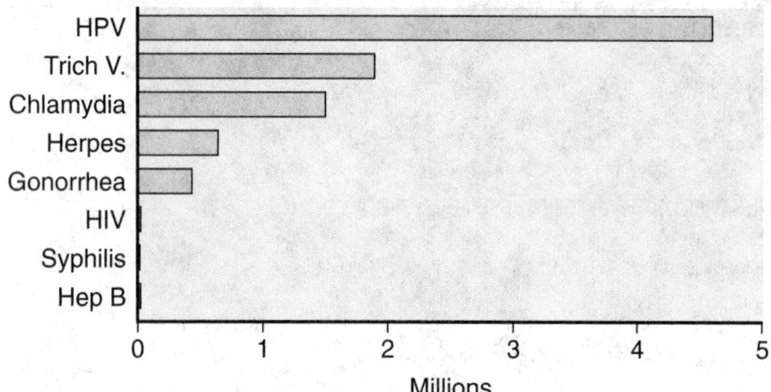

Figure 119-1. Estimated incidence of sexually transmitted infections among American youth ages 15 to 24 years, 2000. (Adapted from Weinstock H, Berman S, Cates W: Sexually transmitted diseases among American youth: Incidence and prevalence estimates, 2000. *Perspect Sex Reprod Health* 2004;36:6–10.)

PATHOGENESIS. During puberty, increasing levels of estrogen cause the vaginal epithelium to thicken and cornify and the cellular glycogen content to rise, the latter causing vaginal pH to fall. These changes increase the resistance of the vaginal epithelium to penetration by certain organisms (including *Neisseria gonorrhoeae*) and increase the susceptibility to others (*Candida albicans* and *Trichomonas*, see Chapter 281). The transformation of the vaginal cells leaves columnar cells on the ectocervix, forming a border of the two cell types on the ectocervix, known as the squamocolumnar junction. The appearance is referred to as **ectopy.** With maturation, this tissue involutes. Prior to involution, it represents a unique vulnerability to infection for adolescent females. A 15 yr old sexually active girl with endocervical colonization has a 1 : 8 chance of developing PID compared to the 1 : 80 chance for a 24 yr old. As a result of these physiologic changes, gonococcal infection becomes primarily cervical and susceptibility to ascending infection is greatest during menses, when the pH is 6.8–7.0. The association of early sexual debut and younger gynecologic age with increased risk of sexually transmitted infections supports this explanation of the pathogenesis of infection in young adolescents.

STI SCREENING. Early detection and treatment are the primary strategies of control for STIs. Some of the most common STIs in adolescents, including HPV (see Chapter 263), HSV (see Chapter 249), and chlamydia, are often asymptomatic and if undetected can be spread inadvertently by the infected host. Screening initiatives for chlamydial infections have demonstrated reductions in PID cases by 40–60%. The lack of a dialogue about STIs or the provision of STI services at annual preventive service visits to adolescents who were sexually experienced are missed opportunities for screening and education. Comprehensive reproductive health services including STI screening should be offered to all sexually experienced adolescents.

CLINICAL MANIFESTATIONS. STI syndromes are generally characterized by the location of the manifestation (vaginitis) or the type of lesion (genital ulcer). Certain constellations of presenting symptoms suggest the inclusion of a possible STI in the differential diagnosis (Table 119-2).

Urethritis. Urethritis is an inflammation of the urethra classically presenting as a urethral discharge or dysuria, or both (Fig. 119-2). Urgency, frequency of urination, erythema of the urethral meatus, and scrotal pain are less common clinical presentations. Asymptomatic or minimally symptomatic presentations are common in males. Adolescent males, in particular, are likely to ignore symptoms that improve spontaneously or sometimes ignore obvious physical signs. The genital examination should be thorough, including examination of the scrotum for signs of epididymitis and retraction of the foreskin in uncircumcised males, regardless of the denial of symptoms by the adolescent. Examining a patient prior to a urinary void is an important factor in observing a minimally symptomatic discharge. *C. trachomatis* and *N. gonorrhoeae* are the most common pathogens. *Ureaplasma urealyticum* and *Mycoplasma genitalium* are considered potential pathogens in nongonococcal urethritis, when *Chlamydia* cannot be confirmed (Table 119-3). Diagnostic tests for these pathogens are not readily available. *Trichomonas vaginalis* and HSV are also considered in the differential diagnosis when nongonococcal urethritis is resistant to treatment. There are classic descriptions of discharges, associating pathogens with color and consistency: yellow-green purulent discharge for gonococci and white mucopurulent discharge for chlamydia; **co-infection** and other factors can alter the appearance of discharges. Co-infection with gonococcal and chlamydial urethritis is reported in >25% of men with urethritis. Consequently, laboratory evaluation is key to determining the involved pathogens.

Epididymitis. The inflammation of the epididymis in adolescent males, unlike that in adult males, is most often associated with

TABLE 119-2. Signs, Symptoms, and Presumptive and Definitive Diagnoses of Genital Ulcers

SIGNS/SYMPTOMS	HERPES SIMPLEX VIRUS	SYPHILIS (PRIMARY)	CHANCROID
Ulcers	Vesicles rupture to form shallow ulcers	Ulcer with well-demarcated indurated borders and a clean base (chancre)	Unindurated and undermined borders and a purulent base
Painful	Painful	Painless*	Painful
Number of lesions	Usually multiple	Usually single	Multiple
Inguinal lymphadenopathy	First-time infections may cause constitutional symptoms and lymphadenopathy	Usually mild and minimally tender	Unilateral or bilateral painful adenopathy in >50% Inguinal bubo formation and rupture may occur
Presumptive diagnosis	Typical lesions plus any of the following: a previously known outbreak, a positive Tzanck smear of lesion scraping, exclusion of other causes of ulcers, or a fourfold increase in acute and convalescent antibody titers (in a first-time infection)	Early syphilis: a typical chancre plus a reactive nontreponemal test (RPR, VDRL) and no history of syphilis or a fourfold increase in a quantitative nontreponemal test in a person with a history of syphilis	Exclusion of other causes of ulcers in the presence of (1) typical ulcers and lymphadenopathy, (2) a typical Gram stain and a history of contact with a high-risk individual (prostitute) or living in an endemic area
Definitive diagnosis	Detection of HSV by culture or nonculture methods (DFA) from ulcer scraping or aspiration of vesicle fluid	Identification *T. pallidum*, from a chancre or lymph node aspirate, on dark-field microscopy or by DFA	Detection of *H. ducreyi* by culture

*Primary syphilitic ulcers may be painful if they become co-infected with bacteria or one of the other organisms responsible for genital ulcers.
DFA, direct fluorescent antibody; HSV, herpes simplex virus; RPR, rapid plasma reagin; VDRL, Venereal Disease Research Laboratory.
Data from Centers for Disease Control and Prevention *Sexually Transmitted Disease Clinical Practice Guidelines*, May 1991; Centers for Disease Control and Prevention *1993 Sexually Transmitted Disease Treatment Guidelines;* and Hoffman I, Schmitz J: Genital ulcers management in the HIV era. *Postgrad Med* 1995;98:67.
From Lappa S, Moscicki A: The pediatrician and the sexually active adolescent: A primer for sexually transmitted diseases. *Pediatr Clin North Am* 1997;44:1430.

an STI. The same pathogens associated with urethritis are prevalent. The presentation of scrotal swelling and tenderness, associated with the history of a spontaneously resolving urethral discharge, constitute the presumptive diagnosis of epididymitis. A urethral discharge may still be present at the time of examination. Males who practice insertive anal intercourse are also vulnerable to *Escherichia coli* infection.

Vaginitis (Vulvitis). Vaginitis is a superficial infection of the vaginal mucosa frequently presenting as a vaginal discharge, with or without vulvar involvement (see Chapter 549) (Table 119-4). Pruritus and the presence of an odor may differentiate the cause of the infection. Colonization without infection, as in bacterial vaginosis, can also present as a vaginal discharge. Lactobacilli are the predominant normal vaginal flora, which convert glucose to lactic acid, keeping the vaginal pH acid in a range of 3.8–4.2. Although bacterial vaginosis is no longer categorized strictly as an STI, sexual activity is associated with increased frequency of vaginosis. Trichomoniasis and candidiasis, together with bacterial vaginosis, are the predominant infections associated with vaginal discharge. The clinical observations of the color, consistency (frothy, floccular, homogeneous), odor, extent of vulvar involvement, and cervical changes lead one to a presumptive diagnosis. Laboratory confirmation is recommended in determining the presence of one or more infections that may present in an uncharacteristic manner.

Cervicitis. The inflammatory process in cervicitis involves the deeper structures in the mucous membrane of the cervix uteri. Vaginal discharge can be a manifestation of cervicitis, if the cervical discharge is profuse. Less subtle clinical manifestations of cervicitis are irregular or postcoital bleeding, mucopurulent discharge from the os, and a friable cervix. The cervical changes associated with cervicitis must be distinguished from cervical ectopy in the younger adolescent to avoid the overdiagnosis of inflammation (Fig. 119-3). The pathogens associated most commonly with cervicitis are *C. trachomatis* and *N. gonorrhoeae*, which are responsible for about 50–60% of cases. HSV is a less common pathogen associated with ulcerative and necrotic lesions on the cervix.

Pelvic Inflammatory Disease. A spectrum of inflammatory disorders of the upper genital tract in females is encompassed under the diagnosis of PID. The spectrum includes endometritis, sal-

Figure 119-2. Gonococcal urethral discharge. (From CDC Public Health Image Library #4065.)

TABLE 119-3. Causes of Urethritis in Men

COMMON DIAGNOSES
- Gonorrhea
- Chlamydial infection
- Nonspecific urethritis

LESS COMMON DIAGNOSES
- *Ureaplasma urealyticum* infection
- *Mycoplasma genitalium* infection
- Trichomoniasis
- Herpes simplex virus infection
- *Escherichia coli* infection
- Bacteroides infection
- Cystitis
- Pyelonephritis
- Trauma
- Foreign body
- Reactive arthritis and allied conditions

From Richens J: Main presentation of sexually transmitted infections in men. *Br Med J* 2004;328:1251–1253.

TABLE 119-4. Pathologic Vaginal Discharge

INFECTIVE DISCHARGE	OTHER REASONS FOR DISCHARGE
Common Causes	**Common Causes**
Organisms	Retained tampon or condom
Candida albicans	Chemical irritation
Trichomonas vaginalis	Allergic responses
Chlamydia trachomatis	Ectropion
Neisseria gonorrhoeae	Endocervical polyp
Conditions	Intrauterine device
Bacterial vaginosis	Atrophic changes
Acute pelvic inflammatory disease	**Less Common Causes**
Postoperative pelvic infection	Physical trauma
Postabortal sepsis	Vault granulation tissue
Puerperal sepsis	Vesicovaginal fistula
	Rectovaginal fistula
Less Common Causes	Neoplasia
Human papillomavirus	
Primary syphilis	
Mycoplasma genitalium	
Ureaplasma urealyticum	
Escherichia coli	

From Mitchell H: Vaginal discharge—causes, diagnosis, and treatment. *Br Med J* 2004;328:1306–1308.

pingitis, tubo-ovarian abscess, and pelvic peritonitis, usually in combination rather than as separate entities. *N. gonorrhoeae* and *C. trachomatis* predominate as the involved pathogenic organisms in younger adolescents; maturation and recurrent disease increase the appearance of other anaerobic and aerobic bacteria such as *Mycoplasma hominis*, group B streptococci, streptococci, *Peptostreptococcus* spp., *Gardnerella vaginalis*, *E. coli*, and various *Bacteroides* spp. There is no association between upper genital tract infection and the use of medroxyprogesterone or oral contraceptives.

The clinical diagnosis of PID is based on the minimal criteria of lower abdominal tenderness, adnexal tenderness, or cervical motion tenderness in a sexually active female adolescent with no other causes for illness. The requirement of only one symptom of the three criteria increases the sensitivity of the diagnosis at the expense of specificity, yet reduces the likelihood of missed or delayed diagnosis. There is a mucopurulent cervical discharge or evidence of white blood cells on a wet prep of vaginal fluid. Clinical criteria are accurate at the 65–90% level when compared to laparoscopy. Only about 20% of young women have the classic picture of PID that can be verified by laparoscopy. The presence of a recent increase in dysmenorrhea, onset of symptoms following menses, fever, urinary symptoms, abnormal vaginal bleeding, and abnormal vaginal discharge add support to the clinical diagnosis. Specific but not always practical criteria for PID include evidence of endometritis on biopsy, transvaginal sonography, or MRI evidence of thickened, fluid-filled tubes or Doppler evidence of tubal hyperemia and laparoscopic evidence of PID.

Genital Ulcer Syndromes. An ulcerative lesion in a mucosal area exposed to sexual contact is the unifying characteristic of infections associated with these syndromes. These lesions are most frequently seen on the penis and vulva, but also occur on oral and rectal mucosa depending on the sexual practices of the adolescent. HSV, *Treponema pallidum* (syphilis), and *Haemophilus ducreyi* (chancroid) are the most common organisms associated with genital ulcer syndromes. Although the initial herpetic lesion is a vesicle, by the time the patient presents clinically, the vesicle most often has ruptured spontaneously, leaving a shallow, painful ulcer. HSV-2 predominates as the pathogen in this age group,

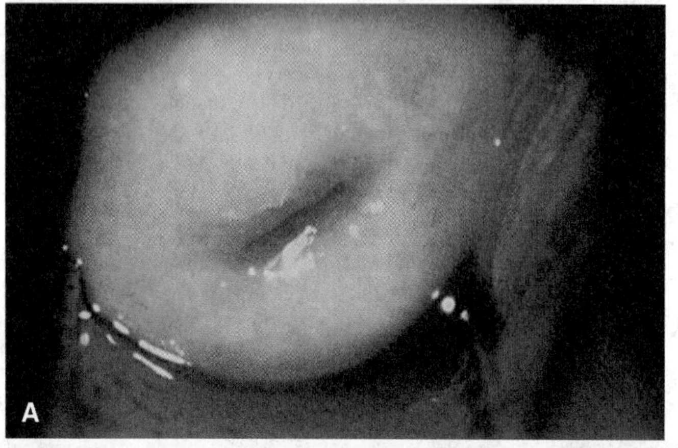

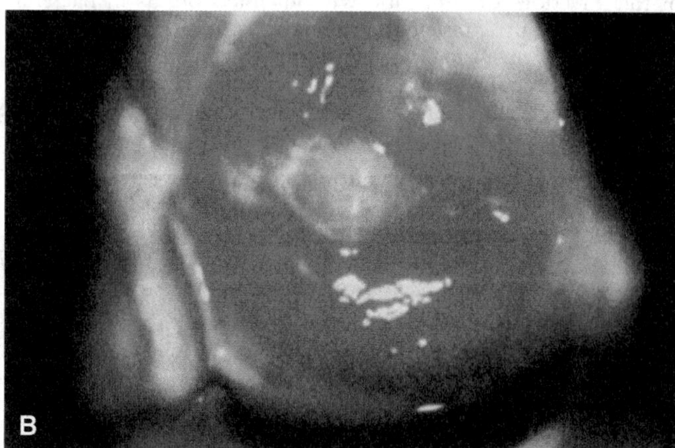

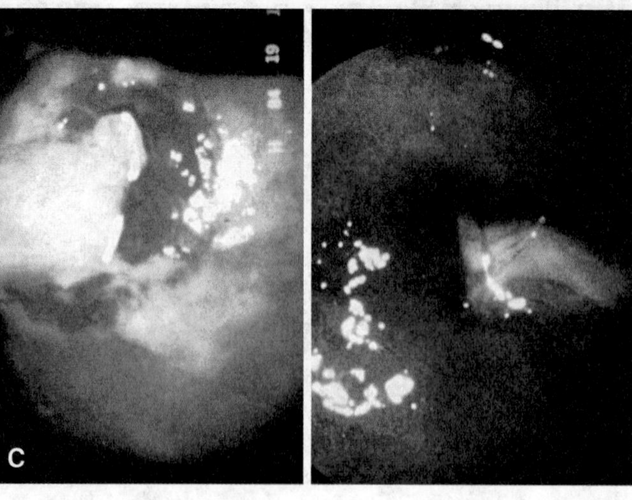

Figure 119-3. Normal and pathologic states of the cervix. *A*, Normal cervix. *B*, Inflamed cervix (cervicitis). *C*, Cervix with ectopy. (From Centers for Disease Control and Prevention. Sexually Transmitted Disease Curriculum for Clinical Educators, 2005.).

with an increasing incidence of HSV-1 recovered in genital lesions, especially in women. Of these syndromes, syphilis and chancroid are less common in adolescents than in adults. Lymphogranuloma venereum due to *C. trachomatis* serovars L1-L3, and donovanosis are rare infections in the United States and other industrialized countries, although outbreaks of lymphogranuloma venereum do occur in men who have sex with men. In these circumstances, genital ulcerations with inflamed inguinal lymph nodes (buboes) are unusual; proctitis or proctocolitis is the usual manifestation. HIV is present in affected men.

Clinical characteristics differentiating the lesions of the most common infections associated with genital ulcers are presented in Table 119-2, along with the required laboratory diagnosis to identify the causative agent accurately.

Genital Lesions and Ectoparasites. Lesions that present as outgrowths on the surface of the epithelium and other limited epidermal lesions are included under this categorization of syndromes. Human papillomavirus types are either low risk, associated with genital warts or mild Pap abnormalities, or high risk, generally asymptomatic, causing mild to severe Pap test abnormalities. Although early age at first intercourse is a risk factor for genital HPV infections, the infections are transient with only 2.4–5% of adolescents with persistent infections progressing to severe Pap test abnormalities. Oncogenic HPV types 16 and 18, if persistent, increase the risk of cervical cancer. Molluscum contagiosum and condyloma lata associated with secondary syphilis complete the classification of genital lesion syndromes. As a result of the close physical contact during sexual contact, common ectoparasitic infestations of the pubic area occur as pediculosis pubis or the papular lesions of scabies.

HIV Disease and Hepatitis B. HIV and hepatitis B infections present as asymptomatic, unexpected occurrences in most infected adolescents. Risk factors identified in the history are much more likely to result in suspicion of disease, leading to the appropriate laboratory screening, than are clinical manifestations in this age group.

DIAGNOSIS. Asymptomatic infections with viral pathogens, such as HIV, HSV, and hepatitis B, are the most common presentations for these infections, whereas asymptomatic presentations for chlamydial and gonorrhea infections range from 17% to 56% and 2% to 33%, respectively. Adolescent males are more likely to be asymptomatic with chlamydia, whereas adolescent females have high rates of asymptomatic infections with chlamydia and gonorrhea. A sexually experienced adolescent who inconsistently uses condoms and/or has multiple partners should be questioned more thoroughly to determine the risk of an asymptomatic or minimally symptomatic infection requiring testing. In addition to the routine history of vaginal or urethral discharge, genital lesions, and lower abdominal pain in women, one should ask about prior treatment of any STI symptoms, including self-treatment using over-the-counter medications. **Dyspareunia** is a consistent symptom in adolescents with PID. A history of oral or anal sex guides the examiner in determining sites from which to obtain specimens. Adolescent men who have sex with men demonstrated high rates of infection for HIV, gonorrhea, chlamydia, syphilis, and hepatitis B. The high prevalence of disease in a community is a risk factor warranting screening, as well as the setting in which an adolescent resides (juvenile detention center, homeless shelter).

Urethritis can be documented in an asymptomatic male with a positive leukocyte esterase test on first voided specimen with >10 white blood cells per high-power field or more than five white blood cells per oil immersion field on a Gram stain of urethral secretions. *Nucleic acid amplification tests* (NAATs) such as polymerase chain reaction, ligase chain reaction, and strand displacement assay are highly recommended for chlamydia screening. Cultures are preferred for *N. gonorrhoeae* when holding and transport conditions are adequate to maintain specimen viability. NAATs are not highly recommended for testing rectal swabs. Availability and cost may limit the use of these tests in some communities. Indirect tests should not be substituted for cultures for STI screening in suspected **sexual abuse** cases because of the possibility of false-positive results from indirect tests. Advances in HIV testing have also increased opportunities for screening asymptomatic adolescents. Rapid HIV testing with the availability of results in 10–60 min can be useful in settings in which the likelihood of adolescents returning for their results is low, although this does not eliminate the need for confirmatory testing. Self-collected vaginal swabs using polymerase chain reaction testing has demonstrated patient acceptability and an increased detection rate in a high-risk transient adolescent population. Self-tests are available to patients via the Internet. Unsupervised self-testing carries with it some risk of poor follow-up of positive tests and of partner identification and treatment. Based on the preceding observations, the recommendations for screening sexually active adolescents are addressed in Chapter 111.

For clinically symptomatic adolescents, further evaluations may be needed to identify the causative agent of the syndrome accurately. For urethritis, a Gram stain when a urethral discharge is present confirms the diagnosis of gonorrhea at the time of the presenting symptom. The wet mount is useful in determining the possible pathogen causing a vaginal discharge (Figs. 119-4 and 119-5). The definitive diagnosis of PID is difficult based on clinical findings alone; even with an experienced clinician, 30% of women are diagnosed incorrectly. Ultrasonography is useful in identifying adnexal masses and ruling out other diagnoses. Transvaginal methods are preferable; however, the sensitivity for the diagnosis of PID is low. Direct visualization through the laparoscopic technique with cultures from the fallopian tube, while infrequently performed in the United States, is the gold standard for definitive diagnosis. The HSV culture is readily available in most clinical settings to identify HSV in genital ulcer syndromes. Dark-field microscopy and fluorescent antibody tests to confirm syphilis are less frequently available, with most clinicians relying on serologic confirmation. Symptomatic or asymptomatic adolescents with STIs should be screened for HIV.

DIFFERENTIAL DIAGNOSES. The differential diagnoses are particular to each of the clinical syndromes (see Tables 119-3 and 119-4). Reactive arthritis is considered an autoimmune response to an STI or enteric pathogen and is characterized by arthritis, nonbacterial urethritis or cervicitis, conjunctivitis, and mucocutaneous lesions. The urinary symptoms associated with urethritis mimic a urinary tract infection, a condition much less common than an STI in adolescent males. Testicular torsion, the main differential diagnosis to consider in scrotal pain, constitutes a surgical emergency, although trauma is a more common occurrence, especially in adolescent males involved in contact sports (see Chapters 546 and 691). Vaginitis and vulvar irritation can result from a foreign body or chemical irritant, for example, bubble bath or spermicide.

The **differential diagnosis** for PID, presenting as acute lower abdominal pain, is extensive, involving the gastrointestinal, reproductive, and urinary systems. The most emergent differential diagnosis in a sexually active adolescent is to distinguish PID from appendicitis or an ectopic pregnancy, both of which require surgical intervention. Given the complexity of the management approach, clinical practice guidelines are extremely useful in moving swiftly and logically to the correct diagnosis (Table 119-5). Most of the conditions in the differential diagnosis of genital ulcerative lesions rarely occur in teenagers in the United States (lymphogranuloma venereum, granuloma inguinale); however, trauma is a common cause that can be detected with a careful history.

TREATMENT. See Part XVI for chapters on the treatment of specific microorganisms and Tables 119-6 to 119-8. Treatment reg-

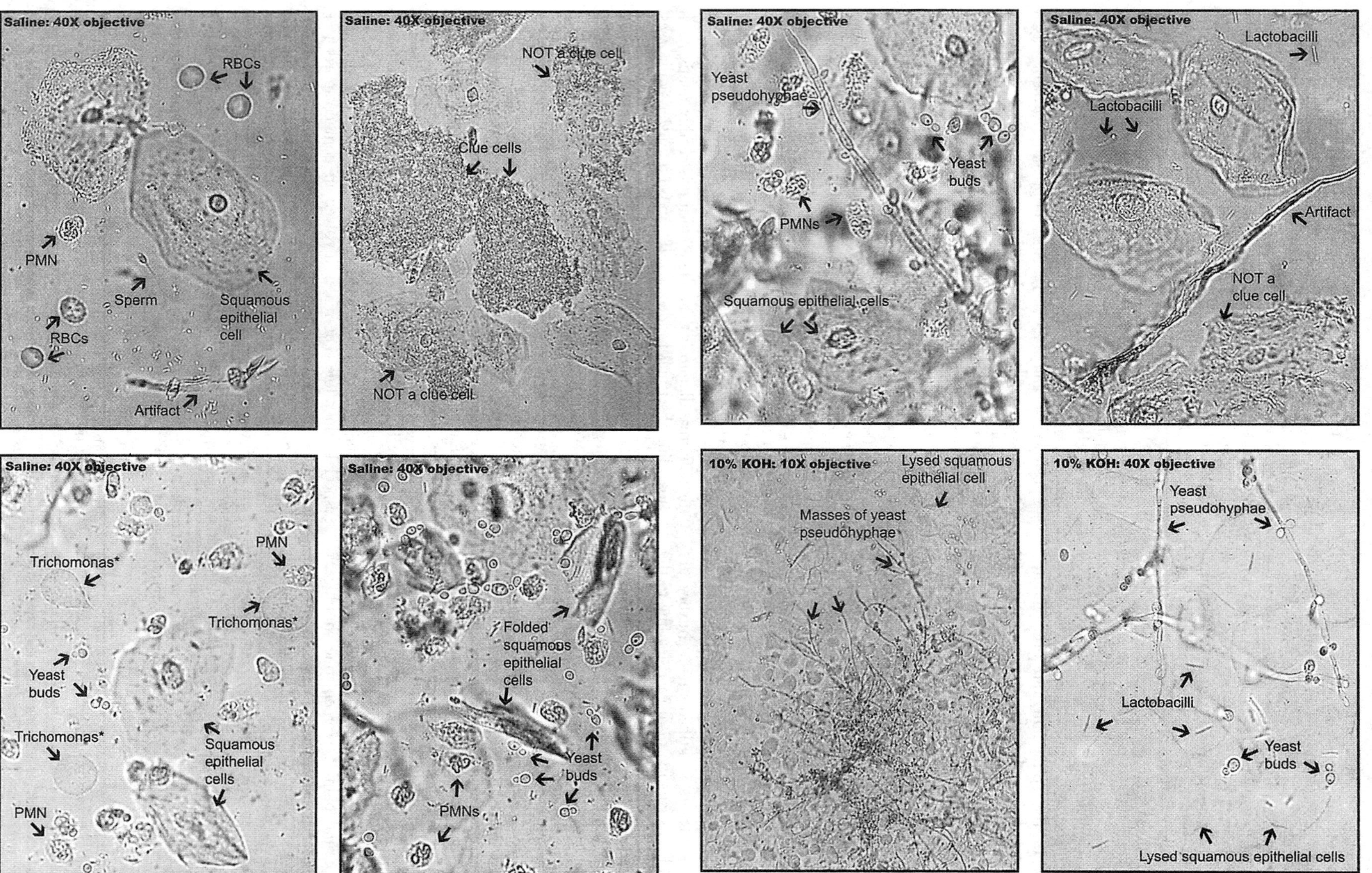

Figure 119-4. Common normal and abnormal microscopic findings during examination of vaginal fluid. (From *Adolescent Medicine: State of the Art Reviews*, Vol. 14, No. 2. Philadelphia, Hanley & Belfus, an affiliate of Elsevier, 2003, pp 350–351.)

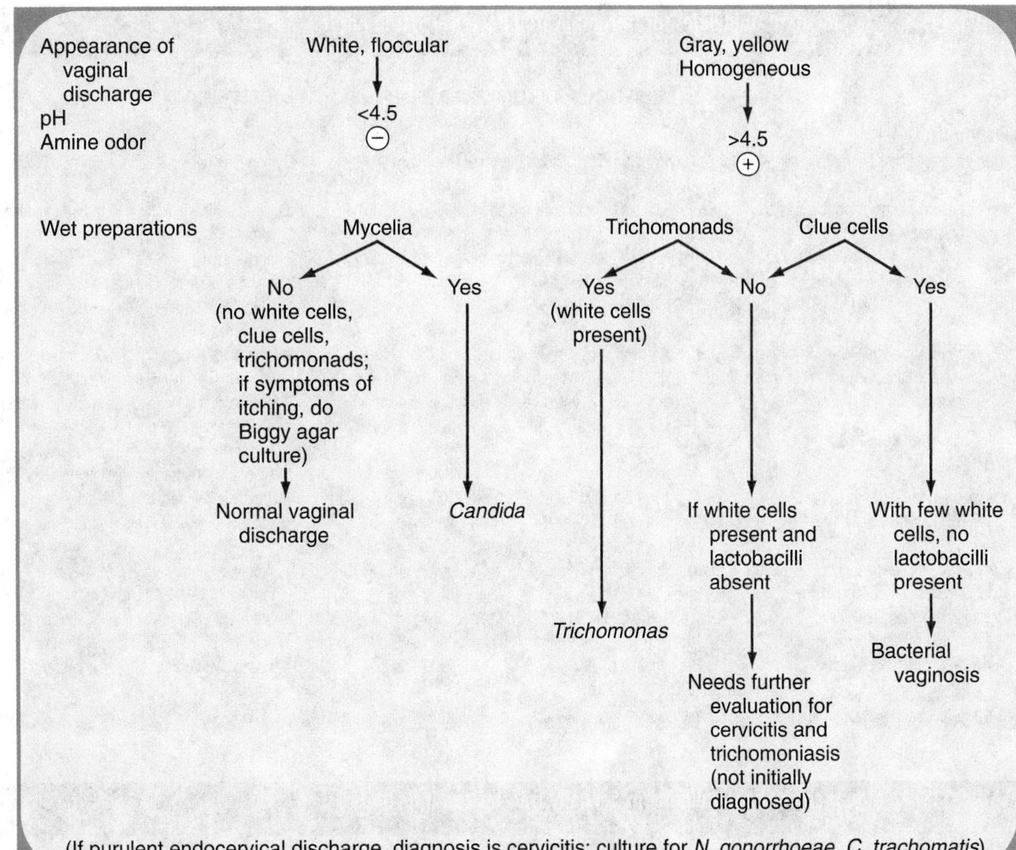

Figure 119-5. Differential diagnosis of vaginitis. (From Emans SJ, Laufer MR, Goldstein DP (editors): *Pediatric and Adolescent Gynecology*, 4th ed. Philadelphia, Lippincott–Raven, 1998, p 427.)

imens using over-the-counter products for candida vaginitis, genital warts, and pediculosis reduce financial and access barriers to rapid treatment for adolescents, but there are potential risks for inappropriate self-treatment and complications from untreated more serious infections that must be considered before using this approach. Minimizing noncompliance with treatment, finding and treating the sexual partner, addressing prevention and contraceptive issues, and making every effort to preserve fertility are additional physician responsibilities. Repeat testing in 3–4 mo is recommended for women with chlamydial infections. Follow-up recommendations for men and for women with other proven infections are less clear. Once an infection is diagnosed, partner evaluation, testing, and treatment are recommended for sexual contacts within 60 days of symptoms or diagnosis or the most recent partner if sexual contact was >60 days, even if the partner is asymptomatic. Abstinence is recommended for at least 7 days after both patient and partner are treated.

Diagnosis and therapy are often necessarily carried out within the context of a confidential relationship between the physician and the patient. Therefore, the need to report certain STIs to

TABLE 119-5. Management of the Patient with Uncomplicated Pelvic Inflammatory Disease (PID)

2002 CENTERS FOR DISEASE CONTROL AND PREVENTION DIAGNOSTIC CRITERIA

Minimal Criteria

Institute empiric treatment for PID if at lease one of the following criteria is present *and* no other cause for the illness (refer to Differential Diagnosis below) can be identified (check all that apply):

☐ Uterine/adnexal tenderness **OR** ☐ Cervical motion tenderness

Additional Criteria to Enhance the Specificity of the Minimal Criteria (Check All That Apply)

☐ Oral temperature >101°F
☐ Abnormal cervical or vaginal mucopurulent discharge
☐ Presence of white blood cells on saline microscopy of vaginal secretions
☐ Elevated ESR
☐ Elevated C-reactive protein
☐ Laboratory documentation of cervical infection with *Neisseria gonorrhoeae* or *Chlamydia trachomatis*

Evaluation (All of the Following are Recommended)

☐ Pelvic examination
☐ Endocervical specimen for *N. gonorrhoeae* (culture)
☐ Endocervical specimen for *C. trachomatis* (culture or DNA probe)
☐ Complete blood count with differential
☐ ESR or C-reactive protein
☐ Rapid plasma reagin
☐ Urine dipstick or urinalysis
☐ Urine culture
☐ Urine β-hCG (pregnancy test)

In Addition, Consider

☐ Pelvic ultrasonography if any one of the following:
☐ Pelvic mass
☐ Adnexal tenderness *and* at least one of the following (check all that apply):
☐ High fever ☐ Elevated WBC Count ☐ Elevated ESR
☐ Other clinical indication
☐ Unable to adequately access gynecologic structures on bimanual examination
☐ Serum β-hCG and type and hold if suspect ectopic pregnancy and urine β-hCG is negative
☐ Gynecology consult if patient is pregnant or ordering an ultrasound for pelvic mass
☐ Surgery consult if suspect appendicitis or other surgical problem

DIFFERENTIAL DIAGNOSIS (PARTIAL LIST)

GI: appendicitis, constipation, diverticulitis, gastroenteritis, inflammatory bowel disease, irritable bowel syndrome

GYN: ovarian cyst (intact, ruptured, or torsed), endometriosis, dysmenorrhea, ectopic pregnancy, mittelschmerz, ruptured follicle, septic or threatened abortion, tubo-ovarian abscess

URINARY TRACT: cystitis, pyelonephritis, urethritis, nephrolithiasis

β-hCG, β subunit human chorionic gonadotropin; ESR, erythrocyte sedimentation rate; GI, gastrointestinal; GYN, gynecologic; WBC, white blood cell.

Adapted from Shrier LA: Bacterial Sexually Transmitted Infections: Gonorrhea, Chlamydia, Pelvic Inflammatory Disease, and Syphilis. *In* Emans SJH, Laufer MR, Goldstein DP (editors): *Pediatric and Adolescent Gynecology*, 4th ed. Philadelphia, Lippincott–Raven, 1998, p 480; updated 5th ed., 2005, p 591.

TABLE 119-6. Management Guidelines for Uncomplicated Bacterial STIs in Adults

INFECTION (DISEASE)	U.S. CENTERS FOR DISEASE CONTROL AND PREVENTION	NOTABLE VARIATIONS	CONTACT-TRACING PRIORITY
Chlamydia trachomatis (urethritis, cervicitis, or proctitis)	Azithromycin 1 g PO in 1 dose or doxycycline 100 mg PO twice daily for 7 days	Erythromycin (not estolate) or amoxicillin PO for 7 days alternatives for pregnant women (HIV positive, treatment unchanged)	High
Neisseria gonorrhoeae (urethritis, cervicitis, proctitis, throat colonization)	Cefixime 400 mg PO in 1 dose or ceftriaxone 125 mg IM in 1 dose or ciprofloxacin 500 mg PO in 1 dose or levofloxacin 250 mg PO in 1 dose (if not ruled out, also treat for *C trachomatis*)	Higher dose of ceftriaxone (250 mg) recommended in Europe and Australia; some think quinolones should be abandoned now (HIV positive, treatment unchanged)	High
Mycoplasma genitalium (urethritis, ?cervicitis)	No recommendation	In vitro and preliminary clinical experience suggests azithromycin (as used for NGU/chlamydia) better than tetracyclines (HIV positive, no recommendation)	To be determined
Treponema pallidum (syphilis: genital ulcers, other mucocutaneous lesions, neurologic, cardiovascular disease)	Benzathine penicillin G 2.4 million units IM in 1 dose (infection <1 yr) or benzathine penicillin G 2.4 million units IM as 3 once-weekly doses (infection >1 yr or unknown duration)	Daily IM procaine penicillin (10–21 days) preferred in some centers. IV penicillin G frequently recommended for neurosyphilis. Doxycycline 200 mg orally each day for 14–30 days an alternative for penicillin-allergic or needle-phobic (HIV positive, treatment generally unchanged). Possibly higher rate of treatment failure and neurologic complications has led some experts to recommend more intensive or longer courses of penicillin	High
Haemophilus ducreyi (chancroid: genital ulcers, lymphadenopathy)	Azithromycin 1 g PO in 1 dose or ceftriaxone 250 mg IM in 1 dose or ciprofloxacin 500 mg PO twice daily for 3 days or erythromycin base 500 mg PO 3 times daily for 7 days	HIV positive: closer follow-up and longer courses of antibiotics should be considered because of higher treatment failure rate	High
C. trachomatis (lymphogranuloma venereum: genital ulcers, lymphadenopathy)	Doxycycline 100 mg PO twice daily for 21 days	Erythromycin base 500 mg PO 4 times daily for 21 days (HIV positive, treatment generally unchanged)	High
Calymmatobacterium granulomatis (donovanosis or granuloma inguinale: genital and extragenital ulcers)	Doxycycline 100 mg PO twice daily for at least 3 wk or trimethoprim-sulfamethoxazole 800 mg/160 mg PO twice daily for at least 3 wk	Azithromycin 1 g PO each week for 4 wk or 500 mg daily for 7 days may improve adherence (HIV positive, treatment generally unchanged; consider adding parenteral gentamycin if severe)	High

NGU, nongonococcal urethritis.
From Donovan B: Sexually transmissible infections other than HIV. *Lancet* 2004;363:545–556.

TABLE 119-7. Management of Miscellaneous Sexually Transmitted Infections

INFECTION (DISEASE)	U.S. CENTERS FOR DISEASE CONTROL AND PREVENTION	NOTABLE VARIATIONS	CONTACT-TRACING PRIORITY
Trichomonas vaginalis (vaginitis, urethritis)	Metronidazole 2 g PO as 1 dose or tinidazole 2 g PO × 1 dose	Metronidazole 500 mg PO twice daily for 7 days (HIV positive, treatment unchanged)	Moderate
Pthirus pubis (pubic lice)	Permethrin 1% rinse applied to affected areas and washed off after 10 min or pyrethrin with piperonyl butoxide for 10 min. Launder clothing and bedding	Other options include malathion 0.5% for 8 to 12 hr or ivermectin 250 μg/kg PO, repeated in 2 wk	Low
Sarcoptes scabiei (scabies)	Permethrin 5% cream applied to all areas from the neck down, washed off after 8–14 hr or ivermectin 200 μg/kg orally, repeated after 2 wk	Lindane (1%) 1 oz of lotion or 30 g of cream in thin layer to all areas of body from neck down; wash off in 8 hr. HIV positive, crusted (Norwegian) scabies more likely if immunodeficient and specialist consultation recommended	Low

Modified from Donovan B: Sexually transmissible infections other than HIV. *Lancet* 2004;363:545–556.

TABLE 119-8. Management of Genital Warts and Herpes

INFECTION (DISEASE)	U.S. CENTERS FOR DISEASE CONTROL AND PREVENTION	NOTABLE VARIATIONS	CONTACT-TRACING PRIORITY
Human papillomaviruses (genital warts)	Podophyllotoxin 0.5% solution or gel self-applied to warts twice daily for 3 consecutive days each week or imiquimod 5% cream self-applied to warts on alternate days 3 times weekly for up to 16 wk, washed off after 6–10 hr, or cryotherapy, laser surgery, or intralesional interferon dependent on practitioner's skills, or trichloroacetic acid or podophyllin resin 10–25% applied weekly by practitioner.	Podophyllotoxin and imiquimod should be avoided in pregnancy. 0.15% podophyllotoxin cream available in Europe and Asia. Podophyllin resin no longer recommended in Europe. No authorities recommend treatment for subclinical human papillomavirus infections. Related neoplasia should be managed according to histology. (HIV positive, treatment generally unchanged, but expect lower treatment response and higher relapse rates; lower threshold for biopsy to exclude neoplasia)	Low
HSV (genital herpes)	First clinical episode (treat for 7–10 days): acyclovir 400 mg PO 3 times daily or acyclovir 200 mg PO 5 times daily or famcyclovir 250 mg PO 3 times daily or valacyclovir 1 g PO twice daily	Patients with >10 recurrences per year may require 1 g/day of valacyclovir for adequate suppression (HIV positive: starting treatment with IV acyclovir (5–10 mg/kg every 8 hr) occasionally necessary for severe disease. Unresponsive lesions should be tested for resistant virus. IV foscarnet or topical cidofovir may be useful for resistant virus)	Moderate
	Episodic therapy for recurrence (for 5 days): acyclovir 400 mg PO 3 times daily or acyclovir 200 mg PO 5 times daily or acyclovir 800 mg PO twice daily for just 2 days or famcyclovir 125 mg PO twice daily or famcyclovir 1,000 mg PO twice daily for 1 day or valacyclovir 500 mg twice daily (3 days as effective as 5 days) or valacyclovir 1,000 mg PO once daily		
	Suppressive therapy (continuous): acyclovir 400 mg PO twice daily or famcyclovir 250 mg PO twice daily or valacyclovir 500 mg PO once daily or valacyclovir 1 g PO once daily		

Modified from Donovan B: Sexually transmissible infections other than HIV. *Lancet* 2004;363:545–556.

health department authorities should be clarified at the outset. Most health departments will not violate confidentiality, if assured that treatment and case finding have been accomplished and that the patient can be expected to follow through in a responsible, mature manner. Expedited partner therapy or having the patient deliver the medication or a prescription to the partner for treatment without a clinical assessment, is being reconsidered as a strategy to reduce further transmission of infection, particularly for male partners of women with gonorrhea and/or chlamydia.

PREVENTION. The prevention messages to be communicated to adolescents regarding the avoidance of STIs are in direct contrast to the known risk factors for contracting the disease: (1) maintaining a healthier sexual behavior, (2) using barrier methods, (3) adopting healthy medical care–seeking behavior, (4) complying with management instruction, and (5) ensuring examination of sexual partners. The elements of maintaining healthier sexual behavior include postponing sexual behavior until at least 2–3 yr after menarche, limiting the number of sexual partners, eliciting information about a partner's STI status, inspecting the genitals of sexual partners, and abstaining from sex if STI symptoms develop. It is highly likely that vaccines will be available for HPV in the near future. Contraceptive counseling and management complete the comprehensive reproductive health service visit for the adolescent patient. Vaccination of all females ages 11 to 12 yr against HPV is recommended.

ACOG Committee on Adolescent Health Care: Sexually transmitted diseases in adolescents. *Sex Transm Dis Adolesc* 2004;104:891–898.

Anderson MR, Klink K, Cohrssen A: Evaluation of vaginal complaints. *JAMA* 2004;291:1368–1379.

Ault KA: Vaccines for the prevention of human papillomavirus and associated gynecologic diseases: a review. *Obstet Gynecol Surv* 2006;61:S26–S31.

Brückner H, Bearman P: After the promise: The STD consequences of adolescent virginity pledges. *J Adolesc Health* 2005;36:271–278.

Burstein GR, Lowry R, Klein JD, et al: Missed opportunities for sexually transmitted diseases, human immunodeficiency virus, and pregnancy prevention services during adolescent health supervision visits. *Pediatrics* 2003;111:996–1001.

Centers for Disease Control and Prevention: Open letter from John M Douglas, Jr., M.D. Director of DSTDP on expedited partner therapy, May 11, 2005, available at: *www.cdc.gov/std/DearColleagueEPT5-10-05.pdf* (accessed June 1, 2005).

Centers for Disease Control and Prevention: Sexually Transmitted Disease Curriculum for Clinical Educators, available at: *www.cdc.gov/stdtraining/readytouse/* (accessed June 1, 2005).

Cherpes TL, Meyn LA, Hillier SL: Cunnilingus and vaginal intercourse are risk factors for herpes simplex virus type 1 acquisition in women. *Sex Transm Dis* 2005;32:84–89.

Collins L, White JA, Bradbeer C: Lymphogranuloma venereum. *Br Med J* 2006;332:66–67.

Dayan L, Donovan B: Chlamydia, gonorrhoea, and injectable progesterone. *Lancet* 2004;364:1387–1388.

Dempsey AF, Zimet GD, Davis RL, et al: Factors that are associated with parental acceptance of human papillomavirus vaccines: a randomized intervention study of information about HPV. *Pediatrics* 2006;117:1486–1493.

Department of Health and Human Services, Centers for Disease Control and Prevention: Sexually transmitted diseases treatment guidelines, 2006. MMWR 2006;55:1–94.

Donovan B: Sexually transmissible infections other than HIV. *Lancet* 2004;363:545–556.

Eckert LO: Acute vulvovaginitis. *N Engl J Med* 2006;355:1244–1252.

Fiscus LC, Ford CA, Miller WC: Infrequency of sexually transmitted disease screening among sexually experienced U.S. female adolescents. *Perspect Sex Reprod Health* 2004;36:233–238.

Fredericks D, Fieler TL, Marrazzo JM: Molecular identification of bacteria associated with bacterial vaginosis. *N Engl J Med* 2005;353:1899–1910.

Gbesso S, Decosas J, Gnahoui-David B, et al: Adolescent sexual health? Let us get real! *Lancet* 2006;367:1221–1222.

Golden MR, Whittington WLH, Handsfield HH: Effect of expedited treatment of sex partners on recurrent or persistent gonorrhea or chlamydial infection. *N Engl J Med* 2005;352:676–684.

Huppert JS, Hiilard PJA: Sexually transmitted disease screening in teens. *Current Womens Health Rep* 2003;3:451–458.

Marrazzo J: Vulvovaginal candidiasis. *Br Med J* 2003;326:993–994.

Mitchell H: Vaginal discharge—causes, diagnosis, and treatment. *Br Med J* 2004;328:1306–1308.

Peipert JF: Genital chlamydial infections. *N Engl J Med* 2003;349:2424–2430.

Richens J: Main presentations of sexually transmitted infections in men. *Br Med J* 2004;328:1251–1253.

Rimsza M: Sexually transmitted infections: New guidelines for an old problem on the college campus. *Pediatr Clin North Am* 2005;52:217–228.

Saslow D, Runowicz CD, Solomon D, et al: American Cancer Society guideline for the early detection of cervical neoplasia and cancer. *CA Cancer J Clin* 2002;52:342–362.

Schiffman M, Castle PE: When to test women for human papillomavirus. *Br Med J* 2006;332:61–62.

Stanberry LR, Rosenthal SL: Progress in vaccines for sexually transmitted diseases. *Infect Dis Clin North Am* 2005;19:477–490.

Steinbrook R: The potential of human papillomavirus vaccines. *N Engl J Med* 2006;354:1109–1112.

Szarewski A, Sasieni P: Cervical screening in adolescents—at least do no harm. *Lancet* 2004;364:1642–1644.

Weinstock H, Berman S, Cates W: Sexually transmitted diseases among American youth: Incidence and prevalence estimates, 2000. *Perspect Sex Reprod Health* 2004;36:6–10.

Winer RL, Hughes JP, Feng Q, et al: Condom use and the risk of genital human papillomavirus infection in young women. *N Engl J Med* 2006;354: 2645–2654.

Chapter 120 ■ Chronic Fatigue Syndrome

Hal B. Jenson and James F. Jones

GENERAL. Numerous terms (chronic mononucleosis, chronic Epstein-Barr virus infection, myalgic encephalomyelitis, immune dysfunction syndrome) have been applied to the syndrome of unusual fatigability associated with mild to debilitating somatic symptoms. This syndrome was formally defined by the Centers for Disease Control and Prevention (CDC) in 1988 as *chronic fatigue syndrome* (CFS) because persistent and unexplained fatigue is the principal and invariable physical symptom. It results in severe impairment of daily functioning and is associated with a variety of physical symptoms. The fatigue is unusual because it does not require exertion by the patient, nor does rest relieve it. The current definition was created in 2003 to exclude psychiatric cases. CFS is a complex illness. It is not a new problem, nor is it the result of enhanced appreciation of a previously unrecognized single clinical illness. An identifiable infectious agent does not cause it, although the differential diagnosis includes many infectious and inflammatory diseases. It is not a single disease with consistent physiologic or pathologic abnormalities but rather the measurable experience of symptoms that occur with various clinical conditions of somatic, psychologic, and mixed causes. Current understanding of this condition is largely from studies among adults and adolescents, with limited descriptions of chronic fatiguing illness among young children.

EPIDEMIOLOGY. CFS includes severe functional impairment and is a diagnostic subset of chronic fatigue, which is a common presenting symptom of adolescents and adults. **Chronic fatigue** encompasses a broader category defined as unexplained fatigue of >6 mo, which in turn is a subset of **prolonged fatigue,** which is defined as fatigue lasting more >1 mo. Fatigue of >1 mo is estimated to occur in 2333/100,000 adolescents. Up to 40% of adults in primary care clinics or in surveys complain of chronic fatigue; the incidence in children is unknown. Prevalence rates vary significantly, but chronic fatiguing illnesses are encountered in all patient populations.

Adults diagnosed with CFS are of various ethnic and racial origins, with a preponderance of those identified in population-based studies being 45–55 yr of age and of lower socioeconomic status. These epidemiologic observations vary from the earlier reports based on patients seen in specialty clinics. The prevalence in the United States among adults older than 18 yr of age who fulfill a strict case definition is estimated to be 250–400/100,000, but the population-based study from which the prevalence figures for adolescents were derived did not identify any cases of CFS per se.

The number of cases of adult **CFS-like cases,** defined as individuals who fulfill a clinical definition of CFS but who have not undergone comprehensive medical and psychiatric evaluation, approaches 1250/100,000. The number of CFS-like cases in adolescents is 338/100,000. Females constitute 75% of adult CFS-like cases, but only 50% of CFS cases.

Most cases of CFS are sporadic and are not associated with secondary cases. There is no evidence supporting transmission of the illness from person to person, in utero to a fetus, or via blood products.

PATHOGENESIS. The cause of CFS is unknown. There is no evidence to support the hypothesis that infection with a known or a new virus is the primary cause of the symptoms of CFS. Some patients correlate the onset with a recent episode of a virus-like illness such as infectious mononucleosis or influenza. In many cases, underlying symptoms of depression such as fatigue, lack of energy and interest, and inability to concentrate merge with or are intensified by the weakness often present during convalescence from a systemic infectious disease, resulting in debilitating fatigue. Persistent fatigue and symptoms consistent with CFS are well recognized following many primary infections, especially infectious mononucleosis and influenza, and occur in up to 10% of persons. Susceptible persons may experience fatigue and exhaustion that is present for months to a few years and may be accompanied by signs of clinical depression. Prolonged illness after infectious mononucleosis is not predicted by control of viremia, an altered host response to Epstein-Barr virus infection, personality style, or psychologic disorders (depression).

Approximately half of adult and adolescent patients with CFS fulfill criteria for co-morbid psychiatric disorders, mainly anxiety and depressive disorders. Patients with CFS have higher rates of somatization and higher anxiety scores. Personality does not affect the predisposition, precipitation, and perpetuation of chronic fatigue. There is strong concordance in CFS patients between subjective complaints of mental fatigue and objective measurements of cognitive impairment, which suggests that mental fatigue is an important component of CFS-related cognitive dysfunction.

Orthostatic intolerance syndromes of circulatory dysfunction including neurally mediated hypotension, instantaneous orthostatic hypotension, and postural tachycardia syndrome have been observed in some patients with CFS, although these findings are not found in population-based studies. The pathophysiology of these manifestations among patients with CFS is unclear. The origin may be as simple as a problem with functional vascular volume or as complex as control of cerebral blood flow and heart-rate variability.

Diverse and conflicting in vitro immunologic alterations (hypo- or hypergammaglobulinemia, immunoglobulin subclass deficiencies, elevated levels of circulating immune complexes, mild increased helper/suppressor lymphocyte ratios, natural killer cell dysfunction, and monocyte dysfunction) have been reported inconsistently in patients with CFS. These findings defy correlation with the majority of patients and fail to provide a unified explanation for CFS. A history of food, inhalant, or drug allergy is reported by 55–80% of patients. No characteristic profile of immune dysfunction has been identified, and the values of the laboratory immunologic changes are usually not outside the normal range. Similarly, imaging studies of the brain have not identified reproducible abnormalities.

CLINICAL MANIFESTATIONS. The dominant symptoms of CFS include fatigue that contributes to loss of activity, cognitive problems, nonrestorative sleep, pain, and an increased level of illness following physical or mental activity. Fatigue as a symptom should not be dismissed as a minor ailment, but consideration needs to be given to the consequences of both the fatigue and the accompanying symptoms. Although the primary symptom of fatigue is perceived as subjective, the presence and magnitude of impairment, as well as the number and magnitude of associated symptoms, can be measured. The syndrome is characterized by fatigue of >6 mo duration associated with significant impairment of the work or school schedule, recreation, and interpersonal relationships. Fatigue is generally manifested as lassitude, profound tiredness, intolerance to exertion with easy fatigability, and general malaise. Nonrestorative nighttime sleeping is common, but there are no common sleep abnormalities. Myalgias and arthralgias may accompany fatigue. Onset of new headache, sore throat, and lymph node tenderness are uncommon but continue to be included as symptom criteria for diagnosis. Cognitive problems and an increase in the magnitude of syndromic symptoms following mental or physical activity complete the definition requirements. There is concern that CFS might be mistaken for readily identifiable psychiatric disorders. Other physical symptoms (chest palpitations, visual blurring, nausea, dizziness, paresthesias, dry eyes and mouth, diarrhea, cough, night sweats, and rash) should suggest a diagnosis other than CFS. Weight loss, as seen in chronic infections or inflammatory conditions, is uncommon in CFS.

Patients diagnosed with CFS in primary-care practices relate an abrupt onset to their symptoms, often as part of an initial virus-like illness characterized by low-grade fever accompanied by sore throat and cough. Individuals identified in population-based studies describe a gradual onset of their illness.

Symptoms among adolescents are similar to those observed in adults. School absenteeism is a major problem, with two thirds missing >2 wk and one third requiring a home tutor. Resolution of symptoms, particularly if the onset follows an infection, as is common among adolescents as well as adults, usually follows within 2 yr of onset of the illness.

Abnormal physical examination findings are conspicuously absent, which provides reassurance to both the patient and the physician.

DIAGNOSIS. There are no pathognomonic signs or diagnostic tests for CFS. The diagnosis is a clinically defined condition based on inclusion and exclusion criteria (Fig. 120-1). The diagnostic criteria are applicable to adults and adolescents >11 yr of age because of the current requirement for a self-generated history. Reliance on parental history for diagnosis is fraught with confusion because of the inaccuracy of the historical information. An empiric definition has been tested in adults that enhances diagnostic reliability. The process relies on results of three readily available questionnaires: Multidimensional Fatigue Inventory, Medical Outcomes Short Form 36, and CDC Symptom Inventory.

CFS is difficult to diagnose in children, who have trouble describing their symptoms and articulating their concerns. Criteria have been developed to address the development of fatigue in relationship to immunization that are applicable to children >5 yr of age. CFS should be diagnosed in children or adults only after a thorough medical and psychiatric evaluation. Careful attention must be directed to the family dynamics to identify and

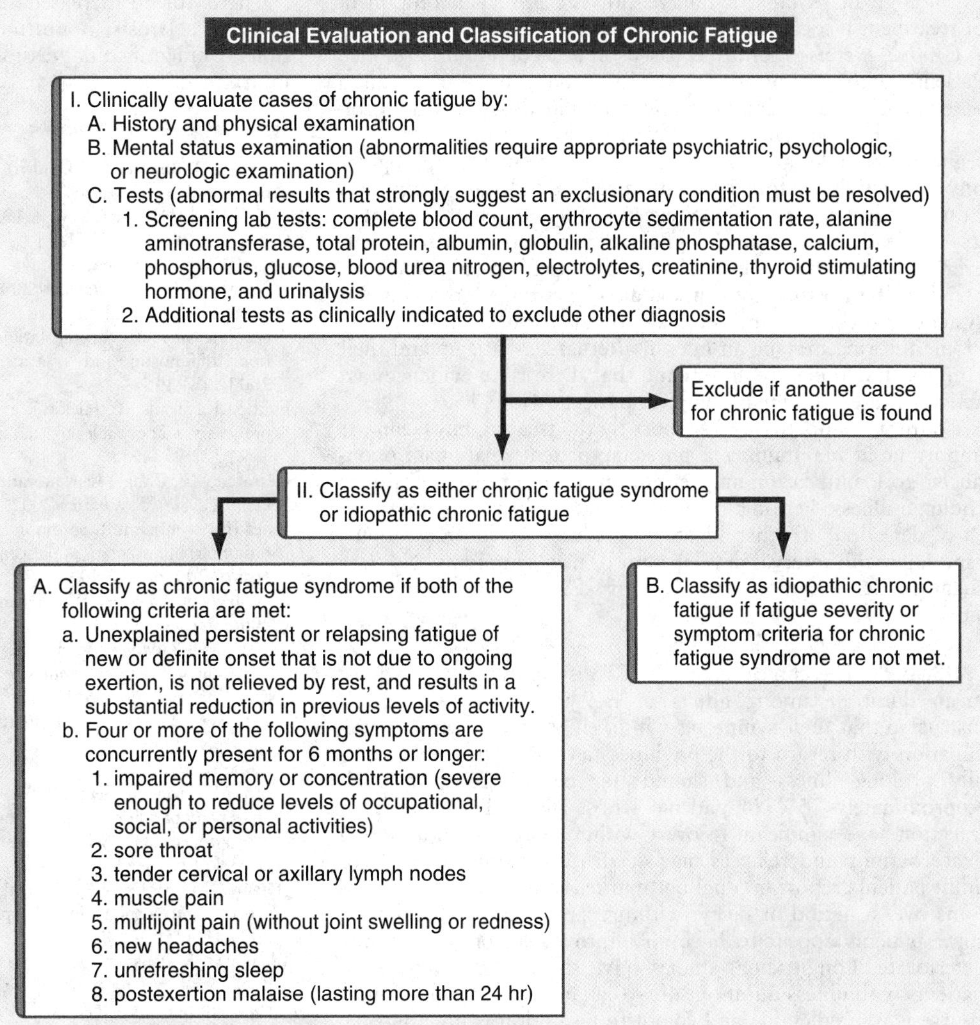

Clinical Evaluation and Classification of Chronic Fatigue
I. Clinically evaluate cases of chronic fatigue by:
A. History and physical examination
B. Mental status examination (abnormalities require appropriate psychiatric, psychologic, or neurologic examination)
C. Tests (abnormal results that strongly suggest an exclusionary condition must be resolved)
1. Screening lab tests: complete blood count, erythrocyte sedimentation rate, alanine aminotransferase, total protein, albumin, globulin, alkaline phosphatase, calcium, phosphorus, glucose, blood urea nitrogen, electrolytes, creatinine, thyroid stimulating hormone, and urinalysis
2. Additional tests as clinically indicated to exclude other diagnosis
Exclude if another cause for chronic fatigue is found
II. Classify as either chronic fatigue syndrome or idiopathic chronic fatigue
A. Classify as chronic fatigue syndrome if both of the following criteria are met:
a. Unexplained persistent or relapsing fatigue of new or definite onset that is not due to ongoing exertion, is not relieved by rest, and results in a substantial reduction in previous levels of activity.
b. Four or more of the following symptoms are concurrently present for 6 months or longer:
1. impaired memory or concentration (severe enough to reduce levels of occupational, social, or personal activities)
2. sore throat
3. tender cervical or axillary lymph nodes
4. muscle pain
5. multijoint pain (without joint swelling or redness)
6. new headaches
7. unrefreshing sleep
8. postexertion malaise (lasting more than 24 hr)
B. Classify as idiopathic chronic fatigue if fatigue severity or symptom criteria for chronic fatigue syndrome are not met.

Figure 120-1. The clinical evaluation and classification of unexplained chronic fatigue. The case definition for chronic fatigue syndrome was proposed by the Centers for Disease Control and Prevention in 1988 (Holmes GP, Kaplan JE, Gantz NM, et al: Chronic fatigue syndrome: A working case definition. *Ann Intern Med* 1988;108:387–389) and refined and simplified by an international working group in 1994 (Fukuda K, Straus SE, Hickie I, et al: The chronic fatigue syndrome: A comprehensive approach to its definition and study. *Ann Intern Med* 1994;121: 953–959).

resolve family problems or psychopathology that may be contributing to a child's perceptions of his or her symptoms. Applying the label of CFS may delay the diagnosis of a treatable medical illness, avoid the detection of psychologic problems or family dysfunction, and perpetuate inappropriate illness behaviors that may have a profound effect on the child's psychosocial development.

The diagnosis of CFS can be established only after alternative medical and psychiatric causes of fatigue, many of which are treatable, have been excluded. These include any medical condition that may explain the presence of chronic fatigue, such as untreated hypothyroidism, sleep apnea, narcolepsy, drug abuse, an adverse effect of medication, or severe obesity as defined by a body mass index [body mass index = weight in kg/(height in meters)^2] of >45. A previously diagnosed medical condition with uncertain resolution that may explain chronic fatigue should be clarified, such as unresolved cases of hepatitis B or C virus infection. CFS should not be diagnosed in persons with prior diagnoses of a major depressive disorder with psychotic or melancholic features, bipolar affective disorders, schizophrenia of any subtype, delusional disorders of any subtype, dementias of any subtype, anorexia nervosa, bulimia nervosa, or alcohol or other substance abuse within 2 yr before the onset of the chronic fatigue or at any time afterward.

Fibromyalgia is a relatively common rheumatic syndrome characterized by widespread musculoskeletal pain in addition to numerous specific tender point sites (see Chapter 167) and symptoms similar to those of CFS. Fibromyalgia and CFS may be diagnosed in the same patient since both are diagnoses by definition and both lack confirmatory laboratory findings.

Although evaluation of each patient should be individualized, initial laboratory evaluation should be limited to screening laboratory tests to provide reassurance of the lack of significant organic dysfunction (see Fig. 120-1). Further tests should be directed primarily toward excluding treatable diseases that may be suggested by the symptoms or physical findings that are present in specific patients. Diagnostic evaluation of chronic fatigue should include psychologic evaluation for anxiety and depression disorders, which should precede exhaustive searches for organic causes.

TREATMENT. Development of definitive treatment for CFS awaits delineation of the causes of the symptoms. No specific therapeutic agents are recommended. Cognitive behavioral therapy and graded exercise therapy are the only interventions that have been shown to be beneficial.

Cognitive behavioral therapy is directed at changing condition-related cognitions and behaviors through explanation, challenging and changing cognition of fatigue-related symptoms, developing coping skills, emotional support for patients and their families, relief of symptoms that actually interfere with function, and minimizing unnecessary and misleading diagnostic and therapeutic tests. Particular attention should be made to identification and specialist treatment of sleep disorders and disturbances.

Psychologic or psychiatric intervention is a principal component of treatment if a co-morbid psychiatric disorder is present.

Graded exercise therapy is based on a deconditioning model. Patients with limitation of activity should be started on a schedule of graded remobilization determined by individual tolerance and, if warranted, physical therapy leading to a regular regimen of moderate exercise. The key element is stopping the physical activity before becoming tired or inducing symptoms. Complete bed rest and lack of exercise only perpetuate immobility and lead to deconditioning; rapid remobilization, for whatever reason, usually exacerbates symptoms and should be avoided. Return to school should also be initiated gradually but systematically to resume normal attendance and socialization. Home tutoring may be an interim alternative. Patients and their families should clearly understand that there is no evidence that activity causes permanent harm in patients with CFS.

Continued empathy and support by the treating physician are important in maintaining a physician-patient relationship conducive to identification and resolution of both organic and psychologic illness. Periodic medical re-evaluation is warranted for early detection of other identifiable causes of chronic fatigue, especially with interval development of new symptoms. No data suggest relief of symptoms or cure of CFS by dietary or vitamin supplements.

PROGNOSIS. The clinical course of CFS is highly variable with a mean duration among adults of 3–9 yr. Patients should be instructed that their symptoms will likely wax and wane. Preoccupation with return to the pre-illness level of activity can actually prolong illness and should not be a short-term goal. Approximately 75% of patients whose illness began with an infection have significant recovery within 2 yr of onset, although exacerbations and relapses may occur. Approximately 60% of adult patients report gradual but marked improvement in symptoms over a period of 2–3 yr without specific therapy, although some patients appear to have no improvement or occasionally deteriorate. Longitudinal studies have shown improvement in patients with illness durations of >10 yr, but the eventual clinical course is unpredictable and complete resolution is not the rule. Patients who deal with stress by somatization and who deny the modulating role of psychosocial factors have a less favorable prognosis.

Children and adolescents with chronic fatiguing illnesses appear to have a more optimistic outcome, typically with an undulating course of gradual but substantial symptomatic improvement, or full recovery, 1–4 yr after diagnosis, and an overall good functional outcome in 80% of cases. Poor prognostic factors include increasing time missed from school, lower socioeconomic status, chronic maternal health problems, and untreated co-morbid individual or family psychiatric disorders.

There are no increased risks of cancer, autoimmune disease, multiple sclerosis, opportunistic infections, or other complications. Unidentified depression, however, can lead to self-inflicted injury or death.

Cameron B, Bharadwaj M, Burrows J, et al: Prolonged illness after infectious mononucleosis is associated with altered immunity but not with increased viral load. *J Infect Dis* 2006;193:664–671.

Capuron L, Welberg L, Heim C, et al: Cognitive dysfunction relates to subjective report of mental fatigue in patients with chronic fatigue syndrome. *Neuropsychopharmacology* 2006;31:1777–1784.

Carruthers BM, Jain AK, De Meirleir KL, et al: Myalgic encephalomyelitis/chronic fatigue syndrome: Clinical working case definition, diagnostic and treatment protocols. *J Chronic Fatigue Syndr* 2003;11:7–115.

Fukuda K, Straus SE, Hickie I, et al: The chronic fatigue syndrome: A comprehensive approach to its definition and study. *Ann Intern Med* 1994;121:953–959.

Gerralda ME, Rangel L: Annotation: Chronic fatigue syndrome in children. *J Child Psychol Psychiatry* 2002;43:169–176.

Jones JF, Nisenbaum R, Solomon L, et al: Chronic fatigue syndrome and other fatiguing illnesses in adolescents: A population-based study. *J Adolesc Health* 2004;35:34–40.

Prins JB, van der Meer JW, Bleijenberg G: Chronic fatigue syndrome. *Lancet* 2006;367:346–355.

Reeves WC, Lloyd A, Vernon SD, et al: Identification of ambiguities in the 1994 chronic fatigue syndrome research case definition and recommendations for resolution. *BMC Health Serv Res* 2003;3:25.

Reeves WC, Wagner D, Nisenbaum R, et al: Chronic fatigue syndrome—a clinically empirical approach to its definition and study. *BMC Med* 2005;3:19.

Smith MS, Martin-Herz SP, Womack WM, et al: Comparative study of anxiety, depression, somatization, functional disability, and illness attrition in adolescents with chronic fatigue or migraine. *Pediatrics* 2003;111:e376–e381.

Stewart JM, McLeod KJ, Sanyal S, et al: Relation of postural vagovagal syncope to splanchnic hypervolemia in adolescents. *Circulation* 2004;110:2575–2581.

Tanaka H, Matsushima R, Tamai H, et al: Impaired postural cerebral hemodynamics in young patients with chronic fatigue with and without orthostatic intolerance. *J Pediatr* 2002;140:412–417.

ter Wolbeek M, van Doornen LJ, Kavelaars A, Heijnen CJ: Severe fatigue in adolescents: a common phenomenon? *Pediatrics* 2006;117:e1078–e1086.

Wagner D, Nisenbaum R, Heim C, et al: Psychometric properties of the CDC symptom inventory for the assessment of chronic fatigue syndrome. *Popul Health Metr* 2005;3:8.

White PD, Thomas JM, Sullivan PF, Buchwald D: The nosology of sub-acute and chronic fatigue syndromes that follow infectious mononucleosis. *Psychol Med* 2004;34:499–507.

Whiting P, Bagnall AM, Sowden AJ, et al: Interventions for the treatment and management of chronic fatigue syndrome: A systematic review. *JAMA* 2001;286:1360–1368.

Part XIII ▪ Immunology

Section 1 — Evaluation of the Immune System — Rebecca H. Buckley

Chapter 121 ▪ Evaluation of Suspected Immunodeficiency

Recurrent infections or fevers in children are among the most frequent clinical dilemmas for primary care physicians. The number of children suspected of having primary or secondary immunodeficiency far exceeds the number of actual cases, as most patients with recurrent infections do not have an identifiable immunodeficiency disorder. A major reason for the apparent high rate of recurrent infections among children is repeated exposure to infectious agents in child care and other group settings.

Primary care physicians must have a high index of suspicion if defects of the immune system are to be diagnosed early enough that appropriate treatment can be instituted before irreversible damage develops. Diagnosis of primary immune defects is difficult in part because these defects are not screened for during the perinatal period or early childhood. Extensive use of antibiotics by physicians has masked the classic presentation of many of the primary immunodeficiency diseases. Evaluation of immune function should be initiated for children with clinical manifestations of a specific immune disorder or with unusual, chronic, or recurrent infections such as (1) one or more systemic bacterial infections (sepsis, meningitis); (2) two or more serious respiratory or documented bacterial infections (cellulitis, draining otitis media, pneumonia, lymphadenitis) within 1 yr; (3) serious infections occurring at unusual sites (liver, brain abscess); (4) infections with unusual pathogens *(Aspergillus, Serratia marcescens, Nocardia, Burkholderia cepacia);* and (5) infections with common childhood pathogens but of unusual severity. Additional clues to immunodeficiency include: ≥8 ear infections per yr; ≥2 serious sinus infections per yr; ≥2 mo treatment with antibiotics with poor results; failure to thrive with or without chronic diarrhea; and the need for intravenous antibiotics to successfully treat an infection usually treated with oral antibiotics. Certain clinical features suggestive of immunodeficiency syndromes are noted in Tables 121-1 and 121-2.

Children with defects in antibody production, phagocytic cells, or complement proteins have recurrent infections with encapsulated bacteria and may grow and develop normally despite their recurring infections, unless they develop bronchiectasis from repeated lower respiratory tract bacterial infections or persistent enteroviral infections of the central nervous system. Patients with only repeated viral infections (with the exception of persistent enterovirus infections) are not as likely to have these types of disorders. By contrast, patients with deficiencies in T-cell function usually develop opportunistic infections early in life and fail to thrive (Table 121-3).

The initial evaluation of immunocompetence includes a thorough history, physical examination, and family history (Table 121-4). Most immunologic defects can be excluded at minimal cost with the proper choice of screening tests, which should be broadly informative, reliable, and cost-effective (Table 121-5 and Fig. 121-1). A complete blood count (CBC), manual differential count, and erythrocyte sedimentation rate (ESR) are among the most cost-effective screening tests. If the ESR is normal, chronic bacterial or fungal infection is unlikely. If an infant's neutrophil count is persistently elevated to extreme levels in the absence of any signs of infection, a leukocyte adhesion deficiency should be suspected. If the absolute neutrophil count is normal, congenital and acquired neutropenias and leukocyte adhesion defects are excluded. If the absolute lymphocyte count is normal, the patient is not likely to have a severe T-cell defect because T cells normally constitute 70% of circulating lymphocytes and their absence results in striking lymphopenia. Normal lymphocyte counts are higher in infancy and early childhood than later in life (Fig. 121-2). Knowledge of the normal values for absolute lymphocyte counts at various ages in infancy and childhood (see Chapter 716) is crucial in the detection of T-cell defects. At 9 mo of age, an age when infants affected with severe T-cell immunodeficiency are likely to present, the lower limit of normal is 4,500 lymphocytes/mm^3. Absence of Howell-Jolly bodies by microscopic examination of erythrocytes rules against congenital asplenia. Normal platelet size or count excludes Wiskott-Aldrich syndrome. If a CBC and a manual differential were performed on the cord blood of all infants, severe combined immunodeficiency (SCID) could be detected at birth by the identification of lymphopenia, and lifesaving immunologic reconstitution could then be provided to all affected infants.

Patients found to have abnormalities on any screening tests should be characterized as fully as possible before any type of immunologic treatment is begun, unless there is a life-threatening illness (Table 121-6). Some "abnormalities" may prove to be laboratory artifacts and, conversely, an apparently straightforward diagnosis may prove to be a much more complex disorder. For patients with recurrent or unusual bacterial infections, evaluation of T-cell and phagocytic cell functions is indicated if results of the initial screening tests including the CBC and manual differential, immunoglobulin levels, and complement levels are normal.

Collectively, congenital immunodeficiency diseases representing antibody deficiencies, T-cell or combined B- and T-cell deficiencies, neutrophil disorders, and complement deficiencies have an estimated incidence of 1 : 10,000 births (Table 121-7). This is higher than some disorders that are part of the newborn metabolic screening program (phenylketonuria [PKU] is 1 : 16,000) (see Chapter 84). The genes for many congenital immunodeficiency diseases are known, which may lead to successful neonatal screening programs. This is valuable because treatments are available, but many affected patients may die before an accurate diagnosis is determined.

B CELLS. Antibody production by B cells is easily evaluated by serum immunoglobulin levels as well as determination of antibodies to specific antigens or after vaccination.

A simple screening test for B-cell defects is the measurement of serum IgA. If the IgA level is normal, selective IgA deficiency, which is the most common B-cell defect, is excluded, as are most of the permanent types of hypogammaglobulinemia since IgA is usually very low or absent in those conditions. If IgA is low, IgG and IgM should also be measured. Patients who are receiving

TABLE 121-1. Characteristic Clinical Patterns in Some Primary Immunodeficiencies

FEATURES	DIAGNOSIS
IN NEWBORNS AND YOUNG INFANTS (0 TO 6 MONTHS)	
Hypocalcemia, heart disease, unusual facies	DiGeorge anomaly
Delayed umbilical cord detachment, leukocytosis, recurrent infections	Leukocyte adhesion defect
Diarrhea, pneumonia, thrush, failure to thrive	Severe combined immunodeficiency
Maculopapular rash, alopecia, lymphadenopathy	Severe combined immunodeficiency with graft-versus-host disease
Bloody stools, draining ears, eczema	Wiskott-Aldrich syndrome
Mouth ulcers, neutropenia, recurrent infections	XL-Hyper IgM syndrome
IN INFANCY AND YOUNG CHILDREN (6 MONTHS TO 5 YEARS)	
Severe progressive infectious mononucleosis	X-linked lymphoproliferative syndrome
Recurrent cutaneous and/or systemic staphylococcal abscesses, coarse facial features	Hyper-IgE syndrome
Persistent thrush, nail dystrophy, endocrinopathies	Chronic mucocutaneous candidiasis
Short stature, fine hair, severe varicella	Cartilage hair hypoplasia with short-limbed dwarfism
Oculocutaneous albinism, recurrent infection	Chédiak-Higashi syndrome
Lymphadenopathy, dermatitis, pneumonia, osteomyelitis	Chronic granulomatous disease
IN OLDER CHILDREN (OLDER THAN 5 YEARS) AND ADULTS	
Progressive dermatomyositis with chronic enterovirus encephalitis	X-linked agammaglobulinemia
Sinopulmonary infections, neurologic deterioration, telangiectasia	Ataxia-telangiectasia
Recurrent neisserial meningitis	C6, C7, or C8 deficiency
Sinopulmonary infections, malabsorption, splenomegaly, autoimmunity	Common variable immunodeficiency
Candidiasis with raw egg ingestion	Biotin-dependent cocarboxylase deficiency

From Stiehm ER, Ochs HD, Winkelstein JA: *Immunologic Disorders in Infants and Children,* 5th ed. Philadelphia, Elsevier/Saunders, 2004.

TABLE 121-2. Common Clinical Features of Immunodeficiency

Usually present	Recurrent upper respiratory infections
	Severe bacterial infections
	Persistent infections with incomplete or no response to therapy
	Paucity of lymph nodes and tonsils
Often present	Persistent sinusitis or mastoiditis *(Streptococcus pneumoniae, Haemophilus, Moraxella catarrhalis, Staphylococcus aureus, Pseudomonas* spp.*)*
	Recurrent bronchitis or pneumonia
	Failure to thrive or growth retardation for infants or children; weight loss for adults
	Intermittent fever
	Infection with unusual organisms
	Skin lesions: rash, seborrhea, pyoderma, necrotic abscesses, alopecia, eczema, telangiectasia
	Recalcitrant thrush
	Diarrhea and malabsorption
	Hearing loss due to chronic otitis
	Chronic conjunctivitis
	Arthralgia or arthritis
	Bronchiectasis
	Evidence of autoimmunity, especially autoimmune thrombocytopenia or hemolytic anemia
	Hematologic abnormalities: aplastic anemia, hemolytic anemia, neutropenia, thrombocytopenia
	History of prior surgery, biopsy
Occasionally present	Lymphadenopathy
	Hepatosplenomegaly
	Severe viral disease (e.g., varicella, herpes simplex)
	Chronic encephalitis
	Recurrent meningitis
	Deep infections: cellulitis, osteomyelitis, organ abscesses
	Chronic gastrointestinal disease, infections, lymphoid hyperplasia, sprue-like syndrome, atypical inflammatory bowel disease
	Autoimmune disease such as autoimmune thrombocytopenia, hemolytic anemia, rheumatologic disease, alopecia, thyroiditis, pernicious anemia
	Pyoderma gangrenosum
	Adverse reaction to vaccines
	Delayed umbilical cord detachment
	Chronic stomatitis or peritonitis

From Goldman L, Ausiello D: *Cecil Textbook of Medicine,* 22nd edition. Philadelphia, WB Saunders, 2004; p. 1598.

corticosteroids or who have protein-losing states (enephrosis, protein-losing enteropathy) often have low serum IgG concentrations but produce antibodies normally. Thus, if immunoglobulins are low, it is crucial before starting intravenous immunoglobulin (IVIG) therapy that antibody titers to specific antigens are obtained to determine whether the levels are low because of inadequate antibody synthesis or due to protein loss. Antibody titers are uninterpretable after the patient has received IVIG, which contains antibodies from a minimum of 60,000 normal donors.

One of the most useful tests for B-cell function is to determine the presence and titer of **isohemagglutinins,** or antibodies to type A and B red blood cell polysaccharide antigens. This test measures predominantly IgM antibodies. Isohemagglutinins may be absent normally in the 1st 2 yr of life and are always absent if the patient is blood type AB.

Because most infants and children are immunized with diphtheria-tetanus-pertussis (DTaP), conjugated *Haemophilus influenzae* type b (Hib), and pneumococcal conjugate vaccine (PCV7), it is often informative to test for specific antibodies to diphtheria, tetanus, *H. influenzae* polyribose phosphate, and pneumococcal antigens. If the titers are low, measurement of antibodies to diphtheria or tetanus toxoids before and 2 wk after a pediatric DTaP or DT booster is helpful in assessing the capacity to form IgG antibodies to protein antigens. To evaluate a patient's ability to respond to polysaccharide antigens, anti-pneumococcal antibodies can be measured before and 3 wk after immunization with pneumococcal polysaccharide vaccine (PPV23) in patients >2–3 yr. Antibodies detected in these tests are of the IgG isotype. These antibody studies can be performed in several different laboratories, but it is important to choose a reliable laboratory and to use the same laboratory for all samples. In children >2 yr of age with low anti-pneumococcal antibody titers, it is useful to boost with conjugate pneumococcal vaccine twice, 1 mo apart, before giving a polysaccharide pneumococcal vaccine 1 mo later and then measuring antibody titers 3 wk later. Patients with significant or permanent B-cell defects do not produce either IgM or IgG antibodies normally. If results of these tests prove to be normal and the immunoglobulins remain low, studies should be performed to evaluate the possible loss of immunoglobulins through the urinary or gastrointestinal tracts (nephrotic syndrome, protein-losing enteropathies, intestinal lymphangiectasia).

TABLE 121-3. Characteristic Features of Primary Immunodeficiency

CHARACTERISTIC	PREDOMINANT T-CELL DEFECT	PREDOMINANT B-CELL DEFECT	GRANULOCYTE DEFECT	COMPLEMENT DEFECT
Age at the onset of infection	Early onset, usually 2–6 mo of age	Onset after maternal antibodies diminish, usually after 5–7 mo of age, later childhood to adulthood	Early onset	Onset at any age
Specific pathogens involved	Bacteria: mycobacteria	Bacteria: streptococci, staphylococci, *Haemophilus, Campylobacter*	Bacteria: staphylococci, *Pseudomonas, Serratia, Klebsiella*	Bacteria: *Neisseria, Escherichia coli*
	Viruses: CMV, EBV, adenovirus, parainfluenza 3, varicella, enterovirus	Viruses: enterovirus*		
	Fungi and parasites: *Candida;* opportunistic infection, PCP	Fungi and parasites: giardia, cryptosporidia	Fungi and parasites: *Candida; Nocardia, Aspergillus*	
Affected organs	Failure to thrive, protracted diarrhea, extensive mucocutaneous candidiasis	Recurrent sinopulmonary infections, chronic gastrointestinal symptoms, malabsorption, arthritis, enteroviral meningoencephalitis*	Skin abscesses: dermatitis, impetigo, cellulitis Lymph nodes: suppurative adenitis Oral cavity: periodontitis, ulcers internal organs, abscesses, osteomyelitis	Infections: meningitis, arthritis, septicemia, recurrent sinopulmonary infections
Special features	Graft-versus-host disease caused by maternal engraftment or nonirradiated blood transfusion; Postvaccination, disseminated BCG or varicella; hypocalcemic tetany in infancy†	Autoimmunity, lymphoreticular malignancy: lymphoma, thymoma; postvaccination paralytic polio	Prolonged attachment of umbilical cord, poor wound healing	Rheumatoid disorders: SLE, vasculitis, dermatomyositis, scleroderma, glomerulonephritis, angioedema

*X-linked (Bruton's) agammaglobulinemia.
†DiGeorge anomaly.
BCG, bacille Calmette-Guérin; CMV, cytomegalovirus; EBV, Epstein-Barr virus; PCP, *Pneumocystis carinii;* SLE, systemic lupus erythematosus.
From Woroniecka M, Ballow M: Office evaluation of children with recurrent infection. *Pediatr Clin North Am* 2000;47:1211–1224.

TABLE 121-4. Special Physical Features Associated with Immunodeficiency Disorders

CLINICAL FEATURES	DISORDERS
DERMATOLOGIC	
Eczema	T-cell defects, T- or B-cell immune deficiency, Wiskott-Aldrich syndrome, IPEX
Sparse and/or hypopigmented hair	Cartilage hair hypoplasia, Chediak-Higashi syndrome, Griscelli's syndrome
Ocular telangiectasia	Ataxia-telangiectasia
Oculocutaneous albinism	Chediak-Higashi syndrome
Severe dermatitis	SCID with acute GVHD, Omenn syndrome
Recurrent abscesses, of lung especially	Hyper-IgE syndrome
Recurrent organ abscesses, liver and rectum especially	Chronic granulomatous disease
Recurrent skin infections, abscesses	Leukocyte adhesion defect, hyper-IgE syndrome
Oral ulcers	Hyper-IgM syndrome, AID (cytokine deaminase)
Peridontitis, gingivitis, stomatitis	Neutrophil defects, hyper-IgM syndrome
Oral or nail candidiasis	T-cell immune defects; combined defects; mucocutaneous candidiasis, hyper-IgE syndrome
Vitiligo	B-cell defects, mucocutaneous candidiasis
Alopecia	B-cell defects, mucocutaneous candidiasis
Chronic conjunctivitis	B-cell defects
EXTREMITIES	
Clubbing of the nails	Chronic lung disease due to antibody defects
Arthritis	Antibody defects, Wiskott-Aldrich syndrome, hyper-IgM
ENDOCRINOLOGIC	
Hypoparathyroidism	DiGeorge's syndrome, mucocutaneous candidiasis
Endocrinopathies (autoimmune)	Mucocutaneous candidiasis
Growth hormone deficiency	X-linked agammaglobulinemia
Gonadal dysgenesis	Mucocutaneous candidiasis
HEMATOLOGIC	
Hemolytic anemia	B- and T-cell immune defects, ALPS
Thrombocytopenia, small platelets	Wiskott-Aldrich syndrome
Neutropenia	Hyper-IgM syndrome, Wiskott-Aldrich variant
Immune thrombocytopenia	B-cell immune defects, ALPS
SKELETAL	
Short-limb dwarfism	Short-limb dwarfism with T- and/or B-cell immune defects
Bony dysplasia	ADA deficiency, SCID

ADA, adenosine deaminase deficiency; AID, activation-induced cytidine deaminase; ALPS, autoimmune lymphoproliferative syndrome; GVHD, graft-versus-host disease; Ig, immunoglobulin; IPEX, X-linked immune dysfunction enteropathy polyendocrinopathy; SCID, severe combined immunodeficiency.
From Goldman L, Ausiello D: *Cecil Textbook of Medicine,* 22nd edition. Philadelphia, WB Saunders, 2004, p. 1599.

Very high serum concentrations of one or more immunoglobulin classes suggest HIV infection, chronic granulomatous disease, or autoimmune lymphoproliferative syndrome (ALPS).

IgG subclass measurements are seldom helpful in assessing immune function in children with recurrent infections. It is difficult to know the biologic significance of the various mild to moderate deficiencies of IgG subclasses, particularly when completely asymptomatic individuals have been described as totally lacking IgG1, IgG2, IgG4, and/or IgA1 owing to immunoglobulin heavy chain gene deletions. Many healthy children have been described as having low levels of IgG2 but normal responses to polysaccharide antigens when immunized. When children with low IgG2 subclass levels and histories of frequent infections were studied in depth, they were found to have broader immunologic dysfunction, including poor responses to protein antigens, suggest-

TABLE 121-5. Initial Immunologic Testing of the Child with Recurrent Infections

COMPLETE BLOOD COUNT, MANUAL DIFFERENTIAL, AND ERYTHROCYTE SEDIMENTATION RATE
Absolute lymphocyte count (normal result [see Chapter 716] rules against T-cell defect)
Absolute neutrophil count (normal result [see Chapter 716] rules against congenital or acquired neutropenia and [usually] both forms of leukocyte adhesion deficiency, in which elevated counts are present even between infections)
Platelet count (normal result excludes Wiskott-Aldrich syndrome)
Howell-Jolly bodies (absence rules against asplenia)
Erythrocyte sedimentation rate (normal result indicates chronic bacterial or fungal infection unlikely)

SCREENING TESTS FOR B-CELL DEFECTS
IgA measurement; if abnormal, IgG and IgM measurement
Isohemagglutinins
Antibody titers to tetanus, diphtheria, *Haemophilus influenzae,* and pneumococcus

SCREENING TESTS FOR T-CELL DEFECTS
Absolute lymphocyte count (normal result indicates T-cell defect unlikely)
Candida albicans intradermal skin test: 0.1 mL of a 1 : 1,000 dilution for patients ≥6 yr, 0.1 mL of a 1 : 100 dilution for patients <6 yr

SCREENING TESTS FOR PHAGOCYTIC CELL DEFECTS
Absolute neutrophil count
Respiratory burst assay

SCREENING TEST FOR COMPLEMENT DEFICIENCY
CH_{50}

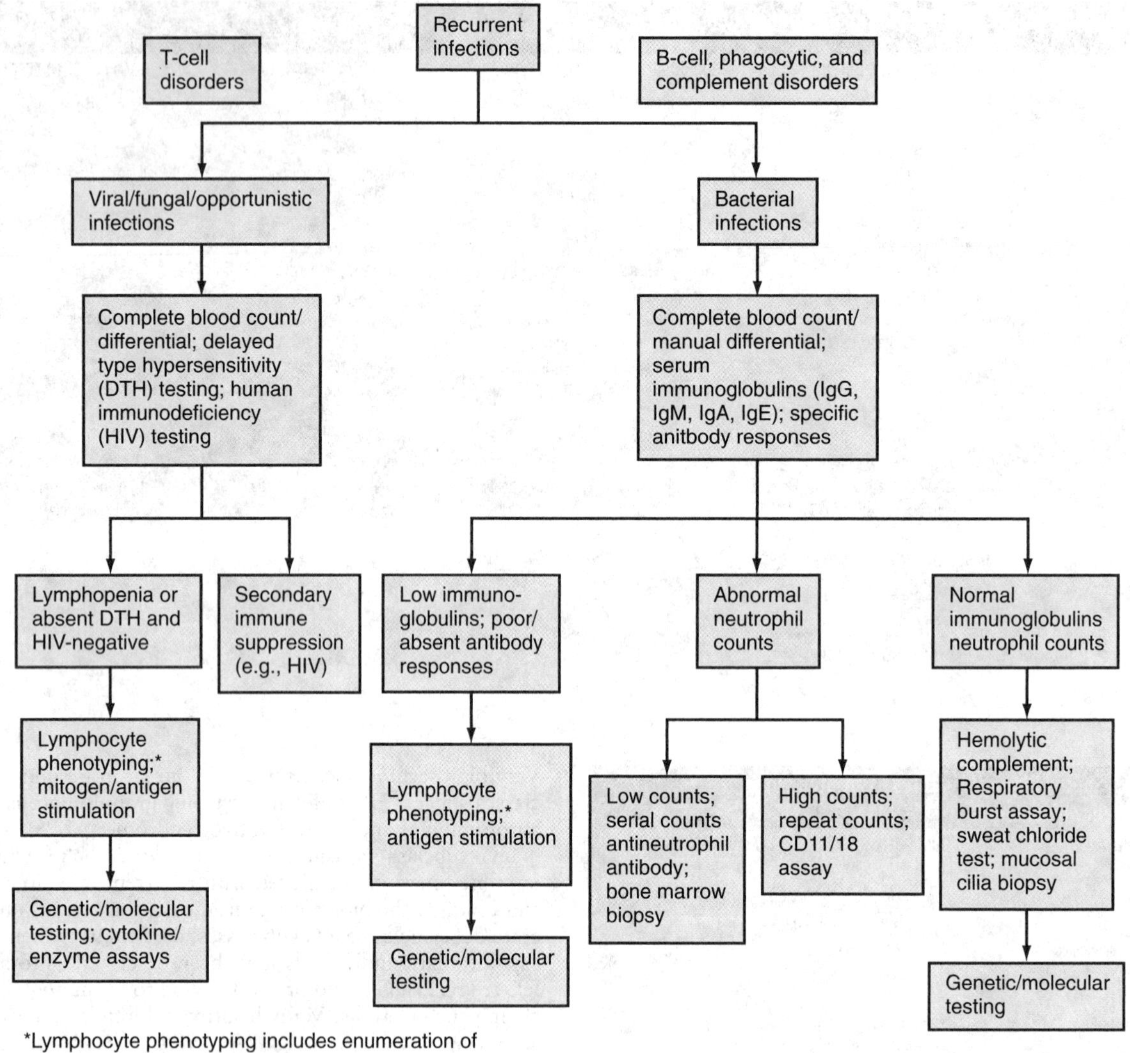

Figure 121-1. A diagnostic testing algorithm for primary immunodeficiency diseases. DTH, delayed type hypersensitivity. (From Lindegren ML, Kobrynski L, Rasmussen SA: Applying public health strategies to primary immunodeficiency diseases: A potential approach to genetic disorders. *MMWR Recomm Rep* 2004;53(RR-1):1–29.)

ing that they may have been in the process of developing into **common variable immunodeficiency (CVID)**. Only when profound antibody deficiencies are detected despite normal levels of immunoglobulins are IgG subclass measurements occasionally helpful. Children who completely lack IgG2 are usually unable to make antibodies to polysaccharide antigens, although this may occur among individuals with normal IgG2. Thus, specific antibody measurements are far more cost-effective than IgG subclass determinations.

Patients found to be **agammaglobulinemic** should have their blood B cells enumerated by **flow cytometry** using dye-conjugated monoclonal antibodies to B-cell–specific CD antigens (usually CD19 or CD20). Normally, approximately 10% of circulating lymphocytes are B cells. B cells are absent in X-linked agammaglobulinemia (XLA), and present in CVID, IgA deficiency, and hyper-IgM syndromes. This distinction is important because children with hypogammaglobulinemia from XLA and CVID can have different clinical problems, and the two conditions clearly have different inheritance patterns. Patients with XLA have a heightened susceptibility to persistent enteroviral infections, whereas those with CVID have more problems with autoimmune diseases and lymphoid hyperplasia. Specific molecular diagnostic tests for XLA (see Chapter 123.1) are necessary in cases without a family history to aid genetic counseling. Molecular testing is also indicated in other B-cell defects.

T CELLS. The ***Candida* skin test** is the most cost-effective test of T-cell function. Adults and children older than 6 yr of age should be tested by intradermal injection with 0.1 mL of a 1 : 1,000 dilution of a known potent *Candida albicans* extract. If the test result is negative at 24 hr, 48 hr, and 72 hr, a 1 : 100 dilution should be used, which can also be used for the initial testing of children <6 yr of age. If the *Candida* skin test result is positive, as defined by erythema and induration of ≥10 mm at 48 hr and that is greater than at 24 hr, all primary T-cell defects are precluded, which obviates the need for more expensive in vitro tests such as lymphocyte phenotyping or assessments of responses to mitogens.

T cells and T-cell subpopulations can be enumerated by **flow cytometry** using dye-conjugated monoclonal antibodies recognizing CD antigens present on T cells (i.e., CD2, CD3, CD4, and CD8). This is a particularly important test to perform on any infant who is lymphopenic, because $CD3^+$ T cells usually constitute 70% of peripheral lymphocytes. Infants with SCID are unable to produce T cells and so are lymphopenic at birth. SCID is a pediatric emergency that can be successfully treated by stem cell marrow transplantation in >95% of cases if diagnosed before

TABLE 121-6. Laboratory Tests in Immunodeficiency

SCREENING TESTS	ADVANCED TESTS	RESEARCH/SPECIAL TESTS
B-CELL DEFICIENCY		
IgG, IgM, IgA levels	B-cell enumeration (CD19 or CD20)	Advanced B-cell phenotyping
Isoagglutinin titers	IgG subclass levels	Biopsies (e.g., lymph nodes)
Ab response to vaccine antigens (e.g., tetanus, diphtheria, rubeola, *Haemophilus influenzae*)	IgD and IgE levels	Ab responses to special antigens (e.g., φX, KLH)
	Natural Ab titers (e.g., anti–streptolysin O, *Escherichia coli*)	Mutation analysis
	Ab responses to new vaccines (e.g., typhoid, pneumococcal vaccines)	
	Lateral pharyngeal x-ray study for adenoidal tissue	
T-CELL DEFICIENCY		
Lymphocyte count and morphology	T-cell subset enumeration (CD3, CD4, CD8)	Advance flow cytometry
Chest x-ray examination for thymic size*	Proliferative responses to mitogens, antigens, allogeneic cells	Cytokine and cytokine receptor analysis
		Cytotoxic assays (e.g., NK, CTL).
Delayed skin tests (e.g., *Candida*, tetanus toxoid)	HLA typing	Enzyme assays (e.g., ADA, PNP)
	Chromosome analysis	Thymic imaging
		T-cell receptor analysis
		T-cell activation studies
		Apoptosis studies
		Biopsies
		Mutation analysis
PHAGOCYTIC DEFICIENCY		
WBC count, morphology	Adhesion molecule assays (e.g., CD11b/CD18, selectin ligand)	
Respiratory burst assay	Bactericidal assays	Enzyme assays (e.g., MPO, G6PD, NADPH oxidase)
IgE level		Mutation analysis
COMPLEMENT DEFICIENCY		
CH_{50} activity	Opsonic assays	Alternative pathway activity
C3 level	Component assays	
C4 level	Activation assays (e.g., C3a, C4a, C4d, C5a)	

*In infants only.

Ab, Antibody; ADA, adenosine deaminase; ADCC, antibody-dependent cellular cytotoxicity; C, complement; CH, hemolytic complement; CTL, cytotoxic T lymphocyte; DR, class II histocompatibility antigen; G6PD, glucose-6-phosphate dehydrogenase; HLA, human leukocyte antigen; IFN, interferon; Ig, immunoglobulin; KLH, keyhole limpet hemocyanin; MIF, migration inhibition factor; MPO, myeloperoxidase; NADPH, nicotinamide adenine dinucleotide phosphate; NBT, nitroblue tetrazolium; NK, natural killer; PNP, purine nucleoside phosphorylase; WBC, white blood cell; φX, phage antigen.

From Stiehm ER, Ochs HD, Winkelstein JA: *Immunologic Disorders in Infants and Children,* 5th ed. Philadelphia, Elsevier/Saunders, 2004.

serious, untreatable infections develop. Normally, there are roughly twice as many $CD4^+$ (helper) T cells as there are $CD8^+$ (cytotoxic) T cells. Because there are examples of severe immunodeficiency in which phenotypically normal T cells are present, tests of T-cell function are far more informative and cost-effective than enumeration of T-cell subpopulations by flow cytometry. T cells are normally stimulated through their T-cell receptors (TCRs) by antigen present in the groove of major histocompatibility complex (MHC) molecules. The TCR can also be stimulated directly with **mitogens** such as phytohemagglutinin (PHA), concanavalin A (Con A), or pokeweed mitogen (PWM). After 3–5 days of incubation with the mitogen, the proliferation of T cells is measured by the incorporation of radiolabeled thymidine into DNA. Other stimulants that can be used to assess T-cell function in the same type of assay include antigens (*Candida*, tetanus toxoid) and allogeneic cells. Additional assays of T-cell function include the measurement of cytokine production by T lymphocytes stimulated with mitogens (see Table 121-6).

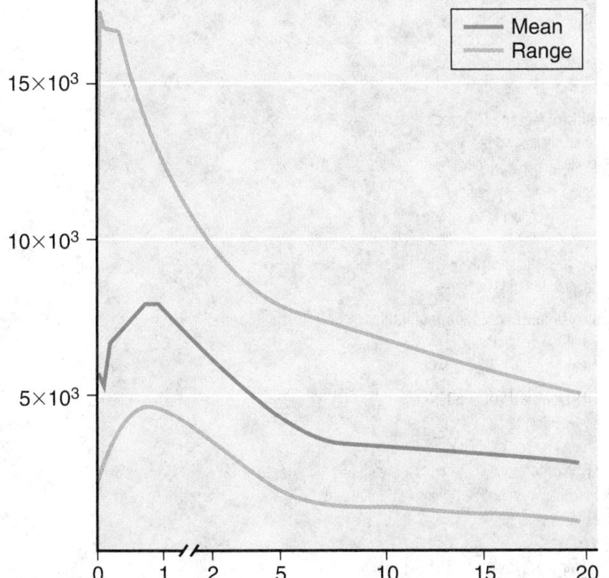

Figure 121-2. Absolute lymphocyte counts in normal individual during maturation. (Data graphed from Altman PL: *Blood and Other Body Fluids.* Prepared under the auspices of the Committee on Biological Handbooks. Washington, DC, Federation of American Societies for Experimental Biology, 1961.)

NK CELLS. Natural killer (NK) cells can be enumerated by flow cytometry using monoclonal antibodies to NK-specific CD antigens, usually CD16 or CD56. NK function is assessed by a radiolabeled chromium-release assay, using the cell line K562, which is readily killed by NK cells.

PHAGOCYTIC CELLS. Killing defects of phagocytic cells, which should be suspected if a patient has recurrent staphylococcal abscesses or gram-negative infections, can be evaluated by screening tests measuring the neutrophil respiratory burst after phorbol ester stimulation. The most reliable and useful test of this type is a flow cytometric assessment of the respiratory burst using rhodamine dye, which has replaced the nitroblue tetrazolium (NBT) dye test, which was plagued by technical problems with reproducibility. Leukocyte adhesion deficiencies can be easily diagnosed by flow cytometric assays of blood lymphocytes or neutrophils, using monoclonal antibodies to CD18 or CD11 (LAD1) or to CD15 (LAD2).

Phagocytic cell defects can be further defined according to their molecular cause. Mutations in the genes encoding four different

TABLE 121-7. 2003 Modified IUIS Classification of Primary and Secondary Immunodeficiencies

GROUPS AND DISEASES	INHERITANCE
A. PREDOMINANTLY ANTIBODY DEFICIENCIES	
XL agammaglobulinemia	XL
AR agammaglobulinemia	AR
Hyper-IgM syndromes	XL
a. XL	
b. AID defect	
c. CD40 defect	AR
d. UNG defect	
e. Other AR defects	AR
Ig heavy-chain gene deletions	AR
κ chain deficiency mutations	AR
Selective IgG class deficiencies	?
Selective IgA deficiency	Variable
Antibody deficiency with normal or elevated Igs	?
Common variable immunodeficiency	Variable
Transient hypogammaglobulinemia of infancy	?
B. COMBINED IMMUNODEFICIENCIES	
T^-B^+ SCID	
a. X-linked (γc deficiency)	XL
b. Autosomal recessive (Jak3 deficiency)	AR
c. IL-7 Rd deficiency	
T^-B^- SCID	
a. RAG-1/2 deficiency	AR
b. ADA deficiency	AR
c. Reticular dysgenesis	AR
d. Artemis defect	AR
T^+B^- SCID	
a. Omenn syndrome	AR
b. IL-2Rα deficiency	AR
Purine nucleoside phosphorylase deficiency	AR
MHC class II deficiency	AR
MHC class I deficiency caused by TAP-2 defect	AR
CD3γ or CD3ε deficiency	AR
CD8 deficiency (ZAP-70 defect)	AR
C. OTHER CELLULAR IMMUNODEFICIENCIES	
Wiskott-Aldrich syndrome	XL
Ataxia-telangiectasia	AR
DiGeorge anomaly	?
Primary CD4 deficiency	
Signal transduction deficiency	
D. DEFECTS OF PHAGOCYTIC FUNCTION	
Chronic granulomatous disease	
a. XL	XL
b. AR	AR
1. p22 phox deficiency	
2. p47 phox deficiency	
3. p67 phox deficiency	
Leukocyte adhesion defect 1	AR
Leukocyte adhesion defect 2	AR
Neutrophil G6PD deficiency	XL
Myeloperoxidase deficiency	AR
Secondary granule deficiency	AR
Schwachman syndrome	AR
Severe congenital neutropenia (Kostmann)	*AR*
Cyclic neutropenia (elastase defect)	*AR*
Leukocyte mycobacterial defects	*AR*
IFN-γR1 or R2 deficiency	AR
IFN-γR1 deficiency	AD
IL-12Rβ1 deficiency	AR
IL-12p40 deficiency	AR
STAT1 deficiency	AD
E. IMMUNODEFICIENCIES ASSOCIATED WITH LYMPHOPROLIFERATIVE DISORDERS	
Fas Deficiency	AD
Fas ligand deficiency	
FLICE or caspase 8 deficiency	
Unknown (caspase 3 deficiency)	
F. COMPLEMENT DEFICIENCIES	
C1q deficiency	AR
C1r deficiency	AR
C4 deficiency	AR
C2 deficiency	AR
C3 deficiency	AR
C5 deficiency	AR
C6 deficiency	AR
C7 deficiency	AR
C8α deficiency	AR
C8β deficiency	AR
C9 deficiency	AR
C1 inhibitor	AD
Factor I deficiency	AR
Factor H deficiency	AR
Factor D deficiency	AR
Properdin deficiency	XL
G. IMMUNODEFICIENCY ASSOCIATED WITH OR SECONDARY TO OTHER DISEASES	
Chromosomal Instability or Defective Repair	
Bloom syndrome	
Fanconi anemia	
ICF syndrome	
Nijmegen breakage syndrome	
Seckel syndrome	
Xeroderma pigmentosum	
Chromosomal Defects	
Down syndrome	
Turner syndrome	
Chromosome 18 rings and deletions	
Skeletal Abnormalities	
Short-limbed skeletal dysplasia	
Cartilage-hair hypoplasia	
Immunodeficiency with Generalized Growth Retardation	
Schimke immuno-osseous dysplasia	
Immunodeficiency with absent thumbs	
Dubowitz syndrome	
Growth retardation, facial anomalies, and immunodeficiency	
Progeria (Hutchinson-Gilford syndrome)	
Immunodeficiency with Dermatologic Defects	
Partial albinism	
Dyskeratosis congenita	
Netherton syndrome	
Acrodermatitis enteropathica	
Anhidrotic ectodermal dysplasia	
Papillon-Lefèvre syndrome	
Hereditary Metabolic Defects	
Transcobalamin 2 deficiency	
Methylmalonic acidemia	
Type 1 hereditary orotic aciduria	
Biotin-dependent carboxylase deficiency	
Mannosidosis	
Glycogen storage disease, type 1b	
Chédiak-Higashi syndrome	
Hypercatabolism of Immunoglobulin	
Familial hypercatabolism	
Intestinal lymphangiectasia	
H. OTHER IMMUNODEFICIENCIES	
Hyper-IgE syndrome	
Chronic mucocutaneous candidiasis	
Chronic mucocutaneous candidiasis with polyendocrinopathy (APECED)	AR
Hereditary or congenital hyposplenia or asplenia	
Ivemark syndrome	
IPEX syndrome	XL
Ectodermal dysplasia (NEMO defect)	XL

AD, autosomal dominant; ADA, adenosine deaminase; AID, activation-induced cytidine deaminase; AR, autosomal recessive; caspase, cysteinyl; aspartate, specific proteinase; FLICE, Fas-associating protein with death domain-like IL-1-converting enzyme; G6PD, glucose 6-phosphate dehydrogenase; ICF, immunodeficiency, centromeric instability, facial anomalies; IFN, interferon; Ig, immunoglobulin; IL, interleukin; IPEX, immune dysregulation, polyendocrinopathy, enteropathy; MHC, major histocompatibility complex; NEMO, IKK-gamma; SCID, severe combined immunodeficiency; TAP-2, transporter associated with antigen presentation; XL, X-linked.

Modified from [no authors listed]: Primary immunodeficiency diseases. Report of an International Union of Immunological Studies Scientific Committee. *Clin Exp Immunol* 1999;118:1–28; and Chapel H, Geha R, Rosen F; IUIS PID (Primary Immunodeficiencies) Classification committee: Primary immunodeficiency diseases: An update. *Clin Exp Immunol* 2003;132:9–15.

From Stiehm ER, Ochs HD, Winkelstein JA: *Immunologic Disorders in Infants and Children,* 5th ed. Philadelphia, Elsevier/Saunders, 2004.

components of the electron transport chain have been discovered in various patients with chronic granulomatous disease (CGD). It is important to identify the specific molecular type of CGD to provide appropriate genetic counseling, as one type is X linked and the other three types are autosomal recessive. Early diagnosis of leukocyte adhesion deficiency (LAD) is of crucial importance because stem cell transplantation can be lifesaving. A confirmatory test for LAD1, if suggested by **flow cytometry,** is absent NK cell function because the lack of adhesion molecules prevents the NK cells of such patients from attaching to the target cells.

COMPLEMENT. The most effective screening test for complement defects is a CH_{50} assay, a bioassay that measures the intactness of the entire complement pathway and yields abnormal results if complement has been consumed from the specimen for any reason. Genetic deficiencies in the complement system are usually characterized by extremely low CH_{50} values. The most common cause of an abnormal CH_{50} result, however, is a delay in or improper transport of the specimen to the laboratory. Specific immunoassays for C3 and C4 are commercially available, but further identification of other complement component deficiencies is usually possible only in research laboratories. Nevertheless, it is extremely important to identify which component is missing, because there are different disease susceptibilities depending on whether there are deficiencies of early or late components (see Chapter 133). Identifying the mode of inheritance is also important for genetic counseling. Properdin deficiency is X linked, but all of the other complement deficiencies are autosomal. Measurement of C4 can be helpful in assessing suspected hereditary angioedema.

Buckley RH: Molecular defects in human severe combined immunodeficiency and approaches to immune reconstitution. *Annu Rev Immunol* 2004;22:625–655.

Buckley RH: Primary immunodeficiency diseases due to defects in lymphocytes. *N Engl J Med* 2000;343:1313–1324.

Fischer A: Human primary immunodeficiency diseases: A perspective. *Nat Immunol* 2004;5:23–30.

Lindegren ML, Kobrynski L, Rasmussen SA: Applying public health strategies to primary immunodeficiency diseases: A potential approach to genetic disorders. *MMWR Recomm Rep* 2004;53:1–29.

McGhee SA, Stiehm R, McCabe RB: Potential costs and benefits of newborn screening for severe combined immunodeficiency. *J Pediatr* 2005;147:603–608.

Notarangelo L, Casanova JL, Conley MS, et al: Primary immunodeficiency diseases: An update. *J Allergy Clin Immunol* 2006;117:883–896.

Woroniecka M, Ballow M: Office evaluation of children with recurrent infection. *Pediatr Clin North Am* 2000;47:1211–1224.

Section 2 — The T-, B-, and NK-Cell Systems — Rebecca H. Buckley

Chapter 122 ■ T Lymphocytes, B Lymphocytes, and Natural Killer Cells

Defense against infectious agents is secured through a combination of anatomic physical barriers including the skin, mucous membranes, mucous blanket, and ciliated epithelial cells, as well as the various components of the immune system. The **immune system** of vertebrates integrates two fundamental response mechanisms. **Innate (natural) immunity** responds to infection regardless of previous exposure to the agent and includes polymorphonuclear leukocytes, dendritic and mononuclear phagocytic cells, various receptors that recognize common pathogen antigens (Toll-like receptors) and the complement system. **Acquired (adaptive) immunity** is a highly specific response that includes T lymphocytes, B lymphocytes, and natural killer (NK) cells. The immune system also helps protect against malignancy and autoimmunity.

LYMPHOPOIESIS IN THE FETUS

ORIGIN OF THE LYMPHOID SYSTEM. The human immune system arises in the embryo from gut-associated tissue. Pluripotential hematopoietic stem cells 1st appear in the yolk sac at 2.5–3 wk of gestational age, migrate to the fetal liver at 5 wk of gestation, and later reside in the bone marrow, where they remain throughout life (Fig. 122-1). Lymphoid stem cells develop from such precursor cells and differentiate into T, B, or NK cells, depending on the organs or tissues to which the stem cells traffic. Development of the **primary lymphoid organs**—thymus and bone marrow—begins during the middle of the 1st trimester of gestation and proceeds rapidly. Development of the **secondary lymphoid organs**—spleen, lymph nodes, tonsils, Peyer patches, and lamina propria—soon follows. These organs serve as sites of differentiation of T, B, and NK lymphocytes from stem cells throughout life. Both the initial organogenesis and the continued cell differentiation occur as a consequence of the interaction of a vast array of lymphocytic and microenvironmental cell surface molecules and proteins secreted by the involved cells. The complexity and number of lymphoid cell surface molecules led to the development of an international nomenclature for **clusters of differentiation (CD)** (Table 122-1).

T and B lymphocytes are the only components of the immune system that have antigen-specific recognition capabilities and are responsible for adaptive immunity. NK cells are lymphocytes that are also derived from hematopoietic stem cells and are thought to have a role in host defense against viral infections, tumor surveillance, and immune regulation. Some of the nonantibody proteins synthesized and secreted by T, B, and NK cells, and by the cells with which they interact, act as intercellular mediators and are referred to as **cytokines** or **interleukins (ILs)** (Table 122-2). Cytokines have the ability to act in an autocrine, paracrine, or endocrine manner to promote and facilitate differentiation and proliferation of the cells of the immune system.

T-CELL DEVELOPMENT AND DIFFERENTIATION. The primitive thymic rudiment is formed from the ectoderm of the 3rd branchial cleft and endoderm of the 3rd branchial pouch at 4 wk gestation. Beginning at 7–8 wk, the right and left rudiments move caudally and fuse in the midline. Blood-borne T-cell precursors from the fetal liver then begin to colonize the perithymic mesenchyme at 8 wk gestation. These precursor **pro–T cells** are identified by surface proteins designated as **CD7** and **CD34.** At 8–

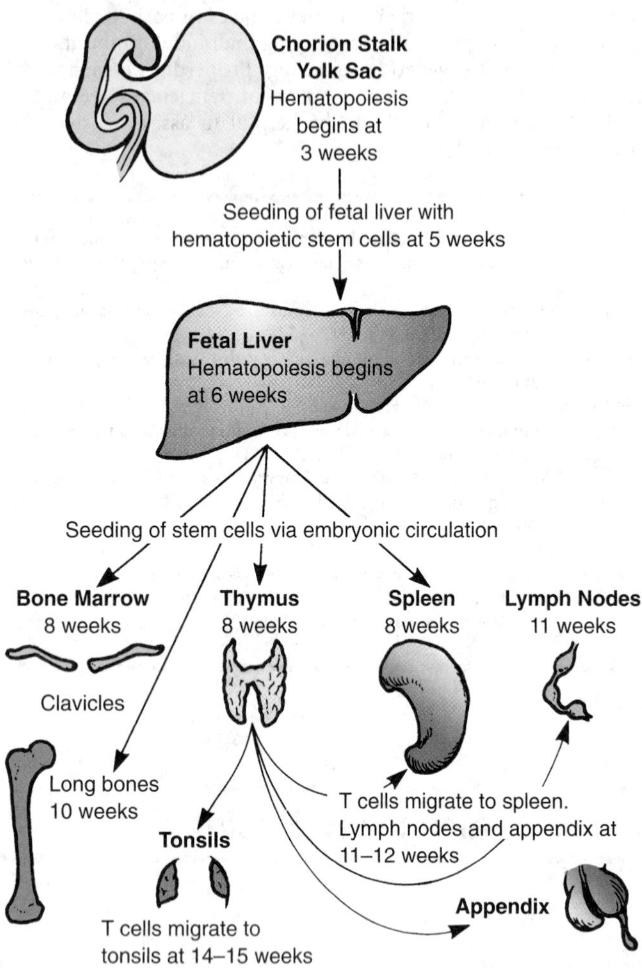

Figure 122-1. Migration patterns of hematopoietic stem cells and mature lymphocytes during human fetal development. (From Haynes BF, Denning SM: Lymphopoiesis. In Stamatoyannopoulis G, Nienhuis A, Majerus P, Varmus H [eds]: *Molecular Basis of Blood Diseases,* 2nd ed. Philadelphia, WB Saunders, 1994.)

8.5 wk gestation, CD7 cells are found intrathymically, with some cells that co-express **CD4,** a protein present on the surfaces of mature T-helper (TH) cells, or **CD8,** a protein found on both mature cytotoxic T cells and NK cells. In addition, some cells bear single T-cell receptor (Ti) chains (β, δ, or γ), but none bear complete T-cell receptors.

The mature **T-cell receptor (TCR)** is a heterodimer of two chains, either α and β or γ and δ, that is co-expressed on the cell surface with **CD3,** a complex of five polypeptide chains (γ, δ, ε, ζ, η). TCR gene rearrangement occurs by a process in which large, noncontiguous blocks of DNA are spliced together. These segments, known as **V (variable), D (diversity),** and **J (joining),** each have a number of variants. VDJ segments are joined to a constant region of the α gene, and VJ segments are joined to the β gene to complete the receptor polypeptide genes. Random combinations of the segments account for much of the enormous diversity of TCRs that enables humans to recognize millions of different antigens. TCR gene rearrangement requires the presence of **recombinase activating genes,** *RAG-1* and *RAG-2,* as well as other recombinase components. This process is flawed in mice with severe combined immunodeficiency (SCID) and in some humans with SCID. Rearrangement of TCR genes signifies commitment of pro–T cells to T-lineage development, becoming **pre–T cells.** TCR gene rearrangement begins shortly after colonization of the thymus with stem cells, and the establishment of the T-cell repertoire begins at 8–10 wk of gestation. By 9.5–10 wk, >95% of thymocytes express CD7, CD2, CD4, CD8, and c (cytoplasmic) CD3, and ≈30% bear the CD1 inner cortical thymocyte antigen. By 10 wk, 25% of thymocytes bear αβ TCRs. Ti αβ T cells gradually increase in number during embryonic life and represent >95% of thymocytes postnatally.

As immature cortical thymocytes begin to express TCRs, the processes of positive and negative selection take place. **Positive selection** occurs through the interaction of immature thymocytes, which express low levels of TCR, with major histocompatibility complex (MHC) antigens present on cortical thymic epithelial cells. As a result, thymocytes with TCR capable of interacting with foreign antigens presented on self HLA molecules are activated and develop to maturity. Mature thymocytes that survive the selection process either express CD4 and are restricted to interacting with self class II HLA antigens or express CD8 and

TABLE 122-1. CD Classification of Some Lymphocyte Surface Molecules

CD NUMBER*	OTHER NAMES	TISSUE/LINEAGE	FUNCTION
CD1	T6	Cortical thymocytes; Langerhans cells	Antigen presentation to TCRγδ cells
CD2	SRBC receptor	T and NK cells	Binds LFA-3 (CD58); alternative pathway of T-cell activation
CD3	T3, Leu 4	T cells	TCR-associated; transduces signals from TCR
CD4	T4, Leu3a	Helper T-cell subset	Receptor for HLA Class II antigens; associated with p56 *lck* tyrosine kinase
CD7	3A1, Leu 9	T and NK cells and their precursors	Co-mitogenic for T lymphocytes
CD8	T8, Leu2a	Cytotoxic T-cell subset; also on 30% of NK cells	Receptor for HLA Class I antigens; associated with p56 *lck* tyrosine kinase
CD10	cALLA	B-cell progenitors	Peptide cleavage
CD11a	LFA-1a ∀ chain	T, B, and NK cells	With CD18, ligand for ICAMS 1, 2 and 3
CD11b,c	MAC-1, CR3; CR4	NK cells	With CD18, receptors for C3bi
CD16	FcRIII	NK cells	FcR for IgG
CD19	B4	B cells	Regulates B-cell activation
CD20	B1	B cells	Mediates B-cell activation
CD21	B2	B cells	C3d, also the receptor for EBV; CR2
CD25	IL-2Rα	T, B, and NK cells	Mediates signaling by IL-2
CD34	My10	Precursor cells	Binds to L-selectin
CD38	T10	T, B, and NK cells and monocytes	Associates with hyaluronic acid
CD40	CD40	B cells and monocytes	Initiates isotype switching when ligated
CD45	Leukocyte common antigen, T200	All leukocytes	Tyrosine phosphatase that regulates lymphocyte activation; CD45RO isoform on memory T cells, CD45RA isoform on naive T cells
CD56	NCAM; NKH-1	NK cells	Mediates NK homotypic adhesion
CD73	Ecto-5′-nucleotidase	T and B cells	Associates with AMP
CD127	IL-7Rα	T cells	Mediates IL-7 signaling
CD132	Common γ chain (γc)	T, B, and NK cells	Mediates signaling by IL-2, IL-4, IL-7, IL-9, IL-15 and IL-21
CD154	CD40 ligand, gp39	Activated CD4+ T cells	Ligates CD40 on B cells and initiates isotype switching
CD278	ICOS	T cells	Interacts with B7-H2

*CD, clusters of determination.

TABLE 122-2. Functional Classification of Cytokines*

1. Cytokines involved in natural immune responses
   - Type I interferons (INF-α and IFN-β): inhibit viral replication, inhibit cell proliferation, activate NK cells, and upregulate class I MHC molecule expression
   - TNF-α: mediates host response to gram-negative bacteria and other infectious agents
   - IL-1α and -β: mediate host inflammatory response to infectious agents
   - IL-1 Ra: a natural antagonist of IL-1, blocks signals delivered by IL-1
   - IL-6: mediates and regulates inflammatory responses
   - Chemokines (IL-8, monocyte chemotactic protein-1 or MCP-1, RANTES, and others): mediate leukocyte chemotaxis and activation
2. Lymphocyte regulatory cytokines
   - a. Immunostimulatory or growth-promoting
     - IL-1: co-stimulates activation of T cells
     - IL-2: growth factor for T, B, NK cells; activates NK and T effector cells
     - IL-4: T- and B-cell growth factor; stimulates IgE production; upregulates class I and II MHC molecule and FcRεII expression on macrophages; expansion of T_H2 subset
     - IL-5: B-cell growth and activation
     - IL-6: growth factor for B cells
     - IL-7: stromal cell factor; growth factor for precursor B and T cells, T-cell homeostatic factor
     - IL-10: growth and differentiation factor for B cells
     - IL-9: growth factor for T cells, B cells, mast cells, eosinophils, neutrophils, endothelial cells
     - IL-12: expansion of T_H1 subset; activates effector cells
     - IL-13: growth and differentiating factor for B cells; stimulates IgE production; upregulates Class I and II MHC molecule and FcRεII expression on macrophages
     - TNF-β: stimulates effector cell function
     - IL-15: regulates NK-cell development and memory cell homeostasis
     - IL-18: induces IFNγ GM-CSF, TNFα in immunocompetent cells
     - IL-21: together with IL-4 regulates IgG and IgE class-switching and Ig synthesis
     - IFNγ: activates macrophages, NK cells; upregulates class I and II MHC molecule expression; inhibits IL-4- or IL-13-induced IgE production
   - b. Immunosuppressive
     - IL-1Rα: regulates IL-1 activities
     - TGF-β: antagonizes lymphocyte responses
     - IL-10: inhibits activities of T_H1 cells
     - IFNα/β: inhibits production of IFNγ
3. Hematopoiesis regulating cytokines
   - GM-CSF, G-CSF, M-CSF: colony stimulating factors
   - Erythropoietin (EPO): differentiation of erythroid precursors
   - IL-3, SCF, *c-kit* receptor: regulate stem cell development
   - IL-4: mast cell development
   - IL-5: eosinophil differentiation and proliferation
   - IL-6: differentiation of B cells
   - IL-7: differentiation of B and T cells
   - IL-8: promotes cell survival in response to hematopoietic cytokines
   - IL-9: mast-cell growth factor
   - IL-11: elevates platelet count in patients given chemotherapy
   - IL-12: expands and activates resting NK cells
   - IL-15: expands and activates resting NK cells
   - IL-21: limits viability of NK cells
4. Pro-inflammatory cytokines
   - IL-1, TNF-α, IL-6: participate in the acute-phase response and synergize to mediate inflammation, shock, and death
   - IL-12: stimulates INF (production by T and NK cells)
   - IL-17: recruitment and activation of airway neutrophils via chemokines
   - IL-18: induces IFNγ, GM-CSF, TNFα; upregulates chemokine receptors
5. Anti-inflammatory cytokines
   - IL-4: reduces endotoxin-induced TNF and IL-1 production
   - IL-6: inhibits TNF production
   - IL-10: suppresses lymphocyte functions and downregulates production of proinflammatory cytokines; anti-atherogenic
   - IL-11: cytoprotective effect on bowel mucosa, skin and joint inflammation
   - IL-13: downregulates functions of macrophages, suppresses production of proinflammatory cytokines
   - TGF-β: has immunosuppressive effects, inhibits IL-1 and TNF gene expression
   - IL-1Rα: competes with the binding of IL-1 to its cell surface receptors and blocks IL-1R
   - TNFsR: soluble TNF receptor; by binding TNF, blocks interaction of TNF with the target cell

*This is not an exhaustive list.
Modified from Whiteside TL: Cytokine measurements and interpretation of cytokine assays in human disease. *J Clin Immunol* 1994;14:327–339.

are restricted to interacting with self class I HLA antigens when foreign antigens are presented by these MHC molecules. **Negative selection** occurs next and is mediated by interaction of the surviving thymocytes, which have much higher levels of TCR expression, with host peptides presented by HLA class I or II antigens present on bone marrow–derived thymic macrophages, dendritic cells, and possibly B cells. This interaction mediates **apoptosis,** or programmed cell death, of such autoreactive thymocytes. Fetal cortical thymocytes are among the most rapidly dividing cells in the body and increase in number by 100,000-fold within 2 wk after stem cells enter the thymus. As these cells mature and the selection process takes place, 97% of all cortical thymocytes die. The surviving cells are no longer doubly positive for both CD4 and CD8, but are singly positive for either one or the other and migrate to the medulla of the thymus.

T-cell functions are acquired concomitantly with the development of single-positive thymocytes, but they are not fully developed until the cells emigrate from the thymus. It has been estimated that one stem cell gives rise to approximately 3,000 mature medullary thymocytes, which are resistant to the lytic effects of corticosteroids. T cells begin to emigrate from the thymus to the spleen, lymph nodes, and appendix at 11–12 wk of embryonic life and to the tonsils by 14–15 wk. They leave the thymus via the bloodstream and are distributed throughout the body, with the heaviest concentrations in the paracortical areas of lymph nodes, the periarteriolar areas of the spleen, and the thoracic duct lymph. Recent thymic emigrants co-express the CD45RA isoforms and CD62L (L-selectin). Rearrangement of the TCR locus during this process leads to the formation of circular episomes as a by-product. These signal joint **TCR recombination excision circles** (**TRECs**) can be detected in T cells that are recent thymic emigrants, whereas T cells that develop extrathymically do not contain these episomes. The homing of lymphocytes to peripheral lymphoid organs is directed by the interaction of a lymphocyte surface adhesion molecule, L-selectin, with carbohydrate moieties on specialized regions of lymphoid organ blood vessels called **high endothelial venules.** By 12 wk gestation, T cells can proliferate in response to plant lectins, such as phytohemagglutinin (PHA) and concanavalin A (Con A), and to allogeneic cells; antigen-binding T cells have been found by 20 wk gestation. **Hassall corpuscles (bodies)**, which are swirls of terminally differentiated medullary epithelial cells, are 1st seen in the thymic medulla at 16–18 wk of embryonic life.

B-CELL DEVELOPMENT AND DIFFERENTIATION. In parallel with T-cell differentiation, B-cell development begins in the fetal liver before 7 wk of gestation. Fetal liver CD34 stem cells are seeded to the bone marrow of the clavicles by 8 wk of embryonic life and to that of the long bones by 10 wk (see Fig. 122-1). **Antigen-independent stages** of B-cell development have been defined according to immunoglobulin gene rearrangement patterns and the surface proteins the cells bear. The **pro–B cell** is the 1st descendent of the pluripotential stem cell committed to B-lineage development that is detected by the presence of both CD34 and CD10 on its surface, although the immunoglobulin genes remain germ line (Fig. 122-2). The next stage is the **pre-pre–B cell,** during which immunoglobulin genes are rearranged but there is no cytoplasmic expression of μ heavy chains or surface IgM (sIgM). These cells are further characterized by the co-expression of membrane CD34, CD10, CD19, and CD40, and somewhat later by the additional presence of CD73, CD22, CD24, and CD38. The **pre–B cell** follows and is distinguished by the expression of cytoplasmic μ heavy chains but no sIgM, because no immunoglobulin light chains are produced yet. These cells also continue to express all CD antigens seen at the pre-pre–B-cell stage except CD34 and CD10, which are lost; in addition, they express CD21. Next is the **immature B-cell** stage, during which sIgM but not sIgD is expressed. The light-chain genes have been rearranged, and CD38 is lost but all other pre–B-cell CD antigens persist. The last stage of antigen-independent B-cell development is the **mature or virgin B cell**, which co-expresses both sIgM and sIgD; CD23 is also acquired at this stage, and all of the other CD antigens present on immature B cells persist. Pre–B cells can be found in fetal liver at 7 wk gestation, sIgM+ and sIgG+ B cells at between 7 and 11 wk, and sIgD+ and sIgA+ B cells by 12–13 wk.

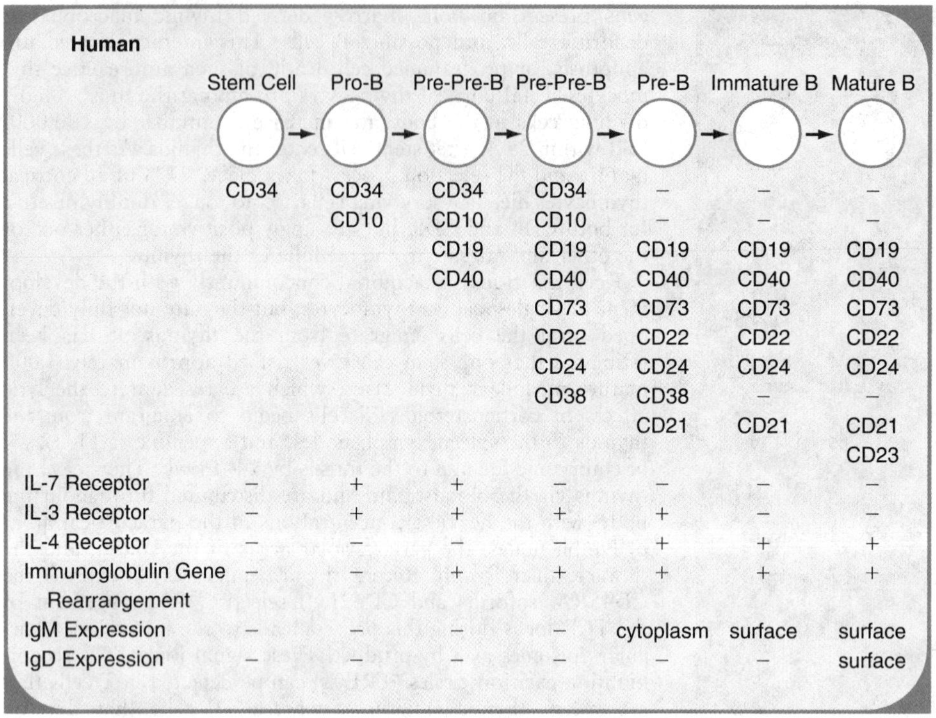

Human

	Stem Cell	Pro-B	Pre-Pre-B	Pre-Pre-B	Pre-B	Immature B	Mature B
	CD34	CD34	CD34	CD34	–	–	–
		CD10	CD10	CD10	–	–	–
			CD19	CD19	CD19	CD19	CD19
			CD40	CD40	CD40	CD40	CD40
				CD73	CD73	CD73	CD73
				CD22	CD22	CD22	CD22
				CD24	CD24	CD24	CD24
				CD38	CD38	–	–
					CD21	CD21	CD21
							CD23
IL-7 Receptor	–	+	+	–	–	–	–
IL-3 Receptor	–	+	+	+	+	–	–
IL-4 Receptor	–	–	–	–	+	+	+
Immunoglobulin Gene Rearrangement	–	–	+	+	+	+	+
IgM Expression	–	–	–	–	cytoplasm	surface	surface
IgD Expression	–	–	–	–	–	–	surface

Figure 122-2. Antigen-independent human B-cell development. (From Haynes BF, Denning SM: Lymphopoiesis. In Stamatoyannopoulis G, Nienhuis A, Majerus P, Varmus H [eds]: *Molecular Basis of Blood Diseases,* 2nd ed. Philadelphia, WB Saunders, 1994.)

By 14 wk of embryonic life, the percentage of circulating lymphocytes bearing sIgM and sIgD is the same as in cord blood and slightly higher than in the blood of adults.

Antigen-dependent stages of B-cell development are those that develop after the mature or virgin B cell is stimulated by antigen through its antigen receptor (sIg); the outcome is the differentiation of the cell and its progeny into sIg+ memory (CD27) B cells (for that particular antigen) and plasma cells, which synthesize and secrete antibody, which is **antigen-specific immunoglobulin.** Deficiency of activation-induced cytidine deaminase (AID) or of uracil DNA glycosylase (UNG), as seen in two forms of autosomal recessive hyper IgM, can result in a failure of isotype switching so that only IgM antibodies are formed. There are five **immunoglobulin isotypes,** which are defined by unique heavy-chains: IgM, IgG, IgA, IgD, and IgE. IgG and IgM, the only complement-fixing isotypes, are the most important immunoglobulins in the blood and other internal body fluids for protection against infectious agents. IgM is confined primarily to the intravascular compartment because of its large size, whereas IgG is present in all internal body fluids. IgA is the major protective immunoglobulin of external secretions—in the gastrointestinal, respiratory, and urogenital tracts—but it is also present in the circulation. IgE, present in both internal and external body fluids, has a major role in host defense against parasites. Because of high-affinity IgE receptors on basophils and mast cells, however, IgE is the principal mediator of allergic reactions of the immediate type. The significance of IgD is still not clear. There are also **immunoglobulin subclasses** including four subclasses of IgG (IgG1, IgG2, IgG3, and IgG4) and two subclasses of IgA (IgA1 and IgA2). These subclasses each have different biologic roles. For example, antipolysaccharide antibody activity is found predominantly in the IgG2 subclass. Secreted IgM and IgE have been found in abortuses as young as 10 wk, and IgG as early as 11–12 wk. Even though these B-cell developmental stages have been described in the context of B-cell ontogeny, it is important to recognize that the process of B-cell development from pluripotential stem cells goes on throughout postnatal life.

Despite the capacity of fetal B lymphocytes to differentiate into immunoglobulin-synthesizing and -secreting cells, plasma cells are not usually found in lymphoid tissues of a fetus until about 20 wk gestation, then only rarely, because of the sterile environment of the uterus. Peyer patches have been found in significant numbers by the 5th intrauterine month, and plasma cells have been seen in the lamina propria by 25 wk gestation. Before birth there may be primary follicles in lymph nodes, but secondary follicles are usually not present.

A human fetus begins to receive significant quantities of maternal IgG transplacentally at around 12 wk gestation, and the quantity steadily increases until, at birth, cord serum contains a concentration of IgG comparable to or greater than that of maternal serum. IgG is the only class to cross the placenta to any significant degree. All four subclasses cross the placenta, but IgG2 does so least well. A small amount of IgM (10% of adult levels) and a few nanograms of IgA, IgD, and IgE are normally found in cord serum. Because none of these proteins crosses the placenta, they are presumed to be of fetal origin. These observations raise the possibility that certain antigenic stimuli normally cross the placenta to provoke responses, even in uninfected fetuses. Some atopic infants occasionally have IgE antibodies to antigens, such as egg white, to which they have had no known exposure during postnatal life, suggesting that synthesis of these antibodies could have been induced in the fetus by antigens ingested by the mother.

NATURAL KILLER (NK)–CELL DEVELOPMENT. NK-cell activity is found in human fetal liver cells at 8–11 wk of gestation. NK lymphocytes are also derived from bone marrow precursors. Thymic processing is not necessary for NK-cell development, although NK cells have been found in the thymus. After release from bone marrow, NK cells enter the circulation or migrate to the spleen, with very few NK cells in lymph nodes. In normal individuals, NK cells represent 8–10% of lymphocytes, which is often slightly lower in cord blood.

Unlike T and B cells, NK cells do not rearrange antigen receptor genes during their development but are defined by their functional capacity to mediate non–antigen-specific cytotoxicity. NK cells have killer inhibitory receptors (KIRs) that recognize certain MHC antigens and inhibit the killing of normal allogeneic cells in four specific patterns of reactivity. The genetic loci controlling these receptors are different from MHC alloantigenic loci, and have been mapped to chromosome 19. Virtually all NK cells express CD56, and >90% bear CD16 (Fcγ RIII) on the cell surface. Other CD antigens found on NK cells include CD57 (50–60%), CD7 and CD2 (70–90%), and CD8 (30–40%) (see Table 122-1). Because NK cells share surface antigens with T and myeloid cells, the lineage relationship of NK cells to the latter is still unclear. Some humans with autosomal recessive SCID who have profound deficiencies in T and B cells have abundant NK cells, whereas those with X-linked and Jak3-deficient SCID have no T or NK cells.

IMMUNE CELL INTERACTIONS. Immune cell interaction is of crucial importance to all phases of the adaptive immune response. Unlike the B-cell antigen receptor (Ig), which can recognize native antigen, the TCR can recognize only processed antigenic peptides presented to it by MHC molecules such as **HLA-A, -B, and -C antigens** (class I) and **HLA-DR, -DP, and -DQ antigens** (class II) present on **antigen-presenting cells (APCs)**, which include macrophages, dendritic cells, and B cells. The MHC molecules have a groove in their protein structure where peptides fit. Class I MHC molecules are found on most nucleated cells in the body. Class II MHC molecules are found on macrophages, dendritic cells, and B cells. The peptides found in the groove of class I HLA molecules come from proteins normally made in the cell that are degraded and inserted into the groove. The peptides include viral peptides if the cell is infected with a virus. The peptides present in the groove of class II molecules come from exogenous native antigens such as vaccine and bacterial proteins. These proteins are taken up by APCs, degraded, and expressed on the cell surface in the groove of class II HLA molecules. The TCR then interacts with the peptide-bearing HLA molecule and, through its functional and physical link to the CD3 complex of signal-transducing molecules, sends a signal to the T cell to produce cytokines that ultimately result in T-cell activation and proliferation.

Two of the main functions of T cells are to signal B cells to make antibody by producing cytokines and membrane molecules that can serve as ligands for B-cell surface molecules and to kill virally infected cells or tumor cells. For a T cell to perform either of these functions, it 1st must bind to an APC or to a target cell. For high-affinity binding of T cells to APCs or target cells, several molecules on T cells, in addition to TCRs, bind to molecules on APCs or target cells. The CD4 molecule present on TH cells binds directly to MHC class II molecules on APCs. CD8 on cytotoxic T cells binds the MHC class I molecule on the target cell. Both CD4 and CD8 molecules are directly involved in the regulation of T-cell activation and are physically linked intracellularly to the p56-lck protein tyrosine kinase. The cytoplasmic tail of CD45, the common leukocyte antigen, is a tyrosine phosphatase capable of regulating T-cell signal-transduction events by virtue of the fact that p56-lck has been shown to be a substrate for CD45 phosphatase activity. Depending on which isoform of CD45 is present on the T cell (CD45RO on memory T cells, CD45RA on naive T cells), mechanisms by which CD45 could upregulate or downregulate T-cell triggering have been proposed. Indeed, one form of human SCID is caused by a deficiency of CD45. LFA-1 on the T cell binds a protein called ICAM-1 (intracellular adhesion molecule 1), now designated CD54, on APCs. CD2 on T cells binds LFA-3 (CD58) on the APCs. With the adhesion of T cells to antigen-presenting cells, TH cells are stimulated to make interleukins and upregulate cell surface molecules, such as the CD40 ligand (CD154), that provide help for B cells, and cytotoxic T cells are stimulated to kill their targets.

In the **primary antibody response**, native antigen is carried to a lymph node draining the site, taken up by specialized cells called **follicular dendritic cells (FDCs)**, and expressed on their surfaces. Virgin B cells bearing sIg specific for that antigen then bind to the antigen on the surfaces of the FDCs. If the affinity of the B-cell sIg antibody for the antigen present on the FDCs is sufficient, and if other signals are provided by activated T-helper cells, the B cell develops into an antibody-producing plasma cell. If the affinity is not high enough or if T-cell signals are not received, the B cell dies through apoptosis. The signals from activated TH cells include several cytokines (IL-4, IL-5, IL-6, IL-10, IL-13, and IL-21) that they secrete (see Table 122-2) and a surface T-cell molecule, CD154, which, on contact of the T cell with the B cell, binds to CD40 on the B-cell surface. CD40 is a type I integral membrane glycoprotein expressed on B cells, monocytes, some carcinomas, and a few other types of cells. It belongs to the tumor necrosis factor (TNF)/nerve growth factor receptor family. Cross linking of CD40 on B cells by CD154 on T cells in the presence of certain cytokines causes the B cells to undergo proliferation and to initiate immunoglobulin synthesis. In the primary immune response, only IgM antibody is usually made, and most of it is of relatively low affinity. Some B cells become memory B cells during the primary immune response. These cells switch their immunoglobulin genes so that IgG, IgA, and/or IgE antibodies of higher affinity are formed on a secondary exposure to the same antigen. The **secondary antibody response** occurs when these memory B cells again encounter that antigen. Plasma cells form, just as in the primary response; however, many more cells are rapidly generated, and IgG, IgA, and IgE antibodies are made. In addition, genetic changes in immunoglobulin genes (somatic hypermutation [SHM]) lead to increased affinity of those antibodies. A lack of SHM is seen in deficiency of AID or UNG. The exact pattern of isotype response to antigen in normal individuals varies, depending on the type of antigen and the cytokines present in the microenvironment.

For NK-mediated lysis, binding to the target is of crucial importance. This is best exemplified by persons with leukocyte adhesion deficiency type I (LADI) who have mutations in the gene encoding CD18, or the β chain of three different adhesion molecules (LFA-1, CR3 and p150,95), and who lack NK function. Thus, binding of NK cells to their targets is facilitated by LFA-1-ICAM interactions. CD56 or NCAM (neural cell adhesion molecule) also mediates homotypic adhesion of NK cells. FcγRIII, or the low-affinity IgG receptor, has a higher affinity for IgG when it is present on NK cells than when it is on neutrophils. FcγRIII also permits NK cells to mediate **antibody-dependent cellular cytotoxicity (ADCC)**, where antibody is bound through its Fc region to the FcγRIII. The antibody-combining portion of the IgG attaches to the target cell, and the NK cell, attached to the target by the Fc portion of the antibody, kills the target cell.

POSTNATAL LYMPHOPOIESIS

T CELLS AND T-CELL SUBSETS. Although the percentage of CD3 T cells in cord blood is somewhat less than in the peripheral blood of children and adults, T cells are actually present in higher number because of a higher absolute lymphocyte count in normal infants. An additional distinction is that the ratio of CD4 to CD8 T cells is usually higher (3.5–4:1) in cord blood than in blood of children and adults (1.5–2:1). Virtually all T cells in cord blood bear the CD45RA (naive) isoform, and a dominance of CD45RA over CD45RO T cells persists during the 1st 2–3 yr of life, after which time the numbers of cells bearing these two isoforms gradually equalize. TH cells can be further subdivided according to the cytokines they produce when activated. **TH1 cells** produce IL-2 and IFN-γ, which promote cytotoxic T-cell or delayed hypersensitivity types of responses, whereas **TH2 cells** produce IL-4, IL-5, IL-6, IL-13, and IL-21 (see Table 122-2), which promote B-cell responses and allergic sensitization. There are important additional subsets of T cells that have regulatory functions. These include CD25 high + T cells (Treg cells), considered to be important in the prevention of autoimmune diseases, and T cells that have phenotypic characteristics of NK cells (NK-T cells). Cord blood T cells have the capacity to respond normally to the **T-cell mitogens** (PHA, Con A, and PWM) and are capable of mounting a normal mixed leukocyte response. Normal newborn infants also have the capacity to develop antigen-specific T cell responses at birth, as evidenced by vigorous tuberculin reactivity a few weeks after BCG vaccination on day 1 of life. Because patients in the 1st few months of life may have unrecognized severe T-cell defects, most hospitals now routinely irradiate all blood products given young infants. T-cell defects can readily be detected even at birth by calculating the absolute lymphocyte count because T cells normally constitute 70% of circulating lymphocytes and their absence results in striking lymphopenia (see Fig. 121-2 and Chapter 716).

B CELLS AND IMMUNOGLOBULINS. Newborn infants have increased susceptibility to infections with gram-negative organisms because IgM antibodies, which are heat-stable opsonins, do not cross the placenta. The level of the heat-labile opsonin, C3b, is also lower in newborn serum than in adults. These factors probably account for impaired phagocytosis of some organisms by newborn polymorphonuclear cells. Maternally transmitted IgG antibodies serve quite adequately as heat-stable opsonins for most gram-positive bacteria, and IgG antibodies to viruses afford adequate protection against those agents. Because there is a relative deficiency of the IgG2 subclass, antibodies to capsular polysaccharide antigens may be deficient. Because premature infants have received less maternal IgG by the time of birth than full-term infants, their serum opsonic activity is low for all types of organisms.

B lymphocytes are present in cord blood in slightly higher percentages but considerably higher numbers than in the blood of children and adults, reflecting the higher absolute lymphocyte counts in all normal infants. Cord blood B cells do not synthesize the range of immunoglobulin isotypes made by B cells from children and adults when stimulated with anti-CD40 plus IL-4 or IL-10, producing primarily IgM and at a much reduced quantity.

Neonates begin to synthesize antibodies of the IgM class at an increased rate very soon after birth in response to the immense antigenic stimulation of their new environment. Premature infants appear to be as capable of doing this as do full-term infants. At about 6 days after birth, the serum concentration of IgM rises sharply. This rise continues until adult levels are achieved by ≈1 yr of age. Cord serum from noninfected normal newborns does not contain detectable IgA. Serum IgA is normally 1st detected at around the 13th day of postnatal life; the level gradually increases during early childhood until adult levels are achieved by 6–7 yr of age. Cord serum contains an IgG concentration comparable to or greater than that of maternal serum. Maternal IgG gradually disappears during the 1st 6–8 mo of life, while the rate of infant IgG synthesis increases (IgG1 and IgG3 faster than IgG2 and IgG4 during the 1st year) until adult concentrations of total IgG are reached and maintained by 7–8 yr of age. IgG1 and IgG4 reach adult levels first, followed by IgG3 at 10 yr and IgG2 at 12 yr of age. The total immunoglobulin level in infants usually reaches a low point at ≈3–4 mo of postnatal life. The rate of development of IgE generally follows that of IgA. After adult concentrations of each of the three major immunoglobulins are reached, these levels remain remarkably constant for a normal individual. The capacity to produce specific antibodies to protein antigens is intact at the time of birth. Normal infants cannot usually produce antibodies to polysaccharide antigens until after 2 yr of age, however, unless the polysaccharide is conjugated to a protein carrier, as is the case for the conjugate *Haemophilus influenzae* type b (Hib) and *Streptococcus pneumoniae* (PCV7) vaccines.

NK CELLS. The percentage of NK cells in cord blood is usually lower than in the blood of children and adults, but the absolute number of NK cells is approximately the same owing to the higher lymphocyte count. The capacity of cord blood NK cells to mediate target lysis in either NK-cell assays or ADCC assays is roughly two thirds that of adults.

LYMPHOID ORGAN DEVELOPMENT. Lymphoid tissue is proportionally small but rather well developed at birth and matures rapidly in the postnatal period. The thymus is largest relative to body size during fetal life and at birth is ordinarily two thirds of its mature weight, which it attains during the 1st year of life. It reaches its peak mass, however, just before puberty, and then gradually involutes thereafter. By 1 yr of age, all lymphoid structures are mature histologically. Absolute lymphocyte counts in the peripheral blood also reach a peak during the 1st yr of life. Peripheral lymphoid tissue increases rapidly in mass during infancy and early childhood. It reaches adult size by approximately 6 yr of age, exceeds those dimensions during the prepubertal years, and then undergoes involution coincident with puberty. The spleen, however, gradually accrues its mass during maturation and does not reach full weight until adulthood. The mean number of Peyer patches at birth is one half the adult number, and gradually increases until the adult mean number is exceeded during adolescent years.

INHERITANCE OF ABNORMALITIES IN T-, B-, AND NK-CELL DEVELOPMENT

More than 120 immunodeficiency syndromes have been described (see Table 121-7). Specific molecular defects have been identified in approximately 100 of these diseases. Most are recessive traits, several of which are caused by mutations in genes on the X chromosome and others by mutations on autosomal chromosomes. The molecular bases of six X-linked immunodeficiency disorders affecting T, B, and/or NK cells are known (see Chapters 123–125): X-linked immunodeficiency with hyper IgM, X-linked lymphoproliferative syndrome, X-linked agammaglobulinemia, X-linked SCID, the Wiskott-Aldrich syndrome, and nuclear factor kappa B essential modulator (NEMO). Autosomal defects for which the molecular basis is known include (1) combined immunodeficiencies due to abnormalities of purine salvage pathway enzymes, either adenosine deaminase (ADA, encoded by a gene on chromosome 20q13-ter) or purine nucleoside phosphorylase (PNP, encoded by a gene on chromosome 14q13.1); (2) combined immunodeficiencies due to mutations in the gene encoding ZAP-70 (localized to chromosome 2q12), a non-src family protein tyrosine kinase important in T-cell signaling; (3) SCID due to mutations in the gene on chromosome 19p13.1 encoding Janus kinase 3 (Jak3), the primary signal transducer from the common cytokine receptor γ chain (γc); (4) mutations in genes on chromosome 11 that encode components of the T-cell receptor, that is, CD3 γ, δ and ε; (5) SCID due to mutations in recombinase activating genes (*RAG1* and *RAG2*); and (6) SCID due to mutations in the gene on chromosome 5p13 that encodes the α chain of the IL-7 receptor. These are only a few of the conditions for which the mutated genes have been discovered and the number is growing, with more than 15 identified in the last 2 yr.

PRENATAL DIAGNOSIS AND CARRIER DETECTION

Intrauterine diagnosis of ADA and PNP deficiencies can be established by enzyme analyses on amnion cells (fresh or cultured) obtained before 20 wk gestation. Diagnosis of several X-linked defects can be established by direct mutation analysis of the X chromosome of cells obtained by chorionic villus sampling or by amniocentesis from male infants whose mothers have been identified as carriers. Diagnosis of enzyme-normal SCID or other severe T-cell deficiencies, MHC class I and/or II antigen deficiencies, chronic granulomatous disease (CGD), or Wiskott-Aldrich syndrome (by platelet size) can be established by appropriate tests of phenotype or function on small samples of blood obtained by fetoscopy at 18–22 wk of gestation, but this procedure carries significant risk. The same diagnostic procedures can be performed on cord blood, but currently, no immunodeficiency disorders are screened for using cord blood of newborns in the United States (see Chapter 121). Carriers of ADA and PNP deficiency can be detected by quantitative enzyme analyses of blood samples. Carriers of X-linked agammaglobulinemia, X-linked SCID, or the Wiskott-Aldrich syndrome can be identified by techniques designed to detect nonrandom X-chromosome inactivation in one or more blood cell lineages or by direct mutation analysis if the family's mutation is known.

Arkwright PD, Abinun M, Cant AJ: Autoimmunity in human primary immunodeficiency diseases. *Blood* 2002;99:2694–2702.

Buckley RH: Primary immunodeficiency diseases due to defects in lymphocytes. *N Engl J Med* 2000;343:1313–1324.

Fischer A: Human primary immunodeficiency diseases: A perspective. *Nat Immunol* 2004;5:23–30.

Fuentes-Panana EM, Bannish G, Monroe JG: Basal B-cell receptor signaling in B lymphocytes: Mechanisms of regulation and role in positive selection, differentiation, and peripheral survival. *Immunol Rev* 2004;197:26–40.

Gill J, Malin M, Sutherland J, et al: Thymic generation and regeneration. *Immunol Rev* 2003;195:28–50.

Haynes BF, Markert ML, Sempowski GD, et al: The role of the thymus in immune reconstitution in aging, bone marrow transplantation, and HIV-1 infection. *Annu Rev Immunol* 2000;18:529–560.

Jiang H, Chess L: An integrated view of suppressor T cell subsets in immunoregulation. *J Clin Invest* 2004;114:1198–1208.

Chapter 123 ■ Primary Defects of Antibody Production

Of all of the primary immunodeficiency diseases, those affecting antibody production are most frequent. Selective absence of serum and secretory IgA is the most common defect, with rates ranging from 1/333 to 1/18,000 persons among different races. By contrast, agammaglobulinemia occurs with a frequency of only 1/10,000 to 1/50,000 persons. Patients with antibody deficiency are usually recognized because they have recurrent infections with encapsulated bacteria or a history of failure of responding to antibiotic treatment; some individuals with selective IgA deficiency or infants with transient hypogammaglobulinemia may have few or no infections (see Table 121-3). The defective gene products for many primary antibody deficiency disorders have been identified (Table 123-1) and localized (Fig. 123-1). Sometimes the defect is not in the B cell itself but in T cells, which are required for complete B-cell function.

X-LINKED AGAMMAGLOBULINEMIA (XLA)

Patients with X-linked agammaglobulinemia (XLA), or **Bruton agammaglobulinemia,** have a profound defect in B-lymphocyte development resulting in severe hypogammaglobulinemia, an absence of circulating B cells, small to absent tonsils, and no palpable lymph nodes.

GENETICS AND PATHOGENESIS. The abnormal gene in XLA maps to q22 on the long arm of the X chromosome and encodes the B-cell protein tyrosine kinase **Btk (Bruton tyrosine kinase).** Btk is a member of the Tec family of cytoplasmic protein tyrosine kinases and is expressed at high levels in all B-lineage cells, including pre–B cells. It appears to be necessary for pre–B-cell expansion and maturation into surface Ig-expressing B cells, but probably has a role at all stages of B-cell development; it has also been found in cells of the myeloid series. To date, more than 554 different mutations in the human *Btk* gene have been recognized; they encompass most parts of the coding portions of the gene. There is not a clear correlation between the location of the mutation and the clinical phenotype (Fig. 123-2). Carriers are detected by identifying nonrandom X-chromosome inactivation in B cells or by direct mutation analysis. Prenatal diagnosis of affected male fetuses is possible by mutation analysis if the defect is known in the family.

The expression of Btk in cells of myeloid lineage is of interest because boys with XLA often have neutropenia at the height of an acute infection. It is conceivable that Btk is only one of the signaling molecules participating in myeloid maturation and that neutropenia is observed in XLA only when rapid production of

TABLE 123-1. Genetic Basis of Primary Antibody Deficiency Disorders

CHROMOSOME AND REGION	GENE PRODUCT	DISORDER	FUNCTIONAL DEFICIENCIES
2p11	κ chain	κ chain deficiency	Absence of immunoglobulins bearing κ chains
2q33	Inducible co-stimulator (ICOS)	ICOS deficient CVID (common variable immunodeficiency)	Low or absent concentrations of all immunoglobulins
6p21.3	Unknown	Selective IgA deficiency; CVID	Low or absent IgA; low concentrations of all immunoglobulins in CVID
12p13	Activation-induced cytidine deaminase (AICDA)*	Autosomal recessive hyper-IgM syndrome (HIGM2)	Failure to produce IgG, IgA, and IgE antibodies
12q23-q24.1	Uracil DNA glycosylase (UNG)	Autosomal recessive hyper-IgM syndrome	Failure to produce IgG, IgA, and IgE antibodies
14q32.3	Immunoglobulin heavy chains*	B-cell-negative agammaglobulinemia; in others, selective isotype deficiencies	Absence of antibody production, lack of B cells, in μ heavy chain mutations; in others, subclasses missing but B cells present
16p11.2	CD19	CD19 deficient CVID	Low or absent concentrations of all immunoglobulins
17p11.2	TACI* (transmembrane activator calcium-modulator, and cyclophilin ligand interactor)	TACI deficient CVID	Low or absent concentrations of all immunoglobulins
20	CD40*	Autosomal recessive hyper IgM syndrome type 3 (HIGM3)	Failure to produce IgG, IgA, and IgE antibodies
22q13.1-q13.31	BAFF-R (B-cell-activating factor of the TNF family receptor)	BAFF-R deficient CVID	Low or absent concentrations of all immunoglobulins
Xq22	Bruton tyrosine kinase (Btk)*	X-linked agammaglobulinemia (XLA, or Bruton agammaglobulinemia)	Absence of antibody production, lack of B cells
Xq25	SLAM-associated protein (SH2D1A)*	X-linked lymphoproliferative disease (XLP)	Lack of anti-EBNA (Epstein-Barr virus nuclear antigen) and long-lived T-cell immunity; low immunoglobulins
Xq26	CD154 (CD40 ligand)*	X-linked hyper-IgM syndrome type 1 (HIGM1)	Failure to produce IgG, IgA, and IgE antibodies
Xq28	Nuclear factor κ B essential modulator (NEMO)*	Anhidrotic ectodermal dysplasia with immunodeficiency	Hyper IgM or IgG subclass and anti-polysaccharide antibody deficiencies

*The gene has been cloned and sequenced.

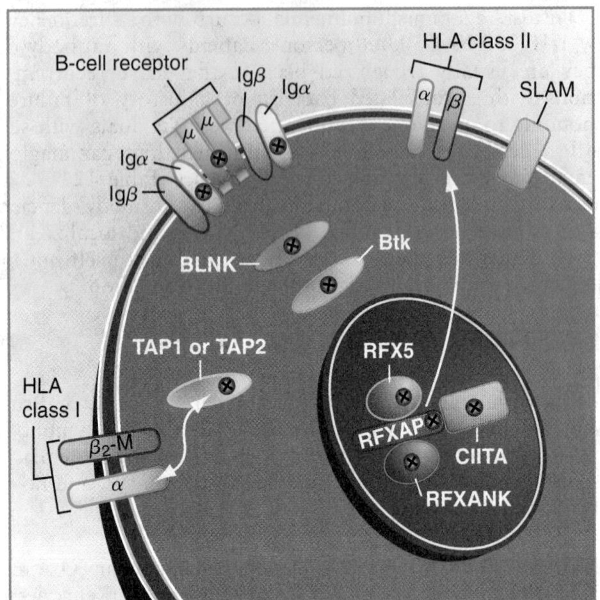

Figure 123-1. Locations of mutant proteins *(X)* in B cells identified in primary immunodeficiency diseases. β_2m, β_2 microglobulin; BLNK, B-cell linker adaptor protein; Btk, Bruton tyrosine kinase; RFX, RFXAP and CIITA transcription factors; SLAM, signaling lymphocyte activation molecule; TAP1 and TAP2, transporters of processed antigen. (From Buckley RH: Primary immunodeficiency diseases due to defects in lymphocytes. *N Engl J Med* 2000;343:1313–1324.)

such cells is needed. Some pre–B cells are found in the bone marrow; the percentage of peripheral blood B lymphocytes is <1%. The percentage of T cells is increased, ratios of T-cell subsets are normal, and T-cell function is intact. The thymus is normal.

Five autosomal recessive defects have also been shown to result in agammaglobulinemia with an absence of circulating B cells (see Fig. 123-2), including mutations in the genes encoding: (1) the μ heavy chain gene; (2) the Igα signaling molecule; (3) B-cell linker adaptor protein (BLNK); (4) the surrogate light chain, λ5/14.1; and (5) in the gene leucine-rich repeat-containing 8 (LRRC8).

CLINICAL MANIFESTATIONS. Most boys afflicted with XLA remain well during the 1st 6–9 mo of life by virtue of maternally transmitted IgG antibodies. Thereafter, they acquire infections with extracellular pyogenic organisms, such as *Streptococcus pneumoniae* and *Haemophilus influenzae,* unless they are given prophylactic antibiotics or immunoglobulin therapy. Infections include sinusitis, otitis media, pneumonia, or, less often, sepsis or meningitis. Infections with *Mycoplasma* are also particularly problematic. Chronic fungal infections are seen; *Pneumocystis carinii* pneumonia rarely occurs. Viral infections are usually handled normally with the exceptions of hepatitis viruses and enteroviruses. Several examples of paralysis after live polio vaccine administration have occurred, and chronic, eventually fatal central nervous system infections with various echoviruses have also occurred. These observations suggest a primary role for antibody, particularly secretory IgA, in host defense against enteroviruses. Viral-associated myositis resembling dermatomyositis has been observed. Growth hormone deficiency has also been reported in association with XLA.

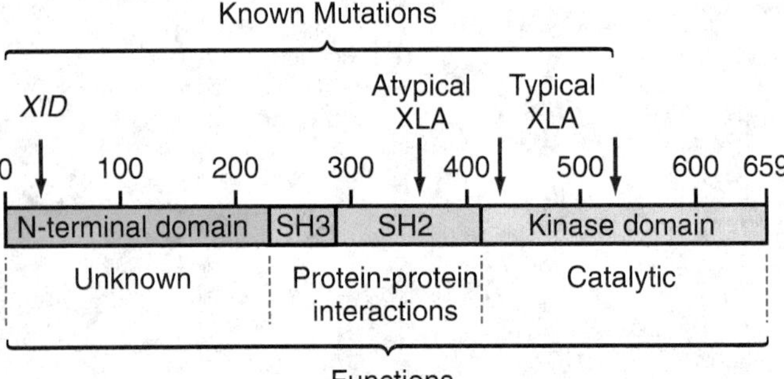

Figure 123-2. Location of mutations in the functional domains of the Bruton tyrosine kinase (Btk) protein. Deletion and point mutations in Btk identified to date in many boys with classic X-linked agammaglobulinemia (XLA) are in the kinase domain, whereas CBA/N XID mice with a less severe B-cell defect have a point mutation at position 28 in the N-terminal domain. More recently, however, boys with classic XLA are also reported to have mutations at the XID mutation site and in the SH2 domain. (From Buckley RH: Breakthroughs in the understanding and therapy of primary immunodeficiency. *Pediatr Clin North Am* 1994;41:665–690.)

DIAGNOSIS. The diagnosis of XLA should be suspected if **lymphoid hypoplasia,** with minimal or no tonsillar tissue and no palpable lymph nodes, is found on physical examination, and serum concentrations of IgG, IgA, IgM, and IgE are far below the 95% confidence limits for appropriate age- and race-matched controls (see Chapter 716), usually with total immunoglobulin <100 mg/dL. Levels of natural antibodies to type A and B red blood cell polysaccharide antigens (isohemagglutinins) and antibodies to antigens given during routine immunizations are abnormally low in this disorder, whereas they are normal in transient hypogammaglobulinemia of infancy. **Flow cytometry** is an important test to demonstrate the absence of circulating B cells, which will distinguish this disorder from common variable immunodeficiency and from transient hypogammaglobulinemia of infancy.

COMMON VARIABLE IMMUNODEFICIENCY

Common variable immunodeficiency (CVID) is a syndrome characterized by hypogammaglobulinemia with phenotypically normal B cells. It has also been called "**acquired hypogammaglobulinemia**" because of a generally later age of onset of infections. CVID patients may appear similar clinically to those with XLA in the types of infections experienced and bacterial etiologic agents involved, except that echovirus meningoencephalitis is rare in patients with CVID. In contrast to XLA, the sex distribution in CVID is almost equal, the age of onset is later (although it may be present in infancy), and infections are less severe.

GENETICS AND PATHOGENESIS. Most patients have no identified molecular diagnosis. CVID is a category of primary immunodeficiency disorders that likely consists of several different genetic defects. The genes currently known to produce the CVID phenotype when mutated include *ICOS* (inducible co-stimulator) deficiency, *SH2DIA* (responsible for X-linked lymphoproliferative disease [XLP]), *CD19, BAFF-R* (B-cell–activating factor of the TNF [tumor necrosis factor] family receptor), and *TACI* (transmembrane activator, calcium-modulator, and cyclophilin ligand interactor).

Because CVID occurs in 1st-degree relatives of patients with selective IgA deficiency, and some patients with IgA deficiency later become panhypogammaglobulinemic, one subtype of CVID may have a common genetic basis with IgA deficiency. The high incidence of abnormal immunoglobulin concentrations, autoantibodies, autoimmune disease, and malignancy in both CVID and IgA deficiency and in other members of their families also suggests a shared hereditary influence. This concept is supported by the discovery of a high incidence of C4-A gene deletions and C2 rare gene alleles in the class III major histocompatibility complex (MHC) region in individuals with either IgA deficiency or CVID, suggesting that a common susceptibility gene is on chromosome

6. Only a few HLA haplotypes are shared by individuals affected with IgA deficiency and CVID, with at least one of two particular haplotypes being present in 77% of those affected. In one large family with 13 members, two had IgA deficiency and three had CVID. All of the immunodeficient patients in the family had at least one copy of an MHC haplotype that is abnormally frequent in IgA deficiency and CVID: HLA-DQB1 *0201, HLA-DR3, C4B-Sf, C4A-deleted, G11-15, Bf-0.4, C2a, HSP70-7.5, TNFa-5, HLA-B8, and HLA-A1. In a study of 83 multiply affected families with IgA deficiency and CVID, increased allele sharing at chromosome 6p21 in the proximal part of the MHC was observed in a susceptibility locus now designated as *IGAD1*. More sensitive genetic analysis in 101 multiple-case and 110 single-case families further localized the defect to the *HLADQ/DR* locus. Environmental factors, particularly drugs such as phenytoin, D-penicillamine, gold, and sulfasalazine are suspected to be triggers for disease expression in individuals with the permissive genetic background.

Most cases of CVID are sporadic or follow an autosomal dominant pattern of inheritance. There have been patients found who had an autosomal recessive pattern of inheritance who lack **inducible co-stimulator (ICOS)**, a surface protein on activated T cells. Binding of ICOS to its ligand induces a significant increase in T-cell proliferation and cytokine production, especially of IL-10, which has been implicated in the differentiation of B cells to plasma cells. Nine such patients from 6 families have been found to have identical homozygous large genomic deletions of the *ICOS* gene, suggesting a founder effect.

Other patients with a clinical presentation of CVID have mutations involving intermediates in B-cell–signaling and developmental pathways. Specifically, defects in *CD19, BAFF-R,* and *TACI* have been identified in such patients. BAFF and APRIL serve as ligands for BAFF-R, TACI, and B-cell maturation antigen (BCMA). Patients with mutations in BAFF-R or TACI most likely lack the necessary B-cell signaling provided through interaction with BAFF and APRIL to promote proper maturation and generation of a diverse antibody repertoire.

Despite normal numbers of circulating immunoglobulin-bearing B lymphocytes and the presence of lymphoid cortical follicles, blood B lymphocytes from CVID patients do not differentiate normally into immunoglobulin-producing cells when stimulated with pokeweed mitogen (PWM) in vitro, even when co-cultured with normal T cells. CVID B cells from some patients can be stimulated both to switch isotype and to synthesize and secrete some immunoglobulin when stimulated with anti-CD40 and IL-4 or IL-10. T cells and T-cell subsets are usually present in normal percentages, although T-cell function is depressed in some patients.

CLINICAL MANIFESTATIONS. The serum immunoglobulin and antibody deficiencies in CVID may be as profound as in XLA. Patients with CVID often have autoantibody formation and normal-sized or enlarged tonsils and lymph nodes, and ≈ 25% of patients have splenomegaly. CVID has also been associated with a sprue-like syndrome with or without nodular follicular lymphoid hyperplasia of the intestine, thymoma, alopecia areata, hemolytic anemia, gastric atrophy, achlorhydria, thrombocytopenia, and pernicious anemia. Lymphoid interstitial pneumonia, pseudolymphoma, B-cell lymphomas, amyloidosis, and noncaseating sarcoid-like granulomas of the lungs, spleen, skin, and liver also occur. There is a 438-fold increase in lymphomas among affected women in the 5th and 6th decades of life. CVID is reported to resolve transiently or permanently in patients who acquire human immunodeficiency virus (HIV) infection.

SELECTIVE IGA DEFICIENCY

An isolated absence or near absence (<10 mg/dL) of serum and secretory IgA is the most common well-defined immunodeficiency disorder, with a disease frequency of 0.33% of the population. This condition is also occasionally associated with ill health.

The basic defect resulting in IgA deficiency is unknown. Phenotypically normal blood B cells are present. IgA deficiency occasionally remits spontaneously or after discontinuation of phenytoin (Dilantin) therapy. The occurrence of IgA deficiency in both males and females and in members of successive generations within families suggests autosomal dominant inheritance with variable expressivity. This defect also occurs commonly in pedigrees containing individuals with CVID. Indeed, IgA deficiency may evolve into CVID, and the finding of rare alleles and deletions of MHC class III genes in both conditions suggests that the susceptibility gene common to these two conditions may reside in the MHC class III region on chromosome 6. IgA deficiency is noted in patients treated with the same drugs associated with producing CVID (phenytoin, D-penicillamine, gold, and sulfasalazine), suggesting that environmental factors may also trigger this disease.

CLINICAL MANIFESTATIONS. Infections occur predominantly in the respiratory, gastrointestinal, and urogenital tracts. Bacterial agents responsible are the same as in other antibody deficiency syndromes. Intestinal giardiasis is common. Children with IgA deficiency vaccinated intranasally with killed poliovirus produce local IgM and IgG antibodies. Serum concentrations of other immunoglobulins are usually normal in patients with selective IgA deficiency, although IgG2 (and other) subclass deficiency is reported, and IgM (usually elevated) may be monomeric.

Patients with IgA deficiency often have IgG antibodies against cow's milk and ruminant serum proteins. These antiruminant antibodies may cause false-positive results in immunoassays for IgA that use goat (but not rabbit) antisera. IgA deficiency is associated with a sprue-like syndrome, which may or may not respond to a gluten-free diet. The incidence of autoantibodies, autoimmune diseases, and malignancy is increased. **Serum antibodies** to IgA are reported in as many as 44% of patients with selective IgA deficiency. If these antibodies are of the IgE isotype, they can cause severe or fatal anaphylactic reactions after intravenous administration of blood products containing IgA. Only five-times washed (in 200-mL volumes) normal donor erythrocytes, or blood products from other IgA-deficient individuals, should be administered to patients with IgA deficiency. Administration of intravenous immunoglobulin (IVIG), which is >99% IgG, is not indicated because most IgA-deficient patients make IgG antibodies normally. Many IVIG preparations contain sufficient IgA to cause anaphylactic reactions.

IgG SUBCLASS DEFICIENCIES

Some patients have deficiencies of one or more of the four subclasses of IgG despite normal or elevated total IgG serum concentration. Most patients with absent or very low concentrations of IgG2 also have IgA deficiency. Other patients with IgG2 deficiency have an evolving pattern of immunodeficiency, such as CVID, suggesting that the presence of IgG subclass deficiency may be a marker for more generalized immune dysfunction. The biologic significance of the numerous moderate deficiencies of IgG subclasses that have been reported is difficult to assess, particularly because commercial laboratory measurement of IgG subclasses is problematic. IgG subclass measurement is not cost-effective in evaluating immune function in the child with recurrent infection. The more relevant issue is a patient's capacity to make specific antibodies to protein and polysaccharide antigens, because profound deficiencies of antipolysaccharide antibodies have been noted even in the presence of normal concentrations of IgG2. IVIG should not be administered to patients with IgG subclass deficiency unless they are shown to have a deficiency of antibodies to a broad array of antigens.

IMMUNOGLOBULIN HEAVY- AND LIGHT-CHAIN DELETIONS

Some completely asymptomatic individuals have been documented to have a total absence of IgG1, IgG2, IgG4, and/or IgA1 due to gene deletions. These abnormalities were discovered fortuitously in 16 individuals, 15 of whom had no history of undue susceptibility to infection, and all of whom produced antibodies of all other isotypes in normal quantities. These patients illustrate the importance of assessing specific antibody formation before deciding to initiate IVIG therapy in IgG subclass–deficient patients.

HYPER-IGM SYNDROME

The hyper-IgM syndrome is genetically heterogeneous and characterized by normal or elevated serum IgM levels associated with low or absent IgG, IgA, and IgE serum levels, indicating a defect in the class-switch recombination (CSR) process. Causative mutations have been identified in two genes on the X chromosome, the CD40 ligand (hyper-IgM syndrome type 1, HIGM1) and NEMO (nuclear factor κB [NF-κB] essential modulator) genes; and three genes on autosomal chromosomes, the AICDA gene (hyper-IgM type 2, HIGM2) on chromosome 12, the uracil DNA glycosylase (UNG) gene on chromosome 12, and the CD40 gene (hyper-IgM type 3, HIGM3) on chromosome 20. Distinctive clinical features permit presumptive recognition of the type of mutation in these patients, thereby aiding proper choice of therapy. All such patients should undergo molecular analysis to ascertain the affected gene for purposes of genetic counseling, carrier detection, and decisions regarding definitive therapy.

X-LINKED HYPER IGM CAUSED BY MUTATIONS IN THE CD40 LIGAND: HYPER IGM TYPE 1 (HIGM1). HIGM1 is caused by mutations in the gene that encodes the CD40 ligand (CD154, CD40L), which is expressed on activated T helper cells. Boys with this syndrome have very low serum concentrations of IgG and IgA, with a usually normal or sometimes elevated concentration of polyclonal IgM, very small tonsils, no palpable lymph nodes, and often profound **neutropenia.**

Genetics and Pathogenesis. B cells from boys with the CD40 ligand defect are capable of synthesizing not only IgM but also IgA and IgG when co-cultured with normal activated T helper cells, indicating that the B cells are actually normal in this condition and that the defect is in the T cells. The abnormal gene is localized to Xq26, and the gene product, CD154 (CD40L), is the ligand for CD40, which is present on B cells and monocytes. CD154 is upregulated on activated T cells. Mutations in CD154 result in an inability to signal B cells to undergo isotype switching, and thus the B cells produce only IgM. The failure of T cells to interact with B cells through this receptor-ligand pair also causes a failure of upregulation of the B cell and monocyte surface molecules CD80 and CD86 that interact with CD28/CTLA4 on T cells, resulting in failure of “cross talk” between immune system cells. The failure of interaction of the molecules of those pathways results in a propensity for tolerogenic T-cell signaling and defective recognition of tumor cells. More than 73 distinct point mutations or deletions in the gene encoding CD154 have been identified in 87 unrelated families, giving rise to frame shifts, premature stop codons, and single amino acid substitutions, most of which are clustered in the domain with homology to TNF, located in the carboxy-terminal region.

Clinical Manifestations. Similar to patients with XLA, boys with the CD40 ligand defect have small tonsils and often no palpable lymph nodes, and become symptomatic during the 1st or 2nd year of life with recurrent pyogenic infections, including otitis media, sinusitis, pneumonia, and tonsillitis. Lymph node histology shows only abortive germinal center formation with severe depletion and phenotypic abnormalities of follicular dendritic cells. These patients have normal numbers of circulating B lymphocytes, marked susceptibility to *P. carinii* pneumonia, and are frequently profoundly neutropenic. Circulating T cells are also present in normal number and in vitro responses to mitogens are normal, but there is decreased antigen-specific T-cell function. In a study of patients with the CD40 ligand defect, 23.3% had died at a mean age at death of 11.7 yr. In addition to opportunistic infections such as *P. carinii* pneumonia, there is an increased incidence of extensive verruca vulgaris lesions, *Cryptosporidium* enteritis, subsequent liver disease, and increased risk of malignancy. Because of the poor prognosis, the treatment of choice is an HLA-identical stem cell transplant at an early age. Alternative treatment for this condition is monthly infusion of IVIG. In patients with severe neutropenia, the use of G-CSF has been beneficial.

X-LINKED HYPER IGM CAUSED BY MUTATIONS IN THE GENE ENCODING NUCLEAR FACTOR κB (NF-κB) ESSENTIAL MODULATOR (NEMO, OR IKKγ). This syndrome in males is characterized most often clinically as **anhydrotic ectodermal dysplasia with associated immunodeficiency (EDA-ID).** The condition results from missense mutations in the IKBKG gene at position 28q on the X chromosome that encodes **nuclear factor κB (NF-κB) essential modulator (NEMO),** a regulatory protein required for the activation of the transcription factor NF-κB. Germ line loss-of-function mutations cause the X-linked dominant condition incontinentia pigmenti in females and are lethal in male fetuses. Mutations in the coding region of IKBKG are associated with EDA-ID. The immunodeficiency is variable, with most patients showing impaired antibody responses to polysaccharide antigens. Some patients with EDA-ID have hyper IgM. Pharmacologic inhibitors of NF-κB activation have been shown to downregulate CD154 mRNA and protein levels, suggesting the mechanism of hyper IgM in this condition. The hyper-IgM patients with this defect should be easily recognizable because of the presence of ectodermal dysplasia, although there is a report of this condition without ectodermal dysplasia.

AUTOSOMAL RECESSIVE HYPER IGM CAUSED BY MUTATIONS IN THE GENE FOR ACTIVATION-INDUCED CYTIDINE DEAMINASE (AICDA): HYPER-IGM TYPE 2 (HIGM2). An autosomal recessive form of hyper-IgM syndrome is caused by mutations in the gene for activation-induced cytidine deaminase (AICDA).

Genetics and Pathogenesis. Patients with autosomal hyper IgM usually have normal numbers of circulating B lymphocytes, but, in contrast to patients with the CD40 ligand defect, B cells from these patients are not able to switch from IgM-secreting to IgG-, IgA-, or IgE-secreting cells, even when co-cultured with monoclonal antibodies to CD40 and a variety of cytokines. When their B cells are cultured in vitro, they spontaneously secrete large amounts of IgM, but this is not further augmented by the addition of IL-4 or anti-CD40 with IL-4 or other cytokines. Thus, in these patients, there is truly an intrinsic B-cell abnormality. The defect in many such patients has been identified as due to mutations in a gene on chromosome 12p13 that encodes AICDA. AICDA is a single-stranded (SS) DNA deaminase required for somatic hypermutation (SHM) and CSR of immunoglobulin genes. Histologic examination of the enlarged lymph nodes reveals the presence of giant germinal centers (5–10 times larger than normal) filled with highly proliferating B cells. Proliferating B cells co-express IgM, IgD, and CD38, a phenotype previously described for a small B-cell subset corresponding to germinal center (GC) founder cells. These cells are thought to correspond to a transitional stage between follicular mantle and GC B cells, at the onset of somatic mutation of the Ig variable region gene and antigen-driven selection. Deficiency of AICDA results in impaired terminal differentiation of B cells, a failure of CSR, and lack of immunoglobulin gene SHM.

Clinical Manifestations. Concentrations of serum IgG, IgA, and IgE are very low in AICDA deficiency. In contrast to the CD40 ligand defect, however, the serum IgM concentration in patients with AICDA deficiency is usually markedly elevated and polyclonal. Patients with this form of hyper IgM have lymphoid hyperplasia, are generally older at age of onset, do not have susceptibility to *P. carinii* pneumonia, often do have isohemagglutinins, and are much less likely to have neutropenia unless it occurs on an autoimmune basis. They have a tendency, however, to develop autoimmune and inflammatory disorders including diabetes mellitus, polyarthritis, autoimmune hepatitis, hemolytic anemia, immune thrombocytopenia, Crohn disease, and chronic uveitis. With early diagnosis and monthly infusions of IVIG, as well as good management of infections with antibiotics, patients with AICDA mutations generally have a more benign course than do boys with the CD40 ligand defect.

AUTOSOMAL RECESSIVE HYPER IGM CAUSED BY MUTATIONS IN THE GENE FOR URACIL DNA GLYCOSYLASE (UNG). Another cause of the hyper-IgM syndrome is a deficiency of uracil DNA glycosylase.

Genetics and Pathogenesis. AICDA deaminates cytosine into uracil in targeted DNA, which is followed by uracil removal by UNG. Profoundly impaired class-switch recombination was found in three hyper-IgM patients reported to have UNG deficiency. Their clinical characteristics were similar to those with AICDA deficiency, with increased susceptibility to bacterial infections and lymphoid hyperplasia. The patients had a markedly elevated serum IgM and profoundly decreased serum IgG and IgA concentrations. Their B cells had an intrinsic defect in CSR when stimulated with anti-CD40 and IL-4 and constitutively produced high quantities of IgM. They had only a partial defect in SHM, however.

AUTOSOMAL RECESSIVE HYPER IGM CAUSED BY MUTATIONS IN CD40: HYPER-IGM TYPE 3 (HIGM3). Patients with autosomal recessive hyper IgM who failed to express CD40 on their B-cell surfaces, resulting from mutations in the CD40 gene, were identified.

Genetics and Pathogenesis. CD40 is a type I integral membrane glycoprotein encoded by a gene on chromosome 20 and belonging to the TNF and nerve growth factor receptor superfamily. It is expressed on B cells, macrophages, dendritic cells, and a few other types of cells. Mutations in the CD40 gene cause an autosomal recessive form of hyper-IgM syndrome that is clinically indistinguishable from HIGM1, resulting from the X-linked CD40 ligand (CD154) defect. In contrast to the CD40 ligand defect, however, the B cells in the autosomal recessive condition are intrinsically abnormal and cannot isotype switch. The T cells are normal except to the extent that they cannot cause upregulation of CD80 and CD86 on B cells and macrophages to interact with CD28/CTLA4 on T cells.

HYPER-IGM TYPE 4 (HIGM4). The defective gene in a fourth autosomal recessive form of hyper-IgM syndrome has not yet been identified, but appears to be in a gene downstream of AICDA. These patients all have defective class-switch recombination with preserved SHM.

X-LINKED LYMPHOPROLIFERATIVE DISEASE

X-linked lymphoproliferative (XLP) disease, also referred to as **Duncan disease** after the original kindred in which it was described, is an X-linked recessive trait characterized by an inadequate immune response to infection with Epstein-Barr virus (EBV).

Genetics and Pathogenesis. The defective gene in XLP was localized to Xq25, cloned, and initially named SAP (for SLAM-associated protein), but is now known officially as SH2D1A. SLAM (signaling lymphocyte activation molecule) is an adhesion molecule that is upregulated on both T and B cells with infection and other stimulation. SH2D1A is highly expressed in thymocytes and peripheral blood T and NK cells, with a prevalent expression on Th1 cells. Its presence on B lymphocytes is unclear. Thus, although antibody deficiency is frequently present, this is really a T and NK cell defect. SH2D1A competes with SHP-2 for binding to SLAM and, as such, is a regulatory molecule (see Fig. 124-1). In XLP patients, the absence of SH2D1A can lead to an uncontrolled cytotoxic T-cell immune response to EBV. The SH2D1A protein associates permissively with 2B4 on NK cells; thus, selective impairment of 2B4-mediated NK-cell activation also contributes to the immunopathology of XLP.

Clinical Manifestations. Affected males are usually healthy until they acquire EBV infection. The mean age of presentation is <5 yr. There are three major clinical phenotypes: (1) fulminant, often fatal, infectious mononucleosis (50% of cases); (2) lymphomas, predominantly involving B-lineage cells (25%); or (3) acquired hypogammaglobulinemia (25%). There is a marked impairment in production of antibodies to the EBV nuclear antigen (EBNA), whereas titers of antibodies to the viral capsid antigen (VCA) have ranged from absent to markedly elevated. XLP has an unfavorable prognosis; 70% of affected boys die by age 10. Only two XLP patients are known to have survived beyond 40 yr of age. Unless there is a family history of XLP, diagnosis prior to the onset of complications is difficult because affected individuals are asymptomatic initially. Using mutation analysis, it is possible to identify affected males within identified kindreds before they develop primary EBV infection. Approximately half of the few patients with XLP given HLA-identical related or unrelated stem cell transplants are currently surviving without signs of the disease.

Two pedigrees have been reported in which boys in one arm of each pedigree were diagnosed with CVID, whereas those in the other arms had fulminant infectious mononucleosis. The family members with CVID never gave a history of infectious mononucleosis. All affected members of each pedigree had the same distinct SH2D1A mutation, however, despite the different clinical phenotypes. Because the SH2D1A mutation was the same but the phenotype varied in these families, XLP should be considered in all males with a diagnosis of CVID, particularly if there is more than one male family member with this phenotype.

123.1 • Treatment of B-Cell Defects

Except for the CD40 ligand defect and XLP, for which stem cell transplantation is recommended, judicious use of antibiotics to treat documented infections and regular administration of intravenous immunoglobulins are the only effective treatments for primary B-cell disorders. The most common form of replacement therapy is with IVIG. Broad antibody deficiency should be carefully documented before such therapy is initiated. The rationale for the use of IVIG is to provide missing antibodies, not to raise the serum IgG or IgG subclass level. The development of safe and effective IVIG is a major advance in the treatment of patients with severe antibody deficiencies, although it is expensive and there have been national shortages. Almost all commercial preparations are isolated from normal plasma by the Cohn alcohol fractionation method or a modification of this method. Cohn fraction II is then further treated to remove aggregated IgG. Additional stabilizing agents such as sugars, glycine, and albumin are added to prevent reaggregation and protect the IgG molecule during lyophilization. The ethanol used in preparation of IVIG and immune serum globulin, used for intramuscular injection, inactivates HIV; an organic solvent/detergent step inactivates hepatitis B and C viruses. Some preparations are also nanofiltered to remove infectious agents. Most commercial lots are produced from plasma pooled from more than 60,000 donors and therefore contain a broad spectrum of antibodies. Each pool must contain adequate levels of antibody to antigens in various vaccines, such as tetanus and measles. However, there is no standardization based on titers of antibodies to more clinically relevant organisms, such as *Streptococcus pneumoniae* and *Haemophilus influenzae* type b.

The IVIG preparations available in the United States have similar efficacy and safety. Rare transmission of hepatitis C virus has occurred in the past, but the potential transmission of hepatitis C virus has been resolved by additional treatment with an organic solvent/detergent mixture. There has been no documented transmission of HIV by any of these preparations. **IVIG (400 mg/kg/mo)** achieves trough IgG levels close to the normal range. Systemic reactions to IVIG may occur, but rarely are these true anaphylactic reactions. Anaphylactic reactions caused by a patient's IgE antibodies to IgA in the IVIG preparation may occur in patients with CVID or IgA deficiency. Newly diagnosed patients with CVID should be screened through the American Red Cross for anti-IgA antibodies. If anti-IgA antibodies are detected, IVIG therapy should consist of the one available IVIG preparation containing almost no IgA (Gammagard S/D, Baxter).

Ballow M: Primary immunodeficiency disorders: Antibody deficiency. *J Allergy Clin Immunol* 2002;109:581–591.

Buckley RH: Primary immunodeficiency diseases due to defects in lymphocytes. *N Engl J Med* 2000;343:1313–1324.

Durandy A, Revy P, Fischer A: Human models of inherited immunoglobulin class switch recombination and somatic hypermutation defects (hyper-IgM syndromes). *Adv Immunol* 2004;82:295–330.

Etzioni A, Ochs HD: The hyper IgM syndrome: An evolving story. *Pediatr Res* 2004;56:519–525.

Jacobsohn DA, Emerick KM, Scholl P, et al: Nonmyeloablative hematopoietic stem cell transplant for x-linked hyper-immunoglobulin M syndrome with cholangiopathy. *Pediatrics* 2004;113:e122–e127.

Kralovicova J, Hammarstrom L, Plebani A, et al: Fine-scale mapping at IGAD1 and genome-wide genetic linkage analysis implicate HLA-DQ/DR as a major susceptibility locus in selective IgA deficiency and common variable immunodeficiency. *J Immunol* 2003;170:2765–2775.

Lindvall JM, Blomberg KE, Valiaho J, et al: Bruton's tyrosine kinase: Cell biology, sequence conservation, mutation spectrum, siRNA modifications, and expression profiling. *Immunol Rev* 2005;203:200–215.

Lougaris V, Badolato R, Ferrari S, et al: Hyper immunoglobulin M syndrome due to CD40 deficiency: Clinical, molecular, and immunological features. *Immunol Rev* 2005;203:48–66.

The Medical Letter: Intravenous immunoglobulin (IVIG). *Med Lett* 2006;48:101–102.

Michel M, Chanet V, Galicier L, et al: Autoimmune thrombocytopenia purpura and common variable immunodeficiency. *Medicine* 2004; 83:254–263.

Nichols KE, Ma CS, Cannons JL, et al: Molecular and cellular pathogenesis of X-linked lymphoproliferative disease. *Immunol Rev* 2005;203:180–199.

Salzer U, Chapel HM, Webster ADB: Mutations in TNFRSF13B encoding TACI are associated with common variable immunodeficiency in humans. *Nat Genetics* 2005;8:820–828.

Salzer U, Maul-Pavicic A, Cunningham-Rundles C, et al: ICOS deficiency in patients with common variable immunodeficiency. *Clin Immunol* 2004;113:234–240.

Schroeder HW Jr, Schroeder HW III, Sheikh SM: The complex genetics of common variable immunodeficiency. *J Investig Med* 2004;52:90–103.

van Zelin MC, Reisli I, vander Burg M, et al: An antibody-deficiency syndrome due to mutations in the CD19 gene. *N Engl J Med* 2006;354:1901–1912.

Winkelstein JA, Marino MC, Lederman HM, et al: X-Linked agammaglobulinemia: report on a United States registry of 201 patients. *Medicine* 2006;85:193–202.

Winkelstein JA, Marono MC, Ochs H, et al: The X-linked hyper-IgM syndrome: Clinical and immunologic features of 79 patients. *Medicine* 2003; 82:373–384.

Chapter 124 ■ Primary Defects of Cellular Immunity

In general, patients with defects in T-cell function have infections or other clinical problems that are more severe than in patients with antibody deficiency disorders (see Table 121-3). The defective gene products for some primary T-cell diseases are identified (Table 124-1). These individuals rarely survive beyond infancy or childhood. Transplantation of thymic tissue, or of major histocompatibility complex (MHC)–compatible sibling or haploidentical (half-matched) parental hematopoietic stem cell, is the treatment of choice for patients with primary T-cell defects (see Chapter 134).

THYMIC HYPOPLASIA (DiGEORGE SYNDROME)

Thymic hypoplasia results from dysmorphogenesis of the 3rd and 4th pharyngeal pouches during early embryogenesis, leading to hypoplasia or aplasia of the thymus and parathyroid glands. Other structures forming at the same age are also frequently affected, resulting in anomalies of the great vessels (right-sided aortic arch), esophageal atresia, bifid uvula, congenital heart disease (conotruncal, atrial, and ventricular septal defects), a short philtrum of the upper lip, hypertelorism, an antimongoloid slant to the eyes, mandibular hypoplasia, and low-set, often notched ears (see Chapters 81 and 108). The diagnosis is often first suggested by hypocalcemic seizures during the neonatal period.

Genetics and Pathogenesis. DiGeorge syndrome occurs in both males and females. Microdeletions of specific DNA sequences from chromosome 22q11.2, the **DiGeorge chromosomal region (DGCR)**, are found in a majority of cases. Several candidate genes have been identified in this region. A T-box transcription family member, *TBX1*, has been implicated as an etiology for most of the major signs of DGS. There appears to be an excess of 22q11.2 deletions of maternal origin. Polymerase chain reaction (PCR)–based genotyping using microsatellite DNA markers located within the commonly deleted region permits rapid detection of such microdeletions. Conotruncal heart defects

TABLE 124-1. Genetic Basis of Primary Cellular Immunodeficiency Diseases

CHROMOSOME AND REGION	GENE PRODUCT	DISORDER	FUNCTIONAL DEFICIENCIES
1p35-p34.3	Lck*	T-cell-activation defect	Impaired T-cell function
2p12	CD8α*	CD8 deficiency	Lack of cytotoxic T cells
2q12	ZAP-70*	CD8 deficiency	Failure of CD4 T cells to respond to usual signals
10p13	Unknown	Thymic hypoplasia (DiGeorge syndrome, velocardiofacial syndrome)	Low number of T cells and impaired T-cell function
11q23	CD3*	CD3 deficiency	Poor T-cell responses to mitogens; lack of cytotoxic T cells; IgG subclass deficiency
21q22.3	Autoimmune regulator (AIRE)	APECED, chronic mucocutaneous candidiasis, parathyroid and adrenal antoimmunity	Poor response to candida antigen; autoimmune responses
22q11.22	?TBX1	Thymic hypoplasia (DiGeorge syndrome, velocardiofacial syndrome)	Low number of T cells and impaired T-cell function

*The gene has been cloned and sequenced.
APECED, autoimmune polyendocrinopathy-candidiasis ectodermal dysplasia; Zap-70, Zeta-associated protein 70.

and 22q deletions are observed in DiGeorge syndrome, velocardiofacial syndrome (VCFS), and conotruncal anomaly face syndrome (CTAFS). The **CATCH 22 syndrome** (*c*ardiac, *a*bnormal facies, *t*hymic hypoplasia, *c*left palate, *h*ypocalcemia) includes the broad clinical spectrum of conditions with 22q11.2 deletions. Other deletions associated with DiGeorge and velocardiofacial syndromes have been identified on chromosome 10p13 (see Chapter 81).

Variable hypoplasia of the thymus and parathyroid glands defines **partial DiGeorge syndrome,** which is more frequent than total aplasia; aplasia is present in <1% of patients with DiGeorge syndrome and defines **complete DiGeorge syndrome.** Slightly less than half of patients with complete DiGeorge syndrome are hemizygous at chromosome 22q11. Approximately one third of infants with complete DiGeorge syndrome have **CHARGE association** (*c*oloboma, *h*eart defect, choanal *a*tresia, growth or developmental *r*etardation, *g*enital hypoplasia, and *e*ar anomalies including deafness). Approximately 15% are born to diabetic mothers. Another 15% of infants have no identified risk factors.

Concentrations of serum immunoglobulins are usually normal, but IgA may be diminished and IgE elevated. Other laboratory findings vary depending on the degree of thymic dysfunction.

Absolute lymphocyte counts are usually only moderately low for age. The CD3 T-cell counts are variably decreased in number, corresponding to the degree of thymic hypoplasia, resulting in an increased percentage of B cells. Lymphocyte responses to mitogen stimulation are absent, reduced, or normal, depending on the degree of thymic deficiency. Thymic tissue, when found, contains Hassall corpuscles, normal density of thymocytes, and corticomedullary distinction. Lymphoid follicles are usually present, but lymph node paracortical areas and thymus-dependent regions of the spleen show variable degrees of depletion.

Clinical Manifestations. Children with partial thymic hypoplasia may have little trouble with infections and grow normally. Patients with complete DiGeorge syndrome resemble patients with severe combined immunodeficiency (SCID) in their susceptibility to infections with low-grade or opportunistic pathogens, including fungi, viruses, and *Pneumocystis carinii (jiroveci),* and to graft versus host disease (GVHD) from nonirradiated blood transfusions. Patients with complete DiGeorge syndrome can develop an atypical phenotype in which oligoclonal T-cell populations appear in the blood associated with rash and lymphadenopathy. These atypical patients appear phenotypically to be similar to patients with Omenn syndrome or maternal lymphocyte engraftment.

It is critical to confirm the diagnosis of complete DiGeorge syndrome in a timely manner because this disease is fatal without treatment. A T-cell count should be obtained on all infants born with primary hypoparathyroidism, CHARGE syndrome, truncus arteriosus, and interrupted aortic arch type B. If a patient has findings consistent with DiGeorge syndrome and also has rash and lymphadenopathy, the patient should be referred to an immunologist for evaluation.

Treatment. The immune deficiency in the complete DiGeorge syndrome is correctable primarily by cultured unrelated thymic tissue transplants or non-irradiated unfractionated bone marrow or peripheral blood transplantation from an HLA-identical sibling (see Chapter 143).

DEFECTIVE EXPRESSION OF THE T-CELL RECEPTOR–CD3 COMPLEX (TI-CD3)

The first type of this disorder was found in two brothers in a Spanish family. The proband presented with severe infections and died at 31 mo of age with autoimmune hemolytic anemia and viral pneumonia. His lymphocytes had responded poorly to mitogens and to anti-CD3 in vitro and could not be stimulated to

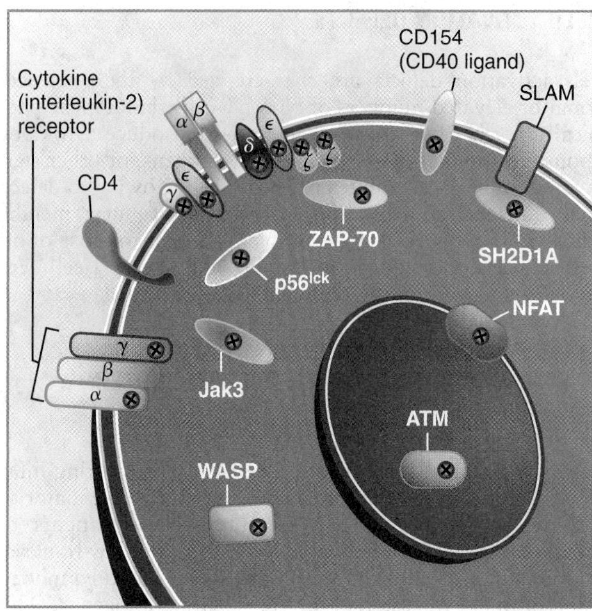

Figure 124-1. Locations of mutant proteins *(X)* in activated CD4 T cells identified in primary immunodeficiency diseases. ZAP-70, zeta-associated protein 70; SLAM, signaling lymphocyte activation molecule; SH2D1A, SLAM-associated protein; ATM, ataxia telangiectasia mutation; NFAT, nuclear factor of activated T cells; Jak3, Janus kinase 3; and WASP, Wiskott-Aldrich syndrome protein. (From Buckley RH: Primary immunodeficiency diseases due to defects in lymphocytes. *N Engl J Med* 2000;343:1313–1324.)

develop cytotoxic T cells. His antibody responses to protein antigens had been normal, indicating normal T-helper-cell function. His 12 yr old brother was healthy, but had almost no CD3-bearing T cells and had IgG2 deficiency similar to his sibling. The defect in this family was due to mutations in the gene encoding the CD3γ chain (Fig. 124-1).

The second type of this disorder was diagnosed in a 4 yr old French boy who had recurrent *Haemophilus influenzae* pneumonia and otitis media in early life but is now healthy. He had a partial defect in expression of Ti-CD3, and thus the percentage of CD3 cells was about half-normal, but the level of expression is markedly decreased. The defect was shown to be due to two independent CD3ε gene mutations, leading to defective CD3ε chain synthesis. There was a splice site mutation on one allele that did not totally abrogate the normal intron 7 splicing, thus there was partial expression of CD3 on the T cells. His T cells did not proliferate normally in response to anti-CD3 or anti-CD2, but did respond normally to stimulation with anti-CD28 or antigens, such as tetanus toxoid. Thus, this mutation did not result in failure of T-cell development, whereas mutations in the portions of the gene that encodes the extracellular component of CD3ε result in a profound deficiency of circulating mature CD3 T cells (see Chapter 125).

DEFECTIVE CYTOKINE PRODUCTION

IL-12, which is produced by activated antigen-presenting cells, promotes the development of Th1 responses and is a powerful inducer of IFN-γ production by T and natural killer (NK) cells. A child with bacille Calmette-Guérin (BCG) and *Salmonella enteritidis* infections had a large homozygous deletion within the IL-12 p40 subunit gene precluding expression of functional IL-12 p70 cytokine by activated dendritic cells and phagocytes. IFN-γ production by the child's lymphocytes was therefore markedly impaired. IL-12 may be essential for protective immunity to intracellular bacteria such as *Mycobacterium* and *Salmonella.*

T-CELL ACTIVATION DEFECTS

T-cell activation defects are characterized by the presence of normal or elevated numbers of blood T cells that appear phenotypically normal but fail to proliferate or produce cytokines in response to stimulation with mitogens, antigens, or other signals delivered to the T-cell antigen receptor (TCR), owing to defective signal transduction from the TCR to intracellular metabolic pathways. These patients have problems similar to those of other T-cell–deficient individuals, and some with severe T-cell activation defects may clinically resemble SCID patients.

CD8 LYMPHOCYTOPENIA DUE TO MUTATIONS IN THE GENE ENCODING ZETA-ASSOCIATED PROTEIN 70 (ZAP-70)

Patients with this T-cell activation defect present during infancy with severe, recurrent, and often fatal infections. The majority of cases are reported among Mennonites. These patients have normal or elevated numbers of blood B cells and low to elevated serum immunoglobulin concentrations. Their blood lymphocytes exhibit normal expression of the T-cell surface antigens CD3 and CD4, but CD8 cells are almost totally absent. These cells fail to respond to mitogens or to allogeneic cells in vitro or to generate cytotoxic T lymphocytes. NK cell activity is normal. The thymus of one patient exhibited normal architecture with normal numbers of CD4:CD8 double-positive thymocytes but an absence of CD8 single-positive thymocytes. This condition is due to mutations in the gene encoding **zeta-associated protein 70 (ZAP-70)**, a non-src family protein tyrosine kinase important in T-cell signaling that is localized to chromosome 2q12 (see Fig. 124-1). The normal number of CD4:CD8 double-positive T cells is because the thymocytes can use the other member of the same tyrosine kinase family, Syk, to facilitate positive selection. Syk is present at fourfold higher levels in thymocytes than in peripheral T cells, possibly accounting for the lack of normal responses by the CD4 blood T cells.

Another condition that can result in CD8 deficiency is a mutation in the gene that encodes CD8α. There is a deficiency of cytotoxic T cells in that condition, but the functional immune defect is mild compared to that of ZAP-70 deficiency.

P56 LCK DEFICIENCY

A 2 mo old male infant who presented with bacterial, viral, and fungal infections was found to be lymphopenic and hypogammaglobulinemic. B and NK cells were present, but there was a low number of CD4 T cells. Mitogen responses were variable. The T cells failed to express the activation marker CD69 when stimulated through the T-cell receptor but did when stimulated with phorbol myristate acetate and a calcium ionophore, suggesting a proximal signaling defect. Molecular studies revealed an alternatively spliced transcript for p56 lck that lacked the kinase domain.

AUTOIMMUNE POLYENDOCRINOPATHY-CANDIDIASIS ECTODERMAL DYSPLASIA (APECED)

Patients with this syndrome present with chronic mucocutaneous candidiasis and autoimmune polyendocrinopathy, usually producing hypoparathyroidism and Addison disease. Additional features include hypogonadism, chronic active hepatitis, alopecia, vitiligo, pernicious anemia, and Sjögren syndrome. APECED, or autoimmune polyendocrinopathy syndrome type I (APS1), is due to a mutation in the autoimmune regulator *(AIRE)* gene. The gene product, AIRE, is expressed at high levels in purified human thymic medullary stromal cells and is thought to regulate the cell surface expression of tissue-specific proteins such as insulin and thyroglobulin. Expression of these self-proteins allows for the negative selection of autoreactive T cells during their development. Failure of negative selection results in organ-specific autoimmune destruction. The overall significance of AIRE in the establishment and maintenance of T-cell self-tolerance is not well understood.

Most pediatric patients are identified by the presence of mucocutaneous candidiasis and later develop insidious signs of Addison disease (see Chapter 572).

Aaltonen J, Björses P, Perheentupa J, et al: An autoimmune disease, APECED, caused by mutations in a novel gene featuring two PHD-type zinc-finger domains. The Finnish-German APECED Consortium. Autoimmune Polyendocrinopathy-Candidiasis-Ectodermal Dystrophy. *Nat Genet* 1997;17:399–403.

Bohn G, Allroth A, Brandes G, et al: A novel human primary immunodeficiency syndrome caused by deficiency of the endosomal adaptor protein p 14. *Nat Med* 2007;13:38–43.

Buckley RH: Primary cellular immunodeficiencies. *J Allergy Clin Immunol* 2002;109:747–757.

Buckley RH: Primary immunodeficiency diseases due to defects in lymphocytes. *N Engl J Med* 2000;343:1313–1324.

Fischer A: Human primary immunodeficiency diseases: A perspective. *Nat Immunol* 2004;5:23–30.

Markert ML, Sarzotti M, Ozaki DA, et al: Thymus transplantation in complete DiGeorge syndrome: Immunologic and safety evaluations in 12 patients. *Blood* 2003;102:1121–1130.

Notarangelo L, Casanova JL, Fischer A, et al: Primary immunodeficiency diseases: An update. *J Allergy Clin Immunol* 2004;114:677–687.

Picard C, Fieschi C, Altare F, et al: Inherited interleukin-12 deficiency: IL-12B genotype and clinical phenotype of 13 patients from six kindreds. *Am J Hum Genet* 2002;70:336–348.

Reichenbach J, Schubert R, Horvath R, et al: Fetal neonatal-onset mitochondrial respiratory chain disease with T cell immunodeficiency. *Pediatr Res* 2006;60:321–326.

Rieux-Laucat F, Hivroz C, Lim A, et al: Inherited and somatic CD3ζ mutations in a patient with T-cell deficiency. *N Engl J Med* 2006;18:1913–1921.

Stoller JZ, Epstein JA: Identification of a novel nuclear localization signal in *TBX1* that is deleted in DiGeorge syndrome patients harboring the 1223delC mutation. *Hum Mol Genet* 2005;14:885–892.

Yagi H, Furutani Y, Hamada H, et al: Role of *TBX1* in human del122q11.2 syndrome. *Lancet* 2003;362:1366–1373.

Chapter 125 ■ Primary Combined Antibody and Cellular Immunodeficiencies

Patients with combined antibody and cellular defects have severe, frequently opportunistic infections that lead to death in infancy or childhood unless they are provided hematopoietic stem cell transplantation early in life. These are thought to be rare defects, although the true incidence is unknown because there is no newborn screening for any of these defects. It is possible that many affected children die of infection during infancy without being diagnosed. The defective gene products for many combined immunodeficiencies are identified (Table 125-1).

125.1 • SEVERE COMBINED IMMUNODEFICIENCY (SCID)

The syndromes of SCID are caused by diverse genetic mutations that lead to absence of all adaptive immune function and, in

TABLE 125-1. Genetic Basis of Combined Immunodeficiency Disorders

CHROMOSOME AND REGION	GENE PRODUCT	DISORDER	FUNCTIONAL DEFICIENCIES
1q	RFX5*	MHC class II antigen deficiency	Low immunoglobulins, lack of T-cell responses to antigens, CD4 deficiency
1q31-q32	CD45*	T-B+NK- SCID	Absence of T- and B-cell functions
5p13	IL-7Rα*	T-B+NK+ SCID	Absence of T- and B-cell functions
6p21.3	TAP1*, TAP2*	MHC class I antigen deficiency	Marked deficiency of CD8 T cells; combined B- and T-cell defects
6q22-q23	IFN-γR1* IFN-γR2* IL-12Rβ1*	Disseminated mycobacterial infections	Failure of macrophages and other cells to produce TNF-α in response to IFN-
9p21-p13	Endoribonuclease RNase MRP*	Cartilage-hair hypoplasia	Combined B- and T-cell defects of varying severity
10p13	Artemis*	T-B-NK+ SCID	Absence of T- and B-cell functions
10p14-p15	IL-2Rα*	Lymphoproliferative syndrome	Poor T-cell responses; impaired apoptosis; increased bcl-2; autoimmunity
11p13	RAG1* or RAG2*	T-B-NK+ SCID	Absence of T- and B-cell functions
11q22.3	DNA-dependent kinase*	Ataxia-telangiectasia	Selective IgA deficiency; T-cell deficiency
11q23	CD3δ or CD3ε*	T-B+NK+ SCID	Absence of T- and B-cell functions
13q	RFXAP*	MHC class II antigen deficiency	Low immunoglobulins, lack of T-cell responses to antigens, CD4 deficiency
14q13.1	Purine nucleosidase*	PNP deficiency	Severe T-cell deficiency; may have immunoglobulins
16p13	CIITA*	MHC class II antigen deficiency	Low immunoglobulins, lack of T-cell responses to antigens, CD4 deficiency
19p13.1	Jak3*	T-B+NK- SCID	Absence of T-, B- and NK-cell functions
20q13.11	ADA*	T-B-NK- SCID	Absence of T- and B-cell functions
Xp11.23	WASP*	Wiskott-Aldrich syndrome	Thrombocytopenia; poor antibody production to polysaccharides; T-cell deficiency
Xq13.1	Common γ chain (γ_c) for several cytokine receptors (including IL-2, IL-4, IL-7, IL-9, IL-15, and IL-21)*	T-B+NK- SCID	Absence of T-, B- and NK-cell functions

*The gene has been cloned and sequenced.

ADA, adenosine deaminase; CIITA, class II transactivator. IFN-γR1, interferon receptor chain 1; IL-2Rα, interleukin 2 receptor α chain; IL-7Rα, interleukin 7 receptor α chain; IL-12Rβ1, interleukin 12 receptor β1 chain; Jak3, Janus kinase 3; MHC, major histocompatibility complex; PNP, purine nucleoside phosphorylase; RAG1 and RAG2, recombinase activating genes 1 and 2; SCID, severe combined immunodeficiency; TAP, transporter of antigenic peptide; TH1, T-helper cell type 1; TH2, T-helper cell type 2; WASP, Wiskott-Aldrich syndrome protein.

some, a lack of natural killer (NK) cells. Patients with this group of disorders have the most severe immunodeficiency.

PATHOGENESIS. SCID results from mutations in any one of 12 known genes that encode components of the immune system crucial for lymphoid cell development (Table 125-2). All patients with SCID have very small thymuses (<1 g) that usually fail to descend from the neck, contain no thymocytes, and lack corticomedullary distinction or Hassall corpuscles. The thymic epithelium appears histologically normal. Both the follicular and paracortical areas of the spleen are depleted of lymphocytes. Lymph nodes, tonsils, adenoids, and Peyer patches are absent or extremely underdeveloped.

CLINICAL MANIFESTATIONS. Affected infants present within the 1st few months of life with recurrent or persistent diarrhea, pneumonia, otitis media, sepsis, and cutaneous infections. Growth may appear normal initially, but extreme wasting usually ensues after diarrhea and infections begin. Persistent infections with opportunistic organisms including *Candida albicans, Pneumocystis carinii (jiroveci),* varicella-zoster virus, measles virus, parainfluenza 3 virus, cytomegalovirus (CMV), Epstein-Barr virus (EBV), adenovirus, and bacillus Calmette-Guérin (BCG) lead to death. Affected infants also lack the ability to reject foreign tissue and are therefore at risk for graft versus host disease (GVHD) from maternal immunocompetent T cells crossing the placenta, or from T lymphocytes in nonirradiated blood products or allogeneic stem cell transplantation.

Because all molecular types of SCID lack T cells, infants with SCID have **lymphopenia** (<2,500/mm^3) that is present at birth, indicating that the condition could be diagnosed in all affected infants if white blood cell counts with manual differential counts were routinely performed on all cord bloods and the absolute lymphocyte count calculated. These infants also have an absence of lymphocyte proliferative responses to mitogens, antigens, and allogeneic cells in vitro. Patients with adenosine deaminase (ADA) deficiency have the lowest absolute lymphocyte counts, usually <500/mm^3. Serum immunoglobulin concentrations are diminished to absent, and no antibodies are formed after immunizations. Analyses of lymphocyte populations and subpopulations demonstrate distinctive phenotypes for the various genetic forms of SCID (see Table 125-2). T cells are extremely low or absent in all types; when detected, they are in most cases transplacentally derived maternal T cells.

TABLE 125-2. 10 Abnormal Genes in Human Severe Combined Immune Deficiency (SCID)

- Cytokine Receptor Genes
  - —*IL-2RG*
  - —*Jak3*
  - —*IL-7Rα*
- Antigen Receptor Genes
  - —*RAG1*
  - —*RAG2*
  - —*Artemis*
  - —*CD3δ*
  - —*CD3ε*
- Other Genes
  - —*ADA*
  - —*CD45*

TREATMENT. SCID is a true pediatric emergency. Unless immunologic reconstitution is achieved through stem cell transplantation, death usually occurs during the 1st year of life and almost invariably before 2 yr of age. If diagnosed at birth or within the 1st 3.5 mo of life, >95% of cases can be treated successfully with HLA-identical or T-cell–depleted haploidentical (half-matched) parental hematopoietic stem cell transplantation without the need for pretransplant chemoablation or post-transplant GVHD prophylaxis. ADA-deficient SCID and X-linked SCID have been treated with somatic gene therapy; although serious adverse events occurred in the case of X-SCID. These successes offer hope for gene therapy becoming the treatment of choice for all forms of SCID for which the gene has been identified. ADA-deficient SCID is also managed with repeated injections of polyethylene glycol conjugated to the bovine-derived enzyme adenosine deaminase (PEG-ADA).

X-LINKED SEVERE COMBINED IMMUNODEFICIENCY (SCIDX1) DUE TO MUTATIONS IN THE GENE ENCODING THE COMMON CYTOKINE RECEPTOR γ CHAIN (γ_c)

X-linked SCID (SCIDX1) is the most common form of SCID in the United States, accounting for 47% of cases (Fig. 125-1). Clinically, immunologically, and histopathologically, affected individuals appear similar to those with other forms of SCID except for having uniformly **low percentages of T and NK cells** and an **elevated percentage of B cells** (T−, B+, NK−), a characteristic feature shared only with Janus kinase 3 (Jak3)–deficient and CD45-deficient patients with SCID. The abnormal gene in SCIDX1 was mapped to Xq13, cloned, and found to encode the common γ chain (γ_c) for several cytokine receptors including IL-2, IL-4, IL-7, IL-9, IL-15, and IL-21. The shared γ_c functions both to increase the affinity of the receptor for the respective cytokine and to enable the receptors to mediate intracellular signaling. Incapacitation of the receptors for all of these developmentally crucial cytokines by genetic mutations in γ_c provides an explanation for the severity of the immunodeficiency in SCIDX1. In the 1st 136 patients studied, 95 distinct mutations spanning all eight IL2RG exons were identified, most of them consisting of small changes at the level of one to a few nucleotides. These mutations resulted in abnormal γ_c chains in two thirds of the cases and absent γ_c protein in the remainder. Carriers can be detected by demonstrating nonrandom X-chromosome inactivation or the deleterious mutation in their T, B, or NK lymphocytes. Unless donor B or NK cells develop, patients with SCID lack B- and NK-cell function after bone marrow transplantation because the abnormal γ_c persists in those host cells, despite excellent reconstitution of T-cell function by donor-derived T cells.

AUTOSOMAL RECESSIVE SEVERE COMBINED IMMUNODEFICIENCY

This pattern of inheritance of SCID is less common in the United States than in Europe. Mutated genes on autosomal chromosomes have been identified in 11 forms of SCID: ADA deficiency, Jak3 deficiency, IL-7 receptor α chain (IL-7Rα) deficiency, RAG1 or RAG2 deficiency, Artemis deficiency, ligase 4 deficiency, CD3δ, CD3ε, CD3ζ deficiency, and CD45 deficiency (see Fig. 125-1).

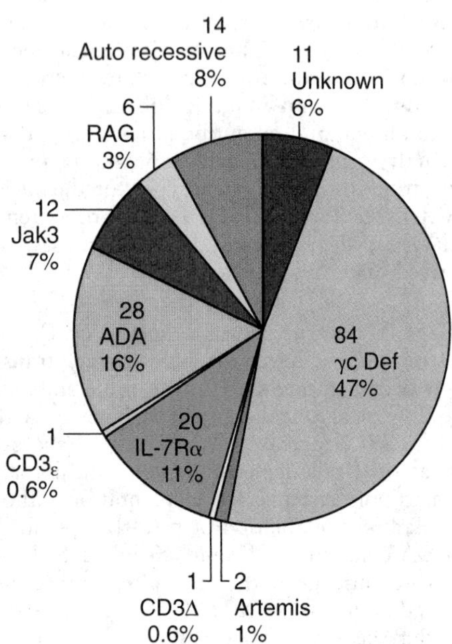

Figure 125-1. Relative frequencies of the different genetic types among 179 patients with severe combined immunodeficiency seen consecutively over 3 decades. RAG, recombinase activating gene; Jak3, Janus kinase 3; ADA, adenosine deaminase; IL-7Rα, interleukin 7 receptor α chain.

ADA DEFICIENCY. An absence of the enzyme adenosine deaminase (ADA) is observed in approximately 15% of patients with SCID, resulting from various point and deletional mutations in the ADA gene on chromosome 20q13-ter. Marked accumulations of adenosine, 2′-deoxyadenosine, and 2′-O-methyladenosine lead directly or indirectly to T-cell apoptosis, which causes the immunodeficiency. ADA-deficient patients usually have a much more profound **lymphopenia** than do infants with other types of SCID, with mean absolute lymphocyte counts of <500/mm^3; the absolute numbers of T, B, and NK cells are very low. NK function is normal. After T-cell function is conferred by hematopoietic stem cell transplantation, without pretransplant chemotherapy, there is generally excellent B-cell function. This is because ADA deficiency affects primarily T-cell function. Milder forms of ADA deficiency have led to delayed diagnosis of immunodeficiency, even to adulthood. Other **distinguishing features** of ADA-deficient SCID include the presence of rib cage abnormalities similar to a rachitic rosary and numerous skeletal abnormalities of chondro-osseous dysplasia, which occur predominantly at the costochondral junctions, at the apophyses of the iliac bones, and in the vertebral bodies where a “bone-in-bone” effect is observed.

As with other types of SCID, ADA deficiency can be cured by HLA-identical or haploidentical T-cell-depleted stem cell transplantation without the need for pre- or post-transplant chemotherapy; this remains the treatment of choice. Enzyme replacement therapy should not be initiated if stem cell transplantation is possible because it confers graft-rejection capability. Enzyme replacement provides protective immunity but over time there is a decline of lymphocyte counts and mitogenic proliferative responses. Eight infants with ADA deficiency have become immune reconstituted by gene therapy; in all cases, PEG-ADA was withheld. Spontaneous reversion to normal of a mutation in the ADA gene has also been reported.

JAK3 DEFICIENCY. Patients with this autosomal recessive defect resemble all other types of SCID patients clinically. They have a lymphocyte phenotype similar only to that of patients with SCIDX1, with an elevated percentage of B cells and very low or no T and NK cells. Because Jak3 is the only signaling molecule known to be associated with γ_c, it was a candidate gene for mutations leading to autosomal recessive SCID. Jak3 deficiency accounts for ≈ 7% of SCID cases. Even after successful T-cell reconstitution by transplantation of haploidentical stem cells, patients with Jak3-deficient SCID fail to develop NK cells or normal B-cell function owing to the defective function of those host cells that bear abnormal cytokine receptors that share γ_c.

IL-7Rα DEFICIENCY. Patients with IL-7Rα-deficient SCID have a distinctive lymphocyte phenotype in that, though lacking T cells, they have normal or elevated numbers of both B and NK cells (T−, B+, NK+). This is the **third most common** form of SCID, accounting for 11% of cases in the United States (see Fig. 125-1). In contrast to patients with γ_c- and Jak3-deficient SCID, the immunologic defect in these patients is completely correctable even by T-cell–depleted haploidentical bone marrow stem cell transplantation, as the host B and NK cells appear to be normal.

RAG1 OR RAG2 DEFICIENCIES. Infants with these causes of SCID have a different lymphocyte phenotype from those of patients with SCID due to γ_c, Jak3, IL-7Rα, or ADA deficiencies in that they lack both B and T lymphocytes and have primarily NK cells in their circulation (T–, B–, NK+). This suggested a problem with their antigen receptor genes, which led to the discovery of mutations in recombinase activating genes, RAG1 or RAG2. Such mutations result in a functional inability to form antigen receptors through genetic recombination. **Omenn syndrome** is an autosomal recessive, fatal condition characterized by profound susceptibility to infection with clonal T-cell infiltration of skin, intestines, liver, and spleen leading to an exfoliative erythroderma, lymphadenopathy, hepatosplenomegaly, and intractable diarrhea. Mutations in the recombinase activating genes, RAG1 and RAG2, have also been found in patients with this condition. These infants have persistent leukocytosis with marked eosinophilia and lymphocytosis; elevated serum IgE; low IgG, IgA, and IgM; and low or absent B cells. There is dominance of clonal TH2-like cells with severely impaired T-cell function due to the restricted heterogeneity of the host T-cell repertoire.

ARTEMIS DEFICIENCY. Another cause of SCID is a deficiency of a novel V(D)J recombination/DNA repair factor that belongs to the metallo-β-lactamase superfamily, which is encoded on chromosome 10p by a gene called Artemis. Deficiency of this factor results in an inability to repair DNA after double-stranded cuts by the RAG1 or RAG2 gene products in rearranging antigen receptor genes from their germ line configuration. Similar to RAG1- and RAG2-deficient SCID, this defect results in failure to develop T and B cells and is, therefore, another form of T–, B–, NK+ SCID, also called **Athabascan SCID.** There is increased radiation sensitivity of both skin fibroblasts and bone marrow cells of those affected with this type of SCID.

CD45 DEFICIENCY. Another molecular defect causing SCID is a mutation in the gene encoding the common leukocyte surface protein CD45. This hematopoietic cell–specific transmembrane protein tyrosine phosphatase functions to regulate src kinases required for T- and B-cell antigen receptor signal transduction. A 2 mo old male infant presented with a clinical picture of SCID and was found to have a very low number of T cells but a normal number of B cells. The T cells failed to respond to mitogens, and serum immunoglobulins diminished with time. He was found to have a large deletion on one CD45 allele and a point mutation causing an alteration of the intervening sequence 13 donor splice site on the other allele. A second case of SCID due to CD45 deficiency has been reported.

CD3δ, CD3ε, AND CD3ζ DEFICIENCIES. Other causes of autosomal recessive SCID are deficiencies of components of the T-cell receptor (CD3δ, CD3ε, and CD3ζ chains). Mutations in the portions of these genes that encode the extracellular components of the proteins result in a profound deficiency of circulating mature CD3 T cells. Thus, CD3δ, CD3ε, and CD3ζ appear to be essential for intrathymic development of T cells. Since only T-cell development is affected in these defects, both B and NK cells are normal. Thus, the lymphocyte phenotype resembles that of SCID infants with IL-7Rα chain deficiency (T–B+NK+).

RETICULAR DYSGENESIS

Reticular dysgenesis was 1st described in identical twin boys who exhibited a total lack of both lymphocytes and granulocytes in their peripheral blood and bone marrow. Seven of eight infants with this defect died between 3 and 119 days of age as a result of overwhelming infections; seven infants have been cured by bone marrow transplantation. The thymus glands have all weighed <1 g, have no Hassall corpuscles, and have few or no thymocytes. Reticular dysgenesis is considered a variant of SCID. The molecular basis of this autosomal recessive disorder is unknown.

125.2 • Combined Immunodeficiency (CID)

CID is distinguished from SCID by the presence of low but not absent T-cell function. Similar to SCID, CID is a syndrome of diverse genetic causes. Patients with CID have recurrent or chronic pulmonary infections, failure to thrive, oral or cutaneous candidiasis, chronic diarrhea, recurrent skin infections, gram-negative bacterial sepsis, urinary tract infections, and severe varicella in infancy. Although they usually survive longer than infants with SCID, they fail to thrive and die early in life. Neutropenia and eosinophilia are common. Serum immunoglobulins may be normal or elevated for all classes, but selective IgA deficiency, marked elevation of IgE, and elevated IgD levels occur in some cases. Although antibody-forming capacity is impaired in most patients, it is not absent.

Studies of cellular immune function show lymphopenia, profound deficiencies of T cells, and extremely low but not absent lymphocyte proliferative responses to mitogens, antigens, and allogeneic cells in vitro. Peripheral lymphoid tissues demonstrate paracortical lymphocyte depletion. The thymus is very small with a paucity of thymocytes and usually no Hassall corpuscles. An autosomal recessive pattern of inheritance is common.

PURINE NUCLEOSIDE PHOSPHORYLASE DEFICIENCY

More than 40 patients with CID have been found to have purine nucleoside phosphorylase (PNP) deficiency. Point mutations identified in the PNP gene on chromosome 14q13.1 account for these deficiencies. In contrast to ADA deficiency, no characteristic physical or skeletal abnormalities have been noted, but serum and urinary uric acid are usually markedly deficient. Deaths result from generalized vaccinia, varicella, lymphosarcoma, or GVHD mediated by allogeneic T cells in nonirradiated blood or bone marrow. Two thirds of patients have neurologic abnormalities, and one third have autoimmune diseases. Lymphopenia is striking, primarily because of a marked deficiency of T cells; T-cell function is decreased to various degrees. The proportion of circulating NK cells is increased. Prenatal diagnosis is possible. Bone marrow transplantation is the only successful form of therapy.

INTERLEUKIN 2 RECEPTOR α CHAIN (IL-2R α [CD25]) MUTATION

An infant boy born of a consanguineous union developed CMV pneumonia, persistent candidiasis, adenoviral gastroenteritis, failure to thrive, lymphadenopathy, hepatosplenomegaly, and chronic inflammation of his lungs and mandible. Biopsy specimens revealed extensive lymphocytic infiltration of his lung, liver, intestines, and bone. Serum IgA level was low. He had T-cell lymphopenia, and the T cells responded poorly to anti-CD3, phytohemagglutinin (PHA) and other mitogens, and IL-2. He was found to have a mutation in the gene encoding the IL-2 receptor α chain (IL-2Rα [CD25]), leading to truncation of the protein. He had no CD1 in his thymus, and an elevation of the antiapoptotic protein bcl-2. This defect reveals that some components of cytokine receptors normally serve a negative regulatory role. Mutations in those components can result in unchecked lymphoproliferation and autoimmunity in addition to immunodeficiency.

CARTILAGE HAIR HYPOPLASIA

Cartilage hair hypoplasia (CHH) is an unusual form of **short-limbed dwarfism** with frequent and severe infections. It occurs predominantly among the Pennsylvania Amish, but non-Amish patients have been described.

GENETICS AND PATHOGENESIS. CHH is an autosomal recessive condition. Numerous mutations that co-segregate with the CHH phenotype have been identified in the untranslated RNase MRP gene, which has recently been mapped to chromosome 9p21–p13 in Amish and Finnish families (see Table 125-1). The RNase MRP endoribonuclease consists of an RNA molecule bound to several proteins and has at least two functions: cleavage of RNA in mitochondrial DNA synthesis and nucleolar cleaving of pre-RNA. Mutations in RMRP cause CHH by disrupting a function of RNase MRP RNA that affects multiple organ systems. In vitro studies show decreased numbers of T cells and defective T-cell proliferation due to an intrinsic defect related to the G1 phase, resulting in a longer cell cycle for individual cells. NK cells are increased in number and function.

CLINICAL MANIFESTATIONS. Clinical features include short, pudgy hands; redundant skin; hyperextensible joints of hands and feet but an inability to extend the elbows completely; and fine, sparse, light hair and eyebrows. Severe and often fatal varicella infections, progressive vaccinia, and vaccine-associated poliomyelitis have been observed. Associated conditions include deficient erythrogenesis, Hirschsprung disease, and an increased risk of malignancies. The bones radiographically show scalloping and sclerotic or cystic changes in the metaphyses and flaring of the costochondral junctions of the ribs. Three patterns of immune dysfunction have emerged: defective antibody-mediated immunity, CID (most common), and SCID. The severity of the immunodeficiency varies; in one series, 11 of 77 patients died before age 20, but two were still alive at age 76. Stem cell transplantation has resulted in immunologic reconstitution in some CHH patients with the SCID phenotype.

DEFECTIVE EXPRESSION OF MAJOR HISTOCOMPATIBILITY COMPLEX ANTIGENS

The two main forms of immunodeficiency and abnormalities of expression of the major histocompatibility complex (MHC) are MHC class I (HLA-A, -B, and -C) antigen deficiency and MHC class II (HLA-DR, -DQ, and -DP) antigen deficiency. The associated defects of both B- and T-cell immunity and of HLA expression emphasize the important biologic role for HLA determinants in effective immune cell cooperation.

MHC CLASS I ANTIGEN DEFICIENCY. Isolated deficiency of MHC class I (HLA-A, -B, and -C) antigens, the **bare lymphocyte syndrome,** is rare. The resulting immunodeficiency is much milder than in SCID, contributing to a later age of presentation. Sera from affected children contain normal quantities of MHC class I antigens and β_2-microglobulin, but MHC class I antigens are not detected on any cells in the body. There is a deficiency of CD8 but not CD4 T cells. Mutations have been found in two genes within the MHC locus on chromosome 6 that encode the peptide transporter proteins TAP1 and TAP2 (see Fig. 123-1). TAP functions to transport antigenic peptides from the cytoplasm across the Golgi apparatus membrane to join the α chain of MHC class I antigens and β_2-microglobulin. All these are then assembled into a MHC class I complex that can then move to the cell surface. If the assembly of the complex cannot be completed because there is no antigenic peptide, the MHC class I complex is destroyed in the cytoplasm.

MHC CLASS II ANTIGEN DEFICIENCY. Many affected with MHC class II (HLA-DR, -DQ, and -DP) deficiency are of North African descent. Patients present in early infancy with persistent diarrhea that is often associated with cryptosporidiosis and enteroviral infections (e.g., poliovirus, coxsackievirus). They also have an increased frequency of infections with herpesviruses and other viruses, oral candidiasis, bacterial pneumonia, *P. carinii (jiroveci)* pneumonia, and septicemia. The immunodeficiency is not as severe as in SCID, as evidenced by their failure to develop disseminated infection after BCG vaccination or GVHD from nonirradiated blood transfusions.

Four different molecular defects resulting in impaired expression of MHC class II antigens have been identified (see Table 125-1 and Fig. 123-1). One form is a mutation in the gene on chromosome 1q that encodes a protein called RFX5, a subunit of RFX, which is a multiprotein complex that binds the X box motif of MHC-II promoters. A second form is caused by mutations in a gene on chromosome 13q that encodes a second 36-kD subunit of the RFX complex, called RFX-associated protein (RFXAP). The most common cause of MHC Class II defects is mutation in RFXANK, the gene encoding a third subunit of RFX. In a fourth type, there is a mutation in the gene on chromosome 16p13 that encodes a novel MHC class II transactivator (CIITA), a non–DNA-binding co-activator that controls the cell-type specificity and inducibility of MHC-II expression. All four of these defects cause impairment in the coordinate expression of MHC class II molecules on the surface of B cells and macrophages.

MHC class II–deficient patients have a very low number of CD4 T cells but normal or elevated numbers of CD8 T cells. Lymphopenia is only moderate. The MHC class II antigens HLA-DP, DQ, and DR are undetectable on blood B cells and monocytes, even though B cells are present in normal number. Patients are hypogammaglobulinemic owing to impaired antigen-specific responses caused by the absence of these antigen-presenting molecules. In addition, MHC antigen-deficient B cells fail to stimulate allogeneic cells in mixed leukocyte culture. Lymphocyte proliferation studies show normal responses to mitogens but no response to antigens. The thymus and other lymphoid organs are severely hypoplastic, and the lack of class II molecules results in abnormal thymic selection with circulating CD4 T cells that have altered CDR3 profiles.

IMMUNODEFICIENCY WITH THROMBOCYTOPENIA AND ECZEMA (WISKOTT-ALDRICH SYNDROME)

Wiskott-Aldrich syndrome, an X-linked recessive syndrome, is characterized by atopic dermatitis, thrombocytopenic purpura with normal-appearing megakaryocytes but small defective platelets, and undue susceptibility to infection.

GENETICS AND PATHOGENESIS. The abnormal gene, on the proximal arm of the X chromosome at Xp11.22–11.23 near the centromere, encodes a 501–amino acid proline-rich cytoplasmic protein restricted in its expression to hematopoietic cell lineages. The Wiskott-Aldrich syndrome protein (WASP) (see Fig. 124-1) binds CDC42H2 and rac, members of the Rho family of guanosine triphosphatases. WASP appears to control the assembly of actin filaments required for microvesicle formation downstream of protein kinase C and tyrosine kinase signaling. Carriers can be detected by nonrandom X-chromosome inactivation in several hematopoietic cell lineages or by demonstration of the deleterious mutation.

CLINICAL MANIFESTATIONS. Patients often have prolonged bleeding from the circumcision site or bloody diarrhea during infancy. The thrombocytopenia is not initially due to antiplatelet antibodies. Atopic dermatitis and recurrent infections usually develop during the 1st year of life. *Streptococcus pneumoniae* and other bacteria having polysaccharide capsules cause otitis media, pneumonia, meningitis, and sepsis. Later, infections with agents such as *P. carinii (jiroveci)* and the herpesviruses become more frequent. Survival beyond the teens is rare; infections, bleeding, and EBV-associated malignancies are major causes of death.

Patients with this defect uniformly have an impaired humoral immune response to polysaccharide antigens, as evidenced by absent or markedly diminished isohemagglutinins, and poor or absent antibody responses after immunization with polysaccharide vaccines. IgG2 subclass concentrations, surprisingly, are normal. Anamnestic responses to protein antigens are poor or absent. There is an accelerated rate of synthesis as well as hypercatabolism of albumin, IgG, IgA, and IgM, resulting in highly variable concentrations of different immunoglobulins, even within the same patient. The predominant immunoglobulin pattern is a low serum level of IgM, elevated IgA and IgE, and a normal or slightly low IgG concentration. Because of their profound antibody deficiencies, these patients should be given monthly infusions of intravenous immunoglobulin (IVIG) regardless of their serum levels of the different immunoglobulin isotypes. Percentages of T cells are moderately reduced, and lymphocyte responses to mitogens are variably depressed.

TREATMENT. Good supportive care includes appropriate nutrition, routine IVIG, use of killed vaccines, aggressive management of eczema and associated cutaneous infections, platelet transfusion for serious bleeding episodes, splenectomy, and high-dose IVIG with systemic steroids for autoimmune complications. Bone marrow or cord blood transplantation is the treatment of choice and may be curative.

ATAXIA-TELANGIECTASIA

Ataxia-telangiectasia is a complex syndrome with immunologic, neurologic, endocrinologic, hepatic, and cutaneous abnormalities.

GENETICS AND PATHOGENESIS. The mutated gene responsible for this defect, ataxia telangiectasia mutation (ATM), was mapped to the long arm of chromosome 11 (11q22–23) and has been cloned (see Fig. 124-1). The gene product is a DNA-dependent protein kinase localized predominantly to the nucleus and involved in mitogenic signal transduction, meiotic recombination, and cell cycle control. Cells from patients as well as those of heterozygous carriers have increased sensitivity to ionizing radiation, defective DNA repair, and frequent chromosomal abnormalities.

In vitro tests of lymphocyte function have generally shown moderately depressed proliferative responses to T- and B-cell mitogens. Percentages of CD3 and CD4 T cells are moderately reduced, with normal or increased percentages of CD8 and elevated numbers of Tiγ/δ T cells. Studies of immunoglobulin synthesis have shown both T-helper-cell and intrinsic B-cell defects. The thymus is very hypoplastic, exhibits poor organization, and lacks Hassall corpuscles.

CLINICAL MANIFESTATIONS. The most prominent clinical features are progressive cerebellar ataxia, oculocutaneous telangiectasias, chronic sinopulmonary disease, a high incidence of malignancy, and variable humoral and cellular immunodeficiency. Ataxia typically becomes evident soon after these children begin to walk and progresses until they are confined to a wheelchair, usually by the age of 10–12 yr. The telangiectasias begin to develop at 3–6 yr of age. The most frequent humoral immunologic abnormality is the selective absence of IgA, which occurs in 50%–80% of these patients. Hypercatabolism of IgA also occurs. IgE concentrations are usually low, and the IgM may be of the low molecular weight variety. IgG2 or total IgG levels may be decreased, and specific antibody titers may be decreased or normal. Recurrent sinopulmonary infections occur in approximately 80% of these patients. Although common viral infections have not usually resulted in untoward sequelae, fatal varicella has occurred. The malignancies associated with ataxia-telangiectasia are usually of the lymphoreticular type, but adenocarcinomas also occur. Unaffected relatives have an increased incidence of malignancy.

125.3 • Defects of Innate Immunity

A number of defects in non–antigen-specific immunity (innate immunity) often affect antigen-specific immune responses, as there is interaction between the adaptive and innate immune systems.

INTERFERON-γ RECEPTOR 1 AND 2 AND IL-12 RECEPTOR β1 MUTATIONS

Disseminated BCG or severe nontuberculosis mycobacterial infections (sepsis, osteomyelitis) occur in patients with severe T-cell defects; however, no specific host defect is identified in approximately half of such cases. The 1st report was a 2.5-mo-old Tunisian girl with fatal idiopathic disseminated BCG infection; four children from Malta had disseminated atypical mycobacterial infections in the absence of a recognized immunodeficiency. There was consanguinity in all; each had a functional defect in the upregulation of tumor necrosis factor α (TNF-α) production by their blood macrophages in response to stimulation with interferon-γ (IFN-γ). Each also had a mutation in the gene on chromosome 6q22–q23 that encodes the IFN-γ receptor 1 (IFN-γR1). IFN-γR1 may be inherited as a complete autosomal recessive (young onset ≈ 3 yr, more episodes, more severe disease, and higher mortality) or partial dominant (onset ≈ 10 yr) disease. Patients with mutations in the IFN-γR2 have also been identified. A third type of defect was found in other patients who had disseminated mycobacterial infections, who have mutations in the β1 chain of the IL-12 receptor (IL-12Rβ1). IL-12 is a powerful inducer of IFN-γ production by T and NK cells, and the mutated receptor chain gene resulted in unresponsiveness of these patients' cells to IL-12 and inadequate IFN-γ production. The children deficient in IFN-γR1, IFN-γR2, or IL-12Rβ1 appeared not to be susceptible to infection with many agents (occasionally salmonella, *Listeria,* histoplasmosis) other than mycobacteria. TH1 responses appeared to be normal in these patients. The susceptibility of these patients to mycobacterial infections thus apparently results from an intrinsic impairment of the IFN-γ pathway response to these particular intracellular pathogens, showing that IFN-γ is obligatory for efficient macrophage antimycobacterial activity.

GERM LINE STAT 1 MUTATION

Interferons induce the formation of two transcriptional activators, gamma-activating factor (GAF) and interferon-stimulated gamma factor 3 (ISGF3). A natural heterozygous dominant germ line *STAT-1* mutation associated with susceptibility to mycobacterial but not viral disease was found in two unrelated patients with unexplained mycobacterial disease. This mutation caused a loss of GAF and ISGF3 activation but was dominant for one cellular phenotype and recessive for the other. It impaired the nuclear accumulation of GAF but not of ISGF3 in cells stimulated by interferons, implying that the antimycobacterial but not the antiviral effects of human interferons are mediated by GAF. More recently, two patients have been identified with homozygous *STAT-1* mutations who developed both post–BCG vaccination disseminated disease and lethal viral infections. The mutations in these patients caused a complete lack of STAT-1 and resulted in a lack of formation of both GAF and ISGF3.

IL-1R–ASSOCIATED KINASE 4 (IRAK4) DEFICIENCY

Members of interleukin-1 receptor (IL-1R) and the Toll-like receptor (TLR) superfamily share an intracytoplasmic Toll-IL-1 receptor (TIR) domain, which mediates recruitment of the interleukin-1 receptor-associated kinase (IRAK) complex via TIR-containing adapter molecules. Three unrelated otherwise healthy children with recurrent pyogenic infections due to pneumococci and staphylococci had normal immunocompetence by standard immune studies. They had normal titers of anti-pneumococcal antibodies. Their blood and fibroblast cells did not activate nuclear factor kB (NFκB) and mitogen-activated protein kinase (MAPK) and failed to induce downstream cytokines in response to any of the known ligands of TIR-bearing receptors. They each were found to have an inherited deficiency of IRAK-4. The TIR-IRAK signaling pathway appears to be crucial for protective immunity against specific bacteria but is redundant against most other microorganisms.

HYPER-IgE SYNDROME

The hyper-IgE syndrome is a relatively rare primary immunodeficiency syndrome characterized by recurrent severe staphylococcal abscesses of the skin, lungs, and other viscera as well as sinusitis mastoiditis, and markedly elevated levels of serum IgE. *Candida albicans* is the second most common pathogen. More than 200 patients with hyper-IgE syndrome have been reported. The inheritance pattern is as a single locus autosomal dominant trait with variable expression.

CLINICAL MANIFESTATIONS. The characteristic clinical features of this condition are staphylococcal abscesses, pneumatoceles, osteopenia, and unusual facial features. There is often history from infancy of recurrent staphylococcal abscesses involving the skin, lungs, joints, and other sites. Persistent pneumatoceles develop as a result of recurrent pneumonia. The pruritic dermatitis that occurs is not typical atopic eczema and does not always persist. Allergic respiratory symptoms are usually absent. The 1st two reported patients were described as having **coarse facial features** including a prominent forehead, deep-set wide-spaced eyes, a broad nasal bridge, a wide fleshy nasal tip, mild prognathism, facial asymmetry, and hemihypertrophy. In older children, delay in shedding primary teeth, recurrent fractures, and scoliosis occur.

These patients demonstrate an exceptionally high serum IgE concentration; an elevated serum IgD concentration; usually normal concentrations of IgG, IgA, and IgM; pronounced blood and sputum eosinophilia; abnormally low anamnestic antibody responses; and poor antibody and cell-mediated responses to neoantigens. In vitro studies show normal percentages of blood T, B, and NK lymphocytes, with the exception of a decreased percentage of T cells with the memory (CD45RO) phenotype. Paradoxically, B cells from these patients demonstrate very low levels of IL-4–stimulated IgE synthesis in vitro, suggesting that they have already been maximally stimulated by a high level of endogenous IL-4. The molecular basis of this disorder remains unknown. Most patients have normal T-lymphocyte proliferative responses to mitogens but very low or absent responses to antigens or allogeneic cells from family members. Blood, sputum, and histologic sections of lymph nodes, spleen, and lung cysts show striking eosinophilia. Hassall corpuscles and thymic architecture are normal. Phagocytic cell ingestion, metabolism and killing, and total hemolytic complement activity are normal in all patients. Results of chemotaxis studies have been mostly normal; thus, defective chemotaxis is not the basic problem in this syndrome.

The most effective **therapy** is long-term administration of therapeutic doses of a penicillinase-resistant antistaphylococcal antibiotic, adding other agents as required for specific infections. IVIG should be administered to antibody-deficient patients, and appropriate thoracic surgery should be provided for superinfected pneumatoceles or those persisting beyond 6 mo.

125.4 • Treatment of Cellular or Combined Immunodeficiency

Good supportive care including prevention and treatment of infections is critical while patients await more definitive therapy (Table 125-3). Having knowledge of the pathogens causing disease with specific immune defects is also useful (see Table 125-3).

Transplantation of MHC-compatible sibling or haploidentical (half-matched) parental hematopoietic stem cells is the treatment of choice for patients with fatal T-cell or combined T- and B-cell

TABLE 125-3. Infection in the Host Compromised by B- and T-cell Immunodeficiency Syndromes

IMMUNODEFICIENCY SYNDROME	OPPORTUNISTIC ORGANISMS ISOLATED MOST FREQUENTLY	APPROACH TO TREATMENT OF INFECTIONS	PREVENTION OF INFECTIONS
B-cell immunodeficiences	Encapsulated bacteria (*Streptococcus pneumoniae, Staphylococcus aureus, Haemophilus influenzae,* and *Neisseria meningitidis*), *Pseudomonas aeruginosa, Campylobacter* sp., enteroviruses rotaviruses, *Giardia lamblia, Crytosporidium* sp., *Pneumocystis jiroveci (carinii), Ureaplasma urealyticum,* and *Mycoplasma pneumoniae*	1. IVIG 200–800 mg/kg 2. Vigorous attempt to obtain specimens for culture before antimicrobial therapy 3. Incision and drainage if abscess present 4. Antibiotic selection on the basis of sensitivity data	1. Maintenance IVIG for patients with quantitative and qualitative defects in IgG metabolism (200–800 mg/kg q3–5 wk) 2. In chronic recurrent respiratory disease, vigorous attention to postural drainage 3; in selected cases (recurrent or chronic pulmonary or middle ear), prophylactic administration of ampicillin, penicillin, or trimethoprim-sulfamethoxazole
T-cell immunodeficiencies	Encapsulated bacteria (*S. pneumoniae, H. influenzae, S. aureus*), facultative intracellular bacteria (*Mycobacterium tuberculosis,* other *Mycobacterium* sp., and *Listeria monocytogenes*); *Escherichia coli; Pseudomonas aeruginosa; Enterobacter* sp.; *Klebsiella* sp.; *Serratia marcescens; Salmonella* sp.; *Nocardia* sp.; viruses (cytomegalovirus, herpes simplex virus, varicella-zoster virus, Epstein-Barr virus, rotaviruses, adenoviruses, enteroviruses, respiratory syncytial virus, measles virus, vaccinia virus, and parainfluenzae viruses); protozoa (*Toxoplasma gondii* and *Cryptosporidium* sp.); and fungi (*Candida* sp., *Cryptococcus neoformans, Histoplasma capsulatum,* and *Pneumocystis jiroveci [carinii]*)	1. Vigorous attempt to obtain specimens for culture before antimicrobial therapy 2. Incision and drainage if abscess present 3. Antibiotic selection on the basis of sensitivity data 4. Early antiviral treatment for herpes simplex, cytomegalovirus, and varicella-zoster viral infections 5. Topical and nonadsorbable antimicrobial agents frequently are useful	1. Prophylactic administration of trimethoprim-sulfamethoxazole for prevention of *P. carinii (jiroveci)* pneumonia 2. Oral nonadsorbable antimicrobial agents to lower concentration of gut flora 3. No live virus vaccines or bacillus Calmette-Guérin vaccine 4. Careful tuberculosis screening

IVIG, intravenous immunoglobulin.
From Stiehm ER, Ochs HD, Winkelstein JA: *Immunologic Disorders in Infants and Children,* 5th ed. Philadelphia, Elsevier/Saunders, 2004.

defects. The major risk to the recipient from transplants of stem cell transplantation is GVHD. The development of techniques to deplete all post-thymic T cells from donor marrow permits safe and successful use of haploidentical related stem cells for the correction of SCID and other fatal immunodeficiency syndromes. Patients with less severe forms of cellular immunodeficiency, including some forms of CID, Wiskott-Aldrich syndrome, cytokine deficiency, and MHC antigen deficiency, reject even HLA-identical marrow grafts unless chemoablative treatment is given before transplantation. Several patients with these conditions have been treated successfully with HLA-identical stem cell transplantation after conditioning.

As many as 90% of patients with primary immunodeficiency transplanted with HLA-identical related marrow will survive with immunologic engraftment. T-cell–depleted haploidentical related marrow transplants in patients with primary immunodeficiency have a 55% survival rate. The greatest success has been in patients with SCID, who do not require pretransplant conditioning or GVHD prophylaxis; up to 90% of patients with SCID will survive with T-cell–depleted parental marrow and without pre-transplant chemotherapy or post-transplant GVHD prophylaxis. Until somatic cell gene therapy is more fully developed, bone marrow transplantation remains the most important and effective therapy for these inborn errors of the immune system. There was remarkable success with gene therapy in immunologically reconstituting nine infants with X-linked SCID. Unfortunately, leukemic-like clonal T cells developed in two of the children and a lymphomatous process in a third. Insertional mutagenesis caused by retroviral insertion of the IL2RG cDNA near the LMO-2 gene produced these serious complications of gene therapy. Efforts are being focused on ways to prevent this problem.

125.5 • Immune Dysregulation with Autoimmunity or Lymphoproliferation

AUTOIMMUNE LYMPHOPROLIFERATIVE SYNDROME (ALPS)

ALPS, also known as Canale-Smith syndrome, is a disorder of abnormal lymphocyte apoptosis leading to polyclonal populations of T cells (double-negative T cells), which express CD3 and α/β antigen receptors but do not have CD4 or CD8 co-receptors (CD3 + T cell receptor α/β^+ $CD4^-$ $CD8^-$). These T cells respond poorly to antigens or mitogens and do not produce growth or survival factors (interleukin 2). The genetic deficit in most patients is a germ line or somatic mutation in the Fas gene, which produces a cell surface receptor of the tumor necrosis factor receptor superfamily (TNFRSF6), which, when stimulated by its ligand, will produce programmed cell death (Table 125-4). Persistent survival of these lymphocytes leads to immune dysregulation and autoimmunity.

CLINICAL MANIFESTATIONS. ALPS is characterized by autoimmunity, chronic persistent or recurrent lymphadenopathy, splenomegaly, hepatomegaly (in 50%), and hypergammaglobinemia (IgG, IgA). Many patients present in the 1st yr of life; most are symptomatic by yr 5. Lymphadenopathy can be striking (Fig. 125-2). Splenomegaly may produce hypersplenism with cytopenias. Autoimmunity also produces anemia (Coombs positive hemolytic anemia) or thrombocytopenia or a mild neutropenia. Lymphoproliferative process (lymphadenopathy, splenomegaly) may regress over time, but autoimmunity does not and is characterized by frequent exacerbations and recurrences. Other autoimmune features include urticaria, uveitis, glomerulonephritis, hepatitis, vasculitis, glomulonephritis, vasculitis, panniculitis, arthritis, and central nervous system involvement (seizures, headaches, encephalopathy).

Malignancies are also more common in patients with ALPS; these include Hodgkin and non-Hodgkin lymphomas and solid tissue tumors of thyroid, skin, heart, or lung.

DIAGNOSIS. Laboratory abnormalities depend on the lymphoproliferative organ response (hypersplenism) or the degree of autoimmunity (anemia, thrombocytopenia). There may be lymphocytosis or lymphopenia. Criteria for the diagnosis are noted in Table 125-4. Flow cytometry helps identify the lymphocyte type (see Fig. 125-2). Functional genetic analysis for the *TNFRSF6* gene often reveals a heterozygous mutation.

TREATMENT. Lymphoproliferative manifestations have been managed with corticosteroids and immunosuppressive agents (Cytoxan [cyclophosphamide], methotrexate, azathioprine); once weaned, the manifestation recurs. Hypersplenism may require splenectomy. Malignancies can be treated with the usual protocols used in patients unaffected by ALPS. Stem cell transplantation is another possible option in treating the autoimmune manifestations of ALPS.

IMMUNE-DYSREGULATION, POLYENDOCRINOPATHY, ENTEROPATHY, X-LINKED (IPEX) SYNDROME

This immune dysregulation syndrome is characterized by onset within the 1st weeks or months of life with watery diarrhea, an eczematous rash, insulin-dependent diabetes mellitus, hyper or hypothyroidism and other autoimmune disorders (Coombs positive hemolytic anemia, thrombocytopenia, neutropenia, alopecia).

IPEX is due to a mutation in the FOXP3 gene, the protein product is a forkhead-winged helix transcription factor *(scurfin)*, which is involved in the function and development of CD4+CD25+ regulatory T cells. Absent regulatory cells may predispose to abnormal activation of effector T cells.

CLINICAL MANIFESTATIONS. Watery diarrhea with intestinal villous atrophy leads to failure to thrive in most patients. Cutaneous lesions (usually eczema) and insulin-dependent diabetes begin in infancy. Lymphadenopathy and splenomegaly are also present.

Serious bacterial infections (meningitis, sepsis, pneumonia, osteomyelitis) may be related to neutropenia, malnutrition, or immune dysregulation.

Laboratory features reflect the associated autoimmune diseases, dehydration, and malnutrition. In addition, serum IgE levels are elevated with normal levels of IgM, IgG, and IgA. The

TABLE 125-4. ALPS Case Criteria and ALPS Classification

REQUIRED
1. Chronic nonmalignant lymphoproliferation
2. Defective lymphocyte apoptosis in vitro
3. ≥1% TCR α/β^+ $CD4^-$ $CD8^-$ T cells (α/β^+-DNT cells) in peripheral blood and/or presence of DNT cells in lymphoid tissue

SUPPORTING
4. Autoimmunity/autoantibodies
5. Mutations in *TNFRSF6*, FasL or caspase 10 genes

ALPS Ia = due to mutation in *TNFRSF6*
ALPS Ib = due to mutation in the gene for Fas ligand
ALPS II = due to mutation in the gene for caspase 10
ALPS III = ALPS without defined genetic cause

From Straus SE, Sneller M, Lenardo MJ, et al: An inherited disorder of lymphocyte apoptosis: The autoimmune lymphoproliferative syndrome. *Ann Intern Med* 1999;130:591–601.
From Bleesing JJH, Straus SE, Fleisher TA: Autoimmune lymphoproliferative syndrome: A human disorder of abnormal lymphocyte survival. *Pediatr Clin North Am* 2000;47:1291–1310.

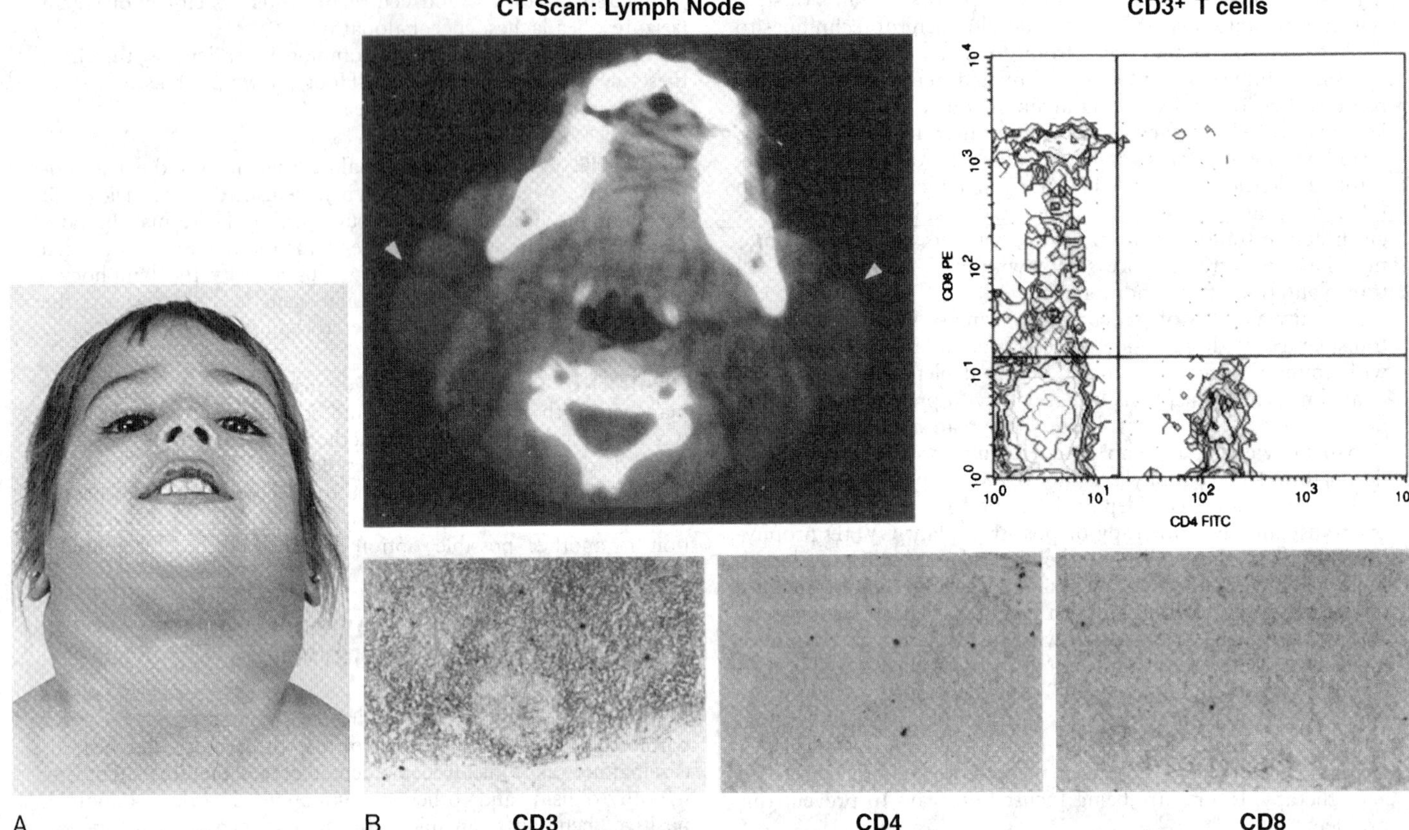

Figure 125-2. Clinical, radiographic, immunologic, and histologic characteristics of the autoimmune lymphoproliferative syndrome. *A,* Front view of the National Institutes of Health patient. *B, Top middle,* a CT scan of the neck is shown demonstrating enlarged preauricular, cervical, and occipital lymph nodes. *Arrowheads* denote the most prominent lymph nodes. The *top right* panels show the flow-cytometric analysis of peripheral blood T cells from a patient with autoimmune lymphoproliferative syndrome (ALPS), with CD8 expression on the vertical axis and CD4 on the horizontal axis. The *lower left quadrant* contains CD4-CD8 (double-negative) T cells, which are usually present at <1% of T cells expressing the αβ TCR. The *bottom panels* show CD3, CD4, and CD8 staining on serial sections of a lymph node biopsy specimen from a patient with ALPS and also shows that large numbers of DNCD3+ CD4-CD8 (double-negative) T cells are present in the interfollicular areas of the lymph node. (Adapted from Siegel RM, Fleisher TA: The role of Fas and related death receptors in autoimmune and other disease states. *J Allergy Clin Immunol* 1999;103:729–738; with permission.)

diagnosis is made clinically and by mutational analysis of the *FOXP3* gene.

TREATMENT. Inhibition of T-cell activation by cyclosporine, tacrolimus, or sirolimus with steroids is the treatment of choice, along with the specific care of the endocrinopathy and other manifestations of autoimmunity. Stem cell transplantation is the only possibility for curing IPEX. Overall, the combination of the risks for serious bacterial infection in the untreated condition and the risks of immunosuppression and bone marrow transplantation gives IPEX a poor prognosis. Untreated, most die by 2 yr of age.

Aiuti A, Slavin S, Aker M, et al: Correction of ADA-SCID by stem cell gene therapy combined with nonmyeloablative conditioning. *Science* 2002;296:2410–2413.

Binder V, Albert MH, Kabus M, et al: The genotype of the original Wiskott phenotype. *N Engl J Med* 2006;355:1790–1793.

Bindl L, Torgerson T, Perroni L, et al: Successful use of the new immune-suppressor sirolimus in IPEX (immune dysregulation, polyendocrinopathy, enteropathy, X-linked syndrome). *J Pediatr* 2005;147:256–259.

Bleesing JJH: Sorting out the causes of ALPS. *J Pediatr* 2005;147:571–574.

Buckley RH: Molecular defects in human severe combined immunodeficiency and approaches to immune reconstitution. *Annu Rev Immunol* 2004; 22:625–655.

Buckley RH: Primary cellular immunodeficiencies. *J Allergy Clin Immunol* 2002;109:747–757.

Buckley RH: The hyper-IgE syndrome. *Clin Rev Allergy Immunol* 2001;20:139–154.

Buckley RH: Primary immunodeficiency diseases due to defects in lymphocytes. *N Engl J Med* 2000;343:1313–1324.

Chan B, Wara D, Bastian J, et al: Long-term efficacy of enzyme replacement therapy for adenosine deaminase (ADA)–deficient severe combined immunodeficiency (SCID). *Clin Immunol* 2005;117:133–143.

Dadi HJ, Simon AJ, Roifman CM: Effect of CD3δ deficiency on maturation of α/β and γ/δ T-cell lineages in severe combined immunodeficiency. *N Engl J Med* 2003;349:1821–1828.

Dorman SE, Picard C, Lammas D, et al: Clinical features of dominant and recessive interferon γ receptor 1 deficiencies. *Lancet* 2004;364: 2113–2120.

Dupuis S, Jouanguy E, Al Hajjar S, et al: Impaired response to interferon-alpha/beta and lethal viral disease in human STAT1 deficiency. *Nat Genet* 2003;33:388–391.

Fischer A, Le Deist F, Hacein-Bey-Abina S, et al: Severe combined immunodeficiency. A model disease for molecular immunology and therapy. *Immunol Rev* 2005;203:98–109.

Gaspar HB, Parsley KL, Howe S, et al: Gene therapy of X-linked severe combined immunodeficiency by use of a pseudotyped gammaretroviral vector. *Lancet* 2004;364:2181–2187.

Grunebaum E, Mazzolari E, Porta F, et al: Bone marrow transplantation for severe combined immune deficiency. *JAMA* 2006;295:508–518.

Hacein-Bey-Abina S, Von Kalle C, Schmidt M, et al: A serious adverse event after successful gene therapy for X-linked severe combined immunodeficiency. *N Engl J Med* 2003;348:255–256.

Hacein-Bey-Abina S, Le Deist F, Carlier F, et al: Sustained correction of X-linked severe combined immunodeficiency by ex vivo gene therapy. *N Engl J Med* 2002;346:1185–1193.

Holzelova E, Vonarbourg C, Stolzenberg MC, et al: Autoimmune lymphoproliferative syndrome with somatic *Fas* mutations. *N Engl J Med* 2004;351:1409–1418.
Ku CL, Yang K, Bustamante J, et al: Inherited disorders of human Toll-like receptor signaling: Immunological implications. *Immunol Rev* 2005; 203:10–20.
Marodi L: Genetic deficiency of signaling via interferon receptors. *Pediatr Res* 2004;55:181–182.
Myers LA, Patel DD, Puck JM, Buckley RH: Hematopoietic stem cell transplantation for severe combined immunodeficiency in the neonatal period leads to superior thymic output and improved survival. *Blood* 2002;99:872–878.
Notarangelo L, Casanova JL, Conley ME, et al: Primary immunodeficiency diseases: An update. *J Allergy Clin Immunol* 2006;117:883–896.
Patel DD, Gooding ME, Parrott RE, et al: Thymic function after hematopoietic stem-cell transplantation for the treatment of severe combined immunodeficiency. *N Engl J Med* 2000;342:1325–1332.
Reith W, Mach B: The bare lymphocyte syndrome and the regulation of MHC expression. *Annu Rev Immunol* 2001;19:331–373.
Rosenzweig SD, Holland SM: Defects in the interferon-gamma and interleukin-12 pathways. *Immunol Rev* 2005;203:38–47.
Rudd CE: Disabled receptor signaling and new primary immunodeficiency disorders. *N Engl J Med* 2006;354:1874–1877.
Snapper SB, Rosen FS: A family of WASPS. *N Engl J Med* 2003;348:350–351.
Tezcan I, Ersoy F, Sanal O, et al: Long-term survival in severe combined immune deficiency: The role of persistent maternal engraftment. *J Pediatr* 2005;146:137–140.
Vihinen M, Arredondo-Vega FX, Casanova JL, et al: Primary immunodeficiency mutation databases. *Adv Genet* 2001;43:103–188.

Section 3 — The Phagocytic System

Chapter 126 ■ Neutrophils

Laurence A. Boxer

THE PHAGOCYTIC INFLAMMATORY RESPONSE. Neutrophils and mononuclear phagocytes share primary functions including the unusual ability to ingest large particles. Neutrophils are of only one type, but there are many varieties of mononuclear phagocytes, including the tissue macrophages, and their circulating precursors, monocytes (see Chapter 127). Neutrophils develop less rapidly in the bone marrow than do monocytes, and remain for only 6 hr in the circulation (Table 126-1).

The hematopoietic progenitor system can be envisioned as a continuum of functional compartments with the most primitive compartment composed of very rare cells known as **pluripotential stem cells,** which have high self-renewal capacity and give rise to more mature stem cells, including cells that are committed to either lymphoid or myeloid development. Lymphoid stem cells give rise to T- and B-cell precursors and their mature progeny (see Chapter 122). Trilineage myeloid stem cells, designated CFU-S for the spleen colony-forming unit described in mice, eventually give rise to committed single-lineage progenitors of the recognizable precursors through a random process of lineage restriction in a stepwise process (Fig. 126-1). The lineage restriction arises from cell-surface expression of lineage-specific growth factor receptors. Single-lineage progenitors, including erythroid burst-forming units (BFU-E), erythroid colony-forming units (CFU-E), megakaryocyte colony-forming units (CFU-Meg), and basophil, granulocyte, monocyte, and eosinophil colony-forming units (CFU-Baso, CFU-G, CFU-M, and CFU-Eo, respectively) proliferate and differentiate into their respective precursors in response to the growth factors that bind to their unique receptors. The capacity of lineage-specific committed progenitors to proliferate and differentiate in response to demand constitutes the most important buffer of the hematopoietic system against increased requirement for mature blood cell production.

TABLE 126-1. Neutrophil and Monocyte Kinetics

NEUTROPHILS	
Average time in mitosis (myeloblast to myelocyte)	7–9 day
Average time in postmitosis and storage (metamyelocyte to neutrophil)	3–7 day
Average half-life in the circulation	6 hr
Average total body pool	6.5×10^8 cells/kg
Average circulating pool	3.2×10^8 cells/kg
Average marginating pool	3.3×10^8 cells/kg
Average daily turnover rate	1.8×10^8 cells/kg
MONONUCLEAR PHAGOCYTES	
Average time in mitosis	30–48 hr
Average half-life in the circulation	36–104 hr
Average circulating pool (monocytes)	1.8×10^7 cells/kg
Average daily turnover rate	1.8×10^9 cells/kg
Average survival in tissues (macrophages)	Months

From Boxer LA: Function of neutrophils and mononuclear phagocytes. In Bennett JC, Plum F (editors): *Cecil Textbook of Internal Medicine,* 20th ed. Philadelphia, WB Saunders, 1996.

HEMATOPOIETIC GROWTH FACTORS. The proliferation, differentiation, and survival of immature hematopoietic progenitor cells are governed by hematopoietic growth factors (HGFs), a family of glycoproteins (Table 126-2). Besides regulating proliferation and differentiation of progenitors, these factors influence the survival and function of mature blood cells. The HGFs include the interleukins and the colony-stimulating factors (CSFs), which are named for their ability to stimulate progenitor cells to form colonies of recognizable mature cells in vitro. The majority of lineage-specific progenitors require the presence of additional growth factors such as interleukin 3 (IL-3) or granulocyte-macrophage CSF (GM-CSF) in addition to a lineage-specific HGF to generate the colonies for which they are programmed. Hence, immature committed progenitors bear receptors for IL-3, stem cell factor (SCF), GM-CSF, and IL-6 (Fig. 126-2). These committed progenitors differ from one another with respect to their lineage-specific receptors; this allows the lineage-specific HGF to produce the colonies for which they are programmed. During granulopoiesis and monopoiesis, several cytokines regulate progenitor cells or mature effector cells at each stage of maturation and differentiation from the primitive pluripotent stem cells to nondividing terminally differentiated cells (monocytes, neutrophils, eosinophils, and basophils). The actions of these growth factors are mediated through lineage-specific receptors. As cells mature, they lose receptors for most cytokines, especially those that influence early cell development, such as SCF. Once the cells

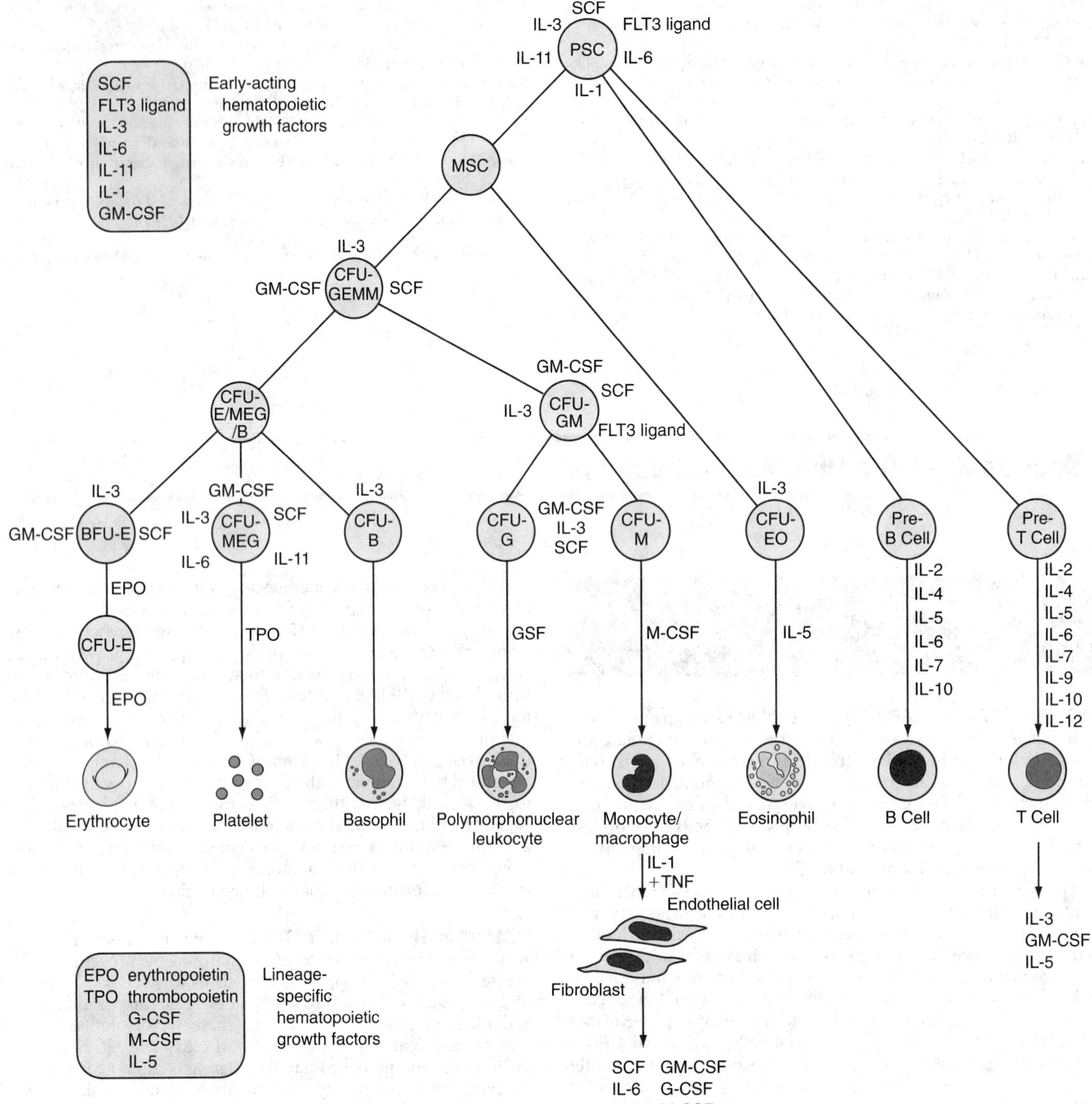

Figure 126-1. Major cytokine sources and actions. Cells of the bone marrow microenvironment such as macrophages (ma), endothelial cells (ec), and reticular fibroblastoid cells (fb) produce macrophage colony–stimulating factor (M-CSF), granulocyte-macrophage colony–stimulating factor (GM-CSF), granulocyte colony–stimulating factor (G-CSF), interleukin 6 (IL-6), and probably stem cell factor (SCF; cellular sources not yet precisely determined) after induction with endotoxin (ma) or IL-1/TNF (ec, fb). T cells produce IL-3, GM-CSF, and IL-5 in response to antigenic and IL-1 stimulation. These cytokines have overlapping actions during hematopoietic differentiation, as indicated, and for all lineages optimal development requires a combination of early- and late-acting factors. MSC, myeloid stem cells; PSC, pluripotent stem cells; TNF, tumor necrosis factor. (Modified from Sieff CA, Nathan DG, Clark SC: The anatomy and physiology of hematopoiesis. In Nathan DG, Orkin SH [editors]: *Hematology of Infancy and Childhood*, 5th ed. Philadelphia, WB Saunders, 1997.)

have matured, however, they express receptors for chemokines, which help direct the cells to sites of inflammation. Chemokine receptors such as CXCR4, along with its ligand SDF-1, play a key role in retention of developing myeloid cells within bone marrow.

NEUTROPHIL MATURATION AND KINETICS. The bone marrow microenvironment supporting the progenitors and precursors must provide for the normal steady-state rates of renewal of the cellular elements of blood through its ability to provide growth and differentiation factors generated by stromal cells themselves. Growth factors such as granulocyte colony–stimulating factor (G-CSF) and GM-CSF not only stimulate cell division, but also affect the synthesis of many cytoplasmic components of the neutrophil as well as expression of transcription factors that are necessary for myeloid cell differentiation and biosynthesis of neutrophil

TABLE 126-2. Human Hematopoietic Growth Factors

FACTOR	SYNONYM	SOURCE	BIOLOGIC ACTIVITIES: PROGENITORS	BIOLOGIC ACTIVITIES: MATURE CELLS
SCF	Steel factor Stem cell factor Kit ligand	Stromal F, Vasc. Endo	Synergistic: IL-3, IL-11, IL-6 on blast CFC; Synergistic: IL- 3, GM-CSF, G-CSF, Epo, TPO, on committed CFC	Mast cell growth
FLT3 ligand		Spleen, lung	Synergistic: SF, IL-3, IL-11 on blast CFC; Synergistic: IL-3, GM-CSF, G-CSF on committed CFC Synergistic: IL-7, SCF on B cell progenitors	
IL-3	Multi CSF	T, mast	ALL CFC	Eo, B, Mo
GM-CSF	CSFα	T, Endo, F, MO	ALL CFC	N, Mo, Eo
G-CSF	CSFβ	MO, Endo, F	CFU-G	N
IL-5		T, mast	CFU-Eo	Eo
M-CSF	CSF-1	F, Endo, F	CFU-M	M
EPO		Kidney	BFU-E, CFU-E	Eb
TPO		Liver, kidney, F, Endo	CFU-Meg	Meg
IL-1α		MO, F, Endo	Synergistic: SCF, IL-3, on blast CFU	Activates cytokine production
IL-1β		MO, F, Endo, Epi, K, SM		
IL-6		MO, T, B, F, Endo, K	Synergistic: SCF, IL-3, on blast CFU	
IL-11		Stromal F	Synergistic: SF, IL-3, SF on CFU-Meg	Meg

B, basophil; B, B cell; BFU-E, erythroid-burst forming unit; CFC, colony-forming cell; CFU, colony-forming unit; CFU-E, erythroid CFU; CFU-EO, eosinophil CFU; CFU-G, granulocyte CFU; CFU-M, monocyte CFU; CFU-Meg, Megakaryocyte CFU; Eb, erythroblast; Endo, endothelial cell; Eo, eosinophil; EPO, erythropoietin; F, fibroblast; G-CSF, granulocyte CSF; GM-CSF, granulocyte-macrophage colony-stimulating factor; IL, interleukin; M-CSF, monocyte CSF; Meg, megakaryocyte; Mo, monocyte; N, neutrophil; SCF, stem cell factor; T, T cell; TPO, thrombopoietin; Vasc., vascular.

Modified from Sieff CA, Nathan DG, Clark SC: The anatomy and physiology of hematopoiesis. In Nathan DG and Orkin SH (editors): *Hematology of Infancy and Childhood,* 5th ed. Philadelphia, WB Saunders, 1997.

granule proteins. The transcription factor PU.1 is essential for myelopoiesis. Other transcription factors such as AML-1, c-myl, CASP, C/EBPα, C/EBPγ, GATA-1, and Elf-1 are expressed in the myeloblast and promyelocyte, and some of these are required for azurophil granule protein expression. As cells enter the myelocyte stage, AML-1, GATA-1, and Elf-1 are downregulated whereas C/EBPε activity rises to initiate specific granule formation. Granulocytes survive for only 6–12 hr in the circulation and, therefore, daily production of 2×10^4 granulocytes/μL of blood is required to maintain a level of circulating granulocytes of 5×10^3/μL. In contrast, lymphocytes can exhibit lifetimes measured in months or years and require daily renewal of lymphocyte progenitors at rates substantially lower than the other hematopoietic progenitors.

The process of intramedullary granulocyte maturation involves changes in nuclear configuration and accumulation of specific intracytoplasmic granules. The relatively small peripheral blood pool is compartmentalized into the circulating pool and the marginating pool. The peripheral blood pool provides entrance into the tissue and is buffered by an immense marrow reserve of identifiable precursors, some of which are undergoing mitosis and some of which are maturing into bands and neutrophils. Proliferation of myeloid cells consisting of approximately five divisions takes place only during the 1st three stages of neutrophil development (myeloblast, promyelocyte, myelocyte). After the myelocyte stage, the cells terminally differentiate into metamyelocytes, bands, and neutrophils. Neutrophil maturation is associated with changes in the nucleus and with the production of azurophilic primary granules and specific or secondary granules. A myeloblast is a relatively undifferentiated cell with a large oval nucleus, a sizeable nucleolus, and a deficiency of granules. Promyelocytes acquire peroxidase-positive azurophilic granules, and myelocytes acquire specific granules. Chromatin condensa-

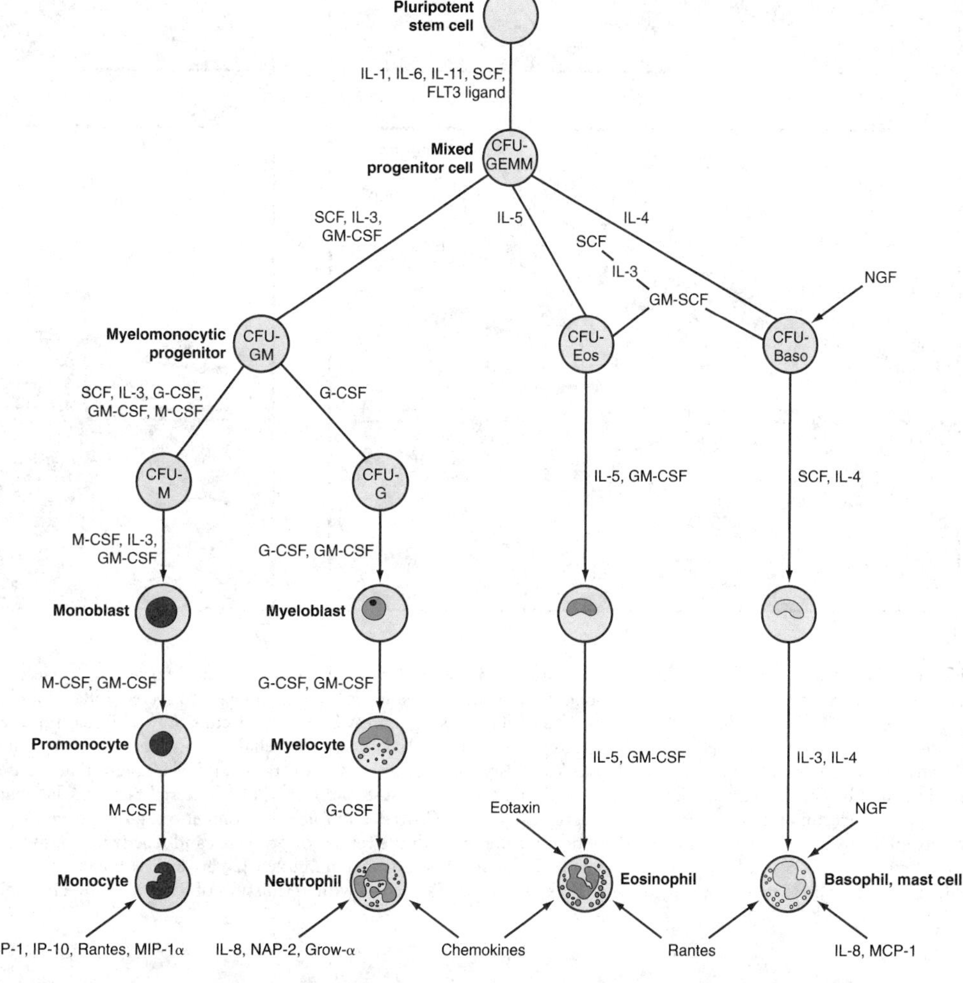

Figure 126-2. Various cytokines and chemokines act at different levels of granulopoiesis and monocytopoiesis. Multiple cytokines regulate progenitor cells or mature effector cells at each stage of maturation/differentiation from the primitive pluripotent stem cell to nondividing terminally differentiated precursors (monocytes, neutrophils, eosinophils, and basophil/mast cells). The cytokines and chemokines also have varying degrees of specificity; some, such as M-CSF and IL-5, act predominantly on the monocytic and eosinophilic pathways, respectively, whereas others, such as CFU, colony-forming unit; CFU-Baso, basophil colony-forming unit; CFU-Eo, eosinophil colony-forming unit; CFU-G, granulocyte colony-forming unit; CFU-M, monocyte colony-forming unit; G-CSF, granulocyte colony–stimulating factor; GM-CSF, act on multiple granulocytic-monocytic (erythroid not shown) cell types. GM-CSF, granulocyte-macrophage colony–stimulating factor; IL, interleukin; M-CSF, macrophage colony–stimulating factor; NGF, nerve growth factor. SCF, stem cell factor. (Modified from Abboud CN, Liesveld JL: Granulopoiesis and monocytopoiesis. In Hoffman R, Benz EB, Shattil SJ, et al [editors]: *Hematology: Basic Principles and Practice,* 2nd ed. New York, Churchill Livingstone, 1995.)

tion, loss of nucleoli, and the shape changes of the nucleus result in the morphometric characteristic of the segmented neutrophil.

NEUTROPHIL FUNCTION. Neutrophil responses are initiated as circulating neutrophils flowing through the postcapillary venules detect low levels of chemokines and other chemotactic substances released from a site of infection. These soluble effectors of inflammation trigger subtle changes in the array and activity of surface molecules on both endothelial cells and neutrophils. The initial associations are low affinity, reversible, and mediated primarily by cell-selectin-carbohydrate interactions. This leads to the phenomenon known as leukocyte rolling, in which loose adhesions are made and broken, causing neutrophils to move hesitantly along the endothelial surface. The rolling of neutrophils allows more intense exposure of neutrophils to activating factors such as tumor necrosis factor (TNF) or IL-1 (Fig. 126-3). This leads to induction of qualitative and quantitative changes in the family of β2 integrin adhesion receptors on the neutrophils (the CD11/CD18 group of surface molecules). The activated integrin receptors mediate tight heterotypic adhesion between neutrophils and endothelial cells and homotypic adhesion of neutrophils with each other. The net result of these interdependent intercellular interactions is that neutrophils flatten onto the endothelial cells, while neutrophil/neutrophil and neutrophil/platelet aggregates partially occlude the venule and reduce blood flow.

The next phase involves loosening of the integrin adhesion through the process of mobilizing integrin receptors to the trailing pseudopod of the neutrophil. The neutrophil is able to displace its integrin receptors and undergo conformational changes, allowing it to migrate between endothelial cell junctions into the extravascular tissue. Once through the endothelium, the neutrophil senses the gradient of chemokines or other chemoattractants and migrates to sites of infection. Neutrophil migration is a complex process involving rounds of receptor engagement,

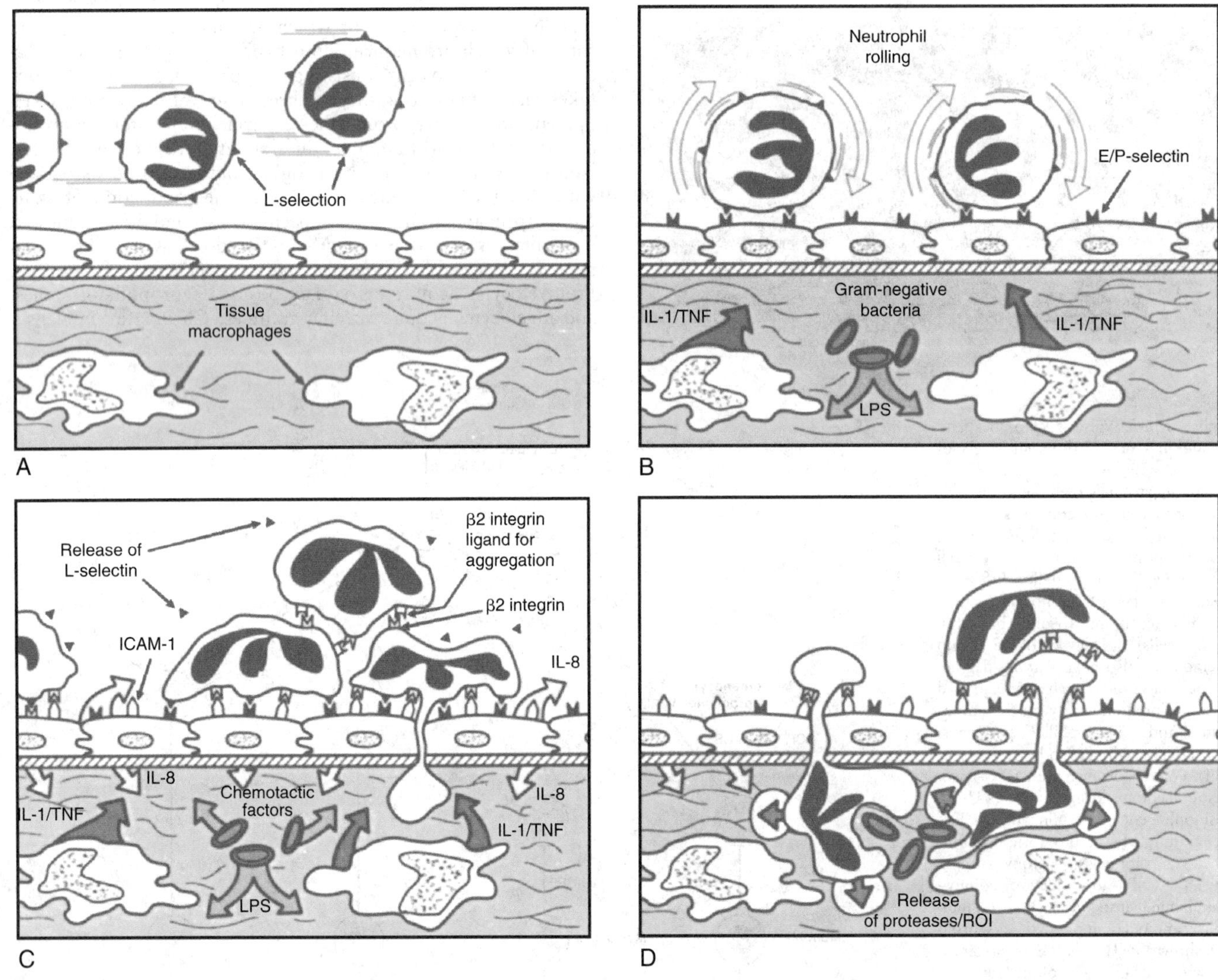

Figure 126-3. The neutrophil-mediated inflammatory response. *A*, Unstimulated neutrophils (expressing L-selectin) entering a postcapillary venule. *B*, Invasion of gram-negative bacteria with release of lipopolysaccharide stimulates tissue macrophages to secrete inflammatory monokines, interleukin 1 (IL-1), and tumor necrosis factor (TNF), which, in turn, activate endothelial cells to express E- and P-selectins. E- and P-selectins serve as counter receptors for neutrophils sialyl Lewis X and Lewis X to cause low-avidity neutrophil rolling. *C*, Activated endothelial cells express ICAM-1, which serves as a counter-receptor for neutrophil β_2 integrin molecules, leading to high-avidity leukocyte spreading and the start of transendothelial migration. Transendothelial migration of activated neutrophils is stimulated by chemotactic factors such as endothelial cell-derived IL-8 and formylated bacterial factors. Chemoattractants promote neutrophil activation with release of L-selectin and an increase in β_2 integrin affinity for ICAM-1 and for other counter-receptors promoting intravascular and neutrophil aggregation. *D*, Neutrophils invade through the vascular basement membrane with the release of proteases and reactive oxidative intermediates, causing local destruction of surrounding tissue at sites of high concentrations of chemotactic factors. (From Smolen JE, Boxer LA: Functions of neutrophils. In Williams WJ, Beutler E, Erslev AJ, et al [editors]: *Hematology,* 5th ed. New York, McGraw-Hill, 1994, with permission of The McGraw-Hill Companies.)

signal transduction, and remodeling of the actin-microfilaments composing in part the cytoskeleton. Additionally, secretion of specific granules or related secretory vesicular elements containing gelatinase, heparinase, and other enzymes allows the neutrophil to cross the basement membrane and transit through connective tissues. When the neutrophil reaches the site of infection, it recognizes pathogens by means of Fc immunoglobulin and complement receptors, fibronectin receptors, and other adhesion molecules.

The neutrophil ingests microbes that are opsonized (prepared for ingestion) by **opsonins,** heat-soluble and heat-labeled factors in human serum, which include immunoglobulin G (IgG) and C3, respectively. These opsonins facilitate phagocytosis of microbes, in which the pathogens are engulfed into a closed vacuole, the **phagosome** (Fig. 126-4).

As phagocytosis proceeds, two cellular responses essential for optimal microbicidal activity occur concomitantly: degranulation and activation of nicotinamide-adenine dinucleotide phosphate (NADPH)–dependent oxidase. Fusion of neutrophil granule membranes with the phagosome membrane occurs, resulting in the delivery of potent antimicrobial proteins into the phagosome. In coordinated succession, the contents of the specific granules and then contents of the azurophil granules are secreted into the phagosome. Occurring concomitantly are assembly and activation of NADPH oxidase at the phagosome membrane (see Fig. 126-4). This enzyme generates large amounts of superoxide (O_2^-) from molecular oxygen that in turn decomposes to produce hydrogen peroxide (H_2O_2) and singlet oxygen. H_2O_2 can react with O_2^- to form hydroxyl radicals. In the presence of **myeloperoxidase,** a major azurophil granule component, a reaction is catalyzed that uses H_2O_2 and ubiquitously present chloride ions to create hypochlorous acid (HOCl) in the phagosome. Although H_2O_2 and HOCl are microbicidal, evidence shows that these agents modulate host defenses. First, these oxidants can denature proteins, making them more susceptible to proteolysis. Additionally, some of the neutrophil proteases are activated by the oxidants. These events jointly serve to enhance breakdown or clearance of pathogens from the site of infection. Also, the oxidants can inactivate chemotactic factors and may serve to terminate the process of neutrophil influx, thereby attenuating the inflammatory process.

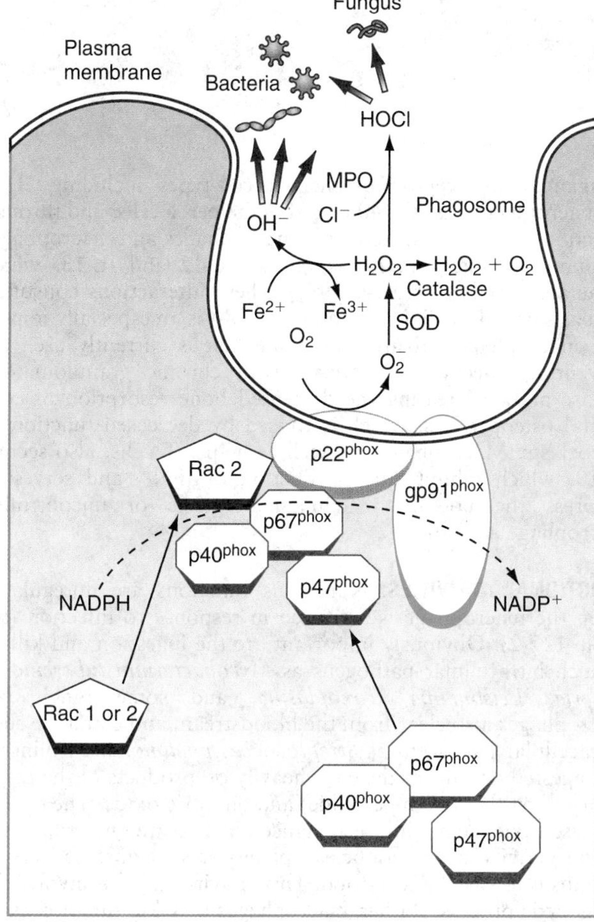

Figure 126-4. NADPH oxidase components and activation. On activation of phagocytic cells, the three cytosolic components of the NADPH oxidase ($p67^{phox}$, $p47^{phox}$, and $p40^{phox}$), plus either Rac1 or Rac2, are translocated to the membrane of the phagocytic vacuole. The $p47^{phox}$ subunit binds to the flavocytochrome$_{b558}$ component of the NADPH oxidase ($gp91^{phox}$ plus $p22^{phox}$). The NADPH oxidase catalyses the formation of superoxide anion by transferring an electron to O_2, thereby forming superoxide. The unstable superoxide anion is converted to hydrogen peroxide, either spontaneously or by superoxide dismutase (SOD). Hydrogen peroxide can follow different metabolic pathways into more potent reactive oxidants (such as OH^- or HOCl) or degradation to $H_2O + O_2 \cdot e^-$, electron; O^-_2, superoxide anion; H_2O_2, hydrogen peroxide; MPO, myeloperoxidase; HOCl, hypochlorous acid; OH^-, hydroxyl anion. (From Stiehm ER, Ochs HD, Winkelstein JA: *Immunologic disorders in Infants and Children,* 5th ed. Philadelphia, Elsevier/Saunders, 2004, p 622.)

Borregaard N, Boxer LA: Disorders of neutrophil function. In Beutler E, Kipps TJ, et al (editors): *Williams Hematology,* 7th ed. New York, McGraw-Hill, 2006.

Fenteany G, Glogauer M: Cytoskeletal remodeling in leukocyte function. *Curr Opin Hematol* 2004;11:15–24.

Papayannopoulou T: Bone marrow homing: The players, the playfield, and their evolving role. *Curr Opin Hematol* 2003;10:214–219.

Chapter 127 ■ Monocytes, Macrophages, and Dendritic Cells

Richard B. Johnston Jr.

Mononuclear phagocytes (monocytes, macrophages) have a central and essential role in innate host defense against infection, in tissue repair and remodeling, and in the antigen-specific adaptive immune response. No human has been identified as having congenital absence of this cell line, probably because macrophages are required to remove primitive tissues during fetal development as new tissues develop to replace them. Monocytes and tissue macrophages in their various forms (Table 127-1) constitute the **mononuclear phagocyte system.** These cells are a system because of their location, common origin, similar morphology, shared surface markers, and common functions, particularly phagocytosis. Bone marrow–derived **myeloid dendritic cells** share these characteristics and may be considered a component of the system.

DEVELOPMENT. Monocytes, the circulating precursors of tissue macrophages, develop more rapidly in the bone marrow and remain longer in the circulation than do neutrophils (see Table 126-1). The 1st recognizable monocyte precursor is the monoblast, followed by the promonocyte, a somewhat larger cell with cytoplasmic granules and an indented nucleus containing finely divided chromatin, and, finally, the fully developed monocyte. A mature monocyte is larger than a neutrophil and has

TABLE 127-1. Principal Sites of Macrophages in Tissues
Liver (Kupffer cells)
Lung (interstitial and alveolar macrophages)
Connective tissue
Serous cavities (pleural and peritoneal macrophages)
Synovial membrane (type A synoviocytes)
Bone (osteoclasts)
Brain and retina (microglial cells)
Spleen, lymph nodes, bone marrow
Intestinal wall
Breast milk
Placenta
Granuloma (multinucleated giant cells)

cytoplasm filled with granules containing hydrolytic enzymes. The transition from monoblast to mature circulating monocyte requires about 6 days. Monocytes retain a limited capacity to divide, and they undergo considerable further differentiation after entering the tissues, where they may live for weeks to months.

Migration of monocytes into the different tissues appears to occur randomly in the absence of localized inflammation. Once in the tissues, monocytes undergo transformation into tissue macrophages with morphologic and sometimes functional properties that are characteristic for the tissue in which they reside (see Table 127-1). Organ-specific factors influence monocyte differentiation and endow each tissue macrophage with particular metabolic and structural features. Monocytes in the liver become **Kupffer cells** that bridge the sinusoids separating adjacent plates of hepatocytes. Those at the lung airway surface become large ellipsoid **alveolar macrophages,** and those in the bone become **osteoclasts.** All macrophages have at least three major functions in common: presentation of antigens to lymphocytes, phagocytosis, and immunomodulation through release of a variety of potent hormone-like factors termed cytokines. At sites of inflammation, monocytes and macrophages can fuse to form multinucleated giant cells, the terminal stage of development in the mononuclear phagocyte line.

ACTIVATION. The most important step in the functional maturation of macrophages is the conversion from a resting to an activated macrophage, a process driven primarily by certain cytokines and microbial products. **Macrophage activation** is a generic term, with the functional characteristics of an activated macrophage population varying with the cytokine, microbial, and other stimuli to which they have been exposed. **Classical activation** is driven by specifically activated T-helper 1 (Th1)–type lymphocytes and natural killer cells through their release of interferon-γ (IFN-γ). Tumor necrosis factor–α (TNF-α) secreted by activated macrophages amplifies their activation, as does bacterial cell wall protein or endotoxin. **Alternative activation** is driven by T-helper 2 (Th2)–type lymphocytes through release of interleukin (IL)-4 and IL-13. These cytokines regulate antibody responses, allergy, and resistance to parasites. They can upregulate macrophage endocytosis, antigen presentation, and expression of certain chemoattractant cytokines (chemokines) and intracellular enzymes. Alternatively activated macrophages may have particular functional advantages, such as in tissue repair. In its most widely accepted sense, the term *activated macrophage* indicates that the cell has an enhanced capacity to kill microorganisms or tumor cells. Activated macrophages are larger, with more pseudopods and pronounced ruffling of the plasma membrane, and they exhibit accelerated activity of many functions (Table 127-2).

Classical macrophage activation is accomplished during infection with intracellular pathogens *(Mycobacterium, Listeria)* through crosstalk between Th1 lymphocytes and antigen-presenting macrophages mediated by the engagement of a series of ligands and receptors on the two cell types, including CD40 on macrophages and CD40 ligand on helper T cells, and through secretion of cytokines. Activated macrophages and macrophages encountering microorganisms release IL-12 and IL-18, which stimulate T cells to release IFN-γ. These interactions constitute the basis of cell-mediated immunity. IFN-γ is an especially important macrophage-activating cytokine that is currently used for preventing infection in patients with chronic granulomatous disease and for treating the decreased bone resorption of congenital osteopetrosis, which is caused by decreased function of osteoclasts. Macrophages, as well as helper T cells, also secrete IL-10, which inhibits the production of IFN-γ and serves to suppress the potentially damaging effects of uncontrolled macrophage activation.

TABLE 127-2. Upregulated Functions in Macrophages Activated in Response to Infection
Microbicidal activity
Tumoricidal activity
Chemotaxis
Phagocytosis (of most particles)
Pinocytosis
Glucose transport and metabolism
Phagocytosis-associated respiratory burst (O_2^-, H_2O_2)
Generation of nitric oxide
Antigen presentation
Secretion
Complement components
Lysozyme
Acid hydrolases
Collagenase
Plasminogen activator
Cytolytic proteinase
Arginase
Fibronectin
Interleukins, including IL-1, IL-12, and IL-15
Tumor necrosis factor-α
Interferon, including IFN-α and IFN-β
Angiogenic factors

H_2O_2, hydrogen peroxide; O_2^-, superoxide anion.

FUNCTIONAL ACTIVITIES. Numerous functions are upregulated when the macrophage is activated in response to infection (see Table 127-2). Obviously important are the ingestion and killing of such intracellular pathogens as *Mycobacterium tuberculosis, Listeria, Leishmania, Toxoplasma,* and some fungi, but macrophages also clear from the bloodstream and eliminate such extracellular pathogens as *Streptococcus pneumoniae.* Killing of the ingested organisms depends heavily on products of the respiratory burst (hydrogen peroxide) and on nitric oxide. The release of these toxic metabolites is enhanced in activated macrophages.

The activity of mononuclear phagocytes against cancers in humans is less well understood. This activity may not involve the phagocytic process. Rather, macrophages may kill tumor cells by means of secreted products including lysosomal enzymes, nitric oxide, oxygen metabolites, cytolytic proteinases, and TNF-α. Proteolytic enzymes and cytocidal factors present on the surface membrane of monocytes may have a role in tumor rejection.

The capacity to undergo diapedesis across the endothelial wall of blood vessels and to migrate to sites of microbial invasion in tissues is essential to monocyte function. Chemotactic factors for monocytes include complement products and chemokines derived from neutrophils, lymphocytes, and other cell types. Phagocytosis of the invading organisms or cells can then occur, influenced by the presence or absence of opsonins for the invader (antibody, complement, mannose-binding and surfactant proteins), the inherent surface properties of the microorganism or tumor, and the state of activation of the macrophage.

Monocytes migrating to intestinal mucosa are modified by stromal factors so that they lose innate receptors for microbial products such as endotoxin, and they do not produce proinflammatory cytokines. They retain, however, the capacity to ingest and kill microbes. They have been modified to promote the absence of inflammation that exists in normal intestinal mucosa in spite of its constant exposure to huge numbers of microbes and their inflammatory by-products.

Macrophages play an essential role in the disposal of damaged and dying cells, which helps resolve the immune response, and in wound healing. Brain microglia demonstrate these functions particularly well. In conditions such as stroke, neurodegenerative disease, and tumor invasion, these cells can become activated, surround damaged and dead cells, and clear cellular debris. Macrophages lining the sinusoids of the spleen are particularly important in ingesting aged erythrocytes. Macrophages in inflammatory sites can recognize changes in phosphatidylserine on the membrane of lymphocytes and neutrophils undergoing programmed cell death (apoptosis), and these can be removed before they become necrotic and spill their toxic contents into the tissue. Macrophages are phylogenetically primitive and can be identified early in fetal development, where they function to remove debris as one maturing embryonic tissue replaces another. They are also important in removing immune complexes, protein fragments, and inorganic particles such as elements of cigarette smoke or dust that enter the alveoli.

Macrophages are integrally involved in the induction and expression of specific immune responses, including antibody formation and cell-mediated immunity. This involvement depends on their capacity to break down foreign material in phagocytic and pinocytic vesicles and then present individual antigens on their surface as peptides or polysaccharides bound to class II major histocompatibility complex (MHC) molecules. B lymphocytes and, especially, myeloid dendritic cells can also present antigen to T cells for the specific immune response. Expression of MHC class II molecules is increased in activated macrophages, and antigen presentation is more effective.

The heightened capacity of activated macrophages to synthesize and release various hydrolytic enzymes and potentially microbicidal materials (see Table 127-2) probably plays a part in their increased killing capacity, although not every macrophage product is secreted in increased amounts when the cell is activated. The macrophage is an extraordinarily active secretory cell; approximately 100 distinct substances have been identified as being secreted by it, placing this cell in a class with the hepatocyte. Because of the profound effect of some of these secretory products on other cells, the large number of macrophages, and their widespread distribution, the mononuclear phagocyte system can be viewed as an important endocrine organ. IL-1 illustrates this point well. Microbes and microbial products, burns, ischemia-reperfusion, and other causes of inflammation or tissue damage stimulate the release of IL-1, mainly by monocytes and macrophages. In turn, IL-1 elicits fever, sleep, and release of IL-6, which induces production of acute phase proteins.

MYELOID DENDRITIC CELLS (DCs). Cells with dendritic (branched) extensions originate from myeloid progenitors in the bone marrow and function as highly efficient **antigen-presenting cells.** They phagocytose, though less well than macrophages. DCs are a heterogeneous population of at least four types: Langerhans cells in the epithelial surfaces of skin and mucosa; dermal or interstitial DCs in subepithelial skin and interstitia of solid organs; monocyte-derived DCs, which can leave the circulation and enter a site of pathogen invasion; and plasmacytoid DCs, believed to be the principal source of IFN-α and IFN-β in response to viral infection. The four types of DCs are distinguished by surface markers expressed after exposure of marrow or blood DCs to cytokines in vitro, and can be identified in tissue, particularly under inflammatory conditions.

DCs migrating from the bloodstream enter skin, epithelial surfaces, and lymphoid organs where, as immature cells, they internalize self- and foreign-antigens. Microbial products, cytokines, or molecules exposed in damaged tissue induce DC maturation, with upregulation of cytokine receptors and MHC class II and co-stimulatory molecules. Stimulated DCs in the periphery migrate to lymphoid organs where they continue to mature. They function there as the most potent of all cells that present antigen to T lymphocytes and induce their proliferation, activities that are central to the antigen-specific immune response.

Myeloid DCs differ from follicular DCs; the latter are probably of mesenchymal origin and do not internalize or process antigens or present antigens in the context of the MHC. Clinical trials have used myeloid DCs from cancer patients; these DCs are amplified and matured from blood monocytes or marrow CD34 progenitor cells by cytokines, exposed to antigens from the patient's tumor, then injected into the patient as a "vaccine" against the cancer.

ABNORMALITIES OF MONOCYTE-MACROPHAGE OR DENDRITIC CELL FUNCTION. Mononuclear phagocytes, as well as neutrophils, from patients with **chronic granulomatous disease** exhibit a profound defect of phagocytic killing (see Chapter 129). The inability of affected macrophages to kill ingested organisms leads to abscess formation and characteristic granulomas at sites of macrophage accumulation beneath the skin and in the liver, lungs, spleen, and lymph nodes. Genetic deficiency of the CD11/CD18 complex of membrane adherence glycoproteins (**leukocyte adhesion defect**), which includes a receptor for opsonic complement component 3, results in impaired phagocytosis by monocytes (see Chapter 129).

The monocyte-macrophage system is prominently involved in several **lipid storage diseases,** the sphingolipidoses (see Chapter 86.3). In these conditions, the expression in macrophages of a systemic enzymatic defect permits the accumulation of cell debris that is normally cleared by macrophages. Resistance to infection can be impaired, at least partly because of impairment in macrophage function. **Gaucher disease** is the prototype for these disorders. In this condition, the enzyme glucocerebrosidase functions abnormally, thus allowing accumulation of glucosylceramide (glucocerebroside) from cell membranes in Gaucher cells throughout the body. In all locations, the Gaucher cell is an altered macrophage. These patients can be treated with infusions of the normal enzyme modified to expose mannose residues, which bind to mannose receptors on macrophages.

The cytokine IL-12 is a powerful inducer of IFN-γ production by T cells and natural killer cells. Individuals with inherited deficiency in macrophage receptors for IFN-γ or lymphocyte receptors for IL-12, or in IL-12 itself, suffer a severe, profound, and selective susceptibility to infection by nontuberculous mycobacteria such as *Mycobacterium avium* complex or bacillus Calmette-Guérin (BCG) (see Chapter 125). About half of these patients have had disseminated *Salmonella* infection. These abnormalities are now grouped under the term **leukocyte mycobactericidal defects.**

Monocyte-macrophage function has been shown to be abnormal in various other clinical conditions. In most of these, however, the abnormality is partial and only a suspected cause of increased infection. Cultured mononuclear phagocytes of newborns are more readily infected than adult cells by human immunodeficiency virus (HIV)–1 and measles virus. Macrophages from newborns release less granulocyte colony–stimulating factor (G-CSF) and IL-6 in culture, and this deficiency is accentuated in cells from preterm infants. This finding supports the observations that levels of G-CSF are significantly decreased in blood from term and preterm infants, and that the bone marrow granulocyte storage pool is diminished in infants, particularly those born before term. Mixed mononuclear cells from newborns produce less IFN-γ and IL-12 than adult cells do, and macrophages cultured from cord blood are not activated normally by IFN-γ. This combination of deficiencies would be expected to blunt the newborn's response to infection by viruses, fungi, and certain bacteria such as *Listeria*.

There are two disorders in which macrophage activation is pathologically excessive. **Familial hemophagocytic lymphohistiocytosis** is characterized by uncontrolled activation of T cells and macrophages, with resultant fever, hepatosplenomegaly, lymphadenopathy, pancytopenia, marked elevation of serum proinflammatory cytokines, and macrophage hemophagocytosis (see Chapter 507). Up to 5% of children with systemic onset juvenile rheumatoid arthritis develop an acute severe complication termed **macrophage activation syndrome,** with persistent fever (rather than typical febrile spikes), hepatosplenomegaly, pancytopenia, macrophage hemophagocytosis, and coagulopathy, which can progress to disseminated intravascular coagulation and death if not recognized (see Chapter 154).

The term histiocyte was originally used to describe cells thought to be macrophages in fixed tissue preparations. Histiocytosis X represents a malignancy-like overgrowth of Langerhans-type dendritic cells (see Chapter 507). Thus, the term **Langerhans cell histiocytosis** better describes this disorder because histiocyte is a histologic term and not cell specific.

Fetler L, Amigorena S: Brain under surveillance: The microglial patrol. *Science* 2005;309:392–393.

Ranjeny T, Arend WP: Antigen-presenting cells. In Harris ED Jr, Budd RC, Firestein GS, et al (eds): *Kelley's Textbook of Rheumatology,* 7th ed. Philadelphia, Elsevier Saunders, 2005, pp 101–119.

Rossi M, Young JW: Human dendritic cells: Potent antigen-presenting cells at the crossroads of innate and adaptive immunity. *J Immunol* 2005;175:1373–1381.

Smythies LE, Sellers M, Clements RH, et al: Human intestinal macrophages display profound inflammatory anergy despite avid phagocytic and bactericidal activity. *J Clin Invest* 2005;115:66–75.

Chapter 128 ■ Eosinophils

Laurence A. Boxer

Eosinophils are distinguished from other leukocytes by their morphology, constituent products, and association with specific diseases. Eosinophils are nondividing fully differentiated cells with a diameter of ≈ 8 µm and a bilobed nucleus. They differentiate from stem cell precursors in the bone marrow under the control of T cell–derived interleukin 3 (IL-3), granulocyte-macrophage colony–stimulating factor (GM-CSF), and, especially, IL-5. Their characteristic membrane-bound specific granules stain reddish brown with eosin and consist of a crystalline core made up of major basic protein (MBP) surrounded by a matrix containing the eosinophil cationic protein (ECP), eosinophil peroxidase (EPO), and eosinophil-derived neurotoxin (EDN). These basic proteins are cytotoxic for the larval stages of helminthic parasites such as *Schistosoma mansoni,* and are also thought to contribute to much of the inflammation associated with asthma, causing sloughing of epithelial cells and contributing to clinical dysfunction (see Chapter 143). Both eosinophil MBP and ECP are also present in large quantities in the airways of patients who have died of asthma and are thought to inflict epithelial cell damage that contributes to airway hyperresponsiveness. MBP has the potential to activate other proinflammatory cells including mast cells, basophils, neutrophils, and platelets. Eosinophils have the capacity to generate large amounts of the lipid mediators platelet-activating factor (PAF) and leukotriene-C4, both of which can cause vasoconstriction and mucus hypersecretion. Eosinophils are a source of a number of proinflammatory cytokines including IL-1, IL-3, IL-4, IL-5, IL-9, IL-13, and GM-CSF. Eosinophils can also present antigens. Eosinophils have considerable potential to initiate and sustain an inflammatory response.

Eosinophil migration from the vasculature into the extracellular tissue is mediated by the binding of leukocyte adhesion receptors to their ligands or counterstructures on the postcapillary endothelium. Similar to neutrophils, transmigration begins as the eosinophil selectin receptor binds to the endothelial carbohydrate ligand in loose association, which promotes eosinophils rolling along the endothelial surface until they encounter a priming stimulus such as a chemotactic mediator. Eosinophils then establish a high-affinity bond between integrin receptors and their corresponding immunoglobulin-like ligand. Unlike neutrophils, which become flattened before transmigrating between the tight junctions of the endothelial cells, eosinophils can use unique integrins, known as VLA-4, to bind to vascular cell adhesion molecule (VCAM)–1, which enhances eosinophil adhesion and transmigration through endothelium. Eosinophils are recruited to tissues in inflammatory states by the chemokine **eotaxin.** These unique pathways account for selective accumulation of eosinophils in allergic and inflammatory disorders. Eosinophils normally dwell primarily in tissues, especially tissues with an epithelial interface with the environment, including the respiratory, gastrointestinal, and lower genitourinary tracts. The life span of eosinophils may extend for weeks within tissues.

In addition to selectively enhancing eosinophil production as well as adhesion to endothelial cells, IL-5 also has a number of important effects on eosinophil function. Considerable evidence shows that IL-5 has a pivotal role in promoting eosinophil accumulation. It is the predominant cytokine in allergen-induced pulmonary late-phase reaction, and antibodies against IL-5 block eosinophil infiltration into the lungs in animal models associated with airway hyperresponsiveness following allergen challenge. Eosinophils also bear unique receptors for several chemokines. These include RANTES, eotaxin, monocyte chemotactic protein (MCP)–3, and MCP-4. These chemokines appear to be key mediators in the induction of tissue eosinophilia.

Blood eosinophil numbers do not always reflect the extent of eosinophil involvement in disease-affected tissues. The **absolute eosinophil count,** calculated as the white blood cell (WBC) count/µL × percent of eosinophils, is usually <450 cells/µL in the blood and varies diurnally, being more abundant in the early morning and diminishing as endogenous glucocorticoid levels rise. Eosinopenia occurs after corticosteroid administration and with some bacterial and viral infections.

DISEASES ASSOCIATED WITH EOSINOPHILIA

The absolute eosinophilia count is used to quantitate eosinophilia. Many diseases are associated with moderately severe (1,500–5,000 cells/µl) or severe (>5,000 cells/µl) eosinophilia (Table 128-1). The genesis of sustained eosinophilia in some patients remains unclear. Patients with sustained blood eosinophilia may develop organ damage, especially cardiac damage as found in the idiopathic hypereosinophilic syndrome, and should be monitored for evidence of cardiac disease. Many cases of moderately severe eosinophilia often have no clear etiology.

ALLERGIC DISEASES. Allergy is the most common cause of eosinophilia in children in the United States. Acute allergic reactions may cause eosinophilic leukemoid responses with absolute eosinophil counts >20,000 cells/µL; chronic allergy is rarely associated with absolute eosinophil counts of >2,000 cells/µL. Hypersensitivity drug reactions can elicit eosinophilia with or without

TABLE 128-1. Causes of Eosinophilia

ALLERGIC DISORDERS
Allergic rhinitis
Asthma
Acute and chronic urticaria
Pemphigoid
Hypersensitivity drug reactions
INFECTIOUS DISEASES
Tissue-Invasive Helminth Infections
Trichinosis
Toxocariasis
Strongyloidosis
Ascariasis
Filariasis
Schistosomiasis
Echinococcosis
Pneumocystis carinii
Toxoplasmosis
Amebiasis
Malaria
Bronchopulmonary aspergillosis
Coccidioidomycosis
Scabies
MALIGNANT DISORDERS
Brain tumors
Hodgkin disease and T-cell lymphoma
Acute myelogenous leukemia
Myeloproliferative disorders
GASTROINTESTINAL DISORDERS
Inflammatory bowel disease
Peritoneal dialysis
Eosinophilic gastroenteritis
Milk precipitin disease
Chronic active hepatitis
RHEUMATOLOGIC DISEASE
Rheumatoid arthritis
Eosinophilic fascitis
IMMUNODEFICIENCY DISEASE
Hyper-IgE syndrome
Wiskott-Aldrich syndrome
Graft vs host reaction
Omenn syndrome
Pulmonary disease
Löffler syndrome
Eosinophilic leukemia
Hypersensitivity pneumonia
MISCELLANEOUS
Thrombocytopenia with absent radii
Vasculitis
Postirradiation of abdomen
Histiocytosis with cutaneous involvement

drug fever or organ dysfunction. Various skin diseases have also been associated with eosinophilia, including atopic dermatitis, eczema, pemphigus, urticaria, and toxic epidermal necrolysis.

INFECTIOUS DISEASES. Eosinophilia is often associated with infection with multicellular helminthic parasites and is the most common cause in developing countries. Severe eosinophilia is commonly due to **visceral larva migrans,** but may rarely be due to **hypereosinophilic syndrome.** The level of eosinophilia tends to parallel the magnitude and extent of tissue invasion, especially by larvae. Eosinophilia often *does not* occur in established parasitic infections that are well contained within tissues or are solely intraluminal in the gastrointestinal tract, such as *Giardia lamblia* and *Enterobius vermicularis.*

In evaluating patients with unexplained eosinophilia, the dietary history and geographic or travel history may indicate potential exposures to helminthic parasites. It is frequently necessary to examine the stool for ova and larvae at least three times. Additionally, the diagnostic parasite stages of many of the helminthic parasites that cause eosinophilia never appear in feces. Thus, normal results of stool examinations do not absolutely preclude a helminthic cause of eosinophilia; diagnostic blood tests or tissue biopsy may be needed. *Toxocara* causes visceral larva migrans usually in toddlers with pica (see Chapter 295). Most young children are asymptomatic, but occasionally some develop fever, pneumonitis, hepatomegaly, and hypergammaglobulinemia accompanied by severe eosinophilia. Isohemagglutinins are frequently elevated. Serology can establish the diagnosis.

Two fungal diseases may be associated with eosinophilia: aspergillosis in the form of allergic bronchopulmonary aspergillosis (see Chapter 234.1) and coccidioidomycosis (see Chapter 237) following primary infection, especially in conjunction with erythema nodosum.

HYPEREOSINOPHILIC SYNDROME. The idiopathic hypereosinophilic syndrome is a **leukoproliferative** disease characterized by sustained overproduction of eosinophils. The three diagnostic criteria for this disorder are (1) eosinophilia >1,500 cells/µL persisting for ≥6 mo, (2) absence of another diagnosis to explain the eosinophilia, and (3) signs and symptoms of organ involvement. The clinical signs and symptoms of hypereosinophilic syndrome can be heterogeneous because of the diversity of potential organ involvement. Eosinophilic leukemia may be distinguished from idiopathic hypereosinophilic syndrome by demonstrating a clonal F1P1L1-PDGFRA fusion gene resulting from a cryptic deletion of part of the long arm of chromosome 4. One of the most serious and life-threatening complications is cardiac disease due to endomyocardial thrombosis and fibrosis. Other organ systems that can be involved can include the skin, liver, spleen, gastrointestinal tract, brain, and lungs. Therapy is aimed at suppressing eosinophilia and is initiated with corticosteroids. Imatinib mesylate, an inhibitor of BCR-ABL, c-kit, and PDGF tyrosine kinases has antileukemic activity and has been effective in patients without elevated IL-5 levels. Hydroxyurea or α-interferon may be beneficial in patients unresponsive to corticosteroids. The underlying causes of hypereosinophilic syndrome remain unknown. For patients with prominent organ involvement who fail to respond to therapy, the mortality is ≈ 75% after 3 yr. Many patients in the past categorized as having the idiopathic hypereosinophilic syndrome had eosinophilic leukemia.

MISCELLANEOUS DISEASES. Eosinophilia is observed in many patients with primary immunodeficiency syndromes, especially hyper-IgE syndrome (see Chapter 116) and Wiskott-Aldrich syndrome. Eosinophilia is also frequently present in syndromes of thrombocytopenia with absent radii and in familial reticuloendotheliosis with eosinophilia. Mild eosinophilia is found in 20% of patients with Hodgkin disease and in gastrointestinal disorders including ulcerative colitis, Crohn disease during symptomatic phases, gastroenteritis that is associated with milk precipitins, and chronic hepatitis.

Bain BJ: Relationship between idiopathic hypereosinophilic syndrome, eosinophilic leukemia, and systemic mastocytosis. *Am J Hematol* 2004; 77:82–85.

Boxer LA: Eosinophilia. In Gills RH (ed): *Practical Algorithms in Pediatric Hematology and Oncology.* New York, Karger, 2003, pp 40–41.

Gleich GJ, Leiferman KM, Pardanani, et al: Treatment of hypereosinophilic syndrome with imatinib mesylate. *Lancet* 2002;359:1577–1578.

Shi H-Z: Eosinophils function as antigen-presenting cells. *J Leuk Biol* 2004; 76:520–527.

Chapter 129 ■ Disorders of Phagocyte Function

Laurence A. Boxer

Neutrophils are particularly important in protecting the skin, mucous membranes, and lining of the respiratory and gastrointestinal tracts as part of the 1st line of defense against microbial invasion. During the critical 2–4 hr after microbial tissue invasion, phagocytic cells must arrive at the site of inflammation if the infection is to be contained. If not, the resulting infection extends to a larger local lesion and potentially disseminates hematogenously.

Immunologic evaluation of patients with suspected immunodeficiency is formidable (see Chapter 121), especially for recurrent or unusual bacterial infections suggesting disorders of phagocyte function (Table 129-1). The differential diagnosis of many diseases can be complicated with symptoms similar to neutrophil defects or antibody or complement deficiency. Disorders of phagocyte function should be considered if results of initial screening tests are normal and the patient has had recurrent or unusual bacterial infections (Fig. 129-1).

Chemotaxis, the direct migration of cells into sites of infection, involves a complex series of events (see Chapter 126). Studies of defective in vitro chemotaxis of neutrophils obtained from children having various clinical conditions have not established whether the increased number of infections arises from a chemotactic abnormality or secondary to medical complications of the underlying disorder. The hyper-IgE syndrome is characterized by reduced neutrophil motility accompanied by markedly elevated levels of IgE leading to chronic dermatitis and recurrent sinopulmonary infections and is associated with coarse facial features, retention of primary teeth, and a propensity for recurrent bone fractures (see Chapter 125).

LEUKOCYTE ADHESION DEFICIENCY

Leukocyte adhesion deficiency 1 (LAD-1) and 2 (LAD-2) are rare autosomal recessive disorders of leukocyte function. LAD-1 affects about one per 10 million individuals and is characterized by recurrent bacterial and fungal infections and depressed inflammatory responses despite striking blood neutrophilia.

GENETICS AND PATHOGENESIS. **LAD-1** results from mutations of the gene on chromosome 21q22.3 encoding CD18, the 95-kD β_2 leukocyte integrin subunit. Normal neutrophils express three heterodimeric adhesion molecules: LFA-1 (CD11a/CD18), Mac-1 (CD11b/CD18, also known as CR3 or iC3b receptor), and p150,95 (CD11c/CD18). These three transmembrane adhesion molecules are composed of unique α_1 subunits of 185, 190, and 150 kD, respectively, encoded on chromosome 16 and sharing a common β_2 subunit. This group of leukocyte integrins is responsible for the tight adhesion of neutrophils to the endothelial cell surface, egress from the circulation, and adhesion to iC3b-coated microorganisms, which promotes phagocytosis and particulate activation of the nicotinamide-adenine dinucleotide phosphate (NADPH) oxidase.

Mutations in the CD18 gene either impair or prevent mRNA production or affect the structure of the synthesized CD18 peptide, leading to abnormal post-translational processing and loss of the abnormal CD11/CD18. The CD11α_1 subunits are not stable as monomers, resulting in deficiency of expression of CD11/CD18 in LAD-1 neutrophils in the 3 CD11α_1 subunits. Some mutations of CD11/CD18 allow a low level of assembly and functional active integrin molecules. These children retain some neutrophil integrin adhesion function and have a moderate phenotype. Failure of neutrophils to bear the β_2-integrins leads to inability to migrate to sites of inflammation outside of the lung because of their inability to adhere firmly to surfaces and undergo transendothelial migration. Failure of the CD11/CD18–deficient neutrophils to undergo transendothelial migration occurs because the β_2-integrins bind to intercellular adhesion molecules 1 (ICAM-1) and 2 (ICAM-2) expressed on inflamed endothelial cells. The neutrophils that do arrive at inflammatory sites in the lungs by CD11/CD18–independent processes fail to recognize microorganisms coated with the opsonin complement fragment iC3b, which is an important stable opsonin formed by the cleavage of C3b by C3b inactivator. Other neutrophil functions such as degranulation and oxidative metabolism normally triggered by iC3b binding are also diminished, and are markedly compromised in neutrophils from patients with LAD-1 resulting in impaired neutrophil function and high risk for serious and recurrent bacterial infections.

Monocyte function is also impaired, with poor fibrinogen-binding function, an activity that is promoted by the CD11/CD18 complex. Consequently, such cells are unable to participate effectively in wound healing.

Children with **LAD-2** share the clinical features of LAD-1 but have normal CD11/CD18 integrins. Features unique to LAD-2 are neurologic defects, cranial facial dysmorphism, and Bombay erythrocyte phenotype. The primary deficiency in LAD-2 is a defect in a specific GDP-L-fucose transporter of the Golgi apparatus that is secondary to distinct mutations in the gene encoding the transporter. This abnormality prevents the incorporation of fucose into various glycoproteins, which are expressed on cell surface membranes. This provides a biochemical basis for both the abnormalities of erythrocyte carbohydrate blood group markers and the defects in neutrophil adhesion. The neutrophils from patients with LAD-2 are deficient in the carbohydrate structure sialyl Lewis X, which renders the cells unable to adhere to activated endothelial cells. The neutrophils from these patients are unable to tether to inflamed venules for subsequent activation and spreading on the endothelium.

CLINICAL MANIFESTATIONS. Patients with the severe clinical form of LAD-1 express <0.3% of the normal amount of the β_2-integrin molecules, whereas patients with the moderate phenotype may express 2–7%. Children with severe disease present in infancy with recurrent, indolent bacterial infections of the skin, mouth, respiratory tract, lower intestinal tract, and genital mucosa. They may have a history of delayed separation of the umbilical cord, usually with associated infection (omphalitis) of the cord stump. Skin infection may progress to large chronic ulcers with polymicrobial infection, including anaerobic organisms. The ulcers heal slowly, require months of antibiotic treatment, and often require plastic surgical grafting. Severe gingivitis similar to what occurs in patients with profound neutropenia is common, with early loss of primary and then secondary teeth.

The pathogens infecting patients with LAD-1 are similar to those affecting patients with severe neutropenia (see Chapter 130) and include *Staphylococcus aureus* and enteric gram-negative organisms such as *Escherichia coli.* These patients are also susceptible to fungal infections such as *Candida* and *Aspergillus.* The typical signs of inflammation such as swelling, erythema, and warmth may be absent. Pus does not form, and few neutrophils are identified microscopically in biopsy specimens of infected tissues. Despite the paucity of neutrophils within the affected tissue, the circulating neutrophil count during infection typically exceeds 30,000/µL and can surpass 100,000/µL. During intervals between infections, the peripheral blood neutrophil count may chronically exceed 12,000/µL. LAD-1 genotypes producing moderate amounts of functional integrins at the surface of the neutrophil significantly reduce the severity and frequency of infections compared to children with the severe form.

The **differential diagnosis** includes patients with endothelial cell E-selectin deficiency, which manifests with delayed separation of

TABLE 129-1. Disorders of Phagocyte Function

DISORDER	ETIOLOGY	IMPAIRED FUNCTION	CLINICAL CONSEQUENCE
DEGRANULATION ABNORMALITIES			
Chédiak-Higashi syndrome	Autosomal recessive; disordered coalescence of lysosomal granules. Responsible gene found at 1q 42–45. The encoded protein has structural features homologous to a vacuolar sorting protein.	Decreased neutrophil chemotaxis, degranulation and bactericidal activity; platelet storage pool defect; impaired NK function, failure to disperse melanosomes	Neutropenia; recurrent pyogenic infections, propensity to develop marked hepatosplenomegaly in the accelerated phase; pigment dilution in the skin and fundus
Specific granule deficiency	Autosomal recessive; abnormal regulation of various myeloid granule genes by a transacting factor	Impaired chemotaxis and bactericidal activity; bilobed nuclei in neutrophils; reduced content of neutrophil defensins, gelatinase, collagenase, vitamin B_{12}–binding protein, lactoferrin	Recurrent deep-seated abscesses
ADHESION ABNORMALITIES			
Leukocyte adhesion deficiency 1	Autosomal recessive; absence of CD11/CD18 surface adhesive glycoprotein (β_2 integrins) on leukocyte membranes most commonly arising from failure to express CD18 mRNA	Decreased binding of C3bi to neutrophils and impaired adhesion to ICAM-1 and ICAM-2	Neutrophilia; recurrent bacterial infection associated with a lack of pus formation
Leukocyte adhesion deficiency 2	Autosomal recessive; absence of neutrophil sialyl Lewis X	Decreased adhesion to activated endothelium expressing ELAM	Neutrophilia; recurrent bacterial infection without pus formation
Neutrophil actin dysfunction	Altered polymerization of neutrophil cytoplasmic actin; perhaps arising from the presence of an inhibitor to F-actin formation	Impaired neutrophil adhesion, chemotaxis, and bacterial killing	Neutrophilia; recurrent bacterial infections without pus formation
DISORDERS OF CELL MOTILITY (with enhanced motile responses)			
Familial Mediterranean fever (FMF)	Autosomal recessive gene responsible for FMF on chromosome 16, which encodes for a protein, called pyrin, that may modify neutrophil activation.	Excessive accumulation of neutrophils at inflamed sites	Recurrent fever, peritonitis, pleuritis, arthritis, and amyloidosis
DEPRESSED MOTILE RESPONSES			
Defects in the generation of chemotactic signals	IgG deficiencies; C3 and properdin deficiency can arise from genetic or acquired abnormalities; mannose-binding protein deficiency predominantly in neonates.	Deficiency of serum chemotaxis and opsonic activities	Recurrent pyogenic infections
Intrinsic defects of the neutrophil, e.g., leukocyte adhesion deficiency, Chédiak-Higashi syndrome, specific granule deficiency, neutrophil actin dysfuntion, neonatal neutrophils	In the neonatal neutrophil, there is diminished ability to express β_2-integrins and there is a qualitative impairment in β_2-integrin function.	Diminished chemotaxis	Propensity to develop pyogenic infections
Direct inhibition of neutrophil mobility, e.g., drugs	Ethanol, glucocorticoids, cyclic AMP	Impaired locomotion and ingestion; impaired adherence	Possible cause for frequent infections; neutrophilia seen with epinephrine is the result of cyclic AMP release from endothelium.
Immune complexes	Bind to Fc receptors on neutrophils in patients with rheumatoid arthritis, systemic lupus erythematosus, other inflammatory states	Impaired chemotaxis	Recurrent pyogenic infections
Hyperimmunoglobulin E syndrome	Autosomal dominant; variable expression of a soluble inhibitor from mononuclear cells affecting neutrophil chemotaxis; high levels of antistaphylococcal IgE	Impaired chemotaxis at times; impaired IgG opsonization of *Staphylococcal aureus*	Recurrent skin and sinopulmonary infections
DEFECTS OF MICROBICIDAL ACTIVITY			
Chronic granulomatous disease (CGD)	X-linked and autosomal recessive; failure to express functional $gp91^{phox}$ in the phagocyte membrane in $p22^{phox}$ (autosomal recessive). Other autosomal recessive forms of CGD arise from failure to express protein $p47^{phox}$ or $p67^{phox}$.	Failure to activate neutrophil respiratory burst leading to failure to kill catalase-positive microbes	Recurrent pyogenic infections with catalase-positive microorganisms
G6PD deficiency	Less than 5% of normal activity of G6PD	Failure to activate NADPH-dependent oxidase	Infections with catalase positive microorganisms
Myeloperoxidase deficiency	Autosomal recessive; failure to process modified precursor protein arising from missense mutation	H_2O_2-dependent antimicrobial activity not potentiated by myeloperoxidase	None
Rac-2 deficiency	Autosomal recessive; dominant negative inhibitor by mutant protein of Rac-2 mediated functions	Absent receptor mediated O_2^- generation and chemotaxis. Impaired neutrophil rolling on endothelium	Neutrophilia; recurrent bacterial infections
Deficiencies of glutathione reductase and glutathione synthetase	Failure to detoxify H_2O_2	Excessive formation of H_2O_2	Minimal problems with recurrent pyogenic infections
IMPAIRED MACROPHAGE FUNCTION			
Defects in the IFN γ-IL-12 axis	IFN-γ-receptor ligand-binding chain, IFN-γ-receptor signaling chain, IL-12-receptor β1 chain, IL-12p40 deficiency. The IFN-γ-receptor abnormalities may be inherited in an autosomal dominant or recessive fashion. The IL γ-12 receptor as well as IL-12 are inherited in an autosomal recessive fashion.	Impaired killing of microorganisms; fatal BCG infection secondary to inability to either produce IL-12 by dendritic cells and macrophages, which is necessary to induce secretion of INF-γ by T-cells and natural killer cells or secondary to depressed bactericidal activity of macrophages lacking normal function of INF-γ receptor	Infection with atypical mycobacteria, *Salmonella*, and *Listeria*
IMPAIRED SPLEEN FUNCTION			
Splenic absence or splenic dysfunction	Congenital absence of spleen, removal of spleen, vascular occlusion of spleen	Removal or impaired function of splenic macrophages	Propensity to infection with encapsulated bacteria

AMP, adenosine phosphate; AR, autosomal recessive; BCG, bacille Calmette-Guérin; C, complement; CGD, chronic granulomatous disease; G6PD, glucose-6-phosphate dehydrogenase; H_2O, hydrogen peroxide; ICAM, intercellular adhesion molecule; IFN, interferon; IL, interleuki; m, messenger; NADPH, nicotinamide-adenine dinucleotide phosphate; NK, natural killer; phox, phagocyte oxidase; X, X-linked;

Modified from Boxer LA: Quantitative abnormalities of granulocytes. In Beutler E, Lichtman MA, Coller BS, et al (eds): *Williams Hematology*, 6th ed. New York, McGraw-Hill, 2001, p 836.

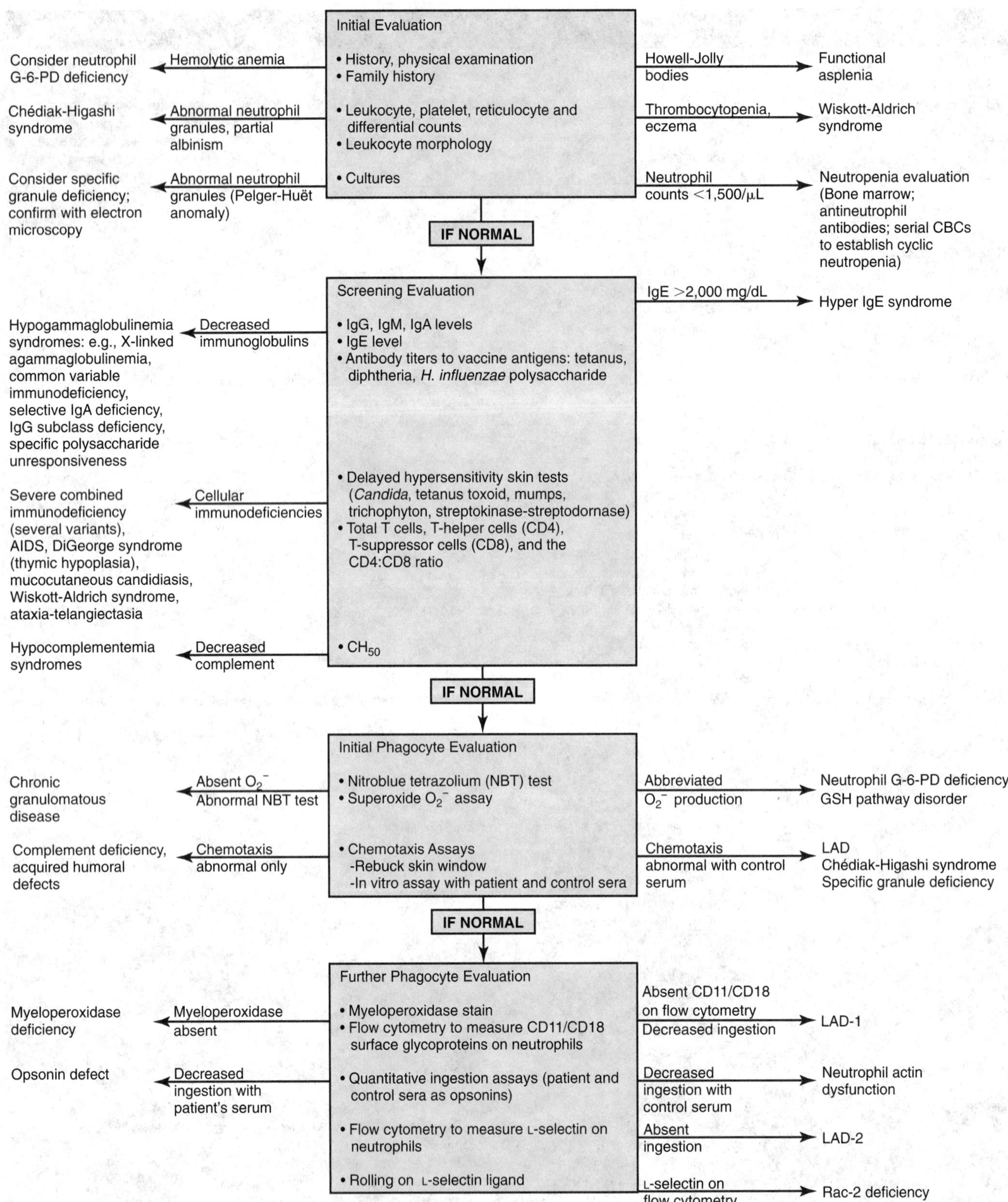

Figure 129-1. Algorithm for the evaluation of the patient with recurrent infections suggesting disorders of phagocyte function. CBC, complete blood count; Ig, immunoglobulin; G6PD, glucose-6-phosphate dehydrogenase; GSH, reduced glutathione; LAD, leukocyte adhesion deficiency. (Modified from Curnutte JT, Boxer LA: Clinically significant phagocyte cell defects. In Remington JS, Swartz MN [eds]: *Current Clinical Topics in Infectious Diseases,* 6th ed. New York, McGraw-Hill, 1985, p 144.)

the umbilical cord and omphalitis, and patients with an autosomal dominant mutation of RAC2 (a number of the Rho family of GTPases needed to regulate actin cytoskeletons and O_2^- production). RAC2 deficiency is characterized by delayed separation of the umbilical cord, leukocytosis, and absence of pus at sites of infection.

LABORATORY FINDINGS. The diagnosis of LAD-1 is established most readily by **flow cytometric** measurements of surface CD11b in stimulated and unstimulated neutrophils using monoclonal antibodies directed against CD11b. Assessment of neutrophil and monocyte adherence, aggregation, chemotaxis, and iC3b-mediated phagocytosis generally demonstrates striking abnormalities that directly correspond to the molecular deficiency. Delayed-type hypersensitivity reactions are normal, and most individuals have normal specific antibody synthesis. Some patients, however, have impaired T lymphocyte–dependent antibody responses that can be demonstrated by suboptimal responses to repeat vaccination with tetanus toxoid, diphtheria toxoid, and poliovirus. The diagnosis of LAD-2 is established by demonstrating the lack of sialyl Lewis X on the neutrophil.

TREATMENT. Treatment of LAD-1 depends on the phenotype as determined by the level of expression of functional CD11/CD18 integrins. Early **allogeneic stem cell transplantation** is the treatment of choice for severe LAD-1 associated with complete absence of the CD11/CD18 integrins. Other treatment is largely supportive. Patients can be maintained on prophylactic trimethoprim-sulfamethoxazole and should have close surveillance to identify infections early. Broad-spectrum antibiotics are indicated for empirical therapy when infection occurs. Determination of the etiologic agent by culture and biopsy is important because of the prolonged antibiotic treatment required for indolent infections.

Some patients but not others responded to fucose supplementation, which induced a rapid reduction in the circulating leukocyte count and appearance of the sialyl Lewis X molecules accompanied by marked improvement in leukocyte adhesion.

PROGNOSIS. The severity of infectious complication correlates with the degree of β_2-integrin deficiency. Patients with severe deficiency may die in infancy, and those surviving infancy have a susceptibility to severe life-threatening systemic infections. Patients with moderate deficiency have infrequent life-threatening infections and relatively long survival.

CHÉDIAK-HIGASHI SYNDROME

Chédiak-Higashi syndrome (CHS) is a rare autosomal recessive disorder characterized by increased susceptibility to infection due to defective degranulation of neutrophils, a mild bleeding diathesis, partial oculocutaneous albinism, progressive peripheral neuropathy, and a tendency to develop a life-threatening lymphoma-like syndrome. CHS is a disorder of generalized cellular dysfunction characterized by increased fusion of cytoplasmic (giant) granules. Pigmentary dilution involving the hair, skin, and ocular fundi results from pathologic aggregation of melanosomes and is associated with a failure of decussation of the optic and auditory nerves. Patients exhibit an increased susceptibility to infection that can be explained in part by defects in neutrophil chemotaxis, degranulation, and bactericidal activity. The presence of giant granules in the neutrophils interferes with the cell's ability to traverse the narrow passages between endothelial cells into tissue.

GENETICS AND PATHOGENESIS. The mutated gene for CHS, LYST (for lysosomal traffic regulator), is located at chromosome 1q2–q44 and has been cloned. The CHS protein is thought to be associated with vesicle transport and to mediate protein-protein interaction and protein-membrane associations. The mutated protein is hypothesized to lead to indiscriminate interactions with lysosomal surface proteins, which regulate fusion of granules with the plasma membrane, yielding uncontrolled fusion of lysosomes with each other.

Almost all cells of patients with CHS show some aspect of the oversized and dysmorphic lysosomes, storage granules, or related vesicular structures. Melanosomes or melanocytes are oversized, and delivery to the keratinocytes and hair follicles is compromised because of the failure to disperse the giant melanosomes properly, resulting in hair shafts devoid of pigment granules. This leads to the macroscopic impression of hair and skin that is lighter than expected from parental coloration. The same abnormality in melanocytes leads to the partial ocular albinism associated with light sensitivity.

Beginning early in neutrophil development there is spontaneous fusion of giant primary granules with each other or with cytoplasmic membrane components, resulting in huge secondary lysosomes that contain reduced content of hydrolytic enzymes including proteinases, elastase, and cathepsin G. In turn, the deficiency of proteolytic enzymes may be responsible for the impaired killing of microorganisms by CHS neutrophils. Because the CHS blood cell membranes are more fluid than cells of normal individuals, it is possible that the altered membrane structure could lead to defective regulation of membrane activation. Changes in membrane fluidity may conceivably affect cell function by altering expression of membrane receptors, which may produce disordered assembly of microtubules, and defective interaction of microtubules with lysosome membranes.

CLINICAL MANIFESTATIONS. Patients with CHS have light skin and silvery hair, and frequently complain of solar sensitivity and photophobia. Other signs and symptoms vary considerably, but frequent infections and neuropathy are common. The infections involve mucous membranes, skin, and respiratory tract. Affected children are susceptible to gram-positive and gram-negative bacteria and fungi, with *S. aureus* being the most common offending organism. The **neuropathy** may be sensory or motor in type, and ataxia may be a prominent feature. Neuropathy often begins in the teenage years and becomes the most prominent problem.

Patients with CHS have prolonged bleeding times with normal platelet counts, resulting in impaired platelet aggregation associated with a deficiency of the dense granules containing adenosine diphosphate and serotonin. Natural killer cell function is also impaired.

The most life-threatening complication of CHS is the development of an accelerated phase of a **lymphoma-like syndrome** characterized by pancytopenia, high fever, and lymphohistiocytic infiltration of liver, spleen, and lymph nodes. The accelerated phase may occur at any age. The onset of this accelerated phase may be related to the inability of these patients to contain and control Epstein-Barr virus infection, which leads to features simulating **virus-associated hemophagocytic syndrome.** The lymphocytic proliferation is associated with recurrent bacterial and viral infections and usually results in death. At autopsy, the lymphohistiocytic infiltrates in the liver, spleen, and lymph nodes are extensive but are not neoplastic by histopathologic criteria.

LABORATORY FINDINGS. The diagnosis of CHS is established by finding large inclusions in all nucleated blood cells. These can be seen on Wright-stained blood films and are accentuated by a peroxidase stain.

TREATMENT. High-dose ascorbic acid (200 mg/day for infants, 2,000 mg/day for adults) improves the clinical status of some children in the stable phase. Although controversy surrounds the efficacy of ascorbic acid, given the safety of the vitamin, it is reasonable to administer ascorbic acid to all patients.

The only cure for the accelerated phase is **hematopoietic stem cell transplantation** from an HLA-compatible donor or an unrelated donor compatible at the D locus. Stem cell transplantation reconstitutes normal hematopoietic and immunologic function and corrects the natural killer cell deficiency in patients entering the accelerated phase, but does not correct or prevent the peripheral neuropathy.

MYELOPEROXIDASE DEFICIENCY

Myeloperoxidase (MPO) deficiency is an autosomal recessive disorder of oxidative metabolism and is one of the most common inherited disorders of phagocytes, occurring at a frequency approaching one per 2,000 individuals. MPO is a green heme protein located in the azurophilic lysosomes of neutrophils and monocytes and is the basis for the greenish tinge to pus accumulated at a site of infection. Most individuals with the trait do not have an increased rate of infection or other clinical manifestations of disease.

GENETICS AND PATHOGENESIS. Mutations in the MPO gene causing this defect provide insight into the post-translational processing of this granule protein. MPO mRNA is transcribed exclusively during the promyelocytic stage of granulopoiesis. The primary translation product of the MPO gene is a single-chain peptide of 80 kD that undergoes co-translational glycosylation followed by a series of modifications of the oligosaccharides. MPO deficiency is caused by a missense mutation in the MPO gene that replaces an arginine with tryptophan and results in an MPO precursor that does not incorporate heme. Although this mutation is the most common cause of MPO deficiency, many patients are compound heterozygotes with one allele bearing the common mutation and the other being normal or possessing a mutation not yet identified. A partial deficiency results if only one allele is normal.

Partial or complete MPO deficiency leads to diminished production of hypochlorous acid (HOCl) and HOCl-derived chloramines. The deficiency in HOCl leads to early depression of gram-positive and gram-negative bacterial rates of killing in vitro that normalizes after 1 hr incubation. These data indicate that deficient cells use an MPO-independent microbicidal system that is slower to kill pathogens than the MPO-H_2O_2-halide system used by normal neutrophils.

CLINICAL MANIFESTATIONS. MPO deficiency is usually clinically silent. Rarely, patients may have disseminated candidiasis, usually in conjunction with diabetes mellitus. Acquired partial MPO deficiency can develop in acute myelogenous leukemia and in myelodysplastic syndromes.

LABORATORY FINDINGS. Deficiency of neutrophil and monocyte MPO can be identified by histochemical analysis.

TREATMENT. There is no specific therapy. Aggressive treatment with antifungal agents should be provided for candidal infections. The prognosis is usually excellent.

CHRONIC GRANULOMATOUS DISEASE

Chronic granulomatous disease (CGD) is characterized by the ability of neutrophils and monocytes to ingest but their inability to kill **catalase-positive microorganisms** because of a defect in the generation of microbial oxygen metabolites. CGD is a rare disease with an incidence of four to five per million individuals, caused by genes affecting one X-linked and three autosomal recessive chromosomes.

GENETICS AND PATHOGENESIS. Activation of the NADPH-dependent oxidase requires stimulation of the neutrophils and involves assembly from cytoplasmic and integral membrane subunits (see Fig. 126-4). Oxidase activation initially arises from phosphorylation of a cationic cytoplasmic protein, $p47^{phox}$ (47kd "phagocyte oxidase" protein). Phosphorylated $p47^{phox}$ together with two other cytoplasmic components of the oxidase, $p67^{phox}$ and a low molecular weight guanine triphosphatase (Rac-2), translocates to the membrane where they interact with the cytoplasmic domains of the transmembrane flavocytochrome b_{558} to form the active oxidase (see Fig. 126-4). The flavocytochrome is a heterodimer of two peptides, $p22^{phox}$ and highly glycosylated $gp91^{phox}$. Current models are consistent with three transmembrane domains within the N-terminus of the flavocytochrome that contain the histidines that coordinate heme binding. The role of $p22^{phox}$ peptide is required for stability of $gp91^{phox}$ and for oxidase activity. The role of $p40^{phox}$ in oxidase activation remains unclear. The $gp91^{phox}$ peptide is required for electron transport through use of an NADPH-binding domain, a flavin-binding domain, and a heme-binding domain. In turn, the $gp91^{phox}$ is stabilized by $p22^{phox}$. Furthermore, $p22^{phox}$ provides a docking site for the cytoplasmic subunits. The cytoplasmic $p47^{phox}$, $p67^{phox}$, and Rac-2 appear to serve as regulatory elements for activation of cytochrome b_{558}.

Approximately 65% of patients with CGD are males who inherit their disorder as a result of mutations in the X-chromosome gene encoding $gp91^{phox}$. About 35% of patients inherit CGD in an autosomal recessive fashion resulting from mutations in the gene encoding $p47^{phox}$ on chromosome 7. Defects in the genes encoding $p67^{phox}$ (chromosome 1) or $p22^{phox}$ (chromosome 16) also occur; these are inherited in an autosomal recessive manner and account for about 5% of cases of CGD.

Effective neutrophil phagocytosis requires activation of NADPH-dependent oxidase (see Chapter 126). After activation of neutrophils, electrons are passed from NADPH to flavin and then to the heme prosthetic group on cytochrome b_{558} and, finally, to molecular oxygen to form O_2^- mutations in the gene for cytochrome b_{558}. Alternatively, the cytosolic factor renders the electron transport system ineffective in generating O_2^-.

The metabolic deficiency of the CGD neutrophil predisposes the host to infection; the CGD phagocytic vacuoles remain acidic, and the bacteria are not digested properly (Fig. 129-2). Hematoxylin-eosin–stained sections from patients' macrophages may contain a golden pigment that reflects this abnormal accumulation of ingested material and contributes to the diffuse granulomas that give CGD its descriptive name.

CLINICAL MANIFESTATIONS. Although the clinical presentation is variable, several features suggest the diagnosis of CGD. Any patient with recurrent or unusual pneumonia, lymphadenitis, hepatic or other abscesses, osteomyelitis at multiple sites, a family history of recurrent infections, or unusual infections with catalase-positive organisms *(S. aureus)* requires evaluation.

The onset of clinical signs and symptoms may occur from early infancy to young adulthood. The attack rate and severity of infections are exceedingly variable. The most common pathogen is *S. aureus,* although any catalase-positive microorganism may be involved. Other organisms frequently causing infections include *Serratia marcescens, Burkholderia cepacia, Aspergillus, Candida albicans, Nocardia,* and *Salmonella.* Pneumonia, lymphadenitis, osteomyelitis, and skin infections are the most common illnesses encountered. Bacteremia or fungemia occur but are much less common than focal infections. Patients may suffer from the sequelae of chronic infection, including anemia of chronic disease, poor growth, lymphadenopathy, hepatosplenomegaly, chronic purulent dermatitis, restrictive lung disease, gingivitis, hydronephrosis, and pyloric outlet narrowing. Perirectal abscesses and recurrent skin infections, including folliculitis, cutaneous granulomas, and discoid lupus erythematosus also suggest

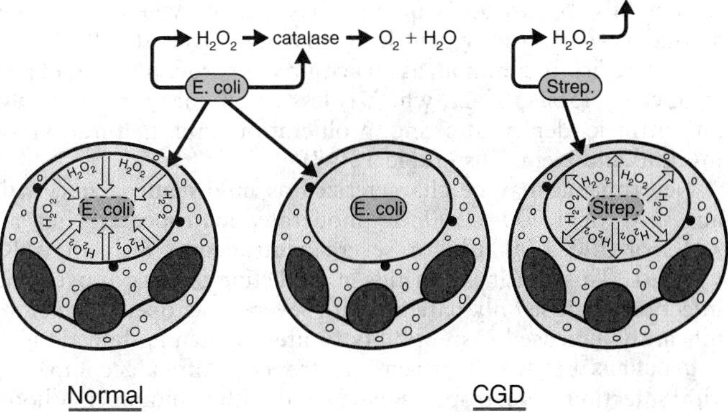

Figure 129-2. The pathogenesis of chronic granulomatous disease (CGD). The manner in which the metabolic deficiency of the CGD neutrophil predisposes the host to infection is shown schematically. Normal neutrophils stimulate hydrogen peroxide in the phagosome containing ingested *Escherichia coli.* Myeloperoxidase is delivered to the phagosome by degranulation, as indicated by the *closed circles.* In this setting, hydrogen peroxide acts as a substrate for myeloperoxidase to oxidize halide to hypochlorous acid and chloramines that kill the microbes. The quantity of hydrogen peroxide produced by the normal neutrophil is sufficient to exceed the capacity of catalase, a hydrogen peroxide–catabolizing enzyme of many aerobic microorganisms, including *Staphylococcus aureus,* most gram-negative enteric bacteria, *Candida albicans,* and *Aspergillus.* When organisms such as *E. coli* gain entry into CGD neutrophils, they are not exposed to hydrogen peroxide because the neutrophils do not produce it, and the hydrogen peroxide generated by microorganisms themselves is destroyed by their own catalase. When CGD neutrophils ingest streptococci, which lack catalase, the organisms generate enough hydrogen peroxide to result in a microbicidal effect. As indicated *(middle),* catalase-positive microbes such as *E. coli* can survive within the phagosome of the CGD neutrophil. (Modified from Boxer LA: Quantitative abnormalities of granulocytes. In Beutler E, Lichtman MA, Coller BS, et al [editors]: *Williams Hematology,* 6th ed. New York, McGraw-Hill, 2001, p 845.)

the possibility of CGD. **Granuloma formation** and inflammatory processes are a hallmark of CGD and may be the presenting symptoms that prompt testing for CGD if they cause pyloric outlet obstruction, bladder outlet or ureter obstruction, and rectal fistulae or intestinal granulomas simulating Crohn disease.

LABORATORY FINDINGS. For screening of CGD, the nitroblue tetrazolium (NBT) dye test is widely used; it is rapidly being replaced by the more accurate **flow cytometry** test using dihydrorhodamine 123 (DHR). DHR detects oxidant production because it increases fluorescence when oxidized by H_2O_2.

Neutrophils from patients with CGD have normal glucose-6-phosphate dehydrogenase (G6PD) activity. A few individuals with apparent CGD have been described as having neutrophils deficient in G6PD activity. The erythrocytes of these patients also lack the enzyme; these patients have chronic hemolysis.

TREATMENT. Hematopoietic stem cell transplantation is the only known **cure** for CGD. Vigorous supportive care along with recombinant interferon (IFN)–γ is used before transplantation. As part of supportive care, patients with CGD should be given daily oral trimethoprim-sulfamethoxazole for prophylaxis of infections. Cultures must be obtained as soon as infection is suspected. Most abscesses require surgical drainage for therapeutic and diagnostic purposes. Prolonged use of antibiotics is often required. Granulocyte transfusions may be necessary if antibiotics are ineffective. If fever occurs without an obvious focus, it is advisable to consider the use of radiographs of the chest and skeleton as well as CT scans of the liver to determine if pneumonia, osteomyelitis, or liver abscesses are present. The cause of fever cannot always be established, and empirical treatment with broad-spectrum parental antibiotics is often required. The erythrocyte sedimentation rate (ESR) may be used to help determine the duration of antibiotic treatment.

Aspergillus infection requires treatment with amphotericin B. Corticosteroids may also be useful for the treatment of children with antral and urethral obstruction. Granulomas may be sensitive to low doses of prednisone (0.5 mg/kg/day); treatment should be tapered over several weeks.

IFN-γ (50 μg/m², 3 times/wk) reduces the number of serious infections. The mechanism of action of IFN-γ therapy in CGD is unknown. **Itraconazole** (200 mg/day for patients >50 kg and 100 mg/day for patients <50 kg and ≥5 yrs of age) administered prophylactically reduces the frequency of fungal infections.

GENETIC COUNSELING. Identifying a patient's specific genetic subgroup is useful primarily for genetic counseling and prenatal diagnosis. In cases of suspected X-linked CGD, further analysis is not necessary if the fetus is initially demonstrated to be a 46,XX female. Fetal blood sampling and NBT slide test analysis of fetal neutrophils can be used for prenatal diagnosis of CGD. DNA analysis of amniotic fluid cells or chorionic villus biopsy is an option for early prenatal diagnosis. Restriction fragment polymorphisms have been identified for $gp91^{phox}$ and $p67^{phox}$ and have proved useful for diagnosis. In families in which the specific mutation is known, prenatal diagnosis is established by analysis of fetal DNA for the presence of mutant alleles using the polymerase chain reaction.

PROGNOSIS. The overall mortality rate for CGD is about two patient deaths/year/100 cases, with the highest mortality among young children. The development of effective infection prophylactic regimens, close surveillance for signs of infections, and aggressive surgical and medical interventions has improved the prognosis.

Bauer TR, Gu YC, Creevy KE, et al: Leukocyte adhesion deficiency in children and Irish setter dogs. *Pediatr Res* 2004;55:363–367.

Borregaard N, Boxer LA: Disorders of neutrophil function. In Beutler E, Lichtman MA, Coller B, et al (editors): *Williams Hematology,* 7th ed. New York, McGraw-Hill. 2006;921–957.

Gallin JI, Alling DW, Malech HL, et al: Itraconazole to prevent fungal infections in chronic granulomatous disease. *N Eng J Med* 2003;348:2416–2422.

Heyworth PG, Cross AR, Cumutte JT: Chronic granulomatous disease. *Curr Opin Immunol* 2003;15:578–584.

Rosenzweig SD, Holland SM: Phagocyte immunodeficiencies and their infections. *J Allergy Clin Immunol* 2004;113:620–626.

Ward DM, Shiflett SL, Kaplan J: Chediak-Higashi syndrome: A clinical and molecular view of a rare lysosomal storage disorder. *Curr Mol Med* 2002;2:469–477.

Winterboum CC, Vissers MC, Kettle AJ: Myeloperoxidase. *Curr Opin Hematol* 2000;7:53–58.

Chapter 130 ■ Leukopenia

Laurence A. Boxer

Marked developmental changes in normal values for the total white blood cell (WBC) count occur during childhood (see Chapter 716). The mean WBC count at birth is high, followed by a rapid fall beginning at 12 hr until the end of the 1st week. Thereafter, values are stable until 1 yr of age. A slow, steady decline in the WBC count continues throughout childhood until reaching the adult value during adolescence. **Leukopenia** in adolescents and adults is defined as a total WBC count <4,000/μL.

Evaluation of patients with leukopenia, neutropenia, or lymphopenia begins with a thorough history, physical examination, family history, and screening laboratory tests (Fig. 130-1).

NEUTROPENIA

Neutropenia is an **absolute neutrophil count (ANC)**, calculated as the WBC count/μL × % of neutrophils and bands, more than two standard deviations below the normal mean. Normal neutrophil counts must be stratified for age and race. For whites, the lower limit of normal for the neutrophil count is 1,500/μL; for blacks, the lower limit of normal is 1,200/μL. The relatively lower limit in blacks probably reflects a relative decrease in neutrophils in the storage compartment of the bone marrow.

ETIOLOGY. **Acute neutropenia** evolving over a few days often occurs when neutrophil use is rapid and production is compromised. **Chronic neutropenia** lasting months or years usually arises from reduced production or excessive splenic sequestration of neutrophils. Neutropenia may be classified by whether it arises secondary to factors extrinsic to marrow myeloid cells (Table 130-1), which is common; as an acquired disorder of myeloid and stem cells (Table 130-2), which is less common; or, more rarely, an intrinsic defect affecting proliferation and maturation of myeloid and stem cells (Table 130-3).

Neutropenia may be characterized as **mild neutropenia,** with an ANC of 1,000–1,500/μL; **moderate neutropenia,** with an ANC of 500–1,000/μL; or **severe neutropenia,** with an ANC <500/μL. This stratification aids in predicting the risk of pyogenic infection because only patients with severe neutropenia have significantly increased susceptibility to life-threatening infections.

Infectious Causes. Transient neutropenia often accompanies viral infections. Neutropenia associated with common childhood viral disease occurs during the 1st 1–2 days of illness and may persist for 3–8 days. It usually corresponds to a period of acute viremia and is related to virus-induced redistribution of neutrophils from the circulating to the marginating pool. Neutrophil sequestration possibly occurs after virus-induced tissue damage. Moderate to severe neutropenia may also be associated with a

TABLE 130-1. Causes of Neutropenia Extrinsic to Marrow Myeloid Cells

CAUSE	ETIOLOGIC FACTORS/AGENTS	ASSOCIATED FINDINGS
Infection	Viruses, bacteria, protozoa, rickettsia, fungi	Redistribution from circulating to marginating pools, impaired production, accelerated destruction
Drug-induced	Phenothiazines, sulfonamides, anticonvulsants, penicillins, aminopyrine	Hypersensitivity reaction (fever, lymphadenopathy, rash, hepatitis, nephritis, pneumonitis, aplastic anemia), antineutrophil antibodies
Immune neutropenia	Alloimmune, autoimmune	Variable arrest from metamyelocyte to segmented neutrophils in bone marrow
Reticuloendothelial sequestration	Hypersplenism	Anemia, thrombocytopenia, neutropenia
Bone marrow replacement	Malignancy (lymphoma, metastatic solid tumor, etc.)	Presence of immature myeloid and erythroid precursors in peripheral blood
Cancer chemotherapy or radiation therapy to bone marrow	Suppression of myeloid cell production	Bone marrow hypoplasia, anemia, thrombocytosis

TABLE 130-2. Acquired Disorders of Myeloid and Stem Cells

CAUSE	ETIOLOGIC FACTORS/AGENTS	ASSOCIATED FINDINGS
Aplastic anemia	Immune suppression of stem cells	Pancytopenia
Vitamin B_{12} or folate deficiency	Malnutrition; congenital deficiency of B_{12} absorption, transport, and storage; vitamin avoidance	Megaloblastic anemia, hypersegmented neutrophils
Acute leukemia, chronic myelogenous; leukemia	Bone marrow replacement with malignant cells	Pancytopenia, leukocytosis
Myelodysplasia	Dysplastic maturation of stem cells	Bone marrow hypoplasia with megaloblastoid red cell precursors, thrombocytopenia
Prematurity leading to birth weight <2 kg	Impaired regulation of myeloid proliferation and reduced size of postmitotic pool	Maternal preeclampsia
Chronic idiopathic neutropenia	Impaired myeloid proliferation and/or maturation	None
Paroxysmal nocturnal hemoglobinuria	Acquired stem cell defect secondary to mutation of PIG-A gene	Pancytopenia, thrombosis

TABLE 130-3. Intrinsic Disorders of Proliferation and Differentiation of Myeloid and Stem Cells

SYNDROME	INHERITANCE (GENE)	CLINICAL FEATURES
Cyclic neutropenia	AD (ELA2)	Periodic oscillation (21-day cycles) in ANC
Severe congenital neutropenia	AD (ELA2) (35–84%)	Static neutropenia, myelodysplasia, AML
	AD (CGf)	Static neutropenia, lymphopenia
	X-linked (WASP)	Neutropenic variant of Wiskott-Aldrich syndrome
Kostmann syndrome	AR (unknown)	Static neutropenia without myelodysplasia or AML
Chronic benign neutropenia	Sporadic (unknown) AD, AR	Variable pattern in the bone marrow, mild neutropenia
Cartilage-hair hyperplasia	AR (RMKP)	Neutropenia, lymphopenia, short-limbed dwarfism, metaphysical chondrodysplasia, fine sparse hair
Shwachman-Diamond syndrome	AR (SBDS)	Pancreatic insufficiency with fatty replacement and atrophy neutropenia, metaphysical dysostosis
Dyskeratosis congenita	X-linked (DKC1)	Nail dystrophy, leukoplakia, reticulated hyperpigmentation of the skin (1/3 develop bone marrow failure)
	AD (hTR)	—
	AR (unknown)	60% will have bone marrow failure
Chédiak-Higashi syndrome	AR (Lyst)	Partial albinism, giant granules in myeloid cells, platelet storage pool defect, impaired natural killer cell function, ineffective myelopoiesis
Glycogen storage disease type 1b	AR (G6PT1)	Hepatic enlargement, growth retardation, impaired neutrophil motility
Barth syndrome	X-linked (Taz1)	Cyclic neutropenia, dilated cardiomyopathy, methylglutaconic aciduria
Griscelli syndrome	AR (Rab27a)	Episodic neutropenia, thrombocytopenia, partial albinism, lymphohistiocytosis
Hyper-IgM syndrome	X-linked (HIGM1)	Absent IgG, elevated IgM, neutropenia, autoimmune cytopenia
WHIM syndrome	AD (CXCR4)	Warts, hypogammaglobulinemia, infections, myelokathexis, neutropenia

AD, autosomal dominant; AML, acute myelogenous leukemia; ANC, absolute neutrophil count; AR, autosomal recessive.

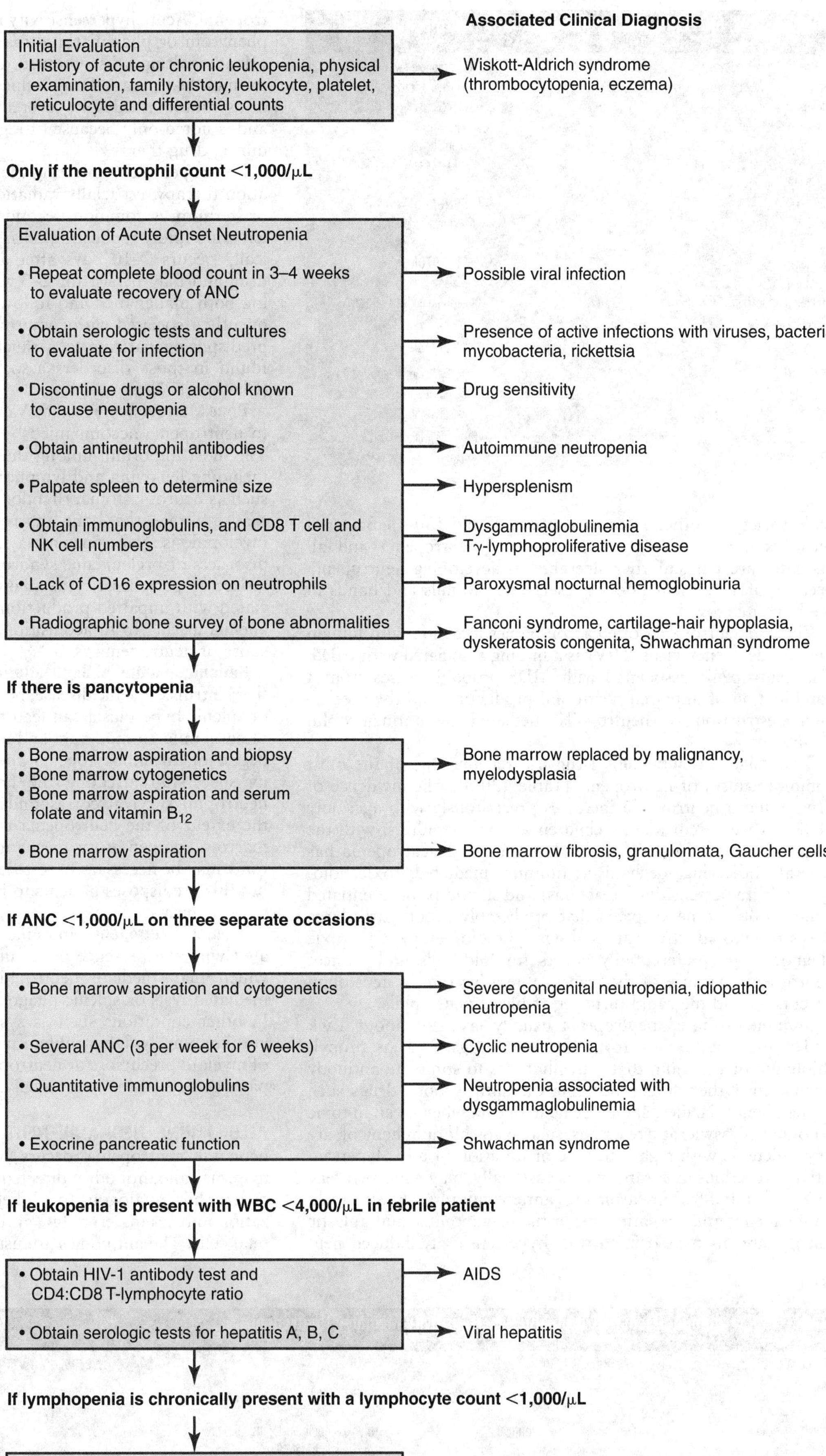
Associated Clinical Diagnosis
Initial Evaluation
• History of acute or chronic leukopenia, physical examination, family history, leukocyte, platelet, reticulocyte and differential counts
Wiskott-Aldrich syndrome (thrombocytopenia, eczema)
Only if the neutrophil count <1,000/μL
Evaluation of Acute Onset Neutropenia
• Repeat complete blood count in 3–4 weeks to evaluate recovery of ANC
Possible viral infection
• Obtain serologic tests and cultures to evaluate for infection
Presence of active infections with viruses, bacteria, mycobacteria, rickettsia
• Discontinue drugs or alcohol known to cause neutropenia
Drug sensitivity
• Obtain antineutrophil antibodies
Autoimmune neutropenia
• Palpate spleen to determine size
Hypersplenism
• Obtain immunoglobulins, and CD8 T cell and NK cell numbers
Dysgammaglobulinemia
Tγ-lymphoproliferative disease
• Lack of CD16 expression on neutrophils
Paroxysmal nocturnal hemoglobinuria
• Radiographic bone survey of bone abnormalities
Fanconi syndrome, cartilage-hair hypoplasia, dyskeratosis congenita, Shwachman syndrome
If there is pancytopenia
• Bone marrow aspiration and biopsy
• Bone marrow cytogenetics
• Bone marrow aspiration and serum folate and vitamin B12
Bone marrow replaced by malignancy, myelodysplasia
• Bone marrow aspiration
Bone marrow fibrosis, granulomata, Gaucher cells
If ANC <1,000/μL on three separate occasions
• Bone marrow aspiration and cytogenetics
Severe congenital neutropenia, idiopathic neutropenia
• Several ANC (3 per week for 6 weeks)
Cyclic neutropenia
• Quantitative immunoglobulins
Neutropenia associated with dysgammaglobulinemia
• Exocrine pancreatic function
Shwachman syndrome
If leukopenia is present with WBC <4,000/μL in febrile patient
• Obtain HIV-1 antibody test and CD4:CD8 T-lymphocyte ratio
AIDS
• Obtain serologic tests for hepatitis A, B, C
Viral hepatitis
If lymphopenia is chronically present with a lymphocyte count <1,000/μL
• Evaluate number and function of T cells
Inherited causes of immunodeficiency

Figure 130-1. Algorithm for evaluation of a patient with leukopenia. ANC, absolute neutrophil count; NK, natural killer cell; WBC, white blood cell count. (From Boxer LA: Approach to the patient with leukopenia. In Humes HD [editor]: *Kelley's Textbook of Internal Medicine,* 4th ed. Philadelphia, Lippincott Williams & Wilkins, 2000.)

TABLE 130-4. Infections that Are Associated with Neutropenia

VIRAL	Paratyphoid fever
Respiratory syncytial virus	Tuberculosis (disseminated)
Dengue fever	Brucellosis
Colorado tick fever	Tularemia
Mumps	Gram-negative sepsis
Viral hepatitis	Psittacosis
Infectious mononucleosis (EBV)	
Influenza	**FUNGAL**
Measles	Histoplasmosis (disseminated)
Rubella	
Varicella	**PROTOZOA**
Cytomegalovirus	Malaria
Human immunodeficiency virus	Leishmaniasis (kala-azar)
Sandfly fever	
	RICKETTSIAL
BACTERIAL	Rocky Mountain spotted fever
Pertussis	Typhus fever
Typhoid fever	Rickettsialpox

From Boxer LA, Blackwood RA: Leukocyte disorders: Quantitative and qualitative disorders of the neutrophil, part 1. *Pediatr Rev* 1996;17:19–28.

wide variety of other infectious causes (Table 130-4). Bacterial sepsis is a particularly serious cause of neutropenia and all neonates are particularly vulnerable to developing neutropenia because of a deficient pool of reserve neutrophils and bands in the bone marrow.

Chronic neutropenia often accompanies infection with human immunodeficiency virus (HIV) as a finding associated with AIDS. The neutropenia associated with AIDS probably arises from a combination of impaired neutrophil production and the accelerated destruction of neutrophils mediated by antineutrophil antibodies.

Drug-Induced Neutropenia. Drug use remains one of the most common causes of neutropenia (Table 130-5). The incidence of drug-induced neutropenia increases precipitously with age; only 10% of cases occur among children and young adults, with the majority of cases among adults. Drug-induced neutropenia has several underlying mechanisms (immune-mediated, toxic, idiosyncratic, hypersensitivity reactions) and should be differentiated from the severe neutropenia that predictably occurs after large doses of cytoreductive cancer drugs or radiotherapy. Cytotoxic chemotherapy preferentially affects myeloid cells and induces neutropenia because of the high proliferative rate of neutrophil precursors and the rapid turnover of blood neutrophils.

Immune-mediated neutropenia usually lasts for about 1 wk and is thought to arise from effects of drugs, such as propylthiouracil or penicillin that act as haptens to stimulate antibody formation. Other drugs, including the antipsychotic drugs such as the phenothiazines, can cause neutropenia when given in toxic amounts. Idiosyncratic reactions, such as to chloramphenicol, are unpredictable with regard to dose or duration of use. Hypersensitivity reactions are rare and occasionally may involve arene oxide metabolites of aromatic anticonvulsants. Fever, rash, lymphadenopathy, hepatitis, nephritis, pneumonitis, and aplastic anemia are often associated with hypersensitivity-induced neutropenia. Acute hypersensitivity reactions such as those caused by phenytoin or phenobarbital may last for only a few days if the offending drug is discontinued. Chronic hypersensitivity may last for months to years. Drug-induced neutropenia may occasionally be asymptomatic despite severely reduced numbers of neutrophils and is noted only because of regular monitoring of WBC counts during drug therapy.

Neutropenia complicating the use of anticancer drugs or radiation therapy, especially radiation therapy directed at the pelvis or sternum, is common, secondary to the effects of the cytotoxicity on rapidly replicating cells. A decline in the WBC count typically occurs 7–10 days after administration of the anticancer drug and may persist for 2–3 wk. The neutropenia accompanying both malignancy and following cancer chemotherapy is frequently associated with compromised cellular immunity, thereby predisposing patients to a much greater risk of infection than found in those disorders associated with isolated neutropenia (Chapter 177).

Bone Marrow Replacement. Various acquired disorders may lead to neutropenia accompanied by anemia and thrombocytopenia. The most important among these are hematologic malignancies including leukemia and lymphoma, and metastatic solid tumors such as neuroblastoma, rhabdomyosarcoma, and Ewing sarcoma that infiltrate the bone marrow, resulting in suppression of myelopoiesis. Neutropenia may also accompany myelodysplastic disorders or preleukemic syndromes, which typically are characterized by peripheral cytopenias and macrocytic blood cells associated with impaired production of myeloid precursors. Aplastic anemia arising from acquisition of damaged stem cells is also a cause of neutropenia.

Reticuloendothelial Sequestration. Splenic enlargement resulting from intrinsic splenic disease, portal hypertension, or other causes of splenic hyperplasia can lead to neutropenia. The neutropenia often is mild to moderate and accompanied by a corresponding degree of thrombocytopenia and anemia, and may be corrected by successfully treating the underlying disease. The reduced neutrophil survival corresponds to the size of the spleen, and the extent of the neutropenia is inversely proportional to bone marrow compensatory mechanisms. In selected cases, splenectomy may be necessary to restore the neutrophil count to normal, but this predisposes patients to infections by encapsulated bacterial organisms.

Immune Neutropenia. Immune neutropenias are usually associated with the presence of circulating antineutrophil antibodies, which may mediate neutrophil destruction by complement-mediated lysis or splenic phagocytosis of opsonized neutrophils. In other conditions such as systemic lupus erythematosus and autoimmune lymphoproliferative disease, accelerated apoptosis of myeloid precursors or neutrophils themselves may underlie the pathogenesis of the neutropenia.

ALLOIMMUNE NEONATAL NEUTROPENIA (ANN). This form of neonatal neutropenia occurs after transplacental transfer of maternal alloantibodies directed against antigens on the infant's neutrophils, analogous to Rh hemolytic disease. Prenatal sensitization induces maternal IgG antibodies to neutrophil antigens on fetal cells. The antibodies are usually complement activating and

TABLE 130-5. Immune-Mediated, Toxic, and Hypersensitivity-Mediated Neutropenia

CHARACTERISTIC	IMMUNOLOGIC FORM	TOXIC FORM	HYPERSENSITIVITY FORM
Paradigm drugs	Aminopyrine, propylthiouracil, penicillin	Phenothiazine	Phenytoin, phenobarbital
Time to onset	Days to weeks	Weeks to months	Weeks to months
Clinical appearance	Acute, often explosive symptoms	Often asymptomatic or insidious onset	May be associated with fever, rash, nephritis, pneumonitis, or aplastic anemia
Rechallenge	Prompt recurrence with small test dose	Latent period; high doses required	Latent period; high doses required
Laboratory findings	Antibody test results positive	Evidence of direct toxicity to cells	Evidence of metabolite-mediated damage to cells

From Boxer LA: Approach to the patient with leukopenia. In Humes H (editor): *Kelley's Textbook of Internal Medicine,* 4th ed. Philadelphia, Lippincott Williams & Wilkins, 2000, p 1579.

are frequently directed to neutrophil-specific antigens. The pathogenesis of ANN usually involves phagocytosis of antibody-coated neutrophils by splenic macrophages. Symptomatic infants may present with delayed separation of the umbilical cord, mild skin infections, fever, and pneumonia within the 1st 2 wk of life; these resolve with antibiotic therapy. The neutropenia is often severe and associated with fever and infections due to the usual microbes that cause neonatal disease. By 7 wk of age, the neutrophil count usually returns to normal, reflecting the duration of maternal antibodies in the infant's circulation. **Treatment** consists of supportive care and appropriate antibiotics for clinical infections.

AUTOIMMUNE NEUTROPENIA. Autoimmune neutropenia is analogous to autoimmune hemolytic anemia and thrombocytopenia. Antibodies causing neutropenia have been detected in patients who have no other signs of autoimmune disease, in patients who have additional antibodies against red blood cells and/or platelets, and in patients who have a connective tissue disorder. Autoimmune neutropenia is distinguished from other forms of neutropenia only by the demonstration of antineutrophil antibodies rather than by abnormal bone marrow histology. Autoimmune neutropenia frequently occurs in children with congenital and acquired forms of immune deficiencies, including dysgammaglobulinemia, immune-mediated thyroiditis, autoimmune hemolytic anemia, and thrombocytopenia.

AUTOIMMUNE NEUTROPENIA OF INFANCY (ANI). This benign condition is diagnosed more frequently as reliable techniques for detection of antineutrophil antibodies are available. The exact incidence of ANI remains unknown, but because of its benign nature, the disorder may be more common than currently appreciated. In one study, ANI occurred with an annual incidence of approximately 1/100,000 among children between infancy and 10 yr. All patients recognized as having ANI have severe neutropenia on presentation, with an ANC usually <500/μL, but the total WBC count is always within normal limits. Monocytosis or eosinophilia may occur but does not seem to affect the rate of infection. The age at diagnosis is usually between 5 and 15 mo, with a female:male ratio of 6:4. None of the affected children has evidence of other autoimmune diseases. Children with ANI present with minor infections such as otitis media, gingivitis, respiratory tract infections, gastroenteritis, and cellulitis. The diagnosis often is considered only after the blood count reveals neutropenia. Occasionally, children may present with more severe infections including pneumonia, sepsis, or abscesses. Longitudinal studies of infants with ANI demonstrate a median duration of disease of ≈ 7–24 mo. The diagnosis is established by the presence of antineutrophil antibodies in serum. **Treatment** with recombinant human granulocyte colony–stimulating factor (rhG-CSF) may be useful in providing temporary remission in infants with severe infections or requiring surgical intervention.

NEONATAL AUTOIMMUNE NEUTROPENIA. Mothers with autoimmune disease may give birth to infants who develop transient neutropenia. The duration of the neutropenia depends on the time required for the infant to clear the maternally transferred circulating IgG antibody. It persists in most cases for a few weeks to a few months. Neonates almost always remain asymptomatic.

Ineffective Myelopoiesis. Ineffective myelopoiesis may result from congenital or acquired vitamin B_{12} deficiency, which may result from resection of the distal ileum, or folic acid deficiency. Megaloblastic pancytopenia also can result from extended use of antibiotics such as trimethoprim-sulfamethoxazole, which inhibit folic acid metabolism, and from the use of phenytoin, which may impair folate absorption in the small intestine. Neutropenia also occurs with starvation and marasmus in infants, anorexia nervosa, and occasionally among patients receiving prolonged parenteral feedings.

Intrinsic Disorders of Proliferation and Maturation of Myeloid Stem Cells. The isolated disorders of proliferation and maturation of myeloid stem cells are rare. These patients frequently benefit from rhG-CSF therapy. Congenital disorders that have severe neutropenia as a clinical feature include the severe combined immunodeficiencies (Chapter 125), hyper IgM (Chapter 125), and common variable immunodeficiency (Chapter 123).

CYCLIC NEUTROPENIA. Cyclic neutropenia, a congenital granulopoietic disorder, is inherited in an autosomal dominant manner in some patients (see Table 130-3). It is characterized by regular, periodic oscillation in the number of peripheral neutrophils from normal to neutropenic values with a mean oscillatory period of 21 ± 3 days. During the neutropenic phase, most patients suffer from oral ulcers, fever, stomatitis, or pharyngitis, occasionally associated with lymph node enlargement. Serious infections occur occasionally and may lead to pneumonia, chronic periodontitis, and recurrent ulcerations of the oral, vaginal, and rectal mucosa. Sepsis, notably with *Clostridium perfringens,* and death may occur. Cyclic neutropenia arises from a regulatory abnormality involving early hematopoietic precursor cells and is associated with mutations in the neutrophil elastase gene. Many patients experience abatement of symptoms with age. The cycles tend to become less noticeable in older patients, and the hematologic picture often begins to resemble that of chronic neutropenia.

Treatment with rhG-CSF elevates the neutrophil counts and improves outcome.

SEVERE CONGENITAL NEUTROPENIA. Severe congenital neutropenia, or Kostmann disease, is characterized by an arrest in myeloid maturation at the promyelocyte stage of the bone marrow, resulting in an ANC of <200/μL (see Table 130-3). This disorder occurs sporadically or as an autosomal dominant or recessive disorder. The dominant form may be due to mutations in the neutrophil elastase gene while the recessive form may be due to mutations in HAX1, which protects cells against apoptosis. Patients typically show monocytosis and eosinophilia and suffer from recurrent, severe pyogenic infections, especially of the skin, mouth, and rectum. Anemia associated with chronic inflammatory disease is often present. Approximately 17% of patients develop acute myelogenous leukemia or myelodysplasia associated with monosomy 7. The neutropenia in the majority of patients is associated with mutations in the neutrophil elastase gene, which, in turn, leads to accelerated apoptosis of bone marrow myeloid cells. Before the use of rhG-CSF, two thirds of these patients died of fatal infections before reaching adolescence.

SHWACHMAN-DIAMOND SYNDROME. Shwachman-Diamond syndrome is an autosomal recessive disorder characterized by pancreatic insufficiency and abnormally low WBC counts (see Table 130-3). (Other selected neutropenic syndromes are also indicated in Table 130-3.) The initial symptoms are usually diarrhea and failure to thrive because of malabsorption, which develops in almost all infants by 4 mo of age. Growth failure and metaphyseal chondrodysplasia associated with dwarfism are especially prominent during the 1st and 2nd yr of life. Puberty is often delayed. Some patients have respiratory problems with pneumonia and frequent otitis media, as well as eczema. Virtually all patients with Shwachman-Diamond syndrome have neutropenia, with the ANC periodically <1,000/μL associated with hypoplastic myelopoiesis. Shwachman-Diamond syndrome is caused by inactivating mutations of the SBDS gene located on chromosome 7. Some children have been reported to have a chemotactic defect that may contribute to the increased susceptibility to pyogenic infection. The illness may progress to bone marrow hypoplasia leading to moderate thrombocytopenia and anemia. Myelodysplasia and acute myelogenous leukemia associated with monosomy 7 have also been reported in this syndrome. The neutropenia responds to treatment with rhG-CSF.

CARTILAGE-HAIR HYPOPLASIA. Cartilage-hair hypoplasia is a multisystem autosomal recessive disorder and is common among the

Finnish and Amish. It is due to mutations in the RMRP gene, which encodes the RNA component of a ribonuclear protein ribonuclease, and the mutations are characterized by short limbs and short stature resulting from abnormal development of long bone cartilage (see Chapter 125). The major symptoms include abnormalities of the spine, hyperextensible fingers, and very fine, thin hair, eyebrows, and eyelashes (see Table 130-3). Cartilage-hair hypoplasia is associated with decreased cell-mediated immunity, neutropenia, macrocytic anemia, and increased rates of malignancy. Stem cell transplantation has been used and restores cellular immunity and corrects the neutropenia.

GLYCOGEN STORAGE DISEASE TYPE Ib. Recurrent infections with neutropenia are a distinctive feature of glycogen storage disease (GSD) type Ib (see Table 130-3). Both classic von Gierke glycogen storage disease (GSDIa) and GSDIb cause massive enlargement of liver and severe growth retardation (see Chapter 87.1). In contrast to GSDIa, glucose-6-phosphatase activity is present by in vitro assays but glucose is not liberated from glucose-6-phosphate in vivo with GSDIb. In the liver, glucose-6-phosphatase requires two microsomal membrane components: a specific transfer system, glucose-6-phosphatase translocase, which shuttles glucose-6-phosphate from the cytoplasm to the lumen of the endoplasmic reticulum where it is hydrolyzed by a second enzyme, glucose-6-phosphalase, into glucose and inorganic phosphate. Neutrophils also appear to have a defective transport system resulting in defective neutrophil motility that is associated with the neutropenia. Patients with GSDIb with severe neutropenia are predisposed to recurrent bacterial infections. **Treatment** with rhG-CSF can correct the neutropenia.

SEVERE CHRONIC NEUTROPENIA. Acquired idiopathic chronic symptomatic neutropenia is characterized by onset of neutropenia after 2 yr of age, and more frequently among adults. It is characterized by neutrophil counts that are occasionally <500/µL. Patients with an ANC persistently <500/µL are afflicted with recurrent pyogenic infections involving the skin, mucous membranes, lungs, and lymph nodes. Bone marrow examination reveals variable patterns of myeloid formation with arrest generally occurring between the myelocyte and band forms (see Table 130-2). Often there is overlap or confusion about the diagnosis of chronic idiopathic neutropenia.

Some forms of chronic neutropenia, such as myelokathexis, arise from an impaired release of neutrophils from the bone marrow into the peripheral blood. **Myelokathexis** is a rare disorder characterized by mild to severe neutropenia with neutrophil hypersegmentation, with the cells showing cytoplasmic vacuoles of thin strands connecting the nuclear lobes. In some cases, these patients also have cellular immune defects and are predisposed to recurrent bacterial infections (see Table 130-3).

CHRONIC BENIGN NEUTROPENIA. In contrast to severe congenital neutropenia, chronic benign neutropenia of childhood represents a common group of disorders characterized by mild to moderate neutropenia that does not lead to an increased risk of pyogenic infections. Spontaneous remissions are often reported, although these may represent misdiagnosis of autoimmune neutropenia of infancy, in which remissions occur commonly during childhood. Chronic benign neutropenia may be inherited in either a dominant or recessive form. An autosomal recessive form of benign neutropenia is encountered in Yemenite Jews. Because of the relatively low risk of serious infection, patients should be not subjected to the potential toxic effects of prolonged administration of corticosteroids, splenectomy, or cytotoxic therapy (see Table 130-3).

Clinical Manifestations. Individuals with neutrophil counts <500/µL are at substantial risk for developing infections, primarily from their endogenous flora as well as from nosocomial organisms. Some patients with isolated chronic neutropenia with an ANC <200/µL may not experience many serious infections, probably because the remainder of the immune system remains intact. In contrast, children whose neutropenia is secondary to acquired disorders of production such as with cytotoxic therapy, immunosuppressive drugs, or radiation therapy, particularly in conjunction with malignancies, are likely to develop serious bacterial infections because many arms of the immune system are markedly compromised.

Leukopenia associated with neutropenia, in addition to monocytopenia and lymphocytopenia, is often more serious than neutropenia alone. The integrity of skin and mucous membranes, the vascular supply to tissues, and the nutritional status of patients influence the risk of infection.

The **clinical presentation** in most patients with **profound neutropenia** is fever >101°F, cellulitis, and furunculosis. Stomatitis, gingivitis, perirectal inflammation, colitis, sinusitis, and otitis media are frequent accompaniments of profound neutropenia in children. Other clinical manifestations of profound neutropenia include hepatic abscesses, recurrent pneumonias, and septicemia. Isolated neutropenia does not heighten a patient's susceptibility to fungal, parasitic, or viral infections or to bacterial meningitis.

The most common pathogens causing infections in neutropenic patients are *Staphylococcus aureus* and gram-negative bacteria. The usual signs and symptoms of local infection and inflammation such as exudate, fluctuance, and regional lymphadenopathy are generally less in the presence of neutropenia because of the inability to form pus. Neutropenic patients experience pain at sites of inflammation.

Laboratory Findings. Isolated absolute neutropenia has a limited number of causes (see Tables 130-1 through 130-3). The duration and severity of the neutropenia greatly influence the extent of laboratory evaluation. Patients with chronic neutropenia since infancy and a history of recurrent fevers and chronic gingivitis should have WBC counts and differential counts determined three times weekly for 6 wk to evaluate the periodicity suggestive of cyclic neutropenia. Bone marrow aspiration and biopsy should be performed on selected patients to assess cellularity. Additional marrow studies such as cytogenetic analysis and special stains for detecting leukemia and other malignant disorders should be obtained for patients with suspected intrinsic defects in the myeloid cells or the progenitors, and for patients with suspected malignancy. Selection of further laboratory tests is determined by the duration and severity of the neutropenia and the associated findings on physical examination (see Fig. 130-1).

Treatment. The management of acquired transient neutropenia associated with malignancies, myelosuppressive chemotherapy, or immunosuppressive chemotherapy differs from that of congenital or chronic forms of neutropenia. In the former situation, infections sometimes are heralded only by fever, and sepsis is a major cause of death. Early recognition and treatment of infections may be lifesaving (see Chapter 177).

Therapy of severe chronic neutropenia is dictated by the clinical manifestations. Patients with benign neutropenia and no evidence of repeated bacterial infections or chronic gingivitis require no specific therapy. Superficial infections in children with mild to moderate neutropenia may be treated with appropriate oral antibiotics. In patients who have life-threatening infections, however, broad-spectrum intravenous antibiotics should be started promptly.

Effective treatment of severe chronic neutropenia including severe congenital neutropenia, chronic symptomatic idiopathic neutropenia, and cyclic neutropenia is available. Subcutaneously administered rhG-CSF at doses ranging from 3.4 to 11.50 µg/kg/day leads to dramatic increases in neutrophil counts, resulting in marked attenuation of infection and inflammation. The long-term effects of rhG-CSF therapy are unknown but include a propensity for the development of moderate splenomegaly, thrombocytopenia, and, occasionally, vasculitis. Autoimmune neutropenia may be responsive to intermittent corticosteroids, especially if it is part of an underlying disease process such as systemic lupus erythematosus. rhG-CSF may also benefit patients who have immune or drug-induced neutropenias.

Those patients with severe congenital neutropenia or Shwachman-Diamond syndrome who develop myelodysplasia or acute myelogenous leukemia respond only to allogeneic stem cell transplantation. Chemotherapy is ineffective.

LYMPHOPENIA

Lymphocytes account for about 30% of the circulating WBCs in a newborn. The proportion of lymphocytes then increases rapidly within the 1st mo, reaching an average of 60% by 2 yr of age. The normal lymphocyte count in children <2 yr of age is 3,000–9,500/µL and in adults is 1,000–4,800/µL. At 6 yr of age, the lower limit of normal is 1,500/µL.

Almost 65% of blood T lymphocytes are CD4 (helper) T lymphocytes. Most patients with lymphocytopenia have a reduction in the absolute number of T lymphocytes, particularly in the number of CD4 T lymphocytes. The average number of CD4 T lymphocytes in adult blood is 1,100/µL (range, 300–1,300/µL), and the average number of CD8 (suppressor) T lymphocytes is 600/µL (range, 100–900/µL), with the normal CD4:CD8 ratio of 1.8–2.0.

Lymphocytopenia by itself usually causes no symptoms and is often detected in the evaluation of other illnesses, particularly recurrent viral, fungal, and parasitic infections. Lymphocyte subpopulations can be measured by multiparameter flow cytometry, which uses the pattern of antigen expression to classify and characterize these cells.

TABLE 130-6. Causes of Lymphocytopenia

ACQUIRED CAUSES
Infectious Diseases
AIDS
Viral hepatitis
Influenza
Tuberculosis
Typhoid fever
Sepsis
Iatrogenic
Immunosuppressive therapy
Corticosteroids
High-dose PUVA therapy
Cytotoxic chemotherapy
Radiation
Thoracic duct drainage
Systemic and Other Diseases
Systemic lupus erythematosus
Myasthenia gravis
Hodgkin disease
Protein-losing enteropathy
Renal failure
Sarcoidosis
Thermal injury
Aplastic anemia
Dietary Deficiency
Dietary deficiency associated with ethanol abuse
INHERITED CAUSES
Aplasia of lymphopoietic stem cells
Severe combined immunodeficiency associated with defect in IL-2 receptor γ-chain, deficiency of ADA or PNP, or unknown
Ataxia-telangiectasia
Wiskott-Aldrich syndrome
Immunodeficiency with thymoma
Cartilage-hair hypoplasia
Idiopathic CD4 T lymphocytopenia

ADA, adenosine deaminase; IL-2, interleukin 2; PNP, purine nucleoside phosphorylase; PUVA, psoralen and ultraviolet A irradiation.

From Boxer LA: Approach to the patient with leukopenia. In Humes HD (editor): *Kelley's Textbook of Internal Medicine*, 4th ed. Philadelphia, Lippincott Williams & Wilkins, 2000, p 1580.

INHERITED CAUSES OF LYMPHOCYTOPENIA. Inherited immunodeficiency disorders may have a quantitative or qualitative stem cell abnormality resulting in ineffective lymphocytopoiesis (Table 130-6). Other disorders such as Wiskott-Aldrich syndrome may have associated lymphocytopenia arising from accelerated destruction of T cells. A similar mechanism is present in patients with adenosine deaminase deficiency and purine nucleoside phosphorylase deficiency.

ACQUIRED LYMPHOCYTOPENIA. Acquired lymphocytopenia is the result of depletion of blood lymphocytes that is not secondary to inherited diseases. AIDS is the most common infectious disease associated with lymphocytopenia, which results from destruction of CD4 T cells infected with HIV-1 or HIV-2. Other viral and bacterial diseases may be associated with lymphocytopenia. In some instances of acute viremia with other viral infections, lymphocytes may undergo accelerated destruction from intracellular viral replication, become trapped in the spleen or nodes, or migrate to the respiratory tract.

Iatrogenic lymphocytopenia is usually caused by cytotoxic chemotherapy, radiation therapy, and long-term administration of antilymphocyte globulin. Long-term treatment of psoriasis with psoralen and ultraviolet irradiation may destroy T lymphocytes. Corticosteroids can cause lymphopenia through increased cell destruction. Systemic autoimmune diseases such as systemic lupus erythematosus are associated with lymphocytopenia. Other conditions such as protein-losing enteropathy and aberrant or surgical drainage of the thoracic duct are associated with lymphocyte depletion, leading to lymphocytopenia.

Boxer L, Dale DC: Neutropenia: Causes and consequences. *Semin Hematol* 2002;39:75–81.

Cham B, Bonilla MA, Winkelstein J: Neutropenia associated with primary immunodeficiency syndromes. *Semin Hematol* 2002;39:107–112.

Dale DC, Bolyard AA, Aprikyan A: Cyclic neutropenia. *Semin Hematol* 2002;39:89–94.

James RM, Kinsey SE: The investigation management of chronic neutropenia in children. *Arch Dis Child* 2006;91:852–858.

Kannourakis G: Glycogen storage disease. *Semin Hematol* 2002;39:103–106.

Klein C, Grudzien M, Appaswamy G, et al: HAX1 deficiency causes autosomal recessive severe congenital neutropenia (Kostmann disease). *Nat Genet* 2007;39:86–92.

Smith OP: Shwachman-Diamond syndrome. *Semin Hematol* 2002;39:95–102.

Zeidler C, Welte K: Kostmann syndrome and severe congenital neutropenia. *Semin Hematol* 2002;39:82–88.

Chapter 131 ■ Leukocytosis

Laurence A. Boxer

Leukocytosis is an elevation in the total leukocyte, or white blood cell (WBC), count that is two standard deviations above the mean count for a particular age (see Chapter 716). The various causes of leukocytosis are categorized by the class of WBCs that is elevated and whether the leukocytosis is acute, chronic, or lifelong.

A WBC count exceeding 50,000/µL is termed a **leukemoid reaction** because of the similarity to features of leukemia. Leukemoid reactions are usually neutrophilic and are most frequently associated with septicemia and severe bacterial infections including shigellosis, salmonellosis, and meningococcemia. Infection in children with leukocyte adhesion deficiency results in WBC counts approaching or exceeding 100,000/µL.

A significant proportion of >5% of immature to mature neutrophil cells is termed a **shift-to-the-left** and indicates rapid release of cells from the bone marrow. This may result in increased circulating band forms, which usually constitute 1–5% of circulating neutrophilic cells, or metamyelocytes and myelocytes, which are not usually found in the peripheral circulation. Higher degrees of shift to the left with more immature neutrophil precursors are indicative of serious bacterial infections but may also be encountered with trauma, burns, surgery, and acute hemolysis or hemorrhage.

NEUTROPHILIA. Neutrophilia is an increase in the total number of blood neutrophils, which for older children and adults is >8,000/µL. During the 1st day of life, the upper limit of the normal neutrophil count ranges from 7,000 to 12,000/µL. In the 1st mo of life, the neutrophil count ranges from 1,800 to 5,400/µL and, by 1 yr of age, the range is 1,500–8,500/µL.

An increase in circulating neutrophils is a result of a disturbance of the normal equilibrium involving bone marrow neutrophil production, movement out of the marrow compartments into the circulation, and neutrophil destruction. Neutrophilia may arise either alone or in combination with enhanced mobilization into the **circulating pool** from either the bone marrow storage compartment or the peripheral blood **marginating pool,** by impaired neutrophil egress into tissues, or after expansion of the circulating neutrophil pool secondary to increased progenitor cell proliferation and terminal differentiation through the myeloid series. Myelocytes are not released to the blood except under extreme circumstances.

To evaluate the patient with leukocytosis, it is critical to determine which class of white blood cells is elevated, and also the duration and extent of the leukocytosis. Each blood count should be evaluated with regard to the absolute number of cells/µL and the age of the patient.

Acute Acquired Neutrophilia. Neutrophilia is usually an acquired disorder and is a common finding with inflammation, infection, injury, and stress. Acute or chronic bacterial infections, trauma, and surgery are among the most common causes encountered in clinical practice. Neutrophilia is often associated with sickle cell disease, some chronic hemolytic anemias, heatstroke, burns, and diabetic ketoacidosis. Drugs commonly associated with neutrophilia include epinephrine, corticosteroids, and recombinant growth factors such as recombinant human granulocyte colony–stimulating factor (rhG-CSF) and recombinant human granulocyte-macrophage colony–stimulating factor (rhGM-CSF). Epinephrine causes release into the circulation of a sequestered pool of neutrophils that normally marginate along the vascular endothelium. Corticosteroids accelerate the release of neutrophils and bands from a large storage pool within the bone marrow and impair the migration of neutrophils from the circulation into tissues. Acute neutrophilia in response to inflammation and infections occurs because of release of neutrophils from the marrow storage pool. The post-mitotic marrow neutrophil pools are approximately 10 times the sizes of the blood neutrophil pool, and about half of these cells are bands and segmented neutrophils. In neutrophil production disorders, such as those associated with malignancies and cancer chemotherapy, the size of this pool may be reduced and the capacity to develop neutrophilia remains impaired. Exposure of blood to foreign substances such as hemodialysis membrane activates the complement system and causes transient neutropenia followed by neutrophilia because of release of bone marrow neutrophils. The colony-stimulating factors G-CSF and GM-CSF cause acute and chronic neutrophilia by mobilizing cells from the marrow reserves and by stimulating neutrophil production.

Chronic Acquired Neutrophilia. Chronic neutrophilia is usually associated with continued stimulation of neutrophil production resulting from persistent inflammatory reactions or chronic infections such as tuberculosis, vasculitis, postsplenectomy states, Hodgkin disease, chronic myelogenous leukemia, chronic blood loss, and prolonged administration of corticosteroids. Chronic neutrophilia can arise after expansion of cell production secondary to stimulation of cell divisions within the mitotic precursor pool, which consists of promyelocytes and myelocytes (Fig. 131-1). Subsequently, the size of the post-mitotic pool increases. These changes lead to an increase in the marrow reserve pool, which can be readily mobilized for release of neutrophils into the circulation. The neutrophil production rate can increase greatly in response to exogenously administered hemopoietic growth factors such as rhG-CSF, with a maximum response taking at least 1 wk to develop.

Lifelong Neutrophilia. Congenital asplenia is associated with lifelong neutrophilia. Uncommon genetic disorders that present with neutrophilia include leukocyte adhesion deficiency, familial myeloproliferative disease, Down syndrome, and Rac-2 mutation (see Chapter 129). In an autosomal dominant form of hereditary neutrophilia, patients maintain an absolute neutrophil count between 1,400 and 150,000/µL, which is associated with hepatosplenomegaly, an increased alkaline phosphatase level, and Gaucher-type histiocytes in the bone marrow.

Evaluation of persistent neutrophilia requires a careful history, physical examination, and laboratory studies to search for infectious, inflammatory, and neoplastic conditions. The leukocyte alkaline phosphatase cytochemical stain of circulating neutrophils is useful to differentiate chronic myelogenous leukemia, in which the level is uniformly near zero, from reactive or secondary neutrophilia, in which normal to elevated levels are found.

MONOCYTOSIS. The average absolute blood monocyte count varies with age, which must be considered in the assessment of monocytosis. Given the role of monocytes in antigen presentation and cytokine secretion and as effectors of ingestion of invading organisms, it is not surprising that many clinical disorders give rise to monocytosis (Table 131-1). Most commonly, mono-

TABLE 131-1. Causes of Monocytosis

INFECTIONS
Bacterial infections
Tuberculosis
Brucellosis
Typhoid fever
Syphilis
Infective endocarditis
Nonbacterial infections
Fungal infections
Rocky Mountain spotted fever
Typhus
Kalz-azar
Malaria
HEMATOLOGIC DISORDERS
Postsplenectomy states
Congenital and acquired neutropenias
Hemolytic anemias
MALIGNANT DISORDERS
Preleukemia
Acute myelogenous leukemia
Chronic myelogenous leukemia
Juvenile chronic myelocytic leukemia
Hodgkin disease
Non-Hodgkin lymphomas
COLLAGEN VASCULAR DISEASES
Systemic lupus erythematosus
Rheumatoid arthritis
Polyarteritis nodosa
GASTROINTESTINAL DISORDERS
Ulcerative colitis
Granulomatous colitis
Cirrhosis
MISCELLANEOUS
Recovery from marrow suppression induced by chemotherapy
Drug reactions
Sarcoidosis

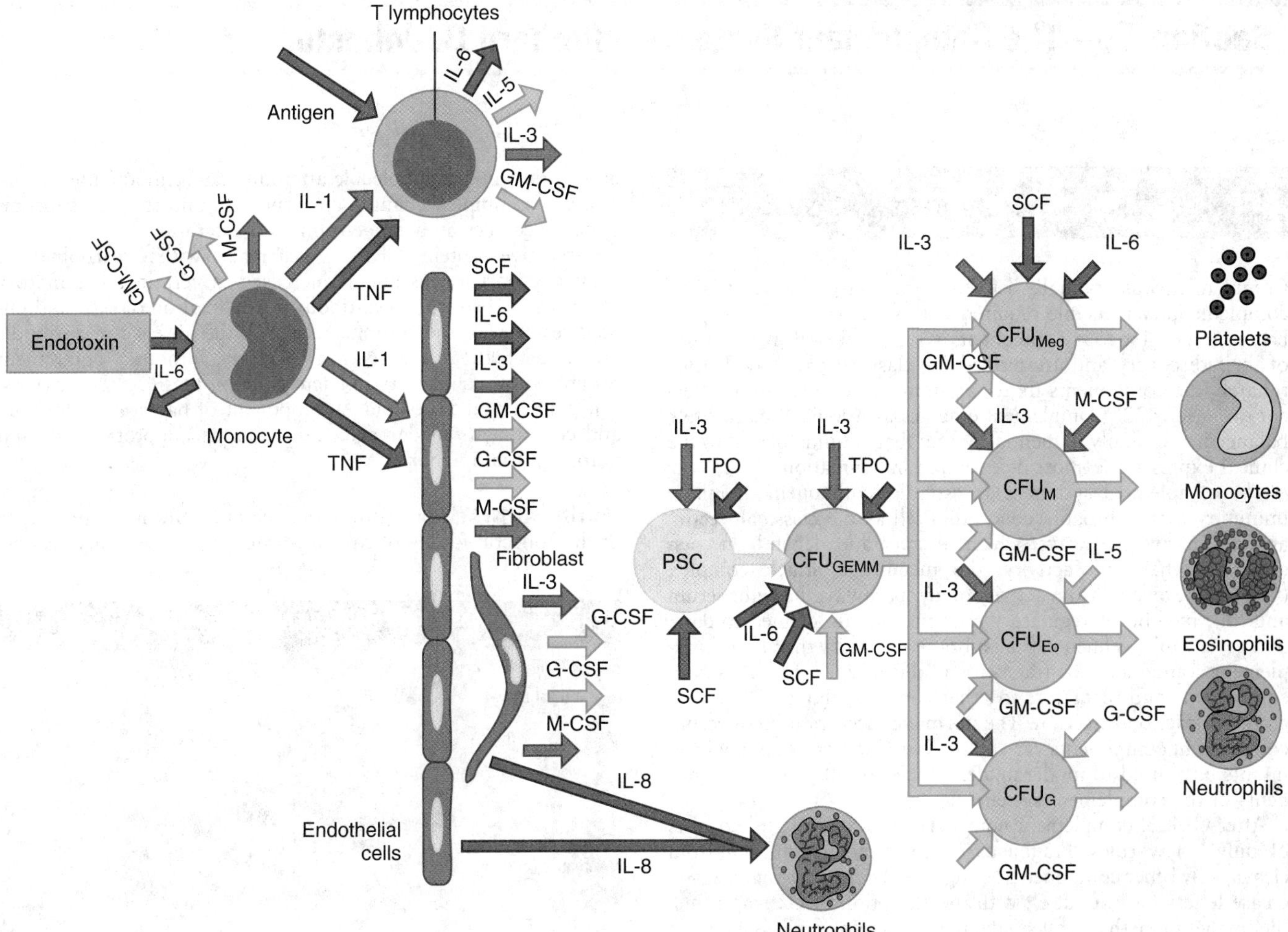

Figure 131-1. Cytokine control of the phagocyte production and activation by release of endotoxin during infection. Both endothelial cells and fibroblasts release substantial quantities of both granulocyte-macrophage colony–stimulating factor (GM-CSF) and granulocyte colony–stimulating factor (G-CSF) in response to tumor necrosis factor (TNF) and interleukin 1 (IL-1). Both TNF and IL-1 are released from endotoxin-activated monocytes and antigen-activated T lymphocytes. Stem cell factor (SCF), interleukin 3 (IL-3), GM-CSF, and interleukin 6 (IL-6) each influence the growth and differentiation of multilineage progenitor cells known as colony forming units (CFU)—granulocytes, eosinophils, monocytes, megakaryocytes (CFU$_{GEMM}$)—to the committed colony forming unit macrophage (CFU$_{M}$), CFU eosinophil (CFU$_{G}$), or CFU granulocyte (CFU$_{G}$). Platelet production can also be augmented by expansion of CFU megakaryocyte (CFU$_{meg}$). Factors that serve as growth and differentiation factors for a specific lineage also act as activation factors for the terminally differentiated forms of the same lineage. Macrophage colony–stimulating factor (M-CSF) enhances antibody-mediated cytotoxicity and phagocyte functions of monocytes. G-CSF promotes neutrophil bactericidal capacity, and interleukin 5 (IL-5) activates eosinophil function. Within hours of an infection, cytokine primed neutrophils move to the invasion site from the circulation under the influence of interleukin 8 (IL-8), which is released from endothelial cells and fibroblasts.

cytosis occurs in patients recovering from myelosuppressive chemotherapy and is a harbinger of the return of the neutrophil count to normal. Monocytosis is often a sign of an acute bacterial, viral, protozoal, or rickettsial infection, and also occurs in some forms of chronic neutropenia and postsplenectomy states. Chronic inflammatory conditions can stimulate sustained monocytosis, including preleukemia, chronic myelogenous leukemia, lymphomas, and occasionally Hodgkin disease.

LYMPHOCYTOSIS. The most common cause of lymphocytosis is an acute viral illness. Lymphocytosis is a normal response to most viral infections because the majority of circulating lymphocytes are T cells. In infectious mononucleosis, the B cells are infected with the Epstein-Barr virus and the T cells react to the viral antigens present in the B cells, resulting in **atypical lymphocytes** with the typical large, vacuolated morphology. Other viral infections classically associated with lymphocytosis are cytomegalovirus and viral hepatitis. Chronic bacterial infections such as tuberculosis and brucellosis may lead to a sustained lymphocytosis. Pertussis is accompanied by lymphocytosis in ≈ 25% of infants infected before 6 mo of age. Thyrotoxicosis and Addison disease are endocrine disorders associated with lymphocytosis. Persistent or profound lymphocytosis suggests acute lymphocytic leukemia.

BASOPHILIA. Basophilia occurs when the basophil count exceeds 100–120 cells/μL. Basophilia is a nonspecific sign of a wide variety of disorders and is usually of limited diagnostic importance. Basophilia is most often present in hypersensitivity reactions.

Boxer LA: Leukocytosis. In Sills RH (editor): *Practical Algorithms in Pediatric Hematology and Oncology.* New York, Karger, 2003, pp 38–39.

Section 4 — The Complement System — Richard B. Johnston, Jr.

Chapter 132 ■ The Complement System

Complement was originally defined as the nonspecific, heat-labile complementary principle required with specific antibody to lyse bacteria. The 1st four components were numbered in the order of their discovery and are termed the classical pathway. Unfortunately the components fix to the immune complex in a different order, C1423. Complement emerges as a logical, exquisitely balanced, and highly influential system that is fundamental to the clinical expression of host defense and inflammation.

The complement system is an essential component of innate immunity that is broadly conceptualized as the **classical, lectin,** and **alternative pathways,** which interact and depend on each other for their full activity; the **membrane attack complex** (C5b6789), formed from activity of any pathway; the eight serum and four membrane regulatory proteins that are defined to date; and seven fully defined cell membrane **receptors** that bind complement components or fragments (Table 132-1). The 27 serum components and regulators together compose about 15% of the globulin fraction of serum. The normal concentrations of serum complement components vary by age (see Chapter 716); newborn infants have mild to moderate deficiencies of all plasma components of the complement system.

After C1423, complement nomenclature is logical and consists of only a few rules. Fragments of components resulting from cleavage by other components acting as enzymes are assigned lowercase letters (a, b, c, d, e); with the exception of C2 fragments, the smaller piece that is released into surrounding fluids is assigned the lowercase letter *a,* and the major part of the molecule, bound to other components or to some part of the immune complex, is assigned letter *b*—for example, C3a and C3b. Components of the alternative pathway, B and D, have been assigned uppercase letters, as have the control proteins I and H, which downregulate both pathways. C3, and especially its major fragment C3b, is a component of both the classical and alternative pathways.

Complement is a system of interacting proteins. The biologic functions of the system depend on the interactions of individual components, which occur in sequential, cascade fashion. Activation of each component, except the 1st, depends on activation of the prior component or components in the sequence. Interaction occurs along three pathways (Fig. 132-1): the **classical pathway,** in the order antigen–antibody–C142356789; **the lectin** (carbohydrate-binding) pathway, in the order microbial carbohydrate–lectin (mannan-binding lectin [MBL] or L- or H-ficolin)/MBL-associated proteases–C42356789; and the **alternative pathway,** in the order activator–C3bBD–C356789. Antibody accelerates the rate of activation of the alternative pathway, but activation can occur on appropriate surfaces in the absence of antibody. The classical and the alternative pathways interact with each other through the ability of both to activate C3.

Activation of the early-acting components of complement (C1423) results in the generation of a series of active enzymes, C1, C42, and C423, on the surface of the immune complex or underlying cell. These enzymes cleave and activate the next component in the sequence. In contrast, the interaction among C5b, C6, C7, C8, and C9 is nonenzymatic and depends on changes in molecular configuration.

CLASSICAL PATHWAY. The classical pathway sequence begins with fixation of C1, by way of C1q, to the Fc, non–antigen-binding part of the antibody molecule after antigen-antibody interaction. The C1 tricomplex changes configuration and the C1s subcomponent becomes an active enzyme, C1 esterase.

C-reactive protein (CRP), which reacts with C carbohydrate from microorganisms and is increased in certain inflammatory states, can substitute for antibody in the fixation of C1q and initiate reaction of the entire sequence in the absence of antibody. Other agents that can activate C1 directly, without a requirement for antibody, include certain bacteria, *Mycoplasma,* RNA viruses, uric acid crystals, the lipid A component of bacterial endotoxin, and components of damaged cells such as apoptotic blebs and mitochondrial membranes.

LECTIN PATHWAY. Mannan-binding lectin (MBL) is the prototype of the collectin family of carbohydrate-binding proteins (lectins)

TABLE 132-1. Constituents of the Complement System

SERUM COMPONENTS
Classical pathway
C1q
C1r
C1s
C4
C2
C3
Alternative Pathway
Factor B
Factor D
Lectin Pathway
Mannose-binding lectin (MBL), L- and H-ficolin
MBL-associated proteases 1, 2, 3
Membrane Attack Complex
C5
C6
C7
C8
C9
Control Protein, Enhancing
Properdin
Control Proteins, Downregulating
C1 inhibitor (C1 INH)
C4-binding protein (C4-bp)
Factor H
Factor I
S protein (vitronectin)
Clusterin
Anaphylatoxin inactivator
Membrane Regulatory Proteins
CR1
Membrane cofactor protein (MCP; CD46)
Decay-accelerating factor (DAF)
CD59 (membrane inhibitor of reactive lysis; protectin)
MEMBRANE RECEPTORS
CR1
CR2 (CD21)
CR3 (CD11b/CD18)
CR4 (CD11c/CD18)
C3a receptor
C5a receptor
C1q receptor

Other downregulating serum factors and membrane receptors have been described but have not been fully defined.
CR, complement receptor.

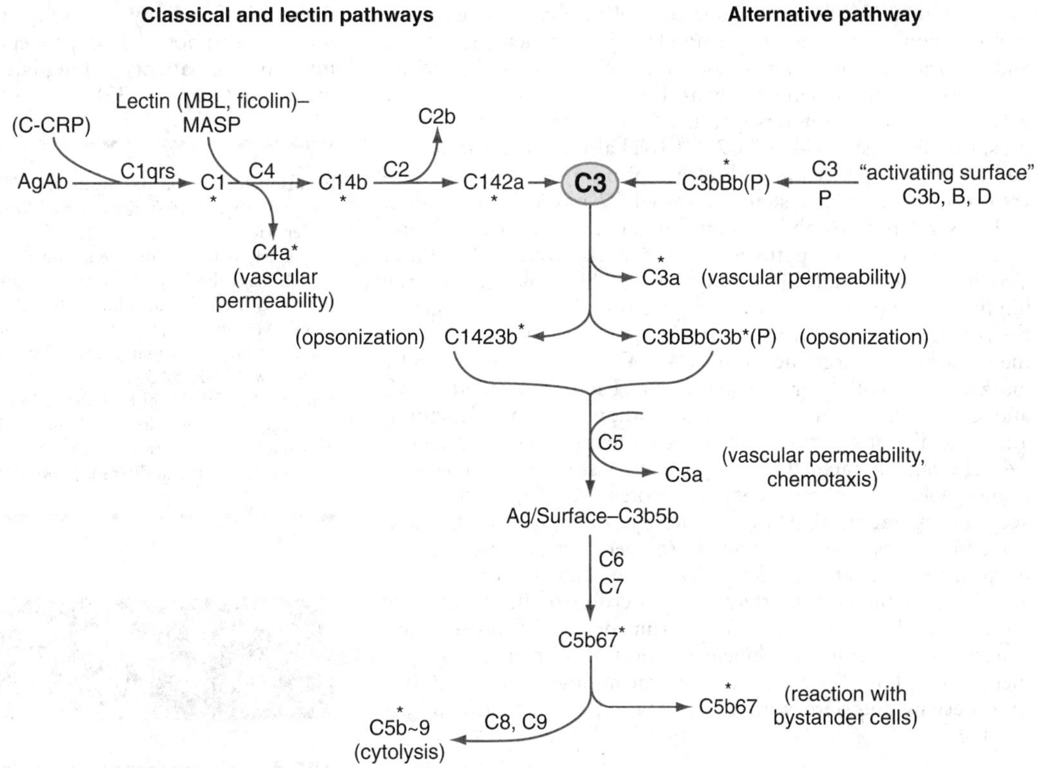

Classical and lectin pathways

Alternative pathway

(C-CRP)
Lectin (MBL, ficolin)–MASP
AgAb → C1qrs → C1* → C4 → C14b* → C2 → C142a* → C3 ← C3bBb(P)* ← C3, P ← "activating surface" C3b, B, D
C2b
C4a* (vascular permeability)
C3a* (vascular permeability)
(opsonization) C1423b* ← → C3bBbC3b*(P) (opsonization)
C5 → C5a (vascular permeability, chemotaxis)
Ag/Surface–C3b5b
C6, C7
C5b67*
→ C5b67* (reaction with bystander cells)
C8, C9 → C5b~9* (cytolysis)

Figure 132-1. Sequence of activation of the components of the classical and lectin (MBL) pathways of complement and interaction with the alternative pathway. Activation of C3 is the functionally essential target. The multiple sites at which inhibitory regulator proteins (not shown) act are indicated by *asterisks,* emphasizing the delicate balance between action and control in this system that is essential for host defense yet capable of mediating profound damage to host tissues. Ab, antibody (IgG or IgM class only); Ag, antigen (bacterium, virus, tumor cell, or erythrocyte); B,D,P, factors B and D, I, and properdin; C-CRP, C carbohydrate–C-reactive protein; C4-bp, C4-binding protein; MASPs, MBL-associated serine proteases; MBL, mannose-binding lectin.

that are believed to play an important part in innate, nonspecific immunity; its structure is homologous to that of C1q. L- and H-ficolin are also in the family. These lectins, in association with MBL-associated serine proteases (MASPs), can bind to mannan, lipoteichoic acid, and other carbohydrates on bacterial and fungal surfaces and function like C1s to cleave C4 and C2 and activate the complement cascade. The peptide C4a has weak anaphylatoxin activity, and reacts with mast cells to release the chemical mediators of immediate hypersensitivity, including histamine. C3a and C5a, released later in the sequence, are potent anaphylatoxins, and C5a is also an important chemotactic factor. Fixation of C4b to the complex permits it to adhere to neutrophils, macrophages, B cells, dendritic cells, and erythrocytes.

Cleavage of C3 and generation of C3b is the next step in the sequence. The serum concentration of C3 is the highest of any component, and its activation is the most crucial step in terms of biologic activity. Cleavage of C3 can be achieved through the **C3 convertase** of the classical pathway, C142, or of the alternative pathway, C3bBb. Once fixed to the complex, C3b permits adherence of the antigen-antibody complex to cells with receptors for C3b (complement receptor 1 [CR1]), including B lymphocytes, erythrocytes, and phagocytic cells (neutrophils, monocytes, and macrophages), leading, in the last case, to phagocytosis. **Phagocytosis** of most microorganisms in vitro, especially by neutrophils, is inefficient without binding of C3 to the microorganism. The severe pyogenic infections that commonly occur in C3-deficient patients indicate that phagocytosis in vivo is also inefficient without C3. The biologic activity of C3b is controlled by cleavage by **factor I (C3b inactivator)** to iC3b, which promotes phagocytosis on binding to the **iC3b receptor (CR3)** on phagocytes. Further degradation of iC3b by factor I and proteases yields C3dg, then C3d; C3d binds to CR2 on B lymphocytes and thereby serves as a co-stimulator of antigen-induced B-cell activation.

ALTERNATIVE PATHWAY. The alternative pathway can be activated by C3b generated through classical pathway activity or proteases from neutrophils or the clotting system. It can also be activated by a form of C3 created by low-grade, spontaneous reaction of native C3 with a molecule of water, a "tickover" that occurs constantly in plasma. Once formed, C3b or the hydrolyzed C3 can bind to any nearby cell or to factor B. Factor B attached to C3b in the plasma or on a surface can be cleaved to Bb by D, which exists as an active proteolytic enzyme. The complex C3bBb becomes an efficient C3 convertase, which generates more C3b through an amplification loop. P can bind to C3bBb, increasing stability of the enzyme and protecting it from inactivation by factors I and H, which modulate the loop and the pathway.

Certain "activating surfaces" promote alternative pathway activation if C3b is fixed to them—for example, bacterial teichoic acid or endotoxin—by protecting the C3bBb enzyme complex from the control otherwise exercised by factors I and H. Rabbit red blood cell membrane is such a surface, which serves as the basis for an assay of serum alternative pathway activity. Endotoxin may alter normally "nonactivating" cell surfaces in vivo so that C3bBb is relatively protected from inactivation, which may partially explain the activation of complement in patients with gram-negative bacteremia. Sialic acid on the surface of microorganisms or cells prevents formation of an effective alternative pathway C3 convertase by promoting activity of factors I and H. Nevertheless, significant activation of C3 can occur through the alternative pathway, and the resultant biologic activities are qualitatively the same as those achieved through activation by C142 (see Fig. 132-1).

MEMBRANE ATTACK COMPLEX. The sequence leading to cytolysis begins with the attachment of C5b to the C5-activating enzyme from the classical pathway, C4b2a3b, or from the alternative pathway, C3bBb3b. C6 is bound to C5b without being cleaved, stabilizing the activated C5b fragment. The C5b6 complex then dissociates from C423 and reacts with C7. C5b67 complexes must attach promptly to the membrane of the parent or a bystander cell or they lose their activity. Next, C8 binds, and the C5b678 complex then promotes the addition of multiple C9 molecules. The C9 polymer of at least 3–6 molecules forms a transmembrane channel, and lysis ensues.

CONTROL MECHANISMS. Without control mechanisms acting at multiple points, there would be no effective complement system, and unbridled consumption of components would generate severe, potentially lethal damage to the host. At the 1st step, C1 inhibitor (C1 INH) inhibits C1r and C1s enzymatic activity and, thus, the cleavage of C4 and C2. C1 INH also regulates the lectin and alternative pathways and release of bradykinin during activation of the contact system. Activated C2 has a short half-life, and this relative instability limits the effective life of C42 and C423. The alternative pathway enzyme that activates C3, C3bBb, also has a short half-life, though it can be prolonged by the binding of **properdin** (P) to the enzyme complex. Serum contains the protein "anaphylatoxin inactivator," an enzyme that cleaves the N-terminus arginine from C4a, C3a, and C5a, thereby markedly reducing their biologic activity. Factor I inactivates C4b and C3b; factor H accelerates inactivation of C3b by factor I, and an analogous factor, C4-binding protein (C4-bp), accelerates C4b cleavage by factor I. Three protein constituents of cell membranes, CR1, membrane cofactor protein (CD46), and decay-accelerating factor (DAF), promote the disruption of C3 and C5 convertases assembled on those membranes. Another cell membrane–associated protein, CD59, can bind C8 or both C8 and C9 and thereby interfere with insertion of the membrane attack complex (C5b6789). The serum proteins S protein and clusterin can inhibit attachment of the C5b67 complex to cell membranes, bind C8 or C9 in a full membrane attack complex, or otherwise interfere with the formation or insertion of this complex.

PARTICIPATION IN HOST DEFENSE. Neutralization of virus by antibody can be enhanced with C1 and C4 and further enhanced by the additional fixation of C3b through the classical or alternative pathway. Complement may, therefore, be particularly important in the early phases of a viral infection when antibody is limited. Antibody and the full complement sequence can also eliminate infectivity of at least some viruses by the production of typical complement "holes," as seen by electron microscopy. Fixation of C1q can opsonize (promote phagocytosis) through binding to the C1q receptor.

C4a, C3a, and C5a can bind to mast cells and thereby trigger release of histamine and other mediators, leading to vasodilatation and the swelling and redness of inflammation. C5a can induce monocytes to release the cytokines tumor necrosis factor and interleukin 1, which amplify the inflammatory response. C5a is a major chemotactic factor for neutrophils, monocytes, and eosinophils, which can efficiently phagocytize microorganisms opsonized with C3b or cleaved C3b (iC3b). Further inactivation of cell-bound C3b by cleavage to C3d removes its opsonizing activity, but it can still bind to B cells. Fixation of C3b to a target cell can enhance its lysis by NK cells or macrophages.

Insoluble immune complexes can be solubilized if they bind C3b, apparently because C3b disrupts the orderly antigen-antibody lattice. Binding C3b to a complex also allows it to adhere to C3 receptors (CR1) on red blood cells, which then transport the complexes to hepatic and splenic macrophages for removal. This phenomenon may at least partially explain the immune complex disease found in patients who lack C1, C4, C2, or C3.

The complement system serves to link the innate and adaptive immune systems. C4b or C3b coupled to immune complexes promotes their binding to antigen-presenting macrophages, dendritic cells, and B cells. Coupling of antigen to C3d allows binding to CR2 on B cells, which reduces the amount of antigen needed to trigger an antibody response by a factor of up to 10,000.

Neutralization of endotoxin in vitro and protection from its lethal effects in experimental animals require later-acting components of complement, at least through C6. Finally, activation of the entire complement sequence can result in lysis of virus-infected cells, tumor cells, and most types of microorganisms. Bactericidal activity of complement has not appeared to be important to host defense, except for the occurrence of *Neisseria* infections in patients lacking later-acting components of complement (see Chapter 133).

Atkinson JP: Complement system. In Harris ED Jr, Budd RC, Firestein GS, et al (editors): *Kelley's Textbook of Rheumatology,* 7th ed. Philadelphia, Elsevier Saunders, 2005, pp 342–355.

Berger M, Frank MM: The serum complement system. In Stiehm ER, Ochs HD, Winkelstein JA (editors): *Immunologic Disorders in Infants and Children,* 5th ed. Philadelphia, WB Saunders, 2005, pp 157–187.

Davis AE, Shenghe C, Liu D: The biological role of the C1 inhibitor in regulation of vascular permeability and modulation of inflammation. *Adv Immunol* 2004;82:331–359.

Gadjeva M, Takahashi K, Thiel S: Mannan-binding lectin—a soluble pattern recognition molecule. *Mol Immunol* 2004; 41:113–121.

Thurman JM, Holers VM: The central role of the alternative complement pathway in human disease. *J Immunol* 2006;176:1305–1310.

Chapter 133 ■ Disorders of the Complement System

133.1 • Evaluation of the Complement System

Testing for **total hemolytic complement activity** (**CH_{50}**) effectively screens for most of the diseases of the complement system. A normal result in this assay depends on the ability of all 11 components of the classical pathway and membrane attack complex to interact and lyse antibody-coated sheep erythrocytes. The dilution of serum that lyses 50% of the cells determines the end-point. In **congenital deficiencies** of C1 through C8, the CH_{50} value is 0 or close to 0; in C9 deficiency, the value is approximately half-normal. Values in the acquired deficiencies vary with the type and severity of the underlying disorder. This assay does not detect deficiency of mannose-binding lectin (MBL), factors D or B of the alternative pathway, or properdin. Deficiency of factors I or H permits consumption of C3, with partial reduction in the CH_{50} value. When clotted blood or serum sits for longer than about an hour or warms, CH_{50} activity begins to decline, which leads to values that are falsely low but not zero.

In **hereditary angioedema,** depression of C4 and C2 during an attack significantly reduces the CH_{50}. Serum concentrations of C4 and C3, and indeed all of the components, can be quantitated using specific antibody. In hereditary angioedema, C4 is characteristically low and C3 normal. Concentrations of C1 inhibitor can be determined with antibody, but a normal result can be anticipated in about 15% of cases. Because C1 acts as an esterase, the specific diagnosis can be established by showing increased capacity of patients' sera to hydrolyze synthetic esters.

A decrease in serum concentration of both C4 and C3 suggests activation of the **classical pathway** by immune complexes. Decreased C3 and normal C4 levels suggest activation of the **alternative pathway.** This difference is particularly useful in distinguishing nephritis secondary to complex deposition from that due to NeF (nephritic factor). In the latter condition and in deficiency of factor I or H, factor B is consumed and C3 serum concentration is low. Alternative pathway activity can be measured with a relatively simple and reproducible hemolytic assay that depends on the capacity of rabbit erythrocytes to serve as both an activating (permissive) surface and a target of alternative pathway activity. This assay detects deficiency of properdin, factor D, and factor B.

A defect of complement function should be considered in any patient with recurrent angioedema, autoimmune disease, chronic nephritis, or partial lipodystrophy, or with recurrent pyogenic infections, disseminated meningococcal or gonococcal infections, or a second episode of bacteremia at any age.

133.2 • Genetic Deficiencies of Complement Components

Congenital deficiencies of all 11 components of the classical-membrane attack pathway and of factor D of the alternative pathway have been described (Table 133-1). All of the components of the classical and alternative pathways except properdin are inherited as autosomal recessive traits of the autosomal co-dominant variety. Each parent transmits a gene that codes for synthesis of half the serum level of the component. Deficiency results from inheritance of one null gene from each parent; the hemizygous parents typically have CH_{50} levels that are low normal. Properdin deficiency is transmitted as an X-linked trait.

Most patients with primary **C1q deficiency** have systemic lupus erythematosus (SLE), an SLE-like syndrome without typical SLE serology, a chronic rash that has shown an underlying vasculitis on biopsy, or membranoproliferative glomerulonephritis (MPGN). Some C1q-deficient children have serious infections, including septicemia and meningitis.

C1rs deficiency occurs as a complete defect of C1r in association with variable deficiency of C1s, presumably due to the close linkage of the genes for these proteins on chromosome 12. Similar to individuals with C1q deficiency, patients with C1r/C1s, **C4, C2,** or **C3 deficiency** have a high incidence of autoimmune syndromes (see Table 133-1), especially SLE or an SLE-like syndrome in which antinuclear antibody level is not elevated.

C4 is encoded by two genes, termed C4A and C4B. **C4 deficiency** represents absence of both gene products. Complete deficiency of only C4A, present in about 1% of the population, also predisposes to SLE, though C4 levels are only partially reduced. Patients with only C4B deficiency may be predisposed to infection. A few patients with **C5, C6, C7,** or **C8 deficiency** have SLE, but recurrent meningococcal infections are much more likely to be the major problem.

The reason for the concurrence of deficiencies of components of complement and these autoimmune diseases is not entirely clear, but deposition of C3 on autoimmune complexes facilitates their removal from the circulation through binding to complement receptor 1 (CR1) on erythrocytes and transport to the spleen and liver. The early components expedite the clearance of necrotic and apoptotic cells, which are sources of autoantigens. Inefficiency of either or both of these processes might explain the particular predisposition to autoimmune disease in individuals with a defect in complement, especially C1, C4, C2, or C3.

Patients with **C2 deficiency** often have repeated life-threatening septicemic illnesses, most commonly due to pneumococci. Most have not had problems with increased susceptibility to infection, presumably because of the protective function of the alternative pathway. The genes for C2, factor B, and C4 are situated close to each other on chromosome 6, and a partial depression of factor B levels can occur in conjunction with C2 deficiency. Persons with a deficiency of both proteins may be at particular risk.

Because C3 can be activated by C142 or by the alternative pathway, a defect in the function of either pathway can be compensated for, at least to some extent. Without C3, however, the chemotactic fragment from C5 (C5a) is not generated, and opsonization of bacteria is inefficient. Some organisms must be well opsonized in order to be cleared, and genetic **C3 deficiency**

TABLE 133-1. Genetic Deficiencies of Plasma Complement Components and Associated Clinical Findings

	INFECTION*			AUTOIMMUNE DISEASE*		
DEFICIENT COMPONENT	Very Common	Common	Occasional	Very Common	Common	Occasional
CLASSICAL PATHWAY						
C1q			Pneumococcal B/M, other pyogenic	SLE	GN	DV/DLE
C1rs		Other pyogenic	Pneumococcal B/M, DGI	SLE		GN
C4		Other pyogenic		SLE	GN, other AD	
C2		Other pyogenic, pneumococcal B/M, meningococcal M			SLE, GN, DV/DLE, other AD	
C3	Other pyogenic	Pneumococcal B/M, meningococcal M			GN, DV/DLE	SLE, other AD
C5	Meningococcal M	DGI	Other pyogenic			SLE, GN
C6	Meningococcal M	DGI	Other pyogenic			SLE, GN, other AD
C7	Meningococcal M		DGI, other pyogenic		SLE, other AD	
C8	Meningococcal M	DGI	Other pyogenic			SLE, GN
C9		Meningococcal M				
LECTIN PATHWAY						
MBL			Other pyogenic, fungal, HIV			SLE
MASP-2			Pneumococcal pneumonia			SLE
ALTERNATIVE PATHWAY						
Factor D	DGI, meningococcal M, other pyogenic					
CONTROL PROTEINS						
C1 INH	Hereditary angioedema[†]					SLE
Factor I	Other pyogenic, meningococcal M	Pneumococcal B/M				
Factor H		Meningococcal B/M	Other pyogenic		GN, HUS	SLE
Properdin		Meningococcal M	Pneumococcal B/M, other pyogenic		DV/DLE	
C4-binding protein						Other AD

*A finding was reported as "very common" if it occurred in 50% or more of reported cases, "common" if reported in about 5–50% of cases, and "occasional" if present in one or two cases or <5% of the more frequent deficiencies.

[†]Hereditary angioedema is a specific entity not typically associated with infection or autoimmunity.

B/M, Bacteremia or meningitis; DGI, disseminated gonococcal infection; DV/DLE, dermal vasculitis or typical discoid lupus erythematosus; GN, glomerulonephritis in various forms, often membranoproliferative; HIV, human immunodeficiency virus; HUS, hemolytic-uremic syndrome; M, meningitis; MASP, MBL-associated serine protease; MBL, mannose-binding lectin; other AD, autoimmune disease (almost all possible diagnoses have been reported); other pyogenic, serious deep or systemic infection due to, or typically caused by, a pyogenic bacterium (abscess, osteomyelitis, pneumonia, bacteremia other than pneumococcal, meningitis other than meningococcal or pneumococcal, cellulitis, myopericarditis, and peritonitis); SLE, typical systemic lupus erythematosus or an SLE-like syndrome without characteristic serologic findings.

Data from Figueroa JE, Densen P: Infectious diseases associated with complement deficiencies. *Clin Microbiol Rev* 1991;4:359–395; Ross SC, Densen P: Complement deficiency states and infection: Epidemiology, pathogenesis and consequences of neisserial and other infections in an immune deficiency. *Medicine* 1984;63:243–273; and other case reports and series.

has been associated with recurrent, severe pyogenic infections due to pneumococci and meningococci.

More than half of the individuals reported to have congenital **C5, C6, C7, or C8 deficiency** have had meningococcal meningitis or extragenital gonococcal infection. Patients with **C9 deficiency** retain about one-third normal CH_{50} titers; some of these patients have also had *Neisseria* disease. In studies of patients ≥10 yr of age with systemic meningococcal disease, 3–15% have had a genetic deficiency of C5, C6, C7, C8, C9, or properdin. Among patients with infections caused by the uncommon *N. meningitidis* serogroups (X, Y, Z, W135, 29E, or nongroupable; not A, B, or C), 33–45% have an underlying complement deficiency. It is not clear why patients with a deficiency of one of the late-acting components suffer a particular predisposition to *Neisseria* infections. It may be that serum bacteriolysis is uniquely important in defense against this organism. Some persons with such a deficiency have no significant illness.

A few individuals have been identified with **deficiency of factor D** of the alternative pathway, all with recurrent infections, which are often caused by *Neisseria*. Hemolytic complement activity and C3 levels in their serum were normal, but alternative pathway activity was markedly deficient or absent. Complete factor B deficiency has not been described.

MBL is a component of the innate immune system. Mutations in the structural gene encoding MBL or polymorphisms in the promoter region of the gene result in pronounced interindividual variation in the level of circulating MBL. More than 90% of MBL-deficient individuals do not express a predisposition to infections. **MBL deficiency** signifies a very low level of MBL with predisposition to recurrent respiratory infections in infants, and serious pyogenic and fungal infections if there is another underlying defect of host defense. MBL-associated serine protease 2 **(MASP-2) deficiency** has been associated with SLE-like symptoms and recurrent pneumococcal pneumonia.

133.3 • Deficiencies of Plasma, Membrane, or Serosal Complement Control Proteins

Congenital deficiencies of five plasma complement control proteins have been described (see Table 133-1). **Factor I deficiency** was reported originally as a deficiency of C3, resulting from hypercatabolism. The 1st patient described had suffered a series of severe pyogenic infections similar to those associated with agammaglobulinemia or congenital deficiency of C3. Further studies indicated that the primary deficiency was that of factor I, an essential regulator of both pathways. This deficiency permits prolonged existence of C3b in the C3 convertase of the alternative pathway, C3bBb, resulting in constant activation of the alternative pathway and cleavage of more C3 to C3b, in circular fashion. Intravenous infusion of plasma or purified factor I induced a prompt rise in serum C3 concentration in the patient and a return to normal of in vitro C3-dependent functions such as opsonization.

The effects of **factor H deficiency** are like those of factor I deficiency because factor H assists in dismantling the alternative pathway C3 convertase. Levels of C3, factor B, total hemolytic activity, and alternative pathway activity have been low or undetectable in all patients tested. Patients have sustained systemic infections due to pyogenic bacteria, particularly *N. meningitidis*. Almost half of the cases have glomerulonephritis, and hemoly-ticuremic syndrome has been relatively common. A common polymorphic variant is associated with age-related macular degeneration. The few patients thus far reported as having **C4-binding protein deficiency** have about 25% of the normal levels of the protein and no typical disease presentation, although one had angioedema and Behçet disease.

Persons with **properdin deficiency** have a striking predisposition to *N. meningitidis* meningitis. All reported patients have been male. The predisposition to infection in these patients demonstrates clearly the need for the alternative pathway in host defense against bacterial infection. Serum hemolytic complement activity is normal in these patients, and if the patient has specific antibacterial antibody, the need for the alternative pathway and properdin is greatly reduced. Several patients have dermal vasculitis or discoid lupus.

Hereditary angioedema occurs in persons unable to synthesize normal levels of C1 inhibitor (C1 INH). In 85% of affected families, the patient has markedly reduced concentrations of inhibitor, averaging 30% of normal; in the other 15%, normal or elevated concentrations of an immunologically cross-reacting but nonfunctional protein occur. Both forms of the disease are transmitted as autosomal dominant traits. C1 INH suppresses the complement proteases C1rs and MASP-1/2, and the activated proteases of the contact and fibrinolysis systems. In doing so, C1 INH, is consumed as a "suicide inhibitor." Thus, in the absence of full C1 INH function, activation of any of these proteases tips the balance toward the protease. This leads to uncontrolled C1 activity with breakdown of C4 and C2, and release of bradykinin, which interacts with vascular endothelial cells to cause vasodilation and localized, nonpitting edema. The biochemical triggers that induce attacks of angioedema in these patients are not clearly defined.

Swelling of the affected part progresses rapidly, without urticaria, itching, discoloration, or redness, and often without severe pain. Swelling of the intestinal wall, however, can lead to intense abdominal cramping, sometimes with vomiting or diarrhea. Concomitant subcutaneous edema is often absent, and patients have undergone abdominal surgery or psychiatric examination before the true diagnosis was established. Laryngeal edema can be fatal. Attacks last 2–3 days and then gradually abate. They may occur at sites of trauma, especially dental, after vigorous exercise, or with menses, fever, or emotional stress. Attacks can begin in the 1st 2 yr of life but are usually not severe until late childhood or adolescence. **Acquired C1 INH deficiency** can occur in association with B-cell cancer or autoantibody to C1 INH. SLE and glomerulonephritis have been reported in patients with the congenital disease.

Three of the membrane complement control proteins—CR1, membrane cofactor protein (CD46), and decay-accelerating factor (DAF)—prevent the formation of the full C3-cleaving enzyme, C3bBb, which is triggered by C3b deposition. CD59 (membrane inhibitor of reactive lysis) prevents the full development of the terminal component membrane attack complex that creates the "hole." **Paroxysmal nocturnal hemoglobinuria** (PNH) is a hemolytic anemia that occurs when DAF and CD59 are not expressed on the erythrocyte surface. The condition is acquired as a somatic mutation in a hematopoietic stem cell of the PIG-A gene on the X chromosome. The product of this gene is required for normal synthesis of a glycosyl-phosphatidylinositol molecule that anchors about 20 proteins to cell membranes, including DAF and CD59. One patient with **genetic isolated CD59 deficiency** had a mild PNH-like disease in spite of normal expression of membrane DAF. In contrast, **genetic isolated DAF deficiency** has not resulted in hemolytic anemia.

133.4 • Secondary Disorders of Complement

Partial deficiency of C1q has occurred in patients with severe combined immunodeficiency disease or hypogammaglobulinemia, apparently secondary to the deficiency of IgG, which normally binds reversibly to C1q and prevents its rapid catabolism.

Plasma from some patients with chronic membranoproliferative glomerulonephritis (MPGN) contains **nephritic factor (NeF)**, an IgG antibody to the C3-cleaving enzyme of the alternative pathway, C3bBb, which protects the enzyme from inactivation and promotes activation of the alternative pathway. The result is increased consumption of C3, although serum C3 concentrations vary widely from patient to patient. Pyogenic infections, including meningitis, may occur if the serum C3 level drops to <10% of normal. This disorder has been found in children and adults with partial lipodystrophy. Adipocytes are the main source of factor D, and synthesize C3 and factor B; exposure to NeF induces their lysis. An IgG nephritic factor that binds to and protects C42, the classical pathway C3 convertase, has been described in acute postinfectious nephritis and in SLE. The consumption of C3 that characterizes poststreptococcal nephritis and SLE could be due to this factor, to complement activation by immune complexes, or to both. A patient has been described with a circulating inhibitor of factor H and hypocomplementemic MPGN, emphasizing the importance of factor H in restraining the uncontrolled conversion of C3.

Newborn infants have mild to moderate deficiencies of all plasma components of the complement system. Opsonization and generation of chemotactic activity in serum from full-term newborns can be markedly deficient through either the classical or the alternative pathway. Complement activity is even lower in preterm infants. Patients with severe chronic cirrhosis of the liver, hepatic failure, malnutrition, or anorexia nervosa may also have significant depletion of components and functional activity of complement. Although synthesis of components is depressed in these conditions, serum from some patients with malnutrition also appears to contain immune complexes that could accelerate depletion.

Patients with sickle cell disease have normal activity of the classical pathway, but some have defective function of the alternative pathway in opsonization of *Streptococcus pneumoniae,* in bacteriolysis and opsonization of *Salmonella,* and in lysis of rabbit erythrocytes. Deoxygenation of erythrocytes from patients with sickle cell disease alters their membranes to increase exposure of phospholipids that can activate the alternative pathway and consume its components. This activation is accentuated during painful crisis. An alternative pathway defect has been described in about 10% of individuals who have undergone splenectomy, and in some patients with β-thalassemia major. The underlying mechanism for this defect in these last two conditions is not known. Children with nephrotic syndrome may have subnormal serum opsonizing activity in association with decreased serum levels of factors B and D.

Immune complexes initiated by microorganisms or their byproducts can induce complement consumption. Activation occurs primarily through fixation of C1 and initiation of the classical pathway. In SLE, immune complexes activate C142, and C3 is deposited at sites of tissue damage, including kidneys and skin; depressed synthesis of C3 is also noted. Formation of immune complexes and consumption of complement have been demonstrated in lepromatous leprosy, bacterial endocarditis, infected ventriculojugular shunts, malaria, infectious mononucleosis, dengue hemorrhagic fever, and acute hepatitis B. Nephritis or arthritis may develop as a result of deposition of immune complexes and activation of complement in these infections. The syndrome of recurrent urticaria, angioedema, eosinophilia, and hypocomplementemia secondary to activation of the classical pathway may be due to autoantibody to C1q and circulating immune complexes. Circulating immune complexes and decreased C3 have been reported in some patients with dermatitis herpetiformis, celiac disease, primary biliary cirrhosis, and Reye syndrome.

In patients with bacteremic shock, bacterial products appear to initiate activation of the classical pathway and direct activation of the alternative pathway. Intravenous injection of iodinated roentgenographic contrast medium can trigger a rapid and significant activation of the alternative pathway, which may explain at least some of the occasional reactions that occur in patients undergoing this procedure.

Burns can induce massive activation of the complement system, especially the alternative pathway, within a few hours after injury. Generation of C3a and C5a occurs, which stimulates neutrophils and induces their sequestration in the lungs. These events may play an important part in the development of shock lung after burn injury. Cardiopulmonary bypass, ECMO, plasma exchange, or hemodialysis using cellophane membranes may be associated with a similar syndrome due to activation of plasma complement, with release of C3a and C5a. In patients with erythropoietic protoporphyria or porphyria cutanea tarda, exposure of the skin to light of certain wavelengths activates complement, generating chemotactic activity. Phototoxicity is associated histologically with lysis of capillary endothelial cells, mast cell degranulation, and the appearance of neutrophils in the dermis.

133.5 • Treatment of Complement Disorders

No specific therapy is available at present for genetic deficiencies of the complement system except hereditary angioedema, but a great deal can be done to protect patients with any of these disorders from serious complications. Management of hereditary angioedema starts with avoidance of precipitating factors, usually trauma. Infusion of C1 INH concentrate, if available, aborts acute attacks and is safe and effective in long-term prophylaxis or in preparation for surgery or dental procedures. Adults with hereditary angioedema respond to danazol, a synthetic androgen with weak virilizing and mild anabolic potential. The drug, given orally, increases the level of C1 INH severalfold and prevents attacks. It has not been recommended for use in children. Antihistamines, adrenalin, and corticosteroids have no effect.

Effective supportive management is available for other primary diseases of the complement system. Identification of a specific defect in the complement system may have an important impact on management. Concern for the associated complications, such as autoimmune disease and infection, should encourage vigorous diagnostic efforts and earlier institution of therapy. Individuals with SLE and a complement defect generally respond as well to therapy as those without complement deficiency. With the onset of unexplained fever, cultures should be obtained and antibiotic therapy instituted more quickly and with less stringent indications than in a normal child. The parent or patient should be given letters describing any predisposition to systemic bacterial infection associated with the patient's deficiency, along with the recommended approach to management, for possible use by school, camp, or emergency room physicians. The patient and close household contacts should be immunized against *H. influenzae, S. pneumoniae,* and *N. meningitidis.* High titers of specific antibody might opsonize effectively without the full complement system, and immunization of household members could reduce the risk of exposing patients to these particularly threatening pathogens. Repeat immunization of patients is probably advisable since complement deficiency can be associated with an antibody response that is blunted or shorter lived than normal.

Casanova JL, Abel L: Human mannose-binding lectin in immunity: Friend, foe, or both? *J Exp Med* 2004;110:1295–1299.

Davis AE III: The pathophysiology of hereditary angioedema. *Clin Immunol* 2005;114:3–9.

Densen P: Complement. In Mandell GL, Bennett JE, Dolin R (editors): *Mandell, Douglas, and Bennett's Principles and Practice of Infectious Diseases,* 6th ed. Philadelphia, Elsevier Churchill Livingstone, 2005, pp 69–93.

Eichenfield LF, Johnston RB Jr: Secondary disorders of the complement system. *Am J Dis Child* 1989;143:595–602.

Fijen CAP, Kuijper EJ, te Bulte MT, et al: Assessment of complement deficiency in patients with meningococcal disease in the Netherlands. *Clin Infect Dis* 1999;28:98–105.

Giclas PC: Choosing complement tests: Differentiating between hereditary and acquired deficiency. In Rose NR, Hamilton RG, Detrick B (editors): *Manual of Clinical Laboratory Immunology*, 6th ed. Washington DC, ASM Press, 2002, pp 111–116.

Johnston RB Jr: Complement disorders. In Burg FD, Ingelfinger JR, Wald ER, Polin RA (editors): *Gellis & Kagan's Current Pediatric Therapy* 16. Philadelphia, WB Saunders, 1999, pp 1077–1079.

Klein RJ, Zeiss C, Chew EY, et al: Complement factor H polymorphism in age-related macular degeneration. *Science* 2005;308:385–389.

Mold C, Tamerius JD, Phillips G Jr: Complement activation during painful crisis in sickle cell anemia. *Clin Immunol Immunopathol* 1995;76:314–320.

Roy S, Knox K, Segal S, et al: MBL genotype and risk of invasive pneumococcal disease: A case-control study. *Lancet* 2002;359:1569–1573.

Stengaard-Pedersen K, Theil S, Gadjeva M, et al: Inherited deficiency of mannan-binding lectin-associated serine protease 2. *N Engl J Med* 2003;349:554–560.

Sullivan KE, Winkelstein JA: Deficiencies of the complement system. In Stiehm ER, Ochs HD, Winkelstein JA (editors): *Immunologic Disorders in Infants and Children*, 5th ed. Philadelphia, WB Saunders, 2004, pp 652–684.

Section 5 — Hematopoietic Stem Cell Transplantation — Andrea Velardi and Franco Locatelli

Chapter 134 ■ Principles and Clinical Indications

Thousands of children have received an infusion of **allogeneic** or **autologous** (from the same individual) hematopoietic stem cells to cure malignant and non-malignant disorders. **Autologous** transplantation is employed as a rescue strategy after delivering otherwise lethal doses of radiotherapy and chemotherapy. **Allogeneic** transplantation is used to treat children with genetic diseases of blood cells, such as thalassemia and primary immunodeficiency diseases, as well as hematologic malignancies, such as leukemia and lymphoma. Bone marrow had represented the only source of hematopoietic progenitors employed. Growth factor (G-CSF)-mobilized peripheral blood hematopoietic stem cells and umbilical cord blood hematopoietic progenitors are also used to perform hematopoietic stem cell transplantation (HSCT). For many years, an HLA-matched sibling was the only type of donor employed. More recently, matched unrelated volunteers, full-haplotype mismatched family members, and unrelated cord blood donors have been largely employed to transplant patients lacking an HLA-identical relative.

Protocols for allogeneic HSCT consist of two parts: the preparative regimen and transplantation itself. During the **preparative conditioning regimen,** chemotherapy, often associated with irradiation, is administered to destroy the patient's hematopoietic system and to suppress the immune system, especially T cells, so that graft rejection is prevented. In patients with malignancies, the preparative regimen also serves to reduce the tumor burden. The patient then receives an intravenous infusion of hematopoietic cells from the donor.

The immunology of HSCT is distinct from that of other types of transplant because, in addition to stem cells, the graft contains mature blood cells of donor origin, including T cells, natural killer (NK) cells, and dendritic cells. These cells repopulate the recipient's lympho-hematopoietic system and give rise to a new immune system, which helps eliminate residual leukemia cells that survive the conditioning regimen. This effect is known as the **graft versus leukemia** (GVL) **effect.**

The donor immune system exerts its GVL effect through T cell–mediated alloreactions directed against recipient histocompatibility antigens displayed on recipient leukemia cells. Because histocompatibility antigens are also displayed on tissues, however, T cell–mediated alloreactions may ensue. Specifically, donor alloreactive cytotoxic $CD8^+$ effector T cells may attack recipient tissues—in particular, the skin, intestinal tract, and liver—causing acute graft versus host disease (GVHD), a condition of varying severity that can be life-threatening (see Chapter 136).

The success of allogeneic HSCT is undermined by diversity between donors and recipients in major and minor histocompatibility antigens. Major histocompatibility complex (MHC) molecules, the HLA-A, HLA-B, and HLA-C MHC class I molecules, present peptides to CD8+ T cells while the HLA-DP, HLA-DQ, and HLA-DR MHC class II molecules present peptides to CD4+ T cells. There are hundreds of variant forms of each class I and class II molecule, and even small differences can provoke alloreactive T-cell responses that mediate graft rejection and/or GVHD. Disparities for HLA-A, -B, -C or -DRB1 alleles are independent risk factors for acute GVHD, and HLA-A or -B allele mismatches are a significant risk factor for chronic GVHD.

Minor histocompatibility antigens derive from differences between the HLA-matched recipient and donor in peptides that are presented by the same HLA allotype. They are due to polymorphisms of non-HLA proteins, to differences in the level of expression of proteins, or to genome differences between males and females such as the H-Y antigens encoded by the Y chromosome, which can stimulate GVHD when a sister donates to an HLA-identical brother. Thus, GVHD can still occur even when the donor and recipient are HLA identical.

The optimal donor for any patient undergoing HSCT is an HLA-identical sibling. Because polymorphic HLA genes are closely linked and usually constitute a single genetic locus, any pair of siblings has a 25% chance of being HLA identical. This allows approximately one third of patients to receive their transplant from an HLA-identical sibling.

HSCT FROM AN HLA-IDENTICAL SIBLING DONOR

Allogeneic HSCT from an HLA-compatible sibling is the treatment of choice for children with hematologic malignancies and congenital diseases (Table 134-1). Best results are achieved in patients with congenital or acquired nonmalignant disorders because the risk of disease recurrence is low and the cumulative transplant-related mortality is lower than in children transplanted for hematologic malignancies.

ACUTE LYMPHOBLASTIC LEUKEMIA (ALL). Allogeneic HSCT is used for pediatric patients with acute lymphoblastic leukemia (ALL),

TABLE 134-1. Indications for Allogeneic Hematopoietic Stem Cell Transplantation for Pediatric Diseases

- Acute lymphoblastic leukemia
  - First complete remission for patients at very high risk of relapse
    - Translocation t(9;22) or t(4;11)
    - Nonresponder after 1 wk of corticosteroid therapy *and*
      - T-immunophenotype *or*
      - >100,000 cells/μL at diagnosis
    - Not in remission at the end of the induction phase
  - Second complete remission
  - Third or later complete remission
- Acute myeloid leukemia in first complete remission *or* in advanced disease phase
- Philadelphia chromosome-positive chronic myeloid leukemia
- Myelodysplastic syndromes
- Hodgkin and non-Hodgkin lymphomas
- Selected solid tumours
  - Metastatic neuroblastoma
  - Rhabdomyosarcoma refractory to conventional treatment
  - Very high risk Ewing sarcoma
- Severe acquired aplastic anemia
- Fanconi anemia
- Congenital dyskeratosis
- Diamond-Blackfan anemia
- Thalassemia major
- Sickle cell disease
- Variants of severe combined immunodeficiency (SCID)
- Hyper-IgM syndrome
- Leukocyte adhesion deficiency
- Omenn syndrome
- Wiskott-Aldrich syndrome
- Chédiak-Higashi syndrome
- Kostmann syndrome (infantile malignant agranulocytosis), chronic granulomatous disease and other severe neutrophil defects
- X-linked lymphoproliferative disease (Duncan syndrome)
- Hemophagocytic lymphohistiocytosis
- Selected severe variants of platelet function disorders (e.g., Glanzmann thromboasthenia or Bernard-Soulier syndrome)
- Selected types of mucopolysaccharidosis or other liposomal/peroxisomal disorders
- Infantile maliganant osteopetrosis
- Life-threatening cytopenia unresponsive to conventional treatments

either in the 1st complete remission but considered to be at high risk of leukemia recurrence, or in complete remission after an episode of marrow relapse. ALL is the most common indicator for HSCT in childhood. Several patient-, donor-, disease-, and transplant-related variables may influence the outcome of patients with ALL given an allogeneic HSCT. The long-term probabilities of event-free survival for patients with ALL transplanted in the 1st or 2nd complete remission is 60–70% and 50%, respectively. Inferior results are obtained in patients transplanted in more advanced phases. The use of radiotherapy, or total body irradiation (TBI), during the preparative regimen offers an advantage in terms of longer event-free survival compared to a regimen consisting of cytotoxic drugs alone (Fig. 134-1). Less intensive GVHD prophylaxis is also associated with a better outcome.

ACUTE MYELOID LEUKEMIA (AML). Allogeneic HSCT from an HLA-identical sibling is employed for postremission treatment of pediatric patients with acute myeloid leukemia, resulting in longer event-free survival for patients with AML in the 1st complete remission given an allogeneic HSCT as compared to those treated with either chemotherapy alone or with autologous transplantation. Results obtained in patients given HSCT from an HLA-identical sibling after either a TBI-containing or a chemotherapy-based preparative regimen are similar, with event-free survival of 60–70%. Children with acute promyelocytic leukemia in molecular remission at the end of treatment with chemotherapy and all-trans retinoic acid, or with AML and either translocation t(8;21) or inversion of chromosome 16 (inv.16) are no longer considered eligible for allogeneic HSCT in the 1st complete remission. Around 40% of pediatric patients with AML in the 2nd complete remission can be rescued by an allograft.

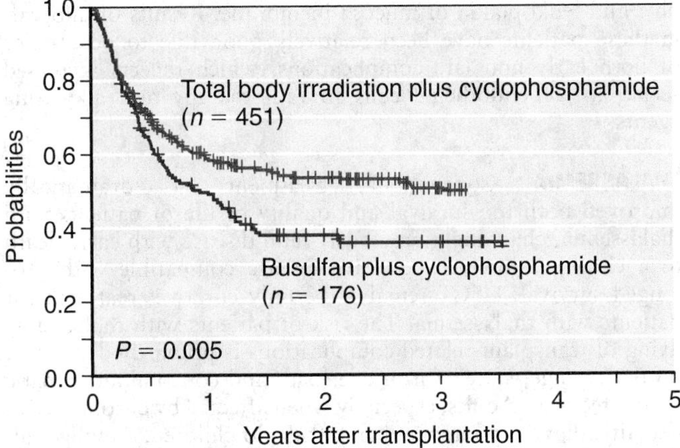

Figure 134-1. Cumulative probability of leukemia-free survival after HLA-identical sibling bone marrow transplantation for childhood acute lymphoblastic leukemia, by pretransplant conditioning regimen of total body irradiation (TBI) plus cyclophosphamide (CY) *(upper line)* or busulfan (Bu) plus cyclophosphamide *(lower line)*. There was superior survival with the total body irradiation plus cyclophosphamide regimen. (From Davies S, Ramsay NK, Klein JP, et al: Comparison of preparative regimens in transplants for children with acute lymphoblastic leukemia. *J Clin Oncol* 2000;18:340–347.)

CHRONIC MYELOGENOUS LEUKEMIA (CML). Allogeneic HSCT is considered to be the only proven curative treatment for children with Philadelphia positive (Ph+) CML. Leukemia-free survival of CML patients after an allograft is 45–80%, with the phase of disease (chronic phase, accelerated phase, blast crisis), recipient age, type of donor (related or unrelated), and time interval between diagnosis and HSCT being the main factors influencing the outcome. The best results are obtained in children transplanted during the chronic phase from an HLA-identical sibling within 1 yr of diagnosis. Treatment with the specific Bcr-Abl tyrosine protein kinase inhibitor imatinib mesylate, which targets the enzymatic activity of the Bcr-Abl fusion protein, could modify the natural history of the disease and, thus, the indications for transplantation.

JUVENILE MYELOMONOCYTIC LEUKEMIA (JMML). This is a rare hematopoietic malignancy of early childhood, representing 2–3% of all pediatric leukemias. JMML is characterized by hepatosplenomegaly and organ infiltration, with excessive proliferation of cells of monocytic and granulocytic lineages. Hypersensitivity to granulocyte-macrophage colony–stimulating factor (GM-CSF) and pathologic activation of the RAS-RAF-MAP (mitogen-activated protein) kinase signaling pathway play an important role in the pathophysiology. JMML usually runs an aggressive clinical course, with a median duration of survival for untreated children <12 mo from diagnosis. HSCT is able to cure approximately 50% of patients with JMML using unrelated donors with comparable results to using HLA-compatible related donors. Leukemia recurrence represents the main cause of treatment failure in children with JMML after HSCT, with the relapse rate as high as 50%. Because children with JMML frequently have massive spleen enlargement, splenectomy has been performed before transplantation. Spleen size at the time of HSCT and splenectomy before HSCT do not appear to affect the posttransplant outcome.

MYELODYSPLASTIC SYNDROMES OTHER THAN JMML. Myelodysplastic syndromes are a heterogeneous group of clonal disorders characterized by ineffective hematopoiesis leading to peripheral blood cytopenia and a propensity to evolve toward AML. HSCT is the treatment of choice for children with refractory anemia with excess of blasts (RAEB) and for those with RAEB in transformation (RAEB-t). The probability of survival without evidence of disease for these children is 50–60% if the donor is an HLA-identical sibling, whereas that of patients transplanted from an alternative donor is slightly lower. It is still unclear whether patients with myelodysplastic syndromes and a blast percentage >20% benefit from pretransplant chemotherapy. HSCT from an HLA-identical sibling is also the preferred treatment for all children with refractory cytopenia, with transplantation from an alternative donor being reserved for children with refractory cytopenia only with either monosomy 7 or life-threatening, transfusion-dependent pancytopenia. For children with refractory cytopenia, the probability of event-free survival after HSCT may be as high as 80%, with disease recurrence rarely observed.

NON-HODGKIN LYMPHOMA AND HODGKIN DISEASE. Childhood non-Hodgkin lymphoma (NHL) and Hodgkin disease (HD) are quite responsive to conventional chemoradiotherapy, but some of these patients are at high risk for relapse. HSCT can cure a proportion of patients with relapsed NHL and HD and should be offered early after relapse, while the disease is still sensitive to therapy. If an HLA-identical sibling is available, allogeneic transplant should be offered to take advantage of the GVL effect. Patients with sensitive disease and little tumor burden have favorable outcomes, with event-free survival rates of 50–60%.

ACQUIRED APLASTIC ANEMIA. HSCT from an HLA-identical sibling is the treatment of choice for children with the severe form of acquired aplastic anemia, defined as two of the following: platelet count <20,000/mm^3, absolute neutrophil count <500/mm^3, or reticulocyte count <1% when anemia is present, together with hypoplastic bone marrow (<20% total cellularity). The probability of survival with sustained donor engraftment for these patients is >80%, with younger patients having even better outcomes. Every child with severe acquired aplastic anemia should undergo HLA-typing as soon as diagnosed in order to identify a suitable HLA-compatible family donor. Graft rejection represents the most important cause of treatment failure. Blood transfusion should be avoided if possible because sensitization to blood products increases the likelihood of graft rejection. GVHD prophylaxis combining cyclosporine and short-term methotrexate is associated with a better outcome as compared to cyclosporine alone (Fig. 134-2). Some uncontrolled studies have suggested that the addition of antithymocyte globulin to the classical conditioning regimen consisting of cyclophosphamide (200 mg/kg) can reduce the risk of graft rejection, particularly in patients with previous heavy sensitization to blood products.

CONSTITUTIONAL APLASTIC ANEMIA. **Fanconi anemia** and **dyskeratosis congenita** are genetic disorders associated with a high risk of developing pancytopenia. Fanconi anemia is an autosomal recessive disease characterized by spontaneous chromosomal fragility, which is increased after exposure of peripheral blood lymphocytes to DNA cross-linking agents, including clastogenic compounds such as mitomycin C and melphalan. Patients with Fanconi anemia, besides being at risk of pancytopenia, show a high propensity to develop clonal disorders of hematopoiesis, such as myelodysplastic syndromes and acute myeloid leukemia. HSCT can rescue aplastic anemia and prevent the occurrence of clonal hematopoietic disorders. In view of their defects in DNA repair mechanisms, which is responsible for the chromosomal

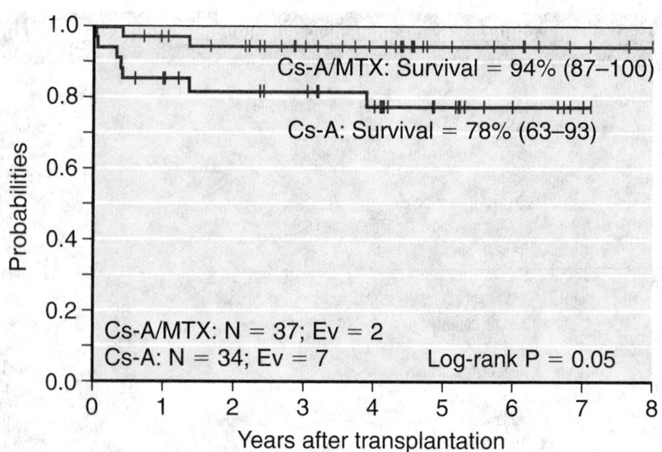

Figure 134-2. Cumulative probability of survival after HLA-identical sibling bone marrow transplantation (BMT) for aplastic anemia, by graft versus host disease (GVHD) prophylaxis with cyclosporin alone *(dotted line)* or cyclosporine plus methotrexate *(continuous line)*. GVHD prophylaxis combining cyclosporin and short-term methotrexate was associated with superior outcome compared to cyclosporin alone. EV, number of events occurring in each arm of randomization; N, number of patients in each arm of randomization. (From Locatelli F, Bruno B, Zecca M, et al: Cyclosporin A and short-term methotrexate versus cyclosporin A as graft versus host disease prophylaxis I patients with severe aplastic anemia given allogeneic bone marrow transplantation from an HLA-identical sibling: Results of a GITMO/EMBT randomized trial. *Blood* 2000;96:1690–1697.)

fragility, Fanconi anemia patients have an exquisite sensitivity to alkylating agents. Thus, they must be prepared to the allograft with reduced doses of cyclophosphamide. Many patients were once successfully transplanted after receiving low-dose cyclophosphamide and thoraco-abdominal irradiation. The use of this regimen is associated with an increased incidence of post-transplant head and neck cancers. Either reduced doses of cyclophosphamide alone or low-dose cyclophosphamide with fludarabine are employed for preparing Fanconi anemia patients to the allograft.

Allogeneic HSCT remains the only potentially curative approach for severe bone marrow failure associated with dyskeratosis congenital, a rare congenital syndrome characterized also by atrophy and reticular pigmentation of the skin, nail dystrophy, and leukoplakia of mucosa membrane. Results of allograft in these patients have been relatively poor, due to occurrence of both early and late complications, which reflects increased sensitivity of endothelial cells to radiotherapy and alkylating agents.

THALASSEMIA. Conventional treatment has dramatically improved both the survival and quality of life of patients with thalassemia, changing a previously fatal disease with early death to a chronic, slowly progressive disease compatible with prolonged survival. HSCT remains the only curative treatment for patients with thalassemia. The risk of patients with thalassemia dying of transplant-related complications is primarily dependent on patient age, state of iron overload, and concomitant hepatic viral infections. Adults, especially when affected by chronic active hepatitis, have a poorer outcome than do children. Among children, three classes of risk have been identified: regularity of previous iron chelation, liver enlargement, and presence of portal fibrosis. In pediatric patients without liver disease who have received regular iron chelation (class 1 patients), the probability of survival with transfusion independence is >90%, whereas for patients with low compliance with iron chelation and signs of severe liver damage (class 3 patients), the probability of survival is 60% (Fig. 134-3).

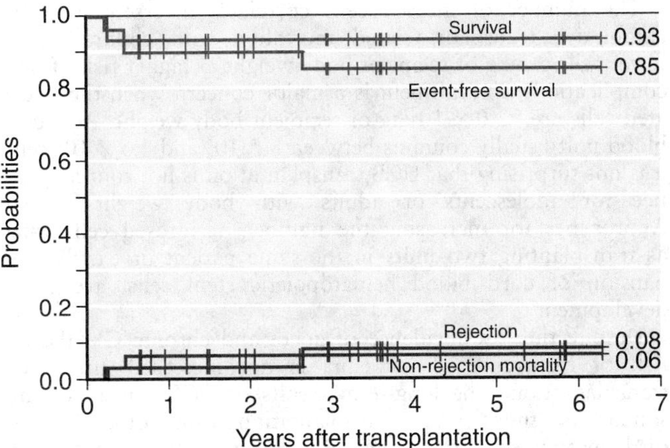

Figure 134-3. Kaplan-Meier estimates of survival and thalassemia-free survival, and cumulative incidences of rejection and nonrejection mortality for 33 thalassemic patients <17 yr of age. Survival was 93%, with incidence of recurrent thalassemia after transplantation of 8%. (From Sodani P, Gaziev D, Polchi P, et al: New approach for bone marrow transplantation in patients with class 3 thalassemia aged younger than 17 years. *Blood* 2004;104:1201–1203).

SICKLE CELL DISEASE. Disease severity varies greatly among patients with sickle cell disease (SCD), with 5–20% of the overall population suffering significant morbidity from vaso-occlusive crises and pulmonary, renal, or neurologic damage. Despite the fact that hydroxyurea, an agent favoring the synthesis of HbF, has been demonstrated to reduce the frequency and severity of vaso-occlusive crises and to improve the quality of life for patients with sickle cell disease, allogeneic HSCT is the only curative treatment for this disease. Although HSCT can cure homozygous HbS disease, selecting appropriate candidates for transplantation is difficult. Patients with SCD may survive for decades, but some patients have a poor quality of life, with repeated hospitalizations for painful vaso-occlusive crises and central nervous system infarcts. The main **indications for** performing HSCT in patients with sickle cell disease are history of strokes, magnetic resonance imaging of central nervous system lesions associated with impaired neuropsychologic function, failure to respond to hydroxyurea as shown by recurrent acute chest syndrome, and/or recurrent vaso-occlusive crises and/or severe anemia and/or osteonecrosis. The results of HSCT are best, with a probability of cure of 80–90%, when performed in children with an HLA-identical sibling.

IMMUNODEFICIENCY DISORDERS. HSCT is the **treatment of choice** for severe combined immunodeficiency (SCID) variants, as well as for other inherited immunodeficiencies (see Table 134-1). With an HLA-identical sibling, the probability of survival approaches 100%, with less favorable results for patients transplanted from an unrelated volunteer or an HLA–partially matched relative. Some children with SCID, mainly those without residual NK activity or maternal T-cell engraftment, may be transplanted without receiving any preparative regimen, with the donor lymphoid cells usually being the only elements that engraft. Sustained donor engraftment is more difficult to achieve in children with Omenn syndrome or hemophagocytic lymphohistiocytosis, or using maternal donor T cells. Life-threatening opportunistic fungal and viral infections occurring before the allograft adversely affect the patient's outcome after HSCT. Patients with the most severe immunodeficiencies must be transplanted as early as possible.

Chapter 135 ■ HSCT from Alternative Sources and Donors

Two thirds of patients do not have an HLA-identical sibling for hematopoietic stem cell transplantation (HSCT). Alternative sources of hematopoietic stem cells are used and include matched unrelated donors (MUDs), unrelated umbilical cord blood (UCB), and haploidentical relatives with one HLA mismatch.

UNRELATED DONOR TRANSPLANTS. The preferred strategy for transplant candidates without an available HLA-identical sibling is to identify an unrelated HLA-matched donor in the general population. Worldwide international registries include more than nine million HLA-typed prospective volunteer donors. HLA-A, -B, -C class I loci, and the DRB1 class II locus are the HLA loci most influencing outcome after HSCT from an unrelated volunteer. Data on serologic typing of class I HLA loci are available for all donors, and there is information on DRB1 typing for approximately one third of donors. The roles played by other class II loci (DQB1, DP1 loci) remain controversial. The chance of finding an HLA-matched donor depends on the frequency of the HLA phenotype, which is closely linked to the ethnic origin of the registry donors, and ranges from 60 to 70% for white patients to <10% for persons of ethnic minority groups.

Identifying a suitable unrelated donor is a complicated and lengthy process, with a median time from the start of search to transplantation of 4–5 mo. During this period, a patient with acute leukemia may relapse and require further therapy, accumulating organ toxicity that unfavorably affects outcome. For various reasons, including poor health, some donors are no longer available or refuse donation. Despite these limitations, many thousands of matched unrelated donor transplants have been performed.

Initially, HLA polymorphism and the restrictions of conventional HLA-typing techniques limited the accuracy of matching, thus increasing rejection rates and the incidence of acute and chronic graft versus host disease (GVHD). Consequently, because the event-free survival of recipients of an unrelated donor allograft is worse than after a compatible sibling transplant, there is no consensus on the use of unrelated donor transplants for nonmalignant diseases, such as thalassemia. DNA-based techniques for HLA typing reveal an impressive number of new alleles within antigens that were previously defined by serology. Matching by these methods reduces the risk of immune complications, namely graft rejection and GVHD, but also the chance of finding a suitable donor. The advent of both high-resolution molecular HLA class I and II antigen-typing coupled with progress in the prophylaxis and treatment of GVHD reduces transplant-related mortality and improves outcomes. Outcomes from a fully matched or a single allelic disparate unrelated volunteer donor are now similar to those of HSCT from an HLA-identical sibling, as indicated by results of unrelated donor transplantation in children with acute lymphoblastic leukemia (ALL) in the 2nd complete remission, juvenile myelomonocytic leukemia, or thalassemia (Fig. 135-1).

The outcome of unrelated donor transplants is poorer for patients with other disorders such as Fanconi anemia, mainly because of a high incidence of transplant-related complications. Disparities of an unrelated donor, such as one antigen disparity with or without allelic disparities at other loci, or multiple allelic disparities at different HLA loci, are associated with worse outcomes. To reduce the risk of acute GVHD, **ex vivo T-cell depletion of the graft** has been employed but has not significantly affected the outcome, which is similar to the outcome

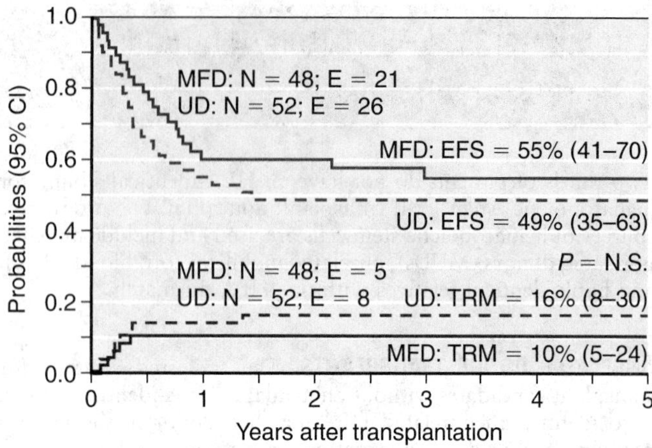

No. of cases at risk:

MFD	48	28	25	19	14	9
UD	52	26	20	16	9	4

Figure 135-1. Kaplan-Meier estimates of event-free survival (EFS) *(upper lines)* and transplantation-related mortality (TRM) *(lower lines)* according to the type of donor used, matched family donor (MFD) or unrelated donor (UD). Matched family donor was superior (55% event-free survival and 10% transplantation-related mortality) compared to unrelated donor (49% event-free survival and 16% transplantation-related mortality). (From Locatelli F, Nöllke P, Zecca M, et al: Hematopoietic stem cell transplantation [HSCT] in children with juvenile myelomonocytic leukemia [JMML]: Results of the EWOG-MDS/EBMT trial. *Blood* 2005;105:410–419.)

of an unmanipulated graft and pharmacologic prophylaxis for GVHD.

The survival rates of unrelated donor HSCT include only patients who are transplanted; these numbers do not take into account those for whom a donor is not found. For patients who urgently need a transplant, the time required to identify a suitable donor from a potential panel, establish eligibility, and harvest the cells may lead to relapse and failure to transplant. For patients who do not have a matched donor or who urgently need a transplant, attention has focused on unrelated cord blood and the haploidentical, three loci mismatched family member.

UMBILICAL CORD BLOOD TRANSPLANTS. UCB transplantation is a viable option for children who require allogeneic HSCT. Several hundred children have been cured by transplant of related or unrelated UCB. It offers the advantages of easy procurement, absence of risks to donors, reduced risk of transmitting infections, and, for transplants from unrelated donors, immediate availability of cryopreserved cells because the median time from start of search to transplantation is 3–4 wk. Mismatches of up to two of the six antigens do not preclude transplant feasibility since the naive T cells in cord blood are less able to cause GVHD than are the mature donor T cells in bone marrow or peripheral blood.

Compared with children transplanted from matched unrelated bone marrow donors, UCB transplant recipients have less probability of sustained donor engraftment, hematopoietic recovery is delayed, the incidence of acute and chronic GVHD is lower, and transplant-related mortality is higher in the early post-transplant period because of infectious complications. The increased risk of fatal infections is primarily due to the slow neutrophil recovery and lack of antigen-experienced (memory) T cells, which are not transferred in UCB. Memory T cells significantly contribute to early immunologic reconstitution of children after unmanipulated allogeneic bone marrow or peripheral blood stem cell transplantation.

The number of infused cells correlates inversely with the cumulative transplant-related mortality, with children given fewer cells per kg of recipient body weight at higher risk of fatal complications. Engraftment is a major concern when the nucleated cells are $<2.0 \times 10^7$/kg of recipient body weight. As a cord blood unit usually contains between 8×10^8 and 1.5×10^9 cells, it is not surprising that UCB transplantation is not routine practice for adolescents or adults with body weight >40 kg. Approaches for increasing the number of infused cells, such as transplanting two units in the same patient or ex vivo expansion of cord blood hematopoietic stem cells, are under development.

Despite the low incidence of acute and chronic GVHD, the risk of recurrence of leukemia is not increased after UCB transplantation. The long-term results of UCB transplants are similar to those after transplantation from other sources of hematopoietic stem cells. Results have been particularly promising in children with acute myeloid leukemia transplanted with cord blood cells from an unrelated donor and in children with hemoglobinopathies given a related UCB transplantation.

HAPLOIDENTICAL TRANSPLANTS. Haploidentical transplantation offers an immediate source of hematopoietic stem cells to almost all leukemia patients who fail to find a matched donor, whether related or unrelated, or a suitable cord blood unit. Nearly all of these children have at least one haploidentical, three loci mismatched family member who is promptly available as donor. The few patients who reject the haploidentical transplant have the advantage of another immediately available donor within the family circle.

Effective T-cell depletion prevents acute and chronic GVHD even when using haploidentical parental bone marrow differing at the three major HLA loci. The benefits of T-cell depletion were first demonstrated in transplantation in patients with severe combined immunodeficiency (SCID), with prevention of GVHD after three log T-cell depletion. More than 300 transplants in SCID patients using haploidentical donors have been performed worldwide, with a high rate of long-term partial or complete immune reconstitution.

As patients with acute leukemia reject a haploidentical bone marrow graft, a megadose of G-CSF-mobilized peripheral blood stem cells is essential for overcoming the HLA barrier. As for patents with SCID, extensive T-cell depletion of the graft prevents GVHD. The conditioning protocol includes total body irradiation (TBI), fludarabine, thiotepa, and antithymocyte globulin (ATG). In a large series of high-risk adult acute leukemia patients, haploidentical transplants were associated with full donor type engraftment in >95%, rapid hematopoietic recovery, and a very low incidence of acute GVHD grade II–IV without the need for any post-transplant immune suppression as prophylaxis. Similar engraftment rates, with no GVHD, have been reported in children with acute leukemia after conditioning with chemotherapy and anti–T cell antibodies.

Several principles emerge from these clinical results. First, the threshold dose of T lymphocytes ($2–4 \times 10^4$/kg) for GVHD as established in haploidentical transplants in SCID patients is valid for leukemia patients. This threshold dose is defined in the context of substantial levels of anti–T cell antibodies, such as ATG or anti-CD3 (anti-OKT3) antibodies, which are part of the highly immuno-myeloablative conditioning regimen. Second, a megadose of purified $CD34^+$ cells is crucial in overcoming the barrier of residual anti-donor cytotoxic T-lymphocyte precursors.

DONOR VS RECIPIENT NK-CELL ALLOREACTIVITY. Donor vs recipient natural killer (NK)–cell alloreactivity is a biologic phenomenon that is unique to the mismatched transplant. It derives from a mismatch between donor NK clones, carrying specific inhibitory receptors for self–MHC class I molecules, and MHC class I ligands on recipient cells. NK cells are primed to kill by several activating receptors. Human NK cells discriminate allelic forms of MHC molecules via **killer cell Ig-like receptors (KIR)**, which are clonally distributed with each cell in the repertoire bearing at least one receptor that is specific for self–MHC class I molecules. Because NK cells co-express inhibitory receptors for self–MHC class I molecules, autologous cells are not killed. When faced with mismatched allogeneic targets, NK cells sense the missing expression of self–class I alleles and mediate alloreactions. In mismatched transplants, there are many donor recipient pairs in which the donor NK inhibitory (KIRs) do not recognize the recipient's class I alleles as self. Consequently, the donor NK cells are not blocked and are activated to lyse the recipient's lymphohematopoietic cells.

Transplantation from NK-alloreactive haploidentical donors controls acute myeloid leukemia (AML) relapse and improves engraftment without causing GVHD. Mismatched HSCT trials demonstrate that MHC class I mismatches, which generate an alloreactive NK-cell response in the graft versus host direction, eradicate myeloid leukemia, improve engraftment, and protect from T cell–mediated GVHD. Lack of an NK-alloreactive donor is the strongest independent risk factor for AML relapse after adjustment for disease status at transplant. In children with acute leukemia, recent studies confirm that transplantation from haploidentical donors with potential for NK cell alloreactivity decreases the risk of relapse. The potential for donor vs recipient NK-cell alloreactivity, which can be predicted by standard HLA typing, is recommended when selecting the donor of choice from among the mismatched family members.

For the approximately 50% of MUD transplants performed in the presence of one or more HLA allele-level mismatches, NK-cell alloreactivity may be expected to occur. Prospective studies are needed to determine whether strategies that harness donor-vs-recipient NK-cell alloreactivity in haploidentical transplantation (high doses of stem cells, T-cell depletion, and no post-transplant immune suppression) can be implemented to improve outcome in MUD transplants.

The search for NK-alloreactive donors, which may require extension beyond the immediate family, increases the chance of finding a "perfect mismatch" from the random 30% to >60%. First, the transplantation candidate is HLA typed. Candidates expressing class I alleles belonging to the three class I groups recognized by KIRs (HLA-C group 1, HLA-C group 2, and HLA-Bw4 alleles) will block all NK cells from every donor and belong to the one third of the population that is resistant to alloreactive NK killing. Patients who express only one or two of these allele groups may find NK-alloreactive donors.

Donor HLA typing identifies family members who do not express the class I group(s) expressed by the patient and, therefore, have the potential for NK alloreactivity. Not all inhibitory KIRs are present in 100% of the population. KIR2DL2/3, the receptor for HLA-C group 1, is present in all persons; KIR2DL1, the receptor for HLA-C group 2, is present in 97% of persons; and KIR3DL1, the receptor for HLA-Bw4 alleles, is present in ≈ 90%. Donor KIR genotyping ensures that the donor expresses the relevant NK cells.

In HLA-Bw4 mismatches, even when the KIR3DL1 gene is present, NK repertoire studies show alloreactive NK cells in approximately two thirds of individuals. This may be because they occur in highly variable frequencies, or because allelic KIR3DL1 variants may not allow receptor expression at the cell membrane. Therefore, for HLA-Bw4 mismatches, direct assessment of the donor NK repertoire is necessary.

TABLE 135-1. Indications to Autologous Hematopoietic Stem Cell Transplantation for Pediatric Diseases

- Acute myeloid leukemia in 1st and 2nd complete remission
- Acute lymphoblastic leukemia after an isolated extramedullary relapse
- Relapsed Hodgkin or non-Hodgkin lymphoma
- Stage IV Neuroblastoma
- Stage IV Rhabdomyosarcoma
- High-risk, relapsed, or resistant brain tumors
- Stage IV Ewing sarcoma
- Life-threatening autoimmune diseases resistant to conventional treatments

AUTOLOGOUS HEMATOPOIETIC STEM CELL TRANSPLANTATION

Autologous transplantation, using the patient's own stored marrow, is associated with a very low risk of life-threatening transplant-related complications, although the main cause of failure is disease recurrence. Bone marrow was once the only source of stem cells employed in patients given an autograft; in the past few years, the vast majority of patients treated with autologous HSCT receive hematopoietic progenitors mobilized in peripheral blood by either cytokines alone (mainly G-CSF) or by cytokines plus cytotoxic agents. When compared to bone marrow, the use of peripheral blood progenitors is associated with a faster hematopoietic recovery and a comparable outcome. A major concern in patients with malignancies given autologous HSCT is represented by the risk of reinfusing malignant cells with the graft; tumor progenitors contained in the graft can contribute to recurrence of the original malignant disease. This observation has provided the rational for **tumor purging** using elaborated strategies aimed at reducing or eliminating tumor contamination of the graft.

Autologous HSCT is employed primarily to prevent relapse in patients with AML who achieve complete remission after induction therapy, and also for selected children with relapsed lymphomas and selected solid tumors (Table 135-1).

Whereas some randomized studies suggest an advantage in terms of event-free survival for patients with AML in the 1st complete remission given an autologous HSCT as compared to those treated with chemotherapy alone, other reports have not confirmed this observation. The probability of event-free survival for children with AML in the 1st complete remission given autologous HSCT has been reported to range from 40 to 60%. Ex vivo purging of bone marrow cells with mafosfamide has been shown to reduce the risk of disease recurrence in children with AML in the 1st complete remission given an autologous transplantation.

Patients with sensitive lymphomas and little tumor burden have favorable outcomes after autologous HSCT, with disease-free survival rates of 50–60%, whereas high-risk patients with bulky tumor or poorly responsive disease have a dismal outcome, with survival rates of 10–20%.

Some studies suggest that, as compared to conventional chemotherapy and radiotherapy, autologous HSCT may offer an advantage in terms of event-free survival to children with ALL in the 2nd complete remission after an isolated extramedullary relapse (CNS, testicular relapse).

Autologous HSCT in patients with high-risk neuroblastoma is associated with a better outcome compared to conventional chemotherapy, especially in patients treated with 13-cis-retinoic acid after the transplant procedure.

For children with brain tumors at high risk of relapse, or resistant to conventional chemotherapy and irradiation, the dose-limiting toxicity for intensifying therapy is myelosuppression, thus providing a role for stem cell rescue. Several studies have provided encouraging results for patients with different histologic types of brain tumors treated with autologous HSCT.

Chapter 136 ■ Graft Versus Host Disease (GVHD) and Rejection

The major cause of mortality and morbidity after allogeneic hematopoietic stem cell transplantation (HSCT) is GVHD, which is caused by engraftment of immunocompetent donor lymphocytes in an immunologically compromised host with histocompatibility differences between the graft and the host that result in donor T-cell activation against host major histocompatibility complex (MHC) antigen. GVHD is classified as acute GVHD, which occurs within 3 mo of transplantation, and chronic GVHD, which, though related, is a different disease.

ACUTE GVHD. Acute GVHD is caused by the alloreactive, donor-derived T cells in the graft attacking nonshared recipient's antigens on target tissues. A two-step circle generates the clinical syndrome. First, conditioning-induced tissue damage activates recipient antigen-presenting cells (APC), which present recipient alloantigens to the donor T cells transferred with the graft. Second, in response to recipient antigens, activated donor $CD4^+$ cells expand and generate cytokines such as tumor necrosis factor-α (TNF-α), interleukin 2 (IL-2), and interferon-γ (IFN-γ) that cause tissue damage and promote differentiation of cytotoxic $CD8^+$ T cells, which, in turn, kill recipient cells and further disrupt tissues.

Acute GVHD usually develops from 2–5 wk post-transplantation. The primary **manifestations** are an erythematous maculopapular rash, persistent anorexia, vomiting and/or diarrhea, and liver disease with increased serum levels of bilirubin, alanine aminotransferase, aspartate aminotransferase, and alkaline phosphatase (Table 136-1). Diagnosis may require skin, liver, or endoscopic biopsy for confirmation. Endothelial damage and lymphocytic infiltrates are seen in all affected organs. The epidermis and hair follicles of the skin are damaged, the hepatic small bile ducts show segmental disruption, and there is destruction of the crypts and mucosal ulceration of the gastrointestinal tract. Grade I acute GVHD (skin rash alone) has a favorable prognosis and often does not require treatment (Fig. 136-1). Grade II GVHD is a moderately severe multiorgan disease requiring therapy. Grade III GVHD is a severe multiorgan disease, and grade IV GVHD is a life-threatening, often fatal condition. The standard **prophylaxis** of GVHD relies mainly on post-transplant administration of immunosuppressive drugs such as cyclosporine or tacrolimus or combinations of either with methotrexate or prednisone, anti–T cell antibodies, mycophenolate mofetyl, and other immunosuppressive agents. An alternative approach, which has been widely used in clinical practice, is the attempt to remove T lymphocytes from the graft (T-cell depletion). Any form of GVHD prophylaxis in itself may impair post-transplant immunologic reconstitution, increasing the risk of infection-related deaths.

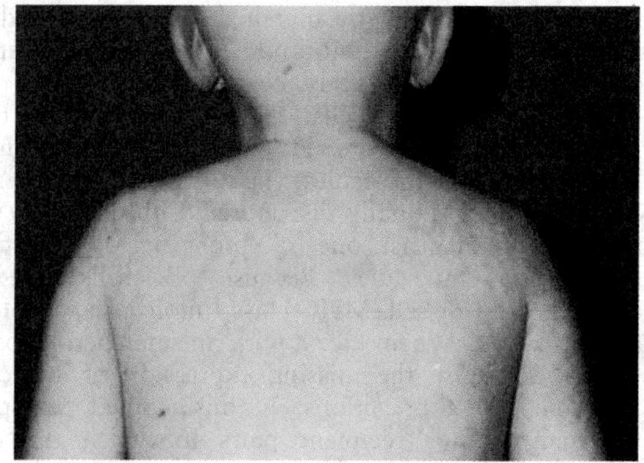

Figure 136-1. Acute graft versus host disease of the skin with ear, arm, shoulder, and trunk involvement. See also color plates. (Courtesy of Evan Farmer, MD.)

Despite prophylaxis, significant acute GVHD develops in ≈30% of recipients of HSCT from matched siblings and in as many as 60% of HSCT recipients from unrelated donors. The risk of acute GVHD is increased by factors such as diagnosis of malignant disease, older donor and recipient ages, and, in patients given an unmanipulated allograft, GVHD prophylaxis with only one drug. Acute GVHD is usually treated with glucocorticoids, antithymocyte globulin, extracorporeal photopheresis, or monoclonal antibodies targeting molecules expressed on T cells or cytokines during the inflammatory cascade, which underlies the physiopathology of GVHD.

CHRONIC GVHD. Chronic GVHD develops or persists >3 mo post-transplant and is the most frequent late complication of allogeneic HSCT with an incidence of ≈25% in pediatric patients. Chronic GVHD is the major cause of nonrelapse mortality and morbidity in long-term HSCT survivors. Acute GVHD has been recognized as the most important factor predicting the development of the chronic form of the disease. The use of matched unrelated volunteers as donors, and of peripheral blood as the stem cell source, has increased the incidence and severity of chronic GVHD. Other factors that predict occurrence of chronic GVHD include older donor and recipient ages, female donor for male recipient, diagnosis of malignancy, and use of total body irradiation (TBI) as part of the preparative regimen.

Chronic GVHD is a disorder of immune regulation characterized by autoantibody production, increased collagen deposition and fibrosis, and clinical symptoms similar to those seen in patients with autoimmune diseases. The predominant cytokines involved in the pathophysiology of chronic GVHD are usually

TABLE 136-1. Clinical Staging and Grading of Graft Versus Host Disease (GVHD)

STAGE	SKIN	LIVER	INTESTINAL TRACT
+	Maculopapular rash <25% of body surface	Bilirubin 2–3 mg/dL	>500 mL diarrhea/day
++	Maculopapular rash 25%–50% of body surface	Bilirubin 3–6 mg/dL	>1,000 mL diarrhea/day
+++	Generalized erythroderma	Bilirubin 6–15 mg/dL	>1,500 mL diarrhea/day
++++	Generalized erythroderma with bullous formation and desquamation	Bilirubin >15 mg/dL	Severe abdominal pain with or without ileus

GVHD GRADE	SKIN STAGE	LIVER STAGE	INTESTINAL TRACT STAGE	DECREASE IN CLINICAL PERFORMANCE
I	+ to ++	0	0	None
II	+ to +++	+	+	Mild
III	++ to +++	++ to ++++	++ to +++	Marked
IV	++ to ++++	++ to ++++	++ to ++++	Extreme

Adapted from Thomas ED, Storb R, Clift RA, et al: Bone marrow transplantation. *N Engl J Med* 1975;292:832–843, 895–902.

type II cytokines such as IL-4, IL-5, and IL-13. IL-4 and IL-5 contribute to eosinophilia, B-cell hyperactivity with elevated IgM, IgG, and IgE titers. Associated monoclonal gammopathies indicate clonal dysregulation. Chronic GVHD is dependent on the development and persistence of donor T cells that are not tolerant to the recipient. They could well derive from the original donor inoculum and/or the recipient thymus that has been damaged by acute GVHD. Maturation of transplanted stem cells within a damaged thymus could lead to errors in negative selection and production of cells that have not been tolerized to recipient antigens and are therefore autoreactive or, more accurately, **recipient reactive.** This ongoing immune reactivity results in clinical features resembling a systemic autoimmune disease with lichenoid and sclerodermatous skin lesions, malar rash, sicca syndrome, arthritis, joint contractures, obliterative bronchiolitis, and bile duct degeneration with cholestasis.

Patients with chronic GVHD involving only the skin and liver have a favorable course (Fig. 136-2). Extensive multiorgan disease may be associated with a very poor quality of life, recurrent infections associated with prolonged immunosuppressive regimens to control GVHD, and a high mortality rate. Morbidity and mortality are highest in patients with a **progressive onset** of chronic GVHD that directly follows acute GVHD, intermediate in those with a **quiescent onset** after resolution of acute GVHD, and lowest in patients with **de novo onset** in the absence of acute GVHD. Single-agent prednisone or cyclosporine is standard treatment at present, although other agents, including thalidomide and extracorporeal photopheresis, have been employed with variable success. As a consequence of prolonged immunosuppression, patients with chronic GVHD are particularly susceptible to infections and should receive appropriate antibiotic prophylaxis, including trimethoprim-sulfamethoxazole. Chronic GVHD resolves in most patients but may require 1–3 yr of immunosuppressive therapy before the drugs can be withdrawn without the disease recurring.

Graft failure is a serious complication exposing patients to a high risk of fatal infection. **Primary graft failure** is defined as failure to achieve a neutrophil count of 0.2×10^9/L by 21 days post-transplant. **Secondary graft failure** is loss of peripheral blood counts following initial transient engraftment of donor cells. Causes of graft failure after autologous and allogeneic transplantation include transplant of an inadequate stem cell dose, and viral infections such as with cytomegalovirus (CMV) or human herpesvirus type 6 (HHV6), which are often associated with activation of recipient macrophages. Graft failure after allogeneic transplantation, however, is mainly caused by immunologically mediated rejection of the graft by residual recipient-type T cells that survive the conditioning regimen. **Diagnosis** of graft failure resulting from immunologic mechanisms is based on examination of peripheral blood and marrow aspirate and biopsy, along with molecular analysis of chimerism status. Persistence of lymphocytes of host origin in allogeneic transplant recipients with graft failure indicates immunologic rejection. The risk of immune-mediated graft rejection is higher in patients given HLA mismatches, T cell–depleted grafts, reduced-intensity conditioning regimens, and transplantation of low numbers of stem cells, and in recipients who are sensitized towards HLA antigens or, less frequently, minor histocompatibility antigens. Allosensitization develops as a consequence of preceding blood product transfusions and it is observed particularly in recipients with aplastic anemia, sickle cell disease, and thalassemia. In HSCT for nonmalignant diseases, such as mucopolysaccharidoses, graft failure is also facilitated by the absence of previous treatment with cytotoxic and immunosuppressive drugs. In thalassemia, graft failure is also facilitated by expansion of hematopoietic cells. GVHD prophylaxis with methotrexate, an antimetabolite, and anti-infective prophylaxis with trimethoprim-sulfamethoxazole or ganciclovir may also delay engraftment.

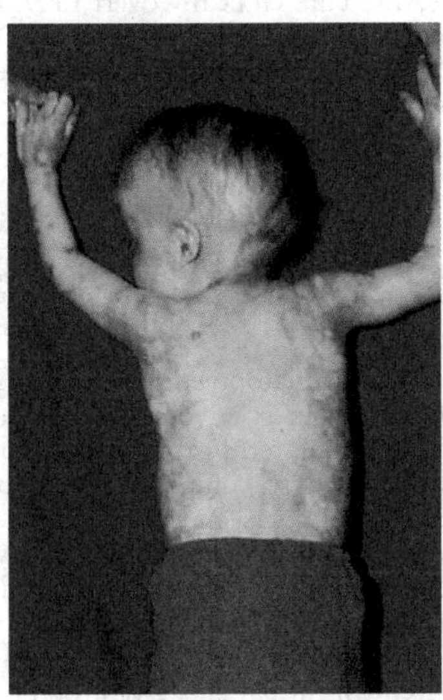

Figure 136-2. Chronic graft versus host disease of the skin with sclerodermoid changes. See also color plates. (Courtesy of Evan Farmer, MD.)

Treatment of graft failure usually requires removing all potentially myelotoxic agents from the treatment regimen and attempting a short trial of hematopoietic growth factors, such as G-CSF. Graft failure due to relapse is managed by either donor lymphocyte infusions (DLI) or cytoreductive chemotherapy followed by DLI and/or a second myeloablative regimen and transplant. When caused by rejection, it is treated with a second myeloablative regimen and transplant. Standard preparative regimens are generally tolerated poorly if administered within 100 days of a 1st transplant because of cumulative toxicities. Use of regimens combining anti-CD3 antibodies with high-dose glucocorticoids has been successful in achieving engraftment in >50% of patients.

Chapter 137 ■ Infectious Complications of HSCT

Hematopoietic stem cell transplantation (HSCT) recipients experience a transient but profound state of immune deficiency. Immediately after transplantation, because neutrophils are absent, patients are particularly susceptible to bacterial and fungal infections. Consequently, most centers start prophylactic antibiotic or antifungal treatment during the conditioning regimen. Despite these prophylactic measures, most patients will develop fever and signs of infection in the early post-transplant period. The common pathogens include enteric bacteria, and fungi such as *Candida* and *Aspergillus*. An indwelling central venous line, routinely employed in all children given HSCT, is a significant risk factor for bacterial and fungal infections, with staphylococcal species and *Candida* being the most frequent pathogens in catheter-related infections (see Chapter 178).

HSCT recipients remain at increased risk of developing severe infections even after the neutrophil count has normalized because T-cell number and function remain below normal for months after transplantation. Unrelated donor transplant recipients are at increased risk of developing graft vs host disease (GVHD), which is itself an additional risk factor for fungal and viral opportunistic infections, as are the associated immunosuppressive treatments. After cord blood transplantation, infections are the consequence of the slow neutrophil engraftment and donor T-cell naïveté. In haploidentical transplantation, the increased risk of infection is the consequence of T-cell depletion of the graft.

Invasive **aspergillosis** remains a significant cause of infectious morbidity and mortality in HSCT recipients. Despite prompt and aggressive administration of potent antifungal agents, proven cases of aspergillosis remain difficult to treat, with case-fatality rates of 80–90%. The annual incidence of invasive aspergillosis has risen with use of stem cells from alternative sources. The incidence is 7.3% in recipients of an HLA-matched related donor transplant and 10.5% in patients with the allograft from either an HLA-mismatched family donor or an unrelated donor volunteer. Most cases of aspergillosis are diagnosed from 40–180 days after HSCT, with 30% diagnosed <40 days and 17% >6 mo after transplantation. The risk of developing aspergillosis is also influenced by GVHD, corticosteroid therapy, post-transplant CMV infection, viral respiratory tract infections, older age, and prolonged neutropenia.

Aspergillus infection often originates from the upper airway mucosa. Early lesions in the nose should be sought in patients with neutropenia who have fever and minimal epistaxis. Rapid extension into the adjacent paranasal sinuses, orbit, or face is usual, with or without the appearance of lung lesions. Invasive aspergillosis generally presents as an acute, rapidly progressive, densely consolidated pulmonary infiltrate. Infection progresses by direct extension across tissue and by hematogenous dissemination to brain and other organs. The earliest CT finding is one or more small pulmonary nodules. As a nodule enlarges, the dense central core of infarcted tissue becomes surrounded by edema or hemorrhage, forming a hazy rim, the **halo sign.** This rim disappears in a few days as the dense core enlarges. In neutropenic patients, when bone marrow function recovers, the infarcted central core cavitates, creating the **crescent sign.** Antifungal prophylaxis and treatment includes isolation of the patient in a laminar air flow or positive pressure room and liposomal amphotericin B and azole compounds (itraconazole) to prevent occurrence or progression of infection. Aspergillosis does not respond satisfactorily to antifungal agents alone, and patients remain at risk until T-cell counts and function recover. This is the rationale for developing strategies to accelerate the recovery of pathogen-specific immune responses.

Cytomegalovirus (CMV) infection remains the most common and potentially severe viral complication in patients given allogeneic HSCT. Seropositivity for CMV is an independent risk factor for mortality, even in recipients of matched sibling or unrelated donor transplants. CMV is itself immunosuppressive as it impairs dendritic cell function. Ganciclovir, the most frequently used anti-CMV agent, may cause leukopenia and T-cell immune suppression.

The period of maximal risk for CMV infection is 1–4 mo after transplantation. Until CMV-specific T-cell responses develop several months after transplant, CMV infection may result in a variety of syndromes including fever, leukopenia, thrombocytopenia, hepatitis, pneumonitis, esophagitis, gastritis, and colitis. CMV pneumonia, the most life-threatening complication related to viral infection, occurs in 15–20% of bone marrow transplant recipients, with a case fatality rate of 85%. The risk is greatest between 5 and 13 wk after transplantation. Risk factors include certain types of immunosuppressive therapy, acute GVHD, older age, viremia, and CMV seropositivity before transplantation.

Gastrointestinal CMV involvement may lead to ulcers of the esophagus, stomach, small intestine, and colon that may result in bleeding or perforation. Tachypnea, hypoxia, and unproductive cough signals respiratory involvement. Chest x-ray often reveals bilateral interstitial or reticulonodular infiltrates, which begin in the periphery of the lower lobes and spread centrally and superiorly. The differential diagnosis includes infection with *Pneumocystis carinii* or other viral, bacterial, or fungal pathogens, pulmonary hemorrhage, and injury secondary to irradiation or to treatment with cytotoxic drugs.

Fatal CMV infections are often associated with persistent viremia and multiorgan involvement. In the 1980s, antiviral treatment was deferred until overt clinical symptoms of CMV infection developed, which led to a high incidence of fatal events. CMV disease has largely been **prevented** through prophylaxis and a preemptive approach. Prophylaxis is based on administration of antiviral drugs to all transplanted patients for a median duration of 3 mo after transplantation. The major drawbacks are drug toxicity, occurrence of late CMV disease, mainly pneumonia, after withdrawal of prophylaxis, treatment of patients at low risk of CMV infection, and low cost-effectiveness. Preemptive, or presymptomatic, therapy aims at treating only CMV-seropositive patients with CMV reactivation who are at risk of developing overt disease, and starts with antiviral drug administration on detection of CMV in blood by any assay. The most widely used assays are CMV antigenemia (pp65) and detection of CMV DNA, which have been used to decide treatment when they either become positive or reach a predetermined threshold. The major drawbacks of this strategy are the continuous monitoring that is required and the sometimes late appearance of HCMV disease. Ganciclovir and foscarnet are usually used for prophylaxis and preemptive treatment of CMV infection.

Epstein-Barr virus (EBV)–related **lymphoproliferative** disease (EBV-LPD) is a major complication in HSCT and solid organ transplantation. In patients given HSCT, selective procedures of T-cell depletion sparing B lymphocytes, as well as the use of HLA partially matched family and unrelated donors, are risk factors for the development of EBV-LPD. These disorders usually present in the 1st 4–6 mo after transplantation as high-grade diffuse large cell B-cell lymphomas, which are oligoclonal or monoclonal, express the full array of EBV antigens, and are of donor origin. High levels of EBV-DNA in blood and in vitro spontaneous growth of EBV-lymphoblastoid cell lines predict development of EBV-LPD.

In immunocompromised hosts, EBV-LPD originates from a deficiency of virus-specific cytotoxic T lymphocytes (CTL), which control outgrowth of EBV-infected B cells. This finding provided the rationale for developing strategies of adoptive cell therapy to restore EBV-specific immune competence. Unselected donor leukocyte infusion (DLI), the first attempt at EBV-directed adoptive immunotherapy in humans, achieves EBV-LPD remission but exposes patients to a high risk of developing clinically relevant GVHD and is not suitable for patients transplanted from an HLA-mismatched donor. A safer approach is infusion of in vitro generated EBV-specific CTL lines of donor origin containing both CD8+ and CD4+ T lymphocytes. These CTL lines prevent lymphoproliferative disorders in patients considered at high risk, such as patients given T-cell depleted HSCT from HLA-disparate donors, and cure clinically overt LPD. In recent years, use of monoclonal antibodies directed against CD20, a molecule expressed on B cells, has significantly reduced the incidence and severity of EBV-related LPD.

Chapter 138 ■ Late Effects of HSCT

Many children given hematopoietic stem cell transplantation (HSCT) become long-term survivors. Besides chronic graft vs host disease (GVHD), long-term complications include impaired growth, neuroendocrine dysfunction, delayed puberty, infertility, second malignancies, cataracts and other ocular complications, leukoencephalopathy, and cardiac and pulmonary dysfunction.

Children given HSCT before puberty may develop **growth impairment,** precluding achievement of the genetic target for adult height. The decrease in growth velocity is similar for boys and girls and is frequent in patients given total body irradiation (TBI) as part of the preparative regimen. Fractionation of irradiation has less adverse impact on height than single-dose TBI, whereas the use of craniospinal radiotherapy before transplantation plays a synergistic detrimental role with TBI in favoring growth impairment. A study of 175 children <6 yr of age, 6–12 yr of age, or 12–15 yr of age receiving TBI-based regimens and not treated with growth hormone reported a mean final adult height of 3.49, 1.92, and 0.37 SD below average, respectively. Chronic GVHD and its treatment with corticosteroids may also contribute to growth impairment. Serial studies of children given a busulfan-based preparative regimen indicate busulfan has much less impact on growth but produces the same gonadal failure as TBI-based regimens. Preparative regimens using only cyclophosphamide for children transplant recipients with aplastic anemia have little, if any, detrimental effect on growth and development.

Growth impairment of patients given TBI is mainly due to direct damage of cartilage plates and the effect of TBI on the hypothalamic-pituitary axis, which leads to an inappropriately low production of growth hormone (GH). GH deficiency is susceptible to at least partial correction through administration of hormonal replacement therapy. Annual growth evaluation should be performed in all children after HSCT. Children showing a decreased growth velocity should be further investigated through evaluation of bone age and secretion of GH in response to pharmacologic stimulus. Current studies are aimed at identifying children with GH deficiencies at an earlier age and administering hormonal replacement therapy. Initial concerns about potential risks of favoring disease recurrence or promoting development of second malignancies in GH substitute therapy have not been confirmed and GH replacement therapy is widely employed.

The use of TBI during the preparative regimen that involves the thyroid gland in the irradiation field may result in **hypothyroidism.** Some children who have received single-dose TBI develop compensated (28–56%) or overt (9–13%) hypothyroidism. The use of fractionated TBI reduces the incidence of both compensated (10–14%) and overt (<5%) hypothyroidism. Children <7 yr at the time of the allograft are at greater risk of developing hypothyroidism. Chemotherapy-only preparative regimens have far fewer adverse effects on normal thyroid function. The site of injury by irradiation is at the level of the thyroid gland rather than at the pituitary or hypothalamus. Therapy with thyroxine is very effective for overt hypothyroidism, but treatment of compensated hypothyroidism is more controversial, although there is evidence that hormonal replacement therapy may reduce the risk of thyroid carcinoma through a suppression of thyroid-stimulating hormone (TSH). Despite treatment of hypothyroidism, the incidence of thyroid carcinoma is not negligible. An annual echo of the thyroid gland is indicated for timely identification of nodules in the thyroid gland suspected to be of neoplastic origin. The cumulative incidence of hypothyroidism increases over time, underscoring the importance of annual thyroid function studies.

Gonadal hormones are essential for normal pubertal growth as well as for development of secondary sexual characteristics. A significant proportion of patients receiving TBI-containing preparative regimens show **delayed development of secondary sexual characteristics,** resulting from primary ovarian or testicular failure. Laboratory evaluation of these patients reveals elevated follicle-stimulating hormone (FSH) and luteinizing hormone (LH) levels with depressed estradiol and testosterone. These patients benefit from careful follow-up with evaluation of annual Tanner scores and endocrine function. Supplementation of gonadal hormones is useful for primary gonadal failure and is administered with growth hormone to promote pubertal growth. The incidence of sex hormone deficiency is lower in patients given a busulfan-based regimen, while infertility during adulthood is a common problem of these children, as well as of those prepared to the allograft with TBI.

The overall risk of developing a **secondary form of cancer** is significantly higher after HSCT than in the general population. Although few studies have specifically analyzed pediatric patients, available evidence indicates that the cumulative incidence of 2nd malignancies show a slight, but continuous, tendency to increase over time. Several types of secondary tumors have been identified in patients given HSCT. The most frequently diagnosed neoplasms are brain tumors, epithelial cancers, and thyroid carcinoma. Young age, male gender, use of TBI during the preparative regimen, chronic GVHD, and an intrinsic genetic predisposition to develop cancer (Fanconi anemia) have been reported to be risk factors for development of secondary malignancies after HSCT.

Cataracts mainly occur in children given a radiotherapy-based preparative regimen. The incidence of cataracts is particularly high if TBI is delivered as a single-fraction (800–1,000 cGy). The introduction of fractionated TBI has led to a marked reduction of this complication to ≈ 10–20% of patients, one third of whom require surgical intervention. Corticosteroids, frequently employed for treating GVHD, have also been demonstrated to promote development of cataracts. A dry eye syndrome, or keratoconjunctivitis sicca, may also affect HSCT recipients. It is often related to chronic GVHD and postradiotherapy fibrosis of the lacrimal gland, and is treated with artificial tears and lubricants.

Adams KM, Nelson JL: Microchimerism: An investigative frontier in autoimmunity and transplantation. *JAMA* 2004;291:1127–1131.

Aggarwal S, Pittenger MF: Human mesenchymal stem cells modulate allogenic immune cell responses. *Blood* 2005;105:1815–1822.

American Academy of Pediatrics Section on Hematology/Oncology and Section on Allergy/Immunology: Cord blood banking for potential future transplantation. *Pediatrics* 2007;119:165–170.

Antoine C, Muller S, Cant A, et al, for the European Group for Blood and Marrow Transplantation, European Society for Immunodeficiency: Long-term survival and transplantation of haemopoietic stem cells for immunodeficiencies: Report of the European experience 1968–1999. *Lancet* 2003;361:553–560.

Atkinson K, Fibbe W, Champlin R, et al (editors): *Clinical Bone Marrow and Blood Stem Cell Transplantation,* 3rd ed. Cambridge University Press, 2004.

Aversa F, Terenzi A, Tabilio A, et al: Full haplotype-mismatched hematopoietic stem-cell transplantation: A phase II study in 104 patients with acute leukemia at high risk of relapse. *J Clin Oncol* 2005;23:3447–3454.

Blume KG, Forman SJ, Appelbaum FR (editors): *Hematopoietic Cell Transplantation,* 3rd ed. Blackwell, 2004.

Burgio GR, Gluckman E, Locatelli F: Ethical reappraisal of 15 years of cord blood transplantation. *Lancet* 2003;361:250–252.

Cohena Y, Nagler A: Hematopoietic stem-cell transplantation using umbilical cord blood. *Leuk Lymphoma* 2003;44:1287–1299.

Cwynarski K, Roberts IA, Iacobelli S, et al: Stem cell transplantation for chronic myeloid leukemia in children. *Blood* 2003;102:1224–1231.

Davies S, Ramsay NK, Klein JP, et al: Comparison of preparative regimens in transplants for children with acute lymphoblastic leukemia. *J Clin Oncol* 2000;18:340–347.

Einsele H, Hamprecht K: Immunotherapy of cytomegalovirus infection after stem-cell transplantation: A new option? *Lancet* 2003;362:1343–1344.

Farag SS, Fehniger TA, Ruggeri L, et al: Natural killer cell receptors: New biology and insights into the graft-versus-leukemia effect. *Blood* 2002;100:1935–1947.

Ferrara JLM, Cooke KR, Deeg J (editors): *Graft vs. Host Disease,* 3rd ed. Marcel Dekker, 2004.

Gluckman E, Rocha V, Arcese W, et al, on behalf of the Eurocord Group: Factors associated with outcomes of unrelated cord blood transplant: Guidelines for donor choice. *Exp Hematol* 2004;32:397–407.

Guardiola P, Pasquini R, Dokal I, et al: Outcome of 69 allogeneic stem cell transplantations for Fanconi anemia using HLA-matched unrelated donors: A study on behalf of the European Group for Blood and Marrow Transplantation. *Blood* 2000;95:422–429.

Horne AC, Janka G, Egeler RM, et al: Hematopoietic stem cell transplantation in Hemophagocytic lymphohistiocytosis. *Br J Haematol* 2005;129:622–630.

Jacobson DA, Duerst R, Tse W, et al: Reduced intensity haemopoietic stem-cell transplantation for treatment of non-malignant diseases in children. *Lancet* 2004;364:156–162.

Kärre K: A perfect mismatch. *Science* 2002;295:2029–2031.

Kolb HJ, Schimd A, Barret J, et al: Graft-versus-leukemia reactions in allogeneic chimeras. *Blood* 2004;103:767–776.

La Nasa G, Giardini G, Argiolu F, et al: Unrelated donor bone marrow transplantation for thalassemia: The effect of extended haplotypes. *Blood* 2002;99:4350–4356.

Le Blanc K, Ringdén O: Mesenchymal stem cells: properties and role in clinical bone marrow transplantation. *Curr Opin Immunol* 2006;18:586–591.

Locatelli F, Bruno B, Zecca M, et al: Cyclosporin A and short-term methotrexate versus cyclosporin A as graft versus host disease prophylaxis in patients with severe aplastic anemia given allogeneic bone marrow transplantation from an HLA-identical sibling: Results of a GITMO/EMBT randomized trial. *Blood* 2000;96:1690–1697.

Locatelli F, Nöllke P, Zecca M, et al: Hematopoietic stem cell transplantation (HSCT) in children with juvenile myelomonocytic leukemia (JMML): Results of the EWOG-MDS/EBMT trial. *Blood* 2005;105:410–419.

Locatelli F, Rocha V, Reed W, et al, for the Eurocord Transplant Group CBT: Related umbilical cord blood transplantation in patients with thalassemia and sickle cell disease. *Blood* 2003;101:2137–2143.

Locatelli F, Zecca M, Rondelli R, et al: Graft versus host disease prophylaxis with low-dose cyclosporine-A reduces the risk of relapse in children with acute leukemia given HLA-identical sibling bone marrow transplantation: Results of a randomized trial. *Blood* 2002;95:1572–1579.

Michel G, Rocha V, Chevret S, et al: Unrelated cord blood transplantation for childhood acute myeloid leukemia: A Eurocord group analysis. *Blood* 2003;102:4290–4297.

Parham P, McQueen KL: Alloreactive killer cells: Hindrance and help for haematopoietic transplants. *Nat Rev Immunol* 2003;3:108–122.

Rocha V, Cornish J, Sievers EL, et al: Comparisons of outcomes of unrelated bone marrow and umbilical cord blood transplants in children with acute leukaemia. *Blood* 2001;97:2962–2971.

Ruggeri L, Capanni M, Urbani E, et al: Effectiveness of donor natural killer cell alloreactivity in mismatched hematopoietic transplants. *Science* 2002;295:2097–2100.

Ruggeri L, Mancusi A, Capanni M, et al: Exploitation of alloreactive natural killer cells in adoptive immunotherapy of cancer. *Curr Opin Immunol* 2005;17:211–217.

Saarinen-Pihkala UM, Gustafsson G, Ringden O, et al: No disadvantages in outcome using matched unrelated donors as compared with matched sibling donors for bone marrow transplantation in children with acute lymphoblastic leukemia in second remission. *J Clin Oncol* 2001;19:3406–3414.

Socie G, Curtis RE, Deeg HJ, et al: New malignant diseases after allogeneic marrow transplantation for childhood acute leukemia. *J Clin Oncol* 2000;18:348–357.

Sodani P, Gaziev D, Polchi P, et al: New approach for bone marrow transplantation in patients with class 3 thalassemia aged younger than 17 years. *Blood* 2004;104:1201–1203.

Souillet G, Rey S, Bertrand Y, et al: Outcome of unrelated bone marrow donor searches in 174 children resulting in 45 patients transplanted in the HLA-matched and -mismatched situation. *Bone Marrow Transplant* 2000;26:31–43.

Steward CG, Jarish A: Haemopoietic stem cell transplantation for genetic disorders. *Arch Dis Child* 2005;90:1259–1263.

Strother D, Ashley D, Kellie SJ, et al: Feasibility of four consecutive high-dose chemotherapy cycles with stem cell rescue for patients with newly diagnosed medulloblastoma or supratentorial primitive neuroectodermal tumor after craniospinal radiation: Results of a collaborative study. *J Clin Oncol* 2001;19:2696–2704.

Velardi A, Ruggeri L, Moretta A, et al: NK cells: A lesson from mismatched hematopoietic transplantation. *Trends Immunol* 2002;23:438–444.

Woods WG, Neudorf S, Gold S, et al. A comparison of allogeneic bone marrow transplantation, autologous bone marrow transplantation, and aggressive chemotherapy in children with acute myeloid leukemia in remission: A report from Children's Cancer Group. *Blood* 2001;97:56–62.

Zecca M, Prete A, Rondelli R, et al: Chronic graft-versus-host disease in children: Incidence, risk factors, and impact on outcome. *Blood* 2002;100:1192–1200.

Part XIV ■ Allergic Disorders

Chapter 139 ■ Allergy and the Immunologic Basis of Atopic Disease

Donald Y. M. Leung

The term allergy refers to patients who express an "altered state of reactivity" to common environmental antigens. Most patients with allergy produce IgE antibodies to the antigens that trigger their illness; the term allergy represents the clinical expression of IgE-mediated allergic disease. Such individuals have a familial predisposition to allergic diseases that manifest as hyperresponsiveness in their target organs such as the lung, skin, or nose. In the past few decades, there has been a remarkable increase in the prevalence of allergic diseases. The increase in allergic disease prevalence is attributed to changes in environmental factors. Understanding the interaction of susceptibility genes, the immune and inflammatory response, and the epithelial cell and environmental interface is critical for the development of effective treatments and management approaches for patients with allergies.

KEY ELEMENTS OF ALLERGIC DISEASES

ALLERGENS. The term *allergen* refers to an antigen that triggers an IgE response in genetically predisposed individuals. Most allergens are proteins that have molecular weights of 10–70 kDa; molecules <10 kDa do not bridge adjacent IgE antibody molecules on the surface of mast cells or basophils; most molecules >70 kDa do not pass through mucosal surfaces needed to reach antigen-presenting cells for stimulation of the immune system. Allergens frequently function in their natural state as proteolytic enzymes, which may contribute to increased mucosal permeability and sensitization. This includes a number of major allergens such as *Dermatophagoides pteronyssinus* allergen I (*Der p* 1) from the house dust mite.

T CELLS. All individuals are exposed to potential allergens. Nonatopic subjects respond with the proliferation of T helper type 1 (Th1) cells, which secrete cytokines, including interferon (IFN)–γ, that are involved in the elicitation of allergen-specific IgG antibodies. Th1 cells are typically involved in the eradication of intracellular organisms such as mycobacteria, because of the ability of Th1 cytokines to activate phagocytes and promote the production of opsonizing and complement-fixing antibodies. Genetically predisposed atopic individuals respond with a brisk expansion of T helper type 2 (Th2) cells that secrete cytokines favoring IgE synthesis and eosinophilia.

Atopic responses include the generation of allergen-specific IgE antibodies that are detectable by serum testing or positive immediate reactions to allergen extracts on prick skin testing (see Chapter 140). The Th2 cytokines interleukin (IL)–4 and IL-13 play a key role in immunoglobulin isotype switching to IgE (Fig. 139-1). IL-5 and IL-9 further enhance IgE synthesis and play an important role in the differentiation and development of eosinophils. The combination of IL-3, IL-4, and IL-9 contributes to mast cell development. Th2 cytokines play an important role in the pathogenesis of asthma and allergic diseases; Th2 cells infiltrate into the affected tissues of acute allergic tissue reactions. Chronic allergic reactions often are characterized by the infiltration of Th1 and Th2 cells. This is important because Th1-type cytokines such as IFN-γ can potentiate the function of allergic inflammatory effector cells such as eosinophils and thereby contribute to disease severity.

A small subset of T cells referred to as **T regulatory (Treg) cells** are thought to play a critical role in allergic and autoimmune diseases. These cells have the ability to suppress effector T cells of either the Th1 or Th2 phenotypes involved in mediating inflammation in a direct cell contact or antigen-specific manner. Treg cells express $CD4^{+}CD25^{+}$ surface molecules and immunosuppressive cytokines such as IL-10 and transforming growth factor (TGF)–β1. The forkhead/winged-helix transcription factor gene FOXP3 is specifically expressed by $CD4^{+}CD25^{+}$ Treg cells and programs their development and function. Adoptive transfer of Treg cells inhibits the development of airway eosinophilia and protects against airway hyperreactivity in animal models of asthma. Patients with mutations in the human FOXP3 gene lack $CD4^{+}CD25^{+}$ Treg cells and develop severe immune dysregulation with polyendocrinopathy and food allergy and high serum IgE levels (XLAAD/IPEX disease) (see Chapter 125). It is thought that $CD4^{+}CD25^{+}$ Treg cells play an important role in controlling the allergic immune response and the lack of such cells may predispose to the development of allergic diseases.

ANTIGEN-PRESENTING CELLS (APC). Dendritic cells, Langerhans cells, monocytes, and macrophages play an important role in the induction of allergic inflammation by presenting allergens to T cells and by contributing to the local recruitment of effector cells. APCs are a heterogeneous group of cells with the common property of presenting antigens in the context of the major histocompatibility complex (MHC). Dendritic cells and Langerhans cells are unique in their ability to prime naïve T cells and are responsible for the primary immune response, which is the **sensitization phase** of allergy. APCs are found primarily in lymphoid organs and the skin. Monocytes and macrophages likely play more of a role in activating memory T-cell responses, which occurs during the **elicitation phase** of allergy.

Dendritic cells residing in peripheral sites such as the skin, intestinal lamina propria, and lung are relatively immature. These immature dendritic cells take up antigens in tissues and then migrate to the T-cell areas in locally draining lymph nodes. During this migration, they undergo phenotypic and functional changes characterized by increased expression of MHC class I, MHC class II, and co-stimulatory molecules that react with CD28 expressed on T cells. In the lymph nodes, they directly present processed antigens to resting T cells to induce their proliferation and differentiation.

Based on their ability to favor Th1 or Th2 differentiation, mature dendritic cells have been designated as DC1 or DC2, respectively. The critical factor for the polarizing mechanism to Th1 cells is the level of IL-12 produced by DC1 cells. Differentiation of T cells in the absence of IL-12 production by DC2 leads to Th2 cells. Histamine and PGE_2 inhibit IL-12 production and contribute to the development of DC2. A unique feature of atopy is the presence of allergen-specific IgE on the cell surface of their APCs. Importantly, the formation of Fc ε receptor I (FcεRI)/IgE/allergen complexes on the APC cell surface markedly facilitates allergen uptake and allergen presentation. The clinical importance of this phenomenon is supported by the observation that FcεRI-positive Langerhans cells bearing IgE molecules is a prerequisite for provocation of eczematous lesions by aeroaller-

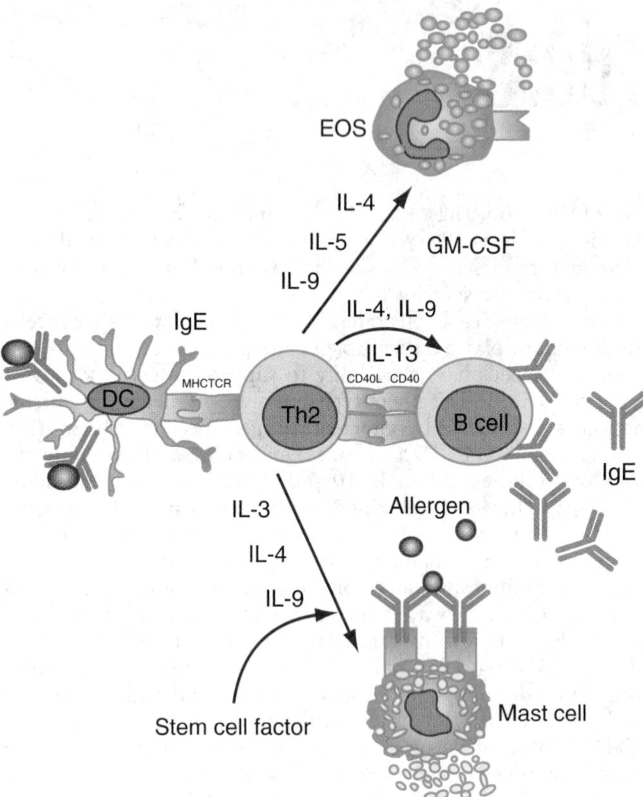

Figure 139-1. Role of Th2 cytokines in allergic cascade. DC, dendritic cell; EOS, eosinophil; GM-CSF, granulocyte-macrophage colony–stimulating factor; IL, interleukin; Th2, T helper type 2.

gens applied to the skin of patients with atopic dermatitis. The role of the low-affinity IgE receptor Fc ε receptor II (FcεRII, CD23) on monocyte-macrophages is less clear, although it appears that under certain conditions it can also facilitate antigen capture. Cross linking of FcεRII as well as FcεRI on monocyte-macrophages leads to the release of inflammatory mediators.

IgE AND ITS RECEPTORS. The acute allergic response is dependent on IgE and its ability to bind selectively to the alpha chain of the high-affinity FcεRI or the low-affinity FcεRII (CD23). Cross linking of receptor-bound IgE molecules on mast cells and basophils by allergen initiates a complex intracellular signaling cascade followed by the release of various mediators of allergic inflammation. The FcεRI molecule is also found on the surface of antigen-presenting dendritic cells (Langerhans cells) but differs from the structure found on mast cells/basophils in that the FcεRI molecule found on dendritic cells lacks the β chain. CD23 is found on mononuclear cells, eosinophils, platelets, and follicular dendritic cells.

The induction of IgE synthesis involves two major signals. The initial signal involves activation of germline transcription at the ε immunoglobulin locus by IL-4 or IL-13, and thus dictates isotype specificity. The second signal involves the engagement of CD40 on B cells by CD40 ligand expressed on T cells. This leads to activation of the recombination machinery, resulting in DNA switch recombination. CD40 engagement can be replaced as a second signal by Epstein-Barr virus infection or glucocorticoid treatment. Interactions between several pairs of co-stimulatory molecules (CD28/B7, LFA-1/ICAM-1, CD2/CD58) can further amplify signal 1 and signal 2 to enhance IgE synthesis. Factors that inhibit IgE synthesis include Th1-type cytokines (IL-12, IFN-α, IFN-γ) and microbial DNA containing CpG repeats.

EOSINOPHILS. Allergic diseases are characterized by peripheral blood and tissue eosinophilia. Eosinophils contain dense intracellular granules that are sources of inflammatory proteins including major basic protein, eosinophil-derived neurotoxin, peroxidase, and cationic protein. Eosinophil granule proteins damage epithelial cells, induce airway hyperresponsiveness, and cause degranulation of basophils and mast cells. Major basic protein released from eosinophils can bind to an acidic moiety on the M2 muscarinic receptor and block its function, thereby leading to increased acetylcholine levels and the development of increased airway hyperreactivity. The eosinophil is also a rich source of leukotrienes, particularly cysteinyl leukotriene C4, which contracts airway smooth muscle and increases vascular permeability. Other secretory products of eosinophils include cytokines (IL-4, IL-5, tumor necrosis factor [TNF]–α), proteolytic enzymes, and reactive oxygen intermediates, all of which can significantly enhance allergic tissue inflammation.

Several cytokines regulate the function of eosinophils in allergic disease. Eosinophils develop and mature in the bone marrow from IL-5–responsive precursor cells. Allergen challenge of allergic patients causes resident bone marrow CD34 cells to express the IL-5 receptor, which stimulates eosinophils to synthesize granule proteins, prolongs their survival, potentiates degranulation of eosinophils, and stimulates the release of eosinophils from the bone marrow. Granulocyte-macrophage colony–stimulating factor (GM-CSF) also enhances proliferation, cell survival, cytokine production, and degranulation of eosinophils. Certain chemokines such as RANTES (regulated upon activation, normal T-cell expressed and secreted), macrophage inflammatory protein 1α (MIP-1α), and eotaxins, play an important role in attracting eosinophils into local allergic tissue inflammatory reactions. Eotaxins mobilize IL-5–dependent eosinophil colony–forming progenitor cells from the bone marrow. These progenitors are rapidly cleared from the blood and either return to the bone marrow or are recruited to inflamed tissue sites.

MAST CELLS. Mast cells are derived from CD34 hematopoietic progenitor cells that arise in the bone marrow, enter the circulation, and travel to peripheral tissue where they undergo tissue-specific maturation. Interactions between the tyrosine kinase receptor c-kit expressed on the surface of mast cells and the fibroblast-derived c-kit ligand stem cell factor (SCF) are essential for mast cell development and survival. Unlike mature basophils, mature mast cells do not usually circulate in the blood but are widely distributed throughout connective tissues, where they often lie adjacent to blood vessels and beneath epithelial surfaces that are exposed to the external environment, such as the respiratory tract, gastrointestinal tract, and skin. Thus, mast cells are positioned anatomically to participate in allergic reactions. There are at least two subpopulations of human mast cells: mast cells with tryptase and mast cells with both tryptase and chymase. Mast cells with tryptase are the predominant type found in the lung and small intestinal mucosa, whereas mast cells with both tryptase and chymase are the predominant type found in the skin, gastrointestinal submucosa, and blood vessels.

Mast cells contain or produce on appropriate stimulation a diverse array of mediators that can have different effects on allergic inflammation and organ function. These include preformed granule-associated mediators (histamine, serine proteases, proteoglycans) and de novo synthesis and release of membrane-derived lipids, cytokines, and chemokines. The most important mast cell–derived lipid mediators are the cyclo-oxygenase and lipoxygenase metabolites of arachidonic acid, which have potent inflammatory activities. The major cyclo-oxygenase product of mast cells is prostaglandin D_2, and the major lipoxygenase products are the sulfidopeptide leukotrienes: LTC_4 and its peptidolytic derivatives LTD_4 and LTE_4. Mast cells also can produce cytokines, including those that promote Th2-type responses (IL-

4, IL-13, GM-CSF) and inflammation (TNF-α, IL-6) and regulate tissue remodeling (transforming growth factor, vascular endothelial cell growth factor). Immunologic activation of mast cells and basophils typically begins by cross linkage of IgE bound to the FcεRI with multivalent allergen. Cell surface FcεRI on mast cells is increased by IL-4 and IgE. Of potential therapeutic interest, surface levels of FcεRI decrease in subjects receiving treatment with anti-IgE antibody that lowers serum IgE.

MECHANISMS OF ALLERGIC TISSUE INFLAMMATION

IgE-mediated immune responses can be classified chronologically according to three patterns of reaction. The **early-phase response** is the immediate response after introduction of allergen into target organs. This response typically results from mast cell degranulation accompanied by the release of preformed mediators, occurring within 10 min after allergen exposure and resolving within 1–3 hr. Acute reactions are associated with increased local vascular permeability leading to leakage of plasma proteins, tissue swelling, increased blood flow, as well as itching, sneezing, wheezing, and acute abdominal cramps in the skin, nose, lung, and gastrointestinal tract, respectively, depending on the target organ in which the allergen challenge takes place.

Second, a **late-phase response** can occur within hours of allergen exposure, reaching a maximum at 6–12 hr and resolving by 24 hr. Cutaneous late-phase responses are characterized by edema, redness, and induration; in the nose, by sustained nasal blockage; and in the lung, by additional wheezing. Late-phase responses are associated with the early infiltration of neutrophils and eosinophils followed by basophils, monocytes and macrophages, and Th2-type cells. The recruitment of inflammatory cells from the circulation requires the upregulation of adhesion molecules on their cell surface and their ligand on endothelial cells, which are under the control of cytokines. Several hours after allergen exposure, TNF-α, which is released by activated mast cells, induces the vascular endothelial expression of cell adhesion molecules, which leads to the transendothelial migration of various inflammatory cells. Preferential accumulation of eosinophils occurs through the interactions between selective adhesion molecules on the eosinophil ($\alpha_4\beta_1$ integrin or VLA-4); VCAM-1 (vascular cell adhesion molecule-1) can be further induced by IL-4 and IL-13 on endothelial cells.

Chemokines are chemotactic cytokines that play a central role in tissue-directed migration of inflammatory cells. RANTES, MIP-1α, monocyte chemotactic protein (MCP)-3, and MCP-4 are chemoattractants for eosinophils and mononuclear cells, whereas the eotaxins are relatively selective for eosinophils. These chemoattractants have been detected in epithelium, macrophages, lymphocytes, and eosinophils at sites of late-phase responses and allergic tissue inflammation. Blockage of their action leads to significant reduction in tissue-directed migration of allergic effector cells.

Third, in patients with **chronic allergic disease,** tissue inflammation can persist for days to years. Several factors contribute to persistent tissue inflammation, including recurrent exposure to allergens and microbial agents with repeated stimulation of allergic effector cells such as mast cells, basophils, eosinophils, and Th2 cells. Th2-type cytokines (IL-3, IL-5, GM-CSF) secreted during allergic reactions can prolong the survival of allergic effector cells because of delayed apoptosis. There is also evidence that local differentiation of tissue-infiltrating eosinophil precursors induced by IL-5 causes self-generation of eosinophils, which contributes to continued damage of local tissue. Tissue remodeling leading to irreversible changes in target organs is also a feature of chronic allergic disease. In asthma, **remodeling** involves thickening of the airway walls, increased submucosal tissue, smooth muscle hypertrophy, and hyperplasia associated with a decline in lung function. In atopic dermatitis, lichenification is an obvious manifestation of skin remodeling.

Th2 cytokines can not only maintain allergic inflammation but also contribute to tissue remodeling by activating resident cells in target organs: IL-4, IL-9, and IL-13 can induce mucus hypersecretion and metaplasia of mucus cells; IL-4 and IL-13 stimulate fibroblast growth and synthesis of extracellular matrix proteins; and IL-5 and IL-9 increase subepithelial fibrosis. Subepithelial fibrosis can result from transforming growth factor-β produced by eosinophils and fibroblasts. IL-11 expressed by eosinophils and epithelial cells also causes subepithelial fibrosis, enhanced deposition of collagen, and the accumulation of myofibroblasts and fibroblasts. This response is further amplified by epithelial injury that results in proinflammatory cytokine release, extracellular matrix deposition in target organs, and angiogenesis. It is thought that genetic predisposition to aberrant injury-repair responses contributes to chronicity of illness. Taken together, once the allergic immune response is established it can be self-perpetuating and lead to chronic disease in genetically predisposed individuals.

GENETIC BASIS OF ATOPY

Allergic diseases are complex genetic conditions that are triggered by environmental factors. There are several major groups of genes likely to contribute to allergic diseases: genes that control systemic expression of atopy (increased IgE synthesis, eosinophili and mast cell responses) that are commonly expressed among various allergic diseases, genes that control local inflammatory and physiologic responses in specific target organs (the skin in atopic dermatitis, the lung in asthma), and genes encoding pattern-recognition receptors of the innate immune system that engage microbial molecules and influence allergic immune responses. Once allergic responses have been initiated, a genetic predisposition to chronic allergic inflammation and aberrant injury-repair responses likely contribute to tissue remodeling and persistent disease.

Atopic diseases have a strong familial predisposition with ≈60% heritability in twin studies of asthma and atopic dermatitis. The 5q23-35 region contains several genes implicated in the pathogenesis of allergic diseases, including the genes coding for Th2 cytokines (IL-3, IL-4, IL-5, IL-9, IL-13, GM-CSF). IL-4 is a well-studied potential candidate gene. A cytosine to thymidine change at position 589 of the IL-4 promoter region is associated with the formation of a unique binding site for the transcription factor, nuclear factor for activated T cells (NF-AT), increased IL-4 gene transcription, higher NF-AT binding affinity, and increased IgE production. Similarly, IL-13 coding region variants have been associated with asthma and atopic dermatitis. An association between atopy and a gain-of-function polymorphism in the α subunit of the IL-4R on chromosome 16 has been found. This is consistent with the important role of IL-4, IL-13, and their receptors in the immunopathogenesis of allergic diseases.

Several genome-wide searches have also linked atopy to chromosome region 11q13. The gene encoding the β subunit of the high-affinity IgE receptor (FcεR1-β), which modifies the activity of the FcεRI on mast cells, has been proposed to be the candidate gene in this region. Several genetic variants of FcεR1-β have been associated with asthma and atopic dermatitis. Chromosome 6 contains the genes that code for human leukocyte antigen (HLA) class I and class II molecules, which regulate the specificity and intensity of immune responses to specific allergens. IgE responses to specific allergens such as ragweed antigen Amb a V and mite allergen *Der p* I have been linked to specific MHC class II loci. TNF-α, a key cytokine that contributes to the influx of inflammatory cells, is also located on chromosome 6. TNF-α polymorphisms have been associated with asthma.

Mutations in SPINK5, the gene encoding a serine protease inhibitor has been shown to cause Netherton disease, a single-gene disorder associated with erythroderma, food allergy, and high serum IgE levels. A common polymorphism in SPINK5 (particularly Glu420Lys) modifies the risk of developing atopic dermatitis and asthma. SPINK5 is expressed in the outer epidermis of the skin and is thought to play an important role in neutralizing the proteolytic activity of *S. aureus* and common allergens such as *Der p* I, which use these proteases to penetrate the skin to induce allergic responses. Genetic linkage studies of atopic dermatitis have also highlighted the importance of chromosome 1q21, which contains genes involved in epidermal and keratinocyte differentiation as well as local inflammatory responses.

Positional cloning of susceptibility genes for asthma has identified other genes: GPRA (G-protein coupled receptor for asthma susceptibility on chromosome 7p14), ADAM 33 (A disintegrin and metalloproteinase 33 on chromosome 20p), and DPP10 (dipeptidyl peptidase 10 on chromosome 2q14). The functions of these genes do not fit into classical pathways of atopy and therefore provide new insights into asthma pathogenesis. GPRA encodes a G-protein coupled receptor with isoforms that are expressed in bronchial epithelial cells and smooth muscle in asthmatics, suggesting an important role for epithelial cells and smooth muscle in asthma. ADAM 33 is expressed in bronchial smooth muscle and is thought to alter the hypertrophic response of bronchial smooth muscle to inflammation. DPP10 encodes a dipeptidyl dipeptidase that can remove the terminal-two peptides from certain proinflammatory chemokines and may therefore modulate allergic inflammation.

Other disease susceptibility genes include the pattern-recognition receptors of the innate immune system, which are expressed by epithelial cells and dendritic cells. These receptors recognize specific microbial components. Polymorphisms in CD14 (engages endotoxin), Toll-like receptor 2 (which engages *Staphylococcus aureus*) and T-cell immunoglobulin domain and mucin domain (which engage hepatitis A virus) have been found to influence susceptibility to asthma and/or atopic dermatitis. These observations support the hygiene hypothesis and a role for microbial stimulation in modulating prevalence of allergic diseases.

Busse WW, Lemanske RF Jr: Asthma. *N Engl J Med* 2001;344:350–362.

Cookson W: The immunogenetics of asthma and eczema. *Nature Immunol Rev* 2004;4:978–988.

Elias JA, Lee CG, Zheng T, et al: New insights into the pathogenesis of asthma. *J Clin Invest* 2003;111:291–297.

Kay AB: Allergy and allergic diseases. *N Engl J Med* 2001;344:30–37.

Leung DYM, Boguniewicz M, Howell MD, et al: New insights into atopic dermatitis. *J Clin Invest* 2004;113:651–657.

Ono SJ, Nakamura T, Miyazaki D, et al: Chemokines: Roles in leukocyte development, trafficking, and effector function. *J Allergy Clin Immunol* 2003;111:1185–1189.

Umetsu DT, Akbari O, Dekruyff RH: Regulatory T cells control the development of allergic disease and asthma. *J Allergy Clin Immunol* 2003;112: 480–487.

Chapter 140 ■ Diagnosis of Allergic Disease

Dan Atkins and Donald Y. M. Leung

Allergic diseases arise from the acute or chronic exposure of a sensitized individual to a specific allergen by inhalation, ingestion, contact, or injection. Symptoms most often involve the nose, eyes, lungs, skin, or gastrointestinal tract either individually or in combination. A carefully obtained history, including environmental exposures, and the appropriate laboratory tests or allergen challenges are critical for an accurate diagnosis.

ALLERGY HISTORY

Obtaining a complete history from the allergic patient involves eliciting a description of all symptoms along with their timing and duration, exposure to common allergens, and responses to previous therapies. Because patients often suffer from more that one allergic disease, the presence or absence of other allergic diseases including allergic rhinitis, allergic conjunctivitis, asthma, food allergy, and atopic dermatitis should be determined. A family history of allergic disease is common and is one of the most important factors predisposing a child to the development of allergies. The risk of allergic disease in a child approaches 50% when one parent is allergic and 66% when both parents are allergic.

Several characteristic behaviors are often seen in allergic children. Because of nasal pruritus and rhinorrhea, children with allergic rhinitis often perform the **allergic salute** by rubbing their nose upward with the palm of their hand. This maneuver gives rise to the **nasal crease,** a horizontal skinfold over the bridge of the nose. Characteristic vigorous **grinding** of the eyes with the thumb and side of the fist is frequently observed in children with allergic conjunctivitis. The **allergic cluck** is produced when the tongue is placed against the roof of the mouth to form a seal and withdrawn rapidly in an effort to scratch the palate. The presence of other symptoms such as fever, unilateral nasal obstruction, and purulent nasal discharge suggests other diagnoses.

The timing of onset and the progression of symptoms are relevant. The onset of recurrent or persistent nasal symptoms coinciding with placement in a daycare center might suggest recurrent infection rather than allergy. When patients present with a history of episodic acute symptoms, it is important to review the setting in which symptoms occur as well as the activities and exposures that immediately precede their onset. Symptoms associated with lawn mowing suggest allergy to grass pollen or fungi, whereas if the symptoms always occur in homes with pets, then animal dander sensitivity is an obvious consideration. Reproducible reactions after the ingestion of a specific food raise the possibility of food allergy. When symptoms wax and wane but evolve gradually and are more chronic in duration, a closer look at whether the timing and progression of symptoms correlate with exposure to a seasonal aeroallergen is warranted.

Aeroallergens such as pollens or fungal spores, the concentration of which in outdoor air fluctuates seasonally, are prominent causes of allergic disease. Correlating symptoms with the seasonal pollination patterns of indigenous plants along with information provided by local pollen counts can aid in identifying the allergen to which the patient is sensitized. Throughout most of the United States, trees pollinate in the early spring. Grasses pollinate in the late spring and early summer, whereas weeds pollinate in late summer through the fall. The presence of fungal spores in the atmosphere follows a seasonal pattern in the northern United States with spore counts increasing with the onset of warmer weather and peaking in the late summer months only to recede again with the onset of colder weather in the late fall through the winter. In warmer regions of the southern United States, fungal spores and grass pollens may cause symptoms on a perennial basis.

Rather than experiencing seasonal symptoms, some patients suffer allergic symptoms year-round. In these patients, sensitization to sources of perennial allergens usually found indoors such as dust mites, animal dander, cockroaches, and fungi warrants consideration. Species of certain fungi such as *Aspergillus* and *Penicillium* are found indoors, whereas *Alternaria* is found in both indoor and outdoor environments. Cockroach allergens are often problematic in inner city environments. Patients sensitive to perennial allergens often also become sensitized to seasonal allergens and experience baseline symptoms year-round with worsening during the spring and fall pollen seasons.

The age of the patient is an important consideration in identifying potential allergens. Infants and young children are 1st sensitized to allergens that are in their environment on a continuous basis, such as dust mites, animal dander, and fungi. Clinically relevant sensitization to seasonal allergens usually takes several seasons of exposure to develop. Food allergies are more common in infants and young children, resulting primarily in cutaneous, gastrointestinal, and, less frequently, respiratory symptoms.

Complete information from all previous evaluations and prior treatments for allergic disease should be reviewed, including the response to all medications that have been used, and the duration and impact of allergen immunotherapy. Improvement in symptoms during treatment with medications or therapies used to treat allergic disease provides additional evidence that the symptoms are the result of an allergic process.

A thorough environmental survey should be performed, with attention to potential sources of allergen and/or irritant exposure. The age and type of the dwelling, how it is heated and cooled, the use of humidifiers or air filtration units (either central or portable), and any history of flooding or water damage should be noted. Forced hot air heating may repeatedly stir up dust mite, fungi, and animal allergens. The irritant effects of wood-burning stoves, fireplaces, and kerosene heaters may provoke respiratory symptoms in allergic patients. Increased humidity or water damage in the home is often associated with increased exposure to dust mites and fungi. Carpeting serves as a reservoir for dust mites, fungi, and animal dander. The number of domestic pets and their movements about the house, including where they sleep, should be ascertained. Special attention should be focused on the bedroom where children spend a significant portion of time. The age and type of bedding, the number of stuffed animals, window treatments, and accessibility of the room to pets should be reviewed. The number of smokers in the home and where they smoke is useful information. Hobbies that might result in exposure to allergens or respiratory irritants such as paint fumes, cleansers, sawdust, latex, or glues should be identified. Similar information should be obtained in regard to other environments where the child spends large portions of time such as a relative's home, the classroom, or daycare center.

PHYSICAL EXAMINATION

In patients with **asthma,** a peak flow analysis or spirometry should be performed for evidence of airway obstruction. If respiratory distress is observed, pulse oximetry should be performed. The child presenting with a chief complaint of rhinitis or rhinoconjunctivitis should be observed for mouth breathing, paroxysms of sneezing, sniffing, or rubbing of the nose and eyes. Infants should be observed during feeding for nasal obstruction severe enough to interfere with feeding as well as for evidence of aspiration or gastroesophageal reflux. The frequency and nature of coughing that occurs during the interview and any positional increase in coughing or wheezing should be noted. Children with asthma should be observed for congested cough, tachypnea at rest, retractions, and audible wheezes. Patients with atopic dermatitis should be monitored for repetitive scratching and the extent of skin involvement.

Because children with severe asthma as well as those receiving oral corticosteroids may suffer growth suppression, an accurate height should be plotted at regular intervals. Poor weight gain in a child with chronic chest symptoms should prompt consideration of cystic fibrosis. The blood pressure should be obtained to evaluate for steroid-induced hypertension. The patient with acute asthma may present with **pulsus paradoxus,** defined as a drop in systolic blood pressure during inspiration >10 mm Hg. Moderate to severe airways obstruction is indicated by a decrease of >20 mm Hg. An increased heart rate may be the result of an asthma flare or the use of a β-agonist or decongestant. Fever is not caused by allergy alone and should prompt consideration of an infectious process, which may exacerbate asthma.

Parents of allergic children are often concerned about a blue-gray to purple discoloration beneath the lower eyelids, attributed to venous stasis and referred to as **allergic shiners.** They are found in up to 60% of allergic patients and almost 40% of patients without allergic disease. They are often accompanied by **Dennie lines (Dennie-Morgan folds),** which are prominent symmetric skinfolds that extend in an arc from the inner canthus beneath and parallel to the lower lid margin.

In most patients with **allergic conjunctivitis,** involvement of the eyes is usually bilateral. Examination of the conjunctiva reveals varying degrees of conjunctival injection and edema. In severe cases, periorbital edema may be observed involving primarily the lower eyelids. The classic discharge associated with allergic conjunctivitis is usually described as "stringy" or "ropy." In children with vernal conjunctivitis, examination of the tarsal conjunctiva may reveal cobblestoning. Children repeatedly receiving large doses of oral corticosteroids for management of severe asthma are at risk for developing posterior subcapsular cataracts. **Keratoconus,** which is protrusion of the cornea, may occur in patients with atopic dermatitis as a result of repeated trauma produced by persistent rubbing of the eyes.

The external ear should be examined for eczematous changes in patients with atopic dermatitis. Because otitis media with effusion is common in children with allergic rhinitis, pneumatic otoscopy should be performed to evaluate for the presence of fluid in the middle ear and to exclude infection.

Examination of the nose in allergic patients often reveals the presence of a transverse nasal crease on top of the nose at the junction of the cartilaginous and bony portions of the nasal bridge caused by frequent rubbing of the nose. Nasal patency should be assessed and the nose examined for structural abnormalities affecting nasal airflow such as a septal deviation, turbinate hypertrophy, septal spurs, or nasal polyps. A decreased or absent sense of smell should raise concern about the presence of nasal polyps, a feature of cystic fibrosis. The nasal mucosa in allergic rhinitis is classically described as pale to purple in comparison to the beefy red mucosa of patients with nonallergic rhinitis. Allergic nasal secretions are typically thin and clear. Purulent secretions suggest another cause of rhinitis. The frontal and maxillary sinuses should be palpated to identify tenderness to pressure that might be associated with sinusitis.

Examination of the lips may reveal cheilitis caused by drying of the lips from continuous mouth breathing and repeated licking of the lips in an attempt to replenish moisture and relieve discomfort. Tonsillar and adenoidal hypertrophy along with a history of impressive snoring suggests the possibility of obstructive sleep apnea. The posterior pharynx should be examined for the presence of postnasal drip and posterior pharyngeal lymphoid hyperplasia.

Chest findings in asthmatic children vary significantly depending on disease duration, severity, and activity. In a child with mild or well-controlled asthma, the chest may appear entirely normal on examination between asthma exacerbations. Examination of the same child during an acute episode of asthma may reveal hyperinflation, tachypnea, cyanosis, use of accessory muscles, wheezing, and decreased air exchange with a prolonged expiratory time. Tachycardia may be caused by the asthma exacerbation or be accompanied by jitteriness and caused by treatment with β_2-agonists. Decreased airflow or rhonchi and wheezes over the right chest may be noted in children with mucus plugging and right middle lobe atelectasis. Unilateral wheezing after an episode of coughing and choking in a small child without a history of previous respiratory illness suggests **aspiration of a foreign body.**

Wheezing limited to the larynx in association with inspiratory stridor is seen in older children and adolescents with **vocal cord dysfunction.** In children with chronic asthma, an increased anteroposterior diameter of the chest suggests significant air trapping. In infants and younger children with significant asthma, a groove along the lower ribs at the site of attachment of the diaphragm may be present. Digital clubbing is rarely seen in patients with uncomplicated asthma and should prompt further evaluation to rule out other potential chronic diagnoses.

The skin of the allergic patient should be examined for evidence of urticaria/angioedema or atopic dermatitis. **Xerosis,** or dry skin, is the most common skin abnormality of allergic children. Keratosis pilaris, often found on the extensor surfaces of the upper arms and thighs, is characterized by roughness of the skin caused by keratin plugs lodged in the openings of hair follicles. Examination of the skin of the palms and feet reveals exaggerated palmar and plantar creases in some allergic children.

DIAGNOSTIC TESTING

The laboratory evaluation of the child suspected of having allergic disease should focus on obtaining objective evidence to support the diagnosis, documenting sensitivity to allergens implicated by the history, and ruling out other potential diagnoses.

IN VITRO TESTS. Allergic diseases are often associated with increased numbers of eosinophils circulating in the peripheral blood and invading the tissues and secretions of target organs. Eosinophilia, defined as the presence of >450 eosinophils/μL in peripheral blood, is the most common hematologic abnormality of allergic patients. Seasonal increases in the number of circulating eosinophils may be observed in sensitized patients after exposure to allergens such as tree, grass, and weed pollens. The number of circulating eosinophils can be suppressed by certain infections and the systemic corticosteroids. In certain pathologic conditions such as drug reactions or eosinophilic pneumonias, significantly increased numbers of eosinophils may be present in the target organ in the absence of peripheral blood eosinophilia. Increased numbers of eosinophils are observed in a wide variety of disorders in addition to allergy (Table 140-1).

TABLE 140-1. Differential Diagnosis of Childhood Eosinophilia

PHYSIOLOGIC
Prematurity
Infants receiving hyperalimentation
Familial
INFECTIOUS
Parasitic (with tissue-invasive helminths, e.g., trichinosis, strongyloidiasis, pneumocystosis, filariasis, cysticercosis, cutaneous and visceral larva migrans, echinococcosis)
Bacterial (brucellosis, tularemia, cat-scratch disease, *Chlamydia*)
Fungal (histoplasmosis, blastomycosis, coccidioidomycosis, allergic bronchopulmonary aspergillosis)
Mycobacterial (tuberculosis, leprosy)
Viral (hepatitis A, hepatitis B, hepatitis C, Epstein-Barr virus)
PULMONARY
Allergic (rhinitis, asthma)
Löeffler syndrome
Hypersensitivity pneumonitis
Eosinophilic pneumonia
Pulmonary interstitial eosinophilia
DERMATOLOGIC
Atopic dermatitis
Pemphigus
Dermatitis herpetiformis
Infantile eosinophilic pustular folliculitis
Episodic angioedema and urticaria
Eosinophilic fasciitis (Schulman syndrome)
Eosinophilic cellulitis (Well syndrome)
Kimura disease
ONCOLOGIC
Neoplasm (lung, gastrointestinal, uterine)
Hodgkin disease
Leukemia
Myelofibrosis
IMMUNOLOGIC
T-cell immunodeficiencies
Hyper IgE (Job) syndrome
Wiskott-Aldrich syndrome
Graft versus host disease
Drug hypersensitivity
Post-irradiation
Post-splenectomy
ENDOCRINE
Post-adrenalectomy
Addison disease
Panhypopituitarism
CARDIOVASCULAR
Löeffler disease (fibroplastic endocarditis)
Congenital heart disease
Hypersensitivity vasculitis
GASTROINTESTINAL
Milk protein allergy
Inflammatory bowel disease
Eosinophilic esophagitis
Eosinophilic gastroenteritis

Nasal and bronchial secretions are often examined for the presence of eosinophils. The presence of eosinophils in the sputum of asthmatic patients is classic. An increased number of eosinophils in a smear of nasal mucus stained with Hansel stain is a more sensitive indicator of nasal allergies than peripheral blood eosinophilia and aids in distinguishing allergic rhinitis from other causes of rhinitis. In young children, nasal eosinophilia is defined as the presence of >4% eosinophils in nasal mucus smears, whereas a finding of >10% eosinophils is required in adolescents and adults. Nasal mucus eosinophilia also has therapeutic implications, predicting a higher probability of responsiveness to topical nasal corticosteroid sprays.

An elevated IgE level is often found in the serum of allergic patients, because IgE is the primary antibody associated with allergic reactions. IgE levels are measured in international units (IU), with 1 IU equal to 2.4 ng of IgE. Maternal IgE does not cross the placenta. Although the fetus is capable of producing IgE as early as the 11th wk of gestation, infants in developed countries produce little IgE in utero owing to the lack of stimulation by allergens. Serum IgE levels gradually rise over the 1st years of life to peak in the teen years and decrease steadily thereafter. A variety of factors in addition to age, such as genetic influences, race, gender, certain diseases, and exposure to cigarette smoke and allergens, affects serum IgE levels. Serum IgE levels may increase two- to fourfold in allergic patients during and immediately after the pollen season, then gradually decline until the next pollen season. Comparison of total serum IgE levels among patients with allergic disease reveals that those with atopic dermatitis tend to have the highest levels, whereas patients with allergic asthma generally have higher levels than those with allergic rhinitis. Although average total serum IgE levels are higher in populations of allergic patients than in comparable populations without allergic disease, the overlap in levels is such that the diagnostic value of a total serum IgE level is poor. Approximately one half of patients with allergic disease have a total serum IgE level in the normal range. Total serum IgE measurement is indicated when the diagnosis of **allergic bronchopulmonary aspergillosis** is suspected; total serum IgE concentration >1,000 ng/mL is a criterion for diagnosis of this disorder (see Chapter 234). Continued monitoring of the total serum IgE in patients with allergic bronchopulmonary aspergillosis is encouraged because serum IgE levels decrease with appropriate therapy and rise again during exacerbations of the disease. The total serum IgE level is also elevated in several nonallergic diseases (Table 140-2).

TABLE 140-2. Nonallergic Diseases Associated with Increased Serum IgE Concentrations

PARASITIC INFESTATIONS
Ascariasis
Capillariasis
Echinococcosis
Fascioliasis
Filariasis
Hookworm
Onchocerciasis
Paragonimiasis
Schistosomiasis
Strongyloidiasis
Trichinosis
Visceral larva migrans
INFECTIONS
Allergic bronchopulmonary aspergillosis
Candidiasis, systemic
Coccidiodomycosis
Cytomegalovirus mononucleosis
Infectious mononucleosis (Epstein-Barr virus)
Leprosy
IMMUNODEFICIENCY
Hyper IgE (Job) syndrome
IgA deficiency, selective
Nezelof syndrome
Thymic hypoplasia (DiGeorge anomaly)
Wiskott-Aldrich syndrome
NEOPLASTIC DISEASES
Hodgkin disease
IgE myeloma
OTHER DISEASES AND DISORDERS
Burns
Cystic fibrosis
Dermatitis, chronic acral
Erythema nodosum, streptococcal infection
Guillain-Barré syndrome
Hemosiderosis, primary pulmonary
Intestinal nephritis, drug-induced
Kawasaki disease
Liver disease
Pemphigus, bullous
Polyarteritis nodosa, infantile
Rheumatoid arthritis

Ig, immunoglobulin.

The presence of IgE specific for a particular allergen can be documented in vivo by skin testing or in vitro by the measurement of allergen-specific IgE levels in the serum (Table 140-3). The most widely employed test for documenting the presence of allergen-specific IgE in the serum is the **radioallergosorbent test (RAST)**, with allergens of an individual allergen extract bound to a solid phase support. A small amount of the patient's serum is incubated with the allergen-coated support, and any IgE in the patient's serum specific for those allergens binds to them on the support. Next, the allergen-coated support to which the patient's allergen-specific IgE is bound is incubated with radiolabeled anti-human-IgE, which then binds to the patient's allergen-specific IgE. Then, the amount of radioactivity associated with the support, to which allergen along with the patient's allergen-specific IgE and radiolabeled antihuman-IgE are attached, is measured. Improvements in the assay for allergen-specific IgE include modification of the solid phase supports to enhance binding of allergen, substituting enzymes for the radiolabels on antihuman-IgE to increase the accuracy of detection while also providing a more stable reagent, and a switch to calibration curves based on known quantities of IgE resulting in quantitative rather than qualitative reporting of results.

The primary advantages of these assays in comparison to allergen skin testing are their safety and that the results are not influenced by skin disease or medications. Overall, the results of these tests correlate well with those obtained by skin testing and provocation challenges. The RAST is not as sensitive as the skin test. In patients with histories of life-threatening reactions to foods, insect stings, drugs, or latex, skin testing is still required because of its higher sensitivity even if the RAST is negative.

TABLE 140-3. Determination of Specific IgE by Skin Testing vs In Vitro Testing*

Variable	Skin Test	Radioallergosorbent Test
Risk of allergic reaction	Yes	No
Relative sensitivity†	High	Less
Affected by antihistamines	Yes	No
Affected by corticosteroids	Usually not	No
Affected by extensive dermatitis or dermographism	Yes	No
Convenience, less patient anxiety	No	Yes
Broad selection of antigens	Yes	No
Immediate results	Yes	No
Expensive	No	Yes
Semiquantitative	No	Yes
Lability of allergens	Yes	No
Results evident to patient	Yes	No

*Radioallergosorbent test as an example of other in vitro tests.
†Because skin tests are more sensitive, they are more reliable than RAST in confirming life-threatening anaphylactic conditions if maximal sensitivity is required such as for penicillin or *Hymenoptera* hypersensitivity.

IN VIVO TESTS. Allergen skin testing is the primary in vivo procedure for the diagnosis of allergic disease. Mast cells with allergen-specific IgE antibodies attached to high-affinity receptors on their surface reside in the skin of allergic patients. The introduction of minute amounts of an allergen to which the patient is allergic into the skin results in cross linking by the allergen of allergen-specific IgE antibodies on the mast cell surface, thereby triggering mast cell activation. Once activated, these mast cells release a variety of preformed and newly generated mediators that act on surrounding tissues. Histamine is the mediator most responsible for the immediate wheal and flare reactions observed in skin testing. Examination of the site of a positive skin test reveals a pruritic wheal surrounded by an area of erythema. The time course of these reactions is rapid in onset, reaching a peak within ≈20 min and usually resolving over the next 20–30 min. In some patients, however, a larger area of less distinctly demarcated edema on an erythematous base develops at the skin test site over the next 6–12 hr. This reaction, the **late-phase response,** usually resolves by 24 hr. Biopsy of the site of a late-phase response reveals the presence of an inflammatory infiltrate consisting of T cells, neutrophils, and eosinophils. These reactions are thought to be similar to the late-phase responses observed in other organs such as the nose and lungs after provocation challenges.

Skin testing in children is usually 1st performed using the **prick/puncture technique.** With this technique, a small drop of allergen is applied to the skin surface and a tiny amount is introduced into the epidermis by lightly pricking or puncturing the skin through the drop of extract with a small needle. When the prick/puncture skin test is negative and the history is suggestive, selective skin testing using the **intradermal technique** may be performed. This technique involves using a 26-gauge needle to inject 0.01–0.02 mL of a dilute allergen extract into the dermis of the arm. This technique is more sensitive than the prick/puncture technique and the allergen extracts used are 1,000- to 100-fold less concentrated than extracts used for prick/puncture testing. Intradermal skin tests are not recommended for use with food allergens because of the risk of triggering anaphylaxis. Irritant rather than allergic reactions can occur with intradermal skin testing if higher concentrations of extracts such as 1:100 weight:volume are used. Although less sensitive than intradermal skin tests, positive prick/puncture skin tests tend to correlate better with symptoms on natural exposure to the allergen.

Panels of skin tests that include the appropriate allergens for a given geographic area in addition to common indoor allergens are often applied; the number of skin tests performed should be individualized, taking into account the allergens suggested by the history. A positive and negative control skin test, using histamine and saline, respectively, is performed with each set of skin tests. A negative control is necessary to ensure that the patient is not dermatographic and that reactions caused merely by applying pressure to overly sensitive skin are not interpreted as due to allergen sensitivity. A positive control is necessary to establish the presence of a cutaneous response to histamine. Medications with antihistaminic properties in addition to adrenergic agents such as ephedrine and epinephrine suppress skin test responses and should be avoided for appropriate intervals before the placement of skin tests. Prolonged courses of systemic corticosteroids may suppress cutaneous reactivity by decreasing the number of tissue mast cells as well as their ability to release mediators.

Under certain circumstances, **provocation testing** is performed to examine the association between allergen exposure and the development of symptoms. Provocation challenges involving exposure of the skin, conjunctiva, nasal mucosa, oral mucosa, gastrointestinal tract, or lungs to allergens are performed in a variety of clinical and research settings. Bronchial provocation challenges are performed by having patients inhale increasingly concentrated solutions of nebulized allergen extracts and monitoring for airways obstruction by clinical observation and the performance of pulmonary function testing. Results of bronchial provocation challenges correlate well with other clinical data obtained by skin testing or in vitro testing. Although a large number of bronchial provocation challenges to allergens have been performed safely, the possibility of a severe reaction and the time, expense, and expertise required for the performance of these tests limit their performance to a research setting.

The bronchial provocation test most frequently performed is to methacholine, which causes potent bronchoconstriction of asthmatic but not of normal airways. **Methacholine challenge testing** is performed to document the presence and degree of bronchial hyperreactivity in a patient suspected of having asthma. After baseline spirometry is obtained, increasing concentrations of nebulized methacholine are inhaled until a specified drop in lung function, such as a 20% decrease in FEV_1, occurs or the patient is able to tolerate the inhalation of a set concentration of methacholine, such as 25 mg/mL, without a significant decrease in lung function.

Oral **food challenges** are performed to determine if a specific food causes symptoms or if a suspected food can be added to the diet. Food challenges are performed to those foods incriminated by the history and results of skin tests and/or in vitro testing. These challenges may be performed in an open, single-blind, double-blind, or double-blind placebo-controlled fashion and involve the ingestion of gradually increasing amounts of the suspected food at set time intervals until the patient either experiences a reaction or tolerates a normal portion of the food openly. Because of the potential for significant allergic reactions, these challenges should only be performed in an appropriately equipped facility with personnel experienced in the performance of food challenges and the treatment of anaphylaxis, including cardiopulmonary resuscitation.

Adkinson NF Jr, Yunginger JW, Busse WW, et al (eds): *Middleton's Allergy: Principles & Practice*, 6th ed. Philadelphia, WB Saunders, 2003.

Beltrani VS: The clinical spectrum of atopic dermatitis. *J Allergy Clin Immunol* 1999;104:S87–S96.

Chusid MJ: Eosinophilia in childhood. *Immunol Allergy Clin North Am* 1999;19:327–346.

Hamilton RG, Adkinson NF Jr: In vitro assays for the diagnosis of IgE-mediated disorders. *J Allergy Clin Immunol* 2004;114:213–225.

Ownby DR: Skin tests in comparison with other diagnostic methods. *Immunol Allergy Clin North Am* 2001;21:355–367.

Tripathi A, Patterson R: Clinical interpretation of skin test results. *Immunol Allergy Clin North Am* 2001;21:291–300.

Chapter 141 ■ Principles of Treatment of Allergic Disease

Dan Atkins and Donald Y. M. Leung

The basic principles of the treatment of allergic disease include the avoidance of exposure to allergens and irritants that trigger symptoms and the pharmacologic management of symptoms caused by inadvertent acute and chronic allergen exposures. In selected patients with allergic disease refractory to avoidance measures and optimal pharmacologic management, allergen immunotherapy may be considered.

ENVIRONMENTAL CONTROL MEASURES

Children spend the majority of their time in indoor environments, including the home. In an effort to save energy, houses and buildings have been built tighter and more insulated with fewer air exchanges. This has led to an increase in indoor humidity and higher concentrations of allergens and irritants in indoor air. Examination of indoor environments suggests that house dust mite, cat, and cockroach allergens are the most common significant triggers of allergic disease in these settings; exposures to allergens from other pets, pests, fungi, and respiratory irritants such as cigarette smoke can also be a problem.

Over 30,000 species of mites have been identified, but the term *dust mites* usually refers to the pyroglyphid mites *Dermatophagoides pteronyssinus, Dermatophagoides farinae,* and *Euroglyphus maynei,* which are the major sources of allergen in house dust. Respiration and water vapor exchange occurs through the skin of dust mites, rendering them sensitive to decreases in humidity and temperature extremes. The regular use of humidifiers and swamp coolers promotes dust mite survival. Mites do not survive with relative humidity <50%. They feed on animal and human skin scales and other debris, which is why they exist in large numbers in mattresses and bedding, carpet, and upholstered furniture. They are also found in flour and mixes for baked goods. Anaphylaxis has been reported following the ingestion of baked goods such as waffles and pancakes prepared with flour infested with dust mites. Dust mite fecal pellets are a major source of allergens. They consist of partially digested food combined with digestive enzymes encased in a permeable membrane, which keeps the fecal pellets intact. These fecal pellets have been likened to pollen grains, given their similarities in size (10–40 μm), the amount of allergen they contain, and their ability to release allergens rapidly on contact with moist mucous membranes. Mites can persist in imported furnishings for at least 2 yr; mite allergens have been shown to remain stable under domestic conditions for periods of at least 4 yr. Dust mite allergens become airborne during normal household activities; a vigorous disturbance such as vacuuming without a vacuum bag or shaking a bed sheet can launch significant amounts of dust mite allergens into the air. Once airborne, dust mite allergen particles settle out of the air relatively rapidly because of their size and weight. Nonetheless, dust mite allergen exposure likely occurs during sleep on mite-infested pillows and mattresses and during normal household activities when dust mite concentrations in the home are high enough. Levels of dust mite allergens as low as 2 μg/g of house dust can lead to sensitization, whereas levels of 10 μg/g of house dust are associated with symptoms.

Appropriate environmental control measures can significantly reduce exposure to dust mite allergens (Table 141-1). Major emphasis should be placed on reducing exposure to dust mite allergens in the bedroom and the bed because of the large amount of time children spend there. Encasements impermeable to dust mite allergens should be placed on all pillows, the mattress, and the box spring. Dust should be removed from the surface of these covers and the bed frame by vacuuming them weekly. The sheets and mattress pad should be washed weekly in hot water at a temperature >130°F. Minimizing the number of items in the room that collect dust, such as books, drapes, toys, stuffed animals, and any clutter, is recommended. Major reservoirs of dust mite allergen often more difficult to deal with include the carpet and upholstered furniture. These should be vacuumed weekly with an efficient double-bagged vacuum cleaner. Although the application of acaricides or denaturing agents to carpets and upholstered furniture has been advised, the actual benefit remains unclear and the amount of effort required may be more than most families are willing to invest. If possible, carpet removal, at least in the bedroom, may prove a better choice for eliminating a large reservoir of dust mite allergen. Other measures for dust mite allergen control include maintaining the indoor relative humidity at <50% and keeping the air conditioning set at the lowest level during the warmer months.

In many countries, more than half of the households have pets, the most common of which are cats and dogs. The major sources of allergens from cats, dogs, horses, and cattle are hair, dander, and saliva, whereas the major source of rodent allergens is their urine. Studies of airborne cat allergen have shown that a significant portion is found on small particles that behave aerodynamically like spheres of <7 μm in diameter. As much as 30% of airborne cat allergen may reside on particles <5 μm. Particles this small may not be adequately filtered by the nose and could potentially be deposited in the airways. Their small size enables these particles to remain airborne for longer periods and to be suspended repeatedly by air currents from heating and ventilation systems or just by walking across the carpet or sitting in an upholstered chair. **Fel d 1**, the major cat allergen, is a highly charged protein that readily sticks to a variety of surfaces, including walls, carpeting, and upholstered furniture. Due to this adhesiveness, cat allergens bind to the cat owner's clothing and are routinely transported to public buildings, including schools, where they have been measured in moderately high amounts. From these sites, significant amounts of cat allergen can subsequently be carried into homes without cats. Analysis of house dust from homes with cats reveals levels of Fel d 1 ranging from 8 μg to 1.5 mg/g of house dust. Levels of Fel d 1 in homes without cats vary from 0.2 to 80 μg/g of house dust. Sensitization to cat allergen has been associated with levels ranging from 1 to 8 μg/g of house dust. Carpets, upholstered furniture, and bedding serve as reservoirs of cat allergens, resulting in the persistence of significant amounts in the home for months after a cat has been removed. Complete avoidance of cat allergen is virtually impossible, although significant reduction in exposure to cat allergens is achievable.

TABLE 141-1. Environmental Control of Allergen Exposure

ALLERGENS	CONTROL MEASURES
Dust mites	Encase bedding in airtight covers
	Wash bedding in water at temperatures >130°F
	Remove wall-to-wall carpeting
	Remove upholstered furniture
Animal dander	Avoid furred pets
	Keep animals out of patient's bedroom
Cockroaches	Control available food supply
	Keep kitchen/bathroom surfaces dry and free of standing water
	Professionally exterminate
Mold	Destroy moisture-prone areas
	Avoid high humidity in patient's bedroom
	Repair water leaks
	Check basements, attics, and crawl spaces for standing water and mold
Pollen	Keep automobile and house windows closed
	Control timing of outdoor exposure
	Restrict camping, hiking, and raking leaves
	Drive in air-conditioned automobile
	Air-condition the home
	Install portable, high-efficiency particular air filters

From Leung DYM, Sampson HA, Geha RS, et al: *Pediatric Allergy Principles and Practice.* St. Louis, Mosby, 2003, p 294.

Removing the pet from the home is obviously the most effective means of reducing exposure to animal allergens, although it has been demonstrated that without other interventions, such as removing carpeting and upholstered furniture and wiping down walls, it takes 6 mo or more for the levels of cat allergen to drop to a level found in houses without a cat. As a result, cat owners who remove their pets from their homes should be informed not to expect immediate results. Unfortunately, advice to remove a pet from the home or keep it outdoors is often ignored. In contrast to dust mite allergens, cat allergen is light and remains suspended in the air for long periods of time. As a result, **HEPA-filtered air cleaners** are helpful in reducing the amount of airborne cat allergen. Other suggested methods include washing the cat regularly and maintaining a cat allergen free bedroom from which the cat is excluded and where mattress covers and air-filtering devices are used. The cat should also be restricted from other living areas where the sensitized child spends large amounts of time, such as the family room or other play areas (see Table 141-1). Regular vacuuming with a HEPA-filtered and double-thickness bag vacuum cleaner is also encouraged. Similar measures are suggested for the control of exposure to other animal allergens, although whether these measures reduce exposure to levels resulting in clinical improvement as demonstrated by decreased symptoms, improved peak flows, or decreases in bronchial hyperreactivity remains to be documented by appropriately controlled studies.

Infestation of the home by insects and other pests such as mice and rats is another potential source of significant allergen exposure in the indoor environment. Studies have identified the importance of exposure to cockroach allergens as a major risk factor for the development of asthma in inner-city children. Once sensitized, inner-city cockroach-sensitive asthmatic children with continued exposure to high levels of cockroach allergens in their bedrooms are at higher risk for urgent care visits and hospitalization than inner-city asthmatic children who are not allergic to cockroaches. Recommended methods to decrease cockroach allergen exposure include reducing access to the home by sealing cracks in the flooring and walls and removing sources of food and water by repairing leaky pipes, putting away food, and frequent cleaning (see Table 141-1). Regular extermination using baits or chemical treatment of infested areas is also advised.

Efforts to improve indoor air quality should also encompass reducing exposure to respiratory irritants. Passive exposure to environmental tobacco smoke worsens asthma and increases nasal symptoms in patients with allergic nasal disease. Smoking cessation should be repeatedly encouraged and smoking indoors should never be permitted. The use of wood-burning stoves and fireplaces and kerosene heaters should be discouraged.

Although exposure to pollens and fungi occurs primarily outdoors, these allergens are detectable indoors during the warmer months when their levels indoors often reflect their prevalence in the outdoor environment. During the winter, when the outdoor levels of other fungi are lowest, the indoor fungi *Aspergillus* and *Penicillium* are the most prevalent. Fungi are often found in damp basements and thrive in conditions associated with increased moisture in the home, such as water leaks, flooding, or increased humidity promoted by the excessive use of humidifiers or swamp coolers. Exposure to indoor fungal allergens can be reduced by maintaining the indoor relative humidity at <50%, removing contaminated carpets, and wiping down washable surfaces prone to fungal growth such as shower stalls, shower curtains, sinks, drip trays, and garbage pails, using solutions of detergent and 5% bleach (see Table 141-1). Dehumidifiers should be placed in damp basements. Standing water at any site in the home should be eliminated and the cause addressed. Removing all items from the home that are prone to fungal contamination and growth is also encouraged. Keeping the windows and doors closed and using air conditioning to filter outdoor air can keep both indoor pollen and fungi levels to a minimum during the warmer months when outdoor levels of these allergens are at their peak. The use of window or attic fans is to be avoided. Laundry should be dried in a dryer rather than on a clothesline. Measures to avoid pollens and fungal spores when out of the house include closing the windows and using the air conditioner when traveling in the car, avoiding moldy vegetation, and wearing a mask when these materials cannot be avoided. Outdoor activities during periods of high pollen counts should be kept to a minimum. Someone other than the sensitized patient should mow the lawn and rake leaves. Frequent handwashing after outdoor play is suggested to avoid transferring pollens from the hands to the eyes and nose. At the end of the day, showering and shampooing is suggested to avoid contamination of the bed with allergens. During the day, the bed should remain covered with a bedspread.

PHARMACOLOGIC THERAPY

ADRENERGIC AGENTS. Adrenergic agents exert their effects through the stimulation of cell surface α- and β-adrenergic receptors in a variety of target tissues. These receptors belong to the G protein–coupled superfamily of receptors. In general, α-adrenergic receptor stimulation results in excitatory responses such as vasoconstriction, whereas β-adrenergic stimulation leads to inhibitory responses such as bronchodilation. The α-adrenergic receptors have been classified into α_1- and α_2-adrenergic receptors. Further studies of these receptors in humans have identified three subtypes of α_1-adrenergic receptors and three subtypes of α_2-adrenergic receptors. The β-adrenergic receptors are further divided into three subtypes: β_1, β_2, and β_3. Each of these adrenergic receptors exhibits a distinctive tissue distribution. The physiologic response in a given tissue to the administration of an adrenergic agent depends on the specific receptor binding characteristics of the drug as well as the number and distribution of the various types of adrenergic receptors in the tissue. Epinephrine remains the drug of choice for the treatment of anaphylaxis because of its combined α- and β-adrenergic effects.

The α-adrenergic agents are effective in the treatment of allergic nasal disease because of their decongestant effects (see Tables 142-2 and 142-4). In the nose, stimulation of α_1-adrenergic receptors on postcapillary venules and α_2-adrenergic receptors on precapillary arterioles leads to vasoconstriction, resulting in a reduction in nasal congestion. The oral decongestants used clinically include pseudoephedrine, phenylephrine, and phenylpropanolamine. These medications are available individually or in combination with antihistamines in liquid and tablet forms, including sustained-release preparations; steps are being taken to discontinue the use of phenylpropanolamine due to concerns about the risk of hemorrhagic stroke. Pseudoephedrine and phenylpropanolamine are rapidly and thoroughly absorbed, whereas phenylephrine, the less effective of the three drugs, is incompletely absorbed, resulting in a significantly lower bioavailability of ≈38%. Peak plasma concentrations of these drugs are reached between 30 min and 2 hr of administration, but the decongestant effect has not been directly correlated to the plasma concentration. Pseudoephedrine and phenylpropanolamine are excreted essentially unchanged by the kidney. The use of oral decongestants should be avoided in patients with hypertension, coronary artery disease, glaucoma, or metabolic disorders such as diabetes or hyperthyroidism. Reported **adverse effects** of oral decongestants include excitability, headache, nervousness, palpitations, tachycardia, arrhythmias, hypertension, nausea, vomiting, and urinary retention. Decongestants available as topical nasal sprays include phenylephrine, oxymetazoline, naphthazoline, tetrahydrozoline, and xylometazoline. Given their efficacy and rapid onset of action, the potential for excessive use of topical nasal decongestants resulting in rebound nasal congestion is high. When this occurs, refraining from the use of these sprays for 2–3 days is necessary for recovery.

Drugs that stimulate β-adrenergic receptors have been used for years in the treatment of asthma because of their potent bronchodilator effects (see Table 143-9). The subclassification of β-adrenergic receptors into β_1 and β_2 subtypes led to the development of drugs selective for the β_2-adrenergic receptor, such as albuterol, that have the advantage of producing significant bronchodilation with less cardiac stimulation. The long-acting inhaled β_2-adrenergic agonists salmeterol and formoterol, with a 12 hr duration of action, are approved for use in children ≥4 yrs of age. Dry powder inhaled preparations that combine a long-acting β_2-adrenergic agonist with an inhaled corticosteroid have had significant impact on the treatment of children with moderate persistent asthma. In addition to their bronchodilating effects, β_2-adrenergic agonists have been reported to improve mucociliary clearance, decrease microvascular permeability, inhibit cholinergic nerve transmission, and reduce mediator release in mast cells, basophils, and eosinophils. The β-adrenergic agonists can be delivered orally, by inhalation, or by injection. The inhaled route is preferred because of the rapid onset of action and fewer adverse effects. Reported **adverse effects** of β-adrenergics agents include tremor, palpitations, tachycardia, arrhythmias, central nervous system stimulation, hyperglycemia, hypokalemia, hypomagnesemia, and a transient increase in hypoxia, which is attributed to an increase in perfusion to inadequately ventilated areas of the asthmatic lung. Levalbuterol, the stereoisomer of albuterol developed to reduce the adverse effects of short-acting β-agonists is clinically comparable to fourfold higher doses of racemic albuterol while exhibiting a preferable safety profile. Levalbuterol is formulated as a nebulized preparation, but a metered dose inhaler preparation is expected soon.

ANTICHOLINERGIC AGENTS. These drugs inhibit vagally mediated reflexes by antagonizing the action of acetylcholine at muscarinic receptors. Of the available anticholinergic agents, **ipratropium bromide** is the most commonly used. It is a quaternary amine that is poorly absorbed across mucosal surfaces and does not readily cross the blood-brain barrier. As a bronchodilator, it has a slower onset of action than short-acting inhaled β_2-agonists and takes longer to reach maximal effect, which makes it less effective as a rescue medication. Ipratropium is available by prescription as a metered-dose inhaler delivering 18 µg/spray and as a 0.02% nebulized solution (500 µg/2.5 mL). Inhaled anticholinergics have very few adverse effects, although they occasionally trigger coughing.

Ipratropium given as a nasal spray (0.03–0.06%) has been shown to be effective in the reduction of rhinorrhea resulting from perennial nonallergic rhinitis, the common cold, or other triggers such as exposure to irritants or cold air. The use of ipratropium is limited in the treatment of moderate to severe allergic rhinitis because it does not alter other common allergic nasal symptoms, such as sneezing, nasal congestion, or pruritus. Nasal dryness and epistaxis are occasionally encountered with use of the nasal spray.

ANTIHISTAMINES. The release of histamine and its effects on surrounding tissues is central to the development of symptoms classically associated with the allergic response. As a result, antihistamines are frequently used for the treatment of allergic disease. Histamine exerts its effects through binding with one of its three receptors, referred to as H_1-, H_2-, or H_3-receptors. Histamine effects triggered through H_1-receptor binding are those most relevant to allergic inflammation and include pain, pruritus, vasodilation, increased vascular permeability, smooth muscle contraction, mucus production, and the stimulation of parasympathetic nerve endings and reflexes. The human H_1-receptor gene has been mapped to the distal short arm of chromosome 3. The antimuscarinic effect of some of the early H_1-type antihistamines may be explained by the reported 45% homology of the H_1-receptor with the human muscarinic receptor. The H_1-type antihistamines prevent the effects of H_1-receptor activation through reversible, competitive inhibition of histamine by binding to the H_1-receptor. As a result, antihistamines work best in preventing rather than reversing the actions of histamine and are most effective when given at doses and dosing intervals resulting in the persistent saturation of target organ tissue histamine receptors.

The H_1-type antihistamines are traditionally divided into six classes based on differences in their chemical structures (Tables 141-2 and 142-2). These antihistamines are further divided into 1st-generation antihistamines, which, because of their lipophilicity, cross the blood-brain barrier to exert effects on the central nervous system, and 2nd-generation antihistamines, which exert minimal, if any, central nervous system effects because of their inability to cross the blood-brain barrier owing to their size, charge, and lipophobicity. The sedative effects and cognitive impairment associated with the use of 1st-generation antihistamines are well documented. Thus, one of the primary advantages of 2nd-generation antihistamines is that they are nonsedating or much less so than 1st-generation antihistamines. Both 1st- and 2nd-generation antihistamines are available in oral preparations. A number of 1st-generation antihistamines are available over the counter, whereas loratadine is currently the only 2nd-generation antihistamine available without a prescription. Other 1st-generation and 2nd-generation antihistamines require a prescription. The only antihistamine available as an intranasal spray is azelastine. The benefit of this form of administration is the potential for a rapid onset of action within 15–30 min. Azelastine, which is systemically absorbed and can cross the blood-brain barrier, causes central nervous system effects in some patients and is not currently approved for use in children <12 yr of age.

Orally administered antihistamines are well absorbed and reach peak serum concentrations within ≈2 hr. High tissue concentrations of antihistamines are usually achieved, which likely accounts for the sustained suppression of wheal and flare reactions even after serum levels have significantly declined. Most antihistamines are metabolized by the hepatic cytochrome P450 enzyme system. Elimination of antihistamines may be reduced in patients with hepatic impairment or by the simultaneous ingestion of inhibitors of this pathway, such as erythromycin and other macrolide antibiotics, ciprofloxacin, ketoconazole, itraconazole, and certain antidepressants such as nefazodone and fluvoxamine. Some antihistamines such as hydroxyzine and loratadine are converted to clinically active metabolites. Clearance of fexofenadine and cetirizine is reduced in patients with impaired renal function. Cetirizine clearance is also reduced in patients with hepatic dysfunction.

The efficacy of antihistamines in the treatment of seasonal and perennial allergic rhinoconjunctivitis is well documented (see Chapter 142). When compared with other medications in regard to the relief of allergic nasal symptoms, antihistamines are more effective than cromolyn sodium but significantly less effective than intranasal corticosteroids. Improvement in symptom relief in patients with allergic rhinitis has been reported when an antihistamine is given in combination with a decongestant or with an intranasal steroid. Numerous formulations combining antihistamines and decongestants are available. Antihistamines have also been shown to be beneficial in the treatment of acute and chronic urticaria/angioedema. With regard to asthma, a significant clinical effect of antihistamines at conventional doses is difficult to document, other than the possible improvement offered by better control of allergic nasal symptoms.

The 2nd-generation antihistamines are often chosen for the treatment of allergic disease in children because of negligible sedative and anticholinergic effects in comparison to 1st-generation antihistamines without a sacrifice in efficacy. Most 2nd-generation antihistamines are effective with once-daily dosing, which, because of the convenience, may improve adherence. The widespread availability of 1st-generation antihistamines and their lower cost result in their continued use. The **adverse effects** most often encountered include the performance impairment and anticholinergic effects noted with the use of 1st-generation antihistamines. The anticholinergic adverse effects encountered may include drying of the mouth and eyes, urinary retention, constipation, excitation, nervousness, palpitations, and tachycardia. Prolongation of the QT interval and ventricular tachycardia (torsades de pointes) was reported in association with the use of two 2nd-generation antihistamines that have since been removed from the market; those currently in use have not been associated with concerning cardiac effects.

TABLE 141-2. Classification of Antihistamines (H_1-antagonists)

CLASS	EXAMPLES
ETHYLENEDIAMINES	
First generation	Antazoline, pyrilamine, tripelennamine
TYPE II ETHANOLAMINES	
First generation	Carbinoxamine, clemastine, diphenhydramine
TYPE III ALKYLAMINES	
First generation	Brompheniramine, chlorpheniramine, triprolidine
Second generation	Acrivastine
TYPE IV PIPERAZINES	
First generation	Cyclizine, hydroxyzine, meclizine
Second generation	Cetirizine
TYPE V PIPERIDINES	
First generation	Azatadine, cyproheptadine
Second generation	Fexofenadine, loratadine
TYPE VI PHENOTHIAZINES	
First generation	Methdilazine, promethazine

CHROMONES. Cromolyn sodium, the disodium salt of 1,3-bis (2-carboxychromon-5-yloxy)-2-hydroxypropane, and nedocromil sodium, a pyranoquinoline dicarboxylic acid, are the two chromones used to treat allergic disorders. Neither cromolyn nor nedocromil is absorbed well orally, with only 1% of the swallowed dose absorbed. Absorbed drug is not metabolized but is rapidly eliminated in approximately equal amounts by the kidneys and liver. These drugs must be applied topically to the mucosal surface of the target organ to be effective. Both drugs inhibit mast cell degranulation and mediator release. They suppress the activation of a variety of cells such as eosinophils, neutrophils, macrophages, and epithelial cells. They also suppress the activity of afferent C–type sensory nerve fibers of the nonadrenergic, noncholinergic nervous system. Both drugs inhibit the intracellular increase in free calcium after mast cell activation and phosphorylate a mast cell protein resembling moesin, which is thought to be involved in terminating mediator release. Despite these findings, the molecular mechanism of action of these drugs remains to be completely defined.

Cromolyn and nedocromil prevent early and late-phase allergic responses when administered before allergen exposure. They block allergen-induced increases in bronchial hyperresponsiveness as well as seasonal increases in nonspecific bronchial hyperresponsiveness. With prolonged use, both drugs are capable of reducing bronchial hyperresponsiveness. These drugs have no bronchodilator properties but can inhibit the bronchoconstrictive effects of a variety of stimuli, such as allergen challenge, exercise, hyperventilation with cold air, ultrasonically nebulized distilled water, and exposure to atmospheric and industrial pollutants.

Cromolyn and nedocromil are used as alternative, but not preferred, therapy for the treatment of mild persistent asthma. Because of their lack of bronchodilator properties, neither drug is useful for the treatment of acute asthma although both may be used as preventive treatment before vigorous exercise or unavoidable known allergen exposure. Nedocromil is the more potent of the two. Cromolyn is available for the treatment of asthma by prescription as a 1% solution (20 mg/2 mL) for nebulization and as a metered-dose inhaler (800 µg/actuation). The suggested dose for the treatment of asthma is 20 mg of cromolyn 2 to 4 times/24 hr by nebulization or 1.6 mg 2 to 4 times/24 hr by metered-dose inhaler. In numerous studies, cromolyn is useful in the treatment of allergic rhinitis and allergic conjunctivitis. Preparations for the nasal and ocular administration of cromolyn are available without a prescription. The suggested dose for the treatment of allergic rhinitis is one spray in each nostril 3 to 4 times daily of a nasal spray containing 5.2 mg of cromolyn per spray (see Table 142-4). For the treatment of allergic conjunctivitis, the suggested dose is 1 drop in each eye 4 to 6 times a day of a 4% ophthalmic solution. Nedocromil is not available in a nebulized form but is available by metered-dose inhaler. The recommended dose for the treatment of asthma is 3.5 mg (1.75 mg/puff) 2 to 4 times/24 hr. A 2% solution of nedocromil is available by prescription for the treatment of allergic conjunctivitis at a suggested dose of 1–2 drops in each eye twice daily.

The safety of these drugs, even with prolonged administration, is well documented. Dry throat and transient bronchoconstriction have been the most frequently reported adverse effects of cromolyn use for the treatment of asthma, with only rare reports of patients becoming sensitized to the drug. Some patients using nedocromil complain about its taste. Infrequently reported adverse effects of nedocromil include coughing, sore throat, rhinitis, headache, and nausea.

GLUCOCORTICOIDS. These are widely used in the treatment of allergic disorders because of their potent anti-inflammatory properties. The diverse anti-inflammatory actions of glucocorticoids are mediated via the glucocorticoid receptor, which is present in all inflammatory effector cells, as well as by direct inhibition of cytokines and mediators. Glucocorticoids are administered topically in ophthalmic preparations, nasal sprays, creams and ointments, metered-dose inhalers, and as a solution for nebulization. Systemic administration is accomplished orally or parenterally. The proper use and efficacy of glucocorticoids in the treatment of allergic disease along with the adverse effects associated with their use are presented in discussions of individual allergic diseases (see Chapters 142–151).

LEUKOTRIENE-MODIFYING AGENTS. Drugs that alter the leukotriene pathway exert their clinical effects either by inhibiting leukotriene production or blocking receptor binding. These agents possess mild anti-inflammatory properties and exhibit bronchodilator effects. In addition to inhibiting the early- and late-phase allergic response to inhaled allergen, they diminish bronchoconstriction induced by exercise and exposure to allergen, aspirin, and cold air. These agents have some use in the treatment of asthma (see Chapter 143) and are modestly effective in the treatment of allergic rhinitis (see Chapter 142).

THEOPHYLLINE. Because of its bronchodilating effects, theophylline (1,3-dimethyxanthine) has been used for years for the treatment of acute and chronic asthma. Nonspecific inhibition of phosphodiesterase isozymes and antagonism of adenosine receptors occur at achievable serum concentrations of the drug. The bronchodilator effect of theophylline is likely caused by its action as a phosphodiesterase inhibitor, whereas its ability to antagonize adenosine receptors may play a role in other effects, such as the attenuation of diaphragmatic muscle fatigue and diminishing adenosine-enhanced mast cell mediator release. Theophylline inhibits the immediate- and late-phase pulmonary response to allergen challenge and exhibits modest protective effects. Selected anti-inflammatory and immunomodulatory effects of this drug are also documented. Theophylline is available by prescription as both rapidly absorbed and slow-release formulations. It is often administered intravenously when used for the treatment of severe acute asthma. The therapeutic and toxic effects of theophylline are related to the serum concentration, with the incidence of toxic effects significantly increasing as the serum levels approach and exceed 20 µg/mL. A variety of conditions and medications are capable of increasing or decreasing theophylline metabolism. The **toxic effects** of theophylline ranging from mild nausea, insomnia, irritability, tremors, and headache to cardiac arrhythmias, seizures, and death necessitate the routine monitoring of theophylline levels. Because of the introduction of other effective therapies for the treatment of acute and chronic asthma, the need to monitor theophylline levels routinely, and the potential for significant toxicity, the role of theophylline in the treatment of asthma has contracted significantly (see Chapter 143).

LODOXAMIDE TROMETHAMINE. This mast cell stabilizer is more effective than topical cromolyn sodium in alleviating signs and symptoms of allergic ocular disease (see Chapter 146). It is used in children >2 yr of age for vernal keratoconjunctivitis, vernal conjunctivitis, and vernal keratitis. Occasional adverse effects have included transient burning or stinging after instillation.

OLOPATADINE HYDROCHLORIDE. This is both a mast cell stabilizer and an H_1-receptor antagonist effective in relieving signs and symptoms of allergic conjunctivitis after topical instillation. It is labeled for use in children at least 3 yr of age. Headaches have occurred in 7% of patients treated; burning and stinging have occurred in <5%.

ANTI-IgE. Monoclonal anti-IgE antibodies (anti-IgE) bind to circulating IgE at a site that prevents its subsequent attachment to the high affinity receptors for IgE on the mast cell surface. The parenteral administration of anti-IgE reduces free serum IgE concentrations, inhibits skin test responses in allergic patients, suppresses early- and late-phase responses to allergens, and decreases sputum eosinophilia in asthmatics. There is a beneficial effect of anti-IgE in the treatment of patients with allergic rhinitis and asthma. An anti-IgE preparation (**omalizumab**) is available for the treatment of children ≥12 yr of age with documented allergen induced asthma and inadequate control with inhaled corticosteroids. Serious adverse effects have not been encountered with this therapy. Anti-IgE may also be beneficial in the treatment of other allergic disorders such as anaphylaxis and food allergy. One monoclonal anti-IgE antibody preparation used in the treatment of adults with peanut allergy resulted in a significant increase in their symptom threshold dose of peanuts. Omalizumab is under study for its efficacy in the treatment of peanut allergy in children and adults. The cost of anti-IgE therapy requires careful patient selection with special consideration for those patients with persistent symptoms despite aggressive pharmacotherapy, significant adverse effects of their current therapy, and more than one allergic disorder.

NEW AND FUTURE THERAPIES. Several strategies for inhibiting the actions of proinflammatory cytokines are under investigation. Approaches include the use of recombinant soluble receptors that attach to a specific cytokine and inhibit subsequent binding to cell surface receptors, the development of specific cytokine receptor antagonists, and the administration of humanized monoclonal anticytokine antibodies. Recombinant soluble IL-4 receptor antagonists exert their effects by binding to and inactivating IL-4 before it can attach to its cell surface receptor. Although initial studies of an inhaled soluble IL-4 receptor in patients with moderate asthma requiring inhaled corticosteroids suggested a beneficial clinical effect, subsequent clinical studies of the effects of anti–IL-4 drugs in the treatment of asthma revealed these therapies to be safe, but clinical efficacy was lacking. A human IL-4 receptor antibody designed to inhibit the signaling of IL-4 and IL-13 is under investigation in preclinical studies. Clinical trials of humanized monoclonal anti–IL-5 antibodies administered by injection to asthmatic patients revealed a decrease in circulating eosinophils and sputum eosinophilia, but a lesser reduction of eosinophils from the bronchial submucosa and this effect was unaccompanied by a reduction in methacholine reactivity or a suppression of the early- or late-phase response to allergen.

The use of cytokines with anti-inflammatory effects in the treatment of allergic disorders is under investigation. Unfortunately, initial studies have not demonstrated a beneficial effect of IL-10 or interferons in the treatment of asthma. Although studies have documented that IL-12 administration is associated with a decrease in eosinophil accumulation in response to allergen challenge, inhibition of early- and late-phase responses to allergen or decreases in bronchial hyperreactivity have not been observed. In addition, the high incidence of significant adverse effects encountered with IL-12 administration limits its potential as a viable therapeutic option.

ALLERGEN IMMUNOTHERAPY

Allergen immunotherapy involves administering gradually increasing doses of allergens to a person with allergic disease for the purpose of reducing or eliminating the patient's adverse clinical response on subsequent natural exposure to those allergens. When properly administered to an appropriate candidate, allergen immunotherapy is a safe, effective form of therapy capable not only of reducing or preventing symptoms, but of potentially altering the natural history of the disease by minimizing disease duration and preventing disease progression.

INDICATIONS AND CONTRAINDICATIONS. Allergen immunotherapy is reserved for patients with an allergic disease demonstrated to respond to this form of therapy, such as seasonal or perennial allergic rhinoconjunctivitis, asthma triggered by allergen exposures, and insect venom sensitivity. Proof of the efficacy of conventional allergen immunotherapy for the treatment of food allergy, latex allergy, or acute or chronic urticaria is lacking and, therefore, allergen immunotherapy is not recommended for the treatment of these disorders. Before considering allergen immunotherapy, sensitivity of the patient to the allergens to be administered should be documented by a positive skin test or an in vitro test revealing an increased serum level of allergen-specific IgE. The clinical relevance of these allergens should be supported by a history of symptoms on known exposure or a timing of symptoms that correlates well with suspected allergen exposure, such as the presence of allergic nasal and ocular symptoms throughout the late summer and fall in a child with a large positive ragweed skin test. The duration and severity of the patient's symptoms should warrant the expense, effort, and risk associated with the administration of allergen immunotherapy. The presence of disabling symptoms in spite of a trial of allergen avoidance and appropriate medications at a suitable dose should be documented. For patients sensitized to seasonal allergens, more than two consecutive seasons of symptoms are usually required before allergen immunotherapy is recommended unless the symptoms are unusually severe or the adverse effects of medication are unacceptable. The obvious exception to this rule is the child with insect sting anaphylaxis who should be started on venom immunotherapy once the sensitivity is correctly diagnosed (see Chapter 145).

Other factors that may affect the decision to institute allergen immunotherapy include quality of life issues such as the amount of school missed or medical resource utilization, the age of the patient, and other logistical factors. With the exception of venom immunotherapy, few data for the efficacy of allergen immunotherapy in children <5 yr of age are available. Allergen immunotherapy is not recommended for children <5 yr of age because of their increased risk of systemic reactions, the special expertise required to treat anaphylaxis in this age group, their potential inability to communicate clearly with their physician in the event of an allergic reaction, and their age-related potential for emotional distress with frequent injections. Other important logistic factors include the willingness of the patient to comply with a schedule of frequent injections over the course of several years, cost considerations, and the availability of an appropriate setting for the administering allergen immunotherapy.

Allergen immunotherapy is **contraindicated** in children on β-blocker therapy as well as those with certain immunologic or autoimmune disorders, allergic bronchopulmonary aspergillosis, hypersensitivity pneumonitis, severe psychiatric disturbance, or a medical condition that would impair the ability to survive an allergic reaction. Pregnancy is a contraindication for the initiation of allergen immunotherapy or dosing increases, although pregnant adolescents can continue to receive their usual maintenance dose. Patients with unstable asthma should not be placed on allergen immunotherapy because of their increased risk for fatal anaphylaxis. Allergen immunotherapy is not used for the treatment of allergic bronchopulmonary aspergillosis or hypersensitivity pneumonitis because it has no benefit. Children on β-blockers should be switched to another form of therapy before allergen immunotherapy is considered because of an increased intensity of allergic reactions and a poor response of conventional therapy to these reactions. Allergen immunotherapy is usually avoided for patients with autoimmune disorders because of the potential for unanticipated stimulation of the immune system, resulting in disease activation.

ALLERGEN EXTRACTS. The potency of the aqueous extracts used in allergen immunotherapy is affected by numerous factors. Allergens from weed and grass pollens are more easily extracted in aqueous solutions and, as a result, are more potent than extracts obtained from other sources, such as molds, tree pollens, and dust mites. Due to their complexity, allergen extracts from fungal allergens are more variable than extracts from pollen allergens. Refrigeration and appropriate handling of allergen extracts used in allergen immunotherapy are important because degradation of many allergen extracts, such as those from tree, grass, and weed pollens and dust mites, may occur at higher temperatures. Dilute extracts are more susceptible to loss of potency resulting from adherence of allergen to the glass vial than are more concentrated extracts. To combat this effect, human serum albumin is sometimes added to dilute allergen extracts. Some allergen extracts, such as those from cockroaches, dust mites, and fungi, contain proteases capable of degrading other allergens in the extract. As a result, it is often recommended that these allergens not be mixed with those from tree, grass, and weed pollens. Insect venoms are never mixed with other allergens. When available, the use of standardized allergen extracts is preferred to ensure consistency in dosing and to avoid the variability in allergen content encountered with allergen extracts that are not standardized.

ALLERGEN EXTRACT ADMINISTRATION. The goal of allergen immunotherapy is to increase gradually the dose of allergen extract administered until the injection of an "optimal" maintenance dose containing 4–12 µg of each major allergen in the extract is reached. The mixture of allergen extracts administered during the course of allergen immunotherapy is individually formulated for each patient based on their documented sensitivities. Although various dosing schedules are used, initial injections are most often given at 5–10 day intervals year-round. Schedules of allergen administration are selected based on the sensitivity of the patient to the allergens in the extract. The most sensitive patients are advanced to maintenance dose more gradually. Doses of allergen immunotherapy are increased according to a set schedule while taking into account the reaction to the previous injection. A systemic reaction to the previous dose would result in a significant reduction in the next dose, whereas reducing the dose based solely on a local reaction does not reduce the rate of systemic reactions. Usually 5–6 mo of weekly injections are required to reach the maintenance dose, although it may take longer in patients with marked sensitivity. Unique schedules for the administration of insect venoms, which differ from those for the administration of other allergens (see Chapter 145), are used. Once the maintenance dose is reached and well tolerated, the time interval between injections is increased to every few weeks to once a month. Because allergen extracts gradually lose potency, the 1st dose from a fresh replacement vial of maintenance allergen extract is reduced from 25–75% and increased in increments weekly until the usual maintenance dose is reached. The recommended length of a course of allergen immunotherapy is 3–5 yr. Insect venom immunotherapy may be continued longer in patients with histories of life-threatening anaphylaxis. Patients who have not improved after 1 yr of receiving maintenance doses of an appropriate allergen extract are unlikely to benefit and should have their allergen immunotherapy discontinued. Most patients enjoy a sustained improvement after allergen immunotherapy, whereas others experience a gradual return of symptoms. Those who experience a relapse may respond to another course of treatment.

Rush immunotherapy is the administration of multiple injections either in a single day or over several days in an attempt to reach maintenance dose more rapidly. The risk of adverse reactions, including systemic reactions, is higher than with traditional allergen immunotherapy schedules. These patients are often pretreated with antihistamines and corticosteroids. Children are at even greater risk for adverse reactions with rush immunotherapy and the benefits vs the risks should be fully considered.

Although allergen immunotherapy is regarded as safe, the potential for anaphylaxis always exists when patients are injected with extracts containing allergens to which they are sensitized. Allergen immunotherapy should only be offered in medical settings where a physician with access to emergency equipment and medications required for the treatment of anaphylaxis is available (see Chapter 148). Allergy shots should never be given at home or by untrained personnel. Patients should remain in the office for 30 min after the injection because most reactions to allergen immunotherapy begin within this time frame. Fatal anaphylaxis triggered by allergen immunotherapy, although rare, is estimated to occur at an incidence of 1 per 2 million injections. The risk of an adverse reaction is increased by dosage errors and the use of rush immunotherapy schedules. Particular caution is warranted when injections from a new vial are given. Patients with exquisite sensitivity, unstable asthma, or those experiencing exacerbations of allergic rhinitis or asthma are also at increased risk for adverse reactions. Allergen immunotherapy is **contraindicated** for patients taking β-blockers. Precautions to reduce significant adverse reactions include using standardized extracts, allowing only trained personnel to administer injections, paying careful attention to detail when giving injections, ensuring beforehand that the patient is medically stable, having appropriate medications and equipment available, and requiring the patient to remain in the office for 30 min after each injection. Checking peak flows or spirometry before an injection is advisable for some asthmatic patients.

Local nasal immunotherapy is administered by having the patient spray allergen solutions into the nose at scheduled intervals. Although symptom amelioration has been noted, a lack of a significant systemic immunologic response has decreased interest in pursuing this form of therapy. Oral immunotherapy involves the sublingual administration of high-dose allergen, which is then swallowed. The use of this form of immunotherapy is likely to increase in the near future. A desire to decrease the likelihood of allergic reactions induced by the administration of aqueous allergens led to the development of alum-precipitated extracts in which the proteins are precipitated with aluminum hydroxide and alum-precipitated pyridine-extracted extracts. Because of the smaller number of available extracts, their use remains limited. Another method developed to reduce allergenicity while maintaining immunogenicity is the polymerization of allergen extracts with glutaraldehyde. When these extracts are used, the maintenance dose can be reached within 2 mo with a markedly reduced incidence of systemic reactions. These extracts have not yet been approved for use in the United States. Other approaches to immunotherapy including chemical or genetic manipulation of the allergen or linking the principle allergenic moiety of a relevant allergen to a highly active adjuvant, such as an immunostimulatory sequence mimicking patterns of bacterial DNA, are under investigation.

EFFICACY. The positive impact of allergen immunotherapy on seasonal or perennial allergic rhinitis or rhinoconjunctivitis is well documented. In regard to the treatment of allergic rhinitis, birch, mountain cedar, grass, ragweed, and *Cladosporium* are allergens for which the efficacy of allergen immunotherapy has been effective. Allergen immunotherapy with other allergens commonly used for the treatment of allergic rhinitis is inconclusive. As with allergic rhinitis, most of the controlled trials examining the effects of allergen immunotherapy on seasonal or perennial allergic asthma also report favorable results. A meta-analysis of 20 trials examining the effects of allergen immunotherapy on allergic asthma revealed a significant increase in the odds for improvement after treatment along with fewer symptoms, improved pulmonary functions, less need for medication, and a reduction in bronchial hyperreactivity. The most convincing data for the benefit of allergen immunotherapy in the treatment of allergic asthma are available for birch, mountain cedar, grass, ragweed, and dust mite, with less conclusive, but suggestive data available for *Cladosporium, Alternaria,* and cat allergens. Studies examining the effects of allergen immunotherapy in the treatment of patients with allergic rhinitis and allergic asthma have usually documented increases in circulating allergen-specific IgG and decreases in allergen-specific IgE after treatment. Reductions in sensitivity to administered allergens have been demonstrated in nasal and bronchial challenges. These studies have often shown that the late-phase response after allergen challenge is ablated or significantly reduced. The protective benefit as well as the safety of venom immunotherapy in patients with sensitivity to Hymenoptera venoms has also been well documented in several large studies. The efficacy of allergen immunotherapy for the treatment of food allergy, atopic dermatitis, urticaria, and latex allergy has not been documented.

Adkinson NF Jr, Yunginger JW, Busse WW, et al (eds): *Middleton's Allergy: Principles & Practice,* 6th ed. Philadelphia, WB Saunders, 2003.

Bernstein DI, Wanner M, Borish L, et al: Twelve-year survey of fatal reactions to allergen injections and skin testing: 1990–2001. *J Allergy Clin Immunol* 2004;113:1129–1136.

Broide DH: Molecular and cellular mechanisms of allergic disease. *J Allergy Clin Immunol* 2001;108:S65–S71.

Creticos PS, Chen YH, Schroeder JT: New approaches in immunotherapy: Allergen vaccination with immunostimulatory DNA. *Immunol Allergy Clin North Am* 2004;24:569–581.

Gentile DA, Friday GA, Skoner PV: Management of allergic rhinitis: Antihistamines and decongestants. *Immunol Allergy Clin North Am* 2000; 20:355–368.

MacDonald SM, Vonakis BM (eds): Emerging therapies for allergic diseases. *Immunol Allergy Clin North Am* 2004;24:551–752.

Moss MH, Bush RK: Patient selection and administration of aeroallergen vaccines. *Immunol Allergy Clin North Am* 2000;20:533–552.

Nelson HS: Advances in upper airway diseases and allergen immunotherapy. *J Allergy Clin Immunol* 2005;115:676–684.

Norman PS: Immunotherapy: 1999–2004. *J Allergy Clin Immunol* 2004;113:1013–1023.

Poole JA, Matangkasombut P, Rosenwasser LJ: Targeting the IgE molecule in allergic and asthmatic diseases: Review of the IgE molecule and clinical efficacy. *J Allergy Clin Immunol* 2005;115:S375–S385.

Simons FER: Advances in H1-antihistimines. *N Engl J Med* 2004;351:2203–2217.

Till SJ, Francis JN, Nouri-Aria K, et al. Mechanisms of immunotherapy. *J Allergy Clin Immunol* 2004;113:1025–1034.

Chapter 142 ■ Allergic Rhinitis

Henry Milgrom and Donald Y. M. Leung

Allergic rhinitis (AR) is an inflammatory disorder of the nasal mucosa characterized by nasal congestion, rhinorrhea, and itching and often accompanied by sneezing and conjunctival irritation. It is a major chronic disease of children based on its high prevalence, co-morbidities, and detrimental effects on the quality of life and school performance.

ETIOLOGY. Two prerequisites for the expression of AR are sensitivity to an allergen and its presence in the environment. AR is currently classified as *seasonal* or *perennial,* terms that may soon be replaced by *intermittent* and *persistent.* Inhalant allergens are the main cause of AR irrespective of classification. **Seasonal (intermittent) AR** (SAR) follows a well-defined course of cyclical exacerbation, while **perennial (persistent) AR** (PAR) causes year-round symptoms. Approximately 20% of cases are strictly seasonal, 40% perennial, and 40% mixed (perennial with seasonal exacerbations). In temperate climates, the **airborne pollens** responsible for SAR appear in distinct phases: trees pollinate in the spring, grasses in the early summer, and weeds in the late summer. Mold spores in temperate climates persist outdoors only in the summer, and in warm climates throughout the year. Symptoms of seasonal allergies cease with the appearance of frost. Knowledge of the occurrence of seasonal symptoms, regional patterns of pollination and mold sporulation, and the patient's specific IgE is necessary to identify the cause of SAR. In contrast, PAR is most often associated with the **indoor allergens:** animal danders, house dust mites, and molds. Cat and dog allergies are of major importance in the United States. The allergens from the saliva and sebaceous secretions may remain airborne for prolonged periods. The ubiquitous major cat allergen, **Fel d 1,** is carried regularly on the owners' clothing into such "cat-free" settings as schools and hospitals.

EPIDEMIOLOGY. In the past 4 decades, there has been a marked increase in the prevalence of AR in urban settings and a smaller rise in rural areas. In prosperous societies, 20–40% of children suffer from AR. The prevalence peaks late in childhood. Symptoms may appear during infancy with the diagnosis generally established by 6 yr of age. Risk factors include family history of atopy and IgE >100 IU/mL before 6 yr of age. The risk increases in children introduced to foods or formula early in infancy; those whose mothers smoke heavily, especially before the child is 1 yr of age; and those with heavy exposure to indoor allergens. Children with food allergy by 4 yr of age are at increased risk for also developing AR. Paradoxically, exposure to dogs, cats, and endotoxin early in childhood decreases the risk of allergic sensitization.

PATHOGENESIS. The exposure of an atopic host to an allergen leads to specific IgE production. Reactions on re-exposure to the allergen have been classified as early-phase responses and late-phase responses. Bridging of the IgE molecules on the surface of mast cells by allergen initiates **early-phase responses,** which are characterized by degranulation of mast cells and the release of preformed and newly generated inflammatory mediators including histamine, prostaglandin 2, and the cysteinyl leukotrienes (see Chapter 139). The **late-phase responses** appear 4–8 hr after allergen exposure and are associated with the cellular infiltration of basophils, eosinophils, neutrophils, mast cells, and mononuclear cells. Eosinophils release proinflammatory mediators including cysteinyl leukotrienes, cationic proteins, eosinophil peroxidase, and major basic protein, and also serve as a source of interleukin (IL)–3, IL-5, IL-13, and granulocyte-macrophage colony–stimulating factor (GM-CSF). Repeated intranasal introduction of allergens causes **priming,** which is a brisk response to reduced provocation. In the course of an allergy season, a multifold increase in epithelial and submucosal mast cells develops. Mast cells, once thought to have a role exclusively in the early-phase response, appear to have an important function in sustaining chronic allergic disease.

CLINICAL MANIFESTATIONS. Symptoms of AR are often ignored or mistakenly attributed to a respiratory infection. Whereas older children are able to blow their noses, younger ones tend to sniff and snort. Nasal itching brings on grimacing, twitching, and picking at the nose that may result in epistaxis. Children with AR often perform the **allergic salute,** an upward rubbing of the nose with an open palm or extended index finger. This maneuver relieves itching and briefly unblocks the airway. It also gives rise to the **nasal crease,** a horizontal skin crease over the bridge of the nose.

Typical complaints include intermittent nasal congestion, itching, sneezing, clear rhinorrhea and conjunctival irritation. Symptoms increase with longer and higher levels of exposure to the responsible allergen. Patients may experience headaches, wheezing, and coughing, and may lose their sense of smell and taste. Nasal congestion is often more severe at night, causing mouth-breathing and snoring, which interferes with sleep, and arousing irritability.

LABORATORY FINDINGS. Epicutaneous skin tests are the best method for detection of allergen-specific IgE. They are sensitive, inexpensive, and fast, and the risks and discomfort are minimal. Response to seasonal respiratory allergens is unlikely before two seasons of exposure, and children <1 yr of age rarely display positive skin tests to these allergens. To avoid false-negative results, before testing, montelukast should be withheld for 1 day, 1st-generation antihistamines for 3–4 days, and 2nd-generation antihistamines for 5–7 days. Serum immunoassays for specific IgE to allergens provide a suitable alternative for patients with dermatographism or extensive dermatitis, taking medications that interfere with mast cell degranulation, at high risk for anaphylaxis, and who cannot cooperate with the procedure. Eosinophils in the nasal smear support the diagnosis of AR, and neutrophils suggest infectious rhinitis. Blood eosinophilia and total serum IgE concentrations have relatively low sensitivity. Better laboratory methods for objective evaluation are still needed to assess the effects of treatment.

DIAGNOSIS AND DIFFERENTIAL DIAGNOSIS. The diagnosis of AR is based on recurrent symptoms of sneezing, rhinorrhea, nasal itching, and congestion that occur most often in the absence of an upper respiratory tract infection or structural abnormalities. The diagnosis is supported by laboratory findings of elevated IgE, specific IgE antibodies, and positive allergy skin tests.

Evaluation of AR calls for a thorough history including details of the patient's environment and diet; family history of allergic conditions such as AR, eczema, and asthma; physical examination; and laboratory evaluation. The history and laboratory findings provide clues to the identity of provoking factors. Signs on physical examination include: abnormalities of facial development; dental malocclusion; the **allergic gape,** which is continuous open-mouth breathing; chapped lips; **allergic shiners,** which are dark circles under the eyes; and the nasal crease. Conjunctival edema, itching, tearing, and hyperemia are frequent findings. A nasal examination performed with a source of light and a speculum may reveal clear nasal secretions; edematous, boggy, and bluish mucous membranes with little or no erythema; and swollen turbinates that may block the nasal airway. It may be necessary to use a topical decongestant to perform an adequate examination. Thick, purulent nasal secretions indicate the presence of infection. Children with AR often have related sinusitis, conjunctivitis, otitis media, serous otitis, and eczema. AR is a risk factor for asthma and often precedes it in the atopic march.

SAR differs from PAR by the time of occurrence and skin test results. Nonallergic rhinitides cause sporadic symptoms that may resemble PAR (Table 142-1). Their causes are often unknown. Nonallergic inflammatory rhinitis with eosinophils (NARES) imitates AR in presentation and response to treatment, but the patients do not have elevated IgE antibodies. Vasomotor rhinitis is characterized by excessive responsiveness of the nasal mucosa to physical stimuli. Other nonallergic conditions that may mimic AR include infectious rhinitis, anatomic abnormalities including nasal polyps and septal deviation, rhinitis medicamentosa (which is caused by overuse of topical vasoconstrictors), hormonal rhinitis associated with pregnancy or hypothyroidism, neoplasms, vasculitides, and granulomatous disorders.

TREATMENT. Safe and effective prevention or relief of symptoms is the goal of treatment. The removal and avoidance of offending allergens is advised. The only effective measure for avoiding animal allergens in the home is the removal of the pet. Sealing the mattress, pillows, and covers in allergen-proof encasings reduces the exposure to mite allergen. Bed linens and blankets should be washed every week in hot water (>130°F). Avoidance of pollen and outdoor molds can be accomplished by staying in a controlled environment. Air-conditioning allows for keeping windows and doors closed to lower the pollen exposure. HEPA and electrostatic air filters reduce the counts of airborne mold spores.

Oral antihistamines (Table 142-2) administered as needed constitute acceptable pharmacotherapy of mild, intermittent symptoms of sneezing and rhinorrhea. First-generation antihistamines and loratadine, all available without prescription, are associated with adverse effects on cognitive function and learning as a result of their sedative properties. Second-generation antihistamines are preferred because they cause less sedation. Four oral 2nd-generation preparations are approved for children: cetirizine and desloratadine for >6 mo of age, loratadine for >2 yr of age, and fexofenadine for >6 yr of age. Azelastine is a topically active antihistamine that is available as a nasal spray for children >5 yr of age. Pseudoephedrine, available without prescription, generally in combination with an antihistamine, is an oral vasoconstrictor that may be used for nasal congestion. It is associated with irritability and insomnia. The anticholinergic nasal spray ipratropium bromide may be used for serous rhinorrhea. Intranasal decongestants should be used for <3–5 days, not to be repeated >1 cycle a month. Sodium cromoglycate, which is available without prescription, is effective but requires frequent administration. Leukotriene modifying agents have a modest effect on rhinorrhea and nasal blockage.

Patients with more persistent, severe symptoms require intranasal corticosteroids, which are the most effective therapy for AR (Table 142-3). These agents reduce all symptoms of AR caused by eosinophilic inflammation, but not of rhinitis associated with neutrophils or free of inflammation. The older drugs beclomethasone, triamcinolone, and flunisolide are absorbed from the gastrointestinal tract as well as the respiratory tract. Mometasone, fluticasone, and budesonide offer greater topical

TABLE 142-1. Causes of Rhinitis

Allergic rhinitis
- Seasonal
- Perennial
- Perennial with seasonal exacerbation

Nonallergic rhinitis
- Structural/mechanical factors
  - Deviated septum/septal wall anomalies
  - Hypertrophic turbinates
  - Adenoidal hypertrophy
  - Foreign bodies
  - Nasal tumors
    - Benign
    - Malignant
  - Choanal atresia
- Infectious
  - Acute
  - Chronic
- Inflammatory/immunologic
  - Wegener granulomatosis
  - Sarcoidosis
  - Midline granuloma
  - Systemic lupus erythematosus
  - Sjögren syndrome
  - Nasal polyposis
- Physiologic
  - Ciliary dyskinesia syndrome
  - Atrophic rhinitis
  - Hormonally induced
    - Hypothyroidism
    - Pregnancy
    - Oral contraceptives
    - Menstrual cycle
    - Exercise
    - Atrophic
- Drug induced
  - Rhinitis medicamentosa
  - Oral contraceptives
  - Antihypertensive therapy
  - Aspirin
  - Nonsteroidal anti-inflammatory drugs
- Reflex induced
  - Gustatory rhinitis
  - Chemical or irritant induced
  - Posture reflexes
  - Nasal cycle
- Environmental factors
  - Odors
  - Temperature
  - Weather/barometric pressure
  - Occupational

Nonallergic rhinitis with eosinophilia syndrome
Perennial nonallergic rhinitis (vasomotor rhinitis)
Emotional factors

From Leung DYM, Sampson HA, Geha RS, et al: *Pediatric Allergy Principles and Practice.* St. Louis, Mosby, 2003, p 290.

TABLE 142-2. Antihistamines and Decongestants for Allergic Rhinitis and Related Conditions

DRUG AND TRADE NAMES	INDICATIONS (MECHANISM OF ACTION) AND ORAL DOSING	CAUTIONS AND ADVERSE EVENTS
Brompheniramine (without prescription) Dimetapp	Allergic rhinitis (H_1 receptor antagonist) <6 yr: 0.125 mg/kg/dose every 6 hr; maximum 12 mg/day 6–12 yr: 2–4 mg/dose every 6–8 hr; maximum 16 mg/day >12 yr: 4–8 mg/dose every 4–6 hr; maximum 24 mg/day. Sustained release: 10 mg/dose every 12 hr; maximum 40 mg/day	Used primarily in combination preparations, most commonly with pseudoephedrine, recommended for cough and colds. For combination preparations with pseudoephedrine, base the dose on pseudoephedrine. Use for treatment of upper respiratory tract infections is unfounded. Has anticholinergic and sedating properties and may cause slight to moderate drowsiness, headache, excitability, fatigue, nervousness, dizziness.
Cetirizine (prescription) Zyrtec	Allergic rhinitis, urticaria (H_1-receptor antagonist) 0.5–2 yr: 2.5 mg once daily 2–5 yr: 2.5–5 mg once daily <6 yr: 5–10 mg once daily	May cause headache, somnolence, insomnia, abdominal pain. Doses >10 mg/day may cause significant drowsiness.
Chlorpheniramine (without prescription) Chlor-Trimeton	Allergic rhinitis, atopic dermatitis, urticaria, nighttime sedation (H_1 receptor antagonist) 2–6 yr: 1 mg every 4–6 hr; maximum 6 mg/day 6–12 yr: 2 mg every 4–6 hr; maximum 12 mg/day. Sustained release: 8 mg at bedtime >12 yr: 4 mg every 4–6 hr; maximum 24 mg/day. Sustained release: 8–12 mg every 8–12 hr	Available in many preparations recommended for cough and colds. Use for treatment of upper respiratory tract infections is unfounded. Has anticholinergic and sedating properties and may cause slight to moderate drowsiness, headache, excitability, fatigue, nervousness, dizziness.
Desloratadine (prescription) Clarinex	Allergic rhinitis, urticaria (a major metabolite of loratadine, a long-acting tricyclic antihistamine with selective H_1-receptor antagonist properties) 6–12 mo: 1 mg once daily 1–5 yr: 1.25 mg once daily 6–12 yr: 2.5 mg once daily >12 yr: 5 mg once daily	May cause headache, fatigue, somnolence, dizziness. Oral disintegrating tablets contain phenylalanine.
Diphenhydramine (without prescription) Benadryl	Allergic rhintis, atopic dermatitis, urticaria, nighttime sedation (H_1-receptor antagonist) 2–6 yr: 6.25 mg every 4–6 hr; maximum 37.5 mg/day 6–12 yr: 12.5–25 mg every 4–6 hr; maximum 150 mg/day >12 yr: 25–50 mg every 4–6 hr; maximum 300 mg/day	Marked anticholinergic and sedating properties and may cause hypotension, tachycardia, drowsiness paradoxical excitement, dry mouth. Chewable tables contain phenylalanine.
Fexofenadine (prescription) Allegra	Allergic rhinitis, urticaria (H_1-receptor antagonist; an active metabolite of terfenadine) 6–12 yr: 30 mg twice daily >12 yr: 60 mg twice daily, or 180 mg once daily	Good safety profile. May cause headache, fever, drowsiness, fatigue, dizziness.
Loratadine (without prescription) Claritin, Alavert, Dimetapp Children's ND	Allergic rhinitis, urticaria (long-acting tricyclic antihistamine with selective H_1-receptor antagonist properties) 2–5 yr: 5 mg once daily >6 yr: 10 mg once daily	Do not exceed recommended dosage. May cause nervousness, fatigue, malaise, excessive dreaming, hyperkinesia, rash, abdominal pain.
Pseudoephedrine (without prescription) Sudafed	Temporary symptomatic relief of nasal congestion due to common cold, allergic rhintis, and sinusitis (α-agonist, used as a decongestant) <2 yr: 4 mg/kg/dose every 6 hr 2–5 yr: 15 mg every 6 hr; maximum 60 mg/day 6–12 yr: 30 mg every 6 hr; maximum 120 mg/day <12 yr: 60 mg every 6 hr. Sustained release: 120 mg twice daily or 240 mg once daily; maximum 240 mg/day.	Use with caution in patients with hyperthyroidism, hypertension, diabetes, arrhythmias, or heart disease. Chewable tablets contain phenylalanine. Antihistamines may be formulated in combination with pseudoephedrine. For combination preparations containing pseudoephedrine and an antihistamine, base the dose on pseudoephedrine. Pseudoephedrine serves as the raw ingredient in the illicit production of methamphetamine. May cause tachycardia, palpitations, arrhythmias, nervousness, excitability, dizziness, insomnia, drowsiness, headache, seizures, hallucinations, nausea, vomiting, tremor, weakness, and diaphoresis.
Phenylephrine (without prescription) Neosynephrine	Tablets >= 6 years to < 12 years: 10 mg orally every 4 hours as needed >= 12 years: 10 to 20 mg orally every 4 hours as needed oral liquid: >= 2 years to < 6 years: 3.75 mg orally every 6 hours not to exceed 15 mg daily	Orally dissolving table contains phenylalanine drug interactions: sympathomimetics, α-receptor antagonists, monoamine oxidase inhibitors
Sudafed PE	>= 6 years to < 12 years: 7.5 mg orally every 6 hours not to exceed 30 mg daily >= 12 years: 15 mg orally every 6 hours not to exceed 60 mg daily oral disintegratng strip: >= 12 years: 10 mg orally every 4 hours not to exceed 6 doses daily	

activity with lower systemic exposure and a better safety profile. Mometasone is approved for children >2 yr of age, fluticasone for >4 yr of age, and budesonide for >6 yr of age. More severely affected patients may benefit from combination treatment with antihistamines, intranasal corticosteroids, and other medications (Table 142-4).

Specific allergen immunotherapy (see Chapter 141) should be considered for children in whom IgE-mediated allergic manifestations cannot be adequately controlled by symptomatic treatment, especially in the presence of co-morbid conditions. Allergen immunotherapy interferes with IgE production and allergen-induced symptoms and is effective in the treatment of AR.

Monoclonal recombinant humanized anti-IgE reduces allergic responses in the nose. Treatment strategies that incorporate anti-IgE and allergen immunotherapy hold promise for the future. Locally applied immunotherapy—oral, sublingual, or nasal—has been used successfully in Europe and South America.

COMPLICATIONS. AR is frequently associated with co-morbid conditions. **Chronic sinusitis** is a common complication of AR, with an inflammatory process that is characterized by marked eosinophilia, mucosal thickening, and nasal polyposis. Allergens, possibly fungal, may be the inciting agents. Bacterial cultures are often negative, although bacterial sinusitis may complicate AR. The sinusitis of **triad asthma** (asthma, sinusitis with nasal polyposis, and aspirin sensitivity) often shows poor response to therapy. Patients who undergo repeated endoscopic sinus surgery derive diminishing benefit with each successive procedure.

TABLE 142-3. Intranasal Inhaled Corticosteroids for Allergic Rhinitis*

DRUG AND TRADE NAME (DOSE/SPRAY)	INTRANASAL DOSING (SPRAYS PER NOSTRIL)
Beclomethasone	
Beconase AQ (42 μg/spray)	≥6 yr: 1–2 sprays twice daily
Budesonide	
Rhinocort AQ (32 μg/spray)	>6 yr: 1 spray once daily; maximum 2 sprays/day >2 yr: 1 spray once daily; maximum: 4 sprays/day
Flunisolide	
Nasarel (25 μg/spray)	≥6 yr: intial dose 1 spray 3 times a day or 2 sprays twice daily. Reduce to lowest effective dose.
Fluticasone	
Flonase (50 μg/spray)	≥4 yr: 1–2 sprays once daily; maximum: 4 sprays/day.
Mometasone	
Nasonex (50 μg/spray)	2–12 yr: 1 spray once daily ≥2 yr: 2 sprays once daily
Triamcinolone	
Nasacort HFA (55 μg/spray)	6–12 yr: 2 sprays once daily
Nasacort AQ (55 μg/spray)	≥12 yr: 4 sprays once daily

*The mechanism of action of intranasal corticosteroids is as an anti-inflammatory immune modulator. Doses given as sprays per nostril. For administration, shake the container before use; blow the nose; occlude one nostril and administer the dose to the other nostril. Repeat for the other nostril. May cause burning and irritation of the nasal mucosa, and epistaxis. Monitor the patient for adverse effects on growth, which are rare.

Rhinitis often coexists with asthma. Up to 78% of asthma patients have AR, and 38% of patients with AR have asthma. Rhinitis patients without asthma often manifest bronchial hyperresponsiveness. The aggravation of AR coincides with exacerbation of asthma; accordingly, treatment of nasal inflammation reduces bronchospasm, asthma-related emergency department visits, and hospitalizations. Postnasal drip associated with AR commonly causes persistent or recurrent cough. Obstruction of the eustachian tube and middle-ear effusion are frequent complications. Chronic allergic inflammation causes hypertrophy of adenoids and tonsils that may be associated with eustachian tube obstruction, serous effusion, otitis media, and obstructive sleep apnea. AR in children is strongly associated with snoring, sleep abnormalities, and daytime fatigue.

Quality of life measures have been developed to explore the effects of disease and therapeutic interventions on children with AR. The Pediatric Rhinoconjunctivitis Quality of Life Questionnaire (PRQLQ) is suitable for children 6–12 yr old and the Adolescent RQLQ for patients 12–17 yr old. Children with AR have increased anxiety and physical, social, and emotional issues that adversely affect learning and the ability to integrate with peers. The symptoms of AR contribute to headaches and fatigue, limit daily activities, interfere with sleep, and contribute to school absenteeism. Children with AR experience frustration over their appearance. Both uncontrolled AR and the adverse effects of sedating medications may diminish cognitive function and learning.

PROGNOSIS. The reported rates of remission of AR among children are 10–23%. Therapy with 2nd-generation antihistamines and intranasal corticosteroids significantly improves health-related quality of life measures in patients of all ages, as long as they continue to take their medication.

Allergic rhinitis after hours: The relevance and consequence of nighttime symptoms. Proceedings of a workshop. *J Allergy Clin Immunol* 2004;114:S133–S153.

Bousquet J, Van Cauwenberge P, Bachert C, et al: Requirements for medications commonly used in the treatment of allergic rhinitis. European Academy of Allergy and Clinical Immunology (EAACI), Allergic Rhinitis and its Impact on Asthma (ARIA). *Allergy* 2003;58:192–197.

Lin H, Boesel KM, Griffith DT, et al: Omalizumab rapidly decreases nasal allergic response and FcεRI on basophils. *J Allergy Clin Immunol* 2004;113:297–302.

Meltzer EO, Berkowitz RB, Grossbard EB: An intranasal Syk-kinase inhibitor (R112) improves the symptoms of seasonal allergic rhinitis in a park environment. *J Allergy Clin Immunol* 2005;115:791–796.

Milgrom H: Anti-IgE therapy in allergic disease. *Curr Opin Pediatr* 2004;16:642–647.

Plaut M, Valentine MD: Allergic rhinitis. *N Engl J Med* 2005;353:1934–1944.

Radcliffe MJ, Lewith GT, Turner RG, et al: Enzyme potentiated desensitation in treatment of seasonal allergic rhinitis: Double blind randomized controlled study. *Br Med J* 2003;327:251–254.

Schapowal A: Randomised controlled trial of butterbur and cetirizine for treating seasonal allergic rhinitis. *Br Med J* 2002;324:144–146.

Sly RM: Epidemiology of allergic rhinitis. *Clin Rev Allergy Immunol* 2002;22:67–103.

Treehorst I, Hak E, Oosting AJ, et al: Evaluation of impermeable covers for bedding in patients with allergic rhinitis. *N Engl J Med* 2003;349:237–246.

TABLE 142-4. Miscellaneous Intranasal Sprays for Allergic Rhinitis and Related Conditions

DRUG AND TRADE NAME	INDICATIONS (MECHANISM OF ACTION) AND DOSING (SPRAYS PER NOSTRIL)	COMMENTS (CAUTIONS, ADVERSE EVENTS, MONITORING)
Ipratropium bromide	Symptomatic relief of rhinorrhea (anticholinergic)	Contraindicated in patients with hypersensitivity to soy lecithin.
Atrovent nasal spray	>6 yr: 0.03% solution 2 sprays 2–3 times a day	May cause epistaxis, nasal dryness, nausea.
Azelastine	Rhinorrhea, sneezing, and nasal pruritus. (H_1-receptor antagonist)	May cause drowsiness, headache, somnolence, bitter taste.
Astelin	6–12 yr: 1 spray twice daily >12 yr: 2 sprays twice daily	
Nasalcrom	Allergic rhinitis (inhibition of mast cell degranulation)	Not effective immediately.
Cromolyn sodium	>2 yr: 1 spray 3–4 times a day; maximum: 6 sprays/day	Requires frequent administration.
Oxymetazoline	Symptomatic relief of nasal mucosal congestion (adrenergic agonist, vasoconstricting agent)	Excessive dosage may cause profound neurological depression. Use for >3 days may result in severe rebound nasal congestion.
Afrin Nostrilla	≥6 yr: 0.05% 2–3 drops, or 1–2 metered sprays twice daily	Do not repeat sequence >1 per month. Use with caution in patients with hyperthyroidism, heart disease, hypertension, and diabetes. May cause hypertension, palpitations, reflex bradycardia, nervousness, dizziness, insomnia, headache, neurological depression, convulsions, hallucinations, nausea, vomiting, mydriasis, elevated intraocular pressure, blurred vision.
Neo-Synephrine	Symptomatic relief of nasal mucosal congestion (adrenergic agonist, vasoconstricting agent)	Use for >3 days may result in severe rebound nasal congestion.
Phenylephrine	>6 mo: 1–2 drops 0.16% solution every 4 hr 1–6 yr: 2–3 drops 0.125% solution every 4 hr 6–12 yr: 2–3 drops 0.25% solution every 4 hr >12 yr: 2–3 drops or 1–2 sprays 0.25% or 0.5% solution every 4 hr	Do not repeat sequence >1 per month. The 0.125% solution is available as Little Noses. May cause reflex bradycardia, excitability, headache, anxiety, and dizziness.

Chapter 143 ■ Childhood Asthma

Andrew H. Liu, Ronina A. Covar, Joseph D. Spahn, and Donald Y. M. Leung

Asthma is a chronic inflammatory condition of the lung airways resulting in episodic airflow obstruction. This chronic inflammation heightens the "twitchiness" of the airways—**airways hyperresponsiveness** (AHR)—to provocative exposures. Asthma management is aimed at reducing airways inflammation by minimizing proinflammatory environmental exposures, using daily "controller" anti-inflammatory medications, and controlling comorbid conditions that can worsen asthma. Less inflammation typically leads to better asthma control, with fewer exacerbations and decreased need for "quick-reliever" asthma medications. Exacerbations can, nevertheless, still occur. Early intervention with systemic corticosteroids greatly reduces the severity of such episodes. Advances in asthma management and especially pharmacotherapy enable all but the uncommon child with severe asthma to live normally.

ETIOLOGY. Although the cause of childhood asthma has not been determined, contemporary research implicates a combination of environmental exposures and inherent biological and genetic vulnerabilities (Fig. 143-1). Respiratory exposures in this causal environment include inhaled allergens, respiratory viral infections, and chemical and biological air pollutants such as environmental tobacco smoke. In the predisposed host, immune responses to these common exposures can be a stimulus for prolonged, pathogenic inflammation and aberrant repair of injured airways tissues. Lung dysfunction (i.e., AHR and reduced airflow) develops. These pathogenic processes in the growing lung during early life adversely affect airways growth and differentiation, leading to altered airways at mature ages. Once asthma has developed, ongoing exposures appear to worsen it, driving disease persistence and increasing the risk of severe exacerbations.

Genetics. More than 22 loci on 15 autosomal chromosomes have been linked to asthma. Although the genetic linkages to asthma have sometimes differed between cohorts, asthma has been consistently linked with loci containing pro-allergic, proinflammatory genes (the interleukin [IL]–4 gene cluster on chromosome 5). Genetic variation in receptors for different asthma medications is associated with variation in biologic response to these medications (polymorphisms in the β_2-adrenergic receptor). Other candidate genes include *ADAM-33* (member of the metalloproteinase family), the gene for the prostanoid DP receptor, and genes located on chromosome 5q31 (possibly IL-12).

Environment. Recurrent wheezing episodes in early childhood are associated with common respiratory viruses, including respiratory syncytial virus, rhinovirus, influenza virus, parainfluenza virus, and human metapneumovirus. This implies that host features affecting immunologic host defense, inflammation, and the extent of airways injury from ubiquitous viral pathogens underlie susceptibility to recurrent wheezing in early childhood. Furthermore, injurious viral infections of the airways manifesting as pneumonia or bronchiolitis requiring hospitalization are risk factors for persistent asthma in childhood. Other airways exposures can also exacerbate ongoing airways inflammation, increase disease severity, and drive asthma persistence. Indoor and home allergen exposures in sensitized individuals can initiate airways inflammation and hypersensitivity to other irritant exposures, and are strongly linked to disease severity and persistence. Consequently, eliminating the offending allergen(s) can lead to resolution of asthma symptoms and can sometimes "cure" asthma.

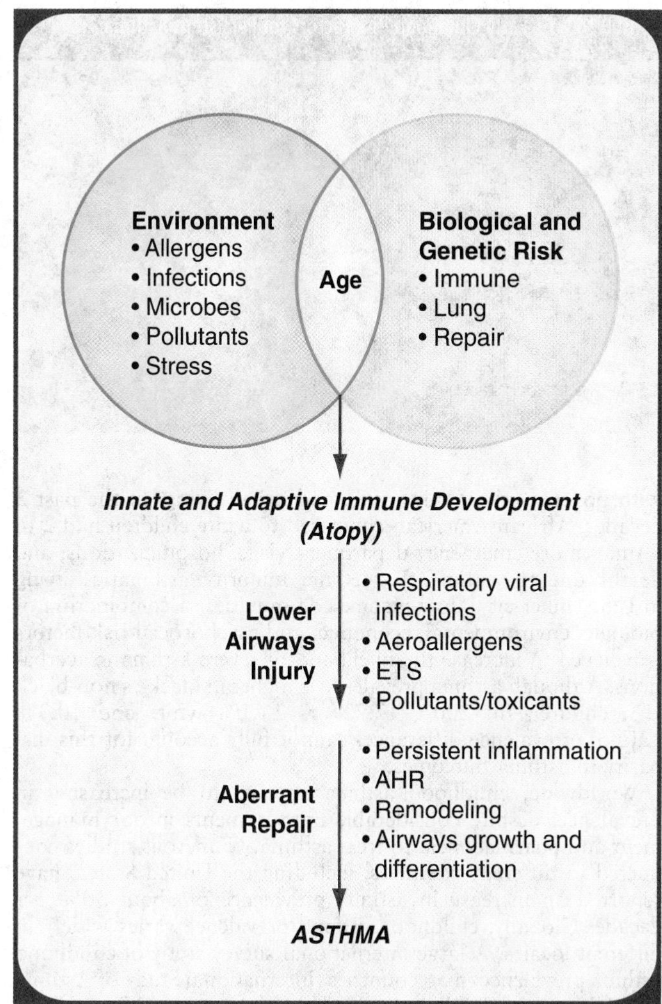

Figure 143-1. Etiology and pathogenesis of asthma. A combination of environmental and genetic factors in early life shape how the immune system develops and responds to ubiquitous environmental exposures. Respiratory microbes, inhaled allergens, and toxins that can injure the lower airways target the disease process to the lungs. Aberrant immune and repair responses to airways injury underlie persistent disease. AHR, airways hyperresponsiveness; ETS, environmental tobacco smoke.

Environmental tobacco smoke and air pollutants (ozone, sulfur dioxide) aggravate airways inflammation and increase asthma severity. Cold dry air and strong odors can trigger bronchoconstriction when airways are irritated, but do not worsen airways inflammation or hyperresponsiveness.

EPIDEMIOLOGY. Asthma is a common chronic disease, causing considerable morbidity. Based on information collected by the National Center for Health Statistics of the Centers for Disease Control and Prevention, in 2002, 8.9 million children (12.2%) had been diagnosed with asthma in their lifetime, and 4.2 million children (5.8%) had an asthma attack in the preceding 12 mo, indicative of current disease. Boys (14% vs 10% girls) and children in poor families (16% vs 10% not poor) are more likely to have asthma.

In the United States, childhood asthma is the most common cause of childhood emergency department visits, hospitalizations, and missed school days, accounting annually for 867,000 emergency department visits, 166,000 hospitalizations, and 10.1 million school days lost. In the United States in 2000, asthma was responsible for 223 childhood deaths. A disparity in asthma outcomes links high rates of asthma hospitalization and death

TABLE 143-1. Early Childhood Risk Factors for Persistent Asthma

Parental asthma
Allergy
Atopic dermatitis
Allergic rhinitis
Food allergy
Inhalant allergen sensitization
Food allergen sensitization
Severe lower respiratory tract infection
Pneumonia
Bronchiolitis requiring hospitalization
Wheezing apart from colds
Male gender
Low birthweight
Environmental tobacco smoke exposure

*Reduced lung function at birth.

with poverty, ethnic minorities, and urban living. In the past 2 decades, African-American compared to white children had 2 to 4 times more emergency department visits, hospitalizations, and deaths due to asthma. For ethnic minority asthmatics living in U.S. "inner-city" low-income communities, a combination of biologic, environmental, economic, and psychosocial risk factors is believed to increase the likelihood of severe asthma exacerbations. Although asthma prevalence is higher in black vs non-black U.S. children (in 2002, 17.7% vs 11.1% white and 10.3% Latino), prevalence differences cannot fully account for this disparity in asthma outcomes.

Worldwide, childhood asthma appears to be increasing in prevalence, despite considerable improvements in our management and pharmacopeia to treat asthma. Numerous studies conducted in different countries, including the United States, have reported an increase in asthma prevalence of about 50% per decade. Globally, childhood asthma prevalence varies widely in different locales. A large international survey study of childhood asthma prevalence in 56 countries (International Study of Asthma and Allergies in Childhood) found a wide range in asthma prevalence, from 1.6 to 36.8%. Furthermore, asthma prevalence correlated well with reported allergic rhinoconjunctivitis and atopic eczema prevalence. Childhood asthma seems particularly common in modern metropolitan locales and is strongly linked with other allergic conditions. In contrast, children living in rural areas of developing countries and farming communities are less likely to develop asthma and allergy.

Approximately 80% of all asthmatics report disease onset prior to 6 yr of age. Of all young children who experience recurrent wheezing, however, only a minority will go on to have persistent asthma in later childhood. Early childhood risk factors for persistent asthma have been identified (Table 143-1). A modified Asthma Predictive Index (Table 143-2) optimizes risk factor assessments of young children to predict the risk for persistent asthma in later childhood. Allergy in young children has emerged as a major risk factor for the persistence of childhood asthma.

TABLE 143-2. Asthma Predictive Index for Children

MAJOR CRITERIA	MINOR CRITERIA
Parent asthma	Allergic rhinitis
Eczema	Wheezing apart from colds
Inhalant allergen sensitization	Eosinophils ≥ 4%
	Food allergen sensitization

Through a statistically optimized model for pre–school-age children with frequent wheezing in the past year, *one major criterion OR two minor criteria* provide a high specificity (97%) and positive predictive value (77%) for persistent asthma into later childhood (Tucson Children's Respiratory Study; Tucson, AZ).

Modified from Castro-Rodriguez JA, Holberg CH, Wright AL, et al: A clinical index to define risk of asthma in young children with recurrent wheezing. *Am J Respir Crit Care* 2000;162:1403–1406; and Guilbert TW, Morgan WJ, Zeiger RS, et al: Atopic characteristics of children with recurrent wheezing at high risk for the development of childhood asthma. *J Allergy Clin Immunol* 2004;114:1282–1287.

Types of Childhood Asthma. Asthma is considered to be a common clinical presentation of intermittent, recurrent wheezing and/or coughing, resulting from different airways pathologic processes underlying different types of asthma. There are 2 main types of childhood asthma: (1) **recurrent wheezing** in early childhood, primarily triggered by common viral infections of the respiratory tract; and (2) **chronic asthma** associated with allergy that persists into later childhood and often adulthood. A 3rd type of childhood asthma typically emerges in females who develop obesity and early-onset puberty (by 11 yr of age). Some children may be hypersensitive to common air pollutants (environmental tobacco smoke, ozone) such that these exposures might not only make existing asthma worse, but they may also have a causal role in the susceptible. Similarly, although asthma mediated by "occupational" exposures is often not considered in children, some are raised in settings where occupational-type exposures can mediate asthma if they are susceptible (on farms or with animals in the home, with increased endotoxin). **Triad asthma,** characteristically associated with hyperplastic sinusitis/nasal polyposis and hypersensitivity to aspirin and nonsteroidal anti-inflammatory medications (ibuprofen), rarely has its onset in childhood. The most common persistent form of childhood asthma is that associated with allergy.

PATHOGENESIS. Airflow obstruction in asthma is the result of numerous pathologic processes. In the small airways, airflow is regulated by smooth muscle encircling the airways lumens; bronchoconstriction of these bronchiolar muscular bands restricts or blocks airflow. A cellular inflammatory infiltrate and exudates distinguished by eosinophils, but also including other inflammatory cell types (neutrophils, monocytes, lymphocytes, mast cells, basophils), can fill and obstruct the airways and induce epithelial damage and desquamation into the airways lumen. Helper T lymphocytes and other immune cells that produce pro-allergic, proinflammatory cytokines (IL-4, IL-5, IL-13) and chemokines (eotaxin) mediate this inflammatory process. Pathogenic immune responses and inflammation may also result from a breach in normal immune regulatory processes (regulatory T lymphocytes that produce IL-10 and transforming growth factor [TGF]–β) that dampen effector immunity and inflammation when they are no longer needed. Airways inflammation is linked to AHR or hypersensitivity of airways smooth muscle to numerous provocative exposures that act as **triggers** (Table 143-3), as well as airways edema, basement membrane thickening, subepithelial collagen deposition, smooth muscle and mucous gland hypertrophy, and mucus hypersecretion—all processes that contribute to airflow obstruction (see Chapter 139).

CLINICAL MANIFESTATIONS AND DIAGNOSIS. Intermittent dry coughing and/or expiratory wheezing are the most common chronic symptoms of asthma. Older children and adults will report associated shortness of breath and chest tightness; younger children are more likely to report intermittent, nonfocal chest "pain." Respiratory symptoms can be worse at night, especially during prolonged exacerbations triggered by respiratory infections or inhalant allergens. Daytime symptoms, often linked with physical activities or play, are reported with greatest frequency in children. Other asthma symptoms in children can be subtle and nonspecific, including self-imposed limitation of physical activities, general fatigue (possibly due to sleep disturbance), and difficulty keeping up with peers in physical activities. Asking about previous experience with asthma medications (bronchodilators) may provide a history of symptomatic improvement with treatment that supports the diagnosis of asthma. Lack of improvement with bronchodilator and corticosteroid therapy is inconsistent with underlying asthma and should prompt more vigorous consideration of asthma-masquerading conditions.

Asthma symptoms can be triggered by numerous common events or exposures: physical exertion and hyperventilation

TABLE 143-3. Asthma Triggers

Common viral infections of the respiratory tract
Aeroallergens in sensitized asthmatics
Animal dander
Indoor allergens
Dust mites
Cockroaches
Molds
Seasonal aeroallergens
Pollens (trees, grasses, weeds)
Seasonal molds
Environmental tobacco smoke
Air pollutants
Ozone
Sulfur dioxide
Particulate matter
Wood- or coal-burning smoke
Endotoxin, mycotoxins
Dust
Strong or noxious odors or fumes
Perfumes, hairsprays
Cleaning agents
Occupational exposures
Farm and barn exposures
Formaldehydes, cedar, paint fumes
Cold air, dry air
Exercise
Crying, laughter, hyperventilation
Co-morbid conditions
Rhinitis
Sinusitis
Gastroesophageal reflux

TABLE 143-4. Differential Diagnosis of Childhood Asthma

UPPER RESPIRATORY TRACT CONDITIONS
Allergic rhinitis*
Chronic rhinitis*
Sinusitis*
Adenoidal or tonsillar hypertrophy
Nasal foreign body
MIDDLE RESPIRATORY TRACT CONDITIONS
Laryngotracheobronchomalacia*
Laryngotracheobronchitis (e.g., pertussis)*
Laryngeal web, cyst, or stenosis
Vocal cord dysfunction*
Vocal cord paralysis
Tracheoesophageal fistula
Vascular ring, sling, or external mass compressing on the airway (e.g., tumor)
Foreign body aspiration*
Chronic bronchitis from environmental tobacco smoke exposure*
Toxic inhalations
LOWER RESPIRATORY TRACT CONDITIONS
Bronchopulmonary dysplasia (chronic lung disease of preterm infants)
Viral bronchiolitis*
Gastroesophageal reflux*
Causes of bronchiectasis:
Cystic fibrosis
Immune deficiency
Allergic bronchopulmonary mycoses (e.g., aspergillosis)
Chronic aspiration
Immotile cilia syndrome, primary ciliary dyskinesia
Bronchiolitis obliterans
Interstitial lung diseases
Hypersensitivity pneumonitis
Pulmonary eosinophilia, Churg-Strauss vasculitis
Pulmonary hemosiderosis
Tuberculosis
Pneumonia
Pulmonary edema (e.g., congestive heart failure)
Medications associated with chronic cough
Acetylcholinesterase inhibitors
β-adrenergic antagonists

*More common asthma masqueraders.

(laughing), cold or dry air, and airways irritants (see Table 143-3). Exposures that induce airways inflammation, such as infections (respiratory syncytial virus, metapneumovirus, torquetenovirus, rhinovirus, parainfluenza virus, influenza virus, adenovirus, *Mycoplasma pneumonia, Chlamydia pneumoniae*), and inhaled allergens, also increase AHR to irritant exposures. Numerous occupational exposures incite asthma in some adults. Similarly, some susceptible children might be chronically exposed to these same airways toxicants in their home or school environments, leading to "occupational"-type asthma in children. Accordingly, an environmental history is essential for optimal asthma diagnosis and management (see Chapter 140).

The presence of risk factors, such as a history of other allergic conditions (allergic rhinitis, allergic conjunctivitis, atopic dermatitis, food allergies), parental asthma, and/or symptoms apart from colds, supports the diagnosis of asthma. During routine clinic visits, children with asthma commonly present without abnormal signs, which stresses the importance of the medical history in diagnosing asthma. Some may exhibit a dry, persistent cough. The chest examination is often normal. Deeper breaths can sometimes elicit otherwise undetectable wheezing. In clinic, quick resolution (within 10 min) or convincing improvement in symptoms and signs of asthma with administration of a short-acting inhaled beta-agonist (SABA [albuterol]) is supportive of the diagnosis of asthma.

During asthma exacerbations, expiratory wheezing and a prolonged expiratory phase can usually be appreciated by auscultation. Decreased breath sounds in some of the lung fields, commonly the right lower posterior lobe, are consistent with regional hypoventilation owing to airways obstruction. Crackles (or rales) and rhonchi can sometimes be heard, resulting from excess mucus production and inflammatory exudate in the airways. The combination of segmental crackles and poor breath sounds can indicate lung segmental atelectasis that is difficult to distinguish from bronchial pneumonia and can complicate acute asthma management. In severe exacerbations, the greater extent of airways obstruction causes labored breathing and respiratory distress manifested as inspiratory and expiratory wheezing, increased prolongation of exhalation, poor air entry, suprasternal and intercostal retractions, nasal flaring, and accessory respiratory muscle use. In extremis, airflow may be so limited that wheezing cannot be heard.

DIFFERENTIAL DIAGNOSIS. Many childhood respiratory conditions can present with symptoms and signs similar to asthma (Table 143-4). Besides asthma, other common causes of chronic, intermittent coughing include rhinosinusitis and gastroesophageal reflux (GER). Both GER and chronic sinusitis can be challenging to diagnose in children. Often, GER is clinically silent in children, and children with chronic sinusitis do not report sinusitis-specific symptoms such as localized sinus pressure or tenderness. In addition, both GER and rhinosinusitis are often co-morbid conditions with childhood asthma and, if not specifically treated, make asthma difficult to manage.

In early life, chronic coughing and wheezing can indicate recurrent aspiration, tracheobronchomalacia, a congenital anatomic abnormality of the airways, foreign body aspiration, cystic fibrosis, or bronchopulmonary dysplasia. In older children and adolescents, **vocal cord dysfunction** (**VCD**) can present as intermittent daytime wheezing. In this condition, the vocal cords close inappropriately, during inspiration and sometimes exhalation, producing shortness of breath, coughing, throat tightness, and often audible laryngeal wheezing and/or stridor. In most VCD cases, spirometric lung function testing will reveal "truncated" and inconsistent inspiratory and expiratory flow-volume loops, a pattern that differs from the reproducible pattern of airflow limitation in asthma that improves with bronchodilators. VCD may also be visualized with laryngoscopy. VCD can coexist with asthma. VCD does not respond to traditional asthma therapy. Speech therapy is the treatment of choice for VCD.

In some locales, hypersensitivity pneumonitis (farming communities, homes of bird owners), pulmonary parasitic infestations (rural areas of developing countries), or tuberculosis may be common causes of chronic coughing and/or wheezing. Rare asthma-masquerading conditions in childhood include bronchiolitis obliterans; interstitial lung diseases; primary ciliary dyskinesias; humoral immune deficiencies; allergic bronchopulmonary mycoses; congestive heart failure; mass lesions in or compressing the larynx, trachea, or bronchi; and medication-induced coughing and/or wheezing as an adverse effect. Chronic pulmonary diseases often produce clubbing; this is a very unusual finding in childhood asthma.

LABORATORY FINDINGS. Lung function tests can help to confirm the diagnosis of asthma and determine disease severity.

Pulmonary Function Testing. Forced expiratory airflow measures are helpful in diagnosing and monitoring asthma and in assessing efficacy of therapy. Lung function testing is particularly helpful in children with asthma who are poor perceivers of airflow obstruction or when physical signs of asthma do not occur until airflow obstruction is severe.

Many asthma guidelines promote spirometric measures of airflow and lung volumes during forced expiratory maneuvers as standard for asthma assessment. **Spirometry** is helpful as an objective measure of airflow limitation (Fig. 143-2). Knowledgeable personnel are needed to perform and interpret spirometry tests. Valid spirometric measures are dependent on a patient's ability to perform properly a full, forceful, and prolonged expiratory maneuver, usually feasible in children >6 yr of age (with some younger exceptions). Reproducible spirometric efforts are an indicator of test validity; if, on 3 attempts, the **FEV_1** (forced expiratory volume in 1 sec) is within 5%, then the *highest* FEV_1 effort of the 3 is used. This standard utilization of the highest of 3 reproducible efforts is indicative of the effort-dependence of reliable spirometric testing.

In asthma, airways blockage results in reduced airflow with forced exhalation and smaller partial-expiratory lung volumes (see Fig. 143-2). Because asthmatics are typically hyperinflated, FEV_1 can be simply adjusted for full expiratory lung volume—the forced vital capacity (FVC)—with an FEV_1/FVC ratio. Generally, an FEV_1/FVC ratio <0.80 indicates significant airflow obstruction (Table 143-5). Normative values for FEV_1 have been determined for children, based on height, gender, and ethnicity. Abnormally low FEV_1 as a percentage of predicted norms is 1 of 4 criteria used to determine asthma severity in the National Institutes of Health (NIH)–sponsored asthma guidelines. The guidelines cutoff criteria of FEV_1 <80% and <60% of predicted for moderate and severe asthma, respectively, are controversial for children with asthma, many of whom can have near-normal or even supra-normal airflow despite having the other hallmarks of moderate to severe disease.

Such measures of airflow alone, however, are not diagnostic of asthma, because numerous other conditions can cause airflow

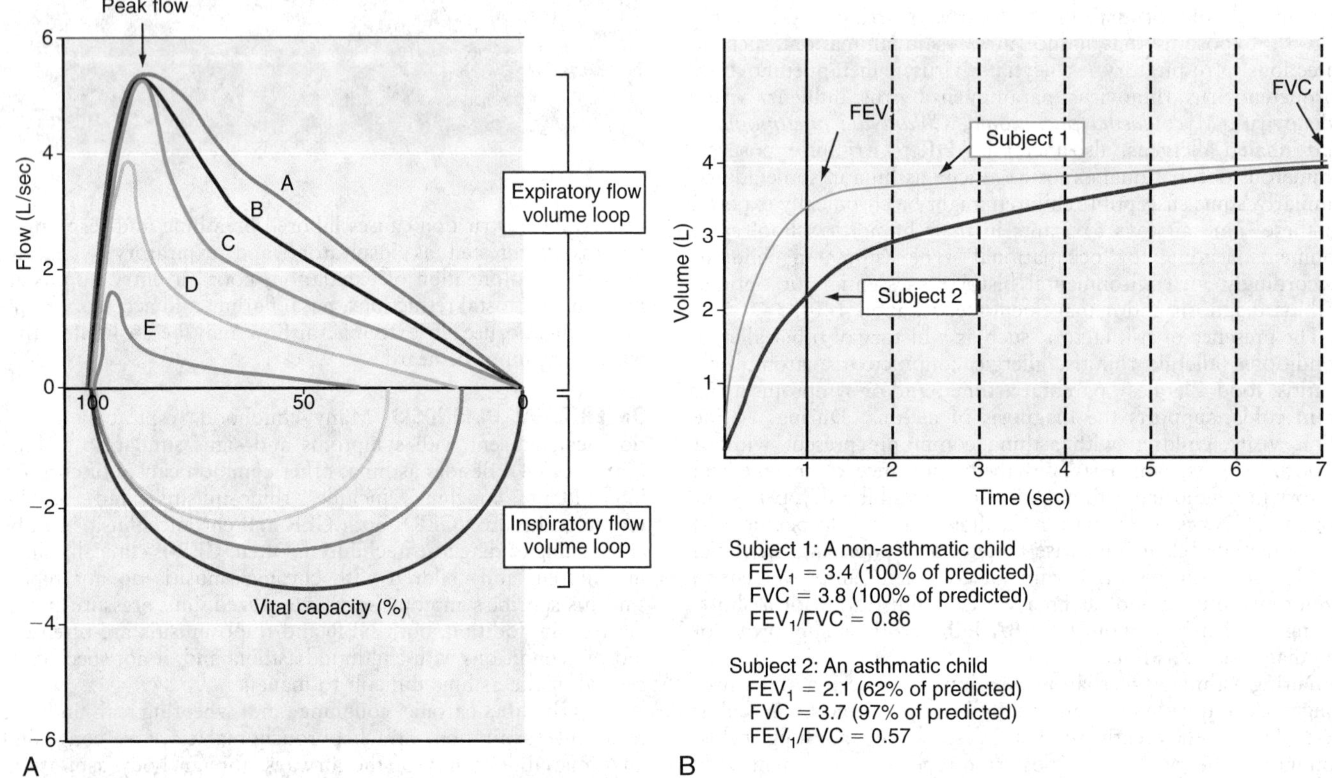

Figure 143-2. Spirometry. *A*, Spirometric flow-volume loops. A is an expiratory flow-volume loop of a nonasthmatic, without airflow limitation. B through E are expiratory flow-volume loops in asthmatic patients with increasing degrees of airflow limitation (B is mild; E is severe). Note the "scooped" or concave appearance of the asthmatic expiratory flow-volume loops; with increasing obstruction, there is greater "scooping." *B*, Spirometric volume-time curves. Subject 1 is a nonasthmatic; subject 2 is an asthmatic. Note how the FEV_1 and FVC lung volumes are obtained. The FEV_1 is the volume of air exhaled in the 1st sec of a forced expiratory effort. The FVC is the total volume of air exhaled during a forced expiratory effort. Note that subject 2's FEV_1 and FEV_1/FVC ratio are smaller than subject 1's, demonstrating airflow limitation. Also, subject 2's FVC is very close to what is expected. FEV_1, forced expiratory volume in 1 sec; FVC, forced vital capacity.

TABLE 143-5. Lung Function Abnormalities in Asthma

Spirometry (in clinic)
Airflow limitation
Low FEV_1 (relative to percentage of predicted norms)
FEV_1/FVC ratio <0.80
Bronchodilator response (to inhaled β-agonist)
Improvement in FEV_1 ≥12% or ≥200 mL*
Exercise challenge
Worsening in FEV_1 ≥15%*
Daily peak flow or FEV_1 monitoring: day to day and/or AM-to-PM variation ≥20%*

*Main criteria consistent with asthma.
FEV_1, forced expiratory volume in 1 sec; FVC, forced vital capacity.

reduction. Bronchodilator response to an inhaled β-agonist (e.g., albuterol) is greater in asthmatics vs non-asthmatics; an improvement in FEV_1 ≥12% or >200 mL is consistent with asthma. **Bronchoprovocation challenges** can be helpful in diagnosing asthma and optimizing asthma management. Asthmatic airways are hyperresponsive and therefore more sensitive to inhaled methacholine, histamine, and cold or dry air. The degree of AHR to these exposures correlates to some extent with asthma severity and airways inflammation. Although bronchoprovocation challenges are carefully dosed and monitored in an investigational setting, their use is rarely practical in a general practice setting. **Exercise challenges** (aerobic exertion or "running" for 6–8 min) can help to identify children with **exercise-induced bron-**

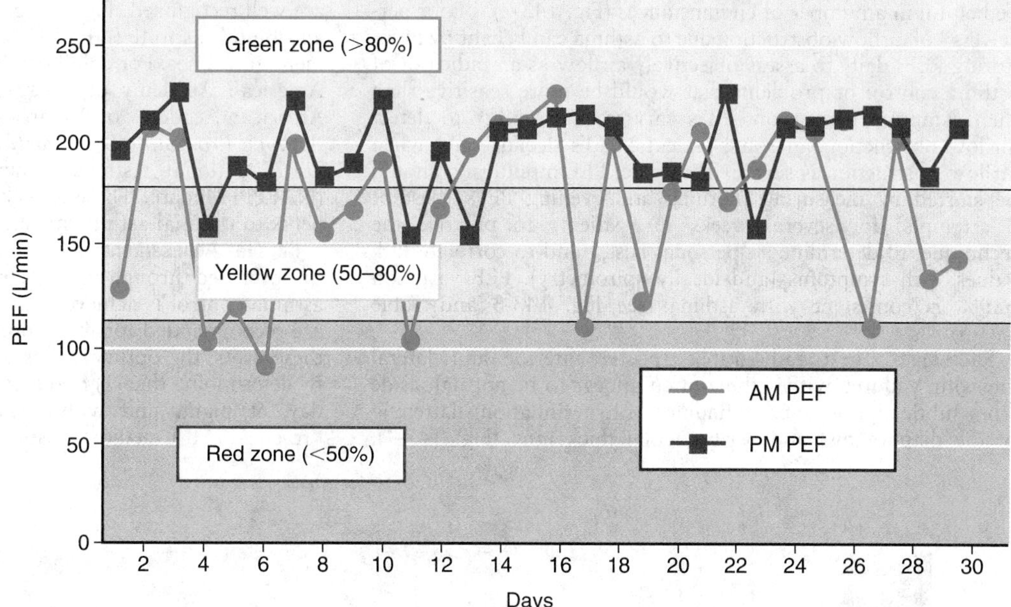

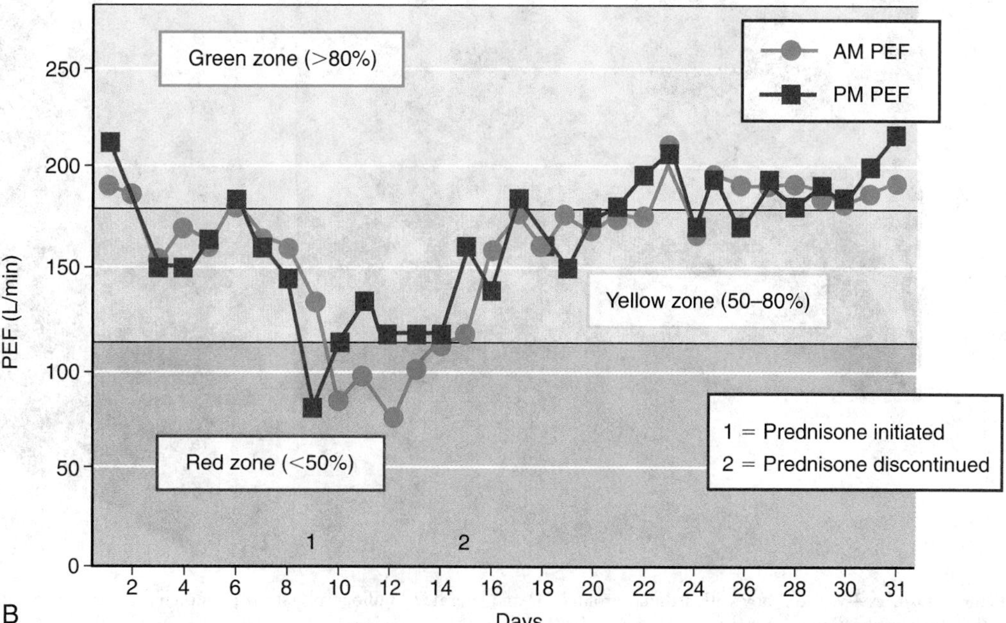

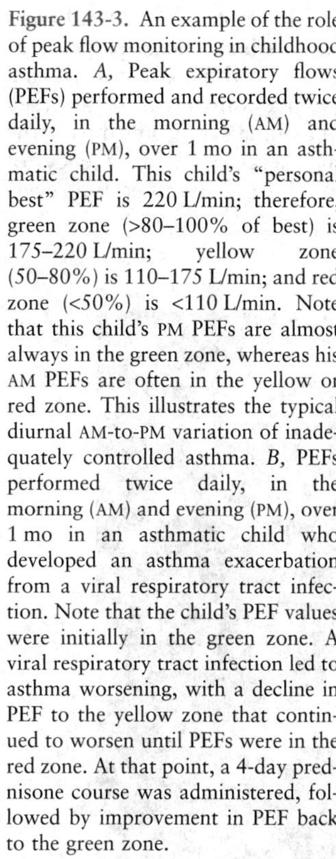

Figure 143-3. An example of the role of peak flow monitoring in childhood asthma. *A,* Peak expiratory flows (PEFs) performed and recorded twice daily, in the morning (AM) and evening (PM), over 1 mo in an asthmatic child. This child's "personal best" PEF is 220 L/min; therefore, green zone (>80–100% of best) is 175–220 L/min; yellow zone (50–80%) is 110–175 L/min; and red zone (<50%) is <110 L/min. Note that this child's PM PEFs are almost always in the green zone, whereas his AM PEFs are often in the yellow or red zone. This illustrates the typical diurnal AM-to-PM variation of inadequately controlled asthma. *B,* PEFs performed twice daily, in the morning (AM) and evening (PM), over 1 mo in an asthmatic child who developed an asthma exacerbation from a viral respiratory tract infection. Note that the child's PEF values were initially in the green zone. A viral respiratory tract infection led to asthma worsening, with a decline in PEF to the yellow zone that continued to worsen until PEFs were in the red zone. At that point, a 4-day prednisone course was administered, followed by improvement in PEF back to the green zone.

chospasm. Although the airflow response of non-asthmatics to exercise is to increase functional lung volumes and improve FEV_1 slightly (5–10%), exercise often provokes airflow obstruction in inadequately treated asthmatics. Accordingly, in asthmatics, FEV_1 typically decreases during or after exercise by >15% (see Table 143-5). The onset of exercise-induced bronchospasm is usually within 15 min after a vigorous exercise challenge and can spontaneously resolve within 30–60 min. Studies of exercise challenges in school-age children typically identify an additional 5–10% with exercise-induced bronchospasm and previously unrecognized asthma. Exercise challenges can induce severe asthma exacerbations in at-risk patients; careful patient selection for exercise challenges and preparedness for severe asthma exacerbations are required.

Measuring **exhaled nitric oxide** (FE_{NO}), a marker of airway inflammation in asthma, can help titrate medications and confirm the diagnosis of asthma.

Peak expiratory flow (PEF) monitoring devices provide a simple and inexpensive home-use tool to measure airflow and can be helpful in a number of circumstances (Fig. 143-3). "Poor perceivers" of airflow obstruction due to asthma can benefit by monitoring PEFs daily to assess objectively airflow as an indicator of asthma control or problems that would be more sensitive than their symptom perception. PEFs vary in their ability to detect airflow obstruction; in some patients, PEFs decline only when airflow obstruction is severe. Therefore, PEF monitoring should be started by measuring morning and evening PEFs (best of 3 attempts) for several weeks for patients to practice the technique, to determine a "personal best," and to correlate PEF values with symptoms (and ideally spirometry). PEF variation >20% is consistent with asthma (see Fig. 143-3 and Table 143-5).

Radiology. Chest radiographs (posteroanterior and lateral views) in children with asthma often appear to be normal, aside from subtle and nonspecific findings of hyperinflation (flattening of the diaphragms) and peribronchial thickening (Fig. 143-4). Chest radiographs can be helpful in identifying abnormalities that are hallmarks of **asthma masqueraders** (aspiration pneumonitis, hyperlucent lung fields in bronchiolitis obliterans), and complications during asthma exacerbations (atelectasis, pneumomediastinum, pneumothorax). Some lung abnormalities can be better appreciated with high-resolution, thin-section chest CT scans. **Bronchiectasis** is sometimes difficult to appreciate on chest radiograph, but is clearly seen on CT scan and implicates an asthma masquerader such as cystic fibrosis, allergic bronchopulmonary mycoses (aspergillosis), ciliary dyskinesias, or immune deficiencies.

Other tests, such as allergy testing to assess sensitization to inhalant allergens, help with the management and prognosis of asthma. In a comprehensive U.S. study of 5–12 yr old asthmatic children (Childhood Asthma Management Program [CAMP]), 88% had inhalant allergen sensitization by allergy prick skin testing.

TREATMENT. The key elements to optimal asthma management are well recognized (Fig. 143-5). The NIH National Heart, Lung and Blood Institute (NHLBI) developed current asthma management guidelines. For childhood asthma, a joint publication of the American Academy of Allergy, Asthma and Immunology, the American Academy of Pediatrics, and the NIH, entitled *Pediatric Asthma: Promoting Best Practice,* has been updated to reflect the 2002 National Asthma Education and Prevention Program (NAEPP) Update. These guidelines describe 4 principle components to optimal asthma management (Table 143-6).

Regular Assessment and Monitoring. Asthma management can be optimized through regular clinic visits every 2–4 wk until good asthma control is achieved. Two to 4 asthma checkups per year are recommended for maintaining good asthma control. During these visits, the optimal goals of asthma control can be assessed by determining the: (1) frequency of asthma symptoms during the day, at night, and with physical exercise; (2) frequency of "rescue" SABA medication use and refills; (3) number and sever-

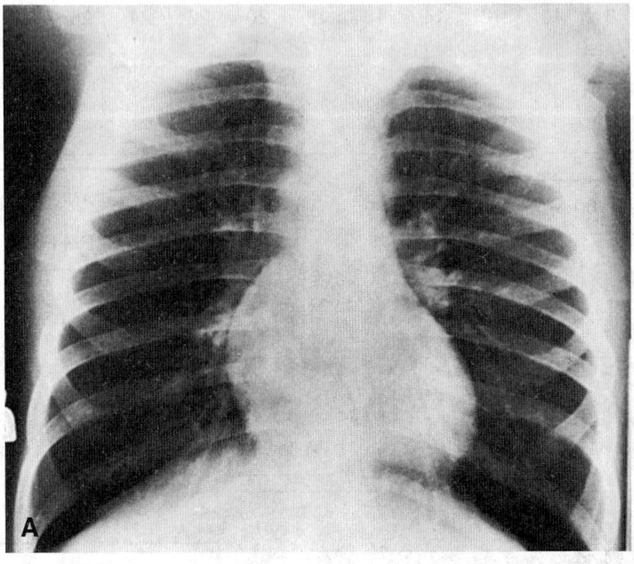

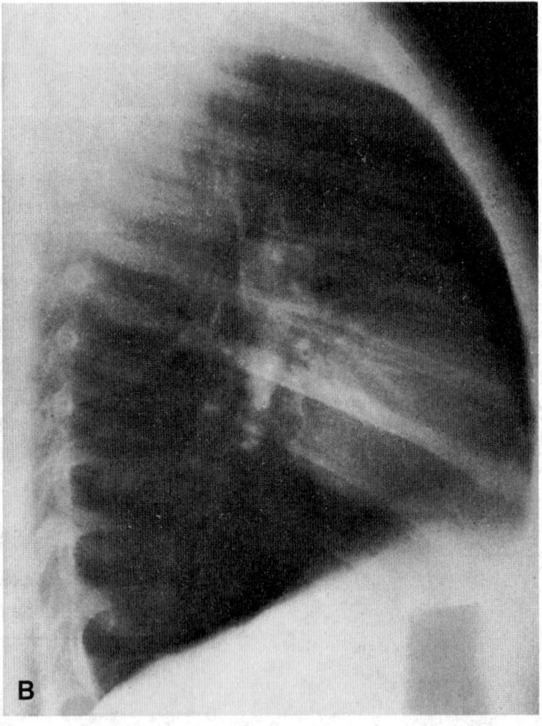

Figure 143-4. A 4-year-old boy with asthma. Frontal *(A)* and lateral *(B)* radiographs show pulmonary hyperinflation and minimal peribronchial thickening. No asthmatic complication is apparent.

Recurrent/chronic cough, wheeze, dyspnea

DIAGNOSIS
- Symptoms
- Exacerbations
- Risk factors (Tables 143-1, 143-2, 143-15)
- Lung function (Table 143-5)
- Differential dx. (Table 143-4)

ASTHMA

MANAGEMENT (Tables 143-6, 143-9,143-10)

• Pharmacotherapy
- Assess severity (Table 143-8)
- Long-term controllers (Tables 143-11, 143-12)
- Quick relievers (Tables 143-9,143-10)

• Exacerbations
- Management (Table 143-14)
- High risk features (Table 143-15)
- Home Action Plan

• Triggers *(Table 143-3)*
- Environmental controls (Table 143-7)

• Co-morbidities
- Rhinitis, sinusitis
- Gastroesophageal reflux
- Steroid adverse effects (Table 143-13)

• Education and follow-up
- Key elements (Table 143-16)

Optimal Goals
- Maintain normal activity
  - Regular school or daycare attendance
  - Full participation in physical exercise, athletics, and other recreational activities
- Prevent sleep disturbance
- Prevent chronic asthma symptoms
- Keep asthma exacerbations from becoming severe
- Maintain normal lung function
- Experience little to no adverse effects of treatment

Figure 143-5. The key elements to optimal asthma management.

ity of asthma exacerbations since the last visit; and (4) participation in school, sports, and other preferred activities (see Fig. 143-5). Lung function testing (spirometry) is recommended at least annually and more often if asthma is inadequately controlled or lung function is abnormally low. PEF monitoring at home can be helpful when assessing asthmatic children with poor symptom

TABLE 143-6. Four Components of Optimal Asthma Management

REGULAR ASSESSMENT AND MONITORING
Asthma checkups
Every 2–4 wk until good control is achieved
2–4 per yr to maintain good control
Lung function monitoring
CONTROL OF FACTORS CONTRIBUTING TO ASTHMA SEVERITIY
Eliminate or reduce problematic environmental exposures
Treat co-morbid conditions: rhinitis, sinusitis, gastroesophageal reflux
ASTHMA PHARMACOTHERAPY
Long-term-control vs quick-relief medications
Classification of asthma severity for anti-inflammatory pharmacotherapy
Step-up, step-down approach
Asthma exacerbation management
PATIENT EDUCATION
Provide a two-part care plan
Daily management
Action plan for asthma exacerbations

TABLE 143-7. Control of Factors Contributing to Asthma Severity

ELIMINATE OR REDUCE PROBLEMATIC ENVIRONMENTAL EXPOSURES
Environmental tobacco smoke elimination or reduction
In home and automobiles
Allergen exposure elimination or reduction in sensitized asthmatics
Animal danders
Pets (cats, dogs, rodents, birds)
Pests (mice, rats)
Dust mites
Cockroaches
Molds
Other airway irritants
Wood- or coal-burning smoke
Strong chemical odors and perfumes (e.g., household cleaners)
Dusts
TREAT CO-MORBID CONDITIONS
Rhinitis
Sinusitis
Gastroesophageal reflux
ANNUAL INFLUENZA VACCINATION (UNLESS EGG-ALLERGIC)

perception, other causes of chronic coughing in addition to asthma, moderate to severe asthma, or a history of severe asthma exacerbations. PEF monitoring is feasible in children as young as 4 yr old and who are able to master this skill. Use of a **stoplight zone system,** tailored to each child's "personal best" PEFs, can optimize effectiveness and interest (see Fig 143-3): The green zone (80–100% of personal best) indicates good control; the yellow zone (50–80%) indicates less than optimal control and necessitates increased awareness and treatment; whereas the red zone (<50%) indicates poor control and increased likelihood of an exacerbation, requiring immediate intervention. In actuality, these ranges are approximate and may need to be adjusted for many asthmatic children by raising the ranges that indicate inadequate control (in the yellow zone from 70 to 90%). The NAEPP guidelines recommend at least once-daily PEF monitoring, preferably in the morning when peak flows are typically lower.

Control of Factors Contributing to Asthma Severity. Controllable factors that can significantly worsen asthma can be generally grouped as (1) environmental exposures and (2) co-morbid conditions (Table 143-7).

ELIMINATING AND REDUCING PROBLEMATIC ENVIRONMENTAL EXPOSURES. The majority of children with asthma have an allergic component to their disease; steps should be taken to investigate and minimize allergen exposures in sensitized asthmatics. For sensitized asthmatics, reduced exposure to perennial allergens in the home decreases asthma symptoms, medication requirements, AHR, and asthma exacerbations. The important home allergens that are linked to asthma worsening differ between locales and even between homes. Common perennial allergen exposures include furred or feathered animals as pets (cats, dogs, ferrets, birds) or as pests (mice, rats) and occult indoor allergens such as dust mites, cockroaches, and molds. Although some sensitized children may report an increase in asthma symptoms on exposure to the allergen source, improvement from allergen avoidance may not become apparent without a sustained period of days to weeks away from the offending exposure. Tobacco, wood and coal smoke, dusts, strong odors, and noxious fumes can all aggravate asthma. These airways irritants should be eliminated or reduced from the homes and automobiles used by asthmatic children. School classrooms and daycare settings can also be sites of asthma-worsening environmental exposures. Eliminating or minimizing these exposures (furred pets in classrooms with sensitized asthmatic children) can reduce asthma symptoms, disease severity, and the amount of medication needed to achieve good asthma control. Annual influenza vaccination continues to be recommended for all asthmatic children (except for those with egg allergy), although influenza is not responsible for the large majority of virus-induced asthma exacerbations experienced by children.

TREAT CO-MORBID CONDITIONS. Rhinitis, sinusitis, and gastroesophageal reflux often accompany asthma and can mimic asthma symptoms and worsen disease severity. Indeed, these conditions with asthma are the 3 most common causes of chronic coughing. Effective management of these co-morbid conditions can often improve asthma symptoms and disease severity, such that less asthma medication is needed to achieve good asthma control.

Gastroesophageal reflux (**GER**) is common in asthmatics, with a reported incidence of up to 64% with GER-related asthma symptoms. GER may worsen asthma through 2 postulated mechanisms: (1) aspiration of refluxed gastric contents (micro- or macro-aspiration); and (2) vagally-mediated reflex bronchospasm. Occult GER should be suspected in individuals with difficult-to-control asthma, especially patients with prominent asthma symptoms while eating or sleeping (in a horizontal position), or who prop themselves up in bed to reduce nocturnal symptoms. GER can be demonstrated by reflux of barium into the esophagus during a barium swallow procedure or by esophageal pH monitoring. Because radiographic studies lack sufficient sensitivity and specificity, extended esophageal pH monitoring is the method of choice for diagnosing GER. If significant GER is noted, reflux precautions should be instituted (no food 2 hr before bedtime, head of the bed elevated 6 in, avoid caffeinated foods and beverages) and medications such as proton pump inhibitors (omeprazole, lansoprazole) or H_2-receptor antagonists (cimetidine, ranitidine) administered for 8 to 12 wk.

Rhinitis is usually co-morbid with asthma, detected in ≈90% of asthmatic children. Rhinitis can be seasonal and/or perennial, with allergic and non-allergic components. Rhinitis complicates and worsens asthma via numerous direct and indirect mechanisms. Nasal breathing may reduce exercise-induced bronchospasm and lower airways dysfunction by humidifying and warming inspired air, and filtering out allergens and irritants that can trigger asthma and increase AHR. Reduction of nasal congestion and obstruction can help the nose to perform these humidifying, warming, and filtering functions. In asthmatics, improvement in rhinitis is also associated with improvement in AHR, lower airways inflammation, asthma symptoms, and asthma medication use. Optimal rhinitis management in children is similar to asthma management in regards to the importance of interventions to reduce nasal inflammation (see Chapter 142).

Radiographic evidence for sinus disease is common in patients with asthma. There is usually significant improvement in asthma control in patients diagnosed and treated for sinus disease. A coronal, "screening" or "limited" CT scan of the sinuses is the gold standard test for sinus disease and is often helpful if recurrent sinusitis has been suspected and treated without such evidence. If the patient with asthma has clinical and radiographic evidence for sinusitis, topical therapy to include nasal saline irrigations and possibly intranasal corticosteroids should be instituted, and a 2–3 wk course of antibiotics administered.

Principles of Asthma Pharmacotherapy. The NAEPP guidelines offer a stepwise approach to management based on asthma severity categorized as mild intermittent, mild persistent, moderate persistent, and severe persistent asthma (Tables 143-8, 143-9, and 143-10). The classification of asthma severity is based on the following parameters: (1) frequency of daytime and (2) nighttime symptoms, (3) degree of airflow obstruction by spirometry, and/or (4) PEF variability (see Table 143-8). For younger children (<5 yr of age), management is primarily based on symptoms since young children cannot perform the maneuvers required for conventional lung function measurements (see Table 143-8). A major objective of this approach is to identify and *treat all "persistent" asthma with anti-inflammatory controller medication.* The type(s) and amount(s) of daily controller medications to be used are determined by the asthma severity rating. The "three strikes" rule is a handy memory aid for determining if an asthmatic child should receive controller therapy. Simply put, if an asthmatic child has asthma symptoms or uses quick-relief medication at least 3 times per wk, awakens at night due to asthma at least 3 times per mo, requires a refill for a quick-relief inhaler prescription at least 3 times per yr, experiences asthma exacerbations at least 3 times per yr, or requires short courses of systemic corticosteroids at least 3 times a yr, then that patient should receive daily controller therapy. In addition, according to the NAEPP guidelines, controller therapy can be considered for children who present with frequent exacerbations (at least 2 exacerbations occurring <6 wk apart). Inhaled corticosteroid (ICS) therapy is recommended as preferred therapy for all levels of asthma severity except for the mild intermittent category. Leukotriene pathway modifiers or sustained-release theophylline (only for patients >5 yr of age) are considered alternative controllers for mild persistent asthmatics. Combination therapy of a low-to-medium dose ICS with a long-acting β-agonist (LABA; preferred) or a leukotriene modifier or theophylline is a mainstay therapy for moderate persistent asthma in older children and adults. While the use of medium-dose ICS alone is an alternative therapy for older children and adults with moderate persistent severity, for infants and young children, it is considered a preferred treatment for moderate persistent asthma. Severe persistent asthmatics should receive high-dose ICS, a long-acting bronchodilator, and routine oral corticosteroids if needed. Daily controller therapy is not recommended for mild intermittent asthma. SABAs are the recommended quick-reliever medications for symptoms and exercise pretreatment for all asthma severity levels.

"STEP-UP, STEP-DOWN" APPROACH. The NAEPP guidelines emphasize initiating higher-level controller therapy at the outset to establish prompt control, with measures to "step down" therapy once good asthma control is achieved. Initially, airflow limitation and the pathology of asthma may limit the delivery and efficacy of ICS such that stepping up to higher doses and/or combination therapy may be needed to gain asthma control. Fur-

TABLE 143-8. Classification of Asthma Severity

				FOR ADULTS AND CHILDREN AGE > 5 YEARS WHO CAN USE A SPIROMETER OR PEAK FLOW METER	
CLASSIFICATION	STEP	DAYS WITH SYMPTOMS	NIGHTS WITH SYMPTOMS	FEV_1 or PEF* % Predicted Normal	PEF Variability (%)
Severe persistent	4	Continual	Frequent	≤60	>30
Moderate persistent	3	Daily	>1/wk	>60–<80	>30
Mild persistent	2	>2/wk, but <1 time/day	>2/mo	≥80	20–30
Mild intermittent	1	≤2/wk	<2/mo	≥80	<20

Based on clinical features before treatment; classification is determined by the patient's most severe feature.

*Percentage of predicted norms for Forced Expiratory Volume in 1 sec (FEV_1); percentage of personal best for Peak Expiratory Flow (PEF).

From National Asthma Education and Prevention Program Expert Panel Report.

Guidelines for the Diagnosis and Management of Asthma – Update on Selected Topics (2002). NIH publication no:02-5075.

TABLE 143-9. Stepwise Approach for Managing Infants and Young Children (≤5 Yr of Age) with Acute or Chronic Asthma; Treatment

CLASSIFY SEVERITY: CLINICAL FEATURES BEFORE TREATMENT OR ADEQUATE CONTROL		MEDICATIONS REQUIRED TO MAINTAIN LONG-TERM CONTROL
	Symptoms/Day **Symptoms/Night**	**Daily Medications**
Step 4 **Severe persistent**	Continual Frequent	• **Preferred treatment** —**High-dose inhaled corticosteroids AND** —**Long-acting inhaled β_2-agonists** **AND,** if needed, —Corticosteroid tablets or syrup long term (2 mg/kg/day, generally do not exceed 60 mg/day). (Make repeat attempts to reduce systemic corticosteroids and maintain control with high-dose inhaled corticosteroids.)
Step 3 **Moderate persistent**	Daily >1 night/wk	• **Preferred treatment** —**Low-dose inhaled corticosteroids and long-acting inhaled β_2-agonists** **OR** —**Medium-dose inhaled corticosteroids.** • Alternative treatment —Low-dose inhaled corticosteroids and either leukotriene receptor antagonist or theophylline. If needed (particularly in patients with recurring severe exacerbations): • **Preferred treatment** —**Medium-dose inhaled corticosteroids and long-acting β_2-agonists.** • Alternative treatment —Medium-dose inhaled corticosteroids and either leukotriene receptor antagonist or theophylline.
Step 2 **Mild persistent**	>2/week but <1 x/day >2 nights/mo	• **Preferred treatment** —**Low-dose inhaled corticosteroid (with nebulizer or MDI with holding chamber with or without face mask or DPI).** • Alternative treatment —Cromolyn (nebulizer is preferred or MDI with holding chamber) OR leukotriene receptor antagonist.
Step 1 **Mild intermittent**	≤2 days/wk ≤2 nights/mo	• No daily medication needed.

Quick Relief All Patients
- Bronchodilator as needed for symptoms. Intensity of treatment will depend on severity of exacerbation.
  - —Preferred treatment: **Short-acting inhaled β_2-agonists** by nebulizer or face mask and space/holding chamber
  - —Alternative treatment: Oral β_2-agonist
- With viral respiratory infection
  - —Bronchodilator q 4–6 hr up to 24 hr (longer with physician consult); in general, repeat no more than once every 6 wk
  - —Consider systemic corticosteroid if exacerbation is severe or patient has history of previous severe exacerbations
- Use of short-acting β_2-agonists >2 times/wk in intermittent asthma (daily, or increasing use in persistent asthma) may indicate the need to initiate (increase) long-term-control therapy.

↓ Step down
Review treatment every 1 to 6 mo; a gradual stepwise reduction in treatment may be possible.

↑ Step up
If control is not maintained, consider step up. First, review patient medication technique, adherence, and environmental control.

GOALS OF THERAPY: ASTHMA CONTROL
- Minimal or no chronic symptoms day or night
- Minimal or no exacerbations
- No limitations on activities; no school/parent's work missed
- Minimal use of short-acting inhaled β_2-agonist
- Minimal or no adverse effects from medications

Note
- The stepwise approach is intended to assist, not replace, the clinical decision-making required to meet individual patient needs.
- Classify severity: assign patient to most severe step in which any feature occurs.
- There are very few studies on asthma therapy for infants.
- Gain control as quickly as possible (a course of short systemic corticosteroids may be required); then step down to the least medication necessary to maintain control.
- Minimize use of short-acting inhaled β_2-agonists. Overreliance on short-acting inhaled β_2-agonists (e.g., use of approximately one canister/mo even if not using it every day) indicates inadequate control of asthma and the need to initiate or intensify long-term-control therapy.
- Provide parent education on asthma management and controlling environmental factors that make asthma worse (e.g., allergies and irritants).
- Consultation with an asthma specialist is recommended for patients with moderate or severe persistent asthma. Consider consultation for patients with mild persistent asthma.

DPI, dry powder inhaler; MDI, metered dose inhaler.
From National Asthma Education and Prevention Program (NAEPP) Expert Panel Report. *Guidelines for the Diagnosis and Management of Asthma-Updated on Selected Topics.* Washington, DC, NIH, 2002 (NIH publication no: 02-5075)

thermore, ICS requires weeks to months of daily administration for optimal efficacy to occur. Combination pharmacotherapy can provide relatively immediate improvement while also providing daily ICS to improve long-term control. Asthma therapy can be stepped down after good asthma control has been achieved and ICS has had time to achieve optimal efficacy, by determining the least number or dose of daily controller medications that can maintain good control, thereby reducing the potential for medication adverse effects. The NAEPP guidelines recommend decreasing ICS dose by about 25% every 2 to 3 mo, as long as good asthma control is maintained. Other "step-down" options include reducing the frequency of controller therapy (bid to qd), discontinuing combination therapy while continuing ICS, or reducing the dose of ICS while maintaining combination therapy.

DELIVERY DEVICES AND INHALATION TECHNIQUE. Inhaled medications are delivered as an aerosolized form in a metered-dose inhaler (MDI), as a dry powder inhaler (DPI) formulation, or in a suspension or solution form delivered via a nebulizer. In the past, MDIs, which require coordination and use of a spacer device, have dominated the market. Spacer devices, recommended for the administration of all MDI medications, are simple and inexpensive tools that: (1) decrease the coordination required to use MDIs, especially in young children; (2) improve the delivery of inhaled drug to the lower airways; and (3) minimize the risk of propellant-mediated adverse effects (thrush). Optimal inhalation technique for each puff of MDI-delivered medication is a slow (5 sec) inhalation, then a 5–10 sec breath-hold. No waiting time between puffs of medication is needed. Young pre–school-age children cannot perform this inhalation technique; MDI medications can then be delivered with a spacer and mask, using a different technique: each puff administered with regular breathing for about 30 sec or 5–10 breaths, a tight seal must be maintained, and talking, coughing, or crying will blow the medication out of the spacer. This technique will not deliver as much medication per puff when compared with the optimal MDI technique used by older children and adults. DPI

TABLE 143-10. Stepwise Approach for Managing Asthma in Adults and Children >5 Yr of Age: Treatment

CLASSIFY SEVERITY: CLINICAL FEATURES BEFORE TREATMENT OR ADEQUATE CONTROL	Symptoms/Day / Symptoms/Night	PEF or FEV_1 / PEF Variability	MEDICATIONS REQUIRED TO MAINTAIN LONG-TERM CONTROL: Daily Medications
Step 4 **Severe persistent**	Continual / Frequent	≤60% / >30%	• **Preferred treatment** —**High-dose inhaled corticosteroids** AND —**Long-acting inhaled β_2-agonists** AND, if needed, —Corticosteroid tablets or syrup long term (2 mg/kg/day, generally do not exceed 60 mg/day). (Make repeat attempts to reduce systemic corticosteroids and maintain control with high-dose inhaled corticosteroids.)
Step 3 **Moderate persistent**	Daily / >1 night/wk	>60%–<80% / >30%	• **Preferred treatment** —**Low-to-medium dose inhaled corticosteroids and long-acting inhaled β_2-agonists.** • Alternative treatment —Increase inhaled corticosteroids within medium-dose range OR —Low-to-medium dose inhaled corticosteroids and either leukotriene modifier or theophylline. If needed (particularly in patients with recurring severe exacerbations): • **Preferred treatment** —**Increase inhaled corticosteroids with medium-dose range and add long-acting inhaled β_2-agonists.** • Alternative treatment —Increase inhaled corticosteroids within medium-dose range and add either leukotriene modifier or theophylline.
Step 2 **Mild persistent**	>2/wk but <1 x/day / >2 nights/mo	≥80% / 20–30%	• **Preferred treatment** —**Low-dose inhaled corticosteroid.** • Alternative treatment (listed alphabetically): cromolyn, leukotriene modifier, nedocromil, OR sustained-release theophylline to serum concentration of 5–15 μ/mL.
Step 1 **Mild intermittent**	≤2 days/wk / ≤2 nights/mo	≥80% / <20%	• No daily medication needed.

Quick Relief All Patients
- Short-acting bronchodilator: 2–4 puffs **short-acting inhaled β_2-agonists** as needed for symptoms.
- Intensity of treatment will depend on severity of exacerbation; up to 3 treatments at 20-minute intervals or a single nebulizer treatment as needed. Course of systemic corticosteroids may be needed.
- Use of short-acting β_2-agonists >2 times/wk in intermittent asthma (daily, or increasing use in persistent asthma) may indicate the need to initiate (increase) long-term-control therapy.

↓ Step down
Review treatment every 1 to 6 mo; a gradual stepwise reduction in treatment may be possible.

↑ Step up
If control is not maintained, consider step up. First, review patient medication technique, adherence, and environmental control.

GOALS OF THERAPY: ASTHMA CONTROL
- Minimal or no chronic symptoms day or night
- Minimal or no exacerbations
- No limitations on activities; no school/work missed
- Maintain (near) normal pulmonary function
- Minimal use of short-acting inhaled β_2-agonist
- Minimal or no adverse effects from medications

Note
- The stepwise approach is meant to assist, not replace, the clinical decision-making required to meet individual patient needs.
- Classify severity: assign patient to most severe step in which any feature occurs (PEF is % of personal best; FEV_1 is % predicted).
- Gain control as quickly as possible (consider a short course of systemic corticosteroids); then step down to the least medication necessary to maintain control.
- Minimize use of short-acting inhaled β_2-agonists. Overreliance on short-acting inhaled β_2-agonists (e.g., use of one canister/mo even if not using it every day) indicates inadequate control of asthma and the need to initiate or intensify long-term-control therapy.
- Provide education on self-management and controlling environmental factors that make asthma worse (e.g., allergens and irritants).
- Refer to an asthma specialist if there are difficulties controlling asthma or if step 4 care is required. Referral may be considered if step 3 care is required.

From National Asthma Education and Prevention Program (NAEPP) Expert Panel Report. *Guidelines for the Diagnosis and Management of Asthma-Update on Selected Topics.* Washington, DC, NIH, 2002 (NIH publication no: 02-5075).

devices (Diskus, Turbuhaler, Autohaler, Aerolizer) are popular because of their simplicity of use, albeit adequate inspiratory flow is needed. They are breath-actuated (the drug comes out only as it is breathed in) and spacers are not needed. Mouth rinsing is recommended after ICS use to rinse out ICS deposited on the oral mucosa and reduce the swallowed ICS and the risk of thrush.

Nebulizers have been the mainstay of aerosol treatment for infants and young children. An advantage of using nebulizers is the simple technique required of relaxed breathing. The preferential nasal breathing, small airways, low tidal volume, and high respiratory rate of infants markedly increase the difficulty of inhaled drug targeting to the lung airways. Disadvantages of nebulizers include need for a power source, inconvenience in that treatments take about 5 min, expense, and potential for bacterial contamination.

ADHERENCE. Asthma is a chronic condition that is often best managed with daily controller medication. Adherence with a daily regimen is commonly suboptimal; ICS are underused 60% of the time. Individuals who require an oral corticosteroid course due to an asthma exacerbation had used their ICS the least (<15% of the time). Adherence is poorer when prescribed frequency of medication administration is greater (3–4 times/24 hr). Controller formulations for twice- and even once-daily dosing can improve patient adherence. Misconceptions about controller medication efficacy and safety often underlie poor adherence and can be addressed by asking about such concerns at each visit.

Long-Term Controller Medications. All levels of persistent asthma should be treated with daily medications to improve long-term control (Tables 143-11 and 143-12). Such medications include ICS, LABAs, leukotriene modifiers, nonsteroidal anti-inflammatory agents, and sustained-release theophylline. An anti-IgE preparation, omalizumab (Xolair), has been approved by the Food and Drug Administration (FDA) for children ≥12 yr as an add-on therapy for patients with moderate to severe allergic asthma. Corticosteroids are the most potent and effective medications used to treat both the acute (administered systemically) and chronic (administered by inhalation) manifestations of asthma. They are available in inhaled, oral, and parenteral forms (see Table 143-12).

INHALED CORTICOSTEROIDS (ICS). The NAEPP guidelines recommend daily ICS therapy as the treatment of choice for all patients with persistent asthma (see Table 143-9). ICS therapy has been shown to reduce asthma symptoms, improve lung function, reduce AHR, reduce "rescue" medication use and, most important, reduce urgent care visits, hospitalizations, and prednisone use for asthma exacerbations by about 50%. ICS therapy

TABLE 143-11. Usual Dosages for Long-Term-Control Medications

MEDICATION	DOSAGE FORM	ADULT DOSE	CHILD DOSE*
INHALED CORTICOSTEROIDS (SEE TABLE 143-12)			
SYSTEMIC CORTICOSTEROIDS			
Methylprednisolone	2, 4, 8, 16, 32 mg tablets	• 7.5–60 mg daily in a single dose in AM or qod as needed for control • Short-course "burst" to achieve control: 40–60 mg/day as single or 2 divided doses for 3–10 days	• 0.25–2 mg/kg daily in single dose in AM or qod as needed for control • Short-course "burst": 1–2 mg/kg/day, maximum 60 mg/day for 3–10 days
Prednisolone	5 mg tablets, 5 mg/5 cc, 15 mg/5 cc,		
Prednisone	1, 2.5, 5, 10, 20, 50 mg tablets; 5 mg/cc, 5 mg/5 cc		
LONG-ACTING INHALED B_2-AGONISTS (SHOULD NOT BE USED FOR SYMPTOM RELIEF OR FOR EXACERBATIONS. USE WITH INHALED CORTICOSTEROIDS.)			
Salmeterol	MDI 21 μg/puff DPI 50 μg/blister	2 puffs q 12 hours 1 blister q 12 hours	1–2 puffs q 12 hours 1 blister q 12 hours
Formoterol	DPI 12 μg/single-use capsule	1 capsule q 12 hours	1 capsule q 12 hours
COMBINED MEDICATION			
Fluticasone/Salmeterol	DPI 100, 250, or 500 μg/50 μg	1 inhalation bid; dose depends on severity of asthma	1 inhalation bid; dose depends on severity of asthma
CROMOLYN AND NEDOCROMIL			
Cromolyn	MDI 1 mg/puff Nebulizer 20 mg/ampule	2–4 puffs tid-qid 1 ampule tid-qid	1–2 puffs tid-qid 1 ampule tid-qid
Nedocromil	MDI 1.75 mg/puff	2–4 puffs bid-qid	1–2 puffs bid-qid
LEUKOTRIENE MODIFIERS			
Montelukast	4 or 5 mg chewable tablet 10 mg tablet	10 mg qhs	4 mg qhs (2–5 yrs) 5 mg qhs (6–14 yrs) 10 mg qhs (>14 yrs)
Zafirlukast	10 or 20 mg tablet	40 mg daily (20 mg tablet bid)	20 mg daily (7–11 yrs) (10 mg tablet bid)
Zileuton	300 or 600 mg tablet	2,400 mg daily (give tablets qid)	
METHYLXANTHINES (SERUM MONITORING IS IMPORTANT [SERUM CONCENTRATION OF 5–15 μG/ML AT STEADY STATE]).			
Theophylline	Liquids, sustained-release tablets, and capsules	Starting dose 10 mg/kg/day up to 300 mg max; usual max 800 mg/day	Starting dose 10 mg/kg/day; usual max: • <1 year of age: 0.2 (age in wk) +5 = mg/kg/day • ≥1 year of age: 16 mg/kg/day

*Children ≤ 12 years of age.
From National Asthma Education and Prevention Program (NAEPP) Expert Panel Report. *Guidelines for the Diagnosis and Management of Asthma—Update on Selected Topics*. Washington, DC, NIH, 2002. (NIH publication no: 02-5075).

may lower the risk of death due to asthma. It can achieve all of the goals of asthma management and, as a result, is viewed as first-line treatment for persistent asthma.

There are currently 5 ICSs that are approved by the FDA, and the NAEPP guidelines provide an equivalence classification (see Table 143-12), although direct comparisons of efficacy and safety outcomes in children are lacking. Newer forms are being developed (mometasone furoate, ciclesonide) that may enhance the efficacy-to-safety profile of ICS therapy while allowing for less frequent dosing. ICSs are available in MDIs, DPIs, or in suspension for nebulization. Fluticasone propionate, mometasone furoate and, to a lesser extent, budesonide are considered "2nd-generation" ICSs in that they have increased anti-inflammatory potency and reduced systemic bioavailability for potential adverse effects, owing to extensive first-pass hepatic metabolism. The selection of the initial ICS dose is based on the determination of disease severity. A fraction of the initial ICS dose is often sufficient to maintain good control after this has been achieved.

Although ICS therapy has been widely used in adults with persistent asthma, its application in children has lagged due to concerns of the potential for adverse effects with chronic use. Generally, clinically significant adverse effects that occur with chronic systemic corticosteroid therapy have not been seen or have been only very rarely reported in children receiving ICSs in recommended doses. The risk of adverse effects from ICS therapy is related to the dose and frequency with which ICSs are given (Table 143-13). High doses (≥1,000 μg/day in children) and frequent administration (4 times/day) are more likely to cause local and systemic adverse effects. Children who are maintained on higher ICS doses are also likely to require systemic corticosteroid courses for asthma exacerbations, further increasing the risk of corticosteroid adverse effects.

The most commonly encountered **adverse effects** from ICSs are local: oral candidiasis (thrush) and dysphonia (hoarse voice). Thrush results from propellant-induced mucosal irritation and local immunosuppression. Dysphonia occurs from vocal cord

TABLE 143-12. Estimated Comparative Daily Dosages for Inhaled Corticosteroids

	LOW DAILY DOSE		MEDIUM DAILY DOSE		HIGH DAILY DOSE	
DRUG	Adult	Child*	Adult	Child*	Adult	Child*
Beclomethasone CFC 42 or 84 μg/puff	168–504 μg	84–336 μg	504–840 μg	336–672 μg	>840 μg	>672 μg
Beclomethasone HFA 40 or 80 μg/puff	80–240 μg	80–160 μg	240–840 μg	160–320 μg	>480 μg	>320 μg
Budesonide DPI 200 μg/inhalation	200–600 μg	200–400 μg	600–1,200 μg	400–800 μg	>1,200 μg	>800 μg
Inhalation suspension for nebulization (child dose)		0.5 μg		1.0 μg		2.0 μg
Flunisolide 250 μg/puff	500–1,000 μg	500–750 μg	1,000–2,000 μg	1,000–1,250 μg	>2,000 μg	>1,250 μg
Fluticasone MDI: 44, 110, or 220 μg/puff	88–264 μg	88–176 μg	264–660 μg	175–440 μg	>660 μg	>440 μg
DPI: 50, 100, or 250 μg/inhalation	100–300 μg	100–200 μg	300–600 μg	200–400 μg	>600 μg	>400 μg
Triamcinolone acetonide 100 μg/puff	400–1,000 μg	400–800 μg	1,000–2,000 μg	800–1,200 μg	>2,000 μg	>1,200 μg

*Children ≤ 12 years of age.
From National Asthma Education and Prevention Program (NAEPP) Expert Panel Report. *Guidelines for the Diagnosis and Management of Asthma—Update on Selected Topics*. (2002). NIH publication no: 02-5075.

TABLE 143-13. Risk Assessment for Corticosteroid Adverse Effects

	CONDITIONS	RECOMMENDATIONS
Low risk	(≤1 risk factor*) Low- to medium-dose ICS (see Table 143-10)	• Monitor blood pressure and weight with each physician visit • Measure height annually (stadiometry); monitor periodically for declining growth rate and pubertal developmental delay • Encourage regular physical exercise • Adequate dietary calcium and vitamin D with additional supplements for daily calcium if needed • Avoid smoking and alcohol • Ensure TSH status if with history of thyroid abnormality
Medium risk	(if >1 risk factor,* consider evaluating as high risk) High-dose ICS (see Table 143-10) At least 4 oral corticosteroid courses/yr	As above, plus: • Yearly ophthalmologic evaluations to monitor for cataracts or glaucoma • Baseline bone densitometry (DEXA scan) • Consider at increased risk for adrenal insufficiency, esp. with physiologic stressors (e.g., surgery, accident, significant illness)
High risk	Chronic systemic corticosteroids (>7.5 mg daily or equivalent for >1 mo) ≥7 oral corticosteroid bursts/year Very high dose ICS (e.g., fluticasone propionate ≥800 μg/day)	As above, plus: • DEXA scan: if DEXA Z score <−1.0, recommend close monitoring (every 12 mo) • Consider referral to a bone or endocrine specialist • Bone age • Complete blood count • Serum calcium, phosphorus, alkaline phosphatase • Urine calcium and creatinine • Testosterone in males, estradiol in amenorrheic premenopausal women, vitamin D (25-OH and 1,25-OH vitamin D), parathyroid hormone, osteocalcin • Urine telopeptides for those on chronic systemic or frequent oral corticosteroid treatment • Assume adrenal insufficiency for physiologic stressors (e.g., surgery, accident, significant illness)

***Risk factors for osteoporosis:** Presence of other chronic illness(es), medications (corticosteroids, anticonvulsants, heparin, diuretics), low body weight, family history of osteoporosis, significant fracture history disproportionate to trauma, recurrent falls, impaired vision, low dietary calcium and vitamin D intake, and lifestyle factors (decreased physical activity, smoking, and alcohol intake).
ICS, inhaled corticosteroid; TSH, thyroid-stimulating hormone.

myopathy. These effects are dose-dependent and are most common in individuals on high-dose ICS and/or oral corticosteroid therapy. The incidence of these local effects can be greatly minimized by using a spacer with MDI ICS because spacers reduce oropharyngeal deposition of the drug and propellant. Mouth rinsing using a "swish and spit" technique after ICS use is also recommended.

The potential for growth suppression with long-term ICS use has been a concern. Complicating this issue is the observation that poorly controlled asthma can adversely affect growth. In the long-term, prospective NIH-sponsored CAMP study, after a mean of 4.3 yr of therapy, children with mild to moderate asthma randomized to budesonide (400 μg/day) had grown 22.7 cm, whereas those randomized to placebo had grown 23.8 cm—a 1.1 cm difference. Of importance, this 1.1 cm difference occurred primarily in the 1st year of ICS therapy, indicating that the growth reduction was a transient, not progressive phenomenon. A controlled study found no difference in the measured vs expected adult heights of asthmatic children who received inhaled budesonide (400 μg/day) for >9 yr. Transient growth suppression was noted in the 1st few years of therapy, with eventual catch-up growth and no effect on final adult height.

Two large pediatric studies that have evaluated the effect of long-term ICS on bone mineral density failed to find a relationship between ICS use and diminished bone mineral density (see Chapter 705). Although these studies cannot predict a significant effect of ICS therapy on osteoporosis in later adulthood, improved asthma control may result in less corticosteroid therapy (oral, inhaled) needed over time. These findings were with budesonide at doses of about 400 μg/day; higher doses of ICSs, especially those with increased potency, have a greater potential for adverse effects. Hence, corticosteroid adverse effects screening and osteoporosis prevention measures are recommended for patients on higher doses of ICSs, as these patients are also likely to require systemic courses for exacerbations (see Table 143-13).

SYSTEMIC CORTICOSTEROIDS. ICS therapy has allowed the large majority of children with asthma to maintain good disease control without maintenance (qod) oral corticosteroids. Oral corticosteroid therapy is used primarily to treat asthma exacerbations and in rare patients with severe disease who remain symptomatic despite optimal use of other asthma medications. In these severe asthmatics, every attempt should be made to exclude any co-morbid conditions and to keep the oral corticosteroid dose at ≤20 mg qod. Doses exceeding this amount are associated with numerous adverse effects (see Chapter 578). To determine the need for continued oral corticosteroid therapy, a taper of the oral corticosteroid dose (over weeks to several months) should be considered, with close monitoring of the patient's symptoms and lung function.

When administered orally, prednisone, prednisolone, and methylprednisolone are rapidly and nearly completely absorbed, with peak plasma concentrations occurring within 1–2 hr. Prednisone is an inactive pro-drug that requires biotransformation via first-pass hepatic metabolism to prednisolone, its active form. Corticosteroids are metabolized in the liver into inactive compounds, with the rate of metabolism influenced by drug interactions and disease states. Anticonvulsants (phenytoin, phenobarbital, carbamazepine) increase the metabolism of prednisolone, methylprednisolone, and dexamethasone, with methylprednisolone most significantly affected. Rifampin also enhances the clearance of corticosteroids and can result in diminished therapeutic effect. Other medications (ketoconazole, oral contraceptives) can significantly delay corticosteroid metabolism. Macrolide antibiotics (erythromycin, clarithromycin, troleandomycin) delay the clearance of only methylprednisolone.

Children who require chronically administered oral corticosteroids are at risk of developing associated adverse effects over time. Essentially all major organ systems can be adversely affected by chronically administered oral corticosteroid therapy (see Chapter 578). Some of these effects occur immediately (metabolic effects). Others can develop insidiously over several months to years (growth suppression, osteoporosis, cataracts). Most adverse effects occur in a cumulative dose- and duration-dependent manner. Children who require routine or frequent short courses of oral corticosteroids, especially with concurrent high-dose ICSs, should receive corticosteroid adverse effects screening (see Table 143-13) and osteoporosis preventive measures (see Chapter 705).

LONG-ACTING INHALED β-AGONIST (LABA). Although LABAs (salmeterol, formoterol) are β-agonists, they are considered to be daily controller medications, **not intended** for use as "rescue" medication for acute asthma symptoms or exacerbations, nor as monotherapy for persistent asthma. Salmeterol has a prolonged onset of action, with maximal bronchodilation about 1 hr after administration, whereas formoterol has an onset of action within 5–10 min. Both medications have a prolonged duration of effect of at least 12 hr. Given their long duration of action, they are well suited for patients with nocturnal asthma and for individuals who require frequent SABA use during the day to prevent exercise-induced bronchospasm. Their major role is as an "add-on" agent in patients who are suboptimally controlled on ICS therapy alone. For those patients, several studies have found the addition of LABA to ICS to be superior to doubling the dose of ICS, especially on day and nocturnal symptoms. There are also controller formulations that combine ICS with LABA (fluticasone/salmeterol, budesonide/formoterol).

LEUKOTRIENE-MODIFYING AGENTS. Leukotrienes are potent pro-inflammatory mediators that can induce bronchospasm, mucus secretion, and airways edema. Two classes of leukotriene modifiers have been developed: inhibitors of leukotriene synthesis and leukotriene receptor antagonists (LTRA). Zileuton, the only leukotriene synthesis inhibitor, is not approved for use in children <12 yr of age. Because zileuton requires administration 4 times daily, can result in elevated liver function enzymes in 2–4% of patients, and interacts with medications metabolized via the cytochrome-P450 system, it is rarely prescribed for children with asthma.

LTRAs have bronchodilator and targeted anti-inflammatory properties and reduce exercise-, aspirin-, and allergen-induced bronchoconstriction. They are recommended as an alternative treatment for mild persistent asthma and as an "add-on" medication to ICS for moderate persistent asthma. Two LTRAs are FDA-approved for use in children: montelukast and zafirlukast. Both medications improve asthma symptoms, decrease need for rescue β-agonist use, and improve lung function. Montelukast, which is FDA-approved for use in children ≥1 yr of age, is administered once daily. Zafirlukast is FDA-approved for use in children ≥5 yr of age and is administered twice daily. Although incompletely studied in children with asthma, LTRAs appear to be less effective than ICSs in patients with moderate persistent asthma. In general, ICS improves lung function by 5–15%, whereas LTRA improves lung function by 2–7.5%. LTRAs are not thought to have significant adverse effects, although case reports described a Churg-Strauss–like vasculitis (pulmonary infiltrates, eosinophilia, cardiomyopathy) in adults with corticosteroid-dependent asthma treated with LTRAs. It remains to be determined whether these patients have a primary eosinophilic vasculitis masquerading as asthma, which was "unmasked" as their oral corticosteroid dose was tapered, or whether the disease is a very rare adverse effect of LTRA.

NONSTEROIDAL ANTI-INFLAMMATORY AGENTS. Cromolyn and nedocromil are non-corticosteroid anti-inflammatory agents that can inhibit allergen-induced asthmatic responses and reduce exercise-induced bronchospasm. According to the NAEPP guidelines, both drugs are considered alternative anti-inflammatory drugs for children with mild persistent asthma. Although largely devoid of adverse effects, these medications must be administered frequently (2–4 times/day) and are not nearly as effective daily controller medications as ICSs and leukotriene-modifying agents. Because they inhibit exercise-induced bronchospasm, they can be used in place of SABAs, especially in children who develop unwanted adverse effects with β-agonist therapy (tremor and elevated heart rate). They can also be used in addition to a SABA as a combination pretreatment for exercise-induced bronchospasm in patients who continue to experience symptoms despite SABA pretreatment alone.

THEOPHYLLINE. In addition to its bronchodilator effects, theophylline has anti-inflammatory properties as a phosphodiesterase inhibitor, although the extent of their clinical relevance has not been clearly established. Theophylline, when used chronically, can reduce asthma symptoms and the need for rescue SABA use. Although it is considered an alternative monotherapy controller agent for older children and adults with mild persistent asthma, it is no longer considered a first-line agent for small children in whom there is significant variability in the absorption and metabolism of different theophylline preparations, necessitating frequent dose monitoring (blood levels) and adjustments. Because theophylline may have some corticosteroid-sparing effects in individuals with oral corticosteroid-dependent asthma, it is still sometimes used in this group of asthmatic children. Theophylline has a narrow therapeutic window; therefore, when used, serum theophylline levels need to be routinely monitored especially if the patient has a viral illness associated with a fever or is placed on a medication known to delay theophylline clearance, such as macrolide antibiotics, cimetidine, oral antifungal agents, oral contraceptives, leukotriene synthesis inhibitor, and ciprofloxacin. Theophylline overdosage and elevated theophylline levels have been associated with headaches, vomiting, cardiac arrhythmias, seizures, and death.

ANTI-IGE (OMALIZUMAB). Omalizumab is a humanized monoclonal antibody that binds IgE, thereby preventing its binding to the high-affinity IgE receptor and blocking IgE-mediated allergic responses and inflammation. Since it is unable to bind IgE that is already bound to high-affinity IgE receptors, the risk of anaphylaxis via direct IgE cross linking by the drug is circumvented. It is FDA-approved for patients >12 yr old with moderate to severe asthma, documented hypersensitivity to a perennial aeroallergen, and inadequate disease control with inhaled and/or oral corticosteroids. It is given every 2–4 wk subcutaneously based on body weight and serum IgE levels. Its clinical efficacy as an "add-on" therapy for patients with moderate to severe allergic asthma has been demonstrated in large clinical trials, with asthmatics receiving omalizumab having fewer asthma exacerbations and symptoms while reducing their ICS and/or oral corticosteroid doses. It is generally well tolerated, although local injection site reactions can occur. Hypersensitivity reactions (including anaphylaxis) and malignancies have been very rarely associated with Omalizumab use.

Quick-Reliever Medications. Quick-relief or "rescue" medications (short-acting inhaled β-agonists, inhaled anticholinergics, and short-course systemic corticosteroids) are used in the management of acute asthma symptoms (Table 143-14).

SHORT-ACTING INHALED β-AGONISTS (SABA). Given their rapid onset of action, effectiveness, and 4–6 hr duration of action, SABAs (albuterol, levalbuterol, terbutaline, pirbuterol) are the first drugs of choice for acute asthma symptoms ("rescue" medication) and for preventing exercise-induced bronchospasm. β-Agonists bronchodilate by inducing airway smooth muscle relaxation, reducing vascular permeability, reducing airways edema, and improving mucociliary clearance. Levalbuterol, or the R-isomer of albuterol, has less tachycardia and tremor, which can be bothersome to some asthmatics. Overuse of β-agonists is associated with an increased risk of death or near-death episodes from asthma. This is a major concern for some patients with asthma who rely on the frequent use of SABAs as a "quick fix" for their asthma, rather than using controller medications in a preventive manner. It is helpful to monitor the frequency of SABA use, in that use of at least 1 MDI/mo or at least 3 MDIs/year (200 inhalations/MDI) indicates inadequate asthma control and necessitates improving other aspects of asthma therapy and management.

ANTICHOLINERGIC AGENTS. As bronchodilators, the anticholinergic agents (ipratropium bromide) are much less potent than the β-agonists. Inhaled ipratropium is primarily used in the treatment of acute severe asthma. When used in combination with albuterol, ipratropium can improve lung function and reduce the rate of hospitalization in children who present to the emergency department with acute asthma. Ipratropium is the

TABLE 143-14. Asthma Exacerbation Management (Status Asthmaticus)

RISK ASSESSMENT ON ADMISSION		
Focused history	• Onset of current exacerbation • Frequency and severity of daytime and nighttime symptoms and activity limitation • Frequency of rescue bronchodilator use • Current medications and allergies • Potential triggers • History of systemic steroid courses, emergency department visits, hospitalization, intubation, or life-threatening episodes	
Clinical assessment	• Physical examination findings: vital signs, breathlessness, air movement, use of accessory muscles, retractions, anxiety level, alteration in mental status • Pulse oximetry • Lung function (defer in patients with moderate to severe distress or history of labile disease)	
Risk factors for asthma morbidity and death	See Table 143-15	
TREATMENT		
DRUG AND TRADE NAME	MECHANISMS OF ACTION AND DOSING	CAUTIONS AND ADVERSE EFFECTS
Oxygen (Mask or nasal cannula)		• Monitor pulse oximetry to maintain oxygen saturation >92% • Cardiorespiratory monitoring
Inhaled short-acting β-agonists Albuterol nebulizer solution (5 mg/mL concentrate; 2.5 mg/3 mL, 1.25 mg/3 mL, 0.63 mg/3 mL) Albuterol MDI (90 μg/puff) Levalbuterol (Xopenex) nebulizer solution (1.25 mg/0.5 mL concentrate; 0.31 mg/3 mL, 0.63 mg/3 mL, 1.25 mg/3 mL)	**Bronchodilator** Nebulizer: 0.15 mg/kg (minimum: 2.5 mg) as often as every 20 min for 3 doses as needed, then 0.15–0.3 mg/kg up to 10 mg every 1–4 hr as needed, or up to 0.5 mg/kg/hr by continuous nebulization 2–8 puffs up to every 20 min for 3 doses as needed, then every 1–4 hr as needed 0.075 mg/kg (minimum: 1.25 mg) every 20 min for 3 doses, then 0.075–0.15 mg/kg up to 5 mg every 1–4 hr as needed, or 0.25 mg/kg/hr by continuous nebulization	• Nebulizer: when giving concentrated forms, dilute with saline to 3 mL total nebulized volume • For MDI: use spacer/holding chamber • During exacerbations, frequent or continuous doses can cause pulmonary vasodilation, V/Q mismatch, and hypoxemia • Adverse effects: palpitations, tachycardia, arrhythmias, tremor, hypoxemia • Levalbuterol 0.63 mg is equivalent to 1.25 mg of standard albuterol for both efficacy and side effects.
Systemic Corticosteroids Prednisone 1, 2.5, 5, 10, 20, 50 mg tablets Methylprednisolone (Medrol) 2, 4, 8, 16, 24, 32 mg tablets; Prednisolone 5 mg tablets; 5 mg/5 mL and 15 mg/5 mL solution Depo-Medrol (IM); Solu-Medrol (IV)	**Anti-inflammatory** 0.5–1 mg/kg every 6–12 hr for 48 hr, then 1–2 mg/kg/day bid (maximum: 60 mg/day) Short-course "burst" for exacerbation: 1–2 mg/kg/day qd or bid for 3–7 days	• If exposed to chickenpox or measles, consider passive immunoglobulin prophylaxis. Also, risk of complications with herpes simplex and tuberculosis. • For daily dosing, 8 AM administration minimizes adrenal suppression • Children may benefit from tapering if course exceeds 7 days • Adverse effects monitoring: Frequent bursts risk numerous corticosteroid adverse effects (see Chapter 579). See Table 143-13 for adverse effects screening recommendations
Anticholinergics Ipratropium Atrovent (nebulizer solution 0.5 mg/2.5 mL; MDI 18 μg/inhalation) Ipratropium with albuterol DuoNeb nebulizer solution (0.5 mg ipratropium + 2.5 mg albuterol/3 mL vial)	**Mucolytic/bronchodilator** Nebulizer: 0.5 mg q6–8 hr (tid-qid) as needed MDI: 2 puffs qid 1 vial by nebulizer qid	• Should not be used as first-line therapy; added to β_2-agonist therapy • Nebulizer: may mix ipratropium with albuterol
Injectable Sympathomimetic **Epinephrine** Adrenalin 1 mg/mL (1 : 1000) EpiPen autoinjection device (0.3 mg; EpiPen Jr 0.15 mg)	**Bronchodilator** SC or IM: 0.01 mg/kg (max dose 0.5 mg); may repeat after 15–30 min	• For extreme circumstances (e.g., impending respiratory failure despite high-dose inhaled SABA, respiratory failure)
Terbutaline Brethine 1 mg/mL	Continuous IV infusion (terbutaline only): 2–10 μg/kg loading dose, followed by 0.1–0.4 μg/kg/min. Titrate in 0.1–0.2 μg/kg/min increments every 30 min, depending on clinical response.	• Terbutaline is β-agonist-selective relative to epinephrine • Monitoring with continuous infusion: cardiorespiratory monitor, pulse oximetry, blood pressure, serum potassium • Adverse effects: tremor, tachycardia, palpitations, arrhythmia, hypertension, headaches, nervousness, nausea, vomiting, hypoxemia
RISK ASSESSMENT FOR DISCHARGE		
Medical Stability	Discharge to home if sustained improvement in symptoms and bronchodilator treatments are at least 3 hr apart, normal physical findings, PEF > 70% of predicted or personal best, oxygen saturation > 92% on room air	
Home Supervision	Capability to administer intervention, and to observe and respond appropriately to clinical deterioration	
Asthma Education	See Table 143-16	

IM, intramuscular; MDI, metered dose inhaler; PEF, peak expiratory flow; SABA, short-acting beta-agonist; SC, subcutaneous; V/Q, ventilation-perfusion.

anticholinergic formulation of choice for children because it has few central nervous system adverse effects and it is available in both MDI and nebulizer formulations. Although widely used in children with asthma exacerbations of all ages, it is approved by the FDA for children >12 yr. of age.

Asthma Exacerbations and Their Management. Asthma exacerbations are acute or subacute episodes of progressively worsening symptoms and airflow obstruction. Airflow obstruction during exacerbations can become extensive, resulting in life-threatening respiratory insufficiency. Often, asthma exacerbations worsen during sleep (between midnight and 8 AM) when airways inflammation and hyperresponsiveness are at their peak. Importantly, SABAs, which are first-line therapy for asthma symptoms and exacerbations, increase pulmonary blood flow through obstructed, unoxygenated areas of the lungs with increasing dosage and frequency. When airways obstruction is not resolved with SABA use, ventilation-perfusion mismatching can cause significant hypoxemia, which can perpetuate bronchoconstriction and further worsen the condition. Severe, progressive asthma exacerbations need to be managed in a medical setting, with administration of supplemental oxygen as first-line therapy and close monitoring for potential worsening. Complications that can occur during severe exacerbations include atelectasis and air leaks in the chest (pneumomediastinum, pneumothorax).

A severe exacerbation of asthma that does not improve with standard therapy is termed **status asthmaticus.** Immediate management of an asthma exacerbation involves a rapid evaluation of the severity of obstruction and assessment of risk for further clinical deterioration (see Table 143-14). For most patients, exacerbations will improve with frequent bronchodilator treatments and a systemic corticosteroid course. The optimal management of a child with an asthma exacerbation should include, however, a more comprehensive assessment of the events leading up to the exacerbation and the underlying disease severity. Indeed, the frequency and severity of asthma exacerbations helps to define the severity of a patient's asthma. Whereas most children who experience life-threatening asthma episodes have moderate to severe asthma by other criteria, some children with asthma appear to have mild disease except when they suffer severe, even near-fatal exacerbations. The biological, environmental, economic, and psychosocial risk factors associated with asthma morbidity and death can further guide this assessment (Table 143-15).

Asthma exacerbations, although characteristically different between individuals, tend to be similar in the same patient. Severe asthma exacerbations, resulting in respiratory distress, hypoxia, hospitalization, and/or respiratory failure are the best predictors of future life-threatening exacerbations or a fatal asthma episode. In addition to distinguishing such high-risk children, some experience exacerbations that come on over days, with airflow obstruction resulting from progressive inflammation, epithelial sloughing, and cast impaction of small airways. When extreme, respiratory failure due to fatigue can ensue and necessitate mechanical ventilation for numerous days. In contrast, some children experience abrupt-onset exacerbations that may result from extreme AHR and physiological susceptibility to airways closure. Such exacerbations, when extreme, are asphyxial in nature, often occur outside of medical settings, are initially associated with very high arterial P_{CO_2} levels, and tend to require only brief periods of supportive ventilation. Recognizing the characteristic differences in exacerbations is important for optimizing early exacerbation management.

TABLE 143-15. Risk Factors for Asthma Morbidity and Mortality

BIOLOGIC
Previous severe asthma exacerbation
Severe airflow obstruction
History of rapidly occurring attacks
Severe airways hyperresponsiveness (AHR)
Increasing and large diurnal variation in peak flows
Decreased chemosensitivity and perception of dyspnea
Poor response to systemic corticosteroid therapy
Male gender
Low birthweight
Nonwhite (especially black) ethnicity
ENVIRONMENTAL
Allergen exposure
Environmental tobacco smoke exposure
Air pollution exposure
Urban environment
ECONOMIC AND PSYCHOSOCIAL
Poverty
Crowding
Mother <20 yr old
Mother with less than high school education
Inadequate medical care
Inaccessible
Unaffordable
No regular medical care (only emergent)
No care sought for chronic asthma symptoms
Delay in care of asthma exacerbations
Inadequate hospital care for asthma exacerbation
Psychopathology in the parent or child
Family problems
Alcohol or substance abuse

Home Management of Asthma Exacerbations. All children with asthma should have a written action plan to guide their recognition and management of exacerbations, along with the necessary medications and tools to manage them. Early recognition of asthma exacerbations in order to intensify treatment early can often prevent further worsening and keep exacerbations from becoming severe. A written home action plan can reduce the risk of asthma death by 70%. The NAEPP guidelines recommend immediate treatment with "rescue" medication (inhaled SABA, up to 3 treatments in 1 hr). A good response is characterized by resolution of symptoms within 1 hr, no further symptoms over the next 4 hr, and improvement in PEF to at least 80% of personal best. The child's physician should be contacted for follow-up, especially if bronchodilators are required repeatedly over the next 24–48 hr. If the child has an incomplete response to initial treatment with rescue medication (persistent symptoms and/or a PEF <80% of personal best), a short course of oral corticosteroid therapy (prednisone 1–2 mg/kg/day [not to exceed 60 mg/day] for 4 days) in addition to inhaled β-agonist therapy should be instituted. The physician should also be contacted for further instructions. Immediate medical attention should be sought for severe exacerbations, persistent signs of respiratory distress, lack of expected response or sustained improvement after initial treatment, further deterioration, or high-risk factors for asthma morbidity or mortality (previous history of severe exacerbations). For patients with severe asthma and/or a history of life-threatening episodes, especially if abrupt-onset in nature, providing an injectable form of epinephrine (EpiPen) and possibly portable oxygen at home should be considered. Use of either of these extreme measures for home management of asthma exacerbations would be an indication to call 911 for emergency support services.

Emergency Department Management of Asthma Exacerbations. In the emergency department, the primary goals of asthma management include correction of hypoxemia, rapid improvement of airflow obstruction, and prevention of progression or recurrence of symptoms. Interventions are based on clinical severity on arrival, response to initial therapy, and presence of risk factors that are associated with asthma morbidity and mortality (see Table 143-15). Indications of a severe exacerbation include breathlessness, dyspnea, retractions, accessory muscle use, tachypnea or labored breathing cyanosis, mental status changes, a silent chest with poor air exchange, and severe airflow limitation (PEF or FEV_1 <50% of personal best or predicted values). Initial treatment includes supplemental oxygen, inhaled β-agonist every 20 min for 1 hr, and, if necessary, systemic corticosteroids given either orally or intravenously (see Table 143-14). Inhaled ipratropium may be added to the β-agonist treatment if no significant response is seen with the 1st inhaled β-agonist treatment. An intramuscular injection of epinephrine or other β-agonist may be administered in severe cases. Oxygen should be administered and continued for at least 20 min after the last injection to compensate for possible ventilation-perfusion abnormalities caused by SABAs.

Close monitoring of clinical status, hydration, and oxygenation are essential elements of immediate management. A poor response to intensified treatment in the 1st hour suggests that the exacerbation will not remit quickly. The patient may be discharged to home if there is sustained improvement in symptoms, normal physical findings, PEF >70% of predicted or personal best, an oxygen saturation >92% on room air for 4 hr. Discharge medications include administration of an inhaled β-agonist up to every 3–4 hr plus a 3–7 day course of an oral corticosteroid. Optimizing controller therapy before discharge is also recommended. The addition of ICS to a course of oral corticosteroid in the emergency department setting reduces the risk of exacerbation recurrence over the subsequent month.

Hospital Management of Asthma Exacerbations. For patients with moderate to severe exacerbations that do not adequately improve within 1–2 hr of intensive treatment, overnight observation and/or admission to the hospital is likely to be needed. Other indications for hospital admission include high-risk features for asthma morbidity or death (see Table 143-15). Admission to an intensive care unit is indicated for patients with severe respiratory distress, poor response to therapy, and concern for potential respiratory failure and arrest.

Supplemental oxygen, frequently or continuously administered inhaled bronchodilator, and systemic corticosteroid therapy are the conventional interventions for children admitted to the hospital for status asthmaticus (see Table 143-14). Supplemental oxygen is administered because many children hospitalized with acute asthma will have or develop hypoxemia, especially at night and with increasing SABA administration. SABAs can be delivered frequently (every 20 min to 1 hr) or continuously (at 5–15 mg/hr). When administered continuously, significant systemic absorption of β-agonist occurs and, as a result, continuous nebulization can obviate the need for intravenous β-agonist therapy. Adverse effects of frequently administered β-agonist therapy include tremor, irritability, tachycardia, and hypokalemia. Patients requiring frequent or continuous nebulized β-agonist therapy should have ongoing cardiac monitoring. Because frequent β-agonist therapy can cause ventilation-perfusion mismatch and precipitate hypoxemia, oximetry is indicated. Inhaled ipratropium bromide is often added to albuterol every 6 hr if patients do not show a remarkable improvement, although there is little evidence to support its use in hospitalized children receiving aggressive inhaled β-agonist therapy and systemic corticosteroids. In addition to its potential to provide a synergistic effect with a β-agonist agent in relieving severe bronchospasm, it may be beneficial in patients with mucous hypersecretion or on β-blockers.

Short-course systemic corticosteroid therapy is recommended for use in moderate to severe asthma exacerbations to hasten recovery and prevent recurrence of symptoms. Corticosteroids are effective as single doses of corticosteroid administered in the emergency department, short courses of oral corticosteroids in the clinic setting, and both oral and intravenous formulations in hospitalized children. Studies in children hospitalized with acute asthma have found corticosteroids administered orally to be as effective as intravenous corticosteroids. Accordingly, oral corticosteroid therapy can often be used, although children with sustained respiratory distress and unable to tolerate oral preparations or liquids are obvious candidates for intravenous corticosteroid therapy.

Patients with persistent severe dyspnea and high-flow oxygen requirements require additional evaluations such as arterial blood gas, complete blood cell counts, serum electrolytes, and chest radiograph to monitor for respiratory insufficiency, co-morbidities, infection, and/or dehydration. Hydration status monitoring is especially important in infants and young children whose increased respiratory rate (insensible losses) and decreased oral intake put them at increased risk for dehydration. Further complicating this situation is the association of increased antidiuretic hormone (ADH) secretion with status asthmaticus. Administration of fluids at or slightly below maintenance fluid requirements is recommended. Chest physical therapy, incentive spirometry, and mucolytics are **not** recommended during the early acute period of asthma exacerbations as they can trigger severe bronchoconstriction.

Despite intensive therapy, some asthmatic children will remain critically ill and at risk for respiratory failure, intubation, and mechanical ventilation. Complications (air leaks) related to asthma exacerbations increase with intubation and assisted ventilation; every effort should be made to relieve bronchospasm and prevent respiratory failure. Several therapies, including parenterally administered epinephrine, β-agonists, methylxanthines, magnesium sulfate (25–75 mg/kg, maximum dose 2.5 g, intravenously over 20 min), and inhaled heliox have demonstrated some benefit as adjunctive therapies in severe status asthmaticus patients. Administration of either methylxanthine or magnesium sulfate requires monitoring of serum levels and cardiovascular status. Parenteral (subcutaneous, intramuscular, or intravenous) epinephrine or terbutaline sulfate may be effective in patients with life-threatening obstruction who are not responding to high doses of inhaled β-agonists, since inhaled medication may not reach the lower airway.

Rarely, a severe asthma exacerbation in children results in respiratory failure, and intubation and mechanical ventilation become necessary. Mechanical ventilation in severe asthma exacerbations requires the careful balance of enough pressure to overcome airways obstruction, while reducing hyperinflation, air trapping, and the likelihood of barotrauma (pneumothorax, pneumomediastinum) (see Chapter 70). To minimize the likelihood of such complications, mechanical ventilation should be anticipated and asthmatic children at risk for the development of respiratory failure should be managed in a pediatric ICU. Elective tracheal intubation with rapid-induction sedatives and paralytic agents is safer than emergency intubation. Mechanical ventilation aims to achieve adequate oxygenation while tolerating mild to moderate hypercapnia (PCO_2 50–70 mm Hg) to minimize barotrauma. Volume-cycled ventilators, using short inspiratory and long expiratory times, 10–15 mL/kg tidal volume, 8–15 breaths/min, peak pressures <60 cm H_2O, and without positive end-expiratory pressure are starting mechanical ventilation parameters that can achieve these goals. As measures to relieve mucous plugs, chest percussion and airways lavage are **not** recommended because they can induce further bronchospasm. Considering the nature of asthma exacerbations leading to respiratory failure, those of rapid or abrupt onset tend to resolve quickly (hours to 2 days); in contrast, those that progress gradually to respiratory failure can require days to weeks of mechanical ventilation. Such prolonged cases are further complicated by muscle atrophy and, when combined with corticosteroid-induced myopathy, can lead to severe muscle weakness requiring prolonged rehabilitation.

In children, management of severe exacerbations in medical centers is usually successful, even when extreme measures are required. Consequently, asthma deaths in children rarely occur in medical centers; most occur at home or in community settings before lifesaving medical care can be administered. This highlights the importance of home and community management of asthma exacerbations, early intervention measures to keep exacerbations from becoming severe, and steps to reduce asthma severity. A follow-up appointment within 1 to 2 weeks of discharge should be used to monitor clinical improvement and to reinforce key educational elements including action plans and controller medications.

SPECIAL MANAGEMENT CIRCUMSTANCES

Management of Infants and Young Children. Recurrent wheezing episodes in pre–school-age children are very common, occurring in as much as $^1/_3$ of this population. Of them, most will improve and even become asymptomatic during the prepubescent school-age years, while others will have lifelong persistent asthma. All require management of their recurrent wheezing problems (see Table 143-9). The updated NAEPP guidelines recommend a modified Asthma Predictive Index (see Table 143-2) to identify pre–school-age children who are likely to have persistent asthma. One implication of this recommendation is that these at-risk children may be candidates for conventional asthma management, including daily controller therapy and early intervention with exacerbations (see Table 143-9). Nebulized budesonide and montelukast appear to be more effective than cromolyn. For young children with a history of moderate to severe exacerbations, nebulized budesonide is FDA-approved and its use as a controller medication could prevent subsequent exacerbations.

Using aerosol therapy in infants and young children with asthma presents unique challenges. There are 2 delivery systems for inhaled medications for this age group: the nebulizer and the MDI with spacer/holding chamber and face mask. Multiple studies have demonstrated the effectiveness of both nebulized albuterol in acute episodes and nebulized budesonide in the treatment of recurrent wheezing in infants and young children. In such young children, inhaled medications via MDI with spacer and face mask may be acceptable although perhaps not preferred due to a current paucity of published information and lack of FDA approval for children <4 yr of age.

Home Management of Asthma Exacerbations. Asthma management in pregnancy essentially follows the NAEPP clinical practice guidelines. The goals of asthma management during pregnancy should include prevention of exacerbations and control of chronic symptoms by using medications that pose minimal risk to the mother and fetus because most drugs cross the placenta. It is considered safer for pregnant asthmatic women to be treated with controller medications than it is to have uncontrolled symptoms and severe exacerbations. Albuterol is the preferred SABA for use during pregnancy. There is reassuring efficacy and safety data from prospective cohort studies supporting ICS use in pregnant women with asthma. Budesonide is currently the preferred ICS for pregnant women, attaining an FDA Pregnancy Category B rating owing to substantial reassuring safety data. Nonmedication approaches to improve asthma control are, as always, encouraged. A multidisciplinary approach with monthly evaluations (including pulmonary function tests when not contraindicated) and ongoing consultation with the obstetrician and asthma specialist is recommended. Frequent fetal and maternal surveillance is especially important for adolescents with suboptimal asthma control, those with moderate to severe asthma, and those with recent exacerbation.

Management of Asthma During Surgery. Patients with asthma are at risk from disease-related complications from surgery such as bronchoconstriction and asthma exacerbation, atelectasis, impaired coughing, respiratory infection, and latex exposure that may induce asthma complications in patients with latex allergy. All patients with asthma should be evaluated before surgery, and those who are inadequately controlled should allow time for intensified treatment in order to improve asthma stability before surgery if possible. A systemic corticosteroid course may be indicated for patients who are having symptoms and/or FEV_1 or PEF <80% of the patient's personal best. In addition, patients who have received more than 2 wk of systemic corticosteroid and/or moderate-to-high dose ICS therapy may be at risk of intraoperative adrenal insufficiency. For these patients, anesthesia should be alerted to provide "stress" replacement doses of systemic corticosteroid for the surgical procedure and possibly the postoperative period if needed.

PATIENT EDUCATION. Specific educational elements in the clinical care of children with asthma are believed to make an important difference in the home management and adherence of families to an optimal plan of care (Table 143-16). With education, the child and family become essential partners in the asthma management process, as the key optimal management depends on their daily assessments and implementation of any management plan. In initial patient visits, a basic understanding of the pathogenesis of asthma (chronic inflammation and AHR underlying a clinically intermittent presentation) can help children with asthma and their parents to understand the importance of recommendations aimed at reducing airways inflammation. The expectations of good asthma control resulting from optimal asthma management should be specified (see Fig. 143-5). Explaining and readdressing the importance of steps to reduce airways inflammation in achieving good asthma control and addressing concerns about potential adverse effects of asthma pharmacotherapy, and especially their risks relative to their benefits, are essential in achieving long-term adherence with asthma pharmacotherapy and environmental control measures.

TABLE 143-16. Key Elements of Productive Clinic Visits for Asthma

Specify goals of asthma management
Explain basic facts about asthma
Contrast normal vs asthmatic airways
Link airways inflammation, "twitchiness," and bronchoconstriction
Long-term-control and quick-relief medications
Address concerns about potential adverse effects of asthma pharmacotherapy
Teach, demonstrate, and have patient show proper technique for:
Inhaled medication use (spacer use with MDI)
Peak flow measures
Investigate and manage factors that contribute to asthma severity
Environmental exposures
Co-morbid conditions
Written two-part asthma management plan
Daily management
Action plan for asthma exacerbations
Regular follow-up visits
Twice yearly (more often if not well controlled)
Monitor lung function annually

Children with asthma and their families benefit from a written asthma management plan with 2 main components: (1) a daily "routine" management plan describing regular asthma medication use and other measures to keep asthma under good control; and (2) an action plan for asthma exacerbations, describing actions to take when asthma worsens, including what medications to take and when to contact the regular physician and/or obtain urgent/emergent medical care. Regular follow-up visits can help to maintain optimal asthma control. In addition to assessing disease severity and revising daily and exacerbation management plans accordingly, follow-up visits should be used to encourage open communication of concerns with asthma management recommendations (daily administration of controller medications). Reassessing the role of different medications in asthma management and the technique used with inhaled medications can be insightful and help to guide teaching to improve adherence to a management plan that might not have been adequately or properly implemented.

PROGNOSIS. Recurrent coughing and wheezing occurs in 35% of pre–school-age children. Of these, $^1/_3$ continue to have persistent asthma into later childhood, while $^2/_3$ improve on their own through the preteen years. Asthma severity by the ages of 7–10 yr of age is predictive of asthma persistence in adulthood. Children with moderate to severe asthma and with lower lung function measures are likely to have persistent asthma as adults. Children with milder asthma and normal lung function are likely to improve over time, with some becoming periodic (disease-free mo to yr); however, complete remission for 5 yr in childhood is uncommon.

PREVENTION. Although chronic airways inflammation may result in pathologic remodeling of lung airways, evidence that conventional anti-inflammatory interventions—the cornerstone of asthma control—in young children with recurrent wheezing can help children "outgrow" their asthma is currently lacking. Investigations into the environmental and lifestyle factors responsible for the lower prevalence of childhood asthma in rural areas and farming communities suggest that early immune modulatory intervention might prevent asthma development. A "hygiene hypothesis" purports that naturally occurring microbial exposures in early life might drive early immune development away from allergen sensitization, persistent airways inflammation, and remodeling. If these natural microbial exposures truly have an asthma-protective effect, without significant adverse health consequences, then these findings may foster new strategies for asthma prevention.

Several nonpharmacotherapeutic measures with numerous positive health attributes—avoidance of environmental tobacco smoke (beginning prenatally), prolonged breastfeeding (>4 mo), an active lifestyle, and a healthy diet—might reduce the likelihood of asthma development. Immunizations are currently not considered to increase the likelihood of developing asthma. Therefore, all standard childhood immunizations are recommended for children with asthma, including varicella and annual influenza vaccines.

Akbari O, Faul JL, Hoyte EG, et al: CD4+ invariant T-cell-receptor+ natural killer T cells in bronchial asthma. *N Engl J Med* 2006;354:1117–1129.

Allen M, Heinzmann A, Noguchi E, et al: Positional cloning of novel gene influencing asthma from chromosome 2q14. *Nat Genet* 2003;35:258–263.

American Academy of Allergy, Asthma & Immunology: *Pediatric Asthma: Promoting Best Practice*. Milwaukee, WI, AAAAI, 2002. Available at www.aaaai.org.

Anderson HR: Prevalence of asthma. *Br Med J* 2005;350:1037–1038.

Anderson HR, Ayres JG, Sturdy PM, et al: Bronchodilator treatment and deaths from asthma: Case-control study. *Br Med J* 2005;330:117–120.

Biscardi S, Lorrot M, Marc E, et al: *Mycoplasma pneumoniae* and asthma in children. *Clin Infect Dis* 2004;38:1341–1346.

Bisgaard H, Szefler S, et al: Long-acting β_2 agonists and paeditric asthma. *Lancet* 2006;367:286–288.

Bleecker ER, Yancey SW, Baitinger LA, et al: Salmeterol response is not affected by β_2-adrenergic receptor genotype in subjects with persistent asthma. *J Allergy Clin Immunol* 2006;118:806–816.

Carl JC, Myers TR, Kirchner HL, Kercsmar CM: Comparison of racemic albuterol and levalbuterol for treatment of acute asthma. *J Pediatr* 2003;143:731–736.

Centers for Disease Control and Prevention: Reducing childhood asthma through community-based service delivery—New York City, 2001–2004. *MMWR* 2005:54:11–14.

Cheuk DKL, Chau TCH, Lee SL: A meta-analysis on intravenous magnesium sulphate for treating acute asthma. *Arch Dis Child* 2005;90:74–77.

Haland G, Lodrup Carlsen KC, Sandvik L, et al: Reduced lung function at birth and the risk of asthma at 10 years of age. *N Engl J Med* 2006;355:1682–1689.

Hartert TV, Edwards K: Antibiotics for asthma? *Clin Infect Dis* 2004;38:1347–1349.

Heaton T, Rowe J, Turner S, et al: An immunoepidemiological approach to asthma: Identification of in-vitro T-cell response patterns associated with different wheezing phenotypes in children. *Lancet* 2005;365:142–148.

Israel E, Chinchilli VM, Ford JG, et al: Use of regularly scheduled albuterol treatment in asthma: Genotype-stratified, randomized, placebo-controlled cross-over trial. *Lancet* 2004;364:1505–1512.

Jenkins C, Costello J, Hodge L: Systematic review of prevalence of aspirin induced asthma and its implications for clinical practice. *Br Med J* 2004;328:434–438.

Khoshoo V, Le T, Haydel RM Jr, et al: Role of gastroesophageal reflux in older children with persistent asthma. *Chest* 2003;123:1008–1013.

Kim K, Phrampus E, Venkataraman S, et al: Helium/oxygen-driven albuterol nebulization in the treatment of children with moderate to severe asthma exacerbations: A randomized, controlled trial. *Pediatrics* 2005;116:1127–1133.

Lau S, Matricardi PM: Worms, asthma, and the hygiene hypothesis. *Lancet* 2006;367:1556–1558.

Li JT, Oppenheimer J, Bernstein L, et al: Attaining optimal asthma control: A practice parameter. *J Allergy Clin Immunol* 2005;116:S3–S11.

Lipworth BJ: Phosphodiesterase-4 inhibitors for asthma and chronic obstructive pulmonary disease. *Lancet* 2005;365:167–175.

Morgan WJ, Crain EF, Gruchalla RS, et al: Results of a home-based environmental intervention among urban children with asthma. *N Engl J Med* 2004;351:1068–1080.

National Asthma Education and Prevention Program: NAEPP guidelines for the diagnosis and management of asthma—update on selected topics, 2002. Washington, DC, NIH, 2002 (NIH publication no. 02-5075).

National Institutes of Health, National Heart, Lung & Blood Institute. National Asthma Education & Prevention Program: Expert Panel report 2: Guidelines for the diagnosis and management of asthma. Washington DC, 1997; and Update on selected topics, 2002. Washington, DC, NIH, 2002. Available at www.nhlbi.nih.gov/guidelines/asthma

[No authors listed]: Omalizumab (Xolair): An anti-IgE antibody for asthma. *Med Lett Drugs Ther* 2003;45:67–68.

O'Byrne PM, Parameswaran K: Pharmacological management of mild or moderate persistent asthma. *Lancet* 2006;368:794–802.

Oguma T, Palmer LJ, Birben E, et al: Role of prostanoid DP receptor variants in susceptibility to asthma. *N Engl J Med* 2004;351:1752–1762.

Paton J, Jardine E, McNeill E, et al: Adrenal responses to low dose synthetic ACTH (Synacthen) in children receiving high dose inhaled fluticasone. *Arch Dis Child* 2006;91:808–881.

Qureshi F, Zaritsky A, Welch C, et al: Clinical efficacy of racemic albuterol versus levalbuterol for the treatment of acute pediatric asthma. *Ann Emerg Med* 2005;46:29–36.

Rodrigo GJ, Castro-Rodriguez JA: Anticholinergics in the treatment of children and adults with acute asthma: A systematic review with meta-analysis. *Thorax* 2005;60:740–746.

Sanford A, Pare P: Homing in on the asthma gene. *Lancet* 2002;360:422–423.

Sayers I, Hall IP: Pharmacogenetic approaches in the treatment of asthma. *Curr Allergy Asthma Rep* 2005;5:101–108.

Schuh S, Dick PT, Stephens D, et al: High-dose inhaled fluticasone does not replace oral prednisolone in children with mild to moderate acute asthma. *Pediatrics* 2006;118:644–650.

Sears MR, Greene JM, Willan AR, et al: A longitudinal, population-based, cohort study of childhood asthma followed to adulthood. *N Engl J Med* 2003;349:1414–1422.

Shapiro SD, Owen CA: *ADAM-33* surfaces as an asthma gene. *N Engl J Med* 2002;347:936–938.

Smith AD, Cowan JO, Brassett KP, et al: Use of exhaled nitric oxide measurements to guide treatment in chronic asthma. *N Engl J Med* 2005;352:2163–2173.

Spanier AJ, Hornung R, Lierl M, Lanphear BP: Environmental exposures and exhaled nitric oxide in children with asthma. *J Pediatr* 2006;149:220–226.

Struck RC, Bloomberg GR: Omalizumab for asthma. *N Engl J Med* 2006;354:2689–2695.

Szefler SJ, Phillips BR, Martinez FD, et al: Characterization of within-subject responses to fluticasone and montelukast in childhood asthma. *J Allergy Clin Immunol* 2005;115:233–242.

United States Environmental Protection Agency: *Clear Your Home of Asthma Triggers*. Available at http://www.epa.gov/iaq/asthma

Vonk JM, Postma DS, Boezen HM, et al: Childhood factors associated with asthma remission after 30 year follow up. *Thorax* 2004;59:925–929.

Williams JV, Crowe JE, Enriquez R, et al: Human metapneumovirus infection plays an etiologic role in acute asthma exacerbations requiring hospitalization in adults. *J Infect Dis* 2005;192:1149–1153.

Williams SG, Schmidt DK, Redd SC, et al: National Asthma Education and Prevention Program: Key clinical activities for quality asthma care. Recommendations of the National Asthma Education and Prevention Program. *MMWR Recomm Rep* 2003;52:1–8.

Wjst M: β_2-adrenoreceptor polymorphisms and asthma. *Lancet* 2006;368:710–711.

Wong GWK, Ko FWS, Hui DSC, et al: Factors associated with difference in prevalence of asthma in children from three cities in China: Multicentre epidemiological survey. *Br Med J* 2004;329:486–488.

Chapter 144 ■ Atopic Dermatitis (Atopic Eczema) Donald Y. M. Leung

Atopic dermatitis (AD) is the most common chronic relapsing skin disease seen in infancy and childhood. It affects 10–20% of children worldwide and frequently occurs in families with asthma, allergic rhinitis, and food allergy. Infants with AD are predisposed to developing allergic rhinitis and/or asthma later in childhood, the so-called "**atopic march.**"

ETIOLOGY. AD is a complex genetic disorder that results in a defective skin barrier, reduced skin innate immune responses, and exaggerated T cell responses to environmental allergens and microbes that lead to chronic skin inflammation.

PATHOLOGY. Clinically unaffected skin of AD patients is not normal but is characterized by mild epidermal hyperplasia and a sparse perivascular T-cell infiltrate. Acute skin lesions are characterized by **spongiosis,** or marked intercellular edema, of the epidermis. In AD, the dendritic antigen-presenting cells (APCs) in skin, the Langerhans cells (LCs), exhibit surface-bound IgE molecules. IgE-bearing LCs play an important role in cutaneous allergen presentation to T helper type 2 (Th2) cells (see Chapter 139). In the acute lesion, there is a marked perivenular T-cell infiltrate with occasional monocyte-macrophages. Mast cells are found in normal numbers but in different stages of degranulation. Chronic lichenified AD is characterized by a hyperplastic epidermis with hyperkeratosis, and minimal spongiosis. There are predominantly IgE-bearing LCs in the epidermis and macrophages in the dermal mononuclear cell infiltrate. The numbers of mast cells and of eosinophils are increased. Eosinophils contribute to allergic inflammation by secreting cytokines and mediators that augment allergic inflammation and induce tissue injury in AD through the production of reactive oxygen intermediates and release of toxic granule proteins.

PATHOGENESIS. Two forms of AD have been identified. **Atopic eczema** is associated with IgE-mediated sensitization and typifies 70–80% of AD patients. **Non-atopic eczema** is not associated with IgE-mediated sensitization and is seen in 20–30% of AD patients. Both forms of AD are associated with eosinophilia. In atopic eczema, memory T cells expressing the skin homing receptor, **cutaneous lymphocyte-associated antigen** (CLA), produce increased levels of Th2 cytokines. These include interleukin (IL)-4 and IL-13, which are known to induce isotype switching to IgE synthesis, as well as IL-5, which plays an important role in eosinophil development and survival. These CLA+ T cells also produce abnormally low levels of interferon-γ (IFN-γ), a Th1 cytokine known to inhibit Th2 cell function. Non-atopic eczema is associated with less IL-4 and IL-13 production than is atopic eczema.

Compared with skin of healthy subjects, unaffected skin and acute skin lesions of AD patients have an increased number of cells expressing IL-4 and IL-13. Acute AD does not contain significant numbers of cells that express IFN-γ or IL-12. Chronic AD skin lesions have significantly fewer cells that express IL-4 and IL-13 but increased numbers of cells that express IL-5, granulocyte-macrophage colony–stimulating factor (GM-CSF), IL-12, and IFN-γ in comparison to acute AD. The increased expression of IL-12 in eosinophils, inflammatory dendritic epidermal cells, and macrophages in chronic AD skin lesions may play a role in initiating the switch to Th1 cell development in chronic AD. The development of AD skin lesions is orchestrated by the local tissue expression of proinflammatory cytokines and chemokines. Cytokines such as tumor necrosis factor-α (TNF-α) and IL-1 from keratinocytes, mast cells, and dendritic cells bind to receptors on vascular endothelium, activating cellular signaling, including the NF-κB pathway, and inducing expression of vascular endothelial cell adhesion molecules. These events initiate the process of tethering, activation, and adhesion to the endothelium followed by extravasation of inflammatory cells. Once the inflammatory cells have infiltrated into the tissue, they respond to chemotactic gradients established by chemokines, which emanate from sites of injury or infection. These molecules play a central role in defining the nature of the inflammatory infiltrate in AD. CCL27 is highly upregulated in AD and preferentially attracts CLA+ T cells to the skin. The C-C chemokines, RANTES, monocyte chemotactic protein-4, and eotaxin are increased in AD skin lesions and likely contribute to the chemotaxis of CCR3-expressing eosinophils, macrophages, and Th2 lymphocytes into AD skin. Selective recruitment of CCR4-expressing Th2 cells into AD skin may also be mediated by MDC and TARC, which are increased in AD. Persistent skin inflammation in chronic lesions may be due to elevated IL-5 and GM-CSF expression in the skin, leading to enhanced survival of eosinophils and monocyte-macrophages as well as LCs. Th1 cells in chronic AD are also thought to potentiate the function of inflammatory effector cells in AD.

CLINICAL MANIFESTATIONS. AD typically begins in infancy. Approximately 50% of patients develop symptoms in the 1st year of life, and an additional 30% are diagnosed between 1 and 5 yr of age. Intense **pruritus** and **cutaneous reactivity** are the cardinal features of AD. Pruritus is usually worse at night. Scratching and excoriation contribute to the development of more pronounced eczematous skin lesions. Foods, inhalant allergens, bacterial infection, reduced humidity, excessive sweating, and irritants (wool, acrylic, soaps, detergents) can exacerbate pruritus and scratching.

Acute AD skin lesions are intensely pruritic with erythematous papules (Figs. 144-1 and 144-2). Subacute dermatitis is characterized by erythematous, excoriated, scaling papules. Chronic AD is characterized by **lichenification** (Fig. 144-3), or thickening of the skin with accentuated surface markings, and **fibrotic papules (prurigo nodularis).** With chronic AD, all 3 stages of skin reactions may coexist in the same individual. Most AD patients have dry, lackluster skin irrespective of their stage of illness. The distribution and skin reaction pattern varies with the patient's age and disease activity. In infancy, the AD is generally more acute and involves the face, scalp, and extensor surfaces of the extremities. The diaper area is usually spared. In older children and those with chronic AD, there is lichenification and localization of the rash to the flexural folds of the extremities. AD often goes into remission as the patient grows older, leaving an adolescent or adult with skin that is prone to itching and inflammation when exposed to exogenous irritants.

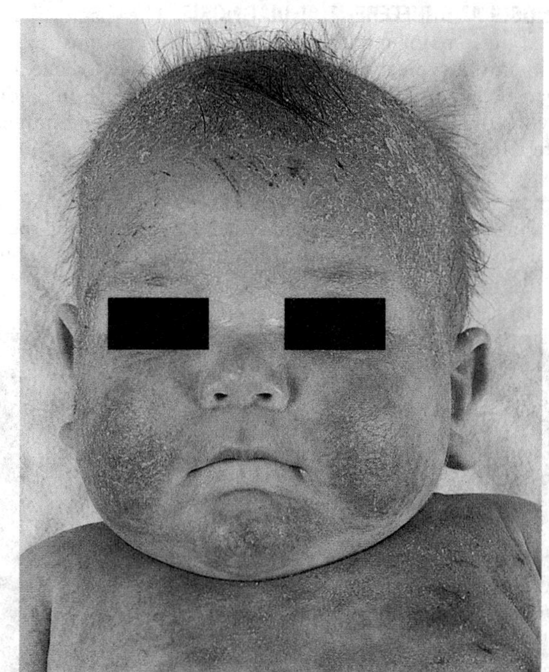

Figure 144-1. Atopic dermatitis typical cheek involvement. (From Eichenfield LF, Friedan IJ, Esterly NB: *Textbook of Neonatal Dermatology.* Philadelphia, WB Saunders, 2001, p 242.)

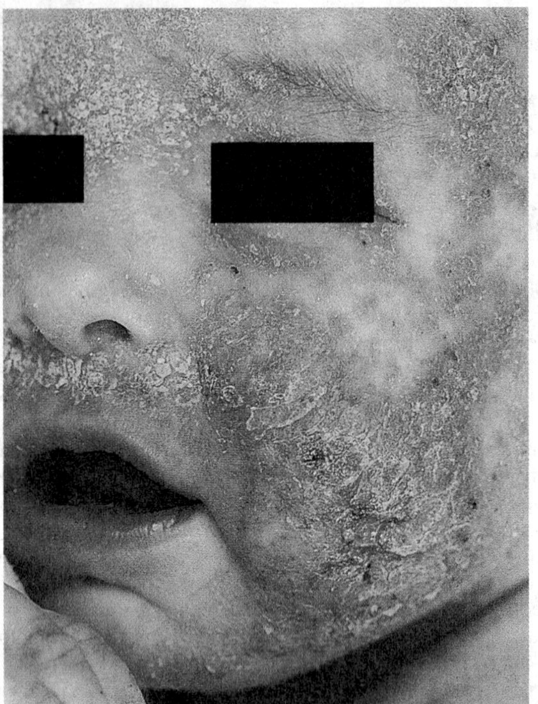

Figure 144-2. Crusted lesions of atopic dermatitis on the face. (From Eichenfield LF, Friedan IJ, Esterly NB: *Textbook of Neonatal Dermatology.* Philadelphia, WB Saunders, 2001, p 242.)

LABORATORY FINDINGS. There are no specific laboratory tests for the diagnosis of AD. Most patients with AD have peripheral blood eosinophilia and increased serum IgE levels. Serum IgE testing can identify the allergens to which patients are sensitized. The diagnosis of clinical allergy to these environmental allergens requires, however, confirmation by history and environmental challenges.

DIAGNOSIS AND DIFFERENTIAL DIAGNOSIS. The diagnosis of AD is based on 3 major features: pruritus, an eczematous dermatitis that fits into a typical distribution, and a chronic or chronically relapsing course (Table 144-1). Associated features including a family history of asthma, hay fever, elevated IgE, and immediate skin test reactivity are variable.

Many inflammatory skin diseases, immunodeficiencies, skin malignancies, genetic disorders, infectious diseases, and infestations share symptoms and signs with AD and should be considered and excluded before a diagnosis of AD is established (Table 144-2). Infants presenting in the 1st year of life with failure to thrive, diarrhea, generalized scaling erythematous rash, and recurrent cutaneous and/or systemic infections should be evaluated for severe combined immunodeficiency syndrome (see Chapter 125.1). Histiocytosis (see Chapter 507) should be excluded in any infant with AD and failure to thrive. Wiskott-Aldrich syndrome (see Chapter 125.2), an X-linked recessive disorder associated with thrombocytopenia, immune defects, and recurrent severe bacterial infections, is characterized by a rash

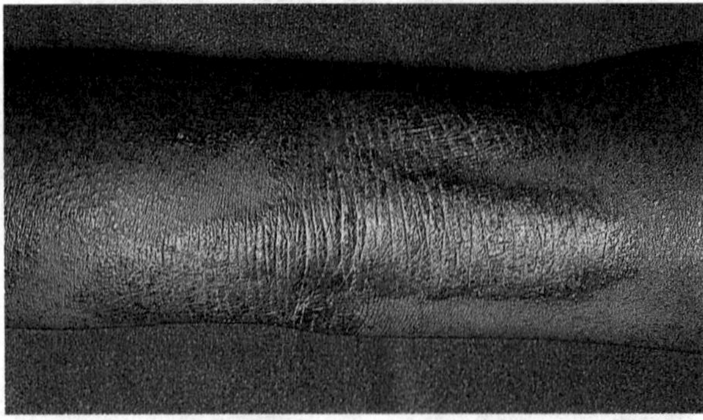

Figure 144-3. Lichenification of the popliteal fossa from chronic rubbing of the skin in atopic dermatitis. (From Weston WL, Lane AT, Morelli JG: *Color Textbook of Pediatric Dermatology,* 2nd ed. St. Louis, Mosby, 1996, p 33.)

TABLE 144-1. Clinical Features of Atopic Dermatitis

MAJOR FEATURES
Pruritus
Facial and extensor eczema in infants and children
Flexural eczema in adolescents
Chronic or relapsing dermatitis
Personal or family history of atopic disease
ASSOCIATED FEATURES
Xerosis
Cutaneous infections (*S. aureus,* group A streptococcus, herpes simplex, vaccinia, molluscum, warts)
Nonspecific dermatitis of the hands or feet
Ichthyosis, palmar hyperlinearity, keratosis pilaris
Nipple eczema
White dermatographism and delayed blanch response
Anterior subcapsular cataracts, keratoconus
Elevated serum IgE levels
Positive immediate-type allergy skin tests
Early age at onset
Dennie lines (Dennie-Morgan infraorbital folds)
Facial erythema or pallor
Course influenced by environmental and/or emotional factors

TABLE 144-2. Differential Diagnosis of Atopic Dermatitis

CONGENITAL DISORDERS
• Netherton syndrome
• Familial keratosis pilaris
CHRONIC DERMATOSES
• Seborrheic dermatitis
• Contact dermatitis (allergic or irritant)
• Nummular eczema
• Psoriasis
• Ichthyoses
INFECTIONS AND INFESTATIONS
• Scabies
• Human immunodeficiency virus–associated dermatitis
• Dermatophytosis
• Insect bites
• Onchocerciasis
MALIGNANCIES
• Cutaneous T cell lymphoma (mycosis fungoides/Sézary syndrome)
• Letterer-Siwe disease
AUTOIMMUNE DISORDERS
• Dermatitis herpetiformis
• Pemphigus foliaceus
• Graft vs host disease
• Dermatomyositis
IMMUNODEFICIENCIES
• Wiskott-Aldrich syndrome
• Severe combined immunodeficiency syndrome
• Hyper-IgE syndrome
METABOLIC DISORDERS
• Zinc deficiency
• Pyridoxine (vitamin B_6) and niacin
• Multiple carboxylase deficiency
• Phenylketonuria

From Leung DYM, Sampson HA, Geha RS, et al: *Pediatric Allergy Principles and Practice* St. Louis, Mosby, 2003, 562.

almost indistinguishable from AD. The hyper-IgE syndrome (see Chapter 125.2) is characterized by markedly elevated serum IgE levels, recurrent deep-seated bacterial infections, chronic dermatitis, and recalcitrant dermatophytosis.

Adolescents who present with an eczematous dermatitis but no history of childhood eczema, respiratory allergy, or atopic family history may have allergic **contact dermatitis.** A contact allergen should be considered in any patient whose AD does not respond to appropriate therapy, because chemicals such as parabens and lanolin are commonly used therapeutic topical agents. Topical glucocorticoid contact allergy has been reported in patients with chronic dermatitis on topical corticosteroid therapy. Eczematous dermatitis has also been reported with HIV infection as well as with a variety of infestations such as scabies. Other conditions that can be confused with AD include psoriasis, ichthyoses, and seborrheic dermatitis.

TREATMENT. The treatment of AD requires a systematic, multifaceted approach that incorporates skin hydration, topical anti-inflammatory therapy, identification and elimination of flare factors, and, if necessary, systemic therapy.

Cutaneous Hydration. Patients with AD have decreased skin barrier function from reduced lipid levels, which results in diffuse, abnormally dry skin, or **xerosis.** Lukewarm soaking baths for at least 20 min followed by the application of an occlusive emollient to retain moisture provides symptomatic relief. Hydrophilic ointments can be obtained in varying degrees of viscosity according to the patient's preference. Occlusive ointments are sometimes not well tolerated because of interference with the function of the eccrine sweat ducts and may induce the development of folliculitis. In these patients, less occlusive agents should be used.

Hydration by baths or wet dressings promotes transepidermal penetration of topical glucocorticoids. Dressings may also serve as an effective barrier against persistent scratching, which promotes healing of excoriated lesions. Wet dressings are recommended for use on severely affected or chronically involved areas of dermatitis refractory to skin care. They have the potential, however, to promote drying and fissuring of the skin if not followed by topical emollient use. Wet dressing therapy can be complicated by maceration and secondary infection and should be closely monitored by a physician.

Topical Corticosteroids. Topical corticosteroids are the cornerstone of anti-inflammatory treatment for acute exacerbations of AD. Patients should be carefully instructed on their use of topical glucocorticoids in order to avoid potential adverse effects. There are 7 classes of topical glucocorticoids, ranked according to their potency based on vasoconstrictor assays (Table 144-3). Because of their potential adverse effects, the ultra-high-potency glucocorticoids should not be used on the face or intertriginous areas and only for very short periods of time on the trunk and extremities. Mid-potency glucocorticoids can be used for longer periods of time to treat chronic AD involving the trunk and extremities. Once control of AD is achieved with a daily regimen of topical corticosteroids, long-term control can be maintained with twice-weekly applications of topical fluticasone or mometasone to areas that have healed but are prone to developing eczema. Compared with creams, ointments have a greater potential to occlude the epidermis, resulting in enhanced systemic absorption. Adverse effects from topical glucocorticoids can be divided into local adverse effects and systemic adverse effects, which result from suppression of the hypothalamic-pituitary-adrenal axis. Local adverse effects include the development of striae and skin atrophy. Systemic adverse effects are related to the potency of the topical corticosteroid, site of application, occlusiveness of the preparation, percentage of the body surface area covered, and length of use. The potential for potent topical corticosteroids to cause adrenal suppression is greatest in infants and young children with severe AD requiring intensive therapy.

TABLE 144-3. Topical Corticosteroids Ranked by Potency

GROUP	GENERIC NAME (SELECTED BRAND NAMES; VEHICLE AND CONCENTRATION)
Group 1 (Most potent)	Clobetasol propionate (Temovate; cream, ointment, lotion 0.05%)
	Betamethasone dipropionate (Diprolene; ointment 0.05%)
	Halobetasol propionate (Ultravate; cream, ointment 0.05%)
Group 2	Fluocinonide (Lidex; cream, ointment, gel, solution 0.05%)
	Mometasone furoate (Elocon; ointment 0.1%)
	Betamethasone diproprionate (Maxivate; ointment 0.05%)
	Amcinonide (Cyclocort; ointment 0.1%)
	Desoximetasone (Topicort; cream, ointment 0.25%; gel 0.5%)
Group 3	Triamcinolone acetonide (Kenalog, Aristocort; ointment 0.1%)
	Amcinonide (Cyclocort; cream, lotion 0.1%)
	Betamethasone diproprionate (Diprosone; cream 0.05%)
	Betamethasone valerate (Valisone; ointment 0.1%)
	Fluticasone propionate (Cutivate; ointment 0.005%)
Group 4	Mometasone furoate (Elocon; cream, lotion 0.1%)
	Triamcinolone acetonide (Kenalog, Aristocort; cream 0.1%)
	Fluocinolone acetonide (Synalar; ointment 0.025%)
	Hydrocortisone valerate (Westcort; ointment 0.2%)
Group 5	Fluticasone propionate (Cutivate; cream 0.05%)
	Fluticasone acetonide (Synalar; cream 0.025%)
	Betamethasone valerate (Valisone; cream 0.1%)
	Hydrocortisone valerate (Westcort; cream 0.2%)
	Betamethasone dipropionate (0.05% lotion)
	Prednicarbate (Dermatop; cream 0.1%)
Group 6	Fluocinolone acetonide (Synalar; solution 0.01%)
	Betamethasone valerate (Diprolene Lotion; lotion 0.05%)
	Triamcinolone acetonide (Aristocort, Kenalog; cream 0.1%)
	Desonide (DesOwen; cream, ointment, lotion 0.05%; Tridesilon; ointment 0.05%)
	Alclometasone dipropionate (Aclovate; cream, ointment 0.05%)
Group 7 (Least potent)	Hydrocortisone (Hytone; cream; ointment, lotion 2.5%; Generic, cream, 0.5%, 1%)
	Pramoxine hydrochloride (HC Pramoxine; cream 1.0%, 2.5%)

Topical Calcineurin Inhibitors. The nonsteroidal topical calcineurin inhibitors are effective in reducing AD skin inflammation. Pimecrolimus cream 1% (Elidel) is indicated for mild to moderate AD. Tacrolimus ointment 0.1% and 0.03% (Protopic) is indicated for moderate to severe AD. Both are approved for the short-term or intermittent long-term treatment of AD in patients ≥2 yr unresponsive to or intolerant of other conventional therapies or for whom these therapies are inadvisable due to potential risks. Other circumstances in which topical calcineurin inhibitors may be advantageous over topical corticosteroids include treatment of patients who are poorly responsive to topical steroids, patients with steroid phobia, and treatment of face and neck dermatitis where ineffective, low-potency topical corticosteroids are usually used due to fears of steroid-induced skin atrophy.

Tar Preparations. Coal tar preparations have antipruritic and anti-inflammatory effects on the skin. The anti-inflammatory properties of tars, however, are usually not as pronounced as those of topical glucocorticoids or calcineurin inhibitors. Tar preparations are useful in reducing the potency of topical glucocorticoids required in chronic maintenance therapy of AD. Tar shampoos can be particularly beneficial for scalp dermatitis. Adverse effects associated with tar preparations include skin irritation, folliculitis, and photosensitivity.

Antihistamines. Systemic antihistamines act primarily by blocking the H_1 receptors in the dermis, thereby reducing histamine-induced pruritus. Histamine is only 1 of many mediators that can induce pruritus of the skin and, therefore, patients may derive minimal benefit from antihistaminic therapy. Because pruritus is usually worse at night, the sedating antihistamines (hydroxyzine, diphenhydramine) may offer an advantage with their soporific adverse effects when used at bedtime. Doxepin hydrochloride has both tricyclic antidepressant and H_1- and H_2-receptor blocking effects. If nocturnal pruritus remains severe, short-term use of a sedative to allow adequate rest may be appropriate. Studies of newer nonsedating antihistamines have shown variable results in the effectiveness of controlling pruritus in AD, although they may be useful in the small subset of AD patients with concomitant urticaria.

Systemic Corticosteroids. The use of systemic corticosteroids is rarely indicated in the treatment of chronic AD. The dramatic clinical improvement that may occur with systemic corticosteroids is frequently associated with a severe rebound flare of AD after discontinuation. Short courses of oral corticosteroids may be appropriate for an acute exacerbation of AD while other treatment measures are being instituted. If a short course of oral corticosteroids is given, it is important to taper the dosage and begin intensified skin care, particularly with topical corticosteroids and frequent bathing followed by application of emollients, to prevent rebound flaring of AD.

Cyclosporine. Cyclosporine is a potent immunosuppressive drug that acts primarily on T cells by suppressing cytokine transcription. It binds to an intracellular protein, cyclophilin, and this complex, in turn, inhibits calcineurin, a phosphatase required for activation of NFAT, a transcription factor necessary for initiation of cytokine gene transcription. Cyclosporin (5 mg/kg/day) for short-term and long-term (1 yr) use has been beneficial for children with severe AD that is refractory to conventional treatments. Adverse effects include renal impairment and hypertension.

Phototherapy. Natural sunlight is frequently beneficial to patients with AD as long as it does not result in sunburn or severe sweating. Many phototherapy modalities are effective for AD including: ultraviolet A-1, ultraviolet B (UVB), narrow-band ultraviolet B, and psoralen plus ultraviolet A (PUVA). Phototherapy is generally reserved for patients who fail standard treatments. For phototherapy to be effective, maintenance treatments are usually required. Short-term adverse effects with phototherapy include erythema, skin pain, pruritus, and pigmentation. Long-term adverse effects include predisposition to cutaneous malignancies.

AVOIDING TRIGGERS OF AD. It is essential to identify and eliminate triggering factors, both during the period of acute symptoms and on an ongoing basis to prevent recurrences.

Irritants. Patients with AD have a low threshold for response to irritants that can trigger their itch-scratch cycle. Common triggers include soaps or detergents, chemicals, smoke, abrasive clothing, and exposure to extremes of temperature and humidity. Patients with AD should use soaps with minimal defatting activity and a neutral pH. New clothing should be laundered before wearing to decrease levels of formaldehyde and other added chemicals. Residual laundry detergent in clothing may be irritating; using a liquid rather than powder detergent and adding a 2nd rinse cycle facilitates removal of the detergent.

Every attempt should be made to allow children with AD to be as normally active as possible. Certain sports such as swimming may be better tolerated than others that involve intense perspiration, physical contact, or heavy clothing and equipment. Chlorine should be rinsed off immediately after swimming and the skin lubricated. Although ultraviolet light may be beneficial to some patients with AD, sunscreens should be used to avoid sunburn.

Foods. Approximately 40% of infants and young children with moderate to severe AD have food allergy (see Chapter 151). Food allergies in AD patients may induce eczematous dermatitis in some patients and urticarial reactions, wheezing, or nasal congestion in others. Increased severity of AD symptoms and younger age correlate directly with the presence of food allergy. Removal of food allergens from the diet leads to significant clinical improvement but requires a great deal of education because most of the common allergens (egg, milk, wheat, soy, peanut) contaminate many foods and are difficult to avoid.

Potential allergens can be identified by a careful history and performing selective skin prick tests or in vitro blood testing for allergen-specific IgE. Negative skin tests and blood tests for allergen-specific IgE have a high predictive value for excluding suspected allergens. Positive skin tests or blood tests to foods often do not correlate with clinical symptoms and should be confirmed with controlled food challenges and elimination diets. Extensive elimination diets, which in some cases can be nutritionally deficient, are rarely required because even with multiple positive skin tests the majority of patients react to fewer than 3 foods on controlled challenge.

Aeroallergens. In older children, exacerbation of AD can occur after intranasal or epicutaneous exposure to aeroallergens such as fungi, animal dander, grass, or ragweed pollen. Avoidance of aeroallergens, particularly dust mites, can result in clinical improvement of AD. In dust mite–allergic patients, avoidance measures include use of dust mite–proof encasings on pillows, mattresses, and box springs; washing bedding in hot water weekly; removal of bedroom carpeting; and decreasing indoor humidity levels with air-conditioning.

Infections. Patients with AD have increased tendency to bacterial, viral, and fungal skin infections. Antistaphylococcal antibiotics are very helpful in the treatment of patients who are heavily colonized or infected with *S. aureus*. Erythromycin and azithromycin are usually beneficial for patients who are not colonized with a resistant *S. aureus* strain. For macrolide-resistant *S. aureus,* however, a 1st-generation cephalosporin (cephalexin) is recommended. Topical mupirocin is useful in the treatment of localized impetiginous lesions, with systemic antibiotic for widespread infections. IL-4–mediated skin inflammation contributes to skin colonization with *S. aureus;* this indicates the importance of combining effective anti-inflammatory therapy with antibiotics in the treatment of patients with moderate to severe AD to avoid the need for repeated courses of antibiotics, which can lead to the emergence of antibiotic-resistant strains of *S. aureus.*

Herpes simplex virus (HSV) can provoke recurrent dermatitis and may be misdiagnosed as *S. aureus* infection. The presence of erosive, punched-out erosions, vesicles, and infected skin lesions that fail to respond to oral antibiotics suggests HSV infection that can be diagnosed by a Giemsa-stained Tzanck smear of cells scraped from the vesicle base or by viral PCR or culture. For suspected HSV infection, topical corticosteroids should be temporarily discontinued. Antiviral treatment for cutaneous HSV infections is of critical importance in the patient with widespread AD because life-threatening dissemination has been reported.

Dermatophyte infections can contribute to exacerbation of AD disease activity. Patients with dermatophyte infection or IgE antibodies to *Malassezia furfur* (formerly known as *Pityrosporum ovale*) may benefit from a trial of topical or systemic antifungal therapy.

COMPLICATIONS. *Staphylococcus aureus* is found in >90% of AD skin lesions. Honey-colored crusting, folliculitis, impetigo, and pyoderma are indicators of *S. aureus* skin infection that requires antibiotic therapy. Regional lymphadenopathy is common in such patients. The importance of *S. aureus* in AD is supported by the observation that patients with severe AD, even those without overt infection, may show clinical response to combined treatment with antistaphylococcal antibiotics and topical corticosteroids.

AD is associated with recurrent viral skin infections. The most serious viral infection is **Kaposi varicelliform eruption,** or **eczema herpeticum,** which is caused by HSV and affects patients of all ages. After an incubation period of 5–12 days, multiple, itchy, vesiculopustular lesions erupt in a disseminated pattern. The vesicular lesions are umbilicated, tend to crop, and often become hemorrhagic and crusted. Patients can also suffer from frequent infection with viruses leading to warts and molluscum contagiosum. Persons with AD are susceptible to **eczema vaccinatum,** which is similar in appearance to eczema herpeticum and historically follows smallpox (vaccinia virus) vaccination (see Chapter 712). Cutaneous warts and molluscum are additional viral infections affecting children with AD.

Patients with AD have an increased prevalence of *Trichophyton rubrum* fungal infections compared to nonatopic controls. There has been particular interest in the role of *M. furfur* in AD because it is a lipophilic yeast commonly present in the seborrheic areas of the skin. IgE antibodies against *M. furfur* have been found in patients with head and neck dermatitis, and a reduction of AD severity has been observed after treatment with antifungal agents.

Patients with extensive skin involvement may develop exfoliative dermatitis that is associated with generalized redness, scaling, weeping, crusting, systemic toxicity, lymphadenopathy, and fever. It is usually caused by superinfection (e.g., with toxin-producing *S. aureus* or HSV infection) or inappropriate therapy. In some cases, the withdrawal of systemic glucocorticoids used to control severe AD precipitate exfoliative erythroderma.

Eyelid dermatitis and chronic blepharitis may result in visual impairment from corneal scarring. **Atopic keratoconjunctivitis** is usually bilateral and can have disabling symptoms that include itching, burning, tearing, and copious mucoid discharge. Vernal conjunctivitis is associated with papillary hypertrophy or cobblestoning of the upper eyelid conjunctiva. It usually occurs in younger patients and has a marked seasonal incidence with exacerbation in the spring. **Keratoconus** is a conical deformity of the cornea believed to result from chronic rubbing of the eyes in patients with AD. Cataracts may be a primary manifestation of AD or from the extensive use of systemic and topical glucocorticoids, particularly around the eyes.

PROGNOSIS. AD generally tends to be more severe and persistent in young children, with periods of remission appearing more frequently as patients grow older. Spontaneous resolution of AD has been reported to occur after age 5 yr in 40–60% of patients affected during infancy, particularly for mild disease. Although earlier studies suggested that approximately 84% of children outgrow their AD by adolescence, more recent studies reported that AD disappears in approximately 20% of children followed from infancy until adolescence and becomes less severe in 65%. In addition, >50% of those adolescents treated for mild dermatitis may experience a relapse of disease as adults, frequently presenting with hand dermatitis, especially if daily activities require repeated hand wetting. Predictive factors of a poor prognosis for AD include widespread AD in childhood, concomitant allergic rhinitis and asthma, family history of AD in parents or siblings, early age at onset of AD, being an only child, and very high serum IgE levels.

PREVENTION. Breast-feeding or a hypoallergic hydrolyzed formula may be beneficial, but if an infant with AD develops food allergy, the mother will need to eliminate the implicated food allergen from her diet. Probiotics may also reduce the incidence or severity of AD. Identification and elimination of triggering factors as part of treatment of AD is also the mainstay for prevention of recurrences.

Arvola T, Moilanen E, Vuento R, et al: Weaning to hypoallergenic formula improves gut barrier function to breast-fed infants with atopic eczema. *J Pediatr Gastroenterol Nutr* 2004;38:92–96.

Ashcroft DM, Dimmock P, Garside R, et al: Efficacy and tolerability of topical pimecrolimus and tacrolimus in the treatment of atopic dermatitis: Meta-analysis of randomized controlled trials. *Br Med J* 2005;330:516–522.

Brown S, Reynolds NJ: Atopic and non-atopic eczema. *BMJ* 2006;332:584–588.

Eichenfield LF, Hanifin JM, Luger TA, et al: Consensus conference on pediatric atopic dermatitis. *J Am Acad Dermatol* 2003;49:1088–1095.

Flohr C, Williams HC: Evidence based management of atopic eczema. *Arch Dis Child Edu Pract Ed* 2006;89:ep35–ep39.

Heine RG, Hill DJ, Hosking CS: Primary prevention of atopic dermatitis in breast-fed infants: What is the evidence? *J Pediatr* 2004;144:564–567.

Ho VC, Gupta A, Kaufmann R, et al: Safety and efficacy of nonsteroid pimecrolimus cream 1% in the treatment of atopic dermatitis in infants. *J Pediatr* 2003;142:155–162.

Leung DY, Bieber T: Atopic dermatitis. *Lancet* 2003;361:151–160.

Leung, DYM, Boguniewicz M, Howell MD, et al: New insights into atopic dermatitis. *J Clin Invest* 2004;113:651–657.

Palmer CNA, Irvine AD, Terron-Kwiatkowski A, et al: Common loss-of-function variants of the epidermal barrier protein filaggrin are a major predisposing factor for atopic dermatitis. *Nat Genetics* 2006;38:441–446.

Rautava S, Kalliomaki M, Isolauri E: Probiotics during pregnancy and breast-feeding might confer immunomodulatory protection against atopic disease in the infant. *J Allergy Clin Immunol* 2002;109:119–121.

Williams HC: Atopic dermatitis. *N Engl J Med* 2005;352:2314–2324.

Williams HC: Evening primrose oil for atopic dermatitis. *Br Med J* 2003;327:1358–1359.

Chapter 145 ■ Insect Allergy

Scott H. Sicherer and Donald Y. M. Leung

The allergic responses to stinging or, more rarely, biting insects vary from localized cutaneous reactions to systemic anaphylaxis. Allergic reactions that are caused by inhalation of airborne particles of insect origin result in acute and chronic respiratory symptoms of seasonal or perennial rhinitis, conjunctivitis, and asthma.

ETIOLOGY. Most reactions to biting and stinging insects such as those induced by mosquitoes, flies, and fleas are limited to a primary lesion isolated to the area of the bite and do not represent an allergic response. Occasionally, insect bites or stings induce pronounced localized reactions or systemic reactions that may be based on immediate or delayed hypersensitivity reactions. Systemic allergic responses to insects are attributed most typically to IgE antibody–mediated responses, which are caused almost entirely by stings from venomous insects of the order Hymenoptera. Members of this order include apids (honeybee, bumblebee), vespids (yellow jacket, wasp, hornet), and formicids (fire and harvester ants) (Fig. 145-1). Among winged stinging insects, yellow jackets are the most notorious for stinging because they are aggressive, ground dwelling, and linger near human activities involving food. Hornets nest in trees, whereas wasps build honeycomb nests in dark areas such as under porches; both are aggressive if disturbed. Honeybees are less aggressive, nest in tree hollows, and, unlike the other flying Hymenoptera, their sting almost always leaves a barbed stinger with venom sac.

In the United States, red or black fire ants are found increasingly in the southeast, living in large mounds of soil. When disturbed, the ants attack in large numbers, anchor themselves to the skin by their mandible, and sting multiple times in a semicircular pattern. Sterile pustules form at the sting sites. Systemic reactions to stinging insects occur in 0.4–0.8% of children and 3% of adults and account for ≈40 deaths each year in the United States.

IgE antibody–mediated allergic responses to airborne particulate matter carrying insect emanations contribute to seasonal and perennial symptoms affecting the upper and lower airway. Seasonal allergy is attributed to exposures to a variety of insects, particularly aquatic insects such as the caddis fly and midge, or lake fly, at a time when larvae pupate and adult flies are airborne.

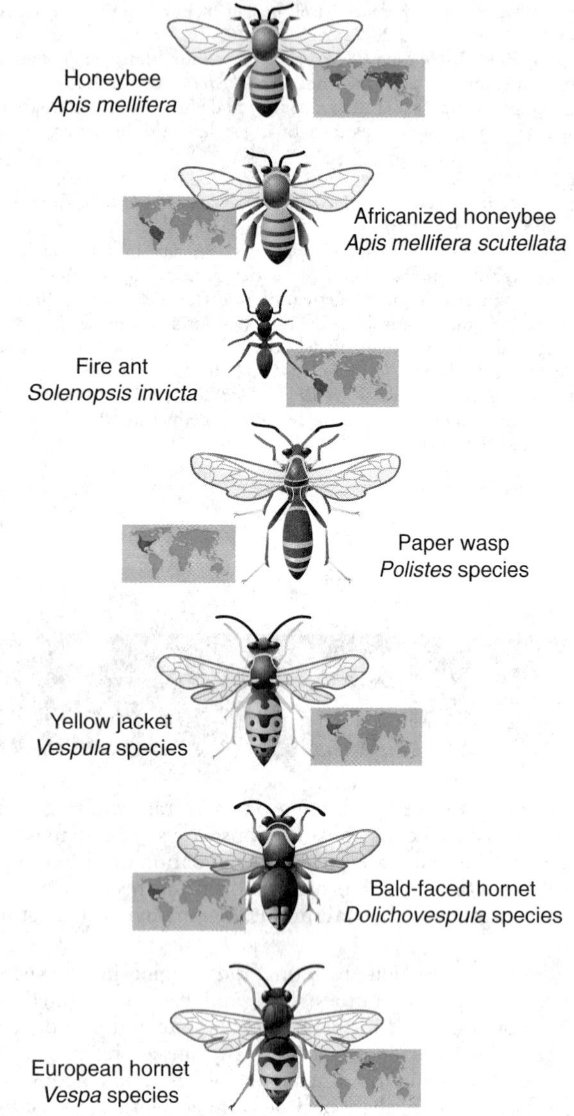

Figure 145-1. Species of Hymenoptera and their geographical distribution. (From Freeman TM: Hypersensitivity to Hymenoptera stings. *N Engl J Med* 2004;351:1978–1984.)

Perennial allergy is attributed to cockroach sensitization, which is associated with increased asthma morbidity for exposed children, and the house dust mite, which is an indoor allergen. The house dust mite, unlike the cockroach, is phylogenetically related to spiders rather than insects and has eight rather than six legs.

PATHOGENESIS. Localized skin responses to biting insects are likely caused by vasoactive or irritant materials derived from insect saliva. There is no evidence for IgE involvement in the local reaction. Systemic IgE-mediated allergic reactions to salivary proteins of biting insects such as mosquitoes are reported but uncommon.

Hymenoptera venoms contain numerous components with toxic and pharmacologic activity and with allergenic potential. These constituents include: vasoactive substances such as histamine, acetylcholine, and kinins; enzymes such as phospholipase and hyaluronidase; apamin; melittin; and formic acid. The majority of patients who experience systemic reactions after Hymenoptera stings have IgE-mediated sensitivity to antigenic substances in the venom. Some venom allergens are homologous among members of the Hymenoptera order; others are family specific. There is substantial cross reactivity among vespid venoms, but these venom allergies are distinct from honeybee.

A variety of proteins derived from insects can become airborne and induce IgE-mediated respiratory responses, causing inhalant allergies. The primary allergen from the caddis fly is a hemocyanin-like protein, and from the midge fly is derived from hemoglobin. Allergens from the cockroach are the best studied and are derived from cockroach saliva, secretions, fecal material, and debris from skin casts. Allergenic proteins from the cockroach include proteases, troponin, tropomyosin, and lipocalin.

CLINICAL MANIFESTATIONS. Insect bites are usually urticarial but may be papular or vesicular. Papular urticaria affecting the lower extremities in children is usually caused by multiple bites. Occasionally, individuals develop large local reactions. IgE antibody–associated immediate- and late-phase allergic responses to mosquito bites sometimes mimic cellulitis.

Clinical reactions to stinging venomous insects are categorized as local, large local, generalized cutaneous, systemic, toxic, and delayed/late. Simple **local reactions** involve limited swelling and pain, and generally last <24 hr. **Large local reactions** develop over hours and days, involve swelling of extensive areas (>10 cm) that are contiguous with the sting site, and may last for days. **Generalized cutaneous reactions** typically progress within minutes and include cutaneous symptoms of urticaria, angioedema, and pruritus beyond the site of the sting. **Systemic reactions** are identical to anaphylaxis from other triggers and may include symptoms of generalized urticaria, laryngeal edema, bronchospasm, and hypotension. Stings from a large number of insects at once may result in **toxic reactions** of fever, malaise, emesis, and nausea owing to the chemical properties of the venom in large doses. Serum sickness, nephrotic syndrome, vasculitis, neuritis, or encephalopathy may occur as **delayed/late reactions** to stinging insects.

Inhalant allergy caused by insects results in clinical disease similar to that induced by other inhalant allergens such as pollens. Depending on individual sensitivity and exposure, reactions may result in seasonal or perennial rhinitis, conjunctivitis, and asthma.

DIAGNOSIS. The diagnosis of allergy from biting and stinging insects is generally evident from the history of exposure, typical symptoms, and physical examination. The diagnosis of Hymenoptera allergy rests in part on the identification of venom-specific IgE by prick skin testing. The primary reasons to pursue testing are to confirm reactivity when venom immunotherapy (VIT) is being considered or when it is clinically necessary to confirm venom hypersensitivity as a cause of a reaction. Venoms of five Hymenoptera (honeybee, yellow jacket, yellow hornet, white-faced hornet, and wasp) as well as the jack jumper ant in Australia and whole-body extract of fire ant are available for skin testing. Although skin tests are considered to be the most sensitive modality for detection of venom-specific IgE, additional evaluation with an in vitro assay for venom-specific IgE is recommended if skin tests are negative in the presence of a convincing history of a severe systemic reaction. With in vitro tests, there is a 20% incidence of both false-positive and false-negative results so it is not appropriate to exclude venom hypersensitivity based on this test alone. If initial skin prick and in vitro tests are negative in the context of a convincing history of a severe reaction, repeat testing is recommended before concluding that treatment is not needed. Skin tests are usually accurate within 1 wk of a sting reaction, but occasionally a refractory period is observed that warrants retesting after 4–6 wk if the initial tests are negative. As many as 40% of skin test–positive subjects may not experience anaphylaxis on sting challenge, so testing without an appropriate clinical history is potentially misleading.

The diagnosis of inhalant insect allergy may be evident by a history of typical symptoms induced seasonally in specific geographic regions. A chronic respiratory symptom during chronic exposure, as may occur with cockroach allergy, is less amenable to identification by history alone. Skin prick or in vitro immunoassay tests for specific IgE to the insect are used to confirm inhalant insect allergy. Allergy tests may be particularly warranted for potential cockroach allergy in patients with persistent asthma and known cockroach exposure.

TREATMENT. For local cutaneous reactions caused by insect bites and stings, treatment with cold compresses, topical medications to relieve itching, and occasionally the use of a systemic antihistamine and oral analgesic are appropriate. Stingers should be removed promptly by scraping, with caution not to squeeze the venom sac because this could inject more venom. Sting sites rarely become infected, possibly owing to the antibacterial actions of venom constituents. Vesicles left by fire ant stings that are scratched open should be cleansed to prevent secondary infection.

Anaphylactic reactions after a Hymenoptera sting are treated in an identical fashion to anaphylaxis from any cause. Therapies may include oxygen, epinephrine, intravenous saline, steroids, antihistamines, and other treatments (see Chapter 148). Referral to an allergist-immunologist should be considered for patients who have experienced a generalized cutaneous or systemic reaction to an insect sting, need education about avoidance and emergency treatment, may be a candidate for VIT, or have a condition that may complicate management of anaphylaxis (use of β-blockers).

Venom Immunotherapy. Hymenoptera VIT is highly effective (95–97%) in decreasing the risk for severe anaphylaxis. The selection of patients for VIT depends on several factors (Table 145-1). Individuals with local reactions regardless of age are not at increased risk for severe systemic reactions on a subsequent sting and are not candidates for VIT. The risk of a systemic reaction for those who experienced a large local reaction is no more than 5–10%; testing or VIT is usually not recommended and prescription of self-injectable epinephrine is considered optional but usually not necessary. Those who experience severe systemic reactions, with airway involvement or hypotension, and have a positive skin test result should receive immunotherapy. Immunotherapy to winged Hymenoptera is not usually indicated for children ≤16 yr of age in whom stings have caused only generalized urticaria or angioedema because their risk for a reaction after a subsequent sting is about 10%, with isolated skin reactions as the most likely event. The risk could be reduced to 1% after treatment with VIT, so it is an option to consider if multiple future stings are anticipated. Immunotherapy to Hymenoptera is indicated in those ≥17 yr of age if skin test results are positive to venom and there is a history of generalized urticaria or a systemic reaction, because the risk for future systemic reactions approaches 60%. VIT is usually not indicated if there is no evidence of IgE to venom. The incidence of adverse effects in the course of treatment is not trivial in adults, as 50% experience large local reactions and about 7% experience systemic reactions. The incidence of both local and systemic reactions is much lower in children. It is uncertain how long immunotherapy with Hymenoptera venom should continue and lifelong treatment has been advocated, particularly for those with very severe reactions. Consideration to discontinue therapy after 3–5 yr has been suggested, however, because >80% of adults who have received 5 yr of therapy tolerate challenge stings without systemic reactions for 5–10 yr after completion of treatment. Long-term responses to treatment are even better for children. Follow-up over a mean of 18 yr of children with moderate to severe insect sting reactions who received VIT for a mean treatment period of 3.5 yrs and were stung again showed a reaction rate of only 5% compared to untreated children who experienced a reaction rate of 32%. Whereas duration of therapy with VIT may be individualized, it is clear that a significant number of untreated children retain their allergy.

Less is known about the natural history of fire ant hypersensitivity and efficacy of immunotherapy for this allergy. The criteria for starting immunotherapy are similar to those for other Hymenoptera, but there is stronger consideration to treat children ≤16 yr of age with VIT if they have only experienced generalized urticaria. Only whole-body fire ant extract is commercially available for diagnostic skin testing and immunotherapy.

Inhalent Allergy. The symptoms of inhalant allergy caused by insects are managed as for other causes of seasonal or perennial rhinitis (see Chapter 142), conjunctivitis (see Chapter 146), and asthma (see Chapter 143).

TABLE 145-1. Indications for Venom Immunotherapy (VIT) to Winged Hymenoptera

SYMPTOMS	AGE	SKIN TEST/IN VITRO TEST	VIT RECOMMENDED
Large local reaction	any	Usually not indicated	Usually not indicated
Generalized cutaneous reaction	≤16 yr	Usually not indicated	Usually not indicated
	≥17 yr	Positive result	Yes
		Negative result	No
Systemic reaction	any	Positive result	Yes
		Negative result	No

PREVENTION. Avoidance of stings and bites is essential. To reduce the risk of stings, sensitized individuals should avoid attractants such as perfumes and bright-colored clothing outdoors, wear gloves when gardening, and wear long pants and shoes with socks when walking in the grass or through fields. Typical insect repellents do not guard against Hymenoptera. Nests should be removed if they are close to the home.

Individuals who have had generalized cutaneous or systemic reactions to Hymenoptera stings should have immediate access to **self-injectable epinephrine.** Adults responsible for allergic children, and older patients who can self-treat, must be carefully taught the indications for and technique of administration of this medication. Particular attention is necessary for children in out-of-home daycare centers, at school, or attending camps to ensure that an emergency action plan is in place. Individuals at risk for anaphylaxis from an insect sting should also wear an identification bracelet indicating their allergy.

Avoidance of the insect is the preferred management of inhalant allergy. This can prove difficult, particularly, for instance, for those living in multiple-dwelling apartments where eradication of cockroaches is problematic. Immunotherapy is occasionally undertaken but beneficial results have not been thoroughly documented.

Bircher AJ: Systemic immediate allergic reactions to arthropod stings and bites. *Dermatology* 2005;210:119–127.

Brown SGA, Wiese MD, Blackman KE, et al: Ant venom immunotherapy: A double-blind, placebo-controlled crossover trial. *Lancet* 2003;361:1001–1006.

Freeman TM: Hypersensitivity to hymenoptera stings. *N Engl J Med* 2004;351:1978–1984.

Golden DB, Kagey-Sobotka A, Norman PS, et al: Outcomes of allergy to insect stings in children, with and without venom immunotherapy. *N Engl J Med* 2004;351:668–674.

Gruchalla RS: Immunotherapy in allergy to insect stings in children. *N Engl J Med* 2004;351:707–709.

Moffitt JE, Golden DB, Reisman RE, et al: Stinging insect hypersensitivity: A practice parameter update. *J Allergy Clin Immunol* 2004;114:869–886.

Morgan WJ, Crain EF, Gruchalla RS et al: Results of a home-based environmental intervention among urban children with asthma. *N Engl J Med* 2004;351:1068–1080.

Peng Z, Simons FE: Mosquito allergy: Immune mechanisms and recombinant salivary allergens. *Int Arch Allergy Immunol* 2004;133:198–209.

Chapter 146 ■ Ocular Allergies

Mark Boguniewicz and Donald Y. M. Leung

The eye is a common target of allergic disorders because of its marked vascularity and direct contact with allergens in the environment. The conjunctiva is the most immunologically active tissue of the external eye. Ocular allergies can occur as isolated target organ disease or more commonly in conjunction with nasal allergies. Ocular symptoms can significantly affect quality of life.

CLINICAL MANIFESTATIONS. There are a few distinct entities that constitute allergic eye disease, all of which have bilateral involvement. Sensitization is necessary for all of these except for giant papillary conjunctivitis. Vernal keratoconjunctivitis and atopic keratoconjunctivitis are potentially sight-threatening.

Allergic Conjunctivitis. Allergic conjunctivitis is the most common hypersensitivity response of the eye, affecting approximately 25% of the general population and 30% of children with atopy. It is caused by direct exposure of the mucosal surfaces of the eye to environmental allergens. Patients complain of variable ocular itching, rather than pain, with increased tearing. Clinical signs include bilateral injected conjunctivae with vascular congestion that may progress to chemosis, or conjunctival swelling, and a watery discharge. Allergic conjunctivitis occurs in a seasonal or, less commonly, perennial form. **Seasonal allergic conjunctivitis** is typically associated with allergic rhinitis (see Chapter 142) and most commonly triggered by ragweed or grass pollens. **Perennial allergic conjunctivitis** is triggered by allergens such as animal danders or dust mites that are present throughout the year. Symptoms are usually less severe than with seasonal allergic conjunctivitis.

Vernal Keratoconjunctivitis. Vernal keratoconjunctivitis is a severe bilateral chronic inflammatory process of the upper tarsal conjunctival surface that occurs in a limbal or palpebral form. It may threaten eyesight if there is corneal involvement. Although vernal keratoconjunctivitis is not IgE mediated, it occurs most frequently in children with seasonal allergies, asthma, or atopic dermatitis. Vernal keratoconjunctivitis affects boys twice as often as girls, and is more common in persons of Asian and African origin. It affects primarily children in temperate areas, with exacerbations in the spring and summer. Symptoms include severe ocular itching exacerbated by exposure to irritants, light, or perspiration. In addition, patients may complain of severe photophobia, foreign-body sensation, and lacrimation. Giant papillae occur predominantly on the upper tarsal plate and are typically described as **cobblestoning.** Other signs include a stringy or thick, ropey discharge, cobblestone papillae, transient yellow-white points in the limbus (Trantas dots) and conjunctiva (Horner points), corneal "shield" ulcers, and Dennie lines (Dennie-Morgan folds), which are prominent symmetric skinfolds that extend in an arc from the inner canthus beneath and parallel to the lower lid margin. Children with vernal keratoconjunctivitis have measurably longer eyelashes, which may represent a reaction to ocular inflammation.

Atopic Keratoconjunctivitis. Atopic keratoconjunctivitis is a **chronic** inflammatory ocular disorder most commonly involving the lower tarsal conjunctiva. It may threaten eyesight if there is corneal involvement. Almost all patients have **atopic dermatitis,** and a significant number have asthma. Atopic keratoconjunctivitis rarely presents before late adolescence. Symptoms include severe ocular itching, burning, and tearing that are much more severe than in allergic conjunctivitis and persist throughout the year. The bulbar conjunctiva is injected and chemotic. Eyelid eczema can extend to the periorbital skin and cheeks with erythema and thick, dry scaling. Secondary staphylococcal blepharitis is common because of eyelid induration and maceration.

TABLE 146-1. Topical Ophthalmic Medications for Allergic Conjunctivitis

DRUG AND TRADE NAMES	MECHANISM OF ACTION AND DOSING	CAUTIONS AND ADVERSE EVENTS
Azelastine hydrochloride 0.05% Optivar	Antihistamine Children ≥3 yr: 1 gtt bid	Not for treatment of contact lens related irritation; the preservative may be absorbed by soft contact lenses. Wait at least 10 min after administration before inserting soft contact lenses.
Emedastine difumarate 0.05% Emadine	Antihistamine Children ≥3 yr: 1 gtt qid	Soft contact lenses should not be worn if the eye is red. Wait at least 10 min after administration before inserting soft contact lenses.
Levocabastine hydrochloride 0.05% Livostin	Antihistamine Children ≥12 yr: 1 gtt bid-qid up to 2 wk	Not for use in patients wearing soft contact lenses during treatment.
Pheniramine maleate 0.3%/naphazoline hydrochloride 0.025% Naphcon-A, Opcon-A	Antihistamine/vasoconstrictor Children >6 yr: 1–2 gtt qid	Avoid prolonged use (>3–4 days) to avoid rebound symptoms. Not for use with contact lenses.
Cromolyn sodium 4% Crolom, Opticrom	Mast cell stabilizer Children >4 yr 1–2 gtt q4–6 hr	Can be used to treat giant papillary conjunctivitis and vernal keratitis. Not for use with contact lenses.
Lodoxamide tromethamine 0.1% Alomide	Mast cell stabilizer Children ≥2 yr: 1–2 gtt qid up to 3 mo	Can be used to treat vernal keratoconjunctivitis. Not for use in patients wearing soft contact lenses during treatment.
Nedocromil sodium 2% Alocril	Mast cell stabilizer Children ≥3 yr 1–2 gtt bid	Avoid wearing contact lenses while exhibiting the signs and symptoms of allergic conjunctivitis.
Pemirolast potassium 0.1% Alamast	Mast cell stabilizer Children >3 yr: 1–2 gtt qid	Not for treatment of contact lens related irritation; the preservative may be absorbed by soft contact lenses. Wait at least 10 min after administration before inserting soft contact lenses.
Epinastine hydrochloride 0.05% Elestat	Antihistamine/mast cell stabilizer Children ≥3 yr 1 gtt bid	Contact lenses should be removed prior to use. Wait at least 10 min after administration before inserting soft contact lenses. Not for the treatment of contact lens irritation.
Ketotifen fumarate 0.025% Zaditor	Antihistamine/mast cell stabilizer Children ≥3 years 1 gtt bid q8–12 hr	Not for treatment of contact lens related irritation; the preservative may be absorbed by soft contact lenses. Wait at least 10 min after administration before inserting soft contact lenses.
Olopatadine hydrochloride 0.1% Patanol	Antihistamine/mast cell stabilizer Children ≥3 yr: 1 gtt bid (8 hr apart)	
Ketorolac tromethamine 0.5% Acular	NSAID Children ≥3 yr: 1 gtt qid	Avoid with aspirin or NSAID sensitivity. Use ocular product with caution in patients with complicated ocular surgeries, corneal denervation or epithelial defects, ocular surface diseases (e.g., dry eye syndrome), repeated ocular surgeries within a short period of time, diabetes mellitus, or rheumatoid arthritis; these patients may be at risk for corneal adverse events that may be sight-threatening. Do not use while wearing contact lenses.

NSAID, nonsteroidal anti-inflammatory drug.

Giant Papillary Conjunctivitis. Giant papillary conjunctivitis has been linked to chronic exposure to foreign bodies, such as contact lenses, both hard and soft, ocular prostheses, and sutures. Symptoms and signs include mild ocular itching, tearing, and excessive ocular discomfort with mild mucoid discharge with white or clear exudate on awakening, which may become thick and stringy. Trantas dots, limbal infiltration, bulbar conjunctival hyperemia, and edema may develop.

Contact Allergy. Contact allergy typically involves the eyelids but can also involve the conjunctivae. It is being recognized more frequently in association with increased exposure to topical medications, contact lens solutions, and preservatives.

DIAGNOSIS. Non-allergic conjunctivitis can be viral, bacterial, or chlamydial in origin. It is typically unilateral but can be bilateral with symptoms initially developing in one eye (Chapter 625). Symptoms include stinging or burning rather than itching, and often a foreign body sensation. Ocular discharge can be watery, mucoid, or purulent. Masqueraders of ocular allergy also include nasolacrimal duct obstruction, foreign body, blepharoconjunctivitis, dry eye, uveitis, and trauma.

TREATMENT. Primary treatment of ocular allergies includes avoidance of allergens, cold compresses, and lubrication. Secondary treatment regimens include the use of oral or topical antihistamines (see Table 142-1) and, if necessary, topical decongestants, mast cell stabilizers, and anti-inflammatory agents (Table 146-1). Drugs with dual antihistamine and mast cell blocking activities provide the most advantageous approach in treating allergic conjunctivitis, with both fast-acting symptomatic relief and disease-modifying action. Children often complain of stinging or burning with use of topical ophthalmic preparations and usually prefer oral antihistamines for allergic conjunctivitis. It is important not to contaminate topical ocular medications by allowing the applicator tip to contact the eye or eyelid. Using refrigerated medications may decrease some of the discomfort associated with their use. Topical decongestants act as vasoconstrictors, reducing erythema, vascular congestion, and eyelid edema, but do not diminish the allergic response. Adverse effects of topical vasoconstrictors include burning or stinging and rebound hyperemia or conjunctivitis medicamentosa with chronic use. Combined use of an antihistamine and a vasoconstrictive agent is more effective than use of either agent alone.

Tertiary treatment of ocular allergy includes topical or, rarely, oral corticosteroids and should be conducted in conjunction with an ophthalmologist. Local administration of topical corticosteroids may be associated with increased intraocular pressure, viral infections, and cataract formation. Allergen immunotherapy can be very effective in seasonal and perennial allergic conjunctivitis, especially when associated with rhinitis, and can decrease the need for oral or topical medications to control allergy symptoms.

Bielory L: Allergic and immunologic disorders of the eye: II. Ocular allergy. J *Allergy Clin Immunol* 2000;106:1019–1032.

Bielory L, Lien KW, Bigelsen S: Efficacy and tolerability of newer antihistamines in the treatment of allergic conjunctivitis. *Drugs* 2005;65:215–228.

Leibowitz HM: The red eye. *N Engl J Med* 2000;343:345–351.

Ono SJ, Abelson MB: Allergic conjunctivitis: Update on pathophysiology and prospects for future treatment. *J Allergy Clin Immunol* 2005;115:118–122.

Pucci N, Novembre E, Lombardi E, et al: Long eyelashes in a case series of 93 children with vernal keratoconjunctivitis. *Pediatrics* 2005;115:e86–e91.

Simons FER: Advances in H_1-antihistamines. *N Engl J Med* 2004;351: 2203–2217.

Stahl JL, Barney NP: Ocular allergic disease. *Curr Opin Allergy Clin Immunol* 2004;4:455–459.

Tanaka M, Dogru M, Takano Y, et al: The relation of conjunctival and corneal findings in severe ocular allergies. *Cornea* 2004;23:464–467.

Chapter 147 ■ Urticaria (Hives) and Angioedema

Donald Y. M. Leung and Stephen C. Dreskin

Urticaria and angioedema affect 20% of individuals at some point in their lives. Episodes of hives that continue for <6 wk are considered acute, and those that persist for >6 wk are designated chronic. The distinction is important because the causes and mechanisms of urticaria formation and the therapeutic approaches are different in each instance.

ETIOLOGY AND PATHOGENESIS. Acute urticaria and angioedema are often caused by an allergic IgE-mediated reaction (Table 147-1). This form of urticaria is a self-limited process that occurs when an allergen activates mast cells in the skin. Systemically absorbed allergens that can induce generalized urticaria include foods, drugs (particularly antibiotics), and stinging insect venoms. If an allergen (latex, animal dander) penetrates the skin locally, hives can develop at the site of exposure. Acute urticaria can also result from non–IgE-mediated stimulation of mast cells caused by radiocontrast agents, viral agents including hepatitis B and Epstein-Barr virus, opiates, and nonsteroidal anti-inflammatory agents. The diagnosis of chronic urticaria is established when an episode has lasted for at least 6 wk and is not physical urticaria or recurrent acute urticaria with repeated exposures to an agent (Table 147-2). Often chronic urticaria is accompanied by angioedema. Rarely, angioedema occurs without urticaria.

Urticaria can also be classified according to the temporal relationship to a stimulus and the duration of a typical hive. Lesions that last 1–2 hr are typically encountered with physically induced hives and an inciting stimulus that is present only briefly. There is prompt mast cell degranulation, and biopsy of such lesions reveals little or no cellular infiltrate. A second form of urticaria can occur spontaneously and last 6–36 hr. These lesions typically have a prominent cellular infiltrate and can be found with food or drug reactions, chronic idiopathic urticaria, chronic autoimmune urticaria, and delayed pressure urticaria. Serum sickness reactions can be seen as a manifestation of drug reactions, and biopsy reveals a small-vessel cutaneous vasculitis. Urticaria in association with systemic lupus erythematosus or other vasculitides appears similar.

Atypical aspects of the gross appearance of the hives or associated symptoms should heighten concern that the urticaria or angioedema may be the manifestation of a systemic disease process. Lesions that burn more than itch, last >24 hr, do not blanch, or are associated with bleeding into the skin (purpura) suggest urticarial vasculitis.

TABLE 147-1. Etiology of Acute Urticaria

Foods	Egg, milk, wheat, peanuts, tree nuts, soy, shellfish, fish, strawberries (direct mast cell degranulation)
Medications	Suspect all medications, even over-the-counter or homeopathic
Insect stings	Hymenoptera (honeybee, yellow jacket, hornets, wasp, fire ants), biting insects (papular urticaria)
Infections	Bacterial (streptococcal pharyngitis, *Mycoplasma*, sinusitis); viral (hepatitis, mononucleosis [EBV], coxsackievirus A and B); parasitic (*Ascaris, Ancylostoma, Echinococcus, Fasciola, Filaria, Schistosoma, Strongyloides, Toxocara, Trichinella*); fungal (dermatophytes, *Candida*)
Contact allergy	Latex, pollen, animal saliva, nettle plants, caterpillars
Transfusion reactions	Blood, blood products, or IV immunoglobulin administration
Idiopathic	

EBV, Epstein-Barr virus.

From Lasley MV, Kennedy MS, Altman LC: Urticaria and angioedema. In Altman LC, Becker JW, Williams PV (eds): *Allergy in Primary Care.* Philadelphia, WB Saunders, 2000, p 232.

TABLE 147-2. Etiology of Chronic Urticaria

Idiopathic	75–90% of cases 35–40% of adult patients have IgG, anti-IgE, and anti-FcεRI (high-affinity IgE receptor α chain) autoantibodies
Physical	Dermatographism
	Cholinergic urticaria
	Cold urticaria
	Delayed pressure urticaria
	Solar urticaria
	Vibratory urticaria
	Aquagenic urticaria
Rheumatologic	Systemic lupus erythematosus
	Juvenile rheumatoid arthritis
Endocrine	Hyperthyroidism
	Hypothyroidism
Neoplastic	Lymphoma
	Mastocytosis
	Leukemia
Angioedema	Hereditary angioedema (autosomal dominant inherited deficiency of C1-esterase inhibitor)
	Acquired angioedema
	Angiotensin-converting enzyme inhibitors

From Lasley MV, Kennedy MS, Altman LC: Urticaria and angioedema. In Altman LC, Becker JW, Williams PV (eds): *Allergy in Primary Care.* Philadelphia, WB Saunders, 2000, p 234.

PHYSICAL URTICARIA. Physically induced urticaria and angioedema share the common property of being induced by environmental factors, such as a change in temperature or by direct stimulation of the skin with pressure, stroking, vibration, or light (Table 147-3).

Cold-Dependent Disorders. Cold urticaria is characterized by the rapid onset of localized pruritus, erythema, and urticaria/angioedema after exposure to a cold stimulus. Total-body exposure such as occurs with swimming can cause massive release of vasoactive mediators, resulting in hypotension and even death if not promptly treated. The diagnosis is confirmed by challenge testing for an isomorphic cold reaction with an ice cube placed on the patient's skin for 10–15 min. Patients with cold urticaria have a positive reaction on rewarming of the chilled skin. Cold urticaria can be associated with the presence of **cryoproteins** such as cold agglutinins, cryoglobulins, cryofibrinogen, and the Donath-Landsteiner antibody seen in secondary syphilis (paroxysmal cold hemoglobinuria). In patients with cryoglobulins, the isolated proteins appear to transfer cold sensitivity and activate the complement cascade on in vitro incubation with normal plasma. The term **idiopathic cold urticaria** generally applies to patients without abnormal circulating plasma proteins such as cryoglobulins. Cold urticaria has also been reported after viral infections. Cold urticaria must be distinguished from the **familial cold autoinflammatory syndrome.**

TABLE 147-3. Diagnostic Testing for Urticaria and Angioedema

DIAGNOSIS	DIAGNOSTIC TESTING
Food and drug reactions	Elimination of offending agent, skin testing, and challenge with suspected foods
Autoimmune urticaria	Autologous serum skin test; anti-thyroid antibodies
Thyroiditis	TSH; anti-thyroid antibodies
Infections	Appropriate cultures or serology
Collagen vascular diseases and cutaneous vasculitis	Skin biopsy, CH_{50}, C1q, C4, C3, factor B, immunofluorescence of tissues, antinuclear antibodies, cryoglobulins
Malignancy with angioedema	CH_{50}, C1q, C4, C1 INH determinations
Cold urticaria	Ice cube test
Solar urticaria	Exposure to defined wavelengths of light, red cell protoporphyrin, fecal protoporphyrin, and coproporphyrin
Dermatographism	Stroking with narrow object, (e.g., tongue blade, fingernail)
Pressure urticaria	Application of pressure for defined time and intensity
Vibratory urticaria	Vibration for 4 min
Aquagenic urticaria	Challenge with tap water at various temperatures
Urticaria pigmentosa	Skin biopsy, test for dermographism
Hereditary angioedema	C4, C2, CH_{50}, C1 INH by protein and function
Familial cold urticaria	Challenge by cold exposure, measurement of temperature, white blood cell count, erythrocyte sedimentation rate, and skin biopsy
C3b inactivator deficiency	C3, factor B, C3b inactivator determinations
Chronic idiopathic urticaria	Skin biopsy, immunofluorescence (negative result), autologous skin test

TSH, thyroid-stimulating hormone.

Cholinergic Urticaria. This form of urticaria is characterized by the onset of small punctate wheals surrounded by a prominent erythematous flare associated with exercise, hot showers, and sweating. When the patient cools down, the rash usually subsides in 30–60 min. Also occasionally seen are symptoms of more generalized cholinergic stimulation such as lacrimation, wheezing, salivation, and syncope. These symptoms are mediated by cholinergic nerve fibers that innervate the musculature via parasympathetic neurons and innervate the sweat glands by cholinergic fibers that travel with the sympathetic nerves. Elevated plasma histamine levels parallel the onset of urticaria triggered by changes in body temperature.

Dermatographism. The ability to write on skin, termed dermatographism (also called dermographism or urticaria factitia), can occur as an isolated disorder or accompany chronic urticaria or other physical urticaria such as cholinergic and cold urticaria. It can be diagnosed by observing the skin after stroking it with a tongue depressor or fingernail. In such patients, a linear response occurs secondary to reflex vasoconstriction, followed by pruritus, erythema, and a linear wheal.

Pressure-Induced Urticaria and Angioedema. Pressure-induced urticaria differs from most types of urticaria or angioedema in that symptoms typically occur 4–6 hr after pressure has been applied. The disorder is clinically heterogeneous in that some patients may complain of swelling secondary to pressure with normal-appearing skin (no urticaria), so that the term *angioedema* is more appropriate. Others are predominantly urticarial and may or may not be associated with significant swelling. When urticaria is present, an infiltrative skin lesion is seen, characterized by a perivascular mononuclear cell infiltrate and dermal edema similar to that seen in chronic idiopathic urticaria. Symptoms occur at sites of tight clothing; foot swelling is common after walking; and buttock swelling may be prominent after sitting for a few hr. This condition can coexist with chronic idiopathic urticaria or can occur separately. The diagnosis is confirmed by challenge testing by pressure applied perpendicular to the skin.

Solar Urticaria. Solar urticaria is a rare disorder in which urticaria develops within 1–3 min of sun exposure. Typically, pruritus occurs 1st, in about 30 sec, followed by edema confined to the light-exposed area and surrounded by a prominent erythematous zone caused by an axon reflex. The lesions usually disappear within 1–3 hr after sun exposure is avoided. When large areas of the body are exposed, systemic symptoms may occur, including hypotension and wheezing. Solar urticaria has been classified into 6 types, depending on (1) the wavelength of light that induces skin lesions and (2) the ability or inability to transfer the disorder passively with serum IgE. The rare inborn error of metabolism erythropoietic protoporphyria can be confused with solar urticaria because of the development of itching and burning of exposed skin immediately after sun exposure. In erythropoietic protoporphyria, fluorescence of UV-irradiated red blood cells can be demonstrated.

Aquagenic Urticaria. Patients with aquagenic urticaria develop small wheals after contact with water, regardless of its temperature, and are therefore distinguishable from patients with cold urticaria or cholinergic urticaria. Direct application of a compress of water to the skin is used to test for its presence.

CHRONIC IDIOPATHIC URTICARIA AND ANGIOEDEMA. This is a common disorder of unknown origin that is often associated with normal routine laboratory studies and no evidence of systemic

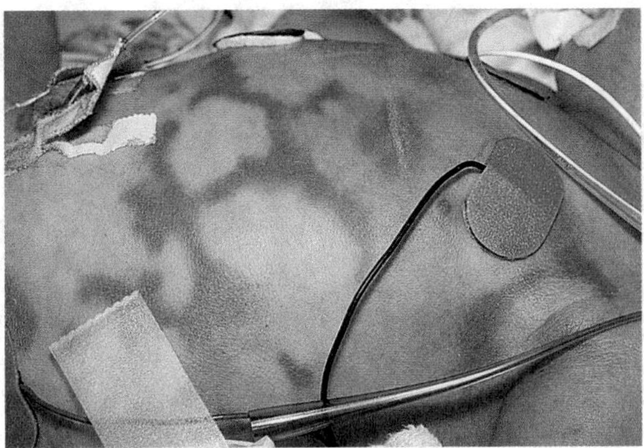

Figure 147-1 Polycyclic lesions of urticaria associated with prostaglandin E_2 infusion. (From Eichenfield LF, Friedan IJ, Esterly NB: *Textbook of Neonatal Dermatology.* Philadelphia, WB Saunders, 2001, p 300.)

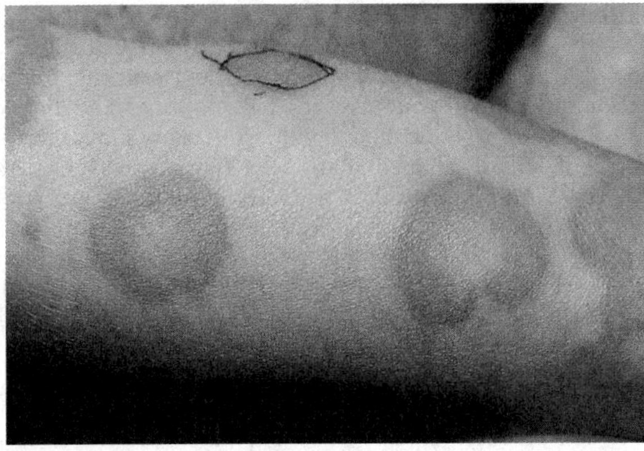

Figure 147-2. Annular urticaria of unknown etiology. (From Eichenfield LF, Friedan IJ, Esterly NB: *Textbook of Neonatal Dermatology.* Philadelphia, WB Saunders, 2001, p 301.)

disease. Chronic urticaria does not appear to be an allergic reaction. It differs from allergen-induced skin reactions or from physically induced urticaria in that histologic studies reveal a cellular infiltrate predominantly about small venules. Skin examination reveals infiltrative hives with palpably elevated borders, sometimes varying greatly in size and/or shape but generally being rounded.

Biopsy of the typical lesion reveals non-necrotizing, perivascular, mononuclear cellular infiltration. Many types of histopathologic processes can occur in the skin and manifest as urticaria. Patients with **hypocomplementemia** and **cutaneous vasculitis** can have urticaria and/or angioedema. Biopsy of these lesions in patients with urticaria, arthralgias, myalgias, and an elevated ESR as manifestations of necrotizing venulitis can reveal fibrinoid necrosis with a predominant neutrophilic infiltrate. Yet the urticarial lesions may be clinically indistinguishable from those seen in the more typical, nonvasculitis cases.

There is an increased association of chronic urticaria with the presence of antithyroid antibodies. Such patients generally have antibodies to thyroglobulin or a microsomal-derived antigen (peroxidase) even if they are euthyroid. The incidence of elevated thyroid antibodies in patients with chronic urticaria is ≈ 12% compared with 3–6% in the general population. Although some patients show clinical reduction of their urticaria on thyroid replacement therapy, others do not. Therefore, many investigators believe that these are associated, parallel, autoimmune events, although some believe that thyroid autoimmunity is driving the urticaria. There is currently no strong evidence to support the latter hypothesis.

Thirty-five to 40% of patients with chronic urticaria have a positive **autologous skin test:** If serum from the patient is intradermally injected into their skin, a significant wheal and flare reaction develops. Such patients frequently have a complement-activating IgG antibody directed to the α subunit of the IgE receptor that can cross link the IgE receptor (α subunit) and degranulate mast cells and basophils. An additional 5–10% of chronic urticaria patients have anti-IgE antibodies rather than anti-IgE receptor antibody. These patients, who are classified as having autoimmune urticaria, tend to have a somewhat more severe clinical course than patients without evidence of autoantibodies, but the difference is not dramatic.

DIAGNOSIS. The diagnosis of both acute and chronic urticaria is primarily clinical and requires that the physician be aware of the various forms of urticaria.

Urticaria is transient, pruritic, erythematous, raised wheals, with flat tops and edema that may become tense and painful. The lesions may coalesce and form polycyclic, serpiginous, or annular lesions (Figs. 147-1 and 147-2). Individual lesions usually last 20 min to 3 hr, and rarely more than 24 hr. The lesions often disappear and reappear. **Angioedema** involves the deeper subcutaneous tissues such as the eyelids, lips, tongue, genitals, and dorsum of the hands or feet.

Drugs and foods are the most common causes of acute urticaria. Allergy skin testing for foods can be helpful in sorting out causes of acute urticaria, especially when supported by historical evidence. The role of an offending food can then be proven by elimination and careful challenge in a controlled setting. In the absence of any clue suggesting an ingestant cause, skin testing for foods and implementation of elimination diets are generally not useful for either acute or chronic urticaria. Skin testing for aeroallergens is not indicated unless there is a concern about contact urticaria (animal dander). Dermatographism is frequent in patients with urticaria and can complicate allergy skin testing by causing false-positive reactions, but this is usually discernable.

An exogenous cause of chronic urticaria is rarely identified, reflecting its autoimmune or idiopathic etiology. An autologous serum skin test is useful to establish the diagnosis of autoimmune urticaria. In vitro testing for antibodies to Fc ε receptor I (FcεRI) may soon be available. The **differential diagnosis** of chronic urticaria includes cutaneous or systemic mastocytosis, complement-mediated disorders, malignancies, mixed connective tissue diseases, and cutaneous blistering disorders (e.g., bullous pemphigoid) (see Table 147-2). In general, laboratory testing should be limited to a complete blood cell count with differential, ESR, urinalysis, thyroid autoantibodies, and liver function tests. Further studies are warranted if the patient has fever, arthralgias, or elevated ESR (see Table 147-3). Hereditary angioedema, a potentially life-threatening form of angioedema associated with deficient C1 inhibitor activity, is the most important familial form of angioedema (see Chapter 133.3) but is not associated with typical urticaria. In patients with eosinophilia, stools for ova and parasites should be obtained because infection with helminthic parasites has been associated with urticaria. A syndrome of episodic angioedema/urticaria and fever with associated eosinophilia has been described in both adults and children. In contrast to other hypereosinophilic syndromes, this entity has a benign course.

Skin biopsy for diagnosis of possible **urticarial vasculitis** is recommended for urticarial lesions that persist at the same location for >24 hr, those with pigmented or purpuric components, and those that burn more than itch. Collagen vascular diseases such as systemic lupus may manifest urticarial vasculitis as a presenting feature. The skin biopsy in urticarial vasculitis typically shows endothelial cell swelling of postcapillary venules with necrosis of the vessel wall, perivenular neutrophil infiltrate, diapedesis of red blood cells, and fibrin deposition associated with deposition of immune complexes.

Mastocytosis is characterized by mast cell hyperplasia in the bone marrow, liver, spleen, lymph nodes, and skin. Clinical effects of mast cell activation are common, including pruritus, flushing, urtication, abdominal pain, nausea, and vomiting. The diagnosis is confirmed by a bone marrow biopsy containing increased numbers of spindle-shaped mast cells that express CD2 and CD25. **Urticaria pigmentosa** is the most common skin manifestation of mastocytosis and may occur as an isolated skin finding. It appears as small, yellow-tan to reddish-brown macules or raised papules that urticate on scratching **(Darier sign).** This sign can be masked by antihistamines. The diagnosis is confirmed by a skin biopsy that shows increased numbers of dermal mast cells.

Physical urticaria should be considered in any patient with chronic urticaria (see Table 147-3). Papular urticaria commonly occurs in small children, generally on the extremities. It presents as grouped or linear highly pruritic wheals or papules mainly on exposed skin at the sites of insect bites.

Exercise-induced anaphylaxis presents as varying combinations of pruritus, urticaria, angioedema, wheezing, laryngeal obstruction, or hypotension after exercise (see Chapter 148). Cholinergic urticaria is differentiated by positive results on heat challenge tests and the rare occurrence of anaphylactic shock. The combination of ingestion of various food allergens (shrimp, celery, or wheat) and postprandial exercise has been associated with urticaria/angioedema and anaphylaxis. In such patients, food or exercise alone may not produce this reaction.

Muckle-Wells syndrome and **familial cold autoinflammatory syndrome (FCAS)** are rare, dominantly inherited conditions associated with recurrent urticarial-like lesions. Muckle-Wells is characterized by arthritis and limb pain that usually appears in adolescence. It is associated with progressive nerve deafness, recurrent fever, elevated ESR, hypergammaglobulinemia, renal amyloidosis, and a poor prognosis. FCAS is characterized by a cold-induced rash that has urticarial features but is rarely pruritic. Cold exposure leads to additional symptoms such as conjunctivitis, sweating, headache, and nausea. Longevity is usually normal.

TABLE 147-4. Treatment of Uticaria and Angioedema

Class/drug	Dose	Frequency
ANTIHISTAMINES, TYPE H1 (2ND GENERATION)		
Fexofenadine	6–11 yr: 30 mg; >12 yr: 60 mg	bid
	Adult: 180 mg	Once daily
Loratadine	2–5 yr: 5 mg >6 yr: 10 mg	qd
Desloratadine	6–11 mo: 1 mg 1–5 yr: 1.25 mg 6–11 yr: 2.5 mg >12 yr: 5 mg	qd
Cetirizine	6–24 mo: 2.5 mg 2–6 yr: 2.5–5 mg >6 yr: 5–10 mg	6–12 mo: once daily 12–24 mo: 1–2 daily 2–12 yr: once daily
ANTIHISTAMINES, TYPE H2		
CIMETIDINE	INFANTS: 10–20 MG/KG/DAY; Children: 20–40 mg/kg/day	DIVIDED Q6–12HR
Ranitidine	1 mo–16 yr: 5–10 mg/kg/day	Divided q12hr
Famotidine	3–12 mo: 1 mg/kg/day 1–16 yr: 1–2 mg/kg/day	Divided q12hr
LEUKOTRIENE PATHWAY MODIFIERS		
Montelukast	12 mo–5 yr: 4 mg 6–14 yr: 5 mg; >14 yr: 10 mg	Once daily
Zafirlukast	5–11 yr: 10 mg	bid
IMMUNOMODULATORY DRUGS		
Cyclosporine	4–6 mg/kg/day	Once daily
Sulfasalazine	>6 yr: 30 mg/kg/day	Divided q6hr‡
IVIG	400 mg/kg/day	5 consecutive days

*Monitor blood pressure, creatinine, potassium, and magnesium monthly.
†Ophthalmologic examinations are required every 6 mo.
‡Monitor complete blood count and liver function tests at baseline, every 2 wk for 3 mo, and then every 1–3 mo.
IVIG, intravenous immunoglobulin.

TREATMENT. Acute urticaria is a self-limited illness requiring little treatment other than antihistamines. Hydroxyzine and diphenhydramine are sedating, but they are effective and commonly used for treatment of urticaria. Loratadine, fexofenadine, and cetirizine are also effective and are preferable because of reduced frequency of drowsiness (Table 147-4). Epinephrine 1 : 1,000, 0.01 mL/kg (maximum: 0.3 mL) usually provides rapid relief of acute, severe urticaria/angioedema. A short burst of corticosteroids should be given only for very severe episodes of urticaria and angioedema.

Most forms of physical urticaria respond to avoidance of triggering stimuli in combination with oral antihistamines. The exception is delayed pressure urticaria, which often requires oral corticosteroids. Cyproheptadine in divided doses is the drug of choice for cold-induced urticaria. Treatment of dermatographism consists of local skin care and antihistamines; for severe symptoms, high doses may be needed. The initial objective of therapy is to decrease pruritus so that the stimulation for scratching is diminished. A combination of antihistamines, sunscreens, and avoidance of sunlight are helpful for most patients.

Chronic urticaria only rarely responds favorably to dietary manipulation. The combined use of H_1- and H_2-type antihistamines is sometimes helpful to control chronic urticaria when H_1-type antihistamines alone, even at higher than standard doses, do not work (see Table 147-4). Doxepin, an antagonist of both H_1 and H_2 receptors, can be helpful, but its usefulness is limited due to adverse effects. H_2-type antihistamines alone may exacerbate urticaria. If hives persist after maximal H_1- and/or H_2-receptor blockade has been achieved, alternate-day therapy with corticosteroids is the most effective treatment. In general, prednisone 20 mg orally as a single morning dose on alternate days is used, with the dosage decreased by 2.5–5.0 mg every 1–3 wk depending on the clinical response. The clinical goal is slow reduction of the use of this drug. Antileukotriene agents in combination with antihistamines may also be helpful. Treatment with cyclosporine 4–6 mg/kg/day has been effective in some adults with chronic urticaria, but is limited by hypertension and/or nephrotoxicity. Removal of urticarial aggravators, such as salicylates, alcohol, or β-blockers, should be considered. Treatment of autoimmune chronic urticaria refractory to medical therapy includes intravenous immunoglobulin, plasmapheresis, or both.

Boguniewicz M: Chronic urticaria in children. *Allergy Asthma Proc* 2005;26:13–17.

Dibbern DA Jr, Dreskin SC: Urticaria and angioedema: An overview. *Immunol Allergy Clin North Am* 2004;24:141–162.

Kaplan AP: Chronic urticaria: Pathogenesis and treatment. *J Allergy Clin Immunol* 2004;114:465–474.

Poon M, Springs A, Reid C: Do steroids help children with acute urticaria? *Arch Dis Child* 2004;89:85–86.

Sackesen C, Sekerel BE, Orhan F, et al: The etiology of different forms of urticaria in childhood. *Pediatr Dermatol* 2004;21:102–108.

Sheikh J: Advances in the treatment of chronic urticaria. *Immunol Allergy Clin North Am* 2004;24:317–334.

Urticaria and angioedema. In Greaves MW, Kaplan AP (eds). New York, Marcel Dekker, 2004.

Chapter 148 ■ Anaphylaxis

Hugh A. Sampson and
Donald Y. M. Leung

Anaphylaxis occurs when there is a sudden release of potent biologically active mediators from mast cells and basophils leading to cutaneous (urticaria, angioedema, flushing), respiratory (bronchospasm, laryngeal edema), cardiovascular (hypotension, dysrhythmias, myocardial ischemia), and gastrointestinal symptoms (nausea, colicky abdominal pain, vomiting, diarrhea).

ETIOLOGY. The most common causes of anaphylaxis in children are different for hospital and community settings. Anaphylaxis occurring in the hospital primarily results from allergic reactions to medications and latex. Food allergy is the most common cause of anaphylaxis occurring outside the hospital, accounting for about $^1/_2$ of the anaphylactic reactions reported in pediatric surveys from the United States, Italy, and South Australia (Table 148-1). Peanut allergy is an important cause of food-induced anaphylaxis accounting for the majority of fatal and near-fatal reactions. In the hospital, latex is a particular problem for children undergoing multiple operations, such as patients with spina bifida and urologic disorders, and has prompted many hospitals to switch to latex-free products. Patients with latex allergy may also experience food allergic reactions from homologous proteins in foods such as bananas, kiwi, avocado, chestnut, and passion fruit.

EPIDEMIOLOGY. The overall annual incidence of anaphylaxis in the United States is estimated at 30 cases/100,000 persons/yr, totaling 81,000 cases/yr). An Australian parental survey found that 0.59% of children 3–17 yr of age experienced at least 1 anaphylactic event.

PATHOGENESIS. Principal pathologic features in fatal anaphylaxis include acute pulmonary hyperinflation, pulmonary edema, intraalveolar hemorrhaging, visceral congestion, laryngeal edema, and urticaria and angioedema. Acute hypotension is attributed to vasomotor dilation and/or cardiac dysrhythmias.

Most cases of anaphylaxis are the result of activation of mast cells and basophils via cell-bound allergen-specific IgE molecules. Patients initially must be exposed to the responsible allergen to generate allergen-specific antibodies. In many cases, the child and the parent are unaware of the initial exposure, which may be due to passage of food proteins in maternal breast milk. When reexposed to the sensitizing allergen, mast cells and basophils and possibly other cells such as macrophages release a variety of mediators (histamine, tryptase) and cytokines that can produce allergic symptoms in any or all target organs. Clinical anaphylaxis may also be caused by mechanisms other than IgE-mediated reactions, sometimes termed **anaphylactoid reactions,** including direct release of mediators from mast cells by medications and physical factors (morphine, exercise, cold), disturbances of leukotriene metabolism (aspirin and nonsteroidal anti-inflammatory drugs), immune aggregates and complement activation (blood products), and probable complement activation (radiocontrast dyes, dialysis membranes).

TABLE 148-1. Common Causes of Anaphylaxis in Children*

Food: peanuts, tree nuts (walnut, hazelnut, cashew, pistachio, Brazil nut), milk, eggs, fish, shellfish (shrimp, crab, lobster, clam, scallop, oyster), seeds (sesame, cottonseed, pine nuts, psyllium), fruits (apples, banana, kiwi, peaches, oranges, melon), grains (wheat)
Drugs: penicillins, cephalosporins, sulfonamides, nonsteroidal anti-inflammatory agents, opiates, muscle relaxants, vancomycin, dextran, thiamine, vitamin B_{12}, insulin, thiopental, local anesthetics
Hymenoptera venom: honeybee, yellow jacket, wasp, hornet, fire ant
Latex
Allergen immunotherapy
Exercise: food-specific exercise, postprandial (non–food-specific) exercise
Vaccinations: tetanus, measles, mumps, influenza
Miscellaneous: radiocontrast media, gammaglobulin, cold temperature, chemotherapeutic agents (asparaginase, cyclosporine, methotrexate, vincristine, 5-fluorouracil), blood products, inhalants (dust and storage mites, grass pollen)
Idiopathic

*In order of frequency.
From Leung DYM, Sampson HA, Geha RS, et al: *Pediatric Allergy Principles and Practice*, St. Louis, Mosby, 2003, p 644.

CLINICAL MANIFESTATIONS AND DIAGNOSIS. The onset of symptoms may vary somewhat depending on the cause of the reaction. Reactions from ingested allergens (foods, medications) are delayed in onset (minutes to 2 hr) compared with injected allergens (insect sting, medications) and tend to have more gastrointestinal symptoms. Initial symptoms will vary depending on the etiology and may include any of the following constellation of symptoms: pruritus about the mouth and face, a sensation of warmth, weakness, and apprehension; flushing, urticaria and angioedema, oral pruritus, tightness in the throat, dry staccato cough and hoarseness, periocular pruritus, nasal congestion, sneezing, dyspnea, deep cough, and wheezing; nausea, abdominal cramping, and vomiting, especially with ingested allergens; uterine contractions (manifesting as lower back pain is not uncommon); and faintness and loss of consciousness in severe cases. Some degree of obstructive laryngeal edema is typically encountered with severe reactions. Cutaneous symptoms may be absent in up to 20% of cases, and the acute onset of severe bronchospasm in a previously well asthmatic should suggest the diagnosis of anaphylaxis. Sudden collapse in the absence of cutaneous symptoms should also raise suspicion of vasovagal collapse, myocardial infarction, aspiration, pulmonary embolism, or seizure disorder. Laryngeal edema, especially with abdominal pain, suggests hereditary angioedema (see Chapter 133.3).

LABORATORY FINDINGS. Laboratory studies may indicate the presence of IgE antibodies to a suspected causative agent, but this is not definitive. Plasma histamine is elevated for a brief period but is unstable and difficult to measure in a clinical setting. **Plasma β-tryptase** is more stable and remains elevated for several hours but often is not elevated, especially in food-induced anaphylactic reactions.

DIAGNOSIS. The diagnosis of anaphylaxis is usually apparent owing to the acute and dramatic nature of the characteristic combination of cutaneous and respiratory manifestations, especially when accompanied by hypotension. The differential diagnosis includes other forms of shock (hemorrhagic, cardiogenic, septic), vasopressor reactions including flush syndromes such as carcinoid syndrome, excess histamine syndromes (systemic mastocytosis), ingestion of monosodium glutamate (MSG), scombroidosis, and heriditary angioedema (see Chapter 133.3).

TREATMENT. Anaphylaxis is a medical emergency requiring aggressive management with **intramuscular** epinephrine, intramuscular or intravenous H_1 and H_2 antihistamine antagonists, oxygen, intravenous fluids, inhaled β-agonists, and corticosteroids (Table 148-2). Patients may experience **biphasic anaphylaxis,** which occurs when anaphylactic symptoms recur after apparent resolution. The mechanism of this phenomenon is unknown, but it appears to be more common when therapy is initiated late and symptoms at presentation are more severe. It does not appear to be affected by the administration of cortico-

TABLE 148-2. Management of a Patient with Anaphylaxis

DRUG CLASSIFICATION	INDICATION AND DOSE	COMMENTS; ADVERSE REACTIONS
PATIENT EMERGENCY MANAGEMENT (DEPENDENT ON SEVERITY OF SYMPTOMS)		
Epinephrine (adrenaline) 0.01 mg/kg up to 0.3 mg	Rx of anaphylaxis, bronchospasm, cardiac arrest EpiPen Jr (0.15 mg) IM 8–25 kg EpiPen (0.3 mg) IM >25 kg	Tachycardia, hypertension, nervousness, headache, nausea, irritability, and tremor
Cetirizine (liquid) (Zyrtec—5 mg/5 mL)	Antihistamine (competitive of H_1 receptor) 0.25 mg/kg up to 10 mg po	Hypotension, tachycardia, and somnolence
Alt: Diphenhydramine (Benadryl—12.5 mg/5 mL)	Antihistamine (competitive of H_1 receptor) 1.25 mg/kg up to 50 mp po	Hypotension, tachycardia, somnolence, and paradoxical excitement
Transport to an Emergency Facility		
EMERGENCY PERSONNEL MANAGEMENT (DEPENDENT ON SEVERITY OF SYMPTOMS)		
Supplemental oxygen and airway management		
Epinephrine (adrenaline) 0.01 mg/kg up to 0.3 mg	Rx of anaphylaxis, bronchospasm, cardiac arrest EpiPen Jr (0.15 mg) IM 8–25 kg EpiPen (0.3 mg) IM >25 kg 0.01 mL/kg/dose of 1 : 1,000 solution up to 0.3 mL IM 0.01 mL/kg/dose of 1 : 10,000 slow IV push	Tachycardia, hypertension, nervousness, headache, nausea, irritability, and tremor May repeat q 10–15 mins For severe hypotension
Volume expanders		
Crystalloids (normal saline or Ringer lactate)	30 mL/kg in first hour	Rate titrated against blood pressure response
Colloids (hydroxyethyl starch)	10 mL/kg rapidly followed by slow infusion	Rate titrated against blood pressure response
Diphenhydramine (Benadryl—12.5 mg/5 mL)	Antihistamine (competitive of H_1 receptor) 1.25 mg/kg up to 50 mg IM	Hypotension, tachycardia, somnolence, and paradoxical excitement
Alt: Cetirizine [liquid] (Zyrtec—5 mg/5 mL)	Antihistamine (competitive of H_1 receptor)	Hypotension, tachycardia, and somnolence
Nebulized albuterol	β-Agonist (0.83 mg/mL [3 mL]) via mask with O_2	Palpitations, nervousness, CNS stimulation, tachycardia; use to supplement epinephrine when bronchospasm appears unresponsive; may repeat
Corticosteroids		
Methylprednisolone	Anti-inflammatory	Hypertension, edema, nervousness, and agitation
Solu-Medrol (IV)	1–2 mg/kg up to 125 mg IV	
Depo-Medrol (IM)	1 mg/kg up to 80 mg IM	
Prednisone	Anti-inflammatory	Hypertension, edema, nervousness, and agitation
For po use	1 mg/kg up to 75 mg po	
Ranitidine (Zantac—25 mg/mL)	Antihistamine (competitive of H_2 receptor) 1 mg/kg up to 50 mg IV	Headache, mental confusion Should be administered slowly
Alt: Cimetidine (Tagamet—25 mg/mL)	Antihistamine (competitive of H_2 receptor) 4 mg/kg up to 200 mg IV	Headache, mental confusion Should be administered slowly
Post-emergency Management		
H_1-antagonist	Cetirizine (5–10 mg qd) or loratidine (5–10 mg qd) for 3 days	
Corticosteroids	Oral prednisone (1 mg/kg up to 75 mg) daily for 3 days	
Preventive Treatment		
Follow-up evaluation to determine/confirm etiology		
Immunotherapy for insect sting allergy		
Prescription for EpiPen and antihistamine		
Provide written plan outlining patient emergency management (may download form from www.foodallergy.org)		
Patient Education		
Instruction on avoidance of causative agent		
Information on recognizing early signs of anaphylaxis		
Stress early treatment of allergic symptoms to avoid systemic anaphylaxis		

IM, intramuscularly

steroids during the initial therapy. More than 90% of biphasic responses occur within 4 hr, so patients should be observed for at least 4 hr before being discharged from the emergency department.

PREVENTION. Patients experiencing anaphylactic reactions to foods must be educated in allergen avoidance, including actively reading food labels and knowledge of potential contamination and high-risk situations, as well as in early recognition of anaphylactic symptoms and ready administration of emergency medications. Any child with food allergy and a history of asthma, peanut or tree nut allergy, or a previous severe anaphylactic reaction should be given an EpiPen (epinephrine), liquid cetirizine (or alternatively, diphenhydramine), and a written emergency plan in case of accidental ingestion. A form can be downloaded from the Food Allergy and Anaphylaxis Network at www.foodallergy.org. Patients with egg allergy should be tested before receiving the influenza or yellow fever vaccines, which contain egg protein. Children experiencing a systemic anaphylactic reaction including respiratory symptoms to an insect sting should be evaluated and treated with immunotherapy, which is more than 90% protective. In cases of food-associated exercise-induced anaphylaxis, children must not exercise within 2–3 hr of ingesting the triggering food and, like children with exercise-induced anaphylaxis, should exercise with a friend, learn to recognize the early signs of anaphylaxis (sensation of warmth and facial pruritus), stop exercising, and seek help immediately if symptoms develop. Any child who is at risk for anaphylaxis should receive emergency medications, education, and a written emergency plan in case of accidental ingestion.

Reactions to medications can be reduced and minimized by using oral medications in preference to injected forms. Hypo-osmolar radiocontrast dyes can be used in cases in which previous reactions are suspected. The use of powder-free, low-allergen latex gloves or nonlatex gloves and materials should be used in children undergoing multiple surgeries.

American Academy of Allergy, Asthma and Immunology Position Statement: Anaphylaxis in schools and other childcare settings. *J Allergy Clin Immunol* 1998;102:173–176.
American Academy of Pediatrics Position Statement: Guidelines for emergency medical care in school. *Pediatrics* 2001;107:435–436.
American Heart Association 2005 Guidelines for CRP and ECC. Part 10.6 Anaphylaxis. *Circulation* 2005;112:IV143–IV145.
Bock SA, Munoz-Furlong A, Sampson HA: Fatalities due to anaphylactic reactions to foods. *J Allergy Clin Immunol* 2001;107:191–193.
Dibs SD, Baker MD: Anaphylaxis in children: A 5-year experience. *Pediatrics* 1997;99:e7.
Lee JM, Greenes DS: Biphasic anaphylactic reactions in pediatrics. *Pediatrics* 2000;106:762–766.
Lieberman P, Kemp SF, Oppenheimer J, et al: The diagnosis and management of anaphylaxis: an updated practice parameter. *J Allergy Clin Immunol* 2005;115:S483–S523.
Sampson HA: Anaphylaxis and emergency treatment. *Pediatrics* 2003;111:1601–1608.
Sampson HA, Munoz-Furlong A, Bock SA, et al: Symposium on the definition and management of anaphylaxis: Summary report. *J Allergy Clin Immunol* 2005;115:571–574.
Sicherer SH, Foreman JA, Noone SA: Use assessment of self-administered epinephrine among food-allergic children and pediatricians. *Pediatrics* 2000;105:359–362.

Chapter 149 ■ Serum Sickness

Scott H. Sicherer and Donald Y.M. Leung

Serum sickness is a systemic, immune complex–mediated hypersensitivity vasculitis classically attributed to the therapeutic administration of foreign serum proteins.

ETIOLOGY. Immune complexes involving heterologous (animal) serum proteins and complement activation are important pathogenic mechanisms in serum sickness. The availability of alternative medical therapies, modified or bioengineered antibodies, and biologicals of human origin have supplanted the use of nonhuman antisera. Reactions originally described as serum sickness–like are now attributed to drug allergy, triggered in particular by antibiotics (penicillin, cefaclor) and rarely to other agents such as human immune globulin, humanized monoclonal antibodies, and insect venom. Antibody therapies derived from the horse are available for treatment of envenomation by the black widow spider and a variety of snakes, treatment of botulism, and for immunosuppression (antithymocyte globulin).

PATHOGENESIS. Serum sickness is a classic example of a type III hypersensitivity reaction caused by antigen-antibody complexes. In the rabbit model using bovine serum albumin as the antigen, symptoms develop with the appearance of antibody against the injected antigen. As free antigen concentration falls and antibody production increases over days, antigen-antibody complexes of various sizes develop in a manner analogous to a precipitin curve. Whereas small complexes usually circulate harmlessly and large complexes are cleared by the reticuloendothelial system, intermediate-sized complexes that develop at the point of slight antigen excess may deposit in blood vessel walls and tissues. There the immune microprecipitates induce vascular and tissue damage through activation of complement and granulocytes.

Complement activation (C3a, C5a) promotes chemotaxis and adherence of neutrophils to the site of immune complex deposition. The process of immune complex deposition and of neutrophil accumulation may be facilitated by increased vascular permeability, owing to the release of vasoactive amines from tissue mast cells. Mast cells may be activated by binding of antigen to IgE or through contact with anaphylatoxins (C3a). Tissue injury results from the liberation of proteolytic enzymes and oxygen radicals from the neutrophils.

CLINICAL MANIFESTATIONS. The symptoms of serum sickness generally begin 7–12 days after injection of the foreign material, but may appear as late as 3 wk afterward. The onset of symptoms may be accelerated if there has been earlier exposure or previous allergic reaction to the same antigen. A few days before the onset of generalized symptoms, the site of injection may become edematous and erythematous. Symptoms usually include fever, malaise, and rashes. Urticaria and morbilliform rashes are the predominant types of skin eruptions, and pruritus is common. In a prospective study of serum sickness induced by administration of equine antithymocyte globulin, an initial rash was noted in most patients. It began as a thin serpiginous band of erythema along the sides of the hands, fingers, feet, and toes at the junction of the palmar or plantar skin with the skin of the dorsolateral surface. In most patients, the band of erythema was replaced by petechiae or purpura, presumably because of low platelet counts. Additional symptoms include edema, myalgia, lymphadenopathy, arthralgia or arthritis involving multiple joints, and gastrointestinal complaints including pain, nausea, diarrhea, and melena. The disease generally runs a self-limited course, with recovery in 1–2 wk. Carditis, glomerulonephritis, Guillain-Barré syndrome, and peripheral neuritis are rare complications.

DIAGNOSIS. Circulating immune complexes are usually detectable, with peak levels at 10–12 days. Serum complement levels (C3 and C4) are generally decreased and reach a nadir at about day 10. C3a anaphylatoxin may be increased. The ESR is usually elevated, and thrombocytopenia is often present. Mild proteinuria, hemoglobinuria, and microscopic hematuria may be seen. In serum sickness caused by horse serum proteins, antibodies of the IgG, IgA, IgM, and IgE classes may be found directed against various horse serum proteins. Direct immunofluorescence studies of skin lesions often reveal immune deposits of IgM, IgA, IgE, or C3.

TREATMENT. Treatment is primarily supportive with antihistamines and analgesics. When the symptoms are especially severe, systemic corticosteroids can be used. High doses are given and rapidly reduced as the patient improves. The utility of extracorporeal removal of circulating immune complexes via plasmapheresis requires further study.

PREVENTION. The primary mode of prevention of serum sickness is to seek alternative therapies, if they are available. In some cases, non–equine-derived formulations may be available in limited supply (human-derived botulinum immune globulin). Other emerging alternatives include partially digested antibodies of animal origin and engineered (humanized) antibodies. The potential of these therapies to elicit serum sickness–like disease appears low. When only equine antitoxin/antivenom is available, skin tests should be performed before administration of serum. The results of allergy skin tests reflect primarily the risk of acute anaphylactic reactions to the serum proteins, with a positive test indicating an increased likelihood and a negative test indicating a small, but not absent, risk of anaphylaxis. Testing generally begins with prick-puncture using a 1:100 dilution of the serum with positive (histamine) and negative (saline) controls and proceeds through several increasingly higher doses until a positive response is seen or a top dose of 0.02 mL of a 1:100 dilution injected intracutaneously is reached. A negative response to the strongest solution indicates that anaphylactic sensitivity to horse serum is unlikely. Unfortunately, skin tests do not predict the likelihood of development of serum sickness.

For patients who have evidence of anaphylactic sensitivity to horse serum, a risk to benefit assessment must be made to determine the need to proceed with treatment. If needed, the serum can usually be successfully administered by a process of rapid desensitization. The suggested desensitization procedure varies slightly by manufacturer, by estimated degree of sensitivity, and by route (intravenous versus intramuscular/subcutaneous). Starting doses are usually quite small (e.g., 0.1 mL of serum diluted to 1:100,000–1:1,000) and administered in gradually increasing increments, as tolerated, until the required cumulative dose is achieved. Generally, the entire amount of antitoxin can be administered safely over a 4–6 hr period. Desensitization is transient, and the patient may regain the previous anaphylactic sensitivity. Serum sickness is not prevented by desensitization or pretreatment with corticosteroids.

Colombel JF, Loftus EV Jr, Tremaine WJ, et al: The safety profile of infliximab in patients with Crohn's disease: The Mayo Clinic experience in 500 patients. *Gastroenterology* 2004;126:19–31.

Kojis FG: Serum sickness and anaphylaxis: Analysis of cases of 6,211 patients treated with horse serum for various infections. *Am J Dis Child* 1942;64:93–143.

Lawley TJ, Bielory L, Gascon P, et al: A prospective clinical and immunological analysis of patients with serum sickness. *N Engl J Med* 1984;311:1407–1413.

Offerman SR, Bush SP, Moynihan JA, et al: Crotaline Fab antivenom for the treatment of children with rattlesnake envenomation. *Pediatrics* 2002;110: 968–971.

Chapter 150 ■ Adverse Reactions to Foods Hugh A. Sampson and Donald Y. M. Leung

Adverse reactions to foods consist of any untoward reaction following the ingestion of a food or food additive and are classically divided into **food intolerances,** which are adverse physiologic responses, and **food hypersensitivities,** which include adverse immunologic responses and allergies (Tables 150-1 and 150-2). Like other atopic disorders, food allergies have increased over the past 3 decades, primarily in "Westernized" countries, and now affect an estimated 3.5% of the U.S. population. Up to 6% of children experience food allergic reactions in the 1st 3 yr of life, including about 2.5% with cow's milk allergy, 1.5% with egg allergy, and 0.6% with peanut allergy. Most children "outgrow" milk and egg allergy, with about $^1/_2$ outgrowing their allergy within 2–3 yr. In contrast, about 80–90% of children with peanut, nut, or seafood allergy retain their allergy for life.

ETIOLOGY. Adverse reactions to foods may result from intolerances, which are based on functional properties of foods, or from physiologic host responses of the host including hypersensitivities and adverse immunologic responses (see Table 150-1). Although food represents the largest antigenic load confronting the body, the gut-associated lymphoid tissue (GALT) is able to readily discriminate between "harmless" foods and pathogenic organisms. Ingestion of food leads to **oral tolerance,** which is the induction of T-cell anergy and T regulatory cells that enable the systemic immune system to "ignore" the roughly 2% of antigenic protein normally entering the systemic circulation at each meal. In young infants, functional barriers (stomach acidity, intestinal enzymes, glycocalyx) and immunologic barriers (secretory IgA) are immature and allow increased penetration of food antigens, and the GALT appears less capable of "tolerizing" compared with the mature system. Consequently, food hypersensitivity reactions most commonly develop during this susceptible age.

TABLE 150-1. Adverse Food Reactions

FOOD INTOLERANCE

Host Factors

Enzyme deficiencies—lactase (primary or secondary), fructase (maturational delay)
Gastrointestinal disorders—inflammatory bowel disease, irritable bowel syndrome
Idiosyncratic reactions—caffeine in soft drinks ("hyperactivity")
Psychologic—food phobias
Migraines (rare)

Food Factors

Infectious organisms—*Escherichia coli, Staphylococcus aureus, Clostridium*
Toxins—histamine (scombroid poisoning), saxitoxin (shellfish)
Pharmacologic agents—caffeine, theobromine (chocolate, tea), tryptamine (tomatoes), tyramine (cheese)
Contaminants—heavy metals, pesticides, antibiotics

FOOD HYPERSENSITIVITIES

IgE-Mediated

Cutaneous—urticaria, angioedema, morbilliform rashes and flushing
Gastrointestinal—oral allergy syndrome, gastrointestinal anaphylaxis
Respiratory—acute rhinoconjunctivitis, bronchospasm (wheezing)
Generalized—anaphylactic shock

Mixed IgE and Cell Mediated

Cutaneous—atopic dermatitis
Gastrointestinal—allergic eosinophilic esophagitis and gastroenteritis
Respiratory—asthma

Cell Mediated

Cutaneous—contact dermatitis, dermatitis herpetiformis
Gastrointestinal—food protein-induced enterocolitis, proctocolitis, and enteropathy syndromes, celiac disease
Respiratory—food-induced pulmonary hemosiderosis (Heiner syndrome)

Unclassified

Cow's milk-induced anemia

TABLE 150-2. Differential Diagnosis of Adverse Food Reactions

GASTROINTESTINAL DISORDERS (WITH VOMITING AND/OR DIARRHEA)

Structural abnormalities (pyloric stenosis, Hirschsprung disease)
Enzyme deficiencies (primary or secondary)
  Disaccharidase deficiency—lactase, fructase, sucrase-isomaltase
  Galactosemia
Malignancy with obstruction
Other: pancreatic insufficiency (cystic fibrosis), peptic disease

CONTAMINANTS AND ADDITIVES

Flavorings and preservatives—rarely cause symptoms
  Sodium metabisulfite, monosodium glutamate, nitrites
Dyes and colorings—very rarely cause symptoms (urticaria, eczema)
  Tartrazine
Toxins
  Bacterial, fungal (aflatoxin), fish related (scombroid, ciguatera)
Infectious organisms
  Bacteria (*Salmonella, Escherichia coli, Shigella*)
  Virus (rotavirus, enterovirus)
  Parasites (*Giardia, Akis simplex* [in fish])
Accidental contaminants
  Heavy metals, pesticides
Pharmacologic agents
  Caffeine, glycosidal alkaloid solanine (potato spuds), histamine (fish), serotonin (banana, tomato), tryptamine (tomato), tyramine (cheese)

PSYCHOLOGIC REACTIONS

Food phobias

PATHOGENESIS. Food intolerances are the result of a variety of mechanisms, whereas food hypersensitivities are predominantly due to IgE-mediated and/or cell-mediated mechanisms. In susceptible individuals exposed to certain allergens, food-specific IgE antibodies are formed that bind to Fcε receptors on mast cells, basophils, macrophages, and dendritic cells. When food allergens penetrate mucosal barriers and reach cell-bound IgE antibodies, mediators are released that induce vasodilatation, smooth muscle contraction, and mucus secretion, which results in symptoms of immediate hypersensitivity. Activated mast cells and macrophages may release several cytokines that attract and activate other cells, such as eosinophils and lymphocytes, leading to prolonged inflammation. Symptoms elicited during acute IgE-mediated reactions can affect the **skin** (urticaria, angioedema, flushing), **gastrointestinal tract** (oral pruritus, angioedema, nausea, abdominal pain, vomiting, diarrhea), **respiratory tract** (nasal congestion, rhinorrhea, nasal pruritus, sneezing, laryngeal edema, dyspnea, wheezing), and **cardiovascular system** (dysrhythmias, hypotension, loss of consciousness). In the other major form of food hypersensitivities, lymphocytes, primarily food allergen–specific T cells, secrete excessive amounts of various cytokines that lead to a "delayed" more chronic inflammatory process affecting the **skin** (pruritus, erythematous rash), **gastrointestinal tract** (cachexia, early satiety, abdominal pain, vomiting, diarrhea), or **respiratory tract** (food-induced pulmonary hemosiderosis). Mixed IgE and cellular responses to food allergens can also lead to chronic disorders such as atopic dermatitis, asthma, and allergic eosinophilic gastroenteritis.

Children developing IgE-mediated food allergies may be sensitized by food allergens penetrating the gastrointestinal barrier, which are **class 1 food allergens,** or by partially homologous allergens such as plant pollens penetrating the respiratory tract, which are **class 2 food allergens.** Any food may serve as a class 1 food allergen but **egg, milk, peanuts, tree nuts, fish, soy, and wheat** account for 90% of food allergies during childhood. Many of the major allergenic proteins of these foods have been characterized (Table 150-3). There is variable but significant cross reactivity with other proteins within an individual food group. Exposure and sensitization to these proteins often occur very early in life, because intact food proteins are passed to the infant through maternal breast milk and, after introduction of solid foods, many parents strive to provide their infant with a highly varied diet. Virtually all milk allergy develops by 12 mo of age and all egg allergy by 18 mo of age, and the median age of 1st peanut allergic reactions is 14 mo. Class 2 food allergens are typically plant or fruit proteins that are partially homologous to pollen proteins (see Table 150-3). With the development of seasonal allergic rhinitis from birch, grass, or ragweed pollens, subsequent ingestion of certain uncooked fruits or vegetables provokes the **oral allergy syndrome.** Intermittent ingestion of allergenic foods may lead to acute symptoms, whereas prolonged exposure may lead to chronic disorders such as atopic dermatitis and asthma. Cell-mediated sensitivity typically develops to class 1 allergens.

TABLE 150-3. Major Food Allergens

CLASS 1 FOOD	PROTEIN	ALLERGEN NAME
Cow's milk	Casein	Bos d8
	β-Lactoglobulin	Bos d5
Egg	Ovomucoid	Gal d1
Peanut	Vicilin	Ara h1
	Conglutin	Ara h2
Fish	Paralbumin	Gad c1
CLASS 2 POLLEN	**PROTEIN**	**CROSS-REACTING FOOD**
Birch	Bet v1	Apple (Mal d1)
		Carrot (Dau c1)
		Potato (Sol t1)
		Cherry (Pru av1)
Ragweed		Watermelon
		Cantaloupe
		Honeydew

CLINICAL MANIFESTATIONS. From a clinical and diagnostic standpoint, it is most useful to subdivide food hypersensitivity disorders by the predominant target organ and immune mechanism (see Table 150-1).

Gastrointestinal Manifestations. Gastrointestinal food allergies are often the 1st form of allergy to affect infants and young children and typically present as irritability, vomiting or "spitting-up," diarrhea, and poor weight gain. Cell-mediated hypersensitivities predominate, making standard allergy tests such as prick skin tests and in vitro tests for food-specific IgE antibodies (RAST) of little diagnostic value.

Food protein–induced enterocolitis syndrome typically presents in the 1st several months of life with irritability and protracted vomiting and diarrhea, and may result in dehydration. Vomiting generally occurs 1–3 hr after feeding, and continued exposure may result in abdominal distention, bloody diarrhea, anemia, and failure to thrive. Symptoms are most commonly provoked by cow's milk or soy protein–based formulas but also occur from food proteins passed in maternal breast milk. A similar enterocolitis syndrome occurs in older infants and children from rice, oat, wheat, egg, peanut, nuts, chicken, turkey, or fish sensitivity. Hypotension occurs in about 15% of cases after allergen ingestion.

Food protein–induced proctocolitis presents in the 1st few months of life as blood-streaked stools in otherwise healthy infants. About 60% of cases occur among breast-fed infants, with the remainder largely among infants fed cow's milk or soy protein–based formula. Blood loss is typically modest, but can occasionally produce anemia.

Food protein–induced enteropathy often presents in the 1st several months of life with diarrhea, not infrequently steatorrhea, and poor weight gain. Symptoms include protracted diarrhea, vomiting in up to $^{2}/_{3}$ of cases, failure to thrive, abdominal distention, early satiety, and malabsorption. Anemia, edema, and hypoproteinemia occur occasionally. **Cow's milk sensitivity** is the most frequent cause of this food protein–induced enteropathy in young infants, but it also has been associated with sensitivity to soy, egg, wheat, rice, chicken, and fish in older children. **Celiac disease** is the most severe form of protein-induced enteropathy and occurs in 1 : 100–1 : 250 of the U.S. population, although it may be "silent" in many patients (see Chapter 335.2). The full-blown form is characterized by extensive loss of absorptive villi and hyperplasia of the crypts leading to malabsorption, chronic diarrhea, steatorrhea, abdominal distention, flatulence, and weight loss or failure to thrive. Oral ulcers and other extraintestinal symptoms secondary to malabsorption are not uncommon. Genetically susceptible individuals (HLA-DQ2 or DQ8) develop a cell-mediated response to tissue transglutaminase (tTGase) deamidated gliadin found in wheat, rye, and barley.

Allergic eosinophilic esophagitis may present from infancy through adolescence. In young children, it is primarily cell mediated and presents as chronic gastroesophageal reflux (GER), intermittent emesis, food refusal, abdominal pain, dysphagia, irritability, sleep disturbance, and failure to respond to conventional reflux medications. Of children <1 yr of age presenting with GER, 40% have cow's milk–induced reflux. **Allergic eosinophilic gastroenteritis** occurs at any age and presents as symptoms similar to esophagitis as well as prominent weight loss or failure to thrive, which are the hallmarks of this disorder. Up to 50% of patients are atopic, and food-induced IgE-mediated reactions have been implicated in a minority of patients. Generalized edema secondary to hypoalbuminemia may occur in some infants with marked protein-losing enteropathy.

Oral allergy syndrome is an IgE-mediated hypersensitivity that occurs in many older children with birch pollen and ragweed-induced allergic rhinitis. Symptoms are usually confined to the oropharynx and consist of the rapid onset of oral pruritus, tingling, and angioedema of the lips, tongue, palate, and throat, and, occasionally, a sensation of pruritus in the ears and tightness in the throat. Symptoms are generally short-lived and are caused by local mast cell activation by fresh fruit and vegetable proteins that cross react with birch pollen (apple, carrot, potato, celery, hazel nuts, kiwi) and ragweed pollen (banana, melons such as watermelon and cantaloupe).

Gastrointestinal anaphylaxis generally presents as acute abdominal pain and vomiting that accompany IgE-mediated allergic symptoms in other target organs.

Skin Manifestations. Cutaneous food allergies are also common in infants and young children.

Atopic dermatitis is a form of eczema that generally begins in early infancy and is characterized by pruritus, a chronically relapsing course, and association with asthma and allergic rhinitis (see Chapter 144). Although not often apparent by history, at least $^1/_3$ of children with moderate to severe atopic dermatitis have food allergies. The younger the child and the more severe the eczema, the more likely food allergy is playing a pathogenic role in the disorder.

Acute urticaria and angioedema are among the most common symptoms of food allergic reactions (see Chapter 147). The onset of symptoms may be very rapid, within minutes after ingesting the responsible allergen. Symptoms result from activation of IgE-bearing mast cells by circulating food allergens that are absorbed and circulated rapidly throughout the body. Foods most commonly incriminated in children include egg, milk, peanuts, and nuts, although reactions to various seeds (sesame, poppy) and fruits (kiwi) are becoming more common. Chronic urticaria and angioedema are rarely due to food allergies.

Respiratory Manifestations. Respiratory food allergies are uncommon as isolated symptoms. Although many parents believe that nasal congestion in infants is often caused by milk allergy, many studies show this not to be the case. **Food-induced rhinoconjunctivitis** symptoms typically accompany allergic symptoms in other target organs, such as skin, and consist of typical allergic rhinitis symptoms (periocular pruritus and tearing, nasal congestion and pruritus, sneezing, rhinorrhea). Wheezing occurs in about 25% of IgE-mediated food allergic reactions, but only about 10% of asthmatic patients have food-induced respiratory symptoms.

Food allergic reactions are the single most common cause of anaphylaxis seen in hospital emergency departments. In addition to the rapid onset of cutaneous, respiratory, and gastrointestinal symptoms, patients may develop cardiovascular symptoms, including hypotension, vascular collapse, and cardiac dysrhythmias, presumably caused by massive mast cell–mediator release. **Food-associated exercise-induced anaphylaxis** is occurring more frequently among teenage athletes, especially females (see Chapter 148).

DIAGNOSIS. A thorough medical history is necessary to differentiate whether a patient's symptomatology represents an adverse reaction (see Table 150-2), whether the adverse food reaction is an intolerance or hypersensitivity reaction, and, if the latter, whether it is likely to be an IgE-mediated or a cell-mediated response (Fig. 150-1). The following facts should be established: (1) the food suspected of provoking the reaction and the quantity ingested, (2) the time interval between ingestion and the development of symptoms, (3) the types of symptoms elicited by the ingestion, (4) whether ingesting the suspected food produced similar symptoms on other occasions, (5) whether other inciting factors, such as exercise, are necessary, and (6) the time interval from the last reaction to the food. Prick skin tests and radioallergosorbent tests are useful for demonstrating IgE sensitization. Many fruits and vegetables require testing with fresh produce because labile proteins are destroyed during commercial preparation. A negative skin test virtually excludes an IgE-mediated form of food allergy. Conversely, the majority of children with positive skin tests to a food will not react when the food is ingested, so more definitive tests, such as quantitative IgE levels or food elimination and challenge, are often necessary to establish a diagnosis of food allergy. Serum food-specific IgE levels ≥15 kU_a/L for milk (≥5 kU_a/L for children ≤1 yr), ≥7 kU_a/L for egg (≥2 kU_a/L for children <3 yr), and ≥14 kU_a/L for peanut are associated with a >95% likelihood of clinical reactivity to these foods. In the absence of a clear history of reactivity to a food and evidence of food-specific IgE antibodies, definitive studies must be performed before recommending avoidance or the use of highly restrictive diets that may be nutritionally deficient, logistically impractical, disruptive to the family, and a potential source of future feeding disorders. IgE-mediated food allergic reactions are generally very food specific, so the use of broad exclusionary diets, such as avoidance of all legumes, cereal grains, or animal products, is not warranted (Table 150-4). Unfortunately, there are no laboratory studies that help identify foods responsible for cell-mediated reactions. Consequently, **elimination diets followed by food challenges** are the only way to establish the diagnosis. Allergists experienced in dealing with food allergic reactions and able to treat anaphylaxis should perform food challenges. Before initiating a food challenge, the suspected food should be eliminated from the diet for 10–14 days for IgE-mediated food allergy and up to 8 wk for some cell-mediated disorders, such as allergic eosinophilic esophagitis. Many children with cell-mediated reactions to cow's milk will not tolerate hydrolysate formulas and must be placed on amino acid–derived products (EleCare or Neocate). If symptoms remain unchanged and appropriate elimination diets have been utilized, it is unlikely that food allergy is responsible for the child's disorder.

TREATMENT. Appropriate identification and elimination of foods responsible for food hypersensitivity reactions are the only validated treatments for food allergies. Complete elimination of common foods (milk, egg, soy, wheat, rice, chicken, fish, peanut, nuts) is very difficult because of their widespread use in a variety of processed food. The Food Allergy and Anaphylaxis Network

TABLE 150-4. Clinical Implications of Cross-Reactive Proteins in IgE-Mediated Allergy

FOOD FAMILY	RISK OF ALLERGY TO ≥1 MEMBER (APPROXIMATE)	FEATURES
Legumes	5%	Main causes of reactions are peanut, soya, lentil, lupine, and garbanzo
Tree nuts (eg, hazel, walnut, brazil)	35%	Reactions are often severe
Fish	50%	Reactions can be severe
Shellfish	75%	Reactions can be severe
Grains	20%	
Mammalian milks	90%	Cow's milk is highly cross reactive with goat's or sheep's milk (92%) but not with mare's (4%)
Rosaceae (rock) fruits	55%	Risk of reactions to more than three related foods is very low (<10%)
Latex-food	35%	For individuals allergic to latex, banana, kiwi, and avocado are the main causes of reactions

From Sicherer SH: Food allergy. *Lancet* 2002;360:701–710.

(www.foodallergy.org or 800-929-4040) provides excellent information to help parents deal with both the practical and emotional issues surrounding these diets. Children with asthma and IgE-mediated food allergy, peanut or nut allergy, or a history of a previous severe reaction should be given self-injectable epinephrine (EpiPen) and a written emergency plan in case of accidental ingestion (see Chapter 148). Since many food allergies are outgrown, arrangements should be made to have children reevaluated periodically by an allergist to determine whether they have lost their clinical reactivity. Anti-IgE immunoglobulin therapy may provide more definitive means of treating food allergies or at least raise the threshold for adverse reactions.

PREVENTION. There is no consensus as to whether food allergies can be prevented. Several authorities, however, recommend delaying introduction of major food allergens to infants from atopic families. Recommendations include promotion of breast-feeding with maternal exclusion of peanut and nut products from the

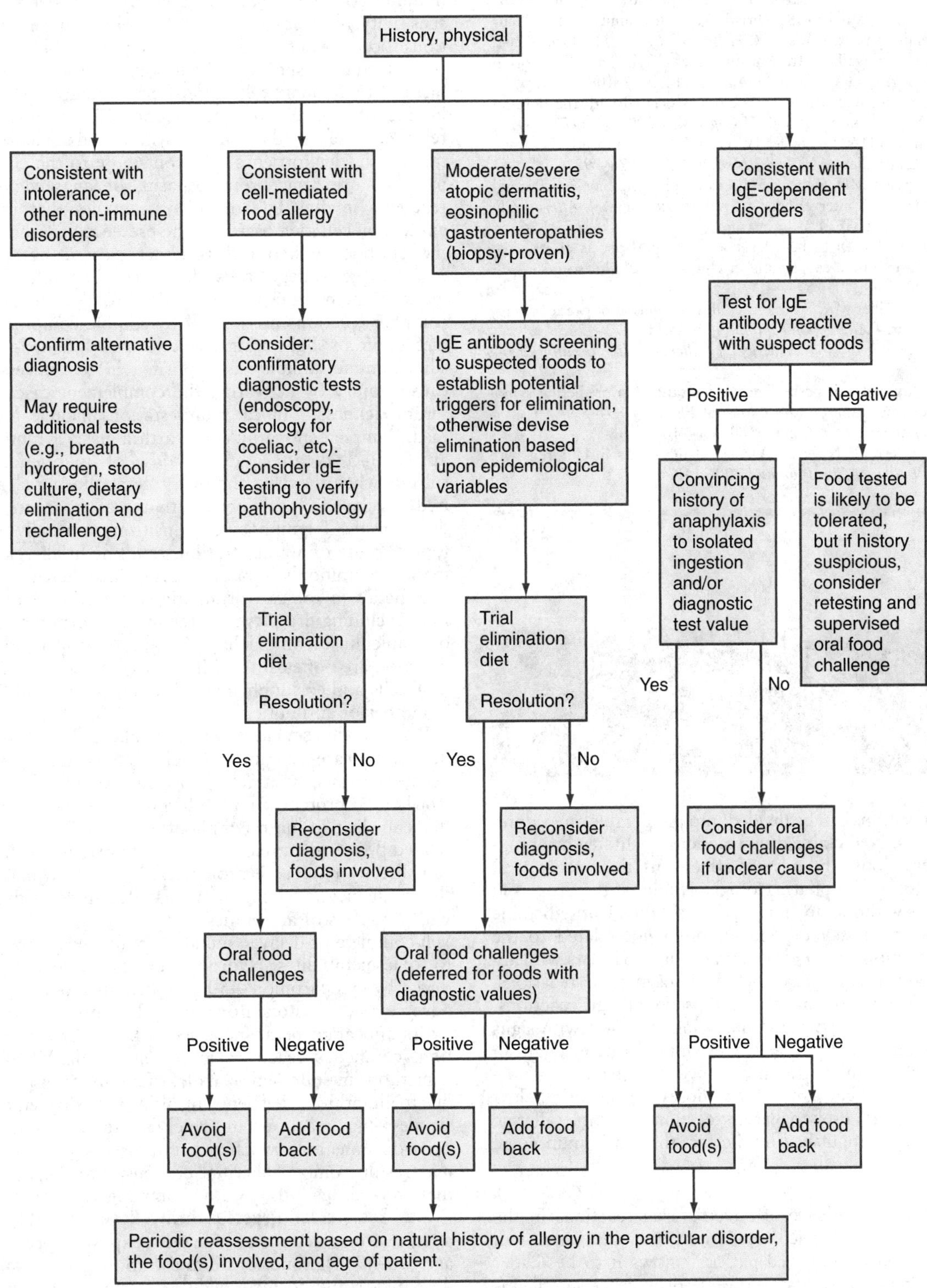

Figure 150-1. General scheme for diagnosis of food allergy. (From Sicherer SH: Food allergy. *Lancet* 2002;360:701–710.)

mother's diet and delay in introducing major allergenic foods: cow's milk until 1 yr of age; egg until 18–24 mo of age; and peanut, tree nuts, and seafood until 3 yr of age. Because some skin preparations contain peanut oil and this may sensitize young infants, especially with cutaneous inflammation, such preparation should be avoided.

American Academy of Pediatrics, Committee on Nutrition: Hypoallergenic infant formulas. *Pediatrics* 2000;106:346–349.

Bischoff SC, Crowe S: Gastrointestinal food allergy: New insights into pathophysiology and clinical perspectives. *Gastroenterol* 2005;128:1089–1113.

Fleischer DM, Conover-Walker MK, Christie L, et al: Peanut allergy: Recurrence and its management. *J Allergy Clin Immunol* 2004;114:1195–1201.

Fleischer DM, Conover-Walker MK, Matsui EC, et al: The natural history of tree nut allergy. *J Allergy Clin Immunol* 2005;116:1087–1093.

Lack G, Fox D, Northstone BA, et al: Factors associated with the development of peanut allergy in childhood. *N Eng J Med* 2003;348:977–984.

Leung DYM, Sampson HA, Yunginger JW, et al: Effect of anti-IgE therapy in patients with peanut allergy. *N Engl J Med* 2003;348:986–992.

Maloney JM, Chapman MD, Sicherer SH: Peanut allergen exposure through saliva: assessment and interventions to reduce exposure. *J Allergy Clin Immunol* 2006;118:719–724.

Markowitz JE, Spergel JM, Ruchelli E, et al: Elemental diet is an effective treatment for eosinophilic esophagitis in children and adolescents. *Am J Gastroenterol* 2003;98:777–782.

Perry TT, Conover-Walker MK, Pomes A, et al: Distribution of peanut allergy in the environment. *J Allergy Clin Immunol* 2004;113:973–976.

Sampson HA: Update of food allergy. *J Allergy Clin Immun* 2004; 113:805–819.

Sampson HA: Utility of food-specific IgE concentrations in predicting symptomatic food allergy. *J Allergy Clin Immunol* 2001;107:891–896.

Sicherer SH: Food allergy. *Lancet* 2002;360:701–710.

Yu JW, Kagan R, Verrault N, et al: Accidental ingestions in children with peanut allergy. *J Allergy Clin Immunol* 2006;118:466–472.

Chapter 151 ■ Adverse Reactions to Drugs

Mark Boguniewicz and Donald Y. M. Leung

Adverse drug reactions can be divided into predictable and unpredictable reactions. **Predictable drug reactions,** including drug toxicity, drug interactions, and adverse effects, are dose dependent, can be related to known pharmacologic actions of the drug, and occur in patients without any unique susceptibility. **Unpredictable drug reactions** are dose independent, often not related to the pharmacologic actions of the drug, and occur in patients who are genetically predisposed. These include idiosyncratic reactions, allergic (hypersensitivity) reactions, and pseudoallergic reactions. Allergic reactions require prior sensitization, manifest with signs or symptoms characteristic of an underlying allergic mechanism such as anaphylaxis or urticaria, and occur in genetically susceptible individuals. They can occur at doses significantly below the therapeutic range. **Pseudoallergic reactions** resemble allergic reactions but are distinguished by the fact that an immunologic mechanism is not involved.

EPIDEMIOLOGY. The incidence of adverse drug reactions in the general as well as pediatric populations remains unknown, although data from hospitalized patients shows it to be 6.7%, with a 0.32% incidence of fatal adverse drug reactions. Cutaneous reactions are the most common form of adverse drug reactions, with ampicillin, amoxicillin, penicillin, and trimethoprim-sulfamethoxazole being the most commonly implicated drugs. Although the majority of adverse drug reactions do not appear to be allergic in nature, 6–10% can be attributed to an allergic or immunologic mechanism.

PATHOGENESIS AND CLINICAL MANIFESTATIONS. Immunologically mediated adverse drug reactions have been classified according to the **Gell and Coombs classification:** immediate hypersensitivity reactions (type I), cytotoxic antibody reactions (type II), immune complex reactions (type III), and delayed-type hypersensitivity reactions (type IV). Immediate hypersensitivity reactions occur when a drug or drug metabolite interacts with preformed drug-specific IgE antibodies that are bound to the surfaces of tissue mast cells and/or circulating basophils. The cross linking of adjacent receptor-bound IgE by antigen causes the release of preformed and newly synthesized mediators such as histamine and leukotrienes that contribute to the clinical development of urticaria, bronchospasm, or anaphylaxis. Cytotoxic reactions involve IgG or IgM antibodies that recognize drug antigen on cell membrane. In the presence of serum complement, the antibody-coated cell is either cleared by the monocyte-macrophage system or is destroyed. Examples include drug-induced hemolytic anemia or thrombocytopenia. Immune complex reactions are caused by soluble complexes of drug or metabolite in slight antigen excess with IgG or IgM antibodies. The immune complex is deposited in blood vessel walls and causes injury by activating the complement cascade as seen in serum sickness. Clinical manifestations include fever, urticaria, rash, lymphadenopathy, and arthralgias. Symptoms typically appear 1–3 wk after the last dose of an offending drug and subside when the drug and/or its metabolite are cleared from the body. Delayed-type hypersensitivity reactions are mediated by drug-specific T lymphocytes. Sensitization usually occurs via the topical route of administration, resulting in allergic contact dermatitis. Commonly implicated drugs include neomycin and local anesthetics in topical formulations. Certain adverse drug reactions including drug fever or the morbilliform rash seen with use of ampicillin or amoxicillin in the setting of Epstein-Barr virus infection are not easily classified. Recent studies point to the role of T cells and eosinophils in delayed maculopapular reactions to a number of antibiotics.

Drug Metabolism and Adverse Reactions. Most drugs and their metabolites are not immunologically detectable until they have become covalently attached to a macromolecule. This multivalent hapten-protein complex forms a new immunogenic epitope that can elicit T- and B-lymphocyte responses. The penicillins and related β-lactam antibiotics are highly reactive with proteins and can directly haptenate protein carriers, which may account for the frequency of immune-mediated hypersensitivity reactions with this class of antibiotics.

Incomplete or delayed metabolism of some drugs can give rise to toxic metabolites. Hydroxylamine, a reactive metabolite produced by cytochrome P-450 oxidative metabolism, may mediate adverse reactions to sulfonamides. Patients who are slow acetylators appear to be at increased risk (see Chapter 56). In addition, cutaneous reactions in patients with AIDS treated with trimethoprim-sulfamethoxazole, rifampin, or other drugs may be due to glutathione deficiency resulting in toxic metabolites. Serum sickness–like reactions in which immune complexes have not been documented, which occur most commonly with cefaclor, may result from an inherited propensity for hepatic biotransformation of drugs into toxic or immunogenic metabolites.

Risk Factors for Hypersensitivity Reactions. Risk factors for adverse drug reactions include prior exposure, previous reactions, age (20–49 yr), route of administration (parenteral or topical), dose (high), and dosing schedule (intermittent), as well as genetic predisposition (slow acetylators). Atopy does not appear to predispose patients to allergic reactions to low molecular weight compounds, but atopic patients who develop an allergic reaction have a significantly increased risk of serious reaction. Atopic patients also appear to be at greater risk for pseudoallergic reactions induced by radiocontrast media. Pharmacogenomics has an important role in identifying individuals at risk for certain drug reactions (see Chapter 56).

DIAGNOSIS. An accurate medical history is an important 1st step in evaluating a patient with a possible adverse drug reaction. Suspected drugs need to be identified with dosages, route of administration, previous exposures, and dates of administration. In addition, underlying hepatic or renal disease may influence drug metabolism. A detailed description of past reactions may yield clues to the nature of the adverse drug reaction. The propensity for a particular drug to cause the suspected reaction can be checked with information in the *Physicians' Desk Reference,* the *Drug Eruption Reference Manual,* or directly from the drug manufacturer. It is important to remember, however, that the history may be unreliable and many patients are inappropriately labeled as being drug allergic. This can result in inappropriate withholding of a needed drug or class of drugs. In addition, relying solely on the history can lead to overuse of drugs reserved for special indications such as vancomycin in patients suspected of penicillin allergy. Approximately 80% of patients with a history of penicillin allergy will not have evidence of penicillin-specific IgE antibodies on testing.

Skin testing is the most rapid and sensitive method of demonstrating the presence of IgE antibodies to a specific allergen. It can be performed with high molecular weight compounds such as foreign antisera, hormones, enzymes, and toxoids. Reliable skin testing can also be performed with penicillin, but not with most other antibiotics. Most immunologically mediated adverse drug reactions are due to metabolites rather than to parent compounds, and the metabolites for most drugs other than penicillin have not been defined. In addition, many metabolites are unstable or must combine with larger proteins to be useful for diagnosis. Testing with nonstandardized reagents requires caution in interpretation of both positive and negative results because some drugs can induce nonspecific irritant reactions. Whereas a wheal-and-flare reaction is suggestive of drug-specific IgE antibodies, a negative skin test does not exclude the presence of such antibodies because the relevant immunogen may not have been used as the testing reagent.

A positive skin test to the major or minor determinants of penicillin has a 60% positive predictive value for an immediate hypersensitivity reaction to penicillin. If skin tests to the major and minor determinants of penicillin are negative, 97–99% of patients (depending on the reagents used) tolerate the drug without an immediate reaction. The positive and negative predictive values of skin testing to antibiotics other than penicillin are not well established. Nevertheless, positive immediate hypersensitivity skin tests to nonirritant concentrations of nonpenicillin antibiotics may be interpreted as a presumptive risk of an immediate reaction to such agents.

Direct and indirect Coombs tests are often positive in drug-induced hemolytic anemia. Assays for specific IgG and IgM have been shown to correlate with a drug reaction in immune cytopenia, but, in most other reactions, such assays are not diagnostic. In general, many more patients express humoral or T-cell immune responses to drug determinants than express clinical disease. Serum tryptase is elevated with systemic mast cell degranulation and can be seen with drug associated mast cell activation, although it is not pathognomonic for drug hypersensitivity and nonelevated tryptase levels can be seen in well-defined anaphylaxis.

TREATMENT. Specific **desensitization,** which involves the progressive administration of an allergen to render effector cells less reactive, is reserved for patients with IgE antibodies to a particular drug for whom an alternative drug is not available or appropriate. Specific protocols for many different drugs have been developed. Desensitization should be performed in a hospital setting, usually in consultation with an allergist with resuscitation equipment available at all times. While mild complications, such as pruritus or rash, are fairly common and often respond to adjustments in the drug dose or dosing intervals and medications to relieve symptoms, more severe systemic reactions can occur. Oral desensitization may be less likely to induce anaphylaxis than parenteral administration. Pretreatment with antihistamines or corticosteroids is not usually recommended.

Graded challenges based on the administration of a drug in an incremental fashion until a therapeutic dose is achieved can be attempted with drugs causing non–IgE-mediated reactions, including trimethoprim-sulfamethoxazole. Graded challenges in aspirin- or nonsteroidal anti-inflammatory drug (NSAID)–intolerant patients, particularly those with respiratory reactions, can also be performed. Gradual introduction of a drug may reveal systemic intolerance early enough to prevent progression to a serious or even life-threatening reaction such as Stevens-Johnson syndrome or toxic epidermal necrolysis.

β-Lactam Hypersensitivity. Penicillin is a frequent cause of anaphylaxis and is responsible for the majority of all drug-mediated anaphylactic deaths in the United States. Although IgE-mediated reactions may occur after administration of penicillin by any route, parenteral administration is more likely to cause anaphylaxis. If a patient requires penicillin and has a past history suggestive of penicillin allergy, it is necessary to skin test the patient for the presence of penicillin-specific IgE with both the major and minor determinants of penicillin. Skin tests to both major and minor determinants of penicillin are necessary because about 20% of patients with documented anaphylaxis do not demonstrate skin reactivity to the major determinant. While the major determinant is available commercially (PrePen), minor determinant mixtures are currently not licensed and are synthesized at select centers. Although penicillin G is often used as a substitute for minor determinant mixture, there is a small but significant risk of false-negative skin test results with this approach. Thus, patients should be referred to an allergist capable of performing appropriate testing. If the skin test is positive to either major or minor determinants of penicillin, the patient should receive an alternative non–cross-reacting antibiotic. If administration of penicillin is deemed necessary, desensitization by an allergist in an appropriate medical setting can be performed. Skin testing for penicillin-specific IgE is not predictive for delayed onset cutaneous, bullous, or immune complex reactions. In addition, penicillin skin testing does not appear to resensitize the patient.

Other β-lactam antibiotics, including semisynthetic penicillins, cephalosporins, carbacephems, and carbapenems, share the β-lactam ring structure. Patients with late-onset morbilliform rashes with amoxicillin are not considered to be at risk for IgE-mediated reactions to penicillin and do not require skin testing before penicillin administration. Patients with Epstein-Barr virus infections treated with ampicillin or amoxicillin can develop a nonpruritic rash in up to 100% of cases. Similar reactions occur in patients with elevated uric acid treated with allopurinol or with chronic lymphocytic leukemia. If the rash to ampicillin or amoxicillin is urticarial or systemic, or the history is unclear, the patient should undergo penicillin skin testing if a penicillin is needed. There have been reports of antibodies specific for semisynthetic penicillin side chains in the absence of β-lactam ring-specific antibodies, although the clinical significance of such side chain–specific antibodies is unclear.

Varying degrees of in vitro cross reactivity have been documented between cephalosporins and penicillins. Although the risk of allergic reactions to cephalosporins in patients with positive skin tests to penicillin appears to be low (<2%), anaphylactic reactions have occurred after administration of cephalosporins in patients with a positive history of penicillin anaphylaxis. If a patient has a history of penicillin allergy and requires a cephalosporin, skin testing to major and minor determinants of penicillin should preferably be performed to determine if the patient has penicillin-specific IgE antibodies. If skin tests are negative, the patient can receive a cephalosporin with no greater risk than found in the general population. If skin tests are positive to penicillin, recommendations may include: administration of an alternative antibiotic; cautious graded challenge with appropriate monitoring, recognizing that there may be a 2% chance of inducing an anaphylactic reaction; or desensitization to the required cephalosporin.

Conversely, patients who require penicillin and have a history of an IgE-mediated reaction to a cephalosporin should also undergo penicillin skin testing. Patients with a negative test can receive penicillin. Patients with a positive test should either receive an alternative medication or undergo desensitization to penicillin. In patients with a history of allergic reaction to one cephalosporin requiring another cephalosporin, skin testing with the required cephalosporin can be performed, recognizing that the negative predictive value is unknown. If the skin test to the cephalosporin is positive, the significance of the test should be checked further in control subjects to determine if the positive response is IgE mediated or an irritant response. The drug can then be administered by graded challenge or desensitization.

Carbapenems (imipenem, meropenem) represent another class of β-lactam antibiotics with a bicyclic nucleus that demonstrate a high degree of cross reactivity with penicillins. In contrast to β-lactam antibiotics, monobactams (aztreonam) have a monocyclic ring structure. Aztreonam-specific antibodies have been shown to be predominantly side-chain specific; data suggest that aztreonam can be safely administered to most penicillin-allergic subjects.

Sulfonamides. The most common type of reaction to sulfonamides is a maculopapular eruption often associated with fever that occurs after 7–12 days of therapy. Immediate reactions including anaphylaxis as well as other immunologic reactions have also been suggested. For those individuals who develop maculopapular rashes after sulfonamide administration, both graded challenge and desensitization protocols have been shown to be effective. These regimens should not be used in individuals with a history of Stevens-Johnson syndrome or toxic epidermal necrolysis. Hypersensitivity reactions to sulfasalazine, for treatment of inflammatory bowel disease, appear to result from the sulfapyridine moiety. Slow desensitization over ≈1 mo permits tolerance of the drug in many patients. In addition, oral and enema forms of 5-ASA, thought to be the pharmacologically active agent in sulfasalazine, are effective alternative therapies.

Stevens-Johnson Syndrome and Toxic Epidermal Necrolysis. Blistering mucocutaneous disorders induced by drugs encompass a spectrum of reactions, including Stevens-Johnson syndrome and toxic epidermal necrolysis (see Chapter 653). Epidermal detachment of less than 10% is suggestive of Stevens-Johnson syndrome, detachment of 30% suggests toxic epidermal necrolysis, and 10–30% detachment suggests overlap of the two syndromes. The features of Stevens-Johnson syndrome include confluent purpuric macules on face and trunk and severe, explosive mucosal erosions, usually at more than one mucosal surface, accompanied by fever and constitutional symptoms. Ocular involvement may be particularly severe, and the liver, kidneys, and lungs may also be involved. Toxic epidermal necrolysis, which appears to be related to keratinocyte apoptosis, manifests with widespread areas of confluent erythema followed by epidermal necrosis and detachment with severe mucosal involvement. The risk of infection and mortality are high. Skin biopsy differentiates subepidermal cleavage characteristic of toxic epidermal necrolysis from intraepidermal cleavage characteristic of the scalded skin syndrome induced by staphylococcal toxins. The effectiveness of corticosteroids in the treatment of Stevens-Johnson syndrome is controversial, but, if used, they should be started as early in the course of the disease as possible. Toxic epidermal necrolysis must be treated in a burn unit. Corticosteroids are contraindicated because they can significantly increase the risk of infection. High intravenous doses of immunoglobulin have been shown to be beneficial in patients with toxic epidermal necrolysis likely due to inhibition of Fas-mediated keratinocyte cell death by naturally occurring Fas-blocking antibodies in the intravenous immunoglobulin preparation.

Perioperative Agents. Anaphylactoid reactions occurring during general anesthesia may be caused by induction agents (thiopental) or muscle-relaxing agents (succinylcholine, pancuronium). Quaternary ammonium muscle relaxants (succinylcholine) can act as bivalent antigens in IgE-mediated reactions. Negative skin tests do not necessarily predict that a drug will be tolerated. Latex allergy should always be considered in the differential diagnosis of a perioperative reaction.

Local Anesthetics. Adverse drug reactions associated with local anesthetic agents are primarily toxic reactions resulting from rapid drug absorption, inadvertent intravenous injection, or overdosage. Local anesthetics are classified as esters of benzoic acid (group I) or amides (group II). Group I includes benzocaine and procaine; group II includes lidocaine, bupivacaine, and mepivacaine. In suspected local anesthetic allergy, skin testing followed by a graded challenge can be performed or an anesthetic agent from a different group can be used.

Insulin. Insulin use has been associated with a spectrum of adverse drug reactions, including local and systemic IgE-mediated reactions, hemolytic anemia, serum sickness reactions, and delayed-type hypersensitivity. In general, human insulin is less allergenic than porcine insulin, which is less allergenic than bovine insulin, but for individual patients, porcine or bovine insulin may be the least allergenic. Patients treated with nonhuman insulin have had systemic reactions to recombinant human insulin even on the 1st exposure. More than 50% of patients who receive insulin develop antibodies against the insulin preparation, although there may not be any clinical manifestations. Local cutaneous reactions usually do not require treatment and resolve with continued insulin administration, possibly owing to IgG-blocking antibodies. More severe local reactions can be treated with antihistamines or by splitting the insulin dose between separate administration sites. Local reactions to the protamine component of neutral protamine Hagedorn (NPH) insulin may be avoided by switching to Lente insulin. Immediate-type reactions to insulin, including urticaria and anaphylactic shock, are unusual and almost always occur after reinstitution of insulin therapy in sensitized patients. Insulin therapy should not be interrupted if a systemic reaction to insulin occurs and continued insulin therapy is essential. Skin testing may identify a less antigenic insulin preparation. The dose following a systemic reaction is usually reduced to one third and successive doses are increased in 2–5 unit increments until the dose resulting in glucose control is attained. Insulin skin testing and desensitization are required if insulin treatment is subsequently interrupted for more than 24–48 hr. Immunologic resistance usually occurs when a patient develops high titers of predominantly IgG antibodies to insulin. A rare form of insulin resistance caused by circulating antibodies to tissue insulin receptors is associated with acanthosis nigricans and lipodystrophy. Coexisting insulin allergy may be present in up to one third of patients with insulin resistance. Approximately half of affected patients benefit from substitution with a less reactive insulin preparation, based on skin testing.

Anticonvulsant Hypersensitivity Syndrome. Anticonvulsant hypersensitivity syndrome (pseudolymphoma) is a potentially life-threatening syndrome that occurs with exposure of variable lengths to anticonvulsant medications. It appears to result from an inherited deficiency of epoxide hydrolase, an enzyme required for the metabolism of arene oxide intermediates produced during hepatic metabolism of anticonvulsant drugs. It is characterized by fever, maculopapular rash, and generalized lymphadenopathy along with visceral organ involvement that resolves with discontinuation of the anticonvulsant. Drug-induced hypersensitivity syndrome has also been described with minocycline, sulfonamides, and dapsone.

Red Man Syndrome. This syndrome is caused by nonspecific histamine release and is most commonly described with administration of intravenous vancomycin. It can be prevented by slowing the vancomycin infusion rate or by preadministration of H_1-blockers.

Radiocontrast Media. Anaphylactoid reactions to radiocontrast media or dye can occur after intravascular administration and during myelograms or retrograde pyelograms. No single pathogenic mechanism has been defined, but it is likely that mast cell activation accounts for the majority of these reactions. Complement activation has also been described. There is no evidence that sensitivity to seafood or iodine predisposes to radiocontrast media reactions. Predictive tests are not available. Patients with atopic profiles, using β-blockers, and with prior anaphylactoid reactions are at increased risk. Other diagnostic alternatives should be considered or patients can be given low osmolality radiocontrast media with a pretreatment regimen including oral prednisone, diphenhydramine, and albuterol, with or without cimetidine or ranitidine.

Narcotic Analgesics. Opiates such as morphine and related narcotics can induce direct mast cell degranulation. Patients may develop generalized pruritus, urticaria, and, occasionally, wheezing. If there is a suggestive history and analgesia is required, a non-narcotic medication should be considered. If this does not control pain, graded challenge with an alternative opiate is an option.

Aspirin and NSAIDs. Aspirin and NSAIDs can cause anaphylactoid reactions or urticaria and/or angioedema in children and, rarely, asthma with or without rhinoconjunctivitis in adolescents. There is no skin or in vitro test to identify patients who may react to aspirin or other NSAIDs. Once aspirin or NSAID intolerance has been established, options include avoidance or pharmacologic desensitization and subsequent continued treatment with aspirin or NSAIDs if indicated. Preliminary studies suggest that cyclooxygenase-2 inhibitors are tolerated by patients with aspirin-induced asthma.

Bernstein IL, Gruchalla RS, Lee RE, et al (eds): Disease management of drug hypersensitivity: A practice parameter. *Ann Allergy Asthma Immunol* 1999;83:678–679.

Campione E, Marulli GC, Carrozzo AM, et al: High-dose intravenous immunoglobulin for severe drug reactions: Efficacy in toxic epidermal necrolysis. *Acta Derm Venereol* 2003;83:430–432.

Carroll MC, Yueng-Yue KA, Esterly NB, et al: Drug-induced hypersensitivity syndrome in pediatric patients. *Pediatrics* 2001;108:485–492.

Gruchalla RS: Drug allergy. *J Allergy Clin Immunol* 2003;111:S548–S559.

Gruchalla RS, Pirmohamed M: Antibiotic allergy. *N Engl J Med* 2006;354: 601–608.

Kelkar PS, Li JT: Cephalosporin allergy. *N Engl J Med* 2001;345:804–809.

Macy E, Mangat R, Burchette RJ: Penicillin skin testing in advance of need: Multiyear follow-up in 568 test result-negative subjects exposed to oral penicillins. *J Allergy Clin Immunol* 2003;111:1111–1115.

Sampson HA, Munoz-Furlong A, Bock SA, et al: Symposium on the definition and management of anaphylaxis: Summary report. *J Allergy Clin Immunol* 2005;115:584–591.

Yawalkar N, Shrikhande M, Hari Y, et al: Evidence for a role for IL-5 and eotaxin in activating and recruiting eosinophils in drug-induced cutaneous eruptions. *J Allergy Clin Immunol* 2000;106:1171–1176.

Part XV ■ Rheumatic Diseases of Childhood (Connective Tissue Diseases, Collagen Vascular Diseases)

Chapter 152 ■ Evaluation of Suspected Rheumatic Disease

Michael L. Miller

Rheumatic diseases result from autoimmune processes that lead to inflammation of target organs. Because many different organs may be affected, rheumatic diseases must be considered for a wide range of presenting complaints. Rarely, children develop **overlap syndromes** with manifestations fulfilling criteria for more than one rheumatic disease. **Mixed connective tissue disease** is sometimes used to describe an overlap syndrome, especially among adult females, characterized by fever, Raynaud phenomenon, skin rash, arthritis, and myositis. Children may also have **undifferentiated connective tissue disease** in which manifestations strongly suggest but do not meet diagnostic criteria for a specific rheumatic disease.

Because specific diagnostic tests are not available, it is essential to exclude nonrheumatic diseases causing similar symptoms. After careful evaluation has excluded nonrheumatic causes, treatment for the suspected rheumatic disease may be considered depending on the risks of morbidity from not providing treatment. Once malignant and infectious etiologies have been excluded, a child with pleuropericarditis and Coombs-positive anemia but negative antinuclear antibodies (ANAs) may be a candidate for presumptive corticosteroid treatment.

Early diagnosis of rheumatic disease may not always be possible because specific diagnostic manifestations may take months or, rarely, even years to develop after the initial presentation. Interval repeated clinical evaluations and review of the differential diagnosis is necessary in these circumstances. A child meeting diagnostic criteria for juvenile rheumatoid arthritis (JRA) may, after several years, develop anemia, diarrhea, and small bowel biopsy findings more consistent with inflammatory bowel disease. Some patients with JRA, particularly those presenting with high titers of ANA, may develop systemic lupus erythematosus (SLE) years after initial presentation. A child presenting with polyarticular arthritis who later develops weakness disproportionate to synovitis may have an inflammatory myositis, such as juvenile dermatomyositis.

ETIOLOGY AND PATHOGENESIS. Rheumatic diseases are characterized by **autoimmune responses.** The immune system normally responds to viruses, bacteria, and other non-self molecules but does not mount reactions to self molecules. This property of **tolerance** to self is lost in rheumatic diseases. Two possible explanations, which are not mutually exclusive, for self-reactivity are (1) similarity between foreign and self molecules that are recognized by immune cells, particularly T lymphocytes, and (2) viral or other infections that incite, exaggerate, or prolong otherwise self-limited immune responses. Certain genetic factors, such as specific HLA alleles, may influence susceptibility to developing disease, whereas other factors, such as those that influence levels of baseline immune activities, may affect disease severity.

Many rheumatic diseases are characterized by a series of abnormal cellular and molecular events. T lymphocytes recognize viruses and other foreign antigens that rest in the groove of the HLA molecule on the surfaces of antigen-presenting cells. Molecular signals are released that activate other cells such as macrophages, which produce inflammatory cytokines including tumor necrosis factor-α (TNF-α), interleukin 1 (IL-1), and IL-6. These cytokines cause tissue damage through direct effects and by attracting additional inflammatory cells to the affected site. Further tissue damage is sometimes mediated by B lymphocytes that are activated by helper T cells to produce excessive antibody, including autoantibodies that bind to self antigens. Normal cells in target organs can be destroyed also by complement-mediated cytolysis, direct or indirect effects of TNF-α, or effects of natural killer or cytolytic T lymphocytes.

The autoimmune response may affect the function of many organs. For example, IL-6 and other cytokines bind to neuronal receptors in the central nervous system, causing fever, and can also interfere with osteoblastic activity, resulting in osteopenia. Molecules produced outside the immune system may, in turn, have an effect on immune responses. During a normal immune response, cytokines appear to induce neuroendocrine pathways to produce cortisol, which suppresses cellular and humoral immunity. It is possible that defects in these pathways amplify autoimmune responses. The increased incidence of some rheumatic diseases in females may be attributable to the property of female sex hormones to augment cellular immune responses.

CLINICAL MANIFESTATIONS. A complete history is important to help distinguish rheumatic conditions from other diseases. Parents of children with school phobias are often anxious about the return of their children to school. In contrast, parents of children with rheumatic diseases are typically more upset with school absences.

Certain classic symptoms and signs, although not specific, strongly suggest rheumatic or other diseases (Table 152-1). Morning stiffness may be reported by children with JRA or postinfectious reactive arthritis. Facial rashes in children with joint complaints or weakness suggest lupus or dermatomyositis. Raynaud phenomenon may be a primary disorder, or it can be a presenting complaint of children with scleroderma, lupus, and overlapping rheumatic syndromes. Weakness can result from muscular dystrophies, viral myositis, and inflammatory myopathies, of which juvenile dermatomyositis is the most common. Monoarticular arthritis near the site of trauma may

TABLE 152-1. Symptoms Suggestive of Rheumatic Diseases

SYMPTOM	RHEUMATIC DISEASES	SOME POSSIBLE NONRHEUMATIC DISEASES CAUSING SIMILAR SYMPTOMS
Fevers	Systemic juvenile rheumatoid arthritis	Malignancies, infections, inflammatory bowel disease, periodic fever syndromes
Arthralgia	Juvenile rheumatoid arthritis, systemic lupus erythematosus, rheumatic fever, juvenile dermatomyositis, scleroderma	Hypothyroidism, trauma, reactive arthritis, endocarditis, other infections
Weakness	Juvenile dermatomyositis	Muscular dystrophies, other myopathies
Malar rash	Systemic lupus erythematosus	Photosensitivity dermatitis, Fifth disease
Chest pain	Juvenile rheumatoid arthritis, systemic lupus erythematosus (with associated pericarditis or costochondritis)	Costochondritis (isolated), rib fracture, viral pericarditis
Back pain	Juvenile rheumatoid arthritis, spondyloarthropathy	Vertebral microfracture, diskitis, intraspinal tumor, spondylolysis, spondylolisthesis

suggest nonrheumatic disease, such as hemarthrosis, a torn meniscus, or osteochondritis. Abnormal gait is associated with many orthopedic problems, such as Legg-Calvé-Perthes disease, as well as JRA. The inability to walk raises the need for immediate attention to exclude conditions such as neuropathy, osteomyelitis, or malignancy. Foreign travel, enteric illness in the family, or exposure to reptile pets may lead to reactive arthritis after an enteric infection. Tick exposure raises the possibility of Lyme arthritis.

Fevers are commonly seen in children with rheumatic diseases, and high, spiking fevers returning to or below baseline are typical of systemic JRA. Fever is not specific for rheumatic diseases, and evaluation for infections or malignancies is necessary. If fevers persist despite an unremarkable evaluation, the autoinflammatory periodic fever syndromes should be considered. **Periodic fever syndromes** have distinct characteristics that are not typical for autoimmune rheumatic diseases (see Chapter 162). These autoinflammatory syndromes are often associated with single gene mutations coding for molecules produced by more primitive immune cells (macrophages) that ordinarily regulate inflammation. Rheumatic diseases are often associated with certain multiple HLA and other genetic alleles resulting in autoimmune activity by T and B lymphocytes.

PHYSICAL EXAMINATION. The physical examination helps identify the organs involved. Because rheumatic diseases may take time to evolve, repeated examinations are important to detect new manifestations. The general appearance may suggest certain diagnoses. A depressed or anxious affect may suggest psychiatric disease. Lack of normal movement on the examination table may be a result of muscle weakness, arthritis, central nervous system disease, or skeletal abnormality. Weight loss or decreased growth velocity may reflect malnutrition from inflammatory bowel disease.

Apparently isolated findings may be important clues to target organ involvement in rheumatic diseases. A pericardial friction rub with orthopnea may occur with pericarditis from lupus or systemic JRA. Persisting oral mucosal lesions are found in lupus and Behçet disease (see Chapter 312). Other mucous membrane involvement, such as swollen tongue or lips, raises the possibility of Kawasaki disease, Stevens-Johnson syndrome, and scarlet fever. Conjunctival injection could be episcleritis of lupus, conjunctival inflammation of Kawasaki disease, or uveitis. Uveitis in children with JRA is an indication for slit-lamp examination. Although persistent joint complaints suggest JRA, other rheumatic diseases, including lupus and dermatomyositis, can also present with arthritis. All children with joint symptoms should be asked about muscle weakness, which is characteristic of dermatomyositis and mixed connective tissue disease.

The joint examination can detect arthritis, which can be infectious, rheumatic, or secondary to trauma. **Arthritis** is evident by either joint swelling or the combination of pain and limited motion. **Arthralgia,** or pain in a joint with full range of motion, is seen in trauma, psychogenic arthralgia, immune complex diseases, or early rheumatic disease that cannot yet be specifically diagnosed. The neurologic examination can identify focal deficits resulting from intracranial or intraspinal lesions as well as muscle weakness. Pain to palpation along the long bones or ribs is not typical for rheumatic diseases, but raises the possibility of leukemia or neuroblastoma.

Growing pains are common in children between 4 and 8 yr of age, are usually bilateral over the anterior thigh or calf or behind the knee, and are intermittent. Children with growing pains have a normal physical examination and normal laboratory tests.

Erythema nodosum, a rash characterized by pretibial tender erythematous nodules found in the deep dermis and subcutaneous tissue (Fig. 152-1), is a hypersensitivity reaction resulting from certain infections, inflammatory diseases, or drugs (see Chapter 659). The finding of erythema nodosum should lead to consideration of possible underlying causes. Common infectious triggers include group A streptococcus pharyngitis, tuberculosis, *Yersinia,* histoplasmosis, and coccidioidomycosis. Erythema nodosum is sometimes the first manifestation of inflammatory bowel disease, sarcoidosis, and spondyloarthropathy. It may also develop after exposure to sulfonamides, phenytoin, or oral contraceptive agents. Lesions evolve from erythematous to bluish, may sometimes be flat, and, in severe cases, may be found along the entire length of the legs and rarely involve the feet or arms. New crops of nodules may develop over several weeks. Erythema nodosum is sometimes accompanied by fever, and must be distinguished from cellulitis, insect bites, thrombophlebitis, and fungal skin

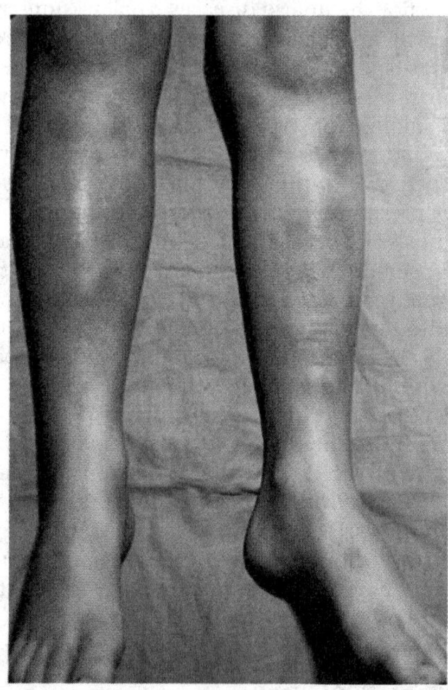

Figure 152-1. The erythematous nodules and plaques of erythema nodosum are present over both shins. The skin overlying the lesions is red, smooth, and shiny. The nodules are usually tender. Erythema nodosum is considered a hypersensitivity reaction and is associated with a variety of diseases including sarcoidosis, ulcerative colitis, and infections including group A streptococcus, tuberculosis, and coccidioidomycosis. (Reprinted from the Clinical Slide Collection on the Rheumatic Diseases; copyright 1991, 1995, 1997. Used by permission of the American College of Rheumatology.)

TABLE 152-2. Specific Antinuclear Antibodies and Associated Diseases

ANTIGEN	DISEASE
Histone	Drug-induced lupus
Ribonucleoprotein	Mixed connective tissue disease
Pm-Sc1	Sclerodermatomyositis
Sc1	Scleroderma
Sm	Systemic lupus erythematosus
Ro/SSA	Sjögren syndrome, congenital heart block, annular erythema
La/SSB	Sjögren syndrome

The antinuclear antibody (ANA) test is a screening test and does not determine against which of various known and unknown nuclear antigens the antinuclear antibody is directed. Nonspecific elevated ANA may be detected in healthy children, usually at low titer, and in persons with various rheumatic and nonrheumatic diseases. These specific ANA patterns are characteristically associated with the corresponding diseases and are sometimes found also in patients without suggestive or diagnostic clinical manifestations.

infections. It resolves with effective treatment of the underlying etiology. Supportive treatment for severe pain includes bed rest, elevation of the legs, and analgesics.

LABORATORY FINDINGS. The erythrocyte sedimentation rate (ESR) and C reactive protein are useful to screen for infectious and rheumatic diseases. A normal ESR value does not exclude rheumatic disease. Infections typically lead to transiently increased ESR. High values persisting for more than several weeks may necessitate further evaluation, depending on the associated symptoms, physical findings, and other laboratory abnormalities.

The ANA test is a screening test for specific antibodies against nuclear constituents, some of which have been characterized (Table 152-2). A positive titer (≥1 : 80) is a nonspecific reflection of increased lymphocyte activity. Positive ANA tests are found in children with rheumatic diseases and other diseases such as idiopathic thrombocytopenic purpura, Crohn disease, chronic autoimmune hepatitis, Graves disease, and, rarely, leukemia or lymphoma. Children with a positive ANA who have nonrheumatic diseases may sometimes develop lupus or overlapping rheumatic syndromes. In such cases, other laboratory findings typically appear (antibodies to DNA in lupus patients). Some drugs, such as anticonvulsant medications (phenytoin, ethosuximide) and antiarrhythmic agents (procainamide) can cause a positive ANA as well as overt lupus. Malaria and some parasitic infections can also cause a positive ANA.

Some children with a positive ANA and no persistent symptoms have normal physical examinations and lack other remarkable laboratory findings. Such children rarely develop a defined rheumatic disease. Others with a positive ANA have arthralgia related to hyperextensible joints; the reason for the association is unknown. These children need to be distinguished from those who develop JRA or other rheumatic disease, which is best detected by periodic re-evaluation to detect changes in physical findings or laboratory abnormalities (anemia, thrombocytopenia, nephritis).

Other immunologic laboratory tests, although not diagnostic of rheumatic disease, are useful in characterizing the extent of immune activation and monitoring response to therapy. Levels of total hemolytic complement (CH_{50}), C3, and C4 are characteristically decreased in active lupus and vasculitis syndromes. Immune activation may be reflected by elevated levels of immune complexes, serum immunoglobulins, neopterin (a macrophage product), and von Willebrand factor antigen (a molecule found on the surface of vascular endothelium).

Other laboratory results may suggest a nonrheumatic diagnosis. Thrombocytopenia, neutropenia, and anemia in a child with limb pain suggest acute lymphocytic leukemia or marrow involvement in neuroblastoma. Lactate dehydrogenase levels may be elevated in rheumatic diseases as a result of cell turnover, and marked elevations raise the possibility of malignancy. Thyroid function studies can exclude hypothyroidism, which may cause musculoskeletal symptoms. Decreased albumin and serum protein may be seen in nephrosis or inflammatory bowel disease.

Imaging studies also contribute to the evaluation. Bone scans or MRI can detect early osteomyelitis or malignancy. MRI studies with gadolinium for joint evaluation and T2 weighted fat suppression for muscle evaluation can reveal abnormalities of JRA, dermatomyositis, and sarcoidosis, and can exclude nonrheumatic abnormalities. Echocardiography can distinguish patients with rheumatic carditis from those with Kawasaki disease or pericarditis resulting from systemic lupus erythematosus or systemic JRA.

Azouz EM, Babyn PS, Mascia AT, et al: MRI of the abnormal pediatric hand and wrist with plain film correlation. *J Comput Assist Tomogr* 1998;22:252–261.

Cabral DA, Tucker LB: Malignancies in children who initially present with rheumatic complaints. *J Pediatr* 1999;134:53–57.

Citera G, Espada G, Maldonado Cocco JA: Sequential development of 2 connective tissue diseases in juvenile patients. *J Rheumatol* 1993;20: 2149–2152.

Deane PM, Liard G, Siegel DM, et al: The outcome of children referred to a pediatric rheumatology clinic with a positive antinuclear antibody test but without an autoimmune disease. *Pediatrics* 1995;95:892–895.

Feldman DS, Hedden DM, Wright JG: The use of bone scan to investigate back pain in children and adolescents. *J Pediatr Orthop* 2000;20:790–795.

Malleson PN, Sailer M, Mackinnon MJ: Usefulness of antinuclear antibody testing to screen for rheumatic diseases. *Arch Dis Child* 1997;77:299–304.

Passo MH, Fitzgerald JF, Brandt KD: Arthritis associated with inflammatory bowel disease in children. Relationship of joint disease to activity and severity of bowel lesion. *Dig Dis Sci* 1986;31:492–497.

Ramsey SE, Cairns RA, Cabral DA, et al: Knee magnetic resonance imaging in childhood chronic monarthritis. *J Rheumatol* 1999;26:2238–2243.

Wallendal M, Stork L, Hollister JR: The discriminating value of serum lactate dehydrogenase levels in children with malignant neoplasms presenting as joint pain. *Arch Pediatr Adolesc Med* 1996;150:70–73.

Zimmerman SA, Ware RE: Clinical significance of the antinuclear antibody test in selected children with idiopathic thrombocytopenic purpura. *J Pediatr Hematol Oncol* 1997;19:297–303.

Chapter 153 ■ Treatment of Rheumatic Diseases

Daniel J. Lovell, Michael L. Miller, and James T. Cassidy

Treatment of children with rheumatic diseases is complex and challenging. The efforts of a team of health care professionals need to be melded into a coordinated system of management that is individualized to meet the needs of each patient and is sensitive to the capabilities and psychosocial resources of the family. Disease manifestations for each child during the course of the disease can vary in severity over time; treatment must be adjusted accordingly. The therapeutic program must provide appropriate therapy for current symptomatic problems, such as arthritis, as well as include appropriate screening methods for often clinically silent complications such as uveitis in children with juvenile rheumatoid arthritis (JRA) and early nephritis in patients with systemic lupus erythematosus (SLE).

Rheumatic disease in a child affects the entire family; management should not be restricted to the affected child. Siblings of a child with a rheumatic disease are often psychosocially affected. Family dynamics have a significant impact on treatment and outcome. The emotional status of the parents at the time of diag-

TABLE 153-1. Multidisciplinary Team for Care of Children with Rheumatic Diseases

CORE TEAM	CONSULTANT TEAM
Parents and child	Orthopedic surgeon
Pediatric rheumatologist	Psychologist/psychiatrist
Pediatrician	Dentist
Nurse	School nurse
Social worker	
Physical therapist	
Occupational therapist	
Nutritionist	
Ophthalmologist	

nosis of their child is one of the strongest predictors of outcome 5–10 yr later. In the context of a complex and ever-changing therapeutic milieu, current approaches to management supervised by a multidisciplinary team (Table 153-1) experienced in the care of children with rheumatic diseases usually result in good clinical outcomes.

Childhood rheumatic diseases are neither benign nor short-lived in the majority of patients. Optimal treatment in this highly specialized area requires the coordinated efforts over months, if not years. The therapeutic program includes physical and psychosocial interventions as well as medications, and requires tailoring to the needs and severity of each particular child's illness that will vary over time. Current therapies are not regarded as curative in most cases, as evidenced by the chronicity of these diseases.

PEDIATRIC RHEUMATOLOGY TEAMS AND PRIMARY CARE PHYSICIANS. The goals for treatment are to maximize the daily functional activities of affected children, relieve discomfort, prevent or reduce organ damage, and avoid or minimize drug toxicity. Nondrug therapy also assumes a large role in the treatment of rheumatic diseases. The responsibility of the physician includes, in addition to prescribing and monitoring medications, coordinating the efforts of the other team members and educating the child and family about management and the nature and expected course of the disease. A key predictor of long-term outcome is early diagnosis and referral to a rheumatology team experienced in the care of children with rheumatic diseases. Significant differences in outcome in patients with JRA 10 yr after onset are evident in patients referred to a pediatric rheumatology center within 6 mo of onset compared with those with referral more than 6 mo after onset.

The pediatric rheumatology team offers coordinated services for these children and their families. By working closely with the team, the primary care physician helps monitor compliance with treatment plans, observe for adverse effects of the medical therapy, evaluate symptoms of intercurrent illnesses, and identify disease exacerbations and concomitant infections. Communicating with subspecialists and teams at tertiary care centers permits timely intervention when poor compliance occurs or symptoms flare.

Each member of the **multidisciplinary pediatric rheumatology team** contributes individually and cooperatively to the child's care (Table 153-2). The pediatric rheumatologist establishes the diagnosis, assesses response to treatment, and monitors for changes in disease manifestations. With assistance from other team members, this leader of the team also monitors the child's psychosocial status including such areas as pain, emotional and behavioral responses to disease, change in roles at home and school, and family response to the child's illness. The nurse provides education about specific chronic illnesses and correct administration of medication. Physical and occupational therapists assess limitations in joint movement and physical function, provide plans for long-term rehabilitation programs, and prescribe and monitor exercise and splinting programs that families perform at home with the child to improve or maintain joint motion in children with arthritis, as well as in patients with myositis to avoid muscle contractures and improve muscle strength. Splints are used to lessen unnecessary mechanical stress on joints that is often associated with routine daily tasks. Splints may also aid in improving muscle or joint contractures and avoiding joint deformities, such as subluxation of the wrist. Ophthalmologists should examine children with JRA every 3–12 mo, depending on the type of JRA, to screen for uveitis and every 6–12 mo for children taking hydroxychloroquine or glucocorticoids to assess for ocular toxicity. Social workers are invaluable to families in helping them confront the significant social and emotional stresses imposed by the illness, deal with the financial maze of insurance coverage and national and state programs, and identify community resources needed to provide support such as the schools and the Bureau of Special Health Care Needs. Children with rheumatic diseases are often undernourished because of disease or medication-related anorexia, or they are obese or overnourished as a result of glucocorticoid therapy. Early and ongoing involvement of a nutritionist can significantly improve the health of these patients.

MEDICATIONS. Medications used for treatment of childhood rheumatic diseases (see Table 153-2) have various mechanisms of action, but all share the ability to suppress inflammation. A key to satisfactory short- and long-term outcomes in these children is early induction of a significant and sustained suppression of the inflammation. **Disease-modifying antirheumatic drugs** address the autoimmune process and include methotrexate and biologic products against tumor necrosis factor (TNF) and other mediators of inflammation.

Nonsteroidal Anti-Inflammatory Drugs (NSAIDs). A large number of NSAIDs are approved by the U.S. Food and Drug Administration (FDA) for use in adults with rheumatoid arthritis, but a much smaller number are approved for use in children. NSAIDs

TABLE 153-2. Cornerstones of Treatment of Children with Rheumatic Diseases

Accurate diagnosis and education of family	Pediatric rheumatologist Pediatrician Nurse Social Worker
Medications	Nonsteroidal anti-inflammatory drugs (NSAIDs) Methotrexate Tumor necrosis factor α (TNF-α) blockers (etanercept) Modulate T-cell activation (abatacept) Anti–CD20(B cell) antibody (rituximab) Interleukin 1–receptor antagonist (anakinra) Hydroxychloroquine Sulfasalazine Intravenous immunoglobulin (IVIG) Cyclophosphamide Cyclosporine Glucocorticoids (oral, intravenous, pulse, ophthalmic, intra-articular) Chaperonin 10 (inhibits Toll-like receptors)
Stem cell transplantation	Experimental approach to treatment-resistant lupus or juvenile rheumatoid arthritis (JRA)
Physical medicine and rehabilitation	Physical therapy Occupational therapy Splints and reconstructive surgery
Physical and psychosocial growth and development	Nutrition School integration Peer group relationships Individual and/or family counseling
Coordination of care	Involvement of patient and family as critical and active team members Communication between the pediatric rheumatologist and pediatrician Involvement of school (school nurse) and community resources (social worker)

are prescribed to decrease acute and chronic inflammation associated with arthritis, pleuritis, pericarditis, uveitis, and some forms of vasculitis. Lower doses, typically those approved for over-the-counter use, or intermittent dosing can result in analgesia but rarely significant anti-inflammatory effect. Reduction of inflammation requires regular administration of adequate doses, dosed on a weight (mg/kg) or body surface area (mg/m^2) basis, and for longer periods than needed for analgesia alone. The mean time to achieve an anti-inflammatory effect in the arthritis associated with JRA is 30 days of consistent administration. NSAIDs work primarily by inhibiting the enzyme **cyclo-oxygenase (COX),** which is critical in the production of **prostaglandins,** a family of substances that have many physiologic effects, including that of promoting inflammation. Two types of COX receptors have been demonstrated; several NSAIDs have been approved for use in adults with rheumatoid arthritis that only inhibit those receptors responsible for promoting inflammation. These **selective COX-2 inhibitors** have similar anti-inflammatory effects with possibly fewer adverse effects. Clinical studies of two selective COX-2 inhibitors, rofecoxib and celecoxib, have been performed in children with JRA. Meloxicam is not as selective as these other COX-2 inhibitors and has also been studied in children with JRA. All three of these drugs were found in children with JRA to be similar in effectiveness to naproxen, with fewer adverse effects. Several of the COX-2 inhibitors that were approved for use in adults (rofecoxib and valdecoxib) have been withdrawn from the market because of increased risk for heart attack and stroke with long-term continuous use.

The most frequent adverse effects of NSAIDs of all classes in children are nausea, decreased appetite, and abdominal pain. Gastritis or gastric or duodenal ulceration occurs less frequently in children than in adults. Other adverse effects, occurring in ≤5% of children on long-term NSAID therapy, include mood change, concentration difficulty that can simulate attention deficit disorder (ADD), sleepiness, irritability, headache, tinnitus, alopecia, anemia, elevated liver enzymes, proteinuria, and hematuria. These NSAID-associated adverse effects reverse quickly once the medication is stopped. Several NSAID-specific adverse reactions may also occur. Ibuprofen can induce aseptic meningitis in some patients with lupus and, rarely, in patients with JRA. Naproxen is far more likely in children than other NSAIDs to cause a unique skin reaction called **pseudoporphyria,** which is characterized by small hypopigmented flat scars occurring in areas of even minor skin trauma (skin fragility), such as fingernail scratches, or after small spontaneous vesicular lesions. Naproxen-induced pseudoporphyria is more likely to occur in fair-skinned individuals and on sun-exposed areas. Confirmation of this skin toxicity should prompt immediate discontinuation of naproxen because the scars can persist for several years or, in some cases, be permanent. NSAIDs should be used cautiously in patients with dermatomyositis or systemic vasculitis because there is an increased frequency of gastrointestinal ulceration with these disorders.

The response to NSAIDs varies greatly among individual patients, but, overall, ≈40–60% of children with JRA experience significant improvement in their arthritis. Patients must often try several different NSAIDs before finding the one that demonstrates the most clinical benefit. NSAIDs with longer half-lives or sustained-release formulations have been developed to allow for once- or twice-daily dosing. For patients with JRA or milder cases of lupus, NSAIDs are often a cornerstone of the treatment program. For ≈20% of patients with JRA, NSAIDs are the only drug therapy required to control the arthritis.

Methotrexate. Methotrexate has been studied for efficacy in almost all of the rheumatic diseases as well as in many nonrheumatic conditions, including inflammatory bowel disease, and uveitis. Studies in adults indicate that the mechanism of action of methotrexate, an analog of folic acid, in arthritis is not suppression of either folic acid metabolism or bone marrow activity. Methotrexate inhibits dihydrofolate reductase, which is important in purine synthesis, resulting in suppression of inflammation.

Methotrexate has a central role in the treatment of arthritis and is used in ≈60% of patients with polyarticular JRA. The response to oral methotrexate (10 mg/m^2 once a wk) is better than placebo (63% vs 36%). A large trial confirmed a response rate of >70% of children to the standard dose of oral methotrexate (8–12.5 mg/m^2 orally once a wk); there is a plateau of efficacy among nonresponders when randomized to parenteral (subcutaneous or intramuscular) methotrexate at 15 mg/m^2/wk (maximum: 20 mg/wk) or 30 mg/m^2/wk (maximum: 40 mg/wk), with 63% vs 58% response rates, respectively. Both doses of parenteral methotrexate are well tolerated. Patients with JRA who demonstrate a clinical response in articular inflammation with methotrexate also have improvement in growth rate, functional ability in daily tasks, and radiologic analysis of joint damage. Subcutaneous administration of methotrexate has similar absorption and pharmacokinetic properties to intramuscular injection, and is much less painful. Methotrexate is commonly used in treatment of juvenile dermatomyositis that has shown no or inadequate response to glucocorticoids. About 70% of patients with dermatomyositis treated with methotrexate demonstrate improvement in their myositis. It has also been successfully used at a dosage of 10–20 mg/m^2/wk in patients with lupus to treat arthritis, serositis, and, in some cases, nephritis.

Methotrexate is well tolerated by children. Because of the lower dose and alternative mechanisms of action, toxicity from methotrexate is much milder and qualitatively different from that observed when methotrexate is used to treat neoplastic diseases. In eight published studies that included 288 patients with JRA on methotrexate therapy, 13% of patients had gastrointestinal toxicity, 3% stomatitis, 15% elevated liver enzymes, 1–2% headache, and <1% leukopenia, interstitial pneumonitis, rash, or alopecia. Hepatotoxicity observed among adults with rheumatoid arthritis treated with methotrexate has raised concern about similar problems occurring in children. In 46 liver biopsies performed in patients with JRA undergoing long-term methotrexate treatment, 95% of specimens were normal and 5% showed mild fibrosis; none demonstrated even moderate liver damage. Children on methotrexate should be counseled on use of alcohol, smoking, and contraception.

Lymphoproliferative disorders have also been reported in adults, usually after primary Epstein-Barr virus infection, and may not be directly related to methotrexate. The relative risk of lymphoproliferative disease while on methotrexate remains low, at ≈1–1.5%.

Methotrexate is one of the cornerstone medications in pediatric rheumatology because of its potential to induce significant improvement in chronic inflammation and to maintain that improvement for long periods because of low toxicity and high patient acceptance.

Glucocorticoids. Glucocorticoids are given by various routes for rheumatic diseases including oral, intravenous, ocular, and intra-articular administration. Oral steroids are the cornerstone of treatment for moderate to severe lupus, dermatomyositis, and most forms of vasculitis. Long-term use, however, always leads to adverse effects of hypercorticism. Glucocorticoid therapy in these chronic diseases must be carefully supervised. A responsible plan requires steroid tapering to acceptable doses over time or the introduction of other anti-inflammatory medications to serve as **steroid-sparing agents.** A negative PPD reaction should be verified, if possible, before initiating steroids.

Intravenous steroids have been used as an alternative to oral administration to treat the severe, acute manifestations of systemic connective tissue diseases such as lupus, dermatomyositis, and vasculitis. The intravenous route allows for higher therapeutic doses to obtain an immediate, profound anti-inflammatory effect. **Methylprednisolone, 10–30 mg/kg/dose** up to a maximum of 1 g, has been the intravenous drug of choice. Although generally associated with fewer adverse effects than oral steroids, intravenous administration has significant and occasionally life-threatening toxicities such as cardiac arrhythmia, acute hypertension, hypotension, and shock.

Ocular steroids are prescribed under the supervision of an ophthalmologist either as drops or injections into the soft tissue surrounding the globe (sub-Tenon injection) for the uveitis associated with JRA. Long-term ocular steroid use can lead to cataract formation and glaucoma. Current ophthalmologic management has significantly decreased the frequency of blindness as a complication of JRA-associated uveitis.

Intra-articular steroids are prescribed with increasing frequency for children with JRA in whom one or several joints have not responded to standard parenteral drug therapy or as the initial therapy in patients with arthritis involving only one or two joints. Almost all patients have significant improvement in both symptoms and physical findings within 2–3 days, which lasts for at least 6 mo in 60% and for at least 12 mo in 45% of patients. Intra-articular administration may result in subcutaneous atrophy and hypopigmentation of the skin in the area surrounding the injection site, as well as subcutaneous calcifications along the needle tract. These complications are rarely clinically significant.

Anti-TNF-α Therapies. Etanercept represents a class of biologic modifiers for the treatment of inflammatory arthritis and is the only one currently approved for use in children. Etanercept is a genetically engineered fusion protein consisting of two identical chains of the recombinant extracellular tumor necrosis factor (TNF) receptor monomer fused with the Fc domain of human IgG1. Etanercept binds both TNF-α and lymphotoxin-α (formerly called TNF-β) and inhibits their activity. Etanercept (0.4 mg/kg subcutaneously twice a week, maximum dose of 25 mg) therapy in children with active polyarticular JRA who fail methotrexate treatment results in 74% of patients demonstrating significant clinical improvement after 3 mo of therapy. Children who respond to etanercept and then continue treatment with etanercept demonstrate a reduced frequency of disease and a delayed time to flare. The overall frequency and type of adverse events are similar for etanercept or placebo except for injection site reactions and frequency of upper respiratory tract infections, which are increased among the etanercept-treated subjects. The FDA approved etanercept for the treatment of children with moderate to severe active polyarticular JRA who have had an inadequate response to one or more second-line agents. Etanercept is perhaps also effective in the control of JRA-associated chronic uveitis that is inadequately responsive to steroid therapy.

The role of TNF blockade in the treatment of a variety of rheumatic diseases in both children and adults is still evolving and requires additional longitudinal experience to establish long-term effectiveness and safety. TNF is known to have a variety of beneficial functions, and the safety of long-term suppression of TNF function is unknown. TNF blockade is associated with an increased frequency of serious systemic infections and should not be initiated in subjects with history of chronic or frequent recurrent infections. **Tuberculosis** should always be excluded before beginning etanercept treatment. TNF blockade has also been shown to be efficacious for treatment of Crohn disease, psoriasis, and psoriatic arthritis, and is being evaluated for treatment of Wegener granulomatosus, spondyloarthropathy, juvenile dermatomyositis, and idiopathic inflammatory myositis in adults.

Two additional anti-TNF therapies, infliximab and adalimumab, have been approved for a variety of chronic inflammatory conditions in adults and both are being evaluated in clinical trials in children with JRA.

Hydroxychloroquine. Hydroxychloroquine sulfate is an antimalarial drug that has an important role in the treatment of lupus and, possibly, dermatomyositis. A 3–6 mo trial of hydroxychloroquine (3–6 mg/kg/day) is necessary to assess the therapeutic response. Hydroxychloroquine is especially helpful in the treatment of the cutaneous aspects of lupus and dermatomyositis. It is used infrequently to treat JRA because a prospective trial in patients with JRA failed to demonstrate increased efficacy of hydroxychloroquine compared with placebo. Potential adverse effects include bone marrow suppression, CNS stimulation, gastric irritation, myasthenia-like weakness, and skin rash. The most significant potential adverse effect is **retinal toxicity,** which occurs very rarely but may result in blindness or loss of central vision. Complete ophthalmologic examinations including peripheral vision and color fields at baseline every 4–6 mo are mandatory during hydroxychloroquine treatment. The frequency of retinal toxicity is very rare (≈1/5,000 patients).

Sulfasalazine. Sulfasalazine has been used for many years in the treatment of inflammatory bowel disease. In children with JRA, sulfasalazine 50 mg/kg/day (maximum: 2,000 mg/day) improves joint inflammation, global assessments, and laboratory parameters when compared with placebo. More than 30% of sulfasalazine-treated patients may withdraw from the treatment because of adverse effects, primarily gastrointestinal irritation and skin rashes. Sulfasalazine is associated with severe systemic hypersensitivity reactions, especially development of the Stevens-Johnson syndrome. These reactions are much more common in patients with active systemic JRA treated with sulfasalazine. Many experts feel that sulfasalazine is contraindicated in children with **active** systemic JRA. In some centers, it is used in polyarticular and pauciarticular JRA and spondyloarthropathy. Sulfasalazine should not be used in patients with porphyria or glucose-6-phosphate dehydrogenase deficiency. The use of sulfasalazine will likely decline with greater use of the far more efficacious anti-TNF therapies.

Intravenous Immunoglobulin (IVIG). IVIG is efficacious in various clinical conditions. IVIG significantly improves the short- and long-term natural history of Kawasaki disease. Open studies have supported benefit for lupus-associated thrombocytopenia, systemic and polyarticular JRA, and dermatomyositis. The doses of IVIG used have generally been large, 1–2 g/kg/dose, and must be given on a regular basis, usually monthly, to maintain benefit. In addition to being expensive and periodically in short supply, IVIG has been occasionally associated with severe systemic allergic-like reactions and postinfusion aseptic meningitis (headache, stiff neck). IVIG seems to hold promise as a treatment for dermatomyositis, although no controlled trials have been performed among children.

Cyclophosphamide. Cyclophosphamide, an alkylating agent, requires metabolic conversion in the liver to its active metabolites, which alkylate the guanine in DNA, leading to the observed immunosuppression by the inhibition of the S2 phase of mitosis. The subsequent decreased numbers of T and B lymphocytes result in diminished humoral and cellular immune responses. Pulse cyclophosphamide IV (500–1,000 mg/m^2) given monthly for 6 mo, then every 3 mo for 12 mo, has been shown to reduce the frequency of renal failure in patients with lupus with diffuse proliferative glomerulonephritis. Open trials also suggest efficacy in severe CNS lupus. Oral cyclophosphamide (2 mg/kg/day) is effective in the treatment of severe Wegener granulomatosis. Cyclophosphamide is a potent cytotoxic drug that is associated with very significant short- and long-term toxicities. Potential short-term adverse events include alopecia, nausea, vomiting, anorexia, oral and gastrointestinal tract ulcerations, cystitis, and bone marrow suppression. Long-term complications include an increased risk for sterility and cancer, especially leukemias, lymphomas, and bladder cancer. In adult women with lupus treated with intravenous cyclophosphamide, the overall frequency of permanent sterility is 30–40%. Ovarian suppression with an inhibitor of gonadotropin-releasing hormone is currently being studied to preserve fertility.

Other Drugs. Cyclosporine has been introduced in the treatment of dermatomyositis and active systemic JRA based on uncontrolled clinical studies. Several drugs commonly used in the past are very seldom used currently, including salicylates, gold compounds, azathioprine, and D-penicillamine.

FUTURE TREATMENTS. Rheumatologists commonly combine several drugs in the treatment of rheumatic diseases to achieve better disease control, often to permit the use of a lower dose of steroids. In adults with rheumatoid arthritis, a combination of methotrexate, hydroxychloroquine, and sulfasalazine has been well tolerated. The combination of these three drugs is more efficacious than any of the drugs individually, or any combination of two of the three drugs. In children with severe systemic JRA, a combination of intravenous methylprednisolone, intravenous cyclophosphamide, and oral methotrexate demonstrates excellent short-term safety and clinical effect.

In addition to inhibitors of TNF, a wide variety of other biologic agents are being studied in adults and many more are in development to modulate individual cell populations or molecular species involved in inflammatory processes. Monoclonal antibodies that can suppress specific T-cell subpopulations, bind particular cytokines or cytokine receptors (IL-1 and IL-6), bind antibody-producing B cells, or inhibit anti–double-stranded DNA autoantibodies are being widely tested in adults with rheumatic diseases, primarily rheumatoid arthritis and lupus. Mycophenolate mofetil has demonstrated remarkable anti-inflammatory and immunosuppression in rheumatic diseases such as lupus in adults. The potential for these therapies in children with rheumatic diseases is great but largely untested at this time.

Binstadt BA, Caldas AMC, Turvey SE, et al: Rituximab therapy for multisystem autoimmune diseases in pediatric patients. *J Pediatr* 2003;143:598–604.

Burgos-Vargas R, Vazquez-Mellado J, Pacheco-Tena C, et al: A 26 week randomized, double blind, placebo controlled exploratory study of sulfasalazine in juvenile onset spondyloarthropathies. *Ann Rheum Dis* 2002;61:941–942.

Burls A, Jobanputra P: The trials of anakinra. *Lancet* 2004;364:827–828.

Frank RG, Hagglund KJ, Schopp LH, et al: Disease and family contributors to adaptation in juvenile rheumatoid arthritis and juvenile diabetes. *Arthritis Care Res* 1998;11:166–176.

Genovese MC, Becker JC, Schiff M, et al: Abatacept for rheumatoid arthritis refractory to tumor necrosis factor β inhibition. *N Engl J Med* 2005; 353:1114–1123.

Giannini EH, Brewer EF, Kuzmina N, et al: Methotrexate in resistant juvenile rheumatoid arthritis. Results of U.S.-U.S.S.R. double-blind, placebo-controlled trial. The Pediatric Rheumatology Collaborative Study Group and the Cooperative Children's Study Group. *N Engl J Med* 1992; 326:1043–1049.

Giannini EH, Cawkwell GD: Drug treatment in children with juvenile rheumatoid arthritis past, present, and future. *Pediatr Clin North Am* 1995; 42:1099–1125.

Ilowite NT: Current treatment of juvenile rheumatoid arthritis. *Pediatrics* 2002;109:109–115.

Lehman TJ: A practical guide to systemic lupus erythematosus. *Pediatr Clin North Am* 1995;42:1223–1238.

Lovell DJ: Juvenile rheumatoid arthritis and juvenile spondyloarthropathy. In Klippel JH (editor): *Primer on the Rheumatic Diseases,* 12th ed. Atlanta, Arthritis Foundation, 2001.

Lovell DJ, Giannini EH, Reiff A, et al: Etanercept in children with polyarticular juvenile rheumatoid arthritis. *N Engl J Med* 2000;342:763–769.

Nicolino Ruperto, Kevin J. Murray, Valeria Gerloni, et al, for the Pediatric Rheumatology International Trials Organization: A randomized trial of parenteral methotrexate comparing an intermediate dose with a higher dose in children with juvenile idiopathic arthritis who failed to respond to standard doses of methotrexate. *Arthritis Rheum* 2004;50:2191–2201.

Rhen T, Cidlowski JA: Antiinflammatory action of glucocorticoids—new mechanisms for old drugs. *N Engl J Med* 2005;353:1711–1723.

Tubach F, Ravaud P, Salmon-Ceron N, et al: Emergence of *Legionella pneumophila* pneumonia in patients receiving tumor necrosis factor-α antagonists. *CID* 2006;43:e95–e200.

Tucker L, Cabral D: Transition of the adolescent patient with rheumatic disease: Issues to consider. *Pediatr Clin North Am* 2005;52:641–652.

Chapter 154 ■ Juvenile Rheumatoid Arthritis

Michael L. Miller and James T. Cassidy

Juvenile rheumatoid arthritis (JRA) is a common, rheumatic disease of children and a major cause of chronic disability. It is characterized by a synovitis of the peripheral joints manifesting in soft tissue swelling and effusion. In the Classification Criteria of the American College of Rheumatology (ACR), JRA is regarded not as a single disease but as a category of diseases with three principal types of onset: (1) oligoarthritis or pauciarticular disease, (2) polyarthritis, and (3) systemic-onset disease (Table 154-1). Nine distinct subtypes are identifiable. The European League Against Rheumatism (EULAR) and the International League of Associations for Rheumatology (ILAR) propose an additional classification schema (Table 154-2). Only the ACR criteria have been statistically validated by extensive, multi-clinic surveys and meet the requirements of evidence-based medicine.

ETIOLOGY. The etiology of this type of chronic arthritis in children is unknown. At least two necessary events are postulated: immunogenetic susceptibility and an external, presumably environmental, trigger. Specific HLA subtypes confer varying degrees of susceptibility, or indeed protection, depending on the age of the child. Possible external triggers include viruses (parvovirus B19, rubella, Epstein-Barr virus), host hyperreactivity to specific self antigens (type II collagen), and enhanced T-cell reactivity to bacterial or mycobacterial heat shock proteins.

EPIDEMIOLOGY. The incidence of JRA is ≈13.9/100,000 children/yr among white children ≤15 yr of age, with a prevalence of ≈113/100,000 children. A report from western Australia, estimates a much higher prevalence of 400/100,000 based on sequential examinations of schoolchildren by a pediatric rheumatologist. Different racial and ethnic groups have varying frequencies of the subtypes of JRA. African-American children may be older at onset and less likely to have elevated antinuclear antibody (ANA) titers or develop chronic uveitis.

PATHOGENESIS. The synovitis of JRA is characterized pathologically by villous hypertrophy and hyperplasia with hyperemia and edema of the subsynovial tissues. Vascular endothelial hyperplasia is prominent and characterized by infiltration of mononuclear and plasma cells (Fig. 154-1). **Pannus formation,** which is an inflammatory exudate over the synovial lining, occurs in advanced uncontrolled disease and results in progressive erosion of articular cartilage and contiguous bone (Fig. 154-2).

Although the etiology of the arthritis is unknown, studies suggest an exaggerated immune reactivity in immunogenetically

TABLE 154-1. Criteria for the Classification of Juvenile Rheumatoid Arthritis

Age at onset: <16 yr
Arthritis (swelling or effusion, or the presence of 2 or more of the following signs: limitation of range of motion, tenderness or pain on motion, increased heat) in ≥1 joints
Duration of disease: ≥ 6 wk
Onset type defined by type of articular involvement in the 1st 6 mo after onset:
Polyarthritis: ≥5 inflamed joints
Oligoarthritis: ≤4 inflamed joints
Systemic disease: arthritis with a characteristic intermittent fever
Exclusion of other forms of juvenile arthritis

Modified from Cassidy JT, Levison JE, Bass JC, et al: A study of classification criteria for a diagnosis of juvenile rheumatoid arthritis. *Arthritis Rheum* 1986;29;174–181.

TABLE 154-2. Characteristics of the ACR, EULAR, and ILAR Classifications of Chronic Arthritis in Children

CHARACTERISTIC	AMERICAN COLLEGE OF RHEUMATOLOGY (ACR)	EUROPEAN LEAGUE AGAINST RHEUMATISM (ELAR)	INTERNATIONAL LEAGUE OF ASSOCIATIONS FOR RHEUMATOLOGY (ILAR)
Onset types	3	6	6
Course subtypes	9	None	1
Age at onset of arthritis	<16 yr	<16 yr	<16 yr
Duration of arthritis	≥6 wk	≥3 mo	≥6 wk
Includes juvenile ankylosing spondylitis	No	Yes	Yes
Includes juvenile psoriatic arthritis	No	Yes	Yes
Includes inflammatory bowel disease	No	Yes	Yes
Exclusion of other diseases	Yes	Yes	Yes

predisposed children, suspected but not proved to be in response to exposure to environmental antigens. Although trauma is often cited by parents as occurring at onset of their child's arthritis, it is more likely the result rather than the cause of the disorder. Studies of T-cell receptor expression confirm recruitment of T cells specific for synovial non-self antigens. These specific populations of T cells may change over time, sometimes with clonal expansion of cells that may be protective (those reactive toward certain heat shock proteins) or associated with improved responsiveness to medical treatment. Resistance to treatment may result in part from migration into the synovium of T cells whose surfaces bear molecules inducing chronic activation of resident cellular components.

It was postulated that HLA typing would identify risk and protective factors. With further studies, however, the association of JRA with HLA alleles has become complex. The recruitment of T cells is facilitated by HLA types that occur with increased frequency in affected children. Polyarthritis is associated with HLA-DR4, particularly the DRB1*0401 and 0404 alleles. Oligoarthritis is associated with HLA alleles at the DR8, particularly DRB1*0801, and DR5, particularly DRB1*1104. The polygenic pathogenesis of JRA seldom results in multiple cases in a family. The exception is twins; there is a 4% concordance in dizygotic births and a 44% concordance in monozygotic twins.

T-cell activation results in a cascade of events leading to tissue damage in joints and other affected tissues, including B-cell activation, complement consumption and immune-complex formation, and, in particular, release of tumor necrosis factor (TNF)–α, interleukin 6 (IL-6), IL-1, and other proinflammatory cytokines, possibly under the control of specific genetic alleles. Inheritance of certain alleles identified by single nucleotide polymorphisms may predispose to upregulation of these cytokine networks, resulting in more severe articular and systemic disease.

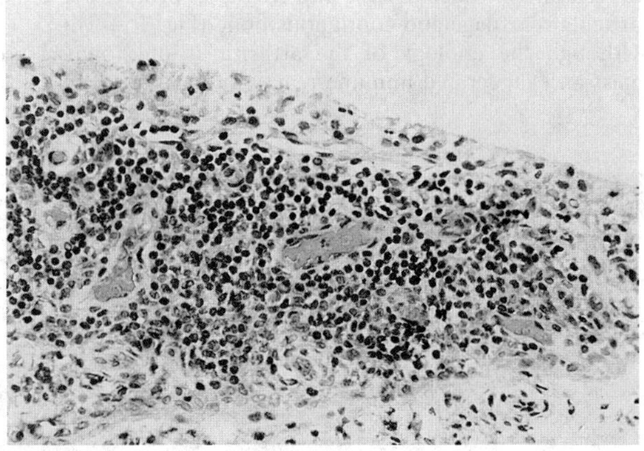

Figure 154-1. Synovial biopsy from a 10 yr old child with pauciarticular juvenile rheumatoid arthritis. There is a dense infiltration of lymphocytes and plasma cells in the synovium.

CLINICAL MANIFESTATIONS. Initial symptoms may be subtle or acute, and often include morning stiffness and gelling, easy fatigability, particularly after school in the early afternoon, joint pain later in the day, and objective joint swelling. The involved joints are often warm, resist full range of motion, are painful on motion, but are not usually erythematous.

Oligoarthritis (pauciarticular disease) predominantly affects the joints of the lower extremities, such as the knees and ankles (Fig. 154-3). Often, only a single joint is involved at onset. Isolated involvement of upper extremity large joints is not characteristic of this type of onset. Involvement of the hip is almost never a presenting sign of JRA. Hip disease may occur later, particularly in polyarticular JRA, and is often a component of a deteriorating functional course (Fig. 154-4).

Polyarthritis (polyarticular disease) is generally characterized by involvement of both large and small joints of both upper and lower extremities (Figs. 154-5 and 154-6). As many as 20–40 joints may be affected in the more severely involved child, although inflammation of only ≥5 joints is required as a criterion

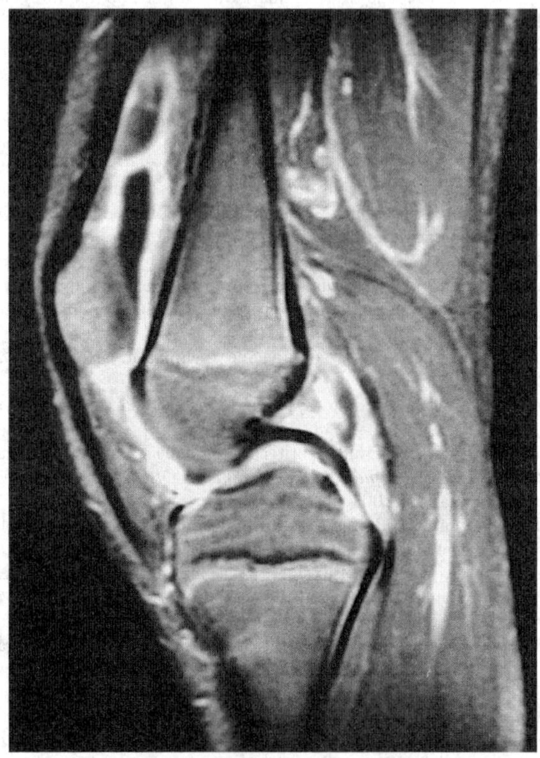

Figure 154-2. MRI scan with gadolinium of a 10 yr old child with juvenile rheumatoid arthritis (same patient as in Fig. 154-1). The dense white signal in the synovium near the distal femur, proximal tibia, and patella reflects inflammation. MRI of the knee is useful to exclude ligamentous injury, chondromalacia of the patella, or tumor.

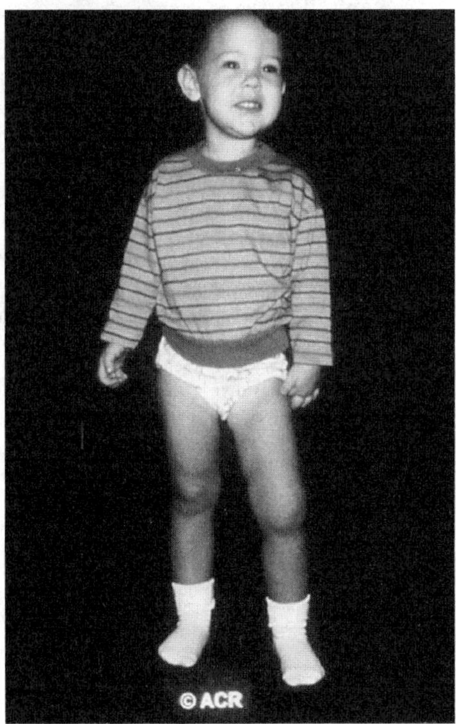

Figure 154-3. Oligoarticular juvenile rheumatoid arthritis with involvement of the left knee and hands. (Reprinted from the Clinical Slide Collection on the Rheumatic Diseases; copyright 1991, 1995, 1997. Used by permission of the American College of Rheumatology.)

for classification of this type of onset. Polyarticular disease may resemble the characteristic presentation of adult rheumatoid arthritis and the HLA profile is often similar. **Rheumatoid nodules** on the extensor surfaces of the elbows and over the Achilles tendons, while unusual, are associated with a more severe course. **Micrognathia** reflects chronic temporomandibular joint disease. Cervical spine involvement of the apophyseal joints (Fig. 154-7) occurs frequently with a risk of atlantoaxial subluxation and potential neurologic sequelae.

Systemic-onset disease is characterized by arthritis and prominent visceral involvement that includes hepatosplenomegaly, lymphadenopathy, and serositis, such as a pericardial effusion. It is characterized by a quotidian fever with temperatures to ≥39°C, sometimes followed by mildly hypothermic temperatures for ≥2 wk. Each febrile episode is frequently accompanied by a characteristic faint, erythematous, macular rash; these evanescent

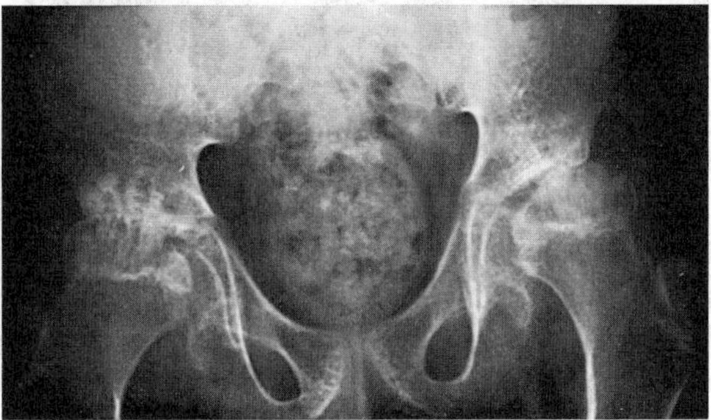

Figure 154-4. Severe hip disease in a 13 yr old boy with active, systemic-onset juvenile rheumatoid arthritis. X-ray shows destruction of the femoral head and acetabula, joint space narrowing, and subluxation of left hip. The patient had received corticosteroids systemically for 9 yr.

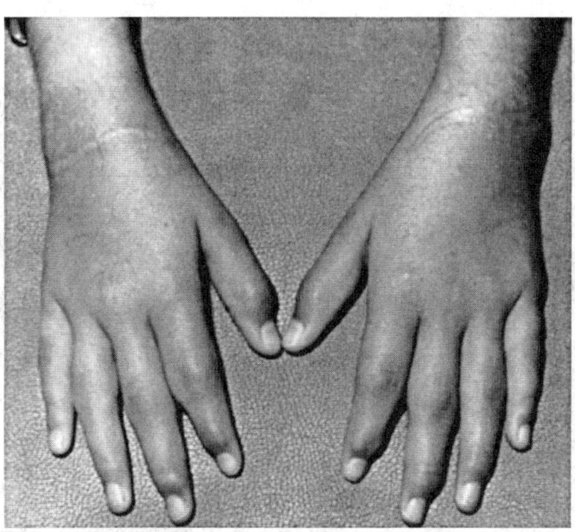

Figure 154-5. Hands and wrists of a girl with rheumatoid factor–negative polyarticular juvenile rheumatoid arthritis. Notice the symmetric involvement of the metacarpophalangeal joints, proximal interphalangeal joints, and distal interphalangeal joints. Both wrists are affected.

salmon-colored lesions may be linear or circular, from 2–5 mm in size, and are often distributed in groups with a linear distribution most commonly over the trunk and proximal extremities (Fig. 154-8). This rash is not pruritic. Its most diagnostic feature is its transient nature, with a group of lesions usually lasting <1 hr. The **Koebner phenomenon,** which is cutaneous hypersensitivity to superficial trauma resulting in a localized recurrence of the rash, is suggestive, but not diagnostic, of systemic-onset disease. Heat, such as a warm bath, also evokes a reappearance of the rash.

DIAGNOSIS. The diagnosis is greatly aided by the ACR Classification Criteria and its subclassification of course of the disease, and by the meticulous clinical exclusion of other articular diseases. There is often no one pathognomonic finding for these disorders. The classic intermittent fever in association with the typical rash and objective arthritis is highly suggestive of systemic-onset JRA. The diagnosis is based on a history compatible with inflammatory joint disease and a physical examination that confirms the presence of arthritis (see Table 154-1). Some children have persistent arthralgia despite repeated normal physical examinations. Although they do not fulfill the diagnostic criteria for JRA initially, that diagnosis may become evident as late as ≥2 yr after the initial presentation. Laboratory abnormalities characteristic of inflammation include elevated erythrocyte sedimentation rate (ESR) and C-reactive protein (CRP), leukocytosis, thrombocytosis, and the anemia of chronic disease, which support the diagnosis.

DIFFERENTIAL DIAGNOSIS. Arthritis can be the presenting manifestation for any of the rheumatic diseases of childhood, including systemic lupus erythematosus (SLE) [see Chapter 157], juvenile dermatomyositis (see Chapter 158), sarcoidosis (see Chapter 164), and the vasculitic syndromes (see Chapter 166) [Table 154-3]. In scleroderma, swelling along the digits early in the disease is not confined to the joints and subsequent loss of motion may occur without any articular swelling. **Acute rheumatic fever** is characterized by exquisite joint pain and tenderness, a remittent fever, and polyarthritis that is usually migratory. Autoimmune hepatitis can be associated with an acute arthritis. **Lyme disease** (see Chapter 219) should be considered in children living in or visiting endemic areas who present with oligoarthritis. Although a history of tick exposure, preceding flu-like illness and subsequent rash should be sought, these are not

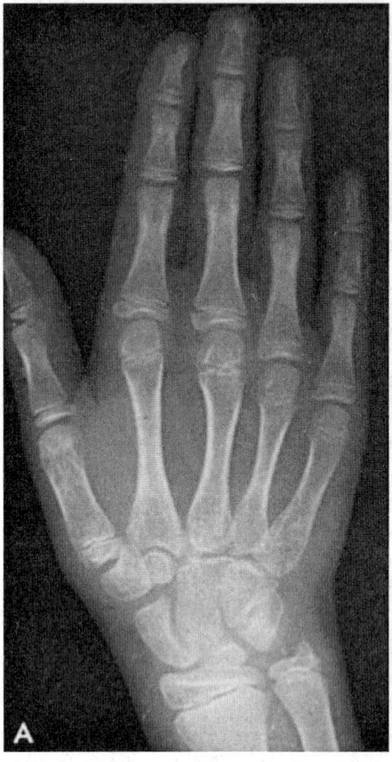

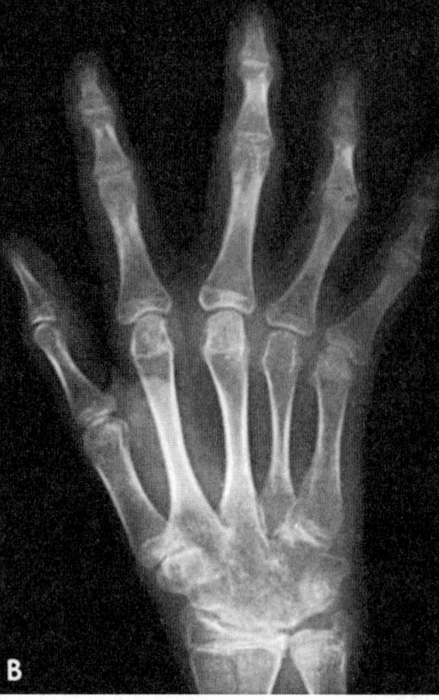

Figure 154-6. Progression of joint destruction in a girl with rheumatoid factor–positive juvenile rheumatoid arthritis despite doses of corticosteroids sufficient to suppress symptoms in the interval between *A* and *B*. *A*, X-ray of the hand at onset. *B*, X-ray 4 yr later, showing a loss of articular cartilage and destruction changes in the distal and proximal interphalangeal and metacarpophalangeal joints and destruction and fusion of wrist bones.

always present. Monarticular arthritis unresponsive to anti-inflammatory treatment may be the result of chronic mycobacterial or other infection; the diagnosis is often established only by synovial biopsy. Joint pain and swelling of a single joint suggests trauma or infection; correlation with history, laboratory, and radiologic findings helps exclude these possibilities.

Physical findings may suggest other diagnoses. Acute onset of a synovial effusion and an inflamed joint suggests bacterial infection. Chondromalacia of the patella or related femoropatellar syndromes can cause knee pain and instability. Tenderness over insertion of ligaments and tendons and lower extremity arthritis, especially in a male, raises the possibility of a spondyloarthropathy. **Psoriatic arthritis** can present with limited joint involvement in an unusual distribution (e.g., small joints of the hand and ankle) prior to onset of cutaneous disease. Until psoriasis develops, which may only occur years after the arthritis, the diagnosis can only be suspected (especially with a positive family history). Isolated hip pain with limited motion raises the possibility of suppurative arthritis (see Chapter 684) or osteomyelitis, Legg-Calvé-Perthes disease, slipped capital femoral epiphysis, or chondrolysis of the hip (see Chapter 677).

Repeated episodes of joint pain and swelling, especially in lower extremity joints, usually lasting <1 wk with complete resolution between episodes, can occur in juvenile episodic arthritis, often attributed to **hypermobility. Inflammatory bowel disease** may present with oligoarthritis, usually affecting joints in the lower extremities, and unexplained anemia. Arthritis can also

Figure 154-7. Radiograph of the cervical spine of a patient with active juvenile rheumatoid arthritis, showing fusion of the neural arch between joints C2 and C3, narrowing and erosion of the remaining neural arch joints, obliteration of the apophyseal space, and loss of the normal lordosis.

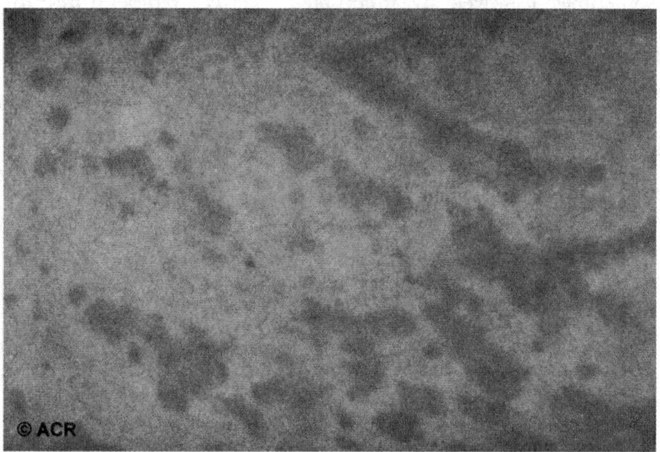

Figure 154-8. The rash of systemic-onset juvenile rheumatoid arthritis. The rash is salmon-colored, macular, and nonpruritic. Individual lesions are transient and occur in crops over the trunk and extremities. (Reprinted from the Clinical Slide Collection on the Rheumatic Diseases; copyright 1991, 1995, 1997. Used by permission of the American College of Rheumatology.)

TABLE 154-3. Conditions Causing Arthritis or Extremity Pain

RHEUMATIC AND INFLAMMATORY DISEASES	Hereditary connective tissue disease (Marfan syndrome, Ehlers-Danlos syndrome)
Juvenile rheumatoid arthritis	Fabry disease
Systemic lupus erythematosus	Farber disease
Juvenile dermatomyositis	Amyloidosis (familial Mediterranean fever)
Polyarteritis	**BONE AND CARTILAGE DISORDERS**
Vasculitis	Trauma
Scleroderma	Patellofemoral syndrome
Sjögren syndrome	Hypermobility syndrome
Behçet disease	Osteochondritis dissecans
Overlap syndromes	Avascular necrosis (including Legg-Calvé-Perthes disease)
Wegener granulomatosis	Hypertrophic osteoarthropathy
Sarcoidosis	Slipped capital femoral epiphysis
Kawasaki syndrome	Osteolysis
Henoch-Schönlein purpura	Benign bone tumors (including osteoid osteoma)
Chronic recurrent multifocal osteomyelitis	Histiocytosis
SERONEGATIVE SPONDYLOARTHROPATHIES	Rickets
Juvenile ankylosing spondylitis	**NEUROPATHIC DISORDERS**
Inflammatory bowel disease	Peripheral neuropathies
Psoriatic arthritis	Carpal tunnel syndrome
Reactive arthritis associated with urethritis, iridocyclitis, and mucocutaneous lesions	Charcot joints
INFECTIOUS ILLNESSES	**NEOPLASTIC DISORDERS**
Bacterial arthritis (septic arthritis, *Staphylococcus aureus*, pneumococcus, gonococcus, *H. influenzae*)	Leukemia
Lyme disease	Neuroblastoma
Viral illness (parvovirus, rubella, mumps, Epstein-Barr virus, hepatitis B)	Lymphoma
Fungal arthritis	Bone tumors (osteosarcoma, Ewing sarcoma)
Mycobacterial infection	Histiocytic syndromes
Spirochetal infection	Synovial tumors
Endocarditis	**HEMATOLOGIC DISORDERS**
REACTIVE ARTHRITIS	Hemophilia
Acute rheumatic fever	Hemoglobinopathies (including sickle cell disease)
Reactive arthritis (post-infectious from *Shigella*, *Salmonella*, *Yersinia*, *Chlamydia*, or meningococcus)	**MISCELLANEOUS DISORDERS**
Serum sickness	Pigmented villonodular synovitis
Toxic synovitis of the hip	Plant-thorn synovitis (foreign body arthritis)
Postimmunization	Myositis ossificans
IMMUNODEFICIENCIES	Eosinophilic fasciitis
Hypogammaglobulinemia	Tendinitis (overuse injury)
Immunoglobulin A deficiency	Raynaud phenomenon
Human immunodeficiency virus	**PAIN SYNDROMES**
CONGENITAL AND METABOLIC DISORDERS	Fibromyalgia
Gout	Growing pains
Pseudogout	Depression (with somatization)
Mucopolysaccharidoses	Reflex sympathetic dystrophy
Thyroid disease (hypothyroidism, hyperthyroidism)	Regional myofascial pain syndromes
Hyperparathyroidism	
Vitamin C deficiency (scurvy)	

follow an enteric infection (see Chapter 156). Unexplained arthralgia accompanied by a fear of returning to school suggests school phobia as a cause for the arthralgia.

Less commonly, other diseases can produce joint symptoms and signs. Children with undiagnosed **leukemia** may have joint pain resulting from metaphyseal expansion of the malignant infiltration of the bone marrow, sometimes months before demonstrating peripheral blood lymphoblasts. Examination of such a child usually reveals a deeper pain to palpation of the bone; bone marrow aspiration confirms the diagnosis. Some diseases, such as cystic fibrosis, diabetes mellitus, and the glycogen storage diseases have associated arthropathies (see Chapter 168). Swelling that extends beyond the joint can be a sign of lymphedema, which may rarely coexist with JRA, or Henoch-Schönlein purpura. A peripheral arthritis indistinguishable from JRA occurs in the humoral immunodeficiencies, such as common variable immunodeficiency and X-linked agammaglobulinemia. Skeletal dysplasias associated with a degenerative arthropathy are diagnosed by characteristic radiologic abnormalities.

LABORATORY FINDINGS. Hematologic abnormalities often reflect the degree of systemic or articular inflammation, with elevated white blood cell and platelet counts and decreased hemoglobin concentration and mean corpuscular volume. The ESR and CRP usually mirror these findings, along with elevated serum immunoglobulins. It is not unusual for the ESR to be normal in some children with chronic arthritis. Because platelets are an acute-phase reactant, a high ESR and neutropenia with a low platelet count may be a clue to leukemia as a cause of periarticular swelling and pain.

Elevated ANA titers are present in at least 40–85% of children with oligoarticular or polyarticular JRA, but are unusual in children with systemic-onset disease. ANA seropositivity is associated with increased risk for the development of **chronic uveitis** in a child with limited joint disease. Rheumatoid-factor (RF) seropositivity may be associated with onset of polyarticular involvement in an older child (≈8%) and the development of rheumatoid nodules, and with a poor overall prognosis with eventual functional disability. Both ANA and RF seropositivity occur in association with transient events during childhood, such as viral infections, particularly Epstein-Barr virus. Seropositivity for both ANA and RF must be defined at a specific titer in relation to accepted positive and negative controls and a laboratory-defined coefficient of variation.

Bone mineral metabolism and skeletal maturation are often abnormal in children with JRA with a history of active synovitis, relatively independent of onset type or course subtype, and predominantly affect appendicular cortical bone, with less effect on the normal age-related development of trabecular bone. Increased levels of cytokines such as IL-6 may decrease bone formation (reflected by decreased serum levels of osteocalcin and bone-specific alkaline phosphatase) to a greater extent than bone resorption (which may also be decreased, as reflected by decreased levels of tartrate-resistant acid phosphatase). Abnormalities of skeletal growth become most prominent during the pubertal growth spurt and in postpubertal children (Tanner stages IV–V) and lead to failure of the child to achieve acceptable peak bone mass (osteopenia).

Early radiographic changes of arthritis include soft tissue swelling, regional osteoporosis, and periosteal new-bone apposition about affected joints (Fig. 154-9). Regional epiphyseal closure may be stimulated, and local bone growth decreased. In large joints, linear growth may be accelerated and limb length discrepancy, especially with involvement of a knee, becomes prominent. Continued active disease may lead to subchondral erosions and narrowing of cartilage space, especially in small tubular bones, with varying degrees of bony destruction and, potentially, fusion. Characteristic radiographic changes in cervical spine, most frequently in the neural arch joints at C2–3 (see Fig. 154-7) may progress to atlantoaxial subluxation. MRI studies may be helpful to evaluate both joint and soft tissues and are more sensitive to early, minimal changes than is plain radiography (see Fig. 154-2).

TREATMENT. The long-term treatment of children with JRA is initiated and subsequently modified if necessary according to disease subtype, severity of the disease, specific manifestations of the illness, and responses to therapy. The objectives of treatment are to establish the child in a pattern of adaptation that is as normal as possible and to accomplish this goal with minimal risk of adverse effects (see Chapter 153).

Most children with oligoarthritis respond to nonsteroidal anti-inflammatory drugs (NSAIDs) with relief of pain and amelioration of the signs of inflammation. Most children with polyarticular disease or with systemic-onset disease, however, require additional anti-inflammatory therapy. One approach is to use combination therapy beginning with the least toxic medications, proceeding through methotrexate and possibly etanercept or infliximab (Figs. 154-10, 154-11, and 154-12). Medications that place the child's present and future health most at risk, such as azathioprine and cyclophosphamide, are reserved for the few children who do not respond to less aggressive therapy. TNF-α blockers may prove to be more specific for synovial inflammatory disease and potentially less toxic than other immunosuppressive medications.

Glucocorticoids are recommended only for management of overwhelming inflammatory or systemic illness, for bridge therapy early in disease in lower doses for the child who has not yet responded to conventional therapy, and for ocular control of uveitis and intra-articular use in persistent limited joint disease. Steroids are effective anti-inflammatory drugs, perhaps the most efficacious in current use for systemic disease, but they impose on the child the risk of severe toxicities, including Cushing syndrome, growth retardation, and osteopenia.

Methotrexate is considered the safest, most efficacious, and least toxic of the currently available second-line agents for initial adjunctive therapy with an NSAID. It is given either orally or subcutaneously once weekly.

A program of management must include periodic slit-lamp ophthalmologic examinations of all patients to monitor for asymptomatic uveitis; dietary evaluation and counseling to ensure appropriate calcium, vitamin D, protein, and caloric intake; and physical and occupational therapy. A social worker and nurse clinician can be an invaluable resource for families to recognize stresses imposed by illness, identify appropriate community resources, and maintain compliance with the treatment protocol.

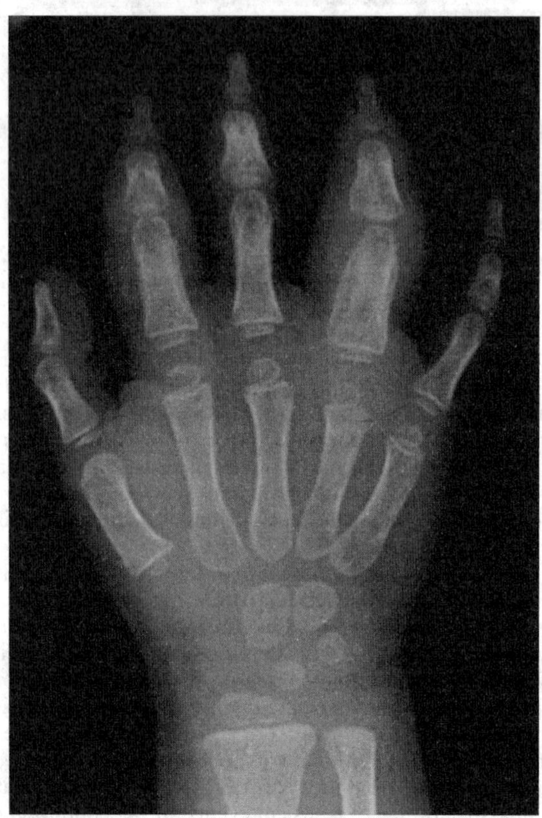

Figure 154-9. Early (6-mo duration) radiographic changes of juvenile rheumatoid arthritis, soft tissue swelling, and periosteal new bone formation appears adjacent to the 2nd and 4th proximal interphalangeal joints.

PROGNOSIS. Although the course of JRA in an individual child is unpredictable, some prognostic generalizations can be made based on the type of onset and course subtype (Table 154-4). Studies from the United States indicate that, based on management in the pre-TNF-α era, ≈45% of JRA patients have active disease persisting into early adulthood, often with severe limitations of physical function.

Children with oligoarthritis, particularly girls with onset of arthritis at an age of <6 yr, are at risk to develop chronic uveitis. There is no association between the activity or severity of the arthritis and the chronic uveitis. Persistent, uncontrolled anterior uveitis (Fig. 154-13) can result in posterior synechiae, cataracts, and band keratopathy, and result in blindness. Currently, however, many of these children do well with expert ophthalmologic therapy.

The child with polyarticular disease often has a more prolonged course of active inflammation of the joints. Functional risk has been associated with older age of onset, RF seropositivity or rheumatoid nodules, and the early development of erosions or disease of the cervical spine or hips.

The child with systemic-onset disease is often the most difficult to control in terms of both articular inflammation and systemic manifestations. Marked systemic disease is usually present only during the 1st few years after onset and tends to regress over

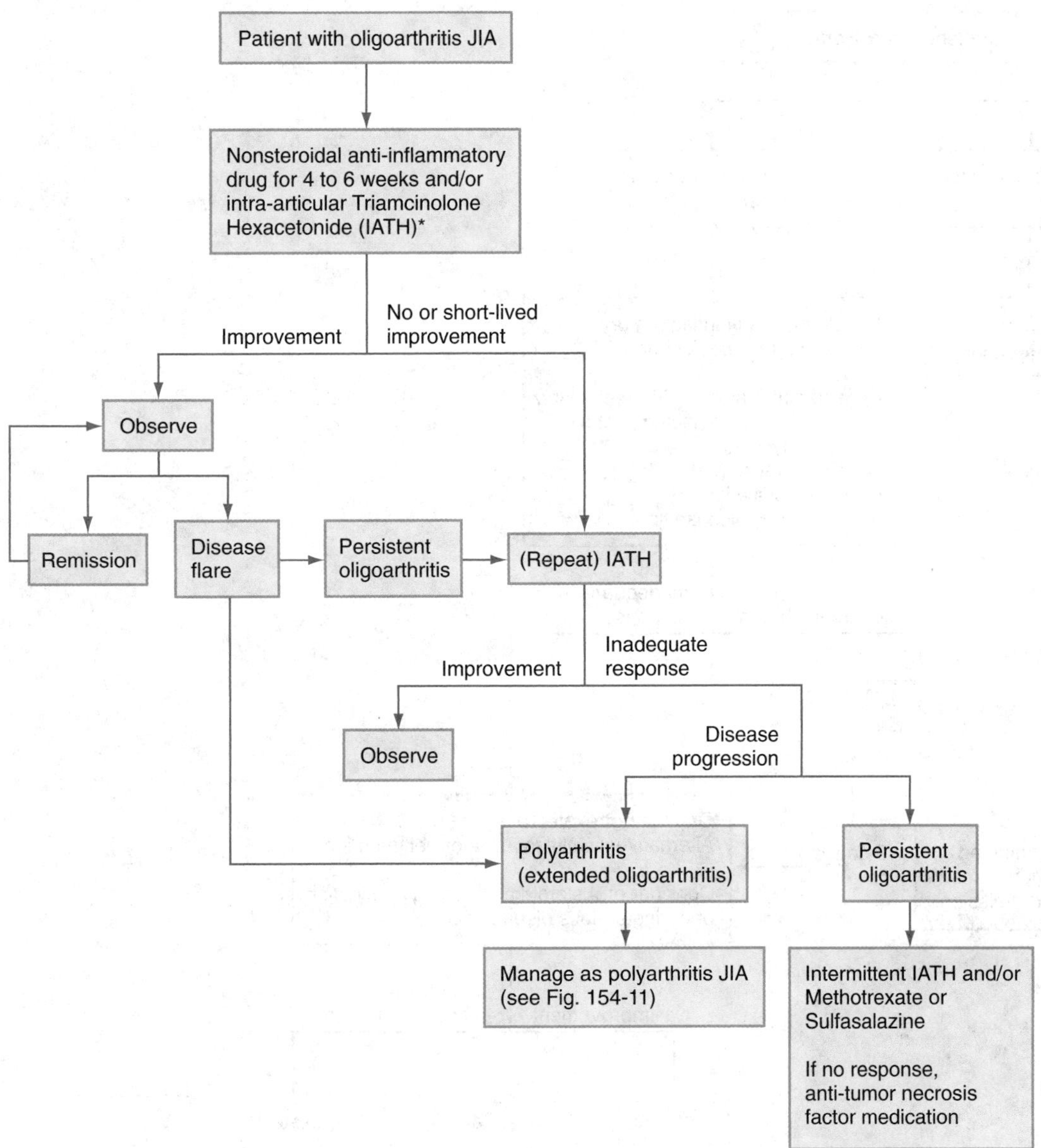

Figure 154-10. Algorithm for medical treatment of oligoarthritis in juvenile idiopathic arthritis (JIA). (From Hashkes PJ, Laxer RM: Medical treatment of juvenile idiopathic arthritis. *JAMA* 2005;294:1671–1684.)

time. Prognosis is dependent on the number of joints involved, duration of active inflammation, and the severity of the arthritis.

The anemia of chronic illness, common in active disease or with a prolonged course, is unresponsive to oral iron administration. Anemia may be exacerbated by gastrointestinal bleeding associated with the use of NSAIDs. Anemia associated with decreases in other blood cell lines raises the possibility of malignancy. Rarely, it is a result of acute hemolysis.

The acute development of a profound anemia associated with thrombocytopenia or leukopenia with a high, spiking fever, lymphadenopathy, and hepatosplenomegaly occurs with the **macrophage activation syndrome,** a rare and occasionally fatal complication of systemic JRA (Table 154-5). This diagnosis is suggested by clinical criteria and confirmed by bone marrow biopsy demonstrating hemophagocytosis. This may be a secondary cause of hemophagocytic lymphohistiocytosis (see Chapter 507). Emergency treatment with high-dose intravenous pulse methylprednisolone, cyclosporine, and, if needed, etanercept, has generally been effective. Severe cases may require therapy similar to that of secondary hemophagocytic lymphohistiocytosis although bone marrow transplantation is not needed (Chapter 507). The development of clinical manifestations of other rheumatic diseases suggests that the initial diagnosis has changed to an overlap syndrome or another specific disease, such as SLE or dermatomyositis.

Orthopedic complications include leg length discrepancy, which can be managed with a shoe lift on the shorter side to prevent secondary scoliosis; popliteal cysts, which require no treatment if small; and flexion contractures, particularly of the knees, hips, and wrists. **Contractures** require aggressive medical control of the arthritis, often in conjunction with intra-articular

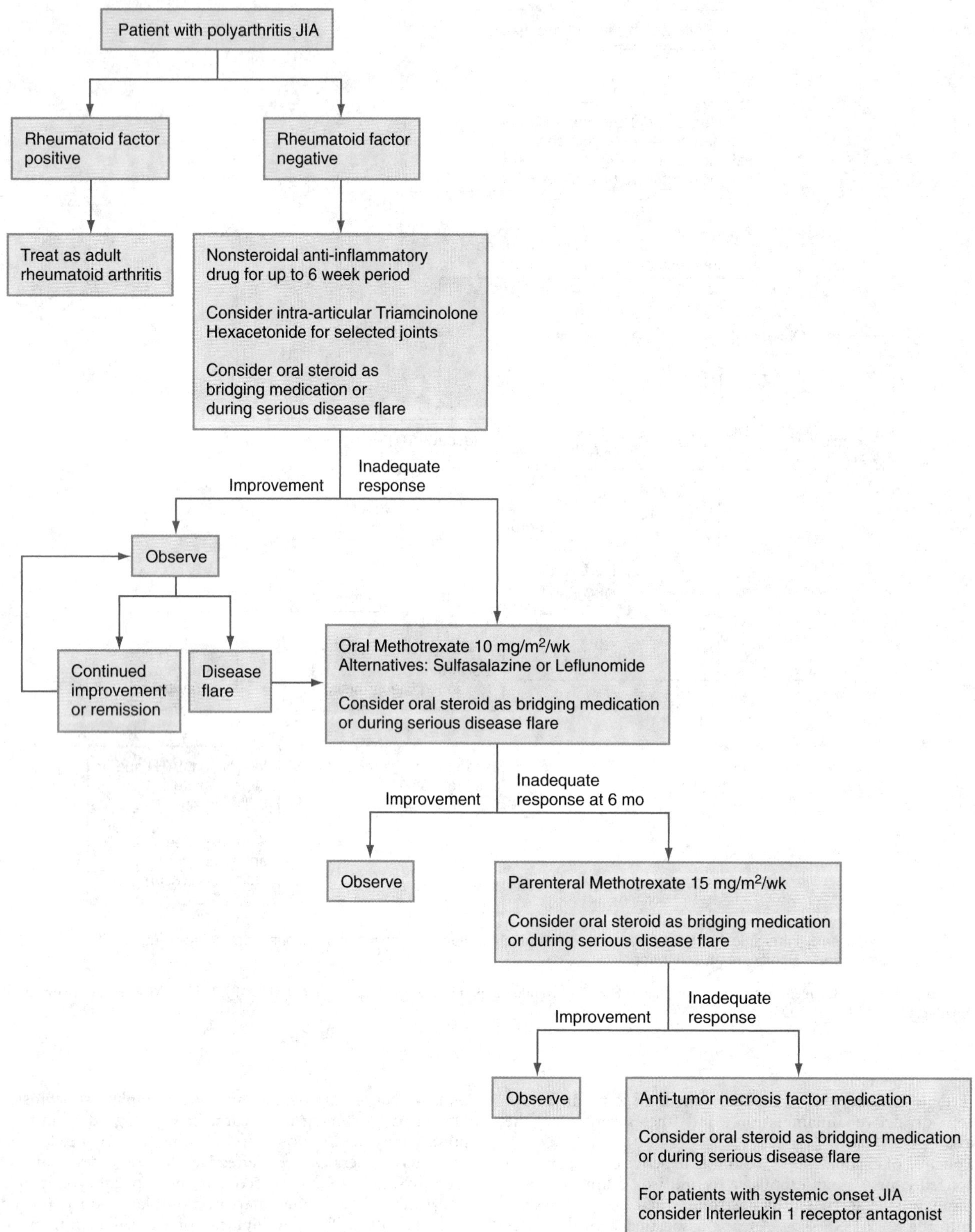

Figure 154-11. Algorithm for medical treatment of polyarthritis in juvenile idiopathic arthritis (JIA). (From Hashkes PJ, Laxer RM: Medical treatment of juvenile idiopathic arthritis. *JAMA* 2005;294:1671–1684.)

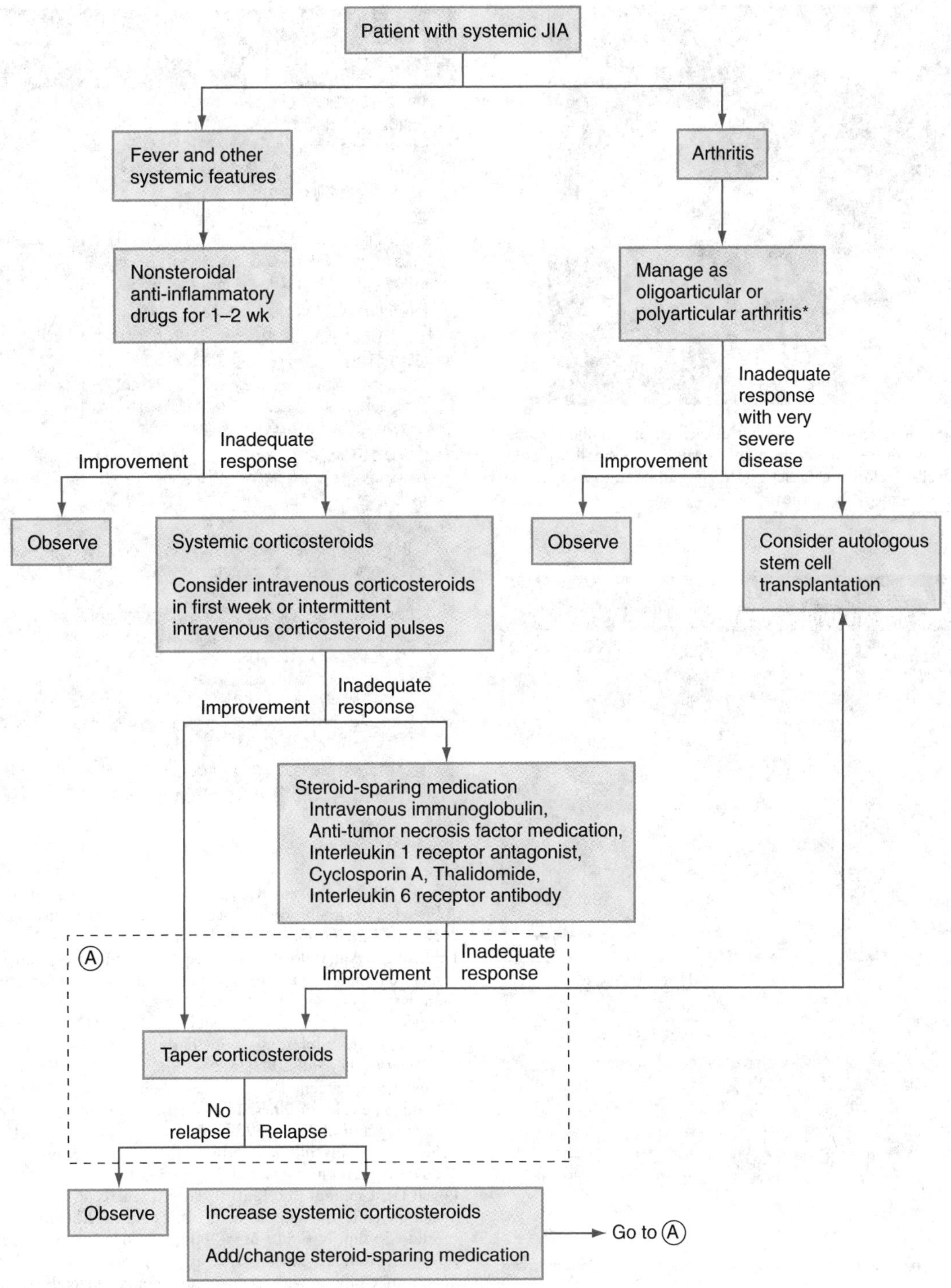

Figure 154-12. Algorithm for medical treatment of systemic arthritis in juvenile idiopathic arthritis (JIA). (From Hashkes PJ, Laxer RM: Medical treatment of juvenile idiopathic arthritis. *JAMA* 2005;294:1671–1684.)

steroid injection, appropriate splinting, and a physical therapy program to allow stretching of affected tendons.

Psychosocial adaptation may be moderately or severely affected. Studies from Scandinavia and the United States indicate that, compared with control subjects, a significant number of these children have problems with lifetime adjustments and employment. Disability not directly associated with arthritis may continue into young adulthood in as many as 20% of patients, together with continuing chronic pain syndromes in a similar frequency. Psychologic complications, including problems with school attendance and socialization, may respond to counseling by mental health professionals. Severe psychosocial disability and family disruption are probably less prevalent than previously thought.

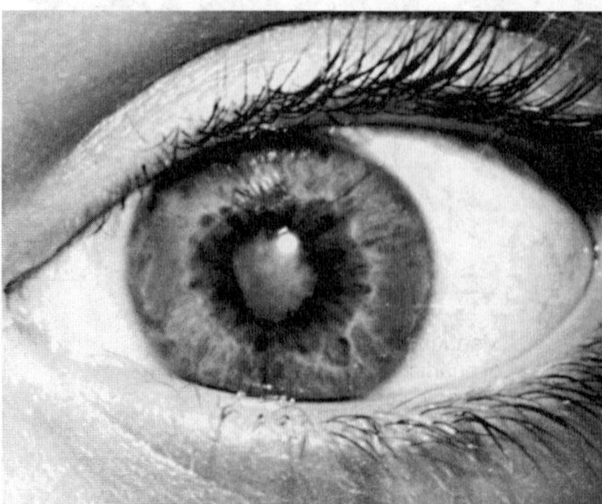

Figure 154-13. Chronic anterior uveitis, or iridocyclitis, of juvenile rheumatoid arthritis. Extensive posterior synechiae have resulted in a small, irregular pupil. There is a well-developed cataract and early band keratopathy at the medial and lateral margins of the cornea.

TABLE 154-4. Characteristic Profile and Prognosis of 250 Children with Juvenile Rheumatoid Arthritis, by Type of Onset and Course Subtype

TYPE OF ONSET (N)	COURSE SUBTYPE (N)	PROFILE	CLINICAL PROGNOSIS
Polyarthritis (78)	RF seropositive (16)	Female Older age Hand-wrist involvement Erosions Nodules Unremitting	Poor
	ANA seropositive (38)	Female Young age	Good
	Seronegative (24)	Variable	Good
Oligoarthritis (121)	ANA seropositive (66)	Female Young age Chronic uveitis (iridocyclitis)	Excellent (except eyes)
	RF seropositive (8)	Polyarthritis Erosions Unremitting	Poor
	HLA-B27-positive (12)	Male Older age	Good
	Seronegative (35)	Variable	Excellent
Systemic disease (51)	Oligoarthritis (30)	Variable	Good
	Polyarthritis (21)	Erosions	Poor

ANA, antinuclear antibody; RF, rheumatoid factor.

From Cassidy JT, Levinson JE, Bass JC, et al: A study of classification criteria for a diagnosis of juvenile rheumatoid arthritis. *Arthritis Rheum* 1986;29:274–278. Reprinted with permission of Wiley-Liss, Inc., a subsidiary of John Wiley & Sons, Inc.

TABLE 154-5. Preliminary Diagnostic Guidelines for Macrophage Activation System (MAS) Complicating Systemic Juvenile Idiopathic Arthritis (S-JIA)

LABORATORY CRITERIA

1. Decreased platelet count (≤262 × 10^9/L)
2. Elevated levels of aspartate aminotransferase (>59 U/L)
3. Decreased white blood cell count (≤4.0 × 10^9/L)
4. Hypofibrinogenemia (≤2.5 g/L)

CLINICAL CRITERIA

1. Central nervous system dysfunction (irritability, disorientation, lethargy, headache, seizures, coma)
2. Hemorrhages (purpura, easy bruising, mucosal bleeding)
3. Hepatomegaly (≥3 cm below the costal arch)

HISTOPATHOLOGICAL CRITERION

Evidence of macrophage hemophagocytosis in the bone marrow aspirate

DIAGNOSTIC RULE

The diagnosis of MAS requires the presence of any 2 or more laboratory criteria or of any 2 or 3 or more clinical and/or laboratory criteria. A bone marrow aspirate for the demonstration of haemophagocytosis may be required only in doubtful cases.

RECOMMENDATIONS

The aforementioned criteria are of value only in patients with active S-JIA. The thresholds of laboratory criteria are provided by way of example only.

COMMENTS

1. The clinical criteria are probably more useful as classification criteria rather than as diagnostic criteria because they often occur late in the course of MAS and may be, therefore, of limited value for the early suspicion of the syndrome.
2. Other abnormal clinical features in S-JIA-associated MAS, not aforementioned, may include: nonremitting high fever, splenomegaly, generalized lymphoadenopathy, and paradoxical improvement of signs and symptoms of arthritis.
3. Other abnormal laboratory findings in S-JIA-associated MAS, not aforementioned, may include: anemia, erythrocyte sedimentation rate fall, elevated levels of alanine aminotransferase, increased bilirubin, presence of fibrin degradation products, elevated lactate dehydrogenase, hypertriglyceridemia, low sodium levels, decreased albumin, and hyperferritinemia.

From Ravelli A, Magni-Manzoni S, Pistorio A, et al: Preliminary diagnostic guidelines for macrophage activation syndrome complicating systemic juvenile idiopathic arthritis. *J Pediatr* 2005;146:598–604.

Avcin T, Tse SML, Schneider R, et al: Macrophage activation syndrome as the presenting manifestation of rheumatic diseases in childhood. *J Pediatr* 2006;148:683–686.

Edwards JCW, Szczepanski L, Szechinski J, et al: Efficacy of B-cell targeted therapy with rituximab in patients with rheumatoid arthritis. *N Engl J Med* 2004;350:2572–2581.

Genovese MC, Becker JC, Schiff M, et al: Abatacept for rheumatoid arthritis refractory to tumor necrosis factor β inhibition. *N Engl J Med* 2005; 353:1114–1123.

Hashkes PJ, Laxer RM: Medical treatment of juvenile idiopathic arthritis. *JAMA* 2005;294:1671–1684.

Ilowite NT: Current treatment of juvenile rheumatoid arthritis. *Pediatrics* 2002;109:109–115.

Klareskog L, van der Heijde D, de Jager JP: Therapeutic effect of the combination of etanercept and methotrexate compared with each treatment alone in patients with pheumatoid arthritis: Double-blind randomized controlled trial. *Lancet* 2004;363:675–680.

Kremer JM, Westhovens R, Leon M, et al: Treatment of rheumatoid arthritis by selective inhibition of T-cell activation with fusion protein CTLA4Ig. *N Engl J Med* 2003;149:1907–1914.

Lahdenne P, Vahasalo P, Honkanen V: Infliximab or etanercept in the treatment of children with refractory juvenile idiopathic arthritis: An open label study. *Ann Rheum Dis* 2003;62:245–247.

LeBovidge JS, Lavigne JV, Donenberg GR, et al: Psychological adjustment of children and adolescents with chronic arthritis: A meta-analytic review. *J Pediatric Psychol* 2003;28:29–39.

LeBovidge JS, Lavigne JV, Miller ML: Adjustment to chronic arthritis of childhood: The roles of illness-related stress and attitude toward illness. *J Pediatric Psychol* 2005; 30:273–286.

Lehman TJA: Juvenile idiopathic arthritis and HSP60 vaccination: Selective down-regulation? *Lancet* 2005;366:9–10.

Lovell DJ, Giannini EH, Reiff A, et al: Etanercept in children with polyarticular juvenile rheumatoid arthritis. Pediatric Rheumatology Collaborative Study Group. *N Engl J Med* 2000;342:763–769.

Lovell DJ, Reiff A, Jones OY, et al: Long-term safety and efficacy of etanercept in children with polyarticular-course juvenile rheumatoid arthritis. *Arth Rheumatol* 2006;54:1987–1994.

Manners PJ, Diepeveen DA: Prevalence of juvenile chronic arthritis in a population of 12-year-old children in urban Australia. *Pediatrics* 1996;98:84–90.

Mason T, Reed AM, Nelson AM, Thomas KB: Radiographic progression in children with polyarticular juvenile rheumatoid arthritis: A pilot study. *Ann Rheum Dis* 64:491–493.

The Medical Letter: Rituximab (*Rituxan*) for rheumatoid arthritis. *Med Lett* 2006;48:34–35.

Modesto C, Woo P, Garcia-Consuegra J, et al: Systemic onset juvenile chronic arthritis, polyarticular pattern and hip involvement as markers for a bad prognosis. *Clin Exp Rheumatol* 2001;19:211–217.

Mouy R, Stephan JL, Pillet P, et al: Efficacy of cyclosporin A in the treatment of macrophage activation syndrome in juvenile arthritis: Report of five cases. *J Pediatr* 1996;129:750–754.

O'Dell JR: Therapeutic strategies for rheumatoid arthritis. *N Engl J Med* 2004;350:2591–2602.

Olson JC: Juvenile idiopathic arthritis: An update. *Wisc Med J* 2003; 102:45–50.

Packham JC, Hall MA: Long-term follow-up of 246 adults with juvenile idiopathic arthritis: Functional outcome. *Rheumatology* 2002;41:1428–1435.

Pepmueller PH, Cassidy JT, Allen SH, et al: Bone mineralization and bone mineral metabolism in children with juvenile rheumatoid arthritis. *Arthritis Rheum* 1996;39:746–757.

Peterson LS, Mason T, Nelson AM, et al: Psychosocial outcomes and health status of adults who have had juvenile rheumatoid arthritis: A controlled, population-based study. *Arthritis Rheum* 1997;40:2235–2240.

Petty RE, Southwood TR, Manners P, et al: International League of Associations for Rheumatology (ILAR) Classification of Juvenile Idiopathic Arthritis: Second revision, Edmonton, 2001. *J Rheumatol* 2004;31:390–392.

Prahalad S, Ryan MH, Shear ES, et al: Twins concordant for juvenile rheumatoid arthritis. *Arthritis Rheum* 2000;43:2611–2612.

Ramanan AV, Rosenblum ND, Feldman BM, et al: Favorable outcome in patients with renal involvement complicating macrophage activation syndrome in systemic onset juvenile rheumatoid arthritis. *J Rheumatol* 2004;31:2068–2070.

Ravelli A: Macrophage activation syndrome. *Curr Opin Rheumatol* 2002;14:548–552.

Ravelli A, Magni-Manizoni S, Pistorio A, et al: Preliminary diagnostic guidelines for macrophage activation syndrome complicating systemic juvenile idiopathic arthritis. *J Pediatr* 2005;146:598–604.

Ravelli A, Martini A: Juvenile idiopathic arthritis. *Lancet* 2007;369:767–778.

Reiff A: The use of anakinra in juvenile arthritis. *Curr Rheum Reports* 2005;434–440.

Schwartz MM, Simpson P, Kerr KL, et al: Juvenile rheumatoid arthritis in African Americans. *J Rheumatol* 1997;24:1826–1829.

Silverman E, Mouy R, Spiegel L, et al: Leflunomide or methotrexate for juvenile rheumatoid arthritis. *N Engl J Med* 2005;352:1655–1666.

Spiegel LR, Schneider R, Lang BA, et al: Early predictors of poor functional outcome in systemic-onset juvenile rheumatoid arthritis: A multicenter cohort study. *Arthritis Rheum* 2000;43:2402–2409.

Villanueva J, Lee S, Giannini EH, et al: Natural killer cell dysfunction is a distinguishing feature of systemic onset juvenile rheumatoid arthritis and macrophage activation syndrome. *Arthritis Res Ther* 2005;7:R30–R37.

Walco GA, Varni JW, Ilowite NT: Cognitive-behavioral pain management in children with juvenile rheumatoid arthritis. *Pediatrics* 1992;89:1075–1079.

Wedderburn LR, Abinun M, Palmer P, et al: Autologous haematopietic stem cell transplantation in juvenile idiopathic arthritis. *Arch Dis Child* 2003; 88:201–205.

Wilkinson N, Jackson G, Gardner-Medwin J: Biologic therapies for juvenile arthritis. *Arch Dis Child* 2003;88:186–191.

Yamazawa K, Kodo K, Maeda J, et al: Hyponatremia, hypophosphatemia, and hypouricemia in a girl with macrophage activation syndrome. *Pediatrics* 2006;118:2557–2560.

Chapter 155 ■ Ankylosing Spondylitis and Other Spondyloarthropathies

Michael L. Miller and Ross E. Petty

The diseases collectively referred to as **spondyloarthropathies** include ankylosing spondylitis, the psoriatic arthritides, arthritis accompanying inflammatory bowel diseases, and chronic reactive arthritis following enteric or genitourinary tract infections. The term **enthesitis-related arthritis** is used to denote what has traditionally been called juvenile ankylosing spondylitis; psoriatic arthritis is considered distinct.

EPIDEMIOLOGY. Estimates of the prevalence of juvenile ankylosing spondylitis (JAS) range from 11 to 86/100,000 children, and of psoriatic arthritis from 10 to 15/100,000 children. JAS occurs most frequently in older boys, adolescents, and young adults. These disorders are frequently familial; the human leukocyte antigen-HLA-B27 is strongly associated with JAS (>90%) and is found in increased frequency in persons having spondyloarthropathies with inflammation of the axial skeleton.

Psoriatic arthritis is particularly common in young girls. The arthropathies of inflammatory bowel diseases and reactive arthritis are much less common in childhood. They can affect children of any age and are somewhat more common in boys.

PATHOGENESIS. The histologic appearance of the synovium in spondyloarthropathies is indistinguishable from that of other idiopathic chronic arthritides. Tenosynovitis may be present, and periostitis may occur. **Enthesitis** (inflammation at the sites of attachments of ligaments, tendons, fascias, and capsules to bone) is characterized by chronic inflammation and, in advanced disease, which is usually found in adults, by calcification of ligaments and fusion of joints.

Chronic reactive arthritis may follow enteric infection with nontyphoidal *Salmonella, Shigella, Yersinia enterocolitica, Campylobacter jejuni, Cryptosporidium parvum,* or *Giardia intestinalis,* or genitourinary tract infection with *Chlamydia trachomatis.* The cause of the other spondyloarthropathies is unknown. It is postulated that **molecular mimicry,** or the similarity between self antigens and bacterial antigens, permits the development of an autoimmune process in genetically predisposed individuals.

CLINICAL MANIFESTATIONS. The spondyloarthropathies are characterized by inflammation of joints of the axial skeleton as well as the limbs, by the presence of enthesitis, and by the absence of rheumatoid factor.

Juvenile Ankylosing Spondylitis. Early JAS is most frequently characterized by oligoarthritis and enthesitis. Joints of the legs are more frequently affected than those of the arms. Abnormalities of the axial skeleton including the sacroiliac joints are usually absent until later in the disease course, although loss of spinal flexibility may eventually be noted (Fig. 155-1). When few joints are affected during the 1st 6 mo of disease, hip joint arthritis is particularly suggestive of early JAS. **Enthesitis,** presenting as localized tenderness at characteristic tendinous locations around the foot and knee, is particularly common and has led to the description of a syndrome of seronegativity (absence of rheuma-

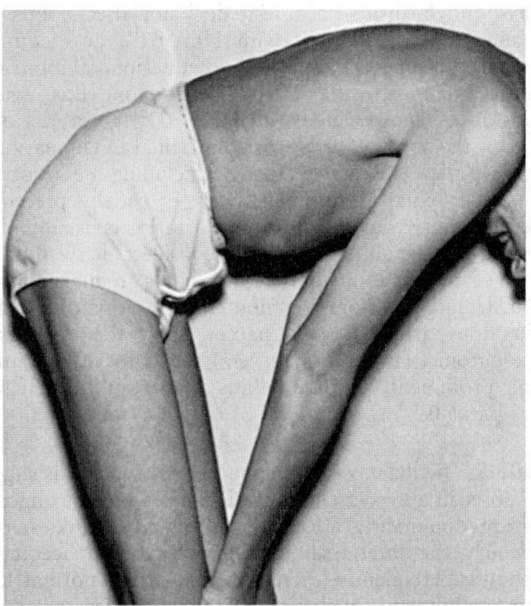

Figure 155-1. Loss of lumbodorsal spine mobility in a boy with ankylosing spondylitis: The lower spine remains straight when the patient bends forward.

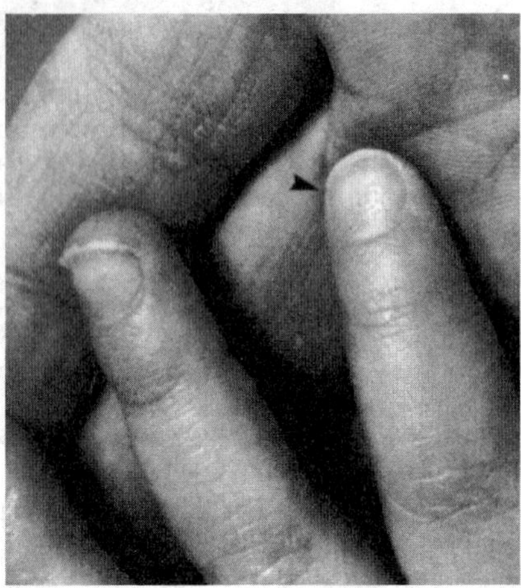

Figure 155-2. Nail pitting *(arrow)* and "sausage digit" (dactylitis) of the left index finger of a girl with juvenile psoriatic arthritis. (From Petty RE, Malleson P: Spondyloarthropathies of childhood. *Pediatr Clin North Am* 1986;33:1079–1096.)

toid factor), enthesitis, and arthritis (**SEA syndrome**), which is probably the most common initial presentation of JAS. The disease course may be characterized by long periods of apparent disease remission. Systemic symptoms such as low-grade fever and weight loss raise the possibility of occult inflammatory bowel disease.

Psoriatic Arthritis. The most common pattern of psoriatic arthritis is an oligoarthritis that affects large and small joints in an asymmetric pattern. Patients with psoriatic arthritis occasionally have symmetric distal interphalangeal joint disease, or HLA-B27-associated sacroiliitis, although most patients are HLA-B27-negative and do not have arthritis of the sacroiliac joints or lumbosacral spine. The presence of nail pitting (Fig. 155-2), dactylitis, onycholysis, or a family history of psoriasis supports the diagnosis of psoriatic arthritis in a child with oligoarthritis or polyarthritis.

Arthritis with Inflammatory Bowel Disease. Two patterns of arthritis complicate Crohn disease and ulcerative colitis. A polyarthritis affecting large and small joints, which reflects the activity of the intestinal inflammation, is most common and is not truly a spondylarthritis because it does not affect joints of the spine and is not associated with HLA-B27. Less commonly, arthritis of the sacroiliac joints and other peripheral joints occurs in a pattern similar to that in ankylosing spondylitis, which, in most instances, is associated with HLA-B27. Its severity is independent of the activity of the gastrointestinal inflammation.

Reactive Arthritis. Reactive arthritis, including the syndrome of arthritis, urethritis, and conjunctivitis, is usually preceded by enteric or urinary tract infection. The arthritis is usually oligoarticular and may be quite severe, with considerable swelling, pain, and even erythema. Joints of the lower limbs are most commonly affected. Unlike the more common clinical forms of self-limited postinfectious arthritis (see Chapter 156), the arthritis may become chronic, lasting from several weeks to years. Enthesitis may be prominent, and sacroiliitis may result in HLA-B27-positive patients.

DIAGNOSIS. The diagnosis of a spondyloarthropathy is suggested by the onset in an older child, particularly a boy, of oligoarthritis that predominantly affects the hips, knees, ankles, or feet (particularly the intertarsal joints), especially if accompanied by enthesitis. Frequently, there is a loss of the normal lumbar lordosis, inability to touch the toes while the legs are straight, and pain on palpating or compressing the pelvis. Ankylosing spondylitis is confirmed if there is radiographic evidence of sacroiliitis. Because radiographic changes seldom occur at onset, it may be difficult to differentiate spondylarthritis from oligoarticular juvenile rheumatoid arthritis (JRA) early in the disease course. The presence of synovitis in the upper extremities tends to be more common in patients with JRA than with spondyloarthropathies. In a child with chronic arthritis, the presence of erythema nodosum, pyoderma gangrenosum, significant fever, weight loss, or anorexia suggests inflammatory bowel disease. The acute onset of arthritis, a recent history of diarrhea, and symptoms of urethritis or conjunctivitis may suggest reactive arthritis. Psoriasis, nail changes (see Fig. 155-2), or a family history of psoriasis suggests the diagnosis of psoriatic arthritis in a child (often a young girl) with oligoarthritis or polyarthritis. Early differentiation among the spondyloarthropathies by laboratory or radiographic means is difficult. Sacroiliac joint change or enthesitis may be seen on technetium-99 bone scan, but results of this examination are often difficult to interpret in children and adolescents.

DIFFERENTIAL DIAGNOSIS. Back pain may occur in children with early ankylosing spondylitis but may also be caused by suppurative arthritis of the sacroiliac joint, osteomyelitis of the pelvis or spine, osteoid osteoma of the posterior elements of the spine, pelvic muscle pyomyositis, or malignancies such as osteogenic sarcoma, Ewing sarcoma, or leukemia (see Chapter 678.5). In addition, mechanical causes such as spondylolysis, spondylolisthesis, and Scheuermann disease should be considered. Back pain secondary to fibromyalgia usually affects the soft tissues of the upper back in a symmetric pattern, as well as other well-localized tender points.

Legg-Calvé-Perthes disease, slipped capital femoral epiphysis, and chondrolysis may also present with pain over the inguinal ligament and loss of internal rotation of the hip joint, similar to spondyloarthropathy.

LABORATORY FINDINGS. Laboratory evidence of systemic inflammation is often present at the onset of disease, with elevated erythrocyte sedimentation rate and mild increase in white blood cell count and platelet count. Rheumatoid factor is absent in all children with spondyloarthropathies. Antinuclear antibodies are absent except in children with psoriatic arthritis, in as many as 50% of whom antinuclear autoantibodies occur. HLA-B27 is present in >90% of children with JAS, but is probably not increased significantly in those with other types of spondylarthritis unless sacroiliitis or acute anterior uveitis is present.

Radiographic changes include periarticular osteoporosis, loss of sharp cortical margins in areas of enthesitis (which may eventually show erosions or bony spurs), indistinct margins and erosions of the sacroiliac joints, with sclerosis on the iliac side of the joint (Fig. 155-3), and, rarely, squaring of the corners of the vertebral bodies. The characteristic **bamboo spine** caused by calcification of ligaments that is so characteristic of advanced ankylosing spondylitis in adults is very rare in childhood.

TREATMENT. The aims of therapy are to control inflammation, minimize pain, and preserve function. These are accomplished by a combination of anti-inflammatory medications, physical therapy, and psychosocial support. Nonsteroidal anti-inflammatory drugs, such as naproxen (15–20 mg/kg/day), may be sufficient. It may be necessary to add sulfasalazine (up to 50 mg/kg/day; maximum: 3 g/day). Intra-articular triamcinolone hexacetonide is useful for controlling localized joint inflammation. In patients not responsive to these medications, oral or subcutaneous methotrexate may be considered. Etanercept or infliximab have been successful in adults with ankylosing spondylitis.

Exercises to maintain range of motion in the back, thorax, and affected joints should be instituted early in the disease course. Custom-fitted insoles are particularly useful in management of painful entheses around the feet.

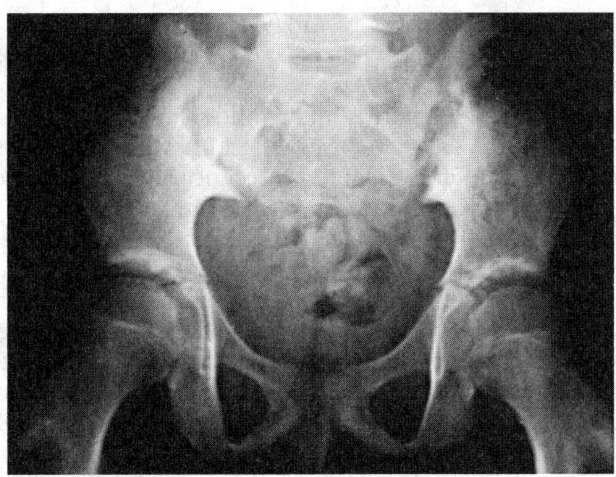

Figure 155-3. Well-developed sacroiliitis in a boy with ankylosing spondylitis. Both sacroiliac joints show extensive sclerosis, erosion of joint margins, and apparent widening of the joint space.

COMPLICATIONS. Acute iridocyclitis, or anterior uveitis, occurs in as many as 25% of patients with JAS. Chronic iridocyclitis similar to that in JRA occurs in approximately 15% of children with psoriatic arthritis. Aortic valve insufficiency is a rare but important complication of ankylosing spondylitis. Atlantoaxial subluxation has also been reported.

PROGNOSIS. There is little reliable information about long-term outcome of the spondyloarthropathies in childhood. These are chronic diseases with highly variable clinical courses. JAS is often characterized by long periods of active disease followed by long periods of inactivity. Most studies have shown that, over many years, the disease progresses to involve joints of the spine and sacroiliac joints and may cause fusion and significant disability. Poor physical function at onset and early hip involvement are predictors of severe chronic disease. Psoriatic arthritis tends to be a chronic unremitting disease. Reactive arthritis may be brief (several weeks or months), but may become chronic and progress to ankylosing spondylitis. In children with inflammatory bowel disease, the peripheral arthritis is usually controlled when the gastrointestinal inflammation is controlled; if the arthritis is associated with HLA-B27, the course tends to be more chronic.

Braun J, Brandt J, Listing J, et al: Treatment of active ankylosing spondylitis with infliximab: A randomized controlled multi centre trial. *Lancet* 2002;359:1187–1193.

Burgos-Vargas R: Juvenile onset spondyloarthropathies: Therapeutic aspects. *Ann Rheum Dis* 2002;61(Suppl 3):33–39.

Burgos-Vargas R, Vazquez-Mellado J: The early clinical recognition of juvenile-onset ankylosing spondylitis and its differentiation from juvenile rheumatoid arthritis. *Arthritis Rheum* 1995;38:835–844.

Dayer JM, Krane SM: Anti-TNF-β therapy for ankylosing spondylitis—a specific or nonspecific treatment? *N Engl J Med* 2002;346:1399–1400.

Foster HE, Cairns RA, Burnell RH, et al: Atlantoaxial subluxation in children with seronegative enthesopathy and arthropathy syndrome: 2 case reports and a review of the literature. *J Rheumatol* 1995;22:548–551.

Gorman JD, Sack KE, Davis JC Jr: Treatment of ankylosing spondylitis by inhibition of tumor necrosis factor β. *N Engl J Med* 2002;346:1349–1356.

McVeigh CM, Cairns AP: Diagnosis and management of alkylosing spondylitis. *BMJ* 2006;333:581–584.

Mielants H, Veys EM, Cuvelier C, et al: Gut inflammation in children with late onset pauciarticular juvenile chronic arthritis and evolution to adult spondyloarthropathy—a prospective study. *J Rheumatol* 1993;20: 1567–1572.

Petty RE, Southwood TR, Baum J et al: Revision of the proposed classification for juvenile idiopathic arthritis. Durban, 1997. *J Rheumatol* 1991;25:1991–1994.

Roberton DM, Cabral DA, Malleson PN, et al: Juvenile psoriatic arthritis: Follow-up and evaluation of diagnostic criteria. *J Rheumatol* 1996; 23:166–170.

Selvaag AM, Lien G, Sorskaar D, et al: Early disease course and predictors of disability in juvenile rheumatoid arthritis and juvenile spondyloarthropathy: A 3 year prospective study. *J Rheumatol* 2005;32:1122–1130.

Sheerin KA, Giannini EH, Brewer EJ Jr, et al: HLA-B27-associated arthropathy in childhood: Long-term clinical and diagnostic outcome. *Arthritis Rheum* 1988;31:1165–1170.

Shore A, Ansell BM: Juvenile psoriatic arthritis—an analysis of 60 cases. *J Pediatr* 1982;100:529–535.

Southwood TR, Petty RE, Malleson PN, et al: Psoriatic arthritis in children. *Arthritis Rheum* 1989;32:1007–1013.

Stamato T, Laxer RM, de Freitas C, et al: Prevalence of cardiac manifestations of juvenile ankylosing spondylitis. *Am J Cardiol* 1995;75:744–746.

Tse SML, Laxer RM: Juvenile spondyloarthropathy. *Curr Opin Rheumatol* 2003;15:374–79.

Chapter 156 ■ Reactive Arthritis

Michael L. Miller and James T. Cassidy

Arthritis associated with infection is classified as suppurative arthritis (see Chapter 684) or reactive arthritis. Although certain infectious organisms have been suspected but not proved to trigger juvenile rheumatoid arthritis (JRA) and other forms of chronic arthritis, bacteria, viruses, or spirochetes are associated with a transient arthritis that does not satisfy the classification criteria for JRA or satisfy criteria for distinct suppurative disease. **Reactive arthritis** follows an infection outside the joint, which is often in the gastrointestinal or genitourinary tract, and characteristically involves immune complexes containing nonviable components of the initiating organism in the inflamed joint. The course of reactive arthritis is variable, dependent on type, and may progress to a chronic spondyloarthropathy (see Chapter 155). **Postinfectious arthritis** is used to distinguish a sterile synovitis that follows curative treatment of suppurative arthritis.

PATHOGENESIS. Reactive arthritis typically follows enteric infection with *Salmonella, Shigella, Yersinia enterocolitica, Campylobacter jejuni, Cryptosporidium parvum,* or *Giardia intestinalis,* or genitourinary tract infection with *Chlamydia trachomatis* or *Ureaplasma.* Other prominent examples of reactive arthritis include the sterile arthritis of acute rheumatic fever caused by the group A streptococcus (see Chapter 168.1) or associated with infective endocarditis (see Chapter 437), and the tenosynovitis associated with *Neisseria gonorrhoeae* (see Chapter 191).

Reactive arthritis may represent an autoimmune response of **molecular mimicry** involving T lymphocytes that cross react with antigens (synovial, cartilaginous, glycosoaminoglycan) in the joints. Studies of synovial fluid from patients with reactive arthritis suggest that T cells may be more engaged pathogenically in promoting inflammation than in eliminating bacteria through cytotoxic mechanisms. The origin of the abnormal cells may be from outside the joint. Another possible mechanism is lymphocytic reactivity to bacterial DNA resident in synovium, perhaps as a by-product of an otherwise successfully cleared suppurative infection. Polymerase chain reaction amplification of joint fluids from patients with reactive arthritis has demonstrated residual bacterial DNA. A relationship to clinical characteristics of specific disorders, however, is not present. Several viruses (rubella, varicella-zoster, herpes simplex, cytomegalovirus) have been isolated from the joints of patients. Antigens from other viruses (hepatitis B, adenovirus 7) have been identified in immune complexes from joint tissue.

Specific HLA types may predispose to development of reactive arthritis, possibly by triggering autoreactive T lymphocytes in response to external antigens. Patients with reactive arthritis following enteric infections have also demonstrated persistent gut inflammation even after resolution of the gastrointestinal involvement, particularly in HLA-B27-positive individuals. Uveitis complicating reactive arthritis to *Yersinia enteritis* has also been associated with HLA-B27. Some children with reactive arthritis, often HLA-B27 positive, eventually develop a spondyloarthropathy, further suggesting that certain HLA specificities predispose to reactive arthritis.

CLINICAL MANIFESTATIONS. Bacterial enteritis caused by *Shigella, Salmonella, Yersinia,* and *Campylobacter* can be followed within days to several weeks by the development of mono- or polyarthritis, and sometimes enthesitis, in a syndrome similar to and overlapping with the spondyloarthropathies (see Chapter 155). Although the erythrocyte sedimentation rate (ESR) may be elevated, fever and leukocytosis are often absent. Urethritis and conjunctivitis occur occasionally in these syndromes. Postinfectious arthritis may follow by 1–2 mo less apparent illness, such as viral upper respiratory tract infections. The pain or joint swelling is usually transient, lasting <6 wk.

Certain viruses associated with arthritis (Table 156-1) may result in particular patterns of joint involvement. Rubella and hepatitis B virus typically affect the small joints; mumps and varicella often involve large joints, especially the knees. The hepatitis B **arthritis-dermatitis syndrome** is characterized by rash and an arthritis resembling that of serum sickness. **Rubella-associated arthropathy** follows natural rubella infection and, infrequently, rubella immunization. It typically occurs in young women, with an increased frequency with advancing age, and is uncommon in preadolescent children and in males. Arthralgias of the knees and hands usually begin within 7 days of onset of the rash or 10–28 days after immunization. **Parvovirus B19**, responsible for erythema infectiosum (fifth disease), can cause arthralgia, symmetric joint swelling, and morning stiffness in adults, particularly women, and less frequently in children. Arthritis occurs occasionally during cytomegalovirus infection, may occur during varicella infections, and is rare after Epstein-Barr virus infection. Varicella may also be complicated by suppurative arthritis, usually due to group A streptococcus. Human immunodeficiency virus is associated with an arthritis that resembles psoriatic arthritis more than JRA.

A nonsuppurative arthritis has been reported in children, usually adolescent boys, with severe truncal acne. Patients often have fever and persistent infection of the pustular skin lesions. Recurrent episodes may also be associated with a sterile myopathy and may last for several months. Infective endocarditis can be associated with arthralgia, arthritis, or signs suggestive of vasculitis, such as Osler nodes, Janeway lesions, and Roth spots. Reactive arthritis perhaps due to immune complexes, also occurs in children with *Neisseria gonorrhoeae, Neisseria meningitidis, Haemophilus influenzae* type b, and *Mycoplasma pneumoniae* infections.

Poststreptococcal arthritis may follow infection with either group A or group G streptococcus. Because valvular lesions have occasionally been documented by echocardiography after the acute illness, some clinicians consider this syndrome to be an incomplete form of acute rheumatic fever (see Chapter 168.1). Certain HLA-DRB1 types may predispose children to develop either poststreptococcal arthritis (*01) or acute rheumatic fever (*16). Poststreptococcal arthritis is oligoarticular, may affect the small and large joints, and persists for months, compared with the typical course of migratory polyarthritis of limited duration of rheumatic fever. The symptoms are usually mild and tend to resolve completely.

Transient synovitis (toxic synovitis) typically affects the hip, often after an upper respiratory tract infection (see Chapter 677.2). Boys from 3 to 10 yr of age are most commonly affected and have an acute onset of severe pain in the hip, with referred pain to the thigh or knee, and a course of ≈1 wk. The ESR and white blood cell count are usually normal. Radiologic or ultrasound examination may confirm widening of the joint space of the hip from an effusion. Aspiration of joint fluid is often necessary to exclude suppurative arthritis, and often results in a dramatic improvement in the pain. The cause of this relatively common syndrome is not known, but it is presumed to be a viral or postinfectious arthritis.

DIAGNOSIS. Acute arthritis affecting a single joint suggests suppurative arthritis; osteomyelitis may cause pain and an effusion in an adjacent joint, but is more often associated with focal bone pain over the site of the infection. The diagnosis of postinfectious arthritis is usually established by exclusion only after the arthritis has resolved. Arthritis associated with gastrointestinal symptoms or abnormal liver functions may be caused by infectious or autoimmune hepatitis. Arthritis or spondyloarthritis may occur in some children with inflammatory bowel disease, either Crohn disease or chronic ulcerative colitis (see Chapter 333). When two or more blood cell lines delineate a progressive decrease in concentration in a child with arthritis, parvovirus infection, macrophage activation (hemophagocytic) syndrome, and leukemia should be considered. Persistent arthritis (>6 wk) suggests the possibility of a rheumatic disease, including JRA, spondyloarthropathy, and systemic lupus erythematosus.

TREATMENT. No specific treatment is necessary for reactive or postinfectious arthritis, except for management of pain and functional limitations with nonsteroidal anti-inflammatory agents. If swelling or arthralgia recurs, further evaluation may be necessary to preclude active infection or evolving rheumatic disease.

COMPLICATIONS AND PROGNOSIS. Postinfectious arthritis following viral infections usually resolves without complications unless it is associated with involvement of other organs, such as encephalomyelitis. Reactive arthritis, especially after bacterial enteric infection or genitourinary tract infection with *Chlamydia trachomatis,* has the potential for evolving over time to a chronic arthritis and spondyloarthropathy (see Chapter 155). Children with reactive arthritis following enteric infections occasionally develop inflammatory bowel disease months to years after onset. Both uveitis and carditis have been reported in children diagnosed with reactive arthritis.

TABLE 156-1. Viruses Associated with Arthritis

Togaviruses	Parvovirus	Paramyxoviruses
Rubivirus	B19	Mumps
Rubella	Hepadnavirus	Enteroviruses
Alphaviruses	Hepatitis B	Echovirus
Ross River	Adenoviruses	Coxsackievirus B
Chikungunya	Adenovirus 7	Orthopoxviruses
O'nyong-nyong	Herpesviruses	Variola virus (smallpox)
Mayaro	Herpes simplex	Vaccinia virus
Sindbis	Cytomegalovirus	
Ockelbo	Epstein-Barr	
Pogosta	Varicella-zoster	

Adapted from Cassidy JT, Petty RE: Arthritis related to infection. In *Textbook of Pediatric Rheumatology*. Philadelphia, WB Saunders, 1995, p 503.

Ahmed S, Ayoub EM, Scornik JC, et al: Poststreptococcal reactive arthritis: Clinical characteristics and association with HLA-DR alleles. *Arthritis Rheum* 1998;41:1096–1102.

Ayoub EM, Majeed HA: Poststreptococcal reactive arthritis. *Curr Opin Rheumatol* 2000;12:306–310.

Chantler JK, Tingle AJ, Petty RE: Persistent rubella virus infection associated with chronic arthritis in children. *N Engl J Med* 1985;313:1117–1123.
Gerard HC, Wang Z, Wang GF, et al: Chromosomal DNA from a variety of bacterial species is present in synovial tissue from patients with various forms of arthritis. *Arthritis Rheum* 2001;44:1689–1697.
Goedvolk CA, von Rosenstiel IA, Bos AP: Immune complex associated complications in the subacute phase of meningococcal disease: Incidence and literature review. *Arch Dis Child* 2003;88:927–930.
Hannu T, Mattila L, Siitonen A, et al: Reactive arthritis attributable to *Shigella* infection: A clinical and epidemiological nationwide study. *Ann Rheum Dis* 2005;64:594–598.
Huppertz HI, Sandhage K: Reactive arthritis due to *Salmonella enteritidis* complicated by carditis. *Acta Paediatr* 1994;83:1230–1231.
Mertz AK, Ugrinovic S, Lauster R, et al: Characterization of the synovial T cell response to various recombinant yersinia antigens in *Yersinia enterocolitica* triggered reactive arthritis. Heat-shock protein 60 drives a major immune response. *Arthritis Rheum* 1998;41:315–326.
Meza-Ortiz F: Giardiasis-associated arthralgia in children. *Arch Med Res* 2001;32:248–250.
Petty RE, Tingle AJ: Arthritis and viral infection. *J Pediatr* 1988;113:948–949.
Poggio TV, Orlando N, Galanternik L, et al: Microbiology of acute arthropathies among children in Argentina: *Mycoplasma pneumoniae* and *hominis* and *Ureaplasma urealyticum*. *Pediatr Infect Dis J* 1998;17:304–308.
Schaad UB: Reactive arthritis associated with *Campylobacter* enteritis. *Pediatr Infect Dis* 1982;1:328–332.
Tingle AJ, Allen M, Petty RE, et al: Rubella-associated arthritis. I. Comparative study of joint manifestations associated with natural rubella infection and RA 27/3 rubella immunization. *Ann Rheum Dis* 1986;45:110–114.
Yin Z, Braun J, Neure L, et al: Crucial role of interleukin-10/interleukin-12 balance in the regulation of the type 2 T-helper cytokine response in reactive arthritis. *Arthritis Rheum* 1997;40:1788–1797.

Chapter 157 ■ Systemic Lupus Erythematosus

Marisa S. Klein-Gitelman and Michael L. Miller

Systemic lupus erythematosus (SLE, or lupus), a rheumatic disease of unknown cause, is characterized by autoantibodies directed against self antigens, leading to inflammatory damage of many target organs including the joints, kidneys, blood-forming cells, and the central nervous system.

ETIOLOGY. The cause and disease mechanisms of lupus remain unknown. Many factors, including genetic predisposition, hormones, and environment, potentially trigger immune dysregulation. The hallmark of lupus is autoantibody production against many self antigens, particularly antinuclear antibodies (ANAs) to DNA and other nuclear antigens, such as ribosomes, small nuclear (anti-Sm) and cytoplasmic (anti-Ro, anti-La) ribonuclear proteins, platelets, coagulation factors, immunoglobulin, erythrocytes, and leukocytes. Elevated levels of autoantibodies, particularly anti–double-stranded DNA (anti-dsDNA) antibodies, are associated with circulating and tissue-bound immune complexes that lead to complement fixation and recruitment of inflammatory cells, culminating in tissue injury. Autoantibodies (ANA, anti-dsDNA, anti-Ro, anti-La, anti-Sm, anti-RNP, antiphospholipid antibody: in descending order of prevalence) may precede the onset of SLE by 9 yr, suggesting a presymptomatic state of autoimmunity.

Genetic predisposition to lupus is suggested by the high frequency (≈10%) in family members of ANA, hypergammaglobulinemia, and lupus or other autoimmune diseases. Depending on the racial and ethnic group, certain HLA types (HLA-B8, HLA-DR2, and HLA-DR3) occur with increased frequency among patients with lupus. Congenital complement deficiencies also predispose to SLE.

EPIDEMIOLOGY. The incidence of lupus is not known but varies by location and ethnicity. Prevalence rates of 4–250/100,000 have been reported, with increased prevalence among Native Americans, Asians, Polynesians, Hispanics, and African-Americans. Disease onset before 8 yr of age is unusual, although lupus has been diagnosed even in the 1st yr of life. Female predominance varies from 4 : 1 before puberty to 8 : 1 afterward.

PATHOGENESIS. Lupus is characterized by production of autoantibodies and polyclonal activation of B lymphocytes that results in elevated immunoglobulin levels, which also contribute to elevated autoantibody levels. The mechanism for polyclonal activation is not understood. Possible causes include nonspecific responses to antigenic stimuli such as viral agents, or following loss of either B-cell immune tolerance to self antigens or suppressor T-cell function. T cells from patients with lupus are hyperreactive, resisting anergy and apoptosis, which is regulated by several proteins including *fas* and *bcl*-2. Dysregulation of apoptosis in lupus may lead to the persistence of self-reactive lymphocytes that normally undergo apoptosis. Abnormalities in macrophages and other cells of the innate immune system include abnormal activation of interferon and toll-like receptors. Studies of families with multiple affected members have identified candidate susceptibility genes, primarily on chromosome 1.

Other mechanisms may have a role in amplifying the manifestations of lupus. Defects in macrophage phagocytosis and processing of immune complexes have been described. The effects of sex hormones may be responsible for the predominance of females with lupus; one study of postpubertal boys and girls with lupus found higher follicle-stimulating hormone and luteinizing hormone levels and lower free androgen levels. Nonetheless, estrogen-containing contraceptives do not produce flares of SLE or other adverse events. Lupus has been associated with complement abnormalities including C1q, C2, and C4 deficiency; a high incidence of C4 null alleles; and abnormal complement receptors. Exposure to ultraviolet rays in sunlight exacerbates lupus manifestations, perhaps through damage to skin cells, resulting in release of nuclear material, such as DNA, which complexes with circulating anti-DNA antibodies.

Fibrinoid deposits resulting from changes in collagen fibers and ground substance are found in blood vessel walls of affected organs. The parenchyma may contain **hematoxylin bodies,** most likely representing degenerated cell nuclei. Rheumatoid nodules and granulomas are sometimes also found in affected tissues.

CLINICAL MANIFESTATIONS. Children with lupus present with diverse and often severe manifestations (Table 157-1). Children

TABLE 157-1. Presenting Manifestations of Systemic Lupus Erythematosus

TARGET ORGAN	MANIFESTATIONS
Constitutional	Fatigue, anorexia, weight loss, prolonged fever, lymphadenopathy
Musculoskeletal	Arthralgias, arthritis
Skin	Malar rash, discoid lesions, livedo reticularis, vasculitis
Renal	Glomerulonephritis, hypertension, nephrotic syndrome, renal failure
Cardiovascular	Pericarditis (cardiac tamponade)
Neurologic	Seizures, psychosis, stroke, cerebral venous thrombosis, pseudotumor cerebri, aseptic meningitis, chorea, global cognitive deficits, mood disorders, transverse myelitis, peripheral neuritis (mononeuritis multiplex)
Pulmonary	Pleuritic pain, pulmonary hemorrhage
Hematologic	Coombs-positive hemolytic anemia, anemia of chronic disease, thrombocytopenia, leukopenia
Laboratory	Elevated ESR and CRP; decreased C3 or C4; positive ANA and anti–double-stranded DNA antibodies

ANA, antinuclear antibody; CRP, C-reactive protein; ESR, erythrocyte sedimentation rate.

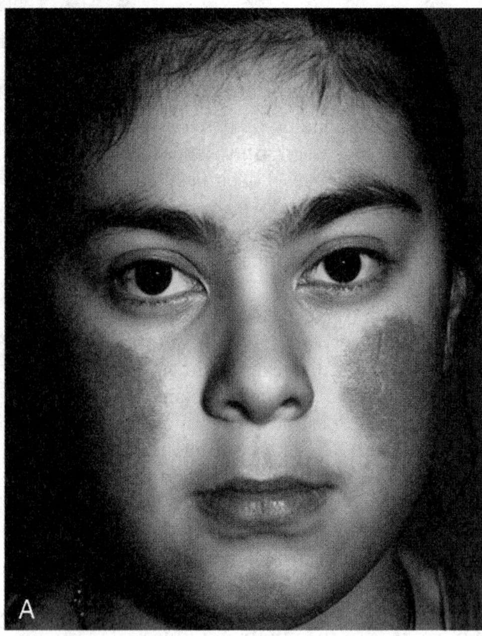

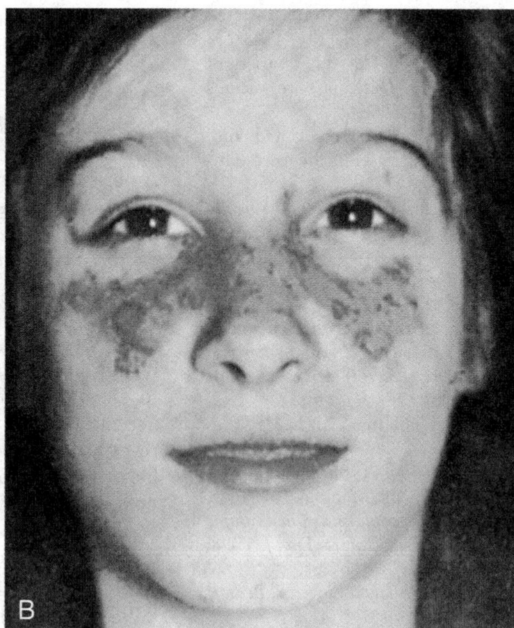

Figure 157-1. The butterfly rash of systemic lupus erythematosus. The rash can vary from an erythematous blush *(A)* to thickened epidermis to scaly patches *(B)*.

most frequently present with fever, fatigue, hematologic abnormalities, arthralgia or arthritis, rash, and renal disease. Symptoms may be intermittent or persistent.

Cutaneous manifestations are frequently present. The characteristic **malar or butterfly rash** involves the cheeks and nasal bridge and varies from an erythematous blush to thickened epidermis to scaly patches (Fig. 157-1). Rashes may be photosensitive and extend to all sun-exposed areas. Mucous membrane changes ranging from vasculitic erythema to ulcers occur, particularly on palatal and nasal mucosa (Fig. 157-2). Discoid lesions are unusual in childhood and occur more frequently as a manifestation of lupus than as **discoid lupus erythematosus (DLE)** alone. Only 2–3% of all DLE occurs in childhood. Other cutaneous manifestations include vasculitic-appearing erythematous macular eruptions (particularly on fingers, palms, and soles), purpura, livedo reticularis (Fig. 157-3), and Raynaud phenomenon. Less common findings include sub-acute psoriasiform or annular skin lesions, bullous or urticarial lesions, and alopecia.

Musculoskeletal findings include arthralgia, arthritis, tendinitis, and myositis. Deforming arthritis is unusual, although hand arthritis can lead to ligament damage and severely lax joints. Osteonecrosis of bone is common and presumed to be secondary to vasculopathy or corticosteroid treatment.

Serositis can affect pleural, pericardial, and peritoneal surfaces. Hepatosplenomegaly and lymphadenopathy are often found. Other gastrointestinal manifestations, most often resulting from vasculitis, include pain, diarrhea, melena, infarction, inflammatory bowel disease, and hepatitis. Serositis may mimic an acute abdomen. Cardiac involvement may affect all cardiac tissues with manifestations that include valvular thickening and verrucous endocarditis (Libman-Sacks disease), cardiomegaly, myocarditis, conduction abnormalities, heart failure, and coronary artery vasculitis and thrombosis. Pulmonary manifestations include acute pulmonary hemorrhage, pulmonary infiltrates (sometimes with superimposed infection), and chronic fibrosis. Early cardiopulmonary disease is often clinically silent and may be detected by annual echocardiogram and pulmonary function tests with diffusing capacities.

Figure 157-2. Erythematous lesion involving the hard palate in a patient with systemic lupus erythematosus. (From Moschella S, Hurley H [eds]: *Dermatology,* 3rd ed. Philadelphia, WB Saunders, 1992.)

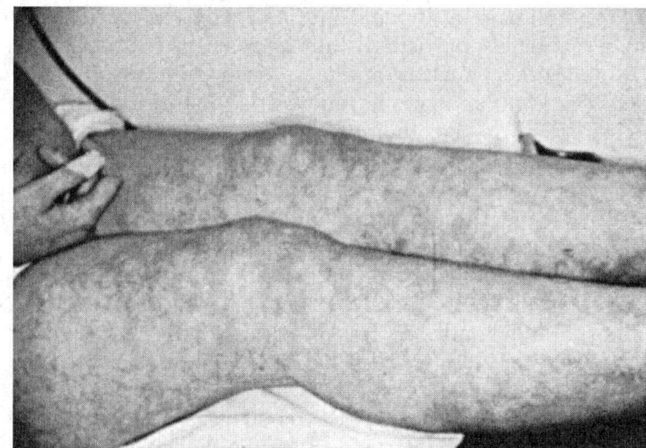

Figure 157-3. Livedo reticularis. Lacelike bluish, purplish, or erythematous discoloration of the skin indicating vascular instability. (From Moschella S, Hurley H [eds]: *Dermatology,* 3rd ed. Philadelphia, WB Saunders, 1992.)

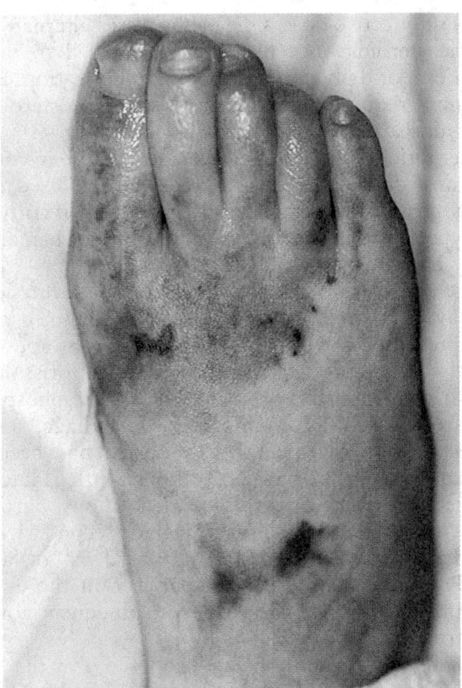

Figure 157-4. A 12 yr old girl with systemic lupus erythematosus and antiphospholipid antibodies with painful cutaneous vasculitis of the right foot. Arterial thrombosis documented by angiography resulted in cyanosis of the large toe. Symptoms resolved with treatment with heparin and corticosteroids.

Neurologic manifestations involve both the central and peripheral nervous system. Many patients with lupus experience memory loss or other cognitive dysfunction in their disease course. Neuropsychiatric manifestations can be severe, and patients may fulfill diagnostic criteria for psychosis. MRI and CT images may be normal although abnormal single-photon emission CT images may be present. The occurrence of arterial or venous thrombosis (Fig. 157-4), suggesting antiphospholipid antibody syndrome, can occur in the brain or any organ and is associated with recurrent fetal loss, livedo reticularis, thrombocytopenia, and Raynaud phenomenon. Thrombotic events can also be associated with the presence of lupus anticoagulant and acquired, activated protein C resistance.

Renal disease is manifest by hypertension, peripheral edema, retinal vascular changes, and other clinical manifestations associated with electrolyte abnormalities, nephrosis, or acute renal failure (see Chapter 514).

DIAGNOSIS. The diagnosis of lupus is confirmed by the combination of clinical and laboratory manifestations revealing multisystem disease. The presence of 4 of 11 criteria (Table 157-2) serially or simultaneously strongly suggests the diagnosis. Patients suspected to have lupus who demonstrate fewer than 4 criteria should receive appropriate medical treatment. In 1997, revised criteria replaced the LE prep with anticardiolipin antibodies or a positive test for lupus anticoagulant. A positive ANA test is not required for diagnosis; absence of ANA in lupus is very rare. Hypocomplementemia is not diagnostic, and extremely low levels or absence of total hemolytic complement suggests the possibility of complement component deficiency (see Chapter 133). Renal biopsy is useful to confirm the diagnosis of lupus nephritis and to guide treatment.

DIFFERENTIAL DIAGNOSIS. Because of its possible manifestations, lupus must be considered in the differential diagnosis of many problems, ranging from fevers of unknown origin to arthralgias, anemia, and nephritis. The differential diagnosis depends on the presenting affected organ and includes systemic-onset juvenile rheumatoid arthritis, acute poststreptococcal glomerulonephritis, acute rheumatic fever, infective endocarditis, leukemia, immune thrombocytopenic purpura, and idiopathic hemolytic anemia. The initial presentation may be atypical such as parotitis, abdominal pain, transverse myelitis, or dizziness. Lupus should be considered in patients with multiorgan symptoms, especially if there are hematologic or urinalysis abnormalities.

Drug-induced lupus is a lupus-like disease that is precipitated by exposure to certain drugs, notably many anticonvulsants, sulfonamides, and antiarrhythmic agents. The finding of antihistone antibodies in many of these patients suggests antigenic similarities between these drugs and histone proteins leading to cross-reactive immune reactions. The typical symptoms of fever, rash, and pleuropericardial disease typically abate with discontinuation of the drug. The serum complement usually remains normal and complications, including renal disease, are rare.

TABLE 157-2. 1997 Revised Classification Criteria for Systemic Lupus Erythematosus

CRITERION*	DEFINITION
Malar rash	Fixed erythema, flat or raised, over the malar eminences, tending to spare the nasolabial folds
Discoid rash	Erythematous raised patches with adherent keratotic scaling and follicular plugging; atrophic scarring may occur in older lesions
Photosensitivity	Rash as a result of unusual reaction to sunlight (elicited by patient history or physician observation)
Oral ulcers	Oral or nasopharyngeal ulceration, usually painless, observed by a physician
Arthritis	Non-erosive arthritis involving two or more peripheral joints, characterized by tenderness, swelling, or effusion
Serositis	Pleuritis: convincing history of pleuritic pain or rub heard by a physician or evidence of pleural effusion
	or
	Pericarditis: documented by ECG or rub or evidence of pericardial effusion
Renal disorder	Persistent proteinuria >0.5 g/day or >3-plus (+++) if quantitation not performed
	or
	Cellular casts: may be red blood cell, hemoglobin, granular, tubular, or mixed
Neurologic disorder	Seizures: in the absence of offending drugs or known metabolic derangements (e.g., uremia, ketoacidosis, or electrolyte imbalance)
	or
	Psychosis: in the absence of offending drugs or known metabolic derangements (e.g., uremia, ketoacidosis, or electrolyte imbalance)
Hematologic disorder	Hemolytic anemia, with reticulocytosis
	or
	Leukopenia: <4,000/mm³ total on two or more occasions
	or
	Lymphopenia: <1,500/mm³ on two or more occasions
	or
	Thrombocytopenia: <100,000/mm³
Immunologic disorder	Anti-DNA antibody to native DNA in abnormal titer
	or
	Anti-Smith: presence of antibody to Smith nuclear antigen
	or
	Positive finding of antiphospholipid antibodies based on (1) an abnormal serum level of IgG or IgM anticardiolipin antibodies; (2) a positive test result for lupus anticoagulant using a standard method, or (3) a false-positive serologic test for syphilis known to be positive for at least 6 mo and confirmed by *Treponema pallidum* immobilization or fluorescent treponemal antibody absorption test (FTA-ABS), Standard methods should be used in testing for the presence of antiphospholipid.
Antinuclear antibody	An abnormal titer of antinuclear antibody by immunofluorescence or an equivalent assay at any time and in the absence of drugs known to be associated with "drug-induced lupus syndrome"

*The proposed classification is based on 11 criteria. For the purpose of identifying patients in clinical studies, a person shall be said to have SLE if any 4 or more of the 11 criteria are present, serially or simultaneously, during any interval of observation. (From Tan EM, Cohen AS, Fries JF, et al: The 1982 revised criteria for the classification of systemic lupus erythematosus. *Arthritis Rheum* 1982;25:1271–1277.)

An approved modification deletes the positive LE cell preparation from the immunologic disorder criteria and substitutes the presence of a biologic false-positive test for syphilis. (From Hochberg MC: Updating the American College of Rheumatology revised criteria for the classification of systemic lupus erythematosus. *Arthritis Rheum* 1997;40:1725. Reprinted with permission of Wiley-Liss, Inc., a subsidiary of John Wiley & Sons, Inc.)

TABLE 157-3. Conditions Associated with Antinuclear Antibodies (ANAs)

Systemic lupus erythematosus	Scleroderma
Drug-induced lupus	Infectious mononucleosis
Juvenile arthritis	Chronic active hepatitis
Juvenile dermatomyositis	Hyperextensibility
Vasculitis syndromes	

LABORATORY FINDINGS. Elevated ANA titers are often present in children with active lupus. This is an excellent screening tool, although ANA can be found without any disease or can be associated with rheumatic and other conditions (Table 157-3). Levels of anti–double-stranded DNA, which are more specific for lupus, often reflect the degree of serologic disease activity. Serum levels of total hemolytic complement (CH_{50}), C3, and C4 are decreased in active disease and provide a second measure of disease activity. Anti-Smith antibody, found specifically in patients with lupus, does not measure disease activity. When present, anti-Ro and anti-La antibodies are rarely associated with Sjögren syndrome in pediatric patients with SLE. Many autoantibodies can be found (Table 157-4). Hypergammaglobulinemia is common but nonspecific.

The **lupus anticoagulant,** found in ⅔ of patients, is associated with antiphospholipid antibodies. It reacts with the cardiolipin used in the serologic test for syphilis and may result in a false-positive test, and also reacts with the phospholipid reagent used in the partial thromboplastin time (PTT), causing an elevated result. It is associated with increased incidence of deep venous thrombosis and neurologic disease including stroke and psychosis.

TREATMENT. The treatment regimen depends on the affected target organs and disease severity. Sun exposure should be minimized and include use of a sunscreen. Patients are treated to promote clinical well-being, using serologic markers of disease activity as guidelines, including serum complement levels. Nonsteroidal anti-inflammatory agents, used to treat arthralgia and arthritis, are used with caution because patients with lupus are more susceptible to hepatotoxicity. Hydroxychloroquine is often used to treat mild manifestations including skin lesions, fatigue, arthritis, and arthralgia. Hydroxychloroquine may also reduce the risk of thromboembolic disease and lowers lipid levels.

Patients with thrombosis and antiphospholipid antibodies or a lupus anticoagulant should receive anticoagulant medication at least until lupus is in remission. The length of therapy is controversial. Low molecular weight heparin is the anticoagulant of choice; warfarin can also be used.

Corticosteroids control symptoms and autoantibody production in lupus. Treatment with corticosteroids has improved kidney disease and the rate of survival. Corticosteroids can make the diagnosis and treatment of tuberculosis difficult; all patients should have PPD and control skin tests, when possible, before corticosteroids are initiated. The optimal dose and route of administration of corticosteroids are controversial. Patients with systemic disease are often started on 1–2 mg/kg/24 hr of oral prednisone in divided daily doses. When complement levels increase to within the normal range, the dose is carefully tapered to the lowest effective dose. One method uses alternate-day high-dose corticosteroids once disease is controlled to prevent the adverse effects of daily corticosteroid administration. Severely ill patients may require pulse intravenous corticosteroid therapy (30 mg/kg/dose, maximum 1 g/day, given over 60 min, for 3 days). Intermittent high-dose intravenous therapy in combination with low-dose daily oral corticosteroids has been used as an alternative regimen in some centers. Adverse effects of corticosteroids include hypertension, gastritis, cataracts, osteopenia, and cushingoid body habitus.

Patients with severe disease may require cytotoxic therapy. Pulse intravenous cyclophosphamide has maintained renal function and prevented progression in patients with lupus nephritis, particularly diffuse proliferative glomerulonephritis; the optimal length of therapy remains controversial. Cyclophosphamide is used to treat vasculitis, pulmonary hemorrhage, and central nervous system involvement. Azathioprine has been used to prevent renal disease progression, although little is known about the long-term sequelae of cytotoxic medications, particularly in children with lupus. Adverse effects include secondary infections, gonadal dysfunction, and possibly increased risk of later malignancies. Prepubertal children, compared with those who have entered puberty, may be at less risk for subsequent gonadal dysfunction from cytotoxic agents.

Other interventions are being proposed for the treatment of lupus. Methotrexate, cyclosporine, and mycophenolate mofetil are used as steroid-sparing agents. Mycophenolate is an alternative to cyclophosphamide for some types of lupus nephritis. Autologous stem cell and allogeneic bone marrow transplantation for patients with severe, persistent disease are undergoing clinical trials in adult and pediatric patients with lupus. Biologic agents that target cytokine production, in particular, anti-CD20/22 monoclonal antibodies, are also being studied. Other potential therapies include rituximab (anti-CD20 monoclonal antibody), as well as blockade of interleukin 6 (IL-6), T cell co-stimulatory molecules and BlyS, a B-cell activating factor.

The extent of renal involvement may be out of proportion to findings on urinalysis; renal biopsy for staging can help determine whether an immunosuppressive agent such as cyclophosphamide needs to be added to a corticosteroid regimen. Biopsy findings according to the World Health Organization classification, which was modified in 2004, correlate with morbidity and mortality. **Class I** is minimal mesangial change without proteinuria or hematuria. **Class II** demonstrates mesangial proliferation. Both Class I and Class II are associated with excellent prognosis. **Class III (focal proliferative glomerulonephritis)** shows involvement of <50% of glomeruli having focal, segmental proliferation of cells near capillaries with necrosis and lymphocytic infiltration, and is often associated with chronic renal disease. **Class IV (diffuse segmental or global proliferative glomerulonephritis)** exhibits a majority of each glomeruli affected by cellular infiltration, mesangial cellular proliferation, and crescent formation corresponding to scarring and has been correlated with increased risk for developing end-stage renal disease in adulthood; intravenous pulse cyclophosphamide can decrease this risk. **Class V disease (membranous glomerulonephritis)** shows thickened capillary walls on light microscopy and subepithelial deposits on electron microscopy along the basement membrane. These changes have been associated with proteinuria, which can occur with the other types of lupus nephritis, and variable chronic renal disease that is often poorly responsive to treatment. **Class VI** is advanced sclerosing nephritis and demonstrates diffuse, chronic damage suggesting progression to renal failure.

The most important aspect of management of lupus is meticulous and frequent re-evaluation of clinical signs and laboratory data, especially for renal and serologic flares of disease. Prompt recognition and treatment of disease flare is essential to patient outcome. Lupus is a lifelong illness, and patients require monitoring indefinitely.

TABLE 157-4. Autoantibodies Often Found in Systemic Lupus Erythematosus

ANTIBODY	MANIFESTATION
Coombs antibodies	Hemolytic anemia
Antiphospholipid antibodies	Antiphospholipid antibody syndrome
Lupus anticoagulant	Coagulopathy (thrombosis)
Antithyroid antibodies	Hypothyroidism
Antiribosomal P antibody	Lupus cerebritis

COMPLICATIONS. The major causes of death in patients with lupus currently include infection, nephritis, central nervous system disease, pulmonary hemorrhage, and myocardial infarction, which may be a result of chronic but not suppressive corticosteroid administration in the setting of immune complex disease. Lupus nephritis is present in most children with lupus; those children with clinically significant nephritis show evidence of progression within 2 yr after onset of symptoms. Persistent leukopenia, anemia, or thrombocytopenia may develop.

PROGNOSIS. Untreated lupus may be followed by spontaneous remission, years of smoldering disease, or rapid death. The natural history of lupus is highly variable, ranging from acute, life-threatening disease to many years of symptoms. Childhood lupus was initially viewed as a uniformly fatal disease. Early diagnosis and treatment tailored to the particular problems of each individual patient greatly improves the course of the disease and, currently, the 5-yr survival rate is >90%. A proportion of patients die of complications of the disease in late adulthood.

157.1 • Neonatal Lupus

Lupus in newborns results from maternal transfer of IgG autoantibodies, usually anti-Ro/SSA or anti-La/SSB, between the 12th and 16th wk of gestation. Only a small percentage of offspring of mothers with autoantibodies to Ro and/or La develop disease. Maternal or fetal factors must have an added role. Symptoms usually derive from a single organ, although multiple organ involvement may occur and include congenital heart block, cutaneous lesions, hepatitis, thrombocytopenia, neutropenia, and pulmonary and neurologic disease. Cutaneous lesions occur after ultraviolet exposure at about 6 wk of life and last 3–4 mo. The rash most frequently occurs on the face and scalp, and 25% of rashes scar. Treatment is supportive. Most manifestations resolve, although congenital heart block is permanent and often requires cardiac pacing, either after birth or, when detected and severe, antenatally. Corticosteroid treatment of the pregnant mother after heart block is detected early in utero and postnatal steroids may be effective. Even infants of asymptomatic mothers with lupus may have slightly prolonged PR intervals. Cardiomyopathy is a rare serious sequela, sometimes requiring heart transplantation.

Neonatal lupus must be distinguished from **neonatal onset multisystem inflammatory disease,** a rare syndrome characterized by fever, rash, arthropathy, chronic meningitis, seizures, uveitis, and lymphadenopathy. This autoinflammatory syndrome, resulting from defective IL-1 regulation in the innate immune system, is difficult to treat and requires long-term immunomodulation (see Chapter 162). Anakinra, an IL-1 antagonist, has been very successful in the treatment of a small cohort of these patients.

Al-Abbad AJ, Cabral DA, Sanatani S, et al: Echocardiography and pulmonary function testing in childhood onset systemic lupus erythematosus. *Lupus* 2001;10:32–37.

Arbuckle MR, McClain MT, Rubertone MV, et al: Development of autoantibodies before the clinical onset of systemic lupus erythematous. *N Engl J Med* 2003;349:1526–1533.

Bader-Meunier B, Armengaud JB, Haddad E, et al: Initial presentation of childhood-onset systemic lupus erythematosus: A French multicenter study. *J Pediatr* 2005;146:648–653.

Burt RK, Traynor A, Statkute L, et al: Nonmyeloablative hematopoietic stem cell transplantation for systemic lupus erythematosus. *JAMA* 2006;295: 527–535.

Cervera R, Khamashita MA, Font J, et al: Morbidity and mortality in systemic lupus erythematosus during a 10-year period. *Medicine* 2003;82:299–308.

Cimaz R, Spence DL, Hornberger L, et al: Incidence and spectrum of neonatal lupus erythematosus: A prospective study of infants born to mothers with anti-Ro autoantibodies. *J Pediatr* 2003;142:678–683.

D'Cruz DP: Systemic lupus erythematosus. *BMJ* 2006;332:890–894.

Fine DM: Pharmacological therapy of lupus nephritis. *JAMA* 2005;293: 3053–3060.

Ginzler EM, Dooley MA, Aranow C, et al: Mycophenolate mofetil or intravenous cyclophosphamide for lupus nephritis. *N Engl J Med* 2005;353:2219–2228.

Hagelberg S, Lee Y, Bargman J, et al: Longterm followup of childhood lupus nephritis. *J Rheumatol* 2002;29:2635–2642.

Hochberg MC: Updating the American College of Rheumatology revised criteria for the classification of systemic lupus erythematosus. *Arthritis Rheum* 1997;40:1725.

Iqbal S, Sher MR, Good RA, et al: Diversity in presenting manifestations of systematic lupus erythematosus in children. *J Pediatr* 1999;135:500–505.

Lovell DJ, Bowyer SL, Solinger AM: Interleukin-1 blockade by anakinra improves clinical symptoms in patients with neonatal-onset multisystem inflammatory disease. *Arthritis Rheum* 2005;52:1283–1286.

Meyer O: Neonatal cutaneous lupus and congenital heart block: It's not all antibodies. *Lancet* 2003;362:1596–1597.

Perfumo F, Martini A: Lupus nephritis in children. *Lupus* 2005;14:83–88.

Ramos-Casals M, Nardi N, Lagrutta M, et al: Vasculitis in systemic lupus erythematosus. *Medicine* 2006;85:95–104.

Ravelli A, Darte-Salazar C, Buratti S, et al: Assessment of damage in juvenile-onset systemic lupus erythematosus: A multicenter cohort study. *Arthritis Rheum* 2003;49:501–507.

Stichweh D, Arce E, Pascual V: Update on pediatric systemic lupus erythematosus. *Curr Opin Rheumatol* 2004;16:577–587.

Weening JJ, D'Agati VD, Schwartz MM, et al: The classification of glomerulonephritis in systemic lupus erythematosus revisited. *J Am Soc Nephrol* 2004;15:241–250. Erratum in *J Am Soc Nephrol* 2004;15:835–836.

Willems M, Haddad E, Niaudet P, et al: Rituximab therapy for childhood-onset systemic lupus erythematosus. *J Pediatr* 2006;148:623–627.

Chapter 158 ■ Juvenile Dermatomyositis

Lauren M. Pachman

Juvenile dermatomyositis (JDM), the most common of the pediatric inflammatory myopathies, is distinguished by a characteristic rash and proximal, symmetric muscle weakness that is often responsive to the immunosuppressive therapy.

ETIOLOGY. Emerging evidence suggests that the inflammatory pathway may be driven by the interaction of genetic predisposition with antigen stimulation and other environmental factors leading to disease. Genetic markers on chromosome 6, DQA1*0501 and DRB1*0301, appear to be associated with JDM susceptibility in the United States, while the DRB1*0501 locus may be more closely linked to cases with JDM in Asia. Maternal T cells positive for DQA1*0501 (microchimerism) have been identified in the muscle of male children with JDM, and also react with the child's lymphocytes by secreting interferon (IFN)–γ, suggesting sensitization. Gene expression profile studies of muscle biopsies from children with untreated JDM as well as studies of circulating lymphocytes document a strong upregulation of genes controlled by IFN-α and IFN-β, providing evidence of an antigen-driven response.

A history of infection in the 3 mo before disease onset is obtained in most affected children. Constitutional signs and upper respiratory symptoms predominate, but ⅓ may have had gastrointestinal symptoms. Some children reported a history of contact with sick animals. Coxsackievirus B and group A streptococcus infections have been associated with the onset of JDM as well as disease flares.

Physical environmental factors may also play a contributing role, as disease onset may be precipitated by excessive sun exposure. Studies in adults have implicated an association with latitude of residence and ultraviolet B (UVB) exposure.

EPIDEMIOLOGY. The incidence of JDM is 3.2 cases/million children/yr, with a preponderance of the disease (73%) among white children. The average age at disease onset (date of recognition of first symptom of rash or weakness) is 6.9 yr, with >25% of children ≤4 yr of age at onset. In the United States, the ratio of girls to boys is 2.3 : 1. Multiple cases of myositis in kindred are rare, but familial autoimmune disease, especially connective tissue disease, is increased in families with JDM compared with families of healthy children. Reports of seasonal association have not been confirmed, although clusters of cases occur. The prevalence of JDM is difficult to determine because persistent symptoms such as mild skin involvement and loss of range of motion are often disregarded.

PATHOGENESIS. Susceptibility to JDM appears to be associated with the class II HLA antigen, DQA1*0501, which is found in >80% of children with JDM in the United States, and may interact with DRB*0301 to define the antigen binding site. Chronicity of JDM is associated with the tumor necrosis factor (TNF)–α-308A allele, which is a substitution of an A for a G in position −308 of the promoter region for the TNF-α gene. Children with JDM who have the TNF-α-308A allele, compared with children with JDM without this allele, frequently have increased cellular production of TNF-α, a chronic disease course requiring immunosuppressive therapy for >36 mo, and increased frequency of pathologic calcifications.

Endothelial cell damage initiated by the putative antigen or immune complexes is accompanied by release of von Willebrand factor antigen from the damaged endothelium. Histologic hallmarks of the muscle biopsy are perifascicular atrophy and occlusion of capillaries and arterioles, which is mediated by a primarily mononuclear cell infiltrate. New-onset, untreated JDM shows an increased proportion of natural killer (NK) cells (CD56) in the muscle as well as in the peripheral blood, suggesting a role for NK cells in the cytotoxic process. Other T-cell subsets are also present in affected muscle. The number of monocytes/macrophages (CD14) present in the muscle, but not the blood, correlates with serum levels of neopterin, a macrophage-derived marker of T-cell activation. Damage to the muscle is indicated by infarcted tissue, muscle fibers with central nuclei, and increased fibrosis composed of type I collagen, which is associated with loss of range of motion. In affected skin, the epidermis thins and the dermis demonstrates edema and vascular inflammation.

CLINICAL MANIFESTATIONS. In the 3 mo before disease onset, presenting children who are <6 yr of age have more fever and upper respiratory symptoms than older children, who have greater arthritis and musculoskeletal complaints, dysphagia, and headaches. Weakness is frequently insidious, with a gradual increase of complaints of fatigue on walking and loss of ability to perform activities of daily living.

The rash often has onset in sun-exposed areas and develops as the first symptom in 50% of cases, and concomitantly with weakness in 25% of cases. The characteristic periorbital violaceous erythema (**heliotrope**) may cross the bridge of the nose, in a mask-like distribution, and involve the ears as well (Fig. 158-1). Edema may be limited to the periorbital area, or generalized, and may involve the scalp with inflammation sufficient to result in partial baldness. The rash is often florid and is usually palpable over joints, especially the metacarpal phalangeal, intercarpal phalangeal (**Gottron papules**), knees, elbows, and medial malleoli of the ankles (Fig. 158-2). Cutaneous involvement can spread to the extensor surfaces of the extremities, the torso in a shawl-like distribution, and be generalized involving the trunk and buttocks. Children with an initial **amyopathic form** of JDM, with rash only, may develop myositis and calcinosis later in their disease course if not appropriately treated. The severity of the rash is reflected by a decreased number of nail-fold capillary loops, which is supporting evidence of a systemic vasculopathy (Fig 158-3). Diffuse severe vasculopathy may be manifest by infarction of the skin on the face in the area of the medial canthi, oral epithelium, or digital or gastrointestinal ulceration. Healing may be accompanied by hyperpigmentation or vitiligo.

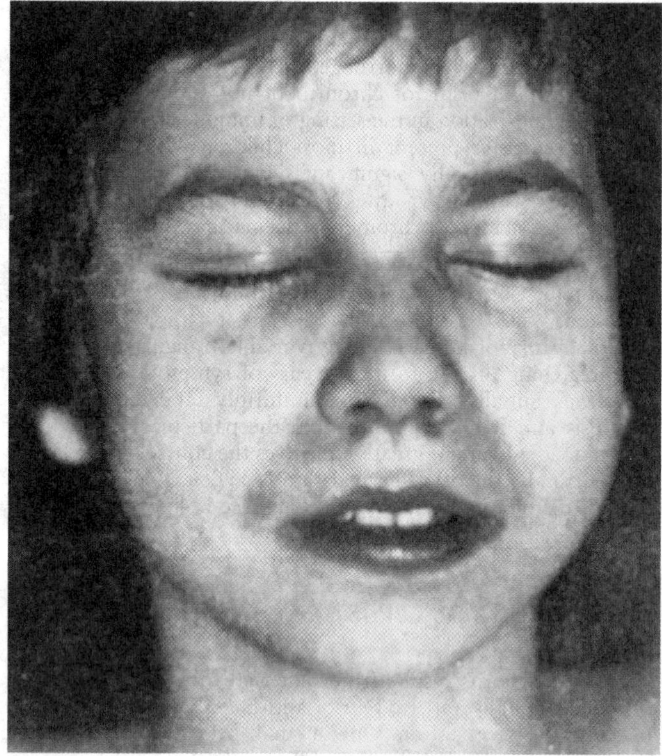

Figure 158-1. The facial rash of juvenile dermatomyositis. There is erythema over the bridge of the nose and malar areas, with violaceous (heliotropic) discolorations of the upper eyelids.

The onset of **proximal weakness** is often difficult to recognize and may be detected by difficulty in climbing stairs, combing hair, or getting in or out of bed, a chair, or the car. Neck flexor weakness, the inability to raise the head from the bed, is often the first symptom to appear and the last to resolve and may be associated with decreased core strength such that the child cannot do a sit-up. Muscles may be tender on compression, so that the child does not want to be hugged. The child may not be able to rise unassisted from the floor without "climbing up the body" (**Gowers sign**). One of the most serious concerns is impairment of upper airway function, which manifests in hoarseness with vocal cord nodules or thickening, a nasal quality of speech, or difficulty in handling secretions. Dysphagia, indicated by difficulty swallowing liquids, is an urgent prognostic sign requiring hospitalization and immediate, aggressive therapy that includes immunosuppression as well as physical care to prevent aspiration pneumonia secondary to impaired swallowing mechanisms. Impairment of the smooth muscles of the gastrointestinal tract can be associated with constipation, abdominal pain, or diarrhea and may indicate gastrointestinal bleeding, which can become life-threatening. Cardiac involvement with conduction abnormality is frequent at diagnosis; dilated cardiomyopathy has been reported. Pulmonary function tests in children negative for myosi-

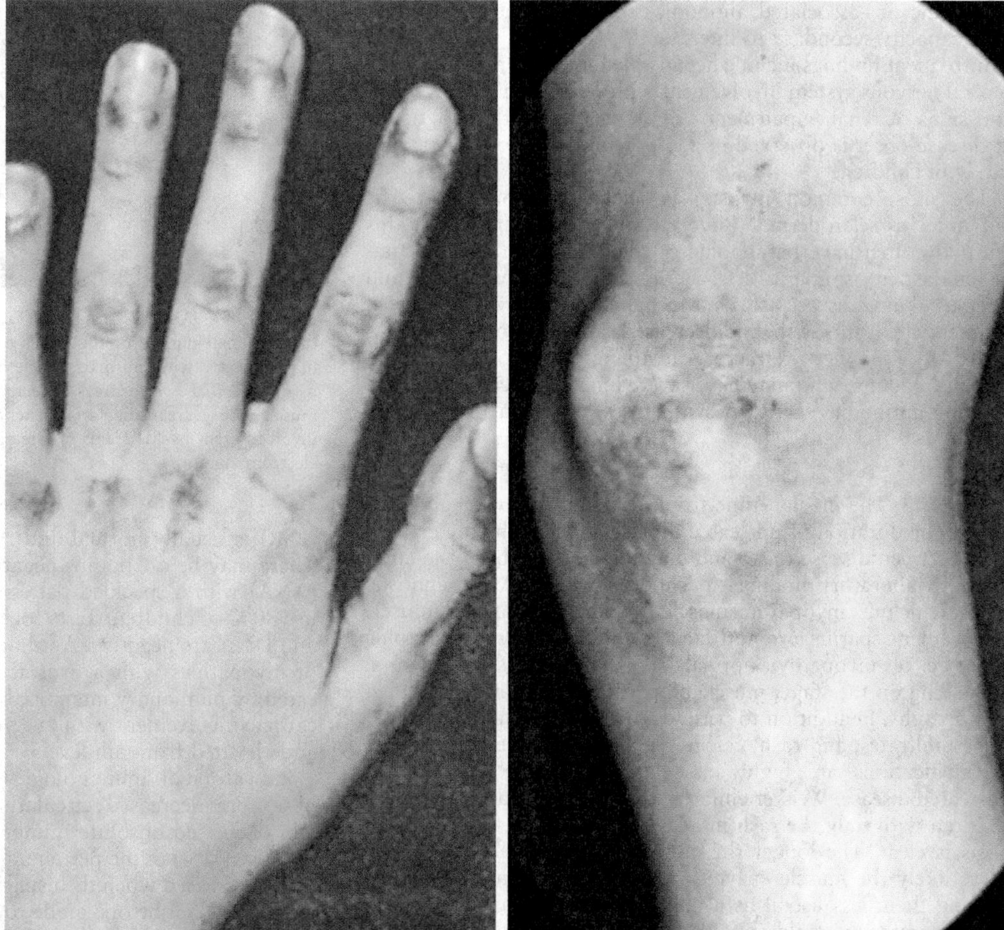

Figure 158-2. The rash of juvenile dermatomyositis. The skin over the metacarpal and proximal interphalangeal joints may be hypertropic and pale red (Gottron papules).

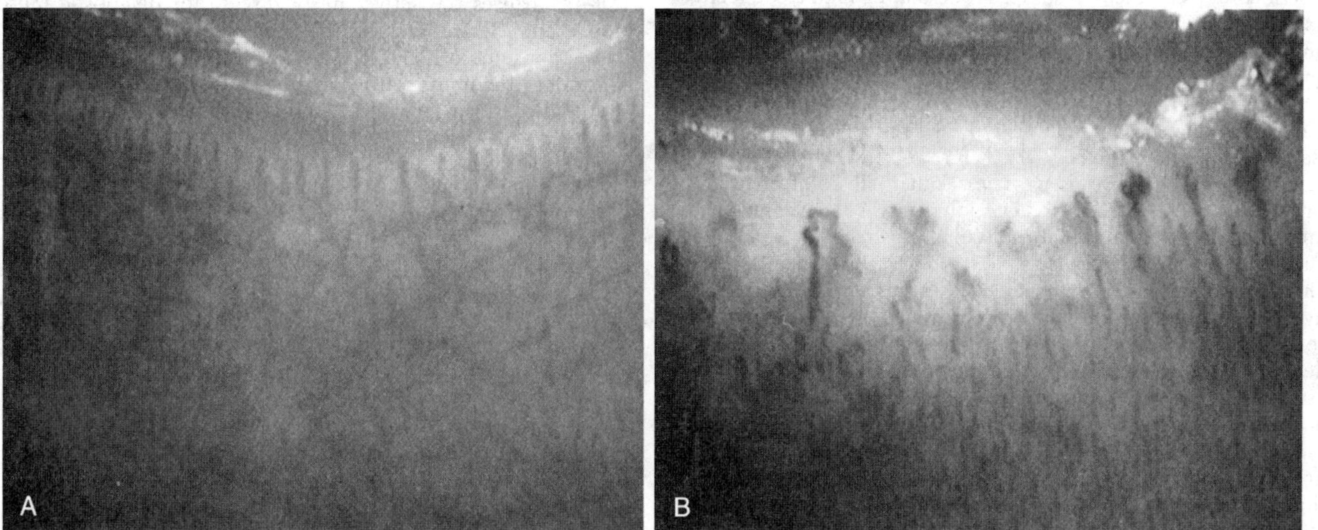

Figure 158-3. Nail-fold capillary pattern in rheumatic diseases. *A*, Normal nail-fold capillary pattern in a healthy child, with a homogeneous distribution and uniform appearance of capillary loops. *B*, The nail-fold capillary pattern in a child with juvenile dermatomyositis that shows dropout of capillary end loops, resulting in a wide band of avascularity. Dilated, tortuous capillaries are also seen, and some with the terminal bush formation found in patterns with juvenile dermatomyositis, with scleroderma, and with Raynaud phenomenon that may progress to scleroderma.

tis-specific or -associated antibodies often document decreased vital capacity secondary to intercostal weakness.

Infrequent findings include hepatosplenomegaly, retinitis, iritis, central nervous system involvement with seizures and depression, and signs of renal impairment. An association with malignancy at disease onset is observed in adults with dermatomyositis, but rarely in children.

The most common myositis-associated antibody is to the **polymyositis/scleroderma (Pm/Scl) antigen.** Children with this antibody often have bambooing of the digits with loss of cutaneous elasticity, similar to scleroderma, and may have cardiac and interstitial lung disease as well. **Mechanic's hands,** with thickened skin, cuticle overgrowth, and decreased range of motion are indicators of a subset of refractory inflammatory myopathies more typical in adults, who may have severe lung involvement and circulating antibodies to tRNA synthetases, of which Jo-1 is most common.

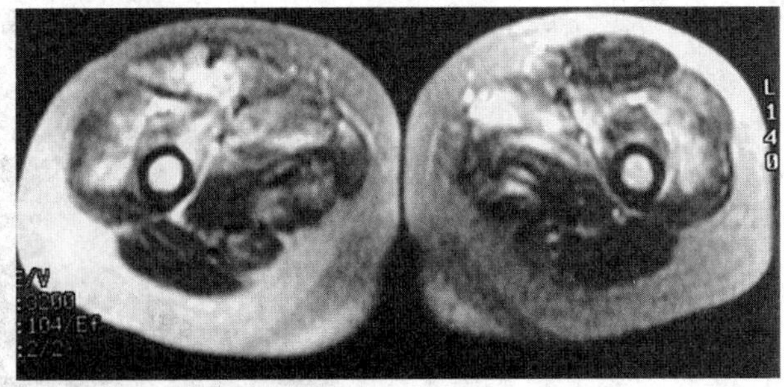

Figure 158-4. An MRI scan with T2-weighted image with fat suppression of the proximal muscle of the lower extremities of a child with juvenile dermatomyositis with normal muscle enzymes. There is focal inflammatory myopathy. The white areas reflect the inflammatory response in involved muscle; those areas that are darker are more normal. Identification of the involved areas by MRI aids in directing the location of the muscle biopsy or electromyogram.

DIAGNOSIS. The median time from disease onset to diagnosis is 4 mo. The duration of untreated disease, reflected by the elapsed time between disease onset and diagnosis, affects both the clinical and laboratory findings in children with JDM. Diagnostic criteria include myopathic muscle weakness (proximal muscle involvement sparing eye and facial muscles); electromyographic evidence of myopathy; normal or elevated muscle enzymes, depending on the stage; muscle biopsy demonstrating perifascicular atrophy, in addition to perifascicular, perimysial, or perivascular infiltrates; and rash, calcinosis, and a positive MRI.

Calcifications are highly associated with the duration of untreated disease. Weaker children are diagnosed earlier, whereas children with only the rash may take many mo before the diagnosis is clear. The longer the interval of untreated disease, the more likely the muscle enzymes are to be in the normal range, making them less useful as a guide to therapy. Bone density is often decreased in children with JDM and is also associated with longer duration of untreated symptoms.

The characteristic rash facilitates early diagnosis but should be differentiated from other connective tissue diseases such as systemic lupus erythematosus, scleroderma, or mixed connective tissue disease by both the specific antibody tests and the clinical findings associated with each of these disorders. Careful examination of the nail-fold capillaries usually documents periungual avascularity with capillary dropout. Those capillaries that remain are usually dilated and have the typical terminal bush formation (see Fig. 158-3).

If the initial symptom is weakness, other causes of myopathy should be considered including polymyositis associated with influenza B infection, the muscular dystrophies (including Duchenne and Becker muscular dystrophies), myasthenia gravis, Guillain-Barré syndrome, endocrinopathies (hyperthyroidism, hypothyroidism, Cushing syndrome, Addison disease, parathyroid disorders), mitochondrial myopathies, and metabolic disorders (glycogen storage diseases, lipid storage diseases). Infections associated with prominent muscular symptoms include trichinosis, toxoplasmosis, and poliomyelitis. Blunt trauma and crush injuries may lead to transient rhabdomyolysis with myoglobinuria. Myositis in children may also be associated with vaccinations, drugs, growth hormone, and bone marrow transplantation in which graft vs host myositis occurs as a component of immune activation (see Chapter 136). Abdominal pain may be associated with celiac disease, which is not infrequent in patients with JDM, or as a consequence of hydroxychloroquine therapy.

LABORATORY FINDINGS. Elevated serum levels of **muscle-derived enzymes** (creatine kinase, aldolase, serum glutamic-oxaloacetic transaminase, lactic acid dehydrogenase) reflect the leaky muscle membranes. Serum levels may be in the normal range for the 1st 4–5 mo after disease onset. The erythrocyte sedimentation rate (ESR) is usually normal and the rheumatoid factor is negative. There may be a Coombs-negative anemia. Antinuclear antibody (ANA) with a speckled pattern (unknown specificity) is present in >80% of children. Tests for antibodies to SSA, SSB, Sm, RNP, and DNA are negative. Antibodies to Pm/Scl identify a subgroup of myopathies with a protracted disease course, often complicated by pulmonary interstitial fibrosis. These children may have cardiac involvement with tachycardia, conduction abnormalities, and elevated troponin levels.

Indicators of immunologic activation in JDM include lymphopenia, decreased circulating ICAM-1 CD8 memory cells, and decreased absolute numbers of natural killer cells ($CD56^+$, $CD3^-$, $CD16^+$) in the peripheral blood. This lymphocyte subset is often decreased when the usual muscle enzymes are in the normal range, and can be one guide to therapy. The percent of $CD19^+$ B cells, which are not activated, may be increased in the circulation secondary to the depletion of other subsets.

Radiographic studies aid both diagnosis and medical management. MRI using T2 weighted images and fat suppression (Fig. 158-4) localizes the active site of disease for diagnostic muscle biopsy and electromyogram, which are each nondiagnostic in 20% of instances if not directed by MRI. Extensive rash and abnormal MRI findings are common despite normal serum levels of muscle-derived enzymes. Muscle biopsy often demonstrates evidence of disease activity and chronicity that is not suspected from the levels of the serum enzymes alone.

A rehabilitation cookie swallow documents significant palatorespiratory dysfunction and identifies an unprotected airway. Pulmonary function testing of the diffusion capacity of the lung for carbon monoxide (DLCO), which can be used for children >6 yr of age, detects decreased respiratory muscle strength as well as alveolar fibrosis associated with other connective tissue diseases. Active disease is frequently associated with decreased bone density with abnormal findings on densitometry and low osteocalcin and vitamin D levels. Calcinosis is detected by plain radiographs (Fig. 158-5).

TREATMENT. The aid of an experienced pediatric rheumatologist is essential in assessing the need for therapeutic intervention. It is important to recognize that the inflammatory pathways for skin and muscle appear to be distinct and are associated with discrete physical and laboratory findings, and that the duration of untreated disease influences both clinical and laboratory findings. Children with only mild cutaneous findings, normal immune and serologic markers of disease activity, and a negative family history of color blindness are administered hydroxychloroquine (maximum: 5 mg/kg/day) with daily oral prednisone (1 mg/kg). Depending on the severity of the nail-fold capillary changes associated with skin involvement, the intensity of therapy may be

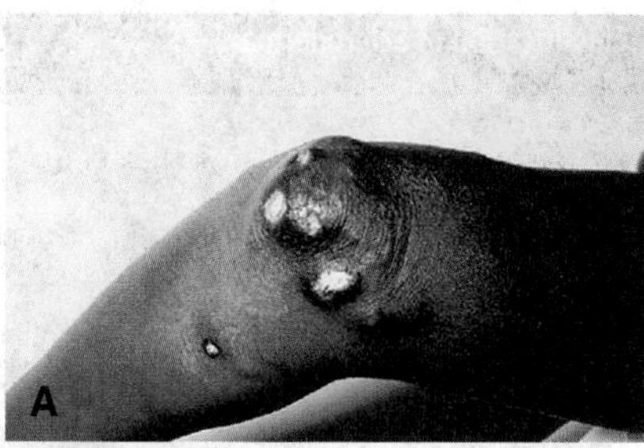

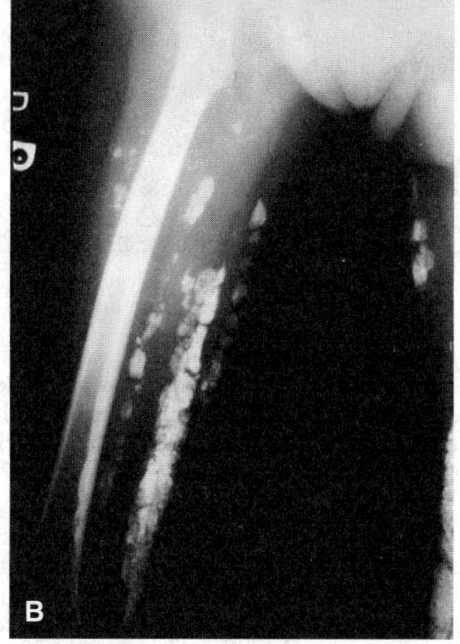

Figure 158-5. Rash and calcifications in dermatomyositis. *A,* Skin effects of calcification. *B,* Radiographic evidence of calcification. (From Dalakas MC, Hohlfeld R: Polymyositis and dermatomyositis. *Lancet* 2003;362:971–982.)

increased. These children should be monitored for the development of muscle involvement by careful physical examination to assess muscle strength, as well as laboratory testing for elevation of immune markers and serum muscle enzymes. If needed, repeat MRI may identify new areas of muscle involvement.

With evidence of minimal inflammation and muscle damage, oral prednisone (1–2 mg/kg/day) may suffice. Children with extensive vasculopathy, reflected by nail-fold capillary dropout, have diminished absorption of oral corticosteroids. High-dose intermittent intravenous methylprednisolone (30 mg/kg/day for 3 days; maximum dose: 1 g/day) rapidly normalizes the muscle enzymes and should be used if the indicators of inflammation (absolute count of $CD56^+$ NK cells, neopterin, vWf:Ag) remain abnormal. Inhibitors of gastric acid secretion are also usually administered to minimize gastric bleeding. After the initial pulse, lower dose methylprednisolone may be required daily in extremely ill children, with a gradual reduction in frequency to once a wk administration until all the indicators of inflammation normalize. Low-dose oral prednisone (0.5 mg/kg/day) is given in the morning with breakfast on nonintravenous methylprednisolone days. Weekly methotrexate (15–20 $mg/m^2/wk$), given preferentially by either the intravenous or subcutaneous route (rather than by mouth) is started at the same time as methylprednisolone, along with oral folic acid (1 mg/day). Cyclosporine (3 mg/kg/day) appears to be helpful for persistent cutaneous involvement, with trough levels maintained at about 100 ng/mL; mycophenolate mofetil may also be effective. This extensive immunosuppression may result in decreased levels of IgG (<500 mg/dL), which may require replacement immunoglobulin (0.4 g/kg/mo) to help prevent infections. Some centers administer high-dose intravenous immunoglobulin (IVIG) [1–2 gm/kg] 1–2 days/mo initially to diminish cutaneous symptoms, but it is not clear that this alters the disease course. Inhibitors of TNF-α have been tried in children with chronic disease with limited success, but may help those with overlap syndrome and chronic arthritis.

Children with dysphagia require a soft diet or nasogastric feedings, if necessary, until treatment restores a functional, protected airway. In rare cases, a respirator and tracheotomy or even extracorporeal membrane oxygenation are required for respiratory failure. Absorption of calories and medication may be impaired by extensive intestinal vasculitis, requiring parenteral hyperalimentation and intravenous administration of drugs. Renal damage secondary to massive creatinine or myoglobin excretion can be averted by appropriate intravenous hydration.

Physical and occupational therapy provide passive stretching early in the disease course and, once active inflammation has resolved, direct reconditioning of muscles to regain strength and range of motion. Bed rest is not indicated. Weight bearing improves bone density. Social work services may help facilitate adjustment to the frustration of physical impairment in a previously active child.

All children with JDM should avoid exposure to sun and also use a sunscreen, even in winter and on cloudy days, that is at least SPF 30 (free of para-aminobenzoic acid), which provides maximal protection against ultraviolet A and B. Vitamin D should be given at a dose appropriate for weight, in addition to exogenous calcium supplements, to repair the osteopenia of JDM and to decrease the frequency of bone fracture.

COMPLICATIONS. Aspiration pneumonia is a frequent major complication associated with unrecognized impairment in swallowing fluids. Progressive bowel infarction can lead to perforation and death. Depression and mood swings are part of the spectrum of central nervous system involvement and may be accentuated by corticosteroid administration, especially in children with family histories of depression.

Pathologic calcifications are a consequence of chronic inflammation and are associated with increased morbidity and mortality. They are present at diagnosis in about 25% of children with JDM. Several factors probably contribute to their development. A genetic predisposition for increased production of proinflammatory cytokines, such as TNF-α, delay in initiation of appropriate therapy, may result in chronic inflammation and promote calcification. The calcium deposits form primarily in subcutaneous tissue and fascia. They may drain a white, cheesy material and resolve, or serve as a nidus for infection, most frequently staphylococcal, which can progress to septicemia and death. Aggressive immunosuppressive therapy at the time of diagnosis appears to be associated with decreased frequency of calcinosis.

Partial lipodystrophy develops in >10% of chronic JDM cases. It is also associated with the TNF-α-308A allele and is characterized by: loss of subcutaneous fat on the extremities, giving a hypermuscular appearance; acanthosis nigricans; weakened abdominal muscles resulting in a potbelly appearance; and abnormal glucose and lipid metabolism. Girls may lose their menses; sterility may result if the onset of JDM is before puberty.

Short stature may be present at diagnosis and further linear growth may be impaired by the administration of corticosteroids. Usually, the child will regain expected stature once the dosage of corticosteroids is safely decreased and the inflammation is controlled. Administration of growth hormone may precipitate a disease flare and is contraindicated.

PROGNOSIS. Prior to the advent of corticosteroids, ⅓ of affected children died and another ⅓ were disabled. The mortality rate is currently about 1%. Although the disease is classified as "chronic," little is known about the consequences of persistent vascular inflammation. The period of active symptoms has decreased from about 3.5 yr to <1.5 yr with more aggressive immunosuppressive therapy. The vascular, skin, and muscle symptoms of children with JDM who are negative for myositis-associated antibodies symptoms respond well to therapy except in children with the TNF-α-308A allele, who have a longer disease course and require immunosuppressive therapy for >36 mo.

Unlike many adults with inflammatory myopathies, children with JDM appear able to repair their vasculature and muscle damage. The impact of partial lipodystrophy on adult morbidity is not known. Overall, with appropriate tests to monitor inflammation and disease activity and to guide the use of more aggressive therapy, the prognosis for this illness has markedly improved.

Compeyrot-Lacassagne S, Feldman BM: Inflammatory myopathies in children. *Pediatr Clin North Am* 2005;52:493–520.

Dalakas MC, Hohlfeld R: Polymyositis and dermatomyositis. *Lancet* 2003;362:971–982.

Danko K, Ponyi A, Constantin T, et al: Long-term survival of patients with idiopathic inflammatory myopathies according to clinical features. A longitudunal study of 162 cases. *Medicine* 2004;83:35–42.

Mendez EP, Lipton R, Ramsey-Goldman R, et al: US incidence of juvenile dermatomyositis, 1995-1998: Results from the National Institute of Arthritis and Musculoskeletal and Skin Diseases Registry. *Arthritis Care Res* 2003;49:300–305.

Pachman LM, Abbott K, Sinecore JM, et al: Duration of illness is an important variable for untreated children with juvenile dermatomyositis. *J Pediatr* 2006;148(2):247–253.

Pachman LM, Lipton R, Ramsey-Goldman R, et al: History of infection before the onset of juvenile dermatomyositis: Results from the National Institute of Arthritis Muscle and Skin Diseases Research Registry. *Arthritis Rheum* 2005;53:166–172.

Reed AM, McNallan K, Wettstein P, et al: Does HLA-dependent chimerism underlie the pathogenesis of juvenile dermatomyositis? *J Immunol* 2004;172:5041–5046.

Rider LG, Miller FW: Classification and treatment of the juvenile idiopathic inflammatory myopathies. *Rheum Dis Clin North Am* 1997;23:619–621.

Smith RL, Sundberg J, Shamiyah E: Skin involvement in juvenile dermatomyositis is associated with loss of end row nailfold capillary loops. *J Rheumatol* 2004;31:1644–1649.

Tezak Z, Hoffman EP, Lutz JL, et al: Gene expression profiling in DQA1*0501+ children with untreated dermatomyositis: A novel model of pathogenesis. *J Immunol* 2002;168:4154–4163.

Troyanov Y, Targoff IN, Tremblay JL, et al: Novel classification of idiopathic inflammatory myopathies based on overlap syndrome features and autoantibodies. *Medicine* 2005;84:231–249.

Chapter 159 ■ Scleroderma and Raynaud Phenomenon

Michael L. Miller

Scleroderma, a chronic disease of unknown cause, is a spectrum of disorders characterized by fibrosis affecting the dermis (scleroderma) and arteries of the lungs, kidneys, and gastrointestinal tract. Scleroderma is classified according to the pattern of skin and internal organ involvement (Table 159-1).

ETIOLOGY. The cause of scleroderma is unknown but appears to involve injury to vascular endothelium. Antinuclear antibodies (ANAs) specific for topoisomerase 1 (Scl-70) and the centromere are present in many patients, which suggests that autoimmune processes play a role in pathogenesis. Rare cases are reported after exposure to polyvinyl chloride, bleomycin, and pentazocine.

TABLE 159-1. Classification of Scleroderma

SYSTEMIC SCLEROSIS
Diffuse: systemic widespread skin fibrosis, including proximal limbs, trunk, and face; early internal organ involvement
Limited (CREST): systemic distal skin involvement, often face, with late, if any, internal organ involvement
Overlap: sclerodermal skin changes with features of other connective tissue disorders
LOCALIZED SCLERODERMA
Morphea
Generalized morphea
Linear scleroderma
On face, forehead, or scalp (coup de sabre)
On extremity
EOSINOPHILIC FASCIITIS
SECONDARY FORMS
Drug induced
Chemically induced
PSEUDOSCLERODERMA

CREST, calcinosis, Raynaud phenomenon, esophageal dysmotility, sclerodactyly, and telangiectasias.
From Uziel Y, Miller ML, Laxer RM: Scleroderma in children, *Pediatr Clin North Am* 1995;42:1171–1203.

EPIDEMIOLOGY. Scleroderma is a rare disease. The peak age at onset for systemic sclerosis is 30–50 yr, with a female:male ratio of 3:1. Children represent <10% of all cases. In children, localized scleroderma is more common than systemic sclerosis. The two forms usually do not overlap.

PATHOGENESIS. Scleroderma is characterized by increased production of extracellular matrix and associated vascular damage and obstruction with decreased vasculogenesis. During the initial stages of disease, lymphocytes, macrophages, mast cells, plasma cells, and eosinophils infiltrate the dermis. Factors released from activated platelets may play a role in Raynaud phenomenon and in triggering fibroblast proliferation that increases collagen synthesis, resulting in fibrosis of the dermis, subcutaneous fat, and sometimes muscle.

Studies suggest that a yet unidentified agent, or possibly subclinical graft versus host reaction from persisting cells of maternal origin (microchimerism), injures vascular endothelial cells resulting in increased expression of adhesion molecules on cell surfaces. These molecules entrap platelets and inflammatory cells, resulting in vascular changes associated with manifestations as Raynaud phenomenon, renovascular hypertension, and pulmonary hypertension. Recruitment of T lymphocytes to areas of vascular damage may be the event that leads to specific autoantibody production in many patients. After these events, macrophages and other inflammatory cells appear to migrate into affected tissues and secrete cytokines such as interleukin 1 (IL-1) causing platelets to release platelet-derived growth factor and transforming growth factor-β. These and other molecules (e.g., IL-2, IL-4) induce fibroblasts to reproduce and synthesize excessive amounts of collagen, resulting in fibrosis. Stimulatory antibodies are also present against the platelet derived growth factor receptor (PDGFR), which in turn may stimulate collagen gene expression.

CLINICAL MANIFESTATIONS. **Raynaud phenomenon** may be primary (idiopathic) or secondary to diseases such as scleroderma, systemic lupus erythematosus (SLE), overlap syndrome, or undifferentiated connective tissue disease and results from arterial spasm, which is induced by exposure to cold and less often to stress. It affects fingers, toes, and occasionally the ears and the tip of the nose with episodes that can vary in duration from minutes to hours. The typical sequence of color change is blanching, cyanosis, and then hyperanemia. Pain and paresthesias are often present. Nonetheless, most patients do not have all three phases; many do not have this sequence. Raynaud phenomenon often begins in adolescents and, in most cases, it is primary, which can be defined by symmetric occurrence, the absence of tissue necrosis or gangrene, no manifestations of a secondary disease, normal nail-fold capillaries, normal erythrocyte sedimentation rate (ESR), and negative ANA or other autoantibodies.

It is often the earliest manifestation of scleroderma and may precede extensive skin and internal organ involvement by months or years. The presence of two of the three stages—pallor, cyanosis, and, finally, erythema—is sufficient for identifying this manifestation. Provocative exposure to ice water is not necessary; photographs may be useful.

Systemic Sclerosis. Systemic sclerosis often presents with a preliminary edematous phase that can last several months before chronic fibrosis develops. These early changes include puffiness around the fingers, on the dorsum of the hands, and sometimes on the face. An eventual decrease in edema is associated with tightening of the skin. Skin changes tend to spread proximally from the hands. Loss of subcutaneous tissue in the face can result in a small oral stoma with decreased distance between the upper and lower teeth when the mouth opens wide (Fig. 159-1). Skin ulceration over pressure points, such as the elbows, may be associated with subcutaneous calcifications. Later, atrophic skin can become shiny and waxy in appearance. Loss of tissue at the fingertips may be associated with ulceration if Raynaud phenomenon is severe (Fig. 159-2). The distal phalanges may exhibit resorption of the distal tufts (**acro-osteolysis**). The fingers assume a tapered appearance associated with tightened skin (**sclerodactyly**) and eventual development of secondary and often severe flexion contractures and limitation of motion (Fig. 159-3). As lesions spread proximally, flexion contractures in the elbows, hips, and knees may be associated with secondary muscle weakness and atrophy. Other chronic changes include epidermal thinning, hair loss, and decreased sweating. Hyperpigmented postinflammatory changes surrounded by atrophic depigmentation may give a salt-and-pepper appearance to some skin lesions. Over a period of years, remodeling of lesions sometimes results in focal improvement in skin thickening at the same time that fibrosis extends elsewhere.

Pulmonary disease includes arterial and interstitial involvement and can vary from minimal disease to a progressive course that eventually results in decreased exercise tolerance, dyspnea at rest, and right-sided heart failure. Chest roentgenograms may appear normal early in the course. Evidence of early involvement may be found only by performing pulmonary function tests, including evaluation of oxygen diffusion by diffusion of carbon monoxide capacity (DLCO). High-resolution CT may also detect changes associated with interstitial disease before they become apparent on chest x-ray.

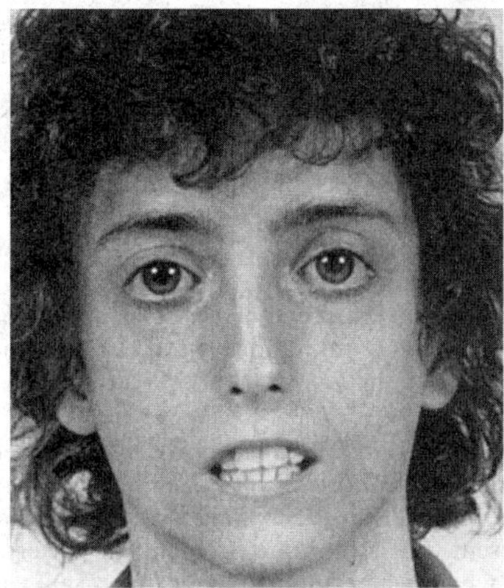

Figure 159-1. Facial changes in a 16 yr old boy with scleroderma. There is a small mouth with puckering of the lips, pinched nose, and hyperpigmentation of the neck. (From Uziel Y, Miller ML, Laxer RM: Scleroderma in children. *Pediatr Clin North Am* 1995;42:1171–1203.)

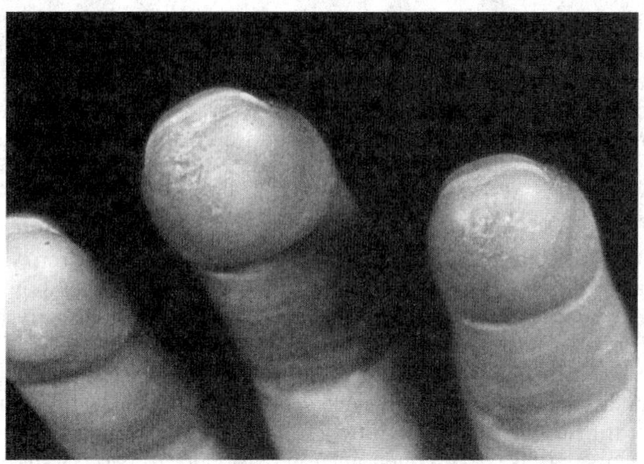

Figure 159-2. Tiny digital pitting scars and loss of pulp space resulting from digital ischemia in a 15 yr old boy with scleroderma. (From Uziel Y, Miller ML, Laxer RM: Scleroderma in children. *Pediatr Clin North Am* 1995;42:1171–1203.)

Scleroderma can also affect other organs. Renal arterial disease can cause chronic or severe episodic hypertension. Esophageal dilatation caused by fibrosis can cause dysphagia. Dilated intestinal loops can result in malabsorption and failure to thrive. Cardiac fibrosis has been associated with arrhythmias, ventricular hypertrophy, and decreased cardiac function.

Scleroderma can present with less extensive involvement. In limited systemic scleroderma, children have less prominent fibrosis that is limited to the distal extremities, face, and neck. Telangiectasias may appear on the fingertips, face, chest wall, and inner surface of lips. The **CREST syndrome** refers to the manifestations of calcinosis, Raynaud phenomenon, esophageal dysmotility, sclerodactyly, and telangiectasias. Severe pulmonary hypertension develops in some patients with CREST syndrome.

Morphea and Linear Scleroderma. In localized scleroderma, the involvement is restricted to the skin; progression to systemic sclerosis is rare. In children with **morphea,** a form of localized scleroderma, lesions are typically discrete and may occur anywhere on the body but particularly on the face. Early inflammation is followed by indurated, hypopigmented, atrophic lesions. Lesions

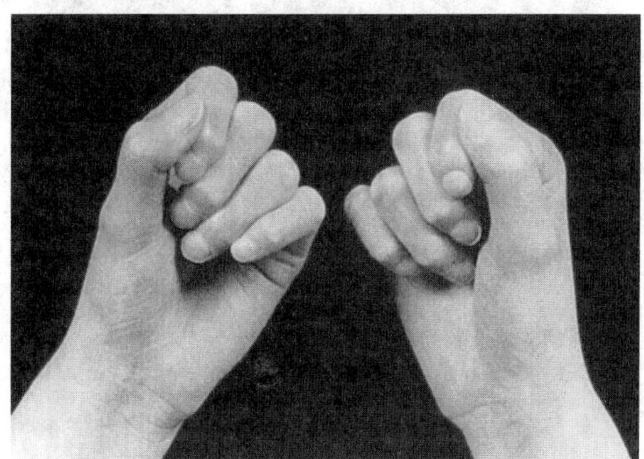

Figure 159-3. Inability to make a full fist due to skin and soft tissue tightening in a 10 yr old girl with scleroderma. (From Uziel Y, Miller ML, Laxer RM: Scleroderma in children. *Pediatr Clin North Am* 1995;42:1171–1203.)

of **linear scleroderma** can vary from a few cm to the entire length of the extremities. Fibrosis in the dermis can extend to muscle, with the potential for total loss of muscle tissue between the dermis and bone. Resulting leg-length discrepancies, joint flexion contractures (Fig. 159-4), or cosmetic deformities of the face, forehead, or scalp with scarring alopecia (**coup de sabre**) may require surgical intervention.

DIAGNOSIS. Scleroderma should be suspected in children who develop Raynaud phenomenon followed by skin changes suggestive of sclerodactyly. If Raynaud phenomenon is present for years before classic disease expression, ANAs (particularly anti-SCL70) are typically found. Subclinical pulmonary fibrosis, suspected if decreased DLCO is found on pulmonary function testing, may be confirmed by high-resolution CT. Nail-fold capillaroscopy of patients with Raynaud phenomenon before progression of disease may reveal a loss of capillaries or abnormal capillary dilatation resulting from vasculopathy (see Fig. 158-3).

According to diagnostic criteria used in adults, the diagnosis of scleroderma requires the presence of the single major criterion (sclerodermatous skin changes proximal to the metacarpophalangeal or metatarsophalangeal joints) or two of the three minor criteria (Table 159-2). The evaluation in these patients should include pulmonary function tests, contrast studies of the upper gastrointestinal tract to evaluate esophageal motility, and echocardiography to identify pulmonary arterial hypertension.

DIFFERENTIAL DIAGNOSIS. Several conditions may present with findings similar to those of scleroderma. Acrocyanosis, in which there is no associated pallor or reflex hyperemia, may be seen with pulmonary arterial hypertension, anorexia nervosa, or frostbite. Diffuse finger swelling extending to the dorsum of the hands can be seen in Henoch-Schönlein purpura and with allergic reactions. Patients with juvenile rheumatoid arthritis usually have swelling in the fingers that is restricted to the joints. Flexion contractures in these patients are a result of chronic tendinitis without dermal involvement; therefore, the skin is not tight, compared with that of patients with scleroderma. Manifestations of graft versus host disease after bone marrow transplantation (see Chapter 136) include erythema affecting the face and distal extremities, sclerodermatous skin changes, hepatitis, and diarrhea.

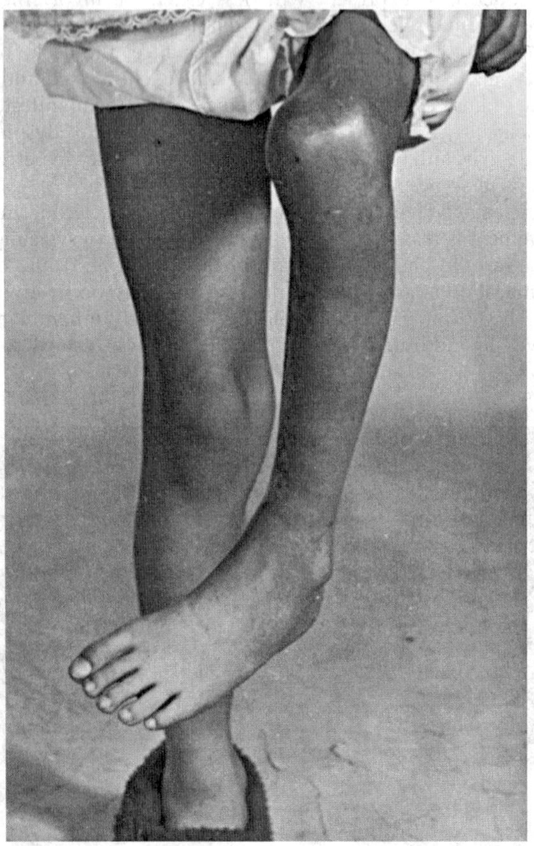

Figure 159-4. Extensive morphea involving the entire left leg, causing shortening and flexion contractures. The skin has a shiny appearance with patches of hyperpigmentation and vitiligo.

TABLE 159-2. Diagnostic Criteria of Scleroderma*

MAJOR CRITERION
Proximal scleroderma: typical sclerodermatous skin changes (tightness, thickening, and nonpitting induration, excluding localized forms of scleroderma) involving areas proximal to the metacarpophalangeal or metatarsophalangeal joints
MINOR CRITERIA
Sclerodactyly: sclerodermatous skin changes limited to digits
Digital pitting scars resulting from digital ischemia
Bibasilar pulmonary fibrosis not attributable to primary lung disease

*The diagnosis of scleroderma requires the presence of the major criterion or two of the three minor criteria.

From Subcommittee for Scleroderma Criteria of the American Rheumatism Association Diagnostic and Therapeutic Criteria Committee: Preliminary criteria for the classification of systemic sclerosis (scleroderma). *Arthritis Rheum* 1980;23:581–590.

Long-term follow-up helps distinguish primary Raynaud phenomenon from secondary Raynaud phenomenon, which occurs prior to the subsequent development of skin or internal organ changes of scleroderma. These patients usually do not have anti-SCL70 or other autoantibodies, and their Raynaud phenomenon does not worsen over time. Weakness, sometimes related to flexion contractures, in patients with skin changes suggestive of early scleroderma raises the possibility of juvenile dermatomyositis or overlap syndromes in which elements of several rheumatic diseases (systemic lupus erythematosus, dermatomyositis, arthritis, and scleroderma) may be present.

Patients with **eosinophilic fasciitis** develop changes similar to those in localized scleroderma. Laboratory evaluation shows a striking eosinophilia, elevated ESR, and occasionally hypergammaglobulinemia. Full-thickness skin biopsy that includes muscle fascia shows a predominantly eosinophilic inflammatory infiltration in the dermis and fascial tissues, which confirms the diagnosis. Progression to systemic sclerosis is rare. Corticosteroid treatment often ameliorates or prevents progression of lesions. Some patients develop severe contracting fibrosis involving the entire length of the extremities. Limited experience suggests that it may be possible in some cases to prevent this complication with the use of methotrexate.

Pseudoscleroderma comprises unrelated diseases characterized by patchy or diffuse cutaneous fibrosis without the other manifestations of scleroderma. Patients with phenylketonuria can develop such lesions as well as eczematous changes. **Scleredema of Buschke** is a transient disease of sudden onset often after a febrile illness (especially streptococcal infections) in which patchy sclerodermatous lesions occur on the neck and shoulders, often extending to the face, trunk, and down the arms. These findings usually resolve spontaneously within several months.

LABORATORY FINDINGS. Inflammation early in systemic disease may be reflected by anemia and sometimes eosinophilia. Immunoglobulin levels may be nonspecifically elevated. ANAs are often present with a speckled or nucleolar pattern. If present, anti-SCL70, which is specific for topoisomerase 1, and anticentromere autoantibodies are strongly suggestive of a diagnosis of scleroderma. Autoantibodies usually found in systemic lupus erythematosus (anti-DNA) or mixed connective tissue disease (anti-ribonucleoprotein) suggest the presence of an overlapping syndrome. In the early phase of the disease, levels of von Willebrand factor antigen, a marker for vascular endothelial damage, may be elevated. In localized scleroderma, laboratory abnormalities are usually restricted to positive ANA (with anti-SCL70 and anticentromere antibodies much less common than in systemic sclerosis) and, on occasion, eosinophilia.

TREATMENT. Although there is no specific treatment, immunosuppressive agents, including methotrexate and corticosteroids, used in the early stages of the disease may help curb inflammation. Corticosteroids later in the course of the disease do not appear to be effective and may exacerbate hypertension. Additional treatment includes physical and occupational therapy to improve flexion contractures and maintain muscle strength, and spring-loaded splints in selected patients.

If **Raynaud phenomenon** persists despite local measures (keeping hands warm during cold exposure with Mylar or sheepskin gloves), therapy with calcium channel blockers (sustained release, nifedipine 30–60 mg, PO, QD; amlodipine besylate), angiotensin-converting enzyme inhibitors (captopril, enalapril), and topical vasodilators (nitroglycerin paste) may be successful in preventing or ameliorating fingertip ulcerations. Vascular compromise threatening to lead to gangrene and autoamputation of the distal digits may respond to parenteral administration of prostaglandin E_1 (alprostadil).

COMPLICATIONS. Raynaud phenomenon can become severe enough to lead to early gangrenous changes with the threat of autoamputation of the digits or osteomyelitis. Arterial disease can also cause esophageal rupture, renovascular hypertensive crises, and pulmonary arterial hypertension. Chronic pulmonary insufficiency can result from pulmonary parenchymal disease and pulmonary arterial hypertension. Gastrointestinal involvement can result in malabsorption and failure to thrive. Renal disease and chronic pulmonary arterial hypertension can lead to death. Patients with overlapping features of myositis may have inflammatory cardiac disease.

PROGNOSIS. The course of scleroderma is variable, and findings at presentation are not predictive. Some patients stabilize after several years and have no new skin or visceral involvement. Others show unrelenting progression of disease, with death, either in childhood or later in life, resulting from end-stage pulmonary, cardiac, or renal vascular disease.

Baroni SS, Santillo M, Bevilacqua F, et al: Stimulatory autoantibodies to the PDGF receptor in systemic sclerosis. *N Engl J Med* 2006;354:2667–2676.

Charles C, Clements P, Furst DE: Systemic sclerosis: hypothesis-driven treatment strategies. *Lancet* 2006;367:1683–1690.

Garty BZ, Athreya BH, Wilmott R, et al: Pulmonary functions in children with progressive systemic sclerosis. *Pediatrics* 1991;88:1161–1167.

Jones GT, Herrick AL, Woodham SE, et al: Occurrence of Raynaud's phenomenon in children ages 12–15 years. *Arthritis Rheum* 2003;48:3518–3521.

Kuwana M, Okazaki Y, Yasuoko H, et al: Defective vasculogenesis in systemic sclerosis. *Lancet* 2004;364:603–610.

Martini G, Foeldvari I, Russo R, et al: Systemic sclerosis in childhood. *Arthritis Rheumatol* 2006;54:3971–3978.

Murray KJ, Laxer RM: Scleroderma in children and adolescents. *Rheum Dis Clin North Am* 2002;28:603–624.

Nigrovic PA, Fuhlbrigge RC, Sundel RP: Raynaud's phenomenon in children: A retrospective review of 123 patients. *Pediatrics* 2003:111:715–721.

Quartier P, Bonnet D, Fournet JC, et al: Severe cardiac involvement in children with systemic sclerosis and myositis. *J Rheumatol* 2002;29:1767–1773.

Seely JM, Jones LT, Wallace C, et al: Systemic sclerosis: Using high-resolution CT to detect lung disease in children. *AJR Am J Roentgenol* 1998;170:691–697.

Tashkin DP, Elashoff R, Clements PJ, et al: Cyclophosphamide versus placebo in scleroderma lung disease. *N Engl J Med* 2006;354:2655–2666.

Wigley FM: Raynaud's phenomenon. *N Engl J Med* 2002;347:1001–1008.

Zulian F, Vallongo C, Woo P, et al: Localized scleroderma in childhood is not just a skin disease. *Arthritis Rheum* 2005;52:2873–2881.

Chapter 160 ■ Behçet Disease

Abraham Gedalia

Behçet disease, a multisystem disorder originally described as recurrent oral and genital ulceration associated with relapsing iritis or uveitis, is often characterized by cutaneous, arthritic, neurologic, vascular, and gastrointestinal manifestations.

EPIDEMIOLOGY. The disease is reported commonly in the Mediterranean basin and Asia and is relatively rare in Europe and the United States. The condition is uncommon in children, who account for an estimated 5% of cases.

ETIOLOGY AND PATHOGENESIS. The etiology of Behçet disease is unknown, although an association with HLA-B5 and HLA-B51 is clear. A few cases of transient neonatal Behçet disease in offspring of mothers with Behçet disease are reported, suggesting that an antibody-mediated immune process may have a role in the pathogenesis. The basic pathologic lesion is vasculitis of small- and medium-sized arteries with cellular infiltrations leading to fibrinoid necrosis and narrowing and obliteration of the vessel lumens. Necrotizing and granulomatous inflammation of large vessels such as the aorta or pulmonary artery may also occur.

CLINICAL MANIFESTATIONS. The clinical course is highly variable, with recurrent exacerbations and disease-free intervals of uncertain duration. The most consistent symptom is painful, shallow oral ulcers, usually 2–10 mm in diameter with surrounding erythema, which develop on the buccal mucosa, gingiva, lips, and tongue, persist for days to weeks, and then heal without scarring in 1–3 wk. These oral necrotic ulcers may occur singly or in crops, with a mean of 13 attacks per year. Genital (labia, scrotum, penis) ulcers occur in most patients and follow a parallel course but may heal with scars. Skin manifestations occur in most patients and include erythema nodosum, papulopustular lesions, pseudofolliculitis, and acneiform nodules. **Cutaneous pathergy** is often present, manifesting as an erythematous sterile pustule that develops 24–48 hr after a needle prick. **Ocular manifestations,** including anterior or posterior uveitis and retinal vasculitis, occur less frequently in children than in adults but are more severe in the pediatric population and may progress to blindness. **Arthritis** is common and is usually acute, recurrent, asymmetric, and polyarticular, involving the large joints. Central nervous system abnormalities such as meningoencephalitis, cranial nerve palsies, and psychosis usually occur later in the course of the disease and indicate a poor prognosis. Fever, orchitis, myositis, pericarditis, nephritis, splenomegaly, and amyloidosis are rare associated manifestations. There is an increases risk for thrombophlebitis and large vessel thrombosis including the superior or inferior vena cava and hepatic veins **(Budd Chiari syndrome).**

DIAGNOSIS. The diagnosis of Behçet disease is not usually confirmed until the mid-twenties or thirties. The International Study Group criteria for diagnosis of Behçet disease include oral aphthae that recur at least 3 times within 12 mo accompanied by 2 of the following: recurrent genital ulcerations, eye lesions (anterior or posterior uveitis, or retinal vasculitis), skin lesions (erythema nodosum, pseudofolliculitis, or acneiforme nodules), and a positive pathergy test. Laboratory tests are not diagnostic, although the finding of HLA-B5 or HLA-B51 supports the diagnosis.

DIFFERENTIAL DIAGNOSIS. The differential diagnosis includes herpes simplex virus infection, inflammatory bowel disease, recurrent aphthous stomatitis, and complex aphthosis, which is recurrent oral and genital aphthous ulcers or ≥3 persistent oral aphthae.

TREATMENT. Treatment is based on anecdotal reports. Many drugs, including corticosteroids, colchicine, chlorambucil, azathioprine, cyclosporine, and tacrolimus, have been used. Colchicine is effective and shows higher efficacy in children than in adults, especially for oral ulcers, skin rash, joint symptoms, and, occasionally, eye disease. Thalidomide has been reported to be a highly effective and useful therapeutic option for severe oral and genital ulcerations that are unresponsive to other therapies. The successful use of anti–tumor necrosis factor-α (TNF-α) therapy or interferon-α-2a in severe or intractable cases of Behçet disease suggests that these agents may also have a role in the management of this disease. Symptomatic treatment of oral ulcerations may include oral rinses with solutions containing tetracycline, topical anesthetics, and chlorhexidine gluconate.

COMPLICATIONS AND PROGNOSIS. Behçet disease has a variable clinical course with exacerbations and remissions, with the serious complications occurring many years after diagnosis. Blindness may result from posterior uveitis. Gastrointestinal lesions resembling orogenital aphthae occur most commonly in the ileocecal region and rarely lead to perforation. Central nervous system complications include venous sinus thrombosis and parenchymal involvement. Mortality is low and is usually attributable to bowel perforation, thrombosis, or central nervous system involvement.

Alpsoy E, Durusoy C, Yilmaz E, et al: Interferon alfa-2a in the treatment of Behçet disease. *Arch Dermatol* 2002;138:467–471.

International Study Group for Behçet's Disease: Criteria for diagnosis of Behçet's disease. *Lancet* 1990;335:1078–1080.

Kari JA, Shah V, Dillon MJ. Behçet's disease in UK children: Clinical features and treatment including thalidomide. *Rheumatology* 2001;40:933–938.

Koné-Paut I, Yurdakul S, Bahabri SA, et al: Clinical features of Behçet's disease in children: An international collaborative study of 86 cases. *J Pediatr* 1998;132: 721–725.

Krause I, Uziel Y, Guedj D, et al: Childhood Behçet's disease: Clinical features and comparison with adult-onset disease. *Rheumatology* 1999;38:457–462.

Kural-Seyahi E, Fresko I, Seyahi N, et al: The long-term mortality and morbidity of Behçet syndrome: A 2 decade outcome survey of 387 patients followed at a dedicated center. *Medicine* 2003;82:60–76.

Marshall SE: Behcet's disease. *Clin Rheumatol* 2004;18:291–311

McCarty MA, Garton RA, Jorizzo JL: Complex aphthosis and Behçet's disease. *Dermatol Clin* 2003;21:41–48.

Siva A, Kantarci OH, Saip S, et al: Behçet's disease: Diagnostic and prognostic aspects of neurological involvement. *J Neurol* 2001;248:95–103.

Chapter 161 ■ Sjögren Syndrome

Abraham Gedalia

Sjögren syndrome is a chronic, inflammatory, autoimmune disease characterized by progressive lymphocytic and plasma cell infiltration of the salivary and lacrimal glands.

EPIDEMIOLOGY. Sjögren syndrome typically presents at 35–45 yr of age, with 90% of cases among women. It is uncommon in the pediatric age group. Sjögren syndrome can occur as an isolated disorder, referred to as primary Sjögren syndrome (sicca complex), or as a secondary form in association with other rheumatic disorders. Most commonly, it accompanies systemic lupus erythematosus, scleroderma, and mixed connective tissue disease, and only rarely is it associated with juvenile rheumatoid arthritis. It precedes the associated autoimmune disease by several years in half the cases.

ETIOLOGY AND PATHOGENESIS. The etiology of Sjögren syndrome is complex and includes genetic predisposition, and possibly an infectious trigger. Lymphocytes and plasma cells infiltrate salivary glands, forming distinct periductal and periacinar foci that become confluent and may replace epithelial structure. This autoimmune exocrinopathy results in xerophthalmia (dry eyes, or keratoconjunctivitis sicca) and xerostomia (dry mouth). Several genes regulating apoptosis influence the chronicity of lymphocytic infiltration.

CLINICAL MANIFESTATIONS. International classification criteria for the diagnosis of Sjögren syndrome in adult patients have been developed (Table 161-1), and diagnostic criteria in children have been proposed. Clinical manifestations are related to exocrine disease of the epithelial surfaces of the eyes, mouth, nose, larynx and trachea, vagina, and skin, leading to the common symptoms of photophobia, burning and itching eyes, blurred vision, painless unilateral or bilateral enlargement of the parotid glands, decreased sense of taste, dental caries, dysphagia, fissured tongue, and angular cheilitis. At the onset of the disease, recurrent parotid gland enlargement and parotitis is the most common manifestation in children, whereas sicca manifestations are most common in adults. Positive antinuclear antibodies (ANAs) and articular manifestations are significantly more frequent in adults. Subjective symptoms of xerostomia are less frequent among juvenile cases, indicating that Sjögren syndrome is a slowly progressive disease. Additional manifestations may include a decreased sense of smell, epistaxis, hoarseness, chronic otitis media, and internal organ exocrine disease involving the lungs, hepatobiliary system, pancreas, gastrointestinal tract, and kidneys.

Non-exocrine disease manifestations of Sjögren syndrome may be related to inflammatory vascular disease (in skin, muscle and

TABLE 161-1. Panel: International Consensus Criteria for Sjögren Syndrome

OCULAR SYMPTOMS (AT LEAST ONE PRESENT)
Persistent, troublesome dry eyes every day for longer than 3 months
Recurrent sensation of sand or gravel in the eyes
Use of a tear substitute more than three times a day
ORAL SYMPTOMS (AT LEAST ONE PRESENT)
Feeling of dry mouth every day for at least 3 months
Recurrent feeling of swollen salivary glands as an adult
Need to drink liquids to aid in swallowing dry foods
OBJECTIVE EVIDENCE OF DRY EYES (AT LEAST ONE PRESENT)
Schirmer I test
Rose-Bengal
Lacrimal-gland biopsy sample with focus score >1
OBJECTIVE EVIDENCE OF SALIVARY-GLAND INVOLVEMENT (AT LEAST ONE PRESENT)
Salivary-gland scintigraphy
Parotid sialography
Unstimulated whole sialometry (≤1.5 mL/15 min)
LABORATORY ABNORMALITY (AT LEAST ONE PRESENT)
Anti-SSA or anti-SSB
Antinuclear antibody (ANA)
IgM rheumatoid factor (anti-IgG Fc)

From Fox RI: Sjogren's syndrome. *Lancet* 2005;366:321–331.

joints, serosae, peripheral and central nervous system), noninflammatory vascular disease (Raynaud phenomenon), mediator-induced disease (hematologic cytopenias, fatigue, and fever), and autoimmune endocrinopathy (thyroiditis).

DIAGNOSIS. The diagnosis is based on clinical features supported by biopsy of the lip or glands demonstrating foci of lymphocytic infiltration, cryoglobulinemia, elevated erythrocyte sedimentation rate (ESR), hypergammaglobulinemia, positive rheumatoid factor, and positive antinuclear antibodies to Ro(SSA) and La(SSB). Anti-β-fodrin autoantibodies, directed against an apoptotic cleavage product of α-fodrin, are a useful diagnostic marker for juvenile Sjögren syndrome. The Schirmer test detects abnormal tear production (≤5 mm of wetting of filter paper strip in 5 min). Imaging studies including MRI, technetium-99 scintigraphy, and sialography are useful in the diagnostic evaluation for Sjögren syndrome.

DIFFERENTIAL DIAGNOSIS. The differential diagnosis of Sjögren syndrome in children includes chronic recurrent parotitis, infectious parotitis, polycystic parotid disease, tumors, and sarcoidosis. In these conditions, sicca complex, rash, arthralgia, and antinuclear antibodies are usually absent.

TREATMENT. Symptomatic treatment includes the use of artificial tears, oral lozenges, and fluids to limit the damaging effects of decreased secretions. Corticosteroids, nonsteroidal anti-inflammatory drugs, and hydroxychloroquine are among the more commonly used agents for treatment. Greater potency immunosuppressive agents such as cyclosporine and cyclophosphamide are reserved for severe functional disorders and life-threatening complications.

COMPLICATIONS AND PROGNOSIS. The symptoms of Sjögren syndrome develop and progress slowly. Diminished salivary flow typically remains constant for years. Because monoclonal B-lymphocyte disease originates chiefly from lymphocytic foci within salivary glands or from parenchymal internal organs, there is increased risk for mucosa-associated lymphoid tissue (MALT) lymphoma. Maternal Sjögren syndrome can be an antecedent to the neonatal lupus syndrome (see Chapter 157.1).

Bartunkova J, Sediva A, Vencovsky J, et al: Primary Sjögren syndrome in children and adolescents: Proposal for diagnostic criteria. *Clin Exp Rheumatol* 1999;17:381–386.

Cimaz R, Casadei A, Rose C, et al: Primary Sjögren's syndrome in paediatric age: A multicentre survey. *Eur J Pediatr* 2003;162:661–665.

Fox RI: Sjögren's syndrome. *Lancet* 2005;366:321–331.

Maeno N, Takei S, Imanaka H, et al: Anti-alpha-fodrin antibodies in Sjögren's syndrome in children. *J Rheumatol* 2001;28:860–864.

Manthrope R, Asmussen K, Oxholm P: Primary Sjögren's syndrome: Diagnostic criteria, clinical features, and disease activity. *J Rheumatol* 1997;24(Suppl 50):8–11.

Chapter 162 ■ Hereditary Periodic Fever Syndromes

Abraham Gedalia

Hereditary periodic fever syndromes, or **human autoinflammatory syndromes**, comprise a group of hereditary disorders with similar clinical features of recurrent short episodes of fever associated with inflammatory manifestations. These are usually self-limited in nature and occur in the absence of infection or autoimmune reaction. Each of these disorders has a distinct genetic defect. Most of these proteins are members of the **Death Domain superfamily** and are involved in inflammation and apoptosis. These proteins mediate the regulation of nuclear factor-κB (NF-κB), cell apoptosis, and interleukin 1β (IL-1β) secretion through cross-regulated and common signaling pathways.

The most common hereditary disorder is familial Mediterranean fever (FMF), followed by tumor necrosis factor (TNF)–receptor-associated periodic syndrome (TRAPS), and hyperimmunoglobulinemia D syndrome (HIDS). Additional syndromes include Muckle-Wells syndrome (MWS); familial cold urticaria (FCU), known also as familial cold autoinflammatory syndrome (FCAS); and chronic infantile neurological cutaneous and articular disease (CINCA), also known as neonatal onset multisystemic inflammatory disease (NOMID). Secondary amyloidosis (AA) was reported as a complication in all of these disorders, although it is less common with HIDS. FMF and HIDS are autosomal recessive diseases, whereas TRAPS and MWS/FCU/CINCA are autosomal dominant diseases. The diagnosis of each of these entities depends on the clinical features and the genetic confirmation (Table 162-1). Another periodic fever syndrome is periodic fever, adenopathy, and pharyngitis with aphthous ulcerations (PFAPA), but it is not classified as a human autoinflammatory syndrome (see Table 162-1).

FAMILIAL MEDITERRANEAN FEVER (FMF)

FMF, the most common entity among the group of periodic fever syndromes, is an inherited disorder characterized by brief, acute, self-limited episodes of fever and polyserositis recurring at irregular intervals, as well as development of AA amyloidosis (see Chapter 163), which, if untreated, leads to end-stage renal failure.

ETIOLOGY. The gene responsible for FMF is mapped to a small interval on the short arm of chromosome 16p13.3. The FMF gene, designated *MEFV* (*ME* for Mediterranean and *FV* for fever), is a member of the *RoRet* gene family. It is approximately 10 kb with 10 exons that express a 3.7-kb transcript encoding a 781 amino acid protein known as **pyrin,** or **marenostrin,** which is expressed in myeloid cells. More than 50 mutations have been discovered, mostly of missense type. It is unclear whether all are truly disease-related mutations. The five most common mutations (M694V, V726A, M694I, M680I, E148Q) are found in more than two thirds of Mediterranean patients with FMF. Haplotypes and mutational analyses show ancestral relationships among carrier chromosomes that have been separated for centuries. Approximately 70% of patients with clinical manifestations of FMF have one of the two mutations that are identifiable by genetic diagnosis. The most common missense mutation is M694V (substitution of methionine with valine at codon 694), which occurs in 20–67% of cases and is associated with full penetrance. Homozygosity for M694V is associated with a greater disease severity and a higher incidence of amyloidosis. The V726A mutation occurs in 7–35% of cases and is associated with milder disease and a lower incidence of amyloidosis. The E148Q mutation is associated with low penetrance and very mild phenotype. These findings suggest that phenotypic differences may reflect different mutations. As with other recessive diseases, it is likely that some heterozygous patients may show attenuated clinical symptoms, with or without increased levels of acute phase reactants.

EPIDEMIOLOGY. FMF appears to be transmitted as an autosomal recessive disease and occurs primarily among ethnic groups of Mediterranean origin, mainly Sephardic Jews, Turks, Armenians, and individuals of Arab descent. In these populations, the carrier frequency is estimated to be as high as 1 in 5 persons. Greeks,

TABLE 162-1. Demographic, Clinical, and Genetic Features of Periodic Fever Syndromes

FEATURES	FAMILIAL MEDITERRANEAN FEVER (FMF)	HYPERIMMUNOGLOBULINEMIA D SYNDROME (HIDS)	TUMOR NECROSIS FACTOR (TNF)-RECEPTOR-ASSOCIATED PERIODIC SYNDROME (TRAPS)	MUCKLE-WELLS SYNDROME (MWS), FAMILIAL COLD URTICARIA (FCU), AND CHRONIC INFANTILE NEUROLOGICAL CUTANEOUS AND ARTICULAR (CINCA) DISEASE	PERIODIC FEVER ADENOPATHY PHARYNGITIS APHTHA (PFAPA)
DEMOGRAPHIC FEATURES					
Age of Onset	Early childhood	First year of life	≤20 yr	Infancy and childhood	≤5 yr
Ethnicity	Sephardic Jews, Turkish Armenian, Arab, Italian	Dutch, French, other European	Irish, Northern European, others	Northern European, other	None specified
CLINICAL FEATURES					
Duration of episodes	1–4 days	3–7 days	>1 wk	Variable (2–3 days)	3–6 days every 4–6 wk
Abdominal pain	Very common (sterile peritonitis)	Common	Common	Rare	Common
Arthritis	Very common (monoarthritis or oligoarthritis)	Common (symmetric polyarthritis)	Rare	Destructive arthritis	Arthralgia
Myalgia	Rare	Rare	Very common migratory	Common	Common
Chest pain	Common	Rare	Common	None	Rare
Rash	<5% with erysipelas-like most common	>90% with erysipelas-like most common	Erysipelas-like most common; migratory	Erythema and urticaria	Uncommon
OTHER CLINICAL FEATURES					
	Pericarditis, Henoch-Schönlein purpura, scrotal involvement, splenomegaly	Cervical lymphadenopathy, hepatosplenomegaly, headaches	Conjunctivitis, periorbital edema	Hearing loss, papillitis, cold sensitivity	Fever, cervical adenopathy, exudative tonsillitis, aphthous stomatitis
GENETICS FEATURES					
Inheritance	Autosomal recessive	Autosomal recessive	Autosomal dominant	Autosomal dominant	Sporadic
Gene responsible	*MEFV*	*MVK*	*TNFRSF1A*	*CIAS1*	Unknown
Chromosomal region	16p13	12q24	12p13	1q44	Unknown
Gene product	Pyrin (marenostrin)	Mevalonate kinase	TNF receptor 1A	Cryopyrin	Unknown
Elevated levels of acute phase reactants	Very common, mainly during the attacks	Very common	Very common	Common, especially with MWS	Common
Increased risk for amyloidosis AA	Common (40–75% of untreated patients)	Not reported	Common (15–25% of patients)	Rare (2% of patients)	No
Treatment	Colchicine	Symptomatic, etanercept, simvastatin	Corticosteroids, etanercept	Symptomatic, anakinra, corticosteroids, etanercept	Single dose prednisone or betamethasone

Hispanics, and Italians are less commonly affected. In addition, cases of FMF are also found among non-Mediterranean persons. It is seen rarely among Ashkenazi Jews, Germans, and Anglo-Saxons and other ethnic groups in which only sporadic cases have been reported.

PATHOGENESIS. The exact pathogenesis of the acute episodes of FMF is unknown. Between episodes, patients with FMF have increased serum levels of interferon-γ and enhanced production of other proinflammatory cytokines such as TNF-α, IL-1β, IL-6, and IL-8 in circulating leukocytes. Pyrin/marenostrin is a member of the Death Domain superfamily and consists of 4 different functional domains that interact with other proteins. Of particular interest is the domain known as the **Pyrin Domain,** a 92-amino-acid N-terminal domain shared by several proteins that are involved in the regulation of the inflammatory response and apoptosis. Pyrin acts as anti-inflammatory factor by inhibiting pro–IL-1β cytokine processing to the active form. This normally takes place through interactions with apoptosis specklike protein with a caspase recruitment domain (ASC) and NF-κB. It is speculated that defective (or mutated) pyrin/marenostrin found in patients with FMF causes defective apoptosis and stimulation of IL-1 processing and secretion, resulting in increased IL-1β levels that are responsible for the uncontrolled inflammation (Fig. 162-1). Another possibility that was previously more popular is based on the finding of C5a inhibitor (inactivating enzyme) deficiency in peritoneal and synovial fluids of patients with FMF. C5a is a fragment of complement, an anaphylatoxin, and a potent chemotactic agent (see Chapter 132). Normally, C5a inhibitor neutralizes the small amounts of C5a released into serosal cavities before it precipitates overt inflammation. The hypothesis is that a deficiency of C5a inhibitor, which is a consequence of pyrin/marenostrin dysfunction in patients with FMF, allows further accumulation of C5a, leading to the acute attack. This theory is less attractive, although it explains the periodicity of FMF. Further understanding of pyrin/marenostrin functions will shed light on aspects of FMF pathogenesis that are not yet fully understood.

CLINICAL MANIFESTATIONS. The onset of clinical manifestations occurs before 5 yr of age in 63–68% of cases and before 20 yr of age in 90% of cases. The onset may be as early as 6 mo of age. Exercise, emotional stress, infection, menses, and surgery may precipitate the acute episodes. The typical acute episode lasts 1–4 days and includes fever and 1 or more symptoms of sterile peritonitis manifested by abdominal pain (90%), arthritis or arthralgia (85%), and pleuritis manifested by chest pain (20%). Other serosal tissues such as the pericardium and tunica vaginalis testis (acute scrotum) are rarely affected. Erysipelas-like skin rash, myalgia, splenomegaly, scrotal involvement in boys, neurologic involvement, Henoch-Schönlein purpura, and hypothyroidism are other less common clinical manifestations.

DIAGNOSIS. Genetic testing for the FMF gene confirms the diagnosis of FMF, which is especially important in areas where the disease is rare and less familiar to physicians. Genetic screening using PCR and restriction analysis systems is available in some commercial clinical genetic laboratories. Genetic laboratories usually screen for the 5 to 10 most common mutations, however, and, thus, rare mutations will be missed. Therefore, the diagnosis of FMF is still based on clinical manifestations, with genetic testing used as a confirmatory test.

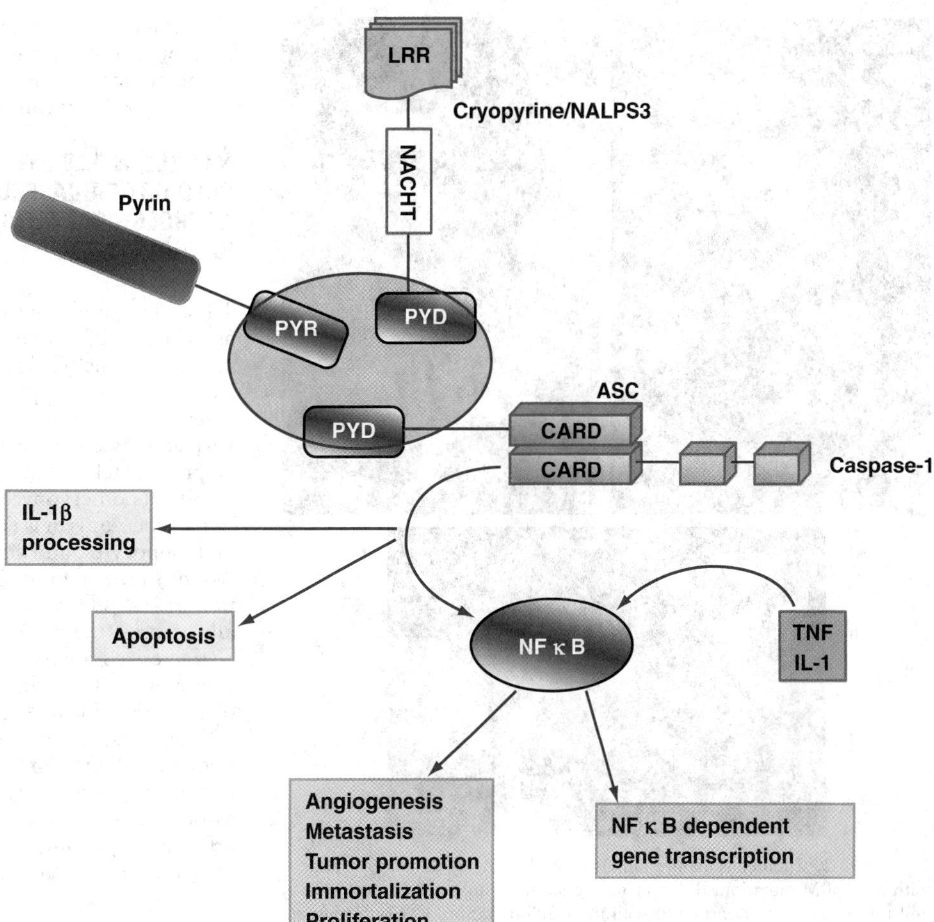

Figure 162-1. Proteins containing PyD domain regulate inflammation through their interaction with apoptotic speck protein (ASC). The assembly of cryopyrin and ASC induces IL-1 processing through caspase-1, whereas pyrin may act as an inhibitor. Loss of function by mutations in the pyrin could potentially lead to autoinflammation by reducing the pyrin inhibitory role. Alternatively, gain-of-function mutations in cryopyrin, as found in MWS/FCU/NOMID patients, could activate this pathway. ASC participates in apoptosis and activation of NF-κB, a transcription factor involved in both initiation and resolution of the inflammatory response. IL-1, interleukin 1; LRR, leucine-rich repeats; TNF, tumor necrosis factor; MWS, Muckle-Wells syndrome; FCU, familial cold urticaria; NOMID, neonatal onset multisystemic inflammatory disease. (From Padeh S: Periodic fever syndromes. *Pediatr Clin North Am* 2005;52:577–609.)

TREATMENT. Attacks of FMF can be prevented by prophylactic colchicine (0.02–0.03 mg/kg/day; maximum: 2 mg/day) in 1 to 2 divided doses. Colchicine therapy reduces the frequency of acute attacks but also greatly decreases the probability of development of amyloidosis; it may produce partial regression of existing amyloidosis. Colchicine therapy for FMF during pregnancy has not been reported to harm either the mother or her fetus.

COMPLICATIONS AND PROGNOSIS. In about $^1/_3$ to $^1/_2$ of untreated children and in $^3/_4$ of adults with FMF, a form of renal amyloidosis develops in which the amyloid derives from a normal serum protein, amyloid A, resulting in **amyloidosis AA.** Renal disease is manifest by proteinuria that progresses to nephrotic syndrome and renal failure over a period of months to several years. Transplantation may be required for renal failure. Amyloidosis is common among Sephardic Jews and Turks and less common in Armenians. Armenians living in Armenia are reported to have a significantly higher incidence of amyloidosis than their counterparts in North America, suggesting that environmental factors may also play a role. Mortality from FMF usually results from complications of renal failure and amyloidosis such as infection, thromboembolism, and uremia.

HYPERIMMUNOGLOBULINEMIA D SYNDROME (HIDS)

HIDS is an inherited periodic fever syndrome with an autosomal recessive mode of transmission. This condition is reported primarily among families of European descent, especially Dutch and French, and is caused by mutations in the mevalonate kinase *(MVK)* gene found on chromosome 12 at 12q24. Mevalonate kinase is an enzyme that enhances the metabolism of mevalonic acid, an intermediary product of cholesterol and isoprenoid synthesis pathways (see Chapter 86). It is speculated that shortage of isoprenoid end products contributes to increased secretion of IL-1β, which subsequently leads to overt inflammation and fever. More than 40 different mutations of the *MVK* gene have been reported. The most common mutation is V377I, likely of Dutch origin. Mutations are associated with decreased activity of mevalonate kinase in lymphocytes, leading to increased plasma levels of mevalonic acid, which is excreted in large amounts in the urine. The majority of patients have onset within the 1st year of life. The manifestations include recurrent, short episodes of fever lasting 3–7 days, with abdominal pain that is often accompanied by diarrhea, nausea, and vomiting. Other clinical manifestations include cervical lymphadenopathy, rash, symmetric poly- or oligo-arthralgia/arthritis, and occasional splenomegaly. In some patients, the attacks may last several weeks. During the attacks, leukocytosis and increased serum levels of acute phase reactants and proinflammatory cytokines are commonly present. The finding of elevated serum levels of IgD (>100 mU/mL) twice in a single month is typical and strongly supports the diagnosis of HIDS. AA amyloidosis has been reported in a 27 yr old male with HIDS, which represents the only case with amyloidosis reported with this disease. The low susceptibility to amyloidosis in HIDS is not fully understood. There is no known therapy for this condition, although treatment with colchicine, nonsteroidal anti-inflammatory drugs (NSAIDs), and glucocorticoids may be associated with partial relief. An incomplete response of HIDS to etanercept has been reported. A trial of simvastatin showed a beneficial clinical effect in 5 of 6 patients with HIDS.

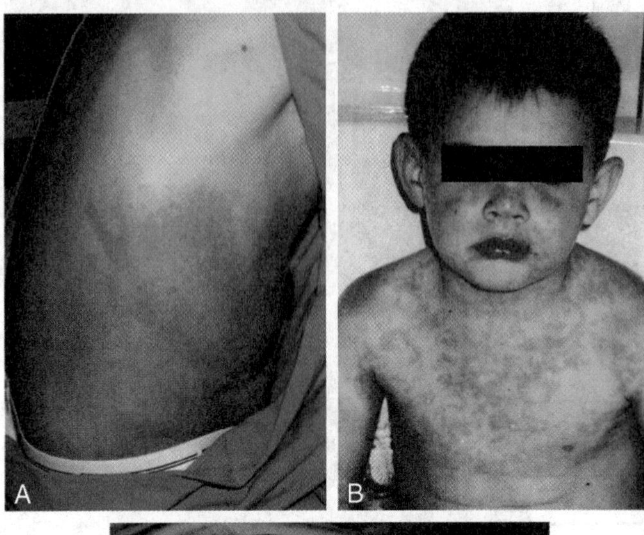

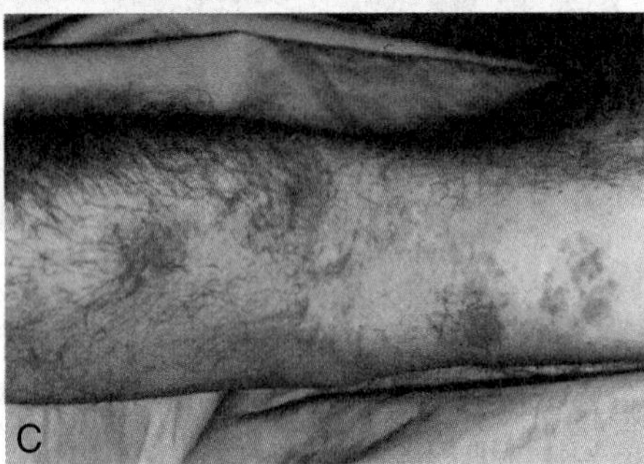

Figure 162-2. Cutaneous manifestations of TRAPS. *A*, right flank of a patient with the T50M mutation. *B*, Serpiginous rash involving the face, neck, torso, and upper extremities of a child with the C30S mutation. *C*, Erythematous, macular patches with crusting on the flexor surface of the right arm of a patient with the T50M mutation. TRAPS, tumor necrosis factor (TNF)–receptor-associated periodic syndrome.

TUMOR NECROSIS FACTOR (TNF)–RECEPTOR ASSOCIATED PERIODIC SYNDROME (TRAPS)

TRAPS is an autosomal dominant inherited periodic fever caused by mutation in the soluble TNF receptor superfamily 1A gene, *TNFRSF1A*. This syndrome was previously known by other names, including **familial Hibernian fever, familial periodic fever,** and **autosomal dominant recurrent fever.** This is a rare disorder that has been reported in a few families of Irish and Scottish ancestry, although other ethnic groups, including African-Americans, may be affected. The *TNFRSF1A* gene is on chromosome 12 at 12p13 and encodes for type 1A TNF receptor protein. More than 40 different mutations of the gene have been reported. Patients with TRAPS usually manifest brief, intermittent febrile episodes, typically lasting 4–6 days, and associated with severe abdominal pain, nausea, and vomiting. Oligoarthritis, myalgias, rash, conjunctivitis, and unilateral periorbital edema are universally present in TRAPS patients (Fig. 162-2). Arthralgias are less common. The acute attacks of TRAPS are slightly longer than the FMF episodes and may persist for up to 3 wk. Amyloidosis develops in up to 25% of the patients, depending on the specific gene mutation and duration of attacks. Increased levels of acute phase reactants may be seen, with the most specific findings being low serum levels of soluble type 1A TNF receptor and increased TNF levels. Colchicine has no effect on the acute attacks or development of amyloidosis in TRAPS patients. Prednisone (1 mg/kg; maximum dose: 20 mg) may be helpful and can attenuate the length and severity of the attacks. Therapy with etanercept (25 mg subcutaneously twice weekly), a recombinant TNF receptor fusion protein, decreases attack frequency, duration, and severity. Etanercept is a steroid-sparing agent and may reverse AA amyloidosis. Although the use of etanercept appears promising, not all patients respond.

MUCKLE-WELLS SYNDROME (MWS), FAMILIAL COLD URTICARIA (FCU), AND CHRONIC INFANTILE NEUROLOGICAL CUTANEOUS AND ARTICULAR (CINCA) DISEASE

These 3 separate entities, which are autosomal dominant, are associated with mutations in the cold-induced anti-inflammatory syndrome gene, *CIAS1,* located on chromosome 1 at 1q44. This gene encodes the protein **cryopyrin** that shares homology in several regions with pyrin (see Fig. 162-1). The term *cryopyrin* was designated because of the association with cold urticaria. Approximately 50 mutations in the CIAS1 gene that have different effects on cryopyrin expression have been described. Similar to pyrin, cryopyrin is expressed in polymorphonuclear leukocytes and monocytes, and activates an adaptor protein known as ASC. As with FMF, mutations in cryopyrin leads to increased production of IL-1β (a common underlying mechanism), which eventually causes these diverse disease entities. All 3 entities are characterized by periodic febrile attacks with urticarial rash, arthralgia and arthritis, ocular involvement, and the development of AA amyloidosis characteristics. Both MWS and CINCA are typically associated with progressive sensorineural hearing loss, optic nerve involvement, and chronic aseptic meningitis. CINCA is a more severe entity, typically with neonatal onset commonly associated with skin rash, neurologic disease, and destructive arthropathy, mainly of the knees, which may lead to major malformation and disability (Fig. 162-3). No known therapy exists

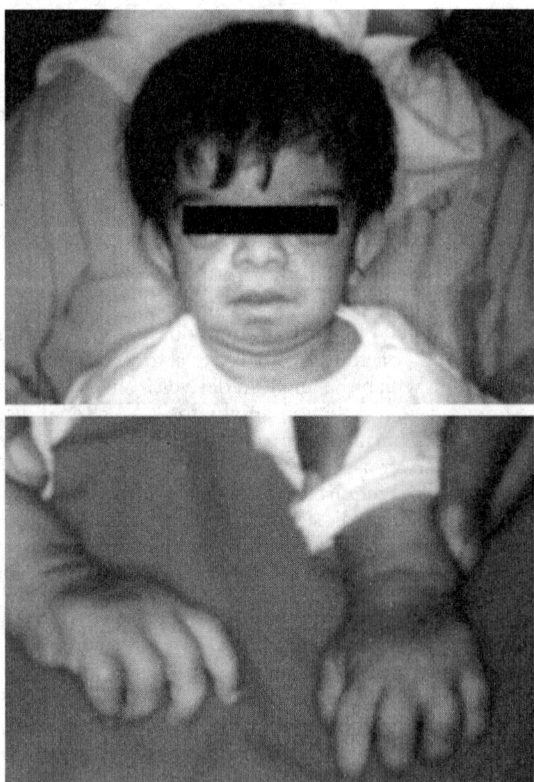

Figure 162-3. A 3 yr old girl with NOMID/CINCA syndrome. Note the markedly deformed hands, rash, frontal bossing, and large head. NOMID, neonatal onset multisystemic inflammatory disease; CINCA, chronic infantile neurological cutaneous and articular disease. (From Padeh S: Periodic fever syndromes. *Pediatr Clin North Am* 2005;52:577–560.)

for these conditions, although treatment with colchicine, NSAIDs, and glucocorticoids may provide some relief. Remarkable responses to anakinra (recombinant IL-1 receptor antagonist) in 3 family members with MWS and 18 patients with CINCA have been reported.

PYOGENIC ARTHRITIS, PYODERMA GANGRENOSUM, AND ACNE (PAPA) AND BLAU SYNDROMES

Further understanding of pyrin functions, especially the interactions with other proteins, has lead to the discovery of two other entities, PAPA and Blau syndromes. **PAPA (pyogenic arthritis, pyoderma gangrenosum, and acne)** is an autosomal dominant disorder with mutations in the gene encoding the adaptor protein proline serine threonine phosphatase-interacting protein (PSTPIP1) located on chromosome 15 at 15q24. **Blau syndrome** is a rare autosomal dominant disorder that manifests with early-onset granulomatous arthritis, uveitis, rash, and flexion contractures at the fingers associated with mutations in the gene encoding CARD15 (caspase recruitment domain 15 protein), known also as NOD2 (nucleotide-binding oligomerization domain 2 protein) located on chromosome 16 at 16q12. These 2 syndromes are additional rare members of the hereditary periodic fever syndromes family.

PERIODIC FEVER, APHTHOUS STOMATITIS, PHARYNGITIS, AND ADENITIS (PFAPA)

Another distinct periodic fever syndrome is manifested by episodes of **periodic fever, aphthous stomatitis, pharyngitis, and adenitis (PFAPA;** also known as **Marshall syndrome)** [see Table 162-1]. PFAPA occurs sporadically with no ethnic predilection. Symptoms begin around 2–6 yr of age and include fever, malaise, exudative appearing tonsillitis with negative throat cultures, cervical lymphadenopathy, and aphthae, and, less commonly, headache, abdominal pain, and arthralgia. The episodes last 4–6 days, regardless of antipyretic or antibiotic treatment, and occur at a frequency of 8–12 episodes/yr. Findings during the episodes may include mild hepatosplenomegaly, mild leukocytosis, and elevated acute phase reactants. Both the frequency and intensity of the episodes diminish over time. The etiology and the pathogenesis of PFAPA remain unknown. It is not clear whether this syndrome represents an infectious or immunogenetic dysregulation entity. The majority of patients respond dramatically to a single dose of prednisone (1–2 mg/kg) or bethamethasone (0.3 mg/kg) with prompt resolution of symptoms within 24 hr. Complete resolution has also been reported after tonsillectomy. Affected children grow normally and have spontaneous resolution within 4–8 yr with no long-term sequelae. One patient developed TRAPS at the age of 22 yr.

Drenth JP, Van der Meer JW: Hereditary periodic fever. *N Engl J Med* 2001;345:1748–1757.

Frenkel J, Houten SM, Waterham HR, et al: Clinical and molecular variability in childhood periodic fever with hyperimmunoglobulinemia D. *Rheumatology* 2001;40:579–584.

Goldbach-Mansky R, Dailey NJ, Canna SW, et al: Neonatal-onset multisystem inflammatory disease responsive to interleukin-1β inhibition. *N Engl J Med* 2006;355:581–592.

Grateau G: Clinical and genetic aspects of hereditary periodic fever syndromes. *Rheumatology* 2004;43:410–415.

Hawkins PN, Lachmann HJ, Aganna E, et al: Spectrum of clinical features in Muckle-Wells syndrome and response to anakinra. *Arthritis Rheum* 2004;50:607–612.

Hull KM, Drewe E, Aksentijevich I, et al: The TNF receptor-associated periodic syndrome (TRAPS): Emerging concepts of an autoinflammatory disorder. *Medicine* 2002;81:349–368.

International FMF Consortium: Ancient missense mutations in a new member of the *RoRet* gene family are likely to cause familial Mediterranean fever. *Cell* 1997;90:797–807.

Kallinich T, Haffner D, Niehues T, et al: Colchicine use in children and adolescents with familial Mediterranean fever: literature review and consensus statement. *Pediatrics* 2007;119:e474–e483.

McDermott MF: A common pathway in periodic fever syndromes. *Trends Immunol* 2004;25:457–460.

Obici L, Manno C, Muda AO, et al: First report of systemic reactive (AA) amyloidosis in a patient with the hyperimmunoglobulinemia D with periodic fever syndrome. *Arthritis Rheum* 2004;50:2966–2969.

Ozkaya N, Yalcinkaya F: Colchicine treatment in children with familial Mediterranean fever. *Clin Rheumatol* 2003;22:314–317.

Padeh S, Brezniak N, Zemer D, et al: Periodic fever, aphthous stomatitis, pharyngitis, and adenopathy syndrome: Clinical characteristics and outcome. *J Pediatr* 1999;135:98–101.

Saulsbury FT, Wispelwey B: Tumor necrosis factor receptor-associated periodic syndrome in a young adult who had features of periodic fever, aphthous stomatitis, pharyngitis, and adenitis as a child. *J Pediatr* 2005:145:283–285.

Shinkai K, Kilcline C, Connolly MK, et al: The pyrin family of fever genes: Unmasking genetic determinants of autoinflammatory disease. *Arch Dermatol* 2005;141:242–247.

Turkish FMF Study Group: The familial Mediterranean fever (FMF) in Turkey. *Medicine* 2005;84:1–11.

Chapter 163 ■ Amyloidosis

Abraham Gedalia

Amyloidosis comprises a group of diseases characterized by extracellular deposition of insoluble, fibrous amyloid proteins in various body tissues.

ETIOLOGY. Amyloid material is composed of microscopic fibrils that are biochemically heterogeneous, with at least 20 different types of protein fibril compositions. All amyloid deposits contain the same nonfibrillar component, serum amyloid P. Amyloid fibril deposition may have no apparent consequences, or it may ultimately interfere with organ function.

The traditional amyloidosis classification system uses the descriptive terms *systemic* and *localized,* which do not designate the etiology or associated clinical manifestations. The systemic, or multisystem, amyloidoses correspond to clinical patterns of primary, secondary, familial, and dialysis-related amyloidosis. The localized, or organ-limited, amyloidoses are associated with aging and diabetes and occur in isolated organs such as endocrine glands without systemic involvement. The newer nomenclature of amyloidoses is based on biochemical analysis and uses *A* for amyloid followed by the abbreviation for the type of fibril protein. The most common type of amyloidosis in the United States, which was known as primary idiopathic amyloidosis or myeloma-associated amyloidosis, has deposition of amyloid composed of pieces of monoclonal immunoglobulin light-chain (abbreviated to *L*) and is now referred to as AL amyloidosis. Amyloidosis in persons with familial Mediterranean fever (FMF), chronic infection, and chronic inflammatory diseases involve amyloid A protein and was formerly known as secondary or reactive amyloidosis, and is now referred to as AA amyloidosis. AA amyloidosis is the most common serious complication of FMF (see Chapter 162). Amyloid conditions associated with aging (Alzheimer disease) as well as several rare autosomal dominant forms of amyloidoses have fibril protein composed of variants of the transport protein transthyretin (TTR) and are now referred to as TTR amyloidosis.

EPIDEMIOLOGY. AL amyloidosis is extremely rare in children and usually occurs in persons of middle age or older. It represents a plasma cell dyscrasia and can occur in isolation or along with multiple myeloma.

Only AA amyloidosis affects children in appreciable numbers, occurring in some persons with FMF, chronic inflammatory diseases including juvenile rheumatoid arthritis (JRA), ankylosing spondylitis, inflammatory bowel disease, chronic infections such as tuberculosis, cystic fibrosis, and, less commonly, systemic lupus erythematosus and juvenile dermatomyositis. The factors that determine the risk for amyloidosis as a complication of inflammation are not clear, as many individuals with long-standing inflammatory disease do not develop tissue amyloid deposition. AA amyloidosis affects as many as 10% of children with JRA in some European countries but is rarely seen as a complication of seemingly similar disease in children in the United States and Canada. Additionally, Armenians with FMF living in Armenia are reported to have a significantly higher incidence of amyloidosis than do their Armenian counterparts in North America. There is also ethnic variability in the frequency of amyloidosis, which among patients with FMF occurs in up to 60% of Turks, 27% of Sephardic Jews, and 1–2% of Armenians living in the United States. Reasons for these differences are unknown, although environmental and genetic factors in addition to the underlying inflammatory disease appear to have a role.

PATHOGENESIS. The AA protein isolated from AA amyloidosis is the 76-amino acid N-terminus fragment of serum amyloid A (SAA). SAA, a polymorphic protein synthesized in the liver, is an acute-phase reactant. Chronic inflammation results in elevated levels of SAA, which is the precursor to the fibril formation of AA amyloidosis. Three protein isoforms of SAA exist. SAA1 is the precursor of AA amyloidosis in majority of cases and has 5 variants that differ from each other by amino acid substitutions.

The factors responsible for determining the site of amyloid deposition in any form of amyloidosis are unknown. AA amyloidosis fibrils have been generated in tissue cultures by incubating SAA with macrophages, which may explain amyloid depositions in tissues such as the liver and spleen. The increased deposition in the kidneys is related to a different mechanism, possibly the glyco-oxidative modification of the AA protein itself.

Amyloid deposits are composed of seemingly homogeneous eosinophilic material that stains with Congo red dye and in polarized light demonstrates the pathognomonic apple-green birefringence. Amyloid can be recognized also by routine hematoxylin and eosin (H&E)–staining.

CLINICAL MANIFESTATIONS. Various patterns of organ dysfunction result from deposition of different types of amyloid fibril protein material. Regardless of the cause of amyloidosis, clinical symptoms usually begin >10 yr after the onset of inflammatory disease. The diagnosis is not usually established until the disease is far advanced. The most common clinical presentation of AA amyloidosis is renal dysfunction, ranging from proteinuria to nephrotic syndrome and eventual renal failure. Involvement of the gastrointestinal system is also frequent and usually manifests as chronic diarrhea, gastrointestinal bleeding, abdominal pain, and malabsorption. Anemia, hepatomegaly, and splenomegaly may be present.

DIAGNOSIS. The diagnosis of amyloidosis is established by biopsy demonstrating amyloid fibril proteins in affected tissues. In the presence of amyloidosis, renal biopsies are contraindicated because of potential bleeding. The liver and spleen are often affected but are not suitable sites for biopsy. Biopsy sites that are more accessible include the rectal mucosa, gingival tissue, and abdominal fat aspirate. A method of microradiographic scintigraphy using serum amyloid P component has been described as a useful tool for the diagnosis as well as for the monitoring of the status of amyloidosis.

LABORATORY FINDINGS. Patients with JRA and AA amyloidosis usually show elevated acute-phase reactants and high levels of immunoglobulins. Specific laboratory testing is only possible for AL amyloidosis. Most of these patients show increased plasma cells in the bone marrow, and serum or urine monoclonal Ig or free light chain. A biopsy showing amyloid deposition along with a monoclonal serum protein distinguishes AL amyloidosis from monoclonal gammopathy of uncertain significance (MGUS), which is common in older adults.

TREATMENT. The primary means of treatment of AA amyloidosis is aggressive management of the underlying inflammatory or infectious disease, which decreases levels of SAA protein. Colchicine is effective in controlling the attacks of FMF and also in preventing the development of amyloidosis associated with FMF. Children with FMF who are homozygous for M694V are at greater risk of developing amyloidosis and should receive colchicine for life.

Unlike AA amyloidosis associated with FMF, AA amyloidosis associated with JRA does not respond to colchicine therapy but instead does respond to chlorambucil, which reverses renal findings and prolongs the life of treated patients. Chlorambucil is associated with chromosome breakage and an unknown risk of subsequent malignancy. There is little experience with other cytotoxic agents or with the therapy for AA amyloidosis associated with other conditions. Anti–tumor necrosis factor-α (TNF-α) therapy, with etanercept or infliximab, is well tolerated and effective in reducing proteinuria in patients with AA amyloidosis secondary to inflammatory arthritides. Drugs that specifically prevent fibril development are in development.

COMPLICATIONS AND PROGNOSIS. End-stage renal failure is the underlying cause of death in 40–60% of cases of amyloidosis, with a median survival time from diagnosis of 2–10 yr.

PREVENTION. The primary means of preventing AA amyloidosis is treatment of the underlying inflammatory or infectious disease, which decreases levels of SAA protein and the risk of amyloid deposition.

David J, Vouyiouka O, Ansell BM, et al: Amyloidosis in juvenile chronic arthritis: A morbidity and mortality study. *Clin Exp Rheumatol* 1993;11:85–90.

Delibas A, Oner A, Balci B, et al: Genetic risk factors of amyloidogenesis in familial Mediterranean fever. *Am J Nephrol* 2005;25:434–440.

Gillmore JD, Lovat LB, Persey MR, et al: Amyloid load and clinical outcome in AA amyloidosis in relation to circulating concentration of serum amyloid A protein. *Lancet* 2001;358:24–29.

Gottenberg JE, Merle-Vincent F, Bentaberry F, et al: Anti–tumor necrosis factor α therapy in 15 patients with AA amyloidosis secondary to inflammatory arthritides. *Arthritis Rheum* 2004;48:2019–2024.

Hirschfield GM: Amyloidosis: A clinico-pathophysiological synopsis. *Semin Cell Dev Biol* 2004;14:39–44

Livneh A, Langevitz P, Shinar Y, et al: *MEFV* mutation analysis in patients suffering from amyloidosis of familial Mediterranean fever. *Amyloid* 1999;6:1–6.

Mimouni A, Magal N, Stoffman N, et al: Familial Mediterranean fever: Effect of genotype and ethnicity on inflammatory attacks and amyloidosis. *Pediatrics* 2000;105:E70.

Saatci U, Bakkaloglu A, Ozen S, et al: Familial Mediterranean fever and amyloidosis in children. *Acta Paediatr* 1993;81:705–706.

Woo P: Amyloidosis in children. *Baillieres Clin Rheumatol* 1994;8:691–697.

Chapter 164 ■ Sarcoidosis

Margaret W. Leigh

Sarcoidosis, a term derived from Greek meaning a "fleshlike condition," is a chronic, multisystem granulomatous disease of unknown cause. It occurs most frequently in young adults but can occur during childhood.

ETIOLOGY. Despite extensive studies, the etiology of sarcoidosis remains obscure. The granulomas of sarcoidosis resemble those associated with certain microbial agents, especially mycobacteria and fungi, and hypersensitivity to organic compounds. These similarities have led to speculation that microbes or organic dusts may be inciting agents of disease in genetically predisposed persons. Several types of exposures, including to insecticides, to microbial bioaerosols, and agricultural employment, are associated with increased risk for sarcoidosis. Specific gene polymorphisms, particularly of class I and II alleles of the major histocompatibility complex (MHC) on chromosome 6, have some impact on age of onset, disease severity, and prognosis.

EPIDEMIOLOGY. Sarcoidosis has a worldwide distribution and affects both sexes and all ethnic groups, with a peak incidence of 25–35 yr of age. Sarcoidosis occurs more frequently in African-Americans, with a tendency to be more acute and more severe, than in whites, with a tendency to present with asymptomatic or chronic disease. Familial clustering of sarcoidosis has been observed and suggests a genetic predisposition; however, the mode of inheritance is unclear.

PATHOLOGY AND PATHOGENESIS. The **noncaseating, epithelioid granulomatous lesions** of sarcoidosis can occur in almost any organ of the body. The lungs and thoracic lymph nodes are involved at some time in almost all patients, with skin, eyes, extrathoracic lymph nodes, bone marrow, heart, and liver variably involved. Sarcoidosis is an interstitial lung disease affecting bronchioles, alveoli, and blood vessels. Granulomas typically are not necrotic and contain epithelioid cells, macrophages, and giant cells in the center surrounded by a mixture of monocytes, lymphocytes, and fibroblasts. Activated T lymphocytes and macrophages within the granulomas release various proinflammatory mediators including interleukin 2 (IL-2), IL-18, interferon-γ, and other cytokines that promote and maintain granulomatous lesions. During active disease, lymphocytes in the granulomas are predominantly CD4 T lymphocytes. These lesions usually heal with complete preservation of the parenchyma. In ≈20% of the lesions, fibroblasts proliferate at the periphery of the granuloma and may produce fibrotic scar tissue, leading to significant and irreversible organ dysfunction. Macrophages within sarcoidosis granulomas produce and secrete 1,25-$(OH)_2$-D_3, the active form of vitamin D typically produced in the kidneys. Excess vitamin D results in hypercalcemia and hypercalciuria in patients with sarcoidosis.

CLINICAL MANIFESTATIONS. The initial clinical presentation is related to sex, race, and age, and is extremely variable, depending on the organ systems involved and extent of granulomatous inflammation. Sarcoidosis may involve only 1 organ at a time, or may be widespread. Manifestations in children usually include fatigue, anorexia, weight loss, bone and joint pain, and anemia. In adults and children, the lung is the most frequently affected organ, but the extent and manifestations of pulmonary involvement are variable and classically include cough, retrosternal chest pain, and dyspnea on exertion. Parenchymal infiltrates, miliary nodules, and hilar and paratracheal lymphadenopathy occur (Fig. 164-1). Pulmonary function tests show primarily restrictive changes. Extrathoracic lymphadenopathy, eye changes consisting of uveitis or iritis, skin lesions, and hepatic and bone marrow involvement occur frequently. Cutaneous involvement occurs in $^1/_4$ of cases, and is usually present on onset of the disease. Red-brown to purple maculopapular lesions <1 cm on the face, neck, upper back, and extremities are the most common skin finding (Fig. 164-2). Neurologic involvement is rare in childhood but may present with seizures, cranial nerve involvement, mass lesions, and hypothalamic dysfunction. Children <4 yr old may have a distinct form of sarcoidosis consisting of a maculopapular erythematous rash, uveitis, and arthritis but minimal or no pulmonary changes. The arthritis, which can be confused with juvenile rheumatoid arthritis, produces large, painless, boggy synovial effusions of the tendon sheaths with little limitation of motion.

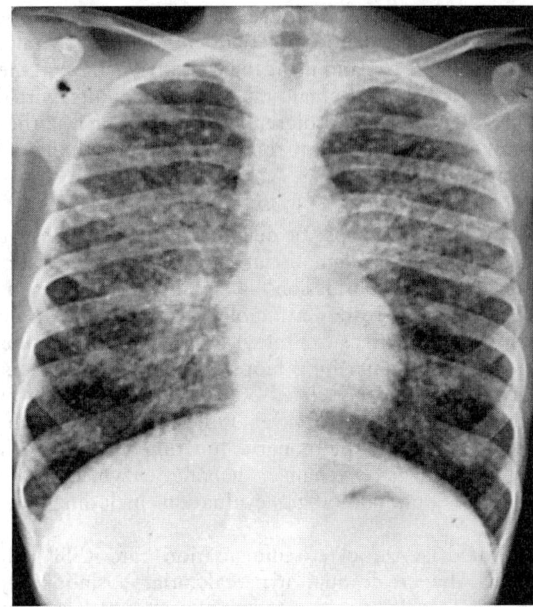

Figure 164-1. Chest x-ray of a white 10 yr old girl with sarcoidosis that shows widely disseminated peribronchial infiltrations, multiple small nodular densities, hyperaeration of the lungs, and hilar lymphadenopathy.

Among adults, most patients present with chronic respiratory symptoms and few constitutional symptoms. African-Americans

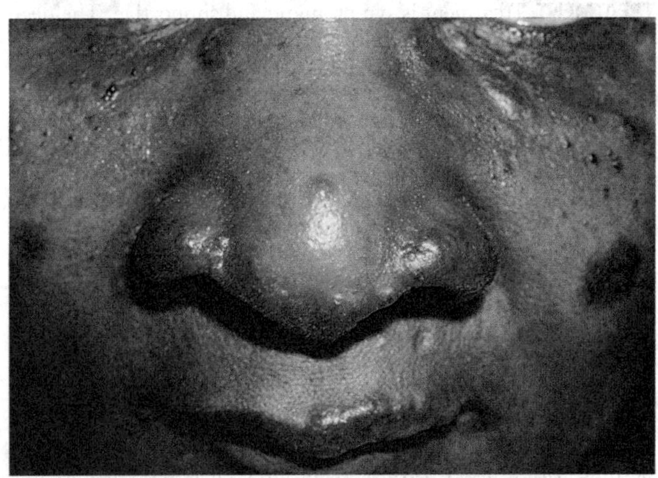

Figure 164-2. Sarcoidosis. Nodules on the face. (From Shah BR, Laude TA: *Atlas of Pediatric Clinical Diagnosis*. Philadelphia, WB Saunders, 2000, p 416.)

are more likely to have skin, eye, hepatic, bone marrow, and extrathoracic lymphadenopathy than are whites. Women are more likely to have eye and neurologic involvement, and men are more likely to have hypercalcemia. Among adults with acute symptoms, 20–50% have **Löfgren syndrome,** which is the combination of erythema nodosum, bilateral hilar lymphadenopathy, and polyarthralgias.

DIAGNOSIS. There is no specific diagnostic laboratory test. Definitive diagnosis requires demonstration of the characteristic noncaseating granulomatous lesions in a biopsy of tissue, usually taken from the most readily available affected organ, and exclusion of other known causes of granulomatous inflammation. Skin and transbronchial lung biopsies have high yield, greater specificity, and fewer associated adverse events than biopsy of mediastinal lymph nodes or liver. Other diagnostic evaluation includes chest x-ray, pulmonary function testing including measurement of gas exchange, hepatic enzymes and renal function, and ophthalmologic evaluation including slit-lamp examination.

An elevated erythrocyte sedimentation rate (ESR), hyperproteinemia, hypercalcemia, hypercalciuria, eosinophilia, and elevated angiotensin-converting enzyme activity are common. Measurement of angiotensin-converting enzyme and gallium-67 scanning has poor diagnostic specificity. Bronchoalveolar lavage fluid reveals excessive lymphocytes with an increased $CD4^+/CD8^+$ ratio of 2 : 1 to 13 : 1. The **Kveim test,** consisting of intradermal injection of homogenated spleen or lymph node tissue from a sarcoid lesion and observation for the formation of a granuloma several weeks later, is used rarely because of the difficulty in obtaining standardized test material and reports of variable sensitivity and specificity.

Significant eye disease and renal damage from hypercalciuria can occur without symptoms; therefore, all patients with sarcoidosis should be evaluated at the initial presentation and monitored at regular intervals for evidence of ocular disease and hypercalciuria.

DIFFERENTIAL DIAGNOSIS. Because of its protean manifestations, the differential diagnosis of sarcoidosis is extremely broad and includes tuberculosis, pulmonary mycoses (histoplasmosis, blastomycosis, and coccidioidomycosis), brucellosis, tularemia, toxoplasmosis, lymphoma, Wegener granulomatosis, hypersensitivity pneumonia, chronic berylliosis or other occupational exposure to metals, and inflammatory ocular lesions such as phlyctenular conjunctivitis.

TREATMENT. Treatment is symptomatic and supportive. The decision to treat with potentially harmful drugs is often difficult because the prognosis and natural history of sarcoidosis in children are uncertain. Corticosteroids may suppress the acute manifestations, especially the inflammatory ocular lesions, progressive pulmonary disease, and hypercalcemia/hypercalciuria. The optimal dose and duration of corticosteroid therapy in children have not been established. Most protocols begin with prednisone or prednisolone (1 mg/kg/day) for 8–12 wk until manifestations improve, then gradually decreasing in 6–12 mo to the minimal effective dose that controls symptoms. Methotrexate may be considered in severe cases that are unresponsive to corticosteroid therapy. Other agents that have been frequently used in adults with active sarcoidosis include chloroquine, azathioprine, cyclophosphamide, thalidomide, and infliximab.

PROGNOSIS. The course of sarcoidosis may be self-limited, or chronic with a progressive or remitting course and chronic lung disease. The overall prognosis is good, but half of patients have some degree of permanent organ dysfunction. All patients are at risk for clinical deterioration or recrudescence following remission. Sarcoidosis associated with Löfgren syndrome has a good prognosis with high rate of spontaneous resolution.

Serial pulmonary function tests with measurement of gas exchange and chest x-rays are useful in following the progress of lung involvement and assessing effects of corticosteroid therapy. Hepatic enzymes and calcium are measured to monitor hepatic and renal function. Eye involvement may lead to blindness; therefore, therapy with topical corticosteroids under careful monitoring by an ophthalmologist is warranted.

Baughman RP: Therapeutic options for sarcoidosis: New and old. *Curr Opin Pulm Med* 2002;8:464–469.

Baughman RP, Lower EE, du Bois RM: Sarcoidosis. *Lancet* 2003; 361:1111–1118.

Baumann RJ, Robertson WC Jr: Neurosarcoid presents differently in children than in adults. *Pediatrics* 2003;112:e480–e486.

Ho LP, Urban BC, Thickett DR, et al: Deficiency of a subset of T cells with immunoregulatory properties in sarcoidosis. *Lancet* 2005;365:1062–1072.

Hoffman AL, Milman N, Byg K-E: Childhood sarcoidosis in Denmark 1979–1994: Incidence, clinical features and laboratory results at presentation in 48 children. *Acta Paediatr* 2004;93:30–36.

Newman LS, Rose CS, Bresnitz EA, et al: A case control etiologic study of sarcoidosis: Environmental and occupational risk factors. *Am J Respir Crit Care Med* 2004;170:1324–1330.

Paramothayan S, Jones PW: Corticosteroid therapy in pulmonary sarcoidosis. *JAMA* 2002;287:1301–1306.

Rybicki BA, Iannuzzi MC, Frederick MM, et al: Familial aggregation of sarcoidosis. A case-control study of saroidosis (ACCESS). *Am J Respir Crit Care Med* 2001;164:2085–2091.

Rybicki BA, Malianik MJ, Poisson LM, et al: The major histocompatibility complex gene region and sarcoidosis susceptibility in African Americans. *Am J Respir Crit Care Med* 2003:167:444–449.

Shetty AK, Gedalia A: Sarcoidosis in children. *Curr Probl Pediatr* 2000;30:149–176.

Chapter 165 ■ Kawasaki Disease

Anne H. Rowley and Stanford T. Shulman

Kawasaki disease (KD), formerly known as **mucocutaneous lymph node syndrome** and **infantile polyarteritis nodosa,** is an acute febrile vasculitis of childhood first described by Dr. Tomisaku Kawasaki in Japan in 1967. The disorder occurs worldwide, with Asians at highest risk. Approximately 20% of untreated patients develop coronary artery abnormalities including aneurysms, with the potential for severely affected patients to develop coronary artery thrombosis or stenosis, myocardial infarction, aneurysm rupture, and sudden death. Kawasaki disease is the leading cause of acquired heart disease in children in the United States and Japan.

ETIOLOGY. The cause of the illness remains unknown, but epidemiologic and clinical features strongly support an infectious origin. These features include the young age group affected, epidemics with wavelike geographic spread of illness, the self-limited nature of the acute febrile illness, and the combination of clinical features of fever, rash, enanthem, conjunctival injection, and cervical lymphadenopathy. Nonetheless, it is unusual to have multiple cases present at the same time from a family or day care center. One hypothesis is that a ubiquitous childhood infectious agent causes Kawasaki disease and that symptomatic illness occurs only in genetically predisposed persons. The infrequent occurrence of the illness in infants <3 mo may be the result of maternal antibody, and the virtual absence of cases in adults may be due to widespread immunity. A KD-associated antigen may be present in cytoplasmic inclusion bodies within ciliated bronchial epithelial cells of acute fatal cases. These inclusions appear consistent with viral protein aggregates, and support the hypothesis of a respiratory portal of entry of the KD agent. Kawasaki disease has recurred in families when previously affected parents have children who develop the disease. Genetic variation of *CCR5*, which encodes a high-affinity receptor for the chemokines CCL3 and CCL3L1, suggests an influential role of gene-gene interactions for susceptibility to Kawasaki disease.

EPIDEMIOLOGY. An estimated 3,000 cases are diagnosed annually in the United States. The incidence of Kawasaki disease in Asian children is substantially higher than in other racial groups, but the illness occurs worldwide in all ethnic groups. Most cases in the United States occur in white and black children, reflecting the racial composition of the population. In Japan, almost 200,000 cases have been reported since the 1960s. Kawasaki disease is not a new illness; infantile periarteritis nodosa was an autopsy diagnosis before the 1960s that appears in retrospect to have represented fatal Kawasaki disease. The disorder bears marked clinical similarities to measles and may have been particularly difficult to identify clinically before widespread immunization with measles vaccine. The illness occurs predominantly in young children; 80% of patients are <5 yr, and, only occasionally, are teenagers or, more rarely, adults affected. More often, affected adolescents or adults may actually meet the criteria for toxic shock syndrome, which has some similar features to Kawasaki disease.

PATHOGENESIS. Kawasaki disease causes severe vasculitis of all blood vessels but predominantly affects the medium-sized arteries, with a striking predilection for the coronary arteries. Pathologic examination of fatal cases in the acute or subacute stages reveals edema of endothelial and smooth muscle cells with intense inflammatory infiltration of the vascular wall, initially by polymorphonuclear cells but rapidly followed by macrophages, lymphocytes (primarily CD8 T cells), and plasma cells. IgA plasma cells are particularly prominent in the inflammatory infiltrate. In the most severely affected vessels, inflammation involves all three layers of the vascular wall with destruction of the internal elastic lamina. The vessel loses its structural integrity and weakens, resulting in dilatation, or saccular or fusiform aneurysm formation. Thrombi may form in the lumen and obstruct blood flow. In the healing phase, the vascular wall can become progressively fibrotic with marked intimal proliferation, which may lead to stenotic occlusion of the vessel over time.

In acute Kawasaki disease, an inflammatory infiltrate, including IgA plasma cells, is present in certain nonvascular tissues including myocardium, upper respiratory tract, pancreas, kidney, and biliary tract, suggesting that the infectious agent may cause a host immune response in a variety of tissues. No significant sequelae appear to occur in any of these nonvascular tissues after resolution of the acute illness.

Elevated serum levels of all immunoglobulins develop during the subacute phase of illness, suggesting that a vigorous antibody response occurs. It is unclear whether the etiologic agent, the host immune response, or both are the major causal factors leading to coronary artery disease.

CLINICAL MANIFESTATIONS. Fever is characteristically high (104°F or higher), remittent, and unresponsive to antibiotics. The duration of fever without treatment is generally 1–2 wk, but it may persist for 3–4 wk. Prolonged fever is prognostic for the development of coronary artery disease. In addition to fever, the **five characteristic features** of Kawasaki disease are: bilateral bulbar conjunctival injection, usually without exudate; erythema of the oral and pharyngeal mucosa with strawberry tongue and dry, cracked lips, and without ulceration; edema and erythema of the hands and feet; rash of various forms (maculopapular, erythema multiforme, or scarlatiniform) with accentuation in the groin area; and nonsuppurative cervical lymphadenopathy, usually unilateral, with node size of ≥1.5 cm (Table 165-1, Figs. 165-1, 165-2, 165-3, and 165-4). Perineal desquamation is common in the acute phase. Periungual desquamation of the fingers and toes begins 1–3 wk after the onset of illness and may progress to involve the entire hand and foot (Fig. 165-5).

Other features include **extreme irritability** that is especially prominent in infants, aseptic meningitis, diarrhea, mild hepatitis, hydrops of the gallbladder, urethritis and meatitis with sterile pyuria, otitis media, and arthritis. Arthritis may occur early in

TABLE 165-1. Clinical and Laboratory Features of Kawasaki Disease

EPIDEMIOLOGIC CASE DEFINITION (CLASSIC CLINICAL CRITERIA)*
Fever persisting at least 5 days†
Presence of at least 4 principal features:
Changes in extremities
Acute: Erythema of palms, soles; edema of hands, feet
Subacute: Periungual peeling of fingers, toes in weeks 2 and 3
Polymorphous exanthem
Bilateral bulbar conjunctival injection without exudate
Changes in lips and oral cavity: Erythema, lips cracking, strawberry tongue, diffuse injection of oral and pharyngeal mucosae
Cervical lymphadenopathy (>1.5 cm diameter), usually unilateral
Exclusion of other diseases with similar findings‡
OTHER CLINICAL AND LABORATORY FINDINGS
Cardiovascular findings
Congestive heart failure, myocarditis, pericarditis, valvular regurgitation
Coronary artery abnormalities
Aneurysms of medium-size noncoronary arteries
Raynaud phenomenon
Peripheral gangrene
Musculoskeletal system
Arthritis, arthralgia
Gastrointestinal tract
Diarrhea, vomiting, abdominal pain
Hepatic dysfunction
Hydrops of gallbladder
Central nervous system
Extreme irritability
Aseptic meningitis
Sensorineural hearing loss
Genitourinary system
Urethritis / meatitis
Other findings
Erythema, induration at BCG inoculation site
Anterior uveitis (mild)
Desquamating rash in groin
LABORATORY FINDINGS IN ACUTE KAWASAKI DISEASE
Leukocytosis with neutrophilia and immature forms
Elevated erythrocyte sedimentation rate (ESR)
Elevated C-reactive protein (CRP)
Anemia
Abnormal plasma lipids
Hypoalbuminemia
Hyponatremia
Thrombocytosis after week 1§
Sterile pyuria
Elevated serum transaminases
Elevated serum gamma glutamyl transpeptidase
Pleocytosis of cerebrospinal fluid
Leukocytosis in synovial fluid

*Patients with fever at least 5 days and <4 principal criteria can be diagnosed with Kawasaki disease when coronary artery abnormalities are detected by 2DE or angiography.

†In the presence of ≥4 principal criteria, Kawasaki disease diagnosis can be made on day 4 of illness. Experienced clinicians who have treated many Kawasaki disease patients may establish diagnosis before day 4.

‡See differential diagnosis.

§Some infants present with thrombocytopenia and disseminated intravascular coagulation.

From Newburger JW, Takahashi M, Gerber MA, et al: Diagnosis, treatment, and long-term management of Kawasaki disease. *Pediatrics* 2004;114:1708–1733.

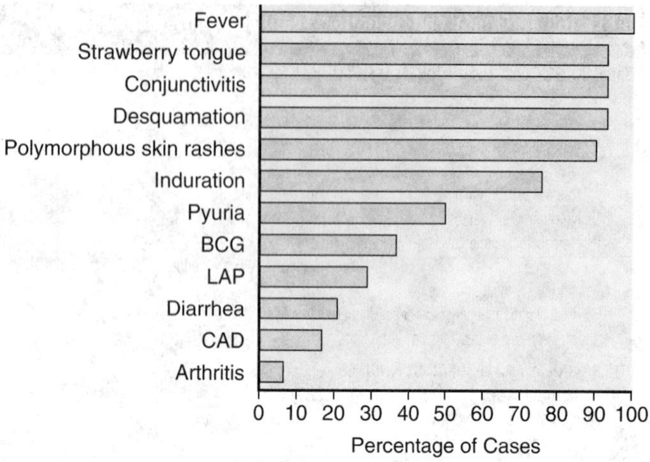

Figure 165-1. Clinical symptoms and signs of Kawasaki disease. A summary of the clinical features from 110 cases of Kawasaki disease seen in Kaohsiung, Taiwan. LAP indicates lymphadenopathy in head and neck area; BCG, reactivation of BCG site; CAD, coronary artery dilatation defined by an internal diameter of >3 mm. (From Wang CL, Wu YT, Liu CA, et al: Kawasaki disease: Infection, immunity and genetics. *Pediatr Infect Dis J* 2005;24:998–1004.)

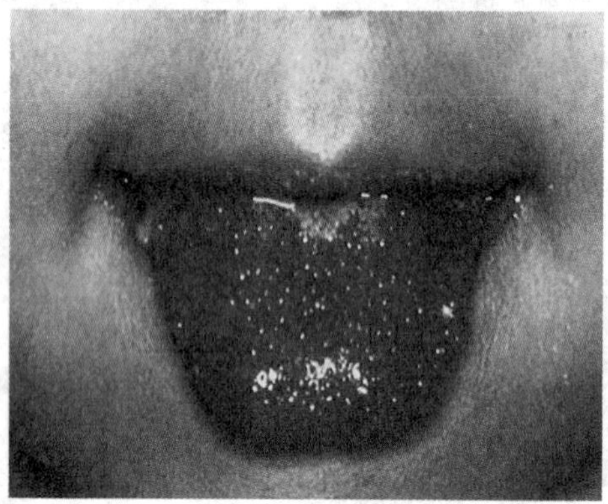

Figure 165-2. Strawberry tongue in mucocutaneous lymph node syndrome (Kawasaki disease). (Courtesy of Tomisaku Kawasaki, MD.) (From Hurwitz S: *Clinical Pediatric Dermatology,* 2nd ed. Philadelphia, WB Saunders, 1993, p 545.)

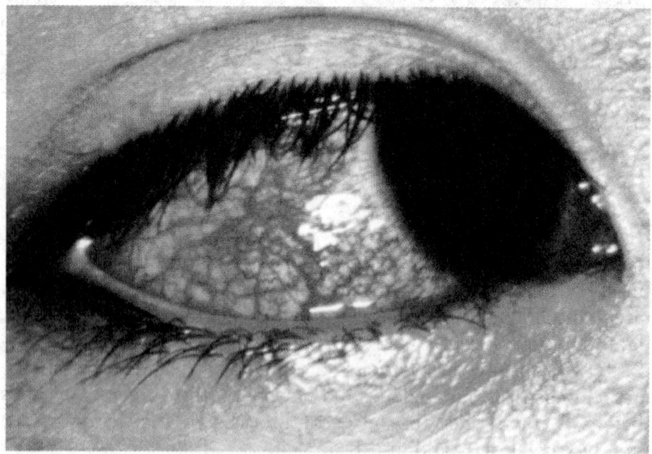

Figure 165-3. Congestion of bulbar conjunctiva in a patient with mucocutaneous lymph node syndrome (Kawasaki disease). (Courtesy of Tomisaku Kawasaki, MD.) (From Hurwitz S: *Clinical Pediatric Dermatology,* 2nd ed. Philadelphia, WB Saunders, 1993, p 545.)

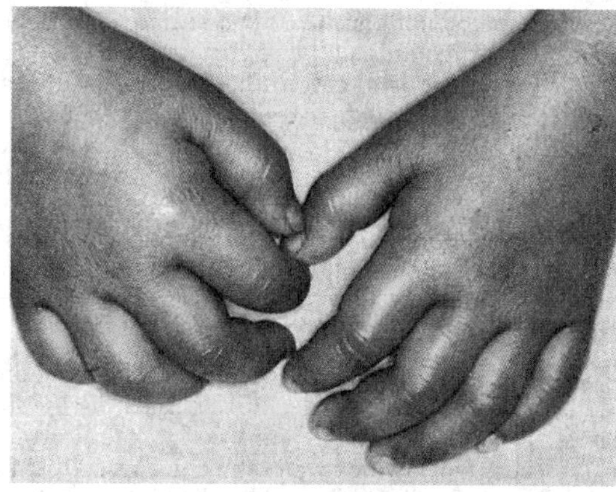

Figure 165-4. Indurative edema of the hands in mucocutaneous lymph node syndrome (Kawasaki disease). (Courtesy of Tomisaku Kawasaki, MD.) (From Hurwitz S: *Clinical Pediatric Dermatology,* 2nd ed. Philadelphia, WB Saunders, 1993, p 545.)

the illness or may develop in the 2nd–3rd week, generally affecting hands, knees, ankles, or hips. It is self-limited but may persist for several weeks.

Cardiac involvement is the most important manifestation of Kawasaki disease. Myocarditis, manifested as tachycardia out of proportion to fever occurs in at least 50% of patients; decreased ventricular function occurs in a smaller number of patients. Pericarditis with a small pericardial effusion is common during the acute illness. Coronary artery aneurysms develop in up to 25% of untreated patients in the 2nd–3rd wk of illness and are best detected by two-dimensional echocardiography. **Giant coronary artery aneurysms** (≥8 mm internal diameter) pose the greatest risk for rupture, thrombosis or stenosis, and myocardial infarction (Fig. 165-6). Significant valvular regurgitation and systemic artery aneurysms may occur but are uncommon. Axillary, popliteal, or other arteries may also be involved and manifest as a localized pulsating mass.

Kawasaki disease is generally divided into three clinical phases. The **acute febrile phase,** which usually lasts 1–2 wk, is characterized by fever and the other acute signs of illness. The dominant cardiac manifestation is myocarditis. In addition, a macrophage activation syndrome may rarely be evident (see Chapter 154). The **subacute phase** begins when fever and other acute signs have abated, but irritability, anorexia, and conjunctival injection may persist. The subacute phase is associated with desquamation, thrombocytosis, the development of coronary aneurysms, and the highest risk of sudden death in those who

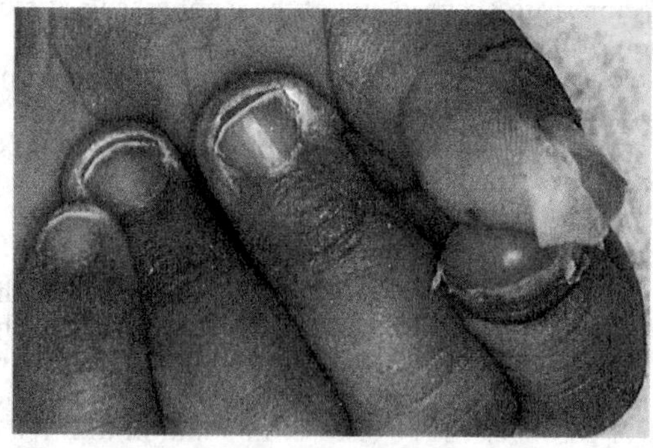

Figure 165-5. Desquamation of the fingers in a patient with mucocutaneous lymph node syndrome (Kawasaki disease). (Courtesy of Tomisaku Kawasaki, MD.) (From Hurwitz S: *Clinical Pediatric Dermatology,* 2nd ed. Philadelphia, WB Saunders, 1993, p 549.)

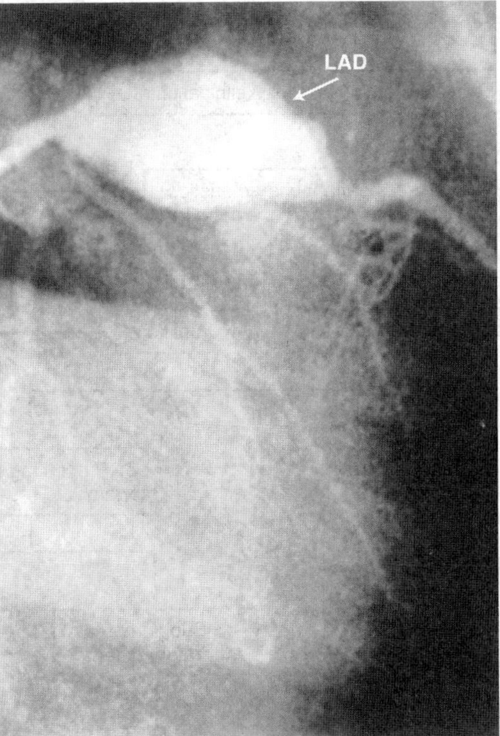

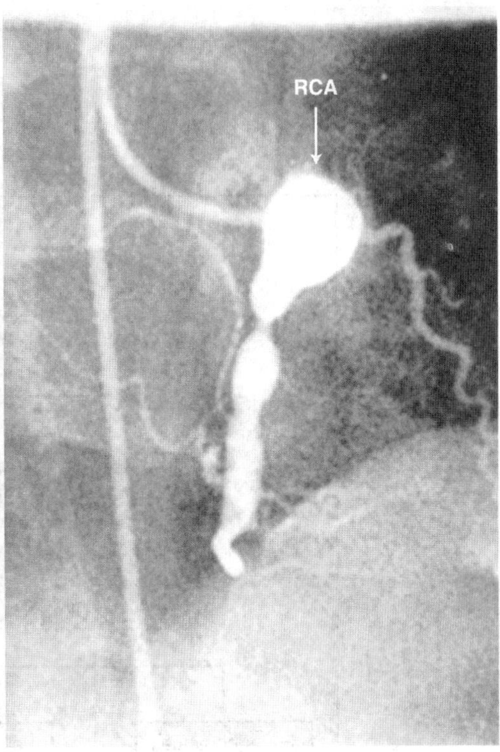

Figure 165-6. Coronary angiogram demonstrating giant aneurysm of the LAD with obstruction and giant aneurysm of the RCA with area of severe narrowing in 6 yr old boy. (From Newburger JW, Takahashi M, Gerber MA, et al: Diagnosis, treatment, and long-term management of Kawasaki disease. *Pediatrics* 2004; 114:1708–1733.)

have developed aneurysms. This phase generally lasts until about the 4th wk. The **convalescent phase** begins when all clinical signs of illness have disappeared and continues until the erythrocyte sedimentation rate (ESR) and C-reactive protein (CRP) return to normal, ≈6–8 wk after the onset of illness.

Certain clinical and laboratory findings may predict a more severe outcome. These include male gender, age <1 yr, prolonged fever, recrudescence of fever after an afebrile period, and the following laboratory values at presentation: low hemoglobin or platelet levels, high neutrophil and band counts, hyponatremia, and low albumin and age-adjusted serum IgG levels. Scoring systems based on these factors, however, have not proven sufficiently sensitive for selective treatment of patients based on risk.

DIAGNOSIS. The diagnosis of Kawasaki disease is based on the presence of characteristic clinical signs. For **classic Kawasaki disease,** the diagnostic criteria require the presence of fever for at least 5 days and at least four of five of the other characteristic clinical features of illness (see Table 165-1). In **atypical or incomplete Kawasaki disease,** the patient has persistent fever but with fewer than four other features of the illness. Accurate identification of incomplete cases is a major clinical challenge (Fig. 165-7). Incomplete cases are most frequent in infants, who, unfortunately, also have the highest likelihood of developing coronary artery disease.

Recognition depends on a high index of suspicion and knowledge of the characteristic clinical features. Unfortunately, if the diagnosis is not established and treatment is not instituted, rare patients may suffer sudden death secondary to myocardial infarction or coronary aneurysm rupture, or may develop serious asymptomatic coronary disease that is unrecognized until symptoms of myocardial ischemia develop later in life.

DIFFERENTIAL DIAGNOSIS. The differential diagnosis of Kawasaki disease includes scarlet fever, toxic shock syndrome, measles, adenovirus infection, drug hypersensitivity reactions including Stevens-Johnson syndrome, juvenile rheumatoid arthritis, and, more rarely, Rocky Mountain spotted fever and leptospirosis. Some features of measles that distinguish it from Kawasaki disease include exudative conjunctivitis, Koplik spots, rash that begins on the face and behind the ears, leukopenia, and a normal ESR and/or CRP. Adenovirus infection is associated with exudative pharyngitis and exudative conjunctivitis, unlike Kawasaki disease. Some features of drug reactions, such as the presence of periorbital edema, oral ulcerations, and a normal or minimally elevaled ESR may help to distinguish these reactions from Kawasaki disease. Toxic shock syndrome is distinguished by the presence of hypotension, renal and hepatic dysfunction, elevated creatine phosphokinase level, and focal *Staphylococcus aureus* infection. A common clinical problem is the differentiation of scarlet fever from Kawasaki disease in a child who is a group A streptococcal carrier. Because patients with scarlet fever have a rapid clinical response to appropriate antibiotic therapy, such treatment for 24–48 hr with clinical reassessment at that time generally clarifies the diagnosis. The presence of lymphadenopathy, hepatosplenomegaly, and an evanescent, salmon-colored rash suggests a diagnosis of juvenile rheumatoid arthritis. Accurate diagnosis of incomplete Kawasaki disease remains a significant challenge for clinicians. Unusual cases should be referred to a center with experience in the diagnosis of Kawasaki disease.

LABORATORY FINDINGS. There is no diagnostic test for Kawasaki disease, but certain laboratory findings are characteristic. The leukocyte count is normal to elevated with a predominance of neutrophils and immature forms. Elevated ESR, CRP, and other acute phase reactants are almost universally present in the acute phase of illness and may persist for 4–6 wk. Normocytic, normochromic anemia is common. The platelet count is generally normal in the 1st week of illness and rapidly increases by the 2nd–3rd wk of illness, sometimes exceeding 1,000,000/mm^3. Tests for antinuclear antibody and rheumatoid factor are negative. Sterile pyuria, mild elevations of the hepatic transaminases, and cerebrospinal fluid pleocytosis may be present.

Two-dimensional echocardiography, which should be performed by a pediatric cardiologist, is the most useful test to monitor potential development of coronary artery abnormalities.

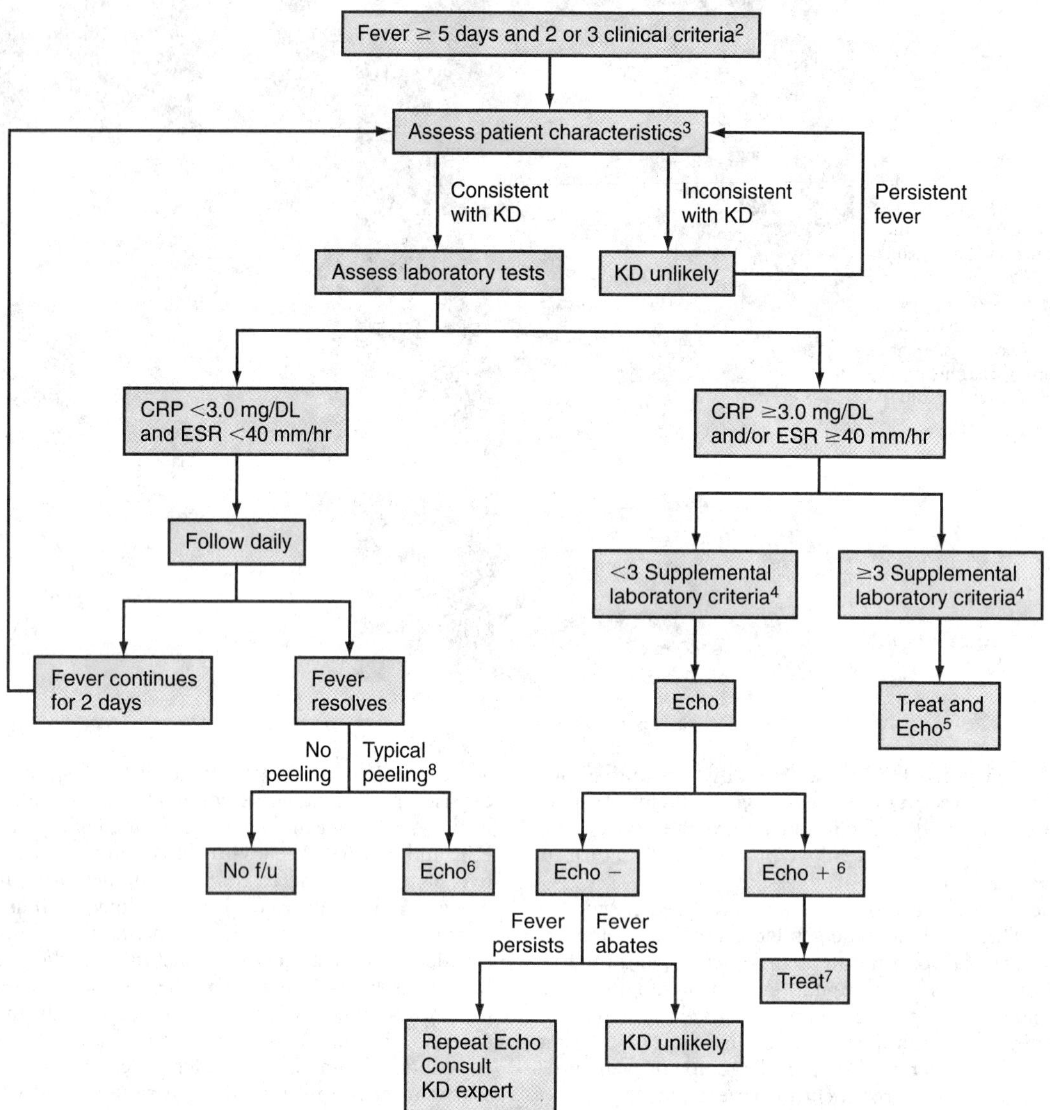

Figure 165-7. Evaluation of suspected incomplete Kawasaki disease (KD). (1) In the absence of gold standard for diagnosis, this algorithm cannot be evidence based but rather represents the informed opinion of the expert committee. Consultation with an expert should be sought anytime assistance is needed. (2) Infants ≤6 months old on day ≥7 of fever without other explanation should undergo laboratory testing and, if evidence of systemic inflammation is found, an echocardiogram, even if the infants have no clinical criteria. (3) Patient characteristics suggesting Kawasaki disease are listed in Table 165-1. Characteristics suggesting disease other than Kawasaki disease include exudative conjunctivitis, exudative pharyngitis, discrete intraoral lesions, bullous or vesicular rash, or generalized adenopathy. Consider alternative diagnoses. (4) Supplemental laboratory criteria include albumin ≤3.0 g/dL, anemia for age, elevation of alanine aminotransferase, platelets after 7 days ≥450,000/mm^3, white blood cell count ≥15,000/mm^3, and urine ≥10 white blood cells/high-power field. (5) Can treat before performing echocardiogram. (6) Echocardiogram is considered positive for purposes of this algorithm if any of 3 conditions are met: z score of LAD or RCA ≥2.5, coronary arteries meet Japanese Ministry of Health criteria for aneurysms, or ≥3 other suggestive features exist, including perivascular brightness, lack of tapering, decreased left ventricle (LV) function, mitral regurgitation, pericardial effusion, or z scores in LAD or RCA of 2–2.5. (7) If the echocardiogram is positive, treatment should be given to children within 10 days of fever onset and to those beyond day 10 with clinical and laboratory signs (CRP, ESR) of ongoing inflammation. (8) Typical peeling begins under nail bed of fingers and then toes. (From Newburger JW, Takahashi M, Gerber MA, et al: Diagnosis, treatment, and long-term management of Kawasaki disease. *Pediatrics* 2004;114:1708–1733.)

Echocardiography should be performed at diagnosis and again after 2–3 wk of illness. If both are normal, a repeat study should be performed 6–8 wk after onset of illness. If coronary abnormalities are not detected by 6–8 wk after onset of illness, and after the ESR has normalized, additional follow-up studies are optional. Some centers routinely perform echocardiography again 6 or 12 mo after onset of illness. Kawasaki disease is an acute vasculitis; there is no convincing evidence of long-term cardiovascular sequelae in children who do not develop coronary abnormalities within 2 mo after the onset of illness.

For patients who develop coronary artery abnormalities, more frequent echocardiographic studies and, potentially, angiography may be indicated. Treatment of such patients should be determined in consultation with a pediatric cardiologist.

TREATMENT. Patients with acute Kawasaki disease should be treated with intravenous immunoglobulin (IVIG) and high-dose aspirin as soon as possible after diagnosis and, ideally, within 10 days of disease onset (Table 165-2). The mechanism of action of IVIG in Kawasaki disease is unknown, but treatment should result in rapid defervescence and resolution of clinical signs of illness in 85–90% of patients. With therapy, the CRP normalizes much more quickly than the ESR, which will often increase immediately after IVIG therapy. IVIG reduces the prevalence of coronary disease from 20–25% in children treated with aspirin alone to 2–4% in those treated with IVIG and aspirin within the 1st 10 days of illness. Consideration should even be given to treatment of patients diagnosed after the 10th illness day if fever has persisted, because the anti-inflammatory effect may be helpful, although the effect of such therapy on the risk of developing coronary aneurysms is unknown. The dose of aspirin is decreased from anti-inflammatory to antithrombotic doses (3–5 mg/kg/day as a single dose) on the 14th illness day or after the patient has been afebrile for at least 3–4 days. Aspirin is continued for its antithrombotic effect until 6–8 wk after onset, when the ESR has normalized in patients that have not developed abnormalities detected by echocardiography.

Occasional patients have **refractory Kawasaki disease** that does not respond to an initial IVIG infusion, or exhibits only a partial or transient response. Strong consideration should be given to retreatment of these patients with an additional infusion of IVIG (2 g/kg). Optimal therapy for patients who do not respond to two infusions of IVIG is uncertain. If there is a poor response to the second dose of IVIG, some patients have responded to IV methylprednisolone at a dose of 30 mg/kg/day for 3 days. The value of infliximab (which binds TNF-α), other immunomodulators (cyclophosphamide, methotrexate), and plasmapheresis in Kawasaki disease is yet to be determined.

Acute thrombosis may occasionally occur in an aneurysmal or stenotic coronary artery. Thrombolytic therapy may be lifesaving in this circumstance (Table 165-3). Abciximab, a glycoprotein IIb/IIIa inhibitor, has been used in some patients with Kawasaki disease who develop giant coronary aneurysms with possible thrombosis. Few data regarding efficacy are available, but the drug may reduce thrombotic complications.

Patients with a small solitary aneurysm should continue aspirin indefinitely. Patients with larger or numerous aneurysms may require the addition of clopidogrel, warfarin, or low molecular weight heparin therapy; such decisions should be made in consultation with a pediatric cardiologist. Long-term follow-up of patients with coronary artery aneurysms should include periodic echocardiography with stress testing, and possibly angiography for those with larger aneurysms. Catheter intervention with percutaneous transluminal coronary rotational ablation, directional coronary atherectomy, and stent implantation have all been used for the management of coronary stenosis caused by Kawasaki disease, with some patients requiring coronary artery bypass grafting.

Patients receiving long-term aspirin therapy are candidates for annual influenza vaccination to reduce the risk of Reye syndrome. Varicella vaccination should be strongly considered, since the risk of Reye syndrome in children who take salicylates and who receive varicella vaccine is likely to be lower than with wild-type varicella. Patients treated with 2 g/kg IVIG should have measles-mumps-rubella and varicella vaccinations delayed for 11 mo because the specific antiviral antibody in IVIG may interfere with the immune response to live-virus vaccines. Other vaccinations do not need to be delayed.

TABLE 165-2. Treatment of Kawasaki Disease

ACUTE STAGE

Intravenous immunoglobulin 2 g/kg over 10–12 hr *with* aspirin 80–100 mg/kg/day divided every 6 hr orally until 14th illness day

CONVALESCENT STAGE

Aspirin 3–5 mg/kg once daily orally until 6–8 wk after illness onset

LONG-TERM THERAPY FOR THOSE WITH CORONARY ABNORMALITIES

Aspirin 3–5 mg/kg once daily orally ± clopidogrel 1 mg/kg/day (max 75 mg/day) (most experts add warfarin for those patients at particularly high risk of thrombosis)

ACUTE CORONARY THROMBOSIS

Prompt fibrinolytic therapy with tissue plasminogen activator, streptokinase, or urokinase under supervision of a pediatric cardiologist

TABLE 165-3. Antiplatelet, Anticoagulant, and Thrombolytic Medications

MEDICATION	ROUTE	DOSAGE
Aspirin	Oral	Antiplatelet dose: 3–5 mg/kg every day
Clopidogrel	Oral	1 mg/kg per day* to max (adult dose) of 75 mg/day
Dipyridamole	Oral	2–6 mg/kg per day in 3 divided doses†
Unfractionated heparin	Intravenous	Load: 50 U/kg Infusion: 20 U/kg/h Adjust dosage to achieve desired therapeutic level, usually plasma heparin level = 0.35–0.7 in antifactor Xa activity or aPTT 60–85 s
Low molecular weight heparin	Subcutaneous	Infants <12 months Treatment: 3 mg/kg per day, divided 12 h Prophylaxis: 1.5 mg/kg per day, divided every 12 h Children/adolescents Treatment: 2 mg/kg per day, divided every 12 h Prophylaxis: 1 mg/kg per day, divided every 12 h Adjust dose to achieve desired therapeutic level, usually antifactor Xa = 0.5–1.0 U/mL
Abciximab	Intravenous	Bolus: 0.25 mg/kg Infusion: 0.125 μg/kg per min for 12 h
Streptokinase	Intravenous	Bolus: 1000–4000 U/kg over 30 min Infusion: 1000–1500 U/kg per h
tPA	Intravenous	Bolus: 1.25 mg/kg Infusion: 0.1–0.5 mg/kg per h for 6 h, then reassess
Urokinase	Intravenous	Bolus: 4400 U/kg over 10 min Infusion: 4400 U/kg per h
Warfarin	Oral	0.1 mg/kg per day, given every day (0.05–0.34 mg/kg per day; adjust dose to achieve desired INR, usually 2.0–2.5)

*No published studies in children.

†Clopidogrel is preferred to dipyridamole, based on adult studies.

From Newburger JW, Takahashi M, Gerber MA, et al: Diagnosis, treatment, and long-term management of Kawasaki disease. *Pediatrics* 2004;114:1708–1733.

COMPLICATIONS AND PROGNOSIS. Recovery is complete and without apparent long-term effects for patients who do not develop coronary disease. Recurrent acute illness occurs in only 1–3% of cases. The prognosis for patients with coronary abnormalities depends on the severity of coronary disease. In Japan, fatality rates are very low, about 0.01%. Overall, 50% of coronary artery aneurysms resolve as assessed by echocardiogram 1–2 yr after the illness. Intravascular ultrasonography has demonstrated, however, that resolved aneurysms are associated with marked myointimal thickening and abnormal functional behavior of the vessel wall. Giant aneurysms are unlikely to resolve and are most likely to lead to thrombosis or stenosis. Coronary artery bypass grafting may be required if myocardial perfusion is significantly impaired, and it is best accomplished with the use of arterial grafts, which grow with the child and are more likely to remain patent long-term than are venous grafts. Heart transplantation has been required in rare cases in which revascularization is not feasible because of distal coronary stenoses, distal aneurysms, or severe myocardial dysfunction. Whether the presence of coronary artery abnormalities resulting from Kawasaki disease predisposes to the development of atherosclerotic heart disease in young adulthood is unknown, although long-term followup studies in Japan, to date, provide little if any evidence of this.

Akagi T, Ogawa S, Ino T, et al: Catheter interventional treatment in Kawasaki disease: A report from the Japanese Pediatric Interventional Cardiology Investigation Group. *J Pediatr* 2000;137:181–186.

Anderson MS, Todd JK, Glodè MP: Delayed diagnosis of Kawasaki syndrome: An analysis of the problem. *Pediatrics* 2005;115:e428–e433.
Baer AZ, Rubin LG, Shapiro CA, et al: Prevalence of coronary artery lesions on the initial echocardiogram in Kawasaki syndrome. *Arch Pediatr Adolesc Med* 2006;160:686–690.
Burns JC, Mason WH, Hauger SB, et al: Infliximab treatment for refractory Kawasaki syndrome. *J Pediatr* 2005;146:662–667.
Burns JC, Shimizu C, Gonzalez E, et al: Genetic variations in the receptor-ligand pair *CCR5* and *CCL3L1* are important determinants of susceptibility to Kawasaki disease. *J Infect Dis* 2005;192:344–349.
Chang FY, Hwang B, Chen SJ, et al: Characteristics of Kawasaki disease in infants younger than six months of age. *Pediatr Infect Dis J* 2006;25:241–244.
Dergun M, Kao A, Hauger SB, et al: Familial occurrence of Kawasaki syndrome in North America. *Arch Pediatr Adolesc Med* 2005;159:876–881.
Durall AL, Phillips JR, Weisse ME, et al: Infantile Kawasaki disease and peripheral gangrene. *J Pediatr* 2006;149:131–133.
Egami K, Muta H, Ishii, et al: Prediction of resistance to intravenous immunoglobulin treatment in patients with Kawasaki disease. *J Pediatr* 2006;149:237–240.
Freeman AF, Shulman ST: Refractory Kawasaki disease. *Pediatr Infect Dis J* 2004;23:463–464.
Minami T, Suzuki H, Takeuchi T, et al: A polymorphism in plasma platelet-activating factor acetylhydrolase is involved in resistance to immunoglobulin treatment in Kawasaki disease. *J Pediatr* 2005;147:78–83.
Miura M, Ohki H, Tsuchihashi T, et al: Coronary risk factors in Kawasaki disease treated with additional gammaglobulin. *Arch Dis Child* 2004;89:776–780.
Muise A, Tallett SE, Silverman ED: Are children with Kawasaki disease and prolonged fever at risk for macrophage activation syndrome? *Pediatrics* 2003;112:e495–e497.
Muta H, Ishii M, Egami K, et al: Early intravenous gamma-globulin treatment for Kawasaki disease: The nationwide surveys in Japan. *J Pediatr* 2004;144:496–499.
Newburger JW, Sleeper LA, McCrindle BW, et al: Randomized trial of pulsed corticosteroid therapy for primary treatment of Kawasaki disease. *New Engl J Med* 2007;356:663–675.
Newburger JW, Takahashi M, Gerber MA, et al: Diagnosis, treatment, and long-term management of Kawasaki disease: A statement for health professionals from the Committee on Rheumatic Fever, Endocarditis, and Kawasaki Disease, Council on Cardiovascular Disease in the Young, American Heart Association. *Pediatrics* 2004;114:1708–1733.
Rowley AH, Baker SC, Shulman ST, et al: Detection of antigen in bronchial epithelium and macrophages in acute Kawasaki Disease by use of synthetic antibody. *J Infect Dis* 2004;190:856–865.
Shulman ST, Rowley AH: Advances in Kawasaki Disease. *Eur J Pediatr* 2004;163:285–291.
Stenberg EV, Windelborg B, Horlyck A, Herlin T: The effect of TNFα blockade in complicated, refractory Kawasaki disease. *Scand J Rheumatol* 2006;35:318–321.
Tsai MH, Huang YC, Yen MH, et al: Clinical responses of patients with Kawasaki disease to different brands of intravenous immunoglobulin. *J Pediatr* 2006;148:38–43.
Uehara R, Yashiro M, Nakamura Y, Yanagawa H: Clinical features of patients with Kawasaki disease whose parents had the same disease. *Arch Pediatr Adolesc Med* 2004;158:1166–1169.
Williams RV, Wilke VM, Tani LY, Minich LL: Does abciximab enhance regression of coronary aneurysms resulting from Kawasaki disease? *Pediatrics* 2002;109:e4.
Yeung RSM: Phenotype and coronary outcome in Kawasaki's disease. *Lancet* 2007;369:85–87.

Chapter 166 ■ Vasculitis Syndromes

Michael L. Miller and Lauren M. Pachman

Vasculitis in childhood is a result of a spectrum of causes ranging from idiopathic conditions with primary vessel inflammation to syndromes after exposure to recognized antigenic triggers such as infectious agents and drugs causing hypersensitivity reactions. Vasculitis is also a component of many autoimmune diseases. The extent of vessel injury can range from moderate, as in most children with Henoch-Schönlein purpura (HSP), to severe, as in children with polyarteritis nodosa. Most classifications of the vasculitic syndromes are based on the size and location of the blood vessels that are primarily involved, as well as the type of inflammatory infiltrate (Table 166-1). The affected target vessels range in size from large afferent vessels with Takayasu arteritis (TA), to capillary and arteriolar occlusion characteristic of juvenile dermatomyositis. The inflammatory infiltrate can include various amounts of polymorphonuclear, mononuclear, and eosinophilic cells.

TABLE 166-1. Classification Scheme of Vasculitides According to Size of Predominant Blood Vessels Involved

PREDOMINANTLY LARGE-VESSEL VASCULITIDES
Takayasu arteritis
Giant cell arteritis
Cogan syndrome
Behçet disease*
PREDOMINANTLY MEDIUM-VESSEL VASCULITIDES
Classic polyarteritis nodosa
Cutaneous polyarteritis nodosa
Rheumatoid vasculitis[†]
Kawasaki disease
Primary angiitis of the central nervous system
PREDOMINANTLY SMALL-VESSEL VASCULITIDES
Immune-complex Mediated
Cutaneous leukocytoclastic angiitis ("hypersensitivity" vasculitis)
Henoch-Schönlein purpura
Urticarial vasculitis
Cryoglobulinemia[†]
Erythema elevatum diutinum
"ANCA-associated" Disorders
Wegener granulomatosis[†]
Microscopic polyangiitis[†]
Churg-Strauss syndrome[†]
Miscellaneous Small-vessel Vasculitides
Connective tissue disorders[†]
Paraneoplastic diseases
Infection
Inflammatory bowel disease

*May involve small-, medium-, and large-sized blood vessels.
[†]Frequent overlap of small- and medium-sized blood vessel involvement.
ANCA, antineutrophil cytoplasmic antibody.
From Goldman L, Ausiello D: *Cecil Textbook of Medicine*, 22nd ed. Philadelphia, WB Saunders, 2004, p 1684.

Immune complexes play a key role in the pathophysiology of many vasculitic syndromes. Immune complexes activate complement, releasing chemotactic fragments (C3a, C5a) that attract inflammatory cells. It is speculated in many vasculitic syndromes that immune complexes, after binding to endothelial cells, increase synthesis of adhesion molecules on the cell surfaces. These adhesion molecules bind to other adhesion molecules on circulating polymorphonuclear leukocytes attracted to the vicinity by chemotactic molecules. Subsequent lysosomal release of digestive enzymes from these leukocytes in many vasculitic syndromes destroys the cellular matrix of the blood vessels and surrounding tissues. In the process of degranulation, the polymorphonuclear leukocytes may disintegrate to the "nuclear dust" typical of leukocytoclastic angiitis (Fig. 166-1).

The signs and symptoms of the vasculitic syndromes are nonspecific and tend to overlap, but certain clinical features are useful in distinguishing the type of vasculature that is primarily affected (Table 166-2). Palpable purpura suggests small vessel vasculitis located deep in the papillary dermis, whereas a circumscribed tender nodule is more likely a result of involvement of medium-sized vessels.

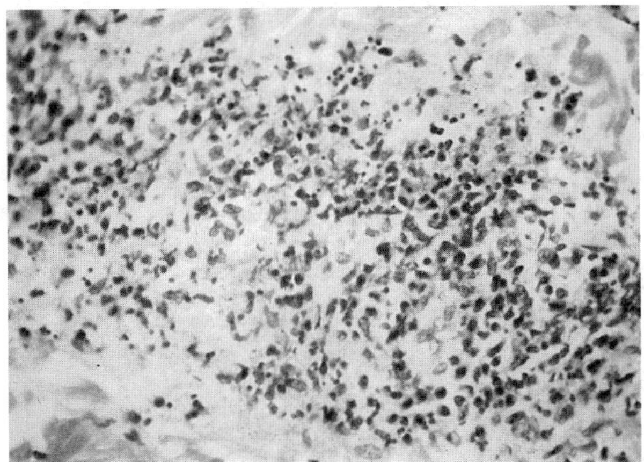

Figure 166-1. Histopathology of a skin biopsy from a patient with Henoch-Schönlein purpura showing leukocytoclastic vasculitis with nuclear degeneration ("nuclear dust").

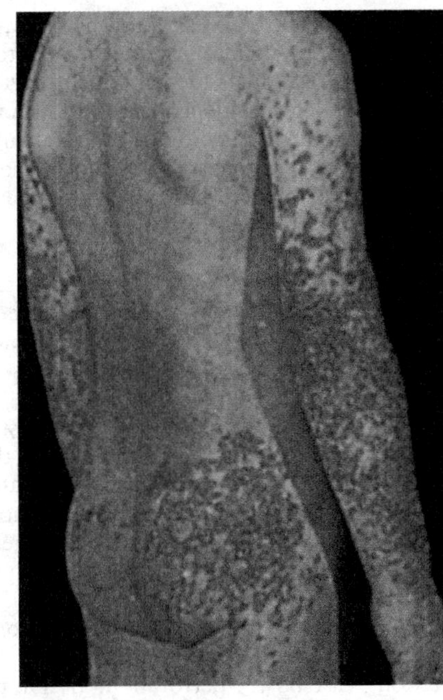

Figure 166-2. Henoch-Schönlein purpura. (From Korting GW: *Hautkrankheiten bei Kindern und Jugendlichen,* 3rd ed. Stuttgart, FK Schattauer Verlag, 1982.)

166.1 • Henoch-Schönlein Purpura

HSP, also known as anaphylactoid purpura, is a common vasculitis of small vessels with cutaneous and systemic complications. It is the most common cause of nonthrombocytopenic purpura in children.

EPIDEMIOLOGY. The etiology is unknown, but HSP often follows an upper respiratory tract infection. The incidence and prevalence of HSP are probably underestimated because cases are not reported to public health agencies. Although HSP accounted for 1% of hospital admissions in the past, changes in medical practice have reduced the frequency of admissions; 0.06% of admissions (62 of 9,083 in 1997) were for HSP at one large Midwestern pediatric center in the United States. HSP is more frequent in children than adults, with most cases occurring between 2 and 8 yr of age, and most frequently in the winter months. The overall incidence is estimated to be 9/100,000 population. Males are affected twice as frequently as females.

PATHOGENESIS. The pathogenesis of HSP is not known, although in specific populations, patients with HSP have a significantly higher frequency of HLA-DRB1*01 and decreased frequency of the *07 haplotype than controls. Active disease is characterized by increased serum concentrations of the cytokines tumor necrosis factor-α (TNF-α) and interleukin (IL)–6. In one study, almost half of the patients had elevated antistreptolysin O (ASO) antibodies, implicating group A streptococcus. HSP is an IgA-mediated vasculitis of small vessels. Immunofluorescence techniques show deposition of IgA and C3 in the small vessels of the skin and the renal glomeruli; the role of complement activation is controversial.

CLINICAL MANIFESTATIONS. The disease onset may be acute, with the appearance of several manifestations simultaneously, or insidious, with sequential occurrence of symptoms over a period of weeks or months. Low-grade fever and fatigue are present in more than half of affected children. The typical rash and the clinical symptoms of HSP are a consequence of the usual location of the acute small vessel damage primarily in the skin, gastrointestinal tract, and kidneys.

The hallmark of the disease is the rash, beginning as pinkish maculopapules that initially blanch on pressure and progress to petechiae or purpura, which are characterized clinically as **palpable purpura** that evolve from red to purple to rusty brown before they eventually fade (Fig. 166-2). The lesions tend to occur in crops, last from 3–10 days, and may appear at intervals that vary from a few days to as long as 3–4 mo. In <10% of children,

TABLE 166-2. Pathologic Characteristics of Selected Forms of Vasculitis

	TAKAYASU ARTERITIS	POLYARTERITIS NODOSA	WEGENER GRANULOMATOSIS	CHURG-STRAUSS SYNDROME	HENOCH-SCHÖNLEIN PURPURA	CUTANEOUS LEUKOCYTOCLASTIC ANGIITIS
Vessels involved	Elastic (large) or muscular (medium-sized) arteries	Medium- and small-sized muscular arteries	Small-sized arteries and veins; sometimes medium-sized vessels	Small-sized arteries and veins; sometimes medium-sized vessels	Capillaries, venules, and arterioles	Capillaries, venules, and arterioles
Organ involvement	Aorta, aortic arch and major branches, and pulmonary arteries	Skin, peripheral nerve, GI tract, and other viscera	Upper respiratory tract, lungs, kidneys, skin, eyes	Upper respiratory tract, lungs, heart, peripheral nerves	Skin, joints, GI tract, kidneys	Skin, joints
Type of vasculitis and inflammatory cells	Granulomatous with some giant cells; fibrosis in chronic stages	Necrotizing, with mixed cellular infiltrate	Necrotizing or granulomatous (or both); mixed cellular infiltrate, plus occasional eosinophils	Necrotizing or granulomatous (or both); prominent eosinophils, and other mixed infiltrate	Leukocytoclastic, with some lymphocytes and variable eosinophils IgA deposits in affected tissues	Leukocytoclastic, with occasional eosinophils

GI, gastrointestinal.
From Goldman L, Ausiello D: *Cecil Textbook of Medicine*, 22nd ed. Philadelphia, WB Saunders, 2004, p 1684.

recurrences of the rash may not end until as late as a yr, and, rarely, several yr, after the initial episode. Damage to cutaneous vessels also results in local angioedema, which may precede the palpable purpura. Edema independent of purpura occurs primarily in dependent areas such as below the waist, over the buttocks (or on the back and posterior scalp in the infant), or in areas of greater tissue distensibility such as the eyelids, lips, scrotum, or dorsum of the hands and feet.

Arthritis, present in more than $^2/_3$ of children with HSP, is usually localized to the knees and ankles and appears to be concomitant with edema. The effusions are serous, not hemorrhagic, in nature and resolve after a few days without residual deformity or articular damage. They may recur during a subsequent reactive phase of the disease.

Edema and damage to the vasculature of the **gastrointestinal tract** may also lead to intermittent abdominal pain that is often colicky in nature. There may be peritoneal exudate, enlarged mesenteric lymph nodes, segmental edema, and hemorrhage into the bowel. More than half of patients have occult heme-positive stools, diarrhea (with or without visible blood), or hematemesis. Intussusception may occur, which is suggested by an empty right lower abdominal quadrant on physical examination or by currant jelly stools, which may rarely be followed by complete obstruction or infarction with bowel perforation. If not resolved by hydrostatic reduction during a contrast study, surgical intervention is necessary.

Renal involvement occurs in 25–50% of children and may manifest with hematuria, proteinuria, or both; nephritis or nephrosis; or acute renal failure. Renal involvement at presentation may lead to chronic hypertension or end-stage renal disease in the future (see Chapter 515). Hepatosplenomegaly and lymphadenopathy may also be present during active disease. A rare but potentially serious outcome of neurological involvement is the development of seizures, paresis, or coma. Other rare complications include rheumatoid-like nodules, cardiac and eye involvement, mononeuropathies, pancreatitis, and pulmonary or intramuscular hemorrhage.

DIAGNOSIS. The pattern of crops of palpable purpuric lesions of similar hue in dependent areas of the body is characteristic of HSP. Diagnostic uncertainty arises when the symptom complex of edema, rash, arthritis with abdominal complaints, and renal findings occurs for a prolonged period. HSP can occur with other forms of vasculitis or autoimmune disease such as familial Mediterranean fever or inflammatory bowel disease. In polyarteritis nodosa, the cutaneous lesions are different, and peripheral neurologic and cardiac manifestations are more common. Palpable purpura can occur in meningococcemia if there are pre-existing coagulation abnormalities such as factor V Leiden, protein S, or protein C deficiency. The presentation of unremitting fever, a maculopapular rash that does not reappear in crops but is prominent on the lower extremities, and peripheral arthritis may suggest Kawasaki disease. HSP must be distinguished from systemic-onset juvenile rheumatoid arthritis, in which the salmon-pink rash is evanescent and maculopapular, with swelling that does not extend beyond the joint.

Acute hemorrhagic edema (**AHE**) is an acute cutaneous benign leukocytoclastic vasculitis seen in children ≤2 yr of age that may be confused with HSP. AHE presents with fever; tender edema of the face, scrotum, hands, and feet; and ecchymosis (usually larger than the purpura of HSP) on the face and extremities (Fig. 166-3). The trunk is spared, but petechiae may be seen in mucous membranes. The patient usually appears well except for the rash. The platelet count is normal or elevated; the urinalysis is normal. The younger age, nature of the lesions, absence of other organ involvement, and biopsy may help distinguish AHE from HSP.

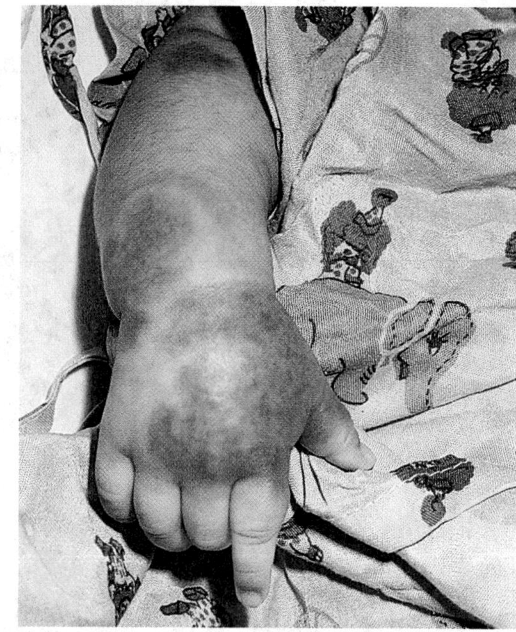

Figure 166-3. Typical lesions of acute hemorrhagic edema on the arm of an infant. (From Eichenfield LF, Frieden IJ, Esterly NB: *Textbook of Neonatal Dermatology.* Philadelphia, WB Saunders, 2001, p 308.)

LABORATORY FINDINGS. Routine laboratory tests are neither specific nor diagnostic. Affected children often have a moderate thrombocytosis and leukocytosis. The erythrocyte sedimentation rate (ESR) may be elevated. Anemia may result from chronic or acute gastrointestinal blood loss. Immune complexes are often present, and 50% of patients have elevated concentrations of IgA as well as IgM but are usually negative for antinuclear antibodies (ANAs), antibodies to nuclear cytoplasmic antigens (ANCAs), and rheumatoid factor (even in the presence of rheumatoid nodules). Anticardiolipin or antiphospholipid antibodies may be present and contribute to the intravascular coagulopathy. Intussusception is usually ileoileal in location; barium enema may be used for both identification and nonsurgical reduction. Renal involvement manifests in red blood cells, white blood cells, casts, or albumin in the urine and azotemia (see Chapter 515).

Definitive diagnosis of vasculitis is confirmed by biopsy, which is obtained when the clinical presentation is atypical, of an involved cutaneous site showing leukocytoclastic angiitis. Renal biopsy may show mesangial deposition of IgA and occasionally IgM, C3, and fibrin.

TREATMENT. Symptomatic treatment including adequate hydration, bland diet, and pain control with acetaminophen is provided for self-limited complaints of arthritis, edema, fever, and malaise. Avoidance of competitive activities and avoidance of maintaining the lower extremities in a dependent position may decrease local edema. If edema involves the scrotum, elevation of the scrotum and local cooling, as tolerated, may decrease discomfort.

Intestinal complications (hemorrhage, obstruction, intussusception) may be life-threatening and managed with corticosteroids and, when necessary, hydrostatic reduction (by air or with contrast) or resection of the intussusception. Therapy with oral or intravenous corticosteroids (1–2 mg/kg/day) is often associated with dramatic improvement of both gastrointestinal and CNS complications. Rarely, children develop chronic or recurrent HSP, which may respond to pulse doses of intravenous methylprednisolone (30 mg/kg/day, maximum 1 g/day, daily for 3 days followed by 1–2 times weekly and tapered in frequency depending on response).

Management of renal involvement is the same as for other forms of acute glomerulonephritis (see Chapter 512). If anticardiolipin or antiphospholipid antibodies are identified and thrombotic events have occurred, aspirin (81 mg) given once may decrease the risks associated with a hypercoagulable state. Rheumatoid nodules may respond to alternate-day colchicine (0.6 mg every other day).

COMPLICATIONS. The major complications of HSP are renal involvement, including nephrotic syndrome, and bowel perforation. In children with normal renal function and urinalysis at presentation, repeated urinalysis should be followed for 6 mo; those with persistent findings require follow-up by a pediatric nephrologist (see Chapter 515). An infrequent complication of scrotal edema is testicular torsion, which is quite painful and must be treated promptly.

PROGNOSIS. HSP is a self-limited vasculitic disease with an excellent overall prognosis. Chronic renal disease may result in morbidity. A population-based study indicated that <1% of patients with HSP develop persistent renal disease and <0.1% develop serious renal disease. Rarely, death may occur during the acute phase of the disease as a result of bowel infarction, CNS involvement, or renal disease. Occasionally, children who present with an HSP-like syndrome acquire characteristics of other connective tissue diseases.

166.2 • Takayasu Arteritis

Takayasu arteritis (TA), also known as **pulseless disease,** is a chronic vasculitis of large vessels.

EPIDEMIOLOGY. TA is infrequently reported in children in the United States. Children of all ethnic backgrounds have been affected, but TA is more common in Asia and India. TA may be the third most common form of childhood vasculitis in the world, after HSP and Kawasaki disease. There is a 2.5 : 1 female : male ratio. About $^1/_3$ of cases have onset before age 20 yr of age, and symptoms usually appear after age 10 yr although children as young as 8 mo have been affected. The interval from initial presentation to diagnosis in children has been reported to be as long as 19 mo, almost 4 times the interval reported for adults.

PATHOGENESIS. TA is a chronic inflammatory and obliterative disease of large vessels, with preference for the aorta and its major branches. In children, a predilection for an abdominal location of the stenotic lesions has been reported. Renal lesions include mesangial proliferative, membranoproliferative, and crescentic glomerulonephritis as well as amyloidosis.

Although the antigen responsible for inciting TA has yet to be defined, exposure to tuberculosis has been reported to be associated with the disease in some studies in Asia. Identification of critical amino acid residues of the HLA-B molecule at position 63(Glu) and 67(Ser) suggests a specific antigen-binding site in some cases. Study of non-Asian populations has provided evidence of similarities of sequence. Immune complex formation and complement activation have been frequently identified as well as antiendothelial antibodies, which upregulate the expression of endothelial adhesion molecules, but it is uncertain why only large vessels are affected.

Cytokines, including IL-6, are increased, and there is a restricted use of T cell receptors, which suggests there is an immune response to an antigen. Studies of inflammatory cytokines by peripheral blood mononuclear cells from adults with TA identified increased TNF and interferon (IFN)–γ mRNA, with lower levels of IL-10.

CLINICAL MANIFESTATIONS. Early disease manifestations, during the prepulseless phase, include night sweats, anorexia, weight loss, fatigue, myalgia, and arthritis, often followed by unexplained hypertension. During the pulseless phase, systemic symptoms are twice as frequent in children compared with adults; splenomegaly may be found. Dermatologic features include erythema nodosum, a malar rash, and erythema induratum. Cardiac involvement includes dilated cardiomyopathy, myocarditis, and pericarditis. Uveitis may be a presenting complaint. Other associated conditions include interstitial lung disease, pneumonic consolidation, ulcerative colitis, rheumatoid arthritis, and polymyositis.

DIAGNOSIS. During the pulseless phase, a characteristic bruit, often over the carotid or subclavian arteries, may be present on auscultation. Children may have diminished or absent radial pulses, although limb claudication appears less frequently than in adults. The presence of intermittent unexplained systemic symptoms of variable duration in conjunction with an elevated ESR should prompt periodic auscultation of large arteries and blood pressure measurements in all 4 limbs. If symptoms develop in the 1st year of life, arterial damage may be accompanied by papular rash, uveitis, symmetric polyarthritis, and granulomatous lesions typical of sarcoid, a condition sometimes termed **juvenile systemic granulomatosis.**

DIFFERENTIAL DIAGNOSIS. TA must be differentiated from acute rheumatic fever and juvenile arthritis. Because aortitis and aortic regurgitation may develop in TA, other disorders with these findings must also be considered, including Behçet disease, Cogan syndrome (a syndrome of ocular inflammation, vestibuloauditory abnormalities, and systemic vasculitis), relapsing polychondritis, ankylosing spondylitis (enthesitis-related arthritis), and seropositive rheumatoid arthritis. Juvenile temporal arteritis is rare, may be associated with a normal ESR, and is not associated with systemic symptoms.

LABORATORY FINDINGS. The ESR is significantly elevated, typically >60 mm/hr (Westergren). A microcytic hypochromic anemia with a leukocytosis is usual, and a polyclonal hypergammaglobulinemia is present in $^1/_3$ of cases. Circulating immune complexes may remain elevated after the ESR has normalized, reflecting continued disease activity. Surgical studies have documented inflammatory vascular lesions in the presence of normalized ESR.

The diagnosis can be confirmed by angiography, which often outlines a massively dilated aortic arch with aneurysmal dilatation and stenosis of various large vessels—carotids, subclavian, abdominal aorta, or, rarely in children, lesions of the coronary artery (Fig. 166-4). Magnetic resonance angiography may be helpful as a noninvasive test for subsequent monitoring of affected vessels.

TREATMENT. Early identification and surgical excision of the predominant lesions are essential, in conjunction with institution of appropriate immunosuppressive therapy. Prednisone (orally or intravenously) is administered in conjunction with other agents. Methotrexate has been useful in some situations, but cyclophosphamide (orally or intravenously) is often necessary to control the intense inflammatory response. Cyclophosphamide increases the risk of *Pneumocystis carinii* pneumonia and, therefore, prophylactic trimethoprim-sulfamethoxazole is recommended. Limited adult studies suggest that treatment with anti-TNF or rituximab may be of use, but data in children are lacking.

COMPLICATIONS. The most dreaded complication of this often fatal illness is an arterial aneurysmal rupture. Therefore, the dilated area is often surgically excised and replaced with an ileal vascular graft. Prevention of chronic hypertension and decreased

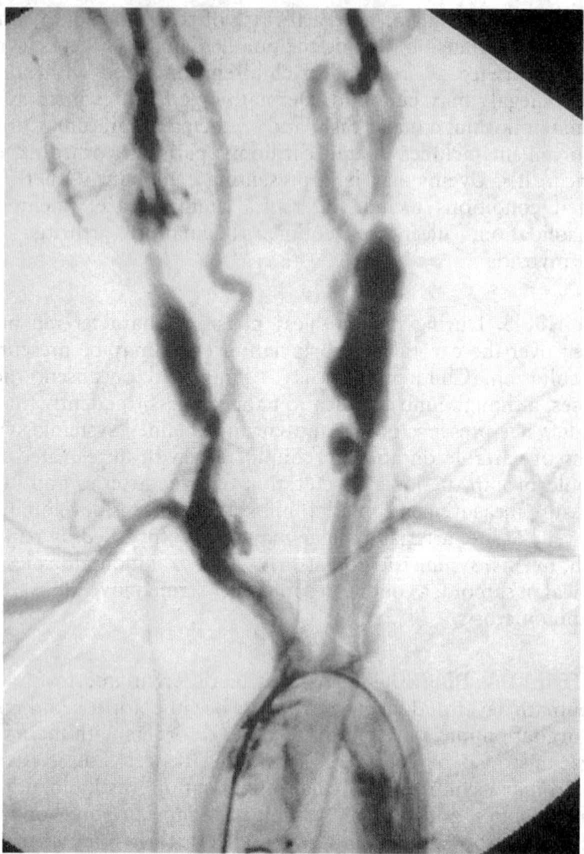

Figure 166-4. Angiogram of a child with Takayasu arteritis showing massive bilateral carotid dilatation, stenosis, and poststenotic dilatation.

perfusion can sometimes be accomplished by excision of a stenotic area with graft replacement or by insertion of an intraluminal stent to forestall the redevelopment of stenosis.

PROGNOSIS. In the past, the mortality rate has been high. Prompt diagnosis with institution of medical and surgical therapy is essential and may prevent progression of vascular lesions. More than 50% of cases achieve remission after the 1st course of therapy, but about 1/4 of cases never achieve remission. The 5-yr mortality has been reported to be as high as 35%, and the outlook for these children remains guarded. Supportive care includes management of hypertension and psychologic support. There is no indication for genetic counseling.

166.3 • Polyarteritis Nodosa

Polyarteritis nodosa (PAN) is a necrotizing vasculitis affecting small- and medium-sized arteries. Aneurysms and nodules may form at irregular intervals throughout affected arteries.

EPIDEMIOLOGY. PAN occurs rarely during childhood. Boys and girls appear to be equally affected, with a mean age of 9 yr of age. The cause is unknown, although the occurrence of PAN after upper respiratory tract infections, group A streptococcus infection, and, more often, chronic hepatitis B infection suggests that PAN represents a postinfectious autoimmune response to these agents in susceptible individuals. Other infections, including infectious mononucleosis, tuberculosis, cytomegalovirus, and parvovirus, have also been associated with PAN.

PATHOGENESIS. Biopsy reveals a necrotizing vasculitis with lymphocytic infiltration affecting all layers of small- and medium-sized muscular arteries (Fig. 166-5). Involvement is usually segmental, including bifurcations of vessels. Different stages of inflammation are found, ranging from mild inflammation to extensive fibrinoid necrosis associated with thrombosis and infarction. Aneurysm formation is common. Vascular occlusion may also occur as a result of postinflammatory fibrosis. Renal arterial involvement is found in the majority of patients, although glomerular involvement is variable.

CLINICAL MANIFESTATIONS. The clinical presentation is variable but generally reflects the location of vessels that have become inflamed. Children may present with fever of unknown origin before other findings develop. Weight loss and severe abdominal pain suggest mesenteric arterial inflammation and possible thrombosis. Renovascular arteritis can result in hypertension, hematuria, or proteinuria. Vasculitis affecting the skin may be manifested by purpura, edema, and linear erythema with palpable, painful nodules along the course of affected arteries. In cutaneous PAN, the findings are limited to the skin. Arteritis affecting the nervous system may result in cerebrovascular accidents, transient ischemic attacks, psychosis, and ischemic peripheral neuropathy in a mononeuritis multiplex pattern, with peripheral paresthesias or weakness. Cardiac involvement characterized by myocarditis may result in myocardial ischemia and heart failure; pericarditis and arrhythmias have been reported. Less common findings include testicular pain that simulates testicular torsion, bone pain, and retinal arteritis, which may cause blindness. Arthralgia, arthritis, or myalgias may be present.

DIAGNOSIS. Diagnosis of PAN requires demonstration of findings characteristic of vasculitis on biopsy or angiography. Biopsy of suggestive cutaneous lesions may reveal vasculitis (see Fig. 166-5). Renal biopsy in patients with renal manifestations may show characteristic necrotizing arteritis. Electromyography in children with peripheral neuropathy may identify affected sites; sural nerve biopsy may show an associated diagnostic vasculitis. Angiography demonstrates areas of aneurysmal dilatation, at branch points of arteries, or segmental stenosis (Fig. 166-6). The renal and mesenteric arteries are often involved. Evidence for previous or active infection should be sought in children with suspected PAN.

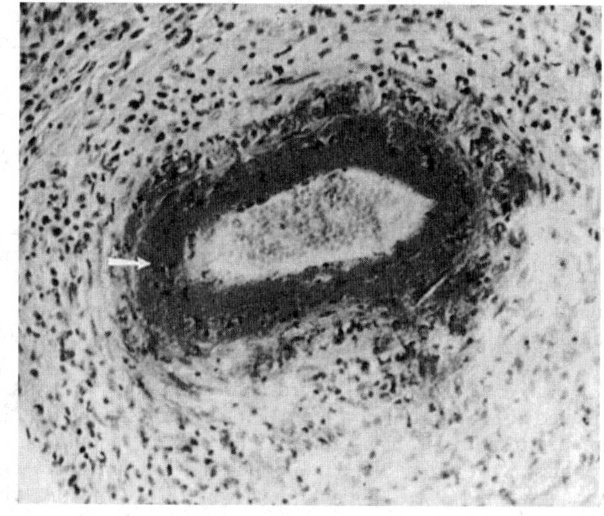

Figure 166-5. Biopsy of a medium-sized muscular artery that exhibits marked fibrinoid necrosis of the vessel wall *(arrow)*. (From Cassidy JT, Petty RE: Juvenile rheumatoid arthritis. In *Textbook of Pediatric Rheumatology*, 3rd ed. Philadelphia, WB Saunders, 1995.)

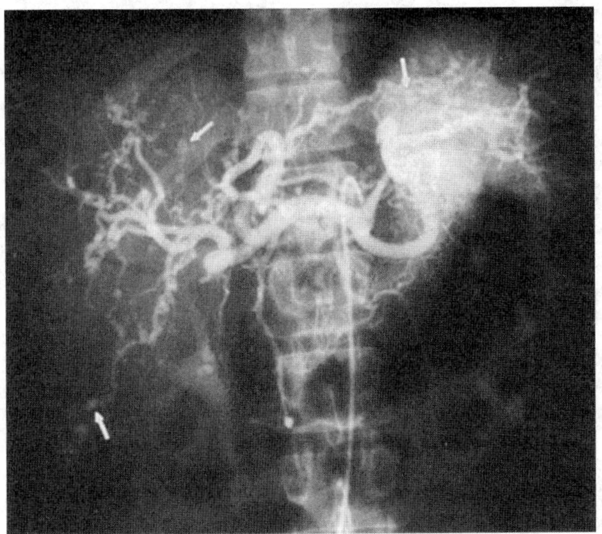

Figure 166-6. Celiac angiography of an 18 yr old boy showing aneurysms in multiple vessels. (From Cassidy JT, Petty RE: Juvenile rheumatoid arthritis. In *Textbook of Pediatric Rheumatology*, 3rd ed. Philadelphia, WB Saunders, 1995.)

DIFFERENTIAL DIAGNOSIS. Early skin lesions may resemble those of HSP, although the finding of nodular lesions and systemic findings distinguish PAN. Pulmonary lesions suggest Wegener granulomatosis (WG) or Goodpasture syndrome. Eosinophilia is noted in Churg-Strauss syndrome and eosinophilic fasciitis. Other rheumatic diseases, including systemic lupus erythematosus, dermatomyositis, and scleroderma have characteristic target organ involvement distinct from PAN. Prolonged fever and weight loss can also characterize inflammatory bowel disease or malignancies.

LABORATORY FINDINGS. An elevated ESR is often the earliest finding. Usually, anemia and leukocytosis are eventually present. Hypergammaglobulinemia reflects polyclonal B-cell activation. Abnormal urine sediment, proteinuria, and hematuria indicate renal disease. Markers of vasculitis may be useful in monitoring response to therapy. Von Willebrand factor antigen, a molecule found in vascular subendothelium, is released in increased amounts from inflamed vessels. Neopterin is released from macrophages that are activated in some patients with vasculitis. Levels of immune complexes, measured by the Raji cell and C1q assay, may also be elevated. Elevated hepatic enzymes suggest hepatitis B infection, which is more common in adults than in children. Hepatitis B surface antigen should be tested in all patients independent of liver function tests.

TREATMENT. Oral and intravenous corticosteroids have been used, sometimes in combination with oral or intravenous cyclophosphamide. Iloprost, a prostacyclin analog, may be used for endarteritis that is associated with vascular compromise in the extremities. If hepatitis B is identified, specific antiviral therapy should be added (see Chapters 355 and 359).

COMPLICATIONS. Cutaneous nodules may ulcerate, posing a risk of infection. Hypertension and chronic renal disease may develop from renal arterial involvement. Cardiac involvement may lead to decreased cardiac function or coronary arterial disease. Hepatic aneurysmal rupture is a rare complication.

PROGNOSIS. The course of PAN varies from mild disease with few complications to a severe, overwhelming, multiorgan disease leading to death. Aggressive immunosuppressive therapy may result in clinical remission. When renal involvement is present, the 1-yr survival rate was 73% and the 5-yr survival rate was 60%.

166.4 • Wegener Granulomatosis

Wegener granulomatosis (WG) is a necrotizing granulomatous small vessel vasculitis that occurs at all ages and often involves the upper airways, lower respiratory tract, and kidneys.

EPIDEMIOLOGY. Although most cases occur in adults, children can develop WG with a mean age at diagnosis of 6 yr, but it may present as early as 2 wk of age. There is a female predominance of 3 : 1. WG predominates among whites, and, in one family, multiple cases have been reported. The cause is unknown, although proteinase 3 (PR3), normally restricted to neutrophil alpha granules, has been found on the surface of neutrophils of patients with WG. Those ANCAs that bind to PR3 are specific for WG, suggesting an etiologic role for abnormal PR3 expression. Interaction of PR3 with the PiZ variant of α_1-antitrypsin has been found in some studies to increase the risk of developing WG.

PATHOGENESIS. Necrotizing granulomas are found in affected organs, including the nasal and sinus mucosa, skin, and lower respiratory tract. In the lungs, infiltrates, alveolar hemorrhage, and vasculitis may also be found. Renal involvement can vary from focal proliferative glomerulonephritis to necrotic crescentic glomerulonephritis.

CLINICAL MANIFESTATIONS. Children initially often complain of nonspecific constitutional symptoms of fever, malaise, weight loss, myalgia, and arthralgia. Many affected children have seasonal allergies. Later symptoms include cough, congestion, and nasal discharge from chronic sinusitis (often with mucosal ulceration and bone destruction from necrotizing granulomas), and hemoptysis and dyspnea from pulmonary lesions (Fig. 166-7).

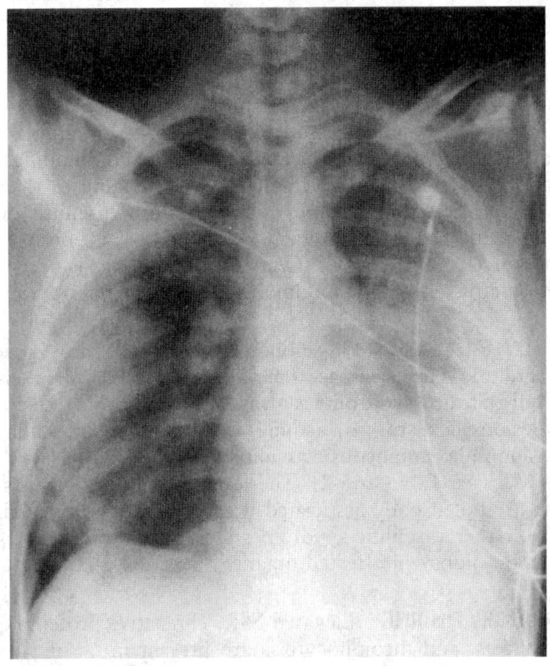

Figure 166-7. Chest radiograph of a 14 yr old girl with Wegener granulomatosis showing widespread infiltrates suggestive of pulmonary hemorrhage. There were considerable day-to-day variability and eventual total resolution of these abnormalities after treatment with prednisone and cyclophosphamide. (From Cassidy JT, Petty RE: Juvenile rheumatoid arthritis. In *Textbook of Pediatric Rheumatology*, 3rd ed. Philadelphia, WB Saunders, 1995.)

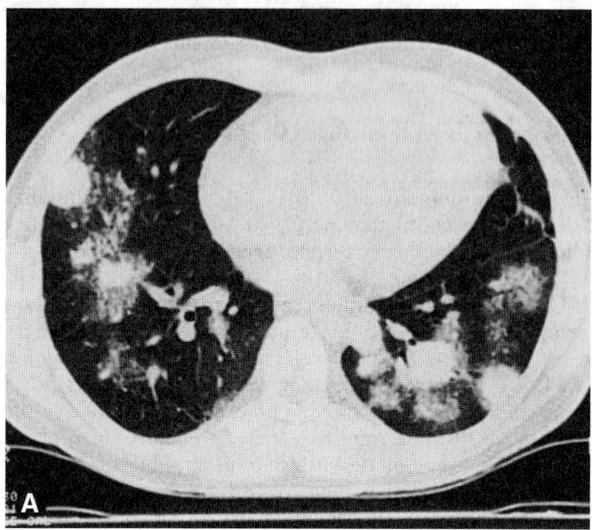

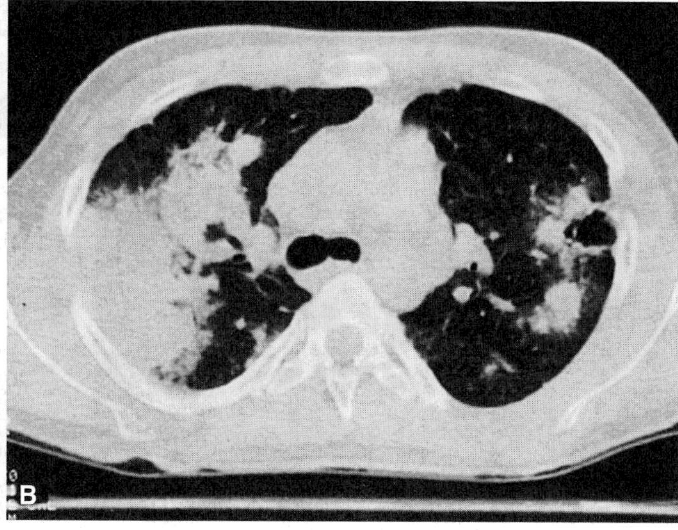

Figure 166-8. Wegener granulomatosis in a 17 yr old boy with renal failure. A chest radiograph (not shown) showed ill-defined bilateral air-space consolidation. High-resolution computed tomography (A and B) reveals air-space consolidation with a halo sign similar to that described in invasive aspergillosis. There is also septal thickening and a single cavitary lesion. Biopsy revealed vasculitis consistent with Wegener granulomatosis. An antineutrophil cytoplasmic autoantibodies test was positive. (From Kuhn JP, Slovis TL, Haller JO: *Caffey's Pediatric Diagnostic Imaging,* vol 1, 10th ed. Philadelphia, Mosby, 2004, p 1063.)

In children, WG is more frequently complicated by subglottic stenosis and nasal deformity. Ophthalmic involvement includes conjunctival and corneal lesions, uveitis, and an invasive orbital pseudotumor. Cranial and peripheral neuropathies due to intracranial granulomas and peripheral granulomatous lesions have been reported. Hematuria and proteinuria due to glomerulonephritis are often later manifestations. Cutaneous lesions may include palpable purpuric nodules and ulcers. The frequency of different system involvement is respiratory tract in 87% of cases, kidneys in 53%, joints in 53%, eyes in 53%, skin in 53%, sinuses 35%, and nervous system in 12%. Initial higher severity of disease activity and baseline organ damage are associated with persistent disease.

DIAGNOSIS. The diagnosis of WG should be suspected in children who have severe sinusitis and who develop radiographic pulmonary findings suggestive of granulomas or renal findings consistent with nephritis. High-resolution CT imaging of the chest may reveal interstitial densities consistent with vasculitis or pulmonary hemorrhage (Fig. 166-8). The diagnosis is confirmed by the presence of anti-PR3 ANCAs and the finding of necrotizing granulomatous angiitis on pulmonary, sinus, or renal biopsy.

DIFFERENTIAL DIAGNOSIS. Antibodies to ANCA are absent in other granulomatous disease such as sarcoidosis and tuberculosis. **Churg-Strauss syndrome** is a vasculitis that can cause chronic sinus lesions; a history of asthma, circulating eosinophilia, and an eosinophilic cutaneous vasculitis distinguish this syndrome from WG (see Table 166-2). The lesions in Churg-Strauss syndrome are not usually associated with destructive upper airway disease. Other vasculitic syndromes lack the characteristic granulomas on biopsy of affected organs.

LABORATORY FINDINGS. Elevated ESR, C-reactive protein (CRP), leukocytosis, and thrombocytosis are present in $^3/_4$ of patients. Anemia may be found. Antibodies to ANCA directed toward PR3 are specific for WG. These antibodies, usually of IgG class, are found on immunofluorescence to be distributed in a diffuse granular staining throughout the cytoplasm (c-ANCA). Staining for myeloperoxidase by ANCA in a perinuclear pattern (p-ANCA) is not specific for WG.

TREATMENT. Oral and intravenous corticosteroids and cyclophosphamide have been effective in many patients. Methotrexate is also used with success. There are scattered reports concerning the successful use of mycophenolate mofetil in children with WG.

COMPLICATIONS. Enlarging granulomas may disrupt local anatomy: Intrasinus lesions can invade the orbit, and lesions in the ear can result in unilateral deafness. Respiratory complications include pulmonary hemorrhage and upper airway obstruction due to subglottic stenosis. Infectious complications include pneumonia and sinusitis, typically complicating granulomatous lesions and obstruction. Chronic glomerulonephritis may progress to end-stage renal disease.

PROGNOSIS. The course is variable. Mortality has been reduced with the introduction of cyclophosphamide and other immunosuppressive agents. Compared to adults, children with WG have fewer treatment-associated morbidities and malignancies.

166.5 • Other Vasculitic Syndromes

Leukocytoclastic vasculitis refers to a spectrum of vasculitic syndromes, including HSP, as well as to specific biopsy findings. It is characterized by cutaneous vessel inflammation affecting both small arteries and postcapillary venules. Purpura and occasionally urticaria are found, particularly on the extremities. The diagnostic term *leukocytoclastic vasculitis* is sometimes used for cases similar to HSP but with atypical distribution and associated symptoms. **Hypersensitivity angiitis** is cutaneous vasculitis occurring after exposure to drugs, such as sulfonamides. Clinical manifestations include fever, myalgia, and arthralgia but rarely visceral involvement. Subsequent development of systemic findings indicating more extensive vasculitis suggests the likelihood of another diagnosis such as PAN. For both leukocytoclastic vasculitis and hypersensitivity angiitis, biopsy of lesions may reveal fibrinoid necrosis of blood vessels, perivascular polymorphonuclear infiltrate, and nuclear debris or dust.

General

Merkel PA: Drug induced vasculitis. *Rheum Dis Clin North Am* 2001;27:849–862.
Nadeau SE: Neurologic manifestations of systemic vasculitis. *Neurol Clin* 2002;20:123–150.
Yalcindag A, Sundel R: Vasculitis in childhood. *Curr Opin Rheumatol* 2001;13:422–427.

Henoch-Schönlein Purpura

Erdström Halling SF, Söderberg MP: Henoch-Schönlein nephritis: Clinical findings related to renal function and morphology. *Pediatr Nephrol* 2005;20:46–51.
Gonzalez-Gay MA, Calvino MC, Vazquez-Lopez ME, et al: Implications of upper respiratory tract infections and drugs in the clinical spectrum of Henoch-Schönlein purpura in children. *Clin Exp Rheumatol* 2004;22:781–784.
Narchi H: Risk of long term renal impairment and duration of follow up recommended for Henoch-Schönlein purpura with normal or minimal urinary findings: A systematic review. *Arch Dis Child* 2005;90:916–920.
Rostoker G: Schönlein-Henoch purpura in children and adults: Diagnosis, pathophysiology and management. *BioDrugs* 2001;15:99–138.
Saulsbury FT: Clinical update: Henoch-Schölein purpura. *Lancet* 2007;369:976–978.

Takayasu Arteritis

Della Rossa, A, Tavoni A, Merlini G, et al: Two Takayasu arteritis patients successfully treated with infliximab: A potential disease-modifying agent? *Rheumatology* 2005;44:1074–1075.
Hoffman GS: Takayasu arteritis: Lessons from the American National Institutes of Health experience. *Int J Cardiol* 1996;54:S99–S102.
Itazawa T, Noguchi K, Ichida F, et al Magnetic resonance imaging for early detection of Takayasu arteritis. *Pediatr Cardiol* 2001;22:163–164.
McCulloch M, Andronikou S, Goddard E, et al: Angiographic features of 26 children with Takayasu's arteritis. *Pediatr Radiol* 2003;33:230–235.
Ozen S, Duzova A, Bakkaloglu A, et al: Takayasu arteritis in children: preliminary experience with cyclophosphamide induction and corticosteroids followed by methotrexate. *J Pediatr* 2007;150:72–76.
Sharma BK, Jain S, Sagar S: Systemic manifestations of Takayasu arteritis: The expanding spectrum. *Int J Cardiol* 1996;54:S149–S154.
Takeda N, Takahashi T, Seko Y, et al: Takayasu myocarditis mediated by cytotoxic T lymphocytes. *Intern Med* 2005;44:256–260.

Polyarteritis Nodosa

Besbas N, Ozen S, Saatci U: Renal involvement in polyarteritis nodosa: Evaluation of 26 Turkish children. *Pediatr Nephrol* 2000;14:325–327.
Guillevin L, Mahr A, Callard P, et al: Hepatitis B virus-associated polyarteritis nodosa. *Medicine* 2005;84:313–322.
Mason A, Theal J, Bain V, et al: Hepatitis B virus replication in damaged endothelial tissues of patients with extrahepatic disease. *Am J Gastroenterol* 2005;100:972–976
Ozen S, Anton J, Arisoy N, et al. Juvenile polyarteritis: results of a multicenter survey of 110 children. *J Pediatr* 2004;145:517–522.
Stone JH: Polyarteritis nodosa. *JAMA* 2002;288:1632–1639.

Wegener Granulomatosis

Belostotsky VM, Shah V, Dillon MJ: Clinical features in 17 pediatric patients with Wegener granulomatosus. *Pediatr Nephrol* 2002;17:754–761.
Frosch M, Foell D: Wegener granulomatosus in childhood and adolescence. *Eur J Pediatr* 2004;163:425–434.
Gottlieb BS, Miller LC, Ilowite NT: Methotrexate treatment of Wegener granulomatosis in children. *J Pediatr* 1996;129:604–607.
Harper L, Savage CO: Leukocyte-endothelial interactions in antineutrophil cytoplasmic antibody-associated systemic vasculitis. *Rheum Dis Clin North Am* 2001;27:887–903.
Valentini RP, Smoyer WE, Sedman AB, et al: Outcome of antineutrophil cytoplasmic autoantibodies-positive glomerulonephritis and vasculitis in children: A single-center experience. *J Pediatr* 1998;132:325–328.

Chapter 167 ■ Musculoskeletal Pain Syndromes

Michael L. Miller

Children with poorly localized pain in the extremities out of proportion to physical or laboratory findings can be considered to have a musculoskeletal pain syndrome (MSPS). MSPS occasionally develops in children with underlying rheumatic diseases, sometimes after trauma; careful follow-up is necessary to distinguish this complication from slowly evolving disease exacerbation. Clinical manifestations of MSPS overlap with other conditions including reflex sympathetic dystrophy (RSD), erythromelalgia, fibromyalgia, and chronic fatigue syndrome (see Chapter 120). Clinical management of these conditions is remarkably similar.

CLINICAL MANIFESTATIONS. A parent may relate a history of pain in the child not confirmed by tenderness during the physical examination. If symptoms have persisted for years, adolescents may also report chronic pain, often with inconsistent details, when compared with the history offered by the parent. Location of pain can vary from a single extremity to generalized. Patients often complain of pain refractory to nonsteroidal anti-inflammatory drugs and analgesic agents. Physical therapy programs may have been tried without success.

Other symptoms associated with pain syndromes include fatigue, sleep problems, and poor school attendance. In contrast to many children with pain resulting from rheumatic diseases, children with MSPS tend to be depressed at the prospect of returning to school instead of staying home from school. Excellent academic performance often precedes prolonged school absences; it is possible that symptoms develop when a child is unable to maintain continuing academic demands. Parents may have a history of organic or functional pain, sometimes in the same anatomic region that is symptomatic in the child.

Physical findings are either normal or too minimal to account for the symptoms. Exquisite tenderness to light touch is often elicited over various parts of the extremities, which may not be reproducible on repeat examination. There are no specific laboratory findings.

DIAGNOSIS. The diagnosis of musculoskeletal pain syndromes is one of exclusion if careful, repeated physical examinations and laboratory testing do not reveal an etiology. Repeated physical examinations over time may reveal eventual development of manifestations suggestive of rheumatic or other diseases. The need for additional testing should be individualized, depending on specific symptoms and physical findings.

DIFFERENTIAL DIAGNOSIS. Cold, clammy, cyanotic distal extremities occasionally suggest autonomic dysfunction, such as in RSD. These findings may improve after a child has exercised. Weakness may result from thyroid disease, inflammatory myositis, muscular dystrophies, or neurologic disease. Chest pain may be a manifestation of costochondritis, pericarditis, coronary arterial abnormality, or aortic stenosis. Proximal leg pain, often occurring at night, may occur with osteoid osteoma. Back pain may indicate local pathology, including spondylolisthesis, diskitis, and vertebral microfractures. When children with poorly localized pain develop tender entheses, ankylosing spondyloarthropathy should be considered (see Chapter 155). Imaging studies, including plain x-rays, MRI, and technetium-99m bone scan, may identify focal pathology resulting from infection, malignancy, or trauma.

Because psychiatric disorders can overlap and present with symptoms of MSPS, psychiatric evaluation should be considered for children, and sometimes their parents, with these syndromes. Prolonged school absence suggests school phobia. When fatigue is more prominent than pain, chronic fatigue syndrome may be considered (see Chapter 120). Physical and sexual abuse may also manifest in pain syndromes. With Munchausen syndrome by proxy (see Chapter 522.4), parental reports of the child's pain are emphasized with the intent of obtaining unnecessary, often interventional, testing and treatments. Intermittent pains in both legs without inflammation that occur at night in children, last several hours, are self-limited or alleviated by massage or mild analgesics, and do not require reduction in activity are sometimes termed **"growing pains"** (see Chapter 152). Laboratory studies for these entities are normal.

TREATMENT. Successful outcome requires that any underlying psychiatric disorder be identified and treated. Therapy should focus on emotional support for the patient and family, relief of symptoms, and minimizing unnecessary and misleading diagnostic tests and therapeutic regimens. Successful behavioral techniques include cognitive restructuring, thought stopping, distraction, relaxation, and self-reward in an approach that combines restoration of a normal sleep pattern and activities of daily living, rehabilitation strategies including exercise for fatigue, and judicious use of nonsteroidal anti-inflammatory or analgesic medications. Children have been found to improve when the physician and other health care providers can overcome parental resistance to a vigorous physical therapy program for stretching and joint protection. Increasing physical activity at home to improve the level of physical fitness can also help. Some centers use bedtime doses of antidepressants for MSPS. If their use is required for more than several weeks, however, psychiatric evaluation may be necessary to evaluate for depression. For children with persisting symptoms, a rehabilitation program by a physiatrist or referral to a pain clinic may be indicated.

COMPLICATIONS. Untreated musculoskeletal pain syndromes can result in impaired physical fitness, decreased socialization leading to isolation, prolonged school absences, and lost opportunities for college or vocational training. When families avoid psychologic evaluation or recommendations, children are at risk for developing or exacerbating depression.

167.1 • Fibromyalgia

A history of sleep disturbances and widespread musculoskeletal pain associated with tenderness over **trigger points** (localized areas of tenderness to palpation) on physical examination suggests fibromyalgia. Treatment is the same as for MSPS. Although classification criteria for fibromyalgia in adults have been used for research studies of children, the clinical characteristics cannot be distinguished from children with MSPS. No study has demonstrated that fibromyalgia is clinically distinct from MSPS, and the elicitation of trigger points on examination in children has not been shown to be reproducible. Nevertheless, juvenile fibromyalgia may be a distinct entity eventually found to have a biologic basis, as has been the case for familial erythromelalgia (see Chapter 167.3). In support of this, previously healthy children can develop fibromyalgia after whiplash and other injuries. Furthermore, many adults with fibromyalgia have reported having symptoms dating from childhood. Children with fibromyalgia experience increased temperamental instability, depression and anxiety, and decreased family cohesion. Whether or not fibromyalgia is a distinct entity in childhood, families concerned with expending time and effort to arrive at a diagnosis of fibromyalgia distinct from MSPS are better served by providing for their affected children the same treatment used to treat children with MSPS.

TABLE 167-1. International Association for the Study of Pain Criteria for Complex Regional Pain Syndrome

An initiating noxious event or a cause of immobilization
Pain, allodynia, or hyperalgesia out of proportion to the event
Edema, changes in skin blood flow, or abnormal sudomotor activity
Exclusion of other diagnosis

Associated nondiagnostic features include hair, nail, or soft tissue atrophy; alterations of hair growth; loss of joint mobility; weakness, tremor, or dystonia; and sympathetically maintained pain.

167.2 • Complex Regional Pain Syndrome (Reflex Sympathetic Dystrophy)

Complex regional pain syndrome (CRPS), a condition of unknown cause, is characterized by diffuse limb pain with color and temperature changes thought to result from autonomic nervous system dysfunction. CRPS is often a response to physical or emotional distress. CRPSI occurs in the absence of nerve energy and was previously called RSD; CRPSII demonstrates evidence of nerve injury and was previously called causalgia. A history of physical activities causing repeated impact on the extremities (ballet dancing) or severe or prolonged emotional trauma (divorce of the parents, death of a sibling) may be elicited. Children complain of pain worsened by touch or movement, often with dysesthesia and a sensation of temperature changes and swelling (Table 167-1). They tend to maintain the hand or foot in a rigid, unusual position, refusing to allow passive motion. Prolonged disuse of the extremity can cause osteopenia; imaging studies (Doppler flow studies, technetium-99m bone scan) may show either increased or decreased blood flow. Assurance, physical therapy, and, when indicated, counseling can result in resolution of symptoms and physical findings. Relaxation techniques provided by a psychologist may also be useful. When these measures are unsuccessful, sympathetic blocks may be considered.

167.3 • Erythromelalgia

Children with erythromelalgia experience episodes of intense pain, erythema, and heat in the distal portion of their legs (rarely, the hands). Mild heat exposure may trigger symptoms that can last for hours and occasionally for days. Although most cases are sporadic, an autosomal dominant hereditary form results from the gene SCN9A on chromosome 2q31-32, responsible for sodium channel function in dorsal root ganglia. Erythromelalgia can also be associated with peripheral neuropathy, frostbite, hypertension, and rheumatic disease. Treatment includes avoidance of heat exposure and application of cold during attacks. Propranolol, carbamazepine, or sodium nitroprusside may be effective.

Anthony KK, Schanberg LE: Pediatric pain syndromes and management of pain in children and adolescents with rheumatic disease. *Pediatr Clin North Am* 2005;52:611–639.

Conte PM, Walco GA, Kimura Y: Temperament and stress response in children with juvenile primary fibromyalgia syndrome. *Arthritis Rheum* 2003;48:2923–2930.

Evans AM, Scutter SD: Prevalence of "growing pains" in young children. *J Pediatr* 2004;145:255–258.

Gedalia A, Garcia CO, Molina JF, et al: Fibromyalgia syndrome in children: Experience in a pediatric rheumatology clinic. *Clin Exp Rheumatol* 2000;18:415–419.

Goldenberg DL, Burckhardt C, Crofford L: Management of fibromyalgia syndrome. *JAMA* 2004;292:2388–2395.

Goodyear-Smith F, Arroll B: Growing pains. *BMJ* 2006;333:456–457.

Maillard SM, Davies K, Khubchandani R, et al: Reflex sympathetic dystrophy: A multidisciplinary approach. *Arthritis Rheum* 2004;51:284–290.
Medcalf P, Bhatia KP: Restless legs syndrome. *BMJ* 2006;333:457–458.
Richards SCM, Scott DL: Prescribed exercise in people with fibromyalgia: Paralled group randomized controlled trial. *Br Med J* 2002;325:185–187.
Schanberg LE, Keefe FJ, Lefebvre JC, et al: Pain coping strategies in children with juvenile primary fibromyalgia syndrome: Correlation with pain, physical function, and psychological distress. *Arthritis Care Res* 1996;9:89–96.
Siegel DM, Janeway D, Baum J: Fibromyalgia syndrome in children and adolescents: Clinical features at presentation and status at follow-up. *Pediatrics* 1998;101:377–382.
Waxman SG, Dib-Hajj SD: Erythromelalgia: A hereditary pain syndrome enters the molecular era. *Ann Neurol* 2005;57:785–788.

Chapter 168 ■ Miscellaneous Conditions Associated with Arthritis

Michael L. Miller

Inflammation of joints or connective tissue may be a manifestation of rare rheumatic diseases as well as nonrheumatic conditions. These should be considered in children with joint complaints especially if the history, clinical findings, or clinical course is not characteristic of common rheumatic diseases.

RELAPSING POLYCHONDRITIS. Relapsing polychondritis is characterized by episodic necrotizing cartilage inflammation that may be so severe that it causes loss of cartilage from the external ears, nose, larynx, and tracheobronchial tree. Antibodies to native type II collagen are present in some patients, suggesting that an autoimmune reaction to this protein plays a role in the pathogenesis. Patients may also develop oligoarthritis or polyarthritis, ocular inflammation, and hearing loss resulting from inflammation near the auditory and vestibular nerves. Children may initially relate only episodes of intense erythema over the outer ears. Diagnostic criteria established for adults are useful guidelines for evaluating children with suggestive symptoms (Table 168-1). The **differential diagnosis** includes Wegener granulomatosis (see Chapter 166.4) and Cogan syndrome, which is characterized by auditory nerve inflammation and keratitis but not chondritis. The clinical course is variable. Many patients respond to nonsteroidal anti-inflammatory drugs, and some require corticosteroids or other immunosuppressive agents. Oral collagen has also been reported to improve symptoms. Severe, progressive, and potentially fatal disease, resulting from destruction of the tracheobronchial tree and airway obstruction, is unusual in childhood.

TABLE 168-1. Empirical Diagnostic Criteria for Relapsing Polychondritis*

MAJOR CRITERIA
Proven inflammatory episodes involving auricular cartilage
Proven inflammatory episodes involving nasal cartilage
Proven inflammatory episodes involving laryngotracheal cartilage
MINOR CRITERIA
Ocular inflammation (conjunctivitis, keratitis, episcleritis, uveitis)
Hearing loss
Vestibular dysfunction
Seronegative inflammatory arthritis

*The diagnosis is established by the presence of 2 major criteria, or 1 major and 2 minor criteria. Histologic examination of affected cartilage is not required.

From Michet CJ Jr, McKenna CH, Luthra HS, et al: Relapsing polychondritis. Survival and predictive role of early disease manifestations. *Ann Intern Med* 1986;104:74–78.

MUCHA-HABERMANN DISEASE. Febrile ulceronecrotic Mucha-Habermann disease, or **pityriasis lichenoides et varioliformis acuta (PLEVA),** is a cutaneous vasculitis characterized by episodes of macules, papules, and papulovesicular lesions that can develop central ulceration, necrosis, and crusting. Arthritis and fever, with an elevated erythrocyte sedimentation rate (ESR), can occur. The diagnosis is confirmed by biopsy of skin lesions, which reveals a perivascular and intramural lymphocytic inflammation affecting capillaries and venules in the upper dermis that may lead to keratinocyte necrosis. When severe, corticosteroids, methotrexate, or other immunosuppressive agents may be necessary to control inflammation.

SWEET SYNDROME. Sweet syndrome, or **acute febrile neutrophilic dermatosis,** occurs most often in young women and is rare in children. It is characterized by recurrent fever and raised, tender erythematous plaques over the face, extremities, and trunk. Some children also have arthritis. The syndrome may be idiopathic or secondary to malignancy, Behçet syndrome (see Chapter 160), or chronic recurrent multifocal osteomyelitis (see Chapter 683). Skin biopsy reveals neutrophilic perivascular infiltrates. The condition usually responds to treatment with corticosteroids.

HYPERTROPHIC OSTEOARTHROPATHY. Some children with chronic disease, especially pulmonary or cardiac disease, develop **clubbing,** which is hypervascularization and soft tissue proliferation about the terminal phalanges, especially of the fingers. There may be associated arthritis of the distal interphalangeal joints, as well as tender periosteal new bone formation along tubular long bones and in bones of the hand. This complication, **hypertrophic osteoarthropathy,** is found in some children with chronic pulmonary disease (cystic fibrosis), congenital heart disease, gastrointestinal diseases (malabsorption syndromes, biliary atresia, and inflammatory bowel disease), and malignancies (nasopharyngeal sarcoma, osteosarcoma, Hodgkin disease). Although the cause is unknown, studies suggest that platelet precursors fail to fragment into platelets within the pulmonary vascular bed before entering the systemic circulation. These clumps are trapped in the peripheral vasculature and interact with peripheral endothelial cells, resulting in release of platelet-derived growth factor and vascular endothelial growth factor, which induces proliferation of vascular endothelial cells, smooth muscle cells, and fibroblasts. Symptoms may improve if the underlying condition can be treated successfully. Evaluation of children with hypertrophic osteoarthropathy should include a chest radiograph to eliminate pulmonary disease or intrathoracic mass.

PLANT THORN SYNOVITIS. Puncture wounds resulting from plant thorns or similar foreign objects that penetrate the synovium can cause acute synovitis that may progress to chronic arthritis. The episode of initial trauma often is forgotten. Plant thorn synovitis should be considered in children with chronic monoarticular arthritis unresponsive to anti-inflammatory medication. Diagnosis may require antibody titers to exclude Lyme disease, MRI, and arthroscopy. Histology often reveals a granulomatous synovitis. Treatment is removal of the foreign body, which may be accomplished by irrigation of the joint during arthroscopy. Chronic synovitis may require synovectomy.

DIABETIC CHEIROARTHROPATHY. Diabetic cheiroarthropathy, or arthropathy of the joints of the hands and fingers, is a complication of juvenile-onset diabetes mellitus. The soft tissues of the hands and fingers undergo progressive thickening and tightening, leading to contractures of the small joints in the hand but without fingertip tapering and loss of digital pulp characteristic of sclerodactyly in scleroderma (see Chapter 159). Occupational therapy can improve loss of motion in affected joints. Diabetic cheiroarthropathy must be distinguished from polyarticular juvenile rheumatoid arthritis, which can coexist with unrelated chronic conditions and in which joint swelling typically precedes flexion contractures.

CYSTIC FIBROSIS. In addition to hypertrophic osteoarthropathy, some patients with cystic fibrosis experience either episodic or persistent arthritis. The cause is unknown but may reflect synovitis resulting from deposition of immune complexes formed in response to recurrent pulmonary infections. It is also possible that persistent arthritis is a result of expression of coexisting, unrelated juvenile rheumatoid arthritis.

ACUTE PANCREATITIS. Periostitis, nodular skin lesions, and synovial fat necrosis may develop as a result of lipases released during pancreatitis. Affected children may have fever, arthritis, and bone pain for several weeks after blunt abdominal trauma (including child abuse) or other causes of pancreatitis. Elevated serum lipase and amylase levels, periosteal new bone formation, and abnormal findings on bone scintigraphy (revealing fat-induced infarcts) may be found. Drainage of pancreatic pseudocysts may alleviate symptoms of arthritis in some patients.

ARTHRITIS ASSOCIATED WITH ORTHOPEDIC CONDITIONS. A degenerative arthritis similar to osteoarthritis found in adults may occur in some children with developmental bone dysplasias or after trauma. Anti-inflammatory or immunosuppressive medication may be helpful, but only after surgical intervention for the underlying problem.

IMMUNODEFICIENCY. Some children with B- and T-lymphocyte immunodeficiencies develop rheumatic diseases. There are several potential mechanisms. Defective mucosal immunity in children with B-cell diseases (IgA deficiency, X-linked agammaglobulinemia, common variable immunodeficiency) may permit entry from the gut into the circulation of viruses that are either cross-reactive with self antigens or capable of causing infective synovitis. T-cell defects may result in the loss of T-lymphocyte control over autoreactive T lymphocytes. Arthritis, both episodic and chronic, has been described in children with various types of hypogammaglobulinemia, IgA deficiency, and DiGeorge syndrome. IgA deficiency has also been associated with other rheumatic diseases, including lupus, dermatomyositis, scleroderma, and spondyloarthropathy. Patients with Wiskott-Aldrich syndrome have been reported to develop arthritis, vasculitis, and other rheumatic manifestations. The differential diagnosis of arthritis in children with immunodeficiencies includes suppurative arthritis and osteomyelitis.

Ansell BM: Hypertrophic osteoarthropathy in the paediatric age. *Clin Exp Rheumatol* 1992;10(Suppl 7):15–18.

Botton E, Saraux A, Laselve H, et al: Musculoskeletal manifestations in cystic fibrosis. *Joint Bone Spine* 2003;70:327–335.

Conley ME, Park CL, Douglas SD: Childhood common variable immunodeficiency with autoimmune disease. *J Pediatr* 1986;108:915–922.

Diren HB, Kutluk MT, Karabent A, et al: Primary hypertrophic osteoarthropathy. *Pediatr Radiol* 1986;16:231–234.

Dupuis-Girod S, Medioni J, Haddad E, et al: Autoimmunity in Wiskott-Aldrich syndrome: risk factors, clinical features, and outcome in a single-center cohort of 55 patients. *Pediatrics* 2003;111:e622–e627.

Maillot F, Goupille P, Valat JP: Plant thorn synovitis diagnosed by magnetic resonance imaging. *Scand J Rheumatol* 1994;23:154–155.

Marhaug G, Hvidsten D: Arthritis complicating acute pancreatitis—a rare but important condition to be distinguished from juvenile rheumatoid arthritis. *Scand J Rheumatol* 1988;17:397–399.

Miyamoto T, Takayama N, Kitada S, et al: Febrile ulceronecrotic Mucha-Habermann disease: A case report and a review of the literature. *J Clin Pathol* 2003;56:795–797.

Navarro MJ, Higgins GC, Lohr KM, et al: Amelioration of relapsing polychondritis in a child treated with oral collagen. *Am J Med Sci* 2002;324: 101–103.

Oddone M, Toma P, Taccone A, et al: Relapsing polychondritis in childhood: A rare observation studied by CT and MRI. *Pediatr Radiol* 1992;22: 537–538.

Scuccimarri R, Azouz EM, Duffy KN, et al: Inflammatory arthritis in children with osteochondrodysplasias. *Ann Rheum Dis* 2000;59:864–869.

Spicknall KE, Zirwas MJ, English JC III: Clubbing: An update on diagnosis, differential diagnosis, pathophysiology, and clinical relevance. *J Am Acad Dermatol* 2005;52:1020–1028.

Sullivan KE, McDonald-McGinn DM, Driscoll DA, et al: Juvenile rheumatoid arthritis-like polyarthritis in chromosome 22q11.2 deletion syndrome (DiGeorge anomalad/velocardiofacial syndrome/conotruncal anomaly face syndrome). *Arthritis Rheum* 1997;40:430–436.

Part XVI ▪ Infectious Diseases

Section 1 — General Considerations

Chapter 169 ▪ Diagnostic Microbiology

Anita K. M. Zaidi and
Donald A. Goldmann

Laboratory diagnosis of infectious diseases is based on 1 or more of the following: (1) direct examination of specimens by microscopic or antigenic techniques, (2) isolation of microorganisms in culture, (3) serologic testing for development of antibodies (**serodiagnosis**), and (4) molecular detection of the pathogen's genome (DNA, RNA). Clinicians must select the appropriate tests and specimens and, when possible, suggest the suspected etiologic agents to the microbiologist, because this facilitates selection of the most cost-effective diagnostic approach. Additional roles of the microbiology laboratory include testing for antimicrobial drug susceptibility and assisting the hospital epidemiologist in detecting and clarifying the epidemiology of nosocomial infections.

LABORATORY DIAGNOSIS OF BACTERIAL AND FUNGAL INFECTIONS

Diagnosis of bacterial and fungal infections relies mainly on direct demonstration of the microorganisms by microscopic examination or antigen detection and on growth of microorganisms on nutrient culture media. Molecular diagnostic methods for direct detection of certain pathogens are available for some pathogens.

MICROSCOPY. The **Gram stain** remains an extremely useful diagnostic technique because it is a rapid, inexpensive method for demonstrating the presence of bacteria and fungi, as well as inflammatory cells. A preliminary assessment of the etiologic agent can be made by noting the morphology of the microorganisms (cocci vs rods) and by noting their color (gram-positive microorganisms stain blue, gram-negative stain red). The presence of inflammatory and epithelial cells can be used to gauge the quality of certain specimens. For example, ≥10 epithelial cells per low-power field in a sputum sample strongly suggest contamination from oral secretions. In many cases, such as in the examination of cerebrospinal fluid (CSF), the Gram stain can provide very rapid and useful results. However, the Gram stain is an insensitive technique, requiring 10^4–10^5 microorganisms/mL for detection. A trained observer may be able to reach a tentative conclusion that there are specific microorganisms in the specimen based on their morphology and Gram reaction (gram-positive cocci in clusters are likely to be staphylococci), but such preliminary interpretations should be made cautiously and must be confirmed by culture. Many different stains are used in clinical microbiology (Table 169-1).

RAPID ANTIGEN DETECTION. Several rapid antigen detection tests for bacterial pathogens are commercially available and widely used. These include **latex agglutination** (LA) tests for detection of *Haemophilus influenzae* type b, *Streptococcus pneumoniae*, group B streptococci, and *Neisseria meningitidis* in CSF, and group A streptococci in the pharynx (see below). Routinely performing LA tests on CSF is expensive and offers no advantage over an adequately performed Gram stain. Their use is best limited to patients with CSF pleocytosis who have received prior antimicrobial therapy.

A rapid and sensitive test for the detection of pneumococcal antigen in the urine of patients with invasive pneumococcal disease (Binax NOW Urinary Antigen Test, Binax, Scarborough, ME) is available in the U.S. However, a major limitation of the Binax urinary test is its inability to distinguish between children who are nasopharyngeal carriers of pneumococci and those with invasive disease, since many well children who are merely colonized with pneumococci also test positive. Utility in the detection of pneumococcal antigen in the CSF of patients with meningitis and in blood of patients with suspected pneumococcal bacteremia is under investigation.

ISOLATION AND IDENTIFICATION. Most medically important bacteria can be cultured on nutrient-rich media such as blood agar and chocolate agar. Specialized agar may be used selectively to grow and differentiate among organisms of different types. For example, MacConkey agar supports growth of gram-negative rods while suppressing gram-positive organisms, and a color change in the media from clear to pink distinguishes lactose-fermenting organisms from other gram-negative rods. Liquid broth media are used for blood cultures and to enhance growth of small numbers of organisms in other clinical specimens. Sabouraud dextrose agar (with antibiotics to inhibit bacterial growth) is used to culture most fungi. Many pathogens, including *Bartonella, Bordetella pertussis, Brucella, Francisella, Legionella*, and mycobacteria, and certain fungal pathogens such as *Malassezia furfur, Mycoplasma*, and *Chlamydia* require specialized growth media or incubation conditions. Consultation with the laboratory is advised when these pathogens are suspected.

After isolation in culture, microbial identity can be confirmed by a series of biochemical tests, by the ability of the organism to grow in the presence of certain substances that inhibit growth of other microorganisms (selective antibiotics, salt, bile), or by antigen detection. Molecular probes can also be used.

Blood Culture. Several different blood culture systems are available. Most use 50–100 mL bottles containing broth that enhances the growth of bacteria and fungi (mainly yeast). Bottles with smaller volumes are also available specifically for pediatric use. Media containing resins are often used to adsorb antibiotics that may be present in a patient's blood and to improve microbial detection. Most laboratories use automated systems that greatly reduce the time to microbial detection; >80% of all cultures containing pathogens become positive within 24 hr of incubation.

Proper skin disinfection before blood collection is essential. Povidone-iodine may be used, but this agent must be allowed to dry completely for maximum activity. Alcohol is rapidly bactericidal and is a suitable alternative agent. Iodine is effective but

TABLE 169-1. Stains Used for Microscopic Examination

TYPE OF STAIN	CLINICAL USE
Gram stain	Stains bacteria, fungi, leukocytes, and epithelial cells.
Potassium hydroxide (KOH)	A 10% solution dissolves cellular and organic debris and facilitates detection of fungal elements.
Calcofluor white stain	Nonspecific fluorochrome that binds to cellulose and chitin in fungal cell walls. Can be combined with 10% KOH to dissolve cellular material.
Ziehl-Neelsen and Kinyoun stains	Acid-fast stains, using basic carbolfuchsin, followed by acid-alcohol decolorization and methylene blue counterstaining. Acid-fast organisms (e.g., *Mycobacterium, Cryptosporidium,* and *Cyclospora*) resist decolorization and stain pink. A weaker decolorizing agent is used for partially acid-fast organisms (e.g., *Nocardia*).
Acridine orange stain	Fluorescent dye that intercalates into DNA. At acid pH, bacteria and fungi stain orange, and background cellular material green.
Auramine-rhodamine stain	Acid-fast stain using fluorochromes that bind to mycolic acid in mycobacterial cell walls, and resist acid-alcohol decolorization. Acid-fast organisms stain orange-yellow against a black background.
India ink stain	Detects *Cryptococcus neoformans,* an encapsulated yeast, by excluding ink particles from the polysaccharide capsule. (Direct testing of specimens for cryptococcal antigen is much more sensitive than India ink preparations.)
Methenamine silver stain	Stains fungal elements, *Pneumocystis* cysts in tissues. Primarily performed in surgical pathology laboratories.
Lugol's iodine stain	Added to wet preparations of fecal specimens for ova and parasites to enhance contrast of the internal structures (nuclei, glycogen vacuoles).
Wright and Giemsa stains	Primarily for detecting blood parasites (*Plasmodium, Babesia,* and *Leishmania*), fungi in tissues (yeasts, *Histoplasma*).
Trichrome stain	Stains stool specimens for identification of protozoa.
Direct fluorescent-antibody stain	Used for direct detection of a variety of organisms in clinical specimens by using specific fluorescein-labeled antibodies, e.g., *Bordetella pertussis, Legionella, Chlamydia trachomatis, Pneumocystis carinii,* many viruses.

must be wiped off with alcohol to avoid skin reactions. The practice of obtaining blood for culture from intravascular catheters without accompanying peripheral venous blood cultures should be discouraged because it is difficult to determine the significance of coagulase-negative staphylococci and other skin flora isolated from blood obtained from "through-the-line" cultures. Differential time to positivity of 120 min or more between paired blood cultures drawn simultaneously from a catheter and peripheral vein is a useful indicator of catheter-related bloodstream infection. For patients with suspected bacteremia or fungemia, 2 or 3 separate blood cultures are preferred. More than 3 blood cultures rarely are indicated, even in endocarditis. Whenever possible, at least 2–3 mL of blood should be obtained for culture before administration of antibiotics. Obtaining a larger volume of blood is necessary to maximize yield from blood cultures, because children may have low-grade bloodstream infections. In 1 recent Kenyan study, the sensitivity of blood cultures fell by almost ⅓ when yield from 1 mL of blood was compared with yield from 3 mL of blood. For most patients, the most effective approach is to culture the entire volume of blood in a single aerobic bottle because anaerobic bacteremia is rare in children. Blood should also be cultured anaerobically for patients at increased risk for anaerobic sepsis, such as children who are immunocompromised or who have head and neck or abdominal infections. Detection of fungi can be aided by lysis-centrifugation techniques, such as the Isolator 1.5 system (Wampole, Cranbury, NJ).

CSF Culture. CSF should be transported quickly to the laboratory, where it is centrifuged to concentrate organisms for microscopic examination. CSF is routinely plated on blood and chocolate agar, which support the growth of common pathogens causing meningitis. If tuberculosis is suspected, cultures for mycobacteria should be specifically requested. Culture of larger volumes of CSF (>5 mL) significantly improves yield of mycobacteria from CSF.

Urine Culture. Urine for culture and colony count can be obtained by collecting clean-voided midstream specimens, by catheterization, or by suprapubic aspiration. Urine samples collected by placing bags on the perineum are unacceptable for culture because of frequent contamination that renders the results uninterpretable. Rapid transport of urine to the laboratory is imperative because gram-negative enteric pathogens have generation times of 20–30 min, and any delay in transport or plating renders colony counts unreliable. Refrigeration can be used when delay is unavoidable. Culture systems using media-coated "paddles" permit prompt inoculation of the specimen, but confluent growth may be difficult to detect; moreover, accurate antibiotic susceptibility testing requires the presence of individual discrete colonies. Urine obtained by suprapubic puncture should normally be sterile. Urine collected by catheterization is likely to reflect infection if there are $\geq 10^3$ organisms/mL. Clean-voided urine is considered abnormal if $\geq 10^5$ organisms/mL are present and possibly abnormal if 10^4–10^5 organisms/mL are present. However, lower counts are sometimes found in urinary tract infections in adolescent girls and young women, especially those with bacterial urethritis, or in patients with fungal infections. A Gram stain of unspun urine with ≥1 bacterium per oil immersion field correlates well with the presence of $\geq 10^5$ organisms/mL.

Genital Culture. Specimens from the genital tract include urethral, cervical, and anorectal swabs. *Neisseria gonorrhoeae* organisms are fragile, and rapid inoculation at the bedside onto Thayer-Martin medium (warmed to room temperature) or 1 of its modifications is crucial. Ordinarily, specimens should be obtained from genital, anorectal, and pharyngeal sources to achieve maximum yield. Specimens for *Chlamydia trachomatis* culture are obtained by cotton-tipped, aluminum-shafted urethral swabs. Endocervical specimens, using swabs with aluminum or plastic shafts, should be collected by rubbing the swab vigorously against the endocervical wall to obtain as much cellular material as possible. *C. trachomatis* is cultured by inoculation into cell culture systems, followed by immunofluorescent staining with monoclonal antibody against the organism. Nonculture methods, such as enzyme immunoassay (EIA) tests, direct immunofluorescent staining by monoclonal antibodies, and DNA amplification methods are widely used and are more cost-effective than culture.

Throat and Respiratory Cultures. Obtaining a throat swab for culture is the most reliable method of diagnosing group A streptococcal pharyngitis and tonsillitis. Vigorous swabbing of the tonsillar area and posterior pharynx is necessary for maximum detection. Even then, a single swab detects only approximately 90% of infections. The pharynx contains many normal flora; thus, most laboratories screen cultures only for the presence of group A β-hemolytic streptococci. Some laboratories do not use selective procedures, however, and may report the presence of meningococci, usually nontypable, nonpathogenic strains, but occasionally typable meningococci and other potential pathogens. Most patients harboring such bacteria are carriers, and the culture report serves only to create needless alarm. The laboratory should be alerted if diphtheria, pertussis, gonococcal pharyngitis, or infection with *Arcanobacterium haemolyticum* is clinically suspected. Cultures for *B. pertussis* are obtained by aspiration or a Dacron or flexible aluminum wire calcium alginate swab (Calgiswab) of the nasopharynx and inoculation onto special charcoal-blood (Regan-Lowe) or Bordet-Gengou media.

The cause of lower respiratory tract disease in children is not easy to confirm microbiologically because of difficulty in obtaining adequate sputum specimens and lack of correlation between upper respiratory tract flora and organisms causing lower respiratory tract disease. Gram-stained smears of specimens with large numbers of epithelial cells or with few neutrophils are unsuitable for culture. Patients with cystic fibrosis can usually provide adequate expectorated sputum, and special media should be used to detect important cystic fibrosis pathogens, such as *Burkholderia cepacia.*

Endotracheal aspirates from intubated patients may be useful if the Gram stain shows abundant neutrophils and bacteria, although pathogens recovered from such specimens may still reflect only contamination from the endotracheal tube or upper airway. Quantitative cultures of bronchoalveolar lavage fluid or bronchial brush specimens may be valuable for distinguishing upper respiratory tract contamination from lower tract disease in special circumstances.

The diagnosis of pulmonary tuberculosis in young children is best made by culture of early morning gastric aspirates, obtained on 3 successive days. Acid-fast stains of gastric aspirates from children are rarely positive. Sputum induction for obtaining specimens for mycobacterial culture has also proved useful in young children but requires skilled personnel and sophisticated containment facilities to prevent exposure to health care workers. Cultures for *Mycobacterium tuberculosis* should be processed only in laboratories equipped with appropriate biologic safety cabinets and containment facilities.

Stool Culture. Most laboratories in North America routinely culture stool for the presence of *Salmonella, Shigella,* and *Campylobacter* by inoculation onto **selective agar** (to decrease the growth of normal fecal flora) and **differential agar** (to help distinguish pathogenic enteric flora from normal enteric flora). Freshly passed stool is preferred, but rectal swabs may be acceptable. Cultures for *Escherichia coli* O157:H7, *Vibrio cholerae, Yersinia enterocolitica, Aeromonas,* and *Plesiomonas* should be specifically requested when these organisms are suspected. Isolation of enterotoxigenic *E. coli,* the most common cause of traveler's diarrhea, and other pathogenic types of *E. coli* except for *E. coli* O157:H7 is not routinely attempted. Bacterial stool cultures in the U.S. rarely yield useful results in patients who have been hospitalized for more than 3 days. Cultures for *Clostridium difficile,* the most common bacterial cause of nosocomial diarrhea, have been replaced by tests that detect toxin production, such as cell culture assays for cytotoxicity, and EIA.

Culture of Other Fluids and Tissues. Abscesses, wounds, pleural fluid, peritoneal fluid, joint fluid, and other purulent fluids are cultured onto routine solid agar and broth media. Whenever possible, fluid rather than swabs from infected sites should be sent to the laboratory because culture of a larger volume of fluid may detect organisms present in low concentration. Anaerobic organisms are involved in many abdominal and wound abscesses. These specimens should be collected and transported rapidly under anaerobic conditions, preferably in anaerobic transport tubes.

ANTIMICROBIAL SUSCEPTIBILITY TESTING. Antimicrobial susceptibility tests are generally performed on all organisms of clinical significance except for a few that have predictable antimicrobial susceptibility patterns (group A streptococci remain universally susceptible to penicillin). The most common technique is the **agar disk diffusion method (Bauer-Kirby method)**, in which a standardized inoculum of the organism is seeded onto an agar plate. Antibiotic-impregnated filter paper disks are then placed on the agar surface. After 18–24 hr of incubation, the zone of inhibition of bacterial growth around each disk is measured and compared with nationally determined standards for susceptibility or resistance.

The other widely used technique for susceptibility testing is **dilution testing.** A standard concentration of a microorganism is inoculated into serially diluted concentrations of antibiotic, and the **minimum inhibitory concentration** (**MIC**) in µg/mL, the lowest concentration of antibiotic required to inhibit growth of the microorganism, is determined. Dilution testing also permits determination of the **minimum bactericidal concentration** (**MBC**), the lowest concentration of antibiotic required to kill the organism. The MBC is sometimes determined to exclude the possibility of bacterial **tolerance** (MBC >4 times the MIC). Automated methods that use microtiter wells with premade dilutions of antibiotics are now used commonly. However, MICs from automated systems should be interpreted with caution for certain pathogen-antibiotic combinations (pneumococci resistant to penicillin, enterococci with low-level resistance to vancomycin). Screening agar plate tests, such as oxacillin disk susceptibility to detect penicillin-resistant pneumococci, followed by confirmatory tests, are recommended. The **E-test** is used to measure the MIC of individual antibiotics on an agar plate. It uses a paper strip impregnated with a known continuous concentration gradient of antibiotic that diffuses across the agar surface, inhibiting microbial growth in an elliptic zone. The MIC is read off the printed strip at the point at which the zone intersects the strip. Major advantages of the E-test are reliable interpretation, reproducibility, and applicability to organisms that require special media or growth conditions, including anaerobic bacteria.

OFFICE BACTERIOLOGY. Many office practices perform rapid antigen testing for detection of group A streptococcal pharyngitis. Susceptibility depends on the type of kit used and on the concentration of streptococci present in the sample. Practitioners should investigate the specific tests available to them. As many as 30% of test results may be false-negative; therefore, all negative results should be confirmed by culture.

Other microbiologic tests may be performed in the office setting, provided the site is certified as meeting appropriate quality assurance standards specified by the Clinical Laboratory Improvement Amendments (CLIA) of 1988. These include procedures listed under the category of "provider-performed microscopy" such as wet mounts, potassium hydroxide (KOH) preparations, pinworm examinations, fecal leukocyte examinations, and urine sediment analysis. Office laboratories licensed for performing **waived tests** are limited to performing these tests and avoid having to undergo inspections and proficiency testing, although they are still subject to CLIA certification requirements specific to these tests. Gram staining, culture inoculation, and isolation of bacteria are considered moderately to highly complex tests under CLIA specifications. Any office laboratory performing Gram stains or cultures must comply with the same requirements and inspections for quality assurance, proficiency testing, and personnel requirements as fully licensed microbiology laboratories.

LABORATORY DIAGNOSIS OF VIRAL INFECTIONS

Specimens for viral diagnosis are selected on the basis of knowledge of the site that is most likely to yield the suspected pathogen. Specimens should be collected early in the course of infection when viral shedding is maximal. Fluids and respiratory secretions should be collected in sterile containers and delivered to the laboratory promptly. Swabs should be rubbed vigorously against mucosal or skin surfaces to obtain as much cellular material as possible, and sent in viral transport media that contain antibiotics to inhibit bacterial growth. Rectal swabs should not be heavily covered with feces because the antibiotics present in viral transport media may be insufficient to kill a large inoculum of bacteria. All specimens should be transported on ice. Freezing specimens can result in a significant decrease in culture sensitivity. Consultation with the laboratory is advised for any unusual specimens or suspected pathogens.

Laboratory diagnosis of viral infections may be by electron microscopy, antigen detection, virus isolation in culture, serologic testing, or quite often by detection of virus genomes by molecular biology techniques. Serologic and molecular tests are the mainstay of diagnosis of viruses such as HIV and Epstein-Barr virus (EBV).

Rapid Antigen Tests. Immunofluorescent-antibody (IFA) techniques or other methods such as EIA that use antibodies to detect viral antigens directly in clinical specimens permit rapid identification of viruses. Smears of cellular material from respiratory secretions stained by immunologic reagents can identify the antigens of respiratory syncytial virus (RSV), adenovirus, influenza virus, and parainfluenza virus within 2–3 hr after the specimen is received. In comparison with isolation in cell culture, IFA is approximately 95% sensitive and 98% specific for the diagnosis of RSV and parainfluenza virus type 3 in reference laboratories; the sensitivity of IFA for influenza viruses and adenoviruses is considerably lower. Sensitive IFA staining techniques are also commercially available for identification of varicella-zoster virus (VZV) and herpes simplex virus (HSV). These specific methods have supplanted the Tzanck smear for multinucleated giant cells characteristic of VZV or HSV infections. A method for detecting cytomegalovirus (CMV) antigen in blood of immunocompromised patients is also available. IFA is not useful for detecting virus in specimens that do not contain an adequate number of infected cells. When possible, an accompanying specimen for virus isolation usually is advisable.

In addition to providing rapid diagnosis, antigen detection EIA tests are commonly used for the diagnosis of viruses that are difficult to culture, such as rotavirus, noroviruses, and hepatitis B virus.

Isolation and Identification. Viruses require living cells for propagation; the cells used most often are human- or animal-derived tissue culture monolayers, such as human embryonic lung fibroblasts or monkey kidney cells. In vivo methods for isolation are sometimes necessary (suckling mice inoculation for culture of arboviruses and rabies virus). Because viruses require various cell culture systems for isolation, it is important for clinicians to provide relevant clinical information to the laboratory to facilitate selection of appropriate cell lines.

Viral growth in susceptible cell cultures can be detected in several ways. Many viruses produce a characteristic **cytopathic effect** (CPE) that is visible by light microscopy under low magnification. For example, RSV and HSV produce multinucleated giant cells and syncytia formation. Other viruses (e.g., influenza and mumps) can be detected by hemadsorption because hemagglutinins on infected cell membranes permit adherence of erythrocytes to infected cells. The most reliable confirmatory method for viral detection in cell culture involves fluorescein- or enzyme-labeled monoclonal antibody staining of infected cell monolayers.

An important technical improvement in respiratory viral cultures is the development of an engineered tissue monolayer (R-mix) for rapid shell vial detection of influenza A and B, respiratory syncytial virus, parainfluenza 1–3, and adenoviruses. Respiratory shell vial cultures have turn-around times of 2 days compared with 2–3 weeks for conventional cultures and are most useful for rapid diagnosis of influenza infections where sensitivity of IFA is low, and rapid detection can result in early institution of appropriate antiviral therapy.

LABORATORY DIAGNOSIS OF PARASITIC INFECTIONS

Most parasites are detected by microscopic examination of clinical specimens. *Plasmodium* and *Babesia* can be detected in stained blood smears, *Leishmania* in bone marrow smears, and helminth eggs, *Entamoeba histolytica, Giardia lamblia* cysts, and trophozoites in fecal smears (see Table 169-1). Serologic tests are important in documenting exposure to certain parasites that are difficult to demonstrate in clinical specimens, such as *Trichinella* and *Toxoplasma.* Serologic testing also has a role in the diagnosis of intestinal strongyloidiasis, given the insensitivity of stool examinations.

Fecal specimens should not be contaminated with water or urine because water may contain free-living organisms that can be confused with human parasites, and urine may destroy motile organisms. Mineral oil, barium, and bismuth interfere with the detection of parasites, and specimen collection should be delayed for 7–10 days after ingestion of these substances. Because *Giardia* and many worm eggs are shed intermittently into feces, a minimum of three specimens are required for an adequate examination. It is recommended that the three specimens be collected on separate days, preferably on alternate days. Because many protozoan parasites are easily destroyed, collection kits with stool preservatives should be used if delay between time of specimen collection and transport to the laboratory is anticipated.

Ova and parasite examination of fecal specimens includes a wet mount (to detect motile organisms if fresh stool is received), concentration (to improve yield), and permanent staining, such as trichrome, for microscopic examination. These techniques may miss parasites such as *Cryptosporidium, Cyclospora,* and microsporidia (*Enterocytozoon bieneusi* and *Encephalitozoon intestinalis*). *Cryptosporidium* and *Cyclospora* are detected by modified acid-fast stain and microsporidia by a modification of the trichrome stain. The laboratory should be alerted if these parasites are suspected. Detection of certain parasites, especially *Giardia* and *Cryptosporidium,* can be simplified by using sensitive EIA antigen detection tests. Combination tests for these 2 pathogens are commercially available. Rapid antigen detection ("dipstick") tests for *Plasmodium falciparum* and *P. vivax* such as those based on detection of *Plasmodium* histidine-rich protein are also available with sensitivities and specificities comparable to expert microscopy. These tests are particularly useful in areas where trained laboratory personnel are not available.

SEROLOGIC DIAGNOSIS

Serologic tests are primarily used in the diagnosis of infectious agents that are difficult to culture in vitro or detect by direct examination, such as *Bartonella, Legionella, Borrelia* (Lyme), *Treponema pallidum, Mycoplasma, Rickettsia, Ehrlichia,* some viruses (HIV, EBV, hepatitis A and B viruses), and parasites *(Toxoplasma, Trichinella).*

Antibody tests may be specific for immunoglobulin G (IgG) or M (IgM) or may measure antibody response regardless of immunoglobulin class. The IgM response occurs earlier in the illness, generally peaking at 7–10 days after infection, and usually disappears within a few weeks but for some infections (e.g., hepatitis A) may persist for months. The IgG response peaks at 4–6 wk and usually persists for life. Because the IgM response is transient, the presence of IgM antibody in most cases correlates with recent infection; therefore, a single positive serum specimen is considered diagnostic. Methods for IgM antibody detection are difficult to standardize, however, and false-positive results frequently occur with some tests. The presence of IgG antibody may indicate new seroconversion or past exposure to the pathogen. To confirm a new infection using IgG testing, it is essential to demonstrate either **seroconversion** or a rising IgG titer. A fourfold increase in a **convalescent titer** obtained 2–3 wk after the **acute titer** is considered diagnostic in most situations. However, for some infections (e.g., *Bartonella, Legionella,* and rickettsiae) a single positive IgG titer is sufficient for diagnosis. Serologic diagnosis of Lyme disease remains problematic because of lack of specificity of the commercial enzyme immunoassays. A confirmatory immunoblot (Western blot) is required for all positive and equivocal EIA results for Lyme disease.

Several rapid enzyme-linked immunospot (ELISPOT) assays that detect interferon production by tuberculosis-specific lymphocytes in the patients' blood are undergoing clinical evaluation and may have useful applicability for diagnosis of tuberculosis in children.

MOLECULAR DIAGNOSTIC TECHNIQUES

Molecular diagnostic techniques are most useful for detecting and identifying pathogens for which culture and serologic tests are difficult, slow, or not available. Molecular diagnostic testing for infectious agents is a rapidly evolving field and is revolutionizing clinical microbiology with full-scale automation, high sensitivities and specificities, and rapid reporting of results. Two of the widely used techniques in clinical microbiology are **DNA probes** for direct detection and **nucleic acid amplification** using polymerase chain reaction (PCR). Microbiologic applications of techniques such as miniaturized DNA chip technology and microarrays based on the ability of DNA to find and spontaneously bind to its complementary sequences (mycobacterial DNA in a patient's blood) are also being developed.

DNA probes detect or identify organisms by hybridization of the probe to complementary sequences in DNA or ribosomal RNA. The principal use of DNA probe technology remains rapid identification of organisms that already have been isolated in culture but require additional time-consuming or complex confirmation procedures. Probes for mycobacterial species can rapidly distinguish *M. tuberculosis* from *M. avium* complex growing in broth cultures. Detection of pathogen nucleic acid directly in clinical specimens is also possible but requires the presence of relatively large numbers of organisms in the specimen. Commercially available probes for direct detection of pathogen from specimens include combination probes for detection of *C. trachomatis* and gonococci from genitourinary specimens.

The high sensitivity and specificity of **PCR amplification** make this the method of choice for **direct** detection of microbial nucleic acid from clinical specimens. The PCR method is based on the ability of thermostable DNA or RNA polymerase to copy targeted gene sequences using complementary nucleotides as primers to amplify a conserved region of the genome. The reaction takes place in a thermal cycler. Each cycle of the reaction theoretically doubles the amount of target nucleic acid, resulting in more than a million-fold amplification after 30 cycles of PCR. The greatest impact of PCR is in clinical virology and mycobacteriology where conventional methods are slow and insensitive. The number of pathogens that can be detected by PCR is increasing rapidly. PCR tests are available using commercial reagents for HIV, hepatitis B and C viruses, CMV, *M. tuberculosis,* and *C. trachomatis.* Multiplex tests such as the Hexaplex assay (Prodesse, Milwaukee, WI) for detection of seven common respiratory viral pathogens in children are also commercially available. Experimental PCR protocols for detection of *Bartonella, B. pertussis, Legionella, M. pneumoniae, Chlamydia pneumoniae,* and HSV are available in some reference laboratories.

Specimens for PCR should be sent in separate sterile containers and rapidly transported. Traditional PCR methods are technically complex and labor intensive. False-positive reactions are a major problem because the extreme sensitivity of the assay can lead to amplification of target nucleic acid from extraneous sources or from crossover contamination from other positive specimens. Technical improvements in thermocycler equipment (quantitative **real-time PCR**) using sealed tubes incorporating fluorescent probes added to the PCR mix to confirm and quantify PCR products as they are generated have significantly reduced processing times and postamplification contamination. Turnaround times of 2–4 hr from receipt of specimen are now possible. Real-time PCR has been used for rapid detection of methicillin-resistant *Staphylococcus aureus* and vancomycin-resistant enterococcal colonization. Clinically relevant diagnostic PCR testing should be performed only in reference laboratories using adequate quality control measures.

Berkley JA, Lowe BS, Mwangi I, et al: Bacteremia among children admitted to a rural hospital in Kenya. *N Engl J Med* 2005;352:39–47.

Committee on Quality Improvement, Subcommittee on Urinary Tract Infection, American Academy of Pediatrics: Practice parameter: The diagnosis, treatment, and evaluation of the initial urinary tract infection in febrile infants and young children. *Pediatrics* 1999;103:843–852.

Dowell SF, Garman RL, Liu G, et al: Evaluation of Binax NOW, an assay for the detection of pneumococcal antigen in urine samples performed among pediatric patients. *Clin Infect Dis* 2001;32:824–825.

Hale YM, Pfyffer GE, Salfinger M: Laboratory diagnosis of mycobacterial infections: New tools and lessons learned. *Clin Infect Dis* 2001;33:834–836.

Henrickson KJ: Cost-effective use of rapid diagnostic techniques in the treatment and prevention of viral respiratory infections. *Pediatr Ann* 2005;34:24–31.

Isaacman DJ, Karasic RB, Reynolds EA, et al: Effect of number of blood cultures and volume of blood on detection of bacteremia in children. *J Pediatr* 1996;128:190–195.

Kaplan RL, Harper MB, Baskin MN, et al: Time to detection of positive cultures in 28- to 90-day-old febrile infants. *Pediatrics* 2000;106:e74.

Liebeschuetz S, Bamber S, Ewer K, et al: Diagnosis of tuberculosis in South African children with a T-cell–based assay: A prospective cohort study. *Lancet* 2004;364:2196–2203.

Marcos MA, Martinez E, Almela M: New rapid antigen test for diagnosis of pneumococcal meningitis. *Lancet* 2001;357:1499–1500.

Maxson S, Lewno MJ, Schutze GE: Clinical usefulness of cerebrospinal fluid bacterial antigen studies. *J Pediatr* 1994;125:235.

McGowan KL, Foster JA, Coffin SE: Outpatient pediatric blood cultures: Time to positivity. *Pediatrics* 2000;106:251–255.

Mein J, Lum G: CSF bacterial antigen detection tests offer no advantage over Gram stain in the diagnosis of bacterial meningitis. *Pathology* 1999;31:67–69.

Navarro D, Garcia-Maset L, Gimeno C, et al: Performance of the Binax NOW *Streptococcus pneumoniae* urinary antigen assay for diagnosis of pneumonia in children with underlying pulmonary diseases in the absence of acute pneumococcal infection. *J Clin Microbiol* 2004;42:4853–4855.

Nicol MP, Pienaar D, Wook K, et al: Enzyme-linked immunospot assay responses to early secretory antigenic target 6, culture filtrate protein 10, and purified protein derivative among children with tuberculosis: Implications for diagnosis and monitoring of therapy. *Clin Infect Dis* 2005;40:1301–1308.

Nissen MD, Sloots TP: Rapid diagnosis in pediatric infectious diseases: The past, the present and the future. *Pediatr Infect Dis J* 2002;21:605–612.

Peters RP, van Agtmael MA, Danner SA, et al: New developments in the diagnosis of bloodstream infections. *Lancet Infect Dis* 2004;4:751–760.

Petti CA, Woods CW, Reller LB: *Streptococcus pneumoniae* antigen test using positive blood culture bottles as an alternative to diagnose pneumococcal bacteremia. *J Clin Microbiol* 2005;43:2510–2512.

Storch GA: Diagnostic virology. *Clin Infect Dis* 2000;31:739–751.

Thwaites GE, Chau TTH, Farrar JJ: Improving the bacteriological diagnosis of tuberculous meningitis. *J Clin Microbiol* 2004;42:378–379.

Weinberg A, Brewster L, Clark J, et al: Evaluation of R-Mix shell vials for the diagnosis of viral respiratory tract infections. *J Clin Virol* 2004;30:100–105.

Zaidi AKM, Knaut AL, Mirrett S, et al: Value of routine anaerobic blood cultures for pediatric patients. *J Pediatr* 1995;127:263–268.

Zar HJ, Hanslo D, Apolles P, et al: Induced sputum versus gastric lavage for microbiological confirmation of pulmonary tuberculosis in infants and young children: A prospective study. *Lancet* 2005;365:130–134. Erratum in *Lancet* 2005;265:1926.

Section 2 — Preventive Measures

Chapter 170 ■ Immunization Practices

Walter A. Orenstein and
Larry K. Pickering

Immunization is one of the most beneficial and cost-effective disease prevention measures. As a result of effective and safe vaccines, smallpox has been eradicated, polio is close to worldwide eradication, and measles and rubella are no longer endemic in the U.S. The incidence of most other vaccine-preventable diseases of childhood has been reduced by ≥99% from the annual morbidity prior to development of the corresponding vaccine (Table 170-1). An analysis of effective prevention measures recommended for widespread use by the U.S. Preventive Services Task Force reported that childhood immunization received a perfect score, based on clinically preventable disease burden and cost-effectiveness.

Immunization is the process of inducing immunity against a specific disease. Immunity can be induced either **passively** through administration of antibody-containing preparations or **actively** by administering a vaccine or toxoid to stimulate the immune system to produce a prolonged humoral and/or cellular immune response. As of 2006, infants, children, and adolescents routinely are vaccinated against 16 diseases in the U.S.: diphtheria, tetanus, pertussis, poliomyelitis, *Haemophilus influenzae* type b (Hib) disease, hepatitis A, hepatitis B (HepB), measles, mumps, rubella, rotavirus, varicella, pneumococcal disease, meningococcal disease, and influenza. Human papillomavirus (HPV) vaccine has been recommended for girls 11–12 yr old.

PASSIVE IMMUNITY. Passive immunity is achieved by administration of preformed antibodies to induce transient protection against an infectious agent. Passive immunity also can be induced naturally through transplacental transfer of antibodies during gestation. Maternally derived antibodies can provide protection during an infant's first months of life. Protection for some diseases may persist for as long as a year after birth.

The major indications for passive immunity are to provide protection to (1) immunodeficient children with B-lymphocyte defects who have difficulties in making antibodies; (2) persons exposed to infectious diseases or who are at imminent risk of exposure where there is not adequate time for them to develop an active immune response to a vaccine; and (3) persons with an infectious disease as part of specific therapy for that disease (Table 170-2).

Immune Globulin. Immune globulin (IG) is a sterile antibody containing solution, usually derived through cold ethanol fractionation of large pools of human plasma. IG contains 15–18% protein, predominantly IgG, and is administered intramuscularly. IG is not known to transmit infectious agents, including viral hepatitis and HIV. The major indications for IG are replacement therapy for children with antibody deficiency disorders, and for passive immunization for measles and hepatitis A. For replacement therapy, the usual dose of IG is 100 mg/kg or 0.66 mL/kg monthly. The usual interval between doses is 2–4 wk depending on trough IgG concentrations. In practice, use of an intravenous preparation of IG (**IGIV**), has replaced IG for this indication. IG can be used to prevent or modify measles if administered to children within 6 days of exposure (usual dose 0.25 mL/kg for immunocompetent children, 0.5 mL/kg for immunocompromised children; maximum dose 15 mL) and to prevent or modify hepatitis A if administered to children within 14 days of exposure (usual dose 0.02 mL/kg). IG also may be administered for prophylaxis of hepatitis A for persons traveling internationally to hepatitis A–endemic areas (0.06 mL/kg), for children too young for vaccination (<1 yr of age), or in conjunction with hepatitis A vaccine when departure to the area must be undertaken <1 mo after receipt of hepatitis A vaccine.

The most common adverse reaction to IG is pain and discomfort at the injection site. More serious reactions are rare and have included chest pain, dyspnea, anaphylaxis, and systemic collapse. Patients with selective IgA deficiency can produce antibodies against the trace amounts of IgA in IG preparations and develop reactions after repeat doses. These reactions can include fever, chills, and a shocklike syndrome. Because these reactions are rare, testing for selective IgA deficiencies is not recommended.

Immune Globulin Intravenous. IGIV is prepared from adult plasma donors using alcohol fractionation and is modified to allow for intravenous use. IGIV is predominantly IgG and is tested to assure minimum antibody titers to diphtheria, HepB, measles, and polio. Liquid and powder preparations are available. The major **recommended indications** for IGIV are replacement therapy for immunodeficiency disorders; treatment of

TABLE 170-1. Representative 20th Century Morbidity, Cases in 2005, and Change

DISEASE	20TH CENTURY ANNUAL CASES PRECEDING VACCINE DEVELOPMENT	2005 CASES	PERCENT DECREASE	HEALTHY PEOPLE 2010 COVERAGE GOAL FOR 19–35 MO OLD CHILDREN	COVERAGE JULY 2005
Smallpox	48,164	0	100†	—	—
Diphtheria	175,885	0	100†	4 doses, ≥90%	86%
Measles	503,282	66	>99	1 dose ≥90%	92%
Mumps	152,209	314	>99	1 dose, ≥90%	92%
Pertussis	147,271	25,616	83	4 doses, ≥90%	86%
Polio (paralytic)	16,316	1	>99	3 doses, ≥90%	92%
Rubella	47,745	11	>99	1 dose, ≥90%	92%
Congenital rubella syndrome	823	1	>99	1 dose, ≥90%	92%
Tetanus	1314	27	98	4 doses, ≥90%	86%
H. influenzae type b and unknown (<5 yr)	20,000	226	99	≥3 doses, ≥90%	94%

†Record lows.

Adapted from Centers for Disease Control and Prevention: Achievements in public health, 1900–1999 impact of vaccines universally recommended for children—United States, 1990–1998. *MMWR* 1999;48:243–248; and Centers for Disease Control and Prevention: Final 2005 reports of notifiable diseases. *MMWR* 2005;54:770–780 and *MMWR* 2006;55:988–993.

TABLE 170-2. Immune Globulins and Animal Antisera Preparations

PRODUCT	MAJOR INDICATIONS
Immune globulin for intramuscular injection	Replacement therapy in antibody deficiency disorders Hepatitis A prophylaxis Measles prophylaxis
Intravenous immune globulin (IGIV)	Replacement therapy in antibody deficiency disorders Kawasaki disease Pediatric HIV infection Hypogammaglobulinemia in chronic B-cell lymphocytic leukemia Bone marrow transplantation May be useful in a variety of other conditions*
Hepatitis B immune globulin	Postexposure prophylaxis Prevention of perinatal infection in infants born to $HBsAg^+$ mothers
Rabies immune globulin	Postexposure prophylaxis
Tetanus immune globulin	Wound prophylaxis Treatment of tetanus
Varicella-Zoster immune globulin (VZIG) or IGIV	Postexposure prophylaxis of susceptible persons at high risk for complications from varicella
Cytomegalovirus IGIV	Prophylaxis of disease in seronegative transplant recipients
Palivizumab (monoclonal antibody)	Prophylaxis for infants and children <2 yr of age with chronic lung disease (CLD) who have required medical therapy for CLD within 6 mo of start of prophylaxis Prophylaxis for infants born at 29–32 wk gestation without CLD up to 6 mo of age at time of respiratory syncytial virus (RSV) season Prophylaxis for infants born at <28 wk gestation up to 12 mo of age at the start of RSV season Prophylaxis of infants born at 32–35 wk gestation who are <6 mo of age at start of RSV season and with at least 2 risk factors
Vaccinia immune globulin	Treatment of serious adverse events following smallpox vaccination due to vaccinia replication
Botulism IGIV	Treatment of infant botulism
Diphtheria antitoxin, equine	Treatment of diphtheria
Trivalent botulinum (A,B,E) and bivalent (A,B) botulinum antitoxin, equine	Treatment of food and wound botulism

*From the American Academy of Pediatrics: Passive immunization. In Pickering LK, Baker CJ, Long SS, McMillan JA (editors): *Red Book 2006: Report of the Committee on Infectious Diseases*, 27th ed. Elk Grove Village, IL, American Academy of Pediatrics, 2006.

Kawasaki disease to prevent coronary artery abnormalities and shorten the clinical course; prevention of serious bacterial infections in children with HIV; prevention of serious bacterial infections in persons with hypogammaglobulinemia in chronic B-cell leukemia; immune-mediated thrombocytopenia; and prophylaxis of infection following bone marrow transplantation. In addition, IGIV may be helpful for patients with severe toxic shock syndrome, Guillain-Barré syndrome, and anemia caused by parvovirus B19. IGIV is used for many other conditions based on clinical experience.

Reactions to IGIV range from 1 to 15%. Some of these reactions appear to be related to the rate of infusion and can be mitigated by decreasing the rate. Such reactions include fever, headache, myalgia, chills, nausea, and vomiting. More serious reactions rarely have been reported, including anaphylactoid events, thromboembolic disorders, aseptic meningitis, and renal insufficiency.

Specific Immune Globulin Preparations. **Hyperimmune globulins** are specific IG preparations that are derived from donors with high titers of antibodies to specific agents and designed to provide protection against those agents (see Table 170-2).

Hyperimmune Animal Antisera Preparations. Animal antisera preparations are derived from horses. The IG fraction is concentrated using ammonium sulfate, and some products are further treated with enzymes to decrease reactions to foreign proteins. As of 2006, there are 2 horse antisera preparations available for humans: diphtheria antitoxin, which is used to treat diphtheria, and botulinum antitoxin, which is used to treat botulism. Great care must be exercised prior to administration of such antisera because of the potential for severe allergic reactions. This includes testing for sensitivity prior to administration, desensitization, if necessary, and treatment of potential reactions, including febrile events, serum sickness, and anaphylaxis.

Monoclonal Antibodies. Monoclonal antibodies are antibody preparations produced against a single antigen. They are mass-produced from a hybridoma, created by fusing an antibody-producing B cell with a fast-growing immortal cell such as a cancer cell. The major monoclonal antibody used in infectious diseases is palivizumab, which can prevent severe disease from respiratory syncytial virus (RSV) among children ≤24 mo of age with chronic lung disease (CLD, also called bronchopulmonary dysplasia) or with a history of premature birth (<35 wk). The American Academy of Pediatrics (AAP) has developed specific recommendations for use of palivizumab (see Chapter 257). Monoclonal antibodies also are used for prevention of transplant rejection and treatment of some types of cancer and autoimmune diseases. Monoclonal antibodies against interleukin 2 (IL-2) and tumor necrosis factor-α (TNF-α) are being used as part of the therapeutic approach to patients with a variety of malignant and autoimmune diseases.

Serious adverse reactions to palivizumab primarily are rare cases of anaphylaxis and hypersensitivity reactions. Adverse reactions to monoclonal antibodies directed at modifying the immune response such as antibodies against IL-2 or TNF can be more serious, such as cytokine release syndrome, fever, chills, tremors, chest pain, immunosuppression, and infection with various organisms, including mycobacterium.

ACTIVE IMMUNIZATION. **Vaccines** are defined as whole or parts of microorganisms administered to prevent an infectious disease. Vaccines can consist of whole inactivated microorganisms (polio and hepatitis A), parts of the organism (acellular pertussis, human papillomavirus [HPV], and HepB), polysaccharide capsules (pneumococcal and meningococcal polysaccharide vaccines), polysaccharide capsules conjugated to protein carriers (Hib, pneumococcal, and meningococcal conjugate vaccines), live attenuated microorganisms (measles, mumps, rubella, varicella, rotavirus, and live attenuated influenza vaccines), and toxoids (tetanus and diphtheria) [Table 170-3]. A **toxoid** is a modified bacterial toxin that is made nontoxic but is still able to induce an active immune response against the toxin.

Immunizing agents may contain a variety of other constituents besides the immunizing antigen. **Suspending fluids** may be sterile water or saline but could be a complex fluid containing small

TABLE 170-3. Currently Available Vaccines in the U.S. by Type*

PRODUCT	TYPE
Anthrax vaccine adsorbed	Cell free filtrate of components including protective antigen
Bacillus Calmette-Guérin (BCG) vaccine	Live attenuated mycobacterial strain used for prevention of tuberculosis in very limited circumstances
Diphtheria and tetanus toxoids and acellular pertussis (DTaP) vaccine	Toxoids of diphtheria and tetanus and purified and detoxified components from *Bordetella pertussis*
DTaP with *Haemophilus influenzae* type b (Hib)	DTaP and Hib polysaccharide conjugated to tetanus toxoid
DTaP–Hepatitis B (HepB) inactivated polio vaccine (IPV)	DTaP with hepatitis B surface antigen produced through recombinant techniques in yeast with inactivated whole polioviruses
Hib conjugate vaccine	Polysaccharide conjugated to either tetanus toxoid or meningococcal type B outer membrane protein
Hepatitis A vaccine	Inactivated whole virus
Hepatitis A–hepatitis B vaccine	Combined hepatitis A and B vaccine
Hepatitis B vaccine	HBsAg produced through recombinant techniques in yeast
Hepatitis B–Hib vaccine	Combined hepatitis B–Hib vaccine. The Hib component is polysaccharide conjugated to meningococcal outer membrane protein.
Influenza virus vaccine inactivated (TIV)	Trivalent (A/H_3N_2, A/H_1N_1, and B) split and purified inactivated vaccine containing the hemagglutinin (H) and neuraminidase (N) of each type and other components
Influenza virus vaccine live, intranasal (LAIV)	Live attenuated, temperature-sensitive, cold-adapted trivalent vaccine containing the H and N genes from the wild strains reassorted to have the 6 other genes from the cold-adapted parent
Japanese encephalitis vaccine	Inactivated whole virus that is purified
Measles, mumps, rubella (MMR) vaccine	Live attenuated viruses
Measles, mumps, rubella, varicella (MMRV) vaccine	Live attenuated viruses
Meningococcal conjugate vaccine against serogroups A, C, W135, and Y (MCV4)	Polysaccharide from each serogroup conjugated to diphtheria toxoid
Meningococcal polysaccharide vaccine against serogroups A, C, W135, and Y (MPS4)	Polysaccharides from each of the serogroups
Papillomavirus	HPV 16, 18, 6, 11 serotypes; prevention of cervical cancer and genital warts Noninfectous HPV-like particles.
Pneumococcal conjugate vaccine (7 valent) (PCV7)	Pneumococcal polysaccharides conjugated to a nontoxic form of diphtheria toxin CRM197. Contains seven serotypes that accounted for >80% of invasive disease in young children prior to vaccine licensure.
Pneumococcal polysaccharide vaccine (23 valent) (PPS23)	Pneumococcal polysaccharides of 23 serotypes responsible for 85–90% of bacteremic disease in the U.S.
Poliomyelitis (inactivated, enhanced potency)	Inactivated whole virus
Rabies vaccines (human diploid and purified chick embryo cell)	Inactivated whole virus
Rotavirus vaccine	Bovine rotavirus pentavalent vaccine; live reassortment attenuated virus
Smallpox vaccine	Vaccinia virus, an attenuated pox virus that provides cross-protection against smallpox
Tetanus and diphtheria toxoids, adsorbed (Td, adult use)	Tetanus toxoid plus a reduced quantity of diphtheria toxoid compared to diphtheria toxoid used for children <7 yr of age
Tetanus and diphtheria toxoids adsorbed plus acellular pertussis (Tdap) vaccine	Tetanus toxoid plus a reduced quantity of diphtheria toxoid plus acellular pertussis vaccine to be used in adolescents and adults
Typhoid vaccine (polysaccharide)	Vi capsular polysaccharide of *Salmonella typhi*
Typhoid vaccine (oral)	Live attenuated Ty21a strain of *Salmonella typhi*
Varicella vaccine	Live attenuated Oka strain
Yellow fever vaccine	Live attenuated 17D strain

*Single vaccines for measles, rubella, and tetanus not included in table.

amounts of proteins or other constituents derived from the biologic system used to grow the immunobiologic. **Preservatives, stabilizers, and antimicrobial agents** are used to inhibit bacterial growth and to prevent degradation of the antigen. Such components may include gelatin, 2-phenoxyethanol, and specific antimicrobial agents. Preservatives are added to multidose vials of vaccines, primarily to prevent bacterial contamination on repeated entry of the vial. In the past, many vaccines for children contained thimerosal, a preservative containing ethyl mercury. Beginning in 1999, removal of thimerosal as a preservative from vaccines for children was begun as a precautionary measure in the absence of any data on harm from the preservative. This was accomplished by switching to single-dose packaging. The only vaccines in the recommended schedule for young children that contain thimerosal as a preservative are some preparations of influenza vaccine. **Adjuvants** are used in some vaccines to enhance the immune response. In the United States, the only adjuvants currently licensed by the Food and Drug Administration (FDA) to be part of vaccines are aluminum salts. Vaccines with adjuvants should be injected deep into muscle masses to avoid local irritation, granuloma formation, and necrosis associated with subcutaneous or intracutaneous administration.

Vaccines can induce immunity through stimulation of antibody formation, cellular immunity, or both. Protection induced by most vaccines is thought to be mediated primarily by B lymphocytes, which produce antibody. Such antibodies can inactivate toxins, neutralize viruses, and prevent their attachment to cellular receptors, facilitate phagocytosis and killing of bacteria, interact with complement to lyse bacteria, and prevent adhesion to mucosal surfaces by interacting with the bacterial cell surface.

Most B-lymphocyte responses require the assistance of T-lymphocyte, CD4 helper cells. These T-lymphocyte or T cell–dependent responses tend to induce high levels of functional antibody with high avidity, mature over time from primarily an IgM response to long-term persistent IgG, and induce immunologic memory that leads to enhanced responses upon boosting. **T lymphocyte–dependent vaccines,** which include protein moieties, induce good immune responses even in young infants. In contrast, polysaccharide antigens induce B-lymphocyte responses in the absence of T-lymphocyte help. These **T lymphocyte–independent vaccines** are associated with poor immune responses in children <2 yr of age, short-term immunity, and absence of an enhanced or booster response on repeat exposure to the antigen. To overcome problems of plain polysaccharide vaccines, polysaccharides have been **conjugated,** or covalently linked, to protein carriers, converting the vaccine to a T lymphocyte–dependent vaccine. In contrast to plain polysaccharide vaccines, conjugate vaccines induce higher avidity antibody, immunologic memory leading to booster responses on repeat exposure to the antigen, long-term immunity, and herd immunity by decreasing carriage of the organism. As of 2006 in the United States, there were licensed conjugate vaccines to prevent Hib, pneumococcal, and meningococcal diseases.

Serum antibodies may be detected as soon as 7–10 days after injection of antigen. Early antibodies are usually of the IgM class that can fix complement. IgM antibodies tend to decline as IgG antibodies increase. The IgG antibodies tend to peak approxi-

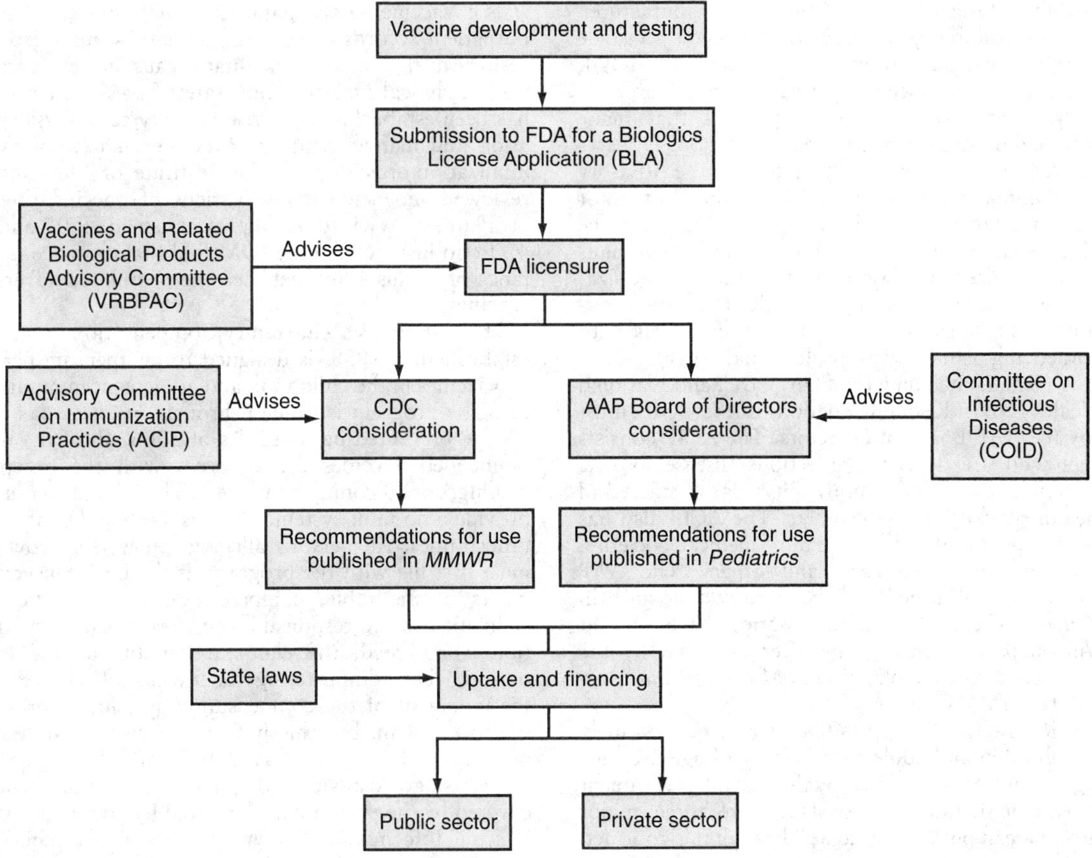

Figure 170-1. Vaccine development and testing. (Modified from Pickering LK, Orenstein WE: Development of pediatric vaccine recommendations and policies. *Semin Pediatr Infect Dis* 2002;13[3]:148–154.)

mately 1 month after vaccination and with most vaccines persist for some time after a primary vaccine course. Secondary or booster responses occur more rapidly and result from rapid proliferation of memory B and T lymphocytes.

Assessment of the immune response to most vaccines is performed through measurement of serum antibodies. While detection of serum antibody at levels considered protective after vaccination may indicate immunity, loss of detectable antibody over time does not necessarily mean susceptibility to disease. Some vaccines may induce immunologic memory leading to a booster or anamnestic response on exposure to the microorganism leading to protection from disease. In some instances, cellular immune response is used to evaluate immune status.

Live attenuated vaccines routinely recommended for children and adolescents include measles, mumps, and rubella (MMR), rotavirus, and varicella. In addition, a cold-adapted live attenuated influenza vaccine (LAIV) is available as an alternative to the trivalent inactivated influenza vaccine (TIV) for children ≥5 yr of age who do not have conditions that place them at high risk for complications from influenza. Live attenuated vaccines tend to induce long-term immune responses. They replicate, often similarly to natural infections, until an immune response shuts down reproduction. Most live vaccines are administered as single-dose schedules. The purpose of repeat doses, such as a second dose of the MMR vaccine, is to induce an initial immune response in persons who failed to respond to the first dose.

The remaining vaccines in the routine schedule for children and adolescents are inactivated vaccines. Inactivated vaccines tend to require multiple doses to induce an adequate immune response and are more likely to need boosters to maintain that immunity than live attenuated vaccines. However, some inactivated vaccines appear to induce long-term immunity, perhaps life-long immunity, after a primary series, including HepB vaccine and inactivated polio vaccine (IPV).

THE VACCINATION SYSTEM IN THE U.S.

Vaccine Development. Basic scientific knowledge about an organism, its pathogenesis, and the immune responses thought to be associated with protection are financed primarily through government sponsorship of academic research, although private industry plays a major role (Fig. 170-1). Private industry usually assumes the lead role for guiding potential vaccine candidates through preclinical testing in humans into human clinical trials. There are three phases of prelicensure clinical trials: **phase I,** involving generally <100 participants to gauge safety and dosing; **phase II,** involving several hundred or more participants to refine safety and dosing; and **phase III** or pivotal trials that can involve thousands or tens of thousands of participants. Phase III trials are the major basis for licensure. Following successful clinical development, the sponsor applies to the FDA for approval. Estimates for the cost of development for each vaccine range to $800 million or more. Following licensure by the FDA, postlicensure monitoring is performed on hundreds of thousands to millions of people to monitor safety and effectiveness.

Vaccine Production. Vaccine production is primarily a responsibility of private industry. Most of the vaccines recommended routinely for children are produced by only one of the vaccine manufacturers. Only Hib, HepB, diphtheria and tetanus toxoids and acellular pertussis (DTaP), and tetanus and diphtheria toxoids and acellular pertussis (Tdap) vaccines for adolescents and adults have multiple manufacturers. IPV as an IPV-only vaccine has only 1 manufacturer, but IPV also is available in a combination DTaP-IPV-HepB from another manufacturer. Influenza vaccine for children <4 yr of age is produced by a single manufacturer. MMR, varicella, rotavirus, HPV, PCV7, MCV4, and Td vaccines also are produced by a single manufacturer.

Vaccine Policy. There are 2 major committees that make vaccine policy for children: the Committee on Infectious Diseases (COID) of the AAP (the Red Book Committee) and the Advisory Committee on Immunization Practices (ACIP) of the Centers for Disease Control and Prevention (CDC). At least annually, the AAP, the ACIP, and the American Academy of Family Physicians (AAFP) issue a **harmonized** childhood and adolescent immunization schedule (www.cdc.gov/nip/acip). The COID consists primarily of academic pediatric infectious disease specialists with liaisons from practicing pediatricians, professional organizations, and government agencies including the FDA, CDC, and National Institutes of Health (NIH). Recommendations of the COID must be approved by the AAP Board of Directors. The ACIP consists of 15 members who are academic infectious disease experts (for both children and adults), family physicians, state and local public health officials, and consumers. The ACIP also has extensive liaison representation from major medical societies, government agencies, managed care, and others. The AAP recommendations are published in the *Red Book* and in issues of *Pediatrics*. The ACIP recommendations, available at www.cdc.gov/nip/acip, are official only after approval by the CDC director. which leads to publication in *Morbidity and Mortality Weekly Report (MMWR)*.

Vaccine Financing. Between 55 and 60% of vaccines routinely administered to children and adolescents <19 yr of age are purchased thorough a contract negotiated by the federal government with licensed vaccine manufacturers. There are three major sources of funds that can purchase vaccines through this contract. The greatest proportion comes from the Vaccines for Children (VFC) program, a federal entitlement program. The VFC program covers children on Medicaid, children without any insurance (uninsured), and American Indians and Alaska Natives. In addition, children who have insurance but whose insurance does not cover immunization (underinsured) can be covered through VFC but only if they go to a federally qualified health center (FQHC) [www.cms.hhs.gov/providers/fghc]. In contrast to other public funding sources that require approval of discretionary funding by legislative bodies, VFC funds are immediately available for new recommendations provided the ACIP votes the vaccine and the recommendation for its use into the VFC, the federal government negotiates a contract, and the Office of Management and Budget (OMB) apportions funds. The VFC program can provide free vaccines to participating private providers. The second major federal funding source is the 317 Discretionary Federal Grant Program to states and selected localities. These funds must be appropriated annually by Congress, but in contrast to VFC, have not had eligibility requirements for use. The third major public source of funds is state appropriations.

Vaccine Safety Monitoring. Monitoring vaccine safety is the responsibility of the FDA, CDC, and vaccine manufacturers. A critical part of that monitoring depends on reports to the Vaccine Adverse Event Reporting System (VAERS). Adverse events following immunization can be reported by calling 1-800-822-7967 or completing a VAERS form that can be obtained from www.vaers.hhs.gov. Individual VAERS case reports may be helpful in generating hypotheses about whether vaccines are causing certain clinical syndromes but in general are not helpful in evaluating the causal role of vaccines in the adverse event. This is because most clinical syndromes that follow vaccination are similar to syndromes that occur in the absence of vaccination. For causality assessment, epidemiologic studies are often necessary comparing the incidence rate of the adverse event after vaccination with the rate in the unvaccinated. A higher rate in the vaccinated would be consistent with causation.

The Vaccine Safety Datalink (VSD) consists of inpatient and outpatient records of some of the largest managed care organizations in the U.S. and facilitates causality evaluation. In addition, a clinical immunization safety assessment network (CISA) has been established to advise primary care physicians on evaluation and management of adverse events (www.partnersforimmunization.org/cisa/pdf). The Institute of Medicine (IOM) has reviewed independently a variety of vaccine safety concerns (available at www.iom.edu/project.asp?id=4705 and Table 170-4). In no instance did the IOM find that evidence favored acceptance of a causal link between the postulated adverse event and vaccines.

The National Vaccine Injury Compensation Program (NVICP), established in 1988, is designed to compensate persons injured by vaccines in the childhood and adolescent immunization schedule. The program is funded through an excise tax of $0.75 per disease prevented per dose. As of 2006, all of the routinely recommended vaccines are covered, with the exception of the meningococcal conjugate vaccine. The NVICP was established to provide a no-fault system. There is a table of related injuries and time frames. All persons alleging injury from covered vaccines must first file with the program. If the injury meets the requirements of the table, compensation is automatic. If not, the claimant has the responsibility to prove causality. If compensation is accepted, the claimant cannot sue the manufacturer or physician administering the vaccine. If the claimant rejects the judgment of the compensation system, he or she can enter the tort system, but this has only occurred rarely. Information on the NVICP is available at 1-800-338-2382 and www.hrsa.gov/osp/vicp. All physicians administering a vaccine covered by the program are required by law to give the approved Vaccine Information Statement (VIS) to the child's parent or guardian at each visit prior to administration of vaccines. Information on the VIS can be obtained from www.cdc.gov/nip/publications/VIS/default.htm.

Vaccine Delivery. To ensure potency, vaccines should be stored at recommended temperatures before and after reconstitution (www.cdc.gov/nip/menus/vaccines.htm#storage). Expiration dates should be noted, and expired vaccine should be discarded. Lyophilized vaccines often have long shelf lives. However, the shelf life of reconstituted vaccines generally is short, ranging from 30 min for the varicella vaccine and some forms of the Hib vaccine to 8 hr for the MMR vaccine and 24 hr for other forms of the Hib vaccine.

All vaccines have a preferred route of administration, which is specified in package inserts and in AAP and ACIP recommendations. Most inactivated vaccines, including DTaP, hepatitis A, HepB, Hib, TIV, PCV7, MCV4, and Tdap, are administered intramuscularly (IM). In contrast, the commonly used live attenuated vaccines, MMR and varicella, should be dispensed subcutaneously (SC). IPV and PPS23 (pneumococcal polysaccharide vaccine) can be given IM or SC. For IM injections, the anterolateral thigh muscle is the preferred site for infants and young

TABLE 170-4. Institute of Medicine Immunization Safety Review Committee Reports and Dates of Release, 2001–2004

Measles-mumps-rubella vaccine and autism—April 2001
Thimerosal-containing vaccines and neurodevelopmental disorders—October 2001
Multiple immunizations and immune dysfunction—February 2002*
Hepatitis B vaccine and demyelinating neurologic disorders—May 2002
SV40 contamination of polio vaccine and cancer—October 2002
Vaccinations and sudden unexpected death in infancy—March 2003
Influenza vaccines and neurologic complications—October 2003
Vaccines and autism—May 2004

*Reviews relationship of vaccines to asthma, diabetes, and heterologous infections.
Data from http://www.iom.edu/project.asp?id=4705
From Cohn AC et al: Immunizations in the US: A Rite of Passage. *Pediatr Clin North Am* 2005;52:669–693.

children. The recommended needle length will vary depending on age and size, ranging from $^5/_8$ inch for newborn infants, 1 inch for infants from 2 to 12 mo of age, and 1 to $1^1/_4$ inches for older children. For adolescents and adults, the deltoid muscle of the arm is the preferred site for IM administration with needle lengths of 1–1½ inches depending on the size of the patient. Most IM injections can be made with 23–25 gauge needles. For SC injections, needle lengths generally range from $^5/_8$ to $^3/_4$ inches with 23–25 gauge needles.

RECOMMENDED IMMUNIZATION SCHEDULE. All children in the U.S. should be vaccinated against 15 diseases (Figs. 170-2 and 170-3) (updated schedule available at www.cdc.gov/nip/acip). Girls 11–12 yr old should also recieve HPV. HepB vaccine is recommended in a 3 dose schedule starting at birth. The birth dose is critical for children born to mothers who are hepatitis B surface antigen positive (HBsAg) or whose immune status is unknown. The DTaP series consists of 5 doses. The 4th dose of DTaP may be administered as early as 12 mo of age, provided 6 mo have elapsed since the 3rd dose and the child is unlikely to return at 15–18 mo of age. A booster, consisting of an adult preparation of Tdap is recommended at 11–12 yr of age. Adolescents 13–18 yr of age who missed the 11–12 year old Td or Tdap booster dose or in whom it has been ≥5 yr since the Td booster dose also should receive a single dose of Tdap if they have completed the diphtheria, tetanus, and pertussis (DTP)/DTaP series. There are 3 licensed preparations of Hib vaccine. The 2 vaccines conjugated to either tetanus toxoid (PRP-T) or CRM197, a nontoxic variant of diphtheria toxin, are given in a 4 dose series, while the Hib vaccine conjugated to meningococcal outer membrane protein (PRP-OMP) is recommended in a 3 dose series. TIV is recommended for all 6–59 mo old children. Children being vaccinated for the 1st time require 2 doses at least 4 wk apart. TIV usually is given in October or November, although there may be benefits even when administered as late as February since influenza seasons typically peak in January or later. IPV should be given at 2, 4, 6–18 mo, and 4–6 yr of age. PCV7 is recommended at 2, 4, 6, and 12–15 mo of age. MMR should be administered at 12–15 mo of age followed by a 2nd dose at 4–6 yr of age. Varicella vaccine should be given at 12–18 mo of age and at 4–6 yrs. The quadrivalent measles, mumps, rubella, and varicella (MMRV) vaccine may be used in place of separate MMR and varicella vaccines both vaccines are indicated. Hepatitis A vaccine, licensed for administration to children ≥12 mo of age, is now recommended for universal administration to all children at 12–23 mo of age and for certain high-risk groups. The 2 doses in the series should be separated by at least 6 mo. A single dose of MCV4 is recommended for all adolescents under one of the following circumstances: (1) at 11–12 yr of age; (2) at high school entry or 15 yr of age, whichever comes first; (3) for unvaccinated persons entering college, particularly for freshman who will live in dormitories; and (4) for high-risk groups. All girls, 11–12 yr old, should receive a 3 dose schedule of HPV. The second dose should be given 2 mo after the first; the third is given 4 mo after the second. Three doses of the rotavirus vaccine are recommended; dose one at 6–12 wk of age; the series is completed by 32 wk of age.

The present schedule can require as many as 37 injections, including 25 injections prior to 2 yr of age. To reduce the injection burdens, several combination vaccines are available: DTaP-IPV-Hep B (Pediarix, GlaxoSmithKline, Research Triangle Park, NC) and Hib (PRP-OMP)-Hep B (Comvax, Merck, West Point, PA) and MMRV (ProQuad, Merck, West Point, PA). Pediarix is indicated for the first 3 doses of the 3 vaccines, reducing the number of injections from 9 to 3. Comvax can be used as a 3 dose series at 2, 4, and 12–15 mo and potentially reduces the number of injections from 6 (or 8 if another Hib preparation is used) to 3. Since a birth dose of single antigen HepB vaccine is recommended when using combinations, which cannot be administered prior to 6 wk of age, a 4 dose series for HepB, counting the birth dose, may be used.

The recommended childhood and adolescent immunization schedule establishes a routine adolescent visit at 11–12 yr of age. MCV4 and a Tdap booster should be administered during this visit and HPV can be started. However, the 11–12 yr old visit is also an opportune time to review all of the immunizations the child has received previously, to provide any doses that were missed, and to review other age-appropriate preventive services. The 11–12 yr visit establishes an important platform for incorporating other vaccines. Information on the current status of new vaccine licensure and recommendations for use can be obtained at http://aapredbook.aappublications.org/news/vaccstatus.shtml and www.fda.gov/cber/vaccine/licvacc.htm.

For children who are at least 1 mo behind in their immunizations, catch-up immunization schedules are available for children 4 mo to 6 yr of age and for children 7–18 yr of age (Fig. 170-4; also available at www.cdc.gov/nip/recs/child-catchup-508.htm).

VACCINES RECOMMENDED IN SPECIAL CIRCUMSTANCES. Several vaccines are recommended for children at increased risk for complications from vaccine-preventable diseases or children who have an increased risk for exposure to these diseases. In addition to annual vaccination of all children 6–59 mo of age with TIV, annual vaccination also is recommended for all children ≥60 mo of age with underlying illnesses that increase their risks from influenza. This includes children with chronic pulmonary disease (including asthma); hemodynamically significant heart disease; immunocompromise, including HIV and AIDS, sickle cell disease, and other hemoglobinopathies; chronic renal dysfunction; chronic metabolic diseases, including diabetes mellitus; and children on long-term salicylate therapy. In addition, TIV is recommended for all household contacts of children with the above conditions and all household contacts of children <5 yr of age to decrease exposure of high-risk children to influenza infection. Healthy contacts 5–49 yr of age may receive LAIV, administered intranasally, as an alternative to TIV.

PCV7 is recommended for all children <5 yr of age who have conditions that place them at high risk for pneumococcal disease. In addition to the conditions listed above for influenza, these conditions include cerebrospinal fluid leaks, functional or anatomic asplenia, and cochlear implants. Children at high risk for pneumococcal disease should also receive PPS23 to provide immunity to serotypes not contained in the 7 valent conjugate vaccine. PPS23 should be administered on or after the 2nd birthday and should follow completion of the PCV7 series by at least 6–8 wk. Two doses of PPS23 are recommended, with an interval of 3–5 yr between doses. Immunization of previously unvaccinated children with high-risk conditions >5 yr of age can be performed with either a dose of PCV7 and/or a dose of PPS23.

MCV4 or MPS4 is recommended for college freshman, children with functional or anatomic asplenia, terminal complement component or properdin deficiencies, and as part of outbreak control programs. MCV4 is preferred but is only licensed for children ≥11 yr of age. MPS4 is an acceptable alternative and is the only vaccine available for children 2–10 yr of age.

A variety of vaccines are available for children who will be **traveling** to areas of the world where certain infectious diseases are common in addition to vaccines in the recommended childhood and adolescent schedule (Table 170-5). Vaccines for travelers include typhoid fever, hepatitis A, HepB, Japanese encephalitis, MCV4 or MPS4, rabies, and yellow fever, depending on the location and circumstances of travel. Measles is endemic in many parts of the world. Children 6–11 mo of age may receive a dose of MMR prior to travel. However, doses of measles vaccine received prior to the first birthday should not be counted in determining compliance with the recommended 2 dose MMR schedule. Additional information on vaccines for international travel can be found at www.cdc.gov/travel.

Recommended immunization schedule for persons aged 0–6 years — United States, 2007

Vaccine ▼ / Age ▶	Birth	1 month	2 months	4 months	6 months	12 months	15 months	18 months	19–23 months	2–3 years	4–6 years
Hepatitis B[1]	HepB	HepB		*See footnote 1*		HepB				HepB Series	
Rotavirus[2]			Rota	Rota	Rota						
Diphtheria, Tetanus, Pertussis[3]			DTaP	DTaP	DTaP		DTaP				DTaP
Haemophilus influenzae type b[4]			Hib	Hib	*Hib*[4]	Hib			Hib		
Pneumococcal[5]			PCV	PCV	PCV	PCV				PCV PPV	
Inactivated Poliovirus			IPV	IPV		IPV					IPV
Influenza[6]								Influenza (Yearly)			
Measles, Mumps, Rubella[7]						MMR					MMR
Varicella[8]						Varicella					Varicella
Hepatitis A[9]							HepA (2 doses)			HepA Series	
Meningococcal[10]										MPSV4	

Range of recommended ages

Catch-up immunization

Certain high-risk groups

This schedule indicates the recommended ages for routine administration of currently licensed childhood vaccines, as of December 1, 2006, for children aged 0–6 years. Additional information is available at http://www.cdc.gov/nip/recs/child-schedule.htm. Any dose not administered at the recommended age should be administered at any subsequent visit, when indicated and feasible. Additional vaccines may be licensed and recommended during the year. Licensed combination vaccines may be used whenever any components of the combination are indicated and other components of the vaccine are not contraindicated and if approved by the Food and Drug Administration for that dose of the series. Providers should consult the respective Advisory Committee on Immunization Practices statement for detailed recommendations. Clinically significant adverse events that follow immunization should be reported to the Vaccine Adverse Event Reporting System (VAERS). Guidance about how to obtain and complete a VAERS form is available at http://www.vaers.hhs.gov or by telephone, 800-822-7967.

1. **Hepatitis B vaccine (HepB).** (Minimum age: birth)
   At birth:
   - Administer monovalent HepB to all newborns before hospital discharge.
   - If mother is hepatitis surface antigen (HBsAg)-positive, administer HepB and 0.5 mL of hepatitis B immune globulin (HBIG) within 12 hours of birth.
   - If mother's HBsAg status is unknown, administer HepB within 12 hours of birth. Determine the HBsAg status as soon as possible and if HBsAg-positive, administer HBIG (no later than age 1 week).
   - If mother is HBsAg-negative, the birth dose can only be delayed with physician's order and mothers' negative HBsAg laboratory report documented in the infant's medical record.

   After the birth dose:
   - The HepB series should be completed with either monovalent HepB or a combination vaccine containing HepB. The second dose should be administered at age 1–2 months. The final dose should be administered at age ≥24 weeks. Infants born to HBsAg-positive mothers should be tested for HBsAg and antibody to HBsAg after completion of ≥3 doses of a licensed HepB series, at age 9–18 months (generally at the next well-child visit).

   4-month dose:
   - It is permissible to administer 4 doses of HepB when combination vaccines are administered after the birth dose. If monovalent HepB is used for doses after the birth dose, a dose at age 4 months is not needed.
2. **Rotavirus vaccine (Rota).** (Minimum age: 6 weeks)
   - Administer the first dose at age 6–12 weeks. Do not start the series later than age 12 weeks.
   - Administer the final dose in the series by age 32 weeks. Do not administer a dose later than age 32 weeks.
   - Data on safety and efficacy outside of these age ranges are insufficient.
3. **Diphtheria and tetanus toxoids and acellular pertussis vaccine (DTaP).** (Minimum age: 6 weeks)
   - The fourth dose of DTaP may be administered as early as age 12 months, provided 6 months have elapsed since the third dose.
   - Administer the final dose in the series at age 4–6 years.
4. **Haemophilus influenzae type b conjugate vaccine (Hib).** (Minimum age: 6 weeks)
   - If PRP-OMP (PedvaxHIB® or ComVax® [Merck]) is administered at ages 2 and 4 months, a dose at age 6 months is not required.
   - TriHiBit® (DTaP/Hib) combination products should not be used for primary immunization but can be used as boosters following any Hib vaccine in children aged ≥12 months.
5. **Pneumococcal vaccine.** (Minimum age: 6 weeks for pneumococcal conjugate vaccine [PCV]; 2 years for pneumococcal polysaccharide vaccine [PPV])
   - Administer PCV at ages 24–59 months in certain high-risk groups. Administer PPV to children aged ≥2 years in certain high-risk groups. See MMWR 2000;49(No. RR-9):1–35.
6. **Influenza vaccine.** (Minimum age: 6 months for trivalent inactivated influenza vaccine [TIV]; 5 years for live, attenuated influenza vaccine [LAIV])
   - All children aged 6–59 months and close contacts of all children aged 0–59 months are recommended to receive influenza vaccine.
   - Influenza vaccine is recommended annually for children aged ≥59 months with certain risk factors, health-care workers, and other persons (including household members) in close contact with persons in groups at high risk. See MMWR 2006;55(No. RR-10):1–41.
   - For healthy persons aged 5–49 years, LAIV may be used as an alternative to TIV.
   - Children receiving TIV should receive 0.25 mL if aged 6–35 months or 0.5 mL if aged ≥3 years.
   - Children aged <9 years who are receiving influenza vaccine for the first time should receive 2 doses (separated by ≥4 weeks for TIV and ≥6 weeks for LAIV).
7. **Measles, mumps, and rubella vaccine (MMR).** (Minimum age: 12 months)
   - Administer the second dose of MMR at age 4–6 years. MMR may be administered before age 4–6 years, provided ≥4 weeks have elapsed since the first dose and both doses are administered at age ≥12 months.
8. **Varicella vaccine.** (Minimum age: 12 months)
   - Administer the second dose of varicella vaccine at age 4–6 years. Varicella vaccine may be administered before age 4–6 years, provided that ≥3 months have elapsed since the first dose and both doses are administered at age ≥12 months. If second dose was administered ≥28 days following the first dose, the second dose does not need to be repeated.
9. **Hepatitis A vaccine (HepA).** (Minimum age: 12 months)
   - HepA is recommended for all children aged 1 year (i.e., aged 12–23 months). The 2 doses in the series should be administered at least 6 months apart.
   - Children not fully vaccinated by age 2 years can be vaccinated at subsequent visits.
   - HepA is recommended for certain other groups of children, including in areas where vaccination programs target older children. See MMWR 2006;55(No. RR-7):1–23.
10. **Meningococcal polysaccharide vaccine (MPSV4).** (Minimum age: 2 years)
    - Administer MPSV4 to children aged 2–10 years with terminal complement deficiencies or anatomic or functional asplenia and certain other high-risk groups. See MMWR 2005;54(No. RR-7):1–21.

Figure 170-2. Childhood Immunization Schedule.

Recommended immunization schedule for persons aged 7–18 years — United States, 2007

Vaccine ▼ / Age ▶	7–10 years	11–12 years	13–14 years	15 years	16–18 years
Tetanus, Diphtheria, Pertussis[1]	*See footnote 1*	Tdap	Tdap		
Human Papillomavirus[2]	*See footnote 2*	HPV (3 doses)	HPV Series		
Meningococcal[3]	MPSV4	MCV4	MCV4	MCV4[3] / MCV4	MCV4
Pneumococcal[4]	PPV				
Influenza[5]	Influenza (Yearly)				
Hepatitis A[6]	HepA Series				
Hepatitis B[7]	HepB Series				
Inactivated Poliovirus[8]	IPV Series				
Measles, Mumps, Rubella[9]	MMR Series				
Varicella[10]	Varicella Series				

Legend: Range of recommended ages; Catch-up immunization; Certain high-risk groups

This schedule indicates the recommended ages for routine administration of currently licensed childhood vaccines, as of December 1, 2006, for children aged 7–18 years. Additional information is available at http://www.cdc.gov/nip/recs/child-schedule.htm. Any dose not administered at the recommended age should be administered at any subsequent visit, when indicated and feasible. Additional vaccines may be licensed and recommended during the year. Licensed combination vaccines may be used whenever any components of the combination are indicated and other components of the vaccine are not contraindicated and if approved by the Food and Drug Administration for that dose of the series. Providers should consult the respective Advisory Committee on Immunization Practices statement for detailed recommendations. Clinically significant adverse events that follow immunization shouldbe reported to the Vaccine Adverse Event Reporting System (VAERS). Guidance about how to obtain and complete a VAERS form is available at http://www.vaers.hhs.gov or by telephone, 800-822-7967.

1. **Tetanus and diphtheria toxoids and acellular pertussis vaccine (Tdap).** (Minimum age: 10 years for BOOSTRIX® and 11 years for ADACEL™)
   - Administer at age 11–12 years for those who have completed the recommended childhood DTP/DTaP vaccination series and have not received a tetanus and diphtheria toxoids vaccine (Td) booster dose.
   - Adolescents aged 13–18 years who missed the 11–12 year Td/Tdap booster dose should also receive a single dose of Tdap if they have completed the recommended childhood DTP/DTaP vaccination series.
2. **Human papillomavirus vaccine (HPV).** (Minimum age: 9 years)
   - Administer the first dose of the HPV vaccine series to females at age 11–12 years.
   - Administer the second dose 2 months after the first dose and the third dose 6 months after the first dose.
   - Administer the HPV vaccine series to females at age 13–18 years if not previously vaccinated.
3. **Meningococcal vaccine.** (Minimum age: 11 years for meningococcal conjugate vaccine [MCV4]; 2 years for meningococcal polysaccharide vaccine [MPSV4])
   - Administer MCV4 at age 11–12 years and to previously unvaccinated adolescents at high school entry (at approximately age 15 years).
   - Administer MCV4 to previously unvaccinated college freshmen living in dormitories; MPSV4 is an acceptable alternative.
   - Vaccination against invasive meningococcal disease is recommended for children and adolescents aged ≥2 years with terminal complement deficiencies or anatomic or functional asplenia and certain other high-risk groups. See MMWR 2005;54(No. RR-7):1–21. Use MPSV4 for children aged 2–10 years and MCV4 or MPSV4 for older children.
4. **Pneumococcal polysaccharide vaccine (PPV).** (Minimum age: 2 years)
   - Administer for certain high-risk groups. See MMWR 1997;46(No. RR-8):1–24, and MMWR 2000;49(No. RR-9):1–35.
5. **Influenza vaccine.** (Minimum age: 6 months for trivalent inactivated influenza vaccine [TIV]; 5 years for live, attenuated influenza vaccine [LAIV])
   - Influenza vaccine is recommended annually for persons with certain risk factors, health-care workers, and other persons (including household members) in close contact with persons in groups at high risk. See MMWR 2006;55 (No. RR-10):1–41.
   - For healthy persons aged 5–49 years, LAIV may be used as an alternative to TIV.
   - Children aged <9 years who are receiving influenza vaccine for the first time should receive 2 doses (separated by ≥4 weeks for TIV and ≥6 weeks for LAIV).
6. **Hepatitis A vaccine (HepA).** (Minimum age: 12 months)
   - The 2 doses in the series should be administered at least 6 months apart.
   - HepA is recommended for certain other groups of children, including in areas where vaccination programs target older children. See MMWR 2006;55 (No. RR-7):1–23.
7. **Hepatitis B vaccine (HepB).** (Minimum age: birth)
   - Administer the 3-dose series to those who were not previously vaccinated.
   - A 2-dose series of Recombivax HB® is licensed for children aged 11–15 years.
8. **Inactivated poliovirus vaccine (IPV).** (Minimum age: 6 weeks)
   - For children who received an all-IPV or all-oral poliovirus (OPV) series, a fourth dose is not necessary if the third dose was administered at age ≥4 years.
   - If both OPV and IPV were administered as part of a series, a total of 4 doses should be administered, regardless of the child's current age.
9. **Measles, mumps, and rubella vaccine (MMR).** (Minimum age: 12 months)
   - If not previously vaccinated, administer 2 doses of MMR during any visit, with ≥4 weeks between the doses.
10. **Varicella vaccine.** (Minimum age: 12 months)
    - Administer 2 doses of varicella vaccine to persons without evidence of immunity.
    - Administer 2 doses of varicella vaccine to persons aged ≤13 years at least 3 months apart. Do not repeat the second dose, if administered ≥28 days after the first dose.
    - Administer 2 doses of varicella vaccine to persons aged ≥13 years at least 4 weeks apart.

Figure 170-3. Childhood and Adolescent Immunization Schedule.

Catch-up immunization schedule for persons aged 4 months–18 years who start late or who are ≥1 month behind — United States, 2007
The table below provides catch-up schedules and minimum intervals between doses for children whose vaccinations have been delayed. A vaccine series does not need to be restarted, regardless of the time that has elapsed between doses. Use the section appropriate for the child's age.

CATCH-UP SCHEDULE FOR PERSONS AGED 4 MONTHS–6 YEARS					
Vaccine	Minimum age for Dose 1	Minimum interval between doses			
		Dose 1 to Dose 2	Dose 2 to Dose 3	Dose 3 to Dose 4	Dose 4 to Dose 5
Hepatitis B[1]	Birth	4 weeks	8 weeks (and 16 weeks after first dose)		
Rotavirus[2]	6 weeks	4 weeks	4 weeks		
Diphtheria, Tetanus, Pertussis[3]	6 weeks	4 weeks	4 weeks	6 months	6 months[3]
Haemophilus influenzae type b[4]	6 weeks	4 weeks if first dose administered at age <12 months 8 weeks (as final dose) if first dose administered at age 12–14 months No further doses needed if first dose administered at age ≥15 months	4 weeks[4] if current age <12 months 8 weeks (as final dose)[4] if current age ≥12 months and second dose administered at age <15 months No further doses needed if previous dose administered at age ≥15 months	8 weeks (as final dose) This dose only necessary for children aged 12 months–5 years who received 3 doses before age 12 months	
Pneumococcal[5]	6 weeks	4 weeks if first dose administered at age <12 months and current age <24 months 8 weeks (as final dose) if first dose administered at age ≥12 months or current age 24–59 months No further doses needed for healthy children if first dose administered at age ≥24 months	4 weeks if current age <12 months 8 weeks (as final dose) if current age ≥12 months No further doses needed for healthy children if previous dose administered at age ≥24 months	8 weeks (as final dose) This dose only necessary for children aged 12 months–5 years who received 3 doses before age 12 months	
Inactivated Poliovirus[6]	6 weeks	4 weeks	4 weeks	4 weeks[6]	
Measles, Mumps, Rubella[7]	12 months	4 weeks			
Varicella[8]	12 months	3 months			
Hepatitis A[9]	12 months	6 months			
CATCH-UP SCHEDULE FOR PERSONS AGED 7–18 YEARS					
Tetanus, Diphtheria/ Tetanus, Diphtheria, Pertussis[10]	7 years[10]	4 weeks	8 weeks if first dose administered at age <12 months 6 months if first dose administered at age ≥12 months	6 months if first dose administered at age <12 months	
Human Papillomavirus[11]	9 years	4 weeks	12 weeks		
Hepatitis A[9]	12 months	6 months			
Hepatitis B[1]	Birth	4 weeks	8 weeks (and 16 weeks after first dose)		
Inactivated Poliovirus[6]	6 weeks	4 weeks	4 weeks	4 weeks[6]	
Measles, Mumps, Rubella[7]	12 months	4 weeks			
Varicella[8]	12 months	4 weeks if first dose administered at age ≥13 years 3 months if first dose administered at age <13 years			

1. **Hepatitis B vaccine (HepB).** (Minimum age: birth)
   - Administer the 3-dose series to those who were not previously vaccinated.
   - A 2-dose series of Recombivax HB® is licensed for children aged 11–15 years.
2. **Rotavirus vaccine (Rota).** (Minimum age: 6 weeks)
   - Do not start the series later than age 12 weeks.
   - Administer the final dose in the series by age 32 weeks. Do not administer a dose later than age 32 weeks.
   - Data on safety and efficacy outside of these age ranges are insufficient.
3. **Diphtheria and tetanus toxoids and acellular pertussis vaccine (DTaP).** (Minimum age: 6 weeks)
   - The fifth dose is not necessary if the fourth dose was administered at age ≥4 years.
   - DTaP is not indicated for persons aged ≥7 years.
4. ***Haemophilus influenzae* type b conjugate vaccine (Hib).** (Minimum age: 6 weeks)
   - Vaccine is not generally recommended for children aged ≥5 years.
   - If current age <12 months and the first 2 doses were PRP-OMP (PedvaxHIB® or ComVax® [Merck]), the third (and final) dose should be administered at age 12–15 months and at least 8 weeks after the second dose.
   - If first dose was administered at age 7–11 months, administer 2 doses separated by 4 weeks plus a booster at age 12–15 months.
5. **Pneumococcal conjugate vaccine (PCV).** (Minimum age: 6 weeks)
   - Vaccine is not generally recommended for children aged ≥5 years.
6. **Inactivated poliovirus vaccine (IPV).** (Minimum age: 6 weeks)
   - For children who received an all-IPV or all-oral poliovirus (OPV) series, a fourth dose is not necessary if third dose was administered at age ≥4 years.
   - If both OPV and IPV were administered as part of a series, a total of 4 doses should be administered, regardless of the child's current age.
7. **Measles, mumps, and rubella vaccine (MMR).** (Minimum age: 12 months)
   - The second dose of MMR is recommended routinely at age 4–6 years but may be administered earlier if desired.
   - If not previously vaccinated, administer 2 doses of MMR during any visit with ≥4 weeks between the doses.
8. **Varicella vaccine.** (Minimum age: 12 months)
   - The second dose of varicella vaccine is recommended routinely at age 4–6 years but may be administered earlier if desired.
   - Do not repeat the second dose in persons aged <13 years if administered ≥28 days after the first dose.
9. **Hepatitis A vaccine (HepA).** (Minimum age: 12 months)
   - HepA is recommended for certain groups of children, including in areas where vaccination programs target older children. See MMWR 2006;55(No. RR-7):1–23.
10. **Tetanus and diphtheria toxoids vaccine (Td) and tetanus and diphtheria toxoids and acellular pertussis vaccine (Tdap).** (Minimum ages: 7 years for Td, 10 years for BOOSTRIX®, and 11 years for ADACEL™)
    - Tdap should be substituted for a single dose of Td in the primary catch-up series or as a booster if age appropriate; use Td for other doses.
    - A 5-year interval from the last Td dose is encouraged when Tdap is used as a booster dose. A booster (fourth) dose is needed if any of the previous doses were administered at age <12 months. Refer to ACIP recommendations for further information. See MMWR 2006;55(No. RR-3).
11. **Human papillomavirus vaccine (HPV).** (Minimum age: 9 years)
    - Administer the HPV vaccine series to females at age 13–18 years if not previously vaccinated.

Figure 170-4. Catch up Immunization Schedule.

TABLE 170-5. Recommended Immunizations for Travelers to Developing Countries*

	LENGTH OF TRAVEL		
Immunizations	**Brief, <2 wk**	**Intermediate, 2 wk to 3 mo**	**Long-term Residential, >3 mo**
Review and complete age-appropriate childhood and adolescent schedule (see text for details)	+	+	+
• DTaP, poliovirus, pneumococcal, and *Haemophilus influenzae* type b vaccines may be given at 4 wk intervals if necessary to complete the recommended schedule before departure			
• Measles: 2 additional doses given if younger than 12 mo of age at first dose			
• Rotavirus			
• Hepatitis A			
• Varicella			
• HPV			
• Hepatitis B[†]			
• Tdap			
• MCV4			
Yellow fever[‡]	+	+	+
Hepatitis A[§]	+	+	+
Typhoid fever[‖]	±	+	+
Meningococcal disease[¶]	±	±	±
Rabies[#]	±	+	+
Japanese encephalitis**	±	±	+

DTaP indicates diphtheria and tetanus toxoids and acellular pertussis; +, recommended; ±, consider.
*See disease-specific chapters in Section 3 for details. For further sources of information, see text.
†If insufficient time to complete 6 mo primary series, accelerated series can be given (see text for details).
‡For regions with endemic infection (see Health Information for International Travel).
§Indicated for travelers to areas with intermediate or high endemic rates of hepatitis A virus infection.
‖Indicated for travelers who will consume food and liquids in areas of poor sanitation.
¶Recommended for regions of Africa with endemic infection and during local epidemics, and required for travel to Saudi Arabia for the Hajj.
#Indicated for people with high risk for animal exposure (especially to dogs) and for travelers to countries with endemic infection.
**For regions with endemic infection (see Health Information for International Travel). For high-risk activities in areas experiencing outbreaks, vaccine is recommended, even for brief travel.
From the American Academy of Pediatrics: In Pickering LK, Baker CJ, Long SS, McMillan JA (editors): *Red Book 2006: Report of the Committee on Infectious Diseases*, 27th ed. Elk Grove Village, IL, American Academy of Pediatrics, 2006, p 99.

Vaccine recommendations for children with **immunocompromise**, either primary (inherited) or secondary (acquired), vary according to the underlying condition, the degree of immune deficit, the risk for exposure to disease, and the vaccine (Table 170-6). Immunization of children with immunocompromise poses the following potential concerns: (1) the incidence or severity of some vaccine-preventable diseases is higher, and therefore certain vaccines are recommended specifically for certain conditions; (2) vaccines may be less effective during the period of altered immunocompetence and may not be deferred or repeated when immune competence is restored; and (3) because of altered immunocompetence, some children and adolescents may be at increased risk for an adverse event following receipt of a live viral vaccine. Live attenuated vaccines generally are contraindicated in immunocompromised persons. The exceptions include MMR, which may be given to a child with HIV infection provided the child is asymptomatic or symptomatic without evidence of severe immunosuppression, and varicella vaccine, which may be given to HIV-infected children if the $CD4^+$ lymphocyte count is at least 15%. Varicella vaccine is available for children with acute lymphoblastic leukemia in remission under special protocol, which requires informed consent and local Institutional Review Board approval. Altered immunocompetence is considered a precaution for rotavirus vaccine because rotavirus disease can be severe in some of these patients, but data on vaccine safety and efficacy are lacking. Inactivated vaccines may be administered to immunocompromised children although, depending on the immune deficit, their effectiveness may not be optimal. Children with complement deficiency disorders can receive all vaccines, including live attenuated vaccines. In contrast, children with phagocytic disorders can receive both inactivated and live attenuated viral vaccines but not live attenuated bacterial vaccines. Corticosteroids can suppress the immune system. Children receiving corticosteroids (≥2 mg/kg/day or ≥20 mg/day of prednisone or equivalent) for 14 or more days should not receive live vaccines until therapy has been discontinued for at least 1 month. Children on the same dose levels but for <2 wk may receive live viral vaccines as soon as therapy is discontinued, although some experts would wait 2 wk post-therapy. Children receiving lower doses of steroids may be vaccinated while on therapy. Children and ado-

TABLE 170-6. Immunization of Children and Adolescents with Primary and Secondary Immune Deficiencies

PRIMARY			
B lymphocyte (humoral)	Severe: X-linked and common variable agammaglobulinemia	OPV,* vaccinia, LAIV,[†] and live-bacteria vaccines;[‡] consider measles and varicella	Effectiveness of any vaccine dependent only on humoral response is doubtful; IGIV interferes with measles and possibly varicella response.
	Less severe: Selective IgA deficiency and selective subclass IgG deficiency	OPV;* other live vaccines seem to be safe, but caution is urged	All vaccines probably effective. Vaccine response may be attenuated.
T lymphocyte (cell-mediated and humoral)	Complete defects	All live vaccines[†,‡]	All vaccines ineffective
	Partial defects		Effectiveness depends on degree of immunosuppression. Inactivated vaccines recommended.
Complement	Deficiency of early components (C1, C4, C2, C3)	None	All routine vaccines probably effective. Pneumococcal and meningococcal vaccines recommended.
	Deficiency of late components (C5–C9), properdin, factor B	None	All routine vaccines probably effective. Meningococcal vaccine recommended.
Phagocytic function	Chronic granulomatous disease Leukocyte adhesion defects Myeloperoxidase deficiency	Live-bacteria vaccines[‡]	All routine vaccines probably effective. Inactivated influenza vaccine recommended to decrease secondary infection.
SECONDARY			
	HIV/AIDS	OPV,* vaccinia, BCG, LAIV[†]; withhold MMR and varicella in severely immunocompromised children	MMR, varicella, and all inactivated vaccines, including influenza, may be effective.[§]
	Malignant neoplasm, transplantation, immunosuppressive or radiation therapy	Live virus and bacteria, depending on immune status[†,‡]	Effectiveness of any vaccine depends on degree of immune suppression.

OPV, oral poliovirus; LAIV, live attenuated influenza vaccine; IGIV, immune globulin intravenous; Ig, immunoglobulin; BCG, bacille Calmette-Guérin; MMR, measles-mumps-rubella.
*OPV vaccine is no longer recommended for routine use in the U.S.
†Live virus vaccines: LAIV, MMR, OPV, varicella, vaccinia (smallpox). Smallpox vaccine is not recommended for children.
‡Live-bacteria vaccines: BCG and Ty21a *Salmonella typhi* vaccine.
§HIV-infected children should receive immune globulin after exposure to measles (see Chapter 243) and may receive varicella vaccine if the $CD4^+$ lymphocyte count is ≥25% of expected for age (see Chapter 250).
From the American Academy of Pediatrics. In Pickering LK, Baker CJ, Long SS, McMillan JA (editors): *Red Book 2006: Report of the Committee on Infectious Diseases*, 27th ed. Elk Grove Village, IL, American Academy of Pediatrics, 2006.

lescents with malignancy, and those who have undergone solid organ or stem cell transplantation and immunosuppressive or radiation therapy, should not receive live virus and live bacterial vaccines depending on their immune status.

Preterm infants generally can be vaccinated at the same chronologic age as full-term infants according to the recommended childhood immunization schedule. An exception is the birth dose of HepB vaccine. Infants weighing ≥2 kg and who are stable may receive a birth dose. However, HepB vaccination should be deferred in infants weighing <2 kg at birth until 30 days of age, if born to an HBsAg-negative mother. All preterm, low birth weight infants born to HBsAg-positive mothers should receive HepB IG and HepB vaccine within 12 hr of birth. However, such infants should receive an additional 3 doses of vaccine starting at 30 days of age.

Some children will present with situations that are not addressed directly in current immunization schedules. There are general rules that physicians can use to guide immunization decisions in some of these instances. In general, vaccines can be given simultaneously on the same day, whether inactivated or live. Different inactivated vaccines can be administered at any interval between doses. However, because of theoretical concerns about viral interference, different live attenuated vaccines (MMR, varicella, LAIV) if not administered on the same day, should be given at least 1 mo apart. An inactivated and a live vaccine can be spaced at any interval from each other.

IG does not interfere with killed vaccines. However, IG can interfere with the immune response to measles vaccine and by inference to varicella vaccine. In general, IG, if needed, should be administered at least 2 wk after measles vaccine. Depending on the dose of IG received, MMR should be deferred for as long as 3–11 mo. IG is not expected to interfere with the immune response to LAIV. Rotavirus vaccine should be deferred for 6 wk following receipt of an antibody-containing product; it should not be deferred before 13 wk of age.

Many agents have been considered for potential use as weapons of bioterrorism. For most of these agents, licensed vaccines are not available in the U.S., although vaccines are being developed for some organisms, including botulinum toxoid, ebola virus, plague, and others. Anthrax vaccine and smallpox (vaccinia) vaccine are available, but they are not recommended for children. Both are indicated in a pre-exposure setting only for selected adults with potential occupational risks of exposure (www.bt.cdc.gov/ provides details on which groups are recommended for vaccination).

PRECAUTIONS AND CONTRAINDICATIONS. Observation of valid precautions and contraindications is critical to assure that vaccines are used in the safest manner possible and to obtain optimal immunogenicity. When a child presents for immunization with a clinical condition considered a precaution, the physician must weigh benefits and risks to that individual child. If benefits are judged to outweigh risks, then the vaccine or vaccines in question may be administered. A contraindication means the vaccine should not be administered under any circumstances. A generic contraindication for all vaccines is anaphylaxis to a prior dose. Anaphylactic hypersensitivity to vaccine constituents is also a contraindication. However, if a vaccine is essential, there are desensitizing protocols for some vaccines. The major constituents of concern are egg proteins for vaccines grown in eggs; gelatin, a stabilizer in many vaccines; and antimicrobial agents. The measles and mumps components of MMR are grown in chick embryo fibroblast tissue culture. However, the amount of egg proteins in MMR is so small as not to require any special procedures prior to administering vaccine to someone with a history of anaphylaxis following egg ingestion. Vaccines usually should be deferred in children with moderate to severe acute illnesses, regardless of the presence of fever, until the child recovers. However, children with mild illnesses may be vaccinated. Studies of undervaccinated children have documented opportunities that were missed because mild illness was used as an invalid contraindication. Complete tables of contraindications and contraindication misperceptions can be found at www.cdc.gov/nip/recs./contraindications.htm.

IMPROVING IMMUNIZATION COVERAGE. Standards for child and adolescent immunization practices have been developed to support achievement of high levels of immunization coverage while providing vaccines in a safe and effective manner, and educating parents about risks and benefits of vaccines (Table 170-7).

Despite the benefits that vaccines have to offer, many children are underimmunized as a result of not receiving recommended vaccines or not receiving them at the recommended ages. Much of the underimmunization problem can be solved through physician actions. Most children have a regular source of health care. However, missed opportunities to provide immunizations at health care visits include failure to provide all recommended vaccines that could be administered at a single visit during that visit, failure to provide immunizations to children outside of well child care when the conditions children may have are not contraindications to immunizations, and referral of children to public health clinics because of inability to pay for vaccines. Simultaneous administration of multiple vaccines generally is safe and effective. Many parents, when the benefits of simultaneous vaccination are explained, would prefer such immunization rather than needing to make an extra visit. Providing all needed vaccines simultaneously should be the standard of practice.

Only valid contraindications and precautions to vaccine administration should be observed. Ideally immunizations should be provided during well child visits, but using other visits to administer vaccines if there are no contraindications, particularly if a child is behind in the schedule, is important. There is no good

TABLE 170-7. Standards for Child and Adolescent Immunization Practices

AVAILABILITY OF VACCINES

1. Vaccination services are readily available.
2. Vaccinations are coordinated with other health care services and provided in a medical home when possible.
3. Barriers to vaccination are identified and minimized.
4. Patient costs are minimized.

ASSESSMENT OF VACCINATION STATUS

5. Health care professionals review the vaccination and health status of patients at every encounter to determine which vaccines are indicated.
6. Health care professionals assess for and follow only medically accepted contraindications.

EFFECTIVE COMMUNICATION ABOUT VACCINE BENEFITS AND RISKS

7. Parents/guardians and patients are educated about the benefits and risks of vaccination in a culturally appropriate manner and in easy-to-understand language.

PROPER STORAGE AND ADMINISTRATION OF VACCINES AND DOCUMENTATION OF VACCINATIONS

8. Health care professionals follow appropriate procedures for vaccine storage and handling.
9. Up-to-date, written vaccination protocols are accessible at all locations where vaccines are administered.
10. Persons who administer vaccines and staff who manage or support vaccine administration are knowledgeable and receive ongoing education.
11. Health care professionals simultaneously administer as many indicated vaccine doses as possible.
12. Vaccination records for patients are accurate, complete, and easily accessible.
13. Health care professionals report adverse events following vaccination promptly and accurately to the Vaccine Adverse Event Reporting System (VAERS) and are aware of a separate program, the National Vaccine Injury Compensation Program (VICP).
14. All personnel who have contact with patients are appropriately vaccinated.

IMPLEMENTATION OF STRATEGIES TO IMPROVE VACCINATION COVERAGE

15. Systems are used to remind parents/guardians, patients, and health care professionals when vaccinations are due and to recall those who are overdue.
16. Office- or clinic-based patient record reviews and vaccination coverage assessments are performed annually.
17. Health care professionals practice community-based approaches.

From the National Vaccine Advisory Committee: Standards for child and adolescent immunization practices. *Pediatrics* 2003;112:958–963.

evidence that providing immunizations outside of well child care ultimately decreases well child visits.

Financial barriers to immunization should be minimized. Participation in the VFC program allows physicians to receive free vaccines for their eligible patients, which helps such patients be immunized in their medical home.

Several interventions have been shown to help physicians increase immunization coverage in their practices. Reminder systems for children prior to an appointment or recall systems for children who fail to keep appointments have been demonstrated repeatedly to improve coverage. Assessment and feedback is also an important intervention. Most physicians overestimate the immunization coverage among patients they serve and, thus, are not motivated to make any changes in their practices to improve performance. Assessing the immunization coverage of patients served by an individual physician and feedback of results can be a major motivator for improvement. Often public health departments can be contacted to provide the assessments and feedback. Alternatively, physicians can perform some self-assessments. Review of approximately 60 consecutive charts of 2 yr old children may provide a reasonable estimate of practice coverage. Another help is to have a staff member review the chart of every patient coming in for a visit and placing immunization needs reminders on the chart for the physician.

Some parents may refuse immunization for their child. Pediatricians should try to open a dialogue with such parents to understand the reasons for refusal and try to work with them to overcome their concerns over time during the course of visits.Discussion should be based on the reason for refusal and the knowledge of the parent. Pediatricians should refer patients to reputable sources for vaccine information (Table 170-8) and discuss risks and benefits of vaccines. Physician concerns about liability should be addressed by appropriate documentation of discussions in the chart. The Committee on Bioethics of the AAP has published guidelines for dealing with parenteral refusal of immunization. Physicians also may wish to consider having parents sign a refusal waiver. A sample of a refusal to vaccinate waiver can be found at www.cispimmunize.org/pro/pdf/refusaltovaccinate_2pageform.pdf.

TABLE 170-8. Vaccine Websites and Resources

HEALTH PROFESSIONAL ASSOCIATIONS
American Academy of Family Physicians (AAFP): **www.familydoctor.org**
American Academy of Pediatrics (AAP): **www.aap.org**
(AAP Childhood Immunization Support Program): **www.cispimmunize.org**
American Medical Association (AMA): **www.ama-assn.org**
American Nurses Association (ANA): **www.nursingworld.org**
Association of State and Territorial Health Officials (ASTHO): **www.astho.org**
Association of Teachers of Preventive Medicine (ATPM): **www.atpm.org/education/education.htm**
National Medical Association (NMA): **www.nmanet.org**
NONPROFIT GROUPS AND UNIVERSITIES
Albert B. Sabin Vaccine Institute: **www.sabin.org**
Allied Vaccine Group (AVG): **www.vaccine.org**
Children's Vaccine Program: **www.childrensvaccine.org**
Every Child By Two (ECBT): **www.ecbt.org**
Global Alliance for Vaccines and Immunization (GAVI): **www.vaccinealliance.org**
Health on the Net Foundation (HON): **www.hon.ch**
National Healthy Mothers, Healthy Babies Coalition (HMHB): **www.hmhb.org**
Immunization Action Coalition (IAC): **www.immunize.org**
Institute of Vaccine Safety (IVS), Johns Hopkins University: **www.vaccinesafety.edu**
Institute of Medicine: **www.iom.edu/IOM/IOMHome.nsf/Pages/immunization+safety+review**
National Alliance for Hispanic Health: **www.hispanichealth.org**
National Network for Immunization Information (NNii): **www.immunizationinfo.org**
Parents of Kids with Infectious Diseases (PKIDS): **www.pkids.org**
The Vaccine Education Center at the Children's Hospital of Philadelphia: **www.vaccine.chop.edu**
The Vaccine Page: **www.vaccines.com**
GOVERNMENT ORGANIZATIONS
Centers for Disease Control and Prevention (CDC)
http://phil.cdc.gov/phil (image library)
www.cdc.gov/travel/vaccinat.htm
National Center for Infectious Diseases (NCID): **www.cdc.gov/ncidod**
National Immunization Program (NIP)
www.cdc.gov/nip
www.cdc.gov/nip/publications
National Vaccine Program Office (NVPO): **www.hhs.gov/nvpo**
National Institute of Allergy and Infectious Diseases (NIAID): **www.niaid.nih.gov/dmid/vaccines**
World Health Organization: **www.who.int/vaccines**

170.1 • International Immunization Practices

Vaccines are used to prevent infectious diseases around the world. However, the types of vaccines in use, the indications and contraindications, and immunization schedules vary substantially. Most developing countries follow a schedule promulgated by the World Health Organization's Expanded Programme on Immunization (EPI) [www.who.int/vaccines-documents/docspdf02/www557.pdf]. According to this schedule, all children should be vaccinated at birth against tuberculosis with bacille Calmette-Guérin (BCG) vaccine. Many children also receive a dose of the live attenuated oral polio vaccine (OPV) at this time. Immunization visits are scheduled for 6, 10, and 14 wk of age when DTP vaccine and OPV are administered. Measles vaccine is given at 9 mo of age. Many developing countries have implemented HepB vaccination. Two schedules may be used depending on whether transmission is primarily perinatally from mother to infant or horizontal from postnatal family or community contacts. To prevent perinatal transmission, doses should be administered at birth and at 6 and 14 wk of age. For prevention of horizontal transmission, doses are recommended at 6, 10, and 14 wk of age. Yellow fever vaccine is recommended for children living in endemic areas at 9 mo of age. Increasing efforts are being made to incorporate Hib and pneumococcal conjugate vaccines into developing country immunization programs. In 1988, the World Health Assembly endorsed the goal of eradicating polio from the world by the end of 2000. While that goal has not been reached, endemic polio transmission has been curtailed to three countries in south Asia—India, Pakistan, and Afghanistan, and one country in Africa. Other countries have had outbreaks from imported cases. The principal strategy has been use of OPV both for routine immunization as well as in mass campaigns, at least twice per year, during which all children <5 yr of age are targeted for immunization, regardless of prior immunization status. The eventual goal, once termination of wild polio virus transmission is achieved, is to stop use of OPV, which can rarely cause vaccine-associated polio and which is capable of mutating and taking on the phenotypic characteristics of the wild viruses.

In Latin America, efforts to eliminate indigenous circulation of measles appear to have been successful. The strategy called for routine immunization at 9 mo of age, a 1-time mass campaign targeting all persons 9 mo through 14 yr of age regardless of prior immunization status, and follow-up campaigns of children born since the prior campaign, generally every 3–5 yr. Latin American countries are attempting to eliminate indigenous rubella with strategies consisting of both routine immunization and mass campaigns.

Immunization schedules in the industrialized world are substantially more variable than in the developing world. Immunization recommendations for Canada are developed by the Canadian National Advisory Committee on Immunization (NACI) but are implemented somewhat differently by each province. The Canadian schedule is similar to the U.S. immunization schedule (www.phac-aspc.gc.ca/naci-ccni/is-si/index.html). Conjugate meningococcal serogroup C vaccine (MCV-C) is recommended in a 3 dose series at 2, 4, and 6 mo of age. A single dose is recommended after 12 mo of age if the child has never been immunized or received <3 doses in infancy. The province of Ontario, Canada, has a recommendation for annual vaccination of all children and adults with TIV.

There is tremendous variation in vaccines used and the immunization schedules recommended in Europe. European immunization schedules can be reviewed at www.who.int/vaccines/globalsummary/immunization/ScheduleSelect.cfm. As an example, the U.K. developed an immunization schedule during the late 1980s that includes visits at 2, 3, and 4 mo of age where a combination DTaP-Hib-IPV is administered along with MCV-C. MMR is recommended in a 2 dose schedule at 13 mo and between 3 yr to 5 yr of age. During the 2nd MMR visit, a booster of DTaP and IPV is provided. A Td/IPV booster is recommended between 13 and 18 yr of age. PCV7 is recommended at 2, 4, 13 mo of age. The U.K. was the first country to use MCV-C vaccine during a massive catch-up campaign for children, adolescents, and young adults. The effectiveness of the vaccine in the 1st year was 88% or greater and herd immunity was induced with reduction in the incidence among unvaccinated children of about ²/₃. MCV-C is administered at 3, 4, and 12 mo. As of October 2006, the U.K. schedule did not include HepB vaccine, varicella vaccine, or influenza vaccine for universal childhood immunization (see www.immunisation.nhs.uk).

The Japanese immunization schedule during January–March 2005 is substantially different from that in the U.S. The Japanese do not use MMR and rely on individual vaccines for measles and rubella. Japanese children also are vaccinated routinely against polio with OPV; against diphtheria, tetanus, and pertussis with DTaP; and against Japanese encephalitis and tuberculosis with BCG (http://idsc.nih.go.jp/vaccine/dschedule/immEN050729rev.gif). The Japanese schedule also does not include any vaccines against encapsulated bacteria.

Some children will come to the U.S. having started or completed international immunization schedules with vaccines produced outside of the U.S. In general, doses administered in other countries should be considered valid if administered at the same ages as recommended in the U.S. For missing doses, age-inappropriate doses, lost immunization records, or other concerns, pediatricians have 2 options: (1) administer or repeat missing or inappropriate doses or (2) perform serologic tests, and if negative, administer vaccines.

American Academy of Pediatrics: In Pickering LK, Baker CJ, Long SS, McMillan JA (editors): *Red Book: 2006 Report of the Committee on Infectious Diseases,* 27th ed. Elk Grove Village, IL, American Academy of Pediatrics, 2006;1–103.

American Academy of Pediatrics Committee on Infectious Diseases: Recommended childhood and adolescent immunization schedule—United States, 2007. *Pediatrics* 2007;119:207–208.

Centers for Disease Control and Prevention: General recommendations on immunization: Recommendations of the Advisory Committee on Immunization Practices. *MMWR* 2007;55:Q1–Q3.

Centers for Disease Control and Prevention: In Atkinson W, Hamborsky J, McIntyre L, Wolfe C (editors): *Epidemiology and Prevention of Vaccine-Preventable Diseases,* 9th ed. Washington, DC, Public Health Foundation, 2006. Also available at www.cdc.gov/nip/publications/default.htm#textbooks.

Centers for Disease Control and Prevention: Recommended adult immunization schedule, United States, October 2006–September 2007. *MMWR* 2006;55:Q1–Q4 available at www.edc.gov/nip/acip.

Centers for Disease Control and Prevention: Update: Guillain-Barré syndrome among recipients of menactra meningococcal conjugate vaccine—United States, June 2005–September 2006. *MMWR* 2006;55:1120–1124.

Centers for Disease Control and Prevention: Vaccine preventable deaths and the global immunization vision and strategy, 2006–2015. *JAMA* 2006;295:2840–2842.

Clark HF, Offit PA, Plotkin SA, Heaton PM: The new pentavalent rotavirus vaccine composed of bovine (strain WC3) human rotavirus reassortments. *Pediatr Infect Dis J* 2006;25:577–582.

Cohn AC, Broder KR, Pickering LK: Immunizations in the US: A rite of passage. *Pediatr Clin North Am* 2005;52:669–693.

Diekema DS, American Academy of Pediatrics Committee on Bioethics: Responding to refusals of immunization of children. *Pediatrics* 2005; 115:1428–1431.

Omer SB, Pan WKY, Halsey NA, et al: Nonmedical exemptions to school immunization requirements: secular trends and association of state policies with pertussis incidence. *JAMA* 2006;296:1757–1763.

O'Brien KL, Levine OS: Effectiveness of pneumococcal conjugate vaccine. *Lancet* 2006;368:1469–1470.

Orenstein WA, Douglas RG, Rodewald LE, Hinman AR: Immunizations in the US: Success, structure and stress. *Health Affairs* 2005;24:559–610.

O'Ryan M, Matson DO: New rotavirus vaccines: renewed optimism. *J Pediatr* 2006;149:448–451.

Plotkin SA, Orenstein WA (editors): *Vaccines,* 5th ed. Philadelphia, Elsevier, 2007.

Varricchio F, Iskander J, Destefano F, et al: Understanding vaccine safety information from the Vaccine Adverse Event Reporting System. *Pediatr Infect Dis J* 2004;23:287–294.

Zimmerman RK: Size of the needle for infant vaccination: longer needles reduce incidence of local reactions. *BMJ* 2006;333:563–564.

Chapter 171 ■ Infection Control and Prophylaxis

Margaret C. Fisher

Infection control is a vital part of pediatric medicine. Such control requires an intact and active public health system, universal immunizations, optimal nutrition, and use of specific methods to prevent transmission of infection from child to child, child to adult, and adult to child. Infection control is the responsibility of every health care provider.

Health care–associated infections are those **acquired** during hospitalization or in other health care settings. An estimated 3–5% of children admitted to hospitals acquire a nosocomial infection; rates are much higher in intensive care units. Infections are also acquired in emergency departments, physicians' offices, and long-term care settings. Medical device–associated infections may also occur in the home. Education of home health care providers as well as of families is essential to prevent or minimize device-associated infections.

Determinants of infection include host factors, prior invasive procedures, use of catheters and other devices, use of antibiotics, and exposure to other patients, visitors, or health care providers with contagious diseases. Host factors that increase the risk for infection include anatomic abnormalities (dermoid sinuses, cleft palate, obstructive uropathy), damage to skin, organ dysfunction, malnutrition, and underlying diseases or co-morbidities. Diseases and therapies that alter immunity are most likely to predispose to infection. Prior procedures may introduce pathogens and damage anatomic host defenses. Intravenous and other catheters bypass host defenses, provide direct access to sterile sites, provide adherence sites for microbes, and may occlude normal ostia such as the eustachian tubes. Antibiotics often alter normal bowel flora and encourage colonization by resistant flora, and they may suppress hematopoiesis. Exposure to adults or children with contagious diseases is a clear risk for nosocomial transmission of disease.

Transmission of infectious agents occurs by various routes, but by far the most common and important route is via the hands. Children are constantly touching things in the environment, touching each other, and placing their hands in their noses, eyes, and mouths. Child-to-child exchange of secretions is common whenever children are together. Bacteria, fungi, viruses, and parasites often travel on hands from one person to another. Medical

TABLE 171-1. Recommendations for Application of Standard Precautions for Care of All Patients in All Health Care Settings

COMPONENT	RECOMMENDATIONS
Hand hygiene	After touching blood, body fluids, secretions, excretions, or contaminated items; immediately after removing gloves; between patient contacts. Alcohol-containing antiseptic hand rubs preferred except when hands visibly are soiled with blood or other proteinaceous materials or if exposure to spores (e.g., *Clostridium difficile, Bacillus anthracis*) is likely to have occurred
Personal protective equipment (PPE)	
Gloves	For touching blood, body fluids, secretions, excretions, or contaminated items; for touching mucous membranes and nonintact skin.
Gown	During procedures and patient-care activities when contact of clothing/exposed skin with blood/body fluids, secretions, and excretions is anticipated.
Mask, eye protection (goggles), face shield	During procedures and patient-care activities likely to generate splashes or sprays of blood, body fluids, or secretions, especially suctioning and endotracheal intubation, to protect health care personnel. For patient protection, use of a mask by the individual inserting an epidural anesthesia needle or performing myelograms when prolonged exposure of the puncture site is likely to occur.
Soiled patient-care equipment	Handle in a manner that prevents transfer of microorganisms to others and to the environment; wear gloves if visibly contaminated; perform hand hygiene.
Environmental control	Develop procedures for routine care, cleaning, and disinfection of environmental surfaces, especially frequently touched surfaces in patient care areas.
Textiles (linens) and laundry	Handle in a manner that prevents transfer of microorganisms to others and the environment.
Injection practices (use of needles and other sharps)	Do not recap, bend, break, or hand manipulate used needles; if recapping is required, use a one-handed scoop technique only; use needle-free safety devices when available; place used sharps in puncture-resistant container. Use a sterile, single-use, disposable needle and syringe for each injection given. Single-dose medication vials are preferred when medications are administered to more than one patient.
Patient resuscitation	Use mouthpiece, resuscitation bag, other ventilation devices to prevent contact with mouth and oral secretions.
Patient placement	Prioritize for single-patient room if patient is at increased risk for transmission, is likely to contaminate the environment, does not maintain appropriate hygiene, or is at increased risk for acquiring infection or developing adverse outcome following infection.
Respiratory hygiene/cough etiquette (source containment of infectious respiratory secretions in symptomatic patients) beginning at the initial point of encounter (e.g., triage and reception areas in emergency departments and physician offices)	Instruct symptomatic people to cover mouth/nose when sneezing/coughing; use tissues and dispose in no-touch receptacle; observe hand hygiene after soiling of hands with respiratory secretions; wear surgical mask if tolerated or maintain spatial separation (>3 feet if possible).

From the American Academy of Pediatrics: In Pickering LK (editor): *Red Book 2006: Report of the Committee on Infectious Diseases*, 27th ed. Elk Grove Village, IL, American Academy of Pediatrics, 2006, p. 155.

equipment, toys, and hospital and office furnishings can be contaminated and thus have a role as fomites for transmission of potential pathogens. Pagers, phones, and computer mice are easily contaminated by health care personnel; these inanimate objects serve as reservoirs for bacteria. Thermometers and other equipment that come into contact with mucous membranes are special risks. Some agents are disseminated by airborne transmission, such as varicella virus, measles virus, and *Mycobacterium tuberculosis*. Food and water can be contaminated and have been involved in hospital outbreaks.

Common causes of health care–associated infections in children are seasonal viruses, staphylococci, and gram-negative bacilli. Fungi and resistant bacteria are frequent causes of infection in immunocompromised children and in those who require intensive care and prolonged hospitalization. Common sites of infection are the respiratory tract, gastrointestinal tract, bloodstream, skin, and urinary tract.

Health care–associated infections cause considerable morbidity and occasional mortality; infections prolong hospital stays and increase health care costs. Surveillance for infection is the 1st step in identifying health care–associated infections and suggesting methods for prevention. Within hospitals, surveillance is the responsibility of the **Infection Control Committee**, a multidisciplinary group that collects and reviews surveillance data, establishes policy, and investigates outbreaks. Surveillance within outpatient settings and during home care is often less well established but no less important. Local, state, and federal health departments play important roles in identifying and controlling outbreaks and in establishing public health policy.

HAND HYGIENE. The most important measure in any infection control program is hand hygiene. Although much attention is directed at the types of soap used, the important component of handwashing is placement of the hands under water and use of friction with or without soap. Studies show that a 15-second scrub removes the majority of transient flora but does not alter the permanent flora. A variety of hand gels and rubs can be used in place of handwashing. **Waterless hand hygiene** products increase compliance and save time; these agents are the preferred agents for routine hand hygiene. These products are effective in killing most microbes; they will not remove dirt or debris. Hands should be cleaned before and after every patient encounter. Studies in developing countries, child-care settings, homes, and schools have determined that handwashing with soap can be taught to families and children and that the rates of infection are decreased when children as well as caregivers regularly clean their hands.

STANDARD PRECAUTIONS. Standard precautions, formerly known as **universal precautions,** are intended to protect health care workers from blood and body fluids and should be used whenever providing care. Infected individuals are often contagious before symptoms of disease develop, and asymptomatic carriers are capable of transmitting the agent. **Standard precautions** involve the use of barriers—gloves, gowns, masks, goggles, and face shields—as needed to prevent transmission of microbes associated with contact with blood or body fluids (Table 171-1).

ISOLATION. Isolation of patients infected with certain pathogens decreases the risk for nosocomial transmission. The type of isolation depends on the infecting agent and the route of transmission. **Contact transmission** is the most frequent mode and involves direct contact or contact with a contaminated intermediate object. **Droplet transmission** is by droplets propelled a short distance through the air and deposited on mucous membranes. **Airborne transmission** occurs by dissemination of droplet nuclei ($\leq 5\ \mu m$) of evaporated droplets or dust particles carrying the infectious agent.

Standard precautions are indicated for all patients and are appropriate in the office as well as the hospital. In addition, for hospitalized patients, transmission-based precautions are indicated for certain diseases (Table 171-2). Contact precautions include gowns and gloves and single room isolation. Droplet precautions include masks for close contact (<3 ft) and single room isolation. For both contact and droplet precautions, a single room is preferred but is not required. Cohorting of children infected with the same pathogen is acceptable. Airborne precautions include masks and single room isolation with negative-pressure ventilation. Transmission-based precautions are continued for as long as a patient is considered to be contagious.

The use of isolation techniques in an outpatient setting has not been studied. Each office must establish policies to ensure that the proper cleaning, disinfection, and sterilization methods are used. Many practices and clinics provide separate waiting areas for sick and well children. Triage of patients is essential to ensure that contagious children or adults are not present in waiting areas. Outbreaks of measles in patients within the waiting area have been reported where airflow allowed the exhaust from the examination room to enter the waiting area. Cleaning the environment is important. Toys and items that are shared between patients should be cleaned between uses; soap and water are sufficient for these items. More complete disinfection or sterilization is required for items that encounter mucous membranes and for all reusable items used for body fluid sampling.

ADDITIONAL MEASURES. Other preventive measures include aseptic technique, catheter care, prudent use of antibiotics, isolation of contagious patients, cleaning of the environment, disinfection and sterilization of medical equipment, reporting of infections, safe handling of needles and other sharp instruments, and establishment of employee health services. Aseptic technique must be used for all invasive procedures; this is especially important during catheter placement and manipulation. Catheter care also includes limiting the duration and number of catheters as much as possible and removing catheters as soon as they become unnecessary. Prudent use of antibiotics is important.

SURGICAL PROPHYLAXIS. Surgical prophylaxis is appropriate when there is a high risk of postoperative infection or when the consequences of infection are catastrophic. The choice of antibiotic depends on the site and type of surgery (Table 171-3). A useful classification of surgical procedures based on this risk recognizes four categories: clean wounds, clean contaminated wounds, contaminated wounds, and dirty and infected wounds. Clinical recommendations are standards of the American College of Surgeons, the Surgical Infection Society, and the American Academy of Pediatrics.

Clean wounds are uninfected operative wounds in which no inflammation is noted and the respiratory, alimentary, and genitourinary tracts and the oropharynx are not entered. In addition, the procedure is elective and is performed as primarily closed or drained with closed drainage. Operative incisional wounds after nonpenetrating trauma are included in this category. For clean wounds, prophylactic antimicrobial therapy is not recommended, except in patients at high risk for infection and in circumstances under which the consequences of infection are potentially life

TABLE 171-2. Selected Diseases and Indications for Transmission-Based Isolation in Addition to Standard Precautions

CLINICAL SYNDROME OR CONDITION	POTENTIAL PATHOGENS	EMPIRICAL PRECAUTIONS
DIARRHEA		
Acute diarrhea with a likely infectious cause in an incontinent or diapered patient	*Salmonella, Shigella, Escherichia coli* 0157:H7, rotavirus, hepatitis A	Contact
Diarrhea in any patient, especially an adult, with a history of recent antibiotic use	*Clostridum difficile*	Contact
MENINGITIS		
	Neisseria meningitidis, Haemophilus influenzae type b	Droplet
	Streptococcus pneumoniae	Standard
RASH OR EXANTHEMS		
Petechial/ecchymotic with fever	*N. meningitidis*	Droplet
Vesicular		
Chickenpox	Varicella-zoster virus	Airborne and contact
Zoster (localized in an immunocompetent patient)	Varicella-zoster virus	Standard
Zoster (disseminated or in an immunocompromised patient)	Varicella-zoster virus	Airborne and contact
Maculopapular with coryza and fever	Measles virus	Airborne
Erythema infectiosum	Parvovirus B19	Standard
Parvovirus B19 in an immunocompromised patient	Parvovirus B19	Droplet
Roseola	Human herpesvirus 6	Standard
Rubella	Rubella virus	Droplet
RESPIRATORY TRACT INFECTIONS		
Paroxysmal or severe persistent cough during periods of pertussis activity	*Bordetella pertussis*	Droplet
Bronchiolitis and croup, other lower respiratory tract infections in infants and young children	Respiratory syncytial or parainfluenza virus	Contact
Influenza	Influenza virus	Droplet
Atypical pneumonia	*Mycoplasma pneumoniae*	Droplet
Afebrile pneumonia in young infants	*Chlamydia trachomatis*	Standard
Diphtheria (pharyngeal)	*Corynebacterium diphtheriae*	Droplet
Pneumonic plague	*Yersinia pestis*	Droplet
Pneumococcal pneumonia	*S. pneumoniae*	Standard
Group A streptococcal pharyngitis, pneumonia, or scarlet fever in infants and young children	Group A streptococcus	Droplet
SKIN DISEASES		
Skin infections that are highly contagious or that may occur on dry skin (cutaneous diphtheria; herpes simplex virus, neonatal or mucocutaneous; impetigo; major or draining abscesses; cellulitis; decubiti; staphylococcal furunculosis; zoster disseminated or in an immunocompromised host)		Contact
URINARY TRACT INFECTIONS		Standard
OTHER INFECTIONS		
Infection or colonization with multidrug-resistant organisms	Resistant bacteria	Contact
Invasive *N. meningitidis* disease (meningitis, pneumonia, and sepsis)	*N. meningitidis*	Droplet
Invasive *H. influenzae* type b disease (meningitis, pneumonia, epiglottitis, and sepsis)	*H. influenzae* type b	Droplet
Viral infections spread by droplet transmission (adenovirus, influenza, mumps, parvovirus B19 in an immunocompromised patient, rubella)		Droplet

Adapted from Garner JS: The Hospital Infection Control Practices Advisory Committee: Guidelines for isolation precautions in hospitals. *Infect Control Hosp Epidemiol* 1996;17:53–80.

TABLE 171-3. Common Surgical Procedures for Which Perioperative Prophylactic Antibiotics Are Recommended

SURGICAL PROCEDURE	LIKELY PATHOGENS	SUGGESTED DRUG
CLEAN WOUNDS		
Cardiac surgery (e.g., open heart surgery)	Skin flora, enteric gram-negative bacilli	Cefazolin or vancomycin
Vascular surgery		
Neurosurgery		
Orthopedic surgery (e.g., joint replacement)		
CLEAN CONTAMINATED WOUNDS		
Head and neck surgery entering the oral cavity or pharynx	Skin flora, oral anaerobes, oral streptococci	Cefazolin or clindamycin
Gastrointestinal and genitourinary surgery	Enteric gram-negative bacilli, anaerobes, gram-positive cocci	Cefazolin; if colon involved, consider oral decontamination with neomycin and erythromycin
CONTAMINATED WOUNDS		
Traumatic wounds (e.g., compound fracture)	Skin flora	Cefazolin
DIRTY WOUNDS		
Appendectomy	Enteric gram-negative bacilli, anaerobes, gram-positive cocci	Cefoxitin, or clindamycin plus gentamicin
Colorectal surgery		

threatening (e.g., implantation of a prosthetic foreign body such as a prosthetic heart valve; open heart surgery for repair of structural defects; surgery in patients who are immunocompromised as a result of an inherited disease or are receiving corticosteroids or chemotherapy for malignancy; and newborn infants). Systemic antimicrobial therapy has been recommended empirically for a clean procedure in the patient with infection at another site.

Clean contaminated wounds are operative wounds in which the respiratory, alimentary, or genitourinary tract is entered under controlled conditions and which do not have unusual contamination preoperatively. These wounds occur in operations that involve the biliary tract, appendix, vagina, and oropharynx and in which no evidence of infection or major break in technique is encountered, as well as in urgent or emergency surgery in an otherwise clean procedure. In clean but potentially contaminated procedures, the risk for contamination is variable. Recommendations for pediatric patients derived from data on adults suggest that prophylaxis be provided for procedures in patients with obstructive jaundice, certain alimentary tract procedures, and urinary tract surgery or instrumentation in the presence of bacteruria or obstructive uropathy.

Contaminated wounds include open, fresh, and accidental wounds; major breaks in otherwise sterile operative technique; gross spillage from the gastrointestinal tract; penetrating trauma occurring less than 4 hr earlier; and incisions in which acute nonpurulent inflammation is encountered.

Dirty and infected wounds include penetrating traumatic wounds longer than 4 hr earlier, those with retained devitalized tissue, and those in which clinical infection is apparent or in which the viscera have been perforated. In contaminated and dirty or infected wound procedures, antimicrobial therapy is indicated and may need to be continued for 5–10 days.

In the truest sense, antimicrobial prophylaxis refers to the use of antibiotics before attachment of contaminating bacteria to the host tissues, as in the clean and potentially contaminated categories. Antibiotics given after the microbial attachment constitute therapy, as in the case of contaminated and dirty wounds.

When used, prophylactic antibiotics should be administered, preferably intravenously, approximately 30 min before the skin incision is made, with the intent of having peak concentrations of the drug at this time. Adequate plasma and tissue concentration of the drugs should be maintained until the incision is closed. Repeat doses are necessary only if the surgery lasts longer than 6 hr. Postoperative therapy is usually not necessary; in cases of contaminated surgery, antibiotics are continued as therapy for infection at the site. Drugs administered postoperatively for prophylaxis do not reduce the infection rate. For patients undergoing colonic procedures, additional oral antibiotics may be used and should also be given on the day before surgery.

The selection of antibiotic regimen for prophylaxis is based on the procedure, the expected contaminating organisms, and safety of the drugs. Because of the vast array of antibiotics available now, more than 1 regimen may be acceptable (see Table 171-2). Knowledge of the susceptibilities of the prevalent bacterial causes of nosocomial infections in each hospital is especially important in choosing drugs.

EMPLOYEE HEALTH. Employee health is important because employees are at risk for acquiring infection from patients and infected employees pose a risk to patients. This risk is minimized by use of standard precautions and hand hygiene before and after all patient contacts. Within hospitals, personnel health services or departments of occupational safety and health manage employee health issues. New employees should be screened for the presence of infectious diseases. Their immunization history should be noted and necessary immunizations offered.

All health care workers (medical or nonmedical, paid or volunteer, full time or part time, student or nonstudent, with or without patient care responsibilities) who work in facilities that provide health care to patients (inpatient or outpatient, public or private) should be immune to measles, rubella, and varicella. All workers who might be exposed to blood or body fluids should be immunized against hepatitis B. Annual influenza immunizations are recommended for all health care workers who have contact with patients at risk for influenza or its complications. This program lessens staff illness and absenteeism during the influenza season and reduces health care–associated infections. Immunizations should be encouraged and whenever possible should be provided free of charge. All health care workers who have duties that involve face-to-face contact with patients with suspected or confirmed tuberculosis (including transport staff) should be included in a tuberculosis screening program. Each office and hospital must comply with the rules developed by the Occupational Safety and Health Administration. Furthermore, each office and hospital should have written policies about exclusion of infected staff. Regular educational sessions should be performed to ensure that the staff is aware of infection control methods and that they adhere to infection control policies.

Abrutyn E, Goldman DA, Scheckler WE (editors): *Saunders Infection Control Reference Service: The Experts' Guide to the Guidelines,* 2nd ed. Philadelphia, WB Saunders, 2001.

Bhutta A, Gilliam C, Honeycutt M, et al: Reduction of bloodstream infections associated with catheters in paediatric intensive care unit: stepwise approach. *BMJ* 2007;334:362–365.

Burke JP: Infection control—A problem for patient safety. *N Engl J Med* 2003;348:651–656.

Centers for Disease Control and Prevention: Recommendations of the Advisory Committee on Immunization Practices (ACIP) and the Hospital Infection Control Practices Advisory Committee (HICPAC): Immunization of health-care workers. *MMWR* 1997;46(RR-18):1–42.

Centers for Disease Control and Prevention: Guideline for hand hygiene in health-care settings: Recommendations of the Healthcare Infection Control Practices Advisory Committee and the HICPAC/SHEA/APIC/ISDA Hand Hygiene Task Force. *MMWR* 2002;51(RR-16):1–56.

Centers for Disease Control and Prevention: Guidelines for preventing the transmission of *Mycobacterium tuberculosis* in health-care settings, 2005. *MMWR* 2005;54(RR-17):1–140.

Committee on Infectious Diseases, and Committee on Practice and Ambulatory Medicine, American Academy of Pediatrics: Infection control in physicians' offices. *Pediatrics* 2000;105:1361–1369.

Hota B: Contamination, disinfection, and cross-colonization: Are hospital surfaces reservoirs for nosocomial infection? *Clin Infect Dis* 2004;39: 1182–1189.

Pronovost P, Needham D, Berenholtz S, et al: An intervention to decrease catheter-related bloodstream infections in the ICU. *N Engl J Med* 2006; 355:2725–2732.

Rutala WA, Weber DJ: Disinfection and sterilization in health care facilities: What clinicians need to know. *Clin Infect Dis* 2004;39:702–709.

Chapter 172 ■ Child Care and Communicable Diseases

Linda A. Waggoner-Fountain

Approximately 15.6 million preschoolers are enrolled in some type of out-of-home care on a routine basis such as nursery school, preschool, and full-day programs based either in centers or in another person's home. Regardless of the age at entry, children entering day care are more prone to infections. Exposure to larger groups of children increases a child's probability of getting sick. Child-care facilities can be classified on the basis of size of enrollment, ages of attendees, health status of the children enrolled, and type of setting. As defined in the United States, **child-care facilities** consist of child-care centers, small and large family child-care homes, and facilities for ill children or for children with special needs. Centers are licensed and regulated by state governments and care for a larger number of children than are cared for in family homes. In contrast, **family child-care homes** are designated as small (1–6 children) or large (7–12 children), may be full day or part day, and designed for either daily or sporadic attendance. Family child-care homes generally are not licensed or registered, depending on state requirements.

Although the majority of children who attend child-care facilities are cared for in child-care home settings, most studies of infectious diseases among children in out-of-home child care have been conducted among infants (birth to 12 mo of age) and toddlers (13-36 mo of age) who are enrolled in a child-care center. Almost any organism has the potential to be spread and to cause disease in a child-care setting. Epidemiologic studies have established that children in child-care facilities are 2–18 times more likely to acquire a variety of infectious diseases than are children not enrolled in child care (Table 172-1). Children in child-care facilities are more likely both to receive more courses of antimicrobial agents for longer periods and to acquire antibiotic-resistant organisms. Transmission of infectious agents in group care depends on the age and immune status of the children, season, hygienic practices, crowding, environmental characteristics of the facilities, and characteristics of the pathogen, including its infectivity, survivability in the environment, and virulence. Rates of infection, duration of illness, and risk for hospitalization tend to decrease among children in child-care facilities after the 1st 6 mo of attendance and decline to levels observed among home-bound children after 3 yr of age. In general, children starting out-of-home care at 2 yr of age handle respiratory tract infections and their complications better than children starting at 6 mo of age. Adult caregivers are also at increased risk for acquiring and transmitting infectious diseases, particularly in the 1st year of contact with children in these settings.

TABLE 172-1. Infectious Diseases in the Child-Care Setting

DISEASE	INCREASED INCIDENCE WITH CHILD CARE
RESPIRATORY TRACT INFECTIONS	
Otitis media	Yes
Sinusitis	Probably
Pharyngitis	Probably
Pneumonia	Yes
GASTROINTESTINAL TRACT INFECTIONS	
Diarrhea (rotavirus, calicivirus, astrovirus, enteric adenovirus, *Giardia lamblia, Cryptosporidium, Shigella, Escherichia coli* 0157:H7, and *Clostridium difficile*)	Yes
Hepatitis A	Yes
SKIN DISEASES	
Impetigo	Probably
Scabies	Probably
Pediculosis	Probably
Tinea (ringworm)	Probably
INVASIVE BACTERIA INFECTIONS	
Haemophilus influenzae type b	No*
Neisseria meningitidis	Probably
Streptococcus pneumoniae	Yes
ASEPTIC MENINGITIS	
Enteroviruses	Probably
HERPESVIRUS INFECTIONS	
Cytomegalovirus	Yes
Varicella-zoster virus	Yes
Herpes simplex virus	Probably
BLOOD-BORNE INFECTIONS	
Hepatitis B	Few case reports
HIV	No cases reported
Hepatitis C	No cases reported
VACCINE-PREVENTABLE DISEASES	
Measles, mumps, rubella, diphtheria, pertussis, tetanus	Not established
Polio	No
H. influenzae type b	No*
Varicella	Yes

*Not in the postvaccine era; yes in the prevaccine era.

EPIDEMIOLOGY. Infectious illnesses among children in child care and their contacts occur in several different patterns. With many viral infections, children often are infectious 2–3 days before they exhibit symptoms of illness. Respiratory tract infections and diarrhea are the most common diseases associated with child care. These infections occur in children, child-care staff, and household contacts and may spread to the community. Both respiratory tract pathogens and enteric pathogens can infect both children and adults in these settings but may have varying degrees of impact, depending on the individual's underlying health, previous exposures, and age. Infections caused by hepatitis A virus may not be clinically apparent in young children who attend child care but may cause major clinical disease among older children and adult contacts, including child-care staff and household contacts. Other diseases, such as otitis media, varicella, and invasive *Haemophilus influenzae* type b disease usually affect children rather than adults. Some common infections, such as cytomegalovirus (CMV) and parvovirus B19, may have serious consequences for the fetuses of pregnant women or for immunocompromised persons. Hepatitis B virus (HBV) transmission has been reported rarely in a child-care setting. Hepatitis C virus (HCV), hepatitis D virus (HDV), and HIV transmission has never been reported in a child-care setting. Both infections and infestations of the skin may be acquired through contact with contaminated linens or through close personal contact.

RESPIRATORY TRACT INFECTIONS. Respiratory tract infections account for the majority of child care–related illnesses. Children <2 yr of age who attend child-care centers have more upper and lower respiratory tract infections than do age-matched children not in child care. The organisms responsible for these illnesses are similar to those that circulate in the community and include respiratory syncytial virus, parainfluenza viruses, influenza viruses, adenoviruses, rhinoviruses, coronaviruses, parvovirus B19, and *Streptococcus pneumoniae.* The risk for developing otitis media is 2–3 times greater among children who attend child-care centers than among children cared for at home. Most prescriptions for antibiotics for children <3 yr of age in child care are to treat otitis media. These children also are at increased risk for recurrent otitis media, which further increases use of antimicrobial agents in this population. Pharyngeal carriage of group A streptococcus occurs earlier among children in child care, although outbreaks of clinical infections with this organism are uncommon. Airborne droplets from the respiratory tract can spread via direct contact with another individual's mucous membranes or by touching surfaces contaminated with secretions. This intimate contact is a routine part of the play and care of young children, regardless of setting. The most common surfaces from which airborne droplets can be spread are the hands; consequently, the most efficient form of infection control in the child-care setting is good hand washing.

GASTROINTESTINAL TRACT INFECTIONS. Acute infectious diarrhea is 2 to 3 times more common among children in child care than among children cared for in their homes. Outbreaks of diarrhea, which occur frequently in child-care centers, usually are caused by enteric viruses such as rotaviruses, enteric adenoviruses, astroviruses, and caliciviruses or by enteric parasites such as *Giardia lamblia* or *Cryptosporidium.* The most common enteropathogens, such as rotavirus and *G. lamblia,* are characterized by low infective doses and high rates of asymptomatic excretion among children in child care. Bacterial enteropathogens such as *Shigella* and *Escherichia coli* O157:H7, and, less commonly, *Campylobacter, Clostridium difficile,* and *Bacillus cereus,* also have caused outbreaks of diarrhea in child-care settings. *Salmonella* rarely is associated with outbreaks of diarrhea in child-care settings, since person-to-person spread of this organism is uncommon. Outbreaks of hepatitis A in children enrolled in child-care facilities have resulted in community-wide outbreaks. Hepatitis A usually is mild or asymptomatic in young children and often is identified only after symptomatic illness becomes apparent among either older children or adult contacts of children in child care. Enteropathogens and hepatitis A virus are transmitted in child-care facilities by the fecal-oral route and only rarely by contaminated food or water. Children in diapers constitute a high risk for the spread of gastrointestinal infections through the fecal-oral route. Enteric illness and hepatitis A are more common in centers that care for children who are not toilet trained and where proper hygienic practices are not followed.

SKIN DISEASES. The most commonly recognized skin infections or infestations in children in child care are impetigo caused by *Staphylococcus aureus* or group A streptococcus, pediculosis, scabies, tinea capitis, and tinea corporis. Many of these diseases are spread by contact with infected linens, clothing, hairbrushes, and hats, and through direct personal contact; they more often affect children >2 yr of age. The magnitude of these infections and infestations in children in child care is not known. Parvovirus B19, which causes fifth disease (erythema infectiosum), is spread through the respiratory route, and outbreaks have occurred in child-care centers. The rash of fifth disease is a systemic manifestation of parvovirus B19 infection; the child is no longer contagious once the rash is present (see Chapter 248). As with CMV, the greatest health hazard is for pregnant women and immunocompromised hosts owing to their respective risks for fetal loss and aplastic crisis.

INVASIVE ORGANISMS. Routine immunization against *H. influenzae* type b has greatly reduced the risk for primary invasive infection. Prior to universal immunization, primary *H. influenzae* type b invasive disease was more common among children in child care, although evidence for increased risk for secondary cases from *H. influenzae* type b in a child-care setting remains less convincing. There is an indication that the risk for primary disease caused by *Neisseria meningitidis* is higher among children in child care than among children cared for at home. Child-care attendance is associated with nasopharyngeal carriage of penicillin-resistant *Streptococcus pneumoniae* and invasive pneumococcal disease, especially among children with a history of recurrent otitis media and use of antibiotics. Secondary spread of *S. pneumoniae* and *N. meningitidis* has been reported, indicating the potential for outbreaks to occur in this setting. Routine use of pneumococcal conjugate vaccine has decreased the incidence of invasive disease and reduced carriage of serotypes of *S. pneumoniae* contained in the vaccine both in the child and in younger siblings. With the recent licensure of a conjugate meningococcal vaccine for routine use in healthy adolescents, the use of conjugate meningococcal vaccine in children <2 yr of age is anticipated in the future. Outbreaks of aseptic meningitis from echovirus 30 have been reported among children in child-care centers as well as among their parents and their teachers.

HERPESVIRUSES. Studies of CMV infection in child-care centers have shown that as many as 70% of diapered children continuously shed CMV in urine and saliva after they become infected. CMV-infected children often transmit the virus to other children with whom they have contact, as well as to their care providers and their mothers at a rate of 8–20% per year. Transmission occurs as a result of contact with either saliva or urine. The overwhelming majority of both primary infection with and reactivation of CMV in otherwise healthy children results in asymptomatic shedding of CMV virus; nonetheless, this can pose a health risk for previously uninfected pregnant child-care providers or immunocompromised persons (see Chapter 252). Varicella frequently has been transmitted in child-care centers, but routine use of varicella vaccine has reduced this risk. Vaccinated children who become infected with varicella often have mild, atypical symptoms and signs of disease that may result in delayed recognition and spread of infection to susceptible contacts. The role of child-care facilities in the spread of herpes simplex virus, especially during episodes of gingivostomatitis, requires further clarification.

BLOOD-BORNE PATHOGENS. Because it is impossible to identify every child who might have a blood-borne infection such as HBV, HCV, HDV, or HIV, it is critical that standard universal precautions be observed routinely to reduce the risk for transmitting these viruses. Transmission of hepatitis B among children in child care has been documented in a few rare instances, but the risk for transmission, which already was low, has declined with implementation of universal immunization of infants with HBV vaccine. Transmission of HCV and HDV in child-care settings has not been reported.

Issues about HIV in child care include the potential risk for HIV transmission within the child-care setting and also concerns of opportunistic infections of HIV-infected children. No cases of HIV transmission in out-of-home child care have been reported. Children with HIV infection enrolled in child-care facilities should be monitored for exposure to infectious diseases, and their health and immune status should be evaluated frequently.

Some infections are spread through contact of contaminated blood with either a mucous membrane or an open wound. While theoretically possible, infection is unlikely to spread via toddler biting in a group setting. Most of these bites do not break the skin, and if a bite does break the skin, the mouth of the biter does not stay on the victim long enough for blood to transfer from the victim to the biter.

ANTIBIOTIC USE AND BACTERIAL RESISTANCE. Antibiotic resistance has become an alarming problem in child-care facilities because the frequency of infection by organisms resistant to frequently used antimicrobial agents has increased dramatically. The estimated annual rate of antibiotic use among children in child care is 2–4 times higher than among age-matched children cared for at home. In addition, the mean duration of antibiotic treatment is 4 times longer among children in child care. This frequency of antibiotic use combined with the propensity for person-to-person transmission of pathogens in a crowded environment has resulted in an increased prevalence of antibiotic-resistant bacteria in the respiratory and intestinal tracts, including *S. pneumoniae, H. influenzae, Moraxella catarrhalis, E. coli* O157:H7, and *Shigella* species.

PREVENTION. Written policies designed to prevent or to control the spread of infectious agents in a child-care center should be available and should be reviewed regularly. It is suggested that all programs utilize a health consultant to help with both development and implementation of infection control policies. Standards for environmental and personal hygiene should include maintenance of current immunization records for both children and staff, appropriate policies for exclusion of ill children and caretakers, targeting of potentially contaminated areas for frequent cleaning, adherence to appropriate procedures for changing diapers, appropriate handling of food, management of pets, and surveillance for and reporting of communicable diseases. Staff whose primary function is the preparation of food should not change diapers. Strategies for improving adherence to these standards should be implemented. Appropriate and thorough hand hygiene is the most important factor for reducing infectious diseases in the child-care setting. Children at risk for introducing an infectious disease should not attend child care until they are no longer contagious (Table 172-2).

In the United States, there are 13 diseases and organisms for which all children should be immunized unless there are contraindications: diphtheria, pertussis, tetanus, measles, mumps, rubella, polio, hepatitis A and B, varicella, *H. influenzae* type b, *S. pneumoniae,* and influenza for children 6–23 mo of age. The Food and Drug Administration has also approved the rotavirus vaccine for children. Rates of immunization among children in licensed child-care facilities are high, in part because of laws in almost all states that require age-appropriate immunizations of children who attend licensed child-care programs. Routine vaccination has had a significant beneficial effect on the health of children in child-care settings. Vaccines against *H. influenzae* type b, HBV, varicella, *S. pneumoniae,* and hepatitis A are of particular benefit to children in child-care centers. Influenza vaccination of younger infants reduces influenza infection and secondary sequelae in both children and the adults that care for them in both their home and in child-care settings. Child-care providers should receive all immunizations that are recommended routinely for adults and have a pre-employment health evaluation, including a 1 or 2 step tuberculin skin test as indicated. Local public health authorities should be notified of cases of reportable communicable disease that occur in children or providers in child-care settings.

TABLE 172-2. Exclusion Criteria from Child-Care Setting

SPECIFIC DISEASES
Diarrhea with blood, mucus, or due to *Escherichia coli* 0157:H7, *Shigella*, *Salmonella* (return depends on pathogen)
Purulent conjunctivitis (may return when cleared by MD)
Tuberculosis (may return when cleared by MD)
Impetigo (may return 24 hr after treatment)
Streptococcal pharyngitis (may return 24 hr after treatment)
Head lice (may return after 1st treatment complete)
Scabies (may return after treatment complete)
Varicella (may return after all lesions dry and crusted)
Rubella (may return 6 days after rash)
Pertussis (may return 5 days after treatment)
Mumps (may return 9 days after parotid swelling)
Measles (may return 4 days after rash)
Hepatitis A (may return 1 wk after jaundice)
NONDIAGNOSTIC MANIFESTATIONS
Unable to participate in activities
Staff unable to care for child
Fever with behavioral or mental status changes
Respiratory distress
Vomiting ≥2 times in 24 hr
Mouth sores and drooling
Rash with fever

STANDARDS. Every state has specific standards for licensing and reviewing child-care centers and family child-care homes. The American Academy of Pediatrics, the American Public Health Association, and the National Resource Center jointly publish comprehensive health and safety performance standards that can be used by pediatricians and other health care professionals to guide decisions about management of infectious diseases and other health-related matters in child-care facilities (available in print form and at nrc.uchsc.edu/CFOC/index.html). Specific standards set by all states also are available at this website as well.

Alder SP, Finney JW, Manganello AM, et al: Prevention of child-to-mother transmission of cytomegalovirus among pregnant women. *J Pediatr* 2004;145:485–491.

American Academy of Pediatrics: In Aronson SS, Shope TR (editors): *Managing Infectious Diseases in Child Care and Schools.* Elk Grove, IL, American Academy of Pediatrics, 2005.

American Academy of Pediatrics and the American Public Health Association: *Caring for Our Children: National Health and Safety Performance Standards: Guidelines for Out-of-Home Child Care,* 2nd ed. Elk Grove, IL, American Academy of Pediatrics, 2002.

Bradley RH: Child care and common communicable illnesses in children aged 37 to 54 months. *Arch Pediatr Adolesc Med* 2003;157:196–200.

Churchill RB, Pickering LK: Infection control challenges in child care centers. *Infect Dis Clin North Am* 1997;11:347–385.

Dagan, R, Sikuler-Cohen M, Zamir O, et al: Effect of a conjugate pneumococcal vaccine on the occurrence of respiratory infections and antibiotic use in day-care center attendees. *Pediatr Infect Dis J* 2001;20:951–958.

Givo-Lavi N, Fraser D, Dagan R: Vaccination of day-care center attendees reduces carriage of *Streptococcus pneumoniae* among their younger siblings. *Pediatr Infect Dis J* 2003;22:524–532.

Hurwitz ES, Haber M, Chang A, et al: Effectiveness of influenza vaccination of day care children in reducing influenza-related morbidity among household contacts. *JAMA* 2000;284:1677–1682.

National Institute of Child Health and Human Development Early Childcare Research Network: Childcare and common communicable illnesses. Results from the National Institute of Child Health and Human Development Study of Early Child Care. *Arch Pediatr Adolesc Med* 2001;155:481–488.

Pass RF: Day care centers and the spread of cytomegalovirus and parvovirus B19. *Pediatr Ann* 1991;20:419–426.

Richardson M, Elliman D, Maguire H, et al: Evidence base of incubation periods, periods of infectiousness and exclusion policies for the control of communicable disease in schools and preschools. *Pediatr Infect Dis J* 2001;20:380–391.

Roberts L, Smith W, Jorm L, et al: Effect of infection control measures on the frequency of upper respiratory infection in childcare: A randomized, controlled trial. *Pediatrics* 2000;105:738–742.

Rossi GA, Medici MC, Arcangeletti MC, et al: Risk factors for severe RSV-induced lower respiratory tract infection over four consecutive opidemics. *Eur J Pediatr* 2007; epub ahead of print. PMID: 17308898.

Thrane N, Olesen C, Mortensen JT, et al: Influence of day care attendance on the use of systemic antibiotics in 0- to 2-year-old children. *Pediatrics* 2001;107:E76.

Chapter 173 ■ Health Advice for Children Traveling Internationally

Chandy C. John and Robert A. Salata

The health risks and pretravel requirements of children traveling internationally, particularly those <2 yr of age, differ from those of adults. In the U.S., recommendations and vaccine requirements for travel to different countries are provided by the Centers for Disease Control and Prevention (CDC) and are available online at www.cdc.gov/travel/.

GENERAL TRAVEL PREPARATION

Parents of traveling children should seek medical consultation at least 4–6 wk before departure to obtain a realistic assessment of health risks, a schedule of vaccinations and list of medications, and instructions on dealing with disease during travel.

HEALTH INSURANCE. Parents should be encouraged to determine whether their health care plan covers health care internationally. If it does, parents should ask about the need for preauthorization for medical treatment, the level of co-payment required, and whether emergency medical evacuation is covered. Additional travel insurance that covers emergency medical evacuation and the costs of local care is available at reasonable rates through various providers, and parents should be made aware of this option.

UNDERLYING MEDICAL ILLNESS. Parents of traveling children should be asked whether the child has any current health problems or has had any problems in the past that have required medical evaluation or medication. Children with medical conditions should take with them a brief medical summary. Parents should be counseled to take a sufficient supply of prescription medications for their children and to ensure that the bottles are clearly identified. For children requiring care by specialists, an international directory for that specialty can be consulted. A directory of physicians worldwide who speak English and who have met certain qualifications is available from the International Association for Medical Assistance to Travelers (www.iamat.org). If medical care is needed urgently when abroad, sources of information include the American embassy or consulate, hotel managers, travel agents catering to foreign tourists, and missionary hospitals. Children with chronic cardiopulmonary disease, diabetes, allergies, and gastrointestinal problems, especially diarrhea associated with malabsorption or inflammatory bowel disease, are at particular risk for health problems when traveling. Children with severe food allergies should take several epinephrine autoinjectors with them. Patients with insulin-dependent diabetes or hemophilia should carry an adequate supply of sterile needles, syringes, and disinfectant swabs. Special arrangements should be made for patients with bleeding disorders, those on anticoagulation therapy, and those who require hemodialysis. Biologic products such as clotting factor concentrates or immune globulin should be avoided if manufactured abroad. A travel health kit consisting of prescription medications and nonprescription items such as acetaminophen, an antihistamine, oral rehydration solution packets, antibiotic ointment, bandages, insect repellent, and sunscreen is highly recommended for all children.

SAFETY. Injuries and motor vehicle accidents are the major causes of serious disability, hospitalization, and loss of life during travel. The use of safety belts for children, preferably sitting in the rear seat, should be emphasized. When possible, child safety-restraint seats should be taken on the trip. Travelers to remote areas should be warned about the risks of venomous animals as snake and scorpion bites can be fatal in infants. Many illnesses that develop in traveling children are related to risks that can be modified with proper advice and supervision by parents.

INFECTIOUS DISEASE PRECAUTIONS. Infectious disease risks to traveling children can generally be divided into four categories: food-borne, insect-borne, transmitted by contact with an infected person or by needle or blood exposure, and transmitted by contact with infected animals or environments.

Food-borne Infections. Ingestion of contaminated food or water makes travel-associated diarrhea the most common health complaint among international travelers. Among the bacterial and protozoan infections children can acquire from contaminated water are shigellosis, salmonellosis, *Escherichia coli* infections, cholera, giardiasis, amebiasis, and cryptosporidiosis. Viral infections, particularly rotavirus infections, are also a major cause of travel-associated diarrhea in children. Boiled water, hot beverages made with boiled water, and canned or bottled carbonated beverages are generally safest. Ice should be avoided, and tap water should not be used when brushing teeth. Boiling water for at least 1 minute is the most reliable method of water disinfection. An acceptable alternative is the use of a micropore filter with an on-demand iodine release system. Unpeeled fruit, uncooked vegetables, unpasteurized milk, milk products such as cheese, and undercooked meat or fish may all be contaminated and should be avoided. Fish, especially reef fish, red snapper, and barracuda, are of particular concern because they may contain toxins. Breast-feeding should be encouraged for young children, especially infants <6 mo of age.

Insect-Borne Infections. Insect-borne infections for which traveling children are at risk include malaria, yellow fever, dengue, Japanese encephalitis, filariasis, trypanosomiasis, and onchocerciasis, depending on the area of travel. Malaria, yellow fever, Japanese encephalitis, and filariasis are typically caused by night-biting mosquitoes, whereas dengue is usually caused by day-biting mosquitoes. Exposure to insect bites can be avoided by restricting high-risk activities, staying indoors in a screened and protected area from dusk to dawn, wearing appropriate attire, and using insect repellents containing permethrin or N,N-diethyl-M-toluamide (DEET). Rare instances of toxic encephalopathy have been reported in young children with exposure to high concentrations of DEET, but use of repellent with no more than 40% DEET and avoidance of repeated applications minimizes the risk of this complication. Concentrations of 25–35% DEET, to be applied every 6–8 hours as needed, are recommended for children. Spraying clothing with permethrin, a synthetic pyrethroid, is a safe and effective method of reducing insect bites in children.

Permethrin-sprayed clothes remain effective for at least 2 weeks, even with laundering. **Bed nets,** particularly permethrin-impregnated bed nets, also decrease the risk of insect bites.

Infections from Contact with Infected Persons or Through Needle Exposure. Many of the infections that may be acquired by children traveling internationally through contact with other individuals are preventable by routine childhood immunizations. Other diseases transmitted through human contact include viral respiratory and gastrointestinal infections, viral hepatitis, and sexually transmitted diseases including HIV infection. Many of these diseases are more prevalent in developing countries than in the United States. Adolescent travelers should be reminded that sexual encounters and needle or blood exposure (including tattooing and body piercing) carry a significant risk of HIV and hepatitis infection. Systematic screening of blood donations for HIV and other blood-borne infections is not yet feasible in many developing countries, so the safety of transfusion services in these countries cannot be ensured. Travelers may wish to have their blood typed before departure to determine whether family members or travel companions have compatible blood types and might be able to donate blood for transfusion in an emergency situation.

Infections from Infected Animals or Environments. Infections potentially acquired from contact with animals include rabies from stray dogs and plague from rodents. Swimming or diving in contaminated water can result in serious injury and increase the risk of infections such as schistosomiasis, leptospirosis, and primary amebic meningoencephalitis.

IMMUNIZATIONS

Parents should allow 4-6 wk before departure for optimal administration of vaccines to their children, because some immunizations require repeated doses for full protection and some vaccines and medications require either simultaneous or staggered dosing for optimal efficacy. The vaccines currently indicated for children traveling internationally, whether part of routine childhood immunization or travel-related, can be given concurrently with no decrease in safety or efficacy. Live-attenuated viral vaccines should be administered concurrently or at least 30 days apart to minimize immunologic interference. Intramuscular immune globulin (IG) interferes with the immune response to measles immunization and possibly to varicella immunization. If a child requires measles or varicella immunization, the vaccines should be given either 2 wk before or 3 mo after IG administration. IG does not interfere with the immune response to oral typhoid, poliovirus, or yellow fever vaccines.

Vaccine products produced in eggs (yellow fever, influenza) may be associated with hypersensitivity responses including anaphylaxis in persons with known severe egg sensitivity. Screening by inquiring about adverse effects when eating eggs is a reasonable way to identify those at risk for anaphylaxis from receiving influenza or yellow fever vaccines. Although measles and mumps vaccines are produced in chick embryo cell cultures, children with egg allergy are at very low risk for anaphylaxis with these vaccines. Most hypersensitivity reactions to measles-containing vaccines have been attributed to trace amounts of gelatin or neomycin.

In general, live-virus vaccines (measles, varicella, live attenuated influenza) and live bacterial vaccines (Bacille Calmette-Guérin [BCG], oral typhoid) are contraindicated in immunocompromised persons. However, HIV-infected children who are not severely immunocompromised should receive measles and varicella vaccines (see Table 170-7). Asymptomatic HIV-infected children may also be vaccinated against yellow fever if the risk is significant, but children with symptomatic HIV infection should not receive yellow fever vaccine. Inactivated vaccines and toxoids are not contraindicated in immunocompromised children but may be associated with diminished immune responses.

TABLE 173-1. Accelerated Schedule of Routine Childhood Immunizations if Necessary for Travel

VACCINE	ACCELERATED SCHEDULE
Diphtheria, tetanus, pertussis	DTaP: 6, 10, 14 wk of age; 4th dose 6 mo after 3rd dose
	DTaP: 4 yr of age (booster)
	dT every 5 yr if at high risk
Haemophilus influenzae type b	HbOC or PRP-T: 6, 10, 14 wk, and 12 mo
	PRP-OMP: 6, 10 wk, and 12 mo
Hepatitis B	Birth, 1, 2 mo; booster at 12 mo
Measles, mumps, rubella	MMR: Two dose at age ≥12 mo, 4 wk apart
	May give first measles dose as early as age 6 mo, with additional two doses age ≥12 mo, 4 wk apart
Poliomyelitis	IPV: 6, 10, 14 wk; booster at 4–6 yr
	A single IPV lifetime booster for adolescents and adults who have completed primary immunization
Pneumococcus	PCV: 6, 10, 14 wk; 4th dose 2 mo after 3rd dose
Varicella	12 mo (2 doses 1 mo apart for persons age ≥13 yr)

DTaP, diphtheria and tetanus toxoids and acellular pertussis; HbOC, diphtheria CRM_{197} protein conjugate; IPV, inactivated poliovirus; MMR, measles, mumps, and rubella; PCV, pneumococcal vaccine; PRP-OMP, polyribosylphosphate outer membrane protein; PRP-T, polyribosylphosphate tetanus toxoid.

ROUTINE CHILDHOOD VACCINES. All children who travel should be immunized according to the routine childhood immunization schedule with all vaccines appropriate for their age (see Chapter 170). The immunization schedule can be accelerated to maximize protection for traveling children, especially for unvaccinated or incompletely vaccinated children (Table 173-1).

Diphtheria, Tetanus, and Pertussis. Diphtheria is endemic in many developing countries. After the disintegration of the Soviet Union in 1991, diphtheria re-emerged in the new independent states. Tetanus is a major cause of worldwide neonatal mortality and is most prevalent in tropical countries. Pertussis is common in developing countries and in some developed nations where pertussis immunization is less widespread than in the U.S. because of earlier concerns about pertussis vaccine adverse effects. The incidence of pertussis also appears to be increasing in the U.S. Children traveling internationally should be up to date on diphtheria and tetanus toxoids and acellular pertussis (DTaP) immunization. A single dose of an **adolescent** preparation of tetanus and diphtheria toxoids and acellular pertussis (TdaP) vaccine is recommended at 11–12 yr of age for those who have completed the recommended diphtheria, tetanus toxoids, and pertussis (DTP)/DTaP series and have not received a tetanus-diphtheria (Td) booster dose. Adolescents 13–18 yr of age who have completed the DTP/DTaP series in whom it has been ≥5 yr or more since the Td booster dose also should receive a single dose of TdaP.

***Haemophilus influenzae* Type b.** *H. influenzae* type b remains the leading cause of meningitis in children 6 mo to 3 yr of age in many developing countries. Before they travel, all unimmunized children <60 mo of age and all children with chronic illness at risk for *H. influenzae* type b infections should be vaccinated (see Chapter 170).

Hepatitis B. Hepatitis B is highly prevalent in eastern and southeastern Asia, sub-Saharan Africa, and the Pacific basin. In certain parts of the world, 8–15% of the population may be chronically infected. Situations in which disease transmission can occur include receipt of blood transfusions not screened for hepatitis B surface antigen, exposure to unsterilized needles, close contact with local children who have open skin lesions, and sexual exposure. Exposure to hepatitis B is more likely for travelers residing for prolonged periods in endemic areas. Partial protection may be provided by 1 or 2 doses.

Measles, Mumps, and Rubella. Measles is still endemic in many developing countries and in some industrialized nations. Measles vaccine, preferably in combination with mumps and rubella vaccines (MMR), should be given to all children at 12–15 mo of age and at 4-6 yr of age, unless there is a contraindication (see Chapter 170). In children traveling internationally, the second vaccination can be given as soon as 4 wk after the 1st. In the accelerated schedule, the 1st MMR vaccination can be given to children as early as 6 mo of age, but if the vaccine is given at earlier than 12 mo of age, the child should be considered unvaccinated and given 2 additional doses at least 4 wk apart after 12 mo of age (see Table 173-1). Infants <6 mo of age are protected by maternal antibodies. HIV-infected children who travel abroad should be vaccinated unless severely immunocompromised (see Table 254-2), because measles in HIV-infected children can be a devastating illness.

Pneumococcus. *Streptococcus pneumoniae* is the leading cause of bacterial pneumonia and among the leading causes of bacteremia and bacterial meningitis in children in developing and industrialized nations. Immunization against *S. pneumoniae* with a protein-conjugated 7-valent pneumococcal vaccine (PCV7) is now part of routine childhood immunization in the U.S. Unimmunized individuals should be immunized if they are at high risk, such as children with sickle cell disease, asplenia, HIV infection, congenital immunodeficiency, nephrotic syndrome, chronic cardiac or pulmonary disease, and those on immunosuppressive medication (see Chapter 170). The Advisory Committee on Immunization Practices (ACIP) recommends that these children receive both the PCV7 vaccine and the 23-valent polysaccharide vaccine. The ACIP also recommends that vaccination with PCV7 be considered in all unimmunized children 24–59 mo of age; PCV7 vaccination of unimmunized children in this age group traveling internationally should be strongly considered.

Poliomyelitis. Poliomyelitis was eradicated from the Western hemisphere in 1991, but it remains endemic in several developing countries, and the 2004 epidemic in Nigeria underscored the importance of vaccination for prevention of this disease. The poliovirus vaccination schedule in the U.S. is now a 4 dose, all inactivated poliovirus (IPV) regimen (see Chapter 170). Oral poliovirus vaccine (OPV) is no longer available in the U.S. Unvaccinated adults who are at increased risk for exposure to poliovirus and who cannot complete the recommended IPV regimen (0, 1–2, and 6–12 mo) should receive 3 doses of IPV given at least 4 wk apart. Length of immunity conferred by IPV immunization is not known; a single booster dose of IPV is recommended for fully vaccinated adults traveling to endemic areas.

Varicella. All children ≥12 mo of age who have no history of varicella vaccination or chickenpox should be vaccinated unless there is a contraindication to vaccination (see Chapter 170). Infants <6 mo of age are generally protected by maternal antibodies. Children <13 yr of age require only 1 dose; children ≥13 yr of age require 2 doses separated by 4–8 wk.

TRAVEL VACCINES. The dosages and age restrictions of vaccines specifically given to children traveling internationally are summarized in Table 173-2.

Cholera. Cholera is present in many developing countries, but the risk for infection among travelers to these countries is very low. No cholera vaccine is currently available in the U.S. No country or territory currently requires cholera vaccination, but rarely a local authority may require documentation of vaccination. A letter of exemption for medical reasons from a physician may suffice. A new oral live cholera vaccine is available in Canada and many European countries for use in children ≥2 yr of age and appears to be safe and effective against most cholera strains. It is not currently available in the U.S.

Hepatitis A. Hepatitis A virus is endemic in most of the world, and travelers are at risk even if their travel is restricted to the usual tourist routes. Hepatitis A infection can occur as a result of eating shellfish harvested from sewage-contaminated waters, eating unwashed vegetables or fruits, or eating food prepared by an asymptomatic carrier of hepatitis A virus. Young children infected with hepatitis A are often asymptomatic, but they may transmit infection to older children and adults, who are more likely to develop clinical hepatitis. Hepatitis A immunization or immune globulin prophylaxis is recommended for children traveling to a developing country and should probably be given to all traveling children regardless of destination, because few areas carry no risk of this infection.

Hepatitis A vaccine is recommended in the U.S. for universal immunization of all children ≥12 mo of age. Vaccination is especially important for children traveling to countries with intermediate or high hepatitis A endemicity (areas other than the U.S., Canada, Australia, New Zealand, Japan, Western Europe, and Scandinavia). Protective immunity develops 2–4 wk after receiving the initial vaccine dose. A combined, 3 dose hepatitis A and hepatitis B vaccine is now available in the U.S. but it is licensed for use only in adults >18 yr of age.

Children <1 yr of age and children who will be traveling to an endemic area within 2 wk should receive intramuscular IG. For

TABLE 173-2. Travel Vaccinations for Children

DISEASE	VACCINE	PRIMARY SERIES	AGE AT VACCINATION	BOOSTER/COMMENTS
Hepatitis A	Havrix	0.5 mL IM at 0 and 6 mo	>1 yr	No booster.
	Vaqta	0.5 mL IM at 0 and 6–8 mo	>1 yr	As for Havrix.
	IG	Travel <2 mo: 0.02 mL/kg IM once Travel >2 mo: 0.06 mL/kg IM once	Birth	See text.
Influenza	Inactivated	6–35 mo: 0.25 mL IM, 1 or 2 doses 3–8 yr: 0.5 mL IM, 1 or 2 doses >9 yr: 0.5 mL IM once	>6 mo	New vaccine yearly. In children <9 yr, 2 doses should be given at least 1 mo apart if no prior vaccination.
	Live attenuated	0.25 mL in each nostril, 1 or 2 doses	>6 yr	New vaccine yearly. In children <9 yr, 2 doses should be given at least 1 mo apart if no prior inactivated or live virus vaccination. Only for healthy children.
Japanese B encephalitis		<3 yr: 0.5 mL SC on days 0, 7, and 14, or 30 >3 yr: 1.0 mL SC on days 0, 7, and 14 or 30	>1 yr	Every 3 yr.
Meningococcal disease	Polysaccharide $ACYW^{135}$	0.5 mL SC once	>2 yr	<4 yr: every 2 yr. >4 yr: every 3–5 yr.
	Conjugate $ACYW^{135}$	0.5 mL IM once	>11 yr	Unknown. Likely >8 yr.
Rabies	HDCV or RVA or CEC	1.0 mL IM on days 0, 7, and 21 or 28	Birth	See text for follow up vaccination if bitten.
Typhoid	Intramuscular Vi	0.5 mL IM once	>2 yr	Every 2 yr.
	Oral Ty21	1 capsule orally every other day, 4 doses	>6 yr	Every 5 yr. See text for administration.
Yellow fever		0.5 mL SC once	>9 mo	Every 10 yr (see text).

$ACYW^{135}$, Serogroup A, C, Y, and W^{135} meningococcal vaccine; CEC, chick embryo cell; HDCV, human diploid cell vaccine; IG, immune globulin; IM, intramuscularly; RVA, rabies vaccine adsorbed; SC, subcutaneously.

short-term protection (1–2 mo), 0.02 mL/kg of IG is given IM; for long-term protection (3–5 mo), 0.06 mL/kg of IG is given IM and repeated every 5 mo while exposure to hepatitis A continues. IG can be administered at the same time as the inactivated vaccine but should be given at a separate site and in a separate syringe. If a child requires MMR or varicella immunization, these live-attenuated viral vaccines should be given either 2 wk before or 3 mo after IG administration.

Influenza. The risk for exposure to influenza during international travel varies depending on the time of year, destination, and intermingling of persons from different parts of the world where influenza may be circulating. In the tropics, such as the Caribbean, influenza can occur throughout the year. In the temperate regions of the Southern hemisphere, including Australia and South America, most activity occurs from April through September. In the Northern hemisphere, including the United States and Canada, influenza generally occurs from November through March. Influenza vaccination is recommended for children ≥6 mo of age at increased risk for complications of influenza, including children of any age with chronic medical conditions such as chronic cardiac, renal, or pulmonary disease, immunosuppressive conditions or therapy, HIV infection, sickle cell disease, and diabetes mellitus (see Chapter 170). Children with any of these conditions should receive only the inactivated vaccine. Healthy children ≥6 yr of age whose parents wish to have them receive influenza vaccination may receive the live attenuated vaccine. However, the list of medical contraindications to this vaccine should be reviewed carefully (see Chapter 170). Currently, there is no available vaccine effective against avian influenza, which has become an increasing concern worldwide.

Japanese Encephalitis. Japanese encephalitis is a disease transmitted by mosquitoes in rural areas of Asia, where people are in close proximity to livestock. Asymptomatic cases outnumber symptomatic cases by at least 200 to 1, but when symptomatic the disease has a 10–70% case fatality rate. The risk in travelers is extremely low, less than 1 case/million travelers, but the risk is highest in children. The disease occurs primarily from June to September in temperate zones and throughout the entire year in tropical zones. Vaccination is recommended for travelers planning visits of greater than 1 mo to rural areas of Asia where the disease is endemic, especially areas of rice or pig farming, or shorter visits to such an area if the traveler will frequently be outdoors (e.g., camping or hiking). Risk for infection can be greatly reduced by following the standard precautions to avoid mosquito bites. Parents of very young children should be discouraged from traveling with their children to high-risk areas.

The inactivated Japanese encephalitis vaccine has an efficacy of more than 95%, but hypersensitivity reactions occur in up to 0.6% of vaccine recipients; 1 in 1,000 vaccinees have urticarial reactions or facial or oropharyngeal angioedema that may occur within minutes or up to 2 wk after vaccination. The series should be completed 2 wk before travel so that any adverse reactions to the vaccine can be observed and treated.

Meningococcus. *Neisseria meningitidis* causes epidemic and endemic disease worldwide (see Chapter 190). Most cases occur in the "meningitis belt" of sub-Saharan Africa between December and June. Epidemics have also occurred in the Indian subcontinent and Saudi Arabia, especially among pilgrims to the Haj. Cases in American travelers are rare, and vaccination is indicated primarily in travelers to an area with an active outbreak or those who may have prolonged contact with the local population in an endemic area, especially in crowded conditions. Saudi Arabia requires all pilgrims to Mecca to have documentation of meningococcal vaccination ≥10 days and within 3 yr before arrival. Serogroup A is the most common cause of epidemics outside the United States, but serogroup C and, rarely, serogroup B have also been associated with epidemics.

There are currently 2 meningococcal vaccines available in the U.S.: a quadrivalent polysaccharide A/C/Y/W-135 vaccine and a quadrivalent conjugate A/C/Y/W-135 vaccine. The quadrivalent polysaccharide vaccine is recommended for children ≥2 yr of age who are at risk for meningococcal disease caused by a vaccine serogroup, as well as for children ≥3 mo of age who are at risk for serogroup A meningococcal disease. The vaccine is ineffective against serogroup A in infants <3 mo of age and may be only partially effective against this serogroup in children 3–11 mo of age, and does not provide protection for children <2 yr of age against the other serogroups. Children vaccinated before 4 yr of age should be revaccinated after 2–3 yr if they remain in an endemic area. The quadrivalent protein conjugate vaccine is recommended for children ≥11 yr of age and may soon be licensed for children 2–10 yr of age. It appears to deliver prolonged high-level antibody titers and may become the vaccine of choice for all children ≥2 yr of age in the future.

Rabies. Rabies is endemic in many countries in Africa, Asia, and Central and South America. Children are at particular risk because facial bites are more common in children. Pre-exposure prophylaxis should be considered if a child will be in an endemic area for longer than 1 mo or will be traveling to an area where rapid, effective postexposure prophylaxis may not be available. An animal bite in a rabies-endemic area is a medical emergency. Immediate medical care should be sought at a facility that can administer appropriate postexposure rabies prophylaxis. If possible, the animal in question should be caught and quarantined for 10 days of observation for signs of rabies. Postexposure prophylaxis is required even for individuals who received pre-exposure vaccination.

Three inactivated rabies vaccines are available in the U.S. for pre-exposure vaccination: human diploid cell vaccine (HDCV), rabies vaccine adsorbed (RVA), and purified chick embryo cell (PCEC) vaccine. Pre-exposure prophylaxis is given either intramuscularly (HDCV, RVA, or PCEC) as 3 doses (1 mL) on days 0, 7, and 28, or intradermally (HDCV) as 3 doses (0.1 mL) on days 0, 7, and 28. Postexposure prophylaxis is given as 5 doses (1 mL) of HDCV, RVA, or PCEC vaccine intramuscularly on days 0, 3, 7, 14, and 28 if previously unvaccinated and 2 doses (1 mL) intramuscularly on days 0 and 3 if previously vaccinated. Previously unvaccinated individuals should receive rabies immune globulin (RIG) (20 IU/kg, with as much of the dose as possible infiltrated around the wound site) at the time of initial postexposure prophylaxis. Previously vaccinated individuals should not receive RIG. Children receiving mefloquine or chloroquine may have limited immune reactions to intradermal rabies vaccine and should be vaccinated intramuscularly. Purified cell culture–derived vaccines are not always available abroad; travelers should be aware that rabies vaccines derived from neural tissue carry an increased risk for adverse reactions, often with neurologic sequelae. Unpurified or purified equine RIG preparations are still used in some developing countries and are also associated with a higher risk for severe reactions, including serum sickness and anaphylaxis. If rabies prophylaxis is initiated abroad, neutralizing titers should be checked on return and immunization completed with a cell culture–derived vaccine.

Tuberculosis. The risk for tuberculosis in the typical traveler is low. All children traveling for prolonged periods to high-risk areas should have tuberculin skin testing done before and after travel. Immunization with bacille Calmette-Guérin (BCG) is controversial. It is not frequently used in the United States, but some authorities believe it should be given to children, especially infants, who will reside for a long time in an area with a high prevalence of tuberculosis or with multidrug-resistant tuberculosis because it appears to be highly protective against meningeal and miliary tuberculosis in children.

Typhoid. *Salmonella typhi* infection, or typhoid fever, is common in many developing countries in Asia, Africa, and Latin

America (see Chapter 195.2). Typhoid vaccination is recommended for children traveling to the Indian subcontinent, the area of highest risk, and for individuals traveling to endemic areas who are at higher risk for infection: long-term travelers (>4 wk), backpackers, and travelers staying with friends or relatives in developing countries. Vaccination should be strongly considered for all children traveling to endemic areas, especially if exposure to contaminated food and water is likely.

Two typhoid vaccines, the intramuscular Vi-polysaccharide vaccine and oral Ty21a strain live-attenuated vaccine, are recommended for use in children in the U.S. The intramuscular Vi-polysaccharide vaccine is licensed for use in children 2 yr of age and older. It can be given any time before departure, but it should ideally be administered 1 mo or more before travel. The oral Ty21a vaccine can only be used in children 6 yr of age and older. The oral vaccine is given in 4 doses over a 1-wk period: 1 enteric-coated capsule is swallowed whole with a cool drink, at least 1 hour before a meal, every other day until the 4 doses are completed. Antibiotics inhibit the immune response to the oral Ty21a vaccine; the vaccine should not be given within 24 hr of antibiotic treatment. Studies have demonstrated that mefloquine, chloroquine, and atovaquone-proguanil can be given concurrently with the oral Ty21a vaccine without affecting the immunogenicity of the vaccine. Oral Ty21a vaccine should not be given to immunocompromised children; these children should receive the intramuscular Vi-polysaccharide vaccine.

Yellow Fever. Yellow fever (see Chapter 267) is a mosquito-borne viral illness resembling other viral hemorrhagic fevers (see Chapter 268) but with more prominent hepatic involvement. Yellow fever is present in tropical areas of South America and Africa.

Yellow fever vaccination is indicated in children >9 mo of age traveling to an endemic area. Some countries require yellow fever vaccination by law for travelers arriving from endemic areas. Some African countries require evidence of vaccination from all entering travelers. Current recommendations can be obtained by contacting state or local health departments or the Division of Vector-Borne Infectious Diseases of the CDC (telephone: 404-332-4555; or website: www.cdc.gov). Most countries accept a medical waiver for children who are too young to be vaccinated (<4 mo of age) and for individuals with a contraindication to vaccination, such as immunodeficiency. Children with asymptomatic HIV infection may be vaccinated if exposure to yellow fever virus cannot be avoided.

Yellow fever vaccine (0.5 mL SC), a live-attenuated vaccine (17D strain) developed in chick embryos, is safe and highly effective in children >9 mo of age, but in young infants it is associated with an increased risk for encephalitis (0.4%) and other severe reactions. Yellow fever vaccine should never be administered to infants <4 mo of age; infants 4–6 mo of age should be vaccinated only in consultation with the CDC; infants 6–9 mo of age should be vaccinated only if they cannot avoid traveling to areas with an ongoing epidemic. Children with a history of anaphylactic reactions to eggs should also not receive yellow fever vaccine. Long-lived, perhaps lifetime immunity develops to this vaccine; however, international travel certificates require proof of immunization within 10 yr.

Traveler's Diarrhea. Traveler's diarrhea, characterized by a 2-fold or greater increase in the frequency of unformed bowel movements, occurs in as many as 40% of all travelers overseas. Children, especially those <3 yr of age, have a higher incidence of diarrhea, more severe symptoms, and more prolonged symptoms than adults. Traveler's diarrhea is usually acquired through ingestion of fecally contaminated food and water. Diverse infectious agents (bacteria, viruses, and parasites) have been associated with traveler's diarrhea; enterotoxigenic *E. coli* is still the most frequent cause. Other bacterial causes include *Shigella, Salmonella, Campylobacter, Vibrio cholerae, Vibrio parahaemolyticus, Aeromonas hydrophilia,* and *Plesiomonas shigelloides.* Protozoan infections such as *Entamoeba histolytica, Giardia lamblia, Cryptosporidium parvum,* and *Isospora* are more common in long-term travelers. Rotavirus has also been associated with traveler's diarrhea. The most important risk factor for traveler's diarrhea is the country of destination. High-risk areas (attack rates of 25–50%) include developing countries of Latin America, Africa, the Middle East, and Asia. Intermediate risk occurs in the Mediterranean, China, and Israel. Low-risk areas include North America, Northern Europe, Australia, and New Zealand. Immunocompromised children, including children with HIV, are at increased risk for complications from bacterial causes of traveler's diarrhea, particularly *Salmonella.* Careful selection and preparation of food and water can significantly reduce the risk for developing traveler's diarrhea. Chemoprophylactic agents for traveler's diarrhea are not recommended for children.

Dehydration is the greatest threat presented by a diarrheal illness in a small child. Parents should be made aware of the symptoms and signs of dehydration. Prepackaged WHO/UNICEF oral rehydration solution (ORS) packets, which are available at stores or pharmacies in almost all developing countries, should be part of a child's travel kit. ORS should be mixed as directed with bottled or boiled water and given slowly, as tolerated, to the child. Antimotility agents such as diphenoxylate (Lomotil) and loperamide (Imodium) should be avoided in young children; loperamide (2 mg tid PO) may be useful for children >8 yr of age if they do not have fever or bloody stools. Bismuth subsalicylate (5 mL for 3–5 yr of age; 10 mL for 6–8 yr of age; 15 mL for 9–11 yr of age; 30 mL for ≥12 yr of age) as often as every 30 min for 8 doses, with no more than 8 doses/day, decreases the rate of stooling and shortens the duration of illness. Higher doses of bismuth subsalicylate should be avoided because of concerns of salicylate toxicity. Bismuth subsalicylate should not be used if the child may have influenza or is in an area experiencing an influenza outbreak because there is an increased risk for Reye syndrome in children with influenza who receive salicylate therapy.

Presumptive self-treatment is usually recommended for adults, and most experts agree that it should also be given to children. For adults ≥18 yr of age the recommended regimen is ciprofloxacin (500 mg), norfloxacin (400 mg), or ofloxacin (300 mg) orally twice daily for 3 days. For children, the drugs of choice are azithromycin (10 mg/kg/day, maximum dose of 500 mg, for 3 days) and ciprofloxacin (25–30 mg/kg/day, divided into 2 doses, maximum dose of 500 mg twice a day, for 3 days). Azithromycin is not specifically approved for the treatment of diarrhea, but it is highly effective against most pathogens that cause traveler's diarrhea and can be prescribed in powder form that can be made into a liquid suspension when needed. Ciprofloxacin is not approved for use in children, but has been used extensively and shown to be safe in children. Antimicrobial therapy for traveler's diarrhea in infants and young children should be administered in consultation with a physician. This is particularly true if the illness is severe, persists for >3 days, or is associated with bloody stools, temperature greater than 102°F, chills, vomiting, or moderate to severe dehydration.

Malaria Chemoprophylaxis. Malaria, a mosquito-borne infection, is the leading parasitic cause of death in children worldwide (see Chapter 285). Of the 4 *Plasmodium* species that infect humans, *P. falciparum* causes the greatest morbidity and mortality. Each year, >8 million U.S. citizens visit parts of the world where malaria is endemic (sub-Saharan Africa, Central and South America, India, Southeast Asia, Oceania). Given the major resurgence of malaria, physicians in developed countries are increasingly required to give advice on prevention, diagnosis, and treatment of malaria. The CDC maintains updated information at www.cdc.gov/travel/, as well as a malaria hotline for physicians (770-488-7788). It is important to check this updated information because recommendations for prophylaxis and treatment are frequently modified due to changes in the risk for developing malaria in different areas of the world, changing *Plasmodium* resistance patterns, and the availability of new antimalarial medications.

Avoidance of mosquitoes and barrier protection from mosquitoes are an important part of malaria prevention for travelers to endemic areas. The *Anopheles* mosquito feeds from dusk to dawn. Travelers should remain in **well-screened areas,** wear clothing that covers most of the body, sleep under a bed net (ideally 1 impregnated with permethrin), and use insect repellents with N,N-diethyl-3-methylbenzamide (DEET) during these hours (see Infectious Disease Precautions). Parents should be discouraged from taking a young child on a trip that will entail evening or nighttime exposure in rural areas of countries with chloroquine- or multidrug-resistant *P. falciparum.*

Chemoprophylaxis is the cornerstone of malaria prevention for nonimmune children and adults who travel to malaria-endemic areas, but it is not a replacement for other protective measures because no chemoprophylaxis regimen guarantees complete protection against malaria. Travelers often do not take malaria prophylaxis as prescribed; frequently they do not take it at all. They are more likely to use prophylactic antimalarial drugs if their physicians provide appropriate recommendations and education before departure. However, in 1 survey, only 14% of persons who sought medical advice obtained correct information about malaria prevention and prophylaxis.

Resistance of *P. falciparum* to the traditional chemoprophylactic agent, chloroquine, is rapidly increasing worldwide, and in most areas of the world other agents must be used (Table 173-3). Factors that must be considered in choosing appropriate chemoprophylaxis medications and dosing schedules include age of the child, travel itinerary (including whether the child will be traveling to areas of risk within a particular country and whether chloroquine-resistant *P. falciparum* is present in the country), vaccinations being given, allergic or other known adverse reactions to antimalarial agents, and the availability of medical care during travel.

Children traveling to areas with chloroquine-resistant *P. falciparum* can be given mefloquine, atovaquone-proguanil, or doxycycline as malaria prophylaxis. For trips under 2 weeks, atovaquone-proguanil is the preferred medication, as it need be given for only a short period before and after travel. Atovaquone-proguanil or doxycycline is also indicated for travel of any duration to western Cambodia and the Thailand-Cambodia and Thailand-Myanmar borders because of mefloquine resistance in these areas. For periods of travel >2 weeks to all other areas with chloroquine-resistant *P. falciparum,* mefloquine is the preferred medication, as it can be taken weekly, as compared to the daily dosing required for atovaquone-proguanil and doxycycline.

Mefloquine is FDA-approved only for children weighing >15 kg, but the CDC recommends mefloquine prophylaxis for all children regardless of weight because the risk for acquiring severe malaria outweighs the risk for potential mefloquine toxicity. Adults have 10–25% incidence of sleep disturbance and dysphoria with mefloquine, but these side effects appear to be less common in children. Other potential side effects of mefloquine therapy include nausea and vomiting. The lack of a liquid or suspension formulation can make chloroquine and mefloquine administration difficult. For children who cannot take tablets, parents should take a chloroquine or mefloquine prescription to a compounding pharmacy, which can pulverize the tablets and place exact dosages into gel capsules. Parents can then open the gel capsules and sprinkle the powder into food. "Disguising" these medications, which have a bitter taste, is important; chocolate syrup has been used successfully as a vehicle for the medication. Individuals with depression, neuropsychiatric disorders, seizure disorders and cardiac conduction defects should not take mefloquine.

Atovaquone/proguanil (fixed combination, trade name Malarone [Glaxo SmithKline, Philadelphia, PA]) is effective and safe chemoprophylaxis for travelers to chloroquine-resistant malaria endemic areas, but it is currently fairly expensive. Adverse effects are infrequent, mild (abdominal pain, vomiting, and headache), and rarely result in discontinuation of the medication. Atovaquone/proguanil prophylaxis must be taken every day, so it is better suited for prophylaxis during short periods of exposure. Daily doxycycline is an alternative chemoprophylaxis regimen for chloroquine-resistant *P. falciparum* malaria that is considerably less expensive than atovaquone/proguanil. Doxycycline has been used extensively and is highly effective, but it cannot be used in children <8 years of age, and adverse effects (nausea, vomiting, photosensitivity, vaginal candidiasis) are not uncommon. Individuals given doxycycline prophylaxis should be warned to decrease exposure to direct sunlight to minimize the possibility of photosensitivity. Primaquine has also been used successfully as chemoprophylaxis, but there are limited data about its use in nonimmune children. Chloroquine, chloroquine-proguanil, and azithromycin do not provide adequate protection for children traveling to a chloroquine-resistant malaria-endemic area.

In those areas of the world where *P. falciparum* remains fully chloroquine sensitive (Haiti, the Dominican Republic, Central America north of the Panama Canal, and some countries in the Middle East), weekly chloroquine is the drug of choice for malaria chemoprophylaxis. Updated information is available at www.cdc.gov/travel.

On leaving an area endemic for *P. vivax* or *P. ovale* after a prolonged visit (usually >3 months), travelers may require "terminal prophylaxis" with primaquine (0.6 mg/kg base or 1.0 mg/kg salt daily, up to a maximum dose of 30 mg base or 52.6 mg salt, for 14 days) to eliminate extraerythrocytic forms of *P. vivax* and *P. ovale* and prevent relapses. Primaquine can cause severe hemolysis in glucose-6-phosphate dehydrogenase (G6PD)–deficient individuals. Individuals must always be screened for G6PD deficiency before primaquine is prescribed.

Small amounts of antimalarial drugs are secreted into breast milk of lactating women. The amounts of transferred drug are not considered to be either harmful or sufficient to provide adequate prophylaxis against malaria. Prolonged infant exposure to doxycycline via breast milk is not advisable.

TABLE 173-3. Chemoprophylaxis of Malaria for Children

AREA	DRUG	DOSAGE (ORAL)
Chloroquine-resistant area	Mefloquine*,†	<15 kg: 4.6 mg base (5 mg salt)/kg/wk 15–19 kg: 1/4 tab/wk 20–30 kg: 1/2 tab/wk 31–45 kg: 3/4 tab/wk >15 kg: 1 tab/wk (228 mg base)
	Doxycyline‡	2 mg/kg daily (max 100 mg)
	Atovaquone/proguanil§ (Malarone)	Pediatric tabs: 62.5 mg atovaquone/25 mg proguanil Adult tabs: 250 mg proguanil/100 mg proguanil 11–20 kg: 1 pediatric tab once daily 21–30 kg: 2 pediatric tabs once daily 31–40 kg: 3 pediatric tabs once daily >40 kg: 1 adult tab once daily
Chloroquine-sensitive area	Chloroquine phosphate	5 mg base/kg/wk (max 300 mg base)

*Chloroquine and mefloquine should be started 1 wk prior to departure and continued for 4 wk after last exposure.
†Mefloquine resistance exists in western Cambodia and along the Thai-Cambodia and Thai-Myanmar borders. Travelers to these areas should take doxycycline or atovaquone-proguanil.
‡Doxycycline should be started 1 day prior to departure and continued for 4 wk after last exposure. Do not use in children <8 yr of age or in pregnant women.
§Atovaquone/proguanil (Malarone) should be started 1–2 days prior to departure and continued for 7 days after last exposure.

TABLE 173-4. Patterns of Illness Among Returning International Travelers

SYSTEMIC FEBRILE ILLNESS
Malaria
Typhoid fever
Dengue
Rickettsial infections (tick-borne spotted fever)
Undetermined fever source
ACUTE DIARRHEA
Giardiasis
Amebiasis
Campylobacter
Shigella
Salmonella
Escherichia coli
Presumed viral
DERMATOLOGIC MANIFESTATIONS
Insect bites
Cutaneous larva migrans
Abscess
Superficial mycosis
Animal bite
Leishmaniasis
Myiasis
Scabies
Impetigo

TABLE 173-5. Common Infectious Diseases of Internationally Adopted Children

DISEASE	COMMENT
Tuberculosis (TB)	Latent TB in 3–20% High rates in Asia, Russia
Hepatitis B virus	Chronic carriers in 5–7% High rates in Asia, Caribbean, Eastern Europe, Africa
Hepatitis C virus	0–2.5% incidence High rates in Eastern Europe, Middle East, Asia
HIV	<1% HIV positive ↑ risk from Russia, Africa, Asia
Syphilis (congenital)	<2% VDRL positive High rates in Eastern Europe, Russia, Asia
Giardia	Very common High rates in Africa, South and Central America, Asia
Ascaris lumbricoides	Common High rates in Asia, Africa, Central and South America
Hookworms	Unknown incidence High rates in Asia, Mediterranean, South America
OTHER PARASITIC DISEASES	
Dientamoeba fragilis	~2% of adoptees
Trichuris trichiura	Unknown prevalence
Enterobius vermicularis	2–30% of adoptees
Strongyloides stercoralis	Most virulent, eosinophilia present

VDRL, Venereal Disease Research Laboratory (test).

THE RETURNING TRAVELER

Post-travel evaluations are part of travel medicine and continuing care. Children who will be traveling abroad for a prolonged period of time (>6 mo) should receive tuberculin skin testing before and after travel and should be tested for asymptomatic gastrointestinal parasitic infections on their return. Physicians unfamiliar with diseases that occur in developing countries often misdiagnose the cause of illness in a child returning from travel abroad.

Three major patterns of illness have been noted (Table 173-4). The etiology of each of these disease presentations is in part dependent on the country visited. Dengue is not common in returning visitors from sub-Saharan Africa or Central America, while tick-borne spotted fever is common in sub-Saharan Africa. Malaria is noted in most developing countries.

Fever is a particularly worrisome symptom: malaria and typhoid are the 2 most common causes of fever in children returning from travel to developing countries, but numerous other illnesses acquired in these countries may cause fever (see Table 173-4). Malaria must be considered in the evaluation of any fever that develops within 1 yr, and particularly within the 1st 2 mo, after travel to malaria-endemic areas. Children returning from international travel who have specific signs and symptoms of illness, such as fever, rash, and acute or chronic diarrhea, should see a pediatric travel medicine or infectious disease specialist (see Table 173-4).

173.1 • Infections in International Adoptees (See also Chapter 33) • R. M. Kliegman

Internationally adopted children have many health problems. Infections or infestations are common and are in part dependent on the international region, nutritional status, and prior immunizations (Table 173-5). Symptoms suggestive of parasitic infections are noted in Table 173-6. Screening tests are noted in Table 173-7. Relevant websites are noted in Table 173-8. The immunization record should be checked and the child immunized against any pathogen not reported in the immunization records. Catch-up immunization should be initiated (see Fig. 170-4).

TABLE 173-6. Clinical Symptoms Suggestive of Specific Parasite Infections

SYMPTOMS	POSSIBLE PARASITE(S)
Diarrhea most common, also behavioral changes, growth arrest, chronic abdominal pain, fecal incontinence	*Giardia*
Large-volume; thick, formless, and odiferous stools; flatulence	*Giardia*
Diarrhea, abdominal pain (often severe), blood and mucus	*Entamoeba histolytica*
Right upper-quadrant abdominal pain, high fever, abdominal distention, irritability, tachypnea	*E. histolytica* liver abscess
Leukocytosis and elevated alkaline phosphatase with normal transaminases	*E. histolytica* liver abscess
Diarrhea and anal pruritis	*Dientamoeba* and *Entamoeba vermicularis*
Acute watery diarrhea	*Dientamoeba fragilis*
Chronic recurrent abdominal pain	*D. fragilis*
Intestinal obstruction	*Entamoeba* or *Ascaris*
Pneumonia and eosinophilia	*Ascaris*, hookworms, *Strongyloides*, *Toxocara*
Hepatic abscess	*Entamoeba* or *Ascaris*
Biliary obstruction	*Ascaris*
Radiographic findings or clinical symptoms resembling inflammatory bowel disease (without elevated ESR)	*Strongyloides* or *Trichuris*
Isolated eosinophilia	*Strongyloides*, *Filaria*, *hookworms*, *Schistosomia*, *Toxocara*
Protein-losing enteropathy	*Strongyloides*
Mucoid diarrhea, vague abdominal pain, distention, voluminous stools	*Strongyloides*
Bloody diarrhea	Parasite ± *Shigella*

ESR, erythrocyte sedimentation rate.

From Miller LC: *The Handbook of International Adoption Medicine: A Guide for Physicians, Parents, and Providers.* New York, Oxford University Press, 2005, p 254.

TABLE 173-7. Screening Tests for Infectious Diseases Recommended for Internationally Adopted Children

TEST	POPULATION TO BE SCREENED	ADDITIONAL TESTING OR CONSIDERATIONS
Tuberculin skin test	All adoptees	Consider repeating in 2–3 mo or when nutritional status is improved if negative on initial screen
Hepatitis serology Hepatitis B surface antigen (HBSAg) Hepatitis B surface antibody (HBSAb) Hepatitis B core antibody (HBcoreAb)	All adoptees	Consider repeating in 6 mo
Complete blood cell count with differential, red blood cell indices, and platelet count	All adoptees	Some findings may suggest, in combination with clinical signs and symptoms, that additional evaluation is necessary as follows: Eosinophilia: parasitic infections Anemia/thrombocytopenia: malaria Thrombocytopenia: CMV Leukopenia: HIV
Syphilis serology Nontreponemal test (RPR, VDRL, ART) Treponemal test (MHA-TP, FTA-ABS)	Nontreponemal tests for all adoptees Treponemal tests if non-treponemal tests are reactive; if clinical signs and/or symptoms of syphilis are present	Children with positive test results and those diagnosed and/or treated in their birth country need additional testing
Stool examination for ova and parasites (3 specimens)	All adoptees	Repeat in those with persistent symptoms Repeat to confirm elimination of parasites after treatment
Stool specimen for antigen for *Giardia lamblia* and *Cryptosporidium parvum* (1 specimen)	All adoptees	
HIV 1 and 2 ELISA (consider DNA PCR in infants)	All adoptees	Consider repeating in 6 mo if negative on initial screen
Hepatitis C	Adoptees from China, Russia, Eastern Europe, and Southeast Asia Adoptees with risk factors for infection	Consider repeating in 6 mo if negative on initial screen

ART, automated reagin test; CMV, cytomegalovirus; ELISA, enzyme-linked immunosorbent assay; FTA-ABS, fluorescent treponemal antibody absorption; MHA-TP, microhemagglutination test for *Treponema pallidum;* PCR, polymerase chain reaction; RPR, rapid plasma reagin; VDRL, Venereal Disease Research Laboratory (test).

From Barnett ED: Immunizations and infectious disease screening for internationally adopted children. *Pediatr Clin North Am* 2005;52:1287–1309.

TABLE 173-8. Online Resources to Guide Families Planning International Adoption

WEBSITE	HIGHLIGHT
http://travel.state.gov/family/adoption/adoption_485.html	International adoption booklet; information on U.S. visa requirements; travel warnings
http://www.cdc.gov/nie/menus/groups.htm#intl	General health information regarding international adoption
http://www.immunize.org/adoption/index.htm	Link to journal articles and recommendations on international adoption; link to numerous resources for parents and providers
http://www.istm.org	Travel clinic directory
http://www.cdc.gov/travel	Travel health warning and precautions; outbreaks; travel health recommendations

From Barnett ED, Chen LH: Prevention of travel-related infectious diseases in families of internationally adopted children. *Pediatr Clin North Am* 2005;52:1271–1286.

Adachi JA, Ostrosky-Zeichner L, DuPont HL, et al: Empirical antimicrobial therapy for traveler's diarrhea. *Clin Infect Dis* 2000;31:1079–1083.

Balkhy HH: Travelling with children. *Int J Antimicrob Agents* 2003;21(2):193–199.

Barnett ED: Immunizations and infectious disease screening for internationally adopted children. *Pediatr Clin North Am* 2005;52:1287–1309.

Barnett ED, Chen LH: Prevention of travel-related infectious diseases in families of internationally adopted children. *Pediatr Clin North Am* 2005;52:1271–1286.

Bottieau E, Clerinx J, Vanden Enden E, et al: Fever after a stay in the tropics. *Medicine* 2007;86:18–25.

Centers for Disease Control and Prevention: Travel-associated dengue—United States, 2005. *MMWR* 2006;55:700–701.

Chen LH, Wilson ME, Schlagonhauf P: Prevention of malaria in long term travelers. *JAMA* 2006;296:2234–2244.

Freedman DO, Weld LH, Kozarsky PE, et al: Spectrum of disease and relation to place of exposure among ill returned travelers. *N Engl J Med* 2006;354:119–130.

Hill DR: The burden of illness in international travelers. *N Engl J Med* 2006;354:115–117.

Kain KC, Shanks GD, Keystone JS: Malaria chemoprophylaxis in the age of drug resistance: I. Currently recommended drug regimens. *Clin Infect Dis* 2001; 33: 226–234.

Katz BZ: Traveling with children. *Pediatr Infect Dis J* 2003;22(3):274–276.

Mackell SM: Vaccinations for the pediatric traveler. *Clin Infect Dis* 2003;37(11):1508–1516.

Miller LC: *The Handbook of International Adoption Medicine: A Guide for Physicians, Parents and Providers.* New York, Oxford University Press, 2005, p 254.

Stauffer WM, Konop RJ, Kamat D: Traveling with infants and young children. Part I: Anticipatory guidance: Travel preparation and preventive health advice. *J Travel Med* 2001;8(5):254–259.

Stauffer WM, Kamat D: Traveling with infants and children. Part II: Immunizations. *J Travel Med* 2002;9(2):82–90.

Stauffer WM, Konop RJ, Kamat D: Traveling with infants and young children. Part III: Travelers' diarrhea. *J Travel Med* 2002;9(3):141–150.

Stauffer WM, Kamat D, Magill AJ: Traveling with infants and children. Part IV: Insect avoidance and malaria prevention. *J Travel Med* 2003; 10(4):225–240.

Chapter 174 ■ Fever

Keith R. Powell

Fever is a controlled increase in body temperature over the normal values for an individual. Body temperature is regulated by **thermosensitive neurons** located in the preoptic or anterior hypothalamus that respond to changes in blood temperature as well as to direct neural connections with cold and warm receptors located in skin and muscle. **Thermoregulatory responses** include redirecting blood to or from cutaneous vascular beds, increased or decreased sweating, extracellular fluid volume regulation (via arginine vasopressin), and behavioral responses, such as seeking a warmer or cooler environmental temperature. Normal body temperature also varies in a regular pattern each day. This circadian temperature rhythm, or **diurnal variation,** results in lower body temperatures in the early morning and temperatures approximately 1°C higher in the late afternoon or early evening.

PATHOGENESIS. Fever is regulated in the same manner as normal temperature is maintained in a cool environment, the difference being that the body's thermostat has been reset at a higher temperature (Fig. 174-1). Regardless of whether fever is associated with infection, rheumatic disease, or malignancy, the thermostat is reset in response to **endogenous pyrogens,** including the cytokines interleukin 1 (IL-1) and IL-6, tumor necrosis factor-α (TNF-α), and interferon-β (IFN-β) and IFN-γ. Stimulated leukocytes and other cells produce lipids that also serve as endogenous pyrogens. The best-studied lipid mediator is prostaglandin E_2 (PGE_2). Most endogenous pyrogen molecules are too large to cross the blood-brain barrier in an efficient manner. However, circumventricular organs in close proximity to the hypothalamus lack a blood-brain barrier and allow for neuronal contact with circulating factors through fenestrated capillaries.

Microbes, microbial toxins, or other products of microbes are the most common "exogenous pyrogens," which are substances that come from outside of the body, stimulate macrophages and other cells to produce endogenous pyrogens, and result in fever. Some substances produced within the body are not pyrogens but are capable of stimulating endogenous pyrogens. Such substances include antigen-antibody complexes in the presence of complement, complement components, lymphocyte products, bile acids, and androgenic steroid metabolites. Endotoxin is 1 of the few substances that can directly affect thermoregulation in the hypothalamus as well as stimulate endogenous pyrogen release. Fever may be caused by infection, vaccines, biologic agents (granulocyte-macrophage colony-stimulating factor, interferons, interleukins), tissue injury (infarction, pulmonary emboli, trauma, intramuscular injections, burns), malignancy (leukemia, lymphoma, hepatoma, metastatic disease), drugs (cocaine, amphotericin B, drug fever), immunologic-rheumatologic disorders (systemic lupus erythematosus, rheumatoid arthritis), inflammatory diseases (e.g., inflammatory bowel disease), granulomatous diseases (sarcoidosis), endocrine disorders (e.g., thyrotoxicosis, pheochromocytoma), metabolic disorders (gout, uremia, Fabry disease, type 1 hyperlipidemia), genetic disorders (familial Mediterranean fever), and unknown or poorly understood entities. **Factitious fever,** or self-induced fever, may be due to intentional manipulation of the thermometer or injection of pyrogenic material.

Increasing body temperature in response to microbial pathogens is a response observed in reptiles, fish, birds, and mammals. When fish are given an exogenous pyrogen, they swim to warmer water to raise their body temperature. In a similar fashion, lizards given exotoxin lie in the sun until they have raised their body temperature to the febrile range. In humans, increased temperatures are associated with decreased microbial reproduction and an increased inflammatory response. Most evidence sug-

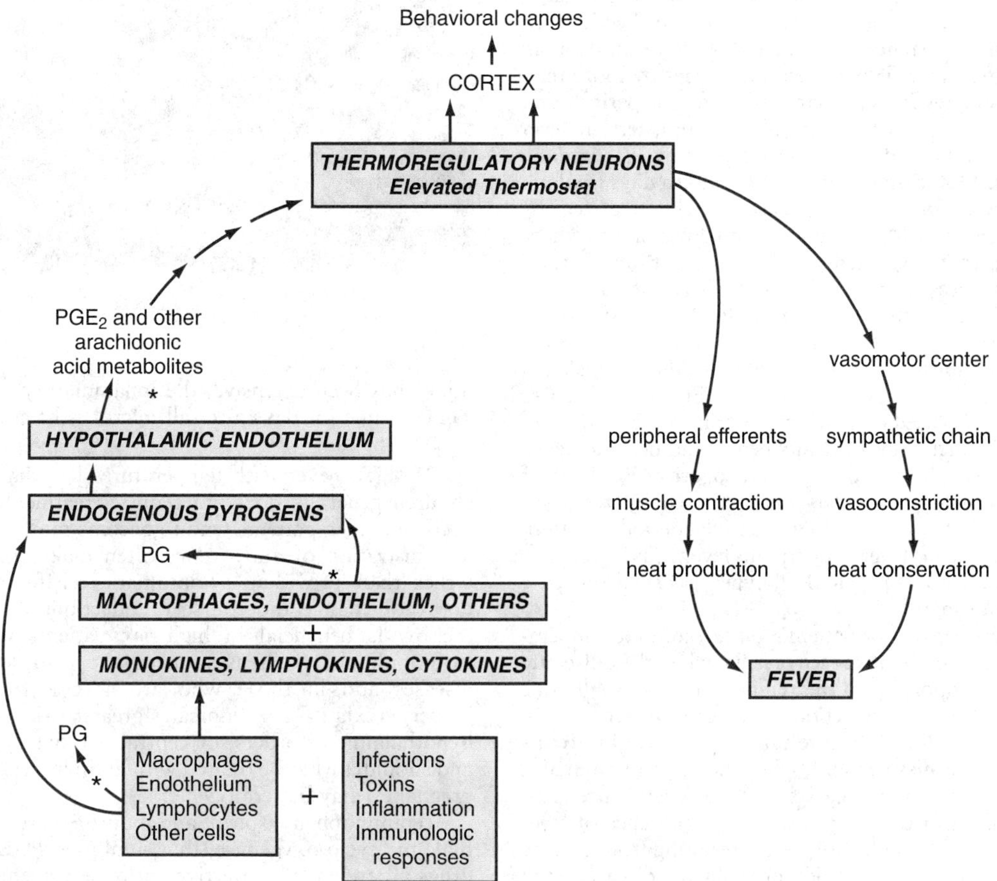

Figure 174-1. The pathogenesis of fever. Various infectious toxins and other mediators induce the production of endogenous pyrogens by host inflammatory cells. Endogenous pyrogens include the cytokines interleukin 1 (IL-1) and IL-6, tumor necrosis factor-α (TNF-α), and interferon-β (IFN-β) and IFN-γ. Endogenous pyrogenic cytokines directly stimulate the hypothalamus to produce prostaglandin E_2 (PGE_2), which then resets the temperature regulatory set point. Neuronal transmission from the hypothalamus leads to conservation and generation of heat, thus raising core body temperature. (From Dinarello CA, Cannon JG, Wolff SM: New concepts on the pathogenesis of fever. *Rev Infect Dis* 1988;10:168–189.)

gests that fever is an adaptive response and should be treated only in selected circumstances. However, fever increases oxygen consumption, carbon dioxide production, and cardiac output, and may exacerbate cardiac insufficiency in patients with heart disease or chronic anemia (e.g., sickle cell disease), pulmonary insufficiency in those with chronic lung disease, and metabolic instability in children with diabetes mellitus or inborn errors of metabolism. Furthermore, children between the ages of 6 mo and 5 yr are at increased risk for benign febrile seizures, whereas those with idiopathic epilepsy may have an increased frequency of seizures associated with a febrile illness (see Chapter 593.1).

CLINICAL MANIFESTATIONS. Although fever patterns per se are not often helpful in determining a specific diagnosis, observing the clinical characteristics of fever can provide useful information. In general, a single isolated fever spike is not associated with an infectious disease. Such a spike can be attributed to the infusion of blood products, some drugs, some procedures, or manipulation of a catheter on a colonized or infected body surface. Similarly, temperatures in excess of 41°C are most often associated with a noninfectious cause. Causes of very high temperatures (>41°C) include **central fever** (resulting from central nervous system dysfunction involving the hypothalamus), malignant hyperthermia, malignant neuroleptic syndrome, drug fever, or heatstroke. Temperatures that are lower than normal (<36°C) can be associated with overwhelming sepsis but are more commonly related to cold exposure, hypothyroidism, or overuse of antipyretics.

Intermittent fever is an exaggerated circadian rhythm that includes a period of normal temperatures on most days; extremely wide fluctuations may be termed **septic or hectic fever. Sustained fever** is persistent and does not vary by more than 0.5°C/day. **Remittent fever** is persistent and varies by more than 0.5°C/day. **Relapsing fever** is characterized by febrile periods that are separated by intervals of normal temperature; **tertian fever** occurs on the 1st and 3rd days (malaria caused by *Plasmodium vivax*), and **quartan fever** occurs on the 1st and 4th days (malaria caused by *Plasmodium malariae*). Diseases characterized by relapsing fevers (Table 174-1) should be distinguished from those infectious diseases that have a tendency to relapse. **Biphasic fever** indicates a single illness with 2 distinct periods (**camelback fever pattern**); poliomyelitis is the classic example. A biphasic course is also characteristic of leptospirosis, dengue fever, yellow fever, Colorado tick fever, spirillary rat-bite fever *(Spirillum minus)*, and the African hemorrhagic fevers (Marburg, Ebola, and Lassa fever). **Periodic fever** is used narrowly to describe fever syndromes with a regular periodicity (cyclic neutropenia, and periodic fever, aphthous stomatitis, pharyngitis, and adenopathy [PFAPA]) or more broadly to include disorders characterized by recurrent episodes of fever that do not follow a strictly periodic pattern (familial Mediterranean fever, Hibernian fever, TNF-receptor-associated periodic syndrome [TRAPS], hyper-IgD syndrome, the Muckle-Wells syndrome).

The relationship between a patient's pulse rate and temperature can be informative. **Relative tachycardia**, when the pulse rate is elevated out of proportion to the temperature, is usually due to noninfectious diseases or infectious diseases in which a toxin is responsible for the clinical manifestations. **Relative bradycardia (temperature-pulse dissociation)**, when the pulse rate remains low in the presence of fever, suggests typhoid fever, brucellosis, leptospirosis, or drug fever. Bradycardia in the presence of fever also may be a result of a conduction defect resulting from cardiac involvement with acute rheumatic fever, Lyme disease, viral myocarditis, or infective endocarditis.

Most infections result in some type of injury that induces an inflammatory response and subsequently results in the release of endogenous pyrogens. Administration of antimicrobial agents can result in a very rapid elimination of bacteria, but if tissue injury has been extensive, the inflammatory response and fever can continue for days after all microbes have been eradicated.

TABLE 174-1. Fevers Prone to Relapse

INFECTIOUS CAUSES
Relapsing fever (*Borrelia recurrentis*)
Trench fever (*Rochalimaea quintana*)
Q Fever (*Coxiella burnetii*)
Typhoid fever (*Salmonella typhi*)
Syphilis (*Treponema pallidum*)
Tuberculosis
Histoplasmosis
Coccidioidomycosis
Blastomycosis
Melioidosis (*Pseudomonas pseudomallei*)
Lymphocytic choriomeningitis (LCM) virus
Dengue fever
Yellow fever
Chronic meningococcemia
Colorado tick fever
Leptospirosis
Brucellosis
Oroya fever (*Bartonella bacilliformis*)
Acute rheumatic fever
Rat-bite fever (*Spirillum minus*)
Visceral leishmaniasis
Lyme disease (*Leptospira burgdorferi*)
Malaria
Babesiosis
Noninfluenza respiratory viruses
Epstein-Barr virus
NONINFECTIOUS CAUSES
Behçet disease
Crohn disease
Weber-Christian disease (panniculitis)
Leukoclastic angiitis
Sweet syndrome
Systemic lupus erythematosus
PERIODIC FEVER SYNDROMES
Familial Mediterranean fever
Cyclic neutropenia
Periodic fever, aphthous stomatitis, pharyngitis, adenopathy (PFAPA)
Hyper IgD syndrome
Hibernian fever (tumor necrosis factor super-family IgA-associated syndrome [TRAPS])
Muckle-Wells syndrome

Modified from Cunha BA: The clinical significance of fever patterns. *Infect Dis Clin North Am* 1996;10:33–44.

TREATMENT. Fever with temperatures less than 39°C in healthy children generally does not require treatment. As temperatures become higher, patients tend to become more uncomfortable and administration of antipyretics often makes patients feel better. Other than providing symptomatic relief, antipyretic therapy does not change the course of infectious diseases. Antipyretic therapy is beneficial in high-risk patients who have chronic cardiopulmonary diseases, metabolic disorders, or neurologic diseases and in those who are at risk for febrile seizures. **Hyperpyrexia** (>41°C) indicates greater risk for severe infection, hypothalamic disorders, or central nervous system hemorrhage, and should always be treated with antipyretics. High fever during pregnancy may be teratogenic.

Acetaminophen, aspirin, and ibuprofen are inhibitors of hypothalamic cyclo-oxygenase, thus inhibiting PGE_2 synthesis. These drugs all are equally effective antipyretic agents. Because aspirin has been associated with Reye syndrome in children and adolescents, it is not recommended for the treatment of fever. Acetaminophen, 10–15 mg/kg orally every 4 hr, is not associated with significant adverse effects; however, prolonged use may produce renal injury, and massive overdose may produce hepatic failure.

Ibuprofen, 5-10 mg/kg orally every 6–8 hr, is also effective and may cause dyspepsia, gastrointestinal bleeding, reduced renal blood flow, and rarely, aseptic meningitis, hepatic toxicity, or aplastic anemia. Serious injury from ibuprofen overdose is unusual. Alternating acetaminophen and ibuprofen Q 4–6 hr or giving both drugs at the same time are also effective. Tepid sponge bathing in warm water (not alcohol) is another recommended method of reducing hyperpyrexia due to infection or hyperthermia resulting from external causes (heatstroke). The decline of body temperature after antipyretic therapy does not distinguish serious bacterial from less serious viral diseases.

Crocetti M, Moghbeli N, Serwint J: Fever phobia revisited: Have parental misconceptions about fever changed in 20 years? *Pediatrics* 2001;107:1241–1246.
Cunha BA: The clinical significance of fever patterns. *Infect Dis Clin North Am* 1996;10:33–44.
Dinarello CA, Cannon JG, Wolff SM: New concepts on the pathogenesis of fever. *Rev Infect Dis* 1988;10:168–189.
Dode C, Andre M, Bienvenu T, et al: The enlarging clinical, genetic, and population spectrum of tumor necrosis factor receptor-associated periodic syndrome. *Arthritis Rheum* 2002;46:2181–2188.
Drenth JP, Van Der Meer JW: Hereditary periodic fever. *N Engl J Med* 2001;345:1748–1757.
Erlewyn-Lajeunesse MDS, Coppens K, Hunt LP, et al: Randomized controlled trial of combined paracetamol and ibuprofen for fever. *Arch Dis Child* 2006;91:414–416.
Kluger MJ, Kozak W, Conn C, et al: The adaptive value of fever. *Infect Dis Clin North Am* 1996;10:1–20.
Mackowiak PA, Boulant JA: Fever's glass ceiling. *Clin Infect Dis* 1996;22: 525–536.
Saper CB, Breder CD: The neurologic basis of fever. *N Engl J Med* 1994;330:1880–1886.
Sarrel EM, Wielunsky E, Cohen HA: Antipyretic treatment in young children with fever: Acetaminophen, ibuprofen, or both alternating in a randomized, double-blind study. *Arch Pediatr Adolesc Med* 2006;160:197–202.
Scholl PR: Periodic fever syndromes. *Curr Opin Pediatr* 2000;12:563–560.

Chapter 175 ■ Fever Without a Focus

Keith R. Powell

Fever is a common manifestation of infectious diseases but is not predictive of severity. Many common viral (rhinitis, pharyngitis, pneumonia) and bacterial (otitis media, pharyngitis, impetigo) infections are usually benign in normal hosts and respond well to appropriate antimicrobial or supportive therapy. Other infections (sepsis, meningitis, pneumonia, osteoarticular infections, pyelonephritis), if untreated, may have significant morbidity or mortality. Most febrile episodes in a normal host can be diagnosed by a careful history and physical examination and require few if any laboratory tests. There are well-defined high-risk groups that, on the basis of age, associated diseases, or immunodeficiency status, require a more extensive evaluation and, in certain situations, prompt antimicrobial therapy before a pathogen is identified (Table 175-1).

FEVER WITHOUT LOCALIZING SIGNS

Fever without localizing signs or symptoms, usually of acute onset and present for <1 wk, is a common diagnostic dilemma for pediatricians caring for children <36 mo of age. Infants <4 wk of age may acquire community pathogens but are also at risk for late-onset neonatal bacterial diseases and perinatally acquired herpes simplex virus infection. Young infants demonstrate limited signs of infection, often making it difficult to clinically distinguish between a serious bacterial infection and self-limited viral illness.

TABLE 175-1. Febrile Patients at Increased Risk for Serious Bacterial Infections

RISK GROUP	DIAGNOSTIC CONSIDERATIONS
IMMUNOCOMPETENT PATIENTS	
Neonates (<28 days)	Sepsis and meningitis caused by group B streptococcus, *Escherichia coli, Listeria monocytogenes*, and herpes simplex virus
Infants <3 mo	Serious bacterial disease in 10–15%, including bacteremia in 5% of febrile infants <3 mo; urinary tract infection common
Infants and children 3–36 mo	Occult bacteremia in <0.5% of children immunized with both *Haemophilus influenzae* type b and pneumococcal conjugate vaccines; urinary tract infections common
Hyperpyrexia (>40°C)	Meningitis, bacteremia, pneumonia, heatstroke, hemorrhagic shock–encephalopathy syndrome
Fever with petechiae	Bacteremia and meningitis caused by *Neisseria meningitides, H. influenzae* type b, and *Streptococcus pneumoniae*
IMMUNOCOMPROMISED PATIENTS	
Sickle cell disease	Sepsis, pneumonia, and meningitis caused by *S. pneumoniae*, osteomyelitis caused by *Salmonella* and *Staphylococcus aureus*
Asplenia	Bacteremia and meningitis caused by *N. meningitidis, H. influenzae* type b, and *S. pneumoniae*
Complement/properdin deficiency	Sepsis caused by *N. meningitidis*
Agammaglobulinemia	Bacteremia, sinopulmonary infections
AIDS	*S. pneumoniae, H. influenzae* type b, and *Salmonella* infections
Congenital heart disease	Infective endocarditis; brain abscess with right-to-left shunting
Central venous line	*Staphylococcus aureus*, coagulase-negative staphylococci, *Candida*
Malignancy	Bacteremia with gram-negative enteric bacteria, *S. aureus*, and coagulase-negative staphylococci; fungemia with *Candida* and *Aspergillus*

INFANTS <3 MO OF AGE. An infectious agent, usually viral, is identified in 70% of infants <3 mo of age with fever; the remainder are presumed to have self-limited but undiagnosed viral infections. However, fever in an infant <3 mo of age should always suggest the possibility of serious bacterial disease. Serious bacterial infections are present in 10–15% of previously healthy full-term infants presenting with rectal temperatures of ≥38°C. These infections include sepsis, meningitis, urinary tract infections, enteritis, osteomyelitis, and suppurative arthritis. Bacteremia is present in 5% of febrile infants <3 mo of age; organisms responsible for bacteremia include group B streptococcus and *Listeria monocytogenes* (late-onset neonatal sepsis and meningitis) and community-acquired pathogens including *Salmonella* (enteritis), *Escherichia coli* (urinary tract infection), *Neisseria meningitidis, Streptococcus pneumoniae,* and *Haemophilus influenzae* type b (sepsis and meningitis), and *Staphylococcus aureus* (osteoarticular infection). Pyelonephritis is more common in uncircumcised infant boys, neonates and infants with urinary tract anomalies, and young girls. Other potential bacterial diseases in this age group include otitis media, pneumonia, omphalitis, mastitis, and other skin and soft tissue infections.

Viral pathogens can be identified in 40–60% of febrile infants <3 mo of age. In contrast to bacterial infections, which have no seasonal pattern, viral diseases have a distinct pattern: respiratory syncytial virus and influenza A virus infections are more common during the winter, whereas enterovirus infections usually occur in the summer and fall.

The approach to febrile patients <3 mo of age includes a careful history and physical examination. **Ill-appearing (toxic)** febrile infants <3 mo of age require prompt hospitalization and immediate parenteral antimicrobial therapy after cultures of blood, urine, and cerebrospinal fluid (CSF) are obtained. Ceftriaxone (50 mg/kg/dose every 24 hr with normal CSF findings, or 80 mg/kg/dose every 24 hr with CSF pleocytosis) or cefotaxime

(50 mg/kg/dose every 6 hr), plus ampicillin (50 mg/kg/dose every 6 hr) to cover for *L. monocytogenes* and enterococcus, is an effective initial antimicrobial regimen for **ill-appearing** infants without focal findings. This regimen is effective against the usual bacterial pathogens causing sepsis, urinary tract infection, and enteritis in young infants. However, if meningitis is suspected because of CSF abnormalities, vancomycin (15 mg/kg/dose every 6 hr) should be given to cover for possible penicillin-resistant *S. pneumoniae,* in addition to the ceftriaxone/cefotaxime and ampicillin, until the results of culture and susceptibility tests are known.

Infants <3 mo of age with fever who appear **generally well;** who have been previously healthy; who have no evidence of skin, soft tissue, bone, joint, or ear infection; and who have a total white blood cell (WBC) count of 5,000–15,000 cells/μL, an absolute band count of <1,500 cells/μL, and normal urinalysis and negative culture results are unlikely to have a serious bacterial infection. The negative predictive value with 95% confidence of these criteria for any serious bacterial infection is >98%, and >99% for bacteremia. Of all serious bacterial infections, pyelonephritis is common and may be seen in well-appearing infants without a focus or in those who appear ill. Bacteremia is present in less than 30% of infants with pyelonephritis. Urinalysis may be negative in infants ≤1–2 mo of age (see Chapters 519.4 and 538).

OCCULT BACTEREMIA IN CHILDREN 3 MO TO 3 YR OF AGE. Approximately 30% of febrile children 3 mo to 3 yr of age have no localizing signs of infection. Occult bacteremia (bacteremia without an apparent focus of infection) due to *S. pneumoniae, N. meningitidis,* and *Salmonella* occurred in approximately 1.5% of relatively well-appearing children between 3 and 36 mo of age with fever (rectal temperature ≥39°C) before conjugated pneumococcal vaccine was recommended for all infants in 2000. The incidence of invasive pneumococcal disease in children <2 yr of age decreased from 188 cases per 100,000 in 1999 to 59 cases per 100,000 in 2000, the year pneumococcal conjugate vaccine was introduced. The observed rate of occult bacteremia at one children's hospital emergency department in 2002 was <1%. The increased incidence of bacteremia among young children may be due in part to a maturational immune deficiency in the production of opsonic IgG antibodies to the polysaccharide antigens present on encapsulated bacteria. *S. pneumoniae* accounts for 90% of cases of occult bacteremia, with *N. meningitidis* and *Salmonella* accounting for most of the remaining positive cultures. *H. influenzae* type b was an important cause of occult bacteremia in young children before the universal use of conjugate *H. influenzae* type b vaccines. Common bacterial infections among children 3–36 mo of age that have localizing signs include otitis media, upper respiratory tract infection, pneumonia, enteritis, urinary tract infection (may have no localizing signs) [see Chapter 538], osteomyelitis, and meningitis (see Chapter 602).

Risk factors indicating increased probability of occult bacteremia include temperature ≥39°C, WBC count ≥15,000/μL, or an elevated absolute neutrophil count, band count, erythrocyte sedimentation rate, or C-reactive protein. The incidence of bacteremia among infants 3–36 mo of age increases as the temperature and WBC count increase. However, no combination of laboratory tests or clinical assessment is completely accurate in predicting the presence of occult bacteremia. Socioeconomic status, race, gender, and age (within the range of 3–36 mo) do not appear to affect the risk for occult bacteremia.

Without therapy, occult bacteremia may resolve spontaneously without sequelae, may persist, or may lead to localized infections, such as meningitis, pneumonia, cellulitis, pericarditis, osteomyelitis, or suppurative arthritis. The pattern of sequelae may be related to both host factors and the offending organism. In some children, the occult bacteremic illness may represent the early signs of serious localized infection rather than merely a transient disease state. *H. influenzae* type b bacteremia is characteristically of higher grade, as determined by quantitative blood culture techniques, and is associated with a higher risk for localized serious infection than is bacteremia due to *S. pneumoniae.* Hospitalized children with *H. influenzae* type b bacteremia often develop focal infections, such as meningitis, epiglottitis, cellulitis, pericarditis, or osteoarticular infection, whereas fewer than 5% of these bacteremias can be considered transient or occult. In contrast, among all patients with pneumococcal bacteremia (occult, symptomatic, or focal), spontaneous resolution occurs in 30–40%, with a higher rate of spontaneous resolution among well-appearing children with occult pneumococcal bacteremia.

Treatment of **toxic-appearing** febrile children 3–36 mo of age who do not have focal signs of infection includes hospitalization and prompt institution of antimicrobial therapy after specimens of blood, urine, and CSF are obtained for culture. Meningitis in patients with occult bacteremia that develops after a lumbar puncture does not represent inoculation of bacteria by the puncture but is coincidental and represents meningeal infection that was developing before the lumbar puncture.

A retrospective review of more than 500 well-appearing febrile children discharged from an emergency department since 1987 and subsequently confirmed to be bacteremic with *S. pneumoniae* found 28% of untreated children to have persistent bacteremia or a focal infection (4% had meningitis) compared with only 5% of children who had received oral or parenteral antimicrobials when 1st seen (1% had meningitis). In addition, children who received antimicrobial therapy were less likely to be febrile upon return. A retrospective study of children with bacterial meningitis showed that children who received antimicrobial therapy before the diagnosis of *S. pneumoniae* meningitis was confirmed had fewer complications attributable to meningitis. These findings argue for empirical antimicrobial therapy for well-appearing children <36 mo of age who have not received *H. influenzae* type b and *S. pneumoniae* conjugate vaccines who have a rectal temperature of ≥39°C and a WBC count of ≥15,000/μL.

Consensus practice guidelines published in 1993 recommended that infants 3–36 mo of age who have a temperature of <39°C and who do not appear toxic can be observed as outpatients without performing diagnostic tests or administering antimicrobial agents. For nontoxic-appearing infants with a rectal temperature of ≥39°C, 2 options were suggested: (1) obtain a blood culture and give empirical antimicrobial therapy (ceftriaxone, a single dose of 50 mg/kg, not to exceed 1 g) or (2) if the WBC count is ≥15,000/μL, obtain a blood culture and begin empirical antimicrobial therapy. A 3rd option, not offered in these guidelines, for selected infants is to obtain a blood culture and observe as outpatients without empirical antimicrobial therapy with return for re-evaluation within 24 hr. Regardless of the management option, the family should be instructed to return immediately if the child's condition deteriorates or new symptoms, such as rash, develop.

Studies of febrile infants 3–36 mo of age conducted in the United States since the introduction of universal immunization of infants with *H. influenzae* type b conjugate vaccines have demonstrated that this pathogen has been virtually eliminated as a cause of occult bacteremia. In 2000, a heptavalent *S. pneumoniae* conjugate vaccine was introduced and recommended for universal administration during infancy. Based on efficacy trials, it is anticipated that there will be a significant (≥90%) decrease in occult bacteremia caused by *S. pneumoniae* in vaccinated infants. Surveillance data from 2000 showed a 69% decrease in the incidence of invasive pneumococcal disease in children <2 yr of age (Fig. 175-1). Guidelines for the management of febrile children 3–36 mo of age who have received both *H. influenzae* type b and *S. pneumoniae* conjugate vaccines have yet to be established, but a stronger case for careful observation without the empirical administration of antimicrobial agents can be made.

If *S. pneumoniae* is isolated from the blood, the child should return to the physician as soon as possible after the culture results

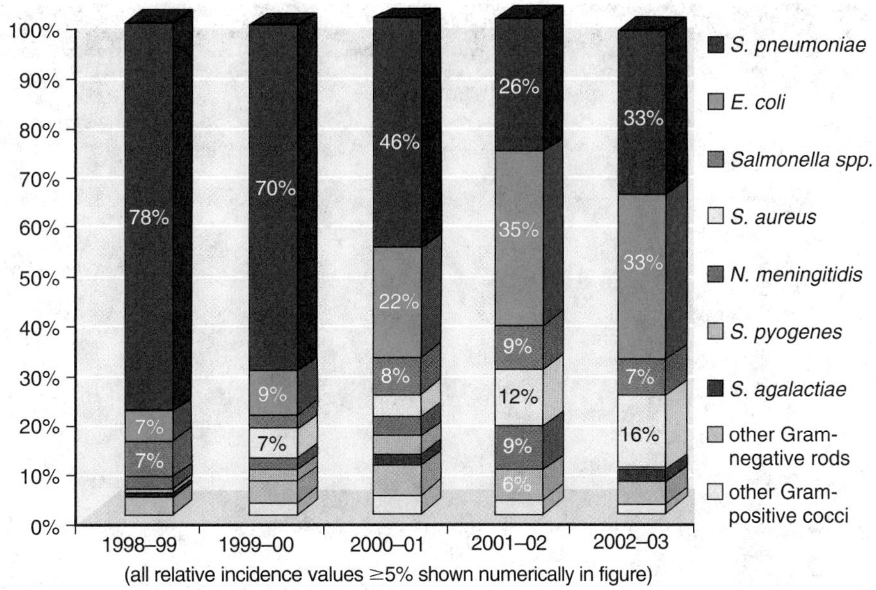

Figure 175-1. Relative incidence of bacteremia by organism from previously healthy children ages 3 mo to 3 yr presenting to outpatient settings at Kaiser Permanente Northern California from 1998 to 2003. All relative incidence values ≥5% shown numerically in figure. (From Herz AM, Greenhow TL, Alcantara J, et al: Changing epidemiology of outpatient bacteremia in 3- to 36-month-old children after the introduction of the heptavalent-conjugated pneumococcal vaccine. *Pediatr Infect Dis J* 2006;25(4):293–300.)

are known. If the child appears well, is afebrile, and the physical findings remain normal, a second blood culture should be obtained if the child did not receive antimicrobial treatment at the 1st visit; all children should then receive a total of 7–10 days of oral antimicrobial therapy. If the child appears ill and continues to have fever with no identifiable focus of infection, or if pneumococcus, *H. influenzae,* or *N. meningitidis* is present in the initial blood culture, the child should have a repeat blood culture, be evaluated for meningitis (including lumbar puncture), and receive treatment in the hospital with appropriate antimicrobial agents. If the initial blood culture remains negative and the child improves in the emergency room with supportive therapy and is no longer ill appearing (normal age-appropriate vital signs, including blood pressure, normal level of consciousness, and age-appropriate behavior), the child may receive ceftriaxone and be managed as an outpatient. If the child develops a localized infection, therapy is directed toward the specific pathogen and the particular site.

FEVER WITH PETECHIAE. Independent of age, fever with petechiae in an ill-appearing patient with or without localizing signs indicates high risk for life-threatening bacterial infections such as bacteremia, sepsis, and meningitis. From 8 to 20% of patients with fever and petechiae have a serious bacterial infection, and 7–10% have meningococcal sepsis or meningitis (see Chapter 190). *H. influenzae* type b disease (see Chapter 192) and Rocky Mountain spotted fever (Chapter 225.1) can also present with fever and petechiae. Management includes prompt hospitalization, culture of blood and CSF, and administration of appropriate parenteral antimicrobial agents. Well-appearing patients with fever and petechiae can be evaluated with a complete blood count and platelet count as well as a blood culture with observation in the office or emergency room. If no further petechiae develop or if they are secondary to emesis or coughing and the patient remains well, the patient can be managed as an outpatient with or without antibiotics depending on the most likely cause of the petechiae.

FEVER IN PATIENTS WITH SICKLE CELL DISEASE. Infection is the most common cause of death among children with sickle cell disease (see Chapter 462.1). The incidence of infection is greatest among children <5 yr of age. The increased risk for infection in these children is due in part to functional asplenia and a defect in the properdin (alternate complement) pathway. Fever without localizing signs in patients with sickle cell disease is a common presentation of infection caused by *S. pneumoniae* (sepsis, pneumonia, meningitis), *H. influenzae* type b (meningitis), *S. aureus* (osteomyelitis), *Salmonella* (osteomyelitis), and *E. coli* (pyelonephritis).

The management of patients with sickle cell hemoglobinopathies requires culture of blood and, if indicated, CSF, stool, and bone, and administration of antimicrobial agents. Children who appear seriously ill, have temperatures of ≥40°C, have a WBC count of <5,000/μL or >30,000/μL, or who have pulmonary infiltrates or complications of sickle cell disease or severe pain should be hospitalized. Other febrile infants with sickle cell disease can be given intramuscular ceftriaxone and cared for as outpatients after appropriate specimens have been obtained for culture. These children should be re-evaluated within 24 hr, or earlier if their condition deteriorates or new symptoms develop.

Prevention of pneumococcal sepsis is possible by instituting long-term penicillin therapy continued until adolescence (oral penicillin V, 125 mg twice daily for children <5 yr of age and 250 mg orally twice daily for children ≥5 yr of age). Pneumococcal and *H. influenzae* vaccines provide some protection but do not supplant long-term antimicrobial therapy.

HYPERPYREXIA. Hyperpyrexia (temperature >41°C) is uncommon and is not associated with higher rates of serious bacterial infections than temperatures of 40°C. Infants and children with hyperpyrexia should be carefully evaluated as for all children with fever.

FEVER OF UNKNOWN ORIGIN

The term **fever of unknown origin** (FUO) is best reserved for children with a fever documented by a health care provider and for which the cause could not be identified after 3 wk of evaluation as an outpatient or after 1 wk of evaluation in hospital. Patients with fever not meeting these criteria, and specifically those admitted to the hospital with neither an apparent site of infection nor a noninfectious diagnosis, may be considered to have **fever without localizing signs.** In most of these children, the development of additional clinical manifestations over a relatively short period confirms the infectious nature of the illness.

TABLE 175-2. Diagnostic Considerations of Fever of Unknown Origin in Children

- Abscesses: abdominal, brain, dental, hepatic, pelvic, perinephric, rectal, subphrenic, psoas
- Infections
  - Bacteria
    - Caused by specific organism
      - Actinomycosis
      - *Bartonella henselae* (cat-scratch disease)
      - Brucellosis
      - *Campylobacter*
      - *Francisella tularensis* (Tularemia)
      - *Listeria monocytogenes* (Listeriosis)
      - Meningococcemia (chronic)
      - *Mycoplasma pneumoniae*
      - Rat-bite fever (*Streptobacillus moniliformis;* streptobacillary form of rat-bite fever)
      - *Salmonella*
      - Tuberculosis
      - Yersiniosis
    - Localized infections
      - Cholangitis
      - Infective endocarditis
      - Mastoiditis
      - Osteomyelitis
      - Pneumonia
      - Pyelonephritis
      - Sinusitis
  - Spirochetes
    - *Borrelia burgdorferi* (Lyme disease)
    - Relapsing fever (*Borrelia recurrentis*)
    - Leptospirosis
    - Rat-bite fever (*Spirillum minus;* spirillary form of rat-bite fever)
    - Syphilis
  - Fungal diseases
    - Blastomycosis (extrapulmonary)
    - Coccidiodomycosis (disseminated)
    - Histoplasmosis (disseminated)
  - *Chlamydia*
    - Lymphogranuloma venereum
    - Psittacosis
  - *Rickettsia*
    - *Ehrlichia canis*
    - Q fever
    - Rocky Mountain spotted fever
    - Tick-borne typhus
  - Viruses
    - Cytomegalovirus
    - Hepatitis viruses
    - HIV
    - Infectious mononucleosis (Epstein-Barr virus)
- Parasitic diseases
  - Amebiasis
  - Babesiosis
  - Giardiasis
  - Malaria
  - Toxoplasmosis
  - Trichinosis
  - Trypanosomiasis
  - Visceral larva migrans (*Toxocara*)
- Rheumatologic diseases
  - Behçet disease
  - Juvenile dermatomyositis
  - Juvenile rheumatoid arthritis
  - Rheumatic fever
  - Systemic lupus erythematosus
- Hypersensitivity diseases
  - Drug fever
  - Hypersensitivity pneumonitis
  - Pancreatitis
  - Serum sickness
  - Weber-Christian disease
- Neoplasms
  - Atrial myxoma
  - Cholesterol granuloma
  - Hodgkin disease
  - Inflammatory pseudotumor
  - Leukemia
  - Lymphoma
  - Neuroblastoma
  - Wilms tumor
- Granulomatous diseases
  - Crohn disease
  - Granulomatous hepatitis
  - Sarcoidosis
- Familial-hereditary diseases
  - Anhidrotic ectodermal dysplasia
  - Fabry disease
  - Familial dysautonomia
  - Familial Mediterranean fever
  - Hypertriglyceridemia
  - Ichthyosis
  - Sickle cell crisis
- Miscellaneous
  - Chronic active hepatitis
  - Diabetes insipidus (non-nephrogenic and nephrogenic)
  - Factitious fever
  - Hemophagocytic syndromes
  - Hypothalamic-central fever
  - Infantile cortical hyperostosis
  - Inflammatory bowel disease
  - Kawasaki disease
  - Kikuchi-Fujimoto disease
  - Pancreatitis
  - Periodic fevers
  - Poisoning
  - Pulmonary embolism
  - Thrombophlebitis
  - Thyrotoxicosis
- Recurrent or relapsing fever
  - See Table 174-1
- Undiagnosed fever
  - Persistent
  - Recurrent
  - Resolved

ETIOLOGY. The principal causes of FUO in children, using these rigorous criteria, are infections and rheumatologic (connective tissue or autoimmune) diseases (Table 175-2). Neoplastic disorders should also be seriously considered, although most children with malignancies do not have fever alone. The possibility of drug fever should be considered if the patient is receiving any drug. Drug fever is usually sustained and not associated with other symptoms. Discontinuation of the drug is associated with resolution of the fever, generally within 72 hr, although certain drugs, such as iodides, are excreted for a prolonged period with fever that may persist for as long as 1 mo after drug withdrawal.

Most fevers of unknown or unrecognized origin result from atypical presentations of common diseases. In some cases, the presentation as an FUO is characteristic of the disease, such as juvenile rheumatoid arthritis (JRA), but the definitive diagnosis can be established only after prolonged observation because initially there are no associated or specific findings on physical examination and all laboratory results are negative or normal.

In the United States, the systemic infectious diseases most commonly implicated in children with FUO (by the rigorous criteria) are salmonellosis, tuberculosis, rickettsial diseases, syphilis, Lyme disease, cat-scratch disease, atypical prolonged presentations of common viral diseases, infectious mononucleosis, cytomegalovirus (CMV) infection, viral hepatitis, coccidioidomycosis, histoplasmosis, malaria, and toxoplasmosis. Less common infectious causes of FUO include tularemia, brucellosis, leptospirosis, and rat-bite fever. AIDS alone is not usually responsible for FUO, although febrile illnesses frequently occur in patients with AIDS as a result of opportunistic infections.

JRA and systemic lupus erythematosus are the connective tissue diseases associated most frequently with FUO. Inflammatory bowel disease, rheumatic fever, and Kawasaki disease are also commonly reported as causes of FUO. If factitious fever (inoculation of pyogenic material or manipulation of the thermometer by the patient or parent) is suspected, the presence and pattern of fever should be documented in the hospital. Prolonged and continuous observation, which may include electronic surveillance, of patients is imperative. FUO lasting more than 6 mo is uncommon in children and suggests granulomatosis or autoimmune disease. Repeat interval evaluation, including history, physical examination, and roentgenographic studies, is required.

DIAGNOSIS. The evaluation of FUO requires a thorough history and physical examination supplemented by a few screening laboratory tests, and additional laboratory and radiographic tests as indicated by the history or abnormalities found on examination or initial screening (Fig. 175-2).

History. The age of the patient is helpful in evaluating FUO. Children <6 yr of age often have a respiratory or genitourinary tract infection, localized infection (abscess, osteomyelitis), JRA, or, rarely, leukemia. Adolescent patients are more likely to have tuberculosis, inflammatory bowel disease, autoimmune processes, or lymphoma, in addition to the causes of FUO found in younger children.

A history of exposure to wild or domestic animals should be solicited. Zoonotic infections in the U.S. are increasing in frequency and are often acquired from pets that are not overtly ill.

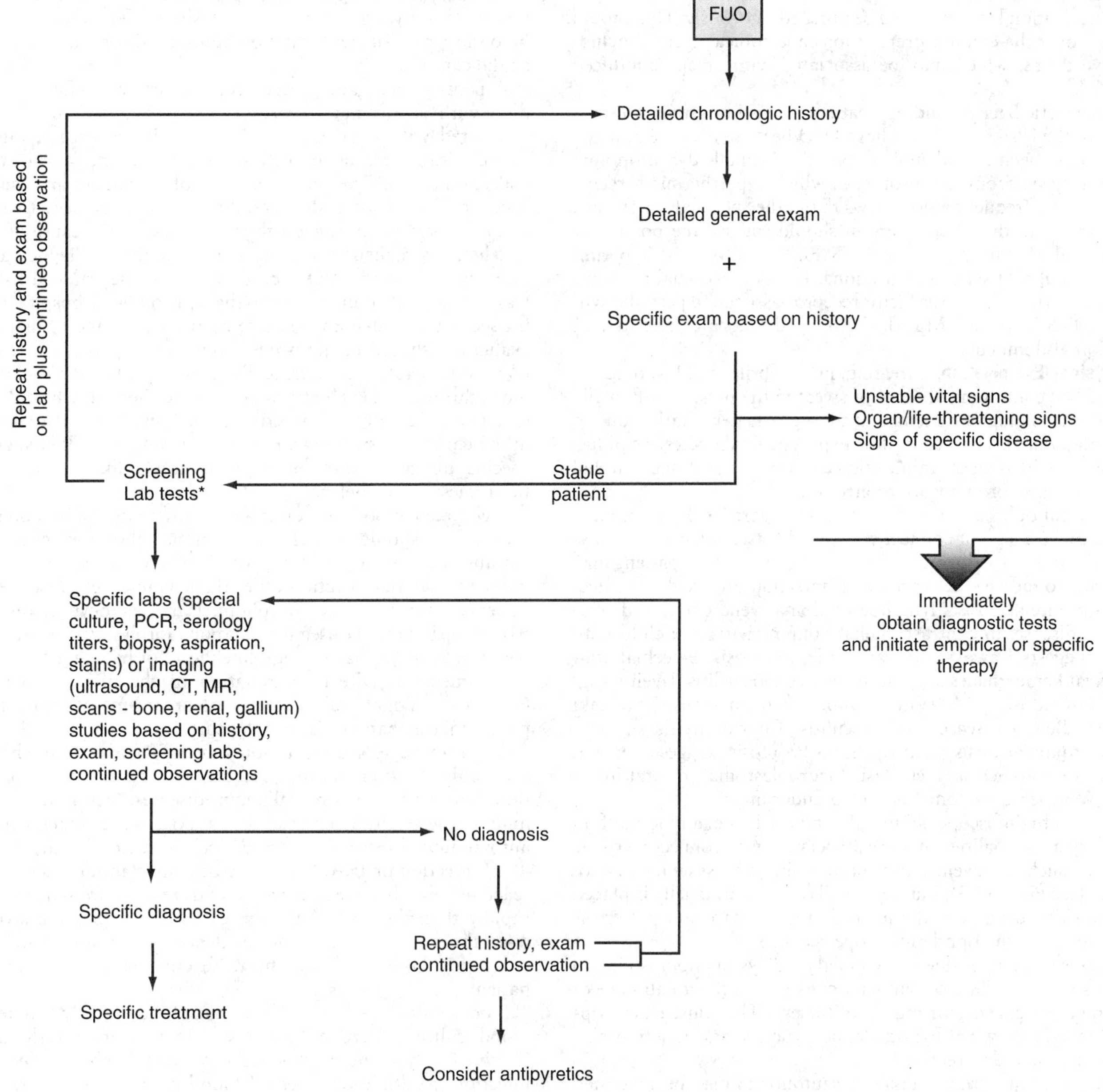

Figure 175-2. Approach to the evaluation of fever of unknown origin (FUO) in children. *Screening laboratory tests (labs) include a complete blood cell count, measurement of erythrocyte sedimentation rate, urinalysis, blood and urine cultures, and a chest radiograph. PCR, polymerase chain reaction. (From Kliegman RM, Greenbaum LA, Lye PS (editors): *Practical Strategies in Pediatric Diagnosis and Therapy,* 2nd ed. Philadelphia, Elsevier/Saunders, 2004, p 990.)

Immunization of dogs against specific disorders such as leptospirosis may prevent canine disease but does not always prevent the animal from carrying and shedding leptospires, which may be transmitted to household contacts. A history of ingestion of rabbit or squirrel meat may provide a clue to the diagnosis of oropharyngeal, glandular, or typhoidal tularemia. A history of tick bite or travel to tick- or parasite-infested areas should be obtained.

Any history of pica should be elicited. Ingestion of dirt is a particularly important clue to infection with *Toxocara* (visceral larva migrans) or *Toxoplasma gondii* (toxoplasmosis).

A history of unusual dietary habits or travel as early as the birth of the child should be sought. Malaria, histoplasmosis, and coccidioidomycosis may re-emerge years after visiting or living in an endemic area. It is important to identify prophylactic immunizations and precautions taken by the individual against ingestion of contaminated water or food during foreign travel. Rocks, dirt, and artifacts from geographically distant regions that have been collected and brought into the home as souvenirs may serve as vectors of disease.

A medication history should be pursued rigorously. This should include over-the-counter preparations and topical agents, including eye drops, which may be associated with atropine-induced fever.

The genetic background of a patient also is important. Descendants of the Ulster Scots may have FUO because they are afflicted with nephrogenic diabetes insipidus. Familial dysautonomia (Riley-Day syndrome), a disorder in which hyperthermia is recurrent, is more frequent among Jews than other population groups. Ancestry from the Mediterranean should suggest the possibility of familial Mediterranean fever (FMF). Both FMF and hyperimmunoglobulin D syndrome are inherited as autosomal-recessive disorders. Tumor necrosis factor receptor-associated periodic syndrome (TRAPS) and Muckle-Wells syndrome are inherited as autosomal-dominant traits.

Physical Examination. Sweating in a febrile child should be noted. The continuing absence of sweat in the presence of an elevated or changing body temperature suggests dehydration due to vomiting, diarrhea, or central or nephrogenic diabetes insipidus. It also should suggest anhidrotic ectodermal dysplasia, familial dysautonomia, or exposure to atropine.

A careful ophthalmic examination is important. Red, weeping eyes may be a sign of connective tissue disease, particularly polyarteritis nodosa. Palpebral conjunctivitis in a febrile patient may be a clue to measles, coxsackievirus infection, tuberculosis, infectious mononucleosis, lymphogranuloma venereum, and cat-scratch disease. In contrast, bulbar conjunctivitis in a child with FUO suggests Kawasaki disease or leptospirosis. Petechial conjunctival hemorrhages suggest infective endocarditis. Uveitis suggests sarcoidosis, JRA, systemic lupus erythematosus, Kawasaki disease, Behçet disease, and vasculitis. Chorioretinitis suggests CMV, toxoplasmosis, and syphilis. Proptosis suggests orbital tumor, thyrotoxicosis, metastasis (neuroblastoma), orbital infection, Wegener granulomatosis, or pseudotumor.

The ophthalmoscope should also be used to examine nailfold capillary abnormalities that are associated with connective tissue diseases such as juvenile dermatomyositis and systemic scleroderma (see Fig. 158-3). Immersion oil or lubricating jelly is placed on the skin adjacent to the nailbed, and the capillary pattern is observed with the ophthalmoscope set on +40.

FUO is sometimes due to hypothalamic dysfunction. A clue to this disorder is failure of pupillary constriction due to absence of the sphincter constrictor muscle of the eye. This muscle develops embryologically when hypothalamic structure and function also are undergoing differentiation.

Fever resulting from familial dysautonomia may be suggested by lack of tears, an absent corneal reflex, or by a smooth tongue with absence of fungiform papillae. Tenderness to tapping over the sinuses or the upper teeth suggests sinusitis. Recurrent oral candidiasis may be a clue to various disorders of the immune system.

Fever blisters are common findings in patients with pneumococcal, streptococcal, malarial, and rickettsial infection. They also are common in children with meningococcal meningitis (which usually does not present as FUO) but rarely are seen in children with meningococcemia. Fever blisters also are rarely seen with *Salmonella* or staphylococcal infections.

Hyperemia of the pharynx, with or without exudate, suggests infectious mononucleosis, CMV infection, toxoplasmosis, salmonellosis, tularemia, Kawasaki disease, or leptospirosis.

The muscles and bones should be palpated carefully. Point tenderness over a bone may suggest occult osteomyelitis or bone marrow invasion from neoplastic disease. Tenderness over the trapezius muscle may be a clue to subdiaphragmatic abscess. Generalized muscle tenderness suggests dermatomyositis, trichinosis, polyarteritis, Kawasaki disease, or mycoplasmal or arboviral infection.

Rectal examination may reveal perirectal lymphadenopathy or tenderness, which suggests a deep pelvic abscess, iliac adenitis, or pelvic osteomyelitis. A guaiac test should be obtained; occult blood loss may suggest granulomatous colitis or ulcerative colitis as the cause of FUO.

Repetitive chills and temperature spikes are common in children with septicemia (regardless of cause), particularly when associated with renal disease, liver or biliary disease, infective endocarditis, malaria, brucellosis, rat-bite fever, or a loculated collection of pus. The general activity of the patient and the presence or absence of rashes should be noted. Hyperactive deep tendon reflexes may suggest thyrotoxicosis as the cause of FUO.

Laboratory Findings. Ordering a large number of diagnostic tests in every child with FUO according to a predetermined list may waste time and money. Alternatively, prolonged hospitalization for sequential tests may be more costly. The tempo of diagnostic evaluation should be adjusted to the tempo of the illness; haste may be imperative in a critically ill patient, but if the illness is more chronic, the evaluation can proceed more slowly and deliberately and, usually, in an outpatient setting. If there are no clues in the patient's history or on physical examination that suggest a specific infection or area of suspicion, it is unlikely that diagnostic studies will be helpful.

A complete blood cell count with a differential WBC count and a urinalysis should be part of the initial laboratory evaluation. An absolute neutrophil count of <5,000/μL is evidence against indolent bacterial infection other than typhoid fever. Conversely, patients with a polymorphonuclear leukocyte count of >10,000/μL or a nonsegmented polymorphonuclear leukocyte count of >500/μL have a high likelihood of having a severe bacterial infection. Direct examination of the blood smear with Giemsa or Wright stain may reveal organisms of malaria, trypanosomiasis, babesiosis, or relapsing fever.

An erythrocyte sedimentation rate (ESR) of >30 mm/hr indicates inflammation and the need for further evaluation for infectious, autoimmune, or malignant diseases. An ESR of >100 mm/hr suggests tuberculosis, Kawasaki disease, malignancy, or autoimmune disease. A low ESR does not eliminate the possibility of infection or JRA. C-reactive protein is another acute-phase reactant that becomes elevated and returns to normal more rapidly than the ESR. Although experts may prefer use of one over the other, there is no evidence that there is value in measuring both the ESR and C-reactive protein in the same patient.

Blood cultures should be obtained aerobically. Anaerobic blood cultures have an extremely low yield and should be obtained only if there are specific reasons to suspect anaerobic infection. Multiple or repeated blood cultures may be required to detect bacteremia associated with infective endocarditis, osteomyelitis, or deep-seated abscesses. Polymicrobial bacteremia suggests factitious self-induced infection or gastrointestinal pathology. The isolation of leptospires, *Francisella,* or *Yersinia* may require selective media or specific conditions not routinely used. Urine culture should be obtained routinely.

Tuberculin skin testing (TST) should be performed with intradermal placement of 5 units of purified protein derivative (PPD) that has been kept appropriately refrigerated.

Radiographic examination of the chest, sinuses, mastoids, or gastrointestinal tract may be indicated by specific historical or physical findings. Radiographic evaluation of the gastrointestinal tract for inflammatory bowel disease may be helpful in evaluating selected children with FUO and no other localizing signs or symptoms.

Examination of the bone marrow may reveal leukemia; metastatic neoplasm; mycobacterial, fungal, or parasitic diseases; and histiocytosis, hemophagocytosis, or storage diseases. If a bone marrow aspirate is performed, cultures for bacteria, mycobacteria, and fungi should be obtained.

Serologic tests may aid in the diagnosis of infectious mononucleosis, CMV infection, toxoplasmosis, salmonellosis, tularemia, brucellosis, leptospirosis, cat-scratch disease, Lyme disease, rickettsial disease, and, on some occasions, JRA. As serologic tests for more diseases become available through commercial laboratories, it is important to ascertain the sensitivity and specificity of each test before relying on these results to make a diagnosis. For example, serologic tests for Lyme disease outside of reference laboratories have been generally unreliable.

Radionuclide scans may be helpful in detecting abdominal abscesses as well as osteomyelitis, especially if the focus cannot be localized to a specific limb or multifocal disease is suspected. Gallium citrate (^{67}Ga) localizes in inflammatory tissues (leukocytes) associated with tumors or abscesses. ^{99m}Tc phosphate is useful for detecting osteomyelitis before plain roentgenograms demonstrate bone lesions. Granulocytes tagged with indium (^{111}In) or iodinated IgG may be useful in detecting localized pyogenic processes. Echocardiograms may demonstrate the presence of vegetation on the leaflets of heart valves, suggesting infective endocarditis. Ultrasonography may identify intra-abdominal abscesses of the liver, subphrenic space, pelvis, or spleen.

Total body CT or MRI permits detection of neoplasms and collections of purulent material without the use of surgical exploration or radioisotopes. CT and MRI are helpful in identifying lesions of the head, neck, chest, retroperitoneal spaces, liver, spleen, intra-abdominal and intrathoracic lymph nodes, kidneys, pelvis, and mediastinum. CT or ultrasound-guided aspiration or biopsy of suspicious lesions has reduced the need for exploratory laparotomy or thoracotomy. MRI is particularly useful for detecting osteomyelitis if there is concern about a specific limb. Diagnostic imaging can be very helpful in confirming or evaluating a suspected diagnosis but rarely leads to an unsuspected cause.

Biopsy is occasionally helpful in establishing a diagnosis of FUO. Bronchoscopy, laparoscopy, mediastinoscopy, and gastrointestinal endoscopy may provide direct visualization and biopsy material when organ-specific manifestations are present.

TREATMENT. Fever and infection in children are not synonymous; antimicrobial agents should not be used as antipyretics, and empirical trials of medication should generally be avoided. An exception may be the use of antituberculous treatment in critically ill children with suspected disseminated tuberculosis. Empirical trials of other antimicrobial agents may be dangerous and can obscure the diagnosis of infective endocarditis, meningitis, parameningeal infection, or osteomyelitis. Hospitalization may be required for laboratory or radiographic studies that are unavailable or impractical in an ambulatory setting, for more careful observation, or for temporary relief of parental anxiety. After a complete evaluation, antipyretics may be indicated to control fever and for symptomatic relief (see Chapter 174).

PROGNOSIS. Children with FUO have a better prognosis than do adults. The outcome in a child is dependent on the primary disease process, which is usually an atypical presentation of a common childhood illness. In many cases, no diagnosis can be established and fever abates spontaneously. In as many as 25% of cases in which fever persists, the cause of the fever remains unclear, even after thorough evaluation.

Bachur R, Harper MB: Reevaluation of outpatients with *Streptococcus pneumoniae* bacteremia. *Pediatrics* 2000;105:502–509.

Bandyopadhyay S, Bergholte J, Blackwell C, et al: Risk of serious bacterial infection in children with fever without a source in the post–*Haemophilus influenzae* era when antibiotics are reserved for culture-proven bacteremia. *Arch Pediatr Adolesc Med* 2004;156:512–517.

Baraff LJ, Bass JW, Fleisher GR, et al: Practice guidelines for the management of infants and children 0–36 months of age with fever without a source. *Ann Emerg Med* 1993;22:1198–1210.

Bleeker-Rovers CP, Vos FJ, de Kleijn EMHA, et al: A prospective multicenter study on fever of unknown origin. *Medicine* 2007;86:26–38.

Bonsu BK, Harper MB: Fever interval before diagnosis, prior antibiotic treatment, and clinical outcome for young children with bacterial meningitis. *Clin Infect Dis* 2001;32:566–572.

Brent AJ, Ahmed I, Ndiritu M, et al: Incidence of clinically significant bacteremia in children who present to hospital in Kenya: Community-based observational study. *Lancet* 2006;367:482–488.

Haddy RI, Perry K, Chacko CE, et al: Comparison of incidence of invasive *Streptococcus pneumoniae* disease among children before and after introduction of conjugated pneumococcal vaccine. *Pediatr Infect Dis J* 2005;24:320–323.

Herz AM, Greenhow TL, Alcantara J, et al: Changing epidemiology of outpatient bacteremia in 3- to 36-month-old children after the introduction of the heptavalent-conjugated pneumococcal vaccine. *Pediatr Infect Dis J* 2006;25(4):293–300.

Hsiao AL, Chen L, Baker D: Incidence and predictors of serious bacterial infections among 57- to 180-day-old infants. *Pediatrics* 2006;117:1695–1701.

Jaskiewicz JA, McCarthy CA, Richardson AC, et al: Febrile infants at low risk for serious bacterial infection—An appraisal of the Rochester criteria and implications for management. *Pediatrics* 1994;94:390–396.

Lee GM, Harper MB: Risk of bacteremia for febrile young children in the post–*Haemophilus influenzae* type b era. *Arch Pediatr Adolesc Med* 1998;152:624–628.

Lohr JA, Hendley JO: Prolonged fever of unknown origin. A record of experiences with 54 childhood patients. *Clin Pediatr* 1977;16:768–773.

Long S: Distinguishing among prolonged, recurrent, and periodic fever syndromes: Approach of a pediatric infectious disease subspecialist. *Pediatr Clin North Am* 2005;52:811–835.

Melendez E, Harper MB: Utility of sepsis evaluation in infants 90 days of age or younger with fever and clinical bronchiolitis. *Pediatr Infect Dis J* 2003;22:1053–1056.

Miller ML, Szer I, Yogev R, et al: Fever of unknown origin. *Pediatr Clin North Am* 1995;42:999–1015.

Palazzi DL, McClain KL, Kaplan SL: Hemophagocytic syndrome in children: An important diagnostic consideration in fever of unknown origin. *Clin Infect Dis* 2003;36:306–312.

Pantell RH, Newman TB, Bernzweig J, et al: Management and outcomes of care of fever in early infancy. *JAMA* 2004;291:1203–1212.

Pizzo PA, Lovejoy FH Jr, Smith DH: Prolonged fever in children: Review of 100 cases. *Pediatrics* 1975;55:468–473.

Roberts KB: Young, febrile infants. A 30-year odyssey ends where it started. *JAMA* 2004;291:1261–1262.

Stoll ML, Rubin LG: Incidence of occult bacteremia among highly febrile young children in the era of the pneumococcal conjugate vaccine. *Arch Pediatr Adolesc Med* 2004;158:671–675.

Trautner BW, Caviness AC, Gerlacher GR, et al: Prospective evaluation of the risk of serious bacterial infection in children who present to the emergency department with hyperpyrexia (temperature of 106°F or higher). *Pediatrics* 2006;118:34–40.

Whitney CG, Farley MM, Hadler J, et al: Decline in invasive pneumococcal disease after the introduction of protein-polysaccharide conjugate vaccine. *N Engl J Med* 2003;348:1737–1746.

Chapter 176 ■ Sepsis, Septic Shock, and Systemic Inflammatory Response Syndrome

Maria Annette Enrione and Keith R. Powell

Despite advances in vaccines and pharmacologic agents, infection triggering sepsis that can progress to septic shock and ultimately death continues to be a major pediatric problem. The **systemic inflammatory response syndrome (SIRS)** is an inflammatory cascade that is initiated by the host in response to infection with bacteria, rickettsiae, fungi, viruses, and protozoa. This inflammatory cascade occurs when the host defense system does not adequately recognize or clear the infection. SIRS can also occur from a number of noninfectious etiologies (Table 176-1). **Sepsis** is defined as SIRS resulting from a suspected or proven infection. The clinical spectrum of sepsis begins when a systemic infection (e.g., bacteremia, fungemia, viremia) or localized infection (e.g., meningitis, pneumonia, pyelonephritis) progresses from sepsis to **severe sepsis** (the presence of sepsis combined with organ dysfunction), **septic shock** (severe sepsis plus the persistence of hypoperfusion or hypotension for >1 hr despite adequate fluid resuscitation or a requirement for inotropic agents or vasopressors), multiple organ dysfunction syndrome (MODS), and ultimately death (Table 176-2). This is a complex clinical problem, and with early recognition and treatment there is a high likelihood of a good outcome.

ETIOLOGY. Sepsis may develop as a complication of a localized infection or may follow colonization and mucosal invasion by virulent pathogens (see Table 176-1). Children 3 mo to 3 yr of age are at risk for occult bacteremia that will occasionally progress to sepsis (see Chapter 175). Patients at risk for sepsis include infants, children with serious injuries, children on chronic antibacterial therapy, malnourished children, and children with chronic medical problems. Also, children who are immune suppressed (transplant recipients on immunosuppressive regimens, patients on chemotherapeutic agents or corticosteroids, patients with acquired or congenital immune deficiencies) are at an increased risk for complications from infection, including sepsis and septic shock.

The infectious agents associated with sepsis in pediatric patients vary with the patient's age and immune status. In the neonatal age group, group B streptococcus, *Escherichia coli, Listeria monocytogenes,* enteroviruses, and herpes simplex virus are the pathogens most commonly associated with sepsis. In older children *Streptococcus pneumoniae, Neisseria meningitidis,* and *Staphylococcus aureus* (methicillin-sensitive or resistant) are more common. Toxic shock syndrome from group A streptococcus or *S. aureus* can also be seen in older children. *Rickettsia rickettsii* causing Rocky Mountain spotted fever occurs in endemic areas and can lead to septic shock. Nosocomial (hospital-acquired) infections pose a special risk to immunocompromised patients (see Chapter 177). Intravenous and arterial catheters, urinary catheters, and endotracheal tubes are portals for the development nosocomial infections (see Chapter 178). Invasive procedures can also lead to nosocomial infections. Infections with gram-negative bacteria (e.g., *Escherichia coli, Pseudomonas, Acinetobacter, Klebsiella, Enterobacter, Serratia*) and fungi (e.g., *Candida, Aspergillus*) most often occur in immunocompromised and hospitalized patients colonized with these organisms. Polymicrobial sepsis occurs in high-risk patients and is associated with catheters, gastrointestinal disease, neutropenia, and malignancy. Unusual pathogens should be suspected in patients who have traveled or been exposed to products or people from distant lands or who are immunocompromised secondary to malignancy, T- or B-cell defects, or asplenia (acquired or congenital). **Pseudobacteremia** may be associated with contaminated heparin flush solutions, intravenous solutions, albumin, cryoprecipitate, and infusion equipment. Contaminants include water-borne organisms such as *Burkholderia cepacia, Pseudomonas aeruginosa,* and *Serratia.*

TABLE 176-1. Differential Diagnosis of SIRS

INFECTION
Bacteremia or meningitis (*Streptococcus pneumoniae, Haemophilus influenzae* type b, *Neisseria meningitidis,* group A streptococcus, *S. aureus*)
Viral illness (influenza, enteroviruses, hemorrhagic fever group, HSV, RSV, CMV, EBV)
Encephalitis (arboviruses, enteroviruses, HSV)
Rickettsiae (Rocky Mountain spotted fever, *Ehrlichia*, Q fever)
Syphilis
Vaccine reaction (pertussis, influenza, measles)
Toxin-mediated reaction (toxic shock, staphylococcal scalded skin syndrome)
CARDIOPULMONARY
Pneumonia (bacteria, virus, mycobacteria, fungi, allergic reaction)
Pulmonary emboli
Heart failure
Arrhythmia
Pericarditis
Myocarditis
METABOLIC-ENDOCRINE
Adrenal insufficiency (adrenogenital syndrome, corticosteroid withdrawal)
Electrolyte disturbances (hyponatremia or hypernatremia; hypocalcemia or hypercalcemia)
Diabetes insipidus
Diabetes mellitus
Inborn errors of metabolism (organic acidosis, urea cycle, carnitine deficiency, mitochondrial disorders)
Hypoglycemia
Reye syndrome
GASTROINTESTINAL
Gastroenteritis with dehydration
Volvulus
Intussusception
Appendicitis
Peritonitis (spontaneous, associated with perforation or peritoneal dialysis)
Necrotizing entercolitis
Hepatitis
Hemorrhage
Pancreatitis
HEMATOLOGIC
Anemia (sickle cell disease, blood loss, nutritional)
Methemoglobinemia
Splenic sequestration crisis
Leukemia or lymphoma
Hemophagocytic syndromes
NEUROLOGIC
Intoxication (drugs, carbon monoxide, intentional or accidental overdose)
Intracranial hemorrhage
Infant botulism
Trauma (child abuse, accidental)
Guillain-Barré syndrome
Myasthenia gravis
OTHER
Anaphylaxis (food, drug, insect sting)
Hemolytic-uremic syndrome
Kawasaki disease
Erythema multiforme
Hemorrhagic shock–encephalopathy syndrome
Poisoning
Toxic envenomation
Macrophage activation syndrome

CMV, cytomegalovirus; EBV, Epstein-Barr virus; HSV, herpes simplex virus; RSV, respiratory syncytial virus; SIRS, systemic inflammatory response syndrome.

PATHOGENESIS. **Shock** is a state of circulatory dysfunction that occurs from (1) decreased cardiac output and/or maldistribution of regional blood flow and (2) increased metabolic demands with or without impaired oxygen utilization at the cellular level despite adequate oxygen delivery (see Chapter 68). Cardiac output may be high, low, or normal. The body has compensatory mechanisms to maintain blood pressure through increased heart rate and peripheral vasoconstriction. Hypotension, a late finding in infants and children, occurs when the compensatory mechanisms are failing and cardiorespiratory arrest is imminent.

Septic shock is a combination of the three classic types of shock: hypovolemic, cardiogenic, and distributive. **Hypovolemia** from intravascular fluid losses occurs through capillary leak. **Cardiogenic shock** results from the myocardial-depressant effects of sepsis. **Distributive shock** is the result of decreased systemic vascular resistance. The degree to which a patient will exhibit each of these responses is variable. Warm shock occurs in some patients with increased cardiac output and decreased systemic vascular resistance. Cold shock occurs in other patients with decreased cardiac output and elevated systemic vascular resistance. In both cases, perfusion to major organ systems may be compromised. Recent data suggest that, unlike adults in septic shock who present with vasodilation and high cardiac output, newborns and children may have fluid refractory shock and develop progressive myocardial dysfunction.

It is important to distinguish between the infection and the host response to the infection, the inflammatory response. The host's immune response, through the actions of the cellular and humoral immune systems, and the reticular endothelium system, prevents the body from developing sepsis in response to breaches in the host defense system. However, this host immune response produces an inflammatory cascade of highly toxic mediators, including hormones, cytokines, and enzymes. If this inflammatory cascade is uncontrolled, SIRS occurs with subsequent organ and cellular dysfunction from derangement of the microcirculatory system.

Microcirculatory dysfunction results in endothelial injury, release of vasoactive substances, changes in cardiovascular tone, mechanical obstruction of the capillary beds from aggregation of cellular elements, and activation of the complement system. At the cellular level there is decreased oxidative phosphorylation secondary to decreased oxygen delivery, anaerobic metabolism secondary to decreased adenosine triphosphate (ATP), glycogen depletion, lactate production, increased cytosolic calcium, activation of membrane phospholipases (further depleting ATP), and release of fatty acids with prostaglandin formation.

The inflammatory cascade (Fig. 176-1) is initiated by toxins or superantigens. Endotoxin (a lipopolysaccharide), mannose, and glycoprotein components of the cell wall of gram-negative bacteria as well as fungi and yeast bind to macrophages leading to activation and expression of inflammatory genes. Superantigens or toxins associated with gram-positive bacteria, mycobacteria, and viruses activate circulating lymphocytes and initiate an inflammatory mediator cascade.

Biochemical responses include the production of arachidonic acid metabolites, release of myocardial depressant factors, release of endogenous opiates, activation of the complement system, as well as the production and release of many other mediators. Arachidonic acid metabolites include (1) thromboxane A2, which causes vasoconstriction and platelet aggregation; (2) prostaglandins, such as $PGF_{2\alpha}$, which causes vasoconstriction, and PGI_2, which causes vasodilation; and (3) leukotrienes that cause vasoconstriction, bronchoconstriction, and increased capillary permeability. Myocardial depressant factors, tumor necrosis factor-α (TNF), and some of the interleukins cause myocardial depression not only via direct myocardial injury but also by an intracardiac increase in inducible nitric oxide synthase. Endogenous opiates, including β-endorphin, decrease sympathetic activity, decrease myocardial contractility, and cause vasodilation. Activation of the complement system leads to release of vasoactive mediators that increase capillary permeability, cause vasodilation, and cause activation and aggregation of platelets and granulocytes.

Endogenous mediators of sepsis continue to be identified and currently include TNF, interleukin 1 (IL-1), IL-2, IL-4, IL-6, IL-8, platelet activating factor (PAF), interferon-γ, eicosanoids (leukotrienes B_4, C_4, D_4, and E_4; thromboxane A_2; prostaglandins E_2 and I_2), granulocyte-macrophage colony-stimulating factor, endothelium-derived relaxing factor, endothelin-1, complement fragments C3a and C5a, toxic oxygen radicals, proteolytic enzymes from polymorphonuclear neutrophils, platelets, transforming growth factor-β, vascular permeability factor, macrophage-derived procoagulant and inflammatory cytokine, bradykinin, thrombin, coagulation factors, fibrin, plasminogen activator inhibitor (PAI-1), myocardial depressant substance, β-endorphin, heat shock proteins, and adhesion molecules (endothelin-derived adhesion molecule [E-selectin]; intercellular adhesion molecule-1 [ICAM]; vascular adhesion molecule-1 [VCAM]).

The **clinical manifestations** of sepsis and shock are mediated through the inflammatory cascade. Hypovolemia, cardiac and vascular failure, acute respiratory distress syndrome, insulin resistance, decreased CYP450 activity (decreased steroid synthesis), coagulopathy, and unresolved or secondary infection are all results of the inflammatory cascade. TNF and other inflammatory mediators increase vascular permeability, leading to diffuse capillary leak, decreased vascular tone, and, at the microcirculatory level, an imbalance between perfusion and metabolic demands of the tissue. TNF and IL-1 stimulate the release of pro-inflammatory and anti-inflammatory mediators causing fever and vasodilatation. Arachidonic acid metabolites lead to the development of fever, tachypnea, ventilation-perfusion abnormalities,

TABLE 176-2. International Consensus Definitions for Pediatric Sepsis

Infection: Suspected or proven infection or a clinical syndrome associated with high probability of infection

SIRS: 2 out of 4 criteria, 1 of which must be abnormal temperature or abnormal leukocyte count

1. Core temperature >38.5°C or <36°C (rectal, bladder, oral, or central catheter)
2. Tachycardia: mean heart rate >2 SD above normal for age in absence of external stimuli, chronic drugs or painful stimuli; OR unexplained persistent elevation over 0.5–4 hr; OR in children <1 yr old persistent bradycardia over 0.5 hr (mean heart rate <10th percentile for age in absence of vagal stimuli, β blocker drugs, or congenital heart disease)
3. Respiratory rate >2 SD above normal for age or acute need for mechanical ventilation not related to neuromuscular disease or general anesthesia
4. Leukocyte count elevated or depressed for age (not secondary to chemotherapy) or >10% immature neutrophils

Sepsis: SIRS plus a suspected or proven infection

Severe Sepsis: Sepsis plus 1 of the following

1. Cardiovascular organ dysfunction defined as
   Despite >40 mL/kg of isotonic intravenous fluid in 1 hr
   Hypotension <5th percentile for age, systolic blood pressure <2 SD below normal for age
   OR
   Need for vasoactive drug to maintain blood pressure
   OR
   2 of the following
   Unexplained metabolic acidosis: base deficit >5 mEq/L
   Increased arterial lactate >2 times upper limit of normal
   Oliguria: urine output <0.5 mL/kg/hr
   Prolonged capillary refill 5 sec
   Core to peripheral temperature gap >3°C
2. Acute respiratory distress syndrome (ARDS) as defined by the presence of a PaO_2/FiO_2 ratio ≤300 mm Hg, bilateral infiltrates on chest radiograph, and no evidence of left heart failure
   OR
   Sepsis plus 2 or more organ dysfunctions (respiratory, renal, neurologic, hematologic, or hepatic)

Septic Shock: Sepsis plus cardiovascular organ dysfunction as defined above

Multiple Organ Dysfunction Syndrome (MODS): Presence of altered organ function such that homeostasis cannot be maintained without medical intervention

SIRS, systemic inflammatory response syndrome; SD, standard deviation.

Adapted from Goldstein B, Giroir B, Randolph A: International pediatric sepsis consensus conference: Definitions for sepsis and organ dysfunction in pediatrics. *Pediatr Crit Care* 2005;6(1):2–8. Copyright 2005, Lippincott Williams & Wilkins.

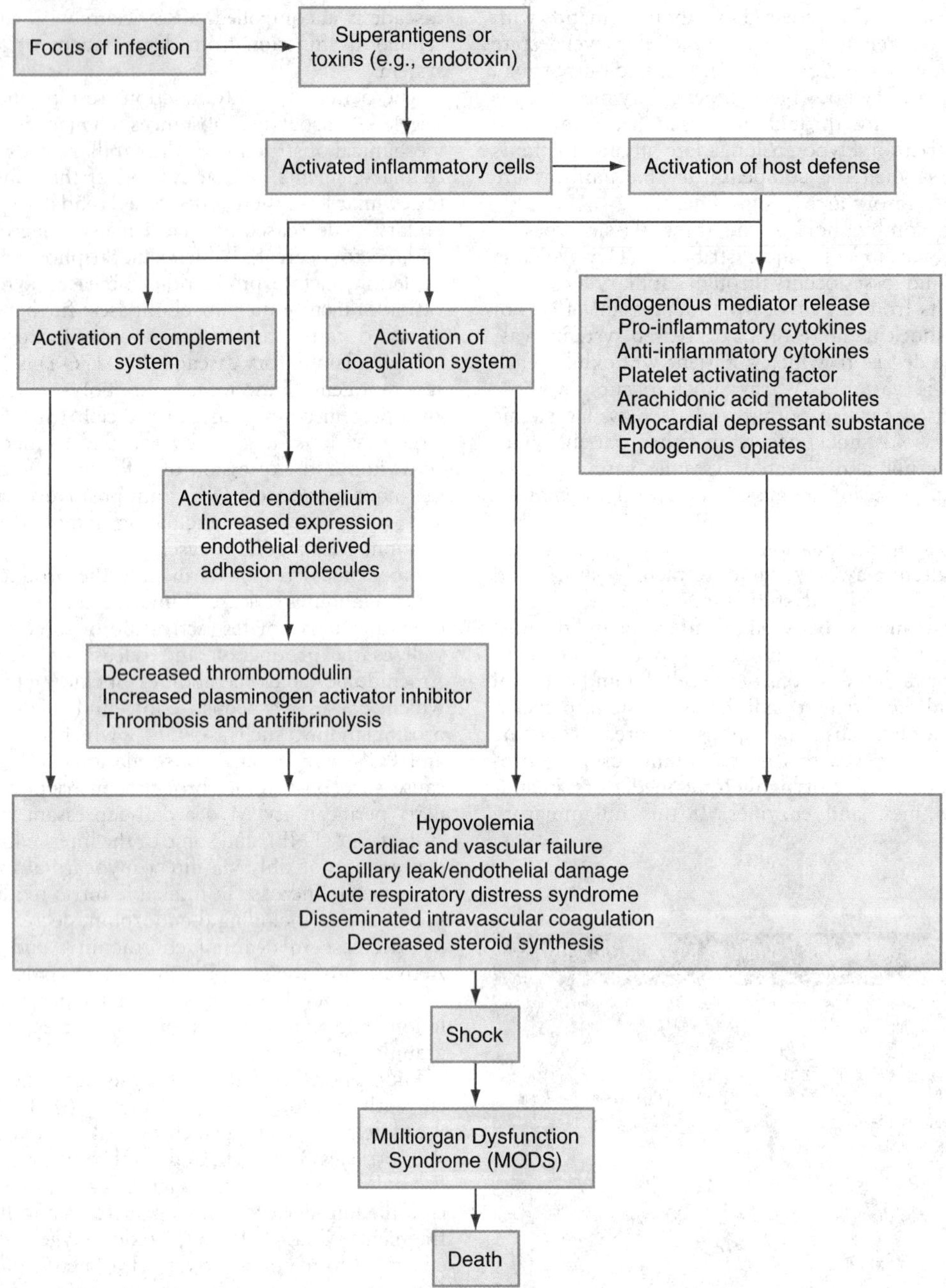

Figure 176-1. Hypothetical pathophysiology of the septic process.

and lactic acidosis. Nitric oxide, released from the endothelium or inflammatory cells, is a major contributor to hypotension. Myocardial depression is caused by myocardial depressant factors, TNF, and some interleukins through direct myocardial injury, depleted catecholamines, increased β-endorphin, and production of myocardial nitric oxide.

In addition to treating the underlying infection, therapies to augment the host defense, block trigger events, prevent leukocyte-endothelial interaction, and inhibit vasoactive substances, cytokines or lipid mediators are being investigated. To date, the results of clinical trials investigating drugs targeting the mediators of SIRS have been disappointing. Trials have been conducted with anti-endotoxin antibodies, antioxidant compounds, an IL-1 receptor antagonist, IL-1 antibodies, bradykinin-receptor antibodies, cyclo-oxygenase inhibitors, thromboxane antagonists, PAF antagonists, inhibitors of leukocyte-adhesion molecules, nitric oxide antagonists, anti-TNF antibody, bactericidal permeability-increasing protein, and recombinant human activated protein C. Recombinant human activated protein C (drotrecogin-α) studies have shown improvement in the 28-day survival in adults, but enrollment in a pediatric trial was closed early because of an unfavorable risk-benefit ratio particularly in neonates. The best treatment is early recognition, early antimicrobial therapy, and early goal-directed therapy.

CLINICAL MANIFESTATIONS. The initial signs and symptoms of sepsis include alterations in temperature regulation (hyperthermia or hypothermia), tachycardia, and tachypnea. In the early stages (hyperdynamic phase), the cardiac output increases in an attempt to maintain adequate oxygen delivery to meet the increased metabolic demands of tissues. As sepsis progresses, cardiac output falls in response to the effects of numerous mediators. Although hypotension (systolic arterial pressure <2 standard deviations below the mean for age) is a late finding in children with sepsis, it is not a criteria for the diagnosis of shock in infants and young children (see Table 176-2). Other signs of poor cardiac output include delayed capillary refill, diminished peripheral and central pulses, cool extremities, and decreased urine output. Alterations in mental status, including confusion, agitation, lethargy, anxiety, obtundation, or coma, can also be signs of poor cardiac output. Capillary leak develops from altered vascular permeability. Lactic acidosis occurs as shock progresses and is the consequence of increased tissue production and decreased hepatic clearance.

Cutaneous lesions seen in septic patients include petechiae, diffuse erythema, ecchymoses, ecthyma gangrenosum, and symmetric peripheral gangrene. Jaundice can be seen either as a sign of infection or as a result of MODS. The patient may also have evidence of focal infection such as meningitis, pneumonia, arthritis, cellulitis, or pyelonephritis.

DIAGNOSIS. The diagnosis of sepsis requires SIRS (see Table 176-2) in the presence of proven infection or a clinical picture consistent with infection. An infectious etiology should be sought by culturing clinically appropriate specimens taken from body fluids (blood, urine, cerebrospinal fluid, abscesses, peritoneal fluid, etc.). Infectious disease and intensive care consults are necessary. Cultures take time for incubation and are not always positive. Additional evidence to identify an infectious etiology as the cause of SIRS includes physical examination findings, imaging (chest radiograph with evidence of pneumonia), presence of white cells in normally sterile body fluids, and suggestive rashes such as petechiae and purpura. Affected children should be admitted to an intensive care unit where continuous, close invasive monitoring can be performed, including central venous pressure and arterial blood pressure (see Chapter 68).

LABORATORY FINDINGS. Laboratory findings often include evidence of hematologic abnormalities and electrolyte disturbances. Hematologic abnormalities include thrombocytopenia, prolonged prothrombin and partial thromboplastin times, reduced serum fibrinogen levels and elevated fibrin split products, and anemia. Also, elevated neutrophil and increased immature forms (bands, myelocytes, promyelocytes), vacuolation of neutrophils, toxic granulations, and Döhle bodies can be seen with infection. Neutropenia is an ominous sign of overwhelming sepsis. Electrolyte abnormalities include hyperglycemia as a stress response or hypoglycemia if glycogen reserves are exhausted. Other electrolyte abnormalities include hypocalcemia, hypoalbuminemia, metabolic acidosis, and low serum bicarbonate. Lactic acidosis can occur if there is significant anaerobic metabolism. Renal and liver function may be abnormal if the patient develops MODS. Patients with acute respiratory distress syndrome or pneumonia will have impaired oxygenation (decreased PaO_2) and ventilation (increased $PaCO_2$). Examination of infected body fluids may reveal neutrophils and bacteria.

TREATMENT. Early administration of antimicrobial agents is associated with a reduction of mortality. The choice of antimicrobial agents is dependent on the predisposing risk factors and the clinical situation. Bacterial resistance patterns in the community should also be considered when selecting optimal antimicrobial therapy.

Broad-spectrum bactericidal synergistic antimicrobial agents should be promptly administered to the patient in septic shock. The choice of antimicrobial agents depends on the specific predisposing risk factors (Table 176-3). Neonates should be treated with ampicillin plus cefotaxime or gentamicin. Acyclovir should be added if herpes simplex virus is suspected. Community-acquired infections with *N. meningitidis, S. pneumoniae,* and *Haemophilus influenzae* can be treated empirically with a 3rd generation cephalosporin (ceftriaxone or cefotaxime) unless resistant *S. pneumoniae* or *S. aureus* is prevalent, which requires the addition of vancomycin. If an intra-abdominal process is suspected, anaerobic coverage should be included with agents such as metronidazole or clindamycin. Nosocomial sepsis should be treated with a 3rd or 4th generation cephalosporin or an extended gram-negative spectrum penicillin (e.g., piperacillin-tazobactam) plus an aminoglycoside. Vancomycin should be added to the regimen if the patient has an indwelling medical device (see Chapter 178) and gram-positive cocci are isolated from the blood, if methicillin-resistant *S. aureus* infection is suspected, and as empiric coverage for *S. pneumoniae* in patients with meningitis. Empirical use of amphotericin B to treat fungal infections should be considered for selected immunocompromised patients (see Chapter 177).

TABLE 176-3. Appropriate Antibiotics for Pediatric Sepsis

Neonate	Ampicillin plus aminoglycoside or cefotaxime Add vancomycin if nosocomial infection Add acyclovir if suspect herpes simplex virus
Child	Cefotaxime or ceftriaxone Add vancomycin for meningitis or in areas of high staphylococcal or pneumococcal resistance to methicillin or cefotaxime, respectively
Immunocompromised patient or nosocomial infection	Vancomycin + antipseudomonal antibacterial agent Ceftazidime or cefepime Aminoglycoside Penicillin β-lactamase inhibitor combination (ticarcillin/clavulanic, piperacillin/tazobactam) Carbapenem (imipenem or meropenem)
Toxic shock syndrome	Penicillin plus clindamycin Vancomycin if methicillin *Staphylococcus aureus* is suspected
Tick-endemic areas	Add doxycycline to above regimens
Suspected anaerobic infections	Add clindamycin or metronidazole to above regimens

SUPPORTIVE CARE. A recommended stepwise approach to pediatric septic shock is based on the consensus statement of the American College of Critical Care Medicine (ACCCM)/Society for Critical Care Medicine Task Force Committee Members (Fig. 176-2).

Early goal-directed therapy is the recommended treatment approach for patients with septic shock. Rapid, aggressive resuscitation with fluids and catecholamines is associated with a reduction in mortality. Every hour of inadequate resuscitation is associated with an increased mortality risk of 40%.

Fluid resuscitation of 60 mL/kg is associated with improved survival without an increased incidence of pulmonary edema. Fluid resuscitation in increments of 20 mL/kg should be titrated to normalize heart rate (using age-based heart rates), urine output (to at least 1 mL/kg/hr), capillary refill (<2 sec), and mental status. Since hypotension is a late ominous finding, blood pressure is not a reliable end-point for assessing resuscitation. Fluid resuscitation may sometimes require as much as 100–200 mL/kg. Although the type of fluid (crystalloid vs colloid) is still an area of debate, there is no question that fluid resuscitation is essential to survival from septic shock (see Chapter 68).

Other fluids to consider include blood products. Oxygen delivery is primarily dependent on the hemoglobin concentration. Thus, maintaining the hemoglobin at 10 g/dL is a reasonable goal in the absence of data from randomized clinical trials. Correction of coagulopathy with fresh frozen plasma, cryoprecipitate, and platelet transfusions should be considered, especially if the patient has active bleeding.

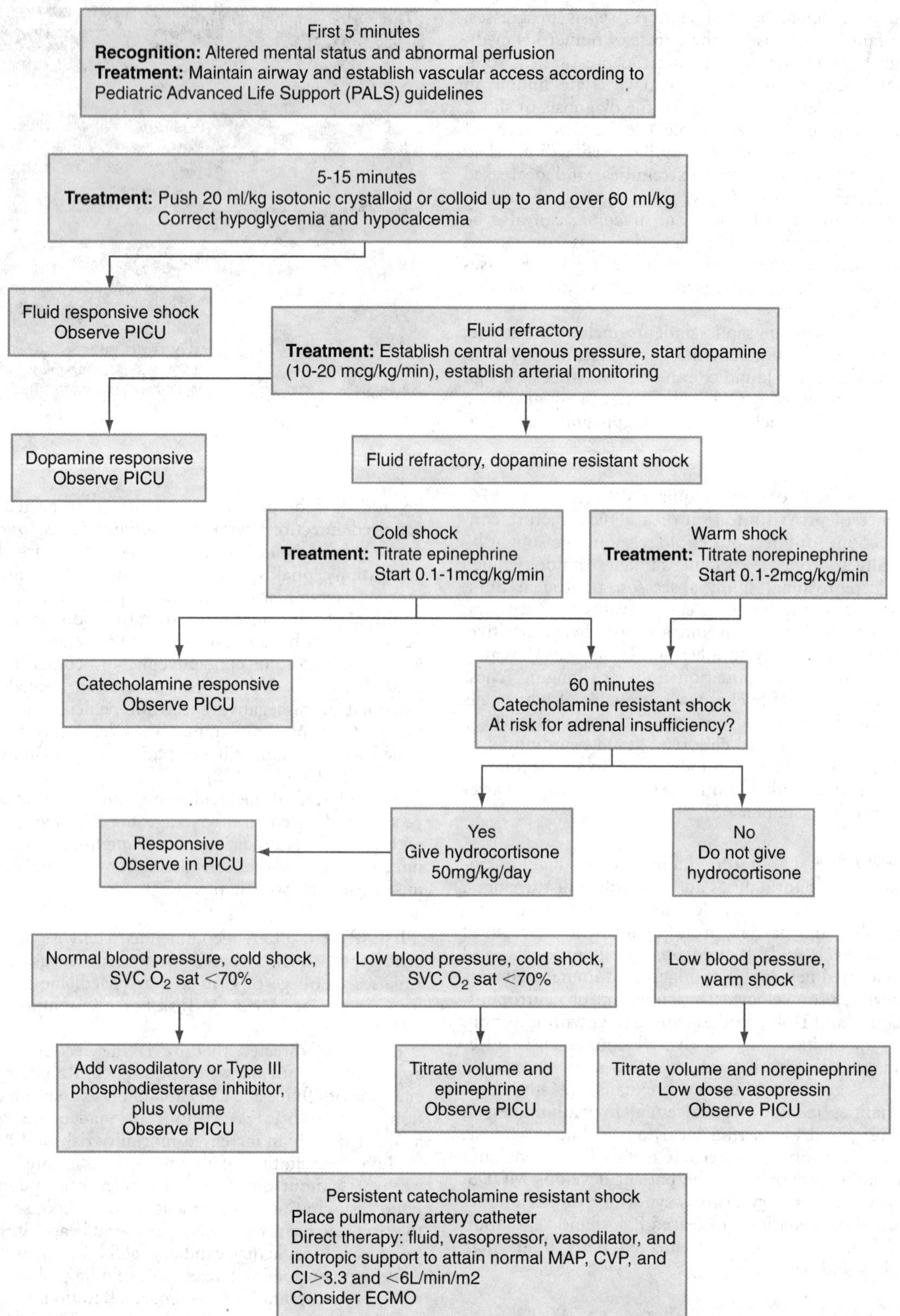

Figure 176-2. American College of Critical Care Medicine and American Heart Association clinical parameters for the hemodynamic support of pediatric patients with septic shock. PICU, pediatric intensive care unit; SVC O_2 sat, superior vena cava oxygen saturation; MAP, mean arterial pressure; CVP, central venous pressure; CI, cardiac index; ECMO, extracorporeal membrane oxygenation. (From Carcillo JA, Fields AI, Task Force Committee Members: Clinical practice parameters for hemodynamic support of pediatric and neonatal patients with septic shock. *Crit Care Med* 2002;30(6):1365–1378. Copyright 2002, Lippincott Williams & Wilkins.)

Evidence suggests that infants and children tend to have low cardiac output with vasoconstriction and that progressive myocardial dysfunction is associated with a higher mortality rate. Thus, goal-directed therapy includes the use of vasopressors and inotropic agents in an attempt to maintain a normal cardiac index. Dopamine is the initial choice for fluid-refractory shock. In dopamine-resistant shock, epinephrine or norepinephrine should be considered. Dobutamine is useful in cases where cardiac output is low. In patients with high systemic vascular resistance and epinephrine-resistant low cardiac output, the use of vasodilators such as nitroprusside or type III phosphodiesterase inhibitors (milrinone) may reverse shock. Arginine vasopressin may be useful in norepinephrine-resistant shock because it does not require the α receptor for action.

Metabolic status should be maintained. Thus, electrolytes should be monitored closely and corrected as needed. Hypoglycemia should be treated with 0.5–1.0 g/kg of glucose. Hypocalcemia, which can contribute to cardiac dysfunction, should be treated with 10–20 mg/kg of calcium chloride through a central venous catheter.

Studies have shown that 50% of children in the intensive care unit have a relative or absolute adrenal insufficiency. Thus, use of stress dose corticosteroids (hydrocortisone 50 mg/kg bolus followed by 50 mg/kg/day) for adrenal insufficiency should be considered, especially if shock is not responsive to catecholamines and fluid resuscitation. Lower dose therapy may also be effective but requires further study. All patients with adrenal suppression secondary to chronic steroid therapy, including patients with asthma, rheumatic diseases, and inflammatory bowel disease, as well as patients with known disorders of the hypothalamic-pituitary axis (hypopituitarism, congenital adrenal hyperplasia) should receive **stress dose corticosteroids.**

Other therapies, including respiratory support and renal replacement therapy, should be used as clinically appropriate. Lung protective strategies (use of positive end-expiratory pressure, low tidal volume ventilation [6–8 mL/kg] plateau pressures less than 30 cm of water, and FiO_2 less than 60%) should be used in patients who have developed acute respiratory distress syndrome or require mechanical ventilation, because overdistended lungs can generate systemic cytokines, worsening the inflammatory cascade. Renal replacement therapy may be useful in children with anuria or oliguria and severe fluid overload. Extracorporeal membrane oxygenation may be considered in selected patients with refractory septic shock.

Monitoring patients with septic shock should minimally include central venous pressure, arterial blood pressure, pulse oximetry, and hourly urine output. Other clinical parameters that should be monitored include heart rate, capillary refill, and mental status. Superior vena cava oxygen saturation may be an indicator of adequate resuscitation. A superior vena cava oxygen saturation of >70% in the 1st 6 hours after shock resuscitation has been associated with improved outcome. There is not enough information to determine whether or not cardiac echocardiography, pulmonary arterial catheterization, and gastric tonography should be used to direct therapy in patients with septic shock. Resuscitation goals include capillary refill <2 sec, normal pulses with no differential between central and peripheral pulses, warm extremities, urine output of >1 mL/kg/hr, normal mental status, and normal blood pressure for age.

PROGNOSIS. The mortality rate for septic shock depends on the initial site of infection, the bacterial pathogen, the presence of MODS, and the host immune response. Severe sepsis remains one of the leading causes of death in children. Recent outcome data show an improvement in neonatal and pediatric sepsis, with mortality rates around 10%. Infants, especially low birth weight infants, and children with chronic medical problems are at highest risk for developing severe sepsis. Pediatric patients who have undergone bone marrow transplantation have an increased rate of mortality compared to other patients with septic shock. Furthermore, patients who survive septic shock demonstrate an improvement in cardiac indices with therapy as compared with nonsurviving patients.

Severe sepsis has an estimated cost of $1.9 billion nationally per year. For children, the mean length of stay was 31 days, with a cost of $40,600. For infants, the mean length of stay was 53 days, with a cost of $56,600. The incidence of severe sepsis is highest among infants (5.2/1,000) and lowest among 5–14 year olds (0.2/1,000).

PREVENTION. Immunization with the conjugate *H. influenzae* type b and *S. pneumoniae* vaccines is recommended for all infants (see Chapter 170). High-risk patients should also receive recommended immunizations. Penicillin prophylaxis to prevent pneumococcal infection is recommended for patients with splenic dysfunction (e.g., sickle cell disease) and those who are asplenic (acquired or congenital). Antibiotic prophylaxis is recommended for household and other close contacts of patients with invasive *N. meningitidis* (see Chapter 190) or *H. influenzae* type b disease (see Chapter 192). There are recommended measures for prevention of nosocomial infections (see Chapter 178) and infection and sepsis in immunocompromised patients (see Chapter 177) and neonates (see Chapter 109).

Annane D, Bellissant E, Bollaert PE, et al: Corticosteroids for severe sepsis and septic shock: A systematic review and meta-analysis. *Br Med J* 2004; 329:480–484.

Baudouin SV, Saunders D, Tiangyou W, et al: Mitochondrial DNA and survival after sepsis: a prospective study. *Lancet* 2005;366:2118–2121.

Bernard GR, Vincent JL, Laterre PF, et al: Efficacy and safety of recombinant human activated protein C for severe sepsis. *N Engl J Med* 2001; 344:699–709.

Brown KA, Brain SD, Pearson JD, et al: Neutrophils in development of multiple organ failure in sepsis. *Lancet* 2006;368:157–169.

Carcillo JA: Pediatric septic shock and multiple organ failure. *Crit Care Clin* 2003;19:413–440.

Carcillo JA, Fields AI, Task Force Committee Members: Clinical practice parameters for hemodynamic support of pediatric and neonatal patients with septic shock. *Crit Care Med* 2002;30(6):1365–1378.

Goldstein B, Giroir B, Randolph A: International pediatric sepsis consensus conference: Definitions for sepsis and organ dysfunction in pediatrics. *Pediatr Crit Care* 2005;6(1):2–8.

Jindal N, Hollenberg SM, Dellinger RP: Pharmacologic issues in the management of septic shock. *Crit Care Clin* 2000;16:233–249.

Nadel S, Goldstein B, Williams MD, et al: Drotrecogin alfa (activated) in children with severe sepsis: a multicentre phase III randomised controlled trial. *Lancet* 2007;369:836–843.

Opal SM: Can we resolve the treatment of sepsis? *Lancet* 2007;369:803–804.

Parker MM, Hazelzet JA, Carcillo JA: Pediatric considerations. *Crit Care Med* 2004;32(Suppl):S591–S594.

Pizarro CF, Troster EJ, Damiani D, Carcillo JA: Absolute and relative adrenal insufficiency in children with septic shock. *Crit Care Med* 2005;33:855–859.

Rivers E, Nguyen B, Havstad S, et al, the Early Goal-Directed Therapy Collaborative Group: Early goal-directed therapy in the treatment of severe sepsis and septic shock. *N Engl J Med* 2001;346(19):1368–1377.

Russell JA: Management of sepsis. *N Engl J Med* 2006;355:1699–1713.

Saez-Llorens X, McCracken GH Jr: Sepsis syndrome and septic shock in pediatrics: Current concepts of terminology, pathophysiology, and management. *J Pediatr* 1993;123:497–508.

Turgeon AF, Hutton B, Fergusson DA, et al: Meta-analysis: Intravenous immunoglobulin in critically ill adult patients with sepsis. *Ann Intern Med* 2007;146:193–203.

Watson RS, Carcillo JA, Linde-Zwirble, et al: The epidemiology of severe sepsis in children in the United States. *Am J Respir Crit Care Med* 2003;167:695–701.

Chapter 177 ■ Infections in Immunocompromised Persons

Marian G. Michaels and Michael Green

Infection and disease develop when the host immune system fails to completely protect against potential pathogens. While infections can occur in individuals with competent immune systems, they usually do so when a person is naive to the microbe and has no previous immunity or because the protective barriers of the body such as the skin have been breached. Healthy children are able to meet the challenge of most infectious agents with an immunologic armamentarium capable of preventing significant disease. Once an infection begins to develop, an array of immune responses is set into action to control the disease and prevent it from reappearing. In contrast, immunocompromised children may not have this same capability. Depending on the level and type of immune defect, the affected child may not be able to contain the pathogen or to develop an immune response to prevent recurrence (see Chapter 121).

General practitioners are likely to see children in their practice with abnormal immune systems because increasing numbers of children survive with primary immunodeficiencies or receive immunosuppressive therapy for treatment of malignancy, autoimmune disorders, or transplantation.

Primary immunodeficiencies are those compromised states that result from genetic defects affecting one or more arms of the immune system (Table 177-1). **Acquired, or secondary, immunodeficiencies** may result from infection, such as with human immunodeficiency virus, malignancy, or as an adverse effect of immunomodulating or immunosuppressing medications. These include medications that affect T cells (steroids, tumor necrosis factor inhibitors, chemotherapy), neutrophils (myelosuppressive agents, idiosyncratic or immune-mediated neutropenia), or all immune cells (chemotherapy). Perturbations of the mucosal and skin barriers or normal microbial flora can also be characterized as secondary immune deficiencies, leaving the host open to infections if only for a temporary period of time.

The major pathogens causing infections among immunocompetent hosts are also the main pathogens causing infections among children with immunodeficiencies. In addition, less virulent organisms, including normal skin flora, commensal bacteria of the oral pharynx or gastrointestinal tract, environmental fungi, and common community viruses of low-level pathogenicity, can cause severe, life-threatening illnesses in immunocompromised patients (Table 177-2). For this reason, close communication with the diagnostic laboratory is critical so that the laboratory does not disregard normal flora and organisms normally considered to be contaminants as being unimportant.

TABLE 177-1. Major Causes of Increased Risk for Infection in Immunocompromised Hosts

PRIMARY IMMUNODEFICIENCIES
Antibody Deficiency (B-cell Defects; see Chapter 123)
X-linked agammaglobulinemia
Common variable immunodeficiency
Selective immunoglobulin A (IgA) deficiency
IgG subclass deficiencies
Hyper-IgM syndrome
Cell-mediated Deficiency (T-cell Defects; see Chapter 124)
Thymic dysplasia (DiGeorge syndrome)
Defective T-cell receptor
Defective cytokine production
T-cell activation defects
CD8 lymphocytopenia
Combined B- and T-cell Defects (see Chapter 125)
Severe combined immunodeficiency
Combined immunodeficiency
Omenn syndrome
Thrombocytopenia and eczema (Wiskott-Aldrich syndrome)
Ataxia telangiectasia
Hyper-IgE syndrome
Phagocyte Defects (see Chapter 129)
Leukocyte adhesion deficiency
Chédiak-Higashi syndrome
Myeloperoxidase deficiency
Chronic granulomatous disease
Leukopenia (see Chapter 130)
Congenital neutropenia (Kostmann syndrome)
Shwachman-Diamond syndrome
Disorders of the complement system (see Chapter 133)
SECONDARY IMMUNODEFICIENCIES
HIV
Malignancies (and cancer chemotherapy)
Transplantation
Bone marrow and stem cell
Solid organ
Burns
Sickle cell disease
Cystic fibrosis
Diabetes mellitus
Immunosuppressive drugs
Asplenia
Implanted foreign body
Malnutrition

177.1 • Infections Occurring With Primary Immunodeficiencies

ABNORMALITIES OF THE PHAGOCYTIC SYSTEM

Children with abnormalities of the phagocytic and neutrophil system have problems with bacteria as well as environmental fungi. Disease manifests as recurrent infections of the skin, mucous membranes, lungs, liver, and bones. Dysfunction of this arm of the immune system can be due to inadequate numbers, abnormal movement properties, or aberrant function of neutrophils (see Chapter 129).

Neutropenia is defined as an absolute neutrophil count of <1,000 cells/mm^3 and can be associated with significant risk for developing severe bacterial and fungal disease, particularly when the absolute count is <500 cells/mm^3 (see Chapter 130). Although acquired neutropenia secondary to bone marrow suppression from a virus or medication is common, genetic causes of neutropenia also exist. Primary congenital neutropenia most often presents during the 1st year of life with cellulitis, perirectal abscesses, or stomatitis from *Staphylococcus aureus* or *Pseudomonas aeruginosa*. Episodes of severe disease, including bacteremia or meningitis, are also possible. Bone marrow evaluation shows a failure of maturation of myeloid precursors. Most forms of congenital neutropenia are autosomal dominant, but some, such as Kostmann syndrome (see Chapter 130) and Shwachman-Diamond syndrome (see Chapter 468) are due to autosomal-recessive mutations. Cyclic neutropenia, which can be associated with autosomal-dominant inheritance or de novo sporadic mutations, manifests as fixed cycles of severe neutropenia between periods of normal granulocyte numbers. Often the neutrophil count has normalized by the time the patient presents with symptoms hampering the diagnosis. The cycles classically occur every 21 days (range, 14–36 days), with neutropenia lasting 3–6 days. Most often the disease is characterized by recurrent aphthous ulcers and stomatitis during the periods of neutropenia. However, life-threatening necrotizing myositis or cellulitis and systemic disease can occur, especially with *Clostridium septicum* or *Clostridium perfringens.* Many of the neutropenic syndromes respond to colony-stimulating factor.

Leukocyte adhesion defects are caused by defects in the β chain of integrin (CD18), which is required for the normal process of neutrophil aggregation and attachment to endothelial surfaces (see Chapter 129). In the most severe form there is a total absence of CD18. Children with this defect may have a history of delayed cord separation and recurrent infections of the skin, oral mucosa, and genital tract beginning early in life. Ecthyma gangrenosum and pyoderma gangrenosum also occur. Because the defect is of leukocyte migration and adherence, the neutrophil count in the peripheral blood is usually extremely elevated and pus is not found at the site of infection. Survival is usually <10 yr in the absence of stem cell transplantation.

TABLE 177-2. Most Common Causes of Infections in Immunocompromised Children

BACTERIA, AEROBIC
Acinetobacter
Bacillus
Burkholderia cepacia
Citrobacter
Corynebacterium
Enterococcus faecalis
Enterococcus faecium
Escherichia coli
Haemophilus influenzae type b
Klebsiella sp
Listeria monocytogenes
Mycobacterium sp
Neisseria meningitidis
Nocardia
Pseudomonas aeruginosa
Staphylococcus aureus
Staphylococcus, coagulase-negative
Streptococcus pneumoniae
Streptococcus, viridans group
BACTERIA, ANAEROBIC
Bacillus
Clostridium
Fusobacterium
Propionibacterium
Peptococcus
Peptostreptococcus
Veillonella
FUNGI
Aspergillus
Candida albicans
Other *Candida*
Cryptococcus neoformans
Zygomycoses *(Absidia, Mucor, Rhizopus, Rhizomucor)*
VIRUSES
Adenoviruses
Cytomegalovirus
Epstein-Barr virus
Herpes simplex virus
Human herpesvirus 6
Respiratory and enteric community-acquired viruses
Varicella-zoster virus
PROTOZOA
Cryptosporidium parvum
Giardia lamblia
Toxoplasma gondii
Pneumocystis carinii

Chronic granulomatous disease is an inherited neutrophil dysfunction syndrome, which can be either X-linked or autosomal recessive (see Chapter 129). Neutrophils have defects in their nicotinamide-adenine dinucleotide phosphate (NADPH) oxidase function, rendering myeloid cells incapable of generating superoxide and thereby impairing intracellular killing. Accordingly, microbes that destroy their own hydrogen peroxide (*S. aureus, Serratia marcescens, Burkholderia cepacia, Aspergillus*) cause recurrent infections in these children. Infections have a predilection to involve the lungs, liver, and bone in these children. Prophylaxis with trimethoprim-sulfamethoxazole and recombinant human interferon-γ (IFN-γ) substantially reduces the incidence of severe infections. In addition, many specialists recommend prophylaxis against *Aspergillus* with itraconazole or voriconazole. Patients with life-threatening infections have also been reported to benefit from aggressive treatment with white cell transfusions in addition to antimicrobial agents directed against the specific pathogen.

DEFECTIVE OPSONIZATION OR COMPLEMENT DEFICIENCY

Children with congenital asplenia, splenic dysfunction due to hemoglobinopathies such as sickle cell disease, or those who have undergone splenectomy are at risk for serious infections from encapsulated bacteria and blood-borne protozoa such as *Plasmodium* and *Babesia.* Prophylaxis against bacterial infection with penicillin should be considered for these patients, particularly children <5 yr of age. The most common causative organisms include *Streptococcus pneumoniae, Haemophilus influenzae* type b, and *Salmonella,* which can cause sepsis, pneumonia, meningitis, and osteomyelitis. Defects in the early pathway of complement components, particularly C2 and C3, can also be associated with severe infection from these bacteria. **Terminal complement defects** (C5, C6, C7, C8, and C9) are associated with recurrent infections with *Neisseria.* Patients with complement deficiency also have an increased incidence of autoimmune disorders. Vaccines for *S. pneumoniae, H. influenzae* type b, and *Neisseria meningitidis* should be administered to all children with abnormalities in opsonization or complement pathways.

B-CELL DEFECTS (HUMORAL IMMUNE DEFICIENCIES)

Antibody deficiencies account for the majority of primary immunodeficiencies among humans (see Chapter 123). Patients with defects in the B-cell arm of the immune system fail to develop appropriate antibody responses, with abnormalities that range from complete agammaglobulinemia to isolated failure to produce antibody against a specific antigen or organism. Antibody deficiencies found in children with diseases such as X-linked agammaglobulinemia or common variable immunodeficiency predispose to infections with encapsulated organisms such as *S. pneumoniae* and *H. influenzae* type b. Other bacteria can also be problematic in these children (see Table 177-2). Even though most other classes of microbes do not cause problems for these patients, some notable exceptions exist. Rotavirus can lead to chronic diarrhea, and enteroviruses can disseminate and cause a chronic meningoencephalitis syndrome. Paralytic polio has developed after immunization with live polio vaccine. Protozoan infections such as giardiasis can be severe and persistent. Children with B-cell defects can develop bronchiectasis over time following chronic or recurrent pulmonary infections.

Children with antibody deficiencies are usually asymptomatic until 5–6 mo of age, when maternally derived antibody levels begin to wane. These children begin to develop recurrent episodes of otitis media, bronchitis, pneumonia, bacteremia, and meningitis. Many of these infections respond quickly to antibiotics, which may delay the recognition of antibody deficiency. Children, especially boys, who require myringotomy tube placement before 2 yr of age because of recurrent episodes of otitis media (≥3 episodes within 6 mo, or ≥4 episodes within 12 mo) should be considered for screening measurement of immunoglobulin levels.

The significance and impact of specific **immunoglobulin G (IgG) subclass deficiencies** is less well understood and remains controversial. Deficiencies of specific IgG subclasses were 1st noted in healthy adult blood donors in whom no increased susceptibility to infections was documented. However, others have identified specific IgG deficiencies to be associated with a predisposition to recurrent bacterial sinopulmonary infection, bacteremia, meningitis, osteomyelitis, and pyoderma. Deficiency of subclass IgG_2 has been associated with poor antibody production after exposure to polysaccharide antigens, either after vaccination or after infection with a polysaccharide-encapsulated organism such as *S. pneumoniae* and *H. influenzae* type b.

Selective IgA deficiency leads to a lack of production of secretory antibody at the mucosal membranes (see Chapter 123). Even though most patients will have no increased risk for infections, some will have mild to moderate disease at sites of mucosal barriers. Accordingly, recurrent sinopulmonary infection and gastrointestinal disease are the major clinical manifestations. These patients also have an increased incidence of allergies and autoimmune disorders compared with the normal population.

Hyper-IgM syndrome is caused by a defect on the CD40 ligand on the T cell and is associated with a deficiency in the production of IgG and IgA antibody (see Chapter 123). In addition, recurrent neutropenia, hemolytic anemia, or aplastic anemia can be present. Similar to patients with agammaglobulinemia, these individuals are at risk for bacterial sinopulmonary infections, *Pneumocystis carinii* pneumonitis, and *Cryptosporidium* intestinal infection.

Replacement of antibody with **intravenous immunoglobulin (IVIG)** is the mainstay of treatment for most of the primary antibody deficiencies. The exception to this is IgA deficiency, because these patients can develop antibody against the minute amounts of IgA found in the standard IVIG preparations with an increased risk for anaphylaxis. Prophylaxis with specific antibiotic regimens is controversial and should be individualized for those patients who do not respond to immunoglobulin replacement.

T-CELL DEFECTS (CELL-MEDIATED IMMUNE DEFICIENCIES)

Children with primary cell-mediated immunodeficiencies, either isolated or more commonly in combination with B-cell defects, present early in life and are susceptible to viral, fungal, and protozoan infections. Clinical manifestations include chronic diarrhea, mucocutaneous candidiasis, and recurrent pneumonia, rhinitis, and otitis media. In thymic hypoplasia (DiGeorge syndrome), hypoplasia or aplasia of the thymus and parathyroid glands occurs during fetal development in association with the presence of other congenital abnormalities (see Chapter 124). Hypocalcemia and cardiac anomalies are usually the presenting features of DiGeorge syndrome, which should prompt evaluation of the T-cell system. **Chronic mucocutaneous candidiasis** is a rare immunodeficiency associated primarily with T-cell dysfunction. These patients may not demonstrate delayed hypersensitivity to skin tests for *Candida* antigen despite having chronic superficial infection with yeast, but do not appear to be at increased risk for systemic yeast infections. Endocrinopathies are commonly associated with chronic mucocutaneous candidiasis.

COMBINED B-CELL AND T-CELL DEFECTS

Patients with defects in both the T-cell and B-cell components of the immune system may manifest a variable disease spectrum depending on the extent of the defect (see Chapter 125). Complete immunodeficiency is found with **severe combined immunodeficiency syndrome (SCID)**, whereas partial defects can be present in such states as ataxia-telangiectasia, Wiskott-Aldrich syndrome, hyper-IgE syndrome, and X-linked immunodeficiency syndrome. Children with SCID present in the 1st 6 mo of life with recurrent, severe infections caused by a variety of bacteria, fungi, and viruses. Failure to thrive, chronic diarrhea, mucocutaneous or systemic candidiasis, *P. carinii* pneumonitis, or cytomegalovirus (CMV) infections are common early in life. Passive maternal antibody is relatively protective against the bacterial pathogens during the 1st few months of life, but thereafter patients are susceptible to both gram-positive and gram-negative organisms. Exposure to live virus vaccines can also lead to disseminated disease. Without stem cell transplantation, most affected children succumb to opportunistic infections within the 1st year of life.

Children with **ataxia-telangiectasia** develop late onset of recurrent sinopulmonary infections from both bacteria and respiratory viruses. In addition, these children experience an increased incidence of malignancies. Wiskott-Aldrich syndrome is an X-linked recessive disease associated with a reduced number of CD3 lymphocytes, moderately suppressed mitogen responses, and impaired antibody response to polysaccharide antigens. Accordingly, infections with *S. pneumoniae* or *H. influenzae* type b are common, as is *P. carinii* pneumonitis. In addition, affected males have thrombocytopenia and eczema. Children with hyper-IgE syndrome have markedly elevated levels of IgE and present with recurrent episodes of *S. aureus* abscesses of the skin, lungs, and musculoskeletal system. While the antibody abnormality is notable, these patients also have marked eosinophilia and poor cell-mediated responses to neoantigens, and they are at increased risk for fungal infections.

177.2 • INFECTIONS OCCURRING WITH ACQUIRED IMMUNODEFICIENCIES

Immunodeficiencies can be secondarily acquired as a result of infections or as a consequence of other underlying disorders such as malignancy, cystic fibrosis, diabetes mellitus, sickle cell disease, or malnutrition. Immunosuppressive medications used to prevent rejection after organ transplantation, graft vs host disease (GVHD) after stem cell transplantation (see Chapter 136), or to treat malignancies also leave the host vulnerable to infections. Similarly, medications used to control collagen vascular or other autoimmune disease may be associated with an increased risk for developing infection. Finally, any process (burns, surgery, or the presence of indwelling catheters) that interrupts or inhibits the normal mucosal and skin barriers can be considered an acquired risk for infection.

ACQUIRED IMMUNODEFICIENCY FROM INFECTIOUS AGENTS

Infection with HIV, the causative agent of AIDS, is the most important infectious cause of acquired immunodeficiency (see Chapter 273). If left untreated, the profound effects of HIV infection on the T-cell arm lead to susceptibility to the same types of infections as with primary T-cell immunodeficiencies.

Other organisms can lead to temporary alterations of the immune system. On rare occasions, transient neutropenia associated with community-acquired viruses can lead to significant disease with bacterial infections. Secondary infections can occur because of impaired immunity or disruption of the normal mucosal immunity, as exemplified by the increased risk for *S.*

pneumoniae pneumonia following influenza infection and group A streptococcus cellulitis and fasciitis following varicella.

MALIGNANCIES

The immune systems of children with malignancies are compromised by the therapies to treat the cancer and, at times, by direct effects of the cancer itself. The type, duration, and intensity of anticancer therapy remain the major risk factors for infections in these children and frequently affect >1 arm of the immune system (see Table 177-2). In addition, the presence of mucous membrane abnormalities, indwelling catheters, malnutrition, prolonged exposure to antibiotics, and frequent hospitalizations add to the risk for infection in these children.

Even though several arms of the immune system can be affected, the major abnormality associated with infection in children with cancer is **neutropenia.** The degree and duration of neutropenia have long been relied upon as accurate predictors of the risk of infection in children being treated for cancer. Patients are at particular risk for bacterial infections if the absolute neutrophil count decreases to <500 cells/mm^3. Counts of >500 cells/mm^3 but <1,000 cells/mm^3 incur some increased risk for infection, but not nearly as great. The lack of neutrophils can lead to a loss of inflammatory response, and fever may be the only manifestation of infection. Accordingly, the absence of physical signs and symptoms is not always reliable and the use of empirical antibiotics is required (Fig. 177-1).

Because patients with **fever and neutropenia** may only have subtle signs and symptoms of infection, the presence of fever warrants thorough physical examination with careful attention to the oropharynx, lungs, perineum and anus, skin, nail beds, and sites along intravascular catheter sites. In addition, a comprehensive laboratory evaluation including a complete blood cell count, serum creatinine, blood urea nitrogen, and transaminases should be obtained. Blood cultures should be obtained from each port of any central venous catheter. Consideration should also be given to obtaining a peripheral venous sample for blood culture. Other microbiologic studies should be done if there are associated clinical symptoms: nasal aspirate for viruses in patients with upper respiratory findings; stool for rotavirus in the appropriate months and *Clostridium difficile* in patients with diarrhea; urine culture in young children, or in older patients with symptoms of urgency, frequency, dysuria, or hematuria; and biopsy and culture of cutaneous lesions. Chest radiographs should be obtained in any individual with respiratory symptoms, although pulmonary infiltrates may be absent in children with severe neutropenia. Sinus films should be obtained if rhinorrhea is prolonged. Abdominal computed tomography scans should also be considered in children with profound neutropenia and abdominal pain to evaluate for the presence of typhlitis. Biopsies for cytology, Gram stain, and culture should be considered if abnormalities are found during endoscopic procedures or if lung nodules are identified radiographically.

Before the routine institution of empirical antimicrobial therapy for fever and neutropenia, 75% of children with fever and neutropenia were ultimately found to have a documented site of infection. Currently, gram-positive cocci are the most common pathogens; however, gram-negative organisms such as *P. aeruginosa*, *Escherichia coli*, and *Klebsiella* can cause life-threatening infection and must be considered in the empirical treatment regimen. Other gram-negative pathogens such as *Enterobacter* and *Acinetobacter* are increasing in prevalence as well. While coagulase-negative staphylococci frequently cause infections in these children in association with central venous catheters, these infections are typically indolent, and a short delay in treatment will usually not lead to a detrimental outcome. Other gram-positive bacteria such as *S. aureus* and *S. pneumoniae* cause more fulminant disease and require prompt institution of therapy. Viridans streptococci are common pathogens in patients with the oral

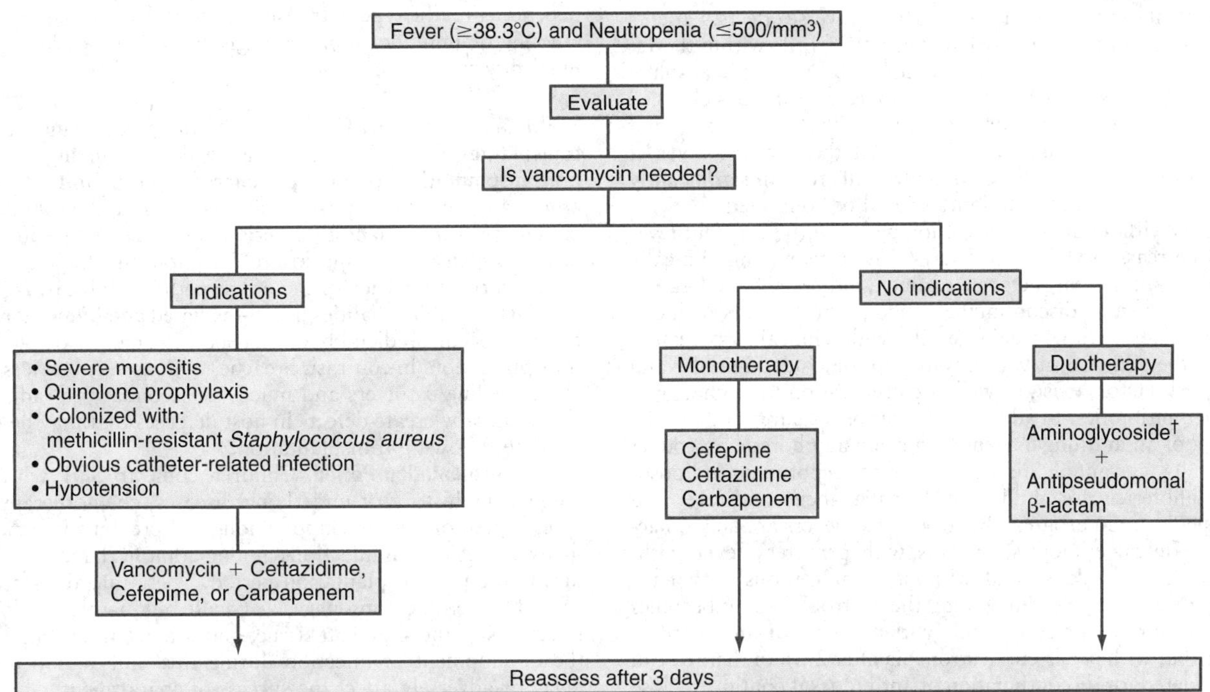

Figure 177-1. Guide to the initial management of the febrile neutropenic patient. Cefepime or meropenem may be as effective as ceftazidime or imipenem as monotherapy. *Aminoglycoside antibiotics should be avoided if the patient is also receiving nephrotoxic, ototoxic, or neuromuscular blocking agents; has renal or severe electrolyte dysfunction; or is suspected of having meningitis (because of poor blood-brain perfusion). (Adapted from Hughes WT, Armstrong D, Bodey GP, et al: 2002 guidelines for the use of antimicrobial agents in neutropenic patients with cancer. *Clin Infect Dis* 2002;34:730–751.)

mucositis that is often associated with the use of cytarabine and selective antibiotics such as quinolones, and can present as an acute septic shock syndrome. Patients with prolonged neutropenia who have received broad antimicrobial therapy are at increased risk for opportunistic fungal infections, especially with *Candida* and *Aspergillus.*

FEVER AND NEUTROPENIA. Management of fever and neutropenia includes empirical antimicrobial treatment, which decreases the risks for sepsis and septic shock and the sequelae of acute respiratory distress syndrome, organ dysfunction, and death. In 2002, the Infectious Diseases Society of America published comprehensive guidelines for the use of antimicrobial agents in neutropenic children and adults with cancer (see Fig. 177-1). First-line antimicrobial therapy should take into consideration the types of microbes anticipated and the local resistance patterns encountered at each institution. In addition, antibiotic choices may be limited by specific circumstances, such as the presence of drug allergy and renal or hepatic dysfunction. The empirical use of oral antibiotics is safe in some low-risk adults who have no evidence of bacterial focus or signs of significant illness (rigors, hypotension, mental status changes) and for whom a quick recovery of the bone marrow is anticipated. However, substantive data for this approach are lacking in children and it is not currently recommended. The decision to use intravenous monotherapy versus an expanded regimen of antibiotics depends on the severity of illness of the patient, history of previous colonization with resistant organisms, and the obvious presence of catheter-related infection. Vancomycin should be added to the empirical initial regimen if the patient has hypotension or other evidence of septic shock, an obvious catheter-related infection, or colonization with methicillin-resistant *S. aureus,* or if the patient is at high risk for viridans streptococci (severe mucositis, acute myelogenous leukemia, or prior quinolone prophylaxis). Monotherapy with cefepime, ceftazidime, a carbapenem (imipenem/cilastatin or meropenem), and piperacillin-tazobactam have been equally effective.

Regardless of the regimen chosen initially, it is critical to carefully and continually evaluate the patient for response to therapy, development of secondary infections, and adverse effects. Patients without an identified etiology who become afebrile within the 1st 3–5 days of therapy and who are clinically well with absolute neutrophil counts of >100 cells/mm^3 can have antibiotics changed to an oral regimen (cefixime or amoxicillin/clavulanate) and should receive a minimum of 7 days of therapy. However, if symptoms persist or evolve or if neutrophils remain significantly depressed, intravenous antibiotics should be continued.

Patients without an identified etiology but with **persistent fever** should be reassessed after 3–5 days. Those remaining clinically well may continue on the same regimen, although consideration should be given to discontinuing vancomycin if it was included initially. Those who remain febrile with clinical progression warrant the addition of vancomycin if not included initially and certain risk factors exist, as well as consideration for a change of the other antibiotics. In addition, if fever persists for >5 days, the addition of an **antifungal agent** such as an amphotericin product is generally warranted. Studies comparing caspofungin to liposomal amphotericin for children with malignancies and fever and neutropenia are in progress. Because not all fevers are due to bacterial or fungal etiologies, patients with persistent fever without an identified cause and without complications may have therapy discontinued 4–5 days after the neutrophil count becomes >500 cells/mm^3. Clinically stable patients without an identified etiology but with persistent neutropenia after 2 wk of therapy can be considered for discontinuation of antibiotics if continued close observation can be assured.

The use of **antiviral agents** in fever and neutropenia is not warranted without specific evidence of viral disease. Active herpes simplex or varicella-zoster lesions merit treatment to decrease the time of healing; even if they are not the source of fever, they are potential portals of entry for bacteria and fungi. CMV is rarely a cause of fever in children with cancer and neutropenia. If CMV infection is strongly suspected, ganciclovir, foscarnet, or cidofovir may be considered, although ganciclovir can cause bone marrow suppression and foscarnet and cidofovir can be nephrotoxic (see Chapter 252). If influenza is identified, specific treatment with zanamivir or oseltamivir should be administered (see Chapter 255).

The use of **hematopoietic growth factors** shortens the duration of neutropenia but has not been proven to reduce morbidity or mortality. Accordingly, the 2002 recommendations from the Infectious Diseases Society of America do not endorse the routine use of hematopoietic growth factors in patients with uncomplicated fever and neutropenia. Infections occur in children with cancer even without neutropenia. Most often these organisms are viral in etiology. However, *P. carinii* can cause pneumonitis regardless of the neutrophil count. Prophylaxis with trimethoprim-sulfamethoxazole against *P. carinii* is an effective preventive strategy and should be provided to all children undergoing active treatment for malignancy (see Chapter 241). Environmental fungi such as *Cryptococcus, Histoplasma,* and *Coccidioides* can also cause disease. *Toxoplasma gondii* is an uncommon but occasional pathogen in children with cancer. Infections encountered in healthy children (*S. pneumoniae,* group A streptococcus) can cause disease in children with cancer regardless of the granulocyte count.

TRANSPLANTATION

Transplantation of stem cells (bone marrow) and solid organs, including heart, liver, kidney, lungs, pancreas, and intestines, is increasingly used as therapy for a variety of disorders. Children with transplants are at risk for infections caused by many of the same microbial agents that cause disease in children with primary immunodeficiencies. Although the type and timing of infections after organ transplantation are in general similar among all recipients of these procedures, some differences exist between patients depending on the type of transplantation performed, the type and amount of immunosuppression given, and the child's previous immunity to specific pathogens.

STEM CELL TRANSPLANTATION. Infections following stem cell transplantation (SCT) can be classified as occurring during the **pretransplantation period, pre-engraftment period** (0–30 days after transplantation), **postengraftment period** (30–100 days), or the **late post-transplantation period** (>100 days). Specific defects in host defenses predisposing to infection and their underlying causes vary within each of these time periods (Table 177-3). Neutropenia and abnormalities in cell-mediated and humoral immune function occur predictably during specific time periods following transplantation. In contrast, breaches of anatomic barriers caused by indwelling catheters and mucositis secondary to radiation or chemotherapy create defects in host defenses that may be present anytime following transplantation.

Pretransplantation Period. Children come to SCT with a heterogeneous history of underlying diseases, chemotherapy exposure, degree of immunosuppression, and previous infections. As many as 12% of all infections among adult SCT recipients occur during the pretransplantation period. These infections are often caused by aerobic gram-negative bacilli and manifest as localized infections of the skin, soft tissue, and urinary tract. Importantly, the development of infection during this time period does not delay or adversely affect the success of engraftment.

Pre-engraftment Period. Bacterial infections predominate in the pre-engraftment period (0–30 days). Bacteremia is the most common documented infection and occurs in as many as 50% of all SCT recipients during the 1st 30 days following transplanta-

TABLE 177-3. Host Defense Defects and Common Pathogens by Time After Bone Marrow Transplantation and Stem Cell Transplantation

TIME PERIOD	HOST DEFENSE DEFECTS	CAUSES	COMMON PATHOGENS
Pretransplant	Neutropenia Abnormal anatomic barriers	Underlying disease Prior chemotherapy	Aerobic gram-negative bacilli
Pre-engraftment	Neutropenia Abnormal anatomic barriers	Chemotherapy Radiation Indwelling catheters	Aerobic gram-positive cocci Aerobic gram-negative bacilli *Candida* *Aspergillus* Herpes simplex virus (in previously infected patients) Community-acquired viral pathogens
Postengraftment	Abnormal cell-mediated immunity Abnormal anatomic barriers	Chemotherapy Immunosuppressive medications Radiation Indwelling catheters Unrelated cord blood donor	Gram-positive cocci Aerobic gram-negative bacilli Cytomegalovirus Adenoviruses Community-acquired viral pathogens *Pneumocystis carinii*
Late post-transplant	Delayed recovery of immune function (cell-mediated, humoral, and abnormal anatomic barriers)	Time required to develop donor-related immune function Graft vs host disease	Varicella-zoster virus *Streptococcus pneumoniae*

tion. Bacteremia is typically secondary to either mucositis or the presence of an indwelling catheter but may be associated with pneumonia. Similarly, more than 40% of children undergoing SCT experienced at least 1 infection in the pre-engraftment period. Gram-positive cocci, gram-negative bacilli, yeast, and, less commonly, other fungi all cause infection during this period. *Aspergillus* has been identified in 4–20% of SCT recipients, most often after ≥3 wk of neutropenia. Infections caused by the emerging fungal pathogens *Fusarium* and *Pseudallescheria boydii* are associated with the prolonged neutropenia during the pre-engraftment period.

Viral infections also occur during the pre-engraftment period. Among adults, reactivation of herpes simplex virus is the most common viral disease observed, but this is less frequent among children, which is likely related to absence of the virus in the recipient before SCT. A history of herpes simplex infection or seropositivity indicates the need for prophylaxis. Nosocomial exposure to community-acquired viral pathogens, including respiratory syncytial virus (RSV), influenza, adenovirus, and rotavirus, represents an important source of infection during this time period. There is growing evidence that community-acquired viruses cause increased morbidity and mortality for SCT recipients during this time period. Adenovirus is a particularly important viral pathogen that may present early, although it typically presents after engraftment.

Postengraftment Period. The predominant defect in host defenses in the postengraftment period is altered cell-mediated immunity. Accordingly, organisms historically categorized as opportunistic pathogens predominate during this time period. The risk is especially accentuated 50–100 days after transplantation when host immunity is lost and donor immunity is not yet established. *P. carinii* pneumonia presents during this time period if patients are not maintained on appropriate prophylaxis. Reactivation of *T. gondii,* a rare cause of disease among SCT recipients, may also present after engraftment. Hepatosplenic candidiasis frequently presents during the postengraftment period, although seeding likely occurred during the neutropenic phase.

CMV is one of the most important causes of morbidity and mortality among SCT recipients. Unlike patients undergoing solid organ transplantation, SCT recipients developing either a primary infection or reactivation of their own latent virus may develop severe CMV disease. **Adenovirus** is another important viral pathogen, having been recovered from up to 5% of adult and pediatric SCT recipients and causing invasive disease in approximately 20% of cases. Children receiving matched unrelated donors or unrelated cord blood cell transplants have as high as 14% incidence of adenovirus infection during this early postengraftment period. **Polyomaviruses,** such as BK virus, have been increasingly recognized as a cause of renal dysfunction and hemorrhagic cystitis after bone marrow transplantation. Infections with other community-acquired pathogens have been associated with excess morbidity and mortality during this time period, similar to the pre-engraftment time.

Late Post-transplantation Period. Infection is unusual after 100 days in the absence of chronic GVHD. The presence of chronic GVHD significantly affects anatomic barriers and is associated with defects in humoral, splenic, and cell-mediated immune function (see Chapter 136). Viral infections, primarily reactivation of varicella-zoster virus (VZV), are responsible for more than 40% of infections during this time period. Bacterial infections, particularly of the upper and lower respiratory tract, account for approximately ⅓ of infections. These may be associated with deficiencies in immunoglobulin production or synthesis, especially IgG_2. Fungal infections account for less than 20% of confirmed infections during the late post-transplantation time period.

SOLID ORGAN TRANSPLANTATION. Factors predisposing to infection after organ transplantation include those that either existed before transplantation or those that are secondary to intraoperative events or post-transplantation therapies (Table 177-4). Some of these additional risks cannot be prevented, and some risks acquired during or after the operation may be dependent on decisions or actions of members of the transplant team. The necessity for substantial immunosuppressive agents is the major factor predisposing to infection following transplantation. Despite efforts to develop optimal immunosuppressive regimens to prevent or treat rejection with minimal impairment of immunity, all current regimens interfere with the ability of the immune system to fight infection. The majority of these immunosuppressive agents are aimed primarily at controlling cell-mediated immunity; regimens may impair many other aspects of the transplant recipient's immune system.

TIMING. The timing of specific types of infections is generally predictable, regardless of which organ is transplanted (Table 177-5). Infectious complications typically develop in 1 of 3 time intervals: early (0–30 days after transplantation), intermediate (30–180 days, or 1–6 mo), and late (>180 days, or >6 mo); most infections develop in the 1st 180 days after transplantation. Table 177-5 should be used as a general guideline to the types of infections encountered but may be modified by newer immunosup-

TABLE 177-4. Risk Factors for Infections Following Solid Organ Transplantation in Children

PRETRANSPLANTATION FACTORS
Age of patient
Underlying disease, malnutrition
Specific organ transplanted
Previous exposures to infectious agents
Previous immunizations
INTRAOPERATIVE FACTORS
Duration of transplant surgery
Exposure to blood products
Technical problems
Organisms transmitted with donor organ
POST-TRANSPLANTATION FACTORS
Immunosuppression
Induction immunosuppression
Maintenance immunosuppression
Augmented treatment for rejection
Indwelling catheters
Nosocomial exposures
Community exposures

pressive therapies and by the use of prophylaxis. Early infections usually result as either a complication of the transplant surgery itself or the presence of indwelling catheters. Infections during the intermediate time period typically result as a complication of the immunosuppression, which tends to be at its greatest intensity during the 1st 6 mo following transplantation. This is the time period of greatest risk for infections due to opportunistic pathogens such as CMV and *P. carinii.* Anatomic abnormalities, such as bronchial stenosis and biliary stenosis, developing as a consequence of the transplant surgery, can also predispose to recurrent infection that presents in this time period. Infections developing late after transplantation typically result as a consequence of uncorrected anatomic abnormalities, chronic rejection, or exposure to community-acquired pathogens. Acquisition of infection due to community-acquired pathogens, such as RSV, may result in severe infection secondary to the immunocompromised state of the transplant recipient during the early and intermediate periods. Compared with the earlier periods, community-acquired infections in the late period are usually benign because levels of immunosuppression are typically maintained at significantly lower levels. However, certain pathogens, such as VZV and Epstein-Barr virus (EBV), may be associated with severe disease even at this late time period.

BACTERIAL AND FUNGAL INFECTIONS. Although there are important graft-specific considerations for bacterial and fungal infections following transplantation, some principles are generally applicable to all transplant recipients. Bacterial and fungal infections following organ transplantation are usually a direct consequence of the surgery, a breach in an anatomic barrier, presence of a foreign body, or an abnormal anatomic narrowing or obstruction. With the exception of infections related to the use of indwelling catheters, sites of bacterial infection tend to occur at or near the transplanted organ. Infections following abdominal transplantation (liver, intestine, or renal) usually occur in the abdomen or at the surgical wound. The pathogens are typically enteric gram-negative bacteria, *Enterococcus,* and occasionally *Candida.* Infections following thoracic transplantation (heart, lung) usually occur in the lower respiratory tract or at the surgical wound. Pathogens associated with these infections include *S. aureus* and gram-negative bacteria. Patients undergoing lung transplantation for cystic fibrosis experience a particularly high rate of infectious complications, because they are frequently colonized with *P. aeruginosa* or *Aspergillus* before transplantation. Even though the infected cystic lungs are removed, the sinuses and upper airways remain colonized with these same pathogens, and subsequent reinfection of the transplanted lungs is not infrequent. Children receiving organ transplants have frequently been hospitalized for long periods and have received many antibiotics; thus, recovery of bacteria with multiple antibiotic resistance is common after all types of organ transplantation. Infections due to *Aspergillus* are less common but occur after all types of organ transplantation and are associated with high rates of morbidity and mortality.

VIRAL INFECTIONS. Viral pathogens, especially herpesviruses, are a major source of morbidity and mortality following solid organ transplantation. The patterns of disease associated with individual viral pathogens generally are similar among all organ transplant recipients. However, the frequency, mode of presentation, and severity differ according to type of organ transplanted and pretransplant serologic status of the recipient.

Viral pathogens can be categorized as reactivated host or donor-associated viruses, such as CMV and EBV, or as community-acquired viruses. For CMV and EBV, primary infection

TABLE 177-5. Timing of Infectious Complications Following Solid Organ Transplantation

EARLY PERIOD (0–30 DAYS)	MIDDLE PERIOD (1–6 MO)	LATE PERIOD (>6 MO)
Bacterial infections	Viral infections	Viral infections
Gram-negative enteric bacilli	Cytomegalovirus	Epstein-Barr virus
Small bowel, liver, neonatal heart	All transplant types	All transplant types, but less risk than middle period
Pseudomonas, Burkholderia, Stenotrophomonas, Alcaligenes	Seronegative recipient of seropositive donor	Varicella-zoster virus
Cystic fibrosis lung	Epstein-Barr virus	All transplant types
Gram-positive organisms	All transplant types (small bowel highest risk group)	Community-acquired viral infections
All transplant types	Seronegative recipient	All transplant types
Fungal infections	Varicella-zoster virus	Bacteria infections
All transplant types	All transplant types	*Pseudomonas, Burkholderia, Stenotrophomonas, Alcaligenes*
Viral infections	Opportunistic infections	Cystic fibrosis lung
Herpes simplex virus	*Pneumocystis carinii*	Lung recipients with chronic rejection
All transplant types	All transplant types	Gram-negative bacillary bacteremia
Nosocomial respiratory viruses	*Toxoplasma gondii*	Small bowel
All transplant types	Seronegative recipient of cardiac transplant from a seropositive donor	Fungal infections
	Bacterial infections	*Aspergillus*
	Pseudomonas, Burkholderia, Stenotrophomonas, Alcaligenes	Lung transplants with chronic rejection
	Cystic fibrosis lung	
	Gram-negative enteric bacilli	
	Small bowel	

Adapted from Green M, Michaels MG: Infections in solid organ transplant recipients. In Long SS, Pickering L, Prober C (editors): *Principles and Practice of Pediatric Infectious Disease.* New York, Churchill Livingstone, 1997.

occurring after transplantation is associated with the greatest degree of morbidity and mortality. The highest risk is in a naive host who receives an organ from a donor who previously was infected with one of these viruses. This "mismatched state" is a frequent cause of severe disease. However, even if the donor is negative for CMV and EBV, these infections can be acquired from a close contact or via blood products. Reactivation of a latent strain within the host or superinfection with a new strain tends to result in milder illness unless the patient is greatly immunosuppressed, which may occur in the setting of treatment of significant rejection. CMV is one of the most commonly recognized transplant viral pathogens and remains a major cause of disease after solid organ transplantation. Clinical manifestations can range from a syndrome of fatigue and fever to disseminated disease that most often affects the liver, lungs, and gastrointestinal tract. Infection due to EBV is increasingly recognized as another important complication of solid organ transplantation ranging from a mild mononucleosis syndrome to disseminated **post-transplantation lymphoproliferative disorder** (PTLD). PTLD is more common among children than adults because primary EBV infection in the immunosuppressed host is more likely to lead to uncontrolled proliferative disorders, including post-transplantation lymphoma. Other viruses such as adenovirus have the capacity to be donor associated but appear to be less common. Donor-associated viral pathogens, including hepatitis B virus, hepatitis C virus, and HIV, are gratefully rare today due to intensive donor screening.

Community-acquired viruses, including respiratory viruses (RSV, influenza, adenovirus, and parainfluenza) and enteric viruses (enteroviruses, rotavirus), may cause important disease in children following organ transplantation. In general, risk factors for more severe infection include young age, acquisition of infection early after transplantation, and augmented immune suppression. Infection in the absence of these risk factors typically results in a clinical illness that is comparable with that seen in immunocompetent children. However, some community-acquired viruses such as adenovirus have been associated with graft dysfunction even when acquired late after transplantation.

OPPORTUNISTIC PATHOGENS. Children undergoing solid-organ transplantation are also at risk for symptomatic infections from pathogens that do not usually cause clinical disease in immunocompetent hosts. Even though most frequently recognized in the intermediate time period, these infections can also occur late in patients requiring prolonged and high levels of immunosuppression. *P. carinii* is a well-recognized cause of pneumonia following solid organ transplantation, although routine prophylaxis has essentially eliminated this problem. *T. gondii* may complicate cardiac transplantations, because of tropism of the organism for cardiac muscle and risk for donor transmission; less commonly it complicates other types of organ transplantation.

177.3 • Prevention Of Infection In Immunocompromised Persons

Infections cannot be completely prevented in children who have defects in 1 or more arms of their immune system, although some measures can decrease the risks for infection. Replacement immunoglobulin is a benefit to children with primary B-cell deficiencies; IFN-γ and trimethoprim-sulfamethoxazole reduce the number of infections occurring in children with chronic granulomatous disease. Likewise, children with depressed cellular immunity from primary diseases, advanced HIV infection, or use of immunosuppressive medications benefit from prophylaxis against *P. carinii*. Immunizations prevent many infections and are particularly important for children with compromised immune systems. Immunizations should ideally be administered before any treatment that would compromise the child's immune system; however, this is not always possible such as with primary immune defects or in children who require transplants early in life.

While immunodeficient children represent a heterogeneic group, some principles of prevention are generally applicable. Inactivated vaccines do not lead to an increased risk for adverse effects, although their efficacy may be reduced due to an impaired immune response. In most cases, children with immunodeficiencies should receive all of the recommended inactivated vaccines. Live, attenuated virus vaccinations can cause disease in some children with immunologic defects, and therefore alternative immunizations should be used whenever possible, such as the use of inactivated polio vaccine rather than live virus oral polio vaccine. In general, live virus vaccines should not be used in children with primary T-cell abnormalities. However, in some instances in which wild-type viral infection can be severe, immunizations, even with live virus vaccine, are warranted. Children with HIV infection and a CD4 percentage of >15% should receive measles vaccination, and also varicella vaccine if the CD4 percentage is ≥15%. Some vaccines should be given to children with immunodeficiencies in addition to routine vaccinations, such as the addition of the meningococcal vaccine and the polysaccharide pneumococcal vaccine to the routinely provided conjugate pneumococcal vaccine for children with newly diagnosed splenic dysfunction or complement deficiency. Influenza vaccination is recommended for immunocompromised children as well as all household contacts to minimize risk for transmission to the immunocompromised child.

American Academy of Pediatrics: Passive and active immunization. In Pickering LK (editor): *Red Book 2006: Report of the Committee on Infectious Diseases,* 27th ed. Elk Grove Village, IL, American Academy of Pediatrics, 2006, pp 1–103.

Benjamin DK Jr, Miller WC, Bayliff S, et al: Infections diagnosed in the first year after pediatric stem cell transplantation. *Pediatr Infect Dis J* 2002;21:227–234.

Buckley RH: Primary immunodeficiency disease due to defects in lymphocytes. *N Engl J Med* 2000;343:1313–1324.

Green M, Avery, RK, Preiksaitis J (editors): Guidelines for the prevention and management of infectious complications of solid organ transplantation. *Am J Transplant* 2004;4(Suppl 10):1–166.

Green M, Michaels MG, Webber SA, et al: The management of Epstein-Barr virus associated post-transplant lymphoproliferative disorders in pediatric solid-organ transplant recipients. *Pediatr Transplant* 1999;3:271–281.

Hernandez de Mezerville M, Tellier R, Richardson S, et al: Adenoviral infections in pediatric transplant recipients: a hospital-based study. *Pediatr Infect Dis J* 2006;25:815–818.

Hughes WT, Armstrong D, Bodey GP, et al: 2002 guidelines for the use of antimicrobial agents in neutropenic patients with cancer. *Clin Infect Dis* 2002;34:730–751.

Kusne S, Dummer JS, Singh N, et al: Infection after liver transplantation. An analysis of 101 consecutive cases. *Medicine* 1988;67:132–143.

Lopez MJ, Thomas S: Immunization of children after solid organ transplantation. *Pediatr Clin North Am* 2003;50:1435–1449.

Mackay IR, Rosen FS: Immunodeficiency diseases caused by defects in phagocytes. Advances in immunology. *N Engl J Med* 2000;343:1703–1714.

Palmer SM, Alexander BD, Sanders LL: Significance of bloodstream infection after lung transplantation: Analysis in 176 consecutive patients. *Transplantation* 2000;69:2360–2366.

Paya C, Fung JJ, Nalesnik MA, et al: Epstein-Barr virus–induced posttransplant lymphoproliferative disorders. *Transplantation* 1999;68:1517–1525.

Sable CA, Donowitz GR: Infections in bone marrow transplant recipients. *Clin Infect Dis* 1994;18:273–281.

Segers P, Speekenbrink RGH, Ubbink DT, et al: Prevention of nonsocomial infection in cardiac surgery by decontamination of the nasopharynx and oropharynx with chlorhexidine gluconate. *JAMA* 2006;296:2460–2466.

Their M, Holmberg C, Lautenschlager I, et al: Infections in pediatric kidney and liver patients after perioperative hospitalization. *Transplantation* 2000;69:1617–1623.

Chapter 178 ■ Infection Associated with Medical Devices

Patricia M. Flynn and Fred F. Barrett

Despite the therapeutic successes and convenience of the many synthetic devices used in pediatric patients, infectious complications are problematic. The pathogenesis of device-related infection is not completely defined, but many factors are important, including the susceptibility of the host, the composition of the device, the ability of microorganisms to adhere to the device itself or to the biofilm that quickly forms on it, and environmental factors that include the insertion technique and maintenance of the device.

INTRAVASCULAR ACCESS DEVICES. Intravascular access devices range from short stainless steel needles to multilumen implantable synthetic plastic catheters that are expected to remain in use for years. Infectious complications include localized infections and systemic infections (catheter-related bacteremia and fungemia). **Exit site infection** denotes infection localized to the exit site often with purulent discharge. **Tunnel tract infection** indicates infection in the subcutaneous tissues tracking along the catheter, which may also include serous or serosanguineous discharge from a draining sinus along the catheter path. This usually mandates removal of the catheter. **Pocket infection** indicates suppurative infection of a subcutaneous pocket containing a reservoir, usually of a totally implanted device. The source of catheter infection is usually contamination by bacteria on the skin rather than bacteremia from another focus seeding the intravascular device. Infection with the microbial skin flora at the insertion site may extend along the external surface of the catheter. This route of infection is most common in intravascular catheters in place for <30 days. Organisms may also gain access to the intraluminal portion of the catheter through improper handling of the catheter hub or contaminated infusate. This route of infection is thought to be more prevalent in catheters in place for >30 days. Gram-positive cocci predominate in both categories, with more than half caused by coagulase-negative staphylococci. Gram-negative enteric bacteria are isolated in approximately 20–30% of episodes, and fungi account for 5–10%.

The **clinical manifestations** of local infection include erythema, tenderness, and purulent discharge at the exit site or along the subcutaneous tunnel tract of the catheter. Catheter-related sepsis may also present as fever without an identifiable focus.

The diagnosis of localized infection is established clinically. A Gram stain and culture of exit site drainage should be performed and may help elucidate the microbiologic cause. The diagnosis of catheter-related bacteremia is confirmed by performing quantitative blood cultures simultaneously from the catheter and the peripheral vein. Evidence of catheter-related bacteremia or fungemia is >4–10 times the number of organisms isolated from blood obtained via the catheter as compared to blood obtained via a peripheral vein. If quantitative blood cultures are not available, a catheter blood culture that becomes positive >2 hr before a peripheral culture, with equal amounts of blood using a radiometric detection system, may also be used for diagnosis. Catheter-related sepsis can also be diagnosed by isolation of the same organism from the blood and the catheter tip. This method, however, requires catheter removal and is not optimal for patients with long-term devices.

Short-term peripheral catheters are most commonly used in pediatric patients, and infectious complications occur infrequently. The rate of peripheral catheter-related bacteremia is <0.15%. Patient age <1 yr, duration of use for >144 hr, and some infusates (e.g., total parenteral nutrition, lipids) are associated with increased risk for catheter-related infection.

Central venous catheters (CVCs) are widely used in both adults and pediatric patients and are responsible for the majority of catheter-related infections. They are commonly used in critically ill patients, including neonates, who often have many risk factors for the development of nosocomial infection. Patients who are in an intensive care unit and who have a CVC in place have a 5-fold greater risk for developing a nosocomial bloodstream infection than those without a CVC. The means for optimal maintenance of these catheters remains controversial. Although prevalence of infection increases with prolonged duration of catheter use, routine replacement of a CVC, either at a new site or over a guide wire, results in significant morbidity and should not be adopted. Catheters should be removed when they are no longer needed. The use of peripherally inserted central catheters (PICCs), which are inserted into a peripheral vein with the distal end in a central vein, has increased in pediatric patients. Published experience with these devices in children is scanty, but studies in adults document a life span of approximately 3 mo and infection rates of 1.9 episodes/1,000 catheter-days, significantly lower than for CVCs.

When prolonged intravenous access is required, a cuffed silicone rubber (Silastic) catheter may be inserted into the right atrium through the subclavian, cephalic, or jugular vein. The extravascular segment of the catheter passes through a subcutaneous tunnel before exiting the skin, usually on the superior aspect of the chest (Broviac or Hickman catheters). Totally implanted devices consist of a reservoir or port placed in a subcutaneous pocket with a self-sealing silicone septum at the distal end that permits repeated percutaneous needle insertions for administration of drugs. The use of central venous devices has improved the quality of life of high-risk patients but has also increased the risk for various infections. The incidence of local (exit site, tunnel, and pocket) infection is 0.2–2.8/1,000 catheter-days. The incidence of Broviac or Hickman catheter-associated sepsis is 0.5–6.8/1,000 catheter days, whereas that for implantable devices is 0.3–1.8/1,000 catheter-days. The risk for catheter infection is increased among premature infants, young children, and those receiving total parenteral nutrition.

If either localized or systemic catheter-related infection is diagnosed in a short-term peripheral catheter or CVC, the device should be removed. Antibiotics should be administered in cases of systemic infection, with the exception of uncomplicated coagulase-negative staphylococcal bacteremia in normal hosts, for which catheter removal is sufficient.

For infections associated with long-term vascular access devices (Hickman, Broviac, totally implantable devices), antibiotic treatment is successful for most systemic bacterial infections without removal of the device. Antibiotic therapy should be directed to the isolated pathogen and given for a total of 10–14 days. Until identification and susceptibility testing are available, empirical therapy with a 3rd generation cephalosporin or aminoglycoside plus vancomycin is indicated. **Antibiotic lock or dwell therapy,** with administration of solutions of high concentrations of antibiotics or ethanol that remain in the catheter for up to 24 hr, may improve outcome. If blood cultures remain positive after 72 hr of appropriate therapy, as confirmed by susceptibility testing, or if a patient deteriorates clinically, the device should be removed. Although new evidence is emerging to support catheter retention, most experts advocate removal of the device as well as therapy with systemic antifungals in cases of catheter-related fungemia. Exit site infections usually respond to local care or systemic antibiotics, but tunnel tract infections require removal of the catheter in approximately ⅔ of patients.

Prevention of Infection. Prevention of infections of long-term vascular access devices includes placement using meticulous surgical aseptic technique in an operating room–like environment, avoidance of bathing or swimming, and careful catheter care. The

Centers for Disease Control and Prevention recommends that short-term peripheral catheters be replaced every 72–96 hr to prevent phlebitis. The use of antimicrobial-impregnated catheters may reduce the risk for catheter-associated bloodstream infections.

CEREBROSPINAL FLUID SHUNTS. Cerebrospinal fluid (CSF) shunting is required for the treatment of many children with hydrocephalus. The usual procedure uses a silicone rubber device with a proximal portion inserted into the ventricle, a unidirectional valve, and a distant segment that diverts the CSF from the ventricles to either the peritoneal cavity (ventriculoperitoneal [VP] shunt) or right atrium (ventriculoatrial [VA] shunt). The incidence of shunt infection ranges from 1 to 20%, with an average of 10%. The highest rates are reported in young infants. Most infections are a result of intraoperative contamination of the surgical wound by skin flora. Accordingly, coagulase-negative staphylococci are isolated in more than half of the cases. *Staphylococcus aureus* is isolated in approximately 20% and gram-negative bacilli in 15%.

Four distinct clinical syndromes have been described: colonization of the shunt, infection associated with wound infection, distal infection with peritonitis, and infection associated with meningitis.

The most common type of infection is colonization of the shunt with symptoms that reflect shunt malfunction as opposed to frank infection. Symptoms associated with colonized VP shunts include lethargy, headache, vomiting, and a full fontanel. Low-grade fever is common. Symptoms usually occur within months of the surgical procedure. Colonization of a VA shunt results in more severe systemic symptoms and often without specific symptoms of shunt malfunction. Septic pulmonary emboli, pulmonary hypertension, and infective endocarditis are frequently reported complications of VA shunt colonization. Chronic VA shunt colonization may cause hypocomplementemic glomerulonephritis due to antigen-antibody complex deposition in the glomeruli, which is commonly called shunt nephritis; clinical findings include hypertension, microscopic hematuria, elevated blood urea nitrogen (BUN) and serum creatinine levels, and anemia. With shunt colonization, CSF obtained from either lumbar or ventricular puncture is often sterile, and the infecting organism is isolated only from the shunt reservoir. Because of this, it is unusual to observe signs of ventriculitis, and CSF findings are only minimally abnormal. Blood culture results are usually negative in cases of VP colonization but positive in VA shunt colonization.

Wound infection presents with obvious infection or dehiscence along the shunt tract and most often occurs within days to weeks of the surgical procedure. *S. aureus* is the most common isolate. In addition to the physical findings, fever is common, and signs of shunt malfunction eventually ensue in most cases.

Distal infection of VP shunts with peritonitis presents with abdominal symptoms, usually without evidence of shunt malfunction. The pathogenesis is likely related to perforation of bowel at the time of VP shunt placement or translocation of bacteria across the bowel wall. Thus, gram-negative isolates predominate and mixed infection is common. The infecting organisms are often isolated from only the distal portion of the shunt.

The usual meningeal pathogens, *Streptococcus pneumoniae, Neisseria meningitidis,* and *Haemophilus influenzae* type b, can also cause bacterial meningitis in patients with shunts in place. The clinical presentation is similar to that for acute bacterial meningitis (see Chapter 602.1).

Treatment of shunt colonization and distal infection with peritonitis includes the use of antibiotics against the specific organisms isolated and, in most situations, removal of the shunt. Intrashunt antibiotics are indicated because of the poor penetration of most antibiotics into the central nervous system across uninflamed meninges. If the isolate is susceptible, a parenteral antistaphylococcal penicillin plus intrashunt vancomycin is the treatment of choice. If the organism is resistant to the penicillins, systemic and intrashunt vancomycin is recommended. In cases of gram-negative infections, a combination of a 3rd generation cephalosporin and intrashunt aminoglycoside is optimal. When using intrashunt antibiotics, monitoring of CSF levels is necessary to avoid toxicity. The best treatment success occurs with initial systemic and intrashunt antibiotics in combination with exteriorization of the distal end of the shunt. After CSF from the reservoir has remained sterile for 48 hr, shunt replacement on the opposite side can be performed. Partial shunt revision with antibiotic therapy or antibiotic therapy alone has been successful in some series, but the relapse rate is higher. When wound infection is diagnosed, the shunt almost always needs to be removed. To allow for continued ventricular drainage, a temporary catheter is often placed, with replacement of a new shunt on the opposite side after the wound infection has healed. Only systemic antibiotics are necessary for treatment of bacterial meningitis in patients with a shunt in place; the shunt itself does not need to be removed.

Prevention of Infection. Prevention of shunt infection includes meticulous cutaneous preparation and surgical technique. Systemic and intraventricular antibiotics, antibiotic-impregnated shunts, and soaking the shunt tubing in antibiotics have been used to reduce the incidence of infection, with varying success. A meta-analysis of 12 clinical trials using various antimicrobial regimens involving 1,359 randomized patients showed that perioperative use of an antimicrobial agent in CSF shunt placement reduced the risk for infection, although only 1 of the 12 studies individually revealed an effect.

URETHRAL CATHETERS. Urinary catheters are a frequent cause of nosocomial infection, with about 14 infections per 1,000 admissions. Like other devices, microorganisms adhere to the catheter surface and establish a biofilm that allows proliferation. The physical presence of the catheter reduces the normal host defenses by preventing complete emptying of the bladder, thus providing a medium for growth, distending the urethra, and blocking periurethral glands. Almost all patients catheterized for >30 days develop bacteriuria. The urinary tract is considered infected if specimens of urine obtained directly from an indwelling catheter harbor ≥100 colony-forming units/mL. Gram-negative bacilli and *Enterococcus* are the predominant organisms isolated in catheter-related urinary tract infection; coagulase-negative staphylococci are implicated in about 15%. Symptomatic urinary tract infections should be treated with antibiotics and catheter removal. Asymptomatic infections can usually be managed with catheter removal alone.

Prevention of Infection. All urinary catheters introduce risk for infection, and their casual use should be avoided. When they are in place, their duration of use should be minimized. Technologic advances have led to development of silver- or antibiotic-impregnated urinary catheters that are associated with lower rates of infection. Prophylactic antibiotics do not reduce the infection rates for long-term indwelling urethral catheters.

PERITONEAL DIALYSIS CATHETERS. During the 1st year of peritoneal dialysis for end-stage renal disease, 65% of children will have 1 or more episodes of peritonitis. Bacterial entry comes from luminal or periluminal contamination of the catheter or by translocation across the intestinal wall. Hematogenous infection is rare. Infections can be localized at the exit site, associated with peritonitis, or both. Organisms responsible for peritonitis include coagulase-negative staphylococci (30–40%), *S. aureus* (10–20%), streptococci (10–15%), *Escherichia coli* (5–10%), *Pseudomonas* (5–10%), other gram-negative bacteria (5–15%), *Enterococcus* (3–6%), and fungi (2–10%). *S. aureus* is more common in localized exit or tunnel tract infections (42%). Most infectious episodes are due to a patient's own flora, and carriers of *S. aureus* have been shown to have increased rates of infection as compared with noncarriers.

The **clinical manifestations** of peritonitis may be subtle and include low-grade fever, mild abdominal pain, and tenderness. Cloudy peritoneal dialysis fluid may be the 1st and predominant sign. With peritonitis, the peritoneal fluid cell count is usually >100 white blood cells/μL. When peritonitis is suspected, the effluent dialysate should be submitted for cell count, Gram stain, and culture. The Gram stain is positive in up to 40% of cases of peritonitis.

Patients with cloudy fluid and clinical symptoms should receive empirical therapy, preferably guided by results of a Gram stain. If no organisms are visualized, vancomycin and either an aminoglycoside or 3rd generation cephalosporin with antipseudomonal activity should be given via the intraperitoneal route. Patients without cloudy fluid and with minimal symptoms may have therapy withheld pending culture results. Once the cause is identified by culture, changes in the therapeutic regimen may be needed. Oral rifampin may be added for *S. aureus* infections. Fungal peritonitis should be treated with a combination of oral flucytosine and intraperitoneal or oral fluconazole alone. The duration of therapy is a minimum of 14 days, with longer treatment of 21–28 days for episodes of *S. aureus* and *Pseudomonas*, and 28–42 days for fungi. Repeat episodes of peritonitis within 4 wk of previous therapy represent "apparently relapsing" peritonitis. If the patient responds to reinstitution of antimicrobial therapy, a course of up to 6 wk should be continued. In all cases, if the infection fails to clear on appropriate therapy or if a patient's condition is deteriorating, the catheter should be removed. Exit site and tunnel infections may occur independently of peritonitis, or may precede it. Appropriate antibiotics should be administered on the basis of Gram stain and culture findings. Some experts recommend that the peritoneal catheter be removed if *Pseudomonas* or fungal organisms are isolated.

Prevention of Infection. In addition to usual hygienic practices, mupirocin, applied either to the nares or at the exit site, reduces exit site infections and bacteremia caused by *S. aureus*.

ORTHOPEDIC PROSTHESES. Orthopedic prostheses are used infrequently in children although their use is increasing in limb salvage procedures for osteosarcoma. Infection most often follows introduction of microorganisms at surgery or via hematogenous spread. Early postoperative infection occurs within 2–4 wk of surgery with typical manifestations that include fever, pain, and local symptoms of wound infection. Rapid assessment, including isolation of the infecting organism, and antimicrobial treatment may allow salvage of the implant. Late chronic infections occur >1 mo after surgery and are often caused by organisms of low virulence that contaminated the implant at the time of surgery. Typical manifestations include pain and deterioration in function. These infections respond poorly to antibiotic treatment and usually require removal of the implant. Hematogenous infections are most often observed ≥2 yr after surgery. As with other long-term implanted devices, the most common organisms are about equally divided between coagulase-negative staphylococci and *S. aureus*.

The use of systemic antibiotic prophylaxis, antibiotic-containing bone cement, and operating rooms fitted with laminar airflow all have been proposed as beneficial in reducing infection. To date, results from clinical studies are conflicting.

Centers for Disease Control and Prevention: Guidelines for the prevention of intravascular catheter-related infections. *MMWR* 2002;51(RR-10):1–29.

Darouiche RO: Device-associated infections: A macroproblem that starts with microadherence. *Clin Infect Dis* 2001;33:1567–1572.

Darouiche RO, Berger DH, Khardori N, et al: Comparison of antimicrobial impregnation with tunneling of long-term central venous catheters: A randomized controlled trial. *Ann Surg* 2005;242:193–200.

Gaur AH, Liu T, Knapp KM, et al: Infections in children and young adults with bone malignancies undergoing limb-sparing surgery. *Cancer* 2005;104:602–610.

McGee DC, Gould MK: Preventing complications of central venous catheterization. *N Engl J Med* 2003;348:1123–1133.

Mermel LA, Farr BM, Sherertz RH, et al: Guidelines for the management of intravascular catheter-related infections. *Clin Infect Dis* 2001;32:1249–1272.

Onland W, Shin CE, Fustar S, et al: Ethanol-lock technique for persistent bacteremia of long-term intravascular devices in pediatric patients. *Arch Pediatr Adolesc Med* 2006;160:1049–1053.

Pronovost P, Needham D, Berenholtz S, et al: An intervention to decrease catheter-related bloodstream infections in the ICU. *J Med* 2006;355:2725–2732.

Schreffler RT, Schreffler AJ, Wittler RR: Treatment of cerebrospinal fluid shunt infections: A decision analysis. *Pediatr Infect Dis* 2002;21:632–636.

Tacconelli E, Carmeli Y, Aizer A, et al: Mupirocin prophylaxis to prevent *Staphylococcus aureus* infection in patients undergoing dialysis: A meta-analysis. *Clin Infect Dis* 2003;37:1629–1638.

Tolzis P: Antibiotic lock technique to reduce central venous catheter-related bacteremia. *Pediatr Infect Dis J* 2006;25:449–450.

Wenzel RP, Edmond MB: Team-based prevention of catheter-related infections. *N Engl J Med* 2006;355:2781–2782.

Widmer AF: New developments in diagnosis and treatment of infection in orthopedic implants. *Clin Infect Dis* 2001;33(Suppl 2):S94–S106.

Zimmerli WE, Trampuz A, Ochsner PE: Prosthetic-joint infections. *N Engl J Med* 2004;351:1645–1654.

Section 3 — Antibiotic Therapy

Chapter 179 ■ Principles of Antibacterial Therapy

Mark R. Schleiss

Antibacterial therapy in infants and children presents many challenges. For some agents there is a paucity of pediatric data regarding pharmacokinetics and optimal dosages; pediatric recommendations are extrapolated from studies in adults. The clinician must consider important differences among various age groups of the pathogenic species responsible for pediatric bacterial infections; age-appropriate antibiotic dosing and toxicities must also be considered. Specific antibiotic therapy is optimally driven by a **microbiologic diagnosis**, such as isolation of the pathogenic organism from a sterile body site, and supported by antimicrobial susceptibility testing. Much of pediatric infectious diseases practice is based on a **clinical diagnosis** with **empirical** use of antibacterial agents before or even without eventual identification of the specific pathogen.

Several key considerations must be incorporated in decisions about the appropriate empirical use of antibacterial agents in infants and children. It is important to know the age-appropriate differential diagnosis with respect to likely pathogens. This affects the choice of antimicrobial agent and also the dose, dosing interval, and route of administration (oral vs parenteral). A complete history and physical examination combined with appropriate laboratory and radiographic studies are necessary to identify specific diagnoses, which in turn affects the choice, dosing, and urgency of administration of antimicrobial agents. The vaccination history may reflect reduced risk, but not necessarily elimination of risk, for diseases for which the vaccination series has been completed. The risk for infections is greatly affected by the immunologic status, which may be compromised by immaturity (neonates), underlying disease, and associated treatments (see Chapter 177). Infections in immunocompromised children often result from bacteria that are not considered pathogenic in immunocompetent children. The presence of foreign bodies also increases the risk of bacterial infections (see Chapter 178). The likelihood of central nervous system (CNS) involvement must be considered because many bacteremic infections in childhood, including *Haemophilus influenzae* type b, pneumococcus, and meningococcus, carry a significant risk for hematogenous spread to the CNS.

The patterns of **antimicrobial resistance** in the community, and for the potential causative pathogen being empirically treated, must also be considered. Resistance to penicillin and cephalosporin antibiotics is now commonplace among strains of *Streptococcus pneumoniae,* often necessitating the use of other classes of antibiotics. The striking emergence of community-acquired methicillin-resistant *Staphylococcus aureus* (MRSA) infections has further complicated antibiotic choices.

Antimicrobial resistance occurs through many modifications of the bacterial genome (Tables 179-1 and 179-2). Mechanisms include enzyme inactivation of the antibiotic, decreased cell membrane permeability to intracellularly active antibiotics, efflux of antibiotics out of the bacteria, protection or alteration of the antibiotic target site, excessive production of the target site, or passing the antimicrobial site of action.

Antibiotic action is related to achieving therapeutic levels at the site of infection. Although measuring the level of antibiotic at the site of infection is not always possible, one may measure the serum level and use it as a surrogate target to achieve the desired effect at the tissue level. Various target serum levels are appropriate for different antibiotic agents and are assessed by the peak and trough serum levels, and the area under the therapeutic drug level curve (Fig. 179-1). These levels are in turn a reflection of the route of administration, drug absorption (IM, PO), volume of distribution, and drug elimination half-life, as well as of drug-drug interactions that might enhance or impede enzymatic inactivation of an antibiotic or result in antimicrobial synergism or antagonism (Fig. 179-2).

TABLE 179-1. Mechanisms of Resistance to β-Lactam Antibiotics

I. Alter target site (PBP, penicillin-binding protein)
  A. Decrease affinity of PBP for β-lactam antibiotic
    1. Modify existing PBP
      a. Create mosaic PBP
        Insert nucleotides obtained from neighboring bacteria, e.g., penicillin-resistant *Streptococcus pneumoniae*
        Mutate structural gene of PBP(s), e.g., ampicillin-resistant β-lactamase-negative *Haemophilus influenzae*
    2. Import new PBP, e.g., mecA in methicillin-resistant *Staphylococcus aureus*
II. Destroy β-lactam antibiotic
  A. Increase production of β-lactamase
    1. Acquire more efficient promoter
      a. Mutate existing promoter
      b. Import new one
    2. Deregulate control of β-lactamase production
      a. Mutate regulator genes, e.g., *ampD* in "stably derepressed" *Enterobacter cloacae*
  B. Modify structure of resident β-lactamase
    1. Mutate its structural gene, e.g., extended-spectrum β-lactamases in *Klebsiella pneumoniae*
  C. Import new β-lactamase(s) with different spectrum of activity
III. Decrease concentration of β-lactam antibiotic inside cell
  A. Restrict its entry (loss of porins)
  B. Pump it out (efflux mechanisms)

TABLE 179-2. Aminoglycoside-Modifying Enzymes

ENZYMES	USUAL ANTIBIOTICS MODIFIED	COMMON GENERA
Phosphorylation		
APH(2″)	K, T, G	SA, SR
APH(3′)-I	K	E, PS, SA, SR
APH(3′)-III	K, ±A	E, PS, SA, SR
Acetylation		
AAC(2′)	G	PR
AAC(3)-I	±T, G	E, PS
AAC(3)-III, -IV, OR-V	K, T, G	E, PS
AAC(6′)	K, T, A	E, PS, SA
Adenylation		
ANT(2″)	K, T, GE, PS	
ANT(4′)	K, T, A	SA

A, amikacin; AAC, aminoglycoside acetyltransferase; ANT, aminoglycoside nucleotidyltransferase; APH, aminoglycoside phosphotransferase; E, Enterobacteriaceae; G, gentamicin; K, karamycin; PR, *Providencia-Proteus*; PS, pseudomonads; SA, staphylococci; SR, streptococci; T, tobramycin.

AGE- AND RISK-SPECIFIC USE OF ANTIBIOTICS IN CHILDREN.

Neonates. The causative pathogens of neonatal infections are typically acquired around the time of delivery. Thus, empiric antibiotic selection must take into account the importance of these pathogens in neonates (see Chapter 109). Among the causes of neonatal sepsis in infants, group B streptococcus is the most common, although intrapartum antibiotic prophylaxis has greatly decreased the incidence of this infection (see Chapter 183). Gram-negative enteric organisms acquired from the maternal birth canal, in particular *Escherichia coli,* are other common causes of neonatal sepsis. Although rare, *Listeria monocytogenes* is also an important pathogen, and is resistant to cephalosporin antibiotics. All of these organisms can be associated with meningitis in the neonate; therefore, if meningitis cannot be excluded, antibiotic management should include agents capable of crossing the blood-brain barrier.

Older Children. Antibiotic choices in toddlers and young children were once driven by the unique susceptibility of this age group to invasive disease caused by *H. influenzae* type b (see Chapter 192). With the advent of conjugate vaccines for *H. influenzae* type b, invasive disease has declined dramatically. It is still appropriate to consider the use of antimicrobials that are active against this pathogen, particularly if meningitis is a consideration. Other particularly important pathogens to be considered in this age group include *S. pneumoniae,* meningococcus, and *S. aureus.* Antimicrobial resistance is commonly exhibited by *S. pneumoniae* and *S. aureus.* Strains of *S. pneumoniae* that are resistant to penicillin and cephalosporin antibiotics are frequently encountered in clinical practice. Similarly, MRSAs are highly prevalent in many regions. Resistance of *S. pneumoniae* as well as MRSA is due to mutations that confer alterations in penicillin binding proteins, the molecular targets of penicillin and cephalosporin activity (see Table 179-1).

Depending on the specific diagnosis, other pathogens that are commonly encountered among older children include *Moraxella catarrhalis,* nontypable strains of *H. influenzae,* and *Mycoplasma pneumoniae,* which cause otorhinolaryngologic infections and pneumonia; group A streptococcus, which causes pharyngitis, skin and soft tissue infections, osteomyelitis, and septic arthritis; *Kingella kingae,* which causes bone and joint infections; viridans streptococci and *Enterococcus,* which cause endocarditis; and *Salmonella,* which causes enteritis, bacteremia, osteomyelitis, and septic arthritis. This complexity underscores the importance of

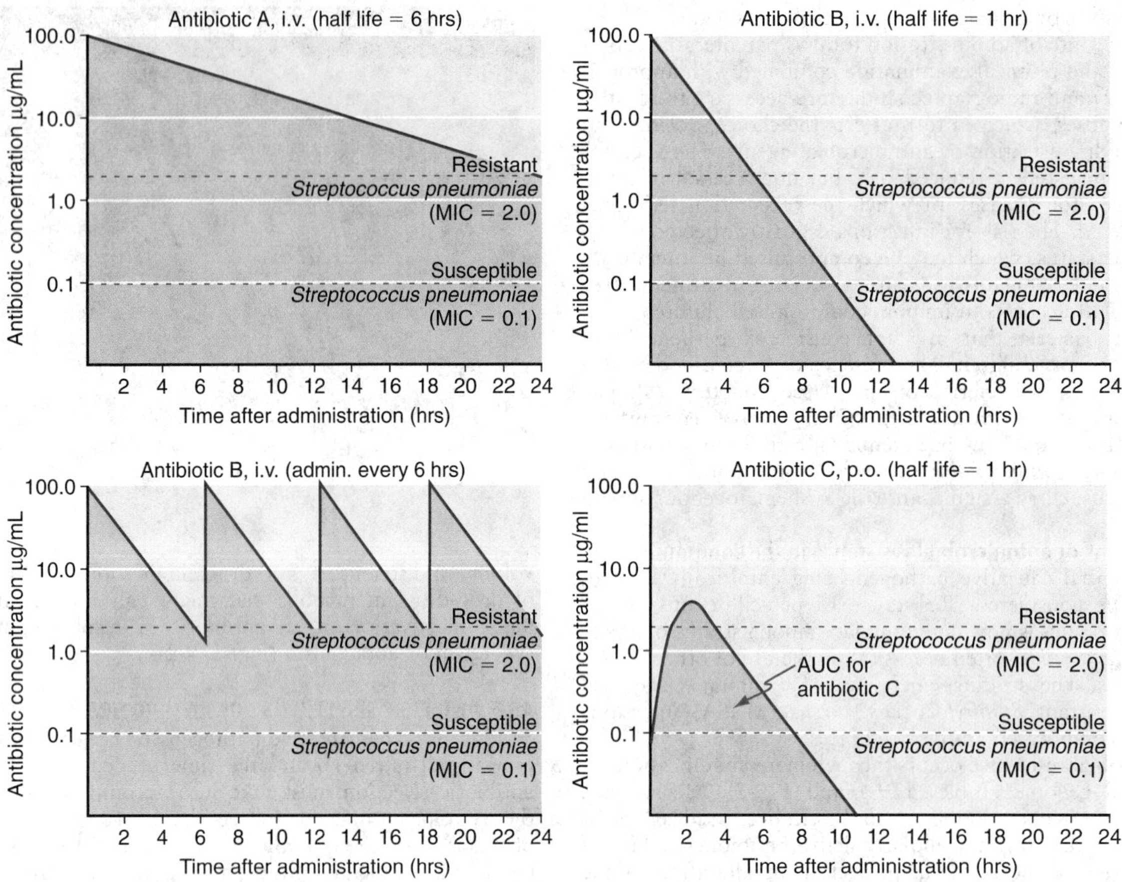

Figure 179-1. The area under the curve *(shaded area)* for different antibiotics. The area under the curve provides a measure of antibiotic exposure to bacterial pathogens. The greatest exposure comes with antibiotics that have a long serum half-life and are administered parenterally (*upper left panel,* antibiotic A). The lowest exposure occurs with oral administration (*lower right panel,* antibiotic C). Dosing of antibiotic B once a day *(upper right panel)* provides far less exposure than dosing the same antibiotic every 6 hr *(lower left panel)*. (From Pong AL, Bradley JS: Guidelines for the selection of antibacterial therapy in children. *Pediatr Clin North Am* 2005;52:869–894.)

formulation of a clear clinical diagnosis, including an assessment of the severity of the infection, in concert with knowledge of local susceptibility patterns in the community.

Immunocompromised and Hospitalized Patients. It is important to consider the risks associated with immunocompromising conditions (malignancy, solid organ, or hematopoietic stem cell transplantation) or with settings where prolonged hospitalization predisposes to nosocomial infections (intensive care, burns). In addition to the usual bacterial pathogens, *Pseudomonas aeruginosa* and enteric organisms, including *Escherichia coli, Klebsiella pneumoniae, Enterobacter,* and *Serratia,* are important considerations as opportunistic pathogens in these settings. Selection of appropriate antimicrobials is challenging because of the diverse causes and scope of antimicrobial resistance exhibited by these organisms. Many strains of enteric organisms have resistance due to extended spectrum β-lactamases (ESBLs) (see Table 179-1). *P. aeruginosa* encodes proteins that function as efflux pumps to eliminate multiple classes of antimicrobials from the cytoplasm or periplasmic space. In addition to these gram-negative pathogens, infections caused by *Enterococcus,* both *E. faecalis*

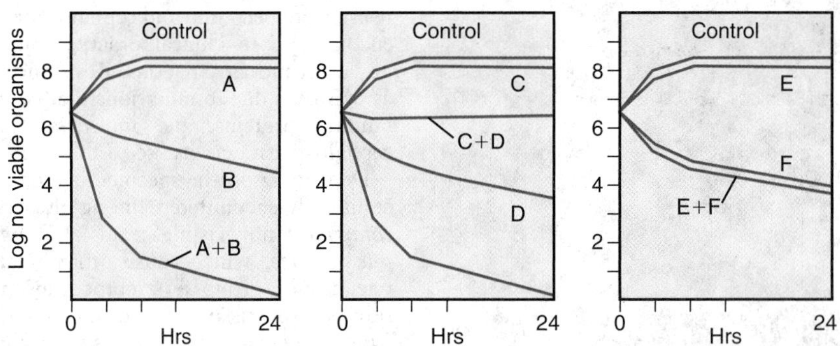

Figure 179-2. Antibacterial effects of antibiotic combinations. *Left:* Curve of A + B illustrates synergism (increased killing). *Center:* Curve of C + D illustrates antagonism (D is less effective when C is added). *Right:* Curve of E + F illustrates indifference, or additive effect (addition of E to F has no effect on F). (From Mandell GL, Bennett JE, Dolin R (editors): *Principles and Practice of Infectious Diseases,* 6th ed, Vol 1. Philadelphia, Elsevier, 2005, p 247.)

and *E. faecium*, are inherently difficult to treat. These organisms may cause urinary tract infection or infective endocarditis in immunocompetent children, and may be responsible for a variety of syndromes in immunocompromised patients, especially in the setting of prolonged intensive care. The occurrence of strains of **vancomycin-resistant** *Enterococcus* (VRE) has further complicated antimicrobial selection in high-risk patients, and has necessitated the development of newer antimicrobials that target these highly resistant gram-positive infections, although experience with many of these newer agents in the management of complex hospitalized pediatric patients is limited.

Infections Associated with Medical Devices. A special situation affecting antibiotic use is the presence of an indwelling medical device, such as a venous catheter, ventriculoperitoneal shunt, stent, or other catheter (see Chapter 178). In addition to *S. aureus*, coagulase-negative staphylococci are also a major consideration. Coagulase-negative staphylococci seldom cause serious disease without a risk factor such as an indwelling catheter. Empiric antibiotic regimens must take this risk into consideration. In addition to appropriate antibiotic therapy, removal or replacement of the colonized prosthetic material is commonly required for cure.

ANTIBIOTICS COMMONLY USED IN PEDIATRIC PRACTICE (TABLE 179-3)

Penicillins. Although there has been ever-increasing emergence of resistance to penicillins, these agents remain valuable and are commonly used for management of many pediatric infectious diseases.

Penicillins remain the drugs of choice for many common pediatric infections caused by group A and group B streptococcus, *Treponema pallidum* (syphilis), *Listeria monocytogenes*, and *Neisseria meningitidis*. The **semisynthetic penicillins** (nafcillin, cloxacillin, dicloxacillin) are useful for management of susceptible staphylococcal infections, although increasing incidence of MRSA has limited the usefulness of these drugs. The **aminopenicillins** (ampicillin, amoxicillin) were developed to provide broad-spectrum activity against gram-negative organisms, including *E. coli* and *H. influenzae*, but the emergence of resistance has limited their utility in many clinical settings. The **carboxypenicillins**

TABLE 179-3. Antibacterial Medications (Antibiotics)

DRUG (TRADE NAMES, FORMULATIONS)	INDICATIONS (MECHANISM OF ACTION) AND DOSING	COMMENTS
Amikacin sulfate Amikin. Injection: 50 mg/mL, 250 mg/ml.	**Aminoglycoside antibiotic active against gram-negative bacilli, especially *Escherichia coli, Klebsiella, Proteus, Enterobacter, Serratia,* and *Pseudomonas.*** Neonates: Postnatal age ≤7 days: 1,200–2,000 g: 7.5 mg/kg q 12–18 hr IV or IM; >2,000 g: 10 mg/kg q 12 hr IV or IM; postnatal age >7 days: 1,200–2,000 g IV or IM: 7.5 mg/kg q 8–12 hr IV or IM; >2,000 g: 10 mg/kg q 8 hr IV or IM. Children: 15–25 mg/kg/24 hr divided q 8–12 hr IV or IM. Adults: 15 mg/kg 24 hr divided q 8–12 hr IV or IM.	*Cautions:* Anaerobes, *Streptococcus* (including *S. pneumoniae*) are resistant. May cause ototoxicity and nephrotoxicity. Monitor renal function. Drug eliminated renally. Administered IV over 30–60 min. *Drug interactions:* May potentiate other ototoxic and nephrotoxic drugs. *Target serum concentrations:* Peak 25–40 mg/L; trough <10 mg/L.
Amoxicillin Amoxil, Polymox. Capsule: 250, 500 mg. Tablet: chewable: 125, 250 mg. Suspension: 125 mg/5 mL, 250 mg/5 mL. Drops: 50 mg/mL.	**Penicillinase-susceptible β-lactam: gram-positive pathogens except *Staphylococcus, Salmonella, Shigella, Neisseria, E. coli,* and *Proteus mirabilis.*** Children: 20–50 mg/kg/24 hr divided q 8–12 hr PO. Higher dose of 80–90 mg/kg 24 hr PO for otitis media. Adults: 250–500 mg q 8–12 hr PO. Uncomplicated gonorrhea: 3 g with 1 g probenecid PO.	*Cautions:* Rash, diarrhea, abdominal cramping. Drug eliminated renally. *Drug interaction:* Probenecid.
Amoxicillin-clavulanate Augmentin. Tablet: 250, 500, 875 mg. Tablet, chewable: 125, 200, 250, 400 mg. Suspension: 125 mg/5 mL, 200 mg/5 mL, 250 mg/5 mL, 400 mg/5 mL.	**β-Lactam (amoxicillin) and β-lactamase inhibitor (clavulanate) enhances amoxicillin activity against pencillinase-producing bacteria. *S. aureus* (not methicillin-resistant organism), *Streptococcus, Haemophilus influenzae, Moraxella catarrhalls, E. coli, Klebsiella, Bacteroides fragilis.*** Neonates: 30 mg/kg/24 hr divided q 12 hr PO. Children: 20–45 mg/kg 24 hr divided q 8–12 hr PO. Higher dose 80–90 mg/kg/24 hr PO for otitis media.	*Cautions:* drug dosed on amoxicillin component. May cause diarrhea, rash. Drug eliminated renally. *Drug interaction:* Probenecid. *Comment:* Higher dose may be active against penicillin tolerant/ resistant *S. pneumoniae.*
Ampicillin Polycillin, Omnipen. Capsule: 250, 500 mg. Suspension: 125 mg/5 mL, 250 mg/5 mL, 500 mg/5 mL. Injection.	**β-Lactam with same spectrum of antibacterial activity as amoxicillin.** Neonates: Postnatal age ≤7 days ≤2,000 g: 50 mg/kg/24 hr IV or IM q 12 hr (meningitis: 100 mg/kg/24 hr divided q 12 hr IV or IM); >2,000 g: 75 mg/kg/24 hr divided q 8 hr IV or IM (meningitis: 150 mg/kg/24 hr divided q 8 hr IV or IM). Postnatal age >7 days <1,200 g: 50 mg/kg/24 hr IV or IM q 12 hr (meningitis: 100 mg/kg/ 24 hr divided q 12 hr IV or IM); 1,200–2,000 g: 75 mg/kg/24 hr divided q 8 hr IV or IM (meningitis: 150 mg/kg/24 hr divided q 8 hr IV or IM); >2,000 g: 100 mg/kg/ 24 hr divided q 6 hr IV or IM (meningitis: 200 mg/kg/24 hr divided q 6 hr IV or IM). Children: 100–200 mg/kg/24 hr divided q 6 hr IV or IM (meningitis: 200–400 mg/kg/ 24 hr divided q 4–6 hr IV or IM). Adults: 250–500 mg q 4–8 hr IV or IM.	*Cautions:* Less bioavailable than amoxicillin causing greater diarrhea. *Drug interaction:* Probenecid.
Ampicillin-sulbactam Unasyn. Injection.	**β-Lactam (ampicillin) β-lactamase inhibitor (sulbactam) enhances ampicillin activity against penicillinase-producing bacteria: *S. aureus, Streptococcus, H. influenzae, M. catarrhalis, E. coli, Klebsiella, B. fragilis.*** Children: 100–200 mg/kg/24 hr divided q 4–8 hr IV or IM. Adults: 1–2 g q 6–8 hr IV or IM (max daily dose: 8 g).	*Cautions:* Drug dosed on ampicillin component. May cause diarrhea, rash. Drug eliminated renally. *Note:* Higher dose may be active against penicillin-tolerant/resistant *S. pneumoniae.* *Drug interaction:* Probenecid.
Azithromycin Zithromax. Tablet: 250 mg. Suspension: 100 mg/5 mL, 200 mg/5 mL.	**Azalide antibiotic with activity against *S. aureus, Streptococcus, H. influenzae, Mycoplasma, Legionella, Chlamydia trachomatis.*** Children: 10 mg/kg PO on day 1 (max: 500 mg) followed by 5 mg/kg PO q 24 hr for 4 days. Group A Streptococcus pharyngitis: 12 mg/kg/24 hr PO (max: 500 mg) for 5 days. Adults: 500 mg PO day 1 followed by 250 mg for 4 days. Uncomplicated *C. trachomatis* infection: single 1 g dose PO.	*Note:* very long half-life permitting once-daily dosing. No metabolic-based drug interactions (unlike erythomycin and clarithromycin), limited gastrointestinal distress. Shorter-course regimens (e.g., 1–3 days) under investigation. Three-day, therapy (10 mg/kg/ 24 hr × 3 days) and single-dose therapy (30 mg/kg): use with increasing frequency (not for streptococcus pharyngitis).

continued

TABLE 179-3. Antibacterial Medications (Antibiotics)—cont'd

DRUG (TRADE NAMES, FORMULATIONS)	INDICATIONS (MECHANISM OF ACTION) AND DOSING	COMMENTS
Aztreonam Azactam. Injection.	**β-Lactam (monobactam) antibiotic with activity against gram-negative aerobic bacteria, *Enterobacteriaceae, and Pseudomonas aeruginosa.*** Neonates: Postnatal age ≤7 days ≤2,000 g: 60 mg/kg/24 hr divided q 12 hr IV or IM; >2,000 g: 90 mg/kg/24 hr divided q 8 hr IV or IM; postnatal age >7 days <1,200 g: 60 mg/kg/24 hr divided q 12 hr IV or IM; 1,200–2,000 g: 90 mg/kg/24 hr divided q 8 hr IV or IM; >2,000 g: 120 mg/kg/24 hr divided q 6–8 hr IV or IM. Children: 90–120 mg/kg/24 hr divided q 6–8 hr IV or IM. For cystic fibrosis up to 200 mg/kg/24 hr IV. Adults: 1–2 g IV or IM q 8–12 hr (max 8 g/24 hr).	*Cautions:* Rash, thrombophlebitis, eosinophilia. Renally eliminated. *Drug interaction:* Probenecid.
Carbenicillin Geopen Injection. Geocillin oral tablet.	**Extended-spectrum penicillin (remains susceptible to penicillinase destruction) active against *Enterobacter,* indole-positive *Proteus,* and *Pseudomonas.*** Neonates: Postnatal age ≤7 days ≤2,000 g: 225 mg/kg/24 hr divided q 8 hr IV or IM; >2,000 g: 300 mg/kg/24 hr divided q 6 hr IV or IM; >7 days: 300–400 mg/kg/24 hr divided q 6 hr IV or IM. Children: 400–600 mg/kg/24 hr divided q 4–6 hr IV or IM.	*Cautions:* Painful given intramuscularly; rash; each gram contains 5.3 mEq sodium. Interferes with platelet aggregation at high doses, increases in liver transaminase levels. Renally eliminated. Oral tablet for treatment of urinary tract infection only. *Drug interaction:* Probenecid.
Cefaclor Ceclor. Capsule: 250, 500 mg. Suspension: 125 mg/5 mL, 187 mg/5 mL, 250 mg/5 mL, 375 mg/5 mL.	**2nd generation cephalosporin active against *S. aureus, Streptococcus* including *S. pneumoniae, H. influenzae, E. coli, Klebsiella,* and *Proteus.*** Children: 20–40 mg/kg/24 hr divided q 8–12 hr PO (max dose: 2 g). Adults: 250–500 mg q 6–8 hr PO.	*Cautions:* β-Lactam safety profile (rash, eosinophilia) with high incidence of serum sickness reaction. Renally eliminated. *Drug interaction:* Probenecid.
Cefadroxil Duricef, Ultracef. Capsule: 500 mg. Tablet: 1,000 mg. Suspension: 125 mg/5 mL, 250 mg/5 mL, 500 mg/5 mL.	**First-generation cephalosporin active against *S. aureus, Streptococcus, E. coli, Klebsiella,* and *Proteus.*** Children: 30 mg/kg/24 hr divided q 12 hr PO (max dose: 2 g). Adults: 250–500 mg q 8–12 hr PO.	*Cautions:* β-Lactam safety profile (rash, eosinophilia). Renally eliminated. Long half-life permits q 12–24 hr dosing. *Drug interaction:* Probenecid.
Cefazolin Ancef, Kefzol. Injection.	**1st generation cephalosporin active against *S. aureus, Streptococcus, E. coli, Klebsiella,* and *Proteus.*** Neonates: Postnatal age ≤7 days 40 mg/kg/24 hr divided q 12 hr IV or IM; >7 days 40–60 mg/kg/24 hr divided q 8 hr IV or IM. Children: 50–100 mg/kg/24 hr divided q 8 hr IV or IM. Adults: 0.5–2 g q 8 hr IV or IM (max dose: 12 g/24 hr).	*Caution:* β-Lactam safety profile (rash, eosinophilia). Renally eliminated. Does not adequately penetrate CNS. *Drug interaction:* Probenecid.
Cefdinir Omnicef. Capsule: 300 mg. Oral suspension: 125 mg/5 mL.	**Extended-spectrum, semi-synthetic cephalosporin.** Children 6 mo–12 yr: 14 mg/kg/24 hr in 1 or 2 doses PO (max: 600 mg/24 hr). Adults: 600 mg q 24 hr PO.	*Cautions:* Reduce dosage in renal insufficiency (creatinine clearance <60 mL/min). Avoid taking concurrently with iron-containing products and antacids because absorption is markedly decreased; take at least 2 hr apart. *Drug interaction:* Probenecid.
Cefepime Maxipime. Injection.	**Expanded-spectrum, 4th generation cephalosporin active against many gram-positive and gram-negative pathogens, including many multi-drug-resistant pathogens.** Children: 100–150 mg/kg/24 hr q 8–12 hr IV or IM. Adults: 2–4 g/24 hr q 12 hr IV or IM.	*Adverse events:* Diarrhea, nausea, vaginal candidiasis *Cautions:* β-Lactam safety profile (rash, eosinophilia). Renally eliminated. *Drug interaction:* Probenecid.
Cefixime Suprax. Tablet: 200, 400 mg. Suspension: 100 mg/5 mL.	**3rd generation cephalosporin active against *Streptococcus, H. influenzae, M. catarrhalis, N. gonorrhoeae, S. marescens,* and *P. vulgaris.* No antistaphylococcal or antipseudomonal activity.** Children: 8 mg/kg/24 hr divided q 12–24 hr PO. Adults: 400 mg/24 hr divided q 12–24 hr PO.	*Cautions:* β-Lactam safety profile (rash, eosinophilia). Renally eliminated. Does not adequately penetrate CNS. *Drug interaction:* Probenecid.
Cefoperazone sodium Cefobid. Injection.	**3rd generation cephalosporin active against many gram-positive and gram-negative pathogens.** Neonates: 100 mg/kg/24 hr divided q 12 hr IV or IM. Children: 100–150 mg/kg/24 hr divided q 8–12 hr IV or IM. Adults: 2–4 g/24 hr divided q 8–12 hr IV or IM (max dose: 12 g/24 hr).	*Cautions:* Highly protein bound cephalosporin with limited potency reflected by weak antipseudomonal activity. Variable gram-positive activity. Primarily hepatically eliminated in bile. *Drug interaction:* Disulfiram-like reaction with alcohol.
Cefotaxime sodium Claforan. Injection.	**3rd generation cephalosporin active against gram-positive and gram-negative pathogens. No antipseudomonal activity.** Neonates: ≤7 days: 100 mg/kg/24 hr divided q 12 hr IV or IM; >7 days: <1,200 g 100 mg/kg/24 hr divided q 12 hr IV or IM; >12,000 g: 150 mg/kg/24 hr divided q 8 hr IV or IM. Children: 150 mg/kg/24 hr divided q 6–8 hr IV or IM (meningitis: 200 mg/kg/24 hr divided q 6–8 hr IV). Adults: 1–2 g q 8–12 hr IV or IM (max: 12 g/24 hr).	*Cautions:* β-Lactam safety profile (rash, eosinophilia). Renally eliminated. Each gram of drug contains 2.2 mEq sodium. Active metabolite. *Drug interaction:* Probenecid.
Cefotetan disodium Cefotan. Injection.	**2nd generation cephalosporin active against *S. aureus, Streptococcus, H. influenzae, E. coli, Klebsiella, Proteus,* and *Bacteroides.* Inactive against *Enterobacter.*** Children: 40–80 mg/kg/24 hr divided IV or IM q 12 hr. Adults: 2–4 g/24 hr divided q 12 hr IV or IM (max: 6 g/24 hr).	*Cautions:* Highly protein-bound cephalosporin, poor CNS penetration; β-Lactam safety profile (rash, eosinophilia), disulfiram-like reaction with alcohol. Renally eliminated (~20% in bile).
Cefoxitin sodium Mefoxin. Injection.	**2nd generation cephalosporin active against *S. aureus, Streptococcus, H. influenzae, E. coli, Klebsiella, Proteus,* and *Bacteroides.* Inactive against *Enterobacter.*** Neonates: 70–100 mg/kg/24 hr divided q 8–12 hr IV or IM. Children: 80–160 mg/kg/24 hr divided q 6–8 hr IV or IM. Adults: 1–2 g q 6–8 hr IV or IM (max dose: 12 g/24 hr).	*Cautions:* Poor CNS penetration; β-Lactam safety profile (rash, eosinophilia). Renally eliminated. Painful given intramuscularly. *Drug interaction:* Probenecid.

TABLE 179-3. Antibacterial Medications (Antibiotics)—cont'd

DRUG (TRADE NAMES, FORMULATIONS)	INDICATIONS (MECHANISM OF ACTION) AND DOSING	COMMENTS
Cefpodoxime proxetil Vantin. Tablet: 100 mg, 200 mg. Suspension: 50 mg/5 mL, 100 mg/5 mL.	**3rd generation cephalosporin active against *S. aureus, Streptococcus, H. influenzae, M. catarrhalis, N. gonorrhoeae, E. coli, Klebsiella,* and *Proteus.* No antipseudomonal activity.** Children: 10 mg/kg/24 hr divided q 12 hr PO. Adults: 200–800 mg/24 hr divided q 12 hr PO (max dose: 800 mg/24 hr). Uncomplicated gonorrhea: 200 mg PO as single-dose therapy.	*Cautions:* β-Lactam safety profile (rash, eosinophilia). Renally eliminated. Does not adequately penetrate CNS. Increased bioavailability when taken with food. *Drug interaction:* Probenecid; antacids and H-2 receptor antagonists may decrease absorption.
Cefprozil Cefzil. Tablet: 250, 500 mg. Suspension: 125 mg/5 mL, 250 mg/5 mL.	**2nd generation cephalosporin active against *S. aureus, Streptococcus, H. Influenzae, E. coli, M. catarrhalis, Klebsiella,* and *Proteus.*** Children: 30 mg/kg/24 hr divided q 8–12 hr PO. Adults: 500–1,000 mg/24 hr divided q 12 hr PO (max dose: 1.5 g/24 hr).	*Cautions:* β-Lactam safety profile (rash, eosinophilia). Renally eliminated. Good bioavailability; food does not affect bioavailability. *Drug interaction:* Probenecid.
Ceftazidime Fortaz, Ceptaz, Tazicer, Tazidime. Injection.	**3rd generation cephalosporin active against gram-positive and gram-negative pathogens including *Pseudomonas aeruginosa.*** Neonates: Postnatal age ≤7 days: 100 mg/kg/24 hr divided q 12 hr IV or IM; >7 dyas ≤1,200 g: 100 mg/kg/24 hr divided q 12 hr IV or IM; >1,200 g: 150 mg/kg/24 hr divided q 8 hr IV or IM. Children: 150 mg/kg/24 hr divided q 8 hr IV or IM (meningitis: 150 mg/kg/24 hr IV divided q 8 hr). Adults: 1–2 g q 8–12 hr IV or IM (max: 8–12 g/24 hr).	*Cautions:* β-Lactam safety profile (rash, eosinophilia). Renally eliminated. Increasing pathogen resistance developing with long-term, widespread use. *Drug interaction:* Probenecid.
Ceftiaoxime Cefizox. Injection.	**3rd generation cephalosporin active against gram-positive and gram-negative pathogens. No antipseudomonal activity.** Children: 150 mg/kg/24 hr divided q 6–8 hr IV or IM. Adults: 1–2 g q 6–8 hr IV or IM (max dose: 12 g/24 hr).	*Cautions:* β-Lactam safety profile (rash, eosinophilia). Renally eliminated. *Drug interaction:* Probenecid.
Ceftriaxone sodium Rocephin. Injection.	**3rd generation cephalosporin active against gram-positive and gram-negative pathogens. No antipseudomonal activity. Very potent and β-lactamase stable.** Neonates: 50–75 mg/kg q 24 hr IV or IM. Children: 50–75 mg/kg q 24 hr IV or IM (meningitis: 75 mg/kg dose 1 then 80–100 mg/kg/24 hr divided q 12–24 hr IV or IM). Adults: 1–2 g q 24 hr IV or IM (max dose: 4 g/24 hr).	*Cautions:* β-Lactam safety profile (rash, eosinophilia). Eliminated via kidney (33–65%) and bile; can cause sludging. Long half-life and dose-dependent protein binding favors q 24 hr rather than q 12 hr dosing. Can add 1% lidocaine for IM injection.
Cefuroxime (cefuroxime axetil for oral administration) Ceftin, Kefurox, Zinacef. Injection. Suspension: 125 mg/5 mL. Tablet: 125, 250, 500 mg.	**2nd generation cephalosporin active against *S. aureus, Streptococcus, H. influenzae, E. coli, M. catarrhalis, Klebsiella,* and *Proteus.*** Neonates: 40–100 mg/kg/24 hr divided q 12 hr IV or IM. Children: 200–240 mg/kg/24 hr divided q 8 hr IV or IM; PO administration: 20–30 mg/kg/24 hr divided q 8 hr PO. Adults: 750–1,500 mg q 8 hr IV or IM (max dose: 6 g/24 hr).	*Cautions:* β-Lactam safety profile (rash, eosinophilia). Renally eliminated. Food increases PO bioavailability. *Drug interaction:* Probenecid.
Cephalexin Keflex, Keftab. Capsule: 250, 500 mg Tablet: 500 mg, 1 g. Suspension: 125 mg/5 mL, 250 mg/5 mL, 100 mg/mL drops.	**1st generation cephalosporin active against *S. aureus, Streptococcus, E. coli, Klebsiella,* and *Proteus.*** Children: 25–100 mg/kg/24 hr divided q 6–8 hr PO. Adults: 250–500 mg q 6 hr PO (max dose: 4 g/24 hr).	*Cautions:* β-Lactam safety profile (rash, eosinophilia). Renally eliminated. *Drug interaction:* Probenecid.
Cephradine Velosef Capsule: 250, 500 mg. Suspension: 125 mg/5 mL, 250 mg/5 mL.	**1st generation cephalosporin active against *S. aureus, Streptococcus, E. coli, Klebsiella,* and *Proteus.*** Children: 50–100 mg/kg/24 hr divided q 6–12 hr PO. Adults: 250–500 mg q 6–12 hr PO (max dose: 4 g/24 hr).	*Cautions:* β-Lactam safety profile (rash, eosinophilia). Renally eliminated. *Drug interaction:* Probenecid.
Chloramphenicol Chloromycetin. Injection. Capsule: 250 mg. Ophthalmic, otic solutions. Ointment.	**Broad-spectrum protein synthesis inhibitor active against many gram-positive and gram-negative bacteria, *Salmonella,* vancomycin-resistant *Enterococcus faecium, Bacteroides,* other anaerobes, *Mycoplasma, Chlamydia,* and *Rickettsia; Pseudomonas* usually resistant.** Neonates: Initial loading dose 20 mg/kg followed 12 hr later by: postnatal age ≤7 days: 25 mg/kg/24 hr q 24 hr IV; >7 days: ≤2,000 g: 25 mg/kg/24 hr q 24 hr IV; >2,000 g: 50 mg/kg/24 hr divided q 12 hr IV. Children: 50–75 mg/kg/24 hr divided q 6–8 hr IV or PO (meningitis: 75–100 mg/kg/24 hr IV divided q 6 hr). Adults: 50 mg/kg/24 hr divided q 6 hr IV or PO (max dose: 4 g/24 hr).	*Cautions:* Gray-baby syndrome (from too-high dose in neonate), bone marrow suppression aplastic anemia (monitor hematocrit, free serum iron). *Drug interactions:* Phenytoin, phenobarbital, rifampin may decrease levels. *Target serum concentrations:* Peak 20–30 mg/L; trough 5–10 mg/L.
Ciprofloxacin Cipro. Tablet: 100, 250, 500, 750 mg. Injection. Ophthalmic solution and ointment. Otic suspension. Oral suspension: 250 and 500 mg/5 mL.	**Quinolone antibiotic active against *P. aeruginosa, Serratia, Enterobacter, Shigella, Salmonella, Campylobacter, Neisseria gonorrhoeae, H. influenzae, M. catarrhalis,* some *S. aureus,* and *Streptococcus.*** Neonates: 10 mg/kg q 12 hr PO or IV. Children: 15–30 mg/kg/24 hr divided q 12 hr PO or IV; cystic fibrosis: 20–40 mg/kg/24 hr divided q 8–12 hr PO or IV. Adults: 250–750 mg q 12 hr; 200–400 mg IV q 12 hr PO (max dose: 1.5 g/24 hr).	*Cautions:* Concerns of joint destruction in juvenile animals not seen in humans; tendonitis, superinfection, dizziness, confusion, crystalluria, some photosensitivity. *Drug interactions:* Theophylline, magnesium-, aluminum-, or calcium-containing antacids, sucralfate, probenecid, warfarin, cyclosporine.
Clarithromycin Biaxin. Tablet: 250, 500 mg. Suspension: 125 mg/5 mL, 250 mg/5 mL.	**Macrolide antibiotic with activity against *S. aureus, Streptococcus, H. influenzae, Legionella, Mycoplasma,* and *C. trachomatis.*** Children: 15 mg/kg/24 hr divided q 12 hr PO. Adults: 250–500 mg q 12 hr PO (max dose: 1 g/24 hr).	*Cautions:* Adverse events less than erythromycin; gastrointestinal upset, dyspepsia, nausea, cramping. *Drug interactions:* Same as erythromycin: astemizole carbamazepine, terfenadine cyclosporine, theophylline, digoxin, tacrolimus.

continued

TABLE 179-3. Antibacterial Medications (Antibiotics)—cont'd

DRUG (TRADE NAMES, FORMULATIONS)	INDICATIONS (MECHANISM OF ACTION) AND DOSING	COMMENTS
Clindamycin Cleocin. Capsule: 75, 150, 300 mg. Suspension: 75 mg/5 mL. Injection. Topical solution, lotion, and gel. Vaginal cream.	**Protein synthesis inhibitor active against most gram-positive aerobic and anaerobic cocci except *Enterococcus*.** Neonates: Postnatal age ≤7 days <200 g; 10 mg/kg/24 hr divided q 12 hr IV or IM; >2,000 g: 15 mg/kg/24 hr divided q 8 hr IV or IM; >7 days <1,200 g: 10 mg/kg/24 hr IV or IM divided q 12 hr; 1,200–2,000 g: 15 mg/kg/24 hr divided q 8 hr IV or IM; >2,000 g: 20 mg/kg/24 hr divided q 8 hr IV or IM. Children: 10–40 mg/kg/24 hr divided q 6–8 hr IV, IM, or PO. Adults: 150–600 mg q 6–8 hr IV, IM, or PO (max dose: 5 g/24 hr IV or IM or 2 g/24 hr PO).	*Cautions:* Diarrhea, nausea, C. difficile-associated colitis, rash. Administer slow IV over 30–60 min. Topically active as an acne treatment.
Cloxacillin sodium Tegopen. Capsule: 250, 500 mg. Suspension: 125 mg/5 mL.	**Penicillinase-resistant penicillin active against *S. aureus* and other gram-positive cocci except *Enterococcus* and coagulase-negative staphylococci.** Children: 50–100 mg/kg/24 hr divided q 6 hr PO. Adults: 250–500 mg q 6 hr PO (max dose: 4 g/24 hr).	*Cautions:* β-Lactam safety profile (rash, eosinophilia). Primarily hepatically eliminated; requires dose reduction in renal disease. Food decreases bioavailabilty. *Drug interaction:* Probenecid.
Co-trimoxazole (trimethoprim-sulfamethoxazole; TMP-SMZ) Bactrim, Cotrim, Septra, Sulfatrim. Tablet: SMZ 400 mg and TMP 80 mg. Tablet DS: SMZ 800 mg and TMP 160 mg. Suspension: SMZ 200 mg and TMP 40 mg/5 mL. Injection.	**Antibiotic combination with sequential antagonism of bacterial folate synthesis with broad antibacterial activity: *Shigella, Legionella, Nocardia, Chlamydia, Pneumocystis carinii.* Dosage based on TMP component.** Children: 6–20 mg TMP/kg/24 hr or IV divided q 12 hr PO. *P. carinii* pneumonia: 15–20 mg TMP/kg/24 hr divided q 12 hr PO or IV. *P. carinii* prophylaxis: 5 mg TMP/kg/24 hr or 3 times/wk PO. Adults: 160 mg TMP q 12 hr PO.	*Cautions:* Drug dosed on TMP (trimethoprim) component. Sulfonamide skin reactions: rash, erythema multiforme, Stevens-Johnson syndrome, nausea, leukopenia. Renal and hepatic elimination; reduce dose in renal failure. *Drug interactions:* Protein displacement with warfarin, possibly phenytoin, cyclosporine.
Demeclocycline Declomycin. Tablet: 150, 300 mg. Capsule: 150 mg.	**Tetracycline active against most gram-positive cocci except Enterococcus, many gram-negative bacilli, anaerobes, *Borrelia burgdorferi* (Lyme disease), *Mycoplasma,* and *Chlamydia*.** Children: 8–12 mg/kg/24 hr divided q 6–12 hr PO. Adults: 150 mg PO q 6–8 hr. Syndrome of inappropriate antidiuretic hormone secretion: 900–1,200 mg/24 hr or 13–15 mg/kg/24 hr divided q 6–8 hr PO with dose reduction based on response to 600–900 mg/24 hr.	*Cautions:* Teeth staining, possibly permanent (if administered <8 yr of age) with prolonged use; photosensitivity, diabetes insipidus, nausea, vomiting, diarrhea, superinfections. *Drug interactions:* Aluminum-, calcium-, magnesium-, zinc- and iron-containing food, milk, dairy products may decrease absorption.
Dicloxacillin Dynapen, Pathocil. Capsule: 125, 250, 500 mg. Suspension: 62.5 mg/5 mL.	**Penicillinase-resistant penicillin active against *S. aureus* and other gram-positive cocci except *Enterococcus* and coagulase-negative staphylococci.** Children: 12.5–100 mg/kg/24 hr divided q 6 hr PO. Adults: 125–500 mg q 6 hr PO.	*Cautions:* β-Lactam safety profile (rash, eosinophilia). Primarily renally (65%) and bile (30%) elimination. Food may decrease bioavailability. *Drug interaction:* Probenecid.
Doxycycline Vibramycin, Doxy. Injection. Capsule: 50, 100 mg. Tablet: 50, 100 mg. Suspension: 25 mg/5 mL. Syrup: 50 mg/5 mL.	**Tetracycline antibiotic active against most gram-positive cocci except *Enterococcus,* many gram-negative bacilli, anaerobes, *Borrelia burgdorferi* (Lyme disease), *Mycoplasma,* and *Chlamydia*.** Children: 2–5 mg/kg/24 hr divided q 12–24 hr PO or IV (max dose: 200 mg/24 hr). Adults: 100–200 mg/24 hr divided q 12–24 hr PO or IV.	*Cautions:* Teeth staining, possibly permanent (<8 yr of age) with prolonged use; photosensitivity, nausea, vomiting, diarrhea, superinfections. *Drug interactions:* Aluminum-, calcium-, magnesium-, zinc-, iron-, kaolin-, and pectin-containing products, food, milk, dairy products may decrease absorption. Carbamazepine, rifampin, barbiturates may decrease half-life.
Erythromycin E-Mycin, Ery-Tab, Ery-C, Ilosone. Estolate 125, 500 mg. Tablet EES: 200 mg. Tablet base: 250, 333, 500 mg. Suspension: estolate 125 mg/5 mL, 250 mg/5 mL, EES 200 mg/5 mL, 400 mg/5 mL. Estolate drops: 100 mg/mL. EES drops: 100 mg/2.5 mL. Available in combination with sulfisoxazole (Pediazole), dosed on erythromycin content.	**Bacteriostatic macrolide antibiotic most active against gram-positive organisms, *Corynebacterium diphtheriae,* and *Mycoplasma pneumoniae.* May also be used to promote gastrointestinal motility and improve feeding intolerance in preterm infants.** Neonates: Postnatal age ≤7 days: 20 mg/kg/24 hr divided q 12 hr PO; >7 days <1,200 g: 20 mg/kg/24 hr divided q 12 hr PO; <1,200 g: 30 mg/kg/24 hr divided q 8 hr PO (give as 5 mg/kg/dose q 6 hr to improve feeding intolerance). Children: Usual max dose 2 g/24 hr. Base: 30–50 mg/kg/24 hr divided q 6–8 hr PO. Estolate: 30–50 mg/kg/24 hr divided q 8–12 hr PO. Stearate: 20–40 mg/kg/24 hr divided q 6 hr PO. Lactobionate: 20–40 mg/kg/24 hr divided q 6–8 hr IV. Gluceptate: 20–50 mg/kg/24 hr divided q 6 hr IV. usual max dose 4 g/24 hr IV. Adults: Base: 333 mg PO q 8 hr; estolate/stearate/base: 250–500 mg q 6 hr PO.	*Cautions:* Motilin agonist leading to marked abdominal cramping, nausea, vomiting, diarrhea. Associated with hypertrophic pyloric stenosis in young infants. Many different salts with questionable tempering of gastrointestinal adverse events. Rare cardiac toxicity with IV use. Dose of salts differ. Topical formulation for treatment of acne. *Drug interactions:* Antagonizes hepatic CYP450 3A4 activity: astemizole, carbamazepine, terfenadine, cyclosporine, theophylline, digoxin, tacrolimus, carbamazepine.
Gentamicin Garamycin. Injection. Ophthalmic solution, ointment, topical cream.	**Aminoglycoside antibiotic active against gram-negative bacilli, especially *E. coli, Klebsiella, Proteus, Enterobacter, Serratia,* and *Pseudomonas*.** Neonates: Postnatal age ≤7 days 1,200–2,000 g: 2.5 mg/kg q 12–18 hr IV or IM; <2,000 g: 2.5 mg/kg q 12 hr IV or IM; postnatal age <7 days 1,200–2,000 g: 2.5 mg/kg q 8–12 hr IV or IM; <2,000 g: 2.5 mg/kg q 8 hr IV or IM. Children: 2.5 mg/kg/24 hr divided q 8–12 hr IV or IM. Alternatively may administer 5–7.5 mg/kg/24 hr IV once daily. Intrathecal: Preservative-free preparation for intraventricular or intrathecal use: neonate: 1 mg/24 hr; children: 1–2 mg/24 hr IT; adults: 4–8 mg/24 hr. Adults: 3–6 mg/kg/24 hr divided q 8 hr IV or IM.	*Cautions:* Anaerobes, *S. pneumoniae,* other *Streptococcus* are resistant. May cause ototoxicity and nephrotoxicity. Monitor renal function. Drug eliminated renally. Administered IV over 30–60 min. *Drug interactions:* May potentiate other ototoxic and nephrotoxic drugs. *Target serum concentrations:* Peak 6–12 mg/L; trough >2 mg/L with intermittent daily dose regimens only.
Imipenem-cilastatin Primaxin. Injection.	**Carbapenem antibiotic active against broad-spectrum gram-positive cocci and gram-negative bacilli including *P. aeruginosa* and anerobes. No activity against *Stenotrophomonas maltophilia*.** Neonates: Postnatal age ≤7 days <1,200 g: 20 mg/kg q 18–24 hr IV or IM; >1,200 g: 40 mg/kg divided q 12 hr IV or IM; postnatal age >7 days 1,200–2,000 g: 40 mg/kg q 12 hr IV or IM; >2,000 g: 60 mg/kg q 8 hr IV or IM. Children: 60–100 mg/kg/24 hr divided q 6–8 hr IV or IM. Adults: 2–4 g/24 hr divided q 6–8 hr IV or IM (max dose: 4 g/24 hr).	*Cautions:* β-Lactam safety profile (rash, eosinophilia), nausea, seizures. Cilastatin possesses no antibacterial activity; reduces renal imipenem metabolism. Primarily renally eliminated. *Drug interaction:* Possibly ganciclovir.

TABLE 179-3. Antibacterial Medications (Antibiotics)—cont'd

DRUG (TRADE NAMES, FORMULATIONS)	INDICATIONS (MECHANISM OF ACTION) AND DOSING	COMMENTS
Linezolid Zyvox. Tablet: 400, 600 mg. Oral suspension: 100 mg/5 mL. Injection: 100 mg/5 mL.	**Oxazolidinone antibiotic active against gram-positive cocci (especially drug-resistant organisms), including *Staphylococcus, Streptococcus, Enterococcus faecium,* and *E. fecalis.* Interferes with protein synthesis by binding to 50S ribosome subunit.** Children: 10 mg/kg q 12 hr IV or PO. Adults: Pneumonia: 600 mg q 12 hr IV or PO; skin infections: 400 mg q 12 hr IV or PO.	*Adverse events:* Myelosuppression, pseudomembranous colitis, nausea, diarrhea, headache. *Drug interaction:* Probenecid.
Loracarbef Lorabid. Capsule: 200 mg. Suspension: 100 mg/5 mL, 200 mg/5 mL.	**Carbacephem very closely related to cefaclor (2nd generation cephalosporin) active against *S. aureus, Streptococcus, H. influenzae, M. catarrhalis, E. coli, Klebsiella,* and *Proteus.*** Children: 30 mg/kg/24 hr divided q 12 hr PO (max dose: 2 g). Adults: 200–400 mg q 12 hr PO (max dose: 800 mg/24 hr).	*Cautions:* β-Lactam safety profile (rash, eosinophilia). Renally eliminated. *Drug interaction:* Probenecid.
Meropenem Merrem. Injection.	**Carbapenem antibiotic active against broad-spectrum gram-positive cocci and gram-negative bacilli including *P. aeruginosa* and anerobes. No activity against *Stenotrophomonas maltophilia.*** Children: 60 mg/kg/24 hr divided q 8 hr IV meningitis: 120 mg/kg/24 hr [max: 6 g/24 hr] q 8 hr IV. Adults: 1.5–3 g q 8 hr IV.	*Cautions:* β-Lactam safety profile; appears to possess less CNS excitation than imipenem. 80% renal elimination. *Drug interaction:* Probenecid.
Metronidazole Flagyl, Metro-IV, generic. Topical gel, vaginal gel. Injection. Tablet: 250, 500 mg.	**Highly effective in the treatment of infections due to anaerobes.** Neonates: <1,200 g: 7.5 mg/kg 48 hr PO or IV; postnatal age ≤7 days 1,200–2,000 g: 7.5 mg/kg/24 hr q 24 hr PO or IV; 2,000 g: 15 mg/kg/24 hr divided q 12 hr PO or IV; postnatal age <7 days 1,200–2,000 g: 15 mg/kg/24 hr divided q 12 hr PO or IV; >2,000 g: 30 mg/kg/24 hr divided q 12 hr PO or IV. Children: 30 mg/kg/24 hr divided q 6–8 hr PO or IV. Adults: 30 mg/kg/24 hr divided q 6 hr PO or IV (max dose: 4 g/24 hr).	*Cautions:* Dizziness, seizures, metallic taste, nausea, disulfiram-like reaction with alcohol. Administer IV slow over 30–60 min. Adjust dose with hepatic impairment. *Drug interactions:* Carbamazepine, rifampin, phenobarbital may enhance metabolism; may increase levels of warfarin, phenytoin, lithium.
Mezlocillin sodium Mezlin. Infection.	**Extended-spectrum penicillin active against *E. coli, Enterobacter, Serratia,* and *Bacteroides;* limited antipseudomonal activity.** Neonates: Postnatal age ≤7 days: 150 mg/kg/24 hr divided q 12 hr IV; >7 days: 225 mg/kg divided q 8 hr IV. Children: 200–300 mg/kg/24 hr divided q 4–6 hr IV; cystic fibrosis 300–450 mg/kg/24 hr IV. Adults: 2–4 g/dose q 4–6 hr IV (max dose: 12 g/24 hr).	*Cautions:* β-Lactam safety profile (rash, eosinophilia); painful given intramuscularly; each gram contains 1.8 mEq sodium. Interferes with platelet aggregation with high doses; increases noted in liver function test results. Renally eliminated. Inactivated by β-lactamase enzyme. *Drug interaction:* Probenecid.
Mupirocin Bactroban. Ointment.	**Topical antibiotic active against *Staphylococcus* and *Streptococcus.*** Topical application: Nasal (eliminate nasal carriage) and to the skin 2–4 times per day.	*Caution:* Minimal systemic absorption as drug metabolized within the skin.
Nafcillin sodium Nafcil, Unipen. Injection. Capsule: 250 mg. Tablet: 500 mg.	**Penicillinase-resistant penicillin active against *S. aureus* and other gram-positive cocci except *Enterococcus* and coagulase-negative staphylococci.** Neonates: Postnatal age ≤7 days 1,200–2,000 g: 50 mg/kg/24 hr divided q 12 hr IV or IM; >2,000 g: 75 mg/kg/24 hr divided q 8 hr IV or IM; postnatal age >7 days 1,200–2,000 g: 75 mg/kg/q 8 hr; >2,000 g: 100 mg/kg divided q 6–8 hr IV (meningitis: 200 mg/kg/24 hr divided q 6 hr IV). Children: 100–200 mg/kg/24 hr divided q 4–6 hr IV. Adults: 4–12 g/24 hr divided q 4–6 hr IV (max dose: 12 g/24 hr).	*Cautions:* β-Lactam safety profile (rash, eosinophilia), phlebitis; painful given intramuscularly; oral absorption highly variable and erratic (not recommended). *Adverse effect:* Neutropenia.
Nalidixic acid NegGram. Tablet: 250, 500, 1,000 mg. Suspension: 250 mg/5 mL.	**1st generation quinolone effective for short-term treatment of lower urinary tract infections caused by *E. coli, Enterobacter, Klebsiella,* and *Proteus.*** Children: 50–55 mg/kg/24 hr divided q 6 hr PO; suppressive therapy 25–33 mg/kg/24 hr divided q 6–8 hr PO. Adults: 1 g q 6 hr PO; suppressive therapy: 500 mg q 6 hr PO.	*Cautions:* Vertigo, dizziness, rash. Not for use in systemic infections. *Drug interactions:* Liquid antacids.
Neomycin sulfate Mycifradin, generic. Tablet: 500 mg. Topical cream, ointment. Solution: 125 mg/5 mL.	**Aminoglycoside antibiotic used for topical application or orally before surgery to decrease gastrointestinal flora (nonabsorbable) and hyperammonemia.** Infants: 50 mg/kg/24 hr divided q 6 hr PO. Children: 50–100 mg/kg/24 hr divided q 6–8 hr PO. Adults: 500–2,000 mg/dose q 6–8 hr PO.	*Cautions:* In patients with renal dysfunction because small amount absorbed may accumulate. *Adverse events:* Primarily related to topical application, abdominal cramps, diarrhea, rash. Aminoglycoside ototoxicity and nephrotoxicity if absorbed.
Nitrofurantoin Furadantin, Furan, Macrodantin. Capsule: 50, 100 mg. Extended-release capsule: 100 mg. Macrocrystal: 50, 100 mg. Suspension: 25 mg/5 mL.	**Effective in the treatment of lower urinary tract infections caused by gram-positive and gram-negative pathogens.** Children: 5–7 mg/kg/24 hr divided q 6 hr PO (max dose: 400 mg/24 hr); suppressive therapy 1–2.5 mg/kg/24 hr divided q 12–24 hr PO (max dose: 100 mg/24 hr). Adults: 50–100 mg/24 hr divided q 6 hr PO.	*Cautions:* Vertigo, dizziness, rash, jaundice, interstitial pneumonitis. Do not use with moderate to severe renal dysfunction. *Drug interactions:* Liquid antacids.
Ofloxacin Ocuflox 0.3% ophthalmic solution: 1, 5, 10 mL. Floxin 0.3% otic solution: 5, 10 mL.	**Quinolone antibiotic for treatment of conjunctivitis or corneal ulcers (ophthalmic solution); and otitis externa and chronic suppurative otitis media (otic solution) caused by susceptible gram-positive, gram-negative, anaerobic bacteria, or *Chlamydia trachomatis.*** Child *>1–12 yr:* Conjunctivitis: 1–2 drops in affected eye(s) q 2–4 hr for 2 days, then 1–2 drops qid for 5 days. Corneal ulcers: 1–2 drops q 30 min while awake and at 4 hours at night for 2 days, then 1–2 drops hourly for 5 days while awake, then 1–2 drops q 6 hr for 2 days. Otitis externa (otic solution): 5 drops into affected ear bid for 10 days. Chronic suppurative otitis media: treat for 14 days.	*Adverse events:* Burning, stinging, eye redness (ophthalmic solution), dizziness with otic solution if not warmed.

continued

TABLE 179-3. Antibacterial Medications (Antibiotics)—cont'd

DRUG (TRADE NAMES, FORMULATIONS)	INDICATIONS (MECHANISM OF ACTION) AND DOSING	COMMENTS
	Child >12 yr and adults: Ophthalmic solution doses same as for younger children. Otitis externa (otic solution): Use 10 drops bid for 10 or 14 days as for younger children.	
Oxacillin sodium Prostaphlin. Injection. Capsule: 250, 500 mg. Suspension: 250 mg/5 mL.	**Penicillinase-resistant penicillin active against *S. aureus* and other gram-positive cocci except *Enterococcus* and coagulase-negative staphylococci.** Neonates: Postnatal age ≤7 days 1,200–2,000 g: 50 mg/kg/24 hr divided q 12 hr IV; >2,000 g: 75 mg/kg/24 hr IV divided q 8 hr IV; postnatal age >7 days <1,200 g: 50 mg/kg/24 hr IV divided q 12 hr IV; 1,200–2,000 g: 75 mg/kg/24 hr divided q 8 hr IV; >2,000 g: 100 mg/kg/24 hr IV divided q 6 hr IV. Infants: 100–200 mg/kg/24 hr divided q 4–6 hr IV. Children: PO 50–100 mg/kg/24 hr divided q 4–6 hr IV. Adults: 2–12 g/24 hr divided q 4–6 hr IV (max dose: 12 g/24 hr).	*Cautions:* β-Lactam safety profile (rash, eosinophilia). Moderate oral bioavailability (35–65%). Primarily renally eliminated. *Drug interaction:* Probenecid. *Adverse effect:* Neutropenia.
Penicillin G Injection. Tablets.	**Penicillin active against most gram-positive cocci; *S. pneumoniae* (resistance is increasing), group A streptococcus, and some gram-negative bacteria (e.g., *N. gonorrhoeae, N. meningitidis*).** Neonates: Postnatal age ≤7 days 1,200–2,000 g: 50,000 units/kg/24 hr divided q 12 hr IV or IM (meningitis: 100,000 units/kg/24 hr divided q 12 hr IV or IM); >2,000 g: 75,000 units/kg/24 hr divided q 8 hr IV or IM (meningitis: 150,000 units/kg/24 hr divided q 8 hr IV or IM); postnatal age >7 days ≤1,200 g: 50,000 units/kg/24 hr divided q 12 hr IV (meningitis: 100,000 units/kg/24 hr divided q 12 hr IV); 1,200–2,000 g: 75,000 units/kg/24 hr q 8 hr IV (meningitis: 225,000 units/kg/24 hr divided q 8 hr IV); >2,000 g: 100,000 units/kg/24 hr divided q 6 hr IV (meningitis: 200,000 units/kg/24 hr divided q 6 hr IV). Children: 100,000–250,000 units/kg/24 hr divided q 4–6 hr IV or IM (max: 400,000 units/kg/24 hr). Adults: 2–24 million units/24 hr divided q 4–6 hr IV or IM	*Cautions:* β-Lactam safety profile (rash, eosinophilia), allergy, seizures with excessive doses particularly in patients with marked renal disease. Substantial pathogen resistance. Primarily renally eliminated. *Drug interaction:* Probenecid.
Penicillin G, benzathine Bicillin. Injection.	**Long-acting repository form of penicillin effective in the treatment of infections responsive to persistent, low penicillin concentrations (1–4 wk), e.g., group A streptococcus pharyngitis, rheumatic fever prophylaxis.** Neonates *>1,200 g:* 50,000 units/kg IM once. Children: 300,000–1.2 million units/kg q 3–4 wk IM (max: 1.2–2.4 million units/dose). Adults: 1.2 million units IM q 3–4 wk.	*Cautions:* β-Lactam safety profile (rash, eosinophilia), allergy. Administer by IM injection only. Substantial pathogen resistance. Primarily renally eliminated. *Drug interaction:* Probenecid.
Penicillin G, procaine Crysticillin. Injection.	**Repository form of penicillin providing low penicillin concentrations for 12 hr.** Neonates >1,200 g: 50,000 units/kg/24 hr IM. Children: 25,000–50,000 units/kg/24 hr IM for 10 days (max: 4.8 million units/dose). Gonorrhea: 100,000 units/kg (max: 4.8 million units/24 hr) IM once with probenecid 25 mg/kg (max dose: 1 g) Adults: 0.6–4.8 million units q 12–24 hr IM.	*Cautions:* β-Lactam safety profile (rash, eosinophilia) allergy. Administer by IM injection only. Substantial pathogen resistance. Primarily renally eliminated. *Drug interaction:* Probenecid.
Penicillin V Pen VK, V-Cillin K. Tablet: 125, 250, 500 mg. Suspension: 125 mg/5 mL, 250 mg/5 mL.	**Preferred oral dosing form of penicillin, active against most gram-positive cocci; *S. pneumoniae* (resistance is increasing), other *Streptococcus,* and some gram-negative bacteria (e.g., *N. gonorrhoeae, N. meningitidis*).** Children: 25–50 mg/kg/24 hr divided q 4–8 hr PO. Adults: 125–500 mg q 6–8 hr PO (max dose: 3 g/24 hr).	*Cautions:* β-Lactam safety profile (rash, eosinophilia), allergy, seizures with excessive doses particularly in patients with renal disease. Substantial pathogen resistance. Primarily renally eliminated. Inactivated by penicillinase. *Drug interaction:* Probenecid.
Piperacillin Pipracil. Injection.	**Extended-spectrum penicillin active against *E. coli, Enterobacter, Serratia, P. aeruginosa,* and *Bacteroides.*** Neonates: Postnatal age ≤7 days 150 mg/kg/24 hr divided q 8–12 hr IV; >7 days; 200 mg/kg divided q 6–8 hr IV. Children: 200–300 mg/kg/24 hr divided q 4–6 hr IV; cystic fibrosis: 350–500 mg/kg/24 hr IV. Adults: 2–4 g/dose q 4–6 hr (max dose: 24 g/24 hr) IV.	*Cautions:* β-Lactam safety profile (rash, eosinophilia); painful given intramuscularly; each gram contains 1.9 mEq sodium. Interferes with platelet aggregation/serum sickness–like reaction with high doses; increases in liver function tests. Renally eliminated. Inactivated by penicillinase. *Drug interaction:* Probenecid.
Piperacillin-tazobactam Zosyn. Injection.	**Extended-spectrum penicillin (piperacillin) combined with a β-lactamase inhibitor (tazobactam) active against *S. aureus, H. influenzae, E. coli, Enterobacter, Serratia, Acinetobacter, P. aeruginosa,* and *Bacteroides.*** Children: 300–400 mg/kg/24 hr divided q 6–8 hr IV or IM. Adults: 3.375 g q 6–8 hr IV or IM.	*Cautions:* β-Lactam safety profile (rash, eosinophilia); painful given intramuscularly; each gram contains 1.9 mEq sodium. Interferes with platelet aggregation, serum sinckness–like reaction with high doses, increases in liver function test results. Renally eliminated. *Drug interaction:* Probenecid.
Quinupristin/dalfopristin Synercid. IV injection: powder for reconstitution, 10 mL contains 150 mg quinupristin, 350 mg dalfopristin.	**Streptogramin antibiotic (quinupristin) active against vancomycin-resistant *E. faecium* (VRE) and methicillin-resistant *S. aureus.* Not active against *E. faecalis.*** Children and adults: VRE: 7.5 mg/kg q 8 hr IV for VRE; skin infections: 7.5 mg/kg q 12 hr IV.	*Adverse events:* Pain, edema, or phlebitis at injection site, nausea, diarrhea. *Drug interactions:* Synercid is a potent inhibitor of CYP3A4.
Sulfadiazine Tablet: 500 mg.	**Sulfonamide antibiotic primarily indicated for the treatment of lower urinary tract infections due to *E. coli, P. mirabilis,* and *Klebsiella.*** Toxoplasmosis: Neonates: 100 mg/kg/24 hr divided q 12 hr PO with pyrimethamine 1 mg/kg/24 hr PO (with folinic acid). Children: 120–200 mg/kg/24 hr divided q 6 hr PO with pyrimethamine 2 mg/kg/24 hr divided q 12 hr PO ≥3 days then 1 mg/kg/24 hr (max dose: 25 mg/24 hr) with folinic acid. Rheumatic fever prophylaxis: ≤30 kg: 500 mg/24 hr q 24 hr PO; >30 kg: 1 g/24 hr q 24 hr PO.	*Cautions:* Rash, Stevens-Johnson syndrome, nausea, leukopenia, crystalluria. Renal and hepatic elimination; avoid use with renal disease. Half-life ~10 hr. *Drug interactions:* Protein displacement with warfarin, phenytoin, methotrexate.

TABLE 179-3. Antibacterial Medications (Antibiotics)—cont'd

DRUG (TRADE NAMES, FORMULATIONS)	INDICATIONS (MECHANISM OF ACTION) AND DOSING	COMMENTS
Sulfamethoxazole Gantanol. Tablet: 500 mg. Suspension: 500 mg/5 mL.	**Sulfonamide antibiotic used for the treatment of otitis media, chronic bronchitis, and lower urinary tract infections due to susceptible bacteria.** Children: 50–60 mg/kg/24 hr divided q 12 hr PO. Adults: 1 g/dose q 12 hr PO (max dose: 3 g/24 hr).	*Cautions:* Rash, Stevens-Johnson syndrome, nausea, leukopenia, crystalluria. Renal and hepatic elimination; avoid use with renal disease. Half-life 12 hr. Initial dose often a loading dose (doubled). *Drug interactions:* Protein displacement with warfarin, phenytoin, methotrexate.
Sulfisoxazole Gantrisin. Tablet: 500 mg. Suspension: 500 mg/5 mL. Ophthalmic solution, ointment.	**Sulfonamide antibiotic used for the treatment of otitis media, chronic bronchitis, and lower urinary tract infections due to susceptible bacteria.** Children: 120–150 mg/kg/24 hr divided q 4–6 hr PO (max dose: 6 g/24 hr). Adults: 4–8 g/24 hr divided q 4–6 hr PO.	*Cautions:* Rash, Stevens-Johnson syndrome, nausea, leukopenia, crystalluria. Renal and hepatic elimination; avoid use with renal disease. Half-life ~7–12 hr. Initial dose often a loading dose (doubled). Drug interactions: Protein displacement with warfarin, phenytoin, methotrexate.
Ticarcillin Ticar. Injection.	**Extended-spectrum penicillin active against *E. coli, Enterobacter, Serratia, P. aeruginosa,* and *Bacteroides.*** Neonates: Postnatal age ≤7 days <2,000 g: 150 mg/kg/24 hr divided q 8–12 hr IV; >7 days: <2,000 g: 225 mg/kg/24 hr divided q 8 hr IV; >7 days <1,200 g: 150 mg/kg/24 hr divided q 12 hr IV; 1,200–2,000 g: 225 mg/kg/24 hr divided q 8 hr IV; >2,000 g: 300 mg/kg/24 hr divided q 6–8 hr IV. Children: 200–400 mg/kg/24 hr divided q 4–6 hr IV; cystic fibrosis: 400—600 mg/kg/24 hr IV. Adults: 2–4 g/dose q 4–6 hr IV (max dose: 24 g/24 hr).	*Cautions:* β-Lactam safety profile (rash, eosinophilia); painful given intramuscularly; each gram contains 5–6 mEq sodium. Interferes with platelet aggregation; increases in liver function tests. Renally eliminated. Inactivated by penicillinase. *Drug interaction:* Probenecid.
Ticarcillin-clavulanate Timentin. Injection.	**Extended-spectrum penicillin (ticarcillin) combined with a β-lactamase inhibitor (clavulanate) active against *S. aureus, H. influenzae, Enterobacter, E. coli, Serratia, P. aeruginosa, Acinetobacter,* and *Bacteroides.*** Children: 280–400 mg/kg/24 hr q 4–8 hr IV or IM. Adults: 3.1 g q 4–8 hr IV or IM (max dose: 18–24 g/24 hr).	*Cautions:* β-Lactam safety profile (rash, eosinophilia); painful given intramuscularly; each gram contains 5–6 mEq sodium. Interferes with platelet aggregation; increases in liver function tests. Renally eliminated. *Drug interaction:* Probenecid.
Tobramycin Nebcin, Tobrex. Injection. Ophthalmic solution, ointment.	**Aminoglycoside antibiotic active against gram-negative bacilli, especially *E. coli, Klebsiella, Enterobacter, Serratia, Proteus,* and *Pseudomonas.*** Neonates: Postnatal age ≤7 days, 1,200–2,000 g: 2.5 mg/kg q 12–18 hr IV or IM; >2,000 g: 2.5 mg/kg q 12 hr IV or IM; postnatal age >7 days, 1,200–2,000 g: 2.5 mg/kg q 8–12 hr IV or IM; >2,000 g: 2.5 mg/kg q 8 hr IV or IM. Children: 2.5 mg/kg/24 hr divided q 8–12 hr IV or IM. Alternatively may administer 5–7.5 mg/kg/24 hr IV. Preservative-free preparation for intraventricular or intrathecal use: neonate: 1 mg/24 hr; children: 1–2 mg/24 hr; adults: 4–8 mg/24 hr. Adults: 3–6 mg/kg/24 hr divided q 8 hr IV or IM.	*Cautions: S. pneumoniae*, other *Streptococcus*, and anaerobes are resistant. May cause ototoxicity and nephrotoxicity. Monitor renal function. Drug eliminated renally. Administered IV over 30–60 min. *Drug interactions:* May potentiate other ototoxic and nephrotoxic drugs. *Target serum concentrations:* Peak 6–12 mg/L; trough <2 mg/L.
Trimethoprim Proloprim, Trimpex. Tablet: 100, 200 mg	**Folic acid antagonist effective in the prophylaxis and treatment of *E. coli, Klebsiella, Proteus mirabilis,* and *Enterobacter* urinary tract infections; *P. carinii* pneumonia.** Children: For urinary tract infection: 4–6 mg/kg/24 hr divided q 12 hr PO. Children >*12 yr and adults:* 100–200 mg q 12 hr PO. *P. carinii* pneumonia (with dapsone): 15–20 mg/kg/24 hr divided q 6 hr for 21 days PO.	*Cautions:* Megaloblastic anemia, bone marrow suppression, nausea, epigastric distress, rash. *Durg interactions:* Possible interactions with phenytoin, cyclosporine, rifampin, warfarin.
Vancomycin Vancocin, Luphocin. Injection. Capsule: 125 mg, 250 mg. Suspension.	**Glycopeptide antibiotic active against most gram-positive pathogens including *Staphylococcus* (including methicillin-resistant *S. aureus* and coagulase-negative staphylococci), *S. pneumoniae* including penicillin-resistant strains, *Enterococcus* (resistance is increasing), and *Clostridium difficile*-associated colitis.** Neonates: Postnatal age ≤7 days, <1,200 g: 15 mg/kg/24 hr divided q 24 hr IV; 1.200–2,000 g: 15 mg/kg/24 hr divided q 12–18 hr IV; >2,000 g: 30 mg/kg/24 hr divided q 12 hr IV; postnatal age >7 days, <1,200 g: 15 mg/kg/24 hr divided q 24 hr IV; 1,200–2,000 g: 15 mg/kg/24 hr divided q 8–12 hr IV; >2,000 g: 45 mg/kg/24 hr divided q 8 hr IV. Children: 45–60 mg/kg/24 hr divided q 8–12 hr IV; *Clostridium difficile*-associated colitis; 40–50 mg/kg/24 hr divided q 6–8 hr PO. Adults: 0.5–1 g IV q 12 hr IV.	*Cautions:* Ototoxicity and nephrotoxicity particularly when co-administered with other ototoxic and nephrotoxic drugs. Infuse IV over 45–60 min. Flushing (red-man syndrome) associated with rapid IV infusions, fever, chills, phlebitis (central line is preferred). Renally eliminated. *Target serum concentrations:* Peak (1 hr after 1 hr infusion) 30–40 mg/L; trough 5–10 mg/L.

(carbenicillin, ticarcillin) and **ureidopenicillins** (piperacillin, mezlocillin, azlocillin) also have bactericidal activity against most strains of *P. aeruginosa*.

Resistance to penicillin is mediated by a variety of mechanisms (see Table 179-1). The production of β-lactamase is a common mechanism exhibited by many organisms that may be overcome, with variable success, by including a β-lactamase inhibitor with the penicillin. These combination products (ampicillin-sulbactam, amoxicillin-clavulanate, piperacillin-tazobactam) are very useful for management of resistant isolates if the resistance is β-lactamase mediated. Notably, *S. aureus* and *S. pneumoniae* mediate β-lactam resistance through mechanisms other than β-lactamase production, rendering these combination agents of little value for the management of these infections.

Adverse reactions to penicillins are noted in Table 179-4.

Cephalosporins. Cephalosporins differ structurally from penicillins by having the β-lactam ring as a 6 member ring, compared to the 5 member ring structure of the penicillins. These agents are widely used in pediatric practice, both in oral and parenteral formulations (Table 179-5). The **1st generation cephalosporins** (cefazolin, a parenteral formulation, and cephalexin, an oral equivalent) are commonly used for management of skin and soft tissue infections caused by susceptible strains of *S. aureus* and group A streptococcus. The **2nd generation cephalosporins**

TABLE 179-4. Adverse Reactions to Penicillins*

TYPE OF REACTION	FREQUENCY (%)	OCCURS MOST FREQUENTLY WITH*
ALLERGIC		
IgE antibody	0.004–0.4	Penicillin G
Anaphylaxis		
Early urticaria (<72 h)		
Cytotoxic antibody	Rare	Penicillin G
Hemolytic anemia		
Antigen-antibody complex disease	Rare	Penicillin G
Serum sickness		
Delayed hypersensitivity	4–8	Ampicillin
Contact dermatitis		
IDIOPATHIC	4–8	Ampicillin
Skin rash		
Fever		
Late-onset urticaria		
GASTROINTESTINAL	2–5	
Diarrhea	2–5	Ampicillin
Enterocolitis	<1	Ampicillin
HEMATOLOGIC		
Hemolytic anemia	Rare	Penicillin G
Neutropenia	1–4	Penicillin G, nafcillin, oxacillin, piperacillin
Platelet dysfunction	3	Carbenicillin, ticarcillin
HEPATIC		
Elevated serum aspartate transaminase level	1–4	Oxacillin, nafcillin, carbenicillin
ELECTROLYTE DISTURBANCE		
Sodium overload	Variable	Ticarcillin
Hypokalemia	Variable	Ticarcillin
Hyperkalemia—acute	Rare	Penicillin G
NEUROLOGIC		
Seizures	Rare	Penicillin G
Bizarre sensations		Procaine penicillin
RENAL		
Interstitial nephritis	1–2	Methicillin
Hemorrhagic cystitis	Rare	Methicillin

*All the reactions can occur with any of the penicillins.
From Mandell GL, Bennett JE, Dolin R (editors): *Principles and Practice of Infectious Diseases*, 6th ed, Vol 1. Philadelphia, Elsevier, 2005, p 286.

TABLE 179-6. Potential Adverse Effects of Cephalosporins

TYPE	SPECIFIC	FREQUENCY
Hypersensitivity	Rash	1–3%
	Urticaria	<1%
	Serum sickness	<1%
	Anaphylaxis	0.01%
Gastrointestinal		
	Diarrhea	1–19%
	Nausea, vomiting	1–6%
	Transient transaminase elevation	1–7%
	Biliary sludge	20–46%*
Hematologic		
	Eosinophilia	1–10%
	Neutropenia	<1%
	Thrombocytopenia	<1–3%
	Hypoprothrombinemia	<1%
	Impaired platelet aggregation	<1%
	Hemolytic anemia	<1%
Renal		
	Interstitial nephritis	<1%
Central nervous system		
	Seizures	<1%
False-positive laboratory		
	Coombs positive	3%
	Glucosuria	Rare
	Serum creatinine	Rare
Other		
	Drug fever	Rare
	Disulfiram-like reaction†	Rare
	Superinfection	Rare
	Phlebitis	Rare

*Ceftriaxone.
†Cephalosporins with thiomethyl tetrazole ring (MTT) side chain.
From Mandell GL, Bennett JE, Dolin R (editors): *Principles and Practice of Infectious Diseases*, 6th ed, Vol 1. Philadelphia, Elsevier, 2005, p 303.

(cefuroxime, cefoxitin) have better activity against gram-negative infections than do 1st generation cephalosporins and are used to treat respiratory tract infections, urinary tract infections, and soft-tissue infections. A variety of orally administered 2nd generation agents (cefaclor, cefprozil, loracarbef, cefpodoxime) are commonly used in the outpatient management of sinopulmonary infections. The **3rd generation cephalosporins** (cefotaxime, ceftriaxone, and ceftazidime) are used for serious pediatric infections, including meningitis and sepsis. Ceftazidime is highly active against most strains of *P. aeruginosa,* making this a useful agent for febrile, neutropenic oncology patients. Another class of **4th generation cephalosporins** (cefepime) is indicated for treatment of pediatric meningitis, has activity against *P. aeruginosa,* and retains good activity against methicillin-susceptible staphylococcal infections.

Adverse reactions to cephalosporins are noted in Table 179-6.

Carbapenems. The carbapenems include imipenem, which is a combination of thienamycin and cilastatin, and the newer agents, meropenem and ertapenem. The basic structure of these agents is similar to that of β-lactam antibiotics, with a similar mechanism of action. The carbapenems provide the broadest spectrum of antibacterial activity of any licensed class of antibiotics, and are active against gram-positive, gram-negative, and anaerobic organisms. Meropenem is licensed for treatment of pediatric meningitis. MRSA and *Enterococcus faecium* are not susceptible to carbapenems. Carbapenems also tend to be poorly active against *Stenotrophomonas maltophilia,* rendering their use for cystic fibrosis patients colonized with this organism problematic.

TABLE 179-5. Classification of Parenteral and Oral Cephalosporins

CEPHALOSPORINS	1ST GENERATION	2ND GENERATION	CEPHAMYCINS	3RD GENERATION	4TH GENERATION
Parenteral	Cefazolin (Ancef, Kefzol) Cephalothin (Keflin, Seffin) Cephapirin (Cefadyl) Cephradine (Velosef)	Cefamandole (Mandol) Cefonicid (Monocid) Cefuroxime (Kefurox, Zinacef)	Cefmetazole (Zefazone) Cefotetan (Cefotan) Cefoxitin (Mefoxin)	Cefoperazole (Cefobid) Cefotaxime (Claforan) Ceftazidime (Fortaz) Ceftizoxime (Cefizox) Ceftriaxone (Rocephin)	Cefepime (Maxipime) Cefpirome
Oral	Cefadroxil (Duricef, Ultracef) Cephalexin (Keflex, Biocef, Keftab) Cephradine (Velosef)	Cefaclor (Ceclor) Cefprozil (Cefzil) Cefuroxime-axetil (Ceftin) Loracarbef (Lorabid)		Cefdinir (Omnicef) Cefditoren (Spectracef) Cefixime (Suprax) Cefpodoxime (Vantin) Ceftibuten (Cedax)	

From Mandell GL, Bennett JE, Dolin R (editors): *Principles and Practice of Infectious Diseases*, 6th ed, Vol 1. Philadelphia, Elsevier, 2005, p 297.

The 1st carbapenem approved for clinical use was imipenem-cilastatin, which has a propensity to cause seizures in children, particularly in the setting of meningitis, and therefore meropenem is more suitable for pediatric use.

Glycopeptides. Glycopeptide antibiotics include vancomycin and teicoplanin, the less commonly available analog. These agents are bacteriocidal and act via inhibition of cell wall biosynthesis. The antimicrobial activity of the glycopeptides is limited to gram-positive organisms, including *S. aureus,* coagulase-negative staphylococci, pneumococcus, *Enterococcus, Bacillus,* and *Corynebacterium.* Vancomycin is frequently employed in pediatric practice and is of particular value for serious infections, including meningitis, caused by MRSA and penicillin- and cephalosporin-resistant *S. pneumoniae.* Vancomycin is also commonly used for infections in the setting of fever and neutropenia, in combination with other antibiotics, in oncology patients (see Chapter 177), and infections associated with indwelling medical devices (see Chapter 178). Oral formulations of vancomycin are occasionally used to treat pseudomembranous colitis due to *Clostridium difficile* infections; intrathecal therapy may also be used for selected CNS infections. Vancomycin must be administered with care due to its propensity to produce red-man syndrome, which is a reversible adverse effect that is rare in young children and can typically be readily managed by slowing the rate of infusion of the drug.

Aminoglycosides. Aminoglycoside antibiotics include streptomycin, kanamycin, gentamicin, tobramycin, netilmicin, and amikacin. The most commonly used aminoglycosides in pediatric practice are gentamicin and tobramycin. They exert their mechanism of action via inhibition of bacterial protein synthesis. Although they are most commonly used to treat gram-negative infections, the aminoglycosides are broad-spectrum agents and have activity against *S. aureus* and provide synergistic activity against group B streptococcus, *L. monocytogenes,* viridans streptococci, corynebacteria JK, *Pseudomonas, Staphylococcus epidermidis,* and *Enterococcus* when co-administered with a β-lactam agent. Aminoglycoside use has decreased with the development of newer alternatives, but they still play a key role in pediatric practice in the management of neonatal sepsis, urinary tract infections, gram-negative sepsis, and complicated intra-abdominal infections; infections in cystic fibrosis patients (including both parenteral and aerosolized forms of therapy); and in oncology patients with fever and neutropenia. Aminoglycosides, in particular streptomycin, are also important in the management of *Francisella tularensis, Mycobacterium tuberculosis,* and atypical mycobacterial infections. Toxicities of aminoglycoside therapy include nephrotoxicity and ototoxicity (cochlear and/or vestibular), and serum levels as well as renal function and hearing should be monitored for patients on long-term therapy. Toxicities of aminoglycosides may be reduced by the use of once-daily dosing regimens based on monitoring serum levels. Hypokalemia, volume depletion, hypomagnesemia, and other nephrotoxic drugs may increase the renal toxicity of aminoglycosides. A rare complication of aminoglycosides is neuromuscular blockade, which may occur in the presence of other neuromuscular blocking agents and with infant botulism.

Tetracyclines. The tetracyclines (tetracycline hydrochloride, doxycycline, and minocycline) are bacteriostatic antibiotics that exhibit their antimicrobial effect by binding to the bacterial 30S ribosomal subunit, inhibiting protein translation. These agents have a broad spectrum of antimicrobial activity against gram-positive and -negative bacteria, rickettsia, and some parasites. The oral bioavailability of these agents facilitates this route of dosing for many infections including Rocky Mountain spotted fever, ehrlichiosis, Lyme disease, and malaria. Tetracyclines must be prescribed judiciously to children <9 yr of age because they can cause staining of teeth, hypoplasia of dental enamel, and abnormal bone growth in this age group. Tigecycline, a semi-synthetic derivative of minocycline, was recently licensed in the United States. It is a parenteral agent of a new class of antibiotics (glycylglycines). It has a broader spectrum of activity (bacteriostatic) than traditional tetracyclines, including activity against tetracycline-resistant gram-positive and -negative pathogens, including MRSA and possibly VRE but not *Pseudomonas.*

Complications of tetracyclines include eosinophilia, leukopenia and thrombocytopenia (tetracycline), pseudotumor cerebri, anorexia, emesis and nausea, candidiasis superinfection, hepatitis, photosensitivity, and a hypersensitivity reaction (urticaria, asthma exacerbation, facial edema, dermatitis) as well as a systemic lupus erythematosus–like syndrome (minocycline).

Sulfonamides. Trimethoprim and the sulfonamides are bacteriostatic agents that inhibit the bacterial folate synthesis pathway, in the process impairing both nucleic acid and protein synthesis. Sulfonamides interfere with the synthesis of dihydropteroic acid from para-aminobenzoic acid, whereas trimethoprim acts at a site further downstream, interfering with synthesis of tetrahydrofolic acid from dihydrofolic acid. The sulfonamides are available in both parenteral and oral formulations. Although there have historically been a large number of sulfonamide antibiotics developed for clinical use, relatively few remain available for pediatric practice. The most important agent is the combination of trimethoprim-sulfamethoxazole, which is commonly used for treatment of urinary tract infections and for *Pneumocystis carinii* infections in immunocompromised patients. Other commonly used sulfonamides include sulfisoxazole, which is used to treat urinary tract infections, and sulfadiazine, which is used to treat toxoplasmosis and as alternative prophylaxis against acute rheumatic fever.

Macrolides. The macrolide antibiotics most commonly employed in pediatric practice include erythromycin and the newer agents clarithromycin and azithromycin. These agents bind to the 50S subunit of the bacterial ribosome and block elongation of bacterial polypeptides. The spectrum of antibiotic activity includes many gram-positive infections, including *S. aureus* and group A streptococcus, although resistance to these agents is now fairly widespread, limiting the usefulness of macrolides for skin and soft tissue infections and streptococcal pharyngitis. The newer macrolides, azithromycin and clarithromycin, have demonstrated efficacy for otitis media. All of the members of this class have an important role in the management of pediatric respiratory infections, including atypical pneumonia caused by *M. pneumoniae, Chlamydia pneumoniae,* and *Legionella pneumophila,* as well as infections caused by *Bordetella pertussis.*

Telithromycin is a ketolide antibiotic derived from the macrolide erythromycin. It is FDA approved in adults for the treatment of mild to moderate community-acquired pneumonia, acute exacerbations of chronic bronchitis, and acute sinusitis, having good activity against the agents causing these infections (pneumococcus, *M. pneumoniae, C. pneumoniae,* and *L. pneumophila* for community-acquired pneumonia; *M. catarrhalis* and *H. influenzae* for sinusitis).

Drug interactions are common with erythromycin and telithromycin, and less so with clarithromycin. These agents can inhibit the CYP3A4 enzyme system, resulting in increased levels of certain drugs such as astemizole, cisapride, the statins, pimozide, and theophylline. Other agents (itraconazole) may increase macrolide levels, while rifampin, carbamazepine, and phenytoin may decrease macrolide levels. There are few reported adverse drug interactions with azithromycin. Cross-resistance may develop between a macrolide and the subsequent use of clindamycin.

Lincosamides. The prototype of the lincosamide class of antibiotics is clindamycin, which acts at the ribosomal level to exert its antimicrobial effect. The spectrum of activity includes gram-positive aerobes and anaerobes. Clindamycin has no significant activity against gram-negative organisms. An important role for clindamycin has emerged in the management of MRSA infections. Because of its outstanding penetration into body fluids (excluding the CNS) and tissues and bone, clindamycin can be utilized for therapy of serious infections caused by MRSA. Clindamycin is also useful, usually in combination with a β-lactam, in the management of invasive group A streptococcus infections, and in the management of many anaerobic infections. There is a form of **inducible clindamycin resistance** exhibited by some strains of MRSA; therefore, consultation with the clinical microbiology laboratory is necessary before treating a serious MRSA infection with clindamycin. Pseudomembranous colitis, a complication of clindamycin therapy commonly encountered in adults, is seldom observed in pediatric patients.

Quinolones. The fluoroquinolones (ciprofloxacin, levofloxacin, moxifloxacin, gemifloxacin) are newer antimicrobials that inhibit bacterial DNA replication by binding to the topoisomerases of the target pathogen, inhibiting the bacterial enzyme, DNA gyrase, and DNA replication. This class has very broad-spectrum activity against both gram-positive and gram-negative organisms. Some of the fluoroquinolones exhibit activity against penicillin-resistant *S. pneumoniae* as well as MRSA. These agents uniformly exhibit excellent activity against gram-negative pathogens, including the Enterobacteriaceae, and respiratory tract pathogens such as *M. catarrhalis* and *H. influenzae*. Quinolones are also very active against pathogens associated with atypical pneumonia, particularly *M. pneumoniae* and *L. pneumophila*.

Although these agents are not approved for use in children, there is a reasonable body of evidence that the fluoroquinolones are safe, well tolerated, and effective against a variety of bacterial infections in children. Parenteral quinolones are appropriate for critically ill patients with gram-negative infections. The use of oral quinolones in stable outpatients is also reasonable for treatment of infections that would otherwise require parenteral antibiotics (*P. aeruginosa* soft tissue infections such as osteochondritis) or selected genitourinary tract infections. However, they should be reserved for situations where no other oral antibiotic alternative is feasible. Where they have been used frequently (typhoid fever) organisms may rapidly develop resistance.

Streptogramins and Oxazolidinones. The emergence of highly resistant gram-positive organisms, in particular VRE, has necessitated development of new classes of antibiotics to treat these infections. One class of antibiotics that is highly useful for resistant gram-positive infections is the streptogramin class. The currently licensed agent in this category, **dalfopristin-quinupristin,** is approved in a parenteral formulation for patients >16 yr of age. It is appropriate for treatment of MRSA, coagulase-negative staphylococcus, penicillin-susceptible and penicillin-resistant pneumococcus, and vancomycin-resistant *E. faecium* but not *E. faecalis*.

Another licensed class of antibiotics for highly resistant gram-positive infections is the oxazolidinone class. The prototype of this group is the **linezolid,** which is available in both oral and parenteral formulations and is approved for use in pediatric patients. Its mechanism of action is through inhibition of ribosomal protein synthesis. It is indicated for MRSA, VRE, coagulase-negative staphylococci, and penicillin-resistant pneumococci. There is little information on dalfopristin-quinupristin and linezolid in treatment of infections involving the CNS, and neither agent is approved for pediatric meningitis. Linezolid can cause anemia and thrombocytopenia and is a monoamine oxidase inhibitor.

Daptomycin. Daptomycin is a cyclic lipopeptide with a spectrum of activity that includes virtually all gram-positive organisms, including *E. faecalis* and *E. faecium* (including VRE) and *S. aureus* (including MRSA). The structure of daptomycin is a 13 member amino acid peptide linked to a 10 carbon lipophilic tail, which results in a novel mechanism of action of disruption of the bacterial membrane through the formation of transmembrane channels. These channels cause leakage of intracellular ions leading to depolarizing the cellular membrane and inhibition of macromolecular synthesis. A theoretical advantage of daptomycin for serious infections is its bactericidal activity against MRSA and *Enterococcus*. It is administered IV. Experience in children is limited. Myopathy and elevations in creatine phosphokinase have been described. Daptomycin is inactivated by surfactant and should not be used to treat pneumonia.

Miscellaneous Agents. Although rarely used today because of safety concerns, chloramphenicol still occasionally plays a role in the management of pediatric infections, particularly those involving the CNS. This agent binds peptidyl transferase, a component of the 50S ribosome, inhibiting bacterial protein synthesis. Metronidazole, which functions by disruption of DNA synthesis, has a unique role as an anti-anaerobic agent as well as possessing antiparasitic and anthelminthic activity. Rifampin, which inhibits bacterial RNA polymerase, has a major role in the management of tuberculosis and is also of value for other bacterial infections in pediatric patients, usually used as a 2nd (synergistic) agent for *S. aureus* infections or to eliminate nasopharyngeal colonization of *H. influenzae* type b and *N. meningitidis*.

Bowlware KL, Stull T: Antibacterial agents in pediatrics. *Infect Dis Clin North Am* 2004;18:513–531.

Bradley JS: Newer antistaphylococcal agents. *Curr Opin Pediatr* 2005;17:71–77.

Buescher ES: Community-acquired methicillin-resistant *Staphylococcus aureus* in pediatrics. *Curr Opin Pediatr* 2005;17:67–70.

Cohen R: Approaches to reduce antibiotic resistance in the community. *Pediatr Infect Dis J* 2006;25:977–980.

Committee on Infectious Diseases: The use of systemic fluoroquinolones. *Pediatrics* 2006;118:1287–1292.

Dagan R, Barkai G, Leibovitz E, et al: Will reduction of antibiotic use reduce antibiotic resistance? *Pediatr Infect Dis* 2006;25:981–986.

Dancer SJ: How antibiotics can make us sick: The less obvious adverse effects of antimicrobial chemotherapy. *Lancet* 2004;4:611–619.

Gendrel D, Chalumeau M, Moulin F, Raymond J: Fluoroquinolones in paediatrics: A risk for the patient or for the community? *Lancet Infect Dis* 2003;3:537–546.

Hancock REW: Mechanisms of action of newer antibiotics for gram-positive pathogens. *Lancet Infect Dis* 2005;5:209–218.

Jacoby GA, Munoz-Price LS: The new β-lactamases. *N Engl J Med* 2005; 352:380–391.

Kline RM, Baorto EP: Treatment of pediatric febrile neutropenia in the era of vancomycin-resistant microbes. *Pediatr Blood Cancer* 2005;44:207–214.

Low DE, Pichichero ME, Schaad UB: Optimizing antibacterial therapy for community-acquired respiratory tract infections in children in an era of bacterial resistance. *Clin Pediatr North Am* 2004;43:135–151.

Malhotra-Kumar S, Lammens C, Coenen S, et al: Effect of azithromycin and clarithromycin therapy on pharyngeal carriage of macrolide-resistant streptococci in healthy volunteers: a randomised, double-blind, placebo-controlled study. *Lancet* 2007;369:482–490.

The Medical Letter: Telithromycine (Ketek) for respiratory infections. *Med Lett* 2004;46:66–68.

The Medical Letter: Tigecycline. *Med Lett* 2005;47:73–74.

Okeke IN, Laxminarayan R, Bhutta ZA, et al: Antimicrobial resistance in developing countries. Part 1: Recent trends and current status. *Lancet Infect Dis* 2005;5:481–492.

Pankey GA, Steele RW: Tigecycline: A single antibiotic for polymicrobial infections. *Pediatr Infect Dis J* 2007;26:77–78.

Pichichero ME: A review of evidence supporting the American Academy of Pediatrics recommendation for prescribing cephalosporin antibiotics for penicillin-allergic patients. *Pediatrics* 2005;115:1048–1057.

Pong AL, Bradley JS: Guidelines for the selection of antibacterial therapy in children. *Pediatr Clin North Am* 2005;52:869–894.

Sabharwal V, Marchant CD: Fluoroquinolone use in children. *Pediatr Infect Dis J* 2006;25:257–258.

Samaha-Kfoury JN, Araj GF: Recent developments in β-lactamases and extended spectrum β-lactamases. *Br Med J* 2003;327:1209–1213.

Wagner T, Burns JL: Anti-inflammatory properties of macrolides. *Pediatr Infect Dis J* 2007;26:75–76.

Wisplinghoff H, Seifert H, Tallent SM, et al: Nosocomial bloodstream infections in pediatric patients in United States hospitals: Epidemiology, clinical features and susceptibilities. *Pediatr Infect Dis J* 2003;22:686–691.

Zaoutis TE, Goyal M, Chu JH, et al: Risk factors for and outcomes of bloodstream infection caused by extended-spectrum beta-lactamase-producing *Escherichia coli* and *Klebsiella* species in children. *Pediatrics* 2005;115: 942–949.

Section 4 — Gram-Positive Bacterial Infections

Chapter 180 ■ *Staphylococcus*

James K. Todd

Staphylococci are hardy, aerobic, gram-positive bacteria that grow in pairs and clusters and are ubiquitous as normal flora of humans and present on fomites and in dust. They are resistant to heat and drying and may be recovered from nonbiologic environments weeks to months after contamination. Strains are classified as *Staphylococcus aureus* if they are coagulase positive or as 1 of the many species of **coagulase-negative staphylococci** *(S. epidermidis, S. saprophyticus, S. haemolyticus)*. Often, *S. aureus* produces a yellow or orange pigment and β-hemolysis on blood agar and *S. epidermidis* produces a white pigment with variable hemolysis results, although definitive species confirmation requires further testing. *S. aureus* has many virulence factors that mediate various serious diseases, whereas coagulase-negative staphylococci tend to be less pathogenic unless an indwelling foreign body (intravascular catheter) is present.

180.1 • *STAPHYLOCOCCUS AUREUS*

S. aureus is the most common cause of pyogenic infection of the skin and soft tissue; causing impetigo, furuncles (boils), cellulitis, abscess, lymphadenitis, paronychia, omphalitis, and wound infection. Bacteremia (primary and secondary) is common and can be associated with or result in osteomyelitis, suppurative arthritis, deep abscesses, pneumonia, empyema, endocarditis, pyomyositis, pericarditis, and rarely meningitis. Toxin-mediated diseases, including food poisoning, staphylococcal scarlet fever, scalded skin syndrome, and toxic shock syndrome (TSS) are caused by certain *S. aureus* strains.

ETIOLOGY. Disease may result from tissue invasion or injury caused by various toxins and enzymes produced by the organism. Strains of *S. aureus* can be identified by the virulence factors they produce and classified classically by means of bacteriophage group typing (groups I–IV, miscellaneous) or by molecular techniques.

Adhesion of *S. aureus* to mucosal cells is mediated by **teichoic acid** in the cell wall; exposure to the submucosa or subcutaneous sites increases adhesion to fibrinogen, fibronectin, collagen, and other proteins. Different strains of *S. aureus* produce many different virulence factors (Table 180-1), which have 1 or more of 4 different roles: protect the organism from host defenses, localize infection, cause local tissue damage, and act as toxins affecting noninfected tissue sites.

Most strains of *S. aureus* possess factors that protect the organism from host defenses. Many staphylococci produce a loose polysaccharide capsule, or **slime layer,** which may interfere with opsonophagocytosis. Production of **coagulase** and/or clumping factor differentiates *S. aureus* from *S. epidermidis* and other coagulase-negative staphylococci. Clumping factor interacts with fibrinogen to cause large clumps of organisms, interfering with effective phagocytosis. Coagulase causes plasma to clot by interacting with fibrinogen; this may have an important role in localization of infection (abscess formation). **Protein A,** which is present in most strains of *S. aureus* but not in *S. epidermidis,* reacts specifically with immunoglobulin G1 (IgG1), IgG2, and IgG4. It is located on the outermost coat of the cell wall and can absorb serum immunoglobulins, preventing antibacterial antibodies from acting as opsonins and thus inhibiting phagocytosis. Other enzymes elaborated by staphylococci include **catalase** (inactivates hydrogen peroxide, promoting intracellular survival), **penicillinase or β-lactamase** (inactivates penicillin at the molecular level), and lipase (associated with skin infection). **Panton-Valentine leukocidin (PVL),** which is produced by many current strains of *S. aureus* and has been associated with invasive skin disease, combines with the phospholipid of the phagocytic cell membrane, producing increased permeability, leakage of protein, and eventual death of the neutrophil and macrophage.

Many strains of *S. aureus* produce substances that cause local tissue destruction. A number of immunologically distinct hemolysins have been identified: α toxin acts on cell membranes and causes tissue necrosis, injures human leukocytes, and produces aggregation of platelets and spasm of smooth muscle; β-hemolysin degrades sphingomyelin, causing hemolysis of red blood cells; δ-hemolysin disrupts membranes by a detergent-like action.

Many strains of *S. aureus* release 1 or more exotoxins. **Exfoliatins A and B** are serologically distinct proteins that produce

TABLE 180-1. Virulence Factors of Community-acquired *Staphylococcus aureus*

VIRULENCE FACTOR	CHARACTERISTIC	CLINICAL SYNDROME
RESISTANCE DETERMINANTS		
SCC*mec* type IV	Resistance to methicillin	
SCC_{476}	Resistance to fusidic acid	
ADHERENCE		
Collagen-adhesin protein (CNA)	Greater adherence to host tissues	EF, NP, arthritis, osteomyelitis
COLONIZATION		
Bacteriocin of SA (*bsa*)	Intraspecies and interspecies competition	EF
Unknown	Greater tolerance to salt	EF
SUPERANTIGENS		
Enterotoxins	Activation of T cells	EF, NP, TSS-like illness
Staphylococcal enterotoxin A (*sea, sak*)		
Staphylococcal enterotoxin B		
Staphylococcal enterotoxin C (*sec4*)		
Staphylococcal enterotoxin G (*seg2*)		
Staphylococcal enterotoxin H	Extremely potent superantigen	
Staphylococcal enterotoxin K (*sek2*)		
Staphylococcal enterotoxin L (*sel2*)		
Staphylococcal enterotoxin O′ (*seo′*)		
EXOTOXINS		
Staphylococcal exotoxin T (*set*16–26)	Possible defence against immunity	
PORE-FORMING TOXINS		
PVL (LukSPV+LukPFV)	Necrosis, edema	EF, NP
LukE+LukD	Destruction of intestinal microvilli	Postantibiotic diarrhea
LukEv+LukDv	Necrosis	EF
α-Haemolysin	Necrosis, vascular leakage, shock	EF, NP
		Bullous impetigo
EXFOLIATIVE TOXINS		
Exfoliative toxin A		
Exfoliative toxin B		

EF, epidemic furunculosis; NP, necrotising pneumonia; SA, *Staphylococcus aureus*; TSS, toxic shock syndrome.

From Zetola N, Francis JS, Nuermberger EL, Bishai WR: Community-acquired methicillin-resistant *Staphylococcus aureus*: An emerging threat. *Lancet Infect Dis* 2005;5:275–286.

localized (bullous impetigo) or generalized (scalded skin syndrome, staphyloccocal scarlet fever) dermatologic complications (see Chapter 658). Exfoliatins produce skin separation by splitting the desmosome and altering the intracellular matrix in the stratum granulosum.

One or more staphylococcal **enterotoxins (types A, B, C_1, C_2, D, E)** are elaborated by most strains of *S. aureus*. Ingestion of preformed enterotoxin A or B is associated with **food poisoning** resulting in vomiting and diarrhea and, in some cases, with the development of profound hypotension. By 10 yr of age, almost all individuals have antibodies to at least 1 enterotoxin.

Toxic shock syndrome toxin-1 (TSST-1) is associated with TSS related to menstruation and focal staphylococcal infection. TSST-1 induces production of interleukin-1 and tumor necrosis factor, resulting in hypotension, fever, and multisystem involvement. Enterotoxin A and enterotoxin B also may be associated with nonmenstrual TSS.

EPIDEMIOLOGY. Most neonates are colonized within the 1st week of life; 20–30% of normal individuals carry at least 1 strain of *S. aureus* in the anterior nares at any given time.

The organisms may be transmitted from the nose to the skin, where colonization seems to be more transient. Persistent umbilical, vaginal, and perianal carriage occurs.

Heavily colonized individual nasal carriers (those with acute nonstaphylococcal respiratory symptoms) are particularly effective disseminators. Inoculation of *S. aureus* generally occurs by auto-inoculation or direct contact with the hands of other colonized individuals. Handwashing between patient contacts is essential to decrease the nosocomial spread of staphylococci. Spread via fomites is rare.

Invasive disease may follow colonization. Antibiotic therapy with a drug to which *S. aureus* is resistant favors colonization and the development of infection. Other factors that increase the likelihood of infection include wounds, skin disease, ventriculoperitoneal shunts, intravenous or intrathecal catheterization, corticosteroid treatment, malnutrition, acidosis, and azotemia. Viral infections of the respiratory tract also may predispose to secondary bacterial infection with staphylococci.

PATHOGENESIS. The development of staphylococcal disease is related to resistance of the host to infection and to virulence of the organism (Fig. 180-1). The intact skin and mucous membranes serve as barriers to invasion by staphylococci. Defects in the mucocutaneous barriers produced by trauma, surgery, foreign surfaces (sutures, shunts, intravascular catheters), and burns increase the risk for infection.

Infants may acquire type-specific humoral immunity to staphylococci transplacentally. Older children and adults develop antibodies to staphylococci as a result of colonization or minor infections. Antibodies acquired after immunization with *S. aureus* capsular material have been shown to temporarily reduce subsequent infection in dialysis patients. Antibody to the various *S. aureus* toxins appears to protect against those specific toxin-mediated diseases but not necessarily focal or disseminated *S. aureus* infection with the same organisms.

Congenital or acquired defects in chemotaxis (Job, Chédiak-Higashi, Wiskott-Aldrich syndromes), defective phagocytosis and killing (neutropenia, chronic granulomatous disease), and defective humoral immunity (antibodies required for opsonization) increase the risk for staphylococcal infections. Impaired mobilization of polymorphonuclear leukocytes has been documented in children with diabetic ketoacidosis and in healthy individuals after ingesting alcohol. Patients with HIV infection have neutrophils that are defective in their ability to kill *S. aureus* in vitro. Patients should be evaluated for immune defects associated with recurrent infection, especially those involving neutrophil dysfunction.

CLINICAL MANIFESTATIONS. The signs and symptoms vary with the location of the infection, which, although most commonly located on the skin, may involve any tissue. Disease states of various degrees of severity are generally a result of local suppuration, systemic dissemination with metastatic infection, or systemic effects of toxin production. Although the nasopharynx and skin of many persons may be colonized with *S. aureus,* disease due to this organism is relatively uncommon. Lesions, especially those of the skin, are considerably more prevalent among persons living in low socioeconomic circumstances and particularly among those in tropical climates.

Newborn. *Staphylococcus* is an important cause of neonatal infections (see Chapter 109).

Skin. *Staphylococcus* is an important cause of pyogenic skin infections, including impetigo contagiosa, ecthyma, bullous impetigo, folliculitis, hydradenitis, furuncles, carbuncles, staphylococcal scalded skin syndrome, and a syndrome resembling the rash of scarlet fever. Infection may also complicate wounds or occur as superinfection of other noninfectious skin disease

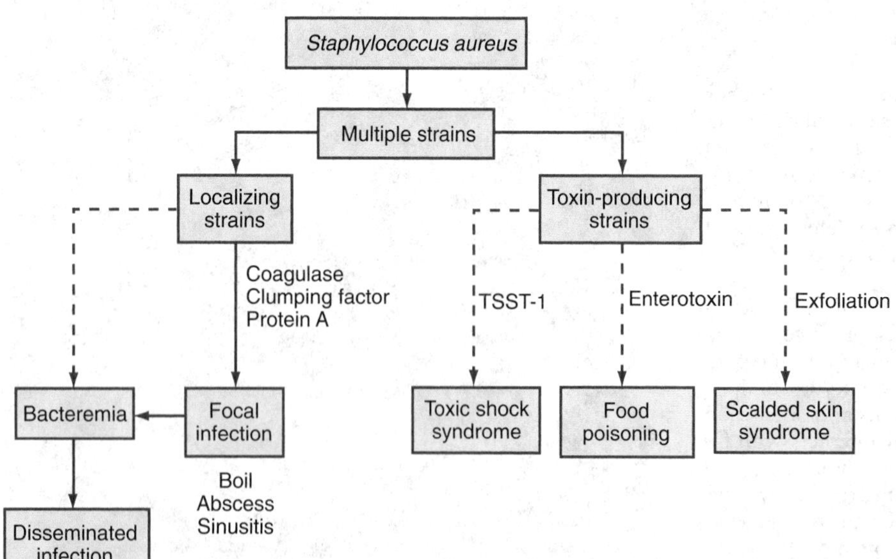

Figure 180-1. Relationship of virulence factors to diseases associated with *Staphylococcus aureus.*

(eczema). Recurrent furunculosis is a disorder of unknown cause and is associated with repeated episodes of pyoderma over months to years. Recurrent skin and soft tissue abscesses is noted with community-associated methicillin resistant *S. aureus* (MRSA). *Staphylococcus* is also an important cause of nosocomial skin infections (see Chapter 171).

Respiratory Tract. Infections of the upper respiratory tract due to *S. aureus* are rare, considering the frequency with which this area (especially the anterior nares) is colonized. Otitis media (see Chapter 641) and sinusitis (see Chapter 377) caused by *S. aureus* occur rarely. Staphylococcal sinusitis is relatively common in children with cystic fibrosis or defects in leukocyte function. Suppurative parotitis is a rare infection, but *S. aureus* is a common cause. A membranous **tracheitis** that complicates viral croup may be infected with *S. aureus* but also by other organisms. Patients typically have high fever, leukocytosis, evidence of severe upper airway obstruction, or a toxic shock–like picture. Direct laryngoscopy or bronchoscopy shows a normal epiglottis with subglottic narrowing and thick, purulent secretions within the trachea. Treatment requires antibiotics and careful airway management.

Pneumonia (see Chapter 397) due to *S. aureus* may be primary (hematogenous) or secondary after a viral infection such as influenza. Hematogenous pneumonia may be secondary to septic emboli, right-sided endocarditis, or the presence of intravascular devices. Inhalation pneumonia is caused by alterations of mucociliary clearance, leukocyte dysfunction, or bacterial adherence initiated by a viral infection. More common are high fever, abdominal pain, tachypnea, dyspnea, and localized or diffuse bronchopneumonia or lobar disease. *S. aureus* often causes a **necrotizing pneumonitis;** empyema, pneumatoceles, pyopneumothorax, and bronchopleural fistulas develop frequently. Staphylococcal pneumonia occasionally produces a diffuse interstitial disease characterized by extreme dyspnea, tachypnea, and cyanosis. Cough may be nonproductive. *S. aureus* is an important pathogen of pneumonia in patients with cystic fibrosis (see Chapter 400).

Sepsis. Staphylococcal bacteremia and sepsis (see Chapter 176) may be primary or associated with any localized infection. The onset may be acute and marked by nausea, vomiting, myalgia, fever, and chills. Organisms may localize subsequently at any site (usually a single deep focus) but are found especially in the heart valves, lungs, joints, and bones.

In some instances, especially in young adolescent males, disseminated staphylococcal disease occurs, characterized by fever, persistent bacteremia despite antibiotics, and focal involvement of 2 or more separate tissue sites (skin, bone, joint, kidney, lung, liver, heart). Endocarditis and septic thrombophlebitis must be ruled out.

Muscle. Localized staphylococcal abscesses in muscle associated with elevation of muscle enzymes but without septicemia have been called **pyomyositis.** This disorder has been reported most frequently from tropical areas; it also occurs in the United States in otherwise healthy children. Multiple abscesses occur in 30–40% of cases. Prodromal symptoms may include coryza, pharyngitis, diarrhea, or prior trauma at the site of the abscess. Surgical drainage and appropriate antibiotic therapy are essential.

Bones and Joints. *S. aureus* is the most common cause of osteomyelitis and suppurative arthritis in children (see Chapters 683 and 684).

Central Nervous System. Meningitis (see Chapter 603.1) caused by *S. aureus* is not common; it is associated with penetrating cranial trauma and neurosurgical procedures (craniotomy, cerebrospinal fluid [CSF] shunt placement) and less frequently with endocarditis, parameningeal foci (epidural or brain abscess), diabetes mellitus, or malignancy. The CSF profile of *S. aureus* meningitis is indistinguishable from that in other bacterial causes of meningitis.

Heart. Infective endocarditis (see Chapter 437) may follow staphylococcal bacteremia. *S. aureus* is a common cause of acute endocarditis on native valves. Perforation of heart valves, myocardial abscesses, heart failure, conduction disturbances, acute hemopericardium, purulent pericarditis, and sudden death may ensue.

Kidney. *S. aureus* is a common cause of renal and perinephric abscess (see Chapter 539) usually of hematogenous origin. Urinary tract infection due to *S. aureus* is unusual.

Toxic Shock Syndrome. *S. aureus* is the principal cause of TSS (see Chapter 180.2).

Intestinal Tract. Staphylococcal enterocolitis rarely follows overgrowth of normal bowel flora by staphylococci. Although uncommon, this can follow use of broad-spectrum oral antibiotic therapy. Diarrhea is associated with blood and mucus. Peritonitis associated with *S. aureus* in patients receiving long-term ambulatory peritoneal dialysis usually involves the catheter tunnel. Removal of the catheter is required to achieve a bacteriologic cure.

Food poisoning (see Chapter 337) may be caused by ingestion of **preformed** enterotoxins produced by staphylococci in contaminated foods. Approximately 2–7 hr after ingestion of the toxin, sudden, severe vomiting begins. Watery diarrhea may develop, but fever is absent or low. Symptoms rarely persist longer than 12–24 hr. Rarely, shock and death may occur.

DIAGNOSIS. The diagnosis of staphylococcal infection depends on isolation of the organisms from nonpermissive sites such as cellulitis aspirates, abscess cavities, blood, or other sites of infection. Isolation from the nose or skin does not necessarily imply causation because these may be normally colonized sites. Because of the increasing prevalence of MRSA, the increasing severity of staphylococcal infections, and the fact that bacteremia is not universally present even in severe staphylococcal infections, it is usually important to obtain a nonpermissive culture of any potential focus of infection as well as a blood culture. The organisms can be grown readily in liquid and on solid media. After isolation, identification is made on the basis of Gram stain and coagulase, clumping factor, and protein A reactivity. Patterns of susceptibility to antibiotics should be assessed in serious cases.

Diagnosis of staphylococcal food poisoning is made on the basis of epidemiologic and clinical findings. Food suspected of contamination should be cultured and can be tested for enterotoxin.

Differential Diagnosis. Skin lesions due to *S. aureus* and those due to group A streptococci may be indistinguishable; the former usually expands slowly while the latter is more prone to spread rapidly. Staphylococcal pneumonia can be suspected on the basis of chest roentgenograms that may reveal pneumatoceles, pyopneumothorax, or lung abscess (Fig. 180-2). Fluctuant skin and soft tissue lesions also can be caused by many organisms, including *Mycobacterium tuberculosis,* atypical mycobacteria, *Bartonella henselae* (cat-scratch disease), *Francisella tularensis,* and various fungi.

TREATMENT. Antibiotic therapy alone is rarely effective in individuals with undrained abscesses or with infected foreign bodies. Loculated collections of purulent material should be relieved by incision and drainage. Foreign bodies should be removed, if possible. Therapy always should be initiated with an antibiotic consistent with the local staphylococcal susceptibility patterns as well as the severity of infection. Penicillin or amoxicillin are not appropriate because more than 90% of all staphylococci isolated, regardless of source, are resistant to penicillin. For serious infections, parenteral treatment is indicated, at least at the outset, until symptoms are controlled. Serious staphylococcal infections, with or without abscesses, tend to persist and recur, necessitating prolonged therapy.

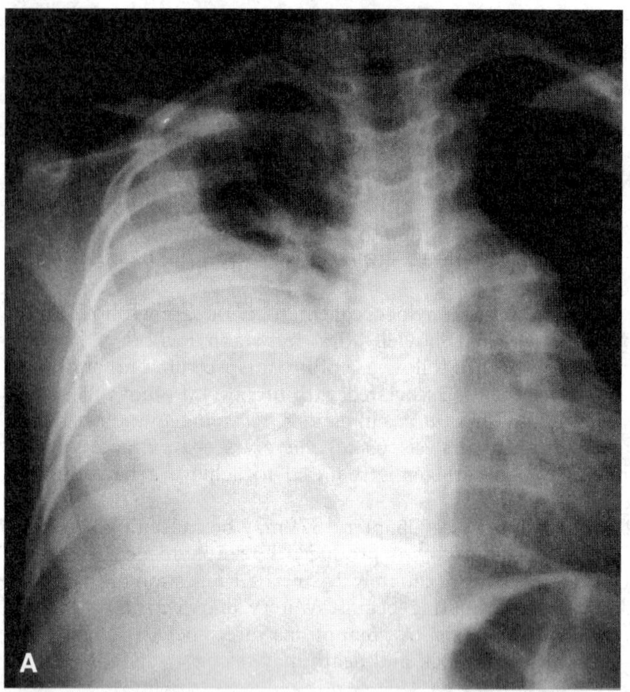

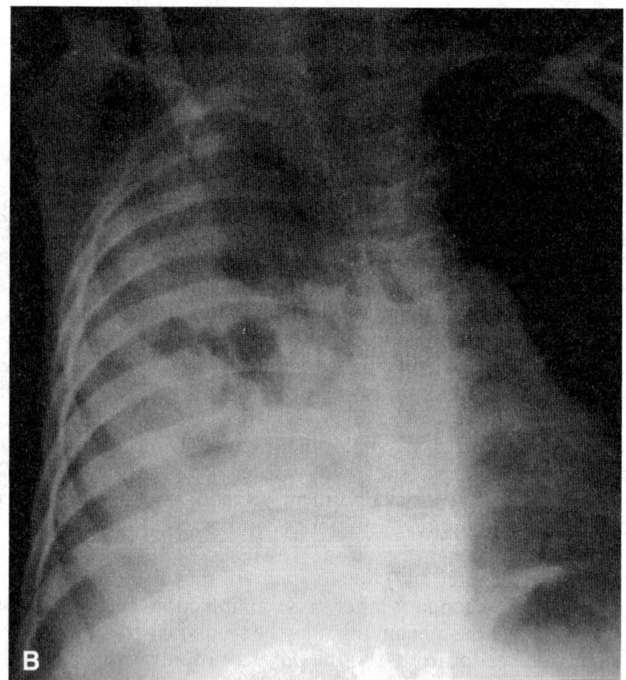

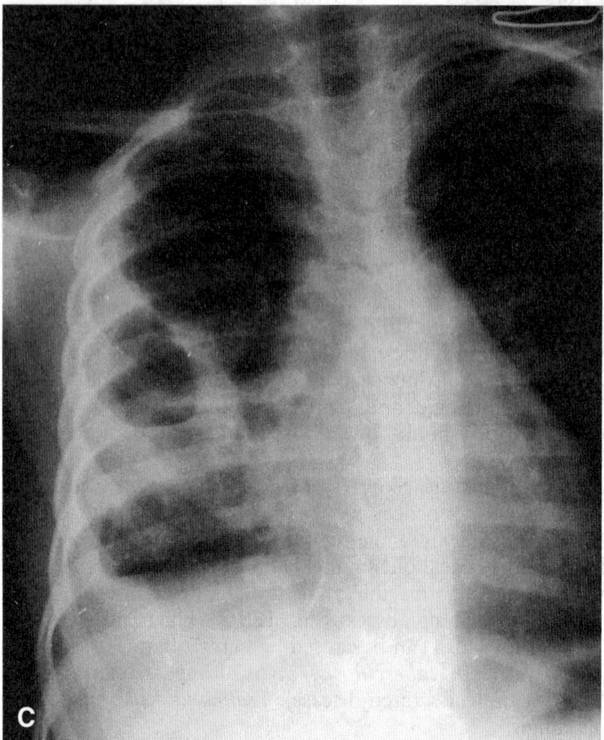

Figure 180-2. Pneumatocele formation. *A through C,* A child, 5 yr of age, with staphylococcal pneumonia initially demonstrated consolidation of the right middle and lower zones *(A)*. *B,* Seven days later, multiple lucent areas are noted as pneumatoceles develop. *C,* Two wk later, significant resolution is evident, with a rather thick-walled pneumatocele persisting in the right midzone associated with significant residual pleural thickening. (From Kuhn JP, Slovis TL, Haller JO: *Caffey's Pediatric Diagnostic Imaging,* 10th ed, Vol 1. Philadelphia, Mosby, 2004, pp 1003–1004.)

The antibiotic used as well as the dose, route, and duration of treatment depend on the site of infection, the response of the patient to treatment, and the susceptibility of the organisms recovered from blood or from local sites of infection. For most patients with serious staphylococcal infection, intravenous treatment is recommended until the patient has been afebrile for 72 hr and other signs of infection have disappeared. Oral therapy is continued for a total of 3 wk, longer in selected cases. Treatment of staphylococcal osteomyelitis (see Chapter 683), meningitis (see Chapter 603.1), and endocarditis (see Chapter 437) are discussed in their respective chapters.

MRSA is an important nosocomial and community-acquired pathogen. Community-acquired MRSA strains are common throughout the United States, even in children without pre-existing risk factors. Resistance to semisynthetic penicillins is related to a novel penicillin-binding protein (PB2A) that is relatively insensitive to antibiotics containing a β-lactam ring. MRSA strains appear to be as virulent as their methicillin-sensitive counterparts. Vancomycin (40–60 mg/kg/24 hr divided every 6 hr IV) can be used as the initial treatment for penicillin-allergic individuals and those with suspected serious *S. aureus* infections. Serum levels of vancomycin should be monitored, with peak concentra-

TABLE 180-2. Parenteral Antimicrobial Agent(s) for Treatment of Bacteremia and Other Serious *Staphylococcus aureus* Infections

SUSCEPTIBILITY	ANTIMICROBIAL AGENTS	COMMENTS
I. Initial empiric therapy (organism of unknown susceptibility)		
Drugs of choice:	Vancomycin + nafcillin or oxacillin ± gentamicin	For life-threatening infections (i.e., septicemia, endocarditis, CNS infection); linezolid could be substituted if the patient has received several recent courses of vancomycin
	Nafcillin or oxacillin*	For non-life-threatening infection without signs of sepsis (e.g., skin infection, cellulitis, osteomyelitis, pyarthrosis) when rates of MRSA colonization and infection in the community are low
	Clindamycin	For non-life-threatening infection without signs of sepsis when rates of MRSA colonization and infection in the community are substantial and prevalence of clindamycin resistance is low
	Vancomycin	For non-life-threatening, hospital-acquired infections
II. Methicillin-susceptible, penicillin-resistant *S. aureus* (MSSA)		
Drugs of choice:	Nafcillin or oxacillin*[,†]	
Alternatives:	Cefazolin*	
	Clindamycin	
	Vancomycin	Only for penicillin- and cephalosporin-allergic patients
	Ampicillin + sulbactam	
III. MRSA (oxacillin MIC, ≥4 µg/mL)		
A. Health care–associated (multidrug-resistant)		
Drugs of choice:	Vancomycin ± gentamicin or ± rifampin[†]	
Alternatives: susceptibility testing results available before alternative drugs are used		
	Trimethoprim-sulfamethoxazole	
	Linezolid[‡]	
	Quinupristin-dalfopristin[‡]	
	Fluoroquinolones	Not recommended for people younger than 18 yr of age or as monotherapy
B. Community (not multidrug-resistant)		
Drugs of choice:	Vancomycin ± gentamicin (or ± rifampin[†])	For life-threatening infections
	Clindamycin (if strain susceptible)	For pneumonia, septic arthritis, osteomyelitis, skin or soft tissue infections
	Trimethoprim-sulfamethoxazole	For skin or soft tissue infections
Alternative:	Vancomycin[†]	
IV. Vancomycin-intermediately susceptible *S. aureus* (MIC, >4 µg/mL and ≤16 µg/mL)[†]		
Drugs of choice:	Optimal therapy is not known	Dependent on in vitro susceptibility test results
	Linezolid[‡]	
	Daptomycin[§]	
	Quinupristin-dalfopristin[‡]	
Alternatives:	Vancomycin + linezolid ± gentamicin	
	Vancomycin + trimethoprim-sulfamethoxazole[†]	

CNS, central nervous system; MRSA, methicillin-resistant *S. aureus*; MIC, minimum inhibitory concentration.
*Penicillin- and cephalosporin-allergic patients should receive vancomycin as initial therapy for serious infections.
[†]One of the adjunctive agents, gentamicin or rifampin, should be added to the therapeutic regimen for life-threatening infections such as endocarditis or CNS infection or infections with a vancomycin-intermediate *S. aureus* strain. Consultation with an infectious diseases specialist should be considered to determine which agent to use and duration of use.
[‡]Linezolid and quinupristin-dalfopristin are 2 agents with activity in vitro and efficacy in adults with multidrug-resistant, gram-positive organisms, including *S. aureus*. Because experience with these agents in children is limited, consultation with an infectious diseases specialist should be considered before use.
[§]Daptomycin is active in vitro against multidrug-resistant, gram-positive organisms, including *S. aureus*, but has not been used in children. Daptomycin is approved by the U.S. Food and Drug Administration only for the treatment of complicated skin and skin structure infections in patients 18 yr of age and older.
From the American Academy of Pediatrics: *Red Book: 2006 Report of the Committee on Infectious Diseases*, 27th ed. Elk Grove Village, IL, American Academy of Pediatrics, 2006, pp 605–606.

tions of 20–40 µg/mL. MRSA is also resistant to cephalosporins and imipenem but may be susceptible to the quinolones. Linezolid, daptomycin, quinupristin-dalfopristin, vancomycin with linezolid and gentamicin, and vancomycin with trimethoprim-sulfamethoxazole may be useful for serious *S. aureus* infections highly resistant to other antibiotics (Table 180-2).

Rare vancomycin-intermediate strains have also been reported, mostly in patients being treated with vancomycin, emphasizing the need for restricting the prescription of unnecessary antibiotics and the importance of isolation of the causative organism and susceptibility testing in serious infections.

Serious staphylococcal infections (septicemia, endocarditis, central nervous system infections, toxic shock syndrome) should be treated initially with intravenous vancomycin and methicillin, nafcillin, or oxacillin until the causative organism is isolated and its susceptibility determined. Rifampin or gentamicin may be added for synergy in serious infections (endocarditis).

In all of these infections, oral treatment may be provided to complete the course of treatment after an initial period of parenteral therapy and once antimicrobial susceptibilities have been determined. Despite in vitro susceptibility of *S. aureus* to ciprofloxacin and other quinolone antibiotics, these agents should not be used in serious staphylococcal infections, because their use has not consistently been associated with high cure rates and the quinolones are not recommended for use in patients younger than 18 yr. Trimethoprim-sulfamethoxazole may be an effective oral antibiotic for both methicillin-susceptible *S. aureus* (MSSA) and MRSA.

Dicloxacillin (50–100 mg/kg/24 hr divided qid PO) and cephalexin (25–100 mg/kg/24 hr divided tid–qid PO) are absorbed well orally and effective for MSSA. Amoxicillin-clavulanate (40–80 mg amoxicillin/kg/24 hr divided tid PO) also is effective. Clindamycin (30–40 mg/kg/24 hr divided tid–qid PO) has proved effective for the treatment of skin, soft tissue, bone, and joint infections due to susceptible *S. aureus* strains. Clindamycin is bacteriostatic and should not be used to treat endocarditis, brain abscess, or meningitis due to *S. aureus*. Many experts add clindamycin (inhibits protein synthesis) to *S. aureus* toxin–mediated illnesses to inhibit toxin production. The duration of oral therapy depends on the response as determined by the clinical, roentgenographic, and laboratory findings.

Skin and soft tissue infection and minor upper respiratory tract infection may often be managed by oral therapy and drainage alone or by an initial brief course of antibiotics provided parenterally, followed by oral medication.

PROGNOSIS. Untreated staphylococcal septicemia is associated with a mortality rate of ≥80%. Mortality rates have been reduced significantly by appropriate antibiotic treatment. Staphylococcal pneumonia can be fatal at any age but is more likely to be associated with high morbidity and mortality in young infants or in patients whose therapy has been delayed. Prognosis also may be influenced by numerous host factors, including nutrition, immunologic competence, and the presence or absence of other debilitating diseases. In most cases with abscess formation, surgical drainage is necessary.

PREVENTION. Staphylococcal infection is transmitted primarily by direct contact. Strict attention to handwashing techniques is the most effective measure for preventing the spread of staphylococci from 1 individual to another (see Chapter 171). Use of a detergent containing an iodophor, chlorhexidine, or hexachlorophene is recommended. In hospitals or other institutional settings, all persons with acute staphylococcal infections should be isolated until they have been treated adequately. There should be constant surveillance for nosocomial staphylococcal infections within hospitals. When MRSA is recovered, strict isolation of affected patients has been shown to be the most effective method for preventing nosocomial spread of infection. Thereafter, control measures should be directed toward identification of new isolates and strict isolation of newly colonized or infected patients. It also may be necessary to identify colonized hospital personnel and eradicate carriage in affected individuals.

Patients with recurrent staphylococcal furunculosis may be treated with hexachlorophene washes and appropriate oral antibiotic and nasal mupirocin to prevent recurrences.

Food poisoning (see Chapter 337) may be prevented by excluding individuals with staphylococcal infections of the skin from the preparation and handling of food. Prepared foods should be eaten immediately or refrigerated appropriately to prevent multiplication of staphylococci with which the food may have been contaminated.

180.2 • Toxic Shock Syndrome

TSS is an acute multisystem disease characterized by high fever, hypotension, vomiting, diarrhea, myalgias, nonfocal neurologic abnormalities, conjunctival hyperemia, strawberry tongue, and an erythematous rash with subsequent desquamation on the hands and feet.

ETIOLOGY. TSS is caused by TSST-1-producing strains of *S. aureus*, which may colonize the vagina or cause focal sites of staphylococcal infection.

EPIDEMIOLOGY. Many cases occur in menstruating women who are 15–25 yr of age and who use tampons or other vaginal devices (diaphragm, contraceptive sponge). TSS also occurs in children, nonmenstruating women, and men. **Nonmenstrual TSS** has occurred with *S. aureus* infection of nasal packing or infections including wound infections, sinusitis, tracheitis, pneumonia, empyema, abscesses, burns, osteomyelitis, and primary bacteremia. Without antimicrobial therapy, menstrual TSS has a 30% recurrence rate, with secondary cases being milder and occurring within 3 mo of the original episode. The overall mortality rate of treated patients is 3%.

TABLE 180-3. Diagnostic Criteria of Staphylococcal Toxic Shock Syndrome

MAJOR CRITERIA (ALL REQUIRED)
Acute fever; temperature >38.8°C
Hypotension (orthostatic, shock; below age-appropriate norms)
Rash (erythroderma with late desquamation)
MINOR CRITERIA (ANY 3)
Mucous membrane inflammation
Vomiting, diarrhea
Liver abnormalities
Renal abnormalities
Muscle abnormalities
Central nervous system abnormalities
Thrombocytopenia
EXCLUSIONARY CRITERIA
Absence of another explanation
Negative blood cultures (except occasionally for *S. aureus*)

From Kuhn JP, Slovis TL, Haller JO: *Caffrey's Pediatric Diagnostic Imaging,* 10th ed, Vol 2. Philadelphia, Mosby, 2004, pp 1003–1004.

PATHOGENESIS. A majority of *S. aureus* strains isolated from confirmed cases are phage group I and produce a number of extracellular toxins. The primary toxin associated with TSS is TSST-1, which causes massive loss of fluid from the intravascular space directly or after production of interleukin 1 and tumor necrosis factor. TSST-1-negative strains have been isolated from patients with TSS, suggesting that other toxins (primarily the enterotoxins) have a role in TSS (especially nonmenstrual). Epidemiologic and in vitro studies suggest that these toxins are selectively produced in a clinical environment consisting of a neutral pH, a high P_{CO_2}, and an "aerobic" P_{O_2}, which are the conditions found in the vagina with tampon use during menstruation. This may explain why 90% of adults have antibody to TSST-1 without a history of clinical TSS; that is, they became colonized with a toxin-producing organism at a site (anterior nares) where low-grade or inactive toxin exposure resulted in an immune response without disease. The risk factors for symptomatic disease require a nonimmune host colonized with a toxin-producing organism, which is exposed to focal growth conditions (menstruation plus tampon use or abscess), which induce toxin production.

CLINICAL MANIFESTATIONS. The diagnosis of TSS is based on clinical manifestations (Table 180-3). The onset is abrupt, with high fever, vomiting, and diarrhea, and is accompanied by sore throat, headache, and myalgias. A diffuse erythematous macular rash (sunburn-like or scarlatiniform) appears within 24 hr and may be associated with hyperemia of pharyngeal, conjunctival, and vaginal mucous membranes. A strawberry tongue is common. Symptoms often include alterations in the level of consciousness, oliguria, and hypotension, which in severe cases may progress to shock and disseminated intravascular coagulation. Complications, including acute respiratory distress syndrome, myocardial dysfunction, and renal failure, are commensurate with the degree of shock. Recovery occurs within 7–10 days and is associated with desquamation, particularly of palms and soles; hair and nail loss have also been observed after 1–2 mo. Many cases of apparent scarlet fever without shock may be caused by TSST-1-producing *S. aureus* strains.

DIAGNOSIS. There is no specific laboratory test; appropriate selective tests reveal involvement of multiple organ systems, including the hepatic, renal, muscular, gastrointestinal, cardiopulmonary, and central nervous systems. Bacterial cultures of the associated focus (vagina, abscess) before administration of antibiotics usually yield *S. aureus,* although this is not a required element of the definition.

Differential Diagnosis. Group A streptococcus can cause a similar TSS-like illness, termed **streptococcal TSS** (see Chapter 182), which is often associated with severe streptococcal sepsis or a focal streptococcal infection such as cellulitis or pneumonia.

Kawasaki disease closely resembles TSS clinically but is usually not as severe or rapidly progressive. Both are associated with fever unresponsive to antibiotics, hyperemia of mucous membranes, and an erythematous rash with subsequent desquamation. Many of the clinical features of TSS, however, are usually absent or rare in Kawasaki disease, including diffuse myalgia, vomiting, abdominal pain, diarrhea, azotemia, hypotension, acute respiratory distress syndrome, and shock (see Chapter 165). Kawasaki disease typically occurs in children younger than 5 yr. Scarlet fever, Rocky Mountain spotted fever, leptospirosis, toxic epidermal necrolysis, sepsis, and measles must also be considered in the differential diagnosis.

TREATMENT. Parenteral administration of a β-lactamase-resistant antistaphylococcal antibiotic (nafcillin or a 1st generation cephalosporin) or vancomycin in areas where MRSA is common is recommended after appropriate cultures have been obtained. The addition of clindamycin in severe or unresponsive cases may terminate toxin production. Drainage of the vagina, by removal of any retained tampons in menstrual TSS, and of focally infected sites in nonmenstrual TSS is important for successful treatment. Antistaphylococcal therapy may also reduce the risk for recurrence in menstrual TSS.

Fluid replacement should be aggressive to prevent or treat hypotension, renal failure, and cardiovascular collapse. Inotropic agents may be needed to treat shock; corticosteroids and intravenous immunoglobulin may be helpful in severe cases.

PREVENTION. The low risk for acquiring TSS (1–2 cases/100,000 menstruating women) may be reduced by not using tampons or by using them intermittently during each menstrual period. If a fever, rash, or dizziness develops during menstruation, any tampon should be removed immediately and medical attention sought.

180.3 • Coagulase-Negative Staphylococci

S. epidermidis is just 1 of many recognized species of coagulase-negative staphylococci (CONS) affecting or colonizing humans. Originally thought to be avirulent commensal bacteria, CONS is now recognized to cause infections in patients with indwelling foreign devices, including intravenous catheters; hemodialysis shunts and grafts, CSF shunts (meningitis), peritoneal dialysis catheters (peritonitis), pacemaker wires and electrodes (local infection), prosthetic cardiac valves (endocarditis), and prosthetic joints (arthritis). CONS is a common cause of nosocomial neonatal infection. *S. haemolyticus,* another CONS species, is an important cause of invasive infection and may develop resistance to vancomycin and teicoplanin.

EPIDEMIOLOGY. CONS consists of normal inhabitants of the human skin, throat, mouth, vagina, and urethra. *S. epidermidis* is the most common and persistent species, representing 65–90% of staphylococci present on the skin and mucous membranes. Colonization, sometimes with strains acquired from hospital staff, precedes infection; alternatively, direct inoculation during surgery may initiate infection of CSF shunts, prosthetic valves, or indwelling vascular lines. For epidemiologic purposes, CONS can be identified on the basis of molecular DNA methods.

PATHOGENESIS. CONS produces an **exopolysaccharide** protective biofilm, or **slime layer,** that surrounds the organism and may enhance adhesion to foreign surfaces, resist phagocytosis, and impair penetration of antibiotics.

CLINICAL MANIFESTATIONS. The low virulence of CONS usually requires the presence of another factor, such as immune compromise or a foreign body, for development of clinical disease.

Bacteremia. CONS, specifically *S. epidermidis,* are the most common cause of nosocomial bacteremia, usually in association with central vascular catheters. In neonates, CONS bacteremia, with or without a central venous catheter, may be manifested as apnea, bradycardia, temperature instability, abdominal distention, hematochezia, meningitis in the absence of CSF pleocytosis, cutaneous abscesses, and persistence of positive blood cultures for as long as 2 wk despite adequate antimicrobial therapy. CONS bacteremia in patients with bone marrow transplantation and malignancy (leukemia, lymphoma) is associated with neutropenia, central venous access (Hickman or Broviac catheters), and gastrointestinal colonization. In most circumstances, CONS bacteremia is indolent and is not usually associated with overwhelming septic shock.

Endocarditis. Infection of native heart valves or the right atrial wall secondary to an infected thrombosis at the end of a central line may produce endocarditis. *S. epidermidis* and other CONS may rarely produce native valve subacute indolent endocarditis in previously normal patients without a central venous catheter. CONS is a common cause of prosthetic valve endocarditis, presumably due to inoculation at the time of surgery. Infection of the valve sewing ring, with abscess formation and dissection, produces valve dysfunction, dehiscence, arrhythmias, or valve obstruction (see Chapter 437).

Central Venous Catheter Infection. Central venous catheters become infected through the exit site and subcutaneous tunnel, which provide a direct path to the bloodstream. *S. epidermidis* is the most common CONS, owing in part to its high rate of cutaneous colonization. **Line sepsis** is usually manifested as fever and leukocytosis; tenderness and erythema may be present at the exit site or along the subcutaneous tunnel. Catheter thrombosis may complicate line sepsis.

Cerebrospinal Fluid Shunts. CONS, introduced at the time of surgery, is the most common pathogen associated with CSF shunt meningitis. Most (70–80%) infections occur within 2 mo of the operation and are manifested by signs of meningeal irritation, fever, increased intracranial pressure (headache), and peritonitis due to the intra-abdominal position of the distal end of the shunt tubing.

Urinary Tract Infection. CONS causes asymptomatic urinary tract infection in hospitalized patients with urinary catheters and after urinary tract surgery or transplantation. *S. saprophyticus* is 1 of the most common causes of primary urinary tract infections in boys and girls. Manifestations are similar to those characteristics of urinary tract infection due to *Escherichia coli* (see Chapter 538).

DIAGNOSIS. Because *S. epidermidis* is a common skin inhabitant and may contaminate poorly collected blood cultures, differentiating bacteremia from contamination is often difficult. True bacteremia should be suspected if blood cultures grow rapidly (within 24 hr), ≥2 blood cultures are positive with the same CONS, the peripheral venous blood culture has a quantitative colony count comparable to that drawn from a central venous catheter, and clinical and laboratory signs and symptoms compatible with CONS sepsis are present and subsequently resolve with appropriate therapy. No blood culture that is positive for CONS in a neonate or patient with intravascular catheter should be considered contaminated without careful assessment of the foregoing criteria and examination of the patient. Before initiating presumptive antimicrobial therapy in such patients, it is always prudent to draw 2 separate blood cultures to facilitate subsequent interpretation if CONS is grown.

TREATMENT. Most CONS strains are resistant to methicillin. Vancomycin is the drug of choice for methicillin-resistant strains. The addition of rifampin or gentamicin to vancomycin may increase antimicrobial efficacy. In many cases of CONS infection associated with foreign bodies, the catheter, valve, or shunt must be removed to ensure a cure. Prosthetic heart valves and CSF shunts usually have to be removed to treat the infection adequately.

Antibiotic therapy given through an infected central venous catheter (through each lumen) may effectively cure CONS line sepsis. If the catheter or reservoir is no longer needed, it should be removed. Unfortunately, this is not always possible owing to the therapeutic requirements of the underlying disease (nutrition for short bowel syndrome, chemotherapy for malignancy). A trial of intravenous vancomycin is indicated to attempt to preserve the use of the central line.

Peritonitis caused by *S. epidermidis* in patients on continuous ambulatory peritoneal dialysis is another infection that may be treated with intravenous or intraperitoneal antibiotics without removing the dialysis catheter. If the organism is resistant to methicillin, vancomycin adjusted for renal function is appropriate therapy.

PROGNOSIS. Most episodes of CONS bacteremia respond successfully to antibiotics and removal of any foreign body that is present. Poor prognosis is associated with malignancy, neutropenia, and infected prosthetic or native heart valves. CONS increases morbidity, the duration of hospitalization, and mortality rates among patients with underlying complicated illnesses.

Staphylococcus aureus

Adem PV, Montgomery CP, Husain AN, et al: *Staphylococcus aureus* sepsis and the Waterhouse-Friderichsen syndrome in children. *N Engl J Med* 2005;353:1245–1251.

Amyes SGB: Treatment of staphylococcal infection. *Br Med J* 2005;330: 976–977.

Bischoff WE, Wallis ML, Tucker BK, Reboussin BA, et al: "Gesundheit!" sneezing, common colds, allergies, and *Staphylococcus aureus* dispersion. *J Infect Dis* 2006;194:119–123.

British Medical Journal: Further lessons from the TGN1412 tragedy. *Br Med J* 2006;333:270.

Centers for Disease Control and Prevention: Community-associated methicillin-resistant *Staphylococcus aureus* infection among healthy newborns—Chicago and Los Angeles county, 2004. *MMWR* 2006;55:329–332.

Chambers HF: Community-associated MRSA—Resistance and virulence converge. *N Engl J Med* 2005;352(14):1485–1487.

Chang FY, Peacock JE Jr, Musher DM, et al: *Staphylococcus aureus* bacteremia recurrence and the impact of antibiotic treatment in a prospective multicenter study. *Medicine* 2003;82:333–339.

Cooper BS, Stone SP, Kibbler CC, et al: Isolation measures in the hospital management of methicillin resistant *Staphylococcus aureus* (MRSA): Systematic review of the literature. *Br Med J* 2004;329(7465):533.

Fortunov RM, Hulten KG, Hammerman WA, et al: Community-acquired *Staphylococcus aureus* infections in term and near-term previously healthy neonates. *Pediatrics* 2006;118:874–881.

Gonzalez BE, Martinez-Aguilar G, Hulten KG, et al: Severe staphylococcal sepsis in adolescents in the era of community-acquired methicillin-resistant *Staphylococcus aureus*. *Pediatrics* 2005;115(3):642–648.

Gorenstein A, Gross E, Houri S, et al: The pivotal role of deep vein thrombophlebitis in the development of acute disseminated staphylococcal disease in children. *Pediatrics* 2000;106:E87.

Gould IM: Community-acquired MRSA: can we control it? *Lancet* 2006;268: 824–825.

Grundmann H, Aires-de-Sousa M, Boyce J, Tiemersma E: Emergence and resurgence of methicillin-resistant *Staphylococcus aureus* as a public-health threat. *Lancet* 2006;368:874–882.

Gubbay AJ, Isaacs D: Pyomyositis in children. *Pediatr Infect Dis J* 2000;19:1009–1012.

Huskins WC, Goldmann DA: Controlling methicillin-resistant *Staphylococcus aureus,* aka "superbug." *Lancet* 2005;365:273–276.

Kaplan SL: Treatment of community-associated methicillin-resistant *Staphylococcus aureus* infections. *Pediatr Infect Dis J* 2005;24(5):457–458.

Kaplan SL, Afghani B, Lopez P, et al: Linezolid for the treatment of methicillin-resistant *Staphylococcus aureus* infections in children. *Pediatr Infect Dis J* 2003;22(9 Suppl):S178–S185.

Martinez-Aguilar G, Hammerman WA, Mason EO Jr, et al: Clindamycin treatment of invasive infections caused by community-acquired, methicillin-resistant and methicillin-susceptible *Staphylococcus aureus* in children. *Pediatr Infect Dis J* 2003;22:593–598.

Miles F, Voss L, Segedin E, Anderson BJ: Review of *Staphylococcus aureus* infections requiring admission to a paediatric intensive care unit. *Arch Dis Child* 2005;90:1274–1278.

Miller LG, Perdreau-Remington F, Rieg G, et al: Necrotizing fasciitis caused by community-associated methicillin-resistant *Staphylococcus aureus* in Los Angeles. *N Engl J Med* 2005;352(14):1445–1453.

Shinefield H, Black S, Fattom A, et al: Use of a *Staphylococcus aureus* conjugate vaccine in patients receiving hemodialysis. *N Engl J Med* 2002;346: 491–496.

Srinivasan A, Dick JD, Perl TM: Vancomycin resistance in staphylococci. *Clin Microbiol Rev* 2002;15(3):430–438.

Valente AM, Jain R, Scheurer M, et al: Frequency of infective endocarditis among infants and children with *Staphylococcus aureus* bacteremia. *Pediatrics* 2005;115(1):e15–e19.

Zetola N, Francis JS, Nuermberger EL, Bishai WR: Community-acquired methicillin-resistant *Staphylococcus aureus:* An emerging threat. *Lancet Infect Dis* 2005;5:275–286.

Toxic Shock Syndrome

Chi CY, Wang SM, Lin HC, Liu CC: A clinical and microbiological comparison of *Staphylococcus aureus* toxic shock and scalded skin syndromes in children. *Clin Infect Dis* 2006;42:181–185.

Todd J, Todd AS: Twenty years of toxic shock syndrome: Evolution of an emerging disease. *Royal Society of Medicine: Int Congress Symp Series* 1998;229:201–204.

Zimbelman J, Palmer A, Todd JK: Improved outcome of clindamycin compared with beta-lactam antibiotics treatment of invasive *Streptococcus pyogenes* infection. *Pediatr Infect Dis J* 1999;18:1096–1100.

Coagulase-Negative Staphylococci

Cordero L, Sananes M, Ayers LW: Bloodstream infections in a neonatal intensive-care unit: 12 years' experience with an antibiotic control program. *Infect Control Hosp Epidemiol* 1999;20:242–246.

Karlowicz MG, Furigay PJ, Croitoru DP, et al: Central venous catheter removal versus in situ treatment in neonates with coagulase-negative staphylococcal bacteremia. *Pediatr Infect Dis J* 2002;21:22–27.

Meskin I: *Staphylococcus epidermidis*. *Pediatr Rev* 1998;19:105–106.

Chapter 181 ■ *Streptococcus Pneumoniae* (Pneumococcus)

Jon S. Abramson and Gary D. Overturf

Streptococcus pneumoniae, or the pneumococcus, frequently colonizes the upper respiratory tract and may cause upper respiratory tract infection (otitis media, sinusitis) or invasive disease (pneumonia, bacteremia, meningitis). *S. pneumoniae* is a common cause of community-acquired bacterial pneumonia and otitis media. With universal immunization with conjugated *Haemophilus influenzae* type b vaccines, *S. pneumoniae* is the second most common cause of bacterial meningitis in children and the most common cause of meningitis in adults. The impact of this microorganism is further increased by worldwide emergence of penicillin- and multi-antibiotic-resistant strains. Introduction of a universal recommendation in 2000 to give all infants the pneumococcal heptavalent conjugate vaccine has substantially modified the epidemiology of this organism by reducing nasopharyngeal carriage, shifting the serotypes, reducing antibiotic resistance of causative pneumococci, and reducing the incidence of pneumococcal disease in vaccinated children and perhaps in unvaccinated adults.

ETIOLOGY. *S. pneumoniae* is a gram-positive, lancet-shaped, polysaccharide-encapsulated diplococcus, occurring occasionally as individual cocci or in chains. Approximately 90 serotypes have been identified by type-specific capsular polysaccharides. Antisera to some pneumococcal polysaccharides cross react with other pneumococcal types defining serogroups (6A and 6B), or other bacteria (*Escherichia coli,* group B streptococcus, *H. influenzae* type b). Smooth or encapsulated strains cause most serious disease in humans. Capsular polysaccharides impede phagocytosis. Virulence is related in part to capsular size, but pneumococcal types with capsules of the same size can vary widely in virulence.

On solid media, *S. pneumoniae* forms unpigmented, umbilicated colonies surrounded by a zone of incomplete (α) hemolysis. *S. pneumoniae* is bile soluble (10% deoxycholate) and Optochin sensitive. *S. pneumoniae* is closely related to the viridans groups of *Streptococcus mitus,* which phenotypically overlap with pneumococci. The conventional laboratory definition of pneumococci continues to rely on bile and/or Optochin sensitivity, although there is considerable confusion of pneumococci and α-streptococci. Pneumococcal capsules can be microscopically visualized and typed by exposing organisms to type-specific antisera that combine with their unique capsular polysaccharide, rendering the capsule refractile (**Quellung reaction**). Specific antibodies to capsular polysaccharides confer protection on the host, promoting opsonization and phagocytosis. **C substance,** a cell wall antigen that is related to the pneumococcal species rather than a specific serotype, consists of a teichoic acid containing phosphocholine and galactosamine-6-phosphate. C substance precipitates with a β-globulin, the C-reactive protein, which activates complement, enhancing phagocytosis.

EPIDEMIOLOGY. Most healthy individuals carry various *S. pneumoniae* serotypes in their upper respiratory tract, with >90% of children 6 mo to 5 yr of age harboring *S. pneumoniae* in the nasopharynx at some point during that time. During the past 4 decades, serotypes 4, 6B, 9V, 14, 18C, 19F, and 23F constituted the majority of invasive isolates in children in the United States and other developed countries. Of these, serotypes 6B, 9V, 14, and 19F frequently have reduced susceptibility to penicillin. A single serotype usually is carried for extended periods (45 days to 6 mo). Carriage does not consistently induce local or systemic immunity sufficient to prevent later reacquisition of the same serotype. Rates of pneumococcal carriage peak during the 1st 2 yr of life and decline gradually thereafter. Carriage rates are highest in institutional settings and during the winter, and rates are lowest in summer. Nasopharyngeal carriage of pneumococci is common among young children attending out-of-home care with rates of 21–59% in point prevalence estimates and 65% in longitudinal studies. Since licensure of the 7 valent pneumococcal conjugate vaccines (PCV7), the prevalence of carriage and infection with vaccine serotypes has declined and a shift to increased carriage or infections with nonvaccine serotypes has occurred (Fig. 181-1).

S. pneumoniae is the most frequent cause of bacteremia, bacterial pneumonia, and otitis media, and the second most common cause of meningitis in children. The decreased ability in children <2 yr of age to produce antibody against the T cell–independent polysaccharide antigens and the high prevalence of colonization may explain an increased susceptibility to pneumococcal infection and the decreased effectiveness of polysaccharide vaccines. Males are more commonly affected than females. Native American and African-American children have rates of invasive disease that are 2- to 10-fold that of other healthy children. Other high-risk groups are noted in Table 181-1. Prior to the introduction of PCV into routine schedules of immunization of children, rates of invasive pneumococcal disease in the U.S. peaked at 6–11 mo of age, with attack rates of >540/100,000 in healthy children before the universal use of PCV7. Following the introduction of PCV, rates of infection have fallen in both high-risk and healthy children. For example, in Tennessee, peak rates have fallen from 235/100,000 prior to routine PCV7 immunization to 46/100,000 in children <2 years of age after introduction of PCV7 and the proportion of penicillin-resistant strains in invasive disease fell

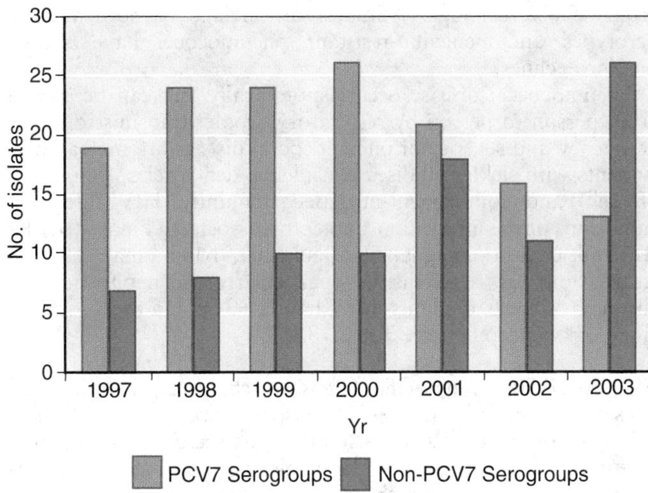

Figure 181-1. Number of isolates from *Streptococcus pneumoniae* serogroups included in the heptavalent pneumococcal conjugate vaccine (PCV7 [Prevnar; Wyeth Lederle Vaccines]) and from nonvaccine serogroups recovered from children treated at Primary Children's Medical Center (Salt Lake City, UT), by year. (From Byington CL, Samore MH, Stoddard GJ, et al: Temporal trends of invasive disease due to *Streptococcus pneumoniae* among children in the intermountain west: Emergence of nonvaccine serogroups. *Clin Infect Dis* 2005; 41:21–29.)

TABLE 181-1. Children at High or Moderate Risk of Invasive Pneumococcal Infection

High risk (incidence of invasive pneumococcal disease ≥150 cases/100,000 people per year)

Children with:
- Sickle cell disease, congenital or acquired asplenia, or splenic dysfunction
- Human immunodeficiency virus infection
- Cochlear implants

Presumed high risk (insufficient data to calculate rates)

Children with:
- Congenital immune deficiency; some B- (humoral) or T-lymphocyte deficiencies, complement deficiencies (particularly C1, C2, C3, and C4), or phagocytic disorders (excluding chronic granulomatous disease)
- Chronic cardiac disease (particularly cyanotic congenital heart disease and cardiac failure)
- Chronic pulmonary disease (including asthma treated with high-dose oral corticosteroid therapy)
- Cerebrospinal leaks from a congenital malformation, skull fracture, or neurologic procedure
- Chronic renal insufficiency, including nephrotic syndrome
- Diseases associated with immunosuppressive therapy or radiation therapy (including malignant neoplasms, leukemias, lymphomas, and Hodgkin disease) and solid organ transplantation
- Diabetes mellitus

Moderate risk (incidence of invasive pneumococcal disease ≥20 cases/100,000 people per year)
- All children 24–35 mo of age
- Children 36–59 mo of age attending out-of-home child care
- Children 36–59 mo of age who are black or of American Indian/Alaska Native descent

From American Academy of Pediatrics: *Red Book: 2006 Report of the Committee on Infectious Diseases,* 27th ed. Elk Grove Village, IL, American Academy of Pediatrics, 2006, p 527.

from 59.8% to 30.4%. Studies of carriage of both vaccine serotypes and penicillin-resistant pneumococci have shown similar declines.

Pneumococcal disease occurs sporadically, but can be spread from person to person by respiratory droplet transmission. The frequency and severity of pneumococcal disease are increased in patients with sickle cell disease, asplenia, deficiencies in humoral (B cell) and complement-mediated immunity, HIV infection, mutations of the interleukin 1 receptor–associated kinase (IRAK-4), and certain malignancies (leukemia, lymphoma); chronic heart, lung, or renal disease (particularly the nephrotic syndrome); cochlear implants (see Chapter 636); and cerebrospinal fluid leak syndromes (see Table 181-1).

PATHOGENESIS. Nonspecific defense mechanisms, including the presence of other bacteria in the nasopharynx, may limit multiplication of pneumococci. Aspiration of secretions containing pneumococci is hindered by the epiglottic reflex and by respiratory epithelial cilia, which move infected mucus toward the pharynx. Similarly, normal ciliary flow of fluid from the middle ear through the eustachian tube and sinuses to the nasopharynx usually prevents infection with nasopharyngeal flora, including pneumococci. Interference with these normal clearance mechanisms by allergy, viral infection, or irritants (e.g., smoke) may allow colonization and subsequent infection with these organisms in otherwise normally sterile sites. The use of cochlear implants for treatment of hearing loss is associated with an increased risk for pneumococcal meningitis (see Chapter 636).

Virulent pneumococci are intrinsically resistant to phagocytosis by alveolar macrophages. Pneumococcal disease frequently is facilitated by viral respiratory tract infection, which may produce mucosal injury, diminish epithelial ciliary activity, and depress the function of alveolar macrophages and neutrophils. Respiratory secretions and alveolar exudate may impede phagocytosis. In tissues, pneumococci multiply and spread through the lymphatics or bloodstream (bacteremia) or, less commonly, by direct extension from a local site of infection (sinuses). The severity of disease is related to the virulence and number of organisms causing bacteremia, and to the integrity of specific host defenses. A poor prognosis correlates with very large numbers of pneumococci and high concentrations of capsular polysaccharide in the circulation and cerebrospinal fluid.

Deficiency of many complement components is associated with recurrent pyogenic infection, including those caused by *S. pneumoniae*. The increased frequency of pneumococcal disease in **asplenic** persons is related to both deficient opsonization of pneumococci as well as to absence of clearance by the spleen of circulating bacteria. Invasive pneumococcal disease is 30- to 100-fold more prevalent in children with **sickle cell disease** and other hemoglobinopathies and in children with congenital or surgical asplenia. This risk is greatest in infants <2 yr of age since antibody production to most serotypes is poor. Children with sickle cell disease have deficits in the antibody-independent properdin (alternative) pathway of complement activation, in addition to functional asplenia. Both pathways contribute to antibody-independent and antibody-dependent opsonophagocytosis of pneumococci. With advancing age (e.g., >5 yr), children with sickle cell disease produce anticapsular antibody, augmenting antibody-dependent opsonophagocytosis and greatly reducing, but not eliminating, the risk for severe pneumococcal disease. The efficacy of phagocytosis also is diminished in patients with B- and T-cell immunodeficiency syndromes (agammaglobulinemia, severe combined immune deficiency) or loss of immune globulin (nephrotic syndrome) and is largely caused by a deficiency of opsonic anticapsular antibody. These observations suggest that opsonization of pneumococci depends on the alternative complement pathway in antibody-deficient persons and that recovery from pneumococcal disease depends on the development of anticapsular antibodies that act as opsonins, enhancing phagocytosis and killing of pneumococci. Children with **HIV infection** also have high rates of invasive pneumococcal infection similar to or greater than that of children with sickle cell disease.

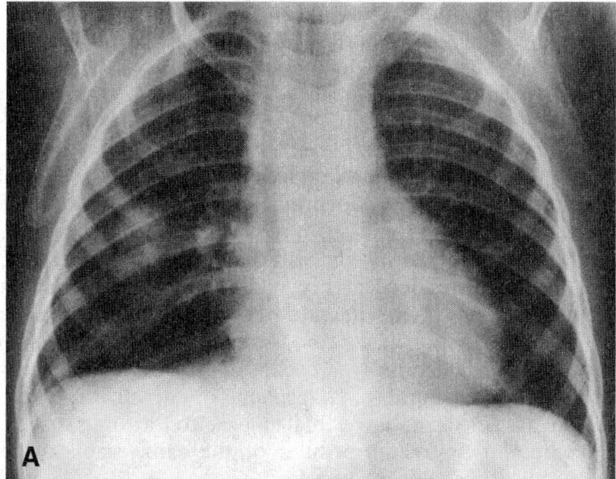

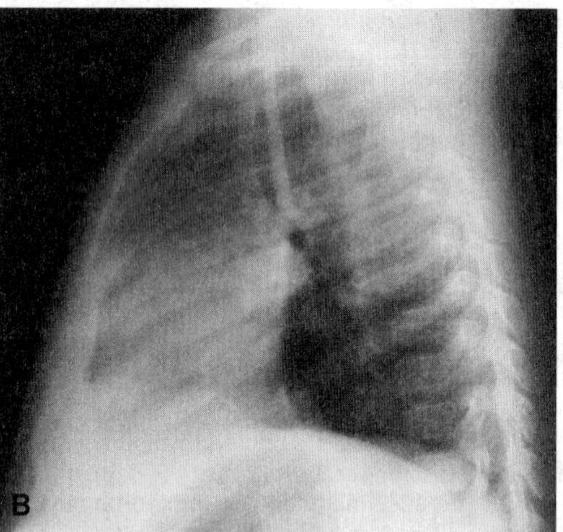

Figure 181-2. Bacterial pneumonia: "round" pneumonia *(S. pneumoniae)* in an 11 mo old girl with a 2 day history of cough and spiking fever. There was leukocytosis with a shift to the left. *A,* The anteroposterior view shows a round, nodular area of consolidation in the right midlung. *B,* On the lateral projection, the nodule lying in the right middle lobe appears somewhat triangular. Such round pneumonias are usually caused by one of the common bacterial pathogens and are most commonly located in the superior segment of a lower lobe. Confusion with a metastatic lesion is possible, but the clinical findings are those of pneumonia. An important radiographic clue is that the consolidation typically appears round on the frontal projection, a shape that does not persist on the lateral view. (Here the infiltrate appears triangular.) (From Hilton SVW, Edwards DK [editors]: *Practical Pediatric Radiology,* 3rd ed. Philadelphia, Elsevier, 2006, p 329.)

In the lungs and other body tissues, the spread of infection is facilitated by the antiphagocytic properties of the pneumococcal capsule. Surface fluids of the respiratory tract contain only small amounts of immunoglobulin G (IgG) and are deficient in complement. During inflammation, there is limited influx of IgG, complement, and neutrophils. Phagocytosis of bacteria by neutrophils may occur, but normal human serum may not opsonize pneumococci and facilitate phagocytosis by alveolar macrophages.

CLINICAL MANIFESTATIONS. The signs and symptoms of pneumococcal infection are related to the anatomic site of disease. Common clinical syndromes include pneumonia (Fig. 181-2) [see Chapter 397], otitis media (see Chapter 641), sinusitis (see

Chapter 377), occult bacteremia in infants and young children (see Chapter 175), and sepsis (see Chapter 176). Before routine use of PCV7, pneumococci caused >80% of bacteremias in children 2–36 mo of age with fever without an identifiable source (occult bacteremia). Pneumococcal abscesses of the upper airway (see Chapter 379), laryngotracheobronchitis (see Chapter 382), and peritonitis (see Chapter 368) occur, but are rare, with the exception of **primary peritonitis** in children with ascites and nephrotic syndrome. Local complications of infection may occur, causing empyema, pericarditis, mastoiditis, epidural abscess, or meningitis. Colonizing pneumococci may spread through the eustachian tube, producing otitis media, and aspiration of infected upper respiratory secretions may produce pneumonia. Epidemic conjunctivitis caused by unencapsulated or encapsulated pneumococci has occurred. Bacteremia may be followed by meningitis (see Chapter 603.1), osteomyelitis (see Chapter 685), suppurative arthritis (see Chapter 686), endocarditis (see Chapter 437), and, rarely, brain abscess (see Chapter 604). **Hemolytic-uremic syndrome** (see Chapter 484.4) and disseminated intravascular coagulation also occur as rare complications of pneumococcal infections.

DIAGNOSIS. The diagnosis of pneumococcal infection is established by recovery of *S. pneumoniae* from the site of infection or the blood. Although pneumococci may be found in the nose or throat of patients with otitis media, pneumonia, septicemia, or meningitis, they may not be related causally to their disease and therefore nasopharyngeal cultures are not helpful for diagnosis. Blood cultures should be obtained in children with pneumonia, meningitis, arthritis, osteomyelitis, peritonitis, pericarditis, or gangrenous skin lesions. Due to the implementation of universal vaccination with PCV7, there has been a substantial decrease in the incidence of occult bacteremia, but blood cultures must be obtained in those with clinical toxicity or significant leukocytosis.

Pneumococci can be identified in body fluids as gram-positive, lancet-shaped diplococci. Early in the course of pneumococcal meningitis, many bacteria may be seen in a relatively acellular cerebrospinal fluid. With current methods of continuously monitored blood culture systems, the average time to isolation of pneumococcal organisms is 14–15 hr and rarely >24 hr. Pneumococcal latex agglutination tests for urine or other body sites suffer from poor sensitivity and add little to standard cultures and Gram-stained fluids. Leukocytosis often is pronounced, with total white blood cell counts frequently >15,000/mm^3, although severe cases (including meningitis) may have a low white count with a shift to the left.

TREATMENT. Before the emergence of penicillin-nonsusceptible organisms, penicillin was the treatment of choice for presumed pneumococcal infection. The incidence of intermediate and high-level penicillin resistance and multidrug resistance (penicillin, tetracycline, chloramphenicol, rifampin, erythromycin, sulfonamides, clindamycin) have increased during the past several decades. In North America, up to 50% of isolates from sterile body sites are nonsusceptible to penicillin G, with a substantial number of these isolates being highly resistant. Multiply resistant strains have been identified throughout the U.S. and worldwide. Resistance to antibiotics is most often noted in pneumococcal serogroups 6, 9, 14, 19, and 23. These serotypes are contained in the conjugated pneumococcal vaccine, and the use of the vaccine appears to have decreased the overall incidence of nonsusceptible pneumococci. However, some serotypes can undergo **capsule switching** (change from 1 serotype to another), which may be associated with development of antibiotic resistance.

Resistance in pneumococcal organisms is defined by the minimal inhibitory concentration (MIC) as **intermediate resistance** to penicillin, with an MIC of 0.1–1.0 μg/L, or **high-grade resistance** to penicillin, with an MIC of ≥2.0 μg/L. Some penicillin-resistant organisms may be resistant to extended spectrum cephalosporins, such as ceftriaxone or cefotaxime. With meningitis, intermediate resistance is defined as an MIC of 1.0 μg/mL, and without meningitis as an MIC is 2.0 μg/mL; high-grade resistance is defined as an MIC of 2.0 μg/mL with meningitis and an MIC of 4.0 μg/mL without meningitis. Some isolates may be multiply resistant, including resistance to erythromycin, clindamycin, tetracycline, trimethoprim-sulfamethoxazole and chloramphenicol. In U.S. surveys, 15–30% of isolates are resistant to erythromycin and 10% are resistant to clindamycin. In cases where the pneumococcus is resistant to erythromycin but sensitive to clindamycin, a **D-test** should be performed to determine whether clindamycin resistance can be induced. If the D-test is positive clindamycin should not be used for treatment. More than 30% of pneumococci are resistant to trimethoprim-sulfamethoxazole. All isolates from children with severe infections should be tested for antibiotic susceptibility. A screening test for susceptibility to penicillin can be performed with a 1 μg oxacillin disk diffusion test, but the use of an E-test or determination of an MIC by a microtiter dilution test is the preferred method for measuring penicillin susceptibility because of greater specificity. Many penicillin-resistant strains are also resistant to the extended spectrum cephalosporins. Resistance to vancomycin has not been reported to date, but vancomycin-tolerant pneumococci that are killed at a slower rate have been reported and may be associated with a worse clinical outcome.

Empirical treatment of pneumococcal disease should be based on knowledge of susceptibility patterns in specific communities. Penicillin G (or ampicillin) is the drug of choice for penicillin-susceptible strains. Recommendations are for oral penicillin V (50–100 mg/kg/day divided every 6–8 hr PO) for minor infections, intravenous penicillin G (200,000–250,000 U/kg/day divided every 4–6 hr IV) for bacteremia or pneumonia, and intravenous penicillin G (300,000 U/kg/day divided every 4–6 hr IV) for meningitis. For serious infections (e.g., meningitis) with strains that are intermediately resistant to penicillin and for all infections with highly penicillin-resistant strains, vancomycin (60 mg/kg/day divided every 6 hr IV) is the treatment of choice until the susceptibilities to other antibiotics are known. Rifampin (20 mg/kg/day divided every 12 hr PO) may be added in severe or unresponsive cases. Resistance to the 3rd-generation cephalosporins, such as cefotaxime and ceftriaxone, is common in penicillin-resistant strains, and treatment failures have been reported when treating meningitis. However, for many intermediately resistant organisms, cefotaxime (225–300 mg/kg/day divided every 8 hr IV) or ceftriaxone (100 mg/kg/day divided every 12–24 hr IV) may be added or substituted for vancomycin, depending on the results of susceptibility testing.

For invasive infections outside the central nervous system (lobar pneumonia with or without bacteremia), high-dose cefotaxime and ceftriaxone are usually effective, even for those infections caused by cephalosporin-intermediate or -resistant strains. For susceptible strains, clindamycin, erythromycin (or related macrolides, such as azithromycin or clarithromycin), cephalosporins, trimethoprim-sulfamethoxazole, and chloramphenicol (available only in a parenteral form in the United States) may provide effective alternative therapy, depending on the site of infection (clindamycin is often effective for pneumococcal infections other than meningitis), for individuals who are allergic to penicillin. Higher doses of amoxicillin-clavulanate (80–90 mg amoxicillin/kg/day divided tid PO), with modified ratios of amoxicillin and clavulanate to permit higher amoxicillin dosing have been successful in the treatment of otitis media caused by resistant strains.

PROGNOSIS. The prognosis depends on the integrity of host defenses, virulence and numbers of the infecting organism, age of the host, site and extent of the infection, and timely initiation and adequacy of treatment.

PREVENTION. Immunologic responsiveness and efficacy following administration of pneumococcal polysaccharide vaccines is unpredictable in children <2 yr of age. Two licensed pneumococcal vaccines contain purified polysaccharide of 23 valent pneumococcal serotypes (PPV23) responsible for >95% of cases of invasive disease. The clinical efficacy of these vaccines is controversial, and studies have yielded conflicting results. Polysaccharide antigens 6A, 14, 19F, and 23F frequently produce childhood disease and are poorly immunogenic in children <5 yr of age.

In contrast, pneumococcal polysaccharide vaccines conjugated to various proteins (heptavalent pneumococcal polysaccharide conjugated to CRM_{197}) provoke "protective" antibody responses in 90% of infants given these vaccines at 2, 4, and 6 mo of age, and greatly enhanced responses (immunologic memory) are apparent after "booster" doses given at 12–15 mo of age. In addition, protein conjugate-polysaccharide vaccines reduce nasopharyngeal carriage of vaccine serotypes by up to 60–70%. The currently available heptavalent vaccine (PCV7) contains conjugated capsular polysaccharides of serotypes 4, 6B, 9V, 14, 19F, 23F, and 18C. In efficacy trials in the U.S., infant immunization with this vaccine decreased invasive infections by >93% and lobar pneumonias by >73%. Its administration was associated with a 6–7% decrease in otitis media, but greater reduction in complications of otitis media such as tympanostomy tube placement. Adverse events after the administration of PCV7 have included local swelling and redness and slightly increased rates of fever, when used in conjunction with other childhood vaccines.

Immunization with PCV7 is recommended for all infants in a schedule of 4 doses administered at 2, 4, 6, and 12–15 mo of age. High-risk children ≥2 yr of age (see Table 181-1), such as those with asplenia, sickle cell disease, some types of immune deficiency (antibody deficiencies), HIV infection, or chronic lung, heart, or kidney disease (including nephrotic syndrome), may benefit also from PPV23 administered after 2 yr of age and following priming with the scheduled doses of PCV7. After the initial immunization, a single supplemental dose of PPV23 may be used 3 yr after the 1st dose for children <10 yr of age at the time of revaccination, or it may be used at 5 yr after the 1st dose for children 10 yr of age or older at the time of revaccination.

Immunization with pneumococcal vaccines also may prevent pneumococcal disease caused by nonvaccine serotypes that are serotypically related to a vaccine strain (6A and 6B). However, because current vaccines do not eliminate all pneumococcal invasive infections, **penicillin prophylaxis** is recommended for children at high risk for invasive pneumococcal disease, including children with asplenia or sickle cell disease. Penicillin V potassium (125 mg bid PO for children <3 yr of age; 250 mg bid PO for children ≥3 yr of age) substantially decreases the incidence of pneumococcal sepsis in children with sickle cell disease. Once monthly intramuscular benzathine penicillin G (600,000 U every 3–4 wk IM for children <60 lb; 1,200,000 U every 3–4 wk IM for children ≥60 lb) may also provide adequate prophylaxis. Erythromycin may be used in children with penicillin allergy, but its efficacy is unproved. Because of the increasing risk for infection with penicillin-nonsusceptible strains, some experts recommend substituting high-dose amoxicillin-clavulanic acid, trimethoprim-sulfamethoxazole, or cefuroxime axetil, but little evidence-based data are available to support such recommendations. Prophylaxis in sickle cell disease has been safely discontinued after the 5th birthday in children who have received all recommended pneumococcal vaccine doses and who had not experienced invasive pneumococcal disease. Prophylaxis is often administered for at least 2 yr after splenectomy or up to 5 yr of age. Efficacy in children >5 yr of age and adolescents is unproved. If oral antibiotic prophylaxis is used, strict compliance must be encouraged. Given the rapid emergence of penicillin-resistant pneumococci, especially in children receiving long-term, low-dose therapy, prophylaxis cannot be relied on to prevent disease. High-risk children with fever should be promptly evaluated and treated regardless of vaccination history or penicillin prophylaxis.

Arbique JC, Poyart C, Trieu-Cuot P, et al: Accuracy of phenotypic and genotypic testing for identification of *Streptococcus pneumoniae* and description of *Streptococcus pseudopneumoniae* sp. *nov. J Clin Microbiol* 2004;42:4868–4896.

Brandt J, Wong C, Mihm S, et al: Invasive pneumococcal disease and hemolytic uremic syndrome. *Pediatrics* 2002;110:371–376.

Brigden ML: Detection, education and management of the asplenic or hyposplenic patient. *Am Fam Physician* 2001;63:499–506.

Buckingham SC, McCullers JA, Lujan-Zilbermann J, et al: Early vancomycin therapy and adverse outcomes in children with pneumococcal meningitis. *Pediatrics* 2006;117:1688–1694.

Byington CL, Korgenski K, Daly J, et al: Impact of pneumococcal conjugate vaccine on pneumococcal parapneumonic empyema. *Pediatr Infect Dis J* 2006;25:250–254.

Byington CL, Samore MH, Stoddard GJ, et al: Temporal trends of invasive disease due to *Streptococcus pneumoniae* among children in the intermountain west: Emergence of nonvaccine serogroups. *Clin Invest Dis* 2005;41:21–29.

Casado-Flores, Aristegui J, de Liria CR, et al: Clinical data and factors associated with poor outcome in pneumococcal meningitis. *Eur J Pediatr* 2005;165:285–289.

Centers for Disease Control and Prevention: Preventing pneumococcal disease among infants and children: Recommendations of the Advisory Committee on Immunization Practices (ACIP). *MMWR* 2000;49(RR-29):1–38.

Dagan R, Barkai G, Leibovitz E, et al: Will reduction of antibiotic use reduce antibiotic resistance? *Pediatric Infect Dis* 2006;25:981–986.

Enders A, Pannicke U, Berner R, et al: Two siblings with lethal pneumococcal meningitis in a family with a mutation in interleukin-1 receptor-associated kinase 4. *J Pediatr* 2004;145:698–700.

Eskola J, Kilpi T, Palmu A, et al: Efficacy of a pneumococcal conjugate vaccine against acute otitis media. *N Engl J Med* 2001;344:403–409.

Gonzalez BE, Hulten KG, Lamberth L, et al: *Streptococcus pneumoniae* serogroups 15 and 33—An increasing cause of pneumococcal infections in children in the United States after the introduction of the pneumococcal 7-valent conjugate vaccine. *Pediatr Infect Dis J* 2006;25:301–305.

Kaplan SL, Mason EO, Barson WJ, et al: Outcome of invasive infections outside the central nervous system caused by *Streptococcus pneumoniae* isolates nonsusceptible to ceftriaxone in children treated with beta-lactam antibiotics. *Pediatr Infect Dis J* 2001;20:392–396.

Kaplan SL, Mason EO, Wald ER, et al: Decrease of invasive pneumococcal infections in children among 8 children's hospitals in the United States after the introduction of the 7-valent pneumococcal conjugate vaccine. *Pediatrics* 2004;113:443–449.

Karlowsky JA, Jones ME, Draghi C, et al: Prevalence and antimicrobial susceptibilities of bacteria isolated from blood cultures of hospitalized patients in the United States in 2002. *Ann Clin Microbiol Antimicrob* 2004;3:7–14.

Kyaw MH, Lynfield R, Schaffner W, et al: Effect of introduction of the pneumococcal conjugate vaccine on drug-resistant *Streptococcus pneumoniae. N Engl J Med* 2006;354:1455–1463.

McIntyre PB, MacIntyre CR, Gilmour R, Wang H: A population based study of the impact of corticosteroid therapy and delayed diagnosis on the outcome of childhood pneumococcal meningitis. *Arch Dis Child* 2005;90:391–396.

Neuman MI, Harper MB: Time to positivity of blood cultures for children with *Streptococcus pneumoniae* bacteremia. *Clin Infect Dis* 2001;33:1324–1328.

O'Brien K, Levine OS: Effectiveness of pneumococcal conjugate vaccine. *Lancet* 2006;368:1469–1470.

Poehling KA, Talbot TR, Griffin MR, et al: Invasive pneumococcal disease among infants before and after introduction of pneumococcal conjugate vaccine. *JAMA* 2006;295:1668–1674.

Reefhuis J, Honein MA, Whitney CG, et al: Risk of bacterial meningitis in children with cochlear implants. *N Engl J Med* 2003;349:335–345.

Rodriquez CA, Atkinson R, Bitar W, et al: Tolerance to vancomycin in pneumococci: Detection with a molecular marker and assessment of clinical impact. *J Infect Dis* 2004;190:1481–1487.

Saha SK, Darmstadt GL, Yamanaka N, et al: Rapid diagnosis of pneumococcal meningitis—Implications for treatment and measuring disease burden. *Pediatr Infect Dis J* 2005;24:1093–1098.

Steenhoff AP, Shah SS, Ratner AJ, et al: Emergence of vaccine-related pneumococcal serotypes as a cause of bacteremia. *Clin Infect Dis* 2006;42:907–914.

Talbot TR, Poehling KA, Hartert T, et al: Reduction in high rates of antibiotic-nonsusceptible invasive pneumococcal disease in Tennessee after introduction of the pneumococcal conjugate vaccine. *Clin Infect Dis* 2004;39:641–651.

Chapter 182 ■ Group A Streptococcus

Michael A. Gerber

Group A streptococcus (GAS), also known as *Streptococcus pyogenes,* is a common cause of infections of the upper respiratory tract (pharyngitis) and the skin (impetigo, pyoderma) in children and is a less common cause of perianal cellulitis, vaginitis, septicemia, pneumonia, endocarditis, pericarditis, osteomyelitis, suppurative arthritis, myositis, cellulitis, and omphalitis. These microorganisms also cause distinct clinical entities (scarlet fever and erysipelas), as well as a toxic shock syndrome and necrotizing fasciitis. GAS is also the cause of 2 potentially serious nonsuppurative complications: rheumatic fever (see Chapters 182.1 and 438) and acute glomerulonephritis (see Chapter 512.1).

ETIOLOGY. Group A streptococci are gram-positive coccoid-shaped bacteria that tend to grow in chains. They are broadly classified by their reactions on mammalian red blood cells. The zone of complete hemolysis that surrounds colonies grown on blood agar distinguishes β-hemolytic (complete hemolysis) from α-hemolytic (green or partial hemolysis) and γ (nonhemolytic) species. The β-hemolytic streptococci can be divided into groups by a group-specific polysaccharide (**Lancefield carbohydrate C**) located in the cell wall. More than 20 serologic groups are identified, designated by the letters A through V. Serologic grouping by the Lancefield method is precise, but group A organisms can be identified more readily by any 1 of a number of latex agglutination, coagglutination, or enzyme immunoassay procedures. Group A strains can also be distinguished from other groups by differences in sensitivity to bacitracin. A disk containing 0.04 U of bacitracin inhibits the growth of most group A strains, whereas other groups are generally resistant to this antibiotic. GAS can be subdivided into >100 serotypes on the basis of the **M protein** antigen, which is located on the cell surface and in fimbriae that project from the outer edge of the cell. M typing has relied primarily on the serologic typing of the surface M protein using available polyclonal sera. However, it is frequently difficult to detect M proteins in this way; a molecular approach to M typing GAS isolates using the polymerase chain reaction is based on sequencing the *emm* gene of GAS that encodes the M protein. More than 180 distinct M types have been identified using *emm* typing, and there has been a good correlation between the known serotypes and the *emm* types.

M serotyping has been valuable for epidemiologic studies; particular GAS diseases tend to be associated with certain M types. Types 1, 12, 28, 3, 4, 2, and 6 (in that order) are the most common causes of uncomplicated streptococcal pharyngitis in the United States. The M types commonly associated with pharyngitis rarely cause skin infections, and the M types commonly associated with skin infections rarely cause pharyngitis. A few of the **pharyngeal** strains (M type 12) have been associated with glomerulonephritis, but far more of the **skin** strains (M types 49, 55, 57, and 60) have been considered nephritogenic. A few of the pharyngeal serotypes, but none of the skin strains, have been associated with acute rheumatic fever. Rheumatogenic potential is not solely dependent on the serotype but is a characteristic of specific strains within several serotypes.

EPIDEMIOLOGY. Humans are the natural reservoir for GAS. These bacteria are highly communicable and can cause disease in normal individuals of all ages who do not have type-specific immunity against the particular serotype involved. Disease in neonates is uncommon, probably because of maternally acquired antibody. The incidence of pharyngeal infections is highest in children 3–15 yr of age, especially in young school-aged children. These infections are most common in the northern regions of the United States, especially during winter and early spring. Children with untreated acute pharyngitis spread GAS by airborne salivary droplets and nasal discharge. Transmission is favored by close proximity; therefore, schools, military barracks, and homes are important environments for spread. The incubation period for pharyngitis is usually 2–5 days. GAS has the potential to be an important upper respiratory tract pathogen and to produce outbreaks of disease in the daycare setting. Foods containing GAS occasionally cause explosive outbreaks of pharyngotonsillitis. Children are usually not infectious 24 hr after appropriate antibiotic therapy has been started. Chronic pharyngeal carriers of GAS rarely transmit this organism to others.

Streptococcal pyoderma (impetigo) occurs most frequently during the summer in temperate climates, or year round in warmer climates, when the skin is exposed and abrasions and insect bites are more likely to occur (see Chapter 664). Colonization of healthy skin by GAS usually precedes the development of impetigo. Because GAS cannot penetrate intact skin, impetigo occurs at the site of open lesions (insect bites, traumatic wounds, burns). Although impetigo serotypes may colonize the throat, spread is from skin to skin, not via the respiratory tract. Fingernails and the perianal region can harbor GAS and play a role in disseminating impetigo. Multiple cases of impetigo in the same family are common. Both impetigo and pharyngitis are more likely to occur among children living in crowded homes and in poor hygienic circumstances.

The incidence of **severe invasive** GAS infections, including bacteremia, streptococcal toxic shock syndrome, and necrotizing fasciitis, has increased in the past decade. The incidence appears to be highest in the very young and in older persons. Varicella is the most commonly identified risk factor in children. Other risk factors include diabetes mellitus, HIV infection, intravenous drug use, and chronic pulmonary or chronic cardiac disease. The portal of entry is unknown in almost 50% of the cases of severe invasive GAS infection; in most cases, it is believed to be skin or mucous membrane. Severe invasive disease rarely follows GAS pharyngitis.

PATHOGENESIS. Virulence of GAS depends primarily on the M protein, and strains rich in M protein resist phagocytosis in fresh human blood, whereas M-negative strains do not. GAS isolated from chronic pharyngeal carriers contain little or no M protein and are relatively avirulent. The M protein antigen stimulates the production of protective antibodies. These antibodies are type specific. They protect against infection with a homologous M type but confer no immunity against other M types. Therefore, multiple GAS infections attributable to different M types are common during childhood and adolescence. By adult life, individuals are probably immune to many of the common M types in the environment, but because of the large number of serotypes it is doubtful that total immunity is ever achieved.

GAS produces a large variety of enzymes and toxins, including erythrogenic toxins (known as streptococcal pyrogenic exotoxins). Streptococcal **pyrogenic exotoxins** A, B, and C are responsible for the **rash of scarlet fever** and are elaborated by streptococci that are infected with a particular bacteriophage. These exotoxins stimulate the formation of specific antitoxin antibodies that provide immunity against the scarlatiniform rash but not against other streptococcal infections. Because GAS can produce three different rash-producing pyrogenic exotoxins (A, B, or C), a second attack of scarlet fever may sometimes occur. Streptococcal pyrogenic exotoxins A, B, and C, as well as several newly discovered exotoxins, appear to be involved in the pathogenesis of invasive GAS disease, including the **streptococcal toxic shock syndrome.**

The roles of most of the other streptococcal toxins and enzymes in human disease have yet to be established. Many of these extracellular substances are antigenic and stimulate antibody production after an infection. However, these antibodies bear no relationship to immunity. Their measurement is useful for evidence of a recent streptococcal infection. The test for antibodies against streptolysin O (antistreptolysin O) is well standardized and is the most commonly used antibody determination. Because the immune response to extracellular antigens varies among individuals as well as with the site of infection, it is sometimes necessary to measure other streptococcal antibodies, such as anti-deoxyribonuclease (anti-DNase).

CLINICAL MANIFESTATIONS. The most common infections caused by GAS involve the respiratory tract and the skin and soft tissues.

Respiratory Tract Infections. GAS is an important cause of acute pharyngitis (see Chapter 378) and pneumonia (see Chapter 397).

Scarlet Fever. Scarlet fever is an upper respiratory tract infection associated with a characteristic rash, which is caused by an infection with **pyrogenic exotoxin (erythrogenic toxin)**–producing GAS in individuals who do not have antitoxin antibodies. It is now encountered less commonly and is less virulent than in the past, but the incidence is cyclic, depending on the prevalence of toxin-producing strains and the immune status of the population. The modes of transmission, age distribution, and other epidemiologic features are otherwise similar to those for GAS pharyngitis.

The rash appears within 24–48 hr after onset of symptoms, although it may appear with the 1st signs of illness (Fig. 182-1A). It often begins around the neck and spreads over the trunk and extremities. It is a diffuse, finely papular, erythematous eruption producing a bright red discoloration of the skin, which blanches on pressure. It is often more intense along the creases of the elbows, axillae, and groin. The skin has a goose-pimple appearance and feels rough. The face is usually spared, although the cheeks may be erythematous with pallor around the mouth. After 3–4 days, the rash begins to fade and is followed by desquamation, 1st on the face, progressing downward, and often resembling that seen subsequent to a mild sunburn. Occasionally, sheetlike desquamation may occur around the free margins of the fingernails, the palms, and the soles. Examination of the pharynx of a patient with scarlet fever reveals essentially the same findings as with GAS pharyngitis. In addition, the tongue is usually coated and the papillae are swollen (Fig. 182-1B). After desquamation, the reddened papillae are prominent, giving the tongue a strawberry appearance (Fig. 182-1C).

Typical scarlet fever is not difficult to diagnose; however, the milder form with equivocal pharyngeal findings can be confused with viral exanthems, Kawasaki disease, and drug eruptions. Staphylococcal infections are occasionally associated with a scar-

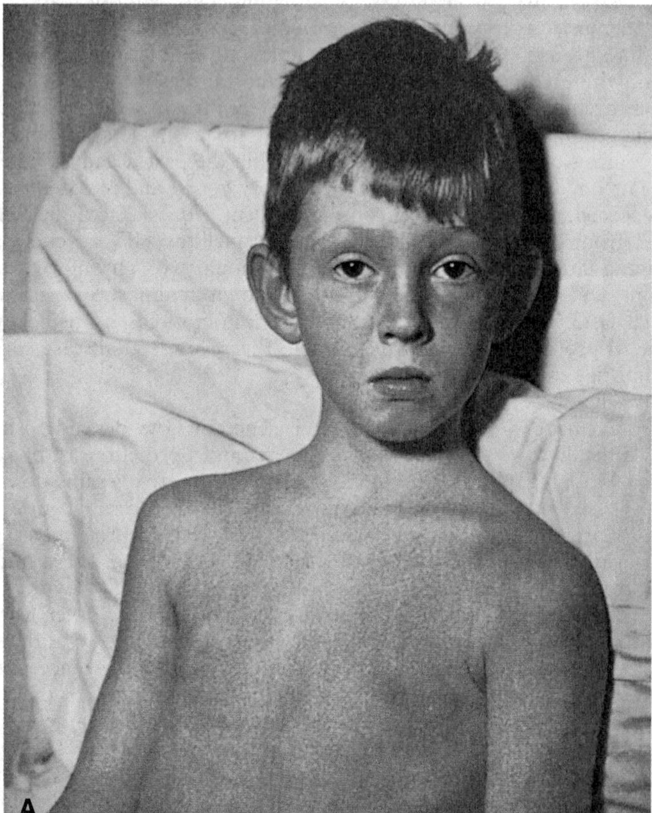

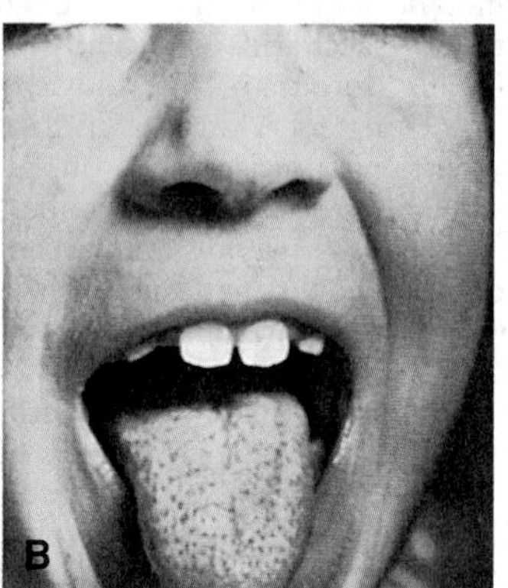

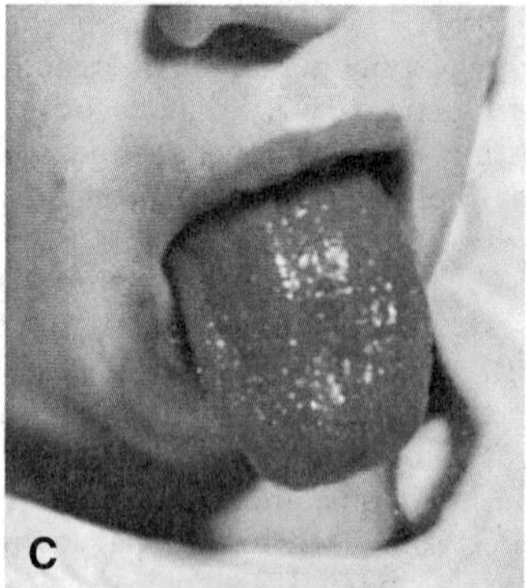

Figure 182-1. Scarlet fever. *A,* Punctate, erythematous rash (2nd day). *B,* White strawberry tongue (1st day). *C,* Red strawberry tongue (3rd day). (Courtesy Dr. Franklin H. Top, Professor and Head of the Department of Hygiene and Preventive Medicine, State University of Iowa, College of Medicine, Iowa City, IA; and Parke, Davis & Company's *Therapeutic Notes.*) (From Gershon AA, Hotez PJ, Katz SL: *Krugman's Infectious Diseases of Children,* 11th ed. Philadelphia, Mosby, 2004, plate 53.)

latiniform rash. A history of recent exposure to a GAS infection is helpful. Identification of GAS in the pharynx confirms the diagnosis, if uncertain.

Impetigo. Impetigo (or pyoderma) has traditionally been classified into 2 clinical forms: bullous and nonbullous (see Chapter 664). Nonbullous impetigo is the more common form and is a superficial infection of the skin that appears 1st as a discrete papulovesicular lesion surrounded by a localized area of redness. The vesicles rapidly become purulent and covered with a thick, confluent, amber-colored crust that gives the appearance of having been stuck on the skin. The lesions may occur anywhere but are more common on the face and extremities. If untreated, nonbullous impetigo is a mild but chronic illness, often spreading to other parts of the body, but occasionally is self-limited. Regional **lymphadenitis** is common. Nonbullous impetigo is generally not accompanied by fever or other systemic signs or symptoms. Impetiginized excoriations around the nares are seen with active GAS infections of the nasopharynx. However, impetigo is not usually associated with an overt streptococcal infection of the upper respiratory tract.

Bullous impetigo is less common and occurs most often in neonates and young infants. It is characterized by flaccid, transparent bullae usually <3 cm in diameter on previously untraumatized skin. The usual distribution involves the face, buttocks, trunk, and perineum. Although *Staphylococcus aureus* has traditionally been accepted as the sole pathogen responsible for bullous impetigo, there has been confusion about the organisms responsible for nonbullous impetigo. In most episodes of nonbullous impetigo, either GAS or *S. aureus,* or a combination of these 2 organisms, is isolated. Earlier investigations suggested that GAS was the causative agent in most cases of nonbullous impetigo and that *S. aureus* was only a secondary invader. However, studies have demonstrated the recent emergence of *S. aureus* as the causative agent in most cases of nonbullous impetigo. Culture of the lesions is the only way to distinguish nonbullous impetigo caused by *S. aureus* from that caused by GAS.

Erysipelas. Erysipelas is a relatively rare acute GAS infection involving the deeper layers of the skin and the underlying connective tissue. The skin in the affected area is swollen, red, and very tender. Superficial blebs may be present. The most characteristic finding is the sharply defined, slightly elevated border. At times, reddish streaks of lymphangitis project out from the margins of the lesion. The onset is abrupt, and signs and symptoms of a systemic infection, such as high fever, are often present. Cultures obtained by needle aspirate of the inflamed area often reveal the causative agent.

Perianal Dermatitis. Perianal dermatitis, also called **perianal streptococcal disease**, is a distinct clinical entity characterized by well-demarcated, perianal erythema associated with anal pruritus, painful defecation, and blood-streaked stools. Physical examination reveals flat, pink to beefy-red perianal erythema with sharp margins extending as far as 2 cm from the anus. Erythema may involve the vulva and vagina. Lesions may be very tender and, particularly when chronic, may fissure and bleed. Systemic symptoms and fever are unusual.

Vaginitis. GAS is a common cause of vaginitis in prepubertal girls (see Chapter 549). Patients usually have a serous discharge with marked erythema and irritation of the vulvar area, accompanied by discomfort in walking and in urination.

Severe Invasive Disease. Invasive GAS infection is defined by isolation of GAS from a normally sterile body site and includes three overlapping clinical syndromes. The 1st is GAS toxic shock syndrome, which is differentiated from other types of invasive GAS infections by the presence of shock and multiorgan system failure early in the course of the infection (Table 182-1). The 2nd is GAS necrotizing fasciitis characterized by extensive local necrosis of subcutaneous soft tissues and skin. The 3rd is the group of focal and systemic infections that do not meet the criteria for toxic shock syndrome or necrotizing fasciitis and includes bacteremia with no identified focus, meningitis, pneumonia, peritonitis, puerperal sepsis, osteomyelitis, suppurative arthritis, myositis, and surgical wound infections.

TABLE 182-1. Definition of Streptococcal Toxic Shock Syndrome

Clinical criteria
Hypotension plus 2 or more of the following:
Renal impairment
Coagulopathy
Hepatic involvement
Adult respiratory distress syndrome
Generalized erythematous macular rash
Soft tissue necrosis
Definite case
Clinical criteria plus group A streptococcus from a normally sterile site
Probable case
Clinical criteria plus group A streptococcus from a nonsterile site

The pathogenic mechanisms responsible for severe, invasive GAS infections, including streptococcal toxic shock syndrome and necrotizing fasciitis, have yet to be defined completely, but an association with streptococcal pyrogenic exotoxins has been suggested. The three original streptococcal pyrogenic exotoxins (A, B, C), the newly discovered streptococcal pyrogenic exotoxins, and potentially other, as yet unidentified toxins produced by GAS act as superantigens, which stimulate an intense activation and proliferation of T lymphocytes and macrophages resulting in the production of large quantities of cytokines. These cytokines are capable of producing shock and tissue injury, and are believed to be responsible for many of the clinical manifestations of severe, invasive GAS infections.

DIAGNOSIS. When attempting to decide whether to perform a microbiologic test on a patient presenting with acute pharyngitis, consideration of the clinical and epidemiologic findings should take place before the test is performed. A history of close contact with a well-documented case of GAS pharyngitis is helpful, as is an awareness of a high prevalence of GAS infections in the community. Testing usually need not be performed on patients with acute pharyngitis whose clinical and epidemiologic features do not suggest a GAS etiology. However the signs and symptoms of streptococcal and nonstreptococcal pharyngitis overlap too broadly to allow the requisite diagnostic precision on clinical grounds alone. The clinical diagnosis of GAS pharyngitis cannot be made with certainty even by the most experienced physicians, and bacteriologic confirmation is required.

Culture of a throat swab on a sheep blood agar plate remains the standard for the documentation of the presence of GAS in the upper respiratory tract and for the confirmation of the clinical diagnosis of acute streptococcal pharyngitis. If performed correctly, a single throat swab cultured on a blood-agar plate has a sensitivity of 90–95% for detecting the presence of GAS in the pharynx.

A disadvantage of culturing a throat swab on a blood-agar plate is the delay (overnight or longer) in obtaining the culture result. **Rapid antigen detection** tests have been developed for the identification of GAS directly from throat swabs. Although these rapid tests are more expensive than the blood-agar culture, the advantage they offer over the traditional procedure is the speed with which they can provide results. Rapid identification and treatment of patients with streptococcal pharyngitis can reduce the risk for the spread of GAS, allowing the patient to return to school or work sooner, and can reduce the acute morbidity of this illness.

The great majority of the rapid antigen detection tests that are currently available have an excellent specificity of >95% when compared with blood-agar plate cultures. False-positive test results are unusual, and, therefore, therapeutic decisions can be made on the basis of a positive test result with confidence. Unfortunately, the sensitivity of most of these tests is 80–90%, possibly lower, when compared with the blood-agar plate culture. Newer tests may be more sensitive than other rapid antigen detection tests and perhaps may even be as sensitive as blood-agar plate cultures. However, in view of conflicting data, physicians who elect to use any rapid antigen detection test in children and adolescents without culture backup of negative test results should do so only after confirming in their own practice that the rapid test is comparable in sensitivity to the throat culture.

GAS infection can also be diagnosed retrospectively on the basis of an elevated or increasing streptococcal antibody titer. The antistreptolysin O assay is the streptococcal antibody test most commonly used. Because streptolysin O also is produced by group C and G streptococcus, the test is not specific for group A infection. The antistreptolysin O response can be feeble in patients with streptococcal impetigo, and its usefulness for this condition is limited. In contrast, the anti-DNase B responses are present after both skin and throat infections. A significant antibody increase is usually defined as an increase in titer of 2 or more dilution increments between the acute phase and convalescent phase specimens, regardless of the actual height of the antibody titer. Interpretation of a single antibody titer for clinical purposes may be difficult and must take several factors into consideration. Antibody titers reported by different clinical laboratories may vary. In addition, the upper limits of normal are higher for children than for adults, and these values, even for the same age groups, are higher in some populations than in others. Frequently, values given by laboratories for upper limits of normal have been determined on adult sera; these values are often much too low to be used in a pediatric population.

Differential Diagnosis. Viruses are the most common cause of acute pharyngitis in children. Respiratory viruses, such as influenza virus, parainfluenza virus, rhinovirus, coronavirus, adenovirus, and respiratory syncytial virus are frequent causes of acute pharyngitis. Other viral causes of acute pharyngitis include coxsackievirus, echovirus, and herpes simplex virus (HSV). Epstein-Barr virus (EBV) is a frequent cause of acute pharyngitis that is often accompanied by other clinical findings of infectious mononucleosis (e.g., splenomegaly, generalized lymphadenopathy). Systemic infections with other viral agents including cytomegalovirus, rubella virus, and measles virus may be associated with acute pharyngitis.

GAS is the most common cause of bacterial pharyngitis, accounting for 15–30% of the cases of acute pharyngitis in children. Groups C and G β-hemolytic streptococcus (see Chapter 184) also produce acute pharyngitis in children. *Arcanobacterium haemolyticum* is a rare cause of acute pharyngitis, particularly in teenagers. *Neisseria gonorrhoeae* can occasionally cause acute pharyngitis in sexually active adolescents. Other bacteria such as *Francisella tularensis* and *Yersinia enterocolitica* as well as mixed infections with anaerobic bacteria (Vincent angina) are rare causes of acute pharyngitis. *Chlamydia pneumoniae* and *Mycoplasma pneumoniae* have been implicated as causes of acute pharyngitis, particularly in adults. *Corynebacterium diphtheriae* (see Chapter 186) can cause pharyngitis but is rare because of universal immunization. Although other bacteria such as *Staphylococcus aureus, Haemophilus influenzae,* and *Streptococcus pneumoniae* are frequently cultured from the throats of children with acute pharyngitis, their etiologic role in pharyngitis has not been established.

GAS pharyngitis is the only common cause of acute pharyngitis for which antibiotic therapy is definitely indicated. Therefore, when confronted with a patient with acute pharyngitis, the clinical decision that usually needs to be made is whether the pharyngitis is attributable to GAS.

TREATMENT. Antibiotic therapy for patients with GAS pharyngitis can prevent acute rheumatic fever, shorten the clinical course of the illness, reduce transmission of the infection to others, and prevent suppurative complications. For the patient with classic scarlet fever, antibiotic therapy should be started immediately, but for the vast majority of patients who present with much less distinctive findings, treatment should be withheld until there is some form of bacteriologic confirmation either by throat culture or rapid antigen detection test. Rapid antigen detection tests, because of their high degree of specificity, have made it possible to initiate antibiotic therapy immediately for someone with a positive test result.

GAS is exquisitely sensitive to penicillin, and resistant strains have never been encountered. Penicillin is, therefore, the drug of choice (except in patients who are allergic to penicillin) for pharyngeal infections as well as for suppurative complications. Treatment with oral penicillin V (250 mg/dose bid–tid for ≤60 lb and 500 mg/dose bid–tid for >60 lb PO) for 10 days is recommended but it must be taken for a full 10 days even though there is symptomatic improvement in 3–4 days. Penicillin V (phenoxyethylpenicillin) is preferred over penicillin G because it may be given without regard to mealtime. The major problem with all forms of oral therapy is the risk that the drug will be discontinued before the 10-day course has been completed. Therefore, when oral treatment is prescribed, the necessity of completing a full course of therapy must be emphasized. If the parents seem unlikely to comply with oral therapy because of family disorganization, difficulties in comprehension, or other reasons, parenteral therapy with a single intramuscular injection of benzathine penicillin G (600,000 IU for ≤60 lb, 1.2 million IU for >60 lb, IM) is the most efficacious and often the most practical method of treatment. Disadvantages include soreness around the site of injection, which may last for several days, and potential for injection into nerves or blood vessels if not administered correctly. The local reaction is diminished when benzathine penicillin G is combined in a single injection with procaine penicillin G, although precautions are necessary to ensure that an adequate amount of benzathine penicillin G is administered.

In some reports, as many as 20% of patients treated with a full course of penicillin continued to harbor GAS. The reasons for these bacteriologic failures are not clear. For patients who have received oral penicillin, poor compliance always has to be considered a possible explanation. It is likely that many of the failures of penicillin therapy occur in children who are merely GAS carriers. Therefore, routine follow-up throat cultures of asymptomatic patients who have completed a full course of therapy are not recommended.

Erythromycin (erythromycin estolate 20–40 mg/kg/day divided bid–qid PO, or erythromycin ethylsuccinate 40 mg/kg/day divided bid–qid PO) for 10 days is the drug of choice for patients allergic to penicillin. Although GAS that is resistant to erythromycin has occasionally been encountered in the United States, erythromycin resistance is a problem in other countries such as Japan and Finland. Investigators in Pittsburgh reported that 48% of the isolates of GAS collected from a single elementary school and 38% of the isolates randomly obtained from the community were resistant to erythromycin. A prospective, multicenter, community-based surveillance of pharyngeal isolates of GAS recovered from children 3–18 yr of age during 3 successive respiratory seasons demonstrated that the erythromycin resistance rate among pharyngeal GAS in the United States was <5% and it was stable. While these results are reassuring, clinicians need to be aware of local resistance rates.

A 10-day course of a narrow-spectrum oral cephalosporin is an acceptable alternative for patients allergic to penicillin. However, because up to 15% of penicillin-allergic patients are also cephalosporin allergic, cephalosporins should not be given to patients with an immediate-type hypersensitivity to penicillin. The additional cost of cephalosporins and their broader spectrum of antibacterial activity compared with penicillin preclude their routine use in patients with GAS pharyngitis who are not penicillin allergic. Sulfonamides and the tetracyclines are not indicated for treatment of GAS infections.

Most oral antibiotics must be administered for the conventional 10 days to achieve maximal pharyngeal eradication rates of GAS, but certain newer agents have been reported to achieve comparable bacteriologic and clinical cure rates when given for 5 days or less. Definitive results from comprehensive studies, however, are not available to allow final evaluation of these proposed shorter courses of oral antibiotic therapy. Therefore, they cannot be recommended at this time. In addition, these antibiotics have a much broader spectrum than penicillin, and most, even when administered for short courses, are more expensive.

Preliminary investigations have demonstrated that once daily amoxicillin therapy is effective in the treatment of GAS pharyngitis. If confirmed by additional investigations, once daily amoxicillin therapy, because of its low cost and relatively narrow spectrum, could become an alternative regimen for the treatment of GAS pharyngitis.

Antibiotic therapy for a patient with nonbullous impetigo can prevent local extension of the lesions, spread to distant infectious foci, and transmission of the infection to others. The ability of antibiotic therapy to prevent poststreptococcal glomerulonephritis, however, has not been demonstrated. Patients with a few superficial, isolated lesions and no systemic signs can be treated with topical antibiotics. Mupirocin is a safe and effective agent that has become the topical treatment of choice. If there are widespread lesions or systemic signs, oral therapy with a β-lactamase-resistant drug (dicloxacillin, cephalexin) will provide coverage for both GAS and *S. aureus*. However, with the rapid emergence of oxacillin-resistant *S. aureus* in many communities, consideration should be given to using clindamycin or trimethoprim-sulfamethoxazole as first-line therapy.

Theoretical considerations and experimental data suggest that intravenous clindamycin is a more effective agent for the treatment of severe, invasive GAS infections than intravenous penicillin. However, because a small proportion of the GAS isolates in the United States are resistant to clindamycin, clindamycin should be used in combination with penicillin for these infections until susceptibility to clindamycin has been established. If **necrotizing fasciitis** is suspected, immediate surgical exploration or biopsy is required to identify a deep soft tissue infection that should be debrided immediately. Patients with **streptococcal toxic shock syndrome** require rapid and aggressive fluid replacement, management of respiratory or cardiac failure, if present, and anticipatory management of multiorgan system failure. Limited data suggest that intravenous gamma globulin may be effective in the management of streptococcal toxic shock syndrome. Intravenous immunoglobulin should be reserved for those patients who do not respond to other therapeutic measures.

COMPLICATIONS. Suppurative complications from the spread of GAS to adjacent structures were very common before antibiotics became available. Cervical lymphadenitis, peritonsillar abscess, retropharyngeal abscess, otitis media, mastoiditis, and sinusitis still occur in children in whom the primary illness has gone unnoticed or in whom treatment of the pharyngitis has been inadequate. GAS pneumonia can rarely occur.

Acute rheumatic fever (see Chapter 182.1) and acute poststreptococcal glomerulonephritis (see Chapter 512.1) are both nonsuppurative sequelae of infections with GAS that occur after an asymptomatic latent period. They are both characterized by lesions remote from the site of the GAS infection. However, acute rheumatic fever and acute glomerulonephritis differ in their clinical manifestations, epidemiology, and potential morbidity. In addition, acute glomerulonephritis can occur after a GAS infection of either the upper respiratory tract or the skin, but acute rheumatic fever can occur only after an infection of the upper respiratory tract.

Poststreptococcal Reactive Arthritis. Poststreptococcal reactive arthritis has been used to describe a syndrome characterized by the onset of acute arthritis following an episode of GAS pharyngitis in a patient whose illness does not otherwise fulfill the Jones criteria for the diagnosis of acute rheumatic fever. There is still considerable debate about whether this entity represents a distinct syndrome or is a manifestation of acute rheumatic fever. Although poststreptococcal reactive arthritis usually involves the large joints, in contrast to the arthritis of acute rheumatic fever, it may involve small peripheral joints as well as the axial skeleton and is typically nonmigratory. The latent period between the antecedent episode of GAS pharyngitis and the poststreptococcal reactive arthritis is considerably shorter (usually <10 days) than that typically seen with acute rheumatic fever. In contrast to the arthritis of acute rheumatic fever, poststreptococcal reactive arthritis does not respond dramatically to therapy with aspirin or other nonsteroidal anti-inflammatory agents. Even though no more than half of the patients with poststreptococcal reactive arthritis who have a throat culture performed have GAS isolated, all have serologic evidence of a recent GAS infection. A small proportion of patients with poststreptococcal reactive arthritis may go on to develop valvular heart disease. Therefore, these patients should be carefully observed for several months for the subsequent development of carditis. Some physicians administer secondary prophylaxis to these patients for a period of up to 1 yr. If carditis is not observed, the prophylaxis can then be discontinued. If carditis is detected, the patient should be classified as having had acute rheumatic fever and should continue to receive secondary prophylaxis.

Pediatric Autoimmune Neuropsychiatric Disorders Associated with *Streptococcus pyogenes* (PANDAS). PANDAS has been used to describe a group of neuropsychiatric disorders (particularly obsessive-compulsive disorders, tic disorders, and Tourette syndrome) for which a possible relationship with GAS infections has been suggested (see Chapter 23). It has been demonstrated that patients with Sydenham chorea (a manifestation of acute rheumatic fever) frequently have obsessive-compulsive symptoms and that a subset of patients with obsessive-compulsive and tic disorders will have chorea as well as acute exacerbations following GAS infections. Therefore, it has been proposed that this subset of patients with obsessive-compulsive and tic disorders produce autoimmune antibodies in response to a GAS infection that cross react with brain tissue similar to the autoimmune response believed to be responsible for the manifestations of Sydenham chorea. It has also been suggested that secondary prophylaxis that prevents recurrences of Sydenham chorea might also be effective in preventing recurrences of obsessive-compulsive and tic disorders in these patients. Because of the proposed autoimmune mechanism, it has also been suggested that these patients may benefit from immunoregulatory therapy such as plasma exchange or intravenous immunoglobulin therapy. The possibility that PANDAS could represent an extension of the spectrum of acute rheumatic fever is intriguing but is yet unproven. Prophylaxis to prevent PANDAS and immunoregulatory therapy to treat PANDAS are under study but are currently not recommended (see Chapter 23).

PROGNOSIS. The prognosis for appropriately treated GAS pharyngitis is excellent and complete recovery is the rule. When therapy is provided within 9 days of onset, acute rheumatic fever is prevented. However, there is no evidence that acute poststreptococcal glomerulonephritis can be prevented once pharyngitis or pyoderma with a nephritogenic strain of GAS has occurred. In rare instances, particularly in neonates or in children whose response to infection is compromised, fulminant pneumonia, septicemia, and death may occur despite usually adequate therapy.

PREVENTION. The only specific indication for long-term use of antibiotics to prevent GAS infections is for patients with a history of acute rheumatic fever or rheumatic heart disease. Mass prophylaxis is generally not feasible except to reduce the number of infections during epidemics of impetigo and to control epidemics of pharyngitis in military populations and in schools. Because the ability of antimicrobial agents to prevent GAS infections is limited, a streptococcal vaccine offers the possibility of a more effective approach. A vaccine was produced using a recombinant fusion protein containing N-terminal fragments from 6 GAS M types of clinical and epidemiologic importance. A phase I trial of this vaccine demonstrated that parenteral vaccine with this alum adjuvant was well tolerated, did not induce cross-reactive antibodies to human tissue, and stimulated bactericidal activity when given as a 3-dose regimen to healthy adults. A similar vaccine containing N-terminal peptides of 26 M types was constructed and is currently undergoing clinical evaluation in adults. Another approach has been to identify a conserved epitope in the c-repeat region of M protein that induces the production of opsonic antibodies. The oral commensal bacterium *Streptococcus gordonii* has been evaluated in humans as a mucosal vector for expressing this conserved fragment of M protein. This vaccine has not as yet entered clinical trials. Several conserved non–M protein antigens have shown promise as protective immunogens in preclinical studies including C5a peptidase, toxoids derived from streptococcal pyrogenic exotoxins, and GAS carbohydrate. However, none of these antigens has been tested in humans.

182.1 • Rheumatic Fever

ETIOLOGY. There is considerable evidence to support the link between GAS upper respiratory tract infections and acute rheumatic fever and rheumatic heart disease. As many as ⅔ of the patients with an acute episode of rheumatic fever have a history of an upper respiratory tract infection several weeks before, and the peak age and seasonal incidence of acute rheumatic fever closely parallel those of GAS infections. Patients with acute rheumatic fever almost always have serologic evidence of a recent GAS infection. Their antibody titers are usually considerably higher than those seen in patients with GAS infections without acute rheumatic fever. Outbreaks of GAS pharyngitis in closed communities, such as boarding schools or military bases, may be followed by outbreaks of acute rheumatic fever. Antimicrobial therapy that eliminates GAS from the pharynx also prevents initial episodes of acute rheumatic fever, and long-term, continuous prophylaxis that prevents GAS pharyngitis also prevents recurrences of acute rheumatic fever.

Not all of the serotypes of GAS can cause rheumatic fever. When some strains (M type 4) were present in a very susceptible rheumatic population, no recurrences of rheumatic fever occurred. In contrast, episodes of pharyngitis with other serotypes prevalent in the same population were associated with frequent recurrences. The concept of rheumatogenicity is further supported by the observation that although serotypes of GAS frequently associated with skin infection are often isolated from the upper respiratory tract, they rarely cause recurrences of rheumatic fever in individuals with a previous history of rheumatic fever. In addition, certain serotypes of GAS (M types 1, 3, 5, 6, 18, 24) are more frequently isolated from patients with acute rheumatic fever than are other serotypes.

EPIDEMIOLOGY. In some developing areas of the world, the annual incidence of acute rheumatic fever is currently as high as 282/100,000 population. Worldwide, rheumatic heart disease remains the most common form of acquired heart disease in all age groups, accounting for as much as 50% of all cardiovascular disease and as much as 50% of all cardiac admissions in many developing countries. However, striking differences are evident in the incidence of acute rheumatic fever and rheumatic heart disease among different ethnic groups within the same country; many, but not all, of these differences appear to be related to differences in socioeconomic status.

In the United States, at the beginning of the 20th century, acute rheumatic fever was a leading cause of death among children and adolescents, with annual incidence rates of 100–200/100,000 population. In addition, rheumatic heart disease was a leading cause of heart disease among adults <40 yr of age. At that time, as many as ¼ of the hospital beds in the United States were occupied by patients with acute rheumatic fever or its complications. By the 1940s, the annual incidence of acute rheumatic fever had decreased to 50/100,000, and over the next 4 decades, the decline in incidence accelerated rapidly. By the early 1980s, the annual incidence in some areas of the United States was as low as 0.5/100,000 population. This sharp decline in the incidence of acute rheumatic fever has been observed in other industrialized countries as well.

The explanation for this dramatic decline in the incidence of acute rheumatic fever and rheumatic heart disease in the United States and other industrialized countries is not clear. Historically, acute rheumatic fever has been associated with poverty, particularly in urban areas. Much of the decline in the incidence of acute rheumatic fever in industrialized countries during the preantibiotic era can probably be attributed to improvements in living conditions. A number of studies have suggested that, of the various manifestations of poverty, crowding, which contributes to the spread of GAS infections, is the one most closely associated with the incidence of acute rheumatic fever. The decline in incidence of acute rheumatic fever in industrialized countries over the past 4 decades has also been attributable in large measure to the greater availability of medical care and to the widespread use of antibiotics. Antibiotic therapy of GAS pharyngitis has been important in preventing initial attacks and, particularly, recurrences of the disease. In addition, the decline can be attributed, at least in part, to a shift in the prevalent strains of GAS from rheumatogenic to nonrheumatogenic strains.

A dramatic outbreak of acute rheumatic fever in the Salt Lake City area began in early 1985, and 198 cases were reported by the end of 1989. Other outbreaks were reported between 1984 and 1988 in Columbus and Akron, OH; Pittsburgh, PA; Nashville and Memphis, TN; New York, NY; Kansas City, MO; Dallas, TX; and among recruits at the San Diego Naval Training Center in California and at the Fort Leonard Wood Army Training Base in Missouri. Evidence suggests that this resurgence of acute rheumatic fever was focal and not nationwide.

Certain rheumatogenic serotypes (types 1, 3, 5, 6, and 18) that were isolated infrequently during the 1970s and early 1980s dramatically reappeared during these focal outbreaks. The appearance of these rheumatogenic strains in selected communities was probably a major factor in these outbreaks of acute rheumatic fever. Another property of GAS that has been associated with rheumatogenicity is the formation of highly mucoid colonies. Mucoid strains of GAS had only rarely been isolated from throat cultures in recent years. However, during these focal outbreaks of acute rheumatic fever, mucoid strains of GAS were commonly isolated from patients, family members, and members of the surrounding community.

In addition to the specific characteristics of the infecting GAS, the risk of a particular person developing acute rheumatic fever is also dependent on various host factors. The incidence of both initial attacks and recurrences of acute rheumatic fever peaks in children 5–15 yr of age, the age of greatest risk for GAS pharyngitis. Patients who have had one attack of acute rheumatic fever tend to have recurrences, and the clinical features of the recurrences tend to mimic those of the initial attack. In addition, there appears to be a genetic predisposition to acute rheumatic fever. Studies in twins have shown a higher concordance rate of acute rheumatic fever in monozygotic than in dizygotic twin pairs.

Some investigators have also demonstrated an association between the presence of both specific human leukocyte antigen (HLA) markers and a specific B-cell alloantigen (D8/17) and susceptibility to acute rheumatic fever. However, others have been unable to confirm these associations.

PATHOGENESIS. The pathogenic link between a GAS infection of the upper respiratory tract and an attack of acute rheumatic fever, characterized by organ and tissue involvement far removed from the pharynx, is still not clear. One of the major obstacles to understanding the pathogenesis of acute rheumatic fever and rheumatic heart disease has been the inability to establish an animal model. Several theories of the pathogenesis of acute rheumatic fever and rheumatic heart disease have been proposed, but only 2 are seriously considered: the cytotoxicity theory and the immunologic theory.

The cytotoxicity theory suggests that a GAS toxin may be involved in the pathogenesis of acute rheumatic fever and rheumatic heart disease. GAS produces several enzymes that are cytotoxic for mammalian cardiac cells, such as streptolysin O, which has a direct cytotoxic effect on mammalian cells in tissue culture. Most of the proponents of the cytotoxicity theory have focused on this enzyme. However, one of the major problems with the cytotoxicity hypothesis is its inability to explain the latent period between GAS pharyngitis and the onset of acute rheumatic fever.

An immune-mediated pathogenesis for acute rheumatic fever and rheumatic heart disease has been suggested by the clinical similarity of acute rheumatic fever to other illnesses produced by immunopathogenic processes and by the latent period between the GAS infection and the acute rheumatic fever. The antigenicity of a large variety of GAS products and constituents, as well as the immunologic cross reactivity between GAS components and mammalian tissues, also lends support to this hypothesis. Common antigenic determinants are shared between certain components of GAS (M protein, protoplast membrane, cell wall group A carbohydrate, capsular hyaluronate) and specific mammalian tissues (e.g., heart, brain, joint). For example, certain M proteins (M1, M5, M6, and M19) share epitopes with human tropomyosin and myosin. Additionally, the involvement of GAS superantigens such as pyrogenic exotoxins in the pathogenesis of acute rheumatic fever has been proposed.

CLINICAL MANIFESTATIONS AND DIAGNOSIS. Because no clinical or laboratory finding is pathognomonic for acute rheumatic fever, T. Duckett Jones in 1944 proposed guidelines to aid in diagnosis and to limit overdiagnosis. The **Jones criteria,** as revised in 1992 by the American Heart Association (Table 182-2), are intended only for the diagnosis of the initial attack of acute rheumatic fever and not for recurrences. There are **5 major** and **4 minor criteria** and an absolute requirement for evidence (microbiologic or serologic) of recent GAS infection. The diagnosis of acute rheumatic fever can be established by the Jones criteria when a patient fulfills 2 major criteria or 1 major and 2 minor criteria and meets the absolute requirement. Even with strict application of the Jones criteria, overdiagnosis as well as underdiagnosis of acute rheumatic fever may occur. There are 3 circumstances in which the diagnosis of acute rheumatic fever can be made without strict adherence to the Jones criteria. Chorea may occur as the only manifestation of acute rheumatic fever. Similarly, indolent carditis may be the only manifestation in patients who 1st come to medical attention months after the onset of acute rheumatic fever. Finally, although most patients with recurrences of acute rheumatic fever fulfill the Jones criteria, some may not.

Major Manifestations. There are 5 major criteria. The presence of 2 major criteria with evidence (microbiologic or serologic) of recent GAS infection fulfills the Jones criteria.

MIGRATORY POLYARTHRITIS. Arthritis occurs in about 75% of patients with acute rheumatic fever and typically involves larger joints, particularly the knees, ankles, wrists, and elbows. Involvement of the spine, small joints of the hands and feet, or hips is uncommon. Rheumatic joints are generally hot, red, swollen, and exquisitely tender; even the friction of bedclothes is uncomfortable. The pain can precede and can appear to be disproportionate to the other findings. The joint involvement is characteristically migratory in nature; a severely inflamed joint can become normal within 1–3 days without treatment, as 1 or more other large joints become involved. Severe arthritis can persist for several weeks in untreated patients. Monoarticular arthritis is unusual unless anti-inflammatory therapy is initiated prematurely, aborting the progression of the migratory polyarthritis. If a child with fever and arthritis is suspected of having acute rheumatic fever, it frequently is useful to withhold salicylates and observe for migratory progression. A dramatic response to even small doses of salicylates is another characteristic feature of the arthritis, and the absence of such a response should suggest an alternative diagnosis. Rheumatic arthritis is typically not deforming. Synovial fluid in acute rheumatic fever usually has 10,000–100,000 white blood cells/mm^3 with a predominance of neutrophils, a protein of about 4 g/dL, a normal glucose, and forms a good mucin clot. Frequently, arthritis is the earliest manifestation of acute rheumatic fever and may correlate temporally with peak antistreptococcal antibody titers. There is an apparent inverse relationship between the severity of arthritis and the severity of cardiac involvement.

CARDITIS. Carditis and resultant chronic rheumatic heart disease are the most serious manifestations of acute rheumatic fever and account for essentially all of the associated morbidity and mortality. Rheumatic carditis is characterized by pancarditis, with active inflammation of myocardium, pericardium, and endocardium (see Chapter 438). Cardiac involvement during acute rheumatic fever varies in severity from fulminant, potentially fatal exudative pancarditis to mild, transient cardiac involvement. Endocarditis (valvulitis), which manifests by 1 or more cardiac murmurs, is a universal finding in rheumatic carditis, whereas the presence of pericarditis or myocarditis is variable. Myocarditis and/or pericarditis without evidence of endocarditis is rarely due to rheumatic heart disease. Most cases consist of either isolated mitral valvular disease or combined aortic and mitral valvular disease. Isolated aortic or right-sided valvular involvement is uncommon. Serious and long-term illness is related entirely to valvular heart disease as a consequence of a single attack or recurrent attacks of acute rheumatic fever. Valvular insufficiency is characteristic of both acute and convalescent stages of acute rheumatic fever, whereas valvular stenosis usually appears several years or even decades after the acute illness. In developing countries, however, where acute rheumatic fever often occurs at a

TABLE 182-2. Guidelines for the Diagnosis of Initial Attack of Rheumatic Fever (Jones Criteria, Updated 1992)

MAJOR MANIFESTATIONS*	MINOR MANIFESTATIONS	SUPPORTING EVIDENCE OF ANTECEDENT GROUP A STREPTOCOCCAL INFECTION
Carditis Polyarthritis	**Clinical features:** Arthralgia Fever	Positive throat culture or rapid streptococcal antigen test Elevated or increasing streptococcal antibody titer
Erythema marginatum Subcutaneous nodules	**Laboratory features:** Elevated acute phase reactants: Erythrocyte sedimentation rate C-reactive protein Prolonged PR interval	
Chorea		

*The presence of 2 major or of 1 major and 2 minor manifestations indicates a high probability of acute rheumatic fever if supported by evidence of preceding group A streptococcal infection.

From Jones criteria, updated 1992. *JAMA* 1992;268:2069–2073. Copyright American Medical Association.

younger age, mitral stenosis and aortic stenosis may develop sooner after acute rheumatic fever than in developed countries, and can occur in young children.

Acute rheumatic carditis usually presents as tachycardia and cardiac murmurs, with or without evidence of myocardial or pericardial involvement. Moderate to severe rheumatic carditis can result in cardiomegaly and congestive heart failure with hepatomegaly and peripheral and pulmonary edema. Echocardiographic findings include pericardial effusion, decreased ventricular contractility, and aortic and/or mitral regurgitation. Mitral regurgitation is characterized by a high-pitched apical holosystolic murmur radiating to the axilla. In patients with significant mitral regurgitation, this may be associated with an apical mid-diastolic murmur of relative mitral stenosis. Aortic insufficiency is characterized by a high-pitched decrescendo diastolic murmur at the upper left sternal border. Echocardiographic demonstration of valvular regurgitation without accompanying auscultatory evidence does not satisfy the Jones criteria for carditis (see Chapter 438).

Carditis occurs in about 50–60% of all cases of acute rheumatic fever. Recurrent attacks of acute rheumatic fever in patients who had carditis with the initial attack are associated with high rates of carditis. The major consequence of acute rheumatic carditis is chronic, progressive valvular disease, particularly valvular stenosis, which can require valve replacement and predispose to infective endocarditis.

CHOREA. Sydenham chorea occurs in about 10–15% of patients with acute rheumatic fever and usually presents as an isolated, frequently subtle, neurologic behavior disorder. Emotional lability, incoordination, poor school performance, uncontrollable movements, and facial grimacing, exacerbated by stress and disappearing with sleep, are characteristic. Chorea occasionally is unilateral. The latent period from acute GAS infection to chorea is usually longer than for arthritis or carditis and can be months. Onset can be insidious, with symptoms being present for several months before recognition. Clinical maneuvers to elicit features of chorea include (1) demonstration of **milkmaid's grip** (irregular contractions of the muscles of the hands while squeezing the examiner's fingers), (2) spooning and pronation of the hands when the patient's arms are extended, (3) wormian darting movements of the tongue upon protrusion, and (4) examination of handwriting to evaluate fine motor movements. Diagnosis is based on clinical findings with supportive evidence of GAS antibodies. However, in patients with a long latent period from the inciting streptococcal infection, antibody levels may have declined to normal. Although the acute illness is distressing, chorea rarely, if ever, leads to permanent neurologic sequelae.

ERYTHEMA MARGINATUM. Erythema marginatum is a rare (<3% of patients with acute rheumatic fever) but characteristic rash of acute rheumatic fever. It consists of erythematous, serpiginous, macular lesions with pale centers that are not pruritic (Fig. 182-2). It occurs primarily on the trunk and extremities, but not on the face, and it can be accentuated by warming the skin.

SUBCUTANEOUS NODULES. Subcutaneous nodules are a rare (≤1% of patients with acute rheumatic fever) and consist of

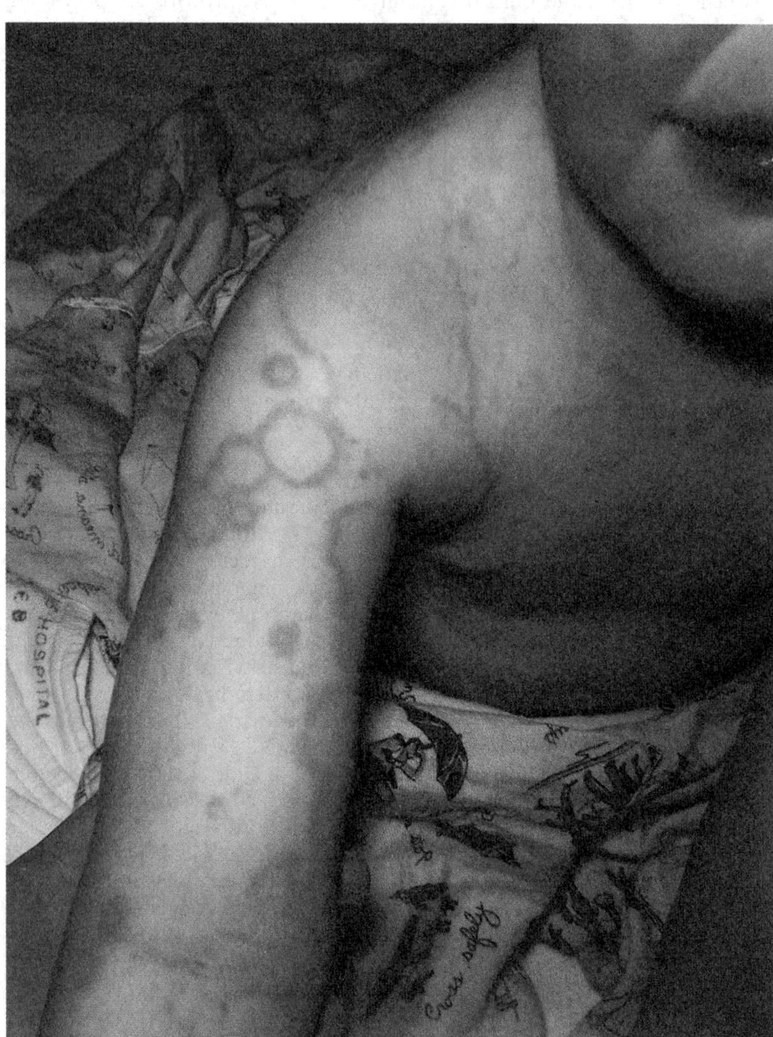

Figure 182-2. Polycyclic red borders of erythema marinatum in a febrile child with acute rheumatic fever. (From Schachner LA, Hansen RC [editors]: *Pediatric Dermatology,* 3rd ed. Philadelphia, Mosby, 2003, p 808.)

firm nodules approximately 1 cm in diameter along the extensor surfaces of tendons near bony prominences. There is a correlation between the presence of these nodules and significant rheumatic heart disease.

Minor Manifestations. The 2 clinical minor manifestations are arthralgia (in the absence of polyarthritis as a major criterion) and fever (typically temperature ≥102°F and occurring early in the course of illness). The 2 laboratory minor manifestations are elevated acute-phase reactants (e.g., C-reactive protein, erythrocyte sedimentation rate) and prolonged PR interval on electrocardiogram (1st degree heart block). However, a prolonged PR interval alone does not constitute evidence of carditis or predict long-term cardiac sequelae.

Recent Group A Streptococcus Infection. An absolute requirement for the diagnosis of acute rheumatic fever is supporting evidence of a recent GAS infection. Acute rheumatic fever typically develops 2–4 wk after an acute episode of GAS pharyngitis at a time when clinical findings of pharyngitis are no longer present and when only 10–20% of the throat culture or rapid streptococcal antigen test results are positive. One third of patients have no history of an antecedent pharyngitis. Therefore, evidence of an antecedent GAS infection is usually based on elevated or increasing serum antistreptococcal antibody titers. A slide agglutination test (Streptozyme) has been introduced, and it is purported to detect antibodies against 5 different GAS antigens. Although this test is rapid, relatively simple to perform, and widely available, it is less standardized and less reproducible than other tests and should not be used as a diagnostic test for evidence of an antecedent GAS infection. If only a single antibody is measured (usually antistreptolysin O), only 80–85% of patients with acute rheumatic fever have an elevated titer; however, 95–100% have an elevation if 3 different antibodies (antistreptolysin O, anti-DNase B, antihyaluronidase) are measured. Therefore, when acute rheumatic fever is suspected clinically, multiple antibody tests are performed. Except for patients with chorea, clinical findings of acute rheumatic fever generally coincide with peak antistreptococcal antibody responses. Most patients with chorea have elevation of antibodies to 1 or more GAS antigens, although these antibodies may be waning. The diagnosis of acute rheumatic fever should not be made in patients with elevated or increasing streptococcal antibody titers who do not fulfill the Jones criteria because such titer changes may be coincidental. This is most often true in younger, school-aged children, many of whom have GAS pyoderma in the summer or unrelated GAS pharyngitis during the winter and spring months.

Differential Diagnosis. The differential diagnoses of rheumatic fever include many infectious as well as noninfectious illnesses (Table 182-3). When children present with arthritis, a collagen vascular disease must be considered. Rheumatoid arthritis in particular must be distinguished from acute rheumatic fever. Children with rheumatoid arthritis tend to be younger and usually have less joint pain relative to their other clinical findings than those with acute rheumatic fever. Spiking fevers, lymphadenopathy, and splenomegaly are more suggestive of rheumatoid arthritis than acute rheumatic fever. The response to salicylate therapy is also much less dramatic with rheumatoid arthritis than with acute rheumatic fever. Systemic lupus erythematosus can usually be distinguished from acute rheumatic fever on the basis of the presence of antinuclear antibodies with systemic lupus erythematosus. Other causes of arthritis, such as gonococcal arthritis, malignancies, serum sickness, Lyme disease, sickle cell disease, and reactive arthritis related to gastrointestinal infections (e.g., *Shigella, Salmonella, Yersinia*) should also be considered.

When carditis is the sole major manifestation of suspected acute rheumatic fever, viral myocarditis, viral pericarditis, Kawasaki disease, and infective endocarditis should also be considered. Patients with infective endocarditis may present with both joint and cardiac manifestations. These patients can usually be distinguished from patients with acute rheumatic fever by blood cultures and the presence of associated findings (e.g., hematuria, splenomegaly, splinter hemorrhages). In general, the absence of auscultatory evidence of a significant cardiac murmur excludes the diagnosis of acute rheumatic carditis.

When chorea is the sole major manifestation of suspected acute rheumatic fever, Huntington chorea, Wilson disease, systemic lupus erythematosus, and various encephalitides should also be considered. These other diseases are usually identified by the history, laboratory studies, and clinical findings.

TABLE 182-3. Differential Diagnosis of Acute Rheumatic Fever

ARTHRITIS	CARDITIS	CHOREA
Rheumatoid arthritis	Viral myocarditis	Huntington chorea
Reactive arthritis (e.g., *Shigella, Salmonella, Yersinia*)	Viral pericarditis	Wilson disease
Serum sickness	Infective endocarditis	Systemic lupus erythematosus
Sickle cell disease	Kawasaki disease	Cerebral palsy
Malignancy	Congenital heart disease	Tics
Systemic lupus erythematosus	Mitral valve prolapse	Hyperactivity
Lyme disease (*Borrelia burgdorferi*)	Innocent murmurs	
Gonococcal infection (*Neisseria gonorrhoeae*)		

TREATMENT. All patients with acute rheumatic fever should be placed on bed rest and monitored closely for evidence of carditis. They can be allowed to ambulate as soon as the signs of acute inflammation have subsided. However, patients with carditis require longer periods of bed rest.

Antibiotic Therapy. Once the diagnosis of acute rheumatic fever has been established and regardless of the throat culture results, the patient should receive 10 days of orally administered penicillin or erythromycin, or a single intramuscular injection of benzathine penicillin to eradicate GAS from the upper respiratory tract. After this initial course of antibiotic therapy, the patient should be started on long-term antibiotic prophylaxis.

Anti-Inflammatory Therapy. Anti-inflammatory agents (e.g., salicylates, corticosteroids) should be withheld if arthralgia or atypical arthritis is the only clinical manifestation of presumed acute rheumatic fever. Premature treatment with 1 of these agents may interfere with the development of the characteristic migratory polyarthritis and thus obscure the diagnosis of acute rheumatic fever. Agents such as acetaminophen can be used to control pain and fever while the patient is being observed for more definite signs of acute rheumatic fever or for evidence of another disease.

Patients with typical migratory polyarthritis and those with carditis without cardiomegaly or congestive heart failure should be treated with oral salicylates. The usual dose of aspirin is 100 mg/kg/day in 4 divided doses PO for 3–5 days, followed by 75 mg/kg/day in 4 divided doses PO for 4 wk. Determination of the serum salicylate level is not necessary unless the arthritis does not respond or signs of salicylate toxicity (tinnitus, hyperventilation) develop. There is no evidence that nonsteroidal anti-inflammatory agents are any more effective than salicylates.

Patients with carditis and cardiomegaly or congestive heart failure should receive corticosteroids. The usual dose of prednisone is 2 mg/kg/day in 4 divided doses for 2–3 wk followed by a tapering of the dose that reduces the dose by 5 mg/24 hr every 2–3 days. At the beginning of the tapering of the prednisone dose, aspirin should be started at 75 mg/kg/day in 4 divided doses for 6 wk. Supportive therapies for patients with moderate to severe carditis include digoxin, fluid and salt restriction, diuretics, and oxygen. The cardiac toxicity of digoxin is enhanced with myocarditis.

Termination of the anti-inflammatory therapy may be followed by the reappearance of clinical manifestations or of laboratory abnormalities. These "rebounds" are best left untreated unless the clinical manifestations are severe; salicylates or steroids should be reinstated in such cases.

Sydenham Chorea. Because chorea often occurs as an isolated manifestation after the resolution of the acute phase of the disease, anti-inflammatory agents are usually not indicated. Sedatives may be helpful early in the course of chorea; phenobarbital (16–32 mg every 6–8 hr PO) is the drug of choice. If phenobarbital is ineffective, then haloperidol (0.01–0.03 mg/kg/24 hr divided bid PO) or chlorpromazine (0.5 mg/kg every 4–6 hr PO) should be initiated.

COMPLICATIONS. The arthritis and chorea of acute rheumatic fever resolve completely without sequelae. Therefore, the long-term sequelae of rheumatic fever are usually limited to the heart (see Chapter 438).

Patients with cardiac valvular disease secondary to acute rheumatic fever are at increased risk for developing infective endocarditis during episodes of transient bacteremia. The antibiotic regimens used to prevent recurrences of acute rheumatic fever are inadequate for protection against infective endocarditis. The current recommendations of the American Heart Association regarding infective endocarditis prophylaxis should be followed (see Chapter 437). Patients with residual rheumatic valvular disease do not always require endocarditis prophylaxis. The importance of good dental hygiene in the prevention of infective endocarditis should also be stressed. Patients who have had rheumatic fever but have no evidence of residual valvular disease do not require endocarditis prophylaxis.

PROGNOSIS. The prognosis for patients with acute rheumatic fever depends on the clinical manifestations present at the time of the initial episode, the severity of the initial episode, and the presence of recurrences. Approximately 70% of the patients with carditis during the initial episode of acute rheumatic fever recover with no residual heart disease; the more severe the initial cardiac involvement, the greater the risk for residual heart disease. Patients without carditis during the initial episode are unlikely to have carditis with recurrences. In contrast, patients with carditis during the initial episode are likely to have carditis with recurrences, and the risk for permanent heart damage increases with each recurrence. Patients who have had acute rheumatic fever are susceptible to recurrent attacks following reinfection of the upper respiratory tract with GAS. Therefore, these patients require long-term continuous chemoprophylaxis.

Before antibiotic prophylaxis was available, 75% of patients who had an initial episode of acute rheumatic fever had 1 or more recurrences during their lifetime. These recurrences were a major source of morbidity and mortality. The risk of recurrence is highest immediately after the initial episode and decreases with time.

Approximately 20% of patients who present with "pure" chorea who are not given secondary prophylaxis develop rheumatic heart disease within 20 yr. Therefore, patients with chorea, even in the absence of other manifestations of rheumatic fever, require long-term antibiotic prophylaxis.

PREVENTION. Prevention of both initial and recurrent episodes of acute rheumatic fever depends on controlling GAS infections of the upper respiratory tract. Prevention of initial attacks (primary prevention) depends on identification and eradication of the GAS that produces episodes of acute pharyngitis. Individuals who have already suffered an attack of acute rheumatic fever are particularly susceptible to recurrences of rheumatic fever with any subsequent GAS upper respiratory tract infection, whether or not they are symptomatic. Therefore, these patients should receive continuous antibiotic prophylaxis to prevent recurrences (secondary prevention).

Primary Prevention. Appropriate antibiotic therapy instituted before the 9th day of symptoms of acute GAS pharyngitis is highly effective in preventing 1st attacks of acute rheumatic fever from that episode. However, about ⅓ of patients with acute rheumatic fever do not recall a preceding episode of pharyngitis.

Secondary Prevention. Secondary prevention is directed at preventing acute GAS pharyngitis in patients at substantial risk of recurrent acute rheumatic fever. Secondary prevention requires continuous antibiotic prophylaxis, which should begin as soon as the diagnosis of acute rheumatic fever has been made and immediately after a full course of antibiotic therapy has been completed. Because patients who have had carditis with their initial episode of acute rheumatic fever are at a relatively high risk for having carditis with recurrences and for sustaining additional cardiac damage, they should receive antibiotic prophylaxis well into adulthood and perhaps for life.

Patients who did not have carditis with their initial episode of acute rheumatic fever have a relatively low risk for carditis with recurrences. Antibiotic prophylaxis may be discontinued in these patients when they reach their early 20s and after at least 5 yr have elapsed since their last episode of acute rheumatic fever. The decision to discontinue prophylactic antibiotics should be made only after careful consideration of potential risks and benefits and of epidemiologic factors such as the risk for exposure to GAS infections.

The regimen of choice for secondary prevention is a single intramuscular injection of benzathine penicillin G (1.2 million IU) every 4 wk (Table 182-4). In certain high-risk patients, and in certain areas of the world where the incidence of rheumatic fever is particularly high, use of benzathine penicillin G every 3 wk may be necessary because levels of penicillin may decrease to marginally effective amounts after 3 wk. In compliant patients, continuous oral antimicrobial prophylaxis can be used. Penicillin V given twice daily and sulfadiazine given once daily are equally effective when used in such patients. For the exceptional patient who is allergic to both penicillin and sulfonamides, erythromycin given twice daily may be used. The duration of secondary prophylaxis is noted in Table 182-5.

TABLE 182-4. Chemoprophylaxis for Recurrences of Acute Rheumatic Fever

DRUG	DOSE	ROUTE
Penicillin G benzathine	1.2 million U, every 4 wk*	Intramuscular
OR		
Penicillin V	250 mg, twice a day	Oral
OR		
Sulfadiazine or sulfisoxazole	0.5 g, once a day for patients ≤27 kg (≤60 lb) 1.0 g, once a day for patients >27 kg (>60 lb)	Oral
FOR PEOPLE WHO ARE ALLERGIC TO PENICILLIN AND SULFONAMIDE DRUGS		
Erythromycin	250 mg, twice a day	Oral

*In high-risk situations, administration every 3 weeks is recommended.
From the American Academy of Pediatrics: *Red Book: 2006 Report of the Committee on Infectious Diseases*, 27th ed. Elk Grove Village, IL, American Academy of Pediatrics, 2006, p 620.

TABLE 182-5. Duration of Prophylaxis for People Who Have Had Acute Rheumatic Fever: Recommendations of the American Heart Association

CATEGORY	DURATION
Rheumatic fever without carditis	5 yr or until 21 yr of age, whichever is longer
Rheumatic fever with carditis but without residual heart disease (no valvular disease*)	10 yr or well into adulthood, whichever is longer
Rheumatic fever with carditis and residual heart disease (persistent valvular disease*)	At least 10 yr since last episode and at least until 40 yr of age; sometimes lifelong prophylaxis

*Clinical or echocardiographic evidence.
From the American Academy of Pediatrics: *Red Book: 2006 Report of the Committee on Infectious Diseases*, 27th ed. Elk Grove Village, IL, American Academy of Pediatrics, 2006, p 619.

Group A Streptococcus

Bisno AL, Stevens DL: Streptococcal infections of skin and soft tissues. *N Engl J Med* 1996;334:240–245.

Blumer JL, Reed MD, Kaplan EL, Drusano GL: Explaining the poor bacteriologic eradication rate of single-dose ceftriaxone in group A streptococcal tonsillopharyngitis: A reverse engineering solution using pharmacodynamic modeling. *Pediatrics* 2005;116:927–932.

Davis HD, McGeer A, Schwartz B, et al: Invasive group A streptococcal infections in Ontario, Canada. *N Engl J Med* 1996;335:547–554.

Gerber MA, Shulman ST: Rapid diagnosis of pharyngitis caused by group A streptococci. *Clin Microbiol Rev* 2004;17:571–580.

Kaul R, McGeer A, Norby-Teglund A, et al: Intravenous immunoglobulin therapy in streptococcal toxic shock syndrome—A comparative observational study. *Clin Infect Dis* 1999;28:800–807.

Kurlan R, Kaplan EL: The pediatric autoimmune neuropsychiatric disorders associated with streptococcal infections (PANDAS) etiology for tics and obsessive-compulsive symptoms: Hypothesis or entity? Practical considerations for the clinician. *Pediatrics* 2004;113:883–886.

Mancini AJ: Bacterial skin infections in children; the common and the not so common. *Pediatr Ann* 2000;29:26–35.

Martin JM, Green M, Barbadora KA, Wald ER: Erthromycin-resistant group A streptococci in school children in Pittsburgh. *N Engl J Med* 2002; 346:1200–1206.

Mell LK, Davis RL, Owens D: Association between streptococcal infection and obsessive-compulsive disorder, Tourette's syndrome, and tic disorder. *Pediatrics* 2005;116:56–60.

Richter SS, Heilman KP, Beekmann SE, et al: Macrolide-resistant *Streptococcus pyogenes* in the United States, 2002-2-3. *Clin Infect Dis* 2005;41: 599–608.

Smith A, Lamagni TL, Oliver I, et al: Invasive group A streptococcal disease: Should close contacts routinely receive antibiotic prophylaxis? *Lancet Infect Dis* 2005;5:494–500.

Stevens DL: Streptococcal toxic shock syndrome associated with necrotizing fasciitis. *Annu Rev Med* 2000;51:271–288.

Tanz RR, Shulman ST, Shortridge VD, et al: Community-based surveillance in the United States of macrolide-resistant pediatric pharyngeal group A streptococci during 3 respiratory disease seasons. *Clin Infect Dis* 2004;39:1794–1801.

The Working Group on Prevention of Invasion Group A Streptococcal Infections: Prevention of invasive group A streptococcal disease among household contacts of case-patients. *JAMA* 1998;279:1206–1210.

Rheumatic Fever

Ayoub EM, Majeed HA: Poststreptococcal reactive arthritis. *Curr Opin Rheumatol* 2000;12:306–310.

Bisno AL: Group A streptococcal infections and acute rheumatic fever. *N Engl J Med* 1991;325:783–793.

Dajani A, Taubert K, Ferrieri P, et al: Treatment of acute streptococcal pharyngitis and prevention of rheumatic fever: A statement for health professionals. *Pediatrics* 1995;96:758–764.

Dajani AS, Ayoub E, Bierman FZ, et al: Guidelines for the diagnosis of rheumatic fever: Jones criteria, 1992 update. *JAMA* 1992;268:2069–2073.

Martin JM, Barbadora KA: Continued high caseload of rheumatic fever in western Pennsylvania: Possible rheumatogenic EMM types of *Streptococcus pyogenes*. *J Pediatr* 2006;149:58–63.

Stollerman GH: Rheumatogenic GABHS and the return of ARF. *Adv Intern Med* 1990;35:1–25.

Stollerman GH: Rheumatic fever. *Lancet* 1997;349:935–942.

Tani LY, Veasy LG, Minich LL, Shaddy RE: Rheumatic fever in children younger than 5 years: Is the presentation different? *Pediatrics* 2003;112:1065–1068.

Taranta A, Markowitz M: *Rheumatic Fever,* 2nd ed. Dordrecht, the Netherlands, Kluwer Academic, 1989.

Veasy LG, Tani LY, Daly JA, et al: Temporal association of the appearance of mucoid strains of *Streptococcus pyogenes* with continuing high incidence of rheumatic fever in Utah. *Pediatrics* 2004;113:e168–e172.

Veasy LG, Tani LY, Hill HR: Persistence of acute rheumatic fever in the intermountain area of the United States. *J Pediatr* 1994;124:9–16.

Veasy LG, Weidmeier SE, Orsmond GS, et al: Resurgence of acute rheumatic fever in the intermountain area of the United States. *N Engl J Med* 1987;316:421–427.

Chapter 183 ■ Group B Streptococcus

Catherine S. Lachenauer and Michael R. Wessels

Group B streptococcus (GBS), or *Streptococcus agalactiae,* has been a major cause of neonatal bacterial sepsis in the United States since the 1960s. While advances in prevention strategies have led to a recent decline in the incidence of neonatal disease, GBS remains a major pathogen for neonates, pregnant women, and immunocompromised nonpregnant adults.

ETIOLOGY. Group B streptococci are facultative anaerobic gram-positive cocci that form chains or diplococci in broth and small gray-white colonies on solid medium. GBS is definitively identified by demonstration of the Lancefield group B carbohydrate antigen, such as with latex agglutination techniques widely used in clinical laboratories. Presumptive identification can be established on the basis of a narrow zone of β-hemolysis on blood agar, resistance to bacitracin and trimethoprim-sulfamethoxazole, lack of hydrolysis of bile esculin, and elaboration of cAMP factor (cyclic adenosine monophosphate, an extracellular protein that, in the presence of the β toxin of *Staphylococcus aureus,* produces a zone of enhanced hemolysis on sheep's blood agar). Individual GBS strains are serologically classified according to the presence of one of the structurally distinct capsular polysaccharides, which are important virulence factors and stimulators of antibody-associated immunity. Nine GBS types have been identified: types Ia, Ib, II, III, IV, V, VI, VII, and VIII.

EPIDEMIOLOGY. GBS emerged as a prominent neonatal pathogen in the late 1960s. For the next 2 decades, the incidence of neonatal GBS disease remained fairly constant, affecting 1.0–5.4/1,000 liveborn infants in the United States. Two patterns of disease were seen: **early-onset disease**, which presents at <7 days of age, and **late-onset disease**, which presents at 7 days of age or later. In the 1990s, widespread implementation of maternal chemoprophylaxis led to a striking 65% decrease in the incidence of early-onset neonatal GBS disease in the United States, from 1.7/1,000 live births to 0.6/1,000 live births, whereas the incidence of late-onset disease remained essentially stable at approximately 0.4/1,000 (Fig. 183-1). In other developed countries, rates of neonatal GBS disease are similar to those in the United States prior to use of GBS chemoprophylaxis. In the developing world, GBS is not a major cause of neonatal sepsis, even though the prevalence of maternal vaginal colonization with GBS (a major risk factor for neonatal disease) among women from developing countries is similar to that reported among women living in the United States The incidence of neonatal GBS disease is higher in premature and low-birthweight infants, although most cases occur in full-term infants.

Colonization by GBS in healthy adults is common. Vaginal or rectal colonization occurs in up to approximately 30% of pregnant women and is the usual source for GBS transmission to newborn infants. In the absence of maternal chemoprophylaxis, approximately 50% of infants born to colonized women acquire GBS colonization, and 1–2% of these infants develop invasive disease. Heavy maternal colonization increases the risk for infant colonization and development of early-onset disease. Additional risk factors for early-onset disease include prolonged rupture of membranes, intrapartum fever, prematurity, maternal bacteriuria during pregnancy, or previous delivery of an infant who developed GBS disease. Risk factors for late-onset disease are less well defined. Whereas late-onset disease may follow vertical transmission, horizontal acquisition from nursery or other community sources has also been described.

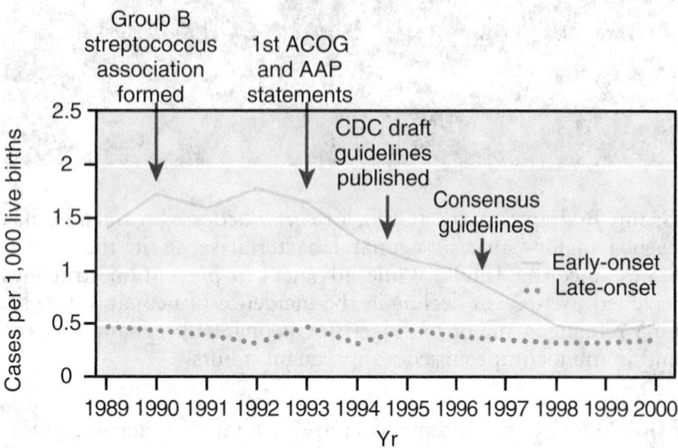

Figure 183-1. Incidence of early-onset and late-onset invasive group B streptococcus disease in three active surveillance areas (California, Georgia, and Tennessee), 1989 through 2000, and activities for the prevention of group B streptococcus disease. Arrows designate the dates when prevention activities occurred. ACOG, American College of Obstetricians and Gynecologists; AAP, American Academy of Pediatrics. (Adapted from Centers for Disease Control and Prevention: Early-onset group B streptococcal disease—United States, 1998–1999. *MMWR* 2000;49:793–796; and Schrag SJ, Zywicki S, Farley MM, et al: Group B streptococcal disease in the era of intrapartum antibiotic prophylaxis. *N Engl J Med* 2000;342:15–20.)

GBS is also an important cause of invasive disease in adults. GBS may cause urinary tract infections, bacteremia, endometritis, chorioamnionitis, and wound infection in pregnant and parturient women. In nonpregnant adults with underlying medical conditions such as diabetes mellitus, cirrhosis, or malignancy, GBS may cause serious infections such as bacteremia, skin and soft tissue infections, endocarditis, pneumonia, and meningitis. In the era of maternal chemoprophylaxis, most invasive GBS infections occur in nonpregnant adults.

The serotypes most commonly associated with neonatal GBS disease are types Ia, III, V, Ib, and II. Strains of serotype III are isolated in up to 80–90% of late-onset disease and of meningitis associated with early- or late-onset disease. The serotype distribution of colonizing and invasive strains from pregnant women is similar to that from infected newborns. In Japan, serotypes VI and VIII have been reported as common maternal colonizing serotypes, and case reports indicate that type VIII strains may cause neonatal disease indistinguishable from that caused by other serotypes.

PATHOGENESIS. A major risk factor for the development of early-onset neonatal GBS infection is maternal vaginal or rectal colonization by GBS. Infants acquire GBS during passage through the birth canal or, in some cases, via ascending infection. Fetal aspiration of infected amniotic fluid may occur. The incidence of early-onset GBS infection increases with the length of rupture of membranes. Infection may also occur through seemingly intact membranes. In cases of late-onset infection, GBS may be vertically transmitted or acquired later from maternal or nonmaternal sources.

Several bacterial factors are implicated in the pathophysiology of invasive GBS disease. Foremost among these is the type-specific capsular polysaccharide. Strains that are associated with invasive disease in humans elaborate more capsular polysaccharide than do colonizing isolates. All GBS capsular polysaccharides are high molecular weight polymers; all contain a short side chain terminating in *N*-acetylneuraminic acid (sialic acid). Studies in type III GBS show that the sialic acid component of the capsular polysaccharide prevents activation of the alternative complement pathway in the absence of type-specific antibody. Thus, the capsular polysaccharide appears to exert a virulence effect by protecting the organism from opsonophagocytosis in the nonimmune host. In addition, type-specific virulence attributes are suggested by the fact that type III strains are implicated in most cases of late-onset neonatal GBS disease and meningitis. Type III strains are taken up by brain endothelial cells more efficiently in vitro than strains of other serotypes, although studies using acapsular mutant strains demonstrate that it is not the capsule itself that facilitates cellular invasion. Other putative GBS virulence factors include GBS surface proteins, which may play a role in adhesion to host cells; C5a peptidase, which is postulated to inhibit the recruitment of polymorphonuclear cells into sites of infection; β-hemolysin, which has been associated with cell injury in in vitro studies; and hyaluronidase, which has been postulated to act as a spreading factor in host tissues.

Mothers colonized with type III GBS who gave birth to healthy infants had higher levels of capsular polysaccharide-specific antibody than women who gave birth to infants who developed invasive disease. In addition, there is a high correlation of antibody to GBS type III in mother-infant paired sera. These observations indicate that transplacental transfer of maternal antibody is critically involved in neonatal immunity to GBS. Optimal immunity to GBS also requires an intact complement system. The classic complement pathway is an important component of GBS immunity in the absence of specific antibody; antibody-mediated opsonophagocytosis may also proceed via the alternative complement pathway. These and other results indicate that anticapsular antibody can overcome the prevention of C3 deposition on the bacterial surface by the sialic acid component of the type III capsule.

The precise steps between GBS colonization and invasive disease remain unclear. In vitro studies showing GBS entry of alveolar epithelium and pulmonary vasculature endothelial cells suggest that GBS may gain access to the bloodstream via invasion from the alveolar space, perhaps following intrapartum aspiration of infected fluid. β-Hemolysin/cytolysin may facilitate GBS entry into the bloodstream following inoculation into the lungs. However, highly encapsulated GBS strains enter eukaryotic cells poorly in vitro compared with capsule-deficient organisms, yet they are associated with virulence clinically and in experimental infection models.

GBS induces the release of proinflammatory cytokines. The group B antigen and the peptidoglycan component of the GBS cell wall are potent inducers of tumor necrosis factor-α release in vitro, whereas purified type III capsular polysaccharide is not. Even though the capsule plays a central role in virulence through avoidance of immune clearance, the capsule does not directly contribute to cytokine release and the resultant inflammatory response.

The complete genome of GBS strains of type III, V, and Ia GBS have been sequenced, and sequencing projects of strains of other serotypes are underway, emphasizing a genomic approach to better understanding GBS. Analysis of these sequences shows that GBS is closely related to *Streptococcus pyogenes* and *Streptococcus pneumoniae*. Many known and putative GBS virulence genes are clustered in **pathogenicity islands** that also contain mobile genetic elements, suggesting that interspecies acquisition of genetic material plays an important role in genetic diversity.

CLINICAL MANIFESTATIONS. Two syndromes of neonatal GBS disease are distinguishable on the basis of age at presentation, epidemiologic characteristics, and clinical features (Table 183-1). **Early-onset neonatal GBS disease** presents within the 1st 7 days of life and is often associated with maternal obstetric complications, including chorioamnionitis, prolonged rupture of membranes, and premature labor. Infants may appear ill at the time of delivery, and most infants become ill within the 1st 24 hr of birth. In utero infection may result in septic abortion. The most

TABLE 183-1. Characteristics of Early- and Late-Onset GBS Disease

	EARLY-ONSET DISEASE	LATE-ONSET DISEASE
Age at onset	0–6 days	7–90 days
Increased risk after obstetric complications	Yes	No
Common clinical manifestations	Sepsis, pneumonia, meningitis	Bacteremia, meningitis, other focal infections
Common serotypes	Ia, III, V, II Ib	III predominates
Case fatality rate	4.7%	2.8%

Adapted from Schrag SJ, Zywicki S, Farley MM, et al: Group B streptococcal disease in the era of intrapartum antibiotic prophylaxis. *N Engl J Med* 2000;342:15–20.

common manifestations of early-onset GBS disease are sepsis (50%), pneumonia (30%), and meningitis (15%). Asymptomatic bacteremia is uncommon but can occur. In symptomatic patients, nonspecific signs such as hypothermia or fever, irritability, lethargy, apnea, and bradycardia may be present. Respiratory symptoms are prominent regardless of the presence of pneumonia and include cyanosis, apnea, tachypnea, grunting, flaring, and retractions. A fulminant course with hemodynamic abnormalities, including tachycardia, acidosis, and shock, may ensue. Persistent fetal circulation may develop. Clinically and radiographically, pneumonia associated with early-onset GBS disease is difficult to distinguish from respiratory distress syndrome (see Chapter 101.4). Patients with meningitis often present with nonspecific findings, as described for sepsis or pneumonia, with more specific signs of central nervous system (CNS) involvement initially being absent.

Late-onset neonatal GBS disease occurs on or after 7 days of life and most commonly manifests as bacteremia (45–60%) and meningitis (25–35%). Focal infections involving bone and joints, skin and soft tissue, the urinary tract, or lungs have been reported in approximately 20% of patients with late-onset disease. Cellulitis and adenitis are often localized to the submandibular or parotid regions. In contrast to early-onset disease, maternal obstetric complications are not risk factors for the development of late-onset GBS disease. Infants with late-onset disease are often less severely ill on presentation than infants with early-onset disease and the disease is often less fulminant.

Invasive GBS disease in children beyond early infancy is uncommon. In a multistate surveillance study in the 1990s, 2% of all cases of invasive GBS disease were identified in children age 90 days to 14 yr. Two of the more common syndromes associated with childhood GBS disease beyond early infancy are bacteremia and endocarditis. HIV infection should be considered in children with invasive GBS disease beyond the neonatal period.

DIAGNOSIS. A major challenge is distinguishing between respiratory distress syndrome and invasive neonatal GBS infection in preterm infants because the 2 illnesses share clinical and radiographic features. Severe apnea, early onset of shock, abnormalities in the peripheral leukocyte count, and greater lung compliance may be more likely in infants with GBS disease. Other neonatal pathogens, including *Escherichia coli* and *Listeria monocytogenes,* may cause illness that is clinically indistinguishable from that due to GBS.

The diagnosis of invasive GBS disease is established by isolation and identification of the organism from a normally sterile site, such as blood, urine, or cerebrospinal fluid (CSF). Isolation of GBS from gastric or tracheal aspirates or from skin or mucous membranes indicates colonization and is not diagnostic of invasive disease. CSF should be examined in all neonates suspected of having sepsis, because specific CNS signs are often absent in the presence of meningitis, especially in early-onset disease. Antigen detection methods that use group B polysaccharide-specific antiserum, such as latex particle agglutination, are available for testing of urine, blood, and CSF, but these tests are less sensitive than culture. Moreover, antigen is often detected in urine samples collected by bag from otherwise healthy neonates who are colonized with GBS on the perineum or rectum.

LABORATORY FINDINGS. Frequently present are abnormalities in the peripheral white blood cell count, including an increased or decreased absolute neutrophil count, an elevated band count, an elevated ratio of bands to total neutrophils, or leukopenia. Elevations in the C-reactive protein level have been investigated as a potential early marker of GBS sepsis but are unreliable. Findings on chest radiograph are often indistinguishable from those of respiratory distress syndrome and may include reticulogranular patterns, patchy infiltrates, generalized opacification, pleural effusions, or increased interstitial markings.

TREATMENT. Penicillin G is the treatment of choice of confirmed GBS infection. Initial empiric therapy of neonatal sepsis should include ampicillin and an aminoglycoside (or cefotaxime), both for the need for broad coverage pending organism identification and for synergistic bactericidal activity. Therapy may be completed with penicillin alone, once GBS has been definitively identified and a good clinical response has occurred. Especially in cases of meningitis, high doses of penicillin (450,000–500,000 U/kg/day) or ampicillin (300–400 mg/kg/day) are recommended because of the relatively high mean inhibitory concentration of penicillin for GBS as well as the potential for a high initial CSF inoculum. The duration of therapy varies according to the site of infection (Table 183-2) and should be guided by clinical circumstances. Extremely ill near-term patients with respiratory failure have been successfully treated with extracorporeal membrane oxygenation (see Chapter 101.8).

In cases of GBS meningitis, some experts recommend that additional CSF be sampled at 24–48 hr to determine whether sterility has been achieved. Persistent GBS growth may indicate an unsuspected intracranial focus or an insufficient antibiotic dose.

For **recurrent neonatal GBS** disease, standard intravenous antibiotic therapy followed by attempted eradication of GBS mucosal colonization has been suggested. This is based on the findings in several studies that invasive isolates from recurrent episodes are often identical to each other and to colonizing strains from the affected infant. Rifampin has most frequently been used for this purpose, but one report demonstrates that eradication of GBS colonization in infants is not reliably achieved by rifampin therapy. Optimal management of this uncommon situation remains unclear.

PROGNOSIS. Studies from the 1970s and 1980s showed that up to 30% of infants surviving GBS meningitis had major long-term neurologic sequelae, including developmental delay, spastic quadriplegia, microcephaly, seizure disorder, cortical blindness, or deafness; less severe neurologic complications may be present in other survivors. Periventricular leukomalacia and severe developmental delay may result from GBS disease and accompanying shock in premature infants, even in the absence of meningitis. The

TABLE 183-2. Recommended Duration of Therapy for Manifestations of GBS Disease

TREATMENT	DURATION
Bacteremia without a focus	10 days
Meningitis	2–3 wk
Ventriculitis	4 wk
Osteomyelitis	4 wk

Adapted from the American Academy of Pediatrics: Group B streptococcal infections. In Pickering LK (editor): *Red Book: 2000 Report of the Committee on Infectious Diseases,* 25th ed. Elk Grove Village, IL, American Academy of Pediatrics, 2000, pp 537–544.

outcome of focal GBS infections outside of the CNS, such as bone or soft tissue infections, is generally favorable.

In the 1990s, the case fatality rates associated with early- and late-onset neonatal GBS disease were 4.7% and 2.8%, respectively. Mortality is higher in premature infants; 1 study reported a case fatality rate of 30% in infants whose gestational age was <33 wk and 2% in infants whose gestational age was 37 wk or older. The case fatality rate in children aged 3 mo to 14 yr was 9%, and in nonpregnant adults was 11.5%.

PREVENTION. Persistent morbidity and mortality from perinatal GBS disease despite advances in neonatal care has spurred intense investigation into modes of prevention. Two basic approaches to GBS prevention have been investigated: (1) elimination of colonization from the mother or infant (chemoprophylaxis), and (2) induction of protective immunity (immunoprophylaxis).

Chemoprophylaxis. Administration of antibiotics to pregnant women **before** the onset of labor does not reliably eradicate maternal GBS colonization and is not an effective means of preventing neonatal GBS disease. Interruption of neonatal colonization is achievable through administration of antibiotics to the mother during labor (Fig. 183-2). Infants born to GBS-colonized women with premature labor or prolonged rupture of membranes who were given intrapartum chemoprophylaxis had a substantially lower risk for GBS colonization (9% vs 51%) and for early-onset disease (0% vs 6%) than did the infants born to women who were not treated. Maternal postpartum febrile illness was also decreased in the treatment group.

Guidelines for chemoprophylaxis specify administration of intrapartum antibiotics to women identified as high-risk by either culture-based or risk factor–based criteria. These guidelines were revised in 2002 after epidemiologic data indicated the superior protective effect of the culture-based approach in the prevention of neonatal GBS disease (see Fig. 183-2). According to current recommendations, vaginorectal GBS screening cultures should be performed for all pregnant women at 35–37 wk gestation. Any woman with a positive prenatal screening culture, GBS bacteriuria during pregnancy, or a previous infant with invasive GBS disease should receive intrapartum antibiotics. Women whose culture status is unknown (culture not done, incomplete, or results unknown) and who deliver prematurely (<37 wk gestation) or experience prolonged rupture of membranes (≥18 hr) or intrapartum fever (≥38.0°C) should also receive intrapartum chemoprophylaxis. If amnionitis is suspected, broad-spectrum antibiotic therapy that includes an agent active against GBS should replace GBS prophylaxis. Routine intrapartum prophylaxis is not recommended for women with GBS colonization undergoing planned cesarean delivery who have not begun labor or had rupture of membranes.

These guidelines also suggest an approach for the management of infants born to mothers who received intrapartum chemoprophylaxis (Fig. 183-3). Data from a large epidemiologic study indicate that the administration of maternal intrapartum antibiotics does not change the clinical spectrum or delay the onset of clinical signs in infants who developed GBS disease despite maternal prophylaxis. Thus, the Centers for Disease Control and Prevention guidelines reserve a full diagnostic evaluation for those infants who appear clinically ill or whose mothers are suspected of having chorioamnionitis.

A significant concern with maternal intrapartum prophylaxis has been that large-scale antibiotic use among parturient women might lead to increased rates of antimicrobial resistance or infection in infants with organisms other than GBS. To date, no GBS strains demonstrating resistance to penicillin have been identified, and increase in the incidence of non-GBS early-onset neonatal infections have been seen only in premature, low-birthweight, and very low birthweight infants, in whom risk factors other than maternal chemoprophylaxis may play a role. At present, the substantial decline in early-onset neonatal GBS disease favors continued broad-scale intrapartum chemoprophylaxis, but continued surveillance is required. Penicillin remains the preferred agent for chemoprophylaxis, because of its narrow spectrum and the universal penicillin susceptibility of GBS isolates. Because of recent reports indicating frequent resistance of GBS to erythromycin (up to 25%) and clindamycin (up to 15%), cefazolin should be used in most cases of intrapartum chemoprophylaxis for penicillin-

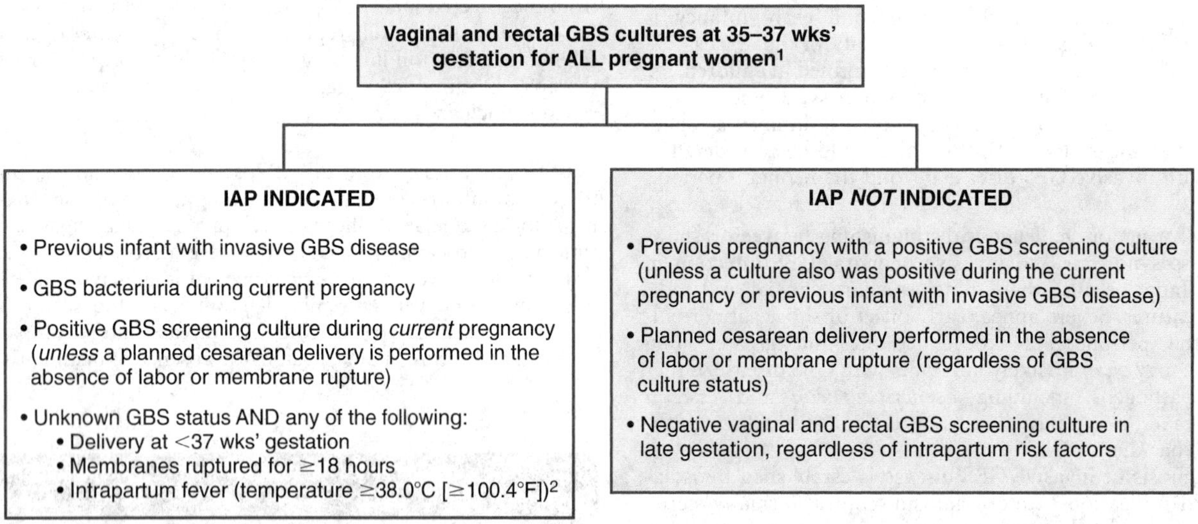

Vaginal and rectal GBS cultures at 35–37 wks' gestation for ALL pregnant women[1]

IAP INDICATED

- Previous infant with invasive GBS disease
- GBS bacteriuria during current pregnancy
- Positive GBS screening culture during *current* pregnancy (*unless* a planned cesarean delivery is performed in the absence of labor or membrane rupture)
- Unknown GBS status AND any of the following:
  - Delivery at <37 wks' gestation
  - Membranes ruptured for ≥18 hours
  - Intrapartum fever (temperature ≥38.0°C [≥100.4°F])[2]

IAP *NOT* INDICATED

- Previous pregnancy with a positive GBS screening culture (unless a culture also was positive during the current pregnancy or previous infant with invasive GBS disease)
- Planned cesarean delivery performed in the absence of labor or membrane rupture (regardless of GBS culture status)
- Negative vaginal and rectal GBS screening culture in late gestation, regardless of intrapartum risk factors

1 Exceptions; women with GBS bacteriuria during the current pregnancy or women with a previous infant with invasive GBS disease.
2 If chorioamnionitis is suspected, broad-spectrum antimicrobial therapy that includes an agent known to be active against GBS should replace GBS IAP.

Figure 183-2. Indications for intrapartum antimicrobial prophylaxis (IAP) to prevent early-onset group B streptococcal (GBS) disease using a universal prenatal culture screening strategy at 35–37 weeks' gestation for all women. (From the American Academy of Pediatrics: *Red Book: 2006 Report of the Committee on Infectious Diseases,* 27th ed. Elk Grove Village, IL, American Academy of Pediatrics, 2006, p 624.)

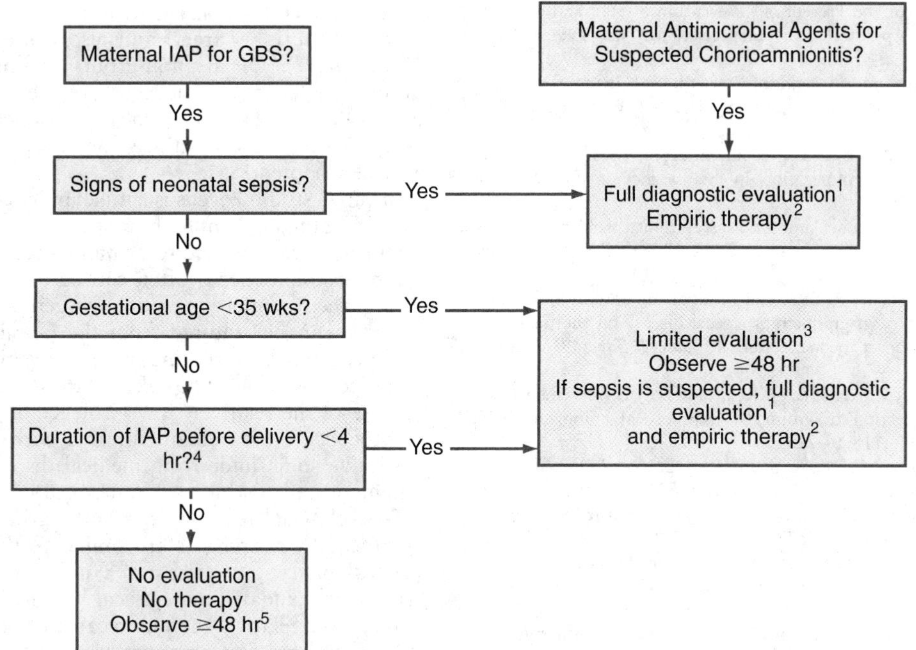

1 Includes complete blood cell (CBC) count with differential, blood culture, and chest radiograph if respiratory abnormalities are present, a lumbar puncture, if feasible, should be performed.
2 Duration of therapy varies depending on results of blood culture, cerebrospinal fluid findings (if obtained), and the clinical course of the infant. If laboratory results and clinical course do not indicate bacterial infection, duration may be as short 48 hr.
3 CBC including white blood cell count with differential and blood culture.
4 Applies only to penicillin, ampicillin, or cefazolin and assumes recommended dosing regimens.
5 A healthy-appearing infant who was ≥38 wk' gestation at delivery and whose mother received ≥4 hr of IAP before delivery may be discharged home after 24 hr if other discharge criteria have been met and a person able to comply fully with instructions for home observation will be present. If any one of these conditions is not met, the infant should be observed in the hospital for at least 48 hr and until criteria for discharge are achieved.

Figure 183-3. Empiric management of a neonate whose mother received intrapartum antimicrobial prophylaxis (IAP) for prevention of early-onset group B streptococcal (GBS) disease or suspected chorioamnionitis. This algorithm is not an exclusive course of management. Variations that incorporate individual circumstances or institutional preferences may be appropriate. (From the American Academy of Pediatrics: *Red Book: 2006 Report of the Committee on Infectious Diseases,* 27th ed. Elk Grove Village, IL, American Academy of Pediatrics, 2006, p 624.)

intolerant women. For penicillin-allergic women at high risk for anaphylaxis, clindamycin or erythromycin should be used, if isolates are demonstrated to be susceptible. Vancomycin should be used if isolates are resistant to clindamycin and erythromycin or if susceptibility to these agents is unknown.

A limitation of the maternal chemoprophylaxis strategy is that intrapartum antibiotic use is unlikely to have an impact on late-onset neonatal disease, miscarriages or stillbirths attributed to GBS, or adult GBS disease.

Maternal Immunization. Human studies demonstrate that transplacental transfer of naturally acquired maternal antibody to the GBS capsular polysaccharide protects newborns from invasive GBS infection and that efficient transplacental passage of vaccine-induced GBS antibodies occurs. Conjugate vaccines composed of the GBS capsular polysaccharides coupled to carrier proteins have been produced for human use. In early clinical trials, conjugate GBS vaccines were well tolerated and induced levels of functional antibodies well above the range believed to be protective in greater than 90% of recipients. A new vaccine containing type III polysaccharide coupled to tetanus toxoid was safely administered to pregnant women and elicited good levels of functionally active type-specific antibody that was efficiently transported to infants. Administration of a multivalent polysaccharide-protein vaccine before or during pregnancy should lead to transplacental passage of vaccine-induced antibody that protects the fetus and newborn against infection by several GBS serotypes. Such a vaccine would eliminate the need for cumbersome cultures during pregnancy, would circumvent the various risks associated with large-scale antibiotic prophylaxis, and would likely have an impact on both early- and late-onset disease. Intrapartum chemoprophylaxis will likely remain an important aspect of prevention, particularly for women in whom opportunities for GBS immunization are missed and for infants born so early that levels of transplacentally acquired antibodies may not be high enough to be protective.

Baker CJ, Kasper DL: Correlation of maternal antibody deficiency with susceptibility to neonatal group B streptococcal infection. *N Engl J Med* 1976;294:753–756.

Baker CJ, Rench MA, McInnes P: Immunization of pregnant women with group B streptococcal type III capsular polysaccharide-tetanus toxoid conjugate vaccine. *Vaccine* 2003:21:3468–3472.

Boyer KM, Gotoff SP: Prevention of early-onset neonatal group B streptococcal disease with selective intrapartum chemoprophylaxis. *N Engl J Med* 1986;314:1665–1669.

Bromberger P, Lawrence JM, Braun D, et al: The influence of intrapartum antibiotics on the clinical spectrum of early-onset group B streptococcal infection in term infants. *Pediatrics* 2000;106:244–250.

Centers for Disease Control and Prevention: Early-onset group B streptococcal disease—United States, 1998–1999. *MMWR* 2000;49:793–796.

Centers for Disease Control and Prevention: Prevention of perinatal group B streptococcal disease: A public health perspective. *MMWR* 1996;45(RR-7):1–24.

Centers for Disease Control and Prevention: Prevention of perinatal group B streptococcal disease. Revised guidelines from CDC. *MMWR* 2002;51(RR-11):1–22.

Fernandez M, Rench MA, Albanyan EA, et al: Failure of rifampin to eradicate group B streptococcal colonization in infants. *Pediatr Infect Dis J* 2001;20:371–376.

Lin F-Y, Azimi P, Weisman LE, et al: Antibiotic susceptibility profiles for group B streptococci isolated from neonates, 1995–1998. *Clin Infect Dis* 2000;31:76–79.

Moore MR, Schrag SJ, Schuchat A: Effects of intrapartum antimicrobial prophylaxis for prevention of group-B-streptococcal disease on the incidence and ecology of early-onset neonatal sepsis. *Lancet Infect Dis* 2003; 3:201–213.

Natarajan G, Johnson YR, Zhang F, et al: Real-time polymerase chain reaction for the rapid detection of group B streptococcal colonization in neonates. *Pediatrics* 2006;118:14–22.

Schrag SJ, Zywicki S, Farley MM, et al: Group B streptococcal disease in the era of intrapartum antibiotic prophylaxis. *N Engl J Med* 2000;342:15–20.

Schuchat A: Group B streptococcal disease: From trials and tribulations to triumph and trepidation. *Clin Infect Dis* 2001;33:751–756.

Stoll BJ, Hansen N, Fanaroff AA, et al: Changes in pathogens causing early-onset sepsis in very-low-birthweight infants. *N Engl J Med* 2002; 347:240–247.

Stoll BJ, Schuchat A: Maternal carriage of group B streptococci in developing countries. *Pediatr Infect Dis J* 1998;17:499–503.

Yow MD, Mason EO, Leeds LJ, et al: Ampicillin prevents intrapartum transmission of group B streptococcus. *JAMA* 1979;241:1245–1247.

Zaleznik DF, Rench MA, Hillier S, et al: Invasive disease due to group B streptococcus in pregnant women and neonates from diverse population groups. *Clin Infect Dis* 2000;30:276–281.

Chapter 184 ■ Non-Group A or B Streptococci

Michael A. Gerber

The genus *Streptococcus* comprises >30 species. *Streptococcus pneumoniae* (see Chapter 181), group A streptococcus (see Chapter 182), and group B streptococcus (see Chapter 183) are the most common causes of human streptococcal infections. The β-hemolytic streptococci of Lancefield groups C to H and K to V and the α-hemolytic streptococci that cannot be classified within a Lancefield group (the viridans streptococci) commonly colonize intact body surfaces (the pharynx, skin, gastrointestinal tract, genitourinary tract) and also cause infections in humans (Table 184-1). Of the non-group A β-hemolytic streptococci, groups C and G streptococcus are the most frequent cause of human disease. The enterococci were once classified among the group D streptococci but are now a separate genus, *Enterococcus* (see Chapter 185).

Group C streptococcus is a much more common cause of infection in animals than in humans. Humans infected with this organism often have had some animal contact. Both group C and group G streptococcus often can be part of the normal human flora of the nasopharynx, skin, and genital tract. Group C streptococcus can be cultured from the umbilicus of asymptomatic newborns and from routine puerperal vaginal cultures. Group G streptococcus also can be cultured from the gastrointestinal tract. Because of the relatively low virulence of group C and group G streptococci, most humans infected with either of these organisms have some underlying medical disorder (diabetes mellitus, malignancy, alcohol abuse, immunosuppression).

The **clinical features** of both group C and group G streptococcal pharyngitis are similar to those of group A streptococcal pharyngitis with fever, mild to moderate sore throat, pharyngeal exudate, and cervical lymphadenitis. Group C streptococcus is a relatively common cause of acute pharyngitis among college students and among adults who come to an emergency department. In addition to endemic pharyngitis, group C streptococcus can cause epidemic food-borne pharyngitis after ingestion of contaminated products, such as unpasteurized cow's milk. Family and school outbreaks of group C streptococcal pharyngitis have also been described. Group C streptococcus has been reported as an uncommon cause of a number of other infections, including skin and soft tissue infections, septic arthritis, osteomyelitis, pneumonitis, infective endocarditis, bacteremia and septicemia, meningitis, epiglottitis, pericarditis, urinary tract infections, and sinusitis. Group C streptococcus also has been associated with epidemic and nonepidemic cases of puerperal sepsis and endometritis; there may be an association between group C streptococcus and reactive arthritis, as well as a toxic shock–like syndrome.

Even though there have been several well-documented food-borne outbreaks of group G streptococcal pharyngitis, the etiologic role of group G streptococcus in acute, endemic pharyngitis remains unclear. A community-wide respiratory outbreak of group G streptococcal pharyngitis in a pediatric population was described in which group G streptococcus was isolated from 56 of 222 (25%) consecutive children with acute pharyngitis seen at a private pediatric office. Results of DNA fingerprinting of the group G streptococcal isolates suggested that 75% of these were

TABLE 184-1. Relationship of Streptococci Identified by Hemolysis and Lancefield Grouping to Sites of Colonization and Disease

	GROUP A STREPTOCOCCUS (*S. PYOGENES*)	GROUP B STREPTOCOCCUS (*S. AGALACTIAE*)	OTHER β-HEMOLYTIC STREPTOCOCCI	VIRIDANS STREPTOCOCCI
Hemolysis	β	β	β	α
Lancefield group	A	B	C–H, K–V	
Species or strains	M types (>180)	Serotypes (Ia, Ib, II, III, IV, V, VI, VII, and VIII)		*S. bovis* *S. mitis* *S. mutans* *S. sanguis* Many others
Normal flora	Pharynx, skin, anus	Gastrointestinal and genitourinary tract	Pharynx, skin, gastrointestinal and genitourinary tracts	Pharynx, nose, skin, genitourinary tract
Common human diseases	Pharyngitis, tonsillitis, erysipelas, impetigo, septicemia, wound infections, necrotizing fasciitis, cellulitis, meningitis, pneumonia, scarlet fever, toxic shock–like syndrome, rheumatic fever, acute glomerulonephritis	Puerperal sepsis chorioamnionitis, endocarditis, neonatal sepsis, meningitis, osteomyelitis, pneumonia	Wound infections, puerperal sepsis, cellulitis, sinusitis, endocarditis, brain abscess, sepsis, nosocomial infections, opportunistic infections	Endocarditis, human bite infections

α, partial hemolysis; β, complete hemolysis; γ, no hemolysis (nonhemolytic).

the same strain. The patients with group G streptococcal pharyngitis were comparable to those with group A streptococcal pharyngitis with respect to clinical findings, antistreptolysin O titer response, and clinical response to antibiotic therapy. These findings suggested that antibiotic therapy may have an impact on the clinical course of group G streptococcal pharyngitis.

Group G streptococcus has been reported to be an uncommon cause of puerperal sepsis and a neonatal infection that is clinically similar to early-onset group B streptococcal disease. Other infections occasionally caused by group G streptococcus include bacteremia, endocarditis, septic arthritis, osteomyelitis, pneumonia, erysipelas and other skin and soft tissue infections, and meningitis. Group G streptococcus has been associated with a toxic shock–like syndrome.

Acute rheumatic fever has not been described as a complication of either group C or group G streptococcal pharyngitis. There have been reports attempting to link acute glomerulonephritis with group G streptococcal pharyngitis; the evidence is anecdotal, and a causal relationship has not been established. Acute glomerulonephritis has been reported as a complication of group C streptococcal pharyngitis; it is extremely unusual. Therefore, the primary reason to identify either group C or group G streptococcus as the etiologic agent of acute pharyngitis is to initiate antibiotic therapy that may reduce the clinical impact of the illness. There is currently no convincing evidence from controlled studies of a clinical response to antibiotic therapy in patients with acute pharyngitis and either group C or group G streptococcus isolated from their upper respiratory tract.

Penicillin is the antibiotic of choice for treating infections due to either group C or group G streptococcal infections. Pharyngitis usually is treated in a similar manner to group A streptococcal upper respiratory infections, whereas more severe infections require parenteral therapy.

Arditi M, Shulman ST, Davis AT, et al: Group C beta-hemolytic streptococcal infections in children: Nine pediatric cases and review. *Rev Infect Dis* 1989;11:34–45.

Gerber MA, Randolph MF, Martin NJ, et al: Community-wide outbreak of group C streptococcal pharyngitis. *Pediatrics* 1991;87:598–603.

Hashikawa S, Iinuma Y, Furushita M, et al: Characterization of group C and group G streptococcal strains that cause streptococcal toxic shock syndrome. *J Clin Microbiol* 2004;42:186–192.

Meier FA, Centor RM, Graham L Jr, et al: Clinical and microbiological evidence for endemic pharyngitis among adults due to group C streptococci. *Arch Intern Med* 1990;150:825–829.

Turner JC, Hayden FG, Lobo MC, et al: Epidemiologic evidence for Lancefield group C beta-hemolytic streptococci as a cause of exudative pharyngitis in college students. *J Clin Microbiol* 1997;35:1–4.

Chapter 185 ■ *Enterococcus*

David B. Haslam

Enterococcus, long recognized as a pathogen in select populations, over the past 2 decades has become a common and particularly troublesome cause of hospital-acquired infection. These organisms, formerly classified with *Streptococcus bovis* and *Streptococcus equinus* as the Lancefield group D streptococcus, are now placed in a separate genus and are notorious for their frequent resistance to antibiotics.

ETIOLOGY. Enterococci are gram-positive, catalase-negative facultative anaerobes that grow in pairs or short chains. Most are nonhemolytic (also called γ-hemolytic) on sheep blood agar, although some isolates have α- or β-hemolytic activity. Enterococci are distinguished from most Lancefield groupable streptococci by their ability to grow in bile and hydrolyze esculin. Enterococci are able to grow in 6.5% NaCl and hydrolyze L-pyrrolidonyl-β-naphthylamide (PYR), features used by clinical laboratories to distinguish *Enterococcus* from group D streptococcus. Identification at the species level is enabled by differing patterns of carbohydrate fermentation.

EPIDEMIOLOGY. Enterococci are normal inhabitants of the gastrointestinal tract of humans and animals. Oral secretions and dental plaque, the upper respiratory tract, skin, and vagina may also be colonized by *Enterococcus. Enterococcus faecalis* is the predominant organism, with colonization commonly occurring in the 1st week of life. By the time of adulthood, *E. faecalis* colonization is nearly ubiquitous. *Enterococcus faecium* colonization is less consistent, although approximately 25% of adults harbor this organism.

E. faecalis accounts for approximately 80% of enterococcal infections, with almost all of the remaining infections caused by *Enterococcus faecium.* Only rarely are other species, such as *Enterococcus gallinarium* and *Enterococcus cassiliflavus,* associated with invasive infection, but these organisms are notable for their intrinsic low-level vancomycin resistance. Typically, the patient's indigenous flora is presumed to be the source of enterococcal infection. However, direct spread from person to person or from contaminated medical devices may occur, particularly within newborn nurseries and intensive care units. Studies have demonstrated the importance of nosocomial spread as a source of hospital outbreaks.

PATHOGENESIS. Enterococci are not aggressively invasive organisms, usually only causing disease in children with damaged mucosal surfaces or impaired immune response. Their dramatic emergence as a cause of nosocomial infection is predominantly due to their resistance to antibiotics commonly used in the hospital setting. Aside from antibiotic resistance genes, few classic virulence factors have been described among enterococci. Adhesion-promoting factors likely account for the propensity of these organisms to cause **endocarditis** and **urinary tract infections** (UTIs). The ability to form biofilms likely facilitates the colonization of urinary and vascular catheters. Many isolates also produce a cytolysin that has a broad range of host cells. Released at high bacterial density in a process called quorum sensing, cytolysin contributes to virulence in experimental models of endocarditis, peritonitis, and endophthalmitis. Other proposed virulence factors include aggregation substance, gelatinase, extracellular superoxide, and extracellular surface protein.

Antimicrobial Resistance. Enterococci are highly resistant to cephalosporins and semisynthetic penicillins such as nafcillin, oxacillin, and methicillin. They are moderately resistant to extended-spectrum penicillins such as ticarcillin and carbenicillin. Ampicillin, imipenem, and penicillin are the most active β-lactams against these organisms. Some strains of *E. faecalis* and *E. faecium* demonstrate decreased resistance to β-lactam antibiotics due to mutations in penicillin binding protein 5. In addition, occasional strains of *E. faecalis* produce a plasmid-encoded β-lactamase similar to that found in *Staphylococcus.* These isolates are completely resistant to penicillins, necessitating the combination of a penicillin plus a β-lactamase inhibitor or the use of imipenem or vancomycin. Any active drug may be insufficient if used alone for serious infections wherein high bactericidal activity is desired.

All enterococci have intrinsic low-level resistance to aminoglycosides because these antibiotics are poorly transported across the *Enterococcus* cell wall (Table 185-1). Concomitant use of a cell wall active agent, such as a β-lactam or glycopeptide antibiotic,

TABLE 185-1. Antimicrobial Resistance of *Enterococcus*

INTRINSIC RESISTANCE (CHROMOSOMALLY ENCODED)
Aminoglycosides (low level)
β-lactams (especially semisynthetic penicillins and cephalosporins)
Trimethoprim-sulfamethoxazole
Clindamycin (low level)
ACQUIRED RESISTANCE
Aminoglycosides (high level)
Chloramphenicol
Erythromycin and high-level clindamycin
Quinolones
Penicillins (β-lactamase)
Tetracyclines
Vancomycin
Teicoplanin
Daptomycin
Streptogramins (quinupristin/dalfopristin)
Oxazolidinones (linezolid)

improves the permeability of the cell wall for the aminoglycosides, resulting in synergistic killing. However, some isolates demonstrate high-level resistance, defined as mean inhibitory concentration (MIC >2,000 µg/mL) due to modification or inactivation of aminoglycoside agents. Strains demonstrating high-level resistance, and even some moderately resistant isolates, are not affected synergistically by aminoglycosides and cell wall–active antibiotics.

Resistance to almost all other antibiotic classes, including tetracyclines, macrolides, and chloramphenicol, has been described among the enterococci, necessitating individual susceptibility testing for these antibiotics when their use is considered. Despite apparent susceptibility in vitro, trimethoprim-sulfamethoxazole has poor activity in vivo, and should not be used as the primary agent against *Enterococcus* infections.

Vancomycin has traditionally been effective against multiresistant isolates, but **resistance to vancomycin**, defined as MIC >32 µg/mL, and other glycopeptides, including teicoplanin and daptomycin, is increasingly common. Both high- and moderate-level resistance are described in *E. faecalis* and *E. faecium*. High-level resistance (MIC ≥64 µg/mL) can be transferred by way of conjugation and is usually due to plasmid-mediated transfer of the *vanA* gene. High-level resistance is most common among *E. faecium* but is increasingly seen among *E. faecalis* isolates. Moderate-level resistance (MIC 8–256 µg/mL) results from a chromosomal homologue of *vanA*, known as *vanB*. Isolates that harbor the *vanB* gene are only moderately resistant to vancomycin and initially demonstrate susceptibility to teicoplanin, although resistance can emerge during therapy.

CLINICAL MANIFESTATIONS. *Enterococcus* infections traditionally occurred predominantly in newborn infants; infection in older children is increasingly common. Most *Enterococcus* infections occur in patients with breakdown of normal physical barriers such as the gastrointestinal tract, skin, or urinary tract. Other risk factors for *Enterococcus* infection include prolonged hospitalization, indwelling vascular catheters, prior use of antibiotics, and compromised immunity.

Neonatal Infections. *Enterococcus* accounts for up to 15% of all neonatal bacteremia and septicemia. Like group B streptococcus infections, *Enterococcus* infections are seen in 2 distinct settings in neonatal patients. Early-onset infection (<7 days of age) may mimic early-onset group B streptococcus septicemia, but tends to be milder. Early-onset *Enterococcus* sepsis most often occurs in full-term infants who are otherwise healthy. Late-onset infection (≥7 days of age) is associated with risk factors such as extreme prematurity, presence of an intravascular catheter, or necrotizing enterocolitis, or it follows an intra-abdominal surgical procedure. Symptoms in late-onset disease are more severe than those in early-onset disease and include apnea, bradycardia, and deteriorating respiratory function. Focal infections such as scalp abscess and catheter infection are commonly associated. Mortality rates range from 6% in early-onset septicemia to 15% in late-onset infections associated with necrotizing enterocolitis.

Enterococci are an occasional cause of meningitis. In neonates in particular, meningitis usually occurs as a complication of septicemia. Alternatively, the organism may gain access to the central nervous system by way of contiguous spread, such as through a neural tube defect or in association with an intraventricular shunt. *Enterococcus* meningitis can be associated with minimal abnormality of cerebrospinal fluid.

Infections in Older Children. *Enterococcus* rarely causes UTIs in healthy children, but accounts for approximately 15% of cases of nosocomially acquired UTIs, both in children and adults. Presence of an indwelling urinary catheter is the major risk factor for nosocomial UTIs. *Enterococcus* is frequently isolated in intra-abdominal infections following intestinal perforation or surgery. Their significance in polymicrobial infections has been questioned, although reported mortality rates are higher when intra-abdominal infections include enterococci. *Enterococcus* is increasingly common as a cause of nosocomial bacteremia; these organisms accounted for 9.4% of nosocomial bloodstream infection in children, ranking second only to coagulase-negative staphylococci. Predisposing factors for enterococcal bacteremia and endocarditis include an indwelling central venous catheter, gastrointestinal surgery, immunodeficiency, and cardiovascular abnormalities.

TREATMENT. Treatment of invasive *Enterococcus* infections must recognize that these organisms are resistant to antimicrobial agents frequently used as empirical therapy. In particular, cephalosporins should not be relied upon in situations where *Enterococcus* is known or suspected to be involved. In general, in the immunocompetent host, minor localized infections due to *Enterococcus* can be treated with ampicillin alone. Antibiotics containing β-lactamase inhibitors (clavulanate or sulbactam) provide advantage only for the few organisms whose resistance is due to production of β-lactamase. In uncomplicated UTIs, nitrofurantoin is efficacious when the organism is known to be sensitive to this antibiotic.

Invasive infections such as sepsis, meningitis, and endocarditis are usually treated with a combination of penicillin or ampicillin and an aminoglycoside when the isolate is susceptible. Vancomycin can be substituted for the penicillins in allergic patients, but should be used with an aminoglycoside, because vancomycin alone is not bactericidal. Endocarditis from strains possessing high-level aminoglycoside resistance may relapse even after prolonged therapy. High-dose or continuous infusion penicillin has been proposed for treatment of these infections in adults, yet ultimately valve replacement may be necessary. In patients with catheter-associated enterococcal bacteremia, the catheter should be removed promptly in most cases, although salvage of infected lines has occurred with the combined use of ampicillin or vancomycin with an aminoglycoside.

Vancomycin-Resistant Enterococcus (VRE). The treatment of serious infections due to multiresistant, vancomycin-resistant strains is particularly challenging. Linezolid, an oxazolidinone antibiotic that inhibits protein synthesis, is bacteriostatic against most *E. faecium* and *E. faecalis*, including vancomycin-resistant isolates. Response rates are generally >90%, including cases of bacteremia and sepsis (see VRSA in Chapter 180.1). Despite being bacteriostatic, linezolid has been successful in the treatment both of endocarditis and meningitis caused by VRE. Linezolid resistance is documented, and nosocomial spread of these resistant organisms can occur.

Quinupristin-dalfopristin is a combined streptogramin antibiotic that inhibits bacterial protein synthesis at 2 different stages. It has activity against most *E. faecium* strains, including those with high-level vancomycin resistance. Approximately 90% of *E. faecium* strains are susceptible to quinupristin-dalfopristin in vitro. Notably, it is inactive against *E. faecalis* and therefore should not be used as the sole agent against gram-positive organisms until culture results exclude the presence of *E. faecalis.* Studies in children suggest that this antibiotic is effective and generally well tolerated. Emergence of resistance to quinupristin-dalfopristin is rare, but has been demonstrated.

PREVENTION. Strategies for preventing enterococcal infections include early removal of urinary and intravenous catheters and debridement of necrotic tissue. Infection control strategies, including surveillance cultures, patient and staff cohorting, and strict gown and glove isolation are effective at decreasing colonization rates with VREs. However, these organisms may persist on inanimate objects, such as stethoscopes, complicating efforts to limit their nosocomial spread. To prevent the emergence and spread of vancomycin-resistant organisms, the Centers for Disease Control and Prevention has developed a series of guidelines for prudent vancomycin use.

Ang JY, Lua JL, Turner DR, Asmar BI: Vancomycin-resistant *Enterococcus faecium* endocarditis in a premature infant successfully treated with linezolid. *Pediatr Infect Dis J* 2003;22:1101–1103.

Centers for Disease Control and Prevention: Recommendations for preventing the spread of vancomycin resistance. Hospital Infection Control Practices Advisory Committee (HICPAC). *MMWR* 1995;44(RR-12):1–130.

Gray JW, George RH: Experience of vancomycin-resistant enterococci in a children's hospital. *J Hosp Infect* 2000;45:11–18.

Linden PK: Treatment options for vancomycin-resistant enterococcal infections. *Drugs* 2002;62:425–441.

Malik RK, Montecalvo MA, Reale MR, et al: Epidemiology and control of vancomycin-resistant enterococci in a regional neonatal intensive care unit. *Pediatr Infect Dis J* 1999;18:352–356.

Moellering RC: Quinupristin/dalfopristin: Therapeutic potential for vancomycin-resistant enterococcal infections. *J Antimicrob Chemother* 1999;44:25–30.

Ostrowsky BE, Trick WE, Sohn AH, et al: Control of vancomycin-resistant *Enterococcus* in health care facilities in a region. *N Engl J Med* 2001;344:1427–1433.

Pintado V, Cabellos C, Moreno S, et al: Enterococcal meningitis: A clinical study of 39 cases and review of the literature. *Medicine* 2003;82:346–364.

Ray AJ, Hoyen CK, Taub TF, et al: Nosocomial transmission of vancomycin resistant enterococci from surfaces. *JAMA* 2002;287:1400–1401.

Rice LB, Bellais S, Carias LL, et al: Impact of specific *pbp5* mutations on expression of β-lactam resistance in *Enterococcus faecium. Antimicrob Agents Chemother* 2004;48:3028–3032.

Sing-Naz N, Rakowsky A, Cantwell E, et al: Nosocomial enterococcal infections in children. *J Infect* 2000;40:145–149.

Sohn AH, Garrett DO, Sinkowitz-Cochran RL, et al: Prevalence of nosocomial infections in neonatal intensive care unit patients: Results from the first national point-prevalence survey. *J Pediatr* 2001;139:821–827.

Treitman AN, Yarnold PR, Warren J, et al: Emerging incidence of *Enterococcus faecium* among hospital isolates (1993 to 2002). *J Clin Microbiol* 2005;43:462–463.

Wisplinghoff H, Seifert H, Tallent S, et al: Nosocomial bloodstream infections in pediatric patients in United States hospitals: Epidemiology, clinical features and susceptibilities. *Pediatr Infect Dis J* 2003;22:686–691.

Zachary KC, Bayne PS, Morrison VJ, et al: Contamination of gowns, gloves, and stethoscopes with vancomycin-resistant enterococci. *Infect Control Hosp Epidemiol* 2001;22:560–567.

Chapter 186 ■ Diphtheria (*Corynebacterium diphtheriae*)

E. Stephen Buescher

Diphtheria is an acute toxic infection caused by *Corynebacterium* species, typically *Corynebacterium diphtheriae* and rarely toxigenic strains of *Corynebacterium ulcerans.* Diphtheria was the 1st infectious disease conquered by the principles of microbiology, immunology, and public health. Although diphtheria was reduced from a major cause of childhood death to a medical rarity in the Western hemisphere in the early 20th century, current reminders of the fragility of this success emphasize the necessity to continue vigorous promotion of those same principles across the global community.

ETIOLOGY. Corynebacteria are aerobic, nonencapsulated, non-spore-forming, mostly nonmotile, pleomorphic, gram-positive bacilli. *C. diphtheriae* is by far the most commonly isolated agent of diphtheria. *C. ulcerans* is more commonly isolated from cattle and can cause similar disease. As corynebacteria are not fastidious in growth requirements, their isolation is enhanced by use of a selective medium (i.e., cystine-tellurite blood agar) that inhibits growth of competing organisms and, when reduced by *C. diphtheriae,* renders colonies gray-black. Differentiation of *C. diphtheriae* from *C. ulcerans* is based on urease activity, as *C. ulcerans* is urease-positive.

Four *C. diphtheriae* biotypes (mitis, intermedius, belfanti, gravis) are capable of causing diphtheria and are differentiated by colonial morphology, hemolysis, and fermentation reactions. The ability to produce diphtheritic toxin results from acquisition of a lysogenic *Corynebacteriophage* by either *C. diphtheriae* or *C. ulcerans,* which encodes the diphtheritic toxin gene and confers diphtheria-producing potential to these strains. Thus, indigenous nontoxigenic *C. diphtheriae* can be rendered toxigenic and disease-producing after importation of a toxigenic *C. diphtheriae* and transmission of the bacteriophage. Demonstration of diphtheritic toxin production or potential for toxin production by an isolate is necessary to confirm disease. The former is performed in vitro by the agar immunoprecipitin technique (Elek test) or by the in vivo toxin neutralization test in guinea pigs, the latter by polymerase chain reaction testing for carriage of the toxin gene. Toxigenic and nontoxigenic strains are indistinguishable by colony type, microscopy, or biochemical tests.

EPIDEMIOLOGY. Unlike other **diphtheroids (coryneform bacteria),** which are ubiquitous in nature, *C. diphtheriae* is an exclusive inhabitant of human mucous membranes and skin. Spread is primarily by airborne respiratory droplets, direct contact with respiratory secretions of symptomatic individuals, or exudate from infected skin lesions. Asymptomatic respiratory tract carriage is important in transmission. Where diphtheria is endemic, 3–5% of healthy individuals can carry toxigenic organisms, but carriage is exceedingly rare if diphtheria is rare. Skin infection and skin carriage are silent reservoirs of *C. diphtheriae,* and organisms can remain viable in dust or on fomites for up to 6 mo. Transmission through contaminated milk and an infected food handler has been proved or suspected.

In the 1920s, more than 125,000 diphtheria cases, with 10,000 deaths, were reported annually in the United States, with the highest fatality rates among the very young and the elderly. The incidence then began to decrease, and, with widespread use of diphtheria toxoid in the United States after World War II, declined steadily through the late 1970s. Since then, ≤5 cases have occurred annually in the United States with no epidemics of respiratory tract diphtheria. Similar decreases occurred in Europe. Despite disease incidence decreasing worldwide, diphtheria remains endemic in many developing countries with poor immunization rates against diphtheria.

When diphtheria was endemic, it primarily affected children <15 yr of age. Since the introduction of toxoid immunization, the disease has shifted to adults who lack natural exposure to toxigenic *C. diphtheriae* in the vaccine era and have low rates of booster immunization. In the 27 sporadic cases of respiratory tract diphtheria reported in the United States in the 1980s, 70% occurred among persons >25 yr of age. The largest outbreak of diphtheria in the developed world since the 1960s occurred from 1990 to 1996 in the newly independent countries of the former Soviet Union, involving >150,000 cases in 14 of 15 countries. Of these, >60% of cases occurred in individuals >14 yr of age. Case fatality rates ranged from 3 to 23% by country. Factors contributing to the epidemic included a large population of underimmunized adults, decreased childhood immunization rates, population migration, crowding, and failure to respond aggressively during early phases of the epidemic. Cases of diphtheria among travelers from these endemic areas were transported to many countries in Europe.

Most proven cases of respiratory tract diphtheria in the United States in the 1990s were associated with **importation** of toxigenic *C. diphtheriae,* although clonally related toxigenic *C. diphtheriae* has persisted in the U.S. and Canada for at least 25 yr.

Cutaneous diphtheria, a curiosity when diphtheria was common, accounted for >50% of reported *C. diphtheriae* isolates in the United States by 1975. This indolent local infection, compared with mucosal infection, is associated with more prolonged bacterial shedding, increased contamination of the environment, and increased transmission to the pharynx and skin of close contacts. Outbreaks are associated with homelessness, crowding, poverty, alcoholism, poor hygiene, contaminated fomites, underlying dermatosis, and introduction of new strains from exogenous sources. No longer a tropical or subtropical disease, 1,100 *C. diphtheriae* infections were documented in a neighborhood in Seattle, WA (the last major U.S. outbreak), from 1971 to 1982; 86% were cutaneous, and 40% involved toxigenic strains. Cutaneous diphtheria is an important source for toxigenic *C. diphtheriae* in the United States, and its importation is frequently the source for subsequent sporadic cases of respiratory tract diphtheria. To focus attention on respiratory tract diphtheria, the condition more likely to cause acute respiratory complications and toxic manifestations, *C. diphtheria* isolates from cutaneous disease were removed from annual diphtheria statistics reported by the Centers for Disease Control and Prevention (CDC) after 1979.

PATHOGENESIS. Both toxigenic and nontoxigenic *C. diphtheriae* cause skin and mucosal infection, and rarely can cause focal infection after bacteremia. The organism usually remains in the superficial layers of skin lesions or respiratory tract mucosa, inducing local inflammatory reaction. The major virulence of the organism lies in its ability to produce the potent 62-kd polypeptide exotoxin, which inhibits protein synthesis and causes local tissue necrosis. Within the 1st few days of respiratory tract infection (usually in the pharynx), a dense necrotic coagulum of organisms, epithelial cells, fibrin, leukocytes, and erythrocytes forms, advances, and becomes a gray-brown, leather-like adherent **pseudomembrane.** (*Diphthera* is Greek for leather.) Removal is difficult and reveals a bleeding edematous submucosa. Paralysis of the palate and hypopharynx is an early local effect of diphtheritic toxin. Toxin absorption can lead to systemic manifestations: kidney tubule necrosis, thrombocytopenia, cardiomyopathy, and/or demyelination of nerves. Because the latter 2 complications can occur 2–10 wk after mucocutaneous infection, the pathophysiology in some cases is suspected to be immunologically mediated.

CLINICAL MANIFESTATIONS. The manifestations of *C. diphtheriae* infection are influenced by the anatomic site of infection, the immune status of the host, and the production and systemic distribution of toxin.

Respiratory Tract Diphtheria. In a classic description of 1,400 cases of diphtheria in California (1954), the primary focus of infection was the tonsils or pharynx (94%), with the nose and larynx the next 2 most common sites. After an average incubation period of 2–4 days, local signs and symptoms of inflammation develop. Infection of the anterior nares, which is more common among infants, causes serosanguineous, purulent, erosive rhinitis with membrane formation. Shallow ulceration of the external nares and upper lip is characteristic. In tonsillar and pharyngeal diphtheria, sore throat is the universal early symptom: only half of patients have fever, and fewer have dysphagia, hoarseness, malaise, or headache. Mild pharyngeal injection is followed by unilateral or bilateral tonsillar membrane formation, which can extend to involve the uvula (which may cause toxin-mediated paralysis), soft palate, posterior oropharynx, hypopharynx, or glottic areas (Fig. 186-1). Underlying soft tissue edema and enlarged lymph nodes can cause a bull-neck appearance. The degree of local extension correlates directly with profound prostration, bull-neck appearance, and fatality due to airway compromise or toxin-mediated complications (Fig. 186-2).

The characteristic adherent membrane, extension beyond the faucial area, dysphagia, and relative lack of fever help differentiate diphtheria from exudative pharyngitis caused by *Streptococcus pyogenes* or Epstein-Barr virus. Vincent angina, infective phlebitis with thrombosis of the jugular veins, and mucositis in patients undergoing cancer chemotherapy are usually differentiated by the clinical setting. Infection of the larynx, trachea, and bronchi can be primary or a secondary extension from the pharyngeal infection. Hoarseness, stridor, dyspnea, and croupy cough are clues. Differentiation from bacterial epiglottitis, severe viral laryngotracheobronchitis, and staphylococcal or streptococcal tracheitis hinges partially on the relative paucity of other signs and symptoms in patients with diphtheria and primarily on visualization of the adherent pseudomembrane at the time of laryngoscopy and intubation.

Patients with laryngeal diphtheria are at significant risk for suffocation because of local soft tissue edema and airway obstruc-

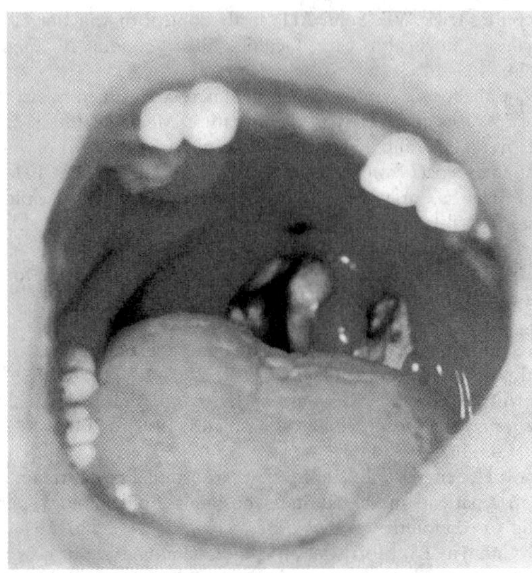

Figure 186-1. Tonsillar diphtheria. (Courtesy Franklin H. Top, MD, Professor and Head of the Department of Hygiene and Preventive Medicine, State University of Iowa, College of Medicine, Iowa City, IA; and Parke, Davis & Company's *Therapeutic Notes.*)

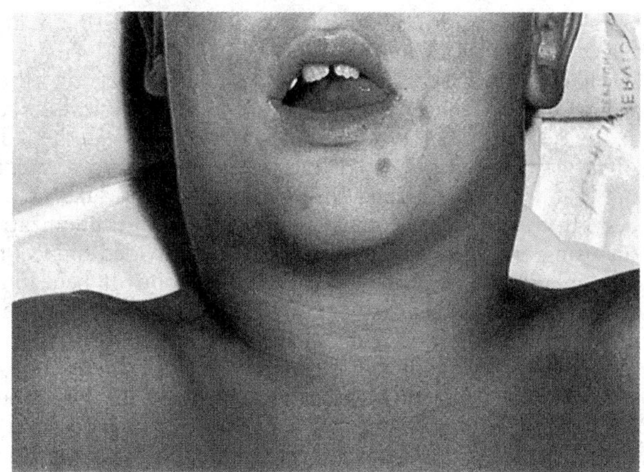

Figure 186-2. Diphtheria. Bull-neck appearance of diphtheritic cervical lymphadenopathy in a 13 yr old boy. (From the American Academy of Pediatrics: *Red Book: 2006 Report of the Committee on Infectious Diseases,* 27th ed. Elk Grove Village, IL, American Academy of Pediatrics, 2006, Atlas 2.)

tion by the diphtheritic membrane, a dense cast of respiratory epithelium, and necrotic coagulum. Establishment of an artificial airway and resection of the pseudomembrane can be lifesaving, but further obstructive complications are common, and systemic toxic complications are inevitable.

Cutaneous Diphtheria. Classic cutaneous diphtheria is an indolent, nonprogressive infection characterized by a superficial, ecthymic, nonhealing ulcer with a gray-brown membrane. Diphtheritic skin infections cannot always be differentiated from streptococcal or staphylococcal impetigo, and they frequently coexist. In most cases, a primary process—dermatosis, laceration, burns, bite, or impetigo—becomes secondarily infected with *C. diphtheriae.* Extremities are more often affected than the trunk or head. Pain, tenderness, erythema, and exudate are typical. Local hyperesthesia or hypesthesia is unusual. Respiratory tract colonization or symptomatic infection with toxic complications occurs in the minority of patients with cutaneous diphtheria. Among infected Seattle adults, 3% with cutaneous infections and 21% with symptomatic nasopharyngeal infection, with or without skin involvement, developed toxic myocarditis, neuropathy, or obstructive respiratory tract complications. All had received at least 20,000 U of equine antitoxin at the time of hospitalization.

Infection at Other Sites. *C. diphtheriae* occasionally causes mucocutaneous infections at other sites, such as the ear (otitis externa), the eye (purulent and ulcerative conjunctivitis), and the genital tract (purulent and ulcerative vulvovaginitis). The clinical setting, ulceration, membrane formation, and submucosal bleeding help differentiate diphtheria from other bacterial and viral causes. Rare cases of septicemia are described and are universally fatal. Sporadic cases of endocarditis occur, and clusters among intravenous drug users have been reported in several countries; skin was the probable portal of entry, and almost all strains were nontoxigenic. Sporadic cases of pyogenic arthritis, mainly due to nontoxigenic strains, have been reported in adults and children. Diphtheroids isolated from sterile body sites should not be routinely dismissed as contaminants without careful consideration of the clinical setting.

DIAGNOSIS. Specimens for culture should be obtained from the nose and throat and any other mucocutaneous lesion. A portion of membrane should be removed and submitted with underlying exudate. The laboratory must be notified to use selective medium. *C. diphtheriae* survives drying. If obtained in a remote area, a swab specimen can be placed in a silica gel pack and sent to the laboratory. Evaluation of a direct smear using Gram stain or specific fluorescent antibody is unreliable. Culture isolates of coryneform organisms should be identified to the species level, and toxigenicity and antimicrobial susceptibility tests should be performed for *C. diphtheriae* isolates.

COMPLICATIONS. Respiratory tract obstruction by pseudomembranes may require bronchoscopy or intubation and mechanical ventilation. Two other tissues usually remote from sites of *C. diphtheriae* infection can be significantly affected by **diphtheritic toxin:** the heart and the nervous system.

Toxic Cardiomyopathy. Toxic cardiomyopathy occurs in 10–25% of patients with respiratory diphtheria and is responsible for 50–60% of deaths. Subtle signs of myocarditis can be detected in most patients, especially the elderly, but the risk for significant complications correlates directly with the extent and severity of exudative local oropharyngeal disease and delay in administration of antitoxin. The 1st evidence of cardiac toxicity characteristically occurs during the 2nd and 3rd weeks of illness as the pharyngeal disease improves, but can appear acutely as early as the 1st wk, a poor prognostic sign, or insidiously as late as the 6th wk of illness. **Tachycardia** out of proportion to fever is common and may be evidence of cardiac toxicity or autonomic nervous system dysfunction. A prolonged PR interval and changes in the ST-T wave on an electrocardiographic tracing are relatively frequent findings; dilated and hypertrophic cardiomyopathy detected by echocardiogram has been described. Single or progressive cardiac **dysrhythmias** can occur, including 1st, 2nd, and 3rd degree heart block. Temporary transvenous pacing may improve outcomes. Atrioventricular dissociation and ventricular tachycardia are also described, the latter having a high associated mortality. Heart failure may appear insidiously or acutely. Elevation of the serum aspartate aminotransferase concentration closely parallels the severity of myonecrosis. Severe dysrhythmia portends death. Histologic postmortem findings are variable: little or diffuse myonecrosis with acute inflammatory response. Recovery from toxic myocardiopathy is usually complete, although survivors of more severe dysrhythmias can have permanent conduction defects.

Toxic Neuropathy. Neurologic complications parallel the severity of primary infection and are multiphasic in onset. Acutely or 2–3 wk after onset of oropharyngeal inflammation, it is common for hypesthesia and local **paralysis** of the soft palate to occur. Weakness of the posterior pharyngeal, laryngeal, and facial nerves may follow, causing a **nasal quality** in the voice, difficulty in swallowing, and risk for aspiration. **Cranial neuropathies** characteristically occur in the 5th wk, leading to oculomotor and ciliary paralysis, which can cause strabismus, blurred vision, or difficulty with accommodation. Symmetric **polyneuropathy** has its onset 10 days to 3 mo after oropharyngeal infection and causes principally motor deficits with diminished deep tendon reflexes. Distal muscle weakness in the extremities that progresses proximally is more commonly described than proximal muscle weakness with distal progression. Clinical and cerebrospinal fluid findings in the former are indistinguishable from those of Guillain-Barré syndrome. Paralysis of the diaphragm may ensue. Complete neurologic recovery is likely, but rarely, 2–3 wk after onset of illness, vasomotor center dysfunction can cause hypotension or cardiac failure.

Recovery from the myocarditis and neuritis is often slow but usually complete. Corticosteroids do not diminish these complications and are not recommended.

TREATMENT. Specific antitoxin is the mainstay of therapy and should be administered on the basis of clinical diagnosis. Because it neutralizes only free toxin, antitoxin efficacy diminishes with elapsed time after the onset of mucocutaneous symptoms. Equine diphtheria antitoxin is available in the United States only from the CDC. Physicians treating a case of suspected diphtheria should contact the CDC diphtheria duty officer (770-488-7100 after hours). Antitoxin is administered as a single empirical dose of 20,000–120,000 U based on the degree of toxicity, site and size of the membrane, and duration of illness. Antitoxin is probably of no value for local manifestations of cutaneous diphtheria, but its use is prudent because toxic sequelae can occur. Commercially available intravenous immunoglobulin preparations contain low titers of antibodies to diphtheria toxin; their use for therapy of diphtheria is not proven or approved. Antitoxin is not recommended for asymptomatic carriers.

The role of antimicrobial therapy is to halt toxin production, treat localized infection, and prevent transmission of the organism to contacts. *C. diphtheriae* is usually susceptible to various agents in vitro, including penicillins, erythromycin, clindamycin, rifampin, and tetracycline. Resistance to erythromycin is common in populations if the drug has been used broadly. Only erythromycin or penicillin is recommended; erythromycin is marginally superior to penicillin for eradication of nasopharyngeal carriage. Appropriate therapy is erythromycin (40–50 mg/kg/day divided every 6 hr PO or IV; maximum 2 g/day), aqueous crystalline penicillin G (100,000–150,000 U/kg/day divided every 6 hr IV or IM), or procaine penicillin (25,000–50,000 U/kg/day divided every 12 hr IM). Antibiotic therapy is not a substitute for antitoxin therapy. Therapy is given for 14 days. Some patients with cutaneous diphtheria have been treated for 7–10 days. Elimination of the organism should be documented by at least 2 successive negative cultures from the nose and throat (or skin) obtained 24 hr apart after completion of therapy. Treatment with erythromycin is repeated if either culture yields *C. diphtheriae.*

SUPPORTIVE CARE. Patients with pharyngeal diphtheria are placed on droplet precautions, and patients with cutaneous diphtheria are placed on contact precautions until the cultures taken after cessation of therapy are negative. Cutaneous wounds are cleaned thoroughly with soap and water. Bed rest is essential during the acute phase of disease, usually for ≥2 wk until the risk for symptomatic cardiac damage has passed, with a return to physical activity guided by the degree of toxicity and cardiac involvement.

PROGNOSIS. The prognosis for patients with diphtheria depends on the virulence of the organism (subspecies gravis has the highest fatality rate), patient age, immunization status, site of infection, and speed of administration of the antitoxin. Mechanical obstruction from laryngeal diphtheria or bull-neck diphtheria and the complications of myocarditis account for most diphtheria-related deaths. The case fatality rate of almost 10% for respiratory tract diphtheria has not changed in 50 yr; the rate was 8% in a Vietnamese series described in 2004. At recovery, administration of diphtheria toxoid is indicated to complete the primary series or booster doses of immunization, because not all patients develop antibodies to diphtheritic toxin after infection.

PREVENTION. Protection against serious disease caused by imported or indigenously acquired *C. diphtheriae* depends on immunization. In the absence of a precisely determined minimum protective level for diphtheria antitoxin, the presumed minimum is 0.01–0.10 IU/mL. In outbreaks, 90% of individuals with clinical disease have had antibody values of <0.01 IU/mL, and 92% of asymptomatic carriers have had values of >0.1 IU/mL. In serosurveys in the United States and Western Europe, where almost universal immunization during childhood has been achieved, 25 to >60% of adults lack protective antitoxin levels, with very low levels common in the elderly.

All suspected diphtheria cases should be reported to local and state health departments. Investigation is aimed at preventing secondary cases in exposed individuals and at determining the source and carriers to halt spread to unexposed individuals. Reported rates of carriage in household contacts of case patients are 0–25%. The risk for developing diphtheria after household exposure to a case is approximately 2%, and the risk is 0.3% after similar exposure to a carrier.

Asymptomatic Case Contacts. All household contacts and those who have had intimate respiratory or habitual physical contact with a patient are closely monitored for illness through the 7 day incubation period. Cultures of the nose, throat, and any cutaneous lesions are performed. Antimicrobial prophylaxis is presumed effective and is administered regardless of immunization status using erythromycin (40–50 mg/kg/day divided qid PO for 7 days; maximum 2 g/day) or a single injection of benzathine penicillin G (600,000 U IM for <30 kg, 1,200,000 U IM for ≥30 kg). Diphtheria toxoid vaccine, in age-appropriate form, is given to immunized individuals who have not received a booster dose within 5 yr. Children who have not received their 4th dose should be vaccinated. Those who have received fewer than 3 doses of diphtheria toxoid or who have uncertain immunization status are immunized with an age-appropriate preparation on a primary schedule.

Asymptomatic Carriers. When an asymptomatic carrier is identified, antimicrobial prophylaxis is given for 7 days and an age-appropriate preparation of diphtheria toxoid is administered immediately if a booster has not been given within 1 yr. Individuals are placed on droplet precautions (respiratory tract colonization) or contact precautions (cutaneous colonization only) until at least 2 subsequent cultures obtained 24 hr apart after cessation of therapy are negative.

Repeat cultures are performed about 2 wk after completion of therapy for cases and carriers, and, if positive, an additional 10 day course of oral erythromycin should be given and follow-up cultures performed. Susceptibility testing of isolates should be performed as erythromycin resistance is reported. Neither antimicrobial agent eradicates carriage in 100% of individuals. In 1 report, 21% of carriers failed a single course of therapy. Antitoxin is not recommended for asymptomatic close contacts or carriers, even if inadequately immunized. Transmission of diphtheria in modern hospitals is rare. Only those with an unusual contact with respiratory or oral secretions should be managed as contacts. Investigation of the casual contacts of patients and carriers or persons in the community without known exposure has yielded extremely low carriage rates and is not routinely recommended.

Vaccine. Universal immunization with diphtheria toxoid throughout life, to provide constant protective antitoxin levels and to reduce severity of *C. diphtheriae* disease, is the only effective control measure. Although immunization does not preclude subsequent respiratory or cutaneous carriage of toxigenic *C. diphtheriae,* it decreases local tissue spread, prevents toxic complications, diminishes transmission of the organism, and provides herd immunity when at least 70–80% of a population is immunized.

Diphtheria toxoid is prepared by formaldehyde treatment of toxin, standardized for potency, and adsorbed to aluminum salts, which enhance immunogenicity. Two preparations of diphtheria toxoids are formulated according to the limit of flocculation (Lf) content, a measure of the quantity of toxoid. The pediatric preparation (i.e., DTaP, DT) contains 6.7–25.0 Lf units of diphtheria toxoid per 0.5 mL dose; the adult preparation (dT) contains no more than 2 Lf units of toxoid per 0.5 mL dose. The higher-potency (D) formulation of toxoid is used for primary series and booster doses for children through 6 yr of age because of superior immunogenicity and minimal reactogenicity. For individuals 7 years of age or older, dT is recommended for the primary series and booster doses because the lower concentration of diphtheria toxoid is adequately immunogenic and because increasing the content of diphtheria toxoid heightens reactogenicity with increasing age.

For children from 6 wk to 7 yr of age, five 0.5-mL doses of diphtheria-containing (D) vaccine are given in a primary series, including 3 doses at 2, 4, and 6 mo of age, with a 4th dose, an integral part of the primary series, 9–12 mo after the third dose. A booster dose is given at 4–6 yr of age (unless the 4th primary dose was administered after the 4th birthday). For persons 7 yr of age and older, three 0.5 mL doses of diphtheria-containing (d) vaccine are given in a primary series of 2 doses 4–8 wk apart and a 3rd dose 6–12 mo after the 2nd dose. The only contraindication to tetanus and diphtheria toxoid is a history of neurologic or severe hypersensitivity reaction after a previous dose. For children <7 yr of age in whom pertussis immunization is contraindicated, DT is used. Those begun with DTaP or DT before 1 yr of age should have a total of five 0.5 mL doses of diphtheria-containing (D) vaccines by 6 yr of age. For those beginning at around 1 yr of age, the primary series is three 0.5 mL doses of diphtheria-containing (D) vaccine, with a booster given at 4–6 yr, unless the 3rd dose was given after the 4th birthday.

A booster dose, consisting of an adult preparation of Tdap, is recommended at 11–12 yr of age. Adolescents 13–18 yr of age who missed the 11–12 year old Td or Tdap booster dose or in whom it has been ≥5 yr since the Td booster dose also should receive a single dose of Tdap if they have completed the DTP/DTaP series.

There is no association of DT or dT with convulsions. Local adverse effects alone do not preclude continued use. Persons who experience Arthus-type hypersensitivity reactions or a temperature >103°F (39.4°C) after a dose of dT, which is rare, usually have high serum tetanus antitoxin levels and should not be given dT more frequently than every 10 yr, even if a significant tetanus-prone injury is sustained. DT or dT preparation can be given concurrently with other vaccines. *Haemophilus influenzae* conjugate vaccines containing diphtheria toxoid (PRP-D) or the variant of diphtheria toxin, CRM_{197} protein (HbOC), are not substitutes for diphtheria toxoid immunization and do not affect reactogenicity.

Centers for Disease Control and Prevention: Fatal respiratory diphtheria in a US traveler to Haiti—Pennsylvania, 2003. *MMWR* 2004;52:1285–1286.

Efstratiou A, Engler KH, Mazurova IK, et al: Current approaches to the laboratory diagnosis of diphtheria. *J Infect Dis* 2000;181(Suppl 1):S134–S138.

Hadfield TL, McEvoy P, Polotshy Y, et al: The pathology of diphtheria. *J Infect Dis* 2000;181(Suppl 1):S116–S120.

Kadirova R, Kartoglu HU, Strebel PM: Clinical characteristics and management of 676 hospitalized diphtheria cases, Kyrgyz Republic, 1995. *J Infect Dis* 2000;181(Suppl 1):S110–S115.

Marston CK, Famieson F, Cahoon F, et al: Persistence of a distinct *Corynebacterium diphtheriae* clonal group within two communities in the United States and Canada where diphtheria is endemic. *J Clin Microbiol* 2001;39:1586–1590.

Chapter 187 ■ *Listeria monocytogenes*

Robert S. Baltimore

Listeriosis in humans is caused principally by *Listeria monocytogenes,* 1 of 7 species of the genus *Listeria* that are widely distributed in the environment and throughout the food chain. Human infections can usually be traced to an animal reservoir. Infection occurs most commonly at the extremes of age. In the pediatric population, perinatal infections predominate and occur usually secondary to maternal infection or colonization. Outside the newborn period, disease is most commonly encountered in immunosuppressed children and adults and in the elderly. In the United States, food-borne outbreaks are caused by improperly processed dairy products and contaminated vegetables, and they principally affect the same individuals at risk for sporadic disease.

ETIOLOGY. Members of the genus *Listeria* are facultatively anaerobic, non-spore-forming, motile, gram-positive bacilli. The 7 *Listeria* species are divided into 2 genomically distinct groups based on DNA-DNA hybridization studies. One group contains the species *L. murrayi* and *L. grayi,* considered nonpathogenic. The 2nd group contains 5 species: the nonhemolytic species *L. innocua* and *L. welshimeri* and the hemolytic species *L. monocytogenes, L. seeligeri,* and *L. ivanovii. L. ivanovii* is pathogenic primarily in animals, and the vast majority of both human and animal disease is due to *L. monocytogenes.*

Subtyping of *L. monocytogenes* isolates for epidemiologic purposes has been attempted using heat-stable somatic O and heat-labile flagellar H antigens, phage typing, ribotyping, and multilocus enzyme electrophoresis. Electrophoretic typing demonstrates the clonal structure of populations of *L. monocytogenes* as well as the sharing of populations between human and animal sources.

Selected biochemical tests together with the demonstration of **tumbling motility, umbrella-type formation below the surface in semisolid medium,** hemolysis, and a typical cyclic adenosine monophosphate (cAMP) test are usually sufficient to establish a presumptive identification of *L. monocytogenes.*

EPIDEMIOLOGY. *L. monocytogenes* is widespread in nature, has been isolated throughout the environment, and is associated with epizootic disease and asymptomatic carriage in more than 42 species of wild and domestic animals and 22 avian species. Epizootic disease in large animals such as sheep and cattle is associated with abortion and "circling disease," a form of basilar meningitis. *L. monocytogenes* is isolated from sewage, silage, and soil where it survives for >295 days. The overall disease rate in the U.S. is approximately 0.7/100,000; however, in infants it is 10/100,000 and in the elderly it is 1.4/100,000. The annual incidence of listeriosis decreased by 44% between 1989 and 1993, and by 38% from 1996 to 2002. However, outbreaks continue to occur. In 2002, an outbreak that resulted in 54 illnesses, 8 deaths, and 3 fetal deaths in 9 states was traced to consumption of contaminated turkey meat. The rate varies between states. Epidemic human listeriosis has been associated with food-borne transmission in several large outbreaks, especially associated with aged soft cheeses; improperly pasteurized milk and milk products; contaminated raw and ready-to-eat beef, pork, poultry, and packaged meats; and vegetables grown on farms where the ground is contaminated with the feces of colonized animals. The incidence of food-transmitted *Listeria* in the U.S. in 2004 was 2.7 cases per million population. The ability of *L. monocytogenes* to grow at temperatures as low as 4°C increases the risk for transmission from aged soft cheeses and stored contaminated food. Small clusters of nosocomial person-to-person transmission have occurred in hospital nurseries and obstetric suites. Sporadic endemic listeriosis is less well characterized. Likely routes include food-borne infection, zoonotic spread, and person-to-person transmission. Zoonotic transmission with cutaneous infections occurs in veterinarians and farmers who handle sick animals.

Reported cases of listeriosis are clustered at the extremes of age. Some studies have shown higher rates in males and a seasonal predominance in the late summer and fall in the Northern hemisphere. Outside the newborn period and during pregnancy, disease is usually reported in patients with underlying immunosuppression, with a 100–300 times increased risk in HIV-infected persons and in the elderly (Table 187-1).

The incubation period is defined only for common-source food-borne disease and is 21–30 days. Asymptomatic carriage and fecal excretion are reported in 1% of healthy persons and 5% of abattoir workers, but duration of excretion, when studied, is short (<1 mo).

PATHOLOGY. One of the major concepts of *Listeria* pathology and pathogenesis is its ability to survive as an intracellular pathogen.

TABLE 187-1. Types of *Listeria monocytogenes* Infections

Listeriosis in pregnancy
Neonatal listeriosis
Early onset
Late onset
Food-borne outbreaks
Listeriosis in normal children and adults (rare)
Focal listeria infections (e.g., meningitis, endocarditis, pneumonia, liver abscess, ostomyelitis, septic arthritis)
Listeriosis in immunocompromised persons
Lymphohematogenous malignancies
Collagen vascular diseases
Diabetes mellitus
HIV infection
Transplant recipients
Renal failure with peritoneal dialysis
Listeriosis in the elderly

Listeria incites a mononuclear response and elaboration of cytokines producing multisystem disease, particularly pyogenic meningitis. Granulomatous reactions and microabscess formation develop in many organs, including liver, lungs, adrenals, kidneys, central nervous system (CNS), and, notably, the placenta. Animal models demonstrate **translocation,** the transfer of intraluminal organisms across intact intestinal mucosa. Histologic examination of tissues including the placenta shows granulomatous inflammation and microabscess formation. Intracellular organisms can often be demonstrated using special stains.

PATHOGENESIS. *Listeria* organisms usually enter the host through the gastrointestinal tract. Studies of intracellular and intercellular spread of *L. monocytogenes* have revealed a complex pathogenesis. Four pathogenic steps are described: internalization, escape from the phagocytic vacuole, **nucleation of actin filaments,** and cell-to-cell spread. Genes involved in each step are known, and isogenic mutants have been shown to reduce virulence. **Listeriolysin,** a hemolysin and the best-characterized virulence factor, probably mediates lysis of vacuoles and is responsible for the zone of hemolysis when grown on blood-containing solid media. In cell-to-cell spread, locomotion proceeds via cytochalasin-sensitive polymerization of actin filaments, which extrude the bacteria in pseudopods, which are phagocytosed by adjacent cells, necessitating escape from a double-membrane vacuole. This mechanism protects intracellular bacteria from the humoral arm of immunity and is responsible for the well-known requirement of T cell–mediated activation of monocytes by lymphokines for clearance of infection and establishment of immunity. The role of opsonizing antibody in protecting against infection is unclear.

CLINICAL MANIFESTATIONS. The clinical presentation of listeriosis is highly dependent on the age of the patient and the circumstances of the infection.

Listeriosis in Pregnancy. *L. monocytogenes* has been grown from placental and fetal cultures of pregnancies ending in spontaneous abortion. The usual presentation in the 2nd and 3rd trimesters is a flulike illness that may result in bacteremia seeding the uterine contents. Rarely is maternal listeriosis severe, but meningitis in pregnancy has been reported. Recognition and treatment at this stage have been associated with normal pregnancy outcomes, but the fetus may not be infected even if listeriosis in the mother is not treated. In other instances, placental listeriosis develops with infection of the fetus that may be associated with stillbirth or premature delivery. Delivery of an infected premature fetus is associated with 50–90% infant mortality. Disseminated disease is apparent at birth, often with a diffuse pustular rash. Infection in the mother usually resolves without specific therapy after delivery, but postpartum fever and infected lochia may occur.

Neonatal Listeriosis. Two clinical presentations are recognized for neonatal listeriosis: **early-onset neonatal disease** (<5 days, usually within 1–2 days), which is a predominantly septicemic form, and **late-onset neonatal disease** (>5 days, mean 14 days), which is a predominantly meningitic form (Table 187-2). The principal characteristics of the 2 presentations resemble the clinical syndromes described for group B streptococcus (see Chapter 183).

Early-onset disease occurs from milder transplacental or ascending infections from the female genital tract. There is a strong association with recovery of *L. monocytogenes* from the maternal genital tract, obstetric complications, prematurity, and neonatal sepsis with multiorgan involvement without CNS localization. The mortality rate is approximately 20–30%.

The epidemiology of late-onset disease is poorly understood. Onset is usually after 5 days but before 30 days of age. Affected infants frequently are full-term, and the mothers are culture negative and asymptomatic. The presenting syndrome is usually of purulent meningitis, which, if adequately treated, has a mortality rate of <20%.

Postneonatal Infections. Listeriosis beyond the newborn period may rarely occur in otherwise healthy children but is most often encountered in association with underlying malignancies or immunosuppression. When associated with food-borne outbreaks, disease may present with gastrointestinal symptoms or any of the *Listeria* syndromes. The clinical presentation is usually meningitis, less commonly sepsis, and rarely other CNS involvement such as cerebritis, meningoencephalitis, brain abscess, spinal cord abscess, or a focus outside the CNS such as suppurative arthritis, osteomyelitis, endocarditis, peritonitis (associated with peritoneal dialysis), or liver abscess. It is not known whether the frequent gastrointestinal signs and symptoms result from enteric infection, because the mode of acquisition is often unknown.

DIAGNOSIS. Listeriosis should be included in the differential diagnosis of infections in pregnancy, neonatal sepsis and meningitis, and of sepsis or meningitis in older children with underlying malignancies, receiving immunosuppressive therapy, or following transplantation. The diagnosis is established by culture of *L. monocytogenes* from blood or cerebrospinal fluid (CSF). Cultures from the maternal cervix, vagina, or lochia and, if possible, placenta should be obtained when intrauterine infections lead to premature delivery or early-onset neonatal sepsis. Cultures from closed space infections may also be helpful. It is helpful to alert the laboratory to suspected cases so that *Listeria* isolates are not discarded as contaminating diphtheroids.

Histologic examination of the placenta is useful. Polymerase chain reaction assays detect *L. monocytogenes*, but commercial assays are not available. Serodiagnostic tests have not proved useful.

TABLE 187-2. Characteristic Features of Early- and Late-Onset Neonatal Listeriosis

EARLY ONSET (<5 DAYS)	LATE ONSET (≥5 DAYS)
Positive maternal *Listeria* culture	Negative maternal *Listeria* culture
Obstetric complications	Uncomplicated pregnancy
Premature delivery	Term delivery
Low birthweight	Normal birthweight
Neonatal sepsis	Neonatal meningitis
Mean age at onset 1.5 days	Mean age at onset 14.2 days
Mortality rate >30%	Mortality rate <10%
	Nosocomial outbreaks

Differential Diagnosis. Listeriosis is indistinguishable clinically from neonatal sepsis and meningitis due to other organisms. The presence of increased peripheral blood monocytes suggests the possibility of listeriosis. Monocytosis or lymphocytosis may be modest or striking. Beyond the neonatal period, *L. monocytogenes* CNS infection is associated with fever, headache, seizures, and signs of meningeal irritation. The brainstem characteristically may be affected. The white blood cell concentration may vary from normal to slightly elevated, and the CSF laboratory findings are variable. Polymorphonuclear leukocytes or mononuclear cells may predominate, with shifts from polymorphonuclear to mononuclear cells in sequential lumbar punctures. A low CSF glucose level that mirrors the severity of disease is usually found. The CSF protein is moderately elevated. *L. monocytogenes* is isolated from the blood in 40–75% of cases of meningitis due to the organism. Deep focal infections, such as endocarditis, osteomyelitis, and liver abscess due to *L. monocytogenes* are also indistinguishable clinically from the more common organisms associated with these sites. Cutaneous infections should be suspected in patients with a history of contact with animals, especially products of conception.

TREATMENT. The emergence of multiple antibiotic resistance mandates routine susceptibility testing of all isolates. The recommended therapy is ampicillin (100–200 mg/kg/day divided every 6 hr IV; 200–400 mg/kg/day divided every 6 hr IV if meningitis is present) alone or in combination with an aminoglycoside (5.0–7.5 mg/kg/day divided every 8 hr IV). The adult dose is ampicillin 4–6 g/day divided every 6 hr plus an aminoglycoside. The ampicillin dose is doubled if meningitis is present. Special attention to dosing is required for neonates, who require longer dosing intervals due to the longer half-lives of the antibiotics. Combination therapy is recommended for severe infections. Isolates usually demonstrate tolerance, with the minimum bactericidal concentration ≥32 times the minimum inhibitory concentration, to ampicillin as well as penicillin, erythromycin, and tetracycline. Addition of gentamicin lowers the minimum bactericidal concentration. *L. monocytogenes* is not susceptible to the cephalosporins, including 3rd generation cephalosporins. If these agents are used for empirical therapy for neonatal sepsis or meningitis in a newborn, ampicillin must be added for the possibility of *L. monocytogenes* infection. Vancomycin, or vancomycin and an aminoglycoside, is an alternative, as are trimethoprim-sulfamethoxazole and erythromycin. The duration of therapy is usually 2–3 wk, with 3 wk recommended for immunocompromised persons or those with meningitis. A longer course is needed for endocarditis, brain abscess, or osteomyelitis.

PROGNOSIS. Early gestational listeriosis may be associated with abortion or stillbirth, although maternal infection with sparing of the fetus has been reported. No convincing evidence shows that *L. monocytogenes* is associated with repeated spontaneous abortions in humans. The mortality rate is >50% for premature infants infected in utero, 30% for early onset neonatal sepsis, 15% for late-onset neonatal meningitis, and <10% in older children with prompt institution of appropriate antimicrobial therapy. Mental retardation, hydrocephalus, and other CNS sequelae are reported in survivors of *Listeria* meningitis.

PREVENTION. Listeriosis can be prevented by pasteurization and thorough cooking of foods. Irradiation of meat products may also be beneficial. Consumption of unpasteurized or improperly processed dairy products, especially aged soft cheeses, uncooked and precooked meat products that have been stored at 4°C for extended periods, and unwashed vegetables should be avoided (Table 187-3). This is particularly important during pregnancy and for immunocompromised persons. Infected domestic animals should be avoided when possible. Careful handwashing is essential to prevent nosocomial spread within obstetric and neonatal units. Immunocompromised patients given prophylaxis with trimethoprim-sulfamethoxazole are protected from *Listeria* infections. Cases and especially outbreaks should be reported immediately to public health authorities so timely investigation can be initiated in order to interrupt transmission from the contaminated source.

TABLE 187-3. Prevention of Food-borne Listeriosis

General recommendations:

- Thoroughly cook raw food from animal sources, such as beef, pork, or poultry.
- Wash raw vegetables thoroughly before eating.
- Keep uncooked meats separate from vegetables and from cooked foods and ready-to-eat foods.
- Avoid unpasteurized (raw) milk or foods made from unpasteurized milk.
- Wash hands, knives, and cutting boards after handling uncooked foods.
- Consume perishable and ready-to-eat foods as soon as possible.

Recommendations for persons at high risk, such as pregnant women and persons with weakened immune systems, in addition to general recommendations (above):

- Do not eat hotdogs, luncheon meats, or deli meats, unless they are reheated until steaming hot.
- Avoid getting fluid from hot dog packages on other foods, utensils, and food preparation surfaces, and wash hands after handling hot dogs, luncheon meats, and deli meats.
- Do not eat soft cheeses (e.g., feta, Brie, and Camembert), blue-veined cheeses, or Mexican-style cheeses (e.g., queso blanco, queso fresco, and Panela) unless they have labels that clearly state they are made from pasteurized milk.
- Do not eat refrigerated pâtés or meat spreads. Canned or shelf-stable pâtés and meat spreads may be eaten.
- Do not eat refrigerated smoked seafood, unless it is contained in a cooked dish, such as a casserole. Refrigerated smoked seafood, such as salmon, trout, whitefish, cod, tuna or mackerel, is most often labeled as "nova-style," "lox," "kippered," "smoked," or "jerky." The fish is found in the refrigerator section or sold at deli counters of grocery stores and delicatessens. Canned or shelf-stable smoked seafood may be eaten.

Adapted from the Centers for Disease Control and Prevention: http://www.cdc.gov/ncidod/dbmd/diseaseinfo/listeriosis_g.htm#prevented. Accessed November 2006.

Borucki MK, Kim SH, Call DR, et al: Selective discrimination of *Listeria monocytogenes* epidemic strains by a mixed-genome DNA microarray compared to discrimination by pulsed-field gel electrophoresis, ribotyping, and multilocus sequence typing. *J Clin Microbiol* 2004;42:5270–5276.

Braden CR: Listeriosis. *Pediatr Infect Dis J* 2003;22:745–746.

Eckburg PB, Montoya JG, Vosti KL: Brain abscess due to *Listeria monocytogenes:* Five cases and a review of the literature. *Medicine* 2001;80:223–235.

Lorber B: Listeriosis. *Clin Infect Dis* 1997;24:1–9.

Mylonakis E, Hohmann EL, Calderwood SB: Central nervous system infection with *Listeria monocytogenes:* 33 years' experience at a general hospital and review of 776 episodes from the literature. *Medicine* 1998;77:313–336.

Mylonakis E, Palious M, Hohmann, EL, et al: Listeriosis during pregnancy. A case series and review of 222 cases. *Medicine* 2002;81:260–269.

Pamer EG: Immune responses to *Listeria monocytogenes*. *Nature Rev Immunol* 2004;4:812–823.

Portnoy DA, Auerbuch V, Glomski IJ: The cell biology of *Listeria monocytogenes* infection: The intersection of bacterial pathogenesis and cell-mediated immunity. *J Cell Biol* 2002;158:409–414.

Posfay-Barbe KM, Wald ER: Listeriosis. *Pediatr Rev* 2004;25:151–159.

Sauders BD, Fortes ES, Morse DL, et al: Molecular subtyping to detect human listeriosis clusters. *Emerg Infect Dis* 2003;9:672–680.

Schlech WF III: Foodborne listeriosis. *Clin Infect Dis* 2000;31:770–775.

Southwick FS, Purich DL: Intracellular pathogenesis of listeriosis. *N Engl J Med* 1996;334:770–776.

Chapter 188 ■ *Actinomyces*

Richard F. Jacobs and Gordon E. Schutze

Actinomyces organisms are slow-growing, gram-positive bacteria that are part of the endogenous oral flora in humans. Their filamentous structure gives them a fungus-like appearance. Infection caused by these bacteria is termed **actinomycosis,** which is a chronic, granulomatous, suppurative disease characterized by direct extension to contiguous tissue across natural anatomic barriers with the formation of numerous draining fistulas and sinus tracts. These infections usually involve the cervicofacial, thoracic, abdominal, or pelvic regions.

ETIOLOGY. *Actinomyces* is a member of the order Actinomycetales, which includes gram-positive filamentous bacteria such as *Nocardia, Streptomyces,* and mycobacteria. *Actinomyces israelii* is the predominant species causing human actinomycosis. Other implicated species, in order of importance, include *Propionibacterium propionicum* (formerly *Arachnia propionicum*), *A. turicensis, A. odontolyticus, A. meyeri, A. naeslundii, A. viscosus, A. europaeus,* and *A. radingae. Arcanobacterium pyogenes* (previously in the *Actinomyces* genus) also causes human actinomycosis.

Actinomyces organisms are non-spore-forming, gram-positive, non-acid-fast, nonmotile, facultative, or strictly anaerobes bacilli with variable morphology ranging from diphtheroid to mycelial with short branching forms. *Actinomyces* organisms are part of the endogenous flora of mucous membranes and are often found in clinical specimens such as sputum, bronchial washes, purulent exudates, and tissues obtained surgically or at necropsy. Staining of crushed tissue specimens rinsed with sterile saline or purulent exudate stained by Gram or acid-fast procedures may reveal organisms within the classic sulfur granules, which are characteristically associated with pulmonary disease caused by *A. israelii* or *A. meyeri.* Cultures on brain-heart infusion agar incubated at 37°C anaerobically (95% nitrogen and 5% carbon dioxide) and a separate set incubated aerobically reveal organisms within the lines of streak at 24–48 hr. *A. israelii* colonies appear as loose masses of delicate, branching filaments with a characteristic spider-like growth. Colonies of *A. naeslundii, A. viscosus,* and *P. propionicum* may have similar growth characteristics. Biochemical testing is frequently used for speciation but is limited by the complexity within this group. Newer speciation methods are based on 16S recombinant RNA sequence analysis.

EPIDEMIOLOGY. Actinomycosis occurs worldwide among all ages, with higher incidence among males, possibly related to increased trauma or poorer dental hygiene. There is no relationship to race, season, or occupation. In a review of 85 cases of actinomycosis, 27% were in persons <20 yr of age, with 7% among children <10 yr of age. The youngest patient in this series was 28 days old. The source of human infection is almost always endogenous flora. The incidence has declined due to improved oral hygiene and early antibiotic treatment of oral infections. Although actinomycosis is not a common opportunistic infection, disease has been associated with corticosteroid use, leukemia, renal failure, congenital immunodeficiency diseases, and HIV infection. In 1 study, antecedent disease and surgery predisposed 81 of 181 subjects to infection.

PATHOGENESIS. The 3 significant sites of *Actinomyces* infection are, in order of frequency, cervicofacial, abdominal and pelvic, and pulmonary, although infection may involve any organ in the body. Infection typically follows introduction of the organism into tissues after trauma or surgery. The use of intrauterine devices (IUDs) may predispose to development of pelvic actinomycosis. Pulmonary actinomycosis occurs after inhalation or aspiration of organisms, introduction of a colonized foreign body, or spread from an existing cervicofacial or abdominal actinomycotic infection.

Infection spreads contiguously and, rarely, hematogenously. Actinomycosis is a chronic, suppurative, scarring inflammatory process. Sites of infection show dense cellular infiltrates and suppuration that form many interconnecting abscesses and sinus tracts. This may be followed by cicatricial healing from which the organism spreads by burrowing along fascial planes, causing deep, communicating scarred sinus tracts. **Sulfur granules** are characteristic of actinomycosis. On hematoxylin-eosin stain, they are an adherent mass of polymorphonuclear neutrophils attached to the radially arranged eosinophilic clubs of the granule, which is the host immune response. They may be microscopic or macroscopic, and are typically yellow, accounting for their name, but may be white, gray, or brown.

Actinomycosis, even in closed infections, is usually, if not always, polymicrobial in nature, involving mixed bacteria. In a large study of more than 650 cases, infection with *Actinomyces* was identified in pure culture in only 1 case and usually was identified with other oral flora, most notably members of the **HACEK group,** which includes *Haemophilus aphrophilus, Actinobacillus actinomycetemcomitans, Cardiobacterium hominis, Eikenella corrodens,* and *Kingella kingae. A. actinomycetemcomitans* is a fastidious, gram-negative bacillus that is part of the oral flora and has been implicated as a pathogen in periodontal disease. Other bacterial species frequently isolated concomitantly in human actinomycosis include *Fusobacterium, Bacteroides, Capnocytophaga, Staphylococcus, Streptococcus, Enterococcus,* and Enterobacteriaceae.

CLINICAL MANIFESTATIONS. The 3 major forms of actinomycosis—cervicofacial, abdominal and pelvic, and pulmonary—arise by different routes but may progress to other forms of the disease. Actinomycosis in children suggests an underlying immunodeficiency, especially chronic granulomatous disease (see Chapter 129).

Cervicofacial Actinomycosis. There is often a history of oral trauma, oral surgery, dental procedures, or caries that facilitates organisms entering cervicofacial tissues. Cervicofacial actinomycosis usually presents as a painless, slow-growing, hard mass and can produce cutaneous fistulas, a condition commonly known as **lumpy jaw** (Fig. 188-1). Less frequently, cervicofacial actinomycosis presents clinically as an acute pyogenic infection with a tender, fluctuant mass with trismus, firm swelling, and fistulas with drainage containing the characteristic sulfur granules. Bone is not involved early in the disease, but periostitis, mandibular osteomyelitis, or perimandibular abscess may develop. Infection may spread by way of sinus tracts to the cranial bones, which may give rise to meningitis. The ability of *Actinomyces* to burrow through tissue planes and even bone is a key difference between actinomycosis and nocardiosis. The cervicofacial form of actinomycosis has the best prognosis, and is usually cured with surgical debridement and excision combined with antibiotic therapy.

Abdominal and Pelvic Actinomycosis. There is characteristically some disruption of the mucosa of the gastrointestinal tract, usually as a result of an acute gastrointestinal perforation or abdominal trauma. Patients often present with a history of gastrointestinal surgery, diverticulitis, or appendicitis. Of all the forms of actinomycosis, delayed diagnosis is most typical for abdominal and pelvic infection. Gastrointestinal disease clinically develops as appendicitis in 25% of cases but can be manifested as various ulcerative diseases. Infection classically appears after appendectomy with a firm, irregular mass in the ileocecal area that softens and then drains externally through a fistula. Hepatic involvement occurs in approximately 15% of abdominal actinomycosis cases, with solitary or multiple liver abscesses or in a

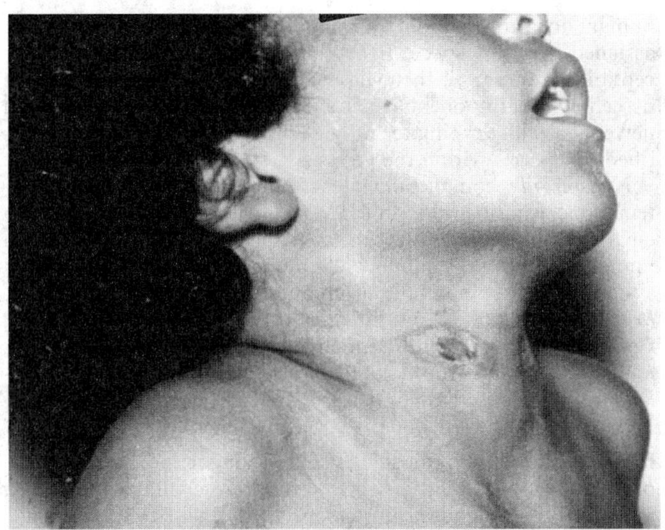

Figure 188-1. A 2 yr old boy with HIV infection who has cervicofacial actinomycosis and a chronic draining fistula.

miliary pattern. The clinical course is indolent, with chills, fever, night sweats, and weight loss, and is similar to the presentation of tuberculous peritonitis. Infection usually spreads by direct extension or, rarely, hematogenously, which may involve any tissue or organ, including muscle, spleen, kidneys, fallopian tubes, ovaries, uterus, testes, bladder, or rectum.

Women using IUDs are at risk for developing pelvic actinomycosis, which classically presents with vaginal discharge, pelvic pain, abdominal pain, menorrhagia, fever, pelvic mass, and a history of pelvic inflammatory disease. The risk is higher if the IUD has been in place for >2–3 yr.

Pulmonary Actinomycosis. Neither the clinical nor the radiographic presentation of pulmonary actinomycosis is specific. Pulmonary actinomycosis may present as an endobronchial infection, a tumor-like lesion, diffuse pneumonia, or a pleural effusion. Principal symptoms include fever, productive cough, chest pain, and weight loss. Infection frequently dissects along tissue planes and may extend through the chest wall or diaphragm, characteristically producing numerous sinus tracts that contain small abscesses and purulent drainage. Other complications include bony destruction of adjacent ribs, sternum, and vertebral bodies. Pyogenic mediastinitis has been attributed to *A. odontolyticus* in lung transplant recipients. Multiple lobe involvement of the lungs is occasionally found. Predisposing conditions include dental caries, aspiration, thermal or chemical inhalation injury, introduction of a colonized foreign body, and pre-existing cervicofacial or abdominal disease. Accurate diagnosis is difficult because of the propensity of *Actinomyces* to infect pre-existing pulmonary cavities. Diagnosis can be confirmed by examining purulent sinus tract drainage for sulfur granules, and by appropriate cultures. The significance of *Actinomyces* in sputum or bronchoscopy specimens is limited because these organisms are normal oral flora.

Other Forms. Laryngeal actinomycosis rarely has been reported in older teenagers. Oropharyngeal colonization with *Actinomyces* may be involved in the development of obstructive tonsillar hypertrophy. *A. pyogenes* only rarely has been implicated as a cause of human infection, although there are reported cases of septicemia, endocarditis, meningitis, arthritis, empyema, pneumonia, otitis media, cystitis, mastoiditis, appendicitis, and cutaneous infection.

Severe forms of periodontitis, particularly localized juvenile periodontitis, are associated with *Actinomyces,* especially in children 10–19 yr of age. *Actinomyces* has a propensity for infecting heart valves and results in an insidious presentation of endocarditis, with fever present in less than half of cases.

DIAGNOSIS AND DIFFERENTIAL DIAGNOSIS. Microscopic examination with appropriate stains and culture of purulent drainage from fistulas, abscesses, draining sinus tracts, bronchoalveolar lavage, and sputum can reveal *Actinomyces.* Except for *A. meyeri,* which is nonbranching, *Actinomyces* organisms appear as branching, filamentous rods. Inoculation of anaerobic and aerobic cultures enhances the yield of cultures. Gram, Gomori methenamine silver, or Giemsa stains of purulent material or tissue reveal diagnostic filamentous, branching bacteria at the periphery of sulfur granules. *Nocardia* is indistinguishable from *Actinomyces* on Gram stain, but *Nocardia* stains with the modified acid-fast stain, unlike *Actinomyces.*

A cranial CT or MRI is important to evaluate the possibility of cerebral actinomycosis in patients with cervicofacial disease or neurologic findings. Infection that invades across tissue planes and ignores anatomic boundaries is highly suggestive of actinomycosis. Abdominal CT scan may be helpful in identifying the presence of a contrast-enhancing, multicystic lesion, which could be approached by CT-guided needle biopsy for culture.

The masslike lesions of actinomycosis may present as a tumor, necessitating invasive approaches for diagnosis. Actinomycosis must be differentiated from other chronic inflammatory infections, including tuberculosis, nocardiosis, polymicrobial bacterial infections, and fungal infections. Actinomycosis may mimic appendicitis, pseudoappendicitis caused by *Yersinia enterocolitica,* amebiasis, hepatic abscess, lung abscess, and osteomyelitis.

TREATMENT. The mainstay of treatment for actinomycosis is an appropriate surgical approach to sinus tracts and abscesses, prolonged antibiotic therapy, and management of complications such as hemoptysis. Large abscesses usually require complete surgical excision. Bone disease may require multiple debridements. Prompt initiation of antibiotics results in a high cure rate. Actinomycosis is treated with penicillin G (250,000 U/kg/day IV divided every 4 hr; maximum, 18–24 million U/day). Other appropriate antibiotics include tetracycline, clindamycin, and carbapenems. Although controversy still exists about the optimal dosage and duration of therapy, appropriate therapy usually includes parenteral antibiotics for 2–6 wk followed by oral antibiotics for 3–12 mo. The oral antibiotic of choice is penicillin V (100 mg/kg/day divided every 6 hr PO). Hepatic abscesses or other deep tissue infections should be treated for 6–12 mo. Although most *A. israelii* strains are sensitive to penicillin with minimum inhibitory concentrations of 0.03–0.5 μg/mL, some resistant strains have been identified. Antibiotic susceptibility testing should be performed on all isolates from patients with significant disease or who are immunocompromised.

A. actinomycetemcomitans is a co-pathogen in at least 30% of actinomycotic infections. It is important to consider also treating this organism empirically, especially in the critically ill patient. Failure to recognize this organism and treat it adequately has resulted in clinical relapse and deterioration in patients with actinomycosis. *A. actinomycetemcomitans* is susceptible to cephalosporins, amoxicillin-clavulanate, rifampin, trimethoprim-sulfamethoxazole, aminoglycosides, ciprofloxacin, tetracycline, and azithromycin. It is susceptible to penicillin and ampicillin in vitro, but test results do not correlate necessarily with clinical outcome. In some patients with periodontitis associated with *A. actinomycetemcomitans,* mechanical periodontal treatment combined with metronidazole plus amoxicillin is effective for subgingival suppression.

PROGNOSIS. The prognosis is excellent with early diagnosis and adequate surgical debridement and antimicrobial therapy. Removal of chronically infected tonsils and treatment of periodontitis or caries may eliminate sources of possible reinfection.

Clarridge JE III, Zhang Q: Genotypic diversity of clinical *Actinomyces* species: Phenotype, source, and disease correlation among genospecies. *J Clin Microbiol* 2002;40:3442–3448.

Feder HM Jr: Actinomycosis manifesting as an acute painless lump of the jaw. *Pediatrics* 1990;85:858–864.

Gahrn-Hansen B, Frederiksen W: Human infections with *Actinomyces pyogenes (Corynebacterium pyogenes). Diagn Microbiol Infect Dis* 1992; 15:349–354.

Olah E, Berger C, Boltshauser E, Nadal D: Cerebral actinomycosis before adolescence. *Neuropediatrics* 2004;35:239–241.

Park JK, Lee HK, Ha HK, et al: Cervicofacial actinomycosis: CT and MR imaging findings in seven patients. *Am J Neuroradiol* 2003;24:331–335.

Reddy I, Ferguson DA Jr, Sarubbi FA: Endocarditis due to Actinomyces pyogenes. *Clin Infect Dis* 1997;25:1476–1477.

Robison JL, Vaudry WL, Dobrovolsky W: Actinomycosis presenting as osteomyelitis in the pediatric population. *Pediatr Infect Dis J* 2005; 24:365–369.

Sabbe LJM, Van De Merwe D, Schouls L, et al: Clinical spectrum of infections due to the newly described *Actinomyces* species *A. turicensis, A. radingae,* and *A. europaeus. J Clin Microbiol* 1999;37:8–13.

Sharma M, Briski LE, Khatib R: Hepatic actinomycosis: An overview of salient features and outcome of therapy. *Scand J Infect Dis* 2002;34:386–391.

Smego RA Jr, Foglia G: Actinomycosis. *Clin Infect Dis* 1998;26:1255–1261.

Tyrrell J, Noone P, Prichard JS: Thoracic actinomycosis complicated by *Actinobacillus actinomycetemcomitans:* Case report and review of literature. *Respir Med* 1992;86:341–343.

Chapter 189 ■ *Nocardia*

Richard F. Jacobs and Gordon E. Schutze

Nocardia organisms cause localized and disseminated disease in children and adults. These organisms are primarily opportunistic pathogens infecting immunocompromised persons. Infection caused by these bacteria is termed **nocardiosis,** which includes acute, subacute, or chronic suppurative infections with a tendency for remissions and exacerbations.

ETIOLOGY. *Nocardia* is a member of the order Actinomycetales, which includes gram-positive filamentous bacteria such as *Actinomyces, Streptomyces,* and mycobacteria. *Nocardia* organisms are environmental saprophytes that are ubiquitous in soil and decaying vegetable matter. These organisms are obligate aerobes and grow on ordinary culture media. Growth is achieved best at 37°C, although many isolates of *Nocardia* are thermophilic and grow at temperatures up to 50°C. At 25°C, the organisms grow very slowly. Colonies appear within 1–2 wk on brain-heart infusion agar and Lowenstein-Jensen media, usually as waxy, folded, or heaped colonies at the edges. With further incubation, these colonies develop aerial hyphae that tend to give them a white, chalky appearance. Using the modified Kinyoun acid-fast staining of biopsy specimens or body fluids, *Nocardia* demonstrates fragmented bacilli with stain concentrated in a **beaded pattern** along portions of the branching filaments.

Numerous taxonomic studies have established the heterogeneity of *Nocardia asteroides,* the most common species causing human nocardiosis, and have led to the description of *N. asteroides* sensu stricto (*N. asteroides* complex). *N. asteroides* is identified by its colony and microscopic morphology, resistance to lysozyme, and inability to hydrolyze casein, tyrosine, xanthine, and hypoxanthine. *N. asteroides, N. farcinica, N. otitidiscaviarum, N. transvalensis,* and *N. nova* share similar features, which has contributed to the apparent heterogeneity of *Nocardia. N. brasiliensis* is the 2nd most frequent etiologic agent of human nocardiosis. Some strains of *N. brasiliensis* have been assigned to a new species, *N. pseudobrasiliensis.* Antibiotic susceptibility testing, biochemical testing, chromatographic analysis of cell wall components including mycolic acid patterns, and newer molecular typing techniques such as ribotyping have identified 12 species within the genus *Nocardia.*

N. asteroides complex includes the most common agents of systemic nocardiosis in the United States. *N. brasiliensis* is the principal cause of localized nocardial cellulitis and lymphadenitis in immunocompetent children and can also cause pulmonary and systemic disease, especially in immunocompromised persons. *N. brasiliensis* is found more commonly in the southern USA, Central America, South America, and Asia. *Actinomadura madurae* (**Madura foot**), *N. farcinica, N. nova,* and *N. transvalensis* also cause human disease.

EPIDEMIOLOGY. Nocardiosis was once thought to be a rare cause of human disease but is being recognized more frequently, and has been diagnosed in persons from 4 wk to 82 yr of age. Almost all patients have compromised cellular immunity from an underlying disease such as organ transplantation, malignancy, corticosteroids, diabetes, HIV infection, or primary immunodeficiency, especially chronic granulomatous disease (see Chapter 129). *Nocardia* infections among stem cell transplant recipients are associated with a high rate of concomitant invasive fungal infection and a notable lack of protection with trimethoprim-sulfamethoxazole prophylaxis.

PATHOGENESIS. Soil is the natural habitat of *Nocardia,* which has been isolated worldwide. The organism is inhaled in aerosolized dust and causes pulmonary infection, with widespread dissemination in susceptible hosts. It can be transmitted by direct cutaneous inoculation, including following arthropod and cat bites. Although human-to-human transmission is rare, a description of *N. farcinica* sternal wound infections among patients undergoing open heart surgery raises concern about *Nocardia* as a nosocomial pathogen.

CLINICAL MANIFESTATIONS. Pulmonary nocardiosis accounts for 75% of cases, almost all of which occur among immunocompromised patients or with underlying pulmonary disease. Demonstration of tissue invasion is important for identifying active pulmonary infection because the organism occasionally exists as a respiratory saprophyte. Clinical manifestations include pneumonia and necrotizing pneumonia with single or multiple abscesses.

Single or multiple metastatic lesions may occur anywhere in the body. The brain is the most common secondary site and is involved in 15–40% of cases of pulmonary nocardiosis. Brain abscess is the most common presentation, with meningitis the 2nd most common that is manifested by pleocytosis (with a lymphocytic or neutrophilic predominance), elevated cerebrospinal fluid protein, and hypoglycorrhachia. Persistent neutrophilic meningitis with sterile cultures is classic for central nervous system (CNS) infection. The onset may be gradual or sudden and includes manifestations varying from headache to coma.

The skin is the 3rd most commonly involved organ and may be manifested by **sporotrichoid nocardiosis** or superficial ulcers (Fig. 189-1). **Mycetoma** is a chronic, progressive infection developing days to months after inoculation, usually on a distal location on the limbs. Renal nocardiosis is the 4th most common site and typically presents with dysuria, hematuria, or pyuria. Lesions may extend from the cortex into the medulla. Gastrointestinal involvement may also be associated with nausea, vomiting, diarrhea, abdominal distention, and melena. Infection may spread to skin, pericardium, myocardium, spleen, liver, or adrenal glands. Bone involvement is rare. Almost all of the involved organs have several abscesses, but in contrast to actinomycosis, granules are

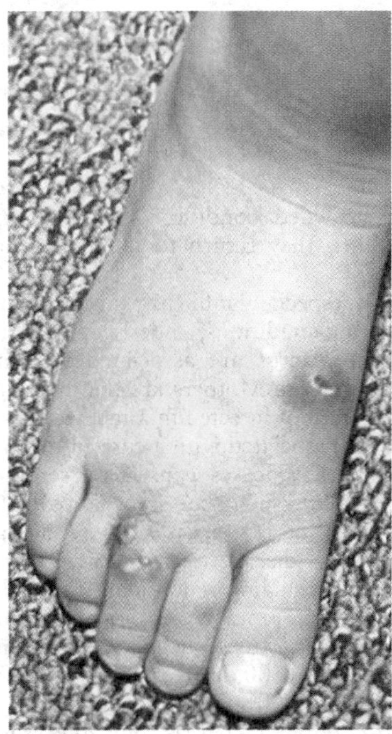

Figure 189-1. A 2 yr old girl with multiple pustules on the dorsum of the right foot caused by *Nocardia brasiliensis.* (Photograph courtesy of Jaime E. Fergie, MD.)

rarely found. Keratitis caused by *N. farcinica* has been associated with the use of semipermeable rigid contact lenses.

DIAGNOSIS. Laboratory diagnosis of nocardiosis requires direct examination of clinical material for characteristic gram-positive, acid-fast organisms and isolation by culture methods. Smears of clinical material are Gram stained or stained by the modified Kinyoun acid-fast stain. *N. asteroides* complex and *N. brasiliensis* appear as delicately branched, gram-positive, coccoid to bacillary bacteria that tend to fragment. In properly stained and decolorized acid-fast smears, the organisms may appear as fragmented bacilli with the stain concentrated in a beaded pattern along the portions of the filaments. Speciation is accomplished by polymerase chain reaction and restriction fragment length polymorphism analysis.

Diagnosis of pulmonary nocardiosis is established in $^1/_3$ of cases in adults by sputum analysis and culture. Bronchoalveolar lavage or lung biopsy may be required to establish the diagnosis in the remaining $^2/_3$ of adults and in children.

Cranial CT or MRI is recommended for all immunocompromised patients with pulmonary nocardiosis, even if asymptomatic, because of the high frequency of CNS involvement, and should be considered for immunocompetent patients with pulmonary nocardiosis.

TREATMENT. Surgical drainage of abscesses is important. The choice, dose, and duration of antimicrobial treatment depend on the site and extent of infection, host immune status, species of *Nocardia,* and initial clinical response. Sulfonamides have been the cornerstone of therapy for the treatment of nocardiosis since the 1940s. Trimethoprim-sulfamethoxazole is the formulation that is recommended, although sulfadiazine and sulfisoxazole demonstrate equal efficacy. A susceptibility study of 78 clinical isolates of the *N. asteroides* complex from the USA found that 95% of strains exhibited 1 of 5 antibiotic resistance patterns. The most common pattern, occurring in 35% of isolates, showed resistance to ampicillin and erythromycin but susceptibility to cefotaxime, ceftriaxone, and carbapenems. Approximately 20% of isolates, which were subsequently identified as *N. farcinica,* were resistant to cefotaxime and ceftriaxone. Another approximately 20% of the isolates, which were subsequently identified as *N. nova,* were susceptible to ampicillin and erythromycin. The remaining isolates had susceptibility patterns that included resistance to cephalosporins and susceptibility to ampicillin and carbenicillin, but intermediate susceptibility to carbapenems. The most active parenteral agents were amikacin (95%), imipenem (88%), ceftriaxone (82%), and cefotaxime (82%). The most active oral agents were sulfonamides (100%) and minocycline (100%). Newer antimicrobial agents with oral bioavailability are desirable because of the increasing reports of sulfonamide resistance and the adverse effects reported among patients with HIV infection. In vitro studies show susceptibility of all strains to linezolid, which appears to be an effective alternative treatment.

Combination therapy with a carbapenem or a 3rd generation cephalosporin with or without amikacin usually is recommended for severely ill patients or with CNS involvement. The mortality rate approaches 50% with sulfonamide used alone for treatment. Based on in vitro susceptibility testing for specific *N. asteroides* complex isolates, alternative drug combinations may include erythromycin and newer macrolides (azithromycin and clarithromycin), carbapenems, streptomycin, minocycline, quinolones, 3rd generation cephalosporins, and linezolid. The issues to be considered for use of linezolid include the limited data of use in children, the unknown adverse affects of long-term use, and the high cost. Clinical trials have shown that ampicillin and amoxicillin-clavulanate are effective in *N. brasiliensis* infections.

Antibiotic resistance has become an important issue in many *Nocardia* infections, with resistance to trimethoprim-sulfamethoxazole, streptomycin, and ampicillin reported. Susceptibility testing of *Nocardia* should be performed by a reference laboratory for isolates from deep-seated or disseminated infections, of strains such as *N. farcinica* or *N. otitidis-caviarum* that are commonly resistant to cephalosporins, if nonsulfonamide treatment regimens are being considered, with poor response to initial therapy, or with relapse.

Superficial cutaneous infection is treated for at least 1–3 mo. Mycetoma, pulmonary, or systemic nocardiosis in immunocompetent persons is treated for at least 6 mo, and CNS infection for at least 12 mo. Relapses have occurred of systemic *Nocardia* infection treated for <3 mo. Parenteral therapy can often be changed to oral therapy, such as high doses of trimethoprim-sulfamethoxazole, after 3–6 wk of parental therapy and good clinical response. Nocardiosis in patients with HIV infection probably should be treated indefinitely.

PROGNOSIS. Despite appropriate therapy, the overall mortality rate is >50%. This high rate may be secondary to delay in diagnosis or to the debilitated state of patients with severely compromised host defenses.

Barton LL: Lymphocutaneous *Nocardia brasiliensis* infection in children. *Pediatr Infect Dis J* 2001;20:232–233.

Chow E, Moore T, Deville J, et al: Nocardia asteroides brain abscesses and meningitis in an immunocompromised 10-year-old child. *Scand J Infect Dis* 2005;37:511–513.

Dorman SE, Guide SV, Conville PS, et al: Nocardia infection in chronic granulomatous disease 2002;35:390–394.

Fergie JE, Purcell K: Nocardiosis in south Texas children. *Pediatr Infect Dis J* 2001;20:711–714.

Moylett EH, Pacheco SE, Brown-Elliott BA, et al: Clinical experience with linezolid for the treatment of Nocardia infection. *Clin Infect Dis* 2003;36:313–318.

Torres OH, Domingo P, Pericas R, et al: Infection caused by *Nocardia farcinica:* Case report and review. *Eur J Clin Microbiol Infect Dis* 2000;19:205–212.

Section 5 — Gram-Negative Bacterial Infections

Chapter 190 ■ *Neisseria Meningitidis* (Meningococcus) Charles R. Woods

Meningococcal disease is a significant health problem worldwide. Most patients with meningococcal infections in developed nations survive, but previously healthy persons continue to succumb to fulminant disease despite advances in critical care medicine. Such cases, especially in the context of community outbreaks of meningococcal infection, create public fear and are not soon forgotten.

ETIOLOGY. *Neisseria meningitidis* is a gram-negative diplococcus. In Gram-stained specimens, the microbes appear as kidney-shaped pairs with adjacent sides flattened. Humans are the only natural reservoir, and meningococci are commensal colonizers of the nasopharynx, although most colonizing strains are unencapsulated commensal strains with little or no virulence. *N. meningitidis* is fastidious. Growth is facilitated in a moist environment at 35–37°C in a 5–10% carbon dioxide atmosphere. Growth is readily supported by chocolate, blood, and Mueller-Hinton media used routinely in clinical laboratories. On solid media, colonies are transparent, nonpigmented, and nonhemolytic. *N. meningitidis* is identified by its ability to ferment glucose and maltose, but not sucrose or lactose. Indole and hydrogen sulfide are not formed. Meningococci produce superoxide dismutase and are oxidase positive due to a cytochrome oxidase in the cell wall.

The meningococcal cell wall has lipid A–containing **lipo-oligosaccharides (LOS)**, including endotoxin, which is covered by a polysaccharide capsule. Antigenic variation of the capsule has led to recognition of 13 serogroups. The vast majority of meningococcal disease worldwide is caused by serogroups A, B, C, W135, and Y. The porin proteins PorB and PorA of the outer membrane complex and LOS are used to subtype strains within serogroups. Meningococcal strains are defined according to a scheme of serogroup (capsule polysaccharide):serotype (PorB):serosubtype (PorA):immunotype (LOS).

EPIDEMIOLOGY. Meningococcal infection occurs as endemic disease punctuated by outbreaks of cases that are clustered temporally and geographically. There is a slight male predominance (55%) among cases. Carriage rates vary by age and are about 2% in infants and young children not in daycare and 24–37% in the 15–24 yr old age group. The carriage rate approaches 100% in closed populations during epidemics.

In the United States, the incidence of reported meningococcal disease ranged from 0.8 to 1.3/100,000 population during the 1990s, with 2100–3500 cases/yr. Invasive disease is most common among young children, with rates of 9 cases/100,000 population in the 1st year of life and >25 cases/100,000 population during the 1st 4 mo of life. Neonatal cases are occasionally seen.

Almost 50% of cases occur among children <2 yr old, with another 25% of cases occurring in people ≥30 yr of age. An increased incidence among young persons 15–19 yr old is observed among younger adolescents and adults. College freshmen living in dormitories have a 3.6-fold higher risk than their noncollegiate peers. Colonization rates increase rapidly during the 1st month of the college academic year, likely due to high social mixing. Persons on religious pilgrimages, such as the Hajj pilgrimage to Mecca, have increased prevalence of colonization resulting from crowded conditions, and subsequently spread meningococci when they return to their households and local communities.

Viral infections, especially influenza, smoking and smoke exposure, crowded living conditions, underlying chronic diseases, and low socioeconomic status are associated with higher risk for meningococcal infection. Mothers are the most common household colonized source of infected infants. Meningococcal disease in children may be associated with a current maternal pregnancy.

In the United States, cases caused by serogroup Y strains increased in the 1990s such that serogroups B, C, and Y now each account for about 1/3 of cases among age groups beyond infancy. Serogroup B disease is still most common in infants. Serogroups B and C remain predominant in much of the rest of the world. Serogroup A remains a major problem in much of the developing world. Many areas, such as in China and Africa, have endemic rates of 10–25/100,000 persons and major periodic epidemics (100–500/100,000). Endemic disease is most common among young children, whereas epidemic disease typically involves older children, adolescents, and young adults. Crowded conditions facilitate epidemic spread.

Endemic disease is caused by heterogeneous meningococcal strains. Analyses with several genotyping methods have shown that outbreaks are caused by single strains (clones). Transcontinental spread of epidemic clones is well documented. **Outbreaks** are defined as >3 cases in a 3 mo period in the same community and an attack rate that exceeds 10 cases/100,000 persons. In the United States from July 1994 to June 2002, 76 meningococcal outbreaks were identified, including 13 in colleges and 19 in elementary and secondary schools, compared to only 6 outbreaks from 1980 to 1989. Vaccination campaigns were conducted in only 34 outbreaks.

Genetic exchange between epidemic and endemic meningococcal strains as well as commensal *Neisseria* species harbored simultaneously in the nasopharynx of colonized persons can lead to serotype and serosubtype changes, and sometimes even capsule switching, as spread of the new clone progresses through susceptible populations. Phase variation in expression of meningococcal surface proteins, including PorA and PorB, and LOS types also occurs. Multilocus sequence typing of 7 meningococcal housekeeping genes is now the standard method for defining such clones.

PATHOGENESIS. *N. meningitidis* is acquired primarily by the respiratory route. Nasopharyngeal colonization usually leads to asymptomatic colonization, which can persist for weeks to months. Invasion is rare, tends to occur soon after acquisition of new strains, and sometimes appears facilitated by concurrent viral respiratory tract infection. Meningococci (and gonococci, but not nonpathogenic *Neisseria*) produce an immunoglobulin A (IgA) protease that may assist in colonization of mucous membranes by cleaving the proline-rich hinge region of secretory IgA.

Meningococci adhere selectively to nonciliated epithelial cells by their type IV pili. Pili attach to CD46 proteins that serve as receptors for C3b, C4b, measles, and other viruses on the epithelial cell surface. This induces host cytoskeletal rearrangements and microvillus production that lead to endocytosis. Opacity-associated proteins (Opa) that extend from the microbial outer membrane interact with the human CD66 family of receptor molecules and facilitate adhesion and endocytosis. Bacteria then traverse the cell in membrane-bound vacuoles. Meningococcal porin proteins play roles in endocytosis, intracellular survival, apoptosis of invaded cells, and escape from complement attack through binding of C4b-binding protein.

Once through the epithelium, meningococci gain entry into the bloodstream. Serum antibody against meningococcal surface antigens, if present, can block this dissemination by initiation of complement-mediated bacterial lysis. Absence of antimeningococcal antibody is associated with development of meningococcemia. If the bacteremia is not cleared, interaction with phagocytes continues, organisms adhere to endothelial cells via pili, Opa, and porin proteins, and the complement system is further activated. Endothelial cell expression of surface adhesion molecules is influenced by LOS and capsular polysaccharide, facilitating attachment of white blood cells. Meningococcal survival is enhanced by the polysaccharide capsule, which helps resist phagocytic killing, and an iron scavenging system that can use host transferrin and lactoferrin. *N. meningitidis* LOS is recognized by Toll-like receptors (TLRs) 2 and 4. Its CpG-rich DNA sequences, which are common among bacteria, likely interact with TLR9. These TLR interactions activate genes via pathways related to nuclear factor-κB (NF-κB) that regulate the adaptive immune response.

The microbial–phagocyte–endothelial cell–complement interactions lead to production of multiple proinflammatory cytokines including tumor necrosis factor-α (TNF-α), interleukin 1β (IL-1β), IL-6, and IL-8, and activation of both the extrinsic (by way of induction of tissue factor expression on endothelial cell and monocytes) and intrinsic pathways of coagulation. Microbial factors other than LOS also are involved in initiating complement activation and inflammation. The degree of activation of the complement and clotting cascades, the concentrations of circulating cytokines, and risk of fatal disease correlate with the concentration of meningococcal LOS in the plasma at presentation. Progression of capillary leak and disseminated intravascular coagulopathy (DIC) can lead to multiple organ system failure, septic shock, and sometimes death. Fatal cases typically have higher concentrations of TNF-α and ILs than do survivors, but the causal relationship remains unclear. LOS and TNF-α levels decrease rapidly once antibiotics are given, correlating with clearance of viable microbes. Activation of the complement and clotting cascades can continue well beyond this point, especially in fulminant cases.

Diffuse vasculitis and DIC are common with meningococcemia. Leukocyte-rich fibrin clots are seen in small vessels, including arterioles and capillaries. The resulting focal hemorrhage and necrosis that initially manifest as purpura in the skin may occur in any organ system. The heart, central nervous system, skin, mucous and serous membranes, and adrenals are affected in most fatal cases, and microbes are often present in these lesions. Myocarditis is present in >50% of patients who die of meningococcal disease. Diffuse adrenal hemorrhage without vasculitis, the **Waterhouse-Friderichsen syndrome,** is common during fulminant meningococcemia. Meningitis is characterized by acute inflammatory cells in the leptomeninges and perivascular spaces. Focal cerebritis is uncommon.

Immunity. Non-LOS antigens appear to drive the dendritic cell maturation required for initiation of the adaptive immune response. IL-12 production, driven by meningococcal LOS, induces a T helper type 1 (Th1) response environment. Bactericidal antibodies are produced against capsular polysaccharide, outer membrane proteins, and LOS antigens. IgM, IgG, and IgA responses are induced within a few weeks after nasopharyngeal colonization. Natural immunity against a wide range of *N. meningitidis* strains seems to develop in most persons after repeated colonization with different serogroups or serosubtypes and from gastrointestinal colonization with enteric bacteria that express cross-reactive antigens. The duration of these antibody responses, and degree of immunologic memory induced even from infection, is unclear. Ongoing natural exposures may help maintain immunity. Mucosal immunity may be more effective in preventing invasion of epithelial cells than colonization. High levels of anticapsular antibodies after vaccination are associated with decreased carriage of vaccine serogroup strains.

Infants also have high carriage rates of the unencapsulated, nonpathogenic *N. lactamica,* which contributes to development of immunity against meningococci. Protective effects of maternally derived IgG wane during the 1st 3 mo of life, with resultant high rates of invasive disease during the remainder of infancy.

Host Factors. Persons with primary deficiencies of complement components have an increased risk for developing meningococcal disease, underscoring the important role of complement in host defense against the meningococcus. Among individuals with properdin, factor D, or terminal component deficiencies, 50–60% will develop serious bacterial infections, caused almost solely by *N. meningitidis.* Some studies suggest disease manifestations with complement deficiencies are less severe than with intact complement function, but this is not certain. Recurrent infection is more common with terminal component deficiencies than with properdin deficiency. Similar increased risk is seen with the acquired complement deficiencies that occur in patients with diseases such as nephrotic syndrome, systemic lupus erythematosus, and hepatic failure. Among persons with meningococcal infections, complement deficiencies are much more prevalent among those >5 yr of age than in younger children. Most cases among complement-deficient persons occur during late childhood or adulthood when carriage rates tend to be higher.

Other host factors that may affect the severity and outcome of meningococcal disease include polymorphisms of IL-1, IL-1 receptor antagonist, mannose-binding lectin, Fc receptor genes (especially Fc γ receptor IIA-R/R131), TLR4, the promoter regions for the genes encoding TNF-α and plasminogen-activator-inhibitor-1, and possibly components of various NF-κB activation pathways. Potential interaction of certain Fc receptor polymorphisms with specific IL-10 alleles suggests that combinations of alleles in different genes may account for variations in disease expression. Presence of factor V Leiden exacerbates meningococcal purpura fulminans but may not affect mortality.

The group B capsule is a homopolymer of sialic acid, which is poorly immunogenic in humans in part because of its structural homology with mammalian neural cell adhesion molecules. The B capsular antigen also does not activate the alternative complement pathway in humans, which is a key part of the innate immune response essential for protection from infections in the absence of specific antibodies. This may explain in part the higher prevalence of serogroup B meningococcal disease in young children.

CLINICAL MANIFESTATIONS. The spectrum of meningococcal disease varies widely from fever and occult bacteremia (see Chapter 175) to sepsis and shock (see Chapter 176) and death. Recognized patterns of disease include bacteremia without sepsis, meningococcemia (sepsis) without meningitis, and meningitis with or without meningococcemia. At least 80% of cases have overt clinical signs. Occult meningococcal bacteremia often presents as fever with or without associated symptoms that suggest minor viral infections. Resolution may occur without antibiotics, but meningitis develops in 58% of disease cases. *N. meningitidis* is isolated from blood in about 2/3 of cases, from cerebrospinal fluid (CSF) in half, and joint fluid in 1% of cases.

Acute meningococcemia initially may mimic viral illness with pharyngitis, fever, myalgias, weakness, vomiting, diarrhea, and/or headache (Table 190-1). A maculopapular rash is evident in about 7% of cases, typically before more serious signs develop. Limb pain, myalgias, or refusal to walk occur in many cases and is the primary complaint in 7% of otherwise clinically unsuspected cases. Cold hands or feet and abnormal skin color are also early signs. In fulminant meningococcemia cases, the disease progresses rapidly over hours to septic shock characterized by prominent petechiae and purpura (**purpura fulminans**), hypotension,

TABLE 190-1. Age-Specific Frequency of Clinical Features of Meningococcal Disease Before Hospital Admission

	<1 YR	1–4 YR	5–14 YR	15–16 YR
EARLY FEATURES %				
Leg pain	5.1	30.6	62.4	53.3
Thirst	3.4	6.4	11.4	12.6
Diarrhea	9.9	7.8	3.1	5.5
Abnormal skin color	20.6	16.8	18.5	19.0
Breathing difficulty	16.2	9.7	7.1	12.1
Cold hands and feet	44.0	46.7	34.9	44.4
CLASSIC FEATURES %				
Hemorrhagic rash	42.3	64.2	69.8	65.9
Neck pain or stiffness	15.5	28.1	45.9	52.9
Photophobia	24.5	24.1	26.4	35.5
Bulging fontanelle	11.5	n/a	n/a	n/a
LATE FEATURES %				
Confusion or delirium	n/a	42.8	49.4	47.6
Seizure	8.9	12.8	7.8	7.3
Unconsciousness	7.0	9.1	5.9	15.1

From Thompson MJ, Ninis N, Perera R, et al: Clinical recognition of meningococcal disease in children and adolescents. *Lancet* 2006;367:397–403.

DIC, acidosis, adrenal hemorrhage, renal failure, myocardial failure, and coma (Fig. 190-1). Meningitis may or may not be present.

The most common clinical manifestation, **meningococcal meningitis,** is distinguishable from other causes of bacterial meningitis (see Chapter 602.1). Headache, photophobia, lethargy, vomiting, and nuchal rigidity and other signs of meningeal irritation typically are present. Seizures and focal neurologic signs occur less frequently than in patients with meningitis caused by pneumococcus or *Haemophilus influenzae* type b. A meningoencephalitis-like picture can occur that may be associated with rapidly progressive cerebral edema, which may be more common with serogroup A infection.

Among 402 children <21 yr old among 3 series of invasive meningococcal disease during the 1980s to early 2000s, about 81% presented with fever, 41% had hypotension or decreased peripheral perfusion, and 50% had petechiae and/or purpura. Purpura fulminans developed in 16%. Other presenting symptoms and signs included emesis (34%), lethargy (30%), irritability (21%), diarrhea (6%), rhinorrhea (10%), seizure (6%), and septic arthritis (8%). Radiographic evidence of pneumonia was present initially in 8% in 1 series. Mechanical ventilation was required in 26% and vasopressor support in 35%. Nonsuppurative arthritis developed in 4–6%. Uncommon manifestations of meningococcal disease include endocarditis, purulent pericarditis, pneumonia, endophthalmitis, mesenteric lymphadenitis, osteomyelitis, sinusitis, otitis media, and periorbital cellulitis. Primary purulent conjunctivitis can lead to invasive disease. Pleural effusion or empyema occurs in 15% of cases with meningococcal pneumonia. *N. meningitidis* infections of the genitourinary tract are rare, but urethritis, cervicitis, vulvovaginitis, and proctitis can occur.

Chronic meningococcemia occurs rarely and is characterized by fever, nontoxic appearance, arthralgias, headache, and a rash similar to that of disseminated gonococcal infection. Symptoms are intermittent, with a mean duration of illness of 6–8 wk. Blood cultures are usually positive but may initially be sterile; meningitis can develop in untreated cases.

DIAGNOSIS. Definitive diagnosis of meningococcal disease is established by isolation of the organism from a normally sterile body fluid such as blood, CSF, or synovial fluid. Isolation from the nasopharynx is not diagnostic for invasive disease. Blood and CSF are the usual sources of the organism. Cultures often are negative if the patient has been treated with antibiotics prior to culture. Meningococci sometimes can be identified in culture or Gram stain of petechial or papular lesions. Bacteria occasionally are seen on Gram stain of the buffy coat layer of a spun blood sample.

With meningitis, the morphologic and clinical characteristics of the CSF are those of acute bacterial meningitis (see Chapter 602.1). CSF cultures sometimes are positive in patients with meningococcemia who do not have CSF pleocytosis or clinical evidence of meningitis. CSF specimens that demonstrate gram negative organisms are sometimes culture negative. Over decolorized pneumococci in Gram stains can be mistaken for meningococci and therefore empirical therapy should not be based on Gram stain alone.

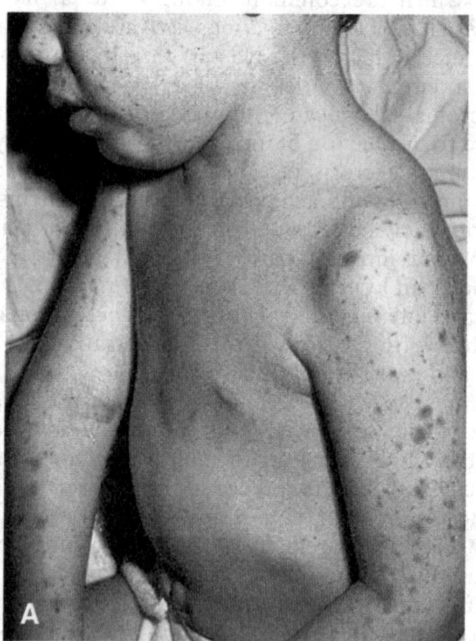

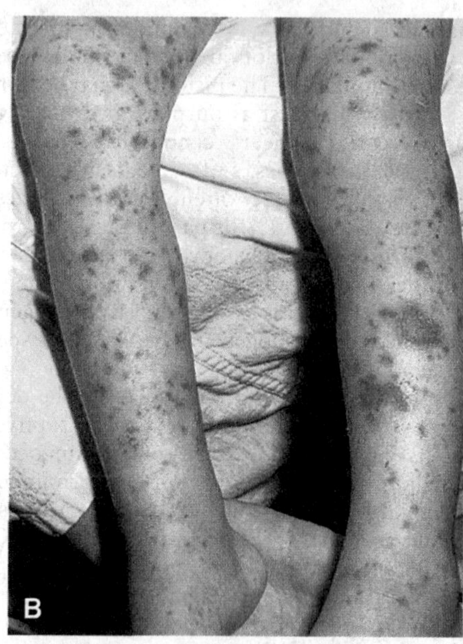

Figure 190-1. Meningococcal infections. *A*, Meningococcemia showing striking involvement of the extremities with relative sparing of the skin of the child's body surface. *B*, This image shows the lower extremities of the patient depicted in A. (From the American Academy of Pediatrics: *Red Book: 2006 Report of the Committee on Infectious Diseases,* 27th ed. Elk Grove Village, IL, American Academy of Pediatrics, 2006, Atlas 7.)

Detection of capsular polysaccharide antigens by rapid latex agglutination tests in CSF can support the diagnosis in cases clinically consistent with meningococcal disease. These tests are most useful when results are positive in the setting of partially treated infections with negative cultures. Antigen tests using serum or urine are not helpful. Rapid antigen tests are not reliable for serogroup B strains due to cross-reactions with other bacterial species (*Escherichia coli* K1 antigen). Polymerase chain reaction–based assays for detection of meningococci in blood and CSF have been developed and are used clinically in the U.K. but not in the United States at this time. These likely will have more widespread use in the near future.

Other laboratory findings include leukocytopenia or leukocytosis, often with increased percentages of neutrophils and band forms, thrombocytopenia, proteinuria, and hematuria. Elevated sedimentation rate and C-reactive protein, hypoalbuminemia, hypocalcemia, and metabolic acidosis often with increased lactate levels are common. Patients with DIC have decreased serum concentrations of prothrombin and fibrinogen and prolonged coagulation studies.

DIFFERENTIAL DIAGNOSIS. Meningococcal disease can appear similar to sepsis or meningitis caused by many other gram-negative bacteria, *Streptococcus pneumoniae, Staphylococcus aureus,* or group A streptococcus; Rocky Mountain spotted fever, ehrlichiosis, or epidemic typhus; and bacterial endocarditis. Viral and other etiologies of encephalitis should be considered in some cases. Autoimmune vasculitides (especially Henoch-Schönlein purpura), serum sickness, hemolytic-uremic syndrome, Kawasaki disease, idiopathic thrombocytopenic purpura, drug eruptions, and ingestion of various poisons can have features that overlap those of meningococcal infection. Infections with echoviruses (particularly types 6, 9, and 16), coxsackieviruses (primarily types A2, A4, A9, and A16), and other viruses also may have severe presentations that initially raise concerns about meningococcal infection.

Benign petechial rashes are common in viral and group A streptococcal infections. The nonpetechial, blanching rash observed in some meningococcal cases may initially be confused with a viral exanthem.

TREATMENT. For hospitalized patients, penicillin G (250,000–400,000 U/kg/day divided every 4–6 hr IV) remains the drug of choice. Cefotaxime (200 mg/kg/day) or ceftriaxone (100 mg/kg/day) are acceptable alternatives and are usually part of initial empiric regimens. Therapy in children is generally continued for 5–7 days.

Early treatment of meningococcal infections may prevent serious sequelae, but timely identification of such patients is often difficult in the absence of skin findings. High fever and leukocytosis with increased neutrophil and band counts are common in older children and adolescents with otherwise unsuspected meningococcal infection. Empiric outpatient treatment of selected patients during meningococcal outbreaks and of nontoxic children with petechial rashes can be considered. Most of the latter will not have meningococcal infection. Blood cultures should be obtained before treatment.

Isolates of *N. meningitidis* with relative resistance to penicillin (minimal inhibitory concentration of penicillin of 0.1–1.0 μg/mL) have been reported from Europe, Africa, Canada, and the United States. Decreased susceptibility is caused, at least in part, by altered penicillin-binding protein 2. In 1991 such strains represented ~4% of isolates in the United States. This degree of penicillin resistance does not appear to impact response to therapy. Strains producing β-lactamase remain exceedingly rare. Routine susceptibility testing of meningococcal isolates is not indicated in the United States at this time, but continued surveillance is necessary.

Optimal supportive care (see Chapter 68) is essential. Many adjunctive therapies have been attempted, but none have shown much benefit in children to date. Recombinant bactericidal/permeability-increasing protein (BPI) may reduce complications in severe cases, but further studies are needed. BPI is present in neutrophils, neutralizes endotoxin, and may attenuate the inflammatory and coagulation cascades. Protein C is a natural anticoagulant that also downregulates the inflammatory response and is depleted in DIC. A clinical trial of activated protein C therapy for severe sepsis in children was terminated in 2005 because of apparent increased risk of intracranial hemorrhage associated with its use. Other anticoagulant or fibrinolytic agents and vasodilators have been used with variable success in anecdotal reports. Combinations of such therapies may be useful in selected cases in the future, but have yet to be evaluated.

Most children who do not require intubation or vasopressor support respond readily to antibiotics plus supportive care and demonstrate clinical improvement within 24–72 hr. Those requiring mechanical ventilation and other critical care interventions often have much more prolonged and complicated courses that can require hospitalization for weeks. Children with severe disease who respond poorly to aggressive fluid and inotropic therapies may have adrenal insufficiency and may benefit from hydrocortisone supplementation. Extracorporeal membrane oxygenation has been used with limited success.

COMPLICATIONS. Acute complications are related to the vasculitis, DIC, and hypotension of severe meningococcal disease. Focal skin infarctions are similar to burns and usually heal but can become secondarily infected, resulting in significant scarring and requiring skin grafting. The gangrene of extremities often seen with purpura fulminans may necessitate amputations. Adrenal hemorrhage, endophthalmitis, arthritis, endocarditis, pericarditis, myocarditis, pneumonia, lung abscess, peritonitis, and renal infarcts can occur during acute infection. Avascular necrosis of epiphyses and epiphyseal-metaphyseal defects can result from the generalized DIC and may lead to growth disturbances and late skeletal deformities.

Deafness is the most frequent neurologic sequela, occurring in 5–10% of children with meningitis in most series. Cerebral arterial or venous thrombosis with resultant cerebral infarction can occur in severe cases. Meningitis is complicated rarely by subdural effusion or empyema or by brain abscess. Other rare neurologic sequelae include ataxia, seizures, blindness, cranial nerve palsies, hemiparesis or quadriparesis, and obstructive hydrocephalus. The latter often presents 3–4 wk after onset of illness.

Nonsuppurative complications of meningococcal disease appear to be **immune complex mediated** and become apparent 4–9 days after the onset of illness. Arthritis and cutaneous vasculitis (erythema nodosum) are most common. The **arthritis** usually is monoarticular or oligoarticular, involves large joints, and has sterile effusions that respond to nonsteroidal anti-inflammatory agents. Long-term sequelae are uncommon. Because most patients with meningococcal meningitis become afebrile by the 7th hospital day, persistence or recrudescence of fever after 5 days of antibiotics warrants evaluation for immune complex–mediated complications.

Reactivation of latent herpes simplex virus infections (primarily herpes labialis) is common during meningococcal infection.

PROGNOSIS. The mortality rate for invasive meningococcal disease remains about 10% in the United States despite modern interventions. Case fatality rates are highest among those 15–24 yr of age. Most deaths occur within 48 hr of hospitalization. Poor prognostic factors on presentation include hypothermia or extreme hyperpyrexia, hypotension or shock, purpura fulminans, seizures, leukopenia, thrombocytopenia (including DIC), acidosis, and high circulating levels of endotoxin and TNF-α. The presence of petechiae for <12 hr before admission, absence of meningitis, and low or normal erythrocyte sedimentation rate indicate rapid, fulminant progression and poorer prognosis.

Screening for complement deficiency after resolution of the acute infection can be considered for any person with meningococcal infection and should be performed for older children and adolescents. Recurrent infections in persons with a complement deficiency also can be severe.

PREVENTION. Close contacts of patients with meningococcal disease are at increased risk for infection and should be carefully monitored and brought to medical attention if fever develops. Antibiotic prophylaxis is indicated as soon as possible for household, daycare, and nursery school contacts and for those who have had contact with the patient's oral secretions during the 7 days before onset of illness. Prophylaxis is not routinely recommended for medical personnel except those with intimate exposure, such as with mouth-to-mouth resuscitation, intubation, or suctioning before antibiotic therapy was begun. Children may be given rifampin (10 mg/kg orally every 12 hr for a total of 4 doses; maximum dose 600 mg; 5 mg/kg/dose for infants <1 mo of age) or ceftriaxone (125 mg in a single dose IM for children <12 yr of age; 250 mg in a single dose IM for those >12 yr of age). Ciprofloxacin (500 mg orally as a single dose) may be given to persons ≥18 yr of age. Penicillin does not eradicate nasopharyngeal carriage; patients treated with penicillin should receive prophylaxis before hospital discharge. Hospitalized patients should be placed on droplet precautions for 24 hr after initiation of effective therapy. All confirmed or probable cases of meningococcal infection must be reported to the local public health department.

Vaccination. A quadrivalent vaccine composed of capsular polysaccharides of meningococcal groups A, C, Y, and W135 (MPSV4) was the primary meningococcal vaccine available in the United States until January 2005, with the approval of a diphtheria toxoid–based protein-conjugate meningococcal vaccine (MCV4) for use in persons 11–55 yr of age. MPSV4 is immunogenic in adults but is unreliable in children <2 yr of age. It remains the only approved vaccine in the United States for children 2–10 yr of age and adults >55 yr of age. About 75% of meningococcal disease among persons ≥11 yrs of age in the United States is caused by serogroups C, Y, or W-135, and thus is potentially vaccine preventable.

MCV4 and MPSV4 produce similar titers of anticapsular bactericidal antibodies against each of the 4 serogroups in the vaccines at 1 mo after vaccination (in age-appropriate patients), with 4-fold increases in titer with both in >90% of vaccinees against serogroups A, C, and W-135 and >80% against serogroup Y. Protective titers (≥1 : 128) are induced in >97% of recipients of either vaccine against all 4 serogroups in age-appropriate patients. MCV4 causes transient fever and local redness, pain, or swelling slightly more frequently than MPSV4, which is attributed to the diphtheria toxoid component of MCV4.

The efficacy of MPSV4 is ≥85% for serogroups A and C and likely similar for serogroups W-135 and Y. Efficacy of MCV4 is expected to be similar to MPSV4 since bactericidal antibodies confer immunity and the titers of these induced by MCV4 are noninferior to those of MPSV4. Use of a serogroup C–diphtheria CRM_{197} conjugate vaccine in the United Kingdom since 1999 has reduced serogroup C disease by about 95% in children in that country, and similar results with use of this vaccine have been reported from Quebec. Reduced nasopharyngeal carriage of serogroup C strains among serogroup C–diphtheria CRM_{197} vaccinees and community immunity (herd immunity) among nonvaccinees have been demonstrated in the U.K.

Duration of immunity from MPSV4 is at most 3–5 yr, such that revaccination of persons with ongoing risk of meningococcal infections can be considered within this time frame for past MPSV4 recipients. Protection from MCV4 is expected to be longer, but the full duration and potential need for revaccination are not yet known. Immune responses to conjugate meningococcal vaccines are boostable (T cell dependent), whereas those to MPSV4 are not (T cell independent). Conjugate vaccines appear to be immunogenic and safe in infants but have not yet been approved or recommended for this age group in the United States.

Strain-specific vaccines can be produced if needed for control of serogroup B outbreaks, but these are not effective against other serogroup B strains because of the high frequency of genetic transformation and resultant antigenic variation within *N. meningitidis*. Genomic and proteomic approaches to identify candidate antigens hold promise for development of vaccines effective against a broad array of serogroup B strains.

MCV4, as a single dose, is the preferred vaccine in the United States for persons 11–55 yr of age for whom meningococcal vaccination is recommended. MPSV4 remains an acceptable alternative for this age range when MCV4 is unavailable and is recommended for children 2–10 yr of age and adults >55 yr of age, pending further evaluation and approval of MCV4 in these age groups. The monovalent serogroup C–diphtheria CRM_{197} conjugate vaccine currently is used in much of Europe, Canada, Australia, and Brazil. A 3 dose series of this vaccine can be given to infants starting at 2 mo of age, with 1 dose recommended for persons ≥1 yr of age.

MCV4 is routinely recommended for all adolescents at 11–12 yr at the pre-adolescent visit, and adolescents at age 15 yr or high school entry if not previously vaccinated. The goal is routine vaccination of all 11 yr old adolescents beginning in 2008. MCV4 and the Tdap (tetanus and diphtheria toxoids and acellular pertussis booster) vaccine should be administered to adolescents during the same visit if both vaccines are indicated. If this is not feasible, MCV4 and Tdap can be administered in either sequence with a minimum interval of 1 mo between vaccines. MCV4 is also recommended for all incoming college freshmen living in dormitories. Many colleges and universities, and some states, have mandated meningococcal immunization of all matriculating freshmen. MCV4 is also indicated for other adolescents who wish to decrease their risk for meningococcal disease.

Tetravalent meningococcal vaccines also are recommended for U.S. children ≥2 yr of age who have anatomic or functional asplenia, complement component deficiencies that prevent terminal attack complex formation, or travel plans to areas with hyperendemic or epidemic meningococcal infection rates such as sub-Saharan Africa during the December–June dry season. Specific travel information is available from the Centers for Disease Control and Prevention at http://cdc.gov/travel. Meningococcal vaccines also are used routinely for American military recruits and to control sustained local outbreaks of meningococcal disease caused by a vaccine serogroup.

Guillain-Barré syndrome (GBS) has been reported to be temporally related to administration of meningococcal vaccine, although the rate among vaccine recipients is similar to that among the general population (see Chapter 615). Persons with previously diagnosed GBS should not receive conjugate meningococcal vaccine.

American Academy of Pediatrics Committee on Infectious Diseases: Prevention and control of meningococcal disease: Recommendations for use of meningococcal vaccines in pediatric patients. *Pediatrics* 2005;116:496–505.

Branco RG, Russell RR: Should steroids be used in children with meningococcal shock? *Arch Dis Child* 2005;90:1195–1196.

Centers for Disease Control and Prevention: Update: Guillain-Barré syndrome among recipients of Menactra meningococcal conjugate vaccine–United States, June 2005–September 2006.

Centers for Disease Control and Prevention: Prevention and control of meningococcal disease. Recommendations of the Advisory Committee on Immunization Practices (ACIP). *MMWR* 2005;54(RR-7):1–17.

De Wals P, Ceceuninck G, Boulianne N, et al: Effectiveness of a mass immunization campaign using serogroup C meningococcal conjugate vaccine. *JAMA* 2004;292:2492–2494.

Emonts M, Hazelzet JA, de Groot R, et al: Host genetic determinants of *Neisseria meningitidis* infections. *Lancet Infect Dis* 2003;3:565–577.

Fijen CAP, Kuijper EJ, te Bulte MT, et al: Assessment of complement deficiency in patients with meningococcal disease in the Netherlands. *Clin Infect Dis* 1999;28:98–105.
Gardner P: Prevention of meningococcal disease. *N Engl J Med* 2006;355:1466–1473.
Hart CA, Thompson APJ: Meningococcal disease and its management in children. *BMJ* 2006;333:685–690.
Inkelis SH, O'Leary D, Wang VJ, et al: Extremity pain and refusal to walk in children with invasive meningococcal disease. *Pediatrics* 2002;110:e3.
Kaplan SL, Schutze GE, Leake JAD, et al: Multicenter surveillance of invasive meningococcal infections in children. *Pediatrics* 2006;118:e979–e984.
Levin M, Quint PA, Goldstein B, et al: Recombinant bactericidal/permeability-increasing protein ($rBPI_{21}$) as adjunctive treatment for children with severe meningococcal sepsis: A randomized trial. *Lancet* 2000;356:961–967.
Mathew S, Overturf GD: Complement and properdin deficiencies in meningococcal disease. *Pediatr Infect Dis J* 2006;25:255–256.
Nascimento-Carvalho CM, Moreno-Carvalho OA: Changing the diagnostic framework of meningococcal disease. *Lancet* 2006;367:371–372.
Nathan N, Borel T, Djibo A, et al: Ceftriaxone as effective as long-acting chloramphenicol in short-course treatment of meningococcal meningitis during epidemics: A randomized non-inferiority study. *Lancet* 2005;366:308–313.
Nathan N, Faust SN, Levin M: Pathophysiology of meningococcal meningitis and septicemia. *Arch Dis Child* 2003;88:601–607.
Ramsey ME, Andrews NJ, Trotter CL, et al: Herd immunity from meningococcal serogroup C conjugate vaccination in England: Database analysis. *Br Med J* 2003;326:365–366.
Sharip A, Sorvillo F, Redelings MD, et al: Population-based analysis of meningococcal disease mortality in the United States 1990–2002. *Pediatr Infect Dis J* 2006;25:191–194.
Thompson MJ, Ninis N, Perera R, et al: Clinical recognition of meningococcal disease in children and adolescents. *Lancet* 2006;367:397–403.
Welch SB, Nadel S: Treatment of meningococcal infection. *Arch Dis Child* 2003;88:608–614.
Yazdankhah S, Caugant DA: *Neisseria meningitidis*: An overview of the carriage state. *J Med Microbiol* 2004;54:821–832.

Chapter 191 ■ *Neisseria Gonorrhoeae* (Gonococcus) Toni Darville

Neisseria gonorrhoeae produces various forms of **gonorrhea,** an infection of the genitourinary tract mucous membranes and rarely of the mucosa of the rectum, oropharynx, and conjunctiva. Gonorrhea transmitted by sexual contact or perinatally is 2nd only to chlamydial infections in the number of cases reported to the Centers for Disease Control and Prevention (CDC) in the United States. This high prevalence and the development of antibiotic-resistant strains have produced significant morbidity in adolescents.

ETIOLOGY. *N. gonorrhoeae* is a nonmotile, aerobic, non-spore-forming, gram-negative intracellular diplococcus with flattened adjacent surfaces. Optimal growth occurs at 35–37°C and at pH 7.2–7.6 in an atmosphere of 3–5% carbon dioxide. The specimen should be inoculated immediately onto fresh, moist, modified Thayer-Martin or specialized transport media because gonococci do not tolerate drying. Thayer-Martin medium contains antimicrobial agents that inhibit hardier normal flora present in clinical specimens that may otherwise overgrow gonococci. Presumptive identification may be based on colony appearance, Gram stain, and production of cytochrome oxidase. Gonococci are differentiated from other *Neisseria* species by the fermentation of glucose but not maltose, sucrose, or lactose. Gram-negative diplococci are seen in infected material, often within polymorphonuclear leukocytes.

Like all gram-negative bacteria, *N. gonorrhoeae* possess a cell envelope composed of an inner cytoplasmic membrane, a middle layer of peptidoglycan, and an outer membrane. The outer membrane contains lipo-oligosaccharides (endotoxin), phospholipid, and a variety of proteins that contribute to cell adherence, tissue invasion, and resistance to host defenses. The 2 systems primarily used to characterize gonococcal strains are auxotyping and serotyping. Auxotyping is based on genetically stable requirements of strains for specific nutrients or cofactors as defined by an isolate's ability to grow on chemically defined media. The most widely used serotyping system is based on porin, a trimeric outer membrane protein that makes up a substantial part of the gonococcal envelope structure. Antibodies generated to Por have been used to serotype gonococci (e.g., PorIA-4 and PorIB-12), and changes in porin proteins present in a community are believed to occur, at least in part, as a result of selective immune pressure.

EPIDEMIOLOGY. *N. gonorrhoeae* infection occurs only in humans. The organism is shed in the exudate and secretions of infected mucosal surfaces and is transmitted through intimate contact, such as sexual contact or parturition and, rarely, by contact with fomites. Gonococcal infections in the newborn period generally are acquired during delivery. Gonorrhea is the most common sexually transmitted infection found in sexually abused children. Rarely, *N. gonorrhoeae* may be spread by sexual play among children, but the index patient is likely to be a victim of sexual abuse. Gonococcal infections in children are acquired rarely through household exposure to infected caretakers. In such cases, the possibility of sexual abuse should be seriously considered.

The number of reported cases of gonorrhea increased steadily in the USA from 1964 to 1977, fluctuated through the early 1980s, and increased until 1987, when reported rates were 323/100,000. Rates decreased annually from 1987 to 1996, when reported rates were 123/100,000 population, after which rates have fluctuated from year to year with a rate of 125/100,000 reported in 2002. The decline in gonorrhea prevalence may be attributed to recommendations by the CDC that only highly effective antimicrobial agents be used to treat gonorrhea. The incidence of gonorrhea is highest in high-density urban areas among persons under 24 yr of age who have multiple sex partners and engage in unprotected sexual intercourse. Increases in gonorrhea prevalence have been noted recently among men who have sex with men (MSM). Risk factors include nonwhite race, homosexuality, increased number of sexual partners, prostitution, presence of other sexually transmitted infections, unmarried status, poverty, and failure to use condoms. Techniques of auxotyping and serotyping, and, more recently, molecular typing methods have been used to analyze the spread of individual strains of *N. gonorrhoeae* within a community.

Maintenance and subsequent spread of gonococcal infections in a community require a hyperendemic, high-risk core group such as prostitutes or adolescents with multiple sexual partners. This is because most persons who have gonorrhea cease sexual activity and seek care, unless economic need or other factors (e.g., drug addiction) drive persistent sexual activity. Thus, many core transmitters belong to a subset of infected persons who lack or ignore symptoms and continue to be sexually active. This underscores the importance of seeking out and treating the sexual contacts of infected persons who present for treatment.

Gonococcal infection of **neonates** usually results from peripartum exposure to infected exudate from the cervix of the mother. An acute infection begins 2–5 days after birth. The incidence of neonatal infection depends on the prevalence of gonococcal infection among pregnant women, prenatal screening for gonorrhea, and neonatal ophthalmic prophylaxis.

PATHOGENESIS AND PATHOLOGY. *N. gonorrhoeae* infect primarily columnar epithelium; stratified squamous epithelium is relatively resistant to invasion. Mucosal invasion by gonococci results in a local inflammatory response that produces a purulent exudate consisting of polymorphonuclear leukocytes, serum, and desquamated epithelium. The gonococcal lipo-oligosaccharide (endotoxin) exhibits direct cytotoxicity, causing ciliostatis and sloughing of ciliated epithelial cells. Once the gonococcus traverses the mucosal barrier, the lipo-oligosaccharide binds bactericidal immunoglobulin M (IgM) antibody and serum complement, causing an acute inflammatory response in the subepithelial space. Tumor necrosis factor and other cytokines are thought to mediate the cytotoxicity of gonococcal infections.

Gonococci may ascend the urogenital tract and in postpubertal males cause urethritis or epididymitis, and in postpubertal females cause acute endometritis, salpingitis, and peritonitis, which are collectively termed **acute pelvic inflammatory disease (PID)**. Dissemination from the fallopian tubes through the peritoneum to the liver capsule results in **perihepatitis (Fitz-Hugh-Curtis syndrome)**. Gonococci that invade the lymphatics and blood vessels may lead to inguinal lymphadenopathy; perineal, perianal, ischiorectal, and periprostatic abscesses; and disseminated gonococcal infection (DGI).

A number of gonococcal virulence and host immune factors are involved in the penetration of the mucosal barrier and subsequent manifestations of local and systemic infection. Selective pressure from different mucosal environments probably leads to changes in the outer membrane of the organism, including expression of variants of pili, opacity or Opa proteins (formerly protein II), and lipo-oligosaccharides. These changes may enhance gonococcal attachment, invasion, replication, and evasion of the host's immune response.

For infection to occur, the gonococcus must first attach to host cells. A gonococcal IgA protease inactivates IgA1 by cleaving the molecule in the hinge region and may be an important factor in colonization or invasion of host mucosal surfaces. Gonococci adhere to the microvilli of nonciliated epithelial cells by hairlike protein structures (pili) that extend from the cell wall. Pili are thought to protect the gonococcus from phagocytosis and complement-mediated killing. Pili undergo high-frequency antigenic variation that may aid in the organism's escape from the host immune response and may provide specific ligands for different cell receptors. Opacity proteins, most of which confer an opaque appearance to colonies, are also thought to function as ligands to facilitate binding to human cells. Gonococci that express certain Opa proteins adhere and are phagocytosed by human neutrophils in the absence of serum.

Other phenotypic changes that occur in response to environmental stresses allow gonococci to establish infection. Examples include iron-repressible proteins for binding transferrin or lactoferrin, anaerobically expressed proteins, and synthesis of proteins mediated by contact with epithelial cells. Gonococci may grow in vivo under anaerobic conditions or in an environment with a relative lack of iron.

Approximately 24 hr after attachment, the epithelial cell surface invaginates and surrounds the gonococcus in a phagocytic vacuole. This phenomenon is thought to be mediated by the gonococcal outer membrane protein I inserting into the host cell and causing alterations in membrane permeability. Subsequently, phagocytic vacuoles begin releasing gonococci into the subepithelial space by means of exocytosis. Viable organisms may then cause local disease (i.e., salpingitis) or disseminate through the bloodstream or lymphatics.

Serum IgG and IgM directed against gonococcal proteins and lipo-oligosaccharides lead to complement-mediated bacterial lysis. Stable serum resistance to this bactericidal antibody probably results from a particular type of porin protein expressed in gonococci (most contain PorIA), and these strains are often the cause of disseminated disease. *N. gonorrhoeae* differentially subvert the effectiveness of complement and alter the inflammatory responses elicited in human infection. Isolates from cases of DGI typically resist killing by normal serum (i.e., are serum resistant), inactivate more C3b, generate less C5a, and result in less inflammation at local sites. PID isolates are serum sensitive, inactivate less C3b, generate more C5a, and result in more inflammation at local sites. IgG antibody directed against gonococcal reduction modifiable protein (Rmp) blocks complement-mediated killing of *N. gonorrhoeae*. Anti-Rmp blocking antibodies may harbor specificity for outer membrane protein sequences shared with other neisserial species or Enterobacteriaceae or may be directed against unique Rmp upstream cysteine loop specific sequences, or both. Preexisting antibodies directed against Rmp facilitate transmission of gonococcal infection to exposed women; Rmp is highly conserved in *N. gonorrhoeae,* and the blocking of mucosal defenses may be 1 of its functions. Gonococcal adaptation also appears to be important in the evasion of killing by neutrophils. Examples include sialylation of lipo-oligosaccharides, increases in catalase production, and changes in the expression of surface proteins.

Host factors may influence the incidence and manifestations of gonococcal infection. Prepubertal girls are susceptible to vulvovaginitis and, rarely, experience salpingitis. *N. gonorrhoeae* infects noncornified epithelium, and the thin noncornified vaginal epithelium and alkaline pH of the vaginal mucin predispose this age group to infection of the lower genital tract. Estrogen-induced cornification of the vaginal epithelium in neonates and mature females resists infection. Postpubertal females are more susceptible to salpingitis, especially during menses, when diminished bactericidal activity of the cervical mucus and reflux of blood from the uterine cavity into the fallopian tubes facilitate passage of gonococci into the upper reproductive tract.

Populations at risk for DGI include asymptomatic carriers; neonates; menstruating, pregnant, and postpartum women; homosexuals; and immunocompromised hosts. The asymptomatic carrier state implies failure of the host immune system to recognize the gonococcus as a pathogen, the capacity of the gonococcus to avoid being killed, or both. Pharyngeal colonization has been proposed as a risk factor for DGI. The high rate of asymptomatic infection in pharyngeal gonorrhea may account for this phenomenon. Women are at greater risk for developing DGI during menstruation and pregnancy and postpartum, presumably because of the maximal endocervical shedding and decreased peroxidase bactericidal activity of the cervical mucus during these periods. A lack of neonatal bactericidal IgM antibody is thought to account for a neonate's increased susceptibility to DGI. Persons with terminal complement component deficiencies (C5–C9) are at considerable risk for developing recurrent episodes of DGI.

CLINICAL MANIFESTATIONS. Gonorrhea is manifested by a spectrum of clinical presentations from asymptomatic carriage, to the characteristic localized urogenital infections, to disseminated systemic infection (see Chapter 119).

Asymptomatic Gonorrhea. The incidence of this form of gonorrhea in children has not been ascertained. Gonococci have been isolated from the oropharynx of young children who have been abused sexually by male contacts; oropharyngeal symptoms are usually absent. Most genital tract infections produce symptoms in children. However, as many as 80% of sexually mature females with urogenital gonorrhea infections are asymptomatic in settings in which most infections are detected through screening or other case-finding efforts. This is in contrast to men, who are asymptomatic only 10% of the time. Asymptomatic rectal carriage of *N. gonorrhoeae* has been documented in 40–60% of females with urogenital infection. Most persons with positive rectal cultures are asymptomatic. Most pharyngeal gonococcal infections are asymptomatic. The importance of documenting pharyngeal infection is debated. Most cases resolve spontaneously, transmission from the pharynx to other patients is uncommon, and the pharynx is rarely the only site of infection. Nevertheless, asymptomatic pharyngeal infection may lead to systemic infection and is occasionally the source of transmission to sexual partners.

Uncomplicated Gonorrhea. Genital gonorrhea has an incubation period of 2–5 days in men and 5–10 days in women. Primary infection develops in the urethra of males, the vulva and vagina of prepubertal females, and the cervix of postpubertal females. Neonatal ophthalmitis occurs in both sexes.

Urethritis is usually characterized by a purulent discharge and by dysuria without urgency or frequency. Untreated urethritis in males resolves spontaneously in several weeks or may be complicated by epididymitis, penile edema, lymphangitis, prostatitis, or seminal vesiculitis. Gram-negative intracellular diplococci are found in the discharge.

In prepubertal females, **vulvovaginitis** usually is characterized by a purulent vaginal discharge with a swollen, erythematous, tender, and excoriated vulva. Dysuria may occur. In postpubertal females, symptomatic gonococcal cervicitis and urethritis are characterized by purulent discharge, suprapubic pain, dysuria, intermenstrual bleeding, and dyspareunia. The cervix may be inflamed and tender. In urogenital gonorrhea limited to the lower genital tract, pain is not enhanced by moving the cervix, and the adnexa are not tender to palpation. Purulent material may be expressed from the urethra or ducts of the Bartholin gland. Rectal gonorrhea, although often asymptomatic, may cause proctitis with symptoms of anal discharge, pruritus, bleeding, pain, tenesmus, and constipation. Asymptomatic rectal gonorrhea may not be due to anal intercourse but may represent colonization from vaginal infection.

Gonococcal **ophthalmitis** may be unilateral or bilateral. It may occur in any age group after inoculation of the eye with infected secretions. Ophthalmia neonatorum due to *N. gonorrhoeae* usually appears from 1 to 4 days after birth (see Chapter 625). Ocular infection in older patients results from inoculation or autoinoculation from a genital site. The infection begins with mild inflammation and a serosanguineous discharge. Within 24 hr, the discharge becomes thick and purulent, and tense edema of the eyelids with marked chemosis occurs. If the disease is not treated promptly, corneal ulceration, rupture, and blindness may follow.

Disseminated Gonococcal Infection. Hematogenous dissemination occurs in 1–3% of all gonococcal infections, more frequently after asymptomatic primary infections than symptomatic infections. Women account for the majority of cases, with symptoms beginning 7–30 days after infection and within 7 days of menstruation. The most common manifestations are asymmetric arthralgia, petechial or pustular acral skin lesions, tenosynovitis, suppurative arthritis, and, rarely, carditis, meningitis, and osteomyelitis. The most common initial symptoms are acute onset of polyarthralgia with fever. Only 25% of patients complain of skin lesions. Most deny genitourinary symptoms; however, primary mucosal infection is documented by genitourinary cultures. Approximately 80–90% of cervical cultures are positive in women with DGI. In males, urethral cultures are positive in 50–60%, pharyngeal cultures are positive in 10–20%, and rectal cultures are positive in 15% of cases.

DGI has been classified into 2 clinical syndromes that have some overlapping features. The 1st and more common is the **tenosynovitis-dermatitis syndrome,** which is characterized by fever, chills, skin lesions, and polyarthralgia predominantly involving the wrists, hands, and fingers. Blood culture results are positive in approximately 30–40% of cases, and synovial fluid cultures are almost uniformly negative. The 2nd syndrome is the **suppurative arthritis syndrome,** in which systemic symptoms and signs are less prominent and monarticular arthritis, often involving the knee, is more common. A polyarthralgia phase may precede the monarticular infection. In cases of monarticular involvement, synovial fluid culture results are positive in approximately 45–55% and synovial fluid findings are consistent with septic arthritis. Blood culture results are usually negative. DGI in neonates usually occurs as a polyarticular suppurative arthritis.

Dermatologic lesions usually begin as painful, discrete, 1–20 mm pink or red macules that progress to maculopapular, vesicular, bullous, pustular, or petechial lesions. The typical necrotic pustule on an erythematous base is distributed unevenly over the extremities, including the palmar and plantar surfaces, usually sparing the face and scalp. The lesions number between 5 and 40, and 20–30% may contain gonococci. Although immune complexes may be present in DGI, complement levels are normal, and the role of the immune complexes in pathogenesis is uncertain.

Acute endocarditis is an uncommon (1–2%) but often fatal manifestation of DGI that usually leads to rapid destruction of the aortic valve. Acute pericarditis is a rarely described entity in patients with disseminated gonorrhea. Meningitis with *N. gonorrhoeae* has been documented. Signs and symptoms are similar to those of any acute bacterial meningitis.

DIAGNOSIS. It is not possible to distinguish gonococcal from nongonococcal urethritis on the basis of symptoms and signs alone. Gonococcal urethritis and vulvovaginitis must be distinguished from other infections that produce a purulent discharge, including β-hemolytic streptococci, *C. trachomatis, Mycoplasma hominis, Trichomonas vaginalis,* and *Candida albicans.* Rarely, infection with human herpes simplex virus type 2 may produce symptoms similar to those of gonorrhea.

In males with symptomatic urethritis, a presumptive diagnosis of gonorrhea can be made by identification of gram-negative intracellular diplococci (within leukocytes) in the urethral discharge. A similar finding in females is not sufficient because *Mima polymorpha* and *Moraxella,* which are normal vaginal flora, have a similar appearance. The sensitivity of the Gram stain for diagnosing gonococcal cervicitis and asymptomatic infections is also low. The presence of commensal *Neisseria* species in the oropharynx prevents the use of the Gram stain for diagnosis of pharyngeal gonorrhea. Nonpathogenic *Neisseria* organisms are not found intracellularly.

Diagnosis of gonococcal disease depends on isolation of *N. gonorrhoeae.* Antibiotic susceptibility testing necessitates isolation by culture. Male urethral specimens are obtained by placing a small swab 2–3 cm into the urethra. Material for cervical cultures is obtained after wiping the exocervix and placing a swab in the cervical os and rotating it gently for several seconds. Rectal swabs are best obtained by passing a swab 2–4 cm into the anal canal; specimens that are heavily contaminated by feces should be discarded. For optimal culture results, specimens should be obtained with noncotton swabs (e.g., a urethrogenital Calgiswab), inoculated directly onto culture plates, and incubated immediately. The choice of anatomic sites to culture depends on the sites exposed and the clinical manifestations. Samples from the urethra should be cultured for heterosexual men, and samples from the endocervix and rectum should be cultured for all females, regardless of a history of anal intercourse. A pharyngeal culture should be obtained from both men and women if symptoms of pharyngitis are present or in the case of oral exposure to a person known to have genital gonorrhea. In a suspected case of child sexual abuse, rectal, pharyngeal, and urethral (males) or vaginal (females) swabs should be cultured. Culture of the endocervix should not be attempted until after puberty.

Specimens from sites (e.g., cervix, rectum, pharynx) that normally are colonized by other organisms should be inoculated on a selective culture medium, such as modified Thayer-Martin medium (fortified with vancomycin, colistin, nystatin, and trimethoprim to inhibit growth of indigenous flora). Specimens from sites that are normally sterile or minimally contaminated (i.e., synovial fluid, blood, cerebrospinal fluid) should be inoculated on a nonselective chocolate agar medium. If DGI is suspected, blood, pharynx, rectum, urethra, cervix, and synovial fluid (if involved) should be cultured. Cultured specimens should be incubated promptly at 35–37°C in 3–5% carbon dioxide.

When specimens must be transported to a central laboratory for culture plating, a reduced, non-nutrient holding medium (i.e., Amies modified Stuart medium) preserves specimens with minimal loss of viability for up to 6 hr. When transport may delay culture plating by more than 6 hr, it is preferable to inoculate the sample directly onto a culture medium and transport it at an ambient temperature in a candle jar. The Transgrow and JEMBEC systems of modified Thayer-Martin medium are alternative transport systems.

When microbiology laboratory facilities are not readily available or when patients may be unavailable for follow-up, rapid diagnostic techniques may prove efficacious. Care must be taken in selecting and interpreting results because many rapid tests are less specific than cultures. Nonculture tests include enzyme immunoassay (EIA; polyclonal antigonococcal antibodies for detection of gonococcal antigen), enzyme-linked immunosorbent assay (ELISA; monoclonal antibodies), DNA probes, and nucleic acid amplification tests (NAATs). These tests appear to be less reliable than culture in low-risk asymptomatic patients, for nongenital specimens, and for specimens obtained from children. DNA probes are approved by the Food and Drug Administration for diagnosis of gonorrhea from endocervical swabs where they have proved to be comparable with culture in sensitivity and specificity. Nucleic acid amplification tests are more sensitive than culture, and more rapid to perform, but more expensive. Nonculture tests cannot replace bacteriologic cultures for definitive diagnosis of *N. gonorrhoeae* or for antimicrobial susceptibility testing. They may serve as useful adjuvant diagnostic tools in high-prevalence, transient populations (i.e., in sexually transmitted disease [STD] clinics for adolescents), in which a rapid and accurate presumptive diagnosis is required for prompt institution of therapy. The ability of NAATs to detect organisms in urine specimens has allowed for noninvasive screening of large populations.

Gonococcal arthritis must be distinguished from other forms of septic arthritis as well as from rheumatic fever, rheumatoid arthritis, inflammatory bowel disease, and arthritis secondary to rubella or rubella immunization. Gonococcal conjunctivitis in the newborn period must be differentiated from chemical conjunctivitis caused by silver nitrate drops as well as from conjunctivitis caused by *C. trachomatis*, *Staphylococcus aureus*, group A or B streptococcus, *Pseudomonas aeruginosa*, *Streptococcus pneumoniae*, or human herpes simplex virus type 2.

TREATMENT. All patients who are presumed or proven to have gonorrhea should be evaluated for concurrent syphilis, hepatitis B, HIV, and *C. trachomatis* infection. The incidence of *Chlamydia* co-infection is 15–25% among males and 35–50% among females. Patients beyond the neonatal period should be treated presumptively for *C. trachomatis* infection (see Chapter 223.2). Sexual partners exposed in the preceding 60 days should be examined, cultures should be taken, and presumptive treatment started.

Because of the prevalence of penicillin-resistant *N. gonorrhoeae*, a 3rd generation cephalosporin, specifically ceftriaxone, is recommended as initial therapy for all ages. Antimicrobial resistance in *N. gonorrhoeae* occurs as plasmid-mediated resistance to penicillin and tetracycline, and chromosomally mediated resistance to penicillins, tetracyclines, spectinomycin, and recently to fluoroquinolones.

Adolescent and Adult Infections. A single dose of ceftriaxone (125 mg IM) eradicates pharyngeal and uncomplicated urogenital gonococcal infections. Ceftriaxone is safe and effective in pregnant women, and it probably aborts incubating syphilis. Alternative regimens include cefixime (400 mg PO), ciprofloxacin (500 mg PO), ofloxacin (400 mg PO), or levofloxacin (250 mg PO) in a single dose. The efficacy of cefixime against incubating syphilis is uncertain. Quinolones are not approved for persons <18 yr of age in the USA and will not abort incubating syphilis. Quinolones should not be used for infections acquired in Asia or the Pacific, including Hawaii. In addition, use of quinolones is inadvisable for treating infections acquired in California and in other areas with increased prevalence of quinolone resistance. Additionally, recent national data suggest that the prevalence of quinolone resistance among MSM is substantial (probably >5%), prompting recommendations by the CDC against the use of quinolones in MSM with suspected or proven gonococcal infection. Besides the fluoroquinolones, cefixime, whose manufacture was suspended in 2002, is the only CDC-recommended oral agent for treating gonorrhea. Spectinomycin (40 mg/kg, maximum dose 2 g) in a single IM dose remains highly effective for genital and rectal gonorrhea in the USA, but is ineffective for pharyngeal infection and does not inhibit *T. pallidum*. Regardless of the regimen chosen, treatment should be followed by a regimen active against *C. trachomatis*. The recommended regimens are doxycycline (100 mg PO twice daily for 7 days) or azithromycin (1 g PO in a single dose). Adolescents and adults who are asymptomatic after treatment need not be cultured for a test of cure.

Pregnant women should not be treated with quinolones or tetracyclines. Those infected with *N. gonorrhoeae* should be treated with a recommended or alternate cephalosporin. Women who cannot tolerate a cephalosporin should be administered spectinomycin (2 g IM as a single dose). Either erythromycin or amoxicillin is recommended for treatment of presumptive or diagnosed *C. trachomatis* infection during pregnancy.

The initial management of DGI includes hospitalization and parenteral administration of ceftriaxone (1 g/day). Patients should be examined for clinical evidence of endocarditis and meningitis. Alternatives for adults and older adolescents include cefotaxime (1 g IV every 8 hr) or ceftizoxime (1 g IV every 8 hr), or for patients allergic to β-lactam drugs, ciprofloxacin (400 mg IV every 12 hr), ofloxacin (400 mg IV every 12 hr), levofloxacin (250 mg IV every 24 hr), or spectinomycin (2 g IM every 12 hr). Treatment may be switched to oral regimens after 24–48 hr and as clinical improvement is obvious. Oral regimens include cefixime (400 mg PO bid), ciprofloxacin (500 mg PO bid), or ofloxacin (400 mg PO bid) to complete 7 days of therapy. Gonococcal conjunctivitis should be treated with ceftriaxone (1 g IM in a single dose) with lavage of the infected eye with saline. Meningitis is treated with ceftriaxone (1–2 g IV every 12 hr) for 10–14 days. Endocarditis is treated for >4 wk with ceftriaxone (1–2 g IV every 12 hr). Concurrent therapy for treatment of genital *Chlamydia* infection is important.

Infant and Pediatric Infections. Uncomplicated gonococcal infections in children should be treated with ceftriaxone in a single dose (50 mg/kg IM, not to exceed 125 mg). Children who cannot tolerate ceftriaxone may be treated with spectinomycin 40 mg/kg IM as a single injection (maximum dose is 2 g). Children who have bacteremia or arthritis should be treated with ceftriaxone (50 mg/kg/day, maximum 1 g/day) for a minimum of 7 days if they are <45 kg and for a minimum of 10–14 days if they are >45 kg. Meningitis should be treated for 10–14 days and endocarditis for a minimum of 28 days with ceftriaxone (50 mg/kg/dose every 12 hr with maximum of 1–2 g IV every 12 hr). Neonatal gonococcal ophthalmia is treated effectively with a single dose of ceftriaxone (50 mg/kg IM, not to exceed 125 mg); a single dose of cefotaxime (100 mg/kg IM) is an acceptable alternative. The conjunctivae should be irrigated frequently with physiologic saline solution. Infants born to mothers who have gonococcal infection also should receive a single dose of ceftriaxone (50 mg/kg IM, not to exceed 125 mg). Neonatal sepsis should be treated parenterally for a minimum of 7 days, and meningitis for a minimum of 10 days. Cefotaxime is recommended for infants with hyperbilirubinemia because ceftriaxone competes for bilirubin binding sites on albumin. Neonates with gonococcal ophthalmitis must be hospitalized and evaluated for DGI.

Pelvic Inflammatory Disease. PID encompasses a spectrum of infectious diseases of the upper genital tract due to *N. gonorrhoeae, C. trachomatis,* and endogenous flora (streptococci, anaerobes, gram-negative bacilli). Therapy must cover a broad spectrum and must be given to adolescents as inpatients. A commonly recommended therapeutic regimen is cefoxitin (2 g IV every 6 hr) or cefotetan (2 g IV every 12 hr) plus doxycycline (100 mg PO or IV every 12 hr). Therapy is continued for at least 48 hr after a patient shows improvement. Thereafter, oral doxycycline is given for a total of 10–14 days. An alternative recommended regimen is clindamycin (900 mg IV every 8 hr) plus a loading dose of gentamicin (2 mg/kg IV) followed by maintenance gentamicin (1.5 mg/kg every 8 hr). Therapy is then continued for 48 hr after a patient improves and is followed by oral clindamycin (450 mg orally PO qid) or oral doxycycline (100 mg PO every 12 hr) to complete 10–14 days of therapy. If an intrauterine device is present, it must be removed and an alternative form of birth control used. Sexual partners should be examined and treated for uncomplicated gonorrhea. Follow-up culture (test of cure) of cephalosporin-doxycycline therapy of gonococcal STD is not recommended owing to the low treatment failure rate. A follow-up examination and culture are recommended in 1–2 mo to evaluate the possibility of reinfection or, rarely, treatment failure.

COMPLICATIONS. Complications of gonorrhea result from the spread of gonococci from a local site of invasion. The interval between primary infection and development of a complication is usually days to weeks. In postpubertal females, endometritis may occur, especially during menses. This may progress to salpingitis and peritonitis (PID). Manifestations of PID include signs of lower genital tract infection (e.g., vaginal discharge, suprapubic pain, cervical tenderness) and upper genital tract infection (e.g., fever, leukocytosis, elevated erythrocyte sedimentation rate, and adnexal tenderness or mass). The differential diagnosis includes gynecologic (ovarian cyst, ovarian tumor, ectopic pregnancy) and intra-abdominal (appendicitis, urinary tract infection, inflammatory bowel disease) disease.

Once inside the peritoneum, gonococci may seed the liver capsule, causing a perihepatitis with right upper quadrant pain (Fitz-Hugh-Curtis syndrome), with or without signs of salpingitis. Perihepatitis may also be caused by *Chlamydia trachomatis.* Progression to PID occurs in about 20% of cases of gonococcal cervicitis, and *N. gonorrhoeae* is isolated in approximately 40% of cases of PID in the United States. Untreated cases may lead to hydrosalpinx, pyosalpinx, tubo-ovarian abscess, and eventual sterility. Even with adequate treatment of PID, the risk for sterility caused by bilateral tubal occlusion approaches 20% after 1 episode of salpingitis and exceeds 60% with 3 or more episodes. The risk for ectopic pregnancy is increased approximately 7-fold after 1 or more episodes of salpingitis. Additional sequelae of PID include chronic pain, dyspareunia, and increased risk for recurrent PID.

Urogenital gonococcal infection acquired during the 1st trimester of pregnancy carries a high risk for septic abortion. After 16 wk, infection causes chorioamnionitis, a major cause of premature rupture of the membranes and premature delivery.

PROGNOSIS. Prompt diagnosis and correct therapy ensure complete recovery from uncomplicated gonococcal disease. Complications and permanent sequelae may be associated with delayed treatment, recurrent infection, metastatic sites of infection (meninges, aortic valve), and delayed or topical therapy of gonococcal ophthalmia.

PREVENTION. Efforts to develop a gonococcal pilus vaccine have been unsuccessful thus far. The high degree of inter- and intrastrain antigenic variability of pili poses a formidable deterrent to the development of a single effective pilus vaccine. Other gonococcal surface structures such as the porin protein, stress proteins, and lipo-oligosaccharides may prove more promising as vaccine candidates. In the absence of a vaccine, prevention of gonorrhea can be achieved through education, use of barrier contraceptives (especially condoms and spermicides), intensive epidemiologic and bacteriologic surveillance (screening sexual contacts), and early identification and treatment of infected contacts.

Gonococcal ophthalmia neonatorum can be prevented by instilling 2 drops of a 1% solution of silver nitrate into each conjunctival sac shortly after birth (see Chapter 625). Erythromycin (0.5%) or tetracycline (1%) ophthalmic ointment may also be used.

Centers for Disease Control and Prevention: 2002 sexually transmitted diseases treatment guidelines for treatment of sexually transmitted diseases. *MMWR* 2002;51(RR-6):1–80.

Cohen MS, Sparling PF: Mucosal infection with *Neisseria gonorrhoeae,* bacterial adaptation and mucosal defenses. *J Clin Invest* 1992;89:1699–1705.

Fox KK, Knapp JS, Holmes KK, et al: Antimicrobial resistance in *Neisseria gonorrhoeae* in the United States, 1988–1994: The emergence of decreased susceptibility to the fluoroquinolones. *J Infect Dis* 1997;175:1396–1403.

Hook EW, Holmes KK: Gonococcal infections. *Ann Intern Med* 1985;102: 229–243.

Mathews C, Coetzee D: Partner notification for the control of STIs. *BMJ* 2007;334:323.

O'Brien JP, Goldenberg DL, Rice PA: Disseminated gonococcal infection: A prospective analysis of 49 patients and a review of pathophysiology and immune mechanisms. *Medicine (Baltimore)* 1983;62:395–406.

Plummer FA, Chubb H, Simonsen JN, et al: Antibody to Rmp (outer membrane protein 3) increases susceptibility to gonococcal infection. *J Clin Invest* 1993;91:339–343.

Rice PA, McQuillen DP, Gulati S, et al: Serum resistance of *Neisseria gonorrhoeae.* Does it thwart the inflammatory response and facilitate the transmission of infection? *Ann NY Acad Sci* 1994;730:7–14.

Tapsall JW: Antibiotic resistance in *Neisseria gonorrhoeae. Clin Infect Dis* 2005;41(Suppl 4):S263–S268.

Chapter 192 ■ *Haemophilus Influenzae*

Susan E. Crawford and Robert S. Daum

An effective vaccine to prevent *Haemophilus influenzae* type b disease introduced in the USA and many other countries has resulted in a dramatic decrease in the incidence of infections caused by this organism. However, mortality and morbidity from *H. influenzae* type b infection remain a problem worldwide, primarily in developing countries. Occasional cases of invasive disease caused by non–type b organisms continue to occur but infrequently. Untypable members of the species are important causes of otitis media and sinusitis.

ETIOLOGY. *H. influenzae* is a fastidious, gram-negative, pleomorphic coccobacillus that requires **factor X (hematin)** and **factor V (phosphopyridine nucleotide)** for growth. Some *H. influenzae* isolates are surrounded by a polysaccharide capsule and can be serotyped into 6 antigenically and biochemically distinct types designated by letters a–f.

EPIDEMIOLOGY. Before the advent of effective type b conjugate vaccine use in 1988, *H. influenzae* type b was a major cause of serious disease among children in all countries. There was a striking age distribution of cases, with >90% in children <5 yr of age, and the majority in children <2 yr of age. The annual attack rate of invasive disease was 64–129 cases/100,000 children <5 yr of age per year. Invasive disease caused by other capsular serotypes has been much less frequent but continues to occur. The incidence of invasive disease caused by non–type b serotypes has been estimated at about 0.7 cases/100,000 children <5 yr of age per year. Nonencapsulated (nontypable) *H. influenzae* organisms also infrequently cause invasive disease, especially in neonates, immunocompromised children, and children in certain developing countries. Nontypable isolates are common etiologic agents in otitis media, sinusitis, and chronic bronchitis in adults.

Humans are the only natural hosts for *H. influenzae,* which is part of the normal respiratory flora in 60–90% of healthy children. Most isolates are nontypable. Before the advent of conjugate immunization, *H. influenzae* type b could be isolated from the pharynx of 2–5% of healthy preschool and school-aged children, with lower rates among infants and adults. Asymptomatic colonization with *H. influenzae* type b occurs at a much lower rate in immunized populations.

The continued circulation of the type b organism despite current vaccine coverage levels suggests that elimination of type b disease may be a formidable task. The few cases of type b invasive disease in the United States now occur in both unvaccinated and fully vaccinated children; about half occur in infants <6 mo of age, too young to have received a 2 or 3 dose primary vaccine series. Among those patients who are age eligible to have received such a series, about $^1/_3$ had received at least a 3 dose primary series, and about $^1/_2$ of these had also received a booster dose. Continued efforts will be required to provide currently available conjugate vaccines to children in developing countries where affordability remains an important issue.

Certain groups and individuals have an increased incidence of invasive type b disease, including Alaskan Eskimos, Apaches, Navajos, and blacks. Persons with certain chronic medical conditions are also known to be at increased risk for invasive disease, including those with sickle cell disease, asplenia, congenital and acquired immunodeficiencies, and malignancies. Unvaccinated infants with invasive infection remain at increased risk for recurrence.

Socioeconomic risk factors for invasive *H. influenzae* type b disease include child-care outside the home, the presence of siblings of elementary school age or younger, short duration of breast-feeding, and parental smoking. A history of otitis media is associated with an increased risk for invasive disease. Much less is known about the epidemiology of *H. influenzae* infections other than for type b.

Among age-susceptible household contacts who have been exposed to a case of invasive *H. influenzae* type b disease, there is increased risk for secondary cases of invasive disease in the 1st 30 days, especially in susceptible children <24 mo of age. Whether a similar increased risk occurs for contacts of non-b disease is unknown.

The mode of transmission is most commonly by direct contact or inhalation of respiratory tract droplets containing *H. influenzae.* The incubation period for invasive disease is variable, and the exact period of communicability is unknown. Most children with invasive *H. influenzae* type b disease are colonized in the nasopharynx before initiation of antimicrobial therapy; 25–40% may remain colonized during the 1st 24 hr of therapy.

With the decline of disease caused by type b organisms, disease caused by other serotypes (a, c, d, e, f) and untypable organisms has been recognized more clearly. There is no evidence that these non–type b infections have increased in frequency. However, clusters of type a, and less often type f, infections have occurred. The age distribution and clinical spectrum of type a infections appear to be similar to those of type b in the prevaccine era.

PATHOGENESIS. The precise mechanisms that facilitate successful colonization of the respiratory epithelium have not been identified. Following bacterial attachment to the respiratory mucosa, the events that result in entry into the intravascular compartment by type b organisms are unclear. Once there, however, *H. influenzae* type b and perhaps other encapsulated strains resist intravascular clearance mechanisms. Whether it was the type b capsule itself that conferred the potential for invasive disease or another closely linked virulence factor is not certain. Once established, the magnitude of *H. influenzae* type b bacteremia and its duration determined the likelihood of dissemination of bacteria into sites such as the meninges or joints.

Noninvasive *H. influenzae* infections such as otitis media, sinusitis, and bronchitis are usually caused by nontypable strains. These organisms gain access to sites such as the middle ear and sinus cavities by direct extension from the nasopharynx. The factors facilitating spread from the pharynx include eustachian tube dysfunction and antecedent viral infections of the upper respiratory tract.

Antibiotic Resistance. Most *H. influenzae* isolates are susceptible to ampicillin or amoxicillin, but about 1/3 produce a β-lactamase and are therefore resistant. A **β-lactamase-negative ampicillin-resistant isolate (BLNAR)** manifests resistance by production of a β-lactam-insensitive cell wall synthesis enzyme called PBP3. These strains may be increasing in frequency.

Amoxicillin-clavulanate was once considered uniformly active against *H. influenzae* clinical isolates. However, about 3% of β-lactamase-positive isolates are resistant to amoxicillin-clavulanate. Amoxicillin-clavulanate offers no apparent synergy against BLNAR isolates. Among macrolides, 99% of *H. influenzae* isolates are susceptible to azithromycin, whereas the activity of erythromycin and clarithromycin against *H. influenzae* clinical isolates is poor. The ketolide telithromycin is less active than azithromycin and not considered useful for *H. influenzae* infection. Resistance to 3rd generation cephalosporins has not been documented. Resistance to trimethoprim-sulfamethoxazole is low (<10%), and resistance to quinolones is believed to be infrequent.

Immunity. The most important known element of host defense is antibody directed against the type b capsular polysaccharide **polyribosylribitol phosphate (PRP).** In the prevaccination era, anti-PRP antibody was acquired in an age-related fashion; its mechanism of action is to facilitate clearance of *H. influenzae* type b from blood. This is related in part to its opsonic activity; other antibodies directed against antigens such as outer membrane proteins or lipopolysaccharides may also have a role in opsonization. Both the classic and alternative complement pathways are important in the opsonization of *H. influenzae* type b.

Before the introduction of vaccination and among recipients of unconjugated PRP vaccines, protection from *H. influenzae* type b infection was presumed to correlate with the concentration of circulating anti-PRP antibody at the time of exposure. A serum antibody concentration of 0.15–1.0 μg/mL was considered protective against invasive infection; the higher concentration in vaccines may predict maintenance of a level of >0.15 μg/mL over time. Unimmunized infants usually lack an anti-PRP antibody concentration of this magnitude and are susceptible to disease after encountering *H. influenzae* type b. This lack of antibody in young infants may reflect a maturational delay in the immunologic response to thymus-independent type 2 (TI-2) antigens such as unconjugated PRP, and it was thought to explain the high incidence of type b infections in young infants in the prevaccination era.

Unlike the unconjugated PRP vaccine, the conjugate vaccines—with the exception of PRP-OMP, which also has TI-1 properties—act as thymus-dependent antigens (Table 192-1). They elicit serum antibody responses in young infants, although repeat doses may be required, and are believed to prime memory antibody responses on subsequent encounters with PRP. The concentration of circulating anti-PRP antibody in a child primed by a conjugate vaccine may not correlate precisely with protection, presumably

TABLE 192-1. ***Haemophilus influenzae*** **Type b Conjugate Vaccines Available in the USA**

ABBREVIATION	TRADE NAME	MANUFACTURER	PROTEIN CARRIER
PRP-OMP*	PedvaxHIB	Merck	OMP (an outer membrane protein complex of *Neisseria meningitidis*)
PRP-T†	ActHIB	Sanofi Pasteur	Tetanus toxoid

*PRP-OMP is also available as a combination vaccine with hepatitis B vaccine (Comvax). This should not be used for hepatitis B immunization at birth.

†PRP-T can be reconstituted with Sanofi Pasteur DTaP vaccine, to produce a combination marketed as TriHIBit, which is acceptable only for the booster (4th) dose in infants ≥15 mo of age.

because a memory response may occur rapidly on exposure to PRP and provide protection.

Much less is known about immunity to other encapsulated *H. influenzae* strains or to nontypable isolates. For untypable isolates, evidence suggests that antibodies directed against 1 or more outer membrane proteins are bactericidal and protect against experimental challenge. A variety of antigens have been evaluated in an attempt to identify vaccine candidates for nontypable *H. influenzae,* including outer membrane proteins (P1, P2, P4, P5, P6, D15, and Tbp A/B), lipopolysaccharide, various adhesins, and lipoprotein D.

DIAGNOSIS. Presumptive identification of *H. influenzae* is established by direct examination of the collected specimen by Gram staining. Because of its small size, pleomorphism, poor uptake of stain by some isolates, and the tendency for fluids, particularly when proteinaceous, to have a red background, *H. influenzae* is sometimes difficult to visualize. Because identification of microorganisms on smear by either technique requires at least 10^5 bacteria/mL, failure to visualize them does not preclude their presence.

Culture of *H. influenzae* requires prompt transport and processing of specimens because the organism is fastidious. Specimens should not be exposed to drying or temperature extremes. Primary isolation of *H. influenzae* can be accomplished on chocolate agar or on blood agar plates using the staphylococcus streak technique.

Serotyping of *H. influenzae* is accomplished by slide agglutination with type-specific antisera. Accurate serotyping is essential to monitor progress toward elimination of type b invasive disease. Timely reporting of cases to public health authorities should be ensured.

CLINICAL MANIFESTATIONS AND TREATMENT. The initial antibiotic therapy of invasive infections possibly due to *H. influenzae* should be a parenterally administered antimicrobial agent effective in sterilizing all foci of infection and effective against ampicillin-resistant strains, usually an extended-spectrum cephalosporin such as cefotaxime or ceftriaxone. These compounds have achieved popularity because of their relative lack of serious adverse effects and ease of administration. After the antimicrobial susceptibility of the isolate has been determined, an appropriate agent can be selected to complete the therapy. Ampicillin remains the drug of choice for the therapy of infections caused by susceptible isolates. If the isolate is resistant to ampicillin, ceftriaxone can be administered once daily in selected circumstances for outpatient therapy.

Oral antimicrobial agents are sometimes used to complete a course of therapy initiated by the parenteral route and as initial therapy for noninvasive infections such as otitis media and sinusitis. If the organism is susceptible to ampicillin, amoxicillin is the drug of choice. An oral 3rd generation cephalosporin (cefixime, cefdinir) or amoxicillin-clavulanate may be used when the isolate is resistant to ampicillin.

Meningitis. In the prevaccine era, meningitis accounted for more than half of invasive *H influenzae* disease. Clinically, meningitis caused by *H. influenzae* type b cannot be differentiated from *Neisseria meningitidis* or *Streptococcus pneumoniae* (see Chapter 603.1). It may be complicated by other foci of infection such as the lungs, joints, bones, or pericardium.

Antimicrobial therapy should be administered intravenously for 7–14 days for uncomplicated cases. Cefotaxime, ceftriaxone, and ampicillin cross the blood-brain barrier during acute inflammation in adequate concentrations to treat *H. influenzae* meningitis. Intramuscular therapy with ceftriaxone is an alternative in patients with normal organ perfusion.

The prognosis of *H. influenzae* type b meningitis depends on the age at presentation, duration of illness before appropriate antimicrobial therapy, cerebrospinal fluid (CSF) capsular polysaccharide concentration, and rapidity with which it is cleared from CSF, blood, and urine. Clinically manifested inappropriate secretion of antidiuretic hormone and evidence of focal neurologic deficits at presentation are poor prognostic features. About 6% of patients with *H. influenzae* type b meningitis are left with some hearing impairment, probably because of inflammation of the cochlea and the labyrinth. Dexamethasone (0.6 mg/kg/day divided every 6 hr for 2 days), particularly when given shortly before or concurrent with the initiation of antimicrobial therapy, decreases the incidence of hearing loss. Major neurologic sequelae of *H. influenzae* type b meningitis include behavior problems, language disorders, delayed development of language, impaired vision, mental retardation, motor abnormalities, ataxia, seizures, and hydrocephalus.

Cellulitis. Children with *H. influenzae* cellulitis often have an antecedent upper respiratory tract infection. They usually have no prior history of trauma, and the infection is thought to represent seeding of the organism to the involved soft tissues during bacteremia. The head and neck, particularly the cheek and preseptal region, are the most common sites of involvement. The involved region generally has indistinct margins and is tender and indurated. Buccal cellulitis is classically erythematous with a violaceous hue, although this sign may be absent. *H. influenzae* may often be recovered directly from an aspirate of the leading edge. The blood culture may also reveal the causative organism. Other foci of infection may be present concomitantly, particularly in children <18 mo of age or with fever. A diagnostic lumbar puncture should be considered at the time of diagnosis for these children.

Parenteral antimicrobial therapy is indicated until patients become afebrile, after which an appropriate orally administered antimicrobial agent may be substituted. A 7–10 day course is customary.

Preseptal Cellulitis. Infection involving the superficial tissue layers anterior to the orbital septum is termed preseptal cellulitis, which may be caused by *H. influenzae.* Uncomplicated preseptal cellulitis does not imply a risk for visual impairment or direct central nervous system extension. However, concurrent bacteremia may be associated with the development of meningitis. *H. influenzae* preseptal cellulitis is characterized by fever, edema, tenderness, warmth of the lid, and, occasionally, purple discoloration. Evidence of interruption of the integument is usually absent. Conjunctival drainage may be associated. *S. pneumoniae, Staphylococcus aureus,* and group A streptococcus cause clinically indistinguishable preseptal cellulitis. The latter 2 pathogens are more likely when fever is absent and the integument is interrupted (e.g., an insect bite).

Children with preseptal cellulitis in whom *H. influenzae* or *S. pneumoniae* are etiologic considerations (young age, high fever, intact integument) should have a blood culture, and a diagnostic lumbar puncture should be considered.

Parenteral antibiotics are indicated for preseptal cellulitis. Because *S. aureus, S. pneumoniae,* and group A β-hemolytic streptococci are other causes, empirical therapy should include agents active against these pathogens. Patients with preseptal cellulitis without concurrent meningitis should receive parenteral therapy for about 5 days until fever and erythema have abated. In uncomplicated cases, antimicrobial therapy should be given for a total of 10 days.

Orbital Cellulitis. Infections of the orbit are infrequent and usually complicate acute ethmoid and sphenoid sinusitis. Orbital cellulitis may present with lid edema but is distinguished by the presence of proptosis, chemosis, impaired vision, limitation of the extraocular movements, decreased mobility of the globe, or pain on movement of the globe. The distinction between preseptal and orbital cellulitis may be difficult and is best delineated by CT.

Orbital infections are treated with parenteral therapy for at least 14 days. Underlying sinusitis or orbital abscess may require surgical drainage and more prolonged antimicrobial therapy.

Supraglottitis or Acute Epiglottitis. Epiglottitis is a cellulitis of the tissues comprising the laryngeal inlet (see Chapter 382). It has become exceedingly rare since the introduction of vaccine. Direct bacterial invasion of the involved tissues is probably the initiating pathophysiologic event. This dramatic, potentially lethal condition can occur at any age. Because of the risk of sudden, unpredictable airway obstruction, supraglottitis is a medical emergency. Other foci of infection, such as meningitis, are rare. Antimicrobial therapy directed against *H. influenzae* type b and other etiologic agents should be administered parenterally but only after the airway is secured, and therapy should be continued until patients are able to take fluids by mouth. The duration of antimicrobial therapy typically is 7 days.

Pneumonia. The true incidence of *H. influenzae* pneumonia in children is unknown because invasive procedures are required to obtain cultures and are seldom performed (see Chapter 397). In the prevaccine era, type b bacteria were the usual cause. The signs and symptoms of pneumonia due to *H. influenzae* cannot be differentiated from those of pneumonia caused by many other microorganisms. Other foci of infection may be present concomitantly.

Children <12 mo of age suspected of having *H. influenzae* pneumonia should receive parenteral antimicrobial therapy initially because of their increased risk for bacteremia and its complications. Older children who do not appear severely ill may be managed with an orally administered antimicrobial. Therapy is continued for 7–10 days.

Uncomplicated pleural effusion associated with *H. influenzae* pneumonia requires no special intervention. However, if empyema develops, surgical drainage is indicated.

Suppurative Arthritis. Large joints, such as the knee, hip, ankle, and elbow, are affected most commonly (see Chapter 686). Other foci of infection may be present concomitantly. Although single joint involvement is the rule, multiple joint involvement occurs in about 6% of cases. The signs and symptoms of septic arthritis caused by *H. influenzae* are indistinguishable from those of arthritis caused by other bacteria.

Uncomplicated septic arthritis should be treated with an appropriate antimicrobial administered parenterally for at least 5–7 days. If the clinical response is satisfactory, the remainder of the course of antimicrobial treatment may be given orally. Therapy is typically given for 3 wk for uncomplicated septic arthritis, but it may be continued beyond 3 wk until the C-reactive protein concentration is normal.

Pericarditis. *H. influenzae* is a rare cause of pericarditis (see Chapter 440). Affected children often have had an antecedent upper respiratory tract infection. Fever, respiratory distress, and tachycardia are consistent findings. Other foci of infection may be present concomitantly.

The diagnosis may be established by recovery of the organism from blood or pericardial fluid. Gram stain or detection of PRP in pericardial fluid, blood, or urine (when type b organisms are the cause) may aid the diagnosis. Antimicrobials should be provided parenterally in a regimen similar to that used for meningitis (see Chapter 603.1). Pericardiectomy is useful for draining the purulent material effectively and preventing tamponade and constrictive pericarditis.

Bacteremia Without an Associated Focus. Bacteremia due to *H. influenzae* type b may be associated with fever without any apparent focus of infection (see Chapter 175). In this situation, risk factors for "occult" bacteremia include the magnitude of fever (≥39°C) and the presence of leukocytosis (≥15,000 cells/μL). About 25% of children with occult *H. influenzae* type b bacteremia develop meningitis if left untreated. In the vaccine era, this *H. influenzae* infection has become exceedingly rare. When it does occur, the child should be re-evaluated for a focus of infection and a 2nd blood culture obtained. In general, the child should be hospitalized and given parenteral antimicrobial therapy after a diagnostic lumbar puncture and chest radiograph are obtained.

Miscellaneous Infections. Urinary tract infection, epididymo-orchitis, cervical adenitis, acute glossitis, infected thyroglossal duct cysts, uvulitis, endocarditis, endophthalmitis, primary peritonitis, osteomyelitis, and periappendiceal abscess are rarely caused by *H. influenzae*.

Invasive Disease in Neonates. Neonates rarely have invasive *H. influenzae* infection. With illness within the 1st 24 hr of life, especially in association with maternal chorioamnionitis or prolonged rupture of membranes, transmission of the organism to the infant is likely to have occurred through the maternal genital tract, which may be (<1%) colonized with nontypable *H. influenzae*. Manifestations of neonatal invasive infection include bacteremia with sepsis, pneumonia, respiratory distress syndrome with shock, conjunctivitis, scalp abscess or cellulitis, or meningitis. Less commonly, mastoiditis, septic arthritis, or a congenital vesicular eruption may occur.

Otitis Media. Acute otitis media is 1 of the most common infectious diseases of childhood (see Chapter 641). It results from the spread of bacteria from the nasopharynx through the eustachian tube into the middle-ear cavity. Usually because of a preceding viral upper respiratory tract infection, the mucosa in the area becomes hyperemic and swollen, resulting in obstruction and an opportunity for bacterial multiplication in the middle ear.

The most common bacterial pathogens are *S. pneumoniae, H. influenzae,* and *Moraxella catarrhalis*. Most *H. influenzae* isolates causing otitis media are nontypable. Ipsilateral conjunctivitis may also be present. Amoxicillin (80–90 mg/kg/day) is a suitable 1st line oral antimicrobial agent as the probability of the causative isolate being resistant to amoxicillin and risk for invasive potential is sufficiently low to justify this approach. Alternatively, in certain cases a single dose of ceftriaxone constitutes adequate therapy.

In the case of treatment failure or if a β-lactamase-producing isolate is obtained by tympanocentesis or from drainage fluid, amoxicillin-clavulanate and erythromycin-sulfisoxazole are among the available alternatives. Erythromycin-sulfisoxazole is useful for patients allergic to β-lactam antibiotics.

Conjunctivitis. Acute infection of the conjunctiva is a common infection in childhood (see Chapter 627). In neonates, *H. influenzae* is an infrequent cause. However, it is an important pathogen in older children, as are *S. pneumoniae* and *S. aureus*. Most *H. influenzae* isolates associated with conjunctivitis are nontypable, although type b isolates and other serotypes are occasionally found. Empirical treatment of conjunctivitis beyond the neonatal period usually consists of topical antimicrobial therapy with sulfacetamide. Topical fluoroquinolone therapy is to be avoided because of its broad spectrum, high cost, and high rate of emergent resistance among many bacterial species. Ipsilateral otitis media caused by the same organism may be present and requires oral antibiotic therapy.

Sinusitis. *H. influenzae* is an important cause of acute sinusitis in children, 2nd in frequency only to *S. pneumoniae* (see Chapter 377). Chronic sinusitis lasting >1 yr or severe sinusitis requiring hospitalization is often caused by *S. aureus* or anaerobes such as *Peptococcus, Peptostreptococcus,* or *Bacteroides.* Nontypable *H. influenzae* and viridans group streptococci are also frequently recovered.

For uncomplicated sinusitis, amoxicillin is acceptable initial therapy. However, if clinical improvement does not occur, a broader-spectrum regimen, such as amoxicillin-clavulanate, may be appropriate. A 10 day course is sufficient for uncomplicated sinusitis. Hospitalization for parenteral therapy is rarely required, usually if progression to orbital cellulitis is suspected.

PREVENTION. Universal immunization with *H. influenzae* type b conjugate vaccine is recommended for all infants. Prophylaxis is indicated if close contacts of an index patient with type b disease are unvaccinated. The contagiousness of non–type b *H. influenzae* infections is not known and prophylaxis is not recommended.

Vaccine. Three *H. influenzae* type b conjugate vaccines are available, which differ in the carrier protein used and the method of conjugating the saccharide to the protein (see Table 192-1 and Chapter 170). One available combination vaccine is PRP-OMP combined with hepatitis B vaccine (Comvax). Additionally, PRP-T can be combined with the DTaP vaccine (diphtheria and tetanus toxoids and acellular pertussis) for the 4th dose only.

Prophylaxis. Unvaccinated children <48 mo of age in close contact are at increased risk for invasive infection if exposed to an index case of invasive *H. influenzae* type b infection. The risk for secondary disease for children >3 mo of age is inversely related to age. About half of the secondary cases among susceptible household contacts occur in the 1st wk after hospitalization of the index case. Because many children are now protected against *H. influenzae* type b by prior immunization, the need for prophylaxis has greatly decreased. When used, rifampin prophylaxis is indicated for all members of the household or close contact group, including the index patient, if the group includes >1 child <48 mo of age who is not fully immunized.

Parents of children hospitalized for invasive *H. influenzae* type b disease should be informed of the increased risk for secondary infection in other young children in the same household if they are not fully immunized. Parents of children exposed to a single case of invasive *H. influenzae* type b disease in a child-care center or nursery school should be similarly informed, although there is disagreement about the need for rifampin prophylaxis for these children.

For prophylaxis, children should be given rifampin orally (0–1 mo of age, 10 mg/kg/dose; >1 mo of age, 20 mg/kg/dose, not to exceed 600 mg/dose) once a day for 4 consecutive days. The adult dose is 600 mg once daily. Rifampin prophylaxis is not recommended for pregnant women.

Adderson, EE, Byington CL, Spencer L, et al: Invasive serotype a *Haemophilus influenzae* infections with a virulence genotype resembling *Haemophilus influenzae* type b: Emerging pathogen in the vaccine era? *Pediatrics* 2001;108:18–24.

Adegbola RA, Secka O, Lahai G, et al: Elimination of *Haemophilus influenzae* type b (BHb) disease from the Gambia after the introduction of routine immunization with a Hib conjugate vaccine: A prospective study. *Lancet* 2005;366:144–150.

Centers for Disease Control and Prevention: Progress toward elimination of *Haemophilus influenzae* type b invasive disease among infants and children—United States, 1998–2000. *MMWR* 2002;51:234–236.

Gessner BD, Sutanto A, Linehan M, et al: Incidences of vaccine-preventable *Haemophilus influenzae* type b pneumonia and meningitis in Indonesian children: Hamlet-randomised vaccine-probe trial. *Lancet* 2005;365:43–52.

McIntyre PB, Berkey CS, King SM, et al: Dexamethasone as adjunctive therapy in bacterial meningitis. A meta-analysis of randomized clinical trials since 1988. *JAMA* 1997;278:925–931.

Prymula P, Peeters P, Chrobok V, et al: Pneumococcal capsular polysaccharides conjugated to protein D for prevention of acute otitis media caused by both *Streptococcus pneumoniae* and non-typeable *Haemophilus influenzae:* A randomized double-blind efficacy study. *Lancet* 2006;367:740–748.

Saha SK, Baqui AH, Darmstadt GL, et al: Invasive *Haemophilus influenzae* type b diseases in Bangladesh, with increased resistance to antibiotics. *J Pediatr* 2005;146:227–233.

Yaro S, Lourd M, Naccro B, et al: The epidemiology of *Haemophilus influenzae* type b meningitis in Burkina Faso. *Pediatr Infect Dis J* 2006;25: 415–419.

Chapter 193 ■ Chancroid *(Haemophilus Ducreyi)*

Parvin Azimi

Chancroid is a sexually transmitted disease characterized by painful genital ulceration and inguinal lymphadenopathy that is caused by *Haemophilus ducreyi,* a fastidious gram-negative bacillus. Chancroid is prevalent in many developing countries and occurs sporadically in the developed world, usually in persons who have recently returned from endemic areas or occasionally in localized urban outbreaks associated with commercial sex workers. It is a risk factor for transmission of HIV. Diagnosis of chancroid in infants and children is strong evidence of sexual abuse.

Illness begins after an incubation period of 4–7 days with a small inflammatory papule on the preputial orifice or frenulum in men and on the labia, fourchette, or perineal region in women. The lesion becomes pustular, eroded, and ulcerative within 2–3 days. The ulcer edge is classically ragged and undermined. Without treatment, the ulcers may persist for weeks to months. Painful, tender inguinal lymphadenitis occurs in >50% of cases, more often among men. The lymphadenopathy can become fluctuant to form **buboes,** which can spontaneously rupture.

Diagnosis is usually established by the clinical presentation and the exclusion of both syphilis *(Treponema pallidum)* and herpes simplex virus infections. Gram stain of ulcer secretions may show gram-negative coccobacilli in parallel clusters (school of fish). Culture requires expensive, special media and has a sensitivity of only 80%. Polymerase chain reaction or indirect immunofluorescence using monoclonal antibodies remain research tools and may become the best means for diagnosis. The ulcer of chancroid is accompanied by concurrent **lymphadenopathy** that is usually unilateral, unlike lymphogranuloma venereum (see Chapter 223.4). Genital herpes is characterized by vesicular lesions with a history of recurrence (see Chapter 249).

Most *H. ducreyi* organisms are resistant to penicillin and ampicillin because of plasmid-mediated β-lactamase production. Spread of plasmid-mediated resistance among *H. ducreyi* has resulted in lack of efficacy of previously useful drugs such as sulfonamides and tetracyclines. The recommended treatment of chancroid is azithromycin (1 g as a single dose PO) or ceftriaxone (250 mg as a single dose IM). Alternative regimens include erythromycin (500 mg tid PO for 7 days), which is most often used in developing countries, and ciprofloxacin (500 mg bid PO for 3 days, for persons ≥18 yr of age). Fluctuant nodes may require drainage. Symptoms usually resolve within 3–7 days. Relapses can usually be treated successfully with the original treatment regimen. Patients with HIV infection may require longer duration of treatment.

Patients with chancroid should be evaluated for other sexually transmitted infections; an estimated 10% have concomitant syphilis or genital herpes. In developing countries, patients with a compatible genital ulcer are treated for both chancroid and syphilis. All sexual contacts of patients with chancroid should be evaluated and treated. Complications include phimosis in men and secondary bacterial infection. Genital ulceration as a syndrome increases the risk for transmission of HIV. Male circumcision appears to lower the risk for chancroid.

Centers for Disease Control and Prevention: Sexually transmitted diseases treatment guidelines, 2006. *MMWR* 2006;55:15.

Lewis DA: Chancroid: Clinical manifestations, diagnosis, and management. *Sex Transm Infect* 2003;79:68–71.

Mackay IM, Harnett G, Jeoffreys N, et al: Detection and discrimination of herpes simplex viruses, *Haemophilus ducreyi, Treponema pallidum,* and *Calymmatobacterium (Klebsiella) granulomatis* from genital ulcers. *Clin Infect Dis* 2006;42:1431–1438.

Mertz KJ, Weiss JB, Webb RM, et al: An investigation of genital ulcers in Jackson, Mississippi, with use of a multiplex polymerase chain reaction assay: High prevalence of chancroid and human immunodeficiency virus infection. *J Infect Dis* 1998;178:1060–1066.

Spinola SM, Bauer ME, Munson RS Jr: Immunopathogenesis of *Haemophilus ducreyi* infection (chancroid). *Infect Immun* 2002;70:1667–1676.

Weiss HA, Thomas SL, Munagi SK, et al: Male circumcision and risk of syphilis, chancroid, and genital herpes: A systematic review and meta-analysis. *Sex Transm Infect* 2006;82:101–109.

Chapter 194 ■ Pertussis *(Bordetella Pertussis and Bordetella Parapertussis)*

Sarah S. Long

Pertussis is an acute respiratory tract infection that was well described initially in the 1500s. Sydenham first used the term *pertussis,* meaning intense cough, in 1670; it is preferable to **whooping cough** because most infected individuals do not "whoop."

ETIOLOGY. *Bordetella pertussis* is the sole cause of epidemic pertussis and the usual cause of sporadic pertussis. *Bordetella parapertussis* is an occasional cause of sporadic pertussis that contributes significantly to total cases of pertussis in eastern and western Europe, but accounts for <5% of *Bordetella* isolates in the United States. *B. pertussis* and *B. parapertussis* are exclusive pathogens of humans and some primates.

B. bronchiseptica is a common animal pathogen. Occasional case reports in humans may involve any body site and typically occur in immunocompromised persons or young children with intense exposure to animals. Protracted coughing can be caused by *Mycoplasma,* parainfluenza or influenza viruses, enteroviruses, respiratory syncytial virus, or adenoviruses. None of these is an important cause of pertussis.

EPIDEMIOLOGY. There are 60 million cases of pertussis each year worldwide, resulting in >500,000 deaths. Before vaccination was available, pertussis was the leading cause of death due to communicable disease among children <14 yr of age in the United States, with 10,000 deaths annually. Widespread use of pertussis vaccine led to a >99% decline in cases. The pivotal role of vaccination in disease control is reflected in the continued high incidence of pertussis in developing countries, and resurgence in other countries where vaccine coverage is low or where less potent vaccine may have been used.

After the low number of 1,010 cases in the United States reported in 1976, there was an increase in annual pertussis incidence to 1.2 cases/100,000 population from 1980 through 1989 with epidemic pertussis in many states in 1989–1990, 1993, and 1996. Pertussis is increasingly endemic, with less cycling or seasonality than previously occurred. In 2004, incidence of reported pertussis in the United States increased for the 3rd year in a row, to 8.9 cases per 100,000 population, more than twice the rate reported in 2003 and an increase from 1.8 in 1994. The number of cases (25,827) was the highest reported since 1959. Of these, 10% occurred among infants <6 mo of age who were too young to have received the 1st 3 of the 5 doses of vaccine that are recommended by 6 yr of age. This age group had the highest reported rate, 136.5/100,000 population. Infants have the highest morbidity associated with pertussis, although adolescents and adults now account for the majority (67%) of reported cases as vaccine-induced immunity wanes and they become susceptible to infection. Approximately 60% of cases are in adolescents and adults. Pertussis is the only vaccine-preventable disease for which universal immunization in the United States is recommended that continues to show rising incidence. There is good evidence that the diagnosis of pertussis is underconsidered, underproven, and underreported.

Pertussis is extremely contagious, with attack rates as high as 100% in susceptible individuals exposed to aerosol droplets at close range. *B. pertussis* does not survive for prolonged periods in the environment. Chronic carriage by humans is not documented. After intense exposure as in households, the rate of subclinical infection is as high as 80% in fully immunized or previously infected individuals. When carefully sought, however, a symptomatic source case can be found for most patients.

Neither natural disease nor vaccination provides complete or lifelong immunity against reinfection or disease. Protection against typical disease begins to wane 3–5 yr after vaccination and is unmeasurable after 12 yr. Subclinical reinfection undoubtedly has contributed significantly to immunity against disease ascribed previously to both vaccine and prior infection. Adolescents and adults in the United States have inadequate antibody to *B. pertussis.* Despite history of disease or complete immunization, outbreaks of pertussis have occurred in the elderly, in nursing homes, in residential facilities with limited exposures, in highly immunized suburbia, and in preadolescents, adolescents, and adults with lapsing time since immunization. Coughing adolescents and adults (usually not recognized as having pertussis) currently are the major reservoir for *B. pertussis* and are the usual sources for "index cases" in infants and children.

In the prevaccine era and in countries such as Germany, Sweden, and Italy, where immunization was limited, the peak incidence of pertussis is in children 1–5 yr of age; infants account for <15% of cases. In the USA in 2003, the highest incidence of pertussis was in infants <6 mo of age (approximately 2,000 cases; 80 cases per 100,000 population), but the largest number of cases occurred among children and adolescents 10–14 yr of age (2,600 cases) and 15–19 yr of age (1,800 cases). A number of studies have documented pertussis in 13–32% of adolescents and adults with cough illness for >7 days. It is estimated that at least 1 million individuals have such *B. pertussis* infections annually in the USA.

Possible explanations for change in epidemiology include waning immunity postimmunization, an aging cohort who received less effective vaccine, and increased awareness and diagnosis. Without natural reinfection with *B. pertussis* or repeated booster vaccinations, adolescents and adults are susceptible to clinical disease if exposed, and mothers provide little if any passive protection to young infants.

PATHOGENESIS. *Bordetella* organisms are tiny, fastidious, gram-negative coccobacilli that only colonize ciliated epithelium. Exact mechanism of disease symptomatology remains unknown. *Bordetella* species share a high degree of DNA homology among virulence genes. Only *B. pertussis* expresses **pertussis toxin** (PT), the major virulence protein. PT has numerous proven biologic activities (e.g., histamine sensitivity, insulin secretion, leukocyte dysfunction), some of which may account for systemic manifestations of disease. PT causes lymphocytosis immediately in experimental animals by rerouting lymphocytes to remain in the circulating blood pool. PT appears to have a central but not a singular role in pathogenesis. *B. pertussis* produces an array of other biologically active substances, many of which are postulated to have a role in disease and immunity. After aerosol acquisition, **filamentous hemagglutinin** (FHA), some **agglutinogens** (especially fimbriae [Fim] types 2 and 3), and a 69 kd nonfimbrial surface protein called **pertactin** (Pn) are important for attachment to ciliated respiratory epithelial cells. **Tracheal cytotoxin,** adenylate cyclase, and PT appear to inhibit clearance of organisms. Tracheal cytotoxin, dermonecrotic factor, and adenylate cyclase are postulated to be predominantly responsible for the local epithelial damage that produces respiratory symptoms and facilitates absorption of PT.

CLINICAL MANIFESTATIONS. Classically, pertussis is a prolonged disease, divided into catarrhal, paroxysmal, and convalescent stages. The **catarrhal stage** (1–2 wk) begins insidiously after an incubation period ranging from 3–12 days with nondistinctive symptoms of congestion and rhinorrhea variably accompanied by low-grade fever, sneezing, lacrimation, and conjunctival suffusion. As initial symptoms wane, coughing marks the onset of the **paroxysmal stage** (2–6 wk). The cough begins as a dry, intermittent, irritative hack and evolves into the inexorable paroxysms that are the hallmark of pertussis. A well-appearing, playful toddler with insignificant provocation suddenly expresses an anxious aura and may clutch a parent or comforting adult before beginning a machine-gun burst of uninterrupted coughs, chin and chest held forward, tongue protruding maximally, eyes bulging and watering, face purple, until coughing ceases and a loud whoop follows as inspired air traverses the still partially closed airway. Post-tussive emesis is common, and exhaustion is universal. The number and severity of paroxysms escalate over days to a week and remain at that plateau for days to weeks. At the peak of the paroxysmal stage, patients may have more than 1 episode hourly. As the paroxysmal stage fades into the **convalescent stage** (≥2 wk), the number, severity, and duration of episodes diminish.

Infants <3 mo of age do not display classical stages. The catarrhal phase lasts only a few days or is unnoticed when after the most insignificant startle from a draft, light, sound, sucking, or stretching, a well-appearing young infant begins to choke, gasp, gag, and flail extremities, with face reddened. Cough (expiratory grunt) may not be prominent. Whoop infrequently occurs in infants <3 mo of age who at the end of a paroxysm lack stature or muscular strength to create sudden negative intrathoracic pressure. Cyanosis can follow a coughing paroxysm, or apnea can occur without a cough. Apnea may be the only symptom. The paroxysmal and convalescent stages in young infants are lengthy.

Paradoxically, in infants, cough and whooping may become louder and more classic in convalescence. Convalescence includes intermittent paroxysmal coughing throughout the 1st year of life, including "exacerbations" with subsequent respiratory illnesses; these are not due to recurrent infection or reactivation of *B. pertussis*.

Immunized children have foreshortening of all stages of pertussis. Adults have no distinct stages. Classically, adults describe a sudden feeling of strangulation followed by uninterrupted coughs, feeling of suffocation, bursting headache, diminished awareness, and then a gasping breath, usually without a whoop. Post-tussive emesis and intermittency of paroxysms separated by hours of well-being are specific clues to the diagnosis in adolescents and adults. In prospective studies, at least $^{1}/_{3}$ of older individuals with pertussis have nonspecific cough illness, distinguished only by duration, which is usually >21 days.

Findings on physical examination generally are uninformative. Signs of lower respiratory tract disease are not expected unless complicating secondary bacterial pneumonia is present. Conjunctival hemorrhages and petechiae on the upper body are common.

DIAGNOSIS. Pertussis should be suspected in any individual who has pure or predominant complaint of cough, especially if the following are absent: fever, malaise or myalgia, exanthem or enanthem, sore throat, hoarseness, tachypnea, wheezes, and rales. For sporadic cases, a clinical case definition of cough of ≥14 days' duration with at least 1 associated symptom of paroxysms, whoop, or post-tussive vomiting has a sensitivity of 81% and specificity of 58% for culture confirmation. Pertussis should be suspected in older children whose cough illness is escalating at 7–10 days and whose coughing episodes are not continuous. Pertussis should be suspected in infants <3 mo of age with apnea, cyanosis, or an acute life-threatening event (ALTE). *B. pertussis* is an occasional cause of sudden infant death.

Adenoviral infections are usually distinguishable by associated features, such as fever, sore throat, and conjunctivitis. *Mycoplasma* causes protracted episodic coughing, but patients usually have a history of fever, headache, and systemic symptoms at the onset of disease as well as more continuous cough and frequent finding of rales on auscultation of the chest. Epidemics of *Mycoplasma* and *B. pertussis* in young adults can be difficult to distinguish on clinical grounds. Although pertussis is often included in the laboratory evaluation of young infants with afebrile pneumonia, *B. pertussis* is not associated with staccato cough (breath with every cough), purulent conjunctivitis, tachypnea, rales or wheezes that typify infection due to *Chlamydia trachomatis,* or predominant lower respiratory tract signs that typify infection due to respiratory syncytial virus. Unless an infant with pertussis has secondary pneumonia (and is then ill appearing), the findings on examination between paroxysms are entirely normal, including respiratory rate.

Leukocytosis (15,000–100,000 cells/mm^3) due to absolute lymphocytosis is characteristic in the catarrhal stage. Lymphocytes are of T- and B-cell origin and are normal small cells, rather than the large atypical lymphocytes seen with viral infections. Adults, partially immune children, and occasionally young infants have less impressive lymphocytosis. Absolute increase in neutrophils suggests a different diagnosis or secondary bacterial infection. Eosinophilia is not a manifestation of pertussis. A severe course and death are correlated with extreme leukocytosis (median peak white blood cell count fatal vs nonfatal cases, 94 vs 18 × 10^9 cells/L) and thrombocytosis (median peak platelet count fatal vs nonfatal cases, 782 vs 556 × 10^9/L). Mild hyperinsulinemia and reduced glycemic response to epinephrine have been demonstrated, although hypoglycemia is reported only occasionally. The chest x-ray is only mildly abnormal in the majority of hospitalized infants, showing perihilar infiltrate or edema (sometimes with a butterfly appearance) and variable atelectasis. Parenchymal consolidation suggests secondary bacterial infection. Pneumothorax, pneumomediastinum, and air in soft tissues can be seen occasionally.

All current methods for confirmation of infection due to *B. pertussis* have limitations in sensitivity, specificity, or practicality. Isolation of *B. pertussis* in culture remains the gold standard for diagnosis. Careful attention must be directed to specimen collection, transport, and isolation technique. The specimen is obtained by deep nasopharyngeal aspiration or by use of a flexible swab, preferably a dacron or calcium alginate swab, held in the posterior nasopharynx for 15–30 sec (or until coughing). A 1.0% casamino acid liquid is acceptable for holding a specimen up to 2 hr; Stainer-Scholte broth or Regan-Lowe semisolid transport medium is used for longer periods, up to 4 days. Regan-Lowe charcoal agar with 10% horse blood and 5–40 µg/mL cephalexin or Stainer-Scholte media with cyclodextrin resins are the preferred isolation media. Cultures are incubated at 35–37°F in a humid environment and examined daily for 7 days for slow-growing, tiny, glistening colonies. Direct fluorescent antibody

(DFA) testing of potential isolates using specific antibody for *B. pertussis* and *B. parapertussis* maximizes recovery. Direct testing of nasopharyngeal secretions by DFA is a rapid test, but is reliable only in laboratories with continuous experience. Polymerase chain reaction (PCR) to test nasopharyngeal wash specimens has a sensitivity similar to that of culture, averts difficulties of isolation, but is not standardized or available universally. Results of DFA, culture, and PCR are all expected to be positive in unimmunized, untreated children during the catarrhal and early paroxysmal stage of disease. Less than 10% of any of these test results are positive in partially or remotely immunized individuals tested in the paroxysmal stage. Serologic tests for detection of antibodies to *B. pertussis* antigens in acute and convalescent samples are the most sensitive tests in immunized individuals and are useful epidemiologically. A single serum sample showing immunoglobulin G (IgG) antibody to pertussis toxin elevated >2 standard deviations above the mean of the immunized population indicates recent infection. Standardization of tests and cut point for a positive result are currently being investigated. IgA and IgM pertussis antibody tests are not reliable methods for diagnosis.

TREATMENT. Goals of therapy are to limit the number of paroxysms, to observe the severity of the cough, to provide assistance when necessary, and to maximize nutrition, rest, and recovery without sequelae (Table 194-1). Infants <3 mo of age are admitted to hospital almost without exception, as are those between 3–6 mo unless witnessed paroxysms are not severe, and those of any age if significant complications occur. Prematurely born young infants and children with underlying cardiac, pulmonary, muscular, or neurologic disorders have a high risk for severe disease.

The specific, limited goals of hospitalization are to (1) assess progression of disease and likelihood of life-threatening events at peak of disease, (2) prevent or treat complications, and (3) educate parents in the natural history of the disease and in care that will be given at home. Heart rate, respiratory rate, and pulse oximetry are monitored continuously with alarm settings so that paroxysms can be witnessed and recorded by health care personnel. Detailed cough records and documentation of feeding, vomiting, and weight change provide data to assess severity. Typical paroxysms that are not life threatening have the following features: duration <45 sec; red but not blue color change; tachycardia, bradycardia (not <60 beats/min in infants), or oxygen desaturation that spontaneously resolves at the end of the paroxysm; whooping or strength for self-rescue at the end of the paroxysm; self-expectorated mucus plug; and post-tussive exhaustion but not unresponsiveness. Assessing the need to provide oxygen, stimulation, or suctioning requires skilled personnel who can document an infant's ability for self-rescue but who will intervene rapidly and expertly when necessary. Infants whose paroxysms repeatedly lead to life-threatening events despite passive delivery of oxygen or whose fatigue leads to hypercarbia require intubation, paralysis, and ventilation. Subsequent management is complex, with frequent need to suction the airway and intervene when bradycardia or secondary pulmonary processes occur. Mist by tent can be useful in some infants with thick, tenacious secretions and excessively irritable airways. The benefit of a quiet, dimly lighted, undisturbed, comforting environment cannot be overestimated or forfeited in a desire to monitor and intervene. Feeding children with pertussis is challenging. The risk for precipitating cough by nipple feeding does not warrant nasogastric, nasojejunal, or parenteral alimentation in most infants. The composition or thickness of formula does not affect the quality of secretions, cough, or retention. Large-volume feedings are avoided.

Within 48–72 hr, the direction and severity of disease usually are obvious by analysis of recorded information. Many infants have marked improvement upon hospitalization and antibiotic therapy, especially if they are early in the course of disease or have been removed from aggravating environmental smoke, excessive stimulation, or a dry or polluting heat source. Hospital discharge is appropriate if over a 48-hr period disease severity is unchanged or diminished, no intervention is required during paroxysms, nutrition is adequate, no complication has occurred, and parents are adequately prepared for care at home. Apnea and seizures occur in the incremental phase of illness and in those with complicated disease. Portable oxygen, monitoring, or suction apparatus should not be needed at home.

Antibiotics. An antimicrobial agent is always given when pertussis is suspected or confirmed primarily to limit the spread of infection and secondarily for possible clinical benefit. Macrolides are preferred agents, which have similar efficacy in vitro (Table 194-2). Resistance has been reported rarely. A 7- to 10-fold relative risk for infantile hypertrophic pyloric stenosis (IHPS) has been reported in neonates treated with orally administered erythromycin. Azithromycin is the preferred agent for use in neonates. Limited use in neonates has not signaled increased risk for IHPS. All infants <1 mo of age treated with any macrolide should be monitored for symptoms of pyloric stenosis.

Adjunct Therapies. No rigorous clinical trial has demonstrated a beneficial effect of β_2-adrenergic stimulants such as salbutamol or albuterol. Fussing associated with aerosol treatment triggers paroxysms. No randomized, blinded clinical trial of sufficient size has been performed to evaluate the usefulness of corticosteroids in the management of pertussis; their clinical use is not warranted.

Isolation. Patients with suspected pertussis are placed in respiratory isolation with use of masks by all health care personnel entering the room. Screening for cough should be performed upon entrance of patients to emergency departments, offices, and clinics to begin isolation immediately and until 5 days after initiation of macrolide therapy. Children and staff with pertussis in child-care facilities or schools should be excluded until macrolide prophylaxis has been taken for 5 days.

Care of Household and Other Close Contacts. A macrolide agent should be given promptly to all household contacts and other close contacts, such as those in daycare, regardless of age, history of immunization, or symptoms (Table 194-2). The same age-related drugs and doses for prophylaxis are used for treatment. Visitation and movement of coughing family members in the hospital must be assiduously controlled until erythromycin has been taken for 5 days. Close contacts <7 yr of age who have received fewer than 4 doses of pertussis-containing vaccines should have vaccination initiated or continued to complete the recommended series. Children <7 yr of age who received a 3rd dose >6 mo before exposure or a 4th dose ≥3 yr before exposure should receive a booster dose. Individuals ≥9 yr should be given a Tdap (adolescent/adult formulation of tetanus and diphtheria toxoids and acellular pertussis) booster if they have not previously received Tdap and >2 yr have passed since receipt of a diphtheria-containing vaccine. Coughing health care workers, with or without known exposure to pertussis, should be promptly evaluated for pertussis (see Chapter 171).

TABLE 194-1. Caveats in Assessment and Care of Infants with Pertussis

Infants with potentially fatal pertussis may appear well between episodes.
A paroxysm must be witnessed before deciding between hospital and home care.
Only analysis of carefully compiled cough record permits assessment of severity and progression of illness.
Suctioning of nose, oropharynx, or trachea should not be performed on a "preventive" schedule.
Feeding in the period following a paroxysm may be more successful than following napping.
Family support begins at the time of hospitalization with empathy for the child's and family's experience to date, transfer of the burden of responsibility for the child's safety to the health care team, and delineation of assessments and treatments to be performed.
Family education, recruitment as part of the team, and continued support after discharge are essential.

TABLE 194-2. Recommended Antimicrobial Treatment and Postexposure Prophylaxis for Pertussis, by Age Group

	PRIMARY AGENTS			ALTERNATE AGENT*
AGE GROUP	Azithromycin	Erythromycin	Clarithromycin	TMP-SMZ
<1 mo	Recommended agent. 10 mg/kg/day in a single dose for 5 days (only limited safety data available)	Not preferred. Erythromycin is associated with infantile hypertrophic pyloric stenosis. Use if azithromycin is unavailable; 40–50 mg/kg/day in 4 divided doses for 14 days.	Not recommended (safety data unavailable)	Contraindicated for infants aged <2 mo (risk for kernicterus)
1–5 mo	10 mg/kg/day in a single dose for 5 days	40–50 mg/kg/day in 4 divided doses for 14 days.	15 mg/kg/day in 2 divided doses for 7 days	Contraindicated at age <2 mo For infants aged ≥2 mo TMP 8 mg/kg/day, SMZ 40 mg/kg/day in 2 divided doses for 14 days
Infants (aged ≥6 mo) and children	10 mg/kg in a single dose on day 1 then 5 mg/kg/day (maximum 500 mg) on days 2–5	40–50 mg/kg/day (maximum 2 g/day) in 4 divided doses for 14 days.	15 mg/kg/day in 2 divided doses (maximum 1 g/day) for 7 days	TMP 8 mg/kg/day, SMZ 40 mg/kg/day in 2 divided doses for 14 days
Adults	500 mg in a single dose on day 1 then 250 mg/day on days 2–5	2 g/day in 4 divided doses for 14 days.	1 g/day in 2 divided doses for 7 days	TMP 320 mg/day, SMZ 1,600 mg/day in 2 divided doses for 14 days

*Trimethoprim-sulfamethoxazole (TMP-SMZ) can be used as an alternative agent to macrolides in patients aged ≥2 mo who are allergic to macrolides, who cannot tolerate macrolides, or who are infected with a rare macrolide-resistant strain of *Bordetella pertussis*.

From Centers for Disease Control and Prevention: Recommended antimicrobial agents for treatment and postexposure prophylaxis of pertussis. 2005 CDC Guidelines. *MMWR* 2005;54:1–16.

COMPLICATIONS. Infants <6 mo of age have excessive mortality and morbidity, with infants <2 mo of age having the highest reported rates of pertussis-associated hospitalization (82%), pneumonia (25%), seizures (4%), encephalopathy (1%), and death (1%). Infants <4 mo of age account for 90% of cases of fatal pertussis. Preterm birth and young maternal age are significantly associated with fatal pertussis.

The principal complications of pertussis are apnea, secondary infections (such as otitis media and pneumonia), and physical sequelae of forceful coughing. The need for intensive care and artificial ventilation is usually limited to infants <3 mo of age. Respiratory failure due to apnea or secondary bacterial pneumonia are events precipitating intubation and ventilation. Progressive pulmonary hypertension or hemorrhage (especially in very young infants) and secondary bacterial pneumonia are usual causes of death. Fever, tachypnea or respiratory distress between paroxysms, and absolute neutrophilia are clues to pneumonia. Expected pathogens include *Staphylococcus aureus, Streptococcus pneumoniae,* and bacteria of oropharyngeal flora. Bronchiectasis has been reported rarely after pertussis. Children who have pertussis before the age of 2 yr may have abnormal pulmonary function into adulthood. Increased intrathoracic and intra-abdominal pressure during coughing can result in conjunctival and scleral hemorrhages, petechiae on the upper body, epistaxis, hemorrhage in the central nervous system (CNS) and retina, pneumothorax and subcutaneous emphysema, and umbilical and inguinal hernias. Laceration of the lingual frenulum is not uncommon.

CNS abnormalities occur at a relatively high frequency and are almost always a result of hypoxemia or hemorrhage associated with coughing or apnea in young infants. Apnea or bradycardia or both may result from apparent laryngospasm or vagal stimulation just before a coughing episode, from obstruction during an episode, or from hypoxemia following an episode. Lack of associated respiratory signs in some young infants with apnea raises the possibility of a primary effect of PT on the CNS. Seizures are usually a result of hypoxemia, but hyponatremia from excessive secretion of antidiuretic hormone during pneumonia can occur. The only neuropathology documented in humans is parenchymal hemorrhage and ischemic necrosis. Particular association of pulmonary hypertension with pertussis is unexplained. Despite extracorporeal membrane oxygenation, this complication portends a mortality rate of >80%.

PREVENTION. Universal immunization of children with pertussis vaccine, beginning in infancy with periodic reinforcing doses, is central to the control of pertussis (see Chapter 170). There is no serologic correlate of protection.

Three diphtheria and tetanus toxoids combined with acellular pertussis (DTaP) vaccines currently are licensed in the USA for children <7 yr of age. DTaP vaccines have fewer adverse effects than the vaccines containing whole-cell pertussis (DTP), which continues to be given to infants and children in many other countries. Acellular pertussis vaccines all contain inactivated PT and contain 2 or more other bacterial components (FHA, Pn, and Fim 2 and 3). Clinical efficacy against severe pertussis, defined as paroxysmal cough >21 days, is 80–85%. Mild local and systemic adverse events as well as more serious events (including high fever, persistent crying of ≥3 hr duration, hypotonic hyporesponsive episodes, and seizures) occur significantly less frequently among infants who receive DTaP compared with DTP vaccine. DTaP-containing vaccines can be administered simultaneously with any other vaccines used in standard schedules for children.

Three (primary) doses of DTaP should be administered during the 1st year of life, generally at ages 2, 4, and 6 mo of age. A 4th dose (1st booster) is recommended for children at 15–18 mo of age, at least 6 mo after the 3rd dose, to maintain adequate immunity during the preschool years. The 4th dose may be administered as early as 12 mo of age, provided 6 mo have elapsed since the 3rd dose and the child is unlikely to return at 15–18 mo of age. The 5th dose (2nd booster) is recommended for children at 4–6 yr of age to confer continued protection against disease during the early years of schooling. A 5th dose is not necessary if the 4th dose in the series is administered on or after the 4th birthday.

Pertussis-containing vaccines and combination vaccines should be used only in the dosing series and age group for which each is licensed, and when all components are indicated. When feasible, the same DTaP product is recommended for the 1st 3 doses of the vaccination series. Local reactions increase in rate and severity with successive doses of DTaP, although never reaching the magnitude of reactions following similar doses of DTP. Up to 2% of 4th and 5th doses of DTaP are associated with entire limb swelling, with concurrent pain and erythema in approximately $^1/_2$ of children affected. Swelling subsides spontaneously without sequelae.

Exempting children from pertussis immunization should be considered only in the narrow limits as recommended. Exemptors have been shown to have significantly increased risk for pertussis as well as a role in outbreaks of pertussis among immunized populations. If infection with *B. pertussis* is proved, the individual should complete the immunization series with at least diphtheria and tetanus toxoids; some experts recommend including the pertussis component as well.

In 2005, 2 tetanus toxoid, reduced diphtheria toxoid and acellular pertussis vaccine, adsorbed (Tdap) products were licensed for use in older individuals as single-dose booster vaccines to provide protection against tetanus, diphtheria, and pertussis. The preferred age for Tdap vaccination is 11–12 yr. All adolescents 11–18 yr of age who received Td, but not Tdap, should receive a single dose of Tdap to provide protection against pertussis if they have completed the recommended childhood DTP/DTaP vaccination series. An interval of at least 5 yr between Td and Tdap is encouraged in routine situations to reduce the risk for local and systemic reactions after Tdap vaccination. However, an interval of <5 yr between Td and Tdap can be used. Both Tdap and tetravalent meningococcal conjugate vaccine should be administered to adolescents 11–18 yr of age during the same visit if both vaccines are indicated and available. Adults 19–64 yr of age should receive a single dose of Tdap to replace their next Td booster dose. Priority for Tdap vaccine should be given for health care workers who have contact with children and for eligible family contacts of neonates. An important objective of administering the adolescent pertussis booster is to protect adolescents and adults against pertussis to control endemic and epidemic spread to young infants who have not completed primary immunization and are at high risk for pertussis and its complications.

American Academy of Pediatrics, Committee on Infectious Diseases: Prevention of pertussis among adolescents: Recommendations for use of tetanus toxoid, reduced diphtheria toxoid, and acellular pertussis (Tdap) vaccine. *Pediatrics* 2006;117:965–978.

Bisgard KM, Pascual FB, Ehresmann KR, et al: Infant pertussis: Who was the source? *Pediatr Infect Dis J* 2004;23:985–990.

Bisgard KM, Rhodes P, Connelly BL, et al: Pertussis vaccine effectiveness among children 6 to 59 months of age in the United States, 1998–2001. *Pediatrics* 2005;116:e285–e294.

Butler C, Francis N, Dinant GJ: Whooping cough in general practice. *BMJ* 2006;333:159–160.

Centers for Disease Control and Prevention: Pertussis—United States, 2001–2003. *MMWR* 2005:54:1283–1286.

Centers for Disease Control and Prevention: Preventing tetanus, diphtheria, and pertussis among adolescents: Use of tetanus toxoid, reduced diphtheria toxoid and acellular pertussis vaccines. Recommendations of the Advisory Committee on Immunization Practices (ACIP). *MMWR* 2006;55(RR-3):1–34.

Centers for Disease Control and Prevention: Recommended antimicrobial agents for treatment and postexposure prophylaxis of pertussis. 2005 CDC guidelines. *MMWR* 2005;54:1–16.

Halasa NB, Barr FE, Johnson JE, et al: Fatal pulmonary hypertension associated with pertussis in infants: Does extracorporeal membrane oxygenation have a role? *Pediatrics* 2003;112:1274–1278.

Halperin SA: Recommendation for an adolescent dose of tetanus and diphtheria toxoids and acellular pertussis vaccine: reassurance for the future. *J Pediatrics* 2006;149:589–591.

Halperin SA: The control of pertussis—2007 and beyond. *N Engl J Med* 2007;356:110–113.

Hewlett EL, Edwards KM: Pertussis—Not just for kids. *N Engl J Med* 2005;352:1215–1222.

Langley JM, Halperin SA, Boucher FD, et al: Azithromycin is as effective as and better tolerated than erythromycin estolate for the treatment of pertussis. *Pediatrics* 2004;114:e96–e101.

Mikelova LK, Halperin SA, Scheifele D, et al: Predictors of death in infants hospitalized with pertussis: A case-control study of 16 pertussis deaths in Canada. *J Pediatr* 2003;143:576–580.

Pichichero ME, Blatter MM, Kennedy WA, et al: Acellular pertussis vaccine booster combined with diphtheria and tetanus toxoids for adolescents. *Pediatrics* 2006;117:1084–1093.

Purdy KW, Hay JW, Botteman MF, Ward JI: Evaluation of strategies for use of acellular pertussis vaccine in adolescents and adults: A cost-benefit analysis. *Clin Infect Dis* 2004;39:20–28.

Tanaka M, Vitek CR, Pascual FB, et al: Trends in pertussis among infants in the United States, 1980–1999. *JAMA* 2003;290:2968–2975.

Tozzi AE, Ravà L, Marta L, et al: Clinical presentation of pertussis in unvaccinated and vaccinated children in the first six years of life. *Pediatrics* 2003;112:1069–1075.

Ward JI, Cherry JD, Chang SJ, et al: Efficacy of an acellular pertussis vaccine among adolescents and adults. *N Engl J Med* 2005;353:1555–1563.

Chapter 195 ■ *Salmonella*

Zulfiqar Ahmed Bhutta

Salmonellosis is a common and widely distributed food-borne disease that is a global major public health problem affecting millions of individuals with significant mortality. Salmonellae live in the intestinal tracts of warm- and cold-blooded animals. Some species are ubiquitous, whereas others are specifically adapted to a particular host.

The recent sequencing of the *Salmonella enterica* serovar Typhi (previously called *Salmonella typhi*) and *Salmonella typhimurium* genomes has indicated almost 95% genetic homology between the organisms. However, the clinical diseases caused by the 2 organisms differ considerably, which appears to be related to several unique clusters of genes known as pathogenicity islands. *Salmonella* causes 2 clinical syndromes in humans: a gastroenteritis that is usually self-limited, and typhoid fever that is a relatively severe systemic illness classically caused by *S. typhi*. Nontyphoidal strains of *Salmonella* can also cause a severe bacteremic illness in some circumstances.

The nomenclature of *Salmonella* reflects the species name *Salmonella enterica* with a number of serovars. *Salmonella* nomenclature has undergone considerable alterations. The original taxonomy was based on clinical syndromes *(S. typhi, S. choleraesuis, S. paratyphi)*. With adoption of serologic analysis, a *Salmonella* species was defined subsequently as "a group of related fermentation phage-type" with the result that each *Salmonella* serovar was considered as a species in itself. Although simplistic, using this classification until 2004 resulted in identification of 2,501 serovars of *Salmonella*, which led to the need for further categorization to aid communication between scientists, public health officials, and the public.

All *Salmonella* serovars form a single DNA hybridization group: a single species composed of 7 subspecies. The current nomenclature with the species name *Salmonella enterica* was adopted with several subspecies, I–VI (Table 195-1). Each subspecies contains various serotypes defined by the O and H antigens. To further simplify the nomenclature for physicians and epidemiologists, the common serovars' names are kept for subspecies I strains, which represent >99.5% of the *Salmonella* strains isolated from humans and other warm-blooded animals.

TABLE 195-1. *Salmonella* Nomenclature

TRADITIONAL USAGE	FORMAL NAME	CDC DESIGNATION
S. typhi	*S. enterica** subsp. enterica ser. Typhi	S. ser. Typhi
S. dublin	*S. enterica* subsp. enterica ser. Dublin	S. ser. Dublin
S. typhimurium	*S. enterica* subsp. enterica ser. Typhimurium	S. ser. Typhimurium
S. choleraesuis	*S. enterica* subsp. enterica ser. Choleraesuis	S. ser. Choleraesuis
S. marina	*S. enterica* subsp. houtenae ser. Marina	S. ser. Marina

CDC, Centers for Disease Control and Prevention; subsp, subspecies; ser., serovar.
*Some authorities prefer *S. choleraesuis* or *S. enteritidis* rather than enterica to describe the species.

195.1 • Nontyphoidal Salmonellosis

ETIOLOGY. Salmonellae are motile, nonsporulating, nonencapsulated, gram-negative rods that grow aerobically and are capable of facultative anaerobic growth. They are resistant to many physical agents but can be killed by heating to 130°F (54.4°C) for 1 hr or 140°F (60°C) for 15 min. They remain viable at ambient or reduced temperatures for days and may survive for weeks in sewage, dried foodstuffs, pharmaceutical agents, and fecal material. Like other members of the family Enterobacteriaceae, *Salmonella* possesses somatic O antigens and flagellar H antigens.

With the exception of a few serotypes that affect only 1 or a few animal species, such as *S. dublin* in cattle and *S. choleraesuis* in pigs, most serotypes have a broad host spectrum. Typically, such strains cause gastroenteritis that is often uncomplicated and does not need treatment, but can be severe in the young, the elderly, and patients with weakened immunity. The causes are typically S. Enteritidis (*S. enterica* serotype Enteritidis) and S. Typhimurium (*S. enterica* serotype Typhimurium), the 2 most important serotypes for salmonellosis transmitted from animals to humans.

EPIDEMIOLOGY. Salmonellosis constitutes a major public health burden and represents a significant cost to society in many countries. It is estimated that, in the United States alone, an estimated 1.4 million nontyphoidal *Salmonella* infections results in 168,000 physician visits, 15,000 hospitalizations, and 580 deaths annually. The total cost associated with *Salmonella* infections is estimated at $3 billion annually in the United States. While there is little information on its epidemiology and the burden of *Salmonella* gastroenteritis from developing countries, *Salmonella* infections are recognized as major causes of childhood diarrheal illness. With the growing burden of HIV infections and malnutrition in Africa, there is a growing interest in the importance of nontyphoidal *Salmonella* bacteremias in children and adults.

Nontyphoidal *Salmonella* infections have a worldwide distribution with an incidence proportional to the standards of hygiene, sanitation, availability of safe water, and food preparation practices. In the developed world, the incidence of *Salmonella* infections and outbreaks has increased several-fold over the past few decades, which may be related to modern practices of mass food production that increase the potential for epidemics. *Salmonella* gastroenteritis accounts for over half of all episodes of bacterial diarrhea in the United States, with incidence peaks at the extreme of ages, among young infants and the elderly. While most human infections have been caused by *S. enterica* serovar Enteritidis, its prevalence has reduced over the past decade, with *S. enterica* serovar Typhimurium overtaking it in some countries.

This rise in *Salmonella* infections in many parts of the world over the past 3 decades may also be related to intensive animal husbandry practices, which selectively promote the rise of certain strains, especially drug-resistant varieties that emerge in response to antimicrobial usage in food animals. Although this may be related to selective pressure from the use of antimicrobials, there may be other factors such as the rise of strains with a selective propensity to develop resistance and virulence. It appears that multidrug-resistant strains of *Salmonella* are more virulent than susceptible strains, and that poorer outcome does not simply relate to the empirical choice of an ineffective antibiotic delaying treatment response. Strains of multidrug-resistant *Salmonella* such as S. Typhimurium phage type DT104 harbor a genomic island that contains many of the drug resistance genes. It is feasible that these integrons also contain genes that express virulence factors. The global spread of multidrug-resistant S. Typhimurium phage type DT104 in animals and humans in recent years may be related to the growing use of antimicrobials and also facilitated by international and national trade of infected animals.

There are several **risk factors** associated with **outbreaks** of *Salmonella* infections. Animals constitute the principal source of human nontyphoidal *Salmonella* disease, and cases have occurred where individuals have had contact with infected animals, including domestic animals such as cats, dogs, reptiles, pet rodents, and amphibians. Specific serotypes may be associated with particular animal hosts; children with *S. enterica* serovar Marina typically have exposure to pet lizards. Domestic animals probably acquire the infection in the same way as humans through consumption of contaminated raw meat, poultry, or poultry-derived products. Animal feeds containing fishmeal or bone meal contaminated with **Salmonella** are an important source of infection for animals. Moreover, subtherapeutic concentrations of antibiotics are often added to animal feed to promote growth. Such practices promote the emergence of antibiotic-resistant bacteria, including *Salmonella,* in the gut flora of the animals, with subsequent contamination of their meat. There is strong evidence to link resistance of S. Typhimurium to fluoroquinolones to its use in animal feeds. While animal-to-animal transmission can occur, most infected animals are asymptomatic.

Salmonella infections in chickens increase the risk for contamination of eggs, and both poultry and eggs are associated with almost half of the common-source outbreaks. Food product–related outbreaks are often caused by contaminated equipment in processing plants or infected food handlers. While almost 80% of **Salmonella** infections are discrete, outbreaks can pose an inordinate burden on public health systems. This may be a particular risk in schools. In an evaluation of a consecutive 604 outbreaks of food-borne disease in schools, *Salmonella* was the most commonly identified pathogen, accounting for 36% of outbreak reports with a known etiology. In 55% of outbreaks, specific food vehicles of transmission were epidemiologically identified and included foods containing poultry (18.6%), salads (6.0%), Mexican-style food (6.0%), beef (5.7%), and dairy products excluding ice cream (5.0%). The most commonly reported food preparation practices that contributed to these school-related outbreaks were improper food storage and holding temperatures and food contaminated by a food handler.

In addition to the effect of antibiotic use in animal feeds, the relationship of *Salmonella* infections to prior antibiotic use among children in the previous month is well recognized. This increased risk for infection in people who have received antibiotics for an unrelated reason may be related to alterations in gut microbial ecology, predisposing them to colonization and infection with antibiotic-resistant *Salmonella* isolates. These resistant strains of *Salmonella* are also more virulent. It is estimated that antimicrobial resistance in *Salmonella* may result in about 30,000 additional *Salmonella* infections, leading to about 300 hospitalizations and 10 deaths.

Given the ubiquitous nature of the organism, nosocomial infections with nontyphoidal *Salmonella* strains can also occur through contaminated equipment and diagnostic or pharmacologic preparations, particularly those of animal origin (pancreatic extracts, pituitary extracts, bile salts). Hospitalized children are at increased risk for severe and complicated ***Salmonella*** infections, especially with drug-resistant organisms.

PATHOGENESIS. The estimated number of bacteria that must be ingested to cause symptomatic disease in healthy adults is 10^6–10^8 *Salmonella* organisms. The gastric acidity inhibits multiplication of the salmonellae, and most organisms are rapidly killed at gastric pH ≤2.0. Achlorhydria, buffering medications, rapid gastric emptying after gastrectomy or gastroenterostomy, and a large inoculum enable viable organisms to reach the small intestine. Neonates and young infants have hypochlorhydria and rapid gastric emptying, which contribute to their increased vulnerability to symptomatic salmonellosis. In infants who typically take fluids, the inoculum size that can produce disease is also comparatively smaller because of faster transit through the stomach.

Once they reach the small and large intestine, the ability of *Salmonella* organisms to multiply and cause infection depends on the infecting dose as well as competition with normal flora. Prior antibiotic therapy may alter this relationship, as might factors such as co-administration of antimotility agents. The typical intestinal mucosal response to nontyphoidal *Salmonella* infection is an enterocolitis with diffuse mucosal inflammation and edema, sometimes with erosions and microabscesses. *Salmonella* organisms are capable of penetrating the intestinal mucosa, although destruction of epithelial cells and ulcers are usually not found. Intestinal inflammation, with polymorphonuclear leukocytes and macrophages, usually involves the lamina propria. Underlying intestinal lymphoid tissue and mesenteric lymph nodes enlarge and may develop small areas of necrosis. Such lymphoid hypertrophy may cause interference with the blood supply to the gut mucosa. Hyperplasia of the reticuloendothelial system is also found within the liver and spleen. If bacteremia develops, it may lead to localized infection and suppuration in almost any organ.

Salmonella species invade epithelial cells in vitro by a process of bacterial-mediated endocytosis, involving cytoskeletal rearrangement, disruption of the epithelial cell brush border, and the subsequent formation of membrane ruffles. An adherent and invasive phenotype of *S. enterica* is activated under conditions similar to those found in the human small intestine (high osmolarity, low oxygen). The invasive phenotype is mediated, in part, by *Salmonella* pathogenicity island 1 (SPI-1), a 40 kb region that encodes regulator proteins (HilA), a type III secretion system (TTSS) that delivers bacterial proteins from the salmonella cytosol into the host cell, and several effector proteins that induce changes within the host cell and promote bacterial uptake.

Although *S.* Typhimurium can cause systemic disease in humans, intestinal infection usually results in a localized enteritis that is associated with a secretory response in the intestinal epithelium, as well as induction of the secretion of interleukin 8 (IL-8) from the basolateral surface and other epithelial pathogen-elicited chemo-attractants toward the apical surface, which direct the recruitment and transmigration of neutrophils into the gut lumen, thus preventing the systemic spread of the bacteria (Fig. 195-1).

Shortly following invasion of the gut epithelium, invasive *Salmonella* organisms encounter macrophages within the gut-associated lymphoid tissue. The interaction between *Salmonella* and macrophages results in alteration in the expression of a number of host genes, including those encoding proinflammatory mediators (inducible nitric oxide synthase [iNOS], chemokines, IL-1b), receptors or adhesion molecules (tumor necrosis factor-α receptor [TNF-αR], CD40, intercellular adhesion molecule 1 [ICAM-1]), and anti-inflammatory mediators (transforming growth factor-β1 and -β2 [TGF-β1 and -β2]). Other upregulated genes include those involved in cell death or apoptosis (intestinal epithelial cell protease, TNF-R1, Fas) and transcription factors (Egr-1, IRF-1). *S.* Typhimurium can induce rapid macrophage death in vitro, which is dependent on the host cell protein caspase-1 and mediated by the SPI-1 effector SipB. Intracellular *S.* Typhimurium is found within specialized *Salmonella* organisms containing vacuoles that have diverged from the normal endocytic pathway. This ability to survive within monocytes/macrophages is essential for *S.* Typhimurium to establish a systemic infection in the mouse. The mucosal pro-inflammatory response to *S.* Typhimurium infection and the subsequent recruitment of phagocytic cells to the site may also facilitate systemic spread of the bacteria.

Some virulence traits are shared by all salmonellae, but others are serotype restricted. These virulence traits have been defined in tissue culture and murine models, and it is likely that clinical features of human *Salmonella* infection will eventually be related to specific DNA sequences. With most diarrhea-associated non-typhoidal salmonelloses, the infection does not extend beyond the lamina propria and the local lymphatics. Specific virulence genes are related to the ability to cause bacteremia. These genes are found significantly more often in strains of *S.* Typhimurium isolated from the blood than in the feces of humans. **Both *S. dublin* and *S. choleraesuis* have a greater propensity to rapidly invade the bloodstream with little or no intestinal involvement.** The development of disease after infection with *Salmonella* depends on the number of infecting organisms, their virulence traits, and several host defense factors. Various host factors may also affect the development of specific complications or clinical syndromes (Table 195-2).

Bacteremia, however, is possible with any *Salmonella* serotype, especially in individuals with reduced host defenses, and especially in those with altered reticuloendothelial or cellular immune function. Thus, children with HIV infection, chronic granulomatous disease, and leukemia are more likely to develop bacteremia after *Salmonella* infection, although the majority of children with *Salmonella* bacteremia in Africa are HIV negative. Children with *Schistosoma mansoni* infection and hepatosplenic involvement as well as chronic malarial anemia are also at a greater risk for developing chronic salmonellosis. Children with sickle cell disease are at increased risk for *Salmonella* septicemia and osteomyelitis. This may be related to the presence of numerous infarcted areas

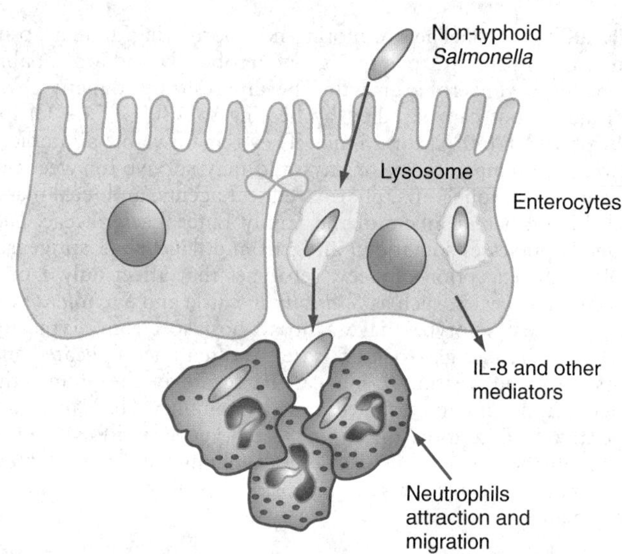

Figure 195-1. Pathogenesis of *Salmonella* gastroenteritis. (Adapted from Santos RL, Tsolis RM, Bäumler AJ, et al: Pathogenesis of *Salmonella*-induced enteritis. *Braz J Med Biol Res* 2003;36[1]:3–12.)

TABLE 195-2. Host Factors and Conditions Predisposing to the Development of Systemic Disease with Non-typhoidal *Salmonella* Strains
Neonates and young infants (≤3 mo of age)
HIV/AIDS
Other immune deficiencies and chronic granulomatous disease
Immunosuppressive and corticosteroid therapy
Malignancies, especially leukemia and lymphoma
Hemolytic anemia, including sickle cell disease, malaria, and bartonellosis
Collagen vascular disease
Inflammatory bowel disease
Achlorhydria or antacid medication use
Impaired intestinal motility
Schistosomiasis, malaria
Malnutrition

in the gastrointestinal tract, bones, and reticuloendothelial system as well as reduced phagocytic and opsonizing capacity of patients, which allows the organism to flourish.

Some inherited defects such as IL-12 deficiency (IL-12 receptor β1 chain deficiency, IL-12 p40 subunit deletion) are associated with increased risk for *Salmonella* infections, suggesting a key role for IL-12 in the clearance of *Salmonella.* IL-12 is produced by activated macrophages and is a potent inducer of interferon-γ by natural killer cells and T lymphocytes. Given the putative protective role of IL-12 against malarial infection, *Salmonella* infection of phagocytes may secondarily affect IL-12 production and thus produce a vicious cycle of chronic malaria and salmonella co-infection.

CLINICAL MANIFESTATIONS.

Acute Enteritis. The most common clinical presentation of salmonellosis is with acute enteritis. After an incubation period of 6–72 hr (mean, 24 hr), there is an abrupt onset of nausea, vomiting, and crampy abdominal pain, primarily in the periumbilical area and right lower quadrant, followed by mild to severe watery diarrhea and sometimes by diarrhea containing blood and mucus. A large proportion of children are febrile, although younger infants may exhibit a normal or subnormal temperature. Symptoms usually subside within 2–7 days in healthy children and fatalities are rare. However, some children develop severe disease with a septicemia-like picture (high fever, headache, drowsiness, confusion, meningismus, seizures, abdominal distention). The stool typically contains a moderate number of polymorphonuclear leukocytes and occult blood. Mild leukocytosis may be detected.

Bacteremia. Although the precise incidence of bacteremia following *Salmonella* gastroenteritis is unclear, transient bacteremia can occur in 1–5% of children with *Salmonella* diarrhea. While bacteremia can occur with minimal associated symptoms in newborns and very young infants, in older infants it typically follows gastroenteritis and can be associated with fever, chills, and septic shock. In patients with AIDS, recurrent septicemia appears despite antibiotic therapy, often with a negative stool culture for *Salmonella* and sometimes with no identifiable focus of infection.

Nontyphoidal *Salmonella* gastrointestinal infections commonly cause bacteremia in developing countries. High rates of invasive disease with *S.* Typhimurium and *S.* Enteritides reported from Africa (38–70% of isolates) suggest an association with HIV infections and malaria.

Extraintestinal Focal Infections. Following bacteremia, salmonellae have the propensity to seed and cause focal suppurative infection of many organs. The most common focal infections involve the skeletal system, meninges, and intravascular sites and sites of pre-existing abnormalities; areas of bone infarction as in sickle cell disease; or bone prostheses. Although meningeal infection is less common than bacteremia, *Salmonella* infections are also associated with focal intracranial infections. The peak incidence of ***Salmonella* meningitis** is in infancy and may be associated with a florid clinical course, high mortality, and neurologic sequelae.

COMPLICATIONS.

Salmonella gastroenteritis can be associated with acute dehydration and complications resulting from delayed presentation and inadequate treatment. Bacteremia in younger infants and immunocompromised individuals can have serious consequences and potentially fatal outcomes. *Salmonella* organisms can seed many organ systems, leading to intracranial infections (meningitis, focal brain abscesses) as well as osteomyelitis in children with sickle cell disease. Reactive arthritis may follow *Salmonella* gastroenteritis, usually in adolescents with HLA-B27 antigen.

In certain high-risk groups, especially those with impaired immunity, the course of *Salmonella* gastroenteritis may be more complicated. Neonates, infants <6 mo of age, and children with primary or secondary immune deficiency may have symptoms persisting for several weeks. The course of illness and complications may also be affected by coexisting pathologies. In children with AIDS, the infection frequently becomes widespread and overwhelming, causing multisystem involvement, septic shock, and death. In patients with inflammatory bowel disease, especially active ulcerative colitis, *Salmonella* gastroenteritis may be potentially fatal, with rapid development of toxic megacolon, bacterial translocation, and sepsis. In children with schistosomiasis, the *Salmonella* may persist and multiply within schistosomes, leading to chronic infection unless the schistosomiasis is effectively treated. Prolonged or intermittent bacteremia is associated with low-grade fever, anorexia, weight loss, diaphoresis, and myalgias, and may occur in children with underlying problems and reticulo-endothelial system dysfunction such as hemolytic anemia or malaria.

DIAGNOSIS.

There are few clinical features that are specific to *Salmonella* gastroenteritis and allow differentiation from other bacterial causes of diarrhea. Definitive diagnosis of *Salmonella* infection is based on clinical correlation of the presentation and culturing and subsequent identification of *Salmonella* organisms from feces or other body fluids. In children with gastroenteritis, cultures of stools have higher yields than rectal swabs. In children with nontyphoidal *Salmonella* gastroenteritis, prolonged fever lasting 5 days or more and young age should be recognized as risk factors closely associated with development of bacteremia. In patients with sites of local suppuration, aspirated specimens should be Gram stained and cultured. *Salmonella* organisms grow well on nonselective or enriched media, such as blood agar, chocolate agar, or nutrient broth, but stool specimens containing mixed bacterial flora require selective media such as MacConkey, xylose-lysine-deoxycholate (XLD), bismuth sulfite (BBL), or *Salmonella-Shigella* (SS) agar for isolation.

Although other rapid diagnostic methods, such as latex agglutination and immunofluorescence, have been developed for rapid diagnosis of *Salmonella* in cultures, there are few comparable tests for rapid serologic detection. Polymerase chain reaction (PCR) techniques may offer a rapid alternative to classic cultures but are as yet not in widespread use in clinical settings.

TREATMENT.

Appropriate therapy relates to the specific clinical presentation of *Salmonella* infection. In children with gastroenteritis, rapid clinical assessment, correction of dehydration and electrolyte disturbances, and supportive care are key (see Chapters 55 and 337). Antibiotics are not generally recommended for the treatment of *Salmonella* gastroenteritis because they may suppress normal intestinal flora and prolong the excretion of *Salmonella* and the remote risk for creating the chronic carrier state (usually in adults). However, given the risk for bacteremia in infants (<3 mo of age) and that of disseminated infection in high-risk groups with immune compromise (HIV, malignancies, immunosuppressive therapy, immunodeficiency states), these children must receive an appropriate antibiotic empirically until culture results are available (Table 195-3). The strain of *S.* Typhimurium phage type DT104 is usually resistant to 5 drugs:

TABLE 195-3. Treatment of *Salmonella* Gastroenteritis

ORGANISM AND INDICATION	DOSE AND DURATION OF TREATMENT
Salmonella infections in infants <3 mo of age, immunocompromised persons	Cefotaxime 100–200 mg/kg/day every 6 hr for 5–14 days *or* Ceftriaxone 75 mg/kg/day once daily for 7 days *or* Ampicillin 100 mg/kg/day every 6 hr for 7 days *or* Chloramphenicol 15 mg/kg/day divided every 6 hr PO for 5–10 days

ampicillin, chloramphenicol, streptomycin, sulfonamides, and tetracycline. An increasing proportion of *S.* Typhimurium phage type DT104 isolates also have reduced susceptibility to fluoroquinolones. Given the higher mortality associated with multidrug-resistant *Salmonella* infections, it is necessary to perform susceptibility tests on all human isolates. Infections with suspected drug-resistant *Salmonella* should be closely monitored and treated with appropriate antimicrobial therapy.

PROGNOSIS. Most healthy children with *Salmonella* gastroenteritis recover fully. However, malnourished children and those who do not receive optimal supportive treatment (see Chapters 55 and 337) are at risk for developing prolonged diarrhea and complications. Young infants and immunocompromised patients often have systemic involvement, a prolonged course, and extraintestinal foci. In particular, children with HIV infection and *Salmonella* infections can have a florid course.

After infection, nontyphoidal salmonellae are excreted in feces for a median of 5 wk. However, after clinical recovery from *Salmonella* gastroenteritis, asymptomatic fecal excretion of the organism may occur for several months, particularly in younger children or those treated with antibiotics. A prolonged carrier state after nontyphoidal salmonellosis is rare (<1%), but may be seen in children with biliary tract disease and cholelithiasis following chronic hemolysis. Prolonged carriage of *Salmonella* organisms is rare in healthy children but has been reported in those with underlying immune deficiency. During the period of *Salmonella* excretion, the individual may infect others, directly by the fecal-oral route or indirectly by contaminating foods.

PREVENTION. Control of the transmission of *Salmonella* infections to humans requires control of the infection in the animal reservoir, judicious use of antibiotics in dairy and livestock farming, prevention of contamination of foodstuffs prepared from animals, and use of appropriate standards in food processing in commercial and private kitchens (Table 195-4). Because large outbreaks are often related to mass food production, it should be recognized that contamination of just 1 piece of machinery used in food processing may cause an outbreak; meticulous cleaning of equipment is essential. Clean water supply and education in handwashing and food preparation and storage is critical to reducing person-to-person transmission. *Salmonella* may remain viable when cooking practices prevent food from reaching a temperature greater than 150°F (65.5°C) for >12 min. Parents should be advised of the risk of reptiles as pets in households with young infants.

In contrast to developed countries, relatively little is known about the transmission of nontyphoidal *Salmonella* infections in developing countries, and it is likely that person-to-person transmission may be relatively more important in some settings. Although some vaccines have been used in animals, no human vaccine against nontyphoidal *Salmonella* infections is currently available. Infections should be reported to public health authorities so that outbreaks can be recognized and investigated. Given the rapid rise of antimicrobial resistance among *Salmonella* isolates, it is imperative that there is rigorous regulation of the use of antimicrobials in animal feeds.

TABLE 195-4. Recommendations for Preventing Transmission of *Salmonella* from Reptiles and Amphibians to Humans

Pet store owners, health care providers, and veterinarians should provide information to owners and potential purchasers of reptiles and amphibians about the risks for and prevention of salmonellosis from these pets.
Persons at increased risk for infection or serious complications from salmonellosis (e.g., children aged <5 yr and immunocompromised persons) should avoid contact with reptiles and amphibians and any items that have been in contact with reptiles and amphibians.
Reptiles and amphibians should be kept out of households that include children aged <5 yr or immunocompromised persons. A family expecting a child should remove any pet reptile or amphibian from the home before the infant arrives.
Reptiles and amphibians should not be allowed in child-care centers.
Persons always should wash their hands thoroughly with soap and water after handling reptiles and amphibians or their cages.
Reptiles and amphibians should not be allowed to roam freely throughout a home or living area.
Pet reptiles and amphibians should be kept out of kitchens and other food preparation areas. Kitchen sinks should not be used to bathe reptiles and amphibians or to wash their dishes, cages, or aquariums. If bathtubs are used for these purposes, they should be cleaned thoroughly and disinfected with bleach.
Reptiles and amphibians in public settings (e.g., zoos and exhibits) should be kept from direct or indirect contact with patrons except in designated animal contact areas equipped with adequate handwashing facilities. Food and drink should not be allowed in animal contact areas.

From the Centers for Disease Control and Prevention: Reptile-associated salmonellosis—Selected states, 1998–2002. *MMWR* 2003;52:1206–1210.

195.2 • Enteric Fever (Typhoid Fever)

Enteric fever (more commonly termed typhoid fever) remains endemic in many developing countries. Given the ease of modern travel, cases are regularly reported from most developed countries, usually from returning travelers.

ETIOLOGY. Typhoid fever is caused by *Salmonella enterica* serovar Typhi (*S.* Typhi), a gram-negative bacterium. A very similar but often less severe disease is caused by *S.* Paratyphi A and rarely by *S.* Paratyphi B (Schotmulleri) and *S.* Paratyphi C (Hirschfeldii). The ratio of disease caused by *S.* Typhi to that caused by *S.* Paratyphi is about 10 to 1, although the proportion of *S.* Paratyphi infections is increasing in some parts of the world. Although *S.* Typhi shares many genes with *Escherichia coli* and at least 95% with *S.* Typhimurium, there are several unique gene clusters known as pathogenicity islands and others that have been acquired during evolution. The inactivation of single genes, as well as the acquisition or loss of single genes or large islands of DNA, may have contributed to host adaptation and restriction of *S.* Typhi.

One of the most specific genes is for the polysaccharide capsule Vi. This is present in about 90% of all freshly isolated *S.* Typhi and has a protective effect against the bactericidal action of the serum of infected patients.

EPIDEMIOLOGY. It is currently estimated that over 21.7 million typhoid cases occur annually, with the vast majority of cases in Asia, with over 200,000 deaths. Additionally, an estimated 5.4 million cases occur due to paratyphoid. Given the paucity of microbiological facilities in developing countries, these figures may be more representative of the clinical syndrome rather than culture-proven disease. In most developing countries, the incidence of typhoid fever is <15 cases per 100,000 population, with most cases occurring in travelers or isolated cases of exposure to carriers. In contrast, the incidence may vary considerably in the developing world, with estimated rates ranging from 100–1,000 cases per 100,000 population. There may also be differences in the age distribution and population at risk. Population-based studies from south Asia also indicate that, contrary to previous views, the age-specific incidence of typhoid may be highest in children <5 yr of age, with comparatively higher rates of complications and hospitalization.

Typhoid fever has been notable for the emergence of drug resistance. Following sporadic outbreaks of chloramphenicol-resistant typhoid, many strains of *S.* Typhi have developed plasmid-mediated multidrug resistance to all 3 of the primary antimicrobials: ampicillin, chloramphenicol, and trimethoprim-sulfamethoxazole. Chromosomally acquired quinolone resistance in *S.* Typhi has been described in various parts of Asia and may be a consequence of widespread and indiscriminate use of these agents.

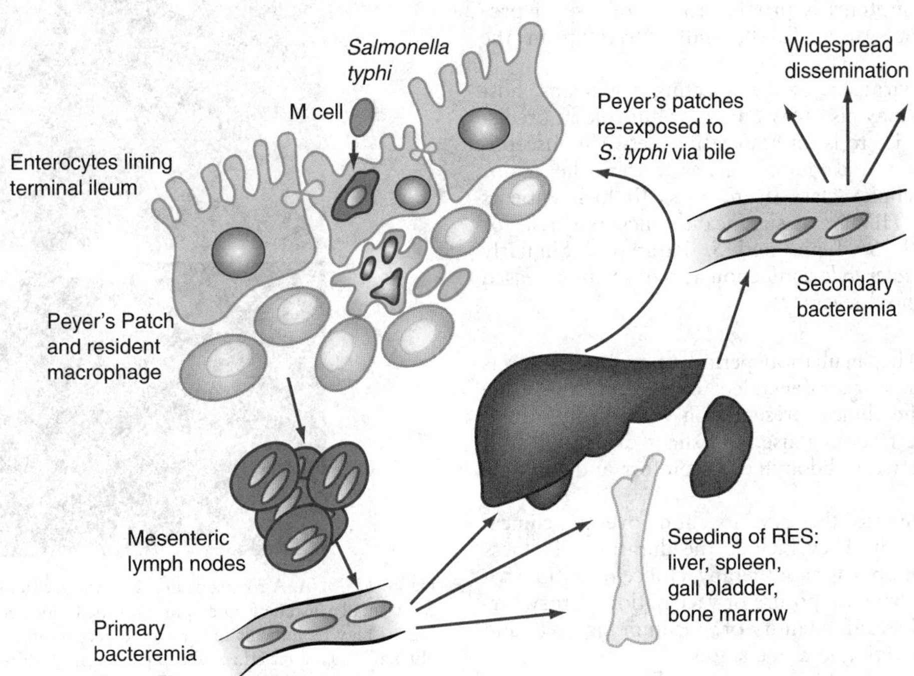

Figure 195-2. Pathogenesis of typhoid fever. (Adapted from Richens J: Typhoid fever. In Cohen J, Powderly WG, Opal SM [editors]: *Infectious Diseases,* 2nd ed. London, Mosby, 2004, pp 1561–1566.)

S. Typhi is highly adapted to infection of human beings to the point that it has lost the ability to cause transmissible disease in other animals. The discovery of the large number of pseudogenes in *S.* Typhi suggests that the genome of this pathogen has undergone degeneration to facilitate a specialized association with human beings. Thus, direct or indirect contact with an infected person (sick or chronic carrier) is a prerequisite for infection. Ingestion of foods or water contaminated with *S.* Typhi from human feces is the most common mode of transmission, although water-borne outbreaks due to poor sanitation or contamination can occur in developing countries. In other parts of the world, oysters and other shellfish cultivated in water contaminated by sewage or the use of night soil as fertilizer may also cause infection.

PATHOGENESIS. The disease occurs by the ingestion of the organism, and a variety of sources of fecal contamination have been reported, including street foods and contamination of water reservoirs.

Human volunteer experiments established an infecting dose of about 10^5–10^9 organisms with an incubation period ranging from 4 to 14 days, depending on the inoculating dose of viable bacteria. After ingestion, *S.* Typhi organisms are thought to invade the body through the gut mucosa in the terminal ileum, possibly through specialized antigen-sampling cells, known as M cells, that overlie gut-associated lymphoid tissues, through enterocytes, or via a paracellular route. *S.* Typhi crosses the intestinal mucosal barrier after attachment to the microvilli by an intricate mechanism involving membrane ruffling, actin rearrangement, and internalization in an intracellular vacuole. After passing through the intestinal mucosa, *S.* Typhi organisms enter the mesenteric lymphoid system, and then pass into the bloodstream via the lymphatics. This primary bacteremia is usually symptomless, and blood cultures are frequently negative at this stage of the disease. The blood-borne bacteria are disseminated throughout the body and are thought to colonize the organs of the reticuloendothelial system, where they may replicate within macrophages. After a period of bacterial replication, *S.* Typhi organisms are shed back into the blood, causing a secondary bacteremia, which coincides with the onset of clinical symptoms and marks the end of the incubation period (Fig. 195-2).

In vitro studies with human cell lines have shown qualitative and quantitative differences in the epithelial cell response to *S.* Typhi and *S.* Typhimurium with regard to cytokine and chemokine secretion. Thus, by avoiding the triggering of an early inflammatory response in the gut, *S.* Typhi could instead colonize deeper tissues and organ systems. Infection with *S.* Typhi produces an inflammatory response in the deeper mucosal layers and underlying lymphoid tissue with hyperplasia of Peyer patches, and subsequent necrosis and sloughing of overlying epithelium with ulceration. The ulcers can bleed but usually heal without scarring or stricture formation. The inflammatory lesion may occasionally penetrate the muscularis and serosa of the intestine and produce perforation. The mesenteric lymph nodes, liver, and spleen are hyperemic and generally reveal areas of focal necrosis as well. A mononuclear response may be seen in the bone marrow in association with areas of focal necrosis. The morphologic changes of *S.* Typhi infection are less prominent in infants compared with older children and adults. In particular, in contrast to adults with typhoid, despite bacterial multiplication in the gall bladder wall, inflammation is both focal and mild.

It is thought that several virulence genes, including the SPI-2 TTSS, may be necessary for the virulence properties and ability to cause systemic infection. The surface Vi (virulence) polysaccharide capsular antigen found in *S.* Typhi interferes with phagocytosis by preventing the binding of C3 to the surface of the bacterium. The ability of organisms to survive within macrophages after phagocytosis is an important virulence trait encoded by the phoP regulon; it may be related to metabolic effects on host cells. The occasional occurrence of diarrhea may be explained by the presence of a toxin related to cholera toxin and *E. coli* heat-labile enterotoxin. The clinical syndrome of fever and systemic symptoms is produced by a release of proinflammatory cytokines (IL-6, IL-1β, and TNF-α) from the infected cells.

In addition to the virulence of the infecting organisms, host factors and immunity may also play an important role in predisposition to infection. There is an association between susceptibility to typhoid fever and human genes within the major histocompatability complex class II and class III loci. Patients who are infected with HIV are at significantly increased risk for clinical infection with *S.* Typhi and *S.* Paratyphi. Similarly patients with *Helicobacter pylori* infection also have an increased risk for acquiring typhoid fever.

CLINICAL FEATURES. The incubation period of typhoid fever is usually 7–14 days but is also dependent on the infecting dose (range 3–30 days). The clinical presentation varies from a mild illness with low-grade fever, malaise, and slight dry cough to a severe clinical picture with abdominal discomfort and multiple complications.

Many factors influence the severity and overall clinical outcome of the infection. They include the duration of illness before the initiation of appropriate therapy, choice of antimicrobial treatment, age, previous exposure or vaccination history, virulence of the bacterial strain, quantity of inoculum ingested, and several host factors affecting immune status.

The presentation of typhoid fever may also differ according to age. Although data from South America and other parts of Africa suggest that typhoid may present as a mild illness in young children, this may vary in different parts of the world. There is emerging evidence from south Asia that the presentation of typhoid may be more dramatic in children <5 yr of age, with comparatively higher rates of complications and hospitalization. Diarrhea, toxicity, and complications such as disseminated intravascular complications are also more common in infancy, with higher case fatality rates. However, some of the other features and complications of typhoid fever seen in adults, such as relative bradycardia, neurologic manifestations, and gastrointestinal bleeding, are rare.

Typhoid fever usually presents with high-grade fever with a wide variety of associated features such as generalized myalgia, abdominal pain, hepatosplenomegaly, abdominal pain, and anorexia (Table 195-5). In children, diarrhea may be present in the earlier stages of the illness and may be followed by constipation. In the absence of localizing signs, the early stage of the disease may be difficult to differentiate from other endemic diseases such as malaria or dengue fever. The fever may rise gradually, but the classic stepladder rise of fever is relatively rare. In about 25% of cases, a macular or maculopapular rash (rose spots) may be visible around the 7th–10th day of the illness, and lesions may appear in crops of 10–15 on the lower chest and abdomen and last 2–3 days (Fig. 195-3). These lesions may be difficult to see in dark-skinned children. Patients managed as outpatients will present with fever (99%) but have less emesis, diarrhea, hepatomegaly, splenomegaly, and myalgias than hospitalized patients.

TABLE 195-5. Common Clinical Features of Typhoid Fever in Children*

High-grade fever	95%
Coated tongue	76%
Anorexia	70%
Vomiting	39%
Hepatomegaly	37%
Diarrhea	36%
Toxicity	29%
Abdominal pain	21%
Pallor	20%
Splenomegaly	17%
Constipation	7%
Headache	4%
Jaundice	2%
Obtundation	2%
Ileus	1%
Intestinal perforation	0.5%

*Karachi, Pakistan, from 2,000 children.

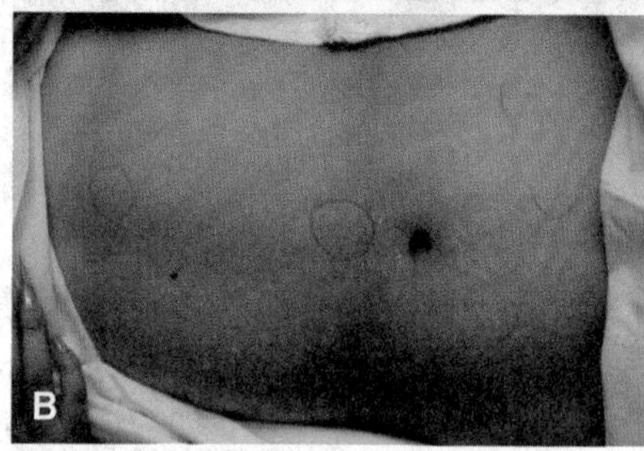

Figure 195-3. *A,* A rose spot in a volunteer with experimental typhoid fever. *B,* A small cluster of rose spots is usually located on the abdomen. These lesions may be difficult to identify, especially in dark-skinned people. (From Huang DB, DuPont HL: Problem pathogens: Extra-intestinal complications of Salmonella enterica serotype Typhi infection. *Lancet Infect Dis* 2005;5: 341–348.)

The presentation of typhoid fever may be tempered by coexisting morbidities and early administration of antibiotics. In malaria-endemic areas and in parts of the world where schistosomiasis is common, the presentation of typhoid may also be atypical. It is also recognized that multidrug-resistant *S.* Typhi infection is a more severe clinical illness with higher rates of toxicity, complications, and case fatality rates, which may be related to the increased virulence as well as higher number of circulating bacteria. These findings may have implications for treatment algorithms, especially in endemic areas with high rates of multidrug-resistant typhoid.

If no complications occur, the symptoms and physical findings gradually resolve within 2–4 wk; however, the illness may be associated with malnutrition in a number of affected children. Although enteric fever caused by *S.* Paratyphi organisms has been classically regarded as a milder illness, recent reports of infections with drug-resistant isolates indicate that paratyphoid fever may also be severe, with significant morbidity and complications.

COMPLICATIONS. Although altered liver function is found in many patients with enteric fever, clinically significant hepatitis, jaundice, and cholecystitis are relatively rare and may be associated with higher rates of adverse outcome. Intestinal hemorrhage (<1%) and perforation (0.5–1%) is infrequent among children. Intestinal perforation may be preceded by a marked increase in abdominal pain (usually in the right lower quadrant), tenderness, vomiting, and features of peritonitis. Intestinal perforation and peritonitis may be accompanied by a sudden rise in pulse rate, hypotension, marked abdominal tenderness and guarding, and

TABLE 195-6. Extraintestinal Infectious Complications of Typhoid Fever Caused by *Salmonella enterica* Serotype Typhi

ORGAN SYSTEM INVOLVED	PREVALENCE	RISK FACTORS	COMPLICATIONS
Central nervous system	3–35%	Residence in endemic region, malignancy, endocarditis, congenital heart disease, paranasal sinus infections, pulmonary infections, meningitis, trauma, surgery, and osteomyelitis of the skull	Encephalopathy, cerebral edema, subdural empyema, cerebral abscess, meningitis, ventriculitis, transient parkinsonism, motor neuron disorders, ataxia, seizures, Guillain-Barré syndrome, psychosis
Cardiovascular system	1–5%	Cardiac abnormalities—e.g., existing valvular abnormalities, rheumatic heart disease, or congenital heart defects	Endocarditis, myocarditis, pericarditis, arteritis, congestive heart failure
Pulmonary system	1–6%	Residence in endemic region, past pulmonary infection, sickle cell anaemia, alcohol abuse, diabetes, HIV infection	Pneumonia, empyema, bronchopleural fistula
Bone and joint	<1%	Sickle cell anaemia, diabetes, systemic lupus erythematosus, lymphoma, liver disease, previous surgery or trauma, those at extremes of age, and steroid use	Osteomyelitis, septic arthritis
Hepatobiliary system	1–26%	Residence in endemic region, pyogenic infections, intravenous drug use, splenic trauma, HIV, haemoglobinopathy	Cholecystitis, hepatitis, hepatic abscesses, splenic abscess, peritonitis, paralytic ileus
Genitourinary system	<1%	Urinary tract, pelvic pathology, and systemic abnormalities	Urinary tract infection, renal abscess, pelvic infections, testicular abscess, prostatitis, epididymitis
Soft tissue infections	At least 17 cases reported in the English-language literature	Diabetes	Psoas abscess, gluteal abscess, cutaneous vasculitis
Haematologic	At least 5 cases reported in the English-language literature		Haemophagocytosis syndrome

From Huang DB, DuPont HL: Problem pathogens: Extra-intestinal complications of *Salmonella enterica* serotype Typhi infection. *Lancet Infect Dis* 2005;5:341–348.

subsequent abdominal rigidity. A rising white blood cell count with a left shift and free air on abdominal radiographs may be seen in such cases.

Rare complications include toxic myocarditis, which may manifest by arrhythmias, sinoatrial block, or cardiogenic shock (Table 195-6). Neurologic complications are also relatively uncommon among children and may include delirium, psychosis, increased intracranial pressure, acute cerebellar ataxia, chorea, deafness, and Guillain-Barré syndrome. Although case fatality rates may be higher with neurologic manifestations, recovery usually occurs with no sequelae. Other reported complications include fatal bone marrow necrosis, disseminated intravascular coagulation (DIC), hemolytic uremic syndrome, pyelonephritis, nephrotic syndrome, meningitis, endocarditis, parotitis, orchitis, and suppurative lymphadenitis.

The propensity to become a carrier follows the epidemiology of gall bladder disease, increasing with age and antibiotic resistance of the prevalent strains. Although limited data are available, in general, rates of chronic carriage are lower in children than adults.

DIAGNOSIS. The mainstay of the diagnosis of typhoid fever is a positive culture from the blood or another anatomic site. Results of blood cultures are positive in 40–60% of the patients seen early in the course of the disease, and stool and urine cultures become positive after the 1st wk. The stool culture result is also occasionally positive during the incubation period. However, the sensitivity of blood cultures in diagnosing typhoid fever in many parts of the developing world is limited as widespread antibiotic prescribing may render bacteriologic confirmation difficult. Although bone marrow cultures may increase the likelihood of bacteriologic confirmation of typhoid, these are difficult to obtain and relatively invasive.

Other laboratory investigations are nonspecific. While blood leukocyte counts are frequently low in relation to the fever and toxicity, but there is a wide range in counts; in younger children leukocytosis is a common association and may reach 20,000–25,000/mm^3. Thrombocytopenia may be a marker of severe illness and accompany DIC. While liver function test results may be deranged, significant hepatic dysfunction is rare.

The classic Widal test measures antibodies against O and H antigens of *S.* Typhi but lacks sensitivity and specificity in endemic areas. Because many false-positive and false-negative results occur, diagnosis of typhoid fever by Widal test alone is prone to error. Other relatively newer diagnostic tests using monoclonal antibodies have been developed that directly detect *S.* Typhi–specific antigens in the serum or *S.* Typhi Vi antigen in the urine. However, few have proved sufficiently robust in large-scale evaluations. A nested PCR using *H1-d* primers has been used to amplify specific genes of *S.* Typhi in the blood of patients, and given the low level of bacteremia in enteric fever, is a promising means of making a rapid diagnosis. Despite these new developments, in much of the developing world the mainstay of diagnosis of typhoid remains clinical, and several diagnostic algorithms have been evaluated in endemic areas.

DIFFERENTIAL DIAGNOSIS. In endemic areas, typhoid fever may mimic many common febrile illnesses without localizing signs. In children with multisystem features, the early stages of enteric fever may be confused with alternative conditions such as acute gastroenteritis, bronchitis, or bronchopneumonia. Subsequently, the differential diagnosis includes malaria; sepsis with other bacterial pathogens; infections caused by intracellular microorganisms, such as tuberculosis, brucellosis, tularemia, leptospirosis, and rickettsial diseases; and viral infections such as Dengue fever, acute hepatitis, and infectious mononucleosis.

TREATMENT. An early diagnosis of typhoid fever and institution of appropriate treatment is essential. The vast majority of children with typhoid can be managed at home with oral antibiotics and close medical follow-up for complications or failure to respond to therapy. Patients with persistent vomiting, severe diarrhea, and abdominal distension may require hospitalization and parenteral antibiotic therapy.

There are general principles of management of typhoid. Adequate rest, hydration, and attention are important to correct fluid-electrolyte imbalance. Antipyretic therapy (acetaminophen 120–750 mg every 4–6 hr PO) should be provided as required. A soft, easily digestible diet should be continued unless the patient has abdominal distention or ileus. Antibiotic therapy is critical to minimize complications (Table 195-7). It has been suggested that traditional therapy with either chloramphenicol or amoxicillin is associated with relapse rates of 5–15% and 4–8%, respectively, whereas the quinolones and 3rd generation cephalosporins are associated with higher cure rates. The antibiotic treatment of typhoid fever in children is also influenced by the prevalence of antimicrobial resistance. Over the past 2 decades, emergence of multidrug-resistant strains of *S.* Typhi (i.e., isolates fully resis-

TABLE 195-7. Treatment of Typhoid Fever in Children

SUSCEPTIBILITY	OPTIMAL THERAPY Antibiotic	Daily Dose (mg/kg/day)	Days	ALTERNATIVE EFFECTIVE DRUGS Antibiotic	Daily Dose (mg/kg/day)	Days
UNCOMPLICATED TYPHOID FEVER						
Fully sensitive	Chloramphenicol	50–75	14–21	Fluoroquinolone, e.g., ofloxacin or ciprofloxacin	15	5–7*
	Amoxicillin	75–100	14			
Multidrug resistant	Fluoroquinolone or	15	5–7	Azithromycin	8–10	7
	cefixime	15–20	7–14	Cefixime	15–20	7–14
Quinolone resistant†	Azithromycin or	8–10	7	Cefixime	20	7–14
	ceftriaxone	75	10–14			
SEVERE TYPHOID FEVER						
Fully sensitive	Ampicillin or	100	14	Fluoroquinolone, e.g., ofloxacin or ciprofloxacin	15	10–14
	ceftriaxone	60–75	10–14			
Multidrug resistant	Fluoroquinolone	15	10–14	Ceftriaxone or	60	10–14
				cefotaxime	80	
Quinolone resistant	Ceftriaxone	60–75	10–14	Fluoroquinolone	20–30	14

*A 3 day course is also effective, particularly for epidemic containment.

†The optimum treatment for quinolone-resistant typhoid fever has not been determined. Azithromycin, 3rd generation cephalosporins, or high-dose fluoroquinolones for 10–14 days are effective.

Modified from World Health Organization: Treatment of typhoid fever. Background document: the diagnosis, prevention and treatment of typhoid fever. Communicable Disease Surveillance and Response Vaccines and Biologicals: World Health Organization. Geneva, 2003. pp. 19–23. [Available from URL: www.who.int/entity/vaccine_research/documents/en/typhoid_diagnosis.pdf]

tant to amoxicillin, trimethoprim-sulfamethoxazole, and chloramphenicol) has necessitated treatment with fluoroquinolones, which are the antimicrobial drug of choice for treatment of salmonellosis in adults, or cephalosporins. The emergence of resistance to quinolones has placed tremendous pressure on public health systems, as therapeutic options are limited.

While it has been suggested that, like adults, children with typhoid should also be treated with fluoroquinolones, others have questioned this approach on the basis of the potential development of further resistance to fluoroquinolones and the fact that quinolones are still not approved for widespread use in children. A Cochrane review of the treatment of typhoid fever also indicates that there is little evidence to support the carte blanche administration of fluoroquinolones to all cases of typhoid. Relapse with all antibiotics may occur in 15% of previously treated patients.

In addition to antibiotics, the importance of supportive treatment and maintenance of appropriate fluid and electrolyte balance must be underscored. Although additional treatment with dexamethasone (3 mg/kg for the initial dose, followed by 1 mg/kg every 6 hr for 48 hr) has been recommended among severely ill patients with shock, obtundation, stupor, or coma, this must only be done under strict controlled conditions and supervision, and signs of abdominal complications may be masked.

PROGNOSIS. The prognosis for a patient with enteric fever depends on the rapidity of diagnosis and institution of appropriate antibiotic therapy. Other factors include the age of the patient, general state of health and nutrition, causative *Salmonella* serotype, and appearance of complications. Infants and children with underlying malnutrition and those infected with multidrug-resistant isolates are at higher risk for adverse outcomes.

Despite appropriate therapy, 2–4% of infected children may relapse after initial clinical response to treatment. Individuals who **excrete *S.* Typhi for ≥3 mo** after infection are regarded as **chronic carriers.** However, the risk for becoming a carrier is low in children and increases with age, but in general is <2% for all infected children. Children with schistosomiasis can develop a chronic urinary carrier state.

PREVENTION. Of the major risk factors for outbreaks of typhoid, contamination of water supplies with sewage is the most important. During outbreaks, therefore, a combination of central chlorination as well as domestic water purification are important. In endemic situations, consumption of street foods, especially ice cream and cut fruit has been recognized as an important risk factor. The human-to-human spread by chronic carriers is also important, and attempts should therefore be made to target food handlers and high-risk groups for *S.* Typhi carriage screening. Once identified, chronic carriers must be counseled as to the risk for disease transmission and given advice on handwashing and preventive strategies.

The classic heat-inactivated whole cell vaccine is associated with an unacceptably high rate of side effects and has been largely withdrawn from public health use. Globally, 2 vaccines are currently available for potential use in children. An oral, live-attenuated preparation of the Ty21a strain of *S.* Typhi has been shown to have good efficacy (67–82%) for up to 5 years. Significant adverse effects are rare. The Vi capsular polysaccharide can be used in people ≥2 yr of age. It is given as a single intramuscular dose, with a booster every 2 yr and has a protective efficacy of 70–80%. The vaccines are currently recommended for traveling into endemic areas, but a few countries have introduced large-scale vaccination strategies. Given the age spectrum and distribution of cases in south Asia, it is important that strategies for vaccinating preschool children be explored. The recent Vi-conjugate vaccine has been shown to have a protective efficacy exceeding 90% in younger children and may offer protection in parts of the world where a large proportion of preschool children are at risk for the disease.

Salmonella Gastroenteritis

Centers for Disease Control and Prevention: Human salmonellosis associated with animal-derived pet treats—United States and Canada, 2005. *MMWR* 2006;55:702–705.

Centers for Disease Control and Prevention: Outbreak of multidrug-resistant Salmonella typhimurium associated with rodents purchased at retail pet stores—United States, December 2003–October 2004. *MMWR* 2005;54:429–434.

Centers for Disease Control and Prevention: Multistate outbreak of Salmonella typhimurium infections associated with eating ground beef, United States, 2004. *MMWR* 2006;55:180–182.

Centers for Disease Control and Prevention: Salmonellosis associated with pet turtles—Wisconsin and Wyoming, 2004. *MMWR* 2005;54:223–226.

Centers for Disease Control and Prevention: Reptile-associated salmonellosis—Selected states, 1998–2002. *MMWR* 2003;52:1206–1210.

Chiu CH, Chuang CH, Chiu S, et al: *Salmonella enterica* serotype choleraesuis infections in pediatric patients. *Pediatrics* 2006;117:e1193–e1196.

Graham SM: Salmonellosis in children in developing and developed countries and populations. *Curr Opin Infect Dis* 2000;15:507–512.

Helms M, Simonsen J, Molbak K: Quinolone resistance is associated with increased risk of invasive illness or death during infection with Salmonella serotype Typhimurium. *J Infect Dis* 2004;190:1652–1654.

Helms M, Vastrup P, Gerner-Smidt P, Molbak K: Excess mortality associated with antimicrobial drug-resistant Salmonella typhimurium. *Emerg Infect Dis* 2002;8:490–495.

Hohmann EL: Nontyphoidal salmonellosis. *Clin Infect Dis* 2001;32:263–269.

International Food Safety Authorities Network: Antimicrobial-resistant Salmonella. Retrieved July 14, 2006, from http://www.who.int/foodsafety/fs_management/en/No_03_Salmonella_Apr05_en.pdf

Jones TF, Ingram LA, Fullerton KE, et al: A case-control study of the epidemiology of sporadic salmonella infection in infants. *Pediatrics* 2006;118: 2380–2387.

McEwen SA, Fedorka-Cray PJ. Antimicrobial use and resistance in animals. *Clin Infect Dis* 2002;34(Suppl 3):S93–S106.

Santos RL, Tsolis RM, Baumler AJ, et al: Pathogenesis of *Salmonella*-induced enteritis. *Braz J Med Biol Res* 2003;36:3–12.

Sirinavin S, Chiemchanya S, Vorachit M: Systemic nontyphoidal *Salmonella* infection in normal infants in Thailand. *Pediatr Infect Dis J* 2001;20: 581–587.

Walsh AL, Phiri AJ, Graham SM, et al: Bacteremia in febrile Malawian children: Clinical and microbiologic features. *Pediatr Infect Dis J* 2000;19: 312–318.

Enteric Fever

Bhutta ZA: Current concepts in the diagnosis and treatment of typhoid fever. *Br Med J* 2006;333:78–82.

Chandel DS, Chaudhry R:. Enteric fever treatment failures: A global concern. *Emerg Infect Dis* 2001;7:762–763.

Crump JA, Luby SP, Mintz ED: The global burden of typhoid fever. *Bull WHO* 2004;82:346–353.

Gasem MH, Keuter M, Dolmans WM, et al: Persistence of salmonellae in blood and bone marrow: Randomized controlled trial comparing ciprofloxacin and chloramphenicol treatments against enteric fever. *Antimicrob Agents Chemother* 2003;47:1727–1731.

House D, Bishop A, Parry C, et al: Typhoid fever: pathogenesis and disease. *Curr Opin Infect Dis* 2001;14:573–578.

Huang DB, DuPont HL: Problem pathogens: Extra-intestinal complications of *Salmonella enterica* serotype Typhi infection. *Lancet Infect Dis* 2005;5: 341–348.

Luby SP, Faizan MK, Fisher-Hoch SP, et al: Risk factors for typhoid fever in an endemic setting, Karachi, Pakistan. *Epidemiol Infect* 1998;120:129–138.

Parry CM, Hien TT, Dougan G, et al: Typhoid fever. *N Engl J Med* 2002; 347:1770–1782.

Prakash P, Mishra OP, Singh AK, et al: Evaluation of nested PCR in diagnosis of typhoid fever. *J Clin Microbiol* 2005;43:431–432.

Sinha A, Sazawal S, Kumar R, et al: Typhoid fever in children aged less than 5 years. *Lancet* 1999;354:734–737.

Thaver D, Zaidi AK, Critchley J, et al: Fluoroquinolones for treating typhoid and paratyphoid fever (enteric fever). *Cochrane Database Syst Rev* 2005;2: CD004530.pub2.

Wain J, House D, Parkhill J, et al: Unlocking the genome of the human typhoid bacillus. *Lancet Infect Dis* 2002;2:163–170.

World Health Organization: Background document: The diagnosis, prevention and treatment of typhoid fever. In: *Communicable Disease Surveillance and Response Vaccines and Biologicals*. Geneva, World Health Organization, 2003, pp 19–23. Available from www.who.int/entity/vaccine_research/documents/en/typhoid_diagnosis.pdf

Chapter 196 ■ *Shigella*

Theresa J. Ochoa and Thomas G. Cleary

Although dysenteric syndromes have long been recognized as a scourge of humans, it is only in the past century that the bacteriology of the most common form of epidemic dysentery, shigellosis, has been appreciated.

ETIOLOGY. Four species of *Shigella* are responsible for bacillary dysentery: *S. dysenteriae* (serogroup A), *S. flexneri* (serogroup B), *S. boydii* (serogroup C), and *S. sonnei* (serogroup D). There are 13 serotypes in group A, 6 serotypes and 15 subserotypes in group B, 18 serotypes in group C, and 1 serotype in group D. Species classification has important therapeutic implications because the species differ in both geographic distribution and antimicrobial susceptibility.

EPIDEMIOLOGY. Infection with *Shigella* occurs most often during the warm months in temperate climates and during the rainy season in tropical climates. Both sexes are affected equally. Although infection can occur at any age, it is most common in the 2nd and 3rd year of life. Approximately 70% of all episodes and 60% of all *Shigella*-related deaths involve children younger than 5 yr. Infection in the 1st 6 mo of life is rare for reasons that are not clear. Breast milk, which in endemic areas contains antibodies to both virulence plasmid–coded antigens and lipopolysaccharides, may partially explain the age-related incidence. Asymptomatic infection of children and adults occurs commonly in endemic areas.

In industrialized societies, *S. sonnei* is the most common cause of bacillary dysentery, with *S. flexneri* second in frequency; in preindustrial societies, *S. flexneri* is most common, with *S. sonnei* second in frequency. *S. dysenteriae* serotype 1 tends to occur in massive epidemics, although it is also endemic in Asia and Africa.

TRANSMISSION. Contaminated food (often a salad or other item requiring extensive handling of the ingredients) and water are important vectors. Person-to-person transmission is probably the major mechanism of infection in most areas of the world. Rapid spread within families, custodial institutions, and child-care centers demonstrate the ability of low numbers of organisms to be transmitted from 1 individual to the next.

Shigellae require very low inocula to cause illness. Ingestion of as few as 10 *S. dysenteriae* serotype 1 organisms can cause dysentery in some susceptible individuals. This is in contrast to organisms such as *Vibrio cholerae*, which require ingestion of 10^8–10^{10} organisms to cause illness. The inoculum effect explains the ease of person-to-person transmission of shigellae in contrast to *V. cholerae*.

PATHOGENESIS. The basic virulence trait shared by all shigellae is the ability to invade intestinal epithelial cells. This characteristic is encoded on a large (220 kb) plasmid that is responsible for synthesis of a group of polypeptides involved in cell invasion and killing. Shigellae that lose the virulence plasmid are no longer pathogenic. *Escherichia coli* organisms that harbor this plasmid, enteroinvasive *E. coli* (see Chapter 197), behave clinically like shigellae. The virulence plasmid encodes approximately 25 proteins secreted by the type III secretion system. This secretion system translocates effector molecules from the bacterial cytoplasm to the membrane and cytoplasm of the host cell. Among these secreted proteins, the invasion plasmid antigens Ipa A, B, C, and D are necessary for invasion. Other proteins (encoded by the genes *icsA* and *sopA*) play a role in the ability of *Shigella* to move within the cytoplasm of infected cells and to spread to other cells. In addition to the major plasmid-encoded virulence traits, chromosomally encoded factors are also required for full virulence. Some shigellae make toxins: Shiga toxin or enterotoxins ShET-1 and ShET-2. Shiga toxin, a potent protein synthesis–inhibiting exotoxin, is produced in significant amounts by *S. dysenteriae* serotype 1, by certain *E. coli*, which are known as Shiga toxin–producing *E. coli* (see Chapter 197), and occasionally by other organisms. This toxin causes the severe complication of hemolytic-uremic syndrome. It is unclear whether the watery diarrhea phase of shigellosis is caused by 1 of the enterotoxins; paradoxically, deleting the genes for both enterotoxins

(ShET 1 and ShET 2) decreased the frequency of fever and dysentery in volunteers during vaccine development studies. Lipopolysaccharides are virulence factors for all shigellae; other traits are important for only a few serotypes (Shiga toxin synthesis by *S. dysenteriae* serotype 1 and ShET-1 by *S. flexneri* 2a).

The pathologic changes of shigellosis take place primarily in the colon, the target organ for shigellae. The changes are most intense in the distal colon, although pancolitis may occur. Shigellae cross the colonic epithelium through M cells in the follicle-associated epithelium overlying the Peyer patches. Grossly, localized or diffuse mucosal edema, ulcerations, friable mucosa, bleeding, and exudate may be seen. Microscopically, ulcerations, pseudomembranes, epithelial cell death, infiltration extending from the mucosa to the muscularis mucosae by polymorphonuclear and mononuclear cells, and submucosal edema occur.

IMMUNITY. Secretory immunoglobulin A and serum antibodies develop within days to weeks after infection with *Shigella*. Both antilipopolysaccharide and antivirulence plasmid polypeptide antibodies have been described; protection is serotype specific. Induction of multiple cytokines and brisk inflammatory responses is followed by healing. Interferon-γ produced by natural killer cells is critically important to resistance.

CLINICAL MANIFESTATIONS. Bacillary dysentery is clinically similar regardless of infecting serotype; however, there are some clinical differences, particularly relating to the greater severity and risk for complications with *S. dysenteriae* serotype 1 infection.

Ingestion of shigellae is followed by an incubation period of 12 hr to several days before symptoms ensue. Severe abdominal pain, high fever, emesis, anorexia, generalized toxicity, urgency, and painful defecation characteristically occur. Physical examination at this point may show abdominal distention and tenderness, hyperactive bowel sounds, and a tender rectum on digital examination.

The diarrhea may be watery and of large volume initially, evolving into frequent small-volume, bloody mucoid stools; most children (>50%) never progress to the stage of bloody diarrhea, whereas in others the 1st stools are bloody. Significant dehydration related to the fluid and electrolyte losses in both feces and emesis can occur. Untreated diarrhea may last 1–2 wk; only about 10% of patients have diarrhea persisting for more than 10 days. Persistent diarrhea occurs in malnourished infants, those with AIDS, and occasionally previously normal children. Even nondysenteric disease can be complicated by persistent illness.

Neurologic findings are among the most common extraintestinal manifestations of bacillary dysentery, occurring in as many as 40% of hospitalized infected children. Enteroinvasive *E. coli* can cause similar neurologic toxicity. Convulsions, headache, lethargy, confusion, nuchal rigidity, or hallucinations may be present before or after the onset of diarrhea. The cause of these neurologic findings is not understood. In the past, these symptoms were attributed to the neurotoxicity of Shiga toxin, but it is clear that that explanation is wrong since the organisms isolated from children with *Shigella*-related seizures are usually not Shiga toxin producers. Seizures sometimes occur when little fever is present, suggesting that simple febrile convulsions do not explain their appearance. Hypocalcemia or hyponatremia may be associated with seizures in a small number of patients. Although symptoms often suggest central nervous system infection, and cerebrospinal fluid pleocytosis with minimally elevated protein levels can occur, *Shigella* meningitis is rare.

The most common complication of shigellosis is dehydration. Inappropriate secretion of antidiuretic hormone with profound hyponatremia may complicate dysentery, particularly when *S. dysenteriae* is the etiologic agent. Hypoglycemia and protein-losing enteropathy may occur. Other major complications, particularly in very young, malnourished children, include sepsis and disseminated intravascular coagulation. Given that shigellae penetrate the intestinal mucosal barrier, these events are surprisingly uncommon. Shigellae and sometimes other gram-negative enteric bacilli are recovered from blood cultures in 1–5% of patients in whom blood cultures are taken; because patients selected for blood cultures represent a biased sample, the risk for bacteremia in unselected cases of shigellosis is presumably lower. Bacteremia is more common with *S. dysenteriae* serotype 1 than with other shigellae; the mortality rate is high (~20%) when sepsis occurs.

Neonatal shigellosis is rare. Newborns may have only low-grade fever with mild nonbloody diarrhea. However, complications occur more commonly than in older children and include septicemia, meningitis, dehydration, colonic perforation, and toxic megacolon.

S. dysenteriae serotype 1 infection is commonly complicated by hemolysis, anemia, and **hemolytic-uremic syndrome.** This syndrome is caused by Shiga toxin–mediated endothelial injury; *E. coli* that produce Shiga toxin (*E. coli* 0157 : H7, *E. coli* 0111 : NM, *E. coli* 026 : H11) also cause hemolytic-uremic syndrome (see Chapter 518).

Rectal prolapse, toxic megacolon or pseudomembranous colitis (usually associated with *S. dysenteriae*), cholestatic hepatitis, conjunctivitis, iritis, corneal ulcers, pneumonia, arthritis (usually 2–5 wk after enteritis), reactive arthritis with uveitis, urethritis and rash, cystitis, myocarditis, and vaginitis (typically with a blood-tinged discharge associated with *S. flexneri*) are uncommon events. Although rare, surgical complications of shigellosis can be severe; the most common are intestinal obstruction, appendicitis, and perforation. Death is a rare outcome in well-nourished older children; malnutrition, illness in the 1st year of life, hypothermia, severe dehydration, thrombocytopenia, hyponatremia, renal failure, and bacteremia are common in children who die during bacillary dysentery. The rare syndrome of severe toxicity, convulsions, extreme hyperpyrexia, and headache associated with brain edema and a rapidly fatal outcome without sepsis or significant dehydration (**Ekiri syndrome** or "lethal toxic encephalopathy") is not well understood.

DIAGNOSIS. Although clinical features suggest shigellosis, they are insufficiently specific to allow confident diagnosis. Infection by *Campylobacter jejuni, Salmonella,* enteroinvasive *E. coli,* Shiga toxin–producing *E. coli* such as *E. coli* 0157 : H7, *Yersinia enterocolitica, Clostridium difficile,* and *Entamoeba histolytica,* as well as inflammatory bowel disease, may cause confusion. Presumptive data supporting a diagnosis of bacillary dysentery include the finding of fecal leukocytes (confirming the presence of colitis), fecal blood, and demonstration in peripheral blood of leukocytosis with a dramatic left shift (often with more bands than segmented neutrophils). The total peripheral white blood cell count is usually 5,000–15,000 cells/mm^3, although leukopenia and leukemoid reactions occur.

Cultures of both stool and rectal swab specimens optimize the diagnosis of *Shigella* infections. Culture media should include MacConkey agar as well as selective media such as xylose-lysine deoxycholate (XLD) and SS agar. Transport media should be used if specimens cannot be cultured promptly. Appropriate media should be used to exclude *Campylobacter* and other agents. Studies of outbreaks and illness in volunteers show that the laboratory is often not able to confirm the clinical suspicion of shigellosis even when the pathogen is present. Although additional tools to improve diagnosis (gene probes) are being developed, the diagnostic inadequacy of cultures makes it incumbent on the clinician to use judgment in the management of clinical syndromes consistent with shigellosis. In children who appear to be toxic, blood cultures should be obtained; this is particularly important in very young or malnourished infants because of their increased risk for bacteremia.

TREATMENT. As with gastroenteritis from other causes, the 1st concern about a child with suspected shigellosis should be for fluid and electrolyte correction and maintenance (see Chapters 55 and 337). Nutrition is a key concern in areas where malnutrition is common. A high-protein diet during convalescence enhances growth in the following 6 mo. A single large dose of vitamin A (200,000 IU) lessens severity of shigellosis in areas where vitamin A deficiency is common. Drugs that retard intestinal motility (diphenoxylate hydrochloride with atropine [Lomotil] or loperamide [Imodium]) **should not be used** because of the risk for prolonging the illness.

Although some authorities recommend withholding antibacterial therapy because of the self-limited nature of the infection, cost of drugs, and risk for emergence of resistant organisms, there is a persuasive logic in favor of empirical treatment of all children in whom shigellosis is strongly suspected. Even if not fatal, the untreated illness may cause a child to be quite ill for weeks with chronic or recurrent diarrhea. Malnutrition may develop or worsen during prolonged illness, particularly in children in developing countries. The risk for continued excretion and subsequent infection of family contacts further argues against the strategy of withholding antibiotics.

There are major geographic variations in antibiotic susceptibility of shigellae. In the United States, shigellae are so frequently resistant to ampicillin that it is not appropriate for empirical therapy. However, oral ampicillin (100 mg/kg/day divided qid PO) may be used if the strain is known to be susceptible. Amoxicillin, because of better gastrointestinal absorption, is less effective than ampicillin for treatment of ampicillin-sensitive strains. In the United States, strains are commonly resistant to trimethoprim-sulfamethoxazole, making it also a poor empirical choice. Ceftriaxone (50 mg/kg/day as a single daily dose IV or IM) can be used for empirical therapy. Oral 1st and 2nd generation cephalosporins are inadequate as alternative drugs despite in vitro susceptibility. Nalidixic acid (55 mg/kg/day divided qid PO), where available, is also an acceptable alternative drug. Azithromycin (12 mg/kg/day PO for the 1st day followed by 6 mg/kg/day for the next 4 days) has proven to be an effective alternative drug for shigellosis. Quinolones such as ciprofloxacin, norfloxacin, or ofloxacin, which have been recommended for use in persons ≥18 yr of age, are not routinely used for children because of the putative risk for arthropathy. Use of these agents is reserved for seriously ill children with bacillary dysentery due to an organism that is suspected or known to be resistant to other agents. Treatment is typically for a 5 day course. Zinc (20 mg/day for 14 days) improves immune response to *Shigella* infection, at least in settings where malnutrition is common. It should probably be included in therapy of dysenteric patients in such settings.

Treatment of patients suspected on clinical grounds of having *Shigella* infection should be initiated when they are first evaluated. Stool culture is obtained to exclude other pathogens and to assist in antibiotic changes should a child fail to respond to empirical therapy. A child who has typical dysentery and who responds to initial empirical antibiotic treatment should be continued on that drug for a full 5 day course, even if the stool culture is negative. The logic of this recommendation is based on the difficulty of culturing *Shigella* from stools. In a child who fails to respond to therapy of a dysenteric syndrome in the presence of initially negative stool culture results, cultures should be retaken and the child re-evaluated for other possible diagnoses.

PREVENTION. Two simple measures decrease the risk for shigellosis in children. The 1st is to encourage prolonged breast-feeding of infants. Breast-feeding decreases the risk for symptomatic shigellosis and lessens its severity in those infants who acquire infection despite breast-feeding. The 2nd measure is to educate families and child-care center personnel in handwashing techniques, especially after defecation and before food preparation and consumption.

Ashkenazi S: *Shigella* infections in children: New insights. *Semin Pediatr Infect Dis* 2004;5:246–252.

Kotloff KL, Pasetti MF, Barry EM, et al: Deletion in the *Shigella* enterotoxin genes further attenuates *Shigella flexneri* 2a bearing guanine auxotrophy in a phase I trial of CVD 1204 and CVD 1208. *J Infect Dis* 2004;190:1745–1754.

Miron D, Torem M, Merom R, Colodner R: Azithromycin as an alternative to nalidixic acid in the therapy of childhood shigellosis. *Pediatr Infect Dis J* 2004;23:367–368.

Munoz C, Baqar S, van de Verg L, et al: Characteristics of *Shigella sonnei* infection of volunteers: Signs, symptoms, immune responses, changes in selected cytokines and acute-phase substances. *Am J Trop Med Hyg* 1995;53:47–54.

Rahman MJ, Sarker P, Roy SK, et al: Effect of zinc supplementation as adjunct therapy on the systemic immune response in shigellosis. *Am J Clin Nutr* 2005;81:495–502.

Replogle ML, Fleming DW, Cieslak PR: Emergence of antimicrobial-resistant shigellosis in Oregon. *Clin Infect Dis* 2000;30:515–519.

Chapter 197 ■ *Escherichia Coli*

Theresa J. Ochoa and Thomas G. Cleary

Escherichia coli organisms are important causes of enteric infections, as well as of urinary tract infections (see Chapter 538), sepsis and meningitis in the newborn (see Chapter 109), and bacteremia and sepsis in immunocompromised patients (see Chapter 177) and patients with intravascular devices (see Chapter 178).

E. coli species are members of the Enterobacteriaceae family and are facultatively anaerobic, gram-negative bacilli that usually ferment lactose. Most fecal *E. coli* organisms are nonpathogens. However, 5 major groups of diarrheagenic *E. coli* have been characterized on the basis of clinical, biochemical, and molecular-genetic criteria: (1) **enterotoxigenic *E. coli*** (ETEC); (2) **enteroinvasive *E. coli*** (EIEC); (3) **enteropathogenic *E. coli*** (EPEC); (4) **Shiga toxin–producing *E. coli*** **(STEC)**, also known as **enterohemorrhagic *E. coli*** (EHEC) or **verotoxin producing *E. coli*** (VTEC); and (5) **enteroaggregative *E. coli*** **(EAEC)**. There are other groups of *E. coli* that probably cause diarrhea but have combinations of virulence genes that do not fit easily within the classification system outlined above. Additional evidence of pathogenicity will be required before they can be generally accepted as bona fide pathogens. Another group most likely to achieve the status of a recognized pathogen is the **diffusely adherent *E. coli*** (DAEC), which is defined by its adherence to the HEp2 cell and presence of specific genes.

Because *E. coli* organisms are normal fecal flora, demonstration of virulence characteristics is the usual way by which the diarrheagenic *E. coli* organisms are defined. The mechanism by which *E. coli* produces diarrhea typically involves adherence of organisms to a glycoprotein or glycolipid receptor, followed by production of some noxious substance that injures gut cells or disturbs their function. The genes for virulence properties and for antibiotic resistance are often carried on transferable plasmids, pathogenicity islands, or bacteriophages. In the developing world, the various diarrheagenic serogroups of *E. coli* cause frequent infections in the 1st few years of life. They occur with increased frequency during the warm months in temperate climates and during rainy season months in tropical climates. Most *E. coli* strains (except STEC and perhaps some EPEC) require a large inoculum of organisms to induce disease. Infection is most likely when food-handling or sewage disposal practices are suboptimal. The diarrheagenic *E. coli* organisms are also important in North America and Europe, although their epidemiology is less well

TABLE 197-1. Clinical Characteristics, Pathogenesis, and Diagnosis of Diarrheagenic *Escherichia coli*

		CHARACTERISTICS OF DIARRHEA			MAIN VIRULENCE FACTORS		DIAGNOSIS
	POPULATIONS AT RISK	Watery	Bloody	Duration	Adherence Factors	Toxins	Target Genes for PCR
ETEC	>1 yr old and travelers	+++	—	Acute	Colonization factor antigens (CFA I, II, IV)	Heat-labile enterotoxin (LT) Heat-stable enterotoxin (ST)	LT, ST
EIEC	>1 yr old	+	++ Dysentery with fever	Acute	Invasion plasmid antigen (IpaABCD)	*Shigella* enterotoxins	IpaH or IAL
EPEC	<2 yr old, especially infants <6 mo	+++	—	Acute or persistent	A/E lesion, intimin/Tir, EspABD BFP	EspF	Eae, BfpA
STEC	6 mo to 10 yr and the elderly	+	+++ Afebrile hemorrhagic colitis; hemolytic uremic syndrome	Acute	A/E lesion	Shiga toxins (Stx1, Stx2, and variants of Stx2)	Eae, Stx1, Stx2
EAEC	<1 yr old and travelers	+++	—	Acute or persistent	Aggregative adherence fimbria (AAF)	ShET1, EAST1, Pet	AggR or AA plasmid

EAEC, enteroaggregative *E. coli*; EIEC, enteroinvasive *E. coli*; EPEC, enteropathogenic *E. coli*; ETEC, enterotoxigenic *E. coli*; PCR, polymerase chain reaction; STEC, Shiga toxin–producing *E. coli*.

defined than in the developing world. Recent data in North America suggest that the various diarrheagenic *E. coli* organisms could be the cause of as much as 30% of infectious diarrhea in children <5 yr of age.

EPIDEMIOLOGY, PATHOGENESIS, AND CLINICAL MANIFESTATIONS. The 5 major subgroups of diarrheagenic *E. coli* are distinguished by different pathophysiologic mechanisms of diarrhea (Table 197-1).

Enterotoxigenic *E. coli*. ETEC organisms are a major cause of dehydrating infantile diarrhea in the developing world as well as important agents of traveler's diarrhea. The typical signs and symptoms include explosive watery, nonmucoid, nonbloody diarrhea, abdominal pain, nausea, vomiting, and little or no fever. The illness is usually self-limited in 3–5 days, but occasionally lasts >1 wk. ETEC organisms account for as much as 20–30% of diarrhea episodes in the developing world.

ETEC organisms cause few or no structural alterations in the gut mucosa. Diarrhea is caused by colonization of the small intestine and subsequent elaboration of enterotoxins. ETEC strains secrete a **heat-labile enterotoxin (LT)** or a **heat-stable enterotoxin (ST)**; some strains make both ST and LT. LT, a large molecule consisting of 5 receptor-binding (B) subunits and 1 enzymatically active (A) subunit, is structurally, functionally, and immunologically related to cholera toxin produced by *Vibrio cholerae*. LT stimulates adenylate cyclase, resulting in increased cyclic adenosine monophosphate. ST is a small molecule not related to LT or cholera toxin. ST stimulates guanylate cyclase, resulting in increased cyclic guanosine monophosphate. A large proportion of ETEC strains also produce EAST1, a heat-stable toxin similar to ST, which was originally identified in EAEC strains.

Colonization of the intestine requires fimbrial **colonization factor antigens (CFAs)**, which promote adhesion to the intestinal epithelium. The most prevalent colonization factors are CFA/I, CFA/II, and CFA/IV. CFAs are composed of distinct *E. coli* surface antigens (CS), expressed in different combinations. A large proportion of ETEC strains produce a type IV pilus called longus, which functions as a colonization factor and is found among several gram-negative bacterial pathogens. The binding of enterotoxigenic invasion protein A (Tia), a 25 kd outer membrane protein, to host epithelial cells is mediated at least in part through heparan sulfate proteoglycans; ETEC organisms belong on the growing list of pathogens that use cell surface glycoconjugates as receptors.

Of the >180 *E. coli* serogroups, only a relatively small number typically are ETEC. These serogroups (06, 08, 015, 020, 025, 027, 063, 078, 080, 085, 0115, 0128ac [but not subgroups 0128ab or 0128ad], 0139, 0148, 0153, 0159, and 0167) are generally different from those found in other diarrhea-associated *E. coli.*

Enteroinvasive *E. coli*. Clinically EIEC infections present either with watery diarrhea or a dysentery syndrome, manifested as blood, mucus, and leukocytes in the stools, with fever, systemic toxicity, crampy abdominal pain, tenesmus, and urgency. They resemble bacillary dysentery because they share virulence genes with *Shigella*. EIEC organisms are mostly described in outbreaks; however, endemic disease occurs in developing countries where these bacteria can be isolated with relatively high frequency. In the developing world, as many as 5% of sporadic diarrhea episodes and 20% of bloody diarrhea cases may be caused by EIEC strains.

EIEC organisms cause colonic lesions with ulcerations, hemorrhage, mucosal and submucosal edema, and infiltration by polymorphonuclear leukocytes. EIEC strains behave like shigellae in their capacity to invade gut epithelium and produce a dysentery-like illness. The invasive process involves (1) initial entry into cells, (2) intracellular multiplication, (3) intracellular and intercellular spread, and (4) host cell death. All bacterial genes necessary for entry into the host cell are clustered within a 30 kb region of a large virulence plasmid, also found in *Shigella*. This region carries genes encoding the entry-mediating proteins, which code for proteins forming a type III secretion apparatus required for secretion of the **invasins (IpaA-D and IpgD)**. IpaB and IpaC have been identified as the primary effector proteins of epithelial cell invasion. The type III secretion apparatus is found in many other pathogenic gram-negative bacteria. It is a system triggered by contact with host cells that bacteria use to transport proteins from their cytoplasm into the host cell plasma membrane and cytoplasm.

EIEC organisms encompass a small number of serogroups (028ac, 029, 0124, 0136, 0143, 0144, 0152, 0164, 0167, and some nontypable strains). These serogroups have lipopolysaccharide (LPS) antigens related to *Shigella* LPS, and, like shigellae, are nonmotile (they lack H or flagellar antigens) and are usually nonlactose fermenting.

Enteropathogenic *E. coli*. EPEC organisms are a major cause of infant acute and persistent diarrhea in developing countries, primarily in children <2 yr of age. In developed countries, EPEC organisms are responsible for occasional outbreaks in daycare centers and pediatric wards. EPEC organisms generally cause acute or protracted disease. In addition to profuse watery, nonbloody diarrhea with mucus, vomiting and low-grade fever are common symptoms. Persistent diarrhea (>14 days) can lead to malnutrition; this is an important outcome of EPEC infection in infants in the developing world. Several studies have shown that breast-feeding is protective against diarrhea due to EPEC.

EPEC colonization causes blunting of villi, inflammatory changes, and sloughing of superficial mucosal cells; these lesions are found from the duodenum through the colon. EPEC organisms induce a characteristic attaching and effacing (A/E) histopathologic lesion, which is defined by the intimate attachment of bacteria to the epithelial surface and effacement of host cell microvilli. Factors responsible for the A/E lesion formation are encoded by the locus of enterocyte effacement (LEE), which is a pathogenicity island that contains the genes for (1) the type III secretion system, (2) the translocated intimin receptor (Tir) and intimin, and (3) effector proteins such as the *E. coli*–secreted proteins (EspA-B-D).

EPEC pathogenesis involves several stages. The initial adherence of the bacteria to the host's intestinal epithelium in a pattern known as localized adherence is mediated in part by the type IV bundle-forming pilus (BFP) encoded on a plasmid (the EAF plasmid). Next, bacterial proteins are translocated through a type III secretion system "needle complex." Filamentous appendages made of EspA form a physical bridge between the bacteria and the host cell for the translocations of bacterial effectors (EspB, EspD, Tir). EspB and EspD form pores in the host's cell membrane. Tir is injected into host cells by way of this conduit. Tir moves to the surface of host cells where it is bound by a bacterial outer membrane protein intimin, which is encoded by the *eae* gene. Intimin-Tir binding triggers polymerization of actin and other cytoskeletal components at the site of attachment. The result of these cytoskeletal changes is intimate bacterial attachment to the host cell, enterocyte effacement, and pedestal formation. Other bacterial effectors include a mitochondrial-associated protein (Map) with membrane-potential disrupting activity and EspF, a protein that disrupts the intestinal barrier function and induces host cell death.

Some serogroups are associated with localized adherence and are EAF probe positive (055, 086, 0111, 0119, 0125, 0126, 0127, 0128ab, and 0142), whereas others (atypical EPEC) are nonadherent or diffusely adherent to HEp-2 cells and are usually EAF probe negative (018, 044, 0112, and 0114). There is more evidence that EPEC organisms with localized adherence are true enteropathogens, although, as noted above, evidence is mounting that at least some of the atypical EPEC organisms are also pathogens.

Shiga Toxin–Producing *E. coli*. STEC organisms have been shown to cause a wide spectrum of diseases. STEC infections may be asymptomatic. Patients develop intestinal symptoms ranging from mild diarrhea to severe hemorrhagic colitis. The gastrointestinal illness is characterized by abdominal pain with diarrhea that is initially watery but within a few days becomes blood streaked or grossly bloody. Although this pattern resembles that of shigellosis or EIEC disease, it differs in that fever is an uncommon manifestation. Most individuals infected with STEC recover from the infection without further complication. However, 5–10% of children go on within a few days to develop systemic complications such as hemolytic-uremic syndrome (HUS), characterized by acute renal failure, thrombocytopenia, and hemolytic anemia (see Chapter 518). Very young children are not a target group of STEC; rather, severe and complicated illness occurs most often among children from 6 mo to 10 yr of age. The elderly may also develop HUS or thrombotic thrombocytopenic purpura.

STEC organisms are transmitted person to person as well as by food and water; ingestion of a low number of these organisms is sufficient to cause disease. Poorly cooked hamburger is a common cause of food-borne outbreaks, although many other foods (apple cider, lettuce, mayonnaise, salami, dry fermented sausage, unpasteurized dairy products) have also been incriminated. Most outbreaks of STEC-associated diarrhea in the Northern hemisphere have been attributed to strains of serotype 0157 : H7, and many other serotypes have been associated with outbreaks and sporadic cases of severe disease.

STEC organisms affect the colon most severely. STEC organisms adhere to intestinal cells, and most strains that affect humans produce attaching-effacing lesions like those seen with EPEC. Most STEC strains also carry a large plasmid encoding proteins such as enterohemolysin (EhyA), an extracellular serine protease (EspP), and a STEC autoagglutinating adhesin (Saa), which may be accessory virulence factors. These organisms cause edema, fibrin deposits, hemorrhage in the submucosa, mucosal ulceration, neutrophil infiltration, and microvascular thrombi. Pseudomembranous colitis may be seen.

Shiga toxins are considered to be the key virulence factor of STEC. There are 2 major toxin types, Stx1 and Stx2. Some STEC organisms produce only Stx1 and others only Stx2, but most STEC organisms produce both toxins. There are strains that produce multiple toxin variants. Stx1 is essentially identical to Shiga toxin, the protein synthesis–inhibiting exotoxin of *Shigella dysenteriae* serotype 1, whereas Stx2 and variants of Stx2 are more distantly related. Each toxin is composed of a single A subunit noncovalently associated with a pentamer composed of identical B subunits. The B subunits bind to globotriaosylceramide (Gb_3), a glycosphingolipid receptor on host cells. The A subunit is taken up by endocytosis. The toxin target is the 28S recombinant RNA, which is depurinated by the toxin at a specific adenine residue, causing protein synthesis to cease and affected cells to die. These toxins are carried on bacteriophages that are normally inactive when inserted into the bacterial chromosome; when the phages are induced to replicate (e.g., by the stress induced by many antibiotics), they cause lysis of the bacteria and release of large amounts of toxin. The toxin enters the systemic circulation after translocation across the intestinal epithelium and damages vascular endothelial cells. This causes activation of the coagulation cascade, formation of microthrombi, intravascular hemolysis, and ischemia. STEC organisms induce proinflammatory cytokines. Clinical outcome of STEC infection depends on the stx genotype of the infecting strain. The Stx2 genotype is associated with a higher risk for causing HUS.

The most common STEC serotypes are *E. coli* O157 : H7, *E. coli* 0111 : NM, and *E. coli* 026 : H11, although several hundred other STEC serotypes have also been described.

Enteroaggregative *E. coli*. EAEC organisms are associated with acute and persistent pediatric diarrhea in developing countries, most prominently in children >12 mo of age. EAEC organisms are etiologic agents in AIDS-associated chronic diarrhea and traveler's diarrhea. EAEC typical illness is manifested by watery, mucoid, secretory diarrhea with low-grade fever and little or no vomiting. One third of patients have grossly bloody stools. The watery diarrhea may persist for weeks. EAEC organisms have been associated with growth retardation in infants and malnutrition in the developing world.

EAEC organisms form a characteristic mucous biofilm on the intestinal mucosa and induce shortening of the villi, hemorrhagic necrosis, and inflammatory responses. The proposed model of pathogenesis of EAEC involves three phases: adherence to the intestinal mucosa by way of the aggregative adherence fimbriae (AAF); enhanced mucus production; and production of toxins and inflammation that result in damage of the mucosa and intestinal secretion. Diarrhea caused by EAEC is predominantly secretory. The intestinal inflammatory response (elevated fecal lactoferrin, interleukin 8 [IL-8] and IL-1β) may be related to growth impairment and malnutrition.

Putative EAEC virulence factors include aggregative adherence fimbriae (AAF-I, AAF-II, and AAF-III), hemolysins, various outer membrane and secreted proteins (dispersin), and several toxins: an oligomeric enterotoxin called *Shigella* enterotoxin 1 (ShET1); an enteroaggregative *E. coli* heat-stable toxin 1 (EAST1), homologous to the Enterotoxigenic *E. coli* heat-stable toxin; and an autotransporter toxin called Pet. A transcriptional activator called AggR controls expression of plasmid-borne and chromosomal virulence factors. Identification of AggR or members of the AggR regulaton may identify typical pathogenic EAEC strains.

Strains of *E. coli* categorized as EAEC belong to a diverse range and combination of O and H serotypes. Definition of these pathogens is in flux. The original diagnostic criteria (HEp2 cell adherence pattern) identified many strains that are probably not true pathogens; genetic criteria appear to more reliably define true pathogens.

DIAGNOSIS. The clinical features of illness are seldom distinctive enough to allow confident diagnosis, and routine laboratory studies are of very limited value. Diagnosis currently depends primarily on laboratory studies that are not readily available. Practical, non-DNA-dependent methods for routine diagnosis of diarrheagenic *E. coli* have been developed primarily for STEC. Serotype O157 : H7 is suggested by isolation of an *E. coli* that fails to ferment sorbitol on MacConkey sorbitol medium; latex agglutination confirms that the organism contains O157 LPS. Other STEC organisms can be detected in routine hospital laboratories using commercially available enzyme immunoassay or latex agglutination to detect Shiga toxins. The diagnosis of other diarrheagenic *E. coli* infection is typically made based on tissue culture (e.g., HEp2 cell assays for EPEC and EAEC), or identification of specific virulence factors of the bacteria by phenotype (e.g., toxins) or genotype. DNA probes for genes encoding the various virulence traits are the best diagnostic tests, but are currently available only as a research tool. Therefore, suspected organisms should be forwarded to reference or research laboratories for definitive evaluation. Such efforts are seldom necessary, but they may be helpful for correct diagnosis when a child has severe or life-threatening complications, persistent diarrhea, or for outbreak investigation. Polymerase chain reaction and DNA probes for genes encoding the various virulence factors are now available for the major diarrheagenic *E. coli* strains. Typical targets include LT and ST for ETEC; IpaH or IaL for EIEC; Eae and BfpA for EPEC; Eae, Stx1, and Stx2 for STEC; and AggR or the AA plasmid for EAEC.

Other laboratory data are at best nonspecific indicators of etiology. Fecal leukocyte examination of the stool is frequently positive with EIEC but negative with other diarrheagenic *E. coli.* With EIEC and STEC there may be an elevated polymorphonuclear leukocyte count with a left shift. Fecal lactoferrin, IL-8, and IL-1β can be used as inflammatory markers. Electrolyte changes are nonspecific, reflecting only fluid loss.

TREATMENT. The cornerstone of management is appropriate fluid and electrolyte therapy (see Chapters 55 and 337). In general, this therapy should include oral replacement and maintenance with rehydration solutions such as those specified by the World Health Organization. Pedialyte and other readily available oral rehydration solutions are acceptable alternatives. After refeeding, continued supplementation with oral rehydration fluids is appropriate to prevent recurrence of dehydration. Early refeeding (within 8–12 hr of initiation of rehydration) with breast milk or infant formula should be encouraged. Prolonged withholding of feeding frequently leads to chronic diarrhea and malnutrition.

Specific antimicrobial therapy of diarrheagenic *E. coli* is problematic because of the difficulty of making an accurate diagnosis of these pathogens and the unpredictability of antibiotic susceptibilities. ETEC organisms respond to antimicrobial agents such as trimethoprim-sulfamethoxazole (TMP-SMZ) when the *E. coli* strains are susceptible. However, other than for a child recently returning from travel in the developing world, empirical treatment of severe watery diarrhea with antibiotics is seldom appropriate. EIEC infections may be treated before the availability of culture results because the clinician suspects shigellosis and has begun empirical therapy. If the organisms are susceptible, TMP-SMZ is an appropriate choice. Although treatment of EPEC infection with TMP-SMZ intravenously or orally for 5 days is effective in speeding resolution, the lack of a rapid diagnostic test makes treatment decisions difficult. Ciprofloxacin or rifaximin are useful for EAEC traveler's diarrhea; pediatric data are sparse. STEC organisms represent a particularly difficult therapeutic dilemma; antibiotic treatment can induce toxin production and phage-mediated bacterial lysis with toxin release. Current data suggest that antibiotics should not be given for STEC infection because they may increase the risk for HUS (see Chapter 518).

PREVENTION. In the developing world, prevention of disease caused by diarrheagenic *E. coli* is probably best done by maintaining prolonged breast-feeding, paying careful attention to personal hygiene, and following proper food- and water-handling procedures. People traveling to these places can be best protected by consuming only processed water, bottled beverages, breads, fruit juices, fruits that can be peeled, or foods that are served steaming hot.

Prophylactic antibiotic therapy, although effective in adult travelers, has not been studied in children and is not recommended. Public health measures, including sewage disposal and food-handling practices, have made pathogens that require large inocula to produce illness relatively uncommon in industrialized countries. Food-borne outbreaks of STEC are a problem for which no adequate solution has been found. During the occasional hospital outbreak of EPEC disease, attention to enteric isolation precautions and cohorting may be critical.

The nature of protective immunity is not fully understood, and no vaccines are available for clinical use. There are several vaccine candidates based on bacterial toxins or colonization factors that are being studied.

Chen HD, Frankel G: Enteropathogenic Escherichia coli: Unraveling pathogenesis. *FEMS Microbiol Rev* 2005;29:83–98.

Cohen MB, Nataro JP, Bernstein DI, et al: Prevalence of diarrheagenic *E. coli* in acute childhood enteritis; a prospective controlled study. *J Pediatr* 2005;146:54–61.

Donnenberg MS, Whittam TS: Pathogenesis and evolution of virulence in enteropathogenic and enterohemorrhagic *Escherichia coli. J Clin Invest* 2001;107:539–548.

Knutton S, Shaw R, Phillips Ad, et al: Phenotypic and genetic analysis of diarrhea-associated *E. coli* isolated from children in the United Kingdom. *J Pediatr Gastroenterol Nutr* 2001;33:32–46.

Nataro JP: Enteroaggregative *Escherichia coli* pathogenesis. *Curr Opin Gastroenterol* 2005;21:4–8.

Nataro JP, Kaper JB: Diarrheagenic *Escherichia coli. Clin Microbiol Rev* 1998;11:142–201.

Robins-Browne RM, Hartland EL: *Escherichia coli* as a cause of diarrhea. *J Gastroenterol Hepatol* 2002;17:467–475.

Chapter 198 ■ Cholera *(Vibrio Cholerae)*

Jacqueline L. Deen

Cholera is a dreaded diarrheal illness because of its severity and potential to cause outbreaks. The disease remains a burden in many underdeveloped countries that cannot afford to establish or to maintain essential infrastructure for safe water supply and sanitation. Seasonal disease occurs in resource-poor endemic settings; epidemics arise during natural disasters and complex emergencies resulting in significant mortality and economic damage. In industrialized countries, cholera is a rare, episodic problem.

ETIOLOGY. *Vibrio cholerae* is a slightly curved, gram-negative, aerobic bacillus (1.5–3.0 × 0.5 μm) with a polar flagellum. Its antigenic structure consists of a flagellar H antigen and a somatic O antigen. Differentiation of the O antigen allows for identification of serogroups known to cause cholera, *V. cholerae* O1 and

O139. On the basis of phenotypic characteristics, *V. cholerae* O1 is subdivided into 2 biotypes, classic and El Tor. *V. cholerae* O1 El Tor is currently the predominant strain. The classic biotype is believed to be extinct, although genetic hybrids between the *V. cholerae* O1 classic and El Tor biotypes have been reported among isolates from Bangladesh and Mozambique. Organisms in both biotypes are further classified according to the presence of somatic antigens into 2 major serotypes, Inaba and Ogawa, and an unstable intermediate type, Hikojima. Strains of *V. cholerae* belonging to serogroups other than O1 and O139 have been incriminated as the causative agents of noncholera gastroenteritis, sometimes with extraintestinal manifestations but without epidemic potential.

EPIDEMIOLOGY. Cholera is an ancient disease with cases in the Bramaputra and Ganges river deltas dating back at least 1,000 years. The 1st 6 cholera pandemics from 1817 to 1923, most likely caused by the classic biotype, originated from this area, spreading to Europe and the Americas. The etiologic organism of the 7th pandemic is *V. cholerae* O1 El Tor, named for the location in Egypt where the strain was first isolated in 1905. This biotype was associated only with sporadic cases until 1961, when the current pandemic began in Celebes (Sulawesi), Indonesia. The disease spread rapidly to other Asian countries and in 1970 invaded West Africa, which had not experienced cholera for >100 yr. Outbreaks occurred in a number of African countries and eventually became endemic in most of the continent. The last extension of this pandemic was to Latin America in 1991, where cholera had also been absent for more than a century. Within the year it spread to 11 countries and subsequently throughout the continent. The 7th pandemic has been the longest lasting, affecting more countries and continents than the other 6 pandemics. In 2002, 13 Asian, 27 African, and 2 Latin American countries reported cholera cases to the World Health Organization (WHO).

Previously, only *V. cholerae* serogroup O1 caused epidemic cholera. In late 1992, large outbreaks of the disease began in India and Bangladesh that were caused by a previously unrecognized serogroup of *V. cholerae,* designated O139, synonym Bengal. Isolation of this organism has now been reported from 11 countries in Southeast Asia. For unknown reasons, O139 has not continued its epidemic spread.

Cholera exists in sporadic, endemic, epidemic, and pandemic forms. The transition from epidemic to endemic, usually seasonal disease, may be due to a population acquiring immune resistance. Immunity is thought to be primary related to mucosal secretory antibodies directed against the organism's lipopolysaccharide. There appears to be at least partial cross-protection between biotypes (El Tor and classical) and serotypes (Ogawa and Inaba) of the O1 serogroup but none between the O1 and O139 serogroups. However, natural disease does not appear to confer life-long immunity, so recurrent attacks are possible.

V. cholerae is found in the aquatic environment and is part of the normal flora of brackish water and estuaries. It is often associated with algae blooms, which are influenced by the temperature of the water. Cholera is introduced to humans through contaminated water and food, with very high attack rates in nonimmune populations and frequent intra-household transmission. Infected humans then shed the organism into the environment.

PATHOGENESIS. A large inoculum of bacteria (>~10^8 viable units) is required to cause clinical disease in part because the organisms are killed by normal gastric acidity. Thus, use of antacids, histamine receptor blockers, and proton pump inhibitors increases the risk for cholera infection and predisposes to more severe disease. Following colonization of the upper small intestine, *V. cholerae* O1 and O139 produce an enterotoxin that promotes the secretion of fluid and electrolytes into the lumen of the small intestine. The enterotoxin consists of 5 binding (B) subunits and 1 active (A) subunit. The B subunits bind to the GM1 ganglioside receptors in the small intestinal mucosa, allowing the A subunit to enter into the cell where it activates adenylate cyclase, leading to an increase in cyclic adenosine monophosphate (AMP). Cyclic AMP blocks the absorption of sodium chloride by the microvilli and promotes the secretion of chloride and water by the crypt cells. The result is massive outpouring of electrolyte-rich isotonic fluid into the small intestine. The large volume of fluid produced in the upper intestine overwhelms the absorptive capacity of the lower bowel, resulting in severe diarrhea. The diarrheal fluid contains large amounts of sodium, chloride, bicarbonate, and potassium. Since the enterotoxin acts locally and does not invade the intestinal wall, few red blood cells and neutrophils are found in the stool. The loss of electrolyte-rich isotonic fluid leads to blood volume depletion with resulting low blood pressure and shock. Loss of bicarbonate and potassium leads to metabolic acidosis and hypokalemia.

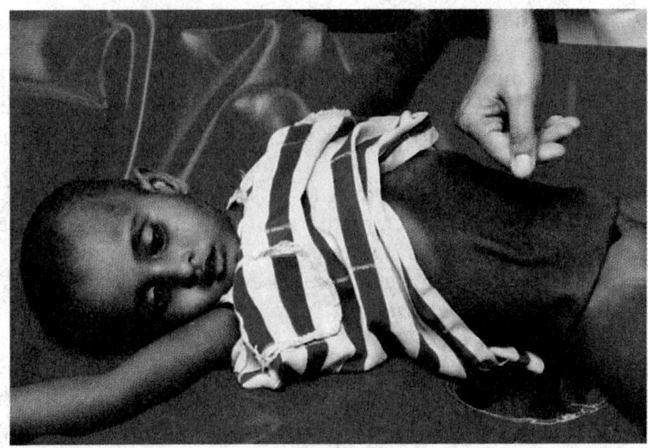

Figure 198-1. A child, lying on a cholera cot, showing typical signs of severe dehydration from cholera. The patient has sunken eyes, lethargic appearance, and poor skin turgor, but within 2 hr was sitting up, alert, and eating normally. (From Sack DA, Sack RB, Nair GB, Siddique AK: Cholera. *Lancet* 2004;363:223–233.)

CLINICAL MANIFESTATIONS. Cholera is characterized by an acute onset of copious watery diarrhea and vomiting **without abdominal cramps or fever.** The stools are colorless with small flecks of mucus ("rice-water") and are sometimes described as having a fishy odor. At first, children may be restless or extremely thirsty, but if fluid and electrolyte losses are not replaced, they may become lethargic or unconscious. Other signs of dehydration may rapidly manifest, including poor skin turgor, sunken eyes, dry mouth and tongue, no urine output, delayed capillary refill, rapid or weak pulse, and low blood pressure (Fig. 198-1). Severe dehydration, metabolic acidosis, and hypokalemia can occur in 4–12 hr. The fluid losses may be so rapid that the child quickly develops hypovolemic shock, hypoglycemia, coma, and seizures and is at risk of dying within a few hours of onset.

The incubation period between ingestion of the organism and onset of manifestations is 18 hr to 5 days. Although the typical clinical picture is severe diarrhea, most infected individuals have no symptoms or only mild diarrhea, indistinguishable from other diarrheal diseases. The ratio of cases to infections ranges from 1 : 3 to 1 : 100, depending on local intestinal immunity, size of the inoculum, adequacy of the gastric acid barrier, and other factors.

LABORATORY FINDINGS. Laboratory findings of hemoconcentration and increased serum specific gravity reflect the degree of isotonic dehydration. Electrolyte and acid-base abnormalities typical of severe dehydration include normal or low serum potassium levels, normal or slightly low sodium and chloride levels, and metabolic acidosis.

DIAGNOSIS. The diagnosis of individual cases of cholera remains primarily on clinical grounds. Laboratory confirmation is required for surveillance and epidemiologic investigations. In endemic areas, a child with severe watery diarrhea should be considered a possible case of cholera pending laboratory confirmation (if available) and treatment should be started immediately. In industrialized countries, the diagnosis should be suspected in any child with severe watery diarrhea and a history of recent travel to an endemic area. Other enteric diseases characterized by acute, watery diarrhea such as those caused by rotavirus or enterotoxigenic *Escherichia coli* may be difficult to differentiate from cholera.

Rapid tests include dark-field microscopy in which a wet mount of liquid stool is examined for "darting" organisms that are halted by the addition of O1 or O139 antiserum. Rapid immunoassays are also available. Diagnosis is confirmed by isolation of the organism on stool culture. Cary-Blair transport medium may be used for transport of a stool specimen or rectal swab to the laboratory. Feces, either fresh or in the transport media, should be plated onto thiosulfate-citrate-bile-sucrose (TCBS) media. *V. cholerae* appears as smooth yellow colonies with slightly raised centers after 18–24 hr of incubation. Presumptive identification of *V. cholerae* O1 or O139 can be established on the basis of typical colonies, which are oxidase positive and agglutinate with O1 or O139 antiserum.

COMPLICATIONS. Lethargy, seizures, altered consciousness, fever, hypoglycemia, and death occur more frequently in children than in adults. Inadequate fluid and electrolyte replacement may lead to acute tubular necrosis. Children with low potassium levels can develop paralytic ileus and abdominal distention that can make oral rehydration impossible. In severely ill children with potassium depletion and acidosis, hypokalemic arrhythmia can cause sudden death. In as many as 10% of small children, prolonged drowsiness, coma, or seizures occur. When the seizures are associated with hypoglycemia, they are often followed by coma and death; in 1 study, 14.3% of children with cholera complicated by hypoglycemia died, compared with 0.7% of children without hypoglycemia. After dehydration, hypoglycemia is the most common life-threatening consequence of cholera in children. Hyperglycemia can also occur due to the secretion of epinephrine, norepinephrine, cortisol, and glucagon in response to the stress of hypovolemia. Pulmonary edema occurs in some children, probably because of fluid overload during rehydration. Transient tetany may occur during correction of electrolyte imbalances. In children treated with excessive sugar and salt, hypernatremia can be observed.

TREATMENT. The mainstay of treatment for cholera is fluid and electrolyte replacement (Table 198-1). Rehydration therapy should be initiated as soon as the diagnosis is suspected (see Chapters 55.1 and 337). For several decades, the most widely recommended formulation of oral rehydration salts (ORS) contained 90 mmol of sodium, 20 mmol of potassium, 80 mmol of chloride, 111 mmol of glucose, and 10 mmol of citrate per liter, with a total osmolarity of 311 mOsm/L. In 2002, a new ORS formula with sodium and glucose lowered to 5 mmol/L and total osmolarity decreased to 245 mOsm/L was launched by the WHO. The reduced-osmolarity ORS appears to be as safe and at least as effective as standard ORS for use in children with cholera. In adults with cholera, its use has been associated with an increased incidence of transient, asymptomatic hyponatremia.

TABLE 198-1. Management of Patients with Suspected Cholera

Assess for dehydration.
Rapidly rehydrate the patient with intravenous Ringer solution for severely dehydrated patients or oral rehydration salts (ORS) for those with less severe dehydration; use rice-based ORS if possible.
Severely dehydrated patients require replacement of 10% of their body weight within 2–4 hr.
Use cholera cot (if possible) to monitor stool output; monitor status of hydration and monitor severity of purging frequently.
Maintain hydration by replacing continuing fluid losses until diarrhea stops.
Give an oral antibiotic (e.g., doxycycline) to dehydrated patients as soon as vomiting stops.
Provide food as soon as patient is able to eat (within a few hours).

From Sack DA, Sack RB, Nair GB, Siddique AK: Cholera. *Lancet* 2004;363:223–233.

Oral rehydration given ad libitum is the treatment of choice unless the child is obtunded, has an ileus, or is in shock; in these circumstances, intravenous saline or lactated Ringer solution rather than oral rehydration is appropriate. Vomiting is not a contraindication to oral rehydration. Although all patients with cholera should be carefully monitored, attention to intake and output is especially important for infants. Food should be restarted as soon as deficits are replaced to minimize the nutritional impact of the illness; refeeding does not affect purging rates or the duration of diarrhea.

Rehydration is the most important treatment. However, antibiotics are useful in shortening the duration of illness, reducing the period of excretion of the organisms, and decreasing the requirements for fluid replacement. Antimicrobial therapy should be considered for patients with moderate or severe disease. Oral tetracycline (50 mg/kg/day divided qid PO for 3 days; maximum 2 g/day) or doxycycline (5 mg/kg PO as a single dose, maximum 200 mg/day) are the drugs of choice for cholera due to *V. cholera* O1 and O139. For children <9 yr of age, the use of tetracycline is not recommended. In resistant strains or children <9 yr of age, trimethoprim-sulfamethoxazole (8–10 mg/kg/day trimethoprim and 40 mg/kg/day sulfamethoxazole, divided bid PO), erythromycin (40 mg/kg/day, maximum 2 g/day), or furazolidone (5–8 mg/kg/day, maximum 400 mg) may be used. Resistance to tetracycline and other antimicrobials is increasing. Antibiotic resistance evaluations should be performed on isolates from sporadic cases and representative cases from an epidemic.

PREVENTION. Ensuring safe water and food, adequate sanitation, and personal and community hygiene constitute the main strategies against cholera. In endemic sites, these interventions cannot be implemented fully in the near future. In acute emergency situations, any existing public health measures worsen or collapse. Thus, a safe, effective, and affordable vaccine would be a potentially useful tool for cholera prevention and control.

At the present time, the manufacture and sale of the only licensed cholera vaccine in the United States, which was the parenteral preparation made of phenol-killed organisms, has been discontinued (Table 198-2). Since the vaccine offered limited protection for only a short duration and was highly reactogenic (i.e.,

TABLE 198-2. Summary of Data on Internationally Licensed Cholera Vaccines

	AVAILABILITY	AGE	DOSE SCHEDULE	ROUTE	PROTECTIVE EFFICACY	ADVERSE EVENT PROFILE
Parenteral phenol-inactivated vaccine	No longer recommended	≥6 mo	2 doses 1–4 wk apart	IM	30–50% for 3–6 mo	High
Oral recombinant–B subunit and *V. cholerae* O1 killed whole cell (rBs-WC, Dukoral™, SBL) vaccine	Europe	≥2 yr	2 doses 1–6 wk apart	Oral	85% during first 6 mo; then 50% for at least 3 yr	Low
Oral live-attenuated *V. cholerae* CVD 103 HgR vaccine (Mutachol, Orachol, Berna)	Canada, Latin America, Europe	≥2 yr	Single dose	Oral	80% for at least 6 mo	Low

pain, erythema, local induration, fever, headaches), it is no longer recommended. No cholera vaccination requirements exist for entry or exit in any country. Travelers to areas endemic for cholera should take appropriate water and food precautions. Visitors to countries reporting cholera who follow common tourist itineraries and who use standard accommodations are at low risk for infection.

Considerable progress has been made during the past decade in the development of modern generation oral vaccines against cholera. These new vaccines promise substantial protection against O1 cholera without side effects. However, neither of these 2 vaccines is available in the USA. One is a recombinant B subunit and *V. cholerae* O1 killed whole cell (rBs-WC) vaccine and the other is a live-attenuated *V. cholerae* CVD 103 HgR vaccine. Both the killed and live-attenuated vaccines are licensed in some countries and are now being considered for wider public health applications. In 2002, the WHO changed its existing policy and recommended that the use of oral cholera vaccination be considered in certain endemic and epidemic situations, complementary to other control strategies.

Ali M, Emch M, von Seidlein L, et al: Herd immunity conferred by killed oral cholera vaccines in Bangladesh: A reanalysis. *Lancet* 2005;366:44–49.

Colwell RR: Infectious disease and environment: Cholera as a paradigm for waterborne disease. *Int Microbiol* 2004;7:285–289.

Heidelberg JF, Eisen JA, Nelson WC, et al: DNA sequence of both chromosomes of the cholera pathogen Vibrio cholerae. *Nature* 2000;406:477–483.

Lucas M, Deen JL, von Seidlein L, et al: High-level effectiveness of a mass oral cholera vaccination in Beira, Mozambique. *N Engl J Med* 2005;352: 757–767.

Reidl J, Klose KE: Vibrio cholerae and cholera: Out of the water and into the host. *FEMS Microbiol Rev* 2002;26:125–139.

Ryan ET, Calderwood S: Cholera vaccines. *Clin Infect Dis* 2000;31:561–565.

Sack DA, Sack RB, Nair GB, Siddique AK: Cholera. *Lancet* 2004;363: 223–233.

Saha D, Karim MM, Khan WA, et al: Single-dose azithromycin for treatment of cholera in adults. *N Engl J Med* 2006;354:2452–2462.

Sur D, Deen JL, Manna B, et al: The burden of cholera in the slums of Kolkata, India: Data from a prospective, community based study. *Arch Dis Child* 2005;90:1175–1181.

World Health Organization: Cholera 2002. *Wkly Epidemiol Rec* 2003;78: 269–276.

World Health Organization: *Cholera Vaccines: A New Public Health Tool?* Geneva, Switzerland, World Health Organization, 2002.

Chapter 199 ■ *Campylobacter*

Gloria P. Heresi, Shahida Baqar, and James R. Murphy

Campylobacter jejuni and *Campylobacter coli* are global zoonoses and are one of the most frequent causes of human intestinal infections. Infection may be followed by severe immunoreactive diseases and possibly immunoproliferative disorders.

ETIOLOGY. The family Campylobacteriaceae includes >20 species. Those known or considered pathogenic for humans include *C. jejuni, C. fetus, C. coli, C. hyointestinalis, C. lari, C. upsaliensis, C. concisus, C. sputorum, C. rectus, C. mucosalis, C. jejuni* subspecies *doylei, C. curvus, C. gracilis,* and *C. cryaerophila*. Additional *Campylobacter* species have been isolated from clinical specimens, but their roles as pathogens have not been proved. *C. jejuni* and *C. coli* are the most important pathogens of the genus. More than 100 serotypes of *C. jejuni* have been identified.

TABLE 199-1. *Campylobacter* **Species Associated with Human Disease**

SPECIES	DISEASES IN HUMANS	COMMON SOURCES
C. jejuni	Gastroenteritis, bacteremia, Guillain-Barré syndrome	Poultry, raw milk, cats, dogs, cattle, swine, monkeys, water
C. coli	Gastroenteritis, bacteremia	Poultry, raw milk, cats, dogs, cattle, swine, monkeys, oysters, water
C. fetus	Bacteremia, meningitis, endocarditis, mycotic aneurysm, diarrhea	Sheep, cattle, birds
C. hyointestinalis	Diarrhea, bacteremia, proctitis	Swine, cattle, deer, hamster, raw milk, oysters
C. lari	Diarrhea, colitis, appendicitis, bacteremia, urinary tract infection	Seagulls, water, poultry, cattle, dog, cat, monkey, oysters, mussels
C. upsaliensis	Diarrhea, bacteremia, abscesses, enteritis, colitis, hemolyticuremic	Cats, other domestic pets
C. concisus	Diarrhea, gastritis, enteritis, periodontitis	Human oral cavity
C. sputorum	Diarrhea, bedsores, abscesses, periodontitis	Human oral cavity, cattle, swine
C. rectus	Periodontitis	
C. mucosalis	Enteritis	Swine
C. jejuni subspecies *doylei*	Diarrhea, colitis, appendicitis, bacteremia, urinary tract infection	Swine
C. curvus	Gingivitis, alveolar abscess	Poultry, raw milk, cats, dogs, cattle, swine, monkeys, water, human oral cavity
C. gracilis	Head and neck abscess, abdominal abscess, empyema	
C. cryaerophila	Diarrhea	Swine

Campylobacter organisms are thin (0.2–0.4 μm wide), curved, gram-negative, non-spore-forming rods (1.5–3.5 μm long) that usually have tapered ends. The morphology is varied and includes short comma- or S-shaped organisms, or long, multispiraled, filamentous, and seagull shaped. The organisms are usually motile with a flagellum at 1 or both poles. *Campylobacter* organisms form small (0.5–1 mm), slightly raised, smooth colonies on solid media. Coccal forms may be seen in older cultures. Visible growth from blood culture is often not apparent until 5–14 days after inoculation. Most *Campylobacter* organisms are microaerophilic and do not oxidize or ferment carbohydrates. Selective culture media developed to enhance isolation of *C. jejuni* may not support, and actually may inhibit, the growth of other *Campylobacter* species. *C. jejuni* has a circular chromosome of 1.64 million base pairs (30.6% G + C) that is predicted to encode 1,654 proteins and 54 stable RNA species. The genome is unusual in that there are virtually no insertion sequences or phage-associated sequences and very few repeat sequences.

Clinical presentations differ, in part, by species (Table 199-1). Intestinal disease is usually associated with *C. jejuni* and *C. coli*, and extraintestinal and systemic infections are most often associated with *C. fetus*. However, *C. jejuni* septicemia is increasingly recognized, which may occur without gastrointestinal signs or symptoms. Less frequently, enteritis is recognized in association with isolation of *C. lari, C. fetus,* and other *Campylobacter* species.

EPIDEMIOLOGY. Human campylobacterioses most commonly result from ingestion of contaminated drinking water or food such as poultry (chicken, turkey) and raw milk, or transmission from pets (cats, dogs, hamsters) and farm animals. Infections are more frequent in resource-limited settings, are prevalent year-round in tropical areas, and may exhibit seasonal peaks in temperate regions (late summer and early fall in most of the United States). In industrialized countries, *Campylobacter* infections peak in early childhood and in adults 15–44 yr of age. Each year in the United States there are an estimated 2.4 million cases of *Campylobacter* infections that result in over 100 deaths.

Although chickens are a classic source of *Campylobacter*, many animal sources of human food, including seafood, can harbor *Campylobacter*. Additionally, many animals kept as pets carry *Campylobacter*, and insects inhabiting contaminated environments may acquire the organism. Direct or indirect exposure to this plethora of environmental sources is the origin of most human infections. Airborne transmission of *Campylobacter* may occur in farm workers. There is increasing evidence that the use of antimicrobials in animal foods increases the prevalence of antimicrobial-resistant *Campylobacter* isolated from humans.

Human infection may result from exposure to as few as a few hundred colony-forming units. At times, *C. jejuni* and *C. coli* may spread person to person, perinatally, and at child-care centers where diapered toddlers are present. Individuals infected with *C. jejuni* usually shed the organism for weeks but may shed for months.

PATHOGENESIS. Most *C. jejuni* colonizations do not cause symptoms. The frequency of asymptomatic colonizations with other *Campylobacter* species is less well known. When disease follows colonization, the pathology generally reflects the site at which the bacteria localize, whether or not septicemia occurs, and whether immunoreactive complications are triggered. *Campylobacter* species differ in preferred sites of colonization and propensity to cause bacteremia.

The conceptual model for *C. jejuni* enteritis comprises requirements for mechanisms to transit the stomach, adhere to intestinal mucosal cells, and initiate intestinal lumen fluid accumulation. Most *Campylobacter* organisms are acid sensitive. Host conditions associated with reduced gastric acidity and foods capable of shielding organisms in transit through the stomach are postulated as mechanisms allowing *Campylobacter* to reach the intestine. Bacterial surface proteins and glycans then enable adhesion to intestinal mucosal cells. Lumen fluid accumulation is associated with toxins including cholera-like toxin, and cytotoxins and direct damage to mucosal cells resulting from bacterial invasion. Additionally, *C. jejuni* may have mechanisms that enable transit away from the mucosal surface. This armamentarium appears to be differentially deployed by various *C. jejuni* organisms.

As a result of analysis of the genome of *C. jejuni* NCTC 11168, an unexpected capacity to produce a variety of carbohydrates was discovered. Many have surface features that may, with further study, allow better understanding of *Campylobacter* pathogenesis and immunity.

C. fetus possesses a high molecular weight S layer protein that endows a high-level resistance to serum-mediated killing and phagocytosis and is thus thought to be responsible for its propensity to bacteremia. *C. jejuni* and *C. coli* are mostly sensitive to serum-mediated killing, but variants of greater resistance exist. It has been suggested that these serum-killing-resistant variants may be more capable of systemic dissemination.

There is a strong association between **Guillain-Barré syndrome** and preceding infection with some serotypes of *C. jejuni* (see Chapter 615). Molecular mimicry between nerve tissue and these agents may be the triggering factor in *Campylobacter*-associated Guillain-Barré syndrome and Miller-Fisher syndrome, a variant of Guillain-Barré syndrome characterized by ataxia, areflexia, and ophthalmoplegia. Reactive arthritis and erythema nodosum may also occur. Most *Campylobacter* infections are not followed by immunoreactive complications, indicating that factors in addition to molecular mimicry are required for these complications.

CLINICAL MANIFESTATIONS. There are several clinical presentations of *Campylobacter* infections that link to the species involved and host factors, such as age, immunocompetence, and underlying conditions. The most common presentation is acute enteritis.

Acute Gastroenteritis. Diarrhea is usually caused by *C. jejuni* (90–95%) or *C. coli* and rarely by *C. lari, C. hyointestinalis,* or *C. upsaliensis*. The incubation period is 1–7 days. Patients typically have loose, watery stools or less frequently bloody and mucus-containing stools that are characteristic of dysentery. Blood appears in the stools 2–4 days after the onset of symptoms. Fever, vomiting, malaise, and myalgia are common. Fever may be the only initial manifestation, but 60–90% of older children also complain of abdominal pain. The abdominal pain is periumbilical; cramping may precede other symptoms or persist after the stools return to normal. Abdominal pain may mimic appendicitis or intussusception.

Mild infection lasts only 1–2 days and resembles viral gastroenteritis. Most patients recover in less than 1 wk, although 20–30% of patients remain ill for 2 wk and 5–10% longer. Fatalities are rare. Persistent or recurrent *Campylobacter* gastroenteritis and emergence of erythromycin resistance during therapy have been reported in immunocompetent persons, patients with hypogammaglobulinemia (congenital or acquired), and patients with AIDS. Persistent infection may mimic chronic inflammatory bowel disease. Fecal shedding of the organisms in untreated patients usually lasts for 2–3 wk. The range may be from a few days to several months. Young children tend to shed the organisms for longer periods. Acute appendicitis, mesenteric lymphadenitis, and ileocolitis have been reported in patients who have had appendectomies during *C. jejuni* infection.

Bacteremia. With the exception of *C. fetus* infections, bacteremia with *Campylobacter* occurs most often among malnourished children, patients with chronic illnesses or immunodeficiency, and at the extremes of age. *C. fetus* causes bacteremia in adults with or without identifiable focal infection. Most have underlying conditions such as malignancy or diabetes mellitus. Bacteremia, when symptomatic, is associated with fever, headache, and malaise. Relapsing or intermittent fever is associated with night sweats, chills, and weight loss when the illness is prolonged. Lethargy and confusion can occur, but focal neurologic signs are unusual without cerebrovascular disease or meningitis. Abdominal pain is frequent; diarrhea, jaundice, and hepatomegaly are less common. A cough may occur, but pulmonary parenchymal involvement is unusual. Results of the physical examination are unimpressive, except for the ill appearance of the patient. Moderate leukocytosis may be found. Both transient asymptomatic bacteremia and rapidly fatal septicemia have been described. A prolonged bacteremia of 8–13 wk has been described, with spontaneous remissions and relapses, especially in immunocompromised hosts. In HIV-infected patients, bacteremia is more frequent, with increased morbidity and mortality. Occasional reports describe bacteremia with *C. upsaliensis*. The rates of *Campylobacter* bacteremia may be substantially underestimated.

Focal Extraintestinal Infections. Focal infections caused by *C. jejuni* occur mainly among neonates and immunocompromised patients, causing infections that include meningitis, pancreatitis, cholecystitis, ileocecitis with right lower quadrant pain mimicking appendicitis, urinary tract infection, arthritis, peritonitis, myocarditis, pericarditis, and endocarditis. *C. fetus* shows a predilection for vascular endothelium, causing endocarditis, pericarditis, thrombophlebitis, and mycotic aneurysms; focal infections include meningitis, septic arthritis, osteomyelitis, urinary tract infections, lung abscess, and cholangitis. *C. hyointestinalis* has been associated with proctitis, *C. upsaliensis* with breast abscesses, and *C. rectus* with periodontitis.

Perinatal Infections. Severe perinatal infections, although uncommon, are usually caused by *C. fetus* and, rarely, by *C. jejuni*. Maternal *C. fetus* and *C. jejuni* infections, which may be asymptomatic, may result in abortion, stillbirth, premature delivery, or neonatal infection with sepsis and meningitis. Newborn infection with *C. jejuni* is associated with diarrhea that may be bloody; *C. fetus* rarely causes diarrhea.

DIAGNOSIS. The clinical presentation of *Campylobacter* enteritis is similar to that of enteritis caused by other bacterial enteropathogens. The differential diagnosis includes *Shigella, Salmonella,* invasive *Escherichia coli, E. coli* O157 : H7, *Yersinia enterocolitica, Aeromonas, Vibrio parahaemolyticus,* and amebiasis. Fecal leukocytes are found in as many as 75% of cases and fecal blood in 50% of cases.

The diagnosis of *Campylobacter* is usually confirmed by identification of the organism in culture. Selective media, such as Skirrow or Butzler media, and microaerophilic conditions (5–10% oxygen) are commonly used. Some *C. jejuni* grow best at 42°C. Filtration methods are available and can preferentially enrich for *Campylobacter* by selecting for their smaller size. These methods allow for subsequent culture of the enriched sample on antibiotic free media. This enhances rates of isolation of those *Campylobacter* organisms inhibited by the antibiotics included in standard selective media.

For rapid diagnosis of *Campylobacter* enteritis, direct carbolfuchsin stain of fecal smear, indirect fluorescence antibody test, dark-field microscopy, or latex agglutination can be used. Antigen detection by enzyme immunoassay is nearly as sensitive and specific as culture. Species-specific DNA probes and specific gene amplification by polymerase chain reaction have been described. Serologic diagnoses may be made.

Extraintestinal infection caused by *Campylobacter* requires parenteral antibiotic therapy with an aminoglycoside, imipenem, or both. In patients with *C. fetus* bacteremia, prolonged therapy is advised. *C. fetus* isolates resistant to erythromycin have been reported.

COMPLICATIONS. Severe, prolonged *C. jejuni* infection can occur in patients with immunodeficiencies, including hypogammaglobulinemia and malnutrition. In patients with AIDS, an increased frequency and severity of *C. jejuni* infection have been reported; severity correlates inversely with CD4 count.

Reactive Arthritis. Reactive arthritis may accompany *Campylobacter* enteritis in adolescents and adults, especially patients who are positive for HLA-B27. It appears 5–40 days after the onset of diarrhea, involves mainly large joints, and resolves without sequelae. The arthritis typically is migratory, and without fever. Synovial fluid is always sterile. Reactive arthritis with conjunctivitis, urethritis, and rash as well as erythema nodosum are less common. IgA nephropathy and immune complex glomerulonephritis with *C. jejuni* antigens in the kidneys have been reported. Other complications are hemolytic anemia and rectal bleeding.

Guillain-Barré Syndrome. Guillain-Barré syndrome is an acute demyelinating disease of the peripheral nervous system characterized clinically by acute flaccid paralysis and is the most common cause of neuromuscular paralysis worldwide (see Chapter 615). Guillain-Barré syndrome carries a mortality rate of ~2%, and ~20% of Guillain-Barré syndrome patients will have major neurologic sequelae. *C. jejuni* is an important causal factor for Guillain-Barré syndrome, which has been reported 1–12 wk after culture-proven *C. jejuni* gastroenteritis in 1 of every 3,000 *C. jejuni* infections. Stool cultures obtained from patients with Guillain-Barré syndrome at the onset of neurologic symptoms have yielded *C. jejuni* in >25% of the cases. Serologic studies suggest that 20–45% of patients with Guillain-Barré syndrome have evidence of recent *C. jejuni* infection. The management of Guillain-Barré syndrome includes supportive care, plasma exchange, and intravenous immunoglobulin.

TREATMENT. Fluid replacement, correction of electrolyte imbalance, and supportive care are the mainstays of treatment of children with *Campylobacter* gastroenteritis (see Chapter 337). Antimotility agents may cause prolonged or fatal disease and should not be used.

The need for antibiotic therapy in patients with uncomplicated gastroenteritis is controversial. Data suggest a shortened duration of symptoms and intestinal shedding if erythromycin ethylsuccinate or azithromycin is initiated early in the disease in patients with the dysenteric form of *Campylobacter* enteritis.

Most *Campylobacter* organisms are susceptible to macrolides, aminoglycosides, chloramphenicol, imipenem, and clindamycin and are resistant to cephalosporins, tetracyclines, rifampin, penicillins, trimethoprim, and vancomycin. Antibiotic resistance among *C. jejuni* has become a serious worldwide problem. Quinolone resistance has developed and is related to the use of quinolones in veterinary medicine. Erythromycin-resistant *Campylobacter* isolates remain uncommon, and erythromycin or azithromycin is the drug of choice if therapy is required. Antibiotics are recommended for patients with the dysenteric form of the disease, high fever, or a severe course and for children who are immunosuppressed or have underlying diseases. Sepsis is treated with parenteral antibiotics such as an aminoglycoside, meropenem, or imipenem.

PROGNOSIS. Although *Campylobacter* gastroenteritis is usually self-limited, immunosuppressed children, including those with AIDS, may experience a protracted or severe course. Septicemia in newborns and immunocompromised hosts has a poor prognosis, with an estimated mortality rate of 30–40%.

PREVENTION. Most human campylobacterioses are sporadic and are acquired indirectly or directly from infected animals or contaminated foods. Interventions to minimize transmission include preparing food under conditions that kill *Campylobacter* and that prevent recontamination after cooking (not using the same surfaces, utensils, or containers for both uncooked and cooked food), ensuring that water sources are not contaminated and that water is kept in clean containers, and taking steps to prevent direct transmission from infected persons or infected domestic pets. Breast-feeding appears to decrease symptomatic *Campylobacter* disease but does not reduce colonization.

Several approaches at immunization are being studied, including the use of live-attenuated organisms, subunit vaccines, and killed whole cell vaccines.

Amieva MR: Important bacterial gastrointestinal pathogens in children: A pathogenesis perspective. *Pediatr Clin North Am* 2005;52(3):749–777.

Angulo FJ, Nargund VN, et al: Evidence of an association between use of anti-microbial agents in food animals and anti-microbial resistance among bacteria isolated from humans and the human health consequences of such resistance. *J Vet Med B Infect Dis Vet Public Health* 2004;51(8–9):374–379.

Friedman CR, Hoekstra RM, Samuel M, et al: Risk factors for sporadic *Campylobacter* infection in the United States: A case-control study in FoodNet sites. *Clin Infect Dis* 2004;38(Suppl 3):S285–S296.

Fullerton KE, Ingram LA, Jones TF, et al: Sporadic campylobacter infection in infants: a population-based surveillance case-control study. *Pediatr Infect Dis J* 2007;26:19–24.

Hannu T, Mattila L, Rautelin H, et al: Three cases of cardiac complications associated with *Campylobacter jejuni* infection and review of the literature. *Eur J Clin Microbiol Infect Dis* 2005;24:1–4.

Hughes R: *Campylobacter jejuni* in Guillain-Barré syndrome. *Lancet Neurol* 2004;3(11):644.

Karlyshev AV, Ketley JM, Wren BW: The *Campylobacter jejuni* glycome. *FEMS Microbiol Rev* 2005;29(2):377–390.

Lukinmaa S, Nakari UM, Eklund M, et al: Application of molecular genetic methods in diagnostics and epidemiology of food-borne bacterial pathogens. *APMIS* 2004;112:908–929.

Moore JE, Corcoran D, Dooley S, et al: *Campylobacter*. *Vet Res* 2005;36:351–382.

Nataro JP: Vaccines against diarrheal diseases. *Semin Pediatr Infect Dis* 2004;15:272–279.

Samuel MC, Vugia DJ, Shallow S, et al: Epidemiology of sporadic *Campylobacter* infection in the United States and declining trend in incidence, FoodNet 1996–1999. *Clin Infect Dis* 2004;36(Suppl 3):S165–S174.

Yuki N, Odaka M: Ganglioside mimicry as a cause of Guillain-Barré syndrome. *Curr Opin Neurol* 2005;18(5):557–561.

Chapter 200 ■ *Yersinia* James R. Murphy and Gloria P. Heresi

The genus *Yersinia* members of the Enterobacteriaceae family comprise >10 named species, 3 of which are established as human pathogens that cause different diseases that will be described separately. *Yersinia enterocolitica,* by far the most frequent *Yersinia* causing human disease, produces fever, abdominal pain, and diarrhea that may **mimic appendicitis.** *Yersinia pseudotuberculosis* is most often associated with **mesenteric lymphadenitis.** *Yersinia pestis,* the agent of **plague,** most commonly causes an acute febrile lymphadenitis (bubonic plague) and less frequently presents as septicemic, pneumonic, or meningeal plague. Untreated plague has a significant mortality rate. Other *Yersinia* organisms are infrequent causes of infections of humans and their identification is often an indicator of **immune deficit.** Yersinioses are zoonoses and can colonize pets, and they are found in most areas of the world. Infection of humans most often results from contact with infected animals or their tissues, ingestion of contaminated water, milk, or meat, or, for *Y. pestis,* the bite of infected fleas. Association with human disease is less clear for *Y. frederiksenii, Y. intermedia, Y. kristensenii* (the 3 preceding were recently separated from *Y. enterocolitica*), *Y. bercovieri, Y. mollaretii,* and *Y. rohedi.*

200.1 • *Yersinia Enterocolitica*

ETIOLOGY. *Y. enterocolitica* is a large, gram-negative coccobacillus that exhibits little or no bipolarity when stained with methylene blue and carbolfuchsin. These facultative anaerobes grow well on common culture media and are motile at 22°C but not at 37°C. *Y. enterocolitica* comprises pathogenic and nonpathogenic members.

EPIDEMIOLOGY. This agent is transmitted to humans through food, water, animal contact, and contaminated blood products. Transmission can occur from mother to newborn. *Y. enterocolitica* appears to have a global distribution but is seldom a cause of tropical diarrhea. There is approximately 1 culture-proved *Y. enterocolitica* infection per 100,000 population/yr in the United States, and infection may be more frequent in northern Europe. Cases are more frequent in colder months and among younger individuals and males. Most infections in children are among those <7 yr of age, with the majority among children <1 yr of age.

Natural reservoirs of *Y. enterocolitica* include rodents, rabbits, pigs, sheep, cattle, horses, dogs, and cats. Contact with feral animals or colonized pets is a common source of human infections. Culture and molecular techniques have found the organism in a variety of foods and in water. A source of sporadic *Y. enterocolitica* infections is pig offal (**chitterlings**). In 1 study, 71% of human isolates were indistinguishable from the strains isolated from pigs. *Y. enterocolitica* is an occupational threat to butchers. In part because of its capacity to multiply at refrigerator temperatures, *Y. enterocolitica* is at times transmitted by intravenous injection of contaminated fluids, including blood products.

Y. enterocolitica infections have increased while *Y. pseudotuberculosis* infections have declined, leading to the suggestion that the former organism is replacing the latter in an ecologic niche. In part, the mass production of animals, development of meat factories based on chains of cold storage, and international trade of meat products and animals are believed to be the reasons for the increasing prevalence of yersiniosis in humans.

PATHOGENESIS. The organisms most often enter by the alimentary tract and cause mucosal ulcerations in the ileum. Necrotic lesions of Peyer patches and mesenteric lymphadenitis occur. If septicemia develops, suppurative lesions can be found in infected organs. Infection may trigger reactive arthritis and erythema nodosum.

Adherence, invasion, and toxin production are established as essential mechanisms of pathogenesis. Bacterial components, some associated with the bacterial type III secretion apparatus, can actively suppress immunologic capacities, suggesting that immunosuppression may contribute to pathogenesis. Motility appears to be required for *Y. enterocolitica* pathogenesis. Serogroups that predominate in human illness are 0 : 3, 0 : 8, 0 : 9, and 0 : 5,27. Virulence traits are both chromosomal and plasmid encoded. Possibly because pathogenic strains require iron, individuals with **iron overload** as in hemochromatosis, thalassemia, and sickle cell disease are at high risk for infection.

CLINICAL MANIFESTATIONS. Disease presents most often as enterocolitis with diarrhea, fever, and abdominal pain. Acute enteritis is more common among younger children, and mesenteric lymphadenitis that may mimic appendicitis may be found in older children and adolescents. Stools may be watery or contain leukocytes and less frequently frank blood and mucus. *Y. enterocolitica* is excreted in stool for 1–4 wk. Family contacts of a case may frequently be found to be asymptomatically colonized with *Y. enterocolitica. Y. enterocolitica* septicemia is less common and most often found in very young children (<3 mo of age) and immunocompromised persons. Systemic infection is associated with splenic and hepatic abscesses, osteomyelitis, meningitis, endocarditis, and mycotic aneurysms. Exudative pharyngitis, pneumonia, empyema, lung abscess, and acute respiratory distress syndrome may infrequently occur. *Y. enterocolitica* infection in immunocompromised persons may present with physical and CT findings suggesting colon cancer with liver metastases.

Reactive complications include erythema nodosum, polyarthritis, arthritis, and the uveitis rash syndrome. These may be more frequent in selected populations (northern Europeans), in association with HLA-B27, and are more frequent in females.

DIAGNOSIS. Culture of *Y. enterocolitica* is the primary method of diagnosis. The organism is easily cultured from normally sterile sites but requires special procedures for isolation from stool where other bacteria may outgrow *Y. enterocolitica.* Cold enrichment where a sample is held in buffered saline can result in preferential growth of *Yersinia,* but the procedure takes weeks. Many laboratories do not routinely perform the procedures required to isolate *Y. enterocolitica* and cultures targeted to this organism must be specifically requested. A history indicating contact with environmental sources of *Yersinia* and detection of fecal leukocytes are helpful indicators of a need to culture for *Y. enterocolitica.* The culture isolation of a *Yersinia* from stool should be followed by tests to confirm that the isolate is a pathogen.

DIFFERENTIAL DIAGNOSIS. The clinical presentation is similar to other bacterial causes of enterocolitis. The most common differential diagnosis is among *Shigella, Salmonella, Campylobacter, Clostridium difficile,* enteroinvasive *Escherichia coli,* and inflammatory bowel disease (see Chapters 333 and 337).

TREATMENT. Enterocolitis occurring in an immunocompetent individual is a self-limiting disease and no benefit to antibiotic therapy is established. Patients with systemic infection and very young children in whom septicemia is common should be treated. Many *Yersinia* organisms are susceptible to trimethoprim-sulfamethoxazole (TMP-SMZ), aminoglycosides, 3rd generation cephalosporins, and quinolones. TMP-SMZ is the recommended empirical treatment in children because most strains are sensitive and it is well tolerated. In severe infections such as bacteremia, 3rd generation cephalosporins with or without aminoglycosides are effective. *Y. enterocolitica* produces lactamases a and b, which are responsible for resistance to penicillins and cephalosporins. Patients on deferoxamine should discontinue iron chelation therapy during treatment for *Y. enterocolitica,* especially if they have complicated gastrointestinal infection or extraintestinal infection.

COMPLICATIONS. Reactive arthritis, erythema nodosum, erythema multiforme, hemolytic anemia, thrombocytopenia, and systemic dissemination of bacteria have been reported in association with *Y. enterocolitica* infection. Septicemia is more frequent in younger children and reactive arthritis in older patients. Arthritis seems mediated by immune complexes, and viable organisms are not present in involved joints.

PREVENTION. Prevention centers on reducing contact with environmental sources of *Yersinia.* Breaking or sterilization of the chain from animal reservoirs to humans holds the greatest potential to reduce infections, and the techniques applied must be tailored to the reservoirs in each area. There is no vaccine.

200.2 • *Yersinia Pseudotuberculosis*

Y. pseudotuberculosis is so named because it causes tuberculosis-like lesions in guinea pigs. The agent has a worldwide distribution, and *Y. pseudotuberculosis* disease is less frequent than *Y. enterocolitica* disease. The most common form of disease is a mesenteric lymphadenitis that produces an appendicitis-like syndrome. *Y. pseudotuberculosis* is associated with a Kawasaki syndrome–like illness in about 8% of cases (see Chapter 165).

ETIOLOGY. *Y. pseudotuberculosis* shares many morphologic and culture characteristics with *Y. enterocolitica* and is differentiated biochemically from *Y. enterocolitica* on the basis of ornithine decarboxylase activity, fermentation of sucrose, sorbitol, cellobiose, and other tests, although some overlap between species occurs. Antisera to somatic O antigens and sensitivity to *Yersinia* phages may also be used to differentiate the 2 species. Subspecies-specific DNA sequences that allow direct probe- and primer-specific differentiation of *Y. pestis, Y. pseudotuberculosis,* and *Y. enterocolitica* have been described. *Y. pseudotuberculosis* is more closely related to *Y. pestis* than to *Y. enterocolitica.*

EPIDEMIOLOGY. *Y. pseudotuberculosis* is a zoonotic agent with reservoirs in wild rodents, rabbits, deer, farm animals, various birds, and domestic animals, including cats and canaries. Transmission to humans is by consumption of contaminated animals, contact with these, or contact with an environmental source, often water, contaminated by animals. Infections are more commonly reported from Europe, in males, and in the winter. Direct evidence of transmission of *Y. pseudotuberculosis* to humans by consumption of lettuce has recently been published. *Y. pseudotuberculosis* bacteremia is an increasingly recognized problem in HIV-infected individuals.

PATHOGENESIS. Ileal and colonic mucosal ulceration and mesenteric lymphadenitis are hallmarks of the infection. Necrotizing epithelioid granulomas may be seen in the mesenteric lymph nodes, but the appendix is frequently grossly and microscopically normal. The mesenteric nodes are often the only source of isolation of the organisms. *Y. pseudotuberculosis* antigens bind directly to HLA class II molecules and may function as superantigens, which may account for the clinical illness resembling Kawasaki syndrome.

CLINICAL MANIFESTATIONS. Pseudoappendicitis with abdominal pain, right lower quadrant tenderness, fever, and leukocytosis is the most common clinical presentation. Enterocolitis and extraintestinal spread are uncommon. Iron overload, diabetes mellitus, and chronic liver disease are often found concomitantly with extraintestinal *Y. pseudotuberculosis* infection. Renal involvement with tubulointerstitial nephritis, azotemia, pyuria, and glucosuria may occur.

DIAGNOSIS. Involved mesenteric lymph nodes removed at appendectomy may yield the organism by culture. Ultrasound examination of children with unexplained fever and abdominal pain may reveal a characteristic picture of enlarged mesenteric lymph nodes, thickening of the terminal ileum, and no image of the appendix. *Y. pseudotuberculosis* is rarely recovered from stool.

DIFFERENTIAL DIAGNOSIS. Appendicitis (most commonly), inflammatory bowel disease, and other intra-abdominal infections should be considered. Kawasaki syndrome, staphylococcal or streptococcal disease, leptospirosis, Stevens-Johnson syndrome, and collagen vascular diseases including acute-onset juvenile rheumatoid arthritis can mimic the syndrome with prolonged fever and rash.

TREATMENT. Uncomplicated mesenteric lymphadenitis due to *Y. pseudotuberculosis* is a self-limited disease, and antimicrobial therapy is not required. Culture-confirmed bacteremia should be treated with an aminoglycoside, ampicillin, chloramphenicol, or a 3rd generation cephalosporin.

COMPLICATIONS. An illness with presentation similar to Kawasaki disease may occur. There may be fever of 1–2 days' duration, strawberry tongue, pharyngeal erythema, a scarlatiniform rash, cracked red swollen lips, conjunctivitis, sterile pyuria, periungual desquamation, and thrombocytosis. Coronary aneurysm has been described. Erythema nodosum and reactive arthritis may follow infection.

PREVENTION. Avoiding exposure to potentially infected animals and good food handling practices can prevent infection. The sporadic nature of the disease makes application of targeted prevention measures difficult.

200.3 • Plague (*Yersinia Pestis*)

ETIOLOGY. *Y. pestis* is a gram-negative, nonmotile, non-spore-forming coccobacillus. The bacterium has several chromosomal and plasmid-associated factors that are essential to its virulence and survival in mammalian hosts and fleas. It shares bipolar staining appearance with *Y. pseudotuberculosis. Y. pestis* can be differentiated from *Y. pseudotuberculosis* by biochemical reactions, serology, phage sensitivity, and molecular techniques. The genome of *Y. pestis* is published. It is a potential agent of bioterrorism (see Chapter 711).

EPIDEMIOLOGY. Plague is endemic in at least 24 countries, and about 3,000 cases are reported worldwide per year. In the USA, plague is most common west of a line from east Texas to east Montana. Plague is infrequent in the United States (0–40 reported cases/yr), with 80% of cases in New Mexico, Arizona, and Colorado. Transmission to humans is most commonly from wild animal sources, although most cases of inhalation plague reported recently to the Centers for Disease Control and Prevention (CDC) were associated with exposure to infected free-roaming domestic cats. The epidemic form of disease killed about 1/4 of the population of Europe in the Middle Ages in 1 of a number of epidemics and pandemics. The epidemiology of epidemic plague involves extension of infection from the zoonotic reservoirs to urban rats, *Rattus ratus* and *Rattus norvegicus,* and from fleas of urban rats to man. Epidemics are no longer seen. Selective pressure exerted by Middle Age pandemics in Europe is hypothesized for enrichment of a deletion mutation in the gene encoding CCR5 (CCR5-delta32). The enhanced frequency of this mutation in European populations has contemporary importance in that it endows about 10% of European descendants with resistance to HIV-1.

The most common mode of transmission of *Y. pestis* to humans is by the bite of infected fleas. Historically most human infections are thought to have resulted from bites of fleas that acquired infection from feeding on infected urban rats. Less frequently, infection is caused by contact with infectious body fluids or tissues or inhaling infectious droplets. Sylvatic plague may exist as a stable enzootic infection or as an epizootic disease with high host mortality. Ground squirrels, rock squirrels, prairie dogs, rats, mice, bobcats, cats, rabbits, and chipmunks may be infected. Transmission among animals is usually by flea bite or by ingestion of contaminated tissue. *Xenopsylla cheopis* is the flea most commonly associated with transmission to humans, but >30 species of fleas have been demonstrated as vector competent, and *Pulex irritans,* the human flea, can transmit plague and may have been an important vector in some historical epidemics. Males and females are similarly affected by plague, and transmission is more common in colder regions and seasons, possibly because of temperature differences in *Y. pestis* infections in vector fleas.

The lack of nucleotide diversity in the *Y. pestis* genome supports the view that *Y. pestis* has emerged relatively recently in evolutionary history from the closely related gastrointestinal pathogen *Y. pseudotuberculosis,* probably from serotype 0 : 1b.

PATHOGENESIS. In the most common form of plague, infected fleas regurgitate organisms into a patient's skin during feeding. The bacteria translocate to regional lymph nodes, where *Y. pestis* replicates, resulting in bubonic plague. In the absence of rapidly implemented specific therapy, bacteremia may occur, resulting in purulent, necrotic, and hemorrhagic lesions in many organs. Both plasmid and chromosomal genes are required for full virulence. Pneumonic plague occurs when infected material is inhaled. The organism is highly transmissible from persons with pneumonic plague and from domestic cats with pneumonic infection. This high transmissibility and high morbidity and mortality have provided an impetus for attempts to use *Y. pestis* as a biological weapon.

CLINICAL MANIFESTATIONS. *Y. pestis* infection can present as several clinical syndromes or infection may be subclinical. The 3 principal clinical presentations of plague are bubonic, septicemic, and pneumonic. **Bubonic plague** is the most frequent form and accounts for 80–90% of cases in the USA. From 2–8 days after a flea bite, 1–10 cm lymph nodes, or **buboes,** which are remarkable for tenderness, develop in draining lymph nodes located in the inguinal (most common), axillary, or cervical region depending on the inoculation site. Fever, chills, weakness, prostration, headache, and the development of septicemia are common. The skin may show insect bites or scratch marks. Purpura and gangrene of the extremities may develop as a result of disseminated intravascular coagulation. These lesions may be the origin of the name Black Death. Untreated plague results in death in >50% of symptomatic individuals. Death may occur within 2–4 days after onset of symptoms.

Occasionally, *Y. pestis* may establish systemic infection and induce the systemic symptoms seen with bubonic plague without causing a bubo (**primary septicemic plague**). Because of the delay in diagnosis linked to the lack of the bubo, septicemic plague carries a higher case fatality rate than bubonic plague. In some regions, bubo-free septicemic plague may comprise 1/4 of cases.

Pneumonic plague is the least common but most dangerous and fatal form of the disease. Pneumonic plague may result from hematogenous dissemination, or rarely as primary pneumonic plague after inhalation of the organism from a human or animal with plague pneumonia or potentially from a biological attack. Signs of pneumonic plague include severe pneumonia with high fever, dyspnea, and hemoptysis.

Plague meningitis, tonsillitis, or gastroenteritis may occur. Meningitis tends toward a late complication following inadequate treatment. Tonsillitis and gastroenteritis may occur with or without apparent bubo formation or lymphadenopathy.

DIAGNOSIS. Patients with fever and history of exposure to small animals in endemic areas should be suspected of having plague. Thus, bubonic plague is suspected in a patient with a painful swollen lymph node, fever, and prostration who has been exposed to fleas or rodents in the western United States. A history of camping or the presence of flea bites increases the index of suspicion.

Y. pestis is readily transmitted to humans by some routine laboratory manipulations. Thus, it is imperative to clearly notify a laboratory if a sample suspected of containing *Y. pestis* is submitted. Laboratory diagnosis is based on bacteriologic culture or direct visualization using Gram, Giemsa, or Wayson stains of lymph node aspirates, blood, sputum, or exudates. *Y. pestis* grows slowly under routine culture conditions and best at temperatures that differ from those used for routine cultures in many clinical laboratories. Suspected isolates of *Y. pestis* should be forwarded to a reference laboratory for confirmation. Special containment shipping precautions are required. Cases of plague should be reported immediately to local and state health departments and the CDC.

DIFFERENTIAL DIAGNOSIS. The Gram stain of *Y. pestis* may be confused with *Enterobacter agglomerans.* Mild and subacute forms of bubonic plague may be confused with other disorders causing localized lymphadenitis and lymphadenopathy. Septicemic plague may be indistinguishable from other forms of overwhelming bacterial sepsis like tularemia and cat scratch disease.

Pulmonary manifestations of plaque are similar to those of anthrax, Q fever, and tularemia, all agents with bioterrorism/warfare potential. Thus, the presentation of a suspected case and especially any cluster of cases require immediate reporting. Additional information on this aspect of plague and procedures can be found at www.bt.cdc.gov.

TREATMENT. Patients suspected of having bubonic plague should be placed in isolation until 2 days after starting antibiotic treatment to prevent the potential spread of the disease if the patient develops pneumonia. The treatment of choice for bubonic plague historically has been streptomycin (30 mg/kg/day, maximum 2 g/day, divided every 12 hr IM for 10 days). However, intramuscular streptomycin is inappropriate for septicemia because absorption may be erratic when perfusion is poor. The poor central nervous system penetration of streptomycin makes this an inappropriate drug for meningitis. In addition, streptomycin may not be widely and immediately available. Septicemia and meningitis are usually treated with other aminoglycosides, doxycycline, or chloramphenicol. In the USA, gentamicin (children, 7.5 mg/kg

IM or IV divided tid; adults, 5 mg/kg IM or IV once daily. Alternative treatments include doxycycline (<45 kg, 4.4 mg/kg/day every 12 hr IV, maximum 200 mg/day; ≥45 kg, 100 mg every 12 hr IV or 200 mg IV once daily), ciprofloxacin (30 mg/kg/day divided every 12 hr, maximum 400 mg every 12 hr IV), and chloramphenicol (100 mg/kg/day divided every 6 hr IV). Gentamicin is preferred for pregnant women. Resistance to these agents and relapses are rare. *Y. pestis* is susceptible to fluoroquinolones in vitro, which is effective in treating experimental plague in animals. *Y. pestis* is susceptible to penicillin in vitro, but this is ineffective in treatment of human disease. Mild disease may be treated with oral chloramphenicol or tetracycline in children >9 yr of age. Clinical improvement is noted within 48 hr of initiating treatment.

Postexposure prophylaxis should be given to close contacts of patients with pneumonic plague. Antimicrobial prophylaxis is recommended within 7 days of exposure for persons with direct, close contact with a pneumonic plague patient, or those exposed to an accidental or terrorist-induced aerosol. Recommended regimens include a 7-day course of tetracycline, doxycycline, or TMP-SMZ. Contacts of cases of uncomplicated bubonic plague do not require prophylaxis. *Y. pestis* is a potential agent of bioterrorism that may require mass casualty prophylaxis (see Chapter 711).

PREVENTION. Avoidance of exposure to infected animals and fleas is the best method of prevention of infection. In the USA, special care is required when in environments inhabited by rodent reservoirs of *Y. pestis* and their ectoparasites. Patients with plague should be isolated if they have pulmonary symptoms, and infected materials should be handled with extreme care. A vaccine is available for individuals at high risk.

Yersinia Enterocolitica

Abdel-Haq NM, Asmar BI, Abuhammour WM, et al: *Yersinia enterocolitica* infection in children. *Pediatr Infect Dis J* 2000;19:954–958.

Bottone EJ: *Yersinia enterocolitica:* Overview and epidemiologic correlates. *Microbes Infect* 1999;1:323–333.

Centers for Disease Control and Prevention: *Yersinia enterocolitica* gastroenteritis among infants exposed to chitterlings—Chicago, Illinois, 2002. *MMWR* 2003;52:956–958.

Crosbie J, Varma J, Mansfield J: *Yersinia enterocolitica* infection in a patient with hemachromatosis masquerading as proximal colon cancer with liver metastases: Report of a case. *Dis Colon Rectum* 2005;48:390–392.

Jones TF, Buckingham SC, Bopp CA, et al: From pig to pacifier: Chitterling-associated yersiniosis outbreak among black infants. *Emerg Infect Dis* 2003;9:1007–1009.

Nelson KM, Young GM, Miller VL:. Identification of a locus involved in systemic dissemination of *Yersinia enterocolitica. Infect Immun* 2001;69(10): 6201–6208.

Ray SM, Ahuja SD, Blake PA, et al: Population-based surveillance for *Yersinia enterocolitica* infections in FoodNet sites, 1996–1999: Higher risk of disease in infants and minority populations. *Clin Infect Dis* 2004;15(38;Suppl 3):S181–S189.

Schulte R, Grassl GA, Preger S, et al: *Yersinia enterocolitica* invasin protein triggers IL-8 production in epithelial cells via activation of Rel p65-p65 homodimers. *FASEB J* 2000;14:1471–1484.

Yersinia Pseudotuberculosis

Nuorti JP, Niskanen T, Hallanvuo S, et al: A widespread outbreak of *Yersinia pseudotuberculosis* O:3 infection from iceberg lettuce. *J Infect Dis* 2000;89(5):766–774.

Press N, Fyfe M, Bowie W, et al: Clinical and microbiological follow-up of an outbreak of *Yersinia pseudotuberculosis* serotype Ib. *Scand J Infect Dis* 2001;33:523–526.

Sieper J: Disease mechanisms in reactive arthritis. *Curr Rheumatol Rep* 2004;6(2):110–116.

Wren BW: The yersiniae—a model genus to study the rapid evolution of bacterial pathogens. *Nat Rev Microbiol* 2003;1(1):55–64.

Plague (Yersinia Pestis)

Barde R: Plague in San Francisco: An essay review. *J Hist Med Allied Sci* 2004;59(3):463–470.

Brubaker RR: The recent emergence of plague: A process of felonious evolution. *Microb Ecol* 2004;47(3):293–299.

Centers for Disease Control and Prevention: Imported plague—New York City, 2002. *MMWR* 2003;52:725–727.

Daya M, Nakamura Y: Pulmonary disease from biological agents: Anthrax, plague, Q fever, and tularemia. *Crit Care Clin* 2005;21(4):747–763.

Dennis DT, Chow CC: Plague. *Pediatr Infect Dis J* 2004;23(1):69–71.

Duncan CJ. Scott S: What caused the Black Death? *Postgrad Med J* 2005; 81(955):315–320.

Hinnebusch BJ: The evolution of flea-borne transmission in *Yersinia pestis. Curr Issues Mol Biol* 2005;7(2):197–212.

Marketon MM, DePaolo RW, DeBord KL, et al: Plague bacteria target immune cells during infection. *Science* 2005;309(5741):1739–1741.

Chapter 201 ■ *Aeromonas* and *Plesiomonas*

Norma Pérez, Gloria P. Heresi, and James R. Murphy

Aeromonas and *Plesiomonas* organisms cause enteritis and less frequently skin and soft tissue infections and septicemia. These organisms are common in fresh and brackish water and in and on animals and plants that are in contact with water.

201.1 • *Aeromonas*

ETIOLOGY. *Aeromonas* organisms are members of the Aeromonadaceae family, and were formerly classified in the family Vibrionaceae. They are oxidase-positive, facultatively anaerobic, gram-negative bacilli that ferment glucose. DNA hybridization recognizes >15 genospecies, with 7 that are recognized as human pathogens. The species most often associated with human infection are *A. hydrophila*, *A. veronii* biotype sobria, and *A. caviae*.

Aeromonas infects many cold- and warm-blooded animals. Aeromonas strains are divided into 2 major groups: the nonmotile psychrophilic organisms that infect cold-blooded animals, and the motile mesophilic organisms that infect humans and other warm-blooded animals.

EPIDEMIOLOGY. *Aeromonas* organisms are ubiquitous and are found in numerous environmental fresh and brackish aquatic sources, including rivers and streams, well water, and sewage. They are most often cultivated from aquatic sources during warm weather months. The prevalence of human infection may or may not exhibit seasonality, apparently depending on local conditions. Some species can resist chlorination water treatment. *Aeromonas* organisms have been isolated from meats, milk, seafood, seaweed, and vegetables consumed by humans. Most human infections are associated with exposure to contaminated water. Asymptomatic colonization with *Aeromonas* occurs in humans and is more common in inhabitants of tropical regions. In the United States it is estimated that *Aeromonas* causes up 13% of reported gastroenteritis cases and up to 18% of cases of traveler's diarrhea. *Aeromonas* infections acquired at sites of natural disasters and presenting at far distant sites of evacuee medical care are recently recognized phenomena. *A. hydrophila* has been isolated from ticks. Prophylaxis against *A. hydrophila* should be used with medicinal leech therapy.

PATHOGENESIS. Clinical and epidemiologic data demonstrate that many *Aeromonas* organisms are enteric pathogens. However, adult volunteers fed 10^4–10^{10} colony-forming units of *Aeromonas* did not develop diarrhea or become colonized. *Aeromonas* possesses various potential virulence factors, including α- and β-hemolysin, adherence fimbriae and other adherence proteins, enterotoxin, cytotoxin, aerolysin, protease, chitinase, and a type III secretion system. The α-hemolysin has been shown to be cytotoxic to various cell lines. Enterotoxin causes fluid accumulation in rabbit ileal loops, increases intracellular cyclic adenosine monophosphate in rabbit intestinal epithelium, and cross-reacts immunologically with cholera toxin. *A. sombria* is the most enterotoxic among clinical isolates. Cytotoxic activity with cytopathic and intracellular effects is found with 89% of *Aeromonas* isolates. Cytopathic effects involve rounding of host cells, nuclear condensation, loss of adhesion, and death. Intracellular effects are cytoplasmic vacuolation with loss of nuclear definition followed by cell destruction. **Aerolysin** is a cytotoxic enterotoxin that has enterotoxic, cytotoxic, and hemolytic activities. It is found in 15% of isolates and is described as an extremely powerful virulence factor associated with *Aeromonas*-mediated intestinal illness. The protease may have a role in extraintestinal manifestations of *Aeromonas* infections. A few strains produce Shiga toxin.

Human serum generally promotes phagocytosis and intracellular killing of *Aeromonas*. Lack of this serum action has been associated with a poor prognosis.

CLINICAL MANIFESTATIONS. Colonization with *Aeromonas* may be asymptomatic or cause illness, including enteritis, focal invasive infection, and septicemia. Apparently immunologically normal individuals may present with each manifestation, but invasive disease is more common among immunocompromised persons. In humans, infection with *Aeromonas* is associated with 3 distinct syndromes: enteritis, skin and soft tissue infections, and septicemia.

Enteritis. The most common clinical manifestation of infection with *Aeromonas* is enteritis, which occurs primarily among children <3 yr of age. *Aeromonas* is the 3rd or 4th most common cause of childhood bacterial diarrhea and has been isolated from 2–10% of patients with diarrhea and 1–5% of asymptomatic control subjects. The diarrheal illness is often watery and self-limited, although a dysentery-like syndrome with blood and mucus in the stool has also been described. Fever, abdominal pain, and vomiting are common in children. Enteritis caused by *A. hydrophila* and *A. sobria* tends to be acute and self-limited, whereas 1/3 of the patients with *A. caviae* enteritis have chronic or intermittent diarrhea that may last 4–6 wk. *A. sobria* and *A. caviae* are most frequently associated with traveler's diarrhea. Complications of *Aeromonas* enteritis include intussusception, failure to thrive, hemolytic-uremic syndrome, bacteremia, and strangulated intestinal hernia. *A. caviae* infection may mimic inflammatory bowel disease.

Skin and Soft Tissue Infections. *A. hydrophila* is the predominant species associated with skin and soft tissue infections, with peak incidence during the summer months. Skin and soft tissue infection is the 2nd most common presentation of *Aeromonas*. Predisposing factors include local trauma and exposure to contaminated fresh water. *Aeromonas* soft tissue infections have been reported to result from alligator bites, sports injuries, tick bites, and medicinal leech therapy. The spectrum of skin and soft tissue infections is broad, ranging from a localized skin nodule to life-threatening necrotizing fasciitis, myonecrosis, and gas gangrene. *Aeromonas* cellulitis is indistinguishable from that due to other bacterial pathogens that cause cellulitis but should be suspected in wounds following contact with a water source, especially during the summer.

Septicemia. *Aeromonas* septicemia, the 3rd most frequent presentation of infection, is associated with a high mortality rate of 27–73%. *Aeromonas* septicemia usually occurs in patients with underlying conditions such as hepatobiliary disease or malignancy but may occur in apparently immunocompetent persons. *Aeromonas* may be the only organism isolated or may be part of a polymicrobial bacteremic syndrome. *A. hydrophila* septicemia tends to occur in patients with less serious underlying disease. *A. caviae* tends to associate with polymicrobial septicemia and is isolated more often from patients with underlying illnesses. *A. sobria* bacteremia has resulted in disseminated intravascular gas production and subsequent acute death in a previously healthy teenage girl.

Other Infections. *Aeromonas* is a rare cause of necrotizing gastroenteritis, endocarditis, meningitis, osteomyelitis, pyogenic arthritis, endophthalmitis, ear infections, urinary tract infection, peritonitis, myositis, cellulitis, necrotizing fasciitis, cholecystitis, lung abscess, liver abscess, septic embolism, and pneumonia. *Aeromonas* has been associated with aspiration pneumonia after near-drowning.

DIAGNOSIS. Diagnosis is established by culture isolation of *Aeromonas*. The organism is easily grown on standard media when the source material is normally sterile. However, isolation of the organism from samples containing numerous bacteria is more difficult, presumably because competing bacteria outgrow *Aeromonas*. Use of selective media such as a blood agar supplemented with ampicillin or MacConkey agar containing Tween 80 and ampicillin enhances isolation. Most (~90%) strains produce β-hemolysis on blood agar. Lactose-fermenting strains of *Aeromonas* may be overlooked in stool specimens if the clinical laboratory does not routinely perform oxidase tests on lactose fermenters isolated on MacConkey or does not routinely use selective media for the isolation of *Aeromonas*. Virulence and toxin gene factors continue to be discovered, posing a challenge in identification and classification of *Aeromonas* species. Biochemical criteria as well as multiple molecular tests including DNA hybridization, polymerase chain reaction (PCR), random amplified polymorphic DNA (RAPD)-PCR, and restriction fragment length polymorphism analysis are being used for gene identification. There is not a consensus as to which is the best method of detection.

TREATMENT. *Aeromonas* enteritis is usually self-limited and antimicrobial therapy may not be indicated. Data from uncontrolled trials suggest that antimicrobial therapy shortens the course of the illness. Antimicrobial therapy is reasonable to consider in patients with protracted diarrhea, dysentery-like illness, or underlying conditions such as hepatobiliary disease or an immunocompromised state. There is uniform resistance by *Aeromonas* to ampicillin. Septicemia should be treated with an aminoglycoside or a 3rd generation cephalosporin. Other options include aztreonam, imipenem, chloramphenicol, trimethoprim-sulfamethoxazole (TMP-SMZ), and quinolones. Many species have developed multidrug resistance, especially to quinolones.

PREVENTION. Reducing contact with contaminated environmental fresh and brackish water and also contaminated foods, especially by immunocompromised persons, should reduce the risk for *Aeromonas* infections. *Aeromonas* in vitro expresses LamB-like proteins that allow bacteria to adhere to host cell surfaces. These are potential target antigens for vaccine development.

201.2 • *PLESIOMONAS SHIGELLOIDES*

ETIOLOGY. *Plesiomonas shigelloides* is the only species in the genus, which includes at least 107 serotypes. *P. shigelloides* is a facultative, anaerobic, gram-negative rod, and is non–spore forming, catalase and oxidase positive, and motile, with 2–5 polar flagella. *P. shigelloides* is associated with acute enteritis and very rarely with extraintestinal infections. The genus has been placed traditionally within the family Vibrionaceae and considered closely related to *Vibrio cholerae* and *Aeromonas.* Both genetic analyses and antigenic profiling, however, indicate a closer relationship to the family Enterobacteriaceae, and *P. shigelloides* has recently reclassified from Vibrionaceae to Enterobacteriaceae.

EPIDEMIOLOGY. *P. shigelloides* is ubiquitous in fresh water and historically has been most often found in warmer and tropical waters, although there are increasing reports of isolation in colder regions. *P. shigelloides* colonizes numerous cold- and warm-blooded animals and may cause disease in cats. Infection of humans is thought to be the result of consumption of contaminated water or food and possibly through contact with colonized animals. The role that colonized animals play in the ecology of human infection is poorly understood. Asymptomatic colonization with *P. shigelloides* is common in some tropical and subtropical regions and more infrequent in colder climates. A majority of symptomatic patients in North America have either traveled abroad or report exposure to potentially contaminated water or food. Clinical disease in humans begins 24 hr to about 4 days after contact with the organism. Exposure to *P. shigelloides* serotype 17 may immunize populations to *Shigella sonnei* because they share the same cell wall lipopolysaccharide.

PATHOGENESIS. Epidemiologic evidence indicates that *P. shigelloides* is an enteropathogen. However, the diarrheagenic capacity of *P. shigelloides* was not confirmed when volunteers were fed the organism. The mechanism of enteritis is not known, but it appears that the species can cause both secretory and invasive disease. Most strains of *P. shigelloides* secrete a β-hemolysin, which is thought to be the major virulence factor associated with intestinal infection. In vitro data show that isolates of *P. shigelloides* interact with cells of enteric origin, Caco-2 cells. The pattern of bacterial internalization differs, suggesting different pathogenic phenotypes, which could explain the diverse clinical spectrum.

CLINICAL MANIFESTATIONS. In pediatric populations, *Plesiomonas* enteritis is usually secretory (up to 84% of cases) but occasionally may be dysenteric (~16%), with blood and mucus. The frequency of secretory vs dysenteric diarrhea clusters by outbreak report, suggesting that either human populations or bacterial populations associate with type of presentation. Symptoms include diarrhea (100%), fever (50%), headache, abdominal cramping (more common with increased age), nausea, vomiting (~70%), and transient arthralgias. Frequently the diarrhea is mild and watery without significant dehydration. Blood, mucus, or both may be passed with stool, and white blood cells may be visualized in stained preparations of stool. The illness usually resolves in about 2 wk, but reports describe diarrhea lasting ≥4 wk (up to 13% in 1 case series).

Extraintestinal infections are rare and usually occur in patients with underlying conditions, such as immunodeficiency, malignancy, sickle cell disease, and cirrhosis, or in those who have other identifiable risks (peritoneal dialysis, exposure to contaminated environment). Rarely, bacteremia accompanying enteritis has been documented in apparently otherwise normal children. Extraintestinal disease includes septicemia, meningitis, osteomyelitis, septic arthritis, reactive arthritis, cellulitis, endophthalmitis, cholecystitis, pseudoappendicitis, pseudomembranous colitis, proctitis, epididymo-orchitis and pyosalpinx. Early-onset neonatal sepsis and meningitis are rare but comprise most of the reported cases of *P. shigelloides* meningitis; it has a very high mortality rate (80%). Septicemia has a high mortality rate in adults.

DIAGNOSIS. A history of foreign travel, ingestion of raw seafood, or exposure to contaminated water or an animal with diarrhea suggests possible *P. shigelloides* infection. Mixed infection with *Salmonella, Aeromonas,* and rotavirus is a typical feature, especially among pediatric patients. Culture and isolation of the organism from stool or sterile body fluids is essential for diagnosis. *P. shigelloides* grows well on traditional enteric media, although selective techniques may be required to isolate the organism from mixed cultures and to differentiate *P. shigelloides* from *Shigella* species. It may be underrecognized by clinical laboratories that do not routinely perform an oxidase test. Molecular methodology is under development for diagnostic purposes but is not yet in routine use.

TREATMENT. Enteritis due to *P. shigelloides* is usually self-limited. In cases associated with dehydration, patients respond favorably to oral rehydration solution. Antimicrobial therapy is reserved for those patients with prolonged or bloody diarrhea. Data from uncontrolled trials suggest that antimicrobial therapy decreases the duration of symptoms. Most strains of *P. shigelloides* are susceptible to TMP-SMZ, cephalosporins, carbapenems, and quinolones, which are not approved for use in the USA in children <18 yr of age. *P. shigelloides* is commonly resistant to broad-spectrum penicillins, streptomycin, and azithromycin. Recently resistance has been found in some strains to TMP-SMZ, quinolones, and tetracyclines.

Antibiotics are essential for therapy of extraintestinal disease. Empirical therapy with a 3rd generation cephalosporin is reasonable because most isolates are susceptible in vitro. Definitive therapy should be guided by the susceptibility of the individual isolate.

Aeromonas

Lau SM, Peng MY, Chang FY: Outcomes of *Aeromonas* bacteremia in patients with different types of underlying disease. *J Microbiol Immunol Infect* 2000;33:241–247.

O'Ryan M, Prado V, Pickering LK: A millennium update on pediatric diarrheal illness in the developing world. *Semin Pediatr Infect Dis* 2005; 16(2):125–136.

Shiina Y, Ii K, Iwanaga M: An *Aeromonas veronii biovar sobria* infection with disseminated intravascular gas production. J Infect Chemother 2004;10: 37–41.

Vila J, Marco F, Soler L, et al: In vitro antimicrobial susceptibility of clinical isolates of *Aeromonas* caviae, *Aeromonas hydrophila* and *Aeromonas veronii* biotype *sobria. J Antimicrob Chemother* 2002;49:701–702.

Vila J, Ruiz J, Gallardo F, et al: *Aeromonas* species and traveler's diarrhea: Clinical features and antimicrobial resistance. *Emerg Infect Dis* 2003; 9(5):552–555.

Plesiomonas Shigelloides

Ampofo K, Graham P, Ratner A, et al: *Plesiomonas shigelloides* sepsis and splenic abscess in an adolescent with sickle-cell disease. *Pediatr Infect Dis J* 2001;20:1178–1179.

González-Rey C, Svenson SB, Bravo L, et al: Serotypes and anti-microbial susceptibility of *Plesiomonas shigelloides* isolates from humans, animals and aquatic environments in different countries. *Comp Immunol Microbiol Infect Dis* 2004;27:129–139.

Khan AM, Furuque SG, Hossain MS, et al: *Plesiomonas shigelloides*-associated diarrhoea in Bangladeshi children: A hospital-based surveillance study. *J Trop Pediatr* 2004;50(6):354–356.

Maluping RP, Lavilla-Pitogo CR, DePaola A, et al: Antimicrobial susceptibility of *Aeromonas* spp., *Vibrio* spp. and *Plesiomonas shigelloides* isolated in the Philippines and Thailand. *Int J Antimicrob Agents* 2005;25(4):348–350.

Woo PC, Lau SK, Yuen K-Y: Biliary tract disease as a risk factor for *Plesiomonas* shigelloides bacteraemia: A nine-year experience in a Hong Kong hospital and review of the literature. *New Microbiol* 2005;28(1):45–55.

Chapter 202 ■ *Pseudomonas, Burkholderia,* and *Stenotrophomonas*

Robert S. Baltimore

Pseudomonas and *Burkholderia* are widespread throughout nature and live abundantly in soil and water and on plants. Most human infections due to these species are opportunistic and occur among low birthweight infants and in older infants and children with impaired host defenses, such as those with traumatic wounds, cystic fibrosis, malignancies, extensive burns, malnutrition (especially in impoverished populations), and primary immunodeficiencies as well as those receiving immunosuppressive therapy. *Pseudomonas aeruginosa* is an important cause of nosocomial infections, including postsurgical infections.

Many species formerly considered under the genus *Pseudomonas* were reclassified on the basis of ribosomal RNA homology. Species formerly classified as *P. cepacia, P. mallei, and P. pseudomallei* are now *Burkholderia cepacia, B. mallei, and B. pseudomallei. P. maltophilia* is now *Stenotrophomonas maltophilia.*

Only a few of the many species of *Pseudomonas* and *Burkholderia* that have been identified are pathogenic for humans; of these, *P. aeruginosa* is by far the most common. Other species occasionally recognized as human pathogens include *B. cepacia, S. maltophilia, P. fluorescens, B. putrefaciens, B. pseudomallei, and B. mallei.*

202.1 • *Pseudomonas Aeruginosa*

ETIOLOGY. *P. aeruginosa* is a gram-negative rod and is a strict aerobe. It can multiply in a great variety of environments that contain minimal amounts of organic compounds because it can use any source of carbon. Strains from clinical specimens may produce β-hemolysis on blood agar, and many produce pigments including pyocyanin, pyoverdin, and others that diffuse into and color the medium surrounding the colonies. Strains of *Pseudomonas* can be differentiated for epidemiologic purposes by serologic, phage, and pyocin typing and by genome restriction fragment length polymorphisms using pulsed-field gel electrophoresis.

EPIDEMIOLOGY. The rate of *P. aeruginosa* bacteremia in children is 3.8/1,000 patients over 10 yr with a 20% mortality rate; rates vary according to the prevalent underlying diseases. *P. aeruginosa* and other pseudomonads frequently enter the hospital environment on the clothes, skin, or shoes of patients or hospital personnel, with plants or vegetables brought into the hospital, and in the gastrointestinal tracts of patients. Colonization of any moist or liquid substance may ensue; the organisms may be found growing in any water reservoir, including distilled water, and in hospital kitchens and laundries, some antiseptic solutions, and equipment used for respiratory therapy. Colonization of patients' skin, throat, stool, and nasal mucosa is low at admission to the hospital but increases to as high as 50–70% with prolonged hospitalization and with the use of broad-spectrum antibiotics, chemotherapy, mechanical ventilation, and urinary catheters. Patients' intestinal microbial flora may be altered by the use of broad-spectrum antibiotics, which reduces resistance to colonization and permits *P. aeruginosa* in the environment to populate the gastrointestinal tract. Intestinal mucosal breakdown associated with medications, especially cytotoxic agents, and nosocomial enteritis may provide a pathway by which *P. aeruginosa* spreads to the lymphatics or bloodstream.

PATHOLOGY. The pathologic manifestations of *Pseudomonas* infections depend on the site and type of infection. Due to its elaboration of toxins and invasive factors, the organism can often be seen invading blood vessels and causing vascular necrosis. In some infections there is spread through tissues with necrosis and microabscess formation. In patients with cystic fibrosis, focal and diffuse bronchitis/bronchiolitis leading to bronchiolitis obliterans has been reported.

PATHOGENESIS. *P. aeruginosa* is a classic opportunist. It rarely causes disease in people who do not have a predisposing risk factor. The requirement of oxygen for growth may account for its lack of invasiveness after it has colonized or even infected the skin. Invasiveness of *P. aeruginosa* is mediated by a host of virulence factors. It produces endotoxin that is involved in invasiveness in acute infection and induces an inflammatory response. It also produces numerous exotoxins, including **exotoxin A,** which causes local necrosis and facilitates systemic bacterial invasion, and **exoenzyme S,** which acts as both an adhesin and a cellular toxin and also appears to impair host defenses. Thus, *Pseudomonas* produces disease in 3 stages. Bacterial colonization and attachment are facilitated by pili or fimbriae and by opportunistic adhesion to epithelium damaged by prior injury or infection. A mucopolysaccharide may inhibit phagocytosis, whereas extracellular proteins, proteases, elastases, and cytotoxin (formerly leukocidin) digest cell membranes, and antibodies produce capillary vascular permeability and inhibit leukocyte function. Dissemination and bloodstream invasion follow extension of local tissue damage and are facilitated by the antiphagocytic properties of endotoxin, the mucoid exopolysaccharide, and protease cleavage of immunoglobulin G. The **mucoid exopolysaccharide** encases the organism and may envelop colonies within a biofilm that protects the organism from host defenses such as antibody and complement as well as from antibiotics. The host responds to infection by producing antibodies to *Pseudomonas* exotoxin (**exotoxin A**) and endotoxin. Compromised host defense mechanisms owing to trauma, neutropenia, mucositis, immunosuppression, or impaired mucociliary transport explain the predominant role of this organism in producing opportunistic infections.

CLINICAL MANIFESTATIONS. Most clinical patterns (Table 202-1) are related to opportunistic infections (see Chapter 177) or are associated with shunts and indwelling catheters (see Chapter 178). *P. aeruginosa* may be introduced into a minor wound of a healthy person as a secondary invader, and cellulitis and a localized abscess that exudes green or blue pus may follow. The characteristic skin lesions of *Pseudomonas,* **ecthyma gangrenosum,** whether caused by direct inoculation or metastatic secondary to septicemia, begin as pink macules and progress to hemorrhagic nodules and eventually to ulcers with ecchymotic and gangrenous centers with eschar formation, surrounded by an intense red areola.

Outbreaks of dermatitis and urinary tract infections caused by *P. aeruginosa* have been reported in healthy persons after use of community swimming pools, wading pools, recreational whirlpools, or family-owned hot tubs. Skin lesions of folliculitis develop several hours to 2 days after contact with these water sources. Skin lesions may be erythematous, macular, papular, or pustular. Illness may vary from a few scattered lesions to extensive truncal involvement. In some children, malaise, fever, vomiting, sore throat, conjunctivitis, rhinitis, and swollen breasts may be associated with dermal lesions.

Pseudomonads other than *P. aeruginosa* rarely cause disease in healthy children, but pneumonia and abscesses due to *B. cepacia,* otitis media due to *P. putrefaciens* or *P. stutzeri,* abscesses due to *P. fluorescens,* and cellulitis and septicemia and osteomyelitis due to *S. maltophilia* have been reported. Septicemia and

TABLE 202-1. *Pseudomonas aeruginosa* Infections

INFECTION	COMMON CLINICAL CHARACTERISTICS
Endocarditis	Native right-sided (tricuspid) valve disease with intravenous drug abuse
Pneumonia	Compromised local (lung) or systemic host defense mechanisms. Nosocomial (respiratory), bacteremic (malignancy), or abnormal mucociliary clearance (cystic fibrosis) may be pathogenetic. Cystic fibrosis is associated with mucoid *Pseudomonas aeruginosa* organisms producing capsular slime.
Central nervous system infection	Meningitis, brain abscess; contiguous spread (mastoiditis, dermal sinus tracts, sinusitis); bacteremia or direct inoculation (trauma, surgery).
External otitis	Swimmer's ear; humid warm climates, swimming pool contamination.
Malignant otitis externa	Invasive, indolent, febrile toxic, destructive necrotizing lesion in young infants, immunosuppressed neutropenic patients, or diabetic patients; associated with 7th nerve palsy and mastoiditis.
Chronic mastoiditis	Ear drainage, swelling, erythema; perforated tympanic membrane.
Keratitis	Corneal ulceration; contact lens keratitis.
Endophthalmitis	Penetrating trauma, surgery, penetrating corneal ulceration; fulminant progression.
Osteomyelitis/septic arthritis	Puncture wounds of foot and osteochondritis; intravenous drug abuse; fibrocartilaginous joints, sternum, vertebrae, pelvis; open fracture osteomyelitis; indolent; pyelonephritis and vertebral osteomyelitis.
Urinary tract infection	Iatrogenic, nosocomial; recurrent urinary tract infections in children, instrumented patients, and those with obstruction or stones.
Intestinal tract infection	Immunocompromise, neutropenia, typhlitis, rectal abscess, ulceration, rarely diarrhea; peritonitis in peritoneal dialysis.
Ecthyma gangrenosum	Metastatic dissemination; hemorrhage, necrosis, erythema, eschar, discrete lesions with bacterial invasion of blood vessels; also subcutaneous nodules, cellulitis, pustules, deep abscesses.
Primary and secondary skin infections	Local infection; burns, trauma, decubitus ulcers, toe web infection, green nail (paronychia); whirlpool dermatitis; diffuse, pruritic, folliculitis, vesiculopustular or maculopapular, erythematous lesions.

endocarditis due to *S. maltophilia* have also been associated with intravenous abuse of drugs.

Burns and Wound Infection. The surfaces of burns or wounds are frequently populated by *Pseudomonas* and other gram-negative organisms; this initial colonization with a low number of adherent organisms is a necessary prerequisite to invasive disease. *P. aeruginosa* colonization of a burn site may develop into burn wound sepsis, which has a high mortality rate when the density of organisms reaches a critical concentration. Administration of antibiotics may diminish the susceptible microbiologic flora, permitting strains of relatively resistant *Pseudomonas* to flourish. Multiplication of organisms in devitalized tissues or associated with prolonged use of intravenous or urinary catheters increases the risk for septicemia with *P. aeruginosa,* a major problem in burned patients (see Chapter 74).

Cystic Fibrosis. *P. aeruginosa* is common in children with cystic fibrosis, with a prevalence that increases with increasing age and severity of pulmonary disease (see Chapter 400). Initial infection may be caused by nonmucoid strains of *P. aeruginosa,* but after a variable period of time, mucoid strains of *P. aeruginosa,* which are rarely encountered in other conditions, predominate. The infection begins insidiously or even asymptomatically, and the progression has a highly variable pace. In children with cystic fibrosis, antibody does not eradicate the organism and antibiotics are only partially effective; thus, after infection becomes chronic it cannot be completely eradicated. Repeated courses of antibiotics select for *P. aeruginosa* strains that are highly antibiotic resistant.

Immunocompromised Persons. Children with leukemia or other debilitating malignancies, particularly those who are receiving immunosuppressive therapy and who are neutropenic, are extremely susceptible to septicemia due to invasion of the bloodstream by *Pseudomonas* with which the patient is already colonized, usually in the respiratory or gastrointestinal tract. Signs of sepsis are often accompanied by a generalized vasculitis, and hemorrhagic necrotic lesions may be found in all organs, including the skin, where they appear as purple nodules or ecchymotic areas that become gangrenous (**ecthyma gangrenosum**). Hemorrhagic or gangrenous perirectal cellulitis or abscesses may occur, associated with ileus and profound hypotension.

Nosocomial Pneumonia. Although not a frequent cause of community-acquired pneumonia in children, *P. aeruginosa* is an increasingly important cause of community-acquired pneumonia in adults and of nosocomial pneumonia, especially ventilator-associated pneumonia in patients of all ages. *P. aeruginosa* has historically been found to contaminate ventilators, tubing, and humidifiers, but this is uncommon today with appropriate disinfection and routine changing of equipment. Nevertheless, colonization of the upper respiratory tract and the gastrointestinal tract may be followed by aspiration of *P. aeruginosa*–contaminated secretions, resulting in severe pneumonia. It appears that prior use of broad-spectrum antibiotics is a risk factor for colonization with antibiotic-resistant strains of *P. aeruginosa.* One of the most challenging situations is distinguishing between colonization and pneumonia in intubated patients. This can often only be resolved by using invasive culture techniques such as bronchoscopy with bronchial brushing or quantitative bronchoalveolar lavage.

Infants. *P. aeruginosa* is an occasional cause of nosocomial bacteremia in newborns and accounts for 2–5% of positive blood culture results in neonatal intensive care units. A frequent focus preceding bacteremia is **conjunctivitis.** Older infants may occasionally present with community-acquired sepsis due to *P. aeruginosa,* but this is uncommon. In the few reports describing this sepsis, preceding conditions included ecthyma-like skin lesions, virus-associated transient neutropenia, and prolonged contact with contaminated bath water or a hot tub.

DIAGNOSIS. *P. aeruginosa* infection is rarely clinically distinctive. Diagnosis depends on recovery of the organism from the blood, cerebrospinal fluid, urine, or needle aspirate of the lung, or from purulent material obtained by aspiration of subcutaneous abscesses or areas of cellulitis. An exception is **ecthyma gangrenosum,** which is characteristic of *Pseudomonas* infection of the skin. Rarely, similar skin lesions may follow septicemia due to *Aeromonas hydrophila,* other gram-negative bacilli, and *Aspergillus.* When *P. aeruginosa* is recovered from nonsterile sites such as skin, mucous membranes, voided urine, and the upper respiratory tract, quantitative cultures are useful to differentiate colonization from invasive infection. In general, ≥100,000 colony forming units/mL of fluid or gram of tissue is evidence suggestive of invasive infection.

TREATMENT. Systemic infections with *Pseudomonas* should be treated promptly with an antibiotic to which the organism is susceptible in vitro. Response to treatment may be limited, and prolonged treatment may be necessary for systemic infection in immunocompromised hosts.

Septicemia and other aggressive infections should be treated with either 1 or 2 bactericidal agents. While the number of agents required is controversial, little evidence shows that more than 1 agent is needed for individuals with normal immunity or when treating urinary tract infections, but dual therapy is often used for a synergistic effect in immunocompromised patients or when the susceptibility of the organism is in doubt. Whether the use of 2 agents delays the development of resistance is also controversial, with evidence both for and against. Appropriate antibiotics for single-agent therapy include ceftazidime, cefepime, ticarcillin-clavulanate, and piperacillin-tazobactam. Gentamicin or another aminoglycosides may be used concomitantly for synergistic effect.

Ceftazidime has proved to be extremely effective in patients with cystic fibrosis (150–250 mg/kg/day divided every 6–8 hr IV). Azlocillin, mezlocillin, or piperacillin-tazobactam (300–450 mg/

kg/day divided every 6–8 hr IV) also have proved to be effective therapy for susceptible strains of *P. aeruginosa* when combined with an aminoglycoside. Additional effective antibiotics include imipenem-cilastatin, meropenem, and aztreonam. Ciprofloxacin is effective but not approved in the USA for persons <18 yr of age except for treatment of urinary tract infections or when there are not other agents to which the organism is susceptible. It is important to base continued treatment on the results of susceptibility tests because antibiotic resistance of *P. aeruginosa* to 1 or more antibiotics is increasing.

P. aeruginosa displays intrinsic and acquired resistance to antibiotics. It may develop many modes of resistance through genetic mutation and the development of new enzymes and other properties, allowing it to elude the activity of multiple antibiotics. Critical care units throughout the USA have documented a rising rate of resistance of *P. aeruginosa* to all of the major classes of antibiotics.

Meningitis can occur from spread from a contiguous focus, as a secondary focus when there is bacteremia, or after invasive procedures. *Pseudomonas* meningitis is best treated with ceftazidime in combination with an aminoglycoside such as gentamicin, both given intravenously. Concomitant intraventricular or intrathecal treatment with gentamicin may be required when intravenous therapy fails but is not recommended for routine use.

SUPPORTIVE CARE. *Pseudomonas* infections vary in severity from superficial to intense septic presentations. With severe infections there is often multisystem involvement and systemic inflammatory response. Supportive care is similar to severe sepsis caused by other gram-negative bacilli and requires support of blood pressure, oxygenation, and appropriate fluid management.

PROGNOSIS. The prognosis is dependent primarily on the nature of the underlying factors that predisposed the patient to *Pseudomonas* infection. In severely immunocompromised patients, the prognosis for patients with *P. aeruginosa* sepsis is poor unless susceptibility factors such as neutropenia or hypogammaglobulinemia can be reversed. Resistance of the organism to 1st line antibiotics also decreases the chance of survival. The outcome may be improved by combined antimicrobial therapy, and is improved when there is a urinary tract portal of entry, absence of neutropenia or recovery from neutropenia, and drainage of local sites of infection. *Pseudomonas* is recovered from the lungs of most children who die of cystic fibrosis and may be responsible for the slow deterioration of these patients. The prognosis for normal development is poor in the few infants who survive *Pseudomonas* meningitis.

PREVENTION. Prevention of infections due to *P. aeruginosa* is not a concern for healthy individuals outside of the hospital but is dependent on limiting contamination of the health care environment and preventing transmission to patients. Effective hospital infection control programs are necessary to identify and eradicate sources of the organism as quickly as possible. *Pseudomonas* may grow in distilled water, some disinfectants, parenteral alimentation solutions, and medications. In newborn nurseries, infection can be transmitted to the infants by the hands of personnel, from washbasin surfaces, from catheters, and from solutions used to rinse suction catheters.

Strict attention to handwashing, particularly with an iodophor-containing solution or alcohol-based hand rubs, before and between contacts with neonates may prevent or interdict epidemic disease. Meticulous care and sterile procedures in suctioning of endotracheal tubes, insertion and care of indwelling catheters, preparation of intravenous solutions and especially for total parenteral nutrition, and regular replacement of intravenous administration tubing greatly reduce the hazard of extrinsic contamination by *Pseudomonas* and other gram-negative organisms.

Prevention of follicular dermatitis caused by *Pseudomonas* contamination of whirlpools or hot tubs is possible by maintaining pool water at a pH of 7.2–7.8 and free chlorine concentration at 70.5 mg/L.

Infections in burned patients may be minimized by protective isolation, debridement of devitalized tissue, and topical application of sulfadiazine or 10% mafenide acetate cream. Administration of intravenous immunoglobulin may be used. Approaches under investigation to prevent infection include development of *Pseudomonas* vaccine and development of hyperimmune globulin. No vaccine is currently licensed.

Pseudomonas infection of dermal sinuses communicating with the cerebrospinal space can be prevented by early identification and surgical repair. *Pseudomonas* infection of the urinary tract may be minimized or prevented by early identification and corrective surgery of obstructive lesions.

202.2 • *BURKHOLDERIA*

BURKHOLDERIA CEPACIA. *B. cepacia* is a filamentous gram-negative rod. It is ubiquitous in the environment but may be difficult to isolate from respiratory specimens in the laboratory, requiring an enriched, selective media oxidation fermentation base supplemented with polymyxin B-bacitracin-lactose agar (OFPBL) and as long as 3 days of incubation.

B. cepacia is a classic opportunist that rarely infects normal tissue but can be a pathogen for individuals with pre-existing damage to respiratory epithelium, especially persons with cystic fibrosis. Resistance to many antibiotics appears to be a factor in its emergence as a nosocomial pathogen. In critical care units it may colonize the tubing used to ventilate patients with respiratory failure. In some this may lead to invasive pneumonia and septic shock. Although it is found throughout the environment, human-to-human spread among patients with cystic fibrosis occurs either directly by inhalation of aerosols or indirectly from contaminated equipment or surfaces. This has led to cohorting of patients with cystic fibrosis in some clinics, hospital wards, and social gatherings on the basis of *B. cepacia* colonization. *B. cepacia* infections in persons with cystic fibrosis may only represent colonization in many patients but in many it is associated with an acute respiratory syndrome of fever, leukocytosis, and progressive respiratory failure, as well as progressive lung deterioration and more rapid decline in pulmonary function and lower survival rate. This is in contradistinction to *P. aeruginosa* infections in persons with cystic fibrosis, which is insidious and less communicable.

Treatment in hospitals should include standard precautions and avoidance of placing colonized and uncolonized patients in the same room. Persons who have cystic fibrosis and who visit or provide care and are not infected or colonized with *B. cepacia* may elect to wear a mask when within 3 ft of a colonized patient. The use of antibiotics is guided by susceptibility studies of a patient's isolates because the susceptibility pattern of this species is quite variable and multiple resistant strains are not uncommon. Ureidopenicillins (mezlocillin, piperacillin), aminoglycosides, ceftazidime, ciprofloxacin, and trimethoprim-sulfamethoxazole frequently show good activity. Resistance to aminoglycosides is the rule, and presence of inducible β-lactamase in many strains is probably the cause of clinical failures reported with ureidopenicillins and ceftazidime. Treatment with 2 or 3 agents may be necessary to control the infection and avoid the development of resistance. No vaccine is currently available.

***BURKHOLDERIA MALLEI* (GLANDERS).** Glanders is a severe infectious disease of horses and other domestic and farm animals due to *B. mallei,* a nonmotile gram-negative bacillus that is occasionally transmitted to humans. It is acquired by inoculation into the skin, usually at the site of a previous abrasion, or by inhalation of aerosols. Laboratory workers may acquire it from clinical specimens. The disease is relatively common in Asia, Africa, and the Middle East. The clinical manifestations include septicemia, acute or chronic pneumonitis, and hemorrhagic necrotic lesions of the skin, nasal mucous membranes, and lymph nodes. The diagnosis is usually made by recovery of the organism in cultures of affected tissue. Glanders is treated with sulfadiazine, tetracyclines, or chloramphenicol and streptomycin over a period of many months. The disease has been eliminated from the USA, but interest in this organism has increased due to the possibility of its use as a bioterrorism agent (see Chapter 711). While standard precautions are appropriate when caring for hospitalized infected patients, biosafety level 3 precautions are required for laboratory staff working with *B. mallei.* No vaccine is available.

***BURKHOLDERIA PSEUDOMALLEI* (MELIOIDOSIS).** This important disease of Southeast Asia and northern Australia occurs in the USA mainly in persons returning from endemic areas. The causative agent is *B. pseudomallei,* an inhabitant of soil and water in the tropics. It is ubiquitous in endemic areas; infection follows inhalation of dust or direct contamination of abrasions or wounds. Human-to-human transmission has only rarely been reported. Serologic surveys demonstrate that asymptomatic infection occurs in endemic areas. The disease may remain latent and appear when host resistance is reduced, sometimes years after the initial exposure. Diabetes mellitus is a risk factor for severe melioidosis.

Melioidosis may present as a single **primary skin lesion** (vesicle, bulla, or urticaria). Pulmonary infection may be subacute and mimic tuberculosis or it may present as an acute necrotizing pneumonia. Occasionally, septicemia occurs and numerous abscesses are noted in various organs of the body. Myocarditis, pericarditis, endocarditis, intestinal abscess, cholecystitis, acute gastroenteritis, urinary tract infections, septic arthritis, paraspinal abscess, osteomyelitis, mycotic aneurysm, and generalized lymphadenopathy all have been observed. Melioidosis may also present as an encephalitic illness with fever and seizures. It has recently been recognized as an agent of severe wound infections following contact with contaminated water following a tsunami.

Diagnosis is based on visualization of characteristic small gram-negative rods in exudates or growth on laboratory media such as eosin-methylene blue or MacConkey agar. Serologic tests are available, and diagnosis can be established by a 4-fold or greater increase in antibody titer in an individual with an appropriate syndrome. It has been recognized as a possible agent of bioterrorism (see Chapter 711).

B. pseudomallei is susceptible to many antimicrobial agents, including 3rd generation cephalosporins (especially ceftazidime), aminoglycosides, tetracycline, cotrimoxazole, sulfisoxazole, chloramphenicol, and amoxicillin-clavulanate. **Therapy** should be guided by antimicrobial susceptibility tests; 2 or 3 agents such as ceftazidime or chloramphenicol plus either trimethoprim-sulfamethoxazole, sulfisoxazole, or an aminoglycoside are usually chosen for severe or septicemic disease. For severe disease, prolonged treatment of 2–6 mo is recommended to prevent relapses. Appropriate antibiotic therapy generally results in recovery.

202.3 • *STENOTROPHOMONAS*

S. maltophilia (formerly *Xanthomonas maltophilia* or *Pseudomonas maltophilia*) is a short to medium-sized straight gram-negative bacillus. It is ubiquitous in nature and can be found in the hospital environment, especially in tap water, standing water, and nebulizers. Strains isolated in the laboratory may be contaminants, may be a commensal from the colonized surface of a patient, or may represent an invasive pathogen. The species is an opportunist. Serious infections usually occur among those requiring intensive care, including neonatal intensive care, typically patients with ventilator-associated pneumonia or catheter-associated infections. Prolonged antibiotic exposure appears to be a frequent factor in nosocomial *S. maltophilia* infections, probably due to its endogenous antibiotic resistance pattern. Common types of infection include pneumonia following airway colonization and aspiration, urinary tract infection, endocarditis, and osteomyelitis. Strains vary as to antibiotic susceptibility. **Treatment** should be based on the results of susceptibility testing. Trimethoprim-sulfamethoxazole, minocycline, doxycycline, ticarcillin-clavulanate, and chloramphenicol frequently show good activity. Trimethoprim-sulfamethoxazole is usually the drug of choice for *Stenotrophomonas* infections. Aminoglycosides, cephalosporins, and carbapenems are usually inactive. Among the quinolone antibiotics, ciprofloxacin often has good activity and has been used clinically, and the newer agents sparfloxacin and levofloxacin usually show good activity in vitro.

Pseudomonas Aeruginosa

Butbul-Aviel Y, Miron D, Halevy R, et al: Acute mastoiditis in children: *Pseudomonas aeruginosa* as a leading pathogen. *Int J Pediatr Otorhinolaryngol* 2003;67:277–281.

Chusid MJ, Hillmann SM: Community-acquired *Pseudomonas* sepsis in previously healthy infants. *Pediatr Infect Dis J* 1987;6:681–684.

Garau J, Gomez L: *Pseudomonas aeruginosa* pneumonia. *Curr Opin Infect Dis* 2003;16:135–143.

Grisaru-Soen G, Lerner-Geva L, Keller N, et al: *Pseudomonas aeruginosa* bacteremia in children: Analysis of trends in prevalence, antibiotic resistance and prognostic factors. *Pediatr Infect Dis J* 2000;19:959–963.

Hilf M, Yu VL, Sharp JS, et al: Antibiotic therapy for *Pseudomonas aeruginosa* bacteremia: Outcome correlations in a prospective study of 200 patients. *Am J Med* 1989;87:540–546.

Keene WE, Markum AC, Samadpour M: Outbreak of *Pseudomonas aeruginosa* infections caused by commercial piercing of upper ear cartilage. *JAMA* 2004;291:981–985.

Lyczak JB, Cannon CL, Pier GB: Lung infections associated with cystic fibrosis. *Clin Microbiol Rev* 2002;15:194–222.

Obritsch MD, Fish DN, MacLaren R, et al: National surveillance of antimicrobial resistance in *Pseudomonas aeruginosa* isolates obtained from intensive care units patients from 1993 to 2002. *Antimicrob Agents Chemother* 2004;48:4606–4610.

Burkholderia Cepacia

Hancock REW: Resistance mechanisms in *P. aeruginosa* and other nonfermentative gram negative bacteria. *Clin Infect Dis* 1998;27(Suppl 1);S93–S99.

Walsh NM, Casano AA, Manangan LP, et al: Risk factors for *Burkholderia cepacia* complex colonization and infection among patients with cystic fibrosis. *J Pediatr* 2002;141:512–517.

Burkholderia Mallei

Centers for Disease Control and Prevention: Laboratory-acquired human glanders—Maryland, May 2000. *MMWR* 2000;49:532–535.

Srinivasan A, Kraus CN, DeShazer D, et al: Glanders in a military research microbiologist. *N Engl J Med* 2001;345:256–258.

Burkholderia Pseudomallei

Apisarnthanarak A, Anthanont P, Kiratisin P, et al: A Thai woman with fever and skin lesions. *Clin Infect Dis* 2005;40:988–989, 1053–1054.

Currie BJ, Fisher DA, Anstey NM, et al: Melioidosis: Acute and chronic disease, relapse and re-activation. *Trans R Soc Trop Med Hyg* 2000; 94:301–304.

Low JGH, Quek AML, Sin YK, et al: Mycotic aneurysm due to *Burkholderia pseudomallei* infection: Case reports and literature review. *Clin Infect Dis* 2005;40:193–198.

Stenotrophomonas Maltophilia

Denton M, Rajgopal A, Mooney L, et al: *Stenotrophomonas maltophilia* contamination of nebulizers used to deliver aerosolized therapy to inpatients with cystic fibrosis. *J Hosp Infect* 2003;55:180–183.

Gulcan H, Kuzucu C, Durmaz R: Nosocomial *Stenotrophomonas maltophilia* cross-infection: Three cases in newborns. *Am J Infect Control* 2004;32: 365–368.

Lanotte P, Cantagrel S, Mereghetti L, et al: Spread of *Stenotrophomonas maltophilia* colonization in a pediatric intensive care unit detected by monitoring tracheal bacterial carriage and molecular typing. *Clin Microbiol Infect* 2003;9:1142–1147.

Chapter 203 ■ Tularemia *(Francisella Tularensis)* Gordon E. Schutze and Richard F. Jacobs

Tularemia is a zoonotic infection caused by the gram-negative bacterium *Francisella tularensis*. Tularemia is primarily a disease of wild animals; human disease is incidental and usually results from contact with blood-sucking insects or live or dead wild animals. The illness caused by *F. tularensis* is manifested by different clinical syndromes, the most common of which consists of an ulcerative lesion at the site of inoculation with regional lymphadenopathy or lymphadenitis. It is also a potential agent of bioterrorism (see Chapter 711).

ETIOLOGY. *F. tularensis,* the causative agent of tularemia, is a small, nonmotile, pleomorphic, gram-negative coccobacillus. The 2 main biovars are *F. tularensis* biovar tularensis (Jellison type A) and *F. tularensis* biovar *holartica* (Jellison type B). Type A produces more serious disease in humans and is most commonly found in North America; type B may be found in North America, Europe, and Asia and produces a less virulent disease. Type A is associated with ticks and lagomorphs (rabbits, hares); type B can be associated with mosquitoes, hamsters, rodents, and water and marine animals.

EPIDEMIOLOGY. During 1990–2000, a total of 1,368 cases of tularemia were reported in the United States from 44 states, averaging 124 cases (range 86–193) per year (Fig. 203-1). Four states accounted for 56% of all reported tularemia cases: Arkansas, 315 cases (23%); Missouri, 265 cases (19%); South Dakota, 96 cases (7%); and Oklahoma, 90 cases (7%).

Transmission. Of all the zoonotic diseases, tularemia is unusual because of the different modes of transmission of disease. A large number of animals serve as a reservoir for this organism, which can penetrate both intact skin and mucous membranes. Transmission can occur through the bite of infected ticks or other biting insects, by contact with infected animals or their carcasses, by consumption of contaminated foods or water, or through inhalation, as might occur in a laboratory setting. This organism is not, however, transmitted from person to person. In the USA, rabbits and ticks are the principal reservoirs. Most disease due to rabbit exposure occurs in the winter, and disease due to tick exposure occurs in the warmer months (April–September). *Amblyomma americanum* (Lone Star tick), *Dermacentor variabilis* (dog tick), and *Dermacentor andersoni* (wood tick) are the most common tick vectors. These ticks usually feed on infected small rodents and later feed on humans. Taking that blood meal through a fecally contaminated field transmits the infection.

PATHOGENESIS. The most common portal of entry for human infection is through the skin or mucous membrane. This may occur through the bite of an infected insect or by way of unapparent abrasions. Inhalation or ingestion of *F. tularensis* can also result in infection. Usually $>10^8$ organisms are required to produce infection if they are ingested, but as few as 10 organisms may cause disease if they are inhaled or injected into the skin.

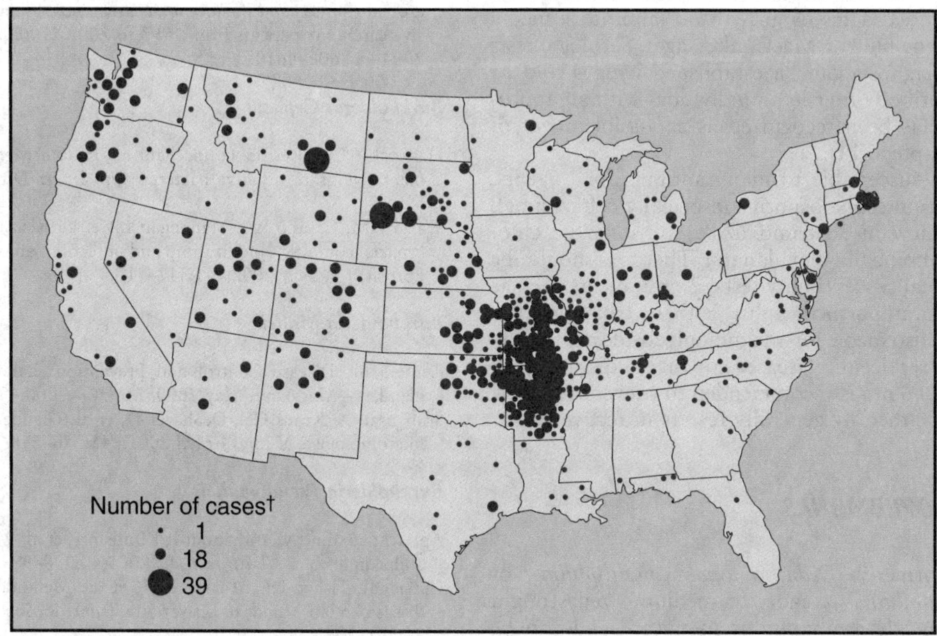

Figure 203-1. Reported cases of tularemia in the United States from 1990–2000, based on 1,347 patients reporting county of residence in the continental United States. Alaska reported 10 cases in 4 counties during 1990–2000. The circle size is proportional to the number of cases, ranging from 1 to 39 cases. (From the Centers for Disease Control and Prevention: Tularemia—United States, 1990–2000. *MMWR* 2002;51:181–184.)

TABLE 203-1. Common Clinical Manifestations of Tularemia in Children

SIGN OR SYMPTOM	FREQUENCY (%)
Lymphadenopathy	96
Fever (>38.3°C)	87
Ulcer/eschar/papule	45
Pharyngitis	43
Myalgias/arthralgias	39
Nausea/vomiting	35
Hepatosplenomegaly	35

Within 48–72 hr after injection into the skin, an erythematous, tender, or pruritic papule may appear at the portal of entry. This papule may enlarge and form an ulcer with a black base, followed by regional lymphadenopathy. Once *F. tularensis* reaches the lymph nodes, the organism may multiply and form granulomas. Bacteremia may also be present, and although any organ of the body may be involved, the reticuloendothelial system is the most commonly affected.

Conjunctival inoculation may result in infection of the eye with preauricular lymphadenopathy. Inhalation, aerosolization, or hematogenous spread of the organisms can result in pneumonia. Chest roentgenograms of such patients may reveal patchy infiltrates rather than areas of consolidation. Pleural effusions may also be present and may contain blood. In pulmonary infections, mediastinal adenopathy may be present; in oropharyngeal disease, patients may develop cervical lymphadenopathy. Typhoidal tularemia may be used to describe severe bacteremic disease, regardless of the mode of transmission or portal of entry.

Infection with tularemia stimulates the host to produce antibodies. This antibody response, however, has only a minor role in fighting this infection. The body is dependent on cell-mediated immunity to contain and eradicate this infection. Infection is usually followed by specific protection; thus, chronic infection or reinfection is unlikely.

CLINICAL MANIFESTATIONS. Although it may vary, the average incubation period from infection until clinical symptoms appear is 3 days (range, 1–21 days). A sudden onset of fever with other associated symptoms is common (Table 203-1). Physical examination may include lymphadenopathy, hepatosplenomegaly, or skin lesions. Various skin lesions have been described, including erythema multiforme and erythema nodosum. Approximately 20% of patients may develop a generalized maculopapular rash that occasionally becomes pustular. These clinical manifestations of tularemia have been divided into various syndromes (Table 203-2).

Ulceroglandular and glandular disease are the 2 most common forms of tularemia diagnosed in children. The most common glands involved are usually the cervical or posterior auricular nodes owing to a tick bite on the head or neck. If an ulcer is present, it is erythematous and painful and may last from 1 to 3 wk. The ulcer is located at the portal of entry. After the ulcer develops, regional lymphadenopathy ensues. These nodes may vary in size from 0.5 to 10 cm and may appear singly or in clusters. These affected nodes may become fluctuant and drain spontaneously, but most usually resolve with treatment. Late suppuration of the involved nodes has been described in 25–30% of patients despite effective therapy. Examination of this material from such lymph nodes usually reveals sterile necrotic material.

TABLE 203-2. Clinical Syndromes of Tularemia in Children

CLINICAL SYNDROME	FREQUENCY (%)
Ulceroglandular	45
Glandular	25
Pneumonia	14
Oropharyngeal	4
Oculoglandular	2
Typhoidal	2
Other*	6

*Includes meningitis, pericarditis, hepatitis, peritonitis, endocarditis, and osteomyelitis.

Pneumonia caused by *F. tularensis* usually presents as variable parenchymal infiltrates that are unresponsive to β-lactam antimicrobial agents. Inhalation-related infection has been described in laboratory workers who are working with the organism; it results in a relatively high mortality rate. Aerosols from farming activities involving rodent contamination (haying, threshing) or animal carcass destruction with lawn mowers have been reported to cause pneumonia as well. Patchy parenchymal infiltrates can also be demonstrated in other forms of tularemia. Patchy segmental infiltrates, hilar adenopathy, and pleural effusions are the most common abnormalities demonstrated on chest roentgenograms. Patients may also complain of a nonproductive cough, dyspnea, or pleuritic chest pain.

Oropharyngeal tularemia results from consumption of poorly cooked meats or contaminated water. This syndrome is characterized by acute pharyngitis, with or without tonsillitis, and cervical lymphadenitis. Infected tonsils may become large and develop a yellowish-white membrane that may resemble the membranes associated with diphtheria. Gastrointestinal disease may also occur and usually presents with mild, unexplained diarrhea but may progress to rapidly fulminant and fatal disease.

Oculoglandular tularemia is uncommon, but when it does occur, the portal of entry is the conjunctiva. Contact with contaminated fingers or debris from crushed insects is the most common way of applying the organisms to the conjunctiva. The conjunctiva is painful and inflamed, with yellowish nodules and pinpoint ulcerations. Purulent conjunctivitis with ipsilateral preauricular or submandibular lymphadenopathy is referred to as **Parinaud oculoglandular syndrome.**

Typhoidal tularemia is usually associated with a large inoculum of organisms and usually presents with fever, headaches, and signs or symptoms of endotoxemia. Patients typically are critically ill, and symptoms mimic those with other forms of sepsis. Clinicians practicing in tularemia-endemic regions must always consider this diagnosis in critically ill children.

DIAGNOSIS. The history and physical examination of the patient may suggest the diagnosis of tularemia, especially if the patient lives in or has visited an endemic region. A history of animal or tick exposure may be especially helpful. Hematologic blood tests are nondiagnostic. Results of routine cultures and smears are positive in only approximately 10% of cases. *F. tularensis* can be cultured in the microbiology laboratory on cysteine-glucose-blood agar, but care should be taken to alert the personnel in the laboratory if this is attempted so that they can take the proper precautions to protect themselves from acquiring infection.

The diagnosis of tularemia is most commonly established through the use of a standard and highly reliable serum agglutination test. In the standard tube agglutination test, a single titer of ≥1 : 160 in a patient with a compatible history and physical findings can establish the diagnosis. A 4-fold increase in titer from paired serum samples collected 2–3 wk apart is also diagnostic. False-negative serologic responses can be obtained early in the infection, and as many as 30% of individuals require longer than 3 wk before testing positive. Once infected, patients may have a positive agglutination test result (1 : 20–1 : 80) that may persist for life.

Other testing techniques available include a microagglutination test, enzyme-linked immunosorbent assay, analysis of urine for tularemia antigen, and polymerase chain reaction. These techniques may become more popular in the future but at this time have a limited role in establishing the diagnosis of tularemia.

Differential Diagnosis. The differential diagnosis of ulceroglandular or glandular tularemia includes cat scratch disease *(Bartonella henselae)*; infectious mononucleosis; Kawasaki syndrome; lymphadenopathy caused by *Staphylococcus aureus,* group A streptococcus, *Mycobacterium tuberculosis, Toxoplasma gondii,* nontuberculous mycobacteria, and *Sporothrix schenckii;* plague; anthrax; melioidosis; and rat-bite fever. Oculoglandular disease may also occur with other infectious agents, such as *B. henselae, Treponema pallidum, Coccidioides immitis,* herpes simplex virus, adenoviruses, and the bacterial agents responsible for purulent conjunctivitis. Oropharyngeal tularemia must be differentiated from the same diseases that cause ulceroglandular/glandular disease and from cytomegalovirus, herpes simplex, adenovirus, and other viral or bacterial etiologies. Pneumonic tularemia must be differentiated from the other non-β-lactam-responsive organisms such as *Mycoplasma, Chlamydia,* mycobacteria, fungi, and rickettsia. Typhoidal tularemia must be differentiated from other forms of sepsis as well as from enteric fever (typhoid and paratyphoid fever) and brucellosis.

TREATMENT. All strains of *F. tularensis* are susceptible to gentamicin and streptomycin. Gentamicin (5 mg/kg/day divided bid or tid IV or IM) is the drug of choice for the treatment of tularemia in children because of the limited availability of streptomycin (30–40 mg/kg/day divided bid IM) and the fewer adverse effects of gentamicin. Therapy is typically continued for 7–10 days, but in mild cases, 5–7 days may be sufficient. Chloramphenicol and tetracyclines have been used, but the high relapse rate has limited their use in children. Early data suggested that *F. tularensis* is susceptible to the 3rd generation cephalosporins (cefotaxime, ceftriaxone), but clinical case reports demonstrate a nearly universal failure rate with these agents. Quinolones are active against *F. tularensis* and have been used for treatment of the milder form of tularemia due to the European biovar *F. tularensis* biovar *holartica.* Further data are required before quinolone therapy can be recommended for the most common biovar encountered in North America, *F. tularensis* biovar *tularensis.*

Patients typically have defervescence within 24–48 hr after starting therapy, and relapses are uncommon if gentamicin or streptomycin is used. Patients who have not started on appropriate therapy early may respond more slowly to antimicrobial therapy. Late suppuration of involved lymph nodes may occur despite adequate therapy but usually contain sterile material.

PROGNOSIS. Poor outcomes are associated with a delay in recognition and treatment, but with rapid recognition and treatment, fatalities are exceedingly rare. The mortality rate for severe untreated disease (e.g., pneumonia, typhoidal disease) can be as high as 30% in these situations, but in general, the overall mortality rate is <1%.

PREVENTION. Prevention of tularemia is based on avoiding exposure. Children living in tick-endemic regions should be taught to avoid tick-infested areas, and families should have a tick control plan for their immediate environment and for their pets. Protective clothing should be worn when entering a tick-infested area, but more importantly, children should undergo frequent tick checks during and after their time in these areas. Skin repellents such as N-N-diethyl-M-toluamide (DEET) can be used but have been described to cause systemic reactions if used incorrectly on small infants. Avoiding taking young infants into tick-endemic regions is the most prudent approach. If DEET-containing compounds are used, they should be used sparingly on the exposed skin, avoiding the hands and face. The repellent should be washed off completely after leaving the high-risk region. Clothing repellents that use permethrin have been demonstrated to be an effective addition to the use of protective clothing. If ticks are found on the child, forceps should be used to pull the tick straight out. The skin should be cleansed before and after this procedure.

Children should also be taught to avoid sick and dead animals. Dogs and cats are most likely to bring these animals to a child's attention. Children should be encouraged to wear gloves while cleaning wild game. A vaccine is available for adults with high-risk vocations (e.g., veterinarians), but there are no recommendations for use in children. Prophylactic antimicrobial agents are not effective in preventing tularemia and should not be used after exposure.

Centers for Disease Control and Prevention: Tularemia—United States, 1990–2000. *MMWR* 2002;51:181–184.

Centers for Disease Control and Prevention: Tularemia associated with a hamster bite, Colorado 2004. *MMWR* 2005;53:1202–1203.

Centers for Disease Control and Prevention: Tularemia transmitted by insect bites, Wyoming, 2001–2003. *MMWR* 2005;54:170–173.

Dennis DT, Inglesby TV, Henderson DA, et al: Tularemia as a biological weapon. *JAMA* 2001;281:2763–2773.

Johansson A, Berglund L, Gothefors L, et al: Ciprofloxacin for treatment of tularemia in children. *Pediatr Infect Dis J* 2000;19:449–453.

Roberst JR, Reigart JR: Does anything beat DEET? *Pediatr Ann* 2004;33:443–453.

Tärnvik A, Priebe HS, Grunow R: Tularemia in Europe: An epidemiological overview. *Scand J Infect Dis* 2004;36:350–355.

Chapter 204 ■ *Brucella*

Gordon E. Schutze and Richard F. Jacobs

Human brucellosis, caused by organisms of the genus *Brucella,* continues to be a major public health problem worldwide. Humans are accidental hosts and acquire this zoonotic disease from direct contact with an infected animal or consumption of products of an infected animal. Although brucellosis is widely recognized as an occupational risk among adults working with livestock, much of the brucellosis in children is food-borne and is associated with consumption of unpasteurized milk products. It is also a potential agent of bioterrorism (see Chapter 711).

ETIOLOGY. *Brucella abortus* (cattle), *B. melitensis* (goat/sheep), *B. suis* (swine), and *B. canis* (dog) are the most common organisms responsible for human disease. These organisms are small, aerobic, non-spore-forming, nonmotile, gram-negative coccobacillary bacteria that are fastidious in their growth but can be grown on various laboratory media including blood and chocolate agars. When brucellosis is suspected, however, the clinical laboratory should be alerted so the cultures can be maintained for ≥21 days to ensure growth if the organism is present.

EPIDEMIOLOGY. Because of improved sanitation, brucellosis has become rare in industrialized countries. Brucellosis exists worldwide and is especially prevalent in the Mediterranean basin, Arabian Gulf, Indian subcontinent, and parts of Mexico and Central and South America. In industrialized countries, recreational or occupational exposure to infected animals is a major risk factor for the development of disease. In the United States, 50% of cases occur in California and Texas. Among children, however, geographic locations that are endemic for *B. melitensis* remain areas of increased risk for the development of infection. In such locations, unpasteurized milk from goats or camels may be used to feed children, thus leading to the development of brucellosis. Consequently, a history of travel to endemic regions or consumption of exotic food or unpasteurized dairy or dairy products may be an important clue to the diagnosis of human brucellosis.

PATHOGENESIS. Routes of infection for these organisms include inoculation through cuts or abrasions in the skin, inoculation of the conjunctival sac of the eye, inhalation of infectious aerosols, or ingestion of contaminated meat or dairy products. The risk for infection depends on the nutritional and immune status of the host, the route of inoculum, and the species of *Brucella.* For reasons that remain unclear, *B. melitensis* and *B. suis* tend to be more virulent than *B. abortus* or *B. canis.*

The major virulence factor for *Brucella* appears to be its cell wall lipopolysaccharide. Strains containing smooth lipopolysaccharide have been demonstrated to have greater virulence and are more resistant to killing by polymorphonuclear leukocytes. These organisms are facultative intracellular pathogens that can survive and replicate within the mononuclear phagocytic cells (monocytes, macrophages) of the reticuloendothelial system. Even though *Brucella* are chemotactic for entry of leukocytes into the body, the leukocytes are less efficient at killing these organisms than other bacteria despite the assistance of serum factors such as complement.

Organisms that are not phagocytosed by the leukocytes are ingested by the macrophages and become localized within the reticuloendothelial system. Specifically, they reside within the liver, spleen, lymph nodes, and bone marrow and result in **granuloma** formation. Antibodies are produced against the lipopolysaccharide and other cell wall antigens. This provides a means of diagnosis and probably has a role in long-term immunity. The major factor in recovery from infection appears to be development of a cell-mediated response resulting in macrophage activation and enhanced intracellular killing. Specifically, sensitized T lymphocytes release cytokines (e.g., interferon-γ and tumor necrosis factor-α), which activate the macrophages and enhance their intracellular killing capacity.

CLINICAL MANIFESTATIONS. Brucellosis is a systemic illness that can be very difficult to diagnose in children without a history of animal or food exposure. Symptoms can be acute or insidious in nature and are usually nonspecific, beginning 2–4 wk after inoculation. Although the clinical manifestations do vary, the classic triad of fever, arthralgia/arthritis, and hepatosplenomegaly can be demonstrated in most patients. Some present as a fever of unknown origin. Other associated symptoms include abdominal pain, headache, diarrhea, rash, night sweats, weakness/fatigue, vomiting, cough, and pharyngitis. A common constellation of symptoms in children is refusal to eat, lassitude, refusal to bear weight, and failure to thrive. Besides hepatosplenomegaly, the physical findings on examination are usually few, with the exception of arthritis. The fever pattern can vary widely, and virtually any organ or tissue can be involved.

If abnormalities are demonstrated on physical examination, the bones and joints frequently are involved, with the sacroiliac joint as well as the hips, knees, and ankles being the most common. Although headache, mental inattention, and depression may be demonstrated in patients with brucellosis, invasion of the nervous system occurs in only about 1% of cases. Neonatal and congenital infections with these organisms have also been described. These have been transmitted transplacentally, from breast milk, and through blood transfusions. The signs and symptoms associated with brucellosis are vague and not pathognomonic.

DIAGNOSIS. Routine laboratory examinations of the blood are not helpful; thrombocytopenia, neutropenia, anemia, or pancytopenia may occur. A history of exposure to animals or ingestion of unpasteurized dairy products may be more helpful. A definitive diagnosis is established by recovering the organisms in the blood, bone marrow, or other tissues. Although automated culture systems and the use of the lysis-centrifugation method have shortened the isolation time from weeks to days, it is prudent to alert the clinical microbiology laboratory that brucellosis is suspected. Isolation of the organism still may require as long as 4 wk from a blood culture sample. Caution is also advised when using automated bacterial identification systems, because isolates have been misidentified as other gram-negative organisms (*Haemophilus influenzae* type b).

In the absence of positive culture results, various serologic tests have been applied to the diagnosis of brucellosis. The serum agglutination test (SAT) is the most widely used and detects antibodies against *B. abortus, B. melitensis,* and *B. suis.* This method does not detect antibodies against *B. canis* because this organism lacks the smooth lipopolysaccharide. No single titer is ever diagnostic, but most patients with acute infections have titers of ≥1 : 160. Low titers may be found early in the course of the illness, requiring the use of acute and convalescent sera testing to confirm the diagnosis. Because patients with active infection have both an immunoglobulin M (IgM) and an IgG response and the SAT measures the total quantity of agglutinating antibodies, the total quantity of IgG is measured by treatment of the serum with 2-mercaptoethanol. This fractionation is important in determining the significance of the antibody titer because low levels of IgM can remain in the serum for weeks to months after the infection has been treated. It is important to remember that all titers must be interpreted in light of a patient's history and physical examination. False-positive results due to cross-reacting antibodies to other gram-negative organisms such as *Yersinia enterocolitica, Francisella tularensis,* and *Vibrio cholerae* can occur. In addition, the prozone effect can give false-negative results in the presence of high titers of antibody. To avoid this issue, serum that is being tested should be diluted to ≥1 : 320.

Among newer tests, the enzyme immunoassay appears to be the most sensitive method for detecting *Brucella* antibodies. Polymerase chain reaction assays are also becoming available but at this time are mostly limited to research facilities.

Differential Diagnosis. Brucellosis may be confused with other infections such as tularemia, cat scratch disease, typhoid fever, and fungal infections due to histoplasmosis, blastomycosis, or coccidioidomycosis. Infections caused by *Mycobacterium tuberculosis,* atypical mycobacteria, rickettsiae, and *Yersinia* can present in a similar fashion to brucellosis.

TREATMENT. Many antimicrobial agents are active in vitro against the *Brucella* species, but the clinical effectiveness does not always correlate with these results. Doxycycline is the most useful antimicrobial agent and, when combined with an aminoglycoside, is associated with the fewest relapses (Table 204-1). Treatment failures with β-lactam antimicrobial agents, including the 3rd generation cephalosporins, may be due to the intracellular nature of the organism. Agents that provide intracellular killing are required for eradication of this infection. Similarly, it is apparent that prolonged treatment is the key to preventing disease relapse. Relapse is confirmed by isolation of *Brucella* within weeks to months after therapy has ended and is usually not associated with antimicrobial resistance.

The onset of initial antimicrobial therapy may precipitate a Jarisch-Herxheimer-like reaction, presumably due to a large antigen load. It is rarely severe enough to require corticosteroid therapy.

PROGNOSIS. Before the use of antimicrobial agents, the course of brucellosis was often prolonged and may have led to death. Since the institution of specific therapy, most deaths are due to specific organ system involvement (e.g., endocarditis) in complicated cases. The prognosis after specific therapy is excellent if patients are compliant with the prolonged therapy (see Table 204-1).

TABLE 204-1. Recommended Therapy for the Treatment of Brucellosis

AGE AND CONDITION	ANTIMICROBIAL AGENT	DOSE	ROUTE	DURATION
≥8 yr	Doxycycline	2–4 mg/kg/day; maximum 200 mg/day	PO	4–6 wk
	+			
	Rifampin	15–20 mg/kg/day; maximum 600–900 mg/day	PO	4–6 wk
	Alternative:			
	Doxycycline	2–4 mg/kg/day; maximum 200 mg/day	PO	4–6 wk
	+			
	Streptomycin	20–30 mg/kg/day; maximum 1 g/day	IM	1–2 wk
	or			
	Gentamicin	3–5 mg/kg/day	IM/IV	1–2 wk
<8 yr	Trimethoprim-sulfamethoxazole (TMP-SMZ)	TMP (10 mg/kg/day; maximum 480 mg/day) and SMZ (50 mg/kg/day; maximum 2.4 g/day)	PO	4–6 wk
	+			
	Rifampin	15–20 mg/kg/day	PO	4–6 wk
Meningitis, osteomyelitis, endocarditis				
	Doxycycline	2–4 mg/kg/day; maximum 200 mg/day	PO	4–6 mo
	+			
	Gentamicin	3–5 mg/kg/day	IV	1–2 wk
	±			
	Rifampin	15–20 mg/kg/day; maximum 600–900 mg/day	PO	4–6 mo

PREVENTION. Prevention of brucellosis is dependent on effective eradication of the organism from cattle, goats, and swineherds as well as from other animals. Pasteurization of milk and dairy products for human consumption remains an important aspect of prevention. No vaccine currently exists for use in children and, therefore, education of the public continues to have a prominent role in prevention of this disease.

Al-Kharfy TM: Neonatal brucellosis and blood transfusion: Case report and review of the literature. *Ann Trop Pediatr* 2001;21:349–352.

Pappas G, Akritidis N, Bosilkovski M, et al: Brucellosis. *N Engl J Med* 2005;352:2325–2336.

Patt HA, Feigin RD: Diagnosis and management of suspected cases of bioterrorism: A pediatric perspective. *Pediatrics* 2002;109:685–692.

Solera J, Geijo P, Largo J, et al: A randomized, double-blind study to assess the optimal duration of doxycycline treatment for human brucellosis. *Clin Infect Dis* 2004;39:1776–1782.

Troy SB, Rickman LS, Davis CE: Brucellosis in San Diego—Epidemiology and species-related differences in acute clinical presentations. *Medicine* 2005;84:174–187.

Tsolia M, Drakonaki S, Messaritaki A, et al: Clinical features, complications and treatment outcome of childhood brucellosis in central Greece. *J Infect* 2002;44:257–262.

Yildirmak Y, Palanduz A, Telhan L, et al: Bone marrow hypoplasia during *Brucella* infection. *J Pediatr Heme Oncol* 2003;25:63–64.

Chapter 205 ■ *Legionella*

Lucy Tompkins

Legionellosis comprises **Legionnaires disease** (*Legionella* pneumonia), other invasive extrapulmonary infections, and an acute flulike illness known as **Pontiac fever.** In contrast to the syndromes associated with invasive disease, Pontiac fever is a self-limiting illness that develops after aerosol exposure and may represent a toxic or hypersensitivity response to *Legionella.*

ETIOLOGY. Legionellaceae are aerobic, non-spore-forming unencapsulated gram-negative bacilli that stain poorly with Gram stain when performed on smears from clinical specimens. Microorganisms in tissue can be better visualized with the Gimenez or silver stains (Dieterle or Warthin-Starry). Stained smears of *Legionella pneumophila* taken from colonial growth resemble *Pseudomonas.* Unlike other *Legionella* species, *L. micdadei* stains acid fast. Although >30 species of the genus have now been identified, the majority (90%) of clinical infections are caused by *L. pneumophila,* and most of the remainder are caused by *L. micdadei, L. bozemanii, L. dumoffii,* and *L. longbeachae.*

The organisms are fastidious and require L-cysteine, ferric ion, and α-keto acids for growth. Colonies develop within 3–5 days on buffered charcoal yeast extract agar, which may contain selected antibiotics to inhibit overgrowth by other microorganisms; *Legionella* rarely grows on routine laboratory media.

EPIDEMIOLOGY. The environmental reservoir of *Legionella* in nature is fresh water (lakes, streams, thermally polluted waters, potable water), and invasive pneumonia (Legionnaires disease) is related to exposure to potable water or to aerosols containing the bacteria. Growth of *Legionella* occurs more readily in warm water, and exposure to warm water sources is an important risk factor for disease. *Legionella* organisms are facultative intracellular parasites and grow inside protozoans present in biofilms consisting of organic and inorganic material found in plumbing and water storage tanks and various other bacterial species. Sporadic cases of community-acquired Legionnaires disease can be attributed to potable water in the local environment of the patient. Risk factors for acquisition of sporadic community-acquired pneumonia include nonmunicipal water supply, residential plumbing repairs, and lower water heater temperatures, which facilitate growth of bacteria or lead to release of a bolus of biofilm containing *Legionella* into potable water. The mode of transmission may be by way of inhalation of aerosols or by aspiration. Outbreaks of Legionnaires disease have been associated with protozoans in the implicated water source; replication within these eukaryotic cells presumably amplifies and maintains *Legionella* within the potable water distribution system. Outbreaks of community-acquired pneumonia and some nosocomial outbreaks have been linked to common sources, including potable hot water heaters, evaporative condensers cooling towers, whirlpool baths, humidifiers, and nebulizers. Travel-associated Legionnaires disease and Pontiac fever are increasingly recognized in major outbreaks.

Hospital-acquired infections are most often linked to potable water. Exposure may occur through 2 general mechanisms: (1) aspiration of ingested microorganisms, including those in gastric feedings, that are mixed with contaminated tap water; and (2) aerosols from showers and sinks. Extrapulmonary legionellosis may occur through topical application of contaminated tap water into surgical or traumatic wounds. In contrast to Legionnaires disease, Pontiac fever outbreaks have occurred through exposure to aerosols from whirlpool baths, ultrasonic humidifiers, and ventilation systems.

The incidence of community-acquired Legionnaires disease caused by *L. pneumophila* occurring sporadically in adults is estimated at 7–20 cases/100,000 per year and demonstrates geographic differences. *Legionella* infections have no seasonal pattern. Approximately 0.5–5.0% of those exposed to a common source develop pneumonia, whereas the attack rate in Pontiac fever outbreaks is very high (85–100%). In 1 large community-based study of adults, *Legionella* was associated with 3% of pneumonia cases. Taken together, *Mycoplasma pneumoniae, Chlamydia pneumoniae,* and *L. pneumophila* account for 10–38% of all community-acquired pneumonia, and therefore the current clinical guidelines for community-acquired pneumonia recommend empirical therapy with macrolides or quinolones.

As estimated by seroconversion to *L. pneumophila* among children hospitalized with pneumonia, the Legionnaires disease rate was found to be quite low. Community-acquired pneumonia occurs most often in children >4 yr of age. Most nosocomial infections have been reported as case reports; therefore, the true incidence of disease in children is unknown. Nosocomial infection rates in adults are difficult to determine because many hospital laboratories do not attempt to isolate *Legionella* by culture. Hospital-acquired legionellosis in children is associated with clinical risk factors and with environmental exposure. Acquisition of antibodies to *L. pneumophila* in healthy children occurs progressively over time, although this presumably reflects subclinical infection or mild respiratory disease or antibodies that cross react with other bacterial species.

PATHOGENESIS. Although *Legionella* can be grown on artificial media, the intracellular environment of eukaryotic cells provides the definitive site of growth. *Legionella* organisms are facultative intracellular parasites of eukaryotic cells. In nature, *Legionella* replicate within protozoans found in fresh water. In humans, the main target cell for *Legionella* is the alveolar macrophage, although other cell types may also be invaded. After entry, virulent strains of *L. pneumophila* stimulate the formation of a special phagosome that permits bacterial replication to proceed. The phagosome is composed of components of the endoplasmic reticulum and escapes the degradative lysosomal pathway. Growth in macrophages occurs to the point of cell death, followed by reinfection of new cells, until these cells are activated and can subsequently kill intracellular microorganisms. Acute, severe infection of the lung provokes an acute inflammatory response and necrosis; early on, more bacteria are found in extracellular spaces as a result of intracellular replication, lysis, and release of bacteria. Subsequently, macrophage activation and other immune responses produce intense infiltration of tissue by macrophages that contain intracellular bacteria, ultimately leading to control of bacterial replication and killing. Corticosteroid therapy poses a high risk for infection by interfering with T-cell and macrophage function. Although community-acquired Legionnaires' disease may occur in healthy, immunocompetent patients, those who have defects in cellular-mediated immunity are at high risk for infection. As in other diseases caused by facultative intracellular microorganisms, the outcome is critically dependent on the specific and nonspecific immune responses of the host, particularly macrophage and T-cell responses.

CLINICAL MANIFESTATIONS. Legionnaires disease was originally believed to cause atypical pneumonia that was associated with extrapulmonary signs and symptoms including diarrhea, hyponatremia, hypophosphatemia, abnormal results of liver function tests, confusion, and renal dysfunction. Although a subset of patients may exhibit these classic manifestations, *Legionella* infection typically causes pneumonia that is indistinguishable from disease produced by other infectious agents. Fever, cough, and chest pain are common presenting symptoms; the cough may be productive of purulent sputum or may be nonproductive. Although the classic chest radiographic appearance demonstrates rapidly progressive alveolar filling infiltrates, in usual cases of pneumonia the chest radiographic appearance is widely variable, appearing as tumor-like shadows, evidence of nodular infiltrates, unilateral or bilateral infiltrates, or cavitation, although cavitation is rarely seen in immunocompetent patients. This picture overlaps substantially with disease caused by *Streptococcus pneumoniae.* Although pleural effusion is less commonly associated with Legionnaires disease, its frequency varies so widely that neither the presence nor absence of effusion is helpful in differential diagnosis. If present, pleural fluid should be obtained for culture.

A few clinical features may help to differentiate *Legionella* pneumonia from other causes. *Legionella* pneumonia produces an acute-onset febrile illness, the radiograph shows alveolar filling infiltrates, and there is no clinical response to broad-spectrum β-lactam (penicillins and cephalosporins) or aminoglycoside antibiotics.

Concomitant infection with other pathogens occurs in 5–10% of cases of Legionnaires disease; therefore, culture of another potential pulmonary pathogen does not preclude the diagnosis of legionellosis.

Reports of nosocomial *Legionella* pneumonia in children demonstrate that rapid onset, temperature greater than 38.5°C, cough, pleuritic chest pain, and dyspnea are present in most. Abdominal pain, headache, and diarrhea are also common. Chest radiographs reveal lobar consolidations or diffuse bilateral infiltrates, and pleural effusions are noted. Symptoms do not respond to treatment with β-lactam antibiotics or aminoglycosides.

Risk factors for Legionnaires disease in adults include chronic diseases of the lung (smoking, bronchitis), older age, diabetes and renal failure, immunosuppression associated with organ transplantation, corticosteroid therapy, and episodes of aspiration. The number of reported cases of community-acquired Legionnaires disease in children is small. Among these, immunocompromised status, especially corticosteroid treatment, coupled with exposure to contaminated potable water is the major risk factor. Infection in a few children with chronic pulmonary disease without immune deficiency has also been reported, but infection in children lacking any risk factors is very uncommon. The modes of transmission of community-acquired disease in children include exposure to mists, fresh water, water coolers, and other aerosol-generating apparatuses. Nosocomial *Legionella* infection occurs more frequently than community-acquired disease in children, and the modes of acquisition include microaspiration, frequently associated with nasogastric tubes, and aerosol inhalation. Bronchopulmonary *Legionella* infections occur in patients with cystic fibrosis and have been associated with aerosol therapy or mist tents. Legionnaires disease is also reported in pediatric patients with asthma and tracheal stenosis. Chronic corticosteroid therapy for asthma is a reported risk factor for *Legionella* infections in children.

Pontiac fever in adults and children is characterized by high fever, myalgia, headache, and extreme debilitation, lasting for a few days. Cough, breathlessness, diarrhea, confusion, and chest pain may occur, but there is no evidence for invasive infection. The disease is self-limited without sequelae. Virtually all exposed individuals seroconvert to *Legionella* antigens. A very large outbreak in Scotland that affected 35 children was attributed to *L. micdadei,* which was isolated from a whirlpool spa. The onset of illness was 1–7 days (median 3 days), and all exposed children developed significant titers of specific antibodies to *L. micdadei.* The pathogenesis of Pontiac fever is not known. In the absence of evidence of true infection, the most likely hypothesis is that this syndrome is caused by a toxic or hypersensitivity reaction to microbial, or protozoan, antigens.

DIAGNOSIS. Culture of *Legionella* from sputum, other respiratory tract specimens, blood, or tissue is the gold standard against which indirect methods of detection should be compared. Specimens obtained from the respiratory tract that are contaminated with oral flora must be treated and processed to reduce contaminants and plated onto selective media. Because these are costly and time-consuming methods, many laboratories do not process specimens for culture. The urinary antigen assay that detects *L. pneumophila* serogroup I has 80% sensitivity and 99% specificity. The assay is a useful method in the prompt diagnosis of Legionnaires disease caused by this serogroup, which accounts for the majority of symptomatic infections. In the USA, this test is frequently used because it is widely available in reference laboratories. The microorganisms can also be identified presumptively by direct immunofluorescence antibody screening, although the sensitivity of the test is generally low in most laboratories, in part because of the lack of antisera directed against other *Legionella* serogroups and species. This method failed to detect the infection in several well-documented pediatric cases. Retrospective diagnosis can be made serologically using the enzyme-linked immunosorbent assay or enzyme immunoassay to detect specific antibody production. Seroconversion may not occur for several weeks after onset of infection, and the available serologic assays do not detect all strains of *L. pneumophila* or all species. In view of the low sensitivity of direct detection and the slow growth of the microorganism in culture, the diagnosis of legionellosis should be pursued actively when there is suggestive clinical evidence, including the lack of response to usual antibiotics, even when results of other laboratory studies are negative.

TREATMENT. In community-acquired pneumonia in adults who are hospitalized, guidelines recommend empirical treatment with a broad-spectrum cephalosporin plus a macrolide or quinolone in order to treat atypical microorganisms *(Legionella, Chlamydia pneumoniae, Mycoplasma pneumoniae)*. Effective treatment of Legionnaires disease is based, in part, on the intracellular concentration of antibiotics. Erythromycin (40 mg/kg/day PO or IV), with or without rifampin (15 mg/kg/day), was considered effective therapy many years ago. Azithromycin (10 mg/kg on day 1, not to exceed 500 mg/day, then 5 mg/kg daily for 4 days PO) and clarithromycin (15 mg/kg/day PO) and the quinolones (ciprofloxacin, levofloxacin, trovafloxacin, sparfloxacin) have replaced erythromycin as therapy for patients with diagnosed *Legionella* infection. Quinolones are not approved for children <18 yr of age. In serious infections or in high-risk patients, parenteral therapy is recommended initially; a switch to oral therapy can be made when a patient has had a clinical response. The duration of oral azithromycin therapy for Legionnaires disease in adults is 4 days, although therapy may be continued for immunocompromised patients. Acute hearing loss, which is reversible, is associated with high-dose parenteral macrolide therapy. Treatment of extrapulmonary infections, including prosthetic valve endocarditis and sternal wound infections may require prolonged therapy. Trimethoprim-sulfamethoxazole (TMP-SMZ; 15 mg TMP/kg/day and 75 mg SMZ/kg/day) has been used as an alternative.

PROGNOSIS. The mortality rate for community-acquired Legionnaires disease in adults who are hospitalized is approximately 15%. The prognosis depends on underlying host factors and possibly on the duration of the illness before appropriate therapy is begun. Despite appropriate antibiotic therapy, patients may succumb to respiratory complications, such as acute respiratory distress syndrome, associated with artificial ventilation and intubation. A high mortality rate is noted in case reports of premature infants and children, virtually all of whom have been immunocompromised.

Abernathy-Carver KJ, Fan LL, Boguncіewicz M, et al: *Legionella* and *Pneumocystis* pneumonias in asthmatic children on high doses of systemic steroids. *Pediatr Pulmonol* 1994;18:135–138.

Benin AL, Benson RF, Arnold KE, et al: An outbreak of travel-associated Legionnaires disease and Pontiac fever: The need for enhanced surveillance of travel-associated legionellosis in the United States. *J Infect Dis* 2002;185:237–243.

Campins M, Ferrer A, Callis L, et al: Nosocomial Legionnaire's disease in a children's hospital. *Pediatr Infect Dis J* 2000;19:228–234.

Famiglietti RF, Bakerman PR, Saubolle MA, et al: Cavitary legionellosis in two immunocompetent infants. *Pediatrics* 1997;99:899–903.

Garrido RMB, Parra FJE, Frances LA, et al: Antimicrobial chemotherapy for Legionnaires' disease: Levofloxacin versus macrolides. *Clin Infect Dis* 2005;40:800–806.

Gervaix A, Beghetti M, Rimensberger P, et al: Bullous emphysema after *Legionella* pneumonia in a two-year-old. *Pediatr Infect Dis J* 2000;19:86–87.

Goldberg DJ, Emslie JA, Fallon RJ, et al: Pontiac fever in children. *Pediatr Infect Dis J* 1992;11:240–241.

Jones TF, Benson RF, Brown EW, et al: Epidemiologic investigation of a restaurant-associated outbreak of Pontiac fever. *Clin Infect Dis* 2003;37:1292–1297.

Levy I, Rubin LG: *Legionella* pneumonia in neonates: A literature review. *J Perinatol* 1998;18:287–290.

Luttichau HR, Vinther C, Uldum SA, et al: An outbreak of Pontiac fever among children following use of a whirlpool. *Clin Infect Dis* 1998;26:1374–1378.

Chapter 206 ■ *Bartonella*

Barbara W. Stechenberg

The spectrum of disease resulting from human infection with *Bartonella* species has expanded rapidly in the past 2 decades, including the association of bacillary angiomatosis with AIDS and cat scratch disease (CSD), with the fastidious gram-negative rod *B. henselae*. Five major *Bartonella* species are pathogenic for humans: *B. bacilliformis, B. henselae, B. quintana, B. elizabethae,* and most recently *B. clarridgeiae*. Several other *Bartonella* species have been found in animals, particularly rodents and moles (Table 206-1).

Members of the genus *Bartonella* are gram-negative, oxidase-negative, fastidious aerobic rods that ferment no carbohydrates. Only 1 species, *B. bacilliformis,* is motile by means of polar flagella. Optimal growth is obtained on fresh media containing 5% or more sheep or horse blood in the presence of 5% carbon dioxide. The use of lysis-centrifugation for specimens from blood on chocolate agar for extended periods (2–6 wk) enhances recovery.

206.1 • Bartonellosis *(Bartonella bacilliformis)*

The 1st human *Bartonella* infection described was bartonellosis, a geographically distinct disease caused by *B. bacilliformis,* which causes 2 predominant forms of illness: **Oroya fever,** a severe, febrile hemolytic anemia; and **verruca peruana** (verruga peruana), an eruption of hemangioma-like lesions. The organism also causes asymptomatic infection. Bartonellosis is also called

TABLE 206-1. *Bartonella* Causing Human Disease

DISEASE	ORGANISM	VECTOR	PRIMARY RISK FACTOR
Bartonellosis	*B. bacilliformis*	Sandfly (*Lutzomyia verrucarum*)	Living in endemic areas (Andes Mountains)
Cat scratch disease	*B. henselae* *B. clarridgeiae* (1 case)	Cat	Cat scratch or bite
Trench fever	*B. quintana*	Human body louse	Body louse infestation during outbreak
Bacteremia, endocarditis	*B. henselae* *B. quintana* *B. elizabethae*	Cat for *B. henselae*	Severely immunocompromised
Bacillary angiomatosis	*B. henselae* *B. quintana*	Cat for *B. henselae*	Severely immunocompromised
Peliosis hepatis	*B. henselae* *B. quintana*	Cat for *B. henselae*	Severely immunocompromised

Carrión disease in honor of the Peruvian medical student who inoculated himself with blood from a verruca and 21 days later developed Oroya fever. He died 39 days after inoculation, thus proving the unitary etiology of the 2 clinical illnesses.

ETIOLOGY. *B. bacilliformis* is a small, motile, gram-negative organism with a brush of 10 or more unipolar flagella, which appear to be important components for invasiveness. An obligate aerobe, it grows best at 28°C in semisolid nutrient agar containing rabbit serum and hemoglobin.

EPIDEMIOLOGY. Bartonellosis is a zoonosis found only in mountain valleys of the Andes Mountains in Peru, Ecuador, Colombia, Chile, and Bolivia at altitudes and environmental conditions favorable for the vector, which is the sandfly, *Lutzomyia verrucarum*.

PATHOGENESIS. After the sandfly bite, *Bartonella* organisms enter the endothelial cells of blood vessels, where they proliferate. Found throughout the reticuloendothelial system, they then reenter the bloodstream and parasitize the erythrocytes. They bind on the cells, deform the membranes, and then enter intracellular vacuoles. The resultant **hemolytic anemia** may involve as many as 90% of the erythrocytes. Patients who survive this acute phase may or may not develop the cutaneous manifestations, which are nodular hemangiomatous lesions or verrucae ranging in size from a few millimeters to several centimeters.

CLINICAL MANIFESTATIONS. The incubation period is 2–14 wk. Patients may be totally asymptomatic or may have nonspecific symptoms such as headache and malaise without anemia.

Oroya fever is characterized by fever with rapid development of anemia. Clouding of the sensorium and delirium are common symptoms and may progress to overt psychosis. Physical examination demonstrates signs of severe anemia, icterus, and pallor, which may be associated with generalized lymphadenopathy.

In the pre-eruptive stage of **verruca peruana** (Fig. 206-1), patients may complain of arthralgias, myalgias, and paresthesias. Inflammatory reactions such as phlebitis, pleuritis, erythema nodosum, and encephalitis may develop. The appearance of verrucae is pathognomonic of the eruptive phase. They vary greatly in size and number.

DIAGNOSIS. The diagnosis is established on clinical grounds in conjunction with a blood smear demonstrating organisms, or by blood culture. The anemia is macrocytic and hypochromic, with reticulocyte counts as high as 50%. *B. bacilliformis* may be seen on Giemsa stain as red-violet rods in the erythrocytes. In the recovery phase, these organisms change to a more coccoid form and disappear from the blood. In the absence of anemia, the diagnosis depends on blood cultures. In the eruptive phase, the typical verruca confirms the diagnosis. Antibody testing has been used to document infection.

TREATMENT. *B. bacilliformis* is sensitive to many antibiotics, including rifampin, tetracycline, and chloramphenicol. Treatment is very effective in rapidly diminishing fever and eradicating the organism from the blood. Chloramphenicol (50–75 mg/kg/day) is considered the drug of choice, because it also is useful in the treatment of concomitant infections such as *Salmonella*. Blood transfusions and supportive care are critical in patients with severe anemia. Antimicrobial treatment for verruca peruana is considered when there are >10 cutaneous lesions, if the lesions are erythematous or violaceous, or if the onset of the lesions was <1 mo before presentation. Oral rifampin is effective in the healing of lesions. Surgical excision may be needed for large disfiguring lesions or those that interfere with function.

PREVENTION. Prevention depends on avoidance of the vector, particularly at night, by the use of protective clothing and insect repellents (see Chapter 173).

206.2 • Cat Scratch Disease (*Bartonella henselae*)

The most common presentation of *Bartonella* infection is CSD, which is a subacute, regional lymphadenitis caused by *B. henselae*. It is the most common cause of chronic lymphadenitis that persists for >3 wk.

ETIOLOGY. *B. henselae* was cultured from the blood of a healthy cat and was used in serologic studies that indicated *B. henselae* as the cause of CSD. *B. henselae* organisms are also the small pleomorphic gram-negative bacilli visualized by Warthin-Starry stain in affected lymph nodes from patients with CSD. Development of serologic tests that showed prevalence of antibodies in 84–100% of cases of CSD, culturing of *B. henselae* from CSD nodes, and detection of *B. henselae* by polymerase chain reaction (PCR) in the majority of lymph node samples and pus from patients with CSD confirmed the organism as the cause of CSD.

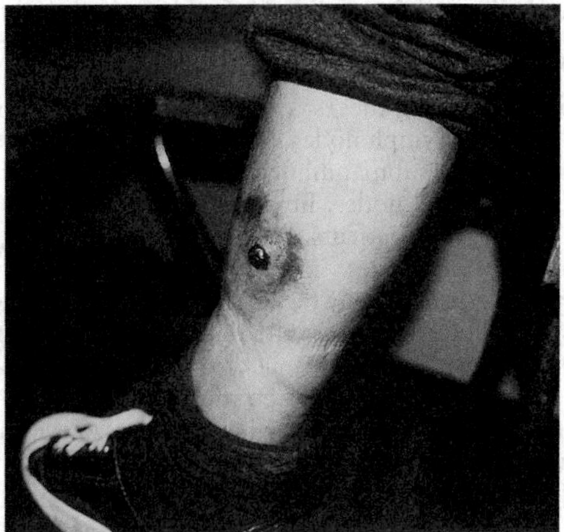

Figure 206-1. A single large lesion of verruca peruana on the leg of an inhabitant of the Peruvian Andes. Such lesions are prone to superficial ulceration, and copious bleeding may occur as a result of their vascular nature. Ecchymosis of the skin surrounding the lesion is also evident. (Courtesy of Dr. J.M. Crutcher, Oklahoma State Department of Health, Oklahoma City.)

Occasional cases of CSD may be caused by other organisms; 1 report described a veterinarian with CSD caused by *B. clarridgeiae*.

EPIDEMIOLOGY. CSD is common, with more than 24,000 estimated cases per year in the United States. It is transmitted by cutaneous inoculation. Most (87–99%) patients have had contact with cats, many of which are kittens <6 mo of age, and >50% have a definite history of a cat scratch or bite. Cats have a high-level *Bartonella* bacteremia for months without any clinical symptoms; kittens are more frequently bacteremic than adult cats. The precise mechanism of cat-to-human transmission remains unclear. Transmission between cats is arthropod borne by the cat flea, *Ctenocephalides felis*. In temperate zones, the majority of cases occur between September and March. This may be related to the seasonal breeding of domestic cats or to close proximity to family pets in the fall and winter. In tropical zones, there is no seasonal prevalence. Distribution is worldwide, and infection occurs in all races.

Cat scratches appear to be more common among children, and boys are affected more often than girls. CSD is a sporadic illness; only 1 family member usually is affected, even though many siblings play with the same kitten. However, clusters do occur with family cases within weeks of one another. Anecdotal reports have implicated other sources such as dog scratches, wood splinters, fishhooks, cactus spines, and porcupine quills.

PATHOGENESIS. The pathologic findings in the primary inoculation **papule** and affected lymph nodes are similar. Both show a central avascular necrotic area with surrounding lymphocytes, giant cells, and histiocytes. Three stages of involvement occur in affected nodes, although they may coexist in the same node. First is generalized enlargement with thickening of the cortex and germinal center hypertrophy. Lymphocytes predominate. Epithelioid granulomas with Langhans giant cells are scattered throughout the node. In the middle stage, granulomas become denser, fuse, and become infiltrated with polymorphonuclear leukocytes. Central necrosis of these granulomas begins in this stage, progressing to the last stage with formation of large pus-filled sinuses. This purulent material may rupture into surrounding tissue. Similar granulomas have been found in the liver and osteolytic lesions of bone when those organs are involved.

CLINICAL MANIFESTATIONS. After an incubation period of 7–12 days (range 3–30 days), 1 or more 3–5 mm red papules develop at the site of cutaneous inoculation, often reflecting a linear cat scratch. Because of their small size, these lesions are often overlooked but with careful search are found in at least $^2/_3$ of patients (Fig. 206-2). Lymphadenopathy generally is evident within a period of 1–4 wk (Fig. 206-3). Chronic regional lymphadenitis is the hallmark, affecting the 1st or 2nd set of nodes draining the entry site. Affected lymph nodes in order of frequency include the axillary, cervical, submandibular, preauricular, epitrochlear, femoral, and inguinal nodes. Involvement of more than 1 group occurs in 10–20% of patients, although at a given site, half the cases involve several nodes.

Nodes involved are usually tender and have overlying erythema but without cellulitis. They usually range between 1 and 5 cm in size, although they can become much larger. Between 10 and 40% eventually suppurate. The duration of enlargement is usually 1–2 mo, with persistence up to 1 yr in rare cases. Fever, usually a temperature of 38–39°C, occurs in about 30% of patients. Other nonspecific symptoms, including malaise, anorexia, fatigue, and headache, affect less than $^1/_3$ of patients. Transient rashes may occur in about 5% of patients. These consist mainly of truncal maculopapular rashes; erythema nodosum, erythema multiforme, and erythema annulare are also reported.

The most common atypical presentation, noted in 2–17% of patients, is **Parinaud oculoglandular syndrome,** which is unilateral conjunctivitis followed by preauricular lymphadenopathy (Fig. 206-4). Direct eye inoculation as a result of rubbing with the hands after cat contact is the presumed mode of spread. A conjunctival granuloma may be found at the inoculation site. The involved eye is usually not painful and has little or no discharge, but it may be quite red and swollen. Submandibular or cervical lymphadenopathy may also occur. CSD is usually a self-limited infection with spontaneous resolution within a few weeks to months.

More severe, disseminated illness occurs in a small percentage of patients. These patients present with high fever often persisting for several weeks. Although systemic symptoms are usually more pronounced than with isolated lymphadenitis, they often seem mild relative to fever, the exception being abdominal pain and weight loss, both of which can be dramatic. **Hepatosplenomegaly** may occur, although hepatic dysfunction is rare (Fig. 206-5). Granulomatous changes may be seen in the liver and spleen. Another common site of dissemination is bone, with the development of **granulomatous osteolytic lesions.** These are usually associated with localized pain, without erythema, tenderness, or swelling. Other uncommon manifestations include

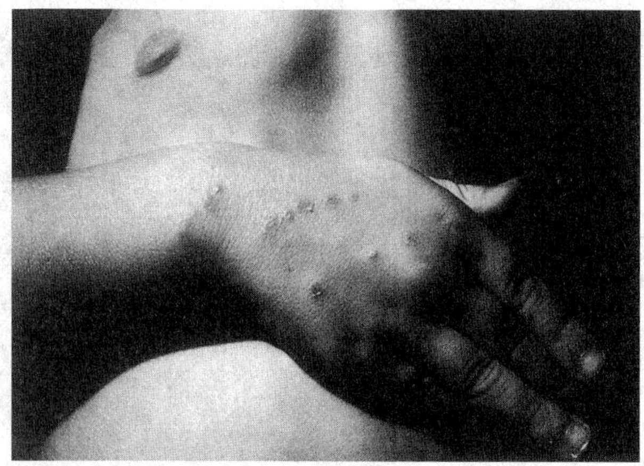

Figure 206-2. A child with typical cat scratch disease demonstrating the original scratch injuries and the primary papule that soon thereafter developed proximal to the middle finger. (Courtesy of Dr. V.H. San Joaquin, University of Oklahoma Health Sciences Center, Oklahoma City.)

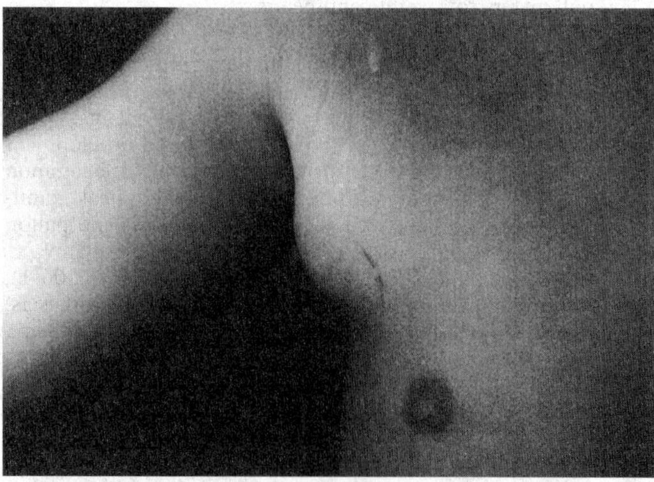

Figure 206-3. Right axillary lymphadenopathy followed the scratches and development of a primary papule in this child with typical cat scratch disease, also shown in Fig. 206-2. (From Mandell GL, Bennett JE, Dolin R [editors]: *Principles and Practice of Infectious Diseases,* 6th ed, Vol 2. Philadelphia, Elsevier, 2006, p 2737.)

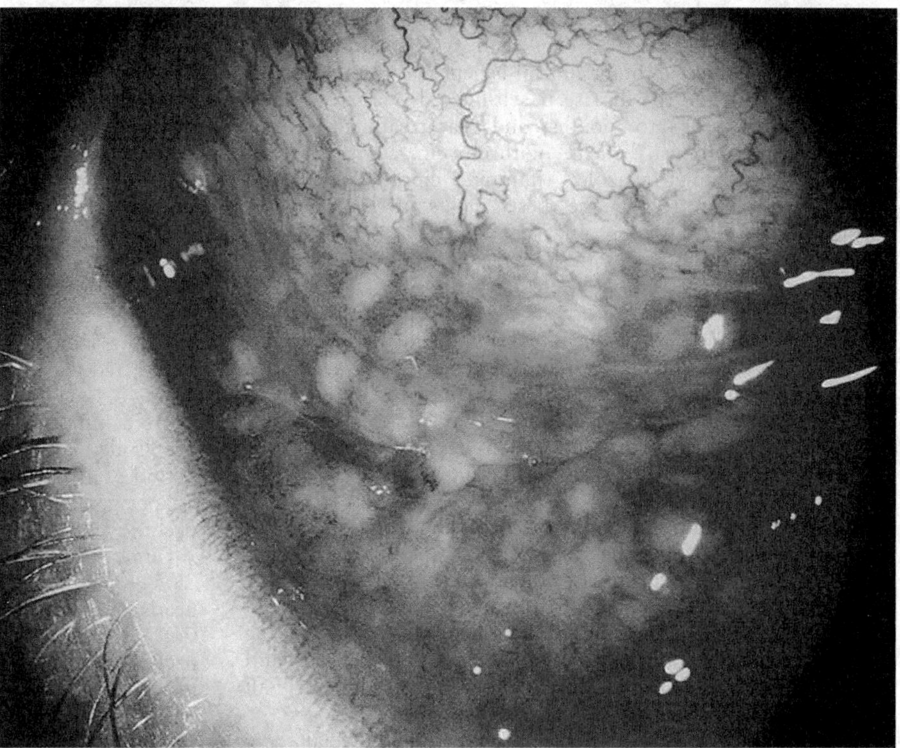

Figure 206-4. The granulomatous conjunctivitis of Parinaud oculoglandular syndrome is associated with ipsilateral local lymphadenopathy, usually preauricular and less commonly submandibular. (From Mandell GL, Bennett JE, Dolin R [editors]: *Principles and Practice of Infectious Diseases,* 6th ed, Vol 2. Philadelphia, Elsevier, 2006, p 2739.)

neuroretinitis with papilledema and stellate macular exudates, encephalitis, fever of unknown origin, and atypical pneumonia.

DIAGNOSIS. In most cases, the diagnosis can be strongly suspected on clinical grounds with the history of exposure to a cat. The Centers for Disease Control and Prevention has developed an indirect immunofluorescent assay (IFA) that has shown good correlation with disease. Other IFA and enzyme-linked immunoassay tests are commercially available, although little comparative data are available. Most patients have elevated antibody titers at presentation; however, the timing of immunoglobulin G (IgG) and IgM response to *B. henselae* can be quite variable. There is cross reactivity among *Bartonella* species, particularly *B. henselae* and *B. quintana.*

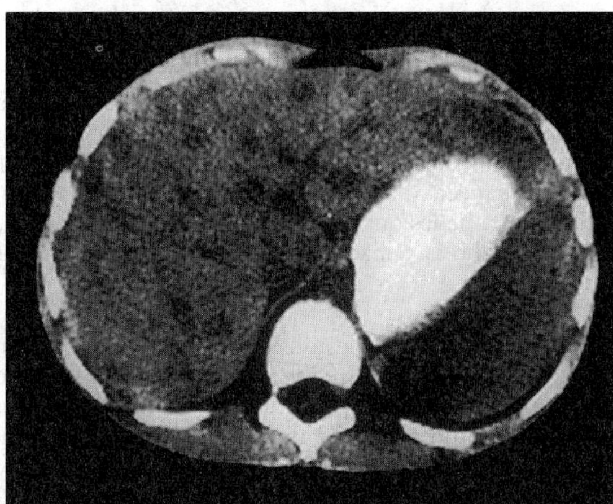

Figure 206-5. In this CT image of a patient with hepatic involvement of cat scratch disease, the absence of enhancement of the multiple lesions after contrast infusion is consistent with the granulomatous inflammation of this entity. Treated empirically with various antibiotics without improvement before establishment of this diagnosis, the patient subsequently recovered fully with no further antimicrobial therapy. (Courtesy of Dr. V.H. San Joaquin, University of Oklahoma Health Sciences Center, Oklahoma City.)

If tissue specimens are obtained, bacilli may be visualized with Warthin-Starry and Brown-Hopp tissue Gram stains. *Bartonella* DNA can be identified by PCR on tissue specimens. Culturing of the organism is not practical for clinical diagnosis.

Use of a skin test antigen prepared by heat-treating purulent aspirate from a CSD node is strongly discouraged because of lack of standardization and potential transmission of infectious agents.

Differential Diagnosis. The differential diagnosis of CSD includes virtually all causes of lymphadenopathy (see Chapter 490). The more common entities include pyogenic lymphadenitis, primarily from staphylococcal or streptococcal infections, atypical mycobacterial infections, and malignancy. Less common entities include tularemia, brucellosis, or sporotrichosis. Epstein-Barr virus, cytomegalovirus, or *Toxoplasma gondii* infections usually cause more generalized lymphadenopathy.

LABORATORY FINDINGS. Routine laboratory tests are not helpful. The erythrocyte sedimentation rate is often elevated. The white blood cell count may be normal or mildly elevated. Hepatic transaminases may be elevated in systemic disease. Ultrasonography or CT may reveal many granulomatous nodules in the liver and spleen, appearing as hypodense round irregular lesions.

TREATMENT. Antibiotic treatment of CSD is not always needed and is not clearly beneficial. For most patients, treatment consists of conservative symptomatic care and observation. Studies show a significant discordance between in vitro activity of antibiotics and clinical effectiveness. For many patients, diagnosis is considered in the context of failure to respond to β-lactam antibiotic treatment of presumed staphylococcal lymphadenitis.

A small prospective study of oral azithromycin (500 mg on day 1, then 250 mg on days 2–5; for smaller children, 10 mg/kg/24 hr on day 1 and 5 mg/kg/24 hr on days 2–5) showed a decrease in initial lymph node volume in 50% of patients during the 1st 30 days, but after 30 days there was no difference in lymph node volume. No other clinical benefit was found. For the majority of patients, the disease is self-limited, with resolution occurring over weeks to months, and that treatment affords minimal, if any, clinical benefit. Azithromycin, clarithromycin, trimethoprim-sulfamethoxazole, rifampin, ciprofloxacin, and gentamicin appear to be the best agents if treatment is considered.

Suppurative lymph nodes that become tense and extremely painful should be drained by needle aspiration, which may need to be repeated. Incision and drainage of nonsuppurative nodes should be avoided because chronic draining sinuses may result. Surgical excision of the node rarely is necessary.

Children with hepatosplenic CSD appear to respond well to rifampin, either alone or in combination with trimethoprim-sulfamethoxazole. These patients usually receive rifampin at a dose of 20 mg/kg for 14 days.

COMPLICATIONS. **Encephalopathy** can occur in as many as 5% of patients, typically occurring 1–3 wk after the onset of lymphadenitis with the sudden onset of neurologic symptoms, which often include seizures, combative or bizarre behavior, and altered level of consciousness. Imaging studies are generally normal. The cerebrospinal fluid is normal or shows minimal pleocytosis and protein elevation. Recovery occurs without sequelae in nearly all patients but takes place slowly over many months.

Other neurologic manifestations include peripheral facial nerve paralysis, myelitis, radiculitis, compression neuropathy, and cerebellar ataxia. One patient with encephalopathy with persistent cognitive impairment and memory loss has been reported.

Stellate macular retinopathy has been associated with several infections, including CSD. Children and young adults present with unilateral or rarely bilateral loss of vision with central scotoma, optic disc swelling, and macular star formation from exudates radiating out from the macula. The findings usually resolve completely, with recovery of vision, usually within 2–3 mo. The optimal treatment for the neuroretinitis is unknown, although adults have been treated with doxycycline and rifampin for 4 to 6 weeks with good results.

Hematologic manifestations include hemolytic anemia, thrombocytopenic purpura, nonthrombocytopenic purpura, and eosinophilia. **Leukocytoclastic vasculitis** similar to Henoch-Schönlein purpura has been reported in association with CSD in 1 child. A systemic presentation of CSD with pleurisy, arthralgia or arthritis, mediastinal masses, enlarged nodes at the head of the pancreas, and atypical pneumonia also has been reported.

PROGNOSIS. The prognosis for CSD in a normal host is generally excellent, with resolution of clinical findings over several months. Recovery occasionally is slower and may take as long as a year.

PREVENTION. Person-to-person spread of *Bartonella* infections is not known. Isolation is not necessary. Prevention would require elimination of cats from households, which is not practical or necessarily desirable. Awareness of the risk of cat (and particularly kitten) scratches should be emphasized to parents.

206.3 • Trench Fever *(Bartonella Quintana)*

ETIOLOGY. The causative agent of trench fever was first designated as *Rickettsia quintana,* then assigned to the genus *Rochalimaea,* which has been reassigned as *B. quintana.*

EPIDEMIOLOGY. Trench fever was first recognized as a distinct clinical entity during World War I, when more than a million troops in the trenches were infected. The disease became quiescent until World War II, when it again was epidemic. It is extremely rare in the United States.

Humans are the only known reservoir. No other animal is naturally infected, nor are the usual laboratory animals susceptible. The human **body louse,** *Pediculus humanus* var. *corporis,* is the vector, capable of transmission to a new host 5–6 days after feeding on an infected person. Lice excrete the organism for life; transovarian passage does not occur. Humans may have prolonged asymptomatic bacteremia for years.

CLINICAL MANIFESTATIONS. The incubation period averages about 22 days (range 4–35 days). The clinical presentation is highly variable. Symptoms can be very mild and brief. About half of infected persons have a single febrile illness with abrupt onset lasting 3–6 days. In others, prolonged, sustained fever may occur. More commonly, patients have periodic febrile illness with 3 to 8 episodes lasting 4–5 days each, sometimes occurring over a period of a year or more. This form is reminiscent of malaria or relapsing fever *(Borrelia recurrentis).* Afebrile bacteremia can occur.

Clinical findings usually include fever (usually temperature of 38.5–40°C), malaise, chills, sweats, anorexia, and severe headache. Common findings include marked conjunctival injection, tachycardia, myalgias, arthralgias, and severe pain in the neck, back, and legs. **Crops of erythematous macules** or **papules** may occur on the trunk in as many as 80% of patients. Splenomegaly and mild liver enlargement may be noted.

DIAGNOSIS. In nonepidemic situations, it is impossible to establish a diagnosis of trench fever on clinical grounds because the findings are not distinctive. A history of body louse infection or having been in an area of epidemic disease should heighten suspicions. *B. quintana* can be cultured from the blood with modification to include culture on epithelial cells. Serologic tests for *B. quintana* are available, but there is cross reaction with *B. henselae.*

TREATMENT. There are no controlled trials of treatment; patients with trench fever have responded dramatically to tetracycline and chloramphenicol with rapid defervescence.

206.4 • Bacillary Angiomatosis and Bacillary Peliosis Hepatis *(Bartonella Henselae and Bartonella Quintana)*

Both *B. henselae* and *B. quintana* cause 2 vascular proliferative diseases, **bacillary angiomatosis (BA)** and **bacillary peliosis,** in severely immunocompromised persons, primarily adult patients with AIDS or cancer and organ transplant recipients. Subcutaneous and lytic bone lesions are strongly associated with *B. quintana,* whereas peliosis hepatis is associated exclusively with *B. henselae.*

BACILLARY ANGIOMATOSIS. Lesions of cutaneous BA, also known as epithelioid angiomatosis, are the most easily identified and recognized form of *Bartonella* infection in immunocompromised hosts. They are found primarily in patients with AIDS with very low CD4 counts. The clinical appearance can be quite diverse. The vasoproliferative lesions of BA may be cutaneous or subcutaneous and resemble the vascular lesions (verruca peruana) of *B. bacilliformis* in immunocompetent persons. They are erythematous papules on an erythematous base with a collarette of scale. They may enlarge to form large pedunculated lesions. Ulceration may occur, as may profuse bleeding after trauma.

BA may be clinically indistinguishable from Kaposi sarcoma. Other considerations in the differential diagnosis are pyogenic granuloma and verruca peruana *(B. bacilliformis)*. Deep soft tissue masses caused by BA may mimic a malignancy.

Osseous BA lesions commonly involve the long bones. These lytic lesions are very painful and highly vascular. Occasionally found is an erythematous plaque over the lesion. The high degree of vascularity, which produces a very positive result on a technetium-99m methylene diphosphonate bone scan, resembles a malignant lesion.

Lesions can be found in virtually any organ, producing similar vascular proliferative lesions. They may appear raised, nodular, or ulcerative when seen on endoscopy or bronchoscopy. They may be associated with enlarged lymph nodes with or without an obvious local cutaneous lesion. Lesions in 1 brain parenchyma have been described.

BACILLARY PELIOSIS. Bacillary peliosis affects the reticuloendothelial system, primarily the liver (**peliosis hepatis**) and less frequently the spleen and lymph nodes. It is a vasoproliferative disorder characterized by random proliferation of venous lakes surrounded by fibromyxoid stroma harboring numerous bacillary organisms. Clinical findings include fever and abdominal pain in association with abnormal results of liver function tests, particularly a markedly increased alkaline phosphatase level. Cutaneous BA or splenomegaly may be associated, with or without thrombocytopenia or pancytopenia. The vascular proliferative lesions in the liver and spleen appear on CT scan as hypodense lesions scattered throughout the parenchyma. The differential diagnosis includes hepatic Kaposi sarcoma, lymphoma, and disseminated infection with *Pneumocystis carinii* or *Mycobacterium avium* complex.

BACTEREMIA AND ENDOCARDITIS. *B. henselae, B. quintana,* and *B. elizabethae* all have been reported to cause bacteremia or endocarditis. They are associated with symptoms of prolonged fevers, night sweats, and profound weight loss. A cluster of cases in Seattle in 1993 occurred in a homeless population with chronic alcoholism. These patients with high fever or hypothermia were thought to represent "urban trench fever," but no body louse infestation was associated. Some cases of culture-negative endocarditis may represent *Bartonella* endocarditis. One report described central nervous system involvement with *B. quintana* in 2 children.

DIAGNOSIS. Diagnosis of BA is made initially by biopsy. The characteristic small vessel proliferation with mixed inflammatory response and the staining of bacilli by Warthin-Starry silver staining distinguish it from pyogenic granuloma or Kaposi sarcoma (see Chapter 254). Travel history can usually preclude verruca peruana.

Culture is impractical for CSD but is the diagnostic procedure for suspected bacteremia or endocarditis. Use of the lysis-centrifugation technique or fresh chocolate or heart infusion agar with 5% rabbit blood with prolonged incubation may increase the yield of culture. PCR also can be a useful tool.

TREATMENT. *Bartonella* infections in immunocompromised hosts caused by both *B. henselae* and *B. quintana* have been treated successfully with antimicrobial agents. BA responds rapidly to erythromycin, azithromycin, or clarithromycin, which are the drugs of choice. Alternative choices are doxycycline or tetracycline. Severely ill patients with peliosis hepatis, endocarditis, or osteomyelitis may be treated initially with intravenous erythromycin or doxycycline with the addition of rifampin or gentamicin. The use of an aminoglycoside for a minimum of 2 wk is associated with improved prognosis in endocarditis. A Jarisch-Herxheimer reaction may occur. Relapses may follow; prolonged treatment for several months may be necessary.

PREVENTION. Immunocompromised persons should consider the potential risks of cat ownership because of the risks for *Bartonella* infections, as well as toxoplasmosis and enteric infections. Those who elect to obtain a cat should adopt or purchase a cat >1 yr of age and in good health. Prompt washing of any wounds from cat bites or scratches is essential.

Arisoy ES, Correa AG, Wagner ML et al: Hepatosplenic cat-scratch disease in children: Selected clinical features and treatment. *Clin Infect Dis* 1999;28:778–784.

Bass JW, Freitas BC, Freitas AD, et al: Prospective randomized double blind placebo-controlled evaluation of azithromycin for treatment of cat-scratch disease. *Pediatr Infect Dis J* 1998;17:447–452.

Bass JW, Vincent JM, Person DA: The expanding spectrum of Bartonella infections: I. Bartonellosis and trench fever. *Pediatr Infect Dis J* 1997;16:2–10.

Bass JW, Vincent JM, Person DA: The expanding spectrum of Bartonella infections: II. Cat scratch disease. *Pediatr Infect Dis J* 1997;16:163–179.

Batts S, Demers DM: Spectrum and treatment of cat-scratch disease. *Pediatr Infect Dis J* 2004;23:1161–1162.

Bryant K, Marshall GS: Hepatosplenic cat scratch disease treated with corticosteroids. *Arch Dis Child* 2003;88:345–346.

Carithers HA, Margileth AM: Cat scratch disease: Acute encephalopathy and other neurologic manifestations. *Am J Dis Child* 1991;145:98–101.

Fournier PE, Lelievre H, Ekyn SJ, et al: Epidemiologic and clinical characteristics of *Bartonella quintana* and *Bartonella henselae* endocarditis: A study of 48 patients. *Medicine* 2001;80:245–251.

Fretzayas A, Papadopoulos NG, Moustaki M, et al: Unsuspected extralymphocutaneous dissemination in febrile cat scratch disease. *Scand J Infect Dis* 2001;33:599–603.

Jacobs R, Schutze G: *Bartonella henselae* as a cause of prolonged fever and fever of unknown origin in children. *Clin Infect Dis* 1998;26:80–84.

Maguiña C, Garcia P, Gotuzzo E, et al: Bartonellosis (Carrión's disease) in the modern era. *Clin Infect Dis* 2001;33:772–779.

Maguiña C, Gotuzzo E: Bartonellosis: New and old. *Infect Dis Clin North Am* 2000;14:1–22.

Metzkor-Cotter E, Kletter Y, Avidor B, et al: Long-term serological analysis and clinical follow-up of patients with cat scratch disease. *Clin Infect Dis* 2003;37:1149–1154.

Ormerod LD, Dailey JP: Ocular manifestations of cat-scratch disease. *Curr Opin Ophthalmol* 1999;10:209–216.

Raoult D, Fournier PE, Vandenesch F, et al: Outcome and treatment of *Bartonella* endocarditis [Original Investigation]. *Arch Intern Med* 2003;163(2):226–230.

Vermeulen MJ, Rutten GJ, Verhagen I, et al: Transient paresis associated with cat-scratch disease. Case report and literature review of vertebral osteomyelitis caused by *Bartonella henselae*. *Pediatr Infect Dis J* 2006;25:1177–1181.

Section 6 — Anaerobic Bacterial Infections

Chapter 207 ■ Botulism *(Clostridium Botulinum)* Stephen S. Arnon

Three naturally occurring forms of human botulism are known: infant (intestinal toxemia) botulism (the most common in the United States), food-borne (classic) botulism, and wound botulism. Two other forms, both manmade, also occur: inhalational botulism from inhaling accidentally aerosolized toxin, and iatrogenic botulism from overdosage of therapeutic or cosmetic use of botulinum toxin.

ETIOLOGY. Botulism is the acute, flaccid paralysis caused by the neurotoxin produced by *Clostridium botulinum* or, rarely, an equivalent neurotoxin produced by atypical strains of *Clostridium butyricum* and *Clostridium baratii. C. botulinum* is a gram-positive, spore-forming, obligate anaerobe whose natural habitat worldwide is soil, dust, and marine sediments. It is found in a wide variety of fresh and cooked agricultural products. Spores of some *C. botulinum* strains endure boiling for several hours, which enables the organism to survive efforts at food preservation. In contrast, botulinum toxin is heat labile and easily destroyed by heating at ≥85°C for 5 min. Neurotoxigenic *C. butyricum* has been isolated from a soybean food and from soils near Lake Weishan in China, the site of food-borne botulism outbreaks associated with this organism. Little is known about the ecology of neurotoxigenic *C. baratii.*

Botulinum toxin is a simple di-chain protein consisting of a 100 kd heavy chain that contains the neuronal attachment sites and a 50 kd light chain that is taken into the cell after binding. Botulinum toxin is the most poisonous substance known, the parenteral human lethal dose being estimated at 10^{-6} mg/kg. The toxin blocks neuromuscular transmission and causes death through airway and respiratory muscle paralysis. Seven antigenic toxin types, designated by letters A–G, are distinguished by the inability of neutralizing antibody against 1 toxin type to protect against a different toxin type. The 7 toxin types serve as convenient clinical and epidemiologic markers. Toxin types A, B, E, and F are well-established causes of human botulism, whereas types C and D cause illness in other animals. Neurotoxigenic *C. butyricum* strains produce a type E toxin, whereas neurotoxigenic *C. baratii* strains produce a type F toxin. Type G has not been established as a cause of either human or animal disease. The phenomenal potency is explained by the fact that its 7 light chains are zinc-endopeptidases, whose substrates are 1 or 2 of 3 proteins of the docking complex by which synaptic vesicles fuse with the terminal cell membrane and release acetylcholine into the synaptic cleft.

EPIDEMIOLOGY. Infant botulism has been reported from all inhabited continents except Africa. Notably, the infant is the only family member who is ill. The most striking epidemiologic feature of infant botulism is its age distribution, in which in 95% of cases the infants are between 3 wk and 6 mo of age, with a broad peak from 2 to 4 mo of age. Cases in infants as young as 1.5 days or as old as 382 days at onset have been recognized. The male : female ratio of cases is 1 : 1, and cases have occurred in most racial and ethnic groups.

Infant botulism is an uncommon and often unrecognized illness. In the USA, about 80–100 cases are diagnosed annually; more than 2,400 cases were reported from 1976 to 2005. Approximately 40% of U.S. cases were reported from California. Consistent with the known asymmetric soil distribution of *C. botulinum* toxin types, most cases west of the Mississippi River have been caused by type A strains, and most cases east of the Mississippi River have been caused by type B strains. One case in each in the states of New Mexico, Washington, Ohio, California, and Iowa have been caused by *C. baratii* and type F toxin, and cases in Italy resulted from *C. butyricum* and type E toxin. Identified risk factors for the illness include breast-feeding, the ingestion of honey, and a slow intestinal transit time (<1 stool/day). Breast-feeding may provide protection against fulminant sudden death from infant botulism. Under rare circumstances of altered intestinal anatomy, physiology, and microflora, older children and adults may contract infant-type botulism.

Food-borne botulism results from the ingestion of a food in which *C. botulinum* has multiplied and produced its toxin. Outbreaks in North America have been associated with baked potatoes, sautéed onions, and chopped garlic served in restaurants; these have revised the traditional view of food-borne botulism as resulting mainly from home-canned foods. Other outbreaks in the United States have occurred from commercial foods sealed in plastic pouches that relied solely on refrigeration to prevent outgrowth of *C. botulinum* spores. Uncanned foods responsible for food-borne botulism cases include peyote tea, the hazelnut flavoring added to yogurt, sweet cream cheese, sautéed onions in "patty melt" sandwiches, potato salad, and fresh and dried fish. A trend toward a single case per outbreak or of cases presenting separately in different cities or hospitals portends that physicians cannot rely on the temporal and geographic clustering of cases to suggest the diagnosis.

Most preserved foods have been implicated in food-borne botulism, but the usual offenders in the United States are the "low-acid" (pH ≥6.0) home-canned foods such as jalapeño peppers, asparagus, olives, and beans. The potential for food-borne botulism exists throughout the world, but outbreaks occur most commonly in the temperate zones rather than the tropics, where preservation of fruits, vegetables, and other foods is less common.

In the past 15 yr, approximately 5–10 outbreaks and 20–25 cases of food-borne botulism have occurred annually in the United States. Most of the continental United States outbreaks resulted from proteolytic type A or type B strains, which produce a strongly putrefactive odor in the food that some people find necessary to verify by tasting. In contrast, in Alaska and Canada, most food-borne outbreaks have resulted from nonproteolytic type E strains in Native American foods, such as fermented salmon eggs and seal flippers, which do not exhibit signs of spoilage. A further hazard of type E strains is their ability to grow at the temperatures (5°C) maintained by household refrigerators.

Wound botulism is an exceptionally rare disease, with <350 cases reported worldwide, but it is important to pediatrics because adolescents and children may be affected. Although many cases have occurred in young, physically active males at greatest risk for traumatic injury, wound botulism also occurs with crush injuries in which no break in the skin is evident. In the past 15 yr, wound botulism from injection has become increasingly common in adult heroin abusers in the western United States and in Europe, not always with evident abscess formation or cellulitis.

A single outbreak of inhalational botulism was reported in 1962 in which 3 laboratory workers in Germany were exposed unintentionally to aerosolized botulinum toxin. Some patients in the United States have been hospitalized by accidental overdose of therapeutic or cosmetic botulinum toxin.

PATHOGENESIS. All forms of botulism produce disease through a final common pathway. Botulinum toxin is carried by the bloodstream to peripheral cholinergic synapses, where it binds irreversibly, blocking acetylcholine release and causing impaired neuromuscular and autonomic transmission. Infant botulism is an infectious disease that results from ingesting the spores of any of the 3 botulinum toxin–producing clostridial strains, with subsequent spore germination, multiplication, and production of botulinum toxin in the large intestine. Food-borne botulism is an intoxication that results when preformed botulinum toxin contained in an improperly preserved or inadequately cooked food is swallowed. Wound botulism results from spore germination and colonization of traumatized tissue by *C. botulinum;* it is the analog of tetanus. Inhalational botulism occurs when aerosolized botulinum toxin is inhaled. A bioterrorist attack could result in large or small outbreaks of inhalational or food-borne botulism (see Chapter 711).

Botulinum toxin is not a cytotoxin and does not causes overt macroscopic or microscopic pathology. Secondary pathologic changes (pneumonia, petechiae on intrathoracic organs) may be found at autopsy. No diagnostic technique is available to identify botulinum toxin bound at the neuromuscular junction. The healing process in botulism consists of sprouting of new terminal unmyelinated motor neurons. Movement resumes when these new twigs locate noncontracting muscle fibers and reinnervate them by inducing formation of a new motor end plate. In experimental animals, this process takes about 4 wk.

CLINICAL MANIFESTATIONS. Botulinum toxin is distributed hematogenously. Because relative blood flow and density of innervation are greatest in the bulbar musculature, all forms of botulism manifest neurologically as a symmetric, descending, flaccid paralysis beginning with the cranial nerve musculature. It is not possible to have botulism without having multiple bulbar palsies, yet in infants such symptoms as poor feeding, weak suck, feeble cry, drooling, and even obstructive apnea are often not recognized as bulbar in origin (Fig. 207-1). Patients with evolving illness may already have generalized weakness and hypotonia in addition to bulbar palsies when first examined. In contrast to botulism caused by *C. botulinum,* a majority of the rare cases caused by intestinal colonization with *C. butyricum* are associated with a Meckel diverticulum accompanying abdominal distention, often leading to misdiagnosis as an acute abdomen. The also rare *C. baratii* type F infant botulism cases have been characterized by very young age at onset, rapidity of onset, and greater severity of paralysis.

In older children with **food-borne** or **wound botulism,** the onset of neurologic symptoms follows a characteristic pattern of diplopia, blurred vision, ptosis, dry mouth, dysphagia, dysphonia, and dysarthria, with deceased gag and corneal reflexes. Importantly, because the toxin acts only on motor nerves, paresthesias are not seen in botulism, except when a patient hyperventilates from anxiety. The sensorium remains clear, but this may be difficult to ascertain because of the slurred speech.

Food-borne botulism begins with gastrointestinal symptoms of nausea, vomiting, or diarrhea in about $^1/_3$ of cases. These symptoms are thought to result from metabolic by-products of growth of *C. botulinum* or from the presence of other toxic contaminants in the food, because gastrointestinal distress is rarely observed in wound botulism. Constipation may occur in food-borne botulism once flaccid paralysis becomes evident. Illness usually begins 12–36 hr after ingestion of the contaminated food but can range from as little as 2 hr to as long as 8 days. The incubation period in wound botulism is 4–14 days. Fever may be present in wound botulism but is absent in food-borne botulism unless a secondary infection (pneumonia) is present. All forms of botulism display a

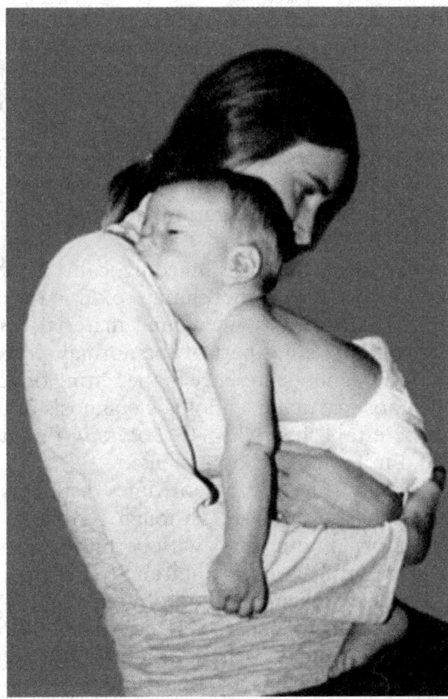

Figure 207-1. A 3 mo old infant with mild infant botulism showing signs of ptosis, an expressionless face, and hypotonia of the neck, trunk, and limbs. The additional bulbar palsies of ophthalmoplegia, weak cry, weak sucking, and dysphagia (drooling) are not apparent in the photograph. (From Arnon SS, Schechter R, Maslanka SE, et al: Human botulism immune globulin for the treatment of infant botulism. *N Engl J Med* 2006;354:462–471.)

wide spectrum in their clinical severity, from the very mild with minimal ptosis, flattened facial expression, minor dysphagia, and dysphonia, to the fulminant with rapid onset of extensive paralysis, frank apnea, and fixed, dilated pupils. Fatigability with repetitive muscle activity is the clinical hallmark of botulism.

Infant botulism differs in apparent initial symptoms of illness only because the infant cannot verbalize them. Usually, the 1st indication of illness is a decreased frequency or even absence of defecation, although this sign is frequently overlooked. Parents typically notice inability to feed, lethargy, weak cry, and diminished spontaneous movement. Dysphagia may be evident as secretions drooling from the mouth. Gag, suck, and corneal reflexes diminish as the paralysis advances. Oculomotor palsies may be evident only with sustained observation. Paradoxically, the pupillary light reflex may be unaffected until the child is severely paralyzed, or it may be initially sluggish. Loss of head control is typically a prominent sign. Respiratory arrest may occur suddenly from airway occlusion by unswallowed secretions or from obstructive flaccid pharyngeal musculature. Occasionally, the diagnosis of infant botulism is suggested by a respiratory arrest that occurs after the infant is curled into position for lumbar puncture.

In mild cases or in the early stages of illness, the physical signs of infant botulism may be subtle and easily missed. Eliciting cranial nerve palsies and fatigability of muscular function requires careful examination. Ptosis may not be seen unless the head of the child is kept erect.

DIAGNOSIS. Clinical diagnosis of botulism is confirmed by specialized laboratory testing that requires hours to days to complete. Therefore, clinical diagnosis is the foundation for early recognition of and response to all forms of botulism. Routine laboratory studies, including those of the cerebrospinal fluid (CSF), are normal in botulism unless dehydration, undernourishment (metabolic acidosis and ketosis), or secondary infection is present.

The **classic triad of botulism** is the acute onset of a symmetric flaccid descending paralysis with clear sensorium, no fever, and no paresthesias. Suspected botulism represents a medical and public health emergency that is immediately reportable by telephone in most U.S. health jurisdictions. State health departments (1st call) and the Centers for Disease Control and Prevention (telephone 770–488–7100 at any time) can arrange for diagnostic testing, epidemiologic investigation, and provision of equine antitoxin.

The diagnosis of botulism is unequivocally established by demonstrating the presence of botulinum toxin in serum or of *C. botulinum* toxin or organisms in wound material, enema fluid, or feces. *C. botulinum* is not part of the normal resident intestinal flora of humans, and its presence in the setting of acute flaccid paralysis is diagnostic. An epidemiologic diagnosis of food-borne botulism can be established when *C. botulinum* organisms and toxin are found in food eaten by patients.

Electromyography (EMG) can sometimes distinguish between causes of acute flaccid paralysis, although results may be variable, including normal, in patients with botulism. The distinctive EMG finding in botulism is facilitation (potentiation) of the evoked muscle action potential at high-frequency (50 Hz) stimulation. In infant botulism, a characteristic pattern, known by the acronym **BSAP** (brief, small, abundant motor unit action potentials), is present only in clinically weak muscles. Nerve conduction velocity and sensory nerve function are normal in botulism.

Infant botulism requires a high index of suspicion for early diagnosis (Table 207-1). "Rule-out sepsis" remains the most common admission diagnosis. If a previously healthy infant, commonly 2–4 mo of age, develops weakness with difficulty in sucking, swallowing, crying, or breathing, infant botulism should be considered a likely diagnosis. A careful cranial nerve examination is then very helpful.

Differential Diagnosis. Botulism is frequently misdiagnosed, most often as a polyradiculoneuropathy (Guillain-Barré or Miller Fisher syndrome), myasthenia gravis, or a disease of the central nervous system (Tables 207-1 and 207-2). In the United States, botulism is more likely than Guillain-Barré syndrome, intoxication, or poliomyelitis to cause a cluster of cases of acute flaccid paralysis. Botulism differs from other flaccid paralyses in its prominent cranial nerve palsies disproportionate to milder weakness and hypotonia below the neck, in its symmetry, and in its absence of sensory nerve damage. Spinal muscular atrophy may closely mimic infant botulism at presentation.

Additional diagnostic procedures may be useful in rapidly excluding botulism as the cause of paralysis. The CSF is unchanged in botulism but is abnormal in many central nervous system diseases. Although the CSF protein level eventually is elevated in Guillain-Barré syndrome, it may be normal early in illness. Imaging of the brain, spine, and chest may reveal hemorrhage, inflammation, or neoplasm. A test dose of edrophonium chloride briefly reverses paralytic symptoms in many patients with myasthenia gravis and, reportedly, in some with botulism. A close inspection of the skin, especially the scalp, may reveal an attached tick that is causing paralysis. Possible organophosphate intoxication should be pursued aggressively because specific antidotes (oximes) are available and because the patient may be part of a commonly exposed group, some of whom have yet to develop illness. Other tests that require days for results include stool culture for *Campylobacter jejuni* as a precipitant of Guillain-Barré syndrome, spinal muscular atrophy and other genetic (including mitochondrial) disorders, and assays for the autoantibodies that cause myasthenia gravis, Lambert-Eaton syndrome, and Guillain-Barré syndrome.

TABLE 207-1. Diagnoses Considered in Infant Botulism

ADMISSION DIAGNOSIS	DIFFERENTIAL DIAGNOSIS
Suspected sepsis, meningitis	Guillain-Barré syndrome
Pneumonia	Myasthenia gravis
Dehydration	Disorders of amino acid metabolism
Viral syndrome	Hypothyroidism
Hypotonia of unknown etiology	Drug ingestion
	Organophosphate poisoning
Constipation	Brainstem encephalitis
Failure to thrive	Heavy metal poisoning (Pb, Mg, As)
Spinal muscular atrophy (Werdnig-Hoffmann disease)	Poliomyelitis
	Viral polyneuritis
	Hirschsprung disease
	Metabolic encephalopathy
	Medium chain acetyl-CoA dehydrogenase (MCAD) deficiency

TABLE 207-2. Diagnoses Considered in Food-borne and Wound Botulism

Acute gastroenteritis	Aminoglycoside-associated paralysis
Myasthenia gravis	Tick paralysis
Guillain-Barré syndrome	Hypocalcemia
Organophosphate poisoning	Hypermagnesemia
Meningitis	Carbon monoxide poisoning
Encephalitis	Hyperemesis gravidarum
Psychiatric illness	Laryngeal trauma
Cerebrovascular accident	Diabetic complications
Poliomyelitis	Inflammatory myopathy
Hypothyroidism	Overexertion

TREATMENT. Human botulism immune globulin (BIG-IV) is licensed for the treatment of infant botulism caused by type A or B botulinum toxin. Treatment with BIG-IV consists of a single intravenous infusion of 50 mg/kg that should be given as soon as possible after infant botulism is suspected. In the USA, BIG-IV may be obtained from the California Department of Health Services (24 hr telephone 510–231–7600; www.infantbotulism.org). In a 5 yr randomized placebo-controlled clinical trial in California, use of BIG-IV shortened mean hospital stay from 5.7 to 2.5 wk; in subsequent nationwide open-label use, comparable mean hospital stay was reduced to 2.0 weeks. Mean hospital costs were reduced by > $100,000 per case (in 2004 dollars).

Older patients with suspected food, wound, or inhalational botulism may be treated with 1 vial of equine botulinum antitoxin, available in the United States through the Centers for Disease Control and Prevention by way of state and local health departments.

Antibiotic therapy is not part of the treatment of uncomplicated infant or food-borne botulism because the toxin is primarily an intracellular molecule that is released into the intestinal lumen with vegetative bacterial cell death and lysis. Antibiotics are reserved for the treatment of secondary infections, and in the absence of antitoxin therapy, a nonclostridiocidal antibiotic such as trimethoprim-sulfamethoxazole is preferred. Aminoglycoside antibiotics should be avoided because they may potentiate the blocking action of botulinum toxin at the neuromuscular junction. Wound botulism requires aggressive treatment with antibiotics and antitoxin in a manner analogous to tetanus (see Chapter 208). The currently licensed botulinum antitoxin used in food-borne and wound botulism is a horse serum–derived product that has adverse effects of serum sickness, anaphylaxis, and potential lifelong sensitization to equine proteins; its use in children requires careful consideration.

SUPPORTIVE CARE. Management of botulism rests on 3 principles: (1) fatigability with repetitive muscle activity is the clinical hallmark of the disease; (2) complications are best avoided by anticipating them; and (3) meticulous supportive care is a necessity. The 1st principle applies mainly to feeding and breathing. *Correct* *positioning is imperative to protect the airway and improve respiratory mechanics.* The patient is placed face up on a rigid-bottomed crib (or bed), the head of which is tilted at 30 degrees. A small cloth roll is placed under the cervical vertebrae to tilt the head back so that secretions drain to the posterior pharynx and away from the airway. In this tilted position, the abdominal viscera pull the diaphragm down, thereby improving respiratory mechanics. The patient's head and torso should not be elevated by bending the middle of the bed; if this is done, the hypotonic thorax will slump into the abdomen and breathing will be compromised.

About half of patients with infant botulism require endotracheal intubation, which is best done prophylactically. The indications include diminished gag and cough reflexes and progressive airway obstruction by secretions. With meticulous management techniques (especially proper tube diameter), monitoring, and positioning, patients have tolerated months of intubation without subglottic stenosis or need for tracheostomy.

Feeding should be done by a nasogastric or nasojejunal tube until sufficient oropharyngeal strength and coordination enable feeding by breast or bottle. Expressed breast milk is the most desirable food for infants, in part because of its immunologic components (e.g., secretory immunoglobulin A [sIgA], lactoferrin, leukocytes). Tube feeding also assists in the restoration of peristalsis, a nonspecific but probably essential part of eliminating *C. botulinum* from the intestinal flora. Intravenous feeding (hyperalimentation) is discouraged because of the potential for infection and the advantages of tube feeding.

Because sensation remains intact, providing auditory, tactile, and visual stimuli is beneficial. Maintaining strong central respiratory drive is essential, so sedatives or central nervous system depressants are discouraged. Full hydration and stool softeners such as lactulose may mitigate the protracted constipation. Cathartics are not recommended. Patients with food-borne and infant botulism excrete *C. botulinum* toxin and organisms in their feces, often for weeks, and care should be taken in handling their excreta. When bladder palsy occurs in severe cases, gentle suprapubic pressure with the patient in the sitting position with the head supported may help attain complete voiding and reduce the risk for urinary tract infection. Families may require emotional and financial support, especially when the paralysis of botulism is prolonged.

COMPLICATIONS. Almost all of the complications of botulism are nosocomial, and a few are iatrogenic (Table 207-3). Some critically ill, paralyzed patients who must spend weeks or months on ventilators in intensive care units will inevitably develop some of these complications. Suspected "relapses" of infant botulism usually reflect premature hospital discharge or an inapparent underlying complication such as pneumonia, urinary tract infection or otitis media.

PROGNOSIS. When the regenerating nerve endings have induced formation of a new motor end plate, neuromuscular transmission is restored. In the absence of complications, particularly those related to hypoxia, the prognosis in infant botulism is for full and complete recovery. Hospital stay in untreated infant botulism averages 5.7 wk but differs significantly by toxin type, with untreated type B patients being hospitalized a mean of 4.2 wk and untreated type A patients 6.7 wk.

In the USA, the case-fatality ratio for hospitalized cases of infant botulism is <1%. After recovery, untreated infant botulism patients appear to have an increased incidence of strabismus that requires timely screening and treatment.

The case-fatality ratio in food-borne and wound botulism varies by age, with younger patients having the best prognosis. Some adults with botulism have reported chronic weakness and fatigue as sequelae.

TABLE 207-3. Complications of Infant Botulism

Acute respiratory distress syndrome	Pneumothorax
Aspiration	Recurrent atelectasis
Clostridium difficile enterocolitis	Seizures secondary to hyponatremia
Hypotension	Sepsis
Inappropriate antidiuretic hormone secretion	Subglottic stenosis
Long bone fractures	Tracheal granuloma
Misplaced or plugged endotracheal tube	Tracheitis
Nosocomial anemia	Transfusion reaction
Otitis media	Urinary tract infection
Pneumonia	

PREVENTION. Food-borne botulism is best prevented by adhering to safe methods of home canning (pressure cooker and acidification), by avoiding suspicious foods, and by heating all home canned foods to 85°C for ≥5 min. Wound botulism is best prevented by not using illicit drugs and by treatment of contaminated wounds with thorough cleansing, surgical debridement, and provision of appropriate antibiotics.

Most infant botulism patients probably inhale and then swallow airborne clostridial spores; these cases cannot be prevented. The 1 identified, avoidable source of botulinum spores for infants is honey. *Honey is an unsafe food for any child younger than 1 yr of age.* Corn syrups were once thought to be a possible source of botulinum spores, but recent evidence indicates otherwise. Breast-feeding appears to slow the onset of infant botulism and to diminish the risk for sudden death in infants in whom the disease develops.

Arnon SS, Schechter R, Inglesby TV, et al: Botulinum toxin as a biological weapon: Medical and public health management. *JAMA* 2001;285:1059–1070.

Arnon SS, Schechter R, Maslanka SE, et al: Human botulism immune globulin for the treatment of infant botulism. *N Engl J Med* 2006;354:462–471.

Barash JR, Tang TWH, Arnon SS: First case of infant botulism caused by *Clostridium baratii* type F in California. *J Clin Microbiol* 2005;43:4280–4282.

Brett MM, Hallas G, Mpamugo O: Wound botulism in the UK and Ireland. *J Med Microbiol* 2004;53(Pt 6):555–561.

Brett MM, McLauchlin J, Harris A, et al: A case of infant botulism with a possible link to infant formula milk powder: Evidence for the presence of more than one strain of *Clostridium botulinum* in clinical specimens and food. *J Med Microbiol* 2005;54:769–776.

Chertow DS, Tan ET, Maslanka SE, et al: Botulism in 4 adults following cosmetic injections with an unlicensed, highly concentrated botulinum preparation. *JAMA* 2006;296:2476–2479.

Cooper JG, Spilke CE, Denton M, Jamieson S: *Clostridium botulinum:* An increasing complication of heroin misuse. *Eur J Emerg Med* 2005;12(5):251–252.

Fernicia L, Da Dalt L, Anniballi F, et al: A case of infant botulism due to neurotoxigenic *Clostridium butyricum* type E associated with *Clostridium difficile* colitis. *Eur J Clin Microbiol Infect Dis* 2002;21:736–738.

Fox CK, Keet CA, Strober JB: Recent advances in infant botulism. *Pediatr Neurol* 2005;32:149–154.

Francisco AMO, Arnon SS: Clinical mimics of infant botulism. *Pediatrics,* 2007;119:826–828.

Keet CA, Fox CK, Margeta M, et al: Infant botulism, type F, presenting at 54 hours of life. *Pediatr Neurol* 2005;32(3):193–196.

Long SS: Infant botulism and treatment with BIG-IV (BabyBIG). *Pediatr Infect Dis J* 2007;26:261–262.

Mitchell WG, Tseng-Ong L: Catastrophic presentation of infant botulism may obscure or delay diagnosis. *Pediatrics* 2005;116:e436–e438.

Nevas M, Lindstrom M, Virtanen A, et al: Infant botulism acquired from household dust presenting as sudden infant death syndrome. *J Clin Microbiol* 2005;43:511–513.

Sobel J: Botulism. *Clin Infect Dis* 2005;41:1167–1173.

Sobel J, Tucker N, Sulka A, et al: Foodborne botulism in the United States, 1990–2000. *Emerg Infect Dis* 2004;10:1606–1611.

Chapter 208 ■ Tetanus *(Clostridium Tetani)*

Stephen S. Arnon

ETIOLOGY. Tetanus, historically called **lockjaw,** is an acute, spastic paralytic illness caused by the neurotoxin produced by *Clostridium tetani,* a motile, gram-positive, spore-forming obligate anaerobe whose natural habitat worldwide is soil, dust, and the alimentary tracts of various animals. It forms spores terminally, producing a drumstick or tennis racket appearance microscopically. Tetanus spores can survive boiling but not autoclaving, whereas the vegetative cells are killed by antibiotics, heat, and standard disinfectants. Unlike many clostridia, *C. tetani* is not a tissue-invasive organism and instead causes illness through the effects of a single toxin, **tetanospasmin,** more commonly referred to as tetanus toxin. Tetanospasmin is the 2nd most poisonous substance known, surpassed in potency only by botulinum toxin. The human lethal dose of tetanus toxin is estimated to be 10^{-5} mg/kg.

EPIDEMIOLOGY. Tetanus occurs worldwide and is endemic in approximately 90 developing countries, although its incidence varies considerably. The most common form, **neonatal (or umbilical) tetanus,** kills approximately 500,000 infants each year, with about 80% of deaths in just 12 tropical Asian and African countries. It occurs because the mother was not immunized. In addition, an estimated 15,000–30,000 unimmunized women worldwide die each year of **maternal tetanus** that results from postpartum, postabortal, or postsurgical wound infection with *C. tetani.* Approximately 50 cases of tetanus are reported each year in the USA, mostly in persons >60 yr of age, although toddler-aged and neonatal cases also occur. Approximately 20% of children in the USA 10–16 yr of age lack a protective antibody level. The majority of recent childhood cases of tetanus in the USA have occurred in unimmunized children whose parents objected to vaccination.

Most non-neonatal cases of tetanus are associated with a traumatic injury, often a penetrating wound inflicted by a dirty object such as a nail, splinter, fragment of glass, or unsterile injection. Tetanus occurring after illicit drug injection is becoming more common. The disease also occurs after the use of contaminated suture material and after intramuscular injection of medicines, most notably quinine for chloroquine-resistant falciparum malaria. The disease may also occur in association with animal bites, abscesses (including dental abscesses), ear and other body piercing, chronic skin ulceration, burns, compound fractures, frostbite, gangrene, intestinal surgery, ritual scarification, infected insect bites, and female circumcision. Rare cases have no history of trauma.

PATHOGENESIS. Tetanus occurs after introduced spores germinate, multiply, and produce tetanus toxin in the low oxidation-reduction potential (E_h) of an infected injury site. A plasmid carries the toxin gene. Toxin is released after vegetative bacterial cell death and lysis. Tetanus toxin (and the botulinum toxins) are 150 kd simple proteins consisting of a heavy (100 kd) and a light (50 kd) chain joined by a single disulfide bond. Tetanus toxin binds at the neuromuscular junction and enters the motor nerve by endocytosis, after which it undergoes retrograde axonal transport to the cytoplasm of the α-motoneuron. In the sciatic nerve, the transport rate was found to be 3.4 mm/hr. The toxin exits the motoneuron in the spinal cord and next enters adjacent spinal inhibitory interneurons, where it prevents release of the neurotransmitters glycine γ-aminobutyric acid (GABA). Tetanus toxin thus blocks the normal inhibition of antagonistic muscles on which voluntary coordinated movement depends; in consequence, affected muscles sustain maximal contraction and cannot relax. The autonomic nervous system is also rendered unstable in tetanus.

The phenomenal potency of tetanus toxin is enzymatic in nature. The light chain of tetanus toxin (and of several botulinum toxins) is a zinc-containing endoprotease whose substrate is synaptobrevin, a constituent protein of the docking complex that enables the synaptic vesicle to fuse with the terminal cell membrane. The heavy chain of the toxin contains its binding and internalization domains.

Because *C. tetani* is not an invasive organism, its toxin-producing vegetative cells remain where introduced into the wound, which may display local inflammatory changes and a mixed bacterial flora.

CLINICAL MANIFESTATIONS. Tetanus may be either generalized, which is more common, or localized. The incubation period typically is 2–14 days, but it may be as long as months after the injury. In **generalized tetanus,** the presenting symptom in about half of cases is **trismus** (masseter muscle spasm, or lockjaw). Headache, restlessness, and irritability are early symptoms, often followed by stiffness, difficulty chewing, dysphagia, and neck muscle spasm. The so-called **sardonic smile of tetanus (risus sardonicus)** results from intractable spasms of facial and buccal muscles. When the paralysis extends to abdominal, lumbar, hip, and thigh muscles, the patient may assume an arched posture of extreme hyperextension of the body, or **opisthotonos,** with the head and the heels bent backward and the body bowed forward with only the back of the head and the heels touching the supporting surface. Opisthotonos is an equilibrium position that results from unrelenting total contraction of opposing muscles, all of which display the typical boardlike rigidity of tetanus. Laryngeal and respiratory muscle spasm can lead to airway obstruction and asphyxiation. Because tetanus toxin does not affect sensory nerves or cortical function, the patient unfortunately remains conscious, in extreme pain, and in fearful anticipation of the next tetanic seizure. These seizures are characterized by sudden, severe tonic contractions of the muscles, with fist clenching, flexion, and adduction of the arms and hyperextension of the legs. Without treatment, the seizures range from a few seconds to a few minutes in length with intervening respite periods, but as the illness progresses, the spasms become sustained and exhausting. The smallest disturbance by sight, sound, or touch may trigger a tetanic spasm. Dysuria and urinary retention result from bladder sphincter spasm; forced defecation may occur. Fever, occasionally as high as 40°C, is common because of the substantial metabolic energy consumed by spastic muscles. Notable autonomic effects include tachycardia, dysrhythmias, labile hypertension, diaphoresis, and cutaneous vasoconstriction. The tetanic paralysis usually becomes more severe in the 1st wk after onset, stabilizes in the 2nd wk, and ameliorates gradually over the ensuing 1–4 wk.

Neonatal tetanus (tetanus neonatorum), the infantile form of generalized tetanus, typically manifests within 3–12 days of birth as progressive difficulty in feeding (sucking and swallowing), associated hunger, and crying. Paralysis or diminished movement, stiffness and rigidity to the touch, and spasms, with or without opisthotonos, are characteristic. The umbilical stump may hold remnants of dirt, dung, clotted blood, or serum, or it may appear relatively benign.

Localized tetanus results in painful spasms of the muscles adjacent to the wound site and may precede generalized tetanus. **Cephalic tetanus** is a rare form of localized tetanus involving the bulbar musculature that occurs with wounds or foreign bodies in the head, nostrils, or face. It also occurs in association with chronic otitis media. Cephalic tetanus is characterized by retracted eyelids, deviated gaze, trismus, risus sardonicus, and spastic paralysis of the tongue and pharyngeal musculature.

DIAGNOSIS. The picture of tetanus is one of the most dramatic in medicine, and the diagnosis may be established clinically. The typical setting is an unimmunized patient (and/or mother) who was injured or born within the preceding 2 wk, who presents with trismus, other rigid muscles, and a clear sensorium.

Routine laboratory studies are usually normal. A peripheral leukocytosis may result from a secondary bacterial infection of the wound or may be stress induced from the sustained tetanic spasms. The cerebrospinal fluid is normal, although the intense muscle contractions may raise intracranial pressure. Neither the electroencephalogram nor the electromyogram shows a characteristic pattern. *C. tetani* is not always visible on Gram stain of wound material, and it is isolated in only about 1/3 of cases.

DIFFERENTIAL DIAGNOSIS. Fully developed, generalized tetanus cannot be mistaken for any other disease. However, trismus may result from parapharyngeal, retropharyngeal, or dental abscesses, or rarely, from acute encephalitis involving the brainstem. Either rabies or tetanus may follow an animal bite, and rabies may present as trismus with seizures. However, rabies may be distinguished from tetanus by hydrophobia, marked dysphagia, predominantly clonic seizures, and pleocytosis (see Chapter 271). Although strychnine poisoning may result in tonic muscle spasms and generalized seizure activity, it seldom produces trismus, and unlike tetanus, general relaxation usually occurs between spasms. Hypocalcemia may produce tetany that is characterized by laryngeal and carpopedal spasms, but trismus is absent. Occasionally, epileptic seizures, narcotic withdrawal, or other drug reactions may suggest tetanus.

TREATMENT. Management of tetanus requires eradication of *C. tetani* and the wound environment conducive to its anaerobic multiplication, neutralization of all accessible tetanus toxin, control of seizures and respiration, palliation and provision of meticulous supportive care, and, finally, prevention of recurrences.

Surgical wound excision and debridement are often needed to remove the foreign body or devitalized tissue that created anaerobic growth conditions. Surgery should be performed promptly after administration of **human tetanus immunoglobulin (TIG)** and antibiotics. Excision of the umbilical stump in neonatal tetanus is no longer recommended.

Tetanus toxin cannot be neutralized by TIG after it has begun its axonal ascent to the spinal cord. TIG should be given as soon as possible in order to neutralize toxin that diffuses from the wound into the circulation before the toxin can bind at distant muscle groups. The optimal dose of TIG has not been determined. A single intramuscular injection of 500 U of TIG is sufficient to neutralize systemic tetanus toxin, but total doses as high as 3,000–6,000 U are also recommended. Infiltration of TIG into the wound is now considered unnecessary. If TIG is unavailable, use of human intravenous immunoglobulin (IVIG), may be necessary. IVIG contains 4–90 U/mL of TIG; the optimal dosage of IVIG for treating tetanus is not known and it is not approved for this indication. Another alternative is equine- or bovine-derived tetanus antitoxin (TAT). The usual dose of TAT is 50,000–100,000 U, with half given intramuscularly and half intravenously, but as little as 10,000 U may be sufficient. TAT is not available in the USA. Approximately 15% of patients given the usual dose of TAT experience serum sickness. When using TAT, it is essential to check for possible sensitivity to horse serum and desensitization may be needed. The human-derived immunoglobulins are much preferred because of their longer half-life (30 days) and the virtual absence of allergic and serum sickness adverse effects. Intrathecal TIG, given to neutralize tetanus toxin in the spinal cord, is not effective.

Penicillin G (100,000 U/kg/day divided every 4–6 hr IV for 10–14 days) remains the antibiotic of choice because of its effective clostridiocidal action and its diffusibility, which is an important consideration because blood flow to injured tissue may be compromised. Metronidazole (500 mg every 8 hr IV for adults) appears to be equally effective. Erythromycin and tetracycline (for persons >8 yr of age) are alternatives for penicillin-allergic patients.

All patients with generalized tetanus need muscle relaxants. Diazepam provides both relaxation and seizure control. The initial dose of 0.1–0.2/kg every 3–6 hr given intravenously is subsequently titrated to control the tetanic spasms, after which it is sustained for 2–6 wk before its tapered withdrawal. Magnesium sulfate, other benzodiazepines (midazolam), chlorpromazine, dantrolene, and baclofen are also used. Intrathecal baclofen produces such complete muscle relaxation that apnea often ensues; like most other agents listed, baclofen should be used only in an intensive care unit setting. The highest survival rates in generalized tetanus are achieved with neuromuscular blocking agents such as vecuronium and pancuronium, which produce a general flaccid paralysis that is then managed by mechanical ventilation. Autonomic instability is regulated with standard α- and β- (or both) blocking agents; morphine has also proved useful.

SUPPORTIVE CARE. Meticulous supportive care in a quiet, dark, secluded setting is most desirable. Because tetanic spasms may be triggered by minor stimuli, the patient should be sedated and protected from all unnecessary sounds, sights, and touch; and all therapeutic and other manipulations must be carefully scheduled and coordinated. Endotracheal intubation may not be required, but it should be done to prevent aspiration of secretions before laryngospasm develops. A tracheostomy kit should be immediately at hand for unintubated patients. Endotracheal intubation and suctioning easily provoke reflex tetanic seizures and spasms, and early tracheostomy should be considered in severe cases not managed by pharmacologically induced flaccid paralysis. Cardiorespiratory monitoring, frequent suctioning, and maintenance of the substantial fluid, electrolyte, and caloric needs are fundamental. Careful nursing attention to mouth, skin, bladder, and bowel function is needed to avoid ulceration, infection, and obstipation. Prophylactic subcutaneous heparin may be of value but must be balanced with the risk for hemorrhage.

COMPLICATIONS. The seizures and the severe, sustained rigid paralysis of tetanus predispose the patient to many complications. Aspiration of secretions and pneumonia may have begun before the 1st medical attention was received. Maintaining airway patency often mandates endotracheal intubation and mechanical ventilation with their attendant hazards, including pneumothorax and mediastinal emphysema. The seizures may result in lacerations of the mouth or tongue, in intramuscular hematomas or rhabdomyolysis with myoglobinuria and renal failure, or in long bone or spinal fractures. Venous thrombosis, pulmonary embolism, gastric ulceration with or without hemorrhage, paralytic ileus, and decubitus ulceration are constant hazards. Excessive use of muscle relaxants, an integral part of care, may produce iatrogenic apnea. Cardiac arrhythmias, including asystole, unstable blood pressure, and labile temperature regulation reflect disordered autonomic nervous system control that may be aggravated by inattention to maintenance of intravascular volume needs.

PROGNOSIS. Recovery in tetanus occurs through regeneration of synapses within the spinal cord and thereby the restoration of muscle relaxation. However, because an episode of tetanus does not result in the production of toxin-neutralizing antibodies, active immunization with tetanus toxoid at discharge with provision for completion of the primary series is mandatory.

The most important factor that influences outcome is the quality of supportive care. Mortality is highest in the very young and the very old. A favorable prognosis is associated with a long incubation period, absence of fever, and localized disease. An unfavorable prognosis is associated with <7 days between the injury and the onset of trismus and <3 days between trismus and the onset of generalized tetanic spasms. Sequelae of hypoxic brain injury, especially in infants, include cerebral palsy, diminished mental abilities, and behavioral difficulties. Most fatalities occur within the 1st wk of illness. Reported case fatality rates for generalized tetanus are 5–35%, and for neonatal tetanus extend from <10% with intensive care treatment to >75% without it. Cephalic tetanus has an especially poor prognosis because of breathing and feeding difficulties.

PREVENTION. Tetanus is an entirely preventable disease. A serum antibody titer of ≥0.01 U/mL is considered protective. Active immunization should begin in early infancy with combined diphtheria toxoid-tetanus toxoid-acellular pertussis (DTaP) vaccine at 2, 4, and 6 mo of age, with a booster at 4–6 yr of age and at 10 yr intervals thereafter throughout adult life (Td or Tdap). Immunization of women with tetanus toxoid prevents neonatal tetanus, and the World Health Organization is engaged currently in a global elimination of neonatal tetanus campaign through maternal immunization with at least 2 doses of tetanus toxoid. For unimmunized persons >7 yr of age, the primary immunization series consists of 3 doses of Td toxoid given intramuscularly, with the 2nd given 4–6 wk after the 1st and the 3rd given 6–12 mo after the 2nd.

Arthus reactions (type III hypersensitivity reactions), a localized vasculitis associated with deposition of immune complexes and activation of complement, are reported rarely after tetanus vaccination. Unanticipated mass immunization campaigns in developing countries have occasionally provoked a widespread hysterical reaction.

Wound Management. Tetanus prevention measures after trauma consist of inducing active immunity to tetanus toxin and of passively providing antitoxic antibody (Table 208-1). Tetanus prophylaxis is an essential part of all wound management, but specific measures depend on the nature of the injury and the immunization status of the patient. Tetanus toxoid should always be given after a dog or other animal bite, even though *C. tetani* is infrequently found in canine mouth flora. All nonminor wounds require human TIG except those in a fully immunized patient. In any other circumstance (e.g., patients with an unknown or incomplete immunization history; crush, puncture, or projectile wounds; wounds contaminated with saliva, soil, or feces; avulsion injuries; compound fractures; or frostbite), TIG 250 U should be given intramuscularly, with 500 U for highly tetanus-prone wounds (i.e., unable to be debrided, with substantial bacterial contamination, or >24 hr since injury). If TIG is unavailable, then use of human IGIV may be considered. If neither of these products is available, then 3,000–5,000 U of equine- or bovine-derived TAT may be given intramuscularly after testing for hypersensitivity. Even at this dose, serum sickness may occur.

The wound should have immediate, thorough surgical cleansing and debridement to remove foreign bodies and any necrotic tissue in which anaerobic conditions might develop. Tetanus toxoid should be given to stimulate active immunity and may be administered concurrently with TIG (or TAT) if given in separate syringes at widely separated sites. A tetanus toxoid booster (preferably Td or Tdap) is administered to all persons with any wound if the tetanus immunization status is unknown or incomplete. A booster is administered to injured persons who have completed their primary immunization series if (1) the wound is clean and minor but ≥10 yr have passed since the last booster or (2) the wound is more serious and ≥5 yr have passed since the last booster. Persons who experienced an Arthus reaction after a dose of tetanus toxoid–containing vaccine should not receive Td more frequently than every 10 yr, even for tetanus prophylaxis as part of wound management. With delayed wound care, active immunization should be started at once. Although fluid tetanus toxoid produces a more rapid immune response than the absorbed or precipitated toxoids, the absorbed toxoid results in a more durable titer.

TABLE 208-1. Tetanus Prophylaxis in Routine Wound Management

HISTORY OF ABSORBED TETANUS TOXOID (DOSES)	CLEAN, MINOR WOUNDS		OTHER WOUNDS*	
	Tdap or Td†	TIG‡	Tdap or Td†	TIG‡
Uncertain, or <3	Yes	No	Yes	Yes
3 or more	No§	No	No‖	No

*Such as, but not limited to, wounds contaminated with dirt, feces, and saliva; puncture wounds; avulsions; wounds resulting from missiles, crushing, burns, and frostbite.

†For children <7 yr of age, DTaP is preferred to tetanus toxoid alone if <3 doses of DTaP have been previously given. If pertussis vaccine is contraindicated, DT is given. For persons ≥7 yr of age, Td (or Tdap for adolescents 11–18 yr of age) is preferred to tetanus toxoid alone. Tdap is preferred to Td for adolescents 11–18 yr of age who have never received Tdap. Td is preferred to tetanus toxoid for adolescents who received Tdap previously or when Tdap is not available.

‡TIG should be administered for tetanus-prone wounds in HIV-infected patients regardless of the history of tetanus immunizations.

§Yes, if ≥10 yr since the last tetanus toxoid-containing vaccine dose.

‖Yes, if ≥5 yr since the last tetanus toxoid-containing vaccine dose. (More frequent boosters are not needed and can accentuate adverse events.)

Adapted from the Centers for Disease Control and Prevention: Preventing tetanus, diphtheria, and pertussis among adolescents: Use of tetanus toxoid, reduced diphtheria toxoid and acellular pertussis vaccines. Recommendations of the Advisory Committee on Immunization Practices (ACIP). *MMWR* 2006;55(RR-3):1–43.

Tdap, tetanus toxoid, reduced diphtheria toxoid, and acellular pertussis vaccine; Td, tetanus toxid and reduced diphtheria toxoid; TIG, tetanus immune globulin.

Brook I: Tetanus in children. *Pediatr Emerg Care* 2004;20:48–51.

Bunch TJ, Thalji MK, Pellikka PA, Aksamit TR: Respiratory failure in tetanus: Case report and review of a 25-year experience. *Chest* 2002;122:1488–1492.

Centers for Disease Control and Prevention: Preventing tetanus, diphtheria, and pertussis among adolescents: Use of tetanus toxoid, reduced diphtheria toxoid and acellular pertussis vaccines. Recommendations of the Advisory Committee on Immunization Practices (ACIP). *MMWR* 2006;55(RR-3):1–43.

Cook TM, Protheroe RT, Handel JM: Tetanus: A review of the literature. *Br J Anaesth* 2001;87:477–487.

Dyce O, Bruno JR, Hong D, et al: Tongue piercing: The new "rusty nail?" *Head Neck* 2000;22:728–732.

Fair E, Murphy TV, Golaz A, et al: Philosophic objection to vaccination as a risk for tetanus among children younger than 15 years. *Pediatrics* 2002;109:E2.

Farrar JJ, Yen LM, Cook T, et al: Tetanus. *J Neurol Neurosurg Psychiatry* 2000;69:292–301.

Kara CO, Cetin CB, Yalcin N: Cephalic tetanus as a result of rooster pecking: An unusual case. *Scand J Infect Dis* 2002;34:64–66.

McQuillan G, Kruszon-Moran D, Deforrest A, et al: Serologic immunity to diphtheria and tetanus in the United States. *Ann Intern Med* 2002;136:660–666.

Miranda-Filho DB, Ximenes RA, Barone AA, et al: Randomised controlled trial of tetanus treatment with antitetanus immunoglobulin by the intrathecal or intramuscular route. *Br Med J* 2004;328:615–617.

Vandalaer J, Birmingham M, Gasse F, et al: Tetanus in developing countries: An update on the Maternal and Neonatal Tetanus Elimination Initiative. *Vaccine* 2003;21:3442–3445.

Chapter 209 ■ Pseudomembranous Colitis *(Clostridium Difficile)*

Margaret C. Fisher

Clostridium difficile–associated diarrhea, also known as **antibiotic-associated diarrhea** or **pseudomembranous colitis,** is the major cause of health care–associated diarrhea. It also occasionally occurs in persons in the community who are not receiving antibiotics.

ETIOLOGY. *C. difficile* is a ubiquitous, spore-forming, gram-positive, anaerobic bacillus. The organism produces 2 toxins: **toxin A (enterotoxin)** acts on the intestinal mucosa to produce diarrhea; **toxin B (cytotoxin)** increases vascular permeability in low doses and is lethal to experimental animals in high doses. Individual strains generally produce either both toxins or no toxin.

EPIDEMIOLOGY. *C. difficile*–associated diarrhea occurs in the setting of altered bowel flora, which is most commonly due to antimicrobial therapy. Ampicillin, 2nd and 3rd generation cephalosporins, and clindamycin are the most frequent offenders, although virtually all antibiotics have been implicated. Some patients have not had any preceding antibiotics.

Newborns are often colonized with *C. difficile* during the 1st weeks of life, with approximately half of healthy infants colonized during the 1st year of life. Many of these strains produce toxin. Carriage decreases to the adult rate of 1–3% by 2 yr of age. Illness is unusual in neonates and infants; the basis for this remains unknown. *C. difficile*–associated diarrhea has been reported in children of all ages. Asymptomatic carriers are not at increased risk for disease unless administered antibiotics. Disease has been acquired from other infected patients in a nosocomial manner. Outbreaks of disease have occurred with a hypervirulent, epidemic *C. difficile* strain with variant toxin genes; this organism is resistant to fluoroquinolones and other antibiotics.

Gastrointestinal surgery and chemotherapy are additional risk factors. The risk for disease increases with enteral feedings, especially if the feedings bypass the stomach. Normal gastric acidity destroys the spores of *C. difficile.*

PATHOGENESIS. Normal gut flora appears to be protective. Administration of antibiotics that impair growth of normal flora but not *C. difficile* is the most common risk factor, but any process that disrupts the normal bowel flora (weaning, chemotherapy) or bowel motility (bowel stasis, bowel surgery) predisposes to *C. difficile*–associated diarrhea.

Toxin A binds to a specific receptor on the intestinal brush border. The binding site for toxin B is still undefined. Both toxins are internalized and act within cells to modify proteins, resulting in cell death. Inflammatory response contributes to the diarrhea and formation of **pseudomembranes.** Antibody to the toxins is protective and appears to prevent binding and modify or abort clinical disease.

CLINICAL MANIFESTATIONS. Clinical symptoms vary widely. Asymptomatic colonization is common in infants and young children. Illness varies from a mild self-limited diarrhea without pseudomembranes, to explosive watery diarrhea with occult blood, to the classic picture of **pseudomembranous colitis** with bloody diarrhea accompanied by fever, cramps, abdominal pain, nausea, and vomiting. Disease may develop during and as long as several weeks after antibiotic therapy. Severe and extensive colitis occurs in children undergoing chemotherapy or those with Hirschsprung disease or inflammatory bowel disease; it has been reported in a few children with cystic fibrosis. *C. difficile* disease occasionally involves the small gut; in some hosts, bacteremia and abscess formation have been reported.

DIAGNOSIS. The diagnosis is confirmed by detecting *C. difficile* or its toxin in the stool of a patient with significant diarrhea or colitis in the setting of prior or current antimicrobial use.

Toxin can be detected by several methods. Inoculation of stool filtrates into cell culture to detect cytotoxicity is considered the reference method. This is a labor-intensive method that requires 24–48 hr for results. Many clinical laboratories use enzyme immunoassay tests that detect toxin A only, or toxin A plus B. Testing for both toxins increases the yield of positive studies. Culture of the stool for *C. difficile* is time consuming and does not differentiate toxin-producing from non-toxin-producing strains. The interpretation of positive *C. difficile* culture or toxin in stool from children <12 mo of age requires clinical correlation.

Findings at sigmoidoscopy or colonoscopy include pseudomembranous nodules and plaques characteristic of toxin-related colitis. Fecal leukocytes are present in approximately half of cases. Occult or frank blood is common.

TREATMENT. The 1st and essential step in treatment is the discontinuation of the current antibiotics, if possible, which is sufficient in most cases in combination with appropriate fluid and electrolyte replacement. If symptoms persist, antibiotics cannot be discontinued, or the illness is severe, then oral metronidazole (20–40 mg/kg/day divided every 6–8 hr PO) or vancomycin (25–40 mg/kg/day divided every 6 hr PO) should be given for 7–10 days. Oral metronidazole is the preferred therapy for most children because it is less expensive, has an excellent response rate, and minimizes the emergence of vancomycin-resistant *Enterococcus*, which is especially important in hospitalized or institutionalized patients (see Chapter 185). Nitazoxanide has been effective in adults with *C. difficile* colitis. Contact isolation of patients is critical to avoid nosocomial spread.

PROGNOSIS. The initial response rate is >95%, but 5–30% of patients have clinical relapse, usually within 1–2 wk of treatment. These patients should be re-evaluated and treated again; most will respond to a 2nd course of the original treatment. A few patients develop multiple recurrences, with short-lived responses to repeated treatment. Treatment strategies for these patients include oral cholestyramine, oral bacitracin, intravenous immunoglobulin, reconstitution of bowel flora with probiotics such as oral lactobacilli or baker's yeast, and instillation of fecal flora by tube feeding or enemas. None of these methods is effective for all cases. A toxoid vaccine has been developed and in pilot studies has been effective in eliminating disease in patients with multiple recurrences.

PREVENTION. *C. difficile* is often acquired during hospitalization or in child-care settings. The spores of the organism are resistant to drying and to some disinfectants (alcohol wash solutions) and frequently contaminate bathrooms and diaper changing areas of hospital rooms or child-care areas. Electronic thermometers are easily contaminated and have been implicated in several hospital outbreaks. Prevention of *C. difficile*–associated diarrhea requires meticulous hand hygiene, use of contact isolation, appropriate environmental cleaning, and appropriate use of antimicrobial agents.

Aas J, Gessert CE, Bakken JS: Recurrent *Clostridium difficile* colitis: Case series involving 18 patients treated with donor stool administered via a nasogastric tube. *Clin Infect Dis* 2003;36:580–585.

Jernigan JA, Siegman-Igra Y, Guerrant RC, et al: A randomized crossover study of disposable thermometers for prevention of *Clostridium difficile* and other nosocomial infections. *Infect Control Hosp Epidemiol* 1998;19:494–499.

Kyne L, Warny M, Qamar A, et al: Association between antibody response to toxin A and protection against recurrent *Clostridium difficile* diarrhoea. *Lancet* 2001;357:189–193.

Musher DM, Logan N, Hamill RJ, et al: Nitazoxanide for the treatment of *Clostridium difficile* colitis. *CID* 2006;43:421–427.

Mylonakis E, Ryan ET, Calderwood SB: *Clostridium difficile*-associated diarrhea. A review. *Arch Intern Med* 2001;161:525–533.

Sebaiha M, Wren B, Mullany P, et al: The multidrug resistant human pathogen *Clostridium difficile* has a highly mobile mosaic genome. *Nat Genet* 2006;38:779–786.

Sougioultzis S, Kyne L, Drudy D, et al: *Clostridium difficile* toxoid vaccine in recurrent *C. difficile*-associated diarrhea. *Gastroenterology* 2005;128:764–770.

Chapter 210 ■ Other Anaerobic Infections Margaret C. Fisher

Anaerobic bacteria are the most numerous organisms colonizing humans. Anaerobes are present in soil and are normal inhabitants of all living animals, but infections caused by anaerobes are relatively uncommon. Anaerobes are relatively or entirely intolerant of exposure to oxygen. Most are **facultative anaerobes** and are able to survive in the presence of oxygen but grow better with reduced oxygen tension. The remainder are **obligate anaerobes** and do not survive any exposure to oxygen.

Infections with anaerobes occur most commonly adjacent to mucosal surfaces and as **mixed infections** with aerobes. Conditions of reduced oxygen tension provide the optimal conditions for proliferation of anaerobes. Traumatized areas, devascularized areas, and areas of crush injury are all ideal sites for anaerobic infections. Often both aerobic and anaerobic organisms are inoculated, with local extension and bacteremia most often caused by the more virulent aerobes. Abscess formation evolves over days to weeks and generally involves both aerobes and anaerobes. Examples of such infections include appendicitis and abscesses such as appendiceal, pelvic, perirectal, peritonsillar, retropharyngeal, parapharyngeal, lung, and dental. Septic thrombophlebitis, which is a consequence of appendicitis, chronic sinusitis, pharyngitis, and otitis media, provides a route for spread of the infection to vital organs such as the liver, brain, or lungs.

Anaerobic infection usually is caused by endogenous flora. Combinations of impaired physical barriers to infection, compromised tissue viability, alterations in normal flora, impaired host immunity, and anaerobic bacterial virulence factors contribute to infection with these normal anaerobic inhabitants of mucous membranes. Virulence factors include capsules, toxins, enzymes, and fatty acids.

CLINICAL MANIFESTATIONS

Anaerobic infections occur in a variety of sites throughout the body (Table 210-1). Anaerobes exist synergistically with aerobes. Infections with anaerobes are almost always polymicrobial and also include aerobes.

CENTRAL NERVOUS SYSTEM. Meningitis is rare, but it has occurred in neonates and as a complication of infections of the ear and neck (**Lemierre syndrome**). Brain abscess and subdural empyema are usually polymicrobial, with anaerobes commonly involved (see Chapter 603). Brain abscess occurs most often as a result of spread of infection from sinuses, middle ear, or lung.

UPPER RESPIRATORY TRACT. The respiratory tract is colonized by both aerobes and anaerobes. Anaerobic bacteria are involved in chronic sinusitis, chronic otitis media, peritonsillar infections, parapharyngeal and retropharyngeal abscesses, and periodontal infections. Anaerobic periodontal disease is most common in patients with poor dental hygiene or who are receiving drugs that cause hypertrophy of the gums. **Vincent angina,** also known as **acute necrotizing ulcerative gingivitis** or **trench mouth,** is an acute, fulminating, mixed bacterial-spirochetal infection of the gingival margin and floor of the mouth. It is characterized by gingival pain, foul breath, and pseudomembrane formation. **Ludwig angina** is an acute, life-threatening cellulitis of dental origin of the sublingual and submandibular spaces. Infection spreads rapidly in the neck and may cause airway obstruction.

Lemierre syndrome, or **postanginal sepsis,** is a suppurative infection of the lateral pharyngeal space that usually begins as pharyngitis. It may complicate infectious mononucleosis. It presents as septic thrombophlebitis of the jugular vein leading to multiple septic pulmonary embolizations. Clinical signs include neck swelling and pain, trismus, and dysphagia culminating with signs of sepsis and respiratory distress. *Fusobacterium necrophorum* is the most commonly involved organism, although polymicrobial infection is frequent.

LOWER RESPIRATORY TRACT. Anaerobic lung abscess, empyema, and anaerobic pneumonia are most common in children with swallowing dysfunction or otherwise at increased risk for aspiration, or with the presence of a foreign body occluding the airway. All children and adults aspirate during sleep and during periods of unconsciousness. In most cases, lung cilia and phagocytes clear particulate matter and microbes. If the aspiration is of increased volume or frequency or a foreign body blocks drainage, the ability of lung clearance mechanisms is overcome and infection ensues.

INTRA-ABDOMINAL INFECTION. The digestive tract is colonized throughout by anaerobes. The density of organisms is highest in the colon, where anaerobes outnumber aerobes 1,000 : 1. Rupture of the gut leads to spillage of gut flora into the peritoneum, resulting in peritonitis that involves both aerobes and anaerobes. Bacteremia caused by aerobes occurs early. As the infection is walled off in the peritoneum, an abscess composed of both aerobes and anaerobes may form. Liver abscesses, which are rare in children, may develop as complications of appendicitis, inflammatory bowel disease, and biliary tract disease. In children with malignancies who are receiving chemotherapy, the gut mucosa is often damaged, leading to translocation of bacteria and focal invasion of bowel flora. **Typhlitis,** or **necrotizing colitis,** is a mixed infection of the gut wall usually beginning in the colon; abdominal pain, diarrhea, fever, and abdominal distention are common features. Empirical antimicrobial therapy of fever and neutropenia may not be optimal against the anaerobes involved in typhlitis (see Chapter 177).

GENITAL TRACT. Pelvic inflammatory disease and tubo-ovarian abscesses are frequently caused by mixed aerobes and anaerobes. Vaginitis can be caused by overgrowth of anaerobic flora. Anaerobes frequently contribute to chorioamnionitis and premature labor and may result in anaerobic bacteremia in the newborn. Although most of these bacteremias are transient, anaerobes occasionally cause invasive disease in the newborn.

SKIN AND SOFT TISSUE. Anaerobic skin infections occur in the setting of bites, foreign bodies, and skin and tissue ulceration caused by pressure necrosis or lack of adequate blood supply. Animal bites and human bites inoculate oral and skin flora into the subcutaneous tissues. Oral flora includes anaerobes, but the more virulent aerobic infections are responsible for most clinical infections (see Chapter 712). The extent of the infection depends on the depth of the bite and the associated crush injury to the tissues.

Clostridial myonecrosis, or **gas gangrene,** is a rapidly progressive infection associated with *Clostridium perfringens.* **Necrotizing fasciitis** is a polymicrobial infection with acute onset and rapid progression, with significant morbidity and mortality. Group A streptococcus and *Staphylococcus aureus* occasionally are the causative pathogens. **Synergistic gangrene** is caused by synergistic infection between *S. aureus* or gram-negative bacilli and anaerobic streptococci. All of these are uncommon infections in healthy children. Early recognition with aggressive surgical debridement and antimicrobial therapy is necessary to limit morbidity and mortality.

OTHER SITES. Occasionally the bone adjacent to anaerobic infection becomes infected by direct extension from contiguous infec-

TABLE 210-1. Infections Associated with Anaerobic Bacteria

SITE AND INFECTION	MAJOR RISK FACTORS	ANAEROBIC BACTERIA*
CENTRAL NERVOUS SYSTEM		
Cerebral abscess Subdural empyema Epidural abscess	Direct extension from contiguous sinusitis, otitis media, mastoiditis	(Polymicrobial) *B. fragilis*[†] *Fusobacterium* *Peptostreptococcus* *Veillonella*
UPPER RESPIRATORY TRACT		
Dental abscess Ludwig angina (cellulitis of sublingual-submandibular space) Necrotizing gingivitis (Vincent stomatitis) Chronic otitis-mastoiditis-sinusitis Peritonsillar abscess Retropharyngeal abscess	Poor periodontal hygiene Drugs that cause gum hypertrophy	*Peptostreptococcus* *Fusobacterium* *P. melaninogenica*
LOWER RESPIRATORY TRACT		
Aspiration pneumonia Necrotizing pneumonitis Lung abscess Pulmonary empyema	Periodontal disease Bronchial obstruction Altered gag or consciousness	(Polymicrobial) *P. melaninogenica* *B. intermedius* *Fusobacterium* *Peptostreptococcus, Eubacterium* *B. fragilis, Veillonella*
INTRA-ABDOMINAL		
Abscess Secondary peritonitis	Appendicitis Penetrating trauma (especially of the colon)	(Polymicrobial) *B. fragilis* Other *Bacteroides* *Clostridium* *Peptostreptococcus* *Eubacterium* *Fusobacterium*
FEMALE GENITAL TRACT		
Bartholin abscess Tubo-ovarian abscess Endometritis Pelvic cellulitis or thrombophlebitis Salpingitis Chorioamnionitis Septic abortion	Vaginosis Intrauterine device	*B. fragilis* *B. bivius* *Peptostreptococcus* *Clostridium* *Mobiluncus* Actinomycosis
SKIN AND SOFT TISSUE		
Cellulitis Perirectal cellulitis Myonecrosis (gas gangrene) Necrotizing fasciitis Synergistic gangrene	Decubitus ulcers Abdominal wounds Pilonidal sinus Trauma Human and animal bites Immunosuppressed or neutropenic patients	(Varies with site and contamination with mouth or enteric flora) *Clostridium perfringens* (myonecrosis) *Bacteroides* *Fusobacterium* *Clostridium tertium* *C. septicum* Anaerobic streptococci
BACTEREMIA	Secondary to intra-abdominal infection, abscess, myonecrosis, or necrotizing fasciitis	*B. fragilis* *Clostridium* Anaerobic streptococci

*Infections may also be due to or involve aerobic bacteria as the sole or part of a mixed infection; brain abscess may contain microaerophilic streptococci; intra-abdominal infections may contain gram-negative enteric organisms and enterococci; and salpingitis may contain *Neisseria gonorrhoeae*, and *Chylamydia trachomatis*.

[†]*Bacteroides fragilis* is usually isolated from infections below the diaphragm except for brain abscesses.

tions or by direct inoculation associated with trauma. Anaerobic infections of the kidneys (renal and perirenal abscesses) and heart (pericarditis) are rare. **Enteritis necroticans (pigbel)** is a rare but often fatal gastrointestinal infection that most commonly follows ingestion of a large meal in a previously starved child or adult.

DIAGNOSIS

The diagnosis of anaerobic infection requires a high index of suspicion and the collection of appropriate and adequate specimens for anaerobic culture (Table 210-2). Cultures should be obtained in a manner that protects the specimen from contamination with mucosal bacteria and from exposure to ambient oxygen. Swab cultures of mucosal surfaces, nasal secretions, respiratory specimens, and stool should not be sent for anaerobic culture because these sites normally harbor many anaerobes. Aspirates of infected sites, abscess material, and biopsy specimens are appropriate. Specimens must be protected from oxygen and transported to the laboratory immediately. A **transport medium** is used to increase the recovery of obligate anaerobes. Gram stains are useful because anaerobic infections are usually polymicrobial. Several laboratory methods for susceptibility testing are available, but susceptibility testing of anaerobes is not always performed because it is labor intensive and time consuming. A rapid and easy screening test is used to detect β-lactamase production.

TREATMENT

Treatment of anaerobic infections requires adequate drainage and appropriate antimicrobial therapy. Antibiotic therapy varies

TABLE 210-2. Clues to Presumptive Diagnosis of Anaerobic Infections*

Infection that is contiguous to or in proximity with a mucosal surface colonized with anaerobic bacteria (oropharynx, intestinal-genitourinary tract)
Foul-smelling, putrid odor (present in half of anaerobic infections)
Severe tissue necrosis, abscesses, gangrene, or fasciitis
Gas formation in tissues (crepitus on exam or visible on plain x-ray)
Failure to recover organisms using conventional aerobic microbiologic methods
Failure of organisms to grow after pretreatment with antibiotics effective against anaerobes
Failure of infection to respond to antibiotics with poor efficacy against anaerobic bacteria (e.g., aminoglycosides)
Toxin-mediated syndromes (botulism, tetanus, gas gangrene, *Clostridium perfringens* food poisoning, *C. difficile* pseudomembranous colitis)
Typical infections associated with anaerobic bacteria (see **Table 210-1**)
Sterile pus
Septic thrombophlebitis
Septicemic syndrome with jaundice or intravascular hemolysis
Mixed polymorphic organisms on Gram stain
Typical Gram stain appearance:
- *Bacteroides* species—small, delicate, pleomorphic, pale, gram-negative bacilli
- *Fusobacterium nucleatum*—thin gram-negative bacilli with fusiform shape, pointed ends
- *F. necrophorum*—pleomorphism gram-negative bacilli with rounded ends
- *Peptostreptococcus*—gram-positive cocci similar to aerobic cocci
- *C. perfringens*—large, short, fat (boxcar-shaped) gram-positive bacilli

*Suspicion of anaerobic infection is critical before specimens are cultured to ensure optimal microbiologic techniques and prompt, appropriate therapy.

depending on the suspected or proven anaerobe involved. Some oral anaerobic flora is susceptible to penicillins, whereas many produce β-lactamase. The drugs that are active against these organisms include metronidazole, penicillins combined with β-lactamase inhibitors (ampicillin-sulbactam, ticarcillin-clavulanate, and piperacillin-tazobactam), carbapenems (imipenem and meropenem), clindamycin, cefoxitin, and chloramphenicol. Penicillin and vancomycin are active against the gram-positive anaerobes.

Aerobes are usually present with the anaerobes, necessitating broad-spectrum antibiotic combinations for empirical therapy. Specific therapy is based on culture results and clinical course.

For soft tissue infections, providing perfusion to the area is key to success; at times, a muscle flap or skin flap procedure is needed to ensure that nutrients and antimicrobial agents are brought to the affected area. Drainage of infected areas is often necessary for cure. Bacteria may survive in abscesses due to high bacterial inoculum, lack of bactericidal activity, and local conditions that facilitate bacterial proliferation. Aspiration is sometimes effective for small collections, whereas incision and drainage may be required for larger abscesses. Extensive debridement and resection of all devitalized tissue is needed to control fasciitis and myonecrosis.

COMMON ANAEROBIC PATHOGENS

CLOSTRIDIUM. Strains of *Clostridium* cause disease by infection, production of toxins, or both. Of the >60 species that have been identified, only a few cause infections in humans. The most commonly recovered organisms are *Clostridium difficile* (see Chapter 209) and *C. perfringens.* Other species encountered in human disease include *C. botulinum* (see Chapter 207), *C. tetani* (see Chapter 208), *C. butyricum, C. septicum, C. sordellii, C. tertium,* and *C. histolyticus.*

C. perfringens produces a variety of toxins and virulence factors. Strains of *C. perfringens* are designated A through E. **Alpha toxin** is a phospholipase that hydrolyzes sphingomyelin and lecithin and is produced by all strains. This toxin causes hemolysis, platelet lysis, increased capillary permeability, and hepatotoxicity. **Beta toxin,** produced by strains B and C, causes hemorrhagic necrosis of the small bowel. **Epsilon toxin,** produced by B and D strains, injures vascular endothelial cells, leading to increased vascular permeability, edema, and organ dysfunction. **Iota toxin,** produced by E strains, causes dermal edema. An enterotoxin is produced by type A and some type C and D strains. Hemolysins and a variety of enzymes are produced by many *C. perfringens* strains.

Clostridium species commonly invade the bloodstream shortly before, during, or just after death, leading to contamination of tissues that may be donated for transplantation. A large outbreak of *Clostridium* infections in tissue graft recipients was reported in 14 patients who received musculoskeletal grafts processed at a single tissue bank. As a result of this outbreak, recommendations for tissue processing now include a processing method that kills bacterial spores.

Myonecrosis (Gas Gangrene). *C. perfringens* is the major cause of myonecrosis, which is a rapidly progressive infection of soft tissue. In immunocompromised persons, especially patients receiving cancer chemotherapy, *C. septicum* is a classic cause of rapidly fatal gas gangrene. A clue to the diagnosis is pain out of proportion to the clinical appearance of the wound. Infection progresses rapidly with edema, swelling, myonecrosis, and sometimes crepitation of soft tissues. Hypotension, mental confusion, shock, and renal failure are common. A characteristic sweet odor is present in the serosanguineous discharge. Gram stain of the exudate reveals gram-positive bacilli and a few leukocytes. Early and complete debridement with excision of necrotic tissue is key to controlling the infection. High-dose penicillin (250,000 U/kg/day divided every 4–6 hr IV) or clindamycin (25–40 mg/kg/day divided every 6–8 hr IV) should be started immediately. The role of hyperbaric oxygen remains unclear but has been beneficial in several studies. The prognosis is poor, even with early, aggressive therapy.

Food Poisoning. *C. perfringens* type A produces an enterotoxin that causes food poisoning (see Chapter 337). The intoxication results in the acute onset of watery diarrhea and crampy abdominal pain. The usual foods containing toxin are improperly prepared meats and gravies. A specific diagnosis is rarely made in children with food poisoning. Therapy consists of rehydration and electrolyte replacement if necessary. The illness resolves spontaneously within 24 hr of onset. Prevention requires the maintenance of hot food at a temperature of ≥74°C.

GASTROENTERITIS. A severe gastroenteritis, termed **enteritis necroticans (pigbel),** is caused by type C strains of *C. perfringens* that produce beta toxin. The disease occurs most commonly in Papua New Guinea and is related to particular dietary habits and malnutrition. Enteritis necroticans was recognized in the USA in a 12 yr old boy with poorly controlled diabetes mellitus, with the source of the infection undercooked pork chitterlings.

Bacteroides and Prevotella. *Bacteroides fragilis* is 1 of the more virulent anaerobic pathogens that is most frequently recovered from blood cultures and cultures of tissue or pus. The most common infection in children is as a complication of appendicitis. The organism is part of normal colonic flora but is not common in the mouth or respiratory tract. *B. fragilis* is usually found as part of a polymicrobial appendiceal and other intra-abdominal abscesses and is involved in genital tract infections such as pelvic inflammatory disease and tubo-ovarian abscess. *Prevotella* organisms are normal oral flora, and infection typically involves gums, teeth, tonsils, and parapharyngeal spaces. Both organisms are sometimes involved in anaerobic pneumonia and lung abscess.

Strains of *B. fragilis* and *P. melaninogenica* produce β-lactamase and are resistant to penicillins. Recommended treatment is with ticarcillin-clavulanate, piperacillin/tazobactam, cefoxitin, metronidazole, clindamycin, imipenem, and meropenem. Because infections involving these organisms are polymicrobial, therapy should include antimicrobial agents active against the likely concomitant aerobic pathogens. Drainage of any abscesses and debridement of necrotic tissue are often required for control of these infections.

Fusobacterium. *Fusobacterium* organisms inhabit the intestine, respiratory tract, and female genital tracts. These organisms are more virulent than most of the normal anaerobic flora and cause bacteremia and a variety of rapidly progressive infections. **Lemierre syndrome,** bone and joint infections, and abdominal and genital tract infections are most common. Some strains produce β-lactamase and are resistant to penicillins.

Veillonella. *Veillonella* organisms are normal flora of the mouth, upper respiratory tract, intestine, and vagina. These anaerobes rarely cause infection. Strains are recovered as part of the polymicrobial flora causing abscess, chronic sinusitis, empyema, peritonitis, and wound infection. *Veillonella* organisms are susceptible to penicillins, cephalosporins, clindamycin, metronidazole, and carbapenems.

ANAEROBIC COCCI

Peptostreptococcus species are normal flora of the skin, respiratory tract, and gut. These organisms are often present in brain abscesses, chronic sinusitis, chronic otitis, and lung abscesses. Such infections are often polymicrobial, and therapy is aimed at the accompanying aerobes as well as the anaerobes. Most of the gram-positive cocci are susceptible to penicillin, cephalosporins, carbapenems, and vancomycin.

Brook I: Anaerobic infections in children. *Adv Pediatr* 2000;47:395–437.

Craig FW, Schunk JE: Retropharyngeal abscess in children: Clinical presentation, utility of imaging, and current management. *Pediatrics* 2003;111:1394–1398.

Hecht DW: Evolution of anaerobe susceptibility testing in the United States. *Clin Infect Dis* 2002;35(Suppl):S28–S35.

Kainer MA, Linden JV, Whaley DN, et al: *Clostridium* infections associated with musculoskeletal-tissue allografts. *N Engl J Med* 2004;350:2564–2571.

Kristensen LH, Prag J: Human necrobacillosis, with emphasis on Lemierre's syndrome. *Clin Infect Dis* 2000;31:524–532.

Petrillo TM, Beck-Sague CM, Songer JG, et al: Enteritis necroticans (pigbel) in a diabetic child. *N Engl J Med* 2000;342:1250–1253.

Nichols RL, Florman S: Clinical presentations of soft-tissue infections and surgical site infections. *Clin Infect Dis* 2001;33(Suppl):S84–S93.

Rautio M, Saxén H, Siitonen A, et al: Bacteriology of histopathologically defined appendicitis in children. *Pediatr Infect Dis J* 2000;19:1078–1083.

Sloas MM, Flynn PM, Kaste SC, et al: Typhlitis in children with cancer: A 30-year experience. *Clin Infect Dis* 1993;17:484–490.

Solomkin JS, Mazuski JE, Baron EJ, et al: Guidelines for the selection of anti-infective agents for complicated intra-abdominal infections. *Clin Infect Dis* 2003;37:997–1005.

Wang C, Schwaitzberg S, Berliner E, et al: Hyperbaric oxygen for treating wounds: A systematic review of the literature. *Arch Surg* 2003;138:272–279.

Section 7 — Mycobacterial Infections

Chapter 211 ■ Principles of Antimycobacterial Therapy

Stacene R. Maroushek

The treatment of mycobacterial infection and disease is often clinically challenging. Patients require therapy with multiple agents, the offending pathogens commonly exhibit complex drug resistance patterns, and patients often have underlying conditions that affect drug choice and monitoring. Several of the drugs have not been well studied in children, and current recommendations are extrapolated from the experience in adults.

As a general rule, single-drug therapy of *Mycobacterium tuberculosis* and nontuberculous mycobacteria is not recommended because of the high likelihood of development of antimicrobial resistance. Susceptibility testing of mycobacterial isolates often can aid in therapeutic decision making.

AGENTS USED AGAINST MYCOBACTERIUM TUBERCULOSIS

COMMONLY USED AGENTS

Isoniazid. Isoniazid (INH) is a hydrazide form of isonicotinic acid and is bactericidal for rapidly growing *M. tuberculosis*. The primary target of INH involves, via poorly understood mechanisms, the INH A gene, which encodes the enoyl ACP (acyl carrier protein) reductase needed for the last step of the mycolic acid biosynthesis pathway of cell wall production. Resistance to INH occurs following mutations in the INH A gene or in other genes encoding enzymes that activate INH such as kat G.

INH is indicated for the treatment of *M. tuberculosis*, *Mycobacterium kansasii*, and *Mycobacterium bovis*. The pediatric dose is 10–15 mg/kg/day PO in a single dose not to exceed 300 mg/day. The adult dose is 5 mg/kg/day PO in a single dose not to exceed 300 mg/day. Alternate pediatric dosing is 20–30 mg/kg PO in a single dose not to exceed 900 mg/dose given twice weekly under **directly observed therapy,** in which patients are observed to ingest each dose of antituberculosis medications, to maximize the likelihood of completion of therapy. The duration of treatment depends on the disease being treated (Table 211-1). INH needs to be taken 1 hr before or 2 hr after meals because food decreases absorption. It is available in liquid, tablet, IV (not approved by the Food and Drug Administration [FDA]), and IM preparations.

Major **adverse events** include hepatotoxicity in 1% of children and ~3% of adults, increasing with age, and dose-related peripheral neuropathy. Pyridoxine can ameliorate the peripheral neu-

TABLE 211-1. Treatment Recommendations for Nonresistant *Mycobacterium tuberculosis* Disease

TYPE OF INFECTION OR DISEASE	TREATMENT REGIMEN	COMMENTS
Latent tuberculosis infection (LTBI)	Isoniazid, daily for 9 mo	Twice weekly dosing of INH not preferred. Use only with strict directly observed therapy (DOT).
Pulmonary or extrapulmonary without meningitis	Isoniazid, rifampin, and pyrazinamide daily for 2 mo, followed by isoniazid and rifampin for 4 mo	If resistance is a concern, a fourth drug such as ethambutol or an aminoglycoside should be added until susceptibilities are known.
Meningitis	Isoniazid, rifampin, pyrazinamide, and an aminoglycoside or ethionamide daily for 2 mo, followed by isoniazid and rifampin for 7–10 mo	Use known geographic and source case resistance patterns to guide choice of fourth drug.

TABLE 211-2. Isoniazid Drug-Drug Interactions

DRUG USED WITH ISONIAZID	EFFECTS
Acetaminophen, alcohol, rifampin	Increased hepatotoxicity of isoniazid or listed drugs
Aluminum salts (antacids)	Decreased absorption of isoniazid
Carbamazepine, phenytoin, theophylline, diazepam, warfarin	Increased level, effect, or toxicity of listed drugs due to decreased metabolism
Itraconazole, ketoconazole, oral hypoglycemic agents	Decreased level/effect of listed drugs due to increased metabolism
Cycloserine, ethionamide	Increased central nervous system adverse effects of cycloserine and ethionamide
Prednisolone	Increased isoniazid metabolism

ropathy and is indicated for breast-feeding infants and their mothers, children and youth on milk- or meat-deficient diets, pregnant adolescents, and symptomatic HIV-infected children. Minor adverse events include rash, worsening of acne, epigastric pain with occasional nausea/vomiting, decreased vitamin D levels, and dizziness. The liquid formulation of INH is mixed in sorbitol, which often causes diarrhea and stomach upset.

INH is accompanied by significant drug-drug interactions (Table 211-2). The metabolism of INH is by acetylation. Acetylation rates have little effect on efficacy, but **slow acetylators** have an increased risk for hepatotoxicity, especially when used in combination with rifampin. Routine baseline liver function testing or monthly monitoring is only indicated for persons with underlying hepatic disease or on concomitant hepatotoxic drugs, including other antimycobacterial agents, acetaminophen, and alcohol. Monthly visits while on INH alone are encouraged to monitor for adherence, adverse effects, and worsening of infection.

Rifamycins. The rifamycins (rifampin, rifabutin, rifapentine) are a class of macrolide antibiotics developed from *Streptomyces mediterranei.* Rifampin is a synthetic derivative of rifamycin B, and rifabutin is a derivative of rifamycin S. Rifapentine is a cyclopentyl derivative. The rifamycins inhibit the DNA-dependent RNA polymerase of mycobacteria, resulting in decreased RNA synthesis. They are generally bactericidal at treatment doses, but may be bacteriostatic at lower doses. Resistance is from a mutation in the DNA-dependent RNA polymerase gene (RpoB) that is often induced by previous incomplete therapy. Cross resistance between rifampin and rifabutin has been demonstrated.

Rifampin is active against *M. tuberculosis, Mycobacterium leprae, M. kansasii,* and *Mycobacterium avium* complex. Rifampin is an integral drug in standard combination treatment of active *M. tuberculosis* disease, and can be used as an alternate to INH in the treatment of latent tuberculosis infection in children unable to tolerate INH. Rifabutin has similar spectrum with increased activity against *M. avium* complex. Rifapentine is undergoing clinical trials in pediatrics and appears to have similar activity as rifampin. The pediatric dose of rifampin is 10–15 mg/kg/day PO in a single dose not to exceed 600 mg/day. The adult rifampin dose is 5–10 mg/kg/day PO in a single dose not to exceed 600 mg/day. Commonly used rifampin preparations include 150 and 300 mg capsules and a suspension, which is usually formulated at a concentration of 10 mg/mL. The shelf life of rifampin suspension is short (~4 wk), so it should not be compounded with other antimycobacterial agents. An intravenous form of rifampin is also available for initial treatment of patients who cannot take oral preparations. Dose adjustment is needed for patients with liver failure. Other rifamycins (rifabutin and rifapentine) have been poorly studied in children and are not recommended for use in children.

Rifampin can be associated with **adverse events** such as transient elevations of liver enzymes, gastrointestinal upset with cramps, nausea, vomiting and anorexia, headache, dizziness, and immunologically mediated fever and flulike symptoms. Thrombocytopenia and hemolytic anemias can also occur. Rifabutin has a similar spectrum of toxicities, except for an increased incidence of rash (4%) and neutropenia (2%). Rifapentine has fewer adverse events but has an association with hyperuricemia and cytopenias, especially lymphopenia and neutropenia. All rifamycins can turn urine and other secretions (tears, saliva, stool, sputum) an orange color, which can stain contact lens. Patients and families should be warned about this common but otherwise innocuous adverse effect.

Rifamycins induce the hepatic cytochrome P450 isoenzyme system and are associated with the increased metabolism/decreased level of several drugs when administered concomitantly. These include digoxin, corticosteroids such as prednisone and dexamethasone, dapsone, fluconazole, phenytoin, oral contraceptives, warfarin, and many antiretroviral agents, especially protease inhibitors and non-nucleoside reverse transcriptase inhibitors. Rifabutin has less of an effect on lowering protease inhibitor levels.

Previous recommendations for the use of pyrazinamide in combination with rifampin for short course latent tuberculosis therapy have been associated with serious liver dysfunction and death. This combination has never been well studied or recommended for pediatric patients and should not to be used.

No routine laboratory monitoring for rifamycins is indicated unless the patient is symptomatic. In patients with signs of toxicity, complete blood counts and renal and liver function tests are indicated.

Pyrazinamide. Pyrazinamide (PZA) is a synthetic pyrazide analog of nicotinamide that is bactericidal against intracellular *M. tuberculosis* organisms in acidic environments, such as within macrophages or inflammatory lesions. A bacterial-specific enzyme (pyrazinamidase) converts PZA to pyrazinoic acid, which leads to low pH levels not tolerated by *M. tuberculosis.* Resistance is poorly understood but may arise from bacterial pyrazinamidase alterations.

PZA is indicated for the initial treatment phase of active tuberculosis disease in combination with other antimycobacterial agents. The pediatric dose is 15–30 mg/kg/day PO in a single dose not to exceed 2,000 mg/day. Twice weekly dosing with directly observed therapy only is with 50 mg/kg/day PO in a single dose not to exceed 4,000 mg/day. It is available in a 500 mg tablet and can be made into a suspension of 100 mg/mL.

Adverse events include gastrointestinal upset (e.g., nausea, vomiting, and poor appetite) in ~4% of children, dose-dependent hepatotoxicity, and elevated serum uric acid levels that may precipitate gout in susceptible adults. Approximately 10% of pediatric patients have elevated uric acid levels, but with no associated clinical sequelae. Minor reactions include arthralgias, fatigue, and, rarely, fever.

Previous recommendations for the use of pyrazinamide in combination with rifampin for short course latent tuberculosis therapy have been associated with serious liver dysfunction and death. This combination has never been well studied or recommended for pediatric patients and should not to be used.

No routine laboratory monitoring for pyrazinamide is required, but monthly visits to reinforce the importance of therapy are desirable.

Ethambutol. Ethambutol is a synthetic form of ethylenedi-imino-di-1-butanol dihydrochloride that inhibits RNA synthesis needed for cell wall formation. At standard doses it is bacteriostatic, but at doses of >25 mg/kg ethambutol has bactericidal activity. The mechanism of resistance is unknown, but resistance is developed rapidly when used as a single agent against *M. tuberculosis.*

Ethambutol is indicated for the treatment of infections caused by *M. tuberculosis, M. kansasii, M. bovis,* and *M. avium* complex. Ethambutol should only be used as part of a combination treatment regimen for *M. tuberculosis.* Daily dosing is 15–20 mg/kg PO in a single dose not to exceed 2,500 mg/day. Twice weekly dosing is with 50 mg/kg PO in a single dose not to exceed

2,500 mg/day. Dose adjustment is needed in renal insufficiency. It is available in 100 and 400 mg tablets.

The **major adverse** effect with ethambutol is optic neuritis. Ethambutol should only be used in children old enough to have visual acuity and color discrimination reliably monitored. Visual changes are usually dose dependent and reversible. Other adverse events include headache, dizziness, confusion, hyperuricemia, gastrointestinal upset, peripheral neuropathy, hepatotoxicity, and cytopenias, especially neutropenia and thrombocytopenia.

Routine laboratory monitoring includes baseline and periodic visual acuity and color discrimination testing, complete blood counts, serum uric acid levels, and renal and liver functions tests.

LESS COMMONLY USED AGENTS

Aminoglycosides. The aminoglycosides used for mycobacterial infections include streptomycin, amikacin, kanamycin, and capreomycin. Streptomycin, isolated from *Streptomyces griseus,* was the 1st drug used to treat *M. tuberculosis.* Capreomycin, a cyclic polypeptide from *Streptomyces capreolus,* and amikacin, a semisynthetic derivative of kanamycin, are newer agents that are recommended when streptomycin is unavailable. Aminoglycosides act by binding irreversibly to the 30S subunit of ribosomes and inhibit subsequent protein synthesis. Streptomycin exhibits concentration-dependent bactericidal activity while capreomycin is bacteriostatic. Resistance is by mutation in the binding site of the 30S ribosome, by decreased transport into cells, or by inactivation by bacterial enzymes. Cross-resistance between aminoglycosides has been demonstrated.

The aminoglycosides are indicated for the treatment of *M. tuberculosis* and *M. avium* complex. All are considered 2nd line drugs in the treatment of *M. tuberculosis* and should be used only when resistance patterns are known. The route is by IM injection as aminoglycosides have poor oral absorption. Pediatric dosing ranges for streptomycin are 20 mg/kg/day if given daily and 20–40 mg/kg/day if given twice weekly, IM in a single daily dose. Capreomycin, amikacin, and kanamycin doses are 15–30 mg/kg/day IM in a single dose not to exceed 1 g/day. Dose adjustment is necessary in renal insufficiency.

Aminoglycosides have **adverse effects** on proximal renal tubules, the cochlea, and vestibular apparatus of the ear. Nephrotoxicity and ototoxicity comprise most of the significant adverse events. Rarely, patients can exhibit fever or rash with the administration of aminoglycosides. Concomitant use of other nephrotoxic or ototoxic agents should be avoided as adverse effects may be additive. An infrequent, but serious, synergistic, dose-dependent, aminoglycoside effect with nondepolarizing neuromuscular blockade agents can result in respiratory depression or paralysis.

Hearing and renal function should be monitored at baseline and periodically. Early signs of ototoxicity include tinnitus, vertigo, and hearing loss. Ototoxicity appears to be nonreversible, but early renal damage may be reversible. As with other aminoglycosides, peak and trough drug levels are helpful in dosing and managing early toxicities.

Cycloserine. Cycloserine, derived from *Streptomyces orchidaceus* or *Streptomyces garyphalus,* is a synthetic analog of the amino acid D-alanine that interferes with bacterial cell wall synthesis via competitive inhibition of D-alanine components to be incorporated into the cell wall. It is bacteriostatic, and the mechanism of resistance is unknown.

Cycloserine is used to treat *M. tuberculosis* and *M. bovis.* The dose is 10–20 mg/kg/day PO divided into 2 doses not to exceed 1 g/day. It is available in a 250 mg capsule.

The major **adverse event** is neurotoxicity with significant psychologic disturbance, including seizures, acute psychosis, headache, confusion, depression, and personality changes. The neurotoxic effects are additive with ethionamide and isoniazid. It has also been associated with megaloblastic anemia. Cycloserine must be dose adjusted with renal impairment. It should be used with caution in patients with underlying psychiatric illness.

Routine laboratory monitoring includes renal and hepatic function, complete blood counts, and cycloserine levels; psychiatric symptoms are less frequent at levels of <30 μg/mL).

Ethionamide. Ethionamide, structurally related to isoniazid, is an ethyl derivative of thioisonicotinamide that inhibits peptide synthesis by an unclear mechanism thought to involve NAD and NADP dehydrogenase disruptions. Ethionamide is bacteriostatic at most therapeutic levels. Resistance develops quickly if used as a single-agent therapy, although the mechanism is unknown.

Ethionamide is used as an alternate to streptomycin or ethambutol in the treatment of *M. tuberculosis,* and has some activity against *M. kansasii* and *M. avium* complex. A metabolite, ethionamide sulfoxide, is bactericidal against *M. leprae.* Ethionamide has been shown to have good central nervous system (CNS) penetration and has been used as a 4th drug in combination with rifampin, isoniazid, and pyrazinamide. The pediatric dosing is 15–20 mg/kg/day PO in 2 divided doses not to exceed 1 g/day. It is available in a 250 mg tablet.

Gastrointestinal upset is common, with other **adverse events** reported including neurologic disturbances (anxiety, dizziness, peripheral neuropathy, seizure, acute psychosis), hepatic enzyme elevations, hypothyroidism, hypoglycemia, and hypersensitivity reaction with rash and fever. It should be used with caution in patients with underlying psychiatric or thyroid disease. The psychiatric adverse effects can be potentiated with concomitant use of cycloserine.

In addition to monitoring mood clinically, routine laboratory monitoring includes thyroid and liver function tests and, in diabetic patients, blood glucose levels.

Fluoroquinolones. The fluoroquinolones are a fluorinated derivative of the quinolone class of antibiotics. Ciprofloxacin is a 1st generation fluoroquinolone, and levofloxacin is the more active L-isomer of ofloxacin. Moxifloxacin and gatifloxacin are newer agents with emerging use in pediatric mycobacterial disease. Fluoroquinolones are not indicated for use in children <18 yr of age, but studies of their use in pediatrics continue to indicate that they may be used in special circumstances. Fluoroquinolones are bactericidal and exert their effect via inhibition of DNA gyrase. The alterations in DNA gyrase result in relaxation of super-coiled DNA and breaks in double-stranded DNA. The mechanism of resistance is not well defined, but likely involves mutations in the DNA gyrase.

Levofloxacin is an important 2nd line drug in the treatment of multidrug-resistant *M. tuberculosis.* Ciprofloxacin has activity against *Mycobacterium fortuitum* complex and against *M. tuberculosis.* The pediatric dose of ciprofloxacin is 20–30 mg/kg/day PO or IV not to exceed 1.5 mg/day PO or 800 mg/day IV. The adult dose is 500–750 mg/dose PO divided into 2 doses or 200–400 mg/dose IV every 12 hr. Ciprofloxacin is available in 100, 250, 500, and 750 mg tablets and can be made in 5% (50 mg/mL) or 10% (100 mg/mL) suspensions. The dose of levofloxacin for children is 5–10 mg/kg/day given once daily either PO or IV not to exceed 1,000 mg/day, and for adults is 500–1,000 mg/day PO or IV not to exceed 1,000 mg/day. Levofloxacin is available in 250, 500, and 750 mg tablets, and a 50 mg/mL suspension can be extemporaneously compounded. The suspension has a shelf life of only 8 wk.

Fluoroquinolones' most frequent **adverse effect** is gastrointestinal upset with nausea, vomiting, abdominal pain, and diarrhea, including pseudomembranous colitis. Other less frequent adverse effects include bone marrow depression, CNS effects (e.g., lowered seizure threshold, confusion, tremor, dizziness, headache); elevated liver transaminases, photosensitivity, and arthropathies. The potential for arthropathies (e.g, tendon ruptures, arthralgias, tendonitis) are the predominant reason why fluoroquinolones are not recommended for pediatric use. The mechanism of injury appears to involve the disruption of extracellular matrix of cartilage and depletion of collagen. This is of special concern in the bone and joint development of children.

Fluoroquinolones induce the cytochrome P450 isoenzymes that can increase the concentrations of dually administered theophylline and warfarin. Nonsteroidal anti-inflammatories can potentiate the CNS effects of fluoroquinolones and should be avoided while taking a fluoroquinolone. Both ciprofloxacin and levofloxacin should be dose adjusted in patients with significant renal dysfunction.

While taking fluoroquinolones, patients should be monitored for hepatic and renal dysfunction, arthropathies, and hematologic abnormalities.

Linezolid. Linezolid, FDA approved for use in 2000, is a synthetic oxazolidinone derivative. Linezolid is not currently approved for use against mycobacterial infection in pediatric or adult patients but has activity against some of these organisms. Studies on efficacy of treatment of mycobacterial infections are underway. Linezolid inhibits translation by binding to the 23S ribosomal component of the 50S ribosome subunit, preventing coupling with the 70S subunit. Resistance is thought to be from a point mutation at the binding site, but is poorly studied as only a few cases of resistance have been reported.

Linezolid's approved indications are for bacterial infections other than mycobacteria, but linezolid has shown preliminary in vitro activity against rapidly growing mycobacterium (*M. fortuitum* complex, *M. chelonae, M. abscessus*), *M. tuberculosis,* and *M. avium* complex. The dose for 0–11 yr old children is 10 mg/kg/day PO or IV in divided doses every 8–12 hr. For persons >12 yr of age, the dose is 600 mg PO or IV every 12 hr. It is available in 400 and 600 mg tablets and a 20 mg/mL suspension.

Adverse events to linezolid include gastrointestinal upset (e.g., nausea, vomiting, diarrhea), CNS disturbances (e.g., dizziness, headache, insomnia, peripheral neuropathy), lactic acidosis, fever, myelosuppression, and pseudomembranous colitis. Linezolid is a weak inhibitor of monoamine oxidase A; therefore, patients are advised to avoid foods with high tyramine content. Linezolid should be used cautiously in patients with pre-existing myelosuppression.

In addition to monitoring for gastrointestinal upset and CNS perturbations, routine laboratory monitoring includes complete blood counts at least weekly.

Para-Amino Salicylic Acid. Para-aminosalicylic acid (PAS) is a structural analog of para-aminobenzoic acid (PABA). It is bacteriostatic and acts by competitively inhibiting the synthesis of folic acid similar to the action of sulfonamides. Resistance mechanisms are poorly understood.

PAS acts against *M. tuberculosis.* The dose is 150 mg/kg/day PO in 2–3 divided doses. PAS is dispensed in 4 g packets, and the granules should be mixed with liquid and swallowed whole.

Common **adverse events** include gastrointestinal upset, and less common events include hypokalemia, hematuria, albuminuria, crystalluria, and elevations of hepatic transaminases. PAS can decrease the absorption of rifampin, and co-administration with ethionamide potentiates the adverse effects of PAS.

In addition to monitoring for weight loss clinically, routine laboratory monitoring includes liver and renal function tests.

AGENTS USED AGAINST MYCOBACTERIUM LEPRAE

DAPSONE. Dapsone is a sulfone antibiotic with characteristics similar to sulfonamides. Similar to other sulfonamides, dapsone acts as a competitive antagonist of PABA, which is needed for the bacterial synthesis of folic acid. Dapsone is bacteriostatic against *M. leprae.* Resistance, not well understood, is thought to occur after alterations at the binding site.

Dapsone is used in the treatment of *M. leprae* in combination with other antileprosy agents (rifampin, clofazimine, ethionamide). The pediatric dose is 1–2 mg/kg/day PO as a single dose not to exceed 100 mg/day for a duration of 3–10 years. The adult dose is 100 mg/day PO as a single dose. Dapsone is available in 25 and 100 mg scored tablets, and an oral suspension of 2 mg/mL (Jacobus Pharmaceutical Company, telephone 609-921-7447). The dose should be adjusted in renal insufficiency.

Dapsone has many reported **adverse events,** including dose-related hemolytic anemia, especially in patients with glucose-6-phosphate dehydrogenase (G6PD) deficiency, pancreatis, renal complications (acute tubular necrosis, acute renal failure, albuminuria), increased liver enzymes, psychosis, tinnitus, peripheral neuropathy, photosensitivity, and a hypersensitivity syndrome with fever, rash, hepatic damage, and malaise. A **"lepra reaction"** may occur with treatment, which is a nontoxic, paradoxical worsening of lepromatous leprosy with the initiation of therapy. This hypersensitivity reaction is not an indication to discontinue therapy. It should be used with caution in patients with G6PD deficiency or taking other folic acid antagonists. Rifampin may decrease dapsone levels, while clotrimazole may increase levels.

Routine laboratory monitoring includes complete blood counts weekly during the 1st month of therapy, weekly through 6 mo of therapy, then every 6 mo thereafter. Other periodic assessments include renal function with creatine levels and urinalysis, and liver function tests.

CLOFAZIMINE. Clofazimine is a synthetic phendimetrazine tartrate derivative that acts by binding to the mycobacterial DNA at guanine sites. It has a slow bactericidal activity against *M. leprae.* Mechanisms of resistance are not well studied. No cross-resistance between clofazimine and dapsone or rifampin has been shown.

Clofazimine is indicated as part of a combination therapy for the treatment of *M. leprae.* It appears there may be some activity against other mycobacteria such as *M. avium* complex, although treatment failures are common. Safety and efficacy of clofazimine are poorly studied in children. The pediatric dose is 1 mg/kg/day PO as a single dose not to exceed 100 mg/day in combination with dapsone and rifampin for 2 yr and then additionally as a single agent for >1 yr. The adult dose is 100 mg/day PO. It should be taken with food to increase absorption.

The most common **adverse event** is a dose-related, reversible pink to tan-brown discoloration of the skin and conjunctiva. Other adverse effects include dry, itchy skin, rash, headache, dizziness, abdominal pain, diarrhea, vomiting, peripheral neuropathy, and elevated liver transaminases.

Routine laboratory monitoring includes periodic liver function tests.

AGENTS USED AGAINST NONTUBERCULOUS MYCOBACTERIA

CEFOXITIN. Cefoxitin, a cephamycin derivative, is a 2nd generation cephalosporin that, like other cephalosporins, inhibits cell wall synthesis by linking with penicillin binding proteins to create an unstable bacterial cell wall. Resistance develops by various alterations in the penicillin binding proteins.

Cefoxitin is often used in combination therapy for mycobacterial disease (Table 211-3). Pediatric dosing is based on disease severity with a range of 80–160 mg/kg/day divided every 4–8 hr not to exceed 12 g/day. Adult doses are 1–2 g/day not to exceed 12 g/day. It is available in IV or IM formulations. Increased dosing intervals are needed with renal insufficiency.

Adverse events are primarily hematologic (eosinophilia, granulocytopenia, thrombocytopenia, hemolytic anemia), gastrointestinal (nausea, vomiting, diarrhea with possible pseudomembranous colitis), and CNS (dizziness, vertigo). Potential additive adverse effects may occur when used with aminoglycosides.

Routine laboratory monitoring with long-term use includes complete blood counts and liver and renal function tests.

TABLE 211-3. Treatment Regimens for Nontuberculous Mycobacteria Infections

MYCOBACTERIA	DISEASE	TREATMENT
Mycobacterium abscessus	Otitis media	Clarithromycin plus cefoxitin plus amikacin, may require surgical intervention.
	Pulmonary infection in patient with cystic fibrosis	Seek expert opinion.
Mycobacterium avian complex	Lymphadenitis	Clarithromycin plus ethambutol with rifampin. (Complete surgical excision alone is often curative.)
	Pulmonary disease	Clarithromycin plus ethambutol with rifampin. If severe disease, consider addition of amikacin or streptomycin.
Mycobacterium fortuitum complex	Catheter infection	Remove catheter, amikacin plus cefoxitin IV initially, followed by oral clarithromycin, ciprofloxacin, or trimethoprim-sulfamethoxazole.
	Cutaneous infection	Excision of lesion, cefoxitin plus amikacin IV, followed by oral clarithromycin, doxycycline, or ciprofloxacin.
Mycobacterium kansasii	Pulmonary disease	Rifampin, ethambutol, and isoniazid.
	Osteomyelitis	Surgical debridement with rifampin, ethambutol, and isoniazid.
Mycobacterium marinum	Cutaneous disease (if moderate to severe)	Rifampin, trimethoprim-sulfamethoxazole, clarithromycin, or doxycycline. Consider surgery for large lesions.

DOXYCYCLINE. Doxycycline is in the tetracycline family of antibiotics and has limited use in pediatrics. Like other tetracyclines, doxycycline acts to decrease protein synthesis by binding to the 30S ribosome and to transfer RNA. It may also cause alterations to the cytoplasmic membrane of susceptible bacteria.

Doxycycline is used to treat *M. fortuitum* (see Table 211-3). Although it can be used to treat *M. marinum,* adult treatment failures have occurred. Pediatric dosing, both PO and IV, is based on age and weight. For children >8 yr of age and <45 kg, the dose is 4.4 mg/kg/day divided twice daily. Dosing for larger children and adults is 100 mg twice daily. Doxycycline is available as 50 and 100 mg capsules or tablets, and in 25 mg/5 mL and 50 mg/5 mL suspensions.

Doxycycline use in children is limited by a permanent tooth discoloration, which is worse with long-term use. Other **adverse events** include photosensitivity, liver and renal dysfunction, and esophagitis, which can be minimized by dosing with large volumes of liquid. Doxycycline may decrease the effectiveness of oral contraceptives. Rifampin, carbamazepine, and phenytoin may decrease the concentration of doxycycline.

Routine laboratory monitoring with long-term use includes renal and liver function tests as well as complete blood counts.

MACROLIDES. Clarithromycin and azithromycin belong to the macrolide family of antibiotics. Clarithromycin is a methoxy derivative of erythromycin. Macrolides act by binding the 50S subunit of ribosomes, subsequently inhibiting protein synthesis. Resistance mechanisms for mycobacteria are not well understood, but may involve binding site alterations. Clarithromycin appears to have synergistic antimycobacterial activity when combined with rifamycins, ethambutol, or clofazimine.

Clarithromycin is widely used for the prophylaxis and treatment *M. avium* complex disease and also has activity against *Mycobacterium abscesses, M. fortuitum,* and *M. marinum.* Azithromycin has significantly different pharmacokinetics compared with other macrolide agents and has not been studied and is not indicated for mycobacterial infections. The pediatric dose of clarithromycin for primary prophylaxis of *M. avium* complex infections is 7.5 mg/kg/dose PO given twice daily not to exceed 500 mg/day. This dose is used for recurrent *M. avium* complex disease but is combined with ethambutol and rifampin. The adult dose is 500 mg PO twice daily to be used as a single agent for primary prophylaxis, or as part of combination therapy with ethambutol and rifampin. Dose adjustment is needed for renal insufficiency but not liver failure. It is available in 250 and 500 mg tablets and suspensions of 125 mg/5 mL and 250 mg/5 mL.

Adverse effects include gastrointestinal upset, which occurs frequently with clarithromycin, including vomiting (6%), diarrhea (6%), and abdominal pain (3%). Other adverse effects include taste disturbances, headache, and QT prolongation if used with inhaled anesthetics, clotrimazole, antiarrhythmic agents, or azoles. It should be used cautiously in patients with renal insufficiency or liver failure.

Routine laboratory monitoring with prolonged use includes periodic liver enzyme tests. Diarrhea is an early sign of pseudomembranous colitis.

TRIMETHOPRIM-SULFAMETHOXAZOLE. Trimethoprim-sulfamethoxazole (TMP-SMZ) is formulated in a fixed ratio of 1 part TMP to 5 parts SMZ. SMZ is a sulfonamide that inhibits synthesis of dihydrofolic acid by competitively inhibiting PABA, similar to dapsone. TMP blocks production of tetrahydrofolic acid and downstream biosynthesis of nucleic acids and protein by reversibly binding to dihydrofolate reductase. The combination of the 2 agents is synergistic and often bactericidal.

TMP-SMZ is often used in combination therapy for mycobacterial disease (see Table 211-3). Oral or IV dosing for pediatrics is 15–20 mg TMP/kg/day divided every 6–8 hr for serious infections and 6–12 mg TMP/kg/day divided every 12 hr for mild infections. The adult dose is 160 mg TMP/800 mg SMZ every 12 hr. Dose reduction may be needed in renal insufficiency. It is available in single-strength tablets (80 mg TMP/400 mg SMZ) and double-strength tablets (160 mg TMP/800 mg SMZ) and in a suspension of 40 mg TMP and 200 mg SMZ/5 mL.

The most common **adverse effect** with TMP-SMZ is myelosuppression. It must be used with caution in patients with G6PD deficiency. Other adverse effects include renal abnormalities, rash, aseptic meningitis, gastrointestinal disturbances (e.g., pancreatitis, diarrhea), and prolonged QT interval if co-administered with inhaled anesthetics, azoles, or macrolides.

Routine laboratory monitoring includes monthly complete blood counts and periodic electrolytes and creatine to monitor renal function.

Blumberg HM, Burman WJ, Chaisson RE, et al: American Thoracic Society/Centers for Disease Control and Prevention/Infectious Diseases Society of America: Treatment of tuberculosis. *Am J Respir Crit Care Med* 2003;167:603–662.

Dooley KE, Sterling TR: Treatment of latent tuberculosis infection: Challenges and prospects. *Clin Chest Med* 2005;26:313–326, vii.

Duncan K, Barry CE: Prospects for new antitubercular drugs. *Curr Opin Microbiol* 2004;7:460–465.

Fortun J, Martin-Davila P, Navas E, et al: Linezolid for the treatment of multidrug-resistant tuberculosis. *J Antimicrob Chemother* 2005;56:180–185.

Hampel B, Hullmann R, Schmidt H: Ciprofloxacin in pediatrics: Worldwide clinical experience based on compassionate use—safety report. *Pediatr Infect Dis J* 1997;16:127–129, 160–162.

Marshall JD, Abdel-Rahman S, Johnson K, et al: Rifapentine pharmacokinetics in adolescents. *Pediatr Infect Dis J* 1999;18:882–888.

McNeill L, Allen M, Estrada C, Cook P: Pyrazinamide and rifampin vs isoniazid for the treatment of latent tuberculosis: Improved completion rates but more hepatotoxicity. *Chest* 2003;123:102–106.

Samigun M, Santoso B: Lowering of theophylline clearance by isoniazid in slow and rapid acetylators. *Br J Clin Pharmacol* 1990;29:570–573.

Van Scoy RE, Wilkowske CJ: Antimycobacterial therapy. *Mayo Clin Proc* 1999;74:1038–1048.

Chapter 212 ■ Tuberculosis (*Mycobacterium Tuberculosis*)

Jeffrey R. Starke and Flor M. Munoz

During the last decade of the 20th century the number of new cases of tuberculosis increased worldwide. Currently, 95% of tuberculosis cases occur in developing countries where HIV/AIDS epidemics have had the greatest impact, and where resources are often unavailable for proper identification and treatment of these diseases (Figs. 212-1 and 212-2). In many industrialized countries, most cases of tuberculosis occur in foreign-born populations (Fig. 212-3). The World Health Organization (WHO) estimates that >8 million new cases of tuberculosis occur and approximately 3 million people die of the disease worldwide each year. Almost 1.3 million cases and 450,000 deaths occur in children each year. More than 1/3 of the world's population is infected with *Mycobacterium tuberculosis*. If present trends continue, 10.5 million new cases are expected to occur annually by 2006, with Africa having more cases than any other region of the world (see Fig. 212-1). In the United States, after a resurgence in the late 1980s, the total number of cases of tuberculosis began to decrease in 1992, but tuberculosis continues to be a public health concern (see Fig. 212-3).

ETIOLOGY. There are 5 closely related mycobacteria in the *M. tuberculosis* complex: *M. tuberculosis, M. bovis, M. africanum, M. microti,* and *M. canetti. M. tuberculosis* is the most important cause of tuberculosis disease in humans. The tubercle bacilli are non-spore-forming, nonmotile, pleomorphic, weakly gram-positive curved rods 2–4 µm long. They may appear beaded or clumped in stained clinical specimens or culture media. They are obligate aerobes that grow in synthetic media containing glycerol as the carbon source and ammonium salts as the nitrogen source (Loewenstein-Jensen culture media). These mycobacteria grow best at 37– 41°C, produce niacin, and lack pigmentation. A lipid-rich cell wall accounts for resistance to the bactericidal actions of antibody and complement. A hallmark of all mycobacteria is **acid fastness**—the capacity to form stable mycolate complexes with arylmethane dyes such as crystal violet, carbolfuchsin, auramine, and rhodamine. Once stained, they resist decoloration with ethanol and hydrochloric or other acids.

Mycobacteria grow slowly, their generation time being 12–24 hr. Isolation from clinical specimens on solid synthetic media usually takes 3–6 wk, and drug susceptibility testing requires an additional 4 wk. Growth can be detected in 1–3 wk in selective liquid medium using radiolabeled nutrients (the BACTEC radiometric system), and drug susceptibilities can be determined in an additional 3–5 days. Once mycobacterial growth is detected, the species of mycobacteria present can be determined within hours using high-pressure liquid chromatography analysis, as each species has a unique fingerprint of mycolic acids. The presence of *M. tuberculosis* in clinical specimens sometimes can be detected directly within hours using **nucleic acid amplification (NAA)** tests, including polymerase chain reaction, that employ a DNA probe complementary to mycobacterial DNA or RNA. Data from children are limited, but the sensitivity of some NAA techniques is similar to that for culture for pulmonary tuberculosis and is better than culture for extrapulmonary disease. Restriction fragment length polymorphism (RFLP) profiling of mycobacteria is a helpful tool to study the epidemiology of tuberculosis.

EPIDEMIOLOGY. Latent tuberculosis infection (LTBI) occurs after the inhalation of infective droplet nuclei containing *M. tuberculosis*. A reactive tuberculin skin test and the absence of clinical and radiographic manifestations are the hallmark of this stage. The word *tuberculosis* refers to disease, which occurs when signs

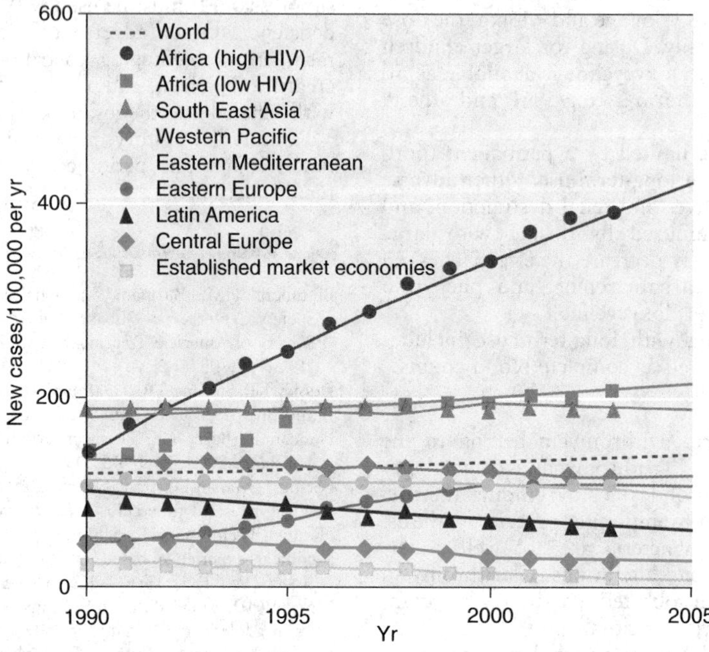

Figure 212-1. Trajectories of tuberculosis epidemic for 9 epidemiologically different regions of the world. Points mark trends in estimated incidence rates, derived from case notifications for 1990–2003. Groupings of countries based on WHO regions. High HIV = incidence >4% in adults aged 15–49 yr in 2003; low HIV = <4%. Established market economies = all 30 OECD (Organization for Economic Co-operation and Development) countries, except Mexico, Slovakia, and Turkey, plus Singapore. Countries in each region listed in full elsewhere. (From Dye C: Global epidemiology of tuberculosis. *Lancet* 2006;367:938–940.)

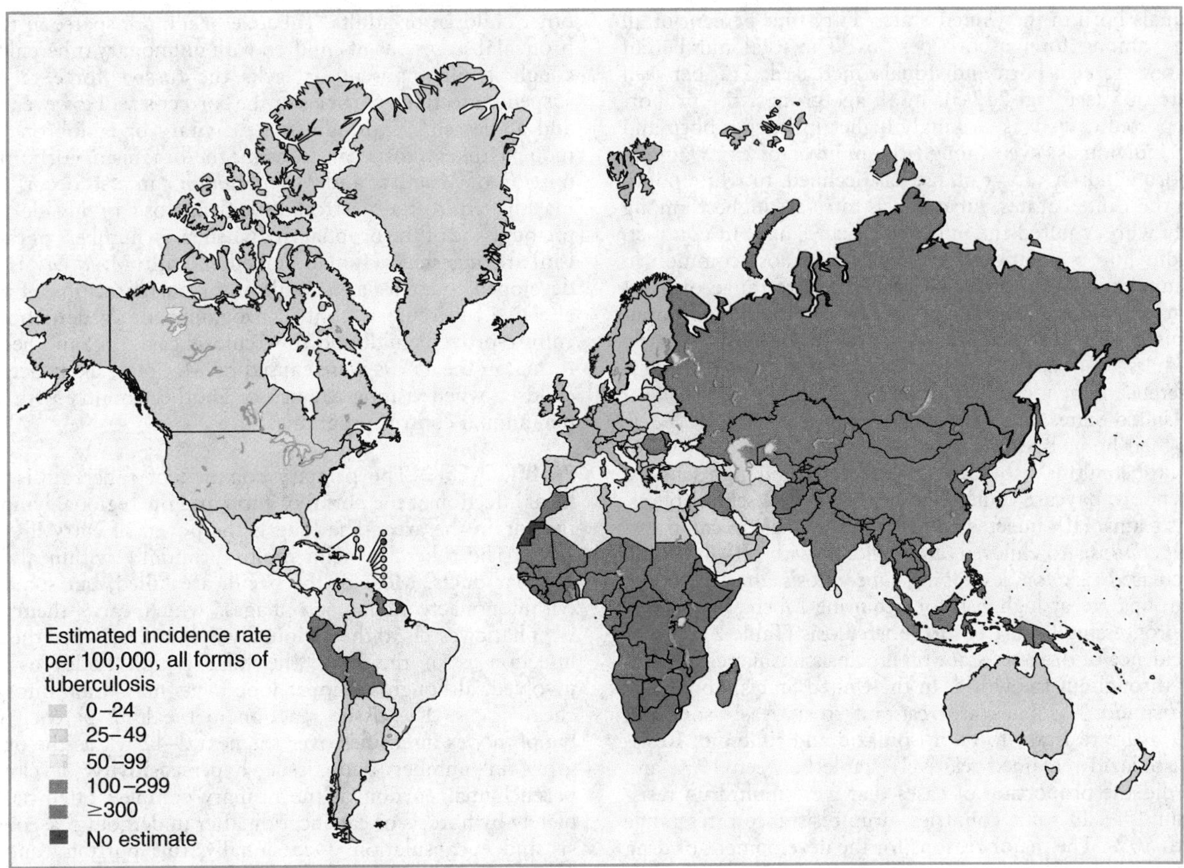

Figure 212-2. Distribution of tuberculosis in the world in 2003. (From Dye C: Global epidemiology of tuberculosis. *Lancet* 2006;367:938–940.)

and symptoms or radiographic changes become apparent. Untreated infants with LTBI have up to a 40% likelihood of developing tuberculosis, with the risk for progression decreasing gradually through childhood to adult lifetime rates of 5–10%. The greatest risk for progression occurs in the 1st 2 yr after infection.

The WHO estimates that 1/3 of the world's population—2 billion people—are infected with *M. tuberculosis*. Infection rates are highest in Africa, Asia, and Latin America (see Fig. 212-2). The global burden of tuberculosis continues to grow due to several factors, including the impact of HIV epidemics, population migration patterns, increasing poverty, social upheaval and crowded living conditions in developing countries and in inner city populations in developed countries, inadequate health coverage and poor access to health services, and inefficient tuberculosis control programs.

Tuberculosis case rates decreased steadily in the USA during the 1st half of the 20th century, long before the advent of antituberculosis drugs, as a result of improved living conditions. A resurgence of tuberculosis in the late 1980s was associated primarily with the HIV epidemic and transmission of the organism in congregate settings, adding to increased immigration and poor tuberculosis control (see Fig. 212-3). Since 1992, the number of reported cases of tuberculosis has decreased each year, reaching a record low of 14,097 cases (rate of 4.9/100,000 population) in the year 2005. Of these, 863 (6.7%) cases occurred in children <15 yr of age (rate 1.5/100,000 population). The decline in overall incidence was mostly due to a substantial decrease in cases

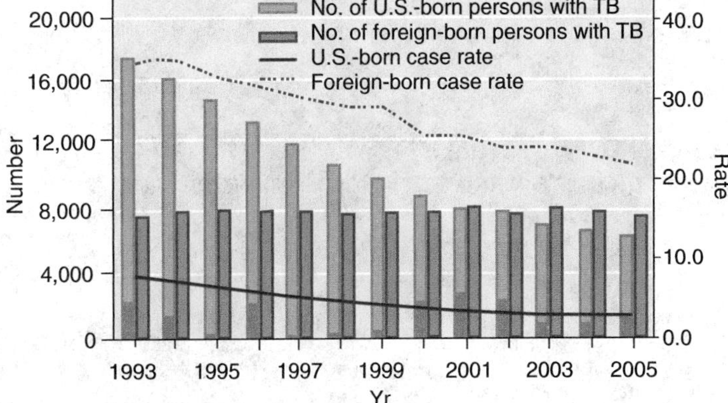

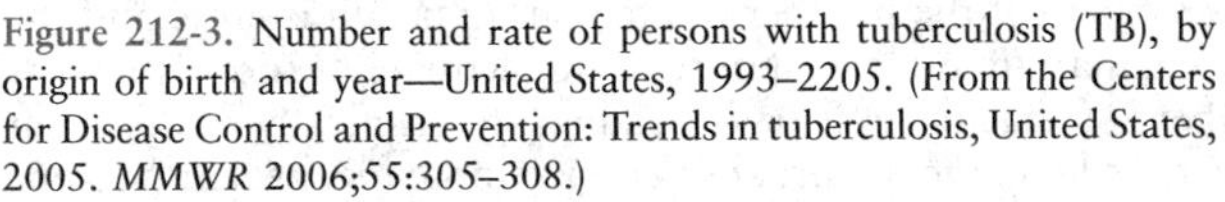
Figure 212-3. Number and rate of persons with tuberculosis (TB), by origin of birth and year—United States, 1993–2205. (From the Centers for Disease Control and Prevention: Trends in tuberculosis, United States, 2005. *MMWR* 2006;55:305–308.)

in individuals born in the United States. Fifty-four percent of all cases were among foreign-born persons. The total number of cases among foreign-born individuals increased 5% between 1992 and 2005 (see Fig. 212-3). In all age groups, the proportion of reported cases was strikingly higher in foreign-born and nonwhite individuals, even though the number of cases among foreign-born children <15 yr of age has declined. In white populations in the United States, tuberculosis rates are highest among the elderly who acquired the infection decades ago. In contrast, among nonwhite populations, tuberculosis is most common in young adults and children <5 yr of age. The age range of 5–14 yr is often called the "favored age" because in all human populations this group has the lowest rate of tuberculosis disease. Among adults, $^{2}/_{3}$ of cases occur in males, but there is no significant difference in gender distribution in childhood.

In the United States, most children are infected with *M. tuberculosis* in their home by someone close to them, but outbreaks of childhood tuberculosis also occur in elementary and high schools, nursery schools, daycare centers, homes, churches, school buses, and sports teams. HIV-infected adults with tuberculosis can transmit *M. tuberculosis* to children, and children with HIV infection are at increased risk for developing tuberculosis after infection. Specific groups are at high risk for acquiring tuberculosis infection and progressing from LTBI to tuberculosis (Table 212-1).

The incidence of **drug-resistant** tuberculosis has increased dramatically throughout the world. In the United States, about 8% of *M. tuberculosis* isolates are resistant to at least isoniazid, whereas 1% are resistant to both isoniazid and rifampin. Resistance to isoniazid remained relatively stable between 1992 and 2004, as did the proportion of cases that were multidrug resistant (about 1%). In some countries, drug resistance rates range from 20 to 50%. The major reasons for the development of drug resistance are poor patient adherence to treatment and provision of inadequate drug regimens by the physician or national tuberculosis program

Transmission. Transmission of *M. tuberculosis* is person to person, usually by airborne mucus droplet nuclei, particles 1–5 μm in diameter that contain *M. tuberculosis*. Transmission rarely occurs by direct contact with an infected discharge or a contaminated fomite. The chance of transmission increases when the patient has an acid-fast smear of sputum, an extensive upper lobe infiltrate or cavity, copious production of thin sputum, and severe and forceful cough. Environmental factors, especially poor air circulation, enhance transmission. Most adults no longer transmit the organism within several days to 2 weeks after beginning adequate chemotherapy, but some patients remain infectious for many weeks. Young children with tuberculosis rarely infect other children or adults. Tubercle bacilli are sparse in the endobronchial secretions of children with pulmonary tuberculosis, and cough is often absent or lacks the tussive force required to suspend infectious particles of the correct size. However, children and adolescents with adult-type cavitary or endobronchial pulmonary tuberculosis can transmit the organism. Airborne transmission of *M. bovis* and *M. africanum* can also occur. *M. bovis* may penetrate the gastrointestinal mucosa or invade the lymphatic tissue of the oropharynx when large numbers of the organism are ingested. Human infection with *M. bovis* is rare in developed countries as a result of the pasteurization of milk and effective tuberculosis control programs for cattle. About $^{1}/_{3}$ of culture-proven childhood tuberculosis cases in San Diego, California, in the 1990s were caused by *M. bovis,* likely acquired by children when visiting Mexico or another country with suboptimal animal control programs.

TABLE 212-1. Groups at High Risk for Acquiring Tuberculosis Infection and Developing Disease in Developed Countries

RISK FACTORS FOR TUBERCULOSIS INFECTION
Children exposed to high-risk adults
Foreign-born persons from high-prevalence countries
Poor and indigent persons, especially in large cities
Homeless persons
Persons who inject drugs
Present and former residents or employees of correctional institutions, homeless shelters, and nursing homes
Health care workers caring for high-risk patients
RISK FACTORS FOR PROGRESSION OF LATENT TUBERCULOSIS INFECTION TO TUBERCULOSIS DISEASE
Infants and children ≤4 yr of age, especially those <2 yr of age
Adolescents and young adults
Persons co-infected with HIV
Persons with skin test conversion in the past 1–2 yr
Persons who are immunocompromised, especially in cases of malignancy and solid organ transplantation, immunosuppressive medical treatments including anti–tumor necrosis factor therapies, diabetes mellitus, chronic renal failure, silicosis, and malnutrition

PATHOGENESIS. The primary complex of tuberculosis includes local infection at the portal of entry and the regional lymph nodes that drain the area. The lung is the portal of entry in >98% of cases. The tubercle bacilli multiply initially within alveoli and alveolar ducts. Most of the bacilli are killed, but some survive within nonactivated macrophages, which carry them through lymphatic vessels to the regional lymph nodes. When the primary infection is in the lung, the hilar lymph nodes usually are involved, although an upper lobe focus may drain into paratracheal nodes. The tissue reaction in the lung parenchyma and lymph nodes intensifies over the next 2–12 wk as the organisms grow in number and tissue **hypersensitivity** develops. The parenchymal portion of the primary complex often heals completely by fibrosis or calcification after undergoing caseous necrosis and encapsulation. Occasionally, this portion continues to enlarge, resulting in focal pneumonitis and pleuritis. If caseation is intense, the center of the lesion liquefies and empties into the associated bronchus, leaving a residual cavity.

The foci of infection in the regional lymph nodes develop some fibrosis and encapsulation, but healing is usually less complete than in the parenchymal lesion. Viable *M. tuberculosis* can persist for decades within these foci. In most cases of initial tuberculosis infection the lymph nodes remain normal in size. However, hilar and paratracheal lymph nodes that enlarge significantly as part of the host inflammatory reaction may encroach on a regional bronchus (Figs. 212-4 and 212-5). Partial obstruction of the bronchus caused by external compression may cause hyperinflation in the distal lung segment. Complete obstruction results in atelectasis. Inflamed caseous nodes can attach to the bronchial wall and erode through it, causing endobronchial tuberculosis or a fistula tract. The caseum causes complete obstruction of the bronchus. The resulting lesion, a combination of pneumonitis and atelectasis, has been called a **collapse-consolidation or segmental lesion** (Fig. 212-6).

During the development of the **primary complex (Ghon complex)**, which is the combination of a parenchymal pulmonary lesion and a corresponding lymph node site, tubercle bacilli are carried to most tissues of the body through the blood and lymphatic vessels. Although seeding of the organs of the reticuloendothelial system is common, bacterial replication is more likely to occur in organs with conditions that favor their growth, such as the lung apices, brain, kidneys, and bones. **Disseminated tuberculosis** occurs if the number of circulating bacilli is large and the host cellular immune response is inadequate. More often the number of bacilli is small, leading to clinically inapparent metastatic foci in many organs. These remote foci usually become encapsulated, but they may be the origin of both extrapulmonary tuberculosis and reactivation tuberculosis in some individuals.

THE TIME BETWEEN INITIAL INFECTION AND CLINICALLY APPARENT DISEASE IS VARIABLE. Disseminated and meningeal tuberculosis are early manifestations, often occurring within 2–6 mo of acqui-

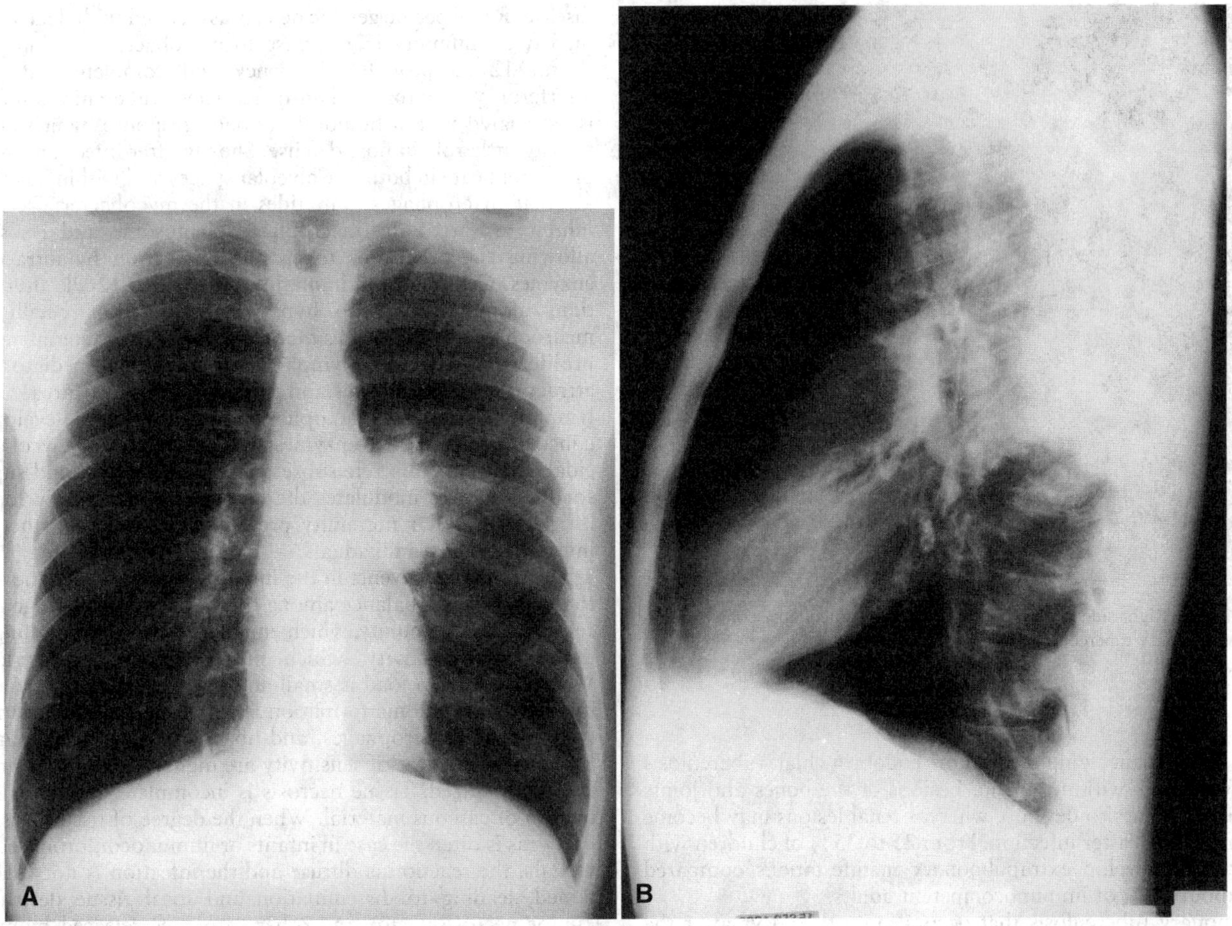

Figure 212-4. A 14 yr old child with proven primary tuberculosis. Frontal *(A)* and lateral *(B)* views of the chest show hyperinflation, prominent left hilar lymphadenopathy, and alveolar consolidation involving the posterior segment of the left upper love as well as the superior segment of the left lower lobe. (From Hilton SVW, Edwards DK [editors]: *Practical Pediatric Radiology,* 3rd ed. Philadelphia, Elsevier, 2003, p 334.)

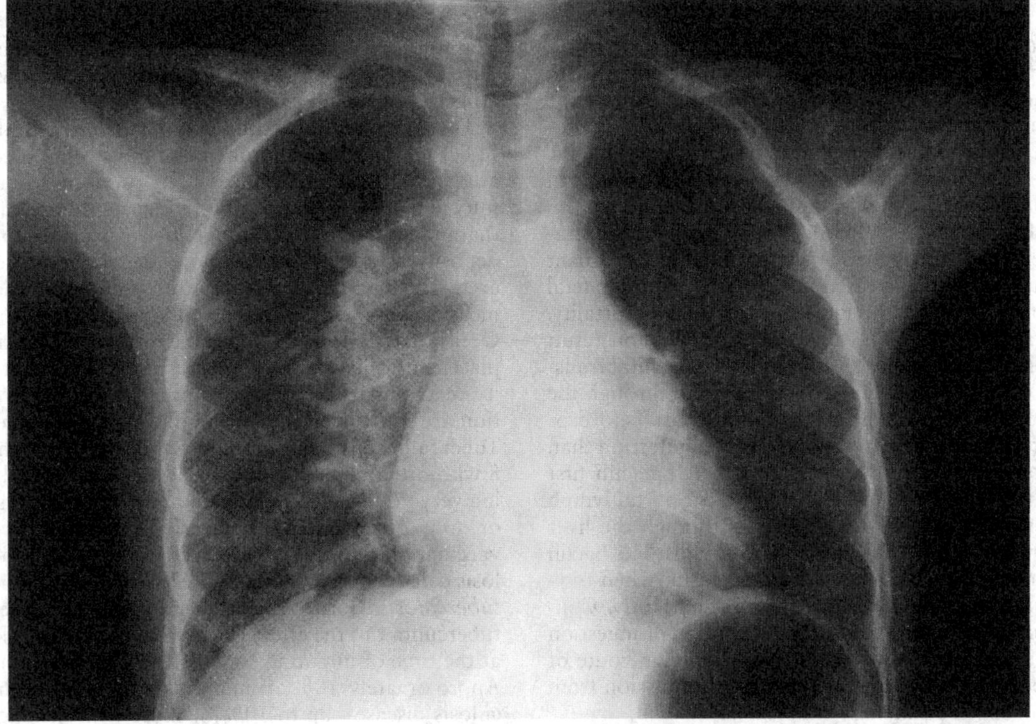

Figure 212-5. An 8 yr old child with a history of cough. A single frontal view of the chest shows marked right hilar and paratracheal lymphadenopathy with alveolar disease involving the right middle and lower lung fields. This was also a case of primary tuberculosis. (From Hilton SVW, Edwards DK [editors]: *Practical Pediatric Radiology,* 3rd ed. Philadelphia, Elsevier, 2003, p 335.)

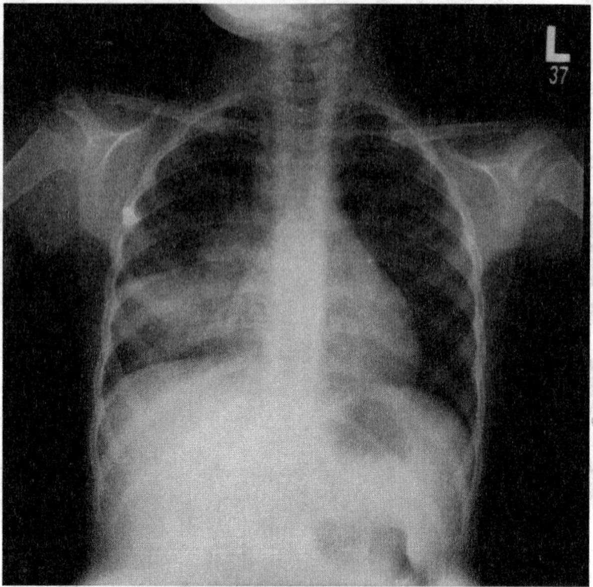

Figure 212-6. Right-sided hilar lymphadenopathy and collapse-consolidation lesions of primary tuberculosis in a 4 yr old child.

sition. Significant lymph node or endobronchial tuberculosis usually appears within 3–9 mo. Lesions of the bones and joints take several years to develop, whereas renal lesions may become evident decades after infection. From 25 to 35% of children with tuberculosis develop extrapulmonary manifestations compared with about 10% of immunocompetent adults.

Pulmonary tuberculosis that occurs more than 1 yr after the primary infection is usually caused by endogenous regrowth of bacilli persisting in partially encapsulated lesions. This **reactivation tuberculosis** is rare in children but is common among adolescents and young adults. The most common form is an infiltrate or cavity in the apex of the upper lobes, where oxygen tension and blood flow are great.

The risk for dissemination of *M. tuberculosis* is very high in HIV-infected persons. Reinfection also can occur in persons with advanced HIV or AIDS. In immunocompetent individuals the response to the initial infection with *M. tuberculosis* usually provides protection against reinfection when a new exposure occurs. However, exogenous reinfection has been reported to occur in adults without immune compromise in highly endemic areas.

Pregnancy and the Newborn. Pulmonary and particularly extrapulmonary tuberculosis other than lymphadenitis in a pregnant woman is associated with increased risk for prematurity, fetal growth retardation, low birthweight, and perinatal mortality. Congenital tuberculosis is rare because the most common result of female genital tract tuberculosis is infertility. Congenital transmission usually occurs from a lesion in the placenta through the umbilical vein. Primary infection in the mother just before or during pregnancy is more likely to cause congenital infection than is reactivation of a previous infection. The tubercle bacilli first reach the fetal liver, where a primary focus with periportal lymph node involvement may occur. Organisms pass through the liver into the main fetal circulation and infect many organs. The bacilli in the lung usually remain dormant until after birth, when oxygenation and pulmonary circulation increase significantly. Congenital tuberculosis may also be caused by aspiration or ingestion of infected amniotic fluid. However, the most common route of infection for the neonate is postnatal airborne transmission from an adult with infectious pulmonary tuberculosis.

Immunity. Conditions that adversely affect cell-mediated immunity predispose to progression from tuberculosis infection to disease. Rare specific genetic defects associated with deficient cell-mediated immunity in response to mycobacteria include interleukin 12 receptor B1 deficiency and complete and partial interferon-γ receptor 1 chain deficiencies. Tuberculosis infection is associated with a humoral antibody response, which appears to play little role in host defense. Shortly after infection, tubercle bacilli replicate in both free alveolar spaces and within inactivated alveolar macrophages. Sulfatides in the mycobacterial cell wall inhibit fusion of the macrophage phagosome and lysosomes, allowing the organisms to escape destruction by intracellular enzymes. **Cell-mediated immunity** develops 2–12 wk after infection, along with tissue hypersensitivity. After bacilli enter macrophages, lymphocytes that recognize mycobacterial antigens proliferate and secrete lymphokines and other mediators that attract other lymphocytes and macrophages to the area. Certain lymphokines activate macrophages, causing them to develop high concentrations of lytic enzymes that enhance their mycobactericidal capacity. A discrete subset of regulator helper and suppressor lymphocytes modulates the immune response. Development of specific cellular immunity prevents progression of the initial infection in most individuals.

The pathologic events in the initial tuberculosis infection seem to depend on the balance among the mycobacterial antigen load; cell-mediated immunity, which enhances intracellular killing; and tissue hypersensitivity, which promotes extracellular killing. When the antigen load is small and the degree of tissue sensitivity is high, granuloma formation results from the organization of lymphocytes, macrophages, and fibroblasts. When both antigen load and the degree of sensitivity are high, granuloma formation is less organized. Tissue necrosis is incomplete, resulting in formation of caseous material. When the degree of tissue sensitivity is low, as is often the case in infants or immunocompromised individuals, the reaction is diffuse and the infection is not well contained, leading to dissemination and local tissue destruction. Tumor necrosis factor and other cytokines released by specific lymphocytes promote cellular destruction and tissue damage in susceptible individuals.

Tuberculin Skin Testing. The development of delayed-type hypersensitivity (DTH) in most individuals infected with the tubercle bacillus makes the tuberculin skin test a useful diagnostic tool. Multipuncture tests (MPTs) are not as accurate as the Mantoux test because the exact dose of tuberculin antigen introduced into the skin cannot be controlled. The MPTs should no longer be used in pediatric practice.

The **Mantoux tuberculin skin test** is the intradermal injection of 0.1 mL containing 5 tuberculin units of purified protein derivative (PPD) stabilized with Tween 80. T cells sensitized by prior infection are recruited to the skin where they release lymphokines that induce induration through local vasodilatation, edema, fibrin deposition, and recruitment of other inflammatory cells to the area. The amount of induration in response to the test should be measured by a trained person 48–72 hr after administration. Occasional patients will have the onset of induration >72 hr after placement; this is also a positive result. Immediate hypersensitivity reactions to tuberculin or other constituents of the preparation are short lived (<24 hr) and not considered a positive result. Tuberculin sensitivity develops 3 wk to 3 mo—most often in 4–8 wk—after inhalation of organisms. Host-related factors, including very young age, malnutrition, immunosuppression by disease or drugs, viral infections (measles, mumps, varicella, influenza), vaccination with live-virus vaccines, and overwhelming tuberculosis can depress the skin test reaction in a child infected with *M. tuberculosis*. Corticosteroid therapy may decrease the reaction to tuberculin, but the effect is variable. Tuberculin skin testing done at the time of initiating corticosteroid therapy is usually reliable. Approximately 10% of immunocompetent children with tuberculosis disease—up to 50% of those with meningitis or disseminated disease—do not react initially to PPD; most become reactive after several months of antituberculosis therapy. Nonreactivity may be specific to tuberculin or more global to a variety of antigens, so positive "control" skin tests with a negative tuberculin test never rule out tuberculosis. The most common reasons for a false-negative skin test are poor technique and misreading of the results.

False-positive reactions to tuberculin can be caused by cross sensitization to antigens of nontuberculous mycobacteria (NTM), which generally are more prevalent in the environment as one approaches the equator. These cross reactions are usually transient over months to years and produce less than 10–12 mm of induration. Previous vaccination with bacille Calmette-Guérin (BCG) also can cause a reaction to a tuberculin skin test. This is especially true if 2 BCG vaccinations have been given. Approximately half of the infants who receive a BCG vaccine never develop a reactive tuberculin skin test, and the reactivity usually wanes in 2–3 yr in those with initially positive skin test results. Older children and adults who receive a BCG vaccine are more likely to develop tuberculin reactivity, but most lose the reactivity by 5–10 yr after vaccination. When skin test reactivity is present, it usually causes <10 mm of induration, although larger reactions occur in some individuals. In general, a tuberculin skin reaction of ≥10 mm in a BCG-vaccinated child or adult indicates infection with *M. tuberculosis*, which necessitates further diagnostic evaluation and treatment. Prior vaccination with BCG is never a contraindication to tuberculin testing.

The appropriate size of induration indicating a positive Mantoux tuberculin skin test result varies with related epidemiologic and risk factors. In children with no risk factors for tuberculosis, skin test reactions are usually false-positive results. The American Academy of Pediatrics (AAP) and Centers for Disease Control and Prevention (CDC) discourage routine testing of children, and recommend targeted tuberculin testing of children at risk identified through periodic screening surveys conducted by the primary care provider (Table 212-2). Possible exposure to an adult with or at high risk for infectious pulmonary tuberculosis is the most crucial risk factor for children. Reaction size limits for determining a positive tuberculin test result vary with the individual's risk for infection (Table 212-3). For adults and children at the highest risk for having infection progress to disease—those with recent contact with infectious persons, clinical illnesses consistent with tuberculosis, or HIV infection or other immunosuppression—a reactive area of ≥5 mm is classified as a positive result, indicating infection with *M. tuberculosis*. For other high-risk groups, a reactive area of ≥10 mm is considered positive. For low-risk persons, especially those residing in communities where the prevalence of tuberculosis is low, the cutoff point for a positive reaction is ≥15 mm. An increase of induration of ≥10 mm within a 2-yr period is considered a tuberculin skin test conversion at any age.

TABLE 212-3. Definitions of Positive Tuberculin Skin Test (TST) Results in Infants, Children, and Adolescents*

INDURATION ≥5 MM

Children in close contact with known or suspected contagious people with tuberculosis disease.

Children suspected to have tuberculosis disease:
- Findings on chest radiograph consistent with active or previously tuberculosis disease
- Clinical evidence of tuberculosis disease[†]

Children receiving immunosuppressive therapy[‡] or with immunosuppressive conditions, including HIV infection.

INDURATION ≥10 MM

Children at increased risk of disseminated tuberculosis disease:
- Children younger than 4 yr of age
- Children with other medical conditions, including Hodgkin disease, lymphoma, diabetes mellitus, chronic renal failure, or malnutrition (see Table 212-2)

Children with increased exposure to tuberculosis disease:
- Children born in high-prevalence regions of the world
- Children frequently exposed to adults who are HIV infected, homeless, users of illicit drugs, residents of nursing homes, incarcerated or institutionalized, or migrant farm workers
- Children who travel to high-prevalence regions of the world

INDURATION ≥15 MM

Children 4 yr of age or older without any risk factors.

*These definitions apply regardless of previous bacille Calmette-Guérin (BCG) immunization; erythema at TST site does not indicate a positive test result. Tests should be read at 48 to 72 hr after placement.

[†]Evidence by physical examination or laboratory assessment that would include tuberculosis in the working differential diagnosis (e.g., meningitis).

[‡]Including immunosuppressive doses of corticosteroids.

From the American Academy of Pediatrics: *Red Book: 2006 Report of the Committee on Infectious Diseases*, 27th ed. Elk Grove Village, IL, American Academy of Pediatrics, 2006, p. 680.

TABLE 212-2. Tuberculin Skin Test (TST) Recommendations for Infants, Children, and Adolescents*

Children for whom immediate TST is indicated[†]
- Contacts of people with confirmed or suspected contagious tuberculosis (contact investigation)
- Children with radiographic or clinical findings suggesting tuberculosis disease
- Children immigrating from countries with endemic infection (e.g., Asia, Middle East, Africa, Latin America, countries of the former Soviet Union) including international adoptees
- Children with travel histories to countries with endemic infection and substantial contact with indigenous people from such countries[‡]

Children who should have annual TST:
- Children infected with HIV
- Incarcerated adolescents

Children at increased risk for progression of LTBI to tuberculosis disease: Children with other medical conditions, including diabetes mellitus, chronic renal failure, malnutrition, and congenital or acquired immunodeficiencies deserve special consideration. Without recent exposure, these people are not at increased risk of acquiring tuberculosis infection. Underlying immune deficiencies associated with these conditions theoretically would enhance the possibility for progression to severe disease. Initial histories of potential exposure to tuberculosis should be included for all of these patients. If these histories or local epidemiologic factors suggest a possibility of exposure, immediate and periodic TST should be considered. **An initial TST should be performed before initiation of immunosuppressive therapy, including prolonged steroid administration, use of tumor necrosis factor-alpha antagonists, or immunosuppressive therapy in any child requiring these treatments.**

*Bacille Calmette-Guérin immunization is not a contraindication to a TST.

[†]Beginning as early as 3 mo of age.

[‡]If the child is well, the TST should be delayed for up to 10 wk after return.

LTBI, latent tuberculosis infection.

From the American Academy of Pediatrics: *Red Book: 2006 Report of the Committee on Infectious Diseases*, 27th ed. Elk Grove Village, IL, American Academy of Pediatrics, 2006, p. 683.

Interferon-γ Release Assays. Two tests (T-SPOT.TB and QuantiFERON-TB Gold) detect interferon-γ generation by the patient's T cells in response to specific *M. tuberculosis* antigens (ESAT-6 and CFP-10). QuantiFERON-TB Gold is approved by the Food and Drug Administration. Both tests have internal controls (similar to placing a *Candida* skin test for the PPD). These tests have several theoretical and practical advantages over the tuberculin skin test, including the need for only 1 patient encounter; lack of cross reaction with BCG vaccination and most other mycobacteria; and absence of boosting (increasing reaction to the tuberculin skin test with serial testing). ELISPOT tests may work best when used in combination with a PPD to increase sensitivity.

CLINICAL MANIFESTATIONS AND DIAGNOSIS. The majority of children with tuberculosis infection develop no signs or symptoms at any time. Occasionally, infection is marked by low-grade fever and mild cough, and rarely by high fever, cough, malaise, and flulike symptoms that resolve within 1 wk. The proportion of extrapulmonary tuberculosis cases has increased over the past 2 decades in the USA. About 15% of adult tuberculosis cases are extrapulmonary, and 25–30% of children with tuberculosis have an extrapulmonary presentation.

Primary Pulmonary Disease. The **primary complex** includes the parenchymal pulmonary focus and the regional lymph nodes. About 70% of lung foci are subpleural, and localized pleurisy is common. The initial parenchymal inflammation usually is not visible on chest radiograph, but a localized, nonspecific infiltrate may be seen before the development of tissue hypersensitivity. All lobar segments of the lung are at equal risk for initial infection.

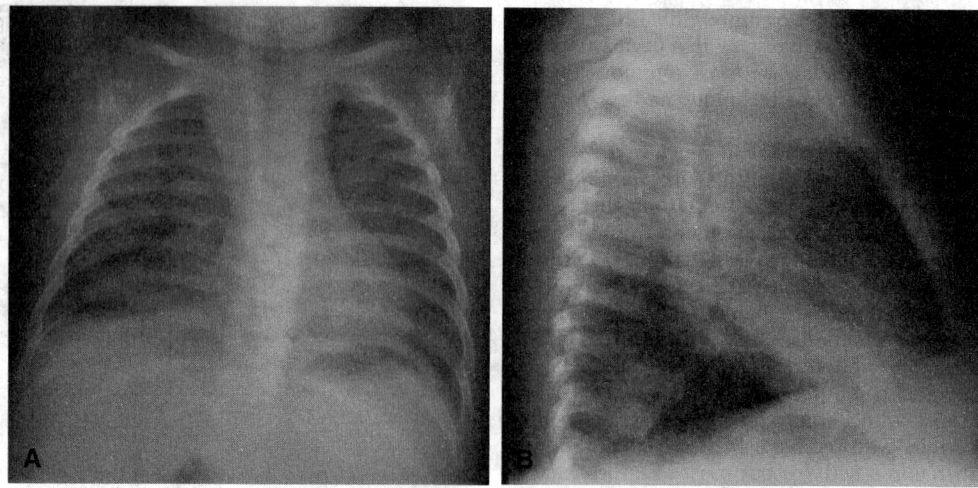

Figure 212-7. Posteroanterior *(A)* and lateral *(B)* chest radiographs of an infant with miliary tuberculosis. The child's mother had failed to complete treatment for pulmonary tuberculosis twice within 3 yr of this child's birth.

Two or more primary foci are present in 25% of cases. The hallmark of primary tuberculosis in the lung is the relatively large size of the regional lymphadenitis compared with the relatively small size of the initial lung focus (see Figs. 212-4 to 212-6). As DTH develops, the hilar lymph nodes continue to enlarge in some children, especially infants, compressing the regional bronchus and causing obstruction. The usual sequence is hilar lymphadenopathy, focal hyperinflation, and then atelectasis. The resulting radiographic shadows have been called collapse-consolidation or segmental tuberculosis (see Fig. 212-6). Rarely, inflamed caseous nodes attach to the endobronchial wall and erode through it, causing endobronchial tuberculosis or a fistula tract. The caseum causes complete obstruction of the bronchus, resulting in extensive infiltrate and collapse. Enlargement of the subcarinal lymph nodes can cause compression of the esophagus and, rarely, a bronchoesophageal fistula.

Most cases of tuberculous bronchial obstruction in children resolve fully with appropriate treatment. Occasionally, there is residual calcification of the primary focus or regional lymph nodes. The appearance of calcification implies that the lesion has been present for at least 6–12 mo. Healing of the segment can be complicated by scarring or contraction associated with cylindrical bronchiectasis, but this is rare.

Children may have lobar pneumonia without impressive hilar lymphadenopathy. If the primary infection is progressively destructive, liquefaction of the lung parenchyma can lead to formation of a thin-walled primary tuberculosis cavity. Rarely, bullous tuberculous lesions can occur in the lungs and lead to pneumothorax if they rupture. Erosion of a parenchymal focus of tuberculosis into a blood or lymphatic vessel may result in dissemination of the bacilli and a **miliary pattern,** with small nodules evenly distributed on the chest radiograph (Fig. 212-7).

The symptoms and physical signs of primary pulmonary tuberculosis in children are surprisingly meager considering the degree of radiographic changes often seen. More than 50% of infants and children with radiographically moderate to severe pulmonary tuberculosis have no physical findings and are discovered only by contact tracing. Infants are more likely to experience signs and symptoms. Nonproductive cough and mild dyspnea are the most common symptoms. Systemic complaints such as fever, night sweats, anorexia, and decreased activity occur less often. Some infants have difficulty gaining weight or develop a true failure-to-thrive syndrome that often does not improve significantly until several months of effective treatment have been taken. Pulmonary signs are even less common. Some infants and young children with bronchial obstruction have localized wheezing or decreased breath sounds that may be accompanied by tachypnea or, rarely, respiratory distress. These pulmonary symptoms and signs are occasionally alleviated by antibiotics, suggesting bacterial superinfection.

The most specific confirmation of pulmonary tuberculosis is isolation of *M. tuberculosis*. Sputum specimens for culture should be collected from adolescents and older children who are able to expectorate. Induce sputum with a jet nebulizer and chest percussion followed by nasopharyngeal suctioning is effective in children as young as 1 mo. Sputum induction provides samples for both culture and smear staining, whereas gastric aspirates are usually cultured. The traditional culture specimen in young children is the early morning gastric acid obtained before the child has arisen and peristalsis has emptied the stomach of the pooled secretions that have been swallowed overnight. Even under optimal conditions, though, 3 consecutive morning gastric aspirates yield the organisms in <50% of cases. The culture yield from bronchoscopy is even lower, but this procedure may demonstrate the presence of endobronchial disease or a fistula. Negative cultures never exclude the diagnosis of tuberculosis in a child. The presence of a positive tuberculin skin test, an abnormal chest radiograph consistent with tuberculosis, and history of exposure to an adult with infectious tuberculosis is adequate proof that the disease is present. Drug susceptibility test results of the isolate from the adult source can be used to determine the best therapeutic regimen for the child. Cultures should be obtained from the child whenever the source case is unknown or the source case has possible drug-resistant tuberculosis.

Progressive Primary Pulmonary Disease. A rare but serious complication of tuberculosis in a child occurs when the primary focus enlarges steadily and develops a large caseous center. Liquefaction may cause formation of a primary cavity associated with large numbers of tubercle bacilli. The enlarging focus may slough necrotic debris into the adjacent bronchus, leading to further intrapulmonary dissemination. Significant signs or symptoms are frequent in locally progressive disease in children. High fever, severe cough with sputum production, weight loss, and night sweats are common. Physical signs include diminished breath sounds, rales, and dullness or egophony over the cavity. The prognosis for full but usually slow recovery is excellent with appropriate therapy.

Reactivation Tuberculosis. Pulmonary tuberculosis in adults usually represents endogenous reactivation of a site of tuberculosis infection established previously in the body. This form of tuberculosis is rare in childhood but may occur in adolescence. Children with a healed tuberculosis infection acquired at <2 yr of age rarely develop chronic reactivation pulmonary disease, which is more common in those who acquire the initial infection at >7 yr of age. The most frequent pulmonary sites are the original parenchymal focus, lymph nodes, or the apical seedings (**Simon foci**) established during the hematogenous phase of the early infection. This form of disease usually remains localized to the lungs because the established immune response prevents further extrapulmonary spread. The most common radiographic presentations of this type of tuberculosis are extensive infiltrates or thick-walled cavities in the upper lobes.

Older children and adolescents with reactivation tuberculosis are more likely to experience fever, anorexia, malaise, weight loss, night sweats, productive cough, hemoptysis, and chest pain than children with primary pulmonary tuberculosis. However, physical examination findings usually are minor or absent, even when cavities or large infiltrates are present. Most signs and symptoms improve within several weeks of starting effective treatment, although the cough may last for several months. This form of tuberculosis may be highly contagious if there is significant sputum production and cough. The prognosis for full recovery is excellent when patients are given appropriate therapy.

Pleural Effusion. Tuberculous pleural effusions, which can be local or general, originate in the discharge of bacilli into the pleural space from a subpleural pulmonary focus or caseated lymph node. Asymptomatic local pleural effusion is so frequent in primary tuberculosis that it is basically a component of the primary complex. Larger and clinically significant effusions occur months to years after the primary infection. Tuberculous pleural effusion is infrequent in children <6 yr of age and rare in children <2 yr of age. Effusions are usually unilateral but can be bilateral. They are virtually never associated with a segmental pulmonary lesion and are rare in disseminated tuberculosis. Often the radiographic abnormality is more extensive than would be suggested by physical findings or symptoms (Fig. 212-8).

Clinical onset of tuberculous pleurisy is often sudden, characterized by low to high fever, shortness of breath, chest pain on deep inspiration, and diminished breath sounds. The fever and other symptoms may last for several weeks after the start of antituberculosis chemotherapy. The tuberculin skin test is positive in only 70–80% of cases. The prognosis is excellent, but radiographic resolution often takes months. Scoliosis is a rare complication from a long-standing effusion.

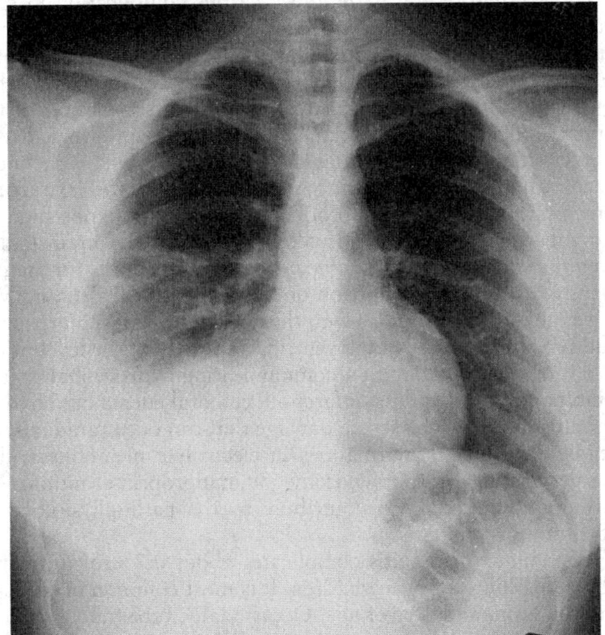

Figure 212-8. Pleural tuberculosis in a 16 yr old girl.

Examination of pleural fluid and the pleural membrane is important to establish the diagnosis of tuberculous pleurisy. The pleural fluid is usually yellow and only occasionally tinged with blood. The specific gravity is usually 1.012–1.025, the protein level is usually 2–4 g/dL, and the glucose concentration may be low, although it is usually in the low-normal range (20–40 mg/dL). Typically there are several hundred to several thousand white blood cells per cubic millimeter with an early predominance of polymorphonuclear cells followed by a high percentage of lymphocytes. Acid-fast smears of the pleural fluid are rarely positive. Cultures of the fluid are positive in only <30% of cases. Biopsy of the pleural membrane is more likely to yield a positive acid-fast stain or culture, and granuloma formation usually can be demonstrated.

Pericardial Disease. The most common form of cardiac tuberculosis is pericarditis. It is rare, occurring in 0.5–4% of tuberculosis cases in children. Pericarditis usually arises from direct invasion or lymphatic drainage from subcarinal lymph nodes. The presenting symptoms are nonspecific, including low-grade fever, malaise, and weight loss. Chest pain is unusual in children. A pericardial friction rub or distant heart sounds with pulsus paradoxus may be present. The pericardial fluid is typically serofibrinous or hemorrhagic. Acid-fast smear of the fluid rarely reveals the organism, but cultures are positive in 30–70% of cases. The culture yield from pericardial biopsy may be higher, and the presence of granulomas often suggests the diagnosis. Partial or complete pericardiectomy may be required when constrictive pericarditis develops.

Lymphohematogenous (Disseminated) Disease. Tubercle bacilli are disseminated to distant sites, including liver, spleen, skin, and lung apices, in all cases of tuberculosis infection. The clinical picture produced by lymphohematogenous dissemination depends on the quantity of organisms released from the primary focus and the adequacy of the host immune response. Lymphohematogenous spread is usually asymptomatic. Rare patients experience protracted hematogenous tuberculosis caused by the intermittent release of tubercle bacilli as a caseous focus erodes through the wall of a blood vessel in the lung. Although the clinical picture may be acute, more often it is indolent and prolonged, with spiking fever accompanying the release of organisms into the bloodstream. Multiple organ involvement is common, leading to hepatomegaly, splenomegaly, lymphadenitis in superficial or deep nodes, and papulonecrotic tuberculids appearing on the skin. Bones and joints or kidneys also may become involved. Meningitis occurs only late in the course of the disease. Early pulmonary involvement is surprisingly mild, but diffuse involvement becomes apparent with prolonged infection.

The most clinically significant form of disseminated tuberculosis is **miliary disease,** which occurs when massive numbers of tubercle bacilli are released into the bloodstream, causing disease in 2 or more organs. Miliary tuberculosis usually complicates the primary infection, occurring within 2–6 mo of the initial infection. Although this form of disease is most common in infants and young children, it is also found in adolescents and older adults, resulting from the breakdown of a previously healed primary pulmonary lesion. The clinical manifestations of miliary tuberculosis are protean, depending on the load of organisms that disseminate and where they lodge. Lesions are often larger and more numerous in the lungs, spleen, liver, and bone marrow than other tissues. Because this form of tuberculosis is most common in infants and malnourished or immunosuppressed patients, the host's immune incompetency probably also plays a role in pathogenesis.

The onset of miliary tuberculosis is sometimes explosive, and the patient may become gravely ill in several days. More often, the onset is insidious with early systemic signs, including anorexia, weight loss, and low-grade fever. At this time, abnormal physical signs are usually absent. Generalized lymphadenopathy and hepatosplenomegaly develop within several weeks in about 50% of cases. The fever may then become higher and more sustained, although the chest radiograph usually is normal and respiratory symptoms are minor or absent. Within several more weeks, the lungs may become filled with tubercles, and dyspnea, cough, rales, or wheezing occur. The lesions of miliary tuberculosis are usually smaller than 2–3 mm in diameter when first visible on chest radiograph (see Fig. 212-7). The smaller lesions coalesce to form larger lesions and sometimes extensive infiltrates. As the pulmonary disease progresses, an alveolar-air block syndrome may result in frank respiratory distress, hypoxia, and pneumothorax, or pneumomediastinum. Signs or symptoms of meningitis or peritonitis are found in 20–40% of patients with advanced disease. Chronic or recurrent headache in a patient with miliary tuberculosis usually indicates the presence of meningitis, whereas the onset of abdominal pain or tenderness is a sign of tuberculous peritonitis. **Cutaneous lesions** include papulonecrotic tuberculids, nodules, or purpura. Choroid tubercles occur in 13–87% of patients and are highly specific for the diagnosis of miliary tuberculosis. Unfortunately, the tuberculin skin test is nonreactive in up to 40% of patients with disseminated tuberculosis.

Diagnosis of disseminated tuberculosis can be difficult, and a high index of suspicion by the clinician is required. Often the patient presents with fever of unknown origin. Early sputum or gastric aspirate cultures have a low sensitivity. Biopsy of the liver or bone marrow with appropriate bacteriologic and histologic examinations more often yields an early diagnosis. The most important clue is usually history of recent exposure to an adult with infectious tuberculosis.

The resolution of miliary tuberculosis is slow, even with proper therapy. Fever usually declines within 2–3 wk of starting chemotherapy, but the chest radiographic abnormalities may not resolve for many months. Occasionally, corticosteroids hasten symptomatic relief, especially when air block, peritonitis, or meningitis is present. The prognosis is excellent if the diagnosis is made early and adequate chemotherapy is given.

Upper Respiratory Tract Disease. Tuberculosis of the upper respiratory tract is rare in developed countries but is still observed in developing countries. Children with laryngeal tuberculosis have a croupy cough, sore throat, hoarseness, and dysphagia. Most children with laryngeal tuberculosis have extensive upper lobe pulmonary disease, but occasional patients have primary laryngeal disease with a normal chest radiograph. Tuberculosis of the middle ear results from aspiration of infected pulmonary secretions into the middle ear or from hematogenous dissemination in older children. The most common signs and symptoms are painless unilateral otorrhea, tinnitus, decreased hearing, facial paralysis, and a perforated tympanic membrane. Enlargement of lymph nodes in the preauricular or anterior cervical chains may accompany this infection. Diagnosis is difficult because stains and cultures of ear fluid are frequently negative, and histology of the affected tissue often shows a nonspecific acute and chronic inflammation without granuloma formation.

Lymph Node Disease. Tuberculosis of the superficial lymph nodes, often referred to as **scrofula,** is the most common form of extrapulmonary tuberculosis in children. Historically, scrofula was usually caused by drinking unpasteurized cow's milk laden with *M. bovis.* Most current cases occur within 6–9 mo of initial infection by *M. tuberculosis,* although some cases appear years later. The tonsillar, anterior cervical, submandibular, and supraclavicular nodes become involved secondary to extension of a primary lesion of the upper lung fields or abdomen. Infected nodes in the inguinal, epitrochlear, or axillary regions result from regional lymphadenitis associated with tuberculosis of the skin or skeletal system. The nodes usually enlarge gradually in the early stages of lymph node disease. They are firm but not hard, discrete, and nontender. The nodes often feel fixed to underlying or overlying tissue. Disease is most often **unilateral,** but bilateral involvement may occur because of the crossover drainage patterns of lymphatic vessels in the chest and lower neck. As infection progresses, multiple nodes are infected, resulting in a mass of matted nodes. Systemic signs and symptoms other than a low-grade fever are usually absent. The tuberculin skin test is usually reactive, but the chest radiograph is normal in 70% of cases. The onset of illness is occasionally more acute, with rapid enlargement of lymph nodes, high fever, tenderness, and fluctuance. The initial presentation is rarely a fluctuant mass with overlying cellulitis or skin discoloration.

Lymph node tuberculosis may resolve if left untreated but more often progresses to caseation and necrosis. The capsule of the node breaks down, resulting in the spread of infection to adjacent nodes. Rupture of the node usually results in a draining sinus tract that may require surgical removal. Tuberculous lymphadenitis can usually be diagnosed by fine-needle aspiration of the node and responds well to antituberculosis therapy, although the lymph nodes do not return to normal size for months or even years. Surgical removal is not always necessary, and must be combined with antituberculous medication because the lymph node disease is but 1 part of a systemic infection.

A definitive diagnosis of tuberculous adenitis usually requires histologic or bacteriologic confirmation, which is best accomplished by fine needle aspiration for culture, stain, and histology. If fine-needle aspiration is not successful in establishing a diagnosis, excisional biopsy of the involved node is indicated. Culture of lymph node tissue yields the organism in only about 50% of cases. Many other conditions can be confused with tuberculous adenitis, including infection due to nontuberculous mycobacteria (NTM), cat scratch disease *(Bartonella henselae),* tularemia, brucellosis, toxoplasmosis, tumor, branchial cleft cyst, cystic hygroma, and pyogenic infection. The most frequent problem is distinguishing infection due to *M. tuberculosis* from lymphadenitis caused by NTM in geographic areas where NTM are common. Both conditions are usually associated with a normal chest radiograph and a reactive tuberculin skin test. An important clue to the diagnosis of tuberculous adenitis is an epidemiologic link to an adult with infectious tuberculosis. In areas where both diseases are common, the only way to distinguish them may be culture of the involved tissue.

Central Nervous System Disease. Tuberculosis of the central nervous system (CNS) is the most serious complication in children and is fatal without prompt and appropriate treatment. Tuberculous meningitis usually arises from the formation of a metastatic caseous lesion in the cerebral cortex or meninges that develops during the lymphohematogenous dissemination of the primary infection. This initial lesion increases in size and discharges small numbers of tubercle bacilli into the subarachnoid space. The resulting gelatinous exudate infiltrates the corticomeningeal blood vessels, producing inflammation, obstruction, and subsequent infarction of cerebral cortex. The brainstem is often the site of greatest involvement, which accounts for the frequently associated dysfunction of cranial nerves III, VI, and VII. The exudate also interferes with the normal flow of cerebrospinal fluid (CSF) in and out of the ventricular system at the level of the basilar cisterns, leading to a communicating hydrocephalus. The combination of vasculitis, infarction, cerebral edema, and hydrocephalus results in the severe damage that can occur gradually or rapidly. Profound abnormalities in electrolyte metabolism, due to salt wasting or the syndrome of inappropriate antidiuretic hormone secretion, also contribute to the pathophysiology of tuberculous meningitis.

Tuberculous meningitis complicates about 0.3% of untreated tuberculosis infections in children. It is most common in children between 6 mo and 4 yr of age. Occasionally, tuberculous meningitis occurs many years after the infection, when rupture of 1 or more of the subependymal tubercles discharges tubercle bacilli into the subarachnoid space. The clinical progression of tuberculous meningitis may be rapid or gradual. Rapid progression tends to occur more often in infants and young children, who may experience symptoms for only several days before the onset of acute hydrocephalus, seizures, and cerebral edema. More commonly, the signs and symptoms progress slowly over several weeks and can be divided into 3 stages. The **1st stage,** which typically lasts 1–2 wk, is characterized by nonspecific symptoms, such as fever, headache, irritability, drowsiness, and malaise. Focal neurologic signs are absent, but infants may experience a stagnation or loss of developmental milestones. The **2nd stage** usually begins more abruptly. The most common features are lethargy, nuchal rigidity, seizures, positive Kernig or Brudzinski signs, hypertonia, vomiting, cranial nerve palsies, and other focal neurologic signs. The accelerating clinical illness usually correlates with the development of hydrocephalus, increased intracranial pressure, and vasculitis. Some children have no evidence of meningeal irritation but may have signs of encephalitis, such as disorientation, movement disorders, or speech impairment. The **3rd stage** is marked by coma, hemiplegia or paraplegia, hypertension, decerebrate posturing, deterioration of vital signs, and eventually death. The prognosis of tuberculous meningitis correlates most closely with the clinical stage of illness at the time treatment is initiated. The majority of patients in the 1st stage have an excellent outcome, whereas most patients in the 3rd stage who survive have permanent disabilities, including blindness, deafness, paraplegia, diabetes insipidus, or mental retardation. The prognosis for young infants is generally worse than for older children. It is imperative that antituberculosis treatment be considered for any child who develops basilar meningitis and hydrocephalus, cranial nerve palsy, or stroke with no other apparent etiology. Often the key to the correct diagnosis is identifying an adult in contact with the child who has infectious tuberculosis. Because of the short incubation period of tuberculous meningitis, the ill adult contact has not yet been diagnosed in many cases.

The diagnosis of tuberculous meningitis can be difficult early in its course, requiring a high degree of suspicion on the part of the clinician. The tuberculin skin test is nonreactive in up to 50% of cases, and 20–50% of children have a normal chest radiograph. The most important laboratory test for the diagnosis of tuberculous meningitis is examination and culture of the lumbar CSF. The CSF leukocyte count usually ranges from 10 to 500 cells/mm^3. Polymorphonuclear leukocytes may be present initially, but lymphocytes predominate in the majority of cases. The CSF glucose is typically <40 mg/dL but rarely <20 mg/dL. The protein level is elevated and may be markedly high (400–5,000 mg/dL) secondary to hydrocephalus and spinal block. Although the lumbar CSF is grossly abnormal, ventricular CSF may have normal chemistries and cell counts because this fluid is obtained from a site proximal to the inflammation and obstruction. During early stage I, the CSF may resemble that of viral aseptic meningitis only to progress to the more severe CSF profile over several weeks. The success of the microscopic examination of acid-fast-stained CSF and mycobacterial culture is related directly to the volume of the CSF sample. Examinations or culture of small amounts of CSF are unlikely to demonstrate *M. tuberculosis.* When 5–10 mL of lumbar CSF can be obtained, the acid-fast stain of the CSF sediment is positive in up to 30% of cases and the culture is positive in 50–70% of cases. Cultures of other fluids, such as gastric aspirates or urine, may help confirm the diagnosis. Radiographic studies may aid in the diagnosis of tuberculous meningitis. CT or MRI of the brain of patients with tuberculous meningitis may be normal during early stages of the disease. As disease progresses, basilar enhancement and communicating hydrocephalus with signs of cerebral edema or early focal ischemia are the most common findings. Some small children with tuberculous meningitis may have 1 or several clinically silent tuberculomas, occurring most often in the cerebral cortex or thalamic regions.

Another manifestation of CNS tuberculosis is the **tuberculoma,** a tumor-like mass resulting from aggregation of caseous tubercles that usually presents clinically as a brain tumor. Tuberculomas account for up to 40% of brain tumors in some areas of the world, but they are rare in North America. In adults tuberculomas are most often supratentorial, but in children they are often infratentorial, located at the base of the brain near the cerebellum. Lesions are most often singular but may be multiple. The most common symptoms are headache, fever, and convulsions. The tuberculin skin test is usually reactive, but the chest radiograph is usually normal. Surgical excision is often necessary to distinguish tuberculoma from other causes of brain tumor. However, surgical removal is not necessary because most tuberculomas resolve with medical management. Corticosteroids are usually administered during the 1st few weeks of treatment or in the immediate postoperative period to decrease cerebral edema. On CT or MRI of the brain, tuberculomas usually appear as discrete lesions with a significant amount of surrounding edema. Contrast medium enhancement is often impressive and may result in a ringlike lesion. Since the advent of CT, the paradoxical development of tuberculomas in patients with tuberculous meningitis who are receiving ultimately effective chemotherapy has been recognized. The cause and nature of these tuberculomas are poorly understood, but they do not represent failure of drug treatment. This phenomenon should be considered whenever a child with tuberculous meningitis deteriorates or develops focal neurologic findings while on treatment. Corticosteroids may help alleviate the occasionally severe clinical signs and symptoms that occur. These lesions may persist for months or even years.

Cutaneous Disease. Cutaneous tuberculosis is rare in the United States but occurs worldwide and accounts for 1–2% of tuberculosis (see Chapter 664).

Bone and Joint Disease. Bone and joint infection complicating tuberculosis is most likely to involve the vertebrae. The classic manifestation of tuberculous spondylitis is progression to Pott disease, in which destruction of the vertebral bodies leads to gibbus deformity and kyphosis (see Chapter 678.4). Skeletal tuberculosis is a late complication of tuberculosis, and although it has become a rare entity since antituberculosis therapy became available, it is more likely to occur in children than in adults. Tuberculous bone lesions may resemble pyogenic and fungal infections, or bone tumors. Multifocal bone involvement can occur. A bone biopsy is essential to confirm the diagnosis.

Abdominal and Gastrointestinal Disease. Tuberculosis of the oral cavity or pharynx is quite unusual. The most common lesion is a painless ulcer on the mucosa, palate, or tonsil with enlargement of the regional lymph nodes. Tuberculosis of the parotid gland has been reported rarely in endemic countries. Tuberculosis of the esophagus is rare in children but may be associated with a tracheoesophageal fistula in infants. These forms of tuberculosis are usually associated with extensive pulmonary disease and swallowing of infectious respiratory secretions. However, they can occur in the absence of pulmonary disease, presumably by spread from mediastinal or peritoneal lymph nodes.

Tuberculous peritonitis, which occurs most often in young men, is uncommon in adolescents and rare in children. Generalized peritonitis may arise from subclinical or miliary hematogenous dissemination. Localized peritonitis is caused by direct extension from an abdominal lymph node, intestinal focus, or genitourinary tuberculosis. Rarely, the lymph nodes, omentum, and peritoneum become matted and can be palpated as a "doughy" irregular nontender mass. Abdominal pain or tenderness, ascites, anorexia, and low-grade fever are typical manifestations. The tuberculin skin test is usually reactive. The diagnosis can be confirmed by paracentesis with appropriate stains and cultures, but this procedure must be performed carefully to avoid entering a bowel that is intertwined with the matted omentum.

Tuberculous enteritis is caused by hematogenous dissemination or by swallowing tubercle bacilli discharged from the patient's own lungs. The jejunum and ileum near Peyer patches and the appendix are the most common sites of involvement. The typical findings are shallow ulcers that cause pain, diarrhea or constipation, and weight loss with low-grade fever. Mesenteric adenitis usually complicates the infection. The enlarged nodes may cause intestinal obstruction or erode through the omentum to cause generalized peritonitis. The clinical presentation of tuberculous enteritis is nonspecific, mimicking other infections and conditions that cause diarrhea. The disease should be suspected in any child with chronic gastrointestinal complaints and a reactive tuberculin skin test. Biopsy, acid-fast stain, and culture of the lesions are usually necessary to confirm the diagnosis.

Genitourinary Disease. Renal tuberculosis is rare in children because the incubation period is several years or longer. Tubercle bacilli usually reach the kidney during lymphohematogenous dissemination. The organisms often can be recovered from the urine in cases of miliary tuberculosis and in some patients with pulmonary tuberculosis in the absence of renal parenchymal disease. In true renal tuberculosis, small caseous foci develop in the renal parenchyma and release *M. tuberculosis* into the tubules. A large mass develops near the renal cortex that discharges bacteria through a fistula into the renal pelvis. Infection then spreads locally to the ureters, prostate, or epididymis. Renal tuberculosis is often clinically silent in its early stages, marked only by sterile pyuria and microscopic hematuria. Dysuria, flank or abdominal pain, and gross hematuria develop as the disease progresses. Superinfection by other bacteria, which often causes more acute symptoms, occurs frequently but may also delay recognition of the underlying tuberculosis. Hydronephrosis or ureteral strictures may complicate the disease. Urine cultures for *M. tuberculosis* are positive in 80–90% of cases, and acid-fast stains of large volumes of urine sediment are positive in 50–70% of cases. The tuberculin skin test is nonreactive in up to 20% of patients. An intravenous pyelogram or CT scan often reveals mass lesions, dilatation of the proximal ureters, multiple small filling defects, and hydronephrosis if ureteral stricture is present. Disease is most often unilateral.

Tuberculosis of the genital tract is uncommon in both males and females before puberty. This condition usually originates from lymphohematogenous spread, although it can be caused by direct spread from the intestinal tract or bone. Adolescent girls may develop genital tract tuberculosis during the primary infection. The fallopian tubes are most often involved (90–100% of cases) followed by the endometrium (50%), ovaries (25%), and cervix (5%). The most common symptoms are lower abdominal pain and dysmenorrhea or amenorrhea. Systemic manifestations are usually absent and the chest radiograph is normal in the majority of cases. The tuberculin skin test is usually reactive. Genital tuberculosis in adolescent males causes epididymitis or orchitis. The condition usually manifests as a unilateral nodular painless swelling of the scrotum. Involvement of the glans penis is extremely rare. Genital abnormalities and a positive tuberculin skin test in an adolescent male or female is suggestive of genital tract tuberculosis.

Disease in HIV-Infected Children. Most cases of tuberculosis in HIV-infected children have been described in developing countries. The rate of tuberculosis disease in HIV-infected children is 30 times higher than in non-HIV-infected children in the USA. Establishing the diagnosis of tuberculosis in an HIV-infected child may be difficult because skin test reactivity can be absent, culture confirmation is difficult, and the clinical features of tuberculosis are similar to many other HIV-related infections and conditions. Tuberculosis in HIV-infected children is often more severe, progressive, and likely to occur in extrapulmonary sites. Radiographic findings are similar to those in children with normal immune systems, but lobar disease and lung cavitation are more common. Nonspecific respiratory symptoms, fever, and weight loss are the most common complaints. Rates of drug-resistant tuberculosis tend to be higher in HIV-infected adults and, probably, are also higher in HIV-infected children. The mortality rate of HIV-infected children with tuberculosis is high, especially as the CD4 lymphocyte numbers decrease. In adults, the host immune response to tuberculosis infection appears to enhance HIV replication and accelerate the immune suppression caused by HIV. Increased mortality rates are attributed to progressive HIV infection rather than tuberculosis. Therefore, HIV-infected children with potential exposures and/or recent infection should be promptly evaluated and treated for tuberculosis. Conversely, all children with tuberculosis disease should be tested for HIV co-infection, because of the potential benefits of early diagnosis and treatment of HIV infection, and because the presence of HIV may necessitate a longer duration of treatment.

Perinatal Disease. Symptoms of congenital tuberculosis may be present at birth but more commonly begin by the 2nd or 3rd wk of life. The most common signs and symptoms are respiratory distress, fever, hepatic or splenic enlargement, poor feeding, lethargy or irritability, lymphadenopathy, abdominal distention, failure to thrive, ear drainage, and skin lesions. The clinical manifestations vary in relation to the site and size of the caseous lesions. Many infants have an abnormal chest radiograph, most often a miliary pattern. Some infants with no pulmonary findings early in the course of the disease later develop profound radiographic and clinical abnormalities. Hilar and mediastinal lymphadenopathy and lung infiltrates are common. Generalized lymphadenopathy and meningitis occur in 30–50% of patients.

The clinical presentation of tuberculosis in newborns is similar to that caused by bacterial sepsis and other congenital infections, such as syphilis, toxoplasmosis, and cytomegalovirus. The diagnosis should be suspected in an infant with signs and symptoms of bacterial or congenital infection whose response to antibiotic and supportive therapy is poor and evaluation for other infections is unrevealing. The most important clue for rapid diagnosis of congenital tuberculosis is a maternal or family history of tuberculosis. Frequently, the mother's disease is discovered only after the neonate's diagnosis is suspected. The infant's tuberculin skin test is negative initially but may become positive in 1–3 mo. A positive acid-fast stain of an early morning gastric aspirate from a newborn usually indicates tuberculosis. Direct acid-fast stains on middle-ear discharge, bone marrow, tracheal aspirate, or biopsy tissue (especially liver) can be useful. The CSF should be examined and cultured, although the yield for isolating *M. tuberculosis* is low. The mortality rate of congenital tuberculosis remains very high because of delayed diagnosis; many children will have a complete recovery if the diagnosis is made promptly and adequate chemotherapy is started.

TREATMENT. The basic principles of management of tuberculosis disease in children and adolescents are the same as those in adults. Several drugs are used to effect a relatively rapid cure and prevent the emergence of secondary drug resistance during therapy (Tables 212-4 and 212-5). The choice of regimen depends on the extent of tuberculosis disease, the host, and the likelihood of drug resistance (Table 212-6). The standard therapy of intrathoracic tuberculosis (pulmonary disease and/or hilar lymphadenopathy) in children recommended by the CDC and AAP is a 6 mo regimen of isoniazid and rifampin supplemented in the 1st 2 mo of treatment by pyrazinamide. Several clinical trials have shown that this regimen yields a success rate approaching 100% with an incidence of clinically significant adverse reactions of <2%. Nine month regimens of isoniazid and rifampin are also highly effective for drug-susceptible tuberculosis, but the necessary length of treatment, the need for good adherence by the patient, and the relative lack of protection against possible initial drug resistance have led to the use of shorter regimens. Most experts recommend that all drug administration be directly observed, meaning that a health care worker is physically present when the medications are administered to the patients. When **directly observed therapy** is used, intermittent (twice weekly) administration of drugs after an

TABLE 212-4. Commonly Used Drugs for the Treatment of Tuberculosis in Infants, Children, and Adolescents

DRUGS	DOSAGE FORMS	DAILY DOSAGE, MG/KG	TWICE A WEEK DOSAGE, MG/KG PER DOSE	MAXIMUM DOSE	ADVERSE REACTIONS
Ethambutol	Tablets 100 mg 400 mg	15–25	50	2.5 g	Optic neuritis (usually reversible), decreased red-green color discrimination, gastrointestinal tract disturbances, hypersensitivity
Isoniazid*	Scored tablets 100 mg 300 mg Syrup 10 mg/mL	10–15[†]	20–30	Daily, 300 mg Twice a week, 900 mg	Mild hepatic enzyme elevation, hepatitis,[†] peripheral neuritis, hypersensitivity
Pyrazinamide*	Scored tablets 500 mg	20–40	50	2 g	Hepatotoxic effects, hyperuricemia, arthralgias, gastrointestinal tract upset
Rifampin*	Capsules 150 mg 300 mg Syrup formulated in syrup from capsules	10–20	10–20	600 mg	Orange discoloration of secretions or urine, staining of contact lenses, vomiting, hepatitis, influenza-like reaction, thrombocytopenia, pruritus; oral contraceptives may be ineffective

*Rifamate is a capsule containing 150 mg of isoniazid and 300 mg of rifampin. Two capsules provide the usual adult (>50 kg) daily doses of each drug. Rifater is a capsule containing 50 mg of isoniazid, 120 mg of rifampin, and 300 mg of pyrazinamide. Isoniazid and rifampin also are available for parenteral administration.

[†]When isoniazid in a dosage exceeding 10 mg/kg per day is used in combination with rifampin, the incidence of hepatotoxic effects may be increased.

From the American Academy of Pediatrics: *Red Book: 2006 Report of the Committee on Infectious Diseases*, 27th ed. Elk Grove Village, IL, American Academy of Pediatrics, 2006, p. 688.

TABLE 212-5. Less Commonly Used Drugs for Treatment of Drug-Resistant Tuberculosis in Infants, Children, and Adolescents*

DRUGS	DOSAGE, FORMS	DAILY DOSAGE, MG/KG	MAXIMUM DOSE	ADVERSE REACTIONS
Amikacin[†]	Vials, 500 mg and 1 g	15–30 (IV or IM administration)	1 g	Auditory and vestibular toxic effects, nephrotoxic effects
Capreomycin[†]	Vials, 1 g	15–30 (IM administration)	1 g	Auditory and vestibular toxicity and nephrotoxic effects
Cycloserine	Capsules, 250 mg	10–20, given in 2 divided doses	1 g	Psychosis, personality changes, seizures, rash
Ethionamide	Tablets, 250 mg	15–20, given in 2–3 divided doses	1 g	Gastrointestinal tract disturbances, hepatotoxic effects, hypersensitivity reactions, hypothyroid
Kanamycin	Vials 75 mg/2 mL 500 mg/2 mL 1 g/3 mL	15–30 (IM or IV administration)	1 g	Auditory and vestibular toxic effects, nephrotoxic effects
Levofloxacin[‡]	Tablets 250 mg 500 mg Vials 25 mg/mL	Adults 500–1000 mg (once daily) Children: not recommended	1 g	Theoretic effect on growing cartilage, gastrointestinal tract disturbances, rash, headache, restlessness, confusion
Para-aminosalicylic acid (PAS)	Packets, 3 g	200–300 (2–4 times a day)	10 g	Gastrointestinal tract disturbances, hypersensitivity, hepatotoxic effects
Streptomycin[†]	Vials 1 g 4 g	20–40 (IM administration)	1 g	Auditory and vestibular toxic effects, nephrotoxic effects, rash

*These drugs should be used in consultation with a specialist in tuberculosis.

[†]Dose adjustment in renal insufficiency.

[‡]Levofloxacin currently is not approved for use in children younger than 18 yr of age; its use in younger children necessitates assessment of the potential risks and benefits.

From the American Academy of Pediatrics: *Red Book: 2006 Report of the Committee on Infectious Diseases*, 27th ed. Elk Grove Village, IL, American Academy of Pediatrics, 2006, p. 689.

TABLE 212-6. Recommended Treatment Regimens for Drug-Susceptible Tuberculosis in Infants, Children, and Adolescents

INFECTION OR DISEASE CATEGORY	REGIMEN	REMARKS
LATENT TUBERCULOSIS INFECTION (POSITIVE TST RESULT, NO DISEASE)		
Isoniazid susceptible	9 mo of isoniazid, once a day	If daily therapy is not possible, DOT twice a week can be used for 9 mo.
Isoniazid resistant	6 mo of rifampin, once a day	If daily therapy is not possible, DOT twice a week can be used for 6 mo.
Isoniazid-rifampin resistant*	Consult a tuberculosis specialist	
PULMONARY AND EXTRAPULMONARY (EXCEPT MENINGITIS)	2 mo of isoniazid, rifampin, and pyrazinamide daily, followed by 4 mo of isoniazid and rifampin[†] by DOT[‡] for drug-susceptible *M. tuberculosis* 9 to 12 mo of isoniazid and rifampin for drug susceptible *M. bovis*	If possible drug resistance is a concern (see text), another drug (ethambutol or an aminoglycoside) is added to the initial 3 drug therapy until drug susceptibilities are determined. DOT is highly desirable. If hilar adenopathy only, a 6 mo course of isoniazid and rifampin is sufficient. Drugs can be given 2 or 3 times/wk under DOT in the initial phase if nonadherence is likely.
MENINGITIS	2 mo of isoniazid, rifampin, pyrazinamide, and an aminoglycoside or ethionamide, once a day, followed by 7–10 mo of isoniazid and rifampin, once a day or twice a week (9–12 mo total) for drug-susceptible *M. tuberculosis* At least 12 mo of therapy without pyrazinamide for drug susceptible *M. bovis*	A fourth drug, such as an aminoglycoside, is given with initial therapy until drug susceptibility is known. For patients who may have acquired tuberculosis in geographic areas where resistance to streptomycin is common, kanamycin, amikacin, or capreomycin can be used instead of streptomycin.

*Duration of therapy is longer for human immunodeficiency virus (HIV)-infected people, and additional drugs may be indicated.

[†]Medications should be administered daily for the first 2 wk to 2 mo of treatment and then can be administered 2–3 times per week by DOT.

[‡]If initial chest radiograph shows cavitary lesions and sputum after 2 mo of therapy remains positive, duration of therapy is extended to 9 mo.

From the American Academy of Pediatrics: *Red Book: 2006 Report of the Committee on Infectious Diseases*, 27th ed. Elk Grove Village, IL, American Academy of Pediatrics, 2006, p. 686.

DOT, directly observed therapy; TST, tuberculin skin test.

initial period as short as 2 wk of daily therapy is as effective in children as daily therapy for the entire course. In locales where the community rate of isoniazid resistance is greater than 5–10%, or when the adult source case is at increased risk for drug-resistant tuberculosis, most experts recommend adding a 4th drug—usually streptomycin, ethambutol, or ethionamide—to the initial regimen. The reason to add the 4th drug is that pyrazinamide is not effective in preventing the emergence of rifampin resistance during therapy when isoniazid resistance already exists.

Controlled clinical trials for treating various forms of extrapulmonary tuberculosis are virtually nonexistent. Extrapulmonary tuberculosis is usually caused by small numbers of mycobacteria. In general, the treatment for most forms of extrapulmonary tuberculosis in children, including cervical lymphadenopathy, is the same as for pulmonary tuberculosis. Exceptions are bone and joint, disseminated, and CNS tuberculosis, for which there are inadequate data to recommend 6 mo therapy. These infections are treated for 9–12 mo. Surgical debridement in bone and joint disease and ventriculoperitoneal shunting in CNS disease are frequently necessary.

The optimal treatment of tuberculosis in HIV-infected children has not been established. HIV-seropositive adults with tuberculosis can be treated successfully with standard regimens that include isoniazid, rifampin, and pyrazinamide. The total duration of therapy should be 6–9 mo, or 6 mo after culture of sputum becomes sterile, whichever is longer. Data for children are limited to isolated case reports and small series. Most experts believe that HIV-seropositive children with drug-susceptible tuberculosis should receive at least 3 drugs such as isoniazid, rifampin, and pyrazinamide for the 1st 2 mo followed by isoniazid and rifampin for a total duration of at least 9 mo. A 4th drug such as ethambutol or streptomycin should be added for disseminated disease and when drug resistance is suspected. Rifampin-resistant tuberculosis is more common in HIV-infected patients. Children with HIV infection appear to have more frequent adverse reactions to antituberculosis drugs and must be monitored closely during therapy. Co-administration of rifampin and some antiretroviral agents results in subtherapeutic blood levels of protease inhibitors and non-nucleoside reverse transcriptase inhibitors, and toxic levels of rifampin. Concomitant administration of these drugs is not recommended. Treatment of HIV-infected children is often empirical based on epidemiologic and radiographic information, because the radiographic appearance of other pulmonary complications of HIV in children, such as lymphoid interstitial pneumonitis and bacterial pneumonia, may be similar to that of tuberculosis. Therapy should be considered when tuberculosis cannot be excluded.

Drug-Resistant Tuberculosis. The incidence of drug-resistant tuberculosis is increasing in many areas of the world, including North America. There are 2 major types of drug resistance. **Primary resistance** occurs when an individual is infected with *M. tuberculosis* that is already resistant to a particular drug. **Secondary resistance** occurs when drug-resistant organisms emerge as the dominant population during treatment. The major causes of secondary drug resistance are poor adherence with the medication by the patient or inadequate treatment regimens prescribed by the physician. Nonadherence with 1 drug is more likely to lead to secondary resistance than failure to take all drugs. Secondary resistance is rare in children because of the small size of their mycobacterial population. Therefore, most drug resistance in children is primary, and patterns of drug resistance among children tend to mirror those found among adults in the same population. The main predictors of drug-resistant tuberculosis among adults are history of previous antituberculosis treatment, co-infection with HIV, and exposure to another adult with infectious drug-resistant tuberculosis.

Treatment of drug-resistant tuberculosis is successful only when at least 2 bactericidal drugs are given to which the infecting strain of *M. tuberculosis* is susceptible. When a child has possible drug-resistant tuberculosis, at least 3 and usually 4 or 5 drugs should be administered initially until the susceptibility pattern is determined and a more specific regimen can be designed. The specific treatment plan must be individualized for each patient according to the results of susceptibility testing on the isolates from the child or the adult source case. Treatment duration of 9 mo with rifampin, pyrazinamide, and ethambutol is usually adequate for isoniazid-resistant tuberculosis in children. When resistance to isoniazid and rifampin is present, the total duration of therapy often must be extended to 12–18 mo, and twice-a-week regimens should not be used. The prognosis of single- or multidrug-resistant tuberculosis in children is usually good if the drug resistance is identified early in the treatment, appropriate drugs are administered under directly observed therapy, adverse reactions from the drugs do not occur, and the child and family are in a supportive environment. The treatment of drug-resistant tuberculosis in children always should be undertaken by a clinician with specific expertise in the treatment of tuberculosis.

Corticosteroids. These are useful in the treatment of some children with tuberculosis disease. They are most beneficial when the host inflammatory reaction contributes significantly to tissue damage or impairment of organ function. There is convincing evidence that corticosteroids decrease mortality rates and long-term neurologic sequelae in some patients with **tuberculous meningitis** by reducing vasculitis, inflammation, and, ultimately, intracranial pressure. Lowering the intracranial pressure limits tissue damage and favors circulation of antituberculosis drugs through the brain and meninges. Short courses of corticosteroids also may be effective for children with **endobronchial tuberculosis** that causes respiratory distress, localized emphysema, or segmental pulmonary lesions. Several randomized clinical trials have shown that corticosteroids can help relieve symptoms and constriction associated with acute tuberculous **pericardial effusion.** Corticosteroids may cause dramatic improvement in symptoms in some patients with tuberculous pleural effusion and shift of the mediastinum. However, the long-term course of disease is probably unaffected. Some children with severe **miliary tuberculosis** have dramatic improvement with corticosteroid therapy if the inflammatory reaction is so severe that alveolocapillary block is present. There is no convincing evidence that 1 corticosteroid preparation is better than another. The most commonly prescribed regimen is prednisone, 1–2 mg/kg/day in 1–2 divided doses orally for 4–6 wk, followed by gradual tapering.

Supportive Care. Children receiving treatment should be followed carefully to promote adherence with therapy, to monitor for toxic reactions to medications, and to ensure that the tuberculosis is being adequately treated. Adequate nutrition is important. Patients should be seen at monthly intervals and should be given just enough medication to last until the next visit. Anticipatory guidance with regard to the administration of medications to children is crucial. The physician should foresee difficulties that the family might have in introducing several new medications in inconvenient dosage forms to a young child. The clinician must report all cases of suspected tuberculosis in a child to the local health department to be sure that the child and family receive appropriate care and evaluation.

Nonadherence to treatment is the major problem in tuberculosis therapy. The patient and family must know what is expected of them through verbal and written instructions in their primary language. From 30 to 50% of patients taking long-term treatment are significantly nonadherent with self-administered medications, and clinicians are usually not able to determine in advance which patients will be nonadherent. Preferably, directly observed therapy should be instituted with the help of the local health department.

PREVENTION. The highest priority of any tuberculosis control program should be case finding and treatment, which interrupts transmission of infection between close contacts. All children and adults with symptoms suggestive of tuberculosis disease and those in close contact with an adult suspected of having infectious pulmonary tuberculosis should be tuberculin skin tested and examined as soon as possible. On average, 30–50% of household contacts to infectious cases will be tuberculin skin test positive, and 1% of contacts already have overt disease. This scheme relies on effective and adequate public health response and resources. Children, particularly young infants, should receive high priority during contact investigations because their risk for infection is high and they are more likely to rapidly develop severe forms of tuberculosis.

Mass testing of large groups of children for tuberculosis infection is an inefficient process. When large groups of children at low risk for tuberculosis are tested, the vast majority of skin test reactions are actually false-positive reactions due to biologic variability or cross sensitization with NTM. However, testing of high-risk groups of adults or children should be encouraged because most of these individuals with positive tuberculin skin test results have tuberculosis infection. Testing should take place only if effective mechanisms are in place to ensure adequate evaluation and treatment of the individuals who test positive.

Bacille Calmette-Guérin Vaccination. The only available vaccine against tuberculosis is the BCG, named for the 2 French investigators responsible for its development. The original vaccine organism was a strain of *M. bovis* attenuated by subculture every 3 wk for 13 yr. This strain was distributed to dozens of laboratories that continued to subculture the organism on different media under various conditions. The result has been production of many BCG vaccines that differ widely in morphology, growth characteristics, sensitizing potency, and animal virulence. The route of administration and dosing schedule for the BCG vaccines are important variables for efficacy. The preferred route of administration is intradermal injection with a syringe and needle because it is the only method that permits accurate measurement of an individual dose. The BCG vaccines are extremely safe in immunocompetent hosts. Local ulceration and regional suppurative adenitis occur in 0.1–1% of vaccine recipients. Local lesions do not suggest underlying host immune defects and do not affect the level of protection afforded by the vaccine. Most reactions are mild and usually resolve spontaneously, but chemotherapy is needed occasionally. Surgical excision of a suppurative draining node is rarely necessary and should be avoided if possible. Osteitis is a rare complication of BCG vaccination that appears to be related to certain strains of the vaccine that are no longer in wide use. Systemic complaints such as fever, convulsions, loss of appetite, and irritability are extraordinarily rare after BCG vaccination. Profoundly immunocompromised patients may develop disseminated BCG infection after vaccination. Children with HIV infection appear to have rates of local adverse reactions to BCG vaccines that are comparable with rates in immunocompetent children. However, the incidence in these children of disseminated infection months to years after vaccination is currently unknown.

Recommended vaccine schedules vary widely among countries. The official recommendation of the WHO is a single dose administered during infancy, including in asymptomatic HIV-infected children in populations where the risk for tuberculosis is high. In some countries repeat vaccination is universal. In others it is based on either tuberculin skin testing or the absence of a typical scar. The optimal age for administration and dosing schedule are unknown because adequate comparative trials have not been performed.

Although dozens of BCG trials have been reported in various human populations, the most useful data have come from several controlled trials. The results of these studies have been disparate. Some demonstrated a great deal of protection from BCG vaccines, but others showed no efficacy at all. A recent meta-analysis of published BCG vaccination trials suggested that BCG is 50% effective in preventing pulmonary tuberculosis in adults and children. The protective effect for disseminated and meningeal tuberculosis appears to be slightly higher, with BCG preventing 50–80% of cases. A variety of explanations for the varied responses to BCG vaccines have been proposed, including methodologic and statistical variations within the trials, interaction with NTM that either enhances or decreases the protection afforded by BCG, different potencies among the various BCG vaccines, and genetic factors for BCG response within the study populations. BCG vaccination administered during infancy has little effect on the ultimate incidence of tuberculosis in adults, suggesting that the effect of the vaccine is time limited.

BCG vaccination has worked well in some situations but poorly in others. Clearly, BCG vaccination has had little effect on the ultimate control of tuberculosis throughout the world because more than 5 billion doses have been administered but tuberculosis remains epidemic in most regions. BCG vaccination does not substantially influence the chain of transmission because those cases of contagious pulmonary tuberculosis in adults that can be prevented by BCG vaccination constitute a small fraction of the sources of infection in a population. The best use of BCG vaccination appears to be prevention of life-threatening forms of tuberculosis in infants and young children.

BCG vaccination has never been adopted as part of the strategy for the control of tuberculosis in the United States. Widespread use of the vaccine would render subsequent tuberculin skin testing less useful. However, BCG vaccination may contribute to tuberculosis control in selected population groups. BCG is recommended for tuberculin skin test–negative infants and children who (1) are at high risk for intimate and prolonged exposure to persistently untreated or ineffectively treated adults with infectious pulmonary tuberculosis and cannot be removed from the source of infection or placed on long-term preventive therapy or (2) are continuously exposed to persons with tuberculosis who have bacilli that are resistant to isoniazid and rifampin. Any child receiving BCG vaccination should have a documented negative tuberculin skin test before receiving the vaccine. After receiving the vaccine, the child should be separated from the possible sources of infection until it can be demonstrated that the child has had a vaccine response, demonstrated by tuberculin reactivity, which usually develops within 1–3 mo. Occasionally, a 2nd BCG vaccination must be given to children who fail to develop skin test reactivity after the 1st dose. In the United States, BCG is contraindicated in children with primary or secondary immunodeficiencies.

Active research to develop new tuberculosis vaccines has led to the creation and preliminary testing of several vaccine candidates based on attenuated strains of mycobacteria, subunit proteins, or DNA. The genome of *M. tuberculosis* has been sequenced, allowing researchers to further study and better understand the pathogenesis and host immune responses to tuberculosis.

Perinatal Tuberculosis. The most effective way of preventing tuberculosis infection and disease in the neonate or young infant is through appropriate testing and treatment of the mother and other family members. High-risk pregnant women should be tested with a tuberculin skin test, and those with a positive test result should receive a chest radiograph with appropriate abdominal shielding. If the mother has a negative chest radiograph and is clinically well, no separation of the infant and mother is needed after delivery. The child needs no special evaluation or treatment if he or she remains asymptomatic. Other household members should undergo tuberculin skin testing and further evaluation as indicated.

If the mother has suspected tuberculosis at the time of delivery, the newborn should be separated from the mother until the chest radiograph is obtained. If the mother's chest radiograph is abnormal, separation should be maintained until the mother has been evaluated thoroughly, including examination of the sputum. If the mother's chest radiograph is abnormal but the history, physical examination, sputum examination, and evaluation of the radiograph show no evidence of current active tuberculosis, it is reasonable to assume that the infant is at low risk for infection. The mother should receive appropriate treatment, and she and her infant should receive careful follow-up care. In addition, all household members should be evaluated for tuberculosis.

If the mother's chest radiograph or acid-fast sputum smear shows evidence of current tuberculosis disease, additional steps are necessary to protect the infant. Isoniazid therapy for newborns has been so effective that separation of the mother and infant is no longer considered mandatory. Separation should occur only if the mother is ill enough to require hospitalization, she has been or is expected to become nonadherent with her treatment, or there is strong suspicion that she has drug-resistant tuberculosis. Isoniazid treatment for the infant should be continued until the mother has been shown to be sputum culture negative for at least 3 mo. At that time, a Mantoux tuberculin skin test should be placed on the child. If positive, isoniazid is continued for a total duration of 9–12 mo; if negative, isoniazid can be discontinued. Because isoniazid resistance is increasing in the United States, it is not always clear that isoniazid therapy will be effective for the neonate. If isoniazid resistance is suspected or the mother's adherence to medication is in question, separation of the infant from the mother should be considered. The duration of separation must be at least as long as is necessary to render the mother noninfectious. An expert in tuberculosis should be consulted if the young infant has potential exposure to the mother or another adult with tuberculosis disease caused by an isoniazid-resistant strain of *M. tuberculosis*.

Although isoniazid is not thought to be teratogenic, the treatment of pregnant women with asymptomatic tuberculosis infection is often deferred until after delivery. However, symptomatic pregnant women or those with radiographic evidence of tuberculosis disease should be appropriately evaluated. Because pulmonary tuberculosis is harmful to both the mother and the fetus, and it represents a great danger to the infant after delivery, tuberculosis in pregnant women always should be treated. The most common regimen for drug-susceptible tuberculosis is isoniazid, rifampin, and ethambutol. The aminoglycosides and ethionamide should be avoided because of their teratogenic effect. The safety of pyrazinamide in pregnancy has not been established.

American Thoracic Society, Centers for Disease Control and Prevention, Infectious Disease Society of America: Treatment of tuberculosis. *Am J Respir Crit Care Med* 2003;167:603–662.

Aziz MA, Wright A, Laszlo A, et al: Epidemiology of antituberculosis drug resistance (the global project on anti-tuberculosis drug resistance surveillance): an updated analysis. *Lancet* 2006;368:2142–2154.

Bozaykut A, Atay E, Sevim H, et al: Effect of BCG vaccine on tuberculin skin tests in 7–11-year-old children. *Acta Paediatr* 2004;93:1033–1035.

Campbell IA, Bah-Sow O: Pulmonary tuberculosis: Diagnosis and treatment. *Br Med J* 2006;332:1194–1197.

Centers for Disease Control and Prevention: Tuberculosis associated with blocking agents against tumor necrosis factor-alpha—California, 2002–03. *MMWR* 2004;53:683–686.

Centers for Disease Control and Prevention: Congenital pulmonary tuberculosis associated with maternal cerebral tuberculosis, Florida, 2002. *JAMA* 2005;293:2710–2711.

Centers for Disease Control and Prevention: Controlling tuberculosis in the United States—Recommendations from the American Thoracic Society, CDC, and the Infectious Diseases Society of America. *MMWR* 2005;54:1–81.

Centers for Disease Control and Prevention: Human tuberculosis caused by *Mycobacterium bovis,* New York City, 2001–2004. *MMWR* 2005;54: 605–608.

Centers for Disease Control and Prevention: *Reported Tuberculosis in the United States, 2004.* Atlanta, GA, U.S. Department of Health and Human Services, CDC, September 2005.

Centers for Disease Control and Prevention: Trends in tuberculosis, United States, 2005. *MMWR* 2006;55:305–308.

Colebunders R, Apers L, Dieltiens G, Worodria W: Tuberculosis in resource poor countries. *BMJ* 2007;334:105–106.

Drobac PC, Mukherjee JS, Joseph JK, et al: Community-based therapy for children with multidrug-resistant tuberculosis. *Pediatrics* 2006;117: 2022–2029.

Dye C: Global epidemiology of tuberculosis. *Lancet* 2006;367:938–940.

Ferrara G, Losi M, D'Amico R, et al: Use in routine clinical practice of two commercial blood tests for diagnosis of infection with *Mycobacterium tuberculosis:* A prospective study. *Lancet* 2006;367: 1328–1334.

Hill PC, Brookes RH, Adetifa MO, et al: Comparison of enzyme-linked immunospot assay and tuberculin skin test in healthy children exposed to *Mycobacterium tuberculosis. Pediatrics* 2006;117:1542–1548.

Lawn SD, Wilkinson R: Extensively drug resistant tuberculosis. *BMJ* 2006; 333:559–560.

Liebeschuetz S, Bamber S, Ewer K, et al: Diagnosis of tuberculosis in South African children with a T-cell-based assay: A prospective cohort study. *Lancet* 2004;364:2196–2203.

Marais BJ, Gie RP, Hesseling AC, et al: A refined symptom-based approach to diagnose pulmonary tuberculosis in children. *Pediatrics* 2006;18:e1350–e1359.

Marais BJ, Gie RP, Hesseling AC, et al: Radiographic signs and symptoms in children treated for tuberculosis. *Pediatr Infect Dis J* 2006;25:237–240.

Marais BJ, Gie RP, Schaaf HS, et al: Childhood pulmonary tuberculosis: Old wisdom and new challenges. *Am J Respir Crit Care Med* 2006;173: 1078–1090.

Moon JW, Chang YS, Kim SK, et al: The clinical utility of polymerase chain reaction for the diagnosis of pleural tuberculosis. *Clin Infect Dis* 2005;41:660–666.

Nelson LJ, Schneider E, Wells CD, et al: Epidemiology of childhood tuberculosis in the United States, 1993–2001: The need for continued vigilance. *Pediatrics* 2004;114:333–341.

Novelli V: BCG vaccination gets a boost. *Lancet* 2006;367:1122–1124.

Pediatric Tuberculosis Collaborative Group: Targeted tuberculin skin testing and treatment of latent tuberculosis infection in children and adolescents. *Pediatrics* 2004;114:1175–1201.

Polesky A, Grove W, Bhatia G: Peripheral tuberculous lymphadenitis: Epidemiology, diagnosis, treatment and outcome. *Medicine* 2005;84:350–362.

Sharma SK, Mohan A, Sharma A, Mitrs DK: Miliary tuberculosis: New insights into an old disease. *Lancet* 2005;5:415–430.

Sharp D: Bovine tuberculosis and badger blame. *Lancet* 2006;367:631–632.

Soysal A, Millington KA, Bakir M, et al: Effect of BCG vaccination on risk of *Mycobacterium tuberculosis* infection in children with household tuberculosis contact: A prospective community-based study. *Lancet* 2005;366: 1443–1450.

Starke JR: Interferon-γ release assays for diagnosis of tuberculosis infection in children. *Pediatr Infect Dis J* 2006;25:941–942.

Starke JR: Transmission of *Mycobacterium tuberculosis* to and from children and adolescents. *Semin Pediatr Infect Dis* 2001;12:115–123.

Swingler GH, du Toit G, Andronikou S, et al: Diagnostic accuracy of chest radiography in detecting mediastinal lymphadenopathy in suspected pulmonary tuberculosis. *Arch Dis Child* 2005;90:1153–1156.

Thwaites GE, Bang ND, Dung NH, et al: Dexamethasone for treatment of tuberculous meningitis in adolescents and adults. *N Engl J Med* 2004;351:1741–1750.

Trunz BB, Fine PEM, Dye C: Effect of BCG vaccination on childhood tuberculous meningitis and miliary tuberculosis worldwide: A meta-analysis and assessment of cost-effectiveness. *Lancet* 2006;367:1173–1180.

Walker V, Selby G, Wacogne I: Does neonatal BCG vaccination protect against tuberculous meningitis? *Arch Dis Child* 2006;91:789–794.

Wang JY, Hsueh PR, Wang SK, et al: Disseminated tuberculosis – a 10-year experience in a medical center. *Medicine* 2007;86:39–46.

Zar HJ, Cotton MF, Strauss S, et al: Effect of isoniazid prophylaxis on mortality and incidence of tuberculosis in children with HIV: randomized controlled trial. *BMJ* 2007;334:136–139.

Zar HJ, Hanslo D, Apolles P, et al: Induced sputum versus gastric lavage for microbiological confirmation of pulmonary tuberculosis in infants and young children: A prospective study. *Lancet* 2005;365:130–134.

Chapter 213 ■ Hansen Disease (*Mycobacterium Leprae*)

Dwight A. Powell

Hansen disease (**leprosy**) is a chronic disease resulting from infection with *Mycobacterium leprae* and moderated by the ensuing host response. The respiratory mucosa, skin, and peripheral nervous system are most prominently affected, with occasional testicular and ocular involvement. Humans were long believed to be the sole host of *M. leprae,* but naturally acquired infection has been documented in armadillos in the southeastern USA, and experimental infection has been established in primates, nude mice, and armadillos.

The sequelae of leprosy include chronic skin lesions, madarosis, sensory neuropathy resulting in the loss of digits or limbs, and paresis secondary to motor nerve dysfunction. The highly visible nature of these debilities led to the historical stigmatization of the "leper." The psychologic and sociologic sequelae of this stigma can be as debilitating as the disease itself and may result in delays in seeking medical attention. To combat this prejudice, the term **leprosy patient** has replaced the word leper, and Hansen disease, after Armauer Hansen who identified *M. leprae* as the cause of leprosy in 1873, is the accepted designation.

ETIOLOGY. *M. leprae* is an acid-fast bacillus of the family Mycobacteriaceae. It is an obligate intracellular pathogen with a generation time of 14 days. *M. leprae* grows optimally at 27–30°C and cannot be cultured in vitro. The incubation period of leprosy in humans ranges from 3 mo to 20 yr (average 3–5 yr). The rare occurrence of leprosy in infants as young as 3 mo of age suggests that in utero transmission may occur or that very short incubation periods may be possible in certain situations.

EPIDEMIOLOGY. After the introduction of multidrug therapy by the World Health Organization (WHO) in 1982, there has been a steady decline in the prevalence of leprosy. In 1991, the WHO called for the elimination of leprosy as defined by a worldwide prevalence of <1/10,000 population. That goal was achieved by the year 2000 in all but 15 of the 122 countries where leprosy was considered a public health problem in 1985. Those countries are mainly in Asia, Africa, and South America. In 1985, there were 10–12 million cases of leprosy worldwide; in 2004, the prevalence was 457,792 cases. However, the new case detection rate has declined less rapidly. In 1998, 750,000 new cases were detected; in 2003, there were 513,798 new cases registered for treatment. By 2004, 80% of the world's leprosy patients resided in India (59%), Brazil (17%), or Indonesia (4%). Approximately 150 cases are reported annually in the USA, of which 85% are in immigrants. Small numbers of endemic cases are reported from Texas, Hawaii, and Louisiana.

Human-to-human transmission is responsible for an overwhelming majority of secondary cases, with the highest risk among family members and other close contacts. Leprosy occurs at all ages, but infections in infants are extremely rare. The incidence rates peak during childhood and early adulthood in endemic areas. HIV infection has not been documented to alter the risk for leprosy in areas of high prevalence for both pathogens.

PATHOGENESIS. Possible modes of transmission include contact with desquamated infected epidermis, ingestion of infected breast milk, and bites of mosquitoes or other vectors. At present, however, the basis for most infections appears to be transmission from untreated lepromatous patients following prolonged contact with infected nasal secretions containing a high bacterial load. Skin testing and serologic studies suggest that up to 90% of infected persons develop immunity without ever manifesting clinical disease. Studies in endemic areas using polymerase chain reaction (PCR) show widespread presence of the organism in nasal secretions from asymptomatic individuals.

M. leprae appears to be transported hematogenously from the nasal mucosa to skin and peripheral nerves. Using the armadillo model of neuritis, *M. leprae* organisms have been shown to colonize the perineural space and gain access to the interstitium of the endoneural space. Once there, organisms are available for phagocytosis by Schwann cells and interstitial macrophages surrounding peripheral nerve axons. Intracellular replication of *M. leprae* follows, with varying degrees depending on the host cellular immune response. *M. leprae* attachment to and ingestion by Schwann cells has been shown to depend on receptors on the lamin-2 glycoprotein in the basal lamina and the α-dystroglycan complex in the Schwann cell basement membrane. *M. leprae*–specific phenolic glycolipid-1 appears to be the ligand mediating this binding.

Once inside the Schwann cell, *M. leprae* replicates slowly over years. At some stage, specific T cells recognize the presence of mycobacterial antigens within the cells and initiate a chronic inflammatory reaction. Genetic susceptibility to leprosy has been linked to the natural resistance associated with macrophage protein-1, which is present only in certain racial groups. Factors that may lead to the development of localized vs disseminated disease are the degree of expression of Toll-like receptors on monocytes and the production of interferon-γ (IFN-γ) by T cells.

Once *M. leprae* colonizes the surface of nerves and infects endoneural macrophages and Schwann cells, several mechanisms of skin and nerve injury may occur, depending on the host immune response. One end of the spectrum is **tuberculoid leprosy (TL)**, in which there is a vigorous and specific cell-mediated immune response to *M. leprae* antigens. In tissue biopsies there are tightly organized granulomas composed of epithelioid cells and lymphocytes, but bacilli are scant or absent. Macrophages, when present, do not contain intracellular organisms. Caseation is rare. Heavy cellular infiltration is found in the dermis with destruction of cutaneous nerve fibers.

At the other end of the spectrum is **lepromatous leprosy (LL)**, in which there is total and specific anergy to *M. leprae* both by skin testing and by in vitro assays of cell-mediated immunity. Large amounts of circulating and tissue-based antibody to mycobacterial antigens is present, but it affords no protective immunity. Bacilli are found in enormous numbers in the skin, nasal mucosa, and peripheral nerves. There is continual bacillemia as well as bacillary invasion of all major organs except the central nervous system. Tissue granulomas are poorly formed and are composed chiefly of loose aggregates of foamy histiocytes. Macrophages teeming with undigested bacilli are common. There is extensive, symmetric involvement of peripheral nerves, although the cutaneous nerve endings are usually spared.

An *M. leprae*–specific suppressor T-cell population is found in the circulation of patients with LL, with increased numbers of suppressor T cells found in the skin granulomas. T cells from lepromatous patients also produce less interleukin 2 and less IFN-γ after stimulation with *M. leprae* antigens than do T cells from tuberculoid patients or normal controls.

Borderline or dimorphous leprosy is subdivided into 3 subclasses that lie between the tuberculoid and lepromatous poles: borderline tuberculoid, borderline, and borderline lepromatous.

CLINICAL MANIFESTATIONS. The manifestations of Hansen disease reflect the host response to the infection.

Indeterminate Leprosy. Indeterminate leprosy (IL) is the earliest clinically detectable form of leprosy. Although it is diagnosed in only 10–20% of infected individuals, most patients with advanced leprosy have passed through this stage. Usually there is

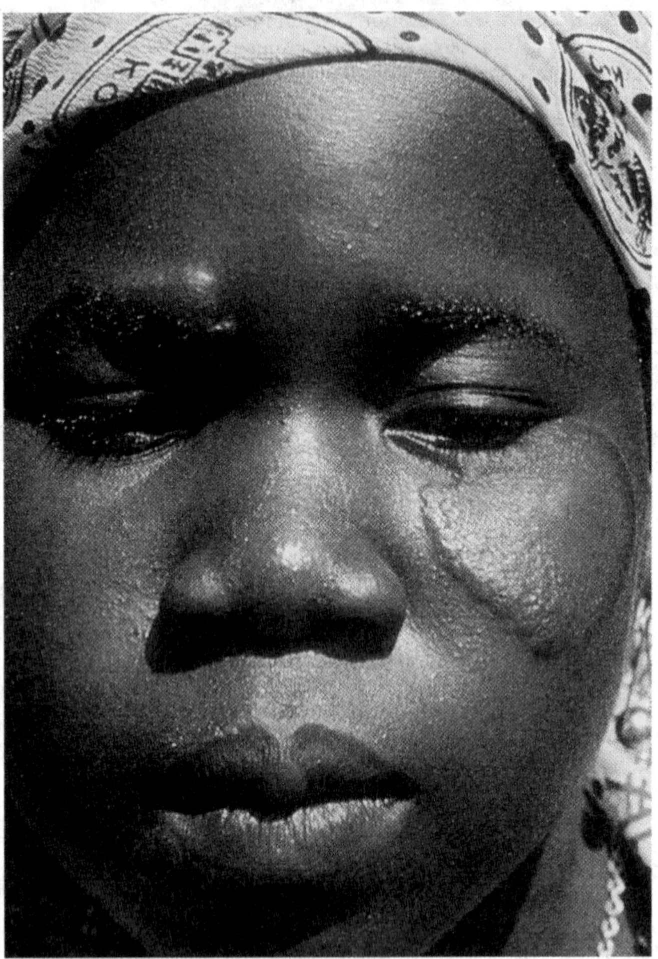

Figure 213-1. A patient with tuberculoid leprosy showing a lesion with a raised border and flattened center.

a single, hypopigmented macule 2–4 cm in diameter with a poorly defined border and without erythema or induration. Anesthesia is minimal or absent, particularly if the lesion is on the face. Tissue samples may show granulomas, but bacilli are rarely demonstrable. The diagnosis is usually made by exclusion of other skin disorders in contacts, especially for children, of leprosy patients. The lesions heal spontaneously in 50–75% of patients with IL, and progress to 1 of the classic forms in the remainder.

Tuberculoid Leprosy. There is usually a single, large (often >10 cm in diameter) lesion with a well-demarcated, elevated erythematous rim (Fig. 213-1). The interior of the lesion is flat, atrophic, hypopigmented, occasionally scaly, and anesthetic. Rarely, there may be as many as 4 lesions. The closest superficial nerve is often impressively thickened. The ulnar, posterior tibial, and great auricular nerves are most commonly affected. Periodic examination of all leprosy patients and their contacts should include palpation of these nerves. Without therapy, the skin lesion tends to enlarge slowly, but documented instances of spontaneous resolution exist. The coloration of the rim slowly fades with therapy and the induration resolves, resulting in a flat lesion with central hypopigmentation and a ring of postinflammatory hyperpigmentation. Loss of hair follicles, sweat glands, cutaneous nerve receptors, and sensation in the central portion of the lesion is irreversible. Marked improvement should be apparent within 1–2 mo after initiating therapy, but complete resolution may take up to 8–12 mo.

There is an entity of **"pure neural" tuberculoid leprosy,** which presents as either pure sensory or combined sensory and motor nerve dysfunction with prominent nerve thickening but no cutaneous lesions. Histopathology is mandatory to establish this diagnosis. Nerve trunk size varies widely, and overdiagnosis of "enlarged" nerves is common among inexperienced histologists. Nodular or fusiform nerve thickening has greater diagnostic value than a palpable nerve that is smooth and symmetric.

Borderline Leprosy. The clinical and histologic criteria for the 3 subdivisions of borderline leprosy are less well defined than are those of the 2 polar categories. In contrast to the tuberculoid and lepromatous patterns, those in the borderline divisions are unstable. Host or bacterial factors can result in immunologic downgrading of the clinical condition toward the lepromatous pattern or upgrading it toward the tuberculoid pattern. Therapy is the most common cause of upgrading reactions; downgrading can be seen in conditions that compromise host immunity (pregnancy). Clinical characteristics of the 3 generally accepted borderline subclasses are as follows.

In the **borderline tuberculoid (BT)** pattern, the lesions are greater in number but smaller in size than in TT. There may be small satellite lesions around older lesions, and the margins of the BT lesions are less distinct. There is usually thickening of 2 or more superficial nerves (Fig. 213-2).

In the **borderline (BB)** pattern, the lesions are more numerous and more heterogeneous in appearance. They may become confluent, and plaques may be present. The borders are poorly defined, and the erythematous rim fades into the surrounding skin (Fig. 213-3). There may be anesthesia, but hypesthesia is more common. Mild to moderate nerve thickening is common, but severe muscle wasting and neuropathy are unusual.

In the **borderline lepromatous (BL)** pattern, a large number of asymmetrically distributed lesions are heterogeneous in appearance. Macules, papules, plaques, and nodules may all coexist. Individual lesions are small unless confluent. Anesthesia is mild and superficial nerve trunks are spared. The initial response to therapy is often dramatic, and nodules and plaques flatten within 2–3 mo. With continued therapy, the lesions become macular and almost invisible.

Lepromatous Leprosy. The lesions are innumerable, often confluent, and symmetric. Initially there may be only vague macules or even uniform, diffuse skin infiltrations without discernible lesions. As the disease progresses, the lesions become increasingly papular and nodular, so that with the diffuse thickening and infiltration of the skin, the characteristic leonine facies accompanied by loss of the eyebrows and distortion of the earlobes becomes apparent. Anesthesia of the lesions is less severe than in TT, but a symmetric peripheral sensory neuropathy usually develops late in the course of the disease. Testicular infiltration leading to azoospermia, infertility, and gynecomastia is common in adults but not in children. Bacilli are demonstrable in most internal organs other than the central nervous system, but tissue damage or interference with function is infrequent. **Glomerulonephritis,** when it occurs, is believed to be secondary to immune complex deposition rather than to infection per se. The initial response to therapy may be encouraging but is often followed by a 2–5 yr period of very slow improvement. In true LL, the specific anergy to the leprosy bacillus persists despite therapy, thus making the patient theoretically susceptible to relapse if even a single viable bacillus remains at the end of therapy.

Reactional States. Acute clinical exacerbations are common in leprosy and are believed to reflect abrupt changes in the host-parasite immunologic balance. Although these reactional states do occur in the absence of therapy, they are especially common during the initial years of treatment. Approximately 30% of patients receiving effective chemotherapy can develop reactions, and, unless adequately treated, they will result in crippling deformities. Two major variants are recognized.

Type 1 (reversal) reactions are observed predominantly in borderline leprosy and result from a sudden increase in effective cell-mediated immunity in response to *M. leprae* antigens in dermis

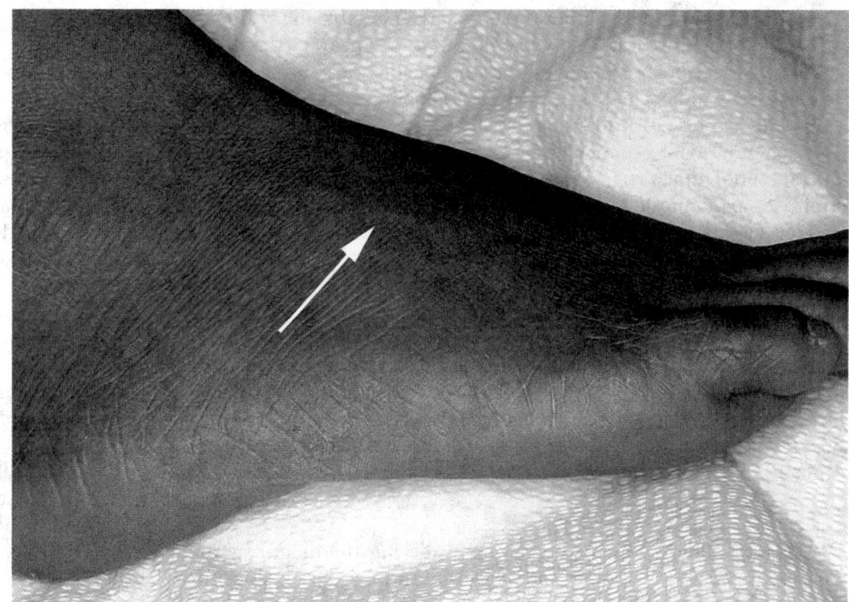

Figure 213-2. Thickened, superficial peroneal nerve of leprosy.

and Schwann cells. Acute tenderness and swelling at the site of existing cutaneous and neural lesions and the development of new lesions are the major manifestations. Existing or new skin lesions often ulcerate to leave hideous scars. The acute neuritis can present either as a severe painful episode or as insidious and painless loss of function that if not treated immediately can lead to irreversible nerve injury with anesthesia, facial paralysis, claw hand, and footdrop. Reversal reactions constitute perhaps the only medical emergency related to leprosy. Patients should be instructed to contact their physicians immediately if signs of a reaction appear.

Type 2 (erythema nodosum leprosum) reactions (ENL) occur in lepromatous and borderline lepromatous cases as a systemic inflammatory response to deposition of extravascular immune complexes of antibody and *M. leprae* antigen. The hallmarks of this syndrome are tender, red dermal papules or nodules that clinically resemble erythema nodosum. These develop in a few hours and last only a few days. High fever, migratory polyarthralgia, painful swelling of lymph nodes or spleen, orchitis, iridocyclitis, and, rarely, nephritis may occur. Leukocytosis and albuminuria may be present. Circulating and tissue-based immune complexes are frequently present and may explain the resemblance to other immune complex disorders, but the underlying mechanism appears to involve the activation of a helper T-cell subset. There is a strong tendency to recurrence, which occurs in 45% of patients, and a risk for amyloidosis and renal failure if treatment is inadequate.

DIAGNOSIS. The critical factor in the diagnosis of leprosy is to consider this in the differential diagnosis of a skin disorder in anyone who has resided in an endemic leprosy region. **Anesthetic skin lesions** with or without **thickened peripheral** nerves are virtually **pathognomonic** of leprosy. A full-thickness skin biopsy from an active lesion (stained with both a standard histologic stain and an acid-fast stain such as Fite-Faraco) is the optimal procedure for confirmation of the diagnosis and accurate disease classification. Acid-fast bacilli are rarely found in patients with indeterminate or tuberculoid disease, but the presence of granulomas and lymphocytic infiltration of nerves in anesthetic skin lesions confirms the diagnosis. For purposes of assigning patients to the appropriate WHO multidrug regimen, slit skin smears are

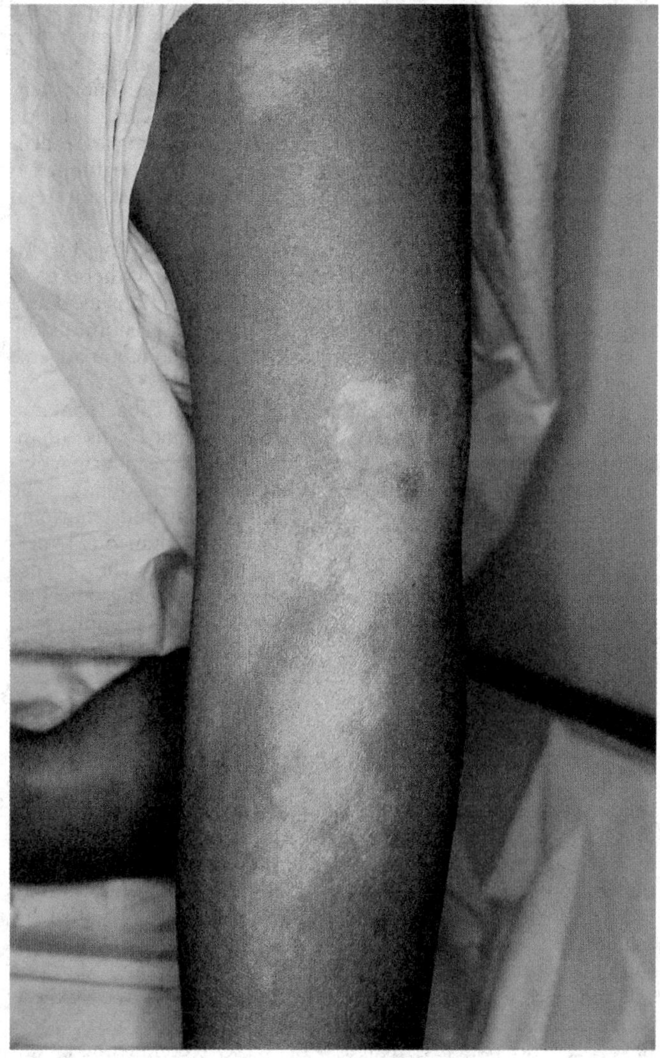

Figure 213-3. Hypopigmented lesions of borderline leprosy.

assessed to determine whether patients have paucibacillary infection (≤5 skin lesions and no bacilli on skin smears) or multibacillary infection (≥6 skin lesions and bacilli on skin smears). The bacterial index can range from 0 (no bacilli in 100 oil-immersion fields) to 6+ (>1,000 bacilli per field). PCR detects *M. leprae* only when biopsy specimens are also positive for acid-fast bacilli.

Differential Diagnosis. Many diseases endemic in developing countries can mimic the appearance of leprosy, including secondary syphilis, cutaneous leishmaniasis, yaws, and cutaneous fungal infections. None of these other disorders involve paresthesia and anesthesia localized to the skin lesions or cause thickening of peripheral nerves. The presence of nerve thickening with skin lesions also differentiates leprosy from primary neurologic disease. IL may present as minimal anesthesia, no nerve thickening, and equivocal histopathology, suggesting a superficial fungal infection, particularly tinea versicolor. The diagnosis of IL should be considered one of exclusion and is rarely established in anyone other than a close contact of a known lepromatous patient.

TREATMENT. Physicians in the USA considering the diagnosis or treatment of leprosy should obtain consultation and assistance in patient management from the National Hansen's Disease Programs (800-642-2477; http://bphc.hrsa.gov/nhdp/default.htm), which maintains an active physician referral list of physicians in all parts of the United States.

Only 3 antimycobacterial agents have proven to be consistently effective in the treatment of leprosy. Dapsone is the cornerstone of therapy because of its low cost, minimal toxicity, and wide availability. Secondary resistance develops when it is used as the sole agent. Dermatitis, hepatitis, and methemoglobinemia are the most common side effects; granulocytopenia is rare but potentially fatal. Dose-related hemolytic anemia, which can be severe, is seen in patients with glucose-6-phosphate dehydrogenase deficiency, methemoglobin reductase deficiency, or hemoglobin M. Pregnancy studies have not shown an increased risk for fetal abnormalities.

Rifampin is the most rapidly mycobactericidal drug for *M. leprae* and achieves excellent levels inside cells, where most leprosy bacilli reside. Resistance develops if rifampin is used as a single agent. The widespread use of rifampin has been limited by cost more than by toxicity. Hepatitis is the most common adverse effect that necessitates discontinuance.

Clofazimine, a phenazine dye with both antimycobacterial and anti-inflammatory activity, has been particularly useful in decreasing the incidence of reactional states. The pharmacokinetics are poorly understood, but the half-life is several days. The drug is avidly taken up by epithelial cells, an attribute that may be important for its activity but also results in cutaneous hyperpigmentation, ichthyosis, xerosis, and enteritis. The intense reddish brown discoloration of the skin is a cosmetic deterrent to use and often results in discontinuation or poor compliance.

Minocycline, some 2nd generation quinolones, and macrolide derivatives such as clarithromycin have shown promise in experimental models but limited human treatment data exist.

Multidrug therapy has been very successful with a high cure rate and a relapse rate of 1%/yr following a full course of therapy. For adults with multibacillary leprosy (all BL and LL patients), therapy is recommended for 12 mo to include rifampin (600 mg once monthly PO, directly observed), dapsone (100 mg once daily PO, self-administered), and clofazimine (300 mg once monthly, directly observed, and 50 mg once daily PO, self-administered). For adults with paucibacillary leprosy (all IL, TT, and most BT patients), therapy is recommended for 6 mo with rifampin (600 mg once monthly PO, directly observed) and dapsone 100 mg once daily PO, self-administered). Patients who experience relapse are retreated with the same regimens. To date there have been no patients treated with WHO-recommended multidrug therapy who have experienced secondary rifampin resistance, which has occurred in persons treated with rifampin monotherapy or multidrug therapy not recommended by WHO.

Patients treated in the United States may be advised to receive regimens that vary from WHO recommendations. Adults with paucibacillary disease receive dapsone (100 mg daily) and rifampin (600 mg daily) for 12 mo; those with multibacillary disease receive dapsone (100 mg daily), rifampin (600 mg daily), and clofazimine (50 mg daily) for 24 mo. Daily pediatric doses are dapsone 1 mg/ kg, rifampin 10 mg/kg, and clofazimine 1 mg/kg, not to exceed the recommended adult doses.

Therapy for reactional states can be complicated and generally requires expert consultation. Management depends on maintenance of antimycobacterial drugs, effective and prolonged anti-inflammatory therapy, and adequate analgesia and physical support during the phase of active neuritis. Mild ENL may respond to nonsteroidal anti-inflammatory agents. **Thalidomide is the drug of choice** for most of the systemic symptoms associated with ENL reactions. Thalidomide accelerates the degradation of messenger RNA encoding TNF-α, resulting in its decreased production by monocytes and macrophages. More severe ENL usually requires corticosteroid therapy (prednisolone 1 mg/kg/day) but often relapses when the drug is discontinued. **Thalidomide is absolutely contraindicated** in women of child-bearing age; otherwise it is much safer than corticosteroids for chronic use. The major adverse effect is fatigue. Pediatric dosages have not been established. Clofazimine 300 mg/day tapering to 100 mg/day or less for 12 mo is also useful in managing chronic ENL. Type 1 reversal reactions are optimally treated with high-dose corticosteroids (prednisolone 40–60 mg/day PO for adults; 1 mg/kg/day PO for children) tapered over several months. Alternate-day regimens may be effective in patients with frequent relapses requiring prolonged treatment.

PROGNOSIS. The prognosis for arresting progression of tissue and nerve damage is good, but recovery of lost sensory and motor function is variable and generally incomplete. Hyperpigmentation, hypopigmentation, and loss of hair follicles or sweat glands persist. Intercurrent reactional states, poor compliance, and emergence of drug resistance can all lead to clinical exacerbations or relapses necessitating close follow-up of patients. Much of the chronic debility results from repeated trauma to anesthetic digits and limbs. Careful counseling of patients and consultation with physical and occupational therapy services are essential for an optimal outcome.

PREVENTION. Two approaches are advocated for interrupting leprosy transmission in endemic areas. The 1st approach is based on the high risk for infection among household and other close contacts of leprosy patients, especially with multibacillary disease. It includes periodic examination of contacts and early treatment at the 1st evidence of leprosy. Contacts 15–19 yr of age or >30 yr of age are at greatest risk for secondary disease. The 2nd approach is the use of bacille Calmette-Guérin (**BCG**) vaccination. One dose of BCG appears to be 50% protective against leprosy; a 2nd dose increases the protective benefit.

The viability of *M. leprae* in skin biopsies decreases sharply within 3 wk of initiating therapy with dapsone and rifampin. This rapid decrease in infectivity combined with the high probability that family members have already had prolonged exposure to the patient before the diagnosis makes physical isolation of leprosy patients unnecessary.

Boggild AK, Keystone JS, Kain KC: Leprosy: A primer for Canadian physicians. *CMAJ* 2004;170:71–78.

Britton WJ, Lockwood DNJ: Leprosy. *Lancet* 2004;363:1209–1219.

Cambau E, Bonnafous P, Perani E, et al: Molecular detection of rifampin and ofloxacin resistance for patients who experience relapse of multibacillary leprosy. *Clin Infect Dis* 2002;34:39–45.

Hartzell JD, Zapor M, Peng S, et al: Leprosy: A case series and review. *South Med J* 2004;97:1252–1256.
Lawn SD, Lockwood DNJ: Leprosy after starting antiretroviral treatment. *BMJ* 2007;334:217–218.
Moet FJ, Pahan D, Schurng RP, et al: Physical distance, genetic relationship, age, and leprosy classification are independent risk factors for leprosy in contacts of patients with leprosy. *J Infect Dis* 2006;193:346–353.
Moschella SL: An update on the diagnosis and treatment of leprosy. *J Am Acad Dermatol* 2004;51:417–426.
Ooi WW, Moschella SL: Update on leprosy in immigrants in the United States: Status in the year 2000. *Clin Infect Dis* 2001;32:930–937.
Ooi WW, Srinivasan J: Leprosy and the peripheral nervous system: Basic and clinical aspects. *Muscle Nerve* 2004;30:393–409.

Chapter 214 ■ Nontuberculous Mycobacteria

Dwight A. Powell

Nontuberculous mycobacteria (NTM), which are also referred to as **atypical mycobacteria, mycobacteria other than tuberculosis (MOTT)**, or potentially pathogenic environmental mycobacteria, are members of the family Mycobacteriaceae. They differ from *Mycobacterium tuberculosis* in their nutritional requirements, ability to produce pigments, enzymatic activity, and susceptibility patterns to antituberculous drugs. NTM are usually acquired from environmental sources rather than by person-to-person spread.

ETIOLOGY. Fourteen strains of NTM are associated with human infections. Phenotypically, they are divided into 4 **Runyon groups** (Table 214-1) based on their colony growth and morphology on solid media. Groups I, II, and III are **slow growing** (>7 days to detect growth). Group IV is **rapid growing** (<7 days to detect growth). **Photochromogens** form pigment after exposure to light, **scotochromogens** form pigment in the dark, and **nonchromogens** fail to produce pigment. Species and serovars of NTM are defined by biochemical reactions, antibody specificity, genetic sequencing using radiolabeled probes and restriction fragment length polymorphisms, or ribosomal-RNA sequencing. Biochemically and immunologically related species that are difficult for clinical laboratories to differentiate are often referred to as "complexes," such as the ***Mycobacterium fortuitum* complex** (*M. fortuitum* and *Mycobacterium chelonae*) and the ***Mycobacterium avium* complex** (*M. avium* and *Mycobacterium intracellulare*).

EPIDEMIOLOGY. NTM are distributed worldwide and are ubiquitous in the environment, existing as saprophytes in soil and water; as pathogens in swine, birds, and cattle; and as part of the normal human pharyngeal flora. Some NTM have well-defined ecologic niches that help explain transmission patterns. The natural reservoir for *Mycobacterium marinum* is fish and other cold-blooded animals, so infections follow injury in an aquatic environment. *M. fortuitum* and *M. chelonae* are ubiquitous in the hospital environment and have caused clusters of nosocomial surgical wound and venous catheter-related infections. *Mycobacterium ulcerans* is recovered only from soils and waters of rain forests and is associated with chronic skin infections in the tropics. *M. avium* complex is found in abundance in the waters, soils, and aerosols of the acid, brown-water swamps of the southeastern United States. In rural counties in this region, asymptomatic infections with *M. avium* complex approach 70% by adulthood.

PATHOGENESIS. The histologic appearances of lesions produced by *M. tuberculosis* and NTM are often indistinguishable. The classic pathologic lesion consists of **caseating granulomas.** Compared with *M. tuberculosis*, NTM infections are more likely to result in granulomas that are **noncaseating,** ill defined (nonpalisading), and irregular or serpiginous. Granulomas may be absent, with only chronic inflammatory changes observed. In patients with **AIDS** and disseminated NTM infection, the inflammatory reaction is usually scant and tissues are filled with large numbers of histiocytes packed with acid-fast bacilli.

TABLE 214-1. Classification of Nontuberculous Mycobacteria Associated with Human Disease

	RUNYON GROUP	MYCOBACTERIA
I.	Photochromogens	
		M. kansasii
		M. marinum
		M. simiae
II.	Scotochromogens	
		M. scrofulaceum
		M. gordonae
		M. szulgai
III.	Nonchromogens	
		M. avium
		M. intracellulare
		M. xenopi
		M. malmoense
		M. terrae
		M. haemophilum
		M. ulcerans
IV.	Rapid growers	
		M. chelonae
		M. fortuitum
		M. abscessus

CLINICAL MANIFESTATIONS. **Lymphadenitis** of the superior anterior cervical or submandibular nodes is the most frequent manifestation of NTM infection in children (Table 214-2). Preauricular, posterior cervical, axillary, and inguinal nodes are involved occasionally. Lymphadenitis is most common in children 1–5 yr of age because of their tendency to put objects contaminated with soil, dust, or standing water into their mouths. Affected children usually lack constitutional symptoms and present with a unilateral subacute and slowly enlarging lymph node or group of closely approximated nodes >1.5 cm that are firm, painless, freely movable, and not erythematous (Fig. 214-1). The involved nodes occasionally resolve without treatment, but most undergo rapid suppuration after several weeks (Fig.

TABLE 214-2. Diseases Caused by Nontuberculous Mycobacterial Species

CLINICAL DISEASE	COMMON SPECIES	LESS COMMON SPECIES IN THE USA
Cutaneous infection	*M. chelonae, M. fortuitum, M. abscessus, M. marinum*	*M. ulcerans**
Lymphadenitis	MAC	*M. kansasii, M. fortuitum, M. malmoense*[†]
Otologic infection	*M. abscessus*	*M. fortuitum*
Pulmonary infection	MAC, *M. kansasii, M. abscessus*	*M. xenopi, M. malmoense,*[†] *M. szulgai, M. fortuitum, M. simiae*
Catheter-associated infection	*M. chelonae, M. fortuitum*	*M. abscessus*
Skeletal infection	MAC, *M. kansasii, M. fortuitum*	*M. chelonae, M. marinum, M. abscessus, M. ulcerans**
Disseminated	MAC	*M. kansasii, M. genavense, M. haemophilum, M. chelonae*

*Not endemic in the USA.
[†]Found primarily in Northern Europe.
MAC, *Mycobacterium avium* complex.
From the American Academy of Pediatrics: *Red Book: 2006 Report of the Committee on Infectious Diseases*, 27th ed. Elk Grove Village, IL, American Academy of Pediatrics, 2006, p 699.

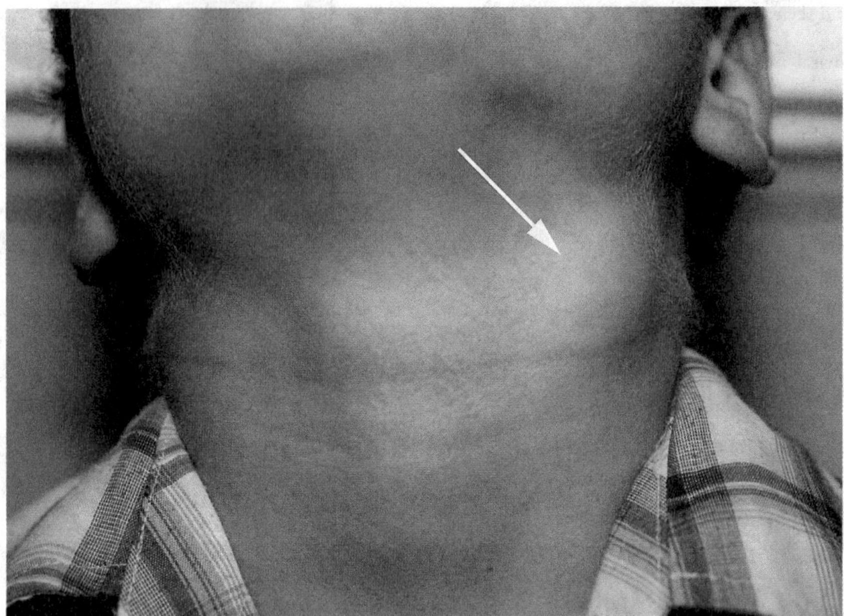

Figure 214-1. An enlarging cervical lymph node infected with *M. avium* complex infection. The node is firm, painless, freely movable, and not erythematous.

214-2). The center of the node becomes fluctuant, and the overlying skin becomes erythematous and thin. Eventually, the nodes rupture and form cutaneous sinus tracts that drain for months or years, resembling the classic scrofula of tuberculosis (Fig. 214-3). In the USA, *M. avium* complex accounts for approximately 80% of NTM lymphadenitis in children. *Mycobacterium scrofulaceum* and *Mycobacterium kansasii* account for most other cases, particularly in the southwestern US. Rarely, *Mycobacterium xenopi, Mycobacterium malmoense, Mycobacterium haemophilum,* and *Mycobacterium szulgai* are described.

Cutaneous disease caused by NTM is rare in children (see Table 214-2). Infection usually follows percutaneous inoculation with fresh or salt water contaminated by *M. marinum*. Within 2–6 wk of exposure, an erythematous papule develops at the site of minor abrasions on the elbows, knees, or feet (**swimming pool granuloma**) and on the hands and fingers of fish fanciers (**fish tank granuloma**). The lesions are usually nontender and enlarge over 3–5 wk to form violaceous plaques. Nodules or pustules may develop and occasionally these may ulcerate, resulting in a serosanguinous discharge. The lesions sometimes resemble sporotrichosis, with satellite lesions near the site of entry extending along the superficial lymphatics. Lymphadenopathy is usually absent. Although most infections remain localized to skin, penetrating *M. marinum* infections may result in tenosynovitis, bursitis, osteomyelitis, or arthritis.

M. ulcerans is the third most common mycobacterial infection in immunocompetent people, after *M. tuberculosis* and *Mycobacterium leprae*. It causes a cutaneous infection most commonly in children living in tropical regions of Africa, Australia, Asia, and South America. In some communities in West Africa up to 16% of people have been affected. Infection follows percutaneous inoculation from minor trauma such as pricks and cuts from

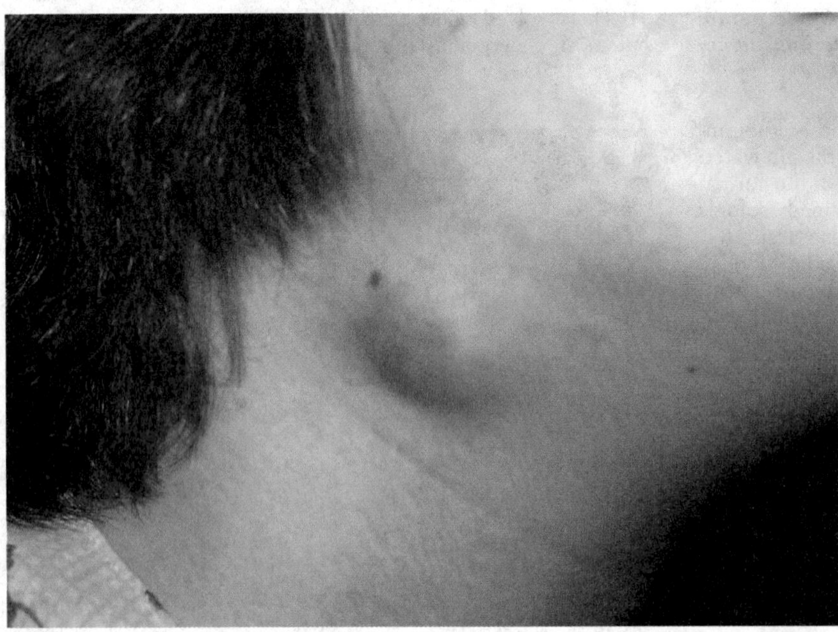

Figure 214-2. A suppurating cervical lymph node infected with *M. avium* complex infection.

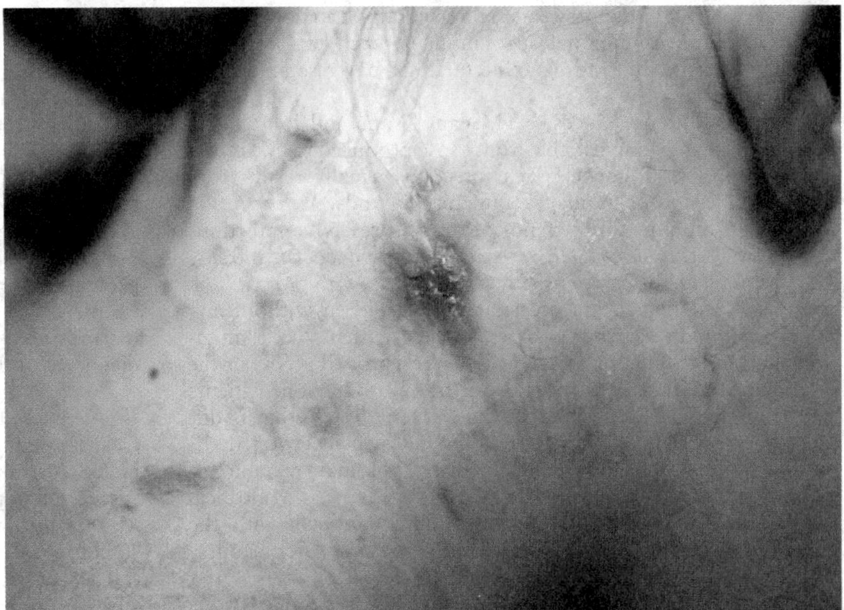

Figure 214-3. A ruptured cervical lymph node infected with *M. avium* complex infection, which resembles the classic scrofula of tuberculosis.

plants and vegetation. After an incubation period of approximately 3 mo, lesions appear as an erythematous nodule, most frequently on legs or arms. The lesion undergoes central necrosis and ulceration. The lesion, often called a **Buruli ulcer** after the region in Uganda where most cases are reported, has a characteristic undermined edge, expands over several weeks, and may result in extensive, deep, soft tissue destruction or bony involvement. Lesions are typically painless, and constitutional symptoms are unusual. Lesions may heal slowly over 6–9 mo or may continue to spread, leading to deformities and contractures.

Skin and soft tissue infections caused by *M. fortuitum, M. chelonae,* or *Mycobacterium abscessus* are rare in children and usually follow percutaneous inoculation from puncture wounds and minor abrasions. Clinical disease usually arises after a 4–6 wk incubation period and presents as localized cellulitis, painful nodules, or a draining abscess. A unique case has been described of mastitis caused by *M. abscessus* following insertion of a nipple ring. *M. haemophilum* can cause painful subcutaneous nodules, which often ulcerate and suppurate in immunocompromised patients, particularly after renal transplantation.

NTM are uncommon sources of **catheter-associated infections,** but are becoming increasingly recognized. These are most commonly caused by *M. fortuitum, M. chelonae,* or *M. abscessus* and may present as bacteremia or localized catheter tunnel infections.

Pulmonary infections, although the most common cause of NTM illness in adults, are uncommon in children. Only 43 cases of pulmonary NTM in immunocompetent children <18 yr of age were reported in the English-language literature between 1930 and 2003. *M. avium* complex, the most frequently identified organism, is a cause of acute pneumonitis, chronic cough, or wheezing associated with paratracheal or peribronchial lymphadenitis and airway compression in normal children. Associated constitutional symptoms such as fever, anorexia, and weight loss occur in 60% of these children. Chest radiographic findings are very similar to those for primary tuberculosis, with unilateral infiltrates and hilar lymphadenopathy (Fig. 214-4). Pleural effusion is uncommon. Rare cases of progression to endobronchial granulation tissue have been reported.

Chronic infections in older patients with cystic fibrosis have been caused by *M. avium* complex, *M. fortuitum, Mycobacterium chelonia, M. kansasii,* and *M. abscessus.* Ten percent of patients with cystic fibrosis have at least 1 sputum culture positive for NTM. *M. abscessus* is a common isolate. NTM infections in patients with cystic fibrosis may be chronic with no resulting change in lung function. One study demonstrated weight gain and improved lung function with antimycobacterial drugs.

M. kansasii, M. xenopi, and *M. szulgai* infections are uncommon in children and usually occur in adults with underlying chronic lung disease. The onset is insidious and consists of low-

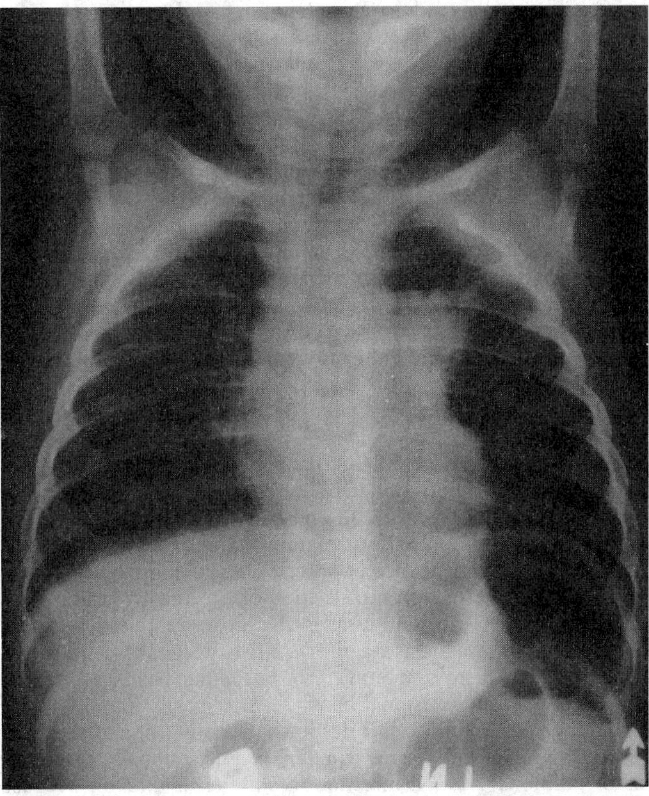

Figure 214-4. Chest radiograph of a 2 yr old child infected with *M. avium* complex demonstrating a left upper lobe infiltrate and left hilar lymphadenopathy.

grade fever, cough, night sweats, and generalized malaise. Thin-walled cavities with minimal surrounding parenchymal infiltrates are characteristic, but radiographic findings may resemble those of tuberculosis.

In unusual circumstances, NTM cause **bone** and **joint infections** that are indistinguishable from those produced by *M. tuberculosis* or bacterial agents. Such infections usually result from operative incision or accidental puncture wounds. *M. fortuitum* infections from puncture wounds of the foot resemble infections caused by *Pseudomonas aeruginosa* and *Staphylococcus aureus.*

Disseminated disease, usually associated with *M. avium* complex infection, occurs occasionally in children without any apparent immunodeficiency. Most of these patients have mutations in genes coding for the interferon-γ receptor (IFNGR) or the interleukin 12 (IL-12) receptor, or for IL-12 production. Patients with complete IFNGR deficiency have severe disease that is difficult to treat. Those with partial IFNGR deficiency or IL-12 pathway mutations have milder disease that may respond to interferon-γ and antimycobacterial therapy. **Multifocal osteomyelitis** is particularly prevalent in individuals with the IFNGR1 818del4 mutation. Recurrence, even years after a course of treatment, has been well documented.

Disseminated disease caused by *M. avium* complex infections is among the most common opportunistic infections in patients with **AIDS,** usually late in the illness when CD4 cell counts are <100 cells/mm^3. Colonization of the respiratory or gastrointestinal tract probably precedes disseminated *M. avium* complex infections, but screening studies of respiratory secretions or stool samples are not useful to predict dissemination. Continuous high-grade bacteremia is usual, and multiple organs are infected, including most commonly lymph nodes, liver, spleen, bone marrow, and gastrointestinal tract. Thyroid, pancreas, adrenal gland, kidney, muscle, and brain may be involved. The most common signs and symptoms of disseminated *M. avium* complex infections in AIDS patients are fever, night sweats, chills, anorexia, marked weight loss, wasting, weakness, generalized lymphadenopathy, and hepatosplenomegaly. Jaundice, elevated alkaline phosphatase level, anemia, and neutropenia may occur. Imaging studies usually demonstrate massive lymphadenopathy of hilar, mediastinal, mesenteric, or retroperitoneal nodes. In children with AIDS, the mean survival period following isolation of *M. avium* complex from a body source is 5–9 mo.

DIAGNOSIS. The differential diagnosis of NTM lymphadenitis includes acute bacterial lymphadenitis, tuberculosis, cat scratch disease (*Bartonella henselae*), mononucleosis, toxoplasmosis, brucellosis, tularemia, and malignancies, especially lymphomas. An intermediate-strength tuberculin skin test (5 tuberculin units) is usually weakly positive with 5–15 mm induration. The Centers for Disease Control and Prevention once produced skin tests representing the different Runyon groups of NTM; these antigens are no longer available. Differentiation between NTM and *M. tuberculosis* may be difficult, but children with NTM lymphadenitis usually have a Mantoux tuberculin skin test reaction of <15 mm induration, unilateral anterior cervical node involvement, a normal chest x-ray, and no history of exposure to adult tuberculosis. Children with tuberculous lymphadenitis may have unilateral or bilateral posterior cervical node involvement, a Mantoux tuberculin skin test reaction of ≥15 mm induration, an abnormal chest x-ray, and history of exposure to adult tuberculosis. Definitive diagnosis requires excision of the involved nodes for culture and histology. Some recommend fine needle aspiration for culture before excisional biopsy.

Diagnosis of cutaneous infections depends on isolating the responsible microorganisms from an excised lesion. The diagnosis of pulmonary NTM infection in children is difficult because many species of NTM, including *M. avium* complex, can be isolated from oral and gastric secretions of healthy children. Definitive diagnosis requires invasive procedures such as bronchoscopy and pulmonary or endobronchial biopsy. Mycolic acids and other lipids in the cell wall of mycobacteria give them their hallmark trait of acid-fastness with the Ziehl-Neelsen or Kinyoun stains. They may also be identified with the fluorochrome stain auramine-rhodamine. The sensitivity of these stains for detecting NTM in tissue samples is less than with *M. tuberculosis.*

Blood cultures are 90–95% sensitive in AIDS patients with disseminated infection. *M. avium* complex may be detected within 7 days of inoculation in nearly all patients with the BACTEC radiometric blood culture system. Commercially available DNA probes differentiate NTM from *M. tuberculosis.* Identification of histiocytes containing numerous acid-fast bacilli from bone marrow and other biopsy tissues provides a rapid presumptive diagnosis of disseminated mycobacterial infection.

TREATMENT. Therapy for NTM infections involves medical, surgical, or combined treatment (Table 214-3). Isolation of the infecting strain followed by susceptibility testing is ideal because susceptibility patterns vary. *M. kansasii, M. marinum, M. xenopi, M. ulcerans,* and *M. malmoense* are usually susceptible to some standard antituberculous drugs. *M. fortuitum, M. chelonae, M. scrofulaceum,* and *M. avium* complex are often resistant to standard antituberculous drugs but have variable susceptibility to other antibiotics such as quinolones and macrolides. Multiple-drug therapy is essential to avoid development of resistance.

The preferred treatment of NTM lymphadenitis is complete surgical excision (see Table 214-3). Nodes should be removed while still firm and encapsulated. Excision is more difficult if extensive caseation with extension to surrounding tissue has occurred, and complications of facial nerve damage or recurrent infection are more likely. Incomplete surgical excision is not advised because chronic drainage may develop. Standard antituberculous medications have little effect on NTM lymphadenitis and are not necessary with complete excision. If there is concern for *M. tuberculosis* infection, therapy with isoniazid, rifampin, and pyrazinamide should be administered until cultures confirm the cause (see Chapter 212). If for some reason surgery of NTM lymphadenitis cannot be performed, removal of infected tissue is incomplete, or recurrence or chronic drainage develops, a 4–6 mo trial of chemotherapy is warranted. Although there are no published controlled trials, several case reports and small series have reported successful treatment with chemotherapy alone or combined with surgical excision. Clarithromycin or azithromycin combined with rifabutin or ethambutol are the most commonly reported therapy regimens (see Table 214-3).

Cutaneous NTM lesions usually heal spontaneously after incision and drainage without other therapy (see Table 214-3). *M. marinum* is susceptible to rifampin, amikacin, ethambutol, sulfonamides, trimethoprim-sulfamethoxazole, and tetracycline. Therapy with a combination of these drugs, particularly rifampin and ethambutol, may be given for 3–4 mo. Corticosteroid injections should not be used. Superficial infections with *M. fortuitum* or *M. chelonae* usually resolve after surgical incision and open drainage, but deep-seated or catheter-related infections require removal of infected central lines and therapy with parenteral amikacin plus cefoxitin or clarithromycin. Pulmonary infections should be treated initially with isoniazid, rifampin, and pyrazinamide pending culture identification and susceptibility testing.

Patients with disseminated *M. avium* complex and IL-12 pathway defects or deficiency of IFNGR should be treated for at least 12 mo with clarithromycin or azithromycin combined with 1 or more 2nd line drugs (rifabutin, clofazimine, ethambutol, or a quinolone). In vitro susceptibility testing is important to guide therapy. Once the clinical illness has resolved, lifelong daily prophylaxis with azithromycin or clarithromycin is advisable to prevent recurrent disease. The use of interferon adjunctive therapy is determined by the specific genetic defect.

In adults with AIDS, daily prophylaxis with azithromycin with or without rifabutin reduces infection with *M. avium* complex by

TABLE 214-3. Treatment of Nontuberculous Mycobacteria Infections in Children

ORGANISM	DISEASE	TREATMENT
SLOWLY GROWING SPECIES		
Mycobacterium avium complex (MAC)	Lymphadenitis	Excision of major nodes; if excision incomplete or disease recurs, clarithromycin or azithromycin plus ethambutol with rifampin or rifabutin.
	Pulmonary infection	Clarithromycin or azithromycin plus ethambutol with rifampin or rifabutin (pulmonary resection in some patients who fail drug therapy). For severe disease, an initial course of amikacin or streptomycin often is included. Clinical data in adults support that 3 times weekly therapy is as effective as daily therapy, with less toxicity.
	Disseminated	See text.
Mycobacterium kansasii	Pulmonary infections	Rifampin plus ethambutol with isoniazid.
	Osteomyelitis	Surgical debridement and prolonged antimicrobial therapy using rifampin plus ethambutol with isoniazid.
Mycobacterium marinum	Cutaneous infection	None, if minor; rifampin, trimethoprim-sulfamethoxazole, clarithromycin, or doxycycline* for moderate disease; extensive lesions may require surgical debridement. Susceptibility testing not required.
Mycobacterium ulcerans	Cutaneous and bone infections	Excision of tissue; rifampicin plus streptomycin under investigation.
RAPIDLY GROWING SPECIES		
Mycobacterium fortuitum group	Cutaneous infection	Excision of tissue; initial therapy for serious disease is amikacin plus meropenem IV, followed by clarithromycin, doxycycline,* or trimethoprim-sulfamethoxazole or ciprofloxacin orally based on in vitro susceptibility testing.
	Catheter infection	Catheter removal and amikacin plus meropenem IV; clarithromycin, trimethoprim-sulfamethoxazole, or ciprofloxacin orally based on in vitro susceptibility testing.
Mycobacterium abscessus	Otitis media	Clarithromycin plus initial course of amikacin plus cefoxitin; may require surgical debridement based on in vitro susceptibility testing (50% are amikacin resistant).
	Pulmonary infection (in cystic fibrosis)	Serious disease, clarithromycin, amikacin, and cefoxitin based on susceptibility testing; may require surgical resection; seek expert advice.
Mycobacterium chelonae	Catheter infection	Catheter removal and tobramycin (initially) plus clarithromycin.
	Disseminated cutaneous infection	Tobramycin and meropenem or linezolid (initially) plus clarithromycin.

*Doxycycline should not be given to children younger than 8 yr unless the benefits of therapy are greater than the risks of dental staining. Only 50% of isolates of *M. marinum* are susceptible to doxycycline.
From the American Academy of Pediatrics: *Red Book: 2006 Report of the Committee on Infectious Diseases*, 27th ed. Elk Grove Village, IL, American Academy of Pediatrics, 2006, pp 702–703.

>50%. Although pediatric studies are lacking, the U.S. Public Health Service recommends either azithromycin (20 mg/kg once weekly PO, maximum 1,200 mg/dose) or clarithromycin (7.5 mg/kg/dose bid PO, maximum 500 mg/dose) for HIV-infected children with significant immune deficiency as defined by the CD4 count (children ≥6 yr, CD4 count <50/µL; 2–6 yr, CD4 count <75/µL; 1–2 yr, CD4 count <500/µL; <1 yr, CD4 count <750 µL).

Albright JT, Pransky SM: Nontuberculous mycobacterial infections of the head and neck. *Pediatr Clin North Am* 2003;50:503–514.

Aubry A, Chosidow O, Caumes E, et al: Sixty-three cases of *Mycobacterium marinum* infection: Clinical features, treatment, and antibiotic susceptibility of causative isolates. *Arch Intern Med* 2002;162:1746–1752.

Centers for Disease Control and Prevention: 2002 USPHSHS/IDSA guidelines for the prevention of opportunistic infections in persons infected with human immunodeficiency virus. *MMWR* 2002;51(RR-8):1–60.

Dorman SE, Picard C, Lammas D, et al: Clinical features of dominant and recessive interferon γ receptor 1 deficiencies. *Lancet* 2004;364:2113–2121.

Forslow U, Geborek A, Hjelte, et al: Early chemotherapy for non-tuberculous mycobacterial infections in patients with cystic fibrosis. *Acta Paediatr* 2003;92:910–915.

Jogi R, Trying SK: Therapy of nontuberculous mycobacterial infections. *Dermatol Ther* 2004;17:491–498.

Lindeboom JA, Prins JM, Bruijnesteijn van Coppenraet LE, et al: Cervicofacial lymphadenitis in children caused by *Mycobacterium haemophilum*. *J Infect Dis* 2005;41:1569–1575.

Nolt D, Michaels MG, Wald ER: Intrathoracic disease from nontuberculous mycobacteria in children: Two cases and a review of the literature. *Pediatrics* 2003;112:e434–e439.

Pszolla N, Sarkar MR, Strecker W, et al: Buruli ulcer: A systemic disease. *Clin Infect Dis* 2003;37:e78–e82.

Sermet-Gaudelus I, LeBourgeois M, Pierre-Audigier C, et al: *Mycobacterium abscessus* and children with cystic fibrosis. *Emerg Infect Dis* 2003;9:1587–1591.

Starke JR: Management of nontuberculous mycobacterial cervical adenitis. *Pediatr Infect Dis J* 2000;199:674–675.

Section 8 — Spirochetal Infections

Chapter 215 ■ Syphilis *(Treponema pallidum)*

Parvin Azimi

ETIOLOGY. Syphilis is a systemic infection caused by *Treponema pallidum*, a long, slender, tightly coiled, motile spirochete with finely tapered ends belonging to the family Spirochaetaceae. The pathogenic members of this genus include *T. pallidum* (venereal syphilis), *Treponema pertenue* (yaws), *Treponema pallidum* subspecies *endemicum* (endemic syphilis), and *Treponema carateum* (pinta). Because these microorganisms stain poorly, detection in clinical specimens requires dark-field microscopy or direct immunofluorescent staining techniques. *T. pallidum* cannot be cultured in vitro and is propagated by intratesticular inoculation in rabbits.

EPIDEMIOLOGY. Two forms of syphilis occur in children. **Acquired syphilis** is transmitted almost exclusively by sexual contact. Less frequent modes of transmission include transfusion of contaminated blood or direct contact with infected tissues. After an epidemic resurgence of primary and secondary syphilis in the 1980s in the United States that peaked in 1989, the annual rate declined 90% by 2000. The total number of cases of primary and secondary syphilis increased each year during 2001–2003. This increase occurred only among men, particularly among men who have sex with men, with an actual decrease among women. Rates in the Southern United States and among non-Hispanic blacks remain disproportionately high (14.1 vs 3.1/100,000) and are increasing in males.

Congenital syphilis results from transplacental transmission of spirochetes. Women with primary and secondary syphilis and spirochetemia are more likely to transmit infection to the fetus than are women with latent infection. Transmission can occur at any stage of pregnancy. The incidence of congenital infection in the offspring of untreated infected women remains highest during the 1st 4 yr after acquisition of primary infection, secondary, and early latent disease. The risk factors most commonly associated with congenital syphilis are lack of prenatal care and cocaine drug abuse, which is associated with prostitution, unprotected sexual contact, and trading of sex for drugs, in addition to inadequate prenatal care and poor treatment of syphilis during pregnancy (Fig. 215-1).

CLINICAL MANIFESTATIONS. **Primary syphilis** is characterized by syphilitic chancre and regional lymphadenitis. A **painless papule** appears at the site of inoculation 2–6 wk after inoculation with *T. pallidum*. The papule soon develops into a clean, painless ulcer with raised borders called a **chancre.** The chancre, usually on the genitals, contains viable *T. pallidum* and is highly contagious. Extragenital chancres can be seen also, depending on the site of primary inoculation. Adjacent lymph nodes are generally enlarged. The chancre heals spontaneously within 4–6 wk, leaving a thin scar.

Untreated patients develop manifestations of **secondary syphilis** 2–10 wk after the chancre heals. Manifestations of secondary syphilis are related to spirochetemia and include a non-

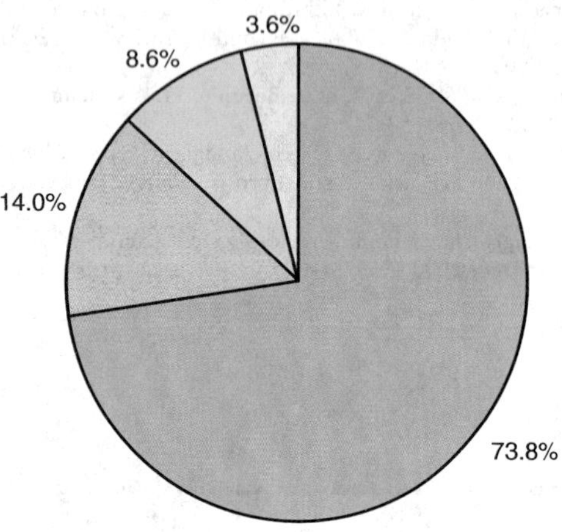

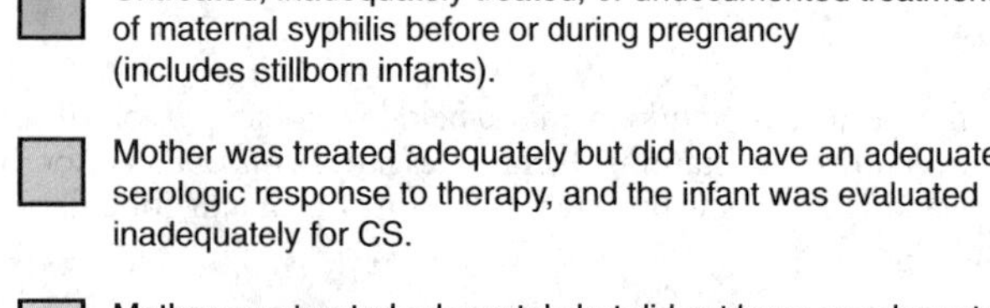

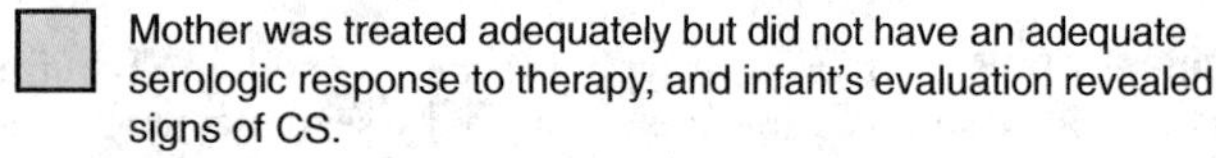

Figure 215-1. Diagnoses of congenital syphilis (CS)—United States, 2002. (From the Centers for Disease Control and Prevention: Primary and secondary syphilis—United States, 2002. *MMWR* 2003;52:1117–1120.)

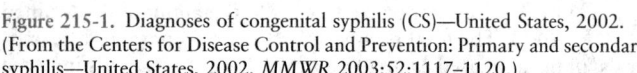

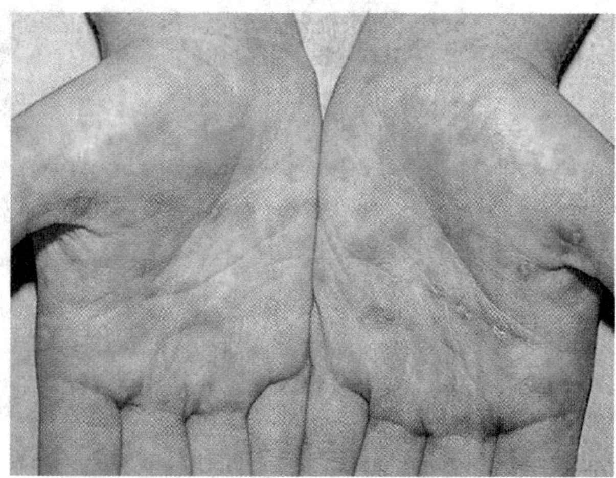

Figure 215-2. Secondary syphilis. Ham-colored palmar acules on an adolescent with secondary syphilis. (From Weston WL, Lane AT, Morelli JG: *Color Textbook of Pediatric Dermatology,* 3rd ed. St. Louis, Mosby, 2002.)

pruritic maculopapular rash, which can cover the entire body, and notably involving the palms and soles (Fig. 215-2). Pustular lesions may also develop. **Condylomata lata,** which are gray-white to erythematous wartlike plaques, can occur in moist areas around the anus and vagina, and white plaques called **mucous patches** may be found in mucous membranes. A **flulike illness** with low-grade fever, headache, malaise, anorexia, weight loss, sore throat, myalgias, arthralgias, and generalized lymphadenopathy is often present. Renal, hepatic, and ophthalmologic manifestations may be present, as may be meningitis, which occurs in 30% of patients with secondary syphilis, manifested by cerebrospinal fluid (CSF) pleocytosis and elevated protein level, although the patient may not show neurologic symptoms. Secondary infection becomes **latent** within 1–2 mo after the onset of the rash. Relapses with secondary manifestations can occur during the 1st year of latency, a period referred to as the **early latent period.** No relapses occur after the 1st year. What follows is **late syphilis,** which may be either asymptomatic (**late latent**) or symptomatic (**tertiary**). At this stage, patients may begin showing the manifestations of tertiary disease, which include neurologic, cardiovascular, and gummatous lesions. The lesions are granulomas of the skin and musculoskeletal system resulting from the host's delayed hypersensitivity reaction.

Congenital Infection. Untreated syphilis during pregnancy has a transmission rate approaching 100%. Fetal or perinatal death occurs in 40% of affected infants. Among survivors, manifestations have traditionally been divided into early and late stages. The **early signs** appear during the 1st 2 yr of life, and **late signs** appear gradually during the 1st 2 decades. Early manifestations result from transplacental spirochetemia and are analogous to the secondary stage of acquired syphilis. Approximately 66% of infected infants are asymptomatic at the time of birth and are identified only by routine prenatal screening; if they are untreated, symptoms develop within weeks or months.

The early manifestations of congenital infection are varied and involve multiple organ systems (Table 215-1). Hepatosplenomegaly, jaundice, and elevated liver enzymes are common. Histologically, liver involvement includes bile stasis, fibrosis, and extramedullary hematopoiesis. Lymphadenopathy tends to be diffuse and to resolve spontaneously, although shotty nodes may persist. Coombs negative hemolytic anemia is characteristic. Thrombocytopenia is often associated with platelet trapping in an enlarged spleen. Characteristic osteochondritis and periostitis (Fig. 215-3) and mucocutaneous rash (Fig. 215-4), pre-

TABLE 215-1. Clues That Suggest a Diagnosis of Congenital Syphilis*

EPIDEMIOLOGIC BACKGROUND	CLINICAL FINDINGS
Untreated early syphilis in the mother	Osteochondritis, periostitis
Untreated latent syphilis in the mother	Snuffles, hemorrhagic rhinitis
An untreated mother who has contact with a known syphilitic during pregnancy	Condylomata lata
Mother treated for syphilis during pregnancy with a drug other than penicillin	Bullous lesions, palmar/plantar rash
Mother treated for syphilis during pregnancy without follow-up to delivery	Mucous patches
	Hepatomegaly, splenomegaly
	Jaundice
	Nonimmune hydrops fetalis
	Generalized lymphadenopathy
	Central nervous system signs; elevated cell count or protein in cerebrospinal fluid
	Hemolytic anemia, diffuse intravascular coagulation, thrombocytopenia
	Pneumonitis
	Nephrotic syndrome
	Placental villitis or vasculitis (unexplained enlarged placenta)
	Intrauterine growth restriction

*Arranged in decreasing order of confidence of diagnosis.
From Remington JS, Klein JO, Wilson CB, Baker CJ (editors): *Infectious Diseases of the Fetus and Newborn Infant*, 6th ed. Philadelphia, Elsevier/Saunders, 2006, p 556.

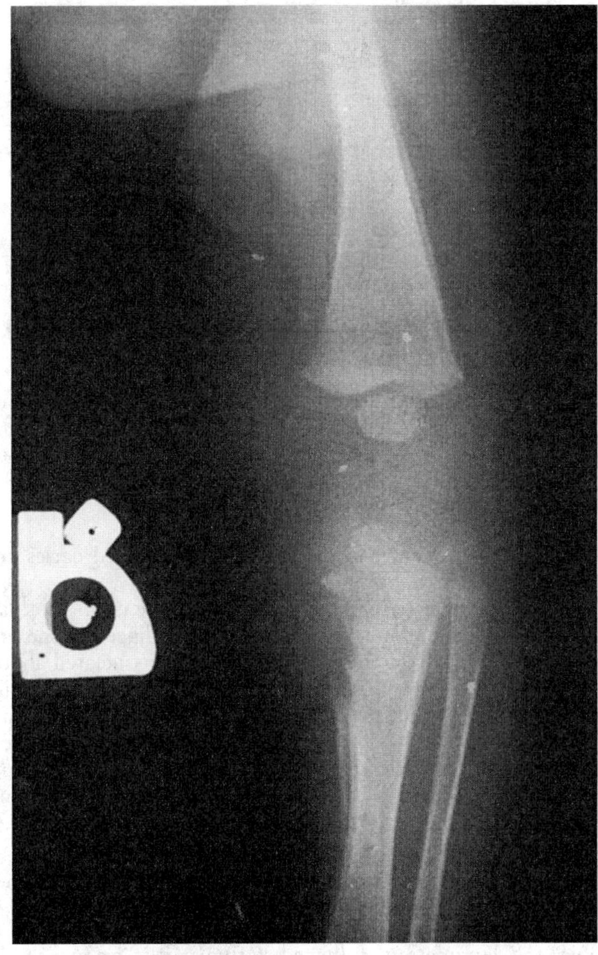

Figure 215-3. Osteochondritis and periostitis in a newborn with congenital syphilis.

senting with erythematous maculopapular or bullous lesions, followed by desquamation involving hands and feet, are common. Mucous patches, rhinitis (**snuffles**), and condylomatous lesions (Fig. 215-5) are highly characteristic features of mucous membrane involvement in congenital syphilis. Bone involvement occurs frequently. Roentgenographic abnormalities include multiple sites of osteochondritis at the wrists, elbows, ankles, and knees, and periostitis of the long bones and rarely the skull. The osteochondritis is painful and often results in irritability and refusal to move the involved extremity (**pseudoparalysis of Parrot**). Central nervous system (CNS) abnormalities, failure to thrive, chorioretinitis, nephritis, and nephrotic syndrome may also be seen. Clinical manifestations of renal involvement include hypertension, hematuria, proteinuria, hypoproteinemia, hypercholesterolemia, and hypocomplementemia. They appear to be related to glomerular deposition of circulating immune complexes. Less common clinical manifestations of early congenital syphilis include gastroenteritis, peritonitis, pancreatitis, pneumonia, eye involvement (glaucoma and chorioretinitis), nonimmune hydrops, and testicular masses.

The late manifestations result primarily from chronic inflammation of bone, teeth, and the CNS. Skeletal changes due to persistent or recurrent periostitis and associated thickening of bone include frontal bossing, a bony prominence of the forehead (**olympian brow**), unilateral or bilateral thickening of the sternoclavicular third of the clavicle (**clavicular or Higouménaki sign**), an anterior bowing of the midportion of the tibia (**saber shins**), and convexity along the medial border of the scapula (**scaphoid scapula**). Dental abnormalities are common and include **Hutchinson teeth** (Fig. 215-6), which are the peg or barrel-shaped upper central incisors that erupt during the 6th yr of life; abnormal enamel, which results in a notch along the biting surface; and **mulberry molars,** the abnormal 1st lower (6 yr) molars characterized by a small biting surface and an excessive number of

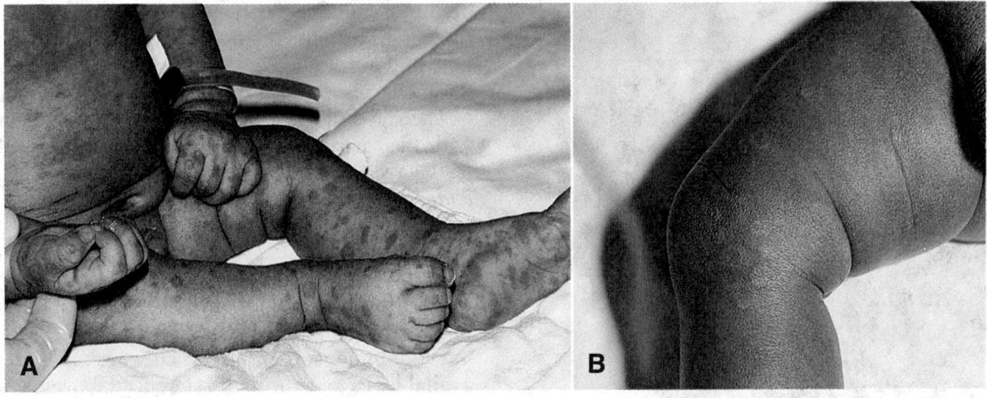

Figure 215-4. Papulosquamous plaques in 2 infants with syphilis. (From Eichenfeld LF, Frieden IJ, Esterly NB [editors]: *Textbook of Neonatal Dermatology.* Philadelphia, WB Saunders, 2001, p 196.)

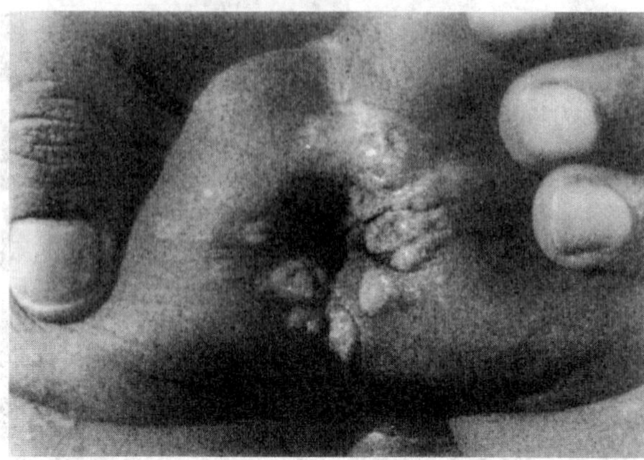

Figure 215-5. Perianal condylomata lata.
(From Karthikeyan K, Thappa DM: Early congenital syphilis in the new millennium. *Pediatr Dermatol* 2002;19:275–276.)

cusps. Defects in enamel formation lead to repeated caries and eventual tooth destruction.

A **saddle nose** (Fig. 215-7), a depression of the nasal root, is a result of syphilitic rhinitis that destroys the adjacent bone and cartilage. A perforated nasal septum may be an associated abnormality. **Rhagades** are linear scars that extend in a spokelike pattern from previous mucocutaneous fissures of the mouth, anus, and genitalia. **Juvenile paresis,** an uncommon latent meningovascular infection, typically presents during adolescence with behavioral changes, focal seizures, or loss of intellectual function. **Juvenile tabes** with spinal cord involvement and cardiovascular involvement with aortitis are extremely rare.

Other late manifestations of congenital syphilis may represent a hypersensitivity phenomenon. These include unilateral or bilateral interstitial keratitis with symptoms such as intense photophobia and lacrimation, followed within weeks or months by corneal opacification and complete blindness. Less common ocular manifestations include choroiditis, retinitis, vascular occlusion, and optic atrophy. Eighth nerve deafness may be unilateral or bilateral, appears at any age, presents initially as vertigo and high-tone hearing loss, and progresses to permanent deafness. The **Clutton joint** represents a unilateral or bilateral synovitis involving the lower extremities (usually the knee), which presents as painless joint swelling with sterile synovial fluid; spontaneous remission usually occurs after a period of several weeks. Soft tissue gummas (identical to those of acquired disease) and paroxysmal cold hemoglobinuria are rare hypersensitivity phenomena.

DIAGNOSIS. Diagnosis of primary syphilis is confirmed when *T. pallidum* is demonstrated by dark-field microscopy or direct fluorescent antibody–*T. pallidum* testing on specimens from skin

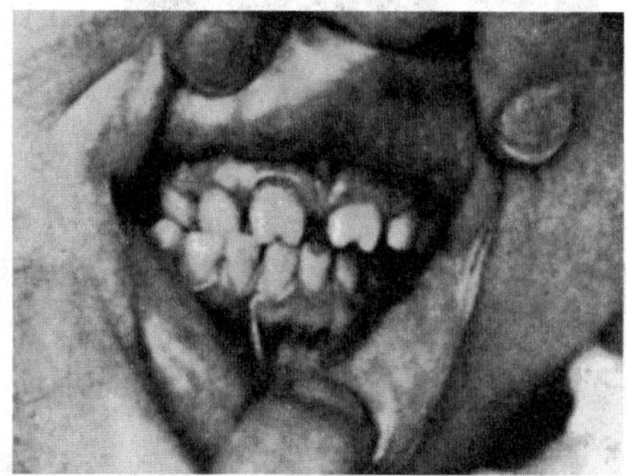

Figure 215-6. Hutchinson teeth as a late manifestation of congenital syphilis.

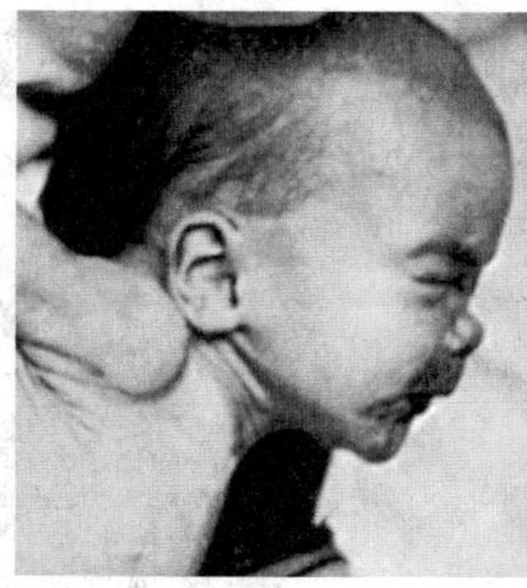

Figure 215-7. Saddle nose in a newborn with congenital syphilis.

lesions, placenta, or umbilicus. Nucleic acid–based amplification assays such as polymerase chain reaction (PCR), are not commercially available. Serologic tests for syphilis remain the principal means for diagnosis.

Nontreponemal tests, which are the **Venereal Disease Research Laboratory (VDRL)** and **rapid plasma reagin (RPR)** tests, detect antibodies against phospholipid antigens on the surface of treponeme that cross react with mammalian cardiolipin antigens. These tests are highly sensitive in early infection. The quantitative results of these nontreponemal tests tend to correlate with disease activity and therefore are helpful in screening. Titers increase with active disease, including treatment failure or reinfection, and decline with adequate treatment (Fig. 215-8). The nontreponemal tests usually become nonreactive within 1 yr of adequate therapy for primary syphilis and within 2 yr of adequate treatment for secondary disease. With congenital infection, these tests become nonreactive within a few months after adequate treatment. Certain conditions such as autoimmune diseases may give false-positive VDRL results in the serum (but not in the CSF), although false-positive results are now much less common because of the use of purified cardiolipin-lecithin-cholesterol antigen. Pregnancy itself does not give a false-positive VDRL result, and therefore all positive maternal serologic tests for syphilis, regardless of the titer, necessitate thorough investigation. Excessively high VDRL titers may give a false-negative reading unless diluted (prozone effect).

Treponemal tests, which measure antibody specific for *T. pallidum,* include the *T. pallidum* hemagglutination assay (TPHA), the fluorescent treponemal antibody absorption (FTA-ABS) test, and the *T. pallidum* particle agglutination (TPPA) test. Treponemal tests are used for confirmatory testing of positive results of the nontreponemal antibody tests. Treponemal antibody titers become positive soon after initial infection and usually remain positive for life, even with adequate therapy (see Fig. 215-8). These antibody titers do not correlate with disease activity and are not quantified. They are useful for diagnosis of a 1st episode of syphilis and for distinguishing false-positive results of nontreponemal antibody tests but are of limited usefulness in the evaluation of response to therapy and possible reinfections.

There is limited cross reactivity of treponemal antibody tests with the causative organisms of Lyme disease (*Borrelia burgdorferi*), yaws (*T. pertenue*), endemic syphilis (*T. pallidum* subspecies *endemicum*), and pinta (*T. carateum*). Only venereal syphilis (*T. pallidum*) and Lyme disease are found in the United States. The nontreponemal tests (VDRL, RPR) are uniformly nonreactive in Lyme disease.

Tests for immunoglobulin M (IgM) antibodies have been developed, including FTA-ABS 19S-IgM, an IgM capture enzyme-linked immunosorbent assay. However, these tests are not widely available, except through reference laboratories.

The interpretation of nontreponemal and treponemal serologic tests in the newborn may be confounded by maternal IgG anti-

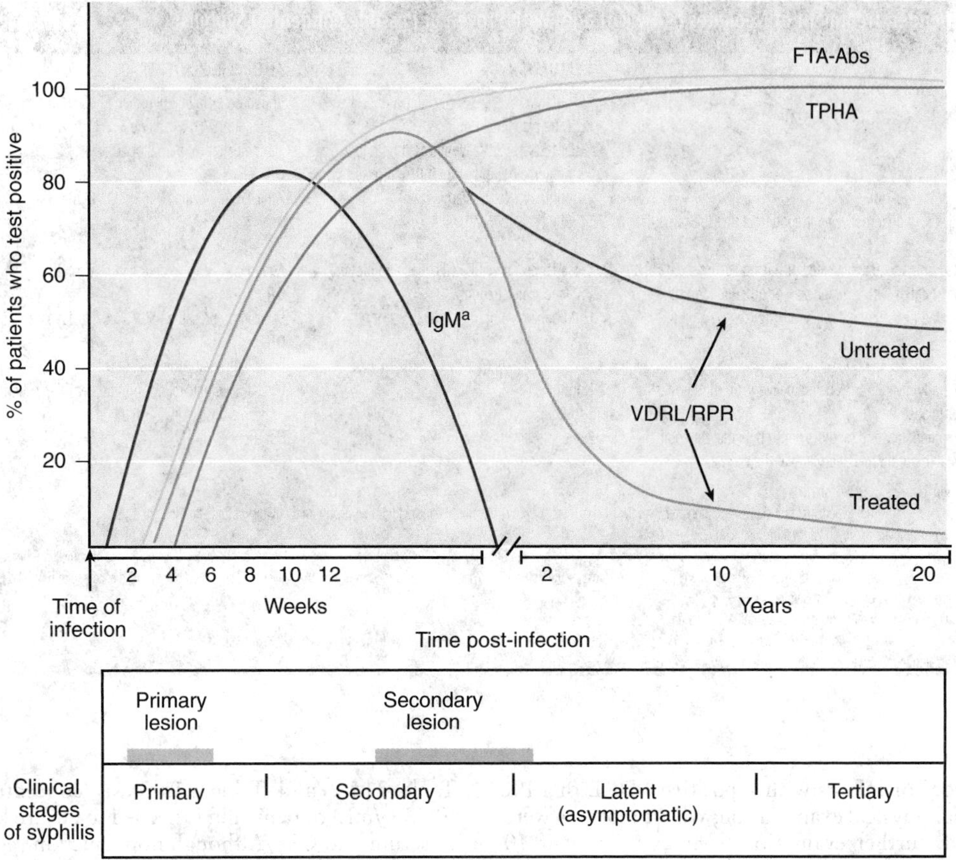

Figure 215-8. Common patterns of serologic reactivity in syphilis patients. FTA-Abs, fluorescent treponemal antibody absorption (test); RPR, rapid plasma reagin (test); TPHA, *Treponema pallidum* hemagglutination assay; VDRL, Venereal Disease Research Laboratory (test).
(From Peeling RW, Ye H: Diagnostic tools for preventing and managing maternal and congenital syphilis: An overview. *Bull WHO* 2004;82:439–446.)

bodies that are transferred to the fetus. Passively acquired antibody is suggested by neonatal titer at least 4-fold (i.e., a 2-tube dilution) less than the maternal titer. This can be verified by gradual decline in antibody in the infant, usually becoming undetectable by 3–6 mo of age.

The diagnosis of neurosyphilis is established by demonstrating pleocytosis and increased protein in the CSF, and a positive CSF VDRL test along with neurologic symptoms. The CSF VDRL test is very specific but relatively insensitive (22–69%) for neurosyphilis.

Dark-field microscopy of scrapings from primary lesions or congenital or secondary lesions can reveal *T. pallidum,* often before serology becomes positive, but this technique is usually not available in clinical practice. Similarly, rabbit infectivity testing, used for measuring the sensitivity of investigational tests such as PCR and Western immunoblotting, is not widely available. Placental examination by gross and microscopic techniques can be useful in the diagnosis of congenital syphilis. The disproportionately large placentas are characterized histologically by focal proliferative villitis, endovascular and perivascular arteritis, and focal or diffuse immaturity of placental villi.

Congenital Syphilis. Symptomatic infants should be thoroughly evaluated (see Table 215-1) and treated. Asymptomatic infants considered at risk for congenital syphilis because the maternal nontreponemal and treponemal serology is positive should be evaluated if (1) maternal treatment was inadequate, unknown, or undocumented; (2) maternal treatment was ≤30 days before delivery; (3) the mother was treated with erythromycin or another nonpenicillin regimen; or (4) the maternal nontreponemal titers did not decrease sufficiently to demonstrate a cure (4-fold or greater). If the maternal treatment was adequate and ≥1 mo before delivery, the infant's positive nontreponemal test result represents passively acquired antibody and the infant does not need treatment at delivery, but follow-up serology should be obtained. If the maternal evaluation is incomplete, these infants are assumed infected and treated (Table 215-2).

The diagnosis of neurosyphilis in the newborn with syphilitic infection is difficult owing to the poor sensitivity of the CSF VDRL test in this age group and the lack of CSF abnormalities. A positive CSF VDRL test result in a newborn warrants treatment for neurosyphilis, even though it might reflect passive transfer of antibodies from serum to CSF. More importantly, it is now accepted that all infants with a presumptive diagnosis of congenital syphilis should be treated with regimens effective for neurosyphilis because this cannot be reliably excluded.

For infants with proven or highly probable disease or abnormal physical findings, complete evaluation including serologic tests (RPR or VDRL), complete blood count with differential and platelet count, long bone radiographs, ophthalmology examination, auditory brainstem response, and other tests as indicated

TABLE 215-2. Recommended Treatment of Neonates (≤4 wk of age) With Proven or Possible Congenital Syphilis

CLINICAL STATUS	EVALUATION	ANTIMICROBIAL THERAPY*
Proven or highly probable disease†	CSF analysis for VDRL, cell count, and protein CBC and platelet count Other tests as clinically indicated (e.g., long bone radiography, liver function tests, ophthalmologic examination)	Aqueous crystalline penicillin G, 100,000–150,000 U/kg/day, administered as 50,000 U/kg/dose IV every 12 hr during the 1st 7 days of life and every 8 hr thereafter for a total of 10 days **OR** Penicillin G procaine,‡ 50,000 U/kg/day IM in a single dose for 10 days
Normal physical examination and serum quantitative nontreponemal titer the same or <4-fold the maternal titer:		
(a) (i) Mother was not treated or inadequately treated or has no documented treatment; (ii) mother was treated with erythromycin or other nonpenicillin regimen; (iii) mother received treatment ≤4 wk before delivery	CSF analysis for VDRL, cell count, and protein CBC and platelet count Long bone radiography	Aqueous crystalline penicillin G IV for 10 days‡ **OR** Penicillin G procaine,‡ 50,000 U/kg/day IM in a single dose for 10 days§ **OR** Penicillin G benzathine, 50,000 U/kg IM in a single dose§
(b) (i) Adequate maternal therapy given >4 wk before delivery; (ii) mother has no evidence of reinfection or relapse	None	Clinical, serologic follow-up, and penicillin G benzathine, 50,000 U/kg IM in a single dose‖
(c) Adequate therapy before pregnancy and mother's nontreponemal serologic titer remained low and stable during pregnancy and at delivery	None	None¶

*If >1 day of therapy is missed, the entire course should be restarted.
†Abnormal physical examination, serum quantitative nontreponemal titer that is 4-fold greater than the mother's titer, or positive result of dark-field or fluorescent antibody test of body fluid(s).
‡Penicillin G benzathine and penicillin G procaine are approved for IM administration *only*.
§A complete evaluation (CSF analysis, bone radiography, CBC) is not necessary if 10 days of parenteral therapy is administered but may be useful to support a diagnosis of congenital syphilis. If a single dose of penicillin G benzathine is used, then the infant must be evaluated fully, the full evaluation must be normal, and follow-up must be certain. If any part of the infant's evaluation is abnormal or not performed or if the CSF analysis is uninterpretable, the 10 day course of penicillin is required.
‖Some experts would not treat the infant but would provide close serologic follow-up.
¶Some experts would treat with penicillin G benzathine, 50,000 U/kg, as a single IM injection if follow-up is uncertain.
From the American Academy of Pediatrics: *Red Book: 2006 Report of the Committee on Infectious Diseases,* 27th ed. Elk Grove Village, IL, American Academy of Pediatrics, 2006, p 638.
CBC, complete blood cell; CSF, cerebrospinal fluid; VDRL, Venereal Disease Research Laboratory (test).

should be performed. For infants with a positive VDRL or RPR test result and normal physical examination, whose mothers were inadequately treated, further evaluation is not necessary if 10 days of parenteral therapy is administered.

TREATMENT. *T. pallidum* is extremely sensitive to penicillin, and there is no evidence of emerging penicillin resistance. Penicillin remains the drug of choice for treatment of syphilis (see Table 215-2 and Table 215-3). A concentration 0.018 µg/mL (0.03 U/mL) of penicillin is needed to ensure killing of spirochetes in serum and CSF. Although nonpenicillin regimens are available to the penicillin-allergic patient, desensitization followed by standard penicillin therapy is the most reliable strategy. An acute systemic febrile reaction, the Jarisch-Herxheimer reaction, with exacerbation of lesions, occurs in 15–20% of all patients with acquired or congenital syphilis who are treated with peni-

TABLE 215-3. Recommended Treatment for Syphilis in People >4 Weeks of Age

	CHILDREN	ADULTS
Congenital syphilis	Aqueous crystalline penicillin G, 200,000–300,000 U/kg/day IV administered as 50,000 U/kg every 4–6 hr for 10 days*	
Primary, secondary, and early latent syphilis†	Penicillin G benzathine,‡ 50,000 U/kg IM up to the adult dose of 2.4 million U in a single dose	Penicillin G benzathine, 2.4 million U IM in a single dose **OR** *If allergic to penicillin and not pregnant,* Doxycycline, 100 mg orally twice a day for 14 days **OR** Tetracycline, 500 mg orally 4 times/day for 14 days
Late latent syphilis§ or latent syphilis of unknown duration	Penicillin G benzathine, 50,000 U/kg IM up to the adult dose of 2.4 million U, administered as 3 single doses at 1 wk intervals (total 150,000 U/kg, up to the adult dose of 7.2 million U)	Penicillin G benzathine, 7.2 million U total, administered as 3 doses of 2.4 million U IM each at 1 wk intervals **OR** *If allergic to penicillin and not pregnant,* Doxycycline, 100 mg orally twice a day for 4 wk **OR** Tetracycline, 500 mg orally 4 times/day for 4 wk
Tertiary	—	Penicillin G benzathine, 7.2 million U total, administered as 3 doses of 2.4 million U IM at 1 wk intervals *If allergic to penicillin and not pregnant, same as for late latent syphilis*
Neurosyphilis‖	Aqueous crystalline penicillin G, 200,000 to 300,000 U/kg/day, given every 4–6 hr for 10–14 days in doses not to exceed the adult dose	Aqueous crystalline penicillin G, 18–24 million U/day, administered as 3–4 million U IV every 4 hr for 10–14 days¶ **OR** Penicillin G procaine,† 2.4 million U IM once daily **PLUS** probenecid, 500 mg orally 4 times/day, both for 10–14 days¶

*If the patient has no clinical manifestations of disease, the CSF examination is normal, and the CSF VCRL result is negative, some experts would treat with up to 3 weekly doses of penicillin G benzathine, 50,000 U/kg IM. Some experts also suggest giving these patients a single dose of penicillin G benzathine, 50,000 U/kg IM after the 10 day course of IV aqueous penicillin.
†Early latent syphilis is defined as being acquired within the preceding year.
‡Penicillin G benzathine and penicillin G procaine are approved for IM administration *only*.
§Late latent syphilis is defined as syphilis beyond 1 year's duration.
‖Patients who are allergic to penicillin should be desensitized.
¶Some experts administer penicillin G benzathine, 2.4 million U IM once per week for up to 3 wk after completion of these neurosyphilis treatment regimens.
From the American Academy of Pediatrics: *Red Book: 2006 Report of the Committee on Infectious Diseases,* 27th ed. Elk Grove Village, IL, American Academy of Pediatrics, 2006, p 640.
CSF, cerebrospinal fluid; VDRL, Venereal Disease Research Laboratory (test).

cillin. It is not an indication for discontinuation of penicillin therapy.

Acquired Syphilis. Primary, secondary, and early latent disease is treated with a single dose of benzathine penicillin G (50,000 units/kg IM, maximum 2.4 million units). Nonpregnant penicillin-allergic patients without neurosyphilis may be treated with either doxycycline (100 mg PO bid for 2 wk) or tetracycline (500 mg PO qid for 2 wk).

Patients who are also infected with HIV are at increased risk for neurologic complications and have higher rates of treatment failures. The Centers for Disease Control and Prevention guidelines recommend the same treatment of primary and secondary syphilis as for non-HIV-infected persons, but some experts recommend 3 weekly doses of benzathine penicillin G. HIV-infected patients with late latent syphilis or latent syphilis of unknown duration should have a CSF evaluation for neurosyphilis before treatment.

Sex partners of infected persons of any stage should be evaluated and treated. Persons exposed ≤90 days preceding the diagnosis in a sex partner should be treated presumptively even if seronegative. Persons exposed >90 days before the diagnosis in a sex partner should be treated if seropositive or if serologic tests are not available. Additionally, follow-up serology should be performed on treated individuals to establish adequacy of therapy, and testing for other sexually transmitted diseases, including HIV, should be performed on all patients.

Syphilis in Pregnancy. When clinical or serologic findings suggest active infection or when the diagnosis of active syphilis cannot be excluded with certainty, treatment is indicated. Patients should be treated with the penicillin regimen appropriate for the woman's stage of syphilis. Women who have been adequately treated in the past do not require additional therapy unless quantitative serology suggests evidence of reinfection (4-fold elevation in titer). Doxycycline and tetracycline should not be administered during pregnancy, and erythromycin does not effectively treat fetal infection. Pregnant patients who are allergic to penicillin should be desensitized and treated with penicillin.

Congenital Syphilis. Adequate maternal therapy should eliminate the risk for congenital syphilis. All infants born to mothers with syphilis should be followed up until nontreponemal serology is negative. The infant should be treated if there is any uncertainty about the adequacy of the mother's treatment.

Congenital syphilis is treated with aqueous penicillin G (100,000–150,000 U/kg/24 hr divided every 12 hr IV for the 1st wk of life, and every 8 hr thereafter) or procaine penicillin G (50,000 U/kg IM once daily) given for 10 days. Higher concentrations of penicillin are achieved in the CSF of infants treated with intravenous aqueous penicillin G than in those treated with intramuscular procaine penicillin. Both penicillin regimens are still recognized as adequate therapy for congenital syphilis. Treated infants should be followed up serologically to confirm decreasing nontreponemal antibody titers. In a very low risk neonate who is asymptomatic and whose mother was treated appropriately, without evidence of relapse or reinfection, but with a low and stable VDRL titer, no evaluation is necessary. Some specialists would treat such an infant with a single dose of benzathine penicillin G 50,000 units/kg IM.

PREVENTION. Testing is indicated at any time for persons with suspicious lesions, a history of recent sexual exposure to a person with syphilis, or diagnosis of another sexually transmitted infection, including HIV infection.

Congenital Syphilis. Routine prenatal screening for syphilis remains the most important factor in the identification of infants at risk for development of congenital syphilis and is legally required at the beginning of prenatal care in all states. In pregnant women without optimal prenatal care, serologic screening for syphilis should be performed at the time pregnancy is diagnosed. Any woman who is delivered of a stillborn infant ≥20 wk of gestation should be tested for syphilis. In communities and populations with a high prevalence of syphilis, or for patients at high risk, testing should be performed at least 2 additional times: at the beginning of the 3rd trimester (28 wk) and at delivery. Some states mandate repeat testing at delivery for all women. Women at high risk for syphilis should possibly be screened more frequently, either monthly or pragmatically because of inconsistent prenatal care, at every medical encounter because they may have repeat infections during pregnancy or reinfection late in pregnancy.

No newborn should leave the hospital without the maternal serologic status having been determined at least once during pregnancy. In states conducting newborn screening for syphilis, both the mother's and infant's serologic results should be known before discharge. Testing of the mother's serum is preferred to testing cord blood or the infant's serum because the titers are frequently lower in the infant and may be nonreactive if the mother was infected late in pregnancy.

Azimi PH, Janner D, Berne P, et al: Concentrations of procaine and aqueous penicillin in the cerebrospinal fluid of infants treated for congenital syphilis. *J Pediatr* 1994;124:649–653.

Beck-Sague C, Alexander ER: Failure of benzathine penicillin G treatment in early congenital syphilis. *Pediatr Infect Dis J* 1987;6:1061–1064.

Centers for Disease Control and Prevention: Sexually transmitted diseases treatment guidelines 2002. *MMWR* 2002;51(RR-6):1–80.

Centers for Disease Control and Prevention: Primary and secondary syphilis—United States, 2002. *MMWR* 2003;51:1117–1120.

Centers for Disease Control and Prevention: Congenital syphilis—United States, 2002. *MMWR* 2004;53:716–719.

Centers for Disease Control and Prevention: *Sexually transmitted disease surveillance, 2003.* Atlanta, GA, U.S. Department of Health and Human Services, CDC, 2004.

Centers for Disease Control and Prevention: Primary and secondary syphilis—United States, 2003–2004. *MMWR* 2006;55:269–272.

French P: Syphilis. *BMJ* 2007;334:143–147.

Hall CS, Klausner JD, Bolan GA: Managing syphilis in the HIV-infected patient. *Curr Infect Dis Rep* 2004;6:72–81.

Hook II EW, Peeling RW: Syphilis control—a continuing challenge. *N Engl J Med* 2004;351:122–124.

Karthikeyan K, Thappa DM: Early congenital syphilis in the new millennium. *Pediatr Dermatol* 2002;19:275–277.

Moyer VA, Schneider V, Yetman R, et al: Contribution of long-bone radiographs to the management of congenital syphilis in the newborn infant. *Arch Pediatr Adolesc Med* 1998;152:353–357.

Peeling RW, Ye H: Diagnostic tools for preventing and managing maternal and congenital syphilis: An overview. *Bull WHO* 2004;82:439–446.

Riedner G, Rusizoka M, Todd J, et al: Single-dose azithromycin versus penicillin G benzathine for the treatment of early syphilis. *N Engl J Med* 2005;353:1236–1244.

Sison CG, Ostrea Jr EM, Reyes MP, et al: The resurgence of congenital syphilis. A cocaine-related problem. *J Pediatr* 1997;130:289–292.

Wicher K, Horowitz HW, Wicher V: Laboratory methods of diagnosis of syphilis for the beginning of the third millennium. *Microbes Infect* 1999;1:1035–1049.

Zenker PN, Berman SM: Congenital syphilis. Trends and recommendations for evaluation and management. *Pediatr Infect Dis J* 1991;10:516–522.

Chapter 216 ■ Nonvenereal Treponemal Infections Parvin Azimi

Nonvenereal treponemal infections—yaws, bejel (endemic syphilis), and pinta—are caused by different subspecies of *Treponema pallidum* and occur in tropical and subtropical areas. The causative agents of nonvenereal treponematoses—*Treponema pertenue, Treponema pallidum* subspecies *endemicum,* and *Treponema carateum*—cannot be distinguished from *T. pallidum* by morphologic or serologic tests. These diseases are characterized by a relapsing clinical course and prominent skin involvement. Penicillin remains the treatment of choice for syphilis and nonvenereal treponemal infections.

216.1 • Yaws (*Treponema pertenue*)

Yaws is a contagious, chronic, relapsing infection involving the skin and bony structures caused by the spirochete *T. pertenue,* which is identical to *T. pallidum* microscopically and serologically. Almost all cases occur in children in tropical and subtropical countries. It is also referred to as "framboesia," "pian," "parangi," and "bouba." A high percentage of the population is infected in endemic areas.

T. pertenue is transmitted by direct contact from an infected lesion through a skin abrasion or laceration. Transmission is facilitated by overcrowding and poor personal hygiene in the rain forest areas of the world. The initial papular lesion, the "**mother yaw,**" occurs 2–8 wk after inoculation. The papule develops into a raised, raspberry-like papilloma and is often accompanied by regional lymphadenopathy. Healing of the mother yaw leaves a hypopigmented scar. The **secondary lesions** may erupt anywhere on the body before or after the healing of the mother yaw, and may be accompanied by lymphadenopathy, anorexia, and malaise. Ulcerated lesions are covered by exudates containing treponemes. Secondary lesions heal without scarring. Recurrent lesions are common within 5 yr after the primary lesion.

The lesions are often associated with bone pain resulting from underlying periostitis or osteomyelitis, especially of the fingers, nose, and tibia. The initial period of clinical activity is followed by a 5–10 yr period of latency. This is followed by the appearance of **tertiary lesions** at puberty, which are often solitary and destructive. These present as painful papillomas on the hands and feet, gummatous skin ulcerations, or osteitis. Bony destruction and deformity are common, as are juxta-articular nodules, depigmentation, and painful hyperkeratosis ("**dry crab yaws**") of the palms and soles.

The diagnosis is based on the characteristic clinical manifestations of the disease in an endemic area. Dark-field examination of cutaneous lesions for treponemes and both treponemal and nontreponemal serologic tests for syphilis, which are positive because of cross reactivity, are used to confirm the diagnosis.

Treatment of yaws consists of a single dose of benzathine penicillin G (1.2 million U IM) for index patients and all contacts. Patients allergic to penicillin may be treated with erythromycin, doxycycline, or tetracycline at appropriate doses for venereal syphilis (see Chapter 215). Treatment cures the lesions of active yaws, renders them noninfectious, and prevents relapse. Eradication of yaws from endemic areas may be accomplished by treating the entire population with penicillin.

216.2 • Bejel (Endemic Syphilis; *Treponema pallidum* Subspecies *Endemicum*)

Bejel, or endemic syphilis, affects children in remote rural communities living in poor hygienic conditions. Bejel, unlike yaws, can occur in temperate as well as dry, hot climates. Infection with *T. pallidum* subspecies *endemicum* follows penetration of the spirochete through traumatized skin or mucous membranes. In experimental infections, a primary papule forms at the inoculation site after an incubation period of 3 wk. A primary lesion is almost never visualized in human infections.

The clinical manifestations of the secondary stage are confined to the skin and mucous membranes and consist of highly infectious mucous patches on the oral mucosa and condyloma-like lesions on the moist areas of the body, especially the axilla and anus. These mucocutaneous lesions resolve spontaneously over a period of several months, but recurrences are common. The secondary stage is followed by a variable latency period before the onset of late or tertiary bejel. The late complications are identical to those of yaws and include gumma formation in skin, subcutaneous tissue, and bone, resulting in painful destructive ulcerations, swelling, and deformity.

The diagnosis is based on the characteristic clinical manifestations of the disease in an endemic area. Dark-field examination of cutaneous lesions for treponemes and both treponemal and nontreponemal serologic tests for syphilis, which are positive because of cross reactivity, are used to confirm the diagnosis.

Differentiation from venereal syphilis is extremely difficult in an endemic area. Bejel is distinguished by the absence of a primary chancre and lack of involvement of the central nervous system and cardiovascular system during the late stage.

Treatment of early infection consists of a single dose of benzathine penicillin G (1.2 million U IM). Late infection is treated with 3 injections of the same dose at intervals of 7 days. Patients allergic to penicillin may be treated with erythromycin or tetracycline.

201.3 • Pinta (*Treponema carateum*)

Pinta is a chronic, nonvenereally transmitted infection caused by *Treponema carateum,* a spirochete morphologically and serologically indistinguishable from other human treponemes. The disease is endemic in Mexico, Central America, South America, and parts of the West Indies. Infection follows direct inoculation of the treponeme through abraded skin. After a variable incubation period of days, the primary lesion appears at the inoculation site as a small asymptomatic erythematous papule resembling localized psoriasis or eczema. The regional lymph nodes are often enlarged. Spirochetes can be visualized on dark-field examination of skin scrapings or from biopsy of the involved lymph nodes. After a period of enlargement, the primary lesion disappears. Secondary lesions follow within 6–8 mo and consist of small macules and papules on the face, scalp, and other sun-exposed portions of the body. These pigmented lesions are scaly and nonpruritic, and may coalesce to form large plaquelike elevations resembling psoriasis. In the late stage, atrophic and depigmented lesions develop on the hands, wrists, ankles, feet, face, and scalp. Hyperkeratosis of palms and soles is uncommon.

The diagnosis is based on the characteristic clinical manifestations of the disease in an endemic area. Dark-field examination of cutaneous lesions for treponemes and both treponemal and nontreponemal serologic tests for syphilis, which are positive because of cross reactivity, are used to confirm the diagnosis.

Treatment consists of a single dose of benzathine penicillin G (1.2 million U IM). Tetracycline and erythromycin are alternatives for patients allergic to penicillin. Treatment campaigns and improvement of standards of living are necessary for reduction and elimination of disease.

Antal GM, Lukehart SA, Meheus AZ: The endemic treponematoses. *Microbes Infect* 2002;4:83–94.

Koff AB, Rosen T: Nonvenereal treponematoses: Yaws, endemic syphilis, and pinta. *J Am Acad Dermatol* 1993;29:519–535.

Scolnik D, Aronson L, Lovinsky R, et al: Efficacy of a targeted, oral-penicillin-based yaws control program among children living in rural South America. *Clin Infect Dis* 2003;36:1232–1238.

Chapter 217 ■ *Leptospira* Parvin Azimi

ETIOLOGY. Leptospirosis is caused by spirochetes of the genus *Leptospira* and is the most widespread zoonosis in the world. The organisms are aerobic bacteria, 6–20 µm long and 0.1 µm wide with a terminal hook at 1 or both ends. They can be visualized by dark-field examination and by silver staining. Leptospires are cultured in liquid media; growth is slow on primary isolation and may require up to 13 wk. Pathogenic leptospires have historically been classified as a single species, *Leptospira interrogans,* which includes >200 distinct serovars that have been useful for characterizing the epidemiology. Nonpathogenic leptospires were classified as *Leptospira biflexa,* which has >60 serovars. Over 200 pathogenic serovars are recognized, making up 23 serogroups. A single serovar may produce a variety of distinct syndromes, and a single clinical manifestation may be caused by multiple serotypes.

EPIDEMIOLOGY. Leptospirosis is a zoonosis of worldwide distribution, with most human cases in tropical and subtropical developing countries. Leptospires infect many species of domestic and feral animals, including pets, livestock, birds, fish, and reptiles. The rat is the principal source of human infection. Other important animal reservoirs include dogs, cats, livestock, and wild animals. Animal infection varies from inapparent to fatal. Once infected, animals excrete spirochetes in urine for an extended period of time. Leptospire survival outside the animal host is dependent on the moisture content, temperature, and pH of the soil or water into which they are shed. The majority of human cases worldwide result from occupational exposure to water or soil contaminated with rat urine. Occupational groups with a high incidence of leptospirosis include those who work or are exposed to flood waters, agricultural workers, veterinarians, abattoir workers, meat inspectors, rodent control workers, laboratory workers, and workers in other occupations that require contact with animals. In the USA, the major animal reservoir is the dog, and contact with spirochetes is often associated with recreational activities that result in contact with contaminated soil or water during the summer months. Transmission via contaminated water, animal bites, and directly from person to person, which is rare, has been reported.

PATHOLOGY AND PATHOGENESIS. Leptospires enter humans through abrasions and cuts in the skin or through mucous membranes. After penetration, leptospires circulate in the bloodstream and spread to all organs of the body. The primary lesion caused by leptospires is damage to the endothelial lining of small blood vessels with resultant ischemic damage to the liver, kidneys, meninges, and muscles.

CLINICAL MANIFESTATIONS. The spectrum of human leptospirosis ranges from asymptomatic infection to a severe syndrome of multiorgan dysfunction with high mortality. The clinical presentation is biphasic. After an incubation period of 7–12 days, the initial or **septicemic phase** begins in which leptospires can be isolated from the blood, cerebrospinal fluid (CSF), and other tissues. Initial symptoms last 2–7 days and may be followed by a brief period of well-being before the onset of the symptomatic immune phase. The **immune or leptospiruric phase** is associated with the appearance of circulating antibody, disappearance of organisms from the blood and CSF, and appearance of additional signs and symptoms associated with localization of leptospires in the tissues. Despite the presence of circulating antibody, leptospires may persist in the kidney, urine, and aqueous humor. The immune phase may last for several weeks.

Most cases of human leptospirosis are subclinical or very mild, with inapparent infection particularly common in high-risk occupational groups such as farmers and their families. Symptomatic infection may present as an acute febrile illness with nonspecific signs and symptoms (70%), as aseptic meningitis (20%), or as hepatorenal dysfunction (10%). The onset is typically sudden, and the illness tends to follow a biphasic course (Fig. 217-1).

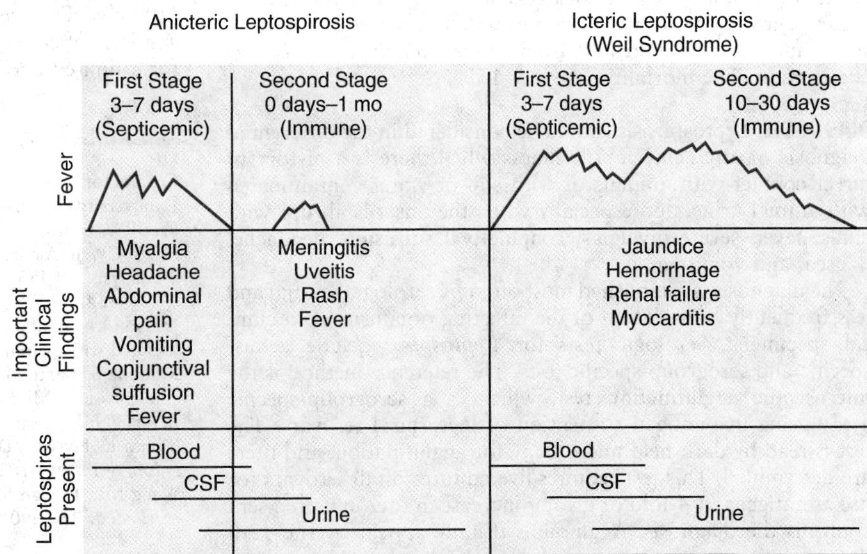

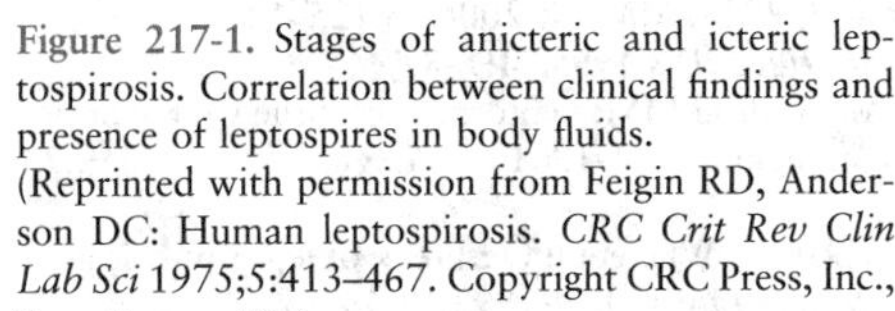

Figure 217-1. Stages of anicteric and icteric leptospirosis. Correlation between clinical findings and presence of leptospires in body fluids.
(Reprinted with permission from Feigin RD, Anderson DC: Human leptospirosis. *CRC Crit Rev Clin Lab Sci* 1975;5:413–467. Copyright CRC Press, Inc., Boca Raton, FL.)

Anicteric Leptospirosis. The onset of the **septicemic phase** is abrupt, with fever, shaking chills, lethargy, severe headache, malaise, nausea, vomiting, and severe, often debilitating myalgia. Some patients have bradycardia and hypotension, but circulatory collapse is uncommon. Additional physical findings include extreme muscle tenderness, which is most prominent in the lower extremities, lumbosacral spine, and abdomen. Conjunctival suffusion with photophobia and orbital pain (in the absence of chemosis and purulent exudate), generalized lymphadenopathy, and hepatosplenomegaly may also be present. A transient rash, lasting <24 hr, may occur in 10% of cases, and usually consists of a truncal erythematous maculopapular rash but may be urticarial, petechial, purpuric, or desquamating. Less common manifestations include pharyngitis, pneumonitis, arthritis, carditis, cholecystitis, and orchitis. The **2nd or immune phase** may follow a brief asymptomatic interlude and is characterized by recurrence of fever and aseptic meningitis. Despite abnormal CSF profiles in 80% of infected children, only 50% have meningeal manifestations. CSF abnormalities include a modest elevation in pressure, a pleocytosis with polymorphonuclear leukocytes initially followed by mononuclear predominance and rarely exceeding 500 cells/mm^3, normal or slightly elevated protein levels, and normal glucose values. Encephalitis, cranial and peripheral neuropathies, papilledema, and paralysis are uncommon. Uveitis may occur during this phase; it can be unilateral or bilateral and is usually self-limited, rarely resulting in permanent visual impairment. Symptoms referable to the central nervous system resolve spontaneously within about 1 wk, with almost no mortality.

Icteric Leptospirosis (Weil Syndrome). This severe form of leptospirosis occurs in <10% of cases and is less common in children and more common in persons older than 30 yr of age. The initial manifestations are similar to those described for anicteric leptospirosis. The immune phase, however, is distinctive, being characterized by clinical and laboratory evidence of hepatic and renal dysfunction. In fulminating cases, hemorrhagic phenomena and cardiovascular collapse also occur. Hepatic abnormalities include right upper quadrant pain, hepatomegaly, direct and indirect hyperbilirubinemia, and modestly elevated serum levels of hepatic enzymes. The jaundice is not the result of hepatocellular necrosis, and liver function usually returns to normal after recovery. Renal manifestations are common; all patients have abnormal findings on urinalysis (hematuria, proteinuria, and casts), and azotemia is common, often associated with oliguria or anuria. Acute renal failure occurs in 16–40% of cases and is the principal cause of death. Abnormal electrocardiograms are present in 90% of cases, but congestive heart failure is uncommon. Hemorrhagic manifestations are rare but when present may include epistaxis, hemoptysis, and gastrointestinal and adrenal hemorrhage. Thrombocytopenia occurs in >50% of cases but is transient and does not result from disseminated intravascular coagulation. The mortality rate is 5–15%.

DIAGNOSIS. Leptospirosis should be considered in the differential diagnosis of any acute febrile illness when there is a history of direct contact with animals or with soil or water contaminated with animal urine, and especially when the onset is abrupt with chills, fever, severe myalgias, conjunctival suffusion, headache, nausea, and vomiting.

The diagnosis is established most often by serologic testing, and less frequently by isolation of the infecting organism from clinical specimens. Serologic tests for *Leptospira* include genus-specific and serogroup-specific tests. The reference method is the **microscopic agglutination test,** which is a serogroup-specific assay using live antigen suspension of leptospiral serovars. The test is read by dark-field microscopy for agglutination, and titers are determined. This test requires live cultures of all serovars for use as antigens. A 4-fold or greater increase in titer in paired sera confirms the diagnosis. Agglutinins usually appear by the 12th day of illness and reach a maximum titer by the 3rd wk. Low titers may persist for years. Approximately 10% of infected persons do not have detectable agglutinins, presumably because available antisera do not identify all *Leptospira* serotypes. An adaptation of the agglutination test is the use of antigens from killed or formalinized organisms; titer results are slightly lower and more cross reactions occur. Enzyme-linked immunosorbent assay (ELISA) methods, including an immunoglobulin M–specific dot-ELISA test, have also been developed.

Warthin-Starry silver staining, polymerase chain reaction, and immunofluorescent and immunohistochemical methods permit identification of leptospires in infected tissue or body fluids. Spirochetes may also be demonstrated by phase-contrast or dark-field microscopy, but these are insensitive.

Unlike other pathogenic spirochetes, leptospires are easily cultured on commercially available media containing rabbit serum or bovine serum albumin and long-chain fatty acids. Repeated blood cultures in the 1st wk of infection with very small inocula of blood are recommended. A small inoculum (i.e., 1 drop of blood in 5 mL of medium) is used to minimize growth inhibitory factors. Leptospires can be recovered from the blood or CSF during the 1st 10 days of illness and from urine after the 2nd wk. The number of leptospires in clinical specimens is small and their growth rate is slow; leptospires may be seen in several days, although prolonged incubation is required and cultures may not become positive for 2–4 mo.

TREATMENT. Despite the in vitro sensitivity of *Leptospira* to penicillin and tetracycline and the efficacy of these agents in treating experimental infection, their effectiveness in human leptospirosis remains controversial. It appears that initiation of treatment before the 7th day will probably shorten the clinical course and decrease the severity of the infection, and therefore treatment with penicillin or tetracycline (in children 9 yr of age or older) should be instituted as soon as the diagnosis is suspected. Parenteral penicillin G (6–8 million U/m^2/day divided every 4 hr IV for 7 days) is recommended, with tetracycline (10–20 mg/kg/day divided every 6 hr PO or IV for 7 days) as an alternative for patients allergic to penicillin. Oral amoxicillin is an alternative therapy for children <9 years of age.

PREVENTION. Prevention of human leptospirosis is facilitated by instituting rodent control measures and avoiding contaminated water and soil. Immunization of livestock and family pets has been recommended as a means of eliminating animal reservoirs. Protective clothing should be worn by persons at risk for occupational exposure. Leptospirosis has been prevented in American servicemen stationed in the tropics by administering doxycycline (200 mg PO once a week) as prophylaxis. This schedule may be similarly effective for the traveler entering a highly endemic area for a limited period of time.

Centers for Disease Control and Prevention: Leptospirosis after flooding of a university campus—Hawaii, 2004. *MMWR* 2006;55:125–127.

Farr RW: Leptospirosis. *Clin Infect Dis* 1995;21:1–8.

Heath CW Jr, Alexander AD, Galton MM: Leptospirosis in the United States. Analysis of 483 cases in man, 1949–1961. *N Engl J Med* 1965;273:857–864.

Jackson LA, Kaufmann AF, Adams WG, et al: Outbreak of leptospirosis associated with swimming. *Pediatr Infect Dis J* 1993;12:48–54.

Karande S, Bhatt M, Kelkar A, et al: An observational study to detect leptospirosis in Mumbai, India, 2000. *Arch Dis Child* 2003;88:1070–1075.

Levett PN: Leptospirosis. *Clin Microbiol Rev* 2001;14:296–326.

Meites E, Jay MT, Deresinski S, et al: Reemerging leptospirosis, California. *Emerg Infect Dis* 2004;10:406–412.

Wong ML, Kaplan S, Dunkle LM, et al: Leptospirosis: A childhood disease. *J Pediatr* 1977;90:532–537.

Chapter 218 ■ Relapsing Fever *(Borrelia)*

Parvin Azimi

ETIOLOGY. Relapsing fever is an arthropod-borne infection characterized by recurrent episodes of fever. It is caused by spirochetes of the genus *Borrelia,* a fastidious microorganism with worldwide distribution that is transmitted to humans by lice or ticks.

Epidemic relapsing fever, or **louse-borne fever,** is caused by *Borrelia recurrentis* and is transmitted from person to person by *Pediculus humanus,* the human body louse. After ingestion of an infective blood meal by the louse, the spirochetes penetrate its midgut, migrate to and multiply within the hemolymph, and remain viable throughout its life span of several weeks. Human infection occurs as a result of crushing lice during scratching, facilitating entry of infected hemolymph through abraded skin.

Endemic relapsing fever, or **tick-borne fever,** is caused by several species of *Borrelia* and is transmitted to humans by *Ornithodoros* ticks. *Borrelia hermsii* and *Borrelia turicatae* are the common species in the western United States, and *Borrelia dugesi* is the major cause of disease in Mexico and Central America. After ingestion of an infective blood meal, spirochetes invade all tissues of their arthropod hosts, including the salivary glands and reproductive tract, which permits transovarian passage of infected spirochetes and perpetuates arthropod infection of successive generations. Human infection occurs when saliva, coxal fluid, or excrement is released by the tick during feeding, thereby permitting spirochetes to penetrate the skin and mucous membranes.

EPIDEMIOLOGY. Louse-borne relapsing fever tends to occur in epidemics, often in association with typhus. Epidemics are associated with war, poverty, famine, and poor personal hygiene. This form of relapsing fever occurs more commonly during the winter. The major endemic focus of the disease is the highlands of Ethiopia.

Ornithodoros ticks, which transmit endemic relapsing fever, are distributed worldwide, including the western United States, prefer warm, humid environments and high altitudes, and are found in rodent burrows, caves, and other nesting sites (Fig. 218-1). Rodents are the principal reservoirs. Infected ticks gain access to human dwellings on the rodent host. Human contact is often unnoticed because these soft ticks, unlike the hard ticks, which attach and feed over a period of days, are nocturnal feeders, have a painless bite, and detach immediately after a short blood meal.

PATHOLOGY AND PATHOGENESIS. The cyclic nature of relapsing fever is explained by the ability of *Borrelia* organisms to continually undergo antigenic (phase) variation. Multiple variants evolve simultaneously during the first relapse, with 1 type becoming predominant. Spirochetes isolated during the primary febrile episode differ antigenically from those recovered during a subsequent relapse. During febrile episodes, spirochetes enter the bloodstream, induce the development of specific immunoglobulin M (IgM) and IgG antibody, and undergo agglutination, immobilization, lysis, and phagocytosis. During remission, *Borrelia* spirochetes may remain in the bloodstream, but spirochetemia is insufficient to produce symptoms. The number of relapses in untreated patients depends on the number of antigenic variants of the infecting strain.

CLINICAL MANIFESTATIONS. Relapsing fever is characterized by periods of fever lasting 2–9 days, separated by afebrile periods of 2–7 days. Louse-borne disease has a longer incubation period, longer periods of pyrexia, fewer relapses, and longer remission periods than tick-borne disease. The incubation period of tick-borne disease is usually 7 days with a range of 2–18 days. Each form of relapsing fever is associated with sudden onset of high fever, lethargy, headache, photophobia, nausea, vomiting, myalgia, and arthralgia. Additional symptoms may appear later and include abdominal pain, a productive cough, and mild respiratory distress. Bleeding manifestations may occur and include epistaxis, hemoptysis, hematuria, and hematemesis. A diffuse, erythematous, macular, or petechial rash may develop over the trunk and shoulders. It is more common in louse-borne fever (25%), occurring almost exclusively during the end of the primary febrile episode, and lasts for 1–2 days. There may also be lymphadenopathy, pneumonia, and splenomegaly. Hepatic tenderness associated with hepatomegaly is a common sign, with jaundice in half of affected children. Central nervous system manifestations may be the principal feature of late relapses in tick-borne disease; they include lethargy, stupor, meningismus, convulsions, peripheral neuritis, focal neurologic deficits, and cranial nerve paralysis. Severe manifestations include myocarditis, hepatic failure, and disseminated intravascular coagulopathy.

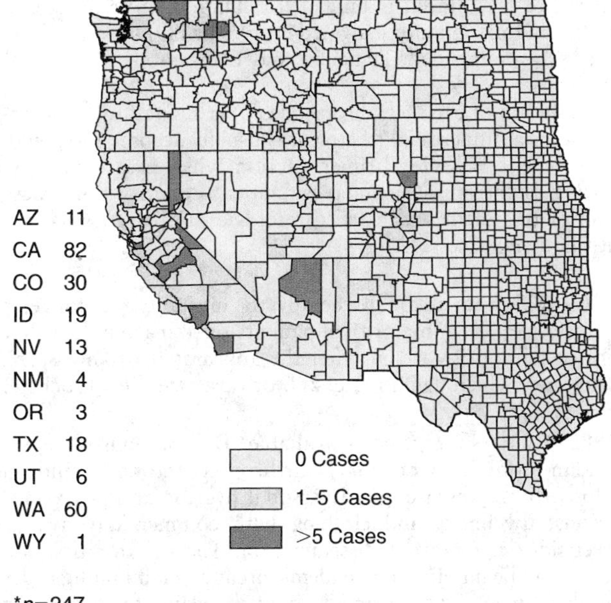

Figure 218-1. Number of cases of tickborne relapsing fever 1990–2000. (Centers for Disease Control and Prevention: Tickborne relapsing fever outbreak after a family gathering—New Mexico, August 2002. *MMWR* 2003;52:809–812.)

The initial symptomatic period characteristically ends with a crisis in 2–9 days, marked by abrupt diaphoresis, hypothermia, hypotension, bradycardia, profound muscle weakness, and prostration. In untreated patients, the first relapse occurs within 1 wk, followed by usually 3 but up to 10 relapses, with symptoms during each relapse becoming milder and shorter as the afebrile remission period lengthens.

DIAGNOSIS. Diagnosis depends on demonstration of spirochetes in thin or thick blood smears stained with Giemsa or Wright's stain and by blood culture. During afebrile remissions, spirochetes are not found in the blood. Serologic tests, such as enzyme immunoassay and Western blotting, are not standardized and generally not available. Tick-borne disease produces a serologic cross reaction with other spirochetes, including *Borrelia burgdorferi,* the agent of Lyme disease.

TREATMENT. Oral or parenteral tetracycline is the drug of choice for louse-borne and tick-borne relapsing fever. For children >8 yr of age and young adults, tetracycline (500 mg PO every 6 hr) for 10 days has been effective. Single-dose treatment with tetracycline (500 mg PO) or erythromycin is efficacious in adults, but experience in children is limited. In children <8 yr of age, erythromycin (50 mg/kg/day divided every 6 hr PO) for a total of 10 days is recommended. Penicillin and chloramphenicol are also effective.

Resolution of each febrile episode either by natural crisis or as a result of antimicrobial treatment is usually accompanied within 2 hr by the Jarisch-Herxheimer reaction, which is associated with clearing of the spirochetemia. Attempts to control this reaction by prior treatment with corticosteroids or antipyretics have met with limited success.

PROGNOSIS. With adequate therapy, the mortality rate for relapsing fever is <5%. A majority of patients recover from their illness with or without treatment after the appearance of anti-*Borrelia* antibodies, which agglutinate, kill, or opsonize the spirochete.

PREVENTION. No vaccine is available. Disease control requires avoidance or elimination of the arthropod vectors. In epidemics of louse-borne disease, good personal hygiene and delousing of persons, dwellings, and clothing with commercially available insecticides can prevent dissemination. The risk for tick-borne disease can be minimized in endemic areas by maintaining rodent-free dwellings. Giving prophylactic doxycycline for 4 days after a tick bite may prevent tick-borne relapsing fever due to *Borrelia persica*.

Butler TC: Relapsing fever: New lessons about antibiotic action. *Ann Intern Med* 1985;102:397–399.
Centers for Disease Control and Prevention: Tickborne relapsing fever outbreak after a family gathering—New Mexico, August 2002. *MMWR* 2003;52:809–812.
Fritz CL, Bronson LR, Smith CR, et al: Isolation and characterization of *Borrelia hermsii* associated with two foci of tick-borne relapsing fever in California. *J Clin Microbiol* 2004;42:1123–1128.
Hasin T, Davidovitch N, Cohen R, et al: Postexposure treatment with doxycycline for the prevention of tick-borne relapsing fever. *N Engl J Med* 2006;355:148–154.
Schwan TG, Policastro PF, Miller Z, et al: Tick-borne relapsing fever caused by *Borrelia hermsii*, Montana. *Emerg Infect Dis* 2003;9:1151–1154.
Vial L, Diatta G, Tall A, et al: Incidence of tick-borne relapsing fever in west Africa: Longitudinal study. *Lancet* 2006;368:37–43.

Chapter 219 ■ Lyme Disease *(Borrelia burgdorferi)* Eugene D. Shapiro

Lyme disease is the most common vector-borne disease in the USA. Although Lyme disease is a public health concern, extensive publicity as well as a very high frequency of misdiagnosis has resulted in a degree of anxiety about Lyme disease that is out of proportion to the actual morbidity that it causes.

ETIOLOGY. Lyme disease is caused by the spirochete *Borrelia burgdorferi*, a fastidious, microaerophilic bacterium that replicates very slowly and requires special media for in vitro growth. *B. burgdorferi* is cylindrically shaped with a cell membrane that is covered by flagella and a loosely associated outer membrane. The 3 major outer-surface proteins—OspA, OspB, and OspC (which are highly charged basic proteins of molecular weights of about 31, 34, and 23 kd, respectively)—as well as the 41 kd flagellar protein, are important targets for the immune response. Differences in the molecular structure of *B. burgdorferi* strains, especially between isolates from Europe and the United States, are well documented. Clinical manifestations of Lyme borreliosis in Europe and the United States, such as the greater frequency of radiculoneuritis in Europe, may be attributable to these differences.

EPIDEMIOLOGY. Lyme disease has been reported from >50 countries. In 2003, a total of 21,273 cases of Lyme disease were reported in the USA. Approximately 95% of all reported cases occurred in Connecticut, Delaware, Maine, Maryland, Massachusetts, Minnesota, New Hampshire, New Jersey, New York, Pennsylvania, Rhode Island, and Wisconsin (Fig. 219-1). In Europe, most cases occur in the Scandinavian countries and in central Europe, especially Germany, Austria, and Switzerland. Estimates of the incidence of Lyme disease are complicated by passive systems for reporting of Lyme disease and the high frequency of misdiagnosis of this illness. In endemic areas, the reported annual incidence ranges from 20 to 100 cases/100,000 population, although this figure may be as high as 1,000 cases/100,000 population in hyperendemic areas such as Lyme, Connecticut. The reported incidence is highest among children 5–10 yr of age, which is almost twice as high as the incidence among older children and adults.

TRANSMISSION. Lyme disease is a zoonosis caused by the transmission of *B. burgdorferi* to humans through the bite of an infected tick of the *Ixodes* species. In the eastern and midwestern United States, the vector is *Ixodes scapularis*, the black-legged tick that is commonly known as the deer tick, which is responsible for most cases of Lyme disease in the United States. The vector on the Pacific Coast is *Ixodes pacificus*, the western black-legged tick. *Ixodes* ticks have a 2 yr, 3 stage life cycle. The larvae hatch in the early summer and are usually uninfected with *B. burgdorferi*. The tick may become infected at any stage of its life cycle by feeding on a host, usually a small mammal such as the white-footed mouse (*Peromyscus leucopus*), which is a natural reservoir for *B. burgdorferi*. The larvae overwinter and emerge the following spring in the nymphal stage, which is the stage of the tick that is most likely to transmit the infection. The nymphs molt to adults in the fall. The females lay their eggs the following spring before they die, and the 2 yr life cycle begins again.

Several factors are associated with increased risk for transmission of *B. burgdorferi* from ticks to humans. The proportion of infected ticks varies by geographic area and by stage of the tick's life cycle. In endemic areas in the northeastern and midwestern United States, 15–25% of nymphal ticks and 35–50% of adult ticks are infected with *B. burgdorferi*. By contrast, *I. pacificus* often feeds on lizards, which are not a competent reservoir for *B. burgdorferi*. Only 1–8% of these ticks, even in the nymphal and adult stages, are infected with *B. burgdorferi*. The risk for transmission of *B. burgdorferi* from infected *Ixodes* ticks is related to the duration of feeding. It takes hours for the mouth parts of ticks to implant fully in the host and much longer (days) for the tick to become fully engorged. Experiments in animals have shown that infected nymphal ticks must feed for ≥36–48 hr, and infected adults must feed for ≥48–72 hr, before the risk for transmission of *B. burgdorferi* becomes substantial. Most individuals who are bitten by a tick will recognize and remove the tick before the transmission of *B. burgdorferi* can occur. Persons with increased occupational, recreational, or residential exposure to tick-infested woods or fields (the preferred habitat of ticks) in endemic areas are at increased risk for developing Lyme disease.

PATHOLOGY AND PATHOGENESIS. The skin is the initial target of infection by *B. burgdorferi*. Inflammation induced by *B. burgdorferi* leads to the development of the characteristic rash, named erythema migrans. Early disseminated Lyme disease is caused by the spread of spirochetes through the bloodstream to tissues throughout the body. The spirochete adheres to the surfaces of a wide variety of different types of cells, which may be responsible for the involvement of many organs. Because the organism may

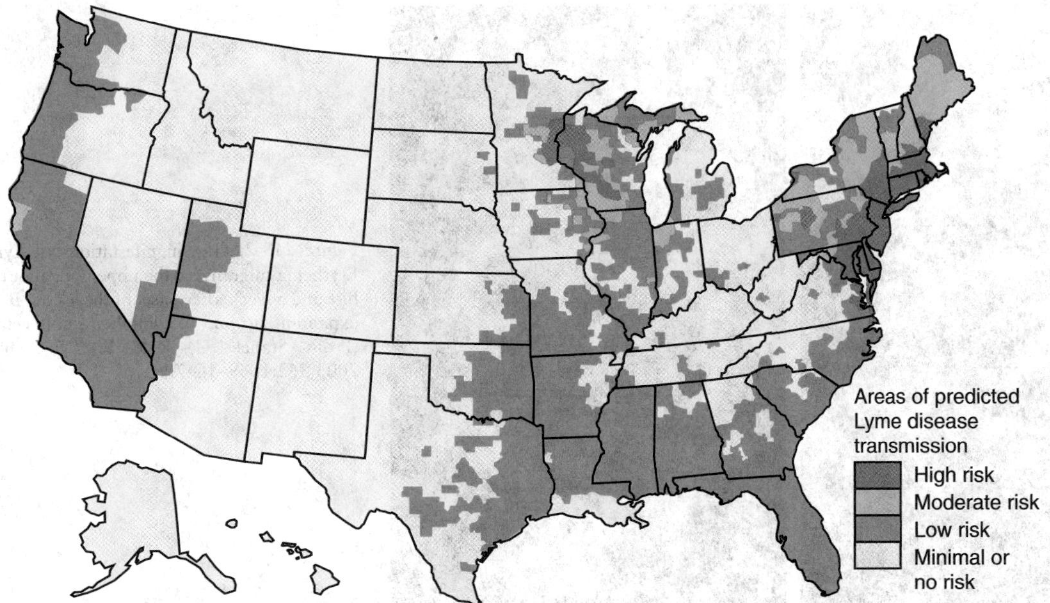

Figure 219-1. The approximate distribution of predicted risk for Lyme disease in the USA. The risk varies by the distribution of *Ixodes scapularis* and *Ixodes pacificus,* the proportion of infected ticks for each species at each stage of the tick's life cycle, and the presence of grassy or wooded locations favored by white-tailed deer.
(From the Centers for Disease Control and Prevention.)

persist in tissues for prolonged periods of time, symptoms may appear very late after initial infection.

The symptoms of early disseminated as well as of late Lyme disease are due to inflammation mediated by interleukin 1 and other lymphokines in response to the presence of the organism. It is likely that relatively few organisms actually invade the host, but cytokines serve to amplify the inflammatory response and lead to much of the tissue damage. The refractory symptoms of late Lyme disease may have an immunogenetic basis. Persons with HLA-DR2, -DR3, and -DR4 allotypes may be genetically predisposed to develop chronic recurrent Lyme arthritis if treatment is delayed substantially. These class II histocompatibility molecules located on macrophages and B cells are involved in the presentation of antigens to T helper cells that initiate the immune response. Although rare, especially in children, *B. burgdorferi* may initiate an autoimmune response in genetically susceptible individuals that causes persistent inflammation of the synovium and clinical symptoms long after the bacteria have been killed.

Lyme disease is characterized by inflammatory lesions that contain both T and B lymphocytes, macrophages, plasma cells, and some mast cells. The erythema migrans rash consists of a moderately dense infiltrate of lymphocytes, plasma cells, and occasional macrophages, located around the small blood vessels of the upper dermis. Lyme myocarditis is a transmural myocarditis with widespread interstitial lymphocytic and plasma cell infiltrate. Similar infiltrates have been seen in the meninges and cerebral cortex. There are few reports of the histology of synovial tissue during the acute stages of Lyme arthritis. At this stage of the illness, the synovial fluid often has a marked predominance of polymorphonuclear cells, suggesting that the synovial tissue also will have a polymorphonuclear inflammatory infiltrate. By contrast, chronic, recurrent arthritis is characterized by a chronic hypertrophic synovitis. This nonspecific abnormality, also found in other disorders such as rheumatoid arthritis, is marked by hyperplasia of the synovial cells with varying degrees of lymphocytic infiltrates that sometimes form abortive germinal centers and follicles. Plasma cells are present at the periphery of the lymphoid aggregates. In advanced disease, neovascularization (a nonspecific response to chronic inflammation) may occur.

CLINICAL MANIFESTATIONS. The clinical manifestations of Lyme disease are divided into early and late stages. Early Lyme disease is further classified as early localized or early disseminated disease. Untreated patients may progressively develop clinical symptoms of each stage of the disease, or they may present with early disseminated or with late disease without apparently having had any symptoms of the earlier stages of Lyme disease.

Early Localized Disease. The 1st clinical manifestation of Lyme disease is the typical annular rash, named **erythema migrans** (Fig. 219-2). Although it usually occurs 7–14 days after the bite, the onset of the rash has been reported from 3 to 32 days later. The initial lesion occurs at the site of the bite. The rash most often is uniformly erythematous, or it may appear as a target lesion with central clearing; rarely, there may be vesicular or necrotic areas in the center of the rash. Occasionally the rash may be itchy or painful, though often it is asymptomatic. The lesion can occur anywhere on the body, although the most common locations are the axilla, periumbilical area, thigh, and groin. It is not unusual for the rash to occur on the neck or face, especially in young children. Erythema migrans may be associated with systemic features including fever, myalgia, headache, or malaise. Without treatment, the rash gradually expands (hence the name migrans) to an average diameter of 15 cm and remains present for at least 1–2 wk. The rash usually resolves without treatment after a median time of 4 wk. A similar rash seen in the southern regions of the United States (southern tick-associated rash illness [STARI]) is not associated with any other manifestation of Lyme disease and is a self-limited illness, caused by *B. lonestari.*

Early Disseminated Disease. In the United States, a substantial proportion (about 20%) of patients with acute *B. burgdorferi* infection develop **secondary erythema migrans** lesions, a common manifestation of early disseminated Lyme disease caused by hematogenous spread of the organisms to multiple skin sites. The secondary lesions, which may develop several days or even weeks after the 1st lesion, usually are smaller than the primary lesion and are often accompanied by fever, myalgia, headache, and malaise; conjunctivitis and lymphadenopathy also may develop. Occasionally, as the erythema migrans rash resolves, new small (1–3 cm), evanescent, erythematous annular lesions that do not

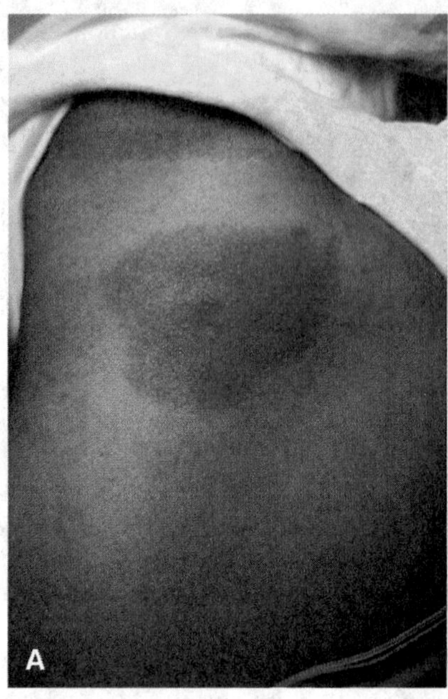

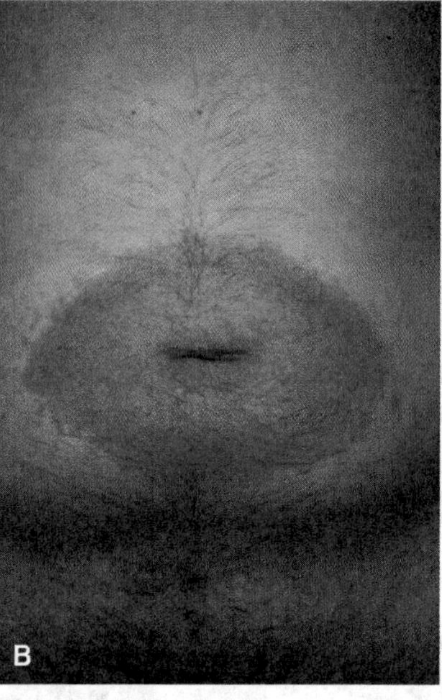

Figure 219-2. Skin manifestations of Lyme borreliosis. *A*, Erythema migrans on the upper leg, about 2 weeks after tick bite and a week after onset of the lesion. *B*, Erythema migrans expanding around the umbilicus; note central clearing. (From Stanek G, Strle F: Lyme borreliosis. *Lancet* 2003;362:1639–1647.)

expand continue to appear for several weeks. Other manifestations may include aseptic meningitis, with signs of meningeal irritation such as nuchal rigidity (and associated with papilledema in about 25–35% of cases); uveitis; focal neurologic findings, especially cranioneuropathies; and, rarely, carditis, with varying degrees of heart block. Paralysis of the facial (7th) cranial nerve is relatively common in children and may be the initial or the only manifestation of Lyme disease. The paralysis usually lasts 2–8 wk and resolves completely in most cases. There is no evidence that the clinical course of the facial palsy is affected by antimicrobial treatment.

Late Disease. Arthritis, beginning weeks to months after the initial infection, is the usual manifestation of late Lyme disease. Arthritis typically involves the large joints, especially the knee, which is affected in >90% of cases, but any joint may be affected. The swollen joint may be only mildly symptomatic or it may be swollen and tender, though patients usually do not experience the exquisite sensitivity and pain that is typical of bacterial arthritis. Although it may last for several weeks, the joint swelling usually resolves within 1–2 wk before recurring, often in other joints. If the disease is not treated, the episodes of arthritis may increase in duration, sometimes lasting for months; but in most cases the disease eventually resolves, even in patients who are untreated and who have had many recurrences of arthritis.

Late manifestations of Lyme disease involving the central nervous system, sometimes termed **tertiary neuroborreliosis,** are rarely reported in children. In adults, chronic demyelinating encephalitis, polyneuritis, and impairment of memory have been attributed to Lyme disease.

Congenital Lyme Disease. Although *B. burgdorferi* has been identified from several abortuses and from a few liveborn children with congenital anomalies, the placentas and the abortuses in which the spirochete was identified usually did not show histologic evidence of inflammation. No consistent pattern of fetal damage has been identified to suggest a clinical syndrome of congenital infection. Furthermore, studies conducted in endemic areas have indicated that there is no difference in the prevalence of congenital malformations among the offspring of women with serum antibodies against *B. burgdorferi* and the offspring of those without such antibodies. A survey of child neurologists in endemic areas found that none had seen a credible case of a child with congenital Lyme disease. If congenital Lyme disease does exist, it must be extremely rare.

DIAGNOSIS. The clinical manifestations of Lyme disease, other than erythema migrans, are not specific. The monoarticular or pauciarticular arthritis may mimic either an acute septic joint or other causes of arthritis in children, such as juvenile rheumatoid arthritis or rheumatic fever. The 7th nerve palsy due to Lyme disease is indistinguishable from idiopathic Bell palsy; Lyme meningitis may mimic enteroviral meningitis. Lyme meningitis usually occurs in older patients (10 vs 5 yr), has a longer duration of symptoms (12 vs 1 day), and has the presence of cranial neuropathies, erythema migrans, as well as papilledema when compared with enteroviral meningitis. The diagnosis of erythema migrans may be difficult because the rash initially may be confused with nummular eczema, tinea, granuloma annulare, an insect bite, or cellulitis. However, the relatively rapid expansion of erythema migrans helps distinguish it from these other conditions.

Although some laboratories use the polymerase chain reaction as a diagnostic test for Lyme disease, its sensitivity may be poor because of the low concentrations of bacteria in many sites. Specificity may also be a problem. Other antigen-based tests, including a test for *B. burgdorferi* antigens in urine, have been unreliable. Consequently, the confirmation of Lyme disease in patients without erythema migrans usually is based on the demonstration of antibodies to *B. burgdorferi* in the patient's serum.

Serology. Specific IgM antibodies appear first, usually at 3–4 wk, peak at 6–8 wk, and subsequently decline, although a prolonged elevation of IgM antibodies sometimes occurs despite effective antimicrobial treatment. Consequently, the results of tests for specific IgM antibodies should not be used as an indicator of either active or recent infection. In addition, because of a high rate of false-positive IgM test results, a positive IgM result alone (in the absence of a positive IgG result) should not be used to support a diagnosis of Lyme disease in patients who have had symptoms for a month or longer. Specific IgG antibodies usually appear at 4–8 wk, peak after 4–6 mo, and may remain elevated indefinitely. The antibody response to *B. burgdorferi* may be abrogated in patients with early Lyme disease who are treated promptly with an effective antimicrobial agent, but in most patients IgG antibodies remain detectable for many years after treatment and clinical resolution of the illness.

Because the immunofluorescent antibody test requires subjective interpretation and is time consuming to perform, it has been replaced by enzyme-linked immunosorbent assays (ELISAs) for

TABLE 219-1. Recommended Treatment of Lyme Disease in Children

DISEASE CATEGORY	DRUG(S) AND DOSE*
EARLY LOCALIZED DISEASE*	
8 yr of age or older	Doxycycline, 100 mg orally twice a day for 14–21 days[†]
All ages	Amoxicillin, 50 mg/kg/day orally divided into 3 doses (maximum 1.5 g/day) for 14–21 days
	OR
	Cefuroxime, 30 mg/kg/day in 2 divided doses (maximum 1,000 mg/day) for 14–21 days
EARLY DISSEMINATED AND LATE DISEASE	
Multiple erythema migrans	Same oral regimen as for early localized disease
Isolated facial palsy	Same oral regimen as for early localized disease[§]
Arthritis	Same oral regimen as for early localized disease, but for 28 days
Persistent or recurrent arthritis[‖]	Ceftriaxone sodium, 75–100 mg/kg IV or IM once a day (maximum 2 g/day), for 14–28 days;
	OR
	Penicillin, 300,000 U/kg/day IV given in divided doses every 4 h (maximum 20 million U/day) for 14–28 days
	OR
	Same oral regimen as for early disease, but for 28 days
Carditis	Ceftriaxone or penicillin: see persistent or recurrent arthritis
Meningitis or encephalitis	Ceftriaxone[¶] or penicillin: see persistent or recurrent arthritis, but for 14–28 days

*For patients who are allergic to penicillin, cefuroxime and erythromycin are alternative drugs.

[†]Tetracyclines are contraindicated in pregnancy.

[‡]Corticosteroids should not be given.

[§]Treatment has no effect on the resolution of facial nerve palsy; its purpose is to prevent late disease; doxycycline is preferred when possible.

[‖]Arthritis is not considered persistent or recurrent unless objective evidence of synovitis exists at least 2 mo after treatment is initiated. Some experts administer a second course of an oral agent before using an IV-administered antimicrobial agent.

[¶]Ceftriaxone should be administered IV for treatment of meningitis or encephalitis.

From the American Academy of Pediatrics: *Red Book: 2006 Report of the Committee on Infectious Diseases,* 27th ed. Elk Grove Village, IL, American Academy of Pediatrics, 2006, p 431.

the detection of antibodies against *B. burgdorferi.* The ELISA method sometimes produces false-positive results because of cross-reactive antibodies to other spirochetal infections (syphilis, leptospirosis, or relapsing fever), to certain viral infections (varicella), against spirochetes that comprise part of the normal oral flora, and with certain autoimmune diseases (systemic lupus erythematosus).

Western blotting (immunoblotting) is also used as a diagnostic test for Lyme disease, although reported results can be confusing since criteria for a positive test require at least 5 positive bands for IgG, and many uninfected individuals have at least some positive bands. Official recommendations for serologic tests for Lyme disease are to perform a quantitative test (such as ELISA) and a confirmatory Western immunoblot test if the ELISA result is either positive or equivocal.

The available serologic tests, especially widely used commercial kits, have only fair specificity. Use of these commercial diagnostic serologic tests results in a high rate of misdiagnosis. In contrast, the serologic tests for Lyme disease performed by reference laboratories are relatively accurate. However, even with these tests, the predictive value of the result still depends primarily on the probability that the patient has Lyme disease based on the clinical and epidemiologic history and the physical examination (the **pretest probability**). With few exceptions, the pretest probability that a patient has Lyme disease will be very low in areas in which Lyme disease is rare. Even in areas with a high prevalence of Lyme disease, patients with only nonspecific signs and symptoms, such as fatigue, headache, or arthralgia, are not likely to have Lyme disease; virtually all positive serologic test results in such patients are false-positive results. Consequently, serologic tests for Lyme disease should not be ordered in such patients. Serologic tests for Lyme disease should only be obtained for patients with a relatively high (≥20%) probability of having Lyme disease—that is, only in patients who have objective physical signs that are suggestive of Lyme disease, in whom the predictive value of a positive test result is high.

Even though a symptomatic patient has antibodies to *B. burgdorferi,* Lyme disease may not be the cause of the patient's symptoms. The test result may be falsely positive, or the patient may have been infected previously. Antibodies to *B. burgdorferi* that develop with infection may persist for many years despite adequate treatment and clinical cure of the disease. Because some people who become infected with *B. burgdorferi* are asymptomatic, the background rate of seropositivity among patients who have never had clinically apparent Lyme disease may be substantial in endemic areas.

Culture. The isolation of *B. burgdorferi* from a symptomatic patient is considered diagnostic of Lyme disease. Although *B. burgdorferi* has been isolated from blood, skin, CSF, myocardium, and the synovium of patients with Lyme disease, the medium in which *B. burgdorferi* is cultured is expensive, it can take as long as 4 wk for the bacteria to grow in culture, and the frequency of isolation of *B. burgdorferi* from patients with active Lyme disease is low. It usually is necessary for patients to undergo an invasive procedure, such as a skin biopsy or a lumbar puncture, to obtain appropriate tissue or fluid for culture. *B. burgdorferi* has been identified with silver stains (Warthin-Starry or modified Dieterle) and with immunohistochemical stains (using monoclonal or polyclonal antibodies) in skin, synovial, and myocardial biopsy specimens. However, *B. burgdorferi* can be confused with normal tissue structures or it can be missed because it usually is present in low concentrations.

Laboratory Findings. Routine laboratory tests rarely are helpful in diagnosing Lyme disease because the associated laboratory abnormalities usually are nonspecific. The peripheral white blood cell count may be either normal or elevated. The erythrocyte sedimentation rate usually is elevated. The white blood cell concentration in joint fluid may range from 25,000 to 125,000/mL, often with a preponderance of polymorphonuclear cells. When the central nervous system is involved, there usually is a mild pleocytosis with a lymphocytic and monocytic predominance. The CSF protein level may be elevated, but the glucose concentration usually is normal.

TREATMENT. Few clinical trials of treatment for Lyme disease have been conducted in children. Recommendations for the treatment of children (Table 219-1) mainly are extrapolated from studies of adults. Children <8 yr of age should not be treated with doxycycline because it may cause permanent discoloration of their teeth. Patients who are treated with doxycycline should be alerted to the risk for developing dermatitis in sun-exposed areas while taking the medication. Cefuroxime is licensed for the treatment of Lyme disease and is an alternative for persons who cannot take doxycycline and who are allergic to penicillin. Preliminary results with azithromycin have been disappointing. There is little need to use newer agents because the results of treatment with either amoxicillin or doxycycline have been excellent.

Some patients may develop a Jarisch-Herxheimer reaction soon after treatment is initiated. The manifestations of this reaction are increased temperature, sweats, and myalgia. These symptoms resolve spontaneously within 24–48 hr, although administration of nonsteroidal anti-inflammatory drugs often is beneficial. Nonsteroidal anti-inflammatory agents also may be useful in treating symptoms of early Lyme disease and of Lyme arthritis.

Fatigue, arthralgia, and myalgia, which may accompany or follow more specific symptoms and signs of Lyme disease but almost never are the sole presenting manifestations of Lyme disease, sometimes persist after treatment but generally resolve over a period of weeks to months. There is little evidence that these symptoms are related to persistence of the organism. Because antibodies against *B. burgdorferi* persist after successful treatment, there is no reason to obtain follow-up serologic tests. There is also no evidence that either repeated or prolonged courses of antimicrobial agents hasten the resolution of such symptoms.

PROGNOSIS. There is a widespread misconception that Lyme disease is difficult to treat successfully and that chronic symptoms and clinical recurrences are common. The most common reason for apparent treatment failure is misdiagnosis in patients who do not have Lyme disease. The impression that Lyme disease requires prolonged treatment, including intravenous antimicrobial therapy, and that treatment is often unsuccessful can be attributed to the treatment of patients whose symptoms were not due to Lyme disease.

The prognosis for children treated for Lyme disease is excellent. Cases in children treated for erythema migrans rarely progress to late Lyme disease. The long-term prognosis for patients who are treated beginning in the late phase of Lyme disease also is excellent. Although recurrences of arthritis do occur rarely, especially among patients with DR2, DR3, or DR4 HLA allotypes (an autoimmune process), most children who are treated for Lyme arthritis are permanently cured. Although there are rare reports of adults who have developed late neuroborreliosis, usually among persons with clinically apparent Lyme disease that either was not treated or in whom treatment was delayed for months or years, similar cases in children have not been documented.

PREVENTION. Children in endemic areas are often bitten by deer ticks, but the overall risk for acquiring Lyme disease after a tick bite is low (1–3%), even in these areas. Even if the patient is bitten by a nymphal stage deer tick infected with *B. burgdorferi*, the risk for acquiring Lyme disease is only 8–10%. If infection develops, treatment of the infection is highly effective. A study of prophylaxis after a tick bite found that a single dose of doxycycline (200 mg PO) was 87% effective in preventing Lyme disease (although the lower limit of the 95% confidence interval for this estimate was only 25%). Because most people who recognize a tick bite remove the tick within 48 hr (before the tick can transmit Lyme disease), the overall risk for Lyme disease after a recognized deer tick bite remains low (1–3%). Most people are not able to identify the species or the stage of the tick (in some instances reported "tick" bites prove not to be from ticks), and therefore administration of antimicrobial **prophylaxis is not recommended** routinely. The routine testing of ticks that have been removed from humans for infection with *B. burgdorferi* also is not recommended because the predictive value of a positive test result in the tick for predicting infection in the human host is unknown.

The most reasonable approach to preventing Lyme disease is to wear appropriate protective clothing (long pants tucked into socks, long sleeve shirts) when entering tick-infested areas and to check for and to remove ticks after spending time in such areas. Insect repellents on the skin (DEET) may provide temporary protection, but they may be absorbed from the skin and, if used in large doses, they may rarely produce toxicity, especially in children.

Permethrins kill ticks but should only be put on clothing. Daily inspection of the scalp, skin, behind the ears, groin, clothing lines, and axilla with removal of ticks is recommended for all children in areas endemic for Lyme disease who are exposed to tick-infested areas (wooded or high grass). Tick removal should be done with a tweezer or, if no tweezer is available, the tick should be covered with a tissue; pulling the tick by grasping its head region in a vertical direction (without twisting) is the only recommended method of tick removal.

Hayes EB, Piesman J: How can we prevent Lyme disease? *N Engl J Med* 2003;348:2424–2430.

Klempner MS, Hu LT, Evans J, et al: Two controlled trials of antibiotic treatment in patients with persistent symptoms and a history of Lyme disease. *N Engl J Med* 2001;345:85–92.

Medical Letter: Treatment of lyme disease. *Med Lett* 2005;47:41–44.

Seltzer EG, Gerber MA, Cartter ML, et al: Long-term outcomes of persons with Lyme disease. *JAMA* 2000;283:609–616.

Seltzer EG, Shapiro ED: Misdiagnosis of Lyme disease: When not to order serologic tests. *Pediatr Infect Dis J* 1996;15:762–763.

Shadick NA, Liang MH, Phillips CB, et al: The cost-effectiveness of vaccination against Lyme disease. *Arch Intern Med* 2001;161:554–561.

Shah SS, Zaoutis TE, Turnquist J, et al: Early differentiation of lyme from enteroviral meningitis. *Pediatr Infect Dis J* 2005;24:542–545.

Shapiro ED: Long-term outcomes of persons with Lyme disease. *Vector Borne Zoonotic Dis* 2002;2:279–281.

Shapiro ED, Gerber MA: Lyme disease. *Clin Infect Dis* 2000;31:533–542.

Shapiro ED, Gerber MA: Lyme disease: Fact versus fiction. *Pediatr Ann* 2002;31:170–177.

Stanek G, Strle F: Lyme borreliosis. *Lancet* 2003;362:1639–1647.

Steere AC: Lyme disease. *N Engl J Med* 2001;345:115–125.

Wormser GP: Early lyme disease. *N Engl J Med* 2006;354:2794–2801.

Wormser GP, Dattwyler RJ, Shapiro ED, et al: The clinical assessment, treatment, and prevention of lyme disease, human granulocytic anaplasmosis, and babesiosis: clinical practice guidelines by the Infectious Disease Society of America. *CID* 2006;43:1089–1134.

Wormser GP, Masters E, Nowakowski J, et al: Prospective clinical evaluation of patients from Missouri and New York with erythema migrans-like skin lesions. *Clin Infect Dis* 2005;41:958–965.

Section 9 — Mycoplasmal Infections

Chapter 220 ■ *Mycoplasma Pneumoniae*

Dwight A. Powell

Among the 5 *Mycoplasma* species isolated from the human respiratory tract, *Mycoplasma pneumoniae* is the only recognized human pathogen. It is a major cause of respiratory infections in school-aged children and young adults.

ETIOLOGY. Mycoplasmas are the smallest self-replicating biologic system and are dependent on attachment to host cells for obtaining essential precursors such as nucleotides, fatty acids, sterols, and amino acids. They are distinguished by the complete absence of a cell wall, double-stranded DNA, and small genomes ranging from 577 to 1,380 kb. *M. pneumoniae* is fastidious, and growth in commercially available culture systems is too slow to be of practical clinical use.

EPIDEMIOLOGY. *M. pneumoniae* infections occur worldwide and throughout the year. In contrast to the acute, short-lived epidemics of some respiratory viral agents, *M. pneumoniae* infection is endemic in larger communities, with epidemic outbreaks occurring every 4–7 yr. In smaller communities, infections are sporadic, with long-lasting and smoldering outbreaks occurring at irregular intervals.

The occurrence of mycoplasmal illness is related, in part, to age and pre-exposure immunity. Overt illness is unusual before 3 yr of age. Younger children appear to have frequent mild or subclinical infections, and reinfections appear to be common. The peak incidence of illness occurs in school-aged children. *M. pneumoniae* accounts for 7–40% of all community-acquired pneumonias among children 3–15 yr of age. Recurrent infections occur infrequently but are well documented to occur in adults at intervals of 4–7 yr.

TRANSMISSION. Infection occurs through the respiratory route by large droplet spread. The incubation period is 1–3 wk. High transmission rates have been documented within families, with a high proportion of secondary cases developing lower respiratory tract infections. Outbreaks can occur in closed settings (military recruits, institutions, summer camps for children) or can occur as community-wide epidemics.

PATHOLOGY AND PATHOGENESIS. Cells of the ciliated respiratory epithelium are the target cells of *M. pneumoniae* infection. The organism is an elongated snakelike structure with an attachment tip characterized by an electron-dense core and a trilaminar outer membrane. Attachment to the ciliary membrane is mediated by a complex network of interactive adhesion and adherence-accessory proteins localized to this specialized attachment tip (P1/B/C, P30, P65, HMW 1–3). These proteins cooperate structurally and functionally to mobilize and concentrate adhesion proteins at the tip and permit mycoplasmal colonization of mucous membranes. Avirulent phenotypes that arise through spontaneous mutations at high frequency cannot synthesize specific cytoadherence-related proteins or are unable to stabilize them at the tip organelle.

Virulent organisms attach to ciliated respiratory epithelial cell surfaces through sialated glycoprotein or sulfated glycolipid receptors and burrow down between cells, resulting in ciliastasis and eventual sloughing of the cells. *M. pneumoniae* can invade certain cell lines in vitro and survive in the cytoplasm or perinuclear regions for prolonged periods of time. *M. pneumoniae* has been detected by polymerase chain reaction (PCR) in many non-respiratory sites. These observations suggest that *M. pneumoniae* causes more extrapulmonary infections and chronic disease than appreciated.

A possible mechanism of *M. pneumoniae* disease is the release of various proinflammatory and anti-inflammatory cytokines. *M. pneumoniae* infection may induce numerous interleukins, interferons, tumor necrosis factor-α, and other cytokines. The disease produced by *M. pneumoniae* is complex; the immunologic response of the host may be responsible for the manifestations of disease itself as well as for protection against infection, depending on the qualitative and quantitative balance of humoral and cellular immunity. Although well documented that specific cell-mediated immunity and antibody titers against *M. pneumoniae* increase with age (and therefore probably follow repeated infections), the immune mechanisms that protect against or resolve infection are not defined. Patients with immunodeficiencies such as hypogammaglobulinemia and sickle cell disease may have more severe mycoplasmal pneumonia than do immunocompetent hosts. *M. pneumoniae* may persist for years in the respiratory tract of patients with hypogammaglobulinemia despite multiple courses of antibiotics. *M. pneumoniae* is a common infectious causes of acute chest syndrome in sickle cell disease, but is not prevalent in patients with AIDS.

CLINICAL MANIFESTATIONS. Bronchopneumonia is the most commonly recognized clinical syndrome associated with *M. pneumoniae* infection. Although the onset of illness may be abrupt, it is usually characterized by gradual onset of headache, malaise, fever, and sore throat, followed by progression of lower respiratory symptoms including hoarseness and cough. Coryza is unusual with *M. pneumoniae* pneumonia and usually suggests a viral etiology. Although the clinical course in untreated individuals is variable, coughing usually worsens during the 1st wk of illness, with all symptoms usually resolving within 2 wk. The cough is initially nonproductive, but older children and adolescents may produce a frothy, white sputum. The severity of symptoms is usually greater than that suggested by the physical signs, which appear later in the disease. Crackles or rales, which are fine and resemble those heard in asthma and bronchiolitis, are the most prominent signs. With progression of the disease, the fever intensifies, the cough becomes more troublesome, and the patient may become dyspneic.

Radiographic findings are not specific. Pneumonia is usually described as interstitial or bronchopneumonic; involvement is most common in the lower lobes, with unilateral, centrally dense infiltrates described in 75% of cases. Lobar pneumonia is seen infrequently. Hilar lymphadenopathy may occur in up to 33% of patients. Significant amounts of pleural fluid are unusual, but patients with large pleural effusions due to *M. pneumoniae* have been described as having severe disease associated with lobar infiltrates and necrotizing pneumonia. The white blood cell and differential counts are usually normal, whereas the erythrocyte sedimentation rate is usually elevated.

Additional respiratory illnesses caused infrequently by *M. pneumoniae* include undifferentiated upper respiratory tract infections, pharyngitis, sinusitis, croup, and bronchiolitis. *M. pneumoniae* may be a common trigger of wheezing in asthmatic children or may cause chronic colonization and resulting lung dysfunction in adolescent and adult asthma patients. Otitis media and bullous myringitis have been described but are rarely seen without associated lower respiratory tract infection.

DIAGNOSIS. No specific clinical, epidemiologic, or laboratory observations permit a definite diagnosis of mycoplasmal infection early in the clinical course. Certain observations, however, are suggestive and can be helpful. Pneumonia in school-aged children and young adults, especially if cough is a prominent finding, is always suggestive of *M. pneumoniae* disease. Cultures on special media of the throat or sputum may demonstrate *M. pneumoniae*, but growth is rarely detected earlier than 1 wk, and few commercial laboratories maintain the capability of culturing *M. pneumoniae*. Positive immunoglobulin M (IgM) *M. pneumoniae* antibody identified by indirect fluorescence or enzyme-linked immune assay (EIA) more specifically supports the diagnosis. IgM antibodies may be positive for 6–12 mo after infection. A 4-fold increase in IgG *M. pneumoniae* antibody titer, by complement fixation or EIA, between acute and convalescent sera obtained 10 days to 3 wk after the onset of illness is diagnostic. PCR of a nasopharyngeal or throat swab (doing both may increase sensitivity) for *M. pneumoniae* DNA is very specific (>97%) in many studies; sensitivity when compared to 4-fold antibody titer rise may only be 50–70%. When *M. pneumoniae* is confirmed in the community in a few patients, the probability of the existence of more widespread mycoplasmal illness is greatly increased.

TREATMENT. *M. pneumoniae* illness is usually mild, and hospitalization is infrequently required. *M. pneumoniae* is exceptionally sensitive to erythromycin, clarithromycin, azithromycin, and the tetracyclines in vitro, which are effective in shortening the course of mycoplasmal illnesses, although they are not mycoplasmacidal. Hence, there may be delay in eradicating the organism from the respiratory tract. Two multicenter studies of pediatric community-acquired pneumonia demonstrated equal efficacy between erythromycin and clarithromycin or azithromycin. These newer macrolides were better tolerated and more effective at eradication of *M. pneumoniae* from the respiratory tract. The recommended treatment is clarithromycin (15 mg/kg/day divided bid PO for 10 days) or azithromycin (10 mg/kg once PO on day 1 and 5 mg/kg once daily PO on days 2–5), which eradicate *M. pneumoniae* in 100% of patients studied. Prophylaxis with azithromycin has been shown to substantially reduce the secondary attack rate in institutional outbreaks.

COMPLICATIONS. Complications, including bacterial superinfection, are unusual. Despite the reportedly rare isolation of *M. pneumoniae* from nonrespiratory sites such as joints, pleural fluid, and cerebrospinal fluid (CSF), the availability of PCR to detect specific segments of *M. pneumoniae* DNA has led to increasing identification of *M. pneumoniae* in nonrespiratory sites, particularly the central nervous system (CNS). Extrarespiratory illness may therefore involve direct invasion with *M. pneumoniae* or may involve autoimmune mechanisms, which is reflected by the frequency with which human antigens cross react with *M. pneumoniae*. Patients with or without respiratory symptoms may manifest illness involving the skin, CNS, blood, heart, gastrointestinal tract, and joints. Skin lesions include a variety of exanthems, most notably maculopapular rashes, erythema multiforme, and Stevens-Johnson syndrome. Stevens-Johnson syndrome associated with *M. pneumoniae* usually develops 3–21 days after initial respiratory symptoms, lasts less than 14 days, and is rarely associated with severe complications (Figs. 220-1 and 220-2).

Neurologic complications include meningoencephalitis, transverse myelitis, aseptic meningitis, cerebellar ataxia, Bell palsy, deafness, brainstem syndrome, acute demyelinating encephalitis, and Guillain-Barré syndrome. Neurologic complications occur 3–28 days (mean 10 days) after respiratory illness but may not be preceded by respiratory illness in 20% of cases. Encephalitis occurring within 5 days of the onset of prodromal symptoms may be caused by direct *M. pneumoniae* infection of the CNS, whereas encephalitis occurring >7 days after onset of prodromal symptoms is more likely to be autoimmune. *M. pneumoniae* accounts for 1–15% of all forms of childhood encephalitis and most commonly manifests as seizures, impaired consciousness, facial motor deficit, ataxia, or meningeal signs. Concomitant infection with viral agents such as herpes simplex virus, human herpesvirus 6, enteroviruses, or respiratory viruses may be common. Involvement of the brainstem may result in severe dystonia and movement disorders. The CSF may be normal or have mild mononuclear pleocytosis. Diagnosis is confirmed with positive CSF PCR, positive PCR from a throat swab, or the presence of definitive serum antibody titers. Findings on MRI include focal ischemic changes, ventriculomegaly, diffuse edema, or multifocal white matter inflammatory lesions consistent with postinfectious demyelinating encephalomyelitis. Neurologic sequelae occur in 20–30% of patients.

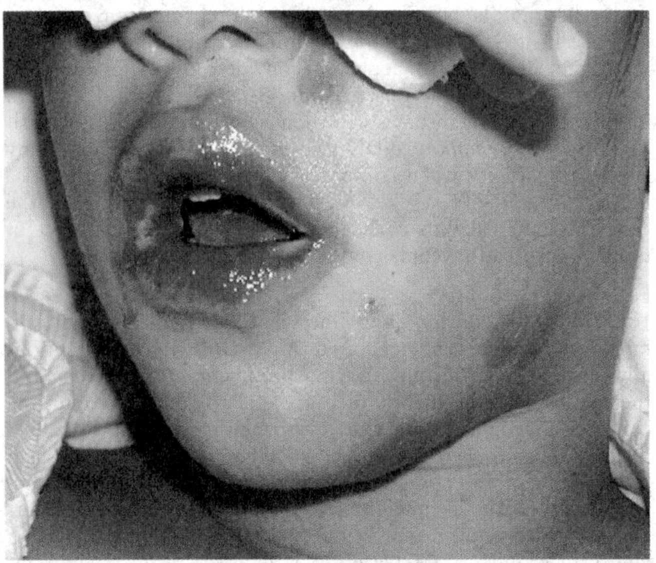

Figure 220-1. Lip changes found in Stevens-Johnson syndrome associated with *Mycoplasma pneumoniae* infection.

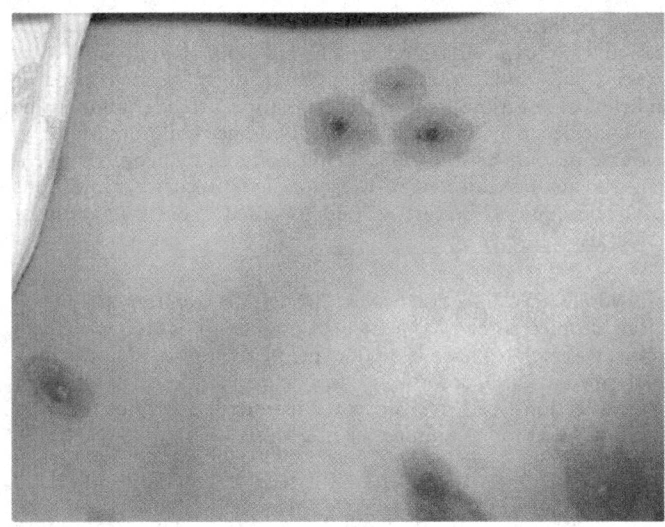

Figure 220-2. Classic erythema multiforme skin lesions found in Stevens-Johnson syndrome associated with *Mycoplasma pneumoniae* infection.

Common **hematologic complications** include mild degrees of hemolysis with positive Coombs test and minor reticulocytosis 2–3 wk after the onset of illness. Severe hemolysis, which is associated with high titers of cold hemagglutinins (≥1:512), is rare, as are thrombocytopenia and coagulation defects. Mild hepatitis, pancreatitis, and protein-losing hypertrophic gastropathy are rarely reported gastrointestinal complications. Myocarditis, pericarditis, and a rheumatic fever–like syndrome are uncommon manifestations, but arrhythmias, ST- and T-wave changes, and cardiac dilation with heart failure may accompany *M. pneumoniae* infection in adults more commonly than children. Transient monoarticular arthritis was described in 1% of patients in 1 large series.

It is unclear from existing literature whether antibiotic treatment of *M. pneumoniae* infection decreases the risk for complications. There is also no specific established therapy for most of the complications. Corticosteroids have been the most frequently used agents in the management of severe *M. pneumoniae* complications, particularly neurologic complications.

PROGNOSIS. Fatal *M. pneumoniae* infections are rare. Anatomic abnormalities such as altered lung perfusion, mild bronchiectasis, and bronchial wall thickening were detected by high-resolution CT in 37% of children 1–2 yr following *M. pneumoniae* pneumonia. Abnormalities in pulmonary gas diffusion have been reported in nearly half of children 6 mo after recovery from *M. pneumoniae*. Patients generally recover without complications, although sequelae of encephalitis may be severe and permanent.

Daxboeck F, Blacky A, Seidl R, et al: Diagnosis, treatment, and prognosis of *Mycoplasma pneumoniae* childhood encephalitis: Systematic review of 58 cases. *J Child Neurol* 2004;19:865–871.

Daxboeck F, Krause R, Wenisch C: Laboratory diagnosis of *Mycoplasma pneumoniae* infection. *Clin Microbiol Infect* 2003;9:263–273.

Korppi M: Community-acquired pneumonia in children. *Pediatr Drugs* 2003;5:821–832.

Korppi M, Heiskanen-Kosma T, Kleemola M: Incidence of community-acquired pneumonia in children caused by *Mycoplasma pneumoniae*: Serological results of a prospective, population-based study in primary health care. *Respirology* 2004;9:109–114.

Kraft M, Cassell GH, Pak J, et al: *Mycoplasma pneumoniae* and *Chlamydia pneumoniae* in asthma. *Chest* 2002;121:1782–1788.

Krause DC, Balish MF: Cellular engineering in a minimal microbe: Structure and assembly of the terminal organelle of *Mycoplasma pneumoniae*. *Mol Microbiol* 2004;51:917–924.

Marrie TJ, Beecroft M, Herman-Gnjidic Z, et al: Symptom resolution in patients with Mycoplasma pneumoniae pneumonia. *Can Respir J* 2004;11:573–577.

McIntosh K: Community-acquired pneumonia in children. *N Engl J Med* 2002;346:429–437.

Michelow IC, Olsen K, Lozano J, et al: Epidemiology and clinical characteristics of community-acquired pneumonia in hospitalized children. *Pediatrics* 2004;113:701–707.

Waites KB, Talkington DF: *Mycoplasma pneumoniae* and its role as a human pathogen. *Clin Microbiol Rev* 2004;17:697–728.

Wang RS, Wang SY, Hsieh KS, et al: Necrotizing pneumonitis caused by Mycoplasma pneumoniae in pediatric patients: Report of five cases and review of literature. *Pediatr Infect Dis J* 2004;23:564–567.

Yang J, Hooper WC, Phillips DJ, et al: Cytokines in *Mycoplasma pneumoniae* infections. *Cytokine Growth Factor Rev* 2004;15:157–168.

Chapter 221 ■ Genital Mycoplasmas (*Mycoplasma Hominis, Mycoplasma Genitalium,* and *Ureaplasma Urealyticum*)

Dwight A. Powell

Three *Mycoplasma* species, *Mycoplasma hominis, Mycoplasma genitalium,* and *Ureaplasma urealyticum,* are human urogenital pathogens. They are often associated with sexually transmitted infections such as nongonococcal urethritis (NGU) or puerperal infections such as endometritis. *M. hominis* and *U. urealyticum* commonly colonize the female genital tract and may cause chorioamnionitis, colonization of neonates, and perinatal infections. *M. genitalium* is a cause of NGU. Two other genital *Mycoplasma* species, *M. fermentans* and *M. penetrans,* are identified in respiratory or genitourinary secretions with greater frequency in HIV-infected patients.

ETIOLOGY. *M. hominis* and *U. urealyticum* require sterols for growth and can grow in cell-free media, and produce characteristic colonies on agar. Colonies of *M. hominis* are 200-300 µm in diameter with a "fried-egg" appearance. (Colonies of *U. urealyticum* are 16–60 µm in diameter.) These organisms are resistant to β-lactams because they lack a cell wall, and resistant to sulfonamides and trimethoprim because they do not produce folic acid. All 7 serovars of *M. hominis* are susceptible to clindamycin, moderately susceptible to chloramphenicol, and resistant to erythromycin and rifampin. Aminoglycosides have limited activity. Increasing numbers of tetracycline-resistant strains are being reported. There are 14 serovars of *U. urealyticum,* and most are susceptible to erythromycin, clarithromycin, and quinolones but resistant to clindamycin. Susceptibility to aminoglycosides and tetracyclines is variable. *M. genitalium* can be isolated with difficulty only in cell culture systems. Identification in most studies has required polymerase chain reaction (PCR).

EPIDEMIOLOGY. *M. hominis* and *U. urealyticum* colonize the genital and urinary tracts of postpubertal females and males. Female colonization is maximal in the vagina and less in the endocervix, urethra, or endometrium. Male colonization occurs primarily in the urethra. Colonization rates are directly related to sexual activity and are highest among persons with multiple sexual partners. Colonization rates are <10% among prepubertal children and sexually inactive adults, and vary from 40 to 90% among pregnant females.

TRANSMISSION. Genital mycoplasmas are transmitted by sexual contact. *M. genitalium* has been identified predominantly in the male urethra and is capable of attaching to human spermatozoa, suggesting a mechanism for sexual transmissibility.

Vertical transmission rates among neonates born to colonized women are 25–60%. The usual route of neonatal acquisition is contamination from colonized amniotic fluid or during vaginal delivery. However, neonatal colonization can occur in the presence of intact amniotic fluid membranes and with delivery by cesarean section. Neonatal colonization rates are higher among infants weighing <1,500 g, being born in the presence of chorioamnionitis, and newborns to mothers of lower socioeconomic status. Organisms are recovered from the newborn's throat, vagina, rectum, and, occasionally, eyes for as long as 3 mo after birth.

PATHOLOGY AND PATHOGENESIS. Genital mycoplasmas can produce chronic inflammation of the genitourinary tract and amniotic fluid membranes. *U. urealyticum* may infect the amniotic sac early in gestation without rupturing the fetal membranes, resulting in a clinically silent, chronic chorioamnionitis characterized by an intense inflammatory response. Attachment to fetal human tracheal epithelium can cause ciliary disarray, clumping, and loss of epithelial cells. *U. urealyticum* induces macrophages in vitro to increase production of interleukin 6 (IL-6) and tumor necrosis factor 2. Very low birthweight infants colonized with *U. urealyticum* have increased levels of monocyte chemoattractant protein and IL-8, which are proinflammatory agents possibly associated with development of bronchopulmonary dysplasia. Immunity appears to require serotype-specific antibody. Thus, a lack of maternal antibody may account for a higher risk for disease in premature newborns.

CLINICAL MANIFESTATIONS. In adults and sexually active adolescents, genital mycoplasmas are associated with sexually transmitted diseases and uncommonly associated with focal infections outside the genital tract. *M. hominis* has been described causing septicemia, endocarditis, wound infection, osteomyelitis, lymphadenitis, pneumonia, meningitis, brain abscess, and arthritis. Life-threatening mediastinitis, sternal wound infections, pleuritis, peritonitis, and pericarditis have been reported with high mortality rates in patients following organ transplantation. Extragenital *U. urealyticum* infections are rarely described but include osteomyelitis, arthritis, meningitis, mediastinitis, infection of aortic grafts, and postcesarean wound infections. Patients with hypogammaglobulinemia appear to be at high risk for chronic arthritis caused by various *Mycoplasma.*

U. urealyticum and *M. genitalium* are recognized pathogens of NGU. Approximately 30% of NGU in males may be caused by these organisms either alone or with *Chlamydia trachomatis* (see Chapter 223). Disease is most common in young adults but is also prevalent in sexually active adolescents. The average incubation period is 2–3 wk, with symptoms typically consisting of scanty, mucoid-white urethral discharge, dysuria, and penile discomfort. The discharge is often evident only in the morning or after the urethra is stripped. Rare complications of NGU are epididymitis and proctitis. Approximately 20–60% of patients with acute NGU develop recurrent or chronic urethritis despite 1–

2 wk of treatment. *U. urealyticum* and *M. genitalium* appear to be the most likely agents of chronic symptomatic urethritis. Females rarely have urethritis, and despite high vaginal colonization rates, vaginitis or cervicitis is uncommon. *M. hominis* is an occasional contributing cause of pelvic inflammatory disease, and both genital mycoplasmas are rarely associated with endometritis and postpartum sepsis.

Neonates. Genital mycoplasmas are associated with a variety of fetal and neonatal infections. *U. urealyticum* may cause clinically inapparent chorioamnionitis resulting in an 8-fold increase in fetal death or premature delivery. Up to 50% of infants <34 wk of gestational age may have *U. urealyticum* recovered from tracheal, blood, cerebrospinal fluid (CSF), or lung biopsy specimens. The role of these organisms causing severe respiratory insufficiency, the need for assisted ventilation, the development of bronchopulmonary dysplasia, or death remains controversial. Early studies demonstrated that infants weighing <1,000 g with *U. urealyticum* isolated from tracheal aspirates within the 1st 24 hr of life were twice as likely to die or develop chronic lung disease compared with uninfected infants of similar birthweight or those weighing >1,000 g. More recent studies, controlling for gestational age and other factors, have shown no correlation between the respiratory isolation of *U. urealyticum* and development of bronchopulmonary dysplasia, duration of ventilatory support, oxygen dependency, or length of hospitalization. Furthermore, 2 small prospective studies of erythromycin therapy in high-risk preterm infants with tracheobronchial colonization of *U. urealyticum* failed to show any difference in treated versus nontreated infants in the development of chronic lung disease.

M. hominis and *U. urealyticum* have been isolated from the CSF of premature and, in a few cases, full-term infants. Simultaneous isolation of other pathogens is unusual, and most infants have no overt signs of central nervous system infection. CSF pleocytosis is not a consistent observation, and spontaneous clearance of mycoplasmas has been documented without specific therapy. *U. urealyticum* meningitis has been associated with intraventricular hemorrhage and hydrocephalus. Meningitis caused by *M. hominis* may be benign. The onset of meningitis varies from 1 to 196 days of life; organisms may persist in the CSF without therapy for days to weeks. *M. hominis* and *U. urealyticum* have been described to cause neonatal conjunctivitis, lymphadenitis, pharyngitis, pneumonitis, osteomyelitis, brain abscess, meningoencephalitis, and scalp abscess.

DIAGNOSIS. Confirmation of genital tract infection is difficult because of high colonization rates in the vagina and urethra. NGU is confirmed by Gram stain of urethral discharge showing at least 3 polymorphonuclear leukocytes per oil-immersion field and the absence of gram-negative diplococci (i.e., *Neisseria gonorrhoeae*). A urethral swab or exudate should be cultured for *C. trachomatis* and *U. urealyticum*. *M. genitalium* can only be identified by PCR testing.

Neonates. *U. urealyticum* and *M. hominis* have been isolated from urine, blood, CSF, tracheal aspirates, pleural fluid, abscesses, and lung tissue. Premature neonates who are clinically ill with pneumonitis, focal abscesses, or central nervous system disease (particularly progressive hydrocephalus with or without pleocytosis) for whom bacterial cultures are negative or in whom there is no improvement with standard antibiotic therapy warrant cultures for genital mycoplasmas. Isolation requires special media, and clinical specimens must be cultured immediately or be frozen at −80°C to avoid loss of organisms. When inoculated into broth containing arginine (for *M. hominis*) or urea (for *U. urealyticum*), growth is indicated by an alkaline pH. Identification of *U. urealyticum* on agar requires 1–2 days of growth and visualization with the dissecting microscope, whereas *M. hominis* is apparent to the eye but may require 1 wk to grow. Cultures from the upper respiratory tract are probably meaningless owing to high colonization rates. Cultures of the lower respiratory tract through endotracheal aspirate or biopsy are essential.

TREATMENT. NGU attributed to genital mycoplasmas in adolescents and adults is treated with azithromycin (1 g PO as a single dose) or doxycycline (100 mg bid PO for 7 days). Sexual partners should also be treated to avoid recurrent disease in the index case. Nongenital mycoplasmal infections may require surgical drainage and prolonged antibiotic therapy. *M. hominis* is resistant to erythromycin and other macrolide antibiotics but usually susceptible to clindamycin, and variably susceptible to quinolones and tetracycline. *U. urealyticum* is susceptible to tetracycline, aminoglycosides, and quinolones. Recurrence rates may be high following treatment of *M. genitalium* with tetracyclines or single-dose azithromycin. An initial azithromycin dose of 500 mg followed by 200 mg daily for 4 days provided excellent cures in 1 study.

Neonates. Therapy for neonatal genital mycoplasma infections is indicated in infections associated with a pure growth of the organism and evidence that the disease manifestations are compatible with an infectious process rather than merely colonization. The role of therapy in preventing chronic lung disease in very low birthweight infants awaits results of further studies. Treatment is based on predictable antimicrobial sensitivities because susceptibility testing is not readily available for individual isolates. For symptomatic central nervous system infections, doxycycline is recommended. The long-term consequences of asymptomatic central nervous system infection with genital mycoplasmas, especially in the absence of pleocytosis, are unknown. Because mycoplasmas may spontaneously clear from the CSF, therapy should involve minimal risks.

Anagius C, Lore B, Jensen JS: *Mycoplasma genitalium*: Prevalence, clinical significance, and transmission. *Sex Transm Infect* 2005;81:458–462.

Horner P, Thomas B, Gilroy CB, et al: Role of Mycoplasma genitalium and Ureaplasma urealyticum in acute and chronic nongonococcal urethritis. *Clin Infect Dis* 2001;32:995–1003.

Jesen JS: *Mycoplasma genitalium*: The etiological agent of urethritis and other sexually transmitted diseases. *J Eur Acad Dermatol Venereol* 2004;18:1–11.

Kotecha S, Hodge R, Schaber JA, et al: Pulmonary *Ureaplasma urealyticum* is associated with the development of acute lung inflammation and chronic lung disease in preterm infants. *Pediatr Res* 2004;55:61–68.

Mabanta CG, Pryhuber GS, Weinberg GA, et al: Erythromycin for the prevention of chronic lung disease in intubated preterm infants at risk for, or colonized or infected with *Ureaplasma urealyticum*. *Cochrane Database Syst Rev* 2003;CD003744.

Mhanna MJ, DeLong LJ, Aziz HF: The value of *Ureaplasma urealyticum* tracheal culture and treatment in premature infants following a acute respiratory deterioration. *J Perinatol* 2003;23:541–544.

Ollikainen J, Korppi M, Heiskanen-Kosma T, et al: Chronic lung disease of the newborn is not associated with Ureaplasma urealyticum. *Pediatr Pulmonol* 2001;32:303–307.

Rao RP, Ghanayem NS, Kaufman BA, et al: *Mycoplasma hominis* and *Ureaplasma* species brain abscess in a neonate. *Pediatric Infect Dis J* 2002;21:1083–1085.

Schlicht MJ, Lovrich SD, Sartin JS et al: High prevalence of genital mycoplasmas among sexually active young adults with urethritis or cervical symptoms in La Crosse, Wisconsin. *J Clin Microbiol* 2004;42:4636–4640.

Taylor-Robinson D: *Mycoplasma genitalium*—an update. *Int J STD AIDS* 2002;13:145–151.

Theilen U, Lyon AJ, Fitzgerald T, et al: Infection with *Ureaplasma urealyticum*: Is there a specific clinical and radiologic course in the preterm infant? *Arch Dis Child Fetal Neonatol Ed* 2004;89:F163–F167.

Section 10 — Chlamydial Infections

Chapter 222 ■ Chlamydophila Pneumoniae Margaret R. Hammerschlag

Chlamydophila (Chlamydia) pneumoniae is a common cause of lower respiratory tract diseases, including pneumonia in children and bronchitis and pneumonia in adults. The 1st isolates of *C. pneumoniae* were obtained during studies of trachoma in the 1960s. Subsequent serologic studies demonstrated that the organism caused an outbreak of mild pneumonia among school children in Finland in 1978. In 1986, the organism was isolated from the respiratory tract of college students with acute respiratory disease.

ETIOLOGY. Chlamydiae are obligate intracellular pathogens that have established a unique niche within the host cell. Chlamydiae cause a variety of diseases in animal species at virtually all phylogenic levels. Recent taxonomic analysis using the 16S and 23S ribosomal RNA genes has supported splitting the genus *Chlamydia* into 2 genera, *Chlamydia* and *Chlamydophila* (Table 222-1). *Chlamydia* includes *C. trachomatis* and 2 new species, *C. muridarum* (MoPn, formerly known as the agent of mouse pneumonitis) and *C. suis*. *Chlamydophila* includes *C. pecorum*, *C. pneumoniae*, *C. psittaci*, and 3 new species split out from *C. psittaci*: *C. abortus*, *C. caviae* (formerly known as *C. psittaci* guinea pig conjunctivitis strain), and *C. felis*. The most significant human pathogens are *C. pneumoniae* and *C. trachomatis* (see Chapter 223). *C. psittaci* is the cause of psittacosis, an important zoonosis (see Chapter 224).

Chlamydiae have a gram-negative envelope without detectable peptidoglycan, although recent genomic analysis has revealed that both *C. pneumoniae* and *C. trachomatis* encode proteins forming a nearly complete pathway for synthesis of peptidoglycan, including penicillin-binding proteins. Chlamydiae also share a group-specific lipopolysaccharide antigen and use host adenosine triphosphate (ATP) for the synthesis of chlamydial proteins.

TABLE 222-1. Classification of Chlamydiae

GENUS	SPECIES	HOST(S)	MAJOR DISEASES
Chlamydia	*C. trachomatis*	Humans	Trachoma, urethritis, cervicitis, pelvic inflammatory disease, neonatal conjunctivitis and pneumonia, lymphogranuloma venereum
	C. suis	Pigs	Gastrointestinal disease
	C. muridarum	Mice	Pneumonia
Chlamydophila	*C. Pneumoniae*	Humans Koalas Bandicoots Amphibians Reptiles	Pneumonia, bronchitis
	C. psittaci	Birds Humans	Gastrointestinal disease, pneumonia
	C. abortus	Cattle Sheep	Abortion
	C. pecorum	Cattle Sheep Koalas	Pneumonia, gastrointestinal disease, genital infections, conjunctivitis
	C. felis	Cats	Keratoconjunctivitis
	C. caviae	Guinea pigs	Conjunctivitis, genital infections

Although chlamydiae are auxotrophic for 3 of 4 nucleoside triphosphates, they do encode functional glucose-catabolizing enzymes that can be used for generation of ATP. As with peptidoglycan synthesis, for some reason these genes are turned off. All chlamydiae also encode an abundant protein called the major outer membrane protein (MOMP, or OmpA) that is surface exposed in *C. trachomatis* and *C. psittaci*, but apparently not in *C. pneumoniae*. The MOMP is the major determinant of the serologic classification of *C. trachomatis* and *C. psittaci* isolates.

EPIDEMIOLOGY. *C. pneumoniae* is primarily a human respiratory pathogen. The organism has also been isolated from nonhuman species, including horse, koalas, reptiles, and amphibians, where it also causes respiratory infection, although the role these infections may play in transmission to humans is unknown. *C. pneumoniae* appears to affect individuals of all ages. The proportion of community-acquired pneumonias associated with *C. pneumoniae* infection is 2–19% varying with geographic location, the age group examined, and the diagnostic methods used. Several studies of the role of *C. pneumoniae* in lower respiratory tract infection in pediatric populations have found evidence of infection from none to more than 18%. Most of these studies have relied entirely on serology for diagnosis. A large multicenter study of community-acquired pneumonia in children 3–12 yr of age found evidence of *C. pneumoniae* infection, based on culture, in 14% and *Mycoplasma pneumoniae* in 22%. The prevalence of *C. pneumoniae* infection is 15% among children <6 yr of age and 18% among children >6 yr of age. Almost 20% of the children with *C. pneumoniae* infection were co-infected with *M. pneumoniae*. *C. pneumoniae* may also be responsible for 10–20% of episodes of **acute chest syndrome in children with sickle cell disease,** 10% of episodes of bronchitis, and 5–10% episodes of pharyngitis in children. Transmission probably occurs from person to person through respiratory droplets. Spread of the infection can occur among members in the same household or individuals in enclosed populations, such as military recruits, and in nursing homes.

PATHOGENESIS. Chlamydiae are characterized by a unique developmental cycle (Fig. 222-1) with morphologically distinct infectious and reproductive forms: the elementary body (EB) and reticulate body (RB). Following infection, the infectious EBs, which are 200–400 μm in diameter, attach to the host cell by a process of electrostatic binding and are taken into the cell by endocytosis that does not depend on the microtubule system. Within the host cell, the EB remains within a membrane-lined phagosome. The phagosome does not fuse with the host cell lysosome. The inclusion membrane is devoid of host cell markers, but lipid markers traffic to the inclusion, which suggests a functional interaction with the Golgi apparatus. The EBs then differentiate into RBs that undergo binary fission. After approximately 36 hr, the RBs differentiate into EBs. At about 48 hr, release may occur by cytolysis or by a process of exocytosis or extrusion of the whole inclusion, leaving the host cell intact. Chlamydiae may also enter a persistent state after treatment with certain cytokines such as interferon-γ, treatment with antibiotics, or restriction of certain nutrients. While chlamydiae are in the persistent state, metabolic activity is reduced. The ability to cause prolonged, often subclinical, infection is 1 of the major characteristics of chlamydiae.

CLINICAL MANIFESTATIONS. Infections caused by *C. pneumoniae* cannot be readily differentiated from those caused by other res-

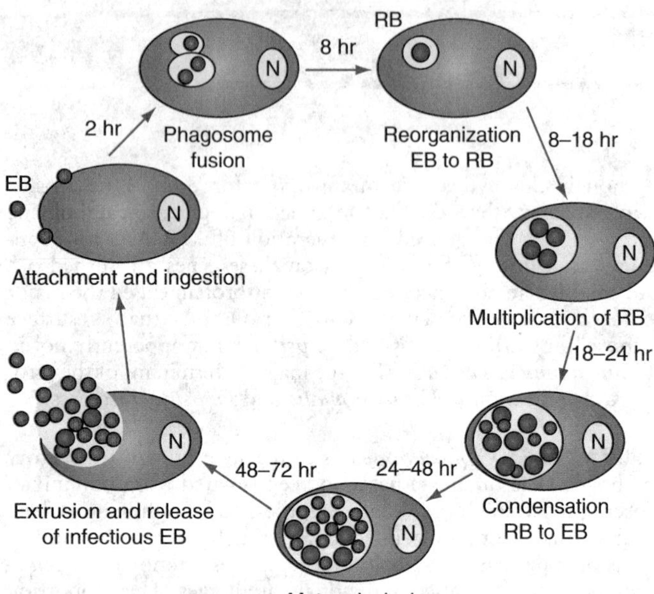

Figure 222-1. Life cycle of chlamydiae in epithelial cells. EB, elementary body; RB, reticulate body. (From Hammerschlag MR: Infections due to *Chlamydia trachomatis* and *Chlamydia pneumoniae* in children and adolescents. *Pediatr Rev* 2004;25:43–50.)

piratory pathogens, especially *M. pneumoniae.* The pneumonia usually presents as a classic atypical (or nonbacterial) pneumonia characterized by mild to moderate constitutional symptoms including fever, malaise, headache, cough, and frequently pharyngitis. However, severe pneumonia with pleural effusions and empyema has been described.

C. pneumoniae may serve as an infectious trigger for asthma and can cause pulmonary exacerbations in patients with cystic fibrosis. *C. pneumoniae* has been isolated from middle ear aspirates of children with acute otitis media, but is usually associated with bacterial otitis media. Asymptomatic respiratory infection has been documented in 2–5% of adults and children and may persist for a year or more.

DIAGNOSIS. It is not possible to differentiate *C. pneumoniae* from other causes of atypical pneumonia on the basis of clinical findings. Auscultation reveals the presence of rales and often wheezing. The chest radiograph often appears worse than the patient's clinical status would indicate and may show mild, diffuse involvement or lobar infiltrates with small pleural effusions. The complete blood count may be elevated with a left shift but is usually unremarkable.

Specific diagnosis of *C. pneumoniae* infection is based on isolation of the organism in tissue culture. *C. pneumoniae* grows best in cycloheximide-treated HEp-2 and HL cells. The optimum site for culture is the posterior nasopharynx; the specimen is collected with wire-shafted swabs in the same manner as that used for *C. trachomatis.* The organism can be isolated from sputum, throat cultures, bronchoalveolar lavage fluid, and pleural fluid, but few laboratories perform such cultures because of technical difficulties.

Polymerase chain reaction (PCR) testing is the most promising technology in the development of a rapid, nonculture method for detection of *C. pneumoniae.* However, no PCR assay is commercially available or has Food and Drug Administration approval and no PCR is standardized or has been extensively validated compared with culture for detection of *C. pneumoniae* in respiratory specimens.

Serologic diagnosis can be accomplished using the microimmunofluorescence (MIF) or the complement fixation (CF) tests. The CF test is genus specific and is also used for diagnosis of lymphogranuloma venereum (see Chapter 223.4) and psittacosis (see Chapter 224). Its sensitivity in hospitalized patients with *C. pneumoniae* infection and children is variable. The Centers for Disease Control and Prevention (CDC) recently proposed modifications in the serologic criteria for diagnosis. Although the MIF test was considered to be the only currently acceptable serologic test, the criteria were made significantly more stringent. Acute infection, using the MIF test, was defined by a 4-fold increase in immunoglobulin G (IgG) titer or an IgM titer of 16 or greater; use of a single elevated IgG titer was discouraged. An IgG titer of 16 or greater was thought to indicate past exposure, but neither elevated IgA titers nor any other serologic marker was thought to be a valid indicator of persistent or chronic infection. Because diagnosis would require paired sera, this would be a retrospective diagnosis. The CDC did not recommend the use of any enzyme-linked immune assay for detection of antibody to *C. pneumoniae* because there is concern about the inconsistent correlation of these results with culture results. Studies of *C. pneumoniae* infection in children with pneumonia and asthma show that more than 50% of children with culture-documented infection have no detectable MIF antibody.

TREATMENT. The optimum dose and duration of antimicrobial therapy for *C. pneumoniae* infections remain uncertain. Most treatment studies have used serology only for diagnosis; thus, the microbiologic efficacy cannot be assessed. Prolonged therapy for ≥2 wk may be desirable because recrudescent symptoms and persistent positive cultures have been described following 2 wk of erythromycin and 30 days of tetracycline or doxycycline.

Tetracyclines, erythromycin, the newer macrolides (azithromycin and clarithromycin), and quinolones show in vitro activity. Like *C. psittaci, C. pneumoniae* is resistant to sulfonamides. The results of recent treatment studies have shown that erythromycin (40 mg/kg/day divided bid PO for 10 days), clarithromycin (15 mg/kg/day divided bid PO for 10 days), and azithromycin (10 mg/kg PO on day 1, then 5 mg/kg/day PO on days 2–5) are effective for eradication of *C. pneumoniae* from the nasopharynx of children with pneumonia in approximately 80% of cases.

PROGNOSIS. Clinical response to antibiotic therapy varies. Coughing often persists for several weeks even after therapy.

Block S, Hedrick J, Hammerschlag MR, et al: *Mycoplasma pneumoniae* and *Chlamydia pneumoniae* in pediatric community-acquired pneumonia. Comparative efficacy and safety of clarithromycin vs. erythromycin ethylsuccinate. *Pediatr Infect Dis J* 1995;14:471–477.

Dowell SF, Peeling RW, Boman J, et al: Standardizing *Chlamydia pneumoniae* assays: Recommendations from the Centers for Disease Control and Prevention (USA) and the Laboratory Centre for Disease Control (Canada). *Clin Infect Dis* 2001;33:492–503.

Hammerschlag MR: Intracellular life of chlamydiae. *Semin Pediatr Infect Dis* 2002;4:239–248.

Hammerschlag MR: Pneumonia due to *Chlamydia pneumoniae* in children: Epidemiology, diagnosis and treatment. *Pediatr Pulmonol* 2003;36: 384–390.

Harris J-A, Kolokathis A, Campbell M, et al: Safety and efficacy of azithromycin in the treatment of community acquired pneumonia in children. *Pediatr Infect Dis J* 1998;17:865–871.

Rockey DD, Lenart J, Stephens RS: Genome sequencing and our understanding of chlamydiae. *Infect Immunol* 2000;68:5473–5479.

Chapter 223 ■ *Chlamydia Trachomatis*

Chlamydia trachomatis is subdivided into 2 biovars: lymphogranuloma venereum (LGV) and trachoma, which is the agent of human oculogenital diseases other than LGV. Although the strains of both biovars have almost complete DNA homology, they differ in growth characteristics and virulence in tissue culture and animals. In developed countries, *C. trachomatis* is the most prevalent sexually transmitted disease, causing urethritis in men, cervicitis and salpingitis in women, and conjunctivitis and pneumonia in infants.

223.1 • Trachoma

Trachoma is the most important preventable cause of **blindness** in the world. It is caused primarily by the A, B, Ba, and C serotypes of *C. trachomatis*. It is endemic in the Middle East and Southeast Asia and among Navajo Indians in the southwestern USA. In areas that are endemic for trachoma, such as Egypt, genital chlamydial infection is caused by the serotypes responsible for oculogenital disease: D, E, F, G, H, I, J, and K. The disease is spread from eye to eye. Flies are a frequent vector.

Trachoma begins as a **follicular conjunctivitis,** usually in early childhood. The follicles heal, leading to conjunctival scarring that may result in an entropion, with the eyelid turning inward so that the lashes abrade the cornea. It is the corneal ulceration secondary to the constant trauma that leads to scarring and blindness. Bacterial superinfection may also contribute to scarring. Blindness occurs years after the active disease.

Trachoma can be diagnosed clinically. The World Health Organization (WHO) suggests that at least 2 of 4 criteria must be present for a diagnosis of trachoma: (1) lymphoid follicles on the upper tarsal conjunctivae, (2) typical conjunctival scarring, (3) vascular pannus, and (4) limbal follicles. The diagnosis is confirmed by culture or staining tests for *C. trachomatis* performed during the active stage of disease. Serologic tests are not helpful clinically because of the long duration of the disease and the high seroprevalence in endemic populations.

Poverty and lack of sanitation are important factors in the spread of trachoma. As socioeconomic conditions improve, the incidence of the disease decreases substantially. Endemic trachoma has been controlled in most instances by administering topical tetracyclines (or, rarely, erythromycin ointment) daily for periods of 6–10 wk or intermittently over a 6 mo period. Oral doxycycline is effective but is contraindicated in children <9 yr of age. Oral erythromycin requires frequent dosing, which is impractical in the control of endemic trachoma. One study reported that 1–6 doses of oral azithromycin were equivalent to 30 days of treatment with topical oxytetracycline/polymyxin ointment. The WHO recommends single-dose azithromycin (20 mg/kg, maximum 1 g) for the treatment of trachoma in children. A recent study from Tanzania demonstrated that mass treatment with a single dose of azithromycin to all the residents of a village dramatically reduced the prevalence and intensity of infection. This effect continued for 2 yr after treatment, probably by interrupting the transmission of ocular *C. trachomatis* infection.

223.2 • Genital Tract Infections

EPIDEMIOLOGY. There are an estimated 3 million new cases of chlamydial sexually transmitted infections each year in the USA. *C. trachomatis* is a major cause of epididymitis and is the cause of 23–55% of all cases of nongonococcal urethritis, although the proportion of chlamydial nongonococcal urethritis has been gradually declining. As many as 50% of men with gonorrhea may be co-infected with *C. trachomatis*. The prevalence of chlamydial cervicitis among sexually active women is 2–35%. Rates of infection among girls 15–19 yr of age exceed 20% in many urban populations but can be as high as 15% in suburban populations as well.

Children who have been sexually abused may acquire anogenital *C. trachomatis* infection, which is usually asymptomatic. Culture is the only method that should be used for diagnosis of *C. trachomatis* from these sites when a prepubertal child is being tested for suspected sexual abuse. However, because perinatally acquired rectal and vaginal *C. trachomatis* infections may persist for ≥3 yr, the detection of *C. trachomatis* in the vagina or rectum of a young child is not absolute evidence of sexual abuse.

CLINICAL MANIFESTATIONS. The trachoma biovar of *C. trachomatis* causes a spectrum of disease in sexually active adolescents and adults. Up to 75% of women with *C. trachomatis* have no symptoms of infection. *C. trachomatis* can cause urethritis (acute urethral syndrome), epididymitis, cervicitis, salpingitis, proctitis, and pelvic inflammatory disease. The symptoms of chlamydial genital tract infections are less acute than those of gonorrhea, consisting of a discharge that is usually mucoid rather than purulent. Asymptomatic urethral infection is frequent in sexually active men. Autoinoculation from the genital tract to the eyes can lead to concomitant inclusion conjunctivitis.

DIAGNOSIS. Definitive diagnosis of genital chlamydial infection is accomplished by isolation of the organism in tissue culture and confirmed by microscopic identification of the characteristic inclusions using fluorescent antibody staining in culture specimens obtained from the urethra in men and the endocervix in women. Care should be taken to obtain epithelial cells, not only discharge. *C. trachomatis* can be cultured in cycloheximide-treated HeLa, McCoy, and HEp-2 cells. Chlamydia culture has been further defined by the Centers for Disease Control and Prevention (CDC) as isolation of the organism in tissue culture and as confirmation of the characteristic intracytoplasmic inclusions by fluorescent antibody staining.

Alternatively, a nonculture method, specifically a nucleic acid amplification test (NAAT) can be used. These tests have high sensitivity, perhaps even detecting 10–20% greater than culture, while retaining high specificity. There are currently three Food and Drug Administration (FDA)-approved, commercially available NAATs for detection of *C. trachomatis*: polymerase chain reaction (PCR; Amplicor Chlamydia test, Roche Molecular Diagnostics, Nutley, NJ); strand displacement amplification (SDA; ProbeTec, BD Diagnostic Systems, Sparks, MD); and transcription-mediated amplification (TMA; Amp CT, Gen-Probe, San Diego, CA). PCR and SDA are DNA amplification tests that use primers that target gene sequences on the cryptogenic *C. trachomatis* plasmid that are present at approximately 10 copies in each infected cell. TMA is a ribosomal RNA amplification assay. All three assays are also available as co-amplification tests for simultaneously detecting *C. trachomatis* and *Neisseria gonorrhoeae*. The currently available commercial NAATs are FDA approved for cervical swabs from adolescent and adult women, urethral swabs from adolescent and adult men, and urine from adolescent and adult men and women. The latest version of TMA was recently approved for use with vaginal swabs in adolescents and adults. Use of urine avoids the necessity for a clinical pelvic examination and may greatly facilitate screening in certain populations, especially adolescents, although using the NAAT on urine is less sensitive than endocervical swabs. As stated above, several studies have now demonstrated that vaginal swabs are superior to urine for NAAT and may be equivalent to endocervical specimens. It was also demonstrated that self-collected vaginal specimens were as good as those obtained by a health care professional.

Data on use of NAATs for vaginal specimens or urine from children are very limited and insufficient to allow making a recommendation for their use. The CDC recommends that NAATs may be used as an alternative to culture only if confirmation is available. Confirmation tests should consist of a 2nd FDA-approved NAAT that targets a different gene sequence from the initial test.

The etiology of most cases of nonchlamydial nongonococcal urethritis is unknown, although *Ureaplasma urealyticum* and possibly *Mycoplasma genitalium* are implicated in up to 1/3 of cases (see Chapter 221). Proctocolitis may develop in individuals who have a rectal infection with an LGV strain (see Subchapter 223.4).

TREATMENT. The 1st line treatment regimens recommended by the CDC for uncomplicated *C. trachomatis* genital infection in men and nonpregnant women are azithromycin (1 g orally PO as a single dose) or doxycycline (100 mg PO bid for 7 days). Alternative regimens are erythromycin base (500 mg PO qid for 7 days), erythromycin ethylsuccinate (800 mg PO qid for 7 days), ofloxacin (300 mg PO bid for 7 days), and levofloxacin (500 mg PO once daily for 7 days). The high erythromycin dosages may not be well tolerated. Doxycycline and ofloxacin or levofloxacin are contraindicated in pregnant women; quinolones are contraindicated in persons younger than 18 yr of age. However, use of ofloxacin and levofloxacin offer no advantages over doxycycline. For pregnant women, the recommended treatment regimen is erythromycin base (500 mg PO bid for 7 days) or amoxicillin (500 mg PO tid for 7 days). Alternative regimens are erythromycin base (250 mg PO qid for 14 days), erythromycin ethylsuccinate (800 mg PO qid for 7 days or 400 mg PO qid for 14 days), and azithromycin (1 g PO in a single dose). Amoxicillin at this dosage is as effective as any of the erythromycin regimens and is much better tolerated. However, experience with all these regimens is still limited.

Empirical treatment without microbiologic diagnosis is recommended only for patients at high risk for infection who are unlikely to return for follow-up evaluation, which includes adolescents with multiple sex partners. These patients should be treated empirically for both *C. trachomatis* and gonorrhea.

Sex partners of patients with nongonococcal urethritis should be treated if they have had sexual contact with the patient during the 60 days preceding the onset of symptoms. The most recent sexual partner should be treated even if the last sexual contact was more than 60 days from onset of symptoms.

COMPLICATIONS. Complications of genital chlamydial infections in women include perihepatitis (Fitz-Hugh-Curtis syndrome) and salpingitis. Of women with untreated chlamydial infection who develop pelvic inflammatory disease, up to 40% will have significant sequelae; approximately 17% will suffer from chronic pelvic pain, approximately 17% will become infertile, and approximately 9% will have an ectopic (tubal) pregnancy. Adolescent girls may be at higher risk for developing complications, especially salpingitis, than older women. Salpingitis in adolescent girls is also more likely to lead to tubal scarring, subsequent obstruction with secondary infertility, and increased risk for ectopic pregnancy. Approximately 50% of neonates born to pregnant women with untreated chlamydial infection will acquire *C. trachomatis* infection (see Subchapter 223.3). Women with *C. trachomatis* infection have a 3–5-fold increased risk for acquiring HIV infection.

PREVENTION. Timely treatment of sex partners is essential for decreasing risk for reinfection. Sex partners should be evaluated and treated if they had sexual contact during the 60 days preceding onset of symptoms in the patient. The most recent sex partner should be treated even if the last sexual contact was >60 days. Patients and their sex partners should abstain from sexual intercourse until 7 days after a single-dose regimen or after completion of a 7-day regimen.

Annual routine screening for *C. trachomatis* is recommended for all sexually active adolescents and females 20–25 yr of age, and older women with risk factors such as new or multiple partners or inconsistent use of barrier contraceptives. Sexual risk assessment may indicate more frequent screening of some women.

223.3 • Conjunctivitis and Pneumonia in Newborns

EPIDEMIOLOGY. Chlamydial genital infection is reported in 5–30% of pregnant women, with a risk for vertical transmission at parturition to newborn infants of about 50%. The infant may become infected at 1 or more sites, including the conjunctivae, nasopharynx, rectum, and vagina. Transmission is rare following cesarean section with intact membranes. The introduction of systematic prenatal screening for *C. trachomatis* infection and treatment of pregnant women has resulted in a dramatic decrease in the incidence of neonatal chlamydial infection in the USA. However, in countries where prenatal screening is not done, such as the Netherlands, *C. trachomatis* remains an important cause of neonatal infection, accounting for >60% of neonatal conjunctivitis.

Inclusion Conjunctivitis. Approximately 30–50% of infants born to mothers with active, untreated, chlamydial infection develop clinical conjunctivitis. Symptoms usually develop 5–14 days after delivery, or earlier with prolonged rupture of membranes. The presentation is extremely variable and ranges from mild conjunctival injection with scant mucoid discharge to severe conjunctivitis with copious purulent discharge, chemosis, and pseudomembrane formation. The conjunctiva may be very friable and may bleed when stroked with a swab. Chlamydial conjunctivitis must be differentiated from gonococcal ophthalmia, which is sight threatening. At least 50% of infants with chlamydial conjunctivitis also have nasopharyngeal infection.

Pneumonia. Pneumonia due to *C. trachomatis* develops in 10–20% of infants born to women with active, untreated chlamydial infection. Only about 25% of infants with nasopharyngeal chlamydial infection develop pneumonia. *C. trachomatis* pneumonia of infancy has a very characteristic presentation. Onset is usually from 1 to 3 mo of age and is often insidious with persistent cough, tachypnea, and absence of fever. Auscultation reveals rales; wheezing is uncommon. The absence of fever and wheezing helps to distinguish *C. trachomatis* pneumonia from respiratory syncytial virus pneumonia. A distinctive laboratory finding is the presence of peripheral eosinophilia (>400 cells/mm^3). The most consistent finding on chest radiograph is hyperinflation accompanied by minimal interstitial or alveolar infiltrates.

Infections at Other Sites. Infants born to mothers with *C. trachomatis* may develop infection in the rectum or vagina. Although infection in these sites appears to be totally asymptomatic, it may cause confusion if identified at a later date. Perinatally acquired rectal, vaginal, and nasopharyngeal infections may persist for ≥3 yr. *C. pneumoniae* can also be confused with *C. trachomatis* infection in nasopharyngeal cultures if a genus-specific monoclonal antibody is used to confirm the culture.

DIAGNOSIS. Definitive diagnosis is achieved by isolation of *C. trachomatis* in cultures of specimens obtained from the conjunctiva or nasopharynx. Several nonculture methods, using direct fluorescent antibody and enzyme immunoassay (EIA), are approved for diagnosis of chlamydial conjunctivitis. These tests have sensitivities of ≥90% and specificities of ≥95% for conjunctival specimens compared with culture. Their accuracy for nasopharyngeal specimens is not as good. Data on use of NAATs for diagnosis of *C. trachomatis* in children are limited. Preliminary data suggest that PCR is equivalent to culture for detection of *C. trachomatis* in the conjunctiva and nasopharynx of infants with conjunctivitis.

Nonculture methods should never be used to test rectal or vaginal specimens obtained from children. Because all available EIAs use genus-specific antibodies, these tests also detect *C. pneumoniae* if used for tests of respiratory specimens.

TREATMENT. The recommended treatment regimen for *C. trachomatis* conjunctivitis or pneumonia in infants is erythromycin (base or ethylsuccinate, 50 mg/kg/day divided qid PO for 14 days). The rationale for using oral therapy for conjunctivitis is that 50% or more of these infants have concomitant nasopharyngeal infection or disease at other sites, and studies have demonstrated that topical therapy with sulfonamide drops and erythromycin ointment is not effective. The failure rate with oral erythromycin remains 10–20%, and some infants require a 2nd course of treatment. The results of 1 small study suggest that a short course of azithromycin (20 mg/kg/day once daily PO for 3 days) was as effective as 14 days of erythromycin. Mothers (and their sexual contacts) of infants with *C. trachomatis* infections should be empirically treated for genital infection. An association between treatment with oral erythromycin and infantile hypertrophic pyloric stenosis has been reported in infants <6 wk of age who were given the drug for prophylaxis after nursery exposure to pertussis.

PREVENTION. Neonatal gonococcal prophylaxis with topical erythromycin or tetracycline ointment, or silver nitrate, does not appear to prevent chlamydial ophthalmia or nasopharyngeal colonization with *C. trachomatis* or chlamydial pneumonia. The most effective method of controlling perinatal chlamydial infection appears to be screening and treatment of pregnant women. For treatment of *C. trachomatis* infection in pregnant women, the CDC currently recommends either azithromycin (1 g PO as a single dose) or amoxicillin (500 mg PO tid for 7 days) as 1st line regimens. Erythromycin base (250 mg PO qid for 14 days), and erythromycin ethylsuccinate (800 mg qid for 7 days, or 400 mg PO qid for 14 days) are listed as alternative regimens. Reasons for failure of maternal treatment to prevent infantile chlamydial infection include poor compliance and reinfection from an untreated sexual partner.

223.4 • Lymphogranuloma Venereum

LGV is a systemic sexually transmitted disease caused by the L_1, L_2, and L_3 serotypes of the LGV biovar of *C. trachomatis*. Unlike strains of the trachoma biovar, LGV strains have a predilection for lymphoid tissue. About 20 cases of LGV have been reported in children, and <1,000 cases are reported in adults in the USA annually. Recently there has been a resurgence of LGV infections among men who have sex with men in Europe and the USA. Many of the individuals were HIV infected and used illicit drugs, specifically methamphetamines.

CLINICAL MANIFESTATIONS. The 1st stage of LGV is characterized by the appearance of the primary lesion, a painless, usually transient papule on the genitals. The 2nd stage is characterized by usually unilaterally femoral or inguinal lymphadenitis with enlarging, painful buboes. The nodes may break down and drain, especially in males. In females, the vulvar lymph drains to the retroperitoneal nodes. Fever, myalgia, and headache are common. In the tertiary stage, a genitoanorectal syndrome occurs with rectovaginal fistulas, rectal strictures, and urethral destruction. Among men who have sex with men, rectal infection with LGV can produce a severe, acute proctocolitis.

DIAGNOSIS. LGV can be diagnosed by culture of *C. trachomatis* or NAAT from a specimen aspirated from a bubo or by serologic testing. Most patients with LGV have complement-fixing antibody titers of >1 : 16. Chancroid and herpes simplex virus can be distinguished clinically from LGV by the concurrent presence of painful genital ulcers. Syphilis can be differentiated by serologic tests. However, co-infections can occur.

TREATMENT. Doxycycline (100 mg PO bid for 21 days) is the recommended treatment. The alternative regimen is erythromycin base (500 mg PO qid for 21 days). Azithromycin (1 g PO once weekly for 3 wk) may also be effective but clinical data are lacking. Sex partners of patients with LGV should be treated if they have had sexual contact with the patient during the 30 days preceding the onset of symptoms.

Blank S, Schillinger JA, Harbatkin D: Lymphogranuloma venereum in the industrialized world. *Lancet* 2005;365:1607–1608.

Centers for Disease Control and Prevention: Screening tests to detect *Chlamydia trachomatis* and *Neisseria gonorrhoeae* infections—2002. *MMWR* 2002;51(RR-15):1–37.

Centers for Disease Control and Prevention: Sexually transmitted diseases treatment guidelines 2006. *MMWR* 2006;55(RR-11):1–100.

Chidambaram JD, Alemayehu W, Melese M, et al: Effect of a single mass antibiotic distribution on the prevalence of infectious trachoma. *JAMA* 2006;295:1142–1146.

Fraser-Hurt N, Bailey RL, Cousens S, et al: Efficacy of oral azithromycin versus topical tetracycline in mass treatment of endemic trachoma. *Bull WHO* 2001;79:632–640.

Gaydos CA, Theodore M, Dalesio N, et al: Comparison of three nucleic acid amplification tests for detection of *Chlamydia trachomatis* in urine specimens. *J Clin Microbiol* 2004;42:3041–3045.

Hammerschlag MR: Appropriate use of nonculture tests for the detection of sexually transmitted diseases in children and adolescents. *Semin Pediatr Infect Dis* 2003;14:54–59.

Hammerschlag MR, Gelling M, Roblin PM, et al: Treatment of neonatal chlamydial conjunctivitis with azithromycin. *Pediatr Infect Dis J* 1998; 17:1049–1050.

Hwang L, Shafer MA: *Chlamydia trachomatis* infection in adolescents. *Adv Pediatr* 2004;51:379–407.

Kent CK, Branzuela A, Fischer L, et al: Chlamydia and gonorrhea screening in San Francisco high schools. *Sex Transm Dis* 2002;29:373–375.

Mabey DCW, Solomon AW, Foster A: Trachoma. *Lancet* 2003;362:223–229.

Michel CECH, Solomon AW, Magbanua JPV, et al: Field evaluation of a rapid point-of-care assay for targeting antibiotic treatment for trachoma control: A comparative study. *Lancet* 2006;376:1585–1590.

Nieuwenhuis RF, Ossewaarde JM, Götz HM, et al: Resurgence of lymphogranuloma venereum in Western Europe: An outbreak of *Chlamydia trachomatis* serovar L_2 proctitis in the Netherlands among men who have had sex with men. *Clin Infect Dis* 2004;39:996–1003.

Schachter J, McCormack WM, Chernesky MA, et al: Vaginal swabs are appropriate specimens for diagnosis of genital tract infection with *Chlamydia trachomatis*. *J Clin Microbiol* 2003;41:3784–3789.

Solomon AW, Holland MJ, Alexander NDE, et al: Mass treatment with single-dose azithromycin for trachoma. *N Engl J Med* 2004;351:1962–1971.

Solomon AW, Peeling RW, Foster A, Mabey DC: Diagnosis and assessment of trachoma. *Clin Microbiol Rev* 2004;17:982–1011.

Taylor HR, Wright HR: Dip-stick test for trachoma control programmes. *Lancet* 2006;367:1553–1554.

West SK, Munoz B, Mkocha H, et al: Infection with Chlamydia trachomatis after mass treatment of a trachoma hyperendemic community in Tanzania: A longitudinal study. *Lancet* 2005;366:1296–1300.

Chapter 224 ■ Psittacosis *(Chlamydophila Psittaci)*

Chlamydophila psittaci, the agent of psittacosis (also known as **parrot fever** and **ornithosis**), is primarily an animal pathogen and causes human disease infrequently. In birds, *C. psittaci* infection is known as avian chlamydiosis.

ETIOLOGY. *C. psittaci* affects psittacine birds (parrots, parakeets, macaws, etc.) and nonpsittacine birds as well (ducks, turkeys); the known host range includes 130 avian species. The life cycle of *C. psittaci* is the same as for *Chlamydophila pneumoniae* (see Chapter 222). Strains of *C. psittaci* have been analyzed by patterns of pathogenicity, inclusion morphology in tissue culture, DNA restriction endonuclease analysis, and monoclonal antibodies, which indicate that there are 7 avian serovars. Two of the avian serovars, psittacine and turkey, are of major importance in the avian population of the USA. Each is associated with important host preferences and disease characteristics.

EPIDEMIOLOGY. From 1988 to 2003 there were 935 reported cases of psittacosis in the United States. Of these, 85% were associated with exposure to birds, including 70% following exposure to caged pet birds, which were usually psittacine birds including cockatiels, parakeets, parrots, and macaws. Chlamydiosis among caged nonpsittacine birds occurs most frequently in pigeons, doves, and mynah birds. Persons at highest risk for acquiring psittacosis include bird fanciers and owners of pet birds (43% of cases) and pet shop employees (10% of cases).

Inhalation of aerosols from feces, fecal dust, and nasal secretions of animals infected with *C. psittaci* is the primary route of infection. Source birds are either asymptomatic or have anorexia, ruffled feathers, lethargy, and watery green droppings. Psittacosis is uncommon in children, in part because children may be less likely to have close contact with infected birds. One high-risk activity is cleaning the cage. Several major outbreaks of psittacosis have occurred in turkey processing plants; workers exposed to turkey viscera are at the highest risk for infection.

CLINICAL MANIFESTATIONS. Infection with *C. psittaci* in humans ranges from clinically inapparent to severe infection involving multiple organ systems as well as pneumonia. The mean incubation period is 15 days after exposure, with a range of 5–21 days. Onset of disease is usually abrupt, with fever, cough, headache, and malaise. The fever is high and often is associated with rigors and sweats. The headache can be so severe that meningitis is considered. The cough is usually nonproductive. Crackles may be heard on auscultation. Chest radiographs are usually abnormal with variable infiltrates, and pleural effusions may be present. The white blood cell count is usually not elevated, but a mild leukocytosis may be present. Elevated levels of aspartate aminotransferase, alkaline phosphatase, and bilirubin are common.

DIAGNOSIS. The diagnosis of psittacosis can be difficult because of the varying clinical presentations. A history of exposure to birds or association with an active case are important clues, but as many as 20% of patients with psittacosis have no known contact. Person-to-person spread has been suggested but not proved. Other infections that cause pneumonia with high fever, unusually severe headache, and myalgia include, most commonly, bacterial and viral respiratory infections as well as *Coxiella burnetii* (Q fever), *Mycoplasma pneumoniae, C. pneumoniae,* tularemia, tuberculosis, fungal infections, and Legionnaires disease.

The mainstay of diagnosis remains serology using the complement fixation (CF) test, which is genus specific. According to the 2000 recommendations from the Centers for Disease Control and Prevention, a confirmed case of psittacosis requires a compatible clinical illness, usually with a reliable history of avian exposure. Laboratory confirmation may be by 1 of the 3 following methods: (1) culture of *C. psittaci* from respiratory secretions; (2) a 4-fold or greater increase in CF or microimmunofluorescence (MIF) titer in sera collected at least 2 wk apart; or (3) a single MIF immunoglobulin M titer of ≥1 : 16. A probable case should be epidemiologically linked to a confirmed case or have a single CF or MIF antibody titer of 1 : 32 or more in at least 1 serum sample obtained after onset of symptoms. As with the use of MIF for diagnosis of *C. pneumoniae* infections, cross reactions with other *Chlamydia* species and bacteria can occur. Early treatment of psittacosis with tetracycline may abrogate the antibody response.

The organism also can be isolated by culture from sputum or pleural fluid. Although *C. psittaci* will grow in the same culture systems used for isolation of *Chlamydia trachomatis* and *C. pneumoniae,* very few laboratories culture for *C. psittaci,* mainly because of the potential biohazard.

TREATMENT. Recommended treatment regimens for psittacosis are doxycycline (100 mg PO bid) or tetracycline (500 mg PO qid) for at least 10–14 days after the fever abates. The initial treatment of severely ill patients is doxycycline hyclate (4.4 mg/kg/day divided every 12 hr IV, maximum 100 mg/dose). Erythromycin (500 mg qid PO) is an alternative drug if tetracyclines are contraindicated (e.g., children <9 yr of age and pregnant women), but may be less effective. Remission is usually evident within 48–72 hr. Initial infection does not appear to be followed by long-term immunity. Reinfection and clinical disease can develop within 2 mo of treatment; 2 well-documented cases of reinfection have been reported.

PROGNOSIS. The mortality rate of untreated psittacosis is 15–20%, but is <1% with appropriate treatment. Severe illness leading to respiratory failure and fetal death has been reported among pregnant women.

PREVENTION. Several control measures are recommended to prevent transmission of *C. psittaci* from birds. Bird fanciers should be cognizant of the potential risk. *C. psittaci* is susceptible to most disinfectants and detergents as well as heat, but is resistant to acid and alkali. Accurate records of all bird-related transactions aid in identifying sources of infected birds and potentially exposed persons. Newly acquired birds, including birds that have been to shows, exhibitions, fairs, or other events, should be isolated for 30–45 days or tested or treated prophylactically before adding them to a group of birds. Care should be taken to prevent transfer of fecal material, feathers, food, or other materials between birdcages. Birds with signs of avian chlamydiosis (e.g., ocular or nasal discharge, watery green droppings, or low body weight) should be isolated and should neither be sold nor purchased. Their handlers should wear protective clothing and a disposable surgical cap and use a respirator with an N95 or higher efficiency rating (not a surgical mask) when handling them or cleaning their cages. Infected birds should be isolated until fully treated, which is generally 45 days.

Moroney JF, Guevara R, Iverson C, et al: Detection of chlamydiosis in a shipment of pet birds, leading to recognition of an outbreak of clinically mild psittacosis in humans. *Clin Infect Dis* 1998;26:1425–1429.

Smith KA, Bradley KK, Stobierski MG, et al: National Association of State Public Health Veterinarians Psittacosis Compendium Committee. Compendium of measures to control *Chlamydophila psittaci* (formerly *Chlamydia psittaci*) infection among humans (psittacosis) and pet birds, 2005. *J Am Vet Med Assoc* 2005;226:532–539.

Yung AP, Grayson ML: Psittacosis: A review of 135 cases. *Med J Aust* 1988;148: 228–233.

Section 11 — Rickettsial Infections

Chapter 225 ■ Spotted Fever Group *Rickettsioses* George K. Siberry and J. Stephen Dumler

Many members of the spotted fever group of rickettsiae are pathogenic for humans (Table 225-1). These include the tick-borne agents *Rickettsia rickettsii,* the cause of Rocky Mountain spotted fever (RMSF); *R. conorii,* the cause of Mediterranean spotted fever (MSF) or boutonneuse fever; *R. sibirica,* the cause of North Asian tick typhus; *R. japonica,* the cause of Oriental spotted fever; *R. australis,* the cause of Queensland tick typhus; *R. honei,* the cause of Flinders Island spotted fever or Thai tick typhus; *R. africae,* the cause of African tick bite fever; the unnamed Israeli spotted fever rickettsia, and possibly others. *R. akari,* the cause of rickettsialpox, is transmitted by the bite of a mite. Infections with the other members of the spotted fever group present with signs similar to those of MSF, including fever, maculopapular rash, and eschar at the initial site of tick attachment. Israeli spotted fever is generally associated with a more severe course, including fatalities in children. African tick typhus is relatively mild, often lacks disseminated rash but may include a vesicular rash, and often presents with multiple eschars. In recent years, new rickettsial agents have been identified as potentially important pathogenic species, including *R. slovaca,* the cause of **TIBOLA (tick-borne lymphadenopathy)**; *R. felis,* the cause of cat flea typhus; and *R. parkeri,* a newly identified cause of eschars in patients bitten by ticks in North America. *R. rickettsii, R. parkeri, R. felis,* and *R. akari* are the only members of the spotted fever group causing disease autochthonous in the United States.

225.1 • Rocky Mountain Spotted Fever (*Rickettsia rickettsii*)

RMSF is the most frequently identified rickettsial disease and the 2nd most common vector-borne disease in the United States, after Lyme disease. RMSF is considered uncommon, but it is probably significantly underdiagnosed. Because it is a potentially rapidly fatal infection, RMSF should be considered in the differential diagnosis of fever, headache, and rash in the summer months, especially after tick exposure.

ETIOLOGY. RMSF is caused by systemic endothelial cell infection by the obligate intracellular bacterium *R. rickettsii.*

EPIDEMIOLOGY. The term *Rocky Mountain spotted fever* is a misnomer because only a small percentage of all documented cases are currently reported from the Rocky Mountain region. The disease occurs throughout the continental USA (except Vermont and Maine), southwestern Canada, Mexico, Central America, and South America. In 2001, most cases were reported from North Carolina, Tennessee, Missouri, Oklahoma, Arkansas, Virginia, Maryland, South Carolina, and Pennsylvania; the changing ecology of tick vectors influences the geographic prevalence over time. The incidence of RMSF varies in a cyclical pattern over decades; the last nadir was between 1993 and 1998. However, the average annual number of cases reported to the Centers for Disease Control and Prevention (CDC) between 1993 and 1998 was 515, whereas that number more than doubled during 2001–2004 at 1,071 per year, and in 2004 there were 1,514 cases of RMSF reported, more than at any time in history. Habitats favored by ticks, including wooded areas or coastal grassland and salt marshes, are associated with disease. Foci of intense infection are also well documented in rural and some urban settings such as the South Bronx. Shared environmental exposures may lead to clusters of cases within families. In the USA, 90% of cases occur between April and September, the peak months of tick and human outdoor activity. The highest age-specific incidence of RMSF is among children <10 yr of age, and boys outnumber girls.

TRANSMISSION. Ticks are the natural hosts, reservoirs, and vectors of *R. rickettsii.* Ticks maintain the infection naturally by transovarial transmission (passage of the organism from infected ticks to their progeny). However, ticks harboring rickettsiae are not as productive as uninfected ticks; thus, horizontal transmission by acquisition of rickettsiae by taking a blood meal from transiently rickettsemic animal hosts such as small mammals or dogs contributes to natural maintenance. Ticks transmit the infectious agent to mammalian hosts (including humans) by regurgitation of infected saliva during feeding. *R. rickettsii* in ticks must be reactivated for virulence by exposure to blood or increased temperature; thus, longer tick attachment times likely increase the risk for transmission. The principal tick hosts of *R. rickettsii* are *Dermacentor variabilis* (the American dog tick) in the eastern United States and Canada, *Dermacentor andersoni* (the wood tick) in the western United States and Canada, *Rhipicephalus sanguineus* (the common brown dog tick) in Mexico and in the southwestern United States, and *Amblyomma cajennense* in Central and South America (Fig. 225-1).

Dogs can also serve as reservoir hosts for *R. rickettsii,* can themselves develop RMSF, and are important vehicles for bringing potentially infected ticks into the environment shared by humans. Serologic studies of patients with RMSF indicate that a high percentage may have contracted the illness from ticks carried by the family dog. Care must be taken during tick removal, since transmission can occur by inoculation of tick fluids or feces into open wounds or conjunctivae from the fingers and hands. Fatalities have occurred in laboratory workers exposed to infectious aerosols.

PATHOLOGY AND PATHOGENESIS. Lesions are most obvious on the skin, but are systemically distributed, affecting nearly all organs and tissues. Following inoculation into the dermis in the tick saliva, the rickettsiae attach to the vascular endothelium via protein ligands and initiate rickettsial phospholipase-mediated host cell membrane injury. The membrane damage induces phagocytosis, and the internalized rickettsia then gains access to the cytosol by continued vacuolar membrane lysis. Members of the spotted fever group actively initiate intracellular actin polymerization to achieve directional movement, and rickettsiae can thus easily invade neighboring cells while inducing minimal initial host cell damage. The rickettsiae proliferate and damage the host cells by peroxidative membrane alterations, protease activation, or continued phospholipase activity.

Initially, a perivascular infiltrate of lymphoid and histiocytic cells and edema without significant endothelial damage are present, coinciding with the development of macules and macu-

TABLE 225-1. Summary of Rickettsial Diseases of Humans, including *Rickettsia*, *Orientia*, *Ehrlichia*, *Anaplasma*, *Neorickettsia*, and *Coxiella*

GROUP/DISEASE	AGENT	ARTHROPOD VECTOR/ TRANSMISSION	HOSTS	GEOGRAPHIC DISTRIBUTION	PRESENTING CLINICAL FEATURES*	COMMON LAB ABNORMALITIES	DIAGNOSTIC TESTS	TREATMENT (PREFERRED IN BOLD)
SPOTTED FEVER								
Rocky Mountain spotted fever	*Rickettsia rickettsii*	Tick bite: *Dermacentor* species (wood tick, dog tick) *Rhipicephalus sanguineus* (brown dog tick)	Dogs Rodents	Western hemisphere	Fever, headache, rash,* emesis, diarrhea, tender calf muscles	↑ AST, ALT ↓ Na (mild) ↓ Platelets ± Leukopenia Left shift	Early: IH, DFA, PCR After 1st wk: IFA	**Doxycycline** Tetracycline Chloramphenicol
Mediterranean spotted fever (Boutonneuse fever)	*Rickettsia conorii*	Tick bite: *R. sanguineus* (brown dog tick)	Dogs Rodents	Africa, Mediterranean, India, Middle East	Painless eschar (tache noir) with regional lymphadenopathy, fever, headache, rash,* myalgias	↑ AST, ALT ↓ Na (mild) ↓ Platelets ± Leukopenia Left shift	Early: IH, DFA, PCR After 1st wk: IFA	**Doxycycline** Tetracycline Chloramphenicol Azithromycin Clarithromycin Fluoroquinolones
African tick-bite fever	*Rickettsia africae*	Tick bite	Cattle Goats?	Sub-Saharan Africa, Caribbean	Fever, single or multiple eschars, regional lymphadenopathy, rash* (often vesicular)	↑ AST, ALT ↓ Platelets	Early: IH, DFA After 1st wk: IFA	**Doxycycline**
Rickettsialpox	*Rickettsia akari*	Mite bite	Mice	North America, Russia, Ukraine, Adriatic, Korea, South Africa	Painless eschar, ulcer or papule; tender regional lymphadenopathy, fever, headache, rash* (varicelliform)	↓ WBC	Early: IH, DFA After 1st wk: IFA	**Doxycycline** Chloramphenicol
Cat flea typhus	*Rickettsia felis*	Flea bite	Opossum Cats Dogs	Western hemisphere, Europe	Fever, rash,* headache	?	Early: PCR After 1st wk: IFA	**Doxycycline**
Tick-borne lymphadenopathy (TIBOLA)	*Rickettsia slovaca*	Tick bite: *Dermacentor*	?	Europe	Eschar (scalp), painful lymphadenopathy	?	PCR	**Doxycycline**
TYPHUS								
Murine typhus	*Rickettsia typhi*	Flea feces	Rats Opossums	Worldwide	Fever, headache, rash,* myalgias, emesis, lymphadenopathy, hepatosplenomegaly	↑ AST, ALT ↓ Na (mild) ↓ WBC ↓ Platelets	Early: DFA After 1st wk: IFA	**Doxycycline** Tetracycline Chloramphenicol
Epidemic (louse-borne) typhus [Recrudescent form: Brill-Zinsser disease]	*Rickettsia prowazekii*	Louse feces	Humans	South America, Central America, Mexico, Africa, Asia, Eastern Europe	Fever, headache, abdominal pain, rash,* CNS involvement	↑ AST, ALT ↓ Platelets	Early: None After 1st wk: IgG/IgM IFA	**Doxycycline** Tetracycline Chloramphenicol
Flying squirrel (sylvatic) typhus	*Riskettsia prowazekii*	Louse feces? Flea feces or bite?	Flying squirrels	Eastern USA	Same as above (often milder)	↑ AST, ALT ↓ Platelets	Early: None After 1st wk: IFA	**Doxycycline** Tetracycline Chloramphenicol
SCRUB TYPHUS								
Scrub typhus	*Orientia tsutsugamushi*	Chigger bite: *Leptotrombidium*	Rodents?	South Asia, Japan, Indonesia, Korea, China, Russia, Australia	Fever, rash,* headache, painless eschar, hepatosplenomegaly, gastrointestinal symptoms	↓ Platelets ↑ AST, ALT	Early: None After 1st wk: IFA	**Doxycycline** Tetracycline Chloramphenicol ***If Doxy resistant:* Rifampicin** Azithromycin
EHRLICHIOSES AND ANAPLASMOSIS								
Human monocytic ehrlichiosis	*Ehrlichia chaffeensis*	Tick bite: *Amblyomma americanum* (lone star tick)	Deer Dogs	USA Europe? Africa? Asia?	Fever, headache, malaise, myalgias, rash* (children†), hepatosplenomegaly†, swollen hands/feet*	↑ AST, ALT ↓ WBC ↓ Platelets ↓ Na (mild)	Early: PCR After 1st wk: IFA	**Doxycycline** Tetracycline
Human granulocytic anaplasmosis	*Anaplasma phagocytophilum*	Tick bite: *Ixodes* species	Rodents Deer Ruminants	USA, Europe, Asia	Fever, headache, malaise, myalgias	↑ AST, ALT ↓ WBC, ↓ ANC ↓ Platelets ↓ Na (mild)	Early: PCR, blood smear After 1st wk: IFA	**Doxycycline** Tetracycline Rifampin
Ewingii ehrlichiosis	*Ehrlichia ewingii*	Tick bite: *Amblyomma americanum* (lone star tick)	Dogs Deer	USA (south-central southeast)	Fever, headache, malaise, Myalgias	↑ AST, ALT ↓ WBC ↓ Platelets ↓ Na (mild)	Early: PCR After 1st wk: IFA	**Doxycycline** Tetracycline
Sennetsu ehrlichiosis	*Neorickettsia sennetsu*	Ingestion of fish helminth?	Unknown	Japan Malaysia	Fever, "mononucleosis" symptoms, postauricular and posterior cervical lymphadenopathy	Atypical Lymphocytosis	Early: None After 1st wk: IFA	**Doxycycline** Tetracycline
Q FEVER								
Q Fever: Acute [Chronic, see chapter text]	*Coxiella burnetti*	Inhale infected aerosols: contact with parturient animals, abattoir, contaminated cheese and milk, ?ticks	Cattle Sheep Goats Cats Rabbits	Worldwide	Fever, headache, arthralgias, myalgias, gastronintestinal symptoms, cough, pneumonia, rash (children)	↑ AST, ALT ↑ WBC ↓ Platelets Interstitial infiltrate	Early: PCR After 1st wk: IFA	**Doxycycline** Tetracycline Fluoroquinolones Trimethoprim-Sulfamethoxazole

*rash is infrequently present at initial presentation but appears during the first week of illness.

†Frequently present in children but not adults.

ALT, alanine aminotransferase; ANC, absolute neutrophil count; AST, aspartate aminotransferase; CNS, central nervous system; DFA, direct fluorescent antibody; IFA, indirect fluorescent antibody; IgG, immunoglobulin G; IgM, immunoglobulin M; IH, immunohistochemistry; PCR, polymerase chain reaction; WBC, white blood cell count.

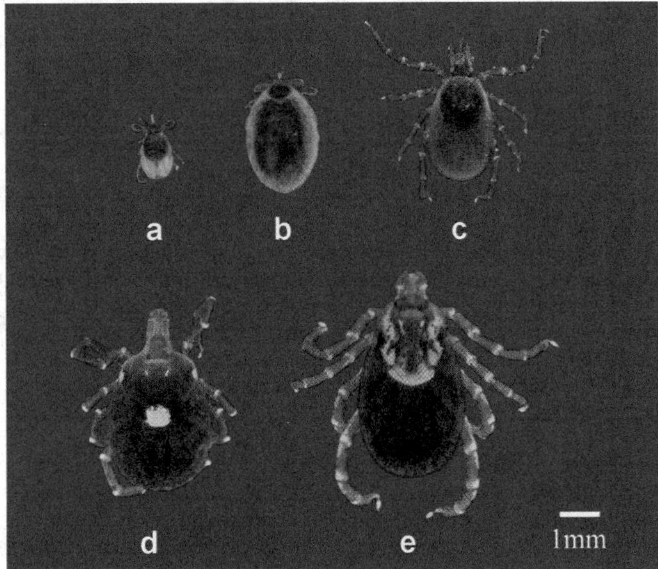

Figure 225-1. Tick vectors of agents of human rickettsial diseases. An unengaged nymph (a), engorged nymph (b), and adult female (c) of *Ixodes scapularis* (deer tick), the vector of *Anaplasma phagocytophilum,* the cause of human granulocytic anaplasmosis. An adult female (d) of *Amblyomma americanum* (lone star tick), the vector of *Ehrlichia chaffeensis* and *Ehrlichia ewingii,* the causes of human monocytic ehrlichiosis and ewingii ehrlichiosis, respectively. An adult female (e) of *Dermacentor variabilis* (American dog tick), the vector of *Rickettsia rickettsii,* the cause of Rocky Mountain spotted fever.

lopapules. Proliferation of rickettsiae within endothelial cell cytoplasm leads to lymphohistiocytic or leukocytoclastic vasculitis of small venules and capillaries that results in petechial skin lesions and microvascular leakage, tissue hypoperfusion, and possibly end-organ ischemic injury. Rickettsiae are localized within endothelial cells of inflamed vessels that may be eccentrically involved, including infrequent nonocclusive thrombi; small and large vessels rarely become completely obliterated by thrombosis, leading to tissue infarction or hemorrhagic necrosis. Interstitial pneumonitis and vascular leakage in the lungs can lead to noncardiogenic pulmonary edema, while meningoencephalitis can cause significant cerebral edema.

The presence of the infectious agent initiates an inflammatory cascade, including release of cytokines such as tumor necrosis factor-α (TNF-α), interleukin 1β, and interferon-γ (IFN-γ). Infection of endothelial cells by *R. rickettsii* induces surface E-selectin expression and procoagulant activity. Chemokine release and vascular selectin expression result in infiltration of the damaged endothelial cells by lymphocytes, macrophages, and occasionally neutrophils. Local inflammatory and immune responses have been suspected as contributors to vascular injury in the rickettsioses; however, the benefits of effective inflammation and immunity outweigh any potential damage mediated by host responses directed toward elimination of local infection. Blockade of TNF-α and IFN-γ action in animal models diminishes survival and increases the morbidity of spotted fever group infections, probably by abrogating upregulation of nitric oxide synthase and arginine-dependent intracellular killing. Important mediators for control of infection include direct contact of infected endothelial cells with CD8 T lymphocytes that produce perforin and natural killer cells that produce IFN-γ. *Rickettsia* infection leads to upregulated expression of procoagulant molecules on the surfaces of infected endothelial cells. This is associated with induction of tissue plasminogen activator inhibitor and reduction in plasminogen activator levels that promote coagulation factor consumption, platelet adhesion, and leukocyte emigration and can result in a clinical syndrome similar to disseminated intravascular coagulation.

CLINICAL MANIFESTATIONS. The incubation period in children varies from 2 to 14 days, with a median of 7 days. There is a history of removal of an attached tick in 60% of patients, although the site of the tick bite is usually inapparent. Exposure in an endemic area, playing or hiking in wooded areas, typical season, similar illness in close contacts, and close contact with a dog (especially a dog who has been sick) are all important epidemiologic clues. Inapparent or mild illness probably occurs only infrequently. In those patients presenting for care, the illness is initially nonspecific, with headache, fever, anorexia, myalgias, and restlessness. Calf muscle pain and tenderness are particularly common in children. Gastrointestinal symptoms including nausea, vomiting, diarrhea, and abdominal pain occur frequently (39–63%) early in the disease. Skin rash is usually not present until after 2–4 days of illness, and approximately 5% of children and up to 20% of adults never develop rash or have atypical cutaneous manifestations. The typical **clinical triad** of headache, fever, and rash is observed in 44% of patients overall but in only 3% of all patients at the time of presentation. Fever and headache persist if the illness is untreated, although headache may occur or may be recognized less consistently in younger children. Fever may exceed 40°C and can be persistently elevated or fluctuate dramatically. Headache is severe, unremitting, and unresponsive to analgesics.

Rash occurs more reliably in children than in adults. Initially, discrete, pale, rose-red blanching macules or maculopapules appear, characteristically on the extremities, including the ankles, wrists, or lower legs (Fig. 225-2). The rash then spreads rapidly to involve the entire body, including the soles and palms. After several days, the rash becomes more petechial or hemorrhagic, sometimes with palpable purpura. In severe disease, the petechiae may enlarge into ecchymoses, which can become necrotic. Severe vascular obstruction secondary to the rickettsial vasculitis and thrombosis is infrequent but can result in gangrene of the digits, earlobes, scrotum, nose, or an entire limb. **Central nervous system** infection often produces meningismus and changes in sensorium. CSF parameters are usually normal, but 1/3 may have mononuclear pleocytosis (<10–300 cells/μL) and 20% may have elevated protein (<200 mg/dL). In addition, patients may manifest ataxia, seizures, coma, or auditory deficits. In the infrequent cases with abnormal CT or MR neuroimaging studies, the findings are gen-

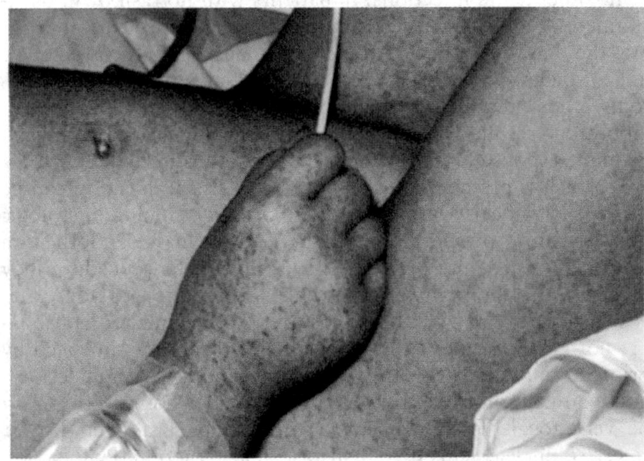

Figure 225-2. Rocky Mountain spotted fever. (Courtesy of Debra Karp Skopocki, MD.)

erally subtle and do not alter treatment. However, in 1 series, 17% of patients with radiologic abnormalities (cerebral edema, meningeal enhancement, and prominent perivascular spaces) died.

Pulmonary disease occurs more commonly in adults than in children, manifesting as rales, infiltrates, and noncardiogenic pulmonary edema. Other findings can include periorbital edema, dorsal hand and foot edema, hepatosplenomegaly, and conjunctival suffusion. Severe disease may include myocarditis, acute renal failure, and vascular collapse.

Persons with **glucose-6-phosphate dehydrogenase (G6PD) deficiency** are at increased risk for fulminant RMSF, defined as *R. rickettsii* infection leading to death in <5 days. The clinical course of fulminant RMSF is characterized by profound coagulopathy and extensive visceral thrombosis with kidney, liver, or respiratory failure. Clinical features associated with a fatal outcome include hepatomegaly, jaundice, stupor, acute renal failure, respiratory distress, and a disseminated intravascular coagulation–like syndrome in the absence of host inflammatory response.

On occasion, rickettsial vascular infection predominates in a single organ or system, erroneously suggesting a localized process such as appendicitis or cholecystitis. A thorough evaluation usually reveals evidence of a systemic process and can avoid unnecessary surgical intervention.

LABORATORY FINDINGS. Laboratory abnormalities are nonspecific but common. Frequently, the total white blood cell count is initially normal or low, but leukocytosis develops as the illness progresses. Other common abnormalities include a left-shifted leukocyte differential, anemia (33%), thrombocytopenia (<150,000 platelets/μL in 33%), hyponatremia (<130 mEq/mL in 20%), and elevated serum aminotransferase activities (50%).

DIAGNOSIS. Delays in diagnosis and treatment are associated with severe and fatal rickettsial infections. Since no reliable diagnostic test is available to confirm RMSF in its acute stage, the initial diagnosis and decision to initiate treatment of RMSF must be based on a clinically suspicious illness with compatible epidemiologic and laboratory features. RMSF should be considered in patients presenting during the spring through fall with an acute febrile illness accompanied by headache and myalgia, particularly following exposure to ticks in endemic regions, in forested or tick-infested rural areas, or after contact with a dog. A history of tick exposure and the appearance of a rash, especially on the palms or soles, together with laboratory findings of normal or low leukocyte count with a marked left shift, a relatively low or decreasing platelet count, and a low serum sodium concentration, are clues that are sometimes helpful in distinguishing RMSF from some other acute infections. In patients with no rash or in dark-skinned individuals in whom a rash can be difficult to appreciate, the diagnosis can be exceptionally elusive and delayed. One half of pediatric fatalities occur within 9 days of onset of symptoms. Thus, treatment should not be withheld pending definitive laboratory results for a patient with clinically suspected illness. Prompt response to early treatment is diagnostically helpful.

If a rash is present, a vasculotropic rickettsial infection can be diagnosed as early as day 3 of illness by immunohistologic demonstration of specific rickettsial antigen in the endothelium in skin biopsy samples of petechial lesions. The procedure may be performed by immunofluorescence or immunoperoxidase and is very specific. However, the sensitivity of this method is probably not greater than 70%, and it can be adversely influenced by prior antimicrobial therapy, suboptimal biopsy of skin lesions, and examination of insufficient tissue because the infection may be very focal. Tissue or blood can also be evaluated for *R. rickettsii* nucleic acids by polymerase chain reaction (PCR) at the CDC and selected public health or reference laboratories; however, blood PCR is less sensitive than tissue PCR and of similar sensitivity to tissue immunohistology, probably because the level of rickettsemia is generally very low (<6 rickettsiae/mL).

Because treatment must be initiated on the clinical diagnosis alone, confirmation is most often accomplished by serologic tests. Unfortunately, serologic responses are usually not present until after the 1st week of illness. Diagnostic serologic criteria include a 4-fold increase in antibody titer, usually by indirect fluorescent antibody (IFA) assay, in acute and convalescent sera (2–4 wk apart) or a single elevated IFA titer of ≥64 in convalescent serum. A case is considered probable if a single titer of ≥128 is found. RMSF antibodies can cross react with other spotted fever and typhus group rickettsiae, but not with ehrlichiae or anaplasmae. Weil-Felix antibody testing should not be performed because it lacks both sensitivity and specificity. *RMSF is a reportable disease nationally.*

DIFFERENTIAL DIAGNOSIS. Other rickettsial infections are easily confused with RMSF, especially all forms of human ehrlichiosis and murine typhus. RMSF can mimic many diseases; among the most important of these are meningococcemia, measles, and enteroviral exanthemas. Negative blood cultures may aid in reaching a correct diagnosis. *R. rickettsii* may cause aseptic meningitis and elicit lymphocytic pleocytosis, suggesting a viral etiology and further confounding the diagnosis. Other diseases sometimes included in the differential diagnosis are typhoid fever, secondary syphilis, Lyme disease, leptospirosis, rat-bite fever, scarlet fever, toxic shock syndrome, rheumatic fever, rubella, parvovirus infection, Kawasaki disease, idiopathic thrombocytopenic purpura, thrombotic thrombocytopenic purpura, Henoch-Schönlein purpura, hemolytic uremic syndrome, aseptic meningitis, acute gastrointestinal illness, acute abdomen, hepatitis, infectious mononucleosis, hemophagocytic syndromes, dengue fever, and drug reactions.

TREATMENT. The time-proven effective therapies for RMSF are tetracyclines and chloramphenicol. The drug of choice for suspected RMSF in patients of all ages is doxycycline, including for young children. Chloramphenicol should be reserved for patients with doxycycline allergy and for pregnant women. Tetracycline and doxycycline may be associated with tooth discoloration in children <8 yr of age, whereas chloramphenicol is rarely associated with aplastic anemia. Doxycycline can be used for RMSF safely in young children because tooth discoloration is dose dependent and it is unlikely that children will require multiple courses. Furthermore, risk factor evaluations demonstrating increased mortality with chloramphenicol alone compared with tetracycline alone, even when other factors such as severity are considered, have led to the preference for doxycycline even in young children. Moreover, chloramphenicol is no longer available as an oral preparation in the United States. The additional benefit of doxycycline over chloramphenicol is its effectiveness against potential concomitant ehrlichial infection. Chloramphenicol is preferred for pregnant women not only because of potential adverse effects of doxycycline on developing fetal teeth and bone, but also because of its increased risk for maternal liver toxicity.

Greater morbidity and excess mortality are associated with sulfonamide therapy, which is discouraged. Other antibiotics, including penicillins, cephalosporins, and aminoglycosides, are not effective. The use of alternative antimicrobial agents such as fluoroquinolones and the macrolides (azithromycin and clarithromycin) for RMSF has not been evaluated.

Recommended treatment regimens for RMSF are doxycycline (2.2 mg/kg/dose bid PO or IV, maximum 200 mg/day), tetracycline (25–50 mg/kg/day divided every 6 hr PO, maximum 2 g/day), or chloramphenicol (50–100 mg/kg/day divided every 6 hr IV, maximum 3 g/day). If used, chloramphenicol should be monitored to maintain serum concentrations of 10–30 µg/mL. Therapy should be continued for a minimum of 5–7 days and until the patient has been afebrile for at least 3 days to avoid relapse, especially in patients who were treated early. Patients treated with 1 of these regimens usually become afebrile within 48 hr, and thus the entire therapy is usually <10 days.

SUPPORTIVE CARE. Most infections resolve rapidly with appropriate antimicrobial therapy and do not require hospitalization or other supportive care. On occasion, severe infections require intensive care. Particular attention to hemodynamic status is required in severely ill children because iatrogenic pulmonary or cerebral edema is easy to precipitate given pre-existing diffuse microvascular lung and meningovascular and cerebrovascular injury. Judicious use of corticosteroids for meningoencephalitis has been advocated by some, although no controlled trials have been conducted.

COMPLICATIONS. Complications of RMSF include noncardiogenic pulmonary edema from pulmonary microvascular leakage, cerebral edema from meningoencephalitis, and multiorgan damage (hepatitis, pancreatitis, cholecystitis, epidermal necrosis, and gangrene) partly mediated by rickettsial vasculitis or the accumulated effects of hypoperfusion and ischemia (acute renal failure). Long-term neurologic sequelae are more likely to occur in patients who have been hospitalized for ≥2 wk and include paraparesis, hearing loss, peripheral neuropathy, bladder and bowel incontinence, cerebellar, vestibular, and motor dysfunction, and language disorders. Learning disabilities and behavioral problems are the most common neurologic sequelae among children who have survived severe disease.

PROGNOSIS. Delays in diagnosis and therapy are significant factors associated with death or severe illness. Before the advent of effective antimicrobial therapy for RMSF, the case fatality rate was 10% for children and 30% for adults. A case fatality rate of 8.5% was documented in Texas from 1986 through 1996. The overall mortality rate is now 2–7%. Diagnosis based on serology alone underestimates the true mortality of RMSF, because patients may die before developing a serologic response. Fatalities occur despite the availability of effective therapeutic agents, indicating the need for vigilant clinical suspicion and a low threshold for early and aggressive therapy in clinically suspected cases. Even with administration of appropriate antimicrobials, delayed therapy may allow irreversible vascular or end-organ damage and long-term sequelae or death. Early therapy in uncomplicated cases ordinarily leads to rapid defervescence within 1–3 days and recovery within 7–10 days. Treatment when the disease is more advanced may have a slower response. In those who survive untreated, the febrile illness will subside in 2–3 wk.

PREVENTION. No vaccines are available. Prevention of RMSF is best accomplished by eliminating tick infestations of dogs, avoiding wooded or grassy areas where ticks reside, using insect repellents containing DEET, wearing protective clothing, and carefully inspecting children who have been playing in the woods or fields. Recovery from infection yields life-long solid immunity.

Prompt and complete **removal of attached ticks** helps reduce the risk for transmission because reactivation to virulence of rickettsiae in the tick requires at least several hours to days of exposure to body heat or blood. Contrary to popular belief, the application of petroleum jelly, 70% isopropyl alcohol, fingernail polish, or using a hot match are not effective in removing ticks. A tick can be safely removed by grasping the mouth parts with a pair of forceps at the site of cutaneous contact and applying gentle and steady retraction without twisting to remove the entire tick and mouth parts. The site of attachment should then be disinfected. Ticks should not be squeezed or crushed because their fluids may be infectious. Tick disposal should be accomplished by soaking the tick in alcohol or flushing it down the toilet, followed by good hand washing. Prophylactic antimicrobial therapy should not be administered because tetracyclines and chloramphenicol are only rickettsiastatic; such therapy simply delays the onset of illness and confuses the clinical picture by prolonging the incubation period.

225.2 • Mediterranean Spotted Fever or Boutonneuse Fever (*Rickettsia conorii*)

The disease caused by *R. conorii* is known by various geographically recognized names, including Mediterranean spotted fever, boutonneuse fever, Kenya tick typhus, Indian tick typhus, Israeli spotted fever, and Astrakhan fever. It is a moderately severe vasculotropic rickettsiosis that is often initially associated with an eschar at the site of the tick bite. Minor differences in clinical presentation may be associated with genetic diversity of the rickettsial subspecies.

ETIOLOGY. MSF is caused by systemic endothelial cell infection by the obligate intracellular bacterium *R. conorii*. Similar illnesses are distributed globally but are caused by distinct yet related species, including *R. sibirica* in Russia, China, Mongolia, and Pakistan, *R. australis* and *R. honei* in Australia, *R. japonica* in Japan, and *R. africae* in South Africa, among other potentially pathogenic *Rickettsia* species (see Table 225-1). These species are closely related to *R. rickettsii* by analysis of antigens and DNA sequences.

EPIDEMIOLOGY. *R. conorii* is distributed over a large geographic region, including India, Pakistan, Russia, Ukraine, Georgia, Israel, Ethiopia, Kenya, South Africa, Morocco, and southern Europe. MSF has demonstrated a steadily increasing incidence since 1980 in southern Europe and has reached seroprevalence rates of 11–26% in some areas. The peak incidence is seen during July and August in the Mediterranean basin, but in other regions it occurs during warm seasons when ticks are active.

TRANSMISSION. Transmission occurs after the bite of the brown dog tick, *R. sanguineus*, or other tick species including *Dermacentor, Haemaphysalis, Amblyomma, Hyalomma,* and *Ixodes*. A strong correlation exists among the incidence of boutonneuse fever, infected ticks, and evidence of infection in both dogs and humans, implicating the household dog as a potential vehicle for transmission.

PATHOLOGY AND PATHOGENESIS. The underlying pathology for MSF is nearly identical to that of RMSF, except that eschars are often identified at the primary site of tick bite and inoculation of the rickettsiae. The histopathology of the tick bite lesion includes necrosis of dermal and epidermal tissues with a superficial crust, and dermal structures are densely infiltrated by lymphocytes, histiocytes, and scattered neutrophils, among damaged capillaries and venules. Immunohistochemical stains confirm that the lesions contain rickettsia-infected endothelial cells, although the remnant structure of the vasculature may not be apparent owing to the extensive inflammation and necrosis. The necrosis results from both direct rickettsia-mediated vasculitis and extensive local inflammation. Rickettsiae released at this site have ready access to lymphatics or venous blood and disseminate to cause a systemic infection.

CLINICAL MANIFESTATIONS AND LABORATORY FINDINGS. Typically symptoms include fever, headache, myalgias, and a maculopapular rash that appears 3–5 days after onset of symptoms. In about 70% of patients, a painless eschar, the **tache noire,** at the initial site of tick attachment and regional lymphadenopathy are present. Although it was previously considered benign and self-limited, this infection may cause severe disease in up to 6% of infected individuals. It is characterized by findings similar to those for RMSF, including purpuric skin lesions, neurologic signs, respiratory distress, acute renal failure, severe thrombocytopenia, and death in 1.4–5.6% of cases. As with RMSF, a particularly malignant form occurs in patients with G6PD deficiency and in individuals with other underlying conditions such as alcoholic liver disease or diabetes mellitus. Fortunately, disease is generally milder in children.

DIAGNOSIS. Laboratory diagnosis of MSF and the other spotted fever group rickettsioses is the same as that for RMSF and may be accomplished by immunohistologic demonstration of rickettsiae on skin biopsy, immunocytologic demonstration of *R. conorii,* in vitro cultivation by means of centrifugation-assisted shell vial tissue culture, or the demonstration of serum antibodies to spotted fever group rickettsiae in convalescent patients. Reagents useful for the diagnosis of RMSF in the United States or MSF in Europe, Africa, and Asia can be used effectively for the diagnosis of infections by most members of the spotted fever group of rickettsiae. Existing serologic tests are not specific for any spotted fever group rickettsia infection, although a 4-fold difference in antibody titer could be used as presumptive evidence.

DIFFERENTIAL DIAGNOSIS. The differential diagnosis is similar to that of RMSF, with the inclusion of conditions associated with single eschars such as anthrax, bacterial ecthyma, brown recluse spider bite, rat-bite fever (caused by *Spirillum minus*), and other rickettsioses such as rickettsialpox, African tick-bite fever, or scrub typhus. The recently described spotted fever rickettsia, *R. africae,* causes a milder illness and is often associated with multiple eschars and sometimes a vesicular rash; it may be observed in African locations where MSF also occurs and is a frequent infection of travelers in sub-Saharan Africa after exposure on safari to the bush or high grasslands.

TREATMENT AND SUPPORTIVE CARE. MSF is effectively treated with tetracycline, doxycycline, chloramphenicol, ciprofloxacin, ofloxacin, pefloxacin, levofloxacin, azithromycin, or clarithromycin. MSF is treated with doxycycline, which is the drug of choice, or tetracycline or chloramphenicol using regimens as for RMSF. Azithromycin (10 mg/kg/day once daily PO for 3 days) and clarithromycin (15 mg/kg/day divided bid PO for 7 days) are alternatives. Specific fluoroquinolone regimens effective for children have not been established. Intensive care may be required for hemodynamic management of severely affected individuals.

COMPLICATIONS. The complications of MSF are similar to those of RMSF. The case fatality rate is approximately 2%. Particularly severe infections have been noted in patients with underlying medical conditions, including G6PD deficiency and diabetes mellitus.

PREVENTION. MSF is transmitted by tick bites, and prevention is the same as recommended for RMSF. No vaccine is currently available.

225.3 • Rickettsialpox (*Rickettsia akari*)

Rickettsialpox is caused by *Rickettsia akari,* which is transmitted by the **mouse mite,** *Allodermanyssus sanguineus.* The mouse host for this mite is widely distributed in cities in the United States, Europe, and Asia. Seroepidemiologic studies suggest a high prevalence for this infection in urban settings. The disease is usually mild and is infrequently diagnosed. Unlike most forms of spotted fever rickettsiosis, the macrophage is an important target cell.

Rickettsialpox is best known because of its association with a varicelliform rash. In fact, this rash is a modified form of an antecedent typical macular or maculopapular rash like those seen in other vasculotropic rickettsioses. At presentation, most patients have fever, headache, and chills. There is a painless papular or ulcerative lesion or eschar at the initial site of inoculation in up to 90% of cases, which may be associated with regional, often tender lymphadenopathy. In some patients, the maculopapular rash, which is distributed over the trunk, head, and extremities, may become vesicular. The infection resolves spontaneously, even without therapy. Doxycycline will hasten resolution but, given the mildness of illness, is often withheld in children <9 yr of age. Alternatively, some experts limit treatment to a brief course (2 days) of doxycycline to young children with more significant illness. Complications and fatalities are rare.

Billings AN, Rawlings JA, Walker DH: Tick-borne disease in Texas: A 10-year retrospective examination of cases. *Tex Med* 1998;94:66–76.

Buckingham SC: Rocky Mountain spotted fever: A review for the pediatrician. *Pediatr Ann* 2002;31:163–168.

Buckingham SC, Marshall GS, Schutze GE, et al: Clinical and laboratory features, hospital course, and outcome of rocky mountain spotted fever in children. *J Pediatr* 2007;150:180–184.

Cascio A, Colomba C, Antinori S, et al: Clarithromycin versus azithromycin in the treatment of Mediterranean spotted fever in children: A randomized controlled trial. *Clin Infect Dis* 2002;34:154–158.

Centers for Disease Control and Prevention: Consequences of delayed diagnosis of Rocky Mountain spotted fever in children—West Virginia, Michigan, Tennessee, and Oklahoma, May–July 2000. *MMWR* 2000;49:885–888.

Centers for Disease Control and Prevention: Diagnosis and management of tickborne rickettsial diseases: Rocky Mountain spotted fever, ehrlichioses, and anaplasmosis—United States. *MMWR* 2006;55:1–29.

Centers for Disease Control and Prevention: Fatal cases of Rocky Mountain spotted fever in family clusters—three states, 2003. *MMWR* 2004;53:407–410.

Comer JA, Tzianabos T, Flynn C, et al: Serologic evidence of rickettsialpox *(Rickettsia akari)* infection among intravenous drug users in inner-city Baltimore, Maryland. *Am J Trop Med Hyg* 1999;60:894–898.

Demma LJ, Traeger MS, Nicholson WL, et al: Rocky Mountain spotted fever from an unexpected tick vector in Arizona. *N Engl J Med* 2005;353:587–594.

Dumler JS, Walker DH: Rocky mountain spotted fever—Changing ecology and persisting virulence. *N Engl J Med* 2005;353:551–553.

Holman RC, Paddock CD, Curns AT, et al: Analysis of risk factors for fatal Rocky Mountain spotted fever: Evidence for superiority of tetracyclines for therapy. *J Infect Dis* 2001;184:1437–1444.

Marshall GS, Stout GG, Jacobs RF, et al: Antibodies reactive to *Rickettsia rickettsii* among children living in the southeast and south central regions of the United States. *Arch Pediatr Adolesc Med* 2003;157:443–448.

Sexton DJ, Kaye KS: Rocky Mountain spotted fever. *Med Clin North Am* 2002;86:351–360.

Thorner AR, Walker DH, Petri WA: Rocky Mountain spotted fever. *Clin Infect Dis* 1998;27:1353–1359.

Treadwell TA, Holman RC, Clarke MJ, et al: Rocky Mountain spotted fever in the United States, 1993–1996. *Am J Trop Med Hyg* 2000;63:21–26.

Walker DH: Tick-transmitted infectious diseases in the United States. *Annu Rev Public Health* 1998;19:237–269.

Chapter 226 ■ Scrub Typhus *(Orientia Tsutsugamushi)*

J. Stephen Dumler and George K. Siberry

Scrub typhus is a common and important febrile infectious disease in many parts of the Eastern hemisphere. Recent reports suggest that natural resistance to doxycycline and other antibiotics make selection of appropriate antimicrobial therapy difficult. Concurrent scrub typhus may inhibit the replication of HIV.

ETIOLOGY. The causative agent of scrub typhus, or Tsutsugamushi fever, is *Orientia tsutsugamushi,* which is distinct from other spotted fever and typhus group rickettsiae (see Table 225-1). *O. tsutsugamushi* lacks both lipopolysaccharide and peptidoglycan in its cell wall. Like other vasculotropic rickettsiae, *O. tsutsugamushi* infects endothelium and causes vasculitis, the predominant clinicopathologic feature of the disease. However, the organism also infects cardiac myocytes and macrophages, raising questions about how these findings may explain the clinical manifestations.

EPIDEMIOLOGY. Approximately 1 million infections occur each year, and it is estimated that more than 1 billion people are at risk. Scrub typhus occurs mostly in the Far East, including areas delimited by Korea, Pakistan, and northern Australia. Outside these tropical and subtropical regions, the disease occurs in Japan, the Primorye of far eastern Russia, Tajikistan, Nepal, and nontropical China, including Tibet. Cases imported to the USA and other parts of the world are reported. Most infections in children are acquired in rural areas. In Thailand, scrub typhus is the cause of 1–8% of acute fevers of unknown origin. Infections are most frequent during rainy months, usually June through November. Among children, infections in boys frequently outnumber those in girls.

TRANSMISSION. *O. tsutsugamushi* is transmitted via the bite of the larval stage (chigger) of a trombiculid mite (*Leptotrombidium*), which serves as both vector and reservoir. Transovarial transmission (passage of the organism from infected ticks to their progeny) and transmission of the organism to mites from infected animals both readily occur. Since only the larval stage takes blood meals, a role for horizontal transmission from infected rodent hosts to uninfected mites has not been proved. Multiple *O. tsutsugamushi* serotypes are recognized, and some share antigenic cross reactivity, but do not stimulate protective cross immunity.

PATHOLOGY AND PATHOGENESIS. The pathogenesis of scrub typhus is uncertain. Recent studies indicate that the process is stimulated by a disseminated rickettsial infection of vascular endothelial cells that corresponds to the distribution of disseminated vasculitic and perivascular inflammatory lesions observed in histopathologic examinations. The major result of the vascular injury appears in autopsy series to be hemorrhage. However, it is very likely that the vascular injury initiated by the rickettsial infection results in significant vascular leakage and compromise and is further confounded by the waxing immune and inflammatory reactions. The net result is significant vascular compromise and ensuing end-organ injury, most often manifested in the brain and lungs, as with other vasculotropic rickettsioses.

CLINICAL MANIFESTATIONS AND LABORATORY FINDINGS. Scrub typhus may be mild or severe in children. Most patients present with fever for 9–11 days (range 1–30 days) before seeking medical care. Regional or generalized lymphadenopathy is reported in 23–93% of patients, hepatomegaly in about 2/3, and splenomegaly in about 1/3 of children with scrub typhus. Gastrointestinal symptoms, including abdominal pain, vomiting, and diarrhea, occur in up to 40% of children at presentation. A single painless eschar with an erythematous rim at the site of the chigger bite is seen in 7–68% of cases, and a maculopapular rash is present in less than 30%. Leukocyte and platelet counts are most frequently within normal ranges, although thrombocytopenia occurs in 1/4 to 1/3 of children, and leukocytosis is observed in about 40%.

DIAGNOSIS AND DIFFERENTIAL DIAGNOSIS. Owing to the potential for severe complications, diagnosis and decision to initiate treatment should be based on clinical suspicion and confirmed by *O. tsutsugamushi* serologic tests such as indirect fluorescent antibody (IFA) or immunoperoxidase assays. The IFA assay is 92% sensitive with ≥11 days of fever. Although the rickettsiae can be cultivated using tissue culture methods and polymerase chain reaction tests appear highly sensitive, these are not widely available. The differential diagnosis includes fever of unknown origin, enteric fever, typhoid fever, dengue hemorrhagic fever, other rickettsioses, tularemia, anthrax, dengue, leptospirosis, malaria, and infectious mononucleosis.

TREATMENT AND SUPPORTIVE CARE. The recommended treatment regimen for scrub typhus is doxycycline (2.2 mg/kg/dose bid PO or IV, maximum 200 mg/day). Alternative regimens include tetracycline (25–50 mg/kg/day divided every 6 hr PO, maximum 2 g/day) or chloramphenicol (50–100 mg/kg/day divided every 6 hr IV, maximum 3 g/24 hr). If used, chloramphenicol should be monitored to maintain serum concentrations of 10–30 µg/mL. Therapy should be continued for a minimum of 5 days and until the patient has been afebrile for at least 3 days to avoid relapse. However, a single dose of oral doxycycline was reported effective for all 38 children treated with this regimen in a report of a large series of children with scrub typhus from Thailand. Most children respond rapidly to doxycycline or chloramphenicol within 1–2 days (range 1–5 days). Highly virulent or potentially doxycycline-resistant *O. tsutsugamushi* strains have emerged in some regions of Thailand. Clinical trials showed that azithromycin may be as effective, and that rifampicin is superior to doxycycline in such cases. Likewise, a retrospective analysis in Korean children with scrub typhus showed that roxithromycin was as effective as either doxycycline or chloramphenicol, suggesting a role as an alternative therapy for children or pregnant women. The use of ciprofloxacin in pregnant women resulted in an adverse outcome in 5 of 5 pregnancies among Indian women. Intensive care may be required for hemodynamic management of severely affected individuals.

COMPLICATIONS. Serious complications include pneumonitis that occurs in 20–35%, meningoencephalitis observed in approximately 10% of children, and, much less frequently, acute renal failure, myocarditis, or a septic shock–like syndrome. Cerebrospinal fluid examinations show a mild mononuclear pleocytosis with normal glucose levels. Chest x-rays reveal transient perihilar or peribronchial interstitial infiltrates in most children who are examined. The case fatality rate in untreated patients may be as high as 30% if left untreated, although deaths in children are infrequent.

PREVENTION. Prevention is based on avoidance of the chiggers that transmit *O. tsutsugamushi.* Protective clothing is the next most useful mode of prevention. Infection provides immunity to reinfection by homologous but not heterologous strains; however, since natural strains are highly heterogeneous, infection does not always provide complete protection against reinfection.

Lee KY, Lee HS, Hong JH, et al: Roxithromycin treatment of scrub typhus (tsutsugamushi disease) in children. *Pediatr Infect Dis J* 2003;22:130–133.
Mathai E, Rolain JM, Verghese L, et al: Case reports: Scrub typhus during pregnancy in India. *Trans R Soc Trop Med Hyg* 2003;97:570–572.
Panpanich R, Garner P: Antibiotics for treating scrub typhus. *Cochrane Database Syst Rev* 2002;(3):CD002150.
Silpapojakul K, Chupuppakam S, Yuthasompob S, et al: Scrub and murine typhus in children with obscure fever in the tropics. *Pediatr Infect Dis J* 1991;10:200–203.
Silpapojakul K, Varachit B, Silpapojakul K: Paediatric scrub typhus in Thailand: A study of 73 confirmed cases. *Trans R Soc Trop Med Hyg* 2004;98:354–359.
Sirisanthana V, Puthanakit T, Sirisanthana T: Epidemiologic, clinical and laboratory features of scrub typhus in thirty Thai children. *Pediatr Infect Dis J* 2003;22:341–345.
Wang CL, Yang KD, Cheng SN, et al: Neonatal scrub typhus: A case report. *Pediatrics* 1992;89:965–968.
Watt G, Kantipong P, de Souza M, et al: HIV-1 suppression during acute scrub-typhus infection. *Lancet* 2000;356:475–479.
Watt G, Kantipong P, Jongsakul K, et al: Doxycycline and rifampicin for mild scrub-typhus infections in northern Thailand: A randomised trial. *Lancet* 2000;356:1057–1061.

Chapter 227 ■ Typhus Group Rickettsioses

J. Stephen Dumler and George K. Siberry

Members of the typhus group of rickettsiae pathogenic for humans (see Table 225-1) include *Rickettsia typhi,* the cause of murine typhus, and *Rickettsia prowazekii,* the cause of epidemic typhus. *R. typhi* is transmitted to humans by fleas, whereas *R. prowazekii* is transmitted in the feces of body lice. Louse-borne or epidemic typhus is widely considered to be the most virulent of all rickettsial diseases, with a high case fatality rate even with treatment. Murine typhus is moderately severe and perhaps 1 of the most under-recognized infections in the world. The genomes of both *R. typhi* and *R. prowazekii* have been sequenced and share considerable genetic identity.

227.1 • Murine Typhus (*Rickettsia typhi*)

ETIOLOGY. Murine typhus is caused by *R. typhi,* a rickettsia transmitted from infected fleas to rats, other rodents, or opossums and back to fleas. Transovarial transmission (passage of the organism from infected fleas to their progeny) in fleas is inefficient. Transmission depends on distribution by the flea to uninfected mammals that become transiently rickettsemic and transmit the organism to uninfected fleas.

Rickettsia felis is a novel agent species identified as a cause of a murine typhus-like illness worldwide. This new rickettsia is genetically a member of the spotted fever group and is capable of highly efficient transovarial transmission in cat fleas. This organism is found in cat fleas obtained from areas endemic for murine typhus in the United States.

EPIDEMIOLOGY. Murine typhus has a worldwide distribution and occurs especially in warm coastal ports where it is maintained in a cycle involving rat fleas (*Xenopsylla cheopis*) and rats (*Rattus* species). Peak incidence occurs when rat populations are highest during spring, summer, and fall. In the United States, the disease is most prevalent in south Texas and southern California, although seroprevalence studies among children indicate a higher than anticipated rate of infection broadly across the southeast and south-central USA, expanding the endemic areas in which pediatricians must be alert for this infection. In the coastal areas of south Texas, the disease is seen predominantly from March through June and is associated with opossums, cats, and cat fleas (*Ctenocephalides felis*).

TRANSMISSION. *R. typhi* normally cycles between rodents or mid-size animals such as opossums and their fleas. Human acquisition of murine typhus occurs when rickettsiae-infected flea feces contaminate flea bite wounds.

PATHOLOGY AND PATHOGENESIS. *R. typhi* is a vasculotropic rickettsia that causes disease in a manner similar to *R. rickettsii* (see Chapter 225.1). *R. typhi* organisms in flea feces deposited on the skin as part of the flea feeding reflex are inoculated into the pruritic flea bite wound. After an interval for local proliferation, the rickettsiae spread systemically to infect the endothelium in many tissues. As with spotted fever group rickettsiae, typhus group rickettsiae infect endothelial cells, but unlike the spotted fever group rickettsiae, they polymerize intracellular actin poorly, have limited intracellular mobility, and probably cause cellular injury by mechanical lysis after accumulating in large numbers within the endothelial cell cytoplasm. Intracellular infection leads to endothelial cell damage, recruitment of inflammatory cells, and vasculitis. The inflammatory cell infiltrates bring in a number of effector cells, including macrophages that produce proinflammatory cytokines, and CD4, CD8, and natural killer lymphocytes, which may produce immune cytokines such as interferon-γ or participate in cell-mediated cytotoxic responses. Intracellular rickettsial proliferation of typhus group rickettsiae is inhibited by cytokine-mediated, nitric oxide–dependent and -independent mechanisms.

Pathologic findings include systemic vasculitis in response to rickettsiae within endothelial cells. This manifests as interstitial pneumonitis, meningoencephalitis, interstitial nephritis, myocarditis, and mild hepatitis with periportal lymphohistiocytic infiltrates. As vasculitis and inflammatory damage accumulate, multiorgan damage may ensue.

CLINICAL MANIFESTATIONS. Murine typhus is a moderately severe infection that is similar to other vasculotropic rickettsioses. The incubation period varies from 1 to 2 wk. The initial presentation is often nonspecific, with fever of undetermined origin the most frequent presentation. Pediatric patients exhibit the typically important clues for murine typhus somewhat less frequently than for the other vasculotropic rickettsioses, including rash (48–80%), myalgias (29–57%), vomiting (29–45%), cough (15–40%), headache (19–77%), and diarrhea or abdominal pain (10–40%). Lymphadenopathy and hepatosplenomegaly are reported frequently among children with murine typhus in Europe. Although neurologic involvement may be a frequent finding in adults with murine typhus, photophobia, confusion, stupor, coma, seizures, meningismus, and ataxia are seen in <17% of hospitalized and <6% of infected children treated as outpatients. A petechial rash is observed in only up to 13% of children, and the usual appearance is that of macules or maculopapules distributed on the trunk and extremities. The rash can involve both the soles and palms.

LABORATORY FINDINGS. Although nonspecific, laboratory findings that may be helpful include mild leukopenia (36–40%) with a moderate left shift, mild to marked thrombocytopenia (43–60%), hyponatremia (20–66%), hypoalbuminemia (46–87%), and elevated aspartate aminotransferase (82%) and alanine aminotransferase (38%). Elevations in serum urea nitrogen are usually due to prerenal mechanisms.

DIAGNOSIS AND DIFFERENTIAL DIAGNOSIS. As for other vasculotropic rickettsioses, delays in diagnosis and therapy are associated with increased morbidity and mortality; thus, diagnosis must be based on clinical suspicion. Occasionally, patients present with findings suggestive of pharyngitis, bronchitis, hepatitis, gastroenteritis, or sepsis; thus, the differential diagnosis may be extensive.

Confirmation of the diagnosis is usually accomplished by comparing acute and convalescent phase antibody titers obtained with the indirect fluorescent antibody assay. Research tools now being evaluated include polymerase chain reaction amplification of rickettsial nucleic acids in acute phase blood, rickettsial culture by the centrifugation-assisted shell vial assay, and immunohistology on skin biopsy.

TREATMENT. Therapy for murine typhus includes the use of tetracyclines or chloramphenicol and is similar to that recommended for Rocky Mountain spotted fever. No controlled trials of other antimicrobial agents have been performed; however, ciprofloxacin has been used effectively to treat murine typhus, and in vitro experiments suggest that minimal inhibitory concentrations of azithromycin and clarithromycin for *R. typhi* should be easily achieved.

The recommended treatment regimen for murine typhus is doxycycline (2.2 mg/kg/dose bid PO or IV, maximum 200 mg/day). Alternative regimens include tetracycline (25–50 mg/kg/day divided every 6 hr PO, maximum 2 g/day) and chloramphenicol (50–100 mg/kg/day divided every 6 hr IV, maximum 3 g/day). Therapy should be continued for a minimum of 5 days and until the patient has been afebrile for at least 3 days to avoid relapse, especially in patients treated early.

SUPPORTIVE CARE. Although usually mild, 7% of children with murine typhus may require intensive care to manage complications such as meningoencephalitis or a disseminated intravascular coagulation-like condition. As for other rickettsial infections with significant systemic vascular injury, careful hemodynamic management is mandatory to avoid pulmonary or cerebral edema.

COMPLICATIONS. Complications of murine typhus in pediatric patients are infrequent; however, relapse, stupor, facial edema, dehydration, splenic rupture, and meningoencephalitis have been reported. Predominance of abdominal pain has led to surgical exploration to exclude a perforated viscus.

PREVENTION. Control of murine typhus was dependent on elimination of the flea reservoir and control of flea hosts, and this remains an important component of control. However, with the recognition of cat fleas as potentially significant reservoirs and vectors, the presence of these flea vectors and their mammalian hosts in suburban and urban areas where close human exposures occur will probably pose increasingly important control problems. It is not known with certainty if infection confers protective immunity; however, reinfection appears to be rare.

227.2 • Epidemic Typhus (*Rickettsia prowazekii*)

ETIOLOGY. Humans are considered the principal or only reservoir of *R. prowazekii,* the causative agent of epidemic or louse-borne typhus, and its recrudescent form, Brill-Zinsser disease. Another reservoir has recently been identified in flying squirrels, implying that a sylvatic cycle with small rodents and their ectoparasites also exists. The rickettsia is the most pathogenic of the genus, and multiplies to very large intracellular quantities before mechanical rupture of infected endothelial cells. *R. prowazekii* and all *Rickettsia* species are recognized as a genetic relative of the eukaryotic mitochondrion.

EPIDEMIOLOGY. The infection is characteristically seen in winter or spring or during times of poor hygienic practices associated with crowding, war, famine, extreme poverty, and civil strife. A cause of some sporadic cases of a mild, typhus-like illness in the United States has been confirmed as *R. prowazekii;* such cases are associated with exposure to flying squirrels harboring infected lice or fleas. *R. prowazekii* organisms isolated from these squirrels appear to be genetically different from isolates obtained during typical outbreaks.

Most cases of louse-borne typhus in the developed world are sporadic, but outbreaks have been identified in Africa (Ethiopia, Nigeria, and Burundi), Mexico, Central America, South America, Eastern Europe, Afghanistan, Russia, northern India, and China within the past 25 years. Following the Burundi Civil War in 1993, there were 35,000–100,000 cases of epidemic typhus diagnosed in displaced refugees, among which it is predicted that about 6,000 deaths occurred.

TRANSMISSION. Human body lice (*Pediculus humanus* subspecies *corporis*) become infected by feeding on rickettsemic persons. The ingested rickettsiae infect the midgut epithelial cells of the lice and are passed into the feces, which in turn are introduced into a susceptible human host through abrasions or perforations in the skin, through the conjunctivae, or rarely through inhalation of dried infected louse excreta present in clothing, bedding, or furniture.

CLINICAL MANIFESTATIONS. Louse-borne typhus can be mild or severe in children. The incubation period is usually <14 days. The typical clinical manifestations include fever, severe headache, abdominal tenderness, and rash in most patients, as well as chills (82%), myalgias (70%), arthralgias (70%), anorexia (48%), nonproductive cough (38%), dizziness (35%), photophobia (33%), nausea (32%), abdominal pain (30%), tinnitus (23%), constipation (23%) meningismus (17%), visual disturbances (15%), vomiting (10%), and diarrhea (7%). However, investigation of recent African outbreaks has shown a lower frequency of rash (25%) and a high frequency of delirium (81%) and cough associated with pneumonitis (70%). The rash is initially pink or erythematous and blanches. In $^1/_3$ of patients, red, nonblanching macules and petechiae appear predominantly on the trunk. Infections identified during the preantibiotic era typically produced a variety of central nervous system findings, including delirium (48%), coma (6%), and seizures (1%). Estimates of case fatality rates range between 3.8% and 20% in outbreaks.

Brill-Zinsser disease is an unusual form of typhus that becomes recrudescent months to years after the primary infection, thus rarely affecting children. When rickettsemic, these infected individuals may transmit the agent to lice that could provide the initial event that triggers an outbreak if hygienic conditions permit.

TREATMENT. Recommended treatment regimens for louse-borne or sylvatic typhus are identical to those used for murine typhus. The treatment of choice is doxycycline (2.2 mg/kg/dose bid PO or IV, maximum 200 mg/day). Alternative treatments include tetracycline (25–50 mg/kg/day divided every 6 hr PO, maximum 2 g/day), or chloramphenicol (50–100 mg/kg/day divided every 6 hr IV, maximum 3 g/day). Therapy should be continued for a minimum of 5 days and until the patient has been afebrile for at least 3 days to avoid relapse, especially in patients treated early. Good evidence exists that doxycycline as a single 200 mg oral dose (4.4 mg/kg if <45 kg) is also efficacious.

PREVENTION. Immediate destruction of vectors with an insecticide is important in the control of an epidemic. For epidemic typhus, antibiotic therapy and delousing measures will interrupt transmission, reduce the prevalence of infection in the human reservoir, and diminish the impact of an outbreak. Dust containing excreta from infected lice is stable and capable of transmitting typhus, and care must be taken to prevent its inhalation. Infection confers solid protective immunity. However, recrudescence may occur years later with Brill-Zinsser disease, implying that immunity is nonsterile.

Bernabeu-Wittel M, Pachon J, Alarcon A, et al: Murine typhus as a common cause of fever of intermediate duration: A 17-year study in the south of Spain. *Arch Intern Med* 1991;159:872–876.

Bitsori M, Galanakis E, Gikas A, et al: *Rickettsia typhi* infection in childhood. *Acta Paediatr* 2002;91:59–61.

Fergie J, Purcell K: Spontaneous splenic rupture in a child with murine typhus. *Pediatr Infect Dis J* 2004;23:1171–1172.

Fergie JE, Purcell K, Wanat D: Murine typhus in South Texas children. *Pediatr Infect Dis J* 2000;19:535–538.

Marshall GS, for the Tick-Borne Infections in Children Study (TICS) Group: *Rickettsia typhi* seroprevalence among children in the southeast United States. *Pediatr Infect Dis J* 2000;9:1103–1104.

Massung RF, Davis LE, Slater K, et al: Epidemic typhus meningitis in the southwestern United States. *Clin Infect Dis* 2001;32:979–982.

Raoult D, Ndihokubwayo JB, Tissot-Dupont H, et al: Outbreak of epidemic typhus associated with trench fever in Burundi. *Lancet* 1998;352:353–358.

Silpapojakul K, Chupuppakam S, Yuthasompob S, et al: Scrub and murine typhus in children with obscure fever in the tropics. *Pediatr Infect Dis J* 1991;10:2000–2003.

Whiteford SF, Taylor JP, Dumler JS: Clinical, laboratory, and epidemiologic features of murine typhus in 97 Texas children. *Arch Pediatr Adolesc Med* 2001;155:396–400.

Chapter 228 ■ Ehrlichioses and Anaplasmosis

George K. Siberry and J. Stephen Dumler

ETIOLOGY. In 1987, clusters of bacteria confined within cytoplasmic vacuoles of circulating leukocytes (morulae), particularly mononuclear leukocytes, were detected in the peripheral blood of a severely ill patient with suspected Rocky Mountain spotted fever (RMSF). The etiologic agent of the infection and of other cases in which serologic tests could not prove RMSF was found to be similar to a canine pathogen in the genus *Ehrlichia.* In 1990, a new species, *Ehrlichia chaffeensis,* was cultivated and identified as the predominant agent of "human ehrlichiosis." Seroepidemiologic investigation has shown that in some geographic areas *E. chaffeensis* infections occur more frequently than RMSF, and the infection is strongly associated with tick bites.

In 1994, another similar species was recognized in human blood with the observation of morulae only in circulating neutrophils. Serologic investigation in these cases revealed the absence of *E. chaffeensis* antibodies, and most had serologic reactions to *Ehrlichia phagocytophila* and *Ehrlichia equi,* previously known only as pathogens of ruminant and horse granulocytes, respectively. DNA of these bacteria was also found in the blood of many infected persons. In 1996, the agent was cultivated in vitro, and based on genetic studies in 2001, the human agent and the 2 veterinary pathogens were unified into a single species and placed into the genus *Anaplasma* under the name *Anaplasma phagocytophilum.*

In 1996, a veterinary pathogen of canine neutrophils, *Ehrlichia ewingii,* was identified as the causative agent of some human infections initially thought to be due to *E. chaffeensis.* The agent is occasionally identified in peripheral blood neutrophils and the infection is generally milder and involves children or adults with pre-existing immunosuppression, including organ transplant recipients or persons with HIV infection. Although not yet cultivated in vitro, it is serologically cross reactive with *E. chaffeensis.*

Although bacteria assigned to various genera cause these infections, the name ehrlichiosis was applied to all. To differentiate among these infections, disease caused by *E. chaffeensis,* which infects predominantly monocytic cells, is called **human monocytic ehrlichiosis (HME)**, and disease caused by *Anaplasma phagocytophilum* is called **human granulocytic anaplasmosis (HGA)**, formerly granulocytic ehrlichiosis (HGE), and disease caused by *E. ewingii* has received various names, including **ewingii ehrlichiosis** (see Table 225-1).

All of these bacteria are now classified in the Anaplasmataceae family, and share many characteristics, including transmission by tick bite. *Neorickettsia* (formerly *Ehrlichia*) *sennetsu* is another related bacterium in this family that is a rare cause of human disease, but is not transmitted by ticks. These are small, pleomorphic, obligate, intracellular bacteria that possess gram-negative-type cell walls. *E. chaffeensis* alters host signaling and transcription to cause the endosome to enter a receptor recycling pathway that avoids phagosome-lysosome fusion and allows the growth of a **morula,** which is a cytoplasmic aggregate of bacteria. Little is known about the vacuoles in which *A. phagocytophilum* and *E. ewingii* grow. These bacteria are pathogens of hematopoietic cells in mammals, and characteristically each species has a specific host cell affinity: *E. chaffeensis* and *N. sennetsu* infect mononuclear phagocytes, and *A. phagocytophilum* and *E. ewingii* infect neutrophils. Infection leads to modifications in function of the host cell, and insufficient levels of infection are usually obtained to account directly for the severity and pathology observed. Thus, an increasing body of data suggests that host immune and inflammatory reactions may in part account for many of the clinical manifestations in all forms of ehrlichiosis.

EPIDEMIOLOGY. Infections with *E. chaffeensis* occur in broad areas across the southeastern, south central, and mid-Atlantic states, in a distribution that parallels that of RMSF. Suspected cases with appropriate serologic and some molecular evidence have been reported in Europe, Africa, and the Far East. HGA is the most frequently recognized of all forms of human ehrlichiosis and is found mostly in the northeast and upper midwestern United States, and infections have now been identified in northern California, the mid-Atlantic, and broadly across Europe, confirming that the agent is widely distributed. Human infections with *E. ewingii* have only been identified in U.S. areas where *E. chaffeensis* also exist, perhaps owing to a shared tick vector.

Although the median age of patients with ehrlichiosis and anaplasmosis is generally older (>42 yr), many infected children have been identified. Little is known about the epidemiologic aspects of *E. ewingii* infection. As expected, all infections are highly associated with tick exposure and tick bites, and are identified predominantly during May through September; a 2nd peak of HGA occurs in late October through December because of activity of the adult stage of *Ixodes scapularis* ticks during this time. Although both nymphal and adult ticks can transmit infection, they are most likely to transmit disease in the nymphal stage since it is most active during summer months.

TRANSMISSION. The predominant tick species that harbors *E. chaffeensis* and *E. ewingii* is *Amblyomma americanum,* the Lone Star tick. Additional vectors such as *Dermacentor variabilis,* the American dog tick, have not been proved but may explain the presence of HME outside the known range of *A. americanum* (see

Fig. 225-1). The tick vectors of *A. phagocytophilum* are *Ixodes,* including *I. scapularis* (black-legged or deer tick) in the eastern United States (see Fig. 225-1), *I. pacificus* (western black-legged tick) in the western United States, *I. ricinus* (sheep tick) in Europe, and potentially *I. persulcatus* in Eurasia. *Ixodes* species ticks also transmit *Borrelia burgdorferi, Babesia microti,* and, in Europe, flaviviruses in the tick-borne encephalitis group. Co-infections with these agents and *A. phagocytophilum* have been documented in children and adults.

Ehrlichia and *Anaplasma* species are maintained in nature predominantly by horizontal transmission (tick to mammal to tick) because the organisms are not transmitted to the progeny of infected adult female ticks (transovarial transmission). The major reservoir host for *E. chaffeensis* is the white-tailed deer (*Odocoileus virginianus*), which is found abundantly in many parts of the United States. A reservoir for *A. phagocytophilum* in the eastern United States appears to be the white-footed mouse, *Peromyscus leucopus,* but increasing evidence also implicates deer or domestic ruminants. This suggests that efficient transmission requires persistent infection of mammals, long recognized in dogs with *Ehrlichia canis,* ruminants with *A. phagocytophilum,* and other hosts of various ehrlichial species. However, while *E. chaffeensis* and *A. phagocytophilum* may cause persistent infections in animals, persistence is exceedingly rarely in humans. Transmission can occur within hours after tick attachment, in contrast to the typical 1–2 day duration of attachment necessary for transmission of *B. burgdorferi.* Similarly, transmission of *A. phagocytophilum* is often via the bite of the small nymphal stage of *I. scapularis* (see Fig. 225-1), which is very active during late spring and early summer in the eastern USA.

PATHOLOGY AND PATHOGENESIS. Although patients with human monocytic ehrlichiosis and anaplasmosis often present with an illness that appears similar to RMSF or typhus, vasculitis is rare. Pathologic findings include diffuse but mild perivascular lymphohistiocytic infiltrates, infrequent hepatocyte apoptoses, Kupffer cell hyperplasia, mild lobular hepatitis, increases in mononuclear phagocyte infiltrates in the spleen, lymph nodes, and bone marrow in which occasional erythrophagocytic cells are present, granulomas of the liver and bone marrow in patients with *E. chaffeensis* infections, and hyperplasia of 1 or more bone marrow hematopoietic lineages.

The exact pathogenetic mechanisms are poorly understood, but histopathologic examinations suggest diffuse mononuclear phagocyte activation and overinduction of host immune and inflammatory reactions. This activation results in moderate to profound leukopenia and thrombocytopenia in the presence of a hypercellular bone marrow, and fatalities are often associated with severe hemorrhage or secondary opportunistic infections. Hepatic or other organ-specific injury occurs by an unknown mechanism that is apparently unrelated to direct infection. An unexplained observation in severe disease is the occurrence of diffuse alveolar damage that results in the clinical picture of adult respiratory distress syndrome (ARDS), which also appears to be unrelated to direct ehrlichial tissue damage. Meningoencephalitis with a mononuclear cell cerebrospinal fluid (CSF) pleocytosis may be present in HME but is rare with HGA.

CLINICAL MANIFESTATIONS. HME, HGA, and ewingii ehrlichiosis are distinct entities caused by infection with different species that result in similar illnesses. Many well-defined cases of pediatric infection of variable severity have been reported, including 1 fatality each from HME and HGA. Population-based studies have shown that mild or subclinical illness is not uncommon in children. Insufficient numbers of children infected with *E. ewingii* have been identified to allow a thorough characterization. The incubation period after the last preceding tick bite or tick exposure ranges from 2 days to 3 wk. No tick bite is documented in nearly $^1/_4$ of all patients. The diseases usually present with nonspecific findings, including fever (~100%) and headache (~75%). A majority of patients also describe myalgias, anorexia, and nausea or vomiting. Nearly $^2/_3$ of children with HME, compared with $^1/_3$ of adults, present with a rash. The rash is usually described as macular or maculopapular, although petechial lesions may occur. Photophobia, conjunctivitis, pharyngitis, arthralgias, and lymphadenopathy occur but are less consistent features.

Hepatomegaly and splenomegaly are detected in nearly half of infected children. Edema of the face, hands, and feet occurs more commonly in children than in adults, but arthritis is uncommon in both. Meningoencephalitis with a lymphocyte-predominant CSF pleocytosis is an infrequently encountered but potentially severe complication of HME that appears to be rare with HGA. CSF protein may be elevated and glucose mildly depressed in adults with HME meningoencephalitis, but CSF protein and glucose in affected children are typically normal. In 1 adult series, brain CT was normal despite central nervous system (CNS) involvement, but 19% of patients with CNS symptoms and abnormal CSF died.

The illness ordinarily lasts 4–12 days, and in most published cases hospitalization was required. Of children with HME in 1 series, 25% required intensive care. Untreated, the illness commonly lasts 3 wk or more in adults. Well-documented cases of seroconversion in the absence of overt clinical manifestations strongly suggest the occurrence of mild or subclinical infections. Clinically evident infections of children with ewingii ehrlichiosis are infrequent; however, the clinical presentation of this illness in adults is very similar to that of adult *E. chaffeensis* infection.

LABORATORY FINDINGS. Characteristically, most children with monocytic ehrlichiosis present with leukopenia (58–72%), lymphopenia (75–78%), and thrombocytopenia (80–92%) that reach their nadir several days into the illness. Lymphopenia is common with HME and HGA, but neutropenia is typical of HGA. Leukocytosis may also occur. Despite the presence of pancytopenia, examination usually reveals a cellular or reactive bone marrow in adults. Interestingly, granulomas and granulomatous inflammation are identified in nearly 75% of bone marrow specimens examined from patients with proven cases of *E. chaffeensis* infection, but this finding is not present in patients with HGA. Mild to severe hepatic injury is documented by the frequent (83–91%) finding of elevated serum transaminase levels. Hyponatremia (<135 mEq/L) is present in a majority of cases. Severely affected children may experience varying degrees of renal failure accompanied by elevated concentrations of serum creatinine and urea nitrogen. A clinical picture similar to disseminated intravascular coagulopathy with prolonged activated partial thromboplastin time and prothrombin time and hypofibrinogenemia has occurred in several patients.

DIAGNOSIS. A delay in diagnosis or treatment may contribute to increased morbidity or mortality; thus, an early clinical diagnosis is important. Because both HME and anaplasmosis have been associated with a fatal outcome, therapy should not be withheld while awaiting confirmatory laboratory test results. In fact, prompt response to therapy can help confirm the diagnosis.

The 1st patient and several subsequent pediatric patients with *E. chaffeensis* infection were identified presumptively on the basis of typical *Ehrlichia* morulae in peripheral blood leukocytes (Fig. 228-1A). This finding has been too infrequent to be considered a useful diagnostic tool. In contrast, HGA presents with a small but significant percentage (1–40%) of circulating neutrophils (Fig. 228-1B) containing typical morulae in 20–60% of patients. The distinction between the 2 infections relies on polymerase chain reaction (PCR) amplification of species-specific DNA sequences or on the demonstration of specific antibodies to *E. chaffeensis* or *A. phagocytophilum* antigen.

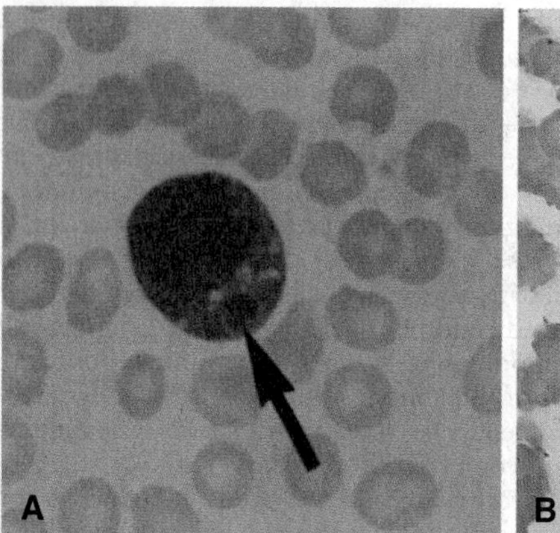

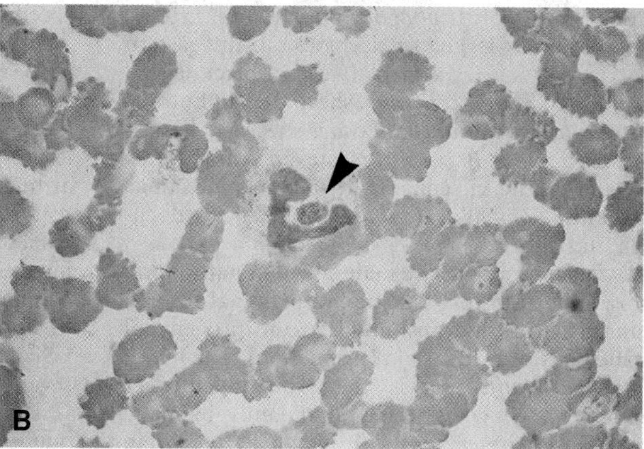

Figure 228-1. Morulae in peripheral blood leukocytes in patients with human monocytic ehrlichiosis and human granulocytic anaplasmosis. *A,* A morula *(arrow)* containing *Ehrlichia chaffeensis* in a monocyte. *B,* A morula *(arrowhead)* containing *Anaplasma phagocytophilum* in a neutrophil. Wright stains, original magnifications ×1,200. *E. chaffeensis* and *A. phagocytophilum* have similar morphologies but are serologically and genetically distinct.

The **diagnostic criteria** for *E. chaffeensis* infection include a seroconversion with a titer of ≥64, or a single serum titer (usually convalescent serum) of ≥128, in the context of a clinically compatible illness. Similarly, **anaplasmosis** may be confirmed by a seroconversion or single high titer of *A. phagocytophilum* antibodies; some laboratories still refer to the causative agent as the HGE agent or *E. equi. E. ewingii* infection induces antibodies that cross react with *E. chaffeensis* in routine serologic tests and can only be differentiated by identification of specific nucleic acids or by the demonstration of morulae in neutrophils where the *E. chaffeensis* titer is at least 4-fold higher than the *A. phagocytophilum* titer. Patients with HGA experience serologic reactions to *E. chaffeensis* in up to 15% of cases, and thus serodiagnosis depends on testing with both *E. chaffeensis* and *A. phagocytophilum* antigens. During the acute phase of illness when antibodies may not be detected, PCR amplification of specific *E. chaffeensis* or *A. phagocytophilum* DNA sequences is sensitive in 50–86% of cases. *E. chaffeensis* and *A. phagocytophilum* have both been cultivated in tissue culture, but neither method provides a timely result.

DIFFERENTIAL DIAGNOSIS. Because of the nonspecific presentation, ehrlichiosis may be mimicked by other arthropod-borne infections such as RMSF, tularemia, babesiosis, Lyme disease, murine typhus, relapsing fever, and Colorado tick fever. Other potential diagnoses considered include otitis media, streptococcal pharyngitis, infectious mononucleosis, Kawasaki disease, endocarditis, viral syndromes, hepatitis, leptospirosis, Q fever, collagen-vascular diseases, and leukemia. If rash and disseminated intravascular coagulopathy predominate, meningococcemia, bacterial sepsis, and toxic shock syndrome should be suspected. Meningoencephalitis may suggest enterovirus or herpes simplex virus infections, bacterial meningitis, or RMSF, whereas severe respiratory disease may be confused with bacterial, viral, or fungal pneumonitis.

TREATMENT. Both HME and HGA are effectively treated with tetracyclines, especially doxycycline, and the majority of patients usually improve within 48 hr. In vitro tests document that both *E. chaffeensis* and *A. phagocytophilum* have minimal inhibitory concentrations to chloramphenicol above safely achieved blood levels. Because of these findings, a short course of doxycycline is the recommended regimen. Doxycycline can be used safely in children <9 yr of age because tooth discoloration is dose dependent and the need for multiple courses is unlikely. Little information exists to recommend alternative therapies; both *E. chaffeensis* and *A. phagocytophilum* are susceptible to rifampin in vitro, and it has been successfully used to treat HGA in pregnant women and children.

The recommended treatment regimen for patients of all ages with severe or complicated HME and HGA is doxycycline (2.2 mg/kg/dose bid PO or IV, maximum dose 200 mg/day). An alternative regimen is tetracycline 25–50 mg/kg/day divided every 6 hr PO, maximum 2 g/day). Therapy should be continued for a minimum of 5 days and until the patient has been afebrile for at least 2–4 days.

Other broad-spectrum antibiotics, including penicillins, cephalosporins, aminoglycosides, and macrolides, are not effective. *A. phagocytophilum* is not susceptible to azithromycin, but in vitro studies suggest a potential role for rifamycins in HME and HGA. In vitro studies show activity for fluoroquinolones against *A. phagocytophilum;* however, *E. chaffeensis* is naturally resistant owing to a single nucleotide change in *gyrA,* suggesting the possibility of resistance rapidly emerging with *A. phagocytophilum.* Increasing evidence suggests that the antecedent treatment with sulfamethoxazole-trimethoprim may result in more severe disease.

COMPLICATIONS AND PROGNOSIS. Fatal monocytic ehrlichiosis has been reported in 1 pediatric patient where the findings were initially dominated by pulmonary involvement with respiratory failure complicated by nosocomial bacterial pneumonia. The pattern of severe pulmonary involvement culminating in diffuse alveolar damage and ARDS and secondary nosocomial or opportunistic infections is now well documented with HME and HGA in adults. One child with HGA died after 3 wk of fever, thrombocytopenia, and lymphadenopathy suspected to be a hematologic malignancy. Other severe complications include a toxic shock–like illness, meningoencephalitis with long-term neurologic sequelae, brachial plexopathy, demyelinating polyneuropathy, myocarditis, rhabdomyolysis, and renal failure. Patients who are immunocompromised (e.g., HIV infection, high-dose corticosteroid therapy, cancer chemotherapy, immunosuppression for organ transplantation) are at high risk for fulminant infection.

PREVENTION. HME, HGA, and ewingii ehrlichiosis are tick-borne diseases, and any activity that allows exposure to the tick vectors increases risk. Avoidance of tick-infested areas, the wearing of appropriate light-colored clothing, tick repellents sprayed on clothing, careful inspection for ticks after exposure, and prompt removal of any attached ticks diminish the risk for acquisition of HME and HGA. The interval after tick attachment and before transmission of the infectious agents may be as short as 4 hr; thus, any attached tick should be promptly removed. The role of prophylactic therapy for ehrlichiosis and anaplasmosis after tick bites has not been investigated. It is not known if infection confers protective immunity. However, reinfection appears to be rare.

Arnez M, Luznik-Bufon T, Avsic-Zupanc T, et al: Causes of febrile illnesses after a tick bite in Slovenian children. *Pediatr Infect Dis J* 2003;22:1078–1083.

Berry DS, Miller RS, Hooke JA, et al: Ehrlichial meningitis with cerebrospinal fluid morulae. *Pediatr Infect Dis J* 1999;18:552–555.

Buller RS, Arens M, Hmiel SP, et al: *Ehrlichia ewingii,* a newly recognized agent of human ehrlichiosis. *N Engl J Med* 1999;341:148–155.

Dumler JS, Dey C, Meier F, et al: Human monocytic ehrlichiosis: A potentially severe disease in children. *Arch Pediatr Adolesc Med* 2000;154:847–849.

Horowitz HW, Kilchevsky E, Haber S, et al: Perinatal transmission of the agent of human granulocytic ehrlichiosis. *N Engl J Med* 1998;339:375–378.

Jacobs RF: Human monocytic ehrlichiosis: Similar to Rocky Mountain spotted fever but different. *Pediatr Ann* 2002;31:180–184.

Jacobs RF, Schutze GE: Ehrlichiosis in children. *J Pediatr* 1997;131:184–192.

Krause PJ, Corrow CL, Bakken JS: Successful treatment of human granulocytic ehrlichiosis in children using rifampin. *Pediatrics* 2003;112:e252–e253.

Lantos P, Krause PJ: Ehrlichiosis in children. *Semin Pediatr Infect Dis* 2002;13:249–256.

Marshall GS, Jacobs RF, Schutze GE, et al: *Ehrlichia chaffeensis* seroprevalence among children in the southeast and south-central regions of the United States. *Arch Pediatr Adolesc Med* 2002;156:166–170.

Moss WJ, Dumler JS: Simultaneous infection with *Borrelia burgdorferi* and human granulocytic ehrlichiosis. *Pediatr Infect Dis J* 2003;22:91–92.

Olano JP, Walker DH: Human ehrlichiosis. *Med Clin North Am* 2002;86:375–392.

Peters TR, Edwards KM, Standaert SM: Severe ehrlichiosis in an adolescent taking trimethoprim-sulfamethoxazole. *Pediatr Infect Dis J* 2000;19:170–172.

Schutze GE: Ehrlichiosis. *Pediatr Infect Dis J* 2006;25:71–72.

Schutze GE, Jacobs RF: Human monocytic ehrlichiosis in children. *Pediatrics* 1997;100:E10.

Stone JH, Dierberg K, Aram G, Dumler JP: Human monocytic ehrlichiosis. JAMA 2004;292:2263–2270.

Chapter 229 ■ Q Fever *(Coxiella Burnetii)*

J. Stephen Dumler and George K. Siberry

Q fever (for **query fever**) is rarely reported in children and is probably underdiagnosed. It is a febrile disease that presents in acute and chronic forms.

ETIOLOGY. The causative organism of Q fever, *Coxiella burnetii,* is genetically distinct from the genera *Rickettsia, Ehrlichia,* and *Anaplasma.* It is no longer classified within the order Rickettsiales, and has been assigned to the order Legionellales of the family Coxiellaceae. *C. burnetii* is highly infectious for humans and animals and is a select agent of concern for bioterrorism since even a single organism can cause infection. The organism can enter a sporogenic differentiation cycle, unlike *Rickettsia,* which renders it highly resistant to chemical and physical treatments.

C. burnetii resides intracellularly within macrophages. The organisms undergo a lipopolysaccharide "phase variation" similar to that described for smooth and rough strains of Enterobacteriaceae. Unlike *Ehrlichia, Anaplasma,* and *Chlamydia, C. burnetii* expressing phase I lipopolysaccharide survives and proliferates within acidified phagosomes to form aggregates often of >100 bacteria. Organisms that express phase II lipopolysaccharide are killed in the phagolysosome.

EPIDEMIOLOGY. The disease is reported worldwide, except in New Zealand. Children have significantly less clinical disease than do adults, although seroepidemiologic studies suggest that infection occurs just as frequently. Approximately 60% of infections are asymptomatic, and when symptomatic, only 5% require hospitalization. Seroprevalence surveys show that between 6 and 70% of children in endemic European and African communities have evidence of past infection, and in France the overall incidence of Q fever is estimated to be 50 cases per 100,000 population. Although only 70 cases of Q fever in the United States were reported to the Centers for Disease Control and Prevention in 2004, the incidence of infection appears to be increasing in Asia and Australia. Most infections are identified during the lamb birthing season in Europe, from January through June, in children following farm visits, or after exposure to the products of conception for dogs, cats, and rabbits. Immunodeficiency or underlying cardiac valve or vascular damage or prostheses are identified as underlying factors in >20% of all patients with acute or chronic Q fever. While men are more likely infected than women, infection is equally likely in boys and girls.

TRANSMISSION. In contrast to other rickettsial infections, humans acquire *C. burnetii* predominantly after inhalation of infectious aerosols or by ingestion of contaminated foods. Ticks are rarely implicated. Domestic livestock, parturient domestic pets and wild animals such as rabbits, and ticks serve as reservoirs. Frequent modes of transmission include aerosols from dust, straw, cloth contaminated with organisms from birth tissues, or processing of animal products (abattoirs, hides, wool), or by ingestion of contaminated raw dairy products (fresh cheese or unpasteurized milk). An increase in incidence is associated with the seasonal Mistral winds in France that coincide with lamb birthing season, while a significant association of acute Q fever and consumption of cheese was observed among children in Greece. In Nova Scotia and Maine, exposure to newborn animals, chiefly kittens, has been associated with small outbreaks of Q fever in family settings. In Europe and Australia, exposure to domestic ruminants is the major risk, although many urban dwellers in France, who presumably lack significant exposure to farm animals, acquire Q fever. Human placental infection is sometimes associated with intrauterine growth retardation, prematurity, or abortion and may result from primary infection or reactivation of maternal infection and subsequent placental insufficiency. Obstetric health care workers are at risk for acquiring infection because of the quantity of *C. burnetii* released from infected products of conception.

PATHOLOGY AND PATHOGENESIS. The pathology of Q fever depends on the mode of transmission, route of dissemination, and specific tissues involved. After inhalation of infectious aerosols, pulmonary infection elicits a mild interstitial lymphocytic pneumonitis with a dense macrophage-rich intra-alveolar exudate heavily infected with *C. burnetii.* Single inflammatory pseudotumors may develop in the pulmonary parenchyma. Occasionally the characteristic fibrin-ring granulomas may be identified in liver, bone marrow, meninges, and other organs, and this finding is generally a sign of an acute, self-limited infection; with hepatic involvement, there is mild to moderate lymphocytic lobular hepatitis. Typically, infected tissues are also infiltrated by lymphoid and histiocytic cells. Chronic Q fever endocarditis and prosthetic valve endocarditis is characterized by macrophage and lymphocyte-rich infiltrates in necrotic fibrinous valvular vegetations and by the absence of granulomas.

Recovery from symptomatic or asymptomatic acute infection can result in persistent subclinical infection and may be maintained by dysregulated cytokine responses. *C. burnetii* persistence in tissue macrophages at sites of pre-existing tissue damage elicits low-grade smoldering inflammation, and eventually leads to irreversible cardiac valve damage, persistent vascular injury, or osteomyelitis.

CLINICAL MANIFESTATIONS AND COMPLICATIONS. Two forms of Q fever occur. **Acute Q fever** is the most frequent and is a self-limited form usually presenting in children as fever only or as an influenza-like illness with interstitial pneumonitis. **Chronic Q fever** usually implies involvement of the native heart valves, prosthetic valves, or other endovascular prostheses in adults, although about half of patients with Q fever osteomyelitis have been children.

Acute Q Fever. Acute Q fever develops about 3 wk (range 14–39 days) after exposure to the causative agent. The severity of illness in children ranges from subclinical infection to a systemic febrile illness characterized by severe frontal headache, arthralgias, and myalgias, often accompanied by respiratory or gastrointestinal (vomiting, abdominal pain, diarrhea) symptoms. Of children with acute Q fever, about 40% present with fever, 25% with pneumonia or an influenza-like illness, >10% with meningoencephalitis, and >10% with myocarditis. The pneumonia in children usually resembles viral or atypical pneumonia with a nonproductive cough. Other manifestations include pericarditis, hepatitis, hemophagocytosis, rhabdomyolysis, and hemolytic uremic syndrome. Skin rash, an unusual finding with adult Q fever, is observed in about 50% of pediatric patients with Q fever, and may vary from maculopapular to purpuric lesions. Rigors and night sweats, common in adults with Q fever, may be less common in children. Other prominent clinical findings that may lead to diagnostic confusion include fatigue, vomiting, abdominal pain, and meningismus. Hepatomegaly and splenomegaly may be detected in some patients.

Laboratory investigations in pediatric acute Q fever are usually normal but may reveal mild leukocytosis and thrombocytopenia. Up to 85% of children will have modestly elevated serum hepatic transaminase levels that usually normalize within 10 days, and hyperbilirubinemia is infrequent in the absence of complications. C-reactive protein is uniformly elevated in childhood Q fever. Chest x-ray films are abnormal in 27% of all patients, and in children the most frequent findings include single or multiple bilateral infiltrates with reticular markings in the lower lobes.

Acute Q fever in children is usually a self-limited illness with fever persisting for only 7–10 days compared with 2–3 wk in adults. However, severe infections, including myocarditis that required cardiac transplantation, meningoencephalitis, pericarditis, and hemophagocytosis, have been reported.

Chronic Q Fever. The risk for development of chronic Q fever is strongly correlated with advancing age and underlying conditions such as cardiac valve damage or immunosuppression. Thus, children are rarely diagnosed with chronic Q fever, including endocarditis. A recent review identified only 5 cases of chronic Q fever endocarditis and 6 cases of osteomyelitis among children, none with known predisposing immune deficiencies. Four of the 5 endocarditis cases occurred in children with underlying congenital heart abnormalities, including vegetations on aortic, pulmonary, and tricuspid valves. Similarly, 4 of the 6 children with Q fever osteomyelitis had a prior diagnosis or clinical courses consistent with idiopathic chronic recurrent multifocal osteomyelitis. Common features to chronic Q fever in children include a long interval before diagnosis and the lack of significant fever. Although Q fever endocarditis often results in death (23–65% of cases), mortality has not been reported for children. Endocarditis can occur months to years after acute Q fever, even in the absence of any history of acute Q fever.

LABORATORY FINDINGS. Laboratory features in children with chronic Q fever are poorly documented; adult patients often display an erythrocyte sedimentation rate of >20 mm/hr (80% of cases), hypergammaglobulinemia (54%), and hyperfibrinogenemia (67%). In children, the presence of rheumatoid factor in >50% of cases and circulating immune complexes in nearly 90%, plus the frequent findings of antiplatelet antibodies, anti-smooth muscle antibodies, antimitochondrial antibodies, circulating anticoagulants, and positive direct Coombs test results, suggests an autoimmune process.

DIAGNOSIS AND DIFFERENTIAL DIAGNOSIS. Although it is infrequently diagnosed, Q fever should be considered in children with fever of unknown origin, atypical pneumonia, myocarditis, meningoencephalitis, culture-negative endocarditis, or recurrent osteomyelitis and who live in rural areas or who are in close contact with domestic livestock, cats, or animal products.

The diagnosis of Q fever is most easily confirmed serologically by testing acute and convalescent sera (2–4 wk apart), which show a 4-fold increase in indirect fluorescent antibody titers to phase I and phase II *C. burnetii* antigens. Predominant, elevated, or increasing titers of phase II antibody are characteristic of acute Q fever, and the appearance and persistence of elevated titers of phase I and phase II antibody are indicative of chronic Q fever. Elevated titers of phase I immunoglobulin A (IgA) antibody are reported to be diagnostic for Q fever endocarditis; however, 1 evaluation showed that a phase II IgG titer of ≥200 is indicative of *C. burnetii* infection and that a phase I IgG titer of <800 is inconsistent with chronic Q fever. Cross reaction with antibodies to *Legionella* and *Bartonella* can occur.

C. burnetii has been cultivated in tissue culture cells, which may become positive within 48 hr, but isolation and antimicrobial susceptibility testing of *C. burnetii* should be attempted only in specialized biohazard facilities. Polymerase chain reaction (PCR) testing has been applied to both blood and tissue samples, but lacks sensitivity and is available in some public health, reference, or research laboratories. Immunohistochemical staining has also been used, but suffers from similar problems as PCR.

The differential diagnosis depends on the clinical presentation. With respiratory disease, *Mycoplasma pneumoniae, Chlamydophila pneumoniae,* legionellosis, psittacosis, and Epstein-Barr virus infection should be considered. With granulomatous hepatitis, tuberculous and nontuberculous mycobacterial infections, salmonellosis, visceral leishmaniasis, toxoplasmosis, Hodgkin disease, monocytic ehrlichiosis, granulocytic anaplasmosis, brucellosis, cat scratch disease (*Bartonella henselae*), or autoimmune disorders including sarcoidosis should be considered. Culture-negative endocarditis suggests infection with *Brucella, Bartonella,* or HACEK organisms, partially treated bacterial endocarditis, or nonbacterial endocarditis.

TREATMENT. Selection of an appropriate antimicrobial regimen for children is difficult owing to the lack of thorough studies, the limited therapeutic window for drugs that are known to be efficacious, and the potential length of therapy required to preclude relapse. Most pediatric patients with Q fever experience a self-limited illness that is identified only on retrospective serologic evaluation. However, to prevent potential complications, patients with acute Q fever should be treated within 3 days of onset of symptoms with doxycycline (2.2 mg/kg/dose bid PO or IV). Chloramphenicol should be reserved for patients with doxycycline allergy and for pregnant women. Tetracycline and doxycycline may be associated with tooth discoloration in children <9 yr of age, whereas chloramphenicol is rarely associated with aplastic anemia. Doxycycline can be used for Q fever safely in young children because tooth discoloration is dose dependent and it is unlikely that children will require multiple courses.

Therapy started >3 days within onset has little effect on the course of the acute infection. Because early laboratory confirmation is not currently available, empirical therapy is warranted in clinically suspected cases. During pregnancy, Q fever is best treated with trimethoprim-sulfamethoxazole. The fluoroquinolones ofloxacin and pefloxacin have proved effective, and success with a combination of pefloxacin and rifampin has also been achieved with prolonged therapy of 16–21 days. Macrolides, including erythromycin, clarithromycin, and roxithromycin, are less effective than doxycycline, but more effective than β-lactams, which are ineffective. However, the efficacy of macrolides in children has not been well studied. Individual reports document success with a wide variety of agents, including chloramphenicol, trimethoprim-sulfamethoxazole, and ceftriaxone. In anecdotal cases of hepatitis associated with "autoimmune" laboratory findings, prednisone was reported to provide additional clinical benefit.

For chronic Q fever, especially endocarditis, therapy for 18–36 mo is mandatory with the bacteriostatic drugs doxycycline or tetracycline in combination with hydroxychloroquine (a lysosomal alkalinizing agent) or with bactericidal drugs such as rifampin, ofloxacin, or pefloxacin. The preferred combination in adults, doxycycline and hydroxychloroquine, has not been specifically evaluated in children. For patients with heart failure, valve replacement may be warranted and should be accompanied by an effective antibiotic regimen to avoid reinfection of the prosthetic valves. Therapy should be monitored by periodic serologic evaluation; phase I titers of <200 for IgG and a negative IgA titer indicate cure. Even with such evaluation, cure of chronic Q fever within 2 yr is unlikely; thus, therapy should be continued for at least 18 mo. Interferon-γ therapy has been used to control intractable Q fever.

PREVENTION. Recognition of the disease in livestock or other domestic animals should alert communities to the risk for human infection. Milk from infected herds must be pasteurized at temperatures sufficient to destroy *C. burnetii. C. burnetii* is resistant to significant environmental conditions but may be inactivated with a solution of 1% Lysol, 1% formaldehyde, or 5% hydrogen peroxide. Special isolation measures are not required because person-to-person transmission is rare, except during exposure to infected products of conception. A vaccine preparation is available and provides protection against Q fever for at least 5 yr in abattoir workers. Because the vaccine is strongly reactogenic and no trials in children have been conducted, it should only be used where extreme risk is judged to exist. Clusters of cases that result from intense local natural exposures are well documented; however, clusters not associated with slaughterhouses, farms, or animal exposures should be investigated as potential sentinel events for bioterrorism.

Fournier PE, Etienne J, Harle JR, et al: Myocarditis, a rare but severe manifestation of Q fever: Report of 8 cases and review of the literature. *Clin Infect Dis* 2001;32:1440–1447.

La Scola B, Maltezou HC: *Legionella* and Q fever community acquired pneumonia in children. *Paediatr Resp Rev* 2004;5(Suppl):S171–S177.

Maltezou HC, Constantopoulou I, Kallergi C, et al: Q fever in children in Greece. *Am J Trop Med Hyg* 2004;70:540–544.

Maltezou HC, Raoult D: Q fever in children. *Lancet Infect* Dis 2002;2:686–691.

Maurin M, Raoult D: Q fever. *Clin Microbiol Rev* 1999;12:518–553.

Nourse C, Allworth A, Jones A, et al: Three cases of Q fever osteomyelitis in children and a review of the literature. *Clin Infect Dis* 2004;39:e61–e66.

Parker NR, Barralet JH, Bell AM: Q fever. *Lancet* 2006;367:679–688.

Raoult D, Marrie TJ, Mege JL: Natural history and pathophysiology of Q fever. *Lancet Infect Dis* 2005;5:219–226.

Raoult D, Tissot-Dupont H, Foucault C, et al: Q fever 1985–1998. Clinical and epidemiologic features of 1,383 infections. *Medicine* (Baltimore) 2000;79:109–123.

Richardus JH, Dumas AM, Huisman J, et al: Q fever in infancy: A review of 18 cases. *Pediatr Infect Dis* 1985;4:369–373.

Ruiz-Contreras J, Montero RG, Amador JT, et al: Q fever in children. *Am J Dis Child* 1993;146:300–302.

Tissot-DuPont H, Raoult D, Brouqui P, et al: Epidemiologic features and clinical presentation of acute Q fever in hospitalized patients: 323 French cases. *Am J Med* 1992;93:427–434.

Section 12 — Fungal Infections

Chapter 230 ■ Principles of Antifungal Therapy

Patricia Ferrieri

Candida and filamentous fungal infections are a serious problem in outpatient and hospitalized pediatric patients. These fungal infections are associated with the aggressive use of chemotherapy and other modalities that profoundly depress the immune system, widespread use of broad-spectrum antibiotics, extensive use of indwelling intravascular catheters, and the immunodeficiency associated with AIDS.

Amphotericin B, which frequently causes serious nephrotoxicity, and 5-fluorocytosine were once the only drugs available to treat serious fungal infections. Newer agents have had a major impact on our ability to treat, more safely and effectively, local and systemic invasive fungal infections. Fluconazole, a triazole agent, has been used to treat >20 million patients with primarily *Candida* and other yeast infections. As might be expected, antifungal resistance has emerged and has led to an increase in the development and marketing of several even newer azole drugs as well as other classes of antifungals (Tables 230-1 and 230-2).

POLYENES. The polyene antifungal agents such as amphotericin B were the standard approach for treating systemic fungal infections. Susceptibility to polyene compounds is dependent on the presence of sterols in the plasmin membrane of the fungal cells. For the larger polyene compounds, such as amphotericin B, the interaction of the antifungal agent with membrane sterol is thought to result in the production of pores or channels consisting of 8 amphotericin B molecules linked hydrophobically to the membrane sterols. In this model the polyene hydroxyl residues face inward in the pore and leads to altered permeability of the membrane and leaking of vital cytoplasmic contents with eventual death of the organism. This simplistic approach does not account for reports of the killing of *Candida albicans,* which is attributed to oxidative damage caused by polyenes.

There are various lipid-associated compounds containing amphotericin B that have been developed, including liposomal amphotericin B, amphotericin B lipid complex (ABLC), and amphotericin B colloidal dispersion (ABCD). Liposomal amphotericin B is as effective as conventional amphotericin B for empirical antifungal therapy in patients with fever and neutropenia while associated with fewer breakthrough fungal infections, less infusion-related toxicity, and less nephrotoxicity. There are newer azole drugs that have been proposed as alternatives for amphotericin B preparations for empirical antifungal therapy in patients with persistent fever and neutropenia. Comparisons of the different lipid formulations of amphotericin B with conventional amphotericin B have revealed no consistent significant differences in treatment efficacy, although differences in serious adverse effects exist with the highest frequency of renal toxicity and infusion-related adverse effects with conventional amphotericin B.

FLUCYTOSINE. Flucytosine (5-flucytosine or 5-FC) is the fluorine analog of a normal body constituent, cytosine. The mechanism of action of flucytosine is interference with pyrimidine metabolism, inhibiting nucleic acids, and disrupting protein synthesis. It is moderately soluble in water and marketed as capsules,

TABLE 230-1. Antifungal Drugs

CLASS AND DRUG	FORMULATION	DOSAGE
POLYENES		
Conventional amphotericin B (amphotericin B deoxycholate)	IV	0.8–1.2 mg/kg/day
Liposomal amphotericin B	IV	1–5 mg/kg/day, usually 3 mg/kg/day
Amphotericin B lipid complex (ABLC)	IV	5 mg/kg/day
Amphotericin B colloidal dispersion (ABCD)	IV	4–6 mg/kg/day
Nystatin	Cream, ointment, oral suspension, vaginal tablet, troche	
IMIDAZOLES		
Clotrimazole	Topical cream, vaginal cream, vaginal tablet, lotion, troche	
Miconazole	Topical cream, vaginal cream, lotion, topical powder and solution, vaginal suppository	
Ketoconazole	Topical cream, shampoo, tablet (for systemic fungal infection although safer azole drugs are available)	
TRIAZOLES		
1st generation triazoles		
Fluconazole	Tablets, suspension, IV	Oral candidiasis: 6 mg/kg/day on day 1 then 3 mg/kg/day one daily Esophageal candidiasis: 6 mg/kg/day on day 1 then 3–12 mg/kg/day once daily Systemic candidiasis: 6–12 mg/kg/day for 28 days Cryptococcal meningitis: 12 mg/kg/day on day 1 then 6–12 mg/kg/day for 10–12 wk
Itraconazole	Capsules, suspension	3–5 mg/kg/day once daily Fungal infection with chronic granulomatous disease: 5–10 mg/kg/day divided every 12–24 hr Disseminated histoplasmosis: 6–8 mg/kg/day
	VI	Adults: 200 mg every 12 hr for 4 doses then 200 mg once daily Children: No established pediatric dosing
2nd generation triazoles		
Voriconazole	Tablets, suspension	<25 kg: 6–10 mg/kg/day divided every 12 hr >25 kg and <40 kg: Load with 200 mg every 12 hr for 2 doses then 100 mg every 12 hr >40 kg: Load 400 mg/dose every 12 hr for 2 doses then 200 mg every 12 hr
	IV	Infants load 8 mg/kg every 12 hr for 2 doses then 6 mg/kg every 12 hr Children load 6 mg/kg/dose every 12 hr for 2 doses then 4 mg/kg/dose every 12 hr
Ravuconazole	Tablets, IV	No established pediatric dosing
Posaconazole	Tablets, suspension	No established pediatric dosing Adults 200 mg every 6 hr or 400 mg every 12 h
ECHINOCANDINS		
Caspofungin	IV	Neonates 1 mg/kg/day for 2 doses then 2 mg/kg/day 2–11 yr: 70 mg/m^2/day on day 1 (maximum 70 mg/day) then 50 mg/m^2/day (maximum 50 mg/day) >12 yr: 70 mg once on day 1 then 50 mg once daily. If not responding or receiving a P450 enzyme inducer, administer 70 mg/day Adults 50–150 mg daily Children ~1–4 mg/kg daily (estimated provisional dosing)
Micafungin	IV	No defined established pediatric dosing
Anidulafungin	IV	No established pediatric dosing Adults load 100–200 mg then 50–100 mg daily

TABLE 230-2. Spectrum of Activity of Selected Antifungal Agents

ANTIFUNGAL	IMPORTANT CLINICAL USES
Amphotericin B	*Blastomyces dermatitidis, coccidioides immitis, Cryptococcus neoformans, Histoplasma capsulatum, Paracoccidioides brasiliensis, Sporotrix schenckii,* most *Candida* species, *Aspergillus,* Zygomycetes (not: *Candida lusitaniae, Scedosporium, Fusarium, Trichosporon*)
5-Fluorocytosine	Only in combination therapy for *Candida, C. neoformans,* dematiaceous molds
Fluconazole	Most *Candida, C. neoformans, B. dermatitidis, H. capsulatum, C. immitis, P. brasiliensis* (not: *Candida krusei, Candida glabrata, Aspergillus*)
Itraconazole	*Candida, Aspergillus, B. dermatitidis, H. capsulatum, C. immitis, P. brasiliensis*
Voriconazole	*Candida, Aspergillus, Fusarium, B. dermatitidis, H. capsulatum, C. immitis, Malassezie* species, *Scedosporium,* dematiaceous molds (not: Zygomycetes; caution: *C. glabrata*)
Caspofungin	*Candida, Aspergillus* (not: *C. neoformans, Fusarium,* Zygomycetes)

From Steinbach WJ: Antifungal agents in children. *Pediatr Clin North Am* 2005;52:895–915.

and a suspension can be formulated for children. Protein binding is barely measurable, and absorption from the gastrointestinal tract is essentially complete with 90% excreted unchanged in the urine. Concentrations in cerebrospinal fluid approximate 74% of simultaneous serum concentrations. Limited data suggest that it may also penetrate into aqueous humor, joints, bronchial secretions, peritoneal fluid, brain, bowel, and bone. The serum half-life with normal kidney function is 3–5 hr but is higher in newborn infants.

Flucytosine is available as capsules and as a liquid. Flucytosine is usually administered in adults and adolescents at 150 mg/kg/day PO in 4 divided doses, in children at 100–150 mg/kg/day PO in 4 divided doses, and in neonates at 50–100 mg/kg/day PO once daily or in 2 divided doses. Patients with elevated serum hepatic enzymes require dose reduction. Various laboratory methods are available to assay flucytosine, even in the presence of amphotericin B; serum levels should be measured and maintained between 20 and 100 µg/mL in adults and between 25 and 80 µg/mL in children. The blood levels should be measured in patients with renal failure 2 hr after the last dose and immediately before the next dose. Adverse effects with flucytosine are infrequent and include rash and diarrhea; hepatic dysfunction occurs in 5% of patients. Indications for flucytosine are as adjunctive therapy with amphotericin B. These 2 drugs may be additive in their effects in vitro and in some animal models of *Candida* and *Cryptococcus* infections. Case reports of combination therapy with flucytosine and amphotericin B describe successful treatment of candidiasis and its complications in newborn infants. Fungal isolates should be tested for susceptibility to flucytosine. Since drug resistance to flucytosine usually arises during monotherapy, it should not be used alone for any fungal infection. Resistance to flucytosine has occurred during combination therapy but this is uncommon.

AZOLES. The azole antifungal agents can be divided into 2 groups, the imidazoles and the triazoles. The imidazoles are older and include miconazole, ketoconazole, and clotrimazole. The triazoles include the 1st generation triazoles fluconazole and itraconazole, as well as the more recently introduced 2nd generation triazoles voriconazole, ravuconazole, and posaconazole. The azole antifungal agents inhibit the cytochrome P450 (CYP)-dependent lanosterol 14-α-demethylase, an important enzyme for the synthesis of ergosterol, the major sterol constituent in the fungal cell membrane that functions as a bioregulator of membrane fluidity and integrity in the fungal cell wall. The newer triazoles were developed to expand the spectrum of antifungal activity of the existing azoles, provide fungicidal activity against molds, and improve on some of the limitations of these drugs.

Voriconazole and ravuconazole are structurally similar to fluconazole, while posaconazole is similar to itraconazole.

Fluconazole. Fluconazole, a 1st generation triazole, is available as tablets, an oral suspension, and an IV formulation. It is well absorbed from the gastrointestinal tract and only 11% of serum drug is protein-bound. Concentrations of fluconazole in cerebrospinal fluid are approximately 70% of simultaneously obtained blood levels, regardless of meningeal inflammation. It also penetrates into the brain and into other organs and body fluids. Elevated hepatic enzymes and hepatotoxicity may occur, although serious adverse effects are uncommon even with chronic therapy. The most common indication is oropharyngeal candidiasis. It is also effective against *Candida* species that do not have fluconazole resistance; patients with candidemia who are not neutropenic or immunosuppressed appear to respond as well to intravenous fluconazole as to amphotericin B. In cryptococcal meningitis, following initial therapy with amphotericin B or amphotericin B plus flucytosine, therapy can be changed to fluconazole for >2 mo. For patients with AIDS, cryptococcal meningitis is treated with life-long maintenance fluconazole therapy after the initial therapy because of frequent relapses. The use of fluconazole as prophylaxis in patients undergoing allogeneic bone marrow transplantation has improved their survival. This is mainly due to the decrease in *Candida* infections and their related mortality without, however, affecting the mortality related to invasive mold infections. Fluconazole is not indicated for *Aspergillus, Mucor,* or *Scedosporium* infections.

Itraconazole. Itraconazole, also a 1st generation triazole, is available as capsules, an oral suspension, and an IV formulation. Oral absorption is significantly enhanced by food when given as a capsule, although absorption of the suspension is best on an empty stomach. A steady state is achieved only after 13–15 days. Tissue and secretion concentrations of itraconazole are generally higher than the plasma concentrations, but cerebrospinal fluid concentrations are usually immeasurable even in patients with meningitis. About 99% of serum itraconazole is bound to plasma proteins.

The most common adverse effects are dose-related nausea and abdominal discomfort, but these symptoms rarely necessitate discontinuation of therapy. Dividing the dose into twice-daily administration improves tolerance and absorption. At higher doses of itraconazole, hypokalemia may occur. Itraconazole does not appear to be hepatotoxic and does not suppress adrenal or testicular function at the recommended dosages. Blood levels are reduced by about half in patients taking drugs that decrease gastric acidity such as H_2 blockers and the gastric proton pump inhibiting agents. Rifampin, rifabutin, isoniazid, phenytoin, carbamazepine, phenobarbital, and cisapride decrease itraconazole blood levels.

Indications for itraconazole include treatment of blastomycosis, histoplasmosis, coccidioidomycosis (including meningeal disease), paracoccidioidomycosis, sporotrichosis, ringworm, including onychomycosis, tinea versicolor, and aspergillosis. Itraconazole is also useful for the prevention of relapse in patients with AIDS and disseminated histoplasmosis.

Voriconazole. Voriconazole is currently the only 2nd generation triazole approved for use in the United States. Compared with 1st generation triazoles, it has an enhanced antifungal spectrum and is more effective in vitro than fluconazole against *Candida,* including *Candida krusei* and *Candida glabrata,* which are intrinsically resistant to fluconazole. Voriconazole has more adverse effects and drug-drug interactions than fluconazole and should not replace fluconazole for treatment of common *Candida* infections. Voriconazole has fungistatic and, at times, even fungicidal activity against several *Aspergillus* species, including *Aspergillus terreus,* which is intrinsically resistant to amphotericin B. It is also effective against several important fungal pathogens that have increased in prevalence, including *Fusarium, Scedosporium apiospermum, Penicillium marneffei,* and *Trichosporon.* Voriconazole has no activity against the Zygomycetes, which include *Absidia, Mucor, Rhizopus,* and *Rhizomucor* species.

The major clinical advantages of voriconazole are broad-spectrum activity against *Candida, Aspergillus,* and *Cryptococcus,* combined with good oral bioavailability and relatively low toxicity. Some *Candida* strains are resistant to voriconazole. In a randomized trial comparing voriconazole with liposomal amphotericin B for empirical therapy in patients with neutropenia and persistent fever, voriconazole did not meet the statistical end point for noninferiority, but had fewer breakthrough invasive fungal infections, particularly aspergillosis. In a randomized, open-label trial comparing voriconazole with amphotericin B deoxycholate for primary therapy of invasive aspergillosis, successful outcome (52.8% vs 31.6%, respectively) and survival rates (70.8% vs 57.9%, respectively) were significantly better in the voriconazole group. There are reports of breakthrough zygomycosis in patients receiving voriconazole, emphasizing the necessity of vigilant evaluation of the possibility of resistant organisms in patients who are at continued risk for fungal infections.

The clinical effectiveness of voriconazole in the pediatric population has not been demonstrated as extensively as in adults, although several case reports have demonstrated successful treatment with voriconazole of pediatric patients with invasive aspergillosis, scedosporiosis, or trichosporonosis. In some of these cases, other antifungal agents were administered along with voriconazole.

Voriconazole is generally well tolerated in adults and children. Common adverse events include elevated liver function tests, skin rash, and visual abnormalities, including photophobia and blurred vision, which are usually transient. Close monitoring is essential since fatal liver failure has been reported.

Voriconazole is available in both oral and IV formulations. It has excellent oral bioavailability, which allows transition from IV to oral administration. Administration with food, especially high-fat meals, reduces drug absorption. It is extensively distributed into tissues, including in cerebrospinal fluid. Pediatric patients have greater capacity for elimination of voriconazole than adults, which may have important implications since optimal dosage is critical for successful treatment of invasive fungal infections in the immunocompromised host.

Voriconazole is metabolized by several CYP isoenzymes with the potential for several drug-drug interactions, which may be life threatening. Rifampin, long-acting barbiturates, and carbamazepine decrease voriconazole concentrations and should be avoided during voriconazole use. Voriconazole results in higher levels of cisapride, cyclosporine, omeprazole, quinidine, tacrolimus, and warfarin. The IV formation of voriconazole accumulates in the presence of renal insufficiency, due to its metabolism, although no adjustment of oral voriconazole is necessary for patients with renal insufficiency.

Ravuconazole. Ravuconazole is an extended-spectrum triazole that is not yet licensed. It exhibits potent in vitro activity against *Candida* and *Aspergillus,* including *A. terreus,* which is usually resistant to fluconazole and amphotericin B. It is also active against *Cryptococcus neoformans, Histoplasma capsulatum,* and *Penicillium* but is less active than voriconazole against *Fusarium, Scedosporium,* and *Trichosporon.* Similar to voriconazole, it is not active against the Zygomycetes. Although ravuconazole is active in vitro against many fluconazole-resistant *Candida* organisms, many strains exhibit reduced susceptibility to ravuconazole with minimum inhibitory concentrations (MICs) of >1 µg/mL. Cross-resistance between fluconazole and ravuconazole is most common among fluconazole-resistant *Candida glabrata* and is variable among the other *Candida* species. Ravuconazole is available in both oral and IV formulations. The safety profile appears excellent, with no hepatotoxicity or nephrotoxicity in animal models. There is minimal efficacy data or pharmacokinetics on ravuconazole in humans.

Posaconazole. The spectrum of activity of posaconazole includes *Candida* (including fluconazole-resistant strains), *Aspergillus, Cryptococcus, Coccidioides, Histoplasma, Trichosporon, Fusarium,* and *Scedosporium.* It also has good activity against the Zygomycetes, with MICs that are considerably lower than those of fluconazole and voriconazole and slightly lower than those of itraconazole. Posaconazole is available as tablets and an oral suspension. There are few published reports of the pharmacokinetics of posaconazole in children. Posaconazole inhibits hepatic CYP3A4 but not other CYP450 enzymes, different from voriconazole and other azoles. Therefore, it may have an improved safety profile compared with the other triazoles.

ECHINOCANDINS. The echinocandins are a novel class of lipopeptide antifungal agents that inhibit β-1,3-D-glucan synthase, an enzyme complex forming glucan polymers in the fungal cell wall. Inhibition leads to disruption of the cell wall followed by osmotic stress, lysis, and death of the fungus. The echinocandins, by targeting the fungal cell wall, have a different mechanism of action than the polyene or azole antifungals, which act by inhibiting synthesis of the fungal cell membrane. Caspofungin was the 1st echinocandin licensed for use in the USA and most of Europe. Micafungin recently received approval in the USA, and anidulafungin is also approved. The pharmacokinetics of these 3 echinocandins is variable. Caspofungin is cleared more rapidly in pediatric patients than adults. For micafungin, drug clearance is higher in children <9 yr of age compared with older children and adults. For anidulafungin, the overall pharmacokinetic profile appears similar for children and adults, with no effect of age.

Caspofungin. Caspofungin was originally approved for patients intolerant of standard therapy or with refractory invasive aspergillosis. It also has been used for *Candida* infections and in vitro is fungicidal against most *Candida* species, including azole-resistant isolates of *C. albicans, C. glabrata,* and *C. krusei.* It is fungistatic against *Aspergillus.* It is also active in vitro against *Coccidioides, Blastomyces dermatitidis,* and *Histoplasma capsulatum,* and has limited or no activity against *Fusarium, Cryptococcus, Scedosporium, Trichosporon,* and the Zygomycetes. Because of low oral bioavailability, caspofungin as well as all echinocandins are available only in an IV formulation. It is highly protein bound and undergoes hepatic metabolism. No dose adjustments are required for renal insufficiency or mild liver disease. Although there are fewer drug-drug interactions than with the azoles, caspofungin interacts with cyclosporine, tacrolimus, and other inducers or inhibitors of hepatic metabolism. Caspofungin reduces the area under the curve for tacrolimus by approximately 20%, but has no effect on cyclosporine levels. Cyclosporine, however, increases the area under the curve for caspofungin by approximately 35%.

Caspofungin is as effective as amphotericin B in adults for treatment of invasive candidiasis, and is as effective as liposomal amphotericin B as empirical antifungal therapy in patients with persistent fever and neutropenia. In patients with invasive aspergillosis refractory or intolerant to standard therapy, complete or partial response is seen in 45% of adults treated with caspofungin. There are few published controlled studies of the clinical efficacy of caspofungin in children. There are many case reports of caspofungin used for treatment of invasive fungal infections in pediatrics with various outcomes. Ordinarily, caspofungin was administered with other antifungal drugs, primarily amphotericin B. One report documents successful caspofungin therapy of 1 full-term infant and 9 premature infants with renal candidiasis, meningitis, and an atrial fungal vegetation. All evidence of clinical infection, including blood cultures, resolved successfully in these infants, who were either unresponsive to or intolerant of amphotericin B deoxycholate.

In a retrospective review of 25 immunocompromised children treated with caspofungin, in dosages ranging from 0.8 to 1.6 mg/kg/day (if <50 kg), only 3 patients had an adverse event that was possibly related to this drug, including hypokalemia, hyperbilirubinemia, and elevated hepatic enzymes. Since these children were also treated with other antifungal agents, no adverse event was definitively related to caspofungin and in no case was therapy discontinued.

Few data in humans have been reported using caspofungin in combination with other antifungal agents such as amphotericin B or any of its lipid formulations.

Micafungin. The spectrum of antifungal activity of micafungin is similar to that of caspofungin, with MICs for *A. terreus* and *Aspergillus niger* that are considerably lower than those of caspofungin. Micafungin is available only in an IV formulation. The pharmacokinetic properties are also similar to those of caspofungin, with no significant differences between adults and children. There are limited data of the safety and tolerability of micafungin in children. Micafungin is as effective as fluconazole for the treatment of esophageal candidiasis in HIV-infected adults. It is also used to prevent *Candida* infections in hematopoietic stem cell recipients. There is some information on the use of micafungin, alone and in combination, for treatment of invasive aspergillosis in pediatric patients, with 35–45% complete or partial responses.

Anidulafungin. The mode of action and structure of anidulafungin is similar to caspofungin and micafungin. There are limited data on the safety, tolerability, and dosing of anidulafungin in children. Like other echinocandins, it is available only in an IV formulation. The spectrum of activity of anidulafungin appears similar to that of caspofungin. It also has been evaluated in several animal models of invasive candidiasis and aspergillosis, demonstrating promising activity and outcome.

COMBINATION ANTIFUNGAL THERAPY. Although there are many animal model studies demonstrating that various combinations of the newer antifungal drugs and amphotericin B or lipid formulations of amphotericin B are effective, the beneficial outcome may be due to either a synergistic or additive antifungal effect. It is not yet possible to make firm recommendations for combined therapy with the newer drugs since appropriately designed and randomized, controlled trials have not been performed to determine the optimal drug combinations for either 1st line or salvage therapy for aspergillosis and other invasive fungal infections. Despite this lack of data, the use of combination antifungal therapy has established itself in many hospitals caring for patients with frequently fatal invasive fungal disease, such as among bone marrow or solid organ transplant patients.

Because of the complexity of the newer antifungal drugs, pediatricians should consult with pediatric infectious disease specialists regarding the use of any of these new single agents, alone or in combination therapy for invasive fungal infections. Since antifungal susceptibility testing is not routine in many laboratories, referral of fungal isolates to reference laboratories experienced in this expanding field of drugs is recommended.

Antachopoulos C, Walsh TJ: New agents for invasive mycoses in children. *Curr Opin Pediatr* 2005;17:78–87.

Blyth CC, Palasanthiran P, O'Brien TA: Antifungal therapy in children with invasive fungal infections: a systematic review. *Pediatrics* 2007;119:772–784.

Cornely OA, Maertens J, Winston DJ, et al: Posaconazole vs. fluconazole or itraconazole prophylaxis in patients with neutropenia. *N Engl J Med* 2007;356:348–359.

Cuenca-Estrella M, Gomez-Lopez A, Mellado E, et al: Head-to-head comparison of the activities of currently available antifungal agents against 3,378 Spanish clinical isolates of yeasts and filamentous fungi. *Antimicrob Agents Chemother* 2006;50:917–921.

Denning DW: Echinocandin antifungal drugs. *Lancet* 2003;362:1142–1151.

Herbrecht R, Denning DW, Patterson TF, et al: Voriconazole versus amphotericin B for primary therapy of invasive aspergillosis. *N Engl J Med* 2002;347:408–415.

Keating GM: Posaconazole. *Drugs* 2005;65:1553–1567.

Mattiuzzi G, Alvarez RH, Giles F: Treatment of invasive *Aspergillus* infections in bone marrow transplant patients. *Antibiotics for Clinicians* 2003;7(Suppl 1):7–12.
The Medical Letter: Micafungin (Mycamine) for fungal infections. *Med Lett* 2005;47:51–52.
The Medical Letter: Posaconazole (noxafil) for invasive fungal infections. *Med Lett* 2006;48:93–94.
Merlin E, Galambrun C, Ribaud P, et al: Efficacy and safety of caspofungin therapy in children with invasive fungal infection. *Pediatr Infect Dis J* 2006;25:1186–1188.
Mukherjee PK, Sheehan DJ, Hitchcock CA, et al: Combination treatment of invasive fungal infections. *Clin Microbiol Rev* 2005;18:163–194.
Odio CM, Araya R, Pinto, LE, et al: Caspofungin therapy of neonates with invasive candidiasis. *Pediatr Infect Dis J* 2004;23:1093–1097.
Pannaraj PS, Walsh TJ, Baker CJ: Advances in antifungal therapy. *Pediatr Infect Dis J* 2005;24:921–922.
Pfaller MA, Diekema DJ, Messer SA, et al: In vitro activities of voriconazole, posaconazole, and four licensed systemic antifungal agents against *Candida* species infrequently isolated from blood. *J Clin Microbiol* 2003;41:78–83.
Sethi A, Antaya R: Systemic antifungal therapy for cutaneous infections in children. *Pediatr Infect Dis J* 2006;25:643–644.
Ullmann AJ, Lipton JH, Vesole DH, et al: Posaconazole or fluconazole for prophylaxis in severe graft-versus-host disease. *N Engl J Med* 2007;356: 335–346.
Walsh TJ, Lutsar I, Driscoll T, et al. Voriconazole in the treatment of aspergillosis, scedosporiosis and other invasive fungal infections in children. *Pediatr Infect Dis J* 2002;21:240–248.
Walsh TJ, Pappas P, Winston DJ, et al: Voriconazole compared with liposomal amphotericin B for empirical antifungal therapy in patients with neutropenia and persistent fever. *N Engl J Med* 2002;346:225–234.
Walsh TJ, Teppler H, Donowitz GR, et al: Caspofungin versus liposomal amphotericin B for empirical antifungal therapy in patients with persistent fever and neutropenia. *N Engl J Med* 2004;351:1391–1402.

Chapter 231 ■ *Candida*

Martin E. Weisse and Stephen C. Aronoff

Candidiasis is the most common fungal infection in the world. The term encompasses many clinical syndromes that may be caused by several species of *Candida*. The term **moniliasis** is based on the former genus name and is used occasionally to describe skin or mucous membrane *Candida* infections.

Candida exists in 3 morphologic forms: oval to round **blastospores or yeast cells** (3–6 mm in diameter); double-walled **chlamydospores** (7–17 mm in diameter), which are usually at the terminal end of a pseudohypha; and **pseudomycelium,** which is a mass of pseudohyphae and represents the tissue phase of *Candida*. **Pseudohyphae** are filamentous processes that elongate from the yeast cell without the cytoplasmic connection of a true hypha. *Candida* grows aerobically on routine laboratory media but may require several days of incubation.

C. albicans accounts for most human infections, but *C. parapsilosis, C. tropicalis, C. krusei, C. lusitaniae, C. glabrata,* and several other species have been reported as pathogens with increasing frequency. Because *C. albicans* is the most frequently isolated pathogen, a rapid **germ tube test** should be performed before further identification tests are performed. *C. albicans* forms a germ tube when suspended in rabbit or human serum and incubated for 1–2 hr. *C. dubliniensis* is the only other clinically significant germ tube–positive *Candida* species. Differentiation and susceptibility testing are important because *C. dubliniensis* is much more frequently resistant to fluconazole. The other clinically important *Candida* species can be identified within 48 hr on the basis of biochemical test results.

Treatment of invasive *Candida* infections is complicated with the emergence of non-albicans strains. Amphotericin is inactive against approximately 20% of strains of *C. lusitaniae.* Fluconazole is useful for many *Candida* infections but is inactive against all strains of *C. krusei* and approximately 20% of strains of *C. glabrata. C. dubliniensis* is often resistant to flucytosine and may develop resistance to fluconazole. These species are usually susceptible to ketoconazole and itraconazole, but cross-resistance to other azoles does occur. Susceptibility testing of these clinical isolates is recommended (Table 231-1).

231.1 • Neonatal Infections

Candida is a common cause of oral mucous membrane infections (**thrush**) and perineal skin infections (**candidal diaper dermatitis**) in newborn infants (see Chapter 665). Disseminated candidiasis and candidemia have become a frequent problem in neonatal intensive care units.

EPIDEMIOLOGY. *C. albicans* is commonly part of the gastrointestinal and vaginal flora of adults. Pregnancy increases the rate of maternal vaginal colonization from <20% to >30%. Maternal colonization rates at time of delivery correlate with the colonization rates of the newborns. Approximately 10% of full-term infants become colonized in the gastrointestinal and respiratory tract in the 1st 5 days of life; the colonization rate in infants weighing <1,500 g approaches 30%. Skin colonization is common after 2 wk of age. H_2 blockers, broad-spectrum cephalosporins, and delayed enteral feedings alter gastrointestinal tract ecology and facilitate colonization.

Neonatal risk factors for invasive candidiasis include very low birthweight status, broad-spectrum antibiotic administration, abdominal surgery, prolonged ventilatory support, prolonged intravenous catheterization, and parenteral alimentation.

PATHOGENESIS. The inability of the newborn infant to localize, control, and eradicate *Candida* infections is related to the relative impairment of specific and nonspecific host defense mechanisms. Overgrowth of *Candida* on mucocutaneous surfaces and

TABLE 231-1. Typical In Vitro Susceptibility of *Candida* Species

SPECIES	FLUCONAZOLE	ITRACONAZOLE	VORICONAZOLE	AMPHOTERICIN	POSACONAZOLE	CANDINS
C-albicans	S	S	S	S	S	S
C-tropicalis	S	S	S	S	S	S
C-parapsilosis	S	S	S	S	S	S (to I?)
C-dubliniensis	S to S-DD	S	S	S	S	S
C-glabrata	S-DD to R	S-DD to R	S to I	S to I	S to I	S
C-krusei	R	S-DD to R	S to I	S to I	S to I	S
C-lusitaniae	S	S	S	S to R	S	S

From Patterson TF: Advances and challenges in management of invasive mycoses. *Lancet* 2005; 366:1013–1025.
I, intermediate; R, resistant; S, susceptible; S-DD, susceptible dose-dependent. Formal breakpoints have not been validated for the newer triazoles or echinocandins, and assessments of susceptibility are based on likely achievable serum concentrations of drug, clinical responses, or both.

colonization of intravenous catheters favor entry and penetration, with development of clinical infection directly related to extent of colonization. Hematogenous spread may lead to vasculitis and miliary nodules in multiple organs, including the skin, liver, spleen, lungs, kidneys, gastrointestinal tract, heart, eyes, and meninges.

CLINICAL MANIFESTATIONS. The manifestations of systemic neonatal candidiasis vary in acuteness and severity from thrush and candidal diaper dermatitis (see subchapter 231.2) to fungemia that may rarely be asymptomatic or may be associated with sepsis and shock indistinguishable from bacterial sepsis. *Candida* causes significant disease in 2–5% of premature infants weighing <1,500 g. Cutaneous evidence of *Candida* infection is present in as many as half of these patients and manifests as a diffuse erythroderma or vesiculopustules from which the organism can be cultured. Renal involvement is found in >50% of patients and may be subclinical with persistent candiduria or may manifest as a flank mass, hypertension, renal failure, renal abscesses, papillary necrosis, or fungal balls in the collecting system, resulting in obstruction and hydronephrosis.

Central nervous system involvement occurs in up to 1/3 of cases and may involve the meninges, ventricles, or cerebral cortex with abscess formation. Since clinical manifestations of central nervous system disease may not be apparent, evaluation of the cerebrospinal fluid in all neonates with disseminated candidiasis is required. **Endophthalmitis** has been noted in as many as 45% of cases, but with earlier effective treatment it is now less than 5%. It remains important to perform retinal examinations in neonates with systemic candidiasis; repeat examinations are necessary to monitor resolution of the retinal lesions. Endophthalmitis begins as chorioretinitis and may extend to the vitreous. Cotton ball exudates are typical of candidal retinal pathologic conditions. Osteoarthritis is a complication in 20% of cases.

Vascular disease ranges from vasculitis of the aorta or vena cava to endocarditis. Infected thrombi in vessels and the right atrium are not uncommon. Candidal endocarditis is an infrequent complication but should be considered in patients with central venous catheters placed into the atrium as well as neonates with persistent candidemia. At autopsy, pneumonia occurs in as many as 70% of patients with disseminated candidemia, although some patients do not have radiographic evidence of pneumonia on initial evaluation. Cultures from the endotracheal tube are not predictive of pulmonary involvement, as *Candida* is a common colonizer of this site.

Congenital Candidiasis. Congenital candidiasis is a rare manifestation. It occurs in otherwise healthy neonates and presents at birth with widespread skin involvement, especially in the intertriginous areas. Congenital candidiasis follows ascending infection from a mother with heavy vaginal colonization or vulvar infection with *Candida*. The newborn rash is maculopapular, vesicular, or pustular with little or no mucous membrane involvement. Nodular lesions may be seen on the umbilical cord and placental membranes. In the absence of systemic manifestations, topical antifungal therapy is the treatment of choice for congenital cutaneous candidiasis in full-term infants. Congenital candidiasis in preterm infants may progress to systemic disease, and therefore systemic therapy with amphotericin or fluconazole may be warranted.

DIAGNOSIS. Definitive diagnosis requires histologic demonstration of the fungus in tissue specimens or recovery of the fungus from normally sterile body fluids. Buffy coat smears of blood may show yeast, allowing a preliminary diagnosis. Skin scrapings of generalized rashes in very low birthweight infants with suspected systemic candidiasis should be examined microscopically for yeast. Because cultures of blood and cerebrospinal fluid are often intermittently positive, multiple samples should be obtained. Cerebrospinal fluid cultures are positive in 1/3 of infants with disseminated infection. Cultures should be obtained from peripheral veins as well as catheters to differentiate systemic infection from contaminated catheters. *Candida* antigen detection in blood samples may increase detection of candidemia. Urine specimens for culture must also be obtained by catheterization or suprapubic tap to differentiate infection from perineal colonization. Polymerase chain reaction (PCR) can be used to diagnose *Candida* bloodstream infection in high-risk patients, as well as for genotyping strains of *Candida* for outbreak investigation.

Radiographs of the chest may reveal pneumonia. Ultrasonography is useful for localizing *Candida* infection in the urinary tract, central nervous system, and cardiovascular system. Ultrasonography, CT, and MRI may also be helpful in identifying foci in the liver and spleen.

TREATMENT. Transient candidemia and disseminated candidiasis associated with a contaminated intravascular catheter requires removal of the catheter. Amphotericin B (0.5–1.0 mg/kg/day IV) had been the mainstay of therapy for systemic candidiasis and is active against both yeast and mycelial forms. The duration of therapy varies widely according to the extent of infection, clinical response, and drug toxicity. The total recommended dose is 20–30 mg/kg. Nephrotoxicity is common in the newborn infant and generally presents with oliguria, azotemia, and hyperkalemia. Lipid-complex formulations of amphotericin B (5 mg/kg/day) are recommended for neonates with compromised renal function (including doubling of the serum creatinine with amphotericin B desoxycholate therapy), also receiving other nephrotoxic therapy, or otherwise intolerant of amphotericin B desoxycholate. The addition of flucytosine (100–150 mg/kg/day divided every 6 hr PO) may be used to treat central nervous system and parenchymal kidney infections. Patients must be observed for bone marrow, gastrointestinal, and hepatic toxicities.

Fluconazole is very useful for treatment of invasive neonatal *Candida* infections, especially urinary tract infections. Fluconazole is inactive against all strains of *C. krusei* and approximately 20% of strains of *C. glabrata*. These strains are usually susceptible to voriconazole and itraconazole, but cross-resistance to other azoles does occur. The susceptibility of these clinical isolates should be tested if treatment with azoles is contemplated. Caspofungin has excellent activity against most *Candida* species and has been used successfully in patients with resistant organisms or in whom other therapies have failed.

Vascular catheters associated with transient fungemia or disseminated infection should be removed, followed by treatment with intravenous antifungal therapy for 2–3 wk. Infected intracardiac and intravascular thrombi usually must be resected, but resolution without surgery has been described.

231.2 • Infections in Immunocompetent Children and Adolescents

ORAL CANDIDIASIS. Oral thrush, or oral pseudomembranous candidiasis, is a superficial mucous membrane infection that affects approximately 2–5% of normal newborns. Infants acquire *Candida* from their mothers at delivery and remain colonized. Thrush may develop as early as 7–10 days of age. The use of antibiotics, especially in the 1st year of life, may lead to recurrent or persistent thrush. The plaques of thrush invade the mucosa superficially and may be found on the lips, buccal mucosa, tongue, and palate. Removal of plaques from these surfaces may cause mild punctate areas of bleeding, which helps to confirm the diagnosis. Thrush may be asymptomatic or may cause pain, fussiness, and decreased feeding. It is uncommon after 12 mo of age but may occur in older children treated with antibiotics. Persistent or recurrent thrush with no obvious predisposing reason, such as recent antibiotic treatment, warrants investigation of an underlying condition such as diabetes mellitus or immunodeficiency, especially vertically transmitted HIV infection.

Treatment of mild cases may not be necessary. When treatment is warranted, the most commonly prescribed antifungal agent is nystatin. Therapeutic agents in decreasing order of efficacy include miconazole gel, amphotericin B suspension, gentian violet, and nystatin suspension. Clotrimazole troches may also be effective, although clinical studies are lacking. Miconazole gel is currently unavailable in the United States. For recalcitrant or recurrent infections, a single dose of fluconazole may be useful. Fluconazole has been shown to be safe in premature infants, and effective in a single dose for HIV-infected children with oral candidiasis. In breast-fed infants, simultaneous treatment of infant and mother with topical nystatin or oral fluconazole may be indicated.

DIAPER DERMATITIS. Diaper dermatitis is the most common infection caused by *Candida* (see Chapter 665). Primary infection generally occurs in the intertriginous areas of the perineum and presents as a confluent papular erythema with erythematous satellite papules. *Candida* diaper dermatitis often complicates other noninfectious diaper dermatitides and occurs as an adverse effect of oral antibiotic treatment.

A common practice is to presumptively treat any diaper rash that has been present for >3 days with topical antifungal therapy such as nystatin cream, powder, or ointment; clotrimazole 1% cream; miconazole 2% ointment; or amphotericin cream or ointment. If significant inflammation is present, the addition of hydrocortisone 1% may be useful for the 1st 1–2 days. Frequent diaper changes and short periods without diapers are important adjunctive treatments. Combination drugs with topical corticosteroids, such as clotrimazole/triamcinolone, should be used cautiously or not at all in infants because the relatively potent topical corticosteroid may lead to unwanted local adverse effects.

UNGUAL AND PERIUNGUAL INFECTIONS. Paronychia and onychomycosis may be caused by *Candida*, although *Trichophyton* and *Epidermophyton* are much more common causes (see Chapter 662). Candidal onychomycosis differs from tinea infections by its propensity to involve the fingernails and not the toenails, and by the associated paronychia. Candidal paronychia often respond to treatment consisting of keeping the hands dry and using a topical antifungal agent. For ungual infections, a short course of systemic therapy with an oral azole antifungal drug may be necessary.

VULVOVAGINITIS. Vulvovaginitis is a common candidal infection of pubertal and postpubertal female patients that affects as many as 75% of female patients at 1 time or another (see Chapter 549). Predisposing factors include pregnancy, oral contraceptive use, poor hygiene, and use of oral antibiotics. Prepubertal girls with candidal vulvovaginitis usually have a predisposing factor such as diabetes mellitus or prolonged antibiotic treatment. Clinical manifestations may include pain or itching, dysuria, vulvar or vaginal erythema, an opaque white or cheesy exudate, and thrushlike mucosal plaques.

Candidal vulvovaginitis can be effectively treated with either vaginal creams or troches of nystatin, clotrimazole, or miconazole. Oral therapy with a single dose of fluconazole has been found to be as effective as topical clotrimazole in women. Persistent vulvovaginal candidiasis can be safely and effectively treated with fluconazole.

231.3 • Infections in Immunocompromised Children and Adolescents

ETIOLOGY. Most cases of candidemia in immunocompromised patients are caused by *C. albicans,* with other *Candida* species accounting for as many as 35% of infections. In decreasing order of frequency, these include *C. tropicalis, C. parapsilosis, C. glabrata, C. lusitaniae, C. krusei, C. dubliniensis,* and *C. guilliermondii.*

CLINICAL MANIFESTATIONS. *Candida* infections in immunocompromised patients vary from superficial mucocutaneous infections to life-threatening sepsis and shock. Evidence of *Candida* of 1 organ system usually points to systemic infection and multiorgan involvement.

HIV-Infected Children. Oral thrush and diaper dermatitis are the most common candidal infections in HIV-infected children, occurring in 50–85% of patients. Infants with symptomatic HIV infection are more than twice as likely to have thrush, which is often much more extensive in these infants than in healthy children. Besides oral candidiasis, 3 other clinical variants of candidal infection may be observed in HIV-infected children: atrophic candidiasis, which presents as a fiery erythema of the mucosa or loss of papilla of the tongue; chronic hyperplastic candidiasis, which presents with oral symmetric white plaques that cannot be rubbed away; and angular cheilitis, in which there is erythema and fissuring of the angles of the mouth. Topical therapy may be effective, but systemic treatment with fluconazole or itraconazole is usually necessary and reduces recurrences. Symptoms of dysphagia or poor oral intake may indicate that the infection has progressed to candidal **esophagitis,** necessitating systemic therapy with either itraconazole or fluconazole.

Candidal dermatitis and onychomycosis are also more common in HIV-infected children. These infections are generally more severe than they are in immunocompetent children and may require oral therapy or more aggressive and prolonged topical therapy.

Cancer and Transplant Patients. Fungal infections, especially *Candida* and *Aspergillus* infections, are a significant problem in oncology patients with chemotherapy-associated neutropenia (see Chapter 177). Although the greatest risk for these patients is from bacterial pathogens, the risk for candidemia increases dramatically after 5–7 days of neutropenia and fever. Accordingly, if fever and neutropenia persist for ≥5–7 days, amphotericin B is usually added as empiric therapy because of the high risk for systemic fungal infection. Fluconazole may be an acceptable alternative to amphotericin B for some patients in hospitals where drug-resistant *Candida* and Aspergillus species are uncommon. Voriconazole and caspofungin have equivalent efficacy and improved safety profiles compared with either amphotericin desoxycholate or lipid-complex formulations of amphotericin.

Bone marrow transplant recipients have a much higher risk for fungal infections because of the dramatically prolonged duration of neutropenia. Prophylactic use of fluconazole decreases the incidence of candidemia in bone marrow transplant recipients but not in leukemia patients undergoing chemotherapy. An increased incidence of infection with *C. krusei,* which is resistant to fluconazole, has been noted. Caspofungin and voriconazole have been successfully used as monotherapy or in combination with each other and amphotericin B. The use of myelopoietic colony-stimulating factor affects the duration of neutropenia after chemotherapy and is associated with decreased risk for candidemia. When *Candida* infection occurs, the lung, spleen, kidney, and liver are involved in >50% of cases.

Solid organ transplant recipients are also at increased risk for superficial and invasive candidal infections. Studies in liver transplant recipients demonstrate the utility of antifungal prophylaxis with amphotericin B, fluconazole, voriconazole, or caspofungin.

Catheter-Associated Infections. Central venous catheter infections occur most often in oncology patients but may affect any patient with a central catheter (see Chapter 178). Neutropenia, use of broad-spectrum antibiotics, and parenteral alimentation are associated with increased risk for candidal central catheter infection. Recovery of *Candida* from the central catheter alone poses the same risk for disseminated infection as culture of the organism from both the central catheter and peripheral blood. Treatment requires removal of the catheter as well as a 2–3 wk course of amphotericin B (1 mg/kg/day, total dose of 20 mg/kg).

DIAGNOSIS. The diagnosis is often presumptive in neutropenic patients with prolonged fever because positive blood fungal cultures occur only in a minority of patients who are later found to have disseminated infection. *Candida* grows readily on routine blood culture media, with ≥90% of positive cultures identified within 72 hr, and ≥97% are identified within 7 days. Candida recovered from urine or tracheal secretions may represent either colonization or infection.

TREATMENT. Amphotericin B remains the treatment of choice for systemic candidal infections, alone or with the addition of flucytosine or fluconazole, which is especially useful for central nervous system infections and parenchymal kidney infections. In 1 study among adults, fluconazole was as effective as amphotericin B for disseminated candidal infections and had fewer adverse effects. Fluconazole may be useful for selected candidal infections but is not effective against *C. krusei* and approximately 20% of strains of *C. glabrata.* Amphotericin is inactive against approximately 20% of strains of *C. lusitaniae,* and therefore susceptibility testing should be performed for all strains. Lipid-complex formulations of amphotericin B (5 mg/kg/day) are recommended for persons with compromised renal function (including doubling of the serum creatinine with amphotericin B desoxycholate therapy), for those who are receiving other nephrotoxic therapy, or for those who are otherwise intolerant of amphotericin B desoxycholate. Voriconazole and caspofungin have not been studied extensively in children.

231.4 • Chronic Mucocutaneous Candidiasis

Chronic mucocutaneous candidiasis is a heterogeneous group of immune disorders with a primary defect of T-lymphocyte responsiveness to *Candida.* Endocrinopathies (e.g., hypoparathyroidism, Addison disease) and autoimmune disorders are often associated with chronic mucocutaneous candidiasis (see Chapter 124). Symptoms may begin in the 1st few months of life or as late as the 2nd decade of life. The disorder is characterized by chronic and severe skin and mucous membrane infections with *Candida* and occasionally other dermatophytes. Systemic candidiasis rarely occurs. Topical antifungal therapy may provide limited improvement early in the course of the disease, but repeated courses of ketoconazole or fluconazole, and occasionally amphotericin B, are usually necessary. The infection usually responds temporarily to treatment but is not eradicated and recurs.

Antoniadou A, Torres HA, Lewis RE, et al: Candidemia in a tertiary care cancer center: In vitro susceptibility and its association with outcome of initial antifungal therapy. *Medicine* 2003;82:309–321.

Bendel CM: Nosocomial neonatal candidiasis. *Pediatr Infect Dis J* 2005;24:831–832.

Feja KN, Wu F, Roberts K, et al: Risk factors for candidemia in critically ill infants: A matched case-control study. *J Pediatr* 2005;147:156–161.

Graybill JR: Voriconazole for candidosis: An important addition? *Lancet* 2005;366:1413–1414.

Kaufman D, Boyle R, Hazen KC, et al: Twice weekly fluconazole prophylaxis for prevention of invasive candida infection in high-risk infants of <1000 grams birth weight. *J Pediatr* 2005;147:172–179.

Kullberh BJ, Sobel JD, Ruhnke M, et al: Voriconazole versus a regimen of amphotericin B followed by fluconazole for candidemia in non-neutropenic patients: A randomized non-inferiority trial. *Lancet* 2005;366:1435–1442.

Long S, Stevenson DK: Reducing candida infections during neonatal intensive care: Management choices, infection control, and fluconazole prophylaxis. *J Pediatr* 2005;147:135–141.

Makhoul IR, Kassis I, Smolkin T: Review of 49 neonates with acquired fungal sepsis: Further characterization. *Pediatrics* 2001;107:61–66.

Maxwell MJ, Messer SA, Hollis RJ, et al: Evaluation of E test method for determining fluconazole and voriconazole MICs for 279 clinical isolates of *Candida* species infrequently isolated from blood. *J Clin Microbiol* 2003;41:1087–1090.

Medical Letter: Anidulafungin (eraxis) for candida infections. *Med Lett* 2006;48:43–44.

Noyola DE, Fernandez M, Moylett EH: Ophthalmologic, visceral and cardiac involvement in neonates with candidemia. *Clin Infect Dis* 2001;32: 1018–1023.

Palma-Carlos AG, Palma-Carlos ML: Chronic mucocutaneous candidiasis revisited. *Allerg Immunol* 2001;33:229–232.

Pappas PS, Rex JH, Sobel JD, et al: Guidelines for treatment of candidiasis. *Clin Infect Dis* 2004;38. Available online at http://www.journals.uchicago.edu/CID/journal/issues/v38n2/32301/32301.html

Patterson TF: Advances and challenges in management of invasive mycoses. *Lancet* 2005;366:1013–1025.

Rodriguez D, Almirante B, Park BJ, et al: Candidemia in neonatal intensive care units, Barcelona, Spain. *Pediatr Infect Dis J* 2006;25:224–229.

Saiman L, Ludington E, Dawson JD, et al: Risk factors for Candida species colonization of neonatal intensive care unit patients. *Pediatr Infect Dis J* 2001;20(12):1119–1124.

Walsh TJ, Pappas P, Winston DJ, et al: Voriconazole compared with liposomal amphotericin B for empirical antifungal therapy in patients with neutropenia and persistent fever. *N Engl J Med* 2002;346:225–234.

Walsh TJ, Teppler H, Donowitz GR, et al: Caspofungin versus liposomal amphotericin B for empirical antifungal therapy in patients with persistent fever and neutropenia. *N Engl J Med* 2004;351(14):1391–1402.

Chapter 232 ■ *Cryptococcus Neoformans*

Robert G. Flood and Stephen C. Aronoff

ETIOLOGY. Cryptococcosis is an invasive fungal disease caused by a monomorphic, encapsulated yeast. *Cryptococcus neoformans* var. *neoformans* is the most common etiologic agent worldwide and is the predominant pathogenic fungal infection among persons infected with human immunodeficiency virus (HIV).

EPIDEMIOLOGY. *C. neoformans* var. *neoformans* (serotypes A, D and AD) is distributed in temperate climates predominantly in soil contaminated with droppings from certain avian species, including pigeons, canaries, and cockatoos. It may also be found on fruits and vegetables, and may be carried by cockroaches. *C. neoformans* var. *gatti* (serotypes B and C) is found in the tropics and subtropics and has been associated with several species of eucalyptus trees. This species causes endemic disease primarily in immunologically competent hosts living in the tropics and is associated with the formation of large granulomas known as **cryptococcomas.**

C. neoformans exposure is much more common than previously thought. Seroprevalence studies in temperate urban environments have shown that most children >2 yr of age, and nearly all adults, have been exposed to this organism. Despite this high prevalence, clinical disease is unusual in immunocompetent persons and is rare in children. Pigeon breeders and laboratory personnel who work with *Cryptococcus* are at greatest risk. Cryptococcosis is also rare (<1%) among HIV-infected children but occurs in 5–10% of HIV-infected adults, with higher rates of infection reported from developing countries. Pediatric cases of cryptococcosis are evenly divided among immunocompetent and immunocompromised individuals.

PATHOGENESIS. In most cases *C. neoformans* is acquired by inhalation of fungal spores. Local inoculation leads to cutaneous or ophthalmic infection rarely. In most immunocompetent individuals, infection is limited to the lung. When the immune system fails to contain the infection, dissemination follows with potential involvement of the brain, meninges, skin, eyes, prostate, and skeletal system.

Pulmonary cryptococcosis produces granulomas that are often subpleural in location and contain yeast forms. Cystic cryptococcomas occur in the central nervous system (CNS) of 20% of non-HIV-infected patients with disseminated disease and may be found in the absence of overt meningitis. Granulomas and microabscesses containing yeast occur in patients with cutaneous and bony infection.

CLINICAL MANIFESTATIONS. The manifestations of cryptococcal infection reflect the route of inoculation and the immunocompetence of the host.

Pneumonia. Pneumonia is the most common form of cryptococcosis. Asymptomatic pulmonary infections occur frequently, especially among pigeon breeders, bird fanciers, and laboratory workers. Asymptomatic carriage may occur in persons with underlying chronic lung disease. Progressive pulmonary disease is symptomatic with fever, cough, pleuritic chest pain, and constitutional symptoms. It often precedes disseminated infection in immunocompromised persons. Chest radiographs may demonstrate a poorly localized bronchopneumonia, nodular changes, or lobar consolidations; cavities and pleural effusions are rare. In adults with HIV infection, cryptococcal pneumonia is usually asymptomatic, although >90% of patients have concomitant CNS infection.

Disseminated Infection. Disseminated infection usually follows primary pulmonary disease, especially among immunocompromised persons. Advanced HIV infection is the most common predisposing factor for disseminated cryptococcosis. Other major predisposing conditions include lymphoproliferative disorders, corticosteroid therapy, primary immunodeficiencies affecting both T- and B-cell lineages, and immunosuppressive therapy for rheumatic disorders, celiac disease, and organ transplantation.

Meningitis. Subacute or chronic meningitis is the most common clinical manifestation of disseminated cryptococcal infection. The clinical presentation is variable and prognostic. Good outcomes are associated with headache as the initial symptom, normal mental status, absence of a predisposing condition, normal cerebrospinal fluid (CSF) opening pressure, normal CSF glucose, CSF white cell count of >20 cells/μL, negative India ink stain, absence of extraneural infection by culture, and cryptococcal antigen titers in CSF and serum of <1 : 32. Overt symptoms of meningitis and HIV infection predict a poor outcome. HIV-infected patients typically present with unexplained fevers, headache, and malaise; cryptococcal antigen titers in these individuals are often >1 : 1,024. CT of the brain identifies cryptococcomas in as many as 30% of patients with disseminated infection even with no clinical signs of CNS involvement. The mortality rate for cryptococcal meningitis is 15–30%, with most deaths occurring within several weeks of diagnosis. The fatality rates are higher among HIV-infected individuals, who, prior to the use of lifelong maintenance antiviral therapy, had relapse rates of >50%. In adults, relapse rates have decreased to <5% with daily fluconazole therapy. Relapse is unusual in adequately treated, immunocompetent persons. Postinfectious sequelae are common and include hydrocephalus, decreased visual acuity, deafness, cranial nerve palsies, seizures, and ataxia.

Sepsis Syndrome. Sepsis syndrome is a rare manifestation of cryptococcosis and occurs almost exclusively among HIV-infected patients. Fever is followed by respiratory distress and multiorgan system disease that is often fatal.

Cutaneous Infection. Cutaneous disease most commonly follows disseminated cryptococcosis and rarely local inoculation. Early lesions are erythematous, may be single or multiple, and are variably indurated and tender. Lesions often become ulcerated with central necrosis and raised borders. Cutaneous cryptococcosis in immunocompromised patients may resemble molluscum contagiosum.

Skeletal Infection. Skeletal infection occurs in approximately 5% of individuals with disseminated infection but rarely in HIV-infected patients. The onset of symptoms is insidious and chronic. Bony involvement is typified by soft tissue swelling and tenderness, and arthritis is characterized by effusion, erythema, and pain on motion. Skeletal disease is unifocal in approximately 75% of cases. The vertebrae are the most common sites of infection, followed by the tibia, ileum, rib, femur, and humerus. Concomitant bone and joint disease results from contiguous spread.

Ocular Infection. Chorioretinitis is rare, occurs primarily in adults, and is usually a manifestation of disseminated disease, although direct inoculation of the eye has been described. Eye infection is characterized by the acute loss of visual acuity, eye pain, visual floaters, and photophobia. Examination usually reveals choroiditis with or without retinitis. Retinal and vitreal masses and anterior uveitis are seen less commonly. Eye disease is often a manifestation of disseminated infection and is associated with a mortality rate of >20%. Only 15% of survivors recover full vision.

Lymph Nodes. Lymphonodular disease has been reported in 2 children, 1 of whom had an underlying immunodeficiency. Lymphonodular cryptococcosis is characterized by disseminated lymphadenopathy including thoracic and abdominal nodes, subcutaneous lesions, liver granulomas, and concomitant pulmonary disease.

DIAGNOSIS. Recovery of the fungus by culture or demonstration of the fungus in histologic sections of infected tissue is definitive. A latex agglutination test, which detects cryptococcal antigen in serum and CSF, is the most useful diagnostic test. Titers of >1 : 4 in bodily fluid are strongly suggestive of infection, and high titers of >1 : 1,024 reflect high burden of yeast, poor host immune response, and greater likelihood of therapeutic failure. India ink preparations of CSF are useful prognostically but are less sensitive than culture and antigen detection. Skin test antigens are poorly characterized, and the sensitivity and specificity of this test are unknown.

TREATMENT. The choice of treatment depends on the sites of involvement and the host immune status. The immunocompetent patient with asymptomatic or mild disease limited to the lungs may be closely observed without therapy or, alternatively, treated with oral fluconazole (200–400 mg/day) or itraconazole (200–400 mg/day) for 3–12 mo, with the duration depending on the clinical response. Patients with cryptococcemia or severe symptoms, and non-HIV-immunocompromised hosts with lung disease, with cryptococcal antigen titers of >1 : 8, or CNS, urinary tract, or cutaneous disease, should be treated in a staged approach since these factors suggest disseminated disease. In general, these patients are treated with induction with amphotericin B (0.7–1 mg/kg/day) plus flucytosine (100 mg/kg/day) for a minimum of 2 wk. Depending on the clinical response, induction therapy may be continued as long as 6–10 wk. Induction is followed by a consolidation phase with fluconazole or itraconazole for 6–12 mo. Lifelong maintenance therapy may be required for children who remain immunocompromised. Lipid-complex amphotericin B (3–6 mg/kg/day) is recommended for individuals intolerant of the desoxycholate amphotericin, although experience with this agent in children with cryptococcosis is limited. Effectiveness of therapy is monitored by serial cryptococcal antigen testing. Serum or CSF values of ≥1 : 8 are predictive of relapse. Ventriculoperitoneal shunts may be required for patients with hydrocephalus, and aggressive medical management of increased intracranial pressure may also be required.

Because of the high rate of relapse, pulmonary, CNS, or disseminated cryptococcal infections in HIV-infected patients require induction, consolidation, and maintenance therapy. Patients with pulmonary disease most often required lifelong therapy with fluconazole (200–400 mg/day) or itraconazole (200–400 mg/day). For those with CNS disease, the most commonly used regimen is amphotericin B (0.7 mg/kg/day) and flucytosine (100 mg/kg/day) for a minimum of 2 wk and as long as 6–10 wk (induction), followed by fluconazole (400 mg/day) for a minimum of 8–10 weeks (consolidation). Fluconazole (200–400 mg/day) should be continued for life (maintenance therapy) after the completion of consolidation therapy. Itraconazole (200–400 mg/day) should be used only in cases where the patient is intolerant or has failed fluconazole therapy due to the higher relapse rates with itraconazole. Cessation of maintenance therapy in those children whose HIV infection is well controlled on antiretroviral therapy has not been well studied to date.

Cutaneous infections are usually treated medically, although surgical biopsy may be required for diagnosis. Skeletal infections generally require surgical debridement in addition to systemic antifungal therapy. Chorioretinitis also requires systemic antifungal therapy with amphotericin B and either fluconazole or flucytosine, both of which achieve high drug concentrations in the vitreous.

PREVENTION. Individuals at high risk should avoid exposures such as bird droppings. Effective antiviral therapy for persons with HIV infection reduces the risk of cryptococcal disease. A cryptococcal glucuronoxylomannan (GXM)-tetanus toxoid conjugate vaccine has been developed that elicits protective antibodies in mice but awaits clinical trials in children. Passive immunization with protective monoclonal antibodies has yet to be studied in children.

Goldman DL, Khine H, Abadi J, et al: Serologic evidence for *Cryptococcus neoformans* infection in early childhood. *Pediatrics* 2001;107(5):E66.

Gonzalez CE, Shetty D, Lewis LL, et al: *Cryptococcus* in human immunodeficiency virus-infected children. *Pediatr Infect Dis J* 1996;15:796–800.

Gumbo T, Kadzirange G, Mielke J, et al: *Cryptococcus neoformans* meningoencephalitis in African children with acquired immunodeficiency syndrome. *Pediatr Infect Dis J* 2002;21:54–57.

Leggiadro RJ, Barrett FF, Hughes WT: Extrapulmonary cryptococcosis in immunocompromised infants and children. *Pediatr Infect Dis J* 1992;11:43–47.

Leggiadro RJ, Kline MW, Hughes WT: Extrapulmonary cryptococcosis in children with acquired immunodeficiency syndrome. *Pediatr Infect Dis J* 1991;10:658–662.

Moncino MD, Gutman LT: Severe systemic cryptococcal disease in a child: Review of prognostic indicators predicting treatment failure and an approach to maintenance therapy with oral fluconazole. *Pediatr Infect Dis J* 1990;9:363–368.

Perfect JR, Casadevall A: Cryptococcosis. *Infect Dis Clin North Am* 2002;16:837–874.

Saag MS, Graybill RJ, Larsen RA, et al: Practice guidelines for the management of cryptococcal disease. *Clin Infect Dis* 2000;30:710–718.

Speed BR, Kaldor J: Rarity of cryptococcal infection in children. *Pediatr Infect Dis J* 1997;16:536–537.

Sweeney DA, Caserta MT, Korones DN, et al: A ten-year-old boy with a pulmonary nodule secondary to *Cryptococcus neoformans*: Case report and review of the literature. *Pediatr Infect Dis J* 2003;2:1089–1093.

Chapter 233 ■ *Malassezia*

Martin E. Weisse

Members of the genus *Malassezia* include the causative agents of **tinea versicolor**, and have been associated with other dermatologic conditions and established as infrequent causes of fungemia in patients with indwelling catheters. *Malassezia* is a commensal lipophilic yeast with a predilection for the sebum-rich areas of skin. There are 7 species and 2 additional recently proposed species. Only *Malassezia pachydermatitis,* a zoophilic yeast that causes dermatitis in dogs, is not lipophilic. Because the yeast forms may be either oval or round, *Malassezia* was earlier designated as *Pityrosporum ovale* and *Pityrosporum orbiculare.* Transformation of the yeast to hyphal forms facilitates invasive disease. The clusters of thick-walled blastospores together with the hyphae produce the characteristic "**spaghetti and meatballs**" appearance of *Malassezia.*

Malassezia globosa, M. sympodialis, M. restricta, and *M. furfur* are the major causes of tinea versicolor (see Chapter 665). *Malassezia* organisms have also been associated increasingly with other dermatologic conditions. *M. sympodialis* and *M. globosa* have been implicated in neonatal acne, and *M. globosa* and *M. restricta* are most closely associated with seborrheic dermatitis and dandruff. Scalp psoriasis, pityrosporum folliculitis, and head and neck atopic dermatitis have also been causally associated with *Malassezia. Malassezia* may be isolated from sebum-rich skin of asymptomatic persons, emphasizing that demonstration of the fungus does not equate with infection.

Effective **therapies for tinea versicolor** include topical therapies such as selenium sulfide, terbinafine, and others, or the oral azoles. *Malassezia*-associated skin diseases of the head and neck can be effectively managed with either 1% ciclopirox, ketoconazole, or zinc pyrithione shampoos.

M. furfur is the species most commonly causing **fungemia,** and *M. pachydermatis* has been implicated in several outbreaks in neonatal intensive care units. The use of lipid emulsions containing medium-chain triglycerides inhibits the growth of *Malassezia* and may prevent infection. Infection is most common in premature infants, although immunocompromised patients, especially those with malignancies, may also be infected. Symptoms of catheter-associated fungemia are indistinguishable from other causes of catheter-associated infections (see Chapter 178) but should be suspected in patients, especially neonates, receiving intravenous lipid infusions. Compared with other causes of fungal sepsis, it is unusual for catheter-related *Malassezia* fungemia to be associated with secondary focal infection.

Malassezia does not grow readily on standard fungal media, and successful culture requires overlaying the agar with olive oil. Recovery of *Malassezia* from blood culture is optimized by supplementing the media with olive oil or palmitic acid.

Fungemia caused by *M. furfur* or other species can be successfully treated in most cases by immediately discontinuing the lipid infusion and removing the involved catheter. For persistent or invasive infections, amphotericin B (desoxycholate or lipid-complex formulations), fluconazole, and itraconazole are effective. Flucytosine has no activity against *Malassezia.*

Bernier V, Weill FX, Hirigoyen V, et al: Skin colonization by Malassezia species in neonates: A prospective study and relationship with neonatal cephalic pustulosis. *Arch Dermatol* 2002;138:215–218.

Gupta AK, Batra R, Bluhm R, et al: Skin diseases associated with *Malassezia* species. *J Am Acad Dermatol* 2004;51:785–798.

Pierard-Franchimont C, Goffin V, Decroix J, Pierard GE: A multicenter randomized trial of ketoconazole 2% and zinc pyrithione 1% shampoos in

severe dandruff and seborrheic dermatitis. *Skin Pharmacol Appl Skin Physiol* 2002;15(6):434–441.
Shuster S, Meynadier J, Kerl H, et al: Treatment and prophylaxis of seborrheic dermatitis of the scalp with antipityrosporal 1% ciclopirox shampoo. *Arch Dermatol* 2005; 141:47–52.

Chapter 234 ■ *Aspergillus*

Macdara Tynan and Stephen C. Aronoff

Aspergillosis refers to a group of diseases caused by monomorphic, mycelial fungi of the genus *Aspergillus.* Most aspergillosis in children is caused by *A. fumigatus,* and less frequently by *A. flavus* and *A. niger.* Infections with *A. nidulans, A. versicolor, A. glaucus,* and *A. terreus* have also been reported in children. *Aspergillus* abounds in the environment, including the hospital environment. **Conidia,** or asexual fungal spores, are readily isolated from stored grain, soil, and decaying plants.

Outbreaks of disease among immunocompromised children may occur after exposure to aerosolized conidia disturbed by construction sites or renovations near hospitals or clinics. Relocation of those at particular risk for infection away from hospital construction has been used to minimize the potential for exposure. Infection is usually acquired from inhalation of airborne spores, which then colonize the upper and lower respiratory tracts. Immunocompromised persons, especially those with impaired neutrophil function or neutropenia, are at risk for hematogenous dissemination and invasive disease. Cutaneous infection usually follows wound or skin contamination and direct contact with traumatized, macerated, or immature skin. Hematogenous or, less commonly, contiguous spread may result in cutaneous infection. Ingestion and aspiration may also produce disease. *Aspergillus*-associated diseases may be immunoglobulin E (IgE) mediated (hypersensitivity syndromes), saprophytic (noninvasive), or invasive.

234.1 • Hypersensitivity Syndromes

ASTHMA. Atopic asthma (see Chapter 143) may be precipitated by inhalation of *Aspergillus* spores, which triggers an IgE-mediated response and bronchospasm. The clinical symptoms are nonspecific and include the acute onset of wheezing in the absence of pulmonary infiltrates or fever.

EXTRINSIC ALVEOLAR ALVEOLITIS. Extrinsic alveolar alveolitis is a hypersensitivity pneumonitis that occurs in nonatopic individuals after repeated exposure to conidia in organic dust. *Aspergillus* is 1 of many organic substances that produce this syndrome, sometimes known as **malt worker's lung** or **farmer's lung.** The pathogenesis is unknown but is similar to the alveolitis caused by other immunogens and may represent an immune complex disease. The clinical manifestations typically follow exposure by 4–6 hr and include fever, cough, and dyspnea. Physical examination often reveals rhonchi without wheezes. Eosinophilia is absent from blood and sputum. Chest radiography often shows diffuse interstitial infiltrates. Chronic exposure gradually leads to irreversible pulmonary fibrosis.

ALLERGIC BRONCHOPULMONARY ASPERGILLOSIS. Allergic bronchopulmonary aspergillosis complicates chronic pulmonary disease in approximately 7–10% of patients with corticosteroid-dependent asthma and 7% of those children with cystic fibrosis. Many patients with cystic fibrosis become colonized with *Aspergillus;* in those who develop allergic aspergillosis, there is increased risk for invasive aspergillosis following lung transplantation. Chronic mucosal colonization with *A. fumigatus* produces an exaggerated IgG and IgE response that results in recurrent bronchospasm and proximal cylindrical bronchiectasis. The diagnosis should be considered in patients with asthma or cystic fibrosis who have recurrent bronchospasm and transient pulmonary infiltrates, seen frequently in the upper lobes and sometimes bilaterally. Chest radiographs may show a **ring sign** or **tram lines** of parallel shadows representing inflamed bronchi. Chest CT may demonstrate bronchiectasis. Expectoration of mucous spirals containing mycelia is a hallmark of this illness. Peripheral eosinophilia is common. The definitive diagnosis of allergic bronchopulmonary aspergillosis requires (1) reversible episodic bronchial obstruction (asthma); (2) immediate scratch test reactivity to *A. fumigatus* antigens; (3) elevated total serum IgE; (4) peripheral blood eosinophilia; (5) precipitating (IgG) serum antibodies against *A. fumigatus;* (6) history of transient or fixed pulmonary infiltrates; and (7) central bronchiectasis. This diagnosis is still likely if all but the last criterion are fulfilled. The disease may progress through 3 stages: steroid-responsive asthma, steroid-dependent asthma; and end-stage pulmonary fibrosis with honeycombed lung.

TREATMENT. Treatment of the hypersensitivity pulmonary syndromes focuses on anti-inflammatory agents, notably systemic corticosteroids, and bronchodilator therapy. Acute exacerbations of disease are characterized by increased episodes of wheezing, diminished pulmonary function, and elevated serum IgE concentrations. These episodes can be treated initially with oral prednisone, 0.5 mg/kg/day for 1 wk followed by 0.5 mg/kg every other day until symptoms abate and serum IgE returns to preillness levels. Corticosteroid therapy usually lasts for 6 wk. If asthma symptoms recur as steroid treatment is withdrawn, inhaled bronchodilators and/or steroids may be required. Disease activity correlates with serum IgE levels. In adults, a 16 wk course of oral itraconazole reduces the immunologic reaction associated with allergic aspergillosis and improves clinical outcome. Adrenal suppression with inhaled corticosteroids and oral itraconazole is a potential concern. No randomized control studies have evaluated the use of antifungal therapies for the treatment of allergic aspergillosis in patients with cystic fibrosis.

234.2 • Saprophytic (Noninvasive) Syndromes

OTOMYCOSIS. Aspergillus may colonize cerumen in the external canal without associated infection. Otomycosis is a chronic condition that is found predominantly in tropical and subtropical regions and is rare in infants and children. It may be associated with habitual wearing of ear-occluding garments. Most infections are caused by *Candida albicans* or *A. niger* or, less commonly, *A. fumigatus.* Coinfection with bacterial agents may often occur. Most cases are unilateral, and patients present with ear pain, itching of the auditory canal, and a sense of fullness. Otorrhea, decreased hearing, and tinnitus are less common. Examination of the auditory canal typically shows conidial "forests" or mycelial mats. Cleaning the affected area followed by application of topical antifungal agents such as nystatin, tolnaftate, or dilute acetic acid, and topical corticosteroids has a beneficial effect. Oral itraconazole has also been effective.

SKIN. Primary cutaneous aspergillosis has been reported primarily as a nosocomially acquired infection occurring predominantly in premature neonates. Immaturity of the immune system, frequent exposure to systemic corticosteroids and broad-spectrum antibiotics, and an impaired skin barrier function of premature and low birthweight infants are predisposing factors among neonates. Early treatment is important to prevent progression to systemic invasive infection. Therapeutic response with amphotericin B for noninvasive infection has been reported.

Skin traumatized by burns, tape removal, or catheter insertion is classically an inoculation site of aspergillosis among immunocompromised patients. Skin maceration from prolonged exposure to a warm, moist environment can also compromise skin integrity and facilitate inoculation.

SINUSITIS. Since conidia are lightweight and easily dispersed, *Aspergillus* is the most common fungal infection of the nose and paranasal sinuses. Noninvasive sinonasal disease may present in 3 forms: sinusitis, sinus aspergilloma, and allergic aspergillosis. Chronic or indolent sinusitis is confined to 1 sinus and presents as a chronic infection that is unresponsive to antibacterial therapy. *A. flavus* is the most common causative organism. Sinus radiograms are nonspecific, showing mucosal thickening without bony changes. Endoscopic surgery is curative in most cases. This may occur without predisposing factors in tropical or desert areas with high environmental levels of spores. However this "indolent" sinusitis will slowly progress over months to years. If left untreated, contiguous involvement of the ethmoid sinuses and orbit may result, with possible cranial bone osteomyelitis and intracranial extension. Surgical debridement and drainage is sufficient in most cases, antifungal therapy is secondary. Sinus aspergilloma, which is rare in children, presents with long-standing nasal symptoms. Sinus radiographs demonstrate a solitary mass in a single cavity, typically the ethmoid or maxillary sinus. Surgical removal of the mass, often endoscopically, is the treatment of choice. Allergic *Aspergillus* sinusitis involves multiple sinuses and occurs in immunocompetent, atopic individuals who usually have a history of nasal congestion, headaches, allergic rhinitis, asthma, nasal polyposis and/or chronic sinusitis. Histology of nasal secretions in these patients reveals thick mucin, eosinophils, and few fungal hyphae. Sinus imaging typically shows involvement of multiple sinuses with hypodense areas and occasional calcifications. Bony expansion or erosions within the sinus are seen in 30–50% of cases; however, invasion is not reported. Criteria for the diagnosis of allergic fungal sinusitis are the same as for allergic bronchopulmonary aspergillosis. Somewhat surprisingly, it is uncommon to see allergic aspergillus sinusitis and allergic aspergillosis in the same patient. Treatment includes surgical drainage and debridement as well as corticosteroid therapy. Antibiotics may be required for secondary bacterial infections.

ASPERGILLOMA. Pulmonary aspergillomas develop in poorly drained bronchi or lung spaces that communicate with the bronchial tree. They may develop in pre-existing pulmonary cavities and may complicate up to 2% of all cases of pulmonary tuberculosis with residual cavities >2.5 cm diameter. Other conditions in children predisposing to aspergillomas include bronchiectasis, congenital heart disease, congenital pulmonary cysts, healed abscess cavities, and histoplasmosis. Rarely, aspergillomas complicate invasive *Aspergillus* pulmonary disease. Colonization and fungal proliferation occur in the cavity, without vascular invasion; an amorphous mycelial mass (mycetoma, fungus ball) results. Affected children are often asymptomatic, although cough, hemoptysis, fever, clubbing, and localized chest findings may be present. Chest radiographs characteristically demonstrate the air shadow of a pulmonary cavity outlining a rounded mass, which may be confirmed by chest CT. There is no consensus regarding the appropriate timing of and interventions for managing aspergillomas. Definitive treatment is surgical resection; however, this has to be weighed against the associated mortality and morbidity, including fungal infection of the postsurgical space, hemorrhage, and bronchopleural fistulas. Life-threatening **hemoptysis** from aspergilloma occurs in a minority of patients. The risk of surgical intervention is influenced by the patient's underlying pulmonary function and clinical condition. In patients experiencing recurrent hemoptysis, bronchial artery embolization (BAL) has been used to occlude vessels supplying the bleeding site. This is only temporarily effective, because collaterals will develop, leading to revascularization. Itraconazole has been used with beneficial effect in adults, although dose and duration of therapy are not standardized. Spontaneous resolution of the aspergilloma has been reported in a few patients.

234.3 • Invasive Disease

Invasive *Aspergillus* infection is characterized by hyphal infiltration of vascular structures, thrombosis, and focal necrosis. Invasive aspergillosis occurs most commonly in **immunocompromised** patients. Risk factors include profound (absolute neutrophil count <500/mm^3) or prolonged (>14 days) neutropenia complicating hematologic malignancies, neutrophil or macrophage dysfunction such as chronic granulomatous disease (CGD) or severe combined immune deficiency, prolonged high-dose corticosteroids or Cushing syndrome with endogenous hypercortisolism, HIV, stem cell transplantation, and, less commonly, solid organ (especially heart-lung) transplantation. The incidence of invasive aspergillosis among stem cell transplant recipients is 5–14%.

Primary invasive disease may occur at any site in which airborne or water-borne conidia may contact, colonize, and germinate, such as the respiratory tract or skin. Sinonasal disease, pulmonary disease, and cutaneous disease are the most common primary invasive infections in children. Otitis media is rare. The central nervous system is the most common **secondary** site of invasive disease. In the neutropenic patient, direct extension from the primary site is followed by hematogenous seeding to distant sites. *Aspergillus* is highly **angiotrophic.** This propensity to invade blood vessels promotes hematogenous spread and also leads to infarction and necrosis of the local tissues.

Blood and tissue culture of *Aspergillus* is difficult and insensitive, and a biopsy or aspirate is often necessary. The diagnosis is established by a clinically compatible illness with culture of *Aspergillus* from a normally sterile site, histologic identification of tissue invasion showing hyphae consistent with *Aspergillus* in a biopsy or aspirate especially with a culture from the site that is positive for *Aspergillus*, or compatible chest radiograph changes with *Aspergillus* recovered from bronchoalveolar lavage.

Visual identification of *Aspergillus* requires careful distinction from several morphologically similar fungal organisms, which confound definitive diagnosis. Histochemical diagnostic techniques using monoclonal antibodies help detect *Aspergillus* in tissue specimens. Reliable data are lacking for serologic testing for galactomannan, a component of the *Aspergillus* cell wall that is secreted from growing hyphae. Antibody detection of mitogillin, an *A. fumigatus* antigen that is highly expressed only during invasive growth, is a new and promising diagnostic tool.

Because diagnostic criteria may not be met, presumptive diagnosis may be necessary. Aspergillosis should be suspected in a persistently febrile neutropenic child receiving broad-spectrum antibiotics with fever and changes on chest radiograph.

SINUSITIS. Acute, invasive sinusitis is a subtype of sinonasal aspergillosis that occurs almost exclusively in patients with profound neutropenia associated with chemotherapy or stem cell transplantation. Early diagnosis is critical. The new onset of local symptoms, particularly epistaxis and sinus pain, warrant otolaryngologic evaluation with careful inspection of the nasal turbinates. A high index of suspicion is justified in high-risk immunocompromised patients. Surveillance nasal cultures are of questionable value. Examination typically shows sinus tenderness, nasal or oral ulceration, and duskiness or necrosis of the nasal septum or inferior turbinates. Mucosal invasion and infarction may progress rapidly in a centrifugal pattern to involve contiguous structures. Sinus CT or radiographs are useful. Biopsy and culture of the nasal or sinus mucosa demonstrate large numbers of hyphae, and fungal cultures typically yield *A. fumigatus, A. flavus,* or, less often, *Rhizopus* or *Candida*. Treatment is not standardized but may include surgical drainage, if the patient's condition permits, as well as extended antifungal therapy. Extensive surgical procedures are often hampered by underlying thrombocytopenia and extensive and often life-threatening hemorrhage. The mortality rate is high.

PNEUMONIA AND PULMONARY ASPERGILLOSIS. Invasive pulmonary aspergillosis is the most common form of *Aspergillus* infection encountered among immunocompromised patients. Symptomatic infection presents acutely with fever, cough, dyspnea, and abnormal chest findings; pleuritic chest pain is an infrequent complaint. Hemoptysis in the neutropenic patient with persistent or recurring fever may herald invasive disease. Chest radiographs commonly show persisting or new nodular infiltrates. Cavitation is not usually observed in children. High resolution CT scanning of the chest is the imaging technique of choice. A characteristic early CT finding in neutropenic patients is the **halo sign,** which is 1 or more nodules with peripheral attenuation lower than the center of the mass. These nodules may evolve into cavitary lesions. An **air crescent sign** is appreciated on CT, typically as the neutropenia resolves. By MRI, a **reverse-target sign** is appreciated and is associated with necrotizing pneumonia. Coexisting sinusitis is a common finding in neutropenic children. In children with chronic granulomatous disease, direct extension from the lungs to the chest wall involving the ribs and intercostal muscles has been reported. Contiguous spread to the pericardium and myocardium from pulmonary tissue has been described among pediatric stem cell transplant recipients.

Diagnosis based on respiratory tract cultures is confounded by the ubiquitous presence of airborne conidia and possible accidental contamination. Culture of *Aspergillus* from normally sterile pulmonary sites, obtained by percutaneous or open lung biopsy, or from pulmonary secretions indicates infection. Sensitivity of testing for *Aspergillus* in BAL secretions varies from 25 to 75%, with higher predictive values among neutropenic patients. Treatment requires aggressive systemic antifungal therapy.

SKIN. Secondary cutaneous aspergillosis results from hematogenous dissemination from another primary site, commonly the lungs. The lesions appear initially as tender erythematous plaques that progress to necrotic eschars or hemorrhagic bullae, **ecthyma gangrenosum.** In children with profound neutropenia, cutaneous manifestations of invasive aspergillosis are a sentinel marker for disseminated disease and indicate a poor outcome. Treatment requires systemic antifungal therapy and immunomodulatory support. Onychomycosis caused by *Aspergillus* has also been described, which may be treated successfully with oral itraconazole alone or combined with topical therapy.

EYE. Fungal endophthalmitis is an important diagnostic finding in immunocompromised children with disseminated *Aspergillus* infection. Endophthalmitis also can occur in patients with *Aspergillus* endocarditis. Pain, photophobia, and diminished visual acuity may occur, although most patients have no ocular symptoms. Examination of the retina shows focal retinitis, an overlying vitreitis, and retinal hemorrhage. Orbital cellulitis rarely complicates invasive sinusitis and follows destruction of the orbital walls and fungal extension into the retro-orbital space. Diplopia, periorbital edema, proptosis, and pain on lateral gaze may occur. Treatment includes management of the underlying immunocompromised state, surgical debridement, and systemic antifungal therapy.

Fungal keratitis and episcleritis are rare problems and follow direct inoculation of spores into the eye. In the absence of significant disseminated disease, topical and intrascleral antifungal therapy is recommended.

CENTRAL NERVOUS SYSTEM. Cerebral aspergillosis is a rare and almost uniformly fatal complication of disseminated disease. In most cases, infection involves single or multiple foci within the cerebral hemispheres or cerebellum. Intracranial abscesses follow hematogenous spread. Angiotrophism results in occlusion of intracranial vessels and tissue infarction. Focal neurologic deficits begin acutely, most often as hemiparesis, anterior cranial nerve palsies, or seizures. Progression to herniation is rapid. Surgical management may provide a tissue diagnosis and allow removal of nonviable tissue.

Aspergillus meningitis is rare and is associated with tuberculosis, prolonged corticosteroid therapy, neutropenia, and intravenous drug abuse. Arachnoiditis may result from contiguous spread from an intracerebral focus or from infected paranasal sinuses. Cerebrospinal fluid (CSF) shows a mild mononuclear pleocytosis, elevated CSF protein, and variable degrees of hypoglycorrhachia. Imaging studies demonstrate focal central nervous system lesions with edema and variable enhancement. The diagnosis can be established by the acute appearance of neurologic symptoms in a patient with proven or suspected invasive aspergillosis or occasionally by CSF or brain biopsy culture. High-dose amphotericin B combined with flucytosine has been effective in a paucity of cases; lipid-complex amphotericin, voriconazole, and itraconazole have also been used. Intraventricular therapy may also be required. Surgical removal of infected tissue may be important.

Epidural abscess is a rare complication of vertebral osteomyelitis caused by *Aspergillus* species. Surgical decompression, with systemic antifungal therapy, may be curative.

BONE. Aspergillosis of the bone is extremely rare and follows direct extension of infection from surgical inoculation, traumatic injury, or hematogenous seeding. Involvement of the vertebrae is most common. Osteomyelitis of the rib is rare and classically occurs in children with chronic granulomatous disease as an extension from a pulmonary focus. Surgical drainage is often required. In patients with CGD, *A. nidulans* is seen more frequently as a cause of osteomyelitis and has a poorer outcome than *A. fumigatus*. Treatment requires prompt systemic antifungal therapy combined with surgery and immunotherapy. Although definitive studies are not available, therapy with amphotericin B plus flucytosine has been used successfully, in spite of the poor bony penetration of amphotericin B. Itraconazole achieves good bone concentrations and has also been used successfully. Voriconazole is an alternate therapy.

HEART. Endocarditis is a rare form of aspergillosis and can follow contamination at the time of surgery or implantation of a contaminated graft, or, uncommonly, it may be a manifestation of disseminated aspergillosis. High-dose amphotericin B therapy coupled with surgical removal of infected grafts or prostheses is recommended.

TREATMENT. The treatment of life-threatening invasive or disseminated aspergillosis is undergoing dynamic change. Amphotericin B deoxycholate has been used as an antifungal agent in the treatment of aspergillosis for >20 yr, with failure rates of 30–80%. Moreover, many children poorly tolerate this agent. Amphotericin B lipid complex has been used in children with *Aspergillus* infections who either failed or were intolerant of amphotericin B deoxycholate. Although better tolerated than amphotericin B deoxycholate, outcomes are not appreciably different.

Voriconazole is a 2nd generation triazole derivative with activity against most *Aspergillus* organisms. Voriconazole is superior to amphotericin B for the treatment of pulmonary and extrapulmonary invasive aspergillosis. In children >12 yr of age, voriconazole is given as a loading dose at 6 mg/kg/dose IV at 12 hr intervals for 2 doses, and then the dose is lowered to 4 mg/kg every 12 hr. Parenteral therapy is usually continued until the patient clinically improves. Maintenance therapy may be given orally (200 mg PO twice daily for a total of 12 wk of therapy). Ocular and renal toxicities have been reported with voriconazole, and also a large number of drug-drug interactions, particularly with immunomodulating agents. In children <12 yr of age with invasive aspergillosis, high dosages of amphotericin B deoxycholate (1.0–1.5 mg/kg/day IV) are recommended for 4–12 wk, depending on the severity and localization of the infection. Amphotericin B lipid complex (4–5 mg/kg/day IV) may be used in place of amphotericin B deoxycholate, especially for patients who fail therapy with or are intolerant of amphotericin B deoxycholate. Voriconazole has been used successfully as rescue therapy when amphotericin B deoxycholate or amphotericin B lipid complex has failed or is not tolerated. Pediatric experience with posaconazole or caspofungin alone, in sequence with amphotericin B or other triazole antifungal agents, or in combination with other agents for invasive aspergillosis is limited. There is limited experience of colony-stimulating factors and cytokines as immunomodulatory therapy as an adjunct to antifungal drugs.

PROGNOSIS. In addition to the use of antifungal drugs, the outcome hinges on resolution of the underlying immunocompromised state. Primary invasive disease, unless considered early and treated aggressively, has a very poor outcome in the immunocompromised host. The mortality of invasive aspergillosis in the pediatric population is 65–85%; half of patients die within 29 days of diagnosis.

PREVENTION. The risk for invasive aspergillosis has led to the practice of fungal prophylaxis for high-risk patients. Aerosolized amphotericin B is currently under investigation for prophylaxis in cancer patients during periods of profound neutropenia. The triazole antifungal agent itraconazole, with appreciable in vitro activity against *Aspergillus,* is often used for prophylaxis (2.5 mg/kg twice daily) of high-risk children undergoing intensive chemotherapy.

Abuhammour W, Hasan RA: Treatment of invasive aspergillosis in children with hematologic malignancies. *Indian J Pediatr* 2004;71:837–843.

Antachopoulos C, Walsh TJ: New agents for invasive mycoses in children. *Curr Opin Pediatr* 2005;17:78–87.

Choi JK, Mauger J, McGowan KL: Immunohistochemical detection of *Aspergillus* species in pediatric tissue samples. *Am J Clin Pathol* 2004;121:18–25.

Denning DW, Ribaud P, Milpied N, et al: Efficacy and safety of voriconazole in the treatment of acute invasive aspergillosis. *Clin Infect Dis* 2002; 34:563–571.

Golan Y: Overview of transplant mycology. *Am J Health Syst Pharm* 2005;62(Suppl 1):S17–S21.

Herbrecht R, Denning DW, Patterson TF, et al: Voriconazole versus amphotericin B for primary therapy of invasive aspergillosis. *N Engl J Med* 2002;347:408–415.

Muller F-MC, Trusen A: Clinical manifestations and diagnosis of invasive aspergillosis in immunocompromised children. *Eur J Pediatr* 2002;161: 563–574.

Steinbach WJ: Pediatric aspergillosis: Disease and treatment differences in children. *Pediatr Infect Dis J* 2005;24:358–364.

Steinbach WJ, Stevens DA: Review of newer antifungal and immunomodulatory strategies for invasive aspergillosis. *Clin Infect Dis* 2003;37(Suppl 3):S157–S187.

Stevens DA, Kan VL, Judson MA, et al: Practice guidelines for diseases caused by *Aspergillus. Clin Infect Dis* 2000;30:696–709.

Wark PA, Gibson PG, Wilson AJ: Azoles for allergic bronchopulmonary aspergillosis associated with asthma. *Cochrane Database Syst Rev* 2003;3:CD001108.

Chapter 235 ■ Histoplasmosis (*Histoplasma Capsulatum*)

Andrea C.S. McCoy and Stephen C. Aronoff

ETIOLOGY. Histoplasmosis is caused by *Histoplasma capsulatum,* a dimorphic fungus found in the environment as a saprophyte in the mycelial (mold) form and in tissues in the parasitic form as yeast.

EPIDEMIOLOGY. The saprophytic form is found in soil throughout the midwestern United States, primarily along the Ohio and Mississippi Rivers. Sporadic cases of human and animal histoplasmosis have been reported from 31 of the 48 contiguous states. In parts of Kentucky and Tennessee, almost 90% of the population >20 yr of age have positive skin test results for histoplasmin. *Histoplasma* is endemic to parts of the Caribbean islands and Central and South America. *H. capsulatum* thrives in soil rich in nitrates such as areas that are heavily contaminated with bird droppings or decayed wood. Fungal spores are often carried on the wings of birds. Focal outbreaks of histoplasmosis have been reported after aerosolization of microconidia resulting from construction in areas previously occupied by starling roosts or chicken coops or by chopping decayed wood. Unlike birds, bats are actively infected with *Histoplasma.* Focal outbreaks of histoplasmosis have also been reported after intense exposure to bat guano in caves and along bridges frequented by bats. Person-to-person transmission does not occur.

PATHOGENESIS. Inhalation of microconidia (fungal spores) is the initial stage of human infection. The conidia reach the alveoli, germinate, and proliferate as yeast. Alternatively, spores may remain as mold with the potential for activation. The initial infection is a bronchopneumonia. As the initial pulmonary lesion ages, giant cells form, followed by formation of granuloma and central necrosis. At the time of spore germination, yeast cells gain access to the reticuloendothelial system via the pulmonary lymphatic system and hilar lymph nodes. Dissemination with splenic involvement typically follows the primary pulmonary infection. In normal hosts, an immune response follows in approximately 2 wk. The initial pulmonary lesion resolves within 2–4 mo but may undergo calcification resembling the Ghon complex of tuberculosis. Alternatively, "buckshot" calcifications involving the lung and spleen may be seen. Unlike tuberculosis, reinfection with *H. capsulatum* occurs and may lead to exaggerated host responses in some cases.

CLINICAL MANIFESTATIONS. There are 3 forms of human histoplasmosis: acute pulmonary infection, chronic pulmonary histoplasmosis, and progressive disseminated histoplasmosis. **Acute pulmonary histoplasmosis** follows initial or recurrent respiratory exposure to microconidia. The majority of patients are asymptomatic. Symptomatic disease occurs more often in young children; in older individuals, symptoms follow exposure to large inocula in closed spaces (e.g., chicken coops or caves) or prolonged exposure (e.g., camping on contaminated soil, chopping decayed wood). The median incubation time is 14 days. The prodrome is not specific and usually consists of flulike symptoms including headache, fever, chest pain, cough, and myalgias. Hepatosplenomegaly occurs more often in infants and young children. Symptomatic infections may be associated with significant respiratory distress and hypoxia and may require intubation, ventilation, and steroid therapy. Acute pulmonary disease may also present with a prolonged illness (10 days to 3 wk) consisting of weight loss, dyspnea, high fever, asthenia, and fatigue. In 10% of patients, infection is a sarcoid-like disease with arthritis or arthralgia, erythema nodosum, keratoconjunctivitis, iridocyclitis, and pericarditis. Most children with acute pulmonary disease have normal chest radiographs. Individuals with symptomatic disease typically have a patchy bronchopneumonia; hilar lymphadenopathy is variably present. In young children, the pneumonia may coalesce. Focal or buckshot calcifications are convalescent findings in patients with acute pulmonary infection.

Exaggerated host responses to fungal antigens within the lung parenchyma or hilar lymph nodes produce thoracic complications of acute pulmonary histoplasmosis. **Histoplasmomas** are of parenchymal origin and are usually asymptomatic. These fibroma-like lesions are often concentrically calcified and single. Rarely, these lesions may produce broncholithiasis associated with "stone spitting," wheezing, and hemoptysis. In endemic regions, these lesions may mimic parenchymal tumors and are occasionally diagnosed at lung biopsy. **Mediastinal granulomas** form when reactive hilar lymph nodes coalesce and mat together. Although these lesions are usually asymptomatic, huge granulomas may compress the mediastinal structures, producing symptoms of esophageal, bronchial, or vena caval obstruction. Local extension and necrosis may produce pericarditis or pleural effusions. **Mediastinal fibrosis** is a rare complication of mediastinal granulomas and represents an uncontrolled fibrotic reaction arising from the hilar nodes. Structures within the mediastinum become encased within a fibrotic mass, producing obstructive symptomatology. Superior vena cava syndrome, pulmonary venous obstruction with a mitral stenosis–like syndrome, and pulmonary artery obstruction with congestive heart failure have been described. Dysphagia accompanies esophageal entrapment, and a syndrome of cough, wheeze, hemoptysis, and dyspnea accompanies bronchial obstruction.

Chronic pulmonary histoplasmosis is an opportunistic infection in adult patients with centrilobular emphysema. This entity is rare in children.

Progressive disseminated histoplasmosis accounts for 10% of histoplasmosis cases and affects young children and **immunocompromised** individuals. Disseminated disease of childhood occurs almost exclusively in children >2 yr of age and follows primary pulmonary infection. Fever is the most common finding and may persist for weeks to months before the condition is diagnosed. The majority of patients have hepatosplenomegaly, anemia, and thrombocytopenia. Pneumonia and pancytopenia are variably present. Half of the infected infants have transient T-cell deficiencies, and many experience transient hyperglobulinemia. Although chest radiographs are normal in over half of these children, the yeast can frequently be identified on bone marrow examination.

Children who are immunosuppressed (oncology patients, organ transplant recipients, those with HIV infection) are at increased risk for disseminated histoplasmosis. In non-HIV-infected individuals, disseminated disease presents with unexplained fevers, weight loss, lymphadenopathy, and interstitial pulmonary disease. **Extrapulmonary** infection is a characteristic of disseminated disease and may include destructive bony lesions, oropharyngeal ulcers, Addison disease, meningitis, multifocal chorioretinitis, cutaneous infection, and endocarditis. Elevated liver function test results and high serum concentrations of angiotensin-converting enzyme may be observed.

Disseminated histoplasmosis in an HIV-infected individual is an AIDS-defining illness. Disseminated disease is often preceded or followed by another opportunistic infection in this patient population. Those HIV-infected individuals at greatest risk for acquiring disseminated histoplasmosis are those with a history of exposure to avian excreta or bat guano, no prior history of antiretroviral therapy, or no history of previous antifungal prophylaxis. Fever and weight loss occur in most individuals. In the majority of patients pulmonary disease develops; hepatosplenomegaly, lymphadenopathy, skin rashes, and meningoencephalitis are variably present. A sepsis-like syndrome has been identified in a small number of HIV-infected patients with disseminated histoplasmosis and is characterized by the rapid onset of shock, multiorgan failure, and coagulopathy. Transplacental transmission of *H. capsulatum* has been reported in immunocompromised mothers.

DIAGNOSIS. Recovery of *H. capsulatum* by culture differs with the form of infection. In normal hosts with symptomatic or asymptomatic acute pulmonary histoplasmosis, sputum cultures are rarely obtained and are variably positive; cultures of bronchoalveolar lavage fluid appear to have a slightly higher yield than sputa. Blood cultures are sterile in patients with acute pulmonary histoplasmosis, and cultures from any source are typically sterile in individuals with the sarcoid form of the disease. Yeast forms may be demonstrated histologically in tissue from patients with complicated forms of acute pulmonary disease (histoplasmoma, mediastinal granuloma, and mediastinal fibrosis). Sputum cultures are positive in 60% of adults with chronic pulmonary histoplasmosis. The yeast can be recovered from blood or bone marrow in >90% of patients with progressive disseminated histoplasmosis. Wright stain of peripheral blood may demonstrate fungal elements within leukocytes. Polymerase chain reaction assay, although not widely available, will enable more accurate and early diagnosis.

Detection of fungal polysaccharide antigen by radioimmunoassay is the most widely available diagnostic study for patients with suspected progressive disseminated histoplasmosis. In HIV-infected patients as well as others at risk for disseminated disease, histoplasma-associated antigen can be demonstrated in the urine, blood, or bronchoalveolar lavage fluid in >90% of cases. False-positive results may occur in individuals with blastomycosis, coccidioidomycosis, and paracoccidioidomycosis. Antigen detection by enzyme immunoassay has comparable sensitivity, improved specificity, but limited availability. Sequential measurement of antigen in patients with disseminated disease is useful for monitoring response to therapy. Serum, urine, and bronchoalveolar lavage fluid from individuals with acute or chronic pulmonary infections are variably antigen positive.

Seroconversion continues to be useful for the diagnosis of acute pulmonary histoplasmosis, its complications, and chronic pulmonary disease. Serum antibody to yeast and mycelium-associated antigens is classically measured by complement fixation. Although titers of >1 : 8 are found in >80% of patients with histoplasmosis, titers of ≥1 : 32 are most significant for the diagnosis of recent infection. Complement fixation antibody titers are often not significant early in the infection and do not become positive until 4–6 wk after exposure. Complement fixation titers may be falsely positive in patients with other systemic mycoses and may be falsely negative in immunocompromised patients. Antibody detection by immunodiffusion is less sensitive but more specific than complement fixation and is used to confirm questionably positive complement fixation titers. Skin testing is useful only for epidemiologic studies because cutaneous reactivity is lifelong, and intradermal injection may elicit an immune response in otherwise seronegative individuals.

TREATMENT. Antifungal therapy is not warranted for persons with asymptomatic or mildly symptomatic acute pulmonary histoplasmosis. Oral itraconazole or fluconazole should be considered in patients with acute pulmonary infections who fail to improve clinically within 1 mo. Itraconazole is superior to fluconazole in treatment of histoplasmosis in adults. Individuals with primary or re-exposure pulmonary histoplasmosis who become hypoxemic or require ventilatory support should receive amphotericin B (0.7 mg/kg/day) or amphotericin B lipid complex (3 mg/kg/day) until improved; continued therapy with oral itraconazole for a minimum of 12 wk is also recommended. Patients with severe obstructive symptoms caused by granulomatous mediastinal disease can be treated sequentially with amphotericin B followed by itraconazole for 6–12 mo. Those individuals with milder mediastinal disease can be treated with oral itraconazole alone. Some experts recommend that surgery be reserved for those patients who fail to improve after 1 mo of intensive amphotericin B therapy. Sarcoid-like disease with or without pericarditis may be treated with nonsteroidal anti-inflammatory agents.

Amphotericin B continues to be the cornerstone of therapy for infants with progressive disseminated histoplasmosis. In 1 study, sequential therapy with amphotericin B and oral ketoconazole for 3 mo was curative in 88% of patients. Alternatively, amphotericin B or its lipid complex may be given acutely for 4–6 wk followed by oral itraconazole as maintenance therapy for 6–18 mo, depending on histoplasma antigen status. In general, amphotericin B lipid complex may be substituted in severely ill children who are intolerant of the classic drug preparation.

Relapses in HIV-infected individuals with progressive disseminated histoplasmosis are common. Currently, induction therapy with amphotericin B (10–15 mg/kg total dose; total dose >500 mg in adults) or lipid complex amphotericin B is recommended. Lifelong suppressive therapy with daily itraconazole (200 mg/day in adults) is also required. For severely immunocompromised HIV-infected children living in endemic regions, itraconazole (2–5 mg/kg every 12–24 hr) may be used prophylactically. Care must be taken to avoid interactions between antifungal azoles and protease inhibitors.

Adderson EE: Histoplasmosis in a pediatric oncology center. *J Pediatr* 2004;144:100–106.

Adderson EE: Histoplasmosis. *Pediatr Infect Dis J* 2006;25:73–74.

Bracca A, Tosello ME, Girardini JE, et al: Molecular detection of Histoplasma capsulatum var. capsulatum in human clinical samples. *J Clin Microbiol* 2003;41:1753–1755.

Goodwin RA, Loyd JE, Des Prez R: Histoplasmosis in normal hosts. *Medicine* 1981;60:231–266.

Guedes HL, Guimaraes AJ, Muniz Mde M, et al: PCR assay for identification of Histoplasma capsulatum based on the nucleotide sequence of the M antigen. *J Clin Microbiol* 2003;41:535–539.

Hajjeh RA, Pappas PG, Henderson H, et al: Multicenter case-control study of risk factors for histoplasmosis in HIV infected persons. *HIV/AIDS* 2001;32: 1215–1220.

Mocheria S, Wheat LJ: Treatment of histoplasmosis. *Semin Respir Infect* 2001;16:141.

Odio CM, Navarrete M, Carillo JM, et al: Disseminated histoplasmosis in infants. *Pediatr Infect Dis J* 1999;18:1065–1068.

Tobon AM, Franco L, Espinal D, et al: Disseminated histoplasmosis in children: The role of itraconazole therapy. *Pediatr Infect Dis J* 1996; 15:1002–1008.

Walsh TJ, Seibel NL, Arndt C, et al: Amphotericin B lipid complex in pediatric patients with invasive fungal disease. *Pediatr Infect Dis J* 1999; 18:702–708.

Wheat J, Hafner R, Wulfsohn M, et al: Prevention of relapse of histoplasmosis with itraconazole in patients with the acquired immunodeficiency syndrome. The NIAID Clinical Trials and Mycoses Study Group Collaborators. *Ann Intern Med* 1993;118:610–616.

Wheat LJ, Kauffman CA: Histoplasmosis. *Infect Dis Clin North Am* 2003; 17:1–19.

Whitt SP, Koch GA, Fender B, et al: Histoplasmosis in pregnancy: Case series and report of transplacental transmission. *Arch Intern Med* 2004;164: 454–458.

Woods JP, Heinecke EL, Leuke JW, et al: Pathogenesis of *Histoplasma capsulatum* infection. *Semin Respir Infect* 2001;16:91–101.

Chapter 236 ■ Blastomycosis (*Blastomyces Dermatitidis*)

David M. Fleece and Stephen C. Aronoff

ETIOLOGY. Blastomycosis is an uncommon fungal disease caused by *Blastomyces dermatitidis,* a thermally dimorphic fungus that exists as a mycelial (mold) form in nature and as a thick-walled yeast cell in tissues.

EPIDEMIOLOGY. Blastomycosis in children is rare; children <15 yr of age constitute 2–10% of reported cases. Sporadic infection in endemic regions accounts for the majority of cases. Blastomycosis is primarily reported in North America and has occasionally been encountered in Africa, India, the Middle East, and Central and South America. The organism is found throughout the midwestern, south-central and southeastern United States, especially the Ohio and Mississippi River valleys and the Great Lakes region. Although difficult to isolate from soil, *B. dermatitidis* is recovered from earth enriched with organic material, particularly near waterways in endemic areas. Epidemics are unusual but have been described after excavation of contaminated soil in endemic regions. Individuals in endemic regions who spend large amounts of time in wooded areas, such as hunters or forestry workers, are at highest risk for infection.

PATHOGENESIS. The pathogenesis of blastomycosis is similar to that of histoplasmosis. The primary site of infection is the lungs. Inhalation of spores results in alveolar inoculation and germination to yeast forms. Although pulmonary macrophages eliminate the majority of spores before infection occurs, those that survive produce pneumonitis and may disseminate hematogenously. The immune response to infection consists of neutrophil and macrophage migration into infected tissues. The resulting pyogranulomatous response with associated necrosis and subsequent fibrosis is characteristic of the disease.

CLINICAL MANIFESTATIONS. The clinical spectrum of disease in human blastomycosis is diverse and ranges from asymptomatic infection to acute, chronic, or disseminated disease. Lack of an inexpensive, reliable diagnostic test prevents identification of infection in most asymptomatic individuals. Initial symptoms may include nonspecific symptoms such as weight loss, unexplained fever, night sweats, and malaise.

Acute pneumonia is the most common form of symptomatic blastomycosis in both adults and children. Symptoms include acute onset of fever, chills, and productive cough, at times with hemoptysis. The most common radiographic findings are nonspecific lobar and segmental consolidation, and thus may be confused with other acute pulmonary infections such as bacterial and tuberculous disease. Acute pneumonia associated with diffuse pulmonary disease and acute respiratory distress syndrome (ARDS) has been described in immunocompetent adults.

Chronic pneumonia is characterized by several months of weight loss, cough, night sweats, and chest pain. Fever is typically low grade, and hemoptysis can occur. Patients with chronic pneumonia are more likely to have masslike lesions on chest x-ray, but diffuse miliary patterns may be present. Cavitary disease is an uncommon complication of this form of infection.

Extrapulmonary or **disseminated disease** is usually preceded by pulmonary symptoms. Dissemination to almost any organ can occur, but the most common sites are skin, bone, central nervous system, and genitourinary system. Cutaneous disease follows hematogenous or direct inoculation of the subcutaneous tissue and presents as either verrucous or ulcerative lesions. **Osteomyelitis** occurs in 25–50% of patients with extrapulmonary infections. The long bones, skull, vertebrae, and ribs are most commonly involved, but almost any bone can be affected. Central nervous system infection occurs in 10% of patients with extrapulmonary infections and is typified by intracranial abscesses or, rarely, meningitis. Prostatitis and orchitis can occur in males but is unusual. Endometrial disease in females is sexually transmitted. Laryngeal blastomycosis generally follows primary infection of the upper airway, and presents as a laryngeal mass. Fungal abscesses may form anywhere, including the heart and its surrounding structures, the orbit, and the sinuses.

DIAGNOSIS. The definitive diagnosis of blastomycosis requires the demonstration of *B. dermatitidis* in body fluids or tissue specimens by staining or culture. A recent advance is the use of specific nucleic acid probes to distinguish *B. dermatitidis* from morphologically similar fungi in cultured material. Serologic diagnosis may be used in clinical situations with diagnostic uncertainty or where it is difficult to obtain culture material. While serologic studies using complement fixation or immunodiffusion have historically been complicated by the high rate of cross reactions, newer commercial tests have demonstrated improved specificity. Serologic tests can be used adjunctively for diagnosis data but should not be used to exclude infection or as a basis for the initiation of therapy. Skin testing is unreliable because reactivity wanes over time at an unpredictable rate.

TREATMENT. Uncomplicated pneumonia may resolve spontaneously, and some patients can be carefully monitored without therapy. Patients should be thoroughly evaluated for extrapulmonary disease if therapy is withheld. Immunocompromised patients and patients with progressive pulmonary disease, disseminated disease, or central nervous system require treatment. Specific treatment regimens are based on the location, severity, and immune status of the patient. Itraconazole (200–400 mg/day) or fluconazole (400–800 mg/day) for ≥6 mo is recommended for adults with isolated mild to moderate pulmonary infection. Itraconazole (5–7 mg/kg/day) has been used successfully to treat a small number of children with non-life-threatening infections. Amphotericin B (total cumulative dose, 1.5–2.5 g in adults and ≥30 mg/kg in children) remains the drug of choice for life-threatening, disseminated, and central nervous system infections in both adults and children, especially for blastomycosis in immunocompromised persons and pregnant women. Immunocompromised persons, especially patients with AIDS, may require chronic suppressive therapy after completing a course of amphotericin B. In selected cases of pulmonary or extrapulmonary disease in immunocompetent persons, initial therapy with amphotericin B can be followed by itraconazole or fluconazole after the patient's condition has stabilized. Data for lipid complex amphotericin B in children with blastomycosis is limited. No data address the use of caspofungin either alone or in combination with amphotericin for the treatment of childhood blastomycosis. The role of surgery in the treatment of blastomycosis is limited.

Areno JP, Campbell GD, George RB: Diagnosis of blastomycosis. *Semin Respir Infect* 1997;12:252–262.

Chapman SW, Bradsher RW, Campbell GD, et al: Practice guidelines for the management of patients with blastomycosis. *Clin Infect Dis* 2000;30:679–683.

Lemos LL, Guo M, Baliga M: Blastomycosis: Organ involvement and etiologic diagnosis. A review of 123 patients from Mississippi. *Ann Diagn Pathol* 2000;4:391–406.

Morris SK, Brophy J, Richardson SE, et al: Blastomycosis in Ontario, 1994–2003. *Emerg Infect Dis* 2006;12:274–279.

Rose NR, Hamilton RG, Detrick B (editors): *Manual of Clinical Laboratory Immunology*, 6th ed. Washington, DC, ASM Press, 2002, pp 563–564.

Schutze GE, Hickerson SL, Fortin EM, et al: Blastomycosis in children. *Clin Infect Dis* 1996;22:496–502.

Wily JM, Seibel NL, Walsh TJ: Efficacy and safety of amphotericin B lipid complex in 548 children and adolescents with invasive fungal infections. *Pediatr Infect Dis J* 2005;24:167–174.

Chapter 237 ■ Coccidioidomycosis (*Coccidioides*)

Demosthenes Pappagianis

ETIOLOGY. Coccidioidomycosis (Valley fever, San Joaquin fever, desert rheumatism, coccidioidal granuloma) is an infection caused by the fungus *Coccidioides immitis*, which is found in the soil. *C. immitis* exhibits dimorphism, existing as a filamentous mycelial form (mold) in nature and usual laboratory cultures and as an endosporulating spherule in human tissues, influenced by body temperature, leukocytes, increased CO_2, and surface active substances. A 2nd species, *Coccidioides posadasii*, has recently been proposed for non-California isolates. The 2 species do not appear to differ with respect to pathogenicity or therapy.

EPIDEMIOLOGY. *Coccidioides* is concentrated in generally arid areas of the Western hemisphere, including California, Arizona, Texas, parts of Nevada, and Utah (including Dinosaur National Monument), Mexico, Central America, and South America (including Brazil). Disease usually occurs among longtime residents, humans, cattle, sheep, dogs, wild rodents, and other animals, although even visitors can develop the disease, which may not be considered in the differential diagnosis when they return to nonendemic areas. Many environmental influences affect the incidence of the disease. Recovery from infection generally confers permanent immunity. The airborne pathogenicity has led to inclusion of *Coccidioides* species in the list of select agents of bioterrorism (see Chapter 711).

PATHOGENESIS. The minute arthroconidia of the *C. immitis* mycelial saprophytic phase that are airborne in dust are inhaled or, rarely, enter the host through injured skin. In the infected host they round up into spherules, which develop endospores. Liberation of the endospores leads to formation of new spherules and endospores, which spread within a host but not to a new host. Viable *C. immitis* occurs in pulmonary cavities, often in the mycelial as well as spherule form. Person-to-person transmission of infection has been documented only through organ transplantation from an infected individual or, rarely, mother to the fetus or newborn. The arthroconidia that occur in nature and on the surface of cultures are highly infectious. Although isolation of the patient is unnecessary, precautions should be taken with dressings and casts over open lesions to preclude the development of infective arthroconidia, which occurs in 4–5 days on surface cultures.

CLINICAL MANIFESTATIONS. Human infection takes 3 forms (Fig. 237-1): (1) a benign, self-limited, primary infection (60% of

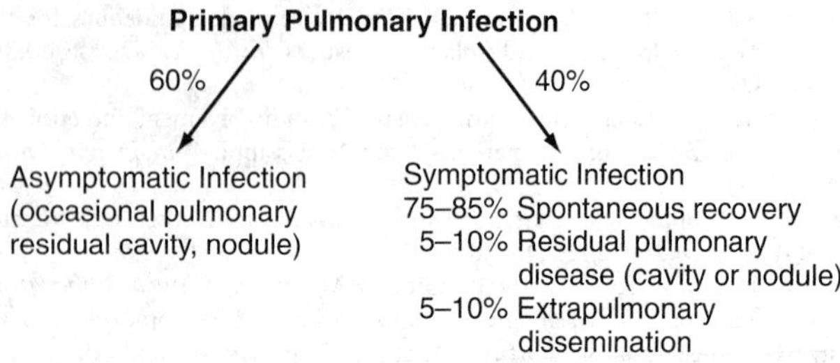

Figure 237-1. Natural history of ciccidioidomycosis.

infected persons show no clinical manifestations); (2) residual pulmonary lesions; and (3) a rare, disseminating, sometimes fatal disease. The disease tends to be milder in children; in children requiring medical attention, dissemination to the bones and meninges is common and approaches the incidence of these complications in adults. Laryngeal coccidioidomycosis, although not frequent, has been detected at a proportionately higher rate in children.

Primary Coccidioidomycosis. The incubation period varies from 1 to 4 wk, with an average of 10–16 days. Symptoms are flulike; the onset may be insidious or abrupt, with malaise, chills, and fever. Chest pain is frequent and may vary from a mere sense of constriction to excruciating pain. Night sweats and anorexia are common. On occasion, there is a persistent dry cough, and the throat may be painful. There also may be headache or backache.

An evanescent, generalized, fine macular erythema or urticarial eruption may appear within the 1st day or so and may be present only in the groin. Rarely, a varicella-like rash has been noted. Most frequently, tibial erythema nodosum occurs, with or without erythema multiforme, usually when sensitivity to coccidioidin is maximal from 3 to 21 days after onset of symptoms. These early rashes do not contain the organism and may result from hypersensitivity to coccidioidal antigen. Skin lesions may occur, however, in persons who are otherwise asymptomatic. Arthritis and phlyctenular conjunctivitis may occur concomitantly.

Auscultation of the lungs may be unrevealing, even though radiography reveals extensive consolidation. Dullness, a friction rub, or fine crackles may be detected. Pleural effusions occasionally occur, even without preceding respiratory symptoms, and may be sufficient to compromise respiratory status. Occasionally, acute respiratory insufficiency may occur. Prominent hilar and mediastinal lymphadenopathy of coccidioidomycosis (Fig. 237-2) may mimic other primary conditions such as lymphoma or sarcoidosis.

Residual Pulmonary Coccidioidomycosis. There are varied manifestations of acute and chronic pulmonary coccidioidomycosis. A transient cavity may develop in an area of pulmonary consolidation during the primary infection. More often, after a variably prolonged period, a persistent cavity may form, more often in patients with diabetes mellitus. There are often no symptoms, and the diagnosis is made radiographically. Occasionally, there is mild to moderate hemoptysis, which may recur and be alarming. Rarely, fatal hemorrhage occurs. Dissemination of the fungus from cavities to other areas is rare. Pulmonary residual "granulomas" sometimes persist. They are not harmful but are difficult to differentiate from tuberculosis or neoplasms. Infrequently, a chronic progressive fibrocavitary pulmonary disease occurs.

Disseminated or Progressive Coccidioidomycosis (Coccidioidal Granuloma). In certain persons, coccidioidal infection does not localize. Dissemination is rare and occurs mainly in male patients, especially Filipinos, other Asians, and African Americans. It usually follows the initial illness within 6 mo, often without any interlude, and is analogous to the course of progressive primary tuberculosis. Specific innate and acquired factors enhance the risk of extrapulmonary dissemination (Table 237-1). Skin lesions and subcutaneous or osseous cold abscesses occur. Infection of the central nervous system may take many forms, including leptomeningitis, ventriculitis and ependymitis, meningeal or cerebral vasculitis, cerebral abscess, or syringomyelia. Meningitis is the most serious of these disseminated lesions and is clinically similar to tuberculous meningitis. Miliary dissemination and peritonitis may be distinguishable from tuberculosis only by demonstration of the causative agent, although coccidioidal peritonitis may present as a very mild disease. The mortality rate of untreated meningitis is practically 100% but varies with other forms of disseminated coccidioidomycosis.

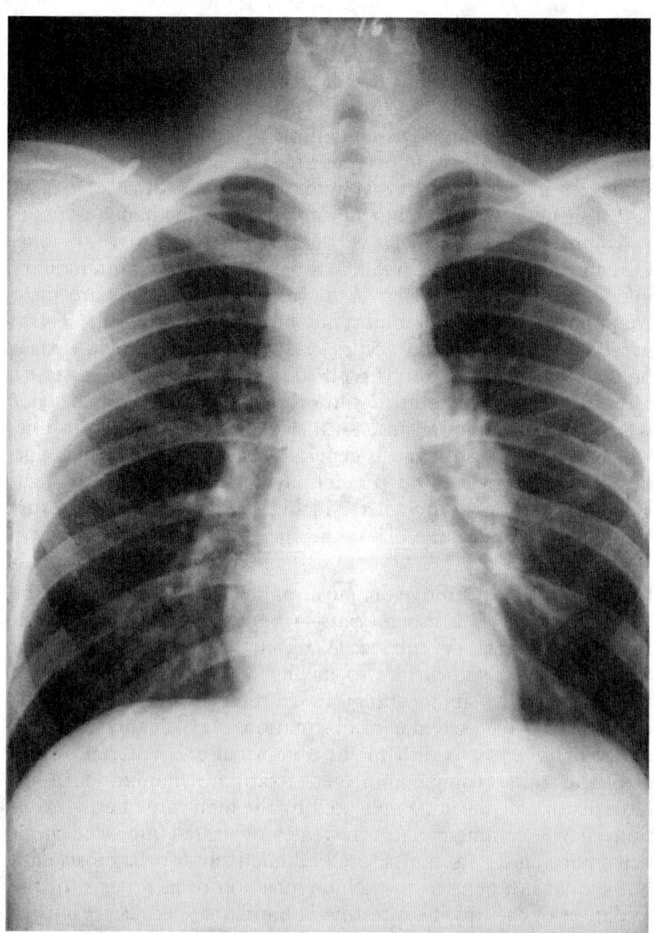

Figure 237-2. Chest radiograph of a 19 yr old man with acute primary coccidioidomycosis. There is prominent hilar lymphadenopathy and mediastinal widening.

DIAGNOSIS. Infection may be confirmed by biopsy or at autopsy. Sputum is often scanty with the primary infection; bronchoalveolar lavage or gastric aspirates, especially in children, may be useful. The diagnosis is confirmed by detection of the character-

TABLE 237-1. Risk factors for extrapulmonary dissemination of Coccidioidomycosis

INNATE	ACQUIRED
Genetic	Lymphoma
Filipino, other Asian	AIDS
African American	Immunosuppression
Blood group B	Diabetes mellitus
HLA class II allele-DRBI∗1301	Pregnancy
	Age (with comorbid condition)

istic endosporulating spherule. Recovery of the fungus by culture and confirmation by DNA probe, exoantigen test, or animal inoculation are also diagnostic. *Cultures are especially hazardous and require special precautions.*

The erythrocyte sedimentation rate is often elevated, and is helpful in evaluating clinical status. Eosinophilia is common and is proportionately higher in patients with more severe infections.

The cerebrospinal fluid (CSF) findings in coccidioidal meningitis are similar to those of tuberculous meningitis (see Chapter 212). Eosinophilic pleocytosis may occur, and in rare instances CSF leukocytes have been reported as "malignant" cells. Lumbar puncture for CSF analysis should be performed in patients with disseminated or progressive coccidioidomycosis. Concomitant coccidioidomycosis and tuberculosis can be confounding.

Skin Test. No coccidioidal skin test reagent has been available in the USA for many years. Such a reagent has historically been used intradermally to detect a remote or recent coccidioidal infection.

Serology. Immunoglobulin M (IgM) antibodies and complement fixation (CF), usually (IgG) antibodies, are detectable in early symptomatic coccidioidomycosis and may persist in those with disseminated coccidioidomycosis. Higher CF antibody titers (>1 : 16) are generally associated with more severe infections. Rarely, serologic test results may be negative in patients with active coccidioidomycosis, especially if they are immunocompromised.

Transplacentally transferred IgG antibodies are detectable by CF in the cord blood and become undetectable by 6 mo of age. Coccidioidal IgM antibodies have been detected in some newborns of mothers with coccidioidomycosis in the absence of the disease in the infants.

C. immitis antibodies in CSF, detectable in 95% of patients with meningitis, are usually diagnostic, although they occasionally are present in patients with juxtadural coccidioidal lesions. CF (IgG) antibody can be detected by immunodiffusion or enzyme immunoassay in the absence of meningitis. CF antibody can be detected in cisternal and lumbar CSF but may be deceptively absent from the ventricular CSF.

Radiography. During the primary infection, chest radiography may not reveal pulmonary changes. There may be single or multiple, sharply circumscribed or soft, feathery, small pulmonary densities or larger consolidated areas. Hilar lymphadenopathy is frequent (see Fig. 237-2). Miliary or reticulonodular lesions are prognostically unfavorable. Pulmonary cavities (Fig. 237-3), which occur less frequently in children than in adults, tend to be thin walled. Pleural effusions vary in extent. Osseous lesions are usually lytic and have a predilection for cancellous bone and can be single or multiple.

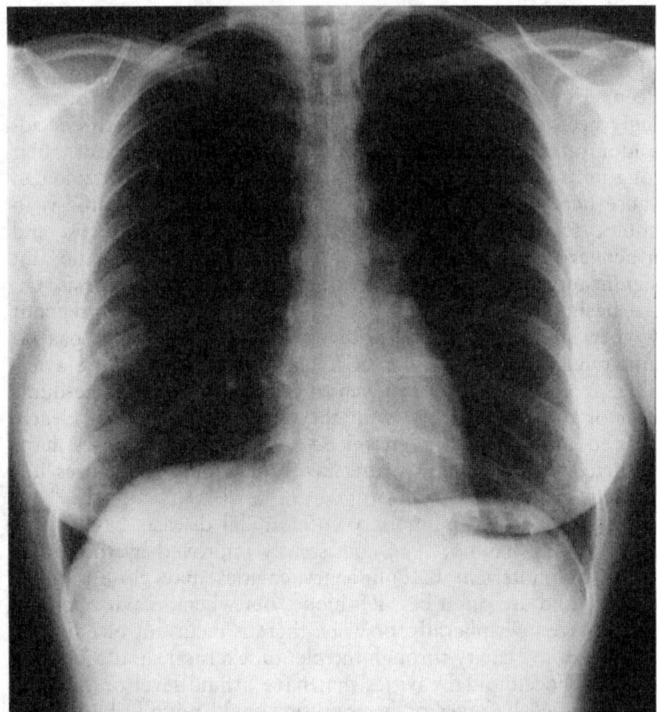

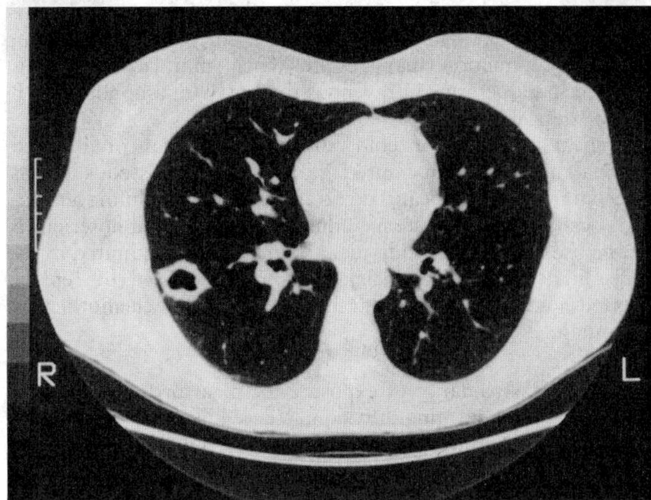

Figure 237-3. *Top panel,* Chest radiograph revealing a chronic cavitary lesion in the right lung of a woman with coccidioidomycosis. *Bottom panel,* CT showing the same cavity in the right lung.

TREATMENT. Because most primary coccidioidal infections resolve spontaneously over a variable time period, they have historically been treated conservatively. The patient's activity and symptomatic measures were restricted until clinical and laboratory findings exhibited improvement. With the advent of the relatively benign oral azoles, physicians have often initiated therapy as soon as coccidioidomycosis is suspected or confirmed. There is limited evidence that such treatment for primary coccidioidomycosis hastens recovery or decreases the risk of extrapulmonary dissemination or development of pulmonary residua (cavity or solitary nodule).

Antifungal chemotherapy is indicated for those at high risk for severe coccidioidomycosis and those who have recognized metapulmonary dissemination. Currently available agents include oral and intravenous fluconazole, itraconazole and voriconazole, and oral ketoconazole, as well as (parenteral) amphotericin B, both desoxycholate and lipid-complex formulations. Amphotericin B (up to 1 mg/kg/day) should be administered for rapidly progressing coccidioidomycosis. Lipid-complex formulations of amphotericin B (5 mg/kg/day) are recommended for persons with compromised renal function (including doubling of the serum creatinine resulting from amphotericin B desoxycholate therapy), those who are receiving other nephrotoxic therapy, or those who are otherwise intolerant of amphotericin B desoxycholate. Once the full daily dose has been achieved, it can be given every other day or 2–3 times a week to minimize renal toxicity.

Systemic amphotericin B desoxycholate does not cross the blood-brain barrier in therapeutic amounts for *C. immitis,* but it may mask the presence of meningitis. Intrathecal (cisternal or lumbar) or intraventricular administration of amphotericin B were previously the mainstay of treatment of coccidioidal meningitis until the availability of azole antifungal agents. Fluconazole, itraconazole, and voriconazole have proved useful in the treatment of coccidioidal meningitis, although lifetime treatment may be required.

Ketoconazole (3–10 mg/kg/day), fluconazole (3–12 mg/kg/day), or itraconazole (3–6 mg/kg/day) administered orally have been useful in treating disseminated coccidioidomycosis outside the central nervous system that is neither extensive nor progressing rapidly. The higher doses may be required for the treatment of meningitis. Voriconazole has been effective in some patients deemed to have failed on fluconazole. The azoles have increasingly been used to treat children as well as adults with coccidioidomycosis, but there is limited information about their long-term adverse effects in younger patients. Ketoconazole can cause hepatic dysfunction and inhibit testosterone synthesis in adults. Fluconazole is primarily excreted by the kidneys, and itraconazole is metabolized in the liver; these drugs do not significantly affect testosterone or adrenocorticoid synthesis. On the basis of limited experience, coccidioidomycosis in pregnant women should be treated with amphotericin B, which has no apparent adverse effect on the fetus. Until more data are available, azoles should not be given to pregnant patients. The duration of therapy required with the azoles has not been clearly defined and must be determined individually. Relapses have occurred in some patients after favorable clinical responses following therapy for >1 yr.

Surgery. Chronic pulmonary coccidioidal disease, cavitary or fibrocavitary, has not been consistently improved by the azoles or by amphotericin B. Pulmonary cavities may close spontaneously and are often best left alone, but when a cavity persists or is located peripherally, or when there is recurrent bleeding or rupture of the cavity through the pleura, excision should be considered. Coccidioidal cavities that have a fluid level or that are accompanied by fever or hemoptysis should initially be treated with antibacterial antibiotics. Infrequently, bronchopleural fistulas or recurrent cavitation occurs as a surgical complication; rarely, dissemination may result. When thoracic surgery is required, perioperative intravenous therapy with amphotericin B may be desirable.

Surgical drainage of cold abscesses, removal of infected synovial membranes, and curettage or excision of osseous lesions is recommended for localized extrapulmonary coccidioidomycosis. Local as well as systemic administration of amphotericin B can be used to treat coccidioidal articular disease. Limited experience indicates that artificial joints may be used to replace infected joints as long as antifungal (triazole) chemotherapy continues.

PREVENTION. Avoidance of exposure to the arthroconidia is the only means of preventing infection. Whole killed cell vaccine did not prevent coccidioidomycosis in humans. Subcellular vaccines have been protective in experimental coccidioidomycosis.

Arsura EL, Johnson R, Penrose J, et al: Neuroimaging as a guide to predict outcomes for patients with coccidioidal meningitis. *Clin Infect Dis* 2005;40:624–627.

Bickel KD, Press BH, Hovey LM: Successful treatment of coccidioidomycosis osteomyelitis in an infant. *Ann Plast Surg* 1993;30:462–465.

Cortez KJ, Walsh TJ, Bennett JE: Successful treatment of coccidioidal meningitis with voriconazole. *Clin Infect Dis* 2003;36:1619–1622.

Crum NF, Lederman ER, Stafford CM, et al: Coccidioidomycosis. A description survey of a reemerging disease. Clinical characteristics and current controversies. *Medicine* 2004;83:149–175.

Herron LD, Kissel P, Smilovitz D: Treatment of coccidioidal spinal infection: Experience in 16 cases. *J Spinal Disord* 1997;10:215–222.

Linsangan LC, Ross LA: *Coccidioides immitis* infection of the neonate: Two routes of infection. *Pediatr Infect Dis J* 1999;18:171–173.

Pappagianis D: Serologic studies in coccidioidomycosis. *Semin Respir Infect* 2001;16:242–250.

Richardson V, Valenciano-Vega JI, Valenzuela-Espinoza A: Bronchoesophageal fistulas secondary to coccidioidomycosis. *Pediatr Infect Dis J* 1994;13: 159–161.

Wright PW, Pappagianis D, Wilson M, et al: Donor-related coccidioidomycosis in organ transplant recipients. *Clin Infect Dis* 2003;37:1265–1269.

Chapter 238 ■ *Paracoccidioides Brasiliensis*

Andrea C.S. Mccoy and Stephen C. Aronoff

ETIOLOGY. Paracoccidioidomycosis (South American or Brazilian blastomycosis, Lutz-Splendore-Almeida disease) is an uncommon fungal infection endemic in South America, with cases reported in Central America and Mexico. The etiologic agent, *Paracoccidioides brasiliensis,* is a thermally dimorphic fungus found in the environment in the mycelial (mold) form and in tissues as yeast.

EPIDEMIOLOGY. *P. brasiliensis* is ecologically unique to Central and South America. Endemic outbreaks occur mainly in the tropical rain forests of Brazil, with cases scattered in Argentina, Colombia, and Venezuela. There is increased incidence in areas with moderately high altitude, high humidity and rainfall, and where coffee and tobacco are grown. Armadillos appear to be a natural reservoir for *P. brasiliensis.* The most common route of infection is by inhalation of conidia. The disease is not usually thought to be contagious, and person-to-person transmission has not been confirmed. Paracoccidioidomycosis is more common among males after puberty due to the role of estrogen in preventing the transition of conidia to the yeast form.

CLINICAL MANIFESTATIONS. There are 2 clinical forms of disease. The **acute** form is rare and occurs almost exclusively in children and persons with impaired immunity, and targets the reticuloendothelial system. Pulmonary symptoms may be absent, although chest radiographs often show patchy, confluent, or nodular densities. Patients typically present acutely with fever, malaise, wasting, lymphadenopathy, and abdominal enlargement from intra-abdominal lymphadenopathy. Hepatomegaly and splenomegaly are nearly constant. Localized bony lesions have been reported in children and may progress to systemic disease. Multifocal osteomyelitis, arthritis, and pericardial effusions can also occur. Nonspecific laboratory findings include anemia, eosinophilia, and hypergammaglobulinemia. Acute paracoccidioidomycosis has a 25% mortality rate.

Adults develop a **chronic,** progressive illness that presents initially with flulike symptoms, fever, and weight loss. Pulmonary infection develops with dyspnea, cough, chest pain, and hemoptysis. Findings on physical examination are scant, although chest radiographs may show infiltrates that are disproportionate with mild clinical findings. Mucositis involving the mouth and its structures as well as the nose may manifest as localized pain, change in voice, or dysphagia. Lesions may extend beyond the oral cavity onto the skin. Generalized lymphadenopathy, hepatosplenomegaly, and adrenal involvement leading to Addison disease may occur. Meningoencephalitis and central nervous system granulomas can occur as presenting or secondary symptoms. Adults with extensive exposure to soil, such as farmers, are most likely to develop the chronic form of the disease.

DIAGNOSIS. Demonstration of the fungus by direct wet mount (potassium hydroxide) preparation of sputum, exudate, or pus supports the diagnosis in many cases. Histopathologic examination of biopsy specimens using special fungal staining techniques is also diagnostic. Culture of the fungus on Sabouraud-dextrose or yeast extract agar confirms the diagnosis. Antibodies to *P. brasiliensis* can be demonstrated in most patients. Serial antibody titers and lymphocyte proliferative responses to fungal antigens are useful for monitoring the response to therapy. The 43,000 kd glycoprotein (gp43) is present in sera of >90% of patients with paracoccidioidomycosis by immunodiffusion and in 100% by immunoblotting. Newer diagnostic methods that may prove to be very useful in the future include polymerase chain reaction detection techniques and capture enzyme-linked immunosorbent assay to detect specific immunoglobulin E in patient sera. Skin testing with paracoccidioidin is not reliable since 1/3 of patients with active disease are nonreactive.

TREATMENT. Itraconazole (50–400 mg/day) orally for 6 mo is the treatment of choice for paracoccidioidomycosis. Fluconazole has also been used, but high doses (600 mg/day or higher) and longer treatment periods are required. Terbinafine, an allylamine, has potent in vitro activity against *P. brasiliensis* and has been used for successful treatment of paracoccidioidomycosis unresponsive to treatment with trimethoprim-sulfamethoxazole (TMP-SMZ). Amphotericin B (total adult dose 3–6 g) is recommended for disseminated disease and if other therapies fail. Therapy with sulfonamide compounds, including sulfadiazine, TMP-SMZ, and dapsone, have been used historically and are generally less expensive than the newer azoles and allylamines. The primary disadvantage is that the treatment course is very long, lasting months to years, depending on the agent selected. Relapse may occur following any form of therapy, including with amphotericin B.

Benard G, Orii NM, Marques HHS, et al: Severe acute paracoccidioidomycosis in children. *Pediatr Infect Dis J* 1994;13:510–515.

Blotta MH, Mamoni RL, Oliveira SJ, et al: Endemic regions of paracoccidioidomycosis in Brazil: A clinical and epidemiologic study of 584 cases in the southeast region. *Am J Trop Med Hyg* 1999;6:390–394.

de Almeida SM, Queiroz-Telles F, Teive HA, et al: Central nervous system paracoccidioidomycosis: Clinical features and laboratorial findings. *J Infection* 2004;48:193–198.

Gomes GM, Cisalpino PS, Taborda CP, et al: PCR for diagnosis of paracoccidioidomycosis. *J Clin Microbiol* 2000;38:3478–3480.

Hahn RC, Fontes CJ, Batista RD, Hamdan JS: In vitro comparison of activities of terbinafine and itraconazole against *Paracoccidioides brasiliensis*. *J Clin Microbiol* 2002;40:2828–2831.

Mamoni RL, Rossi CL, Camargo ZP, et al: Capture enzyme-linked immunosorbent assay to detect specific immunoglobulin E in sera of patients with paracoccidioidomycosis. *Am J Trop Med Hyg* 2001;65:237–241.

Negroni DM, Montero-Gei F, Castro LG, et al: A Pan-American 5-year study of fluconazole therapy for deep mycoses in immunocompetent host. Pan-American Study Group. *Clin Infect Dis* 1992;14(Suppl 1):S68–S76.

Nogueira SA, Guedes AL, Wanke B, et al: Osteomyelitis caused by *Paracoccidioides brasiliensis* in a child from the metropolitan area of Rio de Janeiro. *J Trop Pediatr* 2001;47:311–315.

Ollague JM, de Zurita AM, Calero G: Paracoccidioidomycosis (South American blastomycosis) successfully treated with terbinafine: First case report. *Br J Dermatol* 2000;143:188–191.

Chapter 239 ■ Sporotrichosis *(Sporothrix Schenckii)*

David M. Fleece and Stephen C. Aronoff

ETIOLOGY. Sporotrichosis is a rare fungal infection that occurs worldwide both sporadically and in outbreaks. The etiologic agent, *Sporothrix schenckii,* is a thermally dimorphic fungus found in the environment in the mycelial (mold) form and in tissues as yeast.

EPIDEMIOLOGY. *S. schenckii* is found throughout the world, but most cases of sporotrichosis are reported from North and South America and Japan. The majority of cases in the United States have occurred in the Midwest, particularly in areas along the Mississippi and Missouri Rivers. The fungus occurs in decaying vegetation and has been isolated most commonly from sphagnum moss, rosebushes, barberry, straw, and some types of hay. Sporotrichosis can occur as an occupational disease among farmers, gardeners, veterinarians, and laboratory workers. Transmission from bites and scratches of animals, most frequently cats and armadillos, has occurred. Reports of human-to-human transmission are rare.

PATHOGENESIS. Disease in humans usually follows **cutaneous inoculation** of the fungus into a minor wound. Pulmonary infection may result from the inhalation of large numbers of spores. Disseminated infection is unusual but typically occurs in immunocompromised persons following ingestion or inhalation of spores. The cellular immune response to *S. schenckii* infection is both neutrophilic and monocytic. Histologically, concomitant noncaseating granulomas and microabscess formation are characteristic. Due to the paucity of organisms, it is usually difficult to demonstrate the fungi in biopsy specimens. Antibody does not protect against infection.

CLINICAL MANIFESTATIONS. Cutaneous sporotrichosis is the most common forms of disease in all age groups. Systemic signs and symptoms are uncommon. Cutaneous disease may either be lymphocutaneous or fixed cutaneous, the former being much more frequent. **Lymphocutaneous** sporotrichosis accounts for >75% of reported cases in children and occurs after traumatic subcutaneous inoculation. After a variable and often prolonged incubation period of 1–12 wk, an isolated, painless erythematous papule develops at the inoculation site. The initial lesion is usually on an extremity but may be on the face in children. The original papule enlarges and ulcerates. Satellite lesions follow lymphangitic spread and appear as multiple tender subcutaneous nodules tracking the lymphatic channels that drain the lesion. These secondary nodules are subcutaneous granulomas that adhere to the overlying skin and subsequently ulcerate. Sporotrichosis does not heal spontaneously, and these ulcerative lesions may persist for years if untreated. Alternatively, infection may remain limited to the inoculation site in the fixed cutaneous form.

Extracutaneous sporotrichosis is rare in children and most cases are in adults with underlying medical conditions. The most common form of extracutaneous sporotrichosis is skeletal infection. Pulmonary sporotrichosis usually presents as a chronic pneumonitis similar to the presentation of pulmonary tuberculosis.

DIAGNOSIS. Cutaneous and lymphocutaneous sporotrichosis must be differentiated from other causes of nodular lymphangitis, including atypical mycobacterial infection, nocardiosis, leishmaniasis, tularemia, melioidosis, cutaneous anthrax, and other systemic mycoses, including coccidioidomycosis. Definitive diagnosis requires isolation of the fungus from the site of infection by culture. Special histologic staining, such as periodic acid-Schiff and methenamine silver, is required to identify yeast forms in tissues. In spite of special staining techniques, diagnostic yield from biopsy specimens is low due to the small number of organisms present in the tissues. In cases of disseminated disease, demonstration of serum antibody against *S. schenckii*–related antigens can be diagnostically useful. Currently available serologic tests demonstrate high degrees of specificity and sensitivity. Newer techniques for rapid identification of dimorphic fungal pathogens using specific DNA probes have recently been introduced and may prove to be helpful in the future.

TREATMENT. Itraconazole orally is the recommended treatment of choice for sporotrichosis outside the central nervous system. The usual dosage for children is 100 mg daily or 5 mg/kg daily. The adult dosage is 100–200 mg daily. Alternatively, younger children with cutaneous disease only may be treated with a saturated solution of potassium iodide (SSKI) given orally once daily, beginning at 5–10 drops 3 times per day. The dose is gradually advanced to 25–40 drops 3 times per day for children and 40–50 drops 3 times per day for adolescents and adults. Adverse reactions should be managed with temporary cessation of therapy and reinstitution at a lower dosage. Therapy is continued until the cutaneous lesions have resolved, which usually takes 6–12 wk. Terbinafine, an allylamine, also has been used successfully to treat cutaneous sporotrichosis. Further clinical efficacy data are needed to recommend its use. Therapy with azoles or SSKI should not be used in pregnant women. Pregnant women with cutaneous disease can be treated with local hyperemia, or therapy can be delayed until the pregnancy is completed. Dissemination to the fetus does not occur, nor is the disease worsened by pregnancy. Amphotericin B is the treatment of choice for pulmonary infections, disseminated infection, and infections in immunocompromised persons and pregnant women. Central nervous system infections should be treated with amphotericin B in combination with flucytosine. Surgical debridement has a role in the treatment of some cases of sporotrichosis, particularly in osteoarticular disease.

Burch JM, Morelli JG, Weston WL: Unsuspected sporotrichosis in childhood. *Pediatr Infect Dis J* 2001;20:442–445.
Da Rosa AC, Scrofemeker ML, Bettarato R, et al: Epidemiology of sporotrichosis: A study of 304 cases in Brazil. *J Am Acad Dermatol* 2005;52:451–459.
Kauffman CA: Sporotrichosis. *Clin Infect Dis* 1999;29:231–236.
Kauffman CA, Hajjeh R, Chapman SW, et al: Practice guidelines for the management of patients with sporotrichosis. *Clin Infect Dis* 2000;30:684–687.
Lindsley MD, Hurst SF, Iqbal NJ, et al: Rapid identification of dimorphic and yeast-like fungal pathogens using specific DNA probes. *J Clin Microbiol* 2001;39:3505–3511.
Pappas PG, Tellez I, Deep AE, et al: Sporotrichosis in Peru: Description of an area of hyperendemicity. *Clin Infect Dis* 2000;30:65–70.

Chapter 240 ■ Zygomycosis *(Mucormycosis)*

Macdara Tynan and Stephen C. Aronoff

ETIOLOGY. Zygomycosis refers to a group of opportunistic fungal infections caused by dimorphic fungi of the class Zygomycetes, which are primitive, fast growing fungi that are largely saprophytic and ubiquitous. These organisms are found commonly in soil, decaying plant and animal matter, and on moldy cheese, fruit, and bread.

This class is subdivided into 2 orders, Mucorales and Entomophthorales, each containing human pathogens. The term **mucormycosis** refers only to infections caused by Mucorales, which includes the genera *Absidia, Apophysomyceae, Mucor, Rhizomucor,* and *Rhizopus,* and represent the more common causes of zygomycoses in humans. Infections caused by organisms of the genera *Cunninghamella, Saksenaea,* and *Cokeromyces* are seen less frequently. Mucorales disease in humans is characterized by a rapidly evolving course, tissue necrosis, and blood vessel invasion in addition to subcutaneous infection. These infections are most acute and fulminant in debilitated patients. Genera of the order Entomophthorales causing infection in humans include *Conidiobolus* and *Basidiobolus.* These agents typically cause indolent sinus or subcutaneous infections in immunocompetent persons.

EPIDEMIOLOGY. Zygomycosis is primarily a disease of persons with underlying conditions that impair host immunity. Predisposing factors include diabetes, hematologic malignancies, persistent acidosis, corticosteroid or deferoxamine therapy, organ transplantation, prematurity, and, less frequently, AIDS. Those fungi that are pathogenic in humans grow on almost any carbohydrate substrate and are able to grow at temperatures above 37°C. Acidosis diminishes the phagocytic and chemotactic ability of neutrophils while increasing the availability of unbound iron. Deferoxamine-bound iron can also be used by the fungus to enhance its growth.

PATHOGENESIS. Macrophages and neutrophils are the main host defense against Zygomycetes and other filamentous fungi and provide almost complete immunity against Zygomycetes by phagocytosis and oxidative killing of spores. This may explain the predilection for zygomycosis of patients with neutropenia or neutrophil dysfunction. The primary route of infection from Zygomycetes is inhalation of spores from the environment. In immunocompromised persons, if spores are not cleared by macrophages they will germinate into hyphae, resulting in local invasion and tissue destruction. Cutaneous or percutaneous routes of infection may lead to cutaneous and subcutaneous zygomycosis. Ingestion of contaminated food or drinks has been linked to gastrointestinal disease.

CLINICAL MANIFESTATIONS. There are no unique signs or symptoms of Zygomycosis. It can occur as any of several clinical syndromes, including sinus/rhinocerebral, pulmonary, gastrointestinal, disseminated, or cutaneous/subcutaneous disease.

Sinus and rhinocerebral infection is the most common form of zygomycosis and occurs primarily in persons with diabetes mellitus or who are immunocompromised. Infection typically originates in the paranasal sinuses. Initial symptoms are consistent with sinusitis and include headache, retro-orbital pain, fever, and nasal discharge. Infection may evolve rapidly or be slowly progressive. Orbital involvement manifesting as periorbital edema, proptosis, ptosis, and ophthalmoplegia can occur early in the disease. The nasal discharge is often dark and bloody; examination of the nasal mucosa reveals black, necrotic areas. Extension beyond the nasal cavity into the mouth is common. Involved tissues become red, then violaceous, then black as vessel thrombosis and tissue necrosis occur. Direct bony involvement is common as a result of contiguous pressure effects or because of direct invasion and infarction. Destructive paranasal sinusitis with intracranial extension can be demonstrated by CT or MRI. Cases complicated by cavernous sinus thrombosis and thrombosis of the internal carotid artery have been reported. Brain abscesses can occur in patients with rhinocerebral infection that extends directly from the nasal cavity and sinuses, usually to the frontal or frontotemporal lobes. In patients with disseminated disease, abscesses may involve the occipital lobe or brainstem.

Pulmonary zygomycosis infection usually occurs in severely neutropenic patients and is characterized by fever, tachypnea, and productive cough with pleuritic chest pain and hemoptysis. A wide range of pulmonary radiologic findings, including solitary pulmonary nodule, segmental or lobar consolidation, and cavitary and bronchopneumonic changes, are recognized.

Gastrointestinal zygomycosis is uncommon. It may occur as a complication of disseminated disease or as an isolated intestinal infection in diabetics, immunosuppressed or malnourished children, or preterm infants. Abdominal pain and distention with hematemesis, hematochezia, or melena may occur. Stomach or bowel wall perforation is not uncommon.

Disseminated zygomycosis is associated with a very high mortality rate, especially among immunocompromised persons. Pulmonary involvement is most common, but infection can originate from any of the primary sites of infection.

Cutaneous and soft tissue zygomycosis can complicate burns or surgical wounds. An outbreak occurred among preterm infants following the use of contaminated wooden tongue depressors to immobilize the extremities. Primary cutaneous disease may be invasive locally, progressing through all tissue layers, including muscle, fascia, and bone. Necrotizing fasciitis may occur. Infection presents as an erythematous papule that ulcerates, leaving a black necrotic center. The skin lesions are painful, and affected patients may be febrile. Cutaneous lesions from hematogenous seeding tend to be nodular, with minimal destruction of the epidermis.

DIAGNOSIS. The diagnosis relies on direct morphologic identification of mycotic elements and recovery of Zygomycetes in culture or by biopsy identification in specimens obtained at the site of presumed involvement. To identify the fungus from scrapings, sputum, and exudates under direct microscopy, the use of Calcofluor white or 10% potassium hydroxide and Parker ink is recommended. In lung and other tissue biopsy specimens, demonstration of fungal elements with fungal specific stains is recommended. Mucorales appear as broad, infrequently septate, thin-walled hyphae, branching irregularly at right angles when stained with Gomori methenamine silver or hematoxylin and eosin. Angiotrophism is a hallmark of zygomycosis. The fungi can be cultured on standard laboratory media from sputum, bronchoalveolar lavage fluid, skin lesions, or biopsy material. However, Mucorales are frequent culture contaminants. Serologic tests for detecting zygomycosis are not clinically useful. Diagnosis of disseminated zygomycosis using a polymerase chain reaction assay recently has been reported and may prove to be a useful adjunct to standard diagnostic techniques in the future.

TREATMENT. All forms of the disease can be aggressive and difficult to treat with high fatality rates. The optimal therapy for zygomycosis in children requires early diagnosis and prompt institution of medical therapy combined with extensive surgical debridement of all devitalized tissue. Correction of the underlying disease, if possible, is an essential component of management. Amphotericin B desoxycholate (1–1.5 mg/kg/day to a total dose of 70 mg/kg or 3–4 g over several weeks) or amphotericin B lipid complex (3–5 mg/kg/day) has been successful in treating infection. Anecdotal reports suggest that higher total doses of amphotericin B lipid complex (15–20 mg/kg/day) are associated with better outcomes in invasive infection. Pulmonary and cutaneous disease has been successfully treated with intermediate dosages of amphotericin B (30 mg/kg total dose). Surveillance in the United States suggests an association between use of voriconazole use and the emergence of zygomycosis in transplant patients, which may represent increased patient survival or selection of resistant organisms. Posaconazole together with surgery has been associated with dramatic clinical responses and holds promise as a therapeutic agent for mucormycosis. Caspofungin has limited or no in vitro activity against Zygomycetes. Hyperbaric oxygen and granulocyte-macrophage colony-stimulating factor have been used anecdotally as adjunctive therapies.

Garcia-Diaz JB, Palau L, Pankey GA: Resolution of rhinocerebral zygomycosis associated with adjuvant administration of granulocyte-macrophage colony-stimulating factor. *Clin Infect Dis* 2001;32:145–150.

Gonzalez CE, Rinaldi MG, Sugar AM: Zygomycosis. *Infect Dis Clin North Am* 2002;16(4):895–914.

John BV, Chamilos G, Kontoyiannis DP: Hyperbaric oxygen as an adjunctive treatment for zygomycosis. *Clin Microbiol Infect* 2005;11:515–517.

Loeffler RV, Bohme A, Einsele H, et al: Diagnosis of disseminated zygomycosis using a polymerase chain reaction assay. *Eur J Clin Microbiol Infect Dis* 2001;20:744–745.

Ribes JA, Vanover-Sams CL, Baker DJ: Zygomycetes in human disease. *Clin Microbiol Rev* 2000;13:236–301.

Tobin AM, Arango M, Fernandez D, Restrepo A: Mucormycosis (zygomycosis) in a heart-kidney transplant recipient: Recovery after posaconazole therapy. *Clin Infect Dis* 2003;36:1488–1491.

Walsh TJ, Antachopoulos C: New agents for invasive mycoses in children. *Curr Opin Pediatr* 2005;17:78–87.

Wiley JM, Seibel NL, Walsh TJ: Efficacy and safety of amphotericin lipid complex in 548 children with invasive fungal infections. *Pediatr Infect Dis J* 2005;24:167–174.

Chapter 241 ■ *Pneumocystis Carinii (Pneumocystis Jiroveci)*

Francis Gigliotti and Terry W. Wright

Pneumocystis carinii pneumonia (interstitial plasma cell pneumonitis) in an immunocompromised person is a life-threatening infection. Symptomatic infection in the immunocompetent person is usually subclinical and goes unrecognized. Epidemiologic studies in young children demonstrate that asymptomatic primary infection can result from transmission of the organism. The disease most likely results from new or repeat acquisition of the organism rather than reactivation of latent organisms. Even in the most severe cases, with rare exceptions, the organisms and the disease remain localized to the lungs.

ETIOLOGY. *P. carinii* is a common extracellular parasite found in the lungs of mammals worldwide. The taxonomic placement of this organism has not been unequivocally established, but nucleic acid homologies place it most closely to the fungi despite its morphologic features and susceptibility to drugs that are similar to protozoa. Detailed studies of the basic biology of the organism are not possible due to the inability to maintain *P. carinii* in culture. Both phenotypic and genotypic analysis demonstrates that each mammalian species is infected by a unique strain (or possibly species) of *Pneumocystis.* A biologic correlate for these differences is evidenced by animal experiments that have shown organisms are not transmissible from 1 mammalian species to another. These observations have led to the suggestion that organisms be renamed; with those infecting humans renamed ***Pneumocystis jiroveci.*** Alternative acceptable nomenclature retains the use of *P. carinii* but uses the annotation *forma specialis* (f. sp.) to designate the host of origin such that *P. carinii* infecting humans, rats, or mice would carry the f. sp. designation *hominis, ratti,* or *muris,* respectively. Both nomenclatures appear in the medical literature.

EPIDEMIOLOGY. Serologic surveys show most humans are infected with *P. carinii* before 4 yr of age. In the immunocompetent child, these infections are usually asymptomatic. *P. carinii* DNA can occasionally be detected in nasopharyngeal aspirates of normal infants. Pneumonia caused by *P. carinii* occurs almost exclusively in severely immunocompromised hosts, including those with congenital or acquired immunodeficiency disorders or malignancies, and in organ transplant recipients. Small numbers of *P. carinii* can be found in the lungs of infants dying with a diagnosis of sudden infant death syndrome. This could indicate a cause-and-effect relationship or simply indicate that there is overlap in the timing of the primary infection with *P. carinii* and sudden infant death syndrome.

Without prophylaxis, approximately 40% of infants and children with AIDS, 70% of adults with AIDS, 12% of children with leukemia, and 10% of patients with organ transplant recipients experience *P. carinii* pneumonia. Epidemics that occurred among debilitated infants in Europe during and after World War II are attributed to malnutrition. The addition of tumor necrosis factor-α inhibitors to the management of patients with inflammatory bowel disease has resulted in a demonstrable increase in *P. carinii* pneumonia among this patient population.

The natural habitat and mode of transmission to humans are unknown. Animal transmission is by the airborne route; animal-to-human transmission is unlikely because of the host specificity of *Pneumocystis* species. Person-to-person transmission has been suggested from a few studies but has not been conclusively demonstrated.

PATHOGENESIS. Two forms of *P. carinii* are found in the alveolar spaces: cysts 5–8 μm in diameter that contain up to 8 pleomorphic intracystic sporozoites; and extracystic trophozoites, which are 2–5 μm cells derived from excysted sporozoites. The terminology of sporozoites and trophozoites is based on the morphologic similarities to protozoa since there are not exact correlates for these forms of the organism among the fungi. *P. carinii* attaches to type I alveolar epithelial cells, possibly by adhesive proteins such as fibronectin and or mannose-dependent ligands.

Control of infection depends on intact cell-mediated immunity. Studies in patients with AIDS show increased incidence of *P. carinii* pneumonia with markedly decreased $CD4^+$ T-lymphocyte counts. The $CD4^+$ cell count provides a useful indicator in both older children and adults of the need for prophylaxis for *P. carinii* pneumonia. Although normally functioning $CD4^+$ T cells are central to controlling infection by *P. carinii,* the final effector pathway for destruction of *P. carinii* is poorly understood. A likely role for $CD4^+$ T cells could be to provide help for the production of specific antibody that is then involved in the clearance of organisms through interaction with complement, phagocytes, or T cells or through direct activation of alveolar macrophages.

In the absence of an adaptive immune response, as can be modeled in severe combined immunodeficient (SCID) mice, infection with *P. carinii* produces very little alteration in lung histology or function until very late in the course of the disease. If functional lymphocytes are given to SCID mice infected with *P. carinii,* there is a rapid onset of an inflammatory response that results in an intense cellular infiltrate, markedly reduced lung compliance, and significant hypoxia, which are the characteristic changes of *P. carinii* pneumonia in humans. These inflammatory changes are associated with marked disruption of surfactant function. T-cell subset analysis has shown that $CD4^+$ T cells produce an inflammatory response that clears the organisms but also results in lung injury. $CD8^+$ T cells are ineffective in the eradication of *P. carinii.* $CD8^+$ T cells do help modulate the inflammation produced by $CD4^+$ T cells, but in the absence of $CD4^+$ T cells their ineffectual inflammatory response contributes significantly to lung injury. These various T-cell effects are likely responsible for the variations in presentation and outcome of *P. carinii* pneumonia observed in different patient populations.

PATHOLOGY. The histopathologic features of *P. carinii* pneumonia are of 2 types. The 1st type is **infantile interstitial plasma cell pneumonitis,** which is seen in epidemic outbreaks in debilitated infants 3–6 mo of age. Extensive infiltration with thickening of the alveolar septum occurs, and plasma cells are prominent. The 2nd type is a **diffuse desquamative alveolar pneumonitis** found in immunocompromised children and adults. The alveoli contain large numbers of *P. carinii* in a foamy exudate with alveolar macrophages active in the phagocytosis of organisms. The alveolar septum is not infiltrated to the extent it is in the infantile type, and plasma cells are usually absent.

CLINICAL MANIFESTATIONS. There are at least 3 distinct clinical presentations of *P. carinii* pneumonia. In patients with profound immunodeficiency such as young infants with a congenital immunodeficiency or severe malnutrition or in AIDS patients with very few $CD4^+$ T cells, the onset of hypoxia and symptoms is subtle, with tachypnea, often without fever, progressing to nasal flaring; intercostal, suprasternal, and infrasternal retractions; and cyanosis in severe cases. In the sporadic form of *P. carinii* pneumonia occurring in children and adults with underlying immunodeficiency, the onset of hypoxia and symptoms is usually abrupt, with fever, tachypnea, dyspnea, and cough, progressing to severe respiratory compromise. This type accounts for the majority of cases, although the severity of clinical expression may vary. Rales are usually not detected on physical examination. The 3rd pattern of disease is referred to as **immune restitution disease,** as severely immunocompromised patients with *P. carinii* pneumonia who appear to be responding to therapy have an acute and seemingly paradoxical deterioration associated with return of immune function. This is most commonly seen in newly diagnosed AIDS patients who present with *P. carinii* pneumonia and who have a rapid response to anti-retroviral therapy that is instituted at the same time as anti-pneumocystis therapy. It may also occur in stem cell transplant recipients who engraft while infected with *P. carinii.*

LABORATORY FINDINGS. The chest radiograph reveals bilateral diffuse alveolar disease with a granular pattern. The earliest densities are perihilar, and progression proceeds peripherally, sparing the apical areas until last. The arterial oxygen tension (Pa_{O_2}) is invariably decreased. The major role of the laboratory in establishing a diagnosis of *P. carinii* pneumonia is in identifying organisms in lung specimens by a variety of methods. Once obtained, the specimens are typically stained with 1 of 4 commonly used stains: Grocott-Gomori silver stain and toluidine blue stain for the cyst form, polychrome stains such as Giemsa stain for the trophozoites and sporozoites, and the fluorescein-labeled monoclonal antibody stains for both trophozoites and cysts. Polymerase chain reaction analysis of respiratory specimens offers promise as a rapid diagnostic method, but a standardized system for clinical use has not been established.

DIAGNOSIS. Definitive diagnosis requires demonstration of *P.carinii* in the lung in the presence of clinical signs and symptoms of the infection. Methods for obtaining appropriate specimens for detecting organisms include bronchoalveolar lavage (BAL), tracheal aspirate, transbronchial lung biopsy, bronchial brushings, percutaneous transthoracic needle aspiration, and open lung biopsy. Hypertonic saline–induced sputum samples are helpful if *P. carinii* is found, but the absence of the organisms in induced sputum does not exclude the infection and a BAL should be performed. Open lung biopsy is the most reliable method, although BAL is more practical in most cases. Estimates of the diagnostic yield of the various specimens are 20–40% for induced sputum, 50–60% for tracheal aspirate, 75–95% for BAL, 75–85% for transbronchial biopsy, and 90–100% for open lung biopsy.

TREATMENT. The recommended therapy for *P. carinii* pneumonia is trimethoprim-sulfamethoxazole (TMP-SMZ) (15–20 mg TMP and 75–100 mg SMZ/kg/day divided qid) administered intravenously, or orally if there is mild disease and no malabsorption or diarrhea. The duration of treatment is 3 wk for patients with AIDS and 2 wk for other patients. Unfortunately, adverse reactions frequently occur with TMP-SMZ, especially rash and neutropenia in patients with AIDS, which are less common in patients without AIDS. For patients who cannot tolerate or fail to respond to TMP-SMZ after 5–7 days, pentamidine isethionate (4 mg/kg/day as a single dose IV) may be used. Adverse reactions are frequent and include renal and hepatic dysfunction, hyperglycemia or hypoglycemia, rash, and thrombocytopenia. Atovaquone (750 mg bid with food, for >13 yr of age) is an alternative treatment that has been used primarily in adults with mild to moderate disease. Limited experience is available for younger children. Pharmacokinetic studies of atovaquone show that a dose of 30 mg/kg/day divided bid PO for children >2 yr of age is adequate and safe; a dose of 45 mg/kg/day divided bid PO is needed for children <2 yr of age. Other effective therapies include trimetrexate glucuronate or combinations of trimethoprim plus dapsone, or clindamycin plus primaquine.

Some studies in adults suggest that administration of **corticosteroids** as adjunctive therapy to suppress the inflammatory response increases the chances for survival in moderate and severe cases of *P. carinii* pneumonia. The recommended regimen of corticosteroids for adolescents >13 yr of age and for adults is oral prednisone, 80 mg/day divided bid PO on days 1–5, 40 mg/day once daily PO on days 6–10, and 20 mg/day once daily PO on days 11–21. A reasonable regimen for children is oral prednisone, 2 mg/kg/day for the 1st 7–10 days, followed by a tapering regimen for the next 10–14 days.

SUPPORTIVE CARE. Basic supportive care is dictated by the condition of the patient, with careful attention to maintain appropriate hydration and oxygenation. Only 5–10 % of AIDS patients require mechanical ventilation compared to 50–60% of patients without AIDS, consistent with the hypothesis that the patient's ability to mount an inflammatory response correlates with severity and outcome. There are anecdotal reports of using surfactant replacement in patients with severe *P. carinii* pneumonia, although the use of surfactant for adult-type respiratory distress syndrome is quite controversial.

COMPLICATIONS. Most complications occur as adverse events associated with the drugs used or mechanical ventilation for treatment. The most severe pulmonary complication of *P. carinii* pneumonia is adult-type respiratory distress syndrome. Rarely, *P. carinii* infection affects extrapulmonary sites (e.g., retina, spleen, and bone marrow), but such infections are usually not symptomatic and also respond to treatment.

PROGNOSIS. Without treatment, *P. carinii* pneumonitis is fatal in almost all immunocompromised hosts within 3–4 wk of onset. The mortality rate varies with patient population and is related to inflammatory response rather than organism burden. AIDS patients have a mortality rate of 5–10% while patients with other diseases such as malignancies have mortality rates as high as 20–25%. Patients who go on to need mechanical ventilation have mortality rates of 60–90%. Patients remain at risk for *P. carinii* pneumonia as long as they are immunocompromised. Continuous prophylaxis should be initiated or reinstituted at the end of therapy for patients with AIDS (see Chapter 273).

PREVENTION. Patients at high risk for *P. carinii* pneumonia should be placed on chemoprophylaxis. Prophylaxis of infants born to HIV-infected mothers, and for HIV-infected infants and children, is based on age and CD4 cell counts (see Chapter 273). Patients with severe combined immunodeficiency syndrome, those receiving intensive immunosuppressive therapy for cancer or other diseases, and organ transplant recipients are also candidates for prophylaxis. TMP-SMZ (5 mg TMP and 25 mg SMZ/kg/day once [or divided into two doses] daily PO) is the drug of choice and may be given for 3 consecutive days each week, or, alternatively, each day. Alternatives for prophylaxis, all of which are inferior to TMP-SMZ, include dapsone (2 mg/ kg/day once daily PO, maximum 100 mg/dose; or 4 mg/kg once weekly PO, maximum 200 mg/dose), atovaquone (30 mg/kg/day once daily PO for 1–3 mo for infants >24 mo of age; 45 mg/kg/day for infants 4–23 mo of age), and aerosolized pentamidine (300 mg monthly by Respirgard II nebulizer). The prophylaxis must be continued as long as the patient remains immunocompromised. Some AIDS patients who reconstitute adequate immune response during highly active antiretroviral therapy may have prophylaxis withdrawn.

Hughes WT: *Pneumocystis carinii* pneumonia. *Semin Pediatr Infect Dis* 2001;12:309–314.

Hughes WT, Leoung G, Kramer F, et al: Comparison of atovaquone (566C80) with trimethoprim-sulfamethoxazole to treat *Pneumocystis carinii* pneumonia in patients with AIDS. *N Engl J Med* 1993;328:1521–1527.

Ledergerber B, Mocroft A, Reiss P, et al: Discontinuation of secondary prophylaxis against *Pneumocystis carinii* pneumonia in patients with HIV infection who have a response to antiretroviral therapy. Eight European Study Groups. *N Engl J Med* 2001;344:168–174.

McIntosh K, Cooper E, Xu J, et al: Toxicity and efficacy of daily vs. weekly dapsone for prevention of *Pneumocystis carinii* pneumonia in children infected with human immunodeficiency virus. *Pediatr Infect Dis J* 1999;18:432–439.

Mofenson LM, Oleske J, Serchuck L, et al: Treating opportunistic infections among HIV-exposed and infected children: Recommendations from CDC, the National institutes of Health, and the Infectious Diseases Society of America. *Clin Infect Dis* 2005;40(Suppl 1);S1–S84.

Morgan DJ, Vargas SL, Reyes-Mugica M, et al: Identification of *Pneumocystis carinii* in the lungs of infants dying of sudden infant death syndrome. *Pediatr Infect Dis J* 2001;20:306–309.

Morris A, Lundgren JD, Masur H, et al: Current epidemiology of *Pneumocystis* pneumonia. *Emerg Infect Dis* 2004;10:1713–1720.

Poulsen A, Demeny AK, Bang Plum C, et al: *Pneumocystis carinii* pneumonia during maintenance treatment of childhood acute lymphocytic leukemia. *Med Pediatr Oncol* 2001;37:20–23.

Thomas CF Jr, Limper AH: Pneumocystitis pneumonia. *N Engl J Med* 2004;350:2487–2498.

Torres J, Goldman M, Wheat LJ, et al: Diagnosis of *Pneumocystis carinii* pneumonia in human immunodeficiency virus-infected patients with polymerase chain reaction: A blinded comparison to standard methods. *Clin Infect Dis* 2000;30:141–145.

Vargas SL, Hughes WT, Santolaya ME, et al: Search for primary infection by *Pneumocystis carinii* in a cohort of normal, healthy infants. *Clin Infect Dis* 2001;32:855–861.

Vargas SL, Ponce CA, Hughes WT, et al: Association of primary *Pneumocystis carinii* infection and sudden infant death syndrome. *Clin Infect Dis* 1999;29:1489–1493.

Wright TW, Gigliotti F, Finkelstein JN, et al: Immune-mediated inflammation directly impairs pulmonary function, contributing to the pathogenesis of *Pneumocystis carinii* pneumonia. *J Clin Invest* 1999;104:1307–1317.

Wright TW, Notter RH, Wang Z, et al: Pulmonary inflammation disrupts surfactant function during *Pneumocystis carinii* pneumonia. *Infect Immun* 2001;69:758–764.

Section 13 — Viral Infections

Chapter 242 ■ Principles of Antiviral Therapy

Sharon F. Chen and Mark R. Schleiss

Antiviral chemotherapy typically involves a delicate interplay between host cellular functions and viral targets of action. Many antiviral agents exert significant host cellular toxicity, a limitation that has hindered antiviral drug development. In spite of this limitation, a number of agents are licensed for use against viruses, particularly herpesviruses, respiratory viruses, and hepatitis viruses. In addition to licensed antivirals and recommended regimens (Table 242-1), many national studies are actively enrolling children for evaluation of novel antiviral agents. These studies are funded by the National Institutes of Health and administered through the Collaborative Antiviral Study Group (http://www.casg.uab.edu/).

It is important to obtain appropriate diagnostic specimens, which can help clarify the antiviral of choice. The choice of a specific antiviral is based on the recommended antiviral of choice, pharmacokinetics, toxicities, cost, and potential for development of resistance (Table 242-2). Potential risk factors in the patient should also be considered. Clinicians must monitor antiviral therapy closely for adverse events or toxicities, both anticipated and unanticipated.

TABLE 242-1. Currently Licensed Antiviral Drugs*

ANTIVIRAL	TRADE NAME	MECHANISM OF ACTION
Acyclovir	Zovirax	Inhibits viral DNA polymerase
Adefovir	Hepsera	Nucleotide reverse transcriptase inhibitor
Amantadine	Symmetrel	Blocks M2 protein ion channel
Cidofovir	Vistide	Inhibits viral DNA polymerase
Famciclovir	Famvir	Same as penciclovir
Fomivirsen	Vitravene	Phosphorothioate oligonucleotide inhibits viral replication via antisense mechanism
Foscarnet	Foscavir	Inhibition of viral DNA polymerase and reverse transcriptase at pyrophsphate-binding site
Ganciclovir	Cytovene	Inhibits viral DNA polymerase
Idoxuridine	Herplex	Inhibits viral DNA polymerase
Interferon-α	Intro-A (interferon-α 2b) Roferon-A (interferon-α 2a) Infergen (interferon alfacon-1)	Production of multiple effector proteins that exert antiviral effects; also directly interacts with immune system components
Interferon-α 2b plus ribavirin	Rebetron	Not established
Lamivudine	Epivir	Inhibition viral DNA polymerase and reverse transcriptase
Oseltamivir	Tamiflu	Neuraminidase inhibitor; interference with de-aggregation and release of viral progeny
Pegylated interferon	PEG-Intron (α 2b), Pegasys (α 2a)	Same as interferon
Penciclovir	Denavir	Inhibits viral DNA polymerase
Ribavirin	Virazole, Rebetol, Copegus	Interference with viral messenger RNA
Rimantadine	Flumadine	Blocks M2 protein ion channel
Trifluridine	Viroptic	Inhibits viral DNA polymerase
Valacyclovir	Valtrex	Same as acyclovir
Valganciclovir	Valcyte	Same as ganciclovir
Vidarabine	Ara-A	Inhibits viral DNA polymerase (and to lesser extent, cellular DNA polymerase)
Zanamivir	Relenza	Neuraminidase inhibitor; interference with de-aggregation and release of viral progeny
FDA-APPROVED COMBINATION THERAPIES		
Interferon-α 2b + ribavirin	Rebetron (Intron-A plus Rebetol)	
Interferon-α 2a + ribavirin	Roferon-A + ribavirin	
Pegylated interferon-α 2b + ribavirin	PEG-Intron + Rebetol	
Pegylated interferon-α 2a + ribavirin	Pegasys + Copegus	

*See Chapter 273 for anti-retroviral drugs.

In vitro sensitivity testing of virus isolates to antiviral compounds usually involves a complex tissue culture system. The potency of an antiviral is determined by the **50% inhibitory dose** (**ID_{50}**), which is the antiviral concentration required to inhibit the growth, in cell culture, of a standardized viral inoculum by 50%. Because of the complexity of these assays, the results vary widely, and the actual relationship between antiviral sensitivity testing and antiviral therapy outcomes is sometimes unclear. Unfortunately, these assays are not widely available.

Knowledge of the precise status of a patient's immune system, particularly the cell-mediated immune response, is important in the decision making for using an antiviral agent. Treatment of cytomegalovirus (CMV) infection in an immunocompetent patient is seldom necessary, whereas antiviral therapy may be life-saving when administered to an immunocompromised patient. Antivirals can be employed therapeutically in several different ways. Antivirals can be used as treatment of active disease, as prophylaxis to prevent viral infection or disease, and as preemptive treatment of viral infection to prevent viral disease (CMV infection in bone marrow transplant recipients).

Viruses use host cell components to replicate. Thus, mechanisms of action for antiviral compounds must be selective to virus-specific functions, and antiviral agents may have significant toxicities to the host. Many of the approved antiviral drugs active against the herpesviruses are analogs of deoxynucleosides and subsequently inhibit viral DNA polymerase. Some of the more commonly targeted sites of action for antiviral agents include viral entry, absorption, penetration, and uncoating (amantadine, rimantadine); transcription or replication of the viral genome (acyclovir, valacyclovir, cidofovir, famciclovir, penciclovir, foscarnet, ganciclovir, valganciclovir, ribavirin, trifluridine); viral protein synthesis (interferons); and viral assembly, release, or de-aggregation (oseltamivir, zanamivir, interferons).

Emergence of resistance occurs in the setting of high viral load, high intrinsic viral mutation rate, and prolonged or repeated courses of antiviral therapy. Resistant viruses are more likely to

TABLE 242-2. Antiviral Choices for non-HIV Clinical Conditions

VIRUS	CLINICAL SYNDROME	ANTIVIRAL AGENT OF CHOICE	ALTERNATIVE ANTIVIRAL AGENTS
Influenza A	Treatment	Oseltamivir (>1 yr old)	Rimantadine Amantadine
	Prophylaxis	Oseltamivir (>1 yr old)	Amantadine Rimantadine Zanamivir (>7 yr old)
Influenza B	Treatment	Oseltamivir	Zanamivir (>7 yr old)
Respiratory syncytial virus	Bronchiolitis or pneumonia in high-risk host	Ribavirin aerosol	
Cytomegalovirus	Retinitis in AIDS patients	Valganciclovir	Ganciclovir Cidofovir Foscarnet Ganciclovir ocular insert
	Pneumonitis, colitis; esophagitis in immunocompromised patients	Ganciclovir	Foscarnet Cidofovir Valganciclovir
Herpes simplex virus (HSV)	Neonatal herpes	Acyclovir (IV)	
	HSV encephalitis	Acyclovir (IV)	
	HSV gingivostomatitis	Acyclovir (PO)	Acyclovir (IV)
	1st episode genital infection	Acyclovir (PO)	Valaciclovir Famciclovir Acyclovir (IV) (severe disease)
	Recurrent genital herpes	Acyclovir (PO)	Valaciclovir Famciclovir
	Suppression of genital herpes	Acyclovir (PO)	Valaciclovir Famciclovir
	Whitlow	Acyclovir (PO)	
	Eczema herpeticum	Acyclovir (PO)	Acyclovir (IV) (severe disease)
	Mucocutaneous infection in immunocompromised host (mild)	Acyclovir (IV)	Acyclovir (PO) (if outpatient therapy acceptable)
	Mucocutaneous infection in immunocompromised host (moderate to severe)	Acyclovir (IV)	
	Prophylaxis in bone marrow transplant recipients	Acyclovir (IV)	Valaciclovir Famciclovir
	Acyclovir-resistant HSV	Foscarnet	Cidofovir
	Keratitis or keratoconjunctivitis	Trifluridine	Vidarabine
Varicella-zoster virus	Chickenpox, healthy child	Supportive care	Acyclovir (PO)
	Chickenpox, immunocompromised child	Acyclovir (IV)	
	Zoster (not ophthalmic branch of trigeminal nerve), healthy child	Supportive care	Acyclovir (PO)
	Zoster (ophthalmic branch of trigeminal nerve), healthy child	Acyclovir (IV)	
	Zoster, immunocompromised child	Acyclovir (IV)	Valaciclovir

From Kimberlin DW: Antiviral therapies in children: Has their time arrived? *Pediatr Clin North Am* 2005;52:837–867.

develop or be selected in immunocompromised patients because they are more likely to have multiple or long-term exposures to an antiviral agent in the face of impaired immunity that is unable to facilitate viral clearance.

ANTIVIRALS USED FOR HERPESVIRUSES. The herpesviruses are important pediatric pathogens, particularly in newborns and immunocompromised children. Most of the licensed antivirals are nucleoside analogs that inhibit viral DNA polymerase, inducing premature chain termination during viral DNA synthesis in infected cells.

Acyclovir. Acyclovir has been licensed since the 1980s when it emerged as a safe and effective therapy for herpes simplex virus (HSV) infections. The favorable safety profile of acyclovir derives from its requirement for activation to its active form via phosphorylation by a viral enzyme, thymidine kinase (TK). Acyclovir is most active against HSV and also is active against varicella-zoster virus (VZV); therapy is indicated for these infections under a variety of circumstances. Activity against CMV is less pronounced, and activity against Epstein-Barr virus (EBV) is minimal, both in vitro and clinically. Acyclovir should not be used to treat CMV or EBV infections.

The greatest clinical utility for acyclovir is for the treatment of primary and recurrent genital HSV infections and the management of HSV encephalitis and all manifestations of neonatal HSV infection. Acyclovir is also indicated for the treatment of primary HSV gingivostomatitis. Long-term suppressive therapy, both for genital HSV and recurrent oropharyngeal infections (herpes labialis), is also effective. Long-term suppressive therapy for recurrent episodes of neonatal HSV infection may be useful in preventing recurrences, although this use is investigational. Acyclovir is also recommended for less common HSV infections, including herpetic whitlow, eczema herpeticum, and herpes gladiatorum. Life-threatening HSV disease, including disseminated infection, may occur in immunocompromised or pregnant patients and represents clinical scenarios where acyclovir is warranted.

Acyclovir modifies the course of primary VZV infection, although the effect is modest. Acyclovir or another nucleoside analog should always be utilized in localized or disseminated VZV infections, such as pneumonia, in immunocompromised patients. Primary VZV infection in pregnancy is another setting where acyclovir is indicated, particularly if pneumonia is present.

Acyclovir is available in topical, parenteral, and oral formulations, including a suspension formulation for pediatric use. Topical therapy has little role in pediatric practice and should be avoided in favor of alternative modes of delivery, particularly in infants with vesicular lesions compatible with herpetic infection. The bioavailability of oral formulations is poor, with approximately only 15–30% of the oral formulation being absorbed. There is widespread tissue distribution following systemic administration, and high concentrations of drug are achieved in the kidneys, lungs, liver, myocardium, and skin vesicles. Cerebrospinal fluid (CSF) concentrations are about 50% of plasma concentrations. Acyclovir crosses the placenta, and breast milk concentrations are about 3 times plasma concentrations, although there are no data on efficacy of in utero therapy or impact of therapy on nursing infants. The main route of elimination is renal, and dosage adjustments are necessary for renal insufficiency. Hemodialysis eliminates acyclovir.

Acyclovir has an exceptional safety profile. If administered by rapid infusion to a dehydrated patient or a patient with underlying renal insufficiency, acyclovir can crystallize in renal tubules and produce a reversible obstructive uropathy. High doses of acyclovir have been associated with neurotoxicity, and prolonged use can cause neutropenia. The favorable safety profile of acyclovir is underscored by recent studies of its safe use during pregnancy, and suppressive therapy in pregnant women with histories of recurrent genital HSV infection has been advocated. One uncommon but important complication of long-term use of acyclovir is the selection for acyclovir-resistant HSV strains, which usually occurs from mutations in the HSV TK gene. This is unusual in pediatric practice but should be considered in any patient who has been on long-term antiviral therapy and who has an HSV or VZV infection that fails to clinically respond to acyclovir therapy.

Valacyclovir. Valacyclovir is the L-valyl ester of acyclovir and is rapidly converted to acyclovir following oral administration. This agent has a safety and activity profile similar to acyclovir, but has a bioavailability of >50%, 3–5-fold greater than acyclovir. Plasma concentrations approach those observed with intravenous acyclovir. Valacyclovir is only available for oral administration. A suspension formulation is not available.

Penciclovir and Famciclovir. Penciclovir is an acyclic nucleoside analog that, like acyclovir, inhibits the viral DNA polymerase following phosphorylation to its active form. Compared with acyclovir, penciclovir has a substantially longer intracellular half-life, which may confer superior antiviral activity at the intracellular level. Penciclovir is licensed only as a topical formulation (1% penciclovir cream) that is indicated for therapy of cutaneous HSV infections. Although there are limited data regarding the use of this agent in children, topical therapy for primary or recurrent herpes labialis is an appropriate use of penciclovir.

Famciclovir is the prodrug formulation (diacetyl ester) of penciclovir. In contrast to penciclovir, famciclovir may be administered orally and has bioavailability of approximately 70%. Following oral administration, famciclovir is de-acetylated to the parent drug, penciclovir. The efficacy of famciclovir for HSV and VZV infections appears equivalent to that of acyclovir, although the pharmacokinetic profile is more favorable. Famciclovir is indicated for oral therapy of HSV and VZV infections. There is currently no liquid or suspension formulation available. The toxicity profile is identical to that of acyclovir.

Ganciclovir. Ganciclovir is a nucleoside analog with structural similarity to acyclovir. Like acyclovir, ganciclovir must be phosphorylated for antiviral activity, which is targeted against the viral polymerase. The gene responsible for ganciclovir phosphorylation is not TK but rather a gene known as UL97. Antiviral resistance in CMV can be observed with prolonged use of nucleoside antivirals, which should be considered in patients on long-term therapy who appear to fail to respond clinically. Ganciclovir is broadly active against many herpesviruses, including HSV and VZV, but its greatest value is in its activity against CMV. Ganciclovir was the 1st antiviral agent licensed specifically for the treatment and prevention of CMV infection. It is indicated for prophylaxis against and therapy of CMV infections in high-risk patients, including HIV-infected patients, and solid organ or hematopoietic stem cell transplant recipients. Of particular importance is the use of ganciclovir in the management of CMV retinitis, a sight-threatening complication of HIV infection. Ganciclovir may be of benefit for newborns with symptomatic congenital CMV infection, and may be of particular value in ameliorating the sensorineural hearing loss that is a common complication of congenital CMV infection.

Ganciclovir is supplied as parenteral and oral formulations. Ganciclovir ocular implants are also available for the management of CMV retinitis. The bioavailability of oral ganciclovir is poor, <10%. An oral prodrug, valganciclovir, was recently developed that is well absorbed from the gastrointestinal tract and quickly converted to ganciclovir by intestinal or hepatic metabolism. Bioavailability of ganciclovir (from valganciclovir) is about 60% from tablet and solution formulations. Significant concentrations are found in aqueous humor, subretinal fluid, CSF, and brain tissue (enough to inhibit susceptible strains of CMV). Subretinal concentrations are comparable to plasma concentrations, and intravitreal concentrations are lower. Drug concentrations in the central nervous system (CNS) are about 24–70% of plasma concentrations. The main route of elimination is renal, and dosage adjustments are necessary for renal insufficiency. Dose reduction is proportional to the creatinine clearance reduction. Hemodialysis efficiently eliminates ganciclovir, so administration of additional doses after dialysis is necessary.

Ganciclovir has several important toxicities. Reversible myelosuppression is the most important toxicity associated with ganciclovir therapy and commonly requires discontinuation of therapy or intercurrent administration of granulocyte colony-stimulating factor. There are also the theoretical risks for carcinogenicity and gonadal toxicity, which have been observed in animal models. The decision to administer ganciclovir to a pediatric patient should generally be made in consultation with an infectious diseases specialist.

Foscarnet. Foscarnet has a unique profile as it is not a nucleoside analog but is a pyrophosphate analog that has broad activity against many of the herpesviruses. Foscarnet, like the nucleoside analogs, inhibits viral DNA polymerase, but unlike the nucleoside analogs does not require phosphorylation for antiviral activity. It binds to a different site on the viral DNA polymerase to exert its antiviral effect and therefore retains activity against strains of HSV and CMV that are resistant to nucleoside analogs. Its clinical utility is as a 2nd line agent for management of CMV infections in high-risk patients who cannot tolerate ganciclovir, and as an alternative for patients with persistent or refractory HSV, CMV, or VZV disease with suspected or documented antiviral drug resistance.

Foscarnet is only available as a parenteral formulation and is a toxic agent that must be administered cautiously. Nephrotoxicity is common, and reversible renal insufficiency, evidenced by an increase in serum creatinine, is frequently observed. Abnormalities in calcium and phosphorus homeostasis are common and must be monitored carefully during treatment, along with renal function studies.

Cidofovir. Cidofovir is an acyclic nucleotide analog that requires phosphorylation to the active form, cidofovir diphosphate, to exert its antiviral effect. Analogous to penciclovir, it has an extended intracellular half-life that contributes to its prolonged antiviral activity. Cidofovir is active against HSV, VZV, and CMV. Interestingly, in contrast to most of the other agents, cidofovir also exhibits broad-spectrum activity against other DNA viruses, most notably the poxviruses. Most clinical experience with cidofovir has been in the management of CMV disease caused by strains with ganciclovir resistance.

Cidofovir is administered intravenously and cleared renally by tubular secretion. Extensive prehydration and co-administration of probenecid are recommended. Nephrotoxicity is commonly encountered, even with appropriate prehydration, and co-administration of cidofovir with other nephrotoxic medications must be done with care. Other potential toxicities include reproductive toxicity and carcinogenesis.

Trifluridine. Trifluridine is a pyrimidine nucleoside analog with activity against HSV, CMV, and adenovirus. It is formulated as a 1% ophthalmic solution and approved for topical use in the treatment of HSV keratitis and keratoconjunctivitis. Trifluridine is the treatment of choice for HSV keratitis, a disease that should always be managed in consultation with an ophthalmologist.

Vidarabine (ARA-A, Adenine Arabinoside, VIRA-A). Vidarabine is a nucleoside analog that has activity against HSV. It was the 1st parenteral antiviral agent for HSV infection, although it is no longer available for intravenous administration. A topical preparation remains available for the treatment of HSV keratitis and is considered a 2nd line agent for this indication.

Fomivirsen. Fomivirsen is a novel anti-CMV compound that is used as a 2nd line agent for CMV retinitis by direct injection into the vitreous space. It is an antisense 21-mer DNA oligonucleotide that binds directly to complementary messenger RNA. The standard dose is 330 μg via intravitreal injection every 2 wk for 2 doses followed by maintenance therapy of 330 μg every 4 wk. There is no systemic absorption following intravitreal injection.

ANTIVIRALS USED FOR RESPIRATORY VIRAL INFECTIONS. Antiviral therapies are available for many respiratory pathogens, including respiratory syncytial virus (RSV), influenza A, and influenza B. Antiviral therapy for respiratory viral infections is of particular value for immunocompromised children and newborns.

Ribavirin. Ribavirin is a guanosine analog and has broad-spectrum activity against a variety of viruses, particularly RNA viruses. Its precise mechanism of action is incompletely understood but is probably related to interference with viral messenger RNA processing and translation. Ribavirin is available in oral, parenteral, and aerosolized formulations. Although intravenous ribavirin is highly effective in the management of Lassa fever and other hemorrhagic fevers, this formulation is not licensed for use in the USA, where the only licensed formulations are for aerosolized administration for RSV infection, and for oral formulations that are combined with interferon-α for treatment of hepatitis C. Administration of ribavirin by aerosol route should be considered for serious RSV lower respiratory tract disease in immunocompromised children and infants with increased risk for RSV-associated morbidity and mortality, including infants with chronic lung disease and cyanotic congenital heart disease. In vitro testing and uncontrolled clinical studies also suggest efficacy of aerosolized ribavirin for parainfluenza, influenza, and measles infections.

Ribavirin is generally nontoxic, particularly when administrated by aerosol route. Ribavirin and its metabolites concentrate in red blood cells and can persist for several weeks and, in rare instances, may be associated with anemia. Conjunctivitis and bronchospasm have been reported following exposure to aerosolized drug. Care must be taken when using aerosolized ribavirin in children undergoing mechanical ventilation to avoid precipitation of particles in ventilator tubing. Concerns regarding potential teratogenicity from animal studies have not been borne out in clinical practice, although care should be taken to prevent inadvertent exposure to aerosolized drug among pregnant health care providers.

Amantadine and Rimantadine. Amantadine and rimantadine are tricyclic amines that are highly similar to each other, both structurally and functionally. Both are indicated for the prophylaxis and therapy of influenza A, and neither has discernible activity against influenza B or any other respiratory viruses. For maximal therapeutic efficacy, therapy should begin as soon as possible and within 48 hr of the onset of symptoms. Influenza immunization is a greatly preferred method of disease control, but these agents are useful for prophylaxis, particularly in unimmunized, high-risk persons during annual seasonal epidemics of influenza.

The mechanism of action of the tricyclic amines against influenza A virus is unclear, but they appear to exert their antiviral effect at the level of uncoating of the virus. Both agents are extremely well absorbed after oral administration and are eliminated via the kidneys (90% of the dose is unchanged), necessitating dosage adjustments for renal insufficiency. The toxicities of the tricyclic amines are modest and include CNS adverse effects, including anxiety, difficulty concentrating, and lightheadedness, and gastrointestinal adverse effects, including nausea and loss of appetite. Adverse effects are less common with rimantadine than with amantadine.

Oseltamivir and Zanamivir. Oseltamivir and zanamivir are active against both influenza A and B, although the importance of this broader spectrum of anti-influenzal activity in disease control is modest since influenza B infection is typically a much milder illness. Neither agent has appreciable activity against other respiratory viruses. The mechanism of antiviral activity of these agents is via inhibition of the influenza neuraminidase.

Zanamivir has poor oral bioavailability and is licensed only for inhalational administration. With inhaled administration, >75% of the dose is deposited in the oropharynx and much of it is swallowed. The actual amount distributed to the airways and lungs depends on factors such as the patient's inspiratory flow. About 13% of the dose appears to be distributed to the airways and lungs, with about 10% of the inhaled dose distributed systemically. Local respiratory mucosal drug concentrations greatly exceed the drug concentration needed to inhibit influenza A and B virus. Elimination is via the kidneys, and no dosage adjustment is necessary with renal insufficiency as the amount that is systemically absorbed is low.

Oseltamivir is administered as an esterified prodrug that has high oral bioavailability. It is eliminated by tubular secretion and dosage adjustment is required for patients with renal insufficiency. Gastrointestinal adverse effects including nausea and vomiting are occasionally observed.

ANTIVIRALS USED FOR HEPATITIS VIRUSES AND PAPILLOMAVIRUSES. Antiviral therapy for viral hepatitis and for human papillomavirus (HPV) infections is relatively new because effective agents became available only recently. These are chronic infections that tend to not produce symptoms or disability for many years. The decision to treat viral hepatitis or HPV infections with an antiviral agent should only be undertaken after consultation with an expert in the management of these infections.

Interferons. Interferons are endogenous immunomodulatory proteins elicited by a variety of infectious and inflammatory stimuli. Interferons exert antiviral activity via induction of multiple effector proteins in virus-infected cells. The interferon that has emerged as an effective antiviral agent is interferon-α, a type I interferon. For therapeutic use, interferons are produced using recombinant techniques. Administration of interferons is via subcutaneous or intramuscular administration, with rapid absorption. The attachment of polyethylene glycol moieties to the interferon, known as **pegylation,** is an approach that results in a more sustained plasma concentration, thus allowing a weekly subcutaneous dosage schedule.

Interferons are used in the management of hepatitis B, hepatitis C, and HPV infections. The combination of interferon with oral ribavirin results in additional antiviral activity, particularly against hepatitis C virus. Interferons, either by local injection or systemic delivery, are indicated for anogenital warts caused by HPV, and for laryngeal and respiratory papillomatosis. Interferons can cause significant systemic toxicities that are dose related, including fever, chills, myalgias, gastrointestinal symptoms, and bone marrow suppression.

Lamivudine. Lamivudine is a reverse transcriptase (RT) inhibitor that is used for management of HIV infection (see Chapter 273). Since an RT step is required for replication of hepatitis B virus, it was not surprising that lamivudine was found to have activity against this virus. Lamivudine is useful in the management of hepatitis B infection in children, and is available as an oral suspension for pediatric dosing. It is rapidly absorbed following oral administration with a bioavailability of 80–87%. Lamivudine crosses the placenta and is distributed in breast milk and excreted via the kidneys. A majority of drug is unchanged following oral administration, so dosage adjustment is necessary in the setting of renal insufficiency.

Adefovir Dipivoxil. Adefovir is an acyclic nucleotide analog with activity against human hepatitis B virus. Its mechanism of action appears to be inhibition of the viral DNA polymerase. It is administered orally as a diester prodrug with a bioavailability of approximately 60%. There are few data on the pharmacokinetics of this drug in children. Of concern is the observation of severe exacerbations of liver disease in patients who have discontinued adefovir.

ANTIVIRAL IMMUNE GLOBULINS. Immune globulins are useful adjuncts in the management of viral disease. However, they are more useful as prophylaxis against infection and disease in high-risk patients, and are of less value for therapy of established disease. **Varicella-zoster immune globulin (human) [VariZIG]** is valuable in prophylaxis against VZV in high-risk children, particularly newborns and immunocompromised children (see Chapter 250). **Cytomegalovirus immune globulin (CMV-IG)** is warranted for children at high risk for CMV disease, particularly solid organ and hematopoietic stem cell transplant patients (see Chapter 252). **Palivizumab,** a monoclonal antibody with anti-RSV activity, is effective for prevention of severe RSV lower respiratory tract disease in high-risk premature infants and has replaced use of **respiratory syncytial virus immune globulin** (see Chapter 257). **Hepatitis B immune globulin (HBIG)** is indicated in infants born to hepatitis B surface antigen–positive mothers (see Chapter 355).

Balfour HH Jr: Antiviral drugs. *N Engl J Med* 1999;340(16):1255–1268.

De Clercq E: Antiviral drugs in current clinical use. *J Clin Virol* 2004;30:115–133.

Kimberlin DW: Antiviral therapies in children: Has their time arrived? *Pediatr Clin North Am* 2005;52:837–867.

Littler E, Oberg B: Achievements and challenges in antiviral drug discovery. *Antivir Chem Chemother* 2005;16:155–168.

Chapter 243 ■ Measles

Wilbert H. Mason

Measles is highly contagious and was once an inevitable experience during childhood. Due to widespread vaccination, endemic transmission has been interrupted in the United States; however, indigenous or imported cases have occasionally resulted in epidemics in the United States. In some areas of the world, measles remains a serious threat to children.

ETIOLOGY. Measles virus is a single-stranded lipid enveloped RNA virus in the family Paramyxoviridae and genus *Morbillivirus*. Other members of this genus are rinderpest virus of cattle and distemper virus of dogs, but humans are the only host of measles virus. Of the 6 major structural proteins of measles virus, the 2 most important in terms of induction of immunity are the hemagglutinin (H) protein and the fusion (F) protein. The neutralizing antibodies are directed against the H protein, and antibodies to the F protein limit proliferation of the virus during infection. Small variations in genetic composition have also been identified that result in no effect on protective immunity but provide molecular markers that can distinguish between viral types. These markers have been useful in the evaluation of endemic spread of measles.

EPIDEMIOLOGY. The measles vaccine has changed the epidemiology of measles dramatically. Once worldwide in distribution, endemic transmission of measles has been interrupted in many countries where there is widespread vaccine coverage. Historically, in the United States it caused universal infection in childhood with 90% of children acquiring the infection before 15 yr of age. Morbidity and mortality associated with measles decreased prior to the introduction of the vaccine due to improved health care and nutrition. However, the incidence declined dramatically following the introduction of the measles vaccine 1963. The attack rate fell from 313 cases/100,000 population in 1956–60 to 1.3 cases/100,000 in 1982–88. It is most common in the winter and spring.

A nationwide indigenous measles outbreak occurred in 1989–1991 resulting in >55,000 cases, 11,000 hospitalizations, and 123 deaths, demonstrating that the infection had not yet been conquered. The resurgence was attributed to vaccine failure in a small number of school-aged children and low coverage of preschool-aged children and because of more rapid waning of maternal antibodies in infants born to mothers who never experienced wild-type measles infection. Implementation of the 2 dose vaccine policy and more intensive immunization strategies resulted in interruption of endemic transmission in the United States in 1993. The current rate is <1 case/1,000,000 population.

Measles continues to be imported into the United States from abroad; therefore, continued maintenance of >90% immunity through vaccination is necessary to prevent widespread outbreaks from occurring (Fig. 243-1).

TRANSMISSION. The portal of entry of measles virus is through the respiratory tract or conjunctivae following contact with large droplets or small droplet aerosols in which the virus is suspended. Patients are infectious from 3 days before the rash up to 4–6 days after its onset. Approximately 90% of the exposed susceptible individuals develop measles. Face-to-face contact is not necessary because viable virus may be suspended in air up to 1 hr after a source case leaves a room. Secondary cases have been reported in physicians' offices and in hospitals by spread of aerosolized virus.

PATHOLOGY. Measles infection causes necrosis of the respiratory tract epithelium and an accompanying lymphocytic infiltrate. Measles produces a small vessel vasculitis on the skin and on the oral mucous membranes. Histology of the rash and exanthem reveals intracellular edema and dyskeratosis associated with formation of epidermal syncytial giant cells with up to 26 nuclei. Viral particles have been identified within these giant cells. In lymphoreticular tissue, lymphoid hyperplasia is prominent. Fusion of infected cells results in multinucleated giant cells, the **Warthin-Finkeldey giant cells** that are pathognomonic for measles, with up to 100 nuclei and intracytoplasmic and intranuclear inclusions (Fig. 243-2).

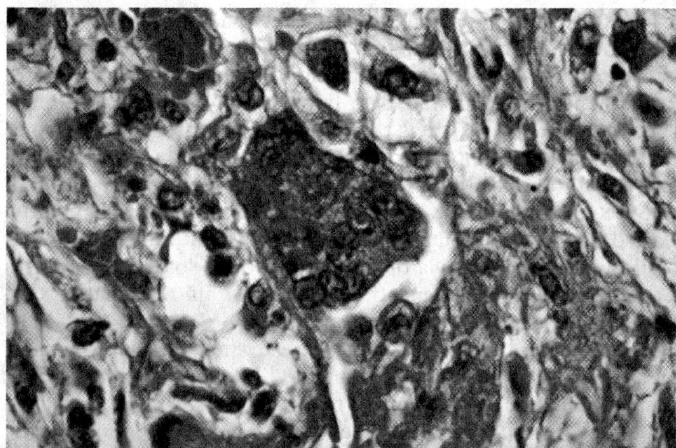

Figure 243-2. Warthin-Finkeldey cell from lung tissue. (Courtesy of Robert M. McAllister, MD, Children's Hospital Los Angeles [retired].)

PATHOGENESIS. Measles consists of 4 phases: incubation period, prodromal illness, exanthematous phase, and recovery. During incubation, measles virus migrates to regional lymph nodes. A primary viremia ensues that disseminates the virus to the reticuloendothelial system. A secondary viremia spreads virus to body surfaces. The prodromal illness begins following the secondary viremia and is associated with epithelial necrosis and giant cell formation in body tissues. Cells are killed by cell-to-cell plasma membrane fusion associated with viral replication that occurs in many body tissues, including cells of the central nervous system (CNS). Virus shedding begins in the prodromal phase. With onset of the rash, antibody production begins and viral replication and symptoms begin to subside. Measles virus also infects $CD4^+$ T cells, resulting in suppression of the Th1 immune response and a multitude of other immunosuppressive effects.

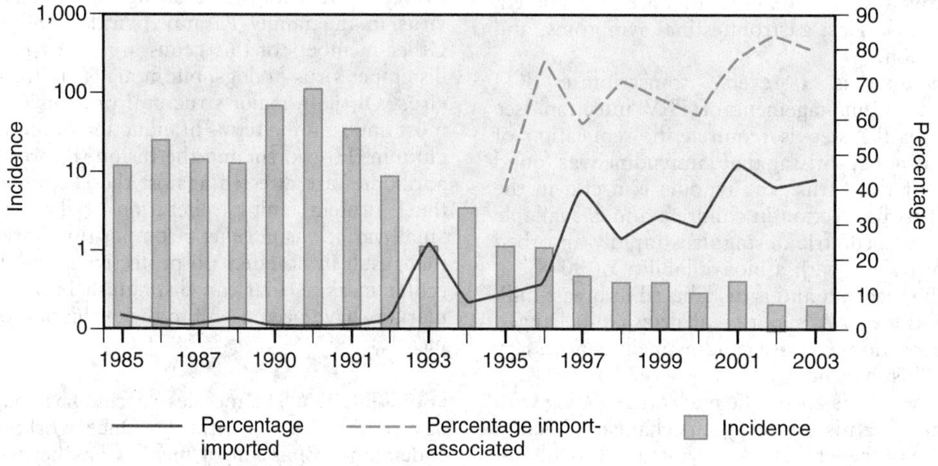

*Per million population.
†Imported, import-linked, and imported virus cases.
§Data for 2003 are provisional.

Figure 243-1. Incidence* and percentage of import-associated† measles cases, by year in the United States, 1985–2003§. (From the Centers for Disease Control and Prevention: Epidemiology of measles—United States, 2001–2003. *MMWR* 2004;53:713–716.)

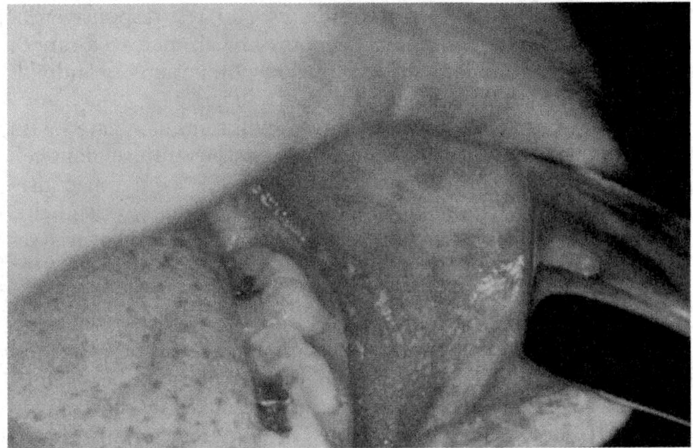

Figure 243-3. Koplik spots on the buccal mucosa during the 3rd day of rash. (From the Centers for Disease Control and Prevention website—Public Health Image Library. Image #4500. Available at http://phil.cdc.gov/phil/details.asp)

CLINICAL MANIFESTATIONS. Measles is a serious infection characterized by high fever, an enanthem, cough, coryza, conjunctivitis, and a prominent exanthem. After an incubation period of 8–12 days, the prodromal phase begins with a mild fever followed by the onset of conjunctivitis with photophobia, coryza, a prominent cough and increasing fever. The enanthem, **Koplik spots,** is the pathognomonic sign of measles and appears 1 to 4 days prior to the onset of the rash (Fig. 243-3). They first appear as discrete red lesions with bluish white spots in the center on the inner aspects of the cheeks at the level of the premolars. They may spread to involve the lips, hard palate, and gingiva. They also may occur in conjunctival folds and in the vaginal mucosa. Koplik spots have been reported in 50–70% of measles cases but probably occur in the great majority.

Symptoms increase in intensity for 2–4 days until the 1st day of the rash. The rash begins around the forehead (around the hairline), behind the ears, and on the upper neck as a red maculopapular eruption. It then spreads downward to the torso and extremities, reaching the palms and soles in up to 50% of cases. The exanthem frequently becomes confluent on the face and upper trunk (Figs. 243-4 and 243-5).

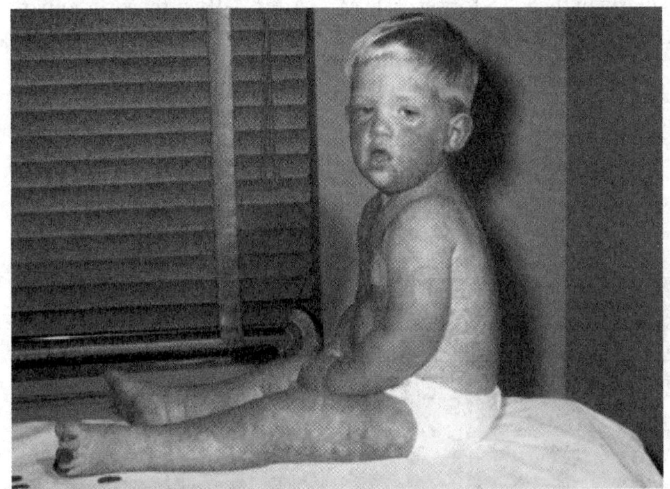

Figure 243-4. A child with measles displaying the characteristic red blotchy pattern on his body during the 3rd day of the rash. (From the Centers for Disease Control and Prevention website—Public Health Image Library. Image #4498. Available at http://phil.cdc.gov/phil/details.asp)

Figure 243-5. Close-up of the maculopapular rash of measles. (From Korting GW: *Hautkrankheiten bei Kindern und Jugendlichen,* 3rd ed. Stuttgart, FK Schattauer Verlag, 1982.)

With the onset of the rash, symptoms begin to subside and the rash fades over about 7 days in the same progression as it evolved, often leaving a fine desquamation of skin in its wake. Of the major symptoms of measles, the cough lasts the longest, often up to 10 days. In more severe cases, generalized lymphadenopathy may be present, with cervical and occipital lymph nodes especially prominent.

INAPPARENT MEASLES INFECTION. In individuals with passively acquired antibody, such as infants or recipients of blood products, a subclinical form of measles may occur. The rash may be indistinct, brief, or, rarely, entirely absent. Likewise, some individuals who have received vaccine when exposed to measles may develop a rash but few other symptoms. Persons with inapparent or subclinical measles do not shed measles virus and do not transmit infection to household contacts.

Children who had received the original formalin-inactivated measles vaccine at times developed a more severe form of disease called **atypical measles.** Patients had onset of high fever and headache followed by the appearance of a maculopapular rash on the extremities that become petechial and purpuric and progressed in a centripetal direction. The illness was frequently complicated by pneumonia and pleural effusions. It is thought that atypical measles was caused by development of circulating immune complexes that formed due to an abnormal immune response to the vaccine.

LABORATORY FINDINGS. The diagnosis of measles is almost always based on clinical and epidemiologic findings. Laboratory findings in the acute phase include reduction in the total white blood cell count, with lymphocytes decreased more than neutrophils. Absolute neutropenia has been known to occur, however. In measles not complicated by bacterial infection, the erythrocyte sedimentation rate and C-reactive protein levels are normal.

DIAGNOSIS. In the absence of a recognized measles outbreak, confirmation of the clinical diagnosis is often recommended. Serologic confirmation is most conveniently made by identification of immunoglobulin M (IgM) antibody in serum. IgM antibody appears 1–2 days after the onset of the rash and remains detectable for about 1 mo. If a serum specimen is collected <72 hours following onset of rash and is negative for measles antibody, a repeat specimen should be obtained. Serologic confirmation may also be made by demonstration of a 4-fold rise in IgG antibodies in acute and convalescent specimens taken 2–4 wk later. Viral isolation from blood, urine, or respiratory secretions can be accomplished by culture at the Centers for Disease Control and Prevention (CDC) or local or state laboratories. Molecular detection by polymerase chain reaction is possible but is a research tool.

DIFFERENTIAL DIAGNOSIS. Typical measles is unlikely to be confused with other illnesses, especially if Koplik spots are observed. Measles in the later stages or inapparent or subclinical cases may be confused with a number of other exanthematous immune-mediated illnesses and infections, including rubella, adenoviruses, enteroviruses, and Epstein-Barr virus. Exanthem subitum (in infants) and erythema infectiosum (in older children) may also be confused with measles. *Mycoplasma pneumoniae* and group A streptococcus may also produce rashes similar to measles. Kawasaki syndrome can manifest many of the same findings as measles but lacks discrete intraoral lesions (Koplik spots) and a severe prodromal cough, and typically has elevated neutrophils and acute-phase reactant levels. In addition, the characteristic thrombocytosis of Kawasaki syndrome is absent in measles (see Chapter 165). Drug eruptions may occasionally be mistaken for measles.

COMPLICATIONS. Complications of measles are largely attributable to the pathogenic effects of the virus on the respiratory tract and immune system (Table 243-1). There are several factors that make complications more likely. Morbidity and mortality from measles are greatest in patients <5 yr of age (especially <1 yr of age) and those >20 yr of age. In developing countries, higher case-fatality rates have been associated with crowding, which is possibly attributable to a larger inoculum dose following household exposure. Severe malnutrition in children results in suboptimal immune response and higher morbidity and mortality with measles infection. Low serum retinol levels in children with measles have been shown to be associated with higher measles morbidity and mortality in developing countries and in the United States. Measles infection lowers serum retinol, so subclinical cases of hyporetinolemia may be made symptomatic during measles. Measles infection in immunocompromised persons is associated with increased morbidity and mortality. Pneumonitis occurs in 58% of patients with malignancy infected with measles, and encephalitis occurs in 20%.

Pneumonia is the most common cause of death in measles. It may manifest as **giant cell pneumonia** caused directly by the viral infection or as superimposed bacterial infection. The most common bacterial pathogens are *S. pneumoniae, H. influenzae,* and *S. aureus*. Following severe measles pneumonia, the final common pathway to a fatal outcome is often the development of bronchiolitis obliterans.

Croup, tracheitis, and bronchiolitis are common complications in infants and toddlers with measles. The clinical severity of these complications frequently requires intubation and ventilatory support until the infection resolves.

Acute otitis media is the most common complication of measles and was of particularly high incidence during the epidemic of the late 1980s and early 1990s because of the relatively young age of affected children. Sinusitis and mastoiditis also occur as complications. Viral and/or bacterial tracheitis are seen and can be life threatening. Retropharyngeal abscess has also been reported.

Measles infection is known to suppress skin test responsiveness to purified tuberculin antigen. There may be an increased rate of activation of pulmonary tuberculoses in populations of individuals infected with *Mycobacterium tuberculosis.*

Diarrhea and vomiting are common symptoms associated with acute measles, and the gastrointestinal tract has diffuse giant cell formation in the epithelium. Dehydration is a common consequence, especially in young infants and children. Appendicitis may occur due to obstruction of the appendiceal lumen by lymphoid hyperplasia.

Febrile seizures occur in <3% of children with measles. Encephalitis following measles has been a long-associated complication, often with an unfavorable outcome. Rates of 1–3/1,000 cases of measles have been reported, with greater numbers occurring in adolescents and adults than in preschool or school-aged children. This is a postinfectious immunologically mediated process rather than due to a direct effect by the virus. Clinical onset begins during the exanthem and presents with seizures (56%), lethargy (46%), coma (28%), and irritability (26%). Findings in cerebrospinal fluid include lymphocytic pleocyosis in 85% and elevated protein concentration. Approximately 15% of patients die, and 20–40% suffer long-term sequelae, including mental retardation, motor disabilities, and deafness.

Measles encephalitis in immunocompromised patients results from direct damage to the brain by the virus. Subacute measles encephalitis presents 1–10 mo following measles in immunocompromised patients, particularly those with AIDS, lymphoreticular malignancies, and immunosuppression. Signs and symptoms include seizures, myoclonus, stupor, and coma. In addition to intracellular inclusions, abundant viral nucleocapsids and viral antigen are seen in brain tissue. Progressive disease and death almost always occurs.

A severe form of measles rarely seen now is **hemorrhagic or "black measles."** It presented with a hemorrhagic skin eruption and was often fatal. Keratitis, appearing as multiple punctate epithelial foci, resolved with recovery from the infection. Thrombocytopenia sometimes occurred following measles.

Myocarditis is a rare complication. Miscellaneous bacterial infections have been reported, including bacteremia, cellulitis, and toxic shock syndrome. Measles during pregnancy has been associated with high maternal morbidity, fetal wastage and stillbirths, and congenital malformations in 3% of live born infants.

Subacute Sclerosing Parencephalitis (SSPE). SSPE is a chronic complication of measles with a delayed onset and an outcome that is nearly always fatal. It appears to result from a persistent infection with an altered measles virus that is harbored intracellularly in the CNS for several years. After 7–10 yr the virus apparently regains virulence and attacks the cells in the CNS that offered the virus protection. This "slow virus infection" results in inflammation and cell death, leading to an inexorable neurodegenerative process.

SSPE is a rare disease and generally follows the prevalence of measles in a population. The incidence rate in the USA in 1960

TABLE 243-1. Complications by Age for Reported Measles Cases, USA 1987–2000

		NO. (%) OF PERSONS WITH COMPLICATION BY AGE GROUP				
COMPLICATION	OVERALL (67,032 CASES WITH AGE INFORMATION)	<5 yr (*n* = 28,730)	5–9 yr (*n* = 6,492)	10–19 yr (*n* = 18,580)	20–29 yr (*n* = 9,161)	>30 yr (*n* = 4,069)
Any	19,480 (29.1)	11,883 (41.4)	1,173 (18.1)	2,369 (12.8)	2,656 (29.0)	1,399 (34.4)
Death	177 (0.3)	97 (0.3)	9 (0.1)	18 (0.1)	26 (0.3)	27 (0.7)
Diarrhea	5,482 (8.2)	3,294 (11.5)	408 (6.3)	627 (3.4)	767 (8.4)	386 (9.5)
Encephalitis	97 (0.1)	43 (0.2)	9 (0.1)	13 (0.1)	21 (0.2)	11 (0.3)
Hospitalization	12,876 (19.2)	7,470 (26.0)	612 (9.4)	1,612 (8.7)	2,075 (22.7)	1,107 (27.2)
Otitis media	4,879 (7.3)	4,009 (14.0)	305 (4.7)	338 (1.8)	157 (1.7)	70 (1.7)
Pneumonia	3,959 (5.9)	2,480 (8.6)	183 (2.8)	363 (2.0)	554 (6.1)	379 (9.3)

From Perry RT, Halsey NA: The clinical significance of measles: A review. *Clin Infect Dis* 2004;189(Suppl 1):S4–S16.

was 0.61 cases per million persons younger than 20 yr. By 1980 the rate had fallen to 0.06 cases per million. Between 1956 and 1982 a total of 634 cases had been reported to the national SSPE registry. After 1982 about 5 cases per year were reported annually in the United States and only 2–3 cases per year in the early 1990s. However, between 1995 and 2000, reported cases in the USA increased and 13 cases were reported in 2000. Nine of the 13 cases occurred in foreign-born individuals. This "resurgence" may be the result of an increased incidence of measles between 1989 and 1991. While the age of onset ranges from <1 to <30 yr, the illness is primarily one of children and adolescents. Measles at an early age favors the development of SSPE: 50% of SSPE patients had primary measles before 2 yr and 75% before 4 yr of age. Males are affected twice as often as females, and there appear to be more cases reported from rural rather than urban populations. Recent observations from the registry indicate a higher prevalence among children of Hispanic origin. The pathogenesis of SSPE remains enigmatic. Factors that seem to be involved include defective measles virus and interaction with a defective or immature immune system. The virus isolated from brain tissue of patients with SSPE is missing 1 of the 6 structural proteins, the matrix or M protein. This protein is responsible for assembly, orientation, and alignment of the virus in preparation for budding during viral replication. Immature virus may be able to reside, and possibly propagate, within neuronal cells for long periods. The fact that most patients with SSPE were exposed at a young age suggests that immune immaturity is involved in pathogenesis. In addition, the intracellular location of the virus sequesters it from the immune system, especially from humoral immunity.

Clinical manifestations of SSPE begin insidiously 7–13 yr after primary measles infection. Subtle changes in behavior or school performance appear, including irritability, reduced attention span, or temper outbursts. This initial phase (stage I) may at times be missed because of brevity or mildness of the symptoms. Fever, headache, or other signs of encephalitis are absent. The hallmark of the 2nd stage is massive myoclonus. This coincides with extension of the inflammatory process site to deeper structures in the brain, including the basal ganglia. Involuntary movements and repetitive myoclonic jerks begin in single muscle groups but give way to massive spasms and jerks involving both axial and appendicular muscles. Consciousness is maintained. In the 3rd stage, involuntary movements disappear and are replaced by choreoathetosis, immobility, dystonia, and lead pipe rigidity that result from destruction of deeper centers in the basal ganglia. Sensorium deteriorates into dementia, stupor, then coma. Stage IV is characterized by loss of critical centers that support breathing, heart rate, and blood pressure. Death soon ensues. Progression through the clinical stages may follow courses characterized as acute, subacute, or chronic progressive.

The **diagnosis** of SSPE can be established through documentation of a compatible clinical course and at least 1 of the following supporting findings: (1) measles antibody detected in CSF, (2) characteristic electroencephalographic findings, or (3) typical histologic findings and/or isolation of virus or viral antigen in brain tissue obtained by biopsy or postmortem examination.

CSF analysis reveals normal cells but elevated IgG and IgM antibody titers in dilutions of >1 : 8. Electroencephalographic patterns are normal in stage I, but in the myoclonic phase suppression-burst episodes are seen that are characteristic of but not pathogenomic for SSPE. Brain biopsy is no longer routinely indicated for diagnosis of SSPE.

Management of SSPE is primarily supportive and similar to care provided to patients with other neurodegenerative diseases. A recent large randomized clinical trial compared the use of oral inosiplex (isoprinosine) alone to oral inosiplex and intraventricular interferon-α2b. The treatment course for both groups was 6 mo. While there were no differences in the rates of stabilization or improvement at 6 mo (34% vs 35%), the study concluded that these rates were substantially better than historically reported spontaneous improvement rates of 5–10%.

Virtually all patients eventually succumb to SSPE. Most die within 1–3 yr of onset from infection or loss of autonomic control mechanisms. Prevention of SSPE depends on prevention of primary measles infection through the use of vaccine. SSPE has been described in patients who have no history of measles infection and only exposure to the vaccine virus. However wild-type virus, not vaccine virus, has been found in brain tissue of at least some of these patients, suggesting they had had subclinical measles previously.

TREATMENT. Management of measles is supportive. Antiviral therapy is not effective in the treatment of measles in otherwise normal patients. Maintenance of hydration, oxygenation, and comfort are goals of therapy. Antipyretics for comfort and fever control are useful. For patients with respiratory tract involvement, airway humidification and supplemental oxygen may be of benefit. Respiratory failure due to croup or pneumonia may require ventilatory support. Oral rehydration is effective in most cases, but severe dehydration may require intravenous therapy. Prophylactic antimicrobial therapy to prevent bacterial infection is not indicated.

Measles infection in immunocompromised patients is highly lethal. Ribavirin is active in vitro against measles virus. Anecdotal reports of ribavirin therapy with or without intravenous gamma globulin suggest some benefit in individual patients. However, no controlled trials have been performed, and ribavirin is not licensed in the United States for treatment of measles.

VITAMIN A. Vitamin A deficiency in children in developing countries has long been known to be associated with increased mortality from a variety of infectious diseases, including measles. In the United States, studies in the early 1990s documented that 22–72% of children with measles had low retinol levels. In addition, 1 study demonstrated an inverse correlation between the level of retinol and severity of illness. Several randomized controlled trials of vitamin A therapy in the developing world and the United States have demonstrated reduced morbidity and mortality from measles. The American Academy of Pediatrics suggests vitamin A therapy for selected patients with measles (Table 243-2).

PROGNOSIS. In the early 20th century, deaths due to measles varied between 2,000 and 10,000, or about 10 deaths per 1,000 cases of measles. With improvements in health care and antimi-

TABLE 243-2. Recommendations for Vitamin A Treatment of Children with Measles

INDICATIONS

- Children 6 mo to 2 yr of age hospitalized with measles and its complications (e.g., croup, pneumonia, and diarrhea). (Limited data are available about the safety and need for vitamin A supplementation for infants <6 mo of age.)
- Children >6 mo of age with measles who are not already receiving vitamin A supplementation and who have any of the following risk factors:
  - immunodeficiency
  - clinical evidence of vitamin A deficiency
  - impaired intestinal absorption
  - moderate to severe malnutrition
  - recent immigration from areas where high mortality rates attributed to measles have been observed

REGIMEN

Parenteral and oral formulations of vitamin A are available in the USA. The recommended dosage, administered as a capsule, is:

- Single dose of 200,000 IU orally for children ≥1 yr of age (100,000 IU for children 6 mo to 1 yr of age)
- The dose should be repeated the next day and again 4 wk later for children with ophthalmologic evidence of vitamin A deficiency

From the American Academy of Pediatrics, Committee on Infectious Disease: Vitamin A treatment of measles. *Pediatrics* 1993;91:1014–1015.

crobial therapy, better nutrition, and decreased crowding, the death to case ratio fell to 1 per 1,000 cases. Between 1982 and 2002, the CDC estimated there were 259 deaths caused by measles in the United States, with a death-to-case ratio of 2.5–2.8/1,000 cases of measles. Pneumonia and encephalitis were complications in most of the fatal cases, and immunodeficiency conditions were identified in 14–16% of deaths.

PREVENTION. Patients shed measles virus from 7 days after exposure to 4–6 days after the onset of rash. Exposure of susceptible individuals to measles patients should be avoided during this period. In hospitals, standard and airborne precautions should be observed for this period. Immunocompromised patients with measles will shed for the duration of the illness, and isolation should be maintained throughout.

VACCINE. Measles vaccine in the United States is available as a monovalent preparation or combined with the rubella (MR) or measles-mumps-rubella (MMR) vaccine, which is the recommended form in most circumstances (Table 243-3). Following the measles resurgence of 1989–1991, a 2nd dose of measles vaccine was added to the schedule. The current recommendations include a 1st dose at 12–15 mo followed by a 2nd at 4–6 yr of age. Seroconversion is slightly lower in children who receive the 1st dose before or at 12 mo of age (87% at 9 mo, 95% at 12 mo, and 98% at 15 mo) because of persisting maternal antibody. For children who have not received 2 doses by 11–12 yr of age, a 2nd dose should be provided. Infants who receive a dose before 12 mo of age should be given 2 additional doses at 12–15 mo and 4–6 yr of age. In any event, this 2nd dose of vaccine may be given anytime 4 wk after the 1st dose.

TABLE 243-3. Recommendations for Measles Immunization*

CATEGORY	RECOMMENDATIONS
Unimmunized, no history of measles (12–15 mo of age)	A 2 dose schedule (with MMR) is recommended. The first dose is recommended at 12–15 mo of age; the 2nd is recommended at 4–6 yr of age
Children 6–11 mo of age in epidemic situations or prior to international travel	Immunize (with monovalent measles vaccine, or if not available, MMR); reimmunization (with MMR) at 12–15 mo of age is necessary, and a 3rd dose is indicated at 4–6 y of age
Children 4–12 yr of age who have received 1 dose of measles vaccine at ≥12 mo of age	Reimmunize (1 dose)
Students in college and other post–high school institutions who have received 1 dose of measles vaccine at ≥12 mo of age	Reimmunize (1 dose)
History of immunization before the 1st birthday	Consider susceptible and immunize (2 doses)
History of receipt of inactivated measles vaccine or unknown type of vaccine, 1963–1967	Consider susceptible and immunize (2 doses)
Further attenuated or unknown vaccine given with IG	Consider susceptible and immunize (2 doses)
Allergy to eggs	Immunize; no reactions likely (see text for details)
Neomycin allergy, nonanaphylactic	Immunize; no reactions likely (see text for details)
Severe hypersensitivity (anaphylaxis) to neomycin or gelatin	Avoid immunization
Tuberculosis	Immunize (see Tuberculosis); if patient has untreated tuberculosis disease, start anti-tuberculosis therapy before immunizing.
Measles exposure	Immunize and/or give IG, depending on circumstances (see text)
HIV-infected	Immunize (2 doses) unless severely immunocompromised (see text)
Personal or family history of seizures	Immunize; advise parents of slightly increased risk of seizures
Immunoglobulin or blood recipient	Immunize at the appropriate interval (see Table 243-4)

*IG, immune globulin; MMR, measles-mumps-rubella vaccine. See text for details and recommendations for use of measles-mumps-rubella-varicella (MMRV) vaccine.

American Academy of Pediatrics: *Red Book: 2006 Report of the Committee on Infectious Diseases,* 27th ed. Elk Grove Village, IL, American Academy of Pediatrics, 2006, p 446.

TABLE 243-4. Suggested Intervals Between Immune Globulin Administration and Measles Immunization (MMR, MMRV, or Monovalent Measles Vaccine)

INDICATION FOR IMMUNOGLOBULIN	ROUTE	DOSE U or mL	DOSE mg IgG/kg	INTERVAL, MO*
Tetanus (as TIG)	IM	250 U	10	3
Hepatitis A prophylaxis (as IG)				
Contact prophylaxis	IM	0.02 mL/kg	3.3	3
International travel	IM	0.06 mL/kg	10	3
Hepatitis B prophylaxis (as HBIG)	IM	0.06 mL/kg	10	3
Rabies prophylaxis (as RIG)	IM	20 IU/kg	22	4
Varicella prophylaxis (as VariZIG)	IM	125 U/10 kg (maximum 625 U)	20–40	5
Measles prophylaxis (as IG)				
Standard	IM	0.25 mL/kg	40	5
Immunocompromised host	IM	0.50 mL/kg	80	6
RSV prophylaxis (palivizumab monoclonal antibody)	IM	—	15 mg/kg (monoclonal)	None
Cytomegalovirus immune globulin	IV	3 mL/kg	150	6
Blood transfusion				
Washed RBCs	IV	10 mL/kg	Negligible	0
RBCs, adenine-saline added	IV	10 mL/kg	10	3
Packed RBCs	IV	10 mL/kg	20–60	5
Whole blood	IV	10 mL/kg	80–100	6
Plasma or platelet products	IV	10 mL/kg	160	7
Replacement (or therapy) of immune deficiencies (as IGIV)	IV	—	300–400	8
ITP (as IGIV)	IV	—	400	8
ITP	IV	—	1,000	10
ITP or Kawasaki disease	IV	—	1,600–2,000	11

*These intervals should provide sufficient time for decreases in passive antibodies in all children to follow for an adequate response to measles vaccine. Physicians should not assume that children are fully protected against measles during these intervals. Additional doses of IG or measles vaccine may be indicated after exposure to measles (see text).

*HBIG, hepatitis B IG; IG, immune globulin; IgG, immunoglobulin G; IGIV, IG intravenous; ITP, immune (formerly termed "idiopathic") thrombocytopenic purpura; MMR, measles-mumps-rubella; MMRV, measles-mumps-rubella-varicella; RBCs, red blood cells; RIG, rabies IG; RSV, respiratory syncytial virus; TIG, tetanus immune globulin.

American Academy of Pediatrics: *Red Book: 2006 Report of the Committee on Infectious Disease,* 27th ed. Elk Grove Village, IL, American Academy of Pediatrics, 2006, p 445.

Adverse events from the MMR vaccine include fever (usually 6–12 days following vaccinations), rash in about 5% of vaccines, and, rarely, transient thrombocytopenia. Children prone to febrile seizures may experience an event following vaccination, so risks and benefits should be discussed with parents. Encephalopathy and autism have not been shown to be causally associated with the MMR vaccine. Specifically, MMR vaccine significantly diminishes the risk for SSPE.

Passively acquired, immunoglobulin may inhibit the immune response to live measles vaccine, and administration should be delayed for variable amounts of time based on the dose of immune globulin (Table 243-4).

Live vaccines should not be administered to pregnant women or immunodeficient or suppressed patients. However, patients with HIV who are not severely immunocompromised should be immunized. Because measles virus may suppress the cutaneous response to tuberculous antigen, skin testing for tuberculosis should be performed before or at the same time as administration of the vaccine. Individuals infected with *M. tuberculosis* should be on appropriate treatment at the time of administration of measles vaccine.

POSTEXPOSURE PROPHYLAXIS. Susceptible individuals exposed to measles may be protected from infection either by vaccine administration or immunization with immunoglobulin. The vaccine is effective in prevention or modification of measles if given within 72 hr of exposure. Immune globulin may be given up to 6 days following exposure to prevent or modify infection. Immunocompetent children should receive 0.25 mL/kg intramuscularly and immunocompromised children should receive 0.5 mL/kg.

Immune globulin is indicated for susceptible household contacts of measles patients, especially infants <6 mo of age, pregnant women, and immunocompromised persons.

American Academy of Pediatrics, Committee on Infectious Diseases: Vitamin A treatment of measles. *Pediatrics* 1993;91:1014–1015.
Asaria P, MacMahon E: Measles in the United Kingdom: Can we eradicate it by 2010? *BMJ* 2006;333:890–895.
Caulfield LE, deOvis M, Blössner M, et al: Undernutrition as an underlying cause of child deaths associated with diarrhea, pneumonia, malaria and measles. *Am J Clin Nutr* 2004;80:193–198.
Centers for Disease Control and Prevention: Epidemiology of measles—United States, 2001–2003. *MMWR* 2004;53:713–716.
Centers for Disease Control and Prevention: Import-associated measles outbreak—Indiana, May–June 2005. *MMWR* 2005;54:1073–1075.
Dyken PR: Nonprogressive disease of post-infectious origin: A review of resurging subacute sclerosing parencephalitis (SSPE). *MRDD Res Rev* 2001;7:217–225.
Elliman D, Bedford H: Achieving the goal for global measles mortality. *Lancet* 2007;369:165–166.
Halsey NA: Measles in developing countries. *BMJ* 2006;333:1234.
Mason WH, Ross LA, Lanson J, et al: Epidemic measles in the post vaccine era: Evaluation of epidemiology, clinical presentation and complications during an urban outbreak. *Pediatr Infect Dis J* 1993;12:42–48.
Meissner HC, Strebel PM, Orenstein WA: Measles vaccine and the potential for worldwide eradication of measles. *Pediatrics* 2004;114:1065–1069.
Otten M, Kezaala R, Fall A, et al: Public-health impact of accelerated measles control in the WHO African region 2000–03. *Lancet* 2005;366:832–838.
Papania MJ, Seward JF, Redd SB, et al: Epidemiology of measles in the United States 1997–2001. *J Infect Dis* 2004;189(Suppl 1):S61–S68.
Parker AA, Staggs W, Dayan GH, et al: Implications of a 2005 measles outbreak in Indiana for sustained elimination of measles in the United States. *N Engl J Med* 2006;355:447–454.
Perry RT, Halsey NA: The clinical significance of measles: A review. *Clin Infect Dis* 2004;189(Suppl 1):S4–S16.
Rosales FJ: Vitamin A supplementation of vitamin deficient measles patients lowers risk of measles-related pneumonia in Zambian children. *J Nutr* 2002;132:3700–3703.
Redd SC, King GE, Heath JL, et al: Comparison of vaccination with measles-mumps-rubella vaccine at 9, 12, and 15 months of age. *J Infect Dis* 2004;189(Suppl 1):S116–S122.
Remington PL, Hall WN, Davis IH, et al: Airborne transmission of measles in a physician's office. *JAMA* 1985;253:1574–1577.
Rivera ME, Mason WH, Ross LA, et al: Nosocomial measles infection in a pediatric hospital during a community-wide epidemic. *J Pediatr* 1991;119:183–186.
Suringa DWR, Bank LJ, Ackerman AB: Role of measles virus in skin lesions and Koplik's spots. *N Engl J Med* 1970;283:1139–1142.

Chapter 244 ■ Rubella

Wilbert H. Mason

Rubella (**German measles** or **3-day measles**) is a mild, often exanthematous disease of infants and children that is typically more severe and associated with more complications in adults. Its major clinical significance is transplacental infection and fetal damage as part of the **congenital rubella syndrome** (**CRS**).

ETIOLOGY. Rubella virus is a member of the family Togaviridae and is the only species of the genus *Rubivirus*. It is a single-stranded RNA virus with a lipid envelope and 3 structural proteins, including a nucleocapsid protein associated with the nucleus and 2 glycoproteins, E1 and E2, associated with the envelope. The virus is sensitive to heat, ultraviolet light, and extremes of pH but is relatively stable at cold temperatures. Humans are the only known host.

EPIDEMIOLOGY. In the prevaccine era, rubella appeared to occur in major epidemics every 6–9 yr with smaller peaks interspersed every 3–4 yr, and was most common in preschool-aged and school-aged children. Following introduction of the vaccine, the incidence fell by >99%, with a relatively higher percentage of infections reported among persons >19 yr of age. After years of decline, a resurgence of rubella and CRS occurred during 1989–1991 (Fig. 244-1). Subsequently, a 2 dose recommendation for rubella vaccine was implemented and the incidence of rubella fell from 0.45/100,000 in 1990 to 0.1/100,000 in 1999, and a corresponding decrease of CRS with an average of 6 infants with CRS reported annually from 1992 to 2004. Mothers of these infants tended to be young, Hispanic, or foreign born. The number of reported cases of rubella continued to decline in the early part of this decade, and in 2004 it was concluded by the Centers for Disease Control and Prevention that the endemic transmission in the United States had been interrupted.

PATHOLOGY. Little information is available on the pathologic findings in rubella occurring postnatally. The few reported studies of biopsy or autopsy material from cases of rubella revealed only nonspecific findings of lymphoreticular inflammation and mononuclear perivascular and meningeal infiltration. The pathologic findings of CRS are often severe and may involve nearly every organ system (Table 244-1).

PATHOGENESIS. The viral mechanisms for cell injury and death in rubella are not well understood for either postnatal or congenital infection. Following infection the virus replicates in the respiratory epithelium then spreads to regional lymph nodes (Fig. 244-2). Viremia ensues and is most intense from 10 to 17 days after infection. Viral shedding from the nasopharynx begins about 10 days after infection and may be detected up to 2 wk following onset of the rash. The period of highest communicability is from 5 days before to 6 days following appearance of the rash.

TABLE 244-1. Pathologic Findings of Congenital Rubella Syndrome

SYSTEM	PATHOLOGIC FINDINGS
Cardiovascular	Patent ductus arteriosus
	Pulmonary artery stenosis
	Ventriculoseptal defect
	Myocarditis
Central nervous system	Chronic meningitis
	Parenchymal necrosis
	Vasculitis with calcification
Eye	Microphthalmia
	Cataract
	Iridocyclitis
	Ciliary body necrosis
	Glaucoma
	Retinopathy
Ear	Cochlear hemorrhage
	Endothelial necrosis
Lung	Chronic mononuclear interstitial pneumonitis
Liver	Hepatic giant cell transformation
	Fibrosis
	Lobular disarray
	Bile stasis
Kidneys	Interstitial nephritis
Andrenal glands	Cortical cytomegaly
Bone	Malformed osteoid
	Poor mineralization of osteoid
	Thinning cartilage
Spleen, lymph nodes	Extramedullary hematopoiesis
Thymus	Histiocytic reaction
	Absence of germinal centers
Skin	Erythropoiesis in dermis

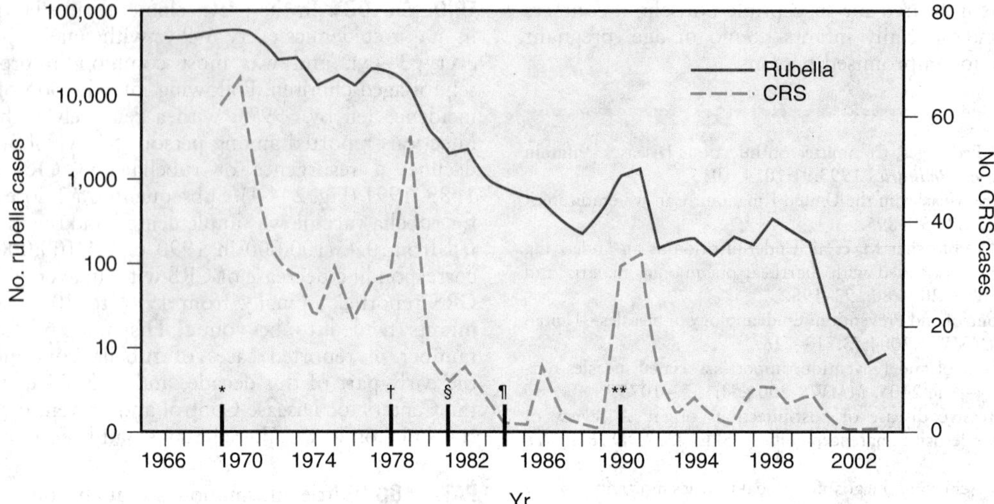

100,000
10,000
1,000
100
10
0
No. rubella cases
80
60
40
20
0
No. CRS cases
Rubella
CRS
1966
1970
1974
1978
1982
1986
1990
1994
1998
2002
Yr
*1969—First official recommendations are published for the use of rubella vaccine. Vaccination is recommended for children aged 1 year to puberty.
†1978—Recommendations for vaccination are expanded to include adolescents and certain adults, particularly females. Vaccination is recommended for adolescent or adult females and males in populations in colleges, certain places of employment (e.g., hospitals), and military bases.
§1981—Recommendations place increased emphasis on vaccination of susceptible persons in training and educational setting (e.g., universities or colleges) and military settings, and vaccination of workers in health-care–settings.
¶1984—Recommendations are published for vaccination of workers in daycare centers, schools, colleges, companies, government offices, and industrial sites. Providers are encouraged to conduct prenatal testing and postpartum vaccination of susceptible women. Recommendations for vaccination are expanded to include susceptible persons who travel abroad.
**1990—Recommendations include implementation of a new 2-dose schedule for measles-mumps-rubella vaccine.

Figure 244-1. Number of reported cases of rubella and congenital rubella syndrome (CRS), by year, and chronology of rubella vaccination recommendations by the Advisory Committee on Immunization Practices, USA, 1996–2004. (From the Centers for Disease Control and Prevention. Achievements in public health: Elimination of rubella and congenital rubella syndrome—United States, 1969–2004. *MMWR* 2005;54:279–282.)

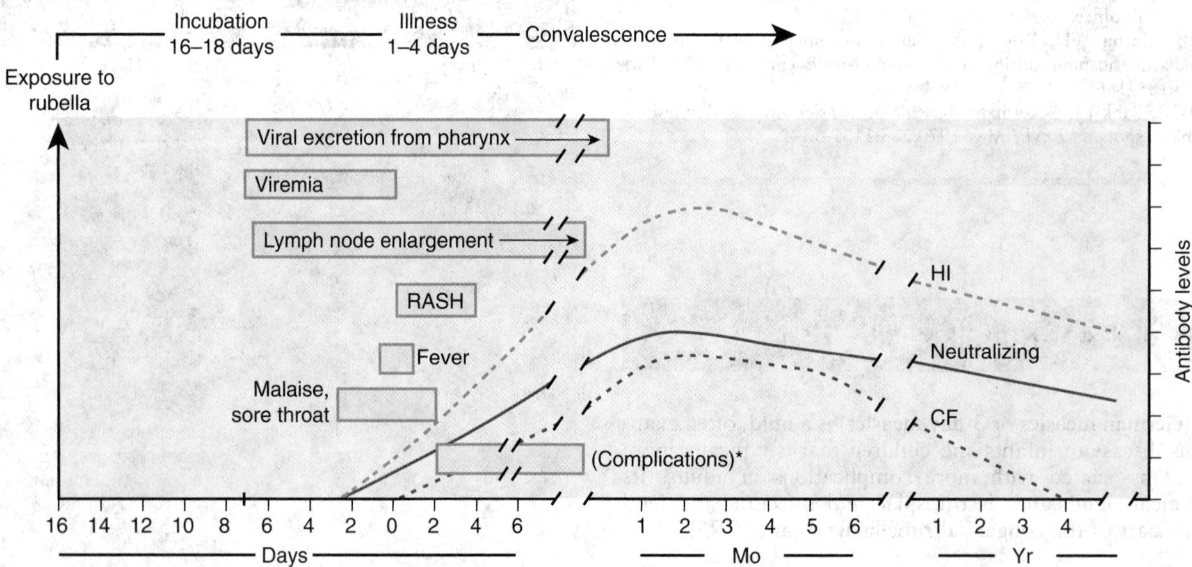

Incubation
16–18 days
Illness
1–4 days
Convalescence
Exposure to rubella
Viral excretion from pharynx
Viremia
Lymph node enlargement
RASH
Fever
Malaise, sore throat
(Complications)*
HI
Neutralizing
CF
Antibody levels
16 14 12 10 8 6 4 2 0 2 4 6
1 2 3 4 5 6
1 2 3 4
Days
Mo
Yr

Figure 244-2. Pathophysiologic events in postnatally acquired rubella virus infection. (*Possible complications inculde arthralgia and/or arthritis, thrombocytopenic purpura, and encephalitis.) (From Lamprecht CL: Rubella virus. In Beshe RB [editor]: *Textbook of Human Virology.* Littleton, MA, PSG Publishing, p 685.)

The most important risk factor for severe congenital defects is the stage of gestation at the time of infection. Maternal infection during the 1st 8 wk of gestation results in the most severe and widespread defects. The risk for congenital defects has been estimated at 90% for maternal infection before 11 wk of gestation, 33% at 11–12 wk, 11% at 13–14 wk, and 24% at 15–16 wk. Defects occurring after 16 wk of gestation are uncommon, even if fetal infection occurs.

Causes of cellular and tissue damage in the infected fetus may include tissue necrosis due to vascular insufficiency, reduced cellular multiplication time, chromosomal breaks, and production of a protein inhibitor causing mitotic arrests in certain cell types. The most distinctive feature of congenital rubella is chronicity. Once the fetus is infected early in gestation, the virus persists in fetal tissue until well beyond delivery. Persistence suggests the possibility of ongoing tissue damage and reactivation, most notably in the brain.

CLINICAL MANIFESTATIONS. **Postnatal infection** with rubella is a mild disease not easily discernible from other viral infections, especially in children. Following an incubation period of 14–21 days, a prodrome of low-grade fever, sore throat, red eyes with or without eye pain, headache, malaise, anorexia, and lymphadenopathy begins. Suboccipital, postauricular, and anterior cervical lymph nodes are most prominent. In children, the 1st manifestation of rubella is usually the rash, which is variable and not distinctive. It begins on the face and neck as small, irregular pink macules that coalesce, and it spreads centrifugally to involve the torso and extremities, where it tends to occur as discrete macules (Fig. 244-3). About the time of onset of the rash, examination of the throat may reveal tiny, rose-colored lesions (**Forchheimer spots**) or petechial hemorrhages on the soft palate. The rash fades from the face as it extends to the rest of the body so that the whole body may not be involved at any 1 time. The duration of the rash is generally 3 days, and it usually resolves without desquamation. Subclinical infections are common, and 25–40% of children may not have a rash.

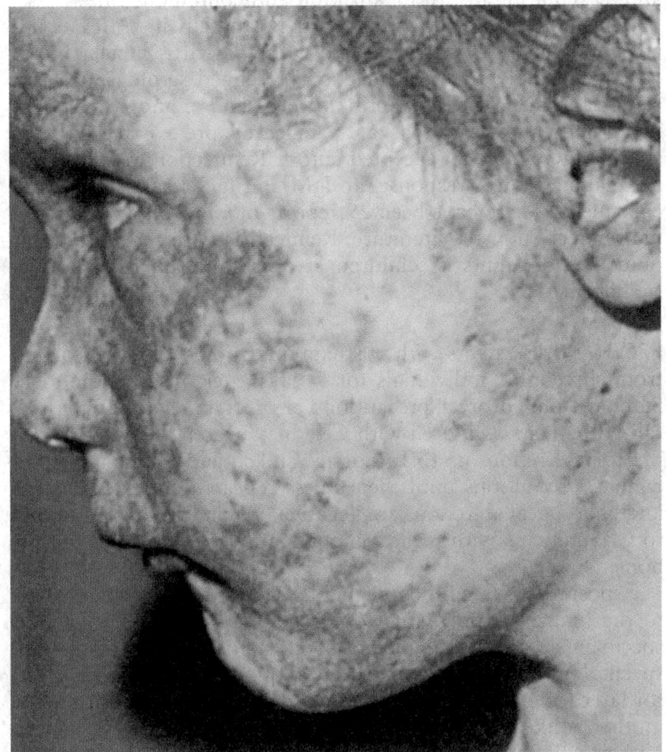

Figure 244-3. Rash of rubella.

LABORATORY FINDINGS. Leukopenia, neutropenia, and mild thrombocytopenia have been described during postnatal rubella.

DIAGNOSES. Specific diagnosis of rubella is important for epidemiologic reasons, for diagnosis of infection in pregnant women, and for confirmation of the diagnosis of congenital rubella. The most common diagnostic test is rubella immunoglobulin M (IgM) enzyme immunosorbent assay. As with any serologic test, the positive predictive value of testing decreases in populations with low prevalence of disease. Tests should be performed in the context of a supportive history of exposure or consistent clinical findings. The relative sensitivity and specificity of commercial kits used in most laboratories range from 96 to 99% and 86 to 97%, respectively. A caveat of testing congenitally infected infants early in infancy is that false-negative results may occur due to competing IgG antibodies circulating in these patients. In such patients, an IgM capture assay, reverse transcriptase polymerase chain reaction test, or viral culture should be performed for confirmation.

DIFFERENTIAL DIAGNOSES. Rubella may present with distinctive features suggesting the diagnosis. It is frequently confused with other infections because it is uncommon, similar to other viral exanthematous diseases, and demonstrates variability in the presence of typical findings. In severe cases it may resemble measles. The absence of both Koplik spots and a severe prodrome as well as a shorter course allow for differentiation from measles. Other diseases frequently confused with rubella include infections caused by adenoviruses, parvovirus B19 (erythema infectiosum), Epstein-Barr virus, enteroviruses, and *Mycoplasma pneumoniae.*

COMPLICATIONS. Complications following postnatal infection with rubella are infrequent and generally not life threatening.

Postinfectious **thrombocytopenia** occurs in about 1 : 3,000 cases of rubella and occurs more frequently among children and in girls. It manifests about 2 wk following the onset of the rash with petechiae, epistaxis, gastrointestinal bleeding, and hematuria. It is usually self-limited.

Arthritis following rubella occurs more commonly among adults, especially women. It begins within 1 wk of onset of the exanthem and classically involves the small joints of the hands. It also is self-limited and resolves within weeks without sequelae. There are anecdotal reports and some serologic evidence linking rubella with rheumatoid arthritis, but a true causal association remains speculative.

Encephalitis is the most serious complication of postnatal rubella. It occurs in 2 forms: a postinfectious syndrome following acute rubella and a rare progressive panencephalitis manifesting as a neurodegenerative disorder years following rubella.

Postinfectious encephalitis is uncommon, occurring in 1/5,000 cases of rubella. It appears within 7 days following onset of the rash with headache, seizures, confusion, coma, focal neurologic signs, and ataxia. Fever may recrudesce with the onset of neurologic symptoms. Cerebrospinal fluid (CSF) may be normal or have a mild mononuclear pleocytosis and/or elevated protein. Virus is rarely, if ever, isolated from CSF or brain, suggesting a noninfectious pathogenesis. Most patients recover completely, but mortality rates of 20% have been reported, as have long-term neurologic sequelae.

Progressive rubella panencephalitis (PRP) is an extremely rare complication of either acquired rubella or CRS. It has an onset and course similar to those of the subacute sclerosing panencephalitis (SSPE) associated with measles (see Chapter 243). Unlike the postinfectious form of rubella encephalitis, with PRP rubella virus may be isolated from brain tissue, suggesting an

TABLE 244-2. Clinical Manifestations of Congenital Rubella Syndrome (CRS) in 376 Children Following Maternal Rubella

Deafness	67%
Ocular	71%
Cataracts	29%
Retinopathy	39%
Heart disease*	48%
Patent ductus arteriosus	78%
Right pulmonary artery stenosis	70%
Left pulmonary artery stenosis	56%
Valvular pulmonic stenosis	40%
Low birthweight	60%
Psychomotor retardation	45%
Neonatal purpura	23%
Death	35%
(Other findings: hepatitis, linear streaking of bone, hazy cornea, congenital glaucoma, delayed growth)	

*Findings in 87 CRS patients with heart disease who underwent cardiac angiography.

From Cooper LZ, Ziring PR, Ockerse AB, et al: Rubella. Clinical manifestations and management. *Am J Dis Child* 1969;118:18–29.

infectious pathogenesis, albeit a "slow" one. The clinical findings and course are undistinguishable from SSPE and other "slow virus" neurodegenerative syndromes (see Chapter 275). Death occurs 2–5 yr after onset.

Other neurologic syndromes rarely reported with rubella include Guillain-Barré syndrome and peripheral neuritis. Myocarditis is a rare complication.

Congenital Rubella Syndrome. In 1941, Norman Gregg, an Australian ophthalmologist, first described a syndrome of cataracts and congenital heart disease with or without mental retardation and microcephaly that he correctly associated with rubella infections in the mothers during early pregnancy (Table 244-2). Shortly after the 1st description, hearing loss was recognized as a common finding. In 1964–1965 a pandemic of rubella occurred, with 20,000 cases reported in the USA leading to >11,000 spontaneous or therapeutic abortions and 2,100 neonatal deaths. From this experience emerged the expanded CRS that included numerous other transient or permanent abnormalities.

Nerve deafness is the single most common finding among infants with CRS. Most infants have some degree of intrauterine growth restriction. Retinal findings described as **salt-and-pepper retinopathy** are the most common ocular abnormality, but it has little early effect on vision. Unilateral or bilateral cataracts are the most serious eye finding, occurring in about 1/3 of infants (Fig. 244-4). Cardiac abnormalities occur in half of the children infected during the 1st 8 wk of gestation. Patent ductus arteriosus is the most frequently reported cardiac defect, followed by lesions of the pulmonary arteries and valvular disease. Interstitial pneumonitis leading to death in some cases has been reported. Neurologic abnormalities are common and may progress following birth. Meningoencephalitis is present in 10–20% of infants with CRS and may persist for up to 12 mo. Longitudinal follow-up through 9–12 yr of infants without initial retardation revealed progressive development of additional sensory, motor, and behavioral abnormalities, including hearing loss and autism. PRP has also been recognized rarely following CRS. Subsequent postnatal growth retardation and ultimate short stature has been reported in a minority of cases. Rare reports of immunologic deficiency syndromes have also been described.

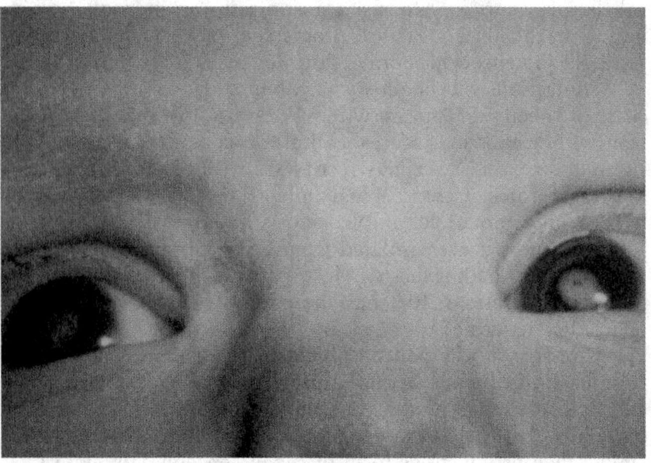

Figure 244-4. Bilateral cataracts in infant with congenital rubella syndrome.

A variety of late-onset manifestations of CRS have been recognized. In addition to PRP, these include diabetes mellitus (20%), thyroid dysfunction (5%), and glaucoma and visual abnormalities associated with the retinopathy, which had previously been considered benign.

TREATMENT. There is no specific treatment available for either acquired rubella or CRS.

SUPPORTIVE CARE. Postnatal rubella is generally a mild illness that requires no care beyond antipyretics and analgesics. Intravenous immunoglobulin or corticosteroids can be considered for severe, nonremitting thrombocytopenia.

Management of children with CRS is more complex and requires pediatric, cardiac, audiologic, ophthalmologic, and neurologic evaluation and follow-up since many manifestations may not be readily apparent initially or may worsen with time. Hearing screening is of special importance since early intervention may improve outcomes.

PROGNOSIS. Postnatal infection with rubella has an excellent prognosis. Long-term outcomes of CRS are less favorable and somewhat variable. In an Australian cohort evaluated 50 yr after infection, many had chronic conditions but most were married and had made good social adjustments. A cohort from New York from the mid-1960s epidemic had less favorable outcomes, with $^1/_3$ leading normal lives, $^1/_3$ in dependent situations but functional, and $^1/_3$ requiring institutionalization and continuous care.

Reinfection with wild virus occurs postnatally in both individuals who were previously infected with wild-virus rubella and in vaccinated individuals. Reinfection is defined serologically as a significant increase in IgG antibody level, and/or an IgM response in an individual who has a documented pre-existing rubella-specific IgG above an accepted cutoff. Reinfection may result in an anamnestic IgG response, an IgM and IgG response, or clinical rubella. There have been 29 reports of CRS following maternal reinfection in the literature. Reinfection with serious adverse outcomes to adults or children are rare and are of unknown significance.

PREVENTION. Patients with postnatal infection should be isolated from susceptible individuals for 7 days after onset of the rash. Standard plus droplet precautions are recommended for hospitalized patients. Children with CRS may excrete the virus in respiratory secretions up to 1 yr of age and should be maintained in contact precautions until then unless repeated cultures of urine and pharyngeal secretions are negative. Similar precautions apply to CRS patients with regard to attendance in school and out-of-home child care.

Exposure of susceptible pregnant women poses a potential risk to the fetus. For pregnant women exposed to rubella, a blood specimen should be obtained as soon as possible for rubella IgG specific antibody testing; a frozen aliquot also should be saved for later testing. If the rubella antibody test result is positive, the mother is likely immune. If negative, a 2nd specimen should be obtained 2–3 wk later and tested concurrently with the saved specimen. If both of these are negative, a 3rd specimen should be obtained 6 wk after exposure and tested concurrently with the saved specimen. If both the 2nd and 3rd specimens test negative, infection has not occurred. A negative 1st specimen and a positive test result in either the 2nd or 3rd specimen indicate the mother has seroconverted, suggesting recent infection. Counseling should be provided about the risks and benefits of termination of pregnancy. The routine use of immune globulin for susceptible pregnant women exposed to rubella is not recommended and is only considered if termination of pregnancy is not an option based on maternal preferences. In such circumstances, immune serum globulin 0.55 mL/kg IM may be given with the understanding that prophylaxis may reduce the risk for clinically apparent infection but does not guarantee prevention of fetal infection.

VACCINATION. Rubella vaccine in the USA is the attenuated RA 27/3 strain that is usually administered combined with measles and mumps (MMR), or also with varicella (MMRV), in a 2 dose regimen at 12–15 mo and 4–6 yr of age. It theoretically may be effective as postexposure prophylaxis if administered within 3 days of exposure. Vaccine should not be administered to severely immunocompromised patients (e.g., transplant patients). Patients with HIV infection who are not severely immunocompromised may benefit from vaccination. Fever is not a contraindication, but if a more serious illness is suspected, immunization should be delayed. Immune globulin preparations may inhibit the serologic response to the vaccine (see Chapter 170). Vaccine should not be administered during pregnancy. If pregnancy occurs within 28 days of immunization, the patient should be counseled on the theoretical risks to the fetus. Studies of over 200 women who had been inadvertently immunized with rubella vaccine during pregnancy showed that none of their offspring developed CRS. Therefore, interruption of pregnancy is probably not warranted.

Adverse reactions to rubella vaccination are uncommon in children. MMR administration is associated with fever in 5–15% of vaccines and rash in about 5%. Arthralgia and arthritis are more common following rubella vaccination in adults. Approximately 25% of postpubertal females experience arthralgia and 10% experience arthritis. Peripheral neuropathies and transient thrombocytopenia may also occur.

Banatvala JE, Brown DWG: Rubella. *Lancet* 2004;363:1127–1137.

Bloom S, Rguig A, Berraho A, et al: Congenital rubella syndrome burden in Morocco: A rapid retrospective assessment. *Lancet* 2005;365:135–140.

Bullens D, Koenraad S, Vanhaesebrouck P: Congenital rubella syndrome after maternal reinfection. *Clin Pediatr* 2000;39:113–116.

Centers for Disease Control and Prevention: Rubella vaccination during pregnancy—United States, 1971–1988. *MMWR* 1989;38:289–292.

Centers for Disease Control and Prevention: Achievements in public health: Elimination of rubella and congenital rubella syndrome—United States, 1969–2004. *MMWR* 2005;54:279–282.

Centers for Disease Control and Prevention: Brief report: Imported case of congenital rubella syndrome—New Hampshire, 2005. *MMWR* 2005;54:1160–1161.

Cooper LZ, Ziring PR, Ockerse AB, et al: Rubella: Clinical manifestations and management. *Am J Dis Child* 1969;118:18–29.

Corcoran C, Hardie DR: Serologic diagnosis of congenital rubella: A cautionary tale. *Pediatr Infect Dis J* 2005;24:286–287.

Dwyer DE, Robertson PW, Field PR: Clinical and laboratory features of rubella. *Pathology* 2001;33:322–328.

Frey RK: Neurological aspects of rubella virus infection. *Intervirology* 1997;40:167–175.

McIntosh ED, Menser MA: A fifty-year follow-up of congenital rubella. *Lancet* 1992;340:414–415.

Miller E, Cradock-Watson JE, Pollock TM: Consequences of confirmed maternal rubella at successive stages of pregnancy. *Lancet* 1982;2:781–784.

Townsend JJ, Stroop WG, Baringer JR, et al: Neuropathology of progressive rubella panencephalitis after childhood rubella. *Neurology* 1982;32:185–190.

Chapter 245 ■ Mumps

Wilbert H. Mason

Mumps is an acute self-limited infection, once commonplace but now unusual in developed countries because of widespread use of vaccination. It is characterized by fever, bilateral or unilateral parotid swelling and tenderness, and the frequent occurrence of meningoencephalitis and orchitis. While no longer common in countries with extensive vaccination programs, it remains endemic in the rest of the world, so continued vaccine protection is warranted.

ETIOLOGY. Mumps virus is in the family Paramyxoviridae and the genus *Rubulavirus*. It is a single-stranded pleomorphic RNA virus encapsulated in a lipoprotein envelope and possessing 7 structural proteins. Two surface glycoproteins, HN (hemagglutinin-neuraminidase) and F (fusion), mediate absorption of the virus to host cells and penetration into cells, respectively. Both stimulate production of protective antibodies. Mumps virus exists as a single immunotype, and humans are the only natural host.

EPIDEMIOLOGY. In the prevaccine era, mumps occurred primarily in young children between the ages of 5 and 9 and in epidemics about every 4 years. Mumps infection occurred more often in the winter and spring months. In 1968, just after the introduction of the mumps vaccine, 185,691 cases were reported in the USA. Following introduction of the mumps vaccine, which was recommended for routine use in 1977, the incidence fell dramatically (Fig. 245-1) and shifted to older children, adolescents, and young adults. Outbreaks continued to occur even in highly vaccinated populations due to vaccine failure and also because of undervaccination of susceptible persons. After implementation of the 2 dose recommendation for the measles-mumps-rubella (MMR) vaccine for measles control in 1989, the number of mumps cases declined further. During 2001–2003, <300 mumps cases were reported each year. A multistate mumps outbreak, with >2,500 cases reported during the 1st half of 2006, was the largest number of mumps cases reported in a single year since 1991. The 1st cases in this outbreak were detected on a college campus in eastern Iowa in December 2005. The source of mumps of the initial cases is unknown. The age group most affected (38% of cases) was young adults 18–24 yr of age and included many college students. The outbreak subsequently spread to all age groups.

Mumps is spread from person to person by respiratory droplets. Virus appears in the saliva from up to 7 days before to as long as 7 days after onset of parotid swelling. The period of maximum infectiousness is 1–2 days before to 5 days after parotid swelling. Viral shedding before onset of symptoms and in asymptomatic infected individuals impairs efforts to contain the infection in susceptible populations.

PATHOLOGY AND PATHOGENESIS. Mumps virus targets the salivary glands, central nervous system (CNS), pancreas, testes, and, to a lesser extent, thyroid, ovaries, heart, kidneys, liver, and joint synovia.

Following infection, initial viral replication occurs in the epithelium of the upper respiratory tract. Infection spreads to the adjacent lymph nodes by the lymphatic drainage, and viremia ensues, spreading the virus to targeted tissues. Mumps virus causes necrosis of infected cells and is associated with a lymphocytic inflammatory infiltrate. Salivary gland ducts are lined with necrotic epithelium, and the interstitium is infiltrated with lymphocytes. Swelling of tissue within the testes may result in focal ischemic infarcts. The cerebrospinal fluid (CSF) frequently contains mononuclear pleocytosis, even in individuals without clinical signs of meningitis.

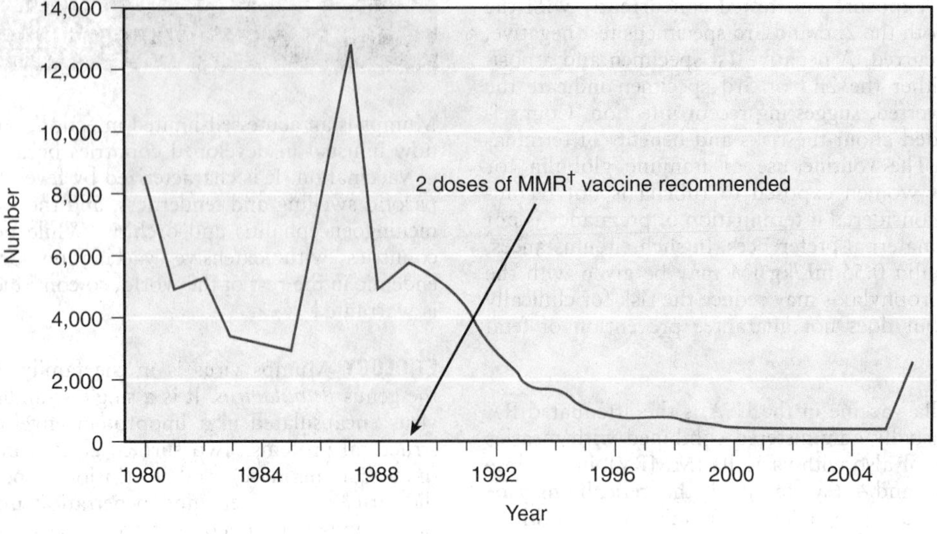

Figure 245-1. Number of reported mumps cases by year in the United States from 1980 to 2006 (data for 2005 and 2006 are provisional). Mumps vaccine was first licensed in 1967 and recommended for routine use in 1977. After expanded recommendation for 2 doses of measles-mumps-rubella (MMR) vaccine in 1989 for measles control, mumps incidence further declined. During 2001–2003 there were <300 mumps cases each year, a 99% decline from the 185,691 cases reported in 1968. Over 2,500 cases were reported in the 1st half of 2006 as part of a multistate outbreak, the largest number of cases in the USA since 1991. (From the Centers for Disease Control and Prevention: Summary of notifiable diseases—United States, 2004. *MMWR* 2006;53:1–79.)

CLINICAL MANIFESTATIONS. The incubation period for mumps ranges from 12 to 25 days, but is usually 16 to 18 days. Mumps virus infection may result in clinical presentation ranging from asymptomatic or nonspecific symptoms to typical illness associated with parotitis with or without complications involving several body systems. The typical case presents with a prodrome lasting 1–2 days consisting of fever, headache, vomiting, and achiness. Parotitis then appears and may be unilateral initially but becomes bilateral in about 70% of cases (Fig. 245-2). The parotid gland is tender, and parotitis may be preceded or accompanied by ear pain on the ipsilateral side. Ingestion of sour or acidic foods or liquids may enhance pain in the parotid area. As swelling progresses, the angle of the jaw is obscured and the ear lobe may be lifted upward and outward. (Figs. 245-2 and 245-3). The opening of the Stensen duct may be red and edematous. The parotid swelling peaks in approximately 3 days then gradually subsides over 7 days. Fever resolves in 3 to 5 days along with the other systemic symptoms. A morbilliform rash is rarely seen. Submandibular salivary glands may also be involved or may be enlarged without parotid

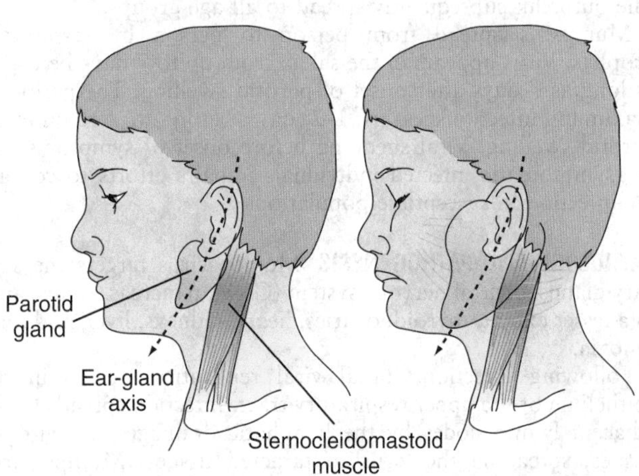

Figure 245-2. Schematic drawing of a parotid gland infected with mumps compared with a normal gland. An imaginary line bisecting the long axis of the ear divides the parotid gland into 2 equal parts, These anatomic relationships are not altered in the enlarged gland. An enlarged cervical lymph node is usually posterior to the imaginary line. (From Mumps [epidemic parotitis]. In Krugman S, Ward R, Katz SL [editors]: *Infectious Diseases in Children*, 6th ed. St. Louis, Mosby, 1977, p 182.)

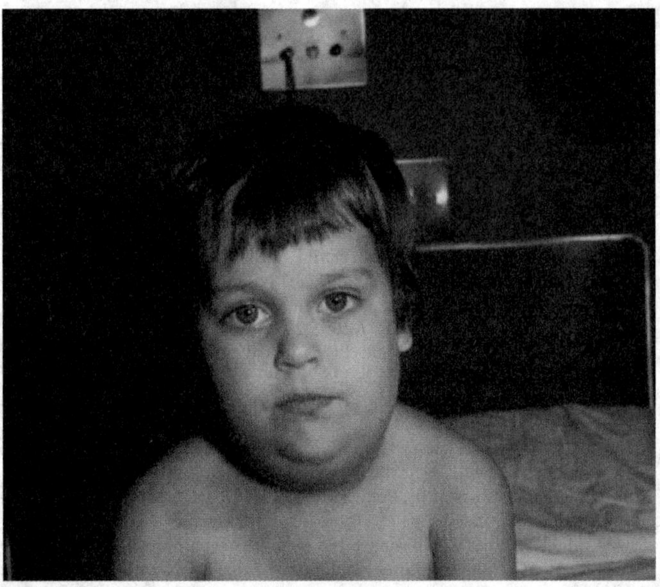

Figure 245-3. A child with mumps showing parotid swelling. (From the Centers for Disease Control and Prevention.)

swelling. Edema over the sternum due to lymphatic obstruction may also occur.

DIAGNOSIS. When mumps was highly prevalent, the diagnosis could be made based on history of exposure to mumps infection, an appropriate incubation period, and development of typical clinical findings. Confirmation of the presence of parotiditis could be made with demonstration of an elevated amylase level. Leukopenia with a relative lymphocytosis was a common finding. Today, in patients with parotiditis of >2 days of unknown cause, a specific diagnosis of mumps should be confirmed or ruled out by virologic or serologic means. This may be accomplished by isolation of the virus in cell culture, detection of viral antigen by direct immunofluorescence, or identification of nucleic acid by reverse transcriptase polymerase chain reaction. Virus can be isolated from upper respiratory tract secretions, CSF, or urine during the acute illness. Serologic testing is usually a more convenient and available mode of diagnosis. A significant increase in serum mumps immunoglobulin G (IgG) antibody between acute and convalescent serum specimens by complement fixation, neutralization hemagglutination, or enzyme immunoassay (EIA) tests establish the diagnosis. However, IgG antibody tests may cross react with antibodies to parainfluenza virus. More commonly, an EIA for mumps IgM antibody is used to identify recent infection. Skin testing for mumps is neither sensitive nor specific and should not be used.

DIFFERENTIAL DIAGNOSIS. Parotid swelling may be caused by many other infections and noninfectious conditions. Viruses that have been shown to cause parotitis include parainfluenza 1 and 3, influenza A, cytomegalovirus, Epstein-Barr virus, enteroviruses, lymphocytic choriomeningitis virus, and HIV. Purulent parotitis, usually caused by *Staphylococcus aureus*, is unilateral, extremely tender, and associated with an elevated white blood cell count, and may have purulent drainage from the Stensen duct. Submandibular or anterior cervical adenitis due to a variety of pathogens may also be confused with parotitis. Other noninfectious causes of parotid swelling include obstruction of the Stensen duct, collagen vascular diseases such as Sjögren syndrome, systemic lupus erythematosis, and tumor.

COMPLICATIONS. The most common complications of mumps are meningitis, with or without encephalitis, and gonadal involvement. Uncommon complications include conjunctivitis, optic neuritis, pneumonia, nephritis, pancreatitis, and thrombocytopenia.

Maternal infection with mumps during the 1st trimester of pregnancy results in increased fetal wastage. No fetal malformations have been associated with intrauterine mumps infection. However, perinatal mumps disease has been reported in infants born to mothers who acquired mumps late in gestation.

Meningitis and Meningoencephalitis. Mumps virus is neurotropic and is thought to enter the CNS via the choroid plexus and infect the choroidal epithelium and ependymal cells, both of which can be found in CSF along with mononuclear leukocytes. Symptomatic CNS involvement occurs in 10–30% of infected individuals, but CSF pleocytosis has been found in 40–60% of patients with mumps parotitis. The meningoencephalitis may occur before, along with, or following the parotitis. It most commonly will present 5 days after the parotitis. Clinical findings vary with age. Infants and young children will have fever, malaise, and lethargy, while older children, adolescents, and adults will complain of headache and demonstrate meningeal signs. In 1 series in children with mumps with meningeal involvement, findings were fever in 94%, vomiting in 84%, headache in 47%, parotitis in 47%, neck stiffness in 71%, lethargy in 69%, and seizures in 18%. In typical cases, symptoms resolve in 7–10 days. CSF in mumps meningitis has a white blood cell pleocytosis of 200–600/mm^3 with a predominance of lymphocytes. The glucose is normal in most patients, but a moderate hypoglycorrhachia (20–40 mg/dL) may be seen in 10–20% of patients. Protein is normal or mildly elevated.

Less common CNS complications of mumps include transverse myelitis, aqueductal stenosis, and facial palsy. Sensorineural hearing loss is rare but has been estimated to occur in 0.5–5.0/100,000 cases of mumps. There is some evidence that it is more likely in patients with meningoencephalitis.

Orchitis and Oophoritis. In adolescent and adult males, epidymo-orchitis is 2nd only to parotitis as a common finding in mumps. Involvement in prepubescent male children is extremely rare, but following puberty it occurs in 30–40% of males. It begins within days following onset of parotitis in the majority of cases and is associated with moderate to high fever, chills, and exquisite pain and swelling of the testes. In $\leq 1/3$ of cases the orchitis is bilateral. Atrophy of the testes may occur, but sterility is rare even with bilateral involvement.

Oophoritis is uncommon in postpubertal females but may cause severe pain and when on the right side it may be confused with appendicitis.

Pancreatitis. Pancreatitis may occur in mumps with or without parotid involvement. Severe disease is rare, but fever, epigastric pain, and vomiting are suggestive. Epidemiologic studies have suggested that mumps may be associated with the subsequent development of diabetes mellitus, but a causal link has not been established.

Cardiac Involvement. Myocarditis has been reported in mumps, and molecular studies have identified mumps virus in heart tissue taken from patients with endocardial fibroelastosis.

Arthritis. Arthralgia, monoarthritis, and migratory polyarthritis have been reported in mumps. It is seen with or without parotitis and usually occurs within 3 weeks of onset of parotid swelling. It is generally mild and self-limited.

Thyroiditis. Thyroiditis is rare following mumps. It has not been reported without parotitis and may occur weeks following the acute infection. Most cases resolve, but some become relapsing and result in hypothyroidism.

TREATMENT. No specific antiviral therapy is available for mumps. Management should be aimed at reducing the pain associated with meningitis or orchitis and maintenance of adequate hydration. Antipyretics may be given for fever.

PROGNOSIS. The outcome of mumps is nearly always excellent, even when complicated by encephalitis, although fatal cases due to CNS involvement or myocarditis have been reported.

PREVENTION. Immunization with the live mumps vaccine is the primary mode of prevention used in the United States. It is given as part of the MMR 2 dose vaccine schedule, at 12–15 mo of age for the 1st dose and 4–6 yr of age for the 2nd dose. If not given at 4–6 yr, the 2nd dose should be given before children enter puberty. Antibody develops in 95% of vaccinees after 1 dose. One study showed vaccine effectiveness of 88% for 2 doses of MMR vaccine compared with 64% for a single dose. Immunity appears to be long lasting, with existing serologic and epidemiologic evidence indicating protection for >25 yr. As a live-virus vaccine, MMR should not be administered to pregnant women or severely immunodeficient or immunosuppressed individuals. HIV-infected patients not severely immunocompromised may receive the vaccine since the risk for severe infection with mumps outweighs the risk for serious reaction to the vaccine. Individuals with anaphylactoid reactions to egg or neomycin may be at risk for immediate-type hypersensitivity reactions to the vaccine. Persons with other types of reactions to egg or reactions to other components of the vaccine are not restricted from receiving the vaccine.

In 2006, in response to the multistate outbreak in the United States, evidence of immunity to mumps through vaccination was redefined. Acceptable presumptive evidence of immunity to mumps now includes 1 of the following: (1) documentation of adequate vaccination, (2) laboratory evidence of immunity, (3) birth before 1957, or (4) documentation of physician-diagnosed mumps. Evidence of immunity through documentation of adequate vaccination is now defined as 1 dose of a live mumps virus vaccine for preschool-aged children and adults not at high risk and 2 doses for school-aged children (i.e., grades K–12) and for adults at high risk (i.e., health care workers, international travelers, and students at post–high school educational institutions).

All persons who work in health care facilities should be immune to mumps. Adequate mumps vaccination for health care workers born during or after 1957 consists of 2 doses of a live mumps virus vaccine. Health care workers with no history of mumps vaccination and no other evidence of immunity should receive 2 doses with >28 days between doses. Health care workers who have received only 1 dose previously should receive a 2nd dose. Because birth before 1957 is only presumptive evidence of immunity, health care facilities should consider recommending 1 dose of a live mumps virus vaccine for unvaccinated workers born before 1957 who do not have a history of physician-diagnosed mumps or laboratory evidence of mumps immunity. During an outbreak, health care facilities should strongly consider recommending 2 doses of a live mumps virus vaccine to unvaccinated workers born before 1957 who do not have evidence of mumps immunity.

Adverse reactions to mumps virus vaccine are rare. Parotitis and orchitis have been reported rarely. Other reactions such as febrile seizures, deafness, rash, purpura, encephalitis, and meningitis may not be causally related to the strain of mumps vaccine virus used for immunization in the USA. Higher rates of aseptic meningitis following vaccination for mumps have been associated with vaccine strains used elsewhere in the world, including the Leningrad 3 and Urabe Am 9 strains. Transient suppression of reactivity to tuberculin skin testing has been reported.

Azimi PH, Cramblett HG, Haynes RE: Mumps meningoencephalitis in children. *JAMA* 1969;207:509–512.

Centers for Disease Control and Prevention: Mumps epidemic—United Kingdom, 2004–2005. *MMWR* 2006;55:173–178.

Centers for Disease Control and Prevention: Mumps epidemic—Iowa, 2006. *MMWR* 2006;55:366–368.

Centers for Disease Control and Prevention: Update: Multistate outbreak of mumps—United States, January 1–May 2, 2006. *MMWR* 2006;55:559–564.

Centers for Disease Control and Prevention: Notice to readers: Updated recommendations of the Advisory Committee on Immunization Practices (ACIP) for the control and elimination of mumps. *MMWR* 2006;55:629–630.

Davidkin I, Jakinen S, Paananen A, et al: Etiology of mumps-like illness in children and adolescents vaccinated for measles, mumps and rubella. *J Infect Dis* 2005;1991:719–723.

Endo A, Izuni H, Miyashita M, et al: Facial palsy associated with mumps parotitis. *Pediatr Infect Dis J* 2001;20:815–816.

Harling R, White JM, Ramsay ME, et al: The effectiveness of the mumps component of the MMR vaccine: A case control study. *Vaccine* 2005;23:4070–4074.

Horel L, Amir J, Reish O, et al: Mumps arthritis in children. *Pediatr Infect Dis J* 1990;9:928–929.

Kanara G, Kara A, Cengiz AB, et al: Mumps meningoencephalitis effect on bearing. *Pediatr Infect Dis J* 2002;1167–1169.

Kupers TA, Petrich JM, Holloway AW, St Gene JW: Depression of tuberculin hypersensitivity by live attenuated mumps virus. *J Pediatr* 1970;76:716–721.

Thompson JA. Mumps: A cause of aqueductal stenosis. *J Pediatr* 1979;94:923–924.

Chapter 246 ■ Polioviruses

Eric A.F. Simoes

ETIOLOGY. The polioviruses are nonenveloped, positive-stranded RNA viruses belonging to the Picornaviridae family, in the genus *Enterovirus,* and include 3 antigenically distinct serotypes (types 1, 2, and 3). Polioviruses spread from the intestinal tract to the central nervous system (CNS), where they cause aseptic meningitis and poliomyelitis, or polio. The polioviruses are extremely hardy and can retain infectivity for several days at room temperature.

EPIDEMIOLOGY. The most devastating result of poliovirus infection is paralysis, although 90–95% of infections are inapparent but induce protective immunity. Clinically apparent but nonparalytic illness occurs in about 5% of all infections, with paralytic polio occurring in about 1/1,000 infections among infants to about 1/100 infections among adolescents. In developed countries prior to universal vaccination, epidemics of paralytic poliomyelitis occurred primarily in adolescents. Conversely, in developing countries with poor sanitation, infection early in life results in infantile paralysis. Improved sanitation explains the virtual eradication of polio from the United States in the early 1960s, when only about $^2/_3$ of the population was immunized with the Salk vaccine, which contributed to the disappearance of circulating wild-type poliovirus in the USA and Europe. Poor sanitation and crowding have permitted the continued transmission of poliovirus in certain poor countries in Africa and Asia, despite massive global efforts to eradicate polio, in some areas with an average of 12–13 doses of polio vaccine administered to children in the 1st 5 yr of life (Fig. 246-1).

Transmission. Humans are the only known reservoir for the polioviruses, which are spread by the fecal-oral route. Poliovirus has been isolated from feces for >2 wk before paralysis to several weeks after the onset of symptoms.

PATHOGENESIS. Polioviruses infect cells by adsorbing to the genetically determined **poliovirus receptor.** The virus penetrates the cell and is uncoated and releases viral RNA. The RNA is translated to produce proteins responsible for replication of the RNA, shut-off of host cell protein synthesis, and synthesis of structural elements that compose the capsid. Mature virus particles are produced in 6–8 hr and are released into the environment by disruption of the cell.

In the contact host, wild-type and vaccine strains of polioviruses gain host entry via the gastrointestinal tract. The primary site of replication is in the M cells lining the mucosa of the small intestine. Regional lymph nodes are infected, and primary viremia occurs after 2–3 days. The virus seeds multiple sites, including the reticuloendothelial system, brown fat deposits, and skeletal muscle. Wild-type poliovirus probably accesses the CNS along peripheral nerves. Vaccine strains of polioviruses do not replicate in the CNS, which accounts for the safety of the live-attenuated vaccine. Occasional **revertants** (by nucleotide substitution) of these vaccine strains develop a neurovirulent phenotype and cause **vaccine-associated paralytic poliomyelitis (VAPP).** Reversion occurs in the small intestine and probably accesses the CNS via the peripheral nerves. Because poliovirus replicates in endothelial cells, the theory of viremic spread to the CNS was favored; however, poliovirus has almost never been cultured from the cerebrospinal fluid (CSF) of patients with paralytic disease, and patients with aseptic meningitis caused by poliovirus never have paralytic disease. With the 1st appearance of non-CNS symptoms, a secondary viremia probably occurs as a result of enormous viral replication in the reticuloendothelial system.

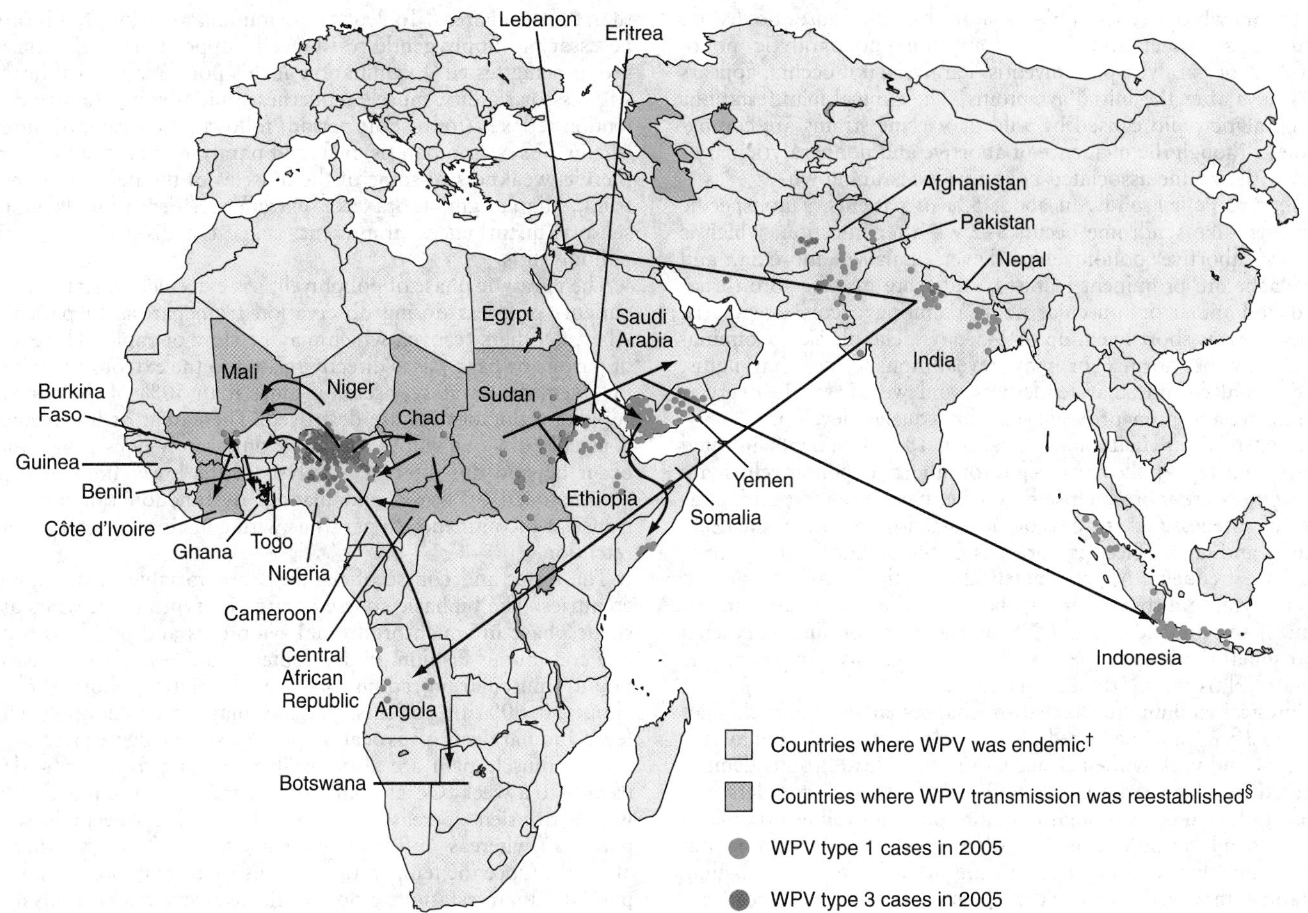

Figure 246-1. Wild poliovirus (WPV) cases in 2005 and WPV importation routes* during 2002–2005 worldwide. (From the Centers for Disease Control and Prevention: Resurgence of wild poliovirus type 1 transmission and consequences of importation—21 countries, 2002–2005. *MMWR* 2006;55:145–150.)

The exact mechanism of entry into the CNS is not known. Once entry is gained, however, the virus may traverse neural pathways, and multiple sites within the CNS are often affected. The effect on motor and vegetative neurons is most striking and correlates with the clinical manifestations. Perineuronal inflammation, a mixed inflammatory reaction with both polymorphonuclear leukocytes and lymphocytes, is associated with extensive neuronal destruction. Petechial hemorrhages and considerable inflammatory edema also occurs in areas of poliovirus infection. The poliovirus primarily infects motor neuron cells in the spinal cord (**the anterior horn cells**) and the medulla oblongata (the cranial nerve nuclei). Because of the overlap in muscle innervation by 2–3 adjacent segments of the spinal cord, clinical signs of weakness in the limbs develop when more than 50% of motor neurons are destroyed. In the medulla, less extensive lesions cause paralysis, and involvement of the reticular formation that contains the vital centers controlling respiration and circulation may have a catastrophic outcome. Involvement of the intermediate and dorsal horn and dorsal root ganglia in the spinal cord results in hyperesthesia and myalgias that are typical of acute poliomyelitis. Other neurons affected are the nuclei in the roof and vermis of the cerebellum, the substantia nigra, and occasionally the red nucleus in the pons; there may be variable involvement of thalamic, hypothalamic, and pallidal nuclei and the motor cortex.

Apart from the histopathology of the CNS, inflammatory changes occur generally in the reticuloendothelial system. Inflammatory edema and sparse lymphocytic infiltration are prominently associated with hyperplastic lymphocytic follicles.

Infants acquire immunity transplacentally from their mothers. Transplacental immunity disappears at a variable rate during the 1st 4–6 mo of life. Active immunity after natural infection is probably lifelong but protects against the infecting serotype only; infections with other serotypes are possible. Poliovirus neutralizing antibodies develop within several days after exposure as a result of replication of the virus in the M cells in the intestinal tract and deep lymphatic tissues. This early production of circulating immunoglobulin G (IgG) antibodies protects against CNS invasion. Local (mucosal) immunity, conferred mainly by secretory IgA, is an important defense against subsequent reinfection of the gastrointestinal tract.

CLINICAL MANIFESTATIONS. The incubation period of poliovirus from contact to initial clinical symptoms is usually considered to be 8–12 days, with a range of 5–35 days. Poliovirus infections with wild-type virus may follow 1 of several courses: **inapparent**

infection, which occurs in 90–95% of cases and causes no disease and no sequelae; abortive poliomyelitis; nonparalytic poliomyelitis; or paralytic poliomyelitis. Paralysis, if it occurs, appears 3–8 days after the initial symptoms. The clinical manifestations of paralytic polio caused by wild or vaccine strains are comparable, although the incidence of abortive and nonparalytic paralysis with vaccine-associated poliomyelitis is unknown.

Abortive Poliomyelitis. In about 5% of patients, a nonspecific influenza-like syndrome occurs 1–2 wk after infection, which is termed abortive poliomyelitis. Fever, malaise, anorexia, and headache are prominent features, and there may be sore throat and abdominal or muscular pain. Vomiting occurs irregularly. The illness is short lived, up to 2–3 days. The **physical examination** may be normal or may reveal nonspecific pharyngitis, abdominal or muscular tenderness, and weakness. Recovery is complete, and no neurologic signs or sequelae develop.

Nonparalytic Poliomyelitis. In about 1% of patients infected with wild-type poliovirus, signs of abortive poliomyelitis are present, as are more intense headache, nausea, and vomiting, as well as soreness and stiffness of the posterior muscles of the neck, trunk, and limbs. Fleeting paralysis of the bladder and constipation are frequent. Approximately 2/3 of these children have a short symptom-free interlude between the 1st phase (**minor illness**) and the 2nd phase (CNS disease or **major illness**). Nuchal and spinal rigidity are the basis for the diagnosis of nonparalytic poliomyelitis during the 2nd phase.

Physical examination reveals nuchal-spinal signs and changes in superficial and deep reflexes. Gentle forward flexion of the occiput and neck will elicit nuchal rigidity. Head drop is demonstrated by placing the hands under the patient's shoulders and raising the trunk. Although normally the head follows the plane of the trunk, in poliomyelitis it often falls backward limply, but this is not due to true paresis of the neck flexors. In struggling infants it may be difficult to distinguish voluntary resistance from clinically important true nuchal rigidity. One may place the infant's shoulders flush with the edge of the table, support the weight of the occiput in the hand, and then flex the head anteriorly. True nuchal rigidity will persist during this maneuver. When open, the anterior fontanel may be tense or bulging.

In the early stages the reflexes are normally active and remain so unless paralysis supervenes. Changes in reflexes, either increased or decreased, may precede weakness by 12–24 hr. The superficial reflexes, the cremasteric and abdominal reflexes, and the reflexes of the spinal and gluteal muscles are usually the 1st to diminish. The spinal and gluteal reflexes may disappear before the abdominal and cremasteric reflexes. Changes in the deep tendon reflexes generally occur 8–24 hr after the superficial reflexes are depressed and indicate impending paresis of the extremities. Tendon reflexes are absent with paralysis. Sensory defects do not occur in poliomyelitis.

Paralytic Poliomyelitis. Paralytic poliomyelitis develops in about 0.1% of persons infected with poliovirus, causing 3 clinically recognizable syndromes that represent a continuum of infection differentiated only by the portions of the CNS most severely affected. These are (1) spinal paralytic poliomyelitis, (2) bulbar poliomyelitis, and (3) polioencephalitis.

Spinal paralytic poliomyelitis may occur as the 2nd phase of a biphasic illness, the 1st phase of which corresponds to abortive poliomyelitis. The patient then appears to recover and feels better for 2–5 days, after which severe headache and fever occur with exacerbation of the previous systemic symptoms. Severe muscle pain is present, and sensory and motor phenomena (e.g., paresthesia, hyperesthesia, fasciculations, and spasms) may develop. On physical examination the distribution of paralysis is characteristically spotty. Single muscles, multiple muscles, or groups of muscles may be involved in any pattern. Within 1–2 days, asymmetric flaccid paralysis or paresis occurs. Involvement of 1 leg is most common, followed by involvement of 1 arm. The proximal areas of the extremities tend to be involved to a greater extent than the distal areas. To detect mild muscular weakness, it is often necessary to apply gentle resistance in opposition to the muscle group being tested. Examination at this point may reveal nuchal stiffness or rigidity, muscle tenderness, initially hyperactive deep tendon reflexes (for a short period) followed by absent or diminished reflexes, and paresis or flaccid paralysis. In the spinal form there is weakness of some of the muscles of the neck, abdomen, trunk, diaphragm, thorax, or extremities. Sensation is intact; sensory disturbances, if present, suggest a disease other than poliomyelitis.

The paralytic phase of poliomyelitis is extremely variable; some patients progress during observation from paresis to paralysis, whereas others recover, which may be slow or rapid. The extent of paresis or paralysis is directly related to the extent of neuronal involvement; paralysis occurs if more than 50% of the neurons supplying the muscles are destroyed. The extent of involvement is usually obvious within 2–3 days; only rarely does progression occur beyond this interval. Paralysis of the lower limbs is often accompanied by bowel and bladder dysfunction ranging from transient incontinence to paralysis with constipation and urinary retention.

The onset and course of paralysis are variable in developing countries. The biphasic course is rare and typically presents as a single phase in which prodromal symptoms and paralysis occur in a continuous fashion. In developing countries, where a history of intramuscular injections precedes paralytic poliomyelitis in about 50–60% of patients, patients may present initially with fever and paralysis (**provocation paralysis**). The degree and duration of muscle pain are also variable, ranging from a few days usually to a week. Occasionally spasm and increased muscle tone with a transient increase in deep tendon reflexes occur in some patients, whereas in most patients flaccid paralysis occurs abruptly. Once the temperature returns to normal, progression of paralytic manifestations stops. Little recovery from paralysis is noted in the 1st days or weeks, but, if it is to occur, is usually evident within 6 mo. The return of strength and reflexes is slow and may continue to improve as long as 18 mo after the acute disease. Lack of improvement from paralysis within the 1st several weeks or months after onset is usually evidence of permanent paralysis. Atrophy of the limb, failure of growth, and deformity is common and is especially evident in the growing child.

Bulbar poliomyelitis may occur as a clinical entity without apparent involvement of the spinal cord. Infection is a continuum, and designation of the disease as bulbar implies only dominance of the clinical manifestations by dysfunctions of the cranial nerves and medullary centers. The clinical findings seen with bulbar poliomyelitis with respiratory difficulty (other than paralysis of extraocular, facial, and masticatory muscles) include (1) nasal twang to the voice or cry caused by palatal and pharyngeal weakness (hard-consonant words such as "cookie" or "candy" bring this out best); (2) inability to swallow smoothly, resulting in accumulation of saliva in the pharynx, indicating partial immobility (holding the larynx lightly and asking the patient to swallow will confirm such immobility); (3) accumulated pharyngeal secretions, which may cause irregular respirations that appear interrupted and abnormal even to the point of falsely simulating intercostal or diaphragmatic weakness; (4) absence of effective coughing, shown by constant fatiguing efforts to clear the throat; (5) nasal regurgitation of saliva and fluids as a result of palatal paralysis, with inability to separate the oropharynx from the nasopharynx during swallowing; (6) deviation of the palate, uvula, or tongue; (7) involvement of vital centers in the medulla, which manifest as irregularities in rate, depth, and rhythm of respiration; as cardiovascular alterations, including blood pressure changes (especially increased blood pressure), alternate flushing and mottling of the skin, and cardiac arrhythmias; and as rapid changes in body temperature; (8) paralysis of 1 or both vocal cords, causing hoarseness, aphonia, and ultimately asphyxia unless this is recognized by laryngoscopy and managed by immediate tracheostomy; and (9) the **rope sign,** an acute angulation between the chin and larynx caused by weakness of the hyoid muscles (the hyoid bone is pulled posteriorly, narrowing the hypopharyngeal inlet).

Uncommonly, bulbar disease may culminate in an ascending paralysis (Landry type), in which there is progression cephalad from initial involvement of the lower extremities. Hypertension and other autonomic disturbances are common in bulbar involvement and may persist for a week or more or may be transient. Occasionally, hypertension is followed by hypotension and shock and is associated with irregular or failed respiratory effort, delirium, or coma. This kind of bulbar disease may be rapidly fatal.

The course of bulbar disease is variable; some patients die as a result of extensive, severe involvement of the various centers in the medulla; others recover partially but require ongoing respiratory support, and others recover completely. Cranial nerve involvement is seldom permanent. Atrophy of muscles may be evident, patients immobilized for long periods may develop pneumonia, and renal stones may form as a result of hypercalcemia and hypercalciuria secondary to bone resorption.

Polioencephalitis is a rare form of the disease in which higher centers of the brain are severely involved. Seizures, coma, and spastic paralysis with increased reflexes may be observed. Irritability, disorientation, drowsiness, and coarse tremors are often present with peripheral or cranial nerve paralysis that coexists or ensues. Hypoxia and hypercapnia caused by inadequate ventilation due to respiratory insufficiency may produce disorientation without true encephalitis. The manifestations are common to encephalitis of any cause and can only be attributed to polioviruses by specific viral diagnosis or if accompanied by flaccid paralysis.

Paralytic poliomyelitis with ventilatory insufficiency results from several components acting together to produce ventilatory insufficiency resulting in hypoxia and hypercapnia. This may produce profound effects on many other systems. Because respiratory insufficiency may develop rapidly, close continued clinical evaluation is essential. Despite weakness of the respiratory muscles, the patient may respond with so much respiratory effort associated with anxiety and fear that overventilation may occur at the outset, resulting in respiratory alkalosis. Such effort is fatiguing and contributes to respiratory failure.

There are certain characteristic patterns of disease. Pure spinal poliomyelitis with respiratory insufficiency involves tightness, weakness, or paralysis of the respiratory muscles (chiefly the diaphragm and intercostals) without discernible clinical involvement of the cranial nerves or vital centers that control respiration, circulation, and body temperature. The cervical and thoracic spinal cord segments are chiefly affected. Pure bulbar poliomyelitis involves paralysis of the motor cranial nerve nuclei with or without involvement of the vital centers. Involvement of the 9th, 10th, and 12th cranial nerves results in paralysis of the pharynx, tongue, and larynx with consequent airway obstruction. Bulbospinal poliomyelitis with respiratory insufficiency affects the respiratory muscles and results in coexisting bulbar paralysis.

The clinical findings associated with involvement of the respiratory muscles include (1) anxious expression; (2) inability to speak without frequent pauses, resulting in short, jerky, "breathless" sentences; (3) increased respiratory rate; (4) movement of the ala nasi and of the accessory muscles of respiration; (5) inability to cough or sniff with full depth; (6) paradoxical abdominal movements caused by diaphragmatic immobility due to spasm or weakness of 1 or both leaves; and (7) relative immobility of the intercostal spaces, which may be segmental, unilateral, or bilateral. When the arms are weak, and especially when deltoid paralysis occurs, there may be impending respiratory paralysis because the phrenic nerve nuclei are in adjacent areas of the spinal cord. Observation of the patient's capacity for thoracic breathing while the abdominal muscles are splinted manually indicates minor degrees of paresis. Light manual splinting of the thoracic cage will help to assess the effectiveness of diaphragmatic movement.

DIAGNOSIS. Poliomyelitis should be considered in any unimmunized or incompletely immunized child with paralytic disease. VAPP should be considered in any child with paralytic disease occurring 7–14 days after receiving the orally administered polio vaccine (OPV). VAPP can occur at later times after administration, and should be considered in any child with paralytic disease in countries or regions where wild-type poliovirus has been eradicated and the OPV has been administered to the child or a contact. The combination of fever, headache, neck and back pain, asymmetric flaccid paralysis without sensory loss, and pleocytosis does not regularly occur in any other illness.

The World Health Organization (WHO) recommends that the laboratory diagnosis of poliomyelitis be confirmed by isolation and identification of poliovirus in the stool, with specific identification of wild-type and vaccine-type strains. In suspected cases of acute flaccid paralysis, 2 stool specimens should be collected 24–48 hr apart, as soon as possible after the diagnosis of poliomyelitis is suspected. Poliovirus concentrations are high in the stool in the 1st week after the onset of paralysis, which is the optimal time for collection of stool specimens. Polioviruses may be isolated from 80–90% of acutely ill patients, whereas <20% may yield virus within 3–4 wk after onset of paralysis. Because most children with spinal or bulbospinal poliomyelitis have constipation, rectal straws may be used to obtain specimens; ideally a minimum of 8–10 g of stool should be collected. In laboratories that can isolate poliovirus, isolates should be sent to either the Centers for Disease Control and Prevention or to 1 of the WHO-certified poliomyelitis laboratories where DNA sequence analysis can be performed to distinguish between wild poliovirus and neurovirulent, revertant OPV strains. With the current WHO plan for global eradication of poliomyelitis, most regions of the world (the Americas, Europe, Australia) have been certified wild-poliovirus free; in these areas, poliomyelitis is most often caused by vaccine strains. Hence it is critical to differentiate between wild-type and revertant vaccine-type strains.

The CSF, while often normal during the minor illness, with CNS involvement demonstrates a pleocytosis of 20–300 cells/mm^3. The cells in the CSF may be polymorphonuclear early during the course of the disease but shift to mononuclear cells soon afterward. By the 2nd week of major illness, the CSF cell count falls to near-normal values. In contrast, the CSF protein is normal or only slightly elevated at the outset of CNS disease but usually rises to 50–100 mg/dL by the 2nd week of illness. In polioencephalitis, the CSF may remain normal or show minor changes. Serologic testing demonstrates seroconversion or a 4-fold or greater increase in antibody titers, when measured during the acute phase of illness and 3–6 wk later.

Differential Diagnosis. Poliomyelitis should be considered in the differential diagnosis of any case of paralysis, and is only 1 of many causes of acute flaccid paralysis in children and adults. There are numerous other causes of acute flaccid paralysis (see Table 246-1). In most conditions, the clinical features are sufficient to differentiate between these various causes, but in some cases nerve conduction studies and electromyograms in addition to muscle biopsies may be required.

The possibility of polio should be considered in any case of acute flaccid paralysis even in countries where polio has been eradicated. The diagnoses most often confused with polio are VAPP, West Nile virus, and other enteroviruses, as well as Guillain-Barré syndrome, transverse myelitis, and traumatic paralysis. In Guillain-Barré syndrome, which is the most difficult to distinguish from poliomyelitis, the paralysis is characteristically symmetric and sensory changes and pyramidal tract signs are common; these are absent in poliomyelitis. Fever, headache, and meningeal signs are less notable, and there are few cells but

TABLE 246-1. Differential Diagnosis of Acute Flaccid Paralysis

SITE, CONDITION, FACTOR, OR AGENT	CLINICAL FINDINGS	ONSET OF PARALYSIS	PROGRESSION OF PARALYSIS	SENSORY SIGNS AND SYMPTOMS	REDUCED OR ABSENT DEEP TENDON REFLEXES	RESIDUAL PARALYSIS	PLEOCYTOSIS
ANTERIOR HORN CELLS OF SPINAL CORD							
Poliomyelitis (wild and VAPP)	Paralysis	Incubation period 7–14 days (4–35 days)	24–48 hr to onset of full paralysis; proximal > distal, asymmetric	No	Yes	Yes	Aseptic meningitis (moderate polymorphonuclear leukocytes at 2–3 days)
Nonpolio enterovirus	Hand-foot-and-mouth disease, aseptic meningitis, AHC	As in poliomyelitis	As in poliomyelitis	No	Yes	Yes	As in poliomyelitis
West Nile virus	Meningitis encephalitis	As in polio	As in polio	No	Yes	Yes	Yes
OTHER NEUROTROPIC VIRUSES							
Rabies virus		Months to years	Acute, symmetric, ascending	Yes	Yes	No	+/–
Varicella-zoster virus	Exanthematous vesicular eruptions	Incubation period 10–21 days	Acute, symmetric, ascending	Yes	+/–	+/–	Yes
Japanese encephalitis virus		Incubation period 5–15 days	Acute, proximal, asymmetric	+/–	+/–	+/–	Yes
GUILLAIN-BARRÉ SYNDROME							
Acute inflammatory polyradiculoneuropathy	Preceding infection, bilateral facial weakness	Hours to 10 days	Acute, symmetric, ascending (days to 4 wk)	Yes	Yes	+/–	No
Acute motor axonal neuropathy	Fulminant, widespread paralysis, bilateral facial weakness, tongue involvement	Hours to 10 days	1–6 days	No	Yes	+/–	No
ACUTE TRAUMATIC SCIATIC NEURITIS							
Intramuscular gluteal injection	Acute, asymmetrical	Hours to 4 days	Complete, affected limb	Yes	Yes	+/–	No
Acute transverse myelitis	Preceding *Mycoplasma pneumoniae Schistosoma*, other parasitic or viral infection	Acute, symmetric hypotonia of lower limbs	Hours to days	Yes	Yes, early	Yes	Yes
Epidural abscess	Headache, back pain, local spinal tenderness, meningismus	Complete		Yes	Yes	+/–	Yes
Spinal cord compression; trauma		Complete	Hours to days	Yes	Yes	+/–	+/–
NEUROPATHIES							
Exotoxin of *Corynebacterium diphtheriae*	In severe cases, palatal paralysis, blurred vision	Incubation period 1–8 wk (paralysis 8–12 wk after onset of illness)		Yes	Yes		+/–
Toxin of *Clostridium botulinum*	Abdominal pain, diplopia, loss of accommodation, mydriasis	Incubation period 18–36 hr	Rapid, descending, symmetric	+/–	No		No
Tick bite paralysis	Ocular symptoms	Latency period 5–10 days	Acute, symmetric, ascending	No	Yes		No
DISEASES OF THE NEUROMUSCULAR JUNCTION							
Myasthenia gravis	Weakness, fatigability, diplopia, ptosis, dysarthria		Multifocal	No	No	No	No
DISORDERS OF MUSCLE							
Polymyositis	Neoplasm, autoimmune disease	Subacute, proximal > distal	Weeks to months	No	Yes		No
Viral myositis		Pseudoparalysis	Hours to days	No	No		No
METABOLIC DISORDERS							
Hypokalemic periodic paralysis		Proximal limb, respiratory muscles	Sudden postprandial	No	Yes	+/–	No
ICU WEAKNESS							
Critical illness polyneuropathy	Flaccid limbs and respiratory weakness	Acute, following SIRS/sepsis	Hours to days	+/–	Yes	+/–	No

AHC, acute hemorrhagic conjunctivitis; ICU, intensive care unit; SIRS, systemic inflammatory response syndrome.
Modified from Marx A, Glass JD, Sutter RW: Differential diagnosis of acute flaccid paralysis and its role in poliomyelitis surveillance. *Epidemiol Rev* 2000;22:298–316.

an elevated protein level in the CSF. Transverse myelitis progresses rapidly over hours to days, causing an acute symmetric paralysis of the lower limbs with concomitant anesthesia and diminished sensory perception. Autonomic signs of hypothermia in the affected limbs are common, and there is bladder dysfunction. The CSF is usually normal. Traumatic neuritis occurs from a few hours to a few days after the traumatic event, is asymmetric, acute, and affects only 1 limb. There is reduced or absent muscle tone and deep tendon reflexes in the affected limb with pain in the gluteus. The CSF is normal.

Conditions causing pseudoparalysis do not present with nuchal-spinal rigidity or pleocytosis. These causes include unrecognized trauma, transient (toxic) synovitis, acute osteomyelitis, acute rheumatic fever, scurvy, and congenital syphilis (pseudoparalysis of Parrot).

TREATMENT. There is no specific antiviral treatment for poliomyelitis. The management is supportive and aimed at limiting progression of disease, prevention of ensuing skeletal deformities, and preparation of the child and family for prolonged treatment required and for permanent disability if this seems likely. Patients with the nonparalytic and mildly paralytic forms of poliomyelitis may be treated at home. All intramuscular injections and surgical procedures are contraindicated during the acute phase of the illness, especially in the 1st week of illness, because these may result in progression of disease.

Abortive Poliomyelitis. Supportive treatment with analgesics, sedatives, an attractive diet, and bed rest until the child's temperature is normal for several days is usually sufficient. Avoidance of exertion for the ensuing 2 wk is desirable, and there should be careful neurologic and musculoskeletal examinations 2 mo later to detect any minor involvement.

Nonparalytic Poliomyelitis. Treatment for the nonparalytic form is similar to that for the abortive form; in particular, relief is indicated for the discomfort of muscle tightness and spasm of the neck, trunk, and extremities. Analgesics are more effective when they are combined with the application of hot packs for 15–30 min every 2–4 hr. Hot tub baths are sometimes useful. A firm bed is desirable and can be improvised at home by placing table leaves or a sheet of plywood beneath the mattress. A footboard or splint should be used to keep the feet at a right angle to the legs. Because muscular discomfort and spasm may continue for some weeks, even in the nonparalytic form, hot packs and gentle physical therapy may be necessary. Such patients should also be carefully examined 2 mo after apparent recovery to detect minor residual effects that might cause postural problems in later years.

Paralytic Poliomyelitis. Most patients with the paralytic form require hospitalization with complete physical rest in a calm atmosphere for the 1st 2–3 weeks. Suitable body alignment is necessary for comfort and to avoid excessive skeletal deformity. A neutral position with the feet at a right angle to the legs, knees slightly flexed, and hips and spine straight is achieved by use of boards, sandbags, and, occasionally, light splint shells. The position should be changed every 3–6 hr. Active and passive movements are indicated as soon as the pain has disappeared. Moist hot packs may relieve muscle pain and spasm. Opiates and sedatives are permissible only if no impairment of ventilation is present or impending. Constipation is common, and fecal impaction should be prevented. When bladder paralysis occurs, a parasympathetic stimulant such as bethanechol may induce voiding in 15–30 min; some patients do not respond, and others respond with nausea, vomiting, and palpitations. Bladder paresis rarely lasts more than a few days. If bethanechol fails, manual compression of the bladder and the psychologic effect of running water should be tried. If catheterization must be performed, care must be taken to prevent urinary tract infections. An appealing diet and a relatively high fluid intake should be started at once unless the patient is vomiting. Additional salt should be provided if the environmental temperature is high or if the application of hot packs induces sweating. Anorexia is common initially. Adequate dietary and fluid intake can be maintained by placement of a central venous catheter. An orthopedist and a physiatrist should see these patients as early in the course of the illness as possible and should assume responsibility for their care before fixed deformities develop.

The management of pure bulbar poliomyelitis consists of maintaining the airway and avoiding all risk of inhalation of saliva, food, or vomitus. Gravity drainage of accumulated secretions is favored by using the head-low (foot of bed elevated 20–25 degrees) prone position with the face to one side. Patients with weakness of the muscles of respiration or swallowing should be nursed in a lateral or semi-prone position. Aspirators with rigid or semirigid tips are preferred for direct oral and pharyngeal aspiration, and soft, flexible catheters may be used for nasopharyngeal aspiration. Fluid and electrolyte equilibrium is best maintained by intravenous infusion because tube or oral feeding in the 1st few days may incite vomiting. In addition to close observation for respiratory insufficiency, the blood pressure should be taken at least twice daily because hypertension is not uncommon and occasionally leads to hypertensive encephalopathy. Patients with pure bulbar poliomyelitis may require tracheostomy because of vocal cord paralysis or constriction of the hypopharynx; most patients who recover have little residual impairment, although some exhibit mild dysphagia and occasional vocal fatigue with slurring of speech.

Impaired ventilation must be recognized early; mounting anxiety, restlessness, and fatigue are early indications for preemptive intervention. Tracheostomy is indicated for some patients with pure bulbar poliomyelitis, spinal respiratory muscle paralysis, and bulbospinal paralysis because these patients are generally unable to cough, sometimes for many months. Mechanical respirators are often needed.

COMPLICATIONS. Paralytic poliomyelitis may be associated with numerous complications. Acute gastric dilatation may occur abruptly during the acute or convalescent stage, causing further respiratory embarrassment; immediate gastric aspiration and external application of ice bags are indicated. Melena severe enough to require transfusion may result from single or multiple superficial intestinal erosions; perforation is rare. Mild hypertension for days or weeks is common in the acute stage and probably related to lesions of the vasoregulatory centers in the medulla and especially to underventilation. In the later stages, because of immobilization, hypertension may occur along with hypercalcemia, nephrocalcinosis, and vascular lesions. Dimness of vision, headache, and a lightheaded feeling associated with hypertension should be regarded as premonitory of a frank convulsion. Cardiac irregularities are uncommon, but electrocardiographic abnormalities suggesting myocarditis are not rare. Acute pulmonary edema occurs occasionally, particularly in patients with arterial hypertension. Hypercalcemia occurs due to skeletal decalcification that begins soon after immobilization and results in hypercalciuria, which in turn predisposes the patient to urinary calculi, especially when urinary stasis and infection are present. High fluid intake is the only effective prophylactic measure.

PROGNOSIS. The outcome of inapparent, abortive poliomyelitis and aseptic meningitis syndromes is uniformly good, with death being exceedingly rare and with no long-term sequelae. The outcome of paralytic disease is determined primarily by degree and severity of CNS involvement. In severe bulbar poliomyelitis, the mortality rate may be as high as 60%, whereas in less severe bulbar involvement and/or spinal poliomyelitis, the mortality rate varies from 5 to 10%, generally from causes other than the poliovirus infection.

Maximum paralysis usually occurs 2–3 days after the onset of the paralytic phase of the illness, with stabilization followed by gradual return of muscle function. The recovery phase lasts usually about 6 mo, beyond which persisting paralysis is permanent. Male children but female adults, generally, are more likely to develop paralysis. Mortality and the degree of disability are greater after the age of puberty. Pregnancy is associated with an increased risk for paralytic disease. Tonsillectomy and intramuscular injections may enhance the risk for acquisition of bulbar or localized disease, respectively. Increased physical activity, exercise, and fatigue during the early phase of illness have been cited as factors leading to an increased risk for paralytic disease. Finally, it has been clearly demonstrated that type 1 poliovirus has the greatest propensity for natural poliomyelitis and type 3 for VAPP.

Postpolio Syndrome. After an interval of 30–40 yr, as many as 30–40% of persons who survived paralytic poliomyelitis in childhood may experience muscle pain and exacerbation of existing weakness, or they may develop new weakness or paralysis. This entity, referred to as postpolio syndrome, has been reported only in persons who were infected in the era of wild-type poliovirus circulation. Risk factors for postpolio syndrome include increasing length of time since acute poliovirus infection, presence of permanent residual impairment after recovery from acute illness, and female sex.

PREVENTION. Vaccination is the only effective method of preventing poliomyelitis. Hygienic measures help limit the spread of the infection among young children, but immunization is necessary to control transmission among all age groups. Both the inactivated polio vaccine (IPV), which is currently produced using improved methods compared with the original vaccine and is sometimes referred to as enhanced IPV, and the live-attenuated OPV have established efficacy in preventing poliovirus infection and paralytic poliomyelitis. Both vaccines induce production of antibodies against the 3 strains of poliovirus. IPV elicits higher serum IgG antibody titers, but the OPV also induces significantly greater mucosal IgA immunity in the oropharynx and gastrointestinal tract that limits replication of the wild poliovirus at these sites. Transmission of wild poliovirus by fecal spread is limited in OPV recipients. The immunogenicity of IPV is not affected by the presence of maternal antibodies, and IPV has no adverse effects. Live vaccine may undergo reversion to neurovirulence as it multiplies in the human intestinal tract and may cause VAPP in vaccinees or in their contacts. The overall risk for recipients is 1 case/6.2 million doses. As of January 2000, the IPV-only schedule is recommended for routine polio vaccination in the USA. All children should receive 4 doses of IPV at 2 mo, 4 mo, 6–18 mo, and 4–6 yr of age.

In 1988, the World Health Assembly resolved to eradicate poliomyelitis globally by 2000, and remarkable progress had been made toward reaching this target. To achieve this, the WHO used 4 basic strategies: routine immunization, National Immunization Days (NIDs), acute flaccid paralysis surveillance, and mopping up immunization. The OPV is the only vaccine recommended by the WHO for eradication. By the end of 1999, at least 1 set of NIDs had been conducted in every polio-endemic country in the world. This strategy has resulted in a greater than 99% decline in poliomyelitis cases; and in early 2002, there were only 10 countries in the world endemic for poliomyelitis. Globally there were 542 cases of polio, of which 478 were confirmed as wild virus in 2001. As of December 8, 2005, 1,598 confirmed wild-virus polio cases and 35 vaccine-associated cases were reported worldwide since the beginning of the year. This is 3 times the number in 2001. As long as the OPV is being used, there is the potential that circulating vaccine-derived poliovirus (VDPV) will acquire the neurovirulent phenotype and transmission characteristics of the wild-type polioviruses. VDPV emerges from the OPV because of continuous replication in immunodeficient persons (iVDPVs) or by circulation in populations with low vaccine coverage (cVDPVs). Outbreaks of cVDPV occurred in Hispaniola, the Philippines, and Madagascar in 2001, while endemic cVDPV circulation occurred in Egypt from 1988 to 1993. The risk appears to be highest with the type 2 strain. The main risk factor for cVDPV circulation appears to be low levels of vaccine coverage. It has also been estimated that the global burden of VAPP varies from 250 to 500 annually, now becoming more common than wild-type poliovirus. The rate of VAPP in the USA was 1 case of paralytic disease per 760,000 1st doses of OPV distributed, with 93% of recipient cases and 76% of VAPP occurring after administration of the 1st or 2nd dose of OPV. The risk for paralysis in the immunodeficient recipient may be as much as 6,800 times that in normal subjects. HIV has not been found to be a cause for long-term excretion of virus.

Currently there are several countries that are global priorities because they face challenges in eradication (see Fig. 246-1). Polioviruses are endemic in India, Pakistan, Afghanistan, Egypt, and Nigeria; transmission has been re-established in Africa: Niger, Chad, Mali, Cameroon, and Sudan, with imported outbreaks in Ethiopia, Eritrea, Somalia, Madagascar, Angola, Yemen, and Indonesia. All of these countries require multilevel eradication activities, but they pose a problem to surrounding countries because wild-type poliovirus can be imported from these countries to countries where immunization rates have dropped (and have been declared poliomyelitis free), such as Yemen and Indonesia. Hence, to achieve global eradication, intensified activities are being conducted in all the remaining identified countries. The WHO has reset the target of 2008 for global eradication of poliomyelitis and the endgame strategy for polio eradication has changed. Global synchronous cessation of the OPV may need to be coordinated by the WHO after coordinated mass campaigns. Transition to IPV in developed countries with high rates of immunization coverage is encouraged. In countries where the risk for VAPP is higher than the risk for transmission of poliomyelitis, the injectable poliovirus vaccines continue to confer immunity and are being used routinely, and in other countries that either cannot afford IPV or where transmission is endemic, the OPV will continue to be used both in routine immunization as well as in the NID strategy.

Centers for Disease Control and Prevention: Poliomyelitis prevention in the United States. Updated recommendations of the Advisory Committee on Immunization Practices (ACIP). *MMWR* 2000;49(RR-5):1–22.

Centers for Disease Control and Prevention: Resurgence of wild poliovirus type 1 transmission and consequences of importation—21 countries, 2002–2005. *MMWR* 2006;55:145–150.

Centers for Disease Control and Prevention: Poliovirus infections in four unvaccinated children—Minnesota, August–October 2005. *MMWR* 2005;54:1053–1055.

Dalakas MC, Elder G, Hallett M, et al: A long-term follow-up study of patients with post-poliomyelitis neuromuscular symptoms. *N Engl J Med* 1986;314:959–963.

Hennessey KA, Lago H, Diomande F, et al: Poliovirus vaccine shedding among persons with HIV in Abidjan, Cote d'Ivoire. *J Infect Dis* 2005;192: 2124–2128.

Kew OM, Wright PF, Agol VI, et al: Circulating vaccine-derived polioviruses: Current state of knowledge. *Bull WHO* 2004;82:16–23.

Marx A, Glass JD, Sutter RW: Differential diagnosis of acute flaccid paralysis and its role in poliomyelitis surveillance. *Epidemiol Rev* 2000;22:298–316.

Pallansch MA, Sandhu HS: The eradication of polio—progress and challenges. *N Engl J Med* 2006;355:2508–2511.

Racaniello VR: One hundred years of poliovirus pathogenesis. *Virology* 2006;344:9–16.

Chapter 247 ■ Nonpolio Enteroviruses

Mark J. Abzug

The genus *Enterovirus* contains a large number of viral agents that produce a broad range of important illnesses. The genus name reflects the importance of the gastrointestinal tract as the primary site of viral invasion and replication and source for transmission. Viremic spread to distant sites accounts for the majority of clinical manifestations.

ETIOLOGY. Enteroviruses are nonenveloped, single-stranded, positive-sense viruses in the Picornaviridae ("small RNA virus") family, which also includes the genera *Rhinovirus, Hepatovirus* (hepatitis A virus), and *Parechovirus* and genera containing related animal viruses. The original human enterovirus subgroups—polioviruses (see Chapter 246), coxsackieviruses, and echoviruses—were differentiated by their replication patterns in tissue culture and animals (Table 247-1). Coxsackieviruses derive their name from Coxsackie, New York, where they were discovered. The name for echoviruses reflects an acronym applied to a group of viruses originally without disease associations (*e*nteric *c*ytopathic *h*uman *o*rphan *viruses*). The human enteroviruses have been recently reclassified based on nucleotide and amino acid sequences into 5 species, polioviruses and human enteroviruses A–D. Enterovirus serotypes are distinguished by antigenic and genetic sequence differences; newer enteroviruses are classified by numbering. Although >70 serotypes have been identified, 10–15 account for the majority of disease. No enterovirus disease is uniquely associated with any specific

TABLE 247-1. Classification of Human Enteroviruses

Family	Picornaviridae
Genus	*Enterovirus*
Subgroups*	Poliovirus serotypes 1–3
	Coxsackie A virus serotypes A1–A22, A24 (A23 reclassified as echovirus 9)
	Coxsackie B virus serotypes B1–B6
	Echovirus serotypes 1–9, 11–27, 29–33 (echoviruses 10 and 28 reclassified as non-enteroviruses; echovirus 34 reclassified as coxsackievirus A24; echoviruses 22 and 23 have been reclassified within the genus *Parechovirus*)
	Numbered enterovirus serotypes (enterovirus 72 reclassified as hepatitis A virus)†

*The human enteroviruses have been alternatively classified based on nucleotide and amino acid sequences into 5 species (polioviruses and human EVs A–D)

†Several new serotypes of enteroviruses have recently been proposed.

serotype, although certain manifestations are preferentially associated with specific serotypes.

EPIDEMIOLOGY. Enterovirus infections are very common and have a worldwide distribution. In temperate climates there is an annual epidemic peak in summer and fall, although some transmission occurs year-round. Enteroviruses are responsible for 33–65% of acute febrile illnesses and 55–65% of hospitalizations for suspected sepsis in infants during the summer and fall in the United States, and 25% year-round. In tropical and semitropical areas, enteroviruses frequently circulate year-round. In general, only a few serotypes circulate simultaneously. Infections by different serotypes in the same child can occur within the same season. Factors associated with increased incidence and/or severity include young age, male sex, poor hygiene, overcrowding, and low socioeconomic status; more than 25% of symptomatic infections occur in children <1 yr of age. Breast-feeding reduces the risk for infection.

Humans are the only known reservoir for human enteroviruses. Virus is primarily spread person to person, by the fecal-oral and respiratory routes, and vertically, from mother to neonate, either prenatally or in the peripartum period. Enteroviruses can survive on environmental surfaces, permitting transmission via fomites. Enteroviruses also can frequently be isolated from water sources and sewage and can survive for months in wet soil. Although environmental contamination (of drinking water, swimming pools) may occasionally be responsible for transmission, it is likely most often the result, rather than the cause, of human infection. Transmission occurs within families with young children (>50% spread to susceptible household contacts), daycare centers, playgrounds, summer camps, orphanages, and hospital nurseries; severe secondary infections may occur in nursery outbreaks. Diaper changing is a risk factor for spread, whereas handwashing decreases transmission.

Large outbreaks of enterovirus infections include epidemics of echovirus 9 or 30 associated with aseptic meningitis in France and the United States; epidemics of hand-foot-and-mouth disease associated with severe central nervous system (CNS) and/or cardiopulmonary disease due to enterovirus 71 in Malaysia, Japan, Taiwan, and Australia; outbreaks of acute hemorrhagic conjunctivitis due to enterovirus 70 and coxsackievirus A24 in India, Malaysia, and other tropical regions and in temperate climates, including the USA; and community outbreaks of enterovirus meningitis and enterovirus-associated uveitis. Reverse transcription polymerase chain reaction (RT-PCR), restriction fragment length polymorphism analysis, single-strand conformation polymorphism analysis, and genomic sequencing help to rapidly identify outbreaks, demonstrate commonality of outbreak strains, and detect differences among epidemic strains and older prototype strains. Such analyses have demonstrated that enteroviruses undergo recombination and genetic drift that can lead to changes in genomic sequence and antigenicity.

The incubation period of enterovirus infections is typically 3–6 days, except for acute hemorrhagic conjunctivitis, which has an incubation period of 1–3 days. Infected children, both symptomatic and asymptomatic, frequently shed enteroviruses from the respiratory tract for <1–3 wk, whereas fecal shedding continues up to 7–11 wk postinfection.

PATHOGENESIS. Following acquisition by the oral or respiratory route, initial viral replication occurs in the pharynx and intestine, possibly within mucosal M cells. The absence of an envelope favors survival in the gastrointestinal tract. Cell surface macromolecules, including poliovirus receptor, integrin very late activation antigen VLA-2, decay accelerating factor complement regulatory protein (DAF/CD55), intercellular adhesion molecule-1 (ICAM-1), and coxsackievirus-adenovirus receptor, serve as receptors. Two or more enteroviruses may invade and replicate in the gastrointestinal tract simultaneously, but replication of 1 type often hinders growth of the heterologous type, a phenomenon known as **interference.**

After an enterovirus attaches to its cell surface receptor, a conformational change in surface capsid proteins facilitates penetration and viral uncoating with release of viral RNA in the cytoplasm. Translation of the positive-sense RNA ensues, resulting in synthesis of a polyprotein that undergoes sequential cleavage by proteinases encoded in the polyprotein. Several proteins produced guide synthesis of negative-sense RNA that serves as a template for replication of new positive-sense RNA. The genome is approximately 7,500 nucleotides long and includes a highly conserved 5′ noncoding region important for replication efficiency and a highly conserved 3′ polyA region, which flank a continuous region encoding viral proteins. The 5′ end is covalently linked to a small viral protein (VPg) necessary for initiation of RNA synthesis. There is significant variation in the genomic regions encoding the structural proteins (with corresponding variability in antigenicity). Replication is followed by further cleavage of proteins and assembly of the genome and the viral capsid into 30 nm icosahedral virions. Of the 4 structural proteins (VP1–4) in the viral capsid (additional regulatory proteins such as an RNA-dependent RNA polymerase and proteases are also present in the virion), VP1 is the most important determinant of serotype specificity. Approximately 10^4–10^5 virions are released from an infected cell by lysis within 5–10 hr of infection.

Initial replication in the pharynx and intestine is followed within days by multiplication in lymphoid tissue such as tonsils, Peyer patches, and regional lymph nodes. A primary, transient viremia (**minor viremia**) results in spread to distant parts of the reticuloendothelial system, including the liver, spleen, bone marrow, and distant lymph nodes. Host immune responses may limit replication and progression beyond the reticuloendothelial system, resulting in subclinical infection. Clinical infection occurs if replication proceeds in the reticuloendothelial system and virus spreads via a secondary, sustained viremia (**major viremia**) to target organs such as the CNS, heart, and skin. Tropism to target organs is determined in part by the infecting serotype.

Enteroviruses can damage a wide variety of organs and systems, including the CNS, heart, liver, lungs, pancreas, kidneys, muscle, and skin. Damage is mediated by local necrosis and the host inflammatory response. CNS infections are often associated with mononuclear pleocytosis of the cerebrospinal fluid (CSF), composed of macrophages and activated T lymphocytes, and a mixed meningeal inflammatory response. Parenchymal involvement may occur at multiple sites, including cerebral white and gray matter, cerebellum, basal ganglia, brainstem, and spinal cord; perivascular and parenchymal mixed or lymphocytic inflammation, gliosis, cellular degeneration, and neuronophagocytosis may be present. Encephalitis during recent outbreaks of enterovirus 71 has been characterized by severe brainstem and spinal cord involvement, frequently complicated by pulmonary edema and/or interstitial pneumonitis and cardiopulmonary failure, presumed to be secondary to brainstem damage, sympathetic hyperactivity, and central nervous system and systemic inflammatory responses, and, only occasionally, myocarditis. Enterovirus myocarditis is characterized by perivascular and interstitial mixed inflammatory infiltrates and myocyte damage, possibly mediated by direct viral cytolytic and immune-mediated mechanisms. Chronic inflammation may persist after viral clearance. Possible persistent infection by enteroviruses, especially coxsackie B viruses, has been implicated in dilated cardiomyopathy. Enteroviral RNA sequences and/or antigens have been demonstrated in a significant percentage of cardiac tissues in some, but not other, series.

Severe **neonatal infections** can manifest as hepatic necrosis, hemorrhage, inflammation, endotheliitis, and veno-occlusive disease; myocardial mixed inflammatory infiltrates, edema, and necrosis; meningeal and brain inflammation, hemorrhage, gliosis, and necrosis; inflammation, hemorrhage, thrombosis, and necrosis in the lungs, pancreas, and adrenal glands; and disseminated intravascular coagulation. In utero infections are characterized by placentitis and infection of multiple fetal organs such as heart, lung, and brain.

Development of circulating type-specific neutralizing antibodies appears to be the most important immune defense, mediating prevention against and recovery from infection. Immunoglobulin M (IgM) antibodies, followed by long-lasting IgA and IgG antibodies, and secretory IgA, mediating mucosal immunity, are produced. Although local reinfection of the gastrointestinal tract can occur, replication is usually limited and not associated with disease. In vitro and animal experiments suggest that heterotypic antibody may enhance disease caused by a different serotype. Cellular defenses (especially macrophage function) may play an important role in recovery from infection. Altered T-lymphocyte responses to enterovirus 71 were associated with severe meningoencephalitis during recent epidemics.

Antibody deficiency states, including hypogammaglobulinemia and agammaglobulinemia, predispose to severe, often chronic enterovirus infections. Similarly, perinatally infected neonates who lack maternal type-specific antibody to the infecting virus are at risk for severe disease. Other risk factors for significant illness include young age, immune suppression (post-transplantation), and, according to animal models and/or epidemiologic observations, exercise, cold exposure, malnutrition, and pregnancy.

CLINICAL MANIFESTATIONS. Clinical manifestations are protean, ranging from asymptomatic infection or undifferentiated febrile or respiratory illnesses in the majority, to, less frequently, severe diseases such as meningoencephalitis, myocarditis, and neonatal sepsis. A majority of individuals shedding virus are asymptomatic or have very mild illness, yet may serve as a significant source for spread of infection. Symptomatic disease is generally more frequent in young children.

Nonspecific Febrile Illness. Nonspecific febrile illnesses are the most common symptomatic manifestations and are especially frequent in infants and young children. These are difficult to clinically differentiate from serious infections such as bacteremia and bacterial meningitis, and necessitate diagnostic testing, presumptive therapy, and hospitalizations for suspected bacterial infection in young infants.

Illness usually begins with abrupt onset of fever, usually 38.5–40°C (101–104°F), malaise, and irritability. Other symptoms may include lethargy, anorexia, diarrhea, nausea, vomiting, abdominal discomfort, rash, sore throat, and respiratory symptoms. In older children, headache and myalgia frequently occur. Findings are generally nonspecific and may include mild conjunctivitis, mild pharyngeal injection, and cervical lymphadenopathy. Meningitis may be present, but, in infants, specific clinical features distinguishing those with meningitis are often lacking. Fever lasts a mean of 3 days. Occasionally, fever is biphasic. Duration of illness is usually 4–7 days but can range from 1 day to >1 wk. White blood cell (WBC) count and results of other routine laboratory tests are generally normal. Concomitant enterovirus and bacterial infection has been observed in a small number of infants.

Enterovirus illnesses may be associated with a wide variety of skin manifestations including macular, maculopapular, urticarial, vesicular, and petechial eruptions. In general, the frequency is inversely related to age. Some serotypes commonly associated with rashes are echoviruses 9, 11, 16, and 25; coxsackie A viruses 2, 4, 9, and 16; and coxsackie B viruses 3–5. Virus can occasionally be recovered from vesicular skin lesions.

Hand-Foot-and-Mouth Disease. Hand-foot-and-mouth disease, 1 of the more distinctive rash syndromes, is most frequently caused by coxsackievirus A16 and can also be caused by enterovirus 71; coxsackie A viruses 5, 7, 9, and 10; and coxsackie B viruses 2 and 5. It is usually a mild illness, with or without low-grade fever. The oropharynx is inflamed and contains scattered vesicles on the tongue, buccal mucosa, posterior pharynx, palate, gingiva, and/or lips (Fig. 247-1). These may ulcerate, leaving 4–8 mm shallow lesions with surrounding erythema. Maculopapular, vesicular, and/or pustular lesions may also occur on the hands and fingers, feet, and buttocks and groin; hands are more commonly involved than the feet (see Fig. 247-1). Lesions on the hands and feet are usually tender vesicles varying in size from 3 to 7 mm and are more common on dorsal surfaces but frequently also occur on palms and soles. Vesicles resolve in about 1 wk. Buttock lesions do not usually progress to vesiculation. Disseminated vesicular rashes may complicate pre-existing eczema. Hand-foot-and-mouth disease caused by enterovirus 71 is frequently more severe than that due to coxsackievirus A16, with high rates of neurologic disease, including, in outbreaks, brainstem encephalomyelitis, neurogenic pulmonary edema, pulmonary hemorrhage, shock, and rapid death, especially in young children.

Herpangina. Herpangina is characterized by sudden onset of fever, sore throat, dysphagia, and lesions in the posterior pharynx. Temperatures can range from normal to 41°C (106°F); fever tends to be greater in younger patients. Headache and backache may occur in older children, and vomiting and abdominal pain occur in 25%. Characteristic lesions, present on the anterior tonsillar pillars, soft palate, uvula, tonsils, posterior pharyngeal wall, and, occasionally, the posterior buccal surfaces, are discrete 1–2 mm vesicles and ulcers that enlarge over 2–3 days to 3–4 mm and are surrounded by erythematous rings that vary in size up to 10 mm. Typically about 5 lesions are present, with a range of 1 to >15. The remainder of the pharynx appears normal or minimally erythematous. Most cases are mild and have no complications; however, some are associated with aseptic meningitis or other more severe illness. Fever generally lasts 1–4 days, and resolution of symptoms occurs in 3–7 days. A variety of enteroviruses can cause herpangina, although coxsackie A viruses are implicated most often. Some cases of herpangina have been noted during recent outbreaks of enterovirus 71 disease.

Respiratory Manifestations. Respiratory symptoms such as sore throat and coryza frequently accompany and sometimes dominate enterovirus illnesses. Findings may include upper respiratory symptoms, wheezing, exacerbation of asthma, apnea, respiratory distress, pneumonia, otitis media, bronchiolitis, croup, parotitis, and pharyngotonsillitis, which may be exudative occasionally.

Pleurodynia (**Bornholm disease**) is an epidemic or sporadic illness characterized by paroxysmal thoracic pain, due to myositis involving chest and abdominal wall muscles. Etiologic agents are most frequently coxsackieviruses B3 and B5, as well as coxsackieviruses B1 and B2 and echoviruses 1 and 6. In epidemics, children and adults are affected, but most cases occur in persons younger than 30 yr. Prodromal symptoms such as malaise, myalgias, and headache are followed by sudden onset of fever and spasmodic, pleuritic pain, typically located in the chest or upper

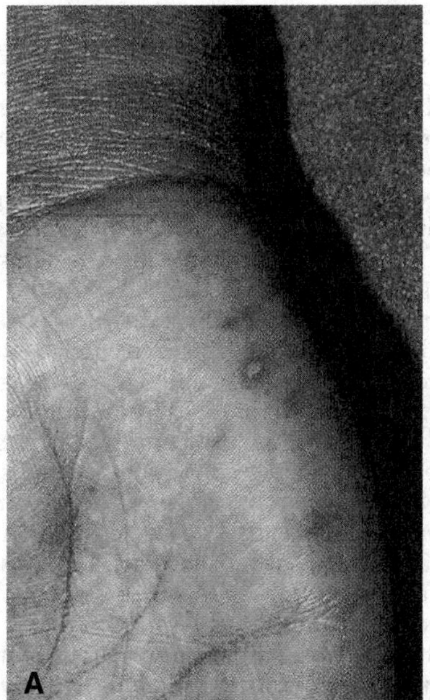

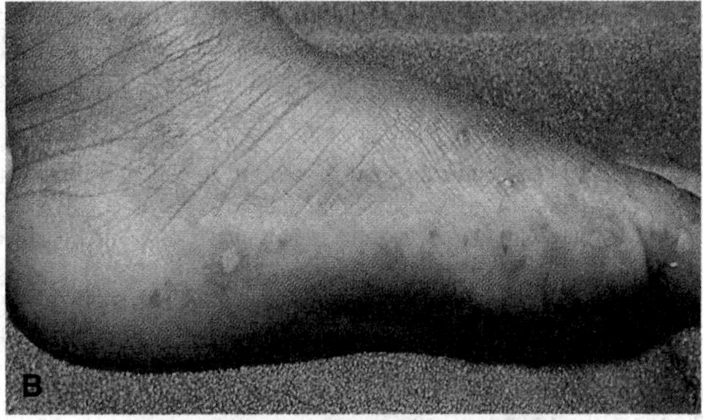

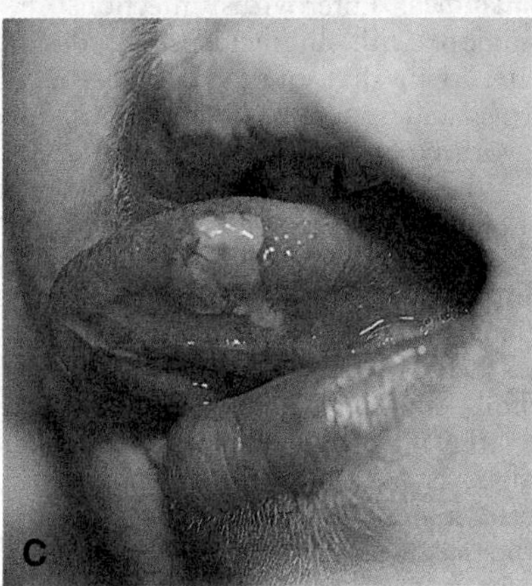

Figure 247-1. *A,* Oval blisters of the palms in a child with hand-foot-and-mouth disease (coxsackie virus A16 infection). *B,* Oval blisters on the feet of a child with hand-foot-and-mouth disease. *C,* Erosion of the tongue in a child with hand-foot-and-mouth disease. (From Weston WL, Lane AT, Morelli JG: *Color Textbook of Pediatric Dermatology,* 3rd ed. St. Louis, MO, Mosby, 2002, p 109.)

abdomen and aggravated by coughing, sneezing, deep breathing, or other movement. During spasms, which last from a few minutes to several hours, pain may be severe and respirations are usually rapid, shallow, and grunting, suggesting pneumonia or pleural inflammation. A pleural friction rub may be noted during pain episodes, although chest radiographs are generally normal. Pain localized to the abdomen is frequently crampy, suggesting colic in the younger child. A pale, sweaty, shocklike appearance may suggest intestinal obstruction; tenderness and guarding may suggest appendicitis and peritonitis. Illness usually lasts 3–6 days, but can last up to a couple of weeks. It is frequently biphasic and, rarely, is associated with several recurrent episodes over a period of a few weeks, with less prominent fever during recurrences. Pleurodynia may be associated with meningitis, orchitis, myocarditis, or pericarditis.

Life-threatening pulmonary edema, hemorrhage, and/or interstitial pneumonitis may occur in patients with enterovirus 71 encephalitis.

Ocular Manifestations. Enterovirus 70 and coxsackievirus A24 are the primary causes of epidemics of **acute hemorrhagic conjunctivitis.** Epidemics are explosive, spread mainly via eye-hand-fomite-eye transmission. School-aged children, teenagers, and adults 20–50 yr of age have the highest attack rates, with young children less often affected. Sudden onset of severe eye pain is associated with photophobia, blurred vision, lacrimation, conjunctival erythema and congestion, lid edema, preauricular lymphadenopathy, and, in some cases, subconjunctival hemorrhages and superficial punctate keratitis. Eye discharge is initially serous but becomes mucopurulent with secondary bacterial infection. Systemic symptoms including fever are rare, although clinical manifestations suggestive of pharyngoconjunctival fever occasionally occur. Recovery is usually complete within 1–2 wk. Polyradiculoneuropathy or paralytic disease following enterovirus 70 acute hemorrhagic conjunctivitis occurs occasionally. Other enteroviruses have occasionally been implicated as causes of keratoconjunctivitis.

Epidemic and sporadic uveitis in infants caused by subtypes of enterovirus 11 and 19 can be associated with severe complications, including destruction of the iris, cataracts, and glaucoma. Enteroviruses have been implicated in cases of chorioretinitis, uveoretinitis, optic neuritis, and unilateral acute idiopathic maculopathy.

Myocarditis and Pericarditis. Enteroviruses account for approximately 25–35% of cases of myocarditis and pericarditis with proven cause (see Chapters 439 and 440). Coxsackie B viruses are the most common etiologic types, although coxsackie A viruses and echoviruses also may be causative. Adolescents and young adults, especially males, are disproportionately affected by enterovirus myocarditis. Myopericarditis may be the dominant feature of illness or it may be part of disseminated disease, as in neonates. Disease ranges from relatively mild to severe. Upper respiratory symptoms frequently precede cardiac manifestations such as fatigue, dyspnea, chest pain, congestive heart failure, and dysrhythmias. Presentations may mimic myocardial infarction; in other cases, patients present with sudden death (including apparent sudden infant death syndrome). A pericardial friction rub indicates pericardial involvement. Chest radiography often demonstrates cardiac enlargement. Electrocardiography frequently reveals ST segment, T wave, and/or rhythm abnormalities, and echocardiography may confirm cardiac dilatation, reduced contractility, and/or pericardial effusion. Myocardial enzymes may be elevated. The acute mortality of enterovirus myocarditis is 0–4%. Recovery is complete without residual disability in the majority. Occasionally, chronic cardiomyopathy, inflammatory ventricular microaneurysms, or constrictive pericarditis may result. The role of persistent enterovirus infection in chronic dilated cardiomyopathy is controversial. Enterovirus infection has been implicated in late adverse cardiac events following heart transplantation. Myocardial dysfunction observed in enterovirus 71 outbreaks most commonly has occurred without evidence of myocarditis and may be of neurogenic origin.

Gastrointestinal and Genitourinary Manifestations. Gastrointestinal symptoms, including emesis (especially with meningitis), diarrhea, which is rarely severe, and abdominal pain, are frequent but generally not dominant features. Diarrhea, hematochezia, pneumatosis intestinalis, and necrotizing enterocolitis have been observed in premature infants during nursery outbreaks. Enterovirus infection has been implicated as a cause of chronic intestinal inflammation in hypogammaglobulinemic patients and as a cause of sporadic hepatitis in normal children. Many coxsackie B virus and echovirus serotypes have been reported to cause pancreatitis, which may result in transient exocrine pancreatic insufficiency. Coxsackie B viruses are 2nd only to mumps as causative agents of orchitis. The illness is frequently biphasic; fever and pleurodynia or meningitis are followed by apparent recovery and then, in about 2 wk, by orchitis, often with epididymitis.

Neurologic Manifestations. Enteroviruses are the most common cause of viral meningitis in mumps-immunized populations, accounting for >90% of cases in which a causative agent is identified. Meningitis is particularly common in infants, especially those <3 mo of age, and disease frequently occurs as part of community epidemics. Frequently implicated serotypes include coxsackieviruses B2–5; echoviruses 4, 6, 7, 9, 11, 16, and 30; and enteroviruses 70 and 71. Most cases in infants and young children are mild and lack specific signs and symptoms. Fever is present in 50–100%; other findings may include irritability, malaise, headache, photophobia, nausea, emesis, anorexia, lethargy, rash, cough, rhinorrhea, pharyngitis, diarrhea, and myalgia. Nuchal rigidity is apparent in more than half of children >1–2 yr of age. Some cases are biphasic, with fever and nonspecific symptoms for a few days, followed by absence of symptoms for several days, then return of fever with meningeal signs. Fever usually resolves in 3–5 days, and other symptoms in infants and young children usually resolve within 1 wk. Symptoms tend to be more severe and longer lasting in adults. **CSF** findings include pleocytosis that generally is <500 WBC/mm^3, but occasionally as high as 1,000–8,000 WBC/mm^3, and often consists predominantly of polymorphonuclear cells in the 1st 48 hr before becoming mostly mononuclear; normal or slightly low glucose, with 10% <40 mg/dL; and normal or mildly increased protein, generally <100 mg/dL. CSF occasionally has normal parameters despite positive viral culture or PCR, particularly in the 1st few months of life. Complications occur in approximately 10% of young children, including simple and complex seizures, obtundation, increased intracranial pressure, syndrome of inappropriate antidiuretic hormone secretion, ventriculitis, transient cerebral arteriopathy, and coma. The prognosis for most children with meningitis is good.

Enteroviruses are also responsible for 10–20% of cases of encephalitis with an identified cause. Frequently implicated serotypes include echoviruses 3, 4, 6, 9, and 11; coxsackieviruses B2, B4, and B5; coxsackievirus A9; and enterovirus 71. After initial nonspecific symptoms, encephalitis becomes apparent by progression to marked confusion, weakness, lethargy, and/or irritability. Depression is usually generalized, although focal findings such as focal motor seizures, hemichorea, acute cerebellar ataxia, aphasia, extrapyramidal symptoms, and/or focal imaging abnormalities may occur. Encephalitis includes a spectrum from altered mental status to coma to decerebrate status; long-term neurologic sequelae or death may follow severe disease. Recurrent cases have been observed rarely.

Neurologic disorders have been prominent in recent epidemics of enterovirus 71 disease. The majority of affected children had hand-foot-and-mouth disease, some had herpangina, and others had no mucocutaneous manifestations. Neurologic syndromes that occurred in a fraction of infected children included meningitis, meningoencephalomyelitis, poliomyelitis-like paralytic disease, Guillain-Barré syndrome, transverse myelitis, cerebellar ataxia, opsoclonus-myoclonus syndrome, benign intracranial hypertension, and brainstem encephalitis (**rhombencephalitis** involving the midbrain, pons, and medulla). The latter is characterized by myoclonus, vomiting, ataxia, nystagmus, tremor, and cranial nerve abnormalities and brainstem lesions on magnetic resonance imaging. Although findings were mild and reversible in some, in others rapid progression to neurogenic pulmonary edema and hemorrhage, cardiopulmonary failure, shock, and coma developed. High mortality rates have been reported, especially in children <5 yr of age. Neurologic deficits such as central hypoventilation, bulbar dysfunction, and limb weakness have been observed among survivors. Similar clinical pictures have been produced by other enterovirus serotypes (echovirus 7).

Patients with **antibody deficiencies** and **combined immunodeficiency** (including human immunodeficiency virus infection and acute lymphocytic leukemia) are at risk for acute or, more commonly, **chronic meningoencephalitis;** the latter is characterized by persistent CSF abnormalities, viral detection by culture or PCR for years, and recurrent encephalitis and/or progressive neurologic deterioration. Clinical findings include insidious intellectual or personality deterioration, altered mental status, seizures, motor weakness, and increased intracranial pressure. Although disease may wax and wane, deficits generally become progressive, and ultimately it is frequently fatal or leads to long-term sequelae. A **dermatomyositis-like syndrome,** hepatitis, arthritis, or myocarditis may supervene in advanced stages. Chronic enterovirus meningoencephalitis has become less common with antibody replacement with high-dose intravenous immunoglobulin.

Nonpoliovirus enteroviruses, especially enteroviruses 70 and 71, coxsackievirus A7, and coxsackie B viruses, can cause poliomyelitis-like acute flaccid paralysis with motor weakness due to anterior horn cell involvement. Disease tends to be milder than that caused by poliovirus, with less bulbar involvement and less persistent weakness. Other neurologic syndromes observed include cerebellar ataxia, transverse myelitis, Guillain-Barré syndrome, peripheral neuritis, optic neuritis, acute disseminated encephalomyelitis, and sudden hearing loss.

Myositis and Arthritis. Although myalgia is common, direct evidence of muscle involvement, including rhabdomyolysis, muscle swelling, focal myositis, and polymyositis, has uncommonly been reported. A dermatomyositis-like syndrome and arthritis can be seen in enterovirus-infected hypogammaglobulinemic patients. Enteroviruses rarely cause arthritis in normal hosts.

Neonatal Infections. Enterovirus infections in neonates are relatively common, with an incidence of disease comparable with or greater than that of neonatal herpes simplex virus, cytomegalovirus, and group B streptococcus disease. Infection frequently is with coxsackieviruses B2–5 and echoviruses 6, 9, 11, and 19, although many serotypes have been implicated. Enteroviruses may be acquired vertically before, during, or after delivery; horizontally from family members; or by transmission in hospital nurseries (sporadic or epidemic). Infection in utero may be associated with fetal demise, nonimmune hydrops fetalis, neonatal illness, and, possibly, congenital anomalies and neurodevelopmental sequelae. Neonatal infection may range from asymptomatic (the majority) to benign febrile illness to severe multisystem disease. Most affected newborns are full term and previously well; maternal history often reveals a recent viral illness, including fever and, frequently, abdominal pain. Symptoms may occur as early as day 1 of life, with onset of severe disease generally within the 1st 2 wk. Frequent findings include fever or hypothermia, irritability, lethargy, anorexia, rash (usually maculopapular, occasionally petechial or papulovesicular), jaundice, respiratory symptoms, apnea, hepatomegaly, abdominal distention, emesis, diarrhea, and decreased perfusion. Most symptomatic neonates have benign courses, with resolution of fever in an average of 3 days and of other symptoms in about 1 wk. A biphasic course may occur occasionally. A minority has severe disease that may be dominated by any combination of sepsis, meningoencephalitis, myocarditis, hepatitis, coagulopathy, and pneumonitis. Meningoencephalitis may be indicated by focal or complex seizures, bulging fontanelle, nuchal rigidity, or reduced level of consciousness. Myocarditis, most often associated with coxsackie B virus infection, may be suggested by tachycardia, dyspnea, cyanosis, and cardiomegaly. Hepatitis and pneumonitis are more associated with echovirus infection, although they may occur with coxsackie B viruses. Laboratory evaluation may reveal leukocytosis, thrombocytopenia, CSF pleocytosis, elevated transaminases and bilirubin, coagulopathy, pulmonary infiltrates, and electrocardiographic changes. Complications include CNS necrosis and generalized or focal neurologic compromise; arrhythmias, congestive heart failure, myocardial infarction, and pericarditis; hepatic necrosis and failure; intracranial or other bleeding; adrenal necrosis and hemorrhage; and rapidly progressive pneumonitis. Myositis, necrotizing enterocolitis, inappropriate antidiuretic hormone secretion, hemophagocytic syndrome, bone marrow failure, and sudden death are rare events. Mortality with severe disease is significant and is most often associated with hepatitis and associated bleeding complications, myocarditis, or pneumonitis. The majority of survivors have gradual resolution of hepatic and cardiac dysfunction, although chronic calcific myocarditis and ventricular aneurysm can occur. CNS infection, especially encephalitis, may be associated with sequelae of speech and language impairment; cognitive deficits; spasticity, hypotonicity, or weakness; seizure disorders; microcephaly or hydrocephaly; and ocular abnormalities. However, most survivors appear not to have long-term sequelae. Risk factors for severe disease include illness onset in the 1st few days of life, maternal illness just prior to or at delivery, prematurity, male sex, infection by echovirus 11 or a coxsackie B virus, positive serum viral culture, absence of neutralizing antibody to the infecting virus, and evidence of severe hepatitis and/or multisystem disease.

Stem Cell Transplant Recipients. Severe and/or prolonged infections have been reported in stem cell transplant recipients including progressive pneumonia, severe diarrhea, pericarditis, heart failure, and disseminated disease. These infections are associated with high fatality rates.

DIAGNOSIS. Clues to enterovirus infection include relatively specific findings such as hand-foot-and-mouth disease or herpangina lesions, consistent seasonality, known community outbreak, and exposure to enterovirus-compatible disease. In the neonate, history of maternal fever, malaise, and/ or abdominal pain near delivery during enterovirus season is suggestive.

Viral culture using a combination of cell lines that support growth of enteroviruses is the gold standard method for confirmation. Sensitivity ranges from 50–75% and can be increased by culturing multiple sites. In children with meningitis, culture yield is enhanced by culturing CSF plus additional sites such as the throat and rectum. In neonates, yields of 30–70% are achieved when blood, urine, and CSF are cultured in addition to mucosal swabs. A major limitation is the inability of most coxsackie A viruses to grow in culture. Culture yield may also be limited by neutralizing antibody in patient specimens, improper specimen handling, or insensitivity of the cell lines used. Culture is relatively slow, with 3–8 days usually required to detect growth. Centrifugation-enhanced antigen detection has been coupled with culture (shell vial techniques) to shorten the time required for detection, but sensitivity has been limiting. Although cultivation of an enterovirus from any site can generally be considered evidence of recent infection, isolation from the rectum or stool can reflect shedding from a more remote infection. Similarly, recovery from a mucosal site may suggest an association with an illness, whereas recovery from a normally sterile site such as CSF, blood, or tissue is more conclusive evidence of causation. Serotype identification, performed in reference laboratories with neutralizing antisera, is generally only required for investigation of an outbreak or an unusual disease manifestation, or to distinguish nonpoliovirus enteroviruses from polioviruses, either vaccine or wild type.

Direct testing of patient specimens for enterovirus nucleic acid overcomes the imperfect sensitivity and delayed results of culture. RT-PCR detection of highly conserved areas of the enterovirus genome can detect the majority of enteroviruses, including coxsackie A viruses (but frequently not the parechoviruses) in a variety of specimens, including CSF; serum; urine; conjunctival, nasopharyngeal, throat, and rectal specimens; and tissues such as myocardium, liver, or brain. Sensitivity and specificity are high, and testing can be accomplished in periods as short as a few hours. Real-time, quantitative PCR assays and nested PCR assays with enhanced sensitivity have been developed, as have enterovirus-containing multiplex PCR assays and nucleic acid sequence–based amplification (NASBA) assays. Results of PCR testing of CSF from children with aseptic meningitis and from hypogammaglobulinemic patients with chronic meningoencephalitis are frequently positive despite negative cultures. In ill neonates and young infants, PCR testing of serum and urine is associated with higher yields than culture. Routine application of PCR to testing of CSF from infants and young children with meningitis decreases diagnostic testing, duration of hospital stay, antibiotic use, and overall costs. Enterovirus RNA may be detected in nasopharyngeal secretions for as long as 2–3 wk after onset of a respiratory infection. Sequence analysis of amplified nucleic acid can be used for serotype identification. Serotype-specific (enterovirus 71) PCR assays have also been developed. In the case of enterovirus 71, the yield of specimens other than CSF (throat and rectal swabs) is greater (by PCR or culture) than the yield of CSF specimens, which uncommonly are virus positive.

Enterovirus infections can be detected serologically by demonstration, in serum or CSF, of a rise in neutralizing, complement fixation, ELISA, or other type-specific antibody or by detection of serotype-specific IgM antibody. However, serologic testing requires presumptive knowledge of the infecting serotype. Sensitivity may also be limited. Except for epidemiologic studies or severe cases with findings characteristic of specific serotypes (e.g., enterovirus 71), serology is generally less useful than culture or nucleic acid detection.

DIFFERENTIAL DIAGNOSIS. The differential diagnosis of enterovirus infections varies with the clinical presentation (Table 247-2).

TREATMENT. Newborns, infants, and children presenting with nonspecific febrile illnesses or meningitis frequently require diagnostic evaluations for bacterial and herpes simplex virus infection and hospitalization for presumptive treatment until tests rule out these diagnoses. Neonates with severe disease and infants and children with myocarditis or concerning neurologic diseases may require intensive supportive care, including cardiorespiratory support and blood products. Liver transplantation has been used for neonates with progressive hepatic failure.

Immune globulin has been used as a therapy for enterovirus infections for several reasons. The humoral immune response is a key defense against enterovirus infection, and lack of neutralizing antibody is a risk factor for symptomatic infection. Immune globulin products contain neutralizing antibodies to many of the commonly circulating serotypes, although titers vary with serotype and among products. Maintenance intravenous immune globulin for hypogammaglobulinemic patients has been associated with a decrease in chronic enterovirus disease. Therefore, anecdotal, uncontrolled use of intravenous immune globulin or infusion of maternal convalescent plasma to treat newborns with severe disease has been reported. The 1 reported randomized, controlled trial was too small to demonstrate significant clinical benefits, although neonates who received immune globulin containing high neutralizing titers to their own isolates had shorter periods of viremia and viruria. Intravenous and intraventricular immune globulin has been used to treat hypogammaglobulinemic patients with chronic enterovirus meningoencephalitis, with variable success. Intravenous immune globulin and corticosteroids have been used for patients with enterovirus 71–associated neurologic disease. A retrospective study suggested that treatment of

TABLE 247-2. Differential Diagnosis of Enterovirus Infections

CLINICAL MANIFESTATION	BACTERIAL PATHOGENS	VIRAL PATHOGENS
Nonspecific febrile illness	*Streptococcus pneumoniae, Haemophilus influenzae* type b, *Neisseria meningitidis*	Influenza viruses, human herpesviruses 6 and 7
Exanthems/enanthems	Group A streptococcus, *Staphylococcus aureus, Neisseria meningitidis*	Herpes simplex virus, adenoviruses, varicella-zoster virus, Epstein-Barr virus, measles virus, rubella virus, human herpesviruses 6 and 7
Respiratory illness/conjunctivitis	*Streptococcus pneumoniae, Haemophilus influenzae* (nontypable and type b), *Neisseria meningitidis Mycoplasma pneumoniae, Chlamydia pneumoniae*	Adenoviruses, influenza viruses, respiratory syncytial virus, parainfluenza viruses, rhinovirus
Myocarditis/pericarditis	*Staphylococcus aureus, Haemophilus influenzae* type b, *Mycoplasma pneumoniae*	Adenoviruses, influenza virus, parvovirus
Meningitis/encephalitis	*Streptococcus pneumoniae, Haemophilus influenzae* type b, *Neisseria meningitidis, Mycobacterium tuberculosis, Borrelia burgdorferi, Mycoplasma pneumoniae, Bartonella henselae, Listeria monocytogenes*	Herpes simplex virus, West Nile virus, Influenza viruses, adenovirus, Epstein-Barr virus, mumps virus, lymphocytic choriomeningitis virus, arboviruses
Neonatal infections	Group B streptococcus, gram-negative enteric bacilli, *Listeria monocytogenes, Enterococcus*	Herpes simplex virus, adenoviruses, cytomegalovirus, rubella virus

presumed viral myocarditis with immune globulin was associated with improved outcome; however, virologic diagnoses were not made. Evaluation of corticosteroids and other immunosuppressive therapy for myocarditis has been inconclusive. Successful treatment of enterovirus myocarditis with interferon-α has been reported anecdotally. Interferon-β was associated with viral clearance and improved cardiac function in a pilot study of chronic cardiomyopathy with persistence of enterovirus or adenovirus genome.

Specific antiviral agents that act at several key steps in the enterovirus life cycle, including attachment, uncoating, translation, protease activity, and replication, are being evaluated. The investigational agent that advanced furthest, pleconaril, inhibits picornavirus (enteroviruses and rhinoviruses) attachment and uncoating. This generally well tolerated, oral medication was associated with modest acceleration of symptom resolution in some trials involving children and adults with enterovirus meningitis and slightly faster clinical resolution of picornavirus upper respiratory tract infections. Uncontrolled experience suggested possible benefits in high-risk enterovirus infections such as severe neonatal disease, myocarditis, encephalitis, paralytic disease, and infections in immunodeficient patients (including chronic meningoencephalitis). Viral resistance was observed in a minority of patients. The Food and Drug Administration denied an application for licensure due to concern for cytochrome P450 3A induction and potential interactions with hormonal contraceptives and other medications. Although a randomized trial in neonates with severe hepatitis, coagulopathy, and/or myocarditis is in progress, commercial development of oral pleconaril has been suspended. Development of a nasal preparation targeting rhinovirus respiratory infections remains a possibility.

COMPLICATIONS AND PROGNOSIS. The prognosis in the vast majority of infections is excellent. Morbidity and mortality are primarily associated with myocarditis, neurologic disease, severe neonatal infections, and infections in immune compromised hosts.

PREVENTION. Vaccines for virulent serotypes such as enterovirus 71 are being investigated but are not currently available. The 1st line of defense against transmission is basic hygiene, such as handwashing to prevent fecal-oral and respiratory spread within families and schools; avoidance of shared utensils and drinking containers and other potential fomites; and disinfection of contaminated surfaces. Appropriate treatment of drinking water and swimming pool water may be important to preventing transmission. Infection control techniques such as cohorting have proven effective in limiting nursery outbreaks. Prophylactic administration of intramuscular or intravenous immunoglobulin or convalescent plasma has been used in nursery epidemics to prevent infection or ameliorate symptomatic disease; simultaneous infection control interventions make it difficult to determine efficacy.

Pregnant women near term should avoid contact with individuals ill with probable enterovirus infections. If a pregnant woman develops an illness likely to be caused by an enterovirus, it is advisable not to proceed with emergent delivery unless there is concern for fetal compromise or obstetric emergencies cannot be excluded. Rather, it may be advantageous to extend pregnancy, allowing the fetus time to passively acquire protective antibodies. A strategy of prophylactically administering immune globulin to neonates born to mothers with enterovirus infections is untested.

Maintenance antibody replacement with high-dose intravenous immune globulin for patients with hypogammaglobulinemia has reduced the incidence of chronic enterovirus meningoencephalitis.

Abzug MJ: Presentation, diagnosis, and management of enterovirus infections in neonates. *Paediatr Drugs* 2004;6:1–10.

Bernit E, de Lamballerie X, Zandotti C, et al: Prospective investigation of a large outbreak of meningitis due to echovirus 30 during summer 2000 in Marseilles, France. *Medicine* 2004;83:245–253.

Bryant PA, Tingay D, Dargaville PA, et al: Neonatal coxsackie B virus infection—a treatable disease? *Eur J Pediatr* 2004;163:223–228.

Centers for Disease Control and Prevention: Outbreaks of aseptic meningitis associated with echoviruses 9 and 30 and preliminary surveillance reports on enterovirus activity—United States, 2003. *MMWR* 2003;52:761–764.

Centers for Disease Control and Prevention: Aseptic meningitis outbreak associated with echovirus 9 among recreational vehicle campers, Connecticut, 2003. *MMWR* 2004;53:710–713.

Chang LY, Huang LM, Gau SSF, et al: Neurodevelopment and cognition in children after enterovirus 71 infection. *N Engl J Med* 2007;356:1226–1234.

Chang L, Tsao K, Hsia S, et al: Transmission and clinical features of enterovirus 71 infections in household contacts in Taiwan. *JAMA* 2004;291:222–227.

Kao SJ, Yang FL, Hsu YH, Chen HI: Mechanism of fulminant pulmonary edema caused by enterovirus 71. *Clin Infect Dis* 2004;38:1784–1788.

Khetsuriani N, LaMonte A, Oberste S, Pallansch M: Neonatal enterovirus infections reported to the National Surveillance System in the United States, 1983–2003. *Pediatr Infect Dis* 2006;25:889–892.

Lin T, Kao H, Hsieh S, et al: Neonatal enterovirus infections: Emphasis on risk factors of severe and fatal infections. *Pediatr Infect Dis* 2003;22:889–894.

Modlin JF: Enterovirus déjà vu. *N Engl J Med* 2007;356:1204–1205.

Ramers C, Billman G, Hartin M, et al: Impact of a diagnostic cerebrospinal fluid enterovirus polymerase chain reaction test on patient management. *JAMA* 2000;283:2680–2685.

Rotbart HA, Webster AD: Treatment of potentially life-threatening enterovirus infections with pleconaril. *Clin Infect Dis* 2001;32:228–235.

Verboon-Maciolek MA, Nijhuis M, van Loon AM, et al: Diagnosis of enterovirus infection in the first 2 months of life by real-time polymerase chain reaction. *Clin Infect Dis* 2003;37:1–6.

Webster ADB: Pleconaril—An advance in the treatment of enteroviral infection in immuno-compromised patients. *J Clin Virol* 2005;32:1–6.

Chapter 248 ■ Parvovirus B19

William C. Koch

Parvovirus B19 is the cause of **erythema infectiosum** or "**fifth disease**," 1 of the classic childhood exanthems.

ETIOLOGY. Parvovirus B19 (B19) was discovered in 1975 and is a member of the genus *Erythrovirus* in the family Parvoviridae. Parvoviruses are small DNA viruses and infect a variety of animal species. As a group, parvoviruses include a number of important animal pathogens such as canine parvovirus and feline panleukopenia virus. B19 is the only parvovirus that is pathogenic in humans. It does not infect other animals, and animal parvoviruses do not infect humans.

B19 is composed of an icosahedral protein capsid without an envelope that contains a single-stranded DNA genome of approximately 5.5 kb. It is relatively heat and solvent resistant. It is antigenically distinct from other mammalian parvoviruses and has only 1 known serotype. Parvoviruses replicate in mitotically active cells and require host cell factors present in late S phase to replicate. B19 can be propagated in tissue culture only in erythropoietin-stimulated erythropoietic cells derived from human bone marrow, umbilical cord blood, or primary fetal liver culture.

EPIDEMIOLOGY. Infections with parvovirus B19 are common and worldwide. Clinically apparent infections, such as the rash illness of erythema infectiosum and transient aplastic crisis, are most prevalent in school-aged children, with 70% of cases occurring between 5 and 15 yr of age. Seasonal peaks occur in the late winter and spring, with sporadic infections throughout the year. Seroprevalence increases with age, with 40–60% of adults having evidence of prior infection.

Transmission of B19 is by the respiratory route, presumably via large droplet spread from nasopharyngeal viral shedding. The transmission rate is 15–30% among susceptible household contacts, and mothers are more commonly infected than fathers. In outbreaks of erythema infectiosum in elementary schools, the secondary attack rates range from 10 to 60%. Nosocomial outbreaks also occur with secondary attack rates of 30% among susceptible health care workers.

Although respiratory spread is the primary mode of transmission, B19 is also transmissible in blood and blood products, which has been documented among children with hemophilia receiving pooled-donor clotting factor. Given the resistance of the virus to solvents, fomite transmission could be important in child-care centers and other group settings, but this mode of transmission has not been documented.

PATHOGENESIS. The primary target of B19 infection is the erythroid cell line, specifically erythroid precursors near the pronormoblast stage. Viral infection produces cell lysis leading to a progressive depletion of erythroid precursors and a transient arrest of erythropoiesis. The virus has no apparent effect on the myeloid cell line. The tropism for erythroid cells is related to the erythrocyte P blood group antigen, which is the cell receptor for the virus that is also found on endothelial cells, placental cells, and fetal myocardial cells. Thrombocytopenia and neutropenia are often observed clinically, but their pathogenesis is unexplained.

Experimental infection of normal volunteers revealed a biphasic illness. From 7 to 11 days after inoculation, subjects had viremia and nasopharyngeal viral shedding with fever, malaise, and rhinorrhea. Reticulocyte counts dropped to undetectable levels but resulted only in a mild, clinically insignificant fall in serum hemoglobin. With the appearance of specific antibodies, symptoms resolved and hemoglobin returned to normal. Several subjects experienced a rash associated with arthralgia 17–18 days after inoculation. Some manifestations of B19 infection, such as transient aplastic crisis, appear to be a direct result of viral infection, whereas others, including the exanthema and arthritis, appear to be **postinfectious phenomena** related to the immune response. Skin biopsy of patients with erythema infectiosum reveals edema in the epidermis and a perivascular mononuclear infiltrate compatible with an immune-mediated process.

Individuals with **chronic hemolytic anemia** and increased red cell turnover are very susceptible to perturbations in erythropoiesis. Infection with B19 leads to a transient arrest in red cell production and a precipitous fall in serum hemoglobin, often requiring transfusion. The reticulocyte count falls to near 0, reflecting the lysis of infected erythroid precursors. Humoral immunity is crucial in controlling infection. Specific immunoglobulin M (IgM) appears within 1–2 days followed by anti-B19 IgG, leading to control of the infection, restoration of reticulocytosis, and a rise in serum hemoglobin.

Individuals with **impaired humoral immunity** are at increased risk for more serious or persistent infection with B19, which usually manifests as chronic red cell aplasia, although neutropenia, thrombocytopenia, and marrow failure are also described. Children on chemotherapy for leukemia or other forms of cancer, those with congenital immunodeficiency states, transplant patients, and those with AIDS are at risk for chronic B19 infections.

Infections in the **fetus** and **neonate** are somewhat analogous to infections in immunocompromised persons. B19 is associated with nonimmune fetal hydrops and stillbirth in women experiencing a primary infection but does not appear to be teratogenic. Like most mammalian parvoviruses, B19 can cross the placenta and cause fetal infection during primary maternal infection. Parvovirus cytopathic effects are seen primarily in erythroblasts of the bone marrow and sites of extramedullary hematopoiesis in the liver and spleen. Fetal infection can presumably occur as early as 6 weeks of gestation, when erythroblasts are first found in the fetal liver; after the 4th month of gestation hematopoiesis switches to the bone marrow. In some cases, fetal infection leads to a profound fetal anemia and subsequent high-output cardiac failure (see Chapter 103). **Fetal hydrops** ensues, often associated with fetal mortality. There may also be a direct effect of the virus on myocardial tissue that contributes to the cardiac failure. However, most infections during pregnancy result in normal deliveries at term. Some of these asymptomatic infants have been reported to have chronic postnatal infection with B19 that is of unknown significance.

CLINICAL MANIFESTATIONS. Many infections are clinically inapparent. Infected children characteristically develop the rash illness of erythema infectiosum. Adults, especially women, frequently develop acute polyarthropathy with or without a rash.

Erythema Infectiosum (Fifth Disease). The most common manifestation of parvovirus B19 is erythema infectiosum, also known as fifth disease, which is a benign, self-limited exanthematous illness of childhood. It was the 5th in a classification scheme of common childhood exanthems. The preceding 4 exanthems were measles, scarlet fever, rubella, and Filatov-Dukes disease (an atypical scarlet fever), with roseola infantum as the "sixth disease."

The incubation period for erythema infectiosum is 4–28 days (average 16–17 days). The prodromal phase is mild and consists of low-grade fever, headache, and symptoms of mild upper respiratory tract infection. The hallmark of erythema infectiosum is the characteristic rash, which occurs in 3 stages that are not always distinguishable. The initial stage is an erythematous facial flushing, often described as a "**slapped-cheek" appearance** (Fig. 248-1). The rash spreads rapidly or concurrently to the trunk and proximal extremities as a diffuse macular erythema in the 2nd stage. Central clearing of macular lesions occurs promptly, giving

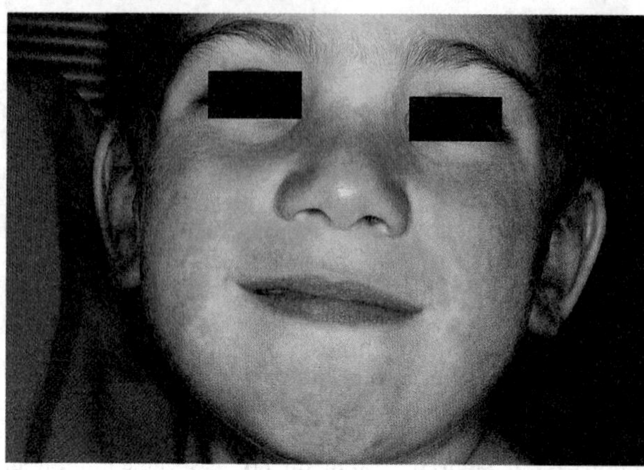

Figure 248-1. Erythema infectiosum. Erythema of the bilateral cheeks, which has been likened to a "slapped cheeks" appearance. (From Paller AS, Macini AJ: *Hurwitz Clinical Pediatric Dermatology,* 3rd ed. Philadelphia, Elsevier Saunders, 2006, p 431.)

the rash a **lacy, reticulated appearance** (Fig. 248-2). The rash tends to be more prominent on extensor surfaces, sparing the palms and soles. Affected children are afebrile and not ill appearing. Older children and adults often complain of mild pruritus. The rash resolves spontaneously without desquamation but tends to wax and wane over 1–3 wk. It can recur with exposure to sunlight, heat, exercise, and stress. Lymphadenopathy and atypical papular, purpuric, vesicular rashes are also described.

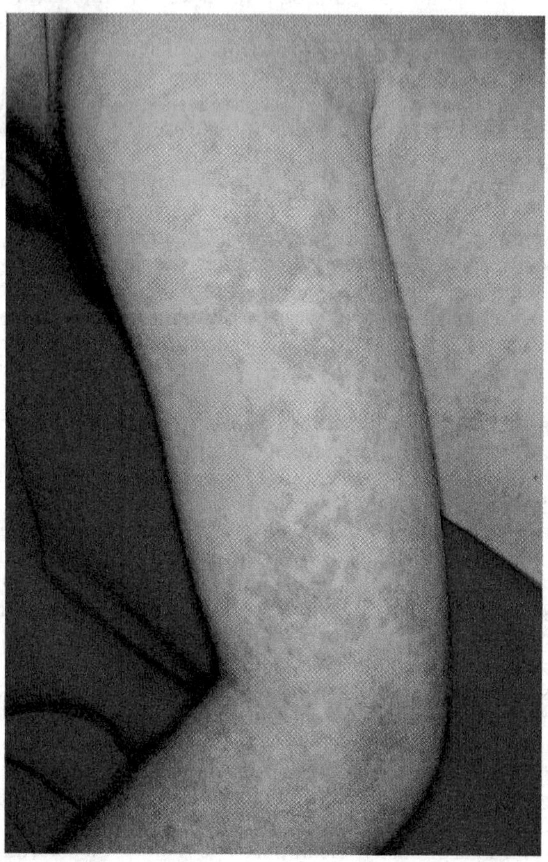

Figure 248-2. Erythema infectiosum. Reticulate erythema on the upper arm of a patient with erythma infectiosum. (From Paller AS, Macini AJ: *Hurwitz Clinical Pediatric Dermatology,* 3rd ed. Philadelphia, Elsevier Saunders, 2006, p 431.)

Arthropathy. Arthritis and arthralgia may occur in isolation or with other symptoms. Joint symptoms are much more common among adults and older adolescents. Females are affected more frequently than males. In 1 large outbreak of fifth disease, 60% of adults and 80% of adult women reported joint symptoms. Joint symptoms range from diffuse polyarthralgia with morning stiffness to frank arthritis. The joints most often affected are the hands, wrists, knees, and ankles, but practically any joint may be affected. The joint symptoms are self-limited and, in the majority of patients, resolve within 2–4 wk. Some patients may have a prolonged course of many months, suggesting rheumatoid arthritis. Transient rheumatoid factor positivity is reported in some of these patients but with no joint destruction.

Transient Aplastic Crisis. The transient arrest of erythropoiesis and absolute reticulocytopenia induced by B19 infection leads to a sudden fall in serum hemoglobin in individuals with chronic hemolytic conditions. This B19-induced red cell aplasia or transient aplastic crisis occurs in patients with all types of chronic hemolysis and/or rapid red cell turnover, including sickle cell disease, thalassemia, hereditary spherocytosis, and pyruvate kinase deficiency. In contrast to children with erythema infectiosum only, these patients are ill with fever, malaise, and lethargy and have signs and symptoms of profound anemia, including pallor, tachycardia, and tachypnea. Rash is rarely present. The incubation period for transient aplastic crisis is shorter than for erythema infectiosum because it occurs coincident with the viremia. Children with sickle cell hemoglobinopathies may also have a concurrent vaso-occlusive pain crisis, further confusing the clinical presentation.

Immunocompromised Persons. Persons with impaired humoral immunity are at risk for chronic parvovirus B19 infection. Chronic anemia is the most common manifestation, sometimes accompanied by neutropenia, thrombocytopenia, or complete marrow suppression. Chronic infections occur in persons receiving cancer chemotherapy or immunosuppressive therapy for transplantation, and persons with congenital immunodeficiencies, AIDS, and functional defects in IgG production who are unable to generate neutralizing antibodies.

Fetal Infection. Primary maternal infection is associated with nonimmune fetal hydrops and intrauterine fetal demise, with the risk for fetal loss after infection estimated at <5%. The mechanism of fetal disease appears to be a viral-induced red cell aplasia at a time when the fetal erythroid fraction is rapidly expanding. This can lead to profound anemia, high-output cardiac failure, and fetal hydrops. Viral DNA has been detected in infected abortuses. The 2nd trimester seems to be the most sensitive period, but fetal losses are reported at every stage of gestation. If maternal infection is suspected, fetal ultrasonography and measurement of the peak systolic flow velocity of the middle cerebral artery are sensitive, noninvasive procedures to diagnose fetal anemia and hydrops. Most infants infected in utero are born normally at term, even some that had ultrasonographic evidence of hydrops. Some of these infants may acquire a chronic or persistent postnatal infection with B19, but its significance is unknown. Congenital anemia associated with intrauterine B19 infection has been reported in a few cases, sometimes following intrauterine hydrops. This process may mimic other forms of congenital hypoplastic anemia (Diamond-Blackfan syndrome). Fetal infection with B19 has not been associated with other birth defects. B19 is only 1 of many causes of hydrops fetalis (see Chapter 103.2).

Myocarditis. B19 infection has been associated with myocarditis in fetuses, infants, children, and a few adults. Diagnosis has often been based on serology suggestive of a concurrent B19 infection, but in many cases B19 DNA has been demonstrated in cardiac tissue. This is plausible because fetal myocardial cells are known to express P antigen, the cell receptor for the virus. In the few cases where histology is reported, a predominantly lymphocytic infiltrate is described. Outcomes have varied from complete recovery to chronic cardiomyopathy to fatal cardiac arrest. Although B19-associated myocarditis seems to be a rare occurrence, there appears to be enough evidence to consider B19 as a potential cause of lymphocytic myocarditis, especially in infants and immunocompromised persons.

Other Cutaneous Manifestations. A variety of atypical skin eruptions have been reported with B19 infection. Most of these are petechial or purpuric in nature, often with evidence of vasculitis on biopsy. Among these rashes, the **papular-purpuric "gloves and socks" syndrome (PPGSS)** is well established in the dermatologic literature as distinctly associated with B19 infection (Fig. 248-3). PPGSS is characterized by fever, pruritus, and painful edema and erythema localized to the distal extremities in a distinct "gloves and socks" distribution, followed by acral petechiae and oral lesions. The syndrome is self-limited and resolves within a few weeks. Initially described in young adults, a number of reports in children have since been published. In those linked to B19 infection, the eruption is accompanied by serologic evidence of acute infection.

DIAGNOSIS. The diagnosis of erythema infectiosum is usually based on clinical presentation of the typical rash. Similarly, the diagnosis of a typical transient aplastic crisis in a child with sickle cell disease rarely requires virologic confirmation.

Serologic tests for the diagnosis of B19 infection are available. B19-specific IgM develops rapidly after infection and persists for 6–8 wk. Anti-B19 IgG serves as a marker of past infection or immunity. Determination of anti-B19 IgM is the best marker of recent/acute infection on a single serum sample; seroconversion of anti-B19 IgG antibodies in paired sera can also be used to confirm recent infection. Demonstration of anti-B19 IgG in the absence of IgM, even in high titer, is not diagnostic of recent infection.

Serologic diagnosis is unreliable in immunocompromised persons; diagnosis in these patients requires methods to detect viral DNA. Since the virus cannot be isolated by standard cell culture, methods to detect viral particles or viral DNA such as polymerase chain reaction or nucleic acid hybridization are necessary to establish the diagnosis. These tests are not widely available outside of research centers or reference laboratories. Prenatal diagnosis of B19-induced fetal hydrops can be accomplished by detection of viral DNA in fetal blood or amniotic fluid by these methods.

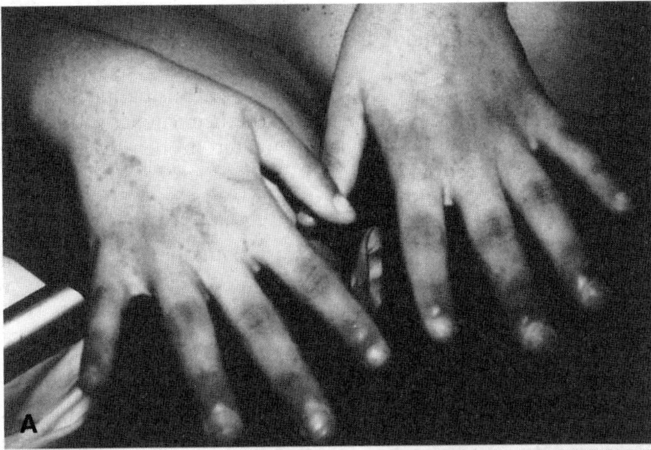

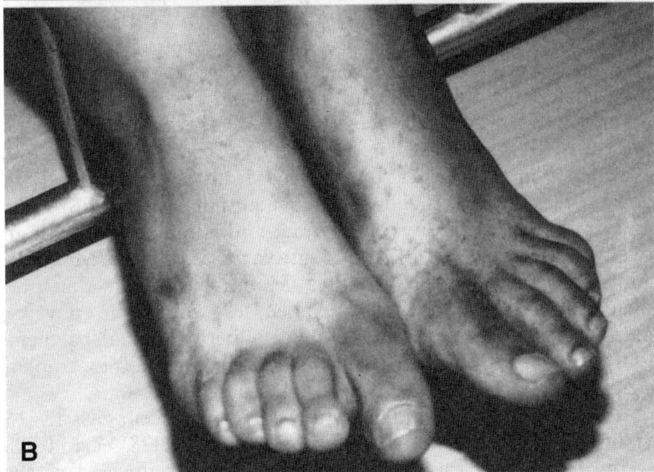

Figure 248-3. Papular-purpuric acrodermatitis with glove and sock-like distribution and edema of the fingers (*A*) and toes (*B*). (From Messina MF, Ruggeri C, Rosano M, et al: Purpuric gloves and socks syndrome caused by parvovirus B19 infection. *Pediatr Infect Dis J* 2003;22:755–756.)

DIFFERENTIAL DIAGNOSIS. The rash of erythema infectiosum must be differentiated from rubella, measles, enteroviral infections, and drug reactions. Rash and arthritis in older children should prompt consideration of juvenile rheumatoid arthritis, systemic lupus erythematosus, serum sickness, and other connective tissue disorders.

TREATMENT. There is no specific antiviral therapy. Commercial lots of intravenous immunoglobulin (IVIG) have been used with some success to treat B19-related episodes of anemia and bone marrow failure in immunocompromised children. Specific antibody may facilitate clearance of the virus; it is not always necessary, however, because cessation of cytotoxic chemotherapy with subsequent restoration of immune function will often suffice. In patients whose immune status is not likely to improve, such as patients with AIDS, administration of IVIG may give only a temporary remission, and periodic re-infusions may be required. In patients with AIDS, clearance of B19 infection has been reported after initiation of highly active antiretroviral therapy without the use of IVIG.

No controlled studies have been published regarding dosing of IVIG for B19-induced red cell aplasia. Doses reported with good results in a limited number of cases include 200 mg/kg/day for 5–10 days or 1 g/kg/day for 3 days. IVIG should not be used for treatment of B19-induced arthropathy.

B19-infected fetuses with anemia and hydrops have been managed successfully with intrauterine transfusions, but this has significant attendant risks. Once fetal hydrops is diagnosed, regardless of the suspected cause, the mother should be referred to a fetal therapy center for further evaluation because of the high risk for serious complications (see Chapter 103.2).

COMPLICATIONS. Erythema infectiosum is often accompanied by arthralgias or arthritis in adolescents and adults, which may persist after resolution of the rash. B19 may cause thrombocytopenic purpura and, rarely, aseptic meningitis in healthy individuals after erythema infectiosum. B19 is also a cause of infection-associated hemophagocytic syndrome, usually in immunocompromised persons.

PREVENTION. Children with erythema infectiosum are not likely to be infectious at presentation because the rash and arthropathy represent immune-mediated, postinfectious phenomena. Isolation and exclusion from school or child care are unnecessary and ineffective after diagnosis.

Children with B19-induced red cell aplasia, including the transient aplastic crisis, are infectious when they present and demonstrate a more intense viremia. Most of these children require transfusions and supportive care until their hematologic status stabilizes. They should be isolated in the hospital to prevent spread to susceptible patients and staff. Isolation should continue for at least 1 wk and until after resolution of fever. Pregnant caregivers should not be assigned to these patients. Exclusion of pregnant women from workplaces where children with erythema infectiosum may be present (e.g., primary and secondary schools) is not recommended as a general policy because it is unlikely to reduce their risk. There are no data to support the use of IVIG for postexposure prophylaxis in pregnant caregivers or immunocompromised children. No vaccine is currently available.

Heegarad ED, Brown KE: Human parvovirus B19. *Clin Microbiol Rev* 2002;15:485–505.
Koch WC: Fifth (human parvovirus) and sixth (herpesvirus 6) diseases. *Curr Opin Infect Dis* 2001;14:343–356.
Koch WC, Harger JH, Barnstein B, et al: Serologic and virologic evidence for frequent intrauterine transmission of human parvovirus B19 with a primary maternal infection during pregnancy. *Pediatr Infect Dis J* 1998;17:489–494.
Lindblom A, Isa A, Norbeck O, et al: Slow clearance of human parvovirus B19 viremia following acute infection. *Clin Infect Dis* 2005;41:1201–1203.
Messina MF, Ruggeri C, Rosana M, et al: Purpuric gloves and socks syndrome caused by parvovirus B19 infection. *Pediatr Infect Dis J* 2003;22:755–756.
Nigro G, Bastianon V, Colloridi V, et al: Human parvovirus B19 infection in infancy associated with acute and chronic lymphocytic myocarditis and high cytokine levels: Report of 3 cases and review. *Clin Infect Dis* 2000;31: 65–69.
Smith SB, Libow LF, Elston DM, et al: Gloves and socks syndrome: Early and late histopathologic features. *J Am Acad Dermatol* 2002;47:749–754.
Smith-Whitley K, Zhao H, Hodinka RL, et al: Epidemiology of human parvovirus B19 in children with sickle cell disease. *Blood* 2004;103:422–427.
Young NS, Brown KE: Parvovirus B19. *N Engl J Med* 2004;350:586–597.
Zimmerman SA, Davis JS, Schultz WH, et al: Subclinical parvovirus B19 infection in children with sickle cell anemia. *J Pediatr Hematol Oncol* 2003; 25387–25389.

Chapter 249 ■ Herpes Simplex Virus

Lawrence R. Stanberry

The 2 closely related herpes simplex viruses (HSVs), HSV type 1 (HSV-1) and HSV type 2 (HSV-2), cause a variety of illnesses depending on the anatomic site where the infection is initiated, the immune state of the host, and whether the symptoms reflect primary or recurrent infection. Common infections involve the skin, eye, oral cavity, and genital tract. Infections tend to be mild and self-limiting, except in the immunocompromised patient and newborn infant, where the infection may be severe and life threatening.

Primary infection occurs in individuals who have not been infected previously with either HSV-1 or HSV-2. Because these individuals are HSV seronegative and have no pre-existing immunity to HSV, primary infections can be severe. **Nonprimary 1st infection** occurs in individuals previously infected with 1 type of HSV (HSV-1) who have become infected for the 1st time with the other HSV type (HSV-2). Because immunity to 1 HSV type provides some cross protection against disease caused by the other HSV type, nonprimary 1st infections tend to be less severe than true primary infections. During primary and nonprimary initial infections HSV establishes latent infection in regional sensory ganglion neurons. Virus is maintained in this latent state for the life of the host but periodically can reactivate and cause **recurrent infection.** Symptomatic recurrent infections tend to be less severe and of shorter duration than 1st infections. Asymptomatic recurrent infections are extremely common. They cause no physical distress, although patients with recurrent infections are contagious and can transmit the virus to susceptible individuals. Reinfection with a new strain of either HSV-1 or HSV-2 at a previously infected anatomic site (the genital tract) can occur but is relatively uncommon, suggesting that host immunity, perhaps site-specific local immunity, resulting from the initial infection affords protection against exogenous reinfection. This observation suggests that it might be feasible to develop effective HSV vaccines.

ETIOLOGY. HSVs contain a double-stranded DNA genome of approximately 152 kb that encodes at least 84 proteins. The DNA is contained within an icosadeltahedral capsid, which is surrounded by an outer envelope that is composed of a lipid bilayer containing at least 12 viral glycoproteins. These glycoproteins are the major targets for humoral immunity, while other nonstructural proteins are important targets for cellular immunity. Two encoded proteins, viral DNA polymerase and thymidine kinase, are targets for antiviral drugs. HSV-1 and HSV-2 have a similar genetic composition with extensive DNA and protein homology. One important difference in the 2 viruses is their glycoprotein G genes, which have been exploited to develop a new generation of commercially available, accurate, type-specific serologic tests that can be used to discriminate whether a patient has been infected with HSV-1, HSV-2, or both.

EPIDEMIOLOGY. HSV infections are ubiquitous and there are no seasonal variations in risk for infection. The only natural host is humans, and the mode of transmission is direct contact between mucocutaneous surfaces. There are no documented incidental transmissions from inanimate objects such as toilet seats.

All infected individuals harbor latent infection with recurrent infections, which may be symptomatic or go unrecognized, and are periodically contagious. This helps explain the widespread prevalence of HSV.

HSV-1 and HSV-2 are equally capable of causing initial infection at any anatomic site but differ in their capacity to cause recurrent infections. HSV-1 has a greater propensity to cause recurrent oral infections, while HSV-2 has a greater proclivity to cause recurrent genital infections. For this reason, HSV-1 infection typically results from contact with contaminated oral secretions, whereas HSV-2 infection most commonly results from anogenital contact.

HSV seroprevalence rates are highest in developing countries and among lower socioeconomic groups, although high rates of HSV-1 and HSV-2 infections are found in developed nations and among persons of the highest socioeconomic strata. Incident HSV-1 infections are more common during childhood and adolescence but are also found throughout later life. Data from the 3rd U.S. population-based National Health and Nutrition Examination Survey (NHANES III) conducted between 1988 and 1994 showed a consistent increase of HSV-1 prevalence with age, increasing from 44% in adolescents 12–19 yr of age to 90% among those >70 yr of age. For persons ≥12 yr of age, the NHANES III study found an overall HSV-2 prevalence of 21.9%. Prevalence increased steadily with age from mid-teens to about age 35. The rate was higher among females than males (26% and 18%, respectively) and varied by race and ethnic group, with an overall seroprevalence of 45.9% in blacks, 22.3% in Mexican-Americans, and 17.8% in whites. Modifiable factors that predicted HSV-2 seropositivity included less education, poverty, cocaine use, and a greater lifetime number of sexual partners. Only 10% of subjects reported a history of genital herpes, emphasizing the asymptomatic nature of most HSV infections.

A 3-yr longitudinal study of Midwestern adolescent girls 12–15 yr of age found that 44% were seropositive for HSV-1 and 7% were seropositive for HSV-2 at enrollment. At the end of the study, 49% were seropositive for HSV-1 and 14% were seropositive for HSV-2. The attack rates, based on the number of cases per 100 person-years, were 3.2 for HSV-1 infection among all girls and 4.4 for HSV-2 infection among girls who reported being sexually experienced. This study indicates that sexually active young women have a high attack rate for genital herpes and suggests that genital herpes should be considered in the differential diagnosis of any young woman who reports recurrent genitourinary complaints. In this study, participants with pre-existing HSV-1 antibodies had a significantly lower attack rate for HSV-2 infection, and those who became infected were less likely to have symptomatic disease than girls who entered the study as HSV seronegative. Prior HSV-1 infection appears to afford adolescent girls with some protection against becoming infected with HSV-2, and, if infected with HSV-2, the pre-existing HSV-1 immunity appears to protect against developing symptomatic genital herpes.

Neonatal herpes is an uncommon but potentially fatal infection of the fetus or more likely the newborn. It is not a reportable disease in most states, and therefore there are not solid epidemiologic data regarding its frequency in the general population. In King County, Washington, the estimated incidence of neonatal herpes per 100,000 live births was 2.6 cases in the late 1960s, 11.9 cases from 1978 to 1981, and 31 cases from 1982 to 1999. This increase in neonatal herpes cases parallels the increase in cases of genital herpes. The estimated rate of neonatal herpes is 1 in 3,000–5,000 live births, which is higher than reported for the reportable perinatally acquired sexually transmitted infections such as congenital syphilis or gonococcal ophthalmia. Greater than 90% of the cases are the result of maternal-fetal transmission. The risk for transmission is greatest during a primary or nonprimary 1st infection (30–50%) and much lower when the exposure is during a recurrent infection (<2%). Infants born to mothers dually infected with HIV and HSV-2 are also at increased risk for acquiring HIV compared with infants born to HIV-positive mothers who are not HSV-2 infected. It is estimated that approximately 25% of pregnant women are HSV-2 infected and that approximately 2% of pregnant women acquire HSV-2 infection during pregnancy.

HSV is a leading cause of sporadic, fatal encephalitis in children and adults. In the USA it is estimated that there are 1,250 cases annually of HSV encephalitis.

PATHOGENESIS. In the immunocompetent host the pathogenesis of HSV infection involves viral replication in skin and mucous membranes followed by replication and spread in neural tissue. Viral infection typically begins at a cutaneous **portal of entry** such as the oral cavity, genital mucosa, ocular conjunctiva, or breaks in keratinized epithelia. Virus replicates locally, resulting in the death of the cell and sometimes produces clinically apparent inflammatory responses that facilitate the development of characteristic herpetic vesicles and ulcers. Virus also enters nerve endings and spreads beyond the portal of entry to sensory ganglia by intraneuronal transport. Virus replicates in some sensory neurons, and the progeny virions are sent via intraneuronal transport mechanisms back to the periphery, where they are released from nerve endings and replicate further in skin or mucosal surfaces. It is virus moving through this neural arc that is primarily responsible for the development of characteristic herpetic lesions, although most HSV infections do not reach a threshold necessary to cause clinically recognizable disease. While many sensory neurons become productively infected during the initial infection, some infected neurons do not initially support viral replication. It is in these neurons that the virus establishes a **latent infection,** a condition where the viral genome persists within the neuronal nucleus in a largely metabolically inactive state. Intermittently throughout the life of the host, undefined changes can occur in latently infected neurons that trigger the virus to begin to replicate. This occurs despite the host having established a variety of humoral and cellular immune responses that successfully controlled the initial infection. With reactivation of the latent neuron, progeny virions are produced and transported within nerve fibers back to cutaneous sites somewhere in the vicinity of the initial infection, where further replication occurs and causes recurrent infections. Recurrent infections may be symptomatic, with typical or atypical herpetic lesions, or the recurrences may be asymptomatic. In either case, virus is shed at the site where cutaneous replication occurs and can be transmitted to susceptible individuals who come in contact with the site or with contaminated secretions. Latency and reactivation are the mechanisms by which the virus is successfully maintained in the human population.

Viremia, or hematogenous spread of the virus, does not appear to play a role in HSV infections in the immunocompetent host but can occur in neonates, individuals with eczema, and severely malnourished children. It is also seen in patients with depressed or defective cell-mediated immunity such as occurs with HIV infection or some immunosuppressive therapies. Viremia can result in dissemination of the virus to visceral organs, including the liver and adrenals. Hematogenous dissemination of virus to the central nervous system appears to only occur in neonates.

The pathogenesis of HSV infection in newborns is complicated by their relative immunologic immaturity. The source of virus in neonatal infections is typically but not exclusively the mother. Transmission generally occurs during delivery, although it is well documented to occur even with cesarean delivery with intact membranes. The most common portals of entry are the conjunctiva, mucosal epithelium of the nose and mouth, and breaks or abrasions in the skin that occur with scalp electrode use or forceps delivery. With prompt antiviral therapy, virus replication may be restricted to the site of inoculation (the skin, eye, or mouth). However, virus may also extend from the nose to the respiratory tract to cause pneumonia, move via intraneuronal transport to the central nervous system to cause encephalitis, or spread by hematogenous dissemination to visceral organs and the brain. Factors that may influence neonatal HSV infection include the virus type, portal of entry, inoculum of virus to which the infant is exposed, gestational age of the infant, and presence of maternally derived antibodies specific to the virus causing infection. Latent infection is established during neonatal infection, and survivors may experience recurrent cutaneous and neural infections.

CLINICAL MANIFESTATIONS. The hallmarks of common HSV infections are skin vesicles and shallow ulcers. Classical infections present with small, 2–4 mm vesicles that may be surrounded by an erythematous base. These may persist for a few days before evolving into shallow, minimally erythematous ulcers. The vesicular phase tends to persist longer when keratinized epithelia is involved and be brief, sometimes fleeting, when moist mucous membranes are the site of infection. Because HSV infections are common and their natural history influenced by many factors, including portal of entry, immune status of the host, and whether it is an initial or recurrent infection, the typical manifestations are seldom classical. Most infections are asymptomatic or unrecognized, and nonclassical presentations such as small skin fissures and small erythematous nonvesicular lesions are common.

Acute Oropharyngeal Infections. Herpes gingivostomatitis most often affects children 6 mo to 5 yr of age, but is seen across the age spectrum. It is an extremely painful condition with sudden onset, pain in the mouth, drooling, refusal to eat or drink, and fever of up to 40.0–40.6°C. The gums become markedly swollen, and vesicles may develop throughout the oral cavity, including on the gums, lips, tongue, palate, tonsils, and pharynx (Fig. 249-1). The vesicles may be more extensively distributed than typically seen with enteroviral herpangina. During the initial phase of the illness there may be tonsillar exudates suggestive of bacterial pharyngitis. The vesicles are generally only present a few days before progressing to form shallow indurated ulcers that may be covered with a yellow-gray membrane. Tender submandibular, submaxillary, and cervical lymphadenopathy are common. The breath may be foul as a result of overgrowth of anaerobic oral bacteria. Untreated, the illness resolves in 7–14 days, although the lymphadenopathy may persist for several weeks.

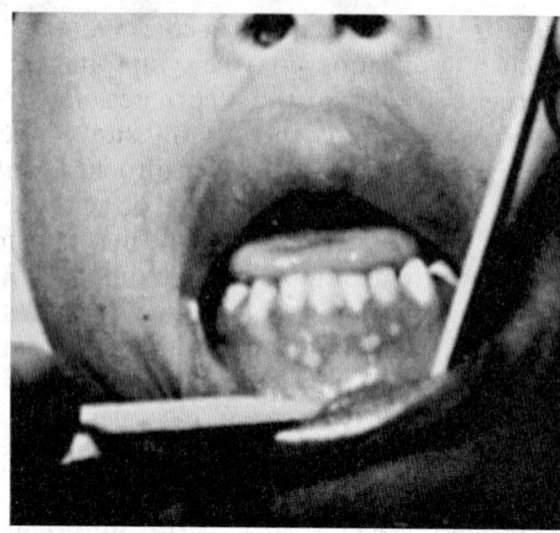

Figure 249-1. Herpetic stomatitis with vesicular-pustular lesions on the gingival mucosa.

In older children, adolescents, and college students, the initial HSV oral infection may manifest as pharyngitis and tonsillitis rather than gingivostomatitis. The vesicular phase is often over by the time the patient presents to a health care provider, and signs and symptoms may be indistinguishable from streptococcal pharyngitis with fever, malaise, headache, sore throat, and white plaques on the tonsils. The course of illness is typically longer than for untreated streptococcal pharyngitis.

Herpes Labialis. **Fever blisters,** or **cold sores,** are the most common manifestation of recurrent HSV-1 infections. The most common site of herpes labialis is the vermilion border of the lip, although lesions sometimes occur on the nose, chin, cheek, or oral mucosa. Older patients report experiencing burning, tingling, itching, or pain 3–6 hr (rarely as long as 24–48 hr) before the development of the herpes lesion. The lesion generally begins as a small grouping of erythematous papules that over a few hours progress to create a small, thin-walled vesicle. The vesicles may form shallow ulcers or become pustular. The short-lived ulcer dries and develops a crusted scab. Complete healing without scarring occurs with re-epithelialization of the ulcerated skin, usually within 6–10 days. Some patients experience local lymphadenopathy but no constitutional symptoms

Cutaneous Infections. In the healthy child or adolescent, cutaneous HSV infections are generally the result of skin trauma with macro- or micro-abrasions and exposure to infectious secretions. This situation most often occurs in play or contact sports such as wrestling (**herpes gladiatorum**) or rugby (**scrumpox**). As with other HSV infections, an initial cutaneous infection establishes a latent infection that can subsequently result in recurrent infections at or near the site of the initial infection. Pain, burning, itching, or tingling often precedes the herpetic eruption by a few hours to a few days. Like herpes labialis, lesions begin as grouped, erythematous papules that progress to vesicles, pustules, ulcers, and crusts and then healing without scarring in 6–10 days. While herpes labialis typically results in a single lesion, a cutaneous HSV infection results in multiple discrete lesions and involves a larger surface area. There can be regional lymphadenopathy, but seldom systemic symptoms. Recurrences are sometimes associated with local edema and lymphangitis or local neuralgia.

Herpes whitlow is a term generally applied to HSV infection of fingers or toes, although strictly speaking it refers to HSV infection of the paronychia. Among children, this is most commonly seen in infants and toddlers who suck their thumb or fingers and who are experiencing either a symptomatic or a subclinical oral HSV-1 infection. Occasionally adolescents develop an HSV-2 herpes whitlow resulting from exposure to infectious genital secretions. The onset of the infection is heralded by itching, pain, and erythema 2–7 days after exposure. The cuticle becomes erythematous and tender and may appear to contain pus, although if incised, little fluid is present. Incising the lesion is discouraged as this typically prolongs recovery and increases the risk for secondary bacterial infection. Lesions and associated pain typically persist for about 10 days, followed by rapid improvement and complete recovery in 18–20 days. Regional lymphadenopathy is common, and lymphangitis and neuralgia may occur. Unlike other recurrent herpes infections, recurrent herpetic whitlows are often as painful as the primary infection, but are generally shorter in duration.

Cutaneous HSV infections can be severe or life threatening in patients with disorders of the skin such as eczema (eczema herpeticum), pemphigus, burns, Darier disease, or following laser skin resurfacing. The lesions are frequently ulcerative and nonspecific in appearance, although typical vesicles may be seen in adjacent normal skin (Fig. 249-2). If untreated, these can progress to disseminated infection and death. Recurrent infections are common but generally less severe than the initial infection.

Genital Herpes. Genital HSV infection is common in sexually experienced adolescents and young adults, but up to 90% of infected individuals are unaware they are infected. Infection may result from genital-genital transmission (usually HSV-2) or oral-genital transmission (usually HSV-1). Symptomatically individuals and also those with asymptomatic or unrecognized infection periodically shed virus from anogenital sites and hence can transmit the infection to sexual partners or, in the case of the pregnant woman, to her newborn. Classical primary genital herpes may be preceded by a short period of local burning and tenderness before vesicles develop on genital mucosal surfaces or keratinized skin and sometimes around the anus or on the buttocks and thighs. Vesicles on mucosal surfaces are short lived and rupture to produce shallow, tender ulcers covered with a yellowish gray exudate and surrounded by an erythematous border. Vesicles on keratinized epithelium persist for a few days before progressing to the pustular stage and then crusting.

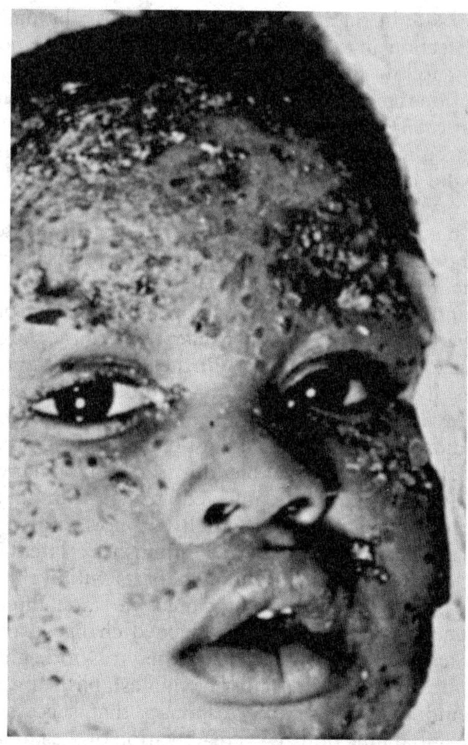

Figure 249-2. Widespread cutaneous herpes infection in a child with underlying eczema (eczema herpeticum).

Patients may develop urethritis and dysuria severe enough to cause urinary retention and bilateral, tender inguinal and pelvic lymphadenopathy. Women may experience a watery vaginal discharge and men a clear mucoid urethral discharge. Significant local pain and systemic symptoms including fever, headache, and myalgia are common. Aseptic meningitis develops in an estimated 15% of cases. The course of classical primary genital herpes, from onset to complete healing, is 2–3 wk.

Most patients with symptomatic primary genital herpes will experience at least 1 recurrent infection in the following year. Recurrent genital herpes is usually less severe and of shorter duration than the primary infection. Some patients experience a sensory prodrome with pain, burning, and tingling at the site where vesicles subsequently develop. Asymptomatic recurrent anogenital HSV infections are common, and all HSV-2 seropositive individuals appear to periodically shed virus from anogenital sites. Most sexual transmissions and maternal-neonatal transmissions of virus result from asymptomatic shedding episodes.

Genital infections caused by HSV-1 and HSV-2 are indistinguishable, but HSV-1 causes significantly fewer subsequent episodes of recurrent infection; hence, knowing which virus is causing the infection has important prognostic value. Genital HSV infection increases the risk for acquiring HIV infection.

Rarely, genital HSV infections are identified in young children and preadolescents. While this should raise concerns about possible sexual abuse, there are documented cases of autoinoculation where a child has inadvertently transmitted virus from contaminated oral secretions to their own genitalia.

Ocular Infections. HSV ocular infections may involve the conjunctiva, cornea, or retina and may be primary or recurrent. Conjunctivitis or keratoconjunctivitis is usually unilateral and often associated with blepharitis and tender preauricular lymphadenopathy. The conjunctiva appears edematous but there is rarely purulent discharge. Vesicular lesions may be seen on the lid margins and periorbital skin. Patients typically have fever. Untreated infection generally resolves in 2–3 weeks. Obvious corneal involvement is rare, but when it occurs it can produce ulcers that are described as appearing dendritic or geographic. Extension to the stroma is uncommon although more likely to occur in patients inadvertently treated with corticosteroids. When it occurs it may be associated with corneal edema, scarring, and corneal perforation. Recurrent infections tend to involve the underlying stroma, and repeated recurrences can cause progressive corneal scarring and injury that can lead to blindness.

Retinal infections are rare and are more likely among infants with neonatal herpes and immunocompromised persons with disseminated HSV infections.

Central Nervous System Infections. HSV encephalitis is the leading cause of sporadic, nonepidemic encephalitis in children and adults in the USA. It is an acute necrotizing infection generally involving the frontal and/or temporal cortex and the limbic system and, beyond the neonatal period, is almost always caused by HSV-1. The infection may present with nonspecific findings, including fever, headache, nuchal rigidity, nausea, vomiting, generalized seizures, and alteration of consciousness. Injury to the frontal or temporal cortex or limbic system may produce findings more indicative of HSV encephalitis, including anosmia, memory loss, peculiar behavior, expressive aphasia and other changes in speech, hallucinations, and focal seizures. The untreated infection progresses to coma and death in 75% of cases. Examination of the cerebrospinal fluid typically shows a moderate number of mononuclear cells and polymorphonuclear leukocytes, a mildly elevated protein concentration, a normal or slightly decreased glucose concentration, and often a moderate number of erythrocytes.

HSV is also a cause of aseptic meningitis and is the most common cause of recurrent aseptic meningitis (**Mollaret meningitis**).

Infections in Immunocompromised Persons. Severe, life-threatening HSV infections can occur in patients with compromised immune functions, including neonates, the severely malnourished, those with primary and secondary immunodeficiencies diseases including AIDS, and those on some immunosuppressive regimens, particularly for cancer and organ transplantation. Mucocutaneous infections, including mucositis and esophagitis, are most common, although their presentations may be atypical and can result in lesions that slowly enlarge, ulcerate, become necrotic, and extend to deeper tissues. Other HSV infections include tracheobronchitis, pneumonitis, and anogenital infections. Disseminated infection can result in a sepsis-like presentation, with liver and adrenal involvement, disseminated intravascular coagulopathy, and shock.

Perinatal Infections. HSV infection may be acquired in utero, during the birth process, or during the neonatal period. Intrauterine and postpartum infections are well described but occur infrequently. Postpartum transmission may be from the mother or another adult with a nongenital (typically HSV-1) infection such as herpes labialis. Most cases of neonatal herpes result from maternal infection and transmission, usually during passage through a contaminated infected birth canal of a mother with asymptomatic genital herpes. Transmission is well documented in infants delivered by cesarean section. Fewer than 30% of mothers of an infant with neonatal herpes have a history of genital herpes. The risk for infection is higher in infants born to mothers with primary genital infection (>30%) compared to recurrent genital infection (<2%). Use of scalp electrodes may also increase risk.

Neonatal HSV infection is almost never asymptomatic. Its clinical presentation reflects timing of infection, portal of entry, and extent of spread. Infants with intrauterine infection typically have skin vesicles or scarring, eye findings including chorioretinitis and keratoconjunctivitis, and microcephaly or hydranencephaly that are present at delivery. Few infants survive without therapy, and those that do generally have severe sequelae. Infants infected during delivery or postpartum present with 1 of 3 patterns of disease: (1) disease localized to the skin, eyes, or mouth; (2) encephalitis with or without skin, eye, or mouth **(SEM) disease;** or (3) disseminated infection involving multiple organs, including the brain, lungs, liver, heart, adrenals, and skin.

Infants with SEM disease generally present at 5–11 days of life and typically develop a few small vesicles, particularly on the presenting part or at sites of trauma such as with scalp electrode placement. If untreated, infants with SEM disease may progress to develop encephalitis or disseminated disease.

Infants with encephalitis typically present at 8–17 days of life with clinical findings suggestive of bacterial meningitis, including irritability, lethargy, poor feeding, poor tone, and seizures. Fever is relatively uncommon, and only about 60% have skin vesicles (Fig. 249-3). If untreated, 50% will die and most survivors have severe neurologic sequelae.

Infants with disseminated HSV infections generally become ill at 5–11 days of life. Their clinical picture is similar to bacterial sepsis with hyper- or hypothermia, irritability, poor feeding, and vomiting. They may also exhibit respiratory distress, cyanosis, apneic spells, jaundice, purpuric rash, and evidence of central nervous system infection; seizures are common. Skin vesicles are seen in about 75% of cases. If untreated, the infection causes shock and disseminated intravascular coagulation; approximately 90% of these infants die, and most survivors have severe neurologic sequelae.

DIAGNOSIS. The clinical diagnosis of an HSV infection, particularly life-threatening infections and genital herpes, should be confirmed by laboratory test, preferably isolation of virus or detection of viral antigen or more often viral DNA by polymerase chain reaction (PCR). Histologic findings or imaging studies may support the diagnosis but should not substitute for virus-specific tests. HSV immunoglobulin M (IgM) tests are notoriously unre-

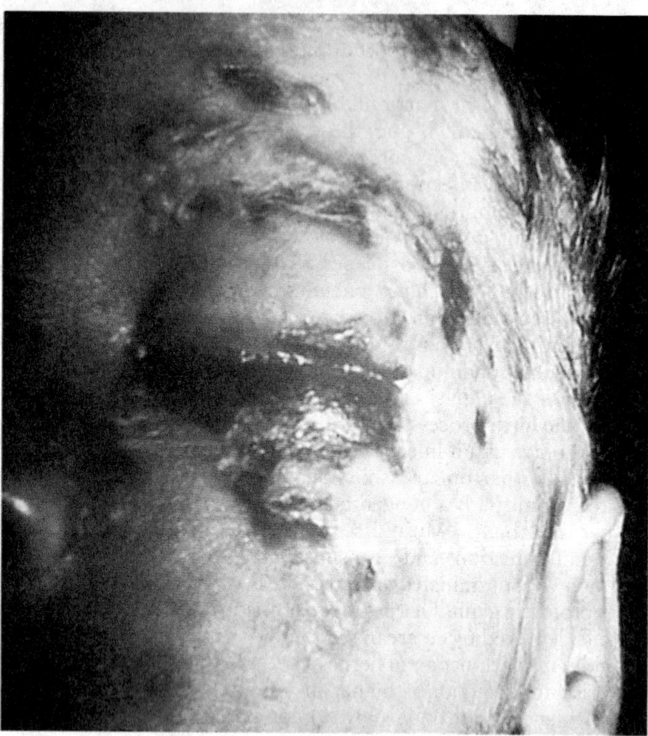

Figure 249-3. Vesicular-pustular lesions on the face of a neonate with herpes simplex virus infection. See also color plates. (From Kohl S: Neonatal herpes simplex virus infection. *Clin Perinatol* 1997;24:129–150.)

liable, and the demonstration of a 4-fold or greater rise in HSV-specific IgG titers between acute and convalescent serum samples is only useful in retrospect.

Virus culture remains the gold standard for diagnosing HSV infections. The highest yield comes from rupturing a suspected herpetic vesicle and vigorously rubbing the base of the lesion to collect fluid and cells. Culturing dried, crusted lesions is generally of low yield. While not as sensitive as viral culture, direct detection of HSV antigens in clinical specimens can be done rapidly and has very good specificity. The use of PCR for detection of HSV DNA is highly sensitive and specific and in some instances can be done rapidly. It is the test of choice in examining cerebrospinal fluid in cases of suspected HSV encephalitis.

Evaluation of the neonate with suspected HSV infection should include cultures of suspicious lesions as well as eye and mouth swabs, and PCR of cerebrospinal fluid. Culture or antigen detection should be used in evaluating lesions associated with suspected acute genital herpes. HSV-2 type-specific antibody tests are useful for evaluating sexually experienced adolescents or young adults who have a history of unexplained recurrent nonspecific urogenital signs and symptoms, but they are less useful for general screening in populations where HSV-2 infections are of low prevalence.

Because most HSV diagnostic tests take at least a few days to complete, treatment should not be withheld but rather initiated promptly in order to ensure the maximum therapeutic benefit.

LABORATORY FINDINGS. Most self-limited HSV infections cause few changes in routine laboratory tests. Mucocutaneous infections may cause a moderate polymorphonuclear leukocytosis. In HSV meningoencephalitis there can be an increase in lymphocytes and protein, the glucose may be normal or reduced, and red blood cells may be present. The electroencephalogram and MRI of the brain may show temporal lobe abnormalities in HSV encephalitis beyond the neonatal period. Encephalitis in the neonatal period tends to be more global, that is, not limited to the temporal lobe. Disseminated infection may cause elevated liver enzymes, thrombocytopenia, and abnormal coagulation.

TREATMENT. Three antiviral drugs—acyclovir, valacyclovir, and famciclovir—are available in the United States for the management of HSV infections. All 3 are available in oral form, but only acyclovir is available in a suspension form. Acyclovir has the poorest bioavailability and hence requires more frequent dosing. Valacyclovir, a prodrug of acyclovir, and famciclovir, a prodrug of penciclovir, both have very good oral bioavailability and are dosed once or twice daily. Acyclovir and penciclovir are also available in a topical form but provide limited or no benefit to patients with recurrent mucocutaneous HSV infections. Only acyclovir has an intravenous formulation. Early initiation of therapy results in the maximal therapeutic benefit. All 3 drugs have an exceptional safety profile and are safe to use in pediatric patients. Doses should be modified in patients with renal impairment.

Acyclovir and penciclovir resistance is rare in immunocompetent persons but does occur in immunocompromised persons. Virus isolates should be tested for drug sensitivities for immunocompromised persons whose HSV infection is not responding or is worsening on acyclovir therapy. Foscarnet and cidofovir have been used in the treatment of HSV infections caused by acyclovir-resistant mutants.

Topical trifluorothymidine, vidarabine, and idoxuridine are used in the treatment of herpes keratitis.

Patients with genital herpes also require counseling to address psychosocial issues, including possible stigma, and to help them understand the natural history and management of this chronic infection.

Acute Mucocutaneous Infections. For gingivostomatitis, oral acyclovir (15 mg/kg/dose 5 times a day PO for 7 days, maximum 1 g/day) started within 72 hr of onset reduces the severity and duration of the illness. Pain associated with swallowing may limit oral intake of infants and children, placing them at risk for dehydration. Intake should be encouraged through the use of cold beverages, ice cream, and yogurt.

For **herpes labialis,** oral treatment is superior to topical antiviral therapy. For treatment of a recurrence in adolescents, oral valacyclovir (2,000 mg bid PO for 1 day), acyclovir (200–400 mg 5 times daily PO for 5 days), or famciclovir (500 mg tid PO for 5 days) shortens the duration of the episode. Chronic daily use of oral acyclovir (400 mg bid PO) or valacyclovir (500 mg qd PO) has been used to prevent recurrences in individuals with frequent or severe recurrences.

Anecdotal reports suggest that treatment of **herpes gladiatorum** with oral acyclovir (200 mg 5 times daily PO for 7–10 days) or valacyclovir (500 mg bid PO for 7–10 days) at the 1st signs of the outbreak can shorten the course of the recurrence. For patients with a history of recurrent herpes gladiatorum, chronic daily prophylaxis with valacyclovir (500–1,000 mg daily) has been reported to prevent recurrences.

There are no clinical trials assessing the benefit of antiviral treatment for **herpetic whitlow.** High-dose oral acyclovir (1,600–2,000 mg/day divided in 2–3 doses PO for 10 days) started at the 1st signs of illness has been reported to abort some recurrences and reduce the duration of others.

A clinical trial has established the effectiveness of oral acyclovir (200 mg 5 times a day PO for 5 days) in the treatment of **eczema herpeticum.** Oral-facial HSV infections can reactivate following cosmetic facial laser resurfacing, causing extensive disease and scarring. Treatment beginning the day before the procedure with either valacyclovir (500 mg twice daily PO for 10–14 days) or famciclovir (250–500 mg bid PO for 10 days) has been reported to be effective in preventing the infections. HSV infections in **burn patients** can be severe or life threatening and have been treated with intravenous acyclovir (10–20 mg/kg/day divided every 8 hr IV).

Antiviral drugs are not effective in the treatment of HSV-associated **erythema multiforme,** but their daily use as for herpes labialis prophylaxis has been shown to prevent erythema multiforme recurrences.

Genital Herpes. Pediatric patients, usually adolescents or young adults, with suspected 1st episode genital herpes should be treated with antiviral therapy. Treatment of the initial infection reduces the severity and duration of the illness but has no effect on the frequency of subsequent recurrent infections. Treatment options for adolescents include acyclovir (400 mg tid PO for 7–10 days), famciclovir (750 mg tid PO for 7–10 days), or valacyclovir (1000 mg bid PO for 7–10 days). The twice daily valacyclovir option avoids treatment during school hours. For smaller children, acyclovir suspension can be used at a dose of 10–20 mg/kg/dose 4 times daily not to exceed the adult dose. The 1st episode of genital herpes can be extremely painful, and use of analgesics is generally indicated. All patients with genital herpes should be offered counseling to help them deal with psychosocial issues and to understand the chronic nature of the illness.

There are 3 strategic options regarding the management of recurrent infections. The choice should be guided by several factors, including the frequency and severity of the recurrent infections, the psychologic impact of the illness on the patient, and concerns regarding transmission to a susceptible sexual partner. Option 1 is no therapy; option 2 is episodic therapy; and option 3 is chronic suppressive therapy. For **episodic therapy,** treatment should be initiated at the 1st signs of an outbreak. Recommended choices for episodic therapy in adolescents include famciclovir (1,000 mg bid PO for 1 day), acyclovir (800 mg tid PO for 2 days), or valacyclovir (500 mg bid PO for 3 days). Chronic suppressive therapy offers the advantage that it prevents most outbreaks, improves patient quality of life pertaining to the psychosocial impact of genital herpes, and, with daily valacyclovir therapy, also reduces (but does not eliminate) the risk for sexual transmission to a susceptible sexual partner. Options for **chronic suppressive therapy** include acyclovir (400 mg bid PO), famciclovir (250 mg bid PO), and valacyclovir (500–1,000 mg qd PO).

Ocular Infections. HSV ocular infections can result in blindness. Management should involve consultation with an ophthalmologist.

Central Nervous System Infections. Patients beyond the neonatal period with herpes encephalitis should be promptly treated with intravenous acyclovir (10 mg/kg every 8 hr given over a 1 hr infusion for 14–21 days). Treatment for increased intracranial pressure, management of seizures, and respiratory compromise may be required.

Infections in Immunocompromised Persons. Severe mucocutaneous and disseminated HSV infections in immunocompromised patients should be treated with intravenous acyclovir (5–10 mg/kg or 250 mg/m^2 every 8 hr) until there is evidence of resolution of the infection. Oral antiviral therapy with acyclovir, famciclovir, or valacyclovir has been used for treatment of less severe HSV infections and for suppression of recurrences during periods of significant immunosuppression. Drug resistance does occur occasionally in immunocompromised patients, and individuals not responding to antiviral drug therapy should have their viral isolates tested to determine their sensitivity. Acyclovir-resistant viruses are often also resistant to famciclovir but may be sensitive to foscarnet or cidofovir.

Perinatal Infections. All infants with proven or suspected neonatal HSV infection should be begun promptly on high-dose intravenous acyclovir (60 mg/kg/day divided every 8 hr IV). Treatment may be discontinued in those infants shown by laboratory testing to not be infected. Infants with HSV disease limited to skin, eyes, and mouth should be treated for 14 days, while those with disseminated or central nervous system disease should receive 21 days of therapy. Patients receiving high-dose therapy should be monitored for neutropenia.

PROGNOSIS. Most HSV infections are self-limiting, last from a few days (for recurrent infections) to 2–3 wk (for primary infections), and heal without scarring. Recurrent oral-facial herpes in a patient who has undergone dermabrasion or laser resurfacing can be severe and lead to scarring. Genital herpes, because it is a sexually transmitted infection, can be stigmatizing and may have psychologic consequences much greater than its physiologic effects. Some HSV infections can be severe and without prompt antiviral therapy may have grave consequences. Life-threatening conditions include neonatal herpes, herpes encephalitis, and HSV infections in immunocompromised patients, burn patients, and severely malnourished infants and children. Recurrent ocular herpes can lead to corneal scarring and blindness.

PREVENTION. Transmission of infection occurs through exposure to virus either as the result of skin-to-skin contact or contact with contaminated secretions. Good handwashing and when appropriate the use of gloves provide health care workers with excellent protection against HSV infection in the workplace. Health care workers with active oral-facial herpes or herpes whitlow should take precautions, particularly when caring for high-risk patients such as newborns, immunocompromised individuals, and those with chronic skin conditions. Patients and parents should be advised about good hygienic practices, including handwashing and avoiding contact with lesions and secretions during active herpes outbreaks. Schools and daycare centers should clean shared toys and athletic equipment such as wrestling mats at least daily following use. Athletes with active herpes infections who participate in contact sports such as wrestling or rugby should be excluded from practice or games until the lesions are completely healed. Genital herpes can be prevented by avoiding genital-genital and oral-genital contact. The risk for acquiring genital herpes can be reduced but not eliminated through the correct and consistent use of condoms. The risk for transmitting genital HSV-2 infection to a susceptible sexual partner can be reduced but not eliminated by the daily use of oral valacyclovir by the infected partner.

For **pregnant women** with **active genital herpes** at the time of delivery, the risk for mother-to-baby transmission can be reduced but not eliminated by delivering the baby via a cesarean section (within 4–6 hr of rupture of membranes). The risk for recurrent genital herpes and therefore the need for cesarean delivery can be reduced but not eliminated in pregnant women with a history of genital herpes by the daily use of oral acyclovir or valacyclovir during the last 4 wk of gestation, which is recommended by the American College of Obstetrics and Gynecology.

Infants delivered vaginally to women with 1st episode genital herpes are at very high risk for acquiring HSV infection. The nasopharynx and umbilicus should be cultured at delivery and at day 2 of life; some recommend that these infants receive anticipatory acyclovir therapy for at least 2 wk. Others treat if signs develop or if the 48 hr cultures are positive. Infants delivered to women with a history of recurrent genital herpes are at low risk for developing neonatal herpes. In this setting parents should be educated about the signs and symptoms of neonatal HSV infection and should be instructed to seek care without delay at the 1st suggestion of infection. When in doubt, infants should be evaluated and the nasopharynx and umbilicus cultured for neonatal herpes and intravenous acyclovir begun until cultures are negative or until another explanation can be found for the signs and symptoms.

Recurrent genital HSV infections can be prevented by the daily use of oral acyclovir, valacyclovir, or famciclovir, and these drugs have been used to prevent recurrences of oral-facial (labialis) and cutaneous (gladiatorum) herpes. Oral and intravenous acyclovir has also been used to prevent recurrent HSV infections in immunocompromised patients. Use of sun blockers has also been reported to be effective in preventing recurrent oral-facial herpes in patients with a history of sun-induced recurrent disease.

Corey L, Wald A, Patel R, et al: Once-daily valacyclovir to reduce the risk of transmission of genital herpes. *N Engl J Med* 2004;350:11–20.
Elbers JM, Bitnum A, Richardson SE, et al: A 12-year prospective study of childhood herpes simplex encephalitis: Is there a broader spectrum of disease. *Pediatrics* 2007;119:e399–e407.
Handsfield HH, Waldo AB, Brown ZA, et al: Neonatal herpes should be a reportable disease. *Sex Transm Dis* 2005;32:521–525.
O'Riordan DP, Golden C, Aucott SW: Herpes simplex virus infections in preterm infants. *Pediatrics* 2006;118:e1612–e1620.
Spruance SL, Kriesel JD: Treatment of herpes simplex labialis. *Herpes* 2002; 3:64–69.
Stanberry LR, Rosenthal SL, Mills L, et al: Longitudinal risk of herpes simplex virus (HSV) type 1, HSV type 2, and cytomegalovirus infections among young adolescent girls. *Clin Infect Dis* 2004;39:1433–1438.
Stanberry LR, Spruance SL, Cunningham AL, et al: Glycoprotein-D-adjuvant vaccine to prevent genital herpes. *N Engl J Med* 2002;347:1652–1661.

Chapter 250 ■ Varicella-Zoster Virus

Martin G. Myers, Jane F. Seward, and Philip S. LaRussa

Varicella-zoster virus (VZV) causes primary, latent, and recurrent infections. The primary infection is manifested as varicella (**chickenpox**) and results in establishment of a lifelong latent infection of sensory ganglion neurons. Reactivation of the latent infection causes herpes zoster (**shingles**). Although often a mild illness of childhood, chickenpox can cause substantial morbidity and mortality in otherwise healthy children; it causes increased morbidity and mortality in adolescents, adults, and immunocompromised persons, and predisposes to severe group A streptococcus and *Staphylococcus aureus* infections. Chickenpox and herpes zoster, if needed, can be treated with antiviral drugs. Initial infection can be prevented by immunization with live-attenuated VZV vaccine and there will soon be another VZV vaccine for older individuals intended to boost their immunity to VZV in order to reduce the rates of herpes zoster and its major complication, painful postherpetic neuralgia.

ETIOLOGY. VZV is a neurotropic human herpesvirus with similarities to herpes simplex virus, which is also α-herpesvirus. These viruses are enveloped with double-stranded DNA genomes that encode more than 70 proteins, including proteins that are targets of cellular and humoral immunity.

EPIDEMIOLOGY. Prior to the introduction of vaccine in 1995, varicella was an almost universal communicable infection of childhood in the United States. Most children were infected by 15 yr of age, with fewer than 5% of adults remaining susceptible. Annual varicella epidemics occurred in winter and spring, accounting for about 4 million cases, 11,000–15,000 hospitalizations, and 100–150 deaths every year. Varicella is a more serious disease with higher rates of complications and deaths among infants, adults, and immunocompromised persons. Within households, transmission of VZV to susceptible individuals occurs at a rate of 65–86%; more casual contact, such as occurs in a school classroom, is associated with lower attack rates among susceptible children. Patients with varicella are contagious from 24 to 48 hr before the rash appears and until vesicles are crusted, usually 3–7 days after onset of rash. Susceptible children may also acquire varicella after close, direct contact with adults or children who have herpes zoster.

Since implementation of the varicella vaccination program, there have been substantial declines in varicella morbidity and mortality. By 2000, varicella cases had declined 71% to 84% in sites where active surveillance was being conducted; further declines have occurred through 2003. By 2001, national varicella hospitalizations had declined 75% compared with hospitalizations from 1993 to 1995, and deaths had decreased by 74% or more among all persons ≤50 yr of age. Morbidity and mortality declined the most among children 1–4 yr of age (>92% decline in deaths) followed by children 5–9 yr of age (89% decline in deaths). However, declines were seen in all age groups, including infants <12 mo of age who are being protected from exposure by indirect vaccination effects. The change in varicella epidemiology—with cases now occurring predominantly in children in upper elementary school rather than in the preschool years—highlights the importance of offering vaccine to every susceptible child, adolescent, and adult. The continued occurrence of breakthrough infections, though most commonly mild, has stimulated discussions regarding the possible need for a 2nd dose of vaccine for children.

Herpes zoster, because it is due to the reactivation of latent VZV, is uncommon in childhood and shows no seasonal variation in incidence. The lifetime risk for herpes zoster for individuals with a history of varicella is 10–15%, with 75% of cases occurring after 45 yr of age. Herpes zoster is very rare in healthy children <10 yr of age except for infants who were infected in utero or in the 1st year of life; herpes zoster in children tends to be milder than disease in adults and is less frequently associated with postherpetic neuralgia. However, herpes zoster occurs more frequently, occasionally multiple times, and may be severe in children receiving immunosuppressive therapy for malignancy or other diseases and in those who have HIV infection. An investigational live-attenuated VZV vaccine given to older adults reduces both the frequency of herpes zoster and its most frequent complication, postherpetic neuralgia.

PATHOGENESIS. VZV is transmitted in respiratory secretions and in the fluid of skin lesions either by airborne spread or through direct contact. Primary infection (varicella) results from inoculation of the virus onto the mucosa of the upper respiratory tract and tonsillar lymphoid tissue. During the early part of the 10–21 day incubation period, virus replicates in the local lymphoid tissue followed by a brief subclinical viremia that spreads the virus to the reticuloendothelial system. Widespread cutaneous lesions occur during a **2nd viremic** phase that lasts 3–7 days. Peripheral blood mononuclear cells carry infectious virus, generating new crops of vesicles during this period of viremia. VZV is also transported back to upper respiratory mucosal sites during the late incubation period, permitting spread to susceptible contacts before the appearance of rash. Host immune responses limit viral replication and facilitate recovery from infection. In the immunocompromised child, the failure of immune responses, especially cell-mediated immune responses, results in continued viral replication that may result in disseminated infection with resultant complications in the lungs, liver, brain, and other organs. Virus is transported in a retrograde manner through sensory axons to the dorsal root ganglia throughout the spinal cord, where the virus establishes latent infection in the neurons associated with these axons. Subsequent **reactivation** of latent virus causes **herpes zoster,** a vesicular rash that usually is dermatomal in distribution. During herpes zoster, necrotic changes may be produced in the associated ganglia. The skin lesions of varicella and herpes zoster have identical histopathology, and infectious VZV is present in both. Varicella elicits humoral and cell-mediated immunity that is highly protective against symptomatic reinfection. Suppression of cell-mediated immunity to VZV correlates with an increased risk for VZV reactivation as herpes zoster.

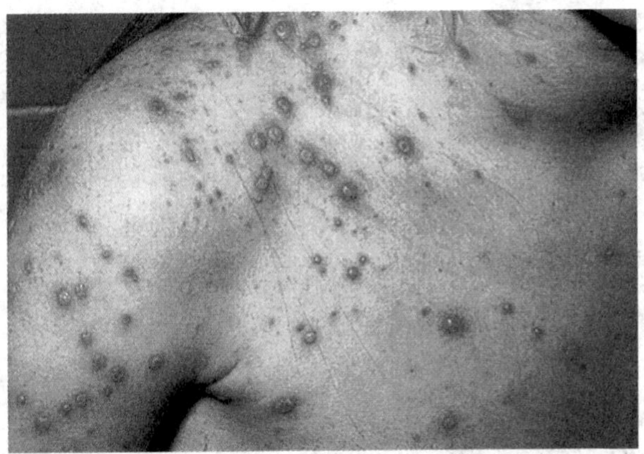

Figure 250-1. Varicella-zoster infections. Adolescent girl with varicella lesions in various stages. (From the American Academy of Pediatrics: *Red Book: 2006 Report of the Committee on Infectious Diseases,* 27th ed. Elk Grove Village, IL, American Academy of Pediatrics, 2006, Atlas 14.)

CLINICAL MANIFESTATIONS. Varicella is an acute febrile rash illness that was common in children prior to the universal childhood vaccination program. It has variable severity but is usually self-limited. It may be associated with severe complications, including bacterial superinfection, pneumonia, encephalitis, bleeding disorders, congenital infection, and life-threatening perinatal infection. Herpes zoster, uncommon in children, causes localized cutaneous symptoms, but may disseminate in immunocompromised patients.

Varicella. The illness usually begins 14–16 days after exposure, although the incubation period can range from 10 to 21 days. Subclinical varicella is rare; almost all exposed, susceptible persons experience a rash. Prodromal symptoms may be present, particularly in older children and adults. Fever, malaise, anorexia, headache, and occasionally mild abdominal pain may occur 24–48 hr before the rash appears. Temperature elevation is usually moderate, usually from 100 to 102°F but may be as high as 106°F; fever and other systemic symptoms persist during the 1st 2–4 days after the onset of the rash.

Varicella lesions often appear first on the scalp, face, or trunk. The initial exanthem consists of intensely pruritic erythematous macules that evolve through the papular stage to form clear, fluid-filled vesicles. Clouding and umbilication of the lesions begin in 24–48 hr. While the initial lesions are crusting, new crops form on the trunk and then the extremities; the simultaneous presence of lesions in various stages of evolution is characteristic of varicella (Fig. 250-1). The distribution of the rash is predominantly central or centripetal, in contrast to smallpox, where the rash is more prominent on the face and distal extremities. Ulcerative lesions involving the mucosa of oropharynx and vagina are also common; many children have vesicular lesions on the eyelids and conjunctivae, but corneal involvement and serious ocular disease is rare. The average number of varicella lesions is about 300, but healthy children may have fewer than 10 to more than 1,500 lesions. In cases resulting from secondary household spread and in older children, more lesions usually occur, and new crops of lesions may continue to develop for a longer period of time. The exanthem may be much more extensive in children with skin disorders, such as eczema or recent sunburn. Hypopigmentation or hyperpigmentation of lesion sites persists for days to weeks in some children, but severe scarring is unusual unless the lesions were secondarily infected.

The **differential diagnosis** of varicella includes vesicular rashes caused by other infectious agents, such as herpes simplex virus, enterovirus, monkey pox, rickettsial pox, or *S. aureus;* drug reactions; contact dermatitis; and insect bites. Severe varicella was the most common illness confused with smallpox before the eradication of smallpox. Because of concerns about smallpox as a potential bioterrorism threat, both smallpox and smallpox vaccine rashes must be considered again in the differential diagnosis of severe chickenpox.

Varicella in Vaccinated Individuals ("Breakthrough Varicella"). Vaccine is >95% effective in preventing severe varicella and is most commonly about 80% (range 70–100%) effective at preventing all disease after exposure to wild-type VZV. This means that following close exposure to VZV, as may occur in a household or an outbreak setting in a school or daycare center, 1 of every 5 vaccinated children may develop breakthrough varicella. Exposure to VZV may also result in asymptomatic infection in the previously immunized child. In contrast, breakthrough disease is varicella that occurs in a person vaccinated >42 days before rash onset and is caused by **wild-type VZV.** In the early stages of the varicella vaccination program, rash occurring within the 1st 2 wk of vaccination was most commonly wild-type VZV, while rash occurring 2–6 weeks after vaccination was due to either the wild or vaccine strains. As varicella disease continues to decline, rashes in the interval 0–42 days postvaccination will be less commonly caused by wild-type VZV. The rash in breakthrough disease is frequently atypical, predominantly maculopapular, vesicles are seen less commonly, and the illness is most commonly mild with <50 lesions and little or no fever. Breakthrough cases are **less contagious** than wild-type infections within household settings. Typical breakthrough cases (<50 lesions) are about 1/3 as contagious as unvaccinated cases, whereas breakthrough cases with ≥50 lesions are as contagious as wild-type cases. Therefore, children with breakthrough disease should be considered potentially infectious and excluded from school until lesions have crusted or, if there are no vesicles present, until no new lesions are occurring. Transmission has been documented to occur from breakthrough cases in household, child-care, and school settings.

Progressive Varicella. Progressive varicella, with visceral organ involvement, coagulopathy, severe hemorrhage, and continued vesicular lesion development, is a dreaded complication of primary VZV infection. Severe abdominal pain, which may reflect involvement of mesenteric lymph nodes or the liver, or the appearance of hemorrhagic vesicles in otherwise healthy adolescents and adults, immunocompromised children, pregnant women, and newborns, may herald this. Although rare in healthy children, the risk for progressive varicella is highest in children with congenital cellular immune deficiency disorders and those with malignancy, particularly if chemotherapy was given during the incubation period and the absolute lymphocyte count is <500 cells/mm^3. The mortality rate for children who acquired varicella while undergoing treatment for malignancy and who were not treated with antiviral therapy approaches 7%; varicella-related deaths usually occur within 3 days after the diagnosis of varicella **pneumonia.** Children who acquire varicella after organ transplantation are also at risk for progressive VZV infection. Children on long-term, low-dose systemic corticosteroid therapy are not considered to be at higher risk for severe varicella, but progressive varicella does occur in patients receiving high-dose corticosteroids and has been reported in patients receiving inhaled corticosteroids as well as in asthmatics receiving multiple short courses of systemic corticosteroid therapy. Unusual clinical findings of varicella, including lesions that develop a unique hyperkeratotic appearance and continued new lesion formation for weeks or months, have been described in children with **HIV infection.** Immunization of HIV-infected children who have a CD4 count greater than 15% as well as children with leukemia and solid organ tumors who are stable on maintenance chemotherapy has reduced this problem. Since the advent of the universal immunization program, immunocompromised children are less likely to be exposed to varicella.

Neonatal Chickenpox. Newborns have particularly high mortality in the circumstances of a susceptible mother contracting varicella around the time of delivery. Infants whose mothers develop varicella in the period from 5 days prior to delivery to 2 days afterward are at high risk for severe varicella. The infant acquires the infection transplacentally as a result of maternal viremia, which may occur up to 48 hr prior to the maternal rash. Depending on when virus crosses the placenta, the infant's rash may occur toward the end of the 1st week to the early part of the 2nd week of life. Because the mother has not yet developed a significant antibody response, the infant receives a large dose of virus without the moderating effect of maternal anti-VZV antibody. If the mother develops varicella more than 5 days prior to delivery, she still may pass virus to the soon-to-be-born child, but infection is attenuated due to transmission of maternal antibody across the placenta. This moderating effect of maternal antibody occurs if delivery occurs after 30 wk of gestation, when maternal immunoglobulin G (IgG) is able to cross the placenta. The recommendations for human varicella-zoster immune globulin (VariZIG) reflect the differing risks to the exposed infant. Newborns whose mothers develop varicella 5 days before to 2 days after delivery should receive 1 vial. Although neonatal varicella may occur in about half of these infants despite administration of VariZIG, it is usually mild. Every premature infant born at <28 wk of gestation to a mother with active chickenpox at delivery (even if the maternal rash has been present for >1 wk) should receive VariZIG. Because perinatally acquired varicella may be life threatening, the infant should be treated with acyclovir (10 mg/kg every 8 hr IV) when lesions develop. Neonatal chickenpox can also follow a postpartum exposure of an infant delivered to a mother who was susceptible to VZV, although the frequency of complications declines rapidly in the weeks after birth. Infants with community-acquired chickenpox who develop severe varicella, especially those who develop a complication such as pneumonia, hepatitis, or encephalitis, should also receive treatment with intravenous acyclovir (10 mg/kg every 8 hr IV).

Congenital Varicella Syndrome. When pregnant women contract chickenpox early in pregnancy, experts estimate that as many as 25% of the fetuses may become infected. Fortunately, clinically apparent disease in the infant is uncommon: up to 2% of fetuses whose mothers had varicella in the 1st 20 wk of pregnancy may demonstrate a VZV embryopathy. The period of greatest risk to the fetus correlates with the gestational period when there is major development and innervation of the limb buds and maturation of the eyes. Fetuses infected at 6–12 wk of gestation appear to have maximal interruption with limb development; fetuses infected at 16–20 wk may have eye and brain involvement. In addition, viral damage to the sympathetic fibers in the cervical and lumbosacral cord may lead to divergent effects such as Horner syndrome and dysfunction of the urethral or anal sphincters. Most of the stigmata can be attributed to virus-induced injury to the nervous system, although there is no obvious explanation why certain regions of the body are preferentially infected during fetal VZV infection. The stigmata involve mainly the skin, extremities, eyes, and brain (Table 250-1). The characteristic cutaneous lesion has been called a cicatrix, a zigzag scarring, in a **dermatomal** distribution, often associated with atrophy of the affected limb. The characteristic cicatricial scarring may represent the cutaneous residua of VZV infection of the sensory nerves, analogous to herpes zoster. The virus may select tissues that are in a rapid developmental stage, such as the limb buds. This may result in 1 or more shortened and malformed extremities (Fig. 250-2). The remainder of the torso may be entirely normal in appearance. Alternatively, there may be neither skin nor limb abnormalities, but the infant may show cataracts or even extensive aplasia of the entire brain. Occasionally, calcifications are evident within a microcephalic head (Fig. 250-3). Histologic examination of the brain demonstrates necrotizing cerebral lesions involving the leptomeninges, cortex, and adjacent white matter.

TABLE 250-1. Stigmata of Varicella-Zoster Virus Fetopathy

DAMAGE TO SENSORY NERVES
Cicatricial skin lesions
Hypopigmentation
DAMAGE TO OPTIC STALK AND LENS VESICLE
Microphthalmia
Cataracts
Chorioretinitis
Optic atrophy
DAMAGE TO BRAIN/ENCEPHALITIS
Microcephaly
Hydrocephaly
Calcifications
Aplasia of brain
DAMAGE TO CERVICAL OR LUMBOSACRAL CORD
Hypoplasia of an extremity
Motor and sensory deficits
Absent deep tendon reflexes
Anisocoria
Horner syndrome
Anal/urinary sphincter dysfunction

Many infants with severe manifestations of congenital varicella syndrome (atrophy and scarring of a limb) have significant neurologic deficiencies, whereas those with only isolated stigmata, amenable to treatment, develop normally throughout childhood. Infants with neonatal chickenpox who receive prompt antiviral therapy have an excellent prognosis.

The diagnosis of VZV fetopathy is based mainly on the history of gestational chickenpox combined with the stigmata seen in the fetus. Virus cannot be cultured from the affected newborn, but viral DNA may be detected in tissue samples by polymerase chain reaction (PCR). Some infants have VZV-specific IgM antibody detectable in the cord blood sample, although the IgM titer drops quickly postpartum and can be nonspecifically positive. Chori-

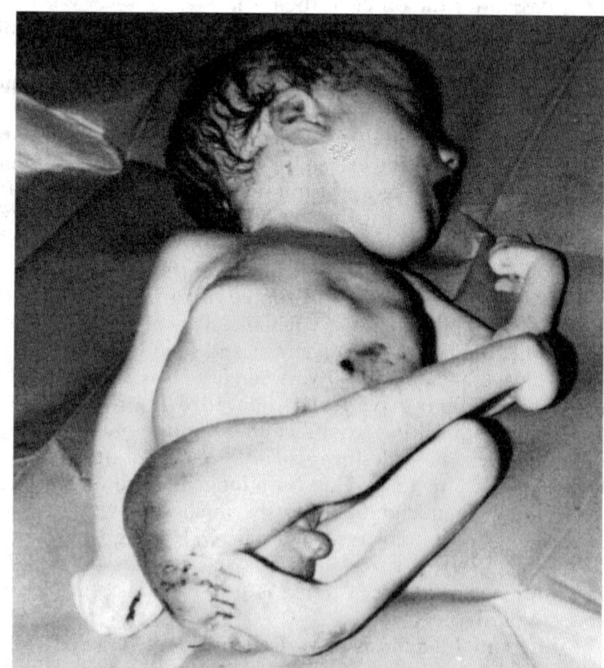

Figure 250-2. Newborn with congenital varicella syndrome. The infant had severe malformations of both lower extremities and cicatricial scarring over his left abdomen.

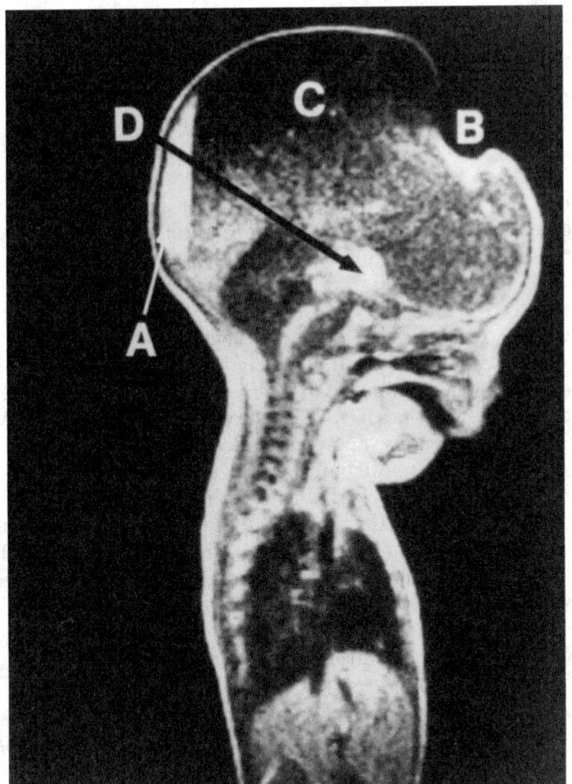

Figure 250-3. MRI of a newborn with encephalitis secondary to congenital varicella syndrome. The intrauterine infection occurred about 3 mo antepartum, at which time there was extensive necrosis of the cerebral hemispheres. The image of the newborn head was taken with the patient supine; therefore, there is a fluid-fluid interface in the dependent occiput (*A*). The hydrocephalus (*C*) and calcifications in the basal ganglia (*D*) are visible; a cranial artifact (*B*) is seen secondary to a scalp vein needle.

onic villus sampling and fetal blood collection for the detection of viral DNA, virus, or antibody have been used in an attempt to diagnose fetal infection and embryopathy. The usefulness of these tests for patient management and counseling has not been defined. Because these tests may not distinguish between infection and disease, their utility may primarily be that of reassurance when the test is negative. A persistently positive VZV IgG antibody titer after 12–18 mo of age is a reliable indicator of prenatal infection in the asymptomatic child, as is the development of zoster in the 1st year of life without evidence of postnatal infection.

Although varicella immune globulin has often been administered to the susceptible mother exposed to chickenpox, it is uncertain as to whether this modifies infection in the fetus. Similarly, acyclovir treatment may be given to the mother with severe varicella. A prospective registry of acyclovir use in the 1st trimester demonstrated that the occurrence of birth defects approximates that found in the general population. The size of the registry, however, is too small ($n = 756$) to conclude that acyclovir is safe for pregnant women and their fetuses. Acyclovir should only be considered when the benefit to the mother outweighs the potential risk to the fetus. The efficacy of acyclovir treatment of pregnant women in preventing or modifying the severity of congenital varicella is not known. Finally, since the damage caused by fetal VZV infection does not progress in the postpartum period, antiviral treatment of infants with congenital VZV syndrome is not indicated.

Herpes Zoster. Herpes zoster manifests as vesicular lesions clustered within 1 or less commonly 2 adjacent dermatomes (Fig.

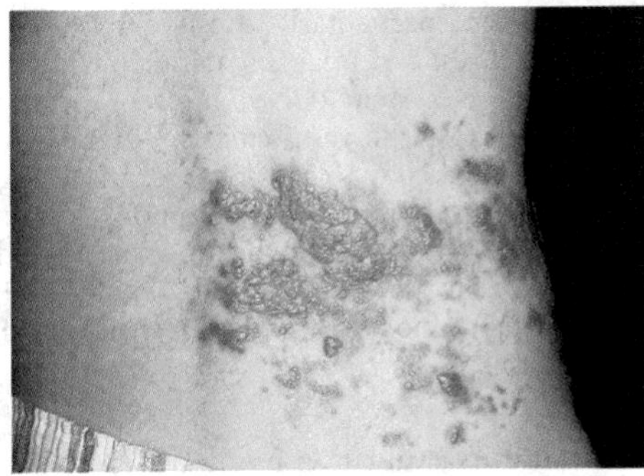

Figure 250-4. Herpes zoster involving the lumbar dermatome. (From Mandell GL, Bennett JE, Dolin R [editors]: *Principles and Practice of Infectious Diseases*, 6th ed, Vol 2. Philadelphia, Elsevier, 2005, p 1783.)

250-4). In the elderly, herpes zoster typically begins with burning pain, with clusters of skin lesions in a dermatomal pattern. Almost half of the elderly with herpes zoster develop complications; the most frequent complication is postherpetic neuralgia, a painful condition that affects the nerves despite resolution of the shingles skin lesions. Unlike herpes zoster in adults, in children it is infrequently associated with localized pain, hyperesthesia, pruritus, and low-grade fever. In children, the rash is mild, with new lesions appearing for a few days; symptoms of acute neuritis are minimal; and complete resolution usually occurs within 1–2 wk. In contrast to adults, postherpetic neuralgia is very unusual in children. Approximately 4% of patients suffer a 2nd episode of herpes zoster; 3 or more episodes are rare. Transverse myelitis with transient paralysis is a rare complication of herpes zoster. An increased risk for herpes zoster early in childhood has been described in children who acquire varicella in the 1st year of life as well as in those whose mothers have a varicella infection in the 3rd trimester of pregnancy (Fig. 250-5).

Immunocompromised children may have more severe herpes zoster, which is similar to that in adults, including postherpetic neuralgia. Immunocompromised patients may also experience disseminated cutaneous disease that mimics varicella, as well as visceral dissemination with pneumonia, hepatitis, encephalitis, and disseminated intravascular coagulopathy. Severely immuno-

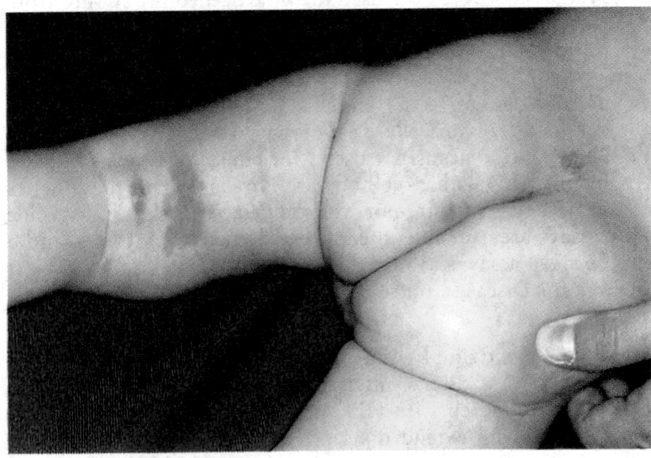

Figure 250-5. Clusters of grouped vesicles on the erythematous bases over the sacrum and popliteal fossa, corresponding to the left S1 dermatome, in a 7 mo old boy who had varicella at age 3 wk after being exposed to his infected sister. (From Kurlan JG, Connelly BL, Lucky AW: Herpes zoster in the first year of life following postnatal exposure to varicella-zoster virus. *Arch Dermatol* 2004;140:1268–1272.)

compromised children, particularly those with HIV infection, may have unusual, chronic or relapsing cutaneous disease, retinitis, or central nervous system (CNS) disease without rash. A lower risk for herpes zoster in vaccinated children with leukemia compared with those who have had varicella disease suggests that varicella vaccine virus reactivates less commonly than wild-type VZV. The risk for herpes zoster in healthy vaccinated children may be lower than in children who had wild-type varicella disease, although many more years of follow-up will be needed to determine that this is the case.

DIAGNOSIS. Laboratory evaluation has not been considered necessary for the diagnosis or management of healthy children with varicella or herpes zoster. However, as disease declines to low levels, laboratory confirmation of all varicella cases may be necessary. The atypical nature of breakthrough varicella, with a higher proportion of rashes being papular rather than vesicular, will pose diagnostic challenges. In addition, severe cases of varicella may need virologic confirmation to distinguish from pox virus infections.

Leukopenia is typical during the 1st 72 hr; it is followed by a relative and absolute lymphocytosis. Results of liver function tests are also usually (75%) mildly elevated. Patients with neurologic complications of varicella or uncomplicated herpes zoster have a mild lymphocytic pleocytosis and a slight to moderate increase in protein in the cerebrospinal fluid; the glucose concentration is usually normal.

Unusual or very severe varicella in otherwise immunocompetent individuals must be distinguished from smallpox, which may occur following deliberate release of smallpox virus (see Chapter 711). A suspected case of smallpox should be reported immediately to the local and state health departments. A protocol for evaluating patients with acute vesicular-pustular rash illness for the possibility of smallpox is available on the CDC website at www.cdc.gov/nip/.

Rapid laboratory diagnosis of VZV is often important in high-risk patients and is sometimes important for infection control. Confirmation of varicella (or herpes simplex virus) can be accomplished by most referral hospital laboratories and all state health laboratories. VZV can be identified quickly by direct fluorescence assay of cells from cutaneous lesions, and by PCR amplification testing. Although multinucleated giant cells can be detected with nonspecific stains (**Tzanck smear**), they have poor sensitivity and do not differentiate VZV from herpes simplex virus infections. Infectious virus may be recovered using tissue culture methods; shell vial assays have decreased the time needed for culture from 7–10 days to 3–4 days. VZV IgG antibodies can be detected by several methods and a 4-fold rise in IgG antibodies is also confirmatory of acute infection. VZV IgG antibody tests can also be valuable to determine the immune status of individuals whose clinical history of varicella is unknown or equivocal. Testing for VZV IgM antibodies is not useful for clinical diagnosis because commercially available methods are unreliable and the kinetics of the IgM response are not well defined. Reliable VZV-specific IgM assays are available in certain reference laboratories, and a capture-IgM assay is available at the national VZV laboratory at Centers for Disease Control.

TREATMENT. Antiviral treatment modifies the course of both varicella and herpes zoster. Antiviral drug resistance is rare but has occurred in children with HIV infection who have been treated with acyclovir for extended periods of time; foscarnet is the only drug available for the treatment of acyclovir-resistant VZV infections.

Varicella. The only antiviral drug available in liquid formulation that is licensed for pediatric use is acyclovir. Given the safety profile of acyclovir and its demonstrated efficacy in the treatment of varicella, treatment of all children, adolescents, and adults with varicella is acceptable. However, acyclovir therapy is not recommended routinely by the American Academy of Pediatrics for treatment of uncomplicated varicella in the otherwise healthy child because of the marginal benefit, the cost of the drug, and the low risk for complications of varicella. Oral therapy with acyclovir (20 mg/kg/dose, maximum 800 mg/dose) given as 4 doses/day for 5 days should be used to treat uncomplicated varicella in nonpregnant individuals >13 yr of age and children >12 mo of age with chronic cutaneous or pulmonary disorders; receiving short-term, intermittent, or aerosolized corticosteroids; receiving long-term salicylate therapy; and possibly 2nd cases in household contacts. To be most effective, treatment should be initiated as early as possible, preferably within 24 hr of the onset of the exanthem. There is dubious clinical benefit if initiation of treatment is delayed more than 72 hr after onset of the exanthem. Acyclovir therapy does not interfere with the induction of VZV immunity. **Intravenous therapy** is indicated for severe disease and for varicella in immunocompromised patients (even after 72 hr duration of rash). Acyclovir has been used to treat varicella in pregnant women; its safety for the fetus has not been established. Some experts recommend the use of famciclovir or valacyclovir in older children who can swallow tablets. While these drugs do not have specific Food and Drug Administration–approved indications for treatment of varicella, they are highly active against VZV by the same mechanism as acyclovir and are better absorbed by the oral route than is acyclovir.

Any patient who has signs of disseminated VZV, including pneumonia, severe hepatitis, thrombocytopenia, or encephalitis, should receive immediate treatment. Intravenous acyclovir (500 mg/m^2 every 8 hr IV) therapy initiated within 72 hr of development of initial symptoms decreases the likelihood of progressive varicella and visceral dissemination in high-risk patients. Treatment is continued for 7 days or until no new lesions have appeared for 48 hr. Delaying antiviral treatment in high-risk individuals until it is obvious that prolonged new lesion formation is occurring is not advisable because visceral dissemination occurs during the same time period.

Herpes Zoster. Antiviral drugs are effective for treatment of herpes zoster. In healthy adults, acyclovir (800 mg 5 times a day PO for 5 days), famciclovir (500 mg tid PO for 7 days), and valacyclovir (1,000 mg tid PO for 7 days) reduce the duration of the illness and the risk for developing postherpetic neuralgia; concomitant corticosteroid usage improves the quality of life in the elderly. In otherwise healthy children, herpes zoster is a less severe disease, and postherpetic neuralgia is rare. Therefore, treatment of uncomplicated herpes zoster in the child with an antiviral agent may not always be necessary, although some experts would treat with oral acyclovir (20 mg/kg/dose, maximum 800 mg/dose) to shorten the duration of the illness. Use of corticosteroids for herpes zoster in otherwise healthy children is not recommended.

In contrast, herpes zoster in **immunocompromised** children can be severe and disseminated disease may be life threatening. Patients at high risk for disseminated disease should receive acyclovir (500 mg/m^2 or 10 mg/kg every 8 hr IV). Oral acyclovir, famciclovir, or valacyclovir are options for immunocompromised patients with uncomplicated herpes zoster and who are considered at low risk for visceral dissemination.

COMPLICATIONS. The complications of VZV infection occur with varicella, or with reactivation of infection, more commonly in immunocompromised patients. In the otherwise healthy child, mild varicella hepatitis is relatively common but rarely clinically symptomatic. Mild thrombocytopenia occurs in 1–2% of children with varicella and may be associated with transient petechiae. Purpura, hemorrhagic vesicles, hematuria, and gastrointestinal bleeding are rare complications that may have serious consequences. **Cerebellar ataxia** occurs in 1 in every 4,000 cases. Other complications of varicella, some of them rare, include encephalitis, pneumonia, nephritis, nephrotic syndrome, hemolytic-uremic syndrome, arthritis, myocarditis, pericarditis, pancreatitis, and orchitis.

Bacterial Infections. Secondary bacterial infections of the skin, usually caused by group A streptococci and *S. aureus,* may occur in up to 5% of children with varicella. These range from superficial impetigo to cellulitis, lymphadenitis, and subcutaneous abscesses. An early manifestation of secondary bacterial infection is erythema of the base of a new vesicle. Recrudescence of fever 3–4 days after the initial exanthem may also herald a secondary bacterial infection. Varicella is a well-described risk factor for serious invasive infections caused by group A streptococcus, which can have a fatal outcome. The more invasive infections, such as varicella gangrenosa, bacterial sepsis, pneumonia, arthritis, osteomyelitis, cellulitis, and necrotizing fasciitis, account for much of the morbidity and mortality of varicella in otherwise healthy children. Bacterial toxin-mediated diseases (toxic shock syndrome) also may complicate varicella. A substantial decline in varicella-related invasive bacterial infections has been associated with the use of the varicella vaccine.

Encephalitis and Cerebellar Ataxia. Encephalitis (1/50,000 cases of varicella) and acute cerebellar ataxia (1/4,000 cases of varicella) are well-described neurologic complications of varicella; morbidity from CNS complications is highest among patients younger than 5 yr or older than 20 yr. Nuchal rigidity, altered consciousness, and seizures characterize meningoencephalitis. Patients with cerebellar ataxia have a gradual onset of gait disturbance, nystagmus, and slurred speech. Neurologic symptoms usually begin 2–6 days after the onset of the rash but may occur during the incubation period or after resolution of the rash. Clinical recovery is typically rapid, occurring within 24–72 hr, and is usually complete. Although severe hemorrhagic encephalitis, analogous to that caused by herpes simplex virus, is very rare in children with varicella, the consequences are similar to herpes encephalitis. Reye syndrome of encephalopathy and hepatic dysfunction associated with varicella has become rare since salicylates are no longer routinely used as antipyretics (see Chapter 358).

Pneumonia. Varicella pneumonia is a severe complication that accounts for most of the increased morbidity and mortality in adults and other high-risk populations, but pneumonia may also complicate varicella in young children. Respiratory symptoms, which may include cough, dyspnea, cyanosis, pleuritic chest pain, and hemoptysis, usually begin within 1–6 days after the onset of the rash. Smoking has been described as a risk factor for severe pneumonia complicating varicella. The frequency of varicella pneumonia may be greater in the parturient and may lead to premature termination of pregnancy.

PROGNOSIS. Primary varicella has a mortality rate of 2–3 per 100,000 cases with the lowest case fatality rates among children 1–9 yr of age (~1 death per 100,000 cases). Compared with these age groups, infants have a 4 times greater risk of dying and adults have a 25 times greater high risk of dying. Approximately 100 deaths occurred in the USA annually before the introduction of the VZV vaccine; the most common complications among people who died from varicella were pneumonia, CNS complications, secondary infections, and hemorrhagic conditions. The mortality rate of untreated primary infection in immunocompromised children is 7–14% and may approach 50% in untreated adults with pneumonia.

Neuritis with herpes zoster should be managed with appropriate analgesics. Postherpetic neuralgia can be a severe problem in adults and may persist for months, requiring care by a specialist in pain management.

PREVENTION. VZV transmission is difficult to prevent because the infection is contagious for 24–48 hr before the rash appears. Infection control practices, including caring for infected patients in isolation rooms with filtered air systems, are essential. All health care workers should have documented VZV immunization or immunity. Susceptible health care workers who have had a close exposure to VZV should not care for high-risk patients during the incubation period.

Vaccine. Varicella is a vaccine-preventable disease. Live virus varicella vaccine is available as a monovalent vaccine and is also available in combination with measles, mumps, and rubella (MMRV) vaccines. Administration of varicella vaccine within 4 wk of MMR vaccine has been associated with a higher risk for breakthrough disease; therefore, it is recommended that the vaccines either be administered simultaneously at different sites or be given at least 4 wk apart. Simultaneous administration of the vaccines may also be accomplished by immunizing with the MMRV vaccine.

Varicella vaccine is recommended for routine administration to children at 12–18 mo and at 4–6 yr of age. Catch-up vaccination with the second dose is recommended for children and adolescents who received only 1 dose. Vaccination with 2 doses, separated by at least 4 wk, is also recommended for children, adolescents, and adults without evidence of immunity. Breakthrough disease may be more common in children vaccinated with a single dose younger than 15 mo.

Varicella vaccine is contraindicated in children with cell-mediated immune deficiencies, although the vaccine may be administered to children with acute lymphoblastic leukemia who are in remission and who meet enrollment criteria under a research protocol, and the vaccine may also be considered for HIV-infected children with a CD4 count greater than 15%. Both these groups should receive 2 doses of vaccine, 3 months apart. Specific guidelines for immunizing these children should be reviewed before vaccination. Children with isolated humoral immune deficiencies may receive VZV vaccine.

Vaccine virus establishes latent infection; however, the risk for developing subsequent herpes zoster is lower after vaccine than after natural VZV infection among immunocompromised children. Postlicensure data also suggest the same trend in healthy vaccinees.

A new VZV vaccine formulation was licensed in 2006 for use as a single immunization of individuals >60 yr of age for prevention of herpes zoster reactivation and to decrease the frequency of postherpetic neuralgia. It is not indicated for the treatment of zoster or postherpetic neuralgia.

Postexposure Prophylaxis. Vaccine given to normal children within 3–5 days after exposure (as soon as possible is preferred) is effective in preventing or modifying varicella, especially in a household setting where exposure is very likely to result in infection. Varicella vaccine is now recommended for postexposure use, for outbreak control. Oral acyclovir administered late in the incubation period may modify subsequent varicella in the normal child; however, its use in this manner is not recommended until it can be further evaluated.

High-titer anti-VZV immune globulin as postexposure prophylaxis is recommended for immunocompromised children, pregnant women, and newborns exposed to maternal varicella. Human varicella-zoster immune globulin (VariZIG) is distributed by FFF Enterprises, California, (1-800-843-7477) to be administered intramuscularly within 96 hr of exposure. The recommended dose is 1 vial (125 units) for each 10 kg increment (maximum 625 units) given intramuscularly as soon as possible but within 96 hr after exposure.

Although licensed pooled intravenous immune globulin (IVIG) preparations contain antivaricella antibodies, the titer varies from lot to lot. The recommended dose of IVIG for postexposure prophylaxis is 400 mg/kg administered once within 96 hr of exposure. Immunocompromised patients who have received high-dose IVIG (100–400 mg/kg) for other indications within 2–3 wk before VZV exposure can be expected to have serum antibodies to VZV.

Newborns whose mothers develop varicella 5 days before to 2 days after delivery should receive 1 vial of VariZIG. VariZIG is also indicated for pregnant women, premature infants <28 wk of gestation (<1,000 g) who were exposed to varicella, and premature infants >28 wk of gestation who are exposed to varicella and whose mother has no evidence of varicella immunity. If possible, adults should be tested for VZV IgG antibodies before VariZIG administration because many adults with no clinical history of varicella are immune. Anti-VZV antibody prophylaxis may ameliorate disease but does not eliminate the possibility of progressive disease, nor does it assure that varicella is not transmitted to close susceptible contacts; patients should be monitored and treated with acyclovir if necessary once lesions develop.

Close contact between a susceptible high-risk patient and a patient with herpes zoster is also an indication for VariZIG prophylaxis. Passive antibody administration or treatment does not reduce the risk for herpes zoster or alter the clinical course of varicella or herpes zoster when given after the onset of symptoms.

Arvin AM: Varicella-zoster virus. *Clin Microbiol Rev* 1996;9:361–368.
Centers for Disease Control and Prevention: Varicella-related deaths among adults—United States, 1997. *MMWR* 1997;46:409–412.
Centers for Disease Control and Prevention: A new product (VariZIG™) for postexposure prophylaxis of varicella available under an investigational new drug application expanded access protocol. *MMWR* 2006;55:1–2.
Chaves SS, Gargiullo P, Zhang JX, et al: Loss of vaccine-induced immunity to varicella over time. *N Engl J Med* 2007;356:1121–1129.
Choo PW, Donahue JG, Manson JE, et al: The epidemiology of varicella and its complications. *J Infect Dis* 1995;172:706–712.
Enders G, Miller E, Cradock-Watson J, et al: Consequences of varicella and herpes zoster in pregnancy. Prospective study of 1739 cases. *Lancet* 1994;343:1548–1551.
Feder HM Jr, Hoss DM: Herpes zoster in otherwise healthy children. *Pediatr Infect Dis J* 2004;23:451–457.
Gershon AA, LaRussa P: Varicella vaccine. *Pediatr Infect Dis J* 1998;17:248–249.
Gershon AA, Mervish N, LaRussa P, et al: Varicella-zoster virus infection in children with underlying human immunodeficiency virus infection. *J Infect Dis* 1997;176:1496–1500.
Guess HA, Broughton DD, Melton LJ II, et al: Population-based studies of varicella complications. *Pediatrics* 1986;78:723–727.
Harris D, Redhead J: Should acyclovir be prescribed for immunocompetent children presenting with chickenpox? *Arch Dis Child* 2005;90:648–650.
Heininger U, Seward JF: Varicella. *Lancet* 2006;368:1365–1376.
Koran G: Congenital varicella syndrome in the third trimester. *Lancet* 2005;366:1591–1592.
Kurlan JG, Connelly BL, Lucky AW: Herpes zoster in the first year of life following postnatal exposure to varicella-zoster virus. *Arch Dermatol* 2004;140:1268–1272.
Kustermann A, Zoppini C, Tassis B, et al: Prenatal diagnosis of congenital varicella infection. *Prenat Diagn* 1996;16:71–74.
The Medical Letter: VariZIG for prophylaxis after exposure to varicella. *Med Lett* 2006;48:69–70.
Meyer PA, Seward JF, Jumaan AO, et al: Varicella mortality: Trends before vaccine licensure in the United States 1970–1994. *J Infect Dis* 2000; 182:383–390.
Mullooly JP, Maher JE, Drew L, et al: Evaluation of the impact of an HMO's varicella vaccination program on incidence of varicella. *Vaccine* 2004;22: 1480–1485.
Oxman MN, Levin MJ, Johnson GR, et al: A vaccine to prevent herpes zoster and postherpetic neuralgia in older adults. *N Engl J Med* 2005;352: 2271–2284.
Patel RA, Binns HJ, Shulman ST: Reduction in pediatric hospitalizations for varicella-related invasive group A streptococcal infections in the varicella vaccine era. *J Pediatr* 2004;144:68–74.
Peterson CL, Mascola L, Chao SM, et al: Children hospitalized for varicella. A pre vaccine review. *J Pediatr* 1996;129:529–536.
Seward JF, Watson BM, Peterson CL, et al: Varicella disease after the introduction of varicella vaccine in the United States, 1995–2000. *JAMA* 2002;287:606–611.
Vazquez M, LaRussa PS, Gershon AA, et al: Effectiveness over time of varicella vaccine. *JAMA* 2004;291:851–855.
Watson BM, Piercy SA, Plotkin SA, et al: Modified chickenpox in children immunized with the Oka/Merck varicella vaccine. *Pediatrics* 1993;91: 17–22.
Zerboni L, Nader S, Aoki K, et al: Analysis of the persistence of humoral and cellular immunity in children and adults immunized with varicella vaccine. *J Infect Dis* 1998;177:1701–1704.

Chapter 251 ■ Epstein-Barr Virus

Hal B. Jenson

Infectious mononucleosis is the best-known clinical syndrome caused by Epstein-Barr virus (EBV). It is characterized by systemic somatic complaints consisting primarily of fatigue, malaise, fever, sore throat, and generalized lymphadenopathy. Originally described as **glandular fever,** it derives its name from the mononuclear lymphocytosis with atypical-appearing lymphocytes that accompany the illness. Other infections may cause infectious mononucleosis-like illnesses.

ETIOLOGY. EBV, a member of the γ-herpesviruses, causes >90% of cases of infectious mononucleosis. Two distinct types of EBV, **type 1 and type 2 (also called type A and type B),** have been characterized and have 70–85% sequence homology. Type 1 is more prevalent worldwide than type 2, although type 2 is more common in Africa than in the United States and Europe. Both types lead to persistent, lifelong, latent infection. Dual infections with both types have been documented among immunocompromised persons. EBV-1 induces in vitro growth transformation of B cells more efficiently then EBV-2, but no type-specific disease manifestations or clinical differences have been identified. Coacquisition of multiple EBV genotypes has been shown by heteroduplex tracking assays to occur commonly in otherwise healthy patients with infectious mononucleosis. However, only a single genotype tends to be cultured. It is unknown if this represents isolation of a predominant strain or if the strains that are not able to be cultured, using the transformation assay, are defective.

As many as 5–10% of infectious mononucleosis-like illnesses are caused by primary infection with cytomegalovirus, *Toxoplasma gondii,* adenovirus, viral hepatitis, HIV, and possibly rubella virus. In the majority of EBV-negative infectious mononucleosis-like illnesses, the exact cause remains unknown.

EPIDEMIOLOGY. The epidemiology of infectious mononucleosis is related to the epidemiology and age of acquisition of EBV infection. EBV infects >95% of the world's population. It is transmitted via penetrative sexual intercourse, and in oral secretions such as "deep kissing." Among children, transmission may occur by exchange of saliva from child to child, such as occurs between children in out-of-home child care. Nonintimate contact, environmental sources, or fomites do not contribute to spread of EBV.

EBV is shed in oral secretions consistently for >6 mo after acute infection and then intermittently for life. As many as 20–30% of healthy EBV-infected persons excrete virus at any particular time. Immunosuppression permits reactivation of latent EBV; 60–90% of EBV-infected immunosuppressed patients shed the virus. EBV is also found in male and female genital secretions and can be spread through sexual contact.

Infection with EBV in developing countries and among socioeconomically disadvantaged populations of developed countries usually occurs during infancy and early childhood. In central Africa, almost all children are infected by 3 yr of age. Primary infection with EBV during childhood is usually inapparent or indistinguishable from other childhood infections; the clinical syndrome of infectious mononucleosis is practically unknown in undeveloped regions of the world. Among more affluent populations in industrialized countries, infection during childhood is also common but occurs less frequently, presumably because of high standards of hygiene, with approximately 1/3 of infections during adolescence and young adulthood. Primary EBV infection in adolescents and adults manifests in >50% of cases as the **classic triad** of fatigue, pharyngitis, and generalized lymphadenopathy, which constitute the major clinical manifestations of infectious mononucleosis. This syndrome may be seen at all ages but is rarely apparent in children <4 yr of age, when most EBV infections are asymptomatic, or in adults >40 yr of age, when most individuals have already been infected by EBV. The true incidence of the syndrome of infectious mononucleosis is unknown but is estimated to occur in 20–70/100,000 persons/yr; in young adults, the incidence increases to about 1/1,000 persons/yr. The prevalence of serologic evidence of past EBV infection increases with age; almost all adults in the United States are seropositive.

PATHOGENESIS. After acquisition in the oral cavity, EBV initially infects oral epithelial cells, which may contribute to the symptoms of pharyngitis. After intracellular viral replication and cell lysis with release of new virions, virus spreads to contiguous structures such as the salivary glands, with eventual viremia and infection of B lymphocytes in the peripheral blood and the entire lymphoreticular system, including the liver and spleen. The atypical lymphocytes that are characteristic of infectious mononucleosis are $CD8^+$ T lymphocytes, which exhibit both suppressor and cytotoxic functions that develop in response to the infected B lymphocytes. This relative as well as absolute increase in $CD8^+$ lymphocytes results in a transient reversal of the normal 2 : 1 $CD4^+/CD8^+$ (helper-suppressor) T-lymphocyte ratio. Many of the clinical manifestations of infectious mononucleosis may result, at least in part, from cytokine release from the host immune response, which is effective in reducing the EBV load to <1 copy/10^5 circulating B lymphocytes, equivalent to <10 copies/µg of DNA from whole blood. The EBV load is more variable among immunocompromised persons and can be >4,000 copies/µg of DNA.

Epithelial cells of the uterine cervix may become infected by sexual transmission of the virus, although local symptoms have been described after sexual transmission. EBV is consistently found intracellularly in smooth muscle cells of leiomyosarcomas of immunocompromised persons.

EBV, like the other herpesviruses, establishes lifelong latent infection after the primary illness. The latent virus is carried in oropharyngeal epithelial cells and systemically in memory B lymphocytes as multiple episomes in the nucleus. The viral episomes replicate with cell division and are distributed to both daughter cells. Viral integration into the cell genome is not typical. Only a few viral proteins, including the EBV-determined nuclear antigens (EBNAs), are produced during latency. These proteins are important in maintaining the viral episome during the latent state. Progression to viral replication begins with production of EBV early antigens (EAs), proceeds to viral DNA replication, is followed by production of viral capsid antigen (VCA), and culminates in cell death and release of mature virions. Reactivation with viral replication occurs at a low rate in populations of latently infected cells and is responsible for intermittent viral shedding in oropharyngeal secretions of infected individuals. Reactivation is apparently asymptomatic and not recognized to be accompanied by distinctive clinical symptoms.

ONCOGENESIS. EBV was the 1st human virus to be associated with malignancy. EBV infection may result in a spectrum of proliferative disorders ranging from self-limited, usually benign disease such as infectious mononucleosis to aggressive, nonmalignant proliferations such as the virus-associated hemophagocytic syndrome to lymphoid and epithelial cell malignancies. Benign EBV-associated proliferations include oral hairy leukoplakia, primarily in adults with AIDS, and lymphoid interstitial pneumonitis, primarily in children with AIDS. Malignant EBV-associated proliferations include nasopharyngeal carcinoma, Burkitt lymphoma, Hodgkin disease, lymphoproliferative disorders, and leiomyosarcoma in immunodeficient states, including AIDS. There is no firm evidence of development of EBV quasispecies that would contribute to the pathogenesis of EBV-positive malignancies.

Nasopharyngeal carcinoma occurs worldwide but is 10 times more common in persons in southern China, where it is the most common malignant tumor among adult men. It is also common among whites in North Africa and Inuits in North America. Patients usually present with cervical lymphadenopathy, eustachian tube blockage, and nasal obstruction with epistaxis. All malignant cells of undifferentiated nasopharyngeal carcinoma contain a high copy number of EBV episomes. Persons with undifferentiated and partially differentiated, nonkeratinizing nasopharyngeal carcinomas have elevated EBV antibody titers that are both diagnostic and prognostic. High levels of immunoglobulin A (IgA) antibody to EA and VCA may be detected in asymptomatic individuals and can be used to follow response to tumor therapy (Table 251-1). Cells of well-differentiated, keratinizing nasopharyngeal carcinoma contain a low number of or no EBV genomes; these persons have EBV serologic patterns similar to those of the general population.

CT and MR images are helpful in both identifying and defining masses in the head and neck. The diagnosis is established by biopsy of the mass or of a suspicious cervical lymph node. Surgery is important for staging and diagnosis. Radiation therapy is effective for control of the primary tumor and regional nodal metastases. Chemotherapy with 5-fluorouracil, cisplatin, and methotrexate is effective but not always curative. The prognosis is good if the tumor is localized.

Endemic (African) Burkitt lymphoma, often found in the jaw, is the most common childhood cancer in equatorial East Africa and New Guinea (see Chapter 496.2). The median age at onset is 5 yr. These regions are holoendemic for *Plasmodium falciparum* malaria and have a high rate of EBV infection early in life. The constant malarial exposure acts as a B-lymphocyte mitogen that contributes to the polyclonal B-lymphocyte proliferation with EBV infection, impairs the T-lymphocyte control of EBV-infected B lymphocytes, and increases the risk for development of Burkitt lymphoma. Approximately 98% of cases of endemic Burkitt lymphoma contain the EBV genome compared with only 20% of nonendemic (sporadic or American) Burkitt lymphoma cases. Individuals with Burkitt lymphoma have unusually and characteristically high levels of antibody to VCA and EA that correlate with the risk for developing tumor (see Table 251-1).

All cases of Burkitt lymphoma, including those that are EBV negative, are monoclonal and demonstrate chromosomal translocation of the c-*myc* proto-oncogene to the constant region of the immunoglobulin heavy-chain locus, t(8;14), to the κ constant light-chain locus, t(2;8), or to the λ constant light-chain locus, t(8;22). This results in the deregulation and constitutive transcription of the c-*myc* gene with overproduction of a normal c-*myc* product that auto-suppresses c-*myc* production on the untranslocated chromosome.

The incidence of **Hodgkin disease** peaks in childhood in developing countries and in young adulthood in developed countries. Levels of EBV antibodies are consistently elevated preceding development of Hodgkin disease; only a small minority of patients are seronegative for EBV. Infection with EBV appears to increase the risk for Hodgkin disease by a factor of 2 to 4. EBV is associated with more than half of cases of mixed cellularity Hodgkin disease and approximately $^1/_4$ of cases of the nodular sclerosing subtype, and is rarely associated with lymphocyte-predominant Hodgkin disease. Immunohistochemical studies have localized EBV to the Reed-Sternberg cells and their variants, the pathognomonic malignant cells of Hodgkin disease.

TABLE 251-1. Correlation of Clinical Status and Serologic Responses to EBV Infection

	SEROLOGIC RESPONSE					
		EBV-SPECIFIC ANTIBODY				
Clinical Status	**Heterophile Antibodies (Qualitative Test)**	**IgM-VCA**	**IgG-VCA**	**EA-D**	**EA-R**	**EBNA**
Negative reaction	–	<1 : 8*	<1 : 10*	<1 : 10*	<1 : 10*	<1 : 2.5*
Susceptible	–	–	–	–	–[†]	–
Acute primary infection: infectious mononucleosis	+	1 : 32 to 1 : 256	1 : 160 to 1 : 640	1 : 40 to 1 : 160	–[†]	– to 1 : 2.5
Recent primary infection: infectious mononucleosis	+/–	– to 1 : 32	1 : 320 to 1 : 1,280	1 : 40 to 1 : 160	–[†]	1 : 5 to 1 : 10
Remote infection	–	–	1 : 40 to 1 : 160	–[‡]	– to 1 : 40	1 : 10 to 1 : 40
Reactivation: immunosuppressed or immunocompromised	–	–	1 : 320 to 1 : 1,280	–[‡]	1 : 80 to 1 : 320	– to 1 : 160
Burkitt lymphoma	–	–	1 : 320 to 1 : 1,280	–[‡]	1 : 80 to 1 : 320	1 : 10 to 1 : 80
Nasopharyngeal carcinoma	–	–	1 : 320 to 1 : 1,280	1 : 40 to 1 : 160	–[§]	1 : 20 to 1 : 160

The data were obtained from numerous studies. Individual responses outside the characteristic range may occur.
*Or the lowest test dilution.
[†]In young children and adults with asymptomatic seroconversion, the anti–early antigen response may be mainly to the EA-R component.
[‡]A minority of individuals will have the anti–early antigen response mainly to the EA-D component.
[§]A minority of individuals will have the anti–early antigen response mainly to the EA-R component.
EA-D, diffuse staining component of early antigen; EA-R, cytoplasmic restricted component of early antigen; EBNA, EBV-determined nuclear antigens; EBV, Epstein-Barr virus; IgG, immunoglobulin G; IgM, immunoglobulin M; VCA, viral capsid antigen; –, negative; +, positive.
Reprinted with permission from Jenson HB: Epstein-Barr virus. In Detrick B, Hamilton RG, Folds JD (editors): *Manual of Molecular and Clinical Laboratory Immunology,* 7th ed. Washington, DC, American Society for Microbiology, 2006.

Failure to control EBV infection may result from host immunologic deficits. The prototype is the **X-linked lymphoproliferative syndrome (Duncan syndrome),** an X chromosome–linked recessive disorder of the immune system associated with severe, persistent, and sometimes fatal EBV infection (see Chapter 123). Approximately $^2/_3$ of these male patients die of disseminated and fulminating lymphoproliferation involving multiple organs at the time of primary EBV infection. Surviving patients acquire hypogammaglobulinemia, B-cell lymphoma, or both. Most patients die within 10 yr.

Numerous congenital and acquired immunodeficiency syndromes are associated with an increased incidence of EBV-associated B-lymphocyte lymphoma, especially central nervous system lymphoma, and leiomyosarcoma. The incidence of lymphoproliferative syndromes parallels the degree of immunosuppression. A decline in T-cell function evidently permits EBV to escape from immune surveillance. Congenital immunodeficiencies predisposing to EBV-associated lymphoproliferation include the X-linked lymphoproliferative syndrome, common-variable immunodeficiency, ataxia-telangiectasia, Wiskott-Aldrich syndrome, and Chédiak-Higashi syndrome. Individuals with acquired immunodeficiencies resulting from anticancer chemotherapy, immunosuppression after solid organ or bone marrow transplantation, or HIV infection have a significantly increased risk for EBV-associated lymphoproliferation. The lymphomas may be focal or diffuse, and they are usually histologically polyclonal but may become monoclonal. Their growth is not reversed on cessation of immunosuppression.

EBV is found intracellularly in all of the smooth muscle cells of leiomyosarcomas occurring in immunocompromised persons, including HIV-infected patients and transplant recipients, but not in leiomyosarcomas occurring in immunocompetent persons.

EBV is also associated with carcinoma of the salivary glands. Other tumors putatively associated with EBV include some T-lymphocyte lymphomas (including lethal midline), angioimmunoblastic lymphadenopathy-like lymphoma, thymomas and thymic carcinomas derived from thymic epithelial cells, supraglottic laryngeal carcinomas, lymphoepithelial tumors of the respiratory tract and gastrointestinal tract, and gastric adenocarcinoma. The precise contribution of EBV to these various malignancies is not well defined.

CLINICAL MANIFESTATIONS. The incubation period of infectious mononucleosis in adolescents is 30–50 days. In children, it may be shorter. The majority of cases of primary EBV infection in infants and young children are clinically silent. In older patients, the onset of illness is usually insidious and vague. Patients may complain of malaise, fatigue, acute or prolonged (>1 wk) fever, headache, sore throat, nausea, abdominal pain, and myalgia. This prodromal period may last 1–2 wk. The complaints of sore throat and fever gradually increase until patients seek medical care. Splenic enlargement may be rapid enough to cause left upper quadrant abdominal discomfort and tenderness, which may be the presenting complaint.

The **physical examination** is characterized by generalized lymphadenopathy (90% of cases), splenomegaly (50% of cases), and hepatomegaly (10% of cases). Lymphadenopathy occurs most commonly in the anterior and posterior cervical nodes and the submandibular lymph nodes and less commonly in the axillary and inguinal lymph nodes. Epitrochlear lymphadenopathy is particularly suggestive of infectious mononucleosis. Symptomatic hepatitis or jaundice is uncommon, but elevated liver enzymes are common. Splenomegaly to 2–3 cm below the costal margin is typical; massive enlargement is uncommon.

The sore throat is often accompanied by moderate to severe pharyngitis with marked tonsillar enlargement, occasionally with exudates (Fig. 251-1). Petechiae at the junction of the hard and soft palate are frequently seen. The pharyngitis resembles that caused by streptococcal infection. Other clinical findings may include rashes and edema of the eyelids.

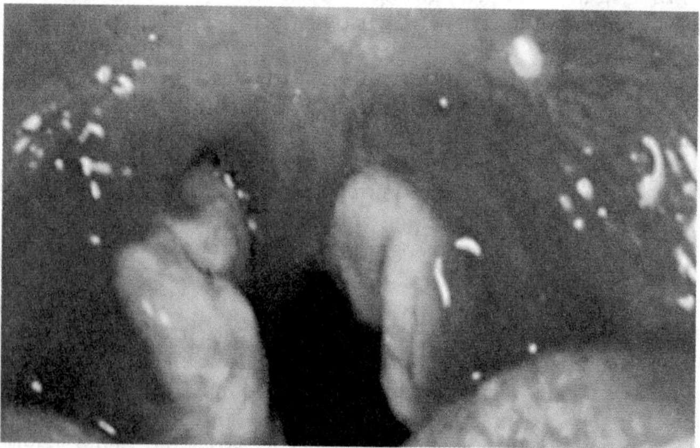

Figure 251-1. Tonsillitis with membrane formation in infectious mononucleosis. See also color plates. (Courtesy of Alex J. Steigman, MD.)

Rashes are usually maculopapular and have been reported in 3–15% of patients. Up to 80% of patients with infectious mononucleosis experience "**ampicillin rash**" if treated with ampicillin or amoxicillin. This vasculitic rash is probably immune mediated and resolves without specific treatment. EBV is also associated with **Gianotti-Crosti syndrome,** a symmetrical rash on the cheeks with multiple erythematous papules, which may coalesce into plaques, and persists for 15–50 days. The rash has the appearance of atopic dermatitis and may appear on the extremities and buttocks.

DIAGNOSIS. The diagnosis of infectious mononucleosis implies primary EBV infection. A presumptive diagnosis may be made by the presence of typical clinical symptoms with atypical lymphocytosis in the peripheral blood. The diagnosis is usually confirmed by serologic testing, either for heterophile antibody or specific EBV antibodies.

Culture of EBV is tedious and requires 4–6 wk. The culture method is the **transformation assay,** which is performed by cocultivating oropharyngeal or genital secretions, peripheral blood (10–30 mL), or tumor with human umbilical cord lymphocytes. The cultures are observed for 6 wk for signs of **cell transformation:** proliferation and rapid growth, mitotic figures, large vacuoles, granular morphology, and cell aggregation. EBV **immortalizes** the umbilical cord cells, resulting in cell lines that can be maintained in perpetuity that harbor EBV isolated from the patient.

Differential Diagnosis. Infectious mononucleosis-like illnesses may be caused by primary infection with cytomegalovirus, *T. gondii,* adenovirus, viral hepatitis, HIV, or possibly rubella virus. Cytomegalovirus infection is a particularly common cause in adults. Streptococcal pharyngitis may cause sore throat and cervical lymphadenopathy indistinguishable from that of infectious mononucleosis but is not associated with hepatosplenomegaly. Approximately 5% of cases of EBV-associated infectious mononucleosis have positive throat cultures for group A streptococcus; this represents pharyngeal streptococcal carriage. Failure of a patient with streptococcal pharyngitis to improve within 48–72 hr should evoke suspicion of infectious mononucleosis. The most serious problem in the diagnosis of acute illness arises in the occasional patient with extremely high or low white blood cell counts, moderate thrombocytopenia, and even hemolytic anemia. In these patients, bone marrow examination and hematologic consultation are warranted to exclude the possibility of leukemia.

LABORATORY TESTS. In >90% of cases there is leukocytosis of 10,000–20,000 cells/mm^3, of which at least 2/3 are lymphocytes; atypical lymphocytes usually account for 20–40% of the total number. The atypical cells are mature T lymphocytes that have been antigenically activated. Compared with regular lymphocytes microscopically, atypical lymphocytes are larger overall, with larger, eccentrically placed indented and folded nuclei with a lower nuclear-to-cytoplasm ratio. Although atypical lymphocytosis may be seen with many of the infections usually causing lymphocytosis, the highest degree of atypical lymphocytes is classically seen with EBV infection. Other syndromes associated with atypical lymphocytosis include acquired cytomegalovirus infection (in contrast to congenital cytomegalovirus infection), toxoplasmosis, viral hepatitis, rubella, roseola, mumps, tuberculosis, typhoid, *Mycoplasma* infection, and malaria, as well as some drug reactions. Mild thrombocytopenia to 50,000–200,000 platelets/mm^3 occurs in >50% of patients but only rarely is associated with purpura. Mild elevation of hepatic transaminases occurs in approximately 50% of uncomplicated cases but is usually asymptomatic without jaundice.

HETEROPHILE ANTIBODY TEST. Heterophile antibodies agglutinate cells from species different from those in the source serum. The transient heterophile antibodies seen in infectious mononucleosis, also known as Paul-Bunnell antibodies, are IgM antibodies detected by the Paul-Bunnell-Davidsohn test for sheep red cell agglutination. The heterophile antibodies of infectious mononucleosis agglutinate sheep or, for greater sensitivity, horse red cells but not guinea pig kidney cells. This adsorption property differentiates this response from the heterophile response found in patients with serum sickness, rheumatic diseases, and some normal individuals. Titers of >1 : 28 or >1 : 40, depending on the dilution system used, after absorption with guinea pig cells are considered positive.

Results of the sheep red cell agglutination test are often positive for several months after infectious mononucleosis; those of the horse red cell agglutination test may be positive for as long as 2 yr. The most widely used method is the qualitative rapid slide test using horse erythrocytes. It detects heterophile antibody in 90% of cases of EBV-associated infectious mononucleosis in older children and adults but in only up to 50% of cases in children <4 yr of age because they typically develop a lower titer. From 5 to 10% of cases of infectious mononucleosis are not caused by EBV and are not uniformly associated with a heterophile antibody response. The false-positive rate is <10%, usually resulting from erroneous interpretation. If the heterophile test result is negative and an EBV infection is suspected, EBV-specific antibody testing is indicated.

SPECIFIC EBV ANTIBODIES. EBV-specific antibody testing is useful to confirm acute EBV infection, especially in heterophile-negative cases, or to confirm past infection and determine susceptibility to future infection. Several distinct EBV antigen systems have been characterized for diagnostic purposes (see Fig. 251-2 and Table 251-1). The EBNA, EA, and VCA antigen systems are most useful for diagnostic purposes. The acute phase of infectious mononucleosis is characterized by rapid IgM and IgG antibody responses to VCA in all cases and an IgG response to EA in most cases. The IgM response to VCA is transient but can be detected for at least 4 wk and occasionally up to 3 mo. The laboratory must take steps to remove rheumatoid factor, which may cause a false-positive IgM VCA result. The IgG response to VCA usually peaks late in the acute phase, declines slightly over the next several weeks to months, and then persists at a relatively stable level for life.

Anti-EA antibodies are usually detectable for several months but may persist or be detected intermittently at low levels for many years. Antibodies to the diffuse-staining component of EA, EA-D, are found transiently in 80% of patients during the acute phase of infectious mononucleosis and reach high titers in patients with nasopharyngeal carcinoma. Antibodies to the cytoplasmic-restricted component of EA, EA-R, emerge transiently in the convalescence from infectious mononucleosis and often attain high titers in patients with EBV-associated Burkitt lymphoma, which in the terminal stage of the disease may be exceeded by antibodies to EA-D. High levels of antibodies to EA-D or EA-R may be found also in immunocompromised patients with persistent EBV infections and active EBV replication. Anti-EBNA antibodies are the last to develop in infectious mononucleosis and gradually appear 3–4 mo after the onset of illness and remain at low levels for life. Absence of anti-EBNA when other antibodies are present implies recent infection, whereas the presence of anti-EBNA implies infection occurring more than 3–4 mo previously. The wide range of individual antibody responses and the various laboratory methods used can occasionally make interpretation of an antibody profile difficult. The detection of IgM antibody to VCA is the most valuable and specific serologic test for the diagnosis of acute EBV infection and is generally sufficient to confirm the diagnosis.

TREATMENT. There is no specific treatment for infectious mononucleosis. Therapy with high doses of acyclovir, with or without

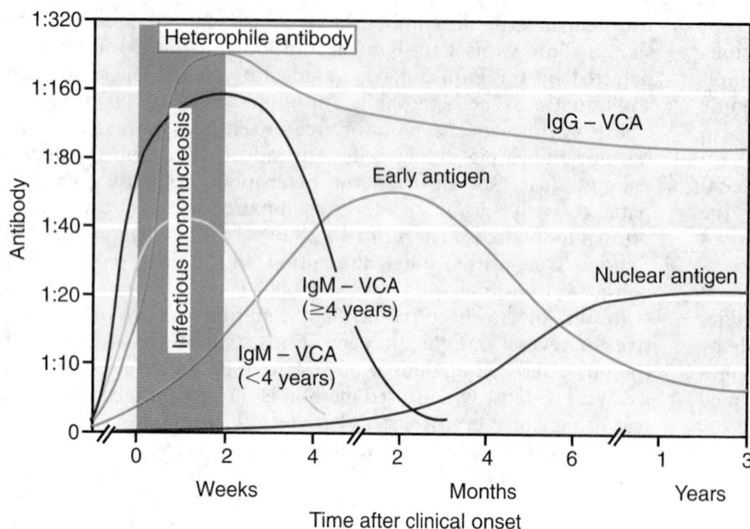

Figure 251-2. Schematic representation of the development of antibodies to various Epstein-Barr virus antigens in patients with infectious mononucleosis. Antibody titers are calculated as geometric mean values expressed as reciprocals of the serum dilution. The immunoglobulin M (IgM) response to viral capsid antigen (VCA) is divided because of the significant differences noted according to age of the patient. IgG, immunoglobulin G. (Reprinted with permission from Jenson HB: Epstein-Barr virus. In Detrick B, Hamilton RG, Folds JD [editors]: *Manual of Molecular and Clinical Laboratory Immunology,* 7th ed. Washington, DC, American Society for Microbiology, 2006.)

corticosteroids, decreases viral replication and oropharyngeal shedding during the period of administration but does not reduce the severity or duration of symptoms or alter the eventual outcome. Rest and symptomatic treatments are the mainstays of management. Bed rest is necessary only when the patient has debilitating fatigue. As soon as there is definite symptomatic improvement, the patient should be allowed to begin resumption of normal activities. Because blunt abdominal trauma may predispose patients to splenic rupture, it is customary and prudent to advise against participation in contact sports and strenuous athletic activities during the 1st 2–3 wk of illness or while splenomegaly is present.

Short courses of corticosteroids (<2 wk) may be helpful for complications of infectious mononucleosis, but this use has not been evaluated critically. Some appropriate indications include incipient airway obstruction, thrombocytopenia with hemorrhaging, autoimmune hemolytic anemia, seizures, and meningitis. A recommended dosage is prednisone 1 mg/kg/day (maximum 60 mg/day) or equivalent for 7 days and tapered over another 7 days. There are no controlled data showing efficacy of corticosteroids in any of these conditions. In view of the potential and unknown hazards of immunosuppression for a virus infection with oncogenic complications, corticosteroids should not be used in uncomplicated cases of infectious mononucleosis.

COMPLICATIONS. Very few patients with infectious mononucleosis experience complications. The most feared complication is subcapsular splenic hemorrhage or splenic rupture, which occurs most frequently during the 2nd week of the disease at a rate of <0.5% of cases in adults; the rate in children is unknown but is probably much lower. Rupture is commonly related to trauma, which often may be mild, and is rarely fatal. Swelling of the tonsils and oropharyngeal lymphoid tissue may be substantial and may cause airway obstruction that manifests as drooling, stridor, and interference with breathing. Airway compromise with progressive symptoms occurs in <5% of cases and is a common indication for hospitalization with infectious mononucleosis. It may be managed by elevating the head of the bed and administration of intravenous hydration, humidified air, and systemic corticosteroids. Respiratory distress with incipient or actual airway occlusion should be managed by tonsillo-adenoidectomy followed by endotracheal intubation for 12–24 hr in an intensive care setting.

Many uncommon and unusual neurologic conditions have been reported to be associated with EBV infectious mononucleosis. Headache is present in about half of cases, with severe neurologic manifestations, such as seizures and ataxia, in 1–5% of cases. Perceptual distortions of sizes, shapes, and spatial relationships, known as the **Alice in Wonderland syndrome (metamorphopsia)**, may be a presenting symptom. There may be meningitis with nuchal rigidity and mononuclear cells in the cerebrospinal fluid, facial nerve palsy, transverse myelitis, and encephalitis.

Guillain-Barré syndrome or Reye syndrome may follow acute illness. Hemolytic anemia, often with a positive Coombs test result and with cold agglutinins specific for red cell antigen i, occurs in 3% of cases. The onset is typically in the 1st 2 wk of illness and lasts for <1 mo. Aplastic anemia is a rare complication that usually presents 3–4 wk after the onset of illness, usually with recovery in 4–8 days, but some cases do require bone marrow transplantation. Mild thrombocytopenia and neutropenia are common, but severe thrombocytopenia (<20,000 platelets/μL) or severe neutropenia (<1,000 neutrophils/μL) are rare. Myocarditis or interstitial pneumonia may occur, both resolving in 3–4 wk. Other rare complications include pancreatitis, parotitis, and orchitis.

PROGNOSIS. The prognosis for complete recovery is excellent if no complications ensue during the acute illness. The major symptoms typically last 2–4 wk, followed by gradual recovery. Second infections with a different type of EBV (type 1 or type 2) have been demonstrated in immunocompromised persons, but symptoms or 2nd attacks of infectious mononucleosis caused by EBV have not been documented. Prolonged and debilitating fatigue, malaise, and some disability that may wax and wane for several weeks to 6 mo are common complaints even in otherwise unremarkable cases. Occasional persistence of fatigue for a few years after infectious mononucleosis is well recognized. There is no convincing evidence linking EBV infection or EBV reactivation to chronic fatigue syndrome (see Chapter 120).

Alpert G, Fleisher GR: Complications of infection with Epstein-Barr virus during childhood. A study of children admitted to the hospital. *Pediatr Infect Dis* 1984;3:304–307.

Balfour HH Jr, Holman CJ, Hokanson KM, et al: A prospective clinical study of Epstein-Barr virus and host interactions during acute infectious mononucleosis. *J Infect Dis* 2005;192:1505–1512.

Crawford DH, Swedlow AJ, Higgins C, et al: Sexual history and Epstein-Barr virus infection. *J Infect Dis* 2002;186:731–736.

Crawford DH, Macsween KF, Higgins CD, et al: A cohort study among university students: Identification of risk factors for Epstein-Barr virus seroconversion and infectious mononucleosis. *Clin Infect Dis* 2006;43:276–282.

Fafi-Kremer S, Morand P, Brion JP, et al: Long-term shedding of infectious Epstein-Barr virus after infectious mononucleosis. *J Infect Dis* 2005;191:985–989.

Horwitz CA, Henle W, Henle G, et al: Clinical and laboratory evaluation of cytomegalovirus-induced mononucleosis in previously healthy individuals. Report of 82 cases. *Medicine* 1986;65:124–134.

Jenson H: Acute complications of Epstein-Barr virus infectious mononucleosis. *Curr Opin Pediatr* 2000;12:263–268.

Jenson H, McIntosh K, Pitt J, et al: Natural history of primary Epstein-Barr virus infection in children of mothers infected with human immunodeficiency virus type 1. *J Infect Dis* 1999;179:1395–1404.

Jenson HB, Leach CT, McClain KL, et al: Benign and malignant smooth muscle tumors containing Epstein-Barr virus in children with AIDS. *Leuk Lymphoma* 1997;27:303–314.

Moormann AM, Chelimo K, Sumba OP, et al: Exposure to holoendemic malaria results in elevated Epstein-Barr virus loads in children. *J Infect Dis* 2005;191:1233–1238.

Sitki-Green DL, Edwards RH, Covington MM, et al: Biology of Epstein-Barr virus during infectious mononucleosis. *J Infect Dis* 2004;189;483–492.

Straus SE, Tosato G, Armstrong G, et al: Persisting illness and fatigue in adults with evidence of Epstein-Barr virus infection. *Ann Intern Med* 1985;102:7–16.

Sumaya CV, Ench Y: Epstein-Barr virus infectious mononucleosis in children I. Clinical and general laboratory findings. *Pediatrics* 1985;75:1003–1010.

Sumaya CV, Ench Y: Epstein-Barr virus infectious mononucleosis in children II. Heterophile antibody and viral-specific responses. *Pediatrics* 1985;75:1011–1019.

Thompson SK, Doerr TD, Hengerer AS: Infectious mononucleosis and corticosteroids. *Arch Otolaryngol Head Neck Surg* 2005;131:900–904.

Tierney RJ, Edwards RH, Sitki-Green D, et al: Multiple Epstein-Barr virus strains in patients with infectious mononucleosis: Comparison of ex vivo samples with in vitro isolates by use of heteroduplex tracking assays. *J Infect Dis* 2006;193:287–297.

Torre D, Tambini R: Acyclovir for treatment of infectious mononucleosis: A meta-analysis. *Scand J Infect Dis* 1999;31:543–547.

Williams H, Macsween K, McAulay K, et al: Analysis of immune activation and clinical events in acute infectious mononucleosis. *J Infect Dis* 2004;190:63–71.

Yoshida M, Tsuda N, Morihata T, et al: Five patients with localized facial eruptions associated with Gianotti-Crosti syndrome caused by primary Epstein-Barr virus infection. *J Pediatr* 2004;145:843–844.

Chapter 252 ■ Cytomegalovirus

Sergio Stagno

Human cytomegalovirus (CMV) is a member of the Herpesviridae family and is widely distributed. Most CMV infections are inapparent, but the virus can cause a variety of clinical illnesses that range in severity from mild to fatal. CMV is the most common cause of congenital infection, which occasionally causes the syndrome of **cytomegalic inclusion disease** (hepatosplenomegaly, jaundice, petechia, purpura, and microcephaly) in neonates. In immunocompetent adults, CMV infection is occasionally characterized by a mononucleosis-like syndrome. In immunocompromised persons, including transplant recipients and patients with AIDS, CMV pneumonitis, retinitis, and gastrointestinal disease are common and can be fatal.

Primary infection occurs in a seronegative, susceptible host. **Recurrent infection** represents reactivation of latent infection or reinfection of a seropositive immune host. Disease may result from primary or recurrent CMV infection, but the former is more commonly associated with severe disease.

ETIOLOGY. CMV is the largest of the herpesviruses, and has a diameter of 200 nm with a double-stranded DNA viral genome of 240 kb in a 64 nm core enclosed by an icosahedral capsid composed of 162 capsomers. The core is assembled in the nucleus of the host cells. The capsid is surrounded by a poorly defined amorphous tegument, which is itself surrounded by a loosely applied, lipid-containing envelope. The envelope is acquired during the budding process through the nuclear membrane into a cytoplasmic vacuole, which contains the protein components of the envelope. Mature viruses exit the cells by reverse pinocytosis. Routine serologic tests do not define specific serotypes. In contrast, restriction endonuclease analysis of CMV DNA shows that, although all known human strains are genetically homologous, none are identical unless obtained from epidemiologically related cases.

EPIDEMIOLOGY. Seroepidemiologic surveys demonstrate CMV infection in every population examined worldwide. The prevalence of infection, which increases with age, is higher in developing countries and among lower socioeconomic strata of the more developed nations.

Transmission sources of CMV include saliva, breast milk, cervical and vaginal secretions, urine, semen, stools, blood, and tissue or organ transplants. The spread of CMV requires very close or intimate contact because it is very labile. Transmission occurs by direct person-to-person contact, but indirect transmission is possible via contaminated fomites.

The incidence of **congenital CMV** infection ranges from 0.2 to 2.4% of all live births, with the higher rates among populations with a lower economic standard of living. The risk for fetal infection is greatest with maternal primary CMV infection (30%) and much less likely with recurrent infection (<1%). In the USA, 1–4% of pregnant women acquire primary CMV infection, with as many as 8,000 newborns with neurodevelopmental sequelae associated with congenital CMV infection.

Perinatal transmission is common, accounting for an incidence of 10–60% through the 1st 6 mo of life. The most important perinatal sources of virus are genital tract secretions at delivery and breast milk. Among CMV-seropositive mothers, virus is detectable in breast milk in 96%, with postnatal transmission occurring in approximately 38% of infants, resulting in symptomatic infection in nearly half of very low birthweight infants. Infected infants excrete virus for years in saliva and urine.

After the 1st year of life, the prevalence of infection is dependent on group activities, with **childcare centers** contributing to rapid spread of CMV among children. Infection rates of 50–80% during childhood are common. For children who are not exposed to other toddlers, the rate of infection increases very slowly throughout the 1st decade of life. A 2nd peak occurs in adolescence as a result of sexual transmission. Seronegative childcare workers and parents of young children shedding CMV have a 10–20% annual risk for acquiring CMV, which contrasts with 1–3% per year for the general population. Health care providers are not at increased risk for acquiring CMV infection from patients.

CMV infection may be transmitted in **transplanted organs** (kidney, heart, bone marrow). Following transplantation, many patients excrete CMV as a result of infection acquired from the donor organ or from reactivation of latent infection caused by immunosuppression. Seronegative transplant recipients of organs from seropositive donors are at greatest risk for severe disease.

Nosocomial infection is a hazard of transfusion of blood and blood products. In a population with a 50% prevalence of CMV infection, the risk has been estimated at 2.7% per unit of whole blood. Leukocyte transfusions pose a much greater risk. Infection is usually asymptomatic, but even in well children and adults there is a risk for disease if the recipient is seronegative and receives multiple units. Immunocompromised patients and seronegative premature infants have a much higher (10–30%) risk for disease.

PATHOGENESIS. Clinical disease generally results from depressed cellular immunity, uncontrolled viral replication with increased virus burden, multiorgan involvement, and end-organ disease secondary to direct viral cytopathic effects. Increased levels of virus replication, as ascertained by genome copy members, are useful in identifying patients at risk for invasive disease and dissemination of infection. CMV induces an inflammatory reaction that is enhanced and prolonged by the presence of viral replication. The presence of CMV in areas of inflammation increases the expression of soluble mediators such as cytokines and chemokines. CMV infects placental cytotrophoblasts and can be transmitted to the fetus.

Infected cells may contain occasionally large intranuclear and smaller intracytoplasmic inclusions, which are pathognomonic for CMV infection. The lung, liver, kidney, gastrointestinal tract, salivary, and other exocrine glands are the most commonly affected organs.

CLINICAL MANIFESTATIONS. The signs and symptoms of CMV infection vary with age, route of transmission, and immunocompetence of the patient. The infection is subclinical in most patients. In infants and young children, primary CMV infection occasionally causes pneumonitis, hepatomegaly, hepatitis, and petechial rashes. In older children, adolescents, and adults, CMV may cause mononucleosis-like syndrome characterized by fatigue, malaise, myalgia, headache, fever, hepatosplenomegaly, elevated liver enzymes, and atypical lymphocytosis. The course of CMV mononucleosis is generally mild, lasting 2–3 wk. Clinical presentations may include occasionally persistent fever, overt hepatitis, or a morbilliform rash. Recurrent infections are asymptomatic in the immunocompetent host.

Immunocompromised Persons. The risk for CMV disease is increased in immunocompromised persons, with both primary and recurrent infections (see Chapter 177). Illness with a primary infection includes pneumonitis (most common), hepatitis, chorioretinitis, gastrointestinal disease, or fever with leukopenia as isolated entities or as manifestations of generalized disease, which may be fatal. The risk is greatest in bone marrow transplant recipients and in patients with AIDS. Pneumonia, retinitis, and involvement of the central nervous system and gastrointestinal tract are usually severe and progressive. Submucosal ulcerations can occur anywhere in the gastrointestinal tract and may lead to hemorrhage and perforation. Pancreatitis and cholecystitis may also occur.

Congenital Infection. Symptomatic congenital CMV infection was originally termed cytomegalic inclusion disease. Only 5% of all congenitally infected infants have severe cytomegalic inclusion disease, another 5% have mild involvement, and 90% are born with subclinical, but still chronic, CMV infection. The characteristic signs and symptoms of clinically manifested infections include intrauterine growth restriction, prematurity, hepatosplenomegaly and jaundice, blueberry muffin–like rash, thrombocytopenia and purpura, and microcephaly and intracranial calcifications. Other neurologic problems include chorioretinitis, sensorineural hearing loss, and mild increases in cerebrospinal fluid protein. Symptomatic newborns are usually easy to identify. The most severe symptomatic congenital infections and those resulting in sequelae are more likely to be caused by primary rather than reactivated infections in pregnant women. Reinfection with a different strain of CMV can lead to symptomatic congenital infection. Asymptomatic congenital CMV infection is likely the leading cause of sensorineural hearing loss, which occurs in approximately 7% of all infants with congenital CMV infection, whether symptomatic at birth or not.

Perinatal Infection. Infections resulting from exposure to CMV in the maternal genital tract at delivery or in breast milk occur despite the presence of maternally derived, passively acquired antibody. Approximately 6–12% of seropositive mothers transmit CMV by contaminated cervical-vaginal secretions and 50% by breast milk to their infants, who usually remain asymptomatic and do not exhibit sequelae. Occasionally, perinatally acquired CMV infection is associated with pneumonitis and sepsis-like syndrome. Premature and ill full-term infants may have neurologic sequelae and psychomotor retardation. However, the risk for hearing loss, chorioretinitis, and microcephaly does not appear to be increased. Premature infants with transfusion-acquired CMV infection have a much greater risk for morbidity.

DIAGNOSIS. Active CMV infection is best confirmed by virus isolation from urine, saliva, bronchoalveolar washings, breast milk, cervical secretions, buffy coat, and tissues obtained by biopsy. Rapid identification within 24 hr is routinely available with the centrifugation-enhanced rapid culture system based on the detection of CMV early antigens using monoclonal antibodies. Several methods are used for rapid quantitative detection of CMV antigens, and quantitative polymerase chain reaction (PCR) assays are also available. The presence of viral shedding and active infection does not distinguish between primary and recurrent infections. A primary infection is confirmed by seroconversion or the simultaneous detection of immunoglobulin M (IgM) and IgG antibodies with low functional avidity. A simple increase in antibody titers in initially seropositive patients must be interpreted with caution because this is occasionally observed years after primary infection. IgG antibodies persist for life. For the 1st weeks after primary infection, the functional avidity of IgG class antibodies is very low and rises to a peak in 4–5 mo. IgM antibodies can be demonstrated transiently in both symptomatic and asymptomatic infection at 4–16 wk, which is during the acute phase of symptomatic disease. IgM antibodies are occasionally found with these assays (0.2–1%) in patients with recurrent infection.

Recurrent infection is defined by the reappearance of viral excretion in a patient known to have been seropositive in the past. The distinction between reactivation of endogenous virus and reinfection with a different strain of CMV requires restriction enzyme analysis of viral DNA or the measurement of antibodies against strain-specific epitopes of CMV, such as glycoprotein H epitopes.

In immunocompromised persons, excretion of CMV, increases in IgG titers, and even the presence of IgM antibodies are common, greatly confounding the ability to distinguish primary and recurrent infections. Demonstrating viremia by buffy coat culture, detection of CMV antigenemia, or CMV DNA implies active disease and worse prognosis regardless of whether the type of infection is primary, recurrent, or uncertain.

Congenital Infection. The definitive method for diagnosis of congenital CMV infection is virus isolation or PCR, which should be performed at or shortly after birth. Urine and saliva are the best specimens for culture. Infants with congenital CMV infection may excrete CMV in the urine for several years. An IgG antibody test is of little diagnostic value because a positive result also reflects maternal antibodies, although a negative result excludes the diagnosis of congenital CMV infection. Demonstration of stable or rising titers in serial specimens during the 1st year of life does not help because acquired infection in the 1st few months of life is common. IgM tests lack sensitivity and specificity and are unreliable for diagnosis of congenital CMV infection.

IgM antibody tests and the measurement of CMV-IgG avidity can identify women at high risk for transmitting CMV in utero. Fetal infection can be confirmed by viral isolation from amniotic fluid. The sensitivity of this method is excellent after the 22nd wk of gestation. The detection of viral genome by PCR in amniotic fluid is equally sensitive and specific; quantitative PCR demonstrating 10^5 genome equivalents per mL of amniotic fluid is a predictor of symptomatic congenital infection.

TREATMENT. There are limited options for treatment of CMV infection. Treatment is not indicated for immunocompetent persons, but is recommended for immunocompromised persons, and remains controversial for infants with symptomatic congenital infection.

Immunocompromised Persons. Ganciclovir combined with immune globulin, either standard intravenous immunoglobulin (IVIG) or hyperimmune CMV IVIG, has been used to treat life-threatening CMV infections in immunocompromised hosts (bone marrow, heart, and kidney transplant recipients and patients with AIDS). Two published regimens are ganciclovir (7.5 mg/kg/day divided every 8 hr IV for 14 days) with CMV IVIG (400 mg/kg on days 1, 2, and 7, and 200 mg/kg on day 14); and ganciclovir (7.5 mg/kg/day divided every 8 hr IV for 20 days with IVIG 500 mg/kg every other day for 10 doses).

CMV retinitis and gastrointestinal disease appear to be clinically responsive to therapy but, like viral excretion, often recur on cessation. Toxicity with ganciclovir is frequent and often severe and includes neutropenia, thrombocytopenia, liver dysfunction, reduction in spermatogenesis, and gastrointestinal and renal abnormalities. Foscarnet is an alternative antiviral agent, although there is limited information on its use in children. CMV prophylaxis with ganciclovir or acyclovir reduces the risk for morbidity in solid organ transplantation. Prophylactic treatment with valacyclovir in adults (900 mg PO once daily for 90 days) is a safe and effective regimen to prevent CMV disease in kidney and pancreas transplant recipients.

Congenital Infection. A randomized controlled phase III study with ganciclovir (6 mg/kg/dose every 12 hr IV for the 1st 6 wk of life) concluded that treatment both prevents hearing deterioration and improves or maintains normal hearing function at 6 mo of age, and may prevent the hearing deterioration that occurs after 1 yr of age. Drug-related toxicity was common, with 63% of ganciclovir-treated patients developing significant neutropenia, compared with 21% in the untreated group. The logistic obstacles of intravenous therapy for the 1st 6 wk of life, limited benefit, and adverse effects have limited enthusiasm for this regimen. A phase I/II study of oral valganciclovir, the orally bioavailable prodrug of ganciclovir, is underway to determine the dose necessary to achieve a safe and effective dose of ganciclovir in the bloodstream.

PROGNOSIS. Patients with CMV mononucleosis usually recover fully, although some have protracted symptoms. Most immunocompromised patients also recover uneventfully, but many experience severe pneumonitis, with a high fatality rate if hypoxemia develops. CMV infection and disease may be fatal in individuals with increased susceptibility to infections such as patients with AIDS.

Congenital Disease. Nearly 90% of children with symptomatic congenital infection demonstrate central nervous system and hearing defects in later years. Infants with subclinical infection have a much more favorable outlook. Principal concerns are the subsequent development of sensorineural hearing loss (5–10%), chorioretinitis (3–5%), and other less frequent manifestations such as developmental abnormalities, microcephaly, and neurologic deficits.

PREVENTION. The use of CMV-free blood products, especially for premature newborns, and, whenever possible, the use of organs from CMV-free donors for transplantation represent important measures to prevent CMV infection and disease in patients at high risk.

Pregnant women who are CMV seropositive are at low risk for delivering a symptomatic newborn. If possible, pregnant women should have a CMV serologic test, especially if they provide care for young children who are potential CMV excreters. Pregnant women who are CMV seronegative should be counseled regarding good handwashing and other hygienic measures and avoidance of contact with oral secretions of others. Those with suspected recent CMV infection may undergo additional diagnostic evaluations to ascertain in utero transmission and fetal disease. Pregnant women with primary CMV who receive CMV hyperimmune globulin may have a reduced risk for delivering a congenitally infected infant.

Passive Immunoprophylaxis. The use of IVIG or CMV IVIG for prophylaxis of infection in solid organ and bone marrow transplant recipients reduces the risk for symptomatic disease but does not prevent infection. The efficacy of prophylaxis is more striking when the hazard of primary CMV infection is greatest, such as in bone marrow transplantation. There is no consensus for a uniform prophylaxis regimen for CMV infection. Recommended regimens include either IVIG (1,000 mg/kg) or CMV IVIG (500 mg/kg) given as a single intravenous dose beginning within 72 hr of transplantation and once weekly thereafter until 90–120 days after transplantation.

Active Immunization. The beneficial role of immunity is substantial, as illustrated by the fact that most severe disease follows primary infection, especially with congenital infection, transfusion-acquired infection, and infection in transplant recipients.

The 1st vaccine tested in humans was developed from the live-attenuated Towne strain of CMV, which proved immunogenic but did not protect renal transplant recipients or normal adult women from becoming infected. However, in renal transplant recipients the vaccine reduced the virulence of primary infection. Other vaccines under study include a chimera between attenuated CMV and wild-type virus; a nonreplicating recombinant vector (canarypox) with either a glycoprotein B envelope or a polypeptide 65 core antigen; a vaccine made by recombinant technology consisting of envelope glycoprotein; and a vaccine consisting of a mixture of synthetic peptides and T-helper and $CD8^+$ cytotoxic T-cell epitopes. Phase I/II trials are under way to generate safety and immunogenicity data, and efficacy testing will soon follow.

Arvin AM, Fast P, Myers M, et al: Vaccine development to prevent cytomegalovirus disease: Report from the National Vaccine Advisory Committee. *Clin Infect Dis* 2004;39:233–239.

Boppana SB, Rivera LB, Fowler KB, et al: Intrauterine transmission of cytomegalovirus to infants of women with preconceptional immunity. *N Engl J Med* 2001;344:1366–1371.

Couchoud C: Cytomegalovirus prophylaxis with antiviral agents for solid organ transplantation. *Cochrane Database Syst Rev* 2000;2:CD001320.

Demmler GJ: Screening for congenital cytomegalovirus infection: A tapestry of controversies. *J Pediatr* 2005;146:162–164.

Fowler KB, Stagno S, Pass RF: Maternal immunity and prevention of congenital cytomegalovirus infection. *JAMA* 2003;289:1008–1011.

Hamprecht K, Maschmann J, Vochem M, et al: Epidemiology of transmission of cytomegalovirus from mother to preterm infant by breastfeeding. *Lancet* 2001;357:513–518.

Kimberlin DW, Lin CY, Sanchez PJ, et al: Effect of ganciclovir therapy on hearing in symptomatic congenital cytomegalovirus disease involving the central nervous system: A randomized, controlled trial. *J Pediatr* 2003;16–25.

Nigro G, Adler SP, La Torre R, et al: Passive immunization during pregnancy for congenital cytomegalovirus infection. *N Engl J Med* 2005;353: 1350–1362.

Noyola DE, Demmler GJ, Nelson CT, et al: Early predictors of neurodevelopmental outcome in symptomatic congenital cytomegalovirus infection. *J Pediatr* 2001;138:325–331.

Pass RF, Fowler KB, Boppana SB, et al: Congenital cytomegalovirus infection following first trimester maternal infection: Symptoms at birth and outcome. *J Clin Virol* 2006;35:216–220.

Rubin RH, Kemmerly SA, Conti D, et al: Prevention of primary cytomegalovirus disease in organ transplant recipients with oral ganciclovir or oral acyclovir prophylaxis. *Transplant Infect Dis* 2000;2:112–117.

Stagno S, Britt W: Cytomegalovirus. In Remington JS, Klein JO (editors): *Infectious Diseases of the Fetus and Newborn Infant,* 6th ed. Philadelphia, WB Saunders, 2005, pp 739–781.

Tanaka-Kitajima N, Sugaya N, Futatani T, et al: Ganciclovir therapy for congenital cytomegalovirus infection in six infants. *Pediatr Infect Dis J* 2005;24:782–785.

Chapter 253 ■ Roseola (Human Herpesviruses 6 and 7) Charles T. Leach

Human herpesvirus 6 (HHV-6) is a dominant cause of roseola infantum (**exanthem subitum** or **sixth disease**), and possibly of other diseases in normal and immunocompromised patients. Disease associations for HHV-7 are fewer, but include a roseola-like illness.

ETIOLOGY. Primary infection with HHV-6, and less frequently HHV-7, causes the majority of cases of roseola. Other viruses (echovirus 16) probably account for the remainder. Nonetheless, most primary infections with HHV-6 and HHV-7 do not result in roseola.

HHV-6 and HHV-7 belong to the β-herpesvirus subfamily of herpesviruses, which includes human cytomegalovirus (CMV). HHV-6 and HHV-7 share physical and biologic characteristics with other herpesviruses, including a large double-stranded DNA genome, the presence of a nucleocapsid, and the establishment of latency after primary infection. HHV-6 is essentially colinear with HHV-7, and both viruses share much homology with CMV. HHV-6 and HHV-7 most efficiently replicate in CD4 T cells; HHV-6 can also infect other T cells, macrophages, epithelial cells, endothelial cells, fibroblasts, hepatic cells, glial cells, fetal astrocytes, and bone marrow progenitor cells. In the laboratory, HHV-6 and HHV-7 are typically cultivated in mitogen-stimulated human mononuclear cells (isolated from cord blood or peripheral blood) and can be identified by the development of large balloon-like cells accompanied by cell lysis. Two distinct types of HHV-6 (types A and B) exist. Type B causes more than 99% of HHV-6-associated roseola cases. Latent type A virus can be found in immunodeficient as well as healthy patients and may reactivate in severely ill adult patients; however, it has not been consistently linked with disease.

EPIDEMIOLOGY. Primary HHV-6 infection occurs early in life. Most (>90%) of newborn infants are HHV-6 seropositive, reflecting transplacental transfer of maternal antibodies. Before 6 mo of age, there is a low rate of primary HHV-6 infection (<10%). However, a rapid increase occurs subsequently, and by 12 mo of age 40% of infants are HHV-6 infected, and 80% acquire infection by 2 yr of age. Peak acquisition of primary HHV-6 infection, from 6 to 15 mo of age, corresponds with peak incidence of roseola. The most common symptoms in infants with HHV-6 infection are fever and fussiness (90%). Only 1/4 of infected children have clinically recognizable roseola. Curiously, much higher rates of roseola symptoms occur in Japanese infants with primary HHV-6 infection. Primary infection with HHV-7 generally occurs slightly later than HHV-6 infection.

Roseola occurs throughout the year. Unlike some of the other childhood exanthems, children with roseola rarely report contact with other affected children, and outbreaks are uncommon. Sex, race, and geography do not play an important role in acquisition of roseola. The incubation period averages 10 days, with a range of 5–15 days.

Most adults excrete HHV-6 and HHV-7 in saliva and may serve as primary sources for virus transmission to children. Although women may uncommonly excrete HHV-6 and HHV-7 in the genital tract, sexual transmissibility has not been demonstrated. HHV-6 can be transmitted in utero at low rates (<2%), with approximately 2/3 associated with type B; only 1 neonate with symptomatic congenital infection has been described. Most congenitally infected patients are asymptomatic, but reactivation may occur after birth. No congenital HHV-7 infections have been identified. There are rare reports of HHV-6 transmission to susceptible infants via donor bone marrow or solid organs. There is no evidence that infection is spread by breast milk, fecal-oral contamination, or blood transfusion.

PATHOGENESIS. Virus is probably acquired from the saliva of healthy persons and enters the host through the oral, nasal, or conjunctival mucosa. Cellular receptors for both viruses have been identified: HHV-6 uses the CD46 receptor (widespread among tissues), and HHV-7 uses the CD4 receptor, which is also used by HIV-1. Following viral replication at an unknown site, a high level of viremia develops in peripheral blood mononuclear cells (PBMCs). After acute infection, HHV-6 and HHV-7 establish latency in blood mononuclear cells and possibly in other sites, including salivary glands, kidneys, lungs, and central nervous system. The basis for the unique pattern of rash **after resolution of fever** in children with roseola is unknown.

HHV-6 can suppress all cellular lineages within the bone marrow; active HHV-6 infection is associated with bone marrow suppression in bone marrow transplant patients. HHV-6 infection also has significant effects on the immune system, including downregulation of the major histocompatibility complex (MHC) type I response, enhancement of natural killer (NK) T-cell activity, suppression of PBMC proliferation, and induction of a proinflammatory cytokine response.

CLINICAL MANIFESTATIONS. Roseola is the prototypical HHV-6 and HHV-7 infection, although nonspecific infections are common.

Roseola Infantum (Exanthem Subitum). Roseola is a mild febrile, exanthematous illness occurring almost exclusively during infancy. More than 95% of roseola cases occur in children younger than 3 yr, with a peak at 6–15 mo of age. Transplacental antibodies likely protect most infants until 6 mo of age.

Infants with classic roseola exhibit a unique constellation of findings displayed over a short period of time. Consequently, classic roseola is infrequently confused with other childhood exanthems.

The prodromal period of roseola is usually asymptomatic but may include mild upper respiratory tract signs, among them minimal rhinorrhea, slight pharyngeal inflammation, and mild conjunctival redness. Mild cervical or, less frequently, occipital lymphadenopathy may be noted. Some children may have mild palpebral edema. Physical findings during the prodromal stage have no clear relationship to roseola, and may simply reflect an accompanying respiratory viral infection. Clinical illness is generally heralded by high temperature, usually ranging from 37.9 to 40°C (101–106°F), with an average of 39°C (103°F). Some children may become irritable and anorexic during the febrile stage, but most behave normally despite high temperatures. Seizures may occur in 5–10% of children with roseola during this febrile period. Infrequent complaints include rhinorrhea, sore throat, abdominal pain, vomiting, and diarrhea. In Asian countries, ulcers at the uvulopalatoglossal junction (**Nagayama spots**) are common in infants with roseola. Fever persists for 3–5 days, and then typically resolves rather abruptly ("crisis"). Occasionally, the fever may gradually diminish over 24–36 hours ("lysis"). A rash appears within 12–24 hr of fever resolution. In many cases, the rash develops during defervescence or within a few hours of fever resolution. The rash of roseola is rose colored, as the name implies, and is fairly distinctive (Fig. 253-1). However, it may be confused with exanthems resulting from rubella, measles, or erythema infectiosum. The roseola rash begins as discrete, small (2–5 mm), slightly raised pink lesions on the trunk and usually spreads to the neck, face, and proximal extremities. The rash is not usually pruritic, and no vesicles or pustules develop. Lesions typically remain discrete but occasionally may become almost confluent. After 1–3 days, the rash fades. Some children experience evanescent rashes that resolve within a few

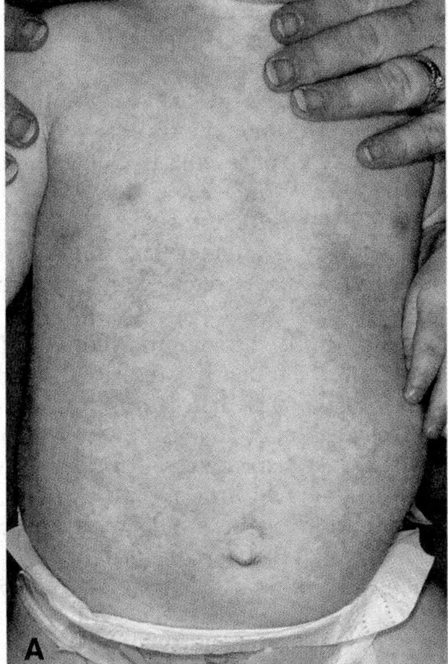

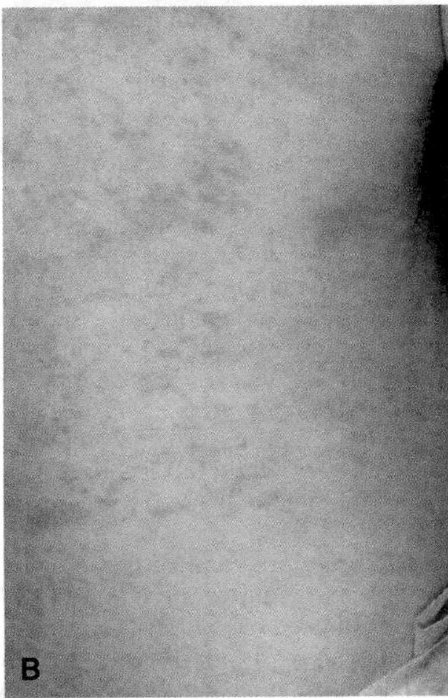

Figure 253-1. Roseola infantum. Erythematous, blanchable macules and papules *(A)* in an infant who had a high fever for 3 days preceding the skin eruption. On closer inspection *(B)*, some lesions reveal a subtle peripheral halo of vasoconstriction. (From Paller AS, Mancinin AJ [editors]: *Hurwitz Clinical Pediatric Dermatology,* 3rd ed. Philadelphia, Elsevier, 2006, p 434.)

hours. Subtle differences in clinical presentation have been noted between roseola associated with HHV-7 compared with HHV-6. These include a slightly older age, lower mean temperature, and shorter duration of fever in HHV-7-associated cases. However, these differences are insufficient to clinically distinguish HHV-6- from HHV-7-associated roseola. There are reports of children experiencing HHV-6-associated roseola followed later by HHV-7-associated roseola.

Fever in Infants Without Classic Roseola. HHV-6 and HHV-7 account for a significant proportion of nonspecific febrile illnesses, without a focus of infection, in infants. Approximately 15% of febrile infants presenting to hospital emergency room have primary HHV-6 or HHV-7 infection.

Central Nervous System Infections. Both HHV-6 and HHV-7 are neurotropic and can invade the CNS. Primary HHV-6 infection is responsible for approximately 10–20% of febrile seizures in infants. Most of these children do not subsequently experience a rash. Smaller studies suggest that HHV-7 is also linked with some febrile seizures. HHV-6 and HHV-7 are associated with rare cases of encephalitis and meningoencephalitis, mostly occurring in immunocompromised patients. HHV-6 DNA is present in cerebrospinal fluid from 6% of children and adults with focal encephalitis of unknown cause.

Mononucleosis-like Illness and Hepatitis. Several heterophile-negative mononucleosis-like infections associated with HHV-6 have been reported in adults. HHV-6 and HHV-7 may rarely cause clinical symptoms of hepatitis. There is controversy regarding the association of HHV-6 with some cases of fulminant liver failure in infants.

Infections in Immunocompromised Patients. Numerous severe and occasionally fatal HHV-6-associated infections (encephalitis, pneumonitis) have occurred in immunocompromised patients, including patients with AIDS or organ transplants. These have occurred predominantly in stem cell transplant recipients and usually reflect **reactivated** HHV-6 infection. Concomitant HHV-6 and HHV-7 infections may augment CMV-associated disease following organ transplantation.

Because HHV-6 shares CD4 cell tropism with HIV, upregulates HIV, and stimulates in vitro replication of HIV, there has been considerable interest in the role of HHV-6 as a cofactor for clinical progression of AIDS. Epidemiologic studies in adults do not support a significant role for HHV-6 as a cofactor. Only 1 small pediatric study suggests more rapid progression of immune deficiency in HIV/HHV-6 co-infected infants. Further prospective studies are necessary to assess the impact of HHV-6 on HIV-infected children.

Other Diseases Possibly Associated with HHV-6 or HHV-7. Rash illness without fever has been described in a small number of infants with primary HHV-6 infection. Small studies or case reports have suggested that HHV-6 may be associated with a wide range of other diseases, including some cases of hemophagocytic syndrome, intussusception, idiopathic thrombocytopenic purpura, recurrent aphthous stomatitis, myocarditis, drug hypersensitivity, Gianotti-Crosti syndrome, progressive multifocal leukoencephalopathy, influenza encephalopathy, large vessel arteritis, Kikuchi's necrotizing lymphadenitis, histiocytosis, and chronic fatigue syndrome. Controversy continues regarding a relationship between HHV-6 and multiple sclerosis. There are conflicting data linking HHV-7 and pityriasis rosea. HHV-6 DNA has been detected in various malignancies, including non-Hodgkin lymphoma, Hodgkin disease, cervical and oral carcinoma, and leukemia. No consistent etiologic relationship has been established with any of these cancers.

DIAGNOSIS. The most important reason for establishing the diagnosis of roseola is to differentiate this generally mild illness from other potentially more serious childhood rash illnesses such as measles. It is also important to identify other, more serious illnesses caused by HHV-6, such as encephalitis and pneumonitis, especially in immunocompromised patients, for timely consideration of antiviral therapy.

The **diagnosis of roseola** can be established primarily on the basis of age, history, and clinical findings. HHV-6- and HHV-7-associated roseola cases cannot be distinguished solely on clinical grounds. Specific testing for HHV-6 or HHV-7 infection may be performed using laboratory methods, including serology, virus culture, and polymerase chain reaction (PCR).

HHV-6 serologic testing is available from many commercial laboratories; few offer HHV-7 serology. An HHV-6 immunoglobulin M (IgM) response typically develops by the 5th–7th day of illness, peaks at 2–3 wk, and resolves within 2 mo. Unfortunately, the accuracy of currently available IgM tests varies widely, and none have been sufficiently evaluated to provide unequivocal evidence of acute HHV-6 infection. Seroconversion of HHV-6 or

-7 IgG antibodies in serum samples collected 2–3 wk apart is a more reliable means of establishing primary infection, but is not timely. Four-fold increases or decreases in HHV-6 or -7 IgG antibodies also suggest active infection (primary or reactivated). Because of the high seroprevalence of these viruses in the general population, a single positive HHV-6 or -7 IgG test is of no significance for diagnosis of acute infection. CMV antibodies can cross react with HHV-6 and HHV-7; therefore, diagnosis of HHV-6 and HHV-7 infections by serologic means requires exclusion of CMV infection.

Identification of HHV-6 or HHV-7 in PBMCs by virus culture firmly establishes the presence of active infection in immunocompetent hosts; association with specific disease is more problematic in immunocompromised patients as a result of a low background rate of viremia. Identification of HHV-6 and HHV-7 by culture requires incubation of PBMCs (with or without co-cultivation with exogenous PBMCs) for days to several weeks, and is presently available only in research laboratories. A commercial HHV-6 rapid (shell-vial) culture is available.

PCR amplification tests for HHV-6 are becoming available and may provide more timely information for diagnosis. Active, replicating infection is indicated if HHV-6 DNA is detected in acellular specimens such as serum or cerebrospinal fluid. It should be noted that detection at other sites (PBMCs, saliva, tissues) does not necessarily indicate active infection, because HHV-6 exists in latent form in many tissues after primary infection. Quantitative PCR and reverse transcriptase PCR may be more useful for diagnosis of active infection using cellular blood specimens, if suitable cutoff thresholds are established. Several commercial laboratories offer quantitative as well as qualitative PCR testing on a variety of specimens. Although not widely available, other diagnostic tests for consideration in selected circumstances include in situ hybridization, immunohistochemistry, and antigen assays.

LABORATORY FINDINGS. White blood cell (WBC) counts of 8,000–9,000 WBCs/μL may be found during the 1st few days of fever in children with roseola, but by the time the exanthem appears, the WBC count falls to 4,000–6,000 WBCs/μL with a relative lymphocytosis (70–90%). The cerebrospinal fluid in children with HHV-6-associated febrile seizures typically is normal. The cerebrospinal fluid from rare cases of HHV-6-associated meningoencephalitis and encephalitis is characterized by a mild pleocytosis with predominance of mononuclear cells, normal glucose, and normal to slightly elevated protein.

DIFFERENTIAL DIAGNOSIS. Children with roseola typically present at 2 different stages of the illness: at the time of fever before the rash (pre-eruptive) and after the rash has appeared. During the pre-eruptive stage, many conditions may be confused with roseola. However, the pattern of fever in a generally well child without significant physical findings, rather precipitous defervescence, and a subsequent rash is unique for roseola.

Roseola historically has been most commonly confused with rubella and measles; with the virtual elimination of these diseases in the United States, there should be little reason to confuse roseola with these diseases, unless there is an exposure history. In contrast to the absence of a distinct prodrome in children with roseola, children with **rubella** invariably have a mildly symptomatic prodromal period, including prominent occipital and postauricular lymphadenopathy (see Chapter 244). Lymphadenopathy is an inconsistent finding in roseola; when present, the occipital lymph nodes are more frequently affected than those in the postauricular region. Rubella usually causes only low-grade fever, which is coincident with the exanthem. The rubella rash is typically more extensive than that seen with roseola, and coalescence is more common. The development of an exanthem at the height of the fever as well as the presence of cough, coryza, conjunctivitis, and Koplik spots on the buccal mucosa in the early stages of **measles** should clearly differentiate measles from roseola (see Chapter 243).

Outbreaks of roseola-like illnesses have been associated with many different viruses, most commonly enteroviruses. In summer and fall months, some cases of roseola-like illnesses may be attributable to enteroviruses.

Scarlet fever may also resemble roseola. Important features of scarlet fever are its rarity in infancy, the simultaneous presence of fever and rash, and the discrete, small, sandpaper-like rash lesions.

Drug hypersensitivity is a common condition resembling roseola. Antibiotics are frequently prescribed to children with roseola during the febrile phase before onset of the rash. A child who acquires a drug rash may do so soon after resolution of the fever, which is the characteristic pattern for children with roseola. However, the usually morbilliform nature, pruritus, and resolution after discontinuation of the implicated drug should distinguish a drug rash.

It may be difficult to distinguish central nervous system disease caused by HHV-6 from other causes. Development of a roseola-like illness in association with febrile seizures, meningoencephalitis, or encephalitis makes HHV-6 infection more likely, yet this occurs infrequently. Hepatitis and heterophile-negative mononucleosis are rarely associated with HHV-6, and other causes for these infections should first be sought.

TREATMENT. HHV-6 is inhibited by ganciclovir, cidofovir, and foscarnet (but not acyclovir) at levels that are achievable in serum; HHV-7 is inhibited by cidofovir and foscarnet. Case reports have indicated successes and failures with these drugs. Adequate prospective trials evaluating the clinical efficacy of antiviral agents for HHV-6 or HHV-7 infections have not been performed. There is not an approved treatment of these infections. *The generally benign nature of roseola precludes consideration of antiviral therapy in immunocompetent persons.* **Treatment** is warranted for **immunocompromised** children with severe disease confirmed to be associated with HHV-6 or HHV-7. Ganciclovir and cidofovir are most commonly used, with duration of therapy typically 2–3 weeks.

Children in the febrile, pre-eruptive phase of roseola usually are quite comfortable and require little supportive therapy. Those children who are uncomfortable and irritable, or in whom histories of febrile convulsions exists, may benefit from treatment with acetaminophen or ibuprofen. Adequate fluid balance should be maintained in all affected children. Referral should be considered in those unusual circumstances in which serious disease develops, such as encephalitis, hepatitis, or pneumonitis.

PROGNOSIS. The prognosis for the great majority of children with roseola is excellent, with no obvious sequelae. Before the discoveries of HHV-6 and HHV-7, rare complications of roseola (hemiparesis, mental retardation) were attributable to brain anoxia during prolonged febrile seizures, though damage resulting from direct viral invasion of the brain, liver, and other organs has been demonstrated for HHV-6. Deaths directly attributable to HHV-6 have been reported in normal as well as immunocompromised patients in whom encephalitis, hepatitis, pneumonitis, disseminated disease, or hemophagocytosis syndrome developed.

PREVENTION. Very little information is available on which to base guidelines for prevention of HHV-6 or HHV-7 infection. Experimental evidence suggests that roseola may be transmitted via blood or saliva, and both HHV-6 and HHV-7 are shed in the saliva. It is likely that healthy immune carriers with latent viral infections transmit infection to susceptible infants and children via saliva.

Caserta MT, Mock DJ, Dewhurst S: Human herpesvirus 6. *Clin Infect Dis* 2001;33:829–833.

De Bolle L, Naesens L, De Clercq E: Update on human herpesvirus 6 biology, clinical features, and therapy. *Clin Microbiol Rev* 2005;18:217–245.

Desachy A, Ranger-Rogez S, Francois B, et al: Reactivation of human herpesvirus type 6 in multiple organ failure syndrome. *Clin Infect Dis* 2001;32:197–203.

Dewhurst S: Human herpesvirus type 6 and human herpesvirus type 7 infections of the central nervous system. *Herpes* 2004;11(Suppl 2);105A–111A.

Hall CV, Caserta MT, Schnabel KC, et al: Congenital infections with human herpesvirus 6 (HHV6) and human herpesvirus 7 (HHV7). *J Pediatr* 2004;145:472–477.

Leach CT: Human herpesvirus-6 and -7 infections in children: Agents of roseola and other syndromes. *Curr Opin Pediatr* 2000;12:269–274.

Leach CT, Pollock BH, McClain KL, et al: Human herpesvirus 6 (HHV-6) and cytomegalovirus (CMV) infections in children with acquired immunodeficiency syndrome (AIDS) and cancer. *Pediatr Infect Dis J* 2002;21:125–132.

Ward KN: The natural history and laboratory diagnosis of human herpesviruses-6 and -7 in the immunocompetent. *J Clin Virol* 2005;32: 183–193.

Ward KN, Andrews NJ, Verity CM, et al: Human herpesviruses-6 and -7 each cause significant neurological morbidity in Britain and Ireland. *Arch Dis Child* 2005;90:619–623.

Yamanishi K, Okuno T, Shiraki K, et al: Identification of human herpesvirus-6 as a causal agent for exanthem subitum. *Lancet* 1988;1:1065–1067.

Yoshikawa T: Human herpesvirus-6 and -7 infections in transplantation. *Pediatr Transplant* 2003;7:11–17.

Zerr DM, Corey L, Kim HW, et al: Clinical outcomes of human herpesvirus 6 reactivation after hematopoietic stem cell transplantation. *Clin Infect Dis* 2005;40:932–940.

Zerr DM, Frenkel LM, Huang ML, et al: Polymerase chain reaction diagnosis of primary human herpesvirus-6 infection in the acute care setting. *J Pediatr* 2006;149:480–485.

Zerr DM, Meier AS, Selke SS, et al: A population-based study of primary human herpesvirus 6 infection. *N Engl J Med* 2005;352:768–776.

Chapter 254 ■ Human Herpesvirus 8

Charles T. Leach

Human herpesvirus 8 (HHV-8), also known as **Kaposi sarcoma (KS)-associated herpesvirus (KSHV)**, is responsible for KS in patients with AIDS. Many studies have revealed its strong association with KS as well as other more uncommon malignancies.

ETIOLOGY. HHV-8 is a member of the γ-herpesviruses, which includes Epstein-Barr virus. HHV-8 is an enveloped DNA virus of approximately 165,000 base pairs and has an overall genomic structure typical of other human herpesviruses. However, unlike most other viruses, the HHV-8 genome contains viral homologues of several human proteins important in the regulation of cellular proliferation. It is postulated that these viral proteins contribute to the pathogenesis of HHV-8-associated malignancies.

EPIDEMIOLOGY. HHV-8 infection is uncommon in healthy children and adults in most developed countries. Rates of HHV-8 infection in HIV-uninfected persons and blood donors in the USA are <10%, but may be higher in specific areas. HHV-8 infection is more common (15–20%) in certain areas of Greece and Italy. HHV-8 seroprevalence rates are much higher in Brazil, Egypt, and Central Africa, where 40–60% of children are infected.

Approximately 1/3 of HIV-infected homosexual males and more than 80% of HIV-infected homosexual males who acquire KS are infected with the virus. Patients with HIV infection acquired in another manner (vertically from an HIV-positive mother or through transfusion of blood or blood products) have low rates (0–5%) of HHV-8 infection that are similar to those observed in HIV-uninfected persons and blood donors.

HHV-8 is shed in the saliva of most HHV-8-infected persons, and probably serves as a major source for intrafamilial transmission. HHV-8 is also detectable in breast milk. Sexual transmission also is important, especially among homosexual males. Rarely, HHV-8 has been transmitted vertically and via blood transfusion. HHV-8-associated disease in transplant recipients can be transmitted via the donor organ or can arise from reactivated recipient virus.

CLINICAL MANIFESTATIONS. Most cases of primary HHV-8 infection appear to be subclinical. Studies outside the United States have indicated that primary HHV-8 infection in children may be associated with fever and rash (Egypt) or mononucleosis (Taiwan). Immunocompromised patients may have more severe symptoms in conjunction with primary HHV-8 infection, including bone marrow failure and disseminated KS.

Three malignancies occurring primarily in adults with AIDS are strongly associated with HHV-8: KS, multicentric Castleman disease, and primary effusion lymphoma. KS is the most common neoplasm associated with AIDS but also occurs in HIV-uninfected persons living in the Mediterranean region (**classic KS**), in equatorial Africa (**endemic KS**), and in organ transplant recipients (**post-transplant KS**). **Multicentric Castleman** disease and primary effusion lymphoma are much rarer lymphoproliferative diseases. HHV-8 contributes to oncogenesis through a variety of mechanisms, including modulation of apoptosis, cell growth, and immune responses.

DIAGNOSIS. HHV-8 infection can be demonstrated by serologic testing (enzyme immunoassay, immunofluorescence, and Western immunoblotting) or detection of HHV-8 DNA sequences by polymerase chain reaction amplification. Combinations of tests are often used to maximize accuracy. However, there are no licensed diagnostic tests, and laboratory testing is presently available only from a limited number of commercial laboratories. The virus is not easily cultivated.

TREATMENT. Several antiviral compounds inhibit HHV-8 in vitro, including ganciclovir, foscarnet, and cidofovir. The benefit of specific antiviral therapy for HHV-8-associated disease has not yet been established. Introduction of highly active anti-retroviral therapy has dramatically improved survival for AIDS patients with KS. Other treatment options for KS include α-interferon, cryotherapy, phototherapy, topical retinoic acid, chemotherapy, radiation therapy, and surgery.

Andreoni M, Sarmati L, Nicastri E, et al: Primary human herpesvirus 8 infection in immunocompetent children. *JAMA* 2002;287:1295–1300.

Baillargeon J, Deng JH, Hettler E, et al: Seroprevalence of Kaposi's sarcoma-associated herpesvirus infection among blood donors from Texas. *Ann Epidemiol* 2002;11:512–518.

Baillargeon J, Leach CT, Deng JH, et al: High prevalence of human herpesvirus 8 (HHV-8) infection in South Texas children. *J Med Virol* 2002;67:542–548.

Bhaduri-McIntosh S: Human herpesvirus-8—Clinical features of an emerging viral pathogen. *Pediatr Infect Dis J* 2005;24:81–82.

Cannon MJ, Laney AS, Pellett PE: Human herpesvirus 8: Current issues. *Clin Infect Dis* 2003;37:82–87.

Chen RL, Lin JC, Wang PJ, et al: Human herpesvirus 8-related childhood mononucleosis—A series of three cases. *Pediatr Infect Dis J* 2004;23: 671–674.

Dedicoat M, Newton R, Alkharsah KR, et al: Mother-to-child transmission of human herpesvirus-8 in South Africa. *J Infect Dis* 2004;190:1068–1075.

Jenson HB: Human herpesvirus 8 infection. *Curr Opin Pediatr* 2003;15: 85–91.

Little RF, Yarchoan R: Treatment of gammaherpesvirus-related neoplastic disorders in the immunosuppressed host. *Semin Hematol* 2003;40:163–171.

Mbuliteye S, Marshall V, Bagni RK, et al: Molecular evidence for mother-to-child transmission of Kaposi sarcoma-associated herpesvirus in Uganda and K1 gene evolution within the host. *J Infect Dis* 2006;19:1250–1257.

Sarmati L, Carlo T, Rossella S, et al: Human herpesvirus-8 infection in pregnancy and labor: Lack of evidence of vertical transmission. *J Med Virol* 2004;72:462–466.

Chapter 255 ■ Influenza Viruses

Peter Wright

Influenza viral infections cause a broad array of respiratory illnesses that are responsible for significant morbidity and mortality in children on a yearly basis. Influenza has the potential for causing periodic global pandemics with even higher penetrance of illness.

ETIOLOGY. Influenza viruses are members of the family Orthomyxoviridae. They are large, single-stranded RNA viruses with a segmented genome encased in a lipid-containing envelope. The 2 major surface proteins that determine the serotype of influenza, hemagglutinin (HA) and neuraminidase (NA), project as spikes through the envelope. Influenza viruses are divided into three types: A, B, and C. Influenza types A and B are the primary influenzal pathogens and cause epidemic disease. Influenza type C is a sporadic cause of predominantly upper respiratory tract disease. Influenza types A and B are further divided into serotypically distinct strains that circulate on a yearly basis through the population.

EPIDEMIOLOGY. Influenza A viruses have a complex epidemiology involving avian and mammalian hosts that serve as reservoirs for diverse strains with the potential for infecting the human population. The segmented nature of the influenza genome allows reassortment to occur between an animal and human virus when co-infection occurs. Thus, potentially any of 15 HAs and 9 NAs residing in animal reservoirs may be introduced into humans; these influenza A viruses behave epidemiologically as though they were immunologically distinct serotypes without cross-protection. Minor changes within a serotype are termed antigenic drift; major changes in serotype are termed antigenic shift. Migratory birds can spread disease, as is being seen with the current H5N1 avian influenza. The introduction of novel HA strains have occurred in the Far East with H5N1 and H9N2 viruses and in the Netherlands with H7N7. The highly virulent **avian H5N1 influenza virus** is a potential threat to spread more broadly in the human population. It has demonstrated its virulence with high mortality in humans in direct contact with infected poultry, although it has not yet acquired the ability to spread readily from person to person. Influenza B has much less capacity for major antigenic change and no identified animal reservoir.

The worldwide epidemiology of influenza viruses demonstrates annual spread between the Northern and Southern hemispheres, with the origins of new strains often traced to Asia. When a virus identified by a novel and serologically distinct HA or NA enters the population, there is potential for a pandemic of influenza with excess morbidity and mortality on a global scale in a largely non-immune population. The most dramatic pandemic in recent history occurred in 1918, when influenza was estimated to have killed more than 20 million people. More common is the almost yearly variation in the antigenic composition of the surface proteins, which confers a selective advantage to a new strain and results in localized epidemics of disease with hospitalization and mortality greatest in infants, the elderly, and those with underlying cardiopulmonary disease. Each year's strain is novel for infants because they have no pre-existing antibody except for maternally transferred antibody in the very young.

The attack rate and frequency of isolation of influenza is highest in young children. In a typical year as many as 30–50% of children have serologic evidence of infection. Influenza is marked by increased school absenteeism and a yearly peak in sick visits to the pediatrician. Children undergoing primary exposure to an influenza strain have higher levels and more prolonged shedding of the virus than adults, making them extremely effective transmitters of infection. Influenza is a disease of the colder months of the year in temperate climates; spread appears to occur by small-particle aerosol. Transmission through a community is rapid; the highest incidence of illness occurs within 2–3 wk of introduction. Influenza has been implicated in hospital spread of infection and may complicate the original illness that required hospitalization.

On a country or global basis, 1 or 2 predominant strains spread to create the annual epidemic. At present, influenza type A strains with the H1N1 and H3N2 serotypes and type B strains are co-circulating, and either type may be predominant in any 1 year, making predictions about the serotype and severity of the upcoming influenza season difficult. Strain variants are identified by their HA and NA serotypes, by the geographic area from which they were originally isolated, by their isolate number, and by year of isolation. Thus, the influenza vaccine for 2005–2006 was trivalent, having strains identified as A/New Caledonia/20/99 (H1N1), A/California/7/04 (H3N2), and B/Shanghi/361/02.

PATHOGENESIS. The virus attaches to sialic acid residues on cells via the HA and, by endocytosis, makes its way into vacuoles, where, with progressive acidification, there is fusion to the endosomal membrane and release of the viral RNA into the cytoplasm. The RNA is transported to the nucleus and transcribed. Newly synthesized RNA is returned to the cytoplasm and translated into proteins, which are transported to the cell membrane. This is followed by budding of virus through the cell membrane. The packaging incorporates the 10 segments of the genome in a manner that is not well understood. A host cell–mediated proteolytic cleavage of the HA occurs at some point in the assembly or release of the virus, which is essential for successful fusion and release from the endosome and amplification of virus titer. In humans, the influenza replicative cycle is confined to the respiratory epithelium. With primary infection, virus replication continues for 10–14 days.

Influenza causes a lytic infection of the respiratory epithelium with loss of ciliary function, decreased mucus production, and desquamation of the epithelial layer. These changes permit secondary bacterial invasion either directly through the epithelium or, in the case of the middle ear space, through obstruction of the normal drainage through the eustachian tube. Influenza types A and B have been reported to cause myocarditis, and influenza type B can cause myositis. Reye syndrome can result with the use of salicylates during influenza type B infection (see Chapter 358).

The exact immune mechanisms involved in termination of primary infection and protection against reinfection are not well understood but may correspond to the induction of cytokines that inhibit viral replication, such as interferon and tumor necrosis factor. The incubation period of influenza to the onset of illness can be as short as 48–72 hr. The extremely short incubation period of influenza and its growth on the mucosal surface pose particular problems for invoking an adaptive immune response. Antigen presentation is primarily at mucosal sites acting through the bronchial-associated lymphoid tract. The most easily detected humoral response is directed against the HA. High serum antibody levels inhibiting HA activity are generated by inactivated vaccine and correlate with protection. Mucosally produced immunoglobulin A (IgA) antibodies are thought to be the most

TABLE 255-1. Relative Frequency of Symptoms and Signs During Classic Influenza in Older Children and Adolescents

VARIABLE	OCCURRENCE
SYMPTOMS	
Chilly sensation	++++
Cough	+++
Headache	+++
Sore throat	+++
Prostration	++
Nasal stuffiness	++
Diarrhea	++
Dizziness	+
Eye irritation or pain	+
Vomiting	+
Myalgia	+
SIGNS	
Fever	++++
Pharyngitis	+++
Conjunctivitis (mild)	++
Rhinitis	++
Cervical lymphadenopathy	+
Pulmonary rales, wheezes, or rhonchi	+

++++, 76–100%; +++, 51–75%; ++, 26–50%; +, 1–25%.

effective and immediate protective response that are generated during influenza infection. Unfortunately, measurable IgA antibodies against influenza persist for a relatively short period. Because of this and strain variation, symptomatic reinfection with influenza can be seen at intervals of 3–4 yr. Although heterotypic immunity can be demonstrated in the mouse through cell-mediated immune mechanisms directed toward common internal proteins, heterotypic immunity has been more difficult to show in humans.

CLINICAL MANIFESTATIONS. Influenza types A and B cause predominantly respiratory illness. The onset of illness is abrupt and is dominated by fever, myalgias, chills, headache, malaise, and anorexia; coryza, pharyngitis, and dry cough are associated features overshadowed by the other systemic signs (Table 255-1). The predominant symptoms may localize anywhere in the respiratory tract, producing an isolated upper respiratory tract illness, croup, bronchiolitis, or pneumonia. More than any other respiratory virus, systemic signs of high temperature, myalgia, malaise, and headache accompany influenza. Many of these symptoms may be mediated through cytokine production by the respiratory tract epithelium, as there is no systemic spread of the virus. The typical duration of the febrile illness is 2–4 days. Cough may persist for longer periods of time, and evidence of small airway dysfunction is often found weeks later. Due to influenza's high transmissibility, other family members or close contacts often have a similar illness. Influenza is a less distinct illness in younger children and infants; manifestations may be localized to any region of the respiratory tract. The young infant or child may be highly febrile and toxic in appearance, prompting a full diagnostic work-up. Despite some distinctive features of influenza, the illness is often indistinguishable from that caused by other respiratory viruses such as respiratory syncytial virus, parainfluenza virus, and adenovirus.

LABORATORY FINDINGS. The clinical laboratory abnormalities associated with influenza are nonspecific. A relative leukopenia is frequently seen. Chest radiographs show evidence of atelectasis or infiltrate in about 10% of children.

DIAGNOSIS AND DIFFERENTIAL DIAGNOSIS. The diagnosis of influenza depends on epidemiologic, clinical, and laboratory considerations. In the context of an epidemic, the clinical diagnosis of influenza in a young child with fever without a focus, malaise, and respiratory symptoms can be made with some certainty. The laboratory confirmation of influenza can be made in 4 ways. If seen early in the illness, virus can be isolated from the nasopharynx by inoculation of the specimen into embryonated eggs or a limited number of cell lines that support the growth of influenza. The presence of influenza in the culture is confirmed by hemadsorption, which depends on the capacity of the HA to bind red cells. Rapid and reliable diagnostic tests for influenza A and B are available that use variations of polymerase chain reaction viral genome detection technology or of antigen capture such as an enzyme-linked immunosorbent assay. The diagnosis can be confirmed serologically with acute and convalescent sera drawn around the time of the illness and tested by hemagglutination inhibition.

TREATMENT. Two classes of antiviral drugs are effective in the treatment of influenza (Table 255-2). Guidelines for the use of the neuraminidase inhibitors zanamivir and oseltamivir include use for children from the ages of 7 yr and 1 yr, respectively. These drugs, given either as an inhalation in the case of zanamivir or orally in the case of oseltamivir, are effective against both influenza A and B strains. The 2nd class of drugs, amantadine and rimantadine, can be used in influenza type A outbreaks. These 2 antivirals are not effective against influenza B and are not approved for use in children <1 yr of age. The emerging avian influenza is often resistant to amantadine and rimantadine. Each class of drug must be given within the 1st 48 hr of symptoms to decrease the severity and duration of influenza. Confusion and inability to concentrate or sleep are seen in some patients given amantadine. Drug resistance develops fairly quickly during a course of amantadine or rimantadine therapy, but it is becoming more widespread among circulating viruses. Partial resistance to the neuraminidase inhibitors may occur but is less common. All of these drugs are only an adjunct to a strong vaccination

TABLE 255-2. Recommended Daily Dosage of Influenza Antiviral Medications for Treatment and Prophylaxis*

				AGE GROUP		
ANTIVIRAL AGENT	ROUTE	TREATMENT	PROPHYLAXIS	1–6 yr	7–9 yr	>10 yr
Zanamivir†	Inhaled	Yes	Not indicated	Not indicated	10 mg bid	10 mg bid
Oseltamivir†	Oral	Yes	Yes§		Dose varies from 30–75 mg bid by child's weight	
Amantadine‡	Oral	Yes	Yes		5 mg/kg/day (maximum dose, 150 mg)	100 mg bid
Rimantadine‡	Oral	Yes	No		5 mg/kg/day (maximum dose, 150 mg)	100 mg bid

*For details, consult annually updated recommendations from the Advisory Committee on Immunization Practices of the Centers for Disease Control and Prevention (http://www.cdc.gov/flu/).
†Effective against both influenza A and B strains.
‡Effective only against influenza A strains.
§For person >12 yr of age, with a single daily dose of 75 mg.

program. The family setting or schoolroom may be appropriate places to try to prevent secondary illness by drug treatment, particularly where individuals have underlying conditions that predispose them to severe or complicated influenza infection.

SUPPORTIVE CARE. Adequate fluid intake and rest are important components in the management of influenza. Acetaminophen or ibuprofen, but not salicylates because of the risk for Reye syndrome (see Chapter 358), should be used as antipyretics to control fever. The most difficult question for parents is the appropriate timing of consultation with a health care provider. Bacterial superinfections are relatively common, and in that case antibiotic therapy should be administered. Bacterial superinfections should be suspected with recrudescence of fever, prolonged fever, or deterioration in clinical status. With uncomplicated influenza, children should feel better after the 1st 48–72 hr.

COMPLICATIONS. Otitis media and pneumonia are common complications of influenza in young children. Acute otitis media may be seen in up to 25% of cases of documented influenza. Pneumonia accompanying influenza may be a primary viral process. An acute hemorrhagic pneumonia may be seen in the most severe cases, as was frequent with the highly virulent strain seen in 1918 and has been seen in patients with the current avian influenza. The more common cause of pneumonia is probably secondary bacterial infection through the damaged epithelial layer. Unusual clinical manifestations of influenza include acute myositis seen with influenza type B, which follows the acute respiratory illness by 5–7 days and is marked by muscle weakness and pain, particularly in the calf muscles, and myoglobinuria. Myocarditis also follows influenza, and toxic shock syndrome can be associated with toxin-producing staphylococcal colonization. Influenza is particularly severe in children with underlying cardiopulmonary disease, including congenital and acquired valvular disease, cardiomyopathy, bronchopulmonary dysplasia, asthma, cystic fibrosis, and neuromuscular diseases affecting the accessory muscles of breathing. Virus is shed for longer periods of time in children receiving cancer chemotherapy and children with immunodeficiency.

PROGNOSIS. The prognosis for recovery is excellent, although full return to normal levels of activity and freedom from cough usually require weeks rather than days.

PREVENTION. Influenza vaccine of targeted populations is the best means of prevention of severe disease from influenza. Recommendations for use of influenza vaccine have become progressively broader as the impact of influenza is appreciated in such groups as pregnant mothers and young children. Chemoprophylaxis with the drugs discussed under the Treatment section is a secondary means of prevention.

Vaccine. An inactivated influenza vaccine becomes available each summer, incorporating changes in formulation that reflect the strains anticipated to circulate in the coming winter. The American Committee on Immunization Practices publishes guidelines for their use each year when the vaccines are formulated and released. Anyone who wants to reduce his or her chances of getting the flu can get vaccinated. Certain persons should get vaccinated each year, including those who are at high risk for having serious flu complications and persons who live with or care for those at high risk for serious complications. Current guidelines for children since 2006 include the administration of inactivated vaccine to all children 6–59 mo of age as well as household contacts and out-of-home caregivers of children 0–23 mo of age (Table 255-3).

Because of the decreased potential for causing febrile reactions, only the split-virus vaccine is recommended for children <12 yr of age. Two doses of vaccine (0.25 mL for 6–36 mo of age; 0.5 mL for 3–8 yr of age) at least 1 mo apart are recommended for primary immunization of children <9 yr of age. Live-attenuated vaccines that are administered intranasally are in clinical trials and have been demonstrated to have an efficacy comparable with that of inactivated vaccine in adults. Trials in children have shown efficacy of 90%. These vaccines are currently licensed for use in ages 5 and above. Their ease of administration could serve to increase influenza vaccination among children.

TABLE 255-3. Indications for Annual Influenza Vaccination

PERSONS AT HIGH RISK FOR COMPLICATIONS FROM THE FLU
All children 6–59 mo of age
Persons ≥65 yr of age
Persons who live in nursing homes and other long-term care facilities that house those with long-term illnesses
Adults and children ≥6 mo of age with chronic heart or lung conditions, including asthma
Adults and children ≥6 mo of age who needed regular medical care or were in a hospital during the previous year because of a metabolic disease (like diabetes), chronic kidney disease, or weakened immune system, including immune system problems caused by medicines or by infection with HIV/AIDS
Children 6 mo to 18 yr of age who are on long-term aspirin therapy because of the increased risk for Reye syndrome (see Chapter 358)
Women who will be pregnant during the influenza season
Persons with any condition that can compromise respiratory function or other handling of respiratory secretions such as a condition that makes it hard to breathe or swallow (e.g., brain injury or disease, spinal cord injuries, seizure disorders, or the nerve or muscle disorders)
PERSONS 50–64 YR OF AGE
Because nearly 1/3 of persons 50–64 yr of age in the USA have 1 or more medical conditions that place them at increased risk for serious flu complications, vaccination is recommended for all persons 50–64 yr of age
PERSONS WHO CAN TRANSMIT FLU TO OTHERS AT HIGH RISK FOR COMPLICATIONS
Any person in close contact with someone in a high-risk group (see above) should get vaccinated. This includes all health care workers, household contacts and out-of-home caregivers of children 0–23 mo of age, and close contacts of persons ≥65 yr of age

CHEMOPROPHYLAXIS. Amantadine and zanamivir are licensed for prophylaxis of influenza A infections (see Table 255-2). They are recommended for prophylaxis for vaccinated and unvaccinated high-risk patients and their unvaccinated health care providers during influenza A outbreaks in closed settings, for unvaccinated persons and health care providers during community influenza A outbreaks and during the period of peak influenza A activity, for immunodeficient persons, and for those for whom the influenza vaccine is contraindicated.

Beigel JH, Farrar J, Han AM, et al: Avian influenza A (H5N1) infection in humans. *N Eng J Med* 2005;353:1374–1385. (Erratum in *N Engl J Med* 2006;354:884.)

Belshe RB, Edwards KM, Vesikari T, et al: Live attenuated versus inactivated influenza vaccine in infants and young children. *N Engl J Med* 2007;356: 685–696.

Belshe RB, Mendelman PM, Treanor J, et al: The efficacy of live attenuated, cold-adapted, trivalent, intranasal influenza virus vaccine in children. *N Engl J Med* 1998;338:1405–1412.

Bhat N, Wright JG, Broder KR, et al: Influenza-associated deaths among children in the United States, 2003–2004. *N Engl J Med* 2005;353:2559–2567.

Centers for Disease Control and Prevention: Prevention and control of influenza: Recommendations of the Advisory Committee on Immunization Practices (ACIP). *MMWR* 2005;54(RR-08):1–40.

Couch RB: Prevention and treatment of influenza. *N Engl J Med* 2000; 343:1778–1787.

de Jong MD, Thanh TT, Khanh TH, et al: Oseltamivir resistance during treatment of influenza A (H5N1) infection. *N Engl J Med* 2005;353:2667–2672.

Ferguson N: Poverty, death, and a future influenza pandemic. *Lancet* 2006; 368:2187–2188.

Glezen PW, Couch RB: Interpandemic influenza in the Houston area (1974–76). *N Engl J Med* 1978;298:587–592.

Hayden FG: Antiviral resistance in influenza viruses—implications for management and pandemic response. *N Engl J Med* 2006;354:785–788.
Moscona A: Oseltamivir-resistant influenza? *Lancet* 2004;364:733–734.
Moscona A: Neuraminidase Inhibitors for Influenza. *N Engl J Med* 2005; 353(13):1363–1373.
Neuzil KM, Mellen BG, Wright PF, et al: The effect of influenza on hospitalizations, outpatient visits, and courses of antibiotics in children. *N Engl J Med* 2001;343:225–231.
Newland JG, Laurich M, Rosenquist AW, et al: Neurologic complications in children hospitalized with influenza: Characteristics, Incidence, and risk factors. *J Pediatr* 2007;150:306–310.
Ohmit SE, Monto AS: Symptomatic predictors of influenza virus positivity in children during the influenza season. *Clin Infect Dis* 2006;43:564–568.
Reichert TA, Sugaya N, Fedson DS, et al: The Japanese experience with vaccinating schoolchildren against influenza. *N Engl J Med* 2002;344:889–896.
Subbarao K, Klimov A, Katz J, et al: Characterization of an avian influenza A (H5N1) virus isolated from a child with a fatal respiratory illness. *Science* 1998;279:393–396.

Chapter 256 ■ Parainfluenza Viruses

Peter Wright

Viruses in the parainfluenza family are common causes of respiratory illness in infants and young children. They cause a spectrum of upper and lower respiratory tract illnesses, but are particularly associated with laryngotracheitis, bronchitis, and croup.

ETIOLOGY. The parainfluenza viruses are members of the Paramyxoviridae family. There are 4 viruses in the parainfluenza group that cause illness in humans; they are designated types 1–4. The viruses have a nonsegmented, single-stranded RNA genome with a lipid-containing envelope derived from budding through the cell membrane. The major antigenic moieties are envelope spike proteins that exhibit hemagglutinating (HN protein) and cell fusion (F protein) properties.

EPIDEMIOLOGY. Parainfluenza viruses are spread from the respiratory tract by aerosolized secretions or direct hand contact with secretions. By 3 yr of age, most children have experienced infection with types 1, 2, and 3. Type 3 is endemic and can cause disease in infants younger than 6 mo of age. Serious illness is seen with parainfluenza type 3 in immunocompromised patients. Types 1 and 2 occur in a seasonal pattern in the summer and fall and usually alternate years in which their serotype is most prevalent. Parainfluenza type 3 is endemic throughout the year, but typically peaks in late spring. Parainfluenza type 4 is more difficult to grow in tissue culture, and thus its epidemiology is less well defined. However, it does not appear to be a major cause of illness.

PATHOGENESIS. Parainfluenza viruses replicate in the respiratory epithelium without evidence of systemic spread. The propensity to cause illness in the upper large airways is presumably related to enhanced replication in the larynx, trachea, and bronchi compared with other viruses. The destruction of cells in the upper airways can lead to secondary bacterial invasion and resultant **bacterial tracheitis.** Eustachian tube obstruction can lead to secondary bacterial invasion of the middle-ear space and acute otitis media.

Illness caused by parainfluenza occurs within 4–5 days after inoculation with the virus. Some parainfluenza viruses induce cell-to-cell fusion. During the budding process, cell membrane integrity is lost, and viruses can induce cell death through the process of apoptosis. Immune destruction of virally infected cells may also occur. The most severe illness coincides with the time of maximal viral shedding. The level of immunoglobulin A antibody is the best predictor of susceptibility to infection. Reinfection is seen, particularly with parainfluenza type 3, as mucosal immunity wanes. The inability of children with serious T-cell defects to clear parainfluenza type 3 suggests a cell-mediated component of immunity critical to termination of infection.

CLINICAL MANIFESTATIONS. Most parainfluenza virus infections are confined to the upper respiratory tract (Table 256-1). The generally mild illness is belied by a spectrum of rarer but more serious illnesses that result in hospitalization. The parainfluenza viruses account for 50% of hospitalizations for croup and 15% of cases of bronchiolitis and pneumonia. Parainfluenza type 1 causes more cases of croup, whereas parainfluenza type 3 causes a broader spectrum of lower respiratory tract diseases.

Parainfluenza virus infections are not usually associated with high fever. Aside from low-grade fever, systemic complaints are rare. The illness usually lasts 4–5 days; however, virus may be recovered in low titers for 2–3 wk. Rarely, parainfluenza viruses have been implicated in parotitis.

DIAGNOSIS. The diagnosis of parainfluenza virus infection in children is usually based only on clinical and epidemiologic criteria. The virus should be specifically sought by viral culture in persistent pneumonias in immunosuppressed children. The radiographic "steeple sign" of progressive narrowing of the subglottic region is characteristic of parainfluenza virus respiratory tract infections.

LABORATORY FINDINGS. There are no distinctive laboratory findings. The laboratory diagnosis of parainfluenza virus infection can be accomplished by inoculation of nasal secretions into tissue

TABLE 256-1. Diagnoses and Signs and Symptoms of Children Younger than 5 Yr of Age with Parainfluenza Infections

DIAGNOSES	TYPE 1 (*n* = 77)	TYPE 2 (*n* = 33)	TYPE 3 (*n* = 157)	OTHER (*n* = 19)
UPPER RESPIRATORY	90%	94%	89%	84%
Common cold	31%	42%	32%	42%
Pharyngitis	21%	18%	10%	11%*
Acute otitis media	38%	30%	52%	32%†
LOWER RESPIRATORY	17%	15%	15%	21%
Croup (laryngotracheobronchitis)	16%	6%	5%	21%‡
Bronchiolitis	1%	9%	6%	0%
SIGNS AND SYMPTOMS				
Coryza	74%	75%	83%	83%
Conjunctivitis	36%	36%	36%	44%
Cough	73%	67%	81%	77%
Hoarseness	28%	18%	11%	39%§
Rales or rhonchi	6%	15%	15%	11%
Wheezing	9%	12%	4%	5%
Temperature >38°C	33%	16%	38%	6%‖
Temperature >39°C	8%	6%	10%	0%
Irritability	47%	30%	54%	72%¶
Anorexia	36%	36%	36%	44%
Vomiting	15%	15%	24%	22%
Diarrhea	21%	15%	14%	22%

Note that p values are for Fisher's exact test for the null hypothesis that all types are alike.
*p = 0.09
†p = 0.03
‡p = 0.01
§p = 0.001
‖p = 0.004
¶p = 0.02
From Reed G, Jewett PH, Thompson J, et al: Epidemiology and clinical impact of parainfluenza virus infections in otherwise healthy infants and young children <5 years old. *J Infect Dis* 1997;175:808. Used with permission.

culture, with presumptive diagnosis based on finding a hemadsorbent agent and final typing based on hemadsorption inhibition with type-specific antisera. Direct immunofluorescent staining is available in some centers for rapid identification of virus antigen in oropharyngeal sections. Many laboratories perform polymerase chain reaction viral genome basal testing.

TREATMENT. The possibility of rapid respiratory compromise during severe croup should influence the acuity of care given (see Chapter 382). Careful attention to symptomatic care is important. A health care provider should provide parents a description of the signs of increasing respiratory distress that would lead to reassessment. Humidification and exposure to cold air are both classically associated with a decrease in mucosal edema and liquefaction of secretions that may help to relieve obstruction; their value has not been shown in controlled trials. Aerosolized racemic epinephrine may temporarily improve aeration, but the patient may experience a rebound in airway constriction. Systemic corticosteroids should be part of the management of croup in the office, hospital, or emergency room setting. The indications for antibiotics are limited to well-documented secondary bacterial infections of the middle ears or lower respiratory tract.

Ribavirin has some antiviral activity against parainfluenza virus and should be considered in the immunocompromised child with persistent parainfluenza viral pneumonia.

COMPLICATIONS. In children with fever or more severe respiratory compromise, the possibility of a bacterial tracheitis with purulent infection below the epiglottis and vocal cords should be considered. The high frequency of otitis media complicating parainfluenza virus indicates that careful pneumatic otoscopy should be performed in all children with suspected parainfluenza virus infection.

PROGNOSIS. The prognosis for full recovery is excellent in the normal child. No long-term pulmonary residua of parainfluenza virus infection have been described.

PREVENTION. Work is progressing on live intranasally administered parainfluenza type 3 vaccines. The live vaccine candidates include a cold-adapted virus of human origin and a bovine parainfluenza virus, which is attenuated because of host range adaptation. The measure of protection afforded by vaccines will be difficult to assess because symptomatic reinfection is seen and the frequency of serious infection in the general population is low. Nonetheless, it is clear that prevention of acute respiratory illness that results from parainfluenza virus is a worthwhile goal.

Belshe RB, Newman FK, Tsai TF, et al: Phase 2 evaluation of parainfluenza type 3 cold passage mutant 45 live attenuated vaccine in health children 6–18 months old. *J Infect Dis* 2004;189(3):462–470.

Belshe RB, Newman FK, Wright PF, et al: Evaluation of combined live, attenuated respiratory Syncytial virus and parainfluenza 3 virus vaccines in infants and young children. *J Infect Dis* 2004;190(12);2096–2103.

Denny FW, Murphy TF, Clyde WA Jr, et al: An 11-year study in a pediatric practice. *Pediatrics* 1983;71:871–876.

Hall CB: Respiratory syncytial virus and parainfluenza virus. *N Engl J Med* 2001;344:1917–1928.

Hall CB, Geiman JM, Breese BB, et al: Parainfluenza infections in children: Correlation of shedding with clinical manifestations. *J Pediatr* 1977;91: 194–198.

Henrickson KJ, Kuhn SM, Savatski LL: Epidemiology and cost of infection with human parainfluenza virus types 1 and 2 in young children. *Clin Infect Dis* 1994;18:770–779.

Landau LI, Geelhoed GC: Aerosolized steroids for croup. *N Engl J Med* 1994;331:322–323.

Orelicek SL: Management of acute laryngotracheobronchitis. *Pediatr Infect Dis J* 1998;17:1164–1165.

Reed G, Jewett PH, Thompson J, et al: Epidemiology and clinical impact of parainfluenza virus infections in otherwise healthy infants and young children <5 years old. *J Infect Dis* 1997;175:807–813.

Chapter 257 ■ Respiratory Syncytial Virus

Kenneth Mcintosh

Respiratory syncytial virus (RSV) is the major cause of bronchiolitis (see Chapter 388) and pneumonia in children <1 yr of age and is the most important respiratory tract pathogen of early childhood.

ETIOLOGY. RSV is a medium-sized, membrane-bound RNA virus that develops in the cytoplasm of infected cells and matures by budding from the cell membrane. It belongs to the family Paramyxoviridae, along with parainfluenza and measles viruses, and is in the subfamily Pneumovirinae, which also contains the human metapneumovirus. It is the only member of the genus *Pneumovirus* that infects humans. There are 2 antigenic subtypes of RSV, based primarily on variation in 1 of the 2 surface proteins, the G glycoprotein that is responsible for attachment. This antigenic variation may contribute to some degree to the frequency with which RSV reinfects children and adults.

RSV grows in many cell cultures and produces characteristic syncytial cytopathology, from which it derives its name.

EPIDEMIOLOGY. RSV is distributed worldwide and appears in yearly epidemics. In temperate climates, these epidemics occur each winter over 4–5 mo. During the remainder of the year, infections are sporadic and much less common. In the Northern hemisphere, epidemics usually peak in January, February, or March, but peaks have been recognized as early as December and as late as June. RSV outbreaks often overlap with outbreaks of influenza and human metapneumovirus but are generally more consistent from year to year and result in more disease overall, especially among infants <6 mo of age. In the tropics, the epidemic pattern is less clear. This pattern of widespread annual outbreaks and the high incidence of infection during the 1st 3–4 mo of life are unique among human viruses.

Placentally transmitted anti-RSV maternal antibody, if present in high concentration, provides partial but incomplete protection. This may account for the lower severity of RSV infections during the 1st 4–6 wk of life, except among infants born prematurely, who receive less maternal immunoglobulin. Children with RSV infection are very contagious, resulting in high attack rates. Infection is almost universal by the 2nd birthday. Reinfection occurs at a rate of 10–20% per epidemic throughout childhood, with a lower frequency among adults. In situations of high exposure such as daycare centers, attack rates are nearly 100% among previously uninfected infants and 60–80% for 2nd and subsequent infections.

Reinfection may occur as early as a few weeks after recovery but usually takes place during subsequent annual outbreaks. The severity of illness during reinfection is usually lower, and appears to be a function of both partial immunity and increased age.

Asymptomatic infection is rare. Most infants experience coryza and pharyngitis, usually with fever and occasionally with otitis media. The lower respiratory tract is involved in 10–40% of children to a varying degree with bronchitis, bronchiolitis, and bronchopneumonia. The hospitalization rate for RSV infection is 1–3%, usually with bronchiolitis, although this is often indistinguishable from RSV pneumonia in infants, and, indeed, the 2 frequently coexist. All RSV diseases of the lower respiratory tract (excluding croup) have their highest incidence at 2–7 mo of age and decrease in frequency thereafter. The syndrome of bronchiolitis is uncommon after the 1st birthday. Acute infective wheezing attacks after that age are often termed "wheezy bronchitis" or asthma attacks. Viral pneumonia is a persistent problem throughout childhood, although RSV becomes less prominent as the etiologic agent after the 1st year. RSV plays a causative role in 40–75% of cases of hospitalized bronchiolitis, 15–40% of childhood pneumonia, and 6–15% of cases of croup.

Bronchiolitis and pneumonia resulting from RSV are more common in boys than in girls by a ratio of about 1.5 : 1. Racial factors make little difference. Lower respiratory tract involvement occurs more often and earlier in life in lower socioeconomic groups and in crowded living conditions.

The incubation period from exposure to 1st symptoms is about 4 days. The virus is excreted for variable periods, probably depending on severity of illness and immunologic status. Most infants with lower respiratory tract illness shed infectious virus for 5–12 days after hospital admission. Excretion for 3 wk and even longer has been documented. Spread of infection occurs when large, infected droplets, either airborne or conveyed on hands, are inoculated in the nose or conjunctiva of a susceptible subject. RSV is probably introduced into most families by schoolchildren undergoing reinfection. Typically, in the space of a few days, older siblings and 1 or both parents acquire colds, but the infant becomes more severely ill with fever, otitis media, or lower respiratory tract disease.

Nosocomial infection during RSV epidemics is an important concern. Virus is usually spread from child to child on the hands of caregivers. Adults undergoing reinfection have also been implicated in spread of the virus.

PATHOGENESIS. Bronchiolitis is characterized by virus-induced necrosis of the bronchiolar epithelium, hypersecretion of mucus, and round cell infiltration and edema of the surrounding submucosa. These changes result in formation of mucous plugs obstructing bronchioles, with consequent hyperinflation or collapse of the distal lung tissue. In interstitial pneumonia the infiltration is more generalized and epithelial necrosis may extend to both the bronchi and the alveoli. Infants are particularly apt to experience small airway obstruction because of the small size of the normal bronchioles.

Several facts suggest immunologic injury as a major factor in the pathogenesis of bronchiolitis caused by RSV. Extensive studies in small animal models show an important role for the immune system in the respiratory pathology induced by RSV infection. Recent studies in infants and in animal models indicate that a large number of soluble factors (e.g., interleukins, leukotrienes, and chemokines) with the potential to stimulate inflammation and tissue damage are liberated during RSV infection. Children who received a highly antigenic, inactivated, parenterally administered RSV vaccine experienced, upon subsequent exposure to wild-type RSV, more severe and more frequent bronchiolitis than did their age-matched controls.

Severe disease requiring hospitalization, including intensive care, occurs primarily in children with underlying risk factors such as prematurity, chronic pulmonary disease (most often bronchopulmonary dysplasia), congenital heart disease, or immune deficiency. Three studies to date implicate coinfection with RSV and human metapneumovirus in a significant proportion of infants requiring assisted ventilation and intensive care. There is also increasing evidence that genetic factors predispose to more severe bronchiolitis.

It is not clear how often superimposed bacterial infection plays a pathogenic role in RSV lower respiratory tract disease. RSV bronchiolitis in infants is probably exclusively viral disease, although there is increasing evidence that bacterial pneumonia is often triggered by respiratory viral infection, including with RSV.

CLINICAL MANIFESTATIONS. The 1st signs of infection of the infant with RSV are rhinorrhea and pharyngitis. Cough may appear simultaneously but more often after an interval of 1–3 days, at which time there may also be sneezing and a low-grade fever. Soon after the cough develops, the child begins to wheeze audibly. If the disease is mild, the symptoms may not progress beyond this stage. Auscultation often reveals diffuse rhonchi, fine rales or crackles, and wheezes. Clear rhinorrhea usually persists throughout the illness, with intermittent fever. Chest x-rays at this stage are frequently normal.

If the illness progresses, cough and wheezing increase and air hunger ensues, with increased respiratory rate, intercostal and subcostal retractions, hyperexpansion of the chest, restlessness, and peripheral cyanosis. Signs of severe, life-threatening illness are central cyanosis, tachypnea of >70 breaths/min, listlessness, and apneic spells. At this stage, the chest may be greatly hyperexpanded and almost silent to auscultation because of poor air movement.

Chest x-rays of infants hospitalized with RSV bronchiolitis are normal in 10–30% of cases, and show hyperexpansion of the chest in 20–40%, peribronchial thickening or central pneumonia in 35–50%, and segmental or lobar consolidation in 8–20%. Pleural effusion is unusual.

In some infants, the course of the illness may resemble pneumonia with the prodromal rhinorrhea and cough followed by dyspnea, poor feeding, and listlessness, with a minimum of wheezing and hyperexpansion. Although the clinical diagnosis is pneumonia, wheezing is often present intermittently and the chest x-ray may show air trapping. In this population, perhaps more prominently in the developing world, superinfection with pneumococcus or other pathogenic bacteria may occur, and the clinical picture merges with that of bacterial pneumonia.

Fever is an inconstant sign in RSV infection. Rash and conjunctivitis each occur in a few cases. In young infants, particularly those who were born prematurely, periodic breathing and apneic spells have been distressingly frequent signs, even with relatively mild bronchiolitis. It is likely that a small portion of deaths included in the category of sudden infant death syndrome are due to RSV infection.

RSV infections in profoundly immunocompromised hosts may be severe at any age. The mortality associated with RSV pneumonia in the 1st few weeks after bone marrow or solid organ transplantation in both children and adults is >50%. RSV infection does not seem to be more severe in HIV-infected patients.

DIAGNOSIS. Bronchiolitis is a clinical diagnosis. RSV can be suspected with varying degrees of certainty based on the season of the year and the presence of a typical outbreak. Other epidemiologic features that may be helpful are the presence of colds in older household contacts and the age of the child, because, aside from RSV, the only respiratory viruses that attack infants frequently during the 1st few months of life are parainfluenza virus type 3 and human metapneumovirus.

Routine laboratory tests are of minimal diagnostic use in most cases of bronchiolitis or pneumonia caused by RSV. The white blood cell count is normal or elevated, and the differential count may be normal with either a neutrophilic or mononuclear predominance. Bacterial cultures of the throat grow only normal flora. Hypoxemia is frequent and tends to be more marked than anticipated on the basis of the clinical findings.

The most important diagnostic concern is to distinguish bacterial or chlamydial involvement. When bronchiolitis is not accompanied by infiltrates on chest x-ray, there is little likelihood of a bacterial component. In infants 1–4 mo of age, interstitial pneumonitis may be caused by *Chlamydia trachomatis* (see Chapter 223.3). With *C. trachomatis* pneumonia there may be a history of conjunctivitis, and the illness tends to be of subacute onset. Coughing and rales are prominent; wheezing is not. Fever is usually absent. There may be eosinophilia.

Consolidation without other signs or with pleural effusion should be considered of bacterial etiology until proved otherwise. Other signs suggesting bacterial pneumonia are neutrophilia, neutropenia in the presence of severe disease, ileus or other abdominal signs, high temperature, and circulatory collapse. In such instances, antibiotics should be initiated.

Definitive diagnosis of RSV infection is based on the detection of virus, viral RNA, or viral antigens in respiratory secretions. An aspirate of mucus or a nasopharyngeal wash from the child's posterior nasal cavity is the optimal specimen. Nasopharyngeal or throat swabs are less preferable but acceptable. A tracheal aspirate is unnecessary. The specimen should be placed on ice, taken directly to the laboratory, and processed for antigen detection or polymerase chain reaction. Both these tests are more sensitive than culture for RSV.

TREATMENT. The treatment of uncomplicated cases of bronchiolitis is symptomatic. Humidified oxygen is usually indicated for hospitalized infants because most are hypoxic. Many infants are slightly to moderately dehydrated, and therefore fluids should be carefully administered in amounts somewhat greater than maintenance. Often intravenous or tube feeding is helpful when sucking is difficult due to tachypnea. Infants may breathe more easily when propped up at an angle of 10–30 degrees.

There is disagreement among experts regarding the usefulness of epinephrine or β_2 agonists in RSV bronchiolitis. Corticosteroids are not indicated except in older children with an established diagnosis of asthma.

In most instances of bronchiolitis, antibiotics are not useful. Interstitial pneumonia in infants 1–4 mo old may be caused by *C. trachomatis,* and erythromycin (40 mg/kg/day) or clarithromycin (7.5 mg/kg every 12 hr) may be indicated.

Ribavirin is an antiviral delivered through an oxygen hood, face mask, or endotracheal tube using the small particle aerosol generator (SPAG-2) for 12–20 hr/day for 3–5 days. Early trials showed a modest beneficial effect on the course of RSV pneumonia with some reduction in the duration of mechanical ventilation and days of hospitalization. Subsequent studies failed to document a clear beneficial effect of ribavirin.

PROGNOSIS. The mortality rate of hospitalized infants with RSV infection of the lower respiratory tract is about 1%. Almost all deaths occur among young, premature infants or those with underlying disease of the neuromuscular, pulmonary, cardiovascular, or immunologic system. High altitude above 2,500 m is a modest predictor for RSV-associated hospitalization.

Many children with asthma have a history of bronchiolitis in infancy. There is recurrent wheezing in 33–50% of children with typical RSV bronchiolitis in infancy. The likelihood of recurrence is increased in the presence of an allergic diathesis (e.g., eczema, hay fever, or a family history of asthma). With a clinical presentation of bronchiolitis in patients >1 yr of age, there is an increasing probability that, although the episode may be virus induced, this is likely the 1st of multiple wheezing attacks that will later be diagnosed as asthma.

PREVENTION. In the hospital, the most important preventive measures are aimed at blocking nosocomial spread. During RSV season, high-risk infants should be separated from all infants with respiratory symptoms. Gowns, gloves, and careful handwashing should be used for the care of all infants with suspected or established RSV infection.

Passive Immunoprophylaxis. Administration of palivizumab (15 mg/kg IM once a month), a monoclonal antibody against RSV, is recommended for protecting high-risk children against serious complications from RSV disease. Immunoprophylaxis reduces the frequency and total days of hospitalization for RSV infections in high-risk infants. Palivizumab is administered monthly from the beginning (October–December) to the end (March–May) of the RSV season.

Candidates for immunoprophylaxis include children with lung disease or who were born very prematurely. Children <2 yr of age with chronic lung disease requiring supplemental oxygen or other medical therapy currently or within the 6 mo before the RSV season should receive prophylaxis for the 1st 2 RSV seasons if they have severe lung disease, and only for the 1st RSV season with less severe lung disease. Children <2 yr of age with hemodynamically significant congenital heart disease (heart failure, cyanosis, pulmonary hypertension) are also candidates for this therapy. Infants born at <28 wk of gestation should receive seasonal RSV prophylaxis up to 12 mo of age, and up to 6 mo of age if they were born at 29–32 wk of gestation. Infants born between 32 and 35 wk of gestation should only receive prophylaxis if they have other risk factors. Adverse events with palivizumab are uncommon.

Vaccine. There is not a vaccine against RSV currently. Vaccine development for RSV has proceeded cautiously since the experience in the 1960s with an alum-precipitated formalin-inactivated vaccine. Children who received this experimental vaccine had paradoxically severe disease after natural RSV infection. Live-attenuated vaccines are under active investigation. The challenge is to produce a vaccine that infects without producing unacceptable symptoms, is genetically stable, and induces immunity to reinfection. The most promising candidates have been engineered in the laboratory from cold-adapted strains of RSV, following the lead of the live influenza vaccines.

Choudhuri JA, Ogden LG, Ruttenber AJ, et al: Effect of altitude on hospitalizations for respiratory syncytial virus infection. *Pediatrics* 2006;17:349–356.

Forster J, Ihorst G, Rieger CHL et al: Prospective population-based study of viral lower respiratory tract infections in children under 3 years of age (the PRI.DE study). *Eur J Pediatr* 2004;163:709–716.

Glezen WP, Paredes A, Allison JE, et al: Risk of respiratory syncytial virus infection for infants from low-income families in relationship to age, sex, ethnic group and maternal antibody level. *J Pediatr* 1981;98:708–715.

Hall CB, Douglas RG Jr, Geiman JM, et al: Nosocomial respiratory syncytial virus infections. *N Engl J Med* 1975;293:1343–1346.

Henderson FW, Collier AM, Clyde WA Jr, et al: Respiratory-syncytial-virus infections, reinfections and immunity: A prospective, longitudinal study in young children. *N Engl J Med* 1979;300:530–534.

Karron RA, Wright PF, Belshe RB, et al: Identification of a recombinant live attenuated respiratory syncytial virus vaccine candidate that is highly attenuated in infants. *J Infect Dis* 2005;191:1093–1104.

Kern S, Uhl M, Berner R, et al: Respiratory syncytial virus infection of the lower respiratory tract: Radiological findings in 108 children. *Eur Radiol* 2001;11:2581–2584.

McNamara PS, Flanagan BF, Hart CA, Smyth RL: Production of chemokines in the lungs of infants with severe respiratory syncytial virus bronchiolitis. *J Infect Dis* 2005;191:1225–1232.

Meissner HC, Long SS: Revised indications for the use of palivizumab and respiratory syncytial virus immune globulin intravenous for the prevention of respiratory syncytial virus infections. *Pediatrics* 2003;112:1447–1452.

Semple MG, Cowell A, Dove W, et al: Dual infection of infants by human metapneumovirus and human respiratory syncytial virus is strongly associated with severe bronchiolitis. *J Infect Dis* 2005;191:382–386.

Ventre K, Randolph AG: Ribavirin for respiratory syncytial virus infection of the lower respiratory tract in infants and young children. *Cochrane Database Syst Rev* 2004;4:CD000181.

Wang EEL, Law BJ, Stephens D, and other members of PICNIC: Pediatric Investigators Collaborative Network on Infections in Canada (PICNIC) prospective study of risk factors and outcomes in patients hospitalized with respiratory syncytial viral lower respiratory tract infection. *J Pediatr* 1995;126:212–219.

Chapter 258 ■ Human Metapneumovirus

James E. Crowe, Jr.

Human metapneumovirus (HMPV), a respiratory virus identified in 2001, is emerging as 1 of the most common causes of serious lower respiratory tract illness in children throughout the world.

ETIOLOGY. HMPV is an enveloped, single-stranded nonsegmented negative-sense RNA genome of the Paramyxoviridae family, which is divided into 2 subfamilies, Pneumovirinae and Paramyxovirinae. The Pneumovirinae subfamily includes the 2 genera *Metapneumovirus* and *Pneumovirus*, which includes respiratory syncytial virus (RSV). HMPV and the avian pneumoviruses (APVs) are highly related and separated into the separate genus *Metapneumovirus* because the gene order in the nonsegmented genome is slightly altered and APV/HMPV lack the 2 nonstructural proteins NS1 and NS2 that are located at the 3′ end of RSV genomes. These proteins are thought to counteract host type I interferons. The absence of NS1/NS2 in the metapneumoviruses may contribute to decreased pathogenicity of HMPV relative to wild-type RSV strains.

Full-length sequences of a number of HMPV genomes have been determined. The genome is predicted to encode 9 proteins in the order 3′-N-P-M-F-M2(orf1 and 2)-SH-G-L-5′. The genome also contains noncoding 3′ leader, 5′ trailer, and intergenic regions, consistent with the organization of most paramyxoviruses, with a viral promoter contained in the 3′ end of the genome. The F (fusion), G (glycosylated), and SH (short hydrophobic) proteins are integral membrane proteins on the surface of infected cells and virion particles. The F protein is a classic type I integral membrane viral fusion protein that contains 2 heptad repeats in the extracellular domain that facilitate membrane fusion. There is a predicted protein cleavage site near a hydrophobic fusion peptide that likely is cleaved by an extracellular protease, activating the F protein for fusion. The predicted attachment (G or glycosylated) protein of HMPV exhibits the basic features of a glycosylated type II mucin-like protein. The HMPV G protein differs from the RSV 6 in that it lacks a cysteine noose structure. The internal proteins of the virus appear similar in function to those of other paramyxoviruses.

EPIDEMIOLOGY. HMPV outbreaks occur in annual epidemics during late winter and early spring in temperate climates, usually overlapping with the annual RSV epidemic (Fig. 258-1). Sporadic infection does occur year round. The usual period of viral shedding is likely to be several weeks following primary infection in infants. The incubation period is about 3–5 days. Humans are the only source of virus. Transmission is thought to occur by close or direct contact with contaminated secretions involving large particle aerosols, droplets, or contaminated surfaces. Nosocomial infections have been reported; contact isolation with excellent

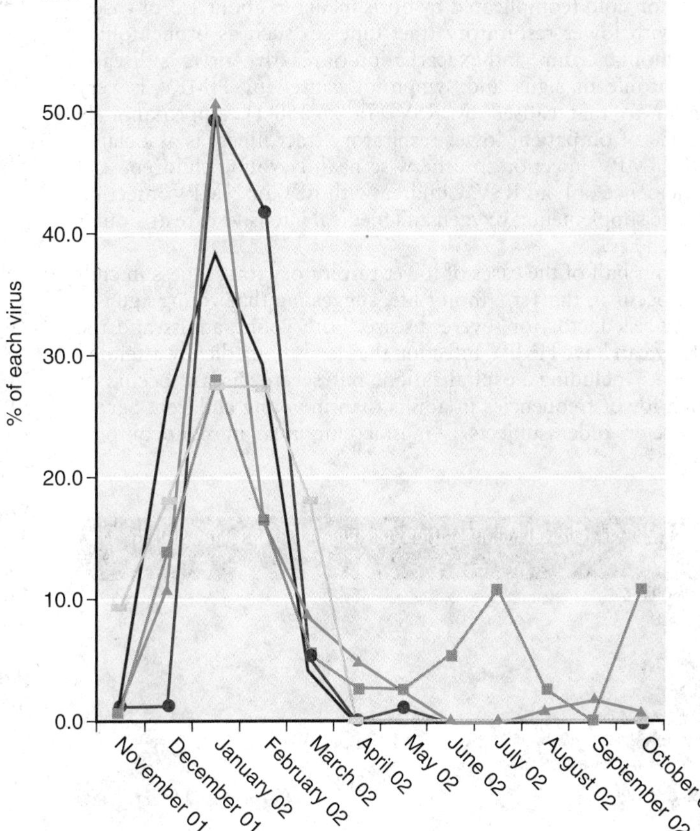

Figure 258-1. Temporal distribution of respiratory viruses among children hospitalized with lower respiratory tract infections from November 2001 through October 2002. Data are displayed as the proportion of each virus detected monthly. (From Wolf DG, Greenberg D, Kalkstein D, et al: Comparison of human metapneumovirus, respiratory syncytial virus and influenza A virus lower reparatory tract infections in hospitalized young children. *Pediatr Infect Dis J* 2006;25:320–324.)

handwashing for health care providers is indicated in medical settings.

PATHOLOGY. Infection is usually limited to the superficial layer of airway epithelial cells. Infection is associated with a local inflammatory infiltrate consisting of lymphocytes and macrophages. Immunocompromised individuals have evidence of both acute and organizing injury during prolonged infection.

PATHOGENESIS. Infection occurs via inoculation of the upper respiratory tract. Infection can spread rapidly to the lower respiratory tract, but it is not clear whether the spread is mediated by cell-to-cell spread or aspiration of infected materials from the upper tract. Severe lower respiratory tract illness, especially wheezing, occurs mainly during the 1st 6 mo of life, at a time when the airways are of a small diameter and high resistance. Maternal serum neutralizing antibodies that cross the placenta may afford a relative protection against severe disease for several weeks or months after birth. Once infection is established, it is suspected that cytotoxic T cells recognize and eliminate virus-infected cells, thus terminating the infection but also causing some cytopathology. Individuals with an underlying predisposition to reactive airways disease (including adults) are susceptible to severe wheezing during reinfection later in life, suggesting that HMPV may cause smooth muscle hyperactivity, inflammation, or increased mucous production in such individuals. Infection in otherwise healthy individuals resolves without apparent long-term consequences in most cases.

CLINICAL MANIFESTATIONS. HMPV is associated with the common cold (complicated by otitis media in about 1/3 of cases) and with lower respiratory tract illnesses such as bronchiolitis, pneumonia, croup, and exacerbation of reactive airways disease. The profile of signs and symptoms caused by HMPV is very similar to that caused by RSV (Table 258-1). Approximately 5–10% of outpatient lower respiratory tract illness is associated with HMPV infection in otherwise healthy young children, 2nd in incidence only to RSV. Children with RSV or HMPV infection require supplemental oxygen and medical intensive care at similar frequencies.

About half of the cases of lower respiratory tract illness in children occur in the 1st 6 mo of life, suggesting that young age is a major risk factor for severe disease. Both young adults and the elderly can have HMPV infection that leads to medically attended illnesses including hospitalization, but severe disease occurs at much lower frequencies in adults than in young children. Severe disease in older subjects is most common in immunocompromised patients, and can be fatal. A significant number of both adult and pediatric patients with asthmatic exacerbation have HMPV infection; it is not clear if the virus causes long-term wheezing. RSV and HMPV coinfections have been reported; coinfections may be more severe resulting in pediatric intensive care unit admissions. It is difficult to define true co-infections since viral genome can be detected by reverse transcriptase polymerase chain reaction (RT-PCR) in respiratory secretions for at least several weeks after illness, even when virus shedding has terminated.

TABLE 258-1. Clinical Manifestations of Human Metapneumovirus in Children
COMMON (>50%)
Fever >38°C
Cough
Rhinitis, coryza
Wheezing
Tachypnea, retractions
Hypoxia (O_2 saturation <94%)
Chest x-ray infiltrates or hyperinflation
LESS COMMON
Otitis media
Pharyngitis
Rales
RARE
Conjunctivitis
Hoarseness
Encephalitis
Fatal respiratory failure in immunocompromised children

LABORATORY FINDINGS. The virus can be seen only by electron microscopy. Conventional bright-field microscopy of infected cell monolayer cultures often reveals cytopathic effect only after multiple passages in cell culture. The characteristics of the cytopathic effect are not sufficiently distinct so that the virus could be identified on this basis alone, even by a trained observer. Direct antigen tests are under development, but none are commercially available. The most sensitive test for identification of HMPV in clinical samples is RT-PCR, usually performed with primers directed to internal genes such as the nucleoprotein. Real-time RT-PCR tests offer enhanced sensitivity and specificity, including assays designed to detect viruses from the 4 known genetic lineages. The virus grows in primary monkey kidney cells or LLC-MK2 cell or Vero cell line monolayer cultures. All current diagnostic tests are experimental and available only in research laboratories.

DIAGNOSIS AND DIFFERENTIAL DIAGNOSIS. In temperate areas, the diagnosis should be suspected during the late winter in infants or young children with wheezing or pneumonia and a negative diagnostic test for RSV. The diseases caused by RSV and HMPV cannot be distinguished clinically. There are currently no licensed diagnostic laboratory tests for HMPV. Many other common respiratory viruses such as parainfluenza viruses, influenza viruses, adenoviruses, rhinoviruses, and coronaviruses can cause similar disease in young children. Some of these viruses can be identified by PCR genetic testing or conventional culture means.

COMPLICATIONS. Coinfection with bacteria is not common, except for the local complication of otitis media.

TREATMENT. There is no specific treatment at this time for HMPV infection. The management is to provide supportive care. The rate of bacterial lung infection or bacteremia associated with HMPV infection is not fully defined but is suspected to be very low. Antibiotics usually are not indicated in treatment of infants hospitalized for HMPV bronchiolitis or pneumonia.

SUPPORTIVE CARE. Treatment is supportive and includes careful attention to hydration, monitoring clinical assessment of respiratory status by physical examination and measurement of oxygen saturation, use of supplemental oxygen, and if necessary, mechanical ventilation.

PROGNOSIS. Most infants and children recover from acute HMPV infection without apparent long-term consequences. Many experts believe an association exists with severe HMPV infections in infancy and risk for recurrent wheezing or the development of asthma; it is not clear whether the virus causes these conditions or precipitates the 1st manifestation.

PREVENTION. The only method of prevention of HMPV infection is reduction of exposure. Contact precautions are recommended for the duration of HMPV-associated illness among hospitalized infants and young children. Patients known to have HMPV infection should be housed in single rooms or with a cohort of HMPV-infected patients. It may be wise to care for patients with RSV infection in a separate cohort from HMPV-infected patients to prevent coinfection. Preventive measures include limiting, where feasible, exposure to contagious settings during annual epidemics (daycare centers) and emphasis on hand hygiene in all settings, including the home, especially during periods when the contacts of high-risk children have respiratory infections. Providers should keep in mind, however, that infection is universal in the 1st several years of life. Reduction of exposure, therefore, makes the most sense during the 1st 6 mo of life, when infants are at highest risk for severe disease.

Crowe JE Jr: Human metapneumovirus as a major cause of human respiratory tract disease. *Pediatr Infect Dis J* 2004;23(Suppl):S215–S221.

Esper F, Martinello RA, Boucher D, et al: A 1-year experience with human metapneumovirus in children aged <5 years. *J Infect Dis* 2004;189:1388–1396.

Foulongne V, Buyon G, Rodiere M, et al: Human metapneumovirus infection in young children hospitalized with respiratory tract disease. *Pediatr Infect Dis J* 2006;25:34–39.

Hamelin ME, Boivin G: Human metapneumovirus—A ubiquitous and long-standing respiratory pathogen. *Pediatr Infect Dis J* 2005;24(Suppl):S203–S207.

Klein MI, Coviello S, Bauer G, et al: The impact of infection with human metapneumovirus and other respiratory viruses in young infants and children at high risk for severe pulmonary disease. *J Infect Dis* 2006;193:1544–1551.

Semple, MG, Cowell, A, Dove, W, et al: Dual infection of infants by human metapneumovirus and human respiratory syncytial virus is strongly associated with severe bronchiolitis. *J Infect Dis* 2005;191:382–386.

Williams JV, Harris PA, Tollefson SJ, et al: Human metapneumovirus and lower respiratory tract disease in otherwise healthy infants and children. *N Engl J Med* 2004;350:443–450.

Williams JV, Martino R, Rabella N, et al: A prospective study comparing human metapneumovirus with other respiratory viruses in adults with hematologic malignancies and respiratory tract infections. *J Infect Dis* 2005;192:1061–1065.

William JV, Wang CK, Yang CF, et al: The role of human metapneumovirus in upper respiratory tract infections in children: A 20-year experience. *J Infect Dis* 2006;193:387–395.

Williams JV, Crowe JE Jr, Enriquez R, et al: Human metapneumovirus infection plays an etiologic role in acute asthma exacerbations requiring hospitalization in adults. *J Infect Dis* 2005;192:1149–1153.

Williams JV, Martino R, Rabella N, et al: A prospective study comparing human metapneumovirus with other respiratory viruses in adults with hematologic malignancies and respiratory tract infections. *J Infect Dis* 2005;192:1061–1065.

Williams JV, Tollefson SJ, Heymann PW, et al: Human metapneumovirus infection in children hospitalized for wheezing. *J Allergy Clin Immunol* 2005;115:1311–1312.

Wolf DG, Greenberg D, Kalkstein D, et al: Comparison of human metapneumovirus, respiratory syncytial virus and influenza A virus lower reparatory tract infections in hospitalized young children. *Pediatr Infect Dis J* 2006;25:320–324.

Chapter 259 ■ Adenoviruses

Kenneth Mcintosh

Adenoviruses cause 5–11% of acute respiratory disease in infants plus a wide array of other syndromes, including pharyngoconjunctival fever, follicular conjunctivitis, epidemic keratoconjunctivitis, myocarditis, hemorrhagic cystitis, acute diarrhea, intussusception, and encephalomyelitis. Only $^1/_3$ of the 51 human serotypes have been associated with disease. Fatal disease is rare and is associated with infection by certain serotypes (particularly type 7) and infection in immunocompromised hosts.

ETIOLOGY. The Adenoviridae are DNA viruses of intermediate size, which are classified into subgenera A to F. The virion has an icosahedral capsid made up of 252 subunits, or capsomers, of which 240 are hexons and 12 are pentons. Hexons have a cross-reacting antigen common to all mammalian adenoviruses. Pentons are the basis of serotype specificity and protective antibody. Adenoviruses can also be classified by their characteristic DNA fingerprints on gels after being digested with restriction endonucleases, which generally conforms to the antigenic types.

All adenovirus types except types 40 and 41, which are the 2 most important serotypes causing enteritis, grow in primary human embryonic kidney cells, and most grow in HEp-2 or HeLa cells, producing a typical destructive cytopathic effect. Types 40 and 41, and other serotypes as well, grow in 293 cells, a line of human embryonic kidney cells into which certain early adenovirus genes have been introduced.

The common adenovirus types, including types 1, 2, and 5, are shed for prolonged periods, particularly from the gastrointestinal tract. These types also establish low-level and chronic infection of the tonsils and adenoids.

EPIDEMIOLOGY. Adenoviral infections are distributed worldwide. They occur year-round but are most prevalent in spring or early summer and again in midwinter in temperate climates. Certain types tend to occur in epidemics, notably types 4 and 7 in outbreaks of febrile respiratory disease; types 3, 7, and 21 in severe pneumonia; type 3 in pharyngoconjunctival fever; type 11 in hemorrhagic cystitis; and types 8, 19, and 37 in epidemic keratoconjunctivitis. For unexplained reasons, adenovirus types 3 and 7 cause severe epidemics of pneumonia in the children of northern China, Taiwan, and Korea, with mortality rates of 5–15%.

More than 60% of school-aged children have antibodies to the common respiratory types, and almost all adults have antibody to types 1–7. Infections with types 1 and 2 tend to occur during the 2nd yr of life, and types 3 and 5 occur a little later. Spread occurs by the respiratory and fecal-oral routes, although it is not clear whether spread is by large- or small-particle aerosol. Hospital outbreaks of respiratory disease and keratoconjunctivitis have been described and may result in severe disease in nurseries or among immunocompromised children.

PATHOGENESIS. Adenoviruses are among the few "respiratory" viruses that grow well in the epithelium of the small intestine. Although mucosal surfaces are the primary target early in infection and typically the site of the most common pathology, viremia can be demonstrated by polymerase chain reaction (PCR) of serum or plasma and occurs relatively frequently, even in immunologically normal children.

Adenoviral pneumonia produces characteristic histologic changes, with dense lymphocytic infiltrates, destruction of the bronchial and bronchiolar epithelium, focal necrosis of mucous glands, hyaline membrane formation, and several types of nuclear inclusion bodies.

CLINICAL MANIFESTATIONS. Adenoviruses cause a wide array of clinical syndromes.

Acute Respiratory Disease. Respiratory tract infections are the most common manifestation of adenovirus infections in children and adults and are usually caused by the **respiratory types,** which are types 1, 2, 3, 5, and 6. Acute adenovirus respiratory tract infections in infants and children are not clinically distinctive. Primary infections in infants are frequently associated with fever and respiratory symptoms and are complicated by otitis media in more than half of cases. Adenovirus respiratory infections are associated with a significant incidence of diarrhea.

Pharyngitis caused by adenovirus typically includes symptoms of coryza, sore throat, and fever. Adenoviruses can be identified in 15–20% of children with isolated pharyngitis, mostly in preschoolers and infants.

About 7–9% of hospitalized children with **acute pneumonia** have adenovirus infection. Adenovirus pneumonia often presents with radiologic features more typical of bacterial disease (lobar infiltrates, high fever, parapneumonic effusions), and children with adenovirus pneumonia often have other systemic signs such as diarrhea, abdominal pain, and even coagulation defects. Any of the "respiratory" types can cause pneumonia, but severe infections are most likely caused by types 3, 7, or 21. These infections have a mortality rate as high as 10%, and survivors may have residual airway damage, manifested by bronchiectasis, bronchiolitis obliterans, or, rarely, pulmonary fibrosis. Neonatal adenovirus pneumonia occurs rarely, but may be severe or fatal.

A **pertussis-like syndrome** has been described in association with adenovirus infections. In these cases, adenoviruses frequently accompany *Bordetella pertussis* as co-infecting agents, but occasionally they may also be causative on their own.

Pharyngoconjunctival fever is a clinically distinct syndrome that occurs typically with type 3 adenovirus. Features include a high temperature that lasts 4–5 days, pharyngitis, conjunctivitis, preauricular and cervical lymphadenopathy, and rhinitis. Nonpurulent conjunctivitis occurs in 75% of patients and is manifested by inflammation of both the bulbar and palpebral conjunctivae of 1 or both eyes, which often persists after the fever and other symptoms have resolved. Headache, malaise, and weakness are common, and there is considerable lethargy after the acute stage.

Conjunctivitis and Keratoconjunctivitis. Adenovirus is 1 of the most common causes of follicular conjunctivitis and keratoconjunctivitis. Follicular conjunctivitis is a relatively mild illness and is highly contagious. Keratoconjunctivitis, which may occur in epidemics, is associated with adenovirus types 8, 19, and 37. Keratitis begins as the conjunctivitis wanes, and may cause corneal opacities that last several years.

Myocarditis. In several series of acute myocarditis or idiopathic cardiomyopathy using PCR to identify the etiology, adenovirus has been found as commonly as or more commonly than nonpolio enteroviruses. It is widely assumed that adenovirus has an important etiologic role in this disease. It has also been associated with heart transplant rejection and with some cases of endocardial fibroelastosis.

Gastrointestinal Infections. Adenoviruses can be found in the stools of 5–9% of children with acute diarrhea. About half of these are the **enteric types,** which are types 40 and 41. It is also clear that enteric infection with any adenovirus serotype is often asymptomatic, so the causative role in these episodes is frequently uncertain.

The pathogenesis of intussusception is thought to include enlarged lymph nodes as an initiating factor. Adenoviruses have been recovered from mesenteric lymph nodes or appendices at surgery and also from surface cultures in a higher percentage of children with intussusception than of controls. Adenoviruses have also been found in the appendices of children with appendicitis.

Hemorrhagic Cystitis. This syndrome has a sudden onset of bacteriologically sterile hematuria, dysuria, frequency, and urgency lasting 1–2 wk. Infection with adenovirus types 11 and 21 has been found in some affected children and young adults.

Reye Syndrome and Reye-like Syndromes. Typical Reye syndrome has followed confirmed adenovirus infection of several serotypes, particularly among very young children. In addition, several cases of a Reye-like syndrome have been reported, all of which are caused by infection with adenovirus type 7 and are frequently fatal. This is characterized by severe bronchopneumonia, hepatitis, seizures, and disseminated intravascular coagulopathy. Circulating adenovirus penton antigen has been found in several patients and has been implicated in the pathogenesis. Adenovirus has also been found in more typical cases of meningoencephalitis, particularly in immunocompromised hosts.

Infections in Immunocompromised Persons. Adenoviruses are increasingly recognized as important pathogens in immunocompromised hosts, particularly children, with abnormalities of B- or T-cell function. In hypogammaglobulinemic patients, a chronic meningoencephalitis similar to that caused by enteroviruses has been described. In children with T-cell dysfunction, regardless of whether this condition is congenital, acquired, or iatrogenic, fulminant hepatitis and pneumonia, frequently with a fatal outcome, have been described. Enterocolitis can also occur and is particularly frequent in intestinal transplants. There is also a close association between adenovirus infection and both hemorrhagic cystitis and tubulointerstitial nephritis in immunocompromised children.

DIAGNOSIS. The laboratory diagnosis of adenovirus infection in children may be made by detection of virus in a clinical specimen by culture, antigen detection, or PCR, demonstration of a rise in antibody titers, or a combination of virus detection and serologic testing. If virus is found in a "privileged" site, such as blood, urine, or cerebrospinal fluid, or in a biopsy of the lung or liver, the implication of infection with disease and organ damage is strong. Likewise, detection of certain adenovirus types in respiratory secretions (type 7 or 21) probably indicates etiologic involvement. The presence of untyped virus or the common childhood types (e.g., 1, 2, and 5) in respiratory secretions or stool does not necessarily indicate clinical adenovirus infection because these viruses may be excreted asymptomatically for long periods. In these instances, discovery of a coincident rise in antibody by complement fixation (group specific) or neutralization or hemagglutination inhibition (type specific) is helpful in assigning a specific adenovirus type to disease. Adenovirus infection often results in a high erythrocyte sedimentation rate and white blood cell count.

PCR is far more sensitive as a diagnostic tool than either culture or antigen detection. Through PCR, the role of adenoviruses in myocarditis and in post-transplantation infections is becoming clearer. After transplantation, serial PCR of blood for viral load has been used to monitor infection and guide decreasing immunosuppressive drugs and initiation of antiviral chemotherapy.

TREATMENT. Ribavirin was the 1st clinically acceptable agent found with some in vitro activity against adenovirus, but there is mounting evidence that it lacks clinical efficacy. Cidofovir is a nucleoside analog with demonstrable in vitro antiviral activity against adenovirus. There is good evidence for a quantitative reduction in virus in immunocompromised patients during cidofovir treatment. Renal toxicity can be dose limiting, however. Newer nucleoside analog agents with promising anti-adenoviral activity in vitro and in animal models are being developed for clinical use.

PREVENTION. Vaccines that contain either killed or live virus were developed to prevent type 4 and 7 infections in military recruits and were used until the late 1990s. These vaccines have not, however, been used in children.

Bowles NE, Ni J, Kearney DL, et al: Detection of viruses in myocardial tissues by polymerase chain reaction: Evidence of adenovirus as a common cause of myocarditis in children and adults. *J Am Coll Cardiol* 2003;42:466–472.

Brandt CD, Kim HW, Jeffries BC, et al: Infections in 18,000 infants and children in a controlled study of respiratory tract disease: II. Adenovirus pathogenicity in relation to serologic type and illness syndrome. *Am J Epidemiol* 1970;90:484–500.

Faden H, Wynn RJ, Campagna L, Ryan RM: Outbreak of adenovirus type 30 in a neonatal intensive care unit. *J Pediatr* 2005;146:447–448.

Hong, JY, Lee HJ, Piedra PA, et al. Lower respiratory tract infections due to adenovirus in hospitalized Korean children: Epidemiology, clinical features, and prognosis. *Clin Infect Dis* 2001;32:1423–1429.

Kelsey DS: Adenovirus meningoencephalitis. *Pediatrics* 1978;61:291–293.

Leruez-Ville M, Minard V, Lacaille F et al: Real-time blood plasma polymerase chain reaction for management of disseminated adenovirus infection. *Clin Infect Dis* 2004;38:45.
Michaels MG, Green M, Wald ER, et al: Adenovirus infection in pediatric liver transplant recipients. *J Infect Dis* 1992;165:170–174.
Nelson KE, Gavitt F, Batt MD, et al: The role of adenoviruses in the pertussis syndrome. *J Pediatr* 1975;86:335–341.
Ruuskanen O, Meurman O, Sarkkinen H: Adenoviral diseases in children: A study of 105 hospital cases. *Pediatrics* 1985;76:79–83.
Seidemanna K, Heim A, Pfister ED, et al: Monitoring of adenovirus infection in pediatric transplant recipients by quantitative PCR: Report of six cases and review of the literature. *Am J Transplant* 2004;4:2102–2108.
Van R, Wun CC, O'Ryan ML, et al: Outbreaks of human enteric adenovirus types 40 and 41 in Houston day care centers. *J Pediatr* 1992;120:516–521.
Walls T, Shankar AG, Shingadia D: Adenovirus: An increasingly important pathogen in paediatric bone marrow transplant patients. *Lancet Infect Dis* 2003;3:79–86.

Chapter 260 ■ Rhinoviruses

Kenneth Mcintosh

Rhinoviruses are collectively the most common cause of the **common cold** in both adults and children. They are difficult to grow in tissue culture, but studies over the past decade using polymerase chain reaction (PCR) applied to samples taken from children indicate that their frequency and importance in both mild and serious respiratory illnesses are considerably greater than was appreciated previously. They are considered the major infectious trigger of asthma exacerbations in children and, probably because of their ubiquity and frequency, are also important contributors to the etiology of bronchiolitis and pneumonia in infants and school-aged children.

ETIOLOGY. There are at least 100 serologically distinct rhinoviruses, members of the Picornaviridae family of small RNA viruses. They are best identified by PCR performed on nasal secretions from infected individuals.

Not all rhinovirus infections are associated with symptoms. In longitudinal studies, only 75% of pediatric rhinovirus infections confirmed by culture are associated with illness, usually rhinitis or pharyngitis. Recent studies using PCR on specimens from children <2 yr of age with bronchiolitis or pneumonia indicate that rhinoviruses ranks 2nd or 3rd in frequency, behind respiratory syncytial virus (RSV). Rhinovirus infections frequently exacerbate asthma in children and chronic bronchitis in adults.

EPIDEMIOLOGY. Rhinoviruses are distributed worldwide with no predictable pattern of infection by serotype. Multiple types may be present in a community at 1 time. In northern temperate climates the incidence of rhinovirus infection peaks in September, with another minor peak in April or May, but infections occur year-round. Rhinoviruses are the principal infectious trigger for asthma among school-aged children, and in many countries there is a sharp increase in asthmatic attacks in this age group when school opens in the fall. The peak incidence in the tropics occurs during the rainy season, from June to October.

Rhinoviruses are recovered in highest concentration in nasal secretions. Virus persists for several hours in secretions on hands or other surfaces. Transmission occurs when infected secretions carried on contaminated fingers are rubbed onto nasal or conjunctival mucosa. Evidence also implicates spread through prolonged contact with aerosols produced by talking, coughing, or sneezing.

PATHOGENESIS. Rhinoviruses, like other picornaviruses, infect cells via specific cell receptors. For most rhinovirus types, this is **ICAM-1,** an intercellular adhesion molecule present on the epithelium covering the adenoids (lymphoepithelium) and on other epithelial cells of the nose after stimulation by various interleukins including interferon-γ (IFN-γ), tumor necrosis factor-α (TNF-α), and interleukin 1 (IL-1). Infection probably begins in the nasopharynx and then, as interleukins are produced, spreads forward to the nasal mucosa. There is also good evidence that rhinovirus spreads into the lower airway and replicates in bronchial epithelium. Experimental infection is most easily accomplished by nasal or conjunctival instillation. The peak nasal inflammatory response occurs 2–4 days after experimental infection, and is accompanied by the production of proinflammatory mediators, principally IL-8, IL-6, IL-1, and TNF-α. Immune responses include specific nasal immunoglobulin A (IgA) and serum IgG antibody, which may modify illness and limit viral shedding. Symptomatic rhinovirus illnesses during infancy appear to be a significant risk factor for the development of preschool childhood wheezing.

CLINICAL MANIFESTATIONS. The primary clinical response to rhinovirus infection is the **common cold** (see Chapter 376). After an incubation period of 1–4 days, symptoms of sneezing, nasal obstruction and discharge, and sore throat ensue. Cough and hoarseness occur in 30–40% of cases. Fever is neither as frequent nor as high as during infections with respiratory syncytial virus, parainfluenza virus, influenza virus, or adenovirus. Symptoms are worse in the 1st 2–3 days of illness and last for 1 wk in the majority of patients. An acute asthma attack may complicate rhinovirus infections in children with atopy or episodes of prior wheezing.

In some fraction of rhinovirus infections in children of all ages, cough and dyspnea may worsen and develop into bronchiolitis or pneumonia. In infants, 21–31% of cases of bronchiolitis are associated with rhinovirus infection. In studies of community-acquired pneumonia where multiple microbial agents were sought including PCR for rhinoviruses, rhinoviruses are found in 25–45% of cases, with about $^1/_3$ of rhinovirus infections in combination with other pathogens such as *Mycoplasma pneumoniae* in school-aged children and *Streptococcus pneumoniae* in infants and toddlers. Rhinoviruses are also found in asymptomatic infants and children, but usually about $^1/_3$ as often as in those with symptoms.

DIAGNOSIS. Because other viral agents can produce the same manifestations, a clinical diagnosis of rhinovirus infection is only presumptive. Laboratory confirmation of rhinovirus infections is neither routinely available nor used. Culture is approximately $^1/_3$ to $^1/_2$ as sensitive as PCR. Serologic testing for detection is not practical because of the numerous serotypes.

Other causes of the common cold include RSV, adenoviruses, and influenza viruses (see Chapter 376). Bacterial antigen testing or cultures can be used to exclude streptococcal pharyngitis (see Chapter 378).

COMPLICATIONS. As with any infection causing edema and inflammation in the nasopharynx, common complications include otitis media and sinusitis. Rhinoviruses are the most common virus recovered from the middle-ear fluids of children with otitis media. Pneumonia might also be considered a complication of rhinoviral infection if there is concomitant infection with *S. pneumoniae* or *M. pneumoniae,* which occurs in about $^1/_3$ of cases of pneumonia.

Rhinoviruses are found in 50–75% of children >2 yrs of age with acute wheezing, far more than other respiratory viruses. RSV is the most common cause of acute wheezing among children <2 yr of age, although rhinoviruses are still frequently found.

TREATMENT. Relief of acute symptoms may be provided by acetaminophen or ibuprofen for antipyresis and mild analgesia, and by saline or decongestant (in children >6 mo of age) nose drops used for a short time for nasal discharge and obstruction.

Several antiviral drugs have been developed with potent activity against rhinoviruses. Tests in volunteers have demonstrated modest reductions in viral excretion, lessened symptoms, and shorter duration of illness. Efforts are now being made to target the host response as well as the virus.

PREVENTION. The best approach to reducing spread includes careful handwashing and avoidance of manual nose and eye manipulation.

Arola M, Ziegler T, Ruuskanen O, et al: Rhinovirus in acute otitis media. *J Pediatr* 1988;113:693–695.

Dick EC, Jennings LC, Mink KA, et al: Aerosol transmission of rhinovirus colds. *J Infect Dis* 1987;156:442–448.

Gwaltney JM Jr, Moskalski PB, Hendley JO: Hand to hand transmission of rhinovirus colds. *Ann Intern Med* 1978;88:463–467.

Hayden, FG: Rhinovirus and the lower respiratory tract. *Rev Med Virol* 2004;14:17–31.

Heymann PW, Carper HT, Murphy DD, et al: Viral infections in relation to age, atopy, and season of admission among children hospitalized for wheezing. *J Allergy Clin Immunol* 2004;114:239–247.

Jartti T, Lehtinen P, Vuorinen T, et al: Respiratory picornaviruses and respiratory syncytial virus as causative agents of acute expiratory wheezing in children. *Emerg Infect Dis* 2004;10:1095–1101.

Johnston SL, Pattemore PK, Sanderson G, et al: Community study of role of viral infections in exacerbations of asthma in 9–11 year old children. *Br Med J* 1995;310:1225–1229.

Juven T, Mertsola J, Waris M, et al: Etiology of community-acquired pneumonia in 254 hospitalized children. *Pediatr Infect Dis J* 2000;19:293–298.

Korppi M, Kotaniemi-Syrjanen A, Waris M, et al: Rhinovirus-associated wheezing in infancy: Comparison with respiratory syncytial virus bronchiolitis. *Pediatr Infect Dis J* 2004;23:995–999.

Lemanske RF Jr, Jackson DJ, Gangnon RE, et al: Rhinovirus illnesses during infancy predict subsequent childhood wheezing. *J Allergy Clin Immunol* 2005;116:571–577.

Loens K, Goossens H, de Laat C, et al: Detection of rhinoviruses by tissue culture and two independent amplification techniques, nucleic acid sequence-based amplification and reverse transcription-PCR, in children with acute respiratory infections during a winter season. *J Clin Microbiol* 2006:44:166–171.

Tsolia MN, Psarras S, Bossios A, et al: Etiology of community-acquired pneumonia in hospitalized school-age children: Evidence for high prevalence of viral infections. *Clin Infect Dis* 2004;39:681–686.

Chapter 261 ■ Coronaviruses Ari Bitnum and Stanley Read

Coronaviruses are a major cause of the common cold. They have also been implicated as a cause of croup, asthma exacerbations, lower respiratory tract infections including bronchiolitis and pneumonia, acute gastroenteritis in infants, and necrotizing enterocolitis in neonates. The severe acute respiratory syndrome (SARS) is caused by a novel coronavirus.

ETIOLOGY. Coronaviruses are pleomorphic, enveloped, positive-sense, single-stranded RNA viruses of medium to large size (80–220 nm). They derive their name from the characteristic widely spaced, petal-shaped surface projections that give the virus a corona or crown-like appearance on electron microscopy. Non-SARS-associated coronaviruses are classified into 3 groups based on antigenic relatedness. Groups I and II include human coronavirus 229E and OC43, respectively, as well as several nonhuman mammalian coronaviruses. Group II includes human coronavirus OC43 and several other nonhuman mammalian coronaviruses. Group III includes avian coronaviruses. Human respiratory and gastrointestinal disease has most often been attributed to human coronavirus 229E and human coronavirus OC43 strains. Several previously unrecognized strains (e.g., NL63, HKU1) have recently been identified in children with upper and lower respiratory tract disease, and with the increasing use of molecular diagnostic methods it is likely that additional strains will be identified.

EPIDEMIOLOGY. Coronavirus infections have a worldwide distribution. Seroprevalence studies indicate that the prevalence of antibodies to human coronaviruses 229E and OC43 increases rapidly during early childhood such that by early adulthood 90–100% of persons are seropositive. While infections occur throughout the year, there is a peak during the winter and early spring. In the United States, outbreaks occur every 2–3 yr. Although some degree of strain-specific protection may be afforded by recent infection, reinfections are common and have been noted to occur despite the presence of strain-specific antibody. Attack rates are similar in different age groups. The virus is transmitted predominantly through the respiratory route; droplet spread appears to be most important, although aerosol transmission may also play a role.

PATHOGENESIS. Coronaviruses replicate in ciliated epithelium and, similar to rhinoviruses, cause minimal cytopathology. Infection is associated with the elaboration of cytokines, including interleukin 8 and interferon-γ, suggesting that symptoms may be at least partially due to the host immune response. In experimentally infected volunteers, serum-specific immunoglobulin A (IgA) and IgG antibodies peak 12–14 days after infection, but decline rapidly thereafter. At 1 yr following experimental infection there is only partial protection against reinfection with the homologous strain.

CLINICAL MANIFESTATIONS. Human coronaviruses have been conclusively demonstrated in human volunteer studies to cause respiratory disease. The role of these viruses in gastrointestinal and neurologic disease is less well delineated.

Respiratory Infections. Approximately 50% of respiratory tract coronavirus infections are asymptomatic. Coronaviruses account for 10–15% of the common cold, which are the most common clinically apparent respiratory tract infection (see Chapter 376). Cold symptoms caused by human coronaviruses are indistinguishable from those caused by rhinoviruses and other respiratory viruses. The average incubation period is 2 days, with symptoms typically lasting 4–7 days. Rhinorrhea, cough, sore throat, malaise, and headache are the most common symptoms. Low-grade fever and chills occur in approximately 20% and 30% of cases, respectively. Coronavirus NL63 is implicated as a cause of croup in children <3 yr of age.

Coronavirus infections have been linked to episodes of wheezing in asthmatic children, albeit at a frequency and severity lower than that observed with rhinovirus and respiratory syncytial virus infections. Lower respiratory tract infections, including bronchiolitis and pneumonia, have also been reported in immunocompetent as well as immunocompromised children and adults. The presence of coronavirus RNA in middle-ear fluid samples of a small proportion of children with acute otitis media suggests that these viruses may predispose or perhaps occasionally cause acute otitis media.

Gastrointestinal Infections. Although the precise role of coronaviruses in human gastrointestinal disease remains controversial, there is some evidence to support such a role, particularly in young children. Coronavirus-like particles have been detected by electron microscopy in the stools of infants with nonbacterial gastroenteritis. In addition, several outbreaks in neonatal intensive care units of gastrointestinal disease characterized by diarrhea, bloody stools, abdominal distention, bilious gastric aspirates, and classic necrotizing enterocolitis have also been associated with the presence of coronavirus-like particles in stools. In older children and adults coronavirus-like viruses have been observed with similar frequency in symptomatic and asymptomatic individuals.

Neurologic Disease. The role of coronaviruses in causing neurologic disease is controversial. They have been detected by culture, in situ hybridization, and reverse transcriptase polymerase chain reaction (RT-PCR) in brain tissue of a few patients with multiple sclerosis. However, coronavirus RNA has also been recovered from the spinal fluid and brain tissue of adults without neurologic disease. Human coronavirus OC43 has been detected by RT-PCR in the spinal fluid and nasopharynx of 1 child with acute disseminated encephalomyelitis.

DIAGNOSIS. Specific diagnostic tests for coronavirus infection are not routinely available in most clinical settings. Rapid diagnosis can be achieved using antigen detection or RT-PCR methodologies. RT-PCR has excellent sensitivity and specificity and appears to be the most promising rapid diagnostic technique at the present time. Viral culture is not readily available and is limited by its relatively poor sensitivity, the need for prolonged incubation, and the variable and stringent growth requirements of different coronavirus strains. Serodiagnosis with complement fixation, neutralization, hemagglutination inhibition, enzyme immunoassay, or the Western blot test has been used in the research setting. Depending on the methodology used, diagnosis requires seroconversion or a 4-fold or greater rise in titer between acute and convalescent sera.

TREATMENT AND PREVENTION. The vast majority of coronavirus infections are self-limited. There are no antiviral agents with proven efficacy against coronaviruses. A coronavirus vaccine is likely to be of limited benefit given the temporary protection afforded by natural infection.

261.1 • Severe Acute Respiratory Syndrome–Associated Coronavirus

The SARS outbreak of 2003 was the 1st major global epidemic of the 21st century. While this outbreak was contained and the spread halted through a remarkable cooperative effort between countries around the world, the occurrence of several laboratory-acquired cases in Singapore, Taiwan, and China as well as sporadic "naturally acquired" infections in southern China in 2004 demonstrates the potential threat posed by species-to-species transmission of coronaviruses.

ETIOLOGY. The causative agent of SARS is a novel coronavirus, referred to as the **SARS-associated coronavirus (SARS-CoV)**, that was discovered in Asia in 2002 and spread rapidly. Phylogenetic analysis has demonstrated that SARS-CoV is distinct from the 3 previously recognized coronavirus groups and likely represents an ancient split-off from group 2 coronaviruses. SARS-CoV infection of humans is zoonotic, although the natural animal reservoir has yet to be identified. The detection of SARS-like coronaviruses in Himalayan palm civets *(Paguma larvata)* and a raccoon dog *(Nyctereutes procyonoides)* housed in a live animal market in Guangdong province in Southern China, along with the finding of serologic evidence of exposure in food handlers and other persons whose occupation increased their exposure to these and other exotic animals held in the same market, suggests that these markets may have facilitated the spread of SARS-CoV from animals to humans. Of potential importance is the observation that the SARS-CoV is capable of infecting a variety of other mammals, including badgers, ferrets, domestic cats, and nonhuman primates.

EPIDEMIOLOGY. The primary mode of SARS-CoV transmission is through direct or indirect contact of mucous membranes with infectious droplets or fomites. Aerosol transmission is less common, but may occur, particularly in the setting of aerosol-generating procedures, such as endotracheal intubation, bronchoscopy, or treatment with aerosolized medications. Fecal-oral transmission does not appear to be an efficient mode of transmission, but may be possible given the profuse diarrhea observed in some patients with SARS-CoV and the large quantities of virus excreted in the stools of such patients. The seasonality of SARS-CoV remains unknown.

The SARS-CoV is not highly infectious. In the absence of infection control precautions, on average only 2–4 secondary cases result from a single infected adult. However, a small number of infected individuals, the so-called "super-spreaders," may transmit the infection to a much larger number of persons. In contrast, persons with mild disease, such as children <12 yr of age, rarely transmit the infection to others. Infectivity correlates with disease stage; transmission has not been observed prior to the onset of symptoms, but rises sharply after the 5th day of illness coincident with a rise in the viral load. During the 2003 outbreak, most individuals with SARS-CoV infection were hospitalized within 3–4 days of symptom onset. Consequently, most subsequent infections occurred within hospitals and involved either health care workers or other hospitalized patients. With the exception of the Amoy Gardens housing complex outbreak in Hong Kong in which opportunistic airborne transmission associated with environmental contamination from the sewage system occurred, the majority of children in Hong Kong and elsewhere were infected through exposure to adult household contacts, often health care workers or international travelers.

PATHOGENESIS. A viral replication phase and immunologic phase are the hallmarks of SARS-CoV infection in teenagers and adults. During the viral replication phase there is a progressive increase in viral load that reaches its peak during the 2nd wk of illness. The appearance of specific antibody coincides with peak viral replication. The clinical deterioration that typifies the 2nd and 3rd wk of illness is characterized by a decline in the viral load and tissue injury resulting from an over-exuberant cytokine-mediated immune response. The explanation for milder clinical disease in children <12 yr of age has not been determined.

CLINICAL MANIFESTATIONS. Seroepidemiologic studies suggest that asymptomatic SARS-CoV infections are uncommon. The incubation period ranges from 1 to 14 days, with a median of 4–6 days. The clinical manifestations are nonspecific; fever, cough, malaise, coryza, chills or rigors, headache, and myalgia are the most common presenting symptoms. Coryza is more common in children <12 yr of age, whereas systemic symptoms such as headache, myalgia, chills, and malaise are more typically seen in teenagers. Some young children have no respiratory symptoms. Gastrointestinal symptoms, including diarrhea and nausea or vomiting, occur in up to ⅓ of cases. Wheezing is rare if it occurs at all, and crackles are relatively uncommon.

The clinical course of SARS-CoV infection varies with age. Adults are most severely affected and classically have a triphasic clinical pattern. The onset of illness is characterized by fever, cough, and systemic symptoms such as chills, myalgia, malaise, and headache. Following an initial improvement toward the end of the 1st week, there is recurrence of fever and development of respiratory distress with dyspnea, hypoxemia, and diarrhea.

Approximately 20% progress into the 3rd phase, characterized by acute respiratory distress syndrome (ARDS) and respiratory failure. Children <12 yr of age have a relatively mild nonspecific illness, with only a minority developing significant lower respiratory tract disease; their illness is typically <5 days in duration. In teenagers, the illness is intermediate in severity; respiratory distress and hypoxemia are observed in 10–20%, and ⅓ of these require ventilatory support.

LABORATORY FINDINGS. The laboratory abnormalities and radiographic findings observed in SARS-CoV-infected children are nonspecific and cannot be differentiated from those associated with other commonly encountered viral illnesses. Lymphopenia is seen in about 70% of children at presentation and 90% during the course of their illness. Other hematologic abnormalities include leukopenia, neutropenia, thrombocytopenia, and mildly prolonged activated partial thromboplastin time. Anemia is not typically observed. Elevated lactate dehydrogenase is seen in 50–70% of children. Other less common biochemical abnormalities include elevated creatine kinase and alanine aminotransferase. Laboratory abnormalities are more common and persist longer in teenagers than in young children.

Early radiographic changes are typified by evidence of airspace disease and include ground-glass opacities or consolidation involving peripheral or mixed central and peripheral lung regions. Interstitial infiltrates, hilar lymphadenopathy, pleural effusion, pneumothorax, and abscess formation are not typically seen. Progression to an ARDS-like pattern with widespread ground-glass opacities and patchy consolidation is characteristic of those who require ventilatory support. In some children, particularly early in the course of illness, plain chest radiographs may be normal. High-resolution CT is highly sensitive and can aid in the detection of pulmonary lesions not apparent on plain chest radiographs.

DIAGNOSIS. The diagnosis of SARS-CoV infection can be confirmed by serologic testing, detection of viral RNA using RT-PCR, or through isolation of the virus in cell culture. Serology is the most reliable diagnostic method, with sensitivity and specificity approaching 100%; detection of IgM antibody, seroconversion from negative to positive, or a 4-fold or greater rise in IgG titer is indicative of recent infection. The disadvantage of serology is that antibody is not detectable until 10 days after the onset of symptoms, and IgG seroconversion may be delayed for up to 4 wk. The mainstay of early diagnosis is RT-PCR. Nasopharyngeal aspirates, plasma or serum, and stool are the preferred samples, although other body fluids and tissues may also contain the virus. Repeated sampling over the course of the illness is recommended because the peak viral load may not occur until the 2nd wk of illness. Nevertheless, with modified RNA extraction protocols and optimized real-time PCR, the virus may be detected in nasopharyngeal aspirates and serum samples of up to 80% of subjects during the 1st wk of illness. Viral culture is not recommended as a 1st line diagnostic test because of its poor sensitivity and the requirement for biosafety level 3 containment.

COMPLICATIONS AND PROGNOSIS. The case fatality rate from SARS-CoV infection during the 2003 outbreak was 10–17%. No pediatric deaths were reported. The estimated case fatality rate according to age varies from <1% for those <20 yr of age to >50% for those >65 yr of age.

The long-term prognosis of children recovering from SARS-CoV infection appears to be favorable. Persistent respiratory or exercise intolerance has not been reported, although, as a group, SARS-CoV-infected children have been noted to have reduced peak oxygen consumption compared with healthy controls. In addition, mild ground-glass opacities and/or air trapping on high-resolution CT and a mild obstructive or restrictive pattern on pulmonary function testing have been observed in a minority of cases. Persistent psychologic problems related to prolonged isolation on a hospital ward and separation from and, in some cases, death of close family members have not been reported, but are of potential concern. Other complications include thinning of hair 2–3 mo after disease onset (acute telogen effluvium) and osteonecrosis secondary to corticosteroid use.

TREATMENT. Treatment of SARS-CoV infection is primarily supportive. Oxygen should be provided to hypoxemic persons. Bronchodilators are generally not needed and their use should be discouraged because of the potential for enhancing aerosolization of the virus. Empiric antibiotic therapy directed at common bacterial causes of community-acquired pneumonia should be considered on an individual basis. The importance of psychologic support for children hospitalized with SARS, whose parents are often hospitalized in other institutions or are restricted from visiting due to infection control requirements, cannot be overemphasized.

The role of antiviral and immune-modulating agents remains inconclusive, largely because none of these therapies have been evaluated in properly conducted randomized controlled trials. Ribavirin was extensively used during the 2003 outbreak, but is of questionable benefit given its poor in vitro activity against SARS-CoV at clinically relevant concentrations. Systemic corticosteroid therapy was temporally associated with clinical improvement in some patients and should be considered in children with moderate to severe hypoxemia. The addition of lopinavir/ritonavir to ribavirin and corticosteroid therapy was associated with significantly fewer cases of acute respiratory distress syndrome or death compared with historic controls in 1 study. In another small open-label nonrandomized pilot study, interferon-α was associated with more rapid resolution of oxygen requirements and radiographic abnormalities. The efficacy of these agents as well as other compounds with in vitro activity against SARS-CoV such as glycyrrhizin, recombinant human interferon-β1a, interferon-β1b and monoclonal antibodies directed at the spike protein of SARS-CoV requires further study.

PREVENTION. An effective vaccine is highly desirable but is not yet available. In the context of an outbreak, quarantine of all potential contacts and adherence to appropriate infection control precautions are effective in controlling the spread of SARS-CoV.

Bastien N, Anderson K, Hart L, et al: Human coronavirus NL63 infection in Canada. *J Infect Dis* 2005;191:503–506.

Bitnun A, Allen U, Heurter H, et al: Children hospitalized with severe acute respiratory syndrome-related illness in Toronto. *Pediatrics* 2003;112:e261–e268.

Bradburne AF, Bynoe ML. Tyrrell DA. Effects of a "new" human respiratory virus in volunteers. *Br Med J* 1967;3:767–769.

Centers for Disease Control and Prevention: Revised U.S. surveillance case definition for severe acute respiratory syndrome (SARS) and update on SARS cases—United States and worldwide, December 2003. *MMWR* 2003:52:1202–1206.

Esper F, Weibel C, Ferguson D, et al: Evidence of a novel human coronavirus that is associated with respiratory tract disease in infants and young children. *J Infect Dis* 2005;191:492–498.

Gerna G, Passarani N, Battaglia M, Rondanelli EG: Human enteric coronaviruses: Antigenic relatedness to human coronavirus OC43 and possible etiologic role in viral gastroenteritis. *J Infect Dis* 1985;51:796–803.

Guan Y, Zheng BJ, He YQ, et al: Isolation and characterization of viruses related to the SARS coronavirus from animals in southern China. *Science* 2003;302:276–278.

Hon KL, Leung CW, Cheng WT, et al: Clinical presentations and outcome of severe acute respiratory syndrome in children. *Lancet* 2003;361:1701–1703.

Kuypers J, Martin ET, Heugel J, et al: Clinical disease in children associated with newly described coronavirus subtypes. *Pediatrics* 2007;119:e70–e76.

Leung CW, Chiu WK: Clinical picture, diagnosis, treatment and outcome of severe acute respiratory syndrome (SARS) in children. *Paediatr Respir Rev* 2004;5:275–288.
Leung CW, Kwan YW, Ko PW, et al: Severe acute respiratory syndrome among children. *Pediatrics* 2004;113:e535–e543.
Lohnston SL, Pattemore PK, Sanderson G, et al: Community study of role of viral infections in exacerbations of asthma in 9–11 year old children. *Br Med J* 1995;310:1225–1228.
Makela MJ, Puhakka T, Ruuskanen O, et al: Viruses and bacteria in the etiology of the common cold. *J Clin Microbiol* 1998;36:539–542.
McIntosh K, Kapikian AZ, Turner HC, et al: Seroepidemiologic studies of coronavirus infection in adults and children. *Am J Epidemiol* 1970;91:585–592.
Peiris JS, Chu CM, Cheng VC, et al: Clinical progression and viral load in a community outbreak of coronavirus-associated SARS pneumonia: A prospective study. *Lancet* 2003;361:1767–1772.
Stockman LJ, Massoudi MS, Helfand R, et al: Severe acute respiratory syndrome in children. *Pediatr Infect Dis J* 2007;26:68–74.
van der Hoek L, Pyrc K, Jebbink MF, et al: Identification of a new human coronavirus. *Nature Med* 2004;10:368–373.
van der Hoek L, Sure K, Ihorst G, et al: Croup is associated with the novel coronavirus NL63. *Adv Exp Med Biol* 2006;581:485–491.
Yeh EA, Collins A, Cohen ME, et al: Detection of coronavirus in the central nervous system of a child with acute disseminated encephalomyelitis. *Pediatrics* 2004;113:e73–e76.

Chapter 262 ■ Rotaviruses, Caliciviruses, and Astroviruses

Dorsey M. Bass

Diarrhea is a leading cause of childhood mortality in the world, accounting for 5–10 million deaths per year. In early childhood, the single most important cause of severe dehydrating diarrhea is rotavirus infection. Rotavirus and other gastroenteritis viruses not only are major causes of pediatric mortality but also lead to significant morbidity. Children in the USA have been estimated to have a risk of hospitalization for rotavirus diarrhea of 1 in 43, corresponding to 80,000 hospitalizations annually.

ETIOLOGY. Rotavirus, astrovirus, caliciviruses such as the **Norwalk agent,** and enteric adenovirus are the medically important pathogens of human viral gastroenteritis.

Rotaviruses, which are in the Reoviridae family, cause disease in virtually all mammals and birds. The virus is a wheel-like, triple-shelled icosahedron containing 11 segments of double-stranded RNA. The diameter of the particles by electron microscopy is approximately 80 nm. Rotaviruses are classified by serogroup (A, B, C, D, E, F, and G) and subgroup (I or II). Rotavirus strains are species specific and do not cause disease in heterologous hosts. Group A includes the common human pathogens as well as a variety of animal viruses. Group B rotavirus is reported as a cause of severe disease in infants and adults in China only. Occasional human outbreaks of group C rotavirus are reported. The other serogroups infect only nonhumans.

Subgrouping of rotaviruses is determined by the antigenic structure of the inner capsid protein, VP6. Serotyping of rotaviruses, described for group A only, is determined by classic cross-neutralization testing and depends on the outer capsid glycoproteins, VP7 and VP4. The VP7 serotype is referred to as the G type (for glycoprotein). There are 10 G serotypes, of which 4 cause most illness and vary from year to year and region to region. The VP4 serotype is referred to as the P type. There are 11 P serotypes. Although both VP4 and VP7 elicit neutralizing immunoglobulin G (IgG) antibodies, the relative role of these systemic antibodies compared with mucosal IgA antibodies and cellular responses in protective immunity remains unclear.

Caliciviruses, which constitute the Caliciviridae family, are small 27–35 nm viruses that are the most common cause of gastroenteritis outbreaks in older children and adults. Caliciviruses also cause a rotavirus-like illness in young infants. They are positive-sense, single-stranded RNA viruses with a single structural protein. Human caliciviruses are divided into 2 genera, the noroviruses and sapoviruses. Caliciviruses have been named for locations of initial outbreaks: Norwalk, Snow Mountain, Montgomery County, Sapporo, and others. Caliciviruses and astroviruses are sometimes referred to as **small, round viruses** on the basis of appearance on electron microscopy.

Astroviruses, which constitute the Astroviridae family, are important agents of viral gastroenteritis in young children, with a high incidence in both the developing and the developed worlds. Astroviruses are positive-sense, single-stranded RNA viruses. They are small, approximately 30 nm diameter particles with a characteristic central 5 or 6 pointed star when viewed by electron microscopy. The capsid consists of 3 structural proteins. There are 8 known human serotypes.

Enteric adenoviruses are a common cause of viral gastroenteritis in infants and children. Although many adenovirus serotypes exist and are found in stool, especially during and after typical upper respiratory tract infections (see Chapter 259), only serotypes 40 and 41 cause gastroenteritis. These strains are very difficult to grow in tissue culture. The virus consists of an 80 nm diameter icosahedral particle with a relatively complex double-stranded DNA genome.

Aichi virus is a picornavirus that has been associated with gastroenteritis and initially described in Asia. Several other viruses that may cause diarrheal disease in animals have been postulated but not well established as human gastroenteritis viruses. These include coronaviruses, toroviruses, and pestiviruses. The **picobirnaviruses** are an unclassified group of small 30 nm, single-stranded RNA viruses that have been found in 10% of patients with HIV-associated diarrhea.

EPIDEMIOLOGY. Worldwide, rotavirus is estimated to cause more than 111 million cases of diarrhea annually in children younger than 5 yr. Of these, 18 million cases are considered at least moderately severe, with approximately 500,000 deaths per year. Rotavirus causes 3 million cases of diarrhea, 80,000 hospitalizations, and 20–40 deaths annually in the United States.

Rotavirus infection is most common in winter months in temperate climates. In the United States, the annual winter peak spreads from west to east (Fig. 262-1). Unlike other winter viruses such as influenza, this wave of increased incidence is not due to a single prevalent strain or serotype. Typically, several serotypes predominate in a given community for 1 or 2 seasons while nearby locations may harbor unrelated strains. Disease tends to be most severe in patients 3–24 mo of age, although 25% of the cases of severe disease occur after 2 yr of age, with serologic evidence of infection developing in virtually all children by 4–5 yr of age. Infants younger than 3 mo are relatively protected by transplacental antibody and possibly breast-feeding. Infections in neonates and in adults in close contact with infected children are generally asymptomatic. Some rotavirus strains have stably colonized newborn nurseries for years, infecting virtually all newborns without any overt illness.

Rotavirus and the other gastroenteritis viruses spread efficiently via a fecal-oral route, and outbreaks are common in children's hospitals and child-care centers. The virus is shed in stool at very high concentration before and for days after the clinical illness. Very few infectious virions are needed to cause disease in a susceptible host.

The epidemiology of **astroviruses** is not as thoroughly studied as rotavirus, but they are a common cause of mild to moderate watery winter diarrhea in children and infants and an uncommon

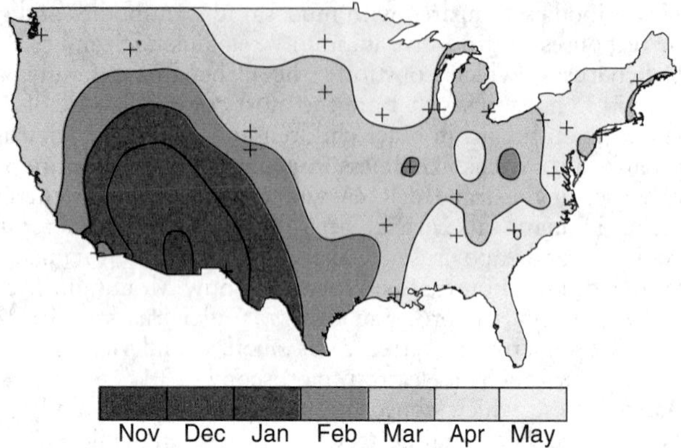

Figure 262-1. Peak rotavirus activity by month in the USA for July 1996 to June 1997. This pattern is typical of the annual rotavirus activity each year. (From the Centers for Disease Control and Prevention: Laboratory-based surveillance for rotavirus—United States, July 1996–June 1997. *MMWR* 1997;46:1092–1094.)

pathogen in adults. Hospital outbreaks are common. **Enteric adenovirus** gastroenteritis occurs year-round, mostly in children younger than 2 yr. Nosocomial outbreaks occur but are less common than with rotavirus and astrovirus. **Calicivirus** is best known for causing large, explosive outbreaks among older children and adults, particularly in settings such as schools, cruise ships, and hospitals. Often a single food, such as shellfish or water used in food preparation, is identified as a source. Caliciviruses are also commonly found in winter infantile gastroenteritis similar to astrovirus and rotavirus.

PATHOGENESIS. Viruses that cause human diarrhea selectively infect and destroy villus tip cells in the small intestine. Biopsies of the small intestines show variable degrees of villus blunting and round cell infiltrate in the lamina propria. Pathologic changes may not correlate with the severity of clinical symptoms and usually resolve before the clinical resolution of diarrhea. The gastric mucosa is not affected despite the commonly used term *gastroenteritis,* although delayed gastric emptying has been documented during Norwalk virus infection.

In the small intestine, the upper villus enterocytes are differentiated cells, which have both digestive functions, such as hydrolysis of disaccharides, and absorptive functions, such as the transport of water and electrolytes via glucose and amino acid co-transporters. Crypt enterocytes are undifferentiated cells that lack the brush border hydrolytic enzymes and are net secretors of water and electrolytes. Selective viral infection of intestinal villus tip cells thus leads to (1) decreased absorption of salt and water and an imbalance in the ratio of intestinal fluid absorption to secretion and (2) diminished disaccharidase activity and malabsorption of complex carbohydrates, particularly lactose. Most evidence supports altered absorption as the more important factor in the genesis of viral diarrhea. It has been proposed that a rotavirus nonstructural protein (NSP4) functions as an enterotoxin.

Symptomatic **extraintestinal infection** is rare in immunocompetent persons, although immunocompromised patients may experience hepatic and renal involvement. The increased vulnerability of infants (compared with older children and adults) to severe morbidity and mortality from gastroenteritis viruses may relate to a number of factors, including decreased intestinal reserve function, lack of specific immunity, and decreased nonspecific host defense mechanisms such as gastric acid and mucus. Viral enteritis greatly enhances intestinal permeability to luminal macromolecules and has been postulated to increase the risk for food allergies.

CLINICAL MANIFESTATIONS. **Rotavirus infection** typically begins after an incubation period of <48 hr (range 1–7 days) with mild to moderate fever as well as vomiting followed by the onset of frequent, watery stools. All 3 symptoms are present in about 50–60% of cases. Vomiting and fever typically abate during the 2nd day of illness, but diarrhea often continues for 5–7 days. The stool is without gross blood or white cells. Dehydration may develop and progress rapidly, particularly in infants. The most severe disease typically occurs among children 4–36 mo of age. Malnourished children and children with underlying intestinal disease such as short-bowel syndrome are particularly likely to acquire severe rotavirus diarrhea. Rarely, immunodeficient children experience severe and prolonged illness. Although most newborns infected with rotavirus are asymptomatic, some outbreaks of necrotizing enterocolitis have been associated with the appearance of a new rotavirus strain in the affected nurseries.

The clinical course of **astrovirus** appears to be similar to that of rotavirus, with the notable exception that the disease tends to be milder, with less significant dehydration. **Adenovirus enteritis** tends to cause diarrhea of longer duration, often 10–14 days. The **Norwalk virus** has a short (12 hr) incubation period. Vomiting and nausea tend to predominate in illness associated with the Norwalk virus, and the duration is brief, usually 1–3 days of symptoms. The clinical and epidemiologic picture of Norwalk virus often closely resembles so-called food poisoning from preformed toxins such as *Staphylococcus aureus* and *Bacillus cereus.*

DIAGNOSIS. In most cases, a satisfactory diagnosis can be made on the basis of the clinical and epidemiologic features. Enzyme-linked immunosorbent assays (ELISAs), which offer >90% specificity and sensitivity, are available for detection of group A rotavirus and enteric adenovirus in stool samples. Latex agglutination assays are also available for group A rotavirus and are less sensitive than ELISA. Research tools include electron microscopy of stools, RNA polymerase chain reaction to identify G and P antigens, and culture. The diagnosis of viral gastroenteritis should always be questioned in patients with persistent or high fever, blood or white cells in the stool, or persistent severe or bilious vomiting, especially in the absence of diarrhea.

LABORATORY FINDINGS. Isotonic dehydration with acidosis is the most common finding in children with severe viral enteritis. The stools are free of blood and leukocytes. Although the white blood cell count may be moderately elevated secondary to stress, the marked left shift seen with invasive bacterial enteritis is absent.

DIFFERENTIAL DIAGNOSIS. The differential diagnosis includes other infectious causes of enteritis such as bacteria and protozoa. Occasionally, surgical conditions such as appendicitis, bowel obstruction, and intussusception may initially mimic viral gastroenteritis.

TREATMENT. Avoiding and treating dehydration are the main goals in treatment of viral enteritis. A secondary goal is maintenance of the nutritional status of the patient (see Chapters 55 and 337).

There is no routine role for antiviral drug treatment of viral gastroenteritis. Controlled studies have shown no benefit from antiemetics or antidiarrheal drugs, and there is a significant risk for serious side effects. Antibiotics are similarly of no benefit. Immunoglobulins have been administered orally to both normal and immunodeficient patients with severe rotavirus gastroenteritis, but this treatment is currently considered experimental. Therapy with probiotic organisms such as *Lactobacillus* species has been shown to be helpful only in mild cases and not in dehydrating disease.

Supportive Treatment. Rehydration via the oral route can be accomplished in most patients with mild to moderate dehydration (see Chapters 55 and 337). Severe rehydration requires immediate intravenous therapy followed by oral rehydration. Modern oral rehydration solutions containing appropriate quantities of sodium and glucose promote optimum absorption of fluid from the intestine (see Table 55.1). There is no evidence that a particular carbohydrate source (rice) or addition of amino acids improves the efficacy of these solutions for children with viral enteritis. Other clear liquids such as flat soda, fruit juice, and sports drinks are inappropriate for rehydration of young children with significant stool loss. Rehydration via the oral (or nasogastric) route should be done over 6–8 hr and feedings begun immediately thereafter. Providing the rehydration fluid at a slow, steady rate, typically 5 mL/min, reduces vomiting and improves the success of oral therapy. Rehydration solution should be continued as a supplement to make up for ongoing excessive stool loss. Initial intravenous fluids are required for the infant in shock or the occasional child with intractable vomiting.

After rehydration has been achieved, resumption of a normal diet for age has been shown to result in a more rapid recovery from viral gastroenteritis. Prolonged (>12 hr) administration of exclusive clear liquids or dilute formula is without clinical benefit and actually prolongs the duration of diarrhea. Breast-feeding should be continued even during rehydration. Selected infants may benefit from lactose-free feedings (such as soy formula or lactose-free cow's milk) for several days, although this is not necessary for most children. Hypocaloric diets low in protein and fat such as **BRAT** (*b*ananas, *r*ice, cereal, *a*pplesauce, and *t*oast) have not been shown to be superior to a regular diet.

PROGNOSIS. Most fatalities occur in infants with poor access to medical care and are attributed to dehydration. Children may be infected with rotavirus each year during the 1st 5 yr of life but with decreasing severity of each subsequent infection. Primary infection results in a predominantly serotype-specific immune response, whereas reinfection, which is usually with a different serotype, induces a broad immune response with cross-reactive heterotypic antibody. After the initial natural infection, children have limited protection against subsequent asymptomatic infection (38%) and greater protection against mild diarrhea (73%) and moderate to severe diarrhea (87%). After the 2nd natural infection, protection increases against subsequent asymptomatic infection (62%) and mild diarrhea (75%) and is complete (100%) against moderate to severe diarrhea. After the 3rd natural infection, there is even higher protection against subsequent asymptomatic infection (74%) and near-complete protection against even mild diarrhea (99%).

PREVENTION. Good hygiene reduces the transmission of viral gastroenteritis, but even in the most hygienic societies virtually all children become infected as a result of the efficiency of infection of the gastroenteritis viruses. Good handwashing and isolation procedures can help control nosocomial outbreaks. The role of breast-feeding in prevention or amelioration of rotavirus infection may be small given the variable protection observed in a number of studies. Vaccines offer the best hope for control of these ubiquitous infections.

Vaccines. A live, oral, pentavalent rotavirus vaccine was approved in 2006 for use in the United States. The vaccine contains 5 reassortant rotaviruses isolated from human and bovine hosts. Four of the reassortant rotaviruses express 1 of the outer proteins (G1, G2, G3, or G4) and the 5th expresses the protein P1A (genotype P[8]) from the human rotavirus parent strain. The pentavalent vaccine protects against rotavirus gastroenteritis when administered as a 3 dose series at 2, 4, and 6 mo of age. The 1st dose should be administered between 6 and 12 wk of age, with all 3 doses completed by 32 wk of age. The vaccine provides substantial protection against rotavirus gastroenteritis with primary efficacy of 98% against severe rotavirus gastroenteritis caused by G1–G4 serotypes, and 74% against any severity, through the 1st rotavirus season after vaccination. It provides a 96% reduction in hospitalizations for rotavirus gastroenteritis through the 1st 2 yr after the 3rd dose. In a study of >70,000 infants, the pentavalent vaccine did not increase the risk for intussusception.

Another new monovalent rotavirus vaccine was recently licensed in Mexico and appears to be safe and effective. Previously, a trivalent rotavirus vaccine was licensed in the United States in 1998 and was subsequently linked to an increased risk for intussusception, especially during the 3–14 day period after the 1st dose and the 3–7 day period after the 2nd dose. It was withdrawn from the market in 1999.

Bresee JS, Parashar UD, Widdowson MA, et al: Update on rotavirus vaccines. *Pediatr Infect Dis J* 2005;24:947–952.

Chandron A, Heinzen RR, Santosham M, et al: Nosocomial rotavirus infections: a systematic review. *J Pediatr* 2006;149:441–447.

Clark B. McKendrick M: A review of viral gastroenteritis. *Curr Opin Infect Dis* 2004;17(5):461–469.

Clark HF, Offit PA, Plotkin SA, Heaton PM: The new pentavalent rotavirus vaccine composed of bovine (strain WC3)—Human rotavirus reassortants. *Pediatr Infect Dis J* 2006;25:577–582.

Coffin SE, Elser J, Marchant C, et al: Impact of acute rotavirus gastroenteritis on pediatric outpatient practices in the United States. *Pediatr Infect Dis J* 2006;25:584–589.

Costa-Ribeiro, H, Ribeiro TC, Mattos AP, et al: Limitations of probiotic therapy in acute, severe dehydrating diarrhea. *J Pediatr Gastroenterol Nutr* 2003;36(1):112–115.

Glass RI, Bresee JS, Parashar UD, et al: The future of rotavirus vaccines: A major setback leads to new opportunities. *Lancet* 2004;363(9420): 1547–1550.

Guandalini S, Pensabene L, Zikri MA, et al: Lactobacillus GG administered in oral rehydration solution to children with acute diarrhea: A multicenter European trial. *J Pediatr Gastroenterol Nutr* 2000;30:54–60.

Guerrero ML, Noel JS, Mitchell DK, et al: A prospective study of astrovirus diarrhea of infancy in Mexico City. *Pediatr Infect Dis J* 1998;17:723–727.

Jiang B, Gentsch JR, Glass RI: The role of serum antibodies in the protection against rotavirus disease: An overview. *Clin Infect Dis* 2002;34:1051–1061.

Lanata CF, Franco M: Nitazoxanide for rotavirus diarrhoea. *Lancet* 2006; 368:100–101.

Lynch M, Shieh WJ, Tatti K, et al: The pathology of rotavirus-associated deaths, using new molecular diagnostics. *Clin Infect Dis* 2003;37:1027–1033.

O'Ryan M, Diaz J, Mamani N, et al: Impact of rotavirus infections on outpatient clinic visits in Chile. *Pediatr Infect Dis J* 2007;26:41–45.

O'Ryan M, Matson DO: New rotavirus vaccines: renewed optimism. *J Pediatr* 2006;149:448–451.

Parashar UD, Holman RC, Clarke MJ, et al: Hospitalizations associated with rotavirus diarrhea in the United States, 1993 through 1995. Surveillance based on the new ICD-9-CM rotavirus-specific diagnostic code. *J Infect Dis* 1998;77:13–17.

Parashar UD, Hummelman EG, Bresee JS, et al: Global illness and deaths caused by rotavirus disease in children. *Emerg Infect Dis* 2003;9(5): 565–572.

Plotkin SA: New rotavirus vaccines. *Pediatr Infect Dis J* 2006;25:575–576.

Rossignol JF, Abu-Zekry M, Hussein A, Santoro MG: Effect of nitazoxanide for treatment of severe rotavirus diarrhoea: Randomized double-blind placebo-controlled trial. *Lancet* 2006;368:124–129.

Ruiz-Palacios GM, Perez-Schael I, Velazquez FR, et al: Safety and efficacy of an attenuated vaccine against severe rotavirus gastroenteritis. *N Engl J Med* 2006;354:11–22.

Soares-Weiser K, Goldberg E, Tamimi G, et al: Rotavirus vaccine for preventing diarrhoea. *Cochrane Database Syst Rev* 2004;1:CD002848.

Staat MA, Azimi PH, Berke T, et al: Clinical presentations of rotavirus infection among hospitalized children. *Pediatr Infect Dis J* 2002;21:221–227.

Tucker AW, Haddix AC, Bresee JS, et al: Cost-effectiveness analysis of a rotavirus immunization program for the United States. *JAMA* 1998;279: 1371–1376.

Vesikari T, Matson DO, Dennehy P, et al: Safety and efficacy of a pentavalent human-bovine (WC3) reassortant rotavirus vaccine. *N Engl J Med* 2006;354:23–33.

Chapter 263 ■ Human Papillomaviruses

Anna-Barbara Moscicki

Human papillomaviruses (HPVs) cause a variety of proliferative cutaneous and mucosal lesions, including common skin warts, benign and malignant anogenital tract lesions, and life-threatening respiratory papillomas. Most HPV-related infections in children and adolescents are benign.

ETIOLOGY. The papillomaviruses are small (55 nm) DNA-containing viruses that are ubiquitous in nature, infecting most mammalian and many nonmammalian animal species. Strains are almost always species specific. More than 100 different types of HPVs have been identified by comparing sequence homologies. The different HPV types typically cause disease in specific anatomic sites; about 30 of the HPV types have been identified from genital tract specimens.

EPIDEMIOLOGY. HPV infections of the skin are common, and most individuals are probably infected with 1 or more HPV types at some time. There are no animal reservoirs for HPV; all transmission is presumably person to person. There is little evidence to suggest that HPV is transmitted by fomites. Common warts, including palmar and plantar warts, are frequently seen in children and adolescents, where they infect the hands and feet, common areas of frequent minor trauma.

Human papillomavirus is the most prevalent viral sexually transmitted infection in the United States. Although up to 70% of sexually active women eventually acquire HPV through sexual transmission, the infection is rare among preadolescent children. The greatest risk for HPV in sexually active adolescents is exposure to new non-condom-using sexual partners, underscoring the ease of transmission of this virus through sexual contact. As with many other genital pathogens, perinatal transmission to newborns also occurs, but the transmission of genital types appears to be relatively inefficient.

The most common manifestation of HPV is latent infection defined by the detection of HPV DNA in the absence of any detectable HPV-associated lesion. Approximately 20% of sexually active adolescents have detectable HPV at any given time, and have normal cytology and no detectable lesions. External genital warts are much less common, occurring in <1% of adolescents. The most common clinically detected lesion in adolescent women is the cervical lesion termed **low-grade squamous intraepithelial lesion (LSIL)** (Table 263-1). This appears to occur in 25–30% of adolescents infected with HPV. LSILs are considered benign cellular changes associated with HPV infection. As with HPV DNA detection, most LSILs regress spontaneously in young women and do not require any intervention or therapy. Less commonly, HPV can induce more severe cellular changes termed **high-grade squamous intraepithelial lesions (HSILs)**. Although HSILs are considered precancerous lesions, these lesions rarely progress to invasive cancer. HSILs occur in approximately 0.4–3% of sexually active women, whereas invasive cervical cancer occurs in <14 cases per 100,000 adult women. In true virginal populations, including children who are not sexually abused, rates of both clinical disease and HPV detection are very low to zero. In the USA, there are approximately 9,000 new cases and 3,700 deaths from cervical cancer each year. Worldwide, cervical cancer is the 2nd most common cause of cancer deaths among women.

Some infants may acquire papillomaviruses during passage through an infected birth canal, leading to recurrent **respiratory papillomatosis.** Cases also have been reported after cesarean section. The maximum incubation period for emergence of clinically apparent lesions (genital warts or laryngeal papillomas) after perinatally acquired infection is unknown, but appears to be 6 mo of age.

TABLE 263-1. Bethesda System for Reporting Cervical/Vaginal Cytology

DESCRIPTIVE DIAGNOSIS OF EPITHELIAL CELL ABNORMALITIES	EQUIVALENT TERMINOLOGY
SQUAMOUS CELL	
Atypical squamous cells of undetermined significance (ASC-US)	Squamous atypia
Atypical squamous cells, cannot exclude HSIL (ASC-H)	
Low-grade squamous intraepithelial lesion (LSIL)	Mild dysplasia, condylomatous atypia, HPV-related changes, koilocytic atypia, cervical epithelial neoplasia (CIN) 1
High-grade squamous intraepithelial lesion (HSIL)	Moderate dysplasia, CIN 2, severe dysplasia, CIN 3, carcinoma in situ
GLANDULAR CELL	
Endometrial cells, cytologically benign, in a postmenopausal woman	
Atypical glandular cells of undetermined significance	
Endocervical adenocarcinoma	
Endometrial adenocarcinoma	
Extrauterine adenocarcinoma	
Adenocarcinoma, not otherwise specified	

Genital warts appearing in later childhood may result from sexual abuse with HPV transmission during the abusive contact. Genital warts may represent a sexually transmitted infection even in some very young children. Their presence is cause to suspect that possibility. A child with genital warts should, therefore, be provided with a complete evaluation for possible abuse (see Chapter 36.1), including the presence of other sexually transmitted infections (see Chapter 119). Presence of genital warts in a child does not confirm sexual abuse since genital warts perinatally transmitted may go undetected until the child is older. Typing for specific genital HPV types in children is not helpful in diagnosis or to confirm sexual abuse status since the same genital types occur in both perinatal transmission and abuse. Nonetheless, the type detected in the infant is not always the same as the mother's type, suggesting other sources of HPV acquisition.

PATHOGENESIS. Initial HPV infection of the cervix is thought to begin by viral invasion of the basal cells of the epithelium, which is enhanced by disruption of the epithelium caused by trauma or inflammation. It is thought that the virus initially remains relatively dormant because virus is present without any evidence of clinical disease. The life cycle of HPV is dependent on the differentiation program of keratinocytes. The pattern of HPV transcription varies throughout the epithelial layer as well as through different stages of disease (LSIL, HSIL, invasive cancer). Understanding of HPV transcription enhances understanding of its ability to behave as an oncovirus. Early region proteins, E6 and E7, function as trans-activating factors that regulate cellular transformation. Complex interactions between E6 and E7 transcribed proteins and host proteins result in the perturbation of normal processes that regulate cellular DNA synthesis. The perturbations caused by E6 and E7 are primarily through disruption of the anti-oncoproteins p53 and retinoblastoma protein (Rb), respectively, contributing to the development of anogenital cancers. Disruption of these proteins results in continued cell proliferation, even under the circumstances of DNA damage, which results in basal cell proliferation, chromosomal abnormalities, and aneuploidy that are hallmarks of SIL development.

Evidence of productive viral infection occurs in benign lesions such as external genital warts and LSILs, with the abundant expression of viral capsid proteins in the superficial keratinocytes. The appearance of the HPV-associated koilocyte is due to the expression of E4, a structural protein that causes collapse of the cytoskeleton. Although not as abundant, mild expression of E6 and E7 proteins results in cell proliferation seen in the basal cell layer of LSILs. LSILs are a manifestation of active viral replication and protein expression. However, as the lesions advance in grade, expression of those products important in the process of cell transformation, such as E6 and E7, now predominate, rather than structural proteins, resulting in the chromosomal abnormalities and aneuploidy characteristic of the higher-grade lesions.

Cutaneous lesions (common and genital warts) are not associated with malignant HPV types, nor do they have any malignant potential except in the rare skin disorder **epidermodysplasia verruciformis.** Genital lesions caused by HPV may be broadly grouped into those with little to no malignant potential (low risk) and those with greater malignant potential (high risk). **Low-risk HPV types** 6 and 11 are most commonly found in genital warts and are rarely if ever found isolated in malignant lesions. **High-risk HPV types,** specifically types 16 and 18 that cause about 70% of cervical cancer, are commonly found in SILs and invasive anogenital cancers. Other HPV types found in invasive cancers but at much lower frequencies include types 31, 33, 35, 39, 45, 51, 52, 56, 58, 59, 68, 73, and 82. HPV 16 is also most commonly found in women without lesions as well, making the connection with cancer confusing. Lesions may also be infected simultaneously with multiple HPV types. Almost all latent infections with low-risk types spontaneously resolve over time. Genital and common warts in general resolve without therapy but may take years. Although 85–90% of latent high-risk type infections resolve as well, they are more likely than low-risk types to persist. This seems to be particularly true for HPV 16, which has a slower rate of regression than other high-risk types. Persistent high-risk type infections are associated with increased risk for developing HSILs and invasive cancer. LSILs have similar regression patterns as latent infection in young women: 92–95% of LSILs in young women will spontaneously regress within 3 yr. Although HSILs are less likely to regress than latent infections or LSILs and therefore warrant treatment, progression to invasive cancer is still rare, with only 5–15% showing progression.

Most infants with recognized genital warts are infected with the low-risk types. In contrast, children with a history of sexual abuse have a picture more like adult genital warts with mixed low- and high-risk types. There are rare reports of HPV-associated genital malignancies occurring in preadolescent children and adolescents. On the other hand, HSILs do occur in sexually active adolescents. There is also a concern that younger age of sexual debut has contributed to the increase of invasive cervical cancer seen in women <50 yr of age in the USA. HPV is considered necessary but not sufficient for the development of invasive cancers. Other risk factors that have relatively strong suggestive evidence of association include smoking, prolonged oral contraceptive use, herpes simplex virus infection, and greater parity.

CLINICAL MANIFESTATIONS. The clinical findings depend on the site of epithelial infection.

Skin Lesions. The typical HPV-induced lesions of the skin are proliferative, papular, and hyperkeratotic. Common warts are raised circinate lesions with a keratinized surface (Fig. 263-1). Plantar and palmar warts are practically flat. Multiple warts are common and may create a mosaic pattern. Flat warts appear as small (1–5 mm), flat, flesh-colored papules.

Genital Warts. Genital warts may be found throughout the perineum around the anus, vagina, and urethra, as well as in the cervical, intravaginal, and intra-anal areas (Fig. 263-2). Intra-anal warts occur predominantly in patients who have had receptive anal intercourse, as contrasted with perianal warts, which may occur in men and women without a history of anal sex. Although rare, lesions caused by genital genotypes can also be found on other mucosal surfaces such as conjunctivae, gingiva, and nasal mucosa. They may be single or multiple lesions and are frequently found in multiple anatomic sites. External genital warts can be flat, dome-shaped, keratotic, pedunculated, and cauliflower shaped; they may occur singly, in clusters, or as plaques. On mucosal epithelium, the lesions are softer. Depending on the size and anatomic location, lesions may be pruritic and painful, cause burning with urination, be friable and bleed, or become superinfected. Children may be very disturbed by the development of genital lesions. Other rarer lesions caused by HPV of the external genital area include Bowen disease, bowenoid papulosis, squamous cell carcinomas, Buschke-Löwenstein tumors, and vulvar intraepithelial neoplasias (VINs).

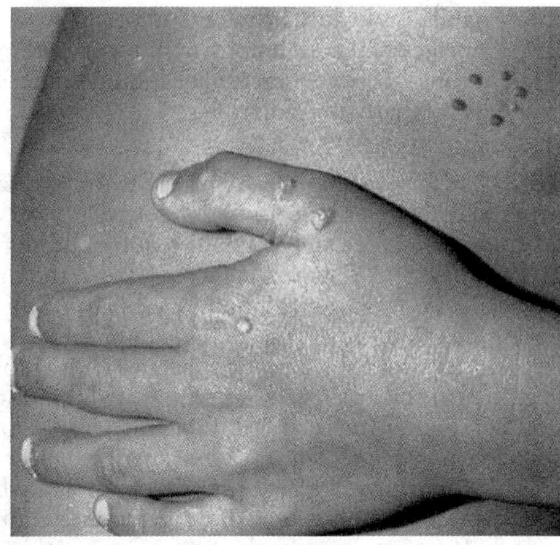

Figure 263-1. Common warts of the left hand and the chest wall. (From Meneghini CL, Bonifaz E: *An Atlas of Pediatric Dermatology.* Chicago, Year Book Medical Publishers, 1986, p 45.)

Squamous intraepithelial lesions detected by cytology are usually invisible to the naked eye and require the aid of colposcopic magnification and acetic acid. With aid, the lesions appear white and show evidence of neovascularity. SIL can occur on the cervix, vagina, vulva, and intra-anus. Invasive cancers tend to be more exophytic, with aberrant-appearing vasculature. These lesions are rarely found in non-sexually active individuals.

Laryngeal Papillomatosis. The median age of onset of recurrent laryngeal papillomatosis is 3 yr. Children present with hoarseness or, in infants, an altered cry and sometimes stridor. Rapid growth

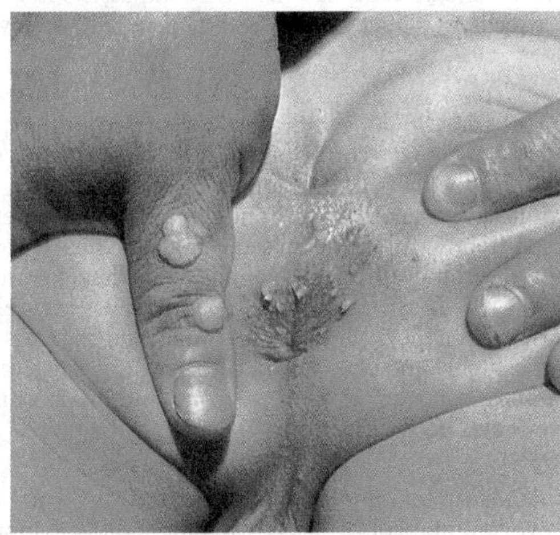

Figure 263-2. Common warts of the hand in a mother and perianal condylomata acuminata in her son. (From Meneghini CL, Bonifaz E: *An Atlas of Pediatric Dermatology.* Chicago, Year Book Medical Publishers, 1986, p 44.)

of respiratory papillomas can occlude the upper airway, causing respiratory compromise. These lesions may recur within weeks of removal, requiring frequent surgery. The lesions do not become malignant unless treated with radiation.

DIAGNOSIS. The diagnosis of external genital warts and common warts may be reliably determined by visual inspection of a lesion by an experienced observer and does not require additional tests for confirmation. A biopsy should be considered if the diagnosis is uncertain, the lesions do not respond to therapy, or the lesions worsen during therapy.

Screening for cervical SILs or cancer begins with cytology by Papanicolaou (Pap) smear, and the recommended terminology is based on the cytologic evaluation (see Table 263-1). Although the purpose of screening is to identify significant precancer HSILs, the majority of confirmed HSILs are found in women who were referred for **atypical squamous cells of undetermined significance (ASCUS)** or LSILs. Cytologic evaluation of cervical cells is a screening test and not confirmatory. Current recommendations for triage to colposcopy and biopsy for women with ASCUS is to repeat a Pap smear in 4–6 mo or to perform reflex HPV testing (HPV testing in a sample obtained at or around the time the ASCUS Pap smear was obtained). Women with persistent abnormal cytology at 4–6 mo or a positive reflex HPV test are referred to colposcopy. The latter recommendation was made based on the observations that women with ASCUS and a positive HPV test result for high-risk types are more likely to have HSILs than women with a negative HPV test result. However, HPV testing in adolescents, whether used for triage or follow-up is not recommended because of the high prevalence of HPV. Because of the high rate of LSIL regression in adolescents and young women, clinicians may also choose to repeat cytology in 12 mo for young women diagnosed with LSILs or ASCUS. For persistent LSILs, at 2 yr referral to colposcopy is recommended. However, once LSILs are confirmed by histology, women can be followed by cytology. All women with cytologically identified HSILs should be referred for colposcopy and biopsy.

Recommendations by the American Cancer Society state that screening may begin within the 1st 3 yr after vaginal intercourse. Screening earlier than 3 yr is more likely to result in unnecessary referrals for colposcopy because most lesions in this group are likely to be LSILs and therefore likely to regress. The upper age limit for screening is 21 yr, which captures those women who have not revealed their sexual activity.

Very sensitive tests for the presence of HPV DNA, RNA, and proteins are becoming generally available, although they are not required for the diagnosis of external genital warts or related conditions. Application of HPV DNA testing assists in the triage of atypical cells of undetermined significance and follow-up of LSILs.

DIFFERENTIAL DIAGNOSIS. A number of other conditions should be considered, including condyloma latum, seborrheic keratoses, dysplastic and benign nevi, molluscum contagiosum, pearly penile papules, and neoplasms. Condyloma latum is due to secondary syphilis and can be diagnosed using dark-field microscopy and standard serologic tests for syphilis. Seborrheic keratoses are common, localized, hyperpigmented lesions that are rarely associated with malignancy. Molluscum contagiosum is caused by a poxvirus, is highly infectious, and is often umbilicated. Pearly penile papules occur at the penile corona and are normal variants that require no treatment.

TREATMENT. Most common (plantar, palmar, skin) warts eventually resolve spontaneously (see Chapter 666). Symptomatic lesions should be removed. Removal includes a variety of self-applied therapies, including salicylic acid preparations and provider-applied therapies (cryotherapy, laser therapy, electrosurgery). Genital warts of children and adolescents are benign and usually remit, but only over an extended period of time. It is recommended that genital lesions be treated if the patient or the parent requests therapy. Similar to common warts, treatment is categorized into self-applied and provider applied. No one therapy has been shown to be more efficacious than any other. Provider-applied therapies include surgical treatments (electrosurgery, surgical excision, laser surgery) and office-based treatment (cryotherapy with liquid nitrogen or a cryoprobe, podophyllin resin 10–25%, and bi- and tri-chloroacetic acid). Podophyllin resins have lost favor to other methods because of the variability in preparations. Intralesional, but not systemic, interferon is no more effective than other therapies and is associated with significant adverse effects. This therapy is reserved for treatment of recalcitrant cases.

Many therapies are painful, and children should not undergo painful genital treatments unless adequate pain control is provided. Parents and patients should not be expected to apply painful therapies themselves. In adolescents and adults, recommended patient-applied treatment regimens for external genital warts include topical podofilox and imiquimod. Podofilox 0.5% solution (using a cotton swab) or gel (using a finger) is applied to visible warts in a cycle of applications twice a day for 3 days followed by 4 days of no therapy, repeated for up to a total of 4 cycles. Imiquimod 5% cream is applied at bedtime, 3 times a week, every other day, for up to 16 wk; the treated area should be washed with mild soap and water 6–10 hr after treatment. Neither podofilox nor imiquimod is recommended during pregnancy. For any of the nonsurgical treatments, prescription is contraindicated when there is any history of hypersensitivity to any product constituents.

If exposure as a result of sexual abuse is suspected or known, the clinician should ensure that the child's safety has been achieved and is maintained.

Ablative treatment including cryotherapy, loop electrosurgical excisional procedure, and laser therapy for HSILs is universally recommended. LSILs, once confirmed by histology, can be observed for an extended period of time before treatment is offered. No recommendations for follow-up have currently been established.

COMPLICATIONS. The presence of these lesions in the genital area may be a cause of profound embarrassment to a child or parent. Complications of therapy are uncommon; chronic pain (vulvodynia) or hypoesthesia may occur at the treatment site. Lesions may heal with hypopigmentation or hyperpigmentation and less commonly with depressed or hypertrophic scars. Surgical therapies can lead to infection and scarring. Repeated procedures of the cervix may lead to problems with infertility.

Although numerous epidemiologic studies of adults, but not children, have demonstrated that infection with HPV, especially types 16 and 18, is a strong risk factor for precancerous lesions and cancer, it is thought that precancers such as HSILs must exist prior to the development of invasive cancers. Respiratory papillomas rarely become malignant, unless they have been treated with radiation.

PROGNOSIS. With all forms of therapy, genital warts commonly recur, and approximately half of children and adolescents require a 2nd or 3rd treatment. Recurrence is also evident in patients with respiratory papillomatosis. Patients and parents should be warned of this likelihood. Combination therapy for genital warts (imiquimod and Podofilox) does not improve response but may increase complications. Prognosis of cervical disease is better, with 85–90% cure rates after a single treatment. Recalcitrant disease should prompt an evaluation and is common in immunocompromised individuals, specifically men and women infected with HIV.

PREVENTION. The only means to prevent infection is to avoid direct contact with lesions. Condoms may reduce the risk for HPV transmission; condoms also prevent other sexually transmitted infections, which are risk factors associated with SIL development. In addition, condoms appear to hasten the regression of LSILs in women. Avoiding smoking cigarettes is important in preventing cervical cancer.

HPV vaccines show efficacy against type-specific persistence and development of type-specific disease. A quadrivalent HPV vaccine against types 6, 11, 16, and 18 was licensed in 2006 in the USA and is based on virus-like particles that are produced in *Saccharomyces cerevisiae*. The efficacy of the vaccine is mediated by the development of humoral immune responses. Vaccination is recommended routinely for all girls at 11–12 yr of age and is administered IM in the deltoid region in a 3 dose series at 0, 2, and 6 mo. It is important that vaccination take place in pre-sexually active children since the rate of HPV acquisition is high shortly after the onset of sexual activity, although females who are sexually active should still be vaccinated. Vaccine can be given to girls as young as 9 yr of age as well as to girls and women 13–26 yr of age at the discretion of the health care provider. Individuals who are already infected with 1 or more vaccine-related HPV types prior to vaccination are protected from clinical disease caused by the remaining vaccine HPV types. Hormonal contraceptives do not affect vaccine efficacy.

American Academy of Pediatrics, Committee on Child Abuse and Neglect: Guidelines for the evaluation of sexual abuse of children. *Pediatrics* 1991;87:254–260.

Beutner KR, Reitano MV, Richwald GA, et al: External genital warts: Report of the American Medical Association Consensus Conference. AMA Expert Panel on External Genital Warts. *Clin Infect Dis* 1998;27:796–806.

Bjorge T, Engeland A, Luostarinen T, et al: Human papillomavirus infection as a risk factor for anal and perianal skin cancer in a prospective study. *Br J Cancer* 2002;87(1):61–64.

Centers for Disease Control and Prevention: Sexually transmitted diseases treatment guidelines 2002. *MMWR* 2002;51(RR-6):1–78.

Harper DM, Franco EL, Wheeler C, et al: Efficacy of a bivalent L1 virus-like particle vaccine in prevention of infection with human papillomavirus types 16 and 18 in young women: A randomised controlled trial. *Lancet* 2004;364(9447):1757–1765.

Ho GYF, Birman R, Beardsley L, et al: Natural history of cervicovaginal papillomavirus infection in young women. *N Engl J Med* 1998;338:423–428.

Koutsky LA, Ault KA, Wheeler CM, et al: A controlled trial of a human papillomavirus type 16 vaccine. *N Engl J Med* 2002;347(21):1645–1651.

Mork J, Lie AK, Glattre E, Hallmans G, et al: Human papillomavirus infection as a risk factor for squamous-cell carcinoma of the head and neck. *N Engl J Med* 2001;344(15):1125–1131.

Moscicki AB, Ellenberg JH, Crowley-Nowick P, et al: Risk of high-grade squamous intraepithelial lesion in HIV-infected adolescents. *J Infect Dis* 2004;190(8):1413–1421.

Moscicki AB, Hills N, Shiboski S, et al: Risks for incident human papillomavirus infection and low-grade squamous intraepithelial lesion development in young females. *JAMA* 2001;285:2995–3002.

Moscicki AB, Shiboski S, Broering J, et al: The natural history of human papillomavirus infection as measured by repeated DNA testing in adolescent and young women. *J Pediatr* 1998;132:277–284.

Moscicki AB, Shiboski S, Hills NK, et al: Regression of low-grade squamous intra-epithelial lesions in young women. *Lancet* 2004;364(9446):1678–1683.

Munoz N, Bosch FX, de Sanjose S, et al: Epidemiologic classification of human papillomavirus types associated with cervical cancer. *N Engl J Med* 2003;348(6):518–512.

Rintala MAM, Grénman SE, Puranen MH, et al: Transmission of high-risk human papillomavirus (HPV) between parents and infant: A prospective study of HPV in families in Finland. *J Clin Microbiol* 2005;43:376–381.

Siegfried E, Rasnick-Conley J, Cook S, et al: Human papillomavirus screening in pediatric victims of sexual abuse. *Pediatrics* 1998;101:43–47.

Sinclair KA, Woods CR, Kirse DJ, Sinal SH: Anogenital and respiratory tract human papillomavirus infections among children: Age, gender, and potential transmission through sexual abuse. *Pediatrics* 2005;116:815–825.

Villa LL, Ault KA, Giuliano AR, et al: Immunologic responses following administration of a vaccine targeting human papillomavirus types 6, 11, 16, and 18. *Vaccine* 2006;24:5571–5583.

Wright TC Jr, Cox JT, Massad LS, et al: 2001 consensus guidelines for the management of women with cervical cytological abnormalities. *JAMA* 2002;287:2120–2129.

Chapter 264 ■ Arboviral Encephalitis in North America

Scott B. Halstead

The arthropod-borne (arbovirus) viral encephalitides are a group of clinically similar severe neurologic infections caused by several different viruses. They are transmitted by mosquitoes during outdoor exposure in warmer weather in overlapping regions across most of the United States and much of southern Canada.

ETIOLOGY. The principal causes of the arthropod-borne encephalitides of North America include West Nile encephalitis (WNE), the St. Louis encephalitides (SLE), the complex of viruses included in the California encephalitis (CE) group of viruses, and, less frequently, western equine encephalitis (WEE), eastern equine encephalitis (EEE), and Colorado tick fever. The etiologic agents belong to different viral taxa: alphaviruses of the family Togaviridae (EEE and WEE), Flaviviridae (WNE, SLE), the California complex of the family Bunyaviridae (CE), and Reoviridae (Colorado tick fever virus). Alphaviruses are 69 nm, enveloped, positive-strand RNA viruses that evolved from a common Venezuelan equine encephalitis-like viral ancestor in the Western hemisphere. Flaviviruses are 40–50 nm, enveloped, positive-strand RNA viruses that evolved from a common ancestor. They are globally distributed and responsible for many important human viral diseases. The California serogroup, 1 of 16 Bunyavirus groups, are 75–115 nm enveloped viruses possessing a 3 segment, negative-strand RNA genome. Reoviruses are 60–80 nm double-stranded RNA viruses.

EPIDEMIOLOGY. Viral encephalitis cases and outbreaks were only recognized during the 20th century, when human population densities across the USA became relatively high, public health disease reporting systems were maturing, and laboratories were able to discriminate viral from bacterial infections. From the mid-19th century, epizootics of equine encephalitis were observed in the United States. In 1931, WEE was isolated from horse cases in the Central Valley of California. In 1938, the same virus was recovered from the central nervous system from fatal human cases. In the summer of 1932, an epidemic of human encephalitis, first regarded as Von Economo's disease, was recognized in Paris, Illinois. The next year, >1,000 cases were reported from St. Louis County, and several SLE viruses were isolated. In 1933, EEE virus was isolated from a horse epizootic, which occurred in Virginia, Maryland, Delaware, and New Jersey. The same virus was isolated from human cases in 1938. The 1st CE virus (La Crosse virus) was isolated in 1960 from a fatal case of encephalitis in a 4 yr old girl in rural Wisconsin. Colorado tick fever was first described as a nosologic entity in 1930.

Eastern Equine Encephalitis. In the USA, EEE is a very low incidence disease, with a median of 3 cases occurring annually in the Atlantic and Gulf states (Fig. 264-1). Transmission occurs often in focal endemic areas of the coast of Massachusetts, the 6 southern counties of New Jersey, and northeastern Florida. In North America, the virus is maintained in freshwater swamps in a zoonotic cycle involving *Culiseta melanura* and birds. Various

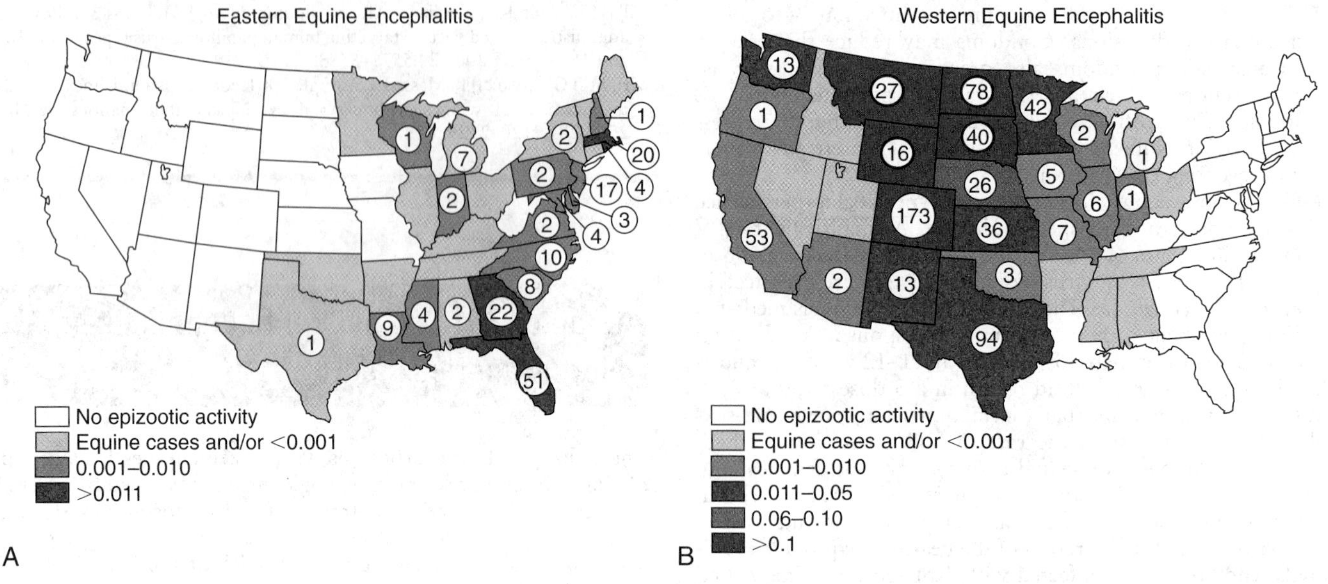

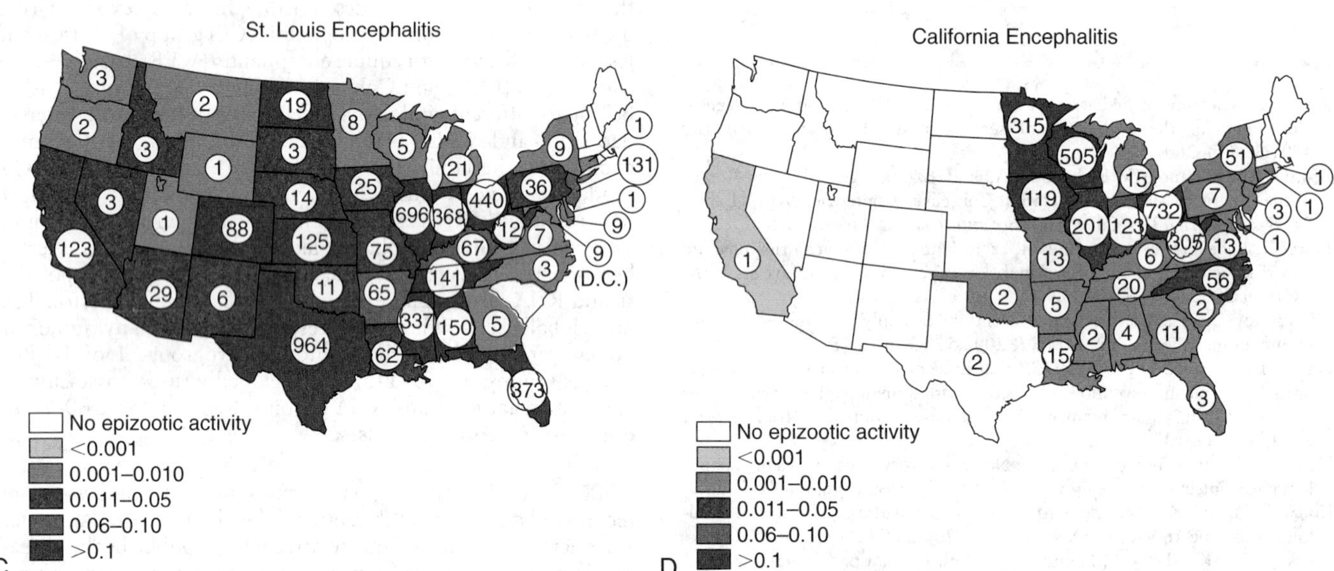

Figure 264-1. The distribution and incidence of reported cases of eastern equine encephalitis *(A)*, western equine encephalitis *(B)*, St. Louis encephalitis *(C)*, and California encephalitis *(D)* reported to the Centers for Disease Control and Prevention in 1997.

other mosquito species obtain viremic meals from birds and transmit the virus to horses and humans. Virus activity varies markedly from year to year in response to still unknown ecologic factors. Most infections in birds are silent, but infections in pheasants are often fatal, and epizootics in these species are used as sentinels for periods of increased viral activity. Cases have been recognized on Caribbean islands. The case-to-infection ratio is lowest in children (1 : 8) and somewhat higher in adults (1 : 29).

Western Equine Encephalitis. Infections occur principally in the USA and Canada west of the Mississippi River (see Fig. 264-1), mainly in rural areas where water impoundments, irrigated farmland, and naturally flooded land provide breeding sites for *Culex tarsalis*. The virus is transmitted in a cycle involving mosquitoes, birds, and other vertebrate hosts. Humans and horses are susceptible to encephalitis. The case-to-infection ratio varies by age, having been estimated at 1 : 58 in children younger than 4 yr and 1 : 1,150 in adults. Infections are most severe at the extremes of life; 1/3 of cases occur in children younger than 1 yr. Recurrent human epidemics have been reported from the Yakima Valley in Washington State and the Central Valley of California; the largest outbreak on record—3,400 cases—occurred in Minnesota, North and South Dakota, Nebraska, and Montana, and Alberta, Manitoba, and Saskatchewan, Canada. Epizootics in horses precede human epidemics by several weeks. For the past 20 years, possibly as a result of successful mosquito abatement, few cases of WEE have been reported.

St. Louis Encephalitis. Cases are reported from nearly all states; the highest attack rates occur in the Gulf and central states (see Fig. 264-1). Epidemics frequently occur in urban and suburban areas; the largest, in 1975, involved 1,800 persons living in Houston, Chicago, Memphis, and Denver. Cases often cluster in areas where there is ground water or septic systems, which support mosquito breeding. The principal vectors are *Culex pipiens* and *Culex quinquefasciatus* in the central Gulf states, *Culex nigripalpus* in Florida, and *Culex tarsalis* in California. SLE virus is maintained in nature in a bird-mosquito cycle. Viral amplification occurs in bird species abundant in residential areas (e.g., sparrows, blue jays, and doves). Virus is transmitted in the late summer and early fall. The case-to-infection ratio may be as high as 1 : 300. Age-specific attack rates are lowest in children and highest in individuals older than 60 yr.

West Nile Encephalitis. During the past decade, WNE virus has been implicated as the cause of sporadic summertime human cases of encephalitis and meningitis in Israel, India, Pakistan, Romania, and Russia. West Nile virus was initially recognized in the United States in September 1999 when it was isolated from a cluster of patients in Queens, New York, following the sentinel deaths of crows and exotic birds at the Bronx Zoo. All American WNE viruses are genetically quite similar and are related to a virus recovered from a goose in Israel in 1998. WNE virus survives in a broad enzootic cycle in the United States and within 4 yr has spread to most states east of the Rocky Mountains plus California (Fig. 264-2). Every state in the continental United States plus 9 provinces in Canada have reported mosquito, bird, mammalian, or human West Nile infection. Through the end of 2005 there have been 19,558 total cases reported, 30–40% of which are encephalitis with 719 deaths. Summer/fall epidemics are common (Fig. 264-3). West Nile virus has entered the blood supply through asymptomatic viremic blood donors. Blood banks now screen for West Nile virus RNA. West Nile virus has also been transmitted to humans via the placenta, breast milk, and organ transplantation. Throughout its range, the virus is maintained in nature by transmission between mosquitoes of the *Culex* genus and various species of birds. In the United States, human infections are largely acquired from *Culex pipiens*. Horses are the non-avian vertebrates most likely to exhibit disease with WNE infection. During the 2002 transmission season, 14,000 equine cases were reported, with a mortality rate of 30%. Disease occurs predominantly in individuals >50 yr of age.

La Crosse/California Encephalitis. La Crosse viral infections are endemic in the United States, occurring annually from July to September, principally in the north-central and central states (see Fig. 264-1). Infections occur in peridomestic environments as the result of bites from *Aedes triseriatus* mosquitoes, which often breed in tree holes. The virus is maintained vertically in nature by transovarial transmission and can be spread between mosquitoes by copulation and amplified in mosquito populations by viremic infections in various vertebrate hosts. Amplifying hosts include chipmunks, squirrels, foxes, and woodchucks. A case-to-infection ratio of 1 : 22–300 has been surmised. La Crosse encephalitis is principally a disease of children, who may constitute up to 75% of cases.

Colorado Tick Fever. Colorado tick fever virus is transmitted by the wood tick *Dermacentor andersoni,* which inhabits high-elevation areas of states extending from the central plains to the Pacific coast. The tick is infected with the virus at the larval stage and remains infected for life. Squirrels and chipmunks serve as primary reservoirs. Human infections typically occur in hikers and campers in indigenous areas during the spring and early summer.

CLINICAL MANIFESTATIONS. With the exception of EEE, these arboviruses produce similar symptoms of encephalitis.

Eastern Equine Encephalitis. Infections result in a fulminant encephalitis with a rapid progression to coma and death in 1/3 of cases. In infants and children, abrupt onset of fever, irritability, and headache are followed by lethargy, confusion, seizures, and coma. High temperature, bulging fontanel, stiff neck, and generalized flaccid or spastic paralysis are observed. There may be a brief prodrome of fever, headache, and dizziness. Unlike most other viral encephalitides, the peripheral white blood cell count usually demonstrates a marked leukocytosis, and the cerebrospinal fluid may show marked pleocytosis. Pathologic changes are found in the cortical and gray matter, with viral antigens localized to neurons. There is necrosis of neurons, neutrophilic infiltration, and perivascular cuffing by lymphocytes.

Western Equine Encephalitis. There may be a prodrome with symptoms of an upper respiratory tract infection. The onset is usually sudden with chills, fever, dizziness, drowsiness, increasing headache, malaise, nausea and vomiting, stiff neck, and disorientation. Infants typically present with the sudden cessation of feeding, fussiness, fever, and protracted vomiting. Convulsions

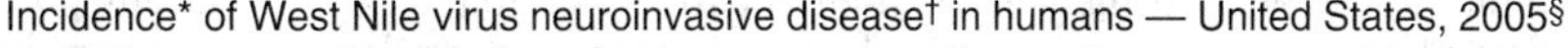

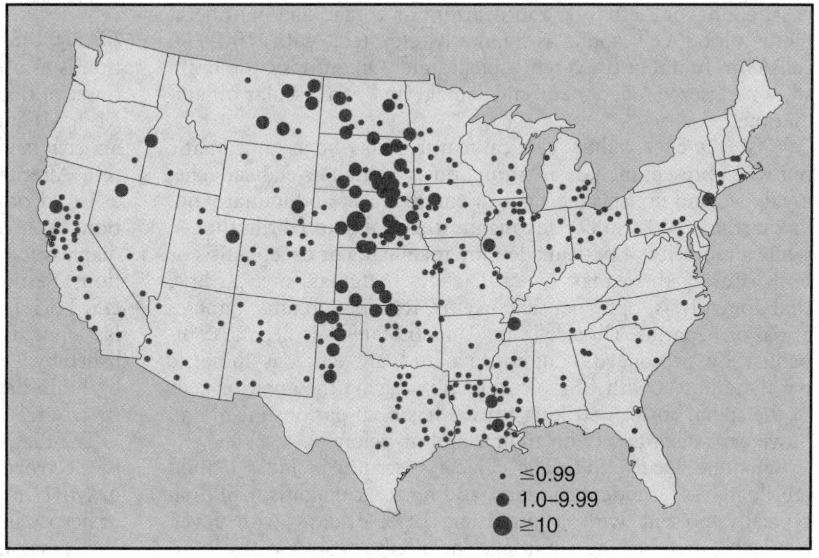

Figure 264-2. Incidence* of West Nile virus neuroinvasive disease† in humans—USA, 2005§. (From the Centers for Disease Control and Prevention: West Nile virus activity—United States, January 1–December 1, 2005. *MMWR* 2005;54:1253–1256.)

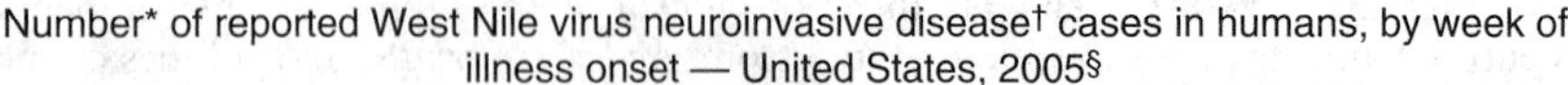

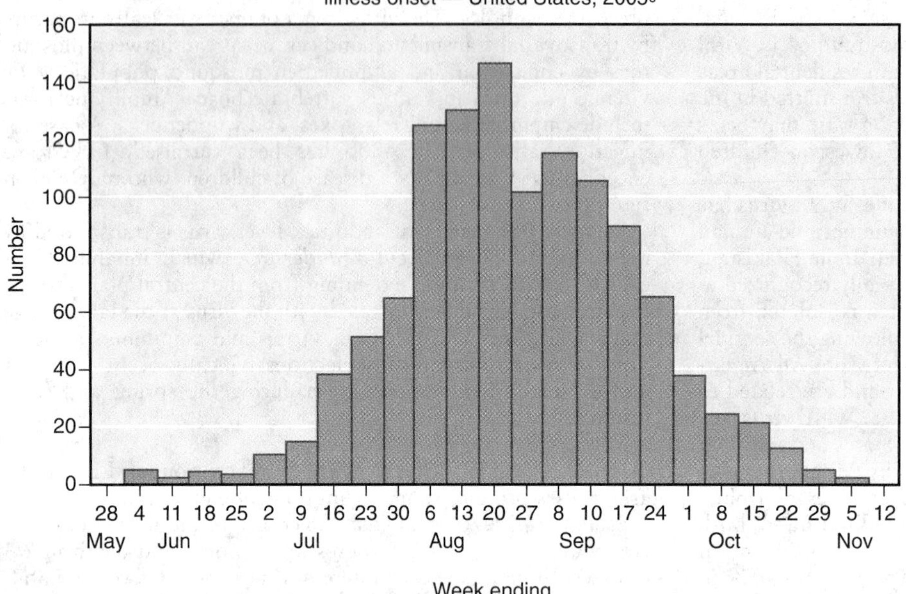

*n = 1,165.
†Meningitis, encephalitis, or acute flaccid paralysis.
§Provisional data as of December 1, 2005.

Figure 264-3. Number of reported West Nile virus neuroinvasive disease† cases in humans, by week of illness onset—USA, 2005§. (From the Centers for Disease Control and Prevention: West Nile virus activity—United States, January 1–December 1, 2005. *MMWR* 2005;54:1253–1256.)

and lethargy develop rapidly. On physical examination, patients are somnolent, exhibit meningeal signs, and have generalized motor weakness and reduced deep tendon reflexes. In infants, a bulging fontanel, spastic paralysis, and generalized convulsions may be observed. On pathologic examination, disseminated small focal abscesses, small focal hemorrhages, and patchy areas of demyelination are distinctive.

St. Louis Encephalitis. Clinical manifestations vary from a mild flulike illness to fatal encephalitis. There may be a prodrome of nonspecific symptoms with subtle changes in coordination or mentation of several days to 1 wk in duration. Early signs and symptoms include fever, photophobia, headache, malaise, nausea, vomiting, and neck stiffness. About half of patients exhibit abrupt onset of weakness, incoordination, disturbed sensorium, restlessness, confusion, lethargy, and delirium or coma. The peripheral white blood cell count is modestly elevated, with 100–200 cells/mm^3 found in the cerebrospinal fluid. On autopsy, the brain shows scattered foci of neuronal damage and perivascular inflammation.

West Nile Encephalitis. Clinical features may be asymptomatic but when present include an abrupt onset of high fever, headache, myalgias, and nonspecific signs of emesis, rash, abdominal pain, or diarrhea. Most infections manifest as a flulike febrile illness, while a minority of patients develop meningitis or encephalitis or both. Rarely there may be cardiac dysrhythmias, myocarditis, rhabdomyolysis, optic neuritis, uveitis, retinitis, orchitis, pancreatitis, or hepatitis. Disease in the United States has been accompanied by prolonged lymphopenia and an acute asymmetric paralytic illness with CSF pleocytosis involving the anterior cells of the spinal cord. A striking feature has been parkinsonism and movement disorders (with tremor and myoclonus).

California Encephalitis. The clinical spectrum includes a mild febrile illness, aseptic meningitis, and fatal encephalitis. Children typically present with a prodrome of 2–3 days with fever, headache, malaise, and vomiting. The disease evolves with clouding of the sensorium, lethargy, and, in severe cases, focal or generalized seizures. On physical examination, children are lethargic but not disoriented. Focal neurologic signs, including weakness, aphasia, and focal or generalized seizures, have been reported in 16–25% of cases. Cerebrospinal fluid shows low to moderate leukocyte counts. On autopsy, the brain shows focal areas of neuronal degeneration, inflammation, and perivascular cuffing.

Colorado Tick Fever. The illness begins with the abrupt onset of a flulike illness, including high temperature, malaise, arthralgias and myalgia, vomiting, headache, and decreased sensorium. Rash is uncommon. The symptoms rapidly disappear after 3 days of illness. However, in approximately half of patients, a 2nd, identical episode recurs 24–72 hr after the 1st, producing the typical "saddle-back" temperature curve of Colorado tick fever. Complications, including encephalitis, meningoencephalitis, or a bleeding diathesis, develop in 3–7% of infected persons and may be more common in children younger than 12 yr.

DIAGNOSIS. The etiologic diagnosis of a specific arboviral infection is established by testing an acute-phase serum ≥5 days after onset of illness for the presence of virus-specific immunoglobulin M (IgM) antibodies using an indirect immunofluorescence test or an enzyme-linked immunosorbent assay (ELISA) IgM capture test. Alternatively, acute and convalescent sera can be tested for a 4-fold or greater increase in ELISA, hemagglutination inhibition, or neutralizing IgG antibody titers. Commercial serologic diagnostic kits are marketed, especially for West Nile viral infections. Serum and CSF should be tested for West Nile virus–specific IgM. IgM may, however, reflect past infection because it may last up to 12 mo after infection. The diagnosis may also be established by isolation in cell cultures of virus in brain tissue, obtained by brain biopsy or at autopsy, or by identification of viral RNA reverse transcriptase polymerase chain reactions.

The diagnosis of encephalitis may be aided by CT or MRI and by electroencephalography. Focal seizures or focal findings on CT or MRI or electroencephalography should suggest the possibility of herpes simplex encephalitis, which should be treated with acyclovir (see Chapter 249).

TREATMENT. There is no specific treatment for arboviral encephalitides. The treatment of acute arboviral encephalitis is intensive supportive care (see Chapter 66), including control of seizures (Chapter 593).

PROGNOSIS. Fatalities occur with all arboviral encephalitides. With the exception of EEE, most resolve without residua.

Eastern Equine Encephalitis. The prognosis is better for patients with a prolonged prodrome; the occurrence of convulsions conveys a poor prognosis. Patient fatality rates are 33–75% and are highest in the elderly. Residual neurologic defects are common, especially in children.

Western Equine Encephalitis. Patient fatality rates are 3–9% and are highest in the elderly. Major neurologic sequelae have been reported in up to 13% of cases and may be as high as 30% in infants. Parkinsonian syndrome has been reported as a residual in adult survivors.

St. Louis Encephalitis. The principal risk factor for fatal outcome is advanced age, with patient fatality rates being as high as 80% in early outbreaks. In children, mortality rates are 2–5%. In adults, underlying hypertensive cardiovascular disease has been a risk factor for fatal outcome. Recovery from SLE is usually complete, but serious neurologic sequelae have been reported to be as high as 10% in children.

West Nile Encephalitis. Cases and deaths occur mainly in the elderly, although many serologic surveys show that person of all ages are infected. During 2002–2004, there were 648 deaths among 16,557 cases, a 3.8% mortality rate. Paralysis may result in permanent weakness.

California Encephalitis. Recovery from CE is usually complete. The case fatality rate is about 1%.

Colorado Tick Fever. Recovery from Colorado tick fever is usually complete. Three deaths have been reported, all in persons with hemorrhagic signs.

PREVENTION. Killed EEE, WEE, and WNE vaccines are available for horses, and an experimental killed vaccine is administered to human laboratory workers who handle EEE virus. Flocks of sentinel chickens or pheasants have been stationed at various locations along the Atlantic coast during the late summer or early fall to obtain early warning of increased transmission of EEE virus.

No human vaccine is licensed for arboviral encephalitides, although WNE vaccines are being developed. Killed WNE vaccines are licensed for veterinary use. Extensive water management and mosquito abatement programs in California have reduced transmission of WEE and the incidence of human infections. Urban WNE and SLE outbreaks in the eastern United States, Texas, and the Midwest have been controlled by the application of ultra-low-volume adulticide chemicals applied from trucks or low-flying aircraft.

Because infections in children may occur as a result of summer daytime mosquito biting in residential areas, sealing mosquito breeding sites, using insect repellents, and instructing children to play in open, sunny areas away from forest fringe may help prevent disease.

Balfour HH Jr, Siem RA, Bauer H, et al: California arbovirus (La Crosse) infections. I. Clinical and laboratory findings in 66 children with meningoencephalitis. *Pediatrics* 1973;52:680–691.

Centers for Disease Control and Prevention: Detection of West Nile virus in blood donations—United States, 2003. *MMWR* 2003;52:769–772.

Centers for Disease Control and Prevention: West Nile virus activity—United States, January 1–December 1, 2005. *MMWR* 2005;54:1253–1256.

Civen R, Villacorte F, Robles DT, et al: West Nile infection in the pediatric population. *Pediatr Infect Dis J* 2006;25:75–78.

Cunha BA, Minnaganti V, Johnson DH, et al: Profound and prolonged lymphocytopenia with West Nile encephalitis. *Clin Infect Dis* 2000;31: 1116–1117.

Earnest MP, Goolishian HA, Calverley JR, et al: Neurologic, intellectual, and psychologic sequelae following western encephalitis: A follow-up study of 35 cases. *Neurology* 1971;21:969–974.

Granwehr BP, Killibridge KM, Higgs S, et al: West Nile virus: Where are we now? *Lancet Infect Dis* 2004;4:647–656.

Hayes EB, O'Leary DR: West Nile virus infection: A pediatric perspective. *Pediatrics* 2004;113:1375–1381.

Hinckley AF, O'Leary DR, Hayes EB: Transmission of West Nile virus through human breast milk seems to be rare. *Pediatrics* 2007;119:e666–e671.

Jeha LE, Sila CA, Lederman RJ, et al: West nile virus infection: A new acute paralytic illness. *Neurology* 2003;61:55–59.

Komar N, Spielman A: Emergence of eastern encephalitis in Massachusetts. *Ann NY Acad Sci* 1995;740:157–168.

Marfin AA, Bleed DM, Lofgren JP, et al: Epidemiological aspects of a St. Louis encephalitis epidemic in Jefferson County, Arkansas. *Am J Trop Med Hyg* 1993;49:30–37.

Mazurek JM, Winpisinger K, Mattson BJ, et al: The epidemiology and early clinical features of West Nile virus infection. *Am J Emerg Med* 2005;23:536–543.

Minke JM, Audonnet JC, Fischer L: Equine viral vaccines: The past, present and future. *Vet Res* 2004;35:425–443.

Monath TP, Tsai TF: St. Louis encephalitis: Lessons from the last decade. *Am J Trop Med Hyg* 1987;37(Suppl):40S–59S.

Przelomski MM, O'Rourke E, Grady GE, et al: Eastern equine encephalitis in Massachusetts: A report of 16 cases, 1970–1984. *Neurology* 1988;38: 736–739.

Sejvar JJ, Hadded MB, Tierney BC, et al: Neurologic manifestations and outcome of West Nile virus infection. *JAMA* 2003;290:511–515.

Solomon T: Flavivirus encephalitis. *N Engl J Med* 2004;351:370–78.

Spruance SL, Bailey A: Colorado tick fever: A review of 115 laboratory confirmed cases. *Arch Intern Med* 1973;131:288–293.

Stramer SL, Fang CT, Foster GA, et al: West Nile virus among blood donors in the United States, 2003 and 2004. *N Engl J Med* 2005;353:451–459.

Tsai TF: Arboviral infections in the United States. *Infect Dis Clin North Am* 1991;5:73–102.

Chapter 265 ■ Arboviral Encephalitis Outside North America

Scott B. Halstead

The principal causes of arboviral encephalitis outside North America are Venezuelan equine encephalitis (VEE) virus, Japanese encephalitis (JE) virus, tick-borne encephalitis (TBE), and West Nile (WN) virus (Table 265-1).

265.1 • Venezuelan Equine Encephalitis

The VEE virus was isolated from an epizootic in Venezuelan horses in 1938. Human cases were first identified in 1943. Hundreds of thousands of equine and human cases have occurred over the past 70 yr. During 1971, epizootics moved through Central America and Mexico to southern Texas. After 2 decades of quiescence, epizootic disease emerged again in Venezuela and Colombia in 1995.

TABLE 265-1. Vectors and Geographic Distribution of Arboviral Encephalitis Outside North America

GENUS	VIRUS AND DISEASE	VECTOR	GEOGRAPHIC DISTRIBUTION
Flavivirus	Japanese encephalitis	*Culex tritaeniorhynchus*	Asia/Japan to Sri Lanka
Flavivirus	Murray Valley encephalitis	*Culex annulirostris*	Eastern Australia
Flavivirus	Rocio	*Psorophora* or *Aedes*	Sao Paulo, Brazil
Flavivirus	West Nile	*Culex* and others	Europe to Australia
Flavivirus	Tick-borne encephalitis	*Ixodes ricinus*	Europe
		Ixodes persulcatus	Russia
Togavirus	Venezuelan equine encephalitis	*Culex* and others	Northern South America

ETIOLOGY. VEE is an alphavirus of the family Togaviridae. VEE circulates in nature in 6 subtypes. Types I and III viruses have multiple antigenic variants. Types IAB and IC have caused epizootics and human epidemics.

EPIDEMIOLOGY. The majority of epizootics resulting from types IAB and IC have occurred in Venezuela and Colombia. The virus resides in ill-defined sylvatic reservoirs in the South American rain forests. Known hosts include rodents and aquatic birds with transmission by *Culex melaconion* species. Vectors for horse-to-horse and horse-to-human transmission include *Aedes taeniorhynchus* and *Psorophora confinnis*. Epizootics move rapidly, up to several miles per day. Human cases are proportional to and follow epizootic occurrences. Viremia levels in human blood are high enough to infect mosquitoes. Because virus can be recovered from human pharyngeal swabs, and household attack rates are often as high as 50%, it is widely believed that person-to-person transmission occurs, although direct evidence is lacking. Type II–VI viruses are restricted to relatively small foci; each has a unique vector-host relationship and rarely results in human infections.

CLINICAL MANIFESTATIONS. The incubation period is 2–5 days, followed by the abrupt onset of fever, chills, headache, sore throat, myalgia, malaise, prostration, photophobia, nausea, vomiting, and diarrhea. In 5–10% of cases, there is a biphasic illness; the 2nd phase is heralded by seizures, projectile vomiting, ataxia, confusion, agitation, and mild disturbances in consciousness. There is cervical lymphadenopathy and conjunctival suffusion. Cases of meningoencephalitis may demonstrate **cranial nerve palsy,** motor weakness, paralysis, seizures, and coma. Microscopic examination of tissues reveals inflammatory infiltrates in lymph nodes, spleen, lung, liver, and brain. Lymph nodes show cellular depletion, necrosis of germinal centers, and lymphophagocytosis. The liver shows patchy hepatocellular degeneration, the lungs demonstrate a diffuse interstitial pneumonia with intra-alveolar hemorrhages, and the brain shows patchy cellular infiltrates.

DIAGNOSIS. The etiologic diagnosis of VEE is established by testing an acute-phase serum collected early in the illness for the presence of virus-specific immunoglobulin M (IgM) antibodies or, alternatively, demonstrating a 4-fold or greater increase in IgG antibody titers by testing paired acute and convalescent sera. The virus can also be identified by polymerase chain reaction (PCR).

TREATMENT. There is no specific treatment for VEE. The treatment is intensive supportive care (see Chapter 66), including control of seizures (see Chapter 593).

PROGNOSIS. In patients with meningoencephalitis, the fatality rate ranges from 10 to 25%. Sequelae include nervousness, forgetfulness, recurrent headache, and easy fatigability.

PREVENTION. Several veterinary vaccines are available to protect equines. VEE virus is highly infectious in laboratory settings, and BL-3 containment should be used. An experimental vaccine is available for use in laboratory workers.

265.2 • Japanese Encephalitis

Epidemics of encephalitis were reported in Japan from the late 1800s. The JE virus was first isolated by Japanese workers by intracerebral inoculation of monkeys in 1934 and subsequently in mice in 1936. The virus was initially called Japanese B encephalitis to distinguish it from an unusual epidemic of von Economo (type A) encephalitis that occurred in Japan in the 1920s.

ETIOLOGY. JE virus is a positive-sense, single-stranded RNA virus of the family Flaviviridae.

EPIDEMIOLOGY. JE is a mosquito-borne viral disease of humans as well as horses, swine, and other domestic animals that causes human infections and acute disease in a vast area of Asia, northern Japan, Korea, China, Taiwan, Philippines, and the Indonesian archipelago and from Indochina through the Indian subcontinent. *Culex tritaeniorhynchus summarosus,* a night-biting mosquito that feeds preferentially on large domestic animals and birds but only infrequently on humans, is the principal vector of zoonotic and human JE in northern Asia. A more complex ecology prevails in southern Asia. From Taiwan to India, *C. tritaeniorhynchus* and members of the closely related *Culex vishnui* group are vectors. Before the introduction of JE vaccine, summer outbreaks of JE occurred regularly in Japan, Korea, China, Okinawa, and Taiwan. Over the past decade, there has been a pattern of steadily enlarging recurrent seasonal outbreaks in Vietnam, Thailand, Nepal, and India, with small outbreaks in the Philippines, Indonesia, and the northern tip of Queensland, Australia. Seasonal rains are accompanied by increases in mosquito populations and increased transmission. Pigs serve as amplifying host.

The annual incidence in endemic areas ranges from 1–10/10,000 population. Children <15 yr of age are principally affected, with nearly universal exposure by adulthood. The case-to-infection ratio for JE virus has been variously estimated at 1 : 25 to 1 : 1,000. Higher ratios have been estimated for populations indigenous to enzootic areas. JE occurs in travelers visiting Asia; therefore, a travel history in the diagnosis of encephalitis is critical.

CLINICAL MANIFESTATIONS. After a 4–14 day incubation period, cases typically progress through 4 stages: prodromal illness (2–3 days), acute stage (3–4 days), subacute stage (7–10 days), and convalescence (4–7 wk). Onset may be characterized by abrupt onset of fever, headache, respiratory symptoms, anorexia, nausea, abdominal pain, vomiting, and sensory changes, including psychotic episodes. Grand mal seizures are seen in 10–24% of children; parkinsonian-like nonintention tremor and cogwheel rigidity are seen less frequently. Particularly characteristic are **rapidly changing central nervous system** signs (e.g., hyperreflexia followed by hyporeflexia or plantar responses that change). The sensory status of the patient may vary from confusion, disorientation, delirium, or somnolence, progressing to coma. There is usually a mild pleocytosis (100–1,000 leukocytes/mm^3) in the cerebrospinal fluid, initially polymorphonuclear but in a few days predominantly lymphocytic. Albuminuria is common. Fatal cases usually progress rapidly to coma, and the patient dies within 10 days.

DIAGNOSIS. JE should be suspected in patients reporting exposure to night-biting mosquitoes in endemic areas during the transmission season. The etiologic diagnosis of JE is established by testing an acute-phase serum collected early in the illness for the presence of virus-specific IgM antibodies or, alternatively, demonstrating a fourfold or greater increase in IgG antibody titers by testing paired acute and convalescent sera. The virus can also be identified by PCR.

TREATMENT. There is no specific treatment for JE. The treatment is intensive supportive care (see Chapter 66), including control of seizures (see Chapter 593).

PROGNOSIS. Patient fatality rates are 24–42% and are highest in children 5–9 yr of age and in persons older than 65 yr. The frequency of sequelae is 5–70% and is directly related to the age of the patient and severity of disease. Sequelae are most common in patients younger than 10 yr at the onset of disease. The more common sequelae are mental deterioration, severe emotional instability, personality changes, motor abnormalities, and speech disturbances.

PREVENTION. Travelers to endemic countries staying ≥1 mo in rural areas of the endemic region during the expected period of seasonal transmission, or those traveling in areas experiencing endemic transmission, should receive JE vaccine. The JE vaccine is given in a 3 dose series (0.5 mL for 1–3 yr of age; 1 mL for >3 yr of age) subcutaneously; the 1st 2 doses are given 1 wk apart and the 3rd dose 30 days later. Booster doses are given every 2 yr while risk for exposure continues. Reactions to vaccination, including headache, malaise, myalgia, tenderness, redness, and swelling, occur in about 20% of vaccines. Serious generalized urticaria, facial angioedema, and respiratory distress have been observed in adults. Because vaccine is prepared in mouse brain, surveillance should be maintained for central nervous system disease after JE vaccination. A highly efficacious live-attenuated vaccine is marketed in some Asian countries. In humans, prior dengue virus infection provides partial protection from clinical JE.

Personal measures should be taken to reduce exposure to mosquito bites, especially for short-term residents in endemic areas. This consists of avoiding evening outdoor exposure, using insect repellents, covering the body with clothing, and using bed nets or house screening.

Commercial pesticides, widely used by rice farmers in Asia, are effective in reducing populations of *C. tritaeniorhynchus*. Fenthion, fenitrothion, and phenthoate are effectively adulticidal and larvicidal. Insecticides may be applied from portable sprayers or from helicopters or light aircraft.

265.3 • Tick-Borne Encephalitis

TBE was identified by Russian scientists in 1937 and was subsequently shown to be widespread in Europe, where it was identified as the cause of milk-borne encephalitis.

ETIOLOGY. TBE virus is a positive-sense, single-stranded RNA virus of the family Flaviviridae.

EPIDEMIOLOGY. Tick-borne encephalitis refers to neurotropic tick-transmitted flaviviral infections occurring across the Eurasian land mass. In the Far East, the disease is called Russian spring-summer encephalitis; the milder, often biphasic form in Europe is simply called tick-borne encephalitis. TBE is found in all countries of Europe except Portugal and the Benelux countries. The incidence is particularly high in Austria, Poland, Hungary, Czech Republic, Slovakia, former Yugoslavia, and Russia. The incidence tends to be very focal. Seroprevalence is as high as 50% in farm and forestry workers. The majority of cases occur in adults, but even young children may be infected while playing in the woods or on picnics or camping trips. The seasonal distribution of cases is midsummer in southern Europe, with a longer season in Scandinavia and the Russian Far East. TBE can be excreted from the milk of goats, sheep, or cows. Before World War II, when milk was consumed unpasteurized, milk-borne cases were common.

Viruses are transmitted principally by hard ticks of *Ixodes ricinus* in Europe and *Ixodes persulcatus* in the Far East. Viral circulation is maintained by a combination of transmission from ticks to birds, rodents, and larger mammals and transtadial transmission from larval to nymphal and adult stages. In some parts of Europe and Russia, ticks feed actively during the spring and early fall, giving rise to the name spring-summer encephalitis.

CLINICAL MANIFESTATIONS. After an incubation period of 7–14 days, the European form begins as an acute nonspecific febrile illness followed in 5–30% of cases by meningoencephalitis. The Far Eastern variety more often results in encephalitis with higher case fatality and sequelae rates. The 1st phase of illness is characterized by fever, headache, myalgia, malaise, nausea, and vomiting for 2–7 days. Fever disappears and after 2–8 days may return accompanied by vomiting, photophobia, and signs of meningeal irritation in children and more severe encephalitic signs in adults. This phase rarely lasts more than 1 wk.

DIAGNOSIS. The diagnosis of TBE should be suspected in patients reporting a tick bite in endemic areas during the transmission season. The etiologic diagnosis of TBE is established by testing an acute-phase serum collected early in the illness for the presence of virus-specific IgM antibodies or, alternatively, demonstrating a 4-fold or greater increase in IgG antibody titers by testing paired acute and convalescent sera. The virus can also be identified by PCR.

TREATMENT. There is no specific treatment for TBE. The treatment is intensive supportive care (see Chapter 66), including control of seizures (see Chapter 593).

PROGNOSIS. The main risk for fatal outcome is advanced age; the fatality rate in adults is about 1%, but sequelae in children are rare. Transient unilateral paralysis of an upper extremity is a common finding in adults. Common sequelae include chronic fatigue, headache, sleep disorders, and emotional disturbances.

PREVENTION. Specific Ig has been given to persons with seasonal tick bite exposure, although efficacy of this preventive therapy is not well studied. Effective inactivated vaccines for human use, made from virus grown in tissue culture, are licensed in Russia and Europe. They are administered in a 3 dose series similar to JE vaccine.

Bista MB, Banerjee MK, Shin SH, et al: Efficacy of a single dose of SA 14–14–2 live-attenuated Japanese encephalitis vaccine: A case-control study. *Lancet* 2001;358:791–795.

Centers for Disease Control and Prevention: Inactivated Japanese encephalitis virus vaccine. Recommendations of the Advisory Committee on Immunization Practices (ACIP). *MMWR* 1993;42(RR-1):1–15.

Innis BL, Nisalak A, Nimmannitya S, et al: An enzyme-linked immunosorbent assay to characterize dengue infections where dengue and Japanese encephalitis co-circulate. *Am J Trop Med Hyg* 1989;40:418–427.

Kluger G, Schottler A, Waldvogel K, et al: Tickborne encephalitis despite specific immunoglobulin prophylaxis. *Lancet* 1995;346:1502.

McNeil JG, Lednar WM, Stansfield SK, et al: Central European tick-borne encephalitis: Assessment of risk for persons in the armed forces and vacationers. *J Infect Dis* 1985;152:650–651.

Paul WS, Moore PS, Karabatsos N, et al: Outbreak of Japanese encephalitis on the island of Saipan, 1990. *J Infect Dis* 1993;167:1053–1058.

Poland JD, Cropp CB, Craven RB, et al: Evaluation of the potency and safety of inactivated Japanese encephalitis vaccine in U.S. inhabitants. *J Infect Dis* 1990;161:878–882.

Rico-Hesse R, Weaver SC, de Siger J, et al: Emergence of a new epidemic/epizootic of Venezuelan equine encephalitis virus in South America. *Proc Natl Acad Sci U S A* 1995;92:5278–5281.

Siegel-Itzkovich J: Twelve die of West Nile virus in Israel. *Br Med J* 2000;321:724.

Tsai TF: Arboviral infections: General considerations for prevention, diagnosis and treatment in travelers. *Semin Pediatr Infect Dis* 1992;3:62–69.

Tsai TF, Popovici F, Cerescu C, et al: West Nile encephalitis epidemic in southeastern Romania. *Lancet* 1998;352:767–771.

Chapter 266 ■ Dengue Fever and Dengue Hemorrhagic Fever

Scott B. Halstead

Dengue fever, a benign syndrome caused by several arthropod-borne viruses, is characterized by biphasic fever, myalgia or arthralgia, rash, leukopenia, and lymphadenopathy. **Dengue hemorrhagic fever** (Philippine, Thai, or Singapore hemorrhagic fever; hemorrhagic dengue; acute infectious thrombocytopenic purpura) is a severe, often fatal, febrile disease caused by dengue viruses. It is characterized by capillary permeability, abnormalities of hemostasis, and, in severe cases, a protein-losing shock syndrome (**dengue shock syndrome**), which is thought to have an immunopathologic basis.

ETIOLOGY. There are at least 4 distinct antigenic types of dengue virus, members of the family Flaviviridae. In addition, 3 other arthropod-borne viruses (arboviruses) cause similar or identical febrile diseases with rash (Table 266-1).

EPIDEMIOLOGY. Dengue viruses are transmitted by mosquitoes of the Stegomyia family. *Aedes aegypti,* a daytime biting mosquito, is the principal vector, and all 4 virus types have been recovered from it. In most tropical areas, *A. aegypti* is highly urbanized, breeding in water stored for drinking or bathing and in rainwater collected in any container. Dengue viruses have also been recovered from *Aedes albopictus,* as in the 2001 Hawaiian epidemic, while outbreaks in the Pacific area have been attributed to several other *Aedes* species. These species breed in water trapped in vegetation. In Southeast Asia and West Africa, dengue may be maintained in a cycle involving canopy-feeding jungle monkeys and *Aedes* species, which feed on monkeys.

Epidemics were common in temperate areas of the Americas, Europe, Australia, and Asia until early in the 20th century. Dengue fever and dengue-like disease are now endemic in tropical Asia, the South Pacific Islands, northern Australia, tropical Africa, the Caribbean, and Central and South America. Dengue fever occurs frequently among travelers to these areas.

Dengue outbreaks in urban areas infested with *A. aegypti* may be explosive; up to 70–80% of the population may be involved. Most disease occurs in older children and adults. Because *A. aegypti* has a limited flight range, spread of an epidemic occurs mainly through viremic human beings and follows the main lines of transportation. Sentinel cases may infect household mosquitoes; a large number of nearly simultaneous secondary infections give the appearance of a contagious disease. Where dengue is endemic, children and susceptible foreigners may be the only persons to acquire overt disease, adults having become immune.

Dengue-Like Diseases. Dengue-like diseases may also occur in epidemics. Epidemiologic features depend on the vectors and their geographic distribution (see Table 266-1). Chikungunya virus is widespread in the most populous areas of the world. In Asia, *A. aegypti* is the principal vector; in Africa, other Stegomyia species may be important vectors. In Southeast Asia, dengue and chikungunya outbreaks occur concurrently. Outbreaks of o'nyong-nyong and West Nile fever usually involve villages or small towns, in contrast to the urban outbreaks of dengue and chikungunya.

Dengue Hemorrhagic Fever. Dengue hemorrhagic fever occurs where multiple types of dengue virus are simultaneously or sequentially transmitted. Currently, it is endemic in all of tropical America and Asia, where warm temperatures and the practices of water storage in homes plus outdoor breeding sites result in large, permanent populations of *A. aegypti.* Under these conditions, infections with dengue viruses of all types are common, and 2nd infections with heterologous types are frequent.

Second dengue infections are relatively mild in the majority of instances, ranging from an inapparent infection through an undifferentiated upper respiratory tract or dengue-like disease, but may also progress to dengue hemorrhagic fever. Nonimmune foreigners, adults and children, exposed to dengue virus during outbreaks of hemorrhagic fever have classic dengue fever or even milder disease. The differences in clinical manifestations of dengue infections between natives and foreigners in Southeast Asia are related more to immunologic status than to racial susceptibility. Dengue hemorrhagic fever can occur during primary dengue infections, most frequently in infants whose mothers are immune to dengue.

Dengue 3 virus strains circulating in mainland Southeast Asia since 1983 are associated with a particularly severe clinical syndrome, characterized by encephalopathy, hypoglycemia, markedly elevated liver enzymes, and, occasionally, jaundice.

PATHOGENESIS. Fatalities with chikungunya and West Nile fever infections have been ascribed to viral encephalitis or hemorrhage.

The pathogenesis is incompletely understood, but epidemiologic studies suggest that it is usually associated with 2nd infections with dengue types 1–4. In the Americas, dengue hemorrhagic fever and dengue shock syndrome have been associated with dengue types 1–4 strains of recent Southeast Asian origin. Recent occurrences of sizable dengue hemorrhagic fever outbreaks in India, Pakistan, and Bangladesh also appear to be related to imported dengue strains. Dengue viruses demonstrate enhanced growth in cultures of human mononuclear phagocytes prepared from dengue-immune donors or in cultures supplemented with non-neutralizing dengue antibodies. Retrospective studies of sera from human mothers whose infants acquired dengue hemorrhagic fever or prospective studies in children acquiring sequential dengue infections have shown that the circulation of infection-enhancing antibodies at the time of infection is the strongest risk factor for development of severe disease. Absence of cross-reactive neutralizing antibodies and presences of enhancing antibodies from passive transfer or active production is the best correlate of risk for dengue hemorrhagic fever. Monkeys infected sequentially or receiving small quantities of enhancing antibodies have enhanced viremias. In humans studied early during the course of secondary dengue infections, viremia levels directly predicted disease severity. Early in the acute stage of secondary dengue infections, there is rapid activation of the complement system. Shortly before or during shock, blood levels of soluble tumor necrosis factor receptor, interferon-γ, and interleukin 2 are elevated. C1q, C3, C4, C5–C8, and C3 proactivators are depressed, and C3 catabolic rates are elevated. These factors may interact at the endothelial cell to produce increased vascular permeability through the nitric oxide final pathway. The blood clotting and fibrinolytic systems are activated, and levels of factor XII (Hageman factor) are depressed. The mechanism of bleeding in dengue hemorrhagic fever is not known, but a mild degree of disseminated intravascular coagulation, liver damage, and thrombocytopenia may operate synergistically. Capillary damage allows fluid, electrolytes, small proteins, and, in some instances, red cells to leak into extravascular spaces. This internal redistribution of fluid, together with deficits caused by fasting,

TABLE 266-1. Vectors and Geographic Distribution of Dengue-like Diseases

VIRUS	GEOGRAPHIC GENUS AND DISEASE	VECTOR	DISTRIBUTION
Togavirus	Chikungunya	*Aedes aegypti* *Aedes africanus*	Africa, India, Southeast Asia
Togavirus	O'nyong-nyong	*Anopheles funestus*	East Africa
Flavivirus	West Nile fever	*Culex molestus* *Culex univittatus*	Europe, Africa, Middle East, India

thirsting, and vomiting, results in hemoconcentration, hypovolemia, increased cardiac work, tissue hypoxia, metabolic acidosis, and hyponatremia.

Usually no pathologic lesions are found to account for death. In rare instances, death may be due to gastrointestinal or intracranial hemorrhages. Minimal to moderate hemorrhages are seen in the upper gastrointestinal tract, and petechial hemorrhages are common in the interventricular septum of the heart, on the pericardium, and on the subserosal surfaces of major viscera. Focal hemorrhages are occasionally seen in the lungs, liver, adrenals, and subarachnoid space. The liver is usually enlarged, often with fatty changes. Yellow, watery, and at times blood-tinged effusions are present in serous cavities in about 3/4 of patients.

Microscopically, there is perivascular edema in the soft tissues and widespread diapedesis of red cells. There may be maturational arrest of megakaryocytes in bone marrow, and increased numbers of them are seen in capillaries of the lungs, in renal glomeruli, and in sinusoids of the liver and spleen.

Dengue virus is frequently absent in tissues at the time of death; viral antigens or RNA have been localized in liver and lymphatic tissues.

CLINICAL MANIFESTATIONS. The incubation period is 1–7 days. The clinical manifestations are variable and are influenced by the age of the patient. In infants and young children, the disease may be undifferentiated or characterized by fever for 1–5 days, pharyngeal inflammation, rhinitis, and mild cough. A majority of infected older children and adults experience sudden onset of fever, with temperature rapidly increasing to 39.4–41.1°C (103–106°F), usually accompanied by frontal or retro-orbital pain, particularly when pressure is applied to the eyes. Occasionally, severe back pain precedes the fever (back-break fever). A transient, macular, generalized rash that blanches under pressure may be seen during the 1st 24–48 hr of fever. The pulse rate may be slow relative to the degree of fever. Myalgia and arthralgia occur soon after the onset and increase in severity. Joint symptoms may be particularly severe in patients with chikungunya or o'nyong-nyong infection. From the 2nd to 6th days of fever, nausea and vomiting are apt to occur, and generalized lymphadenopathy, cutaneous hyperesthesia or hyperalgesia, taste aberrations, and pronounced anorexia may develop.

About 1–2 days after defervescence, a generalized, morbilliform, maculopapular rash appears that spares the palms and soles. It disappears in 1–5 days; desquamation may occur. Rarely there is edema of the palms and soles. About the time this 2nd rash appears, the body temperature, which has previously decreased to normal, may become slightly elevated and demonstrate the characteristic biphasic temperature pattern.

Dengue Hemorrhagic Fever. Differentiation between dengue fever and dengue hemorrhagic fever is difficult early in the course of illness. A relatively mild 1st phase with abrupt onset of fever, malaise, vomiting, headache, anorexia, and cough is followed after 2–5 days by rapid clinical deterioration and collapse. In this 2nd phase, the patient usually has cold, clammy extremities, a warm trunk, flushed face, diaphoresis, restlessness, irritability, and mid-epigastric pain. Frequently, there are scattered petechiae on the forehead and extremities; spontaneous ecchymoses may appear, and easy bruising and bleeding at sites of venipuncture are common. A macular or maculopapular rash may appear, and there may be circumoral and peripheral cyanosis. Respirations are rapid and often labored. The pulse is weak, rapid, and thready and the heart sounds faint. The liver may enlarge to 4–6 cm below the costal margin and is usually firm and somewhat tender. Approximately 20–30% of cases of dengue hemorrhagic fever are complicated by shock (dengue shock syndrome). Fewer than 10% of patients have gross ecchymosis or gastrointestinal bleeding, usually after a period of uncorrected shock. After a 24–36 hr period of crisis, convalescence is fairly rapid in the children who recover. The temperature may return to normal before or during the stage of shock. Bradycardia and ventricular extrasystoles are common during convalescence.

DIAGNOSIS. A clinical diagnosis of dengue fever derives from a high index of suspicion and a knowledge of the geographic distribution and environmental cycles of causal viruses. Because clinical findings vary and there are many possible causative agents, the term *dengue-like disease* should be used until a specific diagnosis is established.

The World Health Organization criteria for dengue hemorrhagic fever are fever, minor or major hemorrhagic manifestations, thrombocytopenia (≤100,000/mm^3), and objective evidence of increased capillary permeability (hematocrit increased by ≥20%), serosal effusion (by chest radiography or ultrasonography), or hypoalbuminemia. Dengue shock syndrome criteria include those for dengue hemorrhagic fever as well as hypotension or narrow pulse pressure (≤20 mm Hg).

Virologic diagnosis can be established by serologic tests or by isolation of the virus from blood leukocytes or serum. In both primary and secondary dengue infections, there is a relatively transient appearance of antidengue immunoglobulin M (IgM) antibodies. These disappear after 6–12 wk, which can be used to time a dengue infection. In 2nd primary dengue infections, most antibody is of the IgG class. Serologic diagnosis depends on a 4-fold or greater increase in IgG antibody titer in paired sera by hemagglutination inhibition, complement fixation, enzyme immunoassay, or neutralization test. Carefully standardized IgM and IgG capture enzyme immunoassays are now widely used to identify acute-phase antibodies from patients with primary or secondary dengue infections in single-serum samples. Usually such samples should be collected not earlier than 5 days nor later than 6 wk after onset. It may not be possible to distinguish the infecting virus by serologic methods alone, particularly when there has been prior infection with another member of the same arbovirus group. Virus can be recovered from acute-phase serum after inoculating tissue culture or living mosquitoes. Viral RNA can be detected in blood or tissues by specific complementary RNA probes or amplified first by the polymerase chain reaction (PCR) or by real-time PCR.

DIFFERENTIAL DIAGNOSIS. The differential diagnosis of dengue fever includes viral respiratory and influenza-like diseases, the early stages of malaria, mild yellow fever, scrub typhus, viral hepatitis, and leptospirosis.

Four arboviral diseases have dengue-like courses but without rash: Colorado tick fever, sandfly fever, Rift Valley fever, and Ross River fever. Colorado tick fever occurs sporadically among campers and hunters in the western USA; sandfly fever in the Mediterranean region, the Middle East, southern Russia, and parts of the Indian subcontinent; and Rift Valley fever in North, East, Central, and South Africa. Ross River fever is endemic in much of eastern Australia, with epidemic extension to Fiji. In adults, Ross River fever often produces protracted and crippling arthralgia involving weight-bearing joints.

Because meningococcemia, yellow fever (see Chapter 267), other viral hemorrhagic fevers (see Chapter 268), many rickettsial diseases, and other severe illnesses caused by a variety of agents may produce a clinical picture similar to dengue hemorrhagic fever, the etiologic diagnosis should be made only when epidemiologic or serologic evidence suggests the possibility of a dengue infection.

LABORATORY FINDINGS. In dengue fever, pancytopenia may occur after the 3–4 days of illness. Neutropenia may persist or reappear during the latter stage of the disease and may continue into convalescence with white blood cell counts of <2,000/mm^3. Platelets rarely fall below 100,000/mm^3. Venous clotting, bleeding and prothrombin times, and plasma fibrinogen values are within normal ranges. The tourniquet test result may be positive. Mild acidosis, hemoconcentration, increased transaminase values, and hypoproteinemia may occur during some primary dengue virus infections. The electrocardiogram may show sinus bradycardia, ectopic ventricular foci, flattened T waves, and prolongation of the P-R interval.

The most common hematologic abnormalities during dengue hemorrhagic fever and dengue shock syndrome are hemoconcentration with an increase of >20% in hematocrit, thrombocytopenia, prolonged bleeding time, and moderately decreased prothrombin level that is seldom <40% of control. Fibrinogen levels may be subnormal and fibrin split products elevated. Other abnormalities include moderate elevations of the serum transaminase levels, consumption of complement, mild metabolic acidosis with hyponatremia, occasionally hypochloremia, slight elevation of serum urea nitrogen, and hypoalbuminemia. Roentgenograms of the chest reveal pleural effusions (left > right) in nearly all patients with dengue shock syndrome.

TREATMENT. Treatment of uncomplicated dengue fever is supportive. Bed rest is advised during the febrile period. Antipyretics should be used to keep body temperature <40°C (104°F). Analgesics or mild sedation may be required to control pain. Aspirin is contraindicated and should not be used because of its effects on hemostasis. Fluid and electrolyte replacement is required for deficits caused by sweating, fasting, thirsting, vomiting, and diarrhea.

Dengue Hemorrhagic Fever. Management of dengue hemorrhagic fever and dengue shock syndrome includes immediate evaluation of vital signs and degrees of hemoconcentration, dehydration, and electrolyte imbalance. Close monitoring is essential for at least 48 hr because shock may occur or recur precipitously early in the disease. Patients who are cyanotic or have labored breathing should be given oxygen. Rapid intravenous replacement of fluids and electrolytes can frequently sustain patients until spontaneous recovery occurs. Normal saline is more effective in treating shock than the more expensive Ringer lactated saline. When pulse pressure is ≤10 mm Hg, or when elevation of the hematocrit persists after replacement of fluids, plasma or colloid preparations are indicated.

Care must be taken to avoid overhydration, which may contribute to cardiac failure. Transfusions of fresh blood or platelets suspended in plasma may be required to control bleeding; they should not be given during hemoconcentration, but only after evaluation of hemoglobin or hematocrit values. Salicylates are contraindicated because of their effect on blood clotting.

Paraldehyde or chloral hydrate may be required for children who are markedly agitated. Use of vasopressors has not resulted in a significant reduction of mortality compared with that observed with simple supportive therapy. Disseminated intravascular coagulation may require treatment (see Chapter 483). Corticosteroids do not shorten the duration of disease or improve prognosis in children receiving careful supportive therapy.

Hypervolemia during the fluid reabsorptive phase may be life threatening and is heralded by a decrease in hematocrit with wide pulse pressure. Diuretics and digitalization may be necessary.

COMPLICATIONS. Primary infections with dengue fever and dengue-like diseases are usually self-limited and benign. Fluid and electrolyte losses, hyperpyrexia, and febrile convulsions are the most frequent complications in infants and young children. Epistaxis, petechiae, and purpuric lesions are uncommon but may occur at any stage. Swallowed blood from epistaxis, vomited or passed by rectum, may be erroneously interpreted as gastrointestinal bleeding. In adults and possibly in children, underlying conditions may lead to clinically significant bleeding. Convulsions may occur during high temperature, especially with chikungunya fever. Infrequently, after the febrile stage, prolonged asthenia, mental depression, bradycardia, and ventricular extrasystoles may occur in children.

In endemic areas, dengue hemorrhagic fever should be suspected in children with a febrile illness suggestive of dengue fever who experience hemoconcentration and thrombocytopenia.

PROGNOSIS. The prognosis of dengue fever may be adversely affected by passively acquired antibody or by prior infection with a closely related virus that predisposes to development of dengue hemorrhagic fever.

Dengue Hemorrhagic Fever. Death has occurred in 40–50% of patients with shock, but with adequate intensive care deaths should occur in <1% of cases. Survival is directly related to early and intense supportive treatment. Infrequently, there is residual brain damage caused by prolonged shock or occasionally by intracranial hemorrhage.

PREVENTION. Several types of dengue type 1–4 vaccines are under development, and a killed vaccine for chikungunya is efficacious but not licensed. Prophylaxis consists of avoiding **mosquito bites** by use of insecticides, repellents, body covering with clothing, screening of houses, and destruction of *A. aegypti* breeding sites. If water storage is mandatory, a tight-fitting lid or a thin layer of oil may prevent egg laying or hatching. A larvicide, such as Abate [O,O′-(thiodi-p-phenylene) O,O,O,O′-tetramethyl phosphorothioate], available as a 1% sand-granule formation and effective at a concentration of 1 ppm, may be added safely to drinking water. Ultra-low-volume spray equipment effectively dispenses the adulticide malathion from truck or airplane for rapid intervention during an epidemic. Only personal antimosquito measures are effective against mosquitoes in the field, forest, or jungle.

The possibility exists that dengue vaccination may sensitize a recipient so that ensuing dengue infection could result in hemorrhagic fever. Vaccination with yellow fever 17D strain has no effect on the severity of dengue illness, although seroconversion rates to a dengue type 2 vaccine were enhanced in persons immune to yellow fever.

Bethell DB, Gamble J, Pham PL, et al: Noninvasive measurement of microvascular leakage in patients with dengue hemorrhagic fever. *Clin Infect Dis* 2001;32:243–253.

Blaney JE Jr, Matro JM, Murphy BR, Whitehead SS: Recombinant, live-attenuated tetravalent dengue vaccine formulations induce a balanced, broad and protective neutralizing antibody response against each of the four serotypes in rhesus monkeys. *J Virol* 2005;79:5516–5528.

Dung NM, Day NP, Tam DT, et al: Fluid replacement in dengue shock syndrome: A randomized, double-blind comparison of four intravenous-fluid regimens. *Clin Infect Dis* 1999;29:787–794.

Guirakhoo F, Pugachev K, Zhang Z, et al: Safety and efficacy of chimeric yellow fever—Dengue virus tetravalent vaccine formulations in nonhuman primates. *J Virol* 2004;78:461–475.

Guzman Mg, Kouri G, Valdes L, et al: Epidemiological studies on dengue in Santiago de Cuba, 1997. *Am J Epidemiol* 2000;152:793–799.

Hales S, van Panhuis W: A new strategy for dengue control. *Lancet* 2005; 365:551–552.

Halstead SB: Dengue—the case definition delemma: a commentary. *Pediatr Infect Dis J* 2007;26:291–292.

Kliks SC, Nisalak A, Brandt WE, et al: Evidence that maternal dengue antibodies are important in the development of dengue hemorrhagic fever in infants. *Am J Trop Med Hyg* 1988;38:411–419.

Kochel T, Watts DG, Halstead SB, et al: Effect of dengue-1 antibodies on American dengue-2 viral infection and dengue haemorrhagic fever. *Lancet* 2002;360:310–312.

Monath TP, McCarthy K, Bedford P, et al: Clinical proof of principle for ChimeriVax: Recombinant live, attenuated vaccines against flavivirus infections. *Vaccine* 2002;20:1004–1018.

Vaughn DW, Green S, Kalayanarooj S, et al: Dengue viremia titer, antibody response pattern and virus serotype correlate with disease severity. *J Infect Dis* 2000;181:2–9.

Watts D, Porter K, Putvatana R, et al: Failure of secondary infections with American genotype dengue 2 viruses to cause dengue haemorrhagic fever. *Lancet* 1999;354:1431–1434.
Wilder-Smith A, Schwartz E: Dengue in travelers. *N Engl J Med* 2005;353: 924–933.
Wills BA, Dung NM, Loon HT, et al: Comparison of three fluid solutions for resuscitation in dengue shock syndrome. *N Engl J Med* 2005;353:877–889.

Chapter 267 ■ Yellow Fever

Scott B. Halstead

Yellow fever is an acute infection characterized in its most severe form by fever, jaundice, proteinuria, and hemorrhage. The virus is mosquito borne and occurs in epidemic or endemic form in South America and Africa. Seasonal epidemics occurred in cities located in temperate areas of Europe and the Americas until 1900, and epidemics continue in West, Central, and East Africa.

ETIOLOGY. Yellow fever is the prototype of the Flavivirus genus of the family Flaviviridae, which are enveloped single-stranded RNA viruses 35–50 nm in diameter.

Yellow fever circulates zoonotically as 3 genotypes: type I in Central Africa, type IIA in West Africa, and type IIB in South America. Type IIA virus is capable of urban transmission between human beings by *Aedes aegypti*. Sometime in the 1600s this virus was brought to the American tropics through the African slave trade. Subsequently, yellow fever caused enormous coastal and riverine epidemics until the 20th century, when the virus and its urban and sylvan mosquito cycles were identified and a vaccine and mosquito control developed.

EPIDEMIOLOGY. Human and nonhuman primate hosts acquire the infection by the bite of infected mosquitoes. After an incubation period of 3–6 days, virus appears in the blood and may serve as a source of infection for other mosquitoes. The virus must replicate in the gut of the mosquito and pass to the salivary gland before the mosquito can transmit the virus. Yellow fever virus is transmitted in an urban cycle—human to *A. aegypti* to human—and a jungle cycle—monkey to jungle mosquitoes to monkey. Classic yellow fever epidemics in the United States, South America, the Caribbean, and parts of Europe were of the urban variety. Since 2000, West Africa has experienced 5 urban epidemics, including the capital cities of Abidjan (Cote d'Ivoire), Conakry (Guinea), and Dakar (Senegal). Most of the approximately 200 cases reported each year in South America are jungle yellow fever. In colonial times, attack rates in white adults were very high, suggesting that subclinical infections are uncommon in this age group. Yellow fever may be less severe in children, with subclinical infection–to–clinical case ratios of ≥2 : 1. In areas where outbreaks of urban yellow fever are common, most cases involve children because many adults are immune. Transmission in West Africa is highest during the rainy season, from July to November. The migration of nonimmune laborers into endemic regions is a significant factor in some outbreaks.

In tropical forests, yellow fever virus is maintained in a transmission cycle involving monkeys and tree hole–breeding mosquitoes (*Haemagogus* in Central and South America, *Aedes africanus* in Africa). In the Americas, most cases involve men who work in forested areas and are exposed to infected mosquitoes. In Africa, the virus is prevalent in moist savanna and savanna transition areas where other tree hole–breeding *Aedes* vectors transmit the virus between monkeys and humans and between humans.

PATHOGENESIS. Pathologic changes seen in the liver include (1) coagulative necrosis of hepatocytes in the midzone of the liver lobule, with sparing of cells around the portal areas and central veins; (2) eosinophilic degeneration of hepatocytes (**Councilman bodies**); (3) microvacuolar fatty change; and (4) minimal inflammation. The kidneys show acute tubular necrosis. In the heart, myocardial fiber degeneration and fatty infiltration are seen. The brain may show edema and petechial hemorrhages. Direct viral injury to the liver results in impaired ability to perform functions of biosynthesis and detoxification; this is the central pathogenic event of yellow fever. Hemorrhage is thought to result from decreased synthesis of vitamin K–dependent clotting factors and, in some cases, disseminated intravascular clotting. Renal dysfunction has been attributed to hemodynamic factors (prerenal failure progressing to acute tubular necrosis). The pathogenesis of shock in patients with yellow fever appears to be similar to that described in dengue shock syndrome and the other viral hemorrhagic fevers.

CLINICAL MANIFESTATIONS. In Africa, inapparent, abortive, or clinically mild infections are frequent; some studies suggest that children experience a milder disease than adults do. Abortive infections, characterized by fever and headache, may be unrecognized except during epidemics.

In its classic form, yellow fever begins with sudden onset of fever, headache, myalgia, lumbosacral pain, anorexia, nausea, and vomiting. Physical findings during the early phase of illness, when virus is present in the blood, include prostration, conjunctival injection, flushing of face and neck, reddening of the tongue at the tip and edges, and relative bradycardia. After 2–3 days, there may be a brief period of remission, followed in 6–24 hr by reappearance of fever with vomiting, epigastric pain, jaundice, dehydration, gastrointestinal and other hemorrhages, albuminuria, hypotension, renal failure, delirium, convulsions, and coma. Death may occur after 7–10 days, with the fatality rate in severe cases approaching 50%. Some patients who survive the acute phase of illness later succumb to renal failure or myocardial damage. Laboratory abnormalities include leukopenia; prolonged clotting, prothrombin, and partial thromboplastin times; thrombocytopenia; hyperbilirubinemia; elevated serum transaminases; albuminuria; and azotemia. Hypoglycemia may be present in severe cases. Electrocardiogram abnormalities of bradycardia and ST-T changes are described.

DIAGNOSIS. Yellow fever should be suspected when fever, headache, vomiting, myalgia, and jaundice appear in residents of endemic areas or in unimmunized visitors who have recently traveled (within 2 wk before onset of symptoms) to endemic areas. Clinically, yellow fever is quite similar to dengue hemorrhagic fever. In contrast to the gradual onset of acute viral hepatitis resulting from hepatitis A, B, C, D, or E viruses, jaundice in yellow fever appears after 3–5 days of high temperature and is often accompanied by severe prostration. Mild yellow fever is dengue-like and cannot be distinguished from a wide variety of other infections. Jaundice and fever may occur in any of several other tropical diseases, including malaria, viral hepatitis, louse-borne relapsing fever, leptospirosis, typhoid fever, rickettsial infections, certain systemic bacterial infections, sickle cell crisis, Rift Valley fever, Crimean-Congo hemorrhagic fever, and other viral hemorrhagic fevers. Outbreaks of yellow fever always include cases with severe gastrointestinal hemorrhage.

Specific diagnosis depends on detection of virus or viral antigen in acute-phase blood samples or antibody assays. The immunoglobulin M enzyme immunoassay is particularly useful. Sera obtained during the 1st 10 days after onset of symptoms should be kept in an ultra-low-temperature freezer (−70°C) and shipped on dry ice for virus testing. Convalescent-phase samples for antibody tests are managed by conventional means. In handling acute-phase blood specimens, medical personnel must take care to avoid contaminating themselves or others on the evacuation trail (laboratory personnel and others). Postmortem diagnosis is based on virus isolation from liver or blood, identification of Councilman bodies in liver tissue, or detection of antigen or viral genome in liver tissue.

TREATMENT. It is customary to keep yellow fever patients in a mosquito-free area, using mosquito nets if necessary. Patients are viremic during the febrile phase of the illness. Although there is no specific treatment for yellow fever, medical care is directed at maintaining physiologic status: (1) sponging and acetaminophen to reduce high temperature, (2) vigorous fluid replacement of losses resulting from fasting, thirsting, vomiting, or plasma leakage, (3) correcting acid-base imbalance, (4) maintaining nutritional intake to lessen the severity of hypoglycemia, and (5) avoiding drugs that are either metabolized by the liver or toxic to the liver, kidney, or central nervous system.

COMPLICATIONS. Complications of acute yellow fever include severe hemorrhage, liver failure, and acute renal failure. Bleeding should be managed by transfusion of fresh whole blood or fresh plasma with platelet concentrates if necessary. Renal failure may require peritoneal dialysis or hemodialysis.

PREVENTION. Yellow fever 17D is a live-attenuated vaccine with a record of safety and efficacy. It is administered as a single 0.5 mL subcutaneous injection at least 10 days before arrival in a yellow fever–endemic area. With exceptions noted below, individuals traveling to endemic areas in South America and Africa should be considered for vaccination, but length of stay, exact locations to be visited, and environmental or occupational exposure may determine the specific risk and individual need for vaccination. Persons traveling from yellow fever–endemic to yellow fever–receptive countries may be required to obtain a yellow fever vaccine (from South America or Africa to India). Usually countries that require travelers to obtain a yellow fever immunization do not issue a visa without a valid immunization certificate. Vaccination is valid for 10 yr for international travel certification, although immunity lasts at least 40 yr and probably for life.

Since 1996, there have been 14 reports of **yellow fever vaccine–associated viscerotropic disease** with higher risk in elderly vaccine recipients and in persons with previous thymectomies. Yellow fever vaccine should not be administered to persons with symptomatic immunodeficiency diseases, those taking immunosuppressant drugs, or persons with a history of thymectomy. Although the vaccine is not known to harm fetuses, its administration during pregnancy is not advised. In very young children, there is a small risk for encephalitis and death after yellow fever 17D vaccination. The 17D vaccine should not be administered to infants younger than 4 mo. Residence or travel to areas of known or anticipated yellow fever activity (e.g., forested areas in the Amazon basin), which places an individual at high risk, warrants immunization of infants 4–9 mo of age. Immunization of children ≥9 mo of age is routinely recommended before entry into endemic areas. Immunization of persons >60 yr of age should be weighed against their risk for sylvatic yellow fever in the American tropics and for urban or sylvatic yellow fever in Africa. Vaccination should be avoided for persons with a history of egg allergy. Alternatively, a skin test can be performed to determine whether a serious allergy exists that would preclude vaccination.

Barrett AD, Monath TP. Epidemiology and ecology of yellow fever virus. *Adv Virus Res* 2003;61:291–315.
Barwick R, Eidex RB: for the Yellow Fever Vaccine Working Safety Group: History of thymoma and yellow fever vaccination. *Lancet* 2004;364:936.
Centers for Disease Control and Prevention: Yellow fever vaccine. Recommendations of the Advisory Committee on Immunization Practices (ACIP), 2002. *MMWR* 2002(RR-17);51:1–11.
Khromava AY, Eidex RB, Weld LH, et al: Yellow fever vaccine and updated assessment of advanced age as a risk factor for serious adverse events. *Vaccine* 2005;23:3256–3263.
Marfin AA, Eidex RS, Kozarsky PE, Cetron MS: Yellow fever and Japanese encephalitis vaccines: Indications and complications. *Infect Dis Clin North Am* 2005;19:151–168.
Martin M, Weld LH, Tsai TF, et al: Advanced age as a risk factor for illness temporally associated with yellow fever vaccination. *Emerg Infect Dis* 2001;7:945–951.
Monath TP: Yellow fever: A medically neglected disease. Report on a seminar. *Rev Infect Dis* 1987;9:165–175.
Monath TP: Yellow fever and dengue: The interactions of virus, vector and host in the re-emergence of epidemic disease. *Semin Virol* 1994;5:133–145.
Mutebi JP, Rijnbrand RC, Wang H, et al: Genetic relationships and evolution of genotypes of yellow fever virus and other members of the yellow fever virus group within the Flavivirus genus based on the 3′ noncoding region. *J Virol* 2004;78:9652–9665.
World Health Organization: Progress in the control of yellow fever in Africa. *Wkly Epidemiol Rec* 2005;80:50–55.

Chapter 268 ■ Other Viral Hemorrhagic Fevers

Scott B. Halstead

Viral hemorrhagic fevers are a loosely defined group of clinical syndromes in which hemorrhagic manifestations are either common or especially notable in severe illness. Both the etiologic agents and clinical features of the syndromes differ, but disseminated intravascular coagulopathy may be a common pathogenetic feature.

ETIOLOGY. Six of the viral hemorrhagic fevers are caused by arthropod-borne viruses (arboviruses) (Table 268-1). Four are togaviruses of the family Flaviviridae, including Kyasanur Forest disease, Omsk, dengue (see Chapter 266), and yellow fever (see Chapter 267) viruses. Three are of the family Bunyaviridae, including Congo, Hantaan, and Rift Valley fever (RVF) viruses. Four are of the family Arenaviridae, including Junin, Machupo, Guanarito, and Lassa viruses. Two are of the family Filoviridae, including Ebola and Marburg viruses. The Filoviridae are enveloped, filamentous RNA viruses that are sometimes branched, unlike any other known virus.

TABLE 268-1. Viral Hemorrhage Fevers

MODE OF TRANSMISSION	DISEASE	VIRUS
Tick borne	Crimean-Congo HF*	Congo
	Kyasanur Forest disease	Kyasanur Forest disease
	Omsk HF	Omsk
Mosquito borne†	Dengue HF	Dengue (four types)
	Rift Valley fever	Rift Valley fever
	Yellow fever	Yellow fever
Infected animals or materials to humans		Argentine HF Junin
	Bolivian HF	Machupo
	Lassa fever*	Lassa
	Marburg disease*	Marburg
	Ebola HF*	Ebola
	Hemorrhagic fever with renal syndrome	Hantaan

*Patients may be contagious; nosocomial infections are common.
†Chikungunya virus is associated infrequently with petechiae and epistaxis. Severe hemorrhagic manifestations have been reported in some cases.
HF, hemorrhagic fever.

EPIDEMIOLOGY AND CLINICAL MANIFESTATIONS. With some exceptions, the viruses causing viral hemorrhagic fevers are transmitted to humans via a nonhuman entity. The specific ecosystem required for viral survival determines the geographic distribution of disease. Although it is commonly thought that all viral hemorrhagic fevers are arthropod borne, 7 may be contracted from environmental contamination caused by animals or animal cells or from infected humans (see Table 268-1). Laboratory and hospital infections have occurred with many of these agents. Lassa fever and Argentine and Bolivian hemorrhagic fevers are reportedly milder in children than in adults.

Crimean-Congo Hemorrhagic Fever. Sporadic human infection in Africa provided the original virus isolation. Natural foci are recognized in Bulgaria, western Crimea, and the Rostov-on-Don and Astrakhan regions; a somewhat similar disease occurs in Kazakhstan and Uzbekistan. Index cases were followed by nosocomial transmission in Pakistan and Afghanistan in 1976, in the Arabian Peninsula in 1983, and in South Africa in 1984. Outbreaks have been reported from Pakistan, Oman, and southern Russia. In the Russian Federation, the vectors are *Hyalomma marginatum* and *Hyalomma anatolicum,* which, along with hares and birds, may serve as viral reservoirs. Disease occurs from June to September, largely among farmers and dairy workers.

Kyasanur Forest Disease. Human cases occur chiefly in adults in an area of Mysore State, India. The main vectors are 2 Ixodidae ticks, *Haemaphysalis turturis* and *Haemaphysalis spinigera.* Monkeys and forest rodents may be amplifying hosts. Laboratory infections are common.

Omsk Hemorrhagic Fever. The disease occurs throughout south-central Russia and northern Romania. Vectors may include *Dermacentor pictus* and *Dermacentor marginatus,* but direct transmission from moles and muskrats to humans seems well established. Human disease occurs in a spring-summer-autumn pattern, paralleling the activity of vectors. This infection occurs most frequently in persons with outdoor occupational exposure. Laboratory infections are common.

Rift Valley Fever. The virus causing RVF is responsible for epizootics involving sheep, cattle, buffalo, certain antelopes, and rodents in North, Central, East, and South Africa. The virus is transmitted to domestic animals by *Culex theileri* and several *Aedes* species. Mosquitoes may serve as reservoirs by transovarial transmission. An epizootic in Egypt in 1977–1978 was accompanied by thousands of human infections, principally among veterinarians, farmers, and farm laborers. Smaller outbreaks occurred in Senegal in 1987, Madagascar in 1990, and Saudi Arabia and Yemen in 2000–2001. Humans are most often infected during the slaughter or skinning of sick or dead animals. Laboratory infection is common.

Argentine Hemorrhagic Fever. Before introduction of vaccine, hundreds to thousands of cases occurred annually from April through July in the maize-producing area northwest of Buenos Aires that reaches to the eastern margin of the Province of Cordoba. Junin virus has been isolated from the rodents *Mus musculus, Akodon arenicola,* and *Calomys laucha laucha.* It infects migrant laborers who harvest the maize and who inhabit rodent-contaminated shelters.

Bolivian Hemorrhagic Fever. The recognized endemic area consists of the sparsely populated province of Beni in Amazonian Bolivia. Sporadic cases occur in farm families who raise maize, rice, yucca, and beans. In the town of San Joaquin, a disturbance in the domestic rodent ecosystem may have led to an outbreak of household infection caused by *Calomys callosus,* ordinarily a field rodent. Mortality rates are high in young children.

Venezuelan Hemorrhagic Fever. In 1989, an outbreak of hemorrhagic illness occurred in the farming community of Guanarito, Venezuela, 200 miles south of Caracas. Subsequently, in 1990–1991, there were 104 cases reported with 26 deaths. Cotton rats *(Sigmodon alstoni)* and cane rats *(Zygodontomys brevicauda)* have been implicated as likely reservoirs.

Lassa Fever. Lassa virus has an unusual potential for human-to-human spread and has resulted in many small epidemics in Nigeria, Sierra Leone, and Liberia. Medical workers in Africa and the United States have also contracted the disease. Patients with acute Lassa fever have been transported by international aircraft, necessitating extensive surveillance among passengers and crews. The virus is probably maintained in nature in a species of African peridomestic rodent, *Mastomys natalensis.* Rodent-to-rodent transmission and infection of humans probably operate via mechanisms established for other arenaviruses.

Marburg Disease. Until recently, the world experience had been limited to 26 primary and 5 secondary cases in Germany and Yugoslavia in 1967, to small outbreaks in Zimbabwe in 1975, Kenya in 1980 and 1988, and South Africa in 1983. But, in 1999 a large outbreak occurred in Congo Republic and a still larger outbreak in Uige Province, Angola, with 351 cases and 312 deaths in 2005. In laboratory and clinical settings, transmission occurs by direct contact with tissues of the African green monkey or with infected human blood or semen. The reservoir and mode of transmission of the virus in nature are unknown.

Ebola Hemorrhagic Fever. Ebola virus was isolated in 1976 from a devastating epidemic involving small villages in northern Zaire and southern Sudan; smaller outbreaks have occurred subsequently. Outbreaks initially have been nosocomial. Attack rates have been highest in the birth to 1 yr and 15–50 yr old age groups. The virus is closely related to Marburg virus. Ebola virus has been particularly active recently, with an outbreak in Kikwit, Zaire, in 1995, followed recently by scattered outbreaks in Uganda and Central and West Africa. The virus has been recovered from chimpanzees and antibodies found in other subhuman primates, but these may not constitute a zoonotic reservoir. The mode of transmission to humans is unknown. Reston virus, related to Ebola, has been recovered from Philippine monkeys and has caused subclinical infections in workers in monkey colonies in the United States.

Hemorrhagic Fever with Renal Syndrome (HFRS). The endemic area of HFRS, also known as epidemic hemorrhagic fever and Korean hemorrhagic fever, includes Japan, Korea, far eastern Siberia, north and central China, European and Asian Russia, Scandinavia, Czechoslovakia, Romania, Bulgaria, Yugoslavia, and Greece. Although the incidence and severity of hemorrhagic manifestations and the mortality are lower in Europe than in northeastern Asia, the renal lesion is the same. Disease in Scandinavia, **nephropathia epidemica,** is caused by a different although antigenically related virus, Puumala virus, associated with the bank vole, *Clethrionomys glareolus.* Cases occur predominantly in the spring and summer. There appears to be no age factor in susceptibility, but because of occupational hazards, young adult men are most frequently attacked. Rodent plagues and evidence of rodent infestation have accompanied endemic and epidemic occurrences. Hantaan virus has been detected in lung tissue and excreta of *Apodemus agrarius coreae.* Antigenically related agents have been detected in laboratory rats and in urban rat populations around the world, including Prospect Hill virus in the wild rodent *Microtus pennsylvanicus* in North America and Sin Nombre virus in the deer mouse in the southern and southwestern USA; these viruses are causes of hantavirus pulmonary syndrome (see Chapter 270). Rodent-to-rodent and rodent-to-human transmission presumably occurs via the respiratory route.

CLINICAL MANIFESTATIONS. Dengue hemorrhagic fever (see Chapter 266) and yellow fever (see Chapter 267) cause similar syndromes in children in endemic areas.

Crimean-Congo Hemorrhagic Fever. The incubation period of 3–12 days is followed by a febrile period of 5–12 days and a prolonged convalescence. Illness begins suddenly with fever, severe headache, myalgia, abdominal pain, anorexia, nausea, and vomiting. After 1–2 days, fever may subside until the patient experiences an erythematous facial or truncal flush and injected conjunctivae. A 2nd febrile period of 2–6 days then develops, with a hemorrhagic enanthem on the soft palate and a fine petechial rash on the chest and abdomen. Less frequently, there are large areas of purpura and bleeding from the gums, nose, intestines, lungs, or uterus. Hematuria and proteinuria are relatively rare. During the hemorrhagic stage, there is usually tachycardia with diminished heart sounds and occasionally hypotension. The liver is usually enlarged, but there is no icterus. In protracted cases, central nervous system signs may include delirium, somnolence, and progressive clouding of consciousness. Early in the disease, leukopenia with relative lymphocytosis, progressively worsening thrombocytopenia, and gradually increasing anemia occur. In convalescence there may be hearing and memory loss. The mortality rate is 2–50%.

Kyasanur Forest Disease and Omsk Hemorrhagic Fever. After an incubation period of 3–8 days, both diseases begin with sudden onset of fever and headache. Kyasanur Forest disease is characterized by severe myalgia, prostration, and bronchiolar involvement; it often presents without hemorrhage but occasionally with severe gastrointestinal bleeding. In Omsk hemorrhagic fever, there is moderate epistaxis, hematemesis, and a hemorrhagic enanthem but no profuse hemorrhage; bronchopneumonia is common. In both diseases, severe leukopenia and thrombocytopenia, vascular dilatation, increased vascular permeability, gastrointestinal hemorrhages, and subserosal and interstitial petechial hemorrhages occur. Kyasanur Forest disease may be complicated by acute degeneration of renal tubules and focal liver damage. In many patients, recurrent febrile illness may follow an afebrile period of 7–15 days. This 2nd phase takes the form of a meningoencephalitis.

Rift Valley Fever. Most infections have occurred in adults with signs and symptoms resembling dengue fever (see Chapter 266). Onset is acute, with fever, headache, prostration, myalgia, anorexia, nausea, vomiting, conjunctivitis, and lymphadenopathy. The fever lasts 3–6 days and is often biphasic. Convalescence is often prolonged. In the 1977–1978 outbreak many patients died after showing signs that included purpura, epistaxis, hematemesis, and melena. RVF affects the uvea and posterior chorioretinal followed by macular scarring, vascular occlusion, and optic atrophy, resulting in permanent visual loss in a high proportion of patients with mild to severe RVF. At autopsy, there was extensive eosinophilic degeneration of the parenchymal cells of the liver.

Argentine, Venezuelan, and Bolivian Hemorrhagic Fever and Lassa Fever. The incubation period is commonly 7–14 days; the acute illness lasts for 2–4 wk. Clinical illnesses range from undifferentiated fever to the characteristic severe illness. **Lassa fever** is most often clinically severe in whites. Onset is usually gradual, with increasing fever, headache, diffuse myalgia, and anorexia (Table 268-2). During the 1st wk, signs frequently include a sore throat, dysphagia, cough, oropharyngeal ulcers, nausea, vomiting, diarrhea, and pains in the chest and abdomen. Pleuritic chest pain may persist for 2–3 wk. In Argentine and Bolivian hemorrhagic fevers, and less frequently in Lassa fever, a petechial enanthem appears on the soft palate 3–5 days after onset and at about the same time on the trunk. The tourniquet test may be positive. The clinical course of Venezuelan hemorrhagic fever has not been well described.

In 35–50% of all patients, these diseases may become severe, with persistent high temperature, increasing toxicity, swelling of the face or neck, microscopic hematuria, and frank hemorrhages from the stomach, intestines, nose, gums, and uterus. A syndrome of **hypovolemic shock** is accompanied by pleural effusion and renal failure. **Respiratory distress** resulting from airway obstruction, pleural effusion, or congestive heart failure may occur. A total of 10–20% of patients experience late neurologic involvement characterized by intention tremor of the tongue and associated speech abnormalities. In severe cases, there may be intention tremors of the extremities, seizures, and delirium. The cerebrospinal fluid is normal. In Lassa fever, nerve deafness occurs in early convalescence in 25% of cases. Prolonged convalescence is accompanied by alopecia, and in Argentine and Bolivian hemorrhagic fevers by signs of autonomic nervous system lability, such as postural hypotension, spontaneous flushing or blanching of the skin, and intermittent diaphoresis.

Laboratory studies reveal marked leukopenia, mild to moderate thrombocytopenia, proteinuria, and, in Argentine hemorrhagic fever, moderate abnormalities in blood clotting, decreased fibrinogen, increased fibrinogen split products, and elevated serum transaminases. There is focal, often extensive eosinophilic necrosis of liver parenchyma, focal interstitial pneumonitis, focal necrosis of the distal and collecting tubules, and partial replacement of splenic follicles by amorphous eosinophilic material. Usually bleeding occurs by diapedesis with little inflammatory reaction. The mortality rate is 10–40%.

Marburg Disease and Ebola Hemorrhagic Fever. After an incubation period of 4–7 days, illness begins abruptly with severe frontal headache, malaise, drowsiness, lumbar myalgia, vomiting, nausea, and diarrhea. A **maculopapular** eruption begins 5–7 days later on the trunk and upper arms. It becomes generalized, often hemorrhagic, and exfoliates during convalescence. The exanthem is accompanied by a dark red enanthem on the hard palate, conjunctivitis, and scrotal or labial edema. Gastrointestinal hemorrhage occurs as the severity of illness increases. Late in the illness, the patient may become tearfully depressed with marked hyperalgesia to tactile stimuli. In fatal cases, patients become hypotensive, restless, and confused and lapse into coma. Convalescent patients may experience alopecia and have paresthesias of the back and trunk. There is a marked leukopenia with necrosis of granulocytes. **Disseminated intravascular coagulation** and thrombocytopenia are universal and correlate with severity of disease; there are moderate abnormalities in clotting proteins and elevated serum transaminases and amylase. The mortality rate of Marburg disease is 25–85% and of Ebola hemorrhagic fever 50–90%. High viral loads in acute-phase blood samples convey a poor prognosis.

Hemorrhagic Fever with Renal Syndrome. In most cases, HFRS is characterized by fever, petechiae, mild hemorrhagic phenomena, and mild proteinuria, followed by relatively uneventful recovery. In 20% of recognized cases, the disease may progress through 4 distinct phases. The febrile phase is ushered in with fever, malaise, and facial and truncal flushing. It lasts 3–8 days and ends with thrombocytopenia, petechiae, and proteinuria. The hypotensive phase of 1–3 days follows defervescence. Loss of fluid from the intravascular compartment may result in marked hemoconcentration. Proteinuria and ecchymoses increase. The oliguric phase, usually 3–5 days in duration, is characterized by a low output of protein-rich urine, increasing nitrogen retention, nausea, vomiting, and dehydration. Confusion, extreme restlessness, and hypertension are common. The diuretic phase, which may last for days or weeks, usually initiates clinical improvement. The kidneys

TABLE 268-2. Clinical Stages of Lassa Fever

STAGE	SYMPTOMS
1 (days 1–3)	General weakness and malaise. High fever, >39°C, constant with peaks of 40–41°C
2 (days 4–7)	Sore throat (with white exudative patches) very common; headache; back, chest, side, or abdominal pain; conjunctivitis; nausea and vomiting; diarrhea; productive cough; proteinuria; low blood pressure (systolic <100 mm Hg); anemia
3 (after 7 days)	Facial edema; convulsions; mucosal bleeding (mouth, nose, eyes); internal bleeding; confusion or disorientation
4 (after 14 days)	Coma and death

From Richmond JK, Baglole DJ: Lassa fever: Epidemiology, clinical features, and social consequences. Br Med J 2003; 327: 1271–1275.

show little concentrating ability, and rapid loss of fluid may result in severe dehydration and shock. Potassium and sodium depletion may be severe. Fatal cases manifest as abundant protein-rich retroperitoneal edema and marked hemorrhagic necrosis of the renal medulla. The mortality rate is 5–10%.

DIAGNOSIS. Diagnosis depends on a high index of suspicion in endemic areas. In nonendemic areas, histories of recent travel, recent laboratory exposure, or exposure to an earlier case should evoke suspicion of a viral hemorrhagic fever.

In all viral hemorrhagic fevers, the viral agent circulates in the blood at least transiently during the early febrile stage. Togaviruses and bunyaviruses can be recovered from acute-phase serum by inoculation into tissue culture or living mosquitoes. Argentine, Bolivian, and Venezuelan hemorrhagic fever viruses can be isolated from acute-phase blood or throat washings by inoculation intracerebrally into guinea pigs, infant hamsters, or infant mice. Lassa virus may be isolated from acute-phase blood or throat washings by inoculation into tissue cultures. For Marburg disease and Ebola hemorrhagic fever, acute-phase throat washings, blood, and urine may be inoculated into tissue culture, guinea pigs, or monkeys. The viruses are readily identified by electron microscopy, with a filamentous structure differentiating them from all other known agents. Specific complement-fixing and immunofluorescent antibodies appear during convalescence. The virus of HFRS is recovered from acute-phase serum or urine by inoculation into tissue culture. A variety of antibody tests using viral subunits are becoming available. Serologic diagnosis depends on demonstrating seroconversion or a 4-fold or greater increase in immunoglobulin G antibody titer in acute and convalescent sera taken 3–4 wk apart. Viral RNA may also be detected in blood or tissues using reverse transcriptase polymerase chain reactions.

Handling blood and other biologic specimens is hazardous and must be performed by specially trained personnel. Blood and autopsy specimens should be placed in tightly sealed metal containers, wrapped in absorbent material inside a sealed plastic bag, and shipped on dry ice to laboratories with biocontainment safety level 4 facilities. Even routine hematologic and biochemical tests should be done with extreme caution.

Differential Diagnosis. Mild cases of hemorrhagic fever may be confused with almost any self-limited systemic bacterial or viral infection. More severe cases may suggest typhoid fever; epidemic, murine, or scrub typhus; leptospirosis; or a rickettsial spotted fever, for which effective chemotherapeutic agents are available. Many of these may be acquired in geographic or ecologic locations endemic for a viral hemorrhagic fever.

TREATMENT. Ribavirin administered intravenously is effective in reducing mortality in Lassa fever and HFRS. Further information and advice about management, control measures, diagnosis, and collection of biohazardous specimens can be obtained from Centers for Disease Control and Prevention, National Center for Infectious Diseases, Special Pathogens Branch, Atlanta, Georgia 30333 (404-639-1115).

The principle involved in all these diseases, especially HFRS, is the reversal of dehydration, hemoconcentration, renal failure, and protein, electrolyte, or blood losses. The contribution of disseminated intravascular coagulopathy to the hemorrhagic manifestations is unknown, and the management of hemorrhage should be individualized. Transfusions of fresh blood and platelets are frequently given. Good results have been reported in a few patients after the administration of clotting factor concentrates. The efficacy of corticosteroids, ε-aminocaproic acid, pressor amines, or α-adrenergic blocking agents has not been established. Sedatives should be selected with regard to the possibility of kidney or liver damage. The successful management of HFRS may require renal dialysis.

PREVENTION. A live-attenuated vaccine (Candid-I) for Argentine hemorrhagic fever is highly efficacious. A form of inactivated mouse brain vaccine is reported to be effective in preventing Omsk hemorrhagic fever. Inactivated RVF vaccines are widely used to protect domestic animals and laboratory workers. HFRS inactivated vaccine is licensed in Korea, and killed and live-attenuated vaccines are widely used in China. A vaccinia-vector glycoprotein vaccine provides protection against Lassa fever in monkeys. VEE replicon Ebola envelope glycoprotein and DNA-adenovirus Ebola glycoprotein vaccines have provided protection in experimental animals. A recombinant vesicular stomatitis virus vaccine containing surface glycoproteins from Ebola and Marburg viruses is effective in preventing both virus hemorrhagic fevers.

Prevention of **mosquito-borne** and **tick-borne infections** includes use of repellents, tight-fitting clothing that fully covers the extremities, and careful examination of the skin after exposure with removal of any vectors found. Diseases transmitted from a rodent-infected environment can be prevented through methods of rodent control; elimination of refuse and breeding sites is particularly successful in urban and suburban areas.

Crimean-Congo hemorrhagic fever, Lassa fever, Marburg disease, and Ebola hemorrhagic fever may be **transmitted in hospital settings.** Patients should be isolated until they are virus-free or for 3 wk after illness. Patients' urine, sputum, blood, clothing, and bedding should be disinfected. Disposable syringes and needles should be used. Prompt and strict enforcement of barrier nursing may be lifesaving. The mortality rate among medical workers contracting these diseases is 50%. A few entirely asymptomatic Ebola infections result in strong antibody production.

Al-Hazmi A, Al-Rajhi AA, Abboud EG, et al: Ocular complications of Rift Valley fever outbreak in Saudi Arabia. *Ophthalmology* 2005;112:313–318.

Becker S: Good news for Marburg virus workers. *Lancet* 2006;367:1373–1374.

Centers for Disease Control and Prevention: Update: Management of patients with suspected viral hemorrhagic fever. *MMWR* 1995;44:475–479.

Centers for Disease Control and Prevention: Update: Outbreak of Rift Valley fever—Saudi Arabia, August–November 2000. *MMWR* 2000;49:982–985.

Fisher-Hoch SP, Platt GS, Neild GH, et al: Pathophysiology of shock and hemorrhage in a fulminating viral infection (Ebola). *J Infect Dis* 1985;152:887–894.

Geisbert TW, Hensley LE, Jahrling PB, et al: Treatment of Ebola virus infection with a recombinant inhibitor of factor VII a tissue factor: A study in rhesus monkeys. *Lancet* 2003;362:1953–1958.

Huggins JW, Hsiang CM, Cosgriff TM, et al: Prospective, double-blind, concurrent, placebo-controlled trial of intravenous ribavirin therapy of hemorrhagic fever with renal syndrome. *J Infect Dis* 1991;164:1119–1127.

Isaacson M: Viral hemorrhagic fever hazards for travelers in Africa. *Clin Infect Dis* 2001;33:1707–1712.

Jones SM, Feldmann H, Strober U, et al: Live attenuated recombinant vaccine protects nonhuman primates against Ebola and Marburg viruses. *Nat Med* 2005;11:786–790.

Leroy EM, Baize S, Volchkov VE, et al: Human asymptomatic Ebola infection and strong inflammatory response. *Lancet* 2000;355:2210–2215.

Leroy EM, Telfer P, Kumulungui B, et al: A serological survey of Ebola virus infection in central African nonhuman primates. *J Infect Dis* 2004;190:1895–1899.

McCormick JB, King IJ, Webb PA, et al: Lassa fever: Effective therapy with ribavirin. *N Engl J Med* 1986;314:20–26.

McCormick JB, King IJ, Webb PA, et al: A case-control study of the clinical diagnosis and course of Lassa fever. *J Infect Dis* 1987;155:445–455.

Peters CJ: Marburg and Ebola—Arming ourselves against the deadly filoviruses. *N Engl J Med* 2005;352:2571–2574.

Pushko P, Bray M, Ludwig GV, et al: Recombinant RNA replicons derived from attenuated Venezuelan equine encephalitis virus protect guinea pigs and mice from Ebola hemorrhagic fever virus. *Vaccine* 2000;19:142–153.

Richmond JK, Baglole DJ: Lassa fever: Epidemiology, clinical features, and social consequences. *Br Med J* 2003;327:1271–1275.

Sanchez A, Lukwiya M, Bausch D, et al: Analysis of human peripheral blood samples from fatal and nonfatal cases of Ebola (Sudan) hemorrhagic fever:

Cellular responses, virus load, and nitric oxide levels. *J Virol* 2004; 78:10370–10377.
Smego RA Jr, Sarwari AR, Siddiqui AR: Crimean-Congo hemorrhagic fever: Prevention and control limitations in a resource-poor country. *Clin Infect Dis* 2004;38:1731–1735.
Sullivan NJ, Sanchez A, Rollin PE, et al: Development of a preventive vaccine for Ebola virus infection in primates. *Nature* 2000;408:605–609.
Towner JS, Rollin PD, Bausch DG, et al: Rapid diagnosis of Ebola hemorrhagic fever by reverse transcription-PCR in an outbreak setting and assessment of patient viral load as a predictor of outcome. *J Virol* 2004;78: 4330–4341.

Chapter 269 ■ Lymphocytic Choriomeningitis Virus (LCMV)

Hal B. Jenson

Lymphocytic choriomeningitis virus (LCMV) infection in immunocompetent humans usually results in either asymptomatic infection or mild, self-limited illness. It can also cause aseptic meningitis, fetal infection with congenital anomalies or fetal demise, and serious and even fatal infection among immunocompromised persons.

ETIOLOGY. LCMV is a member of the family Arenaviridae, which are negative-sense single-stranded RNA viruses. These enveloped viruses are round, oval, or pleomorphic, averaging 110–130 nm in diameter, with a range of 50–300 nm.

The wild house mouse, *Mus musculus,* is the primary reservoir. One study found 9% prevalence among mice. The virus establishes persistent infection in utero from maternal viremia that occurs in chronically infected mice. Their infected offspring do not develop an effective immune response and excrete virus continuously throughout life in saliva, nasal secretions, semen, milk, urine, and feces. Pet hamsters and guinea pigs are not natural reservoirs but can become infected if they have contact with wild house mice, and can shed virus for up to 8 mo without signs of illness.

EPIDEMIOLOGY. The virus is found in temperate regions of Europe and the Americas. Rodent infection is highly focal. Human cases are sporadic and are less common during the summer. Outbreaks have been reported after exposure to infected pet hamsters. Serologic surveys show that up to 5% of adults in the United States had evidence of past infection.

Transmission from rodents to humans is by direct contact with rodents or contaminated food and fluids, aerosolized droplets from rodent secretions or excretions, and infrequently by rodent bites. Clusters have been reported after exposure to infected pet hamsters or laboratory rodents, and associated with solid-organ transplantation. There is no evidence of chronic infection in humans or of direct person-to-person transmission.

PATHOGENESIS. Viral infection of rodents is chronic, with long-term viral shedding but usually no overt disease. Acute infection is associated with viremia and fever, and occasionally with LCMV multiplying in brain and meningeal cells but with no apparent damage. Symptoms result from a CD8 T cell–mediated immunopathologic response. After inhalation of virus by humans, there is viral replication in pulmonary and hilar lymph nodes followed by viremia within 48 hr. The liver, spleen, and lymph nodes are most affected and show lymphoid hyperplasia. The kidneys, heart, skeletal muscle, epididymis, and other organs may show mononuclear infiltration.

CLINICAL MANIFESTATIONS. Infection in humans is inapparent in approximately ⅓ of cases. Symptomatic cases have an incubation period of 5–13 days. Symptoms may include a nonspecific flulike illness that is unrecognized as LCMV infection, or may be characterized by lymphocytic meningitis or meningoencephalitis of varying severity. The classic course is a biphasic illness with usually 3–5 days of nonspecific illness with fever, malaise, myalgias, nausea and vomiting, sore throat and cough, lymphadenopathy, and occasionally a maculopapular rash. There is defervescence for 5–9 days followed by recurrence of fever and headache. In a small proportion of patients, signs of meningitis develop, sometimes without the prodromal symptoms. Rare symptoms include meningoencephalitis, transverse myelitis, and extraneural manifestations of orchitis, parotitis, pneumonitis, arthritis, myocarditis, and alopecia.

There may be papilledema. Thrombocytopenia and leukopenia are typical. The cerebrospinal fluid pressure is elevated with elevated protein (50–300 mg/dL) with up to several hundred lymphocytes per microliter. There are no associated bleeding diatheses, as occur with other arenaviruses (Junin, Machupo, Guanarito, and Lassa) that are associated with viral hemorrhagic fevers (see Chapter 268). Immunosuppression predisposes to hemorrhagic fever–like syndromes.

Infection transmitted from an organ donor results in serious infection in the organ recipient, characterized by abdominal pain, depressed level of consciousness, coagulopathy, hepatitis, graft dysfunction, fever, or leukocytosis. Other manifestations include diarrhea, erythema around the incision site, and seizures.

Fetal Infection. LCMV infection during the 1st or 2nd trimester of pregnancy can cause severe disease or developmental defects in the fetus. Approximately 32 cases of congenital LCMV infection have been reported. Only half of mothers relate illnesses compatible with acute LCMV infection during pregnancy, usually with only flulike symptoms but occasionally compatible with aseptic meningitis. Only ¼ of mothers have known exposure to rodents.

The affected fetus may have chorioretinitis, encephalomalacia, microcephaly, hydrocephalus, and punctate intracranial calcifications associated with psychomotor retardation, blindness, and fetal death. The neonatal presentation is similar to congenital cytomegalovirus and toxoplasmosis but typically without hepatosplenomegaly, and should be considered if there is a history of maternal rodent exposure. Other ophthalmologic manifestations may include optic atrophy, microphthalmia, vitreitis, leukokoria, and cataracts. Unlike congenital cytomegalovirus infection, hearing loss has not been reported.

The cerebrospinal fluid shows a mild pleocytosis (<70 white blood cells/µL) and mildly elevated protein (average of 67 mg/dL; range of 9–477 mg/dL). CT and MRI reveal encephalomalacia, ventricular enlargement, and calcifications (by CT) adjacent to the lateral ventricles or in the periventricular white matter.

DIAGNOSIS. The diagnosis is usually suspected by the clinical manifestations and history of exposure to rodents. There are no licensed diagnostic tests for LCMV infection. Serologic tests using immunofluorescent antibody and enzyme-linked immunosorbent assay methods can confirm the clinical diagnosis. The virus can also be isolated from the blood and cerebrospinal fluid during the 1st week of illness. Polymerase chain reaction testing has also been used for diagnosis.

TREATMENT. There is no specific treatment for LCMV. Ribavirin is active against LCMV and other arenaviruses in vitro. Immunosuppressive therapy if present should be reduced. Supportive care includes analgesia for headache control and intravenous hydration, if necessary.

PROGNOSIS. The illness is usually self-limited and resolves without sequelae. Hydrocephalus, probably resulting from arachnoidal and ependymal inflammation, is a characteristic complication of congenital infection and has been reported rarely after LCMV infection in older children and adults.

PREVENTION. Minimizing direct contact with the rodent hosts, especially excreta, is the best means of prevention. This precaution is especially important for pregnant women and should be emphasized during prenatal counseling. The prevalence of LCMV in laboratory animals and household pets, primarily hamsters, is variable and depends on the breeding and handling conditions. Routine monitoring of rodents for infection is not uniformly practiced or mandated.

Biggar RJ, Woodall JP, Walter PD, et al: Lymphocytic choriomeningitis outbreak associated with pet hamsters. Fifty-seven cases from New York State. *JAMA* 1975;232:494–500.

Centers for Disease Control and Prevention: Update: Interim guidance for minimizing risk for human lymphocytic choriomeningitis virus infection associated with pet rodents. *MMWR* 2005;54:799–801.

Childs J, Glass G, Korch G, et al: Lymphocytic choriomeningitis virus infection and house mouse *(Mus musculus)* distribution in urban Baltimore. *Am J Trop Med* 1992;47:27–34.

Childs JE, Glass GE, Ksiazek TG, et al: Human-rodent contact and infection with lymphocytic choriomeningitis and Seoul viruses in an inner-city population. *Am J Trop Med Hyg* 1991;44:117–121.

Enders G, Barho-Gobel M, Lohler J, et al: Congenital lymphocytic choriomeningitis virus infection: An underdiagnosed disease. *Pediatr Infect Dis J* 1999;18:652–655.

Fischer SA, Graham MB, Kuehnert MJ, et al: Transmission of lymphocytic choriomeningitis virus by organ transplantation. *N Engl J Med* 2006;34:2235–2249.

Mets MB, Barton LL, Khan AS, et al: Lymphocytic choriomeningitis virus: An underdiagnosed cause of congenital chorioretinitis. *Am J Ophthalmol* 2000;130:209–215.

Wright R, Johnson D, Neumann M, et al: Congenital lymphocytic choriomeningitis virus syndrome. A disease that mimics congenital toxoplasmosis or cytomegalovirus infection. *Pediatrics* 1997;100:E9.

Chapter 270 ■ Hantavirus Pulmonary Syndrome

Scott B. Halstead

The hantavirus pulmonary syndrome (HPS), is caused by multiple closely related hantaviruses that have been identified from the western United States, with sporadic cases reported from the eastern United States, Canada, and several countries in South America (Fig. 270-1). HPS is characterized by a febrile prodrome followed by the rapid onset of noncardiogenic pulmonary edema and hypotension or shock. Sporadic cases in the United States caused by related viruses may present with renal involvement. Cases in Argentina and Chile sometimes include severe gastrointestinal hemorrhaging. Nosocomial transmission has been documented in this geographic region only.

ETIOLOGY. Hantaviruses are a genus in the family Bunyaviridae, which are lipid-enveloped viruses with a negative-stranded RNA genome composed of 3 unique segments. Several pathogenic viruses that have been recognized within the genus include Hantaan virus, which causes the most severe form of hemorrhagic fever with renal syndrome (HFRS) seen primarily in mainland Asia; Dobrava virus, which causes the most severe form of HFRS seen primarily in the Balkans; Puumala virus, which causes a milder form of HFRS with a high proportion of subclinical infections and is prevalent in northern Europe; and Seoul virus, which results in moderate HFRS and is transmitted predominantly in Asia by urban rats or worldwide by laboratory rats. Prospect Hill virus, a Hantavirus that is widely disseminated in meadow voles in the United States, is not known to cause human disease.

HPS is associated with Sin Nombre virus, isolated from deer mice, *Peromyscus maniculatus*, in New Mexico. Multiple HPS-like agents isolated to date belong to a single genetic group of hantaviruses and are associated with rodents of the family Muridae, subfamily Sigmodontinae. These rodent species are restricted to the Americas, suggesting that HPS may be a Western hemisphere disease.

EPIDEMIOLOGY. Persons acquiring HPS generally have a history of recent outdoor exposure or live in an area with large populations of deer mice. Clusters of cases have occurred among individuals who have cleaned houses that were rodent infested. *P. maniculatus* is 1 of the most common North American mammals and, where found, is frequently the dominant member of the rodent community. About half of cases occur between the months of May and July. Patients are almost exclusively 12–70 yr of age; 60% of patients are 20–39 yr of age. Rare cases are reported in children <12 yr of age. Two thirds of patients are male, probably reflecting greater outdoor activities. It is not known whether almost complete absence of disease in young children is a reflection of innate resistance or simply lack of exposure. Evidence of human transmission has been obtained in Argentine outbreaks.

Hantaviruses do not cause apparent illness in their reservoir hosts, which remain asymptomatically infected for life. Infected rodents shed virus in saliva, urine, and feces for many weeks, but the duration of shedding and the period of maximum infectivity are unknown. The presence of infectious virus in saliva, the sensitivity of these animals to parenteral inoculation with hantaviruses, and field observations of infected rodents indicate that biting is important for rodent-to-rodent transmission. Aerosols from infective saliva or excreta of rodents are implicated in the transmission of hantaviruses to humans. Persons visiting animal care areas housing infected rodents have been infected after exposure for as little as 5 min. It is possible that hantaviruses are spread through contaminated food and breaks in skin or mucous membranes; transmission to humans has occurred by rodent bites. Person-to-person transmission is distinctly uncommon but has been documented in Argentina.

PATHOGENESIS. HPS is characterized by sudden and catastrophic pulmonary edema, resulting in anoxia and acute heart failure. The virus is detected in pulmonary capillaries, suggesting that pulmonary edema is the consequence of T-cell attack on virus-infected capillaries. Disease severity is predicted by the level of acute-phase viremia titer.

CLINICAL MANIFESTATIONS. HPS is characterized by a prodrome and a cardiopulmonary phase. The mean duration after the onset of prodromal symptoms to hospitalization is 5.4 days. The mean duration of symptoms to death is 8 days (median 7 days; range 2–16 days). The most common **prodromal symptoms** are fever and myalgia (100%); cough or dyspnea (76%); gastrointestinal symptoms, including vomiting, diarrhea, and mid-abdominal pain (76%); and headache (71%). The **cardiopulmonary phase** is heralded by progressive cough and shortness of breath. The most common initial physical findings are tachypnea (100%), tachycardia (94%), and hypotension (50%). Rapidly progressive acute pulmonary edema, hypoxia, and shock develop in most severely ill patients. Pulmonary vascular permeability is complicated by cardiogenic shock associated with increased vascular resistance. The clinical course of the illness in patients who die is characterized by pulmonary edema accompanied by severe hypotension, frequently terminating in sinus bradycardia, electromechanical

Total number of confirmed cases of hantavirus pulmonary syndrome, by state of exposure — United States, 1993–1996*

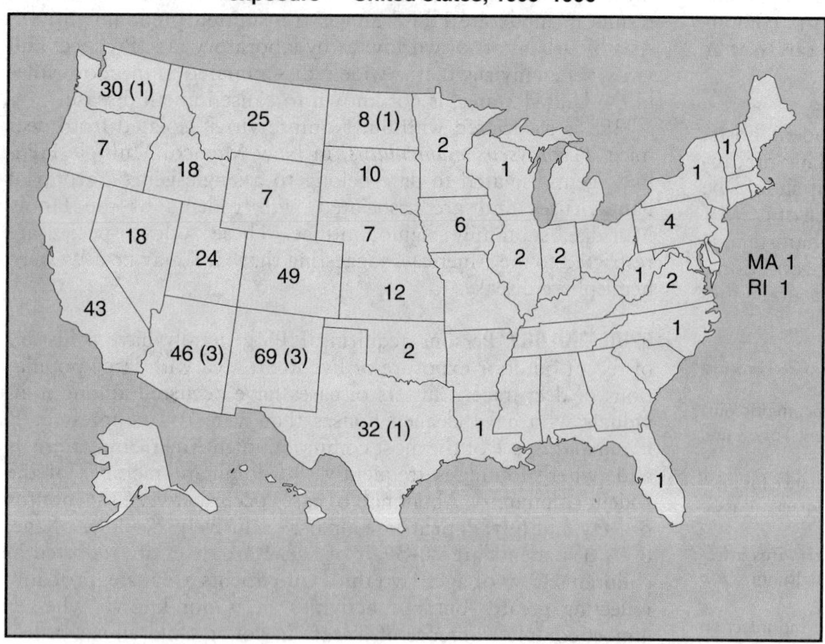

*n = 438 of May 10, 2006. Numbers in parentheses indicate cases confirmed during January–March 2006 (n = nine).

Figure 270-1. Total number of confirmed cases of hantavirus pulmonary syndrome, by state of exposure—United States, 1993–2006.* (From the Centers for Disease Control and Prevention: Hantavirus pulmonary syndrome: Five states, 2006. *MMWR* 2006;55:627–628.)

dissociation, ventricular tachycardia, or fibrillation. Hypotension may be progressive even with adequate oxygenation.

DIAGNOSIS. The diagnosis of HPS should be considered in a previously healthy patient presenting with a febrile prodrome and acute respiratory distress. Occurrence of thrombocytopenia with the febrile prodrome and outdoor exposure in the spring and summer months are strongly suggestive of HPS. Specific diagnosis of HPS is made by serologic tests that detect hantavirus immunoglobulin M antibodies. Hantavirus antigen can be detected in tissue by immunohistochemistry and amplification of hantavirus nucleotide sequences detected by reverse transcriptase polymerase chain reaction. The state health department or the Centers for Disease Control and Prevention should be consulted to assist in diagnosis, epidemiologic investigations, and outbreak control.

Laboratory Findings. Laboratory findings include leukocytosis (median 26,000 cells/μL), elevated hematocrit resulting from hemoconcentration, thrombocytopenia (median 64,000/μL), prolonged prothrombin and partial thromboplastin times, elevated serum lactate dehydrogenase concentration, decreased serum protein concentrations, proteinuria, and microscopic hematuria. Patients who die often experience disseminated intravascular coagulation including frank hemorrhage and exceptionally high leukocyte counts.

Differential Diagnosis. The differential diagnosis includes adult respiratory distress syndrome, pneumonic plague, psittacosis, severe mycoplasmal pneumonia, influenza, leptospirosis, inhalation anthrax, rickettsial infections, pulmonary tularemia, atypical bacterial and viral pneumoniae, legionellosis, meningococcemia, and other sepsis syndromes. The key determinant in the diagnosis of HPS is thrombocytopenia.

TREATMENT. Management of patients with hantavirus infection requires maintenance of adequate oxygenation and careful monitoring and support of cardiovascular function. The pathophysiology of HPS resembles that of dengue shock syndrome (see Chapter 266). Pressor or inotropic agents, such as dobutamine, should be administered in combination with judicious volume replacement to treat symptomatic hypotension or shock while avoiding exacerbating the pulmonary edema. Intravenous ribavirin, which is lifesaving if given early in the course of HFRS, has been shown to be of no value in HPS.

Further information and advice about management, control measures, diagnosis, and collection of biohazardous specimens can be obtained from the Centers for Disease Control and Prevention, National Center for Infectious Diseases, Special Pathogens Branch, Atlanta, Georgia 30333 (404–639–1115).

PROGNOSIS. In some geographic areas fatality rates have been 50%. Severe abnormalities in hematocrit, white blood cell count, lactate dehydrogenase, and partial thromboplastin time, and high viral load predict mortality with high specificity and sensitivity.

PREVENTION. Avoiding contact with rodents is the only preventive strategy. Rodent control in and around the home is important. Barrier nursing is advised and biosafety level 3 facilities and practices are recommended for laboratory handling of blood, body fluids, and tissues from suspect patients or rodents because the virus may be aerosolized.

Armstrong LR, Bryan RT, Sarisky J, et al: Mild hantaviral disease caused by Sin Nombre virus in a four-year-old-child. *Pediatr Infect Dis J* 1995;12:1108–1110.

Bryan RT, Doyle TJ, Moolenaar RL, et al: Hantavirus pulmonary syndrome in children. *Semin Pediatr Infect Dis* 1997;8:44–49.

Centers for Disease Control and Prevention: Hantavirus pulmonary syndrome: United States, 1995 and 1996. *MMWR* 1996;45:291–295.

Centers for Disease Control and Prevention: Hantavirus pulmonary syndrome: Five states, 2006. *MMWR* 2006;55:627–628.

Childs JE, Ksiazek TG, Spiropoulou CF, et al: Serologic and genetic identification of *Peromyscus maniculatus* as the primary rodent reservoir for a new hantavirus in the southwestern United States. *J Infect Dis* 1994;169:1271–1280.

Khan AS, Khabbaz RF, Armstrong LR, et al: Hantavirus pulmonary syndrome: The first 100 U.S. cases. *J Infect Dis* 1996;173:1297–1303.

Peters CJ, Khan AS: Hantavirus pulmonary syndrome: The new American hemorrhagic fever. *Clin Infect Dis* 2002;34:1224–1231.

Peters CJ, Simpson GL, Levy H: Spectrum of hantavirus infection: Hemorrhagic fever with renal syndrome and hantavirus pulmonary syndrome. *Annu Rev Med* 1999;50:531–545.

Chapter 271 ■ Rabies Philip Toltzis

Rabies virus is a bullet-shaped, negative-sense, single-stranded, enveloped RNA virus from the family Rhabodviridae, genus Lyssavirus. There currently are 7 known genotypes of Lyssavirus. Lyssavirus type 1 is the classic rabies virus. This genotype, the only 1 currently identified in the Western hemisphere, is distributed worldwide and naturally infects a large variety of animals. The other 6 genotypes are more geographically confined, and in 5 genotypes bats are the only known reservoir. All 7 Lyssavirus genotypes have been associated with clinical rabies in humans, although type 1 accounts for the marked majority of cases. Within genotype 1 a number of genetic variants have been defined. Each variant is specific to a particular animal reservoir. Consequently, genetic sequence analysis of viruses isolated from human cases enables presumptive identification of the animal source, even when there is no recollection of an animal exposure.

EPIDEMIOLOGY. Rabies is present on all continents except Antarctica. Approximately 50,000 cases of human rabies occur across the globe each year. Theoretically, rabies virus can infect any mammal that then can transmit disease to humans, but true animal reservoirs that maintain the presence of rabies virus in the population are limited to large carnivorous mammals and insectivorous bats. Worldwide, transmission from dogs accounts for >90% of human cases. In Africa and Asia, other animals serve as prominent reservoirs, such as jackals, mongooses, and raccoon dogs. In industrialized nations canine rabies has been largely controlled through the routine immunization of pets. In the United States, raccoons are the most commonly infected animal. Raccoon rabies formerly was identified primarily in animals inhabiting the American Southeast, but spread of rabid raccoons to the middle-Atlantic states occurred during the Carter presidency when members of the administration imported raccoons to the Washington area for hunting purposes. Raccoon rabies subsequently rapidly spread across the entire eastern seaboard and into the midwestern states, promoted in part by the tendency of infected animals to hitch rides on garbage trucks. After raccoons, the most common rabies-infected animals in the USA are skunks, bats, foxes, and coyotes. Rabies also occurs infrequently in livestock. Occasionally rabies is found in American domestic pets; infected cats outnumber infected dogs, probably because cats frequently prowl unsupervised. Notably, rabies in small mammals, including mice, squirrels, and rabbits, is rare; to date no transmission from these animals to humans has been documented.

The epidemiology of human rabies in America is dominated by **cryptogenic bat rabies.** Rabid bats are identified in every state of the union except Hawaii. A review of cases in the United States documented that, of the 32 human cases identified from 1980 to 1996, the largest proportion were infected with a bat variant, and in almost all cases of bat-associated human rabies there was no history of a bat bite. These variants are associated disproportionately with 2 species of bats, namely, the silver haired and eastern pipistrelle bat. These 2 species are found over a broad geographic area but they rarely populate the same space as humans. The reasons underlying their association with human disease in the United States are not known with certainty, but there is experimental evidence that the variants found in silver haired and eastern pipistrelle bats replicate more readily in skin and muscle, the seminal events in human disease, compared with other variants. Moreover, these bats have small fangs possibly resulting in bites that go unnoticed and therefore untreated by the human victim.

TRANSMISSION. Rabies virus is found in large quantities in the saliva of infected animals and transmission occurs almost exclusively through inoculation of the infected saliva through a bite or scratch from a rabid mammal. Approximately 35–50% of people bitten by a known rabies-infected animal and receiving no post-exposure prophylaxis (PEP) contract rabies. The transmission rate is increased if the victim has suffered multiple bites and if the inoculation occurs in highly innervated parts of the body such as the face and the hands. Infection does not occur after exposure of intact skin to infected secretions, but virus may enter the body through intact mucous membranes. Rabies has been transmitted by corneal, lung, liver, and kidney transplantation from tissue harvested from patients dying from unspecified encephalitis or who were misdiagnosed. Patients with unspecified encephalitis are no longer eligible for organ donation. Claims that spelunkers may contract rabies after inhaling bat excreta while exploring caves densely inhabited by bats have come under doubt. While theoretically possible, a cave must host millions of bats in a very confined, humid area to provide the necessary conditions for transmission through inhalation.

Caregivers of a hospitalized patient with rabies are advised to use full barrier precautions with patient contact. The virus is rapidly inactivated in the environment, and contamination of fomites is not a mechanism of spread. Because of the delay in diagnosis that almost invariably is experienced in cases presenting to Western medical centers, the confirmation of rabies in a patient with encephalitis almost always prompts many courses of PEP among medical staff. No case of nosocomial transmission to a health care worker, however, has been documented to date.

PATHOGENESIS. After inoculation, rabies virus replicates slowly in muscle. This slow initial step likely accounts for the disease's long incubation period. Virus then enters the peripheral nerve, utilizing the nicotinic acetylcholine receptor, which also binds to a variety of neurotoxins that share genetic homologies with the rabies surface glycoprotein. The rabies virus probably uses several other receptors for entry into the axon as well. Once in the nerve, the virus travels along the axon by fast axonal transport, jumping from cell to cell across synapses until it enters the central nervous system, where rapid dissemination occurs throughout the brain and spinal cord. Infection includes the brainstem, accounting for autonomic dysfunction and hydrophobia, which is at least partially caused by spasms of the muscles of the upper airway when the patient attempts to swallow. The pathologic hallmark of rabies, the **Negri body,** is composed of clumped viral nucleocapsids that create characteristic cytoplasmic inclusions on routine histology. Negri bodies can, however, be absent in documented rabies virus infection. Despite the profound neurologic dysfunction associated with rabies, histopathologic examination of the infected brain reveals limited damage and neuronal cell death. Some experimental data suggest that the neurologic dysfunction arises more from interference with central neurotransmitters rather than cytolysis of neural cells.

After infection of the central nervous system, the virus then travels anterograde through the peripheral nervous system to virtually all innervated organs. It is through this route that the virus infects the salivary glands. Infection of the heart causes cardiac dysfunction, and many victims of rabies ultimately die from heart failure or uncontrolled dysrhythmia.

CLINICAL MANIFESTATIONS. The incubation period for rabies is 1–3 mo but is variable; in some cases, symptoms first occur within 5 days after exposure, and occasionally the incubation period can extend to >6 mo. Rabies has 2 principal clinical forms. **Encephalitic or "furious" rabies** begins with nonspecific symptoms, including fever, sore throat, malaise, headache, nausea and vomiting, and weakness. These symptoms are accompanied by paresthesias and pruritis at or near the site of the bite that then extend along the affected limb. Soon thereafter the patient begins to demonstrate typical symptoms of severe encephalitis with agitation, depressed mentation, and occasionally seizures. Characteristically patients with rabies encephalitis initially have periods of lucidity intermittent with periods of profound encephalopathy, but ultimately the condition progresses to coma. The cardinal signs of rabies, hydrophobia and aerophobia, are manifested by agitation and fear created by attempting to drink and fanning air in the face, which in turn produces chocking and aspiration through spasms of the larynx, neck, and chest wall. The illness is relentlessly progressive, and death almost always occurs within 2–3 wk after onset.

A 2nd form of rabies known as **paralytic or "dumb" rabies** is seen much less frequently and is characterized principally by ascending motor weakness affecting both the limbs and the cranial nerves. Most patients with dumb rabies also have some element of encephalopathy.

DIFFERENTIAL DIAGNOSIS. The differential diagnosis of rabies encephalitis includes all forms of severe cerebral infections. The diagnosis frequently is delayed in Western countries due to its rarity and the unfamiliarity of the medical staff with the infection. These considerations highlight the need to pursue a history of contact with an animal belonging to 1 of the known reservoirs for rabies or to establish a travel history to a rabies-endemic region. Dumb rabies is most frequently confused with Guillain-Barré syndrome. Unlike rabies, however, this latter illness usually affects the sensory peripheral nerves as well as the motor and is always associated with a clear sensorium.

DIAGNOSIS. A number of tests are available to confirm a clinically suspected case of rabies, including detection of anti-rabies antibody, isolation of virus, and detection of viral protein or RNA. Rabies-specific antibody can be detected in serum or cerebrospinal fluid (CSF) samples. Serum antibody is present only after the onset of symptoms, indicating that incubating virus is protected from immune presentation. Anti-rabies antibodies are present in the sera of patients who have received an incomplete course of the rabies vaccine, precluding a meaningful interpretation in this setting. Antibody in CSF is a reflection of a local humoral response in the central nervous system and is considered diagnostic of rabies regardless of immunization status. Rabies virus can best be isolated for culture from saliva or from brain biopsy material. The virus can be grown both in cell culture and after animal injection, but identification of rabies by these methods is prolonged. Rabies antigen is detected through immunofluorescence of brain biopsy material or infected peripheral tissue. Most frequently this test is applied to a touch preparation of corneal tissue or to a skin biopsy at the nuchal hair line, both of which are highly innervated. Rabies virus RNA has been detected in saliva and brain by the reverse transcription polymerase chain reaction. Early data suggest that this latter test is the most sensitive available assay for the diagnosis of rabies, but experience remains small. All the listed tests can be falsely negative well after the onset of symptoms, recommending that the diagnosis be pursued with more than 1 modality.

TREATMENT AND PROGNOSIS. Rabies is virtually uniformly fatal. There are 6 reported cases of survivors from rabies infection, only 2 of whom had a neurologically satisfactory outcome. Five had received part of the recommended PEP regimen. Although some antiviral treatments, including ribavirin and α-interferon, have been tried in rabies, none has had a consistent beneficial effect. Neither rabies immune globulin (RIG) nor rabies vaccine alters the course of disease once symptoms have appeared. Given the extraordinarily bleak outcome, the approach to the rabies-infected patient is focused on determining the diagnosis to ensure that no in-hospital transmission occurs and to allow an accurate prognosis for the family and appropriate comfort-care for the patient.

The survival of an American teenager who had contracted rabies from a bat and who had received no PEP is the 1st report of its kind, published in 2005. She was treated with ribavirin and amantadine while placed in a drug-induced coma with multiple agents, including ketamine, an antagonist of the *N*-methyl-D-aspartate receptor, which is a putative receptor for rabies virus. Therapy was continued until antibody appeared in the CSF. This patient survived with minimal impairment.

PREVENTION. Primary prevention of rabies infection includes avoiding contact with potentially rabid animals and vaccination of all domestic animals. Special efforts should be made to teach children to avoid wild animals, stray animals, and animals with unusual behavior.

IMMUNIZATION OF ANIMAL RESERVOIRS. The introduction of routine rabies immunization for domestic pets in the United States and Europe during the middle of the 20th century virtually eliminated infection in dogs, which prior to that time had been the principal transmitter of rabies to humans in developed as well as nonindustrialized countries. Since the 1990s, efforts in Europe and North America have shifted to immunization of wildlife reservoirs of rabies. These programs have employed bait laced with either an attenuated rabies vaccine or a recombinant rabies surface glycoprotein inserted into vaccinia, distributed by air or truck into areas inhabited by rabid animals. In Europe, where large reservoirs of rabies have been identified in foxes, bait has been dropped into mountain valleys that serve as bottlenecks to their natural migration. In the United States, efforts have been directed toward immunizing raccoons that, unfortunately, are not as geographically confined. Human contact with vaccine-laden bait has occurred infrequently. Adverse events after such contact have been rare, but the vaccinia vector poses a threat to the same population at risk for vaccinia itself, namely, pregnant women, immunocompromised persons, and people with chronic dermatologic conditions. Unfortunately, rabid bats are widely spread and have eluded immunization strategies, and consequently this reservoir remains uncontrolled.

POSTEXPOSURE PROPHYLAXIS. The relevance of rabies for most pediatricians centers on evaluating whether an animal exposure warrants PEP. Rabies PEP is extremely effective. Indeed, no case of rabies has been documented in a person receiving the fully recommended schedule of PEP.

Algorithms have been devised to aid practitioners in deciding when to initiate rabies PEP (Fig. 271-1). The decision to proceed ultimately depends on the local epidemiology of animal rabies as determined by active surveillance programs, information that can be obtained from local and state health departments (Table 271-1). In general, bats, raccoons, skunks, coyotes, and foxes should be considered rabid unless proven otherwise through euthanasia and testing of brain tissue, whereas bites from small herbivorous animals (squirrels, hamsters, gerbils, chipmunks, rats, mice, and rabbits) can be discounted. The response to bites from pets, particularly dogs, cats, and ferrets, depends on local surveillance statistics and on whether the animal is available for observation. Traditionally practitioners have attempted to discriminate whether an attack by a potentially rabid animal was provoked or unprovoked to help decide whether rabies PEP is warranted, but frequently this distinction is indiscernible.

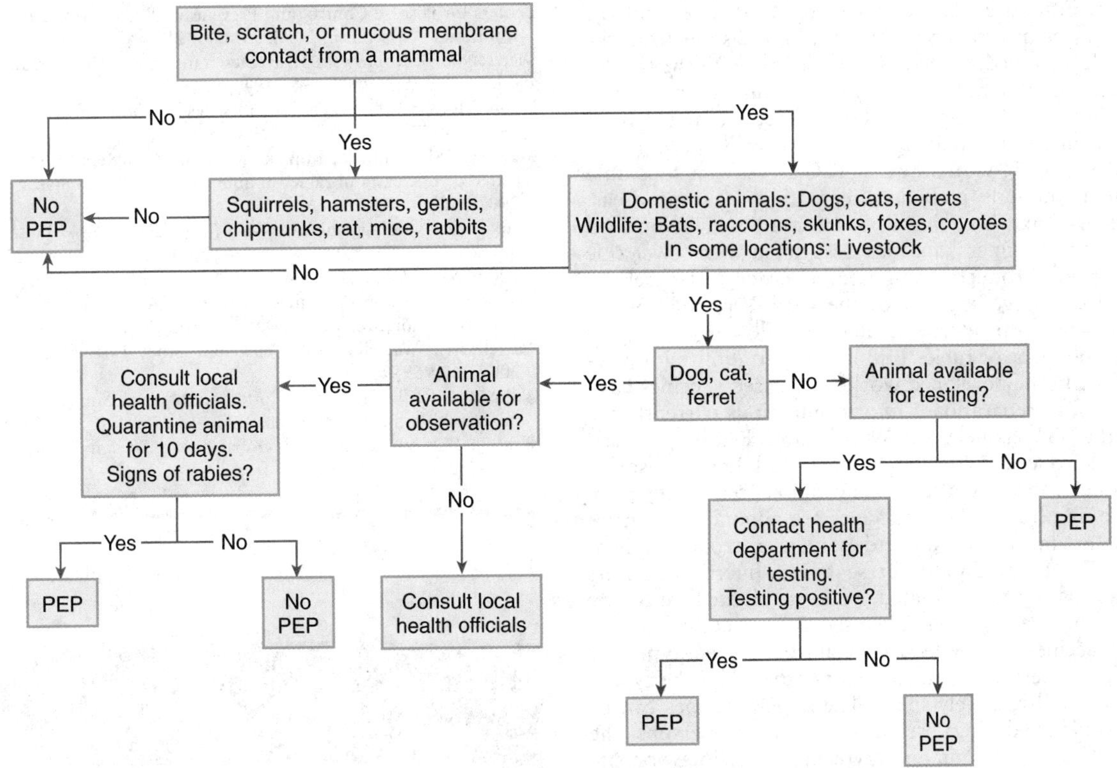

Figure 271-1. Algorithm for evaluating a child for rabies postexposure prophylaxis. This and any other algorithm should be used in concert with local epidemiologic information regarding the incidence of animal rabies in any given location.

The approach to nonbite bat exposures is controversial. In response to the observation that most recent cases of rabies in the USA have been caused by bat variants and that the majority of such patients had no recollection of a bat bite, the Centers for Disease Control and Prevention has recommended that rabies PEP be considered after any nonbite bat exposure (e.g., when a bat is found in the same room) in persons who may not be able to accurately report a bite, assuming that the animal is unavailable for testing. Such people include young children, the mentally disabled, and intoxicated individuals. Bat biologists, on the other hand, insist that bites even from bats with small fangs hurt sufficiently to be noticed. Other nonbite contacts (e.g., handling a carcass or coming into contact with blood or excreta from a potentially rabid animal) usually do not require PEP.

TABLE 271-1. Rabies Postexposure Prophylaxis Guide

ANIMAL TYPE	EVALUATION AND DISPOSITION OF ANIMAL	POSTEXPOSURE PROPHYLAXIS RECOMMENDATIONS
Dogs, cats, and ferrets	Healthy and available for 10 days of observation	Prophylaxis only if animal develops signs of rabies*
	Rabid or suspected of being rabid†	Immediate immunization and RIG
	Unknown (escaped)	
	Consult public health officials for advice	
Bats, skunks, raccoons, foxes, and most other carnivores; woodchucks	Regarded as rabid unless geographic area is known to be free of rabies or until animal proven negative by laboratory tests†	Immediate immunization and RIG
Livestock, rodents, and lagomorphs (rabbits, hares, and pikas)	Consider individually	Consult public health officials. Bites of squirrels, hamsters, guinea pigs, gerbils, chipmunks, rats, mice and other rodents, rabbits, hares, and pikas almost never require antirabies treatment

*During the 10 day holding period, at the first sign of rabies in the biting dog, cat, or ferret, treatment of the exposed person with RIG (human) and vaccine should be initiated. The animal should be euthanatized immediately and tested.

†The animal should be euthanatized and tested as soon as possible. Holding for observation is not recommended. Immunization is discontinued if immunofluorescent test result for the animal is negative.

RIG, rabies immune globulin.

From the American Academy of Pediatrics: *Red Book: 2006 Report of the Committee on Infectious Diseases*, 27th ed. Elk Grove Village, IL, American Academy of Pediatrics, 2006, p 555.

In all instances of a legitimate exposure, effort should be made to recover the animal for quarantine and observation or brain examination after euthanasia. In dogs, cats, and ferrets, symptoms of rabies always occur within several days of viral shedding; therefore, in these animals a 10-day observation period is sufficient to eliminate the possibility of rabies. In most instances PEP can be deferred until the results of observation or brain histology are known. In cases where the risk for rabies contact is high, the vaccine series can be initiated and then discontinued if the results from the animal are negative.

No duration of time between exposure and onset of symptoms should preclude rabies prophylaxis. Rabies PEP is most effective when applied expeditiously and is likely not effective once the virus has entered the peripheral nerve. Nevertheless, the series should be begun in the asymptomatic person as soon as possible regardless of the length of time since the bite.

The 1st step in rabies PEP is to cleanse the wound thoroughly. Soapy water is likely sufficient, and its effectiveness is supported by a broad experience, but other commonly used disinfectants, such as iodine-containing preparations, are virucidal and should be used in addition to soap when available. Probably the most important aspect of this component is that the wound is cleansed with copious volumes of disinfectant. Antibiotics and tetanus prophylaxis (see Chapter 208) should be applied using usual wound care criteria.

The 2nd component of rabies PEP consists of passive immunization with RIG. Human RIG, the formulation used in industrialized countries, is harvested from rabies-immunized individuals and is administered at a dose of 20 IU/kg. As much of the dose is infused around the wound as possible, and the remainder is injected intramuscularly in a limb distant from the 1 injected with the killed vaccine. RIG interferes with the take of live viral vaccines, similar to other immune globulin preparations, for at least 4 mo after receipt of the RIG dose. Human RIG is expensive and in short supply, and it is not available in many parts of the developing world. Equine RIG serves as a substitute for the human immune globulin preparation in some areas. Modern preparations of equine RIG are composed of purified heat-treated Fab2 fragments that are associated with fewer side effects than prior products composed of crude horse serum. Regrettably, for a large segment of the world's population no passive immunization product is available at all.

The 3rd component of rabies PEP is immunization with inactivated vaccine. In the developed world, cell-based vaccines have replaced previous preparations. Two formulations currently are available in the USA, namely, RabAvert (Chiron Behring), a purified chick-embryo cell cultivated vaccine, and Imovax Rabies (Aventis Pasteur), cultivated in human diploid cell cultures. In both children and adults, both vaccines are administered intramuscularly in a 1 mL volume in the deltoid or anterolateral thigh on days 0, 3, 7, 14, and 28 after presentation. Injection into the gluteal area has been associated with a blunted antibody response, and this area should not be used. It is generally believed that these vaccines are effective against all genotypes of Lyssavirus, but experience with exposures other than the type 1 classic rabies is still relatively small. The rabies vaccines can be safely administered during pregnancy. In most persons the vaccine is well tolerated. Pain and erythema at the injection site occur commonly, and local adenopathy, headache, and myalgias occur in 10–20%. Approximately 5% of persons who receive the human diploid cell vaccine experience an immune complex–mediated allergic reaction, including rash, edema, and arthralgias, several days after a booster dose. In the developing world schedules have been devised to induce an effective immune response with smaller amounts of vaccine. These schedules frequently require multiple intradermal injections but with a total dose that is less than that applied in the American schedule. None of these series currently is approved for use in the United States.

Other killed rabies virus vaccines remain available in the developing world. These include avian embryo–cultivated vaccines and vaccines derived from nervous tissue of experimentally infected animals. The latter preparations are particularly dangerous, as they are poorly immunogenic, and cross reactivity with human nervous tissue may occur, producing severe neurologic symptoms even in the absence of rabies infection.

PRE-EXPOSURE PROPHYLAXIS. The killed rabies vaccine can be given to prevent rabies in persons at high risk for exposure to wild-type virus. These include laboratory personnel working with rabies virus, veterinarians, and others likely to be exposed to rabid animals as part of their occupation. Pre-exposure prophylaxis should be considered for persons traveling to a rabies-endemic region where there is a credible risk for a bite or scratch from a rabies-infected animal, particularly if there is likely to be a shortage of RIG or cell-culture based vaccine (see Chapter 173). The schedule for pre-exposure prophylaxis includes 3 intramuscular injections on days 0, 7, and 21 or 28. PEP in the patient who has received pre-exposure prophylaxis or the patient who has received a prior full schedule of PEP consists of 2 doses of vaccine (1 each on days 0 and 3) and does not require RIG. Immunity from pre-exposure prophylaxis wanes after several years and requires boosting if the potential for exposure to rabid animals recurs.

Centers for Disease Control and Prevention: Human rabies prevention—United States, 1999. *MMWR* 1999;48:RR-1.

Centers for Disease Control and Prevention: Recovery of a patient from clinical rabies—Wisconsin, 2004. *MMWR* 2004;53:1171–1173.

Dietzschold B, Koprowski H: Rabies transmission from organ transplants in the USA. *Lancet* 2004;364:648–649.

Lafon M: Bat rabies—The Achilles heel of a viral killer? *Lancet* 2005; 366:876–877.

Messenger SL, Smith JS, Rupprecht CE: Emerging epidemiology of bat-associated cryptic cases of rabies in humans in the United States. *Clin Infect Dis* 2002;35:738–747.

Pounder D: Avoiding rabies. *Br Med J* 2005;331:469–470.

Rupprecht CE, Gibbons RV: Prophylaxis against rabies. *N Engl J Med* 2004;351:2626–2635.

Solomon T, Marston D, Mallewa M, et al: Paralytic rabies after a two-week holiday in India. *Br Med J* 2005;331:501–504.

Warrell MJ, Warrell DA: Rabies and other Lyssavirus diseases. *Lancet* 2004;363:959–968.

Willoughby RE Jr, Tieves KS, Hoffman GM, et al: Survival after treatment of rabies with induction of coma. *N Engl J Med* 2005;352:2508–2514.

Wyatt J: Rabies—update on a global disease. *Pediatr Infect Dis J* 2007;26: 351–352.

Chapter 272 ■ Polyomaviruses (JC virus and BK virus)

Hal B. Jenson

The polyomaviruses, which with the papillomaviruses constitute the Papovaviridae family, are small (45 nm), nonenveloped, double-stranded circular DNA viruses with a genome of 5,000 kbp. The 2 polyomaviruses that infect humans, **JC virus** and **BK virus,** share 75% genome homology but are antigenically distinct. They are named from the initials of the patients from whom the virus isolates were obtained. Both viruses are tropic for renal epithelium; JC virus also infects brain oligodendrocytes and is the etiologic agent of **progressive multifocal leukoencephalopathy (PML),** a rare and fatal demyelinating disease of immunocompromised persons. Several million persons in the United States were exposed to simian virus 40 (SV40), an oncogenic polyomavirus of Asian macaques that shares 70% homology to human polyomaviruses, from contaminated inactivated poliovirus vaccines administered during 1955–1963. There were no recognized sequelae and no demonstrable increased risk for cancer. Viruses that are antigenically indistinguishable from SV40 have been isolated from humans with PML, **SV40-PML viruses,** and may represent another strain of human polyomaviruses.

BK virus and JC virus can induce tumors in mice, and polyomavirus sequences have been identified in human tumors, including osteosarcomas, mesotheliomas, and brain tumors (ependymomas, glioblastomas, oligodendrogliomas, and others). An etiologic role of polyomaviruses in human oncogenesis has not been confirmed.

Infection with polyomaviruses is widespread but usually asymptomatic. Approximately half of children in the USA are infected with BK virus by 3–4 yr of age and with JC virus by 10–14 yr of age, and approximately 60–80% of adults are seropositive for 1 or both viruses. Transmission most likely occurs during close family contact. Polyomaviruses are found in tonsillar tissues, which may be the site of primary infection. Primary BK virus infection in children has been reported with mild upper respiratory tract symptoms, and also with acute cystitis in 3 children. Infection persists throughout life, with the viruses remaining latent in renal epithelium, oligodendrocytes, and peripheral blood mononuclear cells. Approximately 30–50% of healthy persons have detectable BK virus or JC virus in renal tissue at autopsy. Reactivation and viruria occur with increased frequency with advancing age and are more common in immunocompromised persons. BK and JC viruria, as detected by polymerase chain reaction (PCR), occurs in 2.6% and 13.2%, respectively, of persons <30 yr of age and in approximately 9% and 50%, respectively, of persons >60 yr of age.

Reactivation of BK virus and JC virus with asymptomatic viruria occurs in 10–50% of bone marrow transplant patients and in 20% of renal transplant patients. The direct cytopathic effect of reactivated BK virus on donor ureter has caused localized ureteral ulceration and ureteral stenosis in a few renal transplant patients. BK virus has also been associated with prolonged hemorrhagic cystitis in bone marrow transplant recipients. BK virus nephropathy in renal transplant patients results in diminished allograft function in 50% and graft failure in 1–5%.

Virus culture and PCR are used to detect virus. The high seroprevalence in the general population limits the usefulness of serologic testing. There is no specific treatment of BK virus nephropathy in renal transplant patients. Treatment is symptomatic with reduction of immunosuppression, as appropriate.

272.1 • Progressive Multifocal Leukoencephalopathy

PML is a rare central nervous system demyelinating disease resulting from JC virus lytic infection of myelin-producing oligodendrocytes, leading to demyelination, and an abortive infection of astrocytes. It occurs almost exclusively among immunocompromised persons. More than half of the cases of PML are associated with HIV infection, but it is rare among HIV-infected children. PML is found in approximately 5% of autopsied patients with AIDS.

PML characteristically presents with aphasia, ataxia, motor weakness including quadriparesis, visual field deficits (typically a homonymous hemianopsia) including cortical blindness, and speech and cognitive impairment including profound dementia, confusion, and personality change. Less frequent symptoms include cranial nerve deficits, sensory deficits, and extrapyramidal symptoms. Electroencephalography may be normal or reveal only focal slowing. The lesions on CT scan appear as hypodense, nonenhancing focal lesions of the white matter without surrounding edema or inflammation. On MRI the lesions show increased signal intensity on T2-weighted images. The cerebrospinal fluid (CSF) is typically normal, but may show mild elevation of protein and less frequently a mononuclear pleocytosis, usually less than 25 cells/μL. JC virus DNA can be detected by PCR in the CSF. Confirmation of the diagnosis requires brain biopsy for histopathologic examination, which is usually obtained by CT- or MRI-assisted stereotactic biopsy. The histology demonstrates multifocal, asymmetric, coalescing focal demyelination of white matter with a characteristic cytologic appearance of hyperchromatic enlarged oligodendroglial nuclei and bizarre astrocytes with enlarged multilobulated nuclei, usually with minimal inflammatory changes.

There is no recommended treatment for PML. Patients experience rapid neurologic deterioration with death ensuing usually within 6 mo of initial presentation. Case reports have suggested improvement of PML following treatment with interferon, idoxuridine, interleukin 2, or cidofovir. Aggressive antiretroviral therapy is prudent for HIV-infected persons, although neurologic deterioration has been reported, presumably resulting from immune reconstitution syndrome.

Bergsagel DJ, Finegold MJ, Butel JS, et al: DNA sequences similar to those of simian virus 40 in ependymomas and choroid plexus tumors of childhood. *N Engl J Med* 1992;326:988–993.

DeLuca A, Giancola ML, Ammassari A, et al: Potent antiretroviral therapy with or without cidofovir for AIDS-associated progressive multifocal leukoencephalopathy: Extended follow-up of an observational study. *J Neurovirol* 2001;7:364–368.

Elsner C, Dörries K: Evidence of human polyomavirus BK and JC infection in normal brain tissue. *Virology* 1992;191:72–80.

Hirsch HH: Polyomavirus BK nephropathy: A (re-)emerging complication in renal transplantation. *Am J Transplant* 2002;2:25–30.

Hirsch HH, Knowles W, Dickenmann M, et al: Prospective study of polyomavirus type BK replication and nephropathy in renal-transplant patients. *N Engl J Med* 2002;347:488–496.

Limaye AP, Jerome KR, Kuhr CS, et al: Quantitation of BK virus load in serum for the diagnosis of BK virus-associated nephropathy in renal transplant recipients. *J Infect Dis* 2001;183:1669–1672.

Nickeleit V, Klimkait T, Binet I, et al: Testing for polyomavirus type BK DNA in plasma to identify renal-allograft recipients with viral nephropathy. *N Engl J Med* 2000;342:1309–1315.

Randhawa PS, Demetrius AJ: Nephropathy due to polyomavirus type BK. *N Engl J Med* 2000;342:1361–1363.

Sabath BF, Major EO: Traffic of JC virus from sites of initial infection to the brain: The path to progressive multifocal leukoencephalopathy. *J Infect Dis* 2002;186(Suppl):S180–S186.

Strickler HD, Rosenberg PS, Devesa SS, et al: Contamination of poliovirus vaccines with simian virus 40 (1955–1963) and subsequent cancer rates. *JAMA* 1998;279:292–295.

Sundsfjord A, Flaegstad T, Flø R, et al: BK and JC viruses in human immunodeficiency virus type 1-infected persons: Prevalence, excretion, viremia, and viral regulatory regions. *J Infect Dis* 1994;169:485–490.

Chapter 273 ■ Acquired Immunodeficiency Syndrome (Human Immunodeficiency Virus) Ram Yogev and Ellen Gould Chadwick

Advances in research and major improvements in the treatment and management of HIV infection have brought about a substantial decrease in the incidence of new HIV infections and AIDS in children born in the United States and Western Europe. Most HIV-infected children are born in developing countries. It is estimated that in 2004, 640,000 children <15 yr of age were newly infected with HIV. In addition, because HIV-infected mothers are likely to die of AIDS, 13 million children have been orphaned thus far and an estimated 19 million will be orphaned by 2010. HIV infection in children progresses more rapidly than in adults, and some untreated children die within the 1st 2 yr of life. This rapid progression is correlated with higher viral burden and faster depletion of infected CD4 lymphocytes in infants and children than in adults. Accurate diagnostic tests and the availability of potent drugs to inhibit HIV replication have dramatically increased the ability to prevent and control this devastating disease.

ETIOLOGY. HIV-1 and HIV-2 are members of the Retroviridae family and belong to the *Lentivirus* genus, which includes cytopathic viruses causing diverse diseases in several animal species. The HIV-1 genome contains 2 copies of single-stranded RNA that is 9.2 kb in size. At both ends of the genome there are identical regions, called **long terminal repeats,** which contain the regulation and expression genes of HIV. The remainder of the genome includes 3 major sections: the **GAG** region, which encodes the viral core proteins (p24, p17, p9, p6, which are derived from the precursor p55); the **POL** region, which encodes the viral enzymes (i.e., reverse transcriptase [p51], protease [pl0], and integrase

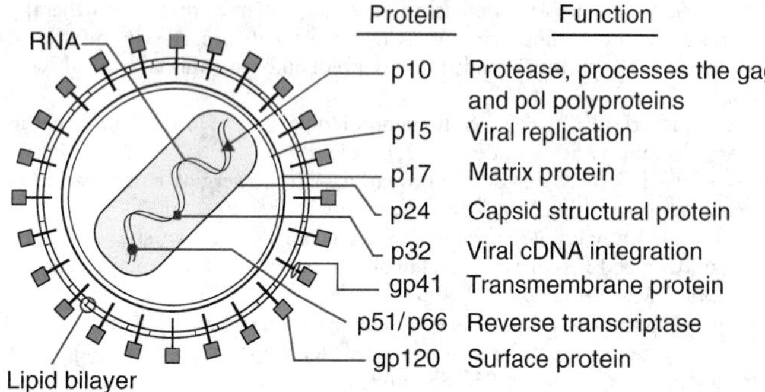

Figure 273-1. The human immunodeficiency virus and associated proteins and their functions.

[p32]); and the **ENV** region, which encodes the viral envelope proteins (gp120 and gp41, which are derived from the precursor gp160). Other regulatory proteins, such as tat (pl4), rev (p19), nef (p27), vpr (pl5), and vif (p23), are involved in transactivation, viral messenger RNA expression, viral replication, induction of cell cycle arrest, promotion of nuclear import of viral reverse transcription complexes, downregulation of cell surface receptors CD4 and class I major histocompatibility complex, proviral DNA synthesis, and virus release (Fig. 273-1).

The major external viral protein of HIV-1 is a heavily glycosylated gp120 protein that is associated with the transmembrane glycoprotein gp41; gp41 is very immunogenic and is used to detect HIV-1 antibodies in diagnostic assays; gp120 is a complex molecule that includes the highly variable **V3 loop.** This region is immunodominant for neutralizing antibodies. The heterogeneity of gp120 presents major obstacles in establishing an effective HIV vaccine. The gp120 glycoprotein also carries the binding site for the CD4 molecule, the most common host cell surface receptor of T lymphocytes. This tropism for $CD4^+$ T cells is beneficial to the virus because it reduces the effectiveness of the host immune system. Other CD4-bearing cells include macrophages and microglial cells. Several chemokines serve as co-receptors for the envelope glycoproteins, permitting membrane fusion and entry into the cell. Most HIV strains have a specific tropism for 1 of the chemokines, including the fusion-inducing molecule **CXCR-4,** which has been shown to act as a co-receptor for HIV attachment to lymphocytes, and **CCR-5,** a β chemokine receptor that facilitates HIV entry into macrophages. Several other chemokine receptors (CCR-3) have also been shown in vitro to serve as virus co-receptors.

Other mechanisms of attachment of HIV to cells use non-neutralizing antiviral antibodies and complement receptors. The Fab portion of these antibodies attaches to the virus surface, and the Fc portion binds to cells that express Fc receptors (macrophages, fibroblasts), thus facilitating virus transfer into the cell. Other cell surface receptors, such as mannose-binding protein on macrophages and **DC-specific C-type lectin (DC-SIGN)** on dendritic cells, also bind to the HIV-1 envelope glycoprotein and increase the efficiency of viral infectivity. Following viral attachment, gp120 and the CD4 molecule undergo conformational changes, and gp41 interacts with the fusion receptor on the cell surface. Viral fusion with the cell membrane allows entry of viral RNA into the cell cytoplasm. This process involves accessory viral proteins (nef, vif) and binding of cyclophilin A (a host cellular protein) to p24. Viral DNA copies are then transcribed from the virion RNA through viral reverse transcriptase enzyme activity, and duplication of the DNA copies produces double-stranded circular DNA. The HIV-1 reverse transcriptase is error prone and lacks error-correcting mechanisms. Thus, many mutations arise, creating wide genetic variation in HIV-1 isolates even within an individual patient. The circular DNA is transported into the cell nucleus, where it is integrated into chromosomal DNA and referred to as the provirus. The provirus has the advantage of latency as it can remain dormant for extended periods. Integration usually occurs near active genes, which allow a high level of viral production in response to various external factors such as an increase in inflammatory cytokines (by infection with other pathogens) and cellular activation. Depending on the relative expression of the viral regulatory genes (tat, rev, nef), the proviral DNA may encode production of the viral RNA genome, which in turn leads to production of viral proteins necessary for viral assembly.

HIV-1 transcription is followed by translation. A capsid polyprotein is cleaved to produce, among others, the virus-specific protease (p10). This enzyme is critical for HIV-1 assembly. Several HIV-1 antiprotease drugs have been developed, targeting the increased sensitivity of the viral protease, which differs from the cellular proteases. The RNA genome is then incorporated into the newly formed viral capsid that requires zinc finger domains (p7) and the matrix protein (p17). As new virus is formed, it buds through specialized membrane areas, known as **lipid rafts,** and is released.

The diversity of HIV (groups M [main], O [outlier], N [non-M, non-O]) probably occurred from multiple zoonotic infections from primates in different geographic regions. Group M diversified to several subtypes (or clades A to H). In each region of the world, certain clades predominate. For example, clade B is found in the United States and South America, clade E in Thailand, and clade C in South Africa. Clades are mixed in some patients due to HIV recombination, and some crossing between groups (i.e., M and O) has been reported.

HIV-2 is known to cause infection in several monkey species. It is a rare cause of infection in children. It is most prevalent in Western Africa, but recently cases from Europe and Southern Asia have been reported. The diagnosis of HIV-2 infection is more difficult because the standard confirmatory assays (immunoblot) are HIV-1 specific and may give indeterminate results with HIV-2 infection. If HIV-2 infection is suspected, a specific immunoblot test that detects antibody to HIV-2 peptides should be used. In addition, the recently approved rapid tests should not be used in patients suspected to be HIV-2 infected because they test only for HIV-1. Third generation standard enzyme-linked immunosorbent assays (ELISA) should be used because they capture both HIV-1 and HIV-2.

EPIDEMIOLOGY. The World Health Organization (WHO) estimated that >39 million persons worldwide were living with HIV infection at the end of 2004, including 2.2 million children <15 yr of age. In 2004, almost 5 million people acquired HIV and 3 million died, including 510,000 children. More than 90% of HIV-infected individuals live in developing nations. Sub-Saharan Africa accounts for the fastest growing epidemic, with almost 90% of the world's total population of HIV-infected children. India and Thailand dominate the epidemic in Southeast Asia, with more recent expansion into Vietnam, China, and Cambodia.

Worldwide, 60% of HIV-infected individuals are women; heterosexual transmission accounts for most HIV spread. In the United States, women account for 27% of AIDS cases reported to the Centers for Disease Control and Prevention (CDC) in 2003. In 2003, the percentage of American women whose exposure category was heterosexual contact rose to 71%, surpassing that of injecting drug use (IDU) (27%). Many of these women have been infected heterosexually by men unrecognized to be infected or to be in a high-risk group. Among mothers giving birth to children with AIDS, almost half reported no identified risk factor. The estimated number of U.S. children with AIDS diagnosed each year increased from 1984 to 1992, then declined by almost 95% by 2003 to <100 cases annually. There were 9,419 children diagnosed with AIDS from the beginning of the epidemic through 2003. This decline most likely reflects the effectiveness of zidovudine (ZDV) and other anti-retroviral drugs in reducing perinatal HIV transmission. While the number of HIV-infected infants is decreasing in industrialized nations, the worldwide number of HIV-infected children is increasing dramatically because of lack of access to medications to prevent perinatal transmission. It is estimated that as of 2004, 12,000 to 15,000 HIV-infected children were living in the United States.

In the United States, virtually all HIV infections in children <13 yr of age are the result of **vertical transmission** from an HIV-infected mother. A vanishing minority of children were infected through receipt of contaminated blood products and/or clotting factors (5%), primarily before 1985, when screening of the blood supply was instituted. Children of racial and ethnic minority groups are disproportionately over-represented, particularly non-Hispanic African-Americans and Hispanics. Race and ethnicity is not a risk factor for HIV infection but more likely reflects other factors that may be predictive of increased risk for HIV infection, such as lack of educational and economic opportunities and higher rates of IDU. New York, Florida, and California account for most U.S. pediatric cases; 85% were diagnosed in metropolitan areas with populations of >500,000 and 9% in metropolitan areas with populations of 50,000–500,000.

Although adolescents (13–24 yr of age) with AIDS represent a minority of U.S. cases (approximately 5%), they constitute 1 of the fastest growing groups of newly infected persons in the country. Considering the long latency period between the time of infection and the development of clinical symptoms, reliance on AIDS case definition surveillance data severely under-represents the impact of the disease in adolescents. Based on a median incubation period of 8–12 yr, it has been estimated that 15–20% of all AIDS cases were acquired between 13 and 19 yr of age. Risk factors for HIV infection vary by gender in adolescents. The majority of teenaged males with AIDS who acquired HIV through sexual contact had male-to-male transmission. In contrast, more than half of adolescent females with AIDS were infected through heterosexual contact and ⅙ through IDU, compared with 8% and 6%, respectively, in teenaged males.

As in the pediatric population, adolescent racial and ethnic minority populations are over-represented, especially among females. In addition, a greater proportion of female adolescents have AIDS (male : female ratio 1.2 : 1) than do female adults >25 yr of age (male : female ratio 4.5 : 1).

Transmission. Transmission of HIV-1 occurs via sexual contact, parenteral exposure to blood, or vertical transmission from mother to child. The primary route of infection in the pediatric population is vertical transmission, accounting for almost all new cases. Rates of transmission of HIV from mother to child have varied in different parts of the United States and among countries. The United States and Europe have documented transmission rates in untreated women between 12–30%. Transmission rates in Africa and Haiti are higher (25–52%). Perinatal treatment of HIV-infected mothers with anti-retroviral drugs has dramatically decreased these rates to <2% in pregnant women on effective therapy.

Vertical transmission of HIV can occur before (**intrauterine**), during (**intrapartum**), or after delivery (through **breast-feeding**). Intrauterine transmission has been suggested by identification of HIV by culture or polymerase chain reaction (PCR) in fetal tissue as early as 10 wk. First trimester placental tissue from HIV-infected women has been demonstrated to contain HIV by in situ hybridization and immunocytochemistry. It is generally accepted that 30–40% of infected newborns are infected in utero, because this percentage of infants has laboratory evidence of infection (positive viral culture or PCR) within the 1st wk of life. Some studies have found that viral detection soon after birth also correlates with early onset of symptoms and rapid progression to AIDS, consistent with more long-standing infection during gestation.

The highest percentage of HIV-infected children acquire the virus intrapartum, evidenced by the fact that 60–70% of infected infants do not demonstrate detectable virus before 1 wk of age. The mechanism of transmission appears to be exposure to infected blood and cervicovaginal secretions in the birth canal, where HIV is found in high titers during late gestation and delivery. The international registry of HIV-exposed twins found that first-born twins were 3 times more likely to be infected, reflecting the longer time that twin A is exposed to the birth canal.

The least common route of vertical transmission in industrialized nations is breast-feeding; this is an important transmission route in developing countries. Both free and cell-associated viruses have been detected in breast milk from HIV-infected mothers. The additional risk for transmission through breast-feeding in women with HIV infection before pregnancy is 14% compared with a 29% increase in breast-feeding women who acquired HIV postnatally. This suggests that the viremia experienced by the mother during primary infection doubles the risk for transmission. It therefore seems reasonable for women to substitute infant formula for breast milk if they are known to be HIV-infected or are at risk for ongoing sexual or parenteral exposure to HIV. However, the WHO recommends that in developing countries where other diseases (diarrhea, pneumonia, malnutrition) substantially contribute to a high infant mortality rate, the benefit of breast-feeding outweighs the risk for HIV transmission, and HIV-infected women in developing countries should breast-feed their infants for the 1st 6 mo of life followed by rapid weaning.

Several risk factors influence the rate of vertical transmission: preterm delivery (<34 wk gestation), a low maternal antenatal CD4 count, and use of illicit drugs during pregnancy. The most important variables appear to be >4 hr duration of ruptured membranes and birthweight <2,500 g, each of which doubles the transmission rate. Elective cesarean delivery decreases transmission by 87% if used in conjunction with zidovudine therapy in the mother and infant. Because these data predated the advent of **highly active anti-retroviral therapy (HAART)**, the additional benefit of cesarean section is probably negligible if the mother's viral load is <1,000 copies/mL. Although several studies have shown an increased rate of transmission in women with advanced disease (i.e., AIDS) or high viral load (>50,000 copies/mL), some transmitting mothers in each group were asymptomatic or had a low, but detectable, viral load. Thus, in the USA it is recommended to consider cesarean section if the viral load is >1,000 copies/mL.

Transfusions of infected blood or blood products have accounted for 3–6% of all pediatric AIDS cases. The period of highest risk was between 1978 and 1985, before the availability of HIV antibody-screened blood products. Whereas the prevalence of HIV infection in individuals with hemophilia treated before 1985 was as high as 70%, heat treatment of factor VIII concentrate and HIV antibody screening of donors has virtually eliminated HIV transmission in this population. Blood donor screening has dramatically reduced, but not eliminated, the risk for transfusion-associated HIV infection. The rate of HIV transmission through antibody-screened blood in the USA is estimated to be approximately 1/60,000 transfused units. In many developing countries, screening of blood donors is not uniform, and the risk for transmitting HIV infection via transfusion is substantial.

Although HIV can be isolated rarely from saliva, it is in very low titers (<1 infectious particle/mL) and has not been implicated as a transmission vehicle. Studies of hundreds of household contacts of HIV-infected individuals have found that the risk for household HIV transmission is practically nonexistent. Only a few cases have been reported in which urine or feces (possibly devoid of visible blood) have been proposed as a possible vehicle of HIV transmission.

In the pediatric population, sexual transmission is infrequent, but a small number of cases resulting from sexual abuse have been reported. Sexual contact is a major route of transmission in the adolescent population, accounting for most of the cases.

PATHOGENESIS. When the mucosa serves as the portal of entry for the HIV, the 1st cells to be infected are the dendritic cells. These cells collect and process antigens introduced from the periphery and transports them to the lymphoid tissue. HIV does not infect the dendritic cell but it binds to its DC-SIGN surface molecule, which allows the virus to survive until it reaches the lymphatic tissue. In the lymph node, the virus selectively binds to cells expressing CD4 molecules on their surface, primarily helper T lymphocytes (CD4 cells) and cells of the monocyte-macrophage lineage. Other cells bearing CD4, such as microglia, astrocytes, oligodendroglia, and placental tissue containing villous Hofbauer cells, may also be infected by HIV. Additional factors (co-receptors) are necessary for HIV fusion and entry into cells. These factors include the chemokines CXCR4 (fusion) and CCR5. Other chemokines (CCR1, CCR3) may be necessary for the fusion of certain HIV strains. Individuals with homozygous CCR5 deletion mutation are highly protected from HIV infection. Usually, CD4 lymphocytes, recruited to respond to viral antigen, migrate to the lymph nodes where they become activated and proliferate, making them highly susceptible to HIV infection. This antigen-driven migration and accumulation of CD4 cells within the lymphoid tissue may contribute to the generalized lymphadenopathy characteristic of the acute retroviral syndrome in adults and adolescents. HIV preferentially infects the very cells that respond to it (HIV-specific memory CD4 cells), which accounts for the progressive loss of these cells' response and the subsequent loss of control of HIV replication. When HIV replication reaches a threshold (usually within 3–6 wk from the time of infection), a burst of plasma viremia occurs. This intense viremia causes **flulike symptoms** (fever, rash, lymphadenopathy, arthralgia) in 50–70% of infected adults. With establishment of a cellular and humoral immune response within 2–4 mo, the viral load in the blood declines substantially, and patients enter a phase characterized by a lack of symptoms and a return of CD4 cells to only moderately decreased levels.

Early HIV-1 replication in children has no apparent clinical manifestations. Whether tested by virus isolation or by PCR for viral nucleic acid sequences, fewer than 50% of HIV-1-infected infants demonstrate evidence of the virus at birth. The virus load increases by 1–4 mo, and almost all HIV-infected infants have detectable HIV-1 in peripheral blood by 4 mo of age.

In adults, the long period of clinical latency (up to 8–12 yr) is not indicative of viral latency. In fact, there is a very high turnover of virus and CD4 lymphocytes (more than a billion cells per day), which gradually causes deterioration of the immune system, evidenced particularly by depletion of CD4 cells. Several mechanisms for the depletion of CD4 cells in adults and children have been suggested, including HIV-mediated single cell killing, formation of multinucleated giant cells of infected and uninfected CD4 cells **(syncytia formation)**, virus-specific immune responses (natural killer cells, antibody-dependent cellular cytotoxicity), superantigen-mediated activation of T cells (rendering them more susceptible to infection with HIV), autoimmunity, and programmed cell death (apoptosis). The viral burden in the lymphoid organs is greater than that in the peripheral blood during the asymptomatic period. As HIV virions and their immune complexes migrate through the lymph nodes, they are trapped in the network of dendritic follicular cells. Because the ability of HIV to replicate in T cells depends on the state of activation of the cells, the immune activation that takes place within the microenvironment of the nodes in HIV disease serves to promote infection of new CD4 cells as well as subsequent viral replication within the cells. Viral replication in monocytes, which can be infected productively yet resist killing, explains their role as reservoirs of HIV and as effectors of tissue damage in organs such as the brain.

Cell-mediated and humoral responses occur early in the infection. CD8 T cells play an important role in containing the infection. These cells produce various ligands (MIP-1α, MIP-1β, RANTES), which suppress HIV replication by blocking the binding of the virus to the co-receptors (CCR5). HIV-specific cytotoxic T lymphocytes (CTLs) develop against both the structural (ENV, POL, GAG) and regulatory (tat) viral proteins. The CTLs appear at the end of the acute retroviral infection as the viral replication is controlled by killing HIV-infected cells before new viruses are produced and by secreting potent antiviral factors that compete with the virus for its receptors (CCR5). Neutralizing antibodies appear later during the infection and seem to help in the continued suppression of viral replication during clinical latency. There are at least 2 possible mechanisms that control the steady-state viral load level during the chronic clinical latency. One mechanism may be the limited availability of activated CD4 cells, which prevent further increase in viral load due to a set point (controlled) replication. The other mechanism, the immune control, suggests that the development of an active immune response (whose magnitude is controlled by the amount of viral antigen) limits viral replication at a steady state. There is no general consensus about which of these 2 mechanisms is more important. The CD4 cell limitation mechanism accounts for the effect of anti-retroviral therapy, whereas the immune control mechanism emphasizes the importance of immune modulation treatment (cytokines, vaccines) to increase the efficiency of the immune response, which, in turn, slows disease progression.

A group of cytokines, such as tumor necrosis factor-α (TNF-α), TNF-β, interleukin 1 (IL-1), IL-2, IL-3, IL-6, IL-8, IL-12, IL-15, granulocyte-macrophage colony-stimulating factor, and macrophage colony-stimulating factor, play an integral role in upregulating HIV expression from a state of quiescent infection to active viral replication. Other cytokines, such as interferon-γ (IFN-γ), IFN-β, and IL-13, exert a suppressive effect on HIV replication. Certain cytokines (IL-4, IL-10, IFN-γ, TGF-β) reduce or enhance viral replication depending on the infected cell type. The interactions among these cytokines influence the concentration of viral particles in the tissues. Plasma concentrations of cytokines need not be elevated for them to exert their effect, because they are produced and act locally in the tissues. Thus, even during states of apparent immunologic quiescence, the complex interaction of cytokines sustains a constant level of viral expression, particularly in the lymph nodes.

Commonly HIV isolated during the clinical latency period grows slowly in culture and produces low titers of reverse transcriptase. These isolates are called **non-syncytium-inducing (NSI) viruses,** which use CCR5 as their co-receptor. By the late stages of clinical latency, the isolated virus is phenotypically different. It grows rapidly and to high titers in culture and it uses CXCR4 as its co-receptor. These isolates are called **syncytium-inducing (SI) viruses.** The switch from NSI to SI increases the capacity of the virus to replicate, to infect a broader range of target cells (CXCR4 is more widely expressed on resting and activated immune cells), and to kill T cells more rapidly and efficiently. As a result, the clinical latency phase is over and progression toward AIDS is noted. The **progression of disease** is related temporally to the gradual disruption of lymph node architecture and degeneration of the follicular dendritic cell network with loss of its ability to trap HIV particles. This frees the virus to recirculate, producing high levels of viremia and an increased disappearance of CD4 T cells during the later stages of disease.

Before HAART was available, 3 **distinct patterns of disease** were described in children. Approximately 15–25% of HIV-infected newborns in developed countries present with a **rapid disease course,** with onset of AIDS and symptoms during the 1st few months of life and, if untreated, a median survival time of 6–9 mo. In resource-poor countries, the majority of HIV-infected newborns will have this rapidly progressing disease. It has been suggested that if intrauterine infection coincides with the period of rapid expansion of CD4 cells in the fetus, it could effectively infect the majority of the body's immunocompetent cells. The normal migration of these cells to the marrow, spleen, and thymus would result in efficient systemic delivery of HIV, unchecked by the immature immune system of the fetus. Thus, infection would be established before the normal ontogenic development of the immune system, causing more severe impairment of immunity. Most children in this group have a positive HIV-1 culture and/or detectable virus in the plasma (median level 11,000 copies/mL) in the 1st 48 hr of life. This early evidence of viral presence suggests that the newborn was infected in utero. The viral load rapidly increases and peaks by 2–3 mo of age (median 750,000 copies/mL) and subsequently declines slowly. In contrast to the viral load in adults, the viral load in infants stays high for at least the 1st 2 yrs of life.

The majority of perinatally infected newborns (60–80%) in developed countries present with a 2nd pattern, that of a much **slower progression** of disease, with a median survival time of 6 yr. Many patients in this group have a negative viral culture or PCR in the 1st wk of life and are therefore considered to be infected intrapartum. In a typical patient, the viral load rapidly increases by 2–3 mo of age (median 100,000 copies/mL) and slowly declines over a period of 24 mo. The slow decline in viral load is in sharp contrast to the rapid decline after primary infection seen in adults. This observation can be explained only partially by the immaturity of the immune system in newborns and infants.

The 3rd pattern of disease (**long-term survivors**) occurs in a small percentage (<5%) of perinatally infected children who have minimal or no progression of disease with relatively normal CD4 counts and very low viral loads for longer than 8 yr. Mechanisms for the delay in disease progression include effective humoral immunity and/or CTL responses, host genetic factors (e.g., HLA profile), and infection with attenuated (defective gene) virus.

HIV-infected children have changes in the immune system that are similar to those in HIV-infected adults. CD4 cell depletion may be less dramatic because infants normally have a relative lymphocytosis. For example, a value of 1,500 CD4 cells/mm^3 in children <1 yr of age is indicative of severe CD4 depletion and is comparable to <200 CD4 cells/mm^3 in adults. Lymphopenia is relatively rare in perinatally infected children and is usually only seen in older children or those with end-stage disease. Although cutaneous anergy is common during HIV infection, it is also frequent in healthy children <1 yr of age, and thus its interpretation is difficult in infected infants.

B-cell activation occurs in most children early in the infection as evidenced by **hypergammaglobulinemia** with high levels of anti-HIV-1 antibody. This response may reflect both dysregulation of T-cell suppression of B-cell antibody synthesis and active CD4 enhancement of B-lymphocyte humoral response. The B-cell dysregulation precedes the CD4 depletion in many children, and may serve as a surrogate marker of HIV infection in symptomatic children in whom specific diagnostic tests (PCR, culture) are not available or are too expensive. Despite the increased levels of immunoglobulins, evidence of specific antibody production does not occur in some children, and in others adequate antibody levels do not confer protection. Hypogammaglobulinemia is very rare (<1%).

Central nervous system (CNS) involvement is more common in pediatric patients than in adults. Macrophages and microglia play an important role in HIV neuropathogenesis, and data suggest that astrocytes may also be involved. Although the specific mechanisms for encephalopathy in children are not yet clear, the developing brain in young infants is affected by at least 2 mechanisms. The virus itself may directly infect various brain cells or cause indirect damage to the nervous system by the release of cytokines (IL-1α, IL-1β, TNF-α, IL-2) or reactive oxygen from HIV-infected lymphocytes or macrophages.

CLINICAL MANIFESTATIONS. The clinical manifestations of HIV infection vary widely among infants, children, and adolescents. In most infants, physical examination at birth is normal. Initial symptoms may be subtle, such as lymphadenopathy and hepatosplenomegaly, or nonspecific, such as failure to thrive, chronic or recurrent diarrhea, interstitial pneumonia, or oral thrush, and may be distinguishable only by their persistence. Whereas systemic and pulmonary findings are common in the USA and Europe, chronic diarrhea, wasting, and severe malnutrition predominate in Africa. Symptoms found more commonly in children than adults with HIV infection include recurrent bacterial infections, chronic parotid swelling, lymphocytic interstitial pneumonitis (LIP), and early onset of progressive neurologic deterioration.

The HIV classification system is used to categorize the stage of pediatric disease by using 2 parameters: clinical status and degree of immunologic impairment (Table 273-1). Among the clinical categories, **category A (mild symptoms)** includes children with at least 2 mild symptoms such as lymphadenopathy, parotitis, hepatomegaly, splenomegaly, dermatitis, and recurrent or persistent sinusitis or otitis media (Table 273-2). **Category B (moderate symptoms)** includes, for example, children with LIP, oropharyngeal thrush persisting for >2 mo, recurrent or chronic diarrhea, persistent fever for >1 mo, hepatitis, recurrent herpes simplex virus (HSV) stomatitis or HSV esophagitis or pneumonitis, disseminated varicella (i.e., with visceral involvement), cardiomegaly, or nephropathy (see Table 273-2). **Category C (severe symptoms)** includes, for example, children with 2 serious bacterial infections (sepsis, meningitis, pneumonia) in a 2 yr

TABLE 273-1. Pediatric HIV Classification for Children Younger Than 13 Years

	IMMUNOLOGIC CATEGORIES: AGE-SPECIFIC CD4$^+$ T-LYMPHOCYTE COUNT AND PERCENTAGE OF TOTAL LYMPHOCYTES*						CLINICAL CLASSIFICATIONS†			
	<12 mo		1–5 yr		6–12 yr					
IMMUNOLOGIC DEFINITIONS	μL	%	μL	%	μL	%	N: No Signs or Symptoms	A: Mild Signs and Symptoms	B: Moderate Signs and Symptoms‡	C: Severe Signs and Symptoms‡
1: No evidence of suppression	≥1500	≥25	≥1000	≥25	≥500	≥25	N1	A1	B1	C1
2: Evidence of moderate suppression	750–1499	15–24	500–999	15–24	200–499	15–24	N2	A2	B1	C2
3: Severe suppression	<750	<15	<500	<15	<200	<15	N3	A3	B3	C3

*To convert values in μL to Système International units ($\times 10^9$/L), multiply by 0.001.

†Children whose HIV infection status is not confirmed are classified by using this grid with a letter E (for perinatally exposed) placed before the appropriate classification code (eg, EN2).

‡Lymphoid interstitial pneumonitis in category B or any condition in category C is reportable to state and local health departments as acquired immunodeficiency syndrome (AIDS-defining conditions) (see Table 273-2 for further definition of clinical categories).

Modified from the Centers for Disease Control and Prevention: 1994 revised classification system for human immunodeficiency virus infection in children less than 13 years of age. Official authorized addenda: Human immunodeficiency virus infection codes and official guidelines for coding and reporting ICD-9-CM. *MMWR Recomm Rep* 1994;43(RR-12):1–19.

From *Red Book: 2006 Report of the Committee on Infectious Diseases*, 27th ed. Elk Grove Village, IL, American Academy of Pediatrics, 2006, p 382.

TABLE 273-2. Clinical Categories for Children Younger Than 13 Years of Age with HIV infection

CATEGORY N: NOT SYMPTOMATIC

Children who have no signs or symptoms considered to be the result of HIV infection or have only 1 of the conditions listed in category A.

CATEGORY A: MILDLY SYMPTOMATIC

Children with 2 or more of the conditions listed but none of the conditions listed in categories B and C.

- Lymphadenopathy (≥0.5 cm at more than 2 sites; bilateral at 1 site)
- Hepatomegaly
- Splenomegaly
- Dermatitis
- Parotitis
- Recurrent or persistent upper respiratory tract infection, sinusitis, or otitis media

CATEGORY B: MODERATELY SYMPTOMATIC

Children who have symptomatic conditions other than those listed for category A or C that are attributed to HIV infection.

- Anemia (hemoglobin <8 g/dL [<80 g/L]), neutropenia (white blood cell count <1,000/μL [<1.0 × 10^9/L]), and/or thrombocytopenia (platelet count <100 × 10^3/μL [<100 × 10^9/L]) persisting for ≥30 days
- Bacterial meningitis, pneumonia, or sepsis (single episode)
- Candidiasis, oropharyngeal (thrush), persisting (>2 mo) in children older than 6 mo of age
- Cardiomyopathy
- Cytomegalovirus infection, with onset before 1 mo of age
- Diarrhea, recurrent or chronic
- Hepatitis
- Herpes simplex virus (HSV) stomatitis, recurrent (>2 episodes within 1 year)
- HSV bronchitis, pneumonitis, or esophagitis with onset before 1 mo of age
- Herpes zoster (shingles) involving at least 2 distinct episodes or more than 1 dermatome
- Leiomyosarcoma
- Lymphoid interstitial pneumonia or pulmonary lymphoid hyperplasia complex
- Nephropathy
- Nocardiosis
- Persistent fever (lasting >1 mo)
- Toxoplasmosis, onset before 1 mo of age
- Varicella, disseminated (complicated chickenpox)

CATEGORY C: SEVERELY SYMPTOMATIC

- Serious bacterial infections, multiple or recurrent (i.e. any combination of at least 2 culture-confirmed infections within a 2 yr period), of the following types: septicemia, pneumonia, meningitis, bone or joint infection, or abscess of an internal organ or body cavity (excluding otitis media, superficial skin or mucosal abscesses, and indwelling catheter-related infections)
- Candidiasis, esophageal or pulmonary (bronchi, trachea, lungs)
- Coccidioidomycosis, disseminated (at site other than or in addition to lungs or cervical or hilar lymph nodes)
- Cryptococcosis, extrapulmonary
- Cryptosporidiosis or isosporiasis with diarrhea persisting >1 mo
- Cytomegalovirus disease with onset of symptoms after 1 mo of age (at a site other than liver, spleen, or lymph nodes)
- Encephalopathy (at least 1 of the following progressive findings present for at least 2 mo in the absence of a concurrent illness other than HIV infection that could explain the findings): (1) failure to attain or loss of developmental milestones or loss of intellectual ability, verified by standard developmental scale or neuropsychologic tests; (2) impaired brain growth or acquired microcephaly demonstrated by head circumference measurements or brain atrophy demonstrated by CT or MRI (serial imaging required for children younger than 2 yr of age); or (3) acquired symmetric motor deficit manifested by 2 or more of the following: paresis, pathologic reflexes, ataxia, or gait disturbance
- HSV infection causing a mucocutaneous ulcer that persists for greater than 1 mo or bronchitis, pneumonitis or esophagitis for any duration affecting a child older than 1 mo of age
- Histoplasmosis, disseminated (at a site other than or in addition to lungs or cervical or hilar lymph nodes)
- Kaposi sarcoma
- Lymphoma, primary, in brain
- Lymphoma, small, noncleaved cell (Burkitt), or immunoblastic; or large-cell lymphoma of B-lymphocyte or unknown immunologic phenotype
- *Mycobacterium tuberculosis* infection, disseminated or extrapulmonary
- *Mycobacterium*, other species or unidentified species infection, disseminated (at a site other than or in addition to lungs, skin, or cervical or hilar lymph nodes)
- *Pneumocystis jiroveci* pneumonia
- Progressive multifocal leukoencephalopathy
- *Salmonella* (nontyphoid) septicemia, recurrent
- Toxoplasmosis of the brain with onset at after 1 mo of age
- Wasting syndrome in the absence of a concurrent illness other than HIV infection that could explain the following findings: (1) persistent weight loss >10% of baseline; (2) downward crossing of at least 2 of the following percentile lines on the weight-for-age chart (e.g., 95th, 75th, 50th, 25th, 5th) in a child 1 yr of age or older; OR (3) <5th percentile on weight-for-height chart on 2 consecutive measurements, ≥30 days apart; PLUS (1) chronic diarrhea (i.e., at least 2 loose stools per day for >30 days); OR (2) documented fever (for >30 days, intermittent or constant)

Modified from the Centers for Disease Control and Prevention. 1994 revised classification system for human immunodeficiency virus infection in children less than 13 years of age. Official authorized addenda: Human immunodeficiency virus infection codes and official guidelines for coding and reporting ICD-9-CM. *MMWR Recomm Rep* 1994;43(RR-12):1–19.
From *Red Book: 2006 Report of the Committee on Infectious Diseases*, 27th ed. Elk Grove Village, IL, American Academy of Pediatrics, 2006, pp 380–381.

period, esophageal or lower respiratory tract candidiasis, cryptococcosis, cryptosporidiosis (>1 mo), encephalopathy, malignancies, disseminated mycobacterial infection, *Pneumocystis* pneumonia, cerebral toxoplasmosis (onset >1 mo of age), and severe weight loss.

The immune classification is based on the absolute CD4 lymphocyte count or the percentage of CD4 cells (see Table 273-1). Age adjustment of the absolute CD4 count is necessary because counts that are relatively high in normal infants decline steadily until 6 yr of age, when they reach adult norms. If there is a discrepancy between the CD4 count and percentage, the disease is classified into the more severe category.

Infections. Approximately 20% of AIDS-defining illnesses in children are recurrent bacterial infections caused primarily by encapsulated organisms such as *Streptococcus pneumoniae* and *Salmonella* (Table 273-3). Other pathogens, including *Staphylococcus, Enterococcus, Pseudomonas aeruginosa,* and *Haemophilus influenzae,* and other gram-positive and gram-negative organisms may also be seen. Most of these infections are the result of HIV-related disturbances in humoral immunity. The most common serious infections are bacteremia, sepsis, and bacterial pneumonia, accounting for >50% of infections in HIV-infected children. Meningitis, urinary tract infections, deep-seated abscesses, and bone/joint infection occur less frequently. Milder recurrent infections, such as otitis media, sinusitis, and skin and soft tissue infections, are very common and may be chronic with atypical presentations.

Opportunistic infections are generally seen in children with severe depression of the CD4 count. In adults, these infections usually represent reactivation of a latent infection acquired early in life. In contrast, young children generally have primary infection and, lacking prior immunity, often have a more fulminant course of disease. This principle is best illustrated by *Pneumocystis carinii (jiroveci)* pneumonia (PCP), the most common opportunistic infection in the pediatric population (see Chapter 241). The peak incidence of PCP occurs at age 3–6 mo, with the highest mortality rate in children <1 yr of age. Aggressive approaches to treatment have improved the outcome substantially.

The classic clinical presentation of **PCP** includes acute onset of fever, tachypnea, dyspnea, and marked hypoxemia; in some children, more indolent development of hypoxemia may precede other clinical or x-ray manifestations. Chest x-ray findings most commonly consist of interstitial infiltrates or diffuse alveolar disease, which rapidly progresses. Nodular lesions, streaky or lobar infiltrates, or pleural effusions may occasionally be seen. Diagnosis is established by demonstration of *P. carinii (jiroveci)* with appropriate staining of bronchoalveolar fluid lavage; rarely, an open lung biopsy is necessary.

The 1st line therapy for PCP is intravenous trimethoprim-sulfamethoxazole (TMP-SMZ) (15–20 mg/kg/day of TMP and 75–100 mg/kg/day of SMZ every 6 hr IV) with adjunctive corticosteroids if the Pao_2 is <70 mm Hg while breathing room air. When the patient has improved, therapy with oral TMP-SMZ

TABLE 273-3. 1993 Revised Case Definition of AIDS-Defining Conditions for Adults and Adolescents 13 Years of Age and Older

Candidiasis of bronchi, trachea, or lungs
Candidiasis, esophageal
Cervical cancer, invasive
Coccidioidomycosis, disseminated or extrapulmonary
Cryptococcosis, extrapulmonary
Cryptosporidiosis, chronic intestinal (>1 mo duration)
Cytomegalovirus disease (other than liver, spleen, or nodes)
Cytomegalovirus retinitis (with loss of vision)
Encephalopathy, HIV related
Herpes simplex: chronic ulcer(s) (>1 mo duration) or bronchitis, pneumonitis, or esophagitis
Histoplasmosis, disseminated or extrapulmonary
Isosporiasis, chronic intestinal (>1 mo duration)
Kaposi sarcoma
Lymphoma, Burkitt (or equivalent term)
Lymphoma, immunoblastic (or equivalent term)
Lymphoma, primary or brain
Mycobacterium avium complex or *Mycobacterium kansasii* infection, disseminated or extrapulmonary
Mycobacterium tuberculosis infection, any site, pulmonary or extrapulmonary
Mycobacterium, other species or unidentified species infection, disseminated or extrapulmonary
Pneumocystic jiroveci pneumonia
Pneumonia, recurrent
Progressive multifocal leukoencephalopathy
Salmonella septicemia, recurrent
Toxoplasmosis of brain
Wasting syndrome attributable to HIV
CD4$^+$ T-lymphocyte count <200/µL (0.20×10^9/L) or CD4$^+$ lymphocyte percentage <15%

Modified from the Centers for Disease Control and Prevention. 1993 revised classification system for HIV infection and expanded surveillance case definition for AIDS among adolescents and adults. *MMWR Recomm Rep* 1992;41(RR-17):1–19.
From *Red Book: 2006 Report of the Committee on Infectious Diseases*, 27th ed. Elk Grove Village, IL, American Academy of Pediatrics, 2006, p 379.

should be continued for a total of 21 days while the corticosteroids are weaned. Historically, up to 1/6 of HIV-infected children have allergic reactions to TMP-SMZ and require desensitization. However, because of the use of adjunctive corticosteroid therapy, this is now considerably less frequent. Alternative therapy for PCP includes intravenous administration of pentamidine (4 mg/kg/day). Other regimens such as TMP plus dapsone, clindamycin plus primaquine, or atovaquone are used as alternatives in adults but have not been widely used in children to date.

Atypical mycobacterial infection, particularly with *Mycobacterium avium-intracellulare* complex (MAC), may cause disseminated disease in HIV-infected children who are severely immunosuppressed. The incidence of MAC infection in children with <100 CD4 cells/mm^3 who were not treated with anti-retroviral drugs has been estimated to be as high as 10%, but effective anti-retroviral combination therapies that result in viral suppression have made MAC infections rare. Disseminated MAC infection is characterized by fever, malaise, weight loss, and night sweats; diarrhea, abdominal pain, and rarely intestinal perforation or jaundice (due to biliary tract obstruction by lymphadenopathy) may also be present. Diagnosis is made by isolation of MAC from blood, bone marrow, or tissue; the isolated presence of MAC in the stool does not confirm a diagnosis of disseminated MAC. Treatment can reduce symptoms and prolong life but is only capable of suppressing the infection if severe CD4 depletion persists. Therapy should include at least 2 drugs: clarithromycin or azithromycin and ethambutol. A 3rd drug (rifabutin, rifampin, ciprofloxacin, levofloxacin, or amikacin) is generally added to decrease the emergence of drug-resistant isolates. Careful consideration of possible drug-drug interactions with anti-retroviral agents is necessary before initiation of disseminated MAC therapy. Drug susceptibilities should be ascertained and the treatment regimen adjusted accordingly in the event of inadequate clinical response to therapy. Because of the great potential for toxicity with most of these medications, surveillance for adverse effects should be ongoing.

Oral candidiasis is the most common fungal infection seen in HIV-infected children. Oral nystatin suspension (2–5 mL qid) is often effective. Clotrimazole troches are an effective alternative. In refractory cases, oral amphotericin suspension should be considered. Oral thrush progresses to involve the esophagus in as many as 20% of children with severe CD4 depletion, presenting with symptoms such as anorexia, dysphagia, vomiting, and fever. Treatment with oral fluconazole (3–6 mg/kg/day) for 7–14 days generally results in rapid improvement in symptoms. Fungemia rarely occurs, usually in the setting of indwelling venous catheters, and up to 50% of cases may be caused by non-albicans species. Disseminated histoplasmosis and coccidioidomycosis or cryptococcosis are rare in pediatric patients but may occur in endemic areas. Parasitic infections such as intestinal cryptosporidiosis and microsporidiosis and rarely isosporiasis or giardiasis are other opportunistic infections that cause significant morbidity. Although usually self-limiting diseases in healthy hosts, they cause severe chronic diarrhea, often leading to malnutrition in HIV-infected children with low CD4 counts; immune reconstitution with HAART often results in clearance of the organism. Early data on nitazoxanide therapy has been promising, with clearance of the infection in some patients and reduction in diarrhea in more patients. Albendazole was reported to be effective against some microsporidia, and TMP-SMZ appears to be effective for isosporiasis.

Viral infections, especially with the herpesvirus group, pose significant problems for HIV-infected children. HSV causes recurrent gingivostomatitis, which may be complicated by local and distant cutaneous dissemination. Primary varicella-zoster virus (VZV) infection (chickenpox) may be prolonged and complicated by bacterial infections or visceral dissemination, including pneumonitis. Recurrent, atypical, or chronic episodes of herpes zoster are often debilitating and require prolonged therapy with acyclovir; in rare instances, VZV has developed resistance to acyclovir, requiring the use of foscarnet. Disseminated cytomegalovirus (CMV) infection can occur with severe CD4 depletion (<50 CD4 cells/mm^3) and may involve single or multiple organs. Retinitis, pneumonitis, esophagitis, gastritis with pyloric obstruction, hepatitis, colitis, and encephalitis have been reported, but these complications are rarely seen if HAART is given. Ganciclovir (5 mg/kg bid IV) or foscarnet (60 mg/kg tid IV) are the drugs of choice; the drugs are often given together in children with sight-threatening CMV retinitis. Measles may occur despite immunization and may present without the typical rash. It often disseminates to the lung or brain with a high mortality rate.

Respiratory viruses such as respiratory syncytial virus (RSV) and adenovirus may present with prolonged symptoms and persistent viral shedding. In parallel with the increased prevalence of genital tract human papillomavirus (HPV) infection, cervical intraepithelial neoplasia (CIN) and anal intraepithelial neoplasia (AIN) also occur with increased frequency among HIV-1-infected adult women compared with HIV-seronegative women. The relative risk for CIN is 5–10 times higher for HIV-1 seropositive women. Multiple modalities are used to treat HPV infection (see Chapter 263), although none are uniformly effective and the recurrence rate is higher among HIV-1-infected persons.

Central Nervous System. The incidence of CNS involvement in perinatally infected children is 50–90% in developing countries but lower in developed countries, with a median onset at 19 mo of age. This may range from subtle developmental delay to progressive encephalopathy with loss or plateau of developmental milestones, cognitive deterioration, impaired brain growth resulting in acquired microcephaly, and symmetric motor dysfunction. **Encephalopathy** may be the initial manifestation of the disease or may present much later when severe immune suppression occurs. With progression, marked apathy, spasticity, hyperreflexia, and gait disturbance may occur, as well as loss of language, oral, fine, and/or gross motor skills. The encephalopathy may progress intermittently, with periods of deterioration followed by transiently stable plateaus. Older children may exhibit behavioral problems and learning disabilities. Associated abnormalities identified by neuroimaging techniques include cerebral atrophy in up to 85% of children with neurologic symptoms, increased ventricular size, basal ganglia calcifications, and, less frequently, leukomalacia.

Focal neurologic signs and seizures are unusual and may imply a comorbid pathologic process such as a CNS tumor, opportunistic infection, or stroke. **CNS lymphoma** may present with a new onset of focal neurologic findings, headache, seizures, and mental status changes. Characteristic findings on neuroimaging studies include a hyperdense or isodense mass with variable contrast enhancement or a diffusely infiltrating contrast-enhancing mass. **CNS toxoplasmosis** is exceedingly rare in young infants, but may occur in HIV-infected adolescents; the overwhelming majority of these cases have the presence of serum IgG antitoxoplasma as a marker of infection. Other opportunistic infections of the CNS are rare and include CMV, JC virus (**progressive multifocal leukoencephalopathy**), HSV, and *Cryptococcus* or *Coccidioides* meningitis. Although the true incidence of cerebrovascular disorders (both hemorrhagic and nonhemorrhagic strokes) is unclear, 6–10% of children from large clinical series have been affected.

Respiratory Tract. Recurrent upper respiratory tract infections such as otitis media and sinusitis are very common. Although the typical pathogens *(S. pneumoniae, H. influenzae, Moraxella catarrhalis)* are most common, unusual pathogens, such as *P. aeruginosa*, yeast, and anaerobes may be present in chronic infections and result in complications such as invasive sinusitis and mastoiditis.

LIP is the most common chronic lower respiratory tract abnormality, historically occurring in approximately 25% of HIV-infected children. LIP is a chronic process with nodular lymphoid hyperplasia in the bronchial and bronchiolar epithelium, often leading to progressive alveolar capillary block over months to years. It has a characteristic chronic diffuse reticulonodular pattern on chest radiography rarely accompanied by hilar lymphadenopathy, which allows a presumptive diagnosis to be made radiographically before the onset of symptoms. There is an insidious onset of tachypnea, cough, and mild to moderate hypoxemia with normal auscultatory findings or minimal rales. Progressive disease may be accompanied by digital clubbing and symptomatic hypoxemia, which usually resolves with oral corticosteroid therapy. Several studies suggest that LIP is associated with a primary Epstein-Barr virus infection in the setting of HIV infection.

Most symptomatic HIV-infected children experience at least 1 episode of pneumonia during the course of their disease. *S. pneumoniae* is the most common bacterial pathogen, but gram-negative bacteria may also be problematic; *P. aeruginosa* pneumonia occurs more commonly in severely symptomatic children (CDC C3 category) and is often associated with acute respiratory failure and death. Rarely, bronchiectasis can develop and cause recurrent secondary infections. PCP is the most common opportunistic infection, but other pathogens, including CMV, *Aspergillus, Histoplasma,* and *Cryptococcus,* can cause pulmonary disease. Infection with common respiratory viruses, including respiratory syncytial virus, parainfluenza, influenza, and adenovirus, may occur simultaneously and have a protracted course and period of viral shedding from the respiratory tract. Pulmonary and extrapulmonary tuberculosis has been reported with increasing frequency in HIV-infected children, although it is considerably more common in HIV-infected adults.

Cardiovascular System. Subclinical cardiac abnormalities in HIV-infected children are common, persistent, and often progressive. A prospective study of young children with symptomatic HIV infection revealed that dilated cardiomyopathy and left ventricular hypertrophy were common; the 2 yr cumulative incidence of congestive heart failure was almost 5%. Children with encephalopathy or other AIDS-defining conditions have the highest rate of adverse cardiac outcomes. Resting sinus tachycardia has been reported in up to 64% and marked sinus arrhythmia in 17% of HIV-infected children. Hemodynamic instability occurs more frequently with advanced HIV disease. Gallop rhythm with tachypnea and hepatosplenomegaly appear to be the best clinical indicators of congestive heart failure in HIV-infected children; anticongestive therapy is generally very effective, especially when initiated early. Electrocardiography and echocardiography are helpful in assessing cardiac function before the onset of clinical symptoms.

Gastrointestinal and Hepatobiliary Tract. Oral manifestations of HIV disease include erythematous or pseudomembranous candidiasis, periodontal disease (e.g., ulcerative gingivitis or periodontitis), salivary gland disease (i.e., swelling, xerostomia), and rarely ulcerations or oral hairy leukoplakia and ulcerations. Gastrointestinal tract involvement is common in HIV-infected children. A variety of pathogens can cause gastrointestinal disease, including bacteria (*Salmonella, Campylobacter,* MAC), protozoa (*Giardia, Cryptosporidium, Isospora,* microsporidia), viruses (CMV, HSV, rotavirus), and fungi *(Candida)*. MAC and the protozoal infections are most severe and protracted in patients with severe CD4 cell depletion. Infections may be localized or disseminated and affect any part of the gastrointestinal tract from the oropharynx to the rectum. Oral or esophageal ulcerations, either viral in origin or idiopathic, are painful and often interfere with eating. Lesions that have negative viral cultures may respond to thalidomide, which is currently investigational, or to short courses of prednisone. AIDS enteropathy, a syndrome of malabsorption with partial villous atrophy not associated with a specific pathogen, has been postulated to be a result of direct HIV infection of the gut. Disaccharide intolerance is common in HIV-infected children with chronic diarrhea.

The most common symptoms of gastrointestinal disease are chronic or recurrent diarrhea with malabsorption, abdominal pain, dysphagia, and failure to thrive (FTT). Prompt recognition of weight loss or poor growth velocity in the absence of diarrhea is critical. Linear growth impairment often correlates with the level of HIV viremia. Supplemental enteral feedings should be instituted, either by mouth or with nighttime nasogastric tube feedings in cases associated with more chronic growth problems; placement of a gastrostomy tube for nutritional supplementation may be necessary. The wasting syndrome, defined as a loss of >10% of body weight, is not as common as FTT in pediatric patients. The resulting malnutrition is associated with a grave prognosis and generally requires parenteral hyperalimentation.

Chronic liver inflammation evidenced by fluctuating serum levels of transaminases with or without cholestasis is relatively common, often without identification of an etiologic agent. Cryptosporidial cholecystitis is associated with abdominal pain, jaundice, and elevated gamma GT. In some patients, chronic hepatitis caused by CMV, hepatitis B or C, or MAC may lead to portal hypertension and liver failure. Several of the anti-retroviral drugs or other drugs such as didanosine, protease inhibitors, and dapsone may also cause reversible elevation of transaminases.

Pancreatitis with increased pancreatic enzymes with or without abdominal pain, vomiting, and fever may be the result of drug therapy (e.g., with pentamidine, didanosine, or lamivudine) or, rarely, opportunistic infections such as MAC or CMV.

Renal Disease. Nephropathy is an unusual presenting symptom of HIV infection, more commonly occurring in older symptomatic children. A direct effect of HIV on renal epithelial cells has been suggested as the cause, but immune complexes, hyperviscosity of the blood (secondary to hyperglobulinemia), and nephrotoxic drugs are other possible factors. A wide range of histologic abnormalities has been reported, including focal glomerulosclerosis, mesangial hyperplasia, segmental necrotizing glomerulonephritis, and minimal change disease. Focal glomerulosclerosis generally progresses to renal failure within 6–12 mo, but other histologic abnormalities in children may remain stable without significant renal insufficiency for prolonged periods. Nephrotic syndrome is the most common manifestation of pediatric renal disease, with edema, hypoalbuminemia, proteinuria, and azotemia with normal blood pressure. Cases resistant to steroid therapy may benefit from cyclosporine therapy. Polyuria, oliguria, and hematuria have also been observed in some patients.

Skin Manifestations. Many cutaneous manifestations seen in HIV-infected children are inflammatory or infectious disorders that are not unique to HIV infection. These disorders tend to be more disseminated and respond less consistently to conventional therapy than in the uninfected child. Seborrheic dermatitis or eczema that is severe and unresponsive to treatment may be an early nonspecific sign of HIV infection. Recurrent or chronic episodes of HSV, herpes zoster, molluscum contagiosum, flat warts, anogenital warts, and candidal infections are common and may be difficult to control.

Allergic drug eruptions are also common, in particular related to sulfonamides, and generally respond to withdrawal of the drug or to desensitization. Epidermal hyperkeratosis with dry, scaling skin is frequently observed, and sparse hair or hair loss may be seen in the later stages of the disease.

Hematologic and Malignant Diseases. Anemia occurs in 20–70% of HIV-infected children, more commonly in children with AIDS. The anemia may be due to chronic infection, poor nutrition, autoimmune factors, virus-associated conditions (hemophagocytic syndrome, parvovirus B19 red cell aplasia), or the adverse effect of drugs (zidovudine). In children with low erythropoietin levels, subcutaneous recombinant erythropoietin may be successful in treating the anemia.

Leukopenia occurs in almost ⅓ of untreated HIV-infected children, and neutropenia often occurs. In some cases, antineutrophil antibodies are the cause, and treatment with intravenous immunoglobulin (IVIG) has been successful. Multiple drugs used for treatment or prophylaxis for opportunistic infections such as PCP, MAC, and CMV or anti-retroviral drugs (zidovudine) may also cause leukopenia and/or neutropenia. In many cases, treatment with subcutaneous granulocyte colony-stimulating factor is successful.

Thrombocytopenia has been reported in 10–20% of patients. The etiology may be immunologic (i.e., circulating immune complexes or antiplatelet antibodies), or due to drug toxicity, or the cause may be unknown. Treatment with IVIG or anti-D offers temporary improvement in most cases. If ineffective, a 2–3 day course of high-dose steroids (30 mg/kg/day) may be an alternative. Anti-retroviral therapy may also reverse thrombocytopenia. Deficiency of clotting factors (factors II, VII, IX) is not rare in children with advanced HIV disease and is often easy to correct (vitamin K). A novel disease of the thymus has been observed in a few HIV-infected children. These patients were found to have characteristic anterior mediastinal multilocular thymic cysts without clinical symptoms. Histologic examination shows focal cystic changes, follicular hyperplasia, and diffuse plasmocytosis and multinucleated giant cells. Spontaneous involution occurred in some cases.

In contrast to the more frequent occurrence in adults, malignant diseases have been reported infrequently in HIV-infected children, representing only 2% of AIDS-defining illnesses. Non-Hodgkin lymphoma, primary CNS lymphoma, and leiomyosarcoma are the most commonly reported neoplasms among HIV-infected children. Epstein-Barr virus is associated with most lymphomas and with all leiomyosarcomas (see Chapter 251). Kaposi sarcoma, which is caused by human herpesvirus 8, occurs frequently among HIV-infected adults but is exceedingly uncommon among HIV-infected children (see Chapter 254).

DIAGNOSIS. All infants born to HIV-infected mothers test antibody-positive at birth because of passive transfer of maternal HIV antibody across the placenta during gestation. Most uninfected infants lose maternal antibody between 6 and 12 mo of age and are known as **seroreverters.** Because a small proportion of uninfected infants continues to test HIV antibody positive for up to 18 mo of age, positive IgG antibody tests, including the rapid tests, cannot be used to make a definitive diagnosis of HIV infection in infants younger than this age. The presence of IgA or IgM anti-HIV in the infant's circulation can indicate HIV infection, because these immunoglobulin classes do not cross the placenta; however, IgA and IgM anti-HIV assays have been both insensitive and nonspecific and therefore are not valuable for clinical use. In any child >18 mo of age, demonstration of IgG antibody to HIV by a repeatedly reactive enzyme immunoassay (EIA) and confirmatory test (immunoblot or immunofluorescence assay) establishes the diagnosis of HIV infection.

Several rapid HIV tests are currently available with sensitivity and specificity better than those of the standard EIA. Many of these new tests require only a single step that allows test results to be reported within less than an hour. Incorporating rapid HIV testing during delivery or immediately after birth is crucial for the care of HIV-exposed newborns whose HIV status was unknown during pregnancy. Viral diagnostic assays, such as HIV DNA or RNA PCR, HIV culture, or HIV p24 antigen immune-dissociated p24 (ICD-p24), are considerably more useful in young infants, allowing a definitive diagnosis in most infected infants by 1–6 mo of age (Table 273-4). By 4–6 mo of age, the HIV culture and/or PCR identify all infected infants. HIV DNA PCR is the preferred virologic assay in developed countries. Almost 40% of infected newborns have positive test results in the 1st 2 days of life, with >90% testing positive by 2 wk of age. Plasma HIV RNA assays, which detect viral replication, may be more sensitive than DNA PCR for early diagnosis, but data are limited. HIV culture has similar sensitivity to HIV DNA PCR; however, it is more technically complex and expensive, and results are often not available for several weeks compared with 2–3 days for PCR. The p24 antigen assay is also highly specific and easy to perform, but it is less sensitive than the other virologic tests. It is not recommended for diagnosis of infection in infants <1 mo of age. In developing countries, the ICD-p24 test may be considered for older infants; however, if results are negative, it does not rule out infection.

Viral diagnostic testing should be performed within the 1st 48 hr of life. Almost 40% of HIV-infected children can be identified at this time. It seems that many of these children have a more rapid progression of their disease and deserve more aggressive therapy. In exposed children with negative virologic testing at 2 days of life, additional testing should be done at 1–2 mo of age and at 4–6 mo of age; some also favor testing at age 14 days to maximize early detection of infected infants, if initiation of anti-retroviral therapy is desired. A positive virologic assay (i.e., detection of HIV by PCR, culture, or p24 antigen) suggests HIV

TABLE 273-4. Laboratory Diagnosis of HIV Infection

TEST	COMMENT
HIV DNA PCR	Preferred test to diagnose HIV-1 subtype B infection in infants and children younger than 18 mo of age; highly sensitive and specific by 2 wk of age and available; performed on peripheral blood mononuclear cells. False negatives can occur in non-B subtype HIV-1 infections
HIV p24 Ag	Less sensitive, false-positive results during 1 mo of life, variable results; not recommended
ICD p24 Ag	Negative test result does not rule out infection; not recommended
HIV culture	Expensive, not easily available, requires up to 4 wk to do test; not recommended
HIV RNA PCR	Not recommended for routine testing of infants and children younger than 18 mo of age, because a negative result cannot be used to exclude HIV infection definitively. Preferred test to identify non-B subtype HIV-1 infections.

From *Red Book: 2006 Report of the Committee on Infectious Diseases*, 27th ed. Elk Grove Village, IL, American Academy of Pediatrics, 2006, p 386.

Ag, antigen; ICD, immune complex dissociated; PCR, polymerase chain reaction.

infection and should be confirmed by a repeat test on a 2nd specimen as soon as possible. A diagnosis of HIV infection can be made with 2 positive virologic test results obtained from different blood samples.

Although the perinatal use of prophylactic zidovudine to prevent vertical transmission has not affected the predictive value of viral diagnostic testing, the effect of more intensive antiviral combinations (protease inhibitors) in pregnant women on the accuracy of the infant's viral tests is unknown. HIV infection can be reasonably excluded if an infant has had at least 2 negative virologic test results with at least 1 test performed at ≥4 mo of age. In some parts of the world where non-subtype B (the predominant type in the United States) are common, interpretation of a negative PCR test result should be done cautiously because the assay may not detect the particular subtype (group O). Close clinical monitoring with serologic testing (by 18 mo of age) or culture (if possible) is recommended. In older infants, 2 or more negative HIV antibody tests performed at least 1 mo apart past 6 mo of age in the absence of hypogammaglobulinemia or clinical evidence of HIV disease can reasonably exclude HIV infection. The infection can be excluded definitively if the same parameters are met when the infant is at least 18 mo of age.

Infants born to HIV-infected mothers should be prescribed zidovudine (ZDV) prophylaxis. A complete blood count, differential leukocyte count, and platelet count should be performed at 4 wk of age to monitor ZDV toxicity. If the child is found to be HIV-infected or if the HIV status is not clear, these tests should be continued every 1–3 mo to assess the hematologic effect of the disease or its treatment (prophylactic TMP-SMZ and antiretroviral therapy). If the child is found to be HIV infected, CD4 and CD8 lymphocyte counts should be performed at 1 and 3 mo of age and repeated every 3 mo. The frequency of the test should be increased (every 4–6 wk) if the CD4 lymphocyte count or percentage declines rapidly.

TREATMENT. The currently available therapy does not eradicate the virus and cure the patient; it only suppresses the virus for extended periods of time and changes the course of the disease to a chronic process. Decisions about anti-retroviral therapy for pediatric HIV-infected patients are based on the magnitude of viral replication (viral load), CD4 lymphocyte count or percentage, and clinical condition. Because anti-retroviral therapy changes as new drugs become available, decisions regarding therapy should be made in consultation with an expert in pediatric HIV infection. Plasma viral load monitoring and measurement of CD4 values have made it possible to implement rational treatment strategies for viral suppression as well as to assess the efficacy of a particular drug combination. The following principles form the basis for anti-retroviral treatment: (1) uninterrupted HIV replication causes destruction of the immune system and progression to AIDS; (2) the magnitude of the viral load predicts the rate of disease progression, and the CD4 cell count reflects the risk of opportunistic infections and HIV infection complications; (3) combinations of HAART, which include at least 3 drugs, should be the initial treatment. Potent combination therapy that suppresses HIV replication to an undetectable level restricts the selection of anti-retroviral-resistant mutants; drug-resistant strains are the major factor limiting successful viral suppression and delay of disease progression; (4) the goal of sustainable suppression of HIV replication is best achieved by the simultaneous initiation of combinations of anti-retroviral agents to which the patient has not been exposed previously and which are not cross-resistant to drugs with which the patient has been treated previously; (5) adherence to the complex drug regimens is crucial for a successful outcome.

Combination Therapy. Anti-retroviral drugs licensed as of 2006 are categorized by their mechanism of action, such as the ability to inhibit the HIV reverse transcriptase or protease enzymes (Table 273-5). Within the reverse transcriptase inhibitors, a further subdivision can be made: **nucleoside (or nucleotide) reverse transcriptase inhibitors (NRTIs)** and **non-nucleoside reverse transcriptase inhibitors (NNRTIs).** The NRTIs have a similar structure to the building blocks of DNA (e.g., thymidine, cytosine). When incorporated into DNA, they act like chain terminators and block further incorporation of nucleosides, which prevents viral DNA synthesis. Among the NRTIs, thymidine analogs (stavudine [d4T], zidovudine [ZDV]) are found in higher concentrations in activated or dividing cells, and nonthymidine analogs (didanosine [ddI], lamivudine [3TC]) have more activity in resting cells. Activated cells are thought to produce >99% of the population of HIV virons. In contrast, resting cells account for <1% of the population, but may serve as a reservoir of HIV. Suppression of replication in both populations is thought to be an important component of long-term viral control. NNRTIs (nevirapine, efavirenz) act differently than the NRTIs. They attach to the reverse transcriptase and restrict its motility, which reduces the activity of the enzyme. The **protease inhibitors** (lopinavir, nelfinavir, saquinavir) are potent agents that act farther along the viral replicative cycle. They bind to the site where the viral long polypeptides are cut to individual, mature, and functional core proteins that produce the infectious virions before they leave the cell. The 1st fusion inhibitor, enfuvirtide, has also been approved. This novel compound binds to viral gp41, which prevents fusion of the virus with the $CD4^+$ cell and entry into the cell.

While the principal site of viral replication is lymphoid tissue, sanctuary sites such as the CNS may harbor residual virions with the potential of being a source of local or persistent disease. Impaired penetration of drugs to these compartments could result in development of resistance. Although data on CNS penetration of antiviral agents are presently limited, ZDV, d4T, and 3TC appear to achieve inhibitory concentrations in the CNS. Indinavir and nevirapine also penetrate the CSF, but other protease inhibitors are actively transported out of the CNS, thereby limiting their potential efficacy at this site.

By targeting different points in the viral life cycle and stages of cell activation, and delivering drug to all tissue sites, maximal viral suppression may be feasible. Combinations of 3 drugs (thymidine analog NRTI [ZDV], a nonthymidine analog NRTI [3TC] to suppress replication in both active and resting cells, and a protease inhibitor [lopinavir/ritonavir or nelfinavir] or an NNRTI [efavirenz]) have been shown to produce prolonged viral suppression. Although not ideal, less potent combinations such as triple NRTIs (abacavir, zidovudine, lamivudine), dual NRTIs, or ritonavir with stavudine may be considered in special situations when there are concerns about adherence to a complex drug regimen or when the patient and/or family prefer a simplified alternative regimen. Combination treatment increases the rate of toxicities (see Table 273-5), and complex drug-drug interactions exist among many of the anti-retroviral drugs. Most NNRTI and protease inhibitor drugs are inducers or inhibitors of the cytochrome P450 system. The protease inhibitors are particularly likely to have serious interactions with multiple drug classes, including nonsedating antihistamines and psychotropic, vasoconstrictor, antimycobacterial, cardiovascular, analgesic, and gastrointestinal drugs (cisapride). Whenever new medications are added to an anti-retroviral treatment, especially a protease inhibitor–containing regimen, a pharmacist and/or HIV specialist should be consulted to address possible drug interactions. The inhibitory effect of ritonavir (a protease inhibitor) on the cytochrome P450 system has been exploited, and small doses of the drug are added to several other protease inhibitors (lopinavir, indinavir, saquinavir) to slow their metabolism by the P450 system and to improve their pharmacokinetic profile. This provides more effective drug levels with less toxicity and, often, less frequent dosing.

Adherence. Assessment of the likelihood of adherence to treatment is an important factor in deciding whether and when to ini-

TABLE 273-5. Summary of Anti-retroviral Therapies (available in 2006)

DRUG (TRADE NAMES, FORMULATIONS)	DOSING	SIDE EFFECTS	COMMENTS
NUCLEOSIDE/NUCLEOTIDE REVERSE TRANSCRIPTASE INHIBITORS (NRTIS)		Class adverse effects: Lactic acidosis with hepatic steatosis	
Abacavir Ziagen, ABC Tablet: 300 mg Oral solution: 20 mg/mL	Children: ≥3 mo to 18 yr: 8 mg/kg PO bid (maximum dose 300 mg PO bid) Adults: 300 mg PO bid or 600 mg PO once daily	Common: Nausea, vomiting, anorexia, fever, headache, diarrhea, rash Less common: Hypersensitivity, lactic acidosis with hepatic steatosis, hepatomegaly, pancreatitis, elevated triglycerides, fatigue	Can be given with food. Serious hypersensitivity reaction occurs rarely; if hypersensitivity is suspected, do not rechallenge.
Didanosine Videx, ddI Chewable buffered tablet: 25, 50, 100, 150, 200 mg Buffered powder packet: 100, 167, 250 mg	Infants 2 wk to 8 mo: 50–100 mg/m² PO bid Children: 120 mg/m² (range 90–150 g/m²) PO bid Adolescents (>13 yr) and adults <60 kg: 125 mg PO bid (buffered oral solution 167 mg PO bid) >60 kg: 200 mg PO bid (buffered oral solution 250 mg PO bid)	Common: Headache, diarrhea, abdominal pain, nausea, vomiting. Less common: Pancreatitis, peripheral neuropathy, electrolyte abnormalities, lactic acidosis with hepatic steatosis, hepatomegaly, retinal depigmentation	Food decreases bioavailability up to 50%. Tablets dissolved in water are stable for 1 hr (4 hr in buffered solution). Drug interactions: Antacids/gastric acid antagonists may increase bioavailability; possible decreased absorption of fluoroquinolones, ganciclovir, ketoconazole, itraconazole, dapsone. Possible decreased efficacy when given with tenofovir.
Videx EC Capsule, delayed release: 125, 200, 250, 400 mg	Children: Not established Adolescent and adults: <60 kg: 250 mg PO once daily ≥60 kg: 400 mg PO once daily	Same as for ddI	Combination with tenofovir increases ddI levels and risk for toxicity. Swallow capsules whole on empty stomach, 30 min before meals or 2 hr after meals
Emtricitabine Emtriva, FTC Capsules: 200 mg Oral solution: 10 mg/mL	Children ≥33 kg, adolescents, and adults: 200 mg capsule PO once daily or 240 mg (24 mL) oral solution q.d.	Common: Headache, diarrhea, nausea, skin discoloration Less common: Lactic acidosis with hepatic steatosis, hepatomegaly	Closely monitor patients with hepatitis B co-infection. Can be given with food.
Lamivudine Epivir, Epivir HBV, 3TC Tablet: 150, 300 mg Solution: 5 mg/mL (Epivir HBV, 10 mg/mL)	Infants, neonates *<30 days:* 2 mg/kg PO bid Infants, children and adolescents: 4 mg/kg PO bid (maximum dose: 150 mg PO bid) Adults: <50 kg: 4 mg/kg/dose PO bid (maximum dose: 150 mg PO bid) ≥50 kg: 150 mg PO bid or 300 mg PO once daily	Common: Headache, nausea, feeding problems, diarrhea, abdominal pain, rash Less common: Pancreatitis, neutropenia, peripheral neuropathy, lactic acidosis with hepatic steatosis, hepatomegaly	May be administered with or without food. Drug interactions: Trimethoprim/sulfamethoxazole increases 3TC levels. Combination with ZDV may prevent ZDV resistance.
Stavudine Zerit, d4T Capsule: 15, 20, 30, 40 mg Solution: 1 mg/mL	Children <30 kg: 1 mg/kg PO bid. Adolescents and adults: 30–60 kg: 30 mg PO bid >60 kg: 40 mg PO bid	Common: Headache, nausea, rash Less common: Peripheral neuropathy, pancreatitis, lactic acidosis with hepatic steatosis, hepatomegaly, elevated liver function tests	Drug interactions: Can be given with food. Should not be administered with ZDV.
Zerit XR Capsule: 75, 100 mg	<60 kg: 75 mg PO once daily >60 mg kg: 100 mg PO once daily		
Tenofovir Viread, TDF Tablet: 300 mg	Children: Not established Adolescents and adults: 300 mg PO once daily	Common: Nausea, vomiting, diarrhea Less common: Lactic acidosis with hepatic steatosis, hepatomegaly, reduced bone density	High fat meal increases absorption. Co-administration with ddI may increase ddI toxicity. Co-administration with atazanavir (ATV) may decrease ATV levels. Boosting with ritonavir (RTV) is required.
Zidovudine Retrovir, AZT, ZDV Capsule: 100 mg Tablet: 300 mg Syrup: 10 mg/mL Injection: 10 mg/mL	Prophylaxis (newborns) Term neonates: 2 mg/kg PO every 6 hr or 2.7 mg/kg PO every 8 hr or 1.5 mg/kg/dose IV every 6 hr (infuse over 30 min) Premature infants (<30 wk gestation): 1.5 mg/kg IV every 12 hr or 2 mg/kg PO every 12 hr for age 0–4 wk, then every 8 hr Premature infants (≥30 wk gestation): 1.5 mg/kg/dose IV every 12 hr or 2 mg/kg PO every 12 hr for age 0–2 wk, then every 8 hr Treatment Children 6 wk to 12 yr: 160 mg/m² PO every 8 hr or 180–240 mg/m² PO every 12 hr or 120 mg/m² IV every 6 hr or Continuous infusion 20 mg/m²/hr IV Adolescents and adults: 200 mg PO tid or 300 mg PO bid	Common: Headache, bone marrow suppression (e.g., anemia, leukopenia) Less common: Liver toxicity, lactic acidosis with hepatic steatosis, myopathy, hepatomegaly	Can be given with food. Infuse IV with 5% dextrose over 1 hr at a final concentration of 4 mg/mL. Drug interactions: Rifampin may increase metabolism Cimetidine, fluconazole, valproic acid may decrease metabolism.

continued

TABLE 273-5. Summary of Anti-retroviral Therapies (available in 2006)—cont'd

DRUG (TRADE NAMES, FORMULATIONS)	DOSING	SIDE EFFECTS	COMMENTS
NON-NUCLEOSIDE REVERSE TRANSCRIPTASE INHIBITORS (NNRTIS)		Class adverse effects: Rash—mild to severe, usually within first 6 wk. Discontinue the drug if severe rash (with blistering, desquamation, muscle involvement or fever)	
Efavirenz Sustiva, EFV Capsule: 50, 100, 200 mg Tablet: 600 mg	Children <3 yr: Not established Children ≥3 yr: Given once daily PO at bedtime Weight 10–<15 kg: 200 mg; 15–<20 kg: 250 mg; 20–<25 kg: 300 mg; 25–<32.5 kg: 350 mg; 32.5–<40 kg: 400 mg; ≥40 kg: 600 mg Adolescents and adults: 600 mg once daily PO at bedtime	Common: Rash, CNS and psychiatric symptoms (e.g., abnormal dreams, impaired concentration, insomnia, depression, hallucination) Less common: Increased liver enzymes; potentially teratogenic	Capsules can be opened for mixing in food. Do not administer with fatty foods because absorption is increased 50%, but may administer with regular meals or without food. Drug interactions: Efavirenz induces CYP3A4 and may increase clearance of drugs metabolized by this pathway (e.g., antihistamines, sedative and hypnotics, cisapride, ergot derivatives, warfarin, ethinyl estradiol) and several other ARVs (i.e., protease inhibitors). Drugs that induce CYP3A4 (e.g., phenobarbital, rifampin, rifabutin) decrease efavirenz levels. Clarithromycin levels decrease with EFV and azithromycin should be considered.
Nevirapine Viramune, NVP Tablet: 200 mg Suspension: 10 mg/mL	Neonates 0–2 mo: 5 mg/kg or 120 mg/m^2 PO once daily for 14 days, then 120 mg/m^2 PO bid for 14 days, then 200 mg/m^2 PO bid. Children 2 mo–8 yr: 4 mg/kg PO once daily for 14 days; if tolerated, increase dose to 7 mg/kg PO bid (maximum dose 200 mg PO bid) ≥8 yr: 4 mg/kg PO once daily for 14 days; if tolerated, increase dose to 4 mg/kg PO bid (maximum dose 200 mg PO bid) Adolescents and adults: 200 mg once daily for 14 days; if tolerated, increase dose to 200 mg PO bid	Common: Rash (can be severe, including Stevens-Johnson syndrome), headache, fever, nausea, abnormal liver function tests Less common: Hepatitis (rarely life threatening), hypersensitivity reactions	May give with or without food. Drug interactions: Induces hepatic CYP450 3A activity and decreases protease inhibitors concentrations such as indinavir, saquinavir, and lopinavir concentrations. Also reduces ketoconazole concentrations (fluconazole should be used as an alternative). Rifampin decreases nevirapine serum levels. Anticonvulsants and psychotropic drugs using same metabolic pathways as NVP should be monitored. Oral contraceptives may also be affected.
PROTEASE INHIBITORS		Class adverse effects: Hyperglycemia, hyperlipidemia (except atazanavir), lipodystrophy, increased transaminases, increased bleeding disorders in hemophiliacs. Can induce metabolism of ethinyl estradiol; use alternate contraception (other than estrogen-containing oral contraceptives). All undergo hepatic metabolism, mostly by CPY3A4, with many drug interactions!	
Amprenavir Agenerase, APV Liquid formulation: 15 mg/mL Capsules: 50 mg	Neonates/infants: Not recommended due to propylene glycol Children 4–16 yr and weighing <50 kg: Oral solution 22.5 mg/kg PO bid; >50 kg: 1,400 mg/dose PO bid; (maximum daily dose: 2,800 mg) Adolescents 13–16 yr and >5 kg, and adults: Use fosamprenavir (fos-APV) rather than APV Adult dose in combination with ritonavir: APV 600 mg + 100 mg RTV PO bid	Common: Vomiting, nausea, diarrhea, rash Less common: Stevens-Johnson syndrome, fat redistribution, insulin resistance	Liquid formulation contains vitamin E; supplemental vitamin E should not be given. Do not use liquid formulation <4 years age or with hepatic failure due to high concentrations of propylene glycol.
Atazanavir Reyataz, ATV Capsules: 100, 150, 200 mg	Children: Not established Adolescents/adults: Antiretroviral naive: 400 mg PO once daily Antiretroviral experienced: ATV 300 mg + RTV 100 mg PO once daily	Common: Asymptomatic elevation of indirect bilirubin; headache, arthralgia, depression, insomnia, nausea, vomiting, diarrhea, paresthesias Less common: Prolongation of PR interval on ECG; rash, rarely progressing to Stevens-Johnson syndrome	Review drug interactions before initiating because ATV interacts with drugs using CYP3A4 for metabolism. Use with caution with cardiac conduction disease or liver impairment
Darunavir Prezista, DRV	Limited data on pediatric dosing or safety Adults: 600 mg DRV PO + 100 mg RTV, bid	Common: Diarrhea, nausea, abdominal pain, fatigue, headache Less common: Skin rash including erythema multiforme and Stevens-Johnson syndrome, lipid elevations	Contraindicated for concurrent therapy with cisapride, ergot alkaloids, benzodiazepines, pimozide or any major CYP3A4 substrates. Use with caution in patients taking anticonvulsants, strong CYP3A4 inhibitors, or moderate/strong CYP3A4 inducers. Adjust dose with concurrent rifamycin therapy. Contains sulfa: potential for cross-sensitivity with sulfonamide class is unknown.
Fosamprenavir Lexiva, fos-APV Tablets: 700 mg	Children: Not established Adolescent/adults: Antiretroviral naive: fos-APV 1,400 mg PO bid or fos-APV 1,400 mg + RTV 200 mg RTV PO once daily or fos-APV 700 mg + RTV 100 mg PO bid Protease inhibitor-experienced: fos-APV 700 mg + RTV 100 mg RTV PO bid	Common: Nausea, vomiting, perioral paresthesias, headache, rash, lipid elevations Less common: Stevens-Johnson syndrome, fat redistribution, neutropenia, elevated creatine kinase Rare: Diabetes mellitus	Use with caution in sulfa-allergic individuals. Interacts with drugs utilizing CYP3A4 metabolism.
Indinavir Crixivan, IDV Capsule: 100, 200, 333, 400 mg	Infants: Not approved Children: Dose not established Investigational dose: 500 mg/m^2 every 8 hr (max single dose: 800 mg) Adolescent and Adults: 800 mg every 8 hr (not tid) Boosted PID dosing: IDV 800 mg + 100–200 RTV bid Dosing with NNRTIs: IDV 1,000 mg PO every 8 hr + EFV or NVP; or IDV 800 mg + RTV 200 mg PO bid with EFV or NVP	Common: Nausea, hyperbilirubinemia, headache, dizziness, lipid abnormalities Less common: Nephrolithiasis, interstitial nephritis, fat redistribution Rare: Diabetes mellitus, hepatitis	Administer on an empty stomach 1 hr before or 2 hr after a meal to decrease food effect. When co-administered with boosting dose of ritonavir, no food restrictions. Reduce dose by ~25% with mild to moderate liver dysfunction. Adequate hydration (48 oz fluid/day in adults) necessary to minimize risk of nephrolithiasis. Chemoprophylaxis is after high-risk exposure given in combination with zidovudine and lamivudine. Drug interactions: Didanosine decreases absorption; rifampin reduces levels; ketoconazole, ritonavir, and other protease inhibitors decrease indinavir metabolism. Do not co-administer astemizole, cisapride, terfenadine.

TABLE 273-5. Summary of Anti-retroviral Therapies (available in 2006)—cont'd

DRUG (TRADE NAMES, FORMULATIONS)	DOSING	SIDE EFFECTS	COMMENTS
Lopinavir/Ritonavir (co-formulated) Kaletra, LPV/RTV, LPV/r Capsules: 133.3 mg LPV/33.3 mg RTV Oral solution: 80 mg LPV-20 mg RTV/mL (contains 42% alcohol by volume)	Infants <6 mo: Not established Children: 7–<15 kg: 12 mg LPV and 3 mg RTV/kg PO bid 15–40 kg: 10 mg LPV and 2.5 mg RTV/kg PO bid >40 kg: 400 mg LPV and 100 mg RTV/kg PO bid or 230 mg and LPV-57.5 mg RTV/m² PO bid (maximum 400 mg LPV and 100 mg RTV/dose) Adolescents and adults: 400 mg LPV and 100 mg RTV PO bid	More common: Diarrhea, headache, nausea and vomiting, lipid elevation Less common: Fat redistribution Rare: Diabetes mellitus, pancreatitis, hepatitis	Adjust dose when used with NNRTIs and other protease inhibitors; interacts with drugs using CYP3A4
Nelfinavir Viracept, NFV Tablet: 250, 625 mg Powder for suspension: 50 mg/level scoop of powder	Neonates: Investigational dose 10 mg/kg every 8 hr; not recommended for children <2 yr of age because of interpatient variability. Children *2–13 yr*: 45–55 mg/kg bid or 25–35 mg/kg tid Adolescents and Adults: 750 mg PO tid or 1,250 mg PO bid	Common: Diarrhea asthenia, abdominal pain, rash, lipid abnormalities Less common: Exacerbation of liver disease, fat redistribution Rare: Diabetes, hepatitis	Administer with a meal to optimize absorption; avoid acidic food or drink (e.g., orange juice). Tablet can be dissolved in water to administer as a solution. Drug interactions: Nelfinavir inhibits CYP3A4 activity, which may cause multiple drug interactions. Rifampin, phenobarbital, and carbamazepine reduce levels. Ketoconazole, ritonavir, indinavir, and other protease inhibitors increase levels. Do not co-administer astemizole, cisapride, terfenadine. May interfere with oral contraceptives.
Ritonavir Norvir, RTV Capsule: 100 mg Solution: 80 mg/mL	Children: 200 mg/m² every 12 hr; titrate upward in 50 mg/m² dose increments (to increase tolerability) to 400 mg/m² every 12 hr Adolescents and adults: 600 mg every 12 hr	Common: Nausea and vomiting, diarrhea, taste aversion, elevated serum lipids, perioral paresthesias Less common: Fat redistribution Rare: Pancreatitis, hepatitis, diabetes mellitus	Administer dose with food to enhance bioavailability Drug interactions: Ritonavir is a substrate and has affinity for many hepatic CYP450 enzymes that may lead to many important drug interactions (e.g., protease inhibitors, antiarrhythmics, antidepressants, cisapride). Ritonavir metabolism is influenced by enzyme inducers and inhibitors. Ritonavir-resistant strains often cross-resistant with other agents.
Saquinavir Invirase, SQV Hard gelatin capsule: 200, 600 mg	Infants and children: Not established ≥16 yr: 1,000 mg plus 100 mg RTV, both bid	Common: Diarrhea, abdominal pain, headache, nausea, rash, lipid abnormalities Rare: Diabetes mellitus, pancreatitis, elevated transaminases	Administration with a high-fat meal enhances bioavailability. Concurrent grapefruit juice may increase bioavailability. Use only in combination with ritonavir boosting dose; lacks potency when given as single protease inhibitor. Drug interactions: Rifampin, phenobarbital, and carbamazepine decrease serum levels; saquinavir may decrease metabolism of calcium channel antagonists; azoles (e.g., ketoconazole), macrolides, and ritonavir increase levels.
Tipranavir Aptivus, TPV	Limited data on pediatric dosing or safety Adults: 500 mg TPV PO + 200 mg RTV PO, bid with a high-fat meal.	Common: Diarrhea, nausea, fatigue, headache, elevated liver enzymes, triglycerides, and cholesterol Less common: Fat redistribution, hepatic decompensation Rare: Fatal and nonfatal intracranial hemorrhage have been reported, but causal relationship is not established	Can inhibit human platelet aggregation: use with caution in patients at risk for increased bleeding (trauma, surgery, etc.) or in patients receiving concurrent medications that may increase the risk of bleeding. Contraindicated in patients with hepatic insufficiency or receiving concurrent therapy with amiodarone, cisapride, ergot alkaloids, benzodiazepines, pimozide.
FUSION INHIBITORS			
Enfuvirtide Fuzeion Injection: Lyophilized powder of 108 mg reconstituted in 1.1 sterile water delivers 90 mg/mL	Children <6 yr: Not established Children >6 yr: 2 mg/kg bid	Common: Local injection site reactions in 98%: erythema, induration nodules, cysts, ecchymoses Less common: Increased incidence of bacterial pneumonia Rare: Hypersensitivity including fever, chills, hypotension; immune-mediated reactions (e.g., glomerulonephritis, respiratory distress)	Give subcutaneously in the upper arm, anterior leg or abdomen (maximum: 90 mg/dose). Severity of adverse effects increased if give intramuscularly Injection sites should be rotated
COMBINATION PRODUCTS		These combinations can be used in adolescents at appropriate Tanner stage (Tanner stages IV and V) and weight (>40 kg).	
Atripla Each tablet contains 600 mg Efavirenz, 200 mg emtricitabine, and 300 mg tenofovir disoproxil fumarate Adult dose: 1 tablet PO once daily			
Combivir Each tablet contains 300 mg AZT + 150 mg 3TC Adult dose: 1 tablet PO bid			
Epzicom Each tablet contains 300 mg 3TC + 600 mg ABC Adult dose: 1 tablet PO once daily			
Trizivir Each tablet contains 300 mg AZT + 150 mg 3TC + 300 mg ABC Adult dose: 1 tablet PO bid			
Truvada Each tablet contains 200 mg FTC + 300 mg TDF Adult dose: 1 tablet PO once daily			

Antiretroviral drugs often have significant drug-drug interactions, with each other and with other classes of medicines, which should be reviewed before initiating any new medication.
The information in this table is not all-inclusive. Updated and additional information on dosing, drug-drug interactions, and toxicities is available on the AIDSinfo website at http://www.aidsinfo.nih.gov.
CNS, central nervous system.

tiate therapy. Numerous studies have shown that compliance of <80–90% results in less successful suppression of the viral load. In addition, poor adherence to prescribed medication regimens results in subtherapeutic drug concentrations and enhances development of resistance, particularly with protease inhibitors and NNRTI drugs. Combination anti-retroviral regimens are often unpalatable, and require extreme dedication on the part of the care provider and child; this makes participation of the family in the decision to initiate therapy essential. Intensive education on the relationship of drug adherence to viral suppression, training on drug administration, frequent follow-up visits, and commitment of the caregiver and the patient (despite the inconvenience of adverse effects, dosing schedule, and so on) are critical for successful antiviral treatment.

Initiation of Therapy. HIV-infected children with symptoms (clinical category A, B, or C) or/with evidence of immune dysfunction (immune category 2 or 3) should be treated with anti-retroviral therapy, regardless of age or viral load (see Tables 273-1 and 273-2). Children <1 yr of age are at high risk for disease progression, and immunologic and virologic tests to identify those likely to develop rapidly progressive disease are less predictive than in older children. Therefore, such infants should be treated with anti-retroviral agents as soon as the diagnosis of HIV infection has been confirmed, regardless of clinical or immunologic status, or viral load. Data suggest that HIV-infected infants who are treated before the age of 3 mo control their HIV infection better than infants whose anti-retroviral therapy started later than 3 mo of age.

Some clinicians advocate treating asymptomatic children ≥1 yr of age to prevent immunologic deterioration. When there are concerns regarding drug adherence, safety, and durability of anti-retroviral response, some providers elect to delay treatment in the immunologically normal child with a viral load of <100,000 copies/mm^3 because the risk for clinical progression is low. Such children should be monitored regularly for evidence of virologic, immunologic, or clinical progression, at which point therapy should be initiated as long as potential adherence issues are addressed.

Inflammatory **immune reconstitution syndromes** have been described for children and adults, and represent the paradoxical emergence of transient to severe inflammation-mediated symptoms as immune function is restored with anti-retroviral therapy. Most of these syndromes are associated with mycobacterial infections, especially *M. tuberculosis,* and have also been reported with *P. carinii, Toxoplasma,* hepatitis B and hepatitis C viruses, CMV, and other pathogens. Immune reconstitution syndromes are characterized by fever and worsening of the clinical manifestations of the opportunistic infection or new manifestations, typically within the 1st few weeks after initiation of anti-retroviral therapy, although they may occur up to several months after the initiation. Determining whether the symptoms represent worsening of a current infection or a new opportunistic infection, an immune reconstitution syndrome, or drug toxicity is often very difficult. If the syndrome does represent an immune reactivation syndrome, adding nonsteroidal anti-inflammatory agents or corticosteroids to alleviate the inflammatory reaction is appropriate. The inflammation may take weeks or months to subside.

Dosing. Data on anti-retroviral drug dosages for neonates are often limited. Because of the immaturity of the neonatal liver, premature infants and newborns often require an increase in the dosing interval of drugs primarily cleared through hepatic glucuronidation.

Adolescents should have anti-retroviral dosages prescribed on the basis of Tanner staging of puberty rather than on the basis of age. During early puberty (Tanner stages I, II, and III), pediatric dosing ranges should be used, whereas adolescents in late puberty (Tanner stages IV and V) should follow adult dosing schedules.

Changing Anti-Retroviral Therapy. Therapy should be changed when the current regimen is judged ineffective as evidenced by increase in viral load, deterioration of the CD4 cell count, or clinical progression. Development of toxicity or intolerance to drugs is another reason to consider a change in therapy. When a change is considered, the patient and family should be reassessed for adherence problems. While considering possible new drug choices, potential cross-resistance should be addressed. In addition, few patients who have virologic failure may still demonstrate elevated CD4 cell counts (discordant response). Impaired replication ability of the resistant virus and enhanced cytotoxic T lymphocyte (CTL) effects are some of the reasons for this discordant response. In these patients, delay in changing therapy should be considered as long as the immunologic benefit is evident. Ideally, when a decision is made to change the anti-retroviral therapy, all drugs should be changed. However, in many situations (previous anti-retroviral experience, intolerance, toxicity) this is not possible, and, therefore, at least 2 drugs should be changed based on the resistance mutation genotype (if available) or previous regimen used.

Monitoring Anti-Retroviral Therapy. Virologic and immunologic surveillance (using HIV RNA copy number and CD4 lymphocyte count or percentage) as well as clinical assessment should be performed regularly in children taking anti-retroviral therapy. Initial virologic response (i.e., at least 5-fold [0.7 $\log_{10}$] reduction in viral load) should be achieved within 4 wk of initiating anti-retroviral therapy. The maximum response to therapy usually occurs within 12–16 wk. Thus, HIV RNA levels should be measured at 4 wk and 3–4 mo after therapy initiation. Once an optimal response has occurred, viral load should then be measured at least every 3–6 mo. If the response is unsatisfactory, another viral load should be performed as soon as possible to verify the results before a change in therapy is considered. The CD4 cells respond more slowly to successful treatment and, therefore, can be monitored less frequently. Potential toxicity should be monitored closely for the 1st 8–12 wk, and if no clinical or laboratory toxicity is documented, a follow-up visit every 2–3 mo is adequate. Several toxicities have caused increasing concern regarding anti-retroviral use (especially protease inhibitors). These toxicities include hematologic complications, hypersensitivity rash, lipodystrophy (e.g., redistribution of body fat), hyperlipidemia (elevation of cholesterol and triglyceride concentrations), hyperglycemia and insulin resistance, mitochondrial toxicity leading to severe lactic acidosis, abnormal bone mineral metabolism, and hepatic toxicity including severe hepatomegaly with steatosis.

Resistance to Anti-Retroviral Therapy. The high mutation rate of HIV (mainly due to the absence of error-correcting mechanisms) severely impairs the success of anti-retroviral therapy. Failure to reduce the viral load to <50 copies/mL increases the risk for developing resistance. Even effectively treated patients do not completely suppress viral replication, and persistence of HIV transcription and evolution of envelope sequences continues in the latent cellular reservoirs. The accumulation of resistance mutation progressively diminishes the potency of the anti-retroviral therapy and challenges the physician to find new regimens. For some drugs (nevirapine, 3TC) a single mutation is associated with resistance, while for other drugs (ZDV, lopinavir) several mutations are needed before resistance develops. Testing for drug resistance, especially when devising a new regimen, is rapidly becoming the standard of care. Two types of tests are available. The **phenotypic assay** measures the virus susceptibility in various concentrations of the drug and the **genotypic assay** predicts the virus susceptibility from mutations identified in the HIV genome isolated from the patient. Several studies have shown that treatment success was higher in patients whose anti-retroviral therapy was guided by genotype or phenotype testing.

Supportive Care. Even before the new anti-retroviral drugs were available, a significant impact on the quality of life and survival of HIV-infected children was achieved when supportive care was given. A multidisciplinary team approach is desirable for successful management. Close attention should be paid to nutrition status, which is often delicately balanced and may require aggressive preemptive intervention (nasogastric or gastric feedings or parenteral nutrition) to achieve adequate caloric and protein intake. Painful oropharyngeal lesions and dental caries are frequent and may interfere with eating; routine dental evaluations and careful attention to oral hygiene should be encouraged. Development should be evaluated regularly with provision of necessary physical, occupational, and/or speech therapy. Recognition of pain in the young child may be difficult, and effective pharmacologic and nonpharmacologic protocols for pain management should be instituted, especially during the terminal phase of the disease.

All HIV-exposed and infected children should receive standard pediatric immunizations. In general, live oral polio vaccine and live bacterial vaccines (BCG) should not be given (Fig. 273-2). Varicella and measles-mumps-rubella (MMR) vaccines are recommended for children in immune categories 1 and 2, but neither varicella nor MMR vaccines should be given to severely immunocompromised children (immune category 3). Of note, prior immunizations do not always provide protection, as evidenced by outbreaks of measles and pertussis in immunized HIV-infected children.

Prophylactic regimens are integral for the care of HIV-infected children. All infants between 6 wk and 1 yr of age who are proven to be HIV infected should receive prophylaxis regardless of the CD4 count or percentage (see Table 273-5). Infants exposed to HIV-infected mothers should receive the same prophylaxis until they are proven to be noninfected. When the HIV-infected child is >1 yr of age, prophylaxis should be given according to the CD4 lymphocyte count (Table 273-6). The best prophylactic regimen is 150/750 mg/m^2/day of TMP/SMZ given as 1–2 daily doses 3 days per week. If the patient experiences a mild allergic reaction (rash), desensitization is usually successful to allow daily TMP/SMZ prophylaxis. For severe adverse reactions to TMP/SMZ, alternative therapies include dapsone, atovaquone, or pentamidine (aerosolized or intravenous).

Prophylaxis against MAC should be offered to HIV-infected children with advanced immunosuppression (i.e., CD4 lymphocyte count <500 cells/mm^3 in children <1 yr of age, <75 cells/ mm^3 in children 1–6 yr of age, and <50 cells/mm^3 in children >6 yr of age). The drugs of choice are clarithromycin (7.5 mg/kg bid PO) or azithromycin (20 mg/kg once a week PO or 5 mg/kg once daily PO).

TABLE 273-6. Recommendations for PCP Prophylaxis and CD4 Monitoring for HIV-Exposed Infants and HIV-Infected Children, by Age and HIV Infection Status

AGE/HIV INFECTION STATUS	PCP PROPHYLAXIS	CD4 MONITORING
Birth to 4–6 wk, HIV exposed	No prophylaxis	1 mo
4–6 wk to 4 mo or HIV exposed 4–12 mo	Prophylaxis	3 mo
HIV-infected or indeterminate	Prophylaxis	6, 9, and 12 mo
HIV infection reasonably excluded*	No prophylaxis	None
1–5 yr, HIV infected	Prophylaxis if: CD4 count is <500 cells/μL or CD4 percentage is <15%‡§	Every 3–4 mo†
6–12 yr, HIV infected	Prophylaxis if: CD4 count is <200 cells/μL or CD4 percentage is <15%§	Every 3–4 mo†

*HIV infection can be reasonably excluded among children who have had 2 or more negative HIV diagnostic tests (i.e., HIV culture or polymerase chain reaction), both of which are performed at ≥1 mo of age and one of which is performed at ≥4 mo of age, or 2 or more negative HIV IgG antibody tests performed at >6 mo of age among children who have no clinical evidence of HIV disease.

†More frequent monitoring (e.g., monthly) is recommended for children whose CD4 counts or percentages are approaching the threshold at which prophylaxis is recommended.

‡Children 1–2 yr of age who were receiving PCP prophylaxis and had a CD4 count of <750 cells/μL or percentage of <15% at <2 mo of age should continue prophylaxis.

§Prophylaxis should be considered on a case-by-case basis for children who might otherwise be at risk for PCP, such as children with rapidly declining CD4 counts or percentages or children with Category C conditions. Children who have had PCP should receive lifelong PCP prophylaxis.

PCP, *Pneumocystis carinii* pneumonia.

From the Centers for Disease Control and Prevention: 1995 revised guidelines for prophylaxis against *Pneumocystis carinii* pneumonia for children infected with or perinatally exposed to human immunodeficiency virus. *MWWR* 1995; 44(RR-4):1–18.

Primary prophylaxis against opportunistic infections may be discontinued if patients have experienced sustained (>6 mo duration) immune reconstitution with HAART. Even if patients have had opportunistic infections such as PCP or disseminated MAC, it may also be possible to discontinue prophylaxis if immune reconstitution has been sustained.

Some experts recommend IVIG to prevent recurrent serious bacterial infections for symptomatic HIV-infected children who (1) have suffered from at least 2 documented serious bacterial infections within 1 yr, (2) have laboratory-documented inability to make antigen-specific antibodies, or (3) are hypogammaglobulinemic. The dose is 400 mg/kg every 4 wk.

All HIV-exposed children should have skin testing (5TU PPD) for tuberculosis at 1 yr of age and be retested every 2 yr. If the child is living in close contact with a person with tuberculosis, he or she should be tested more frequently. To reduce the incidence

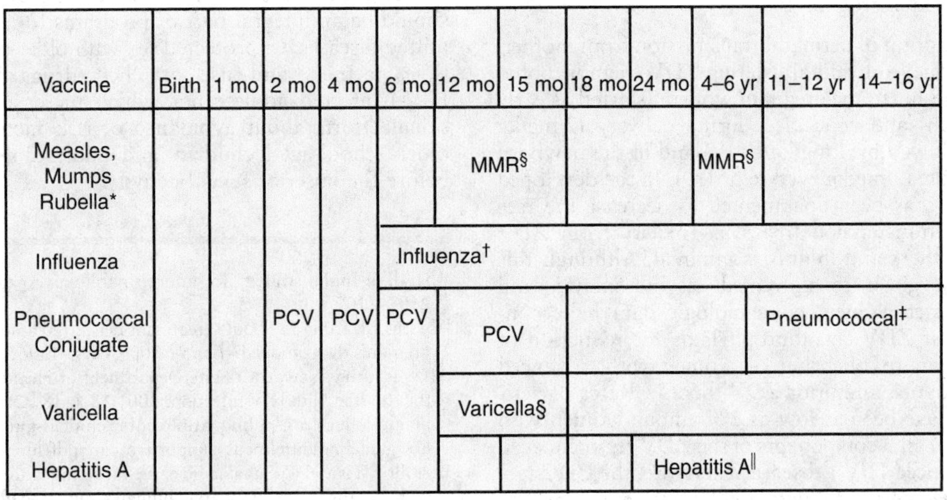

Vaccine	Birth	1 mo	2 mo	4 mo	6 mo	12 mo	15 mo	18 mo	24 mo	4–6 yr	11–12 yr	14–16 yr
Measles, Mumps Rubella*						MMR§				MMR§		
Influenza					Influenza†							
Pneumococcal Conjugate			PCV	PCV	PCV	PCV			Pneumococcal‡			
Varicella						Varicella§						
Hepatitis A									Hepatitis A‖			

* See text.
† Revaccination is recommended every year.
‡ Revaccination with pneumococcal polysaccharide vaccine (PPV) every 5 yr.
§ Contraindicated in children with AIDS or immune category 3 (see Table 273–1).
‖ Recommended routinely for all HIV-infected children.

Figure 273-2. Differences in immunization schedule for HIV-infected children from the routine childhood immunization schedule.

of other potential infections, parents should be counseled about (1) the importance of good handwashing, (2) avoiding raw or undercooked food *(Salmonella)*, (3) avoiding drinking or swimming in lake or river water or being in contact with young farm animals *(Cryptosporidium)*, and (4) the risk of playing with pets (*Toxoplasma* and *Bartonella* from cats, *Salmonella* from reptiles).

Because of the frequent changes in these guidelines, physicians providing care to few HIV-exposed or infected children should periodically consult physicians with expertise in pediatric HIV infection.

PROGNOSIS. The improved understanding of the pathogenesis of HIV infection in children and the availability of more effective anti-retroviral drugs has changed the prognosis considerably. In developed countries where early diagnosis leads to prompt anti-retroviral therapy, progression of the disease to AIDS and the mortality rate have diminished. HIV-infected children live longer with improved quality of life. Even with only partial reduction of viral load, children may have both significant immunologic and clinical benefits. In general, the best prognostic indicators are the sustained suppression of plasma viral load and $CD4^+$ lymphocytes. If determinations of viral load and CD4 lymphocytes are available, the results can be used to evaluate prognosis. It is unusual to see rapid progression in an infant with a viral load <100,000 copies/mL. In addition, a high viral load (>100,000 copies/mL) over time is associated with greater risk for disease progression and death. CD4 lymphocyte percentage is another prognostic indicator, and the mortality rate is higher in patients with a CD4 lymphocyte percentage of <15%. To define prognosis more accurately, the use of changes in both markers (CD4 lymphocyte percentage and plasma viral load) is recommended.

In developing countries where anti-retroviral therapy and sophisticated diagnostic tests are less available, a clinical staging system can be used to predict progression of disease. The suggested clinical staging is similar to the classification recommended in the revised 1994 CDC classification. Children with opportunistic infections (PCP, MAC), encephalopathy, or wasting syndrome have the worst prognosis, with 75% dying before 3 yr of age. Persistent fever and/or oral thrush, serious bacterial infections (meningitis, pneumonia, sepsis), hepatitis, persistent anemia (<8.0 g/dL), and/or thrombocytopenia (<100,000/mm^3) also suggest a poor outcome, with >30% of such children dying before age 3 yr of age. In contrast, lymphadenopathy, splenomegaly, hepatomegaly, lymphoid interstitial pneumonitis, and parotitis are indicators of a better prognosis.

PREVENTION. Interruption of perinatal transmission from mother-to-child has been achieved by administering ZDV chemoprophylaxis (200 mg every 8 hr) to the pregnant woman (started as early as 4 wk of gestation) and continued during delivery (2 mg/kg loading dose IV followed by 1 mg/kg/hr IV) and in the newborn for the 1st 6 wk of life (2 mg/kg every 6 hr PO). In the developed world, such therapy has been documented to decrease the rate of perinatal HIV-1 transmission to <8%. Toxicity from ZDV therapy in both mothers and infants is minimal. Although this treatment was first given to untreated, asymptomatic, and immunologically intact women, epidemiologic data have confirmed the efficacy of ZDV chemoprophylaxis for reduction of perinatal transmission to offspring of women with advanced disease, low CD4 counts, and prior ZDV therapy. Rates of perinatal transmission have been as low as 2% among women who received HAART and all 3 components of the ZDV regimen, even in women with advanced HIV-1 disease. Therefore, the CDC recommends that women be treated with a HAART regimen appropriate for their own health during pregnancy, with collaboration between the HIV-specialist and the obstetrician. Women whose viral load at the time of delivery is >1,000 copies/mL should be counseled about the potential benefit of cesarean section in reducing the risk for vertical transmission.

Retrospective data suggest that even if a mother has received no anti-retroviral therapy during gestation or delivery, the 6-wk component of the ZDV prophylactic regimen instituted for the newborn as soon as possible after delivery (preferably within 12–24 hr of birth) results in a significant reduction of transmission rate. Full-term infants should be given oral ZDV at a dose of 2 mg/kg every 6 hr for 6 wk. Reduced dosages are used for preterm infants (see Table 273-5).

A study evaluating the efficacy of oral nevirapine, a non-nucleoside reverse transcriptase inhibitor, given once to women in labor and once to the infant during the 1st 48–72 hr of life, capitalizes on the prolonged half-life of this drug. In Africa it has been shown to reduce perinatal transmission by 50%, providing a simple and highly cost-effective regimen for resource-poor countries. For women living in resource-constrained settings, the WHO has recommended that pregnant women be treated with an anti-retroviral regimen appropriate for their own health if possible. For those who do not meet indications for or have no access to therapy, a regimen known to prevent vertical HIV-1 transmission should be offered, such as ZDV from 28 wk of pregnancy plus a single dose of nevirapine (SD NVP) during labor and 1 wk of ZDV therapy for the neonate. International studies are under way to determine optimal approaches to interruption of perinatal transmission in breast-fed infants. Studies in non-breast-feeding pregnant women in Thailand have shown that 3rd trimester ZDV with SD NVP in labor with 7 days of ZDV ± SD NVP to the infant was associated with a transmission rate of <3%. These regimens offer simpler, effective, and less expensive approaches to preventing perinatal transmission when longer-term regimens are difficult to implement.

Now that it is clear that perinatal transmission can be reduced dramatically by treating pregnant mothers, a compelling argument can be made for prenatal identification of HIV-1 infection in the mother. The benefit of therapy, both for the mother's health and to prevent transmission to the infant, cannot be overemphasized. The recommended universal prenatal HIV-1 counseling and HIV-1 testing with consent for all pregnant women has reduced the number of new infections dramatically in many areas of the USA. When risk assessment alone is used to decide which women warrant perinatal counseling and testing, a substantial number of women do not receive these services. For women not tested during pregnancy, the use of rapid HIV antibody testing during labor, or in the 1st day of life for the infant, is a way to provide perinatal prophylaxis to an additional group of at-risk infants.

Prevention of sexual transmission involves avoiding the exchange of bodily fluids. In sexually active adolescents, condoms should be an integral part of programs to reduce sexually transmitted diseases. Unprotected sex with older partners or with multiple partners and use of illicit drugs is common among HIV-1-infected adolescents, which increases their risk. Educational efforts about avoidance of risk factors are essential for older school-aged children and adolescents and should begin before the onset of sexual activity.

Abgrall S: Initial strategy for antiretroviral-naive patients. *Lancet* 2006;368:2107–2109.

Abrams EJ, Kuhn L: Should treatment be started among all HIV-infected children and then stopped? *Lancet* 2003;1595–1596.

AIDS Institute New York State Department of Health: Supportive care issues for children with HIV infection, 2001:18-1–18-22. Available at http://www.hivguidelines.org/public_html/center/clinical-guidelines/ped_adolescent_hiv_guidelines/html/peds_supportive_care/pdf/supportive_care.pdf

Bertolli J, Hsu HW, Sukalac T, et al: Hospitalization trends among children and youths with perinatal human immunodeficiency virus infection, 1990–2002. *Pediatr Infect Dis J* 2006;25:628–633.

Bulterys M, Jamieson DJ, O'Sullivan MJ, et al: Rapid HIV-1 testing during labor: A multicenter study. *JAMA* 2004;292:219–233.

Centers for Disease Control and Prevention: Treating opportunistic infections among HIV-exposed and infected children. *MMWR* 2004;53:1–92.

Centers for Disease Control and Prevention: Updated U.S. public health service guidelines for the management of occupational exposures to HIV and recommendations for postexposure prophylaxis. *MMWR* 2005;54:1–17.

Centers for Disease Control and Prevention: Epidemiology of HIV/AIDS—United States, 1981–2005. *MMWR* 2006;55:589–592.
Centers for Disease Control and Prevention: Reduction in perinatal transmission of HIV infection—United States, 1985–2005. *MMWR* 2006;55:592–597.
Committee on Pediatric AIDS: Reducing the risk of HIV infection associated with illicit drug use. *Pediatrics* 2006;117:566–571.
Gona P, Van Dyke RB, Williams PL, et al: Incidence of opportunistic and other infections in HIV-infected children in the HAART era. *JAMA* 2006;296:292–300.
Holmes WR, Savage F: Exclusive breast feeding and HIV. *Lancet* 2007;369:1065–1066.
Jones R, Gazzard B, Halima Y: Preventing HIV infection. *Br Med J* 2005;331:1285–1286.
The Lancet: Newer approaches to HIV prevention. *Lancet* 2007;369:615–616.
Leonard EG, McComsey GA: Metabolic complications of antiretroviral therapy in children. *Pediatr Infect Dis J* 2003;22:77–84.
Lifson AR, Rybicki SL: Routine opt-out HIV testing. *Lancet* 2007;369:539–540.
Lockman S, Shapiro RL, Smeaton LM, et al: Response to antiretroviral therapy after a single, peripartum dose of nevirapine. *N Engl J Med* 2007;356:135–147.
McGrath N, Fawzi WW, Bellinger D, et al: The timing of mother-to-child transmission of human immunodeficiency virus infection and the neurodevelopment of children in Tanzania. *Pediatr Infect Dis J* 2006;25:47–52.
Newell ML, Bärnighausen T: Male circumcision to cut HIV risk in the general population. *Lancet* 2007;369:617–618.
Phillips AN, Gazzard BG, Clumeck N, et al: When should antiretroviral therapy for HIV be started? *BMJ* 2007;334:76–78.
Public Health Service Task Force: Recommendations for use of antiretroviral drugs in pregnant HIV-1-infected women for maternal health and interventions to reduce perinatal HIV-1 transmission in the United States. Available at http://aidsinfo.nih.gov/
Puthanakit T, Oberdorfer P, Akarathum N, et al: Immune reconstruction syndrome after highly active antiretroviral therapy in human immunodeficiency virus-infected Thai children. *Pediatr Infect Dis J* 2006;25:53–58.
Verweel G, Saavedra-Lozano J, van Rossum AMC, et al: Initiating highly active antiretroviral therapy in human immunodeficiency virus type I-infected children in Europe and the United States. *Pediatr Infect Dis J* 2006;25:987–994.
Working Group on Antiretroviral Therapy and Medical Management of HIV-Infected Children: Guidelines for the use of antiretroviral agents in pediatric HIV infection. Available at http://aidsinfo.nih.gov/
World Health Organization: Guidelines for preventing perinatal transmission in resource-constrained settings. Available at http://www.who.int/reproductive-health/rtis/docs/arvdrugsguidelines.pdf

Chapter 274 ■ Human T-Cell Lymphotropic Viruses Types I and II

Hal B. Jenson

ETIOLOGY. Human T-cell lymphotropic viruses type I (HTLV-I) and type II (HTLV-II), members of the Oncovirinae subfamily of the Retroviridae family, are single-stranded RNA viruses that encode reverse transcriptase, an RNA-dependent DNA polymerase that transcribes the single-stranded viral RNA into a double-stranded DNA copy. HTLV-I and II share approximately 65% genome homology and infect T cells, B cells, and synovial cells via the ubiquitous glucose transporter type 1 (GLUT1), which serves as the virus receptor. Circular viral DNA is transported into the nucleus where it is integrated into chromosomal DNA (provirus), evading the usual mechanisms of immune surveillance and resulting in lifelong infection. Serologic assays used in early epidemiologic studies were unable to differentiate between the 2 viruses, but immunoblot assays as well as polymerase chain reaction may be used to discriminate infection with these 2 viruses.

EPIDEMIOLOGY. HTLV-I is endemic in southwestern Japan (where up to 10% of adults are seropositive), areas of the Caribbean including Jamaica and Trinidad (up to 6%), and in parts of sub-Saharan Africa (up to 5%). Lower seroprevalence rates are found in South America (up to 2%). There is microclustering with marked variability within geographic regions.

The seroprevalence of HTLV-I and HTLV-II in the United States in the general population is 0.01–0.03% for each virus, with higher rates with increasing age. HTLV-I infection correlates greatest with birth in endemic areas or sexual contact with persons from endemic areas. HTLV-II infection correlates with intravenous illicit drug use, with an overall prevalence of approximately 18% in 1 study of drug users in the United States, often with concomitant HTLV-I or HIV infection.

HTLV-I and II are transmitted as cell-associated viruses by 3 major routes: from mother to child; sexual contact; and parenterally via contaminated blood products and sharing of needles and syringes associated with intravenous illicit drug use. **Vertical HTLV-I transmission** occurs primarily via breast-feeding from infected mothers, with a 3-fold increased risk for transmission with breast-feeding for >6 mo. Intrauterine and intrapartum transmission account for <5% of vertical transmission. Studies in Japan have shown that approximately 20–25% of children born to infected mothers become infected, and >90% of HTLV-I-infected children have HTLV-I-infected mothers. HTLV-II, like HTLV-I, may also be transmitted via breast-feeding but has a lower breast milk transmission rate of approximately 14%.

CLINICAL MANIFESTATIONS. HTLV-I was the 1st human retrovirus to be associated with cancer, as the cause of adult T-cell leukemia (ATL). HTLV-I is also associated with several nonmalignant conditions, including the neurodegenerative disorder HTLV-I-associated myelopathy (HAM), also known as tropical spastic paraparesis (TSP) and often termed HAM/TSP. The geographic epidemiology of ATL and HAM/TSP are similar. Virus has been reported in tissues from a wide variety of other conditions, including uveitis, polymyositis, bronchioalveolar pneumonitis, autoimmune thyroiditis, and arthritis, although these epidemiologic associations remain weak.

T-Cell Leukemia/Lymphoma. The age distribution of ATL peaks at approximately 50 yr, underscoring the long latent period of HTLV-I infection. HTLV-I-infected persons remain at risk for ATL even if they move to an area of low HTLV-I prevalence, with a lifetime risk for ATL of 2–4%. Most cases of ATL are associated with monoclonal integration of HTLV-I provirus into the cellular genome of CD4 lymphocytes. There is a spectrum of disease that is categorized into 4 forms: acute, chronic, smoldering, and lymphoma-type. The **acute form** of ATL comprises 55–75% of all cases. Smoldering, subclinical lymphoproliferation may spontaneously resolve, in approximately half of cases, or progress to chronic leukemia, lymphoma-type, or culminate in acute ATL. **Chronic, low-grade,** HTLV-I-associated lymphoproliferation (pre-ATL) may persist for years with abnormal lymphocytes with or without peripheral lymphadenopathy before progressing to the acute form. Acute ATL is characterized by hypercalcemia, lytic bone lesions, lymphadenopathy that spares the mediastinum, hepatomegaly, splenomegaly, cutaneous lymphomas, and opportunistic infections. Leukemia may occur with circulating polylobulated malignant lymphocytes, called flower cells, possessing mature T-cell markers. Cyclophosphamide, doxorubicin, vincristine, and prednisolone (CHOP) is often 1st line therapy for ATL, although chemotherapy is not curative and relapses are common. The median survival after diagnosis is 6–13 mo.

Myelopathy. HAM/TSP occurs in up to 4% of persons with HTLV-I infection, usually developing during middle age. It is characterized by infiltration of mononuclear cells into the gray and white matter of the thoracic spinal cord, leading to severe white matter degeneration and fibrosis. The cerebrospinal fluid may have a mildly elevated protein and a mild monocytic pleocytosis. Neuroimaging studies are normal or show periventricular lesions in the white matter. Clinically, there is gradual onset and slowly progressive neurologic degeneration of the corticospinal tracts and, to a lesser extent, the sensory system. HAM/TSP is more common in women than in men, and has a relatively short incubation period after HTLV-1 infection: 1–4 yr compared with 40–60 yr for ATL. Clinical manifestations include slowly progressive evolution of lower extremity spasticity or weakness, lower back pain, and hyperreflexia of the lower extremities with an extensor plantar response. The bladder and intestines may become dysfunctional, and men may become impotent. Some patients may have dysesthesias of the lower extremities with diminished sensation to vibration and pain. Upper extremity function and sensation, cranial nerves, and cognitive function are usually preserved. Treatment regimens have included corticosteroids, danazol, interferon, plasmapheresis, and high-dose vitamin C, although a satisfactory treatment has not been identified.

HTLV-II. HTLV-II was originally identified in patients with hairy cell leukemia, although most patients with hairy cell leukemia are seronegative for HTLV-II infection. HTLV-II has been rarely isolated from patients with leukemias or with myelopathies resembling HAM/TSP, but there is limited evidence of disease specifically associated with HTLV-II infection.

PREVENTION. Routine antibody testing of all blood products using HTLV-I viral lysate began in the USA in 1988, which missed 30–58% of HTLV-II infections. Combination HTLV-I/II antibody testing was implemented in 1997. Formula feeding of infants of HTLV-I-infected mothers is an effective means to control endemic HTLV-I transmission in developed countries. No vaccine is available.

Centers for Disease Control and Prevention: Recommendations for counseling persons infected with human T-lymphotropic virus, types I and II. *MMWR* 1993;42(RR-9):1–13.

Hollsberg P, Hafler DA: Pathogenesis of diseases induced by human lymphotropic virus type I infection. *N Engl J Med* 1993;328:1173–1182.

Kaplan JE, Abrams E, Schaffer N, et al: Low risk of mother-to-child transmission of human lymphotropic virus type II in non-breast-fed infants. *J Infect Dis* 1992;166:892–895.

Levin MC, Jacobson S: HTLV-I associated myelopathy/tropical spastic paraparesis (HAM/TSP): A chronic progressive neurologic disease associated with immunologically mediated damage to the central nervous system. *J Neurovirol* 1997;3:126–140.

Manns A, Hisada M, La Grenade L: Human T-lymphotrophic virus type I infection. *Lancet* 1999;353:1951–1958.

Proietti FA, Carneiro-Proietti BF, Catalan-Soares BC, et al: Global epidemiology of HTLV-I infection and associated diseases. *Oncogene* 2005;24:6058–6068.

Taylor GP, Matsuoka M: Natural history of adult T-cell leukemia/lymphoma and approaches to therapy. *Oncogene* 2005;24:6047–2057.

Van Dyke RB, Heneine W, Perrin ME, et al: Mother-to-child transmission of human T-lymphotropic virus type II. *J Pediatr* 1995;127:924–928.

Chapter 275 ■ Transmissible Spongiform Encephalopathies

David M. Asher

The transmissible spongiform encephalopathies (TSEs) or prion diseases are slow infections of the human nervous system, consisting of at least 4 diseases of humans (Table 275-1): **kuru; Creutzfeldt-Jakob disease** (**CJD**) with its variants-**sporadic CJD** (**sCJD**), **familial CJD** (**fCJD**), **iatrogenic CJD** (**iCJD**), and **new-variant or variant CJD** (**vCJD**); **Gerstmann-Sträussler-Scheinker syndrome** (**GSS**), a familial CJD-like disease; and **fatal familial insomnia** (**FFI**), or the even more rare **sporadic fatal insomnia syndrome.** TSEs also affect animals; the most common and best-known TSEs of animals are **scrapie** in sheep, **bovine spongiform encephalopathy** (**BSE or "mad cow disease"**) in cattle, and a **chronic wasting disease** (**CWD**) of deer and elk found in parts of the United States and Canada. All TSEs have similar clinical manifestations and histopathology, and all are "slow" infections with very long asymptomatic incubation periods of at least a year, durations of several months or more, and overt disease (although not infection) restricted to the nervous system. The most striking neuropathologic change that occurs in each TSE, to a greater or lesser extent, is spongy degeneration of the cerebral cortical gray matter.

ETIOLOGY. The TSEs are all transmissible to susceptible animals by inoculation of tissues from affected subjects. Although the infectious agents replicate in some cell cultures, they do not achieve the high titers of infectivity found in brain tissues or cause recognizable cytopathic effects in cultures. Most studies of TSE agents have relied on in vivo assays, using the appearance of typical neurologic disease in animals as evidence that the agent was present and intact. Inoculation of susceptible recipient animals with small amounts of infectious TSE agent results, months later, in the accumulation in tissues of large amounts of agent with the same physical and biologic properties as the original agent. The TSE agents display a spectrum of extreme resistance to inactivation by a variety of chemical and physical treatments that is unknown among conventional pathogens. This characteristic, as well as their partial sensitivity to protein-disrupting treatments and their consistent association with an abnormal amyloid protein stimulated the hypothesis that the TSE agents are probably subviral in size, composed of protein, and devoid of nucleic acid.

In 1982, S.B. Prusiner suggested the term **prion** (for proteinaceous infectious agent) as an appropriate name for such agents. The prion hypothesis proposes that the molecular mechanism by which the pathogen-specific information of TSE agents is propagated involves a self-replicating change in the folding of a host-encoded protein associated with a transition from an α helix–rich structure in the native protease-sensitive conformation to a β sheet–rich structure in the protease-resistant conformation associated with infectivity. The existence of a 2nd host-encoded protein—termed "protein X"—that participates in the transformation was postulated to explain certain otherwise puzzling findings.

The prion has not been universally accepted; it relies on the postulated existence of a genome-like coding mechanism based on differences in protein folding that have not been satisfactorily explained at a molecular level. In addition, it has yet to account for the many biologic strains of TSE agent that have been observed, although strain-specific differences in the abnormal forms of the prion protein (PrP) have been found and proposed as providing a molecular basis for the coding. Two studies claiming that abnormal PrP uncontaminated with nucleic acid from an infected host has transmitted a typical spongiform encephalopathy to animals await confirmation. If the TSE agents ultimately prove to consist of protein and only protein, without any nucleic acid component, then the term *prion* will indeed be appropriate.

The 1st evidence that abnormal proteins are associated with TSE was morphologic: **Scrapie-associated fibrils** (**SAFs**) were found in extracts of tissues from a variety of patients and animals with spongiform encephalopathies but not in normal tissues. SAFs resemble but are distinguishable from the amyloid fibrils that accumulate in the brains of patients with Alzheimer disease. A group of antigenically related, protease-resistant proteins, now designated **PrP^{Sc} (scrapie-type prion protein)** or **PrP-res (protease-resistant prion protein)**, proved to be components of SAF and to be present in the amyloid plaques found in the brains of patients and animals with TSE.

TABLE 275-1. Clinical and Epidemiologic Features of Human Prion Diseases

DISEASE	CLINICAL FEATURES	SOURCE OF INFECTION	GEOGRAPHIC DISTRIBUTION AND PREVALENCE	USEFUL ANCILLARY TESTS	DURATION OF ILLNESS
sCJD	Dementia, myoclonus, ataxia	Unknown	Worldwide; 1/1 million/yr; 85–95% of CJD cases	EEG—PSWCs; CSF 14-3-3; MRI/DWI	1–24 mo (mean 24 mo)
fCJD	Dementia, myoclonus, ataxia	Genetic (*PRNP* mutations)	Worldwide—geographic clusters; >100 known families; 5–15% of CJD cases	Gene testing; EEG—PSWC rare; MRI/DWI (?)	Mean ≈15 mo
iCJD	Incoordination, dementia (late)	Cadaver dural grafts, human pituitary hormones, corneal transplantation, neurosurgical instruments, EEG depth electrodes	<1% of CJD cases in toto (cadaver dural grafts), >100 cases (human pituitary hormones), >100 cases (corneal transplantation); ≈3 cases (neurosurgical instruments), 6 cases, including 2 from EEG depth electrodes (RBC transfusions), 4 cases (U.K.)		1 mo to 10 yr
vCJD	Mood and behavioral abnormalities, paresthesias, dementia	Linked to BSE in cattle	U.K.; >200 cases	Tonsil biopsy may show PrPSc MRI/FLAIR	8–36 mo (mean 14 mo)
Kuru	Incoordination, ataxia, tremors, dementia (late)	Linked to cannibalism	Fore people of Papua New Guinea (≈2,600 known cases)	EEG—no PSWCs; CSF 14-3-3 often negative; MRI (?)	3–24 mo
GSS	Incoordination, chronic progressive ataxia, corticospinal tract signs, dementia (late), myoclonus (rare)	90% genetic (*PRNP* mutations)	Worldwide; >50 families; 1–10/100 million/yr	Gene testing	2–6 yr (mean ≈57 mo)
FFI	Disrupted sleep > intractable insomnia; autonomic hyperactivation; myoclonus, ataxia; corticospinal tract signs; dementia	*PRNP* gene mutation (D 178L); very rare sporadic cases	≈27 families in Europe, UK., USA, Finland, Australia, China, Japan	EEG—PSWCs only rarely positive; MRI—no DWI abnormalities; CSF 14-3-3 positive in ≈50%	8 mo to 6 yr (mean ≈ 18 mo)

BSE, bovine spongiform encephalopathy; CSF, cerebrospinal fluid; DWI, diffusion-weighted image; EEG, electroencephalography; fCJD, familial Creutzfeldt-Jakob disease; FFI, fatal familial insomnia; FLAIR, fluid attenuation inversion recovery MRI; GSS, Gerstmann-Sträussler-Scheinker syndrome; iCJD, iatrogenic Creutzfeldt-Jakob disease; PrPSc, scrapie-type prion protein; PSWCs, periodic sharp wave complexes; sCJD, sporadic Creutzfeldt-Jakob disease; vCJD, variant Creutzfeldt-Jakob disease.

Modified from Mandell GL, Bennett JE, Dolin R (editors): *Principles and Practice of Infectious Diseases,* 6th ed, Vol 2. Philadelphia, Elsevier, 2005, p 2222.

It is not yet clear whether abnormal PrP constitutes the complete infectious particle of spongiform encephalopathies or a component of those particles, or is simply a pathologic host protein not usually separated from the actual infectious entity by currently used techniques. The demonstration that PrP is encoded by a normal host gene seemed to favor the last possibility. However, several studies have suggested that agent-specific pathogenic information can be transmitted and replicated by different conformations of a protein with the same primary amino acid sequence in the absence of agent-specific nucleic acids. Properties of 2 fungal proteins were found to be heritable without encoding in nucleic acid, although those properties have not been transmitted to recipient fungi as infectious elements. Whatever its relationship to the actual infectious TSE particles, PrP clearly plays a central role in infection, because the normal prion protein must be expressed in mice if they are to acquire a TSE or to sustain replication of the infectious agents.

Normal PrPs are sialoglycoproteins linked to the outer surface of the cell membrane by a glycophosphatidyinositol anchor; protease-resistant PrPs have the physical properties of amyloid proteins. The PrPs of several species of animals are very similar in their amino acid sequences and antigenicity, but are not identical in structure. The primary structure of PrP is encoded by the host and is not altered by the source of the infectious agent provoking its formation. The function of the ubiquitous **protease-sensitive PrP precursor** (designated **PrP^c for cellular PrP** or **PrP-sen for protease-sensitive PrP**) in normal cells is unknown; it binds copper and may play some role in normal synaptic transmission, but it is not required for life or for relatively normal cerebral function. As noted, expression of PrP is clearly required both for development of scrapie disease and for replication of the transmissible agent in mice. The degree of homology between amino acid sequences of PrPs in different animal species may correlate with the "species barrier" that affects susceptibility of animals of 1 species to infection with a TSE agent adapted to grow in another species.

Attempts to find particles resembling those of viruses or virus-like agents in brain tissues of humans or animals with spongiform encephalopathies have generally been unsuccessful. Peculiar tubulovesicles have been seen in thin sections of infected brain tissue. However, it has never been established that those structures are associated with infectivity.

It has been claimed that 2 other human diseases—familial Alzheimer disease of adults and Alpers disease of young children—may be caused by infections with agents similar to those causing the spongiform encephalopathies. The latter is a convulsive disorder associated with hemiatrophy and status spongiosus of the cerebral gray matter. Attempts to confirm these claims failed.

EPIDEMIOLOGY. **Kuru** once affected many children, adolescents, and young adults—mainly women—living in 1 area of Papua New Guinea. Transmission of the infection was interrupted more than 40 yr ago; kuru is now extremely rare and recognized only in older adults born before 1958. The complete disappearance of kuru among young people suggests that the practice of ritual cannibalism was the most important mechanism—probably the only mechanism—by which the infection spread in Papua New Guinea.

CJD, the most common human spongiform encephalopathy, was formerly thought to occur only in older adults; however, iCJD and, much more rarely, sCJD have affected adolescents and young adults. **GSS** and the insomnia syndromes have not been diagnosed in children or adolescents. Variant CJD has a peculiar predilection for younger people; only a few patients with vCJD have been >55 yr of age. CJD has been recognized worldwide, at yearly rates of 0.25–2 cases/million population (not age adjusted), with foci of considerably higher incidence among Libyan Jews in Israel, in isolated villages of Slovakia, and in other limited areas. Epidemiologic surveys have investigated several hypothetical mechanisms of spread of CJD. Person-to-person spread has been confirmed only for iatrogenic cases. The striking resemblance of CJD to scrapie prompted the suggestion that infected sheep tissues might be a source of spongiform encephalopathy in humans. However, no reliable epidemiologic evidence suggests that exposure to potentially scrapie-contaminated animals, meat, meat products, or experimental preparations of the scrapie agent have transmitted a TSE to humans.

The same can no longer be said about BSE. The outbreak of BSE among cattle (probably infected by eating scrapie agent–contaminated meat and bone meal) was first recognized in the U.K. in 1986 and spread to native cattle in at least 25 other countries, including the USA. The finding of a new TSE in ungulate and feline animals in British zoos and then in domestic cats there raised a fear that some strain of the scrapie agent, after crossing the species barrier from sheep to cattle, had acquired a broadened range of susceptible hosts, posing a potential danger for humans. This is the most probable explanation for the occurrence of vCJD, first recognized in adolescents in 1995 and now affecting more than 200 people worldwide (summary available at http://www.cjd.ed.ac.uk/vcjdworld.htm), including 162 in the U.K., 21 in France, 4 in Ireland, 3 in the United States, 2 in the Netherlands, and single cases in Canada, Italy, Japan, Portugal, Saudi Arabia, and Spain. The potential of the CWD agent, now known to have infected wild deer and moose as well as farmed deer and elk in at least 7 states and in Canada, to infect human beings is unknown but is under investigation. Preliminary epidemiologic studies by the Centers for Disease Control and Prevention have not suggested that a history of eating either venison in general or venison from animals in areas where CWD occurs is a risk factor for the later development of CJD. However, it has long seemed prudent to avoid exposing children to meat or other products likely to be contaminated with any TSE agent, including the agents of scrapie and CWD; the BSE agent clearly poses a special danger.

Iatrogenic transmission of CJD has been recognized for >25 yr (Table 275-2). Accidental transmissions of CJD have occurred by means of contaminated neurosurgical instruments or operating facilities, cortical electrodes contaminated during epilepsy surgery, injections of human cadaveric pituitary growth hormone and gonadotropin, and transplantation of contaminated corneas and allografts of human dura mater; most recently, 4 cases of vCJD occurred in elderly recipients of red blood cell concentrate transfusion from donors who later became ill with that disease. Pharmaceuticals and tissue grafts derived from or contaminated with human neural tissues, particularly when obtained from unselected donors and large pools of donors, pose special risks.

Spouses and household contacts of patients are at very low risk for acquiring CJD, although rare instances of conjugal CJD have been reported. However, medical personnel exposed to brains of patients with CJD may be at increased risk, and at least 20 health care workers have been recognized with the disease.

PATHOGENESIS. The probable portal of entry for the kuru agent has been thought to be either through the gastrointestinal tract or lesions in the mouth or integument incidentally exposed to the agent during cannibalism. Most subjects with vCJD (and animals with BSE and related infections) are thought to have been similarly infected with the BSE agent through exposure to some contaminated beef product, probably through the intestinal tract. The 1st site of replication of the TSE agents appears to be in tissues of the reticuloendothelial system.

The TSE agents have been detected in low titers in blood of experimentally infected animals (mice, monkeys, hamsters, and sheep), mainly associated with both nucleated cells and plasma. Circulating lymphoid cells seem to be required to infect mice by peripheral routes. Limited evidence suggests that the scrapie agent also spreads to the central nervous system of mice by ascending peripheral nerves. Several researchers claim to have detected the CJD agent in human blood, although most attempts have failed.

In human kuru, it seems probable that the only portal of exit of the agent from the body, at least in quantities sufficient to infect others, was through infected tissues exposed during cannibalism. In iatrogenically transmitted CJD, the brains and eyes of patients with CJD and blood of clinically healthy donors incubating vCJD have been the probable sources of contamination. Kidney, liver, lung, lymph node, spleen, and cerebrospinal fluid (CSF) may also contain the CJD agent. At no time during the course of any TSE have antibodies or cell-mediated immunity to the infectious agents been convincingly demonstrated in either patients or animals. However, mice must be immunologically competent to be infected with the scrapie agent by peripheral routes of inoculation.

Typical changes in TSE include vacuolation and loss of neurons with hypertrophy and proliferation of glial cells, most pronounced in the cerebral cortex in patients with CJD and in the cerebellum in those with kuru. The CNS lesions are usually most severe in or even confined to gray matter, at least early in the disease. Loss of myelin appears to be secondary to degeneration of neurons. There generally is no inflammation, but usually a marked increase in the number and size of astrocytes is noted. Status spongiosus is not a striking autopsy finding in patients with FFI, and neuronal degeneration is largely restricted to thalamic nuclei.

Amyloid plaques are found in the brains of all patients with GSS and in at least 70% of those with kuru; they are less common in those with CJD. Amyloid plaques are most commonly found in the cerebellum but occur elsewhere in the brain as well. In brains of patients with vCJD, dense plaques surrounded by halos of vacuolated cells (described as **flower-like or florid plaques**) have been a consistent finding. TSE plaques react with antiserum prepared against PrP, and, even in the absence of plaques, extracellular PrP can be detected in the brain parenchyma by immunostaining.

TABLE 275-2. Iatrogenic Transmission of Creutzfeldt-Jakob Disease by Products of Human Origin

		INCUBATION TIME	
PRODUCT	NO. OF PATIENTS	Mean	Range
Cornea	3	17 mo	16–18 mo
Dura mater allograft	>100	7.4 yr	1.3–16 yr
Pituitary extract			
Growth hormone	>100*	12 yr	5–38.5 yr
Gonadotropin	4	13 yr	12–16 yr
Red blood cells	4	?6 yr	6 yr–>5 yr†

*There have been 29 cases reported among approximately 8,000 recipients of human cadaveric growth hormone in the USA; the remaining cases have been reported in other countries.

†The second transfusion-transmitted case of vCJD (Peden AH, Head MW, Ritchie DL, et al: Preclinical vCJD after blood transfusion in a PRNP codon 129 heterozygous patient. *Lancet* 2004;364:527–529) died of unrelated causes about 5 years after transfusion but was found to have accumulations of abnormal PrP in spleen and cervical lymph node—a finding unique to vCJD. The patient is thought to have been in the asymptomatic incubation period of vCJD.

CLINICAL MANIFESTATIONS. Kuru is a progressive degenerative disease of the cerebellum and brainstem with less obvious involvement of the cerebral cortex. The 1st sign of kuru is usually cerebellar ataxia followed by progressive incoordination. Coarse, shivering tremors are characteristic. Variable abnormalities in cranial nerve function appear, frequently with impairment in conjugate gaze and swallowing. Patients die of inanition and pneumonia or of burns from cooking fires, usually ≥1 yr after onset. Although changes in mentation are common, there is no frank dementia or progression to coma, as in CJD. There are no signs of acute encephalitis such as fever, headaches, and convulsions.

CJD occurs throughout the world. Patients initially have either sensory disturbances (most often visual) or confusion and inappropriate behavior, with progression over weeks or months to frank dementia and ultimately coma. Some patients have cerebellar ataxia early in disease, and most experience myoclonic jerking movements. Mean survival of patients with sCJD has been <1 yr from the earliest signs of illness, although about 10% of patients live for approximately 2 yr. Variant CJD (Table 275-3) differs from the more common sCJD: Patients with vCJD are much younger at onset, and they more often present with complaints of dysesthesia and more subtle behavioral changes, often mistaken for psychiatric illness, than those seen in sCJD. Severe mental deterioration occurs later in the course of vCJD. Patients with vCJD have survived substantially longer than those with sCJD.

GSS is a familial disease resembling CJD but with more prominent cerebellar ataxia and amyloid plaques. Dementia may appear only late in the course, and the average duration of illness is longer than that in typical sCJD. FFI and sporadic fatal insomnia are characterized by progressively severe insomnia and dysautonomia as well as ataxia, myoclonus, and other signs resembling those of CJD and GSS. Neither GSS nor an insomnia syndrome has been diagnosed in children or adolescents.

TABLE 275-3. Clinical and Histopathologic Features of Patients with Variant and Typical Sporadic Creutzfeldt-Jakob Disease (CJD)

FEATURE	VARIANT CJD (>10 PATIENTS)	SPORADIC CJD (185 PATIENTS)
Years of age at death* (range)	29 (19–74)	65
Duration of illness, mo (range)	12 (8–23)	4
Presenting signs	Abnormal behavior, dysesthesia	Dementia
Later signs	Dementia, ataxia, myoclonus	Ataxia, myoclonus
Periodic complexes on EEG	Rare	Most
PRNP 129 Met/Met	All tested (except 1 transfusion-transmitted case)	83%
Histopathologic changes	Vacuolation, neuronal loss, astrocytosis, plaques (100%)	Vacuolation, neuronal loss, astrocytosis, plaques (~15%)
Florid PrP plaques[†]	100%	0
PrP glycosylation pattern	BSE-like[‡]	Not BSE-like

*Median age and duration for variant CJD; averages for typical sporadic CJD.
[†]Dense plaques with a pale periphery of surrounding vacuolated cells.
[‡]Characterized by an excess of high molecular mass band and 19 kd nonglycosylated band (type 4) glycoform of PrP-res (Collinge J, Sidle KC, Meads J, et al: Molecular analysis of prion strain variation and the aetiology of "new variant" CJD. *Nature* 1996;383:685–690.)
BSE, bovine spongiform encephalopathy; EEG, electroencephalogram; Met, codon 129 of one *PRNP* gene encoding for methionine; PRNP, prion-protein-encoding gene; PrP, prion protein.
Modified from Will RG, Ironside JW, Zeidler M, et al: A new variant of Creutzfeldt-Jakob disease in the UK. *Lancet* 1996;347:921–925.

DIAGNOSIS. Diagnosis of spongiform encephalopathies is most often determined on clinical grounds after excluding other diseases. The presence of 14-3-3 protein in CSF, while not specific to TSEs, may aid in distinguishing between CJD and Alzheimer disease, although this is not a diagnostic consideration in children. Brain biopsy may be diagnostic of CJD but can be recommended only if a potentially treatable disease remains to be excluded or if there is some other compelling reason to make an antemortem diagnosis. Definitive diagnosis requires microscopic examination of brain tissue obtained at autopsy. The demonstration of protease-resistant PrP proteins in brain extracts has been useful to confirm histopathologic diagnosis. Accumulation of the abnormal PrP in lymphoid tissues, even before the onset of neurologic signs, is typical of vCJD; tonsil biopsy may replace the need for brain biopsy when antemortem diagnosis of vCJD is indicated. Transmission of disease to susceptible animals by inoculation of brain suspension must be reserved for cases of special research interest.

LABORATORY FINDINGS. Virtually all patients with typical sporadic, iatrogenic, and familial forms of CJD have abnormal electroencephalograms (EEGs) as the disease progresses; the background becomes slow and irregular with diminished amplitude. A variety of paroxysmal discharges may also appear—slow waves, sharp waves, spike and wave complexes—and these may sometimes be unilateral or focal as well as bilaterally synchronous. Paroxysmal discharges may be precipitated by loud noise. Many patients have typical periodic suppression-burst complexes of high-voltage slow activity on EEG at some time during the illness. Patients with the vCJD had only generalized slowing, without periodic bursts of high-voltage discharges on EEG. CT or MRI may show cortical atrophy and large ventricles late in the course of CJD; many patients with vCJD have an increase in density of the pulvinar on MRI (especially well seen by fluid attenuation inversion recovery [FLAIR] sequences), something not typical of sCJD.

There may be modest elevation of CSF protein content in patients with TSE. Unusual protein spots were observed in CSF specimens after 2 dimensional separation in gels and silver staining; the spots were identified as 14-3-3 proteins, normal proteins abundant in neurons but not ordinarily detected in CSF. (The 14-3-3 protein is not related to PrP.) However, the finding of 14-3-3 protein in CSF is not specific to CJD; it has also been detected in CSF specimens from some patients with acute viral encephalitides and recent cerebral infarctions. In clinical practice, the usual diagnostic problem is to differentiate between CJD and Alzheimer disease, and the presence of 14-3-3 proteins in CSF, while neither sensitive nor specific, militates against the latter. Finding the 14-3-3 protein in CSF has also been of some help in confirming the diagnosis of vCJD.

TREATMENT. No treatment has proven to be effective. Studies of cell cultures and rodents experimentally infected with TSE agents suggested that treatment with chlorpromazine, quinacrine, tetracyclines, and pentosan polysulfate might be of benefit, especially during the incubation periods of TSEs; early reports of clinical trials based on those studies have not been encouraging, and it seems unlikely that the severe brain damage found in late disease can be reversed by treatment. Appropriate supportive care should be provided as for other progressive fatal neurologic diseases. On the basis of experimental studies in animals, several prophylactic postexposure treatment regimens have been suggested, but none have been widely accepted.

GENETIC COUNSELING. TSE sometimes occurs in families with a pattern of occurrence consistent with an autosomal-dominant mode of inheritance. In patients with a family history of CJD, the clinical and histopathologic findings are similar to those seen in sporadic cases. In the United States, only about 10% of cases of CJD are familial. GSS and FFI are always familial. In some affected families, about 50% of siblings and children of a patient with a familial TSE eventually acquire the disease; in other families, the "penetrance" of illness may be less.

The gene coding for PrP is closely linked if not identical to that controlling the incubation periods of scrapie in sheep and both scrapie and CJD in mice. The gene encoding the PrP in humans, currently designated the PRNP gene, is located on the short arm of chromosome 20. It has an open reading frame of 759 nucleotides (253 codons), in which more than 20 different point mutations, as well as a variety of inserted sequences encoding extra tandem-repeated octapeptides, have been linked to the occurrence of spongiform encephalopathy in families.

Although the interpretation of these findings in regard to the prion hypothesis is in dispute, in affected families with an autosomal-dominant pattern of CJD or GSS, individuals who are heterozygous for linked mutations in the PRNP gene clearly have a high probability of acquiring spongiform encephalopathy. The significance of mutations in the PRNP genes of individuals from families with no history of spongiform encephalopathy is not known. It seems wise to avoid alarming those who have miscellaneous mutations—several of which appear to represent normal polymorphisms—in the PRNP gene and their families because the implications are not yet clear.

The same nucleotide substitution at codon 178 of the PRNP gene associated with CJD in some families has been found in all patients with FFI; however, it is linked to a different amino acid–encoding sequence at codon 129, a site that is polymorphic in normal individuals. Homozygosity for methionine or for valine at codon 129, especially for methionine, seems to increase susceptibility to iCJD and sCJD, although methionine-valine heterozygotes are also susceptible to both diseases. So far, all patients with clinical vCJD to be genotyped have been homozygous for methionine at codon 129 of the PRNP gene. (One of the presumptive transfusion-transmitted cases—diagnosed by the finding of PrP^{Sc} in lymphoid tissue—was in an elderly patient heterozygous for valine and methionine at that locus.) Two possible subclinical vCJD infections have been reported in persons homozygous for valine as well.

PROGNOSIS. The prognosis of spongiform encephalopathies is uniformly poor. About 10% of patients may survive for >1 yr, but the quality of life is poor.

PREVENTION. Standard precautions should be used for handling all human tissues, blood, and body fluids. Materials and surfaces known to be contaminated with tissues or fluids from patients suspected of having CJD must be treated with great care. Whenever possible, contaminated instruments should be discarded by careful packaging and incineration. Contaminated tissues and biologic products probably cannot be completely freed of infectivity without destroying their structural integrity and biologic activity; therefore, the medical and family histories of individual tissue donors should be carefully reviewed to exclude a diagnosis of TSE. Histopathologic examination of brain tissues of donors and testing for abnormal PrP should be performed where feasible. Although no method of sterilization can be relied on to remove all infectivity from contaminated surfaces, exposure to moist heat, sodium hydroxide, chlorine bleach, concentrated formic acid, and guanidine salts markedly reduces infectivity.

Asher DM: Transmissible spongiform encephalopathies. In Yolken R (editor): *Manual of Clinical Microbiology,* 8th ed, Vol. 2. Washington, DC, American Society for Microbiology, 2003, pp 1592–1604.
Brown P: Transfusion medicine and spongiform encephalopathy. *Transfusion* 2001;41:433–436.
Brown P, Will RG, Bradley R, et al: Bovine spongiform encephalopathy and variant Creutzfeldt-Jakob disease: Background, evolution, and current concerns. *Emerg Infect Dis* 2001;7:6–16.
Castilla J, Saa P, Hetz C, Soto C: In vitro generation of infectious scrapie prions. *Cell* 2005;121:195–206.
Colchester ACF, Colchester NTH: The origin of bovine spongiform encephalopathy: The human prion disease hypothesis. *Lancet* 2005;366:856–860.
Collinge J, Sidle KC, Meads J, et al: Molecular analysis of prion strain variation and the aetiology of "new variant" CJD. *Nature* 1996;383:685–690.
Collins SJ, Lawson VA, Masters CL: Transmissible spongiform encephalopathies. *Lancet* 2004;363:51–64.
Couzin J: An end to the prion debate? Don't count on it. *Science* 2004; 305:589.
Gregori L, McCombie N, Palmer D, et al: Effectiveness of leucoreduction for removal of infectivity of transmissible spongiform encephalopathies from blood. *Lancet* 2004;364: 529–531.
Hilton DA, Ghani AC, Conyers L, et al: Prevalence of lymphoreticular prion protein accumulation in UK tissue samples. *J Pathol* 2004;203:733–739.
Hsich G, Kenney K, Gibbs CJ Jr, et al: The 14-3-3 brain protein in cerebrospinal fluid as a marker for transmissible spongiform encephalopathies. *N Engl J Med* 1996;335:924–930.
Legname G, Baskakov IV, Nguyen HO, et al: Synthetic mammalian prions. *Science* 2004;305:673–676.
Llewelyn CA, Hewitt PE, Knight RS, et al: Possible transmission of variant Creutzfeldt-Jakob disease by blood transfusion. *Lancet* 2004;363:417–421.
Manuelidis L: Transmissible encephalopathies: Speculations and realities. *Viral Immunol* 2003;16:123–139.
Otto M, Wiltfang J, Cepek L, et al: Tau protein and 14-3-3 protein in the differential diagnosis of Creutzfeldt-Jakob disease. *Neurology* 2002;58: 192–197.
Peden AH, Head MW, Ritchie DL, et al: Preclinical vCJD after blood transfusion in a PRNP codon 129 heterozygous patient. *Lancet* 2004;364: 527–529.
Sehulster LM: Prion inactivation and medical instrument reprocessing: Challenges facing healthcare facilities. *Infect Control Hosp Epidemiol* 2004;25:276–279.
Spencer MD, Knight RS, Will RG: First hundred cases of variant Creutzfeldt-Jakob disease: Retrospective case note review of early psychiatric and neurological features. *Br Med J* 2002;324:1479–1482.
Taylor DM: Inactivation of transmissible degenerative encephalopathy agents: A review. *Vet J* 2000;159:10–17.
Will RG: Variant Creutzfeldt-Jakob disease. *J Neurol Neurosurg Psychiatry* 2002;72:285–286.
Williams ES, Miller MW: Chronic wasting disease in deer and elk in North America. *Rev Sci Tech* 2002;21:305–316.
Wilson K, Ricketts MN: A third episode of transfusion-derived vCJD. *Lancet* 2006;368:2037–2038.
World Health Organization: Infection control guidelines for transmissible spongiform encephalopathies. Report of a WHO Consultation, Geneva, Switzerland, March 23–26, 1999. WHO Communicable Disease Surveillance and Control. Retrieved June 2005 from http://www.who.int/emc-documents/tse/docs/whocdscsraph 20003.pdf
World Health Organization: WHO guidelines on transmissible spongiform encephalopathies in relation to biological and pharmaceutical products. Report of a WHO Consultation, Geneva, Switzerland, February 3–5, 2003. Retrieved June 2005 from http://www.who.int/bloodproducts/en/index.html

Section 14 — Antiparasitic Therapy

Chapter 276 ■ Principles of Antiparasitic Therapy

Sharon F. Chen

By taxonomy, parasites are divided into 2 main groups: protozoans, which are unicellular, and helminths, which are multicellular. Chemotherapeutic agents for protozoans and helminths are different and not effective for the other group. Not all drugs are readily available. Some drugs are available only from the manufacturer, some are not available in the United States, and some are available under an Investigational New Drug (IND) protocol through the Centers of Disease Control and Prevention Drug Service (telephone: 404-639-3670 weekdays; 404-639-2888 evenings, weekends, and holidays) (Tables 276-1 and 276-2). Pediatric infectious disease consultation may be needed for assistance in use of these antiparasitic drugs and management of the parasitic infection.

SELECTED ANTIPARASITIC DRUGS FOR PROTOZOANS.

Nitazoxanide. Nitazoxanide is a nitrothiazole benzamide, initially developed as a veterinary anthelmintic. In humans, nitazoxanide is effective against many protozoans and helminths. It has been marketed in Latin America since 1996. In December 2002, the U.S. Food and Drug Administration (FDA) approved the use of nitazoxanide for the treatment of diarrhea caused by *Cryptosporidium* species in children 1–11 yr of age and by *Giardia intestinalis* in children ≥1 yr of age. Treatment of adults and immunocompromised persons with *Cryptosporidium* infection is not yet FDA approved. Nitazoxanide is the 1st and only FDA-approved treatment for *Cryptosporidium.*

Nitazoxanide inhibits pyruvate-ferredoxin oxidoreductase, which is an enzyme necessary for anaerobic energy metabolism. This is 1 of the mechanisms of action against protozoans, although it may not be the only mechanism. The other mecha-

Text continued on p. 1456

TABLE 276-1. Drugs for Parasitic Infections

Parasitic infections are found throughout the world. With increasing travel, immigration, use of immunosuppressive drugs, and the spread of AIDS, physicians anywhere may see infections caused by previously unfamiliar parasites. The table below lists first-choice and alternative drugs for most parasitic infections.

INFECTION	DRUG	ADULT DOSAGE	PEDIATRIC DOSAGE
Acanthamoeba keratitis			
Drug of choice:	See footnote 1		
Amebiasis (*Entamoeba histolytica*)			
Asymptomatic			
Drug of choice:	Lodoquinol	650 mg tid × 20 days	30–40 mg/kg/day (max 2 g) in 3 doses × 20 days
OR	Paromomycin	25–35 mg/kg/day in 3 doses × 7 days	25–35 mg/kg/day in 3 doses × 7 days
Alternative:	Diloxanide furoate[2]*	500 mg tid × 10 days	20 mg/kg/day in 3 doses × 10 days
Mild to moderate intestinal disease[3]			
Drug of choice[4]:	Metronidazole	500–750 mg tid × 7–10 days	35–50 mg/kg/day in 3 doses × 7–10 days
OR	Tinidazole[5]	2 g once daily × 3 days	50 mg/kg/day (max 2 g) in 1 dose × 3 days
Severe intestinal and extraintestinal disease[3]			
Drug of choice:	Metronidazole	750 mg tid × 7–10 days	35–50 mg/kg/day in 3 doses × 7–10 days
OR	Tinidazole[5]	2 g once daily × 5 days	50 mg/kg/day (max 2 g) × 5 days
Amebic meningoencephalitis, primary and granulomatous			
Naegleria			
Drug of choice:	Amphotericin B[6,7]	1.5 mg/kg/day in 2 doses × 3 days, then 1 mg/kg/day × 6 days	1.5 mg/kg/day in 2 doses × 3 days, then 1 mg/kg/day × 6 days
Acanthamoeba			
Drug of choice:	See footnote 8		
Balamuthia mandrillaris			
Drug of choice:	See footnote 9		
Sappinia diploidea			
Drug of choice:	See footnote 10		
Ancylostoma caninum (Eosinophilic enterocolitis)			
Drug of choice:	Albendazole[7]	400 mg once	400 mg once
OR	Mebendazole	100 mg bid × 3 days	100 mg bid × 3 days
OR	Pyrantel pamoate[7]	11 mg/kg (max 1 g) × 3 days	11 mg/kg (max 1 g) × 3 days
OR	Endoscopic removal		
Ancylostoma duodenale, see Hookworm			
Angiostrongyliasis (*Angiostrongylus cantonensis, Angiostrongylus costaricensis*)			
Drug of choice:	See footnote 11		
Anisakiasis (*Anisakis* spp.)			
Treatment of choice[12]:	Surgical or endoscopic removal		
Ascariasis (*Ascaris lumbricoides,* roundworm)			
Drug of choice:	Albendazole[7]	400 mg once	400 mg once
OR	Mebendazole	100 mg bid × 3 days or 500 mg once	100 mg bid × 3 days or 500 mg once
OR	Ivermectin[7]	150–200 μg/kg once	150–200 μg/kg once
Babesiosis (*Babesia microti*)			
Drugs of choice[13]:	Clindamycin[7]	1.2 g bid IV or 600 mg tid PO × 7–10 days	20–40 mg/kg/day PO in 3 doses × 7–10 days
	plus quinine[7]	650 mg tid PO × 7–10 days	25 mg/kg/day PO in 3 doses × 7–10 days
OR	Atovaquone[7]	750 mg bid × 7–10 days	20 mg/kg bid × 7–10 days
	plus azithromycin[7]	600 mg daily × 7–10 days	12 mg/kg daily × 7–10 days
Balamuthia mandrillaris, see Amebic meningoencephalitis, primary			
Balantidiasis (*Balantidium coli*)			
Drug of choice:	Tetracycline[7,14]	500 mg qid × 10 days	40 mg/kg/day (max 2 g) in 4 doses × 10 days
Alternatives:	Metronidazole[7]	750 mg tid × 5 days	35–50 mg/kg/day in 3 doses × 5 days
	Iodoquinol[7]	650 mg tid × 20 days	40 mg/kg/day in 3 doses × 20 days
Baylisascariasis (*Baylisascaris procyonis*)			
Drug of choice:	See footnote 15		
Blastocystis hominis infection			
Drug of choice:	See footnote 16		
Capillariasis (*Capillaria philippinensis*)			
Drug of choice:	Mebendazole[7]	200 mg bid × 20 days	200 mg bid × 20 days
Alternatives:	Albendazole[7]	400 mg daily × 10 days	400 mg daily × 10 days
Changes disease, see Trypanosomiasis			
Clonorchis sinensis, see Fluke infection			
Cryptosporidiosis (*Cryptosporidium*)			
Non-HIV infected			
Drug of choice:	Nitazoxanide[4]	500 mg bid × 3 days[7]	1–3 yr: 100 mg bid × 3 days 4–11 yr: 200 mg bid × 3 days
HIV infected			
Drug of choice:	See footnote 17		
Cutaneous larva migrans (creeping eruption, dog and cat hookworm)			
Drug of choice[18]:	Albendazole[7]	400 mg daily × 3 days	400 mg daily × 3 days
OR	Ivermectin[7]	200 μg/kg daily × 1–2 days	200 μg/kg daily × 1–2 days
Alternative:	Thiabendazole	Topically	Topically
Cyclosporiasis (*Cyclospora cayetanensis*)			
Drug of choice[9]:	Trimethoprim-sulfamethoxazole[7]	TMP 160 mg/SMX 800 mg (1 DS tab) bid × 7–10 days	TMP 5 mg/kg, SMX 25 mg/kg bid × 7–10 days

continued

TABLE 276-1. Drugs for Parasitic Infections—cont'd

INFECTION	DRUG	ADULT DOSAGE	PEDIATRIC DOSAGE
Cysticercosis, see Tapeworm infection			
Dientamoeba fragilis infection[20]			
Drug of choice:	Iodoquinol	650 mg tid × 20 days	30–40 mg/kg/day (max 2 g) in 3 doses × 20 days
OR	Paromomycin[7]	25–35 mg/kg/day in 3 doses × 7 days	25–35 mg/kg/day in 3 doses × 7 days
OR	Tetracycline[7,14]	500 mg qid × 10 days	40 mg/kg/day (max 2 g) in 4 doses × 10 days
OR	Metronidazole	500–750 mg tid × 10 days	20–40 mg/kg/day in 3 doses × 10 days
Diphyllobothrium latum, see Tapeworm infection			
Dracunculus medinensis (guinea worm) infection			
Drug of choice:	See footnote 21		
Echinococcus, see Tapeworm Infection			
Entamoeba histolytica, see Amebiasis			
***Enterobius** vermicularis* (pinworm) infection			
Drug of choice[22]:	Pyrantel pamoate	11 mg/kg base once (max 1 g); repeat in 2 wk	11 mg/kg base once (max 1 g); repeat in 2 wk
OR	Mebendazole	100 mg once; repeat in 2 wk	100 mg once; repeat in 2 wk
OR	Albendazole[7]	400 mg once; repeat in 2 wk	400 mg once; repeat in 2 wk
Fasciola hepatica, see Fluke infection			
Filariasis[23]			
Wuchereria bancrofti, Brugia malayi, Brugia timori			
Drug of choice[24]:	Diethylcarbamazine*	6 mg/kg in 3 doses × 14 days[25]	6 mg/kg in 3 doses × 14 days[25]
Loa loa			
Drug of choice[26]:	Diethylcarbamazine*	6 mg/kg in 3 doses × 14 days[25]	6 mg/kg in 3 doses × 14 days[25]
Mansonella ozzardi			
Drug of choice[24]:	See footnote 27		
Mansonella perstans			
Drug of choice[24]:	Albendazole[7]	400 mg bid × 10 days	400 mg bid × 10 days
OR	Mebendazole[7]	100 mg bid × 30 days	100 mg bid × 30 days
Mansonella streptocerca			
Drug of choice[24,28]:	Diethylcarba-mazine*	6 mg/kg/day × 14 days	6 mg/kg/day × 14 days
	Ivermectin[7]	150 μg/kg once	150 μg/kg once
Tropical pulmonary eosinophilia (TPE)[29]			
Drug of choice:	Diethylcarba-mazine*	6 mg/kg/day in 3 doses × 12–21 days	6 mg/kg/day in 3 doses × 12–21 days
Onchocerca volvulus (River blindness)			
Drug of choice:	Invermectin[30]	150 μg/kg once, repeated every 6–12 mo until asymptomatic	150 μg/kg once, repeated every 6–12 mo until asymptomatic
Fluke, hermaphroditic, infection			
Clonorchis sinensis (Chinese liver fluke)			
Drug of choice:	Praziquantel	75 mg/kg/day in 3 doses × 1 day	75 mg/kg/day in 3 doses × 1 day
OR	Albendazole[7]	10 mg/kg × 7 days	10 mg/kg × 7 days
Fasciola hepatica (sheep liver fluke)			
Drug of choice[31]:	Triclabendazole*	10 mg/kg once or twice[32]	10 mg/kg once or twice[32]
Alternative:	Bithionol*	30–50 mg/kg on alternate days × 10–15 doses	30–50 mg/kg on alternate days × 10–15 doses
Fasciolopsis buski, Heterophyes heterophyes, Metagonimus yokogawai (intestinal flukes)			
Drug of choice:	Praziquantel[7]	75 mg/kg/day in 3 doses × 1 day	75 mg/kg/day in 3 doses × 1 day
Metorchis conjunctus (North American liver fluke)[33]			
Drug of choice:	Praziquantel[7]	75 mg/kg/day in 3 doses × 1 day	75 mg/kg/day in 3 doses × 1 day
Nanophyetus salmincola			
Drug of choice:	Praziquantel[7]	60 mg/kg/day in 3 doses × 1 day	60 mg/kg/day in 3 doses × 1 day
Opisthorchis viverrini (Southeast Asian liver fluke)			
Drug of choice:	Praziquantel	75 mg/kg/day in 3 doses × 1 day	75 mg/kg/day in 3 doses × 1 day
Paragonimus westermani (lung fluke)			
Drug of choice:	Praziquantel[7]	75 mg/kg/day in 3 doses × 2 days	75 mg/kg/day in 3 doses × 2 days
Alternative[34]:	Bithionol*	30–50 mg/kg on alternate days × 10–15 doses	30–50 mg/kg on alternate days × 10–15 doses
Giardiasis (*Giardia duodenalis*)			
Drug of choice:	Metronidazole[7]	250 mg tid × 5 days	15 mg/kg/day in 3 doses × 5 days
	Nitazoxanide[4]	500 mg bid × 3 days	1–3 yr: 100 mg every 12 hr × 3 days 4–11 yr: 200 mg every 12 hr × 3 days
	Tinidazole[5]	2 g once	50 mg/kg once (max 2 g)
Alternatives[35]:	Paromomycin[7,36]	25–35 mg/kg/day in 3 doses × 7 days	25–35 mg/kg/day in 3 doses × 7 days
	Furazolidone	100 mg qid × 7–10 days	6 mg/kg/day in 4 doses × 7–10 days
	Quinacrine[2]	100 mg tid × 5 days	2 mg/kg tid × 5 days (max 300 mg/day)
Gnathostomiasis (*Gnathostoma spinigerum*)			
Treatment of choice[37]:	Albendazole[7]	400 mg bid × 21 days	400 mg bid × 21 days
OR	Ivermectin[7]	200 μg/kg/day × 2 days	200 μg/kg/day × 2 days
±	Surgical removal		
Gongylonemiasis (*Gongylonema sp.*)[38]			
Treatment of choice:	Surgical removal		
OR	Albendazole[7]	10 mg/kg/day × 3 days	10 mg/kg/day × 3 days
Hookworm infection (*Ancylostoma duodenale, Necator americanus*)			
Drug of choice:	Albendazole[7]	400 mg once	400 mg once
OR	Mebendazole	100 mg bid × 3 days or 500 mg once	100 mg bid × 3 days or 500 mg once
OR	Pyrantel pamoate[7]	11 mg/kg (max 1 g) × 3 days	11 mg/kg (max 1 g) × 3 days

TABLE 276-1. Drugs for Parasitic Infections—cont'd

INFECTION	DRUG	ADULT DOSAGE	PEDIATRIC DOSAGE
Hydatid cyst, see Tapeworm infection			
Hymenolepis nana, see Tapeworm infection			
Isosporiasis (*Isospora belli*)			
Drug of choice[39]:	Trimethoprim-sulfamethoxazole[7]	TMP 160 mg/SMX 800 mg (1 DS tab) bid × 10 days	TMP 5 mg/kg, SMX 25 mg bid × 10 days
Leishmania infection			
Visceral[40]			
Drugs of choice:	Sodium stibo-gluconate*	20 mg Sb/kg/day IV or IM × 28 days[41]	20 mg Sb/kg/day IV or IM × 28 days[41]
OR	Meglumine antimonate*	20 mg Sb/kg/day IV or IM × 28 days[41]	20 mg Sb/kg/day IV or IM × 28 days[41]
OR	Amphotericin B[7]	0.5–1 mg/kg IV daily or every 2 day for up to 8 wk	0.5–1 mg/kg IV daily or every 2 day for up to 8 wk
OR	Liposomal amphotericin B[42]	3 mg/kg/day IV (days 1–5) and 3 mg/kg/day days 14 and 21[43]	3 mg/kg/day IV (days 1–5) and 3 mg/kg/day days 14 and 21[43]
Alternative[44]:	Pentamidine[7]	4 mg/kg IV or IM daily or every 2 day for 15–30 doses	4 mg/kg IV or IM daily or every 2 day for 15–30 doses
Cutaneous[45]			
Drugs of choice:	Sodium stibo-gluconate*	20 mg Sb/kg/day IV or IM × 20 days[41]	20 mg Sb/kg/day IV or IM × 20 days[41]
OR	Meglumine antimonate*	20 mg Sb/kg/day IV or IM × 20 days[41]	20 mg Sb/kg/day IV or IM × 20 days[41]
Alternatives[46]:	Pentamidine[7]	2–3 mg/kg IV or IM daily or every 2 day × 4–7 doses[47]	2–3 mg/kg IV or IM daily or every 2 day × 4–7 doses[47]
OR	Paromomycin[7,48]	Topically 2×/day × 10–20 days	Topically 2×/day × 10–20 days
Mucosal[49]			
Drugs of choice:	Sodium stibo-gluconate*	20 mg Sb/kg/day IV or IM × 28 days[41]	20 mg Sb/kg/day IV or IM × 28 days[41]
OR	Meglumine antimonate*	20 mg Sb/kg/day IV or IM × 28 days[41]	20 mg Sb/kg/day IV or IM × 28 days[41]
OR	Amphotericin B[7]	0.5–1 mg/kg IV daily or every 2 day for up to 8 wk	0.5–1 mg/kg IV daily or every 2 day for up to 8 wk
Lice infestation (*Pediculus humanus, Pediculus capitis, Phthirus pubis*)[50]			
Drug of choice:	0.5% Malathion[51]	Topically	Topically
OR	1% Permethrin[52]	Topically	Topically
Alternative:	Pyrethrins with piperonyl butoxide[52]	Topically	Topically
OR	Ivermectin[7,53]	200 μg/kg × 3, days 1, 2, and 10	200 μg/kg × 3, days 1, 2, and 10
Loa loa, see Filariasis			
Malaria, treatment of (*Plasmodium falciparum, P. ovale, P. vivax,* and *P. malariae*)			
P. falciparum[54] acquired in areas of **chloroquine-resistance**			
Oral[55]			
Drugs of choice:	Atovaquone/proguanil[56]	2 adult tabs bid[58] or 4 adult tabs once daily × 3 days	<5 kg: not indicated 5–8 kg: 2 pediatric tabs once/day × 3 days 9–10 kg: 3 pediatric tabs once/day × 3 days 11–20 kg: 1 adult tab once/day × 3 days 21–30 kg: 2 adult tabs once/day × 3 days 31–40 kg: 3 adult tabs once/day × 3 days >40 kg: 4 adult tabs once/day × 3 days
OR	Quinine sulfate	650 mg every 8 hr × 3–7 days[57]	30 mg/kg/day in 3 doses × 3–7 days[57]
	plus		
	doxycycline[7,14]	100 mg bid × 7 days	4 mg/kg/day in 2 doses × 7 days
	or plus		
	tetracycline[7,14]	250 mg qid × 7 days	6.25 mg/kg qid × 7 days
	or plus		
	clindamycin[7,59]	20 mg/kg/day in 3 doses × 7 days[60]	20 mg/kg/day in 3 doses × 7 days
Alternatives:	Mefloquine[61]	750 mg followed 12 hr later by 500 mg	15 mg/kg followed 12 hr later by 10 mg/kg
	Artesunate[62]*	4 mg/kg/day × 3 days	4 mg/kg/day × 3 days
	plus		
	mefloquine[61]	750 mg followed 12 hr later by 500 mg	15 mg/kg followed 12 hr later by 10 mg/kg
P. vivax[63] acquired in areas of **chloroquine-resistance**			
Oral[55]			
Drug of choice:	Quinine sulfate	650 mg every 8 hr × 3–7 days[57]	30 mg/kg/day in 3 doses × 3–7 days[57]
	plus		
	doxycycline[7,14]	100 mg bid × 7 days	4 mg/kg/day in 2 doses × 7 days
OR	Mefloquine[61]	750 mg followed 12 hr later by 500 mg	15 mg/kg followed 12 hr later by 10 mg/kg
Alternatives:	Chloroquine	25 mg base/kg in 3 doses over 48 hr	25 mg base/kg in 3 doses over 48 hr
	plus		
	primaquine[64]	30 mg base daily × 14 days	0.6 mg/kg/day × 14 days
All *Plasmodium* except **chloroquine-resistant *P. falciparum***[54] and **chloroquine-resistant *P. vivax***[63]			
Oral[55]			
Drug of choice:	Chloroquine phosphate[65]	1 g (600 mg base), then 500 mg (300 mg base) 6 hr later, then 500 mg (300 mg base) at 24 and 48 hr	10 mg base/kg (max 600 mg base), then 5 mg base/kg 6 hr later, then 5 mg base/kg at 24 and 48 hr
All *Plasmodium*			
Parenteral			
Drug of choice[66]:	Quinidine gluconate[67]	10 mg/kg loading dose (max 600 mg) in normal saline over 1–2 hr, followed by continuous infusion of 0.02 mg/kg/min until PO therapy can be started	10 mg/kg loading dose (max 600 mg) in normal saline over 1–2 hr, followed by continuous infusion of 0.02 mg/kg/min until PO therapy can be started
OR	Quinine dihydrochloride[67]*	20 mg/kg loading dose in 5% dextrose over 4 hr, followed by 10 mg/kg over 2–4 hr every 8 hr (max 1,800 mg/day) until PO therapy can be started	20 mg/kg loading dose in 5% dextrose over 4 hr, followed by 10 mg/kg over 2–4 hr every 8 hr (max 1,800 mg/day) until PO therapy can be started
Alternative:	Artemether[68]*	3.2 mg/kg IM, then 1.6 mg/kg daily × 5–7 days	3.2 mg/kg IM, then 1.6 mg/kg daily × 5–7 days
Prevention of relapses: *P. vivax and P. ovale* only			
Drug of choice:	Primaquine phosphate[64]	30 mg base/day × 14 days	0.6 mg base/kg/day × 14 days

continued

TABLE 276-1. Drugs for Parasitic Infections—cont'd

INFECTION		DRUG	ADULT DOSAGE	PEDIATRIC DOSAGE
Malaria, prevention of[69]				
Chloroquine-sensitive areas[54]				
Drug of choice		Chloroquine phosphate[70,71]	500 mg (300 mg base), once/wk[72]	5 mg/kg base once/wk, up to adult dose of 300 mg base[72]
Chloroquine-resistant areas[54]				
Drug of choice:		Atovaquone/proguanil[56,71]	1 adult tab/day[73]	11–20 kg: 1 pediatric tab/day[56,73] 21–30 kg: 2 pediatric tabs/day[56,73] 31–40 kg: 3 pediatric tabs/day[56,73] >40 kg: 1 adult tab/day[56,73]
	OR	Mefloquine[61,71,74]	250 mg once/wk[72]	5–10 kg: ⅛ tab once/wk[72] 11–20 kg: ¼ tab once/wk[72] 21–30 kg: ½ tab once/wk[72] 31–45 kg: ¾ tab once/wk[72] >45 kg: 1 tab once/wk[72]
	OR	Doxycycline[7,71]	100 mg daily[75]	2 mg/kg/day, up to 100 mg/day[75]
Alternatives:		Primaquine[7,64]	30 mg base daily[76]	0.6 mg/kg base daily
		Chloroquine phosphate	500 mg (300 mg base) once/wk[72]	5 mg/kg base once/wk, up to 300 mg base[72]
		plus proguanil[77]	200 mg once/day	<2 yr: 50 mg once/day 2–6 yr: 100 mg once/day 7–10 yr: 150 mg once/day >10 yr: 200 mg once/day
Malaria, self-presumptive treatment[78]				
Drug of choice:		Atovaquone/proguanil[7,56]	4 adult tabs daily × 3 days	<5 kg: not indicated 5–8 kg: 2 pediatric tabs once/day × 3 days 9–10 kg: 3 pediatric tabs once/day × 3 days 11–20 kg: 1 adult tab once/day × 3 days 21–30 kg: 2 adult tabs once/day × 3 days 31–40 kg: 3 adult tabs once/day × 3 days >40 kg: 4 adult tabs once/day × 3 days
	OR	Quinine sulfate	650 mg every 8 hr × 3–7 days[57]	30 mg/kg/day in 3 doses × 3–7 days[57]
		plus		
		doxycycline[7,14]	100 mg bid × 7 days	4 mg/kg/day in 2 doses × 7 days
	OR	Mefloquine[61]	750 mg followed 12 hr later by 500 mg	15 mg/kg followed 12 hr later by 10 mg/kg
Microsporidiosis				
Ocular (*Encephalitozoon hellem, Encephalitozoon cuniculi, Vittaforma corneae [Nosema corneum]*)				
Drug of choice:		Albendazole[7]	400 mg bid	
		plus fumagillin[79]*		
Intestinal (*Enterocytozoon bieneusi, Encephalitozoon [Septata] intestinalis*)				
E. bieneusi[80]				
Drug of choice:		Fumagillin*	60 mg/day PO × 14 days	
E. intestinalis				
Drug of choice		Albendazole[7]	400 mg bid × 21 days	
Disseminated (*E. hellem, E. cuniculi, E. intestinalis, Pleistophora* sp., *Trachipleistophora* sp., and *Brachiola vesicularum*)				
Drug of choice[81]:		Albendazole[7]	400 mg bid	
Mites, see Scabies				
Moniliformis *moniliformis* infection				
Drug of choice:		Pyrantel pamoate[7]	11 mg/kg once, repeat twice, 2 wk apart	11 mg/kg once, repeat twice, 2 wk apart
***Naegleria* species,** see Amebic meningoencephalitis, primary				
Necator americanus, see Hookworm infection				
Oesophagostomum *bifurcum*				
Drug of choice:		See footnote 82		
Onchocerca volvulus, see Filariasis				
Opisthorchis viverrini, see Fluke infection				
Paragonimus westermani, see Fluke infection				
Pediculus capitis, Pediculus humanus, Phthirus pubis, see Lice				
Pinworm, see *Enterobius*				
Pneumocystis jiroveci (formerly *carinii*) pneumonia (PCP)[83]				
Drug of choice:		Trimethoprim-sulfamethoxazole	TMP 15 mg/kg/day, SMX 75 mg/kg/day, PO or IV in 3 or 4 doses × 14–21 days	TMP 15 mg/kg/day, SMX 75 mg/kg/day, PO or IV in 3 or 4 doses × 14–21 days
Alternatives:		Primaquine[7,64]	30 mg base PO daily × 21 days	
		plus clindamycin[7]	600 mg IV every 6 hr × 21 days, or 300–450 mg PO every 6 hr × 21 days	
	OR	Trimethoprim[7]	5 mg/kg tid × 21 days	
		plus dapsone[7]	100 mg daily × 21 days	
	OR	Pentamidine	3–4 mg/kg IV daily × 14–21 days	3–4 mg/kg IV daily × 14–21 days
	OR	Atovaquone	750 mg bid × 21 days	1–3 mo: 30 mg/kg/day 4–24 mo: 45 mg/kg/day >24 mo: 30 mg/day
Primary and secondary prophylaxis[84]				
Drug of choice:		Trimethoprim-sulfamethoxazole	1 tab (single or double strength) daily	TMP 150 mg/m², SMX 750 mg/m² in 2 doses on 3 consecutive days per wk

TABLE 276-1. Drugs for Parasitic Infections—cont'd

INFECTION		DRUG	ADULT DOSAGE	PEDIATRIC DOSAGE
Alternatives[85]:		Dapsone[7]	50 mg bid, or 100 mg daily	2 mg/kg/day (max 100 mg) or 4 mg/kg (max 200 mg) each wk
	OR	Dapsone[7]	50 mg daily or 200 mg each wk	
		plus pyrimethamine[86]	50 mg or 75 mg each wk	
	OR	Pentamidine aerosol	300 mg inhaled monthly via *Respirgard II* nebulizer	≥5 yr: 300 mg inhaled monthly via *Respirgard II* nebulizer
	OR	Atovaquone[7]	1,500 mg daily	1–3 mo: 30 mg/kg/day 4–24 mo: 45 mg/kg/day >24 mo: 30 mg/kg/day
Roundworm, see Ascariasis				
Sappinia diploidea, see Amebic meningoencephalitis, primary				
Scabies (*Sarcoptes scabiei*)				
Drug of choice:		5% Permethrin	Topically[87]	Topically[87]
Alternatives[88]:		Ivermectin[7,89]	200 μg/kg once[87]	200 μg/kg once[87]
		10% Crotamiton	Topically once/daily × 2 days	Topically once/daily × 2 days
Schistosomiasis (*Bilharziasis*)				
S. haematobium				
Drug of choice:		Praziquantel	40 mg/kg/day in 2 doses × 1 day	40 mg/kg/day in 2 doses × 1 day
S. japonicum				
Drug of choice:		Praziquantel	60 mg/kg/day in 3 doses × 1 day	60 mg/kg/day in 3 doses × 1 day
S. mansoni				
Drug of choice:		Praziquantel	40 mg/kg/day in 2 doses × 1 day	40 mg/kg/day in 2 doses × 1 day
Alternative:		Oxamniquine[90]*	15 mg/kg once[91]	20 mg/kg/day in 2 doses × 1 day[91]
S. mekongi				
Drug of choice:		Praziquantel	60 mg/kg/day in 3 doses × 1 day	60 mg/kg/day in 3 doses × 1 day
Sleeping sickness, see Trypanosomiasis				
Strongyloidiasis (*Strongyloides stercoralis*)				
Drug of choice[92]:		Ivermectin	200 μg/kg/day × 2 days	200 μg/kg/day × 2 days
Alternative:		Albendazole[7]	400 mg bid × 7 days	400 mg bid × 7 days
	OR	Thiabendazole	50 mg/kg/day in 2 doses × 2 days (max 3 g/day)[93]	50 mg/kg/day in 2 doses × 2 days (max 3 g/day)[93]
Tapeworm infection				
Adult (intestinal stage)				
***Diphyllobothrium latum* (fish), *Taenia saginata* (beef), *Taenia solium* (pork), *Dipylidium caninum* (dog)**				
Drug of choice:		Praziquantel[7]	5–10 mg/kg once	5–10 mg/kg once
Alternative:		Niclosamide*	2 g once	50 mg/kg once
***Hymenolepis nana* (dwarf tapeworm)**				
Drug of choice:		Praziquantel[7]	25 mg/kg once	25 mg/kg once
Alternative:		Nitazoxanide[4,7]	500 mg × 3 days[94]	1–3 yr: 100 mg bid × 3 days[94] 4–11 yr: 200 mg bid × 3 days[94]
Larval (tissue stage)				
Echinococcus granulosus (hydatid cyst)				
Drug of choice[95]:		Albendazole	400 mg bid × 1–6 mo	15 mg/kg/day (max 800 mg) × 1–6 mo
Echinococcus multilocularis				
Treatment of choice:		See footnote 96		
Taenia solium (*Cysticercosis*)				
Treatment of choice			See footnote 97	
Alternative:		Albendazole	400 mg bid × 8–30 days; can be repeated as necessary	15 mg/kg/day (max 800 mg) in 2 doses × 8–30 days; can be repeated as necessary
	OR	Praziquantel[7]	50–100 mg/kg/day in 3 doses × 30 days	50–100 mg/kg/day in 3 doses × 30 days
Toxocariasis, see Visceral larva migrans				
Toxoplasmosis (*Toxoplasma gondii*)[98]				
Drugs of choice[99,100]:		Pyrimethamine[101]	25–100 mg/day × 3–4 wk	2 mg/kg/day × 3 days, then 1 mg/kg/day (max 25 mg/day) × 4 wk[102]
		plus		
		sulfadiazine	1–1.5 g qid 3–4 wk	100–200 mg/kg/day × 3–4 wk
Trichinellosis (*Trichinella spiralis*)				
Drugs of choice:		Steroids for severe symptoms		
		plus		
		mebendazole[7]	200–400 mg tid × 3 days, then 400–500 mg tid × 10 days	200–400 mg tid × 3 days, then 400–500 mg tid × 10 days
Alternative:		Albendazole[7]	400 mg bid × 8–14 days	400 mg bid × 8–14 days
Trichomoniasis (*Trichomonas vaginalis*)				
Drug of choice[103]:		Metronidazole	2 g once or 500 mg bid × 7 days	15 mg/kg/day orally in 3 doses × 7 days
	OR	Tinidazole[5]	2 g once	50 mg/kg once (max 2 g)
Trichostrongylus infection				
Drug of choice:		Pyrantel pamoate[7]	11 mg/kg base once (max 1 g)	11 mg/kg once (max 1 g)
Alternative:		Mebendazole[7]	100 mg bid × 3 days	100 mg bid × 3 days
	OR	Albendazole[7]	400 mg once	400 mg once
Trichuriasis (*Trichuris trichiura*, whipworm)				
Drug of choice:		Mebendazole	100 mg bid × 3 days or 500 mg once	100 mg bid × 3 days or 500 mg once
Alternative:		Albendazole[7]	400 mg × 3 days	400 mg × 3 days
		Ivermectin[7]	200 μg/kg daily × 3 days	200 μg/kg daily × 3 days
Trypanosomiasis[104]				
T. cruzi (American trypanosomiasis, Chagas disease)				
Drug of choice:		Benznidazole*	5–7 mg/kg/day in 2 divided doses × 30–90 days	≤12 yr: 10 mg/kg/day in 2 doses × 30–90 days
	OR	Nifurtimox[105]*	8–10 mg/kg/day in 3–4 doses × 90–120 days	1–10 yr: 15–20 mg/kg/day in 4 doses × 90 days 11–16 yr: 12.5–15 mg/kg/day in 4 doses × 90 days

continued

TABLE 276-1. Drugs for Parasitic Infections—cont'd

INFECTION	DRUG	ADULT DOSAGE	PEDIATRIC DOSAGE
T. brucei gambiense (West African trypanosomiasis, sleeping sickness)			
hemolymphatic stage			
Drug of choice[106]:	Pentamidine isethionate[7]	4 mg/kg/day IM × 10 days	4 mg/kg/day IM × 10 days
Alternative:	Suramin*	100–200 mg (test dose) IV, then 1 g IV on days 1, 3, 7, 14, and 21	20 mg/kg on days 1, 3, 7, 14, and 21
Late disease with CNS involvement			
Drug of choice:	Melarsoprol[107]	2.2 mg/kg/day × 10 days	2.2 mg/kg/day × 10 days
OR	Eflornithine[108]*	400 mg/kg/day in 4 doses × 14 days	400 mg/kg/day in 4 doses × 14 days
T. b. rhodesiense (East African trypanosomiasis, sleeping sickness)			
hemolymphatic stage			
Drug of choice:	Suramin*	100–200 mg (test dose) IV, then 1 g IV on days 1, 3, 7, 14, and 21	20 mg/kg on days 1, 3, 7, 14, and 21
Late disease with CNS involvement			
Drug of choice:	Melarsoprol[107]	2–3.6 mg/kg/day × 3 days; after 7 days 3.6 mg/kg/day × 3 days; repeat again after 7 days	2–3.6 mg/kg/day × 3 days; after 7 days 3.6 mg/kg/day × 3 days; repeat again after 7 days
Visceral larva migrans[109] (*Toxocariasis*)			
Drug of choice:	Albendazole[7]	400 mg bid × 5 days	400 mg bid × 5 days
	Mebendazole[7]	100–200 mg bid × 5 days	100–200 mg bid × 5 days
Whipworm, see Trichuriasis			
Wuchereria bancrofti, see Filariasis			

*Availability problems. See Table 276-2.

[1]For treatment of keratitis caused by *Acanthamoeba*, concurrent topical use of 0.1% propamidine isethionate (Brolene) plus neomycin-polymyxin B-gramicidin ophthalmic solution has been successful (SL Hargrave et al, *Ophthalmology* 1999;106:952). In some European countries, propamidine is not available and hexamidine (*Desmodine*) has been used (DV Seal, *Eye* 2003;17:893). In addition, 0.02% topical polyhexamethylene biguanide (PHMB) and/or chlorhexadine has been used successfully in a large number of patients (G Tabin et al, *Cornea* 2001;20:757; YS Wysenbeek et al, *Cornea* 2000;19:464). PHMB is available from Leiter's Park Avenue Pharmacy, San Jose, CA (800-292-6773; www.leiterrx.com). The combination of chlorhexadine, natamycin (pimaricin) and debridement also has been successful (K Kitagawa et al, *Jpn J Ophthalmol* 2003;47:616).

[2]The drug is not available commercially, but as a service can be compounded by Panorama Compounding Pharmacy, 6744 Balboa Blvd, Van Nuys, CA 91406 (800-247-9767) or Medical Center Pharmacy, New Haven, CT (203-688-6816).

[3]Treatment should be followed by a course of iodoquinol or paromomycin in the dosage used to treat asymptomatic amebiasis.

[4]Nitazoxanide is FDA approved as a pediatric oral suspension for treatment of *Cryptosporidium* in immunocompetent children <12 yr old and for *Giardia* (*Med Lett* 2003;45:29). It may also be effective for mild to moderate amebiasis (E Diaz et al, *Am J Trop Med Hyg* 2003;68:384). Nitazoxanide is available in 500 mg tablets and an oral suspension; it should be taken with food.

[5]A nitro-imidazole similar to metronidazole, tinidazole was recently approved by the FDA and appears to be as effective and better tolerated than metronidazole. It should be taken with food to minimize GI adverse effects. For children and patients unable to take tablets, a pharmacist may crush the tablets and mix them with cherry syrup (*Humco*, and others). The syrup suspension is good for 7 days at room temperature and must be shaken before use. Ornidazole, a similar drug, is also used outside the USA.

[6]*Naegleria* infection has been treated successfully with intravenous and intrathecal use of both amphotericin B and miconazole plus rifampin and with amphotericin B, rifampin and ornidazole (J Seidel et al, *N Engl J Med* 1982;306:346; R Jain et al, *Neurol India* 2002;50:470). Other reports of successful therapy are less well documented.

[7]An approved drug, but considered investigational for this condition by the FDA.

[8]Strains of *Acanthamoeba* isolated from fatal granulomatous amebic encephalitis are usually susceptible *in vitro* to pentamidine, ketoconazole, flucytosine, and (less so) to amphotericin B. Chronic *Acanthamoeba* meningitis has been successfully treated in 2 children with a combination of oral trimethoprim-sulfa-methoxazole, rifampin, and ketoconazole (T Singhal et al, *Pediatr Infect Dis J* 2001;20:623) and in an AIDS patient with fluconazole, sulfadiazine, and pyrimethamine combined with surgical resection of the CNS lesion (M Seijo Martinez et al, *J Clin Microbiol* 2000;38:3892). Disseminated cutaneous infection in an immunocompromised patient has been treated successfully with IV pentamidine isethionate, topical chlorhexidine, and 2% ketoconazole cream, followed by oral itraconazole (CA Slater et al, *N Engl J Med* 1994;331:85).

[9]A free-living leptomyxid ameba that causes subacute to fatal granulomatous CNS disease. Several cases of *Balamuthia* encephalitis have been successfully treated with flucytosine, pentamidine, fluconazole, and sulfadiazine plus either azithromycin or clarithromycin (phenothiazines were also used) combined with surgical resection of the CNS lesion (TR Deetz et al, *Clin Infect Dis* 2003;37:1304; S Jung et al, *Arch Pathol Lab Med* 2004;128:466).

[10]A free-living ameba not previously known to be pathogenic to humans. It has been successfully treated with azithromycin, IV pentamidine, itraconazole, and flucytosine combined with surgical resection of the CNS lesion (BB Gelman et al, *J Neuropathol Exp Neurol* 2003;62:990).

[11]Most patients have a self-limited course and recover completely. Analgesics, corticosteroids, and careful removal of CSF at frequent intervals can relieve symptoms from increased intracranial pressure (V Lo Re III and SJ Gluckman, *Am J Med* 2003;114:217). No anthelmintic drug is proven to be effective, and some patients have worsened with therapy (TJ Slom et al, *N Engl J Med* 2002;346:668). In 1 report, however, mebendazole and a corticosteroid appeared to shorten the course of infection (H-C Tsai et al, *Am J Med* 2001;111:109).

[12]A Repiso Ortega et al, *Gastroenterol Hepatol* 2003;26:341. Successful treatment of a patient with *Anisakiasis* with albendazole has been reported (DA Moore et al, *Lancet* 2002;360:54).

[13]Exchange transfusion has been used in severely ill patients and those with high (>10%) parastiemia (JC Hatcher et al, *Clin Infect Dis* 2001;32:1117). In patients who were not severely ill, combination therapy with atovaquone and azithromycin was as effective as clindamycin and quinine and may have been better tolerated (PJ Krause et al, *N Engl J Med* 2000;343:1454).

[14]Use of tetracyclines is contraindicated in pregnancy and in children <8 yr old.

[15]No drugs have been demonstrated to be effective. Albendazole 25 mg/kg/day × 20 days started as soon as possible (up to 3 days after possible infection) might prevent clinical disease and is recommended for children with known exposure (ingestion of racoon stool or contaminated soil) (*MMWR* 2002;50:1153; PJ Gavin and ST Shulman, *Pediatr Infect Dis* 2003;22:651). Mebendazole, thiabendazole, levamisole, or invermectin could be tried if albendazole were not available. Steroid therapy may be helpful, especially in eye and CNS infections. Ocular baylisascariasis has been treated successfully using laser photocoagulation therapy to destroy the intraretinal larvae.

[16]Clinical significance of these organisms is controversial; metronidazole 750 mg tid × 10 days, iodoquinol 650 mg tid × 20 days or trimethoprim-sulfamethoxazole 1 DS tab bid × 7 days have been reported to be effective (DJ Stenzel and PFL Borenam, *Clin Microbiol Rev* 1996;9:563; UZ Ok et al, *Am J Gastroenterol* 1999;94:3245). Metronidazole resistance may be common (K Haresh et al, *Trop Med Int Health* 1999;4:274). Nitazoxanide has been effective in children (E Diaz et al, *Am J Trop Med Hyg* 2003;68:384).

[17]Nitazoxanide has not consistently been shown to be superior to placebo in HIV-infected patients (B Amadi et al, *Lancet* 2002;360;1375). A small randomized, double-blind trial in symptomatic HIV-infected patients who were not receiving HAART found paromomycin similar to placebo (RG Hewitt et al, *Clin Infect Dis* 2000;31:1084).

[18]G Albanese et al, *Int J Dermatol* 2001;40:67.

[19]HIV-infected patients may need higher dosage and long-term maintenance (A Kansouzidou et al, *J Trav Med* 2004;11:61).

[20]A Norberg et al, *Clin Microbiol Infect* 2003;9:65.

[21]Treatment of choice is slow extraction of worm combined with wound care (C Greenaway, *CMAJ* 2004;170:495). 10 days' treatment with metronidazole 250 mg tid in adults and 25 mg/kg/day in 3 doses in children is not curative, but decreases inflammation and facilitates removal of the worm. Mebendazole 400–800 mg/day × 6 days has been reported to kill the worm directly.

[22]Since all family members are usually infected, treatment of the entire household is recommended.

[23]Antihistamines or corticosteroids may be required to decrease allergic reactions due to disintegration of microfilariae from treatment of filarial infections, especially those caused by *Loa loa.* Endosymbiotic *Wolbachia* bacteria may have a role in filarial development and host response, and may represent a new target for therapy. Treatment with doxycycline 100 or 200 mg/day × 4–6 wk in lymphatic filariasis and onchocerciasis has resulted in substantial loss of *Wolbachia* with subsequent block of microfilariae production and absence of microfilaria when followed for 24 mo after treatment (A Hoerauf et al, *Med Microbiol Immunol* 2003;192:211; A Hoerauf et al, *Br Med J* 2003;326:207).

[24]Most symptoms caused by adult worm. Single dose combination of albendazole (400 mg) with either ivermectin (200 μg/kg) or diethylcarbamazine 6 mg/kg is effective for reduction or suppression of *W bancrofti* microfilaria but does not kill the adult forms (D Addiss et al, *Cochrane Database Syst Rev* 2004;CD003753).

[25]For patients with microfilaria in the blood, *Medical Letter* consultants would start with a lower dosage and scale up: day 1, 50 mg; day 2, 50 mg tid; day 3, 100 mg tid; day 4–14, 6 mg/kg in 3 doses (for *Loa Loa* day 4–14, 9 mg/kg in 3 doses). Multidose regimens have been shown to provide more rapid reduction in microfilaria than single-dose diethylcarbamazine, but microfilarla levels are similar 6–12 mo after treatment (LD Andrade et al, *Trans R Soc Trop Med Hyg* 1995;89:319; PE Simonsen et al, *Am J Trop Med Hyg* 1995;53:267). A single dose of 6 mg/kg is used in endemic areas for mass treatment (J Figueredo-Silva et al, *Trans R Soc Trop Med Hyg* 1996;90:192; J Noroes et al, *Trans R Soc Trop Med Hyg* 1997;91:78).

[26]In heavy infections with *Loa loa*, rapid killing of microfilariae can provoke an encephalopathy. Apheresis has been reported to be effective in lowering microfilarial counts in patients heavily infected with *Loa loa* (EA Ottesen, *Infect Dis Clin North Am* 1993;7:619). Albendazole or ivermectin have also been used to reduce microfilaremia; albendazole is preferred because of its slower onset of action and lower risk for encephalopathy (AD Klion et al, *J infect Dis* 1993;168:202; M Kombila et al, *Am J Trop Med Hyg* 1998;58:458). Albendazole may be useful for treatment of loiasis when diethylcarbamazine is ineffective or cannot be used, but repeated courses may be necessary (AD Klion et al, *Clin Infect Dis* 1999;29:680). Diethylcarbamazine, 300 mg once/wk, has been recommended for prevention of loiasis (TB Nutman et al, *N Engl J Med* 1988;319:752).

[27]Diethylcarbamazine has no effect. Ivermectin 200 μg/kg once has been effective.

[28]Diethylcarbamazine is potentially curative due to activity against both adult worms and microfilariae. Ivermectin is only active against microfilariae.

[29]Relapse occurs and can be treated with diethylcarbamazine.

[30]Annual treatment with ivermectin, 150 μg/kg, can prevent blindness due to ocular onchocerciasis (D Mabey et al, *Ophthalmology* 1996;103:1001). Diethylcarbamazine should not be used for treatment of this disease.

[31]Unlike infections with other flukes, *Fasciola hepatica* infections may not respond to praziquantel. Triclabendazole (*Egaten*, Novartis) may be safe and effective but data are limited (CS Graham et al, *Clin Infect Dis* 2001;33:1). It is available from Victoria Pharmacy, Zurich, Switzerland (www.pharmaworld.com; 41-1-211-24-32) and should be given with food for better absorption. A single study has found that nitazoxanide has limited efficacy for treating fascioliasis in adults and children (L Favennec et al, *Aliment Pharmacol Ther* 2003;17:265).

TABLE 276-1. Drugs for Parasitic Infections—cont'd

[32]J Richter et al, *Curr Treat Option Infect Dis* 2002;4:313.

[33]JD MacLean et al, *Lancet* 1996;347:154.

[34]Triclabendazole may be effective in a dosage of 5 mg/kg once/day × 3 days or 10 mg/kb bid + 1 day (M Calvopiña et al, *Trans R Soc Trop Med Hyg* 1998;92:566). See footnote 31 for availability.

[35]Albendazole 400 mg daily × 5 days alone or in combination with metronidazole may also be effective (A Hall and Q Nahar, *Trans R Soc Trop Med Hyg* 1993;87:84; AK Dutta et al, *Indian J Pediatr* 1994;61:689; B Cacopardo et al, *Clin Ter* 1995;146:761). Combination treatment with standard doses of metronidazole and quinacrine given for 3 wk has been effective for a small number of refractory infections (TE Nash et al, *Clin Infect Dis* 2001;33:22). In 1 study, nitazoxanide was used successfully in high doses to treat a case of *Giardia* resistant to metronidazole and albendazole (P Abboud et al, *Clin Infect Dis* 2001;32:1792).

[36]Not absorbed; may be useful for treatment of giardiasis in pregnancy.

[37]M de Gorgolas et al, *J Travel Med* 2003;10:358. All patients should be treated with a medication regardless of whether surgery is attempted.

[38]ML Eberhard and C Busillo, *Am J Trop Med Hyg* 1999;61:51; ME Wilson et al, *Clin Infect Dis* 2001;32:1378.

[39]In immunocompetent patients usually a self-limited illness. Immunosuppressed patients may need higher doses, longer duration (TMP-SMX qid × 10 days, followed by bid × 3 wk) and long-term maintenance. In sulfonamide-sensitive patients, pyrimethamine 50–75 mg daily in divided doses (plus leucovorin 10–25 mg/day) has been effective.

[40]Visceral infection is most commonly due to the Old World species *L. donovani* (kala-azar) and *L. infantum* and the New World species. *L. chagasi.* Treatment duration may vary based on symptoms, host immune status, species, and area of the world where infection was acquired.

[41]May be repeated or continued; a longer duration may be needed for some patients (BL Herwaldt, *Lancet* 1999;354:1191).

[42]Three lipid formulations of amphotericin B have been used for treatment of visceral leishmaniasis. Largely based on clinical trials in patients infected with *L. infantum,* the FDA approved liposomal amphotericin B (*AmBisome*) for treatment of visceral leishmaniasis (A Meyerhoff, *Clin Infect Dis* 1999;28:42). Amphotericin B lipid complex (*Abelcet*) and amphotericin B cholesteryl sulfate (*Amphotec*) have also been used with good results but are considered investigational for this condition by the FDA.

[43]The FDA-approved dosage regimen for immunocompromised patients (e.g., HIV infected) is 4 mg/kg/day (days 1–5) and 4 mg/kg/day on days 10, 17, 24, 31, and 38. The relapse rate is high; maintenance therapy may be indicated, but there is no consensus as to dosage or duration.

[44]For treatment of kala-azar in adults in India, oral miltefosine 100 mg/day (~205 mg/kg/day) for 3–4 wk was 97% effective after 6 mo (TK Jha et al, *N Engl J Med* 1999;341:1795; H Sangraula et al, *J Assoc Physicians India* 2003;51:686). Gastrointestinal adverse effects are common, and the drug is contraindicated in pregnancy. The dose of miltefosine in an open-label trial in children in India was 2.5 mg/kg/day × 28 days (SK Bhattacharya et al, *Clin Infect Dis* 2004;38:217). Miltefosine *(Impavido)* is available from the manufacturer (Zentaris—Frankfurt, Germany at Impavido@zentaris.de).

[45]Cutaneous infection is most commonly due to the Old World species *L. major* and *L. tropica* and the New World species *L. mexicana, L. (Viannia) braziliensis* and others. Treatment duration may vary based on symptoms, host immune status, species, and area of the world where infection was acquired.

[46]In a placebo-controlled trial in patients ≥12 yr old, oral miltefosine was effective for the treatment of cutaneous leishmaniasis due to *L. (V.) panamensis* in Colombia but not *L. (V.) braziliensis* in Guatemala at a dosage of about 2.5 mg/kg/day for 28 days. "Motion sickness," nausea, headache and increased creatinine were the most frequent adverse effects (J Soto et al, *Clin Infect Dis* 2004;38:1266). See footnote 44 regarding miltefosine availability. For treatment of *L. major* cutaneous lesions, a study in Saudi Arabia found that oral fluconazole, 200 mg once/day × 6 wk, appeared to speed healing (AA Alrajhi et al, *N Engl J Med* 2002;346:891).

[47]At this dosage pentamidine has been effective against leishmaniasis in Colombia where the likely organism was *L. (V.) panamensis* (J Soto-Mancipe et al, *Clin Infect Dis* 1993;16:417; J Soto et al, *Am J Trop Med Hyg* 1994;50:107); its effect against other species is not well established.

[48]Topical paromomycin should be used only in geographic regions where cutaneous leishmaniasis species have low potential for mucosal spread. A formulation of 15% paromomycin/12% methylbenzethonium chloride *(Leshcutan)* in soft white paraffin for topical use has been reported to be partially effective in some patients against cutaneous leishmaniasis due to *L. major* in Israel and against *L. mexicana* and *L. (V.) braziliensis* in Guatemala, where mucosal spread is very rare (BA Arana et al, *Am J Trop Med Hyg* 2001;65:466). The methylbenzethonium is irritating to the skin; lesions may worsen before they improve.

[49]Mucosal infection is most commonly due to the New World species *L. (V.) braziliensis, L. (V.) panamensis,* or *L. (V.) guyanensis.* Treatment duration may vary based on symptoms, host immune status, species, and area of the world where infection was acquired.

[50]For infestation of eyelashes with *P. pubis* lice, use petrolatum; TMP-SMX has also been used (TL Meinking, *Curr Probl Dermatol* 1996;24:157). For pubic lice, treat with 5% permethrin or ivermectin as for scabies. TMP-SMX has also been effective together with permethrin for head lice (RB Hipolito et al, *Pediatrics* 2001;107:E30).

[51]KS Yoon et al, *Arch Dermatol* 2003;139:994.

[52]A 2 application is recommended 1 wk later to kill hatching progeny. Some lice are resistant to pyrethrins and permethrin (TL Meinking et al, *Arch Dermatol* 2002;138:220).

[53]Ivermectin is effective against adult lice but has no effect on nits (KN Jones and JC English III, *Clin Infect Dis* 2003;36:1355).

[54]Chloroquine-resistant *P. falciparum* occurs in all malarious areas except Central America west of the Panama Canal Zone, Mexico, Haiti, the Dominican Republic, and most of the Middle East (chloroquine resistance has been reported in Yemen, Oman, Saudi Arabia, and Iran). For treatment of multidrug-resistant. *P. falciparum* in Southeast Asia, especially Thailand, where resistance to mefloquine is frequent, atovaquone/proguanil, artesunate plus mefloquine, or artemether plus mefloquine may be used (JC Luxemburger et al, *Trans R Soc Trop Med Hyg* 1994;88:213; J Karbwang et al, *Trans R Soc Trop Med Hyg* 1995;89:296).

[55]Uncomplicated or mild malaria may be treated with oral drugs.

[56]Atovaquone plus proguanil is available as a fixed-dose combination tablet: adult tablets (*Malarone,* 250 mg atovaquone/100 mg proguanil) and pediatric tablets (*Malarone Pediatric,* 62.5 mg atovaquone/25 mg proguanil). To enhance absorption, it should be taken with food or a milky drink. Atovaquone/proguanil should not be given to pregnant women or patients with severe renal impairment (creatinine clearance <30 mL/min). There have been several isolated reports of resistance in *P. falciparum* in Africa (E Schwartz et al, *Clin Infect Dis* 2003;37:450; A Farnert et al, *Br Med J* 2003;326:628).

[57]In Southeast Asia, relative resistance to quinine has increased and treatment should be continued for 7 days.

[58]Although approved for once daily dosing, *Medical Letter* consultants usually divide the dose in 2 to decrease nausea and vomiting.

[59]For use in pregnancy.

[60]B Lell and PG Kremsner, *Antimicrob Agents Chemother* 2002;46:2315.

[61]At this dosage, adverse effects including nausea, vomiting, diarrhea, dizziness, disturbed sense of balance, toxic psychosis, and seizures can occur. Mefloquine should not be used for treatment of malaria in pregnancy unless there is no other treatment option because of increased risk for stillbirth (F Nosten et al, *Clin Infect Dis* 1999;28:808). It should be avoided for treatment of malaria in persons with active depression or with a history of psychosis or seizures and should be used with caution in persons with psychiatric illness. Mefloquine can be given to patients taking β blockers if they do not have an underlying arrhythmia; it should not be used in patients with conduction abnormalities. Mefloquine should not be given together with quinine, quinidine, or halofantrine, and caution is required in using quinine, quinidine, or halofantrine to treat patients with malaria who have taken mefloquine for prophylaxis. Resistance to mefloquine has been reported in some areas, such as the Thailand-Myanmar and Thailand-Cambodia borders and in the Amazon basin, where 25 mg/kg should be used. In the USA, a 250 mg tablet of mefloquine contains 228 mg mefloquine base. Outside the USA, each 275 mg tablet contains 250 mg base.

[62]F Nosten et al, *Lancet* 2000;356:297; M van Vugt, *Clin Infect Dis* 2002;35:1498.

[63]*P. vivax* with decreased susceptibility to chloroquine is a significant problem is Papua New Guinea and Indonesia. There are also a few reports of resistance from Myanmar, India, the Solomon Islands, Vanuatu, Guyana, Brazil, Colombia, and Peru.

[64]Primaquine phosphate can cause hemolytic anemia, especially in patients whose red cells are deficient in glucose-6-phosphate dehydrogenase (G6PD). This deficiency is most common in African, Asian, and Mediterranean peoples. Patients should be screened for G6PD deficiency before treatment. Primaquine should not be used during pregnancy.

[65]If chloroquine phosphate is not available, hydroxychloroquine sulfate is as effective; 400 mg of hydroxychloroquine sulfate is equivalent to 500 mg of chloroquine phosphate.

[66]Exchange transfusion has been helpful for some patients with high-density (>10%) parasitemia, altered mental status, pulmonary edema, or renal complications (KD Miller et al, *N Engl J Med* 1989;321:65).

[67]Continuous ECG, blood pressure, and glucose monitoring are recommended, especially in pregnant women and young children. For problems with quinidine availability, call the manufacturer (Eli Lilly, 800-545-5979) or the CDC Malaria Hotline (770-488-7788). Quinidine may have greater antimalarial activity than quinine. The loading dose should be decreased or omitted in those patients who have received quinine or mefloquine. If more than 48 hr of parenteral treatment is required, the quinine or quinidine dose should be reduced by 30–50%.

[68]Limited studies of efficacy except with *P. falciparum*; not FDA approved or available in the USA (Artemether-Quinine Meta-Analysis Study Group, *Trans R Soc Trop Med Hyg* 2001;95:637; K Marsh, *East Afr Med J* 2002;79:619).

[69]No drug regimen guarantees protection against malaria. If fever develops within a year (particularly within the first two months) after travel to malarious areas, travelers should be advised to seek medical attention. Insect repellents, insecticide-impregnated bed nets and proper clothing are important adjuncts for malaria prophylaxis (*Med Lett* 2003;45:41). Malaria in pregnancy is particularly serious for both mother and fetus; therefore, prophylaxis is indicated if exposure can not be avoided.

[70]In pregnancy, chloroquine prophylaxis has been used extensively and safely.

[71]For prevention of attack after departure from areas where *P. vivax* and *P. ovale* are endemic, which includes almost all areas where malaria is found (except Haiti), some experts prescribe in addition primaquine phosphate 30 mg base/day or, for children, 0.6 mg base/kg/day during the last 2 wk of prophylaxis. Others prefer to avoid the toxicity of primaquine and rely on surveillance to detect cases when they occur, particularly when exposure was limited or doubtful. See also footnote 64.

[72]Beginning 1–2 wk before travel and continuing weekly for the duration of stay and for 4 wk after leaving.

[73]Beginning 1–2 days before travel and continuing for the duration of stay and for 1 wk after leaving. In 1 study of malaria prophylaxis, atovaquone/proguanil was better tolerated than mefloquine in nonimmune travelers (D Overbosch et al, *Clin Infect Dis* 2001;33:1015).

[74]Mefloquine has not been approved for use during pregnancy. However, it has been reported to be safe for prophylactic use during the 2nd or 3rd trimester of pregnancy and possibly during early pregnancy as well (CDC Health Information for International Travel, 2003–2004, page 111; BL Smoak et al, *J Infect Dis* 1997;176:831). For pediatric doses <½ tablet, it is advisable to have a pharmacist crush the tablet, estimate doses by weighing, and package them in gelatin capsules. There are no data for use in children <5 kg, but based on dosages in other weight groups, a dose of 5 mg/kg can be used. Mefloquine is not recommended for patients with cardiac conduction abnormalities, and patients with a history of depression, seizures, psychosis, or psychiatric disorders should avoid mefloquine prophylaxis. Resistance to mefloquine has been reported in some areas, such as the Thailand-Myanmar and Thailand-Cambodia borders; in these areas, atovaquone/proguanil or doxycycline should be used for prophylaxis.

[75]Beginning 1–2 days before travel and continuing for the duration of stay and for 4 wk after leaving. Use of tetracyclines is contraindicated in pregnancy and in children <8 yr old. Doxycycline can cause gastrointestinal disturbances, vaginal moniliasis, and photosensitivity reactions.

[76]Studies have shown that daily primaquine beginning 1 day before departure and continued until 3–7 days after leaving the malaria area provides effective prophylaxis against chloroquine-resistant *P. falciparum* (JK Baird et al, *Clin Infect Dis* 2003;37:1659). Some studies have shown less efficacy against *P. vivax.* Nausea and abdominal pain can be diminished by taking with food.

[77]Proguanil (*Paludrine*—Wyeth Ayerst, Canada; AstraZeneca, United Kingdom), which is not available alone in the USA but is widely available in Canada and Europe, is recommended mainly for use in Africa south of the Sahara. Prophylaxis is recommended during exposure and for 4 wk afterward. Proguanil has been used in pregnancy without evidence of toxicity (PA Phillips-Howard and D Wood, *Drug Saf* 1996;14:131).

[78]A traveler can be given a course of atovaquone/proguanil, mefloquine, or quinine plus doxycycline for presumptive self-treatment of febrile illness. The drug given for self-treatment should be different from that used for prophylaxis. This approach should be used only in very rare circumstances when a traveler cannot promptly get to medical care.

continued

TABLE 276-1. Drugs for Parasitic Infections—cont'd

[79]Ocular lesions due to *E. hellem* in HIV-infected patients have responded to fumagillin eyedrops prepared from *Fumidil-B* (bicyclohexyl ammonium fumagillin) used to control a microsporidial disease of honey bees (MC Diesenhouse, *Am J Ophthalmol* 1993;115:293), available from Leiter's Park Avenue Pharmacy (see footnote 1). For lesions due to *V. corneae,* topical therapy is generally not effective and keratoplasty may be required (RM Davis et al, *Ophthalmology* 1990;97:953).

[80]Oral fumagillin (Sanofi Recherche, Gentilly, France) has been effective in treating *E. bieneusi* (J-M Molina et al, *N Engl J Med* 2002;346:1963), but has been associated with thrombocytopenia. HAART may lead to microbiologic and clinical response in HIV-infected patients with microsporidial diarrhea (USPHS/IDSA Guidelines for the Treatment of Opportunistic Infections in Adults and Adolescents with HIV, 2004; in press). Octreotide (*Sandostatin*) has provided symptomatic relief in some patients with large-volume diarrhea.

[81]J-M Molina et al, *J Infect Dis* 1995;171:245. There is no established treatment for *Pleistophora.* For disseminated disease due to *Trachipleistophora* or *Brachiola,* itraconazole 400 mg PO once/day plus albendazole may also be tried (CM Coyle et al, *N Engl J Med* 2004;351:42).

[82]Albendazole or pyrantel pamoate may be effective (JB Ziem et al, *Ann Trop Med Parasitol* 2004;98:385).

[83]*Pneumocystis* has been reclassified as a fungus. In severe disease with room air $PO_2 \leq 70$ mm Hg or Aa gradient ≥ 35 mm Hg, prednisone should also be used (S Gagnon et al, *N Engl J Med* 1990;323:1444; E Caumes et al, *Clin Infect Dis* 1994;18:319).

[84]Primary/secondary prophylaxis in patients with HIV can be discontinued after CD4 count increases to $>200 \times 10^6$/L for >3 mo.

[85]An alternative trimethoprim-sulfamethoxazole regimen is one DS tab 3x/wk. Weekly therapy with sulfadoxine 500 mg/pyrimethamine 25 mg/leucovorin 25 mg was effective PCP prophylaxis in liver transplant patients (J Torre-Cisneros et al, *Clin Infect Dis* 1999;29:771).

[86]Plus leucovorin 25 mg with each dose of pyrimethamine.

[87]In some cases, treatment may need to be repeated in 10–14 days.

[88]Lindane (γ-benzene hexachloride; *Kwell*) should be reserved as a 2nd line agent. The FAD has recommended it should not be used for immunocompromised patients, young children, the elderly, and patients <50 kg.

[89]Ivermectin, either alone or in combination with a topical scabicide, is the drug of choice for crusted scabies in immunocompromised patients (P del Giudice, *Curr Opin Infect Dis* 2004;15:123). The safety of oral ivermectin in pregnancy and young children has not been established.

[90]Oxamniquine has been effective in some areas in which praziquantel is less effective (FF Stelma et al, *J Infect Dis* 1997;176:304). Oxamniquine is contraindicated in pregnancy.

[91]In East Africa, the dose should be increased to 30 mg/kg, and in Egypt and South Africa to 30 mg/kg/day × 2 days. Some experts recommend 40–60 mg/kg over 2–3 days in all of Africa (KC Shekhar, *Drugs* 1991;42:379).

[92]In immunocompromised patients or disseminated disease, it may be necessary to prolong or repeat therapy, or to use other agents. Veterinary parenteral and enema formulations of ivermectin have been used in severely ill patients unable to take oral medications (PL Chiodini et al, *Lancet* 2000;355:43; J Orem et al, *Clin Infect Dis* 2003;37:152; PE Tarr *Am J Trop Med Hyg* 2003;68:453).

[93]This dosage is likely to be toxic and may have to be decreased.

[94]JO Juan et al, *Trans R Soc Trop Med Hyg* 2002;96:193.

[95]Patients may benefit from surgical resection or percutaneous drainage of cysts. Praziquantel is useful preoperatively or in case of spillage of cyst contents during surgery. Percutaneous aspiration-injection-reaspiration (PAIR) with ultrasound guidance plus albendazole therapy has been effective for management of hepatic hydatid cyst disease (RA Smego, Jr., et al, *Clin Infect Dis* 2003;37:1073).

[96]Surgical excision is the only reliable means of cure. Reports have suggested that in nonresectable cases use of albendazole or mebendazole can stabilize and sometimes cure infection (P Craig, *Curr Opin Infect Dis* 2003;16:437).

[97]Initial therapy for patients with inflammed parenchymal cysticercosis should focus on symptomatic treatment with anti-seizure medication. Treatment of parenchymal cysticerci with albendazole or praziquantel is controversial (JM Maguire, *N Engl J Med* 2004;350:215). Patients with live parenchymal cysts who have seizures should be treated with albendazole together with steroids (6 mg dexamethasone or 40–60 mg prednisone daily) and an antiseizure medication (HH Garcia et al, *N Engl J Med* 2004;350:249). Patients with subarachnoid cysts or giant cysts in the fissures should be treated for at least 30 days (JV Proaño et al, *N Engl J Med* 2001;345:879). Surgical intervention or CSF diversion is indicated for obstructive hydocephalus; prednisone 40 mg/day may be given with surgery. Arachnoiditis, vasculitis or cerebral edema is treated with prednisone 60 mg/day or dexamethasone 4–6 mg/day together with albendazole or praziquantel (AC White Jr, *Annu Rev Med* 2000;51:187). Any cysticercocidal drug may cause irreparable damage when used to treat ocular or spinal cysts, even when corticosteroids are used. An ophthalmic exam should always precede treatment to rule out intraocular cysts.

[98]In ocular toxoplasmosis with macular involvement, corticosteroids are recommended in addition to antiparasitic therapy for an anti-inflammatory effect.

[99]To treat CNS toxoplasmosis in HIV-infected patients, some clinicians have used pyrimethamine 50–100 mg/day (after a loading dose of 200 mg) with sulfadiazine and, when sulfonamide sensitivity developed, have given clindamycin 1.8–2.4 g/day in divided doses instead of the sulfonamide. Atovaquone plus pyrimethamine appears to be an effective alternative in sulfa-intolerant patients (K Chirgwin et al, *Clin Infect Dis* 2002;34:1243). Treatment is followed by chronic suppression with lower-dosage regimens of the same drugs. For primary prophylaxis in HIV patients with $<100 \times 10^6$/L CD4 cells, either trimethoprim-sulfamethoxazole, pyrimethamine with dapsone, or atovaquone with or without pyrimethamine can be used. Primary or secondary prophylaxis may be discontinued when the CD4 count increases to $>200 \times 10^6$/L for more than 3 mo (USPHS/IDSA Guidelines for the Treatment of Opportunistic Infections in Adults and Adolescents with HIV, 2004; in press).

[100]Women who develop toxoplasmosis during the 1st trimester of pregnancy can be treated with spiramycin (3–4 g/day). After the 1st trimester, if there is no documented transmission to be fetus, spiramycin can be continued until term. If transmission has occurred *in utero*, therapy with pyrimethamine and sulfadiazine should be started (JG Montoya and O Liesenfeld, *Lancet* 2004;363:1965). Pyrimethamine is a potential teratogen and should be used only after the 1st trimester.

[101]Plus leucovorin 10–25 mg with each dose of pyrimethamine.

[102]Congenitally infected newborns should be treated with pyrimethamine every 2 or 3 days and a sulfonamide daily for about 1 yr (JS Remington and G Desmonts, in JS Remington and JO Klein [editors], *Infectious Disease of the Fetus and Newborn Infant*, 5th ed, Philadelphia, Saunders, 2001, 290).

[103]Sexual partners should be treated simultaneously. Metronidazole-resistant strains have been reported and can be treated with higher doses of metronidazole (2–4 g/day × 7–14 days) or with tinidazole (WD Hager, *Sex Transm Dis* 2004;31:343).

[104]MP Barrett et al, *Lancet* 2003;362:1469.

[105]The addition of γ-interferon to nifurtimox for 20 days in experimental animals and in a limited number of patients appears to shorten the acute phase of Chagas disease (RE McCabe et al, *J Infect Dis* 1991;163:912).

[106]For treatment of *T.b. gambiense,* pentamidine and suramin have equal efficacy but pentamidine is better tolerated.

[107]In frail patients, begin with as little as 18 mg and increase the dose progressively. Pretreatment with suramin has been advocated for debilitated patients. Corticosteroids have been used to prevent arsenical encephalopathy (J Pepin et al, *Trans R Soc Trop Med Hyg* 1995;89:92). Up to 20% of patients with *T.b. gambiense* fail to respond to melarsoprol (MP Barrett, *Lancet* 1999;353:1113).

[108]Eflornithine is highly effective in *T.b. gambiense* but not against *T.b. rhodesiense* infections. It is available in limited supply only from the WHO and the CDC.

[109]Optimum duration of therapy is not known; some *Medical Letter* consultants would treat for 20 days. For severe symptoms or eye involvement, corticosteroids can be used in addition.

From Drugs for parasitic infection. *Med Lett* August 2004, pp 1–11. Available at www.medicalletter.org

CDC, Centers for Disease Control and Prevention; CNS, central nervous system; CSF, cerebrospinal fluid; DS, double strength; ECG, electrocardiography; FDA, Food and Drug Administration; GI, gastrointestinal; HAART, highly active anti-retroviral therapy; SMX, sulfamethoxazole; TMP, trimethoprim; WHO, World Health Organization.

nisms against protozoans are unknown; mechanisms against helminths are also unknown.

Nitazoxanide is available as an oral suspension, which has a pink color and strawberry flavor. The bioavailability is doubled with food. The drug is well absorbed from the gastrointestinal tract. One third is excreted in urine and ⅔ is excreted in feces as the active metabolite, tizoxanide. Although in vitro metabolism studies have not demonstrated cytochrome P450 enzyme effects, no pharmacokinetic studies have been done yet in patients with compromised renal or hepatic function. In addition, no studies have been done yet in pregnant or lactating women. Common adverse effects include abdominal pain, diarrhea, and nausea. Rare side effects include anorexia, flatulence, increased appetite, fever, pruritus, and dizziness.

Tinidazole (Tindamax). Tinidazole is a synthetic nitroimidazole with a chemical structure similar to metronidazole. In May 2004, it was FDA approved for treatment of trichomoniasis, and for giardiasis and amebiasis in children ≥3 yr of age. Its mechanism of action against *Trichomonas* may be secondary to the generation of free nitro radicals by the protozoan. The mechanism of action against *Giardia lamblia* and *Entamoeba histolytica* is unknown. After oral administration, tinidazole is rapidly and completely absorbed and distributes into almost all tissues and body fluids, including crossing the blood-brain barrier and placental barrier. It is excreted via urine and feces. Hemodialysis increases clearance of drug. No studies have been performed for patients undergoing peritoneal dialysis nor for patients with compromised hepatic function. Although no studies have been reported for tinidazole, metronidazole has been found to be carcinogenic in mice and rats. Tinidazole carries a pregnancy category C classification, and can be detected in breast milk. Breast-feeding should be interrupted during treatment and for 3 days after treatment.

Atovaquone/Proguanil (Malarone). Atovaquone is a hydroxylnaphthoquinone, which has been used in the past predominantly against *Pneumocystis carinii* pneumonia in AIDS patients. Its mechanism of action is via collapsing the mitochondria membrane potential by interacting with cytochrome B. Atovaquone can effectively inhibit liver stages of all *Plasmodium* species.

Proguanil was approved for use in the United States in 1948 for malaria but ceased to be marketed in the 1970s from decreased use. Its mechanism of action is inhibition of the para-

TABLE 276-2. Manufacturers of Drugs Used to Treat Parasitic Infections

albendazole—Albenza (GlaxoSmithKline)
Albenza (GlaxoSmithKline)—albendazole
Alinia (Romark)—nitazoxanide
amphotericin—Fungizone (Apothecon), others
Ancobon (ICN)—flucytosine
* Antiminth (Pfizer)—pyrantel pamoate
† Aralen (Sanofi)—chloroquine HCl and chloroquine phosphate
* artemether—Artenam (Arenco, Belgium)
* Artenam (Arenco, Belgium)—artemether
* artesunate—(Guilin No. 1 Factory, People's Republic of China)
atovaquone—Mepron (GlaxoSmithKline)
atovaquone/proguanil—Malarone (GlaxoSmithKline)
azithromycin—Zithromax (Pfizer)
† Bactrim (Roche)—TMP/Sulfa
* benznidazole—Rochagan (Roche, Brazil)
Biaxin (Abbott)—clarithromycin
* Biltricide (Bayer)—praziquantel
‡ bithionol—Bitin (Tanabe, Japan)
‡ Bitin (Tanabe, Japan)—bithionol
* Brolene (Aventis, Canada)—propamidine isethionate
chloroquine HCl and chloroquine phosphate—Aralen (Sanofi), others
clarithromycin—Biaxin (Abbott)
† Cleocin (Pfizer)—clindamycin
clindamycin—Cleocin (Pfizer), others
crotamiton—Eurax (Westwood-Squibb)
dapsone—(Jacobus)
Daraprim (GlaxoSmithKline)—pyrimethamine USP
‡ diethylcarbamazine citrate USP—Hetrazan
Diflucan (Roerig)—fluconazole
* diloxanide furoate—Furamide (Boots, U.K.)
doxycycline—Vibramycin (Pfizer), others
‡ eflornithine (Difluoromethylornithine, DFMO)—Ornidyl (Aventis)
* Egaten (Novartis)—triclabendazole
Elimite (Allergan)—permethrin
Ergamisol (Janssen)—levamisole
Eurax (Westwood—Squibb)—crotamiton
fluconazole—Diflucan (Roerig)
† Flagyl (Searle)—metronidazole
flucytosine—Ancobon (ICN)
† Fungizone (Apothecon)—amphotericin
* Furamide (Boots, U.K.)—diloxanide furoate
* furazolidone—Furozone (Roberts)
* Furozone (Roberts)—furazolidone
‡ Germanin (Bayer, Germany)—suramin sodium
* Glucantime (Aventis, France)—meglumine antimonate
‡ Hetrazan—diethylcarbamazine citrate USP
Humatin (Monarch)—paromomycin
* Impavido (Zentaris, Germany)—miltefosine
iodoquinol—Yodoxin (Glenwood), others
itraconazole—Sporanox (Janssen-Ortho)
ivermectin—Stromectol (Merck)
ketoconazole—Nizoral (Janssen), others
‡ Lampit (Bayer, Germany)—nifurtimox
Lariam (Roche)—mefloquine
* Leshcutan (Teva, Israel)—topical paromomycin
levamisole—Ergamisol (Janssen)
Malarone (GlaxoSmithKline)—atovaquone/proguanil
malathion—Ovide (Medicis)
mebendazole—Vermox (McNeil)
mefloquine—Lariam (Roche)
* meglumine antimonate—Glucantime (Aventis, France)
‡ melarsoprol—Mel-B (Specia)
‡ Mel-B (Specia)—melarsoprol
Mepron (GlaxoSmithKline)—atovaquone
metronidazole—Flagyl (Searle), others
* miltefosine—Impavido (Zentaris, Germany)
NebuPent (Fujisawa)—pentamidine isethionate
Neutrexin (US Bioscience)—trimetrexate
* niclosamide—Yomesan (Bayer, Germany)
‡ nifurtimox—Lampit (Bayer, Germany)
nitazoxanide—Alinia (Romark)
† Nizoral (Janssen)—ketoconazole
Nix (GlaxoSmithKline)—permethrin
* ornidazole—Tiberal (Roche, France)
‡ Ornidyl (Aventis)—eflornithine (Difluoromethylornithine, DFMO)
Ovide (Medicis)—malathion
* oxamniquine—Vansil (Pfizer)
* Paludrine (Wyeth Ayerst, Canada; AstraZeneca, U.K.)—proguanil
paromomycin—Humatin (Monarch); Leshcutan (Teva, Israel; (topical formulation not available in USA)
Pentam 300 (Fujisawa)—pentamidine isethionate
pentamidine isethionate—Pentam 300 (Fujisawa), NebuPent (Fujisawa)
‡ Pentostam (GlaxoSmithKline, U.K.)—sodium stibogluconate
permethrin—Nix (GlaxoSmithKline), Elimite (Allergan)
* praziquantel—Biltricide (Bayer)
primaquine phosphate USP
* proguanil—Paludrine (Wyeth Ayerst, Canada; AstraZeneca, U.K.)
proguanil/atovaquone—Malarone (GlaxoSmithKline)
* propamidine isethionate—Brolene (Aventis, Canada)
* pyrantel pamoate—Antiminth (Pfizer)
pyrethrins and piperonyl butoxide—RID (Pfizer), others
pyrimethamine USP—Daraprim (GlaxoSmithKline)
§ quinidine gluconate (Eli Lilly)
* quinine dihydrochloride
quinine sulfate—many manufacturers
† RID (Pfizer)—pyrethrins and piperonyl butoxide
† Rifadin (Aventis)—rifampin
rifampin—Rifadin (Aventis), others
* Rochagan (Roche, Brazil)—benznidazole
§ Rovamycine (Aventis)—spiramycin
‡ sodium stibogluconate—Pentostam (GlaxoSmithKline, U.K.)
§ spiramycin—Rovamycine (Aventis)
Sporanox (Janssen-Ortho)—itraconazole
Stromectol (Merck)—ivermectin
sulfadiazine
‡ suramin sodium—Germanin (Bayer, Germany)
* Tiberal (Roche, France)—ornidazole
Tindamax (Presutti)—tinidazole
tinidazole—Tindamax (Presutti)
TMP/Sulfa—Bactrim (Roche), others
* triclabendazole—Egaten (Novartis)
trimetrexate—Neutrexin (US Bioscience)
* Vansil (Pfizer)—oxamniquine
Vermox (McNeil)—mebendazole
† Vibramycin (Pfizer)—doxycycline
† Yodoxin (Glenwood)—iodoquinol
* Yomesan (Bayer, Germany)—niclosamide
Zithromax (Pfizer)—azithromycin

*Not available in the USA; may be available through a compounding pharmacy.
†Also available generically.
‡Available under an Investigational New Drug (IND) protocol from the CDC Drug Service, Centers for Disease Control and Prevention, Atlanta, Georgia 30333; 404-639-3670 (evenings, weekends, or holidays: 404-639-2888).
§Available in the USA only from the manufacturer.
From Drugs for parasitic infection. *Med Lett* August 2004, p 12. Available at www.medicalletter.org

site dihydrofolate reductase enzyme by the active form, cycloguanil. Alone it has poor efficacy for prophylaxis.

Proguanil acts in synergy with atovaquone on the cytochrome B enzyme in *Plasmodia* mitochondria. The exact mechanism behind the synergy of the 2 drugs is unknown. In 2000, the FDA approved atovaquone/proguanil for the prevention and treatment of acute, uncomplicated *Plasmodium falciparum* malaria. Atovaquone alone and in combination with proguanil is the only drug to completely inhibit the liver stage, which leads to the advantage of only needing to use the drug for 7 days after departing a malaria-endemic area (compared to several weeks).

Two double-blind, randomized clinical trials assessing malaria prophylaxis demonstrated that atovaquone/proguanil was at least comparable with (and perhaps better than) chloroquine plus proguanil and that atovaquone/proguanil was comparable with mefloquine. Atovaquone/proguanil was better tolerated than chloroquine plus proguanil and mefloquine. Atovaquone/proguanil treatment of acute uncomplicated *P. falciparum* infection has demonstrated higher or comparable cure rates when compared with other *P. falciparum* treatment drugs. Compared with other antimalaria treatment therapies, atovaquone/proguanil treatment has the highest cost.

Artemisinin Derivatives (Artemether, Artesunate). Artemisinin is a sesquiterpene lactone isolated from the weed *Artemisia annua.* It was developed in China in the 1960s and is also known as qinghaosu. Artemisinins act very rapidly against *Plasmodium vivax* as well as chloroquine-sensitive and chloroquine-resistant *P. falciparum.* The drug can reduce parasitemia by a factor of 10^4 with each asexual cycle for *Plasmodium.* Artemisinins are also rapidly eliminated. Emerging resistance to artemisinins has been seen in Cambodia, but not all of Southeast Asia. Artemisinin derivatives are not available in the United States.

SELECTED ANTIPARASITIC DRUGS FOR HELMINTHS.

Albendazole (Albenza). Albendazole is a benzimidazole carbamate structurally related to mebendazole and has similar anthelmintic activity. Its absorption from the gastrointestinal tract is poor but improved with a concomitant fatty meal. Albendazole sulfoxide, the principal metabolite with anthelmintic activity, has a plasma half-life of 8.5 hr. It is widely distributed in the body, including the bile and cerebrospinal fluid. It is eliminated by bile. Albendazole is FDA approved for treatment of neurocysticercosis and hydatid diseases *(Echinococcus granulosis).* It is not FDA approved but is used for *Ancylostoma caninum,* ascariasis, Chinese liver fluke, cutaneous larva migrans, pinworms, filariasis, gnathostomiasis, hookworms, microsporidiosis, and visceral larva migrans. Albendazole is generally well tolerated. Common adverse effects include headache, nausea, vomiting, and abdominal pain. Serious adverse effects include elevated liver enzymes and leukopenia, which have occurred in a few patients with treatment of hydatid disease. Rare adverse effects include acute renal failure, pancytopenia, granulocytopenia, and thrombocytopenia.

Ivermectin (Stromectol, Mectizan). Ivermectin is a semi-synthetic derivative of 1 of the avermectins, which is a group of macrocyclic lactones produced by *Streptomyces avermitilis.* After oral administration, ivermectin has peak plasma concentrations after about 4 hr and a plasma elimination half-life of about 12 hr. It is excreted as metabolites over a 2-wk period via feces. It is FDA approved for treatment of onchocerciasis and intestinal strongyloidiasis. It may have some effect in treating cutaneous larva migrans, intestinal nematode infections, loiasis, lymphatic filariasis, *Mansonella* infections, and scabies. Combination therapies of ivermectin with albendazole or diethylcarbamazine are being used to treat lymphatic filariasis. Common adverse events include dizziness, headache, pruritus, and gastrointestinal effects. Serious adverse events include Mazzotti reactions, including arthralgia, synovitis, enlarged lymph nodes, rash, and fever secondary to microfilaria death in patients with onchocerciasis.

Praziquantel (Biltricide). Praziquantel achieves its antiparasitic activity via the pyrazino isoquinoline ring system and was originally synthesized as a potential tranquillizer. After oral administration, praziquantel is rapidly absorbed with peak levels in 1–2 hr and plasma half-life of about 1–3 hr. Elimination via the urine and feces is >80% complete after 24 hr. Praziquantel is metabolized in the liver by the microsomal cytochrome P450 (especially 2B1 and 3A). Bioavailability of praziquantel is increased with concomitant administration of agents that inhibit cytochrome P450. Praziquantel is FDA approved for treatment of Chinese liver fluke, Southeast Asian liver fluke, and schistosomiasis. It is not FDA approved but is used for treatment of intestinal flukes, North American liver fluke, *Nanophyetus salmincola,* lung fluke, and tapeworm infections. Adverse effects can be seen in 30–60% of patients, although most are mild and disappear within 24 hr. Common adverse effects include headache, abdominal pain, dizziness, and malaise. Serious but rare adverse effects include arrhythmias, heart block, and convulsions.

Section 15 — Protozoan Diseases

Chapter 277 ■ Primary Amebic Meningoencephalitis Martin E. Weisse and Stephen C. Aronoff

Naegleria, Acanthamoeba, and *Balamuthia* are small, free-living amebae that cause human amebic meningoencephalitis; skin lesions, sinusitis, or keratitis may be seen with *Acanthamoeba.* Amebic meningoencephalitis has 2 distinct clinical presentations. The more common is an acute, usually fatal **amebic meningitis** that is caused by *Naegleria* and occurs in previously healthy children and young adults. **Granulomatous amebic meningoencephalitis** is caused by *Acanthamoeba, Balamuthia,* and *Sappinia* and is a more indolent infection that is more likely to occur in immunocompromised individuals.

ETIOLOGY. *Naegleria* is an ameboflagellate that can exist as cysts, trophozoites, and transient flagellate forms. Temperature and environmental nutrient and ion concentrations are the major factors that determine the stage of the ameba. Trophozoites are the only stages that are invasive, although cysts are potentially infective because they can convert to the vegetative form very quickly under the proper environmental stimuli. There are several species of *Naegleria,* of which only *N. fowleri* has been shown to be pathogenic for humans.

In contrast to *Naegleria* organisms, *Acanthamoeba* has a cyst and trophozoite form, of which only the trophozoite form is invasive. Cases of *Acanthamoeba* **keratitis** usual follow incidents of trivial corneal trauma followed by flushing with contaminated tap water, as well as in contact lens wearers following contact with contaminated water such as during swimming or using improperly cleaned or stored contact lenses, especially if using tap water. Granulomatous amebic encephalitis from *Acanthamoeba* has been reported worldwide. Most of the cases reported are associated with an immunocompromising condition such as HIV infection, diabetes mellitus, alcoholism, and radiation therapy.

The ameba *Balamuthia mandrillaris* has been implicated in 35 cases of granulomatous amebic encephalitis that had formerly been without definitive diagnosis and were attributed to *Acanthamoeba.* Although the clinical presentation is similar to infection with *Acanthamoeba,* most patients have no known immunocompromising condition.

Sappinia diploidea, a species of free-living protozoa found in animal feces and soil, caused granulomatous encephalitis in an otherwise healthy 38 yr old Texas farmer. He was treated with azithromycin, pentamidine, itraconazole, and flucytosine, and had a complete recovery.

EPIDEMIOLOGY. The free-living amebae have a worldwide distribution. *Naegleria* has been isolated from a variety of freshwater sources, including ponds and lakes, domestic water supplies, hot springs and spas, thermal discharge of power plants, groundwater, and occasionally from the nasal passages of healthy children. *Acanthamoeba* has been isolated from soil, mushrooms and vegetables, brackish water, and seawater, as well as most of the freshwater sources for *Naegleria.* It can also be found in tap water, as chlorination does not kill *Acanthamoeba.*

Naegleria meningoencephalitis has been reported from every continent. Most of the cases have been contracted during the summer months by previously healthy individuals with a history of swimming in or contact with freshwater before their illness. Usually only 1–2 cases are reported per year in the United States, but 8 cases were reported in 2001–2002. Most of the reports have come from the southern and southwestern states, with occasional infections occurring in the Midwest and East.

PATHOGENESIS. The free-living amebae enter the nasal cavity by inhalation or aspiration of dust or water contaminated with trophozoites or cysts. *Naegleria* gains access to the central nervous system through the olfactory epithelium and migration via the olfactory nerve to the olfactory bulbs, which are located in the subarachnoid space bathed by the cerebrospinal fluid (CSF). This space is richly vascularized and is the route of spread to other areas of the central nervous system. In addition to evidence of widespread cerebral edema and hyperemia of the meninges, the olfactory bulbs are necrotic, hemorrhagic, and surrounded by a purulent exudate. Microscopically, the gray matter is the most severely affected, with severe involvement in all cases. Fibrinopurulent exudate may be found throughout the cerebral hemispheres, brainstem, cerebellum, and upper portions of the spinal cord. Pockets of trophozoites may be seen in necrotic neural tissue, usually in the perivascular spaces of arteries and arterioles.

The route of invasion and penetration in cases of granulomatous amebic meningoencephalitis, caused by *Acanthamoeba* and *Balamuthia,* may be through olfactory epithelium or hematogenous, probably originating from a primary focus in the skin or lungs. Pathologic examination reveals granulomatous encephalitis, with multinucleated giant cells mainly in the posterior fossa structures, basal ganglia, bases of the cerebral hemispheres, and cerebellum. Both trophozoites and cysts may be found in the central nervous system lesions, primarily located in the perivascular spaces and invading blood vessel walls. The olfactory bulbs and spinal cord are usually spared. The single case of *Sappinia* encephalitis followed a sinus infection, and evaluation revealed a solitary 2 cm temporal lobe mass with mild ring enhancement.

CLINICAL MANIFESTATIONS. The incubation of ***Naegleria* infection** may be as short as 2 days or as long as 15 days. Symptoms have an acute onset and are rapidly progressive. There is a sudden onset of severe headache, fever, nausea, and vomiting; signs of meningitis; and then encephalitis. Most cases end in death within 1 wk of onset of symptoms.

Granulomatous amebic meningoencephalitis may occur weeks to months after acquiring the organism. The presenting signs and symptoms are often those of single or multiple central nervous system space-occupying lesions and include hemiparesis, personality changes, seizures, and drowsiness. Altered mental status is often a prominent symptom. Headache and fever occur only sporadically, but stiff neck is seen in a majority of cases. Palsies of the cranial nerves may be present. There is also 1 report of acute hydrocephalus and fever with *Balamuthia.* Results of neuroimaging studies of the brain usually demonstrate multiple low-density lesions resembling infarcts or enhancing lesions of granulomas (Fig. 277-1).

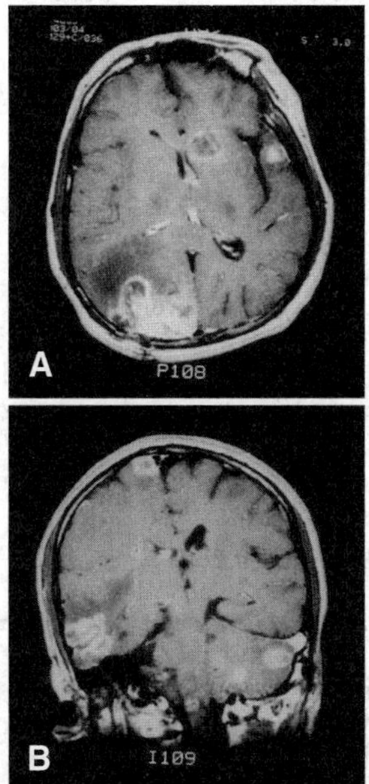

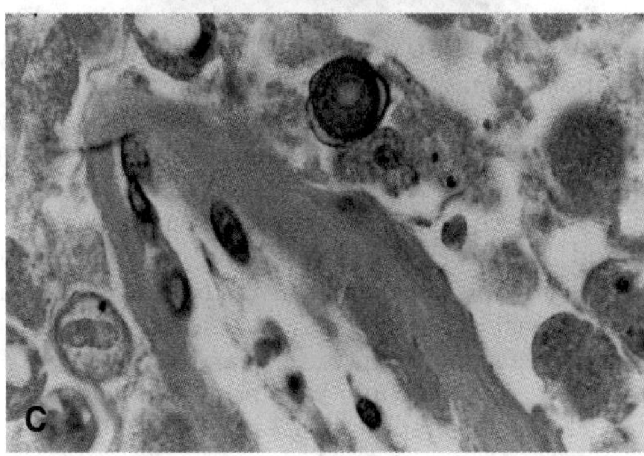

Figure 277-1. *A and B,* MRIs of the brain of a patient with *Balamuthia mandrillaris* granulomatous amebic encephalitis. Multiple enhancing lesions are seen in the right hemisphere, left cerebellum, midbrain, and brainstem. C, Photomicrograph of the brain lesion from the same patient showing perivascular amebic trophozoites. A round amebic cyst with a characteristic double wall is seen in the top center (hematoxylin and eosin, original magnification ×100). (From Deol I, Robledo L, Meza A, et al: Encephalitis due to a free-living amoeba *[Balamuthia mandrillaris]:* Case report with literature review. *Surg Neurol* 2000;53:611–616.)

DIAGNOSIS. The CSF in *Naegleria* infection may mimic that of herpes simplex encephalitis early in the disease, and later of acute bacterial meningitis with a neutrophilic pleocytosis, elevated protein level, and hypoglycorrachia. The amebae, which may be motile, may be seen on a wet mount of the CSF but are often mistaken for lymphocytes. A hanging drop examination of CSF and a strong clinical suspicion early in the course of disease affords the best chance for early treatment and cure. *Naegleria* can be grown on agar enriched with gram-negative bacteria, on which they feed.

The CSF findings of granulomatous meningoencephalitis resemble those of aseptic meningitis. The isolation and identification of *Acanthamoeba* from brain tissue and CSF are the best methods of diagnosis. *Acanthamoeba* may be cultured using the same agar used for growing *Naegleria,* but *Balamuthia* must be grown on mammalian cell cultures. Pediatric cases of *Balamuthia* meningoencephalitis have been diagnosed antemortem by brain biopsy as well as postmortem. Immunofluorescence staining of brain tissue can differentiate *Acanthamoeba* and *Balamuthia.*

TREATMENT. *Naegleria* infection is nearly always fatal, and early recognition and early treatment are crucial to successful therapy. There are several reports of treatment survivors, most of whom recovered fully. *Naegleria* infections have been successfully treated with regimens of amphotericin B, rifampin, and fluconazole or ketoconazole; amphotericin B, rifampin, and chloramphenicol; and amphotericin B alone. The optimal duration of treatment is unknown.

The optimal therapy for granulomatous amebic meningoencephalitis is also uncertain. Strains of *Acanthamoeba* isolated from fatal cases are usually susceptible in vitro to pentamidine, ketoconazole, flucytosine, and less so to amphotericin B. One patient has been successfully treated with sulfadiazine and fluconazole, and another with intravenous pentamidine, topical chlorhexidine, and 2% ketoconazole cream followed by oral itraconazole. *Acanthamoeba* keratitis responds to long courses of topical propamidine—polymyxin B sulfate or topical polyhexamethylene biguanide or chlorhexidine gluconate, and antifungal azoles plus topical steroids. Limited success has been demonstrated in *Balamuthia* infection with systemic azole therapy combined with flucytosine. More recently, the combination of flucytosine, pentamidine, fluconazole, sulfadiazine, a macrolide, and phenothiazines resulted in the survival of 2 patients with *Balamuthia* meningoencephalitis, although both were left with some neuromotor and cognitive impairment. Corticosteroids appear to have a detrimental effect, contributing to rapid progression of disease, and should be avoided.

Centers for Disease Control and Prevention: Primary amebic meningoencephalitis—Georgia, 2002. *MMWR* 2003;52:962–964.

Deetz TR, Sawyer MH, Billman G, et al: Successful treatment of *Balamuthia* amoebic encephalitis: Presentation of 2 cases. *Clin Infect Dis* 2003;37(10): 1304–1312.

Gelman BB, Popov V, Chaljub G, et al: Neuropathological and ultrastructural features of amebic encephalitis caused by *Sappinia diploidea. J Neuropathol Exp Neurol* 2003;62(10):990–998.

Radford CF, Minassian DC, Dart J: Acanthamoeba keratitis in England and Wales: Incidence, outcome, and risk factors. *Br J Ophthalmol* 2002;86(5): 536–542.

Schuster FL, Visvesvara GS: Opportunistic amoebae: Challenges in prophylaxis and treatment. *Drug Resist Update* 2004;7(1):41–51.

Schuster FL, Visvesvara GS: Free-living amoebae as opportunistic and non-opportunistic pathogens of humans and animals. *Int J Parasitol* 2004;34(9): 1001–1027.

Seijo Martinez M, Gonzalez-Medeiro G, Santiago P, et al: Granulomatous amebic encephalitis in a patient with AIDS: Isolation of *Acanthamoeba* sp. Group II from brain tissue and successful treatment with sulfadiazine and fluconazole. *J Clin Microbiol* 2000;38:3892–3895.

Vargas-Zepeda J, Gomez-Alcala AV, Vasquez-Morales JA, et al: Successful treatment of *Naegleria fowleri* meningoencephalitis by using intravenous amphotericin B, fluconazole and rifampicin. *Arch Med Res* 2005;36:83–86.

Yoder JS, Blackburn BG, Craun GF, et al: Surveillance for waterborne-disease—Disease outbreaks associated with recreational water—United States, 2001–2002. In: Surveillance Summaries, October 22, 2004. *MMWR* 2004;53(SS-8):1–20.

Chapter 278 ■ Amebiasis

Chandy C. John and Robert A. Salata

Entamoeba histolytica infects hundred of millions of people worldwide; endemic foci are particularly common in the tropics, especially in areas with low socioeconomic and sanitary standards. In most infected individuals, *E. histolytica* parasitizes the lumen of the gastrointestinal tract and causes few or no symptoms or sequelae. The 2 most common forms of disease caused by *E. histolytica* are **amebic colitis** with parasitic invasion of the intestinal mucosa, and **amebic liver abscess** with dissemination of the parasite to the liver.

ETIOLOGY. Two morphologically identical but genetically distinct species of *Entamoeba* commonly infect humans. *Entamoeba dispar,* the more prevalent species, is associated only with an asymptomatic carrier state. *E. histolytica,* the pathogenic species, can become invasive, causing symptomatic disease. Many patients previously described as asymptomatic carriers of *E. histolytica* based on microscopy findings were probably infected with *E. dispar.* Five other species of nonpathogenic *Entamoeba* infrequently colonize the human gastrointestinal tract: *E. coli, E. hartmanni, E. gingivalis, E. moshkovskii,* and *E. polecki.*

Infection is established by ingestion of parasite cysts, which measure 10–18 mm in diameter and contain 4 nuclei. Cysts are resistant to environmental conditions such as low temperature and the concentrations of chlorine commonly used in water purification but can be killed by heating to 55°C. After ingestion, the cyst, which is resistant to gastric acidity and digestive enzymes, excysts in the small intestine to form 8 trophozoites. These large, actively motile organisms colonize the lumen of the large intestine and may invade the mucosal lining. Infection is not transmitted by trophozoites because of their rapid degeneration outside the body and especially in the low pH of normal gastric contents if swallowed.

EPIDEMIOLOGY. Prevalence of infection with *E. histolytica* varies greatly depending on region and socioeconomic status. Most prevalence studies have not distinguished between *E. histolytica* and *E. dispar,* so the true prevalence of *E. histolytica* infection from these studies is not known. It is estimated that infection with *E. histolytica* leads to 50 million cases of symptomatic disease and 40,000–110,000 deaths annually. Amebiasis is the 3rd leading parasitic cause of death worldwide. Prospective studies have demonstrated that 4–10% of individuals infected with *E. histolytica* develop amebic colitis, and <1% of individuals develop disseminated disease, such as amebic liver abscess. These numbers vary by region: in South Africa and Vietnam, liver abscesses form a disproportionately large number of the cases of invasive disease due to *E. histolytica.* Amebic liver abscesses are rare in children and occur equally frequently in male and female children, whereas in adults, amebic liver abscesses occur predominantly in men.

Amebiasis is highly endemic in Africa, Latin America, India, and Southeast Asia. In the United States, amebiasis is seen most frequently in immigrants from or travelers to developing countries. Residents of institutions for the mentally retarded and men who have sex with men are also at increased risk for invasive amebiasis, although most *Entamoeba* infections in the latter group are *E. dispar.* Food or drink contaminated with *Entamoeba* cysts and direct fecal-oral contact are the most common means of infection. Untreated water and human feces used as fertilizer are important sources of infection. Food handlers carrying amebic cysts can play a role in spreading the infection. Direct contact with infected feces also may be responsible for person-to-person transmission.

PATHOGENESIS. Trophozoites, which are responsible for tissue invasion and destruction, attach to the colonic epithelial cells by a galactose and *N*-acetyl-D-galactosamine (Gal/GalNac)-specific lectin. This lectin is also thought to be responsible for resistance to complement-mediated lysis. Once attached to the colonic mucosa, amebae release a cysteine-rich proteinase that allows for penetration through the epithelial layer. Host cells are destroyed by 2 mechanisms: cytolysis and apoptosis. Cytolysis is mediated by trophozoite release of **amoebapores** (pore-forming proteins), phospholipases, and hemolysins. Amoebapores may also be partially responsible for the induction of apoptosis, or programmed cell death, which has been shown to occur in mice with amebic liver disease and colitis. Early invasive amebiasis produces significant inflammation, due in part to parasite-mediated activation of nuclear factor-κB (NF-κB). Once *E. histolytica* trophozoites invade the intestinal mucosa, the organisms multiply and spread laterally underneath the intestinal epithelium to produce characteristic **flask-shaped ulcers.** Amebae may produce similar lytic lesions if they reach the liver. The hepatic lesions are commonly called abscesses, although they contain no granulocytes. Well-established ulcers and amebic liver abscesses demonstrate little local inflammatory response.

Immunity to infection is associated with a mucosal IgA response against the Gal/GalNac lectin. Neutrophils appear to be important in initial host defense, but *E. histolytica*–induced epithelial cell damage releases neutrophil chemoattractants, and *E. histolytica* is also able to kill neutrophils, which then release mediators that further damage epithelial cells. The disparity between the extent of tissue destruction by amebae and the absence of a local host inflammatory response in the presence of systemic humoral (antibody) and cell-mediated responses may reflect both parasite-mediated apoptosis and the ability of the trophozoite to kill not only epithelial cells but neutrophils, monocytes, and macrophages.

CLINICAL MANIFESTATIONS. Clinical presentations range from asymptomatic cyst passage to amebic colitis, amebic dysentery, ameboma, and extraintestinal disease. *E. histolytica* infection is asymptomatic in about 90% of persons, but it has the potential to become invasive and should be treated. Severe disease is more common in young children, pregnant women, malnourished individuals, and persons taking corticosteroids. Extraintestinal disease usually involves only the liver, but rare extraintestinal manifestations include amebic brain abscess, pleuropulmonary disease, ulcerative skin, and genitourinary lesions.

Amebic Colitis. Amebic colitis may occur within 2 wk of infection or be delayed for months. The onset is usually gradual with colicky abdominal pains and frequent bowel movements (6–8/day). Diarrhea is frequently associated with tenesmus. Stools are blood stained and contain a fair amount of mucus with few leukocytes. Generalized constitutional symptoms and signs are characteristically absent, with fever documented in only 1/3 of patients. Amebic colitis affects all age groups, but its incidence is strikingly high in children 1–5 yr of age. Severe amebic colitis in infants and young children tends to be rapidly progressive with frequent extraintestinal involvement and high mortality rates,

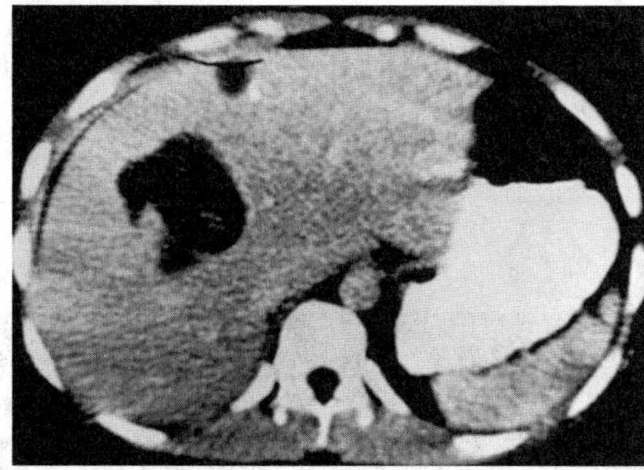

Figure 278-1. Abdominal CT scan of a patient with an amebic liver abscess; the irregular multiple defects present in the right lobe of the liver cannot be differentiated from a pyogenic abscess or hepatocellular carcinoma. (From Mandell GL, Bennett JE, Dolin R [editors]: *Principles and Practice of Infectious Diseases,* 6th ed, Vol 2. Philadelphia, Elsevier, 2006, p 3105.)

particularly in tropical countries. Occasionally, amebic dysentery is associated with sudden onset of fever, chills, and severe diarrhea, which may result in dehydration and electrolyte disturbances.

Amebic Liver Abscess. Amebic liver abscess, a serious manifestation of disseminated infection, is uncommon in children. Although diffuse liver enlargement has been associated with intestinal amebiasis, liver abscess occurs in <1% of infected individuals and may appear in patients with no clear history of intestinal disease. Amebic liver abscess may occur months to years after exposure, so obtaining a careful travel history is critical. In children, fever is the hallmark of amebic liver abscess and is frequently associated with abdominal pain, distention, and enlargement and tenderness of the liver. Changes at the base of the right lung, such as elevation of the diaphragm and atelectasis or effusion, may also occur.

LABORATORY FINDINGS. Laboratory examination findings are often unremarkable in uncomplicated amebic colitis, although mild anemia may be seen. Laboratory findings in amebic liver abscess are a slight leukocytosis, moderate anemia, high erythrocyte sedimentation rate, and elevations of hepatic enzyme (particularly alkaline phosphatase) levels. Stool examination for amebae yields negative results in >50% of patients with documented amebic liver abscess. Ultrasonography, CT, or MRI can localize and delineate the size of the abscess cavity (Fig. 278-1). The most common finding is a single abscess in the right hepatic lobe, in half of cases, although ultrasound and CT studies have shown that left lobe abscess and multiple abscesses are more common than previously recognized.

DIAGNOSIS AND DIFFERENTIAL DIAGNOSIS. A diagnosis of amebic colitis is ideally based on compatible symptoms with detection of *E. histolytica* antigens in stool by commercially available enzyme-linked immunosorbent assays. These assays have demonstrated better sensitivity (>90%) and specificity for detection of *E. histolytica* infection than traditional microscopic examination of stool samples. Microscopic examination of 3 fresh stool samples (within 30 min of passage) by experienced laboratory personnel has a sensitivity of 90% for detecting *Entamoeba,* but microscopy cannot differentiate between *E. histolytica* and *E. dispar* unless phagocytosed erythrocytes, which are specific for *E. histolytica,* are seen. For this reason, microscopy is not acceptable for the diagnosis of *E. histolytica* infection in epidemiologic studies. In a patient with the clinical features of amebic colitis, microscopic demonstration of *Entamoeba* trophozoites with phagocytosed erythrocytes is probably sufficient to establish the diagnosis. However, particularly in highly endemic areas, trophozoites without phagocytosed erythrocytes may reflect co-infection with *E. dispar* in a patient with another cause of colitis, such as shigellosis. Polymerase chain reaction testing of stool is highly sensitive and specific for *E. histolytica* infection, but is at present a research tool. Whenever amebiasis is suspected, an additional stool sample should be preserved in polyvinyl alcohol for further examination. Endoscopy and biopsies of suspicious areas should be performed when stool sample results are negative and the index of suspicion for amebiasis remains high. Patients with invasive amebic colitis have positive test results for fecal occult blood.

Various serum antiamebic antibody tests are available. Serologic results are positive in 70–80% of patients with invasive disease (colitis or liver abscess) at presentation, and in >90% of patients after 7 days of disease symptoms. The most sensitive serologic test, indirect hemagglutination, yields a positive result years after invasive infection. Therefore, many uninfected adults and children in highly endemic areas demonstrate antibodies to *E. histolytica.* Detection of *E. histolytica* antigens in serum is perhaps the ideal test because it is sensitive and specific, can distinguish *E. dispar* from *E. histolytica,* and can distinguish current from past infection. However, serum antigen detection tests are not yet routinely available.

The **differential diagnosis** for amebic colitis includes colitis due to bacterial (*Shigella, Salmonella,* enteropathogenic *Escherichia coli, Campylobacter, Yersinia, Clostridium difficile*) and viral (cytomegalovirus) pathogens, as well as noninfectious causes such as inflammatory bowel disease. Pyogenic liver abscess due to bacterial infection, hepatoma, and echinococcal cysts are in the differential for amebic liver abscess. However, echinococcal cysts are rarely associated with systemic symptoms such as fever.

COMPLICATIONS. Complications of amebic colitis include necrotizing colitis, ameboma, toxic megacolon, extraintestinal extension, or local perforation and peritonitis. Uncommonly, a chronic form of amebic colitis develops, which can mimic inflammatory bowel disease with bouts of abdominal pain and bloody diarrhea, often recurring over several years. An ameboma is a nodular focus of proliferative inflammation sometimes developing in chronic amebiasis, usually in the wall of the colon. Chronic amebiasis should be excluded before initiating corticosteroid treatment for inflammatory bowel disease, as corticosteroid therapy inadvertently given during amebic colitis has been associated with high mortality rates.

Amebic liver abscess may be associated with rupture into the peritoneum, pleural cavity, skin, or, rarely, pericardium when diagnosis and therapy are delayed. Cases of amebic abscesses in extrahepatic sites, including the lung and brain, have been reported.

TREATMENT. Invasive amebiasis is treated with a nitroimidazole, such as metronidazole or tinidazole, followed by treatment with a luminal amebicide (Table 278-1). Tinidazole is available in the United States and may become the preferred agent for amebiasis, as it has similar efficacy to metronidazole with shorter and simpler dosing and less frequent adverse effects, which include nausea, abdominal discomfort, and metallic taste that disappear after completion of therapy. Therapy with a nitroimidazole should be followed by treatment with an agent primarily active in the gut lumen, such as paromomycin, which is preferred, or iodoquinol. Diloxanide furoate may also be used in children >2 yr of age, but it is no longer available in the United States. Paromomycin should not be given at the same time as metronidazole or tinidazole because diarrhea is a common side effect of paromomycin, and this may make it difficult to discern if the patient is responding to initial therapy. Asymptomatic intestinal infection with *E. histolytica* should be treated with paromomycin, which is preferred, or iodoquinol or diloxanide furoate. For fulminant cases of amebic colitis, some experts suggest adding dehy-

TABLE 278-1. Drug Treatment for Amebiasis

MEDICATION	ADULT DOSAGE (ORAL)	PEDIATRIC DOSAGE (ORAL)*
INVASIVE DISEASE		
Metronidazole	Colitis or liver abscess:	Colitis or liver abscess:
or	750 mg tid for 7–10 days	35–50 mg/kg/day in 3 divided doses for 7–10 days
Tinidazole	Colitis: 2 g once daily for 3 days Liver abscess: 2 g once daily for 3–5 days	Colitis: 50 mg/kg/day once daily for 3 days Liver abscess: 50 mg/kg/day once daily for 3–5 days
Followed by:		
Paromomycin (preferred)	25–35 mg/kg/d in 3 divided doses for 7 days	25–35 mg/kg/day in 3 divided doses for 7 days
or		
Diloxanide furoate[†] *or*	500 mg tid for 10 days	20 mg/kg/day in 3 divided doses for 7 days
Iodoquinol	650 mg tid for 20 days	30–40 mg/kg/day in 3 divided doses for 20 days
ASYMPTOMATIC INTESTINAL COLONIZATION		
Paromomycin (preferred)	As for invasive disease	As for invasive disease
or		
Diloxanide furoate[†] *or*		
Iodoquinol		

*All pediatric dosages are up to a maximum of the adult dose.
[†]Not available in the USA.

droemetine (1 mg/kg/day subcutaneously or IM, never IV), which is available only through the Centers for Disease Control and Prevention. Patients should be hospitalized for monitoring if dehydroemetine is administered, and the drug should be discontinued if tachycardia, T-wave depression, arrhythmias, or proteinuria develop.

Broad-spectrum antibiotic therapy may also be indicated in fulminant colitis, to treat spillage of intestinal bacteria into the peritoneum. Intestinal perforation and toxic megacolon are indications for surgery. In amebic liver abscess, image-guided aspiration of large lesions or left lobe abscesses may be necessary if rupture is imminent or if the patient shows a poor clinical response 4–6 days after administration of amebicidal drugs. Chloroquine, which concentrates in the liver, may also be a useful adjunct to nitroimidazoles in the treatment of amebic liver abscess. Stool examination should be repeated every 2 wk until the result is negative after completion of antiamebic therapy to confirm cure.

PROGNOSIS. Most infections evolve to either an asymptomatic carrier state or eradication. Death occurs in about 5% of persons having extraintestinal infection.

PREVENTION. Control of amebiasis can be achieved by exercising proper sanitary measures and avoiding fecal-oral contact. Regular examination of food handlers and thorough investigation of diarrheal episodes may identify the source of infection in some communities. No prophylactic drug or vaccine is currently available for amebiasis.

Blessmann J, Tannich E: Treatment of asymptomatic intestinal *Entamoeba histolytica* infection. *N Engl J Med* 2002;347(17):1384.

Haque R, Duggal P, Ali IM, et al: Innate and acquired resistance to amebiasis in Bangladeshi children. *J Infect Dis* 2002;186(4):547–552.

Haque R, Huston CD, Hughes M, et al: Amebiasis. *N Engl J Med* 2003;348: 1565–1573.

Huston CD, Boettner DR, Miller-Sims V, et al: Apoptotic killing and phagocytosis of host cells by the parasite *Entamoeba histolytica*. *Infect Immun* 2003;71(2):964–972.

Petri WA Jr, Haque R, Mann BJ: The bittersweet interface of parasite and host: Lectin-carbohydrate interactions during human invasion by the parasite *Entamoeba histolytica*. *Annu Rev Microbiol* 2002;56:39–64.

Stanley SL Jr: Amoebiasis. *Lancet* 2003;361(9362):1025–1034.

Stauffer W, Ravdin JI: *Entamoeba histolytica:* An update. *Curr Opin Infect Dis* 2003;16(5):479–485.

Tanyuksel M, Petri WA Jr: Laboratory diagnosis of amebiasis. *Clin Microbiol Rev* 2003;16(4):713–729.

Chapter 279 ■ Giardiasis and Balantidiasis

Chandy C. John

279.1 • Giardia Lamblia

Giardia lamblia is a flagellated protozoan that infects the duodenum and small intestine. Infection results in clinical manifestations that range from asymptomatic colonization to acute or chronic diarrhea and malabsorption. Infection is more prevalent in children than in adults. *Giardia* is endemic in areas of the world with poor levels of sanitation. It is also an important cause of morbidity in developed countries, where it is associated with urban child-care centers, residential institutions for the mentally delayed, and water-borne and food-borne outbreaks. *Giardia* is a particularly significant pathogen in people with malnutrition, certain immunodeficiencies, and cystic fibrosis.

ETIOLOGY. The life cycle of *G. lamblia* (also known as *Giardia intestinalis* or *Giardia duodenalis*) is composed of 2 stages: trophozoites and cysts. *Giardia* infects humans after ingestion of as few as 10–100 cysts. Ingested cysts, which measure 8–10 mm in diameter, each produce 2 trophozoites in the duodenum. After excystation, trophozoites colonize the lumen of the duodenum and proximal jejunum, where they attach to the brush border of the intestinal epithelial cells and multiply by binary fission. The body of the trophozoite is teardrop shaped, measuring 10–20 mm in length and 5–15 mm in width. *Giardia* trophozoites contain 2 oval nuclei anteriorly, a large ventral disk, a curved median body posteriorly, and 4 pairs of flagella. As detached trophozoites pass down the intestinal tract, they encyst to form oval cysts that contain 4 nuclei. Cysts are passed in stools of infected individuals and may remain viable in water for as long as 2 mo. Their viability often is not affected by the usual concentrations of chlorine used to purify water for drinking.

Giardia strains that infect humans are diverse biologically, as shown by differences in antigens, restriction endonuclease patterns, DNA fingerprinting, isoenzyme patterns, and pulsed-field gel electrophoresis. Studies suggest that different *Giardia* genotypes may cause unique clinical manifestations, but these findings appear to vary according to the geographic region tested.

EPIDEMIOLOGY. *Giardia* occurs worldwide and is the most common intestinal parasite identified in public health laboratories in the United States, where it is estimated that up to 2.5 million cases of giardiasis occur annually. *Giardia* infection usually occurs sporadically but is a frequently identified etiologic agent of outbreaks associated with drinking water. The age-specific prevalence of giardiasis is high during childhood and begins to decline after adolescence. The asymptomatic carrier rate of *G. lamblia* in the United States is as high as 20–30% in children younger than 36 mo of age attending child-care centers. Asymptomatic carriage may persist for several months.

Transmission of *Giardia* is common in certain high-risk groups, including children and employees in child-care centers, consumers of contaminated water, travelers to certain areas of the world, men who have sex with men, and persons exposed to certain animals. The major reservoir and vehicle for spread of *Giardia* appears to be water contaminated with *Giardia* cysts, but food-borne transmission occurs. The seasonal peak in age-specific case reports coincides with the summer recreational water season and might be a result of the extensive use of communal swimming venues by young children, the low infectious dose, and the extended periods of cyst shedding that can occur. In addition, *Giardia* cysts are relatively resistant to chlorination and to ultraviolet light irradiation. Boiling is effective for inactivating cysts.

Person-to-person spread also occurs, particularly in areas of low hygiene standards, frequent fecal-oral contact, and crowding. Individual susceptibility, lack of toilet training, crowding, and fecal contamination of the environment all predispose to transmission of enteropathogens, including *Giardia,* in child-care centers. Child-care centers play an important role in transmission of urban giardiasis, with secondary attack rates in families as high as 17–30%. Children in child-care centers may pass cysts for several months. Campers who drink untreated stream or river water, particularly in the western United States, and residents of institutions for the mentally delayed are also at increased risk for infection.

Humoral immunodeficiencies, including common variable hypogammaglobulinemia and X-linked agammaglobulinemia, predispose humans to chronic symptomatic *Giardia* infection, suggesting the importance of humoral immunity in controlling giardiasis. Selective immunoglobulin A (IgA) deficiency is associated with *Giardia* infection, too. Although many individuals with AIDS have relatively mild *Giardia* infections, some reports suggest that severe *Giardia* infection, often refractory to treatment, may occur in a subset of individuals with AIDS. There is a higher incidence of *Giardia* infection in patients with cystic fibrosis, probably owing to local factors such as the increased amount of mucus, which may protect the organism against host factors in the duodenum. Human milk contains glycoconjugates and secretory IgA antibodies that may provide protection to nursing infants.

CLINICAL MANIFESTATIONS. The incubation period of *Giardia* infection usually is 1–2 wk but may be longer. A broad spectrum of clinical manifestations occurs, depending on the interaction between *G. lamblia* and the host. Children who are exposed to *G. lamblia* may experience asymptomatic excretion of the organism, acute infectious diarrhea, or chronic diarrhea with persistent gastrointestinal tract signs and symptoms, including failure to thrive and abdominal pain or cramping. Most infections in both children and adults are asymptomatic. There usually is no extraintestinal spread, but occasionally trophozoites may migrate into bile or pancreatic ducts.

Symptomatic infections occur more frequently in children than in adults. Most symptomatic patients usually have a limited period of acute diarrheal disease with or without low-grade fever, nausea, and anorexia; in a small proportion of patients, an intermittent or more protracted course characterized by diarrhea, abdominal distention and cramps, bloating, malaise, flatulence, nausea, anorexia, and weight loss develops (Table 279-1). Initially, stools may be profuse and watery and later become greasy and foul smelling and may float. Stools do not contain blood, mucus, or fecal leukocytes. Varying degrees of malabsorption may occur. Abnormal stool patterns may alternate with periods of constipation and normal bowel movements. Malabsorption of sugars, fats, and fat-soluble vitamins has been well documented and may be responsible for substantial weight loss. Giardiasis has been associated with growth stunting and repeated *Giardia* infections with a decrease in cognitive function in children in endemic areas.

DIAGNOSIS. Giardiasis should be considered in young children in child care or in any person who has had contact with an index case or a history of recent travel to an endemic area who has persistent diarrhea, intermittent diarrhea and constipation, malabsorption, crampy abdominal pain and bloating, failure to thrive, or weight loss.

TABLE 279-1. Clinical Signs and Symptoms of Giardiasis

SYMPTOM	FREQUENCY (%)
Diarrhea	64–100
Malaise, weakness	72–97
Abdominal distention	42–97
Flatulence	35–97
Abdominal cramps	44–81
Nausea	14–79
Foul-smelling, greasy stools	15–79
Anorexia	41–73
Weight loss	53–73
Vomiting	14–35
Fever	0–28
Constipation	0–27

Traditionally, a diagnosis of giardiasis has been established by microscopy documentation of trophozoites or cysts in stool specimens, but 3 stool specimens are required to achieve a sensitivity of >90%. Stool enzyme immunoassay (EIA) or direct fluorescent antibody tests for *Giardia* antigens are less reader dependent and more sensitive for detection of *Giardia* than microscopy, and are now the tests of choice for giardiasis in most situations. Some studies have reported that a single stool is sufficiently sensitive for detection of *Giardia* by EIA, while others suggest that sensitivity is increased with testing of 2 samples. In patients in whom other parasitic intestinal infections are in the differential diagnosis, microscopy examination of stool allows evaluation for these infections in addition to *Giardia.*

In patients in whom the diagnosis is suspected but in whom testing of stool specimens for *Giardia* yields a negative result, aspiration or biopsy of the duodenum or upper jejunum should be performed. In a fresh specimen, trophozoites usually can be visualized by direct wet mount. An alternate method of directly obtaining duodenal fluid is the commercially available Entero-Test (Hedeco Corp, Mountain View, California), but this method is less sensitive than aspiration or biopsy. The biopsy can be used to make touch preparations and tissue sections for identification of *Giardia* and other enteric pathogens, as well as to visualize changes in histologic features. Biopsy of the small intestine should be considered in patients with characteristic clinical symptoms, negative stool and duodenal fluid specimen findings, and 1 of the following: abnormal radiographic findings, such as edema and segmentation in the small intestine; abnormal lactose tolerance test result; absent secretory IgA level; hypogammaglobulinemia; or achlorhydria.

Laboratories can reduce reagent and personnel costs by pooling specimens submitted for detection of *Giardia* before evaluation by microscopy or EIA. Polymerase chain reaction and gene probe–based detection systems specific for *Giardia* have been used in environmental monitoring but at present remain research tools.

Radiographic contrast studies of the small intestine may show nonspecific findings such as irregular thickening of the mucosal folds. Blood cell counts usually are normal. Giardiasis is not tissue invasive and is not associated with eosinophilia.

TREATMENT. Children with acute diarrhea in whom *Giardia* organisms are identified should receive therapy. In addition, children who manifest failure to thrive or exhibit malabsorption or gastrointestinal tract symptoms such as chronic diarrhea should be treated.

Asymptomatic excreters generally are not treated except in specific instances such as in outbreak control, for prevention of

TABLE 279-2. Drug Treatment for Giardiasis

MEDICATION	ADULT DOSAGE (ORAL)	PEDIATRIC DOSAGE (ORAL)*
RECOMMENDED		
Tinidazole	2 g once daily	>3 yr: 50 mg/kg/day once daily
Nitazoxanide	500 mg bid for 3 days	12–48 mo: 100 mg (5 mL) bid for 3 days 4–12 yr: 200 mg (10 mL) bid for 3 days >12 yr: 500 mg bid for 3 days
Metronidazole	250 mg tid for 5–7 days	15 mg/kg/day in 3 divided doses for 5–7 days
ALTERNATIVE		
Albendazole	400 mg once a day for 5 days	>6 yr: 400 mg once a day for 5 days
Furazolidone	100 mg qid for 10 days	6 mg/kg/day in 4 divided doses for 10 days
Paromomycin	6 mg/kg/day in 3 divided doses for 5 days	Not recommended
Quinacrine†	100 mg tid for 7 days	6 mg/kg/day in 3 divided doses for 5 days

*All pediatric dosages are up to a maximum of the adult dose.
†Can be compounded by Medical Center Pharmacy in New Haven, CT (203-785-6818) or Panorama Compounding Pharmacy in Van Nuys, CA (800-247-9767).

household transmission by toddlers to pregnant women and patients with hypogammaglobulinemia or cystic fibrosis, and in situations requiring oral antibiotic treatment where *Giardia* may have produced malabsorption of the antibiotic.

The Food and Drug Administration (FDA) has approved tinidazole and nitazoxanide for the treatment of *Giardia* in the United States. Both medications have been used to treat *Giardia* in thousands of patients in other countries and have excellent safety and efficacy against *Giardia* (Table 279-2). Tinidazole has the advantage of single-dose treatment and very high efficacy (>90%), while nitazoxanide has the advantage of a suspension form, high efficacy (80–90%), and very few adverse effects. Metronidazole was the treatment of choice for *Giardia* infection in the United States for many years, although it was never approved by the FDA for treatment of *Giardia*. When a full course of therapy is taken, metronidazole is highly effective (80–90% cure rate), and the generic form is considerably less expensive than tinidazole or nitazoxanide. However, frequent adverse effects are seen with metronidazole therapy, and it requires 3 times a day dosing for 5–7 days. Suspension forms of tinidazole and metronidazole must be compounded by a pharmacy; neither drug is sold in suspension form.

Second line alternatives for the treatment of patients with giardiasis include furazolidone, albendazole, paromomycin, and quinacrine (see Table 279-2). Furazolidone, albendazole, and paromomycin are less effective than tinidazole, nitazoxanide, and metronidazole. Furazolidone is approved by the FDA for the treatment of giardiasis and has often been prescribed for children because it is available in liquid form. Albendazole has few adverse effects and is effective against many helminths, making it useful for treatment when multiple intestinal parasites are identified or suspected. Paromomycin, a nonabsorbable aminoglycoside, is less effective than other agents but is recommended for treatment of pregnant women with giardiasis because of potential teratogenic effects of other agents. Quinacrine is effective and inexpensive but is not available from any U.S. manufacturer. Refractory cases of giardiasis have been successfully treated with nitazoxanide, prolonged courses of tinidazole, or a combination of metronidazole and quinacrine.

PROGNOSIS. Symptoms recur in some patients in whom reinfection cannot be documented and in whom an immune deficiency such as an immunoglobulin abnormality is not present, despite use of appropriate therapy. Several studies have demonstrated that variability in antimicrobial susceptibility exists among strains of *Giardia,* and in some instances resistant strains have been demonstrated. Combined therapy may be useful for infection that persists after single-drug therapy, assuming reinfection has not occurred and the medication was taken as prescribed.

PREVENTION. Infected persons and persons at risk should practice strict handwashing after any contact with feces. This is especially important for caregivers of diapered infants in child-care centers, where diarrhea is common and *Giardia* organism carriage rates are high.

Methods to purify public water supplies adequately include chlorination, sedimentation, and filtration. Inactivation of *Giardia* cysts by chlorine requires the coordination of multiple variables such as chlorine concentration, water pH, turbidity, temperature, and contact time. These variables cannot be appropriately controlled in all municipalities and are difficult to control in swimming pools. Individuals, especially children in diapers, should avoid swimming if they have diarrhea. Individuals should also avoid swallowing recreational water and drinking untreated water from shallow wells, lakes, springs, ponds, streams, and rivers.

Travelers to endemic areas are advised to avoid uncooked foods that might have been grown, washed, or prepared with water that was potentially contaminated. Purification of drinking water can be achieved by a filter with a pore size of <1 mm or that has been National Sanitation Foundation rated for cyst removal, or by brisk boiling of water for at least 1 min. Treatment of water with chlorine or iodine is somewhat less effective but may be used as an alternate method when boiling or filtration is not possible.

258.2 • Balantidiasis

Balantidium coli is a ciliated protozoan and is the largest protozoan that parasitizes humans. Both trophozoites and cysts may be identified in feces. Disease caused by this organism is uncommon in the United States and generally is reported where there is a close association of humans with pigs, which are the natural hosts of *B. coli.* Because the organism infects the large intestine, symptoms are consistent with large bowel disease, similar to those associated with amebiasis and trichuriasis, and include nausea, vomiting, lower abdominal pain, tenesmus, and bloody diarrhea. Symptoms associated with chronic infection include abdominal cramps, watery diarrhea with mucus, occasionally bloody diarrhea, and colonic ulcers similar to those associated with *Entamoeba histolytica.* Extraintestinal spread of *B. coli* is rare, and usually occurs only in immunocompromised patients. Most infections are asymptomatic.

Diagnosis using direct saline mounts is established by identification of trophozoites (50–100 mm long) or spherical or oval cysts (50–70 mm in diameter) in stool specimens. Trophozoites usually are more numerous than cysts. The recommended treatment regimen is metronidazole (45 mg/kg/day divided tid PO, maximum 750 mg/dose) for 5 days, or tetracycline (40 mg/kg/day divided qid PO, maximum 500 mg/dose) for 10 days for persons >8 yr of age. An alternative is iodoquinol (40 mg/kg/day divided tid PO, maximum 650 mg/dose) for 20 days. Prevention of contamination of the environment by pig feces is the important means for control.

Ali SA, Hill DR: *Giardia intestinalis. Curr Opin Infect Dis* 2003;16(5):453–460.

Berkman DS, Lescano AG, Gilman RH, et al: Effects of stunting, diarrhoeal disease, and parasitic infection during infancy on cognition in late childhood: A follow-up study. *Lancet* 2002;359(9306):564–571.

Gardner TB, Hill DR: Treatment of giardiasis. *Clin Microbiol Rev* 2001;14(1):114–128.

Hanson KL, Cartwright CP: Use of an enzyme immunoassay does not eliminate the need to analyze multiple stool specimens for sensitive detection of *Giardia lamblia. J Clin Microbiol* 2001;39(2):474–477.

Homan WL, Mank TG: Human giardiasis: Genotype linked differences in clinical symptomatology. *Int J Parasitol* 2001;31(8):822–826.

Johnston SP, Ballard MM, Beach MJ, et al: Evaluation of three commercial assays for detection of *Giardia* and *Cryptosporidium* organisms in fecal specimens. *J Clin Microbiol* 2003;41(2):623–626.

Mank TG, Zaat JO, Deelder AM, et al: Sensitivity of microscopy versus enzyme immunoassay in the laboratory diagnosis of giardiasis. *Eur J Clin Microbiol Infect Dis* 1997;16(8):615–619.

Nash TE: Treatment of *Giardia lamblia* infections. *Pediatr Infect Dis J* 2001;20(2):193–195.

Ortiz JJ, Ayoub A, Gargala G, et al: Randomized clinical study of nitazoxanide compared to metronidazole in the treatment of symptomatic giardiasis in children from Northern Peru. *Aliment Pharmacol Ther* 2001; 15(9):1409–1415.

Pengsaa K, Limkittikul K, Pojjaroen-anant C, et al: Single-dose therapy for giardiasis in school-age children. *Southeast Asian J Trop Med Public Health* 2002;33:711–717.

Chapter 280 ■ *Cryptosporidium, Isospora, Cyclospora,* and Microsporidia

Patricia M. Flynn

The spore-forming intestinal protozoa—*Cryptosporidium, Isospora,* and *Cyclospora*—are important intestinal pathogens in both immunocompetent and immunocompromised hosts. *Cryptosporidium, Isospora,* and *Cyclospora* are coccidian parasites that predominantly infect the epithelial cells lining the digestive tract. Microsporidia, formerly considered spore-forming protozoa, have recently been reclassified as fungi. Microsporidia are ubiquitous, obligate intracellular parasites that infect many other organ systems in addition to the gastrointestinal tract and cause a broader spectrum of disease.

CRYPTOSPORIDIUM. *Cryptosporidium* is recognized as a leading protozoal cause of diarrhea in children worldwide and is a common cause of outbreaks in child-care centers; it is also a significant pathogen in immunocompromised patients.

Etiology. *Cryptosporidium hominis* and *Cryptosporidium parvum* cause cryptosporidiosis in humans. Disease is initiated by ingestion of infectious oocysts that release 4 sporozoites that invade enterocytes, primarily in the small intestine. The infection progresses through 2 stages: the asexual stage, which allows autoinfection at the luminal surface of the epithelium, and the sexual stage, which results in production of oocysts that are shed in the stools. The cysts are immediately infectious to other hosts or can reinfect the same host. Ingestion of very few cysts is required to produce infection, even in immunocompetent hosts.

Epidemiology. Cryptosporidiosis is associated with diarrheal illness worldwide and is more prevalent in developing countries and among children <2 yr of age. It has been implicated as an etiologic agent of persistent diarrhea in the developing world and as a cause of significant morbidity and mortality from malnutrition, including permanent effects on growth.

Transmission of *Cryptosporidium* to humans can occur by close association with infected animals, via person-to-person transmission, or from environmentally contaminated water. Although zoonotic transmission, especially from cows, occurs in persons in close association with animals, person-to-person transmission is probably responsible for cryptosporidiosis outbreaks within hospitals and child-care centers where rates as high as 67% have been reported. Recommendations to prevent outbreaks in child-care centers include strict handwashing, use of protective clothes or diapers capable of retaining liquid diarrhea, and separation of diapering and food-handling areas and responsibilities.

Outbreaks of cryptosporidial infection have been associated with contaminated community water supplies and recreational waters in several states in the United States and U.K. Wastewater, in the form of raw sewage, and runoff from dairies and grazing lands can contaminate both drinking and recreational water sources. It is estimated that *Cryptosporidium* oocysts are present in 65–97% of the surface water in the USA. The organism's small size (4–6 μm in diameter), resistance to chlorination, and ability to survive for long periods outside a host create problems in public water supplies.

Clinical Manifestations. The incubation period is 2–14 days. Infection with *Cryptosporidium* is associated with profuse, watery, nonbloody diarrhea that can be accompanied by diffuse crampy abdominal pain, nausea, vomiting, and anorexia. Although less common in adults, vomiting occurs in >80% of children with cryptosporidiosis. Nonspecific symptoms such as myalgia, weakness, and headache also may occur. Fever occurs in 30–50% of cases. Malabsorption, lactose intolerance, dehydration, weight loss, and malnutrition often occur in severe cases.

In immunocompetent persons, the disease is usually self-limiting, although diarrhea may persist for several weeks and oocyst shedding may persist many weeks after symptoms resolve. Chronic diarrhea is common in individuals with immunodeficiency, such as congenital hypogammaglobulinemia or HIV infection. Symptoms and oocyst shedding can continue indefinitely and may lead to severe malnutrition, wasting, anorexia, and even death.

Cryptosporidiosis in **immunocompromised hosts** is often associated with biliary tract disease, characterized by fever, right upper quadrant pain, nausea, vomiting, and diarrhea. It also has been associated with pancreatitis. Respiratory tract disease, with symptoms of cough, shortness of breath, wheezing, croup, and hoarseness, is very rare.

Diagnosis. Infection can be diagnosed by microscopy using modified acid-fast stain or polymerase chain reaction (PCR), but enzyme-linked immunoassays are the diagnostic method of choice. In stool, oocysts appear as small, spherical bodies (2–6 μm) and stain red with modified acid-fast staining. Because *Cryptosporidium* does not invade below the epithelial layer of the mucosa, fecal leukocytes are not found in stool specimens. Oocyst shedding in feces can be intermittent, and several fecal specimens (at least 3 for an immunocompetent host) should be collected for microscopic examination. Serologic diagnosis is not helpful in acute cryptosporidiosis.

In tissue sections, *Cryptosporidium* organisms can be found along the microvillus region of the epithelia that line the gastrointestinal tract. The highest concentration usually is detected in the jejunum. Histologic section results reveal villus atrophy and blunting, epithelial flattening, and inflammation of the lamina propria.

Treatment. Often the diarrheal illness due to cryptosporidiosis is self-limited in immunocompetent patients and requires no specific antimicrobial therapy. Treatment should focus on supportive care, including rehydration orally or, if fluid losses are severe, intravenously. Nitazoxanide (100 mg bid PO for 3 days for children 1–3 yr of age, 200 mg for children 4–11 yr of age) has been approved for treatment of diarrhea caused by *Cryptosporidium.* Clinical studies, however, have not demonstrated that nitazoxanide is superior to placebo in trials of HIV-infected or immunocompromised patients. In adult patients with AIDS, combination therapy with paromomycin (1 g bid PO) and azithromycin (600 mg/day PO) for 4 wk followed by paromomycin monotherapy for 8 wk has been used with limited success. Treatment with orally administered human serum immunoglobulin or bovine colostrum has been successful in several anecdotal reports.

ISOSPORA. Like *Cryptosporidium, Isospora belli* has been implicated as a cause of diarrhea in institutional outbreaks and in travelers and has also been linked with contaminated water and food.

Isospora appears to be more common in tropical and subtropical climates and in developing areas, including South America, Africa, and Southeast Asia. *Isospora* has not been associated with animal contact. It is also an infrequent cause of diarrhea in patients with AIDS in the United States but may infect up to 15% of AIDS patients in Haiti.

The life cycle and pathogenesis of infection with *Isospora* species are similar to those of *Cryptosporidium* organisms except that oocysts excreted in the stool are not immediately infectious and must undergo further maturation below 37°C. Histologic appearance of gastrointestinal epithelium reveals blunting and atrophy of the villi, acute and chronic inflammation, and crypt hyperplasia.

The **clinical manifestations** are indistinguishable from those of cryptosporidiosis, although fever may be a more common finding. Eosinophilia, not found with other enteric protozoan infections, may be present. The diagnosis is established by detecting the oval, 22–33 µm long by 10–19 µm wide, oocysts by using modified acid-fast staining of the stool. Each oocyst contains 2 sporocysts with 4 sporozoites in each. Fecal leukocytes are not detected.

Unlike cryptosporidiosis, isosporiasis responds promptly to **treatment** with oral trimethoprim-sulfamethoxazole (TMP-SMZ) (5 mg TMP and 25 mg SMZ/kg/dose; maximum 160 mg TMP and 800 mg SMZ/dose qid for 10 days, then bid for 3 wk). In patients with AIDS, relapses are common and often necessitate maintenance therapy. Ciprofloxacin, or a regimen of pyrimethamine alone or with folinic acid, is effective in patients intolerant of sulfonamide drugs.

CYCLOSPORA. *Cyclospora cayetanensis* is a coccidian parasite similar to but larger than *Cryptosporidium.* The organism infects both immunocompromised and immunocompetent individuals and is more common in children <18 mo of age. The pathogenesis and pathologic findings of cyclosporiasis are similar to those of isosporiasis. Asymptomatic carriage of the organism has been found, but travelers who harbor the organism almost always have diarrhea. Outbreaks of cyclosporiasis have been linked with contaminated food and water. Implicated foods include raspberries, lettuce, snow peas, basil, and other fresh food items. After fecal excretion, the oocysts must sporulate to become infectious. This finding explains the lack of person-to-person transmission.

The **clinical manifestations** of cyclosporiasis are similar to those of cryptosporidiosis and isosporiasis and follow an incubation period of approximately 7 days. Moderate *Cyclospora* illness is characterized by a median of 6 stools/day with a median duration of 10 days (range 3–25 days). The duration of diarrhea in immunocompetent persons is characteristically longer in cyclosporiasis than in the other intestinal protozoan illnesses. Associated symptoms frequently include fatigue; abdominal bloating or gas; abdominal cramps or pain; nausea; muscle, joint, or body aches; fever; chills; headache; and weight loss. Vomiting may occur. Bloody stools are uncommon. Biliary disease has been reported. Intestinal pathology includes inflammation with villus blunting.

The diagnosis is established by identification of oocysts in the stool. Oocysts are wrinkled spheres, measure 8–10 µm in diameter, and resemble large *Cryptosporidium* organisms. Each oocyst contains 2 sporocysts, each with 2 sporozoites. The organisms can be seen by using modified acid-fast staining but stain less consistently than *Cryptosporidium.* They can also be detected with phenosafranin stain and by autofluorescence using strong green or intense blue under ultraviolet epifluorescence. New molecular diagnostic testing, including real-time PCR, is currently under investigation. Fecal leukocytes are not present.

The **treatment** of choice for cyclosporiasis, as for isosporiasis, is TMP-SMZ (5 mg TMP and 25 mg SMZ/kg/dose bid PO for 7 days, maximum 160 mg TMP and 800 mg SMZ/dose). Ciprofloxacin is effective in patients intolerant of sulfonamide drugs.

MICROSPORIDIA. Microsporidia are ubiquitous and infect most animal groups, including humans. At least 7 genera and unclassified organisms of the order Microsporida have been linked with human disease in both immunocompetent and immunocompromised hosts. The microsporidian organisms best associated with gastrointestinal disease are *Enterocytozoon bieneusi* and *Encephalitozoon intestinalis.*

Little is known about the epidemiologic characteristics of these organisms, but recent reports suggest they can be transmitted through contaminated water. Unlike *Cryptosporidium* and the other protozoa, spores of microsporidia inject their contents into the host cell to establish infection. Intracellular division produces new spores that can spread to nearby cells, disseminate to other host tissues, or be passed into the environment via feces. Spores also have been detected in urine and respiratory epithelium, suggesting that some body fluids may also be infectious. Once in the environment, microsporidial spores remain infectious for up to 4 mo.

Initially, microsporidial intestinal infection had been almost exclusively reported in patients with AIDS, but there has been recent documentation in immunocompetent individuals. Microsporidia-associated diarrhea is intermittent, copious, watery, and nonbloody. Abdominal cramping and weight loss may be present; fever is unusual. Disseminated disease, involving liver, kidney, bladder, biliary tract, lung, bone, and sinuses, has been reported.

Microsporidia stain with hematoxylin-eosin, Giemsa, Gram, periodic acid-Schiff, and acid-fast stains but are often overlooked because of their small size (1–2 µm) and the absence of associated inflammation in surrounding tissues. Electron microscopy remains the reference method of detection. Multiple research laboratories report success with PCR technology in detecting microsporidia, both in human and environmental samples.

There is no proven **therapy** for microsporidial intestinal infections. *E. intestinalis* infection usually responds to albendazole (adult dose 400 mg bid PO for 3 wk). Fumagillin (adult dose 20 mg tid PO for 2 wk) was effective in a small controlled study. Atovaquone and nitazoxanide have also been reported to decrease symptoms, but controlled clinical trials have not been performed. Improvement in underlying HIV infection with aggressive antiviral therapy also improves microsporidiosis symptoms.

Centers for Disease Control and Prevention: Cryptosporidiosis surveillance—United States 1999–2002 and Giardiasis Surveillance—United States, 1998–2002. *MMWR* 2005;54(SS-1):1–16.

Chen X-M, Keithly JS, Paya CV, et al: Cryptosporidiosis. *N Engl J Med* 2002;346:1723–1731.

Didier ES, Stovall ME, Green LC, et al: Epidemiology of microsporidiosis: Sources and modes of transmission. *Vet Parasitol* 2004;126:145–166.

Herwaldt BL: *Cyclospora cayetanensis:* A review, focusing on the outbreaks of cyclosporiasis in the 1990s. *Clin Infect Dis* 2000;31:1040–1057.

Huang DB, Chappell C, Okhuysen PC: Cryptosporidiosis in children. *Semin Pediatr Infect Dis* 2004;15:253–259.

Molina JM, Tourneur M, Sarfate C, et al: Fumagillin treatment of intestinal microsporidiosis. *N Engl J Med* 2002;346:1963–1969.

Mota P, Rauch CA, Edberg SC: Microsporidia and *Cyclospora:* Epidemiology and assessment of risk from the environment. *Crit Rev Microbiol* 2000;26:69–90.

Ochoa TJ, Salazar-Lindo E, Cleary TG: Management of children with infection-associated persistent diarrhea. *Semin Pediatr Infect Dis* 2004;14: 229–236.

Okhuysen PC: Traveler's diarrhea due to intestinal protozoa. *Clin Infect Dis* 2001;33:110–114.

Tremoulet AH, Avila-Aguero ML, Paris MM, et al: Albendazole therapy for Microsporidium diarrhea in immunocompetent Costa Rican children. *Pediatr Infect Dis J* 2004;23:915–918.

Chapter 281 ■ Trichomoniasis (*Trichomonas Vaginalis*)

Chandy C. John and Robert A. Salata

Trichomonas vaginalis is a sexually transmitted protozoan parasite that primarily causes symptomatic vaginitis in women.

EPIDEMIOLOGY. From 5 to 7 million cases of trichomoniasis occur each year in the United States, primarily in women. The incidence of trichomoniasis is highest among females with multiple sexual partners and in groups with the highest rates of other sexually transmitted infections. *T. vaginalis* is recovered from >60% of female partners of infected men and 30–80% of male sexual partners of infected women. Transmission is thought to occur virtually exclusively by sexual activity. Vaginal trichomoniasis is rare until menarche. Its presence in a younger child should raise the possibility of sexual abuse.

Trichomoniasis may be transmitted to neonates during passage through an infected birth canal. Neonatal infection is usually self-limited, but rare cases of neonatal vaginitis and respiratory infection have been reported.

PATHOGENESIS. Trichomoniasis is caused by *T. vaginalis,* a flagellated parasite. Infected vaginal secretions contain 10^1 to 10^5 or more protozoa/mL. In fresh preparations, *T. vaginalis* are highly motile and pear shaped and are recognized by their characteristic twitching motility. The organisms reproduce by binary fission and exist only as vegetative cells; cyst forms have not been described. *T. vaginalis* damages host cells and tissues by a number of mechanisms: adhesion molecules allow adhesion of *T. vaginalis* to host cells, and hydrolases, proteases, and cytotoxic molecules act to destroy or impair the integrity of host cells. *T. vaginalis* also activates the alternative pathway of complement, attracting polymorphonuclear neutrophils, which in turn can kill the protozoon. Parasite-specific antibodies and lymphocyte priming occur in response to infection, but durable protective immunity does not occur.

CLINICAL MANIFESTATIONS. The incubation period in females is 5–28 days. Symptoms may begin or exacerbate during menses. Up to 50% of infected women are asymptomatic. Signs and symptoms most commonly associated with trichomoniasis include copious malodorous gray, frothy vaginal discharge, vulvovaginal irritation, dysuria, and dyspareunia. Physical examination may reveal a frothy discharge with vaginal erythema and cervical hemorrhages ("strawberry cervix"). The vaginal discharge usually has a pH of >4.5. Unfortunately, none of these signs and symptoms alone or in combination are sensitive or specific enough to establish a diagnosis of trichomoniasis confidently. Abdominal discomfort, although occasionally reported, is unusual and should prompt evaluation for pelvic inflammatory disease (see Chapter 119).

Most males carrying *T. vaginalis* are asymptomatic. The organism can be isolated in 3–20% of men with nongonococcal urethritis; these patients have symptoms that are indistinguishable from those of nongonococcal urethritis of other causes. Symptomatic males usually have dysuria and scant urethral discharge. Trichomonads occasionally cause epididymitis, prostatic involvement, and superficial penile ulceration. Infection in men is often self-limited, spontaneously resolving in 36% of men.

DIAGNOSIS. The accurate diagnosis of trichomoniasis in both sexes is dependent on the demonstration of the protozoan in genital secretions. Trichomonads may be recognized in vaginal secretions by using the wet mount technique, which will identify 60–70% of infected females. Endocervical specimens are unreliable for diagnosis. Wet mount examination of material obtained by platinum loop from the anterior urethra will reveal the organism in 50–90% of infected men. Microscopic examination of urine sediment after prostatic massage is also of high yield in infected men. A negative wet mount finding does not exclude the diagnosis of trichomoniasis. Culture of the organism is the gold standard for detection, and culture media are now commercially available. Enzyme-linked immunosorbent assay and direct fluorescent antigen testing of vaginal secretions are more sensitive than wet mount testing but less sensitive than culture for detection of *T. vaginalis* infection. In women, DNA immunoblot and polymerase chain reaction (PCR) testing of vaginal secretions have similar sensitivity and specificity to culture, but in men, these methods appear to be more sensitive at detection of infection than culture. PCR testing remains primarily a research tool at this time. Patients with *T. vaginalis* should be screened for other sexually transmitted infections, including *Chlamydia* and gonorrhea, which are in the differential diagnosis of a patient with symptoms of trichomoniasis.

COMPLICATIONS. Trichomoniasis is associated with premature delivery, low birthweight, tubal infertility, and vaginal cuff cellulitis. *T. vaginalis* infection is associated with increased acquisition and transmission of HIV.

TREATMENT. In the United States, metronidazole and tinidazole are used; in other countries ornidazole has been used with similar efficacy. The Centers for Disease Control and Prevention (CDC) recommends metronidazole (2 g orally as a single dose for adolescent and adults; alternative regimen, 500 mg orally bid for 7 days). The single-dose regimen is associated with more frequent gastrointestinal adverse effects but ensures compliance. Tinidazole is also given as a single 2 g dose orally in adolescents and adults. All regimens are equally efficacious, eradicating >90% of *T. vaginalis* infections, but adverse effects are less frequent with tinidazole than metronidazole. For children infected prior to adolescence, the recommended regimen is metronidazole 15 mg/kg/day divided in 3 doses orally for 7 days; tinidazole is not approved for dosing in younger children with trichomoniasis. Topical metronidazole gel is not efficacious when used as the sole therapy for *T. vaginalis* infection, but it may decrease symptoms in individuals with severe infection when used in conjunction with oral metronidazole. All sexual partners should be treated simultaneously to prevent reinfection.

Metronidazole therapy is safe in all trimesters of pregnancy. Two studies suggest an increase in premature births with metronidazole treatment of asymptomatic *T. vaginalis* infection in pregnancy, but further studies are needed to confirm these findings. Symptomatic trichomoniasis in any trimester of pregnancy should be treated with the 2 g single-dose regimen of metronidazole.

The number of putative metronidazole failures may be increasing. In some cases, metronidazole-resistant *T. vaginalis* has been documented. In most cases, failure is a consequence of reinfection from an untreated sexual partner or of noncompliance with multidose therapy. Current CDC recommendations for metronidazole treatment failures are retreatment with metronidazole (500 mg orally bid for 7 days) and, if treatment failure occurs again, a higher dose of metronidazole (2 g orally once daily for 3–5 days). Patients who fail this regimen should be managed in consultation with an expert. Options include prolonged tinidazole and topical paromomycin. Topical paromomycin is less effective and has been associated with severe local adverse effects. Consultation for complicated cases is available through the CDC (770-488-4115; http://www.cdc.gov/std/).

PREVENTION. Prevention of *T. vaginalis* infection is best accomplished by treatment of all sexual partners of an infected person and by programs aimed at prevention of all sexually transmitted diseases (see Chapter 119).

Centers for Disease Control and Prevention: Sexually transmitted diseases treatment guidelines 2002. *MMWR* 2002;51(RR-6):1–78.

Cudmore SL, Delgaty KL, Hayward-McClelland SF, et al: Treatment of infections caused by metronidazole-resistant Trichomonas vaginalis. *Clin Microbiol Rev* 2004;17(4):783–793.

Crowell AL, Sanders-Lewis KA, Secor WE: In vitro metronidazole and tinidazole activities against metronidazole-resistant strains of Trichomonas vaginalis. *Antimicrob Agents Chemother* 2003;47:1407–1409.

Klebanoff MA, Carey JC, Hauth JC, et al: Failure of metronidazole to prevent preterm delivery among pregnant women with asymptomatic *Trichomonas vaginalis* infection. *N Engl J Med* 2001;345:487–493.

Schwebke JR, Burgess D: Trichomoniasis. *Clin Microbiol Rev* 2004;17: 794–803.

Chapter 282 ■ Leishmaniasis (*Leishmania*)

Peter C. Melby

The leishmaniases are a diverse group of diseases caused by intracellular protozoan parasites of the genus *Leishmania,* which are transmitted by phlebotomine sandflies. Multiple species of *Leishmania* are known to cause human disease involving the skin and mucosal surfaces and the visceral reticuloendothelial organs. Cutaneous disease is generally mild but may cause cosmetic disfigurement. Mucosal and visceral leishmaniasis is associated with significant morbidity and mortality.

ETIOLOGY. *Leishmania* organisms are members of the Trypanosomatidae family and include 2 subgenera, *Leishmania (Leishmania)* and *Leishmania (Viannia).* The parasite is dimorphic, existing as a flagellate promastigote in the insect vector and as an aflagellate amastigote that resides and replicates only within mononuclear phagocytes of the vertebrate host. Within the sandfly vector the promastigote changes from a noninfective procyclic form to an infective metacyclic stage. Fundamental to this transition are changes that take place in the terminal polysaccharides of the surface lipophosphoglycan (LPG), which allow forward migration of the infective parasites from the sandfly midgut to the mouth parts and inoculation of the host during a blood meal. Metacyclic LPG also plays an important role in the entry and survival of *Leishmania* in the mammalian host by conferring complement resistance and by facilitating entry into the macrophage by way of multiple receptors, including complement receptors 1 and 3. Once within the macrophage, the promastigote transforms to an amastigote and resides and replicates within a phagolysosome. The parasite is resistant to the acidic, hostile environment of the macrophage and eventually ruptures the cell and goes on to infect other macrophages. Infected macrophages have a diminished capacity to initiate and respond to an inflammatory response, thus providing a safe haven for the intracellular parasite.

EPIDEMIOLOGY. The leishmaniases are estimated to affect 10–50 million people in endemic tropical and subtropical regions on all continents except Australia and Antarctica. The different forms of the disease are distinct in their causes, epidemiologic characteristics, transmission, and geographic distribution. The leishmaniases may occur sporadically throughout an endemic region or may occur in epidemic focuses. With only rare exceptions, the *Leishmania* organisms that primarily cause cutaneous disease do not cause visceral disease.

Localized cutaneous leishmaniasis (LCL) is caused by *L. (Leishmania) major* and *L. (L.) tropica* in North Africa, the Middle East, central Asia, and the Indian subcontinent. *L. (L.) aethiopica* is a cause of LCL and diffuse cutaneous leishmaniasis (DCL) in Kenya and Ethiopia. **Visceral leishmaniasis** (VL) in the Old World is caused by *L. (L.) donovani* in Kenya, Sudan, India, Pakistan, and China and by *L. (L.) infantum* in the Mediterranean basin, Middle East, and central Asia. *L. infantum* is also a cause of LCL (without visceral disease) in this same geographic distribution. *L. tropica* also has been recognized as an uncommon cause of visceral disease in the Middle East and India. In the New World, *L. (L.) mexicana* causes LCL in a region stretching from southern Texas through Central America. *L. (L.) amazonensis, L. (L.) pifanoi, L. (L.) garnhami,* and *L. (L.) venezuelensis* cause LCL in South America, the Amazon basin, and northward. Members of the *Viannia* subgenus (*L. [V.] braziliensis, L. [V.] panamensis, L. [V.] guyanensis,* and *L. [V.] peruviana*) cause LCL from the northern highlands of Argentina northward to Central America. Members of the *Viannia* subgenus also cause **mucosal leishmaniasis** (ML) in a similar geographic distribution. VL in the New World is caused by *L. (L.) chagasi* (now considered to be the same organism as *L. infantum*), which is distributed from Mexico (rare) through Central and South America. Like *L. infantum, L. chagasi* can also cause LCL in the absence of visceral disease.

The maintenance of *Leishmania* in most endemic areas is through a zoonotic cycle in which humans are only incidentally infected. In general, the dermotropic strains in both the Old and New Worlds are maintained in rodent reservoirs, and the domestic dog is the usual reservoir for *L. infantum/chagasi.* The transmission between reservoir and sandfly is highly adapted to the specific ecologic characteristics of the endemic region. Human infections occur when human activities bring them in contact with the zoonotic cycle. Anthroponotic transmission, in which humans are the presumed reservoir, occurs with *L. tropica* in some urban areas of the Middle East and with *L. donovani* in India and Sudan. Congenital transmission of *L. donovani* or *L. infantum/chagasi* has been reported.

There have been increased cases reported from many longstanding endemic areas, as well as large numbers of cases in some new areas. Severe epidemics with >100,000 deaths from VL have occurred in India and Sudan. The emergence of the leishmaniases in new areas is the result of (1) movement of a susceptible population into existing endemic areas, usually because of agricultural or industrial development or timber harvesting; (2) increase in vector and/or reservoir populations as a result of agriculture development projects; (3) increase in anthroponotic transmission owing to rapid urbanization in some focuses; and (4) increase in sandfly density resulting from a reduction in vector control programs.

PATHOLOGY. Histopathologic analysis of the LCL lesion shows intense chronic granulomatous inflammation involving the epidermis and dermis. Occasionally, neutrophils and even microabscesses can be seen. The lesions of DCL are characterized by dense infiltration with vacuolated macrophages containing abundant amastigotes. ML is characterized by an intense granulomatous reaction with prominent tissue necrosis, which may include adjacent cartilage or bone. In VL there is prominent reticuloendothelial cell hyperplasia in the liver, spleen, bone marrow, and lymph nodes. Amastigotes are abundant in the histiocytes and Kupffer cells. Late in the course of disease, splenic infarcts are common, centrilobular necrosis and fatty infiltration of the liver occur, the normal marrow elements are replaced by parasitized histiocytes, and erythrophagocytosis is present.

PATHOGENESIS. Cellular immune mechanisms determine resistance or susceptibility to infection with *Leishmania*. Resistance is mediated by expansion of the T helper 1 (Th1) cell population, with interferon-γ production resulting in macrophage activation and parasite killing. Interleukin 12 (IL-12) plays a central role in the development of the protective Th1 response. Susceptibility is associated with expansion of IL-4-producing Th2 cells and/or the production of IL-10 and transforming growth factor-β, which are potent inhibitors of macrophage activation. Patients with ML exhibit a hyperresponsive cellular immune reaction that may contribute to the prominent tissue destruction seen in this form of the disease. Patients with DCL or active VL demonstrate minimal or absent *Leishmania*-specific cellular immune responses, but these responses recover after successful therapy.

Within endemic areas people who have had a subclinical infection can be identified by a positive delayed-type hypersensitivity response to leishmanial antigens (**Montenegro skin test**). Subclinical infection occurs considerably more frequently than does active cutaneous or visceral disease. Host factors (genetic background, concomitant disease, nutritional status), parasite factors (virulence, size of the inoculum), and possibly vector-specific factors (vector genotype, immunomodulatory salivary constituents) influence the expression as either subclinical infection or active disease. Within endemic areas the prevalence of skin test result positivity increases with age and the incidence of clinical disease decreases with age, indicating that immunity is acquired in the population over time. Individuals with prior active disease or subclinical infection are usually immune to a subsequent clinical infection.

CLINICAL MANIFESTATIONS. The different forms of the disease are distinct in their causes, epidemiologic features, transmission, and geographic distribution.

Localized Cutaneous Leishmaniasis. LCL (**Oriental sore**) can affect individuals of any age, but children are the primary victims in many endemic regions. It typically presents as 1 or a few papular, nodular, plaquelike, or ulcerative lesions that are usually located on exposed skin, such as the face and extremities (Fig. 282-1). Rarely, >100 lesions have been recorded. The lesions typically begin as a small papule at the site of the sandfly bite, which enlarges to 1–3 cm in diameter and may ulcerate over the course of several weeks to months. The shallow ulcer is usually nontender and surrounded by a sharp, indurated, erythematous margin. There is no drainage unless a bacterial superinfection develops. Lesions caused by *L. major* and *L. mexicana* usually heal spontaneously after 3–6 mo, leaving a depressed scar. Lesions on the ear pinna caused by *L. mexicana*, called **chiclero ulcer** because they were common in chicle harvesters in Mexico and Central America, often follow a chronic, destructive course. In general, lesions caused by *L. (Viannia)* species tend to be larger and more chronic. Regional lymphadenopathy and palpable subcutaneous nodules or lymphatic cords, the so-called sporotrichoid appearance, are also more common when the patient is infected with organisms of the *Viannia* subgenus. If lesions do not become secondarily infected, there are usually no complications aside from the residual cutaneous scar.

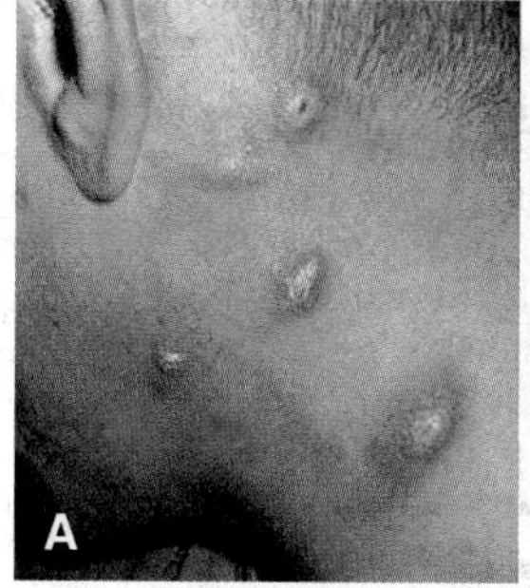

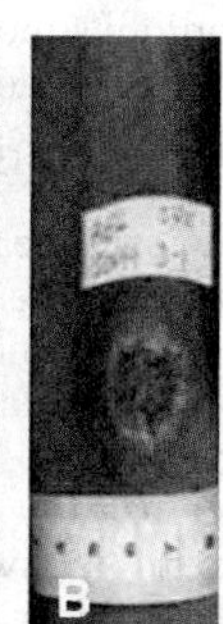

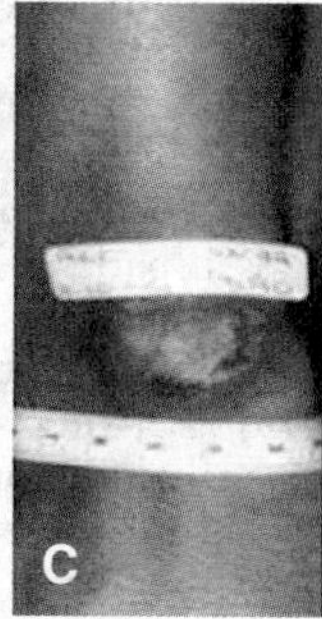

Figure 282-1. Cutaneous and mucosal disease. *A*, Old World infection *(Leishmania major)* acquired in Iraq; note 5 papular and nodular lesions on neck (courtesy of P. Weina). *B*, New World infection *(Leishmania panamensis)* in Colombia; purely ulcerative lesion is characteristic of New World disease (courtesy of J Soto). *C*, Healed infection in patient shown in B 70 days after 20 days of meglumine antimoniate treatment; note paper-thin scar tissue over flat re-epithelialized skin. (Modified from Murray HW, Berman JD, Davies CR, et al: Advances in leishmaniasis. *Lancet* 2005;366:1561–1577.)

Diffuse Cutaneous Leishmaniasis. DCL is a rare form of leishmaniasis caused by organisms of the *L. mexicana* complex in the New World, and *L. aethiopica* in the Old World. DCL manifests as large nonulcerating macules, papules, nodules, or plaques that often involve large areas of skin and may resemble lepromatous leprosy. The face and extremities are most commonly involved. Dissemination from the initial lesion usually takes place over several years. It is thought that an immunologic defect underlies this severe form of cutaneous leishmaniasis.

Mucosal Leishmaniasis. ML (**espundia**) is an uncommon but serious manifestation of leishmanial infection resulting from hematogenous metastases to the nasal or oropharyngeal mucosa from a cutaneous infection. It is usually caused by parasites in the *L. (Viannia)* complex. Approximately half of the patients with mucosal lesions have had active cutaneous lesions within the preceding 2 yr, but ML may not develop until many years after resolution of the primary lesion. ML occurs in <5% of individuals who have, or have had, LCL caused by *L. (V.) braziliensis*. Patients with ML most commonly have nasal mucosal involvement and present with nasal congestion, discharge, and recurrent epistaxis. Oropharyngeal and laryngeal involvement is less common but associated with severe morbidity. Marked soft tissue, cartilage, and even bone destruction occurs late in the course of disease and may lead to visible deformity of the nose or mouth, nasal septal perforation, and tracheal narrowing with airway obstruction.

Visceral Leishmaniasis. VL (**kala-azar**) typically affects children <5 yr of age in the New World *(L. chagasi)* and Mediterranean region *(L. infantum)* and older children and young adults in Africa and Asia *(L. donovani)*. After inoculation of the organism into the skin by the sandfly, the child may have a completely asymptomatic infection or an oligosymptomatic illness that either resolves spontaneously or evolves into active kala-azar. Children with asymptomatic infection are transiently seropositive but show no clinical evidence of disease. Children who are oligosymptomatic have mild constitutional symptoms (malaise, intermittent diarrhea, poor activity tolerance) and intermittent fever; most will have a mildly enlarged liver. In most of these children the illness will resolve without therapy, but in approximately 1/4 it will evolve to active kala-azar within 2–8 mo. Extreme incubation periods of several years have rarely been described. During the 1st few weeks to months of disease evolution the fever is intermittent, there is weakness and loss of energy, and the spleen begins to enlarge. The classic clinical features of high fever, marked splenomegaly, hepatomegaly, and severe cachexia typically develop approximately 6 mo after the onset of the illness, but a rapid clinical course over 1 mo has been noted in up to 20% of patients in some series (Fig. 282-2). At the terminal stages of kala-azar the hepatosplenomegaly is massive, there is gross wasting, the pancytopenia is profound, and jaundice, edema, and ascites may be present. Anemia may be severe enough to precipitate heart failure. Bleeding episodes, especially epistaxis, are frequent. The late stage of the illness is often complicated by secondary bacterial infections, which frequently are a cause of death. A younger age at the time of infection and underlying malnutrition may be risk factors for the development and more rapid evolution of active VL. Death occurs in >90% of patients without specific antileishmanial treatment.

VL has been increasingly recognized as an opportunistic infection associated with HIV infection. Most cases have occurred in

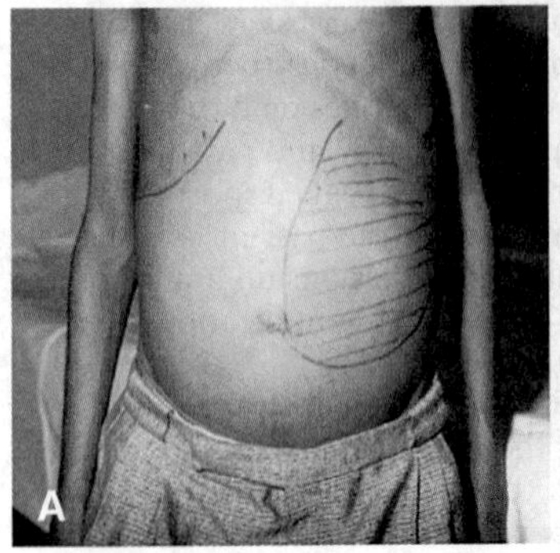

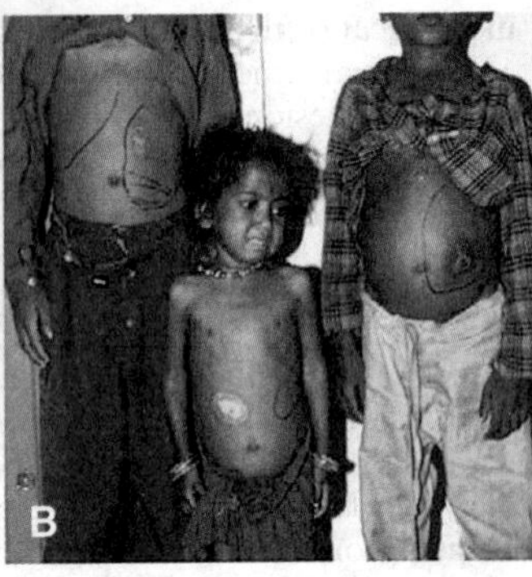

Figure 282-2. Visceral leishmaniasis *(Leishmania donovani)* in Bihar State, India. *A*, Hepatosplenomegaly and wasting in a young man (courtesy of D. Sacks). *B*, Children with burn marks over enlarged spleen or liver—local shaman's unsuccessful remedy (courtesy of R. Kenney). (Modified from Murray HW, Berman JD, Davies CR, et al: Advances in leishmaniasis. *Lancet* 2005;366:1561–1577.)

southern Europe and Brazil, often as a result of needle sharing associated with illicit drug use, with the potential for many more cases as the endemic regions for HIV and VL converge. Leishmaniasis may also result from reactivation of a long-standing subclinical infection. Frequently there is an atypical clinical presentation of VL in HIV-infected individuals with prominent involvement of the gastrointestinal tract and absence of the typical hepatosplenomegaly.

A small percentage of patients previously treated for VL develop diffuse skin lesions, a condition known as **post-kala-azar dermal leishmaniasis (PKDL)**. These lesions may appear during or shortly after therapy (Africa) or up to several years later (India). The lesions of PKDL are hypopigmented, erythematous, or nodular and commonly involve the face and torso. They may persist for several months or for many years.

LABORATORY FINDINGS. Patients with cutaneous or mucosal leishmaniasis generally do not have abnormal laboratory results unless the lesions are secondarily infected with bacteria. Laboratory findings associated with classic kala-azar include anemia (hemoglobin 5–8 mg/dL), thrombocytopenia, leukopenia (2,000–3,000 cells/μL), elevated hepatic transaminase levels, and hyperglobulinemia (>5 g/dL) that is mostly immunoglobulin G (IgG).

DIFFERENTIAL DIAGNOSIS. Diseases that should be considered in the differential diagnosis of LCL include sporotrichosis, blastomycosis, chromomycosis, lobomycosis, cutaneous tuberculosis, atypical mycobacterial infection, leprosy, ecthyma, syphilis, yaws, and neoplasms. Infections such as syphilis, tertiary yaws, histoplasmosis, paracoccidioidomycosis, as well as sarcoidosis, Wegener granulomatosis, midline granuloma, and carcinoma may have clinical features similar to those of ML. VL should be strongly suspected in the patient with prolonged fever, weakness, cachexia, marked splenomegaly, hepatomegaly, cytopenias, and hypergammaglobulinemia who has had potential exposure in an endemic area. The clinical picture may also be consistent with that of malaria, typhoid fever, miliary tuberculosis, schistosomiasis, brucellosis, amebic liver abscess, infectious mononucleosis, lymphoma, and leukemia.

DIAGNOSIS. The development of 1 or several slowly progressive, nontender, nodular, or ulcerative lesions in a patient who had potential exposure in an endemic area should raise suspicion of LCL.

Serologic tests for diagnosis of ML or LCL generally have low sensitivity and specificity and offer little for diagnosis. Serologic testing by enzyme immunoassay, indirect fluorescence assay, or direct agglutination is very useful in VL because of the very high level of antileishmanial antibodies. An enzyme-linked immunosorbent assay using a recombinant antigen (K39) has a sensitivity and specificity for VL that is close to 100%. A negative serologic test result in an immunocompetent individual is strong evidence against a diagnosis of VL. Serodiagnostic tests have positive findings in only about half of the patients who are co-infected with HIV.

Definitive diagnosis of leishmaniasis is established by the demonstration of amastigotes in tissue specimens or isolation of the organism by culture. Amastigotes can be identified in Giemsa-stained tissue sections, aspirates, or impression smears in about half of the cases of LCL but only rarely in the lesions of ML. Culture of a tissue biopsy or aspirate, best performed by using Novy-McNeal-Nicolle (NNN) biphasic blood agar medium, yields a positive finding in only about 65% of cases of CL. Identification of parasites in impression smears, histopathologic sections, or culture medium is more readily accomplished in DCL than in LCL. In patients with VL, smears or cultures of material from splenic, bone marrow, or lymph node aspirations are usually diagnostic. In experienced hands, **splenic aspiration** has a higher diagnostic sensitivity, but it is rarely performed in the USA because of the risk for bleeding complications. A positive culture result allows speciation of the parasite, usually by isoenzyme analysis by a reference laboratory, which may have therapeutic and prognostic significance.

TREATMENT. Specific antileishmanial therapy is not routinely indicated for uncomplicated LCL caused by strains that have a high rate of spontaneous resolution and self-healing *(L. major, L. mexicana)*. Lesions that are extensive, severely inflamed, or located where a scar would result in disability (near a joint) or cosmetic disfigurement (face or ear), that involve the lymphatics, or that do not begin healing within 3–4 mo should be treated. Cutaneous lesions suspected or known to be caused by members of the *Viannia* subgenus (New World) should be treated because of the low rate of spontaneous healing and the potential risk for development of mucosal disease. Similarly, patients with lesions caused by *L. tropica* (Old World), which are typically chronic and nonhealing, should be treated. All patients with VL or ML should receive therapy.

The pentavalent antimony compounds (sodium stibogluconate [Pentostam, GlaxoSmithKline, Uxbridge, U.K.] and meglumine antimoniate [Glucantime, Aventis, Strasbourg, France]) have been the mainstay of antileishmanial chemotherapy for >40 yr. These drugs have similar efficacies, toxicities, and treatment regimens. Currently, for sodium stibogluconate (available in the USA from the Centers for Disease Control and Prevention, Atlanta, Georgia), the recommended regimen is 20 mg/kg/day intravenously or intramuscularly for 20 days (for LCL and DCL) or 28 days (for ML and VL). Repeated courses of therapy may be necessary in patients with severe cutaneous lesions, ML, or VL. An initial clinical response to therapy usually occurs in the 1st week of therapy, but complete clinical healing (re-epithelialization and scarring for LCL and ML and regression of splenomegaly and normalization of cytopenias for VL) is usually not evident for weeks to a few months after completion of therapy. Cure rates with this regimen of 90–100% for LCL, 50–70% for ML, and 80–100% for VL were common in the 1990s, but lower initial cure rates have been noted recently in regions where clinical resistance to antimony therapy is common, such as India, East Africa, and some parts of Latin America. Furthermore, a recent randomized, controlled trial from Colombia showed a very low cure rate in children <5 yr of age. Relapses are common in patients who do not have an effective antileishmanial cellular immune response, such as those who have DCL or are co-infected with HIV. These patients often require multiple courses of therapy or a chronic suppressive regimen. When clinical relapses occur, they are usually evident within 2 mo after completion of therapy. Adverse effects of antimony therapy are dose and duration dependent and commonly include fatigue, arthralgias and myalgias (50%), abdominal discomfort (30%), elevated hepatic transaminase level (30–80%), elevated amylase and lipase levels (almost 100%), mild hematologic changes (slightly decreased leukocyte count, hemoglobin level, and platelet count) (10–30%), and nonspecific T-wave changes on electrocardiography (30%). Sudden death due to cardiac toxicity is extremely rare and usually associated with use of very high doses of pentavalent antimony.

Several other therapies have been used increasingly in the treatment of the leishmaniases. Amphotericin B desoxycholate and the amphotericin lipid formulations are very useful in the treatment of VL or ML, and in some regions have replaced antimony as 1st line therapy. Amphotericin B desoxycholate at doses of 0.5–1.0 mg/kg every day or every other day for 14–20 doses achieved a cure rate for VL of close to 100%, but the renal toxicity commonly associated with amphotericin B was common. The lipid formulations of amphotericin B are especially attractive for treatment of leishmaniasis because the drugs are concentrated in the reticuloendothelial system and are less nephrotoxic. Liposomal amphotericin B (3 mg/kg on days 1–5, and again on day 10) has been shown to be highly effective, with a 90–100% cure rate for VL in immunocompetent children, some of whom were refractory to antimony therapy. Liposomal amphotericin B (Ambisome, Gilead Sciences, Foster City, California) is approved by the Food and Drug Administration for treatment of VL and should be considered for 1st line therapy in the United States. Parenteral treatment of VL with the aminoglycoside paromomycin (aminosidine) has efficacy (~95%) similar to that of amphotericin B in India. Recombinant human interferon-γ has been successfully used as an adjunct to antimony therapy in the treatment of refractory cases of ML and VL. It is not effective alone and has the frequent side effects of fever and flulike symptoms. Miltefosine, a membrane-activating alkylphospholipid, has been recently developed as the 1st oral treatment for VL and has a cure rate of 95% in Indian patients with VL when administered orally at 50–100 mg/day for 28 days. Gastrointestinal adverse effects were frequent but did not require discontinuation of the drug. Treatment of LCL with oral drugs has had only modest success. Ketoconazole has been effective in treating adults with LCL caused by *L. major*, *L. mexicana*, and *L. panamensis* but not *L. tropica* or *L. braziliensis*. Fluconazole 200 mg orally once daily for 6 wk was demonstrated in adults to modestly increase the rate of healing of CL caused by *L. major* in Saudi Arabia. Miltefosine 2.5 mg/kg/day orally for 20 days had a 91% efficacy in treating CL in Colombia *(L. panamensis)* but was significantly less effective in patients from Guatemala *(L. braziliensis)*. Topical treatment of CL with paromomycin plus methylbenzethonium chloride ointment has been effective in selected areas in the both Old and New World. Enhanced drug development efforts and clinical trials of new drugs are clearly needed, especially in children.

PREVENTION. Personal protective measures should include avoidance of exposure to the nocturnal sandflies and, when necessary, the use of insect repellent and permethrin-impregnated mosquito netting. Where peridomiciliary transmission is present, community-based residual insecticide spraying has had some success in reducing the prevalence of leishmaniasis, but long-term effects are difficult to maintain. Control or elimination of infected reservoir hosts (e.g., seropositive domestic dogs) has had limited success. Where anthroponotic transmission is thought to occur, early recognition and treatment of cases are essential. Several vaccines have been demonstrated to have efficacy in experimental models, and vaccination of humans or domestic dogs may have a role in the control of the leishmaniases in the future.

Arana BA, Mendoza CE, Rizzo NR, et al: Randomized, controlled, double-blind trial of topical treatment of cutaneous leishmaniasis with paromomycin plus methylbenzethonium chloride ointment in Guatemala. *Am J Trop Med Hyg* 2001;65:46–70.

Bern C, Hightower AW, Chowdhury R, et al: Risk factors for kala-azar in Bangladesh. *Emerg Infect Dis* 2005;11:655–662.

Bhattacharya SK, Jha TK, Sundar S, et al: Efficacy and tolerability of miltefosine for childhood visceral leishmaniasis in India. *Clin Infect Dis* 2004;38:217–221.

Cascio A, di Martino L, Occorsio P, et al: A 6 day course of liposomal amphotericin B in the treatment of infantile visceral leishmaniasis: The Italian experience. *J Antimicrob Chemother* 2004;54:217–220.

Lockwood DNJ, Sundar S: Serological tests for visceral leishmaniasis. *BMJ* 2006;333:711–712.

Melby PC: Vaccination against cutaneous leishmaniasis: Current status. *Am J Clin Dermatol* 2002;3:557–570.

Murray HW: Treatment of visceral leishmaniasis in 2004. *Am J Trop Med Hyg* 2004;71:787–794.

Murray HW, Berman JD, Davies CR, et al: Advances in leishmaniasis. *Lancet* 2005;366:1561–1577.

Olliaro PL, Guerin PJ, Gerstl S, et al: Treatment options for visceral leishmaniasis: A systematic review of clinical studies done in India, 1980–2004. *Lancet Infect Dis* 2005;5:763–774.

Palacios R, Osorio LE, Grajales LF, et al: Treatment failure in children in a randomized clinical trial with 10 and 20 days of meglumine antimoniate for cutaneous leishmaniasis due to Leishmania Viannia species. *Am J Trop Med Hyg* 2001;64:187–193.

Soto J, Arana BA, Toledo J, et al: Miltefosine for New World cutaneous leishmaniasis. *Clin Infect Dis* 2004;38:1266–1272.

Sundar S, Mehta H, Suresh AV, et al: Amphotericin B treatment for Indian visceral leishmaniasis: Conventional versus lipid formulations. *Clin Infect Dis* 2004;38:377–383.

Chapter 283 ■ African Trypanosomiasis (Sleeping Sickness; *Trypanosoma Brucei* Complex)

Robert A. Bonomo and Robert A. Salata

There are >70 million men, women, and children in close to 40 countries throughout sub-Saharan Africa who suffer from African trypanosomiasis, or sleeping sickness. The burden of this re-emerging disease is highest in the most destitute of countries. The 2 forms of African trypanosomiasis are each caused by a protozoan parasite that causes a specific illness. One form, *Trypanosoma brucei gambiense,* causes a chronic infection lasting years and mostly affecting people who live in western and central Africa (**West African sleeping sickness**). A 2nd form, *Trypanosoma brucei rhodesiense,* is an acute illness lasting several weeks and usually occurring in residents of eastern and southern Africa (**East African sleeping sickness**).

ETIOLOGY. Human trypanosomiasis, or African sleeping sickness, is a vector-borne disease caused by a parasitic trypanosome that is transmitted to humans through the bite of a tsetse fly of the genus *Glossina,* which is found only in Africa. The range of the tsetse fly includes watercourses, lakes, forests, and the savanna.

The tsetse fly feeds on the blood of humans and wild game animals and penetrates intact mucous membranes or skin. Humans usually contract the East African form of disease *(Trypanosoma brucei rhodesiense)* when they venture from towns to rural areas to visit woodlands or livestock. Once inoculated in the skin, the trypanosomes proliferate and gradually invade all organs. The initial bite causes pain and swelling similar to what is seen in Chagas disease.

The West African form *(T. brucei gambiense)* is usually contracted close to settlements. This form only requires a small vector population and thus will be particularly difficult to eradicate. The infective metacyclic forms of the trypanosomes possess no free flagella. After a period of local multiplication in the skin for 1–3 wk, long and slender forms can be seen in the peripheral blood; intermediate and stumpy forms also occur. These are flagellated forms with a well-developed undulating membrane. In the early stages of human infection, the organisms multiply rapidly in the blood and lymph nodes. They appear in waves in the peripheral blood, with each wave followed by a febrile crisis. The reappearance of another population of organisms in the blood heralds the formation of a new antigenic variant. Invasion of the central nervous system (CNS) occurs early in *T. brucei rhodesiense* infection but late in the Gambian form.

The insect intermediate vectors are species of the tsetse flies of the genus *Glossina*. Inside the flies, the organisms localize in the posterior part of the midgut, where they multiply for about 10 days and then gradually migrate anteriorly, where they attach to the walls of the salivary ducts and complete the final stages of development into the infective metacyclic forms. The life cycle within the tsetse fly takes 15–35 days.

Direct transmission to humans has been reported, which occurs either mechanically through contact with the contaminated mouth parts of tsetse flies during feeding or congenitally to infants by way of the placenta of infected mothers (vertical transmission from mother to child).

EPIDEMIOLOGY. Trypanosomiasis is 1 of the major public health problems in sub-Saharan Africa. Human trypanosomiasis in Africa occurs primarily in the region between latitudes 15 degrees north and 15 degrees south, which corresponds roughly to the area where the annual rainfall creates optimal climatic conditions for *Glossina* flies. The greatest risk for contracting disease is in Uganda, Kenya, Tanzania, Malawi, Ethiopia, Zaire, and Botswana. It is at epidemic levels in Angola, the Democratic Republic of the Congo, Sudan, Cameroon, Ivory Coast, Tanzania, and Chad. In the Democratic Republic of the Congo, where 70% of the cases occur, the prevalence of African sleeping sickness has nearly reached that of AIDS. South Sudan, the Democratic Republic of Congo, and Angola have experienced serious epidemics of the Gambian form of the disease.

Each year >20,000–25,000 people are newly infected and 100,000 deaths from sleeping sickness occur, although data regarding the true incidence of the infection are unreliable. Inadequate surveillance, poor health systems, and limited diagnostic testing add to this burden. Political unrest and social change create favorable conditions for the emergence and resurgence of trypanosomiasis. Epidemics in rural areas pose a serious handicap to developing communities.

T. brucei rhodesiense infection is restricted to the eastern 1/3 of the endemic area in tropical Africa, stretching from Ethiopia to the northern boundaries of South Africa. *T. brucei gambiense* occurs mainly in the western half of the continent's endemic region.

T. brucei gambiense infection usually has a chronic protracted course with very low levels of parasitemia. Because of low rates of infection in tsetse flies, the life cycle of the Gambian form necessitates close and repeated contact between humans and insects to permit frequent biting. *T. brucei gambiense* is found in a variety of animal reservoirs that may play an important role in the endemic nature of the Gambian form of infection.

The insect intermediate vector plays a major role in determining the epidemiologic pattern of trypanosomiasis. Several *Glossina* species transmit the infection in different parts of tropical Africa. *Glossina* captured in endemic foci show a low rate of infection, usually <5%. In the Rhodesian form, which usually has an acute and often fatal course, chances of transmission to tsetse flies are greatly reduced. However, the ability of *T. brucei rhodesiense* to multiply enormously in the bloodstream of humans and to infect other species of mammals helps to maintain its life cycle. The length of time the insect vector is able to transmit disease is up to 6 mo. The long duration of infection in human hosts with cycles of intermittent parasitemia and the vector's feeding habits and the intensity of human-fly contact are the major determinants of the dynamics of transmission. East African sleeping sickness has also been diagnosed in the United States in returning travelers.

PATHOGENESIS. The initial entry site of the organisms soon develops into a hard, painful, red nodule known as a **trypanosomal chancre.** Histologically, it contains long, thin trypanosomes multiplying beneath the dermis and is surrounded by a lymphocytic cellular infiltrate. Dissemination into the blood and lymphatic systems follows, with subsequent localization in the CNS. The histopathologic findings in the brain are those of meningoencephalitis, with increased cellularity of the pia-arachnoid owing to lymphocyte infiltration and perivascular cuffing. In chronic cases the appearance of morular cells (large, strawberry-like cells, supposedly derived from plasma cells) is the most characteristic finding.

A key feature of trypanosomiasis is the ability of the parasite to evade the immune system by antigenic variation of **variant surface glycoproteins,** which enables evasion of acquired immunity during infection or in immune host populations. *T. brucei gambiense* regulates internal genetic switches to avoid immunologic attack by the host. Moreover, the mechanisms underlying virulence in human African trypanosomiasis are poorly understood. Disease severity appears to be related to unregulated host inflammatory responses.

CLINICAL MANIFESTATIONS. The clinical presentations vary not only because of the 2 subspecies of organisms but also because of differences in host response in the indigenous population of endemic areas and in newcomers or visitors. Visitors usually suffer more from the acute symptoms, but in untreated cases death is inevitable for natives and visitors alike. Symptoms usually occur within 1–4 wk of infection. Initially, these are nonspecific and include personality changes, weight loss, ataxia, fatigue during the day, and insomnia at night. The clinical syndromes of African trypanosomiasis are best described as the trypanosomal chancre, hemolymphatic stage, and meningoencephalitic stage.

TRYPANOSOMAL CHANCRE. The site of the tsetse fly bite may be the 1st presenting feature. A nodule or chancre develops in 2–3 days and within 1 wk becomes a painful, hard, red nodule surrounded by an area of erythema and swelling. Nodules are commonly seen on the lower limbs but sometimes also on the head. They subside spontaneously in about 2 wk, leaving no permanent scar.

Hemolymphatic Stage. The most common presenting features of acute African trypanosomiasis occur at the time of invasion of the bloodstream by the parasites, 2–3 wk after infection. Irregular episodes of fever, each lasting 1–7 days, are the usual early feature, frequently accompanied by headache, sweating, and generalized lymphadenopathy. Attacks may be separated by symptom-free intervals of days or even weeks. Painless, nonmatted lymphadenopathy, most commonly of the posterior cervical and supraclavicular nodes, is 1 of the most constant signs, particularly in the Gambian form. A common feature of trypanosomiasis in whites is the presence of blotchy, irregular, nonpruritic, erythematous macules, which may appear any time after the 1st febrile episode, usually within 6–8 wk. The majority of macules have a normal central area, giving the rash a circinate outline. This rash is seen mainly on the trunk and is evanescent, fading in 1 place only to appear at another site. Examination of the blood during this stage may show anemia, leukopenia with relative monocytosis, and elevated levels of immunoglobulin M.

Meningoencephalitic Stage. Neurologic symptoms and signs are generally nonspecific, including irritability, insomnia, and irrational and inexplicable anxieties with frequent changes in mood and personality. Neurologic symptoms may precede invasion of the CNS by the organisms. In untreated *T. brucei rhodesiense* infections, CNS invasion occurs within 3–6 wk and is associated with recurrent bouts of headache, fever, weakness, and signs of acute toxemia. Tachycardia may be evidence of myocarditis. Death occurs in 6–9 mo as a result of secondary infection or cardiac failure.

In the Gambian form, cerebral symptoms can be expected to appear within 2 yr after the onset of acute symptoms. A general increase in drowsiness during the day and insomnia at night reflect the continuous progression of infection, which may be further evidenced by increasing anemia, leukopenia, and wasting of body musculature. Patients with chronic Gambian trypanosomiasis have an increased susceptibility to secondary infections.

The chronic, diffuse meningoencephalitis without localizing symptoms is the form commonly known as **sleeping sickness.** Drowsiness and an uncontrollable urge to sleep are the major features of this stage of the disease and may become almost continuous in the terminal stages. Associated signs and symptoms, including tremor or rigidity with stiff and ataxic gait, suggest involvement of the basal ganglia. Psychotic changes occur in almost $^1/_3$ of untreated patients.

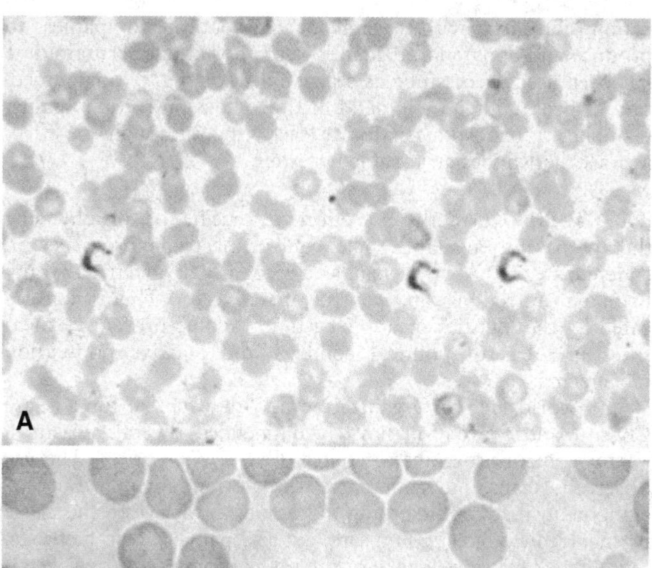

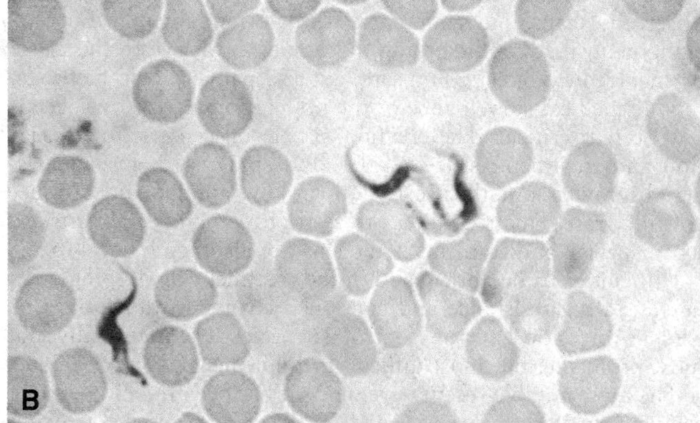

Figure 283-1. Blood films with *(A) Trypanosoma cruzi* trypomastigotes and *(B) Trypanosoma brucei* trypomastigotes. (From Barrett MP, Burchmore RJS, Stich A, et al: The trypanosomiases. *Lancet* 2003;363:1469–1480.)

DIAGNOSIS. There are 3 aspects to case management: screening, diagnosis, and phase diagnosis. Definitive diagnosis can be established during the early stages by examination of a fresh, thick blood smear, which permits visualization of the motile active forms (Fig. 283-1). In the bloodstream, the parasite can be detected using a variety of sensitive techniques: quantitative buffy coat smears and mini anion exchange resins are common examples. The **Card Agglutination Trypanosomiasis Test** (CATT) is of value for epidemiologic purposes and to screen for *T. brucei gambiense*. Dried, Giemsa-stained smears should be examined for the detailed morphologic features of the organisms. If a thick blood or buffy coat smear yields a negative finding, a simple concentration method may help; 10 mL of heparinized blood is added to 30 mL of 0.87% ammonium chloride, the mixture is centrifuged at 1,000 g for 15 min, and the sediment is examined fresh or by staining dried smears. Aspiration of an enlarged lymph node can also be used to obtain material for parasitologic examination. For every patient with a positive result, a sample of cerebrospinal fluid should also be examined for the organisms.

TREATMENT. The choice of chemotherapeutic agents for treatment depends on the stage of the infection and the causative organisms. The hematogenous forms of both Rhodesian and Gambian trypanosomiasis are susceptible to the action of suramin, which is available as a 10% solution for intravenous administration. A test dose (10 mg for children; 100–200 mg for adults) is first administered intravenously to detect the rare idiosyncratic reactions of shock and collapse. The dose for subsequent IV injections is 20 mg/kg (maximum 1 g) administered on days 1, 3, 7, 14, and 21. Suramin is nephrotoxic and therefore urinalysis should be performed before each dose. The presence of marked proteinuria, blood, or casts is a contraindication to continuation of suramin. Pentamidine isethionate (4 mg/kg/day IM for 10 days) is better tolerated than suramin.

If CNS invasion is present, melarsoprol should be used. Melarsoprol is an investigational arsenical compound with trypanosomicidal effects. It has been used outside the United States for the treatment of late hemolymphatic and CNS African trypanosomiasis. Treatment of children is initiated with melarsoprol 0.36 mg/kg/once daily IV, with the dose gradually increased every 1–5 days to 3.6 mg/once daily IV; treatment usually necessitates 10 doses (18–25 mg/kg total dose). Treatment of adults is with melarsoprol 2–3.6 mg/kg once daily IV for 3 days, and after 1 wk, 3.6 mg/kg once daily IV for 3 days, which is repeated after 10–21 days. Recommended guidelines suggest 18–25 mg/kg total over 1 mo. Mild reactions such as fever and pains in the chest or abdomen may rarely occur immediately or very soon after administration. The most important and serious toxic effects are encephalopathy and, less commonly, exfoliative dermatitis.

Eflornithine has been reported to be effective in late-stage West African sleeping sickness or in instances where CNS involvement is suspected or present. It is an alternative to melarsoprol. It is more effective against *T. brucei gambiense* and variably effective against *T. brucei rhodesiense*. It is in short supply and is given as 400 mg/kg/day divided every 6 hr IV. The World Health Organization contracts with several pharmaceutical companies to produce and donate large quantities of eflornithine. Pentamidine has been used successfully as a prophylactic drug. A single injection of pentamidine (3–4 mg/kg IM) provides protection against Gambian trypanosomiasis for at least 6 mo, although the effect against the Rhodesian form is uncertain.

PREVENTION. Currently, an effective vaccine or prophylactic therapy is not available. The control of trypanosomiasis in endemic areas of Africa depends on recognition, effective therapy of human infections, and control of the vector. This is complicated by the logistics of applying the available preventive measures in areas of political conflicts and massive population movements.

The World Health Organization and the Centers for Disease Control and Prevention have recommended several measures. Vector control programs to control *Glossina* is critical. The use of screens, traps, and sanitary measures is fundamental. Encouraging neutral-colored clothing that is not attractive to the tsetse fly may reduce bites. Using serology and parasitologic methods, mobile medical surveillance of the population at risk by specialized staff is critical. The creation of referral centers for evaluation and treatment is needed. Ground spraying of insecticides, aerial spraying, and the use of cloth and live animal baits are successful. Transgenic techniques to restrict the ability of the tsetse fly to survive and transmit pathogens are also being developed.

Difficulties to be anticipated in the treatment of sleeping sickness are drug resistance and continued change in range of antigenic expression. Vector control strategies are potentially the most promising but most difficult to implement.

The most notable recent development has been the full genome sequencing of the *T. brucei* and *T. cruzi* parasites. Sequencing revealed a conserved core proteome of about 6,200 genes in large gene clusters. This advance may help identify genes relevant to the disease and its prevention. Early release of the data allowed groups to identify many new drug targets and pathways (e.g., glycosylated phosphatidyl inositols [GPI] biosynthesis and isoprenoid metabolism). The genome of the bacterium that is essential to the survival and fecundity of the tsetse fly has recently been sequenced also. *Wigglesworthia glossinidia* lives in the tsetse fly's gut, where it produces nutrients required by the fly for its survival and successful reproduction. With the knowledge of this genome, it may be possible to use this bacterium as a vehicle to express foreign gene produces to affect the development of the parasite.

Allsop R: Options for vector control against trypanosomiasis in Africa. *Trends Parasitol* 2001;17:15–19.

Askoy S, Maudlin I, Dale C, et al: Prospects for control of African trypanosomiasis by tsetse vector manipulation. *Trends Parasitol* 2001;17:29–34.

Barrett MP: The rise and fall of sleeping sickness. *Lancet* 2006;367:1377–1378.

Barrett MP, Burchmore RJS, Stich A, et al: The trypanosomiases. *Lancet* 2003;363:1469–1480.

Fèvre EM, Picozzi K, Fyfe C, et al: A burgeoning epidemic of sleeping sickness in Uganda. *Lancet* 2005;366:745–747.

El-Sayed NM, Myler PJ, Blandin G, et al: Comparative genomics of trypanosomatid parasitic protozoa. *Science* 2005;309(5733):404–409.

Inojosa WO, Augusto I, Bisoffi Z, et al: Diagnosing human African trypanosomiasis in Angola using a card agglutination test: Observational study of active and passive case finding strategies. *Br Med J* 2006;332:1479–1481.

Pepin J, Meda H: The epidemiology and control of human African trypanosomiasis. *Adv Parasitol* 2001;49:71–132.

MacLean L, Chrisi JE, Odiit M, et al: Severity of human African trypanosomiasis in East Africa is associated with geographic location, parasite genotype, and host inflammatory cytokine response profile. *Infect Immun* 2004;72:7040–7044.

Chapter 284 ■ American Trypanosomiasis (Chagas Disease; *Trypanosoma Cruzi*)

Robert A. Bonomo and Robert A. Salata

Chagas disease (American trypanosomiasis) is a zoonotic illness caused by the blood-sucking triatomine insects, or "kissing bugs," the reduviid bugs that transmit the parasitic, hemoflagellate protozoan *Trypanosoma cruzi*.

ETIOLOGY. Of the nearly 20 species of *Trypanosoma*, only 4 species infect humans: *Trypanosoma cruzi*, the agent of Chagas disease; *Trypanosoma brucei rhodesiense* and *Trypanosoma brucei gambiense*, the agents of African trypanosomiasis or African sleeping sickness (see Chapter 283); and *Trypanosoma rangeli*. *T. cruzi* has 3 recognizable morphogenetic phases: amastigotes, trypomastigotes, and epimastigotes. **Amastigotes** are intracellular forms found in mammalian tissues that are spherical and have a short flagellum but form clusters of oval shapes (pseudocysts) within infected tissues. **Trypomastigotes** are the extracellular, nondividing forms that are spindle shaped, 20 µm long, and possess a large **kinetoplast**, which is a large complex mitochondrion containing DNA that stains darkly on routine smears. A **flagellum** arises from the **blepharoplast** and extends along the outer edge of the undulating membrane until it reaches the anterior end of the body. Trypomastigotes are found in blood and are responsible for transmission of infection to the insect vector and for cell-to-cell spread of infection. **Epimastigotes** are found in the midgut of the blood-sucking insects *Triatoma infestans*, *Rhodnius prolixus*, and *Panstrongylus megistus*. Epimastigotes multiply in the midgut and rectum of arthropods and differentiate into metacyclic trypomastigotes. Metacyclic trypomastigotes, the infectious form for humans, are released onto the skin of a human when the insect defecates close to the site of a bite. Hence, this is an infection caused by contamination, not inoculation. The trypomastigotes enter via damaged skin or mucous membranes either by infection of host epithelial cells or phagocytosis by macrophages. Once in the host, they multiply intracellularly as amastigotes and are released into the circulation when the cell dies. The blood-borne trypomastigotes circulate until they enter another host cell or are taken up by the bite of another insect, completing the life cycle.

EPIDEMIOLOGY. Chagas disease is found only in the Western hemisphere and is now endemic in 18 countries and in 2 ecological zones in the Americas: Mexico and South America, particularly Brazil, Argentina, Uruguay, Chile, and Venezuela. In South America, many vectors of disease live inside homes, while in Central America, Mexico, and the Andean mountains the vector of disease lives both inside and outside the home. As for African trypanosomiasis (see Chapter 283), millions of persons are infected and at risk for *T. cruzi* disease. The World Health Organization estimates that Chagas disease affects close to 20 million people, primarily children and young adults. Because of its high prevalence, *T. cruzi* is regarded as the most important endemic disease in South America, causing 45,000–70,000 deaths annually.

Infection is frequently asymptomatic and is essentially untreatable, persisting for life. Up to 30% of persons with chronic *T. cruzi* infection eventually develop symptoms. It is still unclear how this parasitic protozoan escapes the immune system because antigenic variation is not reported.

T. cruzi infection is primarily a zoonosis. Humans are not absolutely required to maintain the parasite in nature. *T. cruzi* has a large sylvan reservoir and has been isolated from numerous animal species. The presence of reservoirs and vectors of *T. cruzi* and the socioeconomic and educational levels of the population are the most important risk factors for vector-borne transmission to humans. The arthropod vectors for *T. cruzi* are the **reduviid insects,** or **triatomines,** and variably known as **wild bedbugs, assassin bugs,** or **kissing bugs.** *Triatoma infestans* is 1 of the prominent members of triatomines. The insect vectors are found in rural, wooded areas and become infected by ingesting blood from humans or animals with circulating trypomastigotes. Housing conditions are very important in the transmission chain. The incidence and prevalence of infection depend on the adaptation of the triatomines to human dwellings as well as the vector capacity of the species. The animal reservoirs of reduviid bugs are dogs, cats, rats, opossum, guinea pigs, monkeys, bats, and raccoons. In South America, uncontrolled deforestation, increased migration of infected humans from endemic to nonendemic areas, and the presence of domestic reservoir hosts facilitate spread. Humans often become infected when land in enzootic areas is developed for agricultural or commercial purposes. As the natural reservoir is disrupted, vectors take up residence in domestic areas and establish a cycle of transmission to animals and humans.

Although reduviid insects can be found in warmer regions of the United States as far north as Maryland, Chagas disease is extremely rare owing to the higher standard of domestic housing. Most cases in the United States are associated with laboratory accidents. Approximately 100,000 immigrants from endemic countries living in the USA may be infected with *T. cruzi,* and several cases have been reported among immigrants in American cities.

One of the greatest challenges is vertical transmission; humans can be infected transplacentally, as occurs in 10.5% of infected mothers, causing congenital Chagas disease that is associated with premature birth, fetal wastage, and placentitis. Up to 1,000 neonates infected with *T. cruzi* are born every year in Argentina. Disease transmission may also occur through blood transfusions in endemic areas from asymptomatic blood donors. Seropositivity rates in blood donors from endemic areas are >20%. The risk for transmission through a single blood transfusion from a chagasic donor is 13–23%. Currently, blood in the southern United States is not screened for *T. cruzi.* Percutaneous injection as a result of laboratory accidents is also a documented mode of transmission. Oral transmission through contaminated food has been reported. Although breast-feeding is a very uncommon mode of transmission, women with acute infections should not nurse until they have been treated.

PATHOGENESIS. Although the pathogenesis of chronic Chagas disease is unknown, 2 main mechanisms have been proposed: direct tissue destruction by the parasite; and development of an inflammatory reaction resulting from an allergic response to parasitic antigens absorbed by host cells or an autoimmune reaction resulting from shared antigens between host and parasite.

At the site of entry, or puncture site, polymorphonuclear neutrophils, lymphocytes, macrophages, and monocytes infiltrate. *T. cruzi* organisms are engulfed by macrophages and are sequestered in membrane-bound vacuoles. Parasite attachment and phagocytosis by macrophages are mediated by protease-sensitive receptors on the surface of the macrophage. Trypanosomes lyse the phagosome membrane, escape into the cytoplasm, and replicate. A local tissue reaction, the **chagoma,** develops and the process extends to a local lymph node. Blood forms appear next, and the process disseminates.

T. cruzi strains demonstrate selective parasitism for certain tissues. Most strains are myotropic and invade smooth, skeletal, and heart muscle cells. Attachment is mediated by specific receptors on the trypomastigotes that attach to complementary glycoconjugates on the host cell surface. Attachment to cardiac muscle results in inflammation of the endocardium and myocardium, edema, focal necrosis in the contractile and conducting systems, periganglionitis, and lymphocytic inflammation. The heart becomes enlarged, and endocardial thrombosis or aneurysm may result. Right bundle branch block is also common. Trypanosome parasites also attach to neural cells and reticuloendothelial cells. In patients with gastrointestinal tract involvement, myenteric plexus destruction leads to organ dilatation (e.g., megaesophagus and megacolon).

Immunologic mechanisms for control of parasitism and resistance are not completely understood. Despite strong acquired immunity, there is no parasitologic cure. Antigenic variation that is typical of African trypanosomiasis is not seen with American trypanosomiasis. Antibodies involved with resistance to *T. cruzi* are related to the phase of infection. Immunoglobulin G (IgG) antibodies, probably to several major surface antigens, mediate immunophagocytosis of *T. cruzi* by macrophages. Conditions associated with depression of cell-mediated immunity increase the severity of *T. cruzi* infection. Macrophages probably play a major role in protection against *T. cruzi* infection, especially in the acute phase. Interferon-γ stimulates macrophage killing of amastigotes through oxidative mechanisms. Specific type 1 immune responses (CCR5 and CXCR3) are often seen associated with the development of heart pathology.

CLINICAL MANIFESTATIONS. Chagas disease occurs in acute and chronic forms. **Acute Chagas disease** in children is usually asymptomatic or is associated with a mild febrile illness characterized by malaise, facial edema, and lymphadenopathy. Infants often demonstrate local signs of inflammation at the site of parasite entry, or chagomas. Approximately 50% of children come to medical attention with the **Romaña sign** (unilateral, painless eye swelling), conjunctivitis, and preauricular lymphadenitis. Patients complain of fatigue and headache. Fever can persist for 4–5 wk. More severe systemic presentations can occur in children <2 yr of age and include lymphadenopathy, hepatosplenomegaly, and meningoencephalitis. A cutaneous morbilliform eruption can accompany the acute syndrome. Anemia, lymphocytosis, hepatitis, and thrombocytopenia have been described.

The heart, central nervous system, peripheral nerve ganglia, and reticuloendothelial system are often heavily parasitized. The heart is the primary target organ. The intense parasitism can result in acute inflammation and in 4 chamber cardiac dilatation. Diffuse myocarditis and inflammation of the conduction system lead to the development of fibrosis. Histologic examination reveals the characteristic pseudocysts, which are the intracellular aggregates of amastigotes.

Intrauterine infection in pregnant women can cause spontaneous abortion or premature birth. In children with congenital infection, severe anemia, hepatosplenomegaly, jaundice, and convulsions can mimic congenital cytomegalovirus infection, toxoplasmosis, and erythroblastosis fetalis. *T. cruzi* can be visualized in the cerebrospinal fluid in meningoencephalitis. Children usually undergo spontaneous remission in 8–12 wk and enter an indeterminate phase with lifelong low-grade parasitemia and development of antibodies to many *T. cruzi* cell surface antigens. The mortality rate is 5–10%, with deaths caused by acute myocarditis with resultant heart failure, or meningoencephalitis. Acute Chagas disease must be differentiated from malaria, schistosomiasis, visceral leishmaniasis, brucellosis, typhoid fever, and infectious mononucleosis.

Chronic Chagas disease may be asymptomatic or symptomatic. The most common presentation of chronic *T. cruzi* infection is **cardiomyopathy** manifested by congestive heart failure, arrhythmia, and thromboembolic events. Electrocardiographic abnormalities include partial or complete atrioventricular block and right bundle branch block. Left bundle branch block is unusual. Pathologic examination of infected heart muscle reveals muscle atrophy, myonecrosis, myocytolysis, fibrosis, and lymphocytic infiltration. Myocardial infarction has been reported and may be secondary to left apical aneurysm embolization or necrotizing arteriolitis of the microvasculature. Left ventricular apical aneurysms are pathognomonic of chronic chagasic cardiomyopathy.

Autonomic nervous system abnormalities have also been implicated in Chagas cardiomyopathy. The reduction in acetylcholine and choline acetyltransferase levels in experimental *T. cruzi* infection lends support to this notion.

Autoimmune abnormalities have been reported in Chagas cardiomyopathy. Depletion of CD8 cells accelerates infection. *T. cruzi*–infected human peripheral blood mononuclear and endothelial cells synthesize increased levels of interleukin 1β (IL-1β), IL-6, and tumor necrosis factor (TNF). These cytokines result in increasing leukocyte recruitment and smooth muscle cell proliferation, which may be responsible for some of the manifestations of the disease. Viral myocarditis, rheumatic heart disease, and endomyocardial fibrosis can mimic chronic chagasic cardiomyopathy.

Gastrointestinal manifestations of chronic Chagas disease occur in 8–10% of patients and involve a diminution in Auerbach plexus and Meissner plexus. There are also preganglionic lesions and a reduction in the number of dorsal motor nuclear cells of the vagus nerve. Characteristically, this involvement presents clinically as **megaesophagus** and **megacolon.** Sigmoid dilatation, volvulus, and fecalomas are often found in megacolon. Loss of ganglia in the esophagus results in abnormal dilatation, or megaesophagus; the esophagus can reach up to 26 times its normal weight and hold up to 2 L of excess fluid. Megaesophagus presents as dysphagia, odynophagia, and cough. Esophageal body abnormalities occur independently of lower esophageal dysfunction. Megaesophagus can lead to esophagitis and cancer of the esophagus. Aspiration pneumonia and pulmonary tuberculosis are more common in patients with megaesophagus.

Autonomic dysfunction and peripheral neuropathy can occur. Central nervous system involvement in Chagas disease is uncommon. If granulomatous encephalitis occurs in the acute infection, it is usually fatal.

Immunocompromised Persons. *T. cruzi* infections in immunocompromised persons are caused by transmission from an asymptomatic donor of blood products or activation of prior infection by immunosuppression. Organ donation to allograft recipients can result in a devastating form of the illness. Cardiac transplantation for Chagas cardiomyopathy has resulted in reactivation, despite prophylaxis and postoperative treatment with benznidazole. HIV infection also leads to reactivation; cerebral lesions are more common in these patients and can mimic those of toxoplasmic encephalitis. In immunocompromised patients at risk for reactivation, serologic testing and close monitoring are necessary.

DIAGNOSIS. A careful history with attention to geographic origin and travel is important. Microscopic examination of a fresh preparation of a **peripheral blood smear** or a Giemsa-stained smear during the acute phase of illness will demonstrate motile trypanosomes, which is diagnostic for Chagas disease (see Fig. 283-1). These are only seen in the peripheral blood in the 1st 6–12 wk of the illness. Buffy coat smears may improve yield.

Most persons seek medical attention during the chronic phase of the disease, when parasites are not found in the bloodstream and clinical symptoms are not diagnostic. Serologic testing is also a good means of diagnosis. Complement fixation is considered the most reliable immunodiagnostic method for establishing the diagnosis. Specific IgM antibodies can be detected using an enzyme-linked immunosorbent assay (ELISA) and indirect fluorescent antibody testing. Indirect fluorescent antibody testing is very accurate and can be used to distinguish acute chagasic infection, with IgM antibodies, from chronic infection, with only IgG antibodies. These tests are available from the Centers for Disease Control and Prevention (CDC). Because false-positive reactions can result from other infections (e.g., malaria, syphilis, and leishmaniasis), it is recommended that a minimum of 2 independent serologic tests be performed.

Nonimmunologic methods of diagnosis are also available. Mouse inoculation has been used when repeated peripheral smear results are negative. Xenodiagnosis, allowing uninfected reduviid bugs to feed on a patient's blood and examining the intestinal contents of those bugs 30 days after the meal, detects 100% of cases. Detection assays using polymerase chain reaction (PCR) amplification of nuclear and kinetoplast DNA sequences are in development. Parasites may be cultivated in Nicole-Novy-MacNeal media. PCR has a sensitivity of 96–100% and is able to detect a single parasite in 20 mL of blood. Chemiluminescent ELISAs are being developed and are also reported to be highly sensitive and specific.

TREATMENT. Drug treatment for *T. cruzi* infection is generally limited to 2 drugs: nifurtimox and benznidazole. Both are effective against trypomastigotes and amastigotes and have been used to eradicate parasites in the acute stages of infection. The results vary according to the phase of Chagas disease, duration of treatment, dose, age of the patient, and geographic origin of the patient. Neither drug is safe in pregnancy. There are few trials establishing the effectiveness of preventive therapy or therapy in asymptomatic individuals. Therapy is further complicated in the patient with Chagas disease and infection with HIV.

Nifurtimox has been used most extensively, but whether it is effective in the chronic phase of the illness is uncertain. It is available from the CDC. The treatment regimen for children 1–10 yr of age is 15–20 mg/kg/day divided qid PO for 90 days; for children 11–16 yr of age, 12.5–15 mg/kg/day divided qid PO for 90 days; and for children >16 yr of age, 8–10 mg/kg/day divided tid to qid PO for 90–120 days. Nifurtimox interferes with the carbohydrate metabolism of the parasite by disrupting pyruvic acid synthesis. Because *T. cruzi* is partially deficient in free radical detoxification mechanisms, it is susceptible to such intermediates. Nifurtimox has been associated with weakness, anorexia, gastrointestinal disturbances, toxic hepatitis, tremors, seizures, and hemolysis in patients with glucose-6-phosphate dehydrogenase deficiency. The mode of action of nifurtimox involves generation of nitro-anion radicals by nitroreductases that lead to reactive intermediates.

Benznidazole is a nitroimidazole derivative that is also used and may be more effective than nifurtimox. The mode of action of benznidazole is more complex than that of nifurtimox. The recommended treatment regimen for children <12 yr of age is 10 mg/kg/day divided bid PO for 60 days, and for those >12 yr of age, 5–7 mg/kg/day PO for 60 days. In 1 randomized, double-blind, placebo-controlled trial in a rural area of Brazil, a 60 day course of benznidazole was studied in the treatment of early chronic phase *T. cruzi* infection in schoolchildren 7–12 yr of age. The efficacy of benznidazole was 55.8% in producing negative seroconversion. This drug is also associated with significant toxicities, including rash, photosensitivity, peripheral neuritis, and granulocytopenia and thrombocytopenia. Of some concern are the reports that detail the development of lymphomas in laboratory animals treated with benznidazole. This finding has not been reported in humans.

Regardless of the clinical status or the time elapsed since infection, patients with chronic asymptomatic Chagas disease should be treated with nifurtimox or benznidazole. Nitroimidazolic derivatives substantially reduced and significantly modified parasite-related outcomes compared with placebo. Benznidazole has the greatest effect. It is yet unclear if recombinant interferon-γ should be used in immunocompromised patients.

Biochemical differences between the metabolism of American trypanosomes and that of mammalian hosts may be exploited for chemotherapy. These trypanosomes are very sensitive to oxidative radicals, and they do not possess catalase or glutathione reductase/glutathione peroxidase, which are key enzymes in scavenging free radicals. All trypanosomes also have an unusual reduced nicotinamide-adenine dinucleotide phosphate (NADPH)-dependent disulfide reductase. For this reason, drugs that stimulate H_2O_2 generation or prevent its utilization are potential trypanocidal agents.

Treatment of heart failure and arrhythmia, as well as prevention of thromboembolism, requires the use of diuretics, antiarrhythmics, and anticoagulants. Digitalis toxicity occurs frequently in patients with Chagas cardiomyopathy. Pacemakers may be necessary in cases of severe heart block. According to the Cochrane Database, there is insufficient evidence to support the efficacy of nitrofurans or imidazolic drugs as recommended treatment in *T. cruzi* cardiomyopathy and chronic *T. cruzi* infections. A well-designed randomized controlled trial is necessary to establish if new drugs are suitable for treatment of cardiac patients with cardiomyopathy. Although cardiac transplantation has been successful in chagasic patients, further study is needed.

A light, balanced diet is recommended for megaesophagus. Surgery or dilation of the lower esophageal sphincter treats megaesophagus; pneumatic dilation is the superior mode of therapy. Nitrates and nifedipine have been used to reduce lower esophageal sphincter pressure in patients with megaesophagus. Treatment of megacolon is surgical and symptomatic. Treatment of meningoencephalitis is also supportive.

In accidental infection when parasitic penetration is certain, treatment should be immediately initiated and continued for 10–15 days. Blood is usually collected and serologic samples tested for seroconversion at 15, 30, and 60 days.

PREVENTION. No vaccine or prophylactic therapy is currently available, although vaccine development is under way. An international program has been established in endemic areas (Argentina, Bolivia, Brazil, Uruguay, Paraguay, and Chile) to help eliminate transmission. Screening of emigrants from endemic areas may significantly reduce transmission. Education of residents in endemic areas, use of bed nets, use of insecticides such as dieldrin or lindane, and destruction of adobe houses that harbor reduviid bugs are effective methods to control the bug population. Synthetic pyrethroid insecticides help keep houses free of vectors for 2 yr and have low toxicity for humans. Paints incorporating insecticides have also been used. Vaccine development has been fruitless. Prophylactic therapy with nifurtimox or benznidazole should be considered only for laboratory accidents.

Blood transfusions in endemic areas are a significant risk. Gentian violet, an amphophilic cationic agent that acts photodynamically, has been used to kill the parasite in blood. Photoirradiation of blood containing gentian violet and ascorbate generates free radicals and superoxide anions that are trypanocidal. Mepacrine and maprotiline have also been used to eradicate the parasite in blood transfusions.

Because immigrants can carry this disease to nonendemic areas, serologic testing should be performed in blood and organ donors from endemic areas. Potential seropositive donors can be identified by determining whether they have been or have spent extensive time in an endemic area. Questionnaire-based screening of potentially infected blood and organ donors from areas endemic for infection can reduce the risk for transmission. Seropositivity should be considered a contraindication to organ donation.

In December 2006, the FDA licensed a new screening test for the presence of *T. cruzi* antibodies in blood donations called the Ortho *T. cruzi* ELISA Test System. This is the first batch test approved by the FDA. It is estimated that up to 11,000,000 people in the Americans are infected with *T. cruzi* and up to 100,000 persons infected with *T. cruzi* may be living in the United States. Unfortunately, seven cases of the transfusion-transmitted *T. cruzi* and five cases of organ-transmitted *T. cruzi* have been reported in the United States since 1987. Many other cases may have occurred but have not been recognized. If blood donors test positive, components and other donations from these donors should be quarantines and destroyed or used for research following appropriate labeling. This look-back should use protocols similar to those used for donors seropositive for hepatitis C.

Almeida IC, Covas DT, Soussumi LM, et al: A highly sensitive and specific chemiluminescent enzyme linked immunoabsorbent assay for the diagnosis of acute *Trypanosoma cruzi* infection. *Transfusion* 1997;37:850–857.

de Andrade AL, Zicker F, de Oliveira RM, et al: Randomized trial of the efficacy of benznidazole in the treatment of early *Trypanosoma cruzi* infection. *Lancet* 1996;348:1407–1413.

Docampo R, Moreno SN, Cruz FS: Enhancement of the cytotoxicity of crystal violet against *Trypanosoma cruzi* in blood by ascorbate. *Mol Biochem Parasitol* 1988;27:241–247.

Prata A: Clinical and epidemiological aspects of Chagas' disease. *Lancet Infect Dis* 2001;l:92–100.

Rodrigues Coura JR, de Castro SL: A critical review on Chagas disease chemotherapy. *Mem Inst Oswaldo Cruz* 2002;97:3–24.

Villar JC, Marin-Neto JA, Ebrahim S, et al: Trypanocidal drugs for chronic asymptomatic *Trypanosoma cruzi* infection (Cochrane Review). *Cochrane Database Syst Rev* 2002:CD003463.

Chapter 285 ■ Malaria *(Plasmodium)*

Peter J. Krause

Malaria is an acute and chronic illness characterized by paroxysms of fever, chills, sweats, fatigue, anemia, and splenomegaly. It has played a major role in human history, having arguably caused more harm to more people than any other infectious disease. Malaria is of overwhelming importance in the developing world today, with an estimated 300–500 million cases and >1 million deaths each year. Most malarial deaths occur among infants and young children. Although there is no endemic malaria in the United States, approximately 1,000 imported cases are recognized each year. Physicians practicing in nonendemic areas should consider the diagnosis of malaria in any febrile child who has returned from a malaria-endemic area within the previous year because delay in diagnosis and treatment can result in severe illness or death.

ETIOLOGY. Malaria is caused by intracellular *Plasmodium* protozoa transmitted to humans by female *Anopheles* mosquitoes. Four species of *Plasmodium* cause malaria in humans: *P. falciparum, P. malariae, P. ovale,* and *P. vivax*. Malaria also can be transmitted through blood transfusion, use of contaminated needles, and from a pregnant woman to her fetus. The risk for blood transmission is small and decreasing in the USA but may occur by way of whole blood, packed red blood cells, platelets, leukocytes, and organ transplantation.

EPIDEMIOLOGY. Malaria is a major worldwide problem occurring in >100 countries with a combined population of >1.6 billion people. The principal areas of transmission are Africa, Asia, and South America. *P. falciparum* and *P. malariae* are found in most malarious areas. *P. falciparum* is the predominant species in Africa, Haiti, and New Guinea. *P. vivax* predominates in Bangladesh, Central America, India, Pakistan, and Sri Lanka. *P. vivax* and *P. falciparum* predominate in Southeast Asia, South America, and Oceania. *P. ovale,* the least common species, is transmitted primarily in Africa. Transmission of malaria has been eliminated in most of North America (including the United States), Europe, and the Caribbean, as well as Australia, Chile, Israel, Japan, Korea, Lebanon, and Taiwan. Most cases of malaria in the United States occur among previously infected visitors to the United States from endemic areas and U.S. citizens who travel to endemic areas without appropriate chemoprophylaxis. The most common regions of acquisition of the 10,100 cases of malaria reported to the Centers for Disease Control and Prevention (CDC) among U.S. citizens between 1985 and 2001 were sub-Saharan Africa (58%), Asia (18%), and the Caribbean and Central or South America (16%). Most of the fatal cases were caused by *P. falciparum* (66 of the 70 cases, or 94%), of which 47 (71%) were acquired in sub-Saharan Africa. Since 1957, 63 indigenous cases have been documented in the United States. It is likely that untreated patients with malaria acquired in an endemic country traveled to the United States and infected local mosquitoes that subsequently transmitted the disease to others.

PATHOGENESIS. *Plasmodium* species exist in a variety of forms and have a complex life cycle that enables them to survive in different cellular environments in the human host (asexual phase) and the mosquito vector (sexual phase). A marked amplification of *Plasmodium,* from approximately 10^2 to as many as 10^{14} organisms, occurs during a 2 step process in humans, with the 1st phase in hepatic cells (exoerythrocytic phase) and the 2nd in the red blood cells (erythrocytic phase). The **exoerythrocytic phase** begins with inoculation of sporozoites into the bloodstream by a female *Anopheles* mosquito. Within minutes, the sporozoites enter the hepatocytes where they develop and multiply asexually as a **schizont.** After 1–2 wk, the hepatocytes rupture and release thousands of merozoites into the circulation. The tissue schizonts of *P. falciparum* and *P. malaria* rupture once and do not persist in the liver. There are 2 types of tissue schizonts for *P. ovale* and *P. vivax.* The primary type ruptures in 6–9 days, while a secondary type remains dormant in the liver cell in the **hypnozoite** form for weeks, months, or as long as 5 yr before releasing merozoites, and thereby causing relapses of infection. The **erythrocytic phase** of *Plasmodium* asexual development begins when the merozoites from the liver penetrate erythrocytes. Once inside the erythrocyte, the parasite transforms into the **ring form,** which then enlarges to become a **trophozoite.** These latter 2 forms can be identified with Giemsa stain on blood smear, the primary means of confirming the diagnosis of malaria (Fig. 285-1). The trophozoite multiplies asexually to produce a number of small erythrocytic **merozoites** that are released into the bloodstream when the erythrocyte membrane ruptures, which is associated with fever. Over time, some of the merozoites develop into male and female **gametocytes** that complete the *Plasmodium* life cycle when they are ingested during a blood meal by the female *Anopheline* mosquito. The male and female gametocytes fuse to form a **zygote** in the stomach cavity of the mosquito. After a series of further transformations, sporozoites enter the salivary gland of the mosquito and are inoculated into a new host with the next blood meal.

Four important pathologic processes have been identified in patients with malaria: fever, anemia, immunopathologic events, and tissue anoxia. Fever occurs when erythrocytes rupture and release merozoites into the circulation. Anemia is caused by hemolysis, sequestration of erythrocytes in the spleen and other organs, and bone marrow suppression. Immunopathologic events that have been documented in patients with malaria include polyclonal activation resulting in both hypergammaglobulinemia and the formation of immune complexes, immunodepression, and excessive production of proinflammatory cytokines (tumor necrosis factor) that may produce most of the pathology including tissue hypoxia. Cytoadherence of infected erythrocytes to vascular endothelium occurs with *P. falciparum* malaria that may lead to obstruction of blood flow and capillary damage with resultant vascular leakage of blood, protein and fluid, and tissue hypoxia. Hypoglycemia and lactic acidosis are due to anaerobic metabolism. The cumulative effects of these processes may lead to cerebral, cardiac, pulmonary, intestinal, and hepatic failure.

Immunity after *Plasmodium* infection is incomplete so that severe disease is averted but complete eradication or prevention of future infection is not achieved. In some cases parasites circulate in small numbers for a long time but are prevented from rapidly multiplying and causing severe illness. Repeated episodes of infection occur because the parasite has developed a number of immune evasive strategies, such as intracellular replication, vascular cytoadherence that prevents infected erythrocytes from circulating through the spleen, rapid antigenic variation, and alteration of the host immune system that includes partial immune suppression. The human host response to *Plasmodium* infection includes natural immune mechanisms that prevent infection by other *Plasmodium* species, such as those of birds or rodents, as well as several alterations in erythrocyte physiology that prevent or modify malarial infection. Erythrocytes containing hemoglobin S (sickle erythrocytes) resist malaria parasite growth, erythrocytes lacking Duffy blood group antigen are resistant to *P. vivax,* and erythrocytes containing hemoglobin F (fetal hemoglobin) and ovalocytes are resistant to *P. falciparum.* In hyperendemic areas, newborns rarely become ill with malaria, in part owing to passive maternal antibody and high levels of fetal hemoglobin. Children 3 mo to 2–5 yr of age have little specific immunity to malaria species and therefore suffer yearly attacks of debilitating and potentially fatal disease. Immunity is subsequently acquired, and severe cases of malaria become less common. Severe disease may occur during pregnancy or after extended residence outside the endemic region. In general, extracellular *Plasmodium* organisms are targeted by antibody, whereas intracellular organisms are targeted by cellular defenses such as T lymphocytes, macrophages, polymorphonuclear leukocytes, and the spleen.

CLINICAL MANIFESTATIONS. Children and adults are asymptomatic during the initial phase, the incubation period of malaria infection. The usual incubation periods are *P. falciparum,* 9–14 days; *P. vivax,* 12–17 days; *P. ovale,* 16–18 days; and *P. malariae,* 18–40 days. The incubation period can be as long as 6–12 mo for *P. vivax,* and can also be prolonged for patients with partial immunity or incomplete chemoprophylaxis. A prodrome lasting 2–3 days is noted in some patients before parasites are detected in the blood. Prodromal symptoms include headache, fatigue, anorexia, myalgia, slight fever, and pain in the chest, abdomen, and joints.

The classic presentation of malaria, seldom noted with other infectious diseases, consists of **paroxysms** of fever alternating with periods of fatigue but otherwise relative wellness. Febrile paroxysms are characterized by high fever, rigors, sweats, and headache, as well as myalgia, back pain, abdominal pain, nausea, vomiting, diarrhea, pallor, and jaundice. Paroxysms coincide with the rupture of schizonts that occurs every 48 hr with *P. vivax* and *P. ovale* and result in every other day fever spikes. Rupture of schizonts occurs every 72 hr with *P. malariae* and results in fever spikes every 3rd or 4th day. Periodicity is less apparent with *P. falciparum* and mixed infections. Patients with primary infection, such as travelers from nonendemic regions, also may have irregular symptomatic episodes for 2–3 days before regular paroxysms begin. Children with malaria often have special clinical features that differ from those of adults. In children >2 mo of age who are nonimmune, symptoms of malaria vary widely from low-grade fever and headache to a temperature of >104°F with headache, drowsiness, anorexia, nausea, vomiting, diarrhea, pallor, cyanosis, splenomegaly, hepatomegaly, anemia, thrombocytopenia, a normal or low leukocyte count, or any combination of these manifestations. Severe, high-risk malaria is characterized by a depressed level of consciousness, seizures, irregular respirations or airway obstruction, hypoxia, hypotension, tachycardia, dehydration, hypoglycemia, metabolic acidosis, and hyperkalemia.

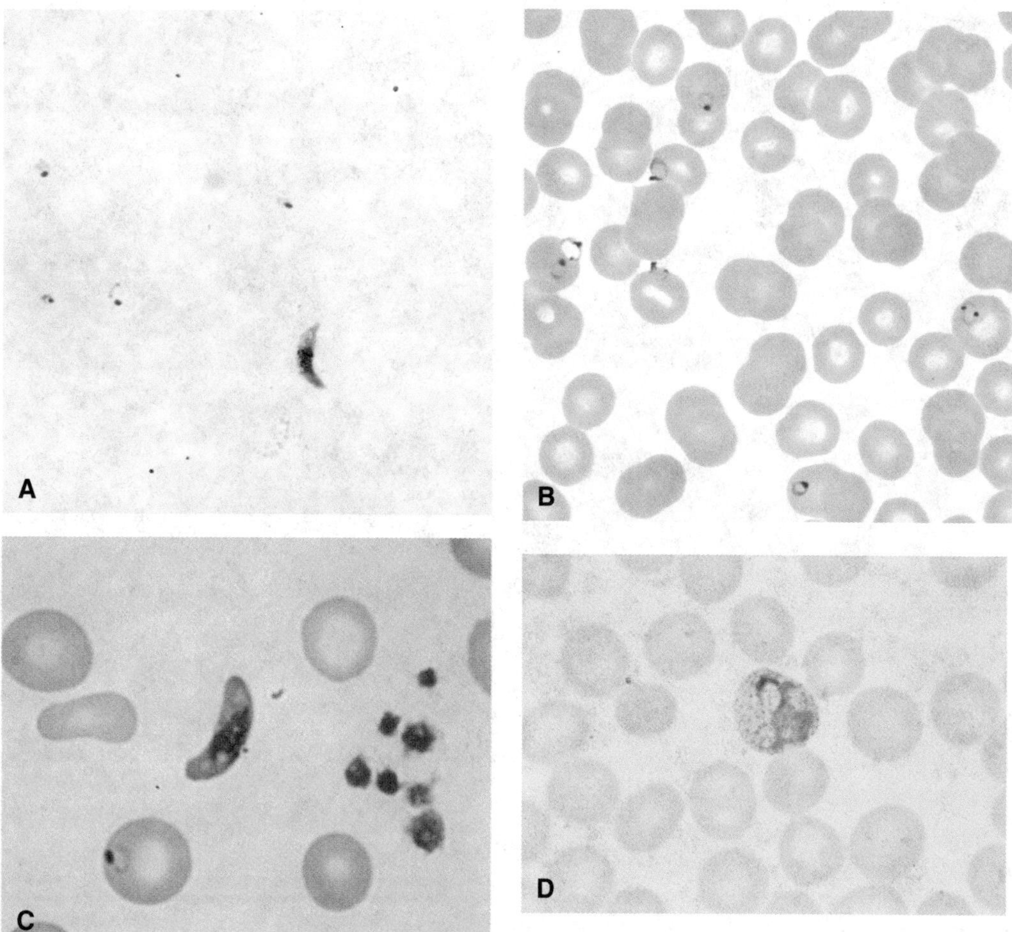

Figure 285-1. Giemsa-stained thick *(A)* and thin *(B–H)* smears used for the diagnosis of malaria and the speciation of *Plasmodium* parasites. *A,* Multiple signet-ring *Plasmodium falciparum* trophozoites, which are visualized outside erythrocytes. *B,* A multiply infected erythrocyte containing signet-ring *P. falciparum* trophozoites, including an accolade form positioned up against the inner surface of the erythrocyte membrane. *C,* Banana-shaped gametocyte unique to *P. falciparum. D,* Ameboid trophozoite characteristic of *Plasmodium vivax.* Both *P. vivax*–and *Plasmodium ovale*–infected erythrocytes exhibit Schuffner dots and tend to be enlarged compared with uninfected erythrocytes.

Recrudescence after a primary attack may occur from the survival of erythrocyte forms in the bloodstream. Long-term relapse is caused by release of merozoites from an exoerythrocytic source in the liver, which occurs with *P. vivax* and *P. ovale,* or persistence within the erythrocyte, which occurs with *P. malariae.* A history of typical symptoms in a person more than a few weeks after return from an endemic area therefore indicates *P. vivax, P. ovale,* or *P. malariae* infection.

P. falciparum is the most severe form of malaria and is associated with more intense parasitemia. The diagnosis of *P. falciparum* malaria constitutes a medical emergency. Fatality rates of up to 25% in nonimmune adults and 30% in nonimmune infants occur if appropriate therapy is not instituted promptly. In contrast to malaria caused by *P. ovale, P. vivax,* and *P. malariae,* which usually results in parasitemia of <2%, malaria caused by *P. falciparum* can reach >60% because *P. falciparum* infects both immature and mature erythrocytes while *P. ovale* and *P. vivax* primarily infect immature erythrocytes, and *P. malariae* infects only mature erythrocytes. *P. falciparum* is most commonly associated with serious complications, although milder or asymptomatic infections occur in persons with partially immunity.

P. vivax malaria generally is less severe than *P. falciparum* malaria but may cause death from ruptured spleen. Relapse of *P. vivax* malaria may occur if antihepatic malaria treatment is not given and is common within 6 mo after an acute attack but may occur as long as 5 yr after initial infection. *P. malariae* is the mildest and most chronic of all malaria infections. **Recrudescence** has been observed 30–50 yr after an acute attack. Although parasitemia is often low, untreated *P. malariae* can cause chronic ill health in addition to acute febrile illness. *P. ovale* malaria is the least common type of malaria. It is similar to *P. vivax* malaria and commonly is found in conjunction with *P. falciparum* malaria.

Congenital malaria is acquired from the mother prenatally or perinatally and is a serious problem in tropical areas but is rarely reported in the United States. In endemic areas, congenital malaria is an important cause of abortions, miscarriages, stillbirths, premature births, intrauterine growth retardation, and neonatal deaths. Congenital malaria usually occurs in the offspring of a nonimmune mother with *P. vivax* or *P. malariae* infection, although it can be observed with any of the human malaria species. The 1st sign or symptom most commonly occurs between 10 and 30 days of age (range 14 hr to several months of age). Signs and symptoms include fever, restlessness, drowsiness, pallor, jaundice, poor feeding, vomiting, diarrhea, cyanosis, and hepatosplenomegaly. Malaria is often severe during pregnancy and may have an adverse effect on the fetus or neonate owing to maternal illness or placental infection even in the absence of transmission from mother to child.

DIAGNOSIS. Any child who presents with fever or unexplained systemic illness who has traveled or resided in a malaria-endemic

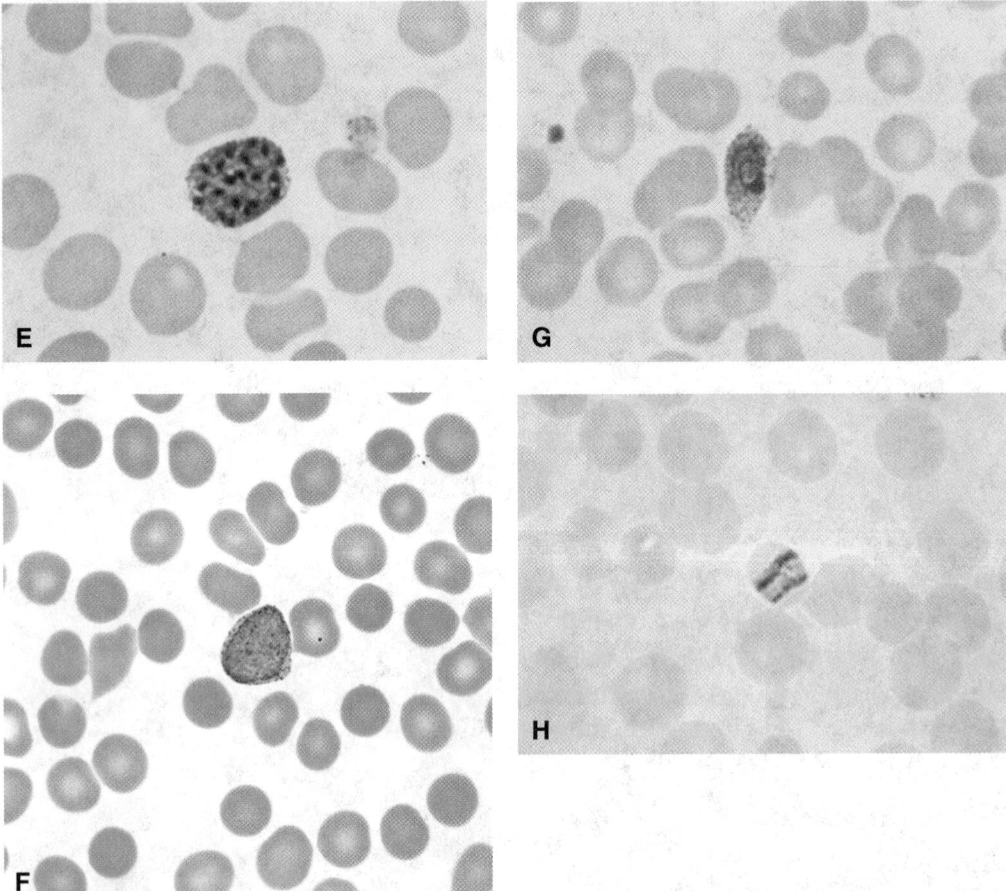

Figure 285-1, cont'd. *E, P. vivax* schizont. Mature *P. falciparum* parasites, by contrast, are rarely seen on blood smears because they sequester in the systemic microvasculature. *F, P. vivax* spherical gametocyte. *G, P. ovale* trophozoite. Note Schuffner dots and ovoid shapes of the infected erythrocyte. *H,* Characteristic band form trophozoite of *Plasmodium malariae,* containing intracellular pigment hemozoin. (Images A, B, and F were kindly provided by DPDx [website of the Centers for Disease Control and Prevention for parasitology identification] at www.dpd.cdc.gov/dpdx/. Images C, D, E, G, and H were contributed by David Wyler, Newton Centre, Massachusetts.)

area within the previous year should be assumed to have life-threatening malaria until proven otherwise. Malaria should be considered regardless of the use of chemoprophylaxis. Important criteria that suggest *P. falciparum* malaria include symptoms occurring <1 mo after return from an endemic area, intense parasitemia (>2%), ring forms with double chromatin dots, and erythrocytes infected with more than 1 parasite.

The diagnosis of malaria is established by identification of organisms on Giemsa-stained smears of peripheral blood (see Fig. 285-1). Giemsa stain is superior to Wright stain or Leishman stain. Both thick and thin blood smears should be examined. The concentration of erythrocytes on a **thick smear** is 20–40 times that on a thin smear and is used to quickly scan large numbers of erythrocytes. The **thin smear** allows for positive identification of the malaria species and determination of the percentage of infected erythrocytes. The latter is useful in following the response to therapy. Identification of the species is best made by an experienced microscopist and checked against color plates of the various *Plasmodium* species (see Fig. 285-1). Although *P. falciparum* is most likely to be identified from blood just after a febrile paroxysm, the timing of the smears is less important than their being obtained several times a day over a period of 3 successive days. A single negative blood smear does not exclude malaria; it may be necessary to repeat the smears as often as every 4–6 hours a day to confirm the diagnosis. Most symptomatic patients with malaria will have detectable parasites on thick blood smears within 48 hr. For nonimmune persons, symptoms typically occur 1–2 days before parasites are detectable on blood smear. A monoclonal antibody test that is incorporated in a test strip for fingerprick blood samples is as sensitive as a thick smear for detection of *P. falciparum.* Polymerase chain reaction is even more sensitive but technically more complex.

DIFFERENTIAL DIAGNOSIS. The differential diagnosis of malaria is broad and includes viral infections such as influenza and hepatitis, sepsis, pneumonia, meningitis, encephalitis, endocarditis, gastroenteritis, pyelonephritis, babesiosis, brucellosis, leptospirosis, tuberculosis, relapsing fever, typhoid fever, yellow fever, amebic liver abscess, Hodgkin disease, and collagen vascular disease.

TREATMENT. Physicians caring for patients with malaria or traveling to endemic areas need to be aware of current information regarding malaria because the problem of resistance to antimalarial drugs is changing and has greatly complicated therapy and prophylaxis. The best source for current information is the CDC Malaria Hotline, which is available to physicians 24 hr a day (770–488–7788 from 8:00 A.M. to 4:30 P.M. Eastern Standard Time (EST) and 770-488-7100 from 4:30 P.M. to 8:00 A.M. EST on weekends and holidays; ask the operator to page the person on call for the Malaria Epidemiology Branch). **Fever without an obvious cause in any patient who has left a *P. falci-***

parum–endemic area within the incubation period of 9–14 days and is nonimmune should be considered a medical emergency. Thick and thin blood smears should immediately be obtained and, if positive, the patient should be hospitalized and begun on therapy. If blood films are negative, they should be repeated every few hours; but if the patient is severely ill, antimalarial therapy should be initiated immediately.

***P. FALCIPARUM* MALARIA.** Malarious regions considered chloroquine-sensitive include Central America west of the Panama Canal, Haiti, the Dominican Republic, and most of the Middle East except Iran, Oman, Saudi Arabia, and Yemen. Malaria acquired in *P. falciparum* areas with chloroquine resistance or where there is any doubt about chloroquine sensitivity after conferring with the CDC should be treated with drugs other than chloroquine (Table 285-1). Intravenous quinidine gluconate (or quinine if outside the USA) should be administered for complicated malaria with impaired consciousness, severe normocytic anemia, renal failure, pulmonary edema, acute respiratory distress syndrome, circulatory shock, disseminated intravascular coagulation, spontaneous bleeding, acidosis, hemoglobinuria, jaundice, repeated generalized convulsions, parasitemia of >5%, or inability to retain oral medications because of vomiting. These patients should be admitted to the intensive care unit for monitoring of complications, plasma quinidine levels, and adverse effects during quinidine administration. During administration of quinidine, blood pressure monitoring for hypotension and cardiac monitoring for widening of the QRS complex or lengthening of the QTc interval should be monitored continuously, and blood glucose monitoring for hypoglycemia should be monitored periodically. Cardiac adverse events may require temporary discontinuation of the drug or slowing of the intravenous infusion. Parenteral therapy should be continued until the parasitemia is <1%, which usually occurs within 48 hr, and the patient can tolerate oral medication. Quinine sulfate (25 mg base/kg/day or 30 mg salt/kg/day divided 3 times a day PO) is then administered for a total of 3 days (Africa or South America) or 7 days (Southeast Asia) of combined quinidine/quinine therapy, with completion of therapy by doxycycline (4 mg/kg/day divided in 2 doses PO for 7 days), tetracycline (25 mg/kg/day divided 4 times a day PO for 7 days), or clindamycin (20 mg/kg/day in 3 doses for 7 days). Parenteral artesunate (2.4 mg/kg bolus IM or IV stat followed by 1.2 mg/kg at 12 and 24 hr and then 2.4 mg/kg daily) or artemether (3.2 mg/kg IM stat followed by 1.6 mg/kg/day) can be substituted for quinine for treatment of severe malaria. Oral or rectal artemisinin drugs are also effective but are not available in the United States.

Patients with mild to moderate infection, parasitemia <5%, and any doubt about chloroquine sensitivity should be given oral quinine sulfate (30 mg/kg/day in 3 doses) for 3–7 days with an additional antimalarial drug consisting of any 1 of the following: doxycycline (4 mg/kg/day PO bid for 7 days), tetracycline (25 mg/kg/day PO qid for 7 days), or clindamycin (20 mg/kg/day PO tid for 7 days). Alternatives include mefloquine given in 2 doses 12 hr apart or artesumate (4 mg/kg/day for 3 days) and mefloquine (see Table 285-1). Exceptions to these regimens include quinine treatment for 7 consecutive days for patients who acquire *P. falciparum* in Thailand. Mefloquine is contraindicated for use in patients with a known hypersensitivity to mefloquine or with a history of epilepsy or severe psychiatric disorders. Mefloquine is not recommended for persons with cardiac conduction abnormalities but may be administered to persons concurrently receiving β blockers if they have no underlying arrhythmia. Quinidine or quinine may exacerbate the adverse effects of mefloquine. Patients not responding to mefloquine therapy or failing mefloquine prophylaxis should be monitored closely if they are treated with quinidine or quinine.

Patients with uncomplicated *P. falciparum* malaria acquired in areas without chloroquine resistance should be treated with oral chloroquine phosphate. If the parasite count does not drop rapidly (within 24–48 hr) and become negative after 4 days, chloroquine resistance should be assumed and the patient begun on a different antimalarial regimen. Supportive therapy is very important and includes red blood cell transfusion(s) to maintain the hematocrit above 20%, exchange transfusion in life-threatening *P. falciparum* malaria with parasitemia >5%, supplemental oxygen and ventilatory support for pulmonary edema or cerebral malaria, careful intravenous rehydration for severe malaria, intravenous glucose for hypoglycemia, anticonvulsants for cerebral malaria with seizures, and dialysis for renal failure. Corticosteroids are no longer recommended for cerebral malaria.

***P. VIVAX, P. OVALE,* OR *P. MALARIAE* MALARIA.** For malaria acquired in areas where *P. falciparum* is not endemic, treatment is with chloroquine even though a few cases of chloroquine-resistant *P. vivax* malaria have been described from Indonesia and New Guinea. Malaria in the independent states of the former Soviet Union has been caused uniformly by *P. vivax* and can be treated as chloroquine sensitive. Clinical and blood smear response to therapy should be monitored. If vomiting precludes oral administration, chloroquine can be given by nasogastric tube, or, in rare cases and with great care, by intramuscular administration. Sudden death has been attributed to parenteral administration of chloroquine to children. Intravenous quinidine or quinine is given in severe cases. Patients with *P. vivax* or *P. ovale* malaria should also be given primaquine once daily for 14 days to prevent relapse from the hypnozoite forms that remain dormant in the liver. Some strains may require 2 courses of primaquine. Testing for glucose-6-phosphate dehydrogenase deficiency must be performed before initiation of primaquine because it can cause hemolytic anemia in such patients. Patients with any type of malaria must be monitored for possible recrudescence with repeat blood smears at the end of therapy because recrudescence may occur >90 days after therapy with low-grade resistant organisms. For children living in endemic areas, mothers should be encouraged to treat fever with an antimalarial drug. If such children are severely ill, they should be given the same therapy as nonimmune children.

COMPLICATIONS. **Cerebral malaria** is a serious complication of *P. falciparum* infection that is most common among children and nonimmune adults. It usually develops after the patient has been ill for several days and may develop precipitously. Cerebral malaria is associated with a fatality rate of 20–40% but rarely causes long-term sequelae if treated appropriately. As with other complications, cerebral malaria is more likely among patients with parasitemia of >5%. The symptoms always include decreased level of consciousness and range in severity from drowsiness and severe headache to confusion, delirium, hallucinations, or deep coma. Physical findings may be normal or may include fever to 106–108°F, seizures, muscular twitching, rhythmic movement of the head or extremities, contracted or unequal pupils, retinal hemorrhages, hemiplegia, absent or exaggerated deep tendon reflexes, and a positive Babinski sign. Lumbar puncture reveals increased pressure and cerebrospinal fluid protein with minimal or no pleocytosis and a normal glucose concentration. There are no specific electroencephalographic findings with cerebral malaria.

Renal failure is a common complication of severe *P. falciparum* malaria and results from deposition of hemoglobin in renal tubules, decreased renal blood flow, and acute tubular necrosis. **Blackwater fever** is a clinical syndrome that consists of severe hemolysis, hemoglobinuria, and renal failure. It is a rare complication that occurs when the combination of antibody directed against parasite-laden erythrocytes and complement result in severe hemolytic anemia, hemoglobinuria, oliguria, and jaundice. Renal failure usually requires peritoneal dialysis or hemodialysis.

Pulmonary edema may occur several days after therapy has begun and is commonly associated with excessive intravenous

TABLE 285-1. Guidelines for Treatment of Malaria*

CLINICAL DIAGNOSIS/ *PLASMODIUM* SPECIES	REGION INFECTION ACQUIRED	RECOMMENDED DRUG AND PEDIATRIC DOSE[1,7] (*PEDIATRIC DOSE SHOULD NEVER EXCEED ADULT DOSE*)	RECOMMENDED DRUG AND ADULT DOSE[1,7]
Uncomplicated malaria/*P. falciparum* or species not identified (if subsequently diagnosed as *P. vivax* or *P. ovale*, treat as below with primaquine)	**Chloroquine-sensitive** (Central America west of Panama Canal, Haiti, the Dominican Republic, and most of the Middle East)	**Chloroquine phosphate** 10 mg base/kg PO immediately followed by 5 mg base/kg PO at 6, 24, and 48 hr; total dose 25 mg base/kg	**Chloroquine phosphate** 600 mg base (1,000 mg salt) PO immediately followed by 300 mg base (500 mg salt) PO at 6, 24, and 48 hr; total dose 1,500 mg base (2,500 mg salt)
	Chloroquine-resistant or unknown resistance[1] (All malarious regions except those specified as chloroquine-sensitive above. Middle Eastern countries with chloroquine-resistant *P. falciparum* include Iran, Oman, Saudi Arabia, and Yemen. Malaria acquired in the states of the former Soviet Union and Korea to date has been caused uniformly by *P. vivax* and should be treated as chloroquine-sensitive infections.)	**A. Quinine sulfate[2] plus one of the following: doxycycline[3], tetracycline,[3] or clindamycin** **Quinine sulfate:** 8.3 mg base/kg (10 mg salt/kg) PO tid × 3–7 days **Doxycycline:** 4 mg/kg/day PO divided bid × 7 days **Tetracycline:** 25 mg/kg/day PO divided qid × 7 days **Clindamycin:** 20 mg/kg/day PO divided tid × 7 days **B. Atovaquone-proguanil[4] (Pediatric tablet: 62.5 mg atovaquone/25 mg proguanil. Adult tablet: 250 mg atovaquone/100 mg proguanil)** 5–8 kg: 2 pediatric tabs PO qd × 3 days 9–10 kg: 3 pediatric tabs PO qd × 3 days 11–20 kg: 1 adult tab PO qd × 3 days 21–30 kg: 2 adult tabs PO qd × 3 days 31–40 kg: 3 adult tabs PO qd × 3 days >40 kg: 4 adult tabs PO qd × 3 days **C. Mefloquine[5]** 13.7 mg base/kg (15 mg salt/kg) PO as initial dose followed by 9.1 mg base/kg (10 mg salt/kg) PO given 6–12 hr after initial dose; total dose 25 mg salt/kg	**A. Quinine sulfate[2] plus 1 of the following: doxycycline, tetracycline, or clindamycin** **Quinine sulfate:** 542 mg base (650 mg salt) PO tid × 3–7 days **Doxycycline:** 100 mg PO bid × 7 days **Tetracycline:** 250 mg PO qid × 7 days **Clindamycin:** 20 mg/kg/day PO divided tid × 7 days **B. Atovaquone-proguanil[4] (Adult tablet: 250 mg atovaquone/100 mg proguanil)** 4 adult tabs PO qd × 3 days **C. Mefloquine[5]** 684 mg base (750 mg salt) PO as initial dose followed by 456 mg base (500 mg salt) PO given 6–12 hr after initial dose; total dose 1,250 mg salt
Uncomplicated malaria/*P. malariae*	**All regions**	**Chloroquine phosphate:** Treatment as above	**Chloroquine phosphate:** Treatment as above
Uncomplicated malaria/*P. vivax* or ***P. ovale***	**All regions**[7] (For suspected chloroquine-resistant *P. vivax*, see below	**Chloroquine phosphate plus primaquine phosphate**[6] **Chloroquine phosphate:** Treatment as above **Primaquine phosphate:** 0.5 mg base/kg PO qd × 14 days	**Chloroquine phosphate plus primaquine phosphate**[6] **Chloroquine phosphate:** Treatment as above **Primaquine phosphate:** 30 mg base PO qd × 14 days
Uncomplicated malaria/*P. vivax*	**Chloroquine-resistant**[7] (Papua New Guinea and Indonesia)	**A. Quinine sulfate[2] plus either doxycycline[3] or tetracycline[3] plus primaquine phosphate[6]** **Quinine sulfate:** Treatment as above **Doxycycline or tetracycline:** Treatment as above **Primaquine phosphate:** Treatment as above **B. Mefloquine plus primaquine phosphate[6]** **Mefloquine:** Treatment as above **Primaquine phosphate:** Treatment as above	**A. Quinine sulfate[2] plus either doxycycline or tetracycline plus primaquine phosphate[6]** **Quinine sulfate:** Treatment as above **Doxycycline or tetracycline:** Treatment as above **Primaquine phosphate:** Treatment as above **B. Mefloquine plus primaquine phosphate[6]** **Mefloquine:** Treatment as above **Primaquine phosphate:** Treatment as above
Uncomplicated malaria: alternatives for pregnant women[8–11]	**Choroquine-sesitive**[11] (see uncomplicated malaria sections above for chloroquine-sensitive *Plasmodium* species by region)	**Not applicable**	**Chloroquine phosphate:** Treatment as above
	Chloroquine resistant *P. falciparum*[8–10] (see uncomplicated malaria sections above for regions with known chloroquine-resistant *P. falciparum*)	**Not applicable**	**Quinine sulfate[2] plus clindamycin** **Quinine sulfate:** Treatment as above **Clindamycin:** Treatment as above
	Chloroquine-resistant *P. vivax*[8–11] (see uncomplicated malaria sections above for regions with chloroquine-resistant *P. vivax*)	**Not applicable**	**Quinine sulfate:** 650 mg salt PO tid × 7 days
Severe malaria[12–15]	**All regions**	**Quinidine gluconate[13] plus 1 of the following: doxycycline[3], tetracycline[3], or clindamycin** **Quinidine gluconate:** 6.25 mg base/kg (10 mg salt/kg) loading dose IV over 1–2 hr then 0.0125 mg base/kg/min (0.02 mg salt/kg/min) continuous infusion for at least 24 hr. An alternative regimen is 15 mg base/kg (24 mg salt/kg) loading dose IV infused over 4 hr, followed by 7.2 mg base/kg (12 mg salt/kg) infused over 4 hr every 8 hr, starting 8 hr after the loading dose. Once parasite density is <1% and patient can take oral medication, complete treatment with oral quinine, dose as above. Quinidine/quinine course is 7 days for infection acquired in Southeast Asia, and 3 days for infection acquired in Africa or South America. **Doxycycline:** Treatment as above. If patient not able to take oral medication, may give IV. For children <45 kg, give 4 mg/kg IV every 12 hr and then switch to oral doxycycline (dose as above) as soon as patient can take oral medication. For children >45 kg, use same dosing as for adults. For IV use, avoid rapid administration. Treatment course is 7 days. **Tetracycline:** Treatment as above	**Quinidine gluconate[13] plus 1 of the following: doxycycline, tetracycline, or clindamycin** **Quinidine gluconate:** Same mg/kg dosing and recommendations as for children. **Doxycycline:** Treatment as above. If patient not able to take oral medication, give 100 mg IV every 12 hr and then switch to oral doxycycline (as above) as soon as patient can take oral medication. For IV use, avoid rapid administration. Treatment course is 7 days. **Tetracycline:** Treatment as above **Clindamycin:** Treatment as above. If patient not able to take oral medication, give 10 mg/kg loading dose IV followed by 5 mg base/kg IV every 8 hr. Switch to oral clindamycin (oral dose as above) as soon as patient can take oral medication. For IV use, avoid rapid administration. Treatment course is 7 days.

TABLE 285-1. Guidelines for Treatment of Malaria*—cont'd

CLINICAL DIAGNOSIS/ *PLASMODIUM* SPECIES	REGION INFECTION ACQUIRED	RECOMMENDED DRUG AND PEDIATRIC DOSE[1,7] (*PEDIATRIC DOSE SHOULD NEVER EXCEED ADULT DOSE*)	RECOMMENDED DRUG AND ADULT DOSE[1,7]
		Clindamycin: Treatment as above. If patient not able to take oral medication, give 10 mg base/kg loading dose IV followed by 5 mg base/kg IV every 8 hr. Switch to oral clindamycin (oral dose as above) as soon as patient can take oral medication. For IV use, avoid rapid administration. Treatment course is 7 days.	

*CDC Malaria Hotline: (770) 488-7788 Monday–Friday 8 A.M. to 4:30 P.M. Eastern time; (770) 488-7100 after hours, weekends, and holidays (ask to page the malaria person on call).

[1]There are three options (A, B, or C) available for treatment of uncomplicated malaria caused by chloroquine-resistant *P. falciparum.* Options A and B are equally recommended. Because of a higher rate of severe neuropsychiatric reactions seen at treatment doses, option C (mefloquine) is not recommended unless options A and B cannot be used. For option A, because there are more data on the efficacy of quinine in combination with doxycycline or tetracycline, these treatment combinations are generally preferred to quinine in combination with clindamycin.

[2]For infections acquired in Southeast Asia, quinine treatment should continue for 7 days. For infections acquired in Africa and South America, quinine treatment should continue for 3 days.

[3]Doxycycline and tetracycline are not indicated for use in children <8 yr of age. For children <8 yr of age with chloroquine-resistant *P. falciparum,* quinine (given alone for 7 days or given in combination with clindamycin) and atovaquone-proguanil are recommended treatment options; mefloquine can be considered if no other options are available. For children <8 yr of age with chloroquine-resistant *P. vivax,* quinine (given alone for 7 days) or mefloquine are recommended treatment options. If none of these treatment options are available or are not being tolerated and if the treatment benefits outweigh the risks, doxycycline or tetracycline may be given to children <8 yr of age.

[4]Give atovaquone-proguanil with food. If patient vomits within 30 min of taking a dose, then he or she should repeat the dose.

[5]Treatment with mefloquine is not recommended in persons who have acquired infections from the Southeast Asian region of Burma, Thailand, and Cambodia due to resistant strains.

[6]Primaquine is used to eradicate any hypnozoite forms that may remain dormant in the liver, and thus prevent relapses, in *P. vivax* and *P. ovale* infections. Because primaquine can cause hemolytic anemia in persons with glucose-6-phosphate dehydrogenase (G6PD) deficiency, patients must be screened for G6PD deficiency prior to starting treatment with primaquine. For persons with borderline G6PD deficiency or as an alternate to the above regimen, primaquine may be given 45 mg orally 1 time per week for 8 wk; consultation with an expert in infectious disease and/or tropical medicine is advised if this alternative regimen is considered in G6PD-deficient persons. Primaquine must not be used during pregnancy.

[7]There are two options (A and B) available for treatment of uncomplicated malaria caused by chloroquine-resistant *P. vivax.* High treatment failure rates due to chloroquine-resistant *P. vivax* have been well documented in Papua New Guinea and Indonesia. Rare case reports of chloroquine-resistant *P. vivax* have also been documented in Burma (Myanmar), India, and Central and South America. Persons acquiring *P. vivax* infections outside of Papua New Guinea or Indonesia should be started on chloroquine. If the patient does not respond, the treatment should be changed to a chloroquine-resistant *P. vivax* regimen and the CDC should be notified using the Malaria Hotline). For treatment of chloroquine-resistant *P. vivax* infections, options A and B are equally recommended.

[8]For pregnant women diagnosed with uncomplicated malaria caused by chloroquine-resistant *P. falciparum* or chloroquine-resistant *P. vivax* infection, treatment with doxycycline or tetracycline is generally not indicated. However, doxycycline or tetracycline may be used in combination with quinine (as recommended for nonpregnant adults) if other treatment options are not available or are not being tolerated, and the benefit is judged to outweigh the risks.

[9]Because there are no adequate, well-controlled studies of atovaquone and/or proguanil hydrochloride in pregnant women, atovaquone-proguanil is generally not recommended for use in pregnant women. For pregnant women diagnosed with uncomplicated malaria caused by chloroquine-resistant *P. falciparum* infection, atovaquone-proguanil may be used if other treatment options are not available or are not being tolerated, and if the potential benefit is judged to outweigh the potential risks. There are no data on the efficacy of atovaquone-proguanil in the treatment of chloroquine-resistant *P. vivax* infections.

[10]Because of a possible association with mefloquine treatment during pregnancy and an increase in stillbirths, mefloquine is generally not recommended for treatment in pregnant women. However, mefloquine may be used if it is the only treatment option available and if the potential benefit is judged to outweigh the potential risks.

[11]For *P. vivax* and *P. ovale* infections, primaquine phosphate for radical treatment of hypnozoites should not be given during pregnancy. Pregnant patients with *P. vivax* and *P. ovale* infections should be maintained on chloroquine prophylaxis for the duration of their pregnancy. The chemoprophylactic dose of chloroquine phosphate is 300 mg base (500 mg salt) orally once per week. After delivery, pregnant patients who do not have G6PD deficiency should be treated with primaquine.

[12]Persons with a positive blood smear OR history of recent possible exposure and no other recognized pathology who have one or more of the following clinical criteria (impaired consciousness/coma, severe normocytic anemia, renal failure, pulmonary edema, acute respiratory distress syndrome, circulatory shock, disseminated intravascular coagulation, spontaneous bleeding, acidosis, hemoglobinuria, jaundice, repeated generalized convulsions, and/or parasitemia of >5%) are considered to have manifestations of more severe disease. Severe malaria is practically always due to *P. falciparum.*

[13]Patients diagnosed with severe malaria should be treated aggressively with parenteral antimalarial therapy. Treatment with IV quinidine should be initiated as soon as possible after the diagnosis has been made. Patients with severe malaria should be given an intravenous loading dose of quinidine unless they have received >40 mg/kg of quinine in the preceding 48 hr or if they have received mefloquine within the preceding 12 hours. Consultation with a cardiologist and a physician with experience treating malaria is advised when treating malaria patients with quinidine. During administration of quinidine, blood pressure monitoring (for hypotension) and cardiac monitoring (for widening of the QRS complex and/or lengthening of the QTc interval) should be monitored continuously and blood glucose (for hypoglycemia) should be monitored periodically. Cardiac complications, if severe, may warrant temporary discontinuation of the drug or slowing of the intravenous infusion.

[14]Consider exchange transfusion if the parasite density (i.e., parasitemia) is >10% or if the patient has altered mental status, non–volume overload pulmonary edema, or renal complications. The parasite density can be estimated by examining a monolayer of red blood cells (RBCs) on the thin smear under oil immersion magnification. The slide should be examined where the RBCs are more or less touching (approximately 400 RBCs per field). The parasite density can then be estimated from the percentage of infected RBCs and should be monitored every 12 hr. Exchange transfusion should be continued until the parasite density is <1% (usually requires 8–10 units). IV quinidine administration should not be delayed for an exchange transfusion and can be given concurrently throughout the exchange transfusion.

[15]Pregnant women diagnosed with severe malaria should be treated aggressively with parenteral antimalarial therapy.

Adapted from the Centers for Disease Control and Prevention (http://www.cdc.gov/malaria/pdf/treatmenttable.pdf).

therapy. It can develop rapidly and may be fatal. Thus, great care should be taken not to overhydrate patients with *P. falciparum* malaria.

Hypoglycemia is a complication of malaria that is more common in children, pregnant women, and patients receiving quinine therapy. Patients may have a decreased level of consciousness that can be confused with cerebral malaria. Hypoglycemia is associated with increased mortality and neurologic sequelae.

Thrombocytopenia is a common complication of *P. falciparum* and *P. vivax* malaria. Although significant bleeding is uncommon without DIC, platelet counts can decrease to 10,000–20,000/mm^3.

Splenic rupture is a rare complication that may occur with acute infection owing to any malaria species. Splenic rupture can occur spontaneously but is usually the result of trauma that includes overly vigorous palpation on physical examination. It causes severe internal hemorrhage and may result in death if removal of the spleen and blood transfusion are not performed in a timely manner.

Algid malaria is a rare form of *P. falciparum* malaria that occurs with overwhelming infection, hypotension, hypothermia, rapid weak pulse, shallow breathing, pallor, and vascular collapse. Death may occur within a few hours.

Among children living in endemic areas, malarial attacks adversely affect the educational attainment of the schoolchild. Prevention of attacks significantly improves educational attainment.

PREVENTION. Malaria prevention consists of reducing exposure to infected mosquitoes and chemoprophylaxis. The most accurate and current information on areas in the world where malaria risk and drug resistance exist can be obtained by contacting local and state health departments or the CDC or consulting *Health Information for International Travel,* which is published by the U.S. Public Health Service.

Travelers to endemic areas should remain in well-screened areas from dusk to dawn when the risk for transmission is highest. They should sleep under permethrin-treated mosquito netting and spray insecticides indoors at sundown. During the day the travelers should wear clothing that covers the arms and legs, with trousers tucked into shoes or boots. Mosquito repellent should be applied to thin clothing and exposed areas of the skin, with applications repeated every 1–2 hours. A child should not be taken outside from dusk to dawn, but, if absolutely necessary, diethyltoluamide (DEET) in a 10–15% solution should be applied to exposed areas except for the eyes, mouth, or hands. Hands are excluded because they are often placed in the mouth.

TABLE 285-2. Malaria Chemoprophylaxis

DRUG	ADULT DOSE	PEDIATRIC DOSE	PRECAUTIONS
P. VIVAX, P. OVALE, P. MALARIAE*, AND CHLOROQUINE-SUSCEPTIBLE *P. FALCIPARUM			
Chloroquine phosphate			
Supplied in 500 mg salt (300 mg base) tablets.	500 mg (300 mg base) once weekly*	8.3 mg/kg (5 mg/kg base) once weekly, up to the adult dose of 300 mg base*	Drug accumulation from prolonged use or inadvertent daily dosing may cause retinopathy.
CHLOROQUINE-RESISTANT *P. FALCIPARUM*			
Mefloquine			
Supplied in 250 mg salt (228 mg base) tablets.	250 mg once weekly†	Dosed according to body weight:* <15 kg: 5 mg/kg once weekly 15–19 kg: 1/4 tablet once weekly 20–30 kg: 1/2 tablet once weekly 31–45 kg: 3/4 tablet once weekly	*Do not* use in individuals with cardiac conduction abnormalities, history of seizures, or serious psychiatric illnesses (e.g., psychosis, major depression). *Do not* use concomitantly with quinidine, quinine, or halofantrine. *Do not* use in first trimester of pregnancy.
CHLOROQUINE- OR MEFLOQUINE-RESISTANT *P. FALCIPARUM*			
Doxycycline			
Supplied in 100 mg tablets.	100 mg once daily‡	For children 8–12 yr old: 2 mg/kg once daily, up to adult dose of 100 mg. For children >13 yr old: 100 mg once daily‡	*Do not* use doxycycline in children <8 yr old or in pregnant women.
Atovaquone *plus* proguanil			
Supplied in fixed combination tablets containing 250 mg atovaquone and 100 mg proguanil (adult tablets) or 62.5 mg/25 mg (pediatric tablets).	250 mg/100 mg (1 tablet) once daily§	Dose per body weight§ 11–20 kg: 62.5 mg/25 mg once daily 21–30 kg: 125 mg/50 mg once daily 31–40 kg: 187.5 mg/75 mg once daily >40 kg: 250 mg/100 mg once daily§	Pregnancy category C.

*Beginning 1–2 wk before travel and continuing weekly for 4 wk after leaving a malarious area.
†For travelers who will be at immediate high risk for malaria, a loading dose of mefloquine is usually well tolerated: 250 mg daily for 3 consecutive days, followed by weekly dosing as shown.
‡Beginning 1–2 days before travel and continuing daily for 4 wk after leaving a malarious area.
§Beginning 1–2 days before travel and continuing daily for 7 days after leaving a malarious area.
Drug regimens adapted from: Advice for travelers. *Med Lett* 2002;1128:38–39.
From Mandell GL, Bennett JE, Dolin R (editors): *Principles and Practice of Infectious Diseases*, 6th ed, Vol 2. Philadelphia, Elsevier, 2005, p 3137.

DEET should then be washed off as soon as the child comes back inside. Adverse reactions to DEET include rashes, toxic encephalopathy, and seizures. Even with these precautions, a child should be taken to a physician immediately if he or she develops illness when traveling to a malarious area.

Chemoprophylaxis is necessary for all visitors to and residents of the tropics who have not lived there since infancy (Table 285-2). Children of nonimmune women should have chemoprophylaxis from birth. Chemoprophylaxis should be started 1–2 wk before entering the endemic area (except for doxycycline administration, which can begin 1–2 days before departure) and continue for at least 4 wk after leaving. Health care providers should consult the latest information on resistance patterns before prescribing prophylaxis for their patients. Chloroquine is given in the few remaining areas of the world free of chloroquine-resistant malaria strains (the Dominican Republic, Haiti, Central America west of the former Panama Canal Zone, Egypt, and some countries in the Middle East). In areas where chloroquine-resistant *P. falciparum* exists, chemoprophylaxis is complicated. Children who travel to areas where chloroquine-resistant strains are transmitted should be given mefloquine. An alternative regimen should be given to children if they have a known hypersensitivity to mefloquine, are receiving cardiotropic drugs, especially β blockers, have a history of convulsive or certain psychiatric disorders, or travel to an area where mefloquine resistance exists (the borders of Thailand with Burma [Myanmar] and Cambodia, in the western provinces of Cambodia, and in the eastern states of Burma [Myanmar]). Such children should be given chloroquine or an alternative antimalarial drug. In addition, if they weigh more than 30 pounds, they should bring Fansidar tablets to be taken if fever develops and medical care is not available within 24 hr. An alternative combination that could be considered for sulfa-sensitive individuals >8 yr of age is chloroquine and, in place of Fansidar, doxycycline. Doxycycline is equivalent to mefloquine for short-term prophylaxis, but for long-term prophylaxis doxycycline is not as good because of side effects associated with its long-term use. There have been several reports of both mefloquine and Fansidar resistance. The combination of atovaquone and proguanil (Malarone) has been approved for prophylaxis of malaria in areas where chloroquine resistance exists, although dosing is uncertain in children who weigh less than 30 pounds. Finally, extensive efforts have been made to develop a malaria vaccine, but results to date have been disappointing.

Aceng JR, Byarugaba JS, Tumwine JK: Rectal artemether versus intravenous quinine for the treatment of cerebral malaria in children in Uganda: Randomized clinical trial. *Br Med J* 2005;330:334–337.

Barennes H, Balima-Koussoube T, Nagot N, et al: Safety and efficacy of rectal compared with intramuscular quinine for the early treatment of moderately severe malaria in children: Randomized clinical trial. *Br Med J* 2006; 332:1055–1057.

Barennes H, Balima-Koussoube T, Nagot N, et al: Safety and efficacy of rectal compared with intramuscular quinine for the early treatment of moderately severe malaria in children: Randomized clinical trial. *Br Med J* 2006;332:1055–1056.

Centers for Disease Control and Prevention: Congenital malaria as a result of *Plasmodium malariae*—North Carolina, 2000. *MMWR* 2002;51:164–165.

Centers for Disease Control and Prevention: Probable transfusion-transmitted malaria—Houston, Texas, 2003. *MMWR* 2003;52:1075–1076.

Centers for Disease Control and Prevention: Congenital malaria—Nassau County, New York, 2004. *MMWR* 2005;54:383–384.

Centers for Disease Control and Prevention: Malaria surveillance—United States, 2003. *MMWR* 2005;54(SS-2):25–39.

Centers for Disease Control and Prevention: Health Information for International Travel, 2005–2006. Atlanta, US Department of Health and Human Services, Public Health Service, 2005–2006. Available at http://www.cdc.gov/travel/yb/index.htm

Centers for Disease Control and Prevention: Malaria in multiple family members—Chicago, Illinois, 2006. *MMWR* 2006;55:645–648.

Chandramohan D, Owusu-Agyei S, Carneiro I, et al: Cluster randomized trial of intermittent preventive treatment for malaria in infants in area of high, seasonal transmission in Ghana. *Br Med J* 2005;331:727–732.

Chen LH, Wilson ME, Schlagenhauf P: Prevention of malaria in long-term travelers. *JAMA* 2006;296:2234–2244.

Desai M, ter Kuile FO, Nosten F, et al: Epidemiology and burden of malaria in pregnancy. *Lancet Infect Dis* 2007;7:93–104.

Greenwood BM, Bojang K, Whitty CJM, Targett GAT: Malaria. *Lancet* 2005;365:1487–1498.

Idro R, Jenkins NE, Newton CR: Pathogenesis, clinical features, and neurological outcome of cerebral malaria. *Lancet Neurol* 2005;4:827–840.

Kain KC, Harrington MA, Tennyson S, et al: Imported malaria: Prospective analysis of problems in diagnosis and management. *Clin Infect Dis* 1998;27:142–149.

Krause G, Schoneberg I, Altmann D, et al: Chemoprophylaxis and malaria death rates. *Emerg Infect Dis* 2006;12:447–451.

Kremsner PG, Krishna S: Antimalarial combinations. *Lancet* 2004;364: 285–294.

Laufer MK, Thesing PC, Eddington ND, et al: Return of chloroquine antimalarial efficacy in Malawi. *N Engl J Med* 2006;355:1959–1966.

Maitland K, Nadel S, Pollard AJ, et al: Management of severe malaria in children: Proposed guidelines for the United Kingdom. *Br Med J* 2005;331: 337–343.

Malenga G, Palmer A, Staedke S, et al: Antimalarial treatment with artemisinin combination therapy in Africa. *Br Med J* 2005;331:706–707.

Maroushek SR, Aguilar EF, Stauffer W, et al: Malaria among refugee children at arrival in the United States. *Pediatr Infect Dis J* 2005;24:450–452.

Ratcliff A, Siswantoro H, Kenangalem E, et al: Two fixed-dose artemisinin combinations for drug-resistant falciparum and vivax malaria in Papua, Indonesia: an open-label randomised comparison. *Lancet* 2007;369:757–765.

Reyburn H, Mbatia R, Drakeley C, et al: Association of transmission intensity and age with clinical manifestations and case fatality of severe *Plasmodium falciparum* malaria. *JAMA* 2005;293:1461–1470.

Schapira A: DDT: A polluted debate in malaria control. *Lancet* 2006;368: 2111–2113.

South East Asian Quinine Artesunate Malaria Trial Group: Artesunate versus quinine for treatment of severe falciparum malaria: A randomized trial. *Lancet* 2005;366:717–724.

Viani RM, Bromberg K: Pediatric imported malaria in New York: Delayed diagnosis. *Clin Pediatr* 1999;38:333–337.

Zurovac D, Ndhlovu M, Rowe AK, et al: Treatment of paediatric malaria during a period of drug transition to artemether-lumefantrine in Zambia: Cross sectional study. *Br Med J* 2005;331:734–738.

Chapter 286 ■ Babesiosis *(Babesia)*

Peter J. Krause

Babesiosis is an emerging malaria-like disease caused by an intraerythrocytic protozoan that is transmitted by ticks. The clinical manifestations of babesiosis range from subclinical illness to fulminant disease resulting in death.

ETIOLOGY. There are >90 species of Babesia that infect a wide variety of wild and domestic animals throughout the world. A *Babesia* organism that also infects mice, *B. microti,* is the most common cause of babesiosis in humans. The primary reservoir for *B. microti* is the white-footed mouse, *Peromyscus leucopus,* and the primary vector is the deer tick, *Ixodes scapularis.* Deer ticks also transmit the causative agents of Lyme disease and human granulocytic ehrlichiosis and may simultaneously transmit all 3 microorganisms. Deer *(Odocoileus virginianus)* serve as the host on which adult ticks most abundantly feed but are incompetent reservoirs.

A parasite very closely related to *Babesia gibsoni* (WA-1) appears to infect humans along the Pacific coast, whereas another that is closely related to *Babesia divergens* (MO-1) has been reported in Missouri.

EPIDEMIOLOGY. Human babesial infections caused by the cattle *Babesia, B. divergens,* have been described in many countries in Europe, while endemic regions of infection with *B. microti* have been identified in Europe and in the northeastern and upper midwestern United States. Human babesiosis cases also have been documented in Asia and Africa. Rarely, babesiosis is acquired through blood transfusions or by transplacental transmission.

In certain sites and in certain years of high transmission, babesiosis constitutes a significant public health burden. Asymptomatic and symptomatic babesial infection rates on Block Island, Rhode Island, total 1,620 cases/100,000 population, with similar rates in parts of southeastern Connecticut. Nantucket Island reported 21 such cases in 1994, which translates to 280 cases/100,000 population, placing the community burden of disease in a category with gonorrhea as "moderately common."

PATHOGENESIS. Erythrocyte lysis is responsible for many of the clinical manifestations and complications of the disease, including fever, hemolytic anemia, jaundice, hemoglobinemia, hemoglobinuria, and renal insufficiency. Obstruction of blood vessels by parasitized erythrocytes causes ischemia and necrosis that may result in splenomegaly, hepatomegaly, hepatic dysfunction, and cerebral abnormalities. The spleen has an important role in clearing parasitemia in addition to T and B cells, antibody, complement, cytokines, macrophages, and polymorphonuclear leukocytes.

CLINICAL MANIFESTATIONS. The clinical severity of babesiosis ranges from subclinical infection to fulminating disease and death. In clinically apparent cases, symptoms of babesiosis begin after an incubation period of 1–9 wk from the beginning of tick feeding or 6–9 wk after transfusion. Typical symptoms in moderate to severe infection include intermittent temperature to as high as 40°C (104°F) accompanied by any combination of chills, sweats, myalgias, arthralgias, nausea, and vomiting. Less commonly noted are emotional lability, hyperesthesia, headache, sore throat, abdominal pain, conjunctival injection, photophobia, weight loss, and nonproductive cough. The findings on physical examination generally are minimal, often consisting only of fever. Splenomegaly, hepatomegaly, or both are noted occasionally, but rash seldom is reported. Abnormal laboratory findings include moderately severe hemolytic anemia, elevated reticulocyte count, thrombocytopenia, proteinuria, and elevated blood urea nitrogen and creatinine levels. The leukocyte count is normal to slightly decreased, with increased bands. Babesiosis usually lasts for a few weeks to several months, with prolonged recovery of up to 18 mo in severe cases. Complications include respiratory failure, DIC, heart failure, renal failure, hepatic failure, and coma.

Risk factors for severe disease include infection with *B. divergens,* anatomic or functional asplenia, immunosuppressive drugs, age >40 yr, and concomitant HIV infection, malignancy, or Lyme disease. Concurrent babesiosis and Lyme disease infection occurs in about 15% of patients experiencing Lyme disease in parts of southern New England and results in more severe illness than with either disease alone. Moderate to severe babesiosis may occur in children, but infection generally is less severe than in adults. Several cases of neonatal babesiosis have been described. Neonates usually are infected from blood transfusion and may develop severe illness.

DIAGNOSIS. Diagnosis of *B. microti* infection in human hosts is by microscopic demonstration of the organism using Giemsa-stained thin blood films. Parasitemia may be exceedingly low, especially early in the course of illness. Thick blood smears may be examined, but the organisms appear as simple chromatin dots that may be mistaken for stain precipitate or iron inclusion bodies. The polymerase chain reaction is a sensitive and specific test for detection of babesia DNA. Subinoculation of blood into hamsters or gerbils and in vitro cultivation are too specialized for all but the most experienced laboratories. Serologic testing is useful, particularly for diagnosing *B. microti* infection. The indirect immunofluorescence serologic assay (for both IgG and IgM antibodies) is sensitive and specific and can quickly confirm a diagnosis of babesiosis when parasites are scarce or undetectable.

TREATMENT. The combination of clindamycin (20–40 mg/kg/day divided tid PO) and quinine (25 mg/kg/day divided tid PO) for 7 to 10 days is the treatment of choice for babesiosis in children. Adverse effects are common, however, especially tinnitus and abdominal distress. In addition, treatment failures have been reported, particularly in persons with HIV infection. The combination of atovaquone (40 mg/kg/day divided bid PO) and azithromycin (12 mg/kg/day as a single dose PO) has been shown in adults to be as effective as clindamycin and quinine but with fewer adverse effects. Atovaquone and azithromycin have been used successfully to treat babesiosis in infants and should be considered for initial use in children with mild to moderate infection. Exchange blood transfusion can decrease parasitemia rapidly and remove toxic by-products of infection and should be used for patients with life-threatening infections.

PROGNOSIS. Moderate to severe disease is frequently observed in some highly endemic areas. The case fatality rate was estimated at 5% in a retrospective study of 136 New York cases. Immunity is sometimes incomplete with low-level parasitemia for as long as 26 mo after symptoms have resolved as well as recrudescence in immunocompromised hosts.

PREVENTION. Prevention of babesiosis can be accomplished by avoiding areas where ticks, deer, and mice are known to thrive. Use of clothing that covers the lower part of the body and that is sprayed or impregnated with diethyltoluamide (DEET), dimethyl phthalate, or permethrin (Permanone) is recommended for those who travel in the foliage of endemic areas. A search for ticks on people and pets should be carried out and the ticks removed using tweezers to grasp the mouth parts without squeezing the body of the tick. Prospective blood donors with a history of babesiosis are excluded from giving blood to prevent transfusion-related cases.

Fox L, Wingerter S, Ahmed A, et al: Neonatal babesiosis: Case report and review of the literature. *Pediatr Infect Dis J* 2006;25:169–173.

Hatcher JC, Greenberg PD, Antigue J, et al: Severe babesiosis in Long Island. Review of 34 cases and their complications. *Clin Infect Dis* 2001;32:1117–1125.

Herwaldt BL, McGovern PC, Gerwel MP, et al: Endemic babesiosis in another eastern state: New Jersey. *Emerg Infect Dis* 2003;9:184–188.

Krause PJ, Lepore T, Sikand VK, et al: Atovaquone and azithromycin for the treatment of babesiosis. *N Engl J Med* 2000;343:1454–1458.

Krause PJ, McKay K, Gadbaw J, et al: Increasing health burden of human babesiosis in endemic sites. *Am J Trop Med Hyg* 2003;68:431–436.

Krause PJ, Telford SR III, Pollack RJ, et al: Babesiosis: An underdiagnosed disease of children. *Pediatrics* 1992;89:1045–1048.

Krause PJ, Telford SR III, Spielman A, et al: Concurrent Lyme disease and babesiosis: Evidence for increased severity and duration of illness. *JAMA* 1996;275:1657–1660.

Chapter 287 ■ Toxoplasmosis (*Toxoplasma Gondii*)

Rima McLeod and Jack S. Remington

Toxoplasma gondii, an obligate intracellular protozoan, is acquired perorally, transplacentally, or, rarely, parenterally in laboratory accidents; by transfusion; or from a transplanted organ. In immunologically normal children, acute acquired infection may be asymptomatic, cause lymphadenopathy, or affect almost any organ. Once acquired, latent encysted organisms persist in the host throughout life. In immunocompromised infants or children, either initial acquisition or recrudescence of latent organisms often causes signs or symptoms related to the central nervous system (CNS). Congenital infection, if untreated, often causes disease either perinatally or later in life, most frequently chorioretinitis and CNS lesions. However, other manifestations such as intrauterine growth, mental and psychosocial retardation, fever, lymphadenopathy, rash, hearing loss, pneumonitis, hepatitis, and thrombocytopenia also occur. Congenital toxoplasmosis in infants with HIV infection may be fulminant.

ETIOLOGY. *T. gondii* is a coccidian protozoan that multiplies only in living cells. The tachyzoites are oval or crescent-like, measuring 2–4 × 4–7 µm. Tissue cysts, which are 10–100 µm in diameter, may contain thousands of parasites and remain in tissues, especially the CNS and skeletal and heart muscle, for the life of the host. *Toxoplasma* can multiply in all tissues of mammals and birds.

Newly infected cats and other Felidae species excrete infectious *Toxoplasma* oocysts in their feces. *Toxoplasma* organisms are transmitted to cats by ingestion of infected meat containing encysted bradyzoites or by ingestion of oocysts excreted by other recently infected cats. The parasites then multiply through schizogonic and gametogonic cycles in the distal ileal epithelium of the cat intestine. Oocysts containing 2 sporocysts are excreted, and, under proper conditions of temperature and moisture, each sporocyst matures into 4 sporozoites. For about 2 wk the cat excretes 10^5–10^7 oocysts/day, which, in a suitable environment, may retain their viability for >1 yr. Oocysts sporulate 1–5 days after excretion and are then infectious. Oocysts are killed by drying or boiling, but not exposure to bleach. Oocysts have been isolated from soil and sand frequented by cats, and outbreaks associated with contaminated water have been reported. Oocysts and tissue cysts are sources of animal and human infections (Fig. 287-1). There are 3 clonal and atypical types of *T. gondii* that have different virulence for mice (and perhaps for humans) and form different numbers of cysts in the brains of outbred mice.

EPIDEMIOLOGY. *Toxoplasma* infection is ubiquitous in animals and is 1 of the most common latent infections of humans throughout the world. Incidence varies considerably among people and animals in different geographic areas. In many areas of the world, approximately 3–35% of pork, 7–60% of lamb, and 0–9% of beef contain *T. gondii* organisms. Significant antibody titers are detected in 50–80% of residents of some localities such as France, Brazil, and Central America, and in <5% in other areas. There is a higher prevalence of infection in warmer, more humid climates.

Human infection is usually acquired orally by eating undercooked or raw meat that contains cysts or food or other material contaminated with oocysts from acutely infected cats. Freezing meat to −20°C or heating it to 66°C renders the cysts noninfectious. Outbreaks of acute acquired infection have occurred in families who have consumed the same infected food. *Toxoplasma* organisms are not transmitted from person to person except for transplacental infection from mother to fetus and, rarely, by organ transplantation or transfusion.

Seronegative transplant recipients who receive an organ or bone marrow from seropositive donors have experienced life-threatening illness requiring therapy. Seropositive recipients may have increased serologic titers without associated disease.

Congenital Toxoplasmosis. Transmission to the fetus usually follows acquisition of infection by an immunologically normal mother during gestation. Congenital transmission from mothers infected before pregnancy is extremely rare except for immunocompromised women who are chronically infected. The incidence

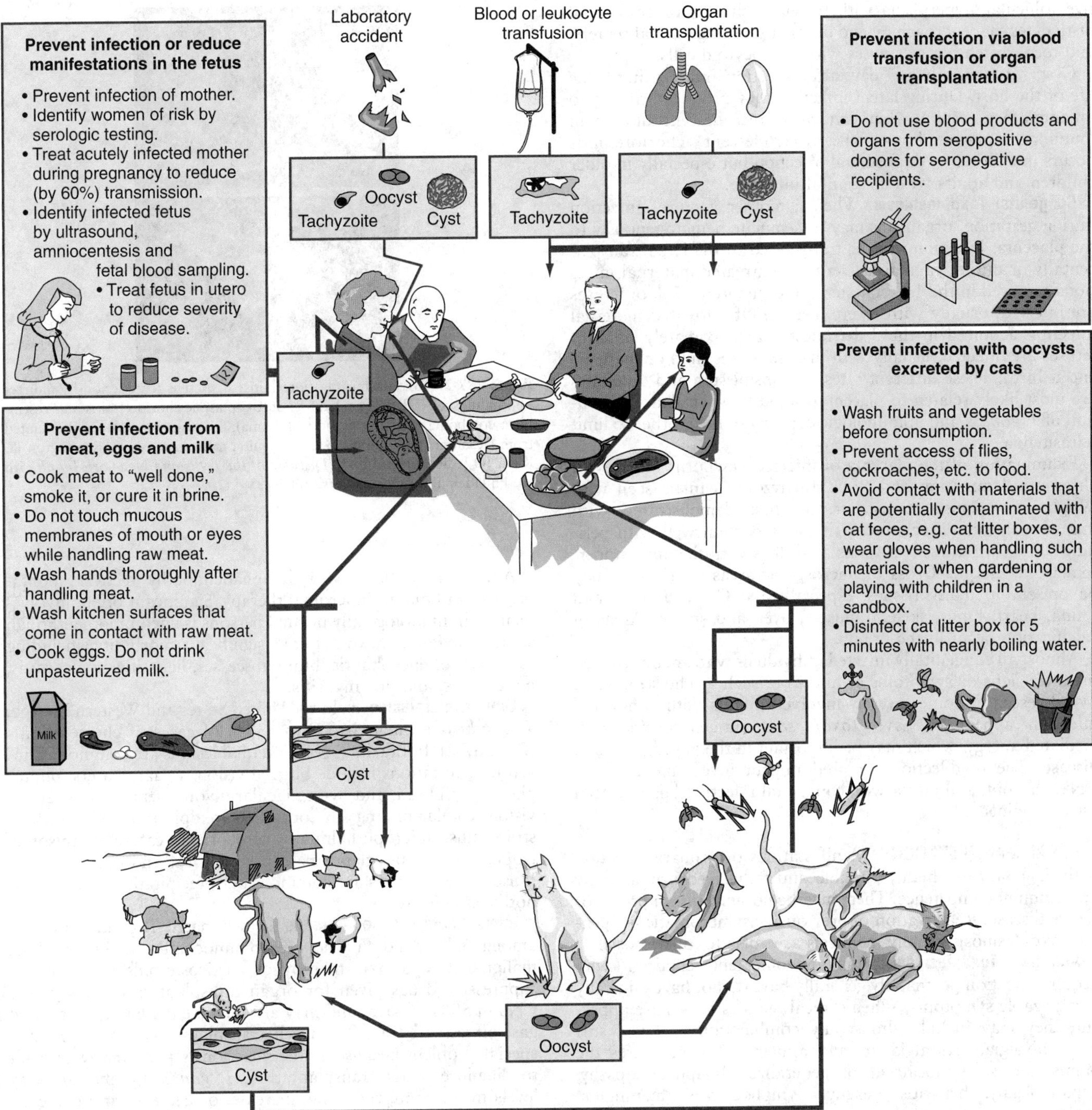

Prevent infection or reduce manifestations in the fetus
• Prevent infection of mother.
• Identify women of risk by serologic testing.
• Treat acutely infected mother during pregnancy to reduce (by 60%) transmission.
• Identify infected fetus by ultrasound, amniocentesis and fetal blood sampling.
• Treat fetus in utero to reduce severity of disease.
Laboratory accident
Blood or leukocyte transfusion
Organ transplantation
Prevent infection via blood transfusion or organ transplantation
• Do not use blood products and organs from seropositive donors for seronegative recipients.
Oocyst
Tachyzoite
Cyst
Tachyzoite
Tachyzoite
Cyst
Tachyzoite
Prevent infection with oocysts excreted by cats
• Wash fruits and vegetables before consumption.
• Prevent access of flies, cockroaches, etc. to food.
• Avoid contact with materials that are potentially contaminated with cat feces, e.g. cat litter boxes, or wear gloves when handling such materials or when gardening or playing with children in a sandbox.
• Disinfect cat litter box for 5 minutes with nearly boiling water.
Prevent infection from meat, eggs and milk
• Cook meat to "well done," smoke it, or cure it in brine.
• Do not touch mucous membranes of mouth or eyes while handling raw meat.
• Wash hands thoroughly after handling meat.
• Wash kitchen surfaces that come in contact with raw meat.
• Cook eggs. Do not drink unpasteurized milk.
Milk
Cyst
Oocyst
Oocyst
Cyst

Figure 287-1. Life cycle of *Toxoplasma gondii* and prevention of toxoplasmosis by interruption of transmission to humans.

of congenital infection in the United States ranges from 1/1,000 to 1/8,000 live births. The incidence of infection among pregnant women depends on the general risk for infection in the specific locale and the proportion of the population that has not been infected previously.

PATHOGENESIS. *T. gondii* is acquired by children and adults from ingesting food that contains cysts or that is contaminated with oocysts usually from acutely infected cats. Oocysts also may be transported to food by flies and cockroaches. When the organism is ingested, bradyzoites are released from cysts or sporozoites from oocysts. The organisms enter gastrointestinal cells where they multiply, rupture cells, infect contiguous cells, enter the lymphatics, and disseminate hematogenously throughout the body. Tachyzoites proliferate, producing necrotic foci surrounded by a cellular reaction. With development of a normal immune response that is both humoral and cell-mediated, tachyzoites disappear from tissues. In immunocompromised persons, and also some apparently immunocompetent persons, acute infection progresses and may cause potentially lethal disease, including pneumonitis, myocarditis, or encephalitis.

Alterations of T-lymphocyte populations during acute *T. gondii* infection are common and include lymphocytosis, increased CD8 count, and decreased CD4 : CD8 ratio. Depletion of CD4 cells in patients with AIDS may contribute to severe manifestations of toxoplasmosis. Characteristic lymph node changes include reactive follicular hyperplasia with irregular clusters of epithelioid histiocytes that encroach on and blur margins of germinal centers, and focal distention of sinuses with monocytoid cells.

Cysts form as early as 7 days after infection and remain for the life of the host. During latent infection they produce little or no inflammatory response but can cause recrudescent disease in immunocompromised persons. Recrudescent chorioretinitis occurs in children with postnatal infection but especially in older children and adults with congenital infection.

Congenital Toxoplasmosis. When a mother acquires infection during gestation, organisms may disseminate hematogenously to the placenta. Infection may be transmitted to the fetus transplacentally or during vaginal delivery. Of untreated maternal infections acquired in the 1st trimester, approximately 17% of fetuses are infected, usually with severe disease. Of untreated maternal infection acquired in the 3rd trimester, approximately 65% of fetuses are infected, usually with disease that is mild or inapparent at birth. These different rates of transmission and outcomes are most likely related to placental blood flow, virulence, inoculum of *T. gondii,* and immunologic capacity of the mother to limit parasitemia.

Examination of the placenta of infected newborns may reveal chronic inflammation and cysts. Tachyzoites can be seen with Wright or Giemsa stains but are best demonstrated with immunoperoxidase technique. Tissue cysts stain well with periodic acid-Schiff and silver stains as well as with the immunoperoxidase technique. Gross or microscopic areas of necrosis may be present in many tissues, especially the CNS, choroid and retina, heart, lungs, skeletal muscle, liver, and spleen. Areas of calcification occur in the brain.

Almost all congenitally infected individuals who are not treated manifest signs or symptoms of infection, such as chorioretinitis, by adolescence. Some severely involved infants with congenital infection appear to have *Toxoplasma* antigen–specific cell-mediated anergy, which may be important in the pathogenesis of disease. The predilection for predominant involvement of the CNS, choroid, and retina with congenital infection has not been fully explained.

CLINICAL MANIFESTATIONS. Manifestations of primary infection with *T. gondii* are highly variable and influenced primarily by host immunocompetence. There may be no signs or symptoms or severe disease. Reactivation of previously asymptomatic congenital toxoplasmosis usually manifests as ocular toxoplasmosis.

Acquired Toxoplasmosis. Immunocompetent children who acquire infection postnatally generally have do not have clinically recognizable symptoms. When clinical manifestations are apparent, they may include almost any combination of fever, stiff neck, myalgia, arthralgia, maculopapular rash that spares the palms and soles, localized or generalized lymphadenopathy, hepatomegaly, hepatitis, reactive lymphocytosis, meningitis, brain abscess, encephalitis, confusion, malaise, pneumonia, polymyositis, pericarditis, pericardial effusion, and myocarditis. Chorioretinitis, usually unilateral, occurs in approximately 1% of cases in the United States. Half the cases of ocular toxoplasmosis in English children are due to acute acquired infection; the appearance does not distinguish acute vs. congenital infection. Symptoms may be present for a few days only or may persist many months. The most common manifestation is enlargement of 1 or a few cervical lymph nodes. Cases of *Toxoplasma* lymphadenopathy rarely resemble infectious mononucleosis (caused by Epstein-Barr virus or cytomegalovirus), Hodgkin disease, or other lymphadenopathies (see Chapter 490). In the pectoral area in older girls and women, enlarged nodes may be confused with breast neoplasms. Mediastinal, mesenteric, and retroperitoneal lymph nodes may be involved. Involvement of intra-abdominal lymph nodes may be associated with fever and mimic appendicitis. Nodes may be tender but do not suppurate. Lymphadenopathy may wax and wane for as long as 1–2 yr.

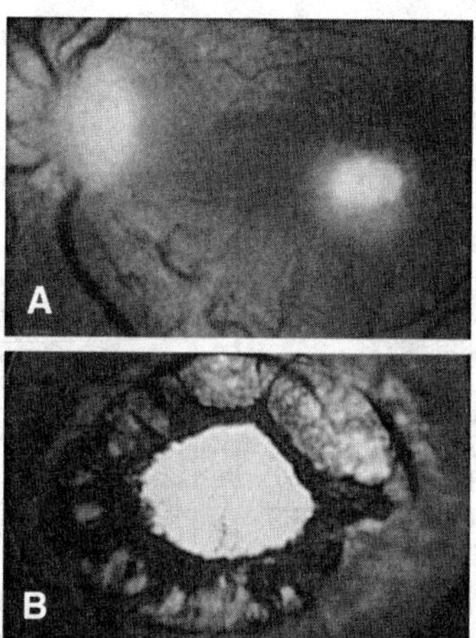

Figure 287-2. Toxoplasmic chorioretinitis. *A,* Active acute lesion by indirect ophthalmoscopy. *B,* The healed foci of toxoplasmic chorioretinitis may resemble a coloboma (macular pseudocoloboma). See also color plates. (B adapted from Desmonts G, Remington J: Congenital toxoplasmosis. In Remington JS, Klein JO [editors]: *Infectious Diseases of the Fetus and Newborn Infant,* 5th ed. Philadelphia, WB Saunders, 2001.)

Almost all patients with lymphadenopathy recover spontaneously without antimicrobial therapy. Significant organ involvement in immunologically normal persons is uncommon, although some individuals have suffered significant morbidity, including rare cases of encephalitis, brain abscesses, hepatitis, myocarditis, pericarditis, and polymyositis.

Ocular Toxoplasmosis. In the United States and Western Europe, *T. gondii* is estimated to cause 35% of cases of chorioretinitis (Fig. 287-2). In Brazil, *T. gondii* retinal lesions are common. Clinical manifestations include blurred vision, visual floaters, photophobia, epiphora, and, with macular involvement, loss of central vision. Ocular findings of congenital toxoplasmosis also include strabismus, microphthalmia, microcornea, cataract, anisometropia, nystagmus, glaucoma, optic neuritis, and optic atrophy. Episodic recurrences are common, but precipitating factors have not been defined.

Immunocompromised Persons. Disseminated *T. gondii* infection among older children who are immunocompromised by AIDS, malignancy, cytotoxic therapy or corticosteroids, or immunosuppressive drugs given for organ transplantation involves the CNS in 50% of cases and may also involve the heart, lungs, and gastrointestinal tract. Stem cell transplant recipients present a special problem because active infection is particularly difficult to diagnose. After transplantation, *T. gondii*–specific antibody levels may remain the same, increase, or decrease and can even become undetectable. Most often immunoglobulin G (IgG) antibody is present; thus, toxoplasmosis in these patients almost always results from transplantation from a seropositive individual to a seronegative recipient. Active infection is often fulminant and rapidly fatal.

Congenital *T. gondii* infection in infants with HIV infection is rare and is often a severe and fulminant disease with substantial CNS involvement, and alternatively may be more indolent in presentation with focal neurologic deficits or systemic manifestations such as pneumonitis.

From 25 to 50% of persons with *T. gondii* antibodies and **HIV infection** eventually experience toxoplasmic encephalitis, which is fatal if not treated. Highly active anti-retroviral therapy and trimethoprim-sulfamethoxazole prophylaxis have diminished the incidence of toxoplasmosis in patients with HIV infection, but toxoplasmic encephalitis remains a presenting manifestation in 20% of adult patients with AIDS. Typical findings include fever, headache, altered mental status, psychosis, cognitive impairment, seizures, and focal neurologic defects, including hemiparesis, aphasia, ataxia, visual field loss, cranial nerve palsies, and dysmetria or movement disorders. In adult patients with AIDS, toxoplasmic retinal lesions are often large with diffuse necrosis and contain many organisms but little inflammatory cellular infiltrate. Diagnosis of presumptive toxoplasmic encephalitis based on neuroradiologic studies in patients with AIDS necessitates a prompt therapeutic trial of medications effective against *T. gondii*. Clear clinical improvement within 7–14 days and improvement of neuroradiologic findings within 3 wk makes the presumptive diagnosis almost certain.

Congenital Toxoplasmosis. Congenital toxoplasmosis usually occurs when a woman acquires primary infection while pregnant. Most often, maternal infection is asymptomatic or without specific symptoms or signs. As with other adults with acute toxoplasmosis, lymphadenopathy is the most common symptom, but this is present in only a small subset of mothers of congenitally infected infants in the United States.

In monozygotic twins the clinical pattern of involvement is most often similar, whereas in dizygotic twins the manifestations often differ, including cases of congenital infection in only 1 twin. The major histocompatibility complex class II gene DQ3 appears to be more frequent among HIV-infected persons seropositive for *T. gondii* who develop toxoplasmic encephalitis, and in children with congenital toxoplasmosis who develop hydrocephalus. These findings suggest that the presence of HLA-DQ3 is a risk factor for severity of toxoplasmosis.

Congenital infection may present as a mild or severe neonatal disease, with onset during the 1st mo of life or with sequelae or relapse of a previously undiagnosed, and untreated, infection presenting during infancy or even later in life. There is a wide variety of manifestations of congenital infection ranging from hydrops fetalis and perinatal death to small size for gestational age, prematurity, peripheral retinal scars, persistent jaundice, mild thrombocytopenia, CSF pleocytosis, and the characteristic triad of chorioretinitis, hydrocephalus, and cerebral calcifications. More than half of congenitally infected infants are considered normal in the perinatal period, but almost all such children develop ocular involvement later in life if they are not treated during infancy. Neurologic signs such as convulsions, setting-sun sign with downward gaze, and hydrocephalus with increased head circumference may be associated with or without substantial cerebral damage, or with relatively mild inflammation obstructing the aqueduct of Sylvius. If affected infants are treated promptly, signs and symptoms may resolve and they may develop normally.

The spectrum and frequency of neonatal manifestations of 210 newborns with congenital *Toxoplasma* infection identified by a serologic screening program of pregnant women are presented in Table 287-1. In this study, 10% had severe congenital toxoplasmosis with CNS involvement, eye lesions, and general systemic manifestations; 34% had mild involvement with normal clinical examination results other than retinal scars or isolated intracranial calcifications; and 55% had no detectable manifestations. These represent an underestimation of the incidence of severe congenital infection for several reasons: the most severe cases, including most of those individuals who died, were not referred; therapeutic abortion was often performed when acute acquired infection of the mother was diagnosed early during pregnancy; in utero spiramycin therapy may have diminished the severity of infection; and only 13 infants had brain CT and 23% did not have a cerebrospinal fluid (CSF) examination. Routine newborn examinations often yield normal findings for congenitally infected infants, but more careful evaluations may reveal significant abnormalities. In 1 study of 28 infants identified by a universal state-mandated serologic screening program for *T. gondii*–specific IgM, 26 had normal findings on routine newborn examination and 14 had significant abnormalities detected with more careful evaluation. The abnormalities included retinal scars (7 infants), active chorioretinitis (3 infants), and CNS abnormalities (8 infants).

TABLE 287-1. Signs and Symptoms in 210 Infants with Proved Congenital *Toxoplasma* Infection*

FINDING	NO. EXAMINED	NO. POSITIVE (%)
Prematurity	210	
Birthweight <2,500 g		8 (3.8)
Birthweight 2,500–3,000 g		5 (7.1)
Intrauterine growth retardation		13 (6.2)
Icterus	201	20 (10)
Hepatosplenomegaly	210	9 (4.2)
Thrombocytopenic purpura	210	3 (1.4)
Abnormal blood count (anemia, eosinophilia)	102	9 (4.4)
Microcephaly	210	11 (5.2)
Hydrocephaly	210	8 (3.8)
Hypotonia	210	12 (5.7)
Convulsions	210	8 (3.8)
Psychomotor retardation	210	11 (5.2)
Intracranial calcification x-ray	210	24 (11.4)
Ultrasound	49	5 (10)
Computed tomography	13	11 (84)
Abnormal electroencephalogram	191	16 (8.3)
Abnormal cerebrospinal fluid	163	56 (34.2)
Microphthalmia	210	6 (2.8)
Strabismus	210	111 (5.2)
Chorioretinitis	210	
Unilateral		34 (16.1)
Bilateral		12 (5.7)

*Infants were identified by prospective study of infants born to women who acquired *Toxoplasma gondii* infection during pregnancy.

Data adapted from Couvreur J, Desmonts G, Tournier G, et al: A homogeneous series of 210 cases of congenital toxoplasmosis in 0–11 mo old infants detected prospectively. *Ann Pediatr (Paris)* 1984;31:815–819.

There is also a wide spectrum of symptoms of untreated congenital toxoplasmosis that presents later in the 1st yr of life (Table 287-2). More than 80% of these children have IQ scores of <70, and many have convulsions and severely impaired vision.

SYSTEMIC SIGNS. From 25% to >50% of infants with clinically apparent disease at birth are born prematurely. Intrauterine growth retardation, low Apgar scores, and temperature instability are common. Other manifestations may include lymphadenopathy, hepatosplenomegaly, myocarditis, pneumonitis, nephrotic syndrome, vomiting, diarrhea, and feeding problems. Bands of metaphyseal lucency and irregularity of the line of provisional calcification at the epiphyseal plate may occur without periosteal reaction in the ribs, femurs, and vertebrae. Congenital toxoplasmosis may be confused with erythroblastosis fetalis resulting from isosensitization, although the Coombs test result is usually negative with congenital *T. gondii* infection.

Skin. Cutaneous manifestations among newborn infants with congenital toxoplasmosis include rashes, petechiae, ecchymoses, and large hemorrhages secondary to thrombocytopenia. Rashes may be fine punctate, diffuse maculopapular, lenticular, deep blue-red, sharply defined macular, or diffuse blue and papular. Macular rashes involving the entire body including the palms and soles; exfoliative dermatitis; and cutaneous calcifications have been described. Jaundice with hepatic involvement and/or hemolysis, cyanosis due to interstitial pneumonitis from congenital infection, and edema secondary to myocarditis or nephrotic syndrome may be present. Jaundice and conjugated hyperbilirubinemia may persist for months.

Endocrine Abnormalities. Endocrine abnormalities may occur secondary to hypothalamic or pituitary involvement or end-organ involvement. Reported endocrinopathies include myxedema, persistent hypernatremia with vasopressin-sensitive diabetes insipidus without polyuria or polydipsia, sexual precocity, and partial anterior hypopituitarism.

TABLE 287-2. Signs and Symptoms Occurring Before Diagnosis or During the Course of Untreated Acute Congenital Toxoplasmosis in 152 Infants (A) and in 101 of These Same Children After They Had Been Followed 4 yr or More (B)

SIGNS AND SYMPTOMS	FREQUENCY OF OCCURRENCE IN PATIENTS WITH "Neurologic" Disease*	"Generalized" Disease†
A. INFANTS	**108 PATIENTS (%)**	**44 PATIENTS (%)**
Chorioretinitis	102 (94)	29 (66)
Abnormal cerebrospinal fluid	59 (55)	37 (84)
Anemia	55 (51)	34 (77)
Convulsions	54 (50)	8 (18)
Intracranial calcification	54 (50)	2 (4)
Jaundice	31 (29)	35 (80)
Hydrocephalus	30 (28)	0 (0)
Fever	27 (25)	34 (77)
Splenomegaly	23 (21)	40 (90)
Lymphadenopathy	18 (17)	30 (68)
Hepatomegaly	18 (17)	34 (77)
Vomiting	17 (16)	21 (48)
Microcephalus	14 (13)	0 (0)
Diarrhea	7 (6)	11 (25)
Cataracts	5 (5)	0 (0)
Eosinophilia	6 (4)	8 (18)
Abnormal bleeding	3 (3)	8 (18)
Hypothermia	2 (2)	9 (20)
Glaucoma	2 (2)	0 (0)
Optic atrophy	2 (2)	0 (0)
Microphthalmia	2 (2)	0 (0)
Rash	1 (1)	11 (25)
Pneumonitis	0 (0)	18 (41)
B. CHILDREN ≥4 YR OF AGE	**70 PATIENTS (%)**	**31 PATIENTS (%)**
Mental retardation	62 (89)	25 (81)
Convulsions	58 (83)	24 (77)
Spasticity and palsies	53 (76)	18 (58)
Severely impaired vision	48 (69)	13 (42)
Hydrocephalus or microcephalus	31 (44)	2 (6)
Deafness	12 (17)	3 (10)
Normal	6 (9)	5 (16)

*Patients with otherwise undiagnosed central nervous system disease in the 1st yr of life.
†Patients with otherwise undiagnosed non-neurologic diseases during the first 2 mo of life.
Adapted from Eichenwald H: A study of congenital toxoplasmosis. In Slim JC (editor): *Human Toxoplasmosis.* Copenhagen, Munksgaard, 1960, pp 41–49. Study performed in 1947. The most severely involved institutionalized patients were not included in the later study of 101 children.

Central Nervous System. Neurologic manifestations of congenital toxoplasmosis vary from massive acute encephalopathy to subtle neurologic syndromes. Toxoplasmosis should be considered as a potential cause of any undiagnosed neurologic disease in children <1 yr of age, especially if retinal lesions are present.

Hydrocephalus may be the sole clinical neurologic manifestation of congenital toxoplasmosis and may either be compensated or require shunt placement. Hydrocephalus may present prenatally and progress during the perinatal period, or, less commonly, may present later in life. Patterns of seizures are protean and have included focal motor seizures, petit and grand mal seizures, muscular twitching, opisthotonus, and hypsarrhythmia, which may resolve with corticotropin (ACTH) therapy. Spinal or bulbar involvement may be manifested by paralysis of the extremities, difficulty swallowing, and respiratory distress. Microcephaly usually reflects severe brain damage, but some children with microcephaly caused by congenital toxoplasmosis who have been treated have normal or superior cognitive function. Untreated congenital toxoplasmosis that is symptomatic in the 1st yr of life can cause substantial diminution in cognitive function and developmental delay. Intellectual impairment also occurs in some children with subclinical infection despite treatment with pyrimethamine and sulfonamides. Seizures and focal motor defects may become apparent after the newborn period, even when infection is subclinical at birth.

CSF abnormalities occur in at least ⅓ of infants with congenital toxoplasmosis. A CSF protein level of >1 g/dL is characteristic of severe CNS toxoplasmosis, which is usually accompanied by hydrocephalus. Local production of *T. gondii*–specific IgG and IgM antibodies may be demonstrated. CT of the brain is useful to detect calcifications, determine ventricular size, and demonstrate porencephalic cystic structures (Fig. 287-3). Calcifications occur throughout the brain, but there is propensity for development of calcifications in the caudate nucleus and basal ganglia, choroid plexus, and subependyma. MRI and contrast-enhanced CT brain scans are useful for detecting active inflammatory lesions. Ultrasonography may be useful for following ventricular size.

Eyes. Almost all untreated congenitally infected infants develop chorioretinal lesions by adulthood, and about 50% will have severe visual impairment. *T. gondii* causes a focal necrotizing retinitis in congenitally infected individuals (see Fig. 287-2). Retinal detachment may occur. Any part of the retina may be involved, either unilaterally or bilaterally, including the maculae. The optic nerve may be involved, and toxoplasmic lesions that involve projections of the visual pathways in the brain or the visual cortex also may lead to visual impairment. In association with retinal lesions and vitritis, the anterior uvea may be intensely inflamed, leading to erythema of the external eye. Other ocular findings include cells and protein in the anterior chamber, large keratic precipitates, posterior synechiae, nodules on the iris, and neovascular formation on the surface of the iris, sometimes with increased intraocular pressure and glaucoma. The extraocular musculature may also be involved directly. Other manifestations include strabismus, nystagmus, visual impairment, and microphthalmia. Enucleation has been required for a blind, phthisic, painful eye. The differential diagnosis of ocular toxoplasmosis includes congenital coloboma and inflammatory lesions caused by cytomegalovirus, *Treponema pallidum, Mycobacterium tuberculosis,* or vasculitis. Ocular toxoplasmosis may be a recurrent and progressive disease that requires multiple courses of therapy. Limited data suggest that occurrence of lesions in the early years of life may be prevented by instituting antimicrobial treatment with pyrimethamine and sulfonamides during the 1st yr of life and that treatment of the infected fetus in utero followed by treatment in the 1st yr of life with pyrimethamine, sulfadiazine, and leukovorin reduces the incidence and the severity of the retinal disease.

Ears. Sensorineural hearing loss, both mild and severe, may occur. It is not known whether this is a static or progressive disorder. Treatment in the 1st yr of life is associated with decreased frequency of hearing loss.

DIAGNOSIS. Diagnosis of acute *Toxoplasma* infection can be established by culture of *T. gondii* from blood or body fluids, identification of tachyzoites in sections or preparations of tissues and body fluids, identification of cysts in the placenta or tissues of a fetus or newborn, and characteristic lymph node histologic features. Serologic tests also are very useful for diagnosis. Polymerase chain reaction (PCR) also is useful to identify *T. gondii* DNA in CSF, amniotic fluid, infant peripheral blood, and urine to definitively establish the diagnosis.

Culture. Organisms are isolated by inoculation of body fluids, leukocytes, or tissue specimens into mice or tissue cultures. Body fluids should be processed and inoculated immediately, but *T. gondii* has been isolated from tissues and blood that have been stored overnight or even for 4–5 days at 4°C. Freezing or treatment of specimens with formalin kills *T. gondii.* From 6 to 10 days after inoculation into mice, or earlier if mice die, peritoneal fluids should be examined for tachyzoites. If inoculated mice survive for 6 wk and seroconvert, definitive diagnosis is made by visualization of *Toxoplasma* cysts in mouse brain. If cysts are not seen, subinoculations of mouse tissue into other mice are performed.

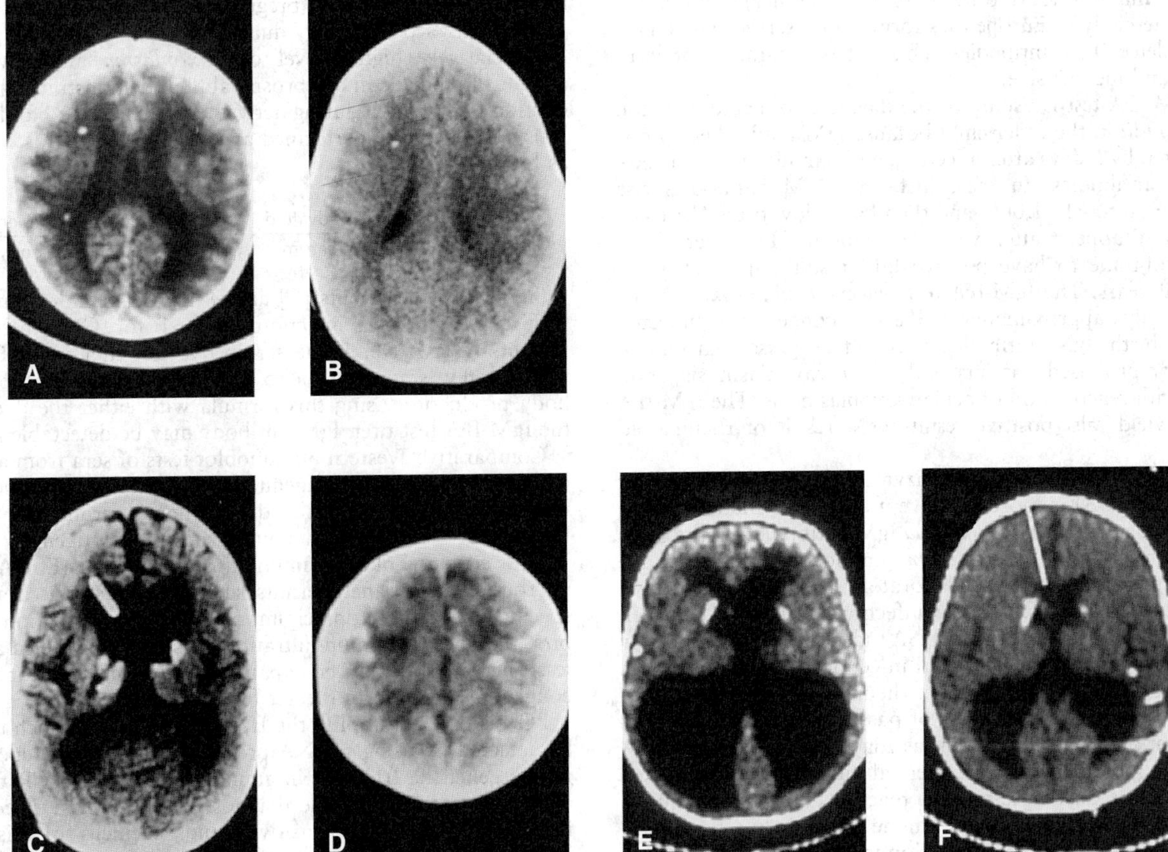

Figure 287-3. Head CT scans of infants with congenital toxoplasmosis. *A*, CT scan at birth that shows areas of hypolucency, mildly dilated ventricles, and small calcifications. *B*, CT scan of the same child at 1 yr of age (after antimicrobial therapy for 1 yr). This scan is normal with the exception of 2 small calcifications. This child's Mental Development Index (MDI) at 1 yr of age was 140 by the Bayley Scale of Infant Development. *C*, CT scan from a 1 yr old infant who was normal at birth. His meningoencephalitis became symptomatic in the 1st weeks of life but was not diagnosed correctly and remained untreated during his 1st 3 mo of life. At 3 mo of age, development of hydrocephalus and bilateral macular chorioretinitis led to the diagnosis of congenital toxoplasmosis, and antimicrobial therapy was initiated. This scan shows significant residual atrophy and calcifications. This child had substantial motor dysfunction, development delays, and visual impairment. *D*, CT scan obtained during the 1st mo of life of a microcephalic child. Note the numerous calcifications. This child's IQ scores using the Stanford-Binet Intelligence Scale for children when she was 3 yr of age and the Wechsler Preschool and Primary Scale Intelligence when she was 5 yr of age were 100 and 102, respectively. She received antimicrobial therapy during her 1st yr of life. *E*, CT scan with hydrocephalus owing to aqueductal stenosis, before shunt. *F*, Scan from the same patient as the scan in E, after shunt. This child's IQ scores using the Stanford-Binet Intelligence Scale for children were approximately 100 when she was 3 and 6 yr of age. (Adapted from McAuley J, Boyer K, Patel D, et al: Early and longitudinal evaluations of treated infants and children and untreated historical patients with congenital toxoplasmosis: The Chicago Collaborative Treatment Trial. *Clin Infect Dis* 1994;18:38–72.)

Microscopic examination of tissue culture inoculated with *T. gondii* shows necrotic, heavily infected cells with numerous extracellular tachyzoites. Isolation of *T. gondii* from blood or body fluids reflects acute infection. Except in the fetus or neonate it is usually not possible to distinguish acute from past infection by isolation of *T. gondii* from tissues such as skeletal muscle, lung, brain, or eye obtained by biopsy or at autopsy.

Diagnosis of acute infection can be established by demonstration of tachyzoites in biopsy tissue sections, bone marrow aspirate, or body fluids such as CSF or amniotic fluid. Immunofluorescent antibody and immunoperoxidase staining techniques may be necessary because it is often difficult to distinguish the tachyzoite using ordinary stains. Tissue cysts are diagnostic of infection but do not differentiate between acute and chronic infection, although the presence of many cysts suggests recent acute infection. Cysts in the placenta or tissues of the newborn infant establish the diagnosis of congenital infection. Characteristic histologic features strongly suggest the diagnosis of toxoplasmic lymphadenitis.

Serologic Testing. Multiple serologic tests may be necessary to confirm the diagnosis of congenital or acutely acquired *Toxoplasma* infection. Each laboratory that reports serologic test results must have established values for their tests that diagnose infection in specific clinical settings, provide interpretation of their results, and ensure appropriate quality control before therapy is based on serologic test results. Serologic test results used as the basis for therapy should be confirmed in a reference laboratory.

The **Sabin-Feldman dye test** is sensitive and specific. It measures primarily IgG antibodies. Results should be expressed in international units (IU/mL), based on international standard reference sera available from the World Health Organization.

The **IgG indirect fluorescent-antibody (IgG-IFA) test** measures the same antibodies as the dye test, and the titers tend to be parallel. These antibodies usually appear 1–2 wk after infection, reach high titers (≥1 : 1,000) after 6–8 wk, and then decline over months to years. Low titers (1 : 4 to 1 : 64) usually persist for life. Antibody titer does not correlate with severity of illness. Approximately half of the commercially available IFA kits for *T. gondii* have been found to be improperly standardized and may yield significant numbers of false-positive and false-negative results.

An **agglutination test** (Bio-Mérieux, Lyon, France) that is available commercially in Europe uses formalin-preserved whole parasites to detect IgG antibodies. This test is accurate, simple to perform, and inexpensive.

The **IgM-IFA test** is useful for the diagnosis of acute infection with *T. gondii* in the older child because IgM antibodies appear earlier, often by 5 days after infection, and diminish more quickly than IgG antibodies. In most instances, IgM antibodies rise rapidly (1 : 50 to <1 : 1,000) and then fall to low titers (1 : 10 or 1 : 20) or disappear after weeks or months. However, some patients continue to have positive IgM results with low titers for several years. The IgM-IFA test detects *Toxoplasma*-specific IgM in only approximately 25% of congenitally infected infants at birth. IgM antibodies may not be present in sera of immunocompromised patients with acute toxoplasmosis or in patients with reactivation of ocular toxoplasmosis. The IgM-IFA test may yield false-positive results as a result of rheumatoid factor.

The **double-sandwich IgM enzyme-linked immunosorbent assay (IgM-ELISA)** is more sensitive and specific than the IgM-IFA test for detection of *Toxoplasma* IgM antibodies. In the older child, serum IgM-ELISA *Toxoplasma* antibodies of >2.0 (a value of 1 reference laboratory; each laboratory must establish its own value) indicates that *Toxoplasma* infection most likely has been acquired recently. The IgM-ELISA identifies approximately 50–75% of infants with congenital infection. IgM-ELISA avoids both the false-positive results from rheumatoid factor and false-negative results from high levels of passively transferred maternal IgG antibody in fetal serum, as may occur in the IgM-IFA test. Results obtained with commercial kits must be interpreted with caution because false-positive reactions are not infrequent. Care must also be taken to determine whether kits have been standardized for diagnosis of infection in specific clinical settings, such as in the newborn infant. The **IgA-ELISA** also is a sensitive test for detection of maternal and congenital infection, and results may be positive when those of the IgM-ELISA are not.

The **immunosorbent agglutination assay (ISAGA)** combines trapping of a patient's IgM, IgA, or IgE to a solid surface and use of formalin-fixed organisms or antigen-coated latex particles. It is read as an agglutination test. There are no false-positive results from rheumatoid factor or antinuclear antibodies. The IgM-ISAGA is more sensitive than the IgM-ELISA and may detect specific IgM antibodies before and for longer periods than the IgM-ELISA.

At present, the IgM-ISAGA as well as the **IgA-ISAGA** and **IgA-ELISA** are the best tests for diagnosis of congenital infection in the newborn. The **IgE-ELISA** and **IgE-ISAGA** are also sometimes useful in establishing the diagnosis of congenital toxoplasmosis or acute acquired *T. gondii* infection. The presence of IgM antibodies in the older child or adult can never be used alone to diagnose acute acquired infection.

The **differential agglutination test (HS/AC)** compares antibody titers obtained with formalin-fixed tachyzoites (**HS antigen**) with titers obtained using acetone- or methanol-fixed tachyzoites (**AC antigen**) to differentiate recent and remote infections in adults and older children. This method may be particularly useful in differentiating remote infection in pregnant women because levels of IgM and IgA antibodies detectable by ELISA or ISAGA may remain elevated for months to years in adults and older children.

The **avidity test** can be helpful to time infection. A high-avidity test result indicates that infection began >16 wk earlier, which is especially useful in determining time of acquisition of infection in the 1st or final 16 wk of gestation. A low-avidity test result may be present for many months and is not diagnostic of recent acquisition of infection.

The **indirect hemagglutination (IHA) test** measures different *T. gondii* antibodies from those measured in IFA and dye tests. They may persist for years. However, the IHA test should not be used in infants with suspected congenital infection or in screening for infection acquired during pregnancy because it may be negative for too long a period early during infection.

A relatively higher level of *Toxoplasma* antibody in the aqueous humor or in cerebrospinal fluid demonstrates local production of antibody during active ocular or CNS toxoplasmosis. This comparison is performed and a coefficient [C] is calculated as follows:

$$C = \frac{\text{Antibody titer in body fluid}}{\text{Antibody titer in serum}} \times \frac{\text{Concentration of IgG in serum}}{\text{Concentration of IgG in body fluid}}$$

Significant coefficients [C] are >8 for ocular infection, >4 for CNS for congenital infection, and >1 for CNS infection in patients with AIDS. If the serum dye test titer is >300 IU/mL, most often it is not possible to demonstrate significant local antibody production using this formula with either the dye test or the IgM-IFA test titer. IgM antibody may be detectable in CSF.

Comparative **Western immunoblot** tests of sera from a mother and infant may detect congenital infection. Infection is suspected when the mother's serum and her infant's serum contain antibodies that react with different *Toxoplasma* antigens.

The **enzyme-linked immunofiltration assay (ELIFA)** using micropore membranes permits simultaneous study of antibody specificity by immunoprecipitation and characterization of antibody isotypes by immunofiltration with enzyme-labeled antibodies. This method may be capable of detecting 85% of cases of congenital infection in the 1st few days of life.

PCR is used to amplify the DNA of *T. gondii,* which then can be detected by using a DNA probe. Detection of a repetitive *T. gondii* gene, the B1 gene, in amniotic fluid is the PCR target of choice for establishing the diagnosis of congenital *Toxoplasma* infection in the fetus. Sensitivity and specificity of this test in amniotic fluid obtained to diagnose infections acquired between 17 and 21 wk of gestation are approximately 95%. Before and after that time, PCR is less sensitive for detection of congenital infection. PCR of vitreous or aqueous fluids also has been used to diagnose ocular toxoplasmosis. PCR of peripheral white blood cells, CSF, and urine has been used to detect congenital infection.

Lymphocyte blastogenesis to *Toxoplasma* antigens has been used to diagnose congenital toxoplasmosis when the diagnosis is uncertain and other test results are negative. However, a negative result does not exclude the diagnosis because many infected newborns do not respond to *T. gondii* antigens.

Acquired Toxoplasmosis. Recent infection is diagnosed by seroconversion from a negative to a positive IgG antibody titer (in the absence of transfusion); a 2 tube increase in *Toxoplasma*-specific IgG titer when serial sera are obtained 3 wk apart and tested in parallel; or the detection of *Toxoplasma*-specific IgM antibody in conjunction with other tests, but never alone.

Ocular Toxoplasmosis. IgG antibody titers of 1 : 4 to 1 : 64 are usual in older children with active *Toxoplasma* chorioretinitis. The diagnosis is likely with characteristic retinal lesions and positive serologic tests. PCR of aqueous or vitreous fluid has been used to diagnose ocular toxoplasmosis but is infrequently performed because of risks associated with obtaining fluid.

Immunocompromised Persons. IgG antibody titers may be low, and *Toxoplasma*-specific IgM is often absent in immunocompromised stem cell transplant recipients, but not kidney or heart transplant recipients with toxoplasmosis. Demonstration of *Toxoplasma* antigens or DNA in serum, blood, and CSF may identify disseminated *Toxoplasma* infection in immunocompromised persons. Resolution of CNS lesions during a therapeutic trial of pyrimethamine and sulfadiazine has been useful to diagnose toxoplasmic encephalitis in patients with AIDS. Brain biopsy has been used to establish the diagnosis if there is no response to a therapeutic trial and to exclude other likely diagnoses such as CNS lymphoma.

Congenital Toxoplasmosis. Fetal ultrasound examination, performed every 2 wk during gestation, beginning at the time acute acquired infection is diagnosed in a pregnant woman, and PCR analysis of amniotic fluid are used for prenatal diagnosis. *T. gondii* may also be isolated from the placenta at delivery.

Serologic tests are also useful in establishing a diagnosis of congenital toxoplasmosis. Either persistent or rising titers in the dye test or IFA test, or a positive IgM-ELISA or IgM-ISAGA result is diagnostic of congenital toxoplasmosis. The half-life of IgM is about 2 days, so if there is a placental leak, the level of IgM antibodies in the infant's serum decreases significantly, usually within 1 wk. Passively transferred maternal IgG antibodies may require many months to a year to disappear from the infant's serum, depending on the magnitude of the original titer. Synthesis of *Toxoplasma* antibody is usually demonstrable by the 3rd mo of life if the infant is untreated. If the infant is treated, synthesis may be delayed for as long as the 9th mo of life and, infrequently, may not occur at all. When an infant begins to synthesize IgG antibody, infection may be documented serologically even without demonstration of IgM antibodies by an increase in the ratio of specific serum IgG antibody titer to the total IgG, whereas the ratio will decrease if the specific IgG antibody has been passively transferred from the mother.

Newborns suspected of having congenital toxoplasmosis should be evaluated by general, ophthalmologic, and neurologic examinations; head CT scan; attempt to isolate *T. gondii* from the placenta and infant's leukocytes from umbilical cord blood and buffy coat; measurement of serum *Toxoplasma*-specific IgG, IgM, IgA, and IgE antibodies, and the levels of total serum IgM and IgG; lumbar puncture including analysis of CSF for cells, glucose, protein, *Toxoplasma*-specific IgG and IgM antibodies, and level of total IgG; and testing of CSF for *T. gondii* by PCR and inoculation into mice. Presence of *Toxoplasma*-specific IgM in CSF that is not contaminated with blood or confirmation of local antibody production of *Toxoplasma*-specific IgG antibody in CSF establishes the diagnosis of congenital *Toxoplasma* infection.

Many manifestations of congenital toxoplasmosis occur in other perinatal infections, especially congenital cytomegalovirus infection. Neither cerebral calcification nor chorioretinitis is pathognomonic. The clinical picture in the newborn infant may also be compatible with sepsis, aseptic meningitis, syphilis, or hemolytic disease. Fewer than 50% of children <5 yr of age with chorioretinitis satisfy the serologic criteria for congenital toxoplasmosis, and some of these are caused by postnatally acquired *T. gondii* infection. The causes of most of the other cases of chorioretinitis are unknown

TREATMENT. Pyrimethamine plus sulfadiazine act synergistically against *Toxoplasma,* and combination therapy is indicated for many of the forms of toxoplasmosis. However, use of pyrimethamine is contraindicated during the 1st trimester of pregnancy. Spiramycin should be used to attempt to prevent vertical transmission of infection to the fetus of acutely infected pregnant women, and to treat congenital toxoplasmosis. Pyrimethamine inhibits the enzyme dihydrofolate reductase (DHFR), and thus the synthesis of folic acid, and therefore produces a dose-related, reversible, and usually gradual depression of the bone marrow, resulting in thrombocytopenia, leukopenia, and anemia. Reversible neutropenia is the most common adverse effect in treated infants. All patients treated with pyrimethamine should have platelet and leukocyte counts twice weekly. Seizures may occur with overdosage of pyrimethamine. Folinic acid, as calcium leukovorin, should always be administered concomitantly and for 1 wk after treatment with pyrimethamine is discontinued to prevent bone marrow suppression. Potential toxic effects of sulfonamides (e.g., crystalluria, hematuria, and rash) should be monitored. Hypersensitivity reactions occur, especially in patients with AIDS.

Acquired Toxoplasmosis. Patients with acquired toxoplasmosis and lymphadenopathy do not need specific treatment unless they have severe and persistent symptoms or evidence of damage to vital organs. If such signs and symptoms occur, treatment with pyrimethamine, sulfadiazine, and leukovorin should be initiated. Patients who appear to be immunocompetent but have severe and persistent symptoms or damage to vital organs (e.g., chorioretinitis, myocarditis) need specific therapy until these specific symptoms resolve, followed by therapy for an additional 2 wk. Therapy is usually administered for at least 4–6 wk. The optimal duration of therapy is unknown. A loading dose of pyrimethamine for older children is 2 mg/kg/day (maximum 50 mg/day), given for the 1st 2 days of treatment. The maintenance dose is 1 mg/kg/day (maximum 50 mg/day). Sulfadiazine is administered to children >1 yr of age at a dosage of 100 mg/kg/day (maximum 4 g/day). Leukovorin is administered orally at a dosage of 5–20 mg 3 times a week (or even daily depending on the leukocyte count).

Ocular Toxoplasmosis. Patients with ocular toxoplasmosis are usually treated with pyrimethamine, sulfadiazine, and leukovorin for approximately 1 wk after the lesion develops a quiescent appearance (i.e., sharp borders and associated inflammatory cells in the vitreous resolve), which usually occurs in 2–4 wk. Within 7–10 days the borders of the retinal lesions sharpen, and visual acuity usually returns to that noted before development of the acute lesion. Systemic corticosteroids have been administered concomitantly with antimicrobial treatment when lesions involve the macula, optic nerve head, or papillomacular bundle. Most new lesions appear contiguous to old ones). Very rarely, vitrectomy and removal of the lens are needed to restore visual acuity.

Immunocompromised Persons. Serologic evidence of acute infection in an immunocompromised patient, regardless of whether signs and symptoms of infection are present or tachyzoites are demonstrated in tissue, are indications for therapy similar to that described for immunocompetent persons with symptoms of organ injury. It is important to establish the diagnosis as rapidly as possible and institute treatment early. In immunocompromised patients other than those with AIDS, therapy should be continued for at least 4–6 wk beyond complete resolution of all signs and symptoms of active disease. Careful follow-up observation of these patients is imperative because relapse may occur, requiring prompt reinstitution of therapy. Relapse is frequent in patients with AIDS, and suppressive therapy with pyrimethamine and sulfonamides, or trimethoprim-sulfamethoxazole, traditionally has been continued for life. Recently, it has been shown to be possible to discontinue maintenance therapy when the CD4 count remains at >200 cells/μL for 4–6 mo and all lesions have resolved. Therapy usually induces a beneficial response clinically, but it does not eradicate cysts. Treatment of *T. gondii*–seropositive patients with AIDS should be continued as long as CD4 counts remain at <200 cells/μL. Prophylactic treatment with trimethoprim-sulfamethoxazole for *Pneumocystis carinii* pneumonia significantly reduces the incidence of toxoplasmosis in patients with AIDS.

Congenital Toxoplasmosis. All newborns infected with *T. gondii* should be treated whether or not they have clinical manifestations of the infection because treatment may be effective in interrupting acute disease that damages vital organs. Infants should be treated for 1 yr with pyrimethamine (2 mg/kg/day for 2 days, then 1 mg/kg/day for 2 or 6 mo, then 1 mg/kg given on Monday, Wednesday, and Friday, or more often, PO), sulfadiazine (100 mg/kg/day divided bid PO), and leukovorin (5–10 mg given on Monday, Wednesday, and Friday, PO). The relative efficacy in reducing sequelae of infection and the safety of treatment with 2 vs 6 mo of the higher dosage of pyrimethamine are being compared in the U.S. National Collaborative Study. Updated information about this study and these regimens is available from Dr. Rima McLeod (773–834–4131). Pyrimethamine and sulfadiazine are available only in tablet form and can be prepared as suspensions. Prednisone (1 mg/kg/day divided bid PO) has been utilized in addition when active chorioretinitis involves the macula or otherwise threatens vision or the CSF protein is >1,000 mg/dL at birth, but the efficacy is not established.

Pregnant Women with *T. gondii* Infection. The immunologically normal pregnant woman who acquired *T. gondii* before conception does not need treatment to prevent congenital infection of her fetus. Although data are not available to allow for a definitive time interval, if infection occurs during the 6 mo prior to conception, it is reasonable to evaluate the fetus by use of PCR with amniotic fluid and ultrasonography and treat to prevent congenital infection in the fetus in the same manner as described for the acutely infected pregnant patient.

Treatment of a pregnant woman who acquires infection at any time during pregnancy reduces the chance of congenital infection in her infant. Spiramycin (1 g every 8 hr PO without food) is recommended for prevention of fetal infection if the mother develops acute *Toxoplasmosis* during pregnancy. Spiramycin is available in the United States through the Food and Drug Administration (301–796–1600, attn. Leo Chan) after the diagnosis of acute infection is confirmed in a reference laboratory (650–326–8120). Adverse reactions are infrequent and include paresthesias, rash, nausea, vomiting, and diarrhea. Pyrimethamine (50 mg once daily PO), sulfadiazine (2 g bid PO), and leukovorin (10 mg once daily PO) are recommended for confirmed or probable fetal infection except in the 1st trimester, when spiramycin is recommended because pyrimethamine is potentially teratogenic. Treatment of the mother of an infected fetus with pyrimethamine and sulfadiazine reduces infection in the placenta and the severity of disease in the newborn. Delay in maternal treatment during gestation results in greater brain and eye disease in the infant. Diagnostic amniocentesis should be performed at >17–18 wk of gestation in pregnancies when there is high suspicion of fetal infection. Overall sensitivity of PCR for amniotic fluid is at 85% between 17 and 21 wk of gestation. The sensitivity of PCR using amniotic fluid is less in early and late gestation than in midgestation.

The approach in France to congenital toxoplasmosis includes systematic serologic screening of all women of childbearing age and again intrapartum. Mothers with acute infection are treated with spiramycin, which decreases the transmission from 60% to 23%. Ultrasonography and amniocentesis for PCR at approximately 18 wk of gestation are used for fetal diagnosis, which have 97% sensitivity and 100% specificity. Confidence intervals for sensitivity are largest early and late in gestation. Fetal infection is treated with pyrimethamine and sulfadiazine, or by termination of pregnancy. This strategy has an excellent outcome with normal development of children. Only 19% have subtle findings of congenital infection, including intracranial calcifications (13%) and chorioretinal scars (6%), although 39% have chorioretinal scars detected at follow-up observation during later childhood.

Chronically infected pregnant women who are immunocompromised have transmitted *T. gondii* to their fetuses. Such women should be treated with spiramycin throughout gestation. The optimal management for prevention of congenital toxoplasmosis in the fetus of a pregnant woman with HIV infection and inactive *T. gondii* infection is unknown. If the pregnancy is not terminated, some investigators suggest that the mother should be treated with spiramycin during the 1st 14 wk of gestation and thereafter with pyrimethamine and sulfadiazine until term. There are no accepted guidelines. In a study of adult patients with AIDS, pyrimethamine (75 mg once daily PO) combined with high dosages of intravenously administered clindamycin (1,200 mg every 6 hr IV) appeared equal in efficacy to sulfadiazine and pyrimethamine in the treatment of toxoplasmic encephalitis. Other currently experimental agents include the macrolides roxithromycin and azithromycin.

PROGNOSIS. Early institution of specific treatment for congenitally infected infants usually cures the active manifestations of toxoplasmosis including active chorioretinitis, meningitis, encephalitis, hepatitis, splenomegaly, and thrombocytopenia. Rarely, hydrocephalus resulting from aqueductal obstruction may develop or become worse during therapy. Treatment appears to reduce the incidence of some sequelae such as diminished cognitive and abnormal motor function. Without therapy and in some treated patients as well, chorioretinitis often recurs. Children with extensive involvement at birth may function normally later in life or have mild to severe impairment of vision, hearing, cognitive function, and other neurologic functions. Delays in diagnosis and therapy, perinatal hypoglycemia, hypoxia, hypotension, repeated shunt infections, and severe visual impairment are associated with a poorer prognosis. The prognosis is guarded but is not necessarily poor for infected babies. Treatment with pyrimethamine and sulfadiazine does not eradicate the encysted parasite.

Studies in Lyon, France, indicated that outcome of treated fetal toxoplasmosis, even when infection is acquired early in gestation, is usually favorable if no hydrocephalus is detected on ultrasound and treatment with pyrimethamine and sulfadiazine is initiated promptly. The Syricot study in Europe indicated that outcome is improved with shorter times between diagnosis and initiation of treatment of fetal toxoplasmosis. Work in Lyon, France has indicated a low incidence of recurrent eye disease in children with congenital toxoplasmosis who had been treated in utero and in their 1st year of life, but most of this cohort is still not in adolescence, a time when recurrences seemed to increase, so longer term outcomes are not yet established. The NCCCTS (1981–2004) in the United States found that neurologic, developmental, audiologic, and ophthalmologic outcomes are considerably better for most, but not all, children who were treated in their 1st year of life with pyrimethamine and sulfadiazine (with leukovorin) when compared to children who had not been treated or were treated for only 1 month in earlier decades. The mean age of the children in this study was 10.8 years at the time of this analysis, and most of the children had not yet entered their teenage years, which is a time when recurrent disease may increase.

PREVENTION. Counseling pregnant women about the methods of preventing transmission of *T. gondii* (see Fig. 287-1) during pregnancy can substantially reduce acquisition of infection during gestation. Women who do not have specific antibody to *T. gondii* before pregnancy should only eat well-cooked meat during pregnancy and avoid contact with oocysts excreted by cats. Cats that are kept indoors, maintained on prepared food, and not fed fresh, uncooked meat should not contact encysted *T. gondii* or shed oocysts. Serologic screening, ultrasound monitoring, and treatment of pregnant women during gestation can also reduce the incidence and manifestations of congenital toxoplasmosis. No protective vaccine is available.

Berrebi A, Bardou M, Bessieres MH, et al: Outcome for children infected with congenital toxoplasmosis in the first trimester and with normal ultrasound findings: A study of 36 cases. *Eur J Obstet Gynecol* 2006;doi 10.1016/j.ejogrb.2006.11.002.

Boyer K, Holfels E, Roizen N, et al: Risk factors for *Toxoplasma gondii* infection in mothers of infants with congenital toxoplasmosis: Implications for prenatal management and screening. *Am J Obstet Gynecol* 2005;192:564–571.

Brezin AP, Thulliez P, Couvreur J, et al: Ophthalmic outcomes after prenatal and postnatal treatment of congenital toxoplasmosis. *Am J Ophthalmol* 2003;135(6):779–784.

Daffos F, Forestier F, Capella-Pavlovsky M, et al: Prenatal management of 746 pregnancies at risk for congenital toxoplasmosis. *N Engl J Med* 1988;318:271–275.

Desmonts G, Couvreur J: Natural history of congenital toxoplasmosis. *Ann Pediatr* 1984;31:799–802.

Foulon W, Villena E, Stray-Pedersen B, et al: Treatment of toxoplasmosis during pregnancy: A multicenter study of impact on fetal transmission and children's sequelae at age 1 year. *Am J Obstet Gynecol* 1999;180;410–415.

Kodjikian L, Wallon M, Fleury J, et al: Ocular manifestations in congenital toxoplasmosis. *Graefes Arch Clin Exp Ophthalmol* 2006;244:14–21.

Liesenfeld O, Montoya JG, Kenney S, et al: Effect of testing for IgG avidity in the diagnosis of *Toxoplasma gondii* infection in pregnant women: Experience in a US reference laboratory. *J Infect Dis* 2001;183:1248–1253.

McAuley J, Boyer K, Patel D, et al: Early and longitudinal evaluations of treated infants and children and untreated historical patients with congenital toxoplasmosis. The Chicago Collaborative Treatment Trial. *Clin Infect Dis* 1994;18:38–72.

McLeod R, Boyer K, Karrison T, et al: Outcome of treatment for congenital toxoplasmosis. 1981–2004: The national collaborative Chicago-based congenital toxoplasmosis study. *Clin Infect Dis* 2006;42:1383–1394.

McLeod R, Boyer K, Roizen N, et al: The child with congenital toxoplasmosis. *Curr Clin Top Infect Dis* 2000;20:189–208.

Mets MB, Holfels E, Boyer KM, et al: Eye manifestations of congenital toxoplasmosis. *Am J Ophthalmol* 1997;123:1–16.

Montoya JG: Laboratory diagnosis of *Toxoplasma gondii* infection and toxoplasmosis. *J Infect Dis* 2002;1855(Suppl):S73–S82.

Montoya JG, Liesenfeld O: Toxoplasmosis. *Lancet* 2004;363:1965–1976.

Remington JS, McLeod R, Thulliez P, et al: Toxoplasmosis. In Remington J, Klein J, Wilson C, Baker C (editors): *Infectious Diseases of the Fetus and Newborn Infant,* 6th ed. Philadelphia, WB Saunders, 2006. pp 947–1092.

Remington JS, Thulliez P, Montoya JG: Recent developments for diagnosis of toxoplasmosis. *J Clin Microbiol* 2004;42:941–945.

Roberts F, Mets MB, Ferguson DJP, et al: Histopathological feature of ocular toxoplasmosis in the fetus and infant. *Arch Ophthalmol* 2001;119: 1–58.

Roizen N, Swisher C, Boyer K, et al: Developmental and neurologic outcome in congenital toxoplasmosis. *Pediatrics* 1995;95:11–20.

Romand S, Wallon J, Franck J, et al: Prenatal diagnosis using polymerase chain reaction on amniotic fluid for congenital toxoplasmosis. *Obstet Gynecol* 2001;97:296–300.

Stanford MR, Tan HK, Gilbert RE: Toxoplasmic retinochoroiditis presenting in childhood: clinical findings in a UK survey. *Br J Ophthalmol* 2006;90: 1464–1467.

The SYROCOT (Systematic Review on Congenital Toxoplasmosis) study group: Effectiveness of prenatal treatment for congenital toxoplasmosis: a meta-analysis of individual patient's data. *Lancet* 2007;369:115–122.

Wallon M, Kodjikian L, Binguiet C, et al: Long-term ocular prognosis in 327 children with congenital toxoplasmosis. *Pediatrics* 2004;113:1567–1572.

Section 16 — Helminthic Diseases

Chapter 288 ■ Ascariasis (*Ascaris Lumbricoides*)

Arlene E. Dent and James W. Kazura

ETIOLOGY. Ascariasis is caused by the nematode, or roundworm, *Ascaris lumbricoides*. Adult worms of *A. lumbricoides* inhabit the lumen of the small intestine and have a life span of 10–24 mo. The reproductive potential of *Ascaris* is prodigious; a gravid female worm produces 200,000 eggs/day. The fertile ova are oval in shape with a thick mammillated covering measuring 45–70 µm in length and 35–50 µm in breadth (Fig. 288-1). After passage in the feces, the eggs embryonate and become infective in 5–10 days under favorable environmental conditions. Adult worms can live for 12–18 mo (Fig. 288-2).

EPIDEMIOLOGY. Ascariasis occurs globally and is the most prevalent human helminthiasis in the world. It is most common in tropical areas of the world where environmental conditions are optimal for maturation of ova in the soil. Approximately 1 billion persons are estimated to be infected, with 4 million cases in the United States. Key factors linked with a higher prevalence of infection include poor socioeconomic conditions, use of human feces as fertilizer, and geophagia. Even though infection can occur at any age, the highest rate is in children of preschool or early school age. Transmission is primarily hand to mouth but may also involve ingestion of contaminated raw fruits and vegetables. Transmission is enhanced by the high output of eggs by fecund female worms and resistance of ova to the outside environment. *Ascaris* eggs can remain viable at 5–10°C for as long as 2 yr.

PATHOGENESIS. *Ascaris* ova hatch in the small intestine after ingestion by the human host. Larvae are released, penetrate the intestinal wall, and migrate to the lungs by way of the venous circulation. The parasites then cause **pulmonary ascariasis** as they enter into the alveoli and migrate through the bronchi and trachea. They are subsequently swallowed and return to the intestines, where they mature into adult worms. Female *Ascaris* begin depositing eggs in 8–10 wk.

CLINICAL MANIFESTATIONS. The clinical presentation depends on the intensity of infection and the organs involved. Most individuals have low to moderate worm burdens and have no symptoms or signs. The most common clinical problems are due to pulmonary disease and obstruction of the intestinal or biliary tract. Larvae migrating through these tissues may cause allergic symptoms, fever, urticaria, and granulomatous disease. The pulmonary manifestations resemble Loeffler syndrome and include transient respiratory symptoms such as cough and dyspnea, pulmonary infiltrates, and blood eosinophilia. Larvae may be observed in the sputum. Vague abdominal complaints have been attributed to the presence of adult worms in the small intestine, although the precise contribution of the parasite to these symptoms is difficult to ascertain. A more serious complication occurs when a large mass of worms leads to acute bowel obstruction. Children with heavy infections may present with vomiting, abdominal distention, and cramps. In some cases, worms may be passed in the vomitus or stools. *Ascaris* worms occasionally migrate into the biliary and pancreatic ducts, where they cause cholecystitis or pancreatitis. Worm migration through the intestinal wall can lead to peritonitis. Dead worms can serve as a nidus for stone formation. It is unclear whether infection with *A. lumbricoides* affects growth and nutrition. Some studies suggest that worm burden and poor growth status are independent, whereas others conclude that children with recurrent heavy infection are at risk for protein-energy malnutrition.

DIAGNOSIS. Microscopic examination of fecal smears can be used for diagnosis because of the high number of eggs excreted by adult female worms (see Fig. 288-1). A high index of suspicion in the appropriate clinical context is needed to diagnose pulmonary ascariasis or obstruction of the gastrointestinal tract.

TREATMENT. Although several chemotherapeutic agents are effective against ascariasis, none have documented utility during the

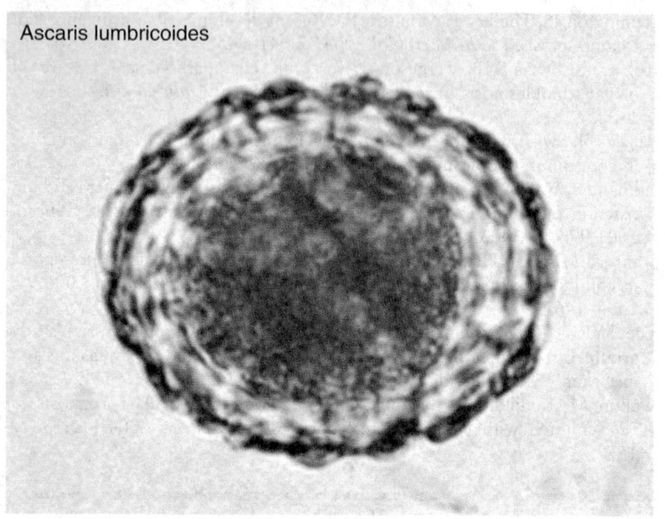

Figure 288-1. Soil-transmitted helminth eggs. (From Bethony J, Brooker S, Albonico M, et al: Soil-transmitted helminth infections: Ascariasis, trichuriasis, and hookworm. *Lancet* 2006;367:1521–1532.)

pulmonary phase of infection. Treatment options for gastrointestinal ascariasis include albendazole (400 mg PO once, for all ages), mebendazole (100 mg bid PO for 3 days or 500 mg PO once for all ages), or pyrantel pamoate (11 mg/kg PO once, maximum 1 g). Piperazine citrate (150 mg/kg PO initially, followed by 6 doses of 65 mg/kg at 12 hr intervals PO), which causes neuromuscular paralysis of the parasite and rapid expulsion of the worms, is the treatment of choice for intestinal or biliary obstruction and is administered as syrup through a nasogastric tube. Surgery may be required for cases with severe obstruction. Nitazoxanide (100 mg bid PO for 3 days for children 1–3 yrs of age, 200 mg bid PO for 3 days for children 4–11 yr, and 500 mg bid PO for 3 days for adolescents and adults) produces cure rates comparable with single-dose albendazole.

PREVENTION. Although ascariasis is the most prevalent worm infection in the world, little attention has been given to its control because of controversy surrounding its public health significance and the likelihood of recurrent infections in epidemiologic settings where transmission rates are high. Short-term preventive measures include chemotherapy. Anthelmintic chemotherapy programs can be implemented in 1 of 3 ways: (1) offering universal treatment to all individuals in an area of high endemicity; (2) offering treatment targeted to groups with high frequency of infection, such as children attending primary school; (3) offering individual treatment based on intensity of current or past infection. Improving sanitary conditions and sewage facilities, discontinuing the practice of using human feces as fertilizer, and education are the most effective long-term preventive measures.

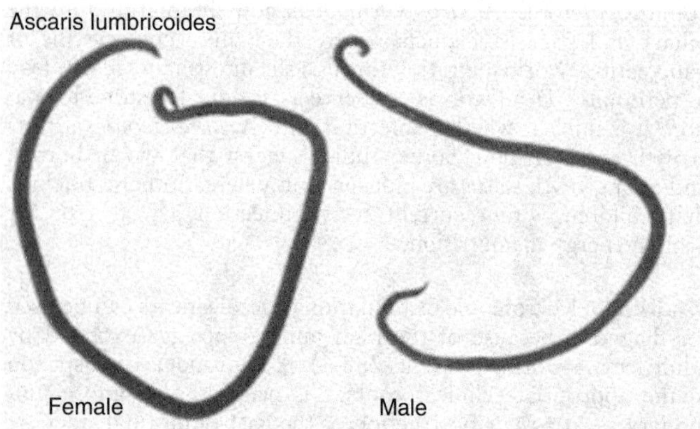

Figure 288-2. Adult male and female soil-transmitted helminths. (From Bethony J, Brooker S, Albonico M, et al: Soil-transmitted helminth infections: Ascariasis, trichuriasis, and hookworm. *Lancet* 2006;367:1521–1532.)

Bethony J, Brooker S, Albonico M, et al: Soil-transmitted helminth infections: Ascariasis, trichuriasis, and hookworm. *Lancet* 2006;367:1521–1532.

Cappello M: Global health impact of soil-transmitted nematodes. *Pediatr Infect Dis J* 2004;23:663–664.

Crompton DW: *Ascaris* and ascariasis. *Adv Parasitol* 2001;48:285–375.

Gilles HM, Hoffman PS. Treatment of intestinal parasitic infections: A review of nitazoxanide. *Trends Parasitol* 2002;18:95–97.

Chapter 289 ■ Hookworms (*Necator Americanus* and *Ancylostoma* spp.)

Peter J. Hotez

ETIOLOGY. Two major genera of hookworms, which are nematodes or roundworms, infect humans. *Necator americanus,* the only representative of its genus, is a major anthropophilic hookworm and is the most common cause of human hookworm infection. Hookworms of the genus *Ancylostoma* includes the major anthropophilic hookworm *Ancylostoma duodenale* that also causes classic hookworm infection and the less common zoonotic species *A. ceylanicum, A. caninum,* and *A. braziliense.* Human zoonotic infection with the dog hookworm, *A. caninum,* is associated with an eosinophilic enteritis syndrome. The larval stage of *A. braziliense,* whose definitive hosts include dogs and cats, is the principal cause of cutaneous larva migrans.

The infective larval stages of the anthropophilic hookworms live in a developmentally arrested state in warm, moist soil. Larvae infect humans either by penetrating through the skin (*N. americanus* and *A. duodenale*) or when they are ingested *(A. duodenale).* Larvae entering the human host by skin penetration undergo **extraintestinal migration** through the venous circulation and lungs before they are swallowed, whereas orally ingested larvae may undergo extraintestinal migration or remain in the gastrointestinal tract. Larvae returning to the small intestine undergo 2 molts to become adult sexually mature male and female worms ranging in length from 5 to 13 mm. The buccal capsule of the adult hookworm is armed with cutting plates *(N. americanus)* or teeth *(A. duodenale)* to facilitate attachment to the mucosa and submucosa of the small intestine. Hookworms can remain in the intestine for 1–5 yr, where they mate and produce eggs. Although approximately 2 mo is required for the larval stages of hookworms to undergo extraintestinal migration and develop into mature adults, *A. duodenale* larvae may remain developmentally arrested for many months before resuming development in the intestine. Mature *A. duodenale* female worms produce about 30,000 eggs/day; daily egg production by *N. americanus* is <10,000/day (Fig. 289-1). The eggs are thin shelled and ovoid, measuring approximately 40–60 μm. Eggs that are deposited on soil with adequate moisture and shade develop into 1st stage larvae and hatch. Over the ensuing several days and under appropriate conditions, the larvae molt twice to the infective stage. Infective larvae are developmentally arrested and nonfeeding. They migrate vertically in the soil until they either infect a new host or exhaust their lipid metabolic reserves and die.

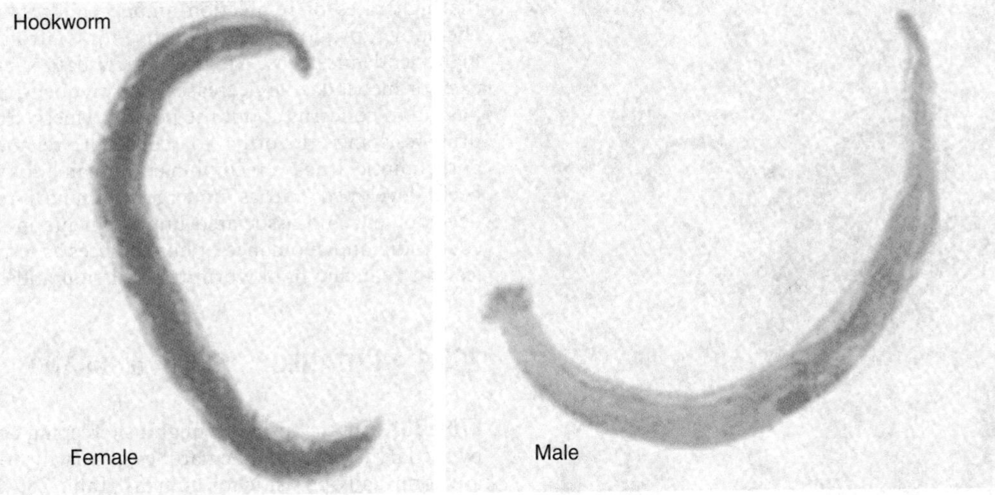

Figure 289-1. Adult male and female soil-transmitted helminths. (From Bethony J, Brooker S, Albonico M, et al: Soil-transmitted helminth infections: Ascariasis, trichuriasis, and hookworm. *Lancet* 2006;367:1521–1532.)

EPIDEMIOLOGY. Hookworm infection is 1 of the most prevalent infectious diseases of humans, affecting an estimated 576 million individuals worldwide. Because of the requirement for adequate soil moisture, shade, and warmth, hookworm infection is usually confined to rural areas, especially where human feces are used for fertilizer or where sanitation is inadequate. Hookworm is an infection associated with economic underdevelopment and poverty throughout the tropics and subtropics. Sub-Saharan Africa, East Asia, and tropical regions of the Americas have the highest prevalence of hookworm infection. High rates of infection are often associated with cultivation of certain agricultural products such as tea in India; sweet potato, corn, cotton, and mulberry trees in China; coffee in Central and South America; and rubber in Africa. It is not uncommon to find dual *N. americanus* and *A. duodenale* infections. *N. americanus* predominates in Central and South America, as well as in South China and southeast Asia, whereas *A. duodenale* predominates in North Africa, in northern India, in China north of the Yangtze River, and among aboriginal people in western Australia. The ability of *A. duodenale* to withstand somewhat harsher environmental and climatic conditions may reflect its ability to undergo arrested development in human tissues. *A. ceylanicum* infection occurs in India and Southeast Asia.

Eosinophilic enteritis caused by *A. caninum* was first described in Queensland, Australia, with 2 reported cases in the United States. Because of its global distribution in dogs, it was initially anticipated that human *A. caninum* infections would be identified in many locales, but this has not been found.

PATHOGENESIS. The major morbidity of human hookworm infection is a direct result of intestinal blood loss. Adult hookworms adhere tenaciously to the mucosa and submucosa of the proximal small intestine by using their cutting plates or teeth and a muscular esophagus that creates negative pressure in their buccal capsules. At the attachment site, host inflammation is downregulated by the release of anti-inflammatory polypeptides by the hookworm. Rupture of capillaries in the lamina propria is followed by blood extravasation, with some of the blood ingested directly by the hookworm. After ingestion, the blood is anticoagulated, the red blood cells are lysed, and the hemoglobin released and digested. Each adult *A. duodenale* hookworm causes loss of an estimated 0.2 mL of blood/day; blood loss is less for *N. americanus*. Individuals with light infections suffer from very little blood loss and, consequently, may have hookworm infection but not hookworm disease. There is a direct correlation between the number of adult hookworms in the gut and the volume of fecal blood loss. Hookworm disease results only when individuals with moderate and heavy infections experience sufficient blood loss to develop iron deficiency and anemia. Hypoalbuminemia and consequent edema and anasarca from the loss of intravascular oncotic pressure can also occur. These features depend heavily on the dietary reserves of the host.

CLINICAL MANIFESTATIONS. Chronically infected children with moderate and heavy hookworm infections suffer from intestinal blood loss resulting in **iron deficiency**, which can lead to **anemia** as well as protein malnutrition. Prolonged iron deficiency associated with hookworms in childhood can lead to physical growth retardation and cognitive and intellectual deficits.

Anthropophilic hookworm larvae elicit dermatitis sometimes referred to as **ground itch** when they penetrate human skin. The vesiculation and edema of ground itch are exacerbated by repeated infection. Infection with a zoonotic hookworm, especially *A. braziliense*, can result in lateral migration of the larvae to cause the characteristic cutaneous tracts of **cutaneous larva migrans** (see Chapter 289.1). Cough subsequently occurs in *A. duodenale* and *N. americanus* hookworm infection when larvae migrate through the lungs to cause laryngotracheobronchitis, usually about 1 wk after exposure. Pharyngitis also can occur.

Intestinal hookworm infection may occur without specific gastrointestinal complaints, although pain, anorexia, and diarrhea have been attributed to the presence of hookworms. Eosinophilia is often first noticed in early gastrointestinal infection. The major clinical manifestations are related to intestinal blood loss. Heavily infected children exhibit all of the signs and symptoms of iron deficiency anemia and protein malnutrition. In some cases, children with chronic hookworm disease acquire a yellow-green pallor known as **chlorosis.**

An infantile form of ancylostomiasis resulting from heavy *A. duodenale* infection has been described. Affected infants experience diarrhea, melena, failure to thrive, and profound anemia. Infantile ancylostomiasis has significant mortality.

Eosinophilic enteritis caused by *A. caninum* is associated with colicky abdominal pain, usually exacerbated by food, which begins in the epigastrium and radiates outward. Extreme cases may mimic acute appendicitis.

DIAGNOSIS. Children with hookworm release eggs that can be detected by direct fecal examination (Fig. 289-2). Quantitative methods are available to determine whether a child has a heavy

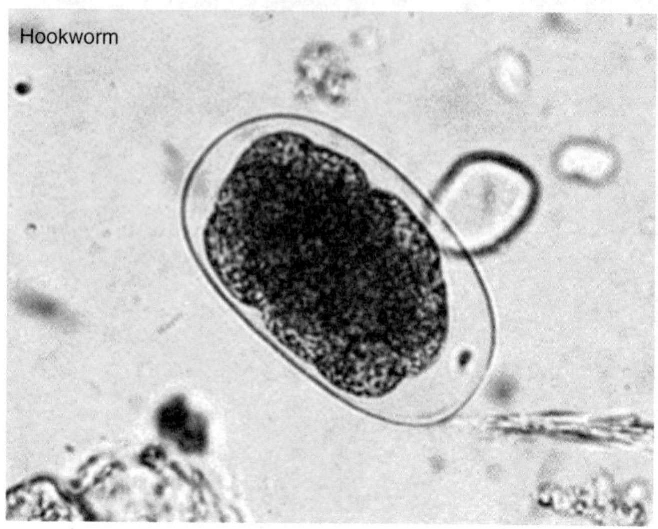

Figure 289-2. Soil-transmitted helminth eggs. (From Bethony J, Brooker S, Albonico M, et al: Soil-transmitted helminth infections: Ascariasis, trichuriasis, and hookworm. *Lancet* 2006;367:1521–1532.)

worm burden that can cause hookworm disease. The eggs of *N. americanus* and *A. duodenale* are morphologically indistinguishable. Species identification typically requires egg hatching and differentiation of 3rd stage infective larvae; newer methods using polymerase chain reaction methods are under development.

In contrast, eggs are generally not present in the feces of patients with eosinophilic enteritis caused by *A. caninum.* Eosinophilic enteritis is often diagnosed by demonstrating ileal and colonic ulcerations by colonoscopy in the presence of significant blood eosinophilia. An adult canine hookworm may occasionally be recovered during colonoscopic biopsy. Patients with this syndrome develop IgG and IgE serologic responses.

TREATMENT. The goal of **deworming** is removal of the adult hookworms with an anthelmintic drug. The benzimidazole anthelmintics, mebendazole and albendazole, are effective at eliminating hookworms from the intestine, although multiple doses are sometimes required. Albendazole (400 mg PO once, for all ages) usually achieves high cure rates, although *N. americanus* adult hookworms are sometimes more refractory and require additional doses. Mebendazole (100 mg bid PO for 3 days, for all ages) is also effective. In many developing countries, mebendazole is administered as a single dose of 500 mg; with this regimen the cure rates can be as low as 20–30%. Mebendazole is recommended for *A. caninum*–associated eosinophilic enteritis, although recurrences are common. Because the benzimidazoles have been reported to be embryotoxic and teratogenic in laboratory animals, their safety during pregnancy and in young children is a potential concern and the risks vs benefits must be carefully considered. The World Health Organization and other international health organizations currently support the use of benzimidazoles in infected children ≥1 yr of age, but at a reduced dose in the youngest age group. Pyrantel pamoate (11 mg/kg PO once daily for 3 days, maximum dose 1 g) is available in liquid form and is an effective alternative to the benzimidazoles. Replacement therapy with oral iron is not usually required to correct hookworm-associated iron deficiency in children.

PREVENTION. In 2001, the World Health Assembly urged its member states to implement programs of periodic deworming in order to control the morbidity of hookworm and other soil-transmitted helminth infections. However, although anthelmintic drugs are effective at eliminating hookworms from the intestine, the high rates of reinfection among children suggest that drug chemotherapy alone is not effective for controlling hookworm in highly endemic areas. Moreover, new data suggest that the efficacy of mebendazole decreases with frequent, periodic use. This has led to concerns about the possible emergence of anthelmintic drug resistance. In order to reduce the reliance exclusively on anthelmintic drugs, a recombinant human hookworm vaccine has been developed and is undergoing clinical testing. Economic development and associated improvements in sanitation, health education, and avoidance of human feces as fertilizer remain critical for reducing hookworm transmission and endemicity.

289.1 • Cutaneous Larva Migrans

ETIOLOGY. Cutaneous larva migrans (**creeping eruption**) is caused by the larvae of several nematodes, primarily hookworms, which are not usually parasitic for humans (Table 289-1). *A. braziliense,* a hookworm of dogs and cats, is the most common cause, but other animal hookworms may also produce the disease.

EPIDEMIOLOGY. Cutaneous larva migrans is usually caused by *A. braziliense,* which is endemic to the southeastern United States and Puerto Rico.

CLINICAL MANIFESTATIONS. After penetrating the skin, larvae localize at the epidermal-dermal junction and migrate in this plane, moving at a rate of 1–2 cm/day. The response to the parasite is characterized by raised, erythematous, serpiginous tracks, which occasionally form bullae (Fig. 289-3). These lesions may be single or numerous and are usually localized to an extremity, although any area of the body may be affected. As the organism migrates, new areas of involvement may appear every few days. Intense localized pruritus, without any systemic symptoms, may be associated with the lesions.

DIAGNOSIS. Cutaneous larva migrans is diagnosed by clinical examination of the skin. Patients are often able to recall the exact time and location of exposure because the larvae produce intense itching at the site of penetration. Eosinophilia may occur but is uncommon.

TREATMENT. If left untreated, the larvae die, and the syndrome resolves within a few weeks to several months. Treatment with

TABLE 289-1. Etiologies of the Cutaneous Larva Migrans Syndrome According to Cutaneous Presentation

CAUSATIVE AGENT	CUTANEOUS TRACK	OTHER CUTANEOUS SIGNS
Animal hookworm	1–10 burrows, on the feet or buttocks, about 3 mm wide and up to 15–20 cm long, slow-moving (2–5 cm/day), chronic (weeks to months).	Highly pruritic, vesiculobullous lesions, impetiginization, hookworm folliculitis
Pelodera strongyloides	10–100 burrows, on abdomen or buttocks, 1–2 cm long, 2–3 mm wide, may persist for months	Pruritus, follicular papules and pustules
Strongyloides stercoralis	Usually 1 burrow, on the abdomen or buttocks; lasts for hours only, may recur, fast-moving (larva currens)	Pruritus, urticaria
Gnathostoma species (*G. hispidum*, etc)	Usually 1 burrow located anywhere, lasts for days, medium-fast-moving	Cutaneous migratory edema (eosinophilic panniculitis), cellulitis, papules, and nodules

From Caumes E, Danis M: From creeping eruption to hookworm-related cutaneous larva migrans. *Lancet Infect Dis* 2004;4:659–660.

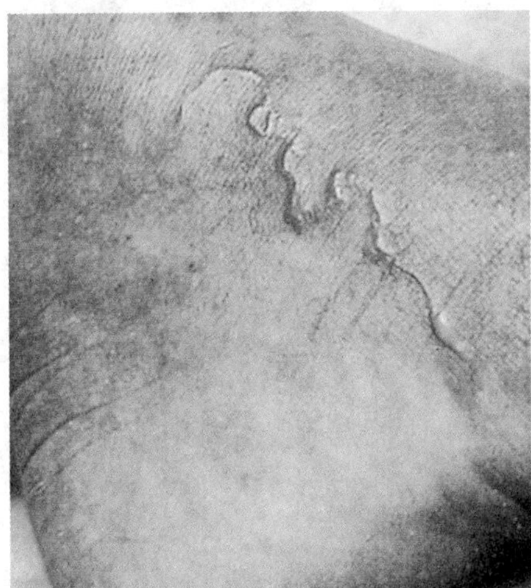

Figure 289-3. Creeping eruption of cutaneous larva migrans. (From Korting GW: *Hautkrankheiten bei Kindern und Jugendlichen*. Stuttgart, Germany, FK Schattauer Verlag, 1969.)

ivermectin (200 µg/kg daily PO for 1–2 days), albendazole (400 mg daily PO for 3 days, for all ages), or topical application of thiabendazole hastens resolution if symptoms warrant treatment. Nausea and vomiting frequently preclude repeated administration of oral thiabendazole.

Bethony J, Brooker S, Albonico M, et al: Soil-transmitted helminth infections: Ascariasis, trichuriasis, and hookworm. *Lancet* 2006;367:1521–1532.

Blackwell V, Vega-Lopez F: Cutaneous larva migrans: Clinical features and management of 44 cases presenting in the returning traveler. *Br J Dermatol* 2001;145:434–437.

Brooker S, Bethony J, Hotez PJ: Human hookworm infection in the 21st century. *Adv Parasitol* 2004;58:197–288.

Caumes E, Danis M: From creeping eruption to hookworm-related cutaneous larva migrans. *Lancet* 2004;4:659–660.

Hotez PJ, Bethony J, Bottazzi ME, et al: Hookworm: "The great infection of mankind." *PLoS Med* 2005;2:e67.

Hotez PJ, Brooker S, Bethony JM, et al: Hookworm infection. *N Engl J Med* 2004;351:799–807.

Chapter 290 ■ Trichuriasis (*Trichuris Trichiura*) Arlene E. Dent and James W. Kazura

ETIOLOGY. Trichuriasis is caused by the **whipworm,** *Trichuris trichiura,* a nematode, or roundworm, that inhabits the cecum and ascending colon of humans. The principal hosts of *T. trichiura* are humans who acquire infection by ingesting embryonated, barrel-shaped eggs (Fig. 290-1). The larvae escape from the shell in the upper small intestine and penetrate the intestinal villi. The worms slowly move toward the cecum, where the anterior 3/4 whiplike portion remains within the superficial mucosa and the short posterior end is free in the lumen (Fig. 290-2). In 1–3 mo, the adult female worm begins producing 5,000–20,000 eggs/day. After excretion in the feces, embryonic development occurs in 2–4 wk with optimal temperature and soil conditions.

EPIDEMIOLOGY. Trichuriasis occurs throughout the world and is especially common in poor rural communities with inadequate sanitary facilities and soil contaminated with human or animal feces. Trichuriasis is 1 of the most prevalent human helminthiases, with an estimated 1 billion infected individuals worldwide. In many parts of the world where protein-energy malnutrition and anemia are common, the prevalence of *T. trichiura* infection can be as high as 95%. It is estimated that 2.2 million people are infected in the rural southeastern United States. The highest rate of infection occurs among children 5–15 yr of age. Infection develops after ingesting embryonated ova by direct contamination of hands, food (raw fruits and vegetables fertilized with human feces), or drink. Transmission can also occur indirectly through flies or other insects.

CLINICAL MANIFESTATIONS. Most persons harbor low worm burdens and do not have symptoms. Some individuals may have a history of right lower quadrant or vague periumbilical pain. Adult *Trichuris* suck approximately 0.005 mL of blood/worm/day. Children, who are most likely to be heavily infected, frequently suffer from disease. Clinical manifestations include chronic dysentery, rectal prolapse, anemia, poor growth, as well as developmental and cognitive deficits. There is no significant eosinophilia, even though a portion of the worm is embedded in the mucosa of the large bowel.

DIAGNOSIS. Because egg output is so high, fecal smears frequently reveal the characteristic barrel-shaped ova of *T. trichiura.*

TREATMENT. Mebendazole (100 mg bid PO for 3 days or 500 mg PO once for all ages) is a safe and effective drug, in part because it is poorly absorbed from the gastrointestinal tract. It reduces egg output by 90–99% and has cure rates of 70–90%. Albendazole (400 mg PO once for all ages) is an alternative, but with heavy infections the daily dose of albendazole may have to be administered for 3 days. A newly licensed therapy for intestinal protozoa infections, nitazoxanide (100 mg bid PO for 3 days for children 1–3 yr of age, 200 mg bid PO for 3 days for children 4–11 yr of age, and 500 mg bid PO for 3 days for adolescents and adults) has been shown to produce higher cure rates than single-dose albendazole.

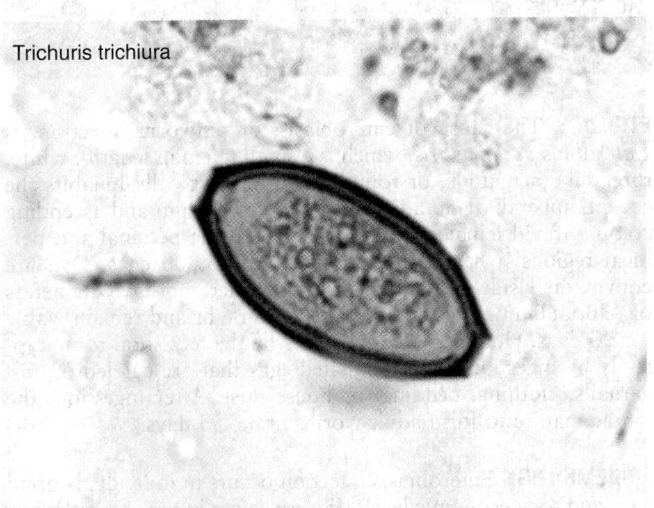

Figure 290-1. Soil-transmitted helminth eggs. (From Bethony J, Brooker S, Albonico M, et al: Soil-transmitted helminth infections: Ascariasis, trichuriasis, and hookworm. *Lancet* 2006;367:1521–1532.)

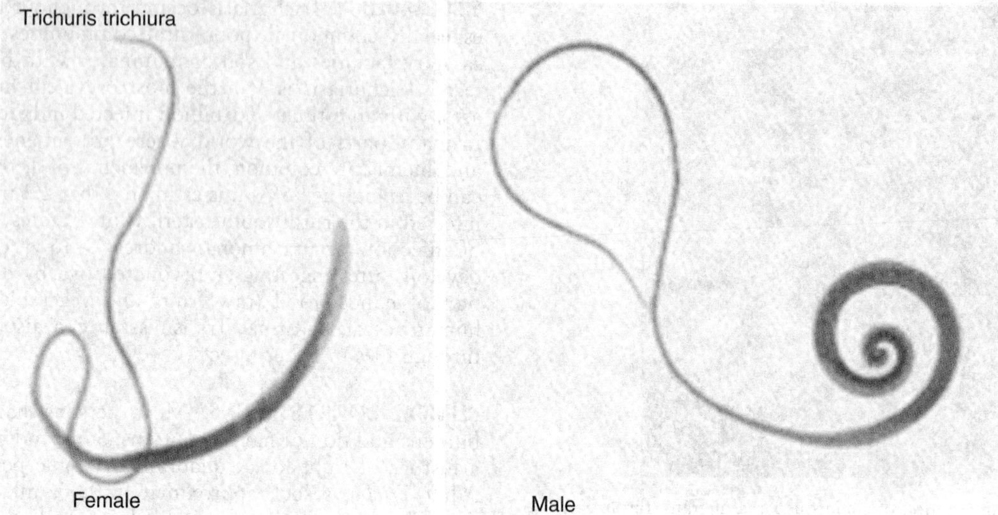

Figure 290-2. Adult male and female soil-transmitted helminths. (From Bethony J, Brooker S, Albonico M, et al: Soil-transmitted helminth infections: Ascariasis, trichuriasis, and hookworm. *Lancet* 2006;367:1521–1532.)

PREVENTION. Disease can be prevented by personal hygiene, improved sanitary conditions, and eliminating the use of human feces as fertilizer.

Bethony J, Brooker S, Albonico M, et al: Soil-transmitted helminth infections: Ascariasis, trichuriasis, and hookworm. *Lancet* 2006;367:1521–1532.
Cappello M: Global health impact of soil-transmitted nematodes. *Pediatr Infect Dis J* 2004;23:663–664.
Gilles HM, Hoffman PS: Treatment of intestinal parasitic infections: A review of nitazoxanide. *Trends Parasitol* 2002;18:95–97.
Stephenson LS, Holland CV, Cooper ES: The public health significance of *Trichuris trichiura*. *Parasitology* 2000;121(Suppl):S73–S95.

Chapter 291 ■ Enterobiasis *(Enterobius Vermicularis)* Arlene E. Dent and James W. Kazura

ETIOLOGY. The cause of enterobiasis, or **pinworm** infection, is *Enterobius vermicularis,* which is a small (1 cm in length), white, threadlike nematode, or roundworm, that typically inhabits the cecum, appendix, and adjacent areas of the ileum and ascending colon. Gravid females migrate at night to the perianal and perineal regions, where they deposit up to 15,000 eggs. Ova are convex on 1 side and flattened on the other and have diameters of ~30 × 60 μm. Eggs embryonate within 6 hr and remain viable for 20 days. Human infection occurs by the fecal-oral route typically by ingestion of embryonated eggs that are carried on fingernails, clothing, bedding, or house dust. After ingestion, the larvae mature to form adult worms in 36–53 days.

EPIDEMIOLOGY. Enterobiasis infection occurs in individuals of all ages and socioeconomic levels. It is prevalent in regions with temperate climates and is the most common helminth infection in the United States. It infects 30% of children worldwide, and humans are the only known host. Infection occurs primarily in institutional or family settings that include children. The prevalence of pinworm infection is highest in children 5–14 yr of age. It is common in areas where children live, play, and sleep close together, thus facilitating egg transmission. Because the life span of the adult worm is short, chronic parasitism is likely due to repeated cycles of reinfection. Autoinoculation can occur in individuals who habitually put their fingers in their mouth.

PATHOGENESIS. *Enterobius* infection may cause symptoms by mechanical stimulation and irritation, allergic reactions, and migration of the worms to anatomic sites where they become pathogenic.

CLINICAL MANIFESTATIONS. Pinworm infection is innocuous and rarely causes serious medical problems. The most common complaints include itching and restless sleep secondary to nocturnal perianal or perineal pruritus. The precise cause and incidence of pruritus are unknown. They may be related to the intensity of infection, psychologic profile of the infected individual and his or her family, or allergic reactions to the parasite. Eosinophilia is not observed in most cases because tissue invasion does not occur. Aberrant migration to ectopic sites occasionally may lead to appendicitis, chronic salpingitis, pelvic inflammatory disease, peritonitis, hepatitis, and ulcerative lesions in the large or small bowel.

DIAGNOSIS. A history of nocturnal perianal pruritus in children strongly suggests enterobiasis. Definitive diagnosis is established by identification of parasite eggs or worms. Microscopic examination of adhesive cellophane tape pressed against the perianal region early in the morning frequently demonstrates eggs (Fig. 291-1). Repeated examinations increase the chance of detecting ova; a single examination detects 50% of infections, 3 examinations 90%, and 5 examinations 99%. Worms seen in the perianal region should be removed and preserved in 75% ethyl alcohol until microscopic examination can be performed. Digital rectal examination may also be used to obtain samples for a wet mount. Routine stool samples rarely demonstrate *Enterobius* ova.

TREATMENT. Anthelmintic drugs should be administered to infected individuals and their family members. A single oral dose of mebendazole (100 mg PO for all ages) repeated in 2 wk results in cure rates of 90–100%. Alternative regimens include a single

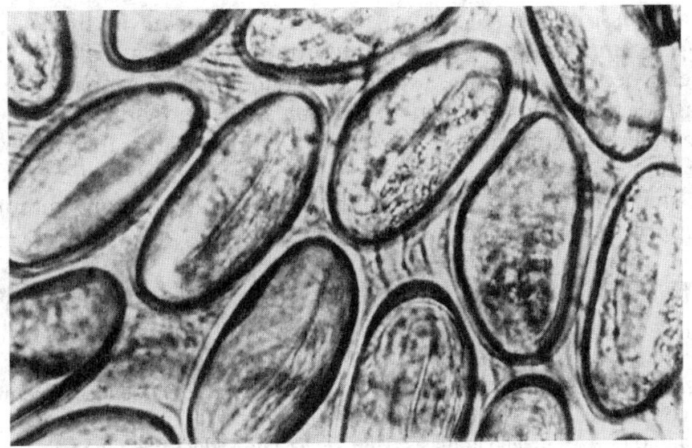

Figure 291-1. Eggs of *Enterobius vermicularis* adherent to cellulose acetate tape. (From Guerrant RL, Walker DH, Weller PF, et al: *Tropical Infectious Diseases.* Philadelphia, Churchill Livingstone, 1999, p 949.)

oral dose of albendazole (400 mg PO for all ages) repeated in 2 wk or a single dose of pyrantel pamoate (11 mg/kg PO, maximum 1 g). Morning bathing removes a large portion of eggs. Frequent changing of underclothes, bed clothes, and bed sheets decreases environmental egg contamination and may decrease the risk for autoinfection.

PREVENTION. Household contacts can be treated at the same time as the infected individual. Repeated treatments every 3–4 mo may be required in circumstances with repeated exposure, such as with institutionalized children. Good hand hygiene is the most effective method of prevention.

Arca MJ, Gates RL, Groner JI, et al: Clinical manifestations of appendiceal pinworms in children: An institutional experience and a review of the literature. *Pediatr Surg Int* 2004;20:372–375.

Kucik CJ, Martin GL, Sortor BV: Common intestinal parasites. *Am Fam Physician* 2004;69:1161–1168.

Sizer AR, Nirmal DM, Shannon J, Davies NJ: A pelvic mass due to infestation of the fallopian tube with *Enterobius vermicularis. J Obstet Gynaecol* 2004;24:462–463.

Tandan T, Pollard AJ, Money DM, et al: Pelvic inflammatory disease associated with *Enterobius vermicularis. Arch Dis Child* 2002;86:439–440.

Weller TH, Sorensen CW: Enterobiasis: Its incidence and symptomatology in a group of 505 children. *N Engl J Med* 1941;224:143–146.

Chapter 292 ■ Strongyloidiasis (*Strongyloides Stercoralis*)

Arlene E. Dent and James W. Kazura

ETIOLOGY. Strongyloidiasis is caused by the nematode, or roundworm, *Strongyloides stercoralis.* Only adult female worms inhabit the small intestine. The nematode reproduces in the human host by parthenogenesis and releases eggs containing mature larvae into the intestinal lumen. Rhabditiform larvae immediately emerge from the ova and are passed in feces, where they can be visualized by stool examination. Rhabditiform larvae either differentiate into free-living adult male and female worms or metamorphose into the infectious filariform larvae. Sexual reproduction occurs only in the free-living stage. Humans are usually infected through skin contact with soil contaminated with infectious larvae. Larvae penetrate the skin, enter the venous circulation and then pass to the lungs, break into alveolar spaces, and migrate up the bronchial tree. They are then swallowed and pass through the stomach, and adult female worms develop in the small intestine. Egg deposition begins about 28 days after initial infection.

The **hyperinfection syndrome** occurs when large numbers of larvae transform into infective organisms during their passage in feces and then reinfect (autoinfect) the host by way of the lower gastrointestinal tract or perianal region. This cycle may be accelerated in immunocompromised persons, particularly those with depressed T-cell function.

EPIDEMIOLOGY. *S. stercoralis* infection is prevalent in tropical and subtropical regions of the world and endemic in several areas of Europe, the southern United States, and Puerto Rico. Transmission requires appropriate environmental conditions, particularly warm, moist soil. Poor sanitation and crowded living conditions are conducive to high levels of transmission. Dogs and cats can act as reservoirs. The highest prevalence of infection in the United States (4% of the general population) is in impoverished rural areas of Kentucky and Tennessee. Infection may be especially common among residents of mental institutions, veterans who were prisoners of war in areas of high endemicity, and refugees and immigrants. Because of internal autoinfection, individuals may remain infected for decades. Individuals with hematologic malignancies, autoimmune diseases, malnutrition, and drug-induced immunosuppression are at high risk for the hyperinfection syndrome. Patients with **AIDS** may experience a rapid course of disseminated strongyloidiasis with a fatal outcome.

PATHOGENESIS. The initial host immune response to infection is production of immunoglobulin E (IgE) and eosinophilia in blood and tissues, which presumably prevents dissemination and hyperinfection in the immunocompetent host. Adult female worms in otherwise healthy and asymptomatic individuals may persist in the gastrointestinal tract for years. If infected persons become immunocompromised, the reduction in cellular and humoral immunity may lead to an abrupt and dramatic increase in parasite load with systemic dissemination.

CLINICAL MANIFESTATIONS. Approximately ⅓ of infected individuals are asymptomatic. The remaining ⅔ have symptoms that correlate with the 3 stages of infection: invasion of the skin, migration of larvae through the lungs, and parasitism of the small intestine by adult worms. **Larva currens** is the manifestation of an allergic reaction to filariform larvae that migrate through the skin, where they leave pruritic, tortuous, urticarial tracks. The lesions may recur and are typically found over the lower abdominal wall, buttocks, or thighs, resulting from larval migration from defecated stool. Pulmonary disease secondary to larval migration through the lung rarely occurs and may resemble **Loeffler syndrome** (cough, wheezing, shortness of breath, transient pulmonary infiltrates accompanied by eosinophilia). Gastrointestinal strongyloidiasis is characterized by indigestion, crampy abdominal pain, vomiting, diarrhea, steatorrhea, protein-losing enteropathy, and weight loss. Edema of the duodenum with irregular mucosal folds, ulcerations, and strictures can be seen radiographically. Infection is associated with **eosinophilia.**

Strongyloidiasis is potentially lethal because of the ability of the parasite to cause overwhelming hyperinfection in immunocompromised persons. The **hyperinfection syndrome** is characterized by an exaggeration of the clinical features that develop in symptomatic immunocompetent individuals. The onset is usually sudden, with generalized abdominal pain, distention, and fever. Multiple organs can be affected as massive numbers of larvae dis-

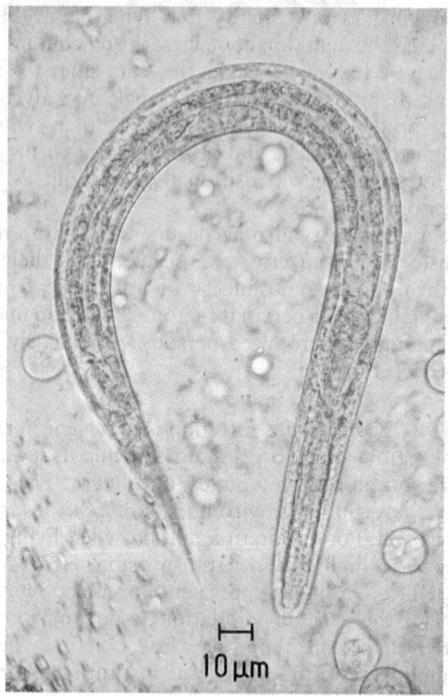

Figure 292-1. Larvae of intestinal strongyloidiasis.

seminate throughout the body and introduce bowel flora. The latter may result in bacteremia and septicemia. Cutaneous manifestations may include petechiae and purpura. Cough, wheezing, and hemoptysis are indicative of pulmonary involvement. Whereas eosinophilia is a prominent feature of strongyloidiasis in immunocompetent persons, this sign may be absent in immunocompromised persons.

DIAGNOSIS. Intestinal strongyloidiasis is diagnosed by examining feces or duodenal fluid for the characteristic larvae (Fig. 292-1). Several stool samples should be examined either by direct smear or a concentration method such as formaldehyde-ether or the Baermann test. Alternatively, duodenal fluid can be sampled by the **enteric string test** (Entero-Test) or aspiration via endoscopy. In children with the hyperinfection syndrome, larvae may be found in sputum, gastric aspirates, and rarely in small intestinal biopsy specimens. An enzyme-linked immunosorbent assay for IgE antibody to *Strongyloides* may be more sensitive than parasitologic methods for diagnosing intestinal infection in the immunocompetent host. The utility of the assay in diagnosing infection in immunocompromised subjects with the hyperinfection syndrome has not been determined. Eosinophilia is common.

TREATMENT. Treatment is directed at eradication of infection. Ivermectin (200 µg/kg/day once daily PO for 1–2 days) is the drug of choice for uncomplicated strongyloidiasis. It is equally effective and associated with fewer adverse effects than thiabendazole (25 mg/kg/dose bid PO for 2 days, maximum 3 g/day), which is the traditional treatment. Patients with the hyperinfection syndrome should be treated with ivermectin for 7–10 days and may require repeated courses. Reducing the dose of immunosuppressive therapy and treatment of concomitant bacterial infections are essential in the management of the hyperinfection syndrome. Close follow-up with repeated stool examination is necessary to ensure complete elimination of the parasite.

PREVENTION. Sanitary practices designed to prevent soil and person-to-person transmission are the most effective control measures. Wearing shoes is a main preventive strategy. Reduction in transmission in institutional settings can be achieved by decreasing fecal contamination of the environment such as by the use of clean bedding. Because infection is uncommon in most settings, case detection and treatment are advisable. Individuals who will be given immunosuppressive drugs before organ transplantation or cancer chemotherapy should have a screening examination for *S. stercoralis*. If infected, they should be treated before immunosuppression is induced.

Burke JA: Strongyloidiasis in childhood. *Am J Dis Child* 1978;132:1130–1138.
Keiser PB, Nutman TB: Strongyloides stercoralis in the immunocompromised population. *Clin Microbiol Rev* 2004;17:208–217.
Mahmoud AA: Strongyloidiasis. *Clin Infect Dis* 1996;23:949–953.
Zaha O, Hirata T, Kinjo F: Strongyloidiasis—Progress in diagnosis and treatment. *Intern Med* 2000;39:695–700.

Chapter 293 ■ Lymphatic Filariasis (*Brugia Malayi, Brugia Timori, Wuchereria Bancrofti*) Arlene E. Dent and James W. Kazura

ETIOLOGY. The filarial worms *Brugia malayi* (**Malayan filariasis**), *Brugia timori,* and *Wuchereria bancrofti* (**bancroftian filariasis**) are threadlike nematodes that cause similar infections. Infective larvae are introduced into humans during blood feeding by the mosquito vector. Over a period of 4–6 mo, the larval forms develop into adult worms. Once an adequate number of male and female worms accumulate in the afferent lymphatic vessels, adult female worms release large numbers of microfilariae that circulate in the bloodstream. The life cycle of the parasite is completed when mosquitoes ingest microfilariae in a blood meal, which molt to form infective larvae over a period of 10–14 days.

EPIDEMIOLOGY. More than 120 million people living in tropical Africa, Asia, and Latin America are infected; approximately 10–20% of these individuals have clinically significant morbidity attributable to filariasis. *W. bancrofti* is transmitted in Africa, Asia, and Latin America and accounts for 90% of lymphatic filariasis. *B. malayi* is restricted to the South Pacific and Southeast Asia, and *B. timori* is restricted to several islands of Indonesia. Travelers from nonendemic areas of the world who spend brief periods of time in endemic areas are rarely infected. Global elimination has been targeted for 2020.

CLINICAL MANIFESTATIONS. The clinical manifestations of *B. malayi, B. timori,* and *W. bancrofti* infection are similar; manifestations of acute infection include transient, recurrent lymphadenitis and lymphangitis, whereas chronic filariasis is characterized by lymphatic obstruction with hydrocele and elephantiasis. The early signs and symptoms include episodic fever, lymphangitis of an extremity, lymphadenitis (especially the inguinal and axillary areas), headaches, and myalgia that last a few days to several weeks. These symptoms are caused by an acute inflammatory response triggered by death of adult worms. Initial damage to lymphatic vessels may remain subclinical for years. The syndrome is most frequently observed in young persons 10–20 yr of age. Manifestations of chronic lymphatic filariasis, such as hydrocele and elephantiasis, occur mostly in

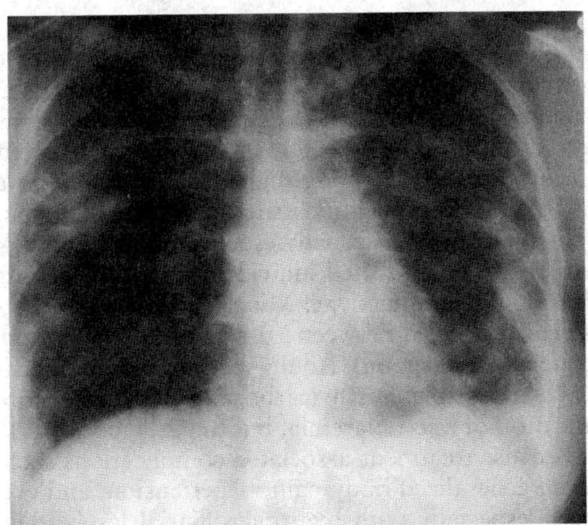

Figure 293-1. Chest radiograph of a woman with tropical pulmonary eosinophilia. Reticulondular opacities are scattered throughout both lungs. (From Mandell GL, Bennett JE, Dolin R [editors]: *Principles and Practice of Infectious Diseases,* 6th ed, Vol 2. Philadelphia, Elsevier, 2006, p 3274.)

adults 30 yr of age or older and result from anatomic and functional obstruction to lymph flow. Elephantiasis may involve 1 or more limbs, the scrotum, the breasts, or the vulva. Bacterial superinfections take advantage of the damaged lymphatic system and contribute to the morbidity of this disease. It is uncommon for children to have overt signs of chronic filariasis.

Tropical Pulmonary Eosinophilia. The presence of microfilariae in the body has no apparent pathologic consequences except in persons with tropical pulmonary eosinophilia, a syndrome of filarial etiology in which microfilariae are found in the lungs and lymph nodes but not the bloodstream. It occurs only in individuals who have lived for years in endemic areas. Men 20–30 yr of age are most likely to be affected, although the syndrome occasionally occurs in children. The presentation includes paroxysmal nocturnal cough with dyspnea, fever, weight loss, and fatigue. Rales and rhonchi are found on auscultation of the chest. The x-ray findings may occasionally be normal, but increased bronchovascular markings, discrete opacities in the middle and basal regions of the lung, or diffuse miliary lesions are usually present (Fig. 293-1). Recurrent episodes may result in interstitial fibrosis and chronic respiratory insufficiency in untreated individuals. Hepatosplenomegaly and generalized lymphadenopathy are often seen in children. The diagnosis is suggested by residence in a filarial endemic area, eosinophilia (>2,000/µL), compatible clinical symptoms, increased serum IgE (>1,000 IU/mL), and high titers of antimicrofilarial antibodies in the absence of microfilaremia. Although microfilariae may be found in sections of lung or lymph node, biopsy of these tissues is unwarranted in most situations. The clinical response to diethylcarbamazine (2 mg/kg/dose tid PO for 12–21 days) is the final criterion for diagnosis; the majority of patients improve with this therapy. If symptoms recur, a 2nd course of the anthelmintic should be administered. Patients with chronic symptoms are less likely to show improvement than those who have been ill for a short time.

DIAGNOSIS. Demonstration of microfilariae in the blood is the primary means for confirming the diagnosis of lymphatic filariasis. Because microfilaremia is **nocturnal** in most cases, blood samples should be obtained between 10 o'clock at night and 2 o'clock in the morning. Anticoagulated blood is passed through a Nuclepore filter that is stained and examined microscopically for microfilariae. Adult worms or microfilariae can be identified in tissue specimens obtained at biopsy. Infection with *W. bancrofti* in the absence of blood-borne microfilariae may be diagnosed by detection of parasite antigen in the serum.

TREATMENT. The use of antifilarial drugs in the management of acute lymphadenitis and lymphangitis is controversial. No controlled studies demonstrate that administration of drugs such as diethylcarbamazine modifies the course of acute lymphangitis. Diethylcarbamazine may be given to asymptomatic microfilaremic persons to lower the intensity of parasitemia. The drug also kills a proportion of the adult worms. Because treatment-associated complications such as pruritus, fever, generalized body pain, hypertension, and even death may occur, especially with high microfilarial levels, the dose of diethylcarbamazine should be increased gradually (children, 1 mg/kg PO as a single dose on day 1, 1 mg/kg tid PO on day 2, 1–2 mg/kg tid PO on day 3, and 6 mg/kg/day divided tid PO on days 4–14; adults, 50 mg PO on day 1, 50 mg tid PO on day 2, 100 mg tid PO on day 3, and 6 mg/kg/day divided tid PO on days 4–14). For patients with no microfilaria in the blood, the full dose (6 mg/kg/day divided tid PO) can be given beginning on day 1. Repeat doses may be necessary to further reduce the microfilaremia and kill lymph-dwelling adult parasites. *W. bancrofti* is more sensitive than *B. malayi* to diethylcarbamazine.

Global programs to control and ultimately eradicate lymphatic filariasis currently recommend a single annual dose of diethylcarbamazine (6 mg/kg PO once) often in combination with albendazole (400 mg PO once) for 5 yr. Recent studies have shown that 4 rounds of mass treatment substantially decreased the rate of transmission and clinical symptoms in Papua New Guinea. In co-endemic areas of filariasis and onchocerciasis, mass drug applications with single-dose ivermectin (150 µg/kg PO once) and albendazole are used because of severe adverse reactions with diethylcarbamazine in onchocerciasis-infected individuals.

Bockarie MJ, Tisch DJ, Kastens W, et al: Mass treatment to eliminate filariasis in Papua New Guinea. *N Engl J Med* 2002;347:1841–1848.

Brown KR, Ricci FM, Ottesen EA: Ivermectin: Effectiveness in lymphatic filariasis. *Parasitology* 2000;121(Suppl):S133–S146.

Fischer P, Supali T, Maizels RM: Lymphatic filariasis and Brugia timori: Prospects for elimination. *Trends Parasitol* 2004;20:351–355.

Kazura JW, Bockarie MJ: Lymphatic filariasis in Papua New Guinea: Interdisciplinary research on a national health problem. *Trends Parasitol* 2003;19:260–263.

Melrose WD, Durrheim DD, Burgess GW: Update on immunological tests for lymphatic filariasis. *Trends Parasitol* 2004;20:255–257.

Molyneux DH: Elimination of transmission of lymphatic filariasis in Egypt. *Lancet* 2006;367:966–968.

Molyneux DH, Bradley M, Hoerauf A, et al: Mass drug treatment for lymphatic filariasis and onchocerciasis. *Trends Parasitol* 2003;19:516–522.

Ramzy RMR, El Setouhy M, Helmy H, et al: Effect of yearly mass drug administration with diethylcarbamazine and albendazole on bancroftian filariasis in Egypt: A comprehensive assessment. *Lancet* 2006;367:992–999.

Stolk WA, de Vlas SJ, Habbema JDF: Anti-Wolbachia treatment for lymphatic filariasis. *Lancet* 2005;365:2067–2068.

Chapter 294 ■ Other Tissue Nematodes

Arlene E. Dent and James W. Kazura

ONCHOCERCIASIS *(ONCHOCERCA VOLVULUS)*. Infection with *Onchocerca volvulus* leads to onchocerciasis or **river blindness.** Onchocerciasis occurs primarily in West Africa but also Central and East Africa and is the world's 2nd leading infectious cause of blindness. There are scattered foci in Central and South America. *O. volvulus* larvae are transmitted to humans by way of the bite of *Simulium* blackflies that breed in fast-flowing streams. The larvae penetrate the skin and migrate through the connective tissue and eventually develop into adult worms that can be found tangled in fibrous tissue. Adult worms can live in the human body for up to 14 yr. Female worms produce large numbers of microfilariae that migrate through the skin and connective tissue. Most infected individuals are asymptomatic. In heavily infected subjects, clinical manifestations are due to localized host inflammatory reactions to dead or dying microfilariae. These reactions produce pruritic dermatitis, punctate keratitis, corneal pannus formation, and chorioretinitis. Adult worms in **subcutaneous nodules** are not painful and tend to occur over bony prominences of the hip. The **diagnosis** can be established by obtaining snips of skin covering the scapulae, iliac crests, buttocks, or calves. The snips are immersed in saline for several hours and examined microscopically for microfilariae that have emerged into the fluid. The diagnosis can also be established by demonstrating microfilariae in the cornea or anterior chamber on slit-lamp examination or finding adult worms on a nodule biopsy specimen. Ophthalmology consultation should be obtained before treatment of eye lesions. A single dose of ivermectin (150 µg/kg PO) is the **drug of choice** and clears microfilariae from the skin for several months, but it has no effect on the adult worm. Treatment with ivermectin should be repeated at 3–6 mo intervals if there are continuing symptoms or evidence of eye infection. Adverse effects of ivermectin therapy include fever, urticaria, and pruritus and are more frequent in individuals not born in endemic areas who acquired the infection following periods of intense exposure, such as Peace Corps volunteers. Patients with concurrent loiasis may develop encephalopathy with ivermectin therapy. Personal protection includes avoiding areas where biting flies are numerous, wearing protective clothing, and using insect repellent. Vector control and mass ivermectin distribution programs have been implemented in Africa in a successful effort to reduce the prevalence of onchocerciasis.

LOIASIS (LOA LOA). Loiasis is caused by infection with the tissue nematode *Loa loa*. The parasite is transmitted to humans via diurnally biting flies *(Chrysops)* that live in the rain forests of West and Central Africa. Migration of adult worms through skin, subcutaneous tissue, and subconjunctivae can lead to transient episodes of pruritus, erythema, localized edema known as **Calabar swellings,** which are nonerythematous areas of subcutaneous edema 10–20 cm in diameter typically found around joints such as the wrist or the knee (Fig. 294-1), or eye pain. They resolve over several days to weeks and may recur at the same or different sites. Although lifelong residents of endemic regions may have microfilaremia and eosinophilia, these individuals are often asymptomatic. In contrast, travelers to endemic regions may have a hyperreactive response to *L. loa* infection characterized by frequent recurrences of swelling, high-level eosinophilia, debilitation, and serious complications such as glomerulonephritis and encephalitis. **Diagnosis** is usually established on clinical grounds, often assisted by the infected individual reporting a worm being seen crossing the conjunctivae. Microfilariae may be detected in blood smears collected between 10 o'clock in the morning and 2 o'clock in the afternoon. Adult worms should be surgically excised when possible. Diethylcarbamazine is the **agent of choice** for eradication of microfilaremia, but the drug does not kill adult worms. Because treatment-associated complications such as pruritus, fever, generalized body pain, hypertension, and even death may occur, especially with high microfilarial levels, the dose of diethylcarbamazine should be increased gradually (children, 1 mg/kg PO on day 1, 1 mg/kg tid PO on day 2, 1–2 mg/kg tid PO on day 3, 6 mg/kg/day divided tid PO on days 4–21; adults, 50 mg PO on day 1, 50 mg tid PO on day 2, 100 mg tid PO on day 3, 6 mg/kg/day divided tid PO on days 4–21). Full doses can be instituted on day 1 in persons without microfilaremia. Individuals concurrently infected with *O. volvulus* are at increased risk for developing encephalopathy with ivermectin treatment. A single dose of ivermectin (150 µg/kg) decreases microfilarial densities in the blood in persons with high-density microfilaremia. A 3 wk course of albendazole can also be used to slowly reduce microfilarial levels as a result of embryotoxic effects on the adult worms. Antihistamines or corticosteroids may be used to limit allergic reactions secondary to killing of microfilariae. Personal protective measures include avoiding areas where biting flies are present, wearing protective clothing, and using insect repellents. Diethylcarbamazine (300 mg PO once weekly) prevents infection in travelers who spend prolonged periods of time in endemic areas.

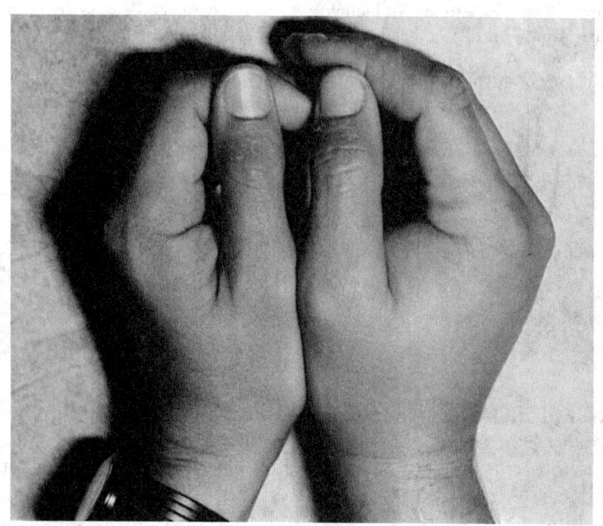

Figure 294-1. Calabar swelling of the right hand. (From Guerrant RL, Walker DH, Weller PF, et al: *Tropical Infectious Diseases*. Philadelphia, Churchill Livingstone, 1999, p 863.)

INFECTION WITH ANIMAL FILARIAE. The most commonly recognized zoonotic filarial infections are caused by members of the genus *Dirofilaria*. The worms are introduced into humans by the bites of mosquitoes containing 3rd stage larvae. The most common filarial zoonosis in the United States is *Dirofilaria tenuis*, a parasite of raccoons. In Europe, Africa, and Southeast Asia, infections are most commonly caused by the dog parasite *Dirofilaria repens*. The **dog heartworm,** *Dirofilaria immitis*, is the 2nd most commonly encountered filarial zoonosis worldwide. Other genera, including *Dipetalonema*-like worms, *Onchocerca*, and *Brugia*, are rare causes of zoonotic filarial infections.

Animal filariae do not undergo normal development in the human host. The clinical manifestations and pathologic findings correspond to the anatomic site of infection and can be categorized into 4 major groups: subcutaneous, lung, eye, and lymphatic. Pathologic examination of affected tissue reveals a localized foreign body reaction around a dead or dying parasite. The lesion consists of granulomas with eosinophils, neutrophils, and tissue necrosis. *D. tenuis* does not leave the subcutaneous tissues, whereas *Brugia beaveri* eventually localizes to superficial lymph nodes. Infections may be present for up to several months. *D. immitis* larvae migrate for several months in subcutaneous tissues and most frequently result in a well-circumscribed coin-like lesion in a single lobe of the lung. The chest x-ray typically reveals a solitary pulmonary nodule 1–3 cm in diameter. Definitive diagnosis and cure depend on surgical excision and identification of the nematode within the surrounding granulomatous response. *D. tenuis* and *B. beaveri* infections present as painful 1–5 cm rubbery nodules in the skin of the trunk, extremities, and around the orbit. Patients often report having been engaged in activities predisposing to exposure to infected mosquitoes, such as working or hunting in swampy areas. Diagnosis and management is by surgical excision. Serologic tests for dirofilariasis are not useful.

ANGIOSTRONGYLUS CANTONENSIS. *Angiostrongylus cantonensis,* the **rat lungworm,** is the most common cause of eosinophilic meningitis worldwide. Rats are the definitive host. Human infection follows ingestion of 3rd stage larvae in raw or undercooked intermediate hosts such as snails and slugs, or transport hosts such as freshwater prawns, frogs, and fish. Most cases are sporadic, but clusters have been reported, including consumption of lettuce contaminated with intermediate or transport hosts. Even though most infections have been described in Southeast Asia, the South Pacific, and Taiwan, shipboard travel of infected rats has spread the parasite to Madagascar, Africa, the Caribbean, and, most recently, Australia and North America. Larvae penetrate the vasculature of the intestinal tract and migrate to the meninges, where they usually die but induce eosinophilic aseptic meningitis. Patients present 2–35 days after ingestion of larvae with severe headache, neck pain or nuchal rigidity, hyperesthesias and paresthesias, fatigue, fever, rash, pruritus, nausea, and vomiting. Neurologic involvement varies from asymptomatic to paresthesias, severe pain, weakness, and focal neurologic findings such as cranial nerve palsies. Symptoms, especially protracted headache, can last for several weeks to months. Coma and death due to hydrocephalus occur rarely in heavy infections. Peripheral blood eosinophilia is not always present on initial examination, but peaks about 5 wk after exposure, often when symptoms are improving. Cerebrospinal fluid (CSF) analysis reveals pleocytosis with >10% eosinophils in more than half of patients, with mildly elevated protein and normal glucose levels, and an elevated opening pressure. The **diagnosis** is established clinically with supporting travel and diet history. A sensitive and specific enzyme-linked immunosorbent assay (ELISA) is available on a limited basis from the Centers for Disease Control and Prevention for testing either CSF or serum. **Treatment** is primarily supportive because the majority of infections are mild and most patients recover within 2 mo without neurologic residua. Analgesics should be given for headache. Careful, repeated lumbar punctures should be performed to relieve hydrocephalus. Anthelmintic drugs have not been shown to influence the outcome and may exacerbate neurologic symptoms. The use of corticosteroids may shorten the duration of symptoms for persistent and severe headaches. There is a higher incidence of permanent neurologic sequelae and mortality among children than among adults. Infection can be avoided by not eating raw or undercooked crabs, prawns, or snails.

ANGIOSTRONGYLUS COSTARICENSIS. *Angiostrongylus costaricensis* is a nematode that infects several species of rodents and causes abdominal angiostrongyliasis, which has been described predominantly in Latin America and the Caribbean. The mode of transmission to humans, who are accidental hosts, is unknown. It is speculated that infectious larvae from a molluscan intermediate host, such as the slug *Vaginulus plebeius,* contaminate water or vegetation that are inadvertently consumed (chopped up in salads or on vegetation contaminated with their mucus secretions). Although this slug is not indigenous to the continental United States, it has been found on imported flowers and produce. A study of 116 Costa Rican children with clinical abdominal angiostrongyliasis reported that the disease was twice as frequent in males as females and occurred predominantly during the rainy season in children 6–13 yr of age and of relatively high socioeconomic status. The incubation period for abdominal angiostrongyliasis is unknown, but limited data suggest it ranges from 2 wk to several months after ingestion of larvae. Third stage larvae migrate from the gastrointestinal tract to the mesenteric arteries, where they mature into adults. These eggs degenerate and elicit an eosinophilic granulomatous reaction. The clinical findings of abdominal angiostrongyliasis **mimic appendicitis,** although the former are typically more indolent. Children can have fever, right lower quadrant pain, a tumor-like mass, abdominal rigidity, and painful rectal examination. Most patients have leukocytosis with eosinophilia. Radiologic examination may show bowel wall edema, spasticity, or filling defects in the ileocecal region and the ascending colon. Examination of stool for ova and parasites is not useful for *A. costaricensis* but is useful for evaluating the presence of other intestinal parasites. An ELISA is available for diagnosis on a limited basis from the Centers for Disease Control and Prevention, but the specificity of the test is low, and it is known to cross react with *Toxocara, Strongyloides,* and *Paragonimus.* Many patients undergo laparotomy for suspected appendicitis and are found to have a mass in the terminal ileum to the ascending colon. No specific treatment is known for abdominal angiostrongyliasis. Even though the use of anthelmintic therapy has not been studied systematically, thiabendazole or diethylcarbamazine has been suggested. The prognosis is generally good. Most cases are self-limited, although surgery may be required in some patients. Cornerstones of prevention include avoidance of slugs and not ingesting raw food and water that may be contaminated with imperceptible slugs or slime from slugs. Rat control is also important in preventing the spread of infection.

DRACUNCULIASIS (DRACUNCULUS MEDINENSIS). Dracunculiasis is caused by the guinea worm, *Dracunculus medinensis.* The World Health Organization has targeted dracunculiasis for eradication. As of 2004, the transmission of the infection was confined to 11 countries in Africa, with Ghana and Sudan each reporting approximately 45% of global cases. Humans become infected by **drinking contaminated stagnant water** containing immature forms of the parasite in the gut of tiny crustaceans (copepods or waterfleas). Larvae are released in the stomach, penetrate the mucosa, mature, and mate. About 1 yr later, the adult female worm (1–2 mm in diameter and up to 1 m long) migrates and partially emerges through the skin, usually of the legs. Thousands of immature larvae are released when the affected body part is immersed in the water. The cycle is completed when larval forms are ingested by the crustaceans. Infected humans have no symptoms until the worm reaches the subcutaneous tissue, causing a **stinging papule** that may be accompanied by urticaria, nausea, vomiting, diarrhea, and dyspnea. The lesion vesiculates, ruptures, and forms a painful ulcer in which a portion of the worm is visible. Diagnosis is established clinically. Larvae can be identified by microscopic examination of the discharge fluid. **Metronidazole** (25 mg/kg/day tid PO for 10 days, maximum dose 750 mg) decreases local inflammation. Although the drug does not kill the worm, it facilitates its removal. The worm must be physically removed by rolling the slowly emerging 1-m long parasite onto a thin stick over a week. Topical corticosteroids shorten the time to complete healing while topical antibiotics decrease the risk for secondary bacterial infection. Dracunculiasis can be prevented by boiling or chlorinating drinking water or passing the water through a cloth sieve before consumption.

GNATHOSTOMA SPINIGERUM. *Gnathostoma spinigerum* is a dog and cat nematode endemic to Southeast Asia, Japan, China, Bangladesh, and India, but has been identified in Mexico and parts of South America. Infection is acquired by ingesting intermediate hosts containing larvae of the parasite such as raw or undercooked freshwater fish, chickens, pigs, snails, or frogs. Penetration of the skin by larval forms and prenatal transmission has also been described. Nonspecific signs and symptoms such as generalized malaise, fever, urticaria, anorexia, nausea, vomiting, diarrhea, and epigastric pain develop 24–48 hr after ingestion of *G. spinigerum.* Ingested larvae penetrate the gastric wall and migrate through soft tissue for up to 10 yr. Moderate to severe eosinophilia can develop. **Cutaneous** gnathostomiasis manifests as intermittent episodes of localized, migratory nonpitting edema associated with pain, pruritus, or erythema. **Central nervous system** involvement in gnathostomiasis is suggested by focal neurologic findings, initially neuralgia followed within a few days by paralysis or changes in mental status. Multiple cranial nerves may be involved, and the cerebrospinal fluid may be xanthochromic but typically shows an eosinophilic pleocytosis. **Diagnosis** of gnathostomiasis is based on clinical presentation and epidemiologic background. Brain and spinal cord lesions may be seen on CT or MRI. Serologic testing varies in sensitivity and specificity and is available through the Centers for Disease Control and Prevention. There is no well-documented effective chemotherapy, although **albendazole** (400 mg PO bid for 21 days) has been suggested to be useful. Corticosteroids have been used to relieve focal neurologic deficits. Surgical resection of the *Gnathostoma* is the major mode of therapy and the treatment of choice. Blind surgical resection of subcutaneous areas of diffuse swelling is not recommended because the worm can rarely be located. Prevention through the avoidance of ingestion of poorly cooked or raw fish, poultry, or pork should be emphasized for individuals living in or visiting endemic areas.

Onchocerciasis (Onchocerca Volvulus)

Burnham G: Onchocerciasis. *Lancet* 1998;351:1341–1346.

Molyneux DH, Bradley M, Hoerauf A, et al: Mass drug treatment for lymphatic filariasis and onchocerciasis. *Trends Parasitol* 2003;19:516–522.

Remme JH: Research for control: The onchocerciasis experience. *Trop Med Int Health* 2004;9:243–254.

Sabrosa NA, Zajdenweber M: Nematode infections of the eye: Toxocariasis, onchocerciasis, diffuse unilateral subacute neuroretinitis, and cysticercosis. *Ophthalmol Clin North Am* 2002;15:351–356.

Loiasis (Loa Loa)

Boussinesq M, Gardon, J: Prevalence of *Loa loa* microfilaremia throughout the area endemic for the infection. *Ann Trop Med Parasitol* 1997;91:573–589.

Hayden MK, Trenholme GM: Photo quiz. Loiasis. *Clin Infect Dis* 1998;27:429, 634–635.

Pion DS, Gardon J, Kamgno J, et al: Structure of the microfilarial reservoir of Loa loa in the human host and its implications for monitoring the programmes of Community-Directed Treatment with Ivermectin carried out in Africa. *Parasitology* 2004;129:613–626.

Infection with Animal Filariae

Litwin CM: Pet-transmitted infections: Diagnosis by microbiologic and immunologic methods. *Pediatr Infect Dis J* 2003;22:768–777.

Orihel TC, Eberhard ML: Zoonotic filariasis. *Clin Microbiol Rev* 1998;11:366–377.

Pampiglione S, Rivasi F, Angeli G, et al: Dirofilariasis due to *Dirofilaria repens* in Italy, an emergent zoonosis: Report of 60 new cases. *Histopathology* 2001;38:344–354.

Angiostrongylus Cantonensis

Chotmongkol V, Sawanyawisuth K, Thavornpitak Y: Corticosteroid treatment of eosinophilic meningitis. *Int J Parasitol* 2000;30:1295–1303.

Lo Re V 3rd, Gluckman SJ: Eosinophilic meningitis. *Am J Med* 2003;114:217–223.

Slom TJ, Crotese MM, Gerber SI, et al: An outbreak of eosinophilic meningitis caused by *Angiostrongylus cantonensis* in travelers returning from the Caribbean. *N Engl J Med* 2002;346:668–675.

Tsai HC, Liu YC, Kunin CM, et al: Eosinophilic meningitis caused by *Angiostrongylus cantonensis:* Report of 17 cases. *Am J Med* 2001;111:109–114.

Angiostrongylus Costaricensis

Hulbert TV, Larsen RA, Chandrasoma PT: Abdominal angiostrongyliasis mimicking acute appendicitis and Meckel's diverticulum: Report of a case in the United States and review. *Clin Infect Dis* 1992;14:836–840.

Kramer MH, Greer GJ, Quinonez JF, et al: First reported outbreak of abdominal angiostrongyliasis. *Clin Infect Dis* 1998;26:365–372.

Loria-Cortes R, Lobo-Sanahuja JF: Clinical abdominal angiostrongyliasis. A study of 116 children with intestinal granulomas caused by *Angiostrongylus costaricensis. Am J Trop Med Hyg* 1980;29:538–544.

Dracunculiasis (Dracunculus Medinensis)

Dracunculiasis eradication. Global surveillance summary, 2004. *Wkly Epidemiol Rec* 2005;80:165–176.

Greenaway C: Dracunculiasis (guinea worm disease). *CMAJ* 2004;170:495–500.

Sing A, Wienert P, Sabisch P, et al: Photo quiz. Infection due to *Dracunculus medinensis. Clin Infect Dis* 1998;27:1361,1508–1509.

Gnathostoma Spinigerum

Lo Re V 3rd, Gluckman SJ: Eosinophilic meningitis. *Am J Med* 2003;114:217–223.

Rusnak JM, Lucey DR: Clinical gnathostomiasis: Case report and review of the English-language literature. *Clin Infect Dis* 1993;16:33–50.

Chapter 295 ■ Toxocariasis (Visceral and Ocular Larva Migrans)

Arlene E. Dent and James W. Kazura

ETIOLOGY. Most cases of human toxocariasis are caused by the **dog roundworm,** *Toxocara canis.* Adult female *T. canis* worms live in the intestinal tracts of young puppies and their lactating mothers. Large numbers of eggs are passed in the feces of dogs and embryonate under optimal soil conditions. *Toxocara* eggs can survive relatively harsh environmental conditions and are resistant to freezing and extremes of moisture and pH. Humans ingest embryonated eggs contaminating soil, hands, or fomites. The larvae hatch and penetrate the intestinal wall and travel via the circulation to the liver, lung, and other tissues. Humans do not excrete *T. canis* eggs because the larvae are unable to complete their maturation to adult worms in the intestine. The **cat roundworm,** *Toxocara cati,* is responsible for far fewer cases of visceral larva migrans (VLM) than *T. canis.* Ingestion of infective larvae of the raccoon ascarid *Baylisascaris procyonis* rarely leads to VLM, but can cause neural larva migrans resulting in eosinophilic meningitis. Ingestion of larvae from the opossum ascarid *Lagochilascaris minor* leads to VLM rarely.

EPIDEMIOLOGY. Human *T. canis* infections have been reported in nearly all parts of the world, primarily in temperate and tropical areas where dogs are popular household pets. Young children are at highest risk because of their unsanitary play habits and tendency to place fingers in the mouth. Other behavioral risk factors include pica, contact with puppy litters, and institutionalization. In North America, the highest prevalences of infection are in the southeastern United States and Puerto Rico, particularly among socially disadvantaged African-American and Hispanic children. In the United States, serosurveys show that 4.6–7.3% of children are infected. Assuming an unrestrained and untreated dog population, toxocariasis is prevalent in settings where other geohelminth infections such as ascariasis, trichuriasis, and hookworm infections are common.

PATHOGENESIS. *T. canis* larvae secrete large amounts of immunogenic glycosylated proteins. These antigens induce immune

TABLE 295-1. Clinical Syndromes of Human Toxocariasis

SYNDROME	CLINICAL FINDINGS	AVERAGE AGE	INFECTIOUS DOSE	INCUBATION PERIOD	LABORATORY FINDINGS	ELISA
Visceral larva migrans	Fevers, hepatomegaly, asthma	5 yr	Moderate to high	Weeks to months	Eosinophilia, leukocytosis, elevated IgE	High (≥1 : 16)
Ocular larva migrans	Visual disturbances, retinal granulomas, endophthalmitis, peripheral granulomas	12 yr	Low	Months to years	Usually none	Low (<1 : 512)
Covert toxocariasis	Abdominal pain, gastrointestinal symptoms, weakness, hepatomegaly, pruritus, rash	School age to adult	Low to moderate	Weeks to years	± Eosinophilia, ± elevated IgE	Low to moderate

ELISA-enzyme-linked immunosorbent assay; IgE, immunoglobulin E; ±, with or without.
Adapted from Liu LX: Toxocariasis and larva migrans syndrome. In Guerrant RL, Walker DH, Weller PF (editors): *Tropical Infectious Diseases: Principles, Pathogens & Practice*. Philadelphia, Churchill-Livingstone, 1999, p 908.

responses that lead to eosinophilia and polyclonal and antigen-specific immunoglobulin E (IgE) production. The characteristic histopathologic lesions are granulomas containing eosinophils, multinucleated giant cells (histiocytes), and collagen. Granulomas are typically found in the liver but may also occur in the lungs, central nervous system, and ocular tissues. Clinical manifestations reflect the intensity and chronicity of infection, anatomic localization of larvae, and host granulomatous responses.

CLINICAL MANIFESTATIONS. There are 3 major clinical syndromes associated with human toxocariasis: VLM, ocular larva migrans (OLM), and covert toxocariasis (Table 295-1). The classic presentation of VLM includes eosinophilia, fever, and hepatomegaly, and occurs most commonly in toddlers with a history of pica and exposure to puppies. The findings include fever, cough, wheezing, bronchopneumonia, anemia, hepatomegaly, leukocytosis, eosinophilia, and positive *Toxocara* serology. OLM tends to occur in older children without signs or symptoms of VLM. Presenting symptoms include unilateral visual loss, eye pain, white pupil, or strabismus that develops over a period of weeks. Granulomas occur on the posterior pole of the retina and may be mistaken for retinoblastoma. Serologic testing for *Toxocara* has allowed the identification of individuals with less obvious or covert symptoms of infection. These children may have nonspecific complaints that do not constitute a recognizable syndrome. Common findings include hepatomegaly, abdominal pain, cough, sleep disturbance, failure to thrive, and headache with elevated *Toxocara* antibody titers. Eosinophilia may be present in only 50–75% of cases. The prevalence of positive *Toxocara* serology in the general population supports the notion that most children with *T. canis* infection are asymptomatic and will not develop overt clinical sequelae over time. A correlation between positive *Toxocara* serology and allergic asthma has also been described.

DIAGNOSIS. A presumptive diagnosis can be established in a young child with **eosinophilia** (>20%), leukocytosis, hepatomegaly, fevers, wheezing, and a history of geophagia and exposure to puppies or unrestrained dogs. Supportive laboratory findings include hypergammaglobulinemia and elevated isohemagglutinin titers to A and B blood group antigens. Most patients with VLM have an absolute eosinophil count of >500/μL. Eosinophilia is less common in subjects with OLM. Biopsy confirms the diagnosis. When biopsies cannot be obtained, an enzyme-linked immunosorbent assay using excretory-secretory proteins harvested from *T. canis* larvae maintained in vitro is the standard serologic test used to confirm toxocariasis. The sensitivity is >91% and specificity >86%. The diagnosis of OLM can be established in patients with typical clinical findings of a retinal or peripheral pole granuloma or endophthalmitis with elevated antibody titers. Vitreous and aqueous humor fluid anti-*Toxocara* titers are usually greater than serum titers. The diagnosis of covert toxocariasis should be considered in individuals with chronic weakness, abdominal pain, or allergic signs with eosinophilia and increased IgE. In temperate regions of the world, nonparasitic causes of eosinophilia that should be considered in the differential diagnosis include allergies, drug hypersensitivity, lymphoma, vasculitis, and the idiopathic hypereosinophilic syndrome (see Chapter 128).

TREATMENT. Most cases do not require treatment because signs and symptoms are mild and subside over a period of weeks to months. Several anthelmintic drugs have been used for symptomatic cases, often with adjunctive corticosteroids to limit inflammatory responses that presumably result from release of *Toxocara* antigens by dying parasites. Albendazole (400 mg bid PO for 5 days for all ages) has demonstrated efficacy in both children and adults. Mebendazole (100–200 mg bid PO for 5 days for all ages) is also useful. Even though there are no clinical trials regarding therapy of OLM, a course of oral corticosteroids such as prednisone (1 mg/kg/day PO for 2–4 wk) has been recommended to suppress local inflammation while treatment with anthelmintic agents is initiated.

PREVENTION. Transmission can be minimized by public health measures that prevent dog feces from contaminating the environment. These include keeping dogs on leashes and excluding pets from playgrounds and sandboxes that toddlers use. Children should be discouraged from putting dirty fingers in their mouth and eating dirt. Vinyl covering of sandboxes reduces the viability of *T. canis* eggs. Widespread veterinary use of broad-spectrum anthelmintics effective against *Toxocara* may lead to a decline in parasite transmission to humans.

Gavin PJ, Shulman ST: Raccoon roundworm *(Baylisascaris procyonis)*. *Pediatr Infect Dis J* 2003;22:651–652.

Gillespie SH: Human toxocariasis. *Communicable Dis Rep CDR Rev* 1993;3:R140–R143.

Litwin CM: Pet-transmitted infections: Diagnosis by microbiologic and immunologic methods. *Pediatr Infect Dis J* 2003;22:768–777.

Mok CH: Visceral larva migrans: A discussion based on review of the literature. *Clin Pediatr* 1968;7:565–573.

Sabrosa NA, Zajdenweber M: Nematode infections of the eye: Toxocariasis, onchocerciasis, diffuse unilateral subacute neuroretinitis, and cysticercosis. *Ophthalmol Clin North Am* 2002;15:351–356.

Schantz PM, Glickman LT: Toxocaral visceral larva migrans. *N Engl J Med* 1978;298:436–439.

Sellman J, Bender J: Zoonotic infections in travelers to the tropics. *Prim Care* 2002;29:907–929.

Chapter 296 ■ Trichinosis *(Trichinella Spiralis)* Arlene Dent and James W. Kazura

ETIOLOGY. Human trichinosis (trichinellosis) is caused by consumption of meat containing encysted larvae of *Trichinella spiralis,* a tissue-dwelling nematode with a worldwide distribution. After ingestion of raw or inadequately cooked meat containing viable *Trichinella* larvae, the organisms are released from the cyst by acid-pepsin digestion of the cyst walls in the stomach and then pass into the small intestine. The larvae invade the small intestine columnar epithelium at the villi base and develop into adult worms. The adult female produces about 500 larvae over 2 wk and is then expelled in the feces. The larvae enter the bloodstream and seed striated muscle by burrowing into individual muscle fibers. Over a period of 3 wk, they coil as they increase about 10 times in length and become capable of infecting a new host if ingested. The larvae eventually become encysted and can remain viable for years.

EPIDEMIOLOGY. Despite veterinary public health efforts to control and eradicate the parasite, reemergence of the disease has been observed in many areas of the world in the past 10–20 yr. Trichinosis is most common in Asia, Latin America, and Central Europe. Swine fed with garbage may become infected when given uncooked trichinous scraps, usually pig meat, or when the carcasses of infected wild animals such as rats are eaten. Prevalence rates of *T. spiralis* in domestic swine range from 0.001% in the United States to ≥25% in China. The resurgence of this disease can be attributed to translocations of animal populations, human travel, and export of food as well as ingestion of sylvatic *Trichinella* (*T. brivoti, T. pseudospiralis,* and *T. murrelli*) through game meat. In the USA from 1997 to 2001, wild game meat (especially bear meat) was the most common source of infection. Most outbreaks occur from the consumption of *T. spiralis*–infected pork (or horse meat in areas of the world where horse is eaten) obtained from a single source.

PATHOGENESIS. During the 1st 2–3 wk after infection, pathologic reactions to infection are limited to the gastrointestinal tract and include a mild, partial villous atrophy with an inflammatory infiltrate of neutrophils, eosinophils, lymphocytes, and macrophages in the mucosa and submucosa. Larvae are released by female worms and disseminate over the next several weeks. Skeletal muscle fibers show the most striking changes with edema and basophilic degeneration. The muscle fiber may contain the typical coiled worm, the cyst wall derived from the host cell, and the surrounding lymphocytic and eosinophilic infiltrate.

CLINICAL MANIFESTATIONS. The development of symptoms depends on the number of viable larvae ingested. Most infections are asymptomatic or mild, and children often show milder symptoms than adults who consumed the same amount of infected meat. Diarrhea is the most common symptom corresponding to maturation of the adult worms in the gastrointestinal tract, which occurs during the 1st 1–2 wk after ingestion. Patients may also complain of abdominal discomfort and vomiting. Fulminant enteritis may develop in individuals with extremely high worm burdens. The classic symptoms of facial and periorbital edema, fever, weakness, malaise, and myalgia peak about 2–3 wk after the infected meat is ingested as the larvae encyst in the muscle. Headache, cough, dyspnea, dysphagia, subconjunctival and splinter hemorrhages, and a macular or petechial rash may occur. Patients with high intensity infection may die from myocarditis, encephalitis, or pneumonia. In symptomatic patients, eosinophilia is common and may be dramatic.

DIAGNOSIS. The Centers for Disease Control and Prevention diagnostic criteria for trichinosis requires positive serology or muscle biopsy for *Trichinella* with 1 or more compatible clinical symptoms (eosinophilia, fever, myalgia, facial or periorbital edema). To declare a discrete outbreak, at least 1 person must have positive serology or muscle biopsy. Antibodies to *Trichinella* are detectable about 3 wk after infection. Severe muscle involvement results in elevated serum creatine phosphokinase and lactic dehydrogenase levels. Muscle biopsy is not usually necessary, but if needed, a sample should be obtained from a tender swollen muscle. A history of eating undercooked meat supports the diagnosis.

TREATMENT. Recommended treatment of trichinosis is mebendazole (200–400 mg tid PO for 3 days then 400–500 mg tid PO for 10 days, for all ages) to eradicate the adult worms if a patient has ingested contaminated meat within the previous 1 wk. An alternative regimen is albendazole (400 mg bid PO for 8–14 days, for all ages). There is no consensus for treatment of muscle stage trichinosis. Systemic corticosteroids along with mebendazole may be used, although evidence for efficacy is anecdotal. Thiabendazole (25 mg/kg bid PO for 10 days) and mebendazole (200 mg bid PO for 10 days) are effective against muscle larvae; mebendazole may have been less active but thiabendazole was poorly tolerated.

PREVENTION. *Trichinella* larvae can be killed by cooking meat (≥55°C) until there is no trace of pink fluid or flesh, or storage in a freezer (−15°C) for ≥3 wk. Freezing to kill larvae should only be applied to pork meat, as larvae in horse, wild boar, or game meat can remain viable even after 4 wk of freezing. Smoking, salting, and drying meat are unreliable methods of killing *Trichinella.* Strict adherence to pubic health measures including garbage feeding regulations, stringent rodent control, prevention of exposure of pigs and other livestock to animal carcasses, constructing barriers between livestock, wild animals, and domestic pets, and proper handling of wild animal carcasses by hunters can reduce infection with *Trichinella.* Current meat inspection for trichinosis is by direct digestion and visualization of encysted larvae in meat samples. Serologic testing does not have a role in meat inspection.

Drugs for parasitic infections. *Med Lett Drugs Ther* 2004;44(1189):1–12. Available at www.medicalletter.org

Kapel CM: Changes in the EU legislation on Trichinella inspection—New challenges in the epidemiology. *Vet Parasitol* 2005;132:189–194.

Murrell KD, Pozio E: Trichinellosis: The zoonosis that won't go quietly. *Int J Parasitol* 2000;30:1339–1349.

Ozdemir D, Ozkan H, Akkoc N, et al: Acute trichinellosis in children compared to adults. *Pediatr Infect Dis J* 2005;24:897–900.

Roy SL, Lopez AS, Schantz PM: Trichinellosis surveillance—United States, 1997–2001. *MMWR Surveill Summ* 2003;52:1–8.

Watt G, Saisorn S, Jongsakul K, et al: Blinded, placebo-controlled trial of antiparasitic drugs for trichinosis myositis. *J Infect Dis* 2000;182:371–374.

Chapter 297 ■ Schistosomiasis *(Schistosoma)* Charles H. King

ETIOLOGY. *Schistosoma* organisms are the trematodes, or flukes, that parasitize the bloodstream. Five schistosome species infect humans: *Schistosoma haematobium, S. mansoni, S. japonicum, S. intercalatum,* and *S. mekongi.* Humans are infected through contact with water contaminated with cercariae, the free-living infective stage of the parasite. These motile, forked-tail organisms emerge from infected snails and are capable of penetrating intact human skin. In the subcutaneous tissues, the cercaria changes into the next developmental stage, the schistosomulum, and migrates to the lungs and finally the liver. As they reach sexual maturity, adult worms migrate to specific anatomic sites characteristic of each schistosome species: *S. haematobium* adults are found in the perivesical and periureteral venous plexus, *S. mansoni* in the inferior mesenteric veins, and *S. japonicum* in the superior mesenteric veins. *S. intercalatum* and *S. mekongi* are usually found in the mesenteric vessels. Adult schistosome worms (1–2 cm long) are clearly adapted for an intravascular existence. Unlike the other flukes, *Schistosoma* organisms are dioecious, and the 2 sexes are dissimilar in appearance. The female accompanies the male in a groove formed by the lateral edges of its body. On fertilization, female worms begin oviposition in the small venous tributaries. The eggs of the 3 main schistosome species have characteristic morphologic features: *S. haematobium* has a terminal spine, *S. mansoni* has a lateral spine, and *S. japonicum* has a smaller size with a short, curved spine (Fig. 297-1). Eggs reach the lumen of the urinary tract or intestines and are carried to the outside environment, where they hatch if deposited in freshwater. Motile miracidia emerge; they infect specific freshwater snail intermediate hosts and divide asexually. In 4–12 wk, the infective cercariae are released in the water.

EPIDEMIOLOGY. Schistosomiasis infects >200 million people worldwide, primarily children and young adults. Prevalence is increasing in many areas as population density increases and new irrigation projects provide broader habitats for vector snails. Humans are the definitive host for the 5 clinically important species of schistosomes, although *S. japonicum* may infect some animals such as dogs and cattle. *S. haematobium* is prevalent in Africa and the Middle East; *S. mansoni* in Africa, the Middle East, the Caribbean, and South America; and *S. japonicum* in China, the Philippines, and Indonesia, with some sporadic foci in parts of Southeast Asia. The other 2 species are less prevalent. *S. intercalatum* is found in West and Central Africa, and *S. mekongi* is found only along the upper Mekong River in the Far East.

Transmission depends on disposal of excreta, the presence of specific intermediate snail hosts, and the patterns of water contact and social habits of the population (Fig. 297-2). The distribution of infection in endemic areas shows that prevalence increases with age to a peak at 10–20 yr of age. Measuring intensity of infection (by quantitative egg count in urine or feces) demonstrates that the heaviest worm loads are found in the younger age groups. Schistosomiasis, therefore, is most prevalent and most severe in children and young adults, who are at maximal risk for suffering from its acute and chronic sequelae.

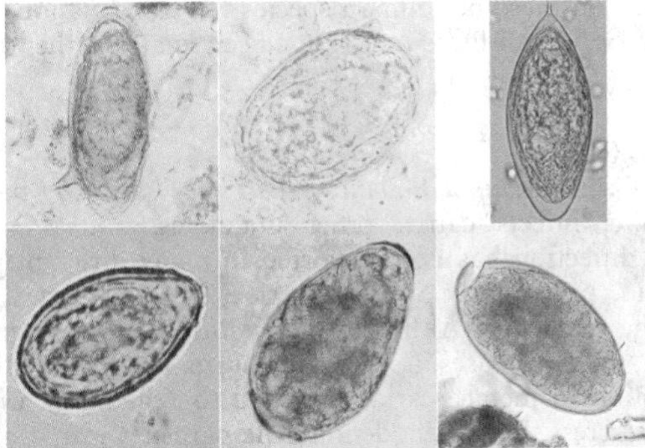

Figure 297-1. Eggs of common human trematodes. Clockwise from upper left: *Schistosoma mansoni, Schistosoma japonicum, Schistosoma haematobium, Clonorchis sinensis, Pargonimus westermani,* and *Fasiola hepatica* (note the partially open operculum). (From DPDx, website for laboratory diagnosis of parasitic diseases of the Division of Parasitic Diseases, National Centers for Infectious Diseases, Centers for Disease Control and Prevention, Atlanta, Georgia [http://www.dpd.cdc.gov/DPDx/].)

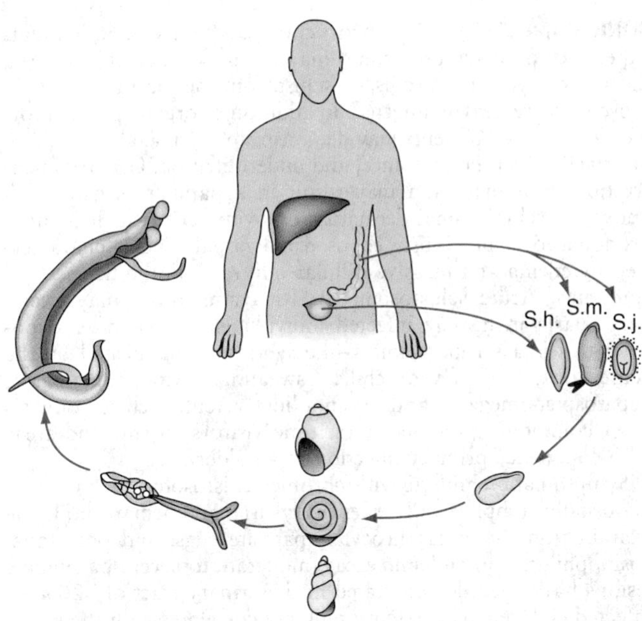

Figure 297-2. Life cycle of schistosomes. Eggs are passed in stools for *Schistosoma mansoni* (S.m.) and *Schistosoma japonicum* (S.j.) and in urine for *Schistosoma haematobium* (S.h.). The eggs hatch in freshwater, miracidia invade specific snail intermediate hosts, and in a few weeks, forked-tail cercariae are liberated. These infective forms penetrate human skin, pass through a migratory phase in the lung and liver, and then pass to their final habitat in the portal venous system (S.m. and S.j.) or the urinary bladder venous plexus (S.h.). Two other species infect humans, although less frequently. *Schistosoma intercalatum* produces terminal spined eggs that may be found in feces, whereas *Schistosoma mekongi* produces eggs similar to but smaller than those of *S. japonicum,* which also may be found in stools. These 2 species of schistosomes have characteristic snail intermediate hosts. (From Mandell GL, Gennett JE, Dolin R [editors]: *Principles and Practice of Infectious Diseases,* 6th ed, Vol 2. Philadelphia, Elsevier, 2006, p. 3278.)

PATHOGENESIS. The early manifestations of schistosomiasis are immunologically mediated. Acute schistosomiasis, known as snail fever or **Katayama fever,** is a febrile illness that represents an immune complex disease associated with early infection and oviposition. The major pathology of infection occurs later, with chronic schistosomiasis, in which retention of eggs in the host tissues is associated with chronic granulomatous injury. Eggs may be trapped at sites of deposition (urinary bladder, ureters, intestine) or be carried by the bloodstream to other organs, most commonly the liver, and less often the lungs and central nervous system. The host response to these eggs involves local as well as systemic manifestations. The cell-mediated immune response leads to granulomas composed of lymphocytes, macrophages, and eosinophils that surround the trapped eggs and add significantly to the degree of tissue destruction. Granuloma formation in the bladder wall and at the ureterovesical junction results in the major disease manifestations of schistosomiasis haematobia: hematuria, dysuria, and obstructive uropathy. Intestinal as well as hepatic granulomas underlie the pathologic sequelae of the other schistosome infections: ulcerations and fibrosis of intestinal wall, hepatosplenomegaly, and portal hypertension due to presinusoidal obstruction of blood flow. Protective immunity against schistosomiasis has been demonstrated in some animal species and may occur in humans.

CLINICAL MANIFESTATIONS. Most chronically infected individuals experience mild symptoms and may not seek medical attention; the more severe symptoms of schistosomiasis occur mainly in those who are heavily infected. In addition to organ-specific morbidities, infected patients may demonstrate anemia, chronic pain, diarrhea, exercise intolerance, and undernutrition. Cercarial penetration of human skin may result in a papular pruritic rash known as schistosomal dermatitis or **swimmer's itch.** It is more pronounced in previously exposed individuals and is characterized by edema and massive cellular infiltrates in the dermis and epidermis. Acute schistosomiasis, **Katayama fever,** may occur, particularly in heavily infected individuals 4–8 wk after exposure; this is a serum sickness–like syndrome manifested by the acute onset of fever, chills, sweating, lymphadenopathy, hepatosplenomegaly, and eosinophilia. Acute schistosomiasis most commonly presents in 1st time visitors to endemic areas who experience primary infection at an older age.

Symptomatic children with chronic schistosomiasis haematobia usually complain of frequency, dysuria, and hematuria. Urine examination shows erythrocytes, parasite eggs, and occasional eosinophiluria. In endemic areas, moderate to severe pathologic lesions have been demonstrated in the urinary tract of >20% of infected children. The extent of disease correlates with the intensity of infection, but significant morbidity can occur even in lightly infected children. The advanced stages of schistosomiasis haematobia are associated with chronic renal failure, secondary infections, and cancer of the bladder.

Children with chronic schistosomiasis mansoni, japonica, intercalatum, or mekongi may have intestinal symptoms; colicky abdominal pain and bloody diarrhea are the most common. The intestinal phase may, however, remain subclinical, and the late syndrome of hepatosplenomegaly, portal hypertension, ascites, and hematemesis may then be the 1st clinical presentation. Liver disease is due to granuloma formation and subsequent fibrosis; no appreciable liver cell injury occurs, and hepatic function may be preserved for a long time. Schistosome eggs may escape into the lungs, causing pulmonary hypertension and cor pulmonale. *S. japonicum* worms may migrate to the brain vasculature and produce localized lesions that cause seizures. Transverse myelitis rarely has been reported in children or young adults with either acute or chronic *S. haematobium* or *S. mansoni* infections.

DIAGNOSIS. Schistosome eggs are found in the excreta of infected individuals; quantitative methods should be used to provide an indication of the intensity of infection. For diagnosis of schistosomiasis haematobia, a volume of 10 mL of urine should be collected around midday, which is the time of maximal egg excretion, and filtered for microscopic examination. Stool examination by the Kato thick smear procedure is the method of choice for diagnosis and quantification of other schistosome infections.

TREATMENT. Treatment of children with schistosomiasis should be based on an appreciation of the intensity of infection and the extent of disease. The recommended treatment for schistosomiasis is praziquantel (40 mg/kg/day divided bid PO for 1 day for schistosomiasis haematobia, mansoni, and intercalatum; 60 mg/kg/day divided tid PO for 1 day for schistosomiasis japonica and mekongi). For *S. mansoni,* oxamniquine has been effective in some areas where praziquantel has been less effective.

PREVENTION. Transmission in endemic areas may be decreased by reducing the parasite load in the human population. The availability of oral, single-dose, effective chemotherapeutic agents may help achieve this goal. Other measures, particularly improved sanitation and focal application of molluscicides, may be useful. Control of schistosomiasis is closely linked to economic and social development.

Case records of the Massachusetts General Hospital: Weekly clinicopathological exercises. Case 31–2000. A 32-year-old man with a lesion of the urinary bladder. *N Engl J Med* 2000;343:1105–1111.

Centers for Disease Control and Prevention: Schistosomiasis. Health Topics A to Z. Available at http://www.cdc.gov/ncidod/dpd/parasites/schistosomiasis/default.htm

Drugs for parasitic infections. *Med Lett Drugs Ther* 2004;44(1189):1–12. Available at www.medicalletter.org

Hatz CF: The use of ultrasound in schistosomiasis. *Adv Parasitol* 2001;48:225–284.

King CH, Dickman K, and Tisch DJ: Reassessment of the cost of chronic helminth infection: Meta-analysis of disability-related outcomes in endemic schistosomiasis. *Lancet* 2005:365:1561–1569.

Saconato H, Atallah A: Interventions for treating schistosomiasis mansoni. *Cochrane Database Syst Rev* 1999:CD000528.

Schistosoma japonicum: Modern tools for an ancient disease. *Lancet* 2004;363:180.

Squires N: Interventions for treating schistosomiasis haematobium. *Cochrane Database Syst Rev* 1997:CD000053.

Wynn TA, Thompson RW, Cheever AW, Mentink-Kane MM: Immunopathogenesis of schistosomiasis. *Immunol Rev* 2004;201:156–167.

Chapter 298 ■ Flukes (Liver, Lung, and Intestinal) Charles H. King

Several different trematodes, or flukes, can parasitize humans and cause disease. Flukes are endemic worldwide but are more prevalent in the less developed parts of the world. They include *Schistosoma,* or the blood flukes (see Chapter 297), as well as fluke species that cause infection in the human biliary tree, lung tissue, and intestinal tract. These latter trematodes are characterized by their complex life cycles. Sexual reproduction of adult worms in the definitive host produces eggs that are passed in the stool. Larvae, called miracidia, develop in freshwater. These, in turn, infect certain species of molluscs (snails or clams), in which asexual multiplication by parasite larvae produces cercariae. Cercariae then seek a 2nd intermediate host such as an insect, crustacean, or fish or attach to vegetation to produce infectious metacercariae. Humans acquire liver, lung, and intestinal fluke infections by eating uncooked, lightly cooked, pickled, or smoked foods containing these infectious parasite cysts. The "alternation of generations" requires that flukes parasitize more than 1 host (often 3) to complete their life cycle. Because parasitic flukes are dependent on these nonhuman species for transmission, the distribution of human fluke infection closely matches their ecologic range.

LIVER FLUKES

Fascioliasis *(Fasciola Hepatica).* *Fasciola hepatica,* the sheep liver fluke, infects cattle, other ungulates, and occasionally humans. Infection has been reported in many different parts of the world, particularly South America, Europe, Africa, China, Australia, and Cuba. Although *F. hepatica* is enzootic in North America, reported cases are extremely rare. Humans are infected by ingestion of metacercariae attached to vegetation, especially wild watercress. In the duodenum, the parasites excyst and penetrate the intestinal wall, liver capsule, and parenchyma. They wander for a few weeks before entering the bile ducts, where they mature. Adult *F. hepatica* (1–2.5 cm) commence oviposition approximately 12 wk after infection; the eggs are large (75–140 μm) and operculated. They pass to the intestines with bile and exit the body in the feces (see Fig. 297-1). On reaching freshwater, the eggs mature and hatch into miracidia, which infect specific snail intermediate hosts to multiply into many cercariae. These then emerge from infected snails and encyst on aquatic grasses and plants.

Clinical manifestations usually occur either during the liver migratory phase of the parasites or after their arrival at their final habitat in bile canaliculi. Fever, right upper quadrant pain, and hepatosplenomegaly characterize the 1st phase of illness. Peripheral blood eosinophilia is usually marked. As the worms enter bile ducts, most of the acute symptoms subside. On rare occasions, patients may suffer from obstructive jaundice or biliary cirrhosis. *F. hepatica* infection is diagnosed by identifying the characteristic eggs in fecal smears or duodenal aspirates.

The recommended **treatment** of fascioliasis is triclabendazole (10 mg/kg once or twice PO) or bithionol (30–50 mg/kg once daily PO on alternate days for a total of 10–15 doses). In the United States, bithionol is available from the Centers for Disease Control and Prevention (telephone: 404–639–3670). The investigational drug triclabendazole (Ciba-Geigy) may also be used as a single oral dose of 10 mg/kg to treat fascioliasis.

Clonorchiasis *(Clonorchis Sinensis)*. Infection of bile passages with *Clonorchis sinensis,* the Chinese or oriental liver fluke, is endemic in China, other parts of East Asia, and Japan. Humans acquire infection by ingestion of raw or inadequately cooked freshwater fish carrying the encysted metacercariae of the parasite under their scales or skin. Metacercariae excyst in the duodenum and pass through the ampulla of Vater to the common bile duct and bile capillaries, where they mature into hermaphroditic adult worms (3–15 mm). *C. sinensis* worms deposit small operculated eggs (14–30 µm), which are discharged by way of the bile duct to the intestine and feces (see Fig. 297-1). The eggs mature and hatch outside the body, releasing motile miracidia into local freshwater streams, rivers, or ponds. If these are taken up by the appropriate snails, they develop into cercariae, which are in turn released from the snail to encyst under the skin or scales of freshwater fish.

Most individuals with *C. sinensis* infection, particularly those with few organisms, are minimally symptomatic. In heavily infected individuals, who tend to be older (>30 yr of age), localized obstruction of a bile duct results from repeated local trauma and inflammation. In these cases, cholangitis and cholangiohepatitis may lead to liver enlargement and jaundice. In Hong Kong, Korea, and other parts of Asia, cholangiocarcinoma is associated with chronic *C. sinensis* infection.

Clonorchiasis is diagnosed by examination of feces or duodenal aspirates for the parasite eggs. The recommended **treatment** of clonorchiasis is praziquantel (75 mg/kg/day divided tid PO for 1 day). An alternative, used in adults, is albendazole (10 mg/kg once daily PO for 7 days).

Opisthorchiasis (Opisthorchis). Infections with species of *Opisthorchis* are clinically similar to those by *C. sinensis. Opisthorchis felineus* and *Opisthorchis viverrini* are liver flukes of cats and dogs that infect humans through ingestion of metacercariae in freshwater fish. Infection with *O. felineus* is endemic in Eastern Europe and Southeast Asia, and *O. viverrini* is found mainly in Thailand. Most individuals are asymptomatic; liver enlargement, relapsing cholangitis, and jaundice may occur in heavily infected individuals. Diagnosis is based on recovering eggs from stools or duodenal aspirates. The recommended **treatment** of opisthorchiasis is praziquantel (75 mg/kg/day divided tid PO for 1 day).

LUNG FLUKES

Paragonimiasis *(Paragonimus)*. Human infection by the lung fluke *Paragonimus westermani,* and less frequently other species of *Paragonimus,* occurs throughout the Far East, in localized areas of West Africa, and in several parts of Central and South America. The highest incidence of paragonimiasis occurs in older children and adolescents 11–15 yr of age. Although *P. westermani* is found in many carnivores, human cases are relatively rare and seem to be associated with specific dietary habits, such as eating raw freshwater crayfish or crabs. These crustaceans contain the infective metacercariae in their tissues. After ingestion, the metacercariae excyst in the duodenum, penetrate the intestinal wall, and migrate to their final habitat in the lungs. Adult worms (5–10 mm) encapsulate within the lung parenchyma and deposit brown operculated eggs (60–100 µm), which pass into the bronchioles and are expectorated by coughing (see Fig. 297-1). Ova can be detected in the sputum of infected individuals or in their feces. If eggs reach freshwater, they hatch and undergo asexual multiplication in specific snails. The cercariae encyst in the muscles and viscera of crayfish and freshwater crabs.

Most individuals infected with *P. westermani* harbor low or moderate worm loads and are minimally symptomatic. The **clinical manifestations** include cough, production of rust-colored sputum, and hemoptysis, which is the principal manifestation and occurs in 98% of symptomatic children. There are no characteristic physical findings, but laboratory examination usually demonstrates marked eosinophilia. Chest x-rays often reveal small patchy infiltrates or radiolucencies in the middle lung fields; however, the radiograph may appear normal in 1/5 of infected individuals. In rare circumstances, lung abscess, pleural effusion, or bronchiectasis may develop. Extrapulmonary localization of *P. westermani* in the brain, peritoneum, intestines, or pleura may rarely occur. Cerebral paragonimiasis occurs primarily in heavily infected individuals living in highly endemic areas of the Far East. The clinical presentation resembles jacksonian epilepsy or the symptoms of cerebral tumors.

Definitive diagnosis of paragonimiasis is established by identification of eggs in fecal or sputum smears. The recommended **treatment** of paragonimiasis is praziquantel (75 mg/kg/day divided tid PO for 2 days).

INTESTINAL FLUKES. Several wild and domestic animal intestinal flukes, including *Fasciolopsis buski, Nanophyetus salmincola,* and *Heterophyes heterophyes,* may accidentally infect humans. *F. buski* is endemic in the Far East. Humans who ingest metacercariae encysted on aquatic plants become infected. These develop into large flukes (1–5 cm) that inhabit the duodenum and jejunum. Mature worms produce operculated eggs that pass with feces; the organism completes its life cycle through specific snail intermediate hosts. Individuals with *F. buski* infection are usually asymptomatic; heavily infected subjects complain of abdominal pain and diarrhea and show signs of malabsorption. Diagnosis of fasciolopsiasis and other intestinal fluke infections is established by fecal examination and identification of the eggs (see Fig. 297-1). As for other fluke infections, **praziquantel** (75 mg/kg/day divided tid PO for 1 day) is the drug of choice.

Drugs for parasitic infections. *Med Lett Drugs Ther* 2004;44(1189):1–12. Available at www.medicalletter.org.

King CH: Pulmonary flukes. In Mahmoud AA (editor): *Parasitic Lung Diseases.* New York, Marcel Dekker, 1997;157–169.

Liu LX, Harinasuta KT: Liver and intestinal flukes. *Gastroenterol Clin North Am* 1996;25:627–636.

Lun ZR, Gasser RB, Lai DH, et al: Clonorchiasis: A key foodborne zoonosis in China. *Lancet Infect Dis* 2005;5:31–41.

MacLean JD, Cross J, Mahanty S: Liver, lung and intestinal fluke infections. In Guerrant RL, Walker DH, Weller PF (editors): *Tropical Infectious Diseases, Principles, Pathogens and Practice,* 2nd ed. Philadelphia, Churchill Livingstone 2006;1349–1369.

Millan JC, Mull R, Freise S, et al: The efficacy and tolerability of triclabendazole in Cuban patients with latent and chronic *Fasciola hepatica* infection. *Am J Trop Med Hyg* 2000;63:264–269.

Price TA, Tuazon CU, Simon GL: Fascioliasis: Case reports and review. *Clin Infect Dis* 1993;17:426–430.

Tshibwabwa ET, Richenberg JL, Aziz ZA: Lung radiology in the tropics. *Clin Chest Med* 2002;23:309–328.
Watanapa P, Watanapa WB: Liver fluke-associated cholangiocarcinoma. *Br J Surg* 2002;89:962–970.

Chapter 299 ■ Adult Tapeworm Infections

Ronald Blanton

Infections with **cestodes,** or **tapeworms,** are prevalent on every continent except Antarctica. The key biology that governs disease is whether humans are infected with the intestinal adult stage or the invasive intermediate stage of the parasite (Table 299-1). No signs or symptoms can clearly be attributed to infection with any adult tapeworm except for *Diphyllobothrium latum*. The intermediate stages of some tapeworms, such as *Taenia solium* (see Chapter 300) and *Echinococcus* (see Chapter 301), are invasive and form cystic structures that produce tissue damage from mass effect or inflammatory reactions. Infection with the adult worm can be easily diagnosed by finding eggs or segments of adult worms in the stool, whereas the invasive stage of the parasite cannot be observed in any easily sampled fluid. Infection with an intermediate stage, therefore, must be diagnosed by serologic tests, imaging, or invasive procedures.

TAENIASIS (TAENIA SAGINATA AND TAENIA SOLIUM)

Etiology. The **beef tapeworm,** *Taenia saginata,* and the **pork tapeworm,** *T. solium,* are large parasites (4–10 m) named for their intermediate hosts. The adult stages are only found in the human intestine. The body of the adult stage is a series of hundreds or thousands of flattened segments (**proglottids**) whose most anterior segment (**scolex**) anchors the parasite to the bowel wall. New segments arise from the tail of the scolex followed by progressively more mature ones. The gravid terminal segments are each packed with 50,000–100,000 eggs, and the eggs or the intact proglottids themselves are passed in the stool. These 2 tapeworms differ most significantly in that the intermediate stage of the pork tapeworm (cysticercus) can also infect humans and cause significant morbidity (see Chapter 300).

Epidemiology. Both *Taenia* species are distributed worldwide, with the highest risk for infection in Central America, Africa, India, Southeast Asia, and China. The prevalence in adults may not reflect the prevalence in young children, because cultural practices may dictate how well meat is cooked and how much is served to children.

Pathogenesis. Uncomplicated infection with the adult beef or pork tapeworm by itself is an infrequent source of symptoms. When children ingest raw or undercooked infected meat, gastric acid and bile facilitate release of the immature scolex that attaches to the lumen of the small intestine. The parasite adds new segments, and after 2–3 mo the terminal segments mature, become gravid, and appear in stool.

Clinical Manifestations. Adult beef and pork tapeworms cause very little overt morbidity apart from nonspecific abdominal symptoms. The proglottids of these tapeworms are visually striking. They are also motile and sometimes produce anal pruritus. They can often be felt as they pass and are thus likely to be noticed and cause a strong emotional reaction in older children and parents when discovered. The adult beef and pork tapeworms are rare causes of intestinal obstruction, cholangitis, and appendicitis.

Diagnosis. It is important to identify the infecting species of tapeworm. Carriers of adult pork tapeworms are at increased risk for transmitting eggs with the pathogenic intermediate stage (cysticercus) to themselves or others, whereas children infected with the beef tapeworm are risk only to livestock. Because proglottids are generally passed intact, visual examination for gravid proglottids in the stool is a sensitive test; these segments may be used to identify species. Eggs, by contrast, are often absent from stool and cannot reliably distinguish between *T. saginata* and *T. solium* (Fig. 299-1). If the parasite is completely expelled, the scolex of each species is diagnostic. The scolex of *T. saginata* has only a set of 4 anteriorly oriented suckers, whereas *T. solium* is armed with a double row of hooks in addition to suckers. The proglottids of *T. saginata* have more than 20 uterine branches from a central uterine structure, and those of *T. solium* have 10 or fewer. When in doubt, more proglottids should be obtained or the sample should be referred to a laboratory with parasitologic expertise.

Differential Diagnosis. Anal pruritus may mimic symptoms of pinworm *(Enterobius vermicularis)* infection. *D. latum* or even *Ascaris lumbricoides* may be mistaken for *T. saginata* or *T. solium* in stools.

Treatment. Infections with all adult tapeworms respond to praziquantel (5–10 mg/kg PO once). An alternative treatment for taeniasis is niclosamide (50 mg/kg PO once for children, 2 g PO once for adults). The parasite is usually expelled on the day of administration.

TABLE 299-1. Common Cestode Parasites of Humans, Their Typical Vectors, and Their Usual Symptoms

PARASITE SPECIES	DEVELOPMENTAL STAGE FOUND IN HUMANS	COMMON NAME	TRANSMISSION SOURCE	SYMPTOMS ASSOCIATED WITH INFECTION
Diphyllobothrium latum	Tapeworm	Fish tapeworm	Plerocercoid cysts in fresh water fish	Usually minimal; with prolonged or heavy infection, vitamin B_{12} deficiency
Hymenolepis nana	Tapeworm, cysticercoids	Dwarf tapeworm	Infected humans	Mild abdominal discomfort
Taenia saginata	Tapeworm	Beef tapeworm	Cysts in beef	Abdominal discomfort, proglottid migration
Taenia solium	Tapeworm	Pork tapeworm	Cysticerci in pork	Minimal
Taenia solium (cysticercus cellulosae)	Cysticerci	Cysticercosis	Eggs from infected humans	Local inflammation, mass effect; if in CNS, seizures, hydrocephalus, arachnoiditis
Echinococcus granulosus	Larval cysts	Hydatid cyst disease	Eggs from infected dogs	Mass effect leading to pain, obstruction of adjacent organs; less commonly, secondary bacterial infection, distal spread of daughter cysts
Echinococcus multilocularis	Larval cysts	Alveolar cyst disease	Eggs from infected canines	Local invasion and mass effect leading to organ dysfunction; distal metastasis possible
Taenia multiceps	Larval cysts	Coenurosis, bladder worm	Eggs from infected dogs	Local inflammation and mass effect
Spirometra mansonoides	Larval cysts	Sparganosis	Cysts from infected copepods, frogs, snakes	Local inflammation and mass effect

CNS, central nervous system.
Form Mandell GL, Bennett JE, Dolin R (editors): *Principles and Practice of Infectious Diseases*, 6th ed, Vol 2. Philadelphia, Elsevier, 2005, p 3286.

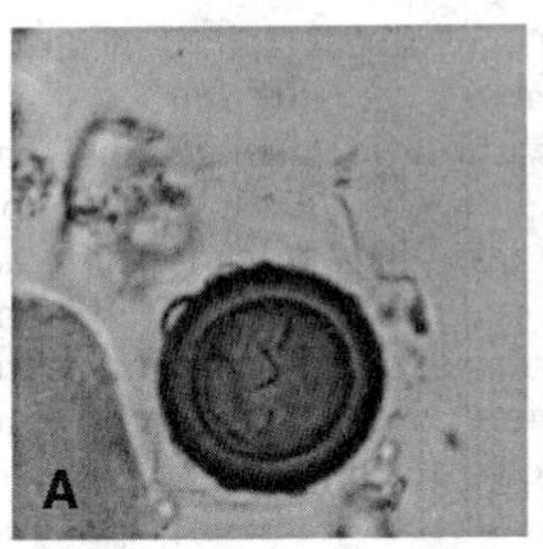

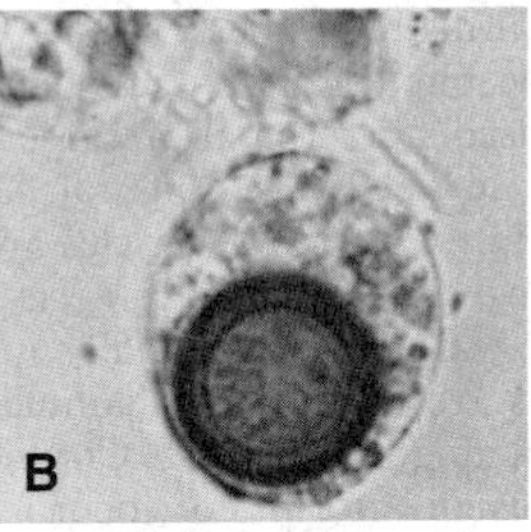

Figure 299-1. Eggs of *Taenia saginata* recovered from feces (original magnification ×400). The eggs are generally bile stained, dark, and prismatic. There is occasionally some surrounding cellular material from the proglottid in which the egg develops, which is more evident in B than in A. The larva within the egg shows three pairs of hooklets *(A)*, which may occasionally be observed in motion.

Prevention. Prolonged freezing or thorough cooking of beef and pork kills the parasite. Appropriate human sanitation can interrupt transmission by preventing infection in livestock.

DIPHYLLOBOTHRIASIS (DIPHYLLOBOTHRIUM LATUM)

Etiology. The **fish tapeworm,** *D. latum,* is the longest human tapeworm (10–20 m) and has an organization similar to that of other adult cestodes. An elongated scolex equipped with slits (**bothria**) along each side, but no suckers or hooks, is followed by thousands of segments looped in the small bowel. The terminal gravid proglottid detaches periodically but tends to disintegrate before expulsion, thus releasing its eggs into the feces. In contrast to taeniids, the life cycle of *D. latum* requires 2 intermediate hosts. Small crustaceans (copepods) take up the embryos hatched from parasite eggs in fresh water. The parasite passes up the food chain as small fish eat the copepods and are in turn eaten by larger fish. In this way, the juvenile parasite becomes concentrated in pike, walleye, perch, salmon, and similar fish. Consumption of raw or undercooked fish leads to human infection with adult fish tapeworms.

Epidemiology. The fish tapeworm is most prevalent in the temperate climates of Europe, North America, and Asia but may be found in cold lakes at high altitudes in South America and Africa. In North America, the prevalence is highest in Alaska, Canada, and the northern United States. The tapeworm is found in fish from those areas brought to market in the continental USA. Persons who prepare raw fish for home or commercial use or who sample fish before cooking are particularly at risk for infection.

Pathogenesis. The adult worm efficiently scavenges vitamin B_{12} for its own use in the constant production of large numbers of segments and as many as 1 million eggs per day. As a result, diphyllobothriasis causes megaloblastic anemia in 2–9% of infections. Children with other causes of vitamin B_{12} or folate deficiency such as chronic infectious diarrhea, celiac disease, or congenital malabsorption are more likely to develop symptomatic infection.

Clinical Manifestations. Infection is largely asymptomatic except in those who develop B_{12} or folate deficiency. Megaloblastic anemia with leukopenia, thrombocytopenia, glossitis, and signs of spinal cord posterior column degeneration (loss of vibratory sense, proprioception, and coordination) can be evidence of advanced nutritional deficiency due to diphyllobothriasis. The hematologic and neurologic signs may present independently or as a cluster. It should be mentioned that an invasive form of infection termed sparganosis results when the intermediate form of this or other members of this group of tapeworm are introduced subcutaneously. Skin, muscle, eye, and brain have been sites of invasion.

Diagnosis. Parasitologic examination of the stool is useful because eggs are abundant in the feces and have a morphology distinct from that of all other tapeworms. The eggs are ovoid and have an operculum, which is a cap structure at 1 end that opens to release the embryo (Fig. 299-2). The worm itself has a distinct scolex and proglottid morphology; however, these are not likely to be passed spontaneously.

Differential Diagnosis. A segment or a whole section of the worm might be confused with *Taenia* or *Ascaris* after it is passed. Pernicious anemia, bone marrow toxins, and dietary restrictions may contribute to or mimic diphyllobothriasis.

Treatment. Infections with all adult tapeworms respond to praziquantel (5–10 mg/kg PO once), which is the recommended treatment for diphyllobothriasis.

Prevention. The intermediate stage is easily eliminated by brief cooking or prolonged freezing. Because humans are the major reservoir for adult worms, health education is 1 of the most important tools for preventing transmission, together with improved human sanitation.

HYMENOLEPIASIS (HYMENOLEPIS). Infection with *Hymenolepis nana,* the **dwarf tapeworm,** is very common in developing countries. It is a major cause of eosinophilia, and although it rarely causes overt disease, the presence of *H. nana* eggs in stool may serve as a marker for exposure to poor hygienic conditions. The intermediate stage develops in various hosts (e.g., rodents, ticks, and fleas), and the entire life cycle can be completed in humans. Hyperinfection with thousands of small adult worms in a single child is thus a potential. Less commonly, a similar infection may occur with the species *H. diminuta.* Eggs but not segments may be found in the stool. *H. nana* infection responds to praziquantel (25 mg/kg PO once) or niclosamide (50 mg/kg PO once for children; 2 gm PO once for adults).

DIPYLIDIASIS (DIPYLIDIUM CANINUM). *Dipylidium caninum* is a common tapeworm of domestic dogs and cats, yet human infection is relatively rare. Direct transmission between pets and humans does not occur; human infection requires ingestion of the parasite's intermediate host, the dog or cat flea. Infants and small children are particularly susceptible because of their level of hygiene, generally more intimate contact with pets, and activities in areas where fleas can be encountered. Eosinophilia may occur, but no symptoms clearly result from infection. Anal pruritus, vague abdominal pain, and diarrhea have at times been associated with dipylidiasis. Dipylidiasis may be confused with pinworm *(E. vermicularis)*. Dipylidiasis responds to treatment with praziquantel (5–10 mg/kg PO once) or niclosamide (50 mg/kg PO once for children; 2 gm PO once for adults). Deworming pets and flea control are the best preventive measures.

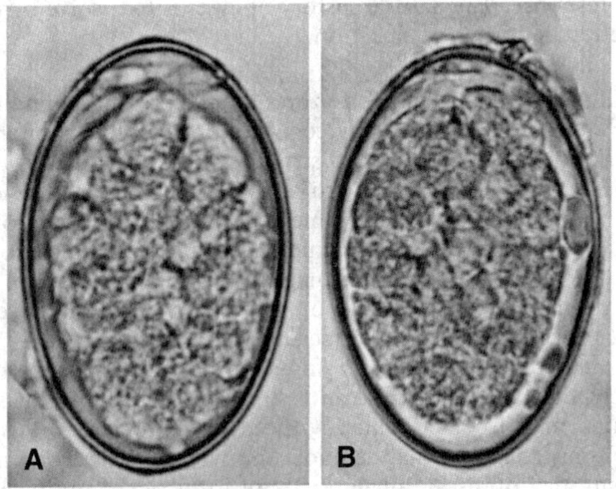

Figure 299-2. Eggs of *Diphyllobothrium latum* as seen in feces (original magnification ×400). The caplike operculum is at the upper end of the egg here.

Schantz PM: Tapeworms (cestodiasis). *Gastroenterol Clin North Am* 1996;25: 637–653.
Weisse ME, Raszka WV Jr: Cestode infection in children. *Adv Pediatr Infect Dis* 1996;12:109–153.

Chapter 300 ■ Cysticercosis

Ronald Blanton

ETIOLOGY. Cysticercosis, the most common and serious parasitic infection of the central nervous system (CNS), is the result of infection with the intermediate stage of *Taenia solium,* the **pork tapeworm.** The intermediate stage of *T. solium,* unlike *Taenia saginata,* is infectious for humans and preferentially invades the CNS, causing **neurocysticercosis.** Cysticercosis may develop even in individuals who do not eat pork, since humans acquire the intermediate form by ingestion of food or water contaminated with the eggs of *T. solium.* By contrast, consumption of infected undercooked pork produces intestinal infection with the adult worm (see Chapter 299). Individuals harboring an adult worm, however, may infect themselves with the eggs by the fecal-oral route. Reverse peristalsis in the small intestine has also been implicated as a means of autoinfection. In the small intestine, the egg releases an **oncosphere** that crosses the gut wall and spreads hematogenously to many tissues, primarily brain and muscle. Wherever the eggs lodge, they produce small (0.2–0.5 cm) fluid-filled bladders containing a single **protoscolex,** the juvenile-stage parasite.

EPIDEMIOLOGY. The pork tapeworm is distributed worldwide wherever pigs are raised. Intense transmission occurs in Central and South America, India, Indonesia, Korea, and China as well as some areas of Africa. In these areas, 20–50% of cases of epilepsy may be due to cysticercosis. Most cases of cysticercosis in the United States are imported; transmission is uncommon but occurs on occasion.

PATHOGENESIS. The cystic stages usually do not provoke a strong immunologic response, while they remain alive and intact. Intact viable cysts can be associated with disease when the initial parasite invasion of the brain is massive or when they obstruct the flow of cerebrospinal fluid (CSF). Most cysts remain viable for 5–10 yr and then begin to degenerate, followed by a vigorous host response. The natural history of cysts is to resolve by complete resorption or calcification.

CLINICAL MANIFESTATIONS. Seizures are the presenting finding in >70% of cases, although any cognitive or neurologic abnormality ranging from psychosis to stroke may be a manifestation of cysticercosis. It is useful to classify neurocysticercosis as parenchymal, intraventricular, meningeal, spinal, or ocular on the basis of anatomic location, clinical presentation, and radiologic appearance. Prognosis and management vary with location.

Parenchymal neurocysticercosis produces seizures as well as focal neurologic deficits. The seizures are generalized in 80% of cases but frequently begin as simple or complex partial seizures. Rarely, cerebral infarction can result from obstruction of small terminal arteries or vasculitis. With extensive frontal lobe disease, symptoms of intellectual deterioration with dementia or parkinsonism may obfuscate diagnosis until focal signs appear. A fulminant encephalitis-like presentation also occurs, most frequently in children who have had a massive initial infection. Intraventricular neurocysticercosis (5–10% of all cases) is associated with hydrocephalus and acute, subacute, or intermittent signs of increased intracranial pressure without localizing signs. The 4th ventricle is the most common site for obstruction and symptoms; cysts in the lateral ventricles are less likely to cause obstruction. Meningeal neurocysticercosis is associated with signs of meningeal irritation and also increased intracranial pressure that results from edema, inflammation, or the presence of a cyst obstructing flow of CSF. Chronic basilar meningitis is associated with many forms of neurocysticercosis, but predominantly meningeal presentations. Racemose neurocysticercosis is a meningeal form of disease in which large, lobulated cysts appear in the basal cisterns. Spinal neurocysticercosis presents with evidence of spinal cord compression, nerve root pain, transverse myelitis, or meningitis. Ocular neurocysticercosis causes decreased visual acuity due to cysticerci floating in the vitreous, retinal detachment, iridocyclitis, or orbital mass effect. Outside of the CNS, cysts can sometimes be palpated under the skin, and very heavy infections in skeletal or heart muscle can result in myositis or carditis.

DIAGNOSIS. Neurocysticercosis should be suspected in a child with onset of any neurologic, cognitive, or personality disorder and who also has a history of residence in an endemic area or a care provider from an endemic area. Seizures, hydrocephalus, unilateral visual impairment, or symptoms of encephalitis are particularly suspicious. Proglottids (segments) or eggs are observed in feces from only 25% of cases of neurocysticercosis; therefore, imaging studies and serologic tests are necessary to confirm a clinical suspicion.

The most useful diagnostic study for parenchymal disease is MRI of the head. MRI provides the most information about cyst viability and associated inflammation. The protoscolex is sometimes visible within the cyst, which provides a pathognomonic sign for cysticercosis (Fig. 300-1A). The MRI also better detects basilar arachnoiditis (Fig. 300-1B), intraventricular cysts (Fig 300-1C), as well as those in the spinal cord. CT is best for identifying calcifications. A solitary parenchymal cyst, with or without contrast enhancement, and numerous calcifications are the most common findings in children (Fig. 300-2). Plain films may reveal calcifications in muscle or brain consistent with cysticercosis, but these are often nondiagnostic in children.

Serologic diagnosis using the enzyme-linked immunotransfer blot (EITB) is available commercially in the USA and through the Centers for Disease Control and Prevention. Serum antibody testing has >90% sensitivity and specificity; testing of CSF is not required. Persons with many parenchymal cysts almost always have a positive serum EITB test result. Cases with solitary lesions or old calcified disease may not have detectable antibodies. Neurocysticercosis is the most important and most frequent cause of **eosinophilia** in CSF, but this is not a reliable finding and if absent does not preclude the diagnosis.

DIFFERENTIAL DIAGNOSIS. Neurocysticercosis can be confused clinically with encephalitis, stroke, meningitis, and many other conditions (Table 300-1). Clinical suspicion is based on travel history or a history of contact with an individual who might carry an adult tapeworm. On imaging studies, cysticerci can be difficult to distinguish from tuberculomas, histoplasmosis, blastomycosis, toxoplasmosis, sarcoidosis, vasculitis, and tumor.

TREATMENT. The inclusion of antiparasitic drugs is controversial. Most associated seizures can be readily controlled using standard anticonvulsants. If seizures are recurrent or associated with calcified lesions, treatment should be continued for 2–3 yr before attempting weaning from anticonvulsants. Evidence of hydrocephalus should be sought and shunting provided if found. Causes other than cysticercosis, especially tuberculoma, must be excluded (see Table 300-1).

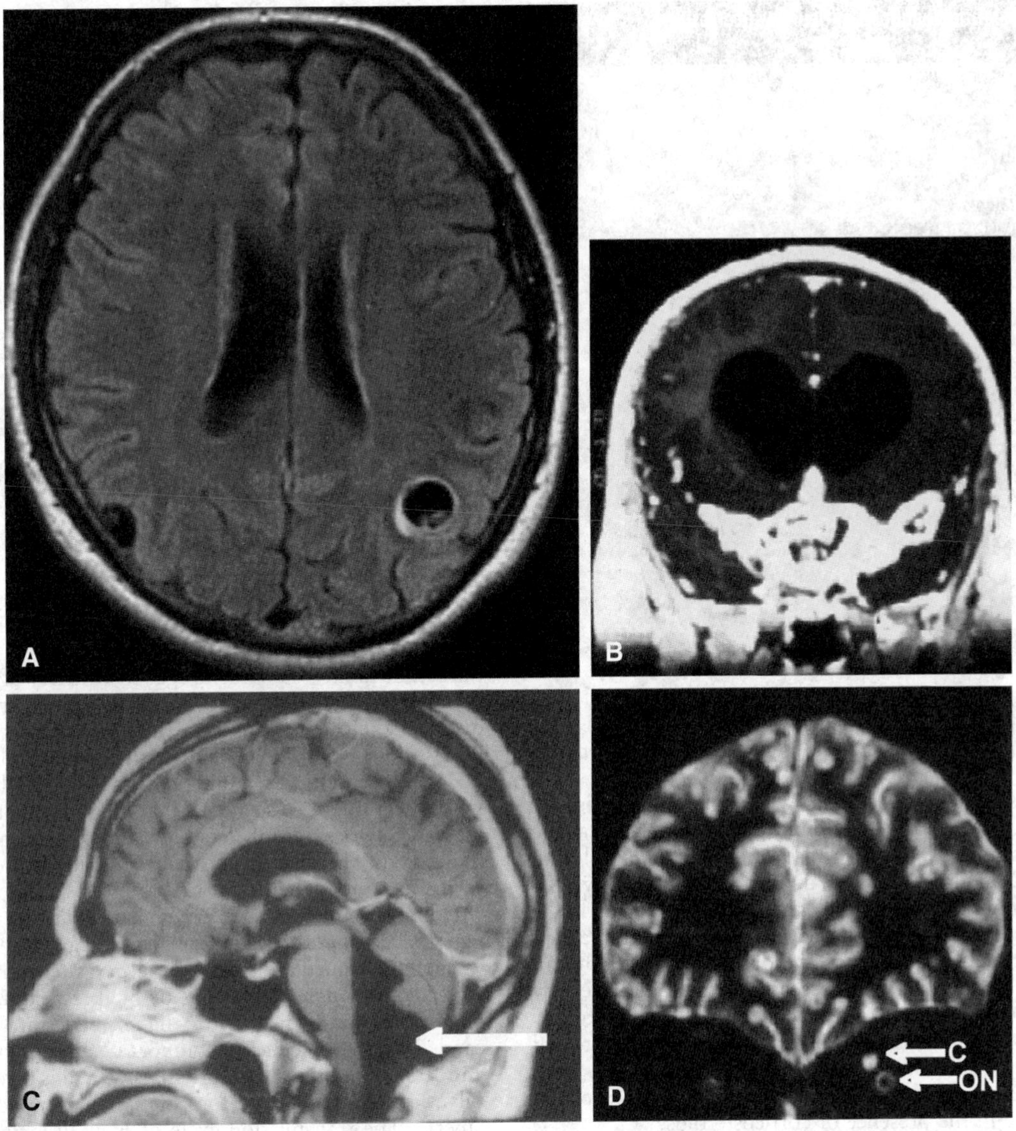

Figure 300-1. *A,* MRI (T1 weighted) demonstrating a parenchymal cyst with protoscolex. *B,* MRI (T1 weighted) of cysticercal basilar arachnoiditis. *C,* MRI (T1 weighted) showing a cyst below the 4th ventricle *(arrow)*. *D,* MRI (T2 weighted) showing cysticercus (C) above the optic nerve (ON).

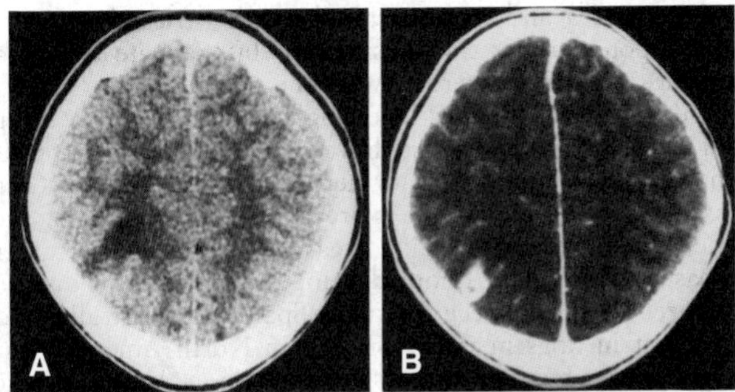

Figure 300-2. CT image of a solitary lesion of neurocysticercosis with *(A)* and without *(B)* contrast, showing contrast enhancement. (Courtesy of Dr. Wendy G. Mitchell and Dr. Marvin D. Nelson, Children's Hospital, Los Angeles.)

The natural history of parenchymal lesions is to resolve spontaneously with or without antiparasitic drugs. Most children present with solitary parenchymal cysts that resolve as readily with as without therapy. Other forms of the disease are uncommon. By contrast, multiple lesions and complex presentations are typical of disease in adults. One double-blind, placebo-controlled study demonstrated a significant decrease in generalized seizures for cysticercosis in adults treated with antiparasitic therapy. Antiparasitic therapy may have some long-term advantages for children with multiple cysts or complicated disease. Antiparasitic therapy with dexamethasone treatment enhances partial or complete resolution of lesions and reduces the risk of recurrent seizures in children with 1–2 ring-enhancing lesions. There is little evidence that the management of acute symptoms improves with these drugs, and they are not indicated where there are only degenerating or calcified lesions.

Subarachnoid disease has a poor prognosis if untreated, but antiparasitic treatment is associated with a better outcome in comparison with historical controls. Ocular cysticercosis is essentially a surgical disease, although there are reports of cure using

TABLE 300-1. Differential Diagnosis of Neurocysticercosis on Neuroimaging

SOLE NON-ENHANCING CYSTIC LESION
Hydatid disease
Arachnoid cysts
Porencephaly
Cystic astrocytoma
Colloid cyst (third ventricle)
SEVERAL NON-ENHANCING CYSTIC LESIONS
Multiple metastases
Hydatid disease (rare)
ENHANCING LESIONS
Tuberculosis
Mycosis
Toxoplasmosis
Abscess
Early glioma
Metastasis
Arteriovenous malformation
CALCIFICATIONS
Tuberous sclerosis
Tuberculosis
Cytomegalovirus infection
Toxoplasmosis

Form Garcia HH, Gonzalez AE, Evans CAW, et al: Taenia solium cysticercosis. *Lancet* 2003;361:547–556.

medical therapy alone. The outcome is not good in most cases, and enucleation is frequently required.

Albendazole is the antiparasitic drug of choice (15 mg/kg/day PO divided bid for 28 days; maximum 800 mg/day). It can be taken with a fatty meal to improve absorption. Praziquantel is an alternative (50–100 mg/kg/day PO divided tid for 28 days). A worsening of symptoms can follow the use of either drug as the host responds to the dying parasite with increased inflammation. Corticosteroids for 2–3 days before and during drug therapy can ameliorate these effects but may decrease praziquantel levels by as much as 50%. An increase of praziquantel (to 100 mg/kg/day divided tid PO) or administration of cimetidine, an inhibitor of the cytochrome P450 system, has been advocated when both praziquantel and corticosteroids are used. Albendazole levels, in contrast, increase in the presence of corticosteroids.

If no anticysticercal drugs are administered, however, it is also necessary to determine whether these patients carry adult worms, which poses a public health risk. Niclosamide used in the treatment of adult worms (see Chapter 299) is not absorbed and does not provoke an inflammatory response to cysticerci.

PREVENTION. All family members of index cases of cysticercosis, as well as persons handling their food, should be examined for signs of disease or evidence of adult worms. Attention to personal hygiene, proper handwashing by food handlers, and avoidance of fresh fruits and vegetables in areas endemic for *T. solium* help prevent ingestion of eggs. All pork should be cooked thoroughly.

Carpio A: Neurocysticercosis: An update. *Lancet Infect Dis* 2002;2:751–762.

Garcia HH, Evans CA, Nash TE, et al: Current consensus guidelines for treatment of neurocysticercosis. *Clin Microbiol Rev* 2002;15:747–756.

Garcia HH, Gonzalez AE, Evans CAW, et al: Taenia solium cysticercosis. *Lancet* 2003;361:547–556.

Garcia HH, Pretell EJ, Gilman RH, et al: Cysticercosis Working Group in Peru: A trial of antiparasitic treatment to reduce the rate of seizures due to cerebral cysticercosis. *N Engl J Med* 2004;350:249–258.

Ito A, Nakao M, Wandra T: Human taeniasis and cysticercosis in Asia. *Lancet* 2003;362:1918–1920.

Kalra V, Dua T, Kumar V: Efficacy of albendazole and short-course dexamethasone treatment in children with 1 or 2 ring-enhancing lesions of neurocysticercosis: A randomized controlled trial. *J Pediatr* 2003;143:111–114.

Proano JV, Madrazo I, Avelar F, et al: Medical treatment for neurocysticercosis characterized by giant subarachnoid cysts. *N Engl J Med* 2001;345:879–885.

Singhi P, Singhi S: Neurocysticercosis in children. *J Child Neurol* 2004;19:482–492.

Sotelo J: Neurocysticercosis—Is the elimination of parasites beneficial? *N Engl J Med* 2004;350:280–282.

Chapter 301 ■ Echinococcosis (*Echinococcus Granulosus* and *Echinococcus Multilocularis*)

Ronald Blanton

ETIOLOGY. Echinococcosis (**hydatid disease** or **hydatidosis**) is the most widespread, serious human cestode infection in the world. It is a zoonosis transmitted from domestic and wild members of the canine family via parasite eggs to a variety of wild and domestic animals. Two major *Echinococcus* species are responsible for distinct clinical presentations, *E. granulosus* (**cystic hydatid disease**) and the more malignant *E. multilocularis* (**alveolar hydatid disease**). The adult parasite is a small (2–7 mm) tapeworm with only 2–6 segments that inhabits the intestines of dogs, wolves, dingoes, jackals, coyotes, and foxes. These animals pass the eggs in their stool and contaminate the soil, pasture, and water, as well as their own fur.

Domestic animals such as sheep, goats, cattle, and camels ingest *E. granulosus* eggs while grazing. Humans are infected with the intermediate stage of the parasite by ingesting food or water contaminated with eggs or by direct contact with infected dogs. The intermediate forms hatch, penetrate the gut, and are carried by the vascular or lymphatic systems to the liver, lungs, and less commonly to other tissues. There is also a less prevalent sylvatic wolf/moose cycle for *E. granulosus* in North America and Siberia. The transmission cycle of *E. multilocularis* is similar to that of *E. granulosus,* except that this species is mainly sylvatic and uses small rodents as its natural intermediate hosts. The rodents are consumed by foxes, their natural predators, and sometimes by dogs and cats.

EPIDEMIOLOGY. *E. granulosus* thrives in environments as diverse as arctic tundra and the deserts of North Africa (Fig. 301-1). There is potential for transmission of this parasite to humans wherever animals are herded with the help of dogs. In urban areas, dogs may be infected by eating entrails after home slaughter of domestic animals. Cysts have been detected in up to 10% of the human population in northern Kenya and Western China. In South America, the disease is prevalent in sheep-herding areas of the Andes, the beef-herding areas of the Brazilian/Argentine Pampas, and Uruguay. Among developed countries, the disease is recognized in Italy, Greece, Portugal, Spain, and Australia, and is reemergent in dogs in Great Britain. In North America, transmission occurs by way of the sylvatic cycle in Alaska, Canada, and Isle Royale on Lake Superior, as well as in foci of the domestic cycle in sheep-raising areas of western United States.

Transmission of *E. multilocularis* occurs primarily in temperate climates of Northern Europe, Siberia, Turkey, and China. Transmission is decreasing among native peoples in Alaska and Canada as dogs are replaced by mechanized forms of transportation. A separate species, *Echinococcus vogeli,* causes polycystic disease similar to alveolar hydatidosis in South America.

PATHOGENESIS. In areas endemic for *E. granulosus,* the parasite is often acquired in childhood, but liver cysts require many years to become large enough to detect or cause symptoms. In children, the lung is a common site, whereas 70% of adults have disease in the right lobe of the liver. Cysts can also develop in bone, the genitourinary system, bowels, subcutaneous tissues, and brain. The host surrounds the primary cyst with a tough, fibrous capsule. Inside this capsule, the parasite produces a thick lamellar layer that supports a thin germinal layer of cells responsible for production of thousands of juvenile-stage parasites (protoscolices) that remain attached to the wall or float free in the cyst fluid. With cystic hydatidosis from *E. granulosus* infection, the established cyst may also produce smaller daughter cysts that are contained within the primary cyst capsule. The fluid in a healthy cyst is colorless, crystal clear, and watery. After medical treatment or with bacterial infection it may become thick and bile stained.

Infection with *E. multilocularis* resembles a malignancy. The secondary reproductive units bud externally and are not confined within a single well-defined structure. Furthermore, the cyst tissues are poorly demarcated from those of the host, which makes these cysts unsuitable for surgical removal. The secondary cysts are also capable of distant metastatic spread. The growing cyst mass eventually replaces a significant portion of the liver and compromises adjacent tissues and structures.

CLINICAL MANIFESTATIONS. In the liver, many cysts never become symptomatic and regress spontaneously or produce relatively nonspecific symptoms. When some cysts do take hold, increased abdominal girth, hepatomegaly, a palpable mass, vomiting, or abdominal pain ensue. The more serious complications, however, result from compression of adjacent structures, spillage of cyst contents, and location of cysts in sensitive areas such as the reproductive tract, brain, and bone. Anaphylaxis can occur with cyst rupture or spillage spontaneously, due to trauma or intraoperatively. Spillage can also be catastrophic long-term, since each protoscolex can form a new cyst. Jaundice due to cystic hydatid disease is rare.

In the lung, cysts produce chest pain, cough, or hemoptysis. Bone cysts may cause pathologic fractures, and in the genitourinary system they can produce hematuria or infertility.

In alveolar hydatid disease, cyst tissue continues to proliferate and may separate and metastasize distantly. The proliferating mass compromises hepatic tissue or the biliary system and causes progressive obstructive jaundice and hepatic failure. Symptoms also occur from expansion of extrahepatic foci.

DIAGNOSIS. On physical examination, subcutaneous nodules, hepatomegaly, or a palpable abdominal mass may be found. The parasite cannot be recovered from any easily accessible body fluid unless a lung cyst ruptures, after which protoscolices or layers of cyst wall may briefly be seen in sputum. Ultrasonography is the most valuable tool for both the diagnosis and treatment of cystic hydatid disease of the liver. The presence of internal membranes and falling echogenic cyst material (hydatid sand) that can be observed in real-time aid in the diagnosis. Alveolar disease is less cystic in appearance and resembles a diffuse solid tumor. CT findings (Fig. 301-2) are similar to those of ultrasonography and can at times be useful in distinguishing alveolar from cystic hydatid disease in geographic regions where both occur. CT or MRI is also important in planning a surgical intervention. Lung hydatid is usually apparent on chest x-ray (Fig. 301-3).

Serologic studies can be useful in confirming a diagnosis of echinococcosis, but the false-negative rate may be as high as 50%. Most patients with alveolar hydatidosis, however, develop detectable antibody responses. Current tests use crude or partially purified antigens that can cross react in individuals infected with other parasites, such as cysticercosis or schistosomiasis.

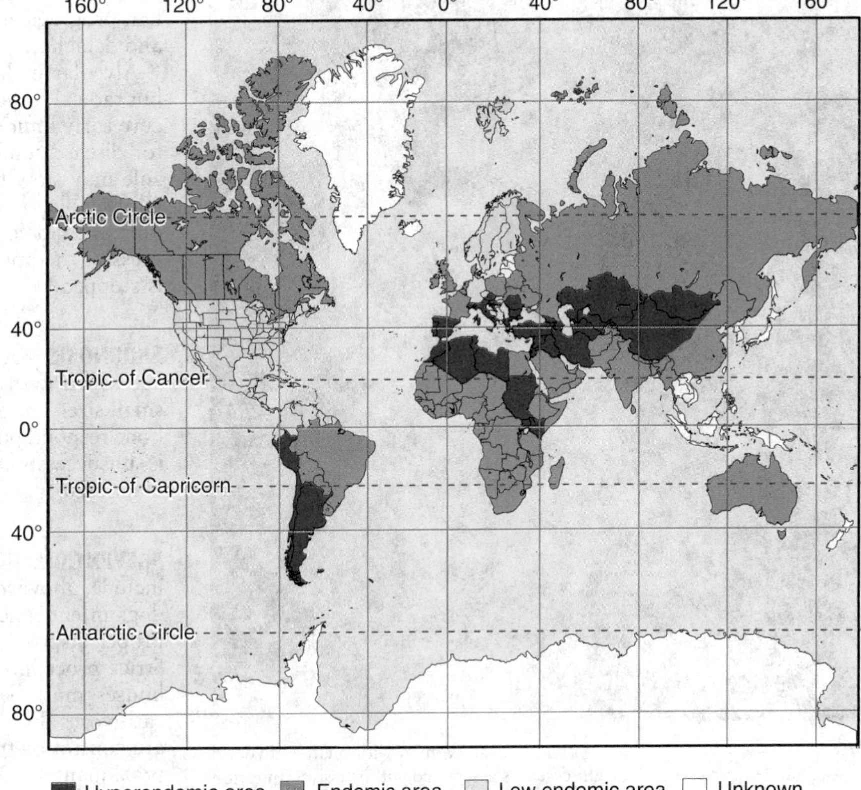

Figure 301-1. Worldwide distribution of cystic echinococcosis. (From McManus DP, Zhang W, Li J, Bartley PB: Echinococcosis. *Lancet* 2003;362:1295–1304.)

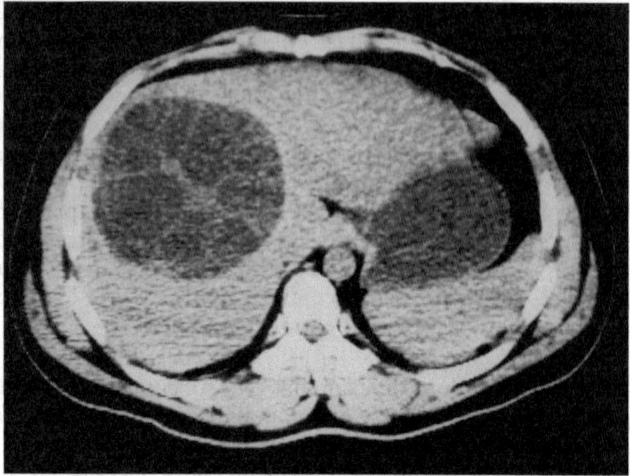

Figure 301-2. CT image of a hepatic *Echinococcus granulosus* hydatid cyst. The membranes of multiple internal daughter cysts are visible within the primary cyst structure. (Courtesy of John R. Haaga, MD, University Hospitals, Cleveland, Ohio.)

DIFFERENTIAL DIAGNOSIS. Benign hepatic cysts are common but can be distinguished by the absence of either internal membranes or hydatid sand. The density of bacterial hepatic abscesses is distinct from the watery cystic fluid characteristic of *E. granulosus* infection, but hydatid cysts may also be complicated by secondary bacterial infection. Alveolar echinococcosis is often confused with hepatoma and cirrhosis and presents features suggestive of pancreatic carcinoma, metastatic liver disease, and cholangitis.

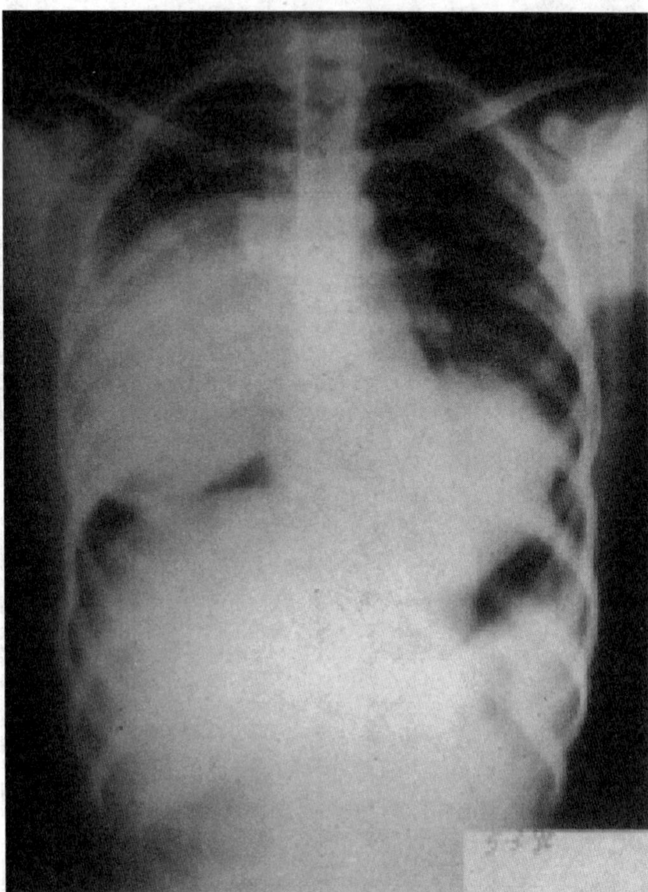

Figure 301-3. Chest x-ray of a young Kenyan woman with bilateral hydatid cysts. Sudden rupture of the right cyst was associated with massive aspiration and acute respiratory distress.

TREATMENT. For simple, accessible cysts, ultrasound- or CT-guided *p*ercutaneous *a*spiration, *i*nstillation of hypertonic saline or another scolicidal agent, and *r*e-aspiration (**PAIR**) is the preferred therapy. Compared with surgical treatment alone, PAIR plus albendazole results in similar cyst disappearance with fewer adverse events and fewer days in the hospital. Compared to albendazole alone, PAIR with or without albendazole provides significantly better cyst reduction and symptomatic relief. Spillage with PAIR is surprisingly uncommon, but prophylactic albendazole therapy is routinely administered 4 hr or even 1 wk prior to PAIR or surgery and continued for 1 mo thereafter. PAIR is contraindicated in pregnancy and for bile-stained cysts, which should not be injected with a scolicidal agent because of increased risk for biliary complications.

For conventional surgery, the inner cyst wall (laminate and germinal layers) can be easily peeled from the fibrous layer, and only these inner layers need be removed. The cavity should then be topically sterilized and either closed or filled with omentum. Considerable care must be taken to avoid spillage of cyst contents, because cyst fluid contains viable protoscolices, each capable of producing secondary cysts wherever it lodges. An additional risk is development of anaphylaxis to spilled cyst fluid. Various specific procedures have been developed to avoid this, so it is useful to employ a surgeon experienced in these techniques.

Nonpregnant patients with cysts not amenable to PAIR or surgery or with contraindications can be managed with albendazole (15 mg/kg/day divided bid PO for 1–6 mo, maximum 800 mg/day). A favorable response occurs in 40–60% of patients. There are few adverse effects except for occasional mild gastrointestinal disturbance and elevated transaminases on prolonged use. Morbid inflammatory response to chemotherapy is not common, as it is in cysticercosis; thus, corticosteroids are not indicated unless patients show signs of immediate hypersensitivity. Ultrasonographic indications of successful therapy are reduction in diameter, a change in shape from spherical to elliptic or flat, progressive increase in echogenicity and density of cyst fluid, and detachment of membranes from the capsule (**water lily sign**).

Alveolar hydatidosis is frequently incurable by any modality, but radical surgery such as partial hepatectomy or lobectomy may cure early limited disease. Liver transplantation is also an option for disease confined to the liver. Medical therapy with albendazole may slow the progression of alveolar hydatidosis, but if at all feasible, removal of the infected tissue provides the best outcome. Some patients have been maintained on long-term suppressive therapy, but the infection generally recurs if albendazole is stopped.

PROGNOSIS. Factors predictive of success with chemotherapy are age of the cyst (<2 yr), low internal complexity of the cyst, and small size. The site of the cyst is not important, although cysts in bone respond poorly. For alveolar hydatidosis, if surgical removal is unsuccessful, the average mortality is 92% by 10 yr after diagnosis.

PREVENTION. Important measures to interrupt transmission include, above all, thorough handwashing, avoiding contact with dogs in endemic areas, boiling or filtering water when camping, proper disposal of animal carcasses, and proper meat inspection. Strict procedures for proper disposal of refuse from slaughterhouses must be instituted and followed so that dogs or wild carnivores do not have access to entrails. Other useful measures are control or treatment of the feral dog population and regular praziquantel treatment of pets and working dogs in endemic areas.

Buishi I, Walters T, Guildea Z, et al: Reemergence of canine *Echinococcus granulosus* infection, Wales. *Emerg Infect Dis* 2005;11:568–571.

Eckert J, Deplazes P: Biological, epidemiological, and clinical aspects of echinococcosis, a zoonosis of increasing concern. *Clin Microbiol Rev* 2004;17:107–135.

McManus DP, Zhang W, Li J, Bartley PB: Echinococcosis. *Lancet* 2003;362: 1295–1304.

Nasseri Moghaddam S, Abrishami A, Malekzadeh R: Percutaneous needle aspiration, injection, and reaspiration with or without benzimidazole coverage for uncomplicated hepatic hydatid cysts. *Cochrane Database Syst Rev* 2006;19:CD003623.

Rausch RL: Cystic echinococcosis in the Arctic and sub-Arctic. *Parasitology* 2003;127(Suppl):S73–S85.

Sayek I, Tirnaksiz MB, Dogan R: Cystic hydatid disease: Current trends in diagnosis and management. *Surg Today* 2004;34:987–996.

Part XVII ▪ The Digestive System

Section 1 — Clinical Manifestations of Gastrointestinal Disease — Robert Wyllie

Chapter 302 ▪ Normal Digestive Tract Phenomena

Gastrointestinal function varies with maturity; what is a physiologic event in a newborn or infant might be a pathologic symptom at an older age. A fetus can swallow amniotic fluid as early as 12 wk gestation, but nutritive sucking in neonates 1st develops at about 34 wk gestation. The coordinated oral and pharyngeal movements necessary for swallowing solids develop within the 1st few months of life. Before this time, the tongue thrust is upward and outward to express milk from the nipple, instead of a backward motion, which propels solids toward the esophageal inlet. By 1 mo of age, infants appear to show preferences for sweet and salty foods. Infants' interest in solids increases at about 4 mo of age. The recommendation to begin solids at 6 mo of age is based on nutritional and cultural concepts rather than maturation of the swallowing process (see Chapter 42). Infants swallow air during feeding and burping is encouraged to prevent gaseous distention of the stomach.

A number of normal anatomic variations may be noted in the mouth. A **short lingual frenulum** ("tongue-tie") may be worrisome to parents but only rarely interferes with eating or speech, generally requiring no treatment. **Surface furrowing** of the tongue (a geographic or scrotal tongue) is usually a normal finding. A **bifid uvula** may be normal or associated with a submucous cleft of the soft palate.

Regurgitation, the result of gastroesophageal reflux, occurs commonly in the 1st year of life. Effortless regurgitation may dribble out of an infant's mouth but also may be forceful. In an otherwise healthy infant with regurgitation, volumes of emesis are commonly ≈15–30 mL but may occasionally be larger. Most often, the infant remains happy, although possibly hungry, after an episode of regurgitation. Episodes may occur from less than one to several times per day. Regurgitation gradually resolves in 80% of infants by 6 mo of age and in 90% by 12 mo. If complications develop or regurgitation persists, gastroesophageal reflux is considered pathologic rather than merely developmental and deserves further evaluation and treatment. Complications of gastroesophageal reflux include failure to thrive, pulmonary disease (apnea or aspiration pneumonitis), and esophagitis with its sequelae (see Chapters 320 and 321).

Infants and young children may be erratic eaters; this may be a worry to parents. A toddler may eat insatiably or refuse to consume food during a meal. There is also a tendency for toddlers and young children to eat only a limited variety of foods. Parents should be encouraged to view nutritional intake over several days and not be overly concerned about individual meals. Infancy and adolescence are periods of rapid growth; high nutrient requirements for growth may be associated with voracious appetites. The reduced appetite of toddlers and preschool children is often a worry to parents who are used to the relatively greater dietary intake during infancy. Demonstration of age-appropriate growth on a growth curve is reassuring.

The number, color, and consistency of stools may vary greatly in the same infant and between infants of similar age without apparent explanation. The earliest stools after birth consist of meconium, a dark, viscous material that is normally passed within the 1st 48 hr of life. With the onset of feeding, meconium is replaced by green-brown transition stools, often containing curds, and, after 4–5 days, by yellow-brown milk stools. **Stool frequency** is extremely variable in normal infants and may vary from none to seven per day. Breast-fed infants may have frequent small, loose stools early (transition stools), and then after 2–3 wk, may have very infrequent soft stools. Some nursing infants may not pass any stool for 1–2 wk and then have a normal soft bowel movement. The color of stool has little significance except for the presence of blood or absence of bilirubin products (white-gray rather than yellow-brown). The presence of vegetable matter, such as peas or corn, in the stool of an older infant or toddler ingesting solids is normal and suggests poor chewing and not malabsorption. A pattern of intermittent loose stools, known as **"toddler's diarrhea,"** occurs commonly between 1 and 3 yr of age. These otherwise healthy growing children often drink excessive carbohydrate-containing beverages. The stools typically occur during the day and not overnight. The volume of fluid intake is often excessive; limiting sugar-containing beverages and increasing fat in the diet often leads to resolution of the pattern of loose stools.

A protuberant abdomen is often noted in infants and toddlers, especially after large feedings. This may result from the combination of weak abdominal musculature, relatively large abdominal organs, and lordotic stance. In the 1st yr of life, it is common to palpate the liver 1–2 cm below the right costal margin. The normal liver is soft in consistency and percusses to normal size for age. A Riedel lobe is a thin projection of the right lobe of the liver that may be palpated low in the right lateral abdomen. A soft spleen tip may also be palpable as a normal finding. In thin young children, the vertebral column is easily palpable and an overlying structure may be mistaken for a mass. Pulsation of the aorta can be appreciated. Normal stool can often be palpated in the left lower quadrant in the descending or sigmoid colon.

Blood loss from the gastrointestinal tract is never normal, but swallowed blood may be misinterpreted as gastrointestinal bleeding. Maternal blood may be ingested at the time of birth or later by a nursing infant if there is bleeding near the mother's nipple. Nasal or oropharyngeal bleeding is occasionally mistaken for gastrointestinal bleeding (see Chapter 103.4). Red dyes in foods or drinks may turn the stool red but do not produce a positive test result for occult blood.

Jaundice is common in neonates, especially among premature infants, and usually results from the inability of an immature liver to conjugate bilirubin, leading to an elevated indirect component (see Chapter 102.3). Persistent elevation of indirect bilirubin levels in nursing infants may be a result of breast milk jaundice, which is usually a benign entity in full-term infants. An elevated direct bilirubin is not normal and suggests liver disease, although in infants it may be a result of extrahepatic infection (urinary tract infection) or pooling of blood with an excessive load of bilirubin being released into the circulation (intracranial hemorrhage). The direct bilirubin fraction should account for no more than 15–20% of the total serum bilirubin. Elevations in direct bilirubin levels can following indirect hyperbilirubinemia as the liver converts excessive indirect to direct bilirubin and the rate-limiting step in bilirubin excretion shifts from the glucuronidation of bilirubin to excretion of direct bilirubin into the bile canaliculus. Indirect hyperbilirubinemia, which occurs commonly in normal newborns, tends to tint the sclerae and skin golden yellow, whereas direct hyperbilirubinemia produces a greenish yellow hue.

Chapter 303 ■ Major Symptoms and Signs of Digestive Tract Disorders

Disorders of organs outside the gastrointestinal tract can produce symptoms and signs that mimic digestive tract disorders and should be considered in the differential diagnosis (Table 303-1). Understanding the potential pathogenesis of symptoms will allow rational diagnosis and management decisions. In children with normal growth and development, treatment may be initiated without a formal evaluation based on a presumptive diagnosis after taking a history and performing a physical examination. Poor weight gain or weight loss is often associated with a significant pathologic process and usually necessitates a more formal evaluation.

DYSPHAGIA. Dysphagia, or difficulty swallowing, may be caused by a structural defect or motility disorder. Structural defects that cause a fixed impediment to the food bolus arise from narrowing within the esophagus, as from a stricture, web, or tumor. Extrinsic obstruction is most often caused by a vascular ring (see Chapter 432). Structural defects typically cause more problems in swallowing solids than liquids. Most nonstructural causes of dysphagia are caused by motility abnormalities of the oropharynx or the esophagus. Swallowing is a complex process that starts in the mouth with mastication and lubrication of food that is formed into a bolus. The bolus is pushed to the pharynx by the tongue. The pharyngeal phase of swallowing is rapid and involves protective mechanisms to prevent food from entering the airway. The epiglottis is lowered over the larynx while the soft palate is elevated against the nasopharyngeal wall; there is a temporary arrest of respiration while the upper esophageal sphincter opens to allow the bolus to enter the esophagus. In the esophagus, peristaltic coordinated muscular contractions push the food bolus toward the stomach. The lower esophageal sphincter relaxes shortly after the upper esophageal sphincter, so liquids that rapidly clear the esophagus enter the stomach without resistance.

Dysphagia during the oropharyngeal phase of swallowing is termed **transfer dysphagia** and is usually associated with neuromuscular disorders (cerebral palsy). The sensation that something is stuck in the upper esophagus is globus (formerly termed *globus hystericus*). **Globus** is typically associated with gastroesophageal reflux.

When dysphagia is associated with a delay in passage through the esophagus, a child may be able to point to the level of the chest where the delay occurs; esophageal symptoms may be referred to the suprasternal notch. When a child points to the suprasternal notch, the impaction can be found anywhere in the esophagus.

Transfer Dysphagia. A complex sequence of neuromuscular events is involved in the transfer of foods to the upper esophagus. Suckling requires the lips to form a tight seal about the nipple while the tongue is displaced posteriorly. As the glottis closes to guard the airway, the soft palate rises to close the nasopharynx, the cricopharyngeal muscles relax, and food passes to the back of the pharynx. Solids similarly require coordinated actions; for large chunks of solid food, jaw movement and teeth become factors to consider. Salivary secretions, stimulated by the anticipation and act of ingestion, lubricate foods as they pass through the mouth. Abnormalities of the muscles involved in the inges-

TABLE 303-1. Some Nondigestive Tract Causes of Gastrointestinal Symptoms in Children

ANOREXIA
Systemic disease (inflammatory, neoplastic)
Cardiorespiratory compromise
Iatrogenic—drug therapy, unpalatable therapeutic diets
Depression
Anorexia nervosa
VOMITING
Inborn errors of metabolism
Medications (erythromycin, chemotherapy)
Increased intracranial pressure
Brain tumor
Infection (urinary tract)
Labyrinthitis
Adrenal insufficiency
Pregnancy
Psychogenic
Abdominal migraine
Toxins
DIARRHEA
Infection (otitis media, urinary)
Uremia
Medications (antibiotics, cisapride)
Tumors (neuroblastoma)
Pericarditis
CONSTIPATION
Hypothyroidism
Spina bifida
Psychomotor retardation
Dehydration (diabetes insipidus, renal tubular lesions)
Medications (narcotics)
Lead poisoning
Infant botulism
ABDOMINAL PAIN
Pyelonephritis, hydronephrosis, renal colic
Pneumonia
Pelvic inflammatory disease
Porphyria
Angioedema
Endocarditis
Abdominal migraine
Familial Mediterranean fever
Sexual or physical abuse
Systemic lupus erythematosus
School phobia
Sickle cell crisis
Vertebral disk inflammation
Medications (NSAIDs)
Pelvic osteomyelitis
ABDOMINAL DISTENTION OR MASS
Ascites (nephrotic syndrome, neoplasm, heart failure)
Discrete mass (Wilms tumor, hydronephrosis, neuroblastoma, mesenteric cyst, hepatoblastoma, lymphoma)
Pregnancy
JAUNDICE
Hemolytic disease
Urinary tract infection
Sepsis
Hypothyroidism
Panhypopituitarism

NSAIDs, nonsteroidal anti-inflammatory drugs.

tion process, their innervation, strength, or coordination, are associated with transfer dysphagia in infants and children. In such cases, an oropharyngeal problem is almost always part of a more generalized neurologic or muscular problem (botulism, diphtheria, neuromuscular disease). Painful oral lesions, such as acute viral stomatitis or trauma, occasionally interfere with ingestion. If the nasal air passage is seriously obstructed, the need for respiration causes severe distress when suckling. Although severe structural, dental, and salivary abnormalities would be expected to create difficulties, ingestion proceeds relatively well in most affected children if they are hungry.

Nontransfer Dysphagia. Primary motility disorders causing impaired peristaltic function and dysphagia are rare in children. Motility of the distal esophagus is disordered after repair of tracheoesophageal fistula. Abnormal motility may accompany collagen vascular disorders. **Achalasia** rarely occurs in children. Esophageal web, tracheobronchial remnant, or vascular ring may cause dysphagia in infancy. An esophageal **stricture** secondary to chronic gastroesophageal reflux and esophagitis occasionally presents with dysphagia as the 1st manifestation. A Schatzki ring, a thin ring of tissue near the lower esophageal sphincter, is another mechanical cause of recurrent dysphagia presenting after infancy. An esophageal **foreign body** or a stricture secondary to a caustic ingestion also causes dysphagia.

REGURGITATION. Regurgitation is the effortless movement of stomach contents into the esophagus and mouth. It is not associated with distress, and infants with regurgitation are often hungry immediately after an episode. The lower esophageal sphincter prevents reflux of gastric contents into the esophagus (see Chapter 320). Regurgitation is a result of gastroesophageal reflux through an incompetent or, in infants, immature lower esophageal sphincter. This is often a developmental process, and regurgitation or "spitting" resolves with maturity. Regurgitation should be differentiated from vomiting, which denotes an active reflex process with an extensive differential diagnosis (Table 303-2).

TABLE 303-2. Differential Diagnosis of Emesis During Childhood

INFANT	CHILD	ADOLESCENT
COMMON		
Gastroenteritis	Gastroenteritis	Gastroenteritis
Gastroesophageal reflux	Systemic infection	GERD
Overfeeding	Gastritis	Systemic infection
Anatomic obstruction	Toxic ingestion	Toxic ingestion
Systemic infection	Pertussis syndrome	Gastritis
Pertussis syndrome	Medication	Sinusitis
Otitis media	Reflux (GERD)	Inflammatory bowel disease
	Sinusitis	Appendicitis
	Otitis media	Migraine
		Pregnancy
		Medication
		Ipecac abuse/bulimia
RARE		
Adrenogenital syndrome	Reye syndrome	Reye syndrome
Inborn error of metabolism	Hepatitis	Hepatitis
Brain tumor (increased intracranial pressure)	Peptic ulcer	Peptic ulcer
	Pancreatitis	Pancreatitis
Subdural hemorrhage	Brain tumor	Brain tumor
Food poisoning	Increased intracranial pressure	Increased intracranial pressure
Rumination	Middle ear disease	Middle ear disease
Renal tubular acidosis	Chemotherapy	Chemotherapy
	Achalasia	Cyclic vomiting (migraine)
	Cyclic vomiting (migraine)	Biliary colic
	Esophageal stricture	Renal colic
	Duodenal hematoma	
	Inborn error of metabolism	

GERD, gastroesophageal reflux disease.

TABLE 303-3. Causes of Gastrointestinal Obstruction

ESOPHAGUS	Malrotation/Ladd bands
Congenital	Ileal atresia
Esophageal atresia	Meconium ileus
Vascular rings	Meckel diverticulum with volvulus or intussusception
Schatzki ring	Inguinal hernia
Tracheobronchial remnant	Intestinal duplication
Acquired	**Acquired**
Esophageal stricture	Postsurgical adhesions
Foreign body	Crohn disease
Achalasia	Intussusception
Chagas disease	Distal ileal obstruction syndrome (cystic fibrosis)
Collagen vascular disease	Duodenal hematoma
STOMACH	Superior mesenteric artery syndrome
Congenital	**COLON**
Antral webs	**Congenital**
Pyloric stenosis	Meconium plug
Acquired	Hirschsprung disease
Bezoars/foreign body	Colonic atresia, stenosis
Pyloric stricture (ulcer)	Imperforate anus
Chronic granulomatous disease of childhood	Rectal stenosis
Eosinophilic gastroenteritis	Pseudo-obstruction
Crohn disease	Volvulus
Epidermolysis bullosa	Colonic duplication
SMALL INTESTINE	**Acquired**
Congenital	Ulcerative colitis (toxic megacolon)
Duodenal atresia	Chagas disease
Annular pancreas	Crohn disease
Malrotation/volvulus	Fibrosing colonopathy (cystic fibrosis)

ANOREXIA. Hunger and satiety centers are located in the hypothalamus; it seems likely that afferent nerves from the gastrointestinal tract to these brain centers are important determinants of the anorexia that characterizes many diseases of the stomach and intestine. Satiety is stimulated by distention of the stomach or upper small bowel, the signal being transmitted by sensory afferents, which are especially dense in the upper gut. Chemoreceptors in the intestine, influenced by the assimilation of nutrients, also affect afferent flow to the appetite centers. Impulses reach the hypothalamus from higher centers, possibly influenced by pain or the emotional disturbance of an intestinal disease. Other regulatory factors include hormones, ghrelin, leptin, and plasma glucose, which, in turn, reflect intestinal function.

VOMITING. Vomiting is a highly coordinated reflex process that may be preceded by increased salivation and begins with involuntary retching. Violent descent of the diaphragm and constriction of the abdominal muscles with relaxation of the gastric cardia actively force gastric contents back up the esophagus. This process is coordinated in the medullary vomiting center, which is influenced directly by afferent innervation and indirectly by the chemoreceptor trigger zone and higher central nervous system (CNS) centers. Many acute or chronic processes can cause vomiting (Tables 303-1 and 303-3).

Vomiting caused by obstruction of the gastrointestinal tract is probably mediated by intestinal visceral afferent nerves stimulating the vomiting center (see Table 303-1). If obstruction occurs below the 2nd part of the duodenum, vomitus is usually bile stained. Emesis may also become bile stained with repeated vomiting in the absence of obstruction when duodenal contents are refluxed into the stomach. Nonobstructive lesions of the digestive tract can also cause vomiting; this includes diseases of the upper bowel, pancreas, liver, or biliary tree. CNS or metabolic derangements may lead to severe, persistent emesis.

Cyclic vomiting is a syndrome with numerous episodes of vomiting interspersed with well intervals. The onset is usually between 2 and 5 yr of age; the frequency of vomiting episodes is variable

TABLE 303-4. Complications of Vomiting

COMPLICATION	PATHOPHYSIOLOGY	HISTORY, PHYSICAL EXAMINATION, AND LABORATORY STUDIES
Metabolic	Fluid loss in emesis	Dehydration
	HCl loss in emesis	Alkalosis; hypochloremia
	Na, K loss in emesis	Hyponatremia; hypokalemia
	Alkalosis →	
	Na into cells	
	HCO_3 loss in urine	Urine pH 7–8
	Na and K loss in urine	Urine Na ↑, K ↑
	Hypochloremia → Cl conserved by kidneys	Urine Cl ↓
Nutritional	Emesis of calories and nutrients	Malnutrition; "failure to thrive"
	Anorexia for calories and nutrients	
Mallory-Weiss tear	Retching → tear at lesser curve of gastroesophageal junction	Forceful emesis → hematemesis
Esophagitis	Chronic vomiting → esophageal acid exposure	Heartburn; hemoccult + stool
Aspiration	Aspiration of vomitus, especially in context of obtundation	Pneumonia; neurologic dysfunction
Shock	Severe fluid loss in emesis or in accompanying diarrhea	Dehydration (accompanying diarrhea can explain acidosis?)
	Severe blood loss in hematemesis	Blood volume depletion

Cl, chloride; HCl, hydrogen chloride; HCO_3, bicarbonate; K, potassium; Na, sodium.
From Kliegman RM, Greenbaum LA, Lye PS (eds): *Practical Strategies in Pediatric Diagnosis and Therapy*, 2nd ed. Philadelphia, Elsevier, 2004, p 318.

(average of 12 episodes per yr) with each episode typically lasting 2–3 days, with four or more emesis episodes per hour. Patients may have a prodrome of pallor, intolerance of noise or light, nausea, lethargy, and headache or fever. Precipitants include infection, stress, and excitement. Idiopathic cyclic vomiting may be a migraine equivalent (**abdominal migraine**), or it may result from altered intestinal motility or mutations in mitochondrial DNA. The **differential diagnosis** includes gastrointestinal anomalies (malrotation, duplication cysts, choledochal cysts), CNS disorders (neoplasm, epilepsy, vestibular pathology), nephrolithiasis, cholelithiasis, hydronephrosis, metabolic-endocrine disorders (urea cycle, fatty acid metabolism, Addison disease, porphyria, hereditary angioedema, familial Mediterranean fever), chronic appendicitis, and inflammatory bowel disease. **Laboratory evaluation** is based on a careful history and physical examination and may include, if indicated, endoscopy, contrast gastrointestinal radiography, brain MRI, and metabolic studies (lactate, organic acids, ammonia). Treatment includes hydration and ondansetron. Prevention may be possible with the antimigraine agent amitriptyline or cyproheptadine.

Potential complications of emesis are noted in Table 303-4. Broad management strategies for vomiting in general and specific causes of emesis are noted in Tables 303-5 and 303-6.

DIARRHEA. Diarrhea is best defined as excessive loss of fluid and electrolyte in the stool. Normally, a young infant has ≈5 g/kg of stool output per day; the volume increases to 200 g/24 hr in an adult. The greatest volume of intestinal water is absorbed in the small bowel; the colon concentrates intestinal contents against a high osmotic gradient. The small intestine of an adult may absorb 10–11 L/day of a combination of ingested and secreted fluid, whereas the colon absorbs ≈0.5 L. Disorders that interfere with absorption in the small bowel tend to produce voluminous diarrhea, whereas disorders compromising colonic absorption produce lower volume diarrhea. **Dysentery** (small-volume, frequent bloody stools with mucus, tenesmus, and urgency) is the predominant symptom of colitis.

The basis for all diarrhea is disturbed intestinal solute transport; water movement across intestinal membranes is passive and is determined by both active and passive fluxes of solutes, particularly sodium, chloride, and glucose. The pathogenesis of most episodes of diarrhea can be explained by secretory, osmotic, or motility abnormalities or a combination of these (Table 303-7).

Secretory diarrhea is often caused by a secretagogue, such as cholera toxin, binding to a receptor on the surface epithelium of the bowel and thereby stimulating intracellular accumulation of cyclic adenosine monophosphate or cyclic guanosine monophosphate. Some intraluminal fatty acids and bile salts cause the colonic mucosa to secrete through this mechanism. Diarrhea not associated with an exogenous secretagogue may also have a secretory component (congenital microvillus inclusion disease). Secretory diarrhea tends to be watery and of large volume; the osmolality of the stool can be accounted for by the presence of electrolytes. Secretory diarrhea generally persists even when no feedings are given by mouth.

Osmotic diarrhea occurs after ingestion of a poorly absorbed solute. The solute may be one that is normally not well absorbed (magnesium, phosphate, lactulose, or sorbitol) or one that is not well absorbed because of a disorder of the small bowel (lactose with lactase deficiency or glucose with rotavirus diarrhea). Malabsorbed carbohydrate is fermented in the colon, and short-chain fatty acids (SCFAs) are produced. Although SCFAs can be absorbed in the colon and used as an energy source, the net effect is to increase the osmotic solute load. This form of diarrhea is usually of lesser volume than a secretory diarrhea and stops with fasting. The osmolality of the stool will not be explained by the electrolyte content, because another osmotic component is present; the difference between electrolyte content (sum of [NA^+], [K^+], and associated anions) and stool osmolality is >50 mOsm (see Chapter 337). Motility disorders can be associated with rapid or delayed transit and are not generally associated with large-volume diarrhea. Slowed motility can be associated with bacterial overgrowth as a cause of diarrhea. The differential diagnosis of common causes of acute and chronic diarrhea is noted in Table 303-8.

CONSTIPATION. Any definition of constipation is relative and depends on stool consistency, stool frequency, and difficulty in passing the stool. A normal child may have a soft stool only every 2nd or 3rd day without difficulty; this is not constipation. A hard stool passed with difficulty every 3rd day should be treated as constipation. Constipation can arise from defects either in filling or emptying the rectum (Table 303-9).

A nursing infant may have very infrequent stools of normal consistency; this is usually a normal pattern. True constipation in the neonatal period is most likely secondary to Hirschsprung disease, intestinal pseudo-obstruction, or hypothyroidism.

Defective rectal filling occurs when colonic peristalsis is ineffective (in cases of hypothyroidism or opiate use and when bowel obstruction is caused either by a structural anomaly or by Hirschsprung disease). The resultant colonic stasis leads to excessive drying of stool and a failure to initiate reflexes from the rectum that normally trigger evacuation. Emptying the rectum by spontaneous evacuation depends on a defecation reflex initiated

TABLE 303-5. Pharmacologic Therapies for Vomiting Episodes

DISEASE/CONDITION	THERAPY-DRUG CLASS: SPECIFIC AGENT/TRADE NAME (DOSE)
Reflux	Dopamine antagonist: metoclopramide (Reglan) (0.1–0.2 mg/kg qid PO/IV)
	Peripheral dopamine antagonist: domperidone (Motilium) (0.2–0.6 mg/kg tid–qid PO)
Gastroparesis	Metoclopramide, domperidone; see above
	Motilin agonist: erythromycin (2–4 mg/kg tid–qid PO/IV)
Intestinal pseudoobstruction	Stimulation of intestinal migratory myoelectric complexes:
	Octreotide (Sandostatin) (1 μg/kg bid–tid SC)
Chemotherapy	Metoclopramide; see above (0.5–1.0 mg/kg qid IV, with antihistamine prophylaxis of extrapyramidal side effects)
	Serotoninergic 5-HT_3 antagonist: ondansetron (Zofran) (0.15–0.3 mg/kg tid IV/PO)
	Phenothiazines: (extrapyramidal, hematologic side effects)
	Prochlorperazine (Compazine) (≈0.3 mg/kg bid–tid PO)
	Chlorpromazine (Thorazine) (>6 mo of age: 0.5 mg/kg tid–qid PO/IV)
	Steroids: dexamethasone (Decadron) (0.1 mg/kg tid PO)
	Cannabinoids: nabilone (tetrahydrocannabinol) (0.05–0.1 mg/kg bid–tid PO)
Postoperative	Ondansetron, phenothiazines: see above
Motion sickness; vestibular disorders	Antihistamine: dimenhydrinate (Dramamine) (1 mg/kg tid–qid PO)
	Anticholinergic: scopolamine (Transderm Scōp) (adults: 1 patch/3 days)
Adrenal crisis	Steroids: cortisol (2 mg/kg bolus IV followed by 0.2–0.4 mg/kg/hr IV [±1 mg/kg IM])
Cyclic vomiting syndrome (CVS)	Supportive:
	Analgesic: meperidine (Demerol) (1–2 mg/kg q4–6h IV/IM)
	Anxiolytic, sedative: Lorazepam (Ativan) (0.05–0.1 mg/kg q6h IV)
	Antihistamine, sedative: diphenhydramine (Benadryl) (1.25 mg/kg q6h IV)
	Abortive:
	Serotoninergic 5-HT_3 antagonist:
	Ondansetron: see above
	Granisetron (Kytril) (10 μg/kg q4–6h IV)
	Nonsteroidal antiinflammatory agent (GI ulceration side effect):
	Ketorolac (Toradol) (0.5–1.0 mg/kg q6–8h IV)
	Serotoninergic 5-HT_{1D} agonist: sumatriptan (Imitres) (>40 kg; 20 mg intranasally/25 mg PO, one time only)
	Prophylactic: (if >1 CVS bout/month; taken daily)
	Antimigraine, β-adrenergic blocker: propranolol (Inderal) (0.5–2.0 mg/kg bid PO)
	Antimigraine, antihistamine: cyproheptadine (Periactin) (0.25–0.5 mg/kg/day ÷ bid–tid PO)
	Antimigraine, tricyclic antidepressant: amitriptyline (Elavil) (0.33–0.5 mg/kg tid PO, and titrate to maximum of 3.0 mg/kg/day as needed; obtain baseline ECG at start of therapy, and consider monitoring drug levels)
	Antimigraine antiepileptic: Phenobarbital (Luminal) (2–3 mg/kg qhs)
	Erythromycin: see above
	Low estrogen oral contraceptives: consider for catamenial CVS episodes

bid, twice daily; ECG, electrocardiogram; GI, gastrointestinal; IM, intramuscularly; IV, intravenously, PO, orally; q4–6h, every 4 to 6 hours; q6h, every 6 hours; q6–8h, every 6 to 8 hour; qhs, each bedtime; SC, subcutaneously; tid, three times daily; qid, four times daily.
From Kliegman RM, Greenbaum LA, Lye PS (eds): *Practical Strategies in Pediatric Diagnosis and Therapy,* 2nd ed. Philadelphia, Elsevier, 2004, p 317.

TABLE 303-6. Supportive and Nonpharmacologic Therapies for Vomiting Episodes

DISEASE	THERAPY
All	Treat cause: obstruction ⟶ operate; allergy ⟶ change diet (±steroids); metabolic error ⟶ Rx defect; acid peptic disease ⟶ H_2RAs, PPIs, etc.
Complications	
Dehydration	IV fluids, electrolytes
Hematemesis	Transfuse, correct coagulopathy
Esophagitis	H_2RAs, PPIs
Malnutrition	NG or NJ drip feeding useful for many chronic conditions
Mecomium ileus	Gastrografin enema
DIOS	Gastrografin enema; balanced colonic lavage solution (e.g., GoLytely)
Intussusception	Barium enema; air reduction enema
Hematemesis	Endoscopic: injection sclerotherapy or banding of esophageal varices; injection therapy, fibrin sealant application, or heater probe electrocautery for selected upper GI tract lesions
Sigmoid volvulus	Colonoscopic decompression
Reflux	Positioning; dietary measures (infants: rice cereal, 1 tbs/oz of formula)
Psychogenic components	Psychotherapy; tricyclic antidepressants; anxiolytics (e.g., diazepam: 0.1 mg/kg/tid–qid PO)

DIOS, distal intestinal obstruction syndrome; GI, gastrointestinal; H_2RAs, histamine$_2$-receptor antagonists; IV, intravenous; NG, nasogastric; NJ, nasojejunal; PO, orally; PPIs, proton pump inhibitors; qid, four times a day; tbs, tablespoon; tid, three times a day.
From Kliegman RM, Greenbaum LA, Lye PS (eds): *Practical Strategies in Pediatric Diagnosis and Therapy,* 2nd ed. Philadelphia, Elsevier, 2004, p 319.

by pressure receptors in the rectal muscle. Stool retention, therefore, can also result from lesions involving these rectal muscles, the sacral spinal cord afferent and efferent fibers, or the muscles of the abdomen and pelvic floor. Disorders of anal sphincter relaxation can also contribute to fecal retention.

Constipation tends to be self-perpetuating, whatever its cause. Hard, large stools in the rectum become difficult and even painful to evacuate; thus, more retention occurs and a vicious circle ensues. Distention of the rectum and colon lessens the sensitivity of the defecation reflex and the effectiveness of peristalsis. Eventually, watery content from the proximal colon may percolate around hard retained stool and pass per rectum unperceived by the child. This involuntary **encopresis** may be mistaken for diarrhea. Constipation itself does not have deleterious systemic organic effects, but urinary tract stasis can accompany severe long-standing cases and constipation can generate anxiety, having a marked emotional impact on the patient and family.

ABDOMINAL PAIN. Individual children differ greatly in their perception of and tolerance for abdominal pain. This is one reason the evaluation of chronic abdominal pain is difficult. A child with functional abdominal pain (no identifiable organic cause) may be as uncomfortable as one with an organic cause. This distinction is an extremely important part of the medical evaluation, guiding how the work-up is approached and the child is treated. The more specific the pain and the more suggestive of a particular diagnosis, the more likely it will have an organic basis. Normal growth

TABLE 303-7. Mechanisms of Diarrhea

PRIMARY MECHANISM	DEFECT	STOOL EXAMINATION	EXAMPLES	COMMENT
Secretory	Decreased absorption, increased secretion, electrolyte transport	Watery, normal osmolality; osmoles = 2 × ($Na^+ + K^+$)	Cholera, toxigenic *E. coli;* carcinoid, VIP, neuroblastoma, congenital chloride diarrhea, *Clostridium difficile,* cryptosporidiosis (AIDS)	Persists during fasting; bile salt malabsorption may also increase intestinal water secretion; no stool leukocytes
Osmotic	Maldigestion, transport defects ingestion of unabsorbable	Watery, acidic, and reducing substances; increased osmolality; osmoles >2 × ($Na^+ + K^+$)	Lactase deficiency, glucose-galactose malabsorption, lactulose, laxative abuse	Stops with fasting; increased breath hydrogen with carbohydrate malabsorption; no stool leukocytes
Increased motility	Decreased transit time	Loose to normal-appearing stool, stimulated by gastrocolic reflex	Irritable bowel syndrome, thyrotoxicosis, postvagotomy dumping syndrome	Infection may also contribute to increased motility
Decreased motility	Defect in neuromuscular unit(s) Stasis (bacterial overgrowth)	Loose to normal appearing stool	Pseudoobstruction, blind loop	Possible bacterial overgrowth
Decreased surface area (osmotic, motility)	Decreased functional capacity	Watery	Short bowel syndrome, celiac disease, rotavirus enteritis	May require elemental diet plus parenteral alimentation
Mucosal invasion	Inflammation, decreased colonic reabsorption, increased motility	Blood and increased WBCs in stool	*Salmonella, Shigella,* infection; amebiasis; *Yersinia, Campylobacter* infections	Dysentery evident in blood, mucus, and WBCs

K^+, potassium; Na^+, sodium; VIP, vasoactive intestinal peptide; WBC, white blood cell.
From Kliegman RM, Greenbaum LA, Lye PS (eds): *Practical Strategies in Pediatric Diagnosis and Therapy,* 2nd ed. Philadelphia, Elsevier, 2004, p 274.

and physical examination (including a rectal examination) are reassuring in a child who is suspected of having functional pain.

A specific cause may be difficult to find, but the nature and location of a pain-provoking lesion can usually be determined from the clinical description. Two types of nerve fibers transmit painful stimuli in the abdomen. In skin and muscle, A fibers mediate sharp localized pain; and C fibers from viscera, peritoneum, and muscle transmit poorly localized, dull pain. These afferent fibers have cell bodies in the dorsal root ganglia, and some axons cross the midline and ascend to the medulla, midbrain, and thalamus. Pain is perceived in the cortex of the postcentral gyrus, which can receive impulses arising from both sides of the body.

Visceral pain tends to be experienced in the dermatome from which the affected organ receives innervation. Painful stimuli originating in the liver, pancreas, biliary tree, stomach, or upper bowel are felt in the epigastrium; pain from the distal small bowel, cecum, appendix, or proximal colon is felt at the umbili-

TABLE 303-8. Differential Diagnosis of Diarrhea

	INFANT	CHILD	ADOLESCENT
ACUTE			
Common	Gastroenteritis Systemic infection Antibiotic associated Overfeeding	Gastroenteritis Food poisoning Systemic infection Antibiotic associated	Gastroenteritis Food poisoning Antibiotic associated
Rare	Primary disaccharidase deficiency Hirschsprung toxic colitis Adrenogenital syndrome Neonatal opiate withdrawal	Toxic ingestion	Hyperthyroidism
CHRONIC			
Common	Postinfectious secondary lactase deficiency Cow's milk/soy protein intolerance Chronic nonspecific diarrhea of infancy Excessive fruit juice (sorbitol) ingestion Celiac disease Cystic fibrosis AIDS enteropathy	Postinfectious secondary lactase deficiency Irritable bowel syndrome Celiac disease Lactose intolerance Excessive fruit juice (sorbitol) ingestion Giardiasis Inflammatory bowel disease AIDS enteropathy	Irritable bowel syndrome Inflammatory bowel disease Lactose intolerance Giardiasis Laxative abuse (anorexia nervosa) Constipation with encopresis
Rare	Primary immune defects Glucose-galactose malabsorption Microvillus inclusion disease (microvillus atrophy) Congenital transport defects (chloride, sodium) Primary bile acid malabsorption Munchausen syndrome by proxy Hirschsprung disease Shwachman syndrome Secretory tumors Acrodermatitis enteropathica Lymphangiectasia Abetalipoproteinemia Eosinophilic gastroenteritis Short bowel syndrome Intractable diarrhea syndrome Autoimmune enteropathy	Acquired immune defects Secretory tumors Pseudoobstruction Sucrase-isomaltase deficiency Eosinophilic gastroenteritis	Secretory tumor Primary bowel tumor Parasitic infections and venereal diseases Appendiceal abscess Addison disease

From Kliegman RM, Greenbaum LA, Lye PS (eds): *Practical Strategies in Pediatric Diagnosis and Therapy,* 2nd ed. Philadelphia, Elsevier, 2004, p 272.

TABLE 303-9. Causes of Constipation

NONORGANIC (FUNCTIONAL)—RETENTIVE	**Drugs**
ORGANIC	Antidepressants
Anatomic	Chemotherapeutic agents (vincristine)
Anal stenosis	Pancreatic enzymes (fibrosing colonopathy)
Imperforate anus	Lead
Anteriorly displaced anus	Vitamin D intoxication
Intestinal stricture (post necrotizing enterocolitis)	**Metabolic Disorders**
Abnormal Musculature	Hypokalemia
Prune-belly syndrome	Hypercalcemia
Gastroschisis	Hypothyroidism
Down syndrome	Diabetes mellitus
Intestinal Nerve or Muscle Abnormalities	**Intestinal Disorders**
Hirschsprung disease	Celiac disease
Pseudo-obstruction (visceral myopathy or neuropathy)	Cow's milk protein intolerance
Intestinal neuronal dysplasia	Cystic fibrosis (meconium ileus equivalent)
Spinal Cord Defects	Inflammatory bowel disease (stricture)
Tethered cord	Tumor
Spinal cord trauma	**Connective Tissue Disorders**
Spina bifida	Systemic lupus erythematosus
Drugs	Scleroderma
Anticholinergics	**Psychiatric Diagnosis**
Narcotics	Anorexia nervosa

cus; and pain from the distal large bowel, urinary tract, or pelvic organs is usually suprapubic. When pain is referred to remote areas supplied by the same neurologic segment as the diseased organ, the phenomenon usually means an increased intensity of the provoking stimuli. **Parietal pain** impulses travel in C fibers of nerves corresponding to dermatomes T6–L1; such pain tends to be more localized and intense than visceral pain.

In the gut, the usual stimulus provoking pain is tension or stretching. Inflammatory lesions can lower the pain threshold, but the mechanisms producing pain of inflammation are not clear. Tissue metabolites released near nerve endings probably account for the pain caused by ischemia. Perception of these painful stimuli can be modulated by input from both cerebral and peripheral sources. Psychologic factors are particularly important. Features of abdominal pain are noted in Tables 303-10 and 303-11.

GASTROINTESTINAL HEMORRHAGE. Bleeding can occur anywhere along the gastrointestinal tract, and identification of the site may be challenging (Table 303-12). Evaluation of the small intestine is facilitated by capsule camera endoscopy. The capsule-sized imaging device is swallowed in older children or placed endoscopically in younger children. Erosive damage to the mucosa of the gastrointestinal tract is the most common cause of bleeding, although variceal bleeding secondary to portal hypertension

TABLE 303-10. Recurrent or Chronic Abdominal Pain in Children

DISORDER	CHARACTERISTICS	KEY EVALUATIONS
NONORGANIC		
Recurrent abdominal pain syndrome (functional abdominal pain)	Nonspecific pain, often periumbilical	Hx and PE; tests as indicated
Irritable bowel syndrome	Intermittent cramps,diarrhea, and constipation	Hx and PE
Nonulcer dyspepsia	Peptic ulcer–like symptoms without abnormalities on evaluation of the upper gastrointestinal tract	Hx; esophagogastroduodenoscopy
GASTROINTESTINAL TRACT		
Chronic constipation	Hx of stool retention, evidence of constipation on examination	Hx and PE; plain x-ray of abdomen
Lactose intolerance	Symptoms may be associated with lactose ingestion; bloating, gas, cramps, and diarrhea	Trial of lactose-free diet; lactose breath hydrogen test
Parasite infection (especially *Giardia*)	Bloating, gas, gramps, and diarrhea	Stool evaluation for O & P; specific immunoassays for Giardia
Excess fructose or sorbitol ingestion	Nonspecific abdominal pain, bloating, gas, and diarrhea	Large intake of apples, fruit juice, or candy/chewing gum sweetened with sorbitol
Crohn disease	See Chapter 333	
Peptic ulcer	Burning or gnawing epigastric pain; worse on awakenig or before meals; relieved with antacids	Esophagogastroduodenoscopy or upper GI contrast x-rays
Esophagitis	Epigastric pain with substernal burning	Esophagogastroduodenoscopy
Meckel's diverticulum	Periumbilical or lower abdominal pain; may have blood in stool	Meckel scan or enteroclysis
Recurrent intussusception	Paroxysmal severe cramping abdominal pain; blood may be present in stool with episode	Identify intussusception during episode or lead point in intestine between episodes with contrast studies of gastrointestinal tract
Internal, inguinal, or abdominal wall hernia	Dull abdomen or abdominal wall pain	PE, CT of abdominal wall
Chronic appendicitis or appendiceal mucocele	Recurrent RLQ pain; often incorrectly diagnosed, may be rare cause of abdominal pain	Barium enema, CT
GALLBLADDER AND PANCREAS		
Cholelithiasis	RUQ pain, may worsen with meals	Ultrasound of gallbladder
Choledochal cyst	RUQ pain, mass ± elevated bilirubin	Ultrasound or CT of RUQ
Recurrent pancreatitis	Persistent boring pain, may radiate to back, vomiting	Serum amylase and lipase ± serum trypsinogen; ultrasound or CT of pancreas
GENITOURINARY TRACT		
Urinary tract infection	Dull suprapubic pain, flank pain	Urinalysis and urine culture; renal scan
Hydronephrosis	Unilateral abdominal or flank pain	Ultrasound of kidneys
Urolithiasis	Progressive, severe pain; flank to inguinal region to testicle	Urinalysis, ultrasound, IVP, CT
Other genitourinary disorders	Suprapubic or lower abdominal pain; genitourinary symptoms	Ultrasound of kidneys and pelvis; gynecologic evaluation
MISCELLANEOUS CAUSES		
Abdominal migraine	See text; nausea, family Hx migraine	Hx
Abdominal epilepsy	May have seizure prodrome	EEG (may require more than one study, including sleep-deprived EEG)
Gilbert syndrome	Mild abdominal pain (causal or coincidental?); slightly elevated unconjugated bilirubin	Serum bilirubin
Familial Mediterranean fever	Paroxysmal episodes of fever, severe abdominal pain, and tenderness with other evidence of polyserositis	Hx and PE during an episode, DNA diagnosis
Sickle cell crisis	Anemia	Hematologic evaluation
Lead poisoning	Vague abdominal pain ± constipation	Serum lead level
Henoch-Schönlein purpura	Recurrent, severe crampy abdominal pain, occult blood in stool, characteristic rash, arthritis	Hx, PE, urinalysis
Angioneurotic edema	Swelling of face or airway, crampy pain	Hx, PE, upper gastrointestinal contrast x-rays, serum C1 esterase inhibitor
Acute intermittent porphyria	Severe pain precipitated by drugs, fasting, or infections	Spot urine for porphyrins

abd, abdominal; EEG, electroencephalogram; Hx, history; IVP, intravenous pyelogrophy; O&P, ova and parasites; PE, physical exam; RLQ, right lower quadrant; RUQ, right upper quadrant.

TABLE 303-11. Distinguishing Features of Acute Gastrointestinal Tract Pain in Children

DISEASE	ONSET	LOCATION	REFERRAL	QUALITY	COMMENTS
Pancreatitis	Acute	Epigastric, left upper quadrant	Back	Constant, sharp, boring	Nausea, emesis, tenderness
Intestinal obstruction	Acute or gradual	Periumbilical–lower abdomen	Back	Alternating cramping (colic) and painless periods	Distention, obstipation, emesis, increased bowel sounds
Appendicitis	Acute	Periumbilical, then localized to lower right quadrant; generalized with peritonitis	Back or pelvis if retrocecal	Sharp, steady	Anorexia, nausea, emesis, local tenderness, fever with peritonitis
Intussusception	Acute	Periumbilical–lower abdomen	None	Cramping, with painless periods	Hematochezia, knees in pulled-up position
Urolithiasis	Acute, sudden	Back (unilateral)	Groin	Sharp, intermittent, cramping	Hematuria
Urinary tract infection	Acute, sudden	Back	Bladder	Dull to sharp	Fever, costochondral tenderness, dysuria, urinary frequency

occurs frequently enough to require consideration. **Prolapse (traumatic) gastropathy** produces subepithelial hemorrhages with prolapse of the stomach into the esophagus during forceful emesis. This may be more commen than Mallory-Weiss lesions secondary to mucosal tears associated with emesis. Vascular malformations are a rare cause in children; they are difficult to identify.

When bleeding originates in the esophagus, stomach, or duodenum, it may cause **hematemesis.** When exposed to gastric or intestinal juices, blood quickly darkens to resemble coffee grounds; massive bleeding is likely to be red. Red or maroon blood in stools, **hematochezia,** signifies either a distal bleeding site or massive hemorrhage above the distal ileum. Moderate to mild bleeding from sites above the distal ileum tends to cause blackened stools of tarry consistency **(melena);** major hemorrhages in the duodenum or above can also cause melena.

Children can develop **iron-deficiency anemia** from chronic enteric blood loss even when occult blood is not found in stools on random testing. Gastrointestinal hemorrhage can produce hypotension and tachycardia but rarely causes gastrointestinal symptoms; brisk duodenal or gastric bleeding can lead to nausea, vomiting, or diarrhea. The breakdown products of intraluminal blood may tip patients into hepatic coma if liver function is already compromised and lead to elevation of serum bilirubin.

ABDOMINAL DISTENTION AND ABDOMINAL MASSES. Enlargement of the abdomen can result from diminished tone of the wall musculature or from increased content: fluid, gas, or solid. **Ascites,** the accumulation of fluid in the peritoneal cavity, distends the abdomen both in the flanks and anteriorly when it is large in volume. This fluid shifts with movement of the patient and conducts a percussion wave.

Ascitic fluid is usually a transudate with a low-protein concentration resulting from reduced plasma colloid osmotic pressure of hypoalbuminemia, from raised portal venous pressure, or from both. In cases of portal hypertension, the fluid leak probably occurs from lymphatics on the liver surface and from visceral peritoneal capillaries, but ascites does not usually develop until the serum albumin level falls. Sodium excretion in the urine decreases greatly as the ascitic fluid accumulates and, thus, additional dietary sodium goes directly to the peritoneal space, taking with it more water. When ascitic fluid contains a high protein concentration, it is usually an exudate caused by an inflammatory or neoplastic lesion.

When fluid distends the gut, either obstruction or imbalance between absorption and secretion should be suspected. The factors causing fluid accumulation in the bowel lumen frequently cause gas to accumulate, too. The result may be audible gurgling noises. The source of gas is usually swallowed air, but endogenous flora can increase considerably in malabsorptive states and produce excessive gas when substrate reaches the lower intestine. Gas in the peritoneal cavity (pneumoperitoneum), perhaps signaled by a tympanitic percussion note even over solid organs such as the liver, indicates a perforated viscus.

An abdominal organ can enlarge diffusely or be affected by a discrete mass. In the digestive tract, such discrete masses can occur in the lumen, in the wall, or in the mesentery. In a constipated child, mobile, nontender fecal masses are often found. Anomalies, cysts, or inflammatory disease can affect the wall of the gut; gut wall neoplasms are extremely rare in children. The liver may enlarge diffusely in response to many disorders. Discrete liver masses may be islands of regenerating liver tissue in a cirrhotic liver or may be inflammatory or neoplastic in origin.

TABLE 303-12. Differential Diagnosis of Gastrointestinal Bleeding in Childhood

INFANT	CHILD	ADOLESCENT
COMMON		
Bacterial enteritis	Bacterial enteritis	Bacterial enteritis
Milk protein allergy	Anal fissure	Inflammatory bowel disease
Intussusception	Colonic polyps	Peptic ulcer/gastritis
Swallowed maternal blood	Intussusception	Prolapse (traumatic) gastropathy 2° emesis
Anal fissure	Peptic ulcer/gastritis	Mallory-Weiss syndrome
Lymphonodular hyperplasia	Swallowed epistaxis	Colonic polyps
	Prolapse (traumatic) gastropathy 2° emesis	
	Mallory-Weiss syndrome	
RARE		
Volvulus	Esophageal varices	Hemorrhoids
Necrotizing enterocolitis	Esophagitis	Esophageal varices
Meckel diverticulum	Meckel diverticulum	Esophagitis
Stress ulcer, stomach	Lymphonodular hyperplasia	Telangiectasia-angiodysplasia
Coagulation disorder (hemorrhagic disease of newborn)	Henoch-Schönlein purpura	Gay bowel disease
	Foreign body	Graft versus host disease
	Hemangioma, arteriovenous malformation	
	Sexual abuse	
	Hemolytic-uremic syndrome	
	Inflammatory bowel disease	
	Coagulopathy	

JAUNDICE. See Chapters 102.3 and 353.

American Academy of Pediatrics Subcommittee on Chronic Abdominal Pain: Chronic abdominal pain in children. *Pediatrics* 2005;115:812–815.

Armon K, Stephenson T, MacFaul R, et al: An evidence and consensus based guideline for acute diarrhoea management. *Arch Dis Child* 2001;85:132–142.

Boey CC, Goh KL: Psychosocial factors and childhood recurrent abdominal pain. *J Gastroenterol Hepatol* 2002;17:1250–1253.

Carty HM: Paediatric emergencies: Non-traumatic abdominal emergencies. *Eur Radiol* 2002;12:2835–2848.

Chong SK: Gastrointestinal problems in the handicapped child. *Curr Opin Pediatr* 2001;13:441–446.

Eccleston C, Morley S, Williams A, et al: Systematic review of randomised controlled trials of psychological therapy for chronic pain in children and adolescents, with a subset meta-analysis of pain relief. *Pain* 2002;99:157–165.

Golden CB, Feusner JH: Malignant abdominal masses in children: Quick guide to evaluation and diagnosis. *Pediatr Clin North Am* 2002;49:1369–1392.

Heuschkel RB, Fletcher K, Hill A, et al: Isolated neonatal swallowing dysfunction: A case series and review of the literature. *Dig Dis Sci* 2003;48:30–35.
Khan S, Di Lorenzo C: Chronic vomiting in children: New insights into diagnosis. *Curr Gastroenterol Rep* 2001;3:248–256.
Li BU, Misiewicz L: Cyclic vomiting syndrome: A brain-gut disorder. *Gastroenterol Clin North Am* 2003;32:997–1019.
Mulvaney S, Lombert EW, Garber J, Walker LS: Trajectories of symptoms and impairment for pediatric patients with functional abdominal pain. *J Am Acad Child Adolesc Psychiatry* 2006;45:737–744.
Rubin G: Constipation in children. *Clin Evid* 2003;10:369–374.
Russell G, Abu-Arafeh I, Symon DN: Abdominal migraine: Evidence for existence and treatment options. *Paediatr Drugs* 2002;4:1–8.

Section 2 — The Oral Cavity — Norman Tinanoff

Chapter 304 ■ Development and Developmental Anomalies of the Teeth

INITIATION

The primary teeth form in dental crypts that arise from a band of epithelial cells incorporated into each developing jaw. By 12 wk of fetal life, each of these epithelial bands (**dental laminae**) has five areas of rapid growth on each side of the maxilla and the mandible, seen as rounded, budlike enlargements. Organization of adjacent mesenchyme takes place in each area of epithelial growth, and the two elements together are the beginning of a tooth.

After the formation of these crypts for the 20 primary teeth, another generation of tooth buds forms lingually (toward the tongue), which will develop into the succeeding permanent incisors, canines, and premolars that eventually replace the primary teeth. This process takes place from ≈5 mo of gestation for the central incisors to about 10 mo of age for the 2nd premolars. The permanent 1st, 2nd, and 3rd molars, on the other hand, arise from extension of the dental laminae distal to the 2nd primary molars; buds for these teeth develop at ≈4 mo of gestation, 1 yr of age, and 4–5 yr of age, respectively.

HISTODIFFERENTIATION-MORPHODIFFERENTIATION. As the epithelial bud proliferates, the deeper surface invaginates and a mass of mesenchyme becomes partially enclosed. The epithelial cells differentiate into the ameloblasts that lay down an organic matrix that forms enamel; the mesenchyme forms the dentin and dental pulp.

CALCIFICATION. After the organic matrix has been laid down, the deposition of the inorganic mineral crystals takes place from several sites of calcification that later coalesce. The characteristics of the inorganic portions of a tooth can be altered by (1) disturbances in formation of the matrix, (2) decreased availability of minerals, or (3) the incorporation of foreign materials. Such disturbances may affect the color, texture, or thickness of the tooth surface. Calcification of primary teeth begins at 3–4 mo in utero and concludes postnatally at ≈12 mo with mineralization of the 2nd primary molars (Table 304-1).

ERUPTION. At the time of tooth bud formation, each tooth begins a continuous movement toward the oral cavity. The times of eruption of the primary and permanent teeth are listed in Table 304-1.

ANOMALIES ASSOCIATED WITH TOOTH DEVELOPMENT

Both failures and excesses of tooth initiation are observed. Developmentally missing teeth can result from environmental insult, a genetic defect involving only teeth, or the manifestation of a syndrome. **Anodontia,** or absence of teeth, occurs when no tooth buds form (ectodermal dysplasia, or familial missing teeth) or when there is a disturbance of a normal site of initiation (the area of a palatal cleft). The teeth that are most commonly absent

TABLE 304-1. Calcification, Crown Completion, and Eruption

TOOTH	FIRST EVIDENCE OF CALCIFICATION	CROWN COMPLETED	ERUPTION
PRIMARY DENTITION			
Maxillary			
Central incisor	3–4 mo in utero	4 mo	7½ mo
Lateral incisor	4½ mo in utero	5 mo	8 mo
Canine	5½ mo in utero	9 mo	16–20 mo
First molar	5 mo in utero	6 mo	12–16 mo
Second molar	6 mo in utero	10–12 mo	20–30 mo
Mandibular			
Central incisor	4½ mo in utero	4 mo	6½ mo
Lateral incisor	4½ mo in utero	4¼ mo	7 mo
Canine	5 mo in utero	9 mo	16–20 mo
First molar	5 mo in utero	6 mo	12–16 mo
Second molar	6 mo in utero	10–12 mo	20–30 mo
PERMANENT DENTITION			
Maxillary			
Central incisor	3–4 mo	4–5 yr	7–8 yr
Lateral incisor	10 mo	4–5 yr	8–9 yr
Canine	4–5 mo	6–7 yr	11–12 yr
First premolar	1½–1¾ yr	5–6 yr	10–11 yr
Second premolar	2–2¼ yr	6–7 yr	10–12 yr
First molar	At birth	2½–3 yr	6–7 yr
Second molar	2½–3 yr	7–8 yr	12–13 yr
Third molar	7–9 yr	12–16 yr	17–21 yr
Mandibular			
Central incisor	3–4 mo	4–5 yr	6–7 yr
Lateral incisor	3–4 mo	4–5 yr	7–8 yr
Canine	4–5 mo	6–7 yr	9–10 yr
First premolar	1¾–2 yr	5–6 yr	10–12 yr
Second premolar	2¼–2½ yr	6–7 yr	11–12 yr
First molar	At birth	2½–3 yr	6–7 yr
Second molar	2½–3 yr	7–8 yr	11–13 yr
Third molar	8–10 yr	12–16 yr	17–21 yr

Modified from Logan WHG, Kronfeld R: Development of the human jaws and surrounding structures from birth to age 15 years. *J Am Dent Assoc* 1993;20:379.

include the 3rd molars, the maxillary lateral incisors, and the mandibular 2nd premolars.

If the dental lamina produces more than the normal number of buds, supernumerary teeth occur, most often in the area between the maxillary central incisors. Because they tend to disrupt the position and eruption of the adjacent normal teeth, their identification by radiographic examination is important. Supernumerary teeth also occur with cleidocranial dysplasia (see Chapter 308) and in the area of cleft palates.

Twinning, in which two teeth are joined together, is most often observed in the mandibular incisors of the primary dentition. It can result from gemination, fusion, or concrescence. **Gemination** is the result of the division of one tooth germ to form a bifid crown on a single root with a common pulp canal; an extra tooth appears to be present in the dental arch. **Fusion** is the joining of incompletely developed teeth that, owing to pressure, trauma, or crowding, continue to develop as one tooth. Fused teeth are sometimes joined along their entire length; in other cases, a single wide crown is supported on two roots. **Concrescence** is the attachment of the roots of closely approximated adjacent teeth by an excessive deposit of cementum. This type of twinning, unlike the others, is found most often in the maxillary molar region.

Disturbances during differentiation can result in alterations in dental morphology, such as **macrodontia** (large teeth) or **microdontia** (small teeth). The maxillary lateral incisors may assume a slender, tapering shape (**peg-shaped laterals**).

Amelogenesis imperfecta represents a group of hereditary conditions that manifest in enamel defects of the primary and permanent teeth without evidence of systemic disorders (Fig. 304-1). The teeth are covered by only a thin layer of abnormally formed enamel through which the yellow underlying dentin is seen. The primary teeth are generally affected more than the permanent teeth. Susceptibility to caries is low, but the enamel is subject to destruction from abrasion. Complete coverage of the crown may be indicated for dentin protection, to reduce tooth sensitivity, and for improved appearance.

Dentinogenesis imperfecta, or hereditary opalescent dentin, is an analogous condition to amelogenesis imperfecta in which the odontoblasts fail to differentiate normally, resulting in poorly calcified dentin (Fig. 304-2). This autosomal dominant disorder may also occur in patients with **osteogenesis imperfecta.** The enamel-dentin junction is altered, causing enamel to break away.

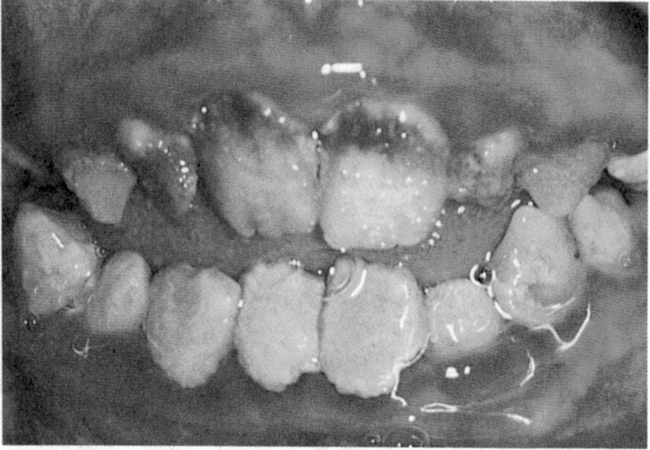

Figure 304-1. Amelogenesis imperfecta, hypocalcified type. The enamel defects result in discoloration and erosion caused by errors in the mineralization stage of tooth development and secondary staining. (From Nazif MM, Martin BS, McKibben DH, et al: Oral disorders. In Zitelli BJ, Davis HW [editors]: *Atlas of Pediatric Physical Diagnosis,* 4th ed. Philadelphia, Mosby, 2002, p 703.)

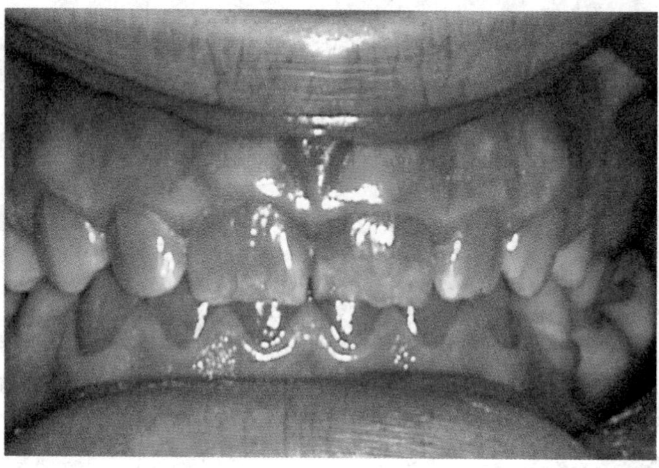

Figure 304-2. Dentinogenesis imperfecta. The bluish, opalescent sheen on several of these teeth results from genetically defective dentin. This condition may be associated with osteogenesis imperfecta. (From Nazif MM, Martin BS, McKibben DH, et al: Oral disorders. In Zitelli BJ, Davis HW [editors]: *Atlas of Pediatric Physical Diagnosis,* 4th ed. Philadelphia, Mosby, 2002, p 703.)

The exposed dentin is then susceptible to abrasion, in some cases worn to the gingiva. The teeth are opaque and pearly, and the pulp chambers are generally obliterated by calcification. Both primary and permanent teeth are usually involved.

Localized disturbances of calcification that correlate with periods of illness, malnutrition, premature birth, or birth trauma are common. **Hypocalcification** appears as opaque white patches or horizontal lines on the tooth; **hypoplasia** is more severe and manifests as pitting or areas devoid of enamel. Systemic conditions, such as renal failure and cystic fibrosis, are associated with enamel defects. Local trauma to the primary incisors can also affect calcification of permanent incisors.

Fluorosis (mottled enamel) can result from systemic fluoride consumption >0.05 mg/kg/day during enamel formation. This high fluoride consumption can be caused by residing in an area of high fluoride content of the drinking water (>2.0 ppm), swallowing excessive fluoridated toothpaste, or inappropriate fluoride prescriptions. Excessive fluoride during enamel formation affects ameloblastic function, resulting in inconspicuous white, lacy patches on the enamel to severe brownish discoloration and hypoplasia. The latter changes are usually seen with fluoride concentrations in the drinking water >5.0 ppm.

Discolored teeth can result from incorporation of foreign substances into developing enamel. Neonatal hyperbilirubinemia can produce blue to black discoloration of the primary teeth. Porphyria produces a red-brown discoloration. Tetracyclines are extensively incorporated into bones and teeth and, if administered during the period of formation of enamel, can result in brown-yellow discoloration and hypoplasia of the enamel. Such teeth fluoresce under ultraviolet light. The period at risk extends from ≈4 mo of gestation to 7 yr of life. Repeated or prolonged therapy with tetracycline carries the highest risk.

Delayed eruption of the 20 primary teeth can be familial or indicate systemic or nutritional disturbances such as hypopituitarism, hypothyroidism, cleidocranial dysplasia, trisomy 21, progeria, Albright osteodystrophy, incontinentia pigmenti, rickets, and multiple syndromes. Failure of eruption of single or small groups of teeth can arise from local causes such as malpositioned teeth, supernumerary teeth, cysts, or retained primary teeth. Premature loss of primary teeth is most commonly caused by premature eruption of the permanent teeth. If the entire dentition is advanced for age and sex, precocious puberty or hyperthyroidism should be considered.

Natal teeth are observed in ≈1/2,000 newborn infants; usually, there are two in the position of the mandibular central incisors. Natal teeth are present at birth, whereas **neonatal teeth** erupt in the 1st mo of life. Attachment of natal/neonatal teeth is generally limited to the gingival margin, with little root formation or bony support. They may be a supernumerary or a prematurely erupted primary tooth. A radiograph can easily differentiate between the two conditions. Natal teeth are associated with cleft palate, Pierre Robin syndrome, Ellis–van Creveld syndrome, Hallermann-Streiff syndrome, pachyonychia congenita, and other anomalies. A family history of natal teeth or premature eruption is present in 15–20% of affected children.

Natal/neonatal teeth can occasionally result in pain and refusal to feed and, at times, can produce maternal discomfort because of abrasion or biting of the nipple during nursing. There is a remote danger of detachment, with aspiration of the tooth. Because the tongue lies between the alveolar processes during birth, it can become lacerated, and, occasionally, the tip is amputated (**Riga-Fede disease**). Decisions regarding extraction of prematurely erupted primary teeth must be made on an individual basis.

Exfoliation failure occurs when a primary tooth is not shed before the eruption of its permanent successor. Most often the primary tooth exfoliates eventually, but in some cases, the primary tooth may need to be extracted. This occurs most commonly in the mandibular incisor region.

Chapter 305 ■ Disorders of the Oral Cavity Associated with Other Conditions

Disorders of the teeth and surrounding structures may occur in isolation or in combination with other systemic conditions (Table 305-1). Most commonly, medical conditions that occur during tooth development may affect tooth formation or appearance. Damage to teeth during their development is permanent.

TABLE 305-1. Dental Problems Associated with Selected Medical Conditions

MEDICAL CONDITION	COMMON ASSOCIATED DENTAL OR ORAL FINDINGS
Cleft lip and palate	Missing teeth, extra (supernumerary) teeth, shifting of arch segments, feeding difficulties, speech problems
Kidney failure	Mottled enamel (permanent teeth), facial dysmorphology
Cystic fibrosis	Stained teeth with extensive medication, mottled enamel
Immunosuppression	Oral candidiasis with potential for systemic candidiasis, cyclosporine-induced gingival hyperplasia
Low birthweight with prolonged oral intubation	Palatal groove, narrow arch
Heart defects with susceptibility for bacterial endocarditis	Bacteremia from dental procedures or trauma
Neutrophil chemotactic deficiency	Juvenile periodontitis (loss of supporting bone around teeth)
Juvenile diabetes (uncontrolled)	Juvenile periodontitis
Neuromotor dysfunction	Oral trauma from falling; malocclusion (open bite); gingivitis from lack of hygiene
Prolonged illness (generalized) during tooth formation	Enamel hypoplasia of crown portions forming during illness
Seizures	Gingival enlargement if phenytoin is used
Maternal infections	Syphilis—abnormally shaped teeth
Vitamin D-dependent rickets	Enamel hypoplasia

Chapter 306 ■ Malocclusion

The oral cavity is essentially a masticatory instrument. The purpose of the anterior teeth is to bite off portions of large amounts of food. The posterior teeth reduce foodstuff to a soft, moist bolus. The cheeks and tongue force the food onto the areas of tooth contact. Establishing a proper relationship between the mandibular and maxillary teeth is important for physiologic and cosmetic reasons.

VARIATIONS IN GROWTH PATTERNS. Growth patterns are classified into three main types of occlusion, determined when the jaws are closed and the teeth are held together (Fig. 306-1). According to the Angle Classification of Malocclusion, in **class I occlusion** (normal), the cusps of the posterior mandibular teeth interdigitate ahead of and inside the corresponding cusps of the opposing maxillary teeth. This relationship provides a normal facial profile. In **class II malocclusion,** "buck teeth," the cusps of the posterior mandibular teeth are behind and inside the corresponding cusps of the maxillary teeth. This common occlusal disharmony is found in ≈45% of the population. The facial profile may give the appearance of a "receding chin" (retrognathia) or protruding front teeth. The resultant increased space between upper and lower anterior teeth encourages finger sucking and tongue-thrust habits. Additionally, children with pronounced class II malocclusions are at greater risk of damage to the incisors due to trauma. In **class III malocclusion,** "underbite," the cusps of the posterior mandibular teeth interdigitate a tooth or more ahead of their opposing maxillary counterparts. The anterior teeth appear in cross bite with the mandibular incisors protruding beyond the maxillary incisors. The facial profile gives the appearance of a "protruding chin" (**prognathia**).

CROSS BITE. Normally, the mandibular teeth are in a position just inside the maxillary teeth, so that the outside mandibular cusps or incisal edges meet the central portion of the opposing maxillary teeth. A reversal of this relation is referred to as a cross bite. Cross bites can be anterior, involving the incisors; can be posterior, involving the molars; or can involve single or multiple teeth.

OPEN AND CLOSED BITES. If the posterior mandibular and maxillary teeth make contact with each other, but the anterior teeth are still apart, the condition is called an open bite. Open bites may be due to skeletal growth pattern or digit sucking. If digit sucking is terminated before skeletal and dental growth is complete, natural resolution of the open bite may occur. If mandibular anterior teeth occlude inside the maxillary anterior teeth in an overclosed position, the condition is referred to as a closed or deep bite. Treatment of open and closed bites consists of orthodontic correction, generally performed in the preteen or teenage years. Some cases require orthognathic surgery to position the jaws optimally in a vertical direction.

DENTAL CROWDING. Overlap of incisors can result when the jaws are too small or the teeth are too large for adequate alignment of the teeth. Growth of the jaws is mostly in the posterior aspects of the mandible and maxilla, and, therefore, inadequate space for the teeth at 7 or 8 yr of age will not resolve with growth of the jaws. Spacing in the primary dentition is normal and favorable for adequate alignment of successor teeth.

DIGIT SUCKING. Various and conflicting etiologic theories and recommendations for correction have been proposed for digit sucking in children. Prolonged digit sucking can cause flaring of

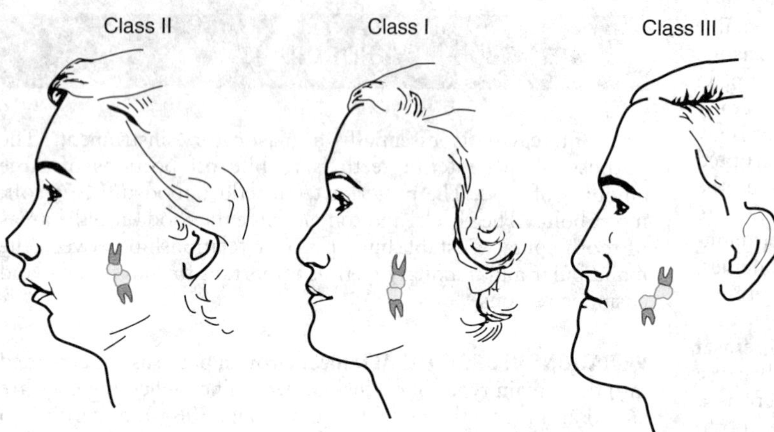

Figure 306-1. Angle classification of occlusion. The typical correspondence between the facial-jaw profile and molar relationship is shown.

the maxillary incisor teeth, an open bite, as well as a posterior cross bite. The prevalence of digit sucking decreases steadily from the age of 2 yr to ≈10% by the age of 5. The earlier the habit is discontinued after the eruption of the permanent maxillary incisors (age 7–8 yr), the greater the likelihood that there will be lessening effects on the dentition. A variety of treatments have been suggested, from behavioral modification to insertion of an appliance with extensions that serves as a reminder when the child attempts to insert the digit. The greatest likelihood of success occurs in cases in which the child desires to stop. Stopping of the habit, however, will not rectify a malocclusion caused by a prior deviant growth pattern.

Chapter 307 ■ Cleft Lip and Palate

Clefts of the lip and palate are distinct entities closely related embryologically, functionally, and genetically. Although there are a variety of theories, it is commonly thought that cleft of the lip appears because of hypoplasia of the mesenchymal layer, resulting in a failure of the medial nasal and maxillary processes to join. Cleft of the palate appears to represent failure of the palatal shelves to approximate or fuse.

INCIDENCE AND EPIDEMIOLOGY. The incidence of cleft lip with or without cleft palate is ≈1/750 white births; the incidence of cleft palate alone is ≈1/2,500 white births. Clefts of the lip are more common in males. Possible causes include maternal drug exposure, a syndrome-malformation complex, or genetic factors. Although both may appear to occur sporadically, the presence of susceptibility genes appears important. There are families in which a cleft lip or palate, or both, is inherited in a dominant fashion *(van der Woude syndrome)*, and careful examination of parents is important to distinguish this type from others, because the recurrence risk is 50%. Ethnic factors also affect the incidence of cleft lip and palate; the incidence is highest among Asians and Native Americans, and lowest among blacks. The incidence of associated congenital malformations (chromosomal aneuploidy, holoprosencephaly) and of impairment in development is increased in children with cleft defects, especially in those with cleft palate alone. The risks of recurrence of cleft defects within families are discussed in Chapters 80 and 83.

CLINICAL MANIFESTATIONS. Cleft lip may vary from a small notch in the vermilion border to a complete separation involving skin, muscle, mucosa, tooth, and bone. Clefts may be unilateral (more often on the left side) or bilateral and may involve the alveolar ridge. Deformed, supernumerary, or absent teeth are associated findings.

Isolated cleft palate occurs in the midline and may involve only the uvula or may extend into or through the soft and hard palates to the incisive foramen. When associated with cleft lip, the defect may involve the midline of the soft palate and extend into the hard palate on one or both sides, exposing one or both of the nasal cavities as a unilateral or bilateral cleft palate. The palate may also present with a submucosal cleft indicated by a bifid uvula, partial separation of muscle with intact mucosa, or a palpable notch at the posterior of the palate.

TREATMENT. A complete program of habilitation for the child with a cleft lip or palate may require years of special treatment by a team consisting of a pediatrician, plastic surgeon, otolaryngologist, oral and maxillofacial surgeon, pediatric dentist, prosthodontist, orthodontist, speech therapist, geneticist, medical social worker, psychologist, and public health nurse. The child's physician should be responsible for seeking the coordinated use of specialists and for parental counseling and guidance.

The immediate problem in an infant born with a cleft lip or palate is feeding. Although some advocate the construction of a plastic obturator to assist in feedings, most believe that with the use of soft artificial nipples with large openings, a squeezable bottle, and proper instruction, feeding of infants with clefts can be achieved with relative ease and effectiveness.

Surgical closure of a cleft lip is usually performed by 3 mo of age, when the infant has shown satisfactory weight gain and is free of any oral, respiratory, or systemic infection. Modification of the Millard rotation-advancement technique is the most commonly used technique; a staggered suture line minimizes notching of the lip from retraction of scar tissue. The initial repair may be revised at 4 or 5 yr of age. Corrective surgery on the nose may be delayed until adolescence. Nasal surgery can also be performed at the time of the lip repair. Cosmetic results depend on the extent of the original deformity, healing potential of the individual, absence of infection, and the skill of the surgeon.

Because clefts of the palate vary considerably in size, shape, and degree of deformity, the timing of surgical correction should be individualized. Criteria such as width of the cleft, adequacy of the existing palatal segments, morphology of the surrounding areas (width of the oropharynx), and neuromuscular function of the soft palate and pharyngeal walls affect the decision. The goals of surgery are the union of the cleft segments, intelligible and pleasant speech, reduction of nasal regurgitation, and avoidance of injury to the growing maxilla.

In an otherwise healthy child, closure of the palate is usually done before 1 yr of age to enhance normal speech development. When surgical correction is delayed beyond the 3rd yr, a contoured speech bulb can be attached to the posterior of a maxillary denture so that contraction of the pharyngeal and velopharyngeal muscles can bring tissues into contact with the bulb to accomplish occlusion of the nasopharynx and help the child develop intelligible speech.

A cleft palate usually crosses the alveolar ridge and interferes with the formation of teeth in the maxillary anterior region. Teeth in the cleft area may be displaced, malformed, or missing. Missing teeth or teeth that are nonfunctional are replaced by prosthetic devices.

POSTOPERATIVE MANAGEMENT. During the immediate postoperative period, special nursing care is essential. Gentle aspiration of the nasopharynx minimizes the chances of the common complications of atelectasis or pneumonia. The primary considerations in postoperative care are maintenance of a clean suture line and avoidance of tension on the sutures. The infant is fed with a Mead Johnson bottle and the arms are restrained with elbow cuffs. A fluid or semifluid diet is maintained for 3 wk; feeding is continued with a Mead Johnson bottle or a cup. The patient's hands, toys, and other foreign bodies must be kept away from the surgical site.

SEQUELAE OF CLEFT LIP AND PALATE. Recurrent otitis media and hearing loss are frequent with cleft palate. Displacement of the maxillary arches and malposition of the teeth usually require orthodontic correction.

Speech defects are often associated with cleft lip and palate and may be present or persist because of inadequate surgical closure of the palate. Such speech is characterized by the emission of air from the nose and by a hypernasal quality with certain sounds. Both before and sometimes after palatal surgery, the speech defect is caused by inadequacies in function of the palatal and pharyngeal muscles. The muscles of the soft palate and the lateral and posterior walls of the nasopharynx constitute a valve that separates the nasopharynx from the oropharynx during swallowing and in the production of certain sounds. If the valve does not function adequately, it is difficult to build up enough pressure in the mouth to make such explosive sounds as *p, b, d, t, h, y,* or the sibilants *s, sh,* and *ch,* and such words as "cats," "boats," and "sisters" are not intelligible. After operation or the insertion of a speech appliance, speech therapy is necessary.

VELOPHARYNGEAL INCOMPETENCE. The speech disturbance characteristic of the child with a cleft palate can also be produced by other osseous or neuromuscular abnormalities where there is an inability to form an effective seal between oropharynx and nasopharynx during swallowing or phonation. The abnormality may be in the structure of the palate or pharynx or in the muscles attached to these structures. In a child who has the potential for abnormal speech, adenoidectomy may precipitate overt hypernasality. A submucous cleft palate may also cause this problem. In such cases, the adenoid mass may have facilitated velopharyngeal closure when contacted by the elevated soft palate. If the neuromuscular function is adequate, compensation in palatopharyngeal movement may take place and the speech defect may improve, although speech therapy is necessary. In other cases, slow involution of the adenoids may allow for gradual compensation in palatal and pharyngeal muscular function. This may explain why a speech defect does not become apparent in some children who have a submucous cleft palate or similar anomaly predisposing to palatopharyngeal incompetence. Velopharyngeal incompetence (VPI) can also occur in children with an inherent palatal abnormality (velocardiofacial syndrome). A craniofacial disorders team and a geneticist should evaluate VPI.

Clinical Manifestation. Although clinical signs vary, the symptoms of VPI are similar to those of a cleft palate. There may be hypernasal speech (especially noted in the articulation of pressure consonants such as *p, b, d, t, h, v, f,* and *s*); conspicuous constricting movement of the nares during speech; inability to whistle, gargle, blow out a candle, or inflate a balloon; loss of liquid through the nose when drinking with the head down; otitis media; and hearing loss. Oral inspection may reveal a cleft palate or a relatively short palate with a large oropharynx; absent, grossly asymmetric, or minimal muscular activity of the soft palate and pharynx during phonation or gagging; or a submucous cleft. The latter is suggested by a bifid uvula, by a translucent membrane in the midline of the soft palate (revealing lack of continuity of muscles), by palpable notching in the posterior border of the hard palate instead of a posterior nasal spinous process, or by forward or V-shaped displacement or grooving on the soft palate during phonation or gagging.

Velopharyngeal incompetence may also be demonstrated radiographically. The head should be carefully positioned to obtain a true lateral view; one film is obtained with the patient at rest and another during continuous phonation of the vowel *u* as in "boom." The soft palate contacts the posterior pharyngeal wall in normal function, whereas in velopharyngeal incompetence such contact is absent. Most accurate evaluations of VPI are accomplished by the use of nasoendoscopy.

In selected cases, the palate may be retropositioned or pharyngoplasty performed using a flap of tissue from the posterior pharyngeal wall. Dental speech appliances have also been used successfully. The type of surgery used is best tailored to the findings on nasoendoscopy.

Chapter 308 ■ Syndromes with Oral Manifestations

Many syndromes have distinct or accompanying facial, oral, and dental manifestations (Apert syndrome, Chapter 592; Crouzon disease, Chapter 592; Down syndrome, Chapter 81).

Osteogenesis imperfecta is often accompanied by effects on the teeth, termed **dentinogenesis imperfecta** (see Chapter 304, Fig. 304-2). Depending on the severity of presentation, treatment of the dentition varies from routine preventive and restorative monitoring to covering affected posterior teeth with stainless steel crowns, to reduce abrasion from chewing. Dentinogenesis imperfecta can also occur in isolation without the bony effects.

Another syndrome, **cleidocranial dysplasia,** has orofacial variations such as frontal bossing, mandibular prognathism, and a broad nasal base. Tooth eruption is often delayed. The primary teeth can be abnormally retained while the permanent teeth remain unerupted. Supernumerary teeth are common, especially in the premolar area. Although the erupted teeth are usually free of hypoplasia, variations in the size and shape of the teeth are common. Restoration of the erupted primary and permanent teeth should be performed when carious lesions are present. Extensive dental rehabilitation therapy may be needed to maintain effective mastication.

Ectodermal dysplasias (see Chapter 648) are a heterogeneous group of conditions in which oral manifestations range from little or no involvement (the dentition is completely normal) to cases in which the teeth can be totally or partially absent or malformed. Because alveolar bone does not develop in the absence of teeth, the alveolar processes can be either totally or partially absent, and the resultant overclosure of the mandible causes the lips to protrude. Facial development is otherwise not disturbed. Teeth, when present, can range from normal to small and conical. If aplasia of the buccal and labial mucous glands is present, dryness and irritation of the oral mucosa can occur. People with ectodermal dysplasia may need either partial or full dentures, even at

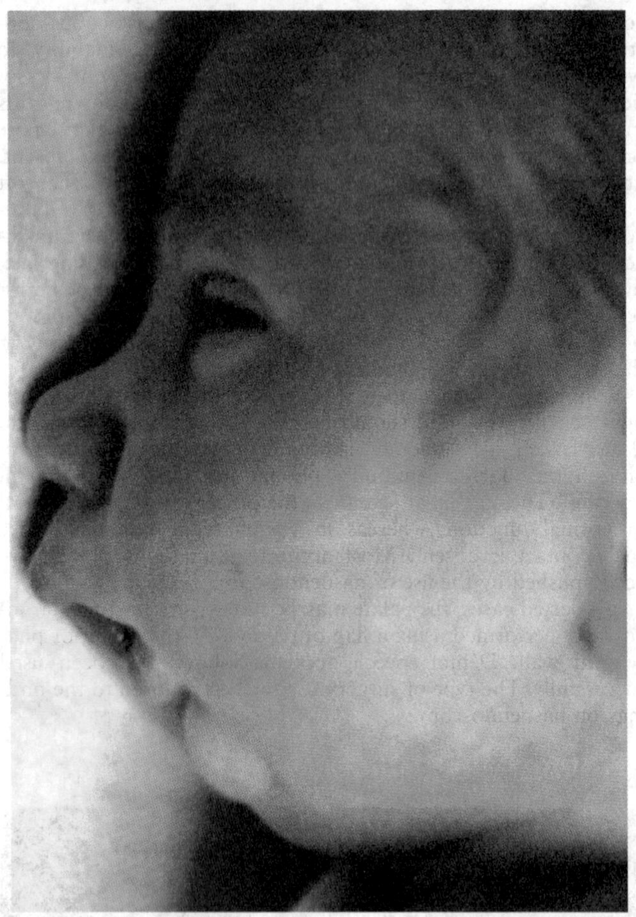

Figure 308-1. Pierre Robin syndrome. (From Clark DA: *Atlas of Neonatology,* 7th ed. Philadelphia, WB Saunders, 2000, p 144.)

a very young age. The vertical height between the jaws is thus restored, improving the position of the lips and facial contours. Masticatory function is restored, and eating habits are therefore improved.

Pierre Robin syndrome consists of micrognathia usually accompanied by a high arched or cleft palate (Fig. 308-1). The tongue is usually of normal size, but the floor of the mouth is foreshortened. Obstruction of the air passages may occur, particularly on inspiration, and usually requires treatment to prevent suffocation. The infant should be maintained in a prone or partially prone position so that the tongue falls forward to relieve respiratory obstruction. Some patients may require endotracheal intubation or, rarely, tracheostomy. Mandibular distraction procedures in the neonate can improve mandibular size, enhance respiration, and facilitate oral feedings. If airway obstruction is present, this is an important alternative to tracheostomy.

Sufficient spontaneous mandibular growth may take place within a few months to relieve the potential airway obstruction. Often the growth of the mandible achieves a normal profile in 4–6 yr. The feeding of infants with mandibular hypoplasia requires great care and patience but can usually be accomplished without resorting to gavage. Dental anomalies usually require individualized treatment. Thirty to 50% of children with Pierre Robin syndrome have Stickler syndrome, an autosomal dominant condition that includes other findings such as early arthritis and ocular problems.

In **mandibulofacial dysostosis** (Treacher Collins syndrome or Franceschetti syndrome), the facial appearance is characterized by downward sloping palpebral fissures, colobomas of the lower eyelids, sunken cheekbones, blind fistulas opening between the angles of the mouth and the ears, deformed pinnae, atypical hair growth extending toward the cheeks, receding chin, and large mouth. Facial clefts, abnormalities of the ears, and deafness are common. The disorder is autosomal dominant, often with incomplete penetrance. The mandible is usually hypoplastic; the ramus may be deficient, and the coronoid and condylar processes are flat or even aplastic. The palatal vault may be either high or cleft. Infrequently, unilateral or bilateral macrostomia, or failure of embryonic fusion of the maxillary and mandibular processes, may occur. Dental malocclusions are frequent. The teeth may be widely separated, hypoplastic, or displaced or have an open bite. Orthodontic and routine dental treatments are indicated.

Hemifacial microsomia is usually characterized by unilateral hypoplasia of the mandible and can be associated with partial paralysis of the facial nerve, macrostomia, blind fistulas between the angles of the mouth and the ears, and deformed external ears. Severe facial asymmetry and malocclusion can develop because of the absence or hypoplasia of the mandibular condyle on the affected side. Congenital condylar deformity tends to increase with age. Early craniofacial surgery may be indicated to minimize the deformity. This disorder can be associated with ocular and vertebral anomalies (oculo-auriculo-vertebral spectrum, including Goldenhar syndrome); therefore, radiographs of the vertebrae and ribs should be considered to determine the extent of skeletal involvement.

Chapter 309 ■ Dental Caries

ETIOLOGY. The development of dental caries depends on interrelationships between the tooth surface, dietary carbohydrates, and specific oral bacteria. Organic acids produced by bacterial fermentation of dietary carbohydrates reduce the pH of dental plaque adjacent to the tooth to a point at which demineralization occurs. The initial carious lesion appears as an opaque white spot on the enamel; and with progressive loss of tooth mineral, cavitation occurs.

A group of microorganisms, **mutans streptococci,** are associated with the development of dental caries. These bacteria have the ability to adhere to enamel, produce abundant acid, and survive at low pH. Once the enamel surface cavitates, other oral bacteria (lactobacilli) colonize the tooth, produce acid, and foster further tooth demineralization. Demineralization from bacterial acid production is determined by the frequency of carbohydrate consumption and by the type of carbohydrate. Sucrose is the most cariogenic sugar because one of its by-products during bacterial metabolism is glucan, a polymer that enables bacteria to adhere more readily to tooth structures. The cariogenic potential of a nursing bottle of a sweetened beverage that is continuously consumed throughout the night or at nap times is much greater than that of the same volume of drink consumed at a single meal. Similarly, sticky candies retained orally for long periods (sucrose in sticky candies) is more cariogenic than the sugar in food products retained for short times.

EPIDEMIOLOGY. The incidence of dental caries has decreased in developed countries in the past 30 yr but remains highly prevalent among low-income children and children from developing countries. The decrease is due to advances in prevention, particularly in the use of fluorides. More than half of the children in the United States have dental caries, with most of those having caries primarily in the pits and fissures of the occlusal (biting) surfaces of the molar teeth.

CLINICAL MANIFESTATIONS. Dental caries of the primary dentition usually begins in the pits and fissures. Small lesions may be

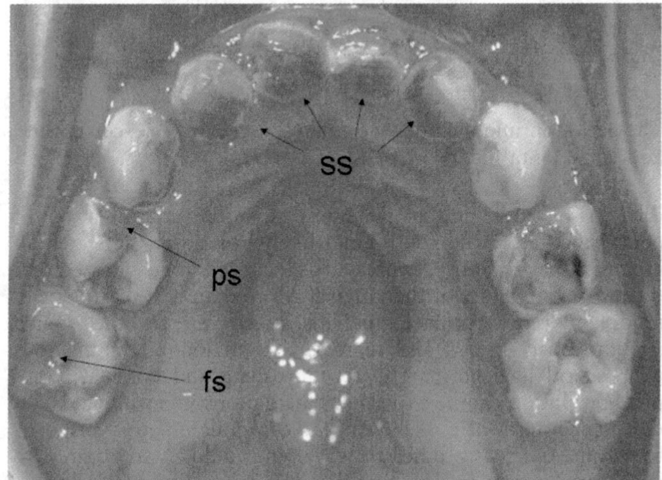

Figure 309-1. Rampant caries (early childhood caries) in 3 yr old child. Note caries on the smooth surfaces of the incisors *(ss)*, proximal surface of the 1st primary molar *(ps)*, and fissure surface of the 2nd primary molar *(fs)*.

difficult to diagnose by visual inspection, but larger lesions present as cavitations of the occlusal surface. The 2nd most frequent location of caries is approximal sites (contact surfaces between the teeth), which in many cases can only be detected by intraoral radiographs. Caries lesions of the exposed smooth (buccal and lingual) surfaces are generally found only in children with rampant caries (Fig. 309-1).

Rampant caries in infants and toddlers, referred to as **early childhood caries** (ECC), nursing bottle caries, or baby bottle tooth decay, is ascribed to inappropriate bottle-feeding. Although the combination of a child infected with cariogenic bacteria and the frequent ingestion of sugar, either in the bottle or in solid foods, is critical, other factors such as enamel hypoplasia of primary teeth because of nutritional deficiencies during pregnancy or because of premature birth may have a role. Reports have also associated "at will" breast-feeding in older infants with early childhood caries. Interestingly, cow's milk is less associated with caries, possibly due to the higher calcium and phosphorus contents of cow's milk relative to breast milk.

Early childhood caries are common, with a reported prevalence of 30–50% in children from low socioeconomic backgrounds and as high as 70% in some Native American groups. It may occur as early as 12 mo of age, long before children visit a dentist. Pediatricians have the responsibility to both examine the child's teeth for caries and to establish a "dental home" (refer to a dentist) before a child at risk for ECC is 1 yr of age. Risk factors include high-frequency sugar consumption (prolonged and frequent drinking from bottle or sippy cup, frequent eating of sugar-containing snacks), children of low socioeconomic status, immigrant children, parents or siblings with high caries rates, and evidence of defects on the teeth.

Children who develop caries at a young age are known to be at high risk for developing further caries as they get older. Therefore, the appropriate prevention of early childhood caries can result in the elimination of major dental problems in toddlers and less decay in later childhood.

COMPLICATIONS. If left untreated, dental caries usually destroy most of the tooth and invade the dental pulp (Fig. 309-2), leading to an inflammation of the pulp (**pulpitis**) and significant pain. Pulpitis can progress to necrosis, with bacterial invasion of the alveolar bone causing a dental abscess (Fig. 309-3). Infection of a primary tooth may disrupt normal development of the successor permanent tooth. In a small percentage of cases, this process may lead to sepsis and facial space infection.

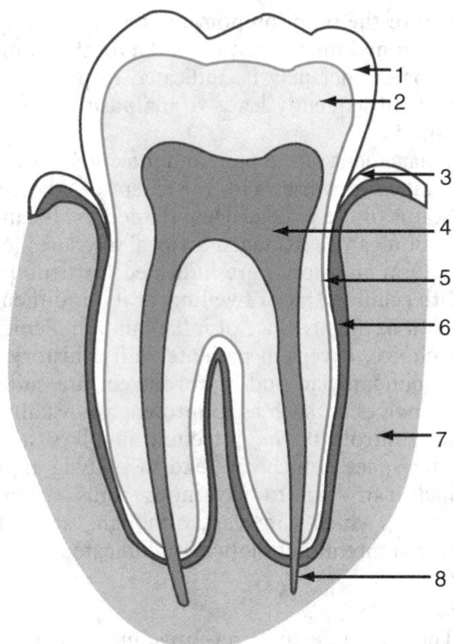

Figure 309-2. Basic dental anatomy: 1 = enamel; 2 = dentin; 3 = gingival margin; 4 = pulp; 5 = cementum; 6 = periodontal ligament; 7 = alveolar bone; 8 = neurovascular bundle.

TREATMENT. The age at which caries occurs is important in dental management. Children <3 yr of age lack the developmental ability to cooperate with dental treatment and often require restraint, sedation, or general anesthesia to repair carious teeth. After age 4, children can generally cope with dental restorative care with the use of local anesthesia.

Dental treatment, using silver amalgam, plastic composite restorations, or stainless steel crowns, can restore most teeth affected with dental caries. If caries involves the dental pulp, a

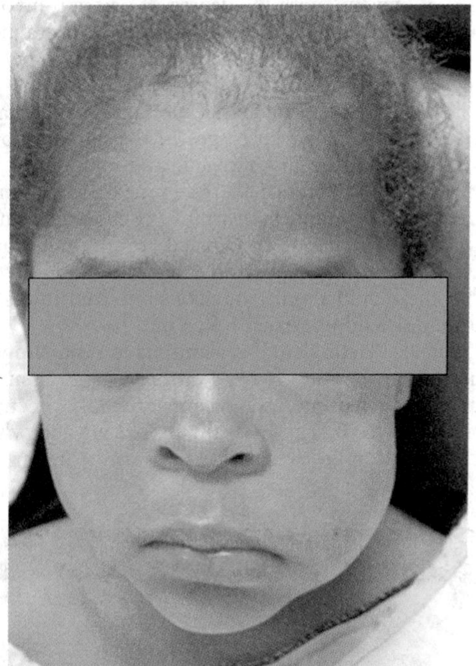

Figure 309-3. Facial swelling from an abscessed primary molar. Resolution of the inflammation can be achieved by a course of antibiotics, followed by either extraction or root canal of the offending tooth.

partial removal of the pulp (pulpotomy) or complete removal of the pulp (pulpectomy) may be required. If a tooth requires extraction, a space maintainer may be indicated to prevent migration of teeth, which subsequently leads to malposition of permanent successor teeth.

Clinical management of the pain and infection associated with untreated dental caries varies with the extent of involvement and the medical status of the patient. Dental infection localized to the dentoalveolar unit can be managed by local measures (extraction, pulpectomy). Oral antibiotics are indicated for dental infections associated with cellulitis, facial swelling, or if it is difficult to anesthetize the tooth in the presence of inflammation. Penicillin is the antibiotic of choice, except in patients with a history of allergy to this agent; clindamycin and erythromycin are suitable alternatives. Oral analgesics, such as ibuprofen, are usually adequate for the pain control. If the infection involves a vital area (submandibular space, which can lead to Ludwig angina; facial triangle, which can lead to cavernous sinus thrombosis; or periorbital space, which can lead, although rarely, to orbital involvement), parenteral antibiotics are indicated.

PREVENTION.

Fluoride. The most effective preventive measure against dental caries is optimizing the fluoride content of communal water supplies to 1 ppm. Children who reside in areas with fluoride-deficient water supplies and are at risk for caries will benefit from dietary fluoride supplements (Table 309-1). The fluoride level of public water supplies can usually be obtained by calling the local health department. If the patient uses a private water supply, it is necessary to get the water tested for fluoride levels before prescribing fluoride supplements. To avoid potential overdoses, no fluoride prescription should be written for more than a total of 120 mg of fluoride. Significant acute overdose of fluoride (>5 mg/kg) needs immediate medical attention. The use of topical fluoride agents, applied professionally or by the patient, is beneficial to children at risk for caries.

Oral Hygiene. Daily brushing, especially with fluoridated toothpaste, will help prevent dental caries. Most children under 8 yr of age do not have the coordination required for adequate tooth brushing. Accordingly, parents should assume responsibility for the child's oral hygiene, with the degree of parental involvement appropriate to the child's changing abilities. Only a pea-sized amount, or less, of fluoridated toothpaste should be used in young children who cannot adequately expectorate.

Diet. Decreasing frequent sugar ingestion prevents dental caries. Therefore, using sweetened beverages in the nursing bottle and bedtime bottle should be discouraged, and children at risk for dental caries should reduce between-meal sugar-containing snacks. Frequent consumption of fruit juice in the nursing bottle and sippy cup is often not recognized for its high cariogenic potential. Therefore, special effort must be made to instruct parents that their child should only consume fruit juices at meal times and they should not exceed 6 oz per day.

Dental Sealant. Plastic dental sealants have been shown to be effective in the prevention of caries on the pit and fissure of the primary and permanent molars. Sealants are most effective when placed soon after teeth erupt (usually in 1–2 yr) and when used in children with deep grooves and fissures in the molar teeth.

TABLE 309-1. Supplemental Fluoride Dosage Schedule

	FLUORIDE IN HOME WATER (PPM)		
AGE	<0.3	0.3–0.6	>0.6
6 mo–3 yr	0.25*	0	0
3–6 yr	0.50	0.25	0
6–16 yr	1.00	0.50	0

*Milligrams of fluoride per day.

Chapter 310 ■ Periodontal Diseases

The periodontium includes the gingiva, alveolar bone, cementum, and periodontal ligament (see Fig. 309-2).

GINGIVITIS. Poor oral hygiene results in the accumulation of dental plaque at the tooth-gingival interface that activates an inflammatory response, expressed as localized or generalized reddening and swelling of the gingiva. More than half of American schoolchildren experience gingivitis. In severe cases, the gingiva spontaneously bleeds and there is oral malodor. Treatment is proper oral hygiene (careful toothbrushing and flossing); complete resolution can be expected. Fluctuations in hormonal levels during the onset of puberty can increase inflammatory response to plaque. Gingivitis in healthy children is unlikely to progress to periodontitis (inflammation of the periodontal ligament resulting in loss of alveolar bone).

AGGRESSIVE PERIODONTITIS IN CHILDREN (PREPUBERTAL PERIODONTITIS). Periodontitis in children before puberty is a rare disease that often begins between the time of eruption of the primary teeth and the age of 4 or 5 yr. The disease occurs in localized and generalized forms. There is rapid bone loss, often leading to premature loss of primary teeth. It is often associated with systemic problems, including neutropenia, leukocyte adhesion or migration defects, hypophosphatasia, Papillon-Lefèvre syndrome, leukemia, and histiocytosis X. In many cases, however, there is no apparent underlying medical problem. Nonetheless, diagnostic work-ups are necessary to rule out underlying systemic disease.

Treatment includes aggressive professional teeth cleaning, strategic extraction of affected teeth, and antibiotic therapy. There are few reports of long-term successful treatment to reverse bone loss surrounding primary teeth.

AGGRESSIVE PERIODONTITIS IN ADOLESCENTS (LOCALIZED JUVENILE PERIODONTITIS). Aggressive periodontitis in adolescents is characterized by rapid alveolar bone loss, especially around the permanent incisors and 1st molars. Overall prevalence in the United States is <1%, but the prevalence among African Americans is reportedly 2.5%. This form of periodontitis is associated with a strain of *Actinobacillus* bacteria. In addition, the neutrophils of patients with aggressive periodontitis may have chemotactic or phagocytic defects. If left untreated, affected teeth lose their attachment and may exfoliate. Treatment varies with the degree of involvement. Patients diagnosed at the onset of the disease are usually managed by surgical or nonsurgical debridement in conjunction with antibiotic therapy. Prognosis depends on the degree of initial involvement and compliance with therapy.

TEETHING. Teething can lead to intermittent localized discomfort in the area of erupting primary teeth, irritability, low-grade fevers, and excessive salivation; however, many children have no apparent difficulties. *Treatment of symptoms includes oral analgesics and ice rings for the child to "gum."* Similar manifestations can also arise when the 1st permanent molars erupt at about age 6 yr.

CYCLOSPORINE- OR PHENYTOIN-INDUCED GINGIVAL OVERGROWTH. The use of cyclosporine to suppress organ rejection or phenytoin for anticonvulsant therapy, and in some cases, calcium channel blockers, is associated with generalized enlargement of the gingiva. Phenytoin and its metabolites have a direct stimulatory action on gingival fibroblasts, resulting in accelerated synthesis of collagen. Phenytoin induces less gingival hyperplasia in patients who maintain meticulous oral hygiene.

Gingival hyperplasia occurs in 10–30% of patients treated with phenytoin. Severe manifestations may include (1) gross enlargement of the gingiva, sometimes covering the teeth; (2) edema and erythema of the gingiva; (3) secondary infection, resulting in abscess formation; (4) migration of teeth; and (5) inhibition of exfoliation of primary teeth and subsequent impaction of permanent teeth. Treatment should be directed toward prevention and, if possible, discontinuation of cyclosporine or phenytoin. Patients undergoing long-term treatment with these drugs should receive frequent dental examinations and oral hygiene care. Severe forms of gingival overgrowth are treated by gingivectomy, but the lesion recurs if drug use is continued.

ACUTE PERICORONITIS. Acute inflammation of the flap of gingiva that partially covers the crown of an incompletely erupted tooth is common in mandibular permanent molars. Accumulation of debris and bacteria between the gingival flap and tooth precipitates the inflammatory response. A variant of this condition is a gingival abscess due to entrapment of bacteria because of orthodontic bands or crowns. Trismus and severe pain may be associated with the inflammation. Untreated cases may result in facial space infections and facial cellulitis.

Treatment includes local debridement and irrigation, warm saline rinses, and antibiotic therapy. When the acute phase has subsided, extraction of the tooth or resection of the gingival flap prevents recurrence. Early recognition of the partial impaction of mandibular 3rd molars and their subsequent extraction prevents these areas from developing pericoronitis.

NECROTIZING PERIODONTAL DISEASE (ACUTE NECROTIZING ULCERATIVE GINGIVITIS). Necrotizing periodontal disease, in the past sometimes referred to as "trench mouth," is a distinct periodontal disease associated with oral spirochetes and fusobacteria. It is not clear, however, whether bacteria initiate the disease or are secondary. It rarely develops in healthy children in developed countries, with a prevalence in the United States of <1%, but is seen more frequently in children and adolescents from developing areas of Africa, Asia, and South America. In certain African countries, where affected children usually have protein malnutrition, the lesion may extend into adjacent tissues, causing necrosis of facial structures (cancrum oris, or noma).

Clinical manifestations of necrotizing periodontal disease include (1) necrosis and ulceration of gingiva between the teeth, (2) an adherent grayish pseudomembrane over the affected gingiva, (3) oral malodor, (4) cervical lymphadenopathy, (5) malaise, and (6) fever. The condition may be mistaken for acute herpetic gingivostomatitis. Dark-field microscopy of debris obtained from necrotizing lesions will demonstrate dense spirochete populations.

Treatment of necrotizing periodontal disease is divided into an acute management with local debridement, oxygenating agents (direct application of 10% carbamide peroxide in anhydrous glycerol qid), and analgesics. Dramatic resolution usually occurs within 48 hr. If a patient is febrile, antibiotics (penicillin or metronidazole) may be an important adjunctive therapy. A 2nd phase of treatment may be necessary if the acute phase of the disease has caused irreversible morphologic damage to the periodontium. The disease is not contagious.

Chapter 311 ■ Dental Trauma

Traumatic oral injuries may be categorized into three groups: (1) injuries to teeth, (2) injuries to soft tissue (contusions, abrasions, lacerations, punctures, avulsions, and burns), and (3) injuries to jaw (mandibular or maxillary fractures or both).

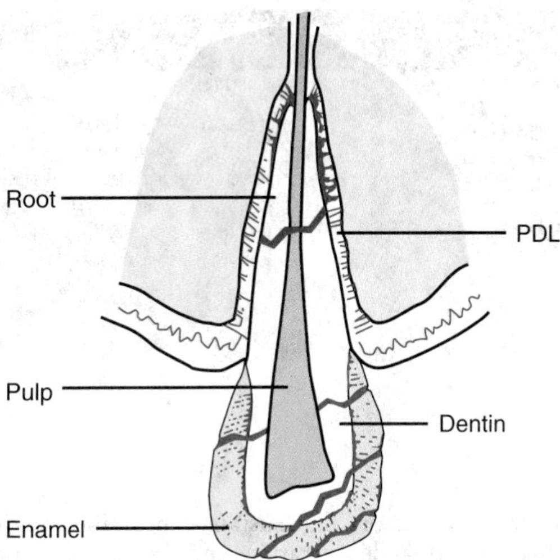

Figure 311-1. Tooth fractures can involve enamel, dentin, or pulp and can occur in the crown or root of a tooth. (From Pinkham JR: *Pediatric Dentistry: Infancy Through Adolescence.* Philadelphia, WB Saunders, 1988, p 172.)

INJURIES TO TEETH. Approximately 10% of children between 18 mo and 18 yr of age will sustain significant tooth trauma. There appear to be three age periods of greatest predilection: (1) toddlers (1–3 yr), usually due to falls or child abuse; (2) school-aged (7–10 yr), usually from bicycle and playground accidents; and (3) adolescents (16–18 yr), often the result of fights, athletic injuries, and automobile accidents. Injuries to teeth are more frequent among children with protruding front teeth. Children with craniofacial abnormalities or neuromuscular deficits are also at increased risk for dental injury. Injuries to teeth may involve the hard dental tissues, the dental pulp (nerve), and injuries to the periodontal structure (surrounding bone and attachment apparatus) [Fig. 311-1 and Table 311-1].

Fractures of teeth may be uncomplicated (confined to the hard dental tissues) or complicated (involving the pulp). Exposure of the pulp will result in its bacterial contamination, which can lead to infection and pulp necrosis. Such pulp exposure complicates therapy and may lower the likelihood of a favorable outcome.

The teeth most often affected are the maxillary incisors. Uncomplicated crown fractures are treated by covering exposed dentin and by placing an aesthetic restoration. Complicated crown fractures usually require **endodontic therapy** (root canal). Crown-root fractures and root fractures usually require extensive dental therapy. Such injuries in the primary dentition can interfere with normal development of the permanent dentition, and, therefore, significant injuries of the primary incisor teeth are usually managed by extraction.

Traumatic oral injuries should be referred to a dentist as soon as possible. Even when the teeth appear intact, a dentist should promptly evaluate the patient. Baseline data (radiographs, mobility patterns, responses to specific stimuli) enable the dentist to assess the likelihood of future complications.

INJURIES TO PERIODONTAL STRUCTURES. Trauma to teeth with associated injury to periodontal structures that hold the teeth usually presents as mobile or displaced teeth. Such injuries are more frequent in the primary than in the permanent dentition. Categories of trauma to the periodontium include (1) concussion, (2) subluxation, (3) intrusive luxation, (4) extrusive luxation, and (5) avulsion.

Concussion. Injuries that produce minor damage to the periodontal ligament are termed concussions. Teeth sustaining such injuries are not mobile or displaced but react markedly to percussion (gentle hitting of the tooth with an instrument). This type of injury usually requires no therapy and resolves without com-

TABLE 311-1. Injuries to Crowns of Teeth

TYPE OF TRAUMA	DESCRIPTION	TREATMENT AND REFERRAL
Enamel infraction (crazing)	Incomplete fracture of enamel without loss of tooth structure	Initially may not require therapy but should be assessed periodically by dentist
Enamel fractures	Fracture of only the tooth enamel	Tooth may be smoothed or treated to replace fragment
Enamel and dentin fracture	Fracture of enamel and dentinal layer of the tooth. Tooth may be sensitive to cold or air. Pulp may become necrotic, leading to periapical abscess.	Refer as soon as possible. Area should be treated to preserve the integrity of the underlying pulp.
Enamel, dentin fracture involving the pulp	Bacterial contamination may lead to pulpal necrosis and periapical abscess. The tooth may have the appearance of bleeding or may display a small red spot.	Refer immediately. The dental therapy of choice depends on the extent of injury, the condition of the pulp, the development of the tooth, time elapsed from injury, and any other injuries to the supporting structures. Therapy is directed toward minimizing contamination in an effort to improve the prognosis.

From Josell SD, Abrams RG: Managing common dental problems and emergencies. *Pediatr Clin North Am* 1991;38:1325–1342.

plication. Primary incisors that sustain concussion may change color, indicating pulpal degeneration, and should be evaluated by a dentist.

Subluxation. Subluxated teeth exhibit mild to moderate horizontal mobility, vertical mobility, or both. Hemorrhage is usually evident around the neck of the tooth at the gingival margin. There is no displacement of the tooth. Many subluxated teeth need to be immobilized by splints to ensure adequate repair of the periodontal ligament. Some of these teeth develop pulp necrosis.

Intrusion. Intruded teeth are pushed up into their socket, sometimes to the point where they are not clinically visible. Intruded primary incisors can give the false appearance of being avulsed (knocked out). To rule out avulsion, a dental radiograph is indicated (Figs. 311-2 and 311-3).

Extrusion. This type of injury is characterized by displacement of the tooth from its socket. The tooth is usually displaced to the lingual (tongue) side, with fracture of the wall of the alveolar socket. These teeth need immediate treatment; the longer the delay, the more likely the tooth will be fixed in its displaced position. Therapy is directed at reduction (repositioning the tooth) and fixation (splinting). In addition, the pulp of such teeth often becomes necrotic and requires endodontic therapy. Extrusive luxation in the primary dentition is usually managed by extraction because complications of reduction and fixation may result in problems with development of permanent teeth.

Avulsion. If avulsed permanent teeth are replanted within 20 min after injury, good success may be achieved; if the delay exceeds 2 hr, however, failure (root resorption, ankylosis) is frequent. The likelihood that normal reattachment will follow replantation of the tooth is related to the viability of the periodontal ligament. Parents confronted with this emergency situation can be instructed to do the following:

1. Find the tooth.
2. Rinse the tooth. (Do not scrub the tooth. Do not touch the root. After plugging the sink drain, hold the tooth by the crown and rinse it under running tap water.)
3. Insert the tooth into the socket. (Gently place it back into its normal position. Do not be concerned if the tooth extrudes slightly. If the parent or child is too apprehensive for replantation of the tooth, the tooth should be placed in cold cow's milk or other cold isotonic solution).
4. Go directly to the dentist. (In transit, the child should hold the tooth in its socket with a finger. The parent should buckle a seatbelt around the child and drive safely.)

After the tooth is replanted, it must be immobilized to facilitate reattachment; endodontic therapy is always required. The initial signs of complications associated with replantation may appear as early as 1 wk post trauma or as late as several years later. Close dental follow-up is indicated for at least 1 yr.

PREVENTION. To minimize the likelihood of dental injuries:

1. Every child or adolescent who engages in contact sports should wear a mouth guard, which may be constructed by a dentist or purchased at any athletic goods store.
2. Helmets with face guards should be worn by children or adolescents with neuromuscular problems or seizure disorders to protect the head and face during falls.
3. Helmets should also be used during biking, roller blading, and skateboarding.
4. All children or adolescents with protruding incisors should be evaluated by a pediatric dentist or orthodontist.

ADDITIONAL CONSIDERATIONS. Children who experience dental trauma may also have sustained head or neck trauma, and, therefore, neurologic assessment is warranted. Tetanus prophylaxis should be considered with any injury that disrupts the integrity of the oral tissues. The possibility of child abuse should always be considered.

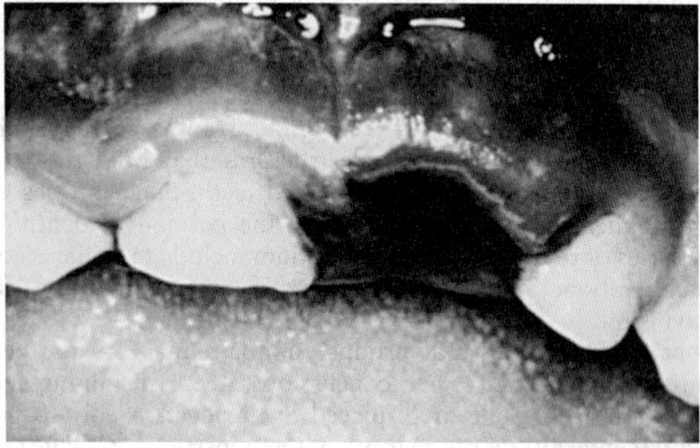

Figure 311-2. Intruded primary incisor that appears avulsed (knocked out).

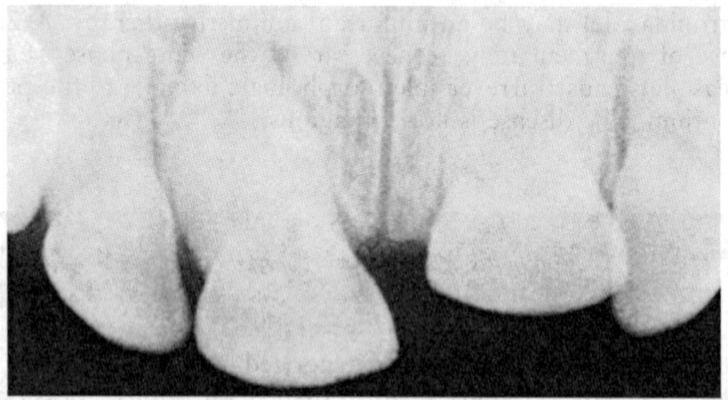

Figure 311-3. Occlusal radiograph documents intrusion of "missing tooth" presented in Figure 311-2.

Chapter 312 ■ Common Lesions of the Oral Soft Tissues

OROPHARYNGEAL CANDIDIASIS (See Chapter 231.1). Oropharyngeal infection with *Candida albicans* (thrush, moniliasis) is common in neonates from contact with the organism in the birth canal or breast. The lesions of oropharyngeal candidiasis (OPC) appear as white plaques covering all or part of the oropharyngeal mucosa. These plaques are removable from the underlying surface, which is characteristically inflamed with pinpoint hemorrhages. The diagnosis is confirmed by direct microscopic examination on potassium hydroxide smears and culture of scrapings from lesions. OPC is usually self-limited in the healthy newborn infant, but treatment with nystatin will hasten recovery and reduce the risk of the infection spreading to other infants. Persistent infections should be treated with fluconazole therapy.

OPC is also a major problem during myelosuppressive therapy. **Systemic candidiasis** (SC), a major cause of morbidity and mortality during myelosuppressive therapy, develops almost exclusively in patients who have had prior oropharyngeal, esophageal, or intestinal candidiasis. This observation implies that prevention of OPC should reduce the incidence of SC. The use of a multiagent regimen, 0.2% chlorhexidine solution and fluconazole, for OPC prophylaxis in children receiving bone marrow transplants may be effective in preventing OPC, SC, or candidal esophagitis.

APHTHOUS ULCERS. The aphthous ulcer (canker sore) is a distinct oral lesion, prone to recurrence. The differential diagnosis is noted in Table 312-1. Aphthous ulcers are reported to develop in 20% of the population. Their etiology is unclear, but infectious causes, such as *Helicobacter pylori,* herpes simplex virus, and even measles, have been implicated. Clinically, these ulcers are characterized by well-circumscribed, ulcerative lesions with a white necrotic base surrounded by a red halo. The lesions last 10–14 days and heal without scarring. Expensive prescription medications appear to offer little advantage over readily available over-the-counter palliative therapies.

HERPETIC GINGIVOSTOMATITIS (See Chapter 249). After an initial incubation period of ≈1 wk, the initial infection with herpes simplex virus manifests as fever and malaise. The oral cavity may show various expressions, including the gingiva becoming erythematous and clusters of small vesicles erupting throughout the mouth. The symptoms usually regress within 2 wk without scarring. Fluids should be encouraged because the child may become dehydrated. Analgesics and anesthetic rinses may make the child more comfortable. Oral acyclovir is beneficial in shortening the duration of symptoms. Caution should be exercised to prevent autoinoculation or transmission of infection to the eyes.

TABLE 312-1. Differential Diagnosis of Oral Ulceration

CONDITION	COMMENT
COMMON	
Aphthous (canker sore)	Painful, circumscribed lesions
Traumatic	Accidents, chronic cheek biter, or after dental local anesthesia
Hand, foot, mouth disease	Painful, lesions on tongue, anterior oral cavity, hands, and feet
Herpangina	Painful, lesions confined to soft palate and oropharynx
Herpetic gingivostomatitis	Vesicles on mucocutaneous borders; painful, febrile
Recurrent herpes labialis	Vesicles on lips; painful
Chemical burns	Alkali, acid, aspirin; painful
Heat burns	Hot food, electrical
UNCOMMON	
Neutrophil defects	Agranulocytosis, leukemia, cyclic neutropenia; painful
Systemic lupus erythematosus	Recurrent, may be painless
Behçet's syndrome	Resembles aphthous lesions; associated with genital ulcers, uveitis
Necrotizing ulcerative gingivostomatitis	Vincent stomatitis; painful
Syphilis	Chancre or gumma; painless
Oral Crohn disease	Aphthous-like; painful
Histoplasmosis	Lingual
Recurrent fever syndromes	See Chapter 162.

RECURRENT HERPES LABIALIS. Approximately 90% of the population develops antibodies to herpes simplex virus. In periods of quiescence, the virus is thought to remain latent in sensory neurons. Unlike primary herpetic gingivostomatitis, which manifests as multiple painful vesicles on the lips, tongue, palate, gingiva, and mucosa, recurrent herpes is generally limited to the lips. Other than the annoyance of causing pain and an unattractive appearance, there are generally no systemic symptoms. Reactivation of the virus is thought to be the result of exposure to ultraviolet light, tissue trauma, stress, or fevers. There is little advantage of antiviral therapy over palliative therapies in an otherwise healthy patient affected by recurrent herpes.

BOHN NODULES. Bohn nodules are small developmental anomalies located along the buccal and lingual aspects of the mandibular and maxillary ridges and in the hard palate of the neonate. These lesions arise from remnants of mucous gland tissue. Treatment is not necessary, as the nodules disappear within a few weeks.

DENTAL LAMINA CYSTS. Dental lamina cysts are small cystic lesions located along the crest of the mandibular and maxillary ridges of the neonate. These lesions arise from epithelial remnants of the dental lamina. Treatment is not necessary; they will disappear within a few weeks.

FORDYCE GRANULES. Almost 80% of adults have multiple yellow-white granules in clusters or plaquelike areas on the oral mucosa, most commonly on the buccal mucosa or lips. They are aberrant sebaceous glands. The glands are present at birth, but they may hypertrophy and 1st appear as discrete yellowish papules during the preadolescent period in ≈50% of children. No treatment is necessary.

PARULIS. The parulis (gum boil) is a soft reddish papule located adjacent to the root of a chronically abscessed tooth. It occurs at the end-point of a draining dental sinus tract. Treatment consists of diagnosing which tooth is abscessed and extracting it or performing root canal on the offending tooth.

CHEILITIS. This dryness of the lips followed by scaling and cracking and accompanied by a characteristic burning sensation is common in children. Cheilitis is usually caused by sensitivity to contact substances (from toys and foods) plus photosensitivity to the sun's rays. It is aggravated by the alternation of wetting with the tongue and drying by the wind, especially in cold weather. Cheilitis often occurs in association with fever. Frequent application of petroleum jelly facilitates healing and is also preventive.

ANKYLOGLOSSIA. Ankyloglossia or "tongue-tie" is characterized by an abnormally short lingual frenum that may hinder the tongue movement but rarely interferes with feeding or speech. The frenum may spontaneously lengthen as the child gets older. If the extent of the ankyloglossia is severe, speech may be affected and surgical correction indicated.

GEOGRAPHIC TONGUE. Geographic tongue (migratory glossitis) is a benign and asymptomatic lesion and is characterized by one or more smooth, bright red patches, often showing a yellow, gray, or white membranous margin on the dorsum of an otherwise normally roughened tongue. The condition has no known cause and no treatment is indicated (see Chapter 663).

FISSURED TONGUE. The fissured tongue (scrotal tongue) is a malformation manifested clinically by numerous small furrows or grooves on the dorsal surface (see Chapter 663). If the tongue is painful, brushing the tongue or irrigating with water can reduce the bacteria in the fissures.

Chapter 313 ■ Diseases of the Salivary Glands and Jaws

With the exception of mumps (see Chapter 245), disease of the salivary glands is rare in children. Bilateral enlargement of the submaxillary glands can occur in AIDS, cystic fibrosis, Epstein-Barr virus infection, and malnutrition and, transiently, during acute asthmatic attacks. Chronic vomiting can be accompanied by enlargement of the parotid glands. Benign salivary gland hypertrophy has been associated with endocrinopathies: thyroid disease, diabetes, and disorders of the pituitary-adrenal axis.

RECURRENT PAROTITIS. Recurrent idiopathic swelling of the parotid gland can occur in otherwise healthy children. The swelling is usually unilateral, but both glands can be involved simultaneously or alternately. There is little pain; the swelling is limited to the gland and usually lasts 2–3 wk. The incidence appears to be higher in the spring.

SUPPURATIVE PAROTITIS. This is usually due to *Staphylococcus aureus* and can be primary or a complication of parotitis from another cause. It is usually unilateral and may be accompanied by fever. The gland becomes swollen, tender, and painful. Suppurative parotitis responds to appropriate antibacterial therapy based on culture obtained from the Stensen duct or by surgical drainage, which is infrequently required.

RANULA. This is a cyst associated with a major salivary gland in the sublingual area. A ranula is a large, soft, mucus-containing swelling in the floor of the mouth. It occurs at any age, including infancy. The cyst should be excised, and the severed duct should be exteriorized.

MUCOCELE. This is a salivary gland lesion caused by a blockage of a salivary gland duct. It is most common on the lower lip and has the appearance of a fluid-filled vesicle or a fluctuant nodule with the overlying mucosa normal in color. Treatment is surgical excision, with removal of the involved accessory salivary gland.

CONGENITAL LIP PITS. These are caused by fistulous tracts that lead to embedded mucous glands in the lower lip. They leak saliva, especially with salivary stimulation. Lip pits can be isolated anomalies, or they can be found in patients with cleft lip or palate. Treatment is surgical excision of the glandular tissue.

ERUPTION CYST. This is a smooth, painless swelling over the erupting tooth. If bleeding occurs in the cyst space, it may appear blue or blue-black. In most cases, no treatment is indicated and the cyst resolves with the full eruption of the tooth.

XEROSTOMIA. Also known as dry mouth, xerostomia may be associated with fever, dehydration, anticholinergic drugs, chronic graft versus host disease, Mikulicz disease (leukemia infiltrates), Sjögren syndrome, or tumoricidal doses of radiation when the salivary glands are within the field. Long-term xerostomia is a high-risk factor for dental caries.

SALIVARY GLAND TUMORS. See Chapter 500.

HISTIOCYTOSIS X (See Chapter 507). The etiology and pathogenesis of histiocytosis remains obscure. In the severe form, there are oral lesions with pain, swelling, gingival necrosis, and destruction of alveolar bone, resulting in premature exfoliation of teeth. Treatment varies according to the extent of the disease, with surgical curettage or radiation therapy being used to treat the focal disease. Multiagent chemotherapy and bone marrow transplantation may be needed to treat disseminated multiorgan disease.

TUMORS OF THE JAW. **Ossifying fibroma** is a common benign tumor of the jaw. It is often asymptomatic, being discovered on routine radiographic examinations. Treatment is enucleation or curettage. **Central giant cell granuloma** is another common lesion thought to be reactive rather than neoplastic. Although usually asymptomatic, it can be expansile, with or without divergence of teeth. Treatment is complete curettage or surgical excision. **Dentigerous cysts** are common lesions associated with the crown of an impacted or unerupted tooth. Although usually asymptomatic, they can become large and destructive. Treatment is surgical removal.

The malignant primary tumors of the jaw in children include Burkitt lymphoma, osteogenic sarcoma, lymphosarcoma, ameloblastoma, and, more rarely, fibrosarcoma.

Chapter 314 ■ Diagnostic Radiology in Dental Assessment

The **panoramic radiograph** provides a single tomographic image of the upper and lower jaw, including all the teeth and supporting structures. The x-ray tube rotates about the patient's head with reciprocal movement of the film or image receptor during the exposure. The panoramic image shows the mandibular bodies, rami, and condyles; maxillary sinuses; and a majority of the facial buttresses. Such images are used to show abnormalities of tooth number, development and eruption pattern, cystic and neoplastic lesions, bone infections, fracture, as well as dental caries and periodontal disease (Fig. 314-1).

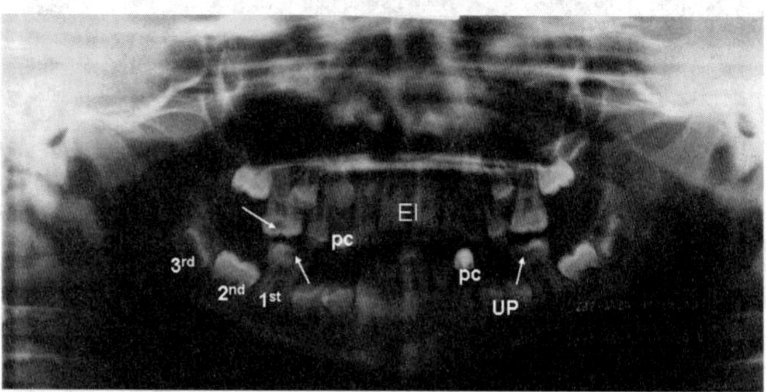

Figure 314-1. A panoramic radiograph of a 10 yr old child showing extensive dental caries of the 1st permanent molars *(arrows)*, as well as normal structures: erupted 1st permanent molar, unerupted 2nd molar, and unerupted 3rd molar; erupted incisors *(EI)*, unerupted permolars *(UP)*, and erupted primary canines *(pc)*.

Cephalometric radiographs are posteroanterior and lateral skull films that are taken using a **cephalostat** (head positioner) and employ techniques that clearly demonstrate the facial skeleton and soft facial tissues. Similar protocols for positioning children are used throughout the world. From these images, cranial and facial points and planes can be determined and compared with standards derived from thousands of images. A child's facial growth can be assessed serially when cephalometric radiographs are taken sequentially. Relationships among the maxilla, mandible, cranial base, and facial skeleton can be determined in a quantitative manner. Additionally, the alignment of the teeth and the relation of the teeth to the supporting bone can be serially measured.

Intraoral dental radiographs are highly detailed, direct exposure films that demonstrate sections of the child's teeth and supporting bone structures. The film or image receptor is placed lingual to the teeth, and the x-ray beam is directed through the teeth and supporting structures. The resulting images are used to detect dental caries, loss of alveolar bone (periodontal disease), abscesses at the roots of the teeth, and trauma to the teeth and alveolar bone and to demonstrate the developmental status of permanent teeth within the bone.

Andreasen JO, Andreasen FM: *Essentials of Traumatic Injuries to the Teeth.* Copenhagen, Munksgaard, 1990.

Bellinger DC, Trachtenberg F, Barregard L, et al: Neuropsychological and renal effects of dental amalgam in children. *JAMA* 2006;295:1775–1782.

Califano JV; American Academy of Periodontology Research, Science and Therapy Committee: Position paper: Periodontal diseases of children and adolescents. *J Periodontol* 2003;74:1696–1704.

Davidkin I, Jokinen S, Paananen A, et al: Etiology of mumps-like illnesses in children and adolescents vaccinated for measles, mumps, and rubella. *J Infect Dis* 2005;191:719–723.

Denny AD, Amm C: New techniques for airway correction in neonates with severe Pierre Robin sequence. *J Pediatr* 2005;147:97–101.

De Rouen TA, Martin MD, Leroux BG, et al: Neurobehavioral effects of dental amalgam in children. *JAMA* 2006;295:1784–1792.

Flaitz CM: Oral pathologic conditions and soft tissue anomalies. In Pinkham JR (editor): *Pediatric Dentistry: Infancy Through Adolescence,* 3rd ed. Philadelphia, WB Saunders, 1999, p 12.

Griffen AL (editor): Pediatric oral health. *Pediatr Clin North Am* 2000; 47.

Hale KJ; American Academy of Pediatrics Section on Pediatric Dentistry: Oral health risk assessment timing and establishment of the dental home. *Pediatrics* 2003;111:1113–1116.

Lin YTJ, Lu PW: Retrospective study of pediatric facial cellulitis of odontogenic origin. *Pediatr Infect Dis J* 2006;25:339–342.

Nelson LP, Shusterman S: Emergency management of oral trauma in children. *Curr Opin Pediatr* 1997;9:242–245.

Scully C: Aphthous ulceration. *N Engl J Med* 2006;355:165–172.

Selwitz RH, Ismail AI, Pitts NB: Dental caries. *Lancet* 2007;369:51–58.

Sonis A, Zaragoza S: Dental health for the pediatrician. *Curr Opin Pediatr* 2001;13:289–295.

Tinanoff N, Kanellis MJ, Vargas CM: Current understanding of epidemiology, mechanisms, and prevention of dental caries in preschool children. *Pediatr Dent* 2002;24:543–551.

Section 3 — The Esophagus

Chapter 315 ■ Embryology, Anatomy, and Function of the Esophagus

Susan Orenstein, John Peters, Seema Khan, Nader Youssef, and Sunny Zaheed Hussain

The esophagus is a hollow muscular tube, separated from the pharynx above and the stomach below by two tonically closed sphincters. Its primary function is to convey ingested material from the mouth to the stomach. Largely lacking digestive glands and enzymes, and exposed only briefly to nutrients, it has no active role in digestion.

EMBRYOLOGY. The esophagus develops from the postpharyngeal foregut and can be distinguished from the stomach in the 4 wk old embryo. At the same time, the trachea begins to bud just anterior to the developing esophagus; the resulting laryngotracheal groove extends and becomes the lung. Disturbance of this stage may result in congenital anomalies such as **tracheoesophageal fistula.** The length of the esophagus is 8–10 cm at birth, and doubles in the 1st 2–3 yr of life, reaching ≈25 cm in an adult. The abdominal portion of the esophagus is as large as the stomach in an 8 wk old fetus but gradually shortens to a few mm at birth, attaining a final length of ≈3 cm by a few years of age. This intra-abdominal location of both the distal esophagus and the lower esophageal sphincter (LES) is an important antireflux mechanism, because increases in intra-abdominal pressure are also transmitted to the sphincter, augmenting its defense. Swallowing can be seen in utero as early as 16–20 wk of gestation, helping to circulate the amniotic fluid; **polyhydramnios** is, thus, a hallmark of lack of normal swallowing or of esophageal or upper gastrointestinal tract obstruction. Sucking and swallowing are not fully coordinated before 34 wk of gestation, a contributing factor for feeding difficulties in premature infants.

ANATOMY. The luminal aspect of the esophagus is covered by thick, protective, nonkeratinized stratified squamous epithelium, which abruptly changes to simple columnar epithelium at the stomach's upper margin at the **gastroesophageal junction (GEJ).** This squamous epithelium is relatively resistant to damage by gastric secretions (in contrast to the ciliated columnar epithelium of the respiratory tract), but chronic irritation by gastric contents may result in morphometric changes and subsequent metaplasia of the cells lining the lower esophagus from squamous to columnar. Deeper layers of the esophageal wall are composed successively of lamina propria, muscularis mucosae, submucosa, and the two layers of muscularis propria (circular surrounded by longitudinal). The two delimiting sphincters of the esophagus, the **upper esophageal sphincter** (UES) at the cricopharyngeus muscle and the **LES** at the **GEJ,** constrict the esophageal lumen at its proximal and distal boundaries. The muscularis propria of the upper third of the esophagus is predominantly striated, and that of the lower two thirds is smooth muscle. Clinical conditions involving striated muscle (cricopharyngeal dysfunction, cerebral palsy) affect the upper esophagus, whereas those involving smooth muscle (achalasia, reflux esophagitis) affect the lower esophagus. The muscular LES and the mucosal "Z-line" of the GEJ may be discrepant up to several cm.

FUNCTION. The esophagus can be divided into three areas: the UES, the esophageal body, and the LES. At rest, the tonic LES pressure is normally ≈20 mm Hg; values <10 mm Hg are usually considered abnormal, although it seems that competence against retrograde flow of gastric material is maintained if the LES pressure is >5 mm Hg. The LES pressure rises during intragastric pressure amplifications, whether caused by gastric contractions, abdominal wall muscle contractions ("straining"), or external pressure applied to the abdominal wall. It also rises in response to cholinergic stimuli, gastrin, gastric alkalization, and certain drugs (bethanechol, metoclopramide, cisapride). The UES pressure is more variable and often higher than that of the LES; it decreases almost to zero during deep sleep but increases markedly during stress and straining.

Swallowing is initiated by elevation of the tongue, propelling the bolus into the pharynx. The larynx elevates and moves anteriorly, pulling open the relaxing UES, while the opposed aryepiglottic folds close. The epiglottis drops back to cover the larynx and direct the bolus over the larynx and into the UES. The soft palate occludes the nasopharynx. The primary peristalsis thus initiated is a contraction originating in the oropharynx that clears the esophagus aborally (Fig. 315-1). The LES, tonically contracted as a barrier against gastroesophageal reflux, relaxes as swallowing is initiated, at nearly the same time as the UES relaxation. The LES relaxation persists considerably longer, until the peristaltic wave traverses it and closes it. The normal esophageal peristaltic speed is ≈3 cm/sec; the wave takes at least 4 sec to traverse the 12 cm esophagus of a young infant and considerably longer in a larger child. Facial stimulation by a puff of air can induce swallowing and esophageal peristalsis in healthy young infants, comprising a reflex termed the **Santmyer swallow.**

In addition to relaxing to move swallowed material past the GEJ into the stomach, the LES normally relaxes to vent swallowed air or to allow retrograde expulsion of material from the stomach. Perhaps as an extension of these functions, the normal LES also permits physiologic reflux episodes, brief events that occur approximately five times in the 1st postprandial hour, particularly in the awake state, but are otherwise uncommon. **Transient LES relaxation,** not associated with swallowing, comprises the major mechanism underlying **pathologic reflux** (see Fig. 315-1).

The close linkage of the anatomy of the upper digestive and respiratory tracts has mandated intricate functional protections of the respiratory tract during retrograde movement of gastric contents as well as during swallowing. The protective functions include the LES tone, the bolstering of the LES by the surrounding diaphragmatic crura, and the "backup protection" of the UES tone. Secondary peristalsis, akin to primary peristalsis but without an oral component, also clears refluxed gastric contents from the esophagus. Another protective reflex is the "pharyngeal swallow" (initiated above the esophagus, but without lingual participation). Multiple levels of protection against aspiration include the rhythmic coordination of swallowing and breathing as well as a series of protective reflexes with esophagopharyngeal afferents and efferents that close the UES or larynx. These reflexes include the esophago-UES contractile reflex, the pharyngo-UES contractile reflex, the esophagoglottal closure reflex, and two pharyngoglottal adduction reflexes. The latter two reflexes have chemoreceptors on the laryngeal surface of the epiglottis and mechanoreceptors on the aryepiglottic folds as their sites of stimulus. It is likely that interactions between the esophagus and the respiratory tract, which cause extraesophageal manifestations of gastroesophageal reflux disease, will be explained by subtle abnormalities in these protective reflexes.

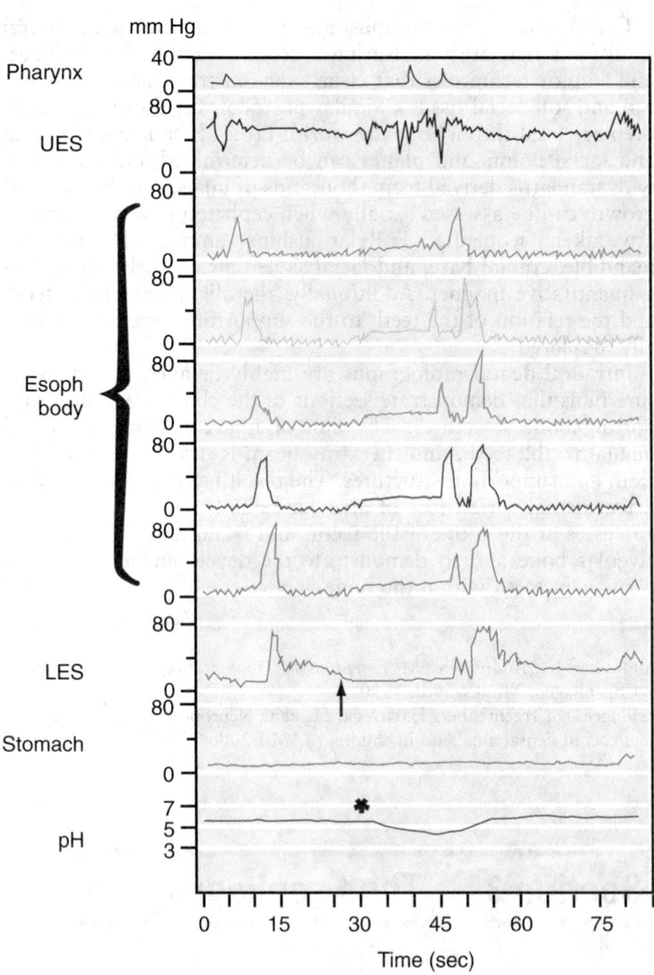

Figure 315-1. A continuous tracing of esophageal motility showing two swallows, as indicated by the pharyngeal contraction associated with relaxation of the upper esophageal sphincter (UES) and followed by peristalsis in the body of the esophagus. The lower esophageal sphincter (LES) also displays a transient relaxation *(arrow)* unassociated with a swallow. There is an episode of gastroesophageal reflux *(*)* recorded by a pH probe at the time of the transient LES relaxation. (Courtesy of John Dent, FRACP, PhD, and Geoffrey Davidson, MD.)

315.1 • Common Clinical Manifestations and Diagnostic Aids

COMMON CLINICAL MANIFESTATIONS. Manifestations of esophageal disease can be categorized as pain, obstruction or difficulty swallowing, abnormal retrograde movement of gastric contents (reflux, regurgitation, or vomiting), or bleeding; esophageal disease can also engender respiratory symptoms. Pain in the chest unrelated to swallowing (**"heartburn"**) can be a sign of esophagitis, but similar pain may also represent cardiac, pulmonary, or musculoskeletal disease. Pain during swallowing (**odynophagia**) localizes the disease more discretely to the pharynx and esophagus and often represents inflammatory mucosal disease. Complete esophageal obstruction can be produced acutely by esophageal foreign bodies, including food impactions; be congenital, as in esophageal atresia; or evolve over time as a peptic stricture occludes the esophagus. Difficulty swallowing (**dysphagia**) can be produced by incompletely occlusive esophageal obstruction (by extrinsic compression, intrinsic narrowing, or foreign bodies) but can also result from dysmotility of the esophagus (whether primary/idiopathic or secondary to systemic disease). Inflammatory lesions of the esophagus without obstruction or dysmotility are a 3rd cause of dysphagia; eosinophilic esophagitis, most often afflicting older male children, is relatively common. The most common esophageal disorder in children is **gastroesophageal reflux disease (GERD)**, which is retrograde return of gastric contents. Esophagitis can be caused by GERD, by eosinophilic disease, by infection, or by caustic substances. Esophageal **bleeding** can result from severe esophagitis that produces erosions or ulcerations and can manifest as anemia or hemoccult-positive stools. More acute or severe bleeding can be due to ruptured **esophageal varices.** The resulting hematemesis must be differentiated from more distal bleeding (gastric ulcer) and from more proximal bleeding (a nosebleed or hemoptysis). Respiratory symptoms of esophageal disease may result from luminal contents incorrectly being directed into the respiratory tract or to reflexive respiratory responses to esophageal stimuli.

DIAGNOSTIC AIDS. The esophagus can be evaluated by radiography, endoscopy, histology, scintigraphy, manometry, pH-metry (linked as indicated with other polysomnography), and intraluminal impedance. Contrast (usually barium) radiographic study of the esophagus usually incorporates fluoroscopic imaging over time so that motility, as well as anatomy, can be assessed. Although most often requested to evaluate for GERD, it is neither sensitive nor specific for this purpose; however, it can detect complications of GERD (stricture or hiatal hernia) or conditions mimicking GERD (pyloric stenosis or malrotation with intermittent volvulus). Barium fluoroscopy is optimal for evaluating for structural anomalies, such as duplications, strictures, or external esophageal compression by an aberrant blood vessel, or for causes of dysmotility, such as achalasia. Modifications of the routine barium fluoroscopic study are used in special situations. When an "H-type" tracheoesophageal fistula is suspected, the test is most sensitive if the radiologist, with the patient prone, distends the esophagus with barium via a nasogastric tube. The videofluoroscopic evaluation of swallowing performed with varying consistencies of barium ("modified barium swallow," oropharyngeal videoesophagogram, or "cookie swallow") optimally evaluates children with dysphagia by demonstrating incoordination of the pharyngeal and esophageal phases of swallowing and any associated aspiration. In some centers, fiberoptic endoscopic evaluation of swallowing (FEES) uses nasopharyngeal endoscopy to visualize the pharynx and larynx during swallowing of dye-enhanced foods when dysphagia, laryngeal penetration, or aspiration are suspected. This is often combined with sensory testing (ST) of the laryngeal adductor reflex in response to a calibrated puff of air through the endoscope to the arytenoids, generating the composite FEESST that examines the mechanisms of any aspiration that is present. Endoscopy allows direct visualization of esophageal mucosa and helps therapeutically in the removal of foreign bodies and treatment of esophageal varices. Endoscopy also allows biopsy samples to be taken, thus improving the diagnosis of "endoscopy-negative" GERD, differentiating GERD from eosinophilic esophagitis, and identifying viral or fungal causes of esophagitis. Radionuclide scintigraphy scans are helpful in evaluating the efficiency of peristalsis and demonstrating reflux episodes. They can be specific, although not very sensitive, for aspiration and can quantify gastric emptying, thus hinting at a cause for GERD. The related radionuclide salivagram can demonstrate aspiration of even minute amounts of saliva. Esophageal manometry evaluates for dysmotility from the pharynx to the stomach; by synchronized quantitative pressure measurements along the esophagus, it detects and characterizes dysfunctions sometimes missed radiographically. Manometry is often challenging in young infants, and sphincters are optimally evaluated with special Dent sleeves, rather than the simple ports available for the esophageal body. Extended pH monitoring of the distal esophagus is a sensitive test for acidic GER episodes that can quantify duration and degree of acidity, but not volume of the reflux episodes. It is linked with polysomnography (a "pneumogram") when GER is suspected to cause apnea or similar symptoms. Intraluminal electric impedance is a method for pH-independent detection of bolus movements in the esophagus; with a pH probe incorporated, it can distinguish between acid and nonacid liquid and gaseous reflux.

Shaker R, Hogan WJ: Reflex-mediated enhancement of airway protective mechanisms. *Am J Med* 2000;108:8S–14S.

Chapter 316 ■ Congenital Anomalies: Esophageal Atresia and Tracheoesophageal Fistula

Susan Orenstein, John Peters, Seema Khan, Nader Youssef, and Sunny Zaheed Hussain

Esophageal atresia (EA) is the most frequent congenital anomaly of the esophagus, affecting ≈1/4,000 neonates. Of these, >90% have an associated tracheoesophageal fistula (TEF). In the most common form of EA, the upper esophagus ends in a blind pouch and the TEF is connected to the distal esophagus. The types of EA and TEF and their relative frequencies are shown in Figure 316-1. This defect has survival rates of >90%, owing largely to improved neonatal intensive care, earlier recognition, and appropriate intervention. Infants weighing <1,500 g at birth have the highest risk for mortality. Fifty percent of infants are nonsyndromic without other anomalies while the rest have associated anomalies, most often associated with the VATER/VACTERL (vertebral, anorectal, [cardiac], tracheal, esophageal, renal,

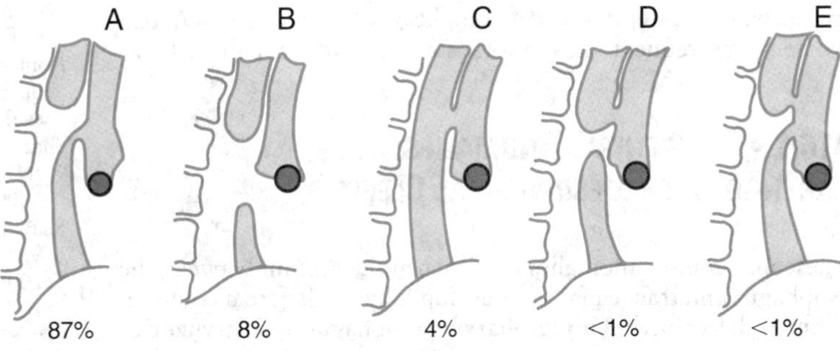

Figure 316-1. Diagrams of the five most commonly encountered forms of esophageal atresia and tracheoesophageal fistula, shown in order of frequency.

radial, [limb]) syndrome. These syndromes should be associated with normal intelligence. Despite low concordance among twins and the low incidence of familial cases, genetic factors have a role in the pathogenesis of TEF in some patients as suggested by discrete mutations in syndromic cases: Feingold syndrome *(N-MYC)*, CHARGE syndrome *(CHD7)* and anophthalmia-esophageal-genital syndrome *(SOX2)*.

PRESENTATION. The neonate with EA typically has frothing and bubbling at the mouth and nose after birth as well as episodes of coughing, cyanosis, and respiratory distress. Feeding exacerbates these symptoms, causes regurgitation, and may precipitate aspiration. Aspiration of gastric contents via a distal fistula causes more damaging pneumonitis than aspiration of pharyngeal secretions from the blind upper pouch. The infant with an isolated TEF in the absence of EA ("H-type" fistula) may come to medical attention later in life with chronic respiratory problems, including refractory bronchospasm and recurrent pneumonias.

DIAGNOSIS. In the setting of early-onset respiratory distress, the inability to pass a nasogastric or orogastric tube in the newborn is suggestive of esophageal atresia. Maternal polyhydramnios may alert the physician to EA. Plain radiography in the evaluation of respiratory distress may reveal a coiled feeding tube in the esophageal pouch and/or an air-distended stomach indicating the presence of a coexisting TEF (Fig. 316-2). Conversely, pure EA may present as an airless, scaphoid abdomen. In isolated TEF, an esophagogram with contrast medium injected under pressure may demonstrate the defect. Alternatively, the orifice may be detected at bronchoscopy or when methylene blue dye injected into the endotracheal tube during endoscopy is observed in the esophagus during forced inspiration.

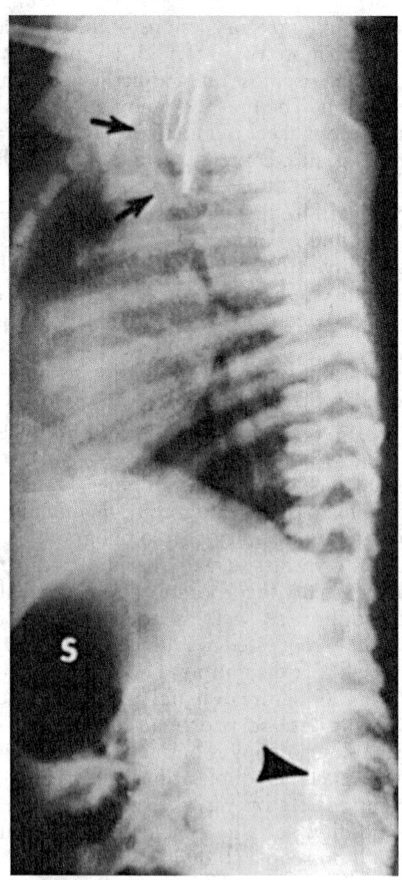

Figure 316-2. Tracheoesophageal fistula. Lateral radiograph demonstrating a nasogastric tube coiled *(arrows)* in the proximal segment of an atretic esophagus. The distal fistula is suggested by gaseous dilatation of the stomach *(S)* and small intestine. The *arrowhead* depicts vertebral fusion, whereas a heart murmur and cardiomegaly suggest the presence of a ventricular septal defect. This patient demonstrated elements of the VATER (vertebral, anorectal, tracheal, esophageal, renal, radial) anomalad. (From Balfe D, Ling D, Siegel M: The esophagus. In Putman CE, Ravin CE [editors]: *Textbook of Diagnostic Imaging*. Philadelphia, WB Saunders, 1988.)

MANAGEMENT. Initially, maintaining a patent airway and preventing aspiration of secretions are paramount. Prone positioning minimizes movement of gastric secretions into a distal fistula, and esophageal suctioning minimizes aspiration from a blind pouch. Endotracheal intubation with mechanical ventilation is to be avoided if possible because it may worsen distention of abdominal viscera. Surgical ligation of the TEF and primary end-to-end anastomosis of the esophagus are performed when feasible. In the premature or otherwise complicated infant, a primary closure may be delayed by temporizing with fistula ligation and gastrostomy tube placement. If the gap between the atretic ends of the esophagus is >3–4 cm, primary repair cannot be done; options include using gastric, jejunal, or colonic segments interposed as a neo-esophagus. Careful search must be undertaken for the common associated cardiac and other anomalies.

OUTCOME. The majority of infants grow up to lead normal lives, but complications are frequently challenging, particularly during infancy. Complications of surgery include anastomotic leak, refistulization, and anastomotic stricture. Gastroesophageal reflux disease (GERD), resulting from intrinsic abnormalities of esophageal function, often combined with delayed gastric emptying, contributes to management challenges in many cases. GERD contributes significantly to the respiratory disease (**reactive airway disease**) that often complicates EA and TEF and also worsens the frequent anastomotic strictures after repair of EA.

316.1 • Congenital Anomalies: Laryngotracheoesophageal Clefts

These uncommon anomalies result when the septum between the esophagus and trachea fails to develop fully, leading to a common channel defect between the pharyngoesophagus and laryngotracheal lumen, thus making the laryngeal closure incompetent during swallowing or reflux. Early in life, the infant presents with stridor, choking, cyanosis, aspiration of feedings, and recurrent chest infections. The diagnosis is difficult and usually requires direct endoscopic visualization of the larynx and esophagus. When contrast radiography is used, material is often seen in the esophagus and trachea. Treatment is surgical repair, which can be complex if the defects are long.

Adzick NS, Nance ML: Pediatric surgery: I. *N Engl J Med* 2000;342:1651–1657.

Carr MM, Clark KD, Webber E, et al: Congenital laryngotracheoesophageal cleft. *J Otolaryngol* 1999;28:112–117.

Romeo C, Bonanno N, Baldari S, et al: Gastric motility disorders in patients operated on for esophageal atresia and tracheoesophageal fistula: Long-term evaluation. *J Pediatr Surg* 2000;35:740–744.

Sharma AK, Shekhawat NS, Agrawal LD, et al: Esophageal atresia and tracheoesophageal fistula: A review of 25 years' experience. *Pediatr Surg Int* 2000;16:478–482.

Shaw-Smith C: Oesophageal atresia, tracheo-oesophageal fistula and the VACTERL association: review of genetics and epidemiology. *J Med Genet* 2006;43:545–554.

Chapter 317 ■ Obstructing and Motility Disorders of the Esophagus

Susan Orenstein, John Peters, Seema Khan, Nader Youssef, and Sunny Zaheed Hussain

Obstructing lesions classically produce **dysphagia** to **solids** earlier and more noticeably than to liquids and may manifest when the infant liquid diet begins to incorporate solids; this is in contrast to **dysphagia** from **dysmotility,** in which swallowing of liquids is affected as early as, or earlier than, solids. In most instances of dysphagia, evaluation begins with fluoroscopy, which may include videofluoroscopic evaluation of swallowing, particularly if aspiration is a primary symptom. Secondary studies are often endoscopic, if intrinsic obstruction is suspected; manometric, if dysmotility is suspected; and other imaging studies in particular cases. Congenital lesions may require surgery, whereas webs and peptic strictures may respond adequately to endoscopic (or bougie) dilation. Peptic strictures, once dilated, should prompt consideration of fundoplication for ongoing prophylaxis.

EXTRINSIC. **Esophageal duplication cysts** comprise the most frequently encountered foregut duplications. These cysts are lined by intestinal epithelium, have a well-developed smooth muscle wall, and are attached to the normal gastrointestinal tract. Two thirds occur on the right side of the esophagus. The most common presentation is respiratory distress caused by compression of the adjacent airways. Dysphagia is a common symptom in older children. Upper gastrointestinal bleeding can occur as a result of acid-secreting gastric mucosa in the duplication wall. **Neuroenteric cysts** may contain glial elements and are associated with **vertebral anomalies.** Diagnosis is made on either barium swallow or chest CT. Treatment is surgical; laparoscopic approach to excision is also possible.

Enlarged mediastinal or subcarinal **lymph nodes,** caused by infection (tuberculosis, histoplasmosis) or neoplasm (lymphoma), are the most common external masses that compress the esophagus and produce obstructive symptoms. **Vascular anomalies** can also compress the esophagus; *dysphagia lusoria* is a term denoting the dysphagia produced by a developmental vascular anomaly, which is often an aberrant right subclavian artery or right-sided or double aortic arch (see Chapter 432.1).

INTRINSIC. Intrinsic narrowing of the esophageal lumen can be congenital or acquired. The etiology is suggested by the location, the character of the lesion, and the clinical situation. The lower esophagus is the most common location for peptic strictures, which are generally somewhat ragged and several cm long. Thin membranous rings, including the Schatzki ring at the squamo-columnar junction, can also occlude this area. In the mid esophagus, congenital narrowing may be associated with the esophageal atresia/tracheoesophageal fistula complex, in which some of the lesions may incorporate cartilage and be impossible to dilate safely; alternatively, reflux esophagitis may induce a ragged and extensive narrowing that appears more proximal than the usual peptic stricture, often because of an associated hiatal hernia. Congenital webs or rings can narrow the upper esophagus. The upper esophagus can also be narrowed by an inflammatory stricture occurring after a caustic ingestion or epidermolysis bullosa. Cricopharyngeal achalasia may manifest radiographically in a cricopharyngeal "bar" posteriorly in the upper esophagus.

Enterline H, Thompson J: *Pathology of the Esophagus.* New York, Springer-Verlag, 1984.

Janssen M, Baggen MG, Veen HF, et al: Dysphagia lusoria: Clinical aspects, manometric findings, diagnosis, and therapy. *Am J Gastroenterol* 2000;95:1411–1416.

Chapter 318 ■ Dysmotility

Susan Orenstein, John Peters, Seema Khan, Nader Youssef, and Sunny Zaheed Hussain

UPPER ESOPHAGEAL AND UPPER ESOPHAGEAL SPHINCTER (UES) DYSMOTILITY (STRIATED MUSCLE). Cricopharyngeal **achalasia** signifies a failure of complete relaxation of the UES, whereas cricopharyngeal **incoordination** implies full relaxation of the UES but incoordination of the relaxation with the pharyngeal contraction. These entities are usually detected on videofluoroscopic evaluation of swallowing (sometimes accompanied by visible cricopharyngeal prominence, termed a *bar*), but often the most precise definition of the dysfunction is obtained with manometry. A self-limited form of cricopharyngeal incoordination occurs in infancy and remits spontaneously in the 1st year of life if nutrition is maintained despite the dysphagia. In older children, idiopathic cricopharyngeal **spasm** is usually treated by myotomy of the UES. It is important, however, to evaluate such children thoroughly, including cranial MRI to detect **Arnold Chiari malformations,** which can present in this way but are best treated by cranial decompression, rather than esophageal, surgery. Cricopharyngeal spasm may be severe enough to produce posterior pharyngeal (Zenker) **diverticulum** above the obstructive sphincter; this entity occurs rarely in children.

Systemic causes of swallowing dysfunction that can affect the oropharynx, UES, and upper esophagus include cerebral palsy, Arnold Chiari malformations, syringomyelia, bulbar palsy or cranial nerve defects (Möbius syndrome, transient infantile paralysis of the superior laryngeal nerve), transient pharyngeal muscle dysfunction, spinal muscular atrophy (including Werdnig-Hoffmann disease), muscular dystrophy, infections (botulism, tetanus, poliomyelitis, diphtheria), inflammatory and connective tissue diseases (dermatomyositis, myasthenia gravis, polyneuritis, scleroderma), and familial dysautonomia. All of these can produce dysphagia. Medications (nitrazepam, benzodiazepines) and tracheostomy can adversely affect the function of the UES and thereby produce dysphagia.

LOWER ESOPHAGEAL AND LOWER ESOPHAGEAL SPHINCTER (LES) DYSFUNCTION (SMOOTH MUSCLE). Causes of dysphagia due to more distal primary esophageal dysmotility include achalasia, diffuse esophageal spasm, nutcracker esophagus, and hypertensive LES; all but achalasia are rare in children.

Achalasia is a primary esophageal motor disorder of unknown etiology characterized by loss of LES relaxation and loss of esophageal peristalsis, both contributing to a functional obstruction of the distal esophagus. Degenerative, autoimmune (antibodies to Auerbach plexus), and infectious (Chagas disease) factors are possible causes. In rare cases, achalasia is familial or part of the achalasia, alacrima, and corticotropin insensitivity syndrome. Pathologically, inflammation surrounds ganglion cells, which are decreased in number. There is selective loss of post-

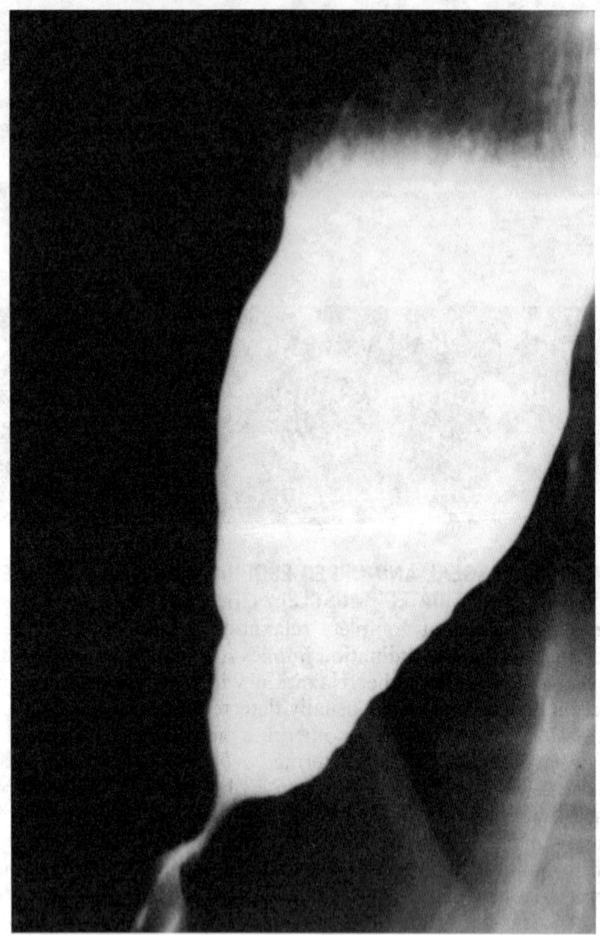

Figure 318-1. Barium esophagogram of a patient with achalasia demonstrating dilated esophagus and narrowing at the lower esophageal sphincter. Note retained secretions layered on top of barium in the esophagus.

ganglionic inhibitory neurons that normally lead to sphincter relaxation, leaving postganglionic cholinergic neurons unopposed. This imbalance produces high basal LES pressures and insufficient LES relaxation. The loss of esophageal peristalsis can be a secondary phenomenon. Achalasia presents as dysphagia for solids and liquids and may be accompanied by undernutrition or respiratory symptoms; retained esophageal food can produce esophagitis. The mean age in children is 8.8 yr with a mean duration of symptoms before diagnosis of 23 mo; it is uncommon before school age. Chest radiograph shows an air-fluid level in a dilated esophagus. **Barium fluoroscopy** reveals a smooth tapering of the lower esophagus leading to the closed LES, resembling a "bird's beak" (Fig. 318-1). Loss of primary peristalsis in the distal esophagus with retained food and poor emptying are often present. **Manometry** confirms the diagnosis and reveals incomplete relaxation of a high-pressure LES during swallowing, often accompanied by nonpropulsive simultaneous contractions in the distal esophagus. The two most effective **treatment options** are pneumatic dilatation and surgical (Heller) myotomy. Surgeons often supplement a myotomy with an antireflux procedure to prevent the gastroesophageal reflux disease that otherwise often ensues when the sphincter is rendered less competent. Calcium channel blockers (nifedipine) and phosphodiesterase inhibitors offer temporary relief of dysphagia. Endoscopic injection of the LES with **botulinum toxin** counterbalances the selective loss of inhibitory neurotransmitters by inhibiting the release of acetylcholine from nerve terminals and may be an effective therapy. Botulinum toxin is expensive; half the patients may require a repeat injection within 1 yr.

Diffuse esophageal spasm causes chest pain and dysphagia and affects adolescents and adults. It is diagnosed **manometrically** and can be treated with nitrates or calcium channel blocking agents.

Gastroesophageal reflux disease constitutes the most common cause of nonspecific abnormalities of esophageal motor function, probably through the effect of the esophageal inflammation on the musculature.

Orenstein SR: Oral, pharyngeal and esophageal motor disorders in infants and children. In Goyal R, Shaker R (editors): *GI Motility Online.* New York, Nature Publishing Group 2006. doi: 10.1038/gimo 38. View at www.nature.com/gimo/index.html

Chapter 319 ■ Hiatal Hernia

Susan Orenstein, John Peters, Seema Khan, Nader Youssef, and Sunny Zaheed Hussain

Herniation of the stomach through the esophageal hiatus can occur as a common sliding hernia, in which the gastroesophageal junction slides into the thorax, or it can be paraesophageal, in which a portion of the stomach (usually the fundus) is insinuated next to the esophagus inside the gastroesophageal junction in the hiatus (Fig. 319-1). Sliding hernias are frequently associated with gastroesophageal reflux, especially in developmentally delayed children. The relationship to hiatal hernias in adults is unclear. Medical treatment is not directed at the hernia but at the gastroesophageal reflux.

Paraesophageal hernias can be encountered after fundoplication for gastroesophageal reflux, especially if the edges of a dilated esophageal hiatus have not been approximated. Fullness after eating and upper abdominal pain are the usual symptoms. Infarction of the herniated stomach is rare.

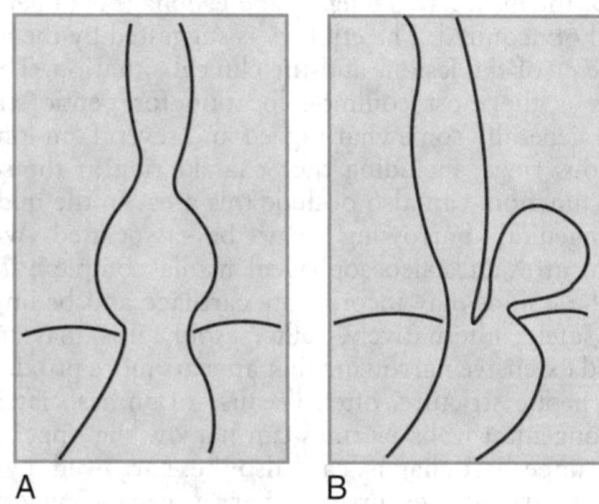

Figure 319-1. Types of esophageal hiatal hernia. *A,* Sliding hiatal hernia, the most common type. *B,* Paraesophageal hiatal hernia.

Chapter 320 ■ Gastroesophageal Reflux Disease (GERD)

Susan Orenstein, John Peters, Seema Khan, Nader Youssef, and Sunny Zaheed Hussain

GERD is the most common esophageal disorder in children of all ages. Gastroesophageal reflux (GER) signifies the retrograde movement of gastric contents across the lower esophageal sphincter (LES) into the esophagus. Although occasional episodes of reflux are physiologic, exemplified by the regurgitation of normal infants, the phenomenon becomes pathologic (GERD) in children who have episodes that are more frequent or persistent, and thus produce esophagitis or esophageal symptoms, or in those who have respiratory sequelae.

PATHOPHYSIOLOGY. Factors determining the esophageal manifestations of reflux include the duration of esophageal exposure (a product of the frequency and duration of reflux episodes), the causticity of the refluxate, and the susceptibility of the esophagus to damage. The LES, supported by the crura of the diaphragm at the gastroesophageal junction, together with valvelike functions of the esophagogastric junction anatomy form the antireflux barrier. In the context of even the normal intra-abdominal pressure augmentations that occur during daily life, the frequency of reflux episodes is increased by insufficient LES tone, by abnormal frequency of LES relaxations, and by hiatal herniation that prevents the LES pressure from being proportionately augmented during abdominal straining. Normal intra-abdominal pressure augmentations may be further exacerbated by straining or respiratory efforts. The duration of reflux episodes is increased by lack of swallowing (during sleep) and by defective esophageal peristalsis. Vicious cycles ensue because chronic esophagitis produces esophageal peristaltic dysfunction (low-amplitude waves, propagation disturbances), decreased LES tone, and inflammatory esophageal shortening that induces hiatal herniation, all worsening reflux.

Transient LES relaxation (TLESR) is the primary mechanism allowing reflux to occur. TLESRs occur independent of swallowing, reducing LES pressure to 0–2 mm Hg (above gastric), and last >10 sec; they appear by 26 wk of gestation. A vagovagal reflex, composed of afferent mechanoreceptors in the proximal stomach, a brainstem pattern generator, and efferents in the LES, regulates TLESRs. Gastric distention (postprandially, or due to abnormal gastric emptying or air swallowing) is the main stimulus for TLESRs. Whether GERD is caused by a higher frequency of TLESRs or by a greater incidence of reflux during TLESRs is debated; each is likely in different individuals. Straining during a TLESR makes reflux more likely, as do positions that place the gastroesophageal junction below the air-fluid interface in the stomach. Other factors influencing gastric pressure-volume dynamics, such as increased movement, straining, obesity, large-volume or hyperosmolar meals, and increased respiratory effort (coughing, wheezing) can have the same effect.

EPIDEMIOLOGY AND NATURAL HISTORY. **Infant reflux** becomes evident in the 1st few months of life, peaks at ≈4 mo, and resolves in most by 12 mo and nearly all by 24 mo. Symptoms in older children tend to be chronic, waxing and waning, but completely resolving in no more than half, which resembles adult patterns. GERD likely has genetic predispositions; family clustering of GERD symptoms, endoscopic esophagitis, hiatal hernia, Barrett esophagus, and adenocarcinoma has been identified. As a continuously variable and common disorder, complex inheritance involving multiple genes and environmental factors is likely. A pediatric autosomal dominant form with otolaryngologic and respiratory manifestations has been proposed on chromosome 13q14.

CLINICAL MANIFESTATIONS. Most of the common clinical manifestations of esophageal disease can signify the presence of GERD. **Infantile reflux** manifests more often with regurgitation (especially postprandially), signs of esophagitis (irritability, arching, choking, gagging, feeding aversion), and resulting failure to thrive; symptoms resolve spontaneously in the majority by 12–24 mo. **Older children,** in contrast, may have regurgitation during the preschool years; complaints of abdominal and chest pain supervene in later childhood and adolescence. Occasional children present with neck contortions (arching, turning of head) designated **Sandifer syndrome.** The respiratory presentations are also age dependent: GERD in infants may manifest as obstructive apnea or as stridor or lower airway disease in which reflux complicates primary airway disease such as laryngomalacia or bronchopulmonary dysplasia. Otitis media, sinusitis, lymphoid hyperplasia, hoarseness, vocal cord nodules, and laryngeal edema have all been associated with GERD. In contrast, airway manifestations in older children are more frequently related to asthma or to otolaryngologic disease such as laryngitis or sinusitis.

DIAGNOSIS. For most of the typical GERD presentations, a thorough history and physical examination suffice to reach the diagnosis initially. This initial evaluation aims to identify the pertinent positives in support of GERD and its complications and the negatives that make other diagnoses unlikely. The history may be facilitated and standardized by questionnaires (the Infant Gastroesophageal Reflux Questionnaire, the I-GERQ, and its derivative, the I-GERQ-R), which also permit quantitative scores to be evaluated for their diagnostic discrimination and for evaluative assessment of improvement or worsening of symptoms. Important other **diagnoses** to consider in the evaluation of an infant or a child with chronic vomiting are milk and other food allergies, pyloric stenosis, intestinal obstruction (especially malrotation with intermittent volvulus), nonesophageal inflammatory diseases, infections, inborn errors of metabolism, hydronephrosis, increased intracranial pressure, rumination, and bulimia. Focused diagnostic testing, depending on the presentation and the differential diagnosis, can then supplement the initial examination.

Most of the esophageal tests are of some use in particular patients suspected of GERD. **Contrast (usually barium) radiographic** study of the esophagus and upper gastrointestinal tract is performed in children with vomiting and dysphagia to evaluate for achalasia, esophageal strictures and stenosis, hiatal hernia, and gastric outlet or intestinal obstruction (Fig. 320-1). Extended **esophageal pH monitoring** of the distal esophagus, no longer considered the sine qua non of a GERD diagnosis, provides a quantitative and sensitive documentation of acidic reflux episodes, the most important type of reflux episodes for pathologic reflux. The distal esophageal pH probe is placed at a level corresponding to 87% of the nares-LES distance, based on regression equations using the patient's height, on fluoroscopic visualization, or on manometric identification of the LES. Normal values of distal esophageal acid exposure (pH <4) are generally established as <5–8% of the total monitored time, but these quantitative normals are insufficient to establish or disprove a diagnosis of pathologic GERD. The most important indications for esophageal pH monitoring are for assessing efficacy of acid suppression during treatment, evaluating apneic episodes in conjunction with a pneumogram and perhaps impedance (see later), and evaluating atypical GERD presentations such as chronic

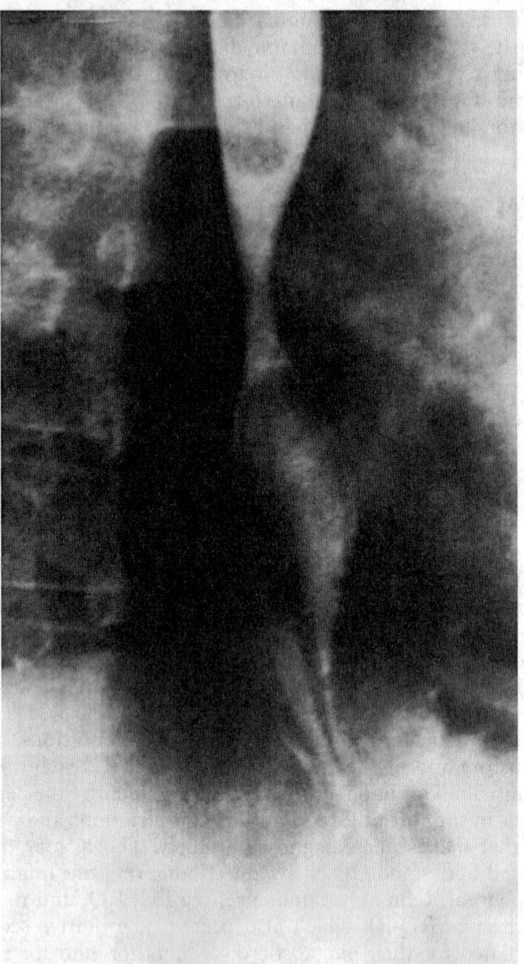

Figure 320-1. Barium esophagogram demonstrating free gastroesophageal reflux. Note stricture caused by peptic esophagitis. Longitudinal gastric folds above the diaphragm indicate the unusual presence of an associated hiatal hernia.

cough, stridor, and asthma. Dual pH probes, adding a proximal esophageal probe to the standard distal one, are used in the diagnosis of extraesophageal GERD, identifying upper esophageal acid exposure times of ≈1% of the total time as threshold values for abnormality. **Endoscopy** allows diagnosis of erosive esophagitis (Fig. 320-2) and complications such as strictures or Barrett esophagus; esophageal biopsies may diagnose histologic reflux esophagitis in the absence of erosions while simultaneously eliminating allergic and infectious causes. Endoscopy is also used therapeutically to dilate reflux-induced strictures. Radionucleotide scintigraphy using technetium may demonstrate aspiration and delayed gastric emptying when these are suspected. The **intraluminal impedance** test is a cumbersome test, infrequently used clinically, but its documentation of nonacid reflux has disclosed the potential importance of neutral reflux in children, particularly in those with respiratory symptoms.

Laryngotracheobronchoscopy evaluates for visible airway signs that are associated with extraesophageal GERD, such as posterior laryngeal inflammation and vocal cord nodules; it may permit diagnosis of silent aspiration (during swallowing or during reflux) by bronchoalveolar lavage with subsequent quantification of lipid-laden macrophages in airway secretions. Esophageal manometry permits evaluation for dysmotility, particularly in preparation for antireflux surgery.

Empirical antireflux therapy, using a time-limited trial of high-dose proton pump inhibitor (PPI), has been demonstrated in adults to be a cost-effective strategy for diagnosis; although not formally evaluated in older children, it has also been applied to this age group. Failure to respond to such empirical treatment, or a requirement for the treatment for prolonged periods, mandates formal diagnostic evaluation.

MANAGEMENT. Conservative therapy and lifestyle modification form the foundation of GERD therapy. Dietary measures for infants include normalization of feeding techniques, volumes, and frequency if abnormal. Thickening of formula with a tbsp of rice cereal per oz of formula results in fewer regurgitation episodes, greater caloric density (30 kcal/oz), and reduced crying time, although it may not modify the number of nonregurgitant reflux episodes. A short trial of a hypoallergenic diet can be used to

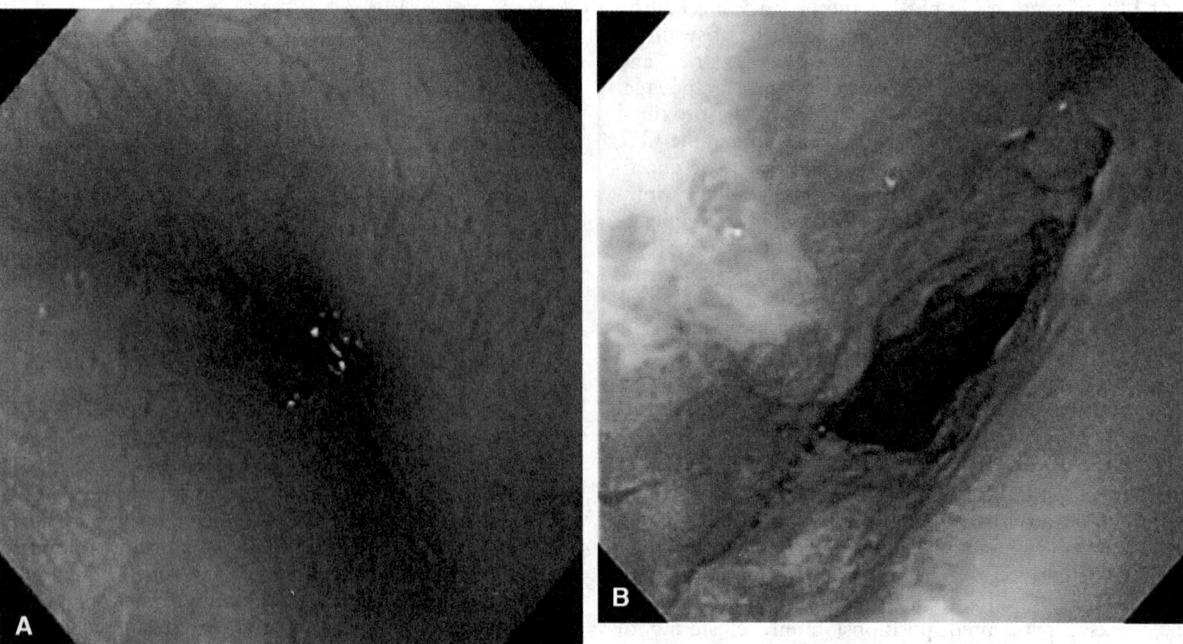

Figure 320-2. Endoscopic image of a normal esophagus *(A)* and erosive peptic esophagitis *(B)*.

exclude milk or soy protein allergy before pharmacotherapy. Older children and adults should be counseled to avoid acidic or reflux-inducing foods (tomatoes, chocolate, mint) and beverages (juices, carbonated and caffeinated drinks, alcohol). Weight reduction for obese patients and elimination of smoke exposure are other crucial measures at all ages.

Positioning measures are particularly important for infants, who cannot control their positions independently. Seated position worsens infant reflux and should be avoided in infants with GERD. Esophageal pH monitoring has shown significantly more reflux episodes in infants in supine and side positions compared with the prone position, but evidence that the supine position reduces the risk of sudden infant death syndrome has led the American Academy of Pediatrics and the North American Society of Pediatric Gastroenterology and Nutrition to recommend supine positioning during sleep. When the infant is awake and observed, prone position and upright carried position can be used to minimize reflux. The efficacy of positioning for older children is unclear, but some evidence suggests a benefit to left side position and head elevation during sleep. Head elevation should utilize elevation of the head of the bed, rather than excess pillows, to avoid abdominal flexion and compression that might worsen reflux.

Pharmacotherapy is directed at ameliorating the acidity of the gastric contents or at promoting their aboral movement. **Antacids** are the most commonly used antireflux therapy and are readily available over the counter. They provide rapid but transient relief of symptoms by acid neutralization. The long-term regular use of antacids cannot be recommended because of side effects of diarrhea (magnesium) and constipation (aluminum) and rare reports of more serious side effects of chronic use.

Histamine-2 receptor antagonists (H2RAs; cimetidine, famotidine, nizatidine, and ranitidine) are widely used antisecretory agents that act by selective inhibition of histamine receptors on gastric parietal cells. There is a definite benefit of H2RAs in treatment of mild-to-moderate reflux esophagitis. H2RAs have been recommended as first-line therapy because of their excellent overall safety profile, but they are being superseded by proton pump inhibitors in this role, as increased experience with pediatric use and safety, Food and Drug Administration approval, and pediatric formulations and dosing are acquired.

Proton pump inhibitors (PPIs; omeprazole, lansoprazole, pantoprazole, rabeprazole, and esomeprazole) provide the most potent antireflux effect by blocking the hydrogen-potassium ATPase channels of the final common pathway in gastric acid secretion. PPIs are superior to H2RAs in the treatment of severe and erosive esophagitis. Doses of omeprazole effective for children have been identified (0.7–3.3 mg/kg/day), higher than those used in adults on a dose per weight basis.

Prokinetic agents available in the United States include metoclopramide (dopamine-2 and 5HT-3 antagonist), bethanechol (cholinergic agonist), and erythromycin (motilin receptor agonist). Most of these increase LES pressure; some improve gastric emptying or esophageal clearance. None affects the frequency of TLESRs. The available controlled trials have not demonstrated much efficacy for GERD. Several new prokinetic agents may prove useful but are as yet inadequately studied for this indication in children.

Surgery, usually **fundoplication,** is effective therapy for intractable GERD in children, particularly those with refractory esophagitis or strictures and those at risk for significant morbidity from chronic pulmonary disease. It may be combined with a gastrostomy for feeding or venting. The availability of potent acid-suppressing medication mandates more rigorous analysis of the relative risks (or costs) and benefits of this relatively irreversible therapy in comparison to long-term pharmacotherapy. Some of the risks of fundoplication include a wrap that is "too tight" (producing dysphagia or gas-bloat) or "too loose" (and thus incompetent). Surgeons may choose to perform a "tight" (360°, Nissen) or "loose" (<360°, Thal, etc.) wrap or to add a gastric drainage procedure (pyloroplasty) to improve gastric emptying, based on their experience and the patient's disease. Preoperative accuracy of diagnosis of GERD and the skill of the surgeon are two of the most important predictors of successful outcome. Long-term studies suggest that fundoplications frequently become incompetent in children, as in adults; this fact currently combines with the potency of PPI therapy that is now available to shift practice toward long-term pharmacotherapy in many cases. Fundoplication procedures may be performed as open operations, by laparoscopy, or by endoluminal (gastroplication) techniques.

Benhamou PH, Francoual C, Glangeaud MC, et al: Risk factors for severe esophageal and gastric lesions in term neonates: A case-control study. Groupe Francophone d'Hepato-Gastroenterologie et Nutrition Pediatrique. *J Pediatr Gastroenterol Nutr* 2000;31:377–380.

Davidson G, Omari TI: Pathophysiological mechanisms of gastroesophageal reflux disease in children. *Curr Gastroenterol Rep* 2001;3:257–262.

Fonkalsrud EW, Ashcraft KW, Coran AG, et al: Surgical treatment of gastroesophageal reflux in children: A combined hospital study of 7,467 patients. *Pediatrics* 1998;101:419–422.

Lehman GA: Endoscopic and endoluminal techniques for the control of gastroesophageal reflux: Are they ready for widespread clinical application? *Gastrointest Endosc* 2000;52:808–811.

Lidums I, Lehmann A, Checklin H, et al: Control of transient lower esophageal sphincter relaxations and reflux by the $GABA_B$ agonist baclofen in normal subjects. *Gastroenterology* 2000;118:7–13.

Orenstein SR: Pediatric gastroesophageal reflux disease. In Orland RC (editor): *Gastroesophageal Reflux Disease.* New York, Marcel Dekker, 2000.

Orenstein SR, Di Lorenzo C: Postfundoplication complications in children. *Curr Treat Options Gastroenterol* 2001;4:441–449.

Orenstein SR, Peters JM: Vomiting and regurgitation. In Kliegman RM (editor): *Practical Strategies in Pediatric Diagnosis and Therapy,* 2nd ed. Philadelphia, Elsevier. 2004, pp 291–321.

Orenstein SR, Shalaby TM, Barmada MM, et al: Genetics of gastroesophageal reflux disease: A review. *J Pediatr Gastroenterol Nutr* 2002;34:506–510.

Orenstein SR, Shalaby TM, Cohn JF: Reflux symptoms in 100 normal infants: Diagnostic validity of the infant gastroesophageal reflux questionnaire. *Clin Pediatr* 1996;35:607–614.

Rothman M, Orenstein SR, Kleinman L, et al: Development of a revised infant gastroesophageal reflux questionnaire. *Acta Gastroenterol Belgica* 2003:73 (presented at the Second European Pediatric Gastrointestinal Motility meeting, Bruges, Belgium, April 23–26, 2003).

Rudolph CD, Mazur LJ, Liptak GS, et al: Pediatric gastroesophageal reflux clinical practice guidelines: Guidelines for evaluation and treatment of gastroesophageal reflux in infants and children. *J Pediatr Gastroenterol Nutr* 2001;32:S1–S31.

Salvia G, De Vizia B, Manguso F, et al: Effect of intragastric volume and osmolality on mechanisms of gastroesophageal reflux in children with gastroesophageal reflux disease. *Am J Gastroenterol* 2001;96:1725–1732.

Thompson M, Fritscher-Ravens A, Hall S, et al: Endoluminal gastroplication in children with significant gastro-oesophageal reflux in disease. *Gut* 2004;53:1745–1750.

Willging JP, Thompson D: Pediatric FEESST: Fiberoptic endoscopic evaluation of swallowing with sensory testing. *Curr Gastroenterol Rep* 2005;7: 240–243.

320.1 • Complications of GERD

ESOPHAGEAL: ESOPHAGITIS AND SEQUELAE—STRICTURE, BARRETT ESOPHAGUS, ADENOCARCINOMA. Esophagitis can manifest as irritability, arching, and feeding aversion in infants; chest or epigastric pain in older children; and, rarely, as hematemesis, anemia, or Sandifer syndrome at any age. Prolonged and severe esophagitis leads to formation of strictures, generally located in the distal esophagus, producing dysphagia, and requiring repeated esophageal dilations and often fundoplication. Long-standing esophagitis predisposes to metaplastic transformation of the normal esophageal squamous epithelium into intestinal columnar epithelium, termed **Barrett esophagus,** a precursor of esophageal adenocarcinoma. Both Barrett esophagus and adenocarcinoma occur more in white males and in those with increased duration, frequency, and severity of reflux symptoms. This transformation increases with age to plateau in the 5th decade; adenocarcinoma is thus rare in childhood. Barrett esophagus, uncommon in children, warrants periodic surveillance biopsies, aggressive pharmacotherapy, and fundoplication for progressive lesions.

NUTRITIONAL. Esophagitis and regurgitation may be severe enough to induce failure to thrive because of caloric deficits. Enteral (nasogastric or nasojejunal, or percutaneous gastric or jejunal) or parenteral feedings are sometimes required to treat such deficits.

EXTRAESOPHAGEAL: RESPIRATORY ("ATYPICAL") PRESENTATIONS. GERD should be included in the differential diagnosis of children with unexplained or refractory otolaryngologic and respiratory complaints. GERD may produce respiratory symptoms by direct contact of the refluxed gastric contents with the respiratory tract (aspiration, laryngeal penetration, or microaspiration) or by reflexive interactions between the esophagus and respiratory tract (inducing laryngeal closure or bronchospasm). Frequently, GERD and a primary respiratory disorder, such as asthma, interact and a vicious cycle between them worsens both diseases. Many children with these extraesophageal presentations do not have typical GERD symptoms, making the diagnosis difficult. These atypical GERD presentations require a thoughtful approach to the differential diagnosis that considers a multitude of primary otolaryngologic (infections, allergies, postnasal drip, voice overuse) and pulmonary (asthma, cystic fibrosis) disorders. Therapy for the GERD must be more intense (usually incorporating a PPI) and prolonged (usually at least 3–6 mo). Subspecialist assistance from the perspective of the airway disease (otolaryngology, pulmonology) and the reflux disease (gastroenterology) is often warranted for specialized diagnostic testing and for optimizing intensive management.

APNEA AND STRIDOR. These upper airway presentations have been linked with GERD in case reports and epidemiologic studies; temporal relationships between them and reflux episodes have been demonstrated in some patients by esophageal pH probe monitoring; and a beneficial response to therapy for GERD provides further support in a number of case series. An evaluation of 1,400 infants with apnea attributed the apnea to GERD in 50%, but other studies have failed to find an association. Apnea due to reflux is generally obstructive, owing to laryngospasm that may be conceived of as an abnormally intense protective reflex. Infants with such apnea are often provocatively positioned (supine or flexed seated), are recently fed, and show signs of obstructive apnea, with unproductive respiratory efforts. Stridor triggered by reflux generally occurs in infants anatomically predisposed toward stridor (laryngomalacia, micrognathia). Spasmodic croup, an episodic frightening upper airway obstruction, can be an analogous condition in older children. Esophageal pH probe studies may fail to demonstrate linkage of these manifestations with reflux owing to the buffering of gastric contents by infant formula and the episodic nature of the conditions. Pneumograms may fail to identify apnea that occurs if they are not designed to identify obstructive apnea by measuring nasal airflow.

Reflux laryngitis and other otolaryngologic manifestations can be attributed to GERD. **Hoarseness,** voice fatigue, throat clearing, chronic cough, pharyngitis, sinusitis, otitis media, and a sensation of globus have been cited. The paucity of well-controlled evaluations of the association contributes to the skepticism with which these associations may be considered. Other risk factors irritating the upper respiratory passages can predispose some patients with GERD to present predominantly with these complaints.

Asthma co-occurs with GERD in ≈50% of children with asthma, which contrasts to the prevalence of each condition independently in ≈10% of children. Children with asthma who are particularly likely to have GERD as a provocative factor are those with symptoms of reflux disease, those with refractory or steroid-dependent asthma, and those with nocturnal worsening of asthma. Endoscopic evaluation that discloses esophageal sequelae of GERD provides an impetus to embark on the aggressive (high dose and many months' duration) therapy of GERD.

Dental erosions constitute the most common oral lesion of GERD, the lesions being distinguished by their location on the lingual surface.

Bauman NM, Bishop WP, Sandler AD, et al: Value of pH probe testing in pediatric patients with extraesophageal manifestations of gastroesophageal reflux disease: A retrospective review. *Ann Otol Rhinol Laryngol* 2000;109:18–24.

El-Serag HB, Gilger MA, Kuebeler M, et al: Extraesophageal associations of gastroesophageal reflux disease in children without neurologic defects. *Gastroenterology* 2001;121:1294–1299.

Fuloria M, Hiatt D, Dillard RG, et al: Gastroesophageal reflux in very low birth weight infants: Association with chronic lung disease and outcomes through 1 year of age. *J Perinatol* 2000;4:235–239.

Goldenhersh MJ, Ament M: Asthma and gastroesophageal reflux in infants and children. *Immunol Allergy Clin North Am* 2001;21:439–448.

Harding SM, Sontag SJ: Asthma and gastroesophageal reflux. *Am J Gastroenterol* 2000;95:S23–S32.

Irwin RS, Madison JM: Anatomical diagnostic protocol in evaluating chronic cough with specific reference to gastroesophageal reflux disease. *Am J Med* 2000;108:126S–130S.

Kimball AL, Carlton DP: Gastroesophageal reflux medications in the treatment of apnea in premature infants. *J Pediatr* 2001;138:355–360.

Linnett V, Seow WK: Dental erosion in children: A literature review. *Pediatr Dent* 2001;23:37–43.

Nostrant TT: Gastroesophageal reflux and laryngitis: A skeptic's view. *Am J Med* 2000;108:149S–152S.

Orenstein SR: Update on gastroesophageal reflux and respiratory disease in children: A review. *Can J Gastroenterol* 2000;14:131–135.

Rosbe KW, Kenna MA, Auerbach AD: Extraesophageal reflux in pediatric patients with upper respiratory symptoms. *Arch Otolaryngol Head Neck Surg* 2003;129:1213–1220.

Sacco O, Fregonese B, Silvestri M, et al: Bronchoalveolar lavage and esophageal pH monitoring data in children with "difficult to treat" respiratory symptoms. *Pediatr Pulmonol* 2000;30:313–319.

Suskind DL, Zeringue GP III, Kluka EA, et al: Gastroesophageal reflux and pediatric otolaryngologic disease: The role of anti-reflux surgery. *Arch Otolaryngol Head Neck Surg* 2001;127:511–514.

Chapter 321 ■ Eosinophilic Esophagits and Non-GERD Esophagitis

Susan Orenstein, John Peters, Seema Khan, Nader Youssef, and Sunny Zaheed Hussain

EOSINOPHILIC ESOPHAGITIS. The esophageal epithelium is infiltrated by eosinophils, typically in a density exceeding 15 per high-power field. Presenting symptoms include vomiting, chest or epigastric pain, and dysphagia with occasional food impactions

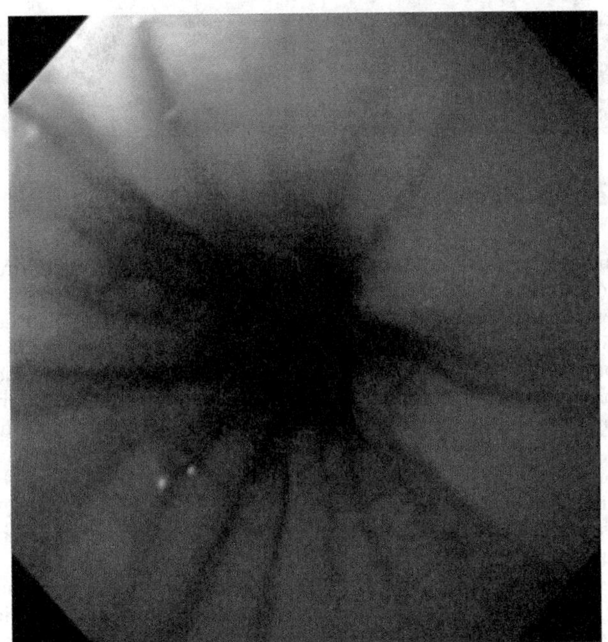

Figure 321-1. Endoscopic image of eosinophilic esophagitis.

or strictures. Most patients are male. The mean age at diagnosis is 7 yr (range 1–17 yr) with the duration of symptoms of 3 yr. Patients often have atopy, associated food allergies, peripheral eosinophilia (≈50% of patients), and elevated immunoglobulin E (IgE) levels. Endoscopically, the esophagus presents a granular, furrowed, or ringed appearance (Fig. 321-1); esophageal histology reveals eosinophilia. Eosinophilic esophagitis is differentiated from gastroesophageal reflux disease (GERD) by its general lack of erosive esophagitis, by its greater eosinophil density, and by its refractoriness to antireflux therapies. **Treatment** involves elimination diets for those with proven allergies, whereas inhaled and systemic corticosteroids have been used successfully for nonresponders and for nonallergic ("primary") eosinophilic esophagitis. Therapies under investigation include leukotriene inhibitors (montelukast) and anti–interleukin 5 (anti–IL-5) antibody (mepolizumab). Little is known about its natural history, but it seems that eosinophilic esophagitis left untreated can result in stricture formation.

INFECTIVE ESOPHAGITIS. Uncommon, and most often affecting immunocompromised children, infective esophagitis is caused by fungal agents, such as *Candida* and *Torulopsis glabrata;* viral agents, such as herpes simplex, cytomegalovirus, and varicella zoster; and, rarely, bacterial infections, including diphtheria and tuberculosis. The typical presenting signs and symptoms are odynophagia, dysphagia, and retrosternal pain; there may also be fever, nausea, and vomiting. Esophageal candidiasis commonly, but not always, presents as concurrent oropharyngeal infection and can affect immunocompetent as well as immunocompromised children. Esophageal viral infections can also present in immunocompetent hosts as an acute febrile illness. Infectious esophagitis, like other forms of esophageal inflammation, occasionally progresses to esophageal stricture. Diagnosis of infectious esophagitis is made by endoscopy and histopathologic examination; adding polymerase chain reaction, tissue-viral culture, and immunocytochemistry enhances the diagnostic sensitivity. Treatment is with appropriate antimicrobial agents, analgesics, and antacids.

"PILL" ESOPHAGITIS. This acute injury is produced by contact with a damaging agent. Medications implicated in "pill" esophagitis include tetracycline, potassium chloride, ferrous sulfate, and nonsteroidal anti-inflammatory medications, with the tablet most often ingested at bedtime with inadequate water. This practice often produces acute discomfort followed by progressive retrosternal pain, odynophagia, and dysphagia; endoscopy shows a focal lesion often localized to one of the anatomic narrowed regions of the esophagus or to an unsuspected pathologic narrowing. Treatment is supportive; lacking much evidence, antacids, topical anesthetics, and bland or liquid diets are often used.

Arora AS, Murray JA: Iatrogenic esophagitis. *Curr Gastroenterol Rep* 2000;2:224–229.

Diaz M, Leal N, Olivares P, et al: Infectious strictures requiring esophageal replacement in children. *J Pediatr Gastroenterol Nutr* 2001;32:611–613.

Khan S, Orenstein SR: Eosinophilic disorders of the gastrointestinal tract. In Feldman M, Friedman LS, Brandt LJ (editors): *Sleisinger & Fordtran's Gastrointestinal & Liver Disease,* 8th ed (in press).

Orenstein SR, Shalaby TM, Di Lorenzo C, et al: The spectrum of pediatric eosinophilic esophagitis beyond infancy: A clinical series of 30 children. *Am J Gastroenterol* 2000;95:1422–1430.

Ramanathan J, Rammouni M, Baran J Jr, et al: Herpes simplex virus esophagitis in the immunocompetent host: An overview. *Am J Gastroenterol* 2000;95:2171–2176.

Sant'Anna AM, Rolland S, Fournet JC, et al: Eosinophilic esophagitis in children: Symptoms, histology and pH probe results. *J Pediatr Gastroenterol Nutr* 2004;39:373–377.

Vodovnik A, Cerar A: Synchronous herpes simplex virus and cytomegalovirus esophagitis. *Z Gastroenterol* 2000;38:491–494.

Chapter 322 ■ Esophageal Perforation

Susan Orenstein, John Peters, Seema Khan, Nader Youssef, and Sunny Zaheed Hussain

The majority of esophageal perforations in children either are from blunt trauma (automobile accidents, gunshot wounds, child abuse) or are iatrogenic. Cardiac massage, the Heimlich maneuver, nasogastric tube placement, traumatic laryngoscopy or endotracheal intubation, excessively vigorous postpartum suctioning of the airway during neonatal resuscitation, difficult upper endoscopy, sclerotherapy of esophageal varices, esophageal compression by a cuffed endotracheal tube, and pneumatic dilatation for therapy of achalasia have all been implicated. Esophageal rupture has also followed forceful vomiting in patients with anorexia or caustic ingestion.

Spontaneous esophageal rupture (**Boerhaave syndrome**) is less frequent and is associated with sudden increases in intraesophageal pressure wrought by situations such as vomiting, coughing, or straining at stool. In children and adults, the tear occurs on the distal left lateral esophageal wall, because the smooth muscle layer here is weakest; in neonates (neonatal Boerhaave syndrome), spontaneous rupture is on the right.

Symptoms of esophageal perforation include pain, neck tenderness, dysphagia, subcutaneous crepitus, fever, and tachycardia; several patients with cervical perforations have displayed cold water polydipsia in an attempt to soothe pain in the throat. Perforations in the proximal thoracic esophagus tend to create signs (pneumothorax, effusions) in the left chest, whereas the signs of distal tears are more often on the right. Cervical spine and chest radiographs are frequently diagnostic, showing mediastinal widening or paracervical free air. If these x-rays are normal, an esophagogram utilizing water-soluble contrast media should be performed, but esophagograms miss >30% of cervical perforations. Therefore, a negative water-soluble contrast esophagogram should be followed by a barium study; the greater density of barium can better demonstrate a small defect, though with a higher risk of inflammatory mediastinitis. Endoscopy may also be useful but carries a 30% false-negative rate. CT of the chest can assist in difficult cases.

Treatment must be individualized. Although small tears and minimal mediastinal contamination can be treated conservatively with broad-spectrum antibiotics, nothing given orally, gastric drainage, and parenteral nutrition, the majority of pediatric esophageal perforations require surgical management.

Chapter 323 ■ Esophageal Varices

Susan Orenstein

Portal hypertension is defined as an elevation of portal venous pressure to levels 10–12 mm Hg higher than pressures present in the inferior vena cava (see Chapter 364). Decompression of this hypertension through portosystemic collateral circulation via the coronary vein, in conjunction with the left gastric veins, gives rise to esophageal varices. Most esophageal varices are "uphill varices"; less commonly, those that arise in the absence of portal hypertension and with superior vena cava (SVC) obstruction are termed "downhill varices." Their treatment is directed at the underlying cause of the SVC abnormality. Hemorrhage from esophageal varices is the major cause of morbidity and mortality due to portal hypertension. Presentation is with significant hematemesis and melena; whereas most patients have liver disease, some children with entities such as extrahepatic portal venous thrombosis may have been previously asymptomatic. Any child with hematemesis and splenomegaly should be presumed to have esophageal variceal bleeding until proven otherwise.

Varices are occasionally seen on fluoroscopic barium contrast studies, but upper endoscopy is preferred because it provides definitive diagnosis as well as therapy for acute bleeding episodes via either sclerotherapy or band ligation.

Treating children with varices with prophylactic sclerotherapy with the goal of preventing an initial hemorrhage can decrease the incidence of esophageal bleeding. Treated patients may bleed from congestive gastropathy, and no improvement in survival rate may be seen. Nonselective β blockade, such as with propranolol, has also been used to prevent variceal bleeding. Endoscopic variceal ligation in adults reduces the risk of first-time variceal bleeding when compared with untreated controls as well as patients treated with β blockade; a decrease in mortality is only noted in comparison to the control group (see Chapter 364).

Goncalves ME, Cardoso SR, Maksoud JG: Prophylactic sclerotherapy in children with esophageal varices: Long-term results of a controlled prospective randomized trial. *J Pediatr Surg* 2000;35:401–405.

Imperiale TF, Chalasani N: A meta-analysis of endoscopic variceal ligation for primary prophylaxis of esophageal variceal bleeding. *Hepatology* 2001; 33:1003–1004.

Chapter 324 ■ Ingestions

Susan Orenstein

324.1 • Foreign Bodies in the Esophagus

The majority (80%) of foreign body ingestions occur in children, most of whom are between 6 mo and 3 yr of age. Youngsters with developmental delays as well as those with psychiatric disorders are also at increased risk. Coins and small toy items are the most commonly ingested foreign bodies. Food impactions are less common in children than in adults and usually occur in children with an underlying structural anomaly or motility disorder, such as repair of esophageal atresia or eosinophilic esophagitis. Most esophageal foreign bodies lodge at either the level of the cricopharyngeus (upper esophageal sphincter [UES]), the aortic arch, or just superior to the diaphragm at the gastroesophageal junction (lower esophageal sphincter [LES]).

At least 30% of children with esophageal foreign bodies may be totally asymptomatic, so any history of foreign body ingestion should be taken seriously and investigated. An initial bout of choking, gagging, and coughing may be followed by excessive salivation, dysphagia, food refusal, emesis, or pain in the neck, throat, or sternal notch regions. Respiratory symptoms such as stridor, wheezing, cyanosis, or dyspnea may be encountered if the esophageal foreign body impinges on the larynx or membranous posterior tracheal wall. Cervical swelling, erythema, or subcutaneous crepitations suggest perforation of the oropharynx or proximal esophagus.

Evaluation of the child with a history of foreign body ingestion starts with plain anteroposterior radiographs of the neck, chest, and abdomen, along with lateral views of the neck and chest. The flat surface of a coin in the esophagus is seen on the anteroposterior view and the edge on the lateral view (Fig. 324-1). The reverse is true for coins lodged in the trachea; here, the edge is seen anteroposteriorly and the flat side is seen laterally. Materials such as plastic, wood, glass, aluminum, and bones may be radiolucent; failure to visualize the object with plain films in a symptomatic patient warrants urgent endoscopy. Although barium contrast studies may be helpful in the occasional asymptomatic patient with negative plain films, their use is to be discouraged because of the potential of aspiration as well as making subsequent visualization and object removal more difficult.

Treatment of esophageal foreign bodies usually merits endoscopic visualization of the object and underlying mucosa and removal of the object; therapeutic endoscopy is most conservatively done with an endotracheal tube protecting the airway. Sharp objects in the esophagus, disc button batteries, or foreign bodies associated with respiratory symptoms mandate urgent removal. Button batteries, in particular, must be expediently removed because they can induce mucosal injury in as little as 1 hr of contact time and involve all esophageal layers within 4 hr. Asymptomatic blunt objects and coins lodged in the esophagus can be observed for up to 24 hr in anticipation of passage into the stomach. If there are no problems in handling secretions, meat impactions can be observed for up to 12 hr. In patients without prior esophageal surgeries, glucagon (0.05 mg/kg intravenously) can sometimes be useful in facilitating passage of distal esophageal food boluses by decreasing the LES pressure. The use of meat tenderizers or gas-forming agents can lead to perforation and are not recommended. An alternative technique for removing esophageal coins impacted for under 24 hr, performed most safely by experienced radiology personnel, consists of passage of a Foley catheter beyond the coin at fluoroscopy, inflating the balloon, and then pulling the catheter and coin back simultaneously with the patient in a prone oblique position. Concerns

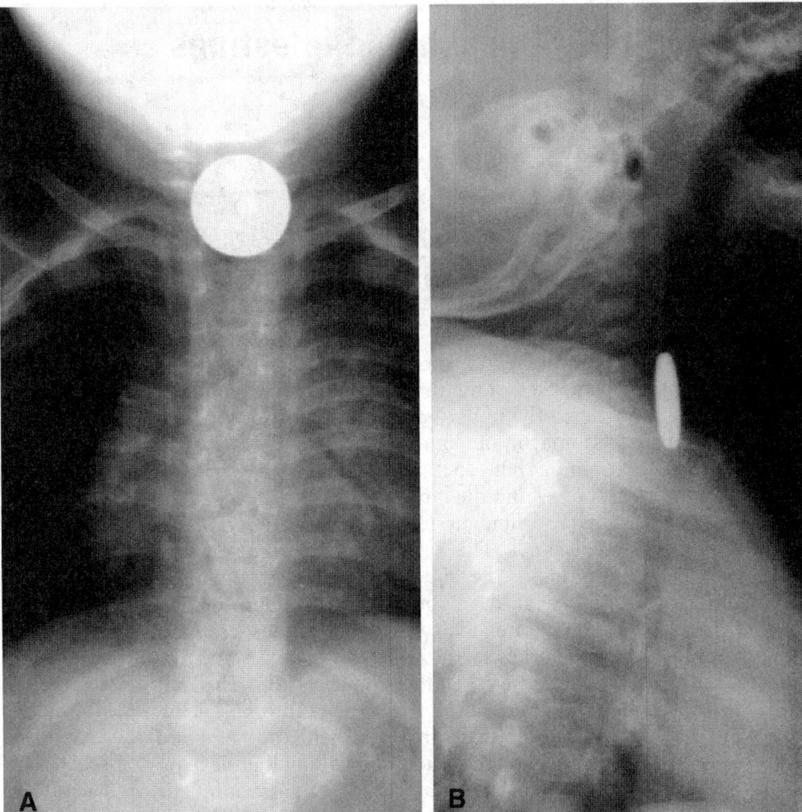

Figure 324-1. Radiographs of a coin in the esophagus. When foreign bodies lodge in the esophagus, the flat surface of the object is seen in the anteroposterior view *(A)* and the edge is seen in the lateral view *(B)*. The reverse is true for objects in the trachea. (Courtesy of Beverley Newman, MD.)

about the lack of direct mucosal visualization and, when tracheal intubation is not used, the lack of airway protection prompt caution in the use of this technique.

Kay M, Wyllie R: Pediatric foreign bodies and their management. *Curr Gastroenterol Rep* 2005;7:212–218.

324.2 • Caustic Ingestions

Ingestion of caustic substances results in esophagitis, necrosis, perforation, and stricture formation (see Chapter 58). Most cases (70%) are accidental ingestions of liquid alkali substances that produce severe, deep liquefaction necrosis; drain decloggers are most common, and because they are tasteless, more is ingested. **Acidic agents** (20% of cases) are bitter, so less may be consumed; they produce coagulation necrosis and a somewhat protective thick eschar. They can produce severe gastritis, and volatile acids can result in respiratory symptoms. Caustic ingestions produce signs and symptoms such as vomiting, drooling, refusal to drink, oral burns, dysphagia, abdominal pain, and stridor. Twenty percent of patients develop esophageal strictures. Absence of oropharyngeal lesions does not exclude the possibility of significant esophagogastric injury, which can lead to perforation or stricture. The absence of symptoms is usually associated with no or minimal lesions; in contrast, hematemesis, respiratory distress, or presence of at least three symptoms predict severe lesions. An upper endoscopy is recommended as the most efficient means of rapid identification of tissue damage and must be undertaken in all symptomatic children. Dilution by water or milk is recommended as acute treatment, but neutralization, induced emesis, and gastric lavage are contraindicated. Treatment depends on the severity and extent of damage. Stricture risk is increased by circumferential ulcerations, white plaques, and sloughing of the mucosa. They may require treatment with dilation, and in some severe cases, surgical resection and colon or small bowel interposition are needed. Silicone stents (self-expanding) placed endoscopically after a dilatation procedure can be an alternate and conservative approach to the management of strictures. Rare late cases of superimposed esophageal carcinoma are reported.

Gupta SK, Croffie JM, Fitzgerald JF: Is esophagogastroduodenoscopy necessary in all caustic ingestions? *J Pediatr Gastroenterol Nutr* 2001;32:50–53.

Broto J, Asensio M, Vernet JMG: Results of a new technique in the treatment of severe esophageal stenosis in children: Poliflex stents. *J Pediatr Gastroenterol Nutr* 2003;37:203–206.

de Jong AL, Macdonald R, Ein S, et al: Corrosive esophagitis in children: A 30-year review. *Int J Pediatr Otorhinolaryngol* 2001;57:203–211.

Section 4 — Stomach and Intestines

Chapter 325 ■ Normal Development, Structure, and Function Robert Wyllie

DEVELOPMENT. The primitive gut is recognizable by the 4th wk of gestation and is composed of the foregut, midgut, and hindgut. The **foregut** gives rise to the upper gastrointestinal tract including the esophagus, stomach, and duodenum to the level of the insertion of the common bile duct. The **midgut** gives rise to the rest of the small bowel and the large bowel to the level of the mid-transverse colon. The **hindgut** forms the remainder of the colon and upper anal canal. The rapid growth of the midgut causes it to protrude out of the abdominal cavity through the umbilical ring during fetal development. The midgut subsequently returns to the peritoneal cavity and rotates counterclockwise until the cecum lies in the right lower quadrant. The process is normally complete by the 8th wk of gestation. The liver derives from the hepatic diverticulum that evolves into parenchymal cells, bile ducts, vascular structures, and hematopoietic and Kupffer cells. The extrahepatic bile ducts and gallbladder develop 1st as solid cords that canalize by the 3rd mo of gestation. The dorsal and ventral pancreatic buds grow from the foregut by the 4th wk of gestation. The two buds fuse by the 6th wk. Exocrine secretory capacity is present by the 5th mo. *Cis*-regulatory genomic sequences govern gene expression during development. Modules of *cis* sequences are linked and allow a cascade of gene regulation that controls functional development. Extrinsic factors have the capacity to influence gene expression. In the gut, several growth factors, including growth factor-β, insulin-like growth factor, and growth factors found in human colostrum (human growth factor and epidermal growth factor), influence gene expression.

Propulsion of food down the gastrointestinal tract relies on the coordinated action of muscles in the bowel wall. The contractions are regulated by the enteric nervous system under the influence of a variety of peptides and hormones. The enteric nervous system is derived from neural crest cells that migrate in a cranial to caudal fashion. Migration of the neural crest tissue is complete by the 24th wk of gestation. Interruption of the migration results in **Hirschsprung disease.** Bowel motor patterns in the newborn differ from adults. Normal fasting upper gastrointestinal motility is characterized by a triphasic pattern known as the migrating motor complex. Migrating motor complexes occur less often in neonates and they have more nonmigrating phasic activity. This leads to ineffective propulsion, particularly in premature infants. Motility in the fed state consists of a series of ring contractions that spread caudad over variable distances.

DIGESTION AND ABSORPTION. The wall of the stomach, small bowel, and colon consists of four layers: the mucosa, submucosa, muscularis, and serosa. Eighty-five percent of the gastric mucosa is lined by oxyntic glands containing cells that secrete hydrochloric acid, pepsinogen, and intrinsic factor, and mucous and endocrine cells that secrete peptides having paracrine and endocrine effects. Pepsinogen is a precursor of the proteolytic enzyme pepsin, and intrinsic factor is required for the absorption of vitamin B_{12}. Pyloric glands are located in the antrum and contain gastrin-secreting cells. Acid production and gastrin levels are inversely related to each other except in pathologic secretory states. Acid secretion is low at birth but increases dramatically by 24 hr. Acid and pepsin secretion peak in the 1st 10 days and decrease from 10 to 30 days after birth. Intrinsic factor secretion rises slowly in the 1st 2 wk of life.

The small bowel is ≈270 cm in length at birth in a term neonate and grows to an adult length of 450–550 cm by 4 yr of age. The mucosa of the small intestine is composed of villi, which are finger-like projections of the mucosa into the bowel lumen that significantly expand the absorptive surface area. The mucosal surface is further expanded by a brush border containing digestive enzymes and transport mechanisms for monosaccharides, amino acids, dipeptides and tripeptides, and fats. The cells of the villi originate in adjacent crypts and become functional as they migrate from the crypt up the villus. The small bowel mucosa is completely renewed in 4–5 days, providing a mechanism for rapid repair after injury; but in young infants or malnourished children, the process may be delayed. Crypt cells also secrete fluid and electrolytes. The villi are present by 8 wk gestation in the duodenum and by 11 wk in the ileum. Disaccharidase activities are measurable at 12 wk, but lactase activity does not reach maximal levels until 36 wk. Even premature infants usually tolerate lactose-containing formulas because of carbohydrate salvage by colonic bacteria. In African and Asian people, lactase levels may begin to fall at 4 yr of age, leading to intolerance to mammalian milk. Mechanisms to digest and absorb protein, including pancreatic enzymes and mucosal mechanisms to transport amino acids, dipeptides, and tripeptides, are in place by the 20th wk of gestation. Carbohydrates, protein, and fat are normally absorbed by the upper half of the small intestine; the distal segments represent a vast reserve of absorptive capacity. Most of the sodium, potassium, chloride, and water are absorbed in the small bowel. Bile salts and vitamin B_{12} are selectively absorbed in the distal ileum, and iron is absorbed in the duodenum and proximal jejunum. Intraluminal digestion depends on the exocrine pancreas. Secretin and cholecystokinin stimulate synthesis and secretion of bicarbonate and digestive enzymes, which are released by the upper intestinal mucosa in response to various intraluminal stimuli, among them components of the diet.

Carbohydrate digestion is normally an efficient process that is completed in the distal duodenum. Starches are broken down to glucose, oligosaccharides, and disaccharides by pancreatic amylase. Residual glucose polymers are broken down at the mucosal level by glucoamylase. Lactose is broken down at the brush border by lactase, forming glucose and galactose, while sucrose is broken down by sucrase isomaltase to fructose and glucose. Galactose and glucose are primarily transported into the cell by a sodium- and energy-dependent process, whereas fructose is transported by facilitated diffusion.

Proteins are hydrolyzed by pancreatic enzymes, including trypsin, chymotrypsin, elastase, and carboxypeptidases, into individual amino acids and oligopeptides. The pancreatic enzymes are secreted as proenzymes, which are activated by release of the mucosal enzyme enterokinase. Oligopeptides are further broken down at the brush border by peptidases into dipeptides, tripeptides, and amino acids. Protein can enter the cell by separate noncompetitive carriers that can transport individual amino acids or dipeptides and tripeptides similar to those in the renal tubule. The human gut is capable of absorbing antigenic intact proteins in the 1st few weeks of life because of "leaky" junctions between enterocytes. Entry of potential protein antigens through the mucosal barrier may have a role in later food- and microbe-induced symptoms.

Fat absorption occurs in two phases. Dietary triglycerides are broken down into monoglycerides and free fatty acids by pancreatic lipase and colipase. The free fatty acids are subsequently emulsified by bile acids forming micelles with phospholipids and other fat-soluble substances and are transported to the cell membrane where they are absorbed. The fats are re-esterified in the enterocyte, forming chylomicrons that are transported through the intestinal lymphatics to the thoracic duct. Medium-chain fats are absorbed more efficiently and can directly enter the cell. They are subsequently transported to the liver via the portal system. Fat absorption can be affected at any stage of the digestion and absorption process. Decreased pancreatic enzymes occur in cystic fibrosis, cholestatic liver disease leads to poor bile salt production and micelle formation, celiac disease affects mucosal surface area, abnormal chylomicron formation occurs in abetalipoproteinemia, and intestinal lymphangiectasia affects transport of the chylomicrons.

Fat absorption is less efficient in the neonate compared with adults. Premature infants can lose up to 20% of their fat calories compared with ≤6% in the adult. Decreased synthesis of bile acids and pancreatic lipase and decreased efficiency of ileal absorption are contributing factors. Fat digestion in the neonate is facilitated by lingual and gastric lipases. Bile salt–stimulated lipase in human milk augments the action of pancreatic lipase. Infants with malabsorption of fat are usually placed on formulas that have a greater percentage of medium-chain triglycerides, which are absorbed independently of bile salts.

The colon is a 75–100 cm sacculated tube due to three strips of longitudinal muscle called *taenia coli* that traverse its length and fold the mucosa into haustra. Haustra and taenia appear by the 12th wk of gestation. The most common motor activity in the colon is nonpropulsive rhythmic segmentation that acts to mix the chyme and expose the contents to the colonic mucosa. Mass movement within the colon typically occurs after a meal. The colon extracts additional water and electrolytes from the luminal contents to render the stools partially or completely solid. The colon also acts to scavenge by-products of bacterial degradation of carbohydrates. Stool is stored in the rectum until distention triggers a defecation reflex that, when assisted by voluntary relaxation of the external sphincter, permits evacuation.

Chapter 326 ■ Pyloric Stenosis and Congenital Anomalies of the Stomach

Robert Wyllie

The hallmark of gastric obstruction is nonbilious vomiting. Other symptoms include abdominal pain and nausea. Signs of gastric outlet obstruction include abdominal distention and bleeding from secondary inflammation of the gastric or esophageal mucosa.

The most common cause of nonbilious vomiting is infantile hypertrophic pyloric stenosis. Similar symptoms may be associated with various other gastric malformations, including pyloric atresia, antral webs, gastric duplications, and gastric volvulus. The differential diagnosis also includes gastroesophageal reflux, peptic ulcer disease, salt-wasting adrenogenital syndrome, eosinophilic gastroenteritis, bezoars, and various other metabolic and motility abnormalities.

326.1 • Hypertrophic Pyloric Stenosis

Hypertrophic pyloric stenosis occurs in 1–3/1,000 infants in the United States. It is more common in whites of northern European ancestry, less common in blacks, and rare in Asians. Males (especially first-borns) are affected approximately four times as often as females. The offspring of a mother and, to a lesser extent, the father who had pyloric stenosis are at higher risk for pyloric stenosis. Pyloric stenosis develops in approximately 20% of the male and 10% of the female descendants of a mother who had pyloric stenosis. The incidence of pyloric stenosis is increased in infants with type B and O blood groups. Pyloric stenosis is associated with other congenital defects, including tracheoesophageal fistula and hypoplasia or agenesis of the inferior labial frenulum.

ETIOLOGY. The cause of pyloric stenosis is unknown, but many factors have been implicated. Pyloric stenosis is usually not present at birth and is more concordant in monozygotic than dizygotic twins. It is unusual in stillbirths and probably develops after birth. Pyloric stenosis has been associated with eosinophilic gastroenteritis, Apert syndrome, Zellweger syndrome, trisomy 18, Smith-Lemli-Opitz syndrome, and Cornelia de Lange syndrome. A variable association has been found with the use of erythromycin in neonates when administered for pertussis postexposure prophylaxis. Abnormal muscle innervation, elevated serum levels of prostaglandins, and infant hypergastrinemia have been implicated. Reduced levels of pyloric nitric oxide synthase have been found with altered expression of the neuronal nitric oxide synthase (nNOS) exon 1c regulatory region, which influences the expression of the nNOS gene. Reduced nitric oxide may contribute to the pathogenesis of pyloric stenosis.

CLINICAL MANIFESTATIONS. Nonbilious vomiting is the initial symptom of pyloric stenosis. The vomiting may or may not be projectile initially but is usually progressive, occurring immediately after a feeding. Emesis may follow each feeding, or it may be intermittent. The vomiting usually starts after 3 wk of age, but symptoms may develop as early as the 1st wk of life and as late as the 5th mo. After vomiting, the infant is hungry and wants to feed again. As vomiting continues, a progressive loss of fluid, hydrogen ion, and chloride leads to hypochloremic metabolic alkalosis. Serum potassium levels are usually maintained, but there may be a total body potassium deficit. Greater awareness of pyloric stenosis has led to earlier identification of patients with fewer instances of chronic malnutrition and severe dehydration.

Jaundice associated with a decreased level of glucuronyl transferase is seen in ≈5% of affected infants. The indirect hyperbilirubinemia usually resolves promptly after relief of the obstruction.

The **diagnosis** has traditionally been established by palpating the pyloric mass. The mass is firm, movable, ≈2 cm in length, olive shaped, hard, best palpated from the left side, and located above and to the right of the umbilicus in the mid epigastrium beneath the liver edge. In healthy infants, feeding can be an aid to the diagnosis. After feeding, there may be a visible gastric peristaltic wave that progresses across the abdomen (Fig. 326-1). After the infant vomits, the abdominal musculature is more relaxed and the "olive" easier to palpate. Sedation can be used to facilitate examination but is usually unnecessary. The diagnosis can be established clinically 60–80% of the time by an experienced examiner.

Ultrasound examination confirms the diagnosis in the majority of cases and allows an earlier diagnosis in infants with suspected disease but no pyloric mass on physical examination. Criteria for diagnosis include pyloric thickness >4 mm or an overall pyloric length >14 mm (Fig. 326-2). Ultrasonography has a sensitivity of ≈95%. When contrast studies are performed, they demonstrate an elongated pyloric channel, a bulge of the pyloric

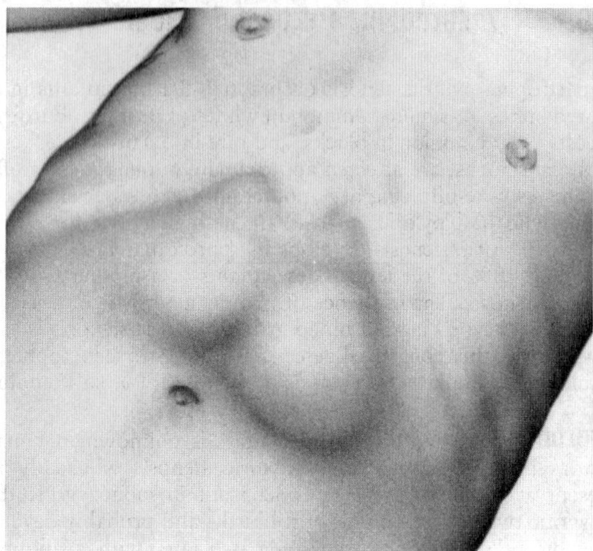

Figure 326-1. Gastric peristaltic wave in an infant with pyloric stenosis.

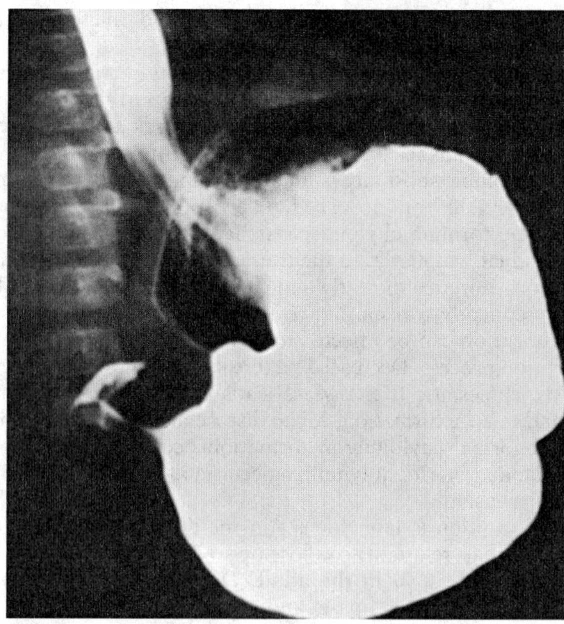

Figure 326-3. Barium in the stomach of an infant with projectile vomiting. The attenuated pyloric canal is typical of congenital hypertrophic pyloric stenosis.

muscle into the antrum (shoulder sign), and parallel streaks of barium seen in the narrowed channel, producing a "double tract sign" (Fig. 326-3).

DIFFERENTIAL DIAGNOSIS. The usual patient can be diagnosed by the characteristic clinical pattern and the identification of a pyloric mass on physical examination or ultrasonography. Infants who are exceptionally reactive to external stimuli, those fed by inexperienced or anxious caretakers, or those for whom an adequate maternal-infant bonding relationship has not been established may vomit frequently in the early weeks of life. Such infants may come to resemble infants with pyloric stenosis; the vomiting may be persistent and even projectile. Gastric waves are occasionally visible in small, emaciated infants who do not have pyloric stenosis. Infrequently, gastroesophageal reflux, with or without a hiatal hernia, may be confused with pyloric stenosis. Gastroesophageal reflux disease can be differentiated from pyloric stenosis by radiographic studies. Adrenal insufficiency can simulate pyloric stenosis, but the absence of a metabolic acidosis and elevated serum potassium and urinary sodium concentrations of adrenal insufficiency aid in differentiation. Inborn errors of metabolism can produce recurrent emesis with alkalosis (urea

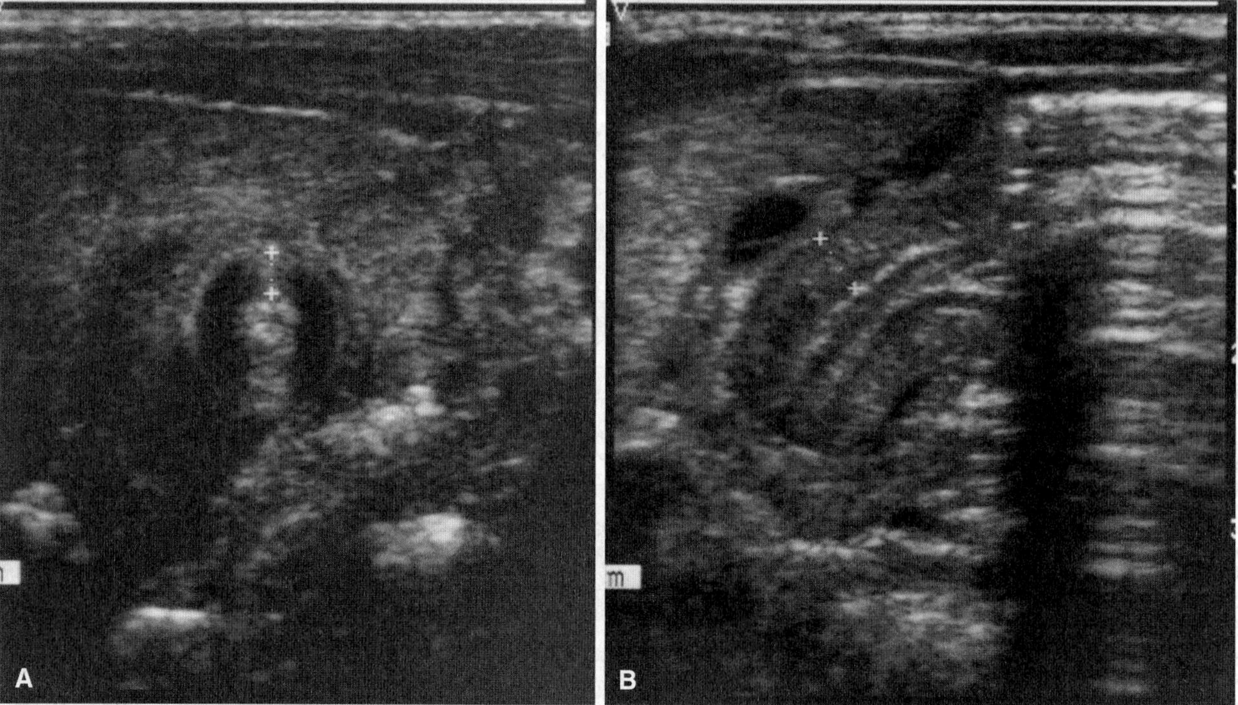

Figure 326-2. *A*, Transverse sonogram demonstrating a pyloric muscle wall thickness of >4 mm (distance between *crosses*). *B*, Horizontal image demonstrating a pyloric channel length >14 mm (wall thickness outlined between *crosses*) in an infant with pyloric stenosis.

cycle) or acidosis (organic acidemia) and lethargy, coma, or seizures. Vomiting with diarrhea suggests gastroenteritis, but patients with pyloric stenosis occasionally have diarrhea. Rarely, a pyloric membrane or pyloric duplication results in projectile vomiting, visible peristalsis, and, in the case of a duplication, a palpable mass. Duodenal stenosis proximal to the ampulla of Vater results in the clinical features of pyloric stenosis but can be differentiated by the presence of a pyloric mass on physical examination or ultrasonography.

TREATMENT. The preoperative treatment is directed toward correcting the fluid, acid-base, and electrolyte losses. Intravenous fluid therapy is begun with 0.45–0.9% saline, in 5–10% dextrose, with the addition of potassium chloride in concentrations of 30–50 mEq/L. Fluid therapy should be continued until the infant is rehydrated and the serum bicarbonate concentration is <30 mEq/dL, which implies that the alkalosis has been corrected. Correction of the alkalosis is essential to prevent postoperative apnea, which may be associated with anesthesia. Most infants can be successfully rehydrated within 24 hr. Vomiting usually stops when the stomach is empty, and only an occasional infant requires nasogastric suction.

The **surgical procedure of choice** is pyloromyotomy. The traditional Ramstedt procedure is performed through a short transverse skin incision. The underlying pyloric mass is split without cutting the mucosa, and the incision is closed. Laparoscopic technique is equally successful. Postoperative vomiting occurs in half the infants and is thought to be secondary to edema of the pylorus at the incision site. In most infants, however, feedings can be initiated within 12–24 hr after surgery and advanced to maintenance oral feedings within 36–48 hr after the surgery. Persistent vomiting suggests an incomplete pyloromyotomy, gastritis, gastroesophageal reflux disease, or another cause of the obstruction.

The surgical treatment of pyloric stenosis is curative, with an operative mortality of 0–0.5%. Conservative medical therapy consisting of small frequent feedings and atropine has been successful in small groups of patients. Endoscopic balloon dilation has been successful in infants with persistent vomiting secondary to incomplete pyloromyotomy.

326.2 • Congenital Gastric Outlet Obstruction

Gastric outlet obstruction resulting from pyloric atresia and antral webs is uncommon and accounts for <1% of all the atresias and diaphragms of the alimentary tract. The cause of the defects is unknown. Pyloric atresia has been associated with **epidermolysis bullosa** and usually presents in early infancy (see Chapter 653). The sex distribution is equal.

CLINICAL MANIFESTATIONS. Infants with pyloric atresia present with nonbilious vomiting, feeding difficulties, and abdominal distention during the 1st day of life. **Polyhydramnios** occurs in the majority of cases, and low birthweight is common. The gastric aspirate at birth is large (>20 mL fluid) and should be removed to prevent aspiration. Rupture of the stomach may occur as early as the 1st 12 hr of life. Infants with antral web may present with less dramatic symptoms, depending on the degree of obstruction. Older children with antral webs present with nausea, vomiting, abdominal pain, and weight loss.

DIAGNOSIS. The diagnosis of congenital gastric outlet obstruction is suggested by the finding of a large, dilated stomach on abdominal plain radiographs or in utero ultrasonography. Upper gastrointestinal contrast series is usually diagnostic and demonstrates a pyloric dimple. An antral web may appear as a thin septum near the pyloric channel. In older children, endoscopy has been helpful in identifying antral webs.

TREATMENT. The treatment of gastric outlet obstruction in neonates starts with the correction of dehydration and hypochloremic alkalosis. Persistent vomiting should be relieved with nasogastric decompression. Surgical or endoscopic repair should be undertaken when a patient is stable.

326.3 • Gastric Duplication

Gastric duplications are uncommon cystic or tubular structures that usually occur within the wall of the stomach. Most are smaller than 12 cm in diameter and do not usually communicate with the stomach lumen. Associated anomalies occur in as many as 35% of patients. Duplications have been attributed to a failure of recanalization after the solid stage of intestinal development.

The most common clinical manifestations are associated with partial or complete gastric outlet obstruction. In 33% of patients, the cyst may be palpable. Communicating duplications may cause gastric ulceration and be associated with hematemesis or melena.

Gastric duplications are visualized on upper gastrointestinal series as an extrinsic defect usually located along the lesser curve of the stomach. CT or ultrasonography may be helpful in defining a cystic structure. Surgical excision is the treatment for symptomatic gastric duplications.

326.4 • Gastric Volvulus

Gastric volvulus presents as a **triad** of a sudden onset of severe epigastric pain, intractable retching with emesis, and inability to pass a tube into the stomach. The stomach is tethered longitudinally by the gastrohepatic, gastrosplenic, and gastrocolic ligaments. In the transverse axis, it is tethered by the gastrophrenic ligament and the retroperitoneal attachment of the duodenum. A volvulus occurs when one of these attachments is absent or stretched, allowing the stomach to rotate around itself. In most children, other associated defects are present, including intestinal malrotation, diaphragmatic defects, or asplenia. Volvulus may occur along the longitudinal axis, producing organoaxial volvulus, or along the transverse axis, producing mesenteroaxial volvulus.

CLINICAL MANIFESTATIONS. The clinical presentation of gastric volvulus is nonspecific and suggests high intestinal obstruction. Gastric volvulus in infancy is usually associated with nonbilious vomiting. Acute volvulus may advance rapidly to strangulation and perforation. Chronic gastric volvulus is more common in older children; the children present with a history of emesis, abdominal pain, and early satiety.

The **diagnosis** is suggested in plain abdominal radiographs by the presence of a dilated stomach. Erect abdominal films demonstrate a double fluid level with a characteristic "beak" near the lower esophageal junction in mesenteroaxial volvulus. In organoaxial volvulus, a single air-fluid level is seen without the characteristic beak. Treatment of acute gastric volvulus is emergent surgery once a patient is stabilized. In selected cases of chronic volvulus in older patients, endoscopic correction has been successful.

326.5 • Hypertrophic Gastropathy

Hypertrophic gastropathy in children is uncommon and, in contrast to that in adults (Ménétrier disease), is usually a transient, benign, and self-limited condition. The condition is most often secondary to cytomegalovirus infection, but other agents, including herpes simplex virus, ***Giardia***, and ***Helicobacter pylori***, have also been implicated. Clinical manifestations include vomiting, anorexia, upper abdominal pain, diarrhea, edema (hypoproteinemic protein-losing enteropathy), ascites, and, rarely, hematemesis if ulceration occurs. Endoscopy with biopsy confirms the diagnosis. The mean age at diagnosis is 5 yr (range 2 days–17 yr); the illness usually lasts 2–4 wk, with complete resolution the rule. The **differential diagnosis** includes eosinophilic gastroenteritis, gastric lymphoma or carcinoma, Crohn disease, and inflammatory pseudotumor.

Hoffer V, Finkelstein Y, Balter J, et al: Ganciclovir treatment in Ménétrier's disease. *Acta Paediatr* 2003;92:983–985.
Kawahara H, Imura K, Nishikawa M, et al: Intravenous atropine treatment in infantile hypertrophic pyloric stenosis. *Arch Dis Child* 2002;87:71–74.
Parrini S, Di Maggio G, Latini G, et al: Abnormal oral mucosal light reflectance in infantile hypertrophic pyloric stenosis. *J Pediatr Gastroenterol Nutr* 2004;39:53–55.
Saur D, Vanderwinden JM, Seidler B, et al. Single-nucleotide promoter polymorphism alters transcription of neuronal nitric oxide synthase exon 1c in infantile hypertrophic pyloric stenosis. *Proc Natl Acad Sci U S A* 2004;101:1662–1667.
To T, Wajja A, Wales PW, Langer JC: Population demographic indicators associated with incidence of pyloric stenosis. *Arch Pediatr Adolesc Med* 2005;159:520–525.
Yagmurlu A, Barnhart DC, Vernon A, et al. Comparison of the incidence of complications in open and laparoscopic pyloromyotomy: A concurrent single institution series. *J Pediatr Surg* 2004;39;292–296.

Chapter 327 ■ Intestinal Atresia, Stenosis, and Malrotation Robert Wyllie

GENERAL CONSIDERATIONS. Intestinal obstruction occurs in ≈1/1,500 live births. Obstruction may be partial or complete and may arise from intrinsic or extrinsic abnormalities of the gut. Obstruction can be further classified as simple or strangulating. Simple obstruction is associated with the failure of progression of aboral flow of luminal contents. Strangulating obstruction is associated with impaired blood flow to the intestine in addition to obstruction of the flow of luminal contents. If strangulating obstruction is not promptly relieved, it can lead to bowel infarction and perforation.

Obstruction is typically associated with an accumulation of ingested food, gas, and intestinal secretions proximal to the point of obstruction, leading to distention of the bowel. As the bowel dilates, intestinal absorption decreases and secretion of fluid and electrolytes increases. The shift in fluid and electrolytes results in isotonic intravascular depletion usually associated with hypokalemia. The gut proximal to the obstruction initially demonstrates an increase in contractile activity, which is followed by a marked decrease with hypoactive bowel sounds. The combination of fluid accumulation (distention) and hypomotility is associated with nausea and vomiting.

Congenital obstructive lesions of the intestines can be viewed as intrinsic (atresia, stenosis, meconium ileus, aganglionic megacolon) or extrinsic (malrotation, constricting bands, intra-abdominal hernias, duplications). An attempt should be made to locate the lesion preoperatively to guide the surgical approach. When the obstruction is complete, there should be little difficulty in clinical recognition, but when it is incomplete or intermittent, the diagnosis may pose considerable difficulty. **Polyhydramnios** frequently accompanies high intestinal obstruction. When polyhydramnios has been noted, the infant's stomach should be aspirated immediately after birth. Aspiration of 15–20 mL or more of gastric fluid, especially if it is bile stained, is suggestive of a high intestinal obstruction.

Meconium stools can be passed initially if the obstruction is in the upper part of the small intestine or if the obstruction developed late in intrauterine life.

When obstruction is incomplete (as with intestinal stenosis, constricting bands, duplications incomplete volvulus), signs (vomiting, abdominal distention, obstipation) may appear shortly after birth or may be delayed an indeterminate time. They may approach the severity of complete obstruction, or they may be sufficiently mild and infrequent as to be overlooked until either an acute episode or diagnostic studies disclose the lesion.

Atresia refers to complete obstruction of the bowel lumen, and stenosis refers to a partial block of luminal contents. Intestinal atresia is common in the duodenum, jejunum, and ileum and rare in the colon. Intestinal atresia accounts for ≈33% of all cases of neonatal intestinal obstruction and affects males and females with equal frequency. Intestinal atresia impairs the development of the myenteric plexus below the level of atresia, which is associated with motility disorders observed after surgical repair.

Blood flow to the obstructed bowel decreases as the bowel dilates. Blood flow is shifted away from the mucosa, with loss of mucosal integrity. Bacteria proliferate in the stagnant bowel, with a predominance of coliforms and anaerobes. The rapid proliferation of bacteria coupled with the loss of mucosal integrity allows bacterial translocation across the bowel wall, potentially resulting in endotoxemia, bacteremia, and sepsis.

The clinical presentation of intestinal obstruction varies with the cause, level of obstruction, and time between the obstructing event and the patient's evaluation. The **classic symptoms** of obstruction include nausea and vomiting, abdominal distention, and obstipation. Obstruction high in the intestinal tract involving the duodenum or proximal jejunum results in large-volume, frequent, bilious emesis. Pain is intermittent and is usually relieved by vomiting. The pain is localized to the epigastrium or periumbilical area, and there is little abdominal distention. Obstruction in the distal small bowel leads to moderate or marked abdominal distention with emesis that is progressively feculent. Pain is usually diffuse over the entire abdomen.

No laboratory studies are diagnostic of obstruction or differentiate simple obstruction from obstruction associated with bowel infarction. Obstruction high in the gastrointestinal tract is often associated with hypochloremic metabolic alkalosis. Marked leukocytosis with or without thrombocytopenia, metabolic acidosis, and hematochezia in a patient with obstruction suggests bowel infarction. Serum amylase and lipase determinations should be performed to rule out pancreatitis.

Bowel obstruction is usually suggested on the basis of history (including prenatal ultrasonography) and physical examination. Imaging is used to confirm the diagnosis and localize the area of obstruction. Plain supine and erect or decubitus radiographs are the initial studies.

Valuable information on the location of congenital obstructive lesions in the intestine may often be obtained from flat and upright radiographs of the abdomen taken without use of contrast media. With completely obstructing lesions, distention of the bowel is noted above the obstruction and a series of fluid levels with superimposed gas in the distended loops may be observed in the upright or cross-table lateral position. **Pneumoperitoneum** may be seen if there is a **perforation** with free air in the subphrenic regions or over the liver in the left lateral decubitus position. **Calcification** within the peritoneal cavity usually indicates **meconium peritonitis.** Rarely, obstruction with intraluminal calcification is associated with rectourinary fistula, colonic aganglionosis, or intestinal atresia. A characteristic ground-glass appearance in the right lower quadrant with trapped bubbles of air within the obstructing meconium may be seen in patients with meconium ileus. Air is usually demonstrable radiographically in the stomach of a normal infant immediately after birth; within 1 hr, air may reach the proximal portion of the small intestine and segments of the colon; air may become visible in the distal parts of the colon as early as the 3rd hr or as late as 18 hr. It may be difficult to differentiate accurately small from large bowel obstruction in children <2 yr.

Ultrasonography is helpful in identifying pyloric stenosis, malrotation, and volvulus or intussusception and in differentiating pyloric stenosis from other causes of proximal obstruction. Contrast studies of the bowel or CT are indicated when plain films or sonograms fail to identify the source of obstruction. Water-soluble contrast studies avoid the risk of barium contamination of the peritoneum when there is a significant chance of perforation not detected by the presence of pneumoperitoneum on plain films. Water-soluble contrast enemas are useful in diagnosing malrotation, meconium ileus, meconium plug, and intussusception. In meconium ileus, meconium plug, and intussusception, the enema may be diagnostic and relieve the obstruction. Oral or nasogastric contrast medium is used to identify obstructing lesions in the proximal bowel (atresia, volvulus, malrotation). Water-soluble agents are used if perforation is suspected. CT scan of the abdomen is also sensitive and specific for diagnosing small bowel obstruction, especially in children >2 yr.

MANAGEMENT. Infants and children with bowel obstruction have mechanical obstruction and loss of fluid and electrolytes. Those with strangulating vascular obstruction may also develop intestinal ischemia with sepsis and shock. Initial treatment must be directed at **fluid resuscitation** and stabilizing the patient. **Nasogastric decompression** usually provides relief of pain and vomiting. After appropriate cultures, broad-spectrum antibiotics are usually started in ill-appearing neonates with bowel obstruction and those with suspected strangulating infarction. Patients with strangulation must have immediate surgical relief before the bowel infarcts, resulting in gangrene and intestinal perforation. Extensive intestinal necrosis results in short bowel syndrome (see Chapter 335.7). Nonoperative conservative management is usually limited to children with suspected adhesions or inflammatory strictures that may resolve with nasogastric decompression or anti-inflammatory medications. If clinical signs of improvement are not evident within 12–24 hr, then operative intervention is usually indicated.

327.1 • Duodenal Obstruction

Duodenal atresia is thought to arise from failure to recanalize the lumen after the solid phase of intestinal development in the 4th and 5th wk of gestation. The incidence of duodenal atresia is 1/10,000 births and accounts for 25–40% of all intestinal atresias. Half the patients are born prematurely. Duodenal atresia can take several forms, including an intact membrane obstructing the lumen, a short fibrous cord connecting two blind duodenal pouches, or a gap between the nonconnecting ends of the duodenum. An unusual cause of obstruction is a "windsock" web, which is a distensible flap of tissue associated with anomalies of the biliary tract. The membranous form of atresia is most common, with obstruction occurring distal to the ampulla of Vater in the majority of patients. Duodenal obstruction can also be a result of an extrinsic compression such as an annular pancreas or from Ladd bands in patients with malrotation. Down syndrome occurs in 20–30% of patients with duodenal atresia. Other congenital anomalies that are associated with duodenal atresia include malrotation (20%), esophageal atresia (10–20%), congenital heart disease (10–15%), and anorectal and renal anomalies (5%).

CLINICAL MANIFESTATIONS. The hallmark of duodenal obstruction is **bilious vomiting** without abdominal distention, which is usually noted on the 1st day of life. Peristaltic waves may be visualized early in the disease process. A history of **polyhydramnios** is present in half the pregnancies and is caused by a failure of absorption of amniotic fluid in the distal intestine. Jaundice is present in one third of the infants. The diagnosis is suggested by the presence of a "**double-bubble sign**" on plain abdominal radiographs (Fig. 327-1). The appearance is caused by a distended and gas-filled stomach and proximal duodenum. Contrast studies are usually not necessary and may be associated with aspiration. Contrast studies may occasionally be needed to exclude malrotation and volvulus because intestinal infarction may occur within 6–12 hr if the volvulus is not relieved. Prenatal diagnosis of duodenal atresia is readily made by fetal ultrasonography.

TREATMENT. The initial treatment of infants with duodenal atresia includes nasogastric or orogastric decompression and intravenous fluid replacement. Echocardiogram and radiology of the chest and spine should be performed to evaluate for associated anomalies. Approximately 30% of infants with duodenal atresia have associated life-threatening congenital anomalies. Definitive correction of the atresia is usually postponed to evaluate and treat these life-threatening anomalies.

The usual surgical repair for duodenal atresia is duodenoduodenostomy. The dilated proximal bowel can be tapered in an attempt to improve peristalsis. A gastrostomy tube can be placed to drain the stomach and protect the airway. Intravenous nutritional support or a transanastomotic jejunal tube is needed until

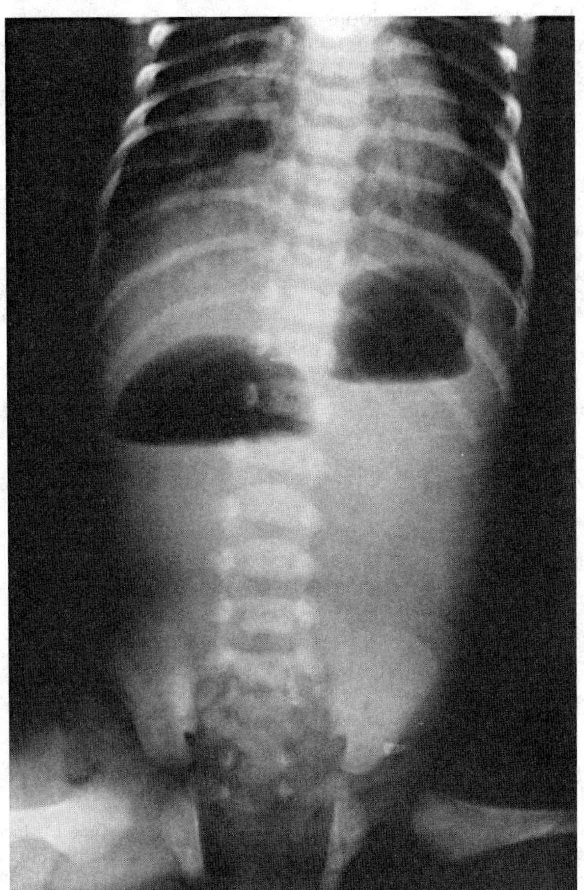

Figure 327-1. Abdominal radiograph of a newborn infant held upright. Note the "double-bubble" gas shadow above and the absence of gas in the distal bowel in this case of congenital duodenal atresia.

infants start to feed orally. The prognosis is primarily dependent on the presence of associated anomalies.

If obstruction is due to Ladd bands with malrotation, an operation is necessary without delay. After division of the abnormal peritoneal folds or bands, the entire large intestine is placed within the left side of the abdomen, after 1st removing the appendix, with the small bowel on the right—the fetal position of nonrotation. Appendectomy is performed to avoid later misdiagnosis of appendicitis. Malrotation can also coexist with an intrinsic duodenal obstruction, such as a membrane or stenosis; passing a balloon-tipped catheter into the jejunum below the site of obstruction, inflating the balloon, and slowly withdrawing the catheter may identify this. Annular pancreas is best treated by duodenoduodenostomy without dividing the pancreas, leaving as short a defunctioned loop as possible. Duodenal diaphragmatic obstruction is managed by duodenoplasty.

327.2 • Jejunal and Ileal Atresia and Obstruction

Jejunoileal atresias have been attributed to intrauterine vascular accidents leading to ischemic necrosis of the sterile bowel and resorption of the affected segments. Four different types of jejunal and ileal atresia are encountered (Fig. 327-2). Type I accounts for 20% of the atresias and is an intraluminal diaphragm that obstructs the lumen while continuity is maintained between the proximal and distal bowel. In type II, a small-diameter solid cord connects the proximal and distal bowel, accounting for about 35% of defects. Type III is divided into two subtypes. Type IIIa accounts for ≈35% of all atresias and occurs when both ends of the bowel end in blind loops accompanied by a small mesenteric defect. Type IIIb is associated with an extensive mesenteric defect and a loss of the normal blood supply to the distal bowel. The distal ileum coils around the ileocolic artery, from which it derives its entire blood supply, producing an **"apple-peel"** appearance. This anomaly is associated with prematurity, an unusually short distal ileum, and significant foreshortening of the bowel. Type IV is multiple segments of bowel atresia and accounts for ≈5% of all bowel atresias. Colon atresia has similarities to jejunoileal atresia but is much less common.

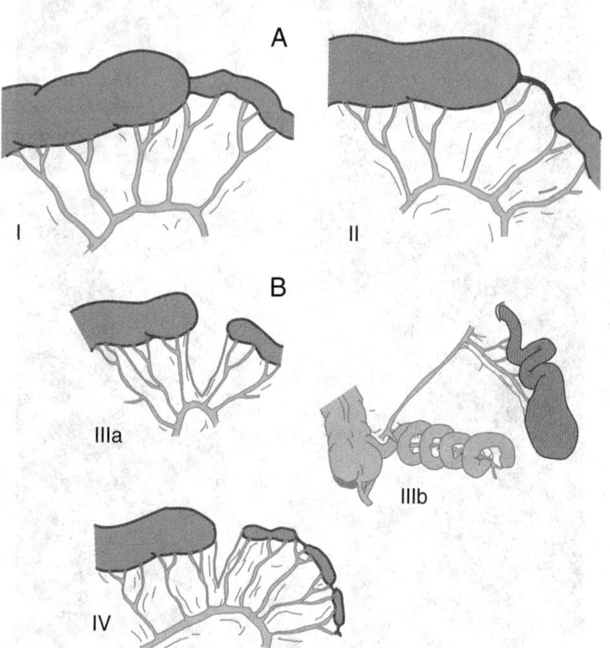

Figure 327-2. *A* and *B,* Classification of intestinal atresia. Type I: Mucosal obstruction caused by an intraluminal membrane with intact bowel wall and mesentery. Type II: Blind ends are separated by a fibrous cord. Type IIIa: Blind ends are separated by a V-shaped mesenteric defect. Type IIIb: "Apple-peel" appearance. Type IV: Multiple atresias. (From Grosfeld J: Jejunoileal atresia and stenosis. In Welch KJ, Randolph JG, Ravitch MM [editors]: *Pediatric Surgery,* 4th ed. Chicago, Year Book Medical Publishers, 1986.)

Meconium ileus occurs primarily in newborn infants with cystic fibrosis. Approximately 10% of infants with cystic fibrosis develop meconium ileus; 80–90% of infants presenting with meconium ileus have cystic fibrosis. In simple meconium ileus, the last 20–30 cm of ileum is collapsed and filled with pellets of pale-colored stool, above which a dilated loop of varying length appears obstructed by meconium of the consistency of thick syrup or glue. Peristalsis fails to propel this very viscid material forward, and it becomes impacted in the ileum. Volvulus, atresia, or perforation of the bowel accompanies complicated meconium ileus. Perforation in utero produces **meconium peritonitis.** Intraperitoneal meconium can cause dense adhesions, leading postnatally to adhesive intestinal obstruction, and can rapidly become **calcified.**

In 5% of patients with **Hirschsprung disease,** the aganglionic segment involves not only the entire colon, but also the terminal ileum. This condition causes a dilated small intestine with ganglionated but somewhat hypertrophied walls, a funnel-shaped transitional hypoganglionic zone, and a collapsed distal aganglionic bowel.

CLINICAL MANIFESTATION. In contrast to duodenal atresia, extragastrointestinal anomalies are less common in atresias of the distal intestine. The diagnosis of jejunoileal atresia can be made by prenatal ultrasonograms. Polyhydramnios occurs in 25% of affected patients. Monozygotic twins are at higher risk for atresias than are dizygotic twins or singletons. Premature birth occurs in 30% of infants. Atresia has also been associated with low birthweight, multiple births, and maternal cocaine use and cigarette smoking.

Most infants become symptomatic in the 1st day of life with abdominal distention and bile-stained emesis or gastric aspirate. Sixty to 75% of the infants fail to pass meconium. Jaundice has been found in 20–30% of the patients. Plain radiographs demonstrate many air-fluid levels (Fig. 327-3) or peritoneal calcification associated with meconium peritonitis. Contrast studies of the upper and lower bowel can delineate the level of obstruction and differentiate atresia from meconium ileus, meconium plug, and Hirschsprung disease. Abdominal ultrasound can distinguish meconium ileus from ileal atresia and identify intestinal malrotation.

In meconium ileus, plain films of the abdomen show a typical hazy or ground-glass appearance in the right lower quadrant. Small bubbles of gas trapped in meconium are dispersed within this area (see Chapter 102.1). Because of their viscid contents, moderately dilated loops of bowel do not have the air-fluid levels usually seen radiographically on the erect projection. If there is meconium peritonitis, patchy calcification may be noted, usually in the flanks. **Pneumoperitoneum** is most readily seen as free air between the liver and the diaphragm on an upright radiograph of the abdomen; if there is a large amount of free air, the entire abdomen may look like a football from distention with air; the ligamentum teres is sometimes clearly visible in the midline.

It is impossible to distinguish consistently small bowel from large bowel by studying plain radiographs of the abdomen in newborns and infants. If plain radiographs are nonspecific, a water-soluble contrast (Gastrografin, Hypaque) study of the colon may be needed to distinguish small from large intestine obstructions. A small colon, "microcolon," suggests disuse and the presence of obstruction proximal to the ileocecal valve. Water-soluble enemas should be used with caution in the diagnosis and treatment of meconium ileus because their hyperos-

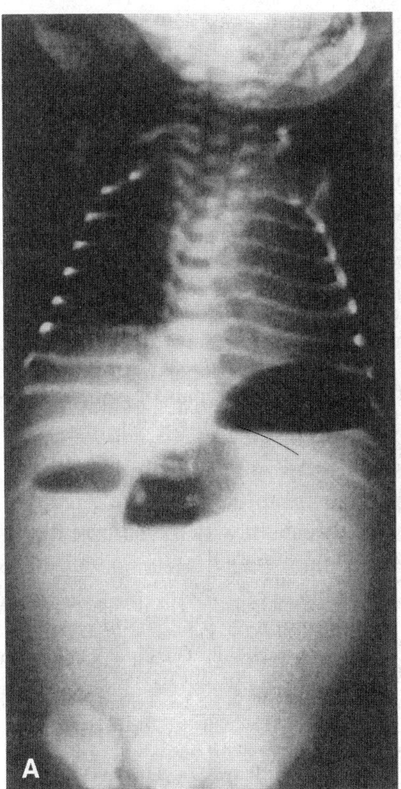

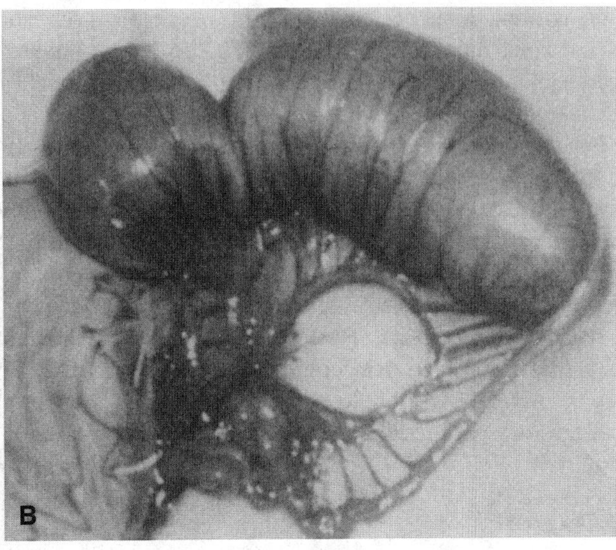

Figure 327-3. *A,* Abdominal radiograph in a neonate with bilious vomiting shows a few loops of dilated intestine with air-fluid levels. *B,* At laparotomy, a type I (mucosal) jejunal atresia was observed. (From O'Neill JA Jr, Grosfeld JL, Fonkalsrud EW, et al [editors]: *Principles of Pediatric Surgery,* 2nd ed. St. Louis, Mosby, 2003, p 493.)

molality may draw fluid into the colon and result in dehydration; the enema pressure may draw fluid into the colon and result in perforation.

TREATMENT. Patients with small bowel obstruction should be stable and in adequate fluid and electrolyte balance before operation or radiographic attempts at disimpaction unless volvulus is suspected. Infections should be treated with appropriate antibiotics. Prophylactic antibiotics are usually given before surgery.

Ileal or jejunal atresia requires resection of the dilated proximal portion of the bowel followed by end-to-end anastomosis. If a simple mucosal diaphragm is present, jejunoplasty or ileoplasty with partial excision of the web is an acceptable alternative to resection. In uncomplicated meconium ileus, Gastrografin enemas will diagnose the obstruction and wash out the inspissated material. Gastrografin is hypertonic and care must be taken to avoid dehydration, shock, and bowel perforation. The enema may have to be repeated after 8–12 hr. Resection after reduction is not needed if there have been no ischemic complications.

About 50% of patients with simple meconium ileus do not adequately respond to water-soluble enemas and need laparotomy. Operative management is indicated when the obstruction cannot be relieved by repeated attempts at nonoperative management and for infants with complicated meconium ileus. The extent of surgical intervention depends on the degree of pathology. In simple meconium ileus, the plug can be relieved by manipulation or direct enteral irrigation with *N*-acetylcysteine following an enterotomy. In complicated cases, bowel resection, peritoneal lavage, abdominal drainage, and stoma formation may be necessary. Total parenteral nutrition will be required.

327.3 • Malrotation

Malrotation is incomplete rotation of the intestine during fetal development. The gut starts as a straight tube from stomach to rectum. The mid bowel (distal duodenum to mid-transverse colon) begins to elongate and progressively protrudes into the umbilical cord until it lies totally outside the confines of the abdominal cavity. As the developing bowel rotates in and out of the abdominal cavity, the superior mesenteric artery, which supplies blood to this section of gut, acts as an axis. The duodenum, on re-entering the abdominal cavity, moves to the region of the ligament of Treitz, and the colon that follows is directed to the left upper quadrant. The cecum subsequently rotates counterclockwise within the abdominal cavity and comes to lie in the right lower quadrant. The duodenum becomes fixed to the posterior abdominal wall before the colon is completely rotated. After rotation, the right and left colon and the mesenteric root become fixed to the posterior abdomen. These attachments provide a broad base of support to the mesentery and the superior mesenteric artery, thus preventing twisting of the mesenteric root and kinking of the vascular supply. Abdominal rotation and attachment are completed by 3 mo of gestation.

Nonrotation occurs when the bowel fails to rotate after it returns to the abdominal cavity. The 1st and 2nd portions of the duodenum are in their normal position, but the remainder of the duodenum, jejunum, and ileum occupy the right side of the abdomen while the colon is located on the left. Malrotation and nonrotation are associated with abdominal heterotaxia and the asplenia-polysplenia congenital heart malformation syndrome anomalad (see Chapter 431.11).

The most common type of malrotation involves failure of the cecum to move into the right lower quadrant (Fig. 327-4). The

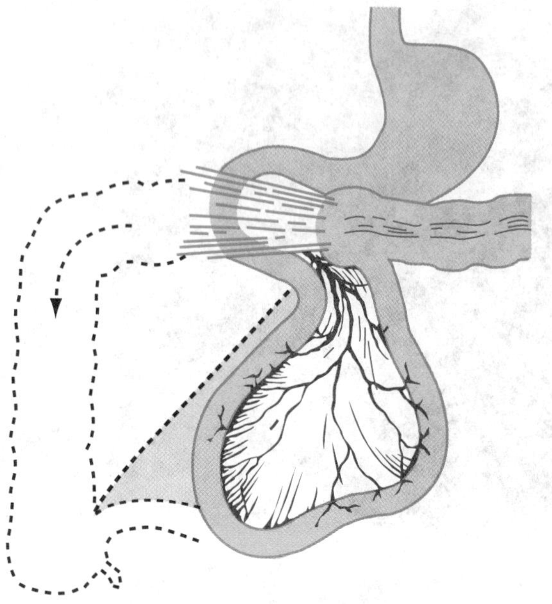

Figure 327-4. The mechanism of intestinal obstruction with incomplete rotation of the midgut (malrotation). The *dotted lines* show the course the cecum should have taken. Failure to rotate has left obstructing bands across the duodenum and a narrow pedicle for the midgut loop, making it susceptible to volvulus. (From Nixon HH, O'Donnell B: *The Essentials of Pediatric Surgery.* Philadelphia, JB Lippincott, 1961.)

usual location of the cecum is in the subhepatic area. Failure of the cecum to rotate properly is associated with failure to form the normal broad-based adherence to the posterior abdominal wall. The mesentery including the superior mesenteric artery is tethered by a narrow stalk, which can twist around itself and produce a midgut volvulus. In addition, bands of tissue (**Ladd bands**) may extend from the cecum to the right upper quadrant, crossing and possibly obstructing the duodenum.

CLINICAL MANIFESTATION. The majority of patients present in the 1st yr of life with symptoms of acute or chronic obstruction. Infants often present in the 1st wk of life with **bilious emesis** and acute bowel obstruction. Older infants present with episodes of recurrent abdominal pain that can mimic colic. Malrotation in older children may present with recurrent episodes of vomiting, abdominal pain, or both. Patients occasionally present with **malabsorption** or **protein-losing enteropathy** associated with bacterial overgrowth. Symptoms are caused by intermittent volvulus or duodenal compression by Ladd bands or other adhesive bands affecting the small and large bowel. Twenty-five to 50% of adolescents with malrotation are asymptomatic. Adolescents who become symptomatic present with acute intestinal obstruction or history of recurrent episodes of abdominal pain with less frequent vomiting and diarrhea. Patients of any age with a rotational anomaly can develop acute bowel threatening volvulus without pre-existing symptoms.

An acute presentation of small bowel obstruction in a patient without previous bowel surgery is usually a result of **volvulus** associated with malrotation. This is a life-threatening complication of malrotation, which resembles an acute abdomen or sepsis and is the main reason that symptoms suggestive of malrotation should always be investigated. The diagnosis is by ultrasound or contrast radiographic studies. The abdominal plain film is usually nonspecific but can demonstrate evidence of duodenal obstruction with a double-bubble sign. Barium enema usually demonstrates malposition of the cecum but is normal in 10% of patients. Upper gastrointestinal series demonstrates malposition of the ligament of Treitz. Ultrasonography demonstrates inversion of the superior mesenteric artery and vein. A superior mesenteric vein located to the left of the superior mesenteric artery is suggestive of malrotation. Malrotation with volvulus is suggested by duodenal obstruction, thickened bowel loops to the right of the spine, and free peritoneal fluid.

Surgical intervention is recommended for any patient with a significant rotational abnormality, regardless of age. If a volvulus is present, surgery is done immediately, the volvulus is reduced, and the duodenum and upper jejunum are freed of any bands and remain in the right abdominal cavity. The colon is freed of adhesions and placed in the right abdomen with the cecum in the left lower quadrant, usually accompanied by incidental appendectomy. Extensive intestinal ischemia from volvulus produces short bowel syndrome (see Chapter 335.7). Persistent symptoms after repair of malrotation should suggest a pseudo-obstruction–like motility disorder.

Basu R, Burge DM: The effect of antenatal diagnosis on the management of small bowel atresia. *Pediatr Surg Int* 2004;20:177–179.

Escobar MA, Ladd AP, Grosfeld JL, et al: Duodenal atresia and stenosis: Long-term follow-up over 30 years. *J Pediatr Surg* 2004;39:867–871.

Forrester MB, Merz RD: Population-based study of small intestinal atresia and stenosis, Hawaii, 1986–2000. *Public Health* 2004;118:434–438.

Karnak I, Ciftci AO, Senocak ME, et al: Colonic atresia: Surgical management and outcome. *Pediatr Surg Int* 2001;17:631–635.

Khen N, Jaubert F, Sauvat F, et al: Fetal intestinal obstruction induces alteration of enteric nervous system development in human intestinal atresia. *Pediatr Res* 2004;56:975–980.

Kumaran N, Shankar KR, Lloyd DA, Losty PD: Trends in the management and outcome of jejuno-ileal atresia. *Eur J Pediatr Surg* 2002;12:163–167.

Mehall JR, Chandler JC, Mehall RL, et al: Management of typical and atypical intestinal malrotation. *J Pediatr Surg* 2002;37:1169–1172.

Millar AJ, Rode H, Cywes S: Malrotation and volvulus in infancy and childhood. *Semin Pediatr Surg* 2003;12:229–236.

Pickhardt PJ, Bhalla S: Intestinal malrotation in adolescents and adults: Spectrum of clinical and imaging features. *AJR Am J Roentgenol* 2002;179:1429–1435.

Werler MM, Sheehan JE, Mitchell AA: Association of vasoconstrictive exposures with risks of gastroschisis and small intestinal atresia. *Epidemiology* 2003;14:349–354.

Chapter 328 ■ Intestinal Duplications, Meckel Diverticulum, and Other Remnants of the Omphalomesenteric Duct Robert Wyllie

328.1 • Intestinal Duplication

Duplications of the intestinal tract are rare anomalies that consist of well-formed tubular or spherical structures firmly attached to the intestine with a common blood supply. The lining of the duplications resembles that of the gastrointestinal tract. Duplications are located on the mesenteric border and may communicate with the intestinal lumen. Duplications can be classified into three categories: localized duplications, duplications associated with spinal cord defects and vertebral malformations, and duplications of the colon. Occasionally (10–15% of cases), multiple duplications are found.

Localized duplications can occur in any area of the gastrointestinal tract but are most common in the ileum and jejunum.

They are usually cystic or tubular structures within the wall of the bowel. The cause is unknown, but their development has been attributed to defects in recanalization of the intestinal lumen after the solid stage of embryologic development. Duplication of the intestine occurring in association with **vertebral and spinal cord anomalies** (hemivertebra, anterior spina bifida, band connection between lesion and cervical or thoracic spine) is thought to arise from splitting of the notochord in the developing embryo. **Duplication of the colon** is usually associated with anomalies of the urinary tract and genitals. Duplication of the entire colon, rectum, anus, and terminal ileum can occur. The defects are thought to be secondary to caudal twinning, with duplication of the hindgut, genital, and lower urinary tracts.

CLINICAL MANIFESTATIONS. Symptoms depend on the size, location, and mucosal lining. Duplications can cause bowel obstruction by compressing the adjacent intestinal lumen, or they can act as the lead point of an intussusception or a site for a volvulus. If they are lined by acid-secreting mucosa, they can cause ulceration, perforation, and hemorrhage of the adjacent bowel. Patients may present with abdominal pain, vomiting, palpable mass, or acute gastrointestinal hemorrhage. Intestinal duplications in the thorax (neuroenteric cysts) can present as respiratory distress. Duplications of the lower bowel can cause constipation or diarrhea or be associated with recurrent prolapse of the rectum.

The diagnosis is suspected on the basis of the history and physical examination. Radiologic studies such as barium studies, ultrasonography, CT, and MRI are helpful but usually nonspecific, demonstrating cystic structures or mass effects. Radioisotope technetium scanning may localize ectopic gastric mucosa. The treatment of duplications is surgical resection and management of associated defects.

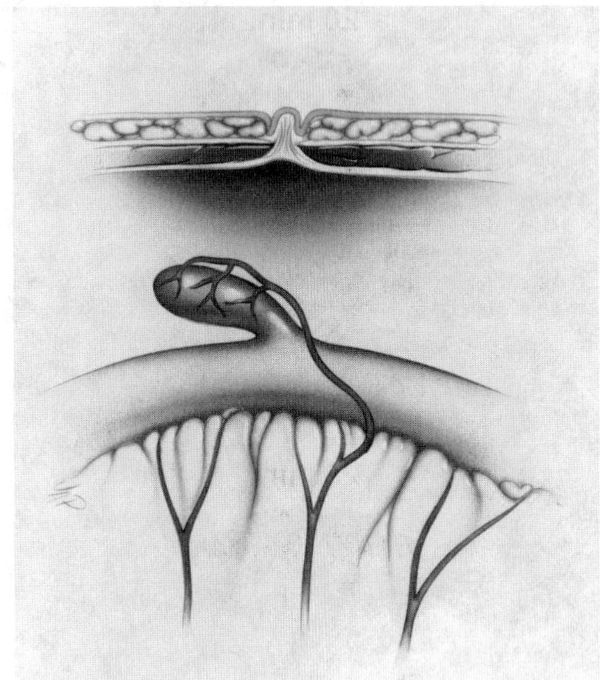

Figure 328-1. Typical Meckel diverticulum located on the antimesenteric border.

328.2 • Meckel Diverticulum and Other Remnants of the Omphalomesenteric Duct

A Meckel diverticulum is a remnant of the embryonic yolk sac, which is also referred to as the omphalomesenteric duct or vitelline duct. The omphalomesenteric duct connects the yolk sac to the gut in a developing embryo and provides nutrition until the placenta is established. Between the 5th and 7th wk of gestation, the duct attenuates and separates from the intestine. Just before this involution, the epithelium of the yolk sac develops a lining similar to that of the stomach. Partial or complete failure of involution of the omphalomesenteric duct results in various residual structures. Meckel diverticulum is the most common of these structures and is the most frequent congenital gastrointestinal anomaly, occurring in 2–3% of all infants. A typical Meckel diverticulum is a 3–6 cm outpouching of the ileum along the antimesenteric border 50–75 cm from the ileocecal valve (Fig. 328-1). The distance from the ileocecal valve depends on the age of the patient. Other omphalomesenteric duct remnants occur infrequently, including a persistently patent duct, a solid cord, or a cord with a central cyst or a diverticulum associated with a persistent cord between the diverticulum and the umbilicus.

CLINICAL MANIFESTATIONS. Symptoms of a Meckel diverticulum usually arise in the 1st 2 yr of life (average 2.5 yr), but initial symptoms can occur in the 1st decade. The majority of symptomatic Meckel diverticula are lined by an ectopic mucosa, including an acid-secreting mucosa that causes intermittent painless rectal bleeding by ulceration of the adjacent normal ileal mucosa. Unlike the upper duodenal mucosa, the acid is not neutralized by pancreatic bicarbonate.

The stool is typically described as brick colored or currant jelly colored. Bleeding can cause significant anemia but is usually self-limited because of contraction of the splanchnic vessels, as patients become hypovolemic. Bleeding from a Meckel diverticulum can also be less dramatic, with melanotic stools.

Less often, a Meckel diverticulum is associated with partial or complete bowel obstruction. The most common mechanism of obstruction occurs when the diverticulum acts as the lead point of an intussusception. The mean age of onset of obstruction is less than that for patients presenting with bleeding. Obstruction can also result from intraperitoneal bands connecting residual omphalomesenteric duct remnants to the ileum and umbilicus. These bands cause obstruction by internal herniation or volvulus of the small bowel around the band. A Meckel diverticulum may occasionally become inflamed (diverticulitis) and present similarly to acute appendicitis. These children are older, with a mean age of 8 yr. Diverticulitis can lead to perforation and peritonitis.

DIAGNOSIS. The diagnosis of omphalomesenteric duct remnants depends on the clinical presentation. If an infant or child presents with significant painless rectal bleeding, the presence of a Meckel diverticulum should be suspected. Confirmation of a Meckel diverticulum can be difficult. Plain abdominal radiographs are of no value, and routine barium studies rarely fill the diverticulum. The most sensitive study is a Meckel radionuclide scan, which is performed after intravenous infusion of technetium-99m pertechnetate. The mucus-secreting cells of the ectopic gastric mucosa take up pertechnetate, permitting visualization of the Meckel diverticulum (Fig. 328-2). The uptake can be enhanced with various agents, including cimetidine, glucagon, and gastrin. The sensitivity of the enhanced scan is approximately 85%, with a specificity of approximately 95%. Other methods of detection include abdominal ultrasound, superior mesenteric angiography, abdominal CT scan, and exploratory laparoscopy. In patients who present with intestinal obstruction or a picture of appendicitis with omphalomesenteric duct remnants, the diagnosis is rarely made before surgery. The treatment of a symptomatic Meckel diverticulum is surgical excision.

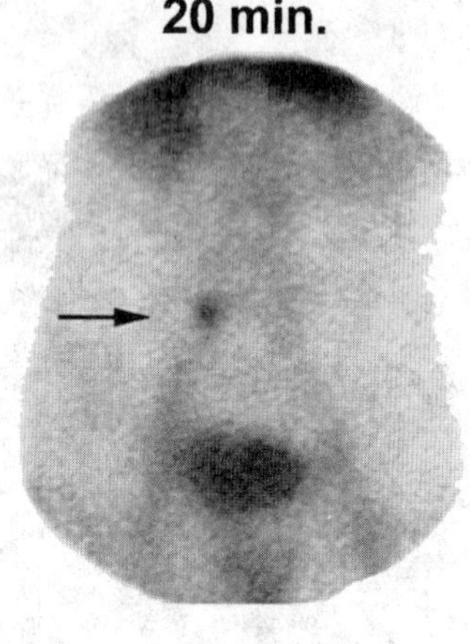

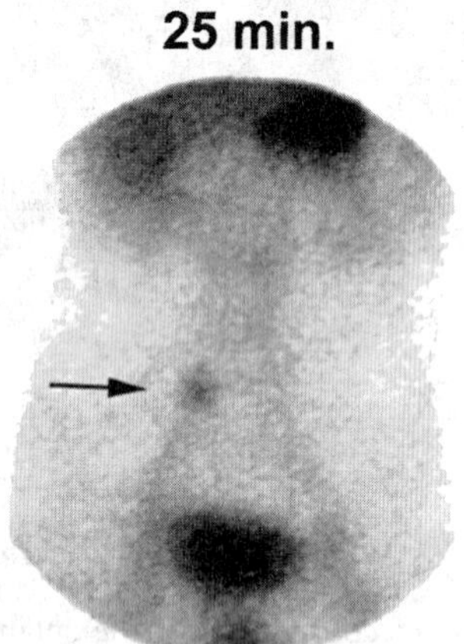

Figure 328-2. Meckel scan demonstrating accumulation of technetium in the stomach superior bladder (inferior) and in the acid-secreting mucosa of a Meckel diverticulum.

Baldisserotto M, Maffazzoni DR, Dora MD: Sonographic findings of Meckel's diverticulitis in children. *AJR Am J Roentgenol* 2003;80:425–428.

Emamian SA, Shalaby-Rana E, Majd M: The spectrum of heterotopic gastric mucosa in children detected by Tc-99m pertechnetate scintigraphy. *Clin Nucl Med* 2001;26:529–535.

Fenton LZ, Buonomo C, Share JC, Chung T: Small intestinal obstruction by remnants of the omphalomesenteric duct: Findings on contrast enema. *Pediatr Radiol* 2000;30:165–167.

Lee KH, Yeung CK, Tam YH, et al: Laparascopy for definitive diagnosis and treatment of gastrointestinal bleeding of obscure origin in children. *J Pediatr Surg* 2000;35:1291–1293.

Swaniker F, Soldes O, Hirschl RB: The utility of technetium-99m pertechnetate scintigraphy in the evaluation of patients with Meckel's diverticulum. *J Pediatr Surg* 1999;34:760–764, discussion 765.

Chapter 329 ■ Motility Disorders and Hirschsprung Disease

Robert Wyllie

329.1 • Chronic Intestinal Pseudo-Obstruction

Chronic intestinal pseudo-obstruction comprises a group of disorders characterized by signs and symptoms of intestinal obstruction in the absence of an anatomic lesion. Pseudo-obstruction can occur as a primary disease or be secondary to a large number of conditions that can transiently or permanently alter bowel motility. Pseudo-obstruction represents a wide spectrum of pathologic disorders from abnormal myoelectric activity to abnormalities of the nerves (**intestinal neuropathy**) or musculature (**intestinal myopathy**) of the gut. The organs involved can include the entire gastrointestinal tract or be limited to certain components, such as the stomach or colon. The distinctive pathologic abnormalities are considered together because of their clinical similarities.

Most congenital forms of pseudo-obstruction occur sporadically. A few clusters of autosomal dominant or recessive individuals have been reported as having cases associated with abnormal gut muscle or nerves. Patients with autosomal dominant forms of pseudo-obstruction have variable expressions of the disease. Acquired pseudo-obstruction may follow episodes of acute gastroenteritis, presumably resulting in injury to the myenteric plexus.

In congenital pseudo-obstruction, abnormalities of the muscle or nerves can be demonstrated in most cases. In muscular disease, the outer longitudinal muscle layer is replaced by fibrous material. In neuronal disease, there may be disorganized ganglia or hypoganglionosis or hyperganglionosis. Abnormalities in the interstitial cells of Cajal have been demonstrated in some children and mitochondrial defects found in others.

CLINICAL MANIFESTATIONS. More than half the children with congenital pseudo-obstruction experience symptoms in the 1st few months of life. Two thirds of the infants presenting in the 1st few days of life are born prematurely, and ≈40% have malrotation of the intestine. In 75% of these children, symptoms occur in the 1st yr of life, and the remainder become symptomatic in the next several years. The **most common symptoms** are abdominal distention and vomiting, which are present in 75% of affected infants. Constipation, growth failure, and abdominal pain occur in ≈60% of patients, and diarrhea occurs in 30–40%. The symptoms wax and wane in the majority of the patients; poor nutrition and intercurrent illness tend to exacerbate symptoms. **Urinary tract involvement** occurs in 40% of children with myopathy and can present as recurrent urinary tract infection, megacystis, or obstructive symptoms. Urinary tract abnormalities are less common in neuronal disease.

The diagnosis of pseudo-obstruction is based on the presence of compatible symptoms in the absence of anatomic obstruction. Plain abdominal radiographs demonstrate air-fluid levels in the small intestine. Neonates with evidence of obstruction at birth have a microcolon. Contrast studies demonstrate slow passage of barium; consideration should be given to using water-soluble agents.

Other studies may provide information on the underlying pathophysiology. Esophageal motility is abnormal in about half the patients. Antroduodenal motility and gastric emptying studies have abnormal results if the upper gut is involved. Manometric evidence of a normal migrating motor complex and postprandial activity should redirect the diagnostic evaluation. Anorectal motility is normal and differentiates pseudo-obstruction from Hirschsprung disease. Full-thickness intestinal biopsy may show involvement of the muscle layers or abnormalities of the intrinsic intestinal nervous system.

The **differential diagnosis** includes Hirschsprung disease, other causes of mechanical obstruction, psychogenic constipation, neurogenic bladder, and superior mesenteric artery syndrome. Secondary causes of ileus or pseudo-obstruction, such as hypothyroidism, opiates, scleroderma, Chagas disease, hypokalemia, diabetic neuropathy, amyloidosis, porphyria, angioneurotic edema, mitochondrial disorders, and radiation, must be excluded.

TREATMENT. Nutritional support is the mainstay of treatment for pseudo-obstruction. Thirty to 50% require partial or complete parenteral nutrition. Some patients can be treated with intermittent enteral supplementation, whereas others may maintain themselves on selective oral diets. Prokinetic drugs are generally not useful. Isolated gastroparesis may follow episodes of viral gastroenteritis and spontaneously resolves, usually in 6–24 mo. Cisapride (a 5-hydroxytryptamine receptor antagonist), erythromycin (a motilin receptor agonist), or tegaserod can enhance gastric emptying and proximal small bowel motility and may be of use in this selected group of patients.

Symptomatic small bowel **bacterial overgrowth** is usually treated with oral antibiotics. Bacterial overgrowth can be associated with steatorrhea and malabsorption. Antibiotics should be used judiciously, however, because they can lead to the emergence of drug-resistant bacteria. Patients with acid peptic symptoms are treated with acid suppressors (see Chapter 332). Some children benefit from decompressive ileostomies or colostomies. Colectomy with ileorectal anastomosis is beneficial if the large bowel is the primary site of the motility abnormality. Bowel transplantation may benefit selected patients (see Chapter 336).

Haftel LT, Lev D, Barash V, et al: Familial mitochondrial intestinal pseudo-obstruction and neurogenic bladder. *J Child Neurol* 2000;15:386–389.

Iyer K, Kaufman S, Sudan D, et al: Long-term results of intestinal transplantation for pseudo-obstruction in children. *J Pediatr Surg* 2001;36:174–177.

329.2 • Functional Constipation

Constipation is defined by a delay or difficulty in defecation that has been present for 2 wk or longer. Functional constipation, also known as idiopathic constipation or fecal withholding, can usually be differentiated from constipation secondary to organic causes on the basis of a history and physical examination. Unlike anorectal malformations and Hirschsprung disease, functional constipation typically starts after the neonatal period. The constipation usually develops after the passage of painful bowel movements with voluntary withholding of feces to avoid the painful stimulus. Perianal inflammation from milk protein allergy may initiate the painful stimuli. When children have the urge to defecate, typical behaviors include contracting the gluteal muscles by stiffening the legs while lying down or holding onto furniture while standing. Some children will squat or hide while passing stool. Caregivers may misinterpret these activities as straining. In functional constipation, daytime encopresis is common, and some children will have a history of blood in the stool noted with the passage of a large bowel movement. Findings suggestive of underlying pathology include failure to thrive, weight loss, abdominal pain, vomiting, or persistent anal fissure or fistula.

The **physical examination** often demonstrates a large volume of stool palpated in the suprapubic area; rectal examination demonstrates a dilated rectal vault filled with guaiac-negative stool. The presence of a hair tuft over the spine or spinal dimple, or failure to elicit a cremasteric reflex or anal wink is suggestive of spinal pathology. A tethered cord is suggested by decreased or absent lower leg reflexes. Spinal cord lesions may occur with overlying skin anomalies. Urinary tract symptoms include recurrent urinary tract infection; evidence of obstruction may occur in constipated children and those with spinal cord disorders. Children with no evidence of abnormalities on physical examination rarely require radiologic evaluation. In refractory patients (intractable constipation), specialized testing should be considered to rule out conditions such as hypothyroidism, hypocalcemia, lead toxicity, and celiac disease. Selected children may benefit from MRI of the spine to identify an intraspinal process, motility studies to identify underlying myopathy or neuropathic bowel abnormalities, or a barium enema to identify structural abnormalities. Rectal motility studies can demonstrate a pattern of paradoxical contraction of the external anal sphincter during defecation, which can be treated by behavior modification. Colonic motility can guide therapy in refractory cases, demonstrating segmental problems that may require surgical intervention.

Therapy for functional constipation includes patient education, relief of impaction, and softening of the stool. The parents must understand that soiling associated with overflow incontinence is associated with loss of normal sensation and not a willful act. A regular bowel training program, including sitting on the toilet for 5–10 min after meals and keeping track of the frequency of bowel movements, is often helpful in establishing a regular bowel habit. If an impaction is present on the initial physical examination, an enema is usually required to clear the impaction while bowel softeners are started as maintenance medications. Typical regimens include the use of **polyethylene glycol** preparations, lactulose, or mineral oil. Prolonged use of stimulants such as senna or bisacodyl should be avoided. Children with behavioral problems that are interfering with successful treatment may benefit from a referral to a mental heath care provider. Maintenance therapy is generally continued until a regular bowel pattern has been established and the association of pain with the passage of stool is abolished. Children with spinal problems can be successfully managed with low volumes of fluid through a cecostomy or sigmoid tube.

Brooks RC, Copen RM, Cox DJ, et al: Review of the treatment literature for encopresis, functional constipation, and stool-toileting refusal. *Ann Behav Med* 2000;22:260–267.

Corazziari E, Badiali D, Bazzocchi G, et al: Long-term efficacy, safety, and tolerability of low daily doses of isosmotic polyethylene glycol electrolyte balanced solution (PMF-100) in the treatment of functional chronic constipation. *Gut* 2000;46:522–526.

Emmanuel AV, Kamm MA: Response to a behavioral treatment, biofeedback, in constipated patients is associated with improved gut transit and autonomic innervation. *Gut* 2001;49:214–219.

Kim HL, Gow KW, Penner JG, et al: Presentation of low anorectal malformations beyond the neonatal period. *Pediatrics* 2000;105:E68.

Rosen R, Buonomo C, Andrade R, Nurko: Incidence of spinal cord lesions in patients with intractable constipation. *J Pediatr* 2004;145:409–411.

Youssef NN, Di Lorenzo C: Childhood constipation: Evaluation and treatment. *J Clin Gastroenterol* 2001;33:199–205.

329.3 • Congenital Aganglionic Megacolon (Hirschsprung Disease)

Hirschsprung disease, or congenital aganglionic megacolon, is caused by abnormal innervation of the bowel, beginning in the internal anal sphincter and extending proximally to involve a variable length of gut. Hirschsprung disease is the most common cause of lower intestinal obstruction in neonates, with an overall incidence of 1/5,000 live births. Males are affected more often than females (4:1); prematurity is uncommon. There is an increased familial incidence in long segment disease. Hirschsprung disease may be associated with other congenital defects, including Down, Smith-Lemli-Opitz, Waardenburg, cartilage-hair hypoplasia, and congenital hypoventilation ("Ondine curse") syndromes and urogenital or cardiovascular abnormalities. Hirschsprung disease has been seen in association with microcephaly, mental retardation, and abnormal facies; with autism; or with cleft palate, hydrocephalus, and micrognathia.

PATHOLOGY. Hirschsprung disease is the result of an absence of ganglion cells in the bowel wall, extending proximally and continuously from the anus for a variable distance. The absence of neural innervation is a consequence of an arrest of neuroblast migration from the proximal to distal bowel. Hirschsprung disease is usually sporadic; dominant and recessive patterns of inheritance have been demonstrated in family groups. Genetic defects have been identified in multiple genes that encode proteins of the RET signaling pathway (*RET, GDNF,* and *NTN*) and that are involved in the endothelin (EDN) type B receptor pathway (*EDNRB, EDN3,* and *EVE-1*). Syndromic forms of Hirschsprung disease have been associated with the *L1CAM, SOX10,* and *SIP1* genes.

The aganglionic segment is limited to the rectosigmoid in 75% of patients; in 10%, the entire colon lacks ganglion cells. Total bowel aganglionosis is rare. Observed histologically is an absence of Meissner and Auerbach plexus and hypertrophied nerve bundles with high concentrations of acetylcholinesterase between the muscular layers and in the submucosa.

CLINICAL MANIFESTATIONS. The clinical symptoms of Hirschsprung disease usually begin at birth with the delayed passage of meconium. In 99% of full-term infants, meconium is passed within 48 hr of birth. Hirschsprung disease should be suspected in any full-term infant (the disease is unusual in preterm infants) with delayed passage of stool. Some infants pass meconium normally but subsequently present with a history of chronic constipation. Failure to thrive, with hypoproteinemia from a protein-losing enteropathy, is a less common presentation because Hirschsprung disease is usually recognized early in the course of the illness. Breast-fed infants may not suffer as severe a disease as formula-fed infants.

Failure to pass stool leads to dilatation of the proximal bowel and abdominal distention. As the bowel dilates, intraluminal pressure increases, resulting in decreased blood flow and deterioration of the mucosal barrier. Stasis allows proliferation of bacteria, which can lead to enterocolitis (*Clostridium difficile, Staphylococcus aureus,* anaerobes, coliforms) with associated sepsis and signs of bowel obstruction. Early recognition of Hirschsprung disease before the onset of enterocolitis is essential in reducing morbidity and mortality.

Hirschsprung disease in older patients must be distinguished from other causes of abdominal distention and chronic constipation (Table 329-1 and Fig. 329-1). The history often reveals increasing difficulty with the passage of stools, starting in the 1st few weeks of life. A large fecal mass is palpable in the left lower abdomen; the rectum is usually empty of feces. The stools, when passed, may consist of small pellets, be ribbon-like, or have a fluid consistency; the large stools and fecal soiling of patients with functional constipation are absent. In neonates, Hirschsprung disease must be differentiated from meconium plug syndrome, meconium ileus, and intestinal atresia. In older patients, the **Currarino triad** must be considered (**anorectal malformations**—ectopic, anus, rectal stenosis; **sacral bone anomalies**—hypoplasia, poor segmentation; or **presacral masses**—anterior meningoceles, teratoma, cysts).

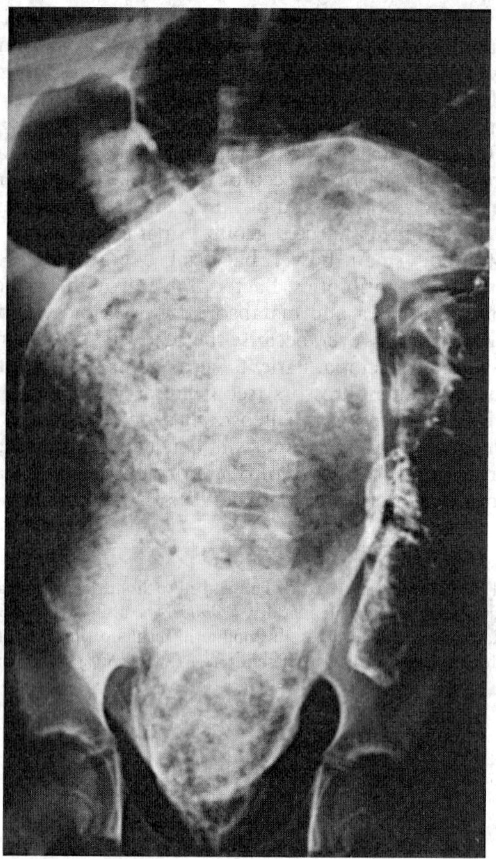

Figure 329-1. Barium enema in a 14 yr old boy with severe constipation. The enormous dilatation of the rectum and distal colon is typical of acquired functional megacolon.

TABLE 329-1. Distinguishing Features of Hirschsprung Disease and Functional Constipation

VARIABLE	FUNCTIONAL (ACQUIRED)	HIRSCHSPRUNG DISEASE
HISTORY		
Onset of constipation	After 2 yr of age	At birth
Encopresis	Common	Very rare
Failure to thrive	Uncommon	Possible
Enterocolitis	None	Possible
Forced bowel training	Usual	None
EXAMINATION		
Abdominal distention	Uncommon	Common
Poor weight gain	Rare	Common
Anal tone	Normal	Normal
Rectal examination	Stool in ampulla	Ampulla empty
Malnutrition	None	Possible
LABORATORY		
Anorectal manometry	Distention of the rectum causes relaxation of the internal sphincter	No sphincter relaxation or paradoxical increase in pressure
Rectal biopsy	Normal	No ganglion cells, increased acetylcholinesterase staining
Barium enema	Massive amounts of stool, no transition zone	Transition zone, delayed evacuation (>24 hr)

Rectal examination demonstrates normal anal tone and is usually followed by an explosive discharge of foul-smelling feces and gas. Intermittent attacks of intestinal obstruction from retained feces may be associated with pain and fever.

DIAGNOSIS. Rectal manometry and rectal suction biopsy are the easiest and most reliable indicators of Hirschsprung disease.

Rectal suction biopsies are the **procedure of choice** and should be performed no closer than 2 cm to the dentate line to avoid the normal area of hypoganglionosis at the anal verge. The biopsy material should contain an adequate sample of submucosa to evaluate for the presence of ganglion cells. The biopsy specimen can be stained for acetylcholinesterase, which may facilitate interpretation. Patients with aganglionosis demonstrate a large number of hypertrophied nerve bundles that stain positively for acetylcholinesterase with an absence of ganglion cells.

Anorectal manometry measures the pressure of the internal anal sphincter while a balloon is distended in the rectum. In normal individuals, rectal distention initiates a reflex decline in internal sphincter pressure. In patients with Hirschsprung disease, the pressure fails to drop or there is a paradoxical rise in pressure with rectal distention. The accuracy of this diagnostic test is >90%, but the test is technically difficult to perform in young infants. A normal response in the course of manometric evaluation precludes a diagnosis of Hirschsprung disease; an equivocal or paradoxical response requires a repeat motility or rectal biopsy.

The radiographic diagnosis of Hirschsprung disease is based on the presence of a transition zone between normal dilated proximal colon and a smaller-caliber obstructed distal colon caused by the nonrelaxation of the aganglionic bowel. The transition zone is not usually present before 1–2 wk of age and, on a radiograph, is a funnel-shaped area of intestine between the proximal dilated colon and the constricted distal bowel. Radiologic evaluation should be performed without preparation to prevent transient dilatation of the aganglionic segment. Twenty-four hr delayed films are helpful (Fig. 329-2). If significant barium is still present in the colon, it increases the suspicion of Hirschsprung disease even if a transition zone is not identified. Barium enema examination is useful in determining the extent of aganglionosis before surgery and in evaluating other diseases that present as lower bowel obstruction in a neonate. Full-thickness rectal biopsy can be performed at the time of surgery to confirm the diagnosis and level of involvement.

TREATMENT. Once the diagnosis is established, the definitive treatment is operative intervention. The operative options are to perform a definitive procedure as soon as the diagnosis is established or perform a temporary colostomy and wait until the infant is 6–12 mo old to perform definitive repair. There are three basic surgical options. The 1st successful surgical procedure, described by Swenson, was to excise the aganglionic segment and anastomose the normal proximal bowel to the rectum 1–2 cm above the dentate line. The operation is technically difficult and led to the development of two other procedures. Duhamel described a procedure to create a neorectum, bringing down normally innervated bowel behind the aganglionic rectum. The neorectum created in this procedure has an anterior aganglionic half with normal sensation and a posterior ganglionic half with normal propulsion. The endorectal pull-through procedure described by Boley involves stripping the mucosa from the aganglionic rectum and bringing normally innervated colon through the residual muscular cuff, thus bypassing the abnormal bowel from within. Advances in techniques have led to successful laparoscopic endorectal pull-through procedures, which are the **treatment of choice.**

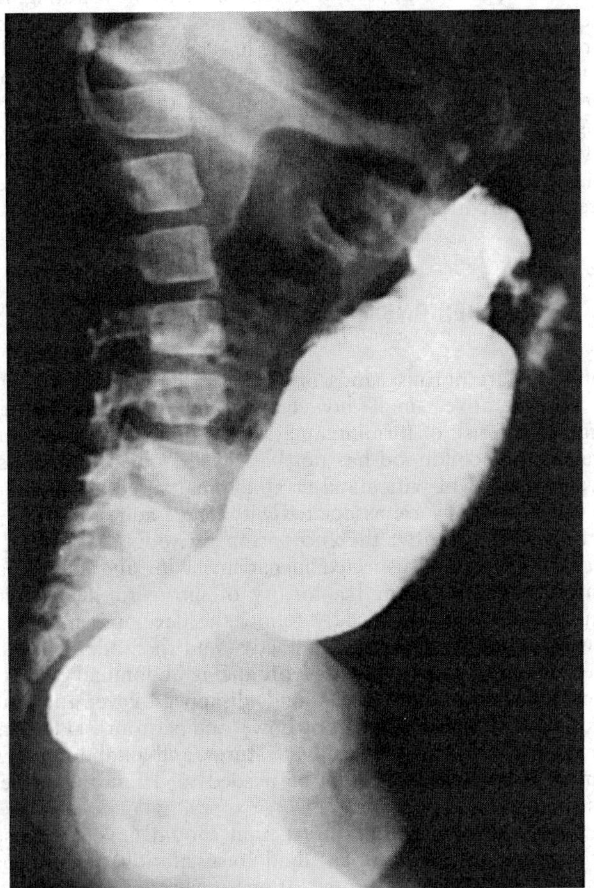

Figure 329-2. Lateral view of a barium enema in a 3 yr old girl with Hirschsprung disease. The aganglionic distal segment is narrow, with distended normal ganglionic bowel above it.

In **ultrashort segmental** Hirschsprung disease or internal sphincter achalasia, the aganglionic segment is limited to the internal sphincter. The clinical symptoms are similar to those of children with functional constipation. Ganglion cells are present on rectal suction biopsy, but the rectal motility is abnormal. Excision of a strip of rectal muscle usually leads to a more regular bowel pattern.

Long-segment Hirschsprung disease involving the entire colon and part of the small bowel presents a difficult problem. Rectal motility studies and rectal suction biopsy demonstrate findings of Hirschsprung disease, but radiologic studies are difficult to interpret because no colonic transition zone can be identified. The extent of aganglionosis can be determined accurately by biopsy at the time of laparotomy. When the entire colon is aganglionic, often together with a length of terminal ileum, ileal-anal anastomosis is the treatment of choice, preserving part of the aganglionic colon to facilitate water absorption, which helps the stools to become firm.

The prognosis of surgically treated Hirschsprung disease is generally satisfactory; the great majority of patients achieve fecal continence. Postoperative problems include recurrent enterocolitis, stricture, prolapse, perianal abscesses, and fecal soiling. Some children will require myectomy or a redo pull-through procedure.

329.4 • Intestinal Neuronal Dysplasia

This disorder may mimic Hirschsprung disease, but in contrast to an absence of intestinal ganglion cells, it demonstrates in **type A** (absent or hypoplasia of sympathetic innervation of myenteric and submucosal plexuses with increased parasympathetic nerve fibers, myenteric plexus hyperplasia, and colonic mucosal inflammation) and in **type B** (dysplastic submucosal plexus with giant ganglia and thickened nerve fibers, increased acetylcholine esterase staining, and isolated ganglion cells in the lamina propria).

Clinical manifestations include abdominal distention, constipation, and enterocolitis. Various lengths of bowel may be affected (segmental to entire intestinal tract). Some patients also have Hirschsprung disease; others have had associated prematurity, small left colon syndrome, and meconium plug syndrome.

Management includes that for functional constipation and, if unsuccessful, surgery is indicated.

Benailly HK, Lapierre JM, Laudier B, et al: *PMX2B*, a new candidate gene for Hirschsprung's disease. *Clin Genet* 2003;64:204–209.

Cucchiara S, Borrelli O, Salvia G, et al: A normal gastrointestinal motility excludes chronic intestinal pseudoobstruction in children. *Dig Dis Sci* 2000;45:258–264.
DeLorijn F, Reitsma JB, Voskuijl WP, et al: Diagnosis of Hirschsprung's disease: A prospective comparative accuracy study of common tests. *J Pediatr* 2005;146:787–792.
Hackam DJ, Reblock K, Barksdale EM, et al: The influence of Down's syndrome on the management and outcome of children with Hirschsprung's disease. *J Pediatr Surg* 2003;38:946–949.
Haftel LT, Lev D, Barash V, et al: Familial mitochondrial intestinal pseudo-obstruction and neurogenic bladder. *J Child Neurol* 2000;15: 386–389.
Keshtgar AS, Ward HC, Clayden GS, de Sousa NM: Investigations for incontinence and constipation after surgery for Hirschsprung's disease in children. *Pediatr Surg Int* 2003;19:4–8.
Langer JC, Durrant AC, de la Torre L, et al: One-stage transanal Soave pullthrough for Hirschsprung disease: A multicenter experience with 141 children. *Ann Surg* 2003;238:569–583, discussion 583–585.
Lapointe SP, Rivet C, Goulet O, et al: Urological manifestations associated with chronic intestinal pseudo-obstructions in children. *J Urol* 2002;168: 1768–1770.
Mousa H, Hyman PE, Cocjin J, et al: Long-term outcome of congenital intestinal pseudoobstruction. *Dig Dis Sci* 2002;47:2298–2305.
Pensabene L, Youssef NN, Griffiths JM, Di Lorenzo C: Colonic manometry in children with defecatory disorders. Role in diagnosis and management. *Am J Gastroenterol* 2003;98:1052–1057.
Teitelbaum DH, Coran AG: Reoperative surgery for Hirschsprung's disease. *Semin Pediatr Surg* 2003;12:124–131.

329.5 • Superior Mesenteric Artery Syndrome (Wilkie Syndrome, Cast Syndrome, Arteriomesenteric Duodenal Compression Syndrome)

The superior mesenteric artery syndrome describes an extrinsic compression of the duodenum in children after rapid weight loss and in a supine position. The compression is thought to occur as the mesentery loses its fat and allows the superior mesenteric artery to collapse on the duodenum, compressing it between the superior mesenteric artery anteriorly and the aorta posteriorly. Alternatively, the cause may be that the loss of supporting fat in the 2nd and 3rd portions of the duodenum allows the duodenum to collapse against the spine.

The **classic example** is an adolescent who starts vomiting after application of a body cast for orthopedic surgery. Other associated factors include anorexia, prolonged bed rest, weight loss, abdominal surgery, and exaggerated lumbar lordosis. The diagnosis is established radiologically with the demonstration of a cutoff of the duodenum just to the right of the midline. The duodenal obstruction may be accompanied by proximal duodenal and gastric dilatation.

Treatment of the acute syndrome involves relief of the obstruction and improved nutrition to alter the anatomic relationships of the duodenum with surrounding structures. Positioning patients in a lateral or prone position shifts the duodenum away from potential obstructing structures and may allow resumption of oral intake. Prokinetic agents such as metoclopramide or cisapride may be helpful. If repositioning is unsuccessful in relieving symptoms, a nasojejunal tube can be placed past the point of obstruction and feedings begun. Some patients require total parenteral nutrition to restore lost body fat, and occasional patients need surgical intervention.

Chapter 330 ■ Ileus, Adhesions, Intussusception, and Closed-Loop Obstructions Robert Wyllie

330.1 • Ileus

Ileus is the failure of intestinal peristalsis without evidence of mechanical obstruction. Lack of normal gut motility interferes with aboral movement of intestinal contents and in children is most often associated with abdominal surgery or infection (pneumonia, gastroenteritis, peritonitis). Ileus also accompanies metabolic abnormalities, such as uremia, hypokalemia, hypercalcemia, hypermagnesemia, or acidosis, and occurs with administration of certain drugs, such as opiates and vincristine. Ileus can also occur when antimotility drugs such as loperamide are used during episodes of gastroenteritis.

Ileus presents as increasing abdominal distention, emesis, and initially minimal pain. Pain increases with increasing distention. Bowel sounds are minimal or absent, in contrast to early mechanical obstruction, when they are hyperactive. Plain abdominal radiographs demonstrate multiple air-fluid levels throughout the abdomen. Serial radiographs usually do not show progressive distention as they do in mechanical obstruction. Contrast radiographs, if performed, demonstrate slow movement of the barium through a patent lumen.

Treatment of ileus involves correction of the underlying abnormality. Nasogastric decompression is used if abdominal distention is associated with pain or to relieve recurrent vomiting. Ileus after abdominal surgical procedures usually results in return of normal intestinal motility in 24–72 hr. Prokinetic agents such as metoclopramide or erythromycin can stimulate the return of normal bowel motility and be of assistance to children with prolonged ileus. Oral administration of drugs that block gastrointestinal opiate receptors but do not block central nervous system opiate action may reduce the ileus in postoperative patients receiving narcotics.

330.2 • Adhesions

Adhesions are fibrous bands of tissue that are a common cause of postoperative small bowel obstruction after abdominal surgery. The risk of forming an adhesion that causes obstructive symptoms in childhood has not been well studied but seems to occur in 2–3% of patients after abdominal surgery. The majority of obstructions are associated with single adhesions and can occur at any time after the 2nd postoperative week.

The **diagnosis** is suspected in patients with abdominal pain, constipation, emesis, and a history of intraperitoneal surgery. Nausea and vomiting quickly follow the development of pain. Bowel sounds are initially hyperactive and the abdomen is flat. The bowel subsequently dilates, producing abdominal distention in most patients, and bowel sounds disappear. Fever and leukocytosis are suggestive of necrotic bowel and peritonitis. Plain radiographs demonstrate obstructive features, and an abdominal CT scan or contrast studies may be needed to define the cause of obstruction.

Patients with suspected obstruction should have nasogastric decompression, intravenous fluid resuscitation, and broad-spectrum antibiotics in anticipation of surgery. Nonoperative intervention is contraindicated unless a patient is stable with clear evidence of clinical improvement. In children with recurrent adhesions and obstruction, fibrin-glued plication of adjacent loops of small bowel has reduced the risk of recurrent problems.

330.3 • INTUSSUSCEPTION

Intussusception occurs when a portion of the alimentary tract is telescoped into an adjacent segment. It is the most common cause of intestinal obstruction between 3 mo and 6 yr of age. Sixty percent of patients are younger than 1 yr, and 80% of the cases occur before 24 mo; it is rare in neonates. The incidence varies from 1 to 4/1,000 live births. The male:female ratio is 4:1. A few intussusceptions reduce spontaneously, but if left untreated, most will lead to intestinal infarction, perforation, peritonitis, and death.

ETIOLOGY AND EPIDEMIOLOGY. The cause of most intussusceptions is unknown. The seasonal incidence has peaks in spring and autumn. Correlation with prior or concurrent respiratory adenovirus (type C) infection has been noted, and the condition may complicate otitis media, gastroenteritis, **Henoch-Schönlein purpura,** or upper respiratory tract infections. The risk of intussusception in infants ≤1 yr of age after receiving a no longer available tetravalent rhesus-human reassortant rotavirus vaccine within 2 wk of immunization was increased. The risk is much greater after the 1st dose of the vaccine compared with the risk after the 2nd dose. The Advisory Committee on Immunization Practices no longer recommends this vaccine. Although rotavirus produces an enterotoxin, there is no association between wild-type human rotavirus and intussusception. The currently approved rotavirus vaccines may not be associated with an increased risk of intussusception (see Chapter 262).

It is postulated that gastrointestinal infection or the introduction of new food proteins results in swollen Peyer patches in the terminal ileum. Lymphoid nodular hyperplasia is another related risk factor. Prominent mounds of lymph tissue lead to mucosal prolapse of the ileum into the colon, thus causing an intussusception. In 2–8% of patients, **recognizable lead points** for the intussusception are found, such as a Meckel diverticulum, intestinal polyp, neurofibroma, intestinal duplication, hemangioma, or malignant conditions such as lymphoma. Intussusception can complicate mucosal hemorrhage, as in Henoch-Schönlein purpura or hemophilia. Cystic fibrosis is another risk factor. Postoperative intussusception is ileoileal and usually occurs within 5 days of an abdominal operation. Lead points are more common in children >2 yr of age. Intrauterine intussusception may be associated with the development of intestinal atresia. Intussusception in premature infants is rare.

PATHOLOGY. Intussusceptions are most often ileocolic, less commonly cecocolic, and rarely exclusively ileal. Very rarely, the appendix forms the apex of an intussusception. The upper portion of bowel, the **intussusceptum,** invaginates into the lower, the **intussuscipiens,** pulling its mesentery along with it into the enveloping loop. Constriction of the mesentery obstructs venous return; engorgement of the intussusceptum follows, with edema, and bleeding from the mucosa leads to a bloody stool, sometimes containing mucus. The apex of the intussusception can extend into the transverse, descending, or sigmoid colon, even to and through the anus in neglected cases. This presentation must be distinguished from rectal prolapse. Most intussusceptions do not strangulate the bowel within the 1st 24 hr but may later eventuate in intestinal gangrene and shock.

CLINICAL MANIFESTATIONS. In typical cases, there is sudden onset, in a previously well child, of severe paroxysmal colicky pain that recurs at frequent intervals and is accompanied by straining efforts with legs and knees flexed and loud cries. The infant may initially be comfortable and play normally between the paroxysms of pain; but if the intussusception is not reduced, the infant becomes progressively weaker and lethargic. At times, the **lethargy** is out of proportion to the abdominal signs. Eventually, a shocklike state, with fever, can develop. The pulse becomes weak and thready, the respirations become shallow and grunting, and the pain may be manifested only by moaning sounds. Vomiting occurs in most cases and is usually more frequent in the early phase. In the later phase, the vomitus becomes bile stained. Stools of normal appearance may be evacuated in the 1st few hours of symptoms. After this time, fecal excretions are small or more often do not occur and little or no flatus is passed. Blood is generally passed in the 1st 12 hr, but at times not for 1–2 days, and infrequently not at all; 60% of infants pass a stool containing red blood and mucus, the currant jelly stool. Some patients have only irritability and alternating or progressive lethargy.

Palpation of the abdomen usually reveals a slightly tender sausage-shaped mass, sometimes ill defined, which may increase in size and firmness during a paroxysm of pain and is most often in the right upper abdomen, with its long axis cephalocaudal. If it is felt in the epigastrium, the long axis is transverse. About 30% of patients do not have a palpable mass. The presence of bloody mucus on the finger as it is withdrawn after rectal examination supports the diagnosis of intussusception. Abdominal distention and tenderness develop as intestinal obstruction becomes more acute. On rare occasions, the advancing intestine prolapses through the anus. This prolapse can be distinguished from prolapse of the rectum by the separation between the protruding intestine and the rectal wall, which does not exist in prolapse of the rectum.

Ileoileal intussusception may have a less typical clinical picture, the symptoms and signs being chiefly those of small intestinal obstruction. **Recurrent intussusception** is noted in 5–8% and is more common after hydrostatic than surgical reduction. Chronic intussusception, in which the symptoms exist in milder form at recurrent intervals, is more likely to occur with or after acute enteritis and can arise in older children as well as in infants.

DIAGNOSIS. When the clinical history and physical findings are suggestive of intussusception, an ultrasound is typically performed. If a plain abdominal radiograph is performed, it may show a density in the area of the intussusception. Screening ultrasounds for suspected intussusception increases the yield of diagnostic/therapeutic enemas and reduces unnecessary radiation exposure in children with negative ultrasound examinations. The diagnostic findings of intussusception on ultrasound include a tubular mass in longitudinal views and a doughnut or target appearance in transverse images (Fig. 330-1). Air, hydrostatic (saline), and, less often, water-soluble contrast enemas have replaced barium examinations. Contrast enemas demonstrate a filling defect or cupping in the head of the contrast media where its advance is obstructed by the intussusceptum (Fig. 330-2). A central linear column of contrast media may be visible in the compressed lumen of the intussusceptum, and a thin rim of contrast may be seen trapped around the invaginating intestine in the folds of mucosa within the intussuscipiens (coiled-spring sign), especially after evacuation. Retrogression of the intussusceptum under pressure and visualized on x-ray or ultrasound documents successful reduction. Air reduction is associated with fewer complications and lower radiation exposure than traditional contrast hydrostatic techniques.

DIFFERENTIAL DIAGNOSIS. It may be particularly difficult to diagnose intussusception in a child who already has gastroenteritis; a change in the pattern of illness, in the character of pain, or in the

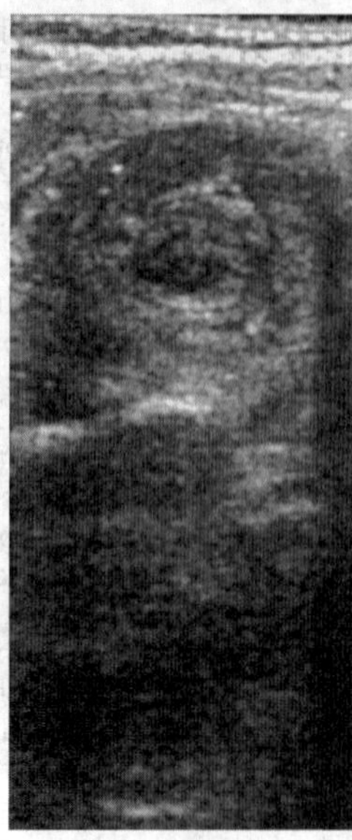

Figure 330-1. Transverse image of an ileocolic intussusception. Note the loops within the loops of bowel.

nature of vomiting or the onset of rectal bleeding should alert the physician. The bloody stools and abdominal cramps that accompany enterocolitis can usually be differentiated from intussusception because in enterocolitis the pain is less severe and less regular, there is diarrhea, and the infant is recognizably ill between pains. Bleeding from Meckel diverticulum is usually painless. Joint symptoms or purpura usually but not invariably accompany the intestinal hemorrhage of Henoch-Schönlein purpura. Because intussusception can be a complication of this disorder, ultrasonography may be needed to distinguish the conditions.

TREATMENT. Reduction of an acute intussusception is an emergency procedure and performed immediately after diagnosis in preparation for possible surgery. In patients with prolonged intussusception with signs of shock, peritoneal irritation, intestinal perforation, or pneumatosis intestinalis, reduction should not be attempted.

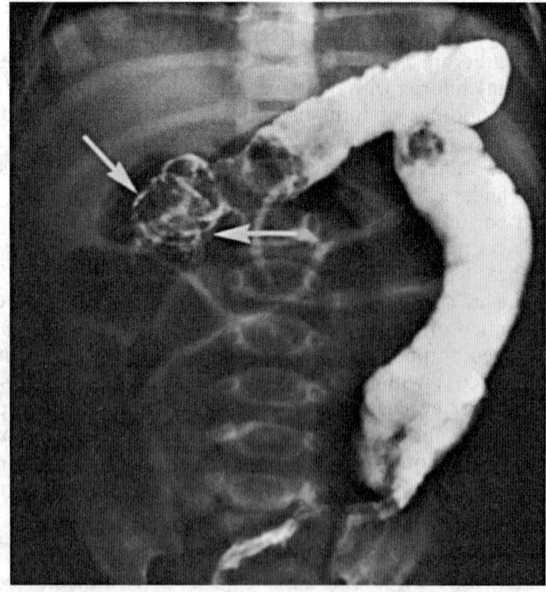

Figure 330-2. Intussusception in an infant. The obstruction is evident in the proximal transverse colon. Contrast material between the intussusceptum and the intussuscipiens is responsible for the coiled-spring appearance.

The success rate of radiologic hydrostatic reduction under fluoroscopic or ultrasonic guidance is ≈50% if symptoms are present longer than 48 hr and 70–90% if reduction is done in the 1st 48 hr. Bowel perforations occur in 0.5–2.5% of attempted barium and hydrostatic (saline) reductions. The perforation rate with air reduction ranges from 0.1 to 0.2%.

An **ileoileal intussusception** is best demonstrated by abdominal ultrasonography. Reduction by instillation of contrast agents, saline, or air may not be possible. Such intussusceptions can develop insidiously after bowel surgery and require reoperation if they do not spontaneously reduce. If manual operative reduction is impossible or the bowel is not viable, resection of the intussusception is necessary, with end-to-end anastomosis.

PROGNOSIS. Untreated intussusception in infants is usually fatal; the chances of recovery are directly related to the duration of intussusception before reduction. Most infants recover if the intussusception is reduced in the 1st 24 hr, but the mortality rate rises rapidly after this time, especially after the 2nd day. Spontaneous reduction during preparation for operation is not uncommon.

The **recurrence rate** after reduction of intussusceptions is ≈10%, and after surgical reduction it is 2–5%; none has recurred after surgical resection. Corticosteroids may reduce the frequency of recurrent intussusception. Recurrent intussusception can usually be reduced radiologically. It is unlikely that an intussusception caused by a lesion such as lymphosarcoma, polyp, or Meckel diverticulum will be successfully reduced by radiologic intervention. With adequate surgical management, operative reduction carries a very low mortality rate in early cases.

330.4 • Closed-Loop Obstructions

Intestinal obstruction can be caused by defects in the mesentery (**"internal hernias"**) through which loops of small bowel may pass and become trapped. Vascular engorgement of the trapped bowel results in intestinal ischemia and gangrene unless promptly relieved. Symptoms include bilious vomiting, abdominal distention, and abdominal pain. Peritoneal signs suggest ischemic bowel. Plain radiographs demonstrate signs of small bowel obstruction or free air if the bowel has perforated. Supportive management includes intravenous fluids, antibiotics, and nasogastric decompression. Prompt surgical relief of the obstruction is indicated if intestinal gangrene is to be prevented. Symptoms can occasionally be transient, chronic, or recurrent if the herniated bowel slides out of the mesenteric defect, spontaneously relieving the obstruction.

Bajaj L, Roback MG: Postreduction management of intussusception in a children's hospital emergency department. *Pediatrics* 2003;112:1302–1307.

Bines JE, Liem NT, Justice FA, et al: Risk factors for intussusception in infants in Vietnam and Australia: Adenovirus implicated, but not rotavirus. *J Pediatr* 2006;149:452–460.

Burke MS, Ragi JM, Karamanoukian HL, et al: New strategies in nonoperative management of meconium ileus. *J Pediatr Surg* 2002;37:760–764.

Centers for Disease Control and Prevention: Postmarketing monitoring of intussusception after Rota Teg vaccination—United States, February 1, 2006–February 15, 2007. *MMWR* 2007;56:218–222.

Crystal P, Hertzanu Y, Farber B, et al: Sonographically guided hydrostatic reduction of intussusception in children. *J Clin Ultrasound* 2002;30:343–348.

Fischer TK, Bihrmann K, Perch M, et al: Intussusception in early childhood: A cohort study of 1.7 million children. *Pediatrics* 2004;114:782–785.

Henrikson S, Blane CE, Koujok K, et al: The effect of screening sonography on the positive rate of enemas for intussusception. *Pediatr Radiol* 2003;33:190–193.

Henry MCW, Brever CK, Tashjian DB, et al: The appendix sign: a radiographic marker for irreducible intussusception. *J Pediatr Surg* 2006;41:487–489.

Koumanidou C, Vakaki M, Pitsoulakis G, et al: Sonographic detection of lymph nodes in the intussusception of infants and young children: Clinical evaluation and hydrostatic reduction. *AJR Am J Roentgenol* 2002;178:445–450.

Kubota A, Imura K, Yagi M, et al: Functional ileus in neonates: Hirschsprung's disease-allied disorders versus meconium-related ileus. *Eur J Pediatr Surg* 1999;9:392–395.

O'Ryan M, Lucero Y, Pena A, Valenzuela MT: Two year review of intestinal intussusception in six large public hospitals of Santiago, Chile. *Pediatr Infect Dis J* 2003;22:717–721.

Shteyer E, Koplewitz BZ, Gross E, Granot E: Medical treatment of recurrent intussusception associated with intestinal lymphoid hyperplasia. *Pediatrics* 2003;111:682–685.

Chapter 331 ■ Foreign Bodies and Bezoars

Robert Wyllie

331.1 • Foreign Bodies in the Stomach and Intestine

Once in the stomach, 95% of all ingested objects pass without difficulty through the remainder of the gastrointestinal tract. Perforation after ingestion of a foreign body is estimated to be <1% of all objects ingested. Perforation tends to occur in areas of physiologic sphincters (pylorus, ileocecal valve), acute angulation (duodenal sweep), congenital gut malformations (webs, diaphragms, diverticula), or areas of previous bowel surgery.

Patients with nonfood foreign bodies often describe a history of ingestion. Young children may have a witness to ingestion. Approximately 90% of foreign bodies are opaque. Radiologic examination is routinely performed to determine the type, number, and location of the suspected objects. Contrast radiographs may be necessary to demonstrate some objects such as plastic parts or toys.

Conservative management is indicated in most foreign bodies that have passed through the esophagus and entered the stomach. Most objects pass though the intestine in 4–6 days, although some may take as long as 3–4 wk. While waiting for the object to pass, parents are instructed to continue a regular diet and to observe the stools for the appearance of the ingested object. Cathartics should be avoided. Exceptionally long or sharp objects are usually monitored radiologically. Parents or patients should be instructed to report abdominal pain, vomiting, persistent fever, and hematemesis or melena immediately to their physician. Failure of the object to progress within a 3 to 4 wk period seldom implies an impeding perforation but may be associated with a congenital malformation or acquired bowel abnormality.

Certain objects pose more risk than others. Small magnets used to secure earrings have been associated with bowel perforation. When the magnets disperse after ingestion, they may be attracted to each other across bowel wall, leading to pressure necrosis and perforation. Inexpensive toy medallions containing lead can lead to **lead toxicity.** Ingestion of batteries rarely leads to problems, but symptoms can arise from leakage of alkali or heavy metal (mercury) from battery degradation in the gastrointestinal tract. Lithium toxicity has also been reported. Newer coins can also decompose when subjected to prolonged acid exposure. Unless multiple coins are ingested, however, the metals released are unlikely to pose a clinical risk.

In older children and adults, oval objects >5 cm in diameter or 2 cm in thickness tend to lodge in the stomach and should be endoscopically retrieved. Thin objects >10 cm in length fail to negotiate the duodenal sweep and should also be removed. In infants and toddlers, objects >3 cm in length or >20 mm in diameter do not usually pass through the pylorus and should be removed. Open safety pins should also be endoscopically retrieved, but other sharp objects can be managed conservatively. Drugs (aggregated iron pills, cocaine packing) may need to be surgically removed; initial management can include oral polyethylene glycol lavage.

Children occasionally place objects in their rectum. Small, blunt objects usually pass spontaneously, but large or sharp objects typically need to be retrieved. Adequate sedation is essential to relax the anal sphincter before attempted endoscopic or speculum removal. If the object is proximal to the rectum, observation for 12–24 hr usually allows the object to descend into the rectum.

331.2 • Bezoars

A bezoar is an accumulation of exogenous matter in the stomach or intestine. Most bezoars have been found in females with underlying personality problems or in neurologically impaired individuals. Patients who have undergone abdominal surgery are at higher risk for the development of bezoars. The peak age at onset of symptoms is the 2nd decade of life. Bezoars are classified on the basis of their composition. **Trichobezoars** are composed of the patient's own hair, and **phytobezoars** are composed of a combination of plant and animal material. **Lactobezoars** were previously found most often in premature infants and can be attributed to the high casein or calcium content of some premature formulas. Swallowed chewing gum can occasionally lead to a bezoar.

Trichobezoars can become large and form casts of the stomach; they can enter into the proximal duodenum. They present as symptoms of gastric outlet or partial intestinal obstruction including vomiting, anorexia, and weight loss. Patients may complain of abdominal pain, distention, and severe halitosis. Physical examination may demonstrate patchy baldness and a firm mass in the left upper quadrant. Patients occasionally have iron-deficiency anemia, hypoproteinemia, or steatorrhea caused by an associated chronic gastritis. Phytobezoars present in a similar manner.

An abdominal plain film may suggest the presence of a bezoar, which can be confirmed on ultrasound or CT examination. Bezoars in the stomach can usually be removed endoscopically. If endoscopy is unsuccessful, surgical intervention may be needed. Lactobezoars usually resolve when feedings are withheld for 24–48 hr.

Aktay AN, Werlin SL: Penetration of the stomach by an accidentally ingested straight pin. *J Pediatr Gastroenterol Nutr* 2002;34:81–82.

Centers for Disease Control and Prevention: Gastrointestinal injuries from magnet ingestion in children—United States, 2003–2006. *MMWR* 2006;55:1296–1300.

Cerri RW, Liacouras CA: Evaluation and management of foreign bodies in the upper gastrointestinal tract. *Pediatr Case Rev* 2003;3:150–156.

Kaneko H, Tomomasa T, Kubota Y, et al: Pharmacobezoar complicating treatment with sodium alginate. *J Gastroenterol* 2004;39:69–71.

Karjoo M, Kader H: A novel technique for closing and removing an open safety pin from the stomach. *Gastrointest Endosc* 2003;57:627–629.

Mallon PT, White JS, Thompson RL: Systemic absorption of lithium following ingestion of a lithium button battery. *Hum Exp Toxicol* 2004;23:193–195.

Puig S, Scharitzer M, Cengiz K, et al: Effects of gastric acid on euro coins: Chemical reaction and radiographic appearance after ingestion by infants and children. *Emerg Med J* 2004;21:553–556.

Schalamon J, Haxhija EQ, Ainoedhofer H, et al: The use of a hand-held metal detector for localisation of ingested metallic foreign bodies—a critical investigation. *Eur J Pediatr* 2004; 163:257–259.
VanArsdale JL, Leiker RD, Kohn M, et al: Lead poisoning from a toy necklace. *Pediatrics* 2004; 114:1096–1099.

Chapter 332 ■ Peptic Ulcer Disease in Children Samra S. Blanchard and Steven J. Czinn

Peptic ulcer disease, the end result of inflammation due to an imbalance between cytoprotective and cytotoxic factors in the stomach and duodenum, presents with varying degrees of gastritis or frank ulceration. The pathogenesis of peptic ulcer disease is multifactorial, but the final common pathway for the development of ulcers is the action of acid and pepsin-laden contents of the stomach on the gastric and duodenal mucosa and the inability of mucosal defense mechanisms to allay those effects. Abnormalities in the gastric and duodenal mucosa can be visualized on endoscopy, with or without histologic changes. Deep mucosal lesions that disrupt the muscularis mucosa of the gastric or duodenal wall define **peptic ulcers.** Gastric ulcers are generally located on the lesser curvature of the stomach, and 90% of duodenal ulcers are found in the duodenal bulb. Despite the lack of large population-based pediatric studies, rates of peptic ulcer disease in childhood appear to be low. Large pediatric centers anecdotally report an incidence of 5–7 children with gastric or duodenal ulcers per 2,500 hospital admissions each year.

Ulcers in children can be classified as **primary** peptic ulcers, which are chronic and more often duodenal, or **secondary,** which are usually more acute in onset and are more often gastric. Primary ulcers are most often associated with *Helicobacter pylori* infection; however, idiopathic primary peptic ulcers account for up to 20% of duodenal ulcers in children. Secondary peptic ulcers can result from stress due to sepsis, shock, or an intracranial lesion (Cushing ulcer) or in response to a severe burn injury (Curling ulcer). Secondary ulcers can also occur as a result of aspirin or nonsteroidal anti-inflammatory drug (NSAID) use, hypersecretory states like Zollinger-Ellison syndrome (see Chapter 332.1), short bowel syndrome, and systemic mastocytosis.

PATHOGENESIS

ACID SECRETION. By 3–4 yr of age, gastric acid secretion approximates adult values. Acid initially secreted by the oxyntic cells of the stomach has a pH of ≈0.8, whereas the pH of the stomach contents is 1–2. Excessive acid secretion is associated with a large parietal cell mass, hypersecretion by antral G cells, and increased vagal tone, resulting in increased or sustained acid secretion in response to meals and increased secretion during the night. Control of acid secretion is achieved through multiple different feedback mechanisms involving endocrine, paracrine, and neural pathways. The secretagogues that promote gastric acid production include acetylcholine released by the vagus nerve, histamine secreted by enterochromaffin cells, and gastrin released by the G cells of the antrum. Mediators that decrease gastric acid secretion and enhance protective mucin production include prostaglandins.

MUCOSAL DEFENSE. A continuous layer of mucous gel that serves as a diffusion barrier to hydrogen ions and other chemicals covers the gastrointestinal mucosa. Mucus production and secretion are stimulated by prostaglandin E_2. Underlying the mucous coat, the epithelium forms a second-line barrier, the characteristics of which are determined by the biology of the epithelial cells and their tight junctions. Another important function of epithelial cells is to secrete chemokines when threatened by microbial attack. Secretion of bicarbonate into the mucous coat, which is regulated by prostaglandins, is important for neutralization of hydrogen ions. If mucosal injury occurs, active proliferation and migration of mucosal cells occurs rapidly, driven by epithelial growth factor, transforming growth factor-α, insulin-like growth factor, gastrin, and bombesin, and covers the area of epithelial damage.

CLINICAL MANIFESTATIONS

The presenting symptoms of peptic ulcer disease varies with the age of patient. Hematemesis or melena is reported in up to half of the patients with peptic ulcer disease. School-aged children and adolescents more commonly present with epigastric pain and nausea, presentations generally seen in adults. Infants and younger children usually present with feeding difficulty, vomiting, crying episodes, hematemesis, or melena. In the neonatal period, gastric perforation can be the initial presentation.

The classic symptom of peptic ulceration, epigastric pain alleviated by the ingestion of food, is present only in a minority of children. Many pediatric patients present with poorly localized abdominal pain, which may be periumbilical. The vast majority of patients with periumbilical or epigastric pain or discomfort do not have a peptic ulcer, but rather a functional gastrointestinal disorder, such as irritable bowel syndrome or functional dyspepsia. Patients with peptic ulceration rarely present with acute abdominal pain from perforation or symptoms and signs of pancreatitis from a posterior penetrating ulcer. Occasionally, bright red blood per rectum may be seen if the rate of bleeding is brisk and the intestinal transit time is short. Vomiting can be a sign of gastric outlet obstruction.

The pain is often described as dull or aching, rather than sharp or burning, as in adults. It can last from minutes to hours; patients have frequent exacerbations and remissions lasting from weeks to months. Nocturnal pain is common in older children. A history of typical ulcer pain with prompt relief after taking antacids is found in <33% of children. Rarely, in patients with acute or chronic blood loss, penetration of the ulcer into the abdominal cavity or adjacent organs produces shock, anemia, peritonitis, or pancreatitis. If inflammation and edema are extensive, acute or chronic gastric outlet obstruction can occur.

DIAGNOSIS

Esophagogastroduodenoscopy is the method of choice to establish the diagnosis of peptic ulcer disease. It can be safely performed in all ages by experienced pediatric gastroenterologists. Endoscopy allows for the direct visualization of esophagus, stomach, and duodenum, identifying the specific lesions. Biopsy specimens must be obtained from the esophagus, stomach, and duodenum for histologic assessment as well as to screen for the presence of *H. pylori* infection. Endoscopy also provides the opportunity for hemostatic therapy including injection and the use of a heater probe or electrocoagulation if necessary.

PRIMARY ULCERS

***HELICOBACTER PYLORI* GASTRITIS.** *H. pylori* is among the most common bacterial infections in humans. *H. pylori* is a gram-negative, S-shaped rod that produces urease, catalase, and oxidase, which may play a role in the pathogenesis of peptic ulcer disease.

The mechanism of acquisition and transmission of *H. pylori* is unclear, although the most likely mode of transmission is fecal-oral or oral-oral. This mode of transmission is supported by studies demonstrating that viable *H. pylori* organisms can be cultured from the stool or vomitus of infected patients. Risk factors such as low socioeconomic status in childhood or affected family members also influence the prevalence. All children infected with *H. pylori* develop histologic chronic active gastritis but are often asymptomatic. In children, *H. pylori* infection can present with abdominal pain or vomiting, and less often, refractory iron deficiency anemia or growth retardation. *H. pylori* can be associated, though rarely, with chronic autoimmune thrombocytopenia. Chronic colonization with *H. pylori* can predispose children to a significantly increased risk of developing a duodenal ulcer, gastric cancer such as adenocarcinoma, or MALT (mucosa-associated lymphoid tissue) lymphomas. The relative risk of gastric carcinoma is 2.3–8.7 times greater in infected adults as compared to uninfected subjects. *H. pylori* has been classified by the World Health Organization as a group I carcinogen.

The **diagnosis** of *H. pylori* infection is made histologically by demonstrating the organism in the biopsy specimens (Fig. 332-1). Although serologic assays using validated immunoglobulin G (IgG) antibody detection may be helpful for screening children for the presence of *H. pylori,* they do not help predict active infection or assess the success of antimicrobial eradication therapy. ^{13}C-urea breath tests and stool antigen tests are also available noninvasive methods of detecting *H. pylori* infection. Nonetheless, for children suspected of having *H. pylori* infection, an initial upper endoscopy is recommended to evaluate and confirm *H. pylori* disease. The range of endoscopic findings in children with *H. pylori* infection varies from being grossly normal to the presence of nonspecific gastritis with prominent rugal folds, nodularity (Fig. 332-2), or ulcers. Because the antral mucosa appears to be endoscopically normal in a significant number of children with primary *H. pylori* gastritis, gastric biopsies should always be obtained from the body and antrum of the stomach regardless of the endoscopic appearance. If *H. pylori* is identified, even in a child with no symptoms, eradication therapy should be offered (Tables 332-1 and 332-2).

IDIOPATHIC ULCERS. *H. pylori*–negative duodenal ulcers in children that have no history of taking NSAIDs represent 15–20% of pediatric duodenal ulcers. These patients do not have nodularity in the gastric antrum, or histologic evidence of gastritis. In idiopathic ulcers, acid suppression alone is the preferred effective treatment. Either proton pump inhibitors or H_2 receptor antagonists may be used. Idiopathic ulcers have a high recurrence rate after discontinuing antisecretory therapy. These children should be followed closely, and if symptoms recur, antisecretory therapy should be restarted. In such cases, if the child is older than 1 yr, proton pump inhibitors are preferred for maintenance therapy, as they have been shown to be superior to H_2 receptor antagonists in preventing recurrent ulcers.

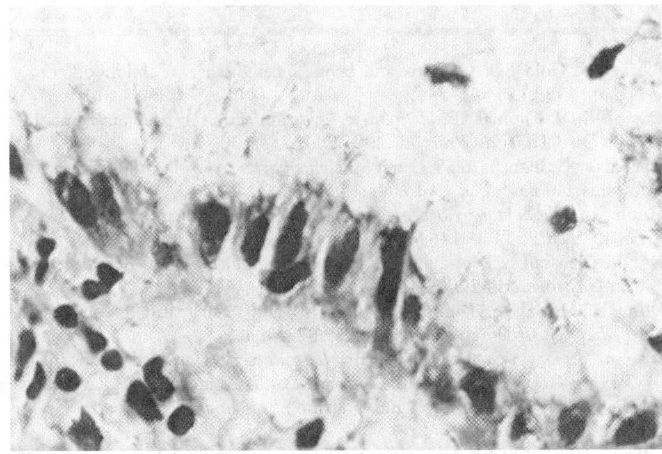

Figure 332-1. Appearance of *Helicobacter pylori* on the gastric mucosal surface with Giemsa stain (high-power view). (From Campbell DI, Thomas JE: *Heliobacter pylori* infection in paediatric practice. *Arch Dis Child Edu Pract Ed* 2005;90:ep25–ep30.)

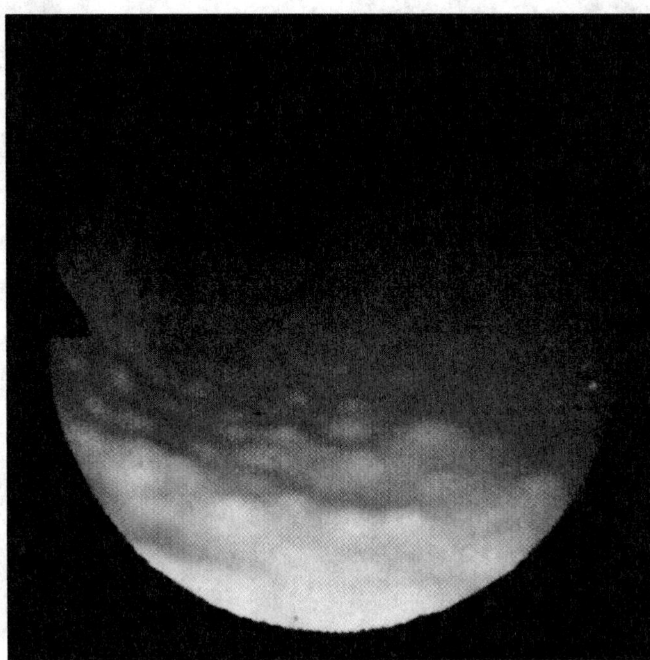

Figure 332-2. Endoscopic view of lymphoid modular hyperplasia of the gastric antrum. (From Campbell DI, Thomas JE: *Heliobacter pylori* infection in paediatric practice. *Arch Dis Child Edu Pract Ed* 2005;90:ep25–ep30.)

SECONDARY ULCERS

ASPIRIN AND OTHER NONSTEROIDAL ANTI-INFLAMMATORY DRUGS (NSAIDS). NSAIDs produce mucosal injury by direct local irritation and by inhibiting cyclooxygenase and prostaglandin formation. Prostaglandins enhance mucosal resistance to injury; therefore, a decrease in prostaglandin production increases the risk of mucosal injury. The severe erosive gastropathy produced by NSAIDs can ultimately result in bleeding ulcers or gastric perforations. The location of these ulcers is more commonly in the stomach than in the duodenum, and usually in the antrum.

TABLE 332-1. Recommended Eradication Therapies for *H. pylori*–associated Disease in Children

MEDICATIONS	DOSE	DURATION OF TREATMENT
Amoxicillin	50 mg/kg/d ÷ bid	14 days
Clarithromycin	15 mg/kg/d ÷ bid	14 days
Proton pump inhibitor	1 mg/kg/d ÷ bid	1 mo
Amoxicillin	50 mg/kg/d ÷ bid	14 days
Metronidazole	20 mg/kg/d ÷ bid	14 days
Proton pump inhibitor	1 mg/kg/d ÷ bid	1 mo
Clarithromycin	15 mg/kg/d ÷ bid	14 days
Metronidazole	20 mg/kg/d ÷ bid	14 days
Proton pump inhibitor	1 mg/kg/d ÷ bid	1 mo

Adapted from Gold BD, et al: Medical position statement: The North American Society for Pediatric Gastroenterology and Nutrition. *Helicobacter pylori* infectious children: Recommendations for diagnosis and treatment. *J Pediatr Gastroenterol Nutr* 2000;31:490–497.

TABLE 332-2. Antisecretory Therapy with Pediatric Dosages

MEDICATION	PEDIATRIC DOSE	HOW SUPPLIED
H_2 RECEPTOR ANTAGONISTS		
Cimetidine	20–40 mg/kg/day Divided twice a day to four times a day	Syrup: 300 mg/mL Tablets: 200, 300, 400, 800 mg
Ranitidine	4–10 mg/kg/day Divided twice or three times a day	Syrup: 75 mg/5 mL Tablets: 75, 150, 300 mg
Famotidine	1–2 mg/kg/day Divided twice a day	Syrup: 40 mg/5 mL Tablets: 20, 40 mg
Nizatidine	10 mg/kg/day Divided twice a day	
PROTON PUMP INHIBITORS		
Omeprazole	1.0–3.3 mg/kg/day <20 kg: 10 mg/day >20 kg: 20 mg/day Approved for use in those >2 yr old	Capsules: 10, 20, 40 mg
Lansoprazole	0.8–4 mg/kg/day <30 kg: 15 mg/day >30 kg: 30 mg/day Approved for use in those >1 yr old	Capsules: 15, 30 mg Powder packet: 15, 30 mg Solu-tab: 15, 30 mg
Rabeprazole	Adult dose: 20 mg/day	Tablet: 20 mg
Pantoprazole	Adult dose: 40 mg/day	Tablet: 40 mg
CYTOPROTECTIVE AGENTS		
Sucralfate	40–80 mg/kg/day	Suspension: 1,000 mg/5 mL Tablet: 1,000 mg

"STRESS" ULCERATION. This usually occurs within 24 hr of onset of a critical illness in which physiologic stress is present. In many cases, the patients bleed from gastric erosions, rather than ulcers. Approximately 25% of the critically ill children in a pediatric intensive care unit (PICU) will have macroscopic evidence of gastric bleeding. Preterm and term infants in the neonatal intensive care unit can also develop gastric mucosal lesions and may present with upper gastrointestinal bleeding or perforated ulcers. Although prophylactic measures to prevent stress ulcers in children are not standardized, drugs that inhibit gastric acid production (see later) are often used in the PICU to reduce the rate of gastric erosions or ulcers.

TREATMENT OF PEPTIC ULCER DISEASE

Ulcer therapy has two goals: ulcer healing and elimination of the primary cause. Other important considerations are relief of symptoms and prevention of complications. The **first-line drugs** for the treatment of gastritis and peptic ulcer disease in children are H_2 receptor antagonists and proton pump inhibitors (see Table 332-2). Proton pump inhibitors are more potent in ulcer healing. Cytoprotective agents can also be used as adjunct therapy if mucosal lesions are present. Antibiotics in combination with a proton pump inhibitor must be used for the treatment of *H. pylori*–associated ulcers (see Table 332-1).

H_2 receptor antagonists (cimetidine, ranitidine, famotidine, nizatidine) competitively inhibit the binding of histamine at the H_2 subtype receptor of the gastric parietal cell. Proton pump inhibitors block the gastric parietal cell H^+/K^+ATPase pump in a dose-dependent fashion, reducing basal and stimulated gastric acid secretion. At least 5 proton pump inhibitors are available in the United States: omeprazole, lansoprazole, pantoprazole, esomeprazole, and rabeprazole. Although not all of them are approved for use in children, they are well tolerated with only minor adverse effects such as: diarrhea (1–4%), headache (1–3%), and nausea (1%). When one considers therapeutic efficacy, the evidence suggests that all proton pump inhibitors have comparable efficacy in treatment of peptic ulcer disease using standard doses and are superior to H_2-receptor antagonists. Proton pump inhibitors have their greatest effect when given before a meal.

TREATMENT OF *H. PYLORI*–RELATED PEPTIC ULCER DISEASE. In pediatrics, antibiotics and bismuth salts have been used in combination with proton pump inhibitors to treat *H. pylori* infection (see Table 332-1). Eradication rates in children range from 68% to 92% when the dual or triple therapy is used for 4–6 wk. The ulcer healing rate ranges from 91% to 100%. Triple therapy yields a higher cure rate than dual therapy. The optimal regimen for the eradication of *H. pylori* infection in children has yet to be established, but the use of a proton pump inhibitor in combination with clarithromycin and amoxicillin or metronidazole for 2 wk is a well-tolerated and recommended triple therapy (see Table 332-1). Although children <5 yr of age may become reinfected, the most common reason for treatment failure is poor compliance or antibiotic resistance.

SURGICAL THERAPY. Since the discovery of *H. pylori* and the availability of modern medical management, peptic ulcer disease requiring surgical treatment has become extremely rare. The indications for surgery remain uncontrolled bleeding, perforation, and obstruction. Since the introduction of H_2 receptor antagonists, the recognition and treatment of *H. pylori*, and the use of proton pump inhibitors, the incidence of surgery for bleeding and perforation has decreased dramatically.

332.1 • Zollinger-Ellison Syndrome

This rare syndrome is characterized by refractory, severe peptic ulcer disease caused by gastric hypersecretion due to the autonomous secretion of gastrin by a neuroendocrine tumor, a gastrinoma. Clinical presentations are similar to those of peptic ulcer disease with the addition of diarrhea. The diagnosis is suspected by the presence of recurrent, multiple, or atypically located ulcers. More than 98% of patients have elevated fasting gastrin levels. Zollinger-Ellison syndrome is a frequent occurrence in patients with **multiple endocrine neoplasia (MEN1)** and a rare occurrence with **neurofibromatosis** and **tuberous sclerosis**. Prompt and effective management of increased gastric acid secretion is essential in the management. Proton pump inhibitors are the drug of choice due to their long duration of action and potency. H_2 receptor antagonists are also effective, but higher doses are required than those used in peptic ulcer disease.

Blecker U, Gold BD: Gastritis and peptic ulcer disease in childhood. *Eur J Pediatr* 1999;158:541–546.

Campbell DI, Thomas JE: *Heliobacter pylori* infection in paediatric practice. *Arch Dis Child Edu Pract Ed* 2005;90:ep25–ep30.

Chelimsky G, Blanchard SS, Czinn SJ: *Helicobacter pylori* in children and adolescents. *Adolesc Med Clin* 2004;15:53–66.

Czinn SJ: *Heliobacter pylori* infection: Detection, investigation, and management. *J Pediatr* 2005;146:S21–S26.

Dohil R, Hassall E: Peptic ulcer disease in children. *Baillieres Best Pract Res Clin Gastroenterol* 2000;14:53–73.

Dohil R, Hassall E, Dimmick J: Gastritis and gastropathy of childhood. *J Pediatr Gastroenterol Nutr* 1999;29:378–394.

Drumm B, Day AS, Gold B, et al: *Helicobacter pylori* and peptic ulcer: Working Group Report of the Second World Congress of Pediatric Gastroenterology, Hepatology, and Nutrition. *J Pediatr Gastroenterol Nutr* 2004;39:S626–S631.

Elitsur Y: *Helicobacter pylori* diagnostic tools: Is it in the stool? *J Pediatr* 2005;146:164–167.

Gibril F, Jensen RT: Zollinger-Ellison syndrome revisited: Diagnosis, biologic markers, associated inherited disorders, and acid hypersecretion. *Curr Gastroenterol Rep* 2004;6:454–463.

Gold BD: Current therapy for *Helicobacter pylori* infection in children and adolescents. *Can J Gastroenterol* 1999;13:571–579.
Kato S, Sherman PM: What is new related to *Heliocobacter pylori* infection in children and teenagers? *Arch Pediatr Adolesc Med* 2005;159:415–421.
Mulberg A, Linz C, Bern E, et al: Identification of non-steroidal anti-inflammatory drug-induced gastroduodenal injury in children with juvenile rheumatoid arthritis. *J Pediatr* 1993;122:647–649.
Sabbi T, De Angelis P, Colistro F, et al: Efficacy of noninvasive tests in the diagnosis of *Helicobacter pylori* infection in pediatric patients. *Arch Pediatr Adolesc Med* 2005;159:238–241.
Shah R: Dyspepsia and helicobacter pylori. *BMJ* 2007;334:41–43.

Chapter 333 ■ Inflammatory Bowel Disease

Jeffrey S. Hyams

The term *inflammatory bowel disease* (IBD) is used to represent two distinctive disorders of idiopathic chronic intestinal inflammation: Crohn disease and ulcerative colitis. Their respective etiologies are poorly understood, and both disorders are characterized by unpredictable exacerbations and remissions. The most common time of onset of IBD is during the preadolescence/adolescence era and young adulthood. A bimodal distribution has been shown with an early onset at 10–20 yr of age and a 2nd, smaller peak at 50–80 yr of age. Twenty-five per cent of patients present before 20 yr of age. Nonetheless, IBD may begin as early as the 1st yr of life, and an increased incidence among young children has been observed over the past decade. Children with early onset IBD are more likely to have colonic involvement. In developed countries, these disorders are the major causes of chronic intestinal inflammation in children beyond the 1st few yr of life. A 3rd, less common category, indeterminate colitis, represents ≈10% of pediatric patients.

Both genetic and environmental influences are involved in the pathogenesis of IBD. The incidence of IBD among whites and nonwhites is similar in the United States; the incidence in blacks in Africa is low. The prevalence of Crohn disease in the United States is much lower for Hispanics and Asians than for whites and blacks. The risk of IBD in family members of an affected individual has been reported in the range of 7–30%; a child whose parents both have IBD has a >35% chance of acquiring the disorder. Relatives of an individual with ulcerative colitis have a greater risk of acquiring ulcerative colitis than Crohn disease, whereas relatives of an individual with Crohn disease have a greater risk of acquiring this disorder; the two diseases can occur in the same family. The risk of occurrence of IBD among relatives of individuals with Crohn disease is somewhat greater than for individuals with ulcerative colitis.

The importance of genetic factors in the development of IBD is noted by a higher chance that both twins will be affected if they are monozygotic rather than dizygotic. The concordance rate in twins is higher in Crohn disease (36%) than in ulcerative colitis (16%). Genetic disorders that have been associated with IBD include Turner syndrome, the Hermansky-Pudlak syndrome, glycogen storage disease type Ib, and various immunodeficiency disorders. Genetic linkage analyses, through genome-wide screens, have identified a number of susceptibility loci, designated IBD1 through IBD6 on chromosome 16, 12, 6, 14, 5, and 19, respectively. The IBD1 locus has shown the greatest association and is termed *NOD2/CARD15*. Three main polymorphisms have been described *(R702W, G908R, 1007fs)*. Additional alleles include *SNP5, JW1,* and *3020insC*. Whereas having one copy of the risk allele confers a small increased risk of developing Crohn disease (two- to fourfold), having two copies (homozygote or compound heterozygote) increases risk by 20- to 40-fold. These genetic variants alter intestinal nuclear factor-κβ (NF-κβ) activation in response to bacterial lipopolysaccharide and peptidoglycan. Other IBD loci may encode for the multidrug resistant gene and genes in the organic cation transporter gene cluster. Only 20% of patients with Crohn disease are homozygous for *NOD2* variants. Carriage of *NOD2/CARD15* risk alleles is associated with ileal and stricturing disease phenotypes. These genes are uncommon in African-American patients but are present in 40–50% of white patients.

A perinuclear antineutrophil antibody (pANCA) is found in ≈70% of individuals with ulcerative colitis compared with <20% of those with Crohn disease and is believed to represent a marker of genetically controlled immunoregulatory disturbance. About 55% of those with Crohn disease are positive for anti–*Saccharomyces cerevisiae* (ASCA) antibody.

Environmental factors are also important and presumably explain discordance between twins and changes in risk among the same race in different geographic regions; the precise factors remain unknown. Individuals migrating to developed countries often appear to acquire the higher rates of IBD associated with these regions. Cigarette smoking is a risk factor for Crohn disease but paradoxically protects against ulcerative colitis. No specific infectious agent has been reproducibly associated with IBD.

An abnormality in intestinal mucosal immunoregulation may be of primary importance in the pathogenesis of IBD. The gut is under constant immunologic stimulation from microbial agents and dietary antigens. In response, the mucosa normally displays "physiologic" inflammation. In IBD, the mechanisms that keep "physiologic" inflammation in check fail and pathologic inflammation ensues. It is not clear if this represents an abnormal response to customary enteric antigens or a normal response to an as yet unidentified microbe. Mediators of inflammation (cytokines, arachidonic acid metabolites, reactive oxygen metabolites, growth factors) are involved, leading to tissue destruction and remodeling with fibrosis. Most therapies are aimed at interfering with these mediators.

It is usually possible to distinguish between ulcerative colitis and Crohn disease by the clinical presentation and radiologic, endoscopic, and histopathologic findings (Table 333-1). It is not

TABLE 333-1. Comparison of Crohn Disease and Ulcerative Colitis

FEATURE	CROHN DISEASE	ULCERATIVE COLITIS
Rectal bleeding	Sometimes	Common
Diarrhea	Variable	Common
Abdominal pain	Common	Variable
Abdominal mass	Common	Not present
Growth failure	Common	Variable
Perianal disease	Common	Unusual
Rectal disease	Occasional	Universal
Pyoderma gangrenosum	Rare	Present
Erythema nodosum	Common	Less common
Mouth ulceration	Common	Rare
Thrombosis	Less common	Present
Colonic disease	50–75%	100%
Ileal disease	Common	None except backwash ileitis
Stomach-esophageal disease	Uncommon	None
Strictures	Common	Unusual
Fissures	Common	None
Fistulas	Common	Unusual
Toxic megacolon	None	Present
Sclerosing cholangitis	Less common	Present
Risk for cancer	Increased	Greatly increased
Discontinuous (skip) lesions	Common	Not present
Transmural involvement	Common	Unusual
Crypt abscesses	Less common	Common
Granulomas	Common	Unusual
Linear ulcerations	Uncommon	Common
Perinuclear antineutrophil	Uncommon	Common cytoplasmic antibodies (pANCA)
Anti-*Saccharomyces cerevisiae*	Common	Uncommon antibodies

possible to make a definitive diagnosis in ≈10% of individuals with chronic colitis; this disorder is called *indeterminate colitis*. Occasionally, a child initially believed to have ulcerative colitis on the basis of clinical findings is subsequently diagnosed with Crohn colitis. The treatments of Crohn disease and ulcerative colitis overlap.

Extraintestinal manifestations occur slightly more commonly with Crohn disease than with ulcerative colitis (Table 333-2). Growth retardation is seen in 15–35% of individuals with Crohn disease at diagnosis. Of the extraintestinal manifestations that occur with IBD, joint, skin, eye, mouth, and hepatobiliary involvement tend to be associated with colitis, whether ulcerative or Crohn. For some manifestations, activity correlates with activity of the bowel disease, including peripheral arthritis, erythema nodosum, and anemia. Activity of pyoderma gangrenosum correlates less well with activity of the bowel disease, whereas activities of sclerosing cholangitis, ankylosing spondylitis, and sacroiliitis do not correlate with intestinal disease. Arthritis occurs in three patterns: migratory peripheral arthritis involving primarily large joints, ankylosing spondylitis, and sacroiliitis. The peripheral arthritis of IBD tends to be nondestructive. Ankylosing spondylitis begins in the 3rd decade and occurs most commonly in individuals with ulcerative colitis who have the human leukocyte antigen B27 phenotype. Symptoms include low back

TABLE 333-2. Extraintestinal Complications of Inflammatory Bowel Disease

MUSCULOSKELETAL
- Peripheral arthritis
- Granulomatous monoarthritis
- Granulomatous synovitis
- Rheumatoid arthritis
- Sacroiliitis
- Ankylosing spondylitis
- Digital clubbing and hypertrophic osteoarthropathy
- Periosteitis
- Osteoporosis, osteomalacia
- Rhabdomyolysis
- Pelvic osteomyelitis
- Recurrent multifocal osteomyelitis
- Relapsing polychondritis

SKIN AND MUCOUS MEMBRANES
- Oral lesions
- Cheilitis
- Apthous stomatitis, glossitis
- Granulomatous oral Crohn disease
- Inflammatory hyperplasia fissures and cobblestone mucosa
- Peristomatitis vegetans

DERMATOLOGIC
- Erythema nodosum
- Pyoderma gangrenosum
- Sweet syndrome
- Metastatic Crohn disease
- Psoriasis
- Epidermolysis bullosa acquisita
- Perianal skin tags
- Polyarteritis nodosa

OCULAR
- Conjunctivitis
- Uveitis, iritis
- Episcleritis
- Scleritis
- Retrobulbar neuritis
- Chorioretinitis with retinal detachment
- Crohn keratopathy
- Posterior segment abnormalities
- Retinal vascular disease

BRONCHOPULMONARY
- Chronic bronchitis with bronchiectasis
- Chronic bronchitis with neutrophilic infiltrates
- Fibrosing alveolitis
- Pulmonary vasculitis
- Small airway disease and bronchiolitis obliterans
- Eosinophilic lung disease
- Granulomatous lung disease
- Tracheal obstruction

CARDIAC
- Pleuropericarditis
- Cardiomyopathy
- Endocarditis
- Myocarditis

MALNUTRITION
- Decreased intake food: IBD, dietary restriction
- Malabsorption: IBD, bowel resection, bile salt depletion, bacterial overgrowth
- Intestinal losses: electrolytes, minerals, nutrients
- Increased caloric needs: inflammation, fever

HEMATOLOGIC
- Anemia: iron deficiency (blood loss)
- Vitamin B_{12} (ileal disease or resection, bacterial overgrowth, folate deficiency)
- Anemia of chronic inflammation
- Anaphylactoid purpura (Crohn disease)
- Hyposplenism
- Autoimmune hemolytic anemia
- Coagulation abnormalities
  - Increased activation of coagulation factors
  - Activated fibronolysis
  - Anticardiolipin antibody
  - Increased risk of arterial and venous thrombosis with cerebrovascular stroke, myocardial infarction, peripheral arterial and venous occlusions

RENAL AND GENITOURINARY
- Metabolic: urinary crystal formation (nephrolithiasis, uric acid, oxylate)
- Hypokalemic nephropathy
- Inflammation: retroperitoneal abscess, fibrosis with ureteral obstruction, fistula formation
- Glomerulitis
- Membranonephritis
- Renal amyloidosis, nephrotic syndrome

PANCREATITIS
- Secondary to medications (sulfasalazine, 6-mercaptopurine, azathioprine, parenteral nutrition)
- Ampullary Crohn disease
- Granulomatous pancreatitis
- Decreased pancreatic exocrine function
- Sclerosing cholangitis with pancreatitis

HEPATOBILIARY
- Primary sclerosing cholangitis (PSC)
- Small duct PSC (pericholangitis)
- Carcinoma of the bile ducts
- Fatty infiltration of the liver
- Cholelithiasis
- Autoimmune hepatitis

ENDOCRINE AND METABOLIC
- Growth failure, delayed sexual maturation
- Thyroiditis
- Osteoporosis, osteomalacia

NEUROLOGIC
- Peripheral neuropathy
- Meningitis
- Vestibular dysfunction
- Pseudotumor cerebri

G6PD, glucose-6-phosphate dehydrogenase; IBD, inflammatory bowel disease.
Modified from Kugathasan S: Diarrhea. In Kliegman RM, Greenbaum LA, Lye PS (editors): *Practical Strategies in Pediatric Diagnosis and Therapy*, 2nd ed. Philadelphia, Elsevier/Saunders, 2004, p. 285.

pain and morning stiffness; back, hips, shoulders, and sacroiliac joints are typically affected. Isolated sacroiliitis is usually asymptomatic but is common when a careful search is performed. Among the skin manifestations, erythema nodosum is most common. Individuals with erythema nodosum or pyoderma gangrenosum have a high likelihood of having arthritis as well. Glomerulonephritis and a hypercoagulable state are other rare manifestations that occur in childhood. Cerebral thromboembolic disease has been described in children with IBD. Uveitis occurs in ≈5% of children with IBD and is usually asymptomatic and transient; its occurrence does not correlate with activity of bowel disease. There is a poor phenotype-genotype correlation between symptoms or complications.

333.1 • Chronic Ulcerative Colitis

Ulcerative colitis, an idiopathic chronic inflammatory disorder, is localized to the colon and spares the upper gastrointestinal tract. Disease usually begins in the rectum and extends proximally for a variable distance. When it is localized to the rectum, the disease is ulcerative proctitis, whereas disease involving the entire colon is pancolitis. Pancolitis is noted in the majority of children. Ulcerative proctitis is less likely to be associated with systemic manifestations, although it may be less responsive to treatment than more diffuse disease. About 30% of children who present with ulcerative proctitis experience proximal spread of the disease. Ulcerative colitis has rarely been noted to present in infancy. Dietary protein intolerance can easily be misdiagnosed as ulcerative colitis in this age group. Dietary protein intolerance (cow's milk protein) is a transient disorder; symptoms are directly associated with the intake of the offending antigen.

The incidence of ulcerative colitis has remained relatively constant, in contrast to an increase in Crohn disease, but varies with country of origin. Incidence rates are highest in northern European countries and the United States (15/100,000) and lowest in Japan and South Africa (1/100,000). The incidence of ulcerative colitis in Israel varies with the country of origin; those born in Asia or Africa have the lowest risk. The prevalence of ulcerative colitis in northern European countries and the United States varies from 100 to 200/100,000 population. Men are slightly more likely to acquire ulcerative colitis than are women; the reverse is true for Crohn disease.

CLINICAL MANIFESTATIONS. Blood in the stool and diarrhea are the typical presentation of ulcerative colitis. Constipation may be observed in those with proctitis. Symptoms such as tenesmus, urgency, cramping abdominal pain (especially with bowel movements), and nocturnal bowel movements are common. The mode of onset may range from insidious with gradual progression of symptoms to acute and fulminant. Fever, severe anemia, hypoalbuminemia, leukocytosis, and more than five bloody stools per day for 5 days, defines fulminant colitis. Chronicity is an important part of the diagnosis; it is difficult to know if a patient has a subacute, transient infectious colitis or ulcerative colitis when a child has had 1–2 wk of symptoms. Symptoms beyond this duration often prove to be secondary to IBD. Anorexia, weight loss, and growth failure may be present, although these complications are more typical of Crohn disease.

Extraintestinal manifestations that tend to occur more commonly with ulcerative colitis than with Crohn disease include pyoderma gangrenosum, sclerosing cholangitis, chronic active hepatitis, and ankylosing spondylitis. Iron deficiency may result from chronic blood loss as well as decreased intake. Folate deficiency is unusual but may be accentuated in children treated with sulfasalazine, which interferes with folate absorption. Chronic inflammation and the elaboration of a variety of inflammatory cytokines can interfere with erythropoiesis and result in the anemia of chronic disease. Secondary amenorrhea is common during periods of active disease in older girls.

The clinical course of ulcerative colitis is marked by remission and relapse, often without apparent explanation. After treatment of initial symptoms, ≈5% of children with ulcerative colitis have a prolonged remission (>3 yr). About 25% of children presenting with severe ulcerative colitis require colectomy within 5 yr of diagnosis, compared with only 5% of those presenting with mild disease. It is important to consider the possibility of enteric infection with recurrent symptoms; these infections may mimic a flare-up or actually provoke a recurrence. The use of nonsteroidal anti-inflammatory drugs is considered by some to predispose to exacerbation.

It is generally believed that the risk of colon cancer begins to increase after 8–10 yr of disease and may then increase by 0.5–1% per yr. The risk is delayed by ≈10 yr in individuals with colitis limited to the descending colon. Proctitis alone is associated with virtually no increase in risk over the general population. Because colon cancer is usually preceded by changes of mucosal dysplasia, it is recommended that patients who have had ulcerative colitis for >10 yr be screened with colonoscopy and biopsy every 1–2 yr. Although this is the current standard of practice, it is not clear if morbidity and mortality are changed by this approach. Two competing concerns about this plan of management remain unresolved: (1) the original studies may have overestimated the risk of colon cancer and, therefore, the need for surveillance has been overemphasized; and (2) screening for dysplasia may not be adequate for the prevention of colon cancer in ulcerative colitis if some cancers are not preceded by dysplasia.

DIFFERENTIAL DIAGNOSIS. The major conditions to exclude are infectious colitis, allergic colitis, and Crohn colitis. Every child with a new diagnosis of ulcerative colitis should have stool cultured for enteric pathogens, stool evaluation for ova and parasites, and perhaps serologic studies for amebae (Table 333-3). In the setting of antibiotic use, pseudomembranous colitis secondary to *Clostridium difficile* should be considered. Cytomegalovirus infection can mimic ulcerative colitis or be associated with an exacerbation of existing disease. The most difficult distinction is from Crohn disease because the colitis of Crohn disease may initially appear identical to that of ulcerative colitis. The gross appearance of the colitis or development of small bowel disease eventually leads to the correct diagnosis; this may occur years after the initial presentation.

At the onset, the colitis of hemolytic-uremic syndrome may be identical to that of early ulcerative colitis. Ultimately, signs of microangiopathic hemolysis (the presence of schistocytes on blood smear), thrombocytopenia, and subsequent renal failure should confirm the diagnosis of hemolytic-uremic syndrome. Although Henoch-Schönlein purpura may present as abdominal pain and bloody stools, it is not usually associated with colitis. Behçet disease can be distinguished by its typical features (see Chapters 160 and 333.3). Other considerations are radiation proctitis, viral colitis in immunocompromised individuals, and ischemic colitis (Table 333-4). In infancy, dietary protein intolerance can be confused with ulcerative colitis, although the former is a transient problem that resolves on removal of the offending protein. Hirschsprung disease may produce an enterocolitis before or within months after surgical correction; this is unlikely to be confused with ulcerative colitis.

DIAGNOSIS. The diagnosis of ulcerative colitis or ulcerative proctitis requires a typical presentation in the absence of an identifiable specific cause (see Tables 333-3 and 333-4) and typical endoscopic and histologic findings (see Table 333-1). One should be hesitant to make a diagnosis of ulcerative colitis in a child who has experienced symptoms for <2–3 wk until infection has been excluded. When the diagnosis is suspected in a child with suba-

TABLE 333-3. Infectious Agents Mimicking Inflammatory Bowel Disease

AGENT	MANIFESTATIONS	DIAGNOSIS	COMMENTS
BACTERIAL			
Campylobacter jejuni	Acute diarrhea, fever, fecal blood, and leukocytes	Culture	Common in adolescents, may relapse
Yersinia enterocolitica	Acute → chronic diarrhea, right lower quadrant pain, mesenteric adenitis—pseudoappendicitis, fecal blood, and leukocytes Extraintestinal manifestations, mimics Crohn disease	Culture	Common in adolescents as FUO, weight loss, abdominal pain
Clostridium difficile	Postantibiotic onset, watery → bloody diarrhea, pseudomembrane on sigmoidoscopy	Cytotoxin assay	May be nosocomial Toxic megacolon possible
Escherichia coli 0157 : H7	Colitis, fecal blood, abdominal pain	Culture and typing	Hemolytic-uremic syndrome
Salmonella	Watery → bloody diarrhea, food borne, fecal leukocytes, fever, pain, cramps	Culture	Usually acute
Shigella	Watery → bloody diarrhea, fecal leukocytes, fever, pain, cramps	Culture	Dysentery symptoms
Edwardsiella tarda	Bloody diarrhea, cramps	Culture	Ulceration on endoscopy
Aeromonas hydrophila	Cramps, diarrhea, fecal blood	Culture	May be chronic Contaminated drinking water
Plesiomonas	Diarrhea, cramps	Culture	Shellfish source
Tuberculosis	Rarely bovine, now *Mycobacterium tuberculosis* Ileocecal area, fistula formation	Culture, PPD, biopsy	May mimic Crohn disease
PARASITES			
Entamoeba histolytica	Acute bloody diarrhea and liver abscess, colic	Trophozoite in stool, colonic mucosal flask ulceration, serologic tests	Travel to endemic area
Giardia lamblia	Foul-smelling, watery diarrhea, cramps, flatulence, weight loss; no colonic involvement	"Owl"-like trophozoite and cysts in stool; rarely duodenal intubation	May be chronic
AIDS-ASSOCIATED ENTEROPATHY			
Cryptosporidium	Chronic diarrhea, weight loss	Stool microscopy	Mucosal findings not like IBD
Isospora belli	As in *Cryptosporidium*		Tropical location
Cytomegalovirus	Colonic ulceration, pain, bloody diarrhea	Culture, biopsy	

FUO, fever of unknown origin; IBD, inflammatory bowel disease; PPD, purified protein derivative.

cute symptoms, the physician should make a firm diagnosis only when there is evidence of chronicity on colonic biopsy. Laboratory studies may demonstrate evidence of anemia (either iron deficiency or the anemia of chronic disease) or hypoalbuminemia. Although the sedimentation rate is often elevated, it may be normal even with fulminant colitis. An elevated white blood cell count is usually seen only with more severe colitis. Barium enema is suggestive but not diagnostic of acute (Fig. 333-1) or chronic burned out disease (Fig. 333-2).

TABLE 333-4. Chronic Inflammatory-like Intestinal Disorders

INFECTION (SEE TABLE 333-3)
- Bacterial
- Parasite

AIDS-ASSOCIATED
- Toxin

IMMUNE-INFLAMMATORY
- Congenital immunodeficiency disorders
- Acquired immunodeficiency diseases
- Dietary protein enterocolitis
- Behçet disease
- Lymphoid nodular hyperplasia
- Eosinophilic gastroenteritis
- Graft versus host disease

VASCULAR-ISCHEMIC DISORDERS
- Systemic vasculitis (SLE, dermatomyositis)
- Henoch-Schönlein purpura
- Hemolytic-uremic syndrome

OTHER
- Prestenotic colitis
- Diversion colitis
- Radiation colitis
- Neonatal necrotizing enterocolitis
- Typhlitis
- Hirschsprung colitis
- Intestinal lymphoma
- Laxative abuse

SLE, systemic lupus erythematosus.

The diagnosis of ulcerative colitis must be confirmed by endoscopic and histologic examination of the colon. Classically, disease starts in the rectum with a gross appearance characterized by erythema, edema, loss of vascular pattern, granularity, and friability. There may be a "cutoff" demarcating the margin between inflammation and normal colon, or the entire colon may be involved. There may be some variability in the intensity of inflammation even in those areas involved. Flexible sigmoidoscopy can confirm the diagnosis; colonoscopy can evaluate the extent of disease and rule out Crohn colitis. A colonoscopy should not be performed when fulminant colitis is suspected because of the risk of provoking *toxic megacolon* or causing a perforation during the procedure. The degree of colitis can be evaluated by the gross appearance of the mucosa. One does not generally see discrete ulcers, which would be more suggestive of Crohn colitis. The endoscopic findings of ulcerative colitis result from microulcers, which give the appearance of a diffuse abnormality. With very severe chronic colitis, pseudopolyps may be seen. Biopsy of involved bowel demonstrates evidence of acute and chronic mucosal inflammation. Typical findings are cryptitis, crypt abscesses, separation of crypts by inflammatory cells, foci of acute inflammatory cells, edema, mucus depletion, and branching of crypts. The last finding is not seen in infectious colitis. Granulomas, fissures, or full-thickness involvement of the bowel wall (usually on surgical rather than endoscopic biopsy) suggest Crohn disease. Rectal biopsy can also distinguish chronic IBD from acute self-limiting colitis.

Perianal disease, with the exception of mild local irritation or anal fissures associated with diarrhea, should make the clinician think of Crohn disease. Plain radiographs of the abdomen may demonstrate loss of haustral markings in an air-filled colon or marked dilatation with toxic megacolon. With severe colitis, the colon may become dilated; a diameter of >6 cm, determined radiographically, in an adult suggests toxic megacolon. If it is necessary to examine the colon radiologically in a child with severe colitis (to evaluate the extent of involvement or to try to rule out

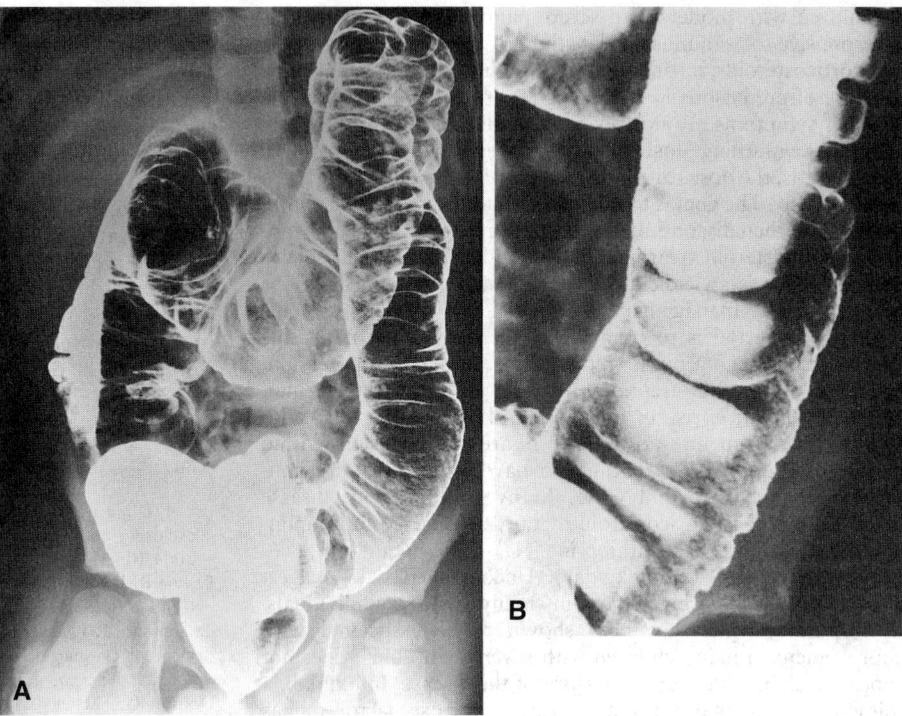

Figure 333-1. Ulcerative colitis: double-contrast barium enema in a 5 yr old boy who had had intermittent intestinal and extraintestinal symptoms since the age of 3 yr. *A,* Small ulcerations are distributed uniformly about the colonic circumference and continuously from the rectum to the proximal transverse colon. This pattern of involvement is typical of ulcerative colitis. *B,* In this coned view of the sigmoid in the same patient, small ulcerations are represented by fine spiculation of the colonic contour in tangent and by fine stippling of the colon surface en face. (From Hoffman AD, Hilton SW, Edwards DK [editors]: The child with diarrhea. In *Practical Pediatric Radiology,* 2nd ed. Philadelphia, WB Saunders, 1994, p 260.)

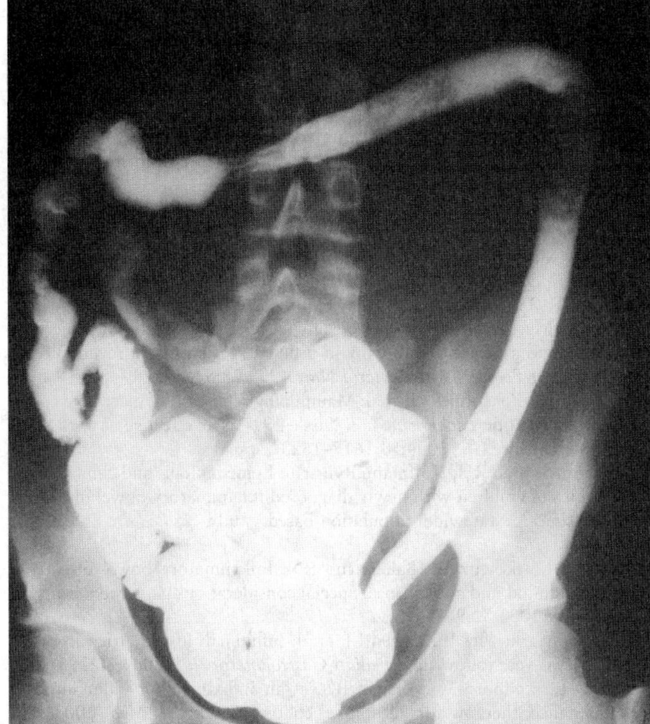

Figure 333-2. Ulcerative colitis: late changes. This single-contrast barium enema shows the late changes of ulcerative colitis in a 15 yr old girl. The colon is featureless, reduced in caliber, and shortened. Dilatation of the terminal ileum (backwash ileitis) is present. (From Hoffman AD, Hilton SW, Edwards DK [editors]: The child with diarrhea. In *Practical Pediatric Radiology,* 2nd ed. Philadelphia, WB Saunders, 1994, p 262.)

Crohn disease), it is sometimes helpful to perform an upper gastrointestinal contrast series with small bowel follow-through and then look at delayed films of the colon. A barium enema is contraindicated in the setting of a potential toxic megacolon.

TREATMENT. A medical cure for ulcerative colitis is not available; treatment is aimed at controlling symptoms and reducing the risk of recurrence. The intensity of treatment varies with the severity of the symptoms. Twenty to 30% of individuals with ulcerative colitis have spontaneous improvement in symptoms. The 1st drug class to be used with mild colitis is an aminosalicylate. Sulfasalazine is composed of a sulfur moiety linked to the active ingredient 5-aminosalicylate. This linkage prevents the premature absorption of the medication in the upper gastrointestinal tract, allowing it to reach the colon, where the two components are separated by bacterial cleavage. The dose of sulfasalazine is 50–75 mg/kg/24 hr (divided into two to four doses). Generally, the dose is not more than 2–3 g/24 hr. It is recommended that the dosage gradually increase to full dose over the 1st wk of treatment to avoid gastrointestinal symptoms (nausea, abdominal pain) and headache and to detect sulfa hypersensitivity. Onset of action can take several weeks. Sulfasalazine treats colitis; recurrences may be prevented with its use. It is recommended that the medication be continued even when the disorder is in remission. Hypersensitivity to the sulfa component is the major side effect of sulfasalazine and occurs in 10–20% of individuals. Other less allergenic preparations of 5-aminosalicylate (mesalamine, 50–70 mg/kg/day) are useful and have been shown to treat ulcerative colitis and prevent recurrences with efficacy equal to that of sulfasalazine.

Perhaps 10–20% of individuals who have an allergic reaction to sulfasalazine will have a similar reaction to another 5-aminosalicylate product. On rare occasions, these medications cause exacerbation of colitis. Aminosalicylate can also be given in enema form and is especially useful for proctitis. Hydrocortisone enemas (100 mg) are used to treat proctitis as well. Either form of enema can be administered to older children once a day (usually bedtime) for 2–3 wk. Many children prefer oral medication to enemas.

Children with moderate to severe pancolitis or colitis that is unresponsive to 5-aminosalicylate therapy should be treated with oral corticosteroids, most commonly, prednisone. The usual starting dose of prednisone is 1–2 mg/kg/24 hr (40–60 mg maximum dose). If symptoms are not severe, this medication can be given in a single morning dose to lessen adrenal suppression. With severe colitis, the dose can be divided twice daily and can be given intravenously. The goal is to taper to an alternate-day dose within 1–3 mo and then discontinue the prednisone. Persistence of symptoms despite steroid treatment for 7–10 days or the inability to taper the dose is an indication for the use of other medications or for surgical management. Prolonged use of daily steroids beyond this period is to be avoided because of the many side effects, including growth retardation, adrenal suppression, cataracts, osteopenia, aseptic necrosis of the head of the femur, glucose intolerance, risk of infection, and cosmetic effects. With medical management, most children are in remission within 3 mo; however, 5–10% continue to have symptoms unresponsive to treatment beyond 6 mo. Many children with disease requiring frequent corticosteroid therapy are started on immunomodulators such as azathioprine (1.5–2.5 mg/kg/day) or 6-mercaptopurine (1–1.5 mg/kg/day). Uncontrolled data suggest a corticosteroid-sparing effect in many treated individuals. Cyclosporine, which has been shown to be associated with improvement in many children with severe symptoms, does not appear to change the natural history of the disease. Infliximab, a chimeric monoclonal antibody to tumor necrosis factor–α, has been used in some cases of fulminant colitis. Infliximab induction and maintenance therapy in adults with moderate to severe disease has been successful in producing positive clinical responses. Probiotic agents may have a role in maintaining remission and may be as effective in preventing relapse as mesalamine.

Colectomy is performed for intractable disease, complications of therapy, and fulminant disease that is unresponsive to medical management. No clear benefit of the use of total parenteral nutrition or a continuous enteral elemental diet in the treatment of severe ulcerative colitis has been noted. Nevertheless, parenteral nutrition is often used if oral intake is insufficient so that the patient will be nutritionally ready for surgery if medical management fails. With any medical treatment for ulcerative colitis, the clinician should always weigh the risk of the medication or therapy against the fact that colitis can be successfully treated surgically.

Surgical treatment for intractable or fulminant colitis is total colectomy. The optimal approach is to combine colectomy with an endorectal pull-through where a segment of distal rectum is retained and the mucosa is stripped from this region. The distal ileum is pulled down and sutured at the internal anus with a J pouch created from ileum immediately above the rectal cuff. This procedure allows the child to maintain continence. Commonly, a temporary ileostomy is created to protect the delicate anastomosis between the sleeve of the pouch and the rectum. The ileostomy is usually closed within several months, restoring bowel continuity. At that time, stool frequency is often increased but may be improved with loperamide. The major complication of this operation is *"pouchitis,"* which is a chronic inflammatory reaction in the pouch, leading to bloody diarrhea, abdominal pain, and, occasionally, low-grade fever. The cause of this complication is unknown, although it is more frequent when the ileal pouch has been constructed for ulcerative colitis than for other indications (familial polyposis coli). Pouchitis is seen in 30–40% of patients who had ulcerative colitis. It commonly responds to treatment with oral metronidazole or ciprofloxacin.

Psychosocial support is an important part of therapy for this disorder. This may include adequate discussion of the disease manifestations and management between patient and physician, psychologic counseling for the child when necessary, and family support from a social worker or family counselor. Patient support groups have proved helpful for some families. Children with ulcerative colitis should be encouraged to participate fully in age-appropriate activities; however, activity may need to be reduced during periods of disease exacerbation.

PROGNOSIS. The course of ulcerative colitis is marked by remissions and exacerbations. Most children with this disorder respond initially to medical management. Many children with mild manifestations continue to respond well to medical management and may stay in remission on a prophylactic 5-aminosalicylate preparation for long periods. An occasional child with mild onset, however, experiences intractable symptoms at a later time. Beyond the 1st decade of disease, the risk of development of colon cancer begins to increase rapidly. The risk of colon cancer may be diminished with surveillance colonoscopies beginning after 8–10 yr of disease. Detection of significant dysplasia on biopsy would prompt colectomy.

Arts J, D'Haens G, et al: Long-term outcome of treatment with intravenous cyclosporine in patients with severe ulcerative colitis. *Inflamm Bowel Dis* 2004;10:73–78.

Beattie RM, Croft NM, Fell JM, et al: Inflammatory bowel disease. *Arch Dis Child* 2006;91:426–432.

de Saussure P, Lavergne-Slove A, Mazeron MC, et al: A prospective assessment of cytomegalovirus infection in active inflammatory bowel disease. *Aliment Pharmacol Ther* 2004;20:1323–1327.

Dobson G, Hickey C, Trinder J: *Clostridium difficile* colitis causing toxic megacolon, severe sepsis and multiple organ dysfunction syndrome. *Intensive Care Med* 2003;29:1030.

Dolgin SE, Shlasko E, Gorfine S, et al: Restorative proctocolectomy in children with ulcerative colitis utilizing rectal mucosectomy with or without diverting ileostomy. *J Pediatr Surg* 1999;34:837–839.

Heyman M, Kirschner BS, Gold BD, et al: Children with early onset inflammatory bowel disease (IBD): Analysis of a pediatric IBD consortium registry. *J Pediatr* 2004;146:35–40.

Ho GT, Mowat C, Goddard CJ, et al: Predicting the outcome of severe ulcerative colitis: Development of a novel risk score to aid early selection of patients for second-line medical therapy or surgery. *Aliment Pharmacol Ther* 2004;19:1079–1087.

Hyams JS: Extraintestinal manifestations of inflammatory bowel disease in children. *J Pediatr Gastroenterol Nutr* 1994;19:7–21.

Hyams JS, Markowitz J, Treem W, et al: Characterization of hepatic abnormalities in children with inflammatory bowel disease. *Inflamm Bowel Dis* 1995;1:27–33.

Kader HA, Mascarehnas MR, Piccoli DA, et al: Experience with 6-mercaptopurine and azathioprine therapy in pediatric patients with severe ulcerative colitis. *J Pediatr Gastroenterol Nutr* 1999;28:54–58.

Kruis W, Fric P, Pokrotnieks J, et al: Maintaining remission of ulcerative colitis with the probiotic *Escherichia coli* Nissle 1917 is as effective as with standard mesalazine. *Gut* 2004;53:1617–1623.

Kugathasan S, Judd RH, Hoffmann RG, et al: Epidemiologic and clinical characteristics of children with newly diagnosed inflammatory bowel disease in Wisconsin: A statewide population-based study. *J Pediatr* 2003;143:525–531.

Mamula P, Markowitz JE, Baldassano RN: Inflammatory bowel disease in early childhood and adolescence: Special considerations. *Gastroenterol Clin North Am* 2003;32:967–995.

Mamula P, Markowitz JE, Cohen LJ, et al: Infliximab in pediatric ulcerative colitis: Two-year follow-up. *J Pediatr Gastroenterol Nutr* 2004;38:298–301.

Rutgeerts P, Sandborn WJ, Feagan BG, et al: Infliximab for induction and maintenance therapy for ulcerative colitis. *N Engl J Med* 2005;353:2462–2476.

333.2 • Crohn Disease (Regional Enteritis, Regional Ileitis, Granulomatous Colitis)

Crohn disease, an idiopathic, chronic inflammatory disorder of the bowel, involves any region of the alimentary tract from the mouth to the anus. Although there are many similarities between ulcerative colitis and Crohn disease, there are also major differences in the clinical course and distribution of the disease in the gastrointestinal tract (see Table 333-1). The inflammatory process tends to be eccentric and segmental, often with skip areas (normal regions of bowel between inflamed areas). Although inflammation in ulcerative colitis is limited to the mucosa (except in toxic megacolon), gastrointestinal involvement in Crohn disease is often transmural. Among children with Crohn disease, the initial presentation most commonly involves ileum and colon (ileocolitis) but involves the small bowel alone in ≈30% (70% of these patients have terminal ileitis alone) or colon alone in 10–15%. Upper gastrointestinal involvement (esophagus, stomach, duodenum) is seen in up to 30% of children. Isolated colonic disease is common in children <8 yr of age. Crohn disease tends to have a bimodal age distribution, with the 1st peak beginning in the teens. Diagnosis before 20 yr of age is associated with a greater chance of small bowel disease, development of stricture, and eventual need for surgery when compared with diagnosis after 40 yr of age.

The incidence of Crohn disease has been increasing, whereas that of ulcerative colitis has been stable. The reported incidence of Crohn disease is ≈3–4/100,000, and the prevalence is 30–100/100,000. The prevalence of Crohn disease in whites and blacks appears to be 3–10 times that of Hispanics and Asians living in the United States.

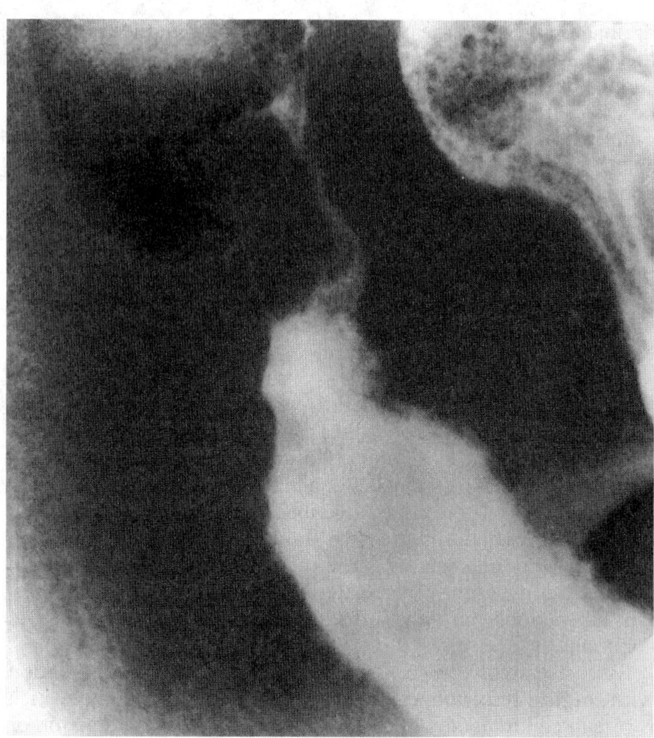

Figure 333-3. Stenotic Crohn disease. Severe stenosis of the terminal ileum is present in this 16 yr old boy. Inflammatory effacement of the mucosal folds and small ulcerations characterize the proximal nonstenotic segment. (From Hoffman AD, Hilton SW, Edwards DK [editors]: The child with diarrhea. In *Practical Pediatric Radiology,* 2nd ed. Philadelphia, WB Saunders, 1994, p 267.)

CLINICAL MANIFESTATIONS. The Vienna classification of subtypes of Crohn disease (variables include age, location, and disease behavior of either inflammatory [nonstricturing/nonpenetrating], stricturing or fibrostenosing, or penetrating) has been proposed but not validated as a prognostic tool in either adults or children. Patients with small bowel disease are more likely to have an obstructive pattern (most commonly with right lower quadrant pain) characterized by fibrostenosis, while those with colonic disease are more likely to have symptoms resulting from inflammation (diarrhea, bleeding, cramping). Disease phenotypes often change as duration of disease lengthens (inflammatory becomes stricturing). Systemic signs and symptoms are more common in Crohn disease than in ulcerative colitis. Fever, malaise, and easy fatigability are common. Growth failure with delayed bone maturation and delayed sexual development may precede other symptoms by 1 or 2 yr and is at least twice as likely to occur with Crohn as with ulcerative colitis. Children may present with growth failure as the only manifestation of Crohn disease. Causes of growth failure include inadequate caloric intake, suboptimal absorption or excessive loss of nutrients, the effects of chronic inflammation on bone metabolism, and the use of corticosteroids during treatment. Primary or secondary amenorrhea is common. In contrast to ulcerative colitis, perianal disease is common (tags, fistula, abscess). Gastric or duodenal involvement may be associated with recurrent vomiting and epigastric pain. Partial small bowel obstruction, usually secondary to narrowing of the bowel lumen from inflammation or stricture, can cause symptoms of cramping abdominal pain (especially with meals), borborygmus, and intermittent abdominal distention (Fig. 333-3). Stricture should be suspected if the child notes relief of symptoms in association with a sudden sensation of gurgling of intestinal contents through a localized region of the abdomen. Ureteral obstruction (usually right-sided) secondary to extension of the inflammatory process is a rare complication of Crohn disease.

Penetrating disease is demonstrated by fistula formation. Enteroenteric or enterocolonic fistulas (between segments of bowel) are often asymptomatic but can contribute to malabsorption if they have high output or result in bacterial overgrowth (Fig. 333-4). Enterovesical fistulas (between bowel and urinary bladder) originate from ileum or sigmoid colon and present as signs of urinary infection, pneumaturia, or fecaluria. Enterovaginal fistulas originate from the rectum, cause feculent vaginal

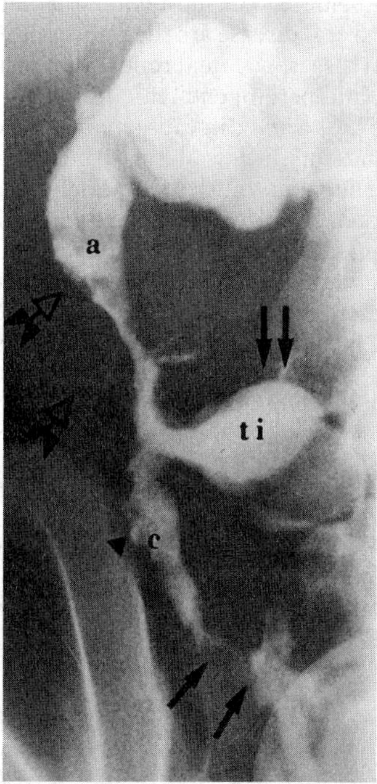

Figure 333-4. Crohn disease: sinuses and fistula. Severe ileocolitis has resulted in an ileocecal fistula *(single arrows, lower)* and sinus formation in the ascending colon (a) *[arrows on platform]*. c, cecum *(arrowhead);* ti, terminal ileum *(paired arrows)*. (From Hoffman AD, Hilton SW, Edwards DK [editors]: The child with diarrhea. In *Practical Pediatric Radiology,* 2nd ed. Philadelphia, WB Saunders, 1994, p 268.)

drainage, and are difficult to manage. Enterocutaneous fistulas (between bowel and abdominal skin) often are caused by prior surgical anastomoses with leakage. Intra-abdominal abscess may be associated with fever and pain but may have relatively few symptoms. Hepatic or splenic abscess can occur with or without a local fistula. Anorectal abscesses often originate immediately above the anus at the crypts of Morgagni. The patterns of perianal fistulas are complex because of the different tissue planes. Perianal abscess is usually painful, but perianal fistulas tend to produce fewer symptoms than anticipated. Purulent drainage is commonly associated with perianal fistulas. *Psoas abscess* secondary to intestinal fistula can present as hip pain, decreased hip extension (psoas sign), and fever.

Extraintestinal manifestations occur more commonly with Crohn disease than with ulcerative colitis; those that are especially associated with Crohn disease include oral aphthous ulcers, peripheral arthritis, erythema nodosum, digital clubbing, episcleritis, renal stones (uric acid, oxalate), and gallstones. Any of the extraintestinal disorders described in the section on IBD can occur with Crohn disease (see Table 333-2). The peripheral arthritis is nondeforming. The occurrence of extraintestinal manifestations usually correlates with the presence of colitis. During periods of active disease, secondary amenorrhea is common.

Extensive involvement of small bowel, especially in association with surgical resection, can lead to short bowel syndrome, which is rare in children. Complications of terminal ileal dysfunction or resection include bile acid malabsorption with secondary diarrhea and vitamin B_{12} malabsorption. Chronic steatorrhea can lead to oxaluria with secondary renal stones. The risk of cholelithiasis is also increased secondary to bile acid depletion.

A disorder with this diversity of manifestations can have a major impact on an affected child's lifestyle. Fortunately, the majority of children with Crohn disease are able to continue with their normal activities, having to limit activity only during periods of increased symptoms.

DIFFERENTIAL DIAGNOSIS. The most common diagnoses to be distinguished from Crohn disease are the infectious enteropathies (in the case of Crohn disease: acute terminal ileitis, infectious colitis, enteric parasites, and periappendiceal abscess) [see Tables 333-3, 333-4, and 333-5]. *Yersinia* can cause many of the radiologic and endoscopic findings in the distal small bowel that are seen in Crohn disease. The symptoms of bacterial dysentery are more likely to be mistaken for ulcerative colitis than for Crohn disease. Celiac disease or *Giardia* infection have been noted to produce a Crohn-like presentation including diarrhea, weight loss, and protein-losing enteropathy. Gastrointestinal tuberculosis is rare but can mimic Crohn disease. Foreign-body perforation of the bowel (toothpick) can mimic a localized region with Crohn disease. Small bowel lymphoma can mimic Crohn disease but tends to be associated with nodular filling defects of the bowel without ulceration or narrowing of the lumen. Bowel lymphoma is much less common in children than is Crohn disease. Recurrent functional abdominal pain can mimic the pain of small bowel Crohn disease. *Lymphoid nodular hyperplasia* of the terminal ileum (a normal finding) may be mistaken for Crohn ileitis. Right lower quadrant pain or mass with fever can be the result of periappendiceal abscess. This entity is occasionally associated with diarrhea as well. Necrotizing jejunitis is a rare condition of transient, acute inflammation of jejunum (or less commonly, ileum or colon), which can recur.

Growth failure may be the only manifestation of Crohn disease; other disorders such as growth hormone deficiency, gluten-sensitive enteropathy (celiac disease), or anorexia nervosa must be considered. If arthritis precedes the bowel manifestations, an initial diagnosis of juvenile rheumatoid arthritis may be made. Refractory anemia may be the presenting feature and may be mistaken as a primary hematologic disorder. Leukemia can present with abdominal pain in association with an abnormal blood cell count and may initially be mistaken for Crohn disease. Chronic granulomatous disease of childhood can cause inflammatory changes in the bowel with granulomas seen at biopsy. Antral narrowing in this disorder may be mistaken for a stricture secondary to Crohn disease.

DIAGNOSIS. Crohn disease can present as a variety of symptom combinations. At the onset, symptoms may be subtle (growth retardation, abdominal pain alone); this explains why the diagnosis may not be made until 1 or 2 yr after the start of symptoms. The diagnosis of Crohn disease depends on finding typical clinical features of the disorder (history, physical examination, laboratory studies, and endoscopic or radiologic findings), ruling out specific entities that mimic Crohn disease, and demonstrating chronicity. The history may include any combination of abdominal pain (especially right lower quadrant), diarrhea, vomiting, anorexia, weight loss, growth retardation, and extraintestinal manifestations. Only 25% initially have the triad of diarrhea, weight loss, and abdominal pain. Most don't have diarrhea and only 25% have gastrointestinal bleeding.

Children with Crohn disease often appear chronically ill. They commonly have weight loss and are often malnourished. Linear growth retardation frequently precedes clinical presentation by as much as 1–2 yr; this manifestation may not have been appreciated until the diagnosis is established. Children with Crohn disease often appear pale, with decreased energy level and poor appetite; the latter finding sometimes results from an association between meals and abdominal pain or diarrhea. There may be abdominal tenderness that is either diffuse or localized to the right lower quadrant. A tender mass or fullness may be palpable in the right lower quadrant. Perianal disease, when present, may be characteristic. Large anal skin tags (1–3 cm diameter) or perianal fistulas with purulent drainage are suggestive of Crohn disease. Digital clubbing, findings of arthritis, and skin mani-

TABLE 333-5. Differential Diagnosis of Presenting Symptoms of Crohn Disease

PRIMARY PRESENTING SYMPTOM	DIAGNOSTIC CONSIDERATIONS
Right lower quadrant abdominal pain, with or without mass	Appendicitis, infection (e.g., *Campylobacter, Yersinia* spp.), lymphoma, intussusception, mesenteric adenitis, Meckel diverticulum, ovarian cyst
Chronic periumbilical or epigastric abdominal pain	Irritable bowel syndrome, constipation, lactose intolerance, peptic disease
Rectal bleeding, no diarrhea	Fissure, polyp, Meckel diverticulum, rectal ulcer syndrome
Bloody diarrhea	Infection, hemolytic-uremic syndrome, Henoch-Schönlein purpura, ischemic bowel, radiation colitis
Watery diarrhea	Irritable bowel syndrome, lactose intolerance, giardiasis, *Cryptosporidium* infection, sorbitol, laxatives
Perirectal disease	Fissure, hemorrhoid (rare), streptococcal infection, condyloma (rare)
Growth delay	Endocrinopathy
Anorexia, weight loss	Anorexia nervosa
Arthritis	Collagen vascular disease, infection
Liver abnormalities	Chronic hepatitis

From Kugathasan S: Diarrhea. In Kliegman RM, Greenbaum LA, Lye P (editors): *Practical Strategies in Pediatric Diagnosis and Therapy*, 2nd ed. Philadelphia, Elsevier/Saunders, 2004, p. 287.

festations may be present. A complete blood cell count commonly demonstrates an anemia, often with a component of iron deficiency. Although the erythrocyte sedimentation rate is often elevated, it may be normal; an elevated platelet count (>600,000/mm^3) is common. The white blood cell count may be normal or mildly elevated. The serum albumin level may be low, and the stool α_1-antitrypsin level may be elevated, consistent with a protein-losing enteropathy. Fecal calprotectin or lactoferrin is usually elevated. Anti–*Saccharomyces cerevisiae* antibodies are identified in 55% of children with Crohn disease but in only 5% of children with ulcerative colitis.

The small and large bowel should be examined in the child with suspected Crohn disease. The initial choice of colonoscopy or a radiologic study depends partly on the anticipated location of disease. For small bowel involvement, an upper gastrointestinal contrast examination with small bowel follow-through would be the initial study. A variety of findings may be apparent on radiologic studies. Plain films of the abdomen may be normal or may demonstrate findings of partial small bowel obstruction or thumbprinting of the colon wall. An upper gastrointestinal contrast study with small bowel follow-through may show aphthous ulceration and thickened, nodular folds as well as narrowing of the lumen anywhere in the gastrointestinal tract. Linear ulcers may give a cobblestone appearance to the mucosal surface. Bowel loops are often separated as a result of thickening of bowel wall and mesentery. Terminal ileum is most commonly involved. Diseased regions tend to be eccentric, and normal regions may be found between diseased segments (skip areas). Video capsule endoscopy has revealed evidence of small bowel mucosal lesions in some patients with normal radiologic evaluation.

Other manifestations on radiographic studies that suggest more severe Crohn disease are fistulas between bowel (enteroenteric or enterocolonic), sinus tracts, and strictures (see Figs. 333-3 and 333-4). Following the flow of barium antegrade into the colon may reveal right-sided colonic disease. Ultrasonography and contrast CT are most useful in identifying intra-abdominal abscess. Thickened bowel wall may be seen on CT. MRI can localize areas of active bowel disease, although this study is probably no better for identifying an abscess. MRI is also useful in evaluating Crohn disease during pregnancy because it does not use ionizing radiation. Radionuclide scans utilizing white blood cells tagged with indium may help locate affected areas.

Colonoscopy with biopsy can be more helpful than radiologic or radionuclide studies in evaluating colon disease and in establishing a diagnosis. Ileal intubation during colonoscopy can be helpful in clarifying an equivocal diagnosis of ileal Crohn disease. Findings on colonoscopy may include patchy, nonspecific inflammatory changes (erythema, friability, loss of vascular pattern), aphthous ulcers, linear ulcers, nodularity, and strictures. Findings on biopsy may be only nonspecific inflammatory changes. Noncaseating granulomas, similar to those of sarcoidosis, are the most characteristic histologic findings, although often they are not present. Transmural inflammation is also characteristic but can be identified only in surgical specimens.

TREATMENT. Crohn disease cannot be cured by either medical or surgical therapy. The aim of treatment is to relieve symptoms and prevent complications of chronic inflammation (anemia, growth failure), prevent relapse, and, if possible, effect mucosal healing. The specific therapeutic modalities used depend on geographic localization of disease, severity of inflammation, age of the patient, and the presence of complications (abscess). For mild terminal ileal disease or mild Crohn disease of the colon, an initial trial of mesalamine (50–70 mg/kg/day, maximum 3–4 g) may be attempted. Specific pharmaceutical preparations have been formulated to release the active 5-ASA compound in the ileum and colon. Sulfasalazine may be effective for mild Crohn colitis but will not be helpful for small bowel disease. Budesonide, a corticosteroid with local anti-inflammatory activity on the bowel mucosa and with high hepatic first-pass metabolism is also used for mild ileal or ileocecal disease (adult dose, 9 mg daily). For more extensive or severe small bowel or colonic disease, most clinicians initiate therapy with corticosteroids (prednisone, 1–2 mg/kg/day, maximum 40–60 mg). The goal is to taper to a single morning, alternate-day dose as soon as the disease becomes quiescent. Typically, tapering can begin by 3–4 wk and continue over several months. Clinicians vary in their tapering schedules, but most decrease the daily dose by 2.5–5.0 mg every 6–8 days until the daily dose is about 0.5 mg/kg, and then a similar decrease is effected on alternate days in 6–8 day cycles (25 mg alternating with 20 mg for 8 days, followed by 25 mg alternating with 15 mg for 8 days, and so forth). Eventually, the prednisone is given on alternate days only and then that dose is tapered as tolerated. This approach is well tolerated, but the disease may flare during the process. Continuing daily or alternate-day prednisone as maintenance therapy to prevent relapse has not been shown to be effective.

Growth is impaired with either active disease or daily corticosteroid therapy. Growth is not impaired by alternate-day therapy. Side effects of daily steroid treatment tend to occur more rapidly and be more severe when the serum albumin level is reduced. Steroid enemas have been used for distal colon disease. Budesonide is often used to mitigate corticosteroid side effects. It appears to be as effective as mesalamine in mild to moderate ileal and right-sided colonic disease but is less effective than prednisone. Whether it has less growth suppressive activity than prednisone has not been established.

Unfortunately, up to 50% of children with Crohn disease will either become refractory to corticosteroid therapy or become dependent on daily dosing and quickly experience flare of the disease when the dose is decreased. Immunomodulators such as azathioprine (1.5–2.5 mg/kg/day) or 6-mercaptopurine (1.0–1.5 mg/kg/day) may be effective in some individuals who have a poor response to prednisone or who are steroid dependent. Because a beneficial effect of these drugs can be delayed for 3–6 mo after starting therapy, they are not helpful acutely. The early use of these agents can decrease cumulative prednisone dosages over the 1st 1–2 yr of therapy. Genetic variations in the enzyme systems responsible for metabolism of these agents (thiopurine S-methyltransferase or TPMT) can affect response rates and potential toxicity. In patients in whom azathioprine resistance is noted, or when toxicity occurs, methotrexate is used (25 mg/1.73 m^2 weekly).

Therapy with antibodies directed against mediators of inflammation is used for patients with Crohn disease. Infliximab (5 mg/kg given intravenously), a chimeric monoclonal antibody to tumor necrosis factor–α, has been approved for the initial treatment and subsequent maintenance therapy of adults with Crohn disease. It is commonly used in children, and noncontrolled published series suggest marked symptom improvement in 50–70% of patients. Its onset of action is quite rapid and it is initially given as three infusions over a 6 wk period (0, 2, and 6 wk). The durability of response to infliximab is variable and can be as short as 4–8 wk, making maintenance therapy necessary. Side effects include infusion reactions, increased incidence of infections (especially reactivation of latent tuberculosis), demyelinating disease, possibly malignancy, and the development of autoantibodies. The development of antibodies to infliximab (ATI) is associated with an increased incidence of infusion reactions and decreased durability of response. The concomitant use of immunomodulators such as azathioprine with infliximab therapy is associated with decreased levels of ATI. Long-term safety of this biologic therapy appears good, but long-term observation is required to assess potential late side effects such as lymphoma. A purified protein derivative (PPD) test for tuberculosis should be done before starting infliximab. Active or latent intra-abdominal infection (abscess) is a contraindication to infliximab therapy. Humanized antibodies against tumor necrosis factor–α, anti-interleukin 12, and leukocyte adhesion molecules (natalizumab against α-integrin) are being tested.

There are several therapies available to treat perirectal fistula. Metronidazole (10–20 mg/dL/day) is often effective, but long-term therapy can cause neuropathy with paresthesias, requiring cessation of therapy. Azathioprine and 6-mercaptopurine have succeeded in this situation. Infliximab is also useful, although recurrence is common.

Nutritional therapy is an effective primary as well as adjunctive treatment. The enteral nutritional approach (elemental or polymeric diets) is both as rapid in onset of response and as effective as the other treatments. Other studies suggest prednisone is more effective for the acute control of disease. Because elemental diets are relatively unpalatable, they are administered via a nasogastric or gastrostomy infusion. With severe, acute disease, they can be given continuously as a 24 hr infusion; the treatment can then be cycled to overnight infusion at home. Repletion should be planned for ideal weight to allow for catch-up growth. Most children are hesitant to use nasogastric infusion, but once it is begun, most find it is not difficult. The advantages are that it (1) is relatively free of side effects, (2) avoids the problems associated with corticosteroid therapy, and (3) simultaneously addresses the nutritional rehabilitation. Children can participate in normal daytime activities. A major disadvantage of this approach is similar to that of other therapies: early relapse on discontinuing treatment. In addition, perianal and colon disease does not respond well. For children with growth failure, this approach may be ideal, however.

High-calorie oral supplements, although effective, are often not tolerated because of early satiety or exacerbation of symptoms (abdominal pain, vomiting, or diarrhea). Nonetheless, they should be offered to children whose weight gain is suboptimal. The continuous administration of nocturnal nasogastric feedings for chronic malnutrition and growth failure has been effective with a much lower risk of complications than parenteral hyperalimentation. Complex formula can be given at 500–1,000 kcal nightly; some clinicians consider treatment with 50–80 kcal/kg/night monthly every 4 mo equally effective.

The initial onset or a recurrence of Crohn disease can be acute, with severe pain, anorexia, fever, abdominal tenderness, and an elevated white blood cell count. In this situation, it is difficult to rule out an infectious process involving the bowel wall (microperforation). In addition to the use of intravenous corticosteroids, broad-spectrum intravenous antibiotic coverage for bowel flora (gram-negative bacteria and anaerobes) should be started initially and discontinued only if it appears that there is not an infectious process. An ultrasonogram or contrast CT study of the abdomen is necessary to rule out an intra-abdominal abscess. The development of an enteroenteric or colonic fistula may be identified on CT, although it is best seen on a conventional small bowel contrast study.

Surgical therapy should be reserved for very specific indications. Recurrence rate after bowel resection is high (>50% by 5 yr); the risk of requiring additional surgery increases with each operation. Potential complications of surgery include development of fistula or stricture, anastomotic leak, postoperative partial small bowel obstruction secondary to adhesions, and short bowel syndrome. Surgery is the treatment of choice for localized disease of small bowel or colon that is unresponsive to medical treatment, bowel perforation, fibrosed stricture with symptomatic partial small bowel obstruction, and intractable bleeding. Intra-abdominal or liver abscess may sometimes be successfully treated by ultrasonographic or CT-guided catheter drainage and concomitant intravenous antibiotic treatment. Open surgical drainage is necessary if this approach is not successful. Perianal abscess often requires drainage unless it drains spontaneously. In general, perianal fistulas should be managed medically. A severely symptomatic perianal fistula may require fistulotomy, however; this procedure should be considered only if the location allows the sphincter to remain undamaged. Growth retardation was once considered an indication for resection; without other indications, this approach has not been shown to be beneficial, and medical or nutritional therapy, or both, is preferred.

The surgical approach for Crohn disease is to remove as limited a length of bowel as possible. There is no evidence that removing bowel up to margins that are free of histologic disease has a better outcome than removing only grossly involved areas. The latter approach reduces the risk of short bowel syndrome. One approach to symptomatic small bowel stricture has been to perform a strictureplasty rather than resection. The surgeon makes a longitudinal incision across the stricture but then closes the incision with sutures in a transverse fashion. This is ideal for short strictures without active disease. The reoperation rate is no higher with this approach than with resection, whereas bowel length is preserved. Postoperative medical therapy with agents such as azathioprine is often given to decrease the likelihood of postoperative recurrence.

Severe perianal disease can be incapacitating and difficult to treat if unresponsive to medical management. Colon diversion can allow the area to be less active; but on reconnection of the colon, disease activity usually recurs. Therefore, surgical treatment of severe perianal disease may require colectomy. Procedures that create a continent ileostomy or endorectal pull-through are generally discouraged in Crohn disease because of the risk of recurrence of the disease in remaining bowel. With colectomy, a conventional ileostomy is performed.

Psychosocial issues for the child with Crohn disease include a sense of being different, concerns about body image, difficulty in not participating fully in age-appropriate activities, and family conflict brought on by the added stress of this disease. Social support is an important component of the management of Crohn disease. Parents are often interested in learning about other children with similar problems, but children may be hesitant to participate. Social support and individual psychologic counseling are important in the adjustment to a difficult problem at an age that by itself often has difficult adjustment issues. Patients who are socially "connected" fare better. Ongoing education about the disease is an important aspect of management because children generally fare better if they understand and anticipate problems. The Crohn and Colitis Foundation of America has local chapters throughout the United States.

PROGNOSIS. Crohn disease is a chronic disorder that is associated with high morbidity but low mortality. Symptoms tend to recur despite treatment and often without apparent explanation. One exception is that symptoms of partial small obstruction may occur after a high-residue meal in the presence of a small bowel stricture. Weight loss and growth failure can usually be improved with treatment and attention to nutritional needs. Up to 15% of individuals with early growth retardation secondary to Crohn disease have a permanent decrease in linear growth. Osteopenia is particularly common in those with chronic poor nutrition and frequent exposure to high doses of corticosteroids. Some of the extraintestinal manifestations can, in themselves, be major causes of morbidity, including sclerosing cholangitis, chronic active hepatitis, pyoderma gangrenosum, and ankylosing spondylitis.

The region of bowel involved may increase with time, although rapid progression typically occurs early and is subsequently slow. Complications of the inflammatory process tend to increase with time and include bowel strictures, fistulas, perianal disease, and intra-abdominal or retroperitoneal abscess. Nearly all individuals with Crohn disease eventually require surgery for one of its many complications; the rate of reoperation is high. The time between the onset of symptoms and the need for surgery appears to be shorter in children than in adults. Surgery is unlikely to be curative and should be avoided except for the specific indications noted previously. Repeated small bowel resection, which may be unavoidable, can lead to malabsorption secondary to short bowel syndrome (see Chapter 335.7). Resection of terminal ileum can result in bile acid malabsorption with diarrhea and vitamin B_{12} malabsorption. The risk of colon cancer in individuals with long-standing Crohn colitis approaches that associated with ulcerative colitis, and screening colonoscopy after 10 years of colonic disease is indicated.

Despite these complications, most children with Crohn disease lead active, full lives with intermittent flare-up in symptoms.

Ardizzone S, Maconi G, Sampietro GM, et al: Azathioprine and mesalamine for prevention of relapse after conservative surgery for Crohn disease. *Gastroenterology* 2004;127:730–740.

Baert F, Noman M, Vermeire S, et al: Influence of immunogenicity on the long-term efficacy of infliximab in Crohn's disease. *N Engl J Med* 2003;348:601–608.

Baldassano RN, Han PD, Jeshion WC, et al: Pediatric Crohn's disease: Risk factors for postoperative recurrence. *Am J Gastroenterol* 2001;196: 2169–2176.

Brown SL, Greene MH, Gershon SK, et al: Tumor necrosis factor antagonist therapy and lymphoma development: Twenty-six cases reported to the Food and Drug Administration. *Arthritis Rheum* 2002;46:3151–3158.

Canani RB, de Horatio LT, Terrin G, et al: Combined use of noninvasive tests is useful in the initial diagnostic approach to a child with suspected inflammatory bowel disease. *J Pediatr Gastro Nutr* 2006;42:9–15.

Cosnes J, Cattan S, Blain A, et al: Long-term evolution of disease behavior of Crohn's disease. *Inflamm Bowel Dis* 2002;8:244–250.

Dietz DW, Laureti S, Strong SA, et al: Safety and long-term efficacy of stricture plasty in 314 patients with obstructing small bowel Crohn's disease. *J Am Coll Surg* 2001;192:330–337.

Dubinsky MC, Yang H, Hassard P: 6-MP metabolite profiles provide a biochemical explanation for 6-MP resistance in patients with inflammatory bowel disease. *Gastroenterology* 2002;122:904–915.

Gaya DR, Russell RK, Nimmo ER, Satsangi J: New genes in inflammatory bowel disease: lessons for complex disease? *Lancet* 2006;367: 1271–1284.

Hampe J, Franke A, Rosensteil P, et al: A genome-wide association scan of nonsynonymous SNPs identifies a susceptibility variant for Crohn disease in ATG16 L1. *Nat Genet* 2007;39:207–211.

Hanauer SB, Feagan BG, Lichtenstein GR, et al: Maintenance infliximab for Crohn's disease: The ACCENT I randomised trial. *Lancet* 2002;359: 1541–1549.

Hanauer SB, Korelitz BI, Rutgeerts P, et al: Postoperative maintenance of Crohn's disease remission with 6-mercaptopurine, mesalamine, or placebo: A 2 year trial. *Gastroenterology* 2004;127:723–729.

Heuschkel RB, Menache CC, Megerian JT, et al: Enteral nutrition and corticosteroids in the treatment of acute Crohn's disease in children. *J Pediatr Gastroenterol Nutr* 2000;31:8–15.

Keane J, Gershon S, Wise RP, et al: Tuberculosis associated with infliximab, a tumor necrosis factor α–neutralizing agent. *N Engl J Med* 2001;345:1098–1104.

Kobayashi KS, Chamaillard M, Ogura Y, et al: *NOD2*-dependent regulation of innate and adaptive immunity in the intestinal tract. *Science* 2005; 307:731–738.

Kugathasan S, Collins N, Maresso K, et al: *CARD15* gene mutations confers an increased risk for early surgery in pediatric-onset Crohn's disease. *Clin Gastroenterol Hepatol* 2004;2:1003–1009.

Levine A, Weizman Z, Broide E, et al: A comparison of budesonide and prednisone for the treatment of active pediatric Crohn disease. *J Pediatr Gastroenterol Nutr* 2003;36:248–252.

Mannon PJ, Fuss IJ, Mayer L, et al: Anti–interleukin-12 antibody for active Crohn's disease. *N Engl J Med* 2004;351:2069–2078.

Markowitz J, Grancher K, Kohn N, et al: A multicenter trial of 6-mercaptopurine and prednisone in children with newly diagnosed Crohn's disease. *Gastroenterology* 2000;119:895–902.

Miele E, Markowitz JE, Mamula P, et al: Human antichimeric antibody in children and young adults with inflammatory bowel disease receiving infliximab. *J Pediatr Gastroenterol Nutr* 2004;38:502–508.

Neurath MF: IL-23: a master regulator in Crohn disease. *Nat Med* 2007;13: 26–28.

Peltekova VD, Wintle RF, Rubin LA, et al: Functional variants of OCTN cation transporter genes are associated with Crohn disease. *Nat Genet* 2005;36:471–475.

Russell RK, Drummond HE, Nimmo ER, et al: The contribution of the DLGS 113A variant in early-onset inflammatory bowel disease. *J Pediatr* 2007;150:268–273.

Sandborn WJ, Hanauer S, Loftus EV Jr, et al: An open-label study of the human anti-TNF monoclonal antibody adalimumab in subjects with prior loss of response or intolerance to infliximab for Crohn's disease. *Am J Gastroenterol* 2004;99:1984–1989.

Sands BE, Anderson FH, Bernstein CN, et al: Infliximab maintenance therapy for fistulizing Crohn's disease. *N Engl J Med* 2004;350:876–885.

Selby WS: Mycobacterium avium subspecies paratuberculosis bacteriemia in patients with inflammatory bowel disease. *Lancet* 2004;364:1013–1014.

Sentongo TA, Semeao EJ, Piccoli DA, et al: Growth, body composition, and nutritional status in children and adolescents with Crohn's disease. *J Pediatr Gastroenterol Nutr* 2002;31:33–40.

Stephens MC, Shepanski MA, Mamula P, et al: Safety and steroid-sparing experience using infliximab for Crohn's disease at a pediatric inflammatory bowel disease center. *Am J Gastroenterol* 2003;98:104–111.

Weiss B, Shamir R, Bujanover Y, et al: *NOD2/CARD15* mutation analysis and genotype-phenotype correlation in Jewish pediatric patients compared with adults with Crohn's disease. *J Pediatr* 2004;145:208–212.

333.3 • Behçet Disease

Behçet disease is a systemic vasculitis that is rare in children (see Chapter 160). Though the precise pathogenesis remains unknown, there is a high prevalence of human leukocyte antigen (HLA) B51, increased expression of heat shock protein 60, and Th1-dominant immune responses. There appears to be significant familial aggregation. Aphthous stomatitis, erythema nodosum, and arthritis are among the most common manifestations. The ulcers are 2–10 mm in diameter and occur anywhere in the mouth or posterior pharynx; intestinal ulceration can mimic Crohn disease. The ulcers are covered by white-yellow membranes, have red borders, and are painful. Other signs are genital ulcers, central nervous system (CNS) involvement, and myositis. Ocular findings (iridocyclitis) are less common in children than in adults. Initial management is usually with nonsteroidal anti-inflammatory drugs, corticosteroids, immunosuppressants, and colchicine. Therapies also include interferon-α/β, anti–tumor necrosis factor antibody, and thalidomide. Low-dose weekly administration of methotrexate has been used for CNS involvement.

Kone-Paut I, Geisler I, Wechsler B, et al: Familial aggregation in Behçet's disease: High frequency in siblings and parents of pediatric probands. *J Pediatr* 1999;135:89–93.

Kone-Paut I, Yurdakul S, Bahabri AS, et al: Clinical features of Behçet's disease in children: An international collaborative study of 86 cases. *J Pediatr* 1998;132:721–725.

Suzuki Kurokowa M, Suzuki N: Behcet's disease. *Clin Exp Med* 2004;4:10–20.

Wechsler B, Sable-Fourtassou R, Bodaghi B, et al: Infliximab in refractory uveitis due to Behçet's disease. *Clin Exp Rheumatol* 2004;22:S14–S16.

Chapter 334 ■ Food Allergy (Food Hypersensitivity)

Jeffrey S. Hyams

Food allergy is a group of disorders in which symptoms result from immunologic responses to specific food antigens (see Chapter 150). Food allergy occurs in as many as 6% of children during the 1st 3 yr of life, including the 2–3% of infants and toddlers with cow's milk allergy. Reactions are classified as IgE mediated and non–IgE mediated. IgE-mediated reactions are caused by inflammatory mediators released when food antigen binds to specific IgE antibody on mast cells and basophils. These reactions are associated with rapid development of symptoms. Non–IgE-mediated reactions are cell mediated and develop over hours to days. For some clinical conditions, there appear to be multiple mechanisms involved.

CLINICAL MANIFESTATIONS. Food antigen may provoke respiratory, skin, or gastrointestinal symptoms. Gastrointestinal manifestations can occur anywhere in the alimentary tract and often dominate. Behavioral manifestations have been described but are controversial.

IGE-MEDIATED FOOD HYPERSENSITIVITY.

Oral Allergy Syndrome. Contact with the allergen on the oropharynx causes itching or tingling and angioedema of the lips, tongue, palate, and throat. These symptoms may precede other IgE-mediated manifestations of food allergy. Allergy to pollen (hay fever) is also common in these patients. Facial erythema from contact with citrus and tomato products is not considered an immune response.

Gastrointestinal Anaphylaxis. Rapid onset of nausea, cramping abdominal pain, vomiting, or diarrhea or a combination of these conditions occurs after ingestion of an allergen. The most common proteins implicated are milk, egg, peanut, soy, cereal, and fish.

Other Nongastrointestinal Manifestations. These include cutaneous—urticaria, angioedema, and atopic dermatitis (eczema); respiratory—asthma and rhinoconjunctivitis; and systemic anaphylaxis. Life-threatening reactions are typically associated with ingestion of peanuts, nuts, fish, and shellfish. These subjects often have a concomitant history of asthma.

MIXED (IGE- AND NON–IGE-MEDIATED) FOOD HYPERSENSITIVITY. These disorders are characterized by intense eosinophilic infiltration of the specific organ involved. The inflammatory infiltrate may involve the mucosa, muscularis, or serosa of the stomach or small intestine. Eosinophilic infiltration of the muscularis leads to thickening and nodularity, causing symptoms of obstruction (pain and vomiting), whereas serosal infiltration leads to eosinophilic ascites. Many patients with these disorders respond to removal of certain dietary antigens from the diet (milk), whereas others require a more drastic whole protein restriction with the concomitant use of hydrolyzed protein or amino acid–based formulas. Occasional patients also require corticosteroid therapy.

Allergic Eosinophilic Esophagitis. This disorder is characterized by intense eosinophilic infiltration of the esophageal mucosa. In infants and toddlers, vomiting is the most common symptom, whereas in older children dysphagia and abdominal pain or heartburn are more common (see Chapter 321). Rarely, esophageal strictures are present in older children and adolescents. Clinicians mistakenly diagnose these patients with gastroesophageal reflux, but the patients do not respond to usual therapies, and intraesophageal pH probe testing is normal. Treatment usually involves dietary modification in younger patients, with the occasional temporary need for an amino acid–based diet; older patients are usually treated with corticosteroids.

Allergic Eosinophilic Gastritis. This disorder is more common in infancy and adolescence and presents as abdominal pain, vomiting, anorexia, hematemesis, poor weight gain, and, rarely, gastric outlet obstruction. It can mimic pyloric stenosis in young infants. Atopic features, elevated serum IgE levels, and peripheral eosinophilia are seen in ≈50% of patients. Gastric biopsy reveals intense eosinophilic infiltration of the mucosa and submucosa, particularly in the antrum.

Allergic Eosinophilic Gastroenterocolitis. These patients have similar symptoms to those described for allergic esophagitis and gastritis. Failure to thrive is common, and the majority of affected individuals have atopic symptoms. Marked protein-losing enteropathy may present as generalized edema and hypogammaglobulinemia.

NON–IGE-MEDIATED DISORDERS.

Allergic Proctocolitis. Infants may present between 1 day and 3 mo of age with spots or streaks of blood and mucus in stool and occasional mild diarrhea. Increased numbers of white blood cells in stool and peripheral eosinophilia may be present. Typically, a patchy, mild colitis is present; nodular lymphoid hyperplasia occurs in ≈25% of cases. Most often, proctocolitis results from hypersensitivity to cow's milk; soy sensitivity is less common. This disorder also occurs in exclusively breast-fed patients and occasionally abates with maternal diet modification with elimination of milk products. Non–breast-fed infants can be treated with protein hydrolysate formulas. Occasionally, an amino acid–based formula may be required.

Food-Induced Enterocolitis. Protracted vomiting and diarrhea begin between 1 wk and 3 mo of age. Less severe reactions can occur in older children and adults. Stools contain occult blood, neutrophils, and eosinophils. Jejunal biopsy demonstrates flattened villi, edema, and inflammatory cells. Symptoms resolve within 72 hr of removal of the offending food and recur within 1–6 hr of reintroduction. The blood neutrophil count increases by at least 3.5×10^9/L at 4–6 hr after a food challenge. Older infants may develop a poorly characterized syndrome of anemia, hypoproteinemia, and failure to thrive when weaned from nursing or formula to ordinary cow's milk. Eosinophilia is common. Casein hydrolysate or amino acid–based formulas successfully treat most patients.

Food-Induced Enteropathy. Malabsorption, protracted diarrhea, vomiting, and failure to thrive caused by food hypersensitivity occur most often in the 1st mo of life. Small bowel biopsy shows patchy villus atrophy with mononuclear cell inflammatory response. Reaction to food challenge as well as resolution of symptoms on removal of the offending food may take several days to weeks.

Celiac Disease (Gluten-Sensitive Enteropathy) and Dermatitis Herpetiformis. Both entities occur as an immunologic response to gluten ingestion, and the two can occur together. See Chapter 335.2.

Pulmonary Hemosiderosis (Heiner Syndrome). A combination of pulmonary infiltrates from pulmonary hemorrhage, gastrointestinal bleeding, iron-deficiency anemia, peripheral eosinophilia, and failure to thrive secondary to food intolerance (often cow's milk protein) resolves on removal of the offending food from the diet.

DIAGNOSIS. Food allergy is suspected when typical symptoms occur with the introduction of specific foods. Other nonallergic mechanisms of food intolerance should be ruled out (compromised digestive or absorptive processes, contamination with microbes or toxins, or pharmacologic activity of foods). Lactose intolerance should be considered when cow's milk allergy is suspected. Elimination diet and subsequent double-blind, placebo-controlled food challenge (DBPCFC) are the gold standard for diagnosis of food allergy. In DBPCFC, suspected foods are administered in capsules in progressively increasing amounts, alternating with placebo, and reactions are evaluated in a blinded fashion. Open food challenges, although commonly performed, are less reliable (except in young infants). Symptoms can be reproduced by DBPCFC in only 40% of children with suspected food allergy. When anaphylaxis has followed ingestion of a food, challenge should not be performed, and an allergist should evaluate the child.

The judicious use of a skin prick test or radioallergosorbent test (RAST) can be very useful in determining whether an IgE allergic reaction is the cause of a food allergy. Children can be tested for IgE reactions to foods at any age because IgE is made by 24 wk of gestation. A negative IgE test, especially if the patient is >1 yr of age, is very accurate in predicting that the reaction is not IgE mediated. The significance of a positive IgE test has to be determined by the history and the age of the patient. A positive skin test is found in nearly 100% of children ≥3 yr of age who have a positive DBPCFC. Total serum IgE is unreliable in diagnosing food allergy.

In infancy, hypersensitivity is most often associated with ingestion of cow's milk or soy protein. Although nursing can prevent the development of food allergy, manifestations of food allergy, especially proctocolitis, can occur with nursing. Cow's milk in the mother's diet is the most common identifiable cause of food-allergic reactions in nursing infants; reaction to peanut, soy, or egg in the mother's diet occurs less often.

Among infants and children with food allergy, 90% of reactions are to egg, milk, peanut, soy, or wheat. Seventy-five per cent of children with proven food allergy react only to a single food. Children with allergic eosinophilic gastroenteritis are the exception, often reacting to multiple foods.

TREATMENT AND PROGNOSIS. The only therapy proved effective for food allergy is an elimination diet. Most gastrointestinal manifestations resolve within several days, although some may take weeks (food-induced enteropathy). A child at risk for a severe and life-threatening IgE-mediated reaction should have access to injectable epinephrine and an antihistamine. Recent progress in the development of anti-IgE therapy may prove useful for children with severe disease. Infants at high risk for developing food allergy may benefit from breast-feeding and the elimination of solids and cow's milk protein from their diet for the 1st 6 mo of life.

At least 30% of infants with cow's milk allergy also demonstrate sensitivity to soy protein. Generally, these infants improve with protein hydrolysate formula; <5% have persistent symptoms and these cases resolve with the use of amino acid–based formulas. Re-lactation is an alternative when cow's milk allergy presents early. About 50% of infants who experience proctocolitis while nursing improve with removal of cow's milk from the mother's diet. In the others, one must decide whether the symptoms are severe enough (anemia and hypoproteinemia) to warrant a change in the infant's diet to a protein hydrolysate formula.

Eighty-five per cent of infants with non–IgE-mediated food hypersensitivity to milk proteins no longer have symptoms on food challenge by 3 yr of age. Resolution of symptoms from cow's milk or soy protein hypersensitivity is common by 1 yr of age. When milk is reintroduced, only a tsp or less should be offered at first and then increased progressively over a few days if tolerated. Even older children and adults may lose their sensitivity to an offending food when it is eliminated from the diet for 1 to 2 yr. Symptoms from IgE-mediated allergy to peanut, nuts, fish, or shellfish are the exception and do not resolve.

Brownell J, Casale TB: Anti-IgE therapy. *Immunol Allergy Clin North Am* 2004;24:551–568.

Hill DJ, Heine RG, Hosking CS: The diagnostic value of skin prick testing in children with food allergy. *Pediatr Allergy Immunol* 2004;15:435–441.

Liacouras CA, Ruchelli E: Eosinophilic esophagitis. *Curr Opin Pediatr* 2004;16:560–566.

Muraro A, Dreborg S, Halken S, et al: Dietary prevention of allergic diseases in infants and small children. Part III: Critical review of published peer-reviewed observational and interventional studies and final recommendations. *Pediatr Allergy Immunol* 2004;15:291–307.

Sampson HA: Update on food allergy. *J Allergy Clin Immunol* 2004; 113:805–819.

Sampson HA, Anderson JA: Summary and recommendations: Classification of gastrointestinal manifestations due to immunologic reactions to foods in infants and young children. *J Pediatr Gastroenterol Nutr* 2000;30: S87–S94.

Scurlock AM, Burks AW: Peanut allergenicity. *Ann Allergy Asthma Immunol* 2004;93:S12–S18.

Sicherer SH, Teuber S: Current approach to the diagnosis and management of adverse reactions to foods. *J Allergy Clin Immunol* 2004;114:1146–1150.

Snyder JD, Rosenblum N, Wershil B, et al: Pyloric stenosis and eosinophilic gastroenteritis in infants. *J Pediatr Gastroenterol Nutr* 1987;6:543–547.

334.1 • Eosinophilic Gastroenteritis

This entity consists of a group of rare and poorly understood disorders that have in common gastric and small intestine infiltration with eosinophils and peripheral eosinophilia. The esophagus and large intestine may also be involved. Tissue eosinophilic infiltration can be seen in mucosa, muscularis, or serosa. Mucosal involvement may produce nausea, vomiting, diarrhea, abdominal pain, gastrointestinal bleeding, protein losing enteropathy, or malabsorption. Involvement of the muscularis may produce obstruction (especially of the pylorus), whereas serosal activity produces eosinophilic ascites.

This condition clinically overlaps the dietary protein hypersensitivity disorders of the small bowel and colon (see Chapter 334). Allergies to multiple foods are often seen, and serum IgE is commonly elevated. Peripheral eosinophilia is present in more than 50% of individuals with this disorder. The mucosal form is most frequent and is diagnosed by identifying large numbers of eosinophils in biopsy specimens of gastric antrum or small bowel.

The disease usually runs a chronic, debilitating course with sporadic severe exacerbations. Rare patients are helped by elimination diets or the use of cromolyn, but most require systemic administration of corticosteroids. Isolated eosinophilic esophagitis, unresponsive to gastroesophageal reflux therapy, may improve with an elimination diet; in the absence of stomach or small bowel involvement, this may be a separate entity.

Heine RG: Pathophysiology, diagnosis and treatment of food protein induced gastrointestinal disease. *Curr Opin Allergy Clin Immunol* 2004;4:221.

Ngo P, Furuta G, Burks W: The pathobiology of esoinophilic gastroenteritis of childhood: Is it really the eosinophil, allergic mediated, or something else? *Curr Gastroenterol Rep* 2004;6:436–440.

Rothenberg ME: Eosinophilic gastrointestinal disorders (EGID). *J Allergy Clin Immunol* 2004;113:11–28.

Chapter 335 ■ Disorders of Malabsorption

Manu R. Sood

Disorders of malabsorption constitute a broad spectrum of diseases with multiple etiologies and varied clinical manifestations. All are associated with diminished intestinal absorption of one or more dietary nutrients. Malabsorption can result from either a defect in the nutrient **digestion** in the intestinal lumen or mucosal **absorption.** Malabsorption disorders can be categorized into generalized mucosal abnormalities usually resulting in multiple nutrient malabsorption (Table 335-1) and specific nutrient malabsorption disorders (carbohydrate, fat, protein, vitamin, mineral malabsorption) [Table 335-2].

TABLE 335-1. Malabsorption Disorders Associated with Generalized Mucosal Defect

FOOD-INDUCED ENTEROPATHY
Gluten-sensitive enteropathy (Celiac disease)
Cow's milk and other protein-sensitive enteropathies
Eosinophilic enteropathy
CONGENITAL BOWEL MUCOSAL DEFECTS
Microvillous inclusion disease
Tufting enteropathy
Carbohydrate-deficient glycoprotein syndrome
Enterocyte heparan sulfate deficiency
Enteric anendocrinosis (*NEUROG 3* mutation)
PROTEIN-LOSING ENTEROPATHY
Lymphangiectasia (congenital and acquired)
Disorders causing bowel mucosal inflammation
INFECTION INDUCED
Parasitic infections (e.g., *Giardia* and cryptosporidium)
Bacterial overgrowth
Tropical sprue
Postinfectious enteropathy
IMMUNODEFICIENCY DISORDERS
Congenital immunodeficiency disorders
Selective IgA deficiency (can be associated with celiac disease)
Severe combined immunodeficiency
Agammaglobulinemia
X-linked hypogammaglobulinemia
Wiskott-Aldrich syndrome
Common variable immunodeficiency disease
Chronic granulomatous disease
Acquired immune deficiency
HIV infection
Immunosuppressive therapy and post bone marrow transplantation
AUTOIMMUNE ENTEROPATHY
MISCELLANEOUS
Immunoproliferative small intestinal disease
Short bowel syndrome
Chronic malnutrition
Radiation enteritis

CLINICAL APPROACH TO A CHILD WITH SUSPECTED MALABSORPTION

The clinical features depend on the extent and type of the malabsorbed nutrient. The common presenting features, especially in toddlers with malabsorption, are diarrhea, abdominal distention, and failure to gain weight, with a fall in growth chart percentiles. Physical findings include the disappearance of the subcutaneous fat, muscle wasting, and the appearance of skin being too loose for the child (Fig. 335-1). The nutritional consequences of malabsorption are more dramatic in toddlers, because of the limited energy reserves and higher proportion of calorie intake being used for weight gain and linear growth. In older children, malnutrition may result in growth retardation, as commonly seen in children with late diagnosis of celiac disease. If untreated, linear growth slows and with prolonged malnutrition death may follow (see Chapter 43). This extreme outcome is usually restricted to children living in the developing world, where resources to provide enteral and parenteral nutrition support may be limited. Specific findings on examination may guide toward a particular disorder; edema is usually associated with protein-losing enteropathy, digital clubbing with cystic fibrosis and celiac disease, perianal excoriation and gaseous abdominal distention with carbohydrate malabsorption, perianal and circumoral rash with acrodermatitis enteropathica, abnormal hair with Menkes syndrome, and the typical facial features diagnostic of the Johannson-Blizzard syndrome.

Many children with malabsorption disorders have very good appetites and try to compensate for the fecal protein and energy losses. In exocrine pancreatic insufficiency, fecal losses of up to 40% of ingested protein and energy do not lead to malnutrition, as long as they are compensated by an increased appetite. In conditions associated with villous atrophy or inflammation (celiac disease, postinfectious enteropathy), fecal protein and energy losses are usually modest, but associated anorexia and reduced food intake results in malnutrition.

The nutritional assessment is an important part of clinical evaluation in children with malabsorptive disorders (see Chapter 43). Long-term calcium and vitamin D malabsorption can lead to reduced bone mineral density and metabolic bone disease with increased risk of bone fractures. Vitamin K malabsorption, irrespective of the underlying mechanism (fat malabsorption, mucosal atrophy), can result in coagulopathy. Severe protein-losing enteropathy is often associated with malabsorption syndromes (celiac disease, intestinal lymphangiectasia) and causes hypoalbuminemia and edema. Other nutrient deficiencies include iron malabsorption causing microcytic anemia and low reticulocyte count, low serum folate levels in conditions associated with

TABLE 335-2. Classification of Malabsorption Disorders Based on the Predominant Nutrient Which Is Malabsorbed

CARBOHYDRATE MALABSORPTION
Lactose malabsorption
Congenital lactase deficiency
Hypolactasia (adult type)
Secondary lactase deficiency
Congenital sucrase-isomaltase deficiency
Glucose galactose malabsorption
FAT MALABSORPTION
Pancreatic exocrine insufficiency
Cystic fibrosis
Shwachman-Diamond syndrome
Chronic pancreatitis
Pearson syndrome
Protein-calorie malnutrition
Liver and biliary disorders
Cholestatic liver disease
Bile acid synthetic defects
Bile acid malabsorption (terminal ileal disease)
Mucosal causes
Abetalipoproteinemia
Homozygous hypobetalipoproteinemia
Chylomicron retention disease (Anderson disease)
AMINO ACID MALABSORPTION
Lysinuric protein intolerance (defect in dibasic amino acid transport, see Chapter 74.3)
Hartnup disease (defect in free neutral amino acids)
Blue diaper syndrome (isolated tryptophan malabsorption)
Oast-house urine disease (defect in methionine absorption)
Lowe syndrome (lysine and arginine malabsorption)
MINERAL AND VITAMIN MALABSORPTION
Congenital chloride diarrhea
Congenital sodium absorption defect
Acrodermatitis enteropathica (zinc malabsorption)
Menke disease (copper malabsorption)
Vitamin D–dependent rickets.
Folate malabsorption
Congenital
Secondary to mucosal damage (celiac disease)
Vitamin B_{12} malabsorption
Autoimmune pernicious anemia
Decreased gastric acid (H_2 blockers or proton pump inhibitors)
Terminal ileal disease (e.g., Crohn disease) or resection
Inborn errors of vitamin B_{12} transport and metabolism
Primary hypomagnesemia
DRUG INDUCED
Sulfasalazine: folic acid malabsorption
Cholestyramine: calcium and fat malabsorption
Phenytoin: calcium malabsorption

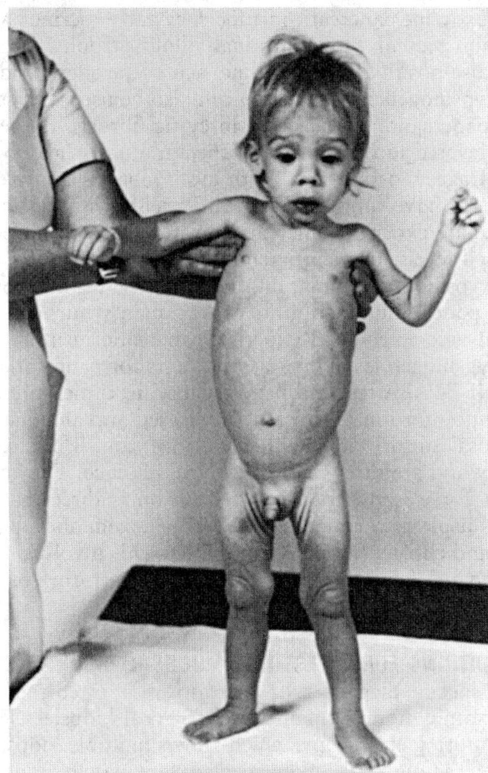

Figure 335-1. An 18-mo-old boy with active celiac disease. Note the loose skinfolds, marked proximal muscle wasting, and full abdomen. The child looks ill.

mucosal atrophy, and low serum vitamin A and vitamin E concentration in fat malabsorption.

Clinical history alone may not be sufficient to make a specific diagnosis, but can direct the pediatrician toward a more structured and rational investigative approach. Diarrhea is the main clinical expression of malabsorption. Onset of diarrhea in early infancy suggests a congenital defect (Table 335-3). In congenital chloride diarrhea and microvillus inclusion disease, the stool is watery and can be mistaken for urine. Onset of symptoms after introduction of a particular food into a child's diet may provide diagnostic clues, such as seen with sucrose in sucrase-isomaltase deficiency. The nature of the diarrhea may be helpful: explosive watery diarrhea suggests carbohydrate malabsorption; loose, bulky stools are associated with celiac disease; and pasty and yellowish offensive stool suggests an exocrine pancreatic insufficiency. Stool color is usually not helpful; green stool with undigested "peas and carrots" may suggest rapid intestinal transit in toddler's diarrhea, which is a self-limiting condition and not associated with failure to thrive.

335.1 • Evaluation of Children with Suspected Intestinal Malabsorption

The choice of investigative studies is usually guided by the history and physical examination. In a child presenting with diarrhea, the initial work-up should include stool occult blood and leukocytes to exclude inflammatory disorders, stool microscopy and antibody tests for parasites such as *Giardia*, stool pH and reducing substance for carbohydrate malabsorption, and quantitative stool fat examination to identify fat malabsorption.

A complete blood count including peripheral smear for microcytic anemia, lymphopenia (lymphangiectasia), neutropenia (Shwachman syndrome), and acanthocytosis (abetalipoproteinemia) is useful. If celiac disease is suspected, serum immunoglobulin A (IgA) and tissue transglutaminase levels should be determined. Depending on the initial investigation results, more specific investigations can be planned.

INVESTIGATIONS FOR CARBOHYDRATE MALABSORPTION. Measurement of carbohydrate in the stool, using a Clinitest reagent, which identifies reducing substances, is a simple screening test. Acidic stool with reducing substance >2+ suggests carbohydrate malabsorption. Sucrose or starch in the stool is not recognized as a reducing sugar until after hydrolysis with hydrochloric acid, which converts them to reducing sugars.

Breath hydrogen test is used to identify the specific carbohydrate that is malabsorbed. After an overnight fast, the suspected sugar (lactose or sucrose) is administered as an oral solution (carbohydrate load 1–2 g/kg, maximum 50 g). In malabsorption, the sugar is not digested or absorbed in the small bowel, passes to the colon, and is metabolized by the normal bacteria flora. One of the products of this process is hydrogen gas, which is absorbed through the colon mucosa and excreted in the breath. Increased hydrogen concentration in the breath samples suggests carbohydrate malabsorption. A rise in breath hydrogen of 20 parts per million (ppm) above the baseline is considered a positive test. The child should not be on antibiotics, as colonic flora is essential for fermenting the sugar.

Small bowel mucosal biopsies can directly measure mucosal disaccharidase (lactase, sucrase, maltase, palatinase) concentration. In primary enzyme deficiencies, the mucosal enzyme levels are low and small bowel mucosal morphology is normal. Partial or total villous atrophy can result in secondary disaccharidase deficiency and transient lactose intolerance in celiac disease and after rotavirus gastroenteritis. Disaccharidase levels revert to normal after mucosal healing.

INVESTIGATIONS FOR FAT MALABSORPTION. The presence of fat globules in the stool suggests fat malabsorption. The ability to assimilate fat varies with age; a premature infant may absorb only 65–75% of dietary fat, a full-term infant absorbs almost 90%, and an older child >95% of fat in a typical diet. Therefore, finding fat globules in the stool of a premature baby or a young infant may not be abnormal but is uncommon in the stool of an older child. Definitive evaluation of fat malabsorption requires 3 day stool collection for evaluation of quantitative fat excretion and determination of the coefficient of fat absorption (coefficient of fat absorption [%] = [fat intake (g) – fecal fat losses (g) / fat intake (g)] × 100). Because fecal fat balance studies are cumbersome, expensive, and unpleasant to perform, simple tests are often preferred. Among these stool tests, the acid steatocrit test is the most reliable. Duodenal fluid aspirate, for the evaluation of bile acid levels in rare cases in which bile acid deficiency causes fat malabsorption, may also be useful.

TABLE 335-3. Diarrheal Diseases Presenting in the Neonatal Period

CONDITION	CLINICAL FEATURES
Congenital microvillus atrophy	Intractable watery diarrhea
Tufting enteropathy	Intractable watery diarrhea
Congenital glucose-galactose malabsorption	Acidic diarrhea
Congenital lactase deficiency	Acidic diarrhea
Congenital chloride diarrhea	Hydramnios, intractable watery diarrhea
Congenital defective jejunal Na^+/H^+ exchange	Hydramnios, intractable watery diarrhea
Congenital bile acid malabsorption	Steatorrhea
Congenital enterokinase deficiency	Failure to thrive, edema
Enteric anendocrinosis (*NEUROG 3* mutation)	Hyperchloremic acidosis, failure to thrive

Adapted from Schmitz J: Maldigestion and malabsorption. In Walker WA, Durie PR, Hamilton JR, et al (editors): *Pediatric Gastrointestinal Disease*, 3rd ed. Hamilton, Ontario, BC Decker, 2000, p 55.

Fat malabsorption and pancreatic exocrine insufficiency are usually associated with fat-soluble vitamin A, D, E, and K deficiencies. Vitamin A, D, and E serum concentration can be measured. A prolonged prothrombin time is an indirect test to assess vitamin K deficiency.

INVESTIGATIONS FOR GASTROINTESTINAL PROTEIN LOSS. Dietary and endogenous proteins secreted into the bowel are almost completely absorbed; <1 g of protein from these sources passes into the colon. The majority of the stool nitrogen is derived from gut bacterial proteins. Excessive bowel protein loss usually manifests as **hypoalbuminemia.** The most common cause of hypoalbuminemia in children is renal disease; therefore, urine protein excretion must be determined. Other potential causes for hypoalbuminemia include liver disease (reduced production) and inadequate protein intake. Measurement of stool **α_1-antitrypsin** is a useful screening test for protein-losing enteropathy. This serum protein has similar molecular weight as albumin and, unlike albumin, is resistant to digestion in the gastrointestinal tract. Excessive α_1-antitrypsin excretion in the stool should prompt further investigations to identify the specific cause of gut protein loss.

INVESTIGATIONS FOR PANCREATIC EXOCRINE FUNCTION (FIG. 335-2). Cystic fibrosis is the most common cause of exocrine pancreatic insufficiency in children; therefore, a sweat chloride test must be performed before embarking on invasive tests to investigate possible exocrine insufficiency. Many cases of cystic fibrosis are detected by neonatal screening genetic testing programs; occasional rare mutations are undetected. **Fecal elastase-1** estimation is a sensitive test to assess exocrine pancreatic function in chronic pancreatitis and cystic fibrosis. Elastase-1 is an endoprotease that is both human and pancreas specific. It is stable during conditions of abnormal intestinal transport and not altered by supplementation of pancreatic enzymes. One disadvantage of the fecal elastase-1 test is the lack of full differentiation between primary exocrine pancreatic insufficiency and exocrine pancreatic dysfunction secondary to intestinal villous atrophy. It may also give a false-positive result during acute episodes of diarrhea. **Serum trypsinogen** concentration can also be used as a screening test for pancreatic insufficiency. In cystic fibrosis, the levels are greatly elevated in early life, and then gradually fall, so that by 5–7 yr of age, most patients with cystic fibrosis and pancreatic insufficiency have subnormal levels. Patients with cystic fibrosis and adequate exocrine pancreatic function tend to have normal or elevated levels. In such patients, observing the trend in serial serum trypsinogen estimation may be useful in monitoring exocrine pancreatic function. In Shwachman syndrome, another condition associated with exocrine pancreatic insufficiency, the serum trypsinogen level is low. Other tests for pancreatic insufficiency (NBT-PABA test and pancreolauryl test) measure urine or breath concentration of substances released and absorbed across the mucosal surface after pancreatic digestion. These tests lack specificity and are rarely used in clinical practice. The gold standard test for exocrine pancreatic function is direct analysis of **duodenal aspirate** for bicarbonate, trypsinogen, and lipase after secretin and cholecystokinin stimulation. This involves duodenal intubation and few centers in United States perform this test (see Chapter 345 for details).

INVESTIGATIONS FOR INTESTINAL MUCOSAL DISORDERS. Establishing a specific diagnosis for malabsorption often requires histologic examination of small bowel mucosal biopsies. These are obtained during endoscopy, which allows multiple biopsies to be performed, as mucosal involvement can be patchy, especially in celiac disease. Bowel mucosal lesions may also be segmental in cases of intestinal lymphangiectasia. In these situations, radiographic small bowel series may identify a region of thickened bowel responsible for protein loss. During endoscopy, mucosal biopsies can be obtained to measure mucosal disaccharidases activities, and duodenal aspirates performed to measure pancreatic enzyme concentration as well as for quantitative bacterial

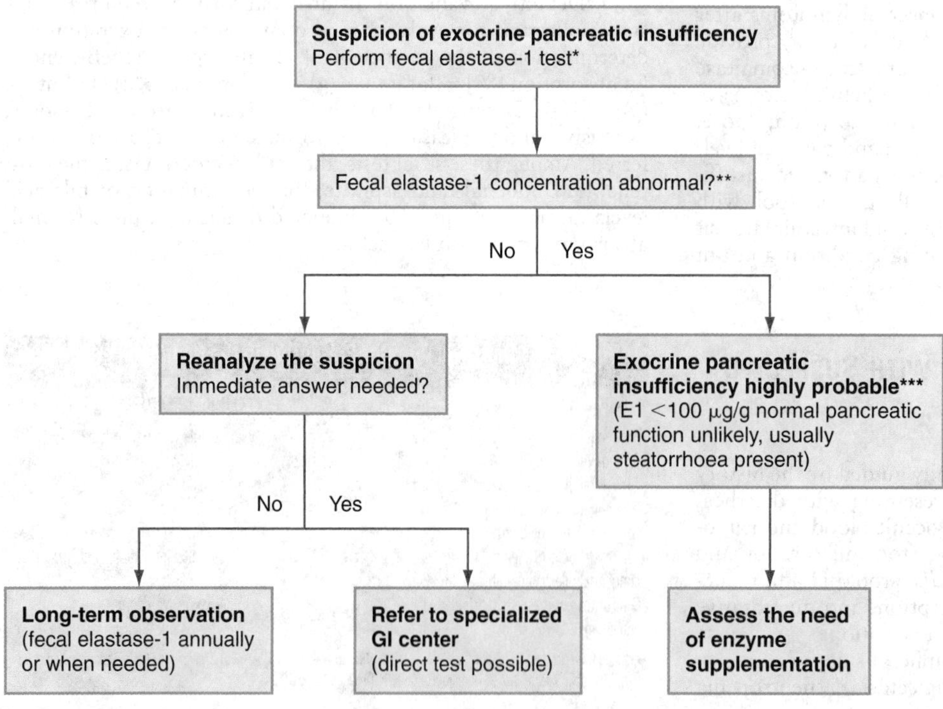

Figure 335-2. Algorithm for assessment of exocrine pancreatic function. *If not available, use other test. Perform appropriate imaging studies of the pancreas. **In case of borderline values, consider repeating the test with three independent samples. ***Consider differential diagnosis (especially consider villous atrophy and dilution effect of watery stool). (Adapted from Walkowiak J, Nousia-Arvanitakis S, Henker J, et al: Indirect pancreatic function tests in children. *J Pediatr Gastroenterol Nutr* 2005;40:107–114.)

cultures. Aspirates to evaluate for other infections such as *Giardia* may be useful.

IMAGING PROCEDURES. Plain radiographs and barium contrast studies may suggest a site and cause of intestinal stasis. Although flocculation of normal barium and dilated bowel with thickened mucosal folds have been attributed to diffuse malabsorptive lesions such as celiac disease, these abnormalities are nonspecific.

335.2 • Gluten-Sensitive Enteropathy (Celiac Disease)

Celiac disease is an immune-mediated enteropathy caused by permanent sensitivity to gluten in genetically susceptible individuals. Although epidemiologic studies in Europe and the United States suggest that it is common and may occur in 0.5–1.0% of the general population, long delays between onset of symptoms and diagnosis often occur. Based on a number of studies from Europe and the United States, it has been estimated that the prevalence of celiac disease in children between 2.5 and 15 yr in the general population ranges from 3 to 13/1,000 children or ≈1/300 to 1/80 children. Therefore, in a pediatric practice of 1,500 children, there are probably between 5 and 20 children with celiac disease either diagnosed or undiagnosed. In the United States, it has been estimated that for every celiac patient there are 53 undiagnosed subjects, due to poor recognition of the variable clinical manifestations of the disease.

PATHOGENESIS. Celiac disease develops only after dietary exposure to the protein gluten, which is found in wheat, rye, and barley. The activity of gluten resides in the gliadin fraction, which contains certain repetitious amino acid sequences (motifs) that lead to sensitization of lamina propria lymphocytes. A 33-mer peptide may be the primary initiator of the inflammatory response in susceptible individuals. It reacts with transglutaminase and is a potent inducer of intestine-derived human T-cell lines. A genetic predisposition is suggested by concordance in monozygotic twins approaching 100%. Two to 5% of first-degree relatives have symptomatic gluten-sensitive enteropathy, and as many as 10% of first-degree relatives have asymptomatic damage to small bowel mucosa consistent with this disorder. The disorder is associated with major histocompatibility complex class II alleles DQA1*0501 and DQB1*0201. This HLA-DQ2 allelic combination is found in 98% of celiac patients in Northern Europe. In Southern Europe, DQ2 is present in 92% of confirmed celiac disease patients. Celiac disease is associated with certain human leukocyte antigen (HLA) types (B8, DR7, DR3, and DQw2). Other genetic influences, not linked to HLA, may be required for the development of the disease, given that the rate of discordance in HLA-identical siblings is reported to be 30–50%. It is estimated that almost 30% of the general population in North America is DQ2-positive. Other gene loci possibly associated with celiac disease have been reported. The development of celiac disease is multigenic, with DQ2 and DQ8 being the essential component. In type 1 diabetes, a positive serologic test for celiac disease is found predominantly in those with the HLA DQ2 or DQ8 genotype. Celiac disease in individuals with Down syndrome is mainly linked to HLA DQ2 heterodimer, with a carriage rate of almost 100%. An additional allele has also been implicated in 20% of Down syndrome patients. Celiac disease occurs at a higher frequency in children with type 1 diabetes and is 50 times more common in children with Down syndrome. An increased frequency is also observed in children with Turner syndrome, William syndrome, thyroiditis, and selective IgA deficiency.

Environmental factors such as viruses may also play a role in the expression of this genetic predisposition. A high degree of amino acid sequence homology is found between gliadin and adenovirus type 12 and 7, rubella, and human herpesvirus 1.

The bowel mucosal immunologic response involves the activation of Th1/Th0 CD4$^+$ gluten-sensitive T cells. The inflammatory response results in villus atrophy, crypt hyperplasia, and damage to the surface epithelium in the small bowel. The injury is greatest in the proximal small bowel and extends distally for a variable distance. The latter observation is undoubtedly the explanation for the variable degree of symptoms and findings of malabsorption among persons with gluten-sensitive enteropathy. The gluten-induced enteropathy results in a decrease in the absorptive and digestive capacity of the small intestinal surface area and a relative increase in immature epithelial cells. Pancreatic secretion is decreased as a result of lowered serum cholecystokinin and secretin levels.

CLINICAL PRESENTATION. The mode of presentation of celiac disease can be quite variable (Table 335-4), but because of the availability of serologic tests, patients with subtle abdominal symptoms are being diagnosed. The **typical presentation** of a toddler with diarrhea, abdominal distention, and failure to thrive is becoming less common. Diarrhea is still the most common symptom and can be acute or insidious in onset. The stools are characteristically pale, loose, and offensive. The child may also have recurrent attacks of more severe diarrhea, sometimes with the stools becoming watery. Poor weight gain and/or poor linear growth may occur, due to malabsorption or decreased appetite (Fig. 335-3). Neurologic symptoms do occur; many children are emotionally withdrawn, irritable, and fretful. Other nongastrointestinal manifestations and associations of celiac disease are noted in Table 335-5. There is often a history of abdominal distention, and some children complain of abdominal pain, although this is not usually severe. Muscle wasting and loss of muscular power with hypotonia may be present, and the child may be delayed in motor milestones.

Many adolescents and young adults have latent disease and do not have weight loss or diarrhea. Manifestations in these patients include fatigue, abdominal pain, bloating, and anemia.

SCREENING AND DIAGNOSIS. Screening for celiac disease has been recommended for specific risk factors (Fig. 335-4). The anti-endomysium IgA antibody and anti-tissue transglutaminase IgA antibody tests are highly sensitive and specific in identifying individuals with celiac disease. The anti-endomysium IgA antibody test is an immunofluorescent technique and is relatively expensive; interpretation is operator dependent and prone to errors so that it has largely been replaced by anti-tissue transglutaminase

TABLE 335-4. Active Childhood Celiac Disease: 42 Cases

	NO. OF PATIENTS
SYMPTOMS	
Failure to thrive	36
Diarrhea	30
Irritability	30
Vomiting	24
Anorexia	24
Foul stools	21
Abdominal pain	8
Excessive appetite	6
Rectal prolapse	3
SIGNS	
Height <25th percentile	30
Body weight <25th percentile	37
Wasted muscles	40
Abdominal distention	33
Edema	14
Finger clubbing	11

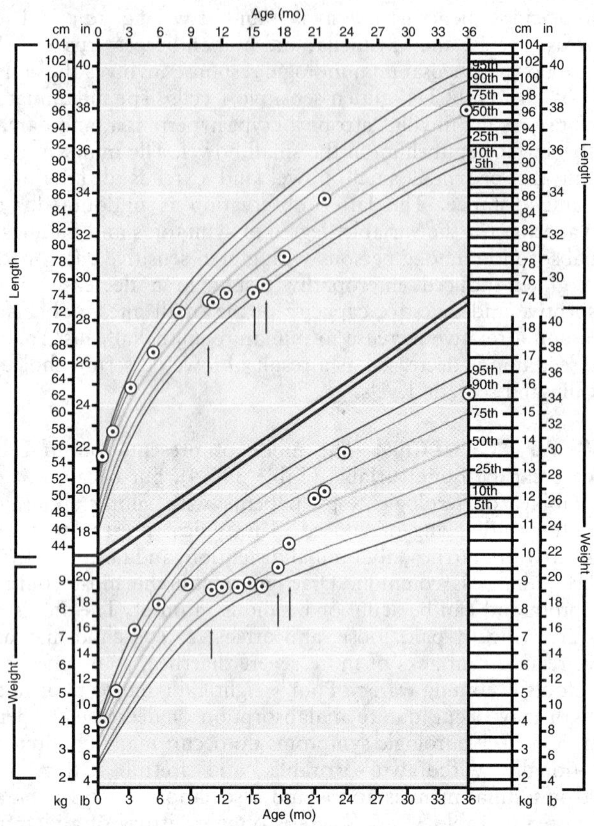

Figure 335-3. Gluten-sensitive enteropathy. Growth curve demonstrates initial normal growth from 0 to 9 mo, followed by onset of poor appetite with intermittent vomiting and diarrhea after initiation of gluten-containing diet *(single arrow)*. After biopsy confirmed diagnosis and treatment with gluten-free diet *(double arrow)*, growth improves.

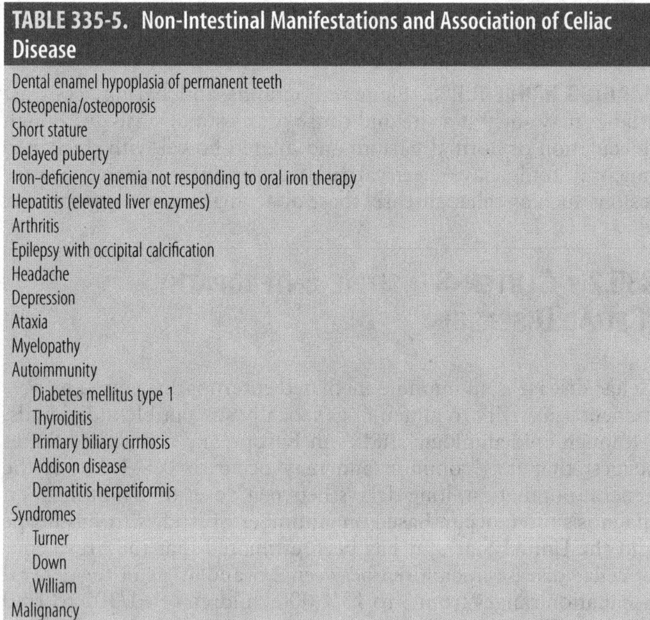

TABLE 335-5. Non-Intestinal Manifestations and Association of Celiac Disease

Dental enamel hypoplasia of permanent teeth
Osteopenia/osteoporosis
Short stature
Delayed puberty
Iron-deficiency anemia not responding to oral iron therapy
Hepatitis (elevated liver enzymes)
Arthritis
Epilepsy with occipital calcification
Headache
Depression
Ataxia
Myelopathy
Autoimmunity
Diabetes mellitus type 1
Thyroiditis
Primary biliary cirrhosis
Addison disease
Dermatitis herpetiformis
Syndromes
Turner
Down
William
Malignancy

IgA antibody tests, which are simpler to perform and have similar sensitivity and specificity. Anti-gliadin IgA and IgG and anti-reticulin IgA antibody tests are no longer recommended tests due to lack of specificity. The anti-endomysium IgA and anti-tissue transglutaminase IgA antibody test can be falsely negative with IgA deficiency, which is associated with an increased incidence of celiac disease. Measurement of serum IgA concentration is mandatory to assure that false-negative results in IgA-deficient individuals are excluded. If celiac disease is suspected in patients

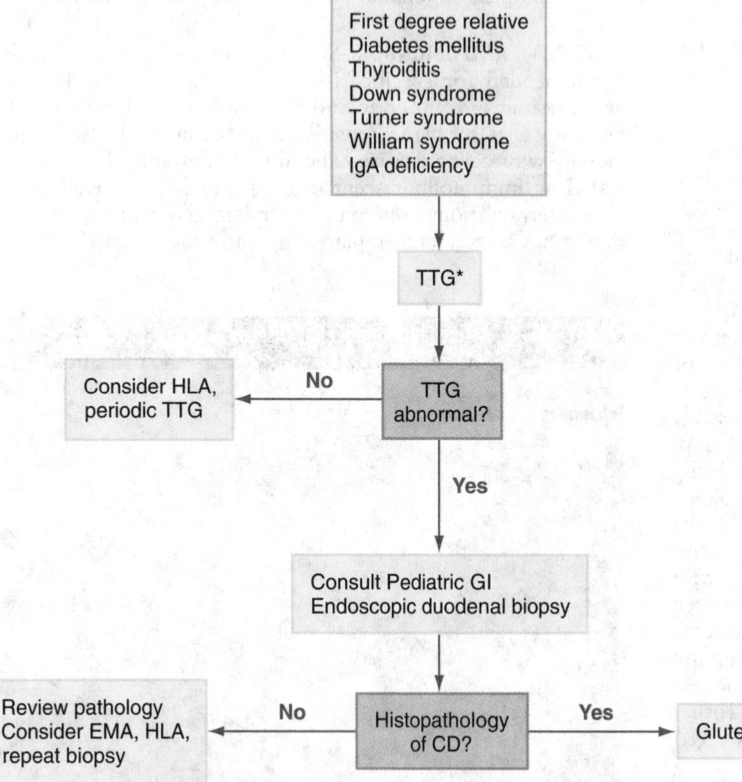

Figure 335-4. Serologic tests such as anti-endomysium IgA antibody test (EMA), anti-tissue transglutaminase IgA antibody test (TTG), and HLA DQ2 or DQ8 genotype testing are useful for evaluation of asymptomatic subjects with diabetes mellitus, thyroiditis, Down syndrome, Turner syndrome, William syndrome, or IgA deficiency who have a higher incidence of celiac disease, and first-degree relatives of patients with celiac disease (CD). (Adapted from Hill ID, Dirks MH, Liptak GS, et al: Guideline for the diagnosis and treatment of celiac disease in children: Recommendation of the North American Society for Pediatric Gastroenterology, Hepatology and Nutrition. *J Pediatr Gastroenterol Nutr* 2005;40:1–19.)

with IgA deficiency, intestinal biopsy may be required. Because screening with antibodies may identify patients without documented celiac disease on biopsy, it is important to set the lower limit of antibody titers high enough to avoid false-positive results.

Small Intestinal Biopsy. **Definitive diagnosis** of celiac disease requires small intestinal biopsy, as none of the available serologic tests are 100% reliable. The characteristic histologic changes include partial or total villous atrophy, crypt elongation and decreased villous/crypt ratio, increased number of intraepithelial lymphocytes, intraepithelial lymphocyte mitotic index >0.2%, decreased height of epithelial cells, and loss of nuclear polarity. The mucosal involvement can be patchy, so multiple biopsies must be obtained. The intestinal biopsy–based criteria for diagnosis of celiac disease were published by the European Society of Pediatric Gastroenterology, Hepatology and Nutrition and revised in 1990. According to the revised criteria, children with characteristic histologic features and unequivocal clinical response to gluten withdrawal can be considered definitive for celiac disease. Reversal of positive serologic tests after gluten withdrawal is considered supportive evidence. In children <2 yr of age, milk protein–sensitive enteropathy can produce changes similar to celiac disease; confirmation of diagnosis after a gluten challenge is sometimes required. This necessitates three biopsies: an initial biopsy at presentation, the 2nd to document healing with gluten withdrawal, and the 3rd to show recurrent damage with reintroduction of gluten.

TREATMENT. *The only treatment for celiac disease is lifelong exclusion of gluten. This requires a wheat-, barley-, and rye-free diet.* Previously, oats had been implicated in gluten-induced enteropathy. Despite evidence that oats are safe for individuals with celiac disease, there remains a concern of contamination of oats with gluten during harvesting and milling. Unless the purity of oats can be guaranteed, their safety remains questionable. After gluten withdrawal, there is rapid remission of symptoms, improved bone mineralization, and reversal of growth failure and nutritional deficiencies. In asymptomatic patients diagnosed after screening tests, improved physical and psychologic well-being occurs after gluten withdrawal. There is evidence that even a small amount of gluten ingested at regular intervals can induce mucosal damage. Previously, products containing <200 ppm were considered gluten free, but the Codex Alimentarius Guidelines now define gluten free as <20 ppm and the National Food Authority has redefined gluten free as no gluten and <200 ppm as low gluten. It is important that an experienced dietician with specific expertise in celiac disease counseling educate the family and the child about dietary restriction. Adherence to a gluten-free diet can be difficult, especially in older children. It is recommended that children with celiac disease be monitored with periodic visits for assessment of symptoms, growth, physical examination, and adherence to the gluten-free diet. Complete lack of adherence to a gluten-free diet has been reported in 6–37% of patients. Measuring tissue transglutaminase levels 6 mo after gluten withdrawal to document reduction in antibody titers, as an indirect evidence of adherence to a gluten-free diet, can be helpful. In asymptomatic patients, the antibodies are checked annually and reappearance of the antibody suggests noncompliance, which may be unintentional due to dietary errors.

PROGNOSIS. The clinical response to a gluten-free diet usually results in improvement of mood, appetite, and lessening of the diarrhea within a week. Reduced bone mineral density also improves with gluten exclusion. No long-term complications from a gluten-free diet have been recognized. Celiac disease is associated with intestinal lymphoma and other forms of cancer, especially adenocarcinoma of the small intestine, of the pharynx, and of the esophagus. Enteropathy-associated T-cell lymphoma is a rare form of high-grade, T-cell non-Hodgkin lymphoma, which arises in patients with either previously or concomitantly diagnosed celiac disease. Several follow-up studies suggest that a gluten-free diet protects from cancer development, especially if started in the 1st years of life. Therefore, early diagnosis and strict dietary restrictions appear to be the only possibility of preventing risk for rare but very aggressive forms of cancer associated with celiac disease.

335.3 • Other Malabsorptive Syndromes

CONGENITAL INTESTINAL MUCOSAL DEFECTS.

Microvillus Inclusion Disease (Congenital Microvillus Atrophy). Microvillus inclusion disease is an autosomal recessive disorder, which presents at birth with **profuse watery secretory diarrhea.** It is the most commonly recognized cause of congenital diarrhea. Light microscopy of the small bowel mucosa demonstrates diffuse thinning of the mucosa, with hypoplastic villus atrophy and no inflammatory infiltrate. Electron microscopy shows enterocytes with absent or sparse microvilli. The apical cytoplasm of the enterocytes contains electron-dense secretory granules; the hallmark is presence of microvilli within involutions of the apical membrane. Antenatal ultrasound scans usually show multiple fluid-filled dilated loops of bowel and polyhydramnios. Neonates usually present with dehydration and failure to thrive. Despite parenteral nutrition, the diarrhea continues and initial fluid management is difficult. The disease is fatal without long-term parenteral nutrition support. Nonetheless, most children die in infancy or early childhood. The somatostatin analog octreotide has been used as **treatment** and may reduce the volume of stool in some infants. Intestinal transplantation is the only definitive treatment for this rare disease (see Chapter 336).

Tufting Enteropathy. Tufting enteropathy (intestinal epithelial dysplasia) presents in the 1st weeks of life with **persistent watery diarrhea** and accounts for a small fraction of infants with protracted diarrhea of infancy. Symptoms typically do not begin immediately after birth, but present in early infancy. The distinctive feature on small intestinal mucosal biopsy is focal epithelial "tufts" (teardrop-shaped groups of closely packed enterocytes with apical rounding of the plasma membrane) involving 80–90% of the epithelial surface. In other known enteropathies, tufts are seen on ≤15% of the epithelial surface. The colonic epithelium shows no abnormality. Shortening but not the absence of the microvilli is seen on electron microscopy. The pathogenesis of this disorder is unknown, but it may be due to disorder of cell-cell and cell matrix interactions, since there is an abnormal distribution of α2-β1-integrin along the crypt-villus axis, increased expression of desmoglein, and ultrastructural changes of desmosomes. No **treatment** has been effective, so management requires permanent parenteral nutrition with possible intestinal transplantation (see Chapter 336).

Enteric Anendocrinosis. Mutations of the *NEUROG3* gene produce generalized mucosal malabsorption, vomiting, diarrhea, failure to thrive, dehydration, and a hyperchloremic metabolic acidosis. Oral alimentation with anything other than water produces diarrhea. Treatment is with total parenteral nutrition and small bowel or hepatic and small bowel transplantation.

CARBOHYDRATE-DEFICIENT GLYCOPROTEIN SYNDROME AND ENTEROCYTE HEPARAN SULFATE DEFICIENCY. **Congenital disorder of glycosylation** (CDG) is a genetic disorder of assembly of N-glycans in the cytosol and endoplasmic reticulum, resulting in a variety of manifestations (see Chapter 87.6). The subtypes of CDG I are all associated with **protein-losing enteropathy. Diagnosis** can be established by isoelectric focusing of serum transferrin, enzyme analysis, and/or DNA analysis. Oral mannose can provide effective **therapy** in CDG Ib, so early identification of children presenting with hypoglycemia, hypothyroidism, and/or thyroid binding globulin deficiency is beneficial.

Congenital enterocyte heparan deficiency (CEHD) is a rare cause of intractable diarrhea with protein-losing enteropathy, which may be an unusual presentation of the carbohydrate-deficient glycoprotein syndrome (CDGS) type 1 (also known as Jaeken syndrome) [see Chapter 87.6]. Heparan sulfate is a glycosaminoglycan with multiple roles in the intestine, including restriction of charged macromolecules, such as albumin, in the vascular lumen.

INTESTINAL LYMPHANGIECTASIA. Obstruction of the lymphatic drainage of the intestine can be due to congenital defects in lymphatic duct formation or to secondary causes (Table 335-6). The **congenital** form is often associated with lymphatic abnormalities elsewhere in the body, as occur with Turner, Noonan, and Klippel-Trenaunay-Weber syndromes. Causes of **secondary** lymphangiectasia include constrictive pericarditis, heart failure, retroperitoneal fibrosis, abdominal tuberculosis, and retroperitoneal malignancies. Lymph rich in proteins and lymphocytes leaks into the bowel lumen, resulting in protein-losing enteropathy and lymphocyte depletion. Hypoalbuminemia, hypogammaglobulinemia, edema, lymphocytopenia, fat and fat-soluble vitamin malabsorption, and chylous ascites often occur. Intestinal lymphangiectasia can also present with ascites, peripheral edema, and a low serum albumin.

The **diagnosis** is suggested by the typical findings in association with an elevated fecal α_1-antitrypsin level. Radiologic findings of uniform, symmetric thickening of mucosal folds throughout the small intestine are characteristic. Small bowel mucosal biopsy shows dilated lacteals with distortion of villi, and no inflammatory infiltrate. **Treatment** of lymphangiectasia requires restricting the amount of long-chain fat ingested by administering a formula containing protein and medium-chain triglycerides (MCTs). Supplementing a low-fat diet with MCT oil in cooking is used in the management of older children with lymphangiectasia. Rarely, parenteral nutrition is required. If only a portion of the intestine is involved, surgical resection may be considered.

AUTOIMMUNE ENTEROPATHY. Symptoms of autoimmune enteropathy usually present after the 1st 6 mo of life. Often the patient is diagnosed with celiac disease, but the lack of response to a gluten-free diet leads to further evaluation. Histologic findings in the small bowel include partial or complete villous atrophy, crypt hyperplasia, and an increase in chronic inflammatory cells in the lamina propria. Specific serum anti-enterocyte antibodies can be identified in ≥50% of patients by indirect immunofluorescent staining of normal small bowel mucosa and the kidney. The colon may also be involved. **Extraintestinal autoimmune disorders** are usual and include arthritis, membranous glomerulonephritis, insulin-dependent diabetes, thrombocytopenia, autoimmune hepatitis, hypothyroidism, and hemolytic anemia. **Treatment** has included prednisone, azathioprine, cyclophosphamide, cyclosporine, tacrolimus, and bone marrow transplantation.

TABLE 335-6. Causes of Protein-Losing Enteropathy

Primary intestinal lymphangiectasia
Secondary intestinal lymphangiectasia
Constrictive pericarditis
Congestive heart failure
Post Fontan procedure
Malrotation
Lymphoma
Sarcoidosis
Radiation therapy
Bowel mucosal inflammation
Infection
Cytomegalovirus (CMV)
Bacterial overgrowth
Invasive bacterial infection
Gastric inflammation
Menetrier disease
Eosinophilic gastroenteritis
Intestinal inflammation
Celiac disease
Crohn disease
Protein-sensitive enteropathy
Tropical sprue
Radiation enteritis
Colonic inflammation
Inflammatory bowel disease
Necrotizing enterocolitis
Congenital disorders of glycosylation

BILE ACID MALABSORPTION. In primary bile acid malabsorption, mutation of the ileal Na1/bile acid cotransporter gene, *SLC10A2*, results in congenital diarrhea, steatorrhea, interruption of enterohepatic circulation of bile acids, and reduced plasma cholesterol levels. Bile acids are synthesized from cholesterol in the liver and secreted into the small intestine, where they facilitate absorption of fat, fat-soluble vitamins, and cholesterol. The bile acids are reabsorbed from the intestine, returned to the liver via the portal venous circulation, and re-secreted into bile. Normally, enterohepatic circulation of bile acids is an extremely efficient process; 10% of the intestinal bile acids escape reabsorption and are eliminated in the feces. Bile acid secretion is largely autoregulated, but there is only a limited capacity to increase bile acid secretion. Reduction in bile acid pool due to bile acid malabsorption causes steatorrhea, which requires restriction of dietary fat. The unabsorbed bile acids stimulate chloride excretion in the colon, resulting in diarrhea, which responds to cholestyramine, an anion-binding resin. Secondary bile acid malabsorption can result from ileal disease such as in Crohn disease or from ileal resection.

ABETALIPOPROTEINEMIA (SEE CHAPTER 86). This rare autosomal recessive disorder of lipoprotein metabolism is associated with severe fat malabsorption from birth. Children fail to thrive during the 1st year of life, and their stools are pale, foul smelling, and bulky. The abdomen is distended, and deep tendon reflexes are absent as a result of peripheral neuropathy, which is secondary to vitamin E deficiency. Intellectual development tends to be slow. After 10 yr of age, intestinal symptoms are less severe, ataxia develops, and there is a loss of position and vibration sensation with the onset of intention tremors. These last symptoms reflect involvement of the posterior columns, cerebellum, and basal ganglia. In adolescence, atypical retinitis pigmentosa develops.

Diagnosis rests on finding acanthocytes in the peripheral blood and extremely low plasma levels of cholesterol (<50 mg/dL); triglycerides are very low (<20 mg/dL). Chylomicrons and very low density lipoproteins are not detectable, and the low-density lipoprotein (LDL) fraction is virtually absent from the circulation; marked triglyceride accumulation in villus enterocytes occurs in the fasting duodenal mucosa. Steatorrhea occurs in younger patients, but other processes of assimilation are intact. Rickets may be an unusual initial manifestation of abetalipoproteinemia and hypobetalipoproteinemia. Rickets is caused by steatorrhea-induced calcium losses. Patients have mutations of the microsomal triglyceride transfer protein (MTP) gene, resulting in absence of MTP function in the small bowel. This protein is required for normal assembly and secretion of very low density lipoproteins and chylomicrons. Specific **treatment** is not available. Large supplements of the fat-soluble vitamins A, D, E, and K should be given. Vitamin E (100–200 mg/kg/24 hr) and vitamin A (10,000–25,000 IU/day) may arrest the neurologic and retinal degeneration. Limiting long-chain fat intake can alleviate intestinal symptoms; medium-chain triglycerides can be used to supplement the fat intake.

HOMOZYGOUS HYPOBETALIPOPROTEINEMIA (SEE CHAPTER 86). This disorder is transmitted as an autosomal dominant trait. The homozygous form is indistinguishable from abetalipoproteinemia. The parents of these patients, as heterozygotes, have reduced plasma LDL and apoprotein-β concentrations, whereas the parents of patients with abetalipoproteinemia have normal levels. On election microscopy of small bowel biopsies, the size of the lipid vacuoles differentiates between abetalipoproteinemia and hypobetalipoproteinemia: many small vacuoles are present in hypobetalipoproteinemia, and large vacuoles are seen in abetalipoproteinemia.

CHYLOMICRON RETENTION DISEASE (ANDERSON DISEASE). In this rare recessive disorder, there is a defect in chylomicron exocytosis from the enterocytes. The Sar1-GTP promotes the formation of endoplasmic reticulum to Golgi transport carriers and Sar1b is defective in Anderson disease. These patients have severe intestinal symptoms with steatorrhea, chronic diarrhea, and failure to thrive. Acanthocytosis is rare, and neurologic manifestations are less severe than those observed in abetalipoproteinemia. Plasma cholesterol levels are moderately reduced (<75 mg/dL); fasting triglycerides are normal; but the fat-soluble vitamins, particularly A and E, are very low. Treatment is early aggressive therapy with fat-soluble vitamins and modification of dietary fat intake, as in abetalipoproteinemia treatment.

WOLMAN DISEASE. This rare lethal lipid storage disease leads to lipid accumulation in many organs, including the small intestine. In addition to vomiting, severe diarrhea, and hepatosplenomegaly, patients may have steatorrhea as the result of lymphatic obstruction. Deficiency of lysosomal acid lipase is the cause of the disease (see Chapter 86). Successful long-term bone marrow engraftment has resulted in the normalization of peripheral leukocyte lysosomal acid lipase enzyme activity with subsequent resolution of the diarrhea and restoration of developmental milestones.

335.4 • Intestinal Infections Associated with Malabsorption

Malabsorption is a rare consequence of primary intestinal infection in immunocompetent children but may occur after infection with *Giardia,* rotavirus, *Campylobacter, Shigella, Salmonella,* and coccidioidosis. These infectious causes of malabsorption are more common in immunocompromised children.

BACTERIAL OVERGROWTH. Bacteria are normally present in large numbers in the colon and have a symbiotic relationship with the host, providing nutrients and protecting the host from pathogenic organisms. Excessive numbers of bacteria in the small bowel or stomach are harmful. Bacteria usually are present only in a small number in the stomach and small bowel. Gastric acid pH prevents the ingested organisms from colonizing the small bowel; small bowel motility and the migrating motor complex cleanse the small bowel between meals and at night; the ileocecal valve prevents colonic bacteria from entering the ileum; and mucosal defenses such as mucins and immunoglobulins prevent bacterial overgrowth in the small bowel. Bacterial overgrowth can result from clinical conditions, which alter the gastric pH or small bowel motility, including disorders such as partial bowel obstruction, diverticulum, short bowel, intestinal duplications, diabetes mellitus, and scleroderma. Prematurity, immunodeficiency, and malnutrition are other factors associated with bacterial overgrowth of the small bowel.

Diagnosis of bacterial overgrowth can be made by culturing small bowel aspirate or by lactulose hydrogen breath test; lactulose is a synthetic disaccharide, which is not digested by mucosal brush border enzymes but can be fermented by bacteria. High baseline hydrogen and a quick rise in hydrogen in expired breath samples support the diagnosis of bacterial overgrowth, but false-positive tests are common.

Bacterial overgrowth leads to inefficient intraluminal processing of dietary fat and to steatorrhea due to bacterial deconjugation of bile salts, vitamin B_{12} malabsorption, and microvillus brush border damage with malabsorption. Overproduction of D-lactate (the enantiomer of L-lactate) can cause stupor, neurologic dysfunction, and shock from D-lactic acidosis. Diagnosis of lactic acidosis should be suspected in children at risk of bacterial overgrowth with neurologic deterioration and a high anion gap metabolic acidosis not explained by measurable acids such as L-lactate. Measurement of D-lactate enantiomer is required since standard lactate assay only measures the L-enantiomer.

Treatment of bacterial overgrowth focuses on correction of underlying causes such as partial obstruction. The oral administration of antibiotics is the mainstay of therapy. Initial treatment with 2–4 wk of metronidazole may provide relief for many months. Cycling of antibiotics including azithromycin, trimethoprim-sulfamethoxazole, ciprofloxacin, and metronidazole is required. Other alternatives are oral non-absorbable antibiotics such as aminoglycosides. Occasionally, antifungal therapy may be required to control fungal overgrowth of the bowel.

TROPICAL SPRUE. Natives and expatriates of certain tropical regions can present with a diffuse lesion of the small intestinal mucosa, tropical sprue, even long after emigration. The endemic regions include South India, the Philippines, and some islands in the Caribbean. It is uncommon in Africa, Jamaica, and Southeast Asia. The etiology of this disorder is unclear; because it follows outbreaks of acute diarrheal disease and improves with antibiotic therapy, an infectious etiology is suspected. The incidence appears to be decreasing, possibly due to frequent use of antibiotics for gastroenteritis in developing countries.

Clinical symptoms include fever and malaise followed by watery diarrhea. After ≈1 wk, the acute features subside and chronic malabsorption, intermittent diarrhea, and anorexia result in severe malnutrition characterized by glossitis, stomatitis, cheilosis, night blindness, hyperpigmentation, and edema. Muscle wasting is often marked, and the abdomen is often distended. Megaloblastic anemia results from folate and vitamin B_{12} deficiencies. **Diagnosis** is made by small bowel biopsy, which shows villous flattening, crypt hyperplasia, and a chronic inflammatory cell infiltrate of the lamina propria with adjacent lipid accumulation in the surface epithelium.

Treatment requires nutritional supplementation, folate, and vitamin B_{12} therapy. To prevent recurrence, 6 mo therapy with oral folic acid (5 mg) and tetracycline or sulfonamides is recommended. Relapses occur in 10–20% of patients who continue to reside in an endemic tropical region; additional courses of antibiotics may be necessary.

335.5 • Immunodeficiency Disorders

Malabsorption can occur with **congenital immunodeficiency** disorders, including selective IgA deficiency, severe combined immunodeficiency, agammaglobulinemia, Wiskott-Aldrich syndrome, common variable immunodeficiency disease, and chronic granulomatous disease. Selective IgA deficiency is usually asymptomatic, but malabsorption due to giardiasis, nonspecific enteropathy with bacterial overgrowth, and disaccharidase deficiency can occur. Celiac disease should be excluded because it is common in patients with IgA deficiency. Chronic rotavirus, giardiasis, bacterial overgrowth and protein-losing enteropathy are well-recognized complications of X-linked agammaglobulinemia that cause malabsorption. Malabsorption occurs in ≈10% of patients with the late-onset common variable hypogammaglobulinemia often secondary to giardiasis. In chronic granulomatous disease, phagocytic function is impaired and granulomas develop throughout the gastrointestinal tract, mimicking Crohn disease. Diarrhea, steatorrhea, and vitamin B_{12} malabsorption have also been reported.

Malnutrition, diarrhea, and failure to thrive are common in untreated children with **HIV infection.** The risk of gastrointestinal infection is related to the depression of the CD4 count. Opportunistic infections include *Cryptosporidium parvum,* cytomegalovirus, *Mycobacterium avium-intracellulare, Isospora belli, Enterocytozoon bieneusi, Candida albicans,* astrovirus, calicivirus, adenovirus, and the usual bacterial enteropathogens. In these patients, *Cryptosporidium* can cause a chronic secretory diarrhea.

Cancer chemotherapy can cause bowel mucosal damage leading to secondary lactose malabsorption. After bone marrow transplantation, mucosal damage from **graft vs host disease** can cause diarrhea and malabsorption. Small bowel biopsy shows nonspecific villous atrophy, mixed inflammatory cell infiltrate, and apoptosis. Cancer chemotherapy and bone marrow transplantation have both been associated with pancreatic damage leading to pancreatic insufficiency.

335.6 • Immunoproliferative Small Intestinal Disease

Immunoproliferative small intestinal disease (**Mediterranean lymphoma**) occurs most often in 10–30 yr olds in the Mediterranean basin, Mideast, Far East, and Africa. This is an IgA lymphoproliferative disorder that can progress to a B-cell lymphoma. Poverty and frequent episodes of gastroenteritis during infancy are antecedent risk factors. In some areas, the incidence of this disorder has decreased with improvement in socioeconomic status. Sporadic cases have been reported from Europe and America, predominantly in immigrants from developing countries. A similar disorder has also been described in patients with AIDS. Initially, presentation is with intermittent diarrhea and abdominal pain. Later, persistent chronic diarrhea, malabsorption, protein-losing enteropathy, weight loss, digital clubbing, and growth failure occur. **Diagnosis** requires multiple duodenal and jejunal mucosal biopsies to demonstrate mucosa-associated lymphoid tissue lymphomas. A serum marker (α heavy-chain paraprotein) of IgA is present in most cases. **Treatment** with prolonged (≈6 mo) tetracycline or metronidazole therapy in early disease may alleviate symptoms in some patients. Prelymphomatous stage and lymphomas require chemotherapy.

335.7 • Short Bowel Syndrome

Short bowel syndrome results from congenital malformations or resection of the small bowel. Causes of short bowel syndrome are listed in Table 335-7. Loss of >50% of the small bowel, with or without a portion of the large intestine, can result in symptoms of generalized malabsorption disorder or in specific nutrient deficiency, depending on the region of the bowel resected. At birth, the length of small bowel is between 200 and 250 cm; by adulthood, it grows to 300–800 cm. Bowel resection in an infant has better prognosis, compared to an adult, because of the potential for intestinal growth. An infant with as little as 15 cm of bowel with an ileocecal valve, or 20 cm without, has the potential to survive and be eventually weaned from total parenteral nutrition (TPN).

TABLE 335-7. Causes of Short Bowel Syndrome

Congenital
Congenital short bowel syndrome
Multiple atresias
Gastroschisis
Bowel resection
Necrotizing enterocolitis
Volvulus with or without malrotation
Long segment Hirschsprung disease
Meconium peritonitis
Crohn disease
Trauma

In addition to the length of the bowel, anatomic location of the resection is also important. The jejunum has more circular folds and longer villi. The proximal 100–200 cm of jejunum is the main site for carbohydrate, protein, iron, and water-soluble vitamin absorption, whereas fat absorption occurs over a larger length of the small bowel. Depending on the region of the bowel resected, specific nutrient malabsorption can result. Vitamin B_{12} and bile salts are only absorbed in the distal ileum (Fig. 335-5). Jejunal resections are generally tolerated better than ileal resection because the ileum can adapt to absorb nutrients and fluids. Net sodium and water absorption is relatively much higher in the ileum. Ileal resection has a profound effect on fluid and electrolyte absorption due to malabsorption of sodium and water by the remaining ileum; ileal malabsorption of bile salts stimulates increased colonic secretion of fluid and electrolytes.

TREATMENT. After bowel resection, treatment of short bowel syndrome is initially focused on repletion of massive fluid and electrolyte losses as the bowel initially accommodates to absorb these losses. Nutritional support is often provided via parenteral nutrition. A central venous catheter should be inserted to provide parenteral fluid and nutrition support. The ostomy or stool output should be measured and fluid and electrolyte losses adequately replaced. Measurement of urinary Na^+ to assess body Na^+ stores is useful to prevent Na^+ depletion. Maintaining urinary Na^+ higher than K^+ assures that Na^+ intake is adequate. Use of oral glucose electrolyte solutions improves sodium reabsorption, particularly in patients without a colon. After the initial few weeks post resection, fluid and electrolyte losses stabilize and the focus of therapy shifts to bowel rehabilitation with the gradual reintroduction of enteral feeds. Continuous small volume trophic enteral feeding should be initiated with a protein hydrolysate and medium-chain triglyceride enriched formula to stimulate gut hormones and promote mucosal growth. Enteral feeding also increases pancreatobiliary flow and reduces parenteral nutrition–induced hepatotoxicity. As soon as possible, the infant should be given a small amount of water, then formula by mouth to maintain an interest in oral feeding and minimize or avoid the development of **oral aversion.** Essential fatty acids must be provided by either a parenteral route or enteral feeds. As intestinal adaptation occurs, enteral feeding increases and parenteral supplementation decreases. The bowel mucosa proliferates and bowel lengthens with growth. After achieving the maximal increase in bowel absorptive capacity, management of specific micronutrient and vitamin deficiencies and treatment of transient problems with mucosal malabsorption after infections are required. Gastrointestinal infections such as rotavirus or small bowel bacterial overgrowth can cause setbacks in the progression to full enteral feeding in patients with marginal absorptive function. A marked increase in stool output or evidence of carbohydrate malabsorption (stool pH <5.5 and reducing substances) contraindicates further increases in enteral feeds. Slow advancement of continuous enteral feeding rates continues until all nutrients are provided enterally. Then the feeds can be altered to

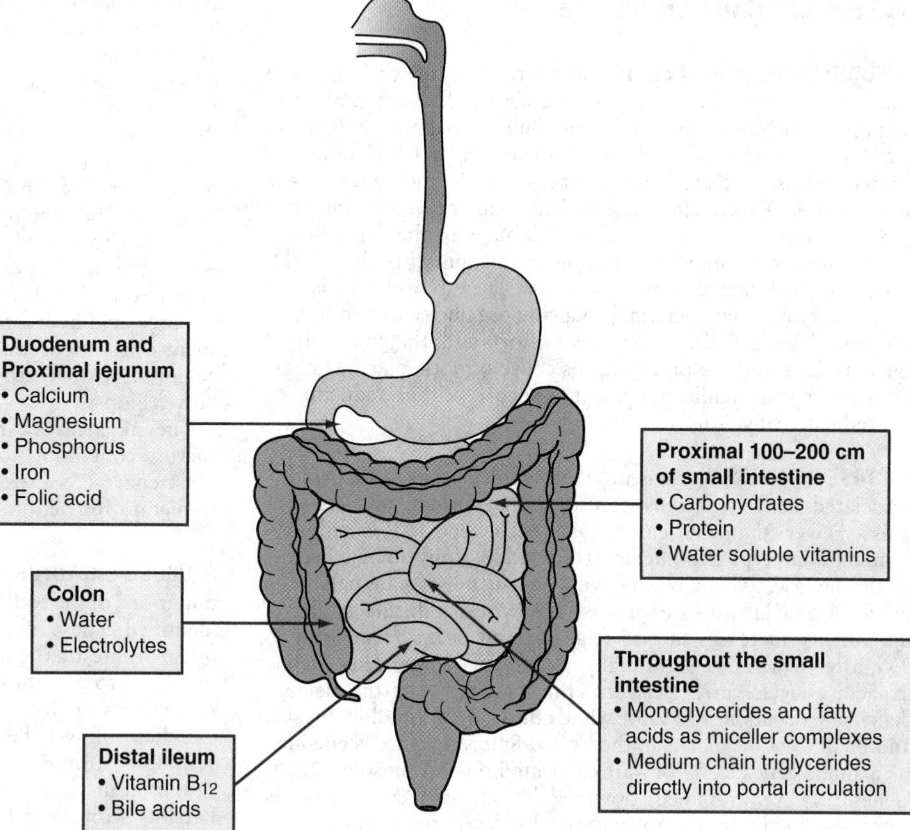

Figure 335-5. Absorption of nutrients in the small bowel varies with the region.

include increased oral or bolus feeding volumes. In those patients with large stool outputs, addition of soluble fiber and antidiarrheal agents such as loperamide and anticholinergics can be beneficial, although these drugs can cause increased risk of bacterial overgrowth. Cholestyramine can be beneficial for patients with distal ileal resection, but its potential depletion of bile acid pool can increase steatorrhea. Bacterial overgrowth is common in infants with a short bowel and may delay progression of enteral feedings. Empiric treatment with metronidazole or nonabsorbable antibiotics is often useful.

Long-term complications of short bowel syndrome include those of parenteral nutrition: central catheter infection, thrombosis, hepatic cholestasis and cirrhosis, and gallstones. Appropriate care of central line to prevent infection and catheter blockage is extremely important. Some of these patients may need long-term parenteral nutrition support, and lack of central line access is potentially life-threatening and an indication for small bowel transplantation. Inappropriate removal or changes of central lines in the neonatal period should be avoided. Other complications with terminal ileal resection include vitamin B_{12} deficiency, which may not appear until 1–2 yr after parenteral nutrition is withdrawn. Long-term monitoring for deficiencies of vitamin B_{12}, folate, iron, fat-soluble vitamins, and trace minerals such as zinc and copper is important. **Renal stones** can occur as a result of hyperoxaluria secondary to steatorrhea (calcium binds to the excess fat and not to oxalate, so more oxalate is reabsorbed and excreted in urine). Venous thrombosis and vitamin deficiency have been associated with hyperhomocystinemia in short bowel syndrome. Bloody diarrhea secondary to patchy, mild colitis can develop during the progression of enteral feedings. The pathogenesis of this "feeding colitis" is unknown, but it is usually benign and may improve with hypoallergenic diet or treatment with sulfasalazine.

In patients who are unable to achieve full enteral feeding after several years of nutritional rehabilitation, bowel lengthening surgical procedure may be considered. In some children with complications of parenteral nutrition or marginal venous access for continued parenteral nutrition, small intestinal transplantation may be considered (see Chapter 336).

335.8 • Chronic Malnutrition

Primary malnutrition is rare in developed countries. A majority of children with malnutrition have an underlying chronic digestive disorder. Child neglect and improper preparation of formulas can result in severe malnutrition. Primary malnutrition remains common in developing countries and is a frequent cause of mortality (see Chapter 43). In protein energy malnutrition, the intestinal structure, nutrient digestion and absorption, as well as the immunologic and bowel mucosal barrier function are affected. A cycle of protracted diarrhea of infancy ensues, probably through small bowel bacterial overgrowth. In kwashiorkor, severe villous atrophy, similar to what is seen in celiac disease, can occur. Mucosal disaccharidase activity is reduced, but severe lactose intolerance is not typically observed. In marasmus, villous structure is relatively well preserved, although microvillous changes and intracellular electron microscopic abnormalities are observed. Exocrine pancreatic function is also impaired, further contributing to fat and fat-soluble vitamin malabsorption.

Clinical and subclinical micronutrient deficiencies can have a major impact on intestinal tract response to gut pathogens. Nutritional rehabilitation corrects abnormalities of gastrointestinal absorption. Vitamin A supplementation reduces diarrhea-related mortality and diarrheal severity in developing countries. Similarly, zinc supplementation during diarrheal illness shortens the illness duration. Nutritional rehabilitation in malnourished children is discussed in Chapter 43.

335.9 • Enzyme Deficiencies

CARBOHYDRATE MALABSORPTION. Symptoms of carbohydrate malabsorption include loose watery diarrhea, flatulence, abdominal distention, and pain. Some children are asymptomatic unless the malabsorbed carbohydrate is consumed in large amounts. Disaccharidases are present on the brush border membrane of the small bowel. Disaccharidase deficiency can be either due to a genetic defect or secondarily due to damage to the small bowel epithelium, as occurs with infection or inflammatory disorders.

Unabsorbed carbohydrate enters the large bowel and is fermented by intestinal bacteria, producing organic acids and hydrogen gas. The gas can cause discomfort and the unabsorbed carbohydrate and the organic acids cause osmotic diarrhea characterized by an acidic pH and presence of either reducing or nonreducing sugars in the stool.

LACTASE DEFICIENCY. **Congenital lactase deficiency** is rare and is associated with symptoms occurring on exposure to lactose in milk. Fewer than 50 cases have been reported worldwide. **Primary adult type hypolactasia** is caused by a physiologic decline in the lactase, which occurs with age in most mammals. The brush border lactase is expressed at low levels during fetal life; the activity increases in late fetal life and peaks from term to 3 yr, after which levels gradually decrease with age. This decline in lactase levels varies between ethnic groups such that lactase deficiency occurs in ≈15% of white adults, 40% of adult Asians, and 85% of adult blacks in the United States. Lactase is encoded by a single gene *(LCT)* of ≈50 kb located on chromosome 2q21. Genetically programmed downregulation of lactase gene is detectable in children as early as the 2nd yr of life. Persistence of lactase in white populations of northern and central European descent and some nomadic African tribes is likely due to there being a survival advantage in these traditionally dairy-based economies. **Secondary lactose intolerance** follows small bowel mucosal damage (celiac disease, rotavirus infection) and is usually transient, improving with mucosal healing.

Lactase deficiency can be **diagnosed** by hydrogen breath test or by measurement of mucosal lactase concentration with small bowel biopsy. Diagnostic testing is not mandatory and often simple dietary changes that reduce or eliminate lactose from the diet result in symptom relief.

Treatment of lactase deficiency consists of a milk-free diet. A lactose-free formula (based on either soy or cow's milk) can be used in infants. In older children, milk in which lactose is predigested by lactase allows modest quantities of milk to be ingested. A tablet with lactase activity can also be ingested with meals. A lactase preparation is available in the market in prepackaged milk with 100% of lactose predigested. Live-culture yogurt contains bacteria that produce lactase enzyme and is therefore tolerated by patients with lactase deficiency. Hard cheeses have a small amount of lactose and are generally well tolerated.

JUICE DRINKING SYNDROME. Children consuming a large quantity of juice rich in fructose corn syrup may present with diarrhea, abdominal distention, and slow weight gain; this can mimic carbohydrate malabsorption disorders. Restricting the amount of juice in the diet resolves the symptoms and helps avoid unnecessary investigations.

SUCRASE-ISOMALTASE DEFICIENCY. Sucrase-isomaltase deficiency is a rare autosomal recessive disorder with a complete absence of sucrase and reduced maltase digestive activity. The sucrase-isomaltase complex is composed of 1,927 amino acids encoded by a 3,364 bp mRNA. The gene locus on chromosome 3 has 30 exons spanning 106.6 kb. The majority of sucrase-isomaltase mutations result in a lack of enzyme protein synthesis (null mutation). Post-translational processing defects are also identified. Approximately 2% of European Americans are mutant heterozygote. Sucrase deficiency is especially common in indigenous Greenlanders (estimated 5%) in whom it is often accompanied by lactase deficiency.

Symptoms of sucrase-isomaltase deficiency usually begin when the infant is exposed to sucrose or a glucose polymer diet. This can occur with ingestion of non–lactose based infant formula or on the introduction of pureed food, especially fruits and sweets. Diarrhea, abdominal pain, and poor growth are observed. Occasional patients may present with symptoms in late childhood or even adult life, but careful history often indicates that symptoms appeared earlier. **Diagnosis** of sucrase-isomaltase malabsorption requires acid hydrolysis of stool for reducing substances because sucrase is a nonreducing sugar. Alternatively, diagnosis can be achieved with hydrogen breath test or enzyme assay of small bowel biopsy.

The mainstay of **treatment** is lifelong dietary restriction of sucrose-containing foods. Enzyme replacement with a purified yeast enzyme, sacrosidase (Sucraid) is a highly effective adjunct to dietary restriction.

GLUCOSE-GALACTOSE MALABSORPTION. More than 30 different mutations of the sodium/glucose co-transporter gene *(SGLT1)* are identified. These mutations cause a rare autosomal recessive disorder of intestinal glucose and galactose/Na^+ co-transport system that leads to osmotic diarrhea. Since most dietary sugars are polysaccharides or disaccharides with glucose or galactose moieties, diarrhea follows the ingestion of glucose, breast milk, or conventional formulas. Dehydration and acidosis can be severe, resulting in death. The stools are acidic and contain sugar. Patients with the defect have normal absorption of fructose and their small bowel function and structure are normal in all other aspects. Intermittent or permanent glycosuria after fasting or after a glucose load is a frequent finding due to the transport defect also being present in the kidney. The finding of positive reducing substances in watery stools and slight glycosuria despite low blood sugar levels is highly suggestive of glucose-galactose malabsorption. Malabsorption of glucose and galactose is easily identified using the breath hydrogen test. It is safe to perform the 1st test with a dose of 0.5 g/kg of glucose; if necessary, a second test can be performed using 2 g/kg. Breath H_2 will rise more than 20 ppm. The small intestinal biopsy is useful to document a normal villous architecture and normal disaccharidase activities. The identification of mutations of *SGLT1* makes it possible to perform prenatal screening in families at risk for the disease.

Treatment consists of rigorous restriction of glucose and galactose. Fructose, the only carbohydrate that can be given safely, should be added to a carbohydrate-free formula at a concentration of 6–8%. Diarrhea immediately ceases when infants are given such a formula. Although the defect is permanent, later in life, limited amounts of glucose (in starches) or sucrose may be tolerated.

EXOCRINE PANCREATIC INSUFFICIENCY. Disorders of exocrine pancreatic insufficiency are discussed in Chapter 346. Cystic fibrosis is the most common congenital disorder associated with exocrine pancreatic insufficiency. Although rare, the next most common cause of pancreatic insufficiency in children is Shwachman syndrome. Other rare disorders causing exocrine pancreatic insufficiency are Johanson-Blizzard syndrome (severe steatorrhea, aplasia of alae nasi, deafness, hypothyroidism, scalp defects), Pearson bone marrow syndrome (sideroblastic anemia, variable degree of neutropenia, thrombocytopenia), and isolated pancreatic enzyme deficiency (lipase, colipase, trypsinogen, amylase, lipase-colipase).

Autoimmune polyendocrinopathy-candidiasis-ectodermal dystrophy (APCED) is a rare autosomal recessive disorder. Chronic mucocutaneous candidiasis is associated with failure of parathyroid glands, adrenal cortex, pancreatic β cells, gonads, gastric parietal cells, and thyroid gland. Pancreatic insufficiency and steatorrhea have been associated with the condition.

335.10 • Liver and Biliary Disorders Causing Malabsorption

In cholestatic liver disease, fat malabsorption results from reduced duodenal bile acid concentration, and there may be associated exocrine pancreatic dysfunction. In addition to steatorrhea, patients with these disorders acquire deficiencies of fat-soluble vitamins (vitamins A, D, E, and K). Most children with chronic liver disease have increased energy requirement, but are unable to meet these because of associated anorexia. The goal of nutritional management of these children is to provide adequate caloric and nitrogen intake with fat-soluble supplementation. Enteral feeding supplements or tube feeding support may be needed.

Vitamin E deficiency in patients with chronic cholestasis is associated with a progressive neurologic syndrome, which includes peripheral neuropathy (presenting as loss of deep tendon reflexes and ophthalmoplegia), cerebellar ataxia, and posterior column dysfunction. Early in the course, findings are partially reversible with treatment; late features may not be reversible. It can be difficult to identify vitamin E deficiency because the elevated blood lipid levels in cholestatic liver disease can falsely elevate the serum vitamin E level. Therefore, it is important to measure the ratio of serum vitamin E to total serum lipids; the normal level for patients <12 yr of age is >0.6, and for patients ≥12 yr, it is >0.8. The neurologic disease can be prevented with the use of an oral water-soluble vitamin E preparation (d-α-tocopherol polyethylene glycol 1,000 succinate [TPGS], Liqui-E) at 25–50 IU/day in neonates and 1 IU/kg/day in children.

Metabolic bone disease can develop secondary to vitamin D deficiency. Simultaneous administration of vitamin D with the water-soluble vitamin E preparation (TPGS) enhances absorption of vitamin D. In young infants, oral vitamin D_3 is given at 1,000 IU/kg/24 hr. After 1 mo, if the serum 25-hydroxyvitamin D level is low, the same dose of oral vitamin D is mixed with TPGS. 25-Hydroxyvitamin D is then monitored every 3 mo, with adjustment of doses as necessary.

Vitamin K deficiency can occur as a result of cholestasis and poor fat absorption. Easy bruising may be the 1st sign. In neonatal cholestasis, coagulopathy due to vitamin K deficiency can present with intracranial bleeds with devastating consequences and, therefore, routine measurement of prothrombin (a more sensitive test) and partial thromboplastin time should be performed to monitor for deficiency in children with cholestasis. All children with cholestasis should receive vitamin K supplements.

Vitamin A deficiency is associated with night blindness, xerophthalmia, and increased mortality when patients contract measles. Serum vitamin A levels should be monitored and adequate supplementation considered.

335.11 • Defects of Absorption or Transport

AMINO ACID TRANSPORT DEFECTS. In several of the specific congenital disorders of amino acid transport, defective intestinal amino acid transport occurs. At least three specific small bowel carriers appear to be involved in active transport of amino acids. Amino acid uptake into the intestinal mucosa is defective in **cystinuria**, but these patients have no gastrointestinal symptoms. In **Hartnup disease**, malabsorption of neutral amino acids including tryptophan leads to ataxia, intellectual deterioration, a pellagra-like rash, and, at times, diarrhea. The clinical manifestations are due to the malabsorption of tryptophan, producing nicotinamide deficiency. Oral administration of nicotinamide leads to a dramatic clinical improvement. **Methionine malabsorption** is associated with episodes of diarrhea in fair-complexioned retarded children whose urine has a sweet odor and contains excess β-hydroxybutyric acid. In the **blue diaper syndrome**, tryptophan absorption is defective.

DISORDERS OF VITAMIN AND MINERAL ABSORPTION.

Vitamin B_{12} Malabsorption. Vitamin B_{12} deficiency can result from decreased intake (breast-fed babies whose mothers have undiagnosed vitamin B_{12} deficiency because of strict vegetarian diets), abnormal absorption (gastric resection, autoimmune pernicious anemia with decreased intrinsic factor), competition for B_{12} in the intestine (bacterial overgrowth), disruption of absorption across the ileal surface (Crohn disease, tropical sprue), or from inborn errors of vitamin B_{12} transport and metabolism.

Several rare congenital defects can affect assimilation of vitamin B_{12}. These conditions are much less common than dietary vitamin B_{12} deficiency or malabsorption secondary to terminal ileal resection or dysfunction. In **juvenile pernicious anemia,** intrinsic factor production in the stomach is defective. Vitamin B_{12} malabsorption results, leading to megaloblastic anemia and growth failure. Gastric structure and function are otherwise normal. **Transcobalamin II deficiency** is an inherited defect of a protein necessary for intestinal transport of vitamin B_{12}. The result is severe megaloblastic anemia, diarrhea, and vomiting. **Imerslund syndrome** occurs in patients in whom ileal absorption of vitamin B_{12} is defective. Ileal structure and function are otherwise normal. Megaloblastic anemia develops toward the end of the 1st yr. Proteinuria is commonly associated.

Treatment of these disorders is to administer vitamin B_{12} by injection: 1,000 μg/twice weekly for transcobalamin II deficiency and 100 μg/mo for the others. Once patients are in hematologic remission after intramuscular vitamin B_{12} therapy, **intranasal** vitamin B_{12} (500 μg in once weekly metered doses) can be substituted.

Congenital Malabsorption of Folic Acid. Isolated congenital folate malabsorption has been described in fewer than 20 patients. It may be the consequence of a selective defect in the intestinal and blood-brain barrier folate transporter. Inheritance studies suggest an autosomal recessive disorder. Severe megaloblastic anemia is observed as early as 3 mo of age. Neurologic symptoms can include ataxia, convulsions, mental retardation, and intracranial calcifications. Gastrointestinal symptoms may present in the 1st week of life and include mouth ulcers, diarrhea, and failure to thrive. Diagnosis is made by lack of an increase in serum or cerebrospinal fluid (CSF) folate after a loading test with oral folic acid (5 mg). Early and aggressive **treatment** with parenteral folinic acid is critical and should be guided with documentation of improvement of CSF folate levels. Subsequent treatment, aimed at maintaining levels of folate in serum, red blood cells, and CSF, requires administration of large (up to 100 mg/day) oral doses of folic, folinic, or methyltetrahydrofolic acid.

Vitamin D–Dependent Rickets. In this autosomal recessive disorder, a specific defect in the metabolism of vitamin D causes malabsorption of calcium. Intestinal function is otherwise normal (see Chapter 48).

Chloride-Losing Diarrhea. This rare recessive inherited disorder is caused by mutations in a chromosome 7 gene, 1st known as *DRA* (downregulated in adenoma). The chloride/bicarbonate transport mechanism in the distal ileum and colon is defective, causing severe watery diarrhea, beginning at birth. Maternal polyhydramnios is common. Watery diarrhea leads to dehydration and a severe electrolyte disturbance characterized by hypokalemia, hypochloremia, and alkalosis, a most unusual pattern for an infant with chronic diarrhea. Other aspects of intestinal absorption are normal. Stools contain chloride in excess of the sum of sodium and potassium (125–150 mEq/L). **Treat-**

ment does not alter diarrhea but diminishes complications. All losses of electrolytes and water are at 1st replaced intravenously; oral solutions are usually tolerated after 1 mo. If the diagnosis is made early in the neonatal period and adequate therapy started immediately, the affected infant will show perfect growth and development.

Congenital Sodium Diarrhea. The apparent basis for this rare syndrome is a defect in sodium-hydrogen exchange in the small intestine and colon. As in congenital chloride diarrhea, patient presents with profuse watery, secretory diarrhea from birth and a history of maternal polyhydramnios. Unlike congenital chloride diarrhea, however, this condition is characterized by acidosis and fecal chloride concentration less than sodium concentration (as high as 145 mEq/L). **Treatment** with oral hydration solution is effective in maintaining normal growth.

Primary Hypomagnesemia. This specific intestinal transport defect in magnesium transport causes severe hypomagnesemia and secondary hypocalcemic tetany in infancy. Other aspects of intestinal function are normal. The findings are reversed by large supplements of magnesium, which must be continued indefinitely.

ACRODERMATITIS ENTEROPATHICA (SEE CHAPTER 670). This presents in early life with rashes around mucocutaneous junctions and on the extremities, alopecia, chronic diarrhea, and sometimes steatorrhea. Serum zinc concentration and alkaline phosphatase activity are low. Acquired zinc deficiency presents in a similar manner. Intestinal mucosal biopsy specimens show Paneth cell inclusions that disappear after treatment. Analysis of maternal breast milk zinc concentrations can help differentiate acrodermatitis enteropathica from acquired zinc deficiency; low breast milk concentration is seen in acquired zinc deficiency. **Treatment** with oral zinc sulfate, 1–2 mg elemental zinc/kg/24 hr, causes rapid healing of the skin lesions and improvement of diarrhea in acrodermatitis enteropathica.

MENKES (KINKY HAIR) SYNDROME (SEE CHAPTER 661). Menkes disease is an X-linked multisystemic lethal disorder of copper metabolism dominated by neurodegenerative symptoms and connective tissue disturbances. The Menkes gene is located on the long arm of the X chromosome at Xq13.3, and the gene product is a P type adenosine triphosphatase (ATPase). There is a widespread defect in cellular copper transport affecting the intestine as well as other tissues. Orally ingested copper accumulates in the intestines, and there is defective copper absorption. Menkes disease is characterized by growth retardation, abnormal hair, cerebellar degeneration, severe vasculopathy, fractures, and early death. Serum copper and ceruloplasmin levels are low, but cellular copper content is increased. The currently accepted **treatment** is the administration of parenteral copper; few patients avoid the neurologic complications.

DRUG-INDUCED ABSORPTIVE DEFECTS. Some drugs have a diffuse impact on the small intestinal epithelium. **Methotrexate** can cause arrest of enterocyte mitoses and can result in a mucosal lesion; large doses of neomycin also affect mucosal structure. **Sulfasalazine** interferes with folic acid absorption. **Cholestyramine** binds bile salts and calcium in the intestinal lumen to cause hypocalcemia and steatorrhea. **Phenytoin** interferes with calcium absorption and can cause rickets.

Malabsorption Syndromes

Branski D, Lerner A, Lebenthal E: Chronic diarrhea and malabsorption. *Pediatr Clin North Am* 1996;43:307–331.

Couper R, Oliver M: Pancreatic function tests. In Walker WA, Goulet O, Kleinman RE. et al (editors): *Pediatric Gastrointestinal Disease,* 4th ed. Hamilton, Ontario, BC, Decker, 2004, pp 1816–1829.

Khouri M, Huang G, Shiau Y: Sudan stain of fecal fat: New insight into an old test. *Gastroenterology* 1989;96:421–427.

Kleinman RE, Klish W, Lebenthal E, et al: Role of juice carbohydrate malabsorption in chronic nonspecific diarrhea in children. *J Pediatr* 1992; 120:825–829.

Riby JE, Fujisawa T, Kretchmer N: Fructose absorption. *Am J Clin Nutr* 1993;58:748S–753S.

Riddlesberger MM: Evaluation of the gastrointestinal tract in the child: CT, MRI, and isotopic studies. *Pediatr Clin North Am* 1988;35:281–310.

Tabrez S, Roberts IM: Malabsorption and malnutrition. *Prim Care* 2001; 28:505–522.

Wang J, Cortina G, Wu SV, et al: Mutant neurogenin-3 in congenital malabsorptive diarrhea. *N Engl J Med* 2006;355:270–280.

Weaver LT, Amarri S, Swart GR: 13C mixed triglyceride breath test. *Gut* 1998;43:S13–S19.

Celiac Disease

Barker CC, Mitton C, Jevon G, Mock T: Can tissue transglutaminase antibody titers replace small-bowel biopsy to diagnose celiac disease in select pediatric populations? *Pediatrics* 2005;115:1341–1346.

Bibgley PJ, Williams AJK, Norcross AJ, et al: Undiagnosed coeliac disease at age seven: Population based prospective birth cohort study. *Br Med J* 2004;328:322–324.

Bostwick H, Berezin S, Halata M, et al: Celiac disease presenting with microcephaly. *J Pediatr* 2001;138:589–592.

Branski D, Fasano A, Troncone R: Latest developments in the pathogenesis and treatment of celiac disease. *J Pediatr* 2006;149:295–300.

Catassi C, Bearzi I, Holmes GK: Association of celiac disease and intestinal lymphomas and other cancers. *Gastroenterology* 2005;128:S79–S86.

Ciclitira PJ, King AL, Fraser JS: AGA technical review on celiac sprue. American Gastroenterological Association. *Gastroenterology* 2001;120:1526–1540.

Farrell R, Kelly C: Current concepts: Celiac sprue. *N Engl J Med* 2002; 346:180–188.

Green PHR, Fleischauer AT, Bhagat G, et al: Risk of malignancy in patients with celiac disease. *Am J Med* 2003;115:191–195.

Hill ID, Dirks MH, Liptak GS, et al: Guideline for the diagnosis and treatment of celiac disease in children: Recommendation of the North American Society for Pediatric Gastroenterology, Hepatology and Nutrition. *J Pediatr Gastroenterol Nutr* 2005;40:1–19.

Hoffenberg E, Haas J, Drescher A, et al: A trial of oats in children with newly diagnosed celiac disease. *J Pediatr* 2000;137:361–366.

Labate A, Gambardella A, Messina D, et al: Silent celiac disease in patients with childhood localization-related epilepsies. *Epilepsia* 2001;42:1153–1155.

Larizza D, Calcaterra V, De Giacomo C, et al: Celiac disease in children with autoimmune thyroid disease. *J Pediatr* 2001;139:738–740.

Liu E, Li M, Bao F, et al: Need for quantitative assessment of transglutaminase autoantibodies for celiac disease in screening-identified children. *J Pediatr* 2005;146:494–499.

[No authors listed]: Revised criteria for diagnosis of coeliac disease. Report of Working Group of European Society of Paediatric Gastroenterology and Nutrition. *Arch Dis Child* 1990;65:909–911.

Norris JM, Barriga K, Hoffenberg EJ, et al: Risk of celiac disease autoimmunity and timing of gluten introduction in the diet of infants at increased risk of disease. *JAMA* 2005;293:2342–2351.

Pellechia M: Idiopathic cerebellar ataxia associated with celiac disease: Lack of distinctive neurological features. *J Neurol Neurosurg Psychiatry* 1999; 66:32–35.

Pueschel S, Romano C, Failla P, et al: A prevalence study of celiac disease in persons with Down's syndrome residing in the United States of America. *Acta Paediatr* 1999;88:953–956.

Swigonski NL, Kuhlenschmidt HL, Bull MJ, et al: Screening for celiac disease in asymptomatic children with Down syndrome: cost-effectiveness of preventing lymphoma. *Pediatrics* 2006;118:594–602.

Van Rijn JCW, Grate FK, Oostdijk W, et al: Short stature and the probability of coeliac disease, in the absence of gastrointestinal symptoms. *Arch Dis Child* 2004;9:882–883.

Watson PGP: Diagnosis of coeliac disease. *Br Med J* 2005;330:739–740.

Zachor DA, Mroczek-Musulman E, Brown P: Prevalence of celiac disease in Down syndrome in the United States. *J Pediatr Gastroenterol Nutr* 2000;31:275–279.

Zelnick N, Pacht A, Obeid R, Lerner A: Range of neurologic disorders in patients with celiac disease. *Pediatrics* 2004;113:1672–1676.

Congenital Bowel Mucosal Defects

Damen G, de Klerk H, Huijmans J, et al: Gastrointestinal and other clinical manifestations in 17 children with congenital disorders of glycosylation type Ia, Ib, and Ic. *J Pediatr Gastroenterol Nutr* 2004;38:282–287.
Kennea N, Norbury R, Anderson G, Tekay A: Congenital microvillous inclusion disease presenting as antenatal bowel obstruction. *Ultrasound Obstet Gynecol* 2001;17:172–174.
Murch SH, Winyard PJ, Koletko S, et al: Congenital enterocyte heparan sulphate deficiency with massive albumin loss, secretory diarrhea, and malnutrition. *Lancet* 1996;347:1299–1301.
Patey N, Scoazec JY, Cuenod-Jabri B, et al: Distribution of cell adhesion molecules in infants with intestinal epithelial dysplasia (tufting enteropathy). *Gastroenterology* 1997;113:833–843.
Reifen RM, Cutz E, Griffiths AM, et al: Tufting enteropathy: A newly recognized clinicopathological entity associated with refractory diarrhea in infants. *J Pediatr Gastroenterol Nutr* 1994;18:379–385.
Walker-Smith J, Murch S: Miscellaneous disorders of the small intestine. In Walker-Smith J and Murch S (editors): *Diseases of the Small Intestine in Childhood,* 4th ed. Oxford, Isis Medical Media, 1999, pp 380–381.

Protein-Losing Enteropathy

Cheong JL, Cowan FM, Modi N. Gastrointestinal manifestations of postnatal cytomegalovirus infection in infants admitted to a neonatal intensive care unit over a five-year period. *Arch Dis Child Fetal Neonatal Ed* 2004; 89:F367–F369.
Salvia G, Cascioli C, Ciccimarra F, et al: A case of protein losing enteropathy caused by intestinal lymphangiectasia in a preterm infant. *Pediatrics* 2001;107:416–417.
Schmider A, Henrich W, Reles A, et al: Isolated fetal ascites caused by primary lymphangiectasia: A case report. *Am J Obstet Gynecol* 2001;184:227–228.
Vardy PA, Lebenthal E, Shwachman H: Intestinal lymphangiectasis: A reappraisal. *Pediatrics* 1975;55:842–851.

Infections Causing Malabsorption

Farthing MJG: The molecular pathogenesis of giardiasis. *J Pediatr Gastroenterol Nutr* 1997;24:79–88.
Liebman WM, Thaler MM, Dehorimier A, et al: Intractable diarrhea of infancy due to intestinal coccidiosis. *Gastroenterology* 1980;78:579–584.
Sood M, Booth I: Is prolonged rotavirus infection a common cause of protracted diarrhoea? *Arch Dis Child* 1999;80:309–310.

Bacterial Overgrowth

Lichtman S: Bacterial overgrowth. In Walker WA, Goulet O, Kleinman RE, et al (editors): *Pediatric Gastrointestinal Disease,* 4th ed. Hamilton, Ontario, BC, Decker, 2004, pp 691–701.
Ruckebusch Y: Development of digestive motor patterns during perinatal life: Mechanism and significance. *J Pediatr Gastroenterol Nutr* 1986;5:523–536.

Tropical Sprue

Gray G: Tropical sprue: Chronic intestinal malabsorption in the tropics. In Blaser M, Smith P, Pavdin J, et al (editors): *Infections of the Gastrointestinal Tract.* New York, Raven Press, 1995, pp 333–341.

Immunodeficiency Disorders

Kotler DP, Francisco A, Clayton F, et al: Small intestinal injury and parasitic diseases in AIDS. *Ann Intern Med* 1990;113:444–449.
Weikel CS, Gaynes BN, Roche JK: Diarrheal disease in the immunocompromised host. In Guerrant R (editor): *Baillière's Clinical Tropical Medicine and Communicable Diseases,* vol 3. London, Baillière Tindall, 1988, p 401.
Winter H, Chang TI: Gastrointestinal and nutritional problems in children with immunodeficiency and AIDS. *Pediatr Clin North Am* 1996;43: 573–590.
Woroniecka M, Ballow M: Office evaluation of children with recurrent infection. *Pediatr Clin North Am* 2000;47:1211–1224.
Yolken RH, Hart W, Oung I, et al: Gastrointestinal dysfunction and disaccharide intolerance in children infected with human immunodeficiency virus. *J Pediatr* 1991;118:359–363.

Autoimmune Enteropathy

Bousvaros A, Leichtner AM, Book L, et al: Treatment of pediatric autoimmune enteropathy with tacrolimus (FK506). *Gastroenterology* 1996;111: 237–243.
Russo PA, Brochu P, Seidman EG, Roy CC: Autoimmune enteropathy. *Pediatr Dev Pathol* 1999;2:65–71.

Immunoproliferative Small Intestinal Disease

Akbulut H, Soykan I, Yakaryilmaz F, et al: Five-year results of the treatment of 23 patients with immunoproliferative small intestinal disease: A Turkish experience. *Cancer* 1997;80:8–14.

Short Bowel Syndrome

Andorsky D, Lund D, Lillehei C, et al: Nutritional and other postoperative management of neonates with short bowel syndrome correlates with outcomes. *J Pediatr* 2001;139:27–31.
Bines J, Francis D, Hill D, et al: Reducing parenteral requirement in children with short bowel syndrome: Impact of an amino acid–based complete infant formula. *J Pediatr Gastroenterol Nutr* 1998;26:123–128.
Fishbein TM, Matsumoto CS: Intestinal replacement therapy: timing and indications for referral of patients to an intestinal rehabilitation and transplant program. *Gastroenterology* 2006;130:5147–5151.
Kauffman SS, Atkinson JB, Bianchi A, et al: Indications for pediatric intestinal transplantation: A position paper of the American Society of Transplantation. *Pediatr Transplant* 2001;5:80–87.
Kaufman SS, Loseke CA, Lupo JV, et al: Influence of bacterial overgrowth and intestinal inflammation on duration of parenteral nutrition in children with short bowel syndrome. *J Pediatr* 1997;131:356–361.
Kocoshis S: Evolving concepts and improving prospects for neonates with short bowel syndrome. *J Pediatr* 2001;139:5–7.
Sigalet DL: Short bowel syndrome in infants and children: An overview. *Semin Pediatr Surg* 2001;10:49–55.
Taylor SF, Sondheimer JM, Sokol RJ, et al: Noninfectious colitis associated with short gut syndrome in infants. *J Pediatr* 1991;119:24–28.
Vanderhoof JA, Young RJ, Thompson JS: New and emerging therapies for short bowel syndrome in children. *Paediatr Drugs* 2003;5:525–531.

Digestive Tract in Chronic Malnutrition

Durie PR, Forstner GG, Gaskin KJ, et al: Elevated serum immunoreactive pancreatic cationic trypsinogen in acute malnutrition: Evidence of pancreatic damage. *J Pediatr* 1985;106:233–238.
Romer H, Urbach R, Gomez MA, et al: Moderate and severe protein-energy malnutrition in childhood: Effects on jejunal mucosal morphology and disaccharidase activities. *J Pediatr Gastroenterol Nutr* 1983;2:459–464.

Disaccharidase Deficiencies

Ament ME, Perera DR, Esther L: Sucrase-isomaltase deficiency: A frequently misdiagnosed disease. *J Pediatr* 1973;83:721–727.
Flatz G: The genetics of lactose digestion in humans. *Adv Hum Genet* 1987;16:1–77.
Heyman MB, Committee on Nutrition: Lactose intolerance in infants, children, and adolescents. *Pediatrics* 2006;118:1279–1286.
Newton T, Murphy MS, Booth IW: Glucose polymer as a cause of protracted diarrhea in infants with unsuspected congenital sucrase-isomaltase deficiency. *J Pediatr* 1996;128:753–756.
Ouwendijk J, Moolenaar CE, Peters WJ, et al: Congenital sucrase-isomaltase deficiency: Identification of a glutamine to proline substitution that leads to a transport block of sucrase-isomaltase in a pre-Golgi compartment. *J Clin Invest* 1996;97:633–641.
Treem WR: Congenital sucrase-isomaltase deficiency. *J Pediatr Gastroenterol Nutr* 1995;21:1–14.
Treem WR, McAdams L, Stanford L, et al: Sacrosidase therapy for congenital sucrase-isomaltase deficiency. *J Pediatr Gastroenterol Nutr* 1999;28: 137–142.

Juice Drinking Syndrome

Hourihane JO, Rolles CJ: Morbidity from excessive intake of high energy fluids: The "squash drinking syndrome." *Arch Dis Child* 1995;72:141–143.

Glucose-Galactose Malabsorption

Evans L, Grasset E, Heyman M, et al: Congenital selective malabsorption of glucose and galactose. *J Pediatr Gastroenterol Nutr* 1985;4:878–886.

Fairclough PD, Clark ML, Dawson AM, et al: Absorption of glucose and maltose in congenital glucose-galactose malabsorption. *Pediatr Res* 1978; 12:1112–1114.

Martin MG, Turk E, Lostao MP: Defects in Na^+/glucose cotransporter *(SGLT1)* trafficking and function cause glucose-galactose malabsorption. *Nat Genet* 1996;12:216–220.

Liver and Biliary Disorders

Argao EA, Heubi JE: Fat-soluble vitamin deficiency in infants and children. *Curr Opin Pediatr* 1993;5:562–566.

Hadorn B, Hess J, Troesch V, et al: Role of bile acids in the activation of trypsinogen by enterokinase: Disturbance of trypsinogen activation in patients with intrahepatic biliary atresia. *Gastroenterology* 1974;66: 548–555.

Kooh SW, Jones G, Reilly BJ, et al: Pathogenesis of rickets in chronic hepatobiliary disease in children. *J Pediatr* 1979;94:870–874.

Primary Bile Acid Malabsorption

Heubi JE, Balistreri WF, Fondacaro JD, et al: Primary bile acid malabsorption: Defective in vitro ileal active bile acid transport. *Gastroenterology* 1982;83:804–811.

Oelkers P, Kirby LC, Heubi JE, et al: Primary bile acid malabsorption caused by mutations in the ileal sodium-dependent bile acid transporter gene *(SLC10A2)*. *J Clin Invest* 1997;99:1880–1887.

Abetalipoproteinemia, Hypobetalipoproteinemia, and Anderson Disease

Levy E, Chouraqui JP, Ray CC: Steatorrhea and disorders of chylomicron synthesis and secretion. *Pediatr Clin North Am* 1988;35:53–67.

Narchi H, Amr SS, Mathew PM, El Jamil MR: Rickets as an unusual initial presentation of abetalipoproteinemia and hypobetalipoproteinemia. *J Pediatr Endocrinol Metab* 2001;14:329–333.

Rader DJ, Brewer B: Abetalipoproteinemia: New insights into lipoprotein assembly and vitamin E metabolism from a rare genetic disease. *JAMA* 1993;270:865–869.

Scott BB, Miller JP, Losowsky MS: Hypobetalipoproteinemia: A variant of the Bassen-Kornzweig syndrome. *Gut* 1979;20:163–168.

Vitamin B_{12} Malabsorption

Hall CA: Congenital disorders of vitamin B12 transport and their contribution to concepts. *Gastroenterology* 1973;65:684–686.

Hitzig WH, Dohmann V, Pluss HJ, et al: Hereditary transcobalamin II deficiency: Clinical findings in a new family. *J Pediatr* 1974;85:622–628.

Imerslund O: Idiopathic chronic megaloblastic anaemia in children. *Acta Paediatr Suppl* 1960;49:1–115.

MacKenzie IL, Donaldson RM, Trier JS, et al: Ileal mucosa in familial selective vitamin B12 malabsorption. *N Engl J Med* 1972;286:1021–1025.

Folate Malabsorption

Malatack J, Moran M, Moughan B: Isolated congenital malabsorption of folic acid in a male infant: Insights into treatment and mechanism of defect. *Pediatrics* 1999;104:1133–1137.

Urbach J, Abrahamov A, Grossowicz N: Congenital isolated folic acid malabsorption. *Arch Dis Child* 1987;62:78–80.

Chloride-Losing Diarrhea

Holmberg C, Perheentupa J, Launiala K, et al: Congenital chloride diarrhea. *Arch Dis Child* 1977;52:255–267.

Kere J, Lohi H, Höglund P: Genetic disorders of membrane transport III. Congenital chloride diarrhea. *Am J Physiol* 1999;276:G7–G13.

Congenital Sodium Diarrhea

Booth IW, Murer H, Strange G, et al: Defective jejunal brush border Na^+/H^+ exchange: A cause of congenital secretory diarrhea. *Lancet* 1985;1: 1066–1069.

Holmberg C, Perheentupa J: Congenital Na^+ diarrhea: A new type of secretory diarrhea. *J Pediatr* 1985;106:56–61.

Primary Hypomagnesemia

Romero R, Meacham LR, Winn KT: Isolated magnesium malabsorption in a 10-year-old boy. *Am J Gastroenterol* 1996;91:611–613.

Stromme JH, Nesbakken R, Normann T, et al: Familial hypomagnesemia. *Acta Paediatr Scand* 1969;58:433–444.

Acrodermatitis Enteropathica

Bohane TD, Cutz E, Hamilton JR, et al: Acrodermatitis enteropathica, zinc and the Paneth cell. *Gastroenterology* 1977;73:587–592.

Moynahan EJ: Acrodermatitis enteropathica: A lethal inherited human zinc-deficiency disorder. *Lancet* 1974;2:399–400.

Menkes Syndrome

Danks DM: Of mice and men, metals and mutations. *J Med Genet* 1986; 23:99–106.

Jankov RP, Boerkoel CF, Hellman J, et al: Lethal neonatal Menkes' disease with severe vasculopathy and fractures. *Acta Paediatr* 1998;87: 1297–1300.

Kodama H, Murata Y, Kobayashi M: Clinical manifestation and treatment of Menkes disease and its variants. *Pediatr Int* 1999;41:423–429.

Drug-Induced Malabsorption

Franklin JL, Rosenberg HH: Impaired folic acid absorption in inflammatory bowel disease: Effects of salicylazosulfapyridine (Azulfidine). *Gastroenterology* 1973;64:517–525.

Morijiri Y, Sato T: Factors causing rickets in institutionalised handicapped children on anticonvulsant therapy. *Arch Dis Child* 1981;56:446–449.

Rogers AL, Vloedman DA, Bloom EC, et al: Neomycin-induced steatorrhea. *JAMA* 1966;197:185–190.

Trier JS: Morphologic alterations induced by methotrexate in the mucosa of human proximal intestine: I. Serial observations by light microscopy. *Gastroenterology* 1962;42:295–305.

Chapter 336 ■ Intestinal Transplantation in Children

Jorges D. Reyes

The practice of intestinal transplantation was enhanced by the introduction of **tacrolimus** in 1989, which resulted in significantly improved patient and graft survivals after liver transplantation in children. The success of this drug was not only due to control of rejection, but also to the subsequent ability to withdraw long-term immunosuppressive drug therapy with a consequent decrease in drug toxicities and infections. The evolution of the **multiorgan procurement** techniques allowed for the procurement and implantation of the intestine in association with other intra-abdominal organs, most importantly, the liver. The understanding that the liver may be protective of the intestine against rejection had been suggested by previous combinations of liver plus other organs such as the kidney. These procedures could be applied to the varied recipient population, with near elimination of the more complex multiorgan operation, thus allowing for easier perioperative care. A critical development was the demonstration of the interaction (host vs graft and graft vs host) between recipient and donor immunocytes (brought with the allograft), which under the cover of immunosuppression allows for varying degrees of graft acceptance and eventual minimization of drug therapy.

INDICATIONS FOR INTESTINAL TRANSPLANT

The success of intestinal transplantation has fostered the concept of **intestinal failure** (IF), whereby patients who have lost the ability to maintain nutritional support with their intestine are permanently dependent on total parenteral nutrition (TPN). The majority of these patients have short bowel as a result of a congenital deficiency or acquired condition (see Chapter 335.7). In others, the cause of IF is a functional disorder of motility or absorption (Table 336-1). Rarely do patients receive intestinal transplants for benign neoplasms; these patients may or may not be receiving TPN. Unlike other types of organ failure, however, IF is a syndrome of "satellite" complications that includes paucity of venous access, life-threatening infections, and TPN-induced cholestatic liver disease. Patients who develop these complications have an ≈70% 1 yr mortality, and thus should be referred for intestinal transplantation.

PAUCITY OF VENOUS ACCESS. The administration of TPN requires the insertion of a centrally placed venous catheter; and there are only six readily accessible sites (bilateral internal jugular, subclavian, and iliac veins). The loss of venous access generally occurs in the setting of recurrent catheter sepsis; loss of 50% of these venous access sites places the patient at risk of not being able to be treated with TPN.

LIFE-THREATENING INFECTIONS. These are usually catheter-related, however, the absence of significant lengths of intestine may be associated with abnormal motility of the residual bowel (producing both delayed or rapid emptying) with varying degrees of bacterial overgrowth and possible bacterial translocation as a consequence to loss of intestinal barrier function and/or loss of gut immunity. This can produce cholestatic liver disease, multisystem organ failure, and metastatic infectious foci in lungs, kidneys, liver, and the brain.

LIVER DISEASE. TPN-induced cholestatic liver disease is understood to be a result of the toxic effects of TPN on hepatocytes. The effects on the liver include fatty transformation, steatohepatitis and necrosis, fibrosis, and then cholestasis. Development of clinical jaundice (total bilirubin >3 mg/dL) is a significant risk factor for poor outcome, since these changes lead to the development of portal hypertensive gastroenteropathy, hypersplenism, coagulopathy, and uncontrollable bleeding.

TRANSPLANT OPERATION

DONOR SELECTION. Intestinal grafts are usually procured from hemodynamically stable, ABO-identical brain-dead donors who did not have clinical or laboratory evidence suggestive of intra-abdominal ischemia. Exclusion criteria include a history of malignancy, as well as intra-abdominal evidence of infection; systemic viral or bacterial infections are not excluded. Donor preparation has been limited to the administration of systemic and enteral antibiotics. Prophylaxis for graft vs host disease (GVHD) with graft pretreatment using irradiation or a monoclonal antilymphocyte antibody has varied over time and among the centers performing this procedure.

TYPES OF INTESTINAL GRAFTS. Intestinal allografts are utilized in various forms, either as an isolated small intestine or as a composite graft when it is included with the liver, duodenum, pancreas, and/or stomach, the most common being the liver with intestine and multivisceral grafts. The procurement of these various types of grafts focuses on the preservation of the arterial vessels of celiac and/or superior mesenteric arteries, as well as appropriate venous outflow, which would include the superior mesenteric vein or the hepatic veins in the composite grafts. The various etiologies precipitating intestinal failure have prompted the development of these various combinations of intestinal allografts, where the component organs can be removed or retained according to the clinical needs of the individual patient. The larger composite grafts inherently retain the celiac and superior mesenteric arteries; this includes multivisceral grafts, liver/small bowel grafts, and modified multivisceral grafts in which the liver is excluded, but the entire gastrointestinal tract is transplanted, including stomach. The isolated intestine graft retains the superior mesenteric artery and vein; this can be accomplished with preservation of the vessels going to the pancreas, when this organ has been allocated to another recipient. The graft that is to be utilized in a particular recipient is dissected out in situ and then removed after cardiac arrest of the donor, with core cooling of the organs, using an infusion of preservation solution (Fig. 336-1).

THE RECIPIENT OPERATION. Intestinal transplantation can be a significant technical challenge that varies according to the degree of illness of the patient (whether or not the child has liver disease and portal hypertension), as well as the history of previous abdominal procedures. Transplantation of an isolated intestinal allograft involves exposure of the lower abdomen, infrarenal aorta, and inferior vena cava. Placement of vascular grafts using donor iliac artery and vein to these vessels allows for arterialization and venous drainage of the intestinal graft. In patients who have retained their intestine and then undergo an enterectomy at the time of transplant, use of the native superior mesenteric vessels is feasible.

Transplantation of a larger composite graft (liver with intestine or multivisceral grafts) requires a bigger operation with more extensive dissection. In a similar fashion, the infrarenal aorta is exposed for placement of an arterial conduit graft (donor thoracic aorta) for arterialization of the graft. When the operation involves removal of the native liver, the venous drainage is achieved through the retained hepatic veins, which are fashioned to a single conduit for anastomosis to the allograft liver.

The intestinal anastomoses to native proximal and distal bowel are performed, leaving an ostomy of distal allograft ileum; this will be used for routine post-transplant surveillance endoscopy and biopsy. This ostomy is closed 3 to 6 mo post transplant (Fig. 336-2).

POSTOPERATIVE MANAGEMENT

IMMUNOSUPPRESSION. Immunosuppression for intestinal transplantation had been based on tacrolimus and corticosteroid induction. This required high levels of tacrolimus (in the nephrotoxic range), and although initial success rates were high, it was

TABLE 336-1. Causes of Intestinal Failure Requiring Transplantation

SHORT BOWEL	INTESTINAL DYSMOTILITY	ENTEROCYTE DYSFUNCTION	TUMORS
Necrotizing enterocolitis	Intestinal pseudo-obstruction	Microvillus inclusion disease	Familial polyposis
Gastroschisis	Intestinal aganglionosis (Hirschsprung disease)	Tufting enteropathy	Inflammatory pseudotumor
Volvulus		Autoimmune enteropathy	
Intestinal atresia			
Trauma			

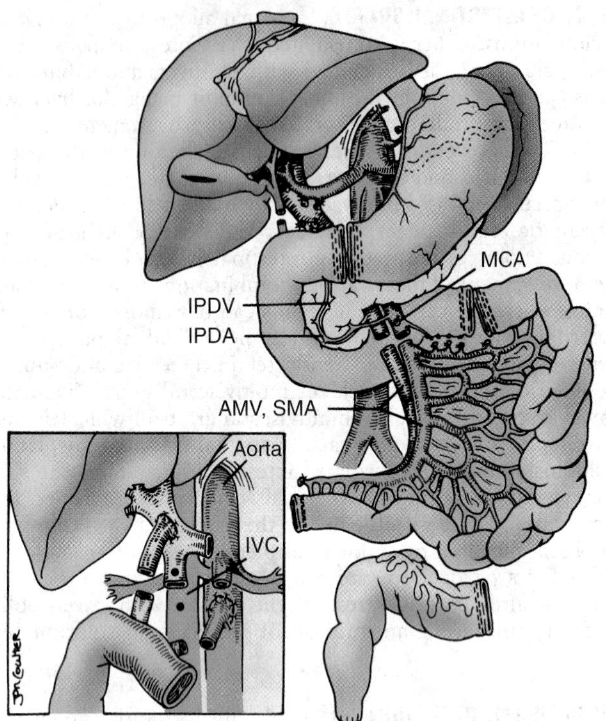

Figure 336-1. The various abdominal organs can be dissected in situ, providing isolated or composite grafts to fit the individual patient needs. Separation of intestine and pancreas is feasible, with preservation of the inferior pancreaticoduodenal artery (IPDA) and vein (IPDV). The use of vascular grafts from the donor allow for connections to the superior mesenteric pedicle (SMA and SMV) to aorta and inferior vena cava (IVC) or portal vein (inset). (Reproduced with permission from Abu-Elmagd K, Fung J, Bueno J, et al: Logistics and technique for procurement of intestinal, pancreatic and hepatic grafts from the same donor. *Ann Surg* 2000;232:680–697.)

followed by rejection rates of >80%, infection, and late drug toxicities. This has resulted in a gradual loss of patients and grafts in the course of 10 yr. The next protocols incorporated the addition of other agents such as azathioprine, cyclophosphamide, mycophenolate mofetil, rapamycin, and induction with an interleukin-2 (IL-2) antibody antagonist. This resulted in a decreased incidence in the severity of initial rejection; however, the ability to decrease immunosuppression later did not allow for stabilization of long-term survival. The introduction of recipient pretreatment using antilymphocyte antibodies and the elimination of recipient therapy with steroids have resulted in improved transplant survival, with a significant decrease in incidence of rejection and infection. This has permitted the gradual decrease of immunosuppressive drug therapy within 3 mo and a decline in drug toxicity events.

ALLOGRAFT ASSESSMENT. There are no simple laboratory tools that allow for assessment of the intestinal allograft. The gold standard for diagnosis of intestinal allograft rejection has been serial endoscopic surveillance and biopsies through the allograft ileostomy. Clinical signs and symptoms of rejection or infection of the allograft may overlap and mimic each other, producing either rapid diarrhea or complete ileus with pseudo-obstruction syndromes, or gastrointestinal bleeding. Any changes in clinical status should warrant thorough evaluation for rejection with endoscopic biopsies, as well as an evaluation for opportunistic infection, malabsorption, and other enteral infections.

The diagnosis of acute rejection is based on seeing destruction of crypt epithelial cells from apoptosis, in association with a mixed lymphocytic infiltrate. These histologic findings may or may not correlate with endoscopic evidence of injury, which varies from diffuse erythema and friability to ulcers and, in cases of severe rejection, exfoliation of the intestinal mucosa. Chronic rejection of the allograft can be diagnosed only through full thickness sampling of the intestine, which shows the typical vasculopathy that can result in progressive ischemia of the allograft.

REJECTION. Rejection rates for the intestinal allograft are significantly higher than with any other organ, in the range of 80–90%, and severe rejection requiring the use of antilymphocyte antibody preparations may be as high as 30%. Triple drug regimens and the utilization of IL-2 antibody inhibitors have resulted in significant decreases in rejection rates; nonetheless, the amount of immunosuppression was incompatible with improvements in long-term patient and graft survival. Rejection rates of 40% are achievable with the utilization of antilymphocyte globulin. These protocols induce varying degrees of "tolerance" and eventually minimize immunosuppression, thus reducing the risk of drug toxicity and infection.

INFECTIONS. The most common infections after intestinal transplantation occur as a result of the continuing need for venous catheter placement for as long as 1 yr post transplant. Infections as a consequence of immunosuppressive drug management are

Small Bowel Transplantation Surgery

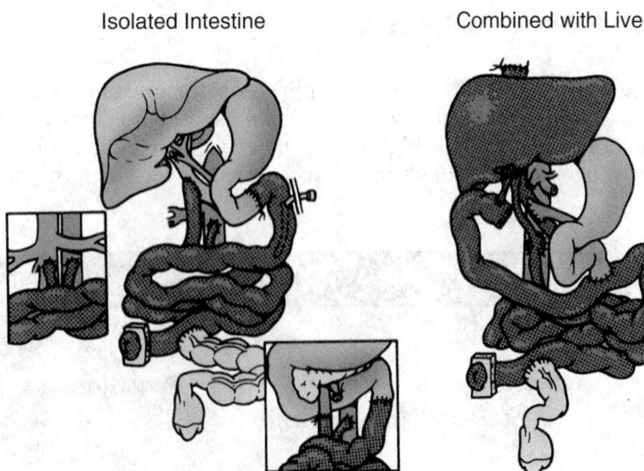

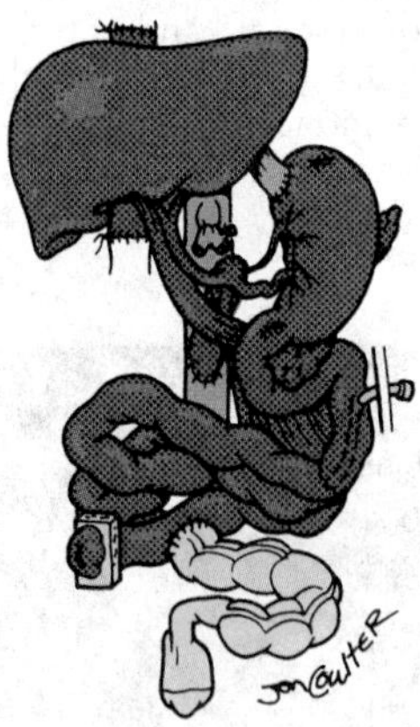

Figure 336-2. The three basic intestinal transplant procedures (the graft is *shaded*). With the isolated intestine, the venous outflow may be to the recipient portal vein *(main figure)*, inferior vena cava *(inset left)*, or superior mesenteric vein *(inset right)*. With the composite grafts, which include the liver, the arterialization is from the aorta with venous drainage out from the liver graft to the recipient inferior vena cava.

due to cytomegalovirus (CMV) infection (22% incidence), Epstein-Barr virus (EBV)–induced infections (21% incidence), and adenovirus enteritis (40% incidence). Successful management of these viral infections is achieved through early detection and preemptive therapy, both for CMV and EBV, before the development of a serious life-threatening infection. This has improved outcomes for CMV, eliminating the mortality in the pediatric patient population (see Chapters 177, 251, and 252).

OUTCOMES. Intestinal transplantation is the standard of care for children with intestinal failure who are suffering complications of total parenteral nutrition. Data from the International Transplant Registry, as well as center-specific data, have documented gradual improvements with short- and long-term survivals for transplantations occurring between 1990 and 2004. Medicare recognizes intestinal transplantation as a clinical standard of care. Intestinal transplantation survival rates are now 97% and 89% for 1 and 3 yrs, respectively. It is hoped that with the minimization strategies presently used, the long-term survival will plateau, as occurs with other organ transplants.

Abu-Elmagd K, Fung J, Bueno J, et al: Logistics and technique for procurement of intestinal, pancreatic and hepatic grafts from the same donor. *Ann Surg* 2000;232:680–697.

Bond G, Reyes J, Mazariegos G, et al: The impact of positive T-cell lymphocytotoxic crossmatch on intestinal allograft rejection and survival. *Transplant Proc* 2000;32:1197–1198.

Fishbein TW, Matsumoto CS: Intestinal replacement therapy: timing and indications for referral of patients to an intestinal rehabilitation and transplant program. *Gastroenterology* 2006;130:S147–S151.

Grant D, Abu-Elmagd K, Reyes J, et al: 2003 report of the Intestine Transplant Registry: A new era has dawned. *Ann Surg* 2005;241:607–613.

Green M, Reyes J, Webber S, Rowe D: The role of antiviral and immunoglobulin therapy in the prevention of Epstein-Barr virus infection and post-transplant lymphoproliferative disease following solid organ transplantation. *Transplant Infect Dis* 2001;3:97–103.

Kauffman SS, Atkinson JB, Bianchi A, et al: Indications for pediatric intestinal transplantation. *Pediatr Transplant* 2001;5:80–87.

Organ Procurement and Transplantation Network data (liver, kidney, and lung) website: http://www.optn.org/latestData/rptData.asp.

Reyes J, Mazariegos GV, Abu-Elmagd K, et al: Intestinal transplantation under tacrolimus monotherapy after perioperative lymphoid depletion with rabbit anti-thymocyte globulin (thymoglobulin). *Am J Transplant* 2005;5:1430–1436.

Reyes J, Mazariegos GV, Bond GM, et al: Pediatric intestinal transplantation: Historical notes, principles and controversies. *Pediatr Transplant* 2002;6:193–207.

Rogers J, Bueno J, Shapiro R, et al: Results of simultaneous and sequential pediatric liver and kidney transplantation. *Transplantation* 2001;72:1666–1670.

Chapter 337 ■ Acute Gastroenteritis in Children

Zulfiqar Ahmed Bhutta

The term *gastroenteritis* denotes infections of the gastrointestinal tract caused by bacterial, viral, or parasitic pathogens (Tables 337-1 to 337-3). Many of these infections are food-borne illnesses. The most common manifestations are diarrhea and vomiting, which may also be associated with systemic features such as abdominal pain and fever. The term **gastroenteritis** captures the bulk of infectious cases of diarrhea. The term **diarrheal disorders** is more commonly used to denote infectious diarrhea in public health settings, although several noninfectious causes of gastrointestinal illness with vomiting and/or diarrhea are well recognized (Table 337-4).

EPIDEMIOLOGY OF CHILDHOOD DIARRHEA

Diarrheal disorders in childhood account for a large proportion (18%) of childhood deaths, with an estimated 1.8 million deaths per year globally. The World Health Organization (WHO) suspects that there are >700 million episodes of diarrhea annually in children <5 yr of age in developing countries. While global mortality may be declining, the overall incidence of diarrhea remains unchanged at about 3.2 episodes per child year (Fig. 337-1). In the United States, there are ≈1.5 million outpatient visits for gastroenteritis, 200,000 hospitalizations, and 300 deaths annually.

Globally, it was estimated in 1999 that *Shigella* infections may lead to 600,000 deaths per year of children <5 yr of age, or a quarter to a third of all diarrhea-related mortality in this age group. Rates of hospitalization and deaths due to *Shigella* infections, especially *S. dysenteriae* type 1, the most severe form of shigellosis, may be declining; recent estimates are 160,000 deaths. Rotavirus infections (the most common identifiable viral cause of gastroenteritis in all children) account for at least 35% of severe and potentially fatal watery diarrhea episodes, with an estimated 500,000 deaths per year worldwide due to rotavirus infections.

The decline in diarrheal mortality, despite the lack of significant changes in incidence, is the result of improved case management of diarrhea, as well as improved nutrition of infants and children. These interventions have included widespread home- and hospital-based oral rehydration therapy, as well as improved nutritional management of children with diarrhea.

Persistently high rates of diarrhea among young children, despite intensive efforts at control, are of particular concern. There is very little information on the long-term consequences of diarrheal diseases, especially persistent or prolonged diarrhea and malnutrition. Diarrheal illnesses may have a significant impact on psychomotor and cognitive development in young children. Early and repeated episodes of childhood diarrhea during periods of critical development, especially when associated with malnutrition, co-infections, and anemia may have long-term effects on linear growth, as well as on physical and cognitive functions.

ETIOLOGY OF DIARRHEA

Gastroenteritis is due to infection acquired through the feco-oral route or by ingestion of contaminated food or water. Gastroenteritis is associated with poverty, poor environmental hygiene, and development indices. Enteropathogens that are infectious in a small inoculum (*Shigella, Escherichia coli,* noroviruses, rotavirus, *Giardia lamblia, Cryptosporidium parvum, Entamoeba histolytica*) can be transmitted by person-to-person contact, whereas others such as cholera are generally a consequence of contamination of food or water supply (see Tables 337-1 to 337-3). In the United States, rotavirus and the noroviruses (small round viruses such as Norwalk-like virus and caliciviruses) are the most common viral agents, followed by enteric adenoviruses and astroviruses (see Table 337-2). Food-borne outbreaks of diarrhea in the United States are most commonly due to *Salmonella* and *Campylobacter* species, followed much less often by *Shigella, Cryptosporidium, E. coli* 0157:H7, *Yersinia, Listeria, Vibrio,* and *Cyclospora* species, in that order. *Salmonella, Shigella,* and, most notably, the various diarrhea-producing *E. coli* organisms are the most common pathogens in developing countries (see Table 337-1). *Clostridium difficile* (by toxin production) is linked to antibiotic-associated diarrhea and pseudomembranous colitis, although most cases of antibiotic-associated diarrhea in children are not due to *C. difficile. C. dif-*

TABLE 337-1. Food-borne Illnesses (Bacterial)

ETIOLOGY	INCUBATION PERIOD	SIGNS AND SYMPTOMS	DURATION OF ILLNESS	ASSOCIATED FOODS	LABORATORY TESTING	TREATMENT
Bacillus anthracis	2 days to weeks	Nausea, vomiting, malaise, bloody diarrhea, acute abdominal pain	Weeks	Insufficiently cooked contaminated meat	Blood	Penicillin is first choice for naturally acquired gastrointestinal anthrax. Ciprofloxacin is second option.
Bacillus cereus (preformed enterotoxin)	1–6 hr	Sudden onset of severe nausea and vomiting. Diarrhea may be present.	24 hr	Improperly refrigerated cooked or fried rice, meats	Normally a clinical diagnosis. Clinical laboratories do not routinely identify this organism. If indicated, send stool and food specimens to reference laboratory for culture and toxin identification.	Supportive care
Bacillus cereus (diarrheal toxin)	10–16 hours	Abdominal cramps, watery diarrhea, nausea.	24–48 hr	Meats, stews, gravies, vanilla sauce	Testing not necessary, self-limiting (consider testing food and stool for toxin in outbreaks).	Supportive care
Brucella abortus, B. melitensis, and *B. suis*	7–21 days	Fever, chills, sweating, weakness, headache, muscle and joint pain, diarrhea, bloody stools during acute phase	Weeks	Raw milk, goat cheese made from unpasteurized milk, contaminated meats	Blood culture and positive serology	*Acute:* Rifampin and doxycycline daily for ≥6 wk. Infections with complications require combination therapy with rifampin, tetracycline, and an aminoglycoside.
Campylobacter jejuni	2–5 days	Diarrhea, cramps, fever, and vomiting; diarrhea may be bloody.	2–10 days	Raw and undercooked poultry, unpasturized milk, contaminated water	Routine stool culture; *Campylobacter* requires special media and incubation at 42°C to grow.	Supportive care. For severe cases, antibiotics such as erythromycin and quinolones may be indicated early in the diarrheal disease. Guillain-Barré syndrome can be a sequela.
Clostridium botulinum—children and adults (preformed toxin)	12–72 hr	Vomiting, diarrhea, blurred vision, diplopia, dysphagia, and descending muscle weakness	Variable (from days to months). Can be complicated by respiratory failure and death.	Home-canned foods with a low acid content, improperly canned commercial foods, home-canned or fermented fish, herb-infused oils, baked potatoes in aluminium foil, cheese sauce, bottled garlic, foods held warm for extended periods of time (e.g., in a warm oven)	Stool, serum, and food can be tested for toxin. Stool and food can also be cultured for the organism. These tests can be performed at some state health department laboratories and CDC.	Supportive care. Botulism antitoxin is helpful if given early in the course of the illness. Contact the state health department. The 24-hour number for state health departments to call is (700) 488-7100.
Clostridium botulinum—infants	3–30 days	In infants <12 mo, lethargy, weakness, poor feeding, constipation, hypotonia, poor head control, poor gag and sucking reflex	Variable	Honey, home-canned vegetables and fruits, corn syrup	Stool, serum, and food can be tested for toxin. Stool and food can also be cultured for the organism. These tests can be performed at some state health department laboratories and CDC.	Supportive care. Botulism immune globulin can be obtained from the Infant Botulism Prevention Program, Health and Human Services, California (510-540-2646), Botulinum antitoxin is generally not recommended for infants.
Clostridium perfringens toxin	8–16 hr	Watery diarrhea, nausea, abdominal cramps; fever is rare.	24–48 hr	Meats, poultry, gravy, dried or precooked foods, time- and/or temperature-abused food	Stools can be tested for enterotoxin and cultured for organism. Because *Clostridium perfringens* can normally be found in stool, quantitative cultures must be done.	Supportive care. Antibiotics not indicated.
Enterohemorrhagic *E. coli* (EHEC) including *E. coli* O157 : H7 and other *Shiga* toxin–producing *E. coli* (STEC)	1–8 days	Severe diarrhea that is often bloody, abdominal pain and vomiting. Usually, little or no fever is present. More common in children <4 yr old.	5–10 days	Undercooked beef especially hamburger, unpasteurized milk and juice, raw fruits and vegetables (e.g., sprouts), salami (rarely), and contaminated water	Stool culture; *E. coli* O157 : H7 requires special media to grow. If *E. coli* O157 : H7 is suspected, specific testing must be requested. *Shiga* toxin testing may be done using commercial kits; positive isolates should be forwarded to public health laboratories for confirmation and serotyping.	Supportive care, monitor renal function, hemoglobin, and platelets closely. *E. coli* O157 : H7 infection is also associated with hemolytic uremic syndrome (HUS), which can cause lifelong complications. Studies indicate that antibiotics may promote the development of HUS.
Enterotoxigenic *E. coli* (ETEC)	1–3 days	Watery diarrhea, abdominal cramps, some vomiting	3 to >7 days	Water or food contaminated with human feces	Stool culture. ETEC requires special laboratory techniques for identification. If suspected, must request specific testing.	Supportive care. Antibiotics are rarely needed except in severe cases. Recommended antibiotics include TMP-SMX and quinolones.
Listeria monocytogenes	9–48 hr for gastrointestinal symptoms, 2–6 wk for invasive disease	Fever, muscle aches, and nausea or diarrhea. Pregnant women may have mild flu-like illness, and infection can lead to premature delivery or stillbirth. Elderly or immunocompromised patients may have bacteremia or meningitis.	Variable	Fresh soft cheeses, unpasteurized milk, inadequately pasteurized milk, ready-to-eat deli meats, hot dogs	Blood or cerebrospinal fluid cultures. Asymptomatic fecal carriage occurs; therefore, stool culture usually not helpful. Antibody to listerolysin O may be helpful to identify outbreak retrospectively.	Supportive care and antibiotics; Intravenous ampicillin, penicillin, or TMP-SMX are recommended for invasive disease.
	At birth and infancy	Infants infected from mother at risk for sepsis or meningitis.				

TABLE 337-1.—*Cont'd.* Food-borne Illnesses (Bacterial)

Salmonella spp.	1–3 days	Diarrhea, fever, abdominal cramps, vomiting. *S. typhi* and *S. paratyphi* produce typhoid with insidious onset characterized by fever, headache, constipation, malaise, chills, and myalgia; diarrhea is uncommon, and vomiting is not usually severe.	4–7 days	Contaminated eggs, poultry, unpasteurized milk or juice, cheese, contaminated raw fruits and vegetables (alfalfa sprouts, melons). *S. typhi* epidemics are often related to fecal contamination of water supplies or street-vended foods.	Routine stool cultures	Supportive care. Other than for *S. typhi* and *S. paratyphi*, antibiotics are not indicated unless there is extra-intestinal spread, or the risk of extra-intestinal spread, of the infection. Consider ampicillin, gentamicin, TMP-SMX, or quinolones if indicated. A vaccine exists for *S. typhi*.
Shigella spp.	24–48 hr	Abdominal cramps, fever, and diarrhea. Stools may contain blood and mucus.	4–7 days	Food or water contaminated with human fecal material. Usually person-to-person spread, fecal-oral transmission. Ready-to-eat foods touched by infected food workers, e.g., raw vegetables, salads, sandwiches.	Routine stool cultures	Supportive care. TMP-SMX recommended in the U.S. if organism is susceptible; nalidixic acid or other quinolones may be indicated if organism is resistant, especially in developing countries.
Staphylococcus aureus (preformed enterotoxin)	1–6 hr	Sudden onset of severe nausea and vomiting. Abdominal cramps. Diarrhea and fever may be present.	24–48 hrs	Unrefrigerated or improperly refrigerated meats, potato and egg salads, cream pastries.	Normally a clinical diagnosis. Stool, vomitus, and food can be tested for toxin and cultured if indicated.	Supportive care.
Vibrio cholerae (toxin)	24–72 hr	Profuse watery diarrhea and vomiting, which can lead to severe dehydration and death within hours	3–7 days. Causes life-threatening dehydration.	Contaminated water, fish, shellfish, street-vended food typically from Latin America or Asia	Stool culture; *Vibrio cholerae* requires special media to grow. If *V. cholerae* is suspected, must request specific testing.	Supportive care with aggressive oral and intravenous rehydration. In cases of confirmed cholera, tetracycline or doxycycline is recommended for adults, and TMP-SMX for children (<8 yr).
Vibrio parahaemolyticus	2–48 hr	Watery diarrhea, abdominal cramps, nausea, vomiting.	2–5 days	Undercooked or raw seafood, such as fish, shellfish	Stool cultures. *Vibrio parahaemolyticus* requires special media to grow. If *V. parahaemolyticus* is suspected, must request specific testing.	Supportive care. Antibiotics are recommended in severe cases: tetracycline, doxycycline, gentamicin, and cefotaxime.
Vibrio vulnificus	1–7 days	Vomiting, diarrhea, abdominal pain, bactermia, and wound infections. More common in the immunocompromised, or in patients with chronic liver disease (presenting with bullous skin lesions). Can be fatal in patients with liver disease and the immunocompromised.	2–8 days	Undercooked or raw shellfish, especially oysters, other contaminated seafood, and open wounds exposed to seawater	Stool, wound, or blood cultures. *Vibrio vulnificus* requires special media to grow. If *V. vulnificus* is suspected, must request specific testing.	Supportive care and antibiotics; tetracycline, doxycycline, and ceftazidime are recommended.
Yersinia enterocolytica and *Y. pseudotuberculosis*	24–48 hr	Appendicitis-like symptoms (diarrhea and vomiting, fever, and abdominal pain) occur primarily in older children and young adults. May have a scarlitiniform rash or erythema nodosum with *Y. pseudotuberculosis*.	1–3 wk, usually self-limiting	Undercooked pork, unpasteurized milk, tofu, contaminated water. Infection has occurred in infants whose caregivers handled chitterlings.	Stool, vomitus, or blood culture. *Yersinia* requires special media to grow. If suspected, must request specific testing. Serology is available in research and reference laboratories.	Supportive care. If septicemia or other invasive disease occurs, antibiotic therapy with gentamicin or cefotaxime (doxycycline and ciprofloxacin also effective).

CDC, Centers for Disease Control and Prevention; TMP-SMX, trimethoprim-sulfamethoxazole.
From: Department of Health and Human Services, Centers for Disease Control and Prevention: Diagnosis and management of foodbourne illnesses. *MMWR* 2004:53:7–9.

ficile negative antibiotic associated hemorrhagic colitis in adults may be due to cytotoxin-producing *Klebsiella oxytoca*.

In developed countries, episodes of infectious diarrhea can occur through seasonal exposure to organisms such as rotavirus or exposure to pathogens in settings of close contact (e.g., daycare centers). Children in developing countries become infected with a diverse group of bacterial and parasitic pathogens, whereas all children in developed as well as developing countries acquire rotavirus and, in many cases, other viral enteropathogens as well as *G. lamblia* and *C. parvum* in their 1st 5 yr of life.

PATHOGENESIS OF INFECTIOUS DIARRHEA

Pathogenesis and severity of bacterial disease depend on whether organisms have preformed toxins *(Staphylococcus aureus, Bacillus cereus)*, produce toxins, or are invasive and on whether they replicate in food. Enteropathogens can lead to either an inflammatory or noninflammatory response in the intestinal mucosa.

Enteropathogens elicit **noninflammatory diarrhea** through **enterotoxin** production by some bacteria, destruction of villus (surface) cells by viruses, adherence by parasites, and adherence and/or translocation by bacteria. **Inflammatory diarrhea** is usually caused by bacteria that directly invade the intestine or produce cytotoxins with consequent fluid, protein, and cells (erythrocytes, leukocytes) that enter the intestinal lumen. Some enteropathogens possess more than one virulence property. Some viruses, such as rotavirus, target the microvillous tips of the enterocytes and can enter the cells by either direct invasion or calcium-dependent endocytosis. This can result in villus shortening and loss of enterocyte absorptive surface through cell shortening and loss of microvilli (Fig. 337-2).

Most bacterial pathogens elaborate enterotoxins; the rotavirus protein NSP4 acts as a viral enterotoxin. Bacterial enterotoxins

TABLE 337-2. Food-borne Illnesses (Viral)

ETIOLOGY	INCUBATION PERIOD	SIGNS AND SYMPTOMS	DURATION OF ILLNESS	ASSOCIATED FOODS	LABORATORY TESTING	TREATMENT
Hepatitis A	28 days average (15–50 days)	Diarrhea, dark urine, jaundice, and flu-like symptoms, i.e., fever, headache, nausea, and abdominal pain	Variable, 2 wk–3 mo	Shellfish harvested from contaminated waters, raw produce, contaminated nated drinking water, uncooked foods and cooked foods that are not reheated after contact with infected food handler	Increase in ALT, billirubin. Positive IgM and anti–hepatitis A antibodies.	Supportive care. Prevention with immunization.
Noroviruses (and other caliciviruses)	12–48 hr	Nausea, vomiting, abdominal cramping, diarrhea, fever, myalgia, and some headache. Diarrhea is more prevalent in adults and vomiting is more prevalent in children. Prolonged asymptomatic excretion possible.	12–60 hr	Shellfish, fecally contaminated foods, ready-to-eat foods touched by infected food workers (salads, sandwiches, ice, cookies, fruit)	Routine RT-PCR and EM on fresh unpreserved stool samples. Clinical diagnosis, negative bacterial cultures. Stool is negative for WBCs.	Supportive care such as rehydration. Good hygiene.
Rotavirus	1–3 days	Vomiting, watery diarrhea, low-grade fever. Temporary lactose intolerance may occur. Infants and children, elderly, and immunocompromised are especially vulnerable.	4–8 days	Fecally contaminated foods. Ready-to-eat foods touched by infected food workers (salads, fruits).	Identification of virus in stool via immunoassay	Supportive care. Severe diarrhea may require fluid and electrolyte replacement.
Other viral agents (astroviruses, adenoviruses, parvoviruses)	10–70 hr	Nausea, vomiting, diarrhea, malaise, abdominal pain, headache, fever	2–9 days	Fecally contaminated foods. Ready-to-eat foods touched by infected food workers. Some shellfish.	Identification of the virus in early acute stool samples. Serology. Commercial ELISA kits are now available for adenoviruses and astroviruses.	Supportive care, usually mild, self-limiting. Good hygiene.

ALT, alanine aminotransferase; ELISA, enzyme linked immunoserbent assay; EM, electron microscopy; IgM, immunoglobulin M; RT-PCR, reverse transcriptose polymerase chain reaction; WBCs, white blood cells.
From: Department of Health and Human Services, Centers for Disease Control and Prevention: Diagnosis and management of foodbourne illnesses. *MMWR* 2004:53:9.

can selectively activate enterocyte intracellular signal transduction, and can also affect cytoskeletal rearrangements with subsequent alterations in the water and electrolyte fluxes across enterocytes. Upregulation of these pathways results in inhibition of NaCl-coupled transport and increased efflux of chloride, resulting, in turn, in net secretion and loss of water into the intestinal lumen (Fig. 337-3). Coupled transport of sodium to glucose and amino acids is largely unaffected. The nitric oxide pathway can also be involved, as endogenous nitric oxide production is significantly higher in infectious compared with noninfectious diarrhea.

Enterotoxigenic *E. Coli* (ETEC) colonizes and adheres to enterocytes of the small bowel via its surface fimbriae (pili) and induces hypersecretion of fluids and electrolytes into the small intestine through one of two toxins: the heat-labile enterotoxin (LT) or the heat-stable enterotoxin. LT is structurally similar to

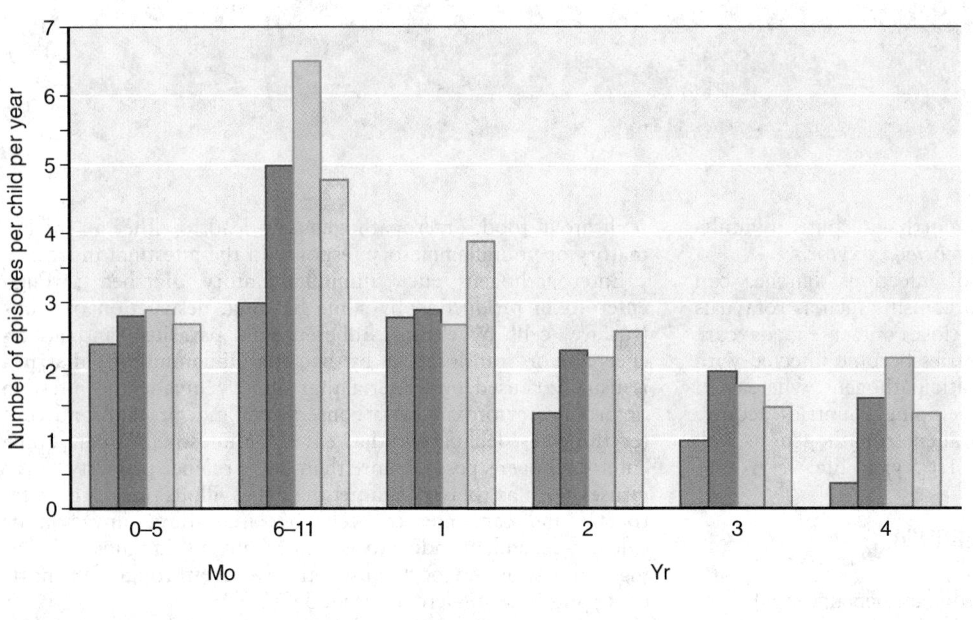

Figure 337-1. Global trends in diarrhea incidence.

TABLE 337-3. Food-borne Illnesses (Parasitic)

ETIOLOGY	INCUBATION PERIOD	SIGNS AND SYMPTOMS	DURATION OF ILLNESS	ASSOCIATED FOODS	LABORATORY TESTING	TREATMENT
Angiostrongylus cantonensis	1 wk to ≥1 mo	Severe headaches, nausea, vomiting, neck stiffness, paresthesias, hyperesthesias, seizures, and other neurologic abnormalities	Several weeks to several months	Raw or undercooked intermediate hosts (e.g., snails or slugs), infected paratenic (transport) hosts (e.g., crabs, freshwater shrimp), fresh produce contaminated with intermediate or transport hosts	Examination of CSF for elevated pressure, protein, leukocytes, and eosinophils; serologic testing using ELISA to detect antibodies to *Angiostrongylus cantonensis*	Supportive care. Repeat lumbar punctures and use of corticosteroid therapy may be used for more severely ill patients.
Cryptosporidium	2–10 days	Diarrhea (usually watery), stomach cramps, upset stomach, slight fever	May be remitting and relapsing over weeks to months	Any uncooked food or food contaminated by an ill food handler after cooking; drinking water	Request specific examination of the stool for *Cryptosporidium*. May need to examine water or food.	Supportive care, self-limited. If severe consider paromomycin for 7 days. For children aged 1–11 yr, consider nitazoxanide for 3 days.
Cyclospora cayetanensis	1–14 days, usually at least 1 wk	Diarrhea (usually watery), loss of appetite, substantial loss of weight, stomach cramps, nausea, vomiting, fatigue	May be remitting and relapsing over weeks to months	Various types of fresh produce (imported berries, lettuce)	Request specific examination of the stool for *Cyclospora*. May need to examine water or food.	TMP-SMX for 7 days.
Entamoeba histolytica	2–3 days to 1–4 wk	Diarrhea (often bloody), frequent bowel movements, lower abdominal pain	May be protracted (several weeks to several months)	Any uncooked food or food contaminated by an ill food handler after cooking; drinking water	Examination of stool for cysts and parasites—may need at least 3 samples. Serology for long-term infections.	Metronidazole and a luminal agent (iodoquinol or paromomycin)
Giardia lamblia	1–2 wk	Diarrhea, stomach cramps, gas, weight loss	Days to weeks	Any uncooked food or food contaminated by an ill food handler after cooking; drinking water.	Examination of stool for ova and parasites—may need at least 3 samples.	Metronidazole
Toxoplasma gondii	5–23 days	Generally asymptomatic, 20% may develop cervical lymphadenopathy and/or a flu-like illness. In immunocompromised patients: central nervous system (CNS) disease, myocarditis, or pneumonitis is often seen.	Months	Accidental ingestion of contaminated substances (e.g., soil contaminated with cat feces on fruits and vegetables), raw or partly cooked meat (especially pork, lamb, or venison)	Isolation of parasites from blood or other body fluids; observation of parasites in patient specimens via microscopy or histology. Detection of organisms is rare; serology (reference laboratory needed) can be a useful adjunct in diagnosing toxoplasmosis. However, IgM antibodies may persist for 6–18 mo and thus may not necessarily indicate recent infection. PCR of bodily fluids. For congenital infection: isolation of *T. gondii* from placenta, umbilical cord, or infant blood. PCR of white blood cells, CSF, or amniotic fluid, or IgM and IgA serology, performed by a reference laboratory.	Asymptomatic healthy, but infected, persons do not require treatment. Spiramycin or pyrimethamine plus sulfadiazine may be used for pregnant women. Pyrimethamine plus sulfadiazine may be used for immunocompromised persons, in specific cases. Pyrimethamine plus sulfadiazine (with or without steroids) may be given for ocular disease when indicated. Folinic acid is given with pyrimethamine plus sulfadiazine to counteract bone marrow suppression.
Toxoplasma gondii (congenital infection)	In infants at birth	Treatment of the mother may reduce severity and/or incidence of congenital infection. Most infected infants have few symptoms at birth. Later, they will generally develop signs of congenital toxoplasmosis (mental retardation, severely impaired eyesight, cerebral palsy, seizures), unless the infection is treated	Months	Passed from mother (who acquired acute infection during pregnancy) to child		
Trichinella spiralis	1–2 days for initial symptoms; others begin 2–8 wk after infection	Acute: nausea, diarrhea, vomiting, fatigue, fever, abdominal discomfort followed by muscle soreness, weakness, and occasional cardiac and neurologic complications	Months	Raw or undercooked contaminated meat, usually pork or wild game meat (e.g., bear or moose)	Positive serology or demonstration of larvae via muscle biopsy. Increase in eosinophils.	Supportive care plus mebendazole or albendazole

CSF, cerebrospinal fluid; ELISA, enzyme linked immunoserbent assay; IgM, immunoglobulin M; PCR, polymerase chain reaction; TMP-SMX, trimethoprim-sulfamethoxazole.
From: Department of Health and Human Services, Centers for Disease Control and Prevention: Diagnosis and management of foodbourne illnesses. *MMWR* 2004:53:9–10.

the *Vibrio cholera* toxin, and activates adenylate cyclase, resulting in an increase in intracellular cyclic guanosine monophosphate (cGMP) (see Fig. 337-3). In contrast, *Shigella* spp. cause gastroenteritis via a superficial invasion of colonic mucosa, which they invade through M cells located over Peyer patches. After phagocytosis, a series of events occurs, including apoptosis of macrophages, multiplication and spread of bacteria into adjacent cells, release of inflammatory mediators (interleukin [IL]-1 and IL-8), transmigration of neutrophils into the lumen of the colon, neutrophil necrosis and degranulation, further breach of the epithelial barrier, and mucosal destruction (Fig. 337-4).

RISK FACTORS FOR GASTROENTERITIS

Major risks include environmental contamination and increased exposure to enteropathogens. Additional risks include young age, immune deficiency, measles, malnutrition, and lack of exclusive

TABLE 337-4. Food-borne Illnesses (Noninfectious)

ETIOLOGY	INCUBATION PERIOD	SIGNS AND SYMPTOMS	DURATION OF ILLNESS	ASSOCIATED FOODS	LABORATORY TESTING	TREATMENT
Antimony	5 min–8 hr usually <1 hr	Vomiting, metallic taste	Usually self-limited	Metallic container	Identification of metal in beverage or food	Supportive care
Arsenic	Few hours	Vomiting, colic, diarrhea	Several days	Contaminated food	Urine. May cause eosinophilia	Gastric lavage, BAL (dimercaprol)
Cadmium	5 min–8 hr usually <1 hr	Nausea, vomiting, myalgia, increase in salivation, stomach pain	Usually self-limited	Seafood, oysters, clams, lobster, grains, peanuts	Identification of metal in food	Supportive care
Ciguatera fish poisoning (ciguatera toxin)	2–6 hr	GI: abdominal pain, nausea, vomiting, diarrhea	Days to weeks to months	A variety of large reef fish: grouper, red snapper, amberjack, and barracuda (most common)	Radioassay for toxin in fish or a consistent history	Supportive care, IV mannitol. Children more vulnerable.
	3 hr	Neurologic: paresthesias, reversal of hot or cold, pain, weakness				
	2–5 days	Cardiovascular: bradycardia, hypotension, increase in T wave abnormalities				
Copper	5 min–8 hr usually <1 hr	Nausea, vomiting, blue or green vomitus	Usually self-limited	Metallic container	Identification of metal in beverage or food	Supportive care
Mercury	1 wk or longer	Numbness, weakness of legs, spastic paralysis, impaired vision, blindness, coma. Pregnant women and the developing fetus are especially vulnerable.	May be protracted	Fish exposed to organic mercury, grains treated with mercury fungicides	Analysis of blood, hair	Supportive care
Mushroom toxins, short-acting (museinol, muscarine, psilocybin, *Coprius artemetaris*, ibotenic acid)	<2 hr	Vomiting, diarrhea, confusion, visual disturbance, salivation, diaphoresis, hallucinations, disulfiram-like reaction, confusion, visual disturbance.	Self-limited	Wild mushrooms (cooking may not destroy these toxins)	Typical syndrome and mushroom identified or demonstration of the toxin	Supportive care
Mushroom toxins, long-acting (amanitin)	4–8 hr diarrhea; 24–48 hr liver failure	Diarrhea, abdominal cramps, leading to hepatic and renal failure	Often fatal	Mushrooms	Typical syndrome and mushroom identified and/or demonstration of the toxin	Supportive care, life-threatening, may need life support
Nitrite poisoning	1–2hr	Nausea, vomiting, cyanosis, headache, dizziness, weakness, loss of consciousness, chocolate-brown colored blood	Usually self-limited	Cured meats, any contaminated foods, spinach exposed to excessive nitrification	Analysis of the food, blood	Supportive care, methylene blue
Pesticides (organophosphates or carbamates	Few min to few hours	Nausea, vomiting, abdominal cramps, diarrhea, headache, nervousness, blurred vision, twitching, convulsions, salivation and meiosis	Usually self-limited	Any contaminated food	Analysis of the food, blood	Atropine; 2-PAM (Pralidoxime) is used when atropine is not able to control symptoms and is rarely necessary in carbamate poisoning.
Puffer fish (tetrodotoxin)	<30 min	Parasthesias, vomiting, diarrhea, abdominal pain, ascending paralysis, respiratory failure	Death usually in 4–6 hr	Puffer fish	Detection of tetrodotoxin in fish	Life-threatening, may need respiratory support
Scombroid (histamine)	1 min–3 hr	Flushing, rash, burning sensation of skin, mouth and throat, dizziness, urticaria, parasthesias	3–6 hr	Fish: bluefin, tuna, skipjack, mackerel, marlin, escolar, and mahi mahi	Demonstration of histamine in food or clinical diagnosis	Supportive care, antihistamines
Shellfish toxins (diarrheic, neurotoxic, amnesic)	Diarrheic shellfish poisoning (DSP)—30 min to 2 hr	Nausea, vomiting, diarrhea, and abdominal pain accompanied by chills, headache, and fever	Hours to 2–3 days	A variety of shellfish, primarily mussels, oysters, scallops, and shellfish from the Florida coast and the Gulf of Mexico	Detection of the toxin in shellfish; high-pressure liquid chromatography	Supportive care, generally self-limiting. Elderly are especially sensitive to ASP
	Neurotoxic shellfish poisoning (NSP)—few min to hours	Tingling and numbness of lips, tongue, and throat, muscular aches, dizziness, reversal of the sensations of hot and cold, diarrhea, and vomiting				
	Amnesic shellfish poisoning (ASP)—24–48 hr	Vomiting, diarrhea, abdominal pain and neurologic problems such as confusion, memory loss, disorientation, seizure, coma				
Shellfish toxins (paralytic shellfish poisoning)	30 min–3 hr	Diarrhea, nausea, vomiting leading to parasthesias of mouth, lips, weakness, dysphasia, dysphonia, respiratory paralysis	Days	Scallops, mussels, clams, cockles	Detection of toxin in food or water where fish are located; high-pressure liquid chromatography	Life-threatening, may need respiratory support
Sodium fluoride	Few min to 2 hr	Salty or soapy taste, numbness of mouth, vomiting, diarrhea, dilated pupils, spasms, pallor, shock, collapse	Usually self-limited	Dry foods (e.g., dry milk, flour, baking powder, cake mixes) contaminated with sodium fluoride–containing insecticides and rodenticides	Testing of vomitus or gastric washings. Analysis of the food.	Supportive care
Thallium	Few hours	Nausea, vomiting, diarrhea, painful parathesias, motor polyneuropathy, hair loss	Several days	Contaminated food	Urine, hair	Supportive care
Tin	5 min–8 hr usually <1 hr	Nausea, vomiting, diarrhea	Usually self-limited	Metallic container	Analysis of the food	Supportive care
Vomitoxin	Few min to 3 hr	Nausea, headache, abdominal pain, vomiting	Usually self-limited	Grains such as wheat, corn, barley	Analysis of the food	Supportive care
Zinc	Few hours	Stomach cramps, nausea, vomiting, diarrhea, myalgias	Usually self-limited	Metallic container	Analysis of the food, blood and feces, saliva or urine	Supportive care

From: Department of Health and Human Services, Centers for Disease Control and Prevention: Diagnosis and management of foodbourne illnesses. *MMWR* 2004:53:11–12.

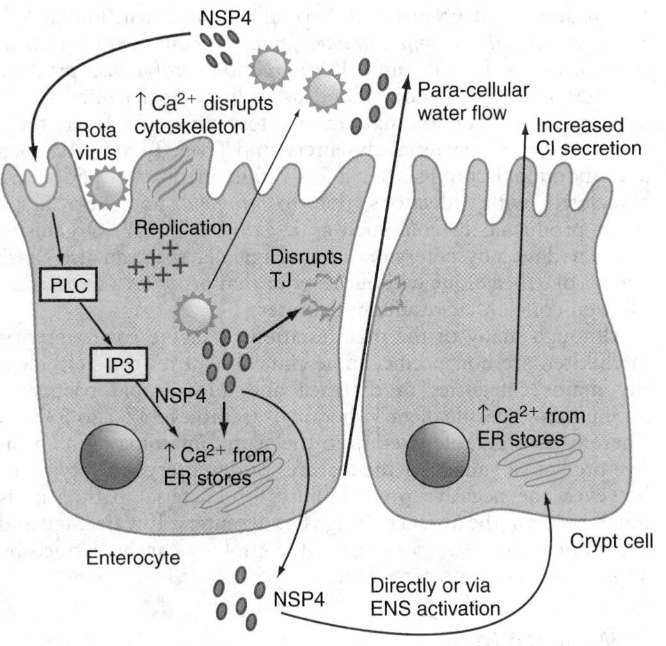

Figure 337-2. Pathogenesis of rotavirus infection and diarrhea. ER, endoplasmic reticulum; TJ, tight junction. (Adapted from Ramig RF: Pathogenesis of intestinal and systemic rotavirus infection. *J Virol* 2004;78:10213–10220.)

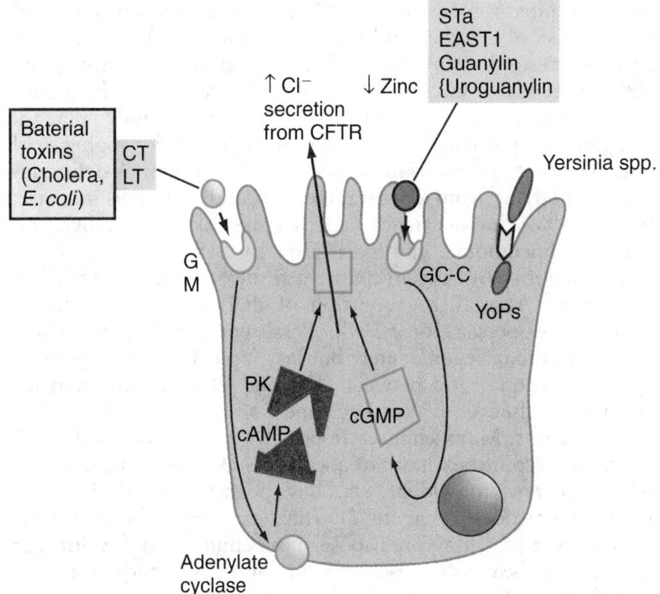

Figure 337-3. Mechanism of cholera toxin. (Adapted from Thapar M, Sanderson IR: Diarrhoea in children: An interface between developing and developed countries. *Lancet* 2004;363:641–653; and Montes M, DuPont HL: Enteritis, enterocolitis and infectious diarrhea syndromes. In Cohen J, Powderly WG, Opal SM, et al [editors]: *Infections Diseases,* 2nd ed. London, Mosby, 2004, pp 31–52.)

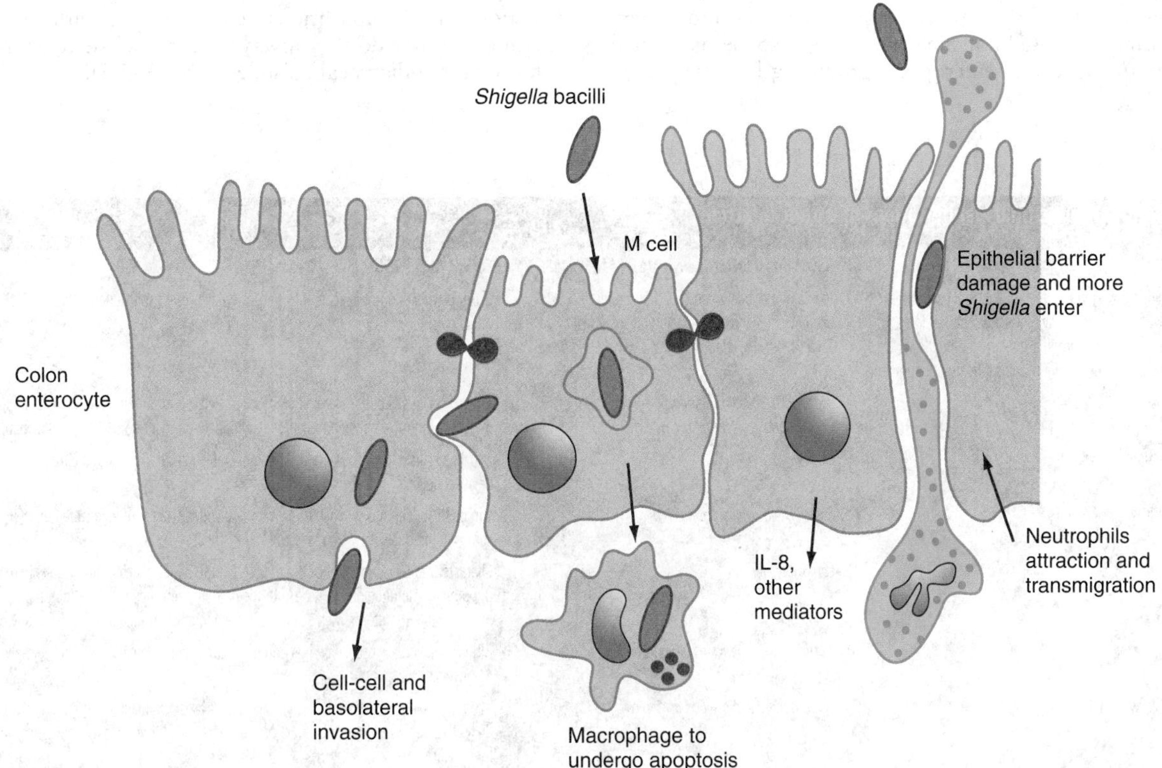

Figure 337-4. Pathogenesis of *Shigella* infection and diarrhea. (Adapted from Opal SM, Keusch GT: Host responses to infection. In Cohen J, Powderly WG, Opal SM, et al [editors]: *Infections Diseases,* 2nd ed. London, Mosby, 2004, pp 31–52.)

or predominant breast-feeding. Malnutrition increases severalfold the risk of diarrhea and associated mortality. The fraction of such infectious diarrhea deaths that are attributable to nutritional deficiencies varies with the prevalence of deficiencies; the highest attributable fractions are in sub-Saharan Africa, south Asia, and Andean Latin America. The risks are particularly higher with micronutrient malnutrition; in children with **vitamin A deficiency,** the risk of dying from diarrhea, measles, and malaria is increased by 20–24%. **Zinc deficiency** increases the risk of mortality from diarrhea, pneumonia, and malaria by 13–21%.

The majority of cases of diarrhea resolve within the 1st wk of the illness. A smaller proportion of diarrheal illnesses fail to resolve and persist for >2 wk. **Persistent diarrhea** is defined as episodes that began acutely but last for at least 14 days. Such episodes account for between 3% and 20% of all diarrheal episodes in children <5 yr of age and up to 50% of all diarrhea-related deaths. Many children (especially infants and toddlers) in developing countries have frequent episodes of acute diarrhea. Although few individual episodes persist beyond 14 days, frequent episodes of acute diarrhea can result in nutritional compromise and may predispose these children to develop persistent diarrhea, protein-calorie malnutrition, and secondary infections.

CLINICAL MANIFESTATION OF DIARRHEA

Most of the clinical manifestations and clinical syndromes of diarrhea are related to the infecting pathogen and the dose/inoculum (see Tables 337-1 to 337-3). Additional manifestations depend on the development of complications (such as dehydration and electrolyte imbalance) and the nature of the infecting pathogen (see Chapter 55.1). Usually the ingestion of preformed toxins (such as those of *Staphylococcus aureus*) is associated with the rapid onset of nausea and vomiting within 6 hr, with possible fever, abdominal cramps, and diarrhea within 8–72 hr. Watery diarrhea and abdominal cramps after an 8–16 hr incubation period are associated with enterotoxin-producing *Clostridium perfringens* and *Bacillus cereus.* Abdominal cramps and watery diarrhea after a 16–48 hr incubation period can be associated with noroviruses, several enterotoxin-producing bacteria, *Cryptosporidium,* and *Cyclospora.* Several organisms, including *Salmonella, Shigella, Campylobacter jejuni, Yersinia enterocolitica,* enteroinvasive *E. coli,* and *Vibrio parahaemolyticus,* produce diarrhea that can contain blood as well as fecal leukocytes in association with abdominal cramps, tenesmus, and fever; these features suggest **bacterial dysentery** and fever. Bloody diarrhea and abdominal cramps after a 72–120 hr incubation period are associated with infections due to *Shigella* and also Shiga toxin–producing *E. coli,* such as *E. coli* 0157 : H7. Organisms associated with dysentery or hemorrhagic diarrhea can also cause watery diarrhea alone without fever or that precedes a more complicated course that results in dysentery.

Although many of the manifestations of acute gastroenteritis in children are nonspecific, some clinical features can help identify major categories of diarrhea and allow rapid triage for antibiotic or specific dietary therapy (see Tables 337-1 to 337-3). There is considerable overlap in the symptomatology. The positive predictive values for the features of dysentery are very poor; however, the negative predictability for bacterial pathogens is much better in the absence of signs of dysentery. If warranted and if facilities and resources permit, the etiology can be verified by appropriate laboratory testing.

COMPLICATIONS

Most of the complications associated with gastroenteritis are related to delays in diagnosis and delays in the institution of appropriate therapy. Without early and appropriate rehydration, many children with acute diarrhea would develop dehydration with associated complications (see Chapters 53, 54, 55, and 68). These can be life-threatening in infants and young children. Inappropriate therapy can lead to prolongation of the diarrheal episodes, with consequent malnutrition and complications such as secondary infections and micronutrient deficiencies (iron, zinc). In developing countries, associated bacteremias are well-recognized complications in malnourished children with diarrhea.

Specific pathogens are associated with extra-intestinal manifestations and complications. These are not pathognomonic of the infection nor do they always occur in close temporal association with the diarrheal episode (Table 337-5).

TABLE 337-5. Extraintestinal Manifestations of Enteric Infections

MANIFESTATION	ASSOCIATED ENTERIC PATHOGEN(S)	ONSET AND PROGNOSIS
Focal infections due to systemic spread of bacterial pathogens, including vulvovaginitis, urinary tract infection, endocarditis, osteomyelitis, meningitis, pneumonia, hepatitis, peritonitis, chorioamnionitis, soft tissue infection, and septic thrombophlebitis	All major pathogens can cause such direct extraintestinal infections, including *Salmonella, Shigella, Yersinia, Campylobacter, Clostridium difficile*	Onset usually during the acute infection, but may present subsequently. Prognosis depends on infection site.
Reactive arthritis	*Salmonella, Shigella, Yersinia, Campylobacter, Cryptosporidium, Clostridium difficile*	Typically occurs about 1–3 wk after infection. Relapses after reinfection may develop in 15–50% of people but most children recover fully within 2–6 mo after the 1st symptoms appear.
Guillain-Barré syndrome	*Campylobacter*	Usually occurs a few weeks after the original infection. Prognosis good although 15–20% may have sequelae.
Glomerulonephritis	*Shigella, Campylobacter, Yersinia*	Can be of sudden onset in acute, referring to a sudden attack of inflammation, or chronic, which comes on gradually. In most cases, the kidneys heal with time.
IgA nephropathy	*Campylobacter*	Characterized by recurrent episodes of blood in the urine, this condition results from deposits of the protein immunoglobulin A (IgA) in the glomeruli. IgA nephropathy can progress for years with no noticeable symptoms. Men seem more likely to develop this disorder than are women.
Erythema nodosum	*Yersinia, Campylobacter, Salmonella*	Although painful, is usually benign and more commonly seen in adolescents. Resolves with 4–6 weeks.
Hemolytic uremia syndrome	*Shigella dysenteriae* 1, *Escherichia coli* 0157:H7, others	Sudden onset, short-term renal failure. In severe cases, renal failure requires several sessions of dialysis to take over the kidney function, but most children recover without permanent damage to their health.
Hemolytic anemia	*Campylobacter, Yersinia*	Relatively rare complication and may have a chronic course.

From: Department of Health and Human Services, Centers for Disease Control and Prevention: Managing acute gastroenteritis among children. *MMWR Recomm Rep* 2004; 53:1–33.

TABLE 337-6. Symptoms Associated with Dehydration

SYMPTOM	MINIMAL OR NO DEHYDRATION (<3% LOSS OF BODY WEIGHT)	MILD TO MODERATE DEHYDRATION (3–9% LOSS OF BODY WEIGHT)	SEVERE DEHYDRATION (>9% LOSS OF BODY WEIGHT)
Mental status	Well; alert	Normal, fatigued or restless, irritable	Apathetic, lethargic, unconscious
Thirst	Drinks normally; might refuse liquids	Thirsty; eager to drink	Drinks poorly; unable to drink
Heart rate	Normal	Normal to increased	Tachycardia, with bradycardia in most severe cases
Quality of pulses	Normal	Normal to decreased	Weak, thready, or impalpable
Breathing	Normal	Normal; fast	Deep
Eyes	Normal	Slightly sunken	Deeply sunken
Tears	Present	Decreased	Absent
Mouth and tongue	Moist	Dry	Parched
Skinfold	Instant recoil	Recoil in <2 sec	Recoil in >2 sec
Capillary refill	Normal	Prolonged	Prolonged; minimal
Extremities	Warm	Cool	Cold; mottled; cyanotic
Urine output	Normal to decreased	Decreased	Minimal

Sources: Adapted from Duggan C, Santosham M, Glass RI: The management of acute diarrhea in children: Oral rehydration, maintenance, and nutritional therapy. *MMWR* 1992;41 (No. RR-16):1–20; and World Health Organization: The treatment of diarrhoea: a manual for physicians and other senior health workers. Geneva, Switzerland: World Health Organization, 1995. Available at http://www.who.int/child-adolescent-health/New_Publications/CHILD_HEALTH/WHO.CDR.95.3.htm.
From: Department of Health and Human Services, Centers for Disease Control and Prevention: Diagnosis and management of foodbourne illnesses. *MMWR* 2004:52;5.

DIAGNOSIS

The diagnosis of gastroenteritis is based on clinical recognition, an evaluation of its severity by rapid assessment, and confirmation by appropriate laboratory investigations, if indicated.

CLINICAL EVALUATION OF DIARRHEA. The most common manifestation of gastrointestinal tract infection in children is diarrhea, abdominal cramps, and vomiting. Systemic manifestations are varied and associated with a variety of causes. The evaluation of a child with acute diarrhea includes:

Assess the degree of dehydration and acidosis and provide rapid resuscitation and rehydration with oral or intravenous fluids as required (Tables 337-6 and 337-7).

Obtain appropriate contact or exposure history. This includes information on exposure to contacts with similar symptoms, intake of contaminated foods or water, child-care center attendance, recent travel to a diarrhea-endemic area, and use of antimicrobial agents.

Clinically determine the etiology of diarrhea for institution of prompt antibiotic therapy, if indicated. Although nausea and vomiting are nonspecific symptoms, they are indicative of infection in the upper intestine. Fever is suggestive of an inflammatory process but also occurs as a result of dehydration or co-infection (e.g., urinary tract infection, otitis media). Fever is common in patients with inflammatory diarrhea. Severe abdominal pain and tenesmus are indicative of involvement of the large intestine and rectum. Features such as nausea and vomiting and absent or low-grade fever with mild to moderate periumbilical pain and watery diarrhea are indicative of small intestine involvement and also reduce the likelihood of a serious bacterial infection.

This clinical approach to the diagnosis and management of diarrhea in young children is a critical component of the **integrated management of childhood illness** (IMCI) package that is being implemented in developing countries with high burden of diarrhea mortality (Fig. 337-5).

STOOL EXAMINATION. Microscopic examination of the stool and cultures can yield important information on the etiology of diarrhea. Stool specimens should be examined for mucus, blood, and leukocytes. Fecal leukocytes are indicative of bacterial invasion of colonic mucosa, although some patients with shigellosis have minimal leukocytes at an early stage of infection, as do patients infected with Shiga toxin–producing *E. coli* and *E. histolytica*. In endemic areas, stool microscopy must include examination for parasites causing diarrhea, such as *G. lamblia* and *E. histolytica*.

Stool cultures should be obtained as early in the course of disease as possible from children with **bloody diarrhea** in whom stool microscopy indicates **fecal leukocytes;** in **outbreaks** with suspected **hemolytic-uremic syndrome** (HUS); and in **immunosuppressed** children with diarrhea. Stool specimens for culture need to be transported and plated quickly; if the latter is not quickly available, specimens may need to be transported in special media. The yield and diagnosis of bacterial diarrhea can be significantly improved by using molecular diagnostic procedures such as PCR. In most previously healthy children with uncomplicated watery diarrhea, no laboratory evaluation is needed except for epidemiologic purposes.

TREATMENT

The broad principles of management of acute gastroenteritis in children include oral rehydration therapy, enteral feeding and diet

TABLE 337-7. Summary of Treatment Based on Degree of Dehydration

DEGREE OF DEHYDRATION	REHYDRATION THERAPY	REPLACEMENT OF LOSSES	NUTRITION
Minimal or no dehydration	Not applicable	<10 kg body weight: 60–120 mL oral rehydration solution (ORS) for each diarrheal stool or vomiting episode; >10 kg body weight: 120–240 mL ORS for each diarrheal stool or vomiting episode	Continue breast-feeding, or resume age-appropriate normal diet after initial hydration, including adequate caloric intake for maintenance*
Mild to moderate dehydration	ORS, 50–100 mL/kg body weight over 3–4 hr	Same	Same
Severe dehydration	Lactated Ringer solution or normal saline in 20 mL/kg body weight intravenous amounts until perfusion and mental status improve; then administer 100 mL/kg body weight ORS over 4 hr or 5% dextrose ½ normal saline intravenously at twice maintenance fluid rates	Same; if unable to drink, administer through nasogastric tube or administer 5% dextrose ¼ normal saline with 20 mEq/L potassium chloride intravenously	Same

*Overly restricted diets should be avoided during acute diarrheal episodes. Breast-fed infants should continue to nurse ad libitum even during acute rehydration. Infants too weak to eat can be given milk or formula through a nasogastric tube. Lactose-containing formulas are usually well tolerated. If lactose malabsorption appears clinically substantial, lactose-free formulas can be used. Complex carbohydrates, fresh fruits, lean meats, yogurt, and vegetables are all recommended. Carbonated drinks or commercial juices with a high concentration of simple carbohydrates should be avoided.
From: Department of Health and Human Services, Centers for Disease Control and Prevention: Diagnosis and management of foodbourne illnesses. *MMWR* 2004;52:1–33.

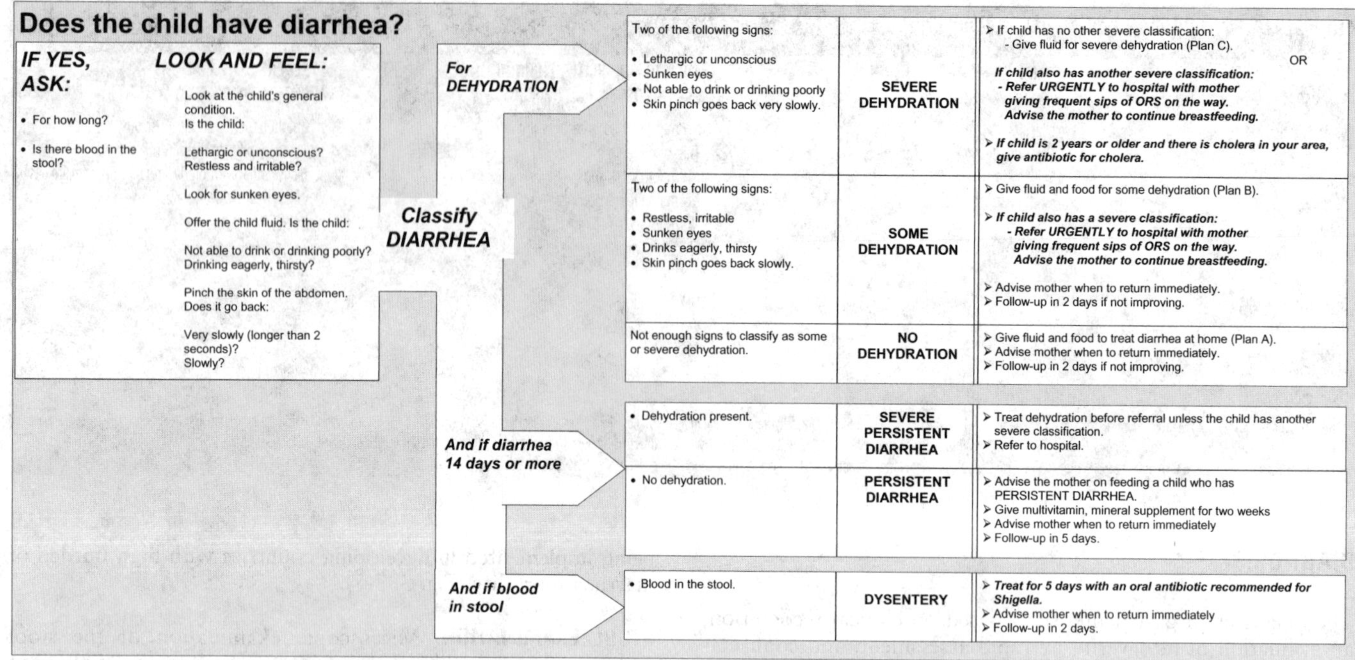

Figure 337-5. Integrated management of the sick child (IMCI) protocol for the recognition and management of diarrhea in developing countries.

selection, zinc supplementation, and additional therapies such as probiotics.

ORAL REHYDRATION THERAPY. Children, especially infants, are more susceptible than adults to dehydration because of the greater basal fluid and electrolyte requirements per kg and because they are dependent on others to meet these demands. **Dehydration** must be evaluated rapidly and corrected in 4–6 hr according to the degree of dehydration and estimated daily requirements. A small minority of children, especially those in shock or unable to tolerate oral fluids, require initial intravenous rehydration, but oral rehydration is the preferred mode of rehydration and replacement of ongoing losses (Tables 337-7 and 337-8). Risks associated with severe dehydration that may necessitate intravenous resuscitation include: age <6 mo, prematurity, chronic illness, fever >38°C if < 3 mo or >39°C if 3–36 mo, bloody diarrhea, persistent emesis, poor urine output, sunken eyes, and a depressed level of consciousness. Although, in general, the standard WHO oral rehydration solution (ORS) is adequate, lower osmolality oral rehydration fluids can be more effective in

TABLE 337-8. Composition of Commercial Oral Rehydration Solutions (ORS) and Commonly Consumed Beverages

SOLUTION	CARBOHYDRATE (G/L)	SODIUM (MMOL/L)	POTASSIUM (MMOL/L)	CHLORIDE (MMOL/L)	BASE* (MMOL/L)	OSMOLARITY (MOSM/L)
ORS						
World Health Organization (WHO) [2005]	13.5	75	20	65	10	245
WHO [2002]	13.5	75	20	65	30	245
WHO (1975)	20	90	20	80	30	311
European Society of Paediatric Gastroenterology, Hepatology and Nutrition	16	60	20	60	30	240
Enfalyte†	30	50	25	45	34	200
Pedialyte§	25	45	20	35	30	250
Rehydralyte¶	25	75	20	65	30	305
CeraLyte**	40	50–90	20	NA††	30	220
COMMONLY USED BEVERAGES (NOT APPROPRIATE FOR DIARRHEA TREATMENT)						
Apple juice§§	120	0.4	44	45	N/A	730
Coca-Cola¶¶ Classic	112	1.6	N/A	N/A	13.4	650

*Actual or potential bicarbonate (e.g., lactate, citrate, or acetate).
†Mead-Johnson Laboratories, Princeton, New Jersey. Additional information is available at http://www.meadjohnson.com/products/cons-infant/enfalyte.html.
§Ross Laboratories (Abbott Laboratories), Columbus, Ohio. Data regarding Flavored and Freezer Pop Pedialyte are identical. Additional information is available at http://www.pedialyte.com.
¶Ross Laboratories (Abbott Laboratories), Columbus, Ohio. Additional information is available at http://rpdcon40.ross.com/pn/PediatricProducts.NSF/web_Ross.com_XML_PediatricNutrition/96A5745B1183947385256A80007546E5?OpenDocument.
**Cera Products, L.L.C., Jessup, Maryland. Additional information is available at http://www.ceralyte.com/index.htm.
††Not applicable.
§§Meeting U.S. Department of Agriculture minimum requirements.
¶¶Coca-Cola Corporation, Atlanta, Georgia. Figures do not include electrolytes that might be present in local water used for bottling. Base = phosphate.
From: Department of Health and Human Services, Centers for Disease Control and Prevention: Diagnosis and management of foodbourne illnesses. *MMWR* 2004;52:1–33.

reducing stool output. Compared with standard ORS, lower sodium and glucose ORS (containing 75 mEq of sodium and 75 mmol of glucose per liter, with total osmolarity of 245 mOsm per liter) reduces stool output, vomiting, and the need for intravenous fluids without substantially increasing the risk of hyponatremia.

Cereal-based oral rehydration fluids can also be advantageous in malnourished children and can be prepared at home. Home remedies including decarbonated soda beverages, fruit juices, and tea are not suitable for rehydration or maintenance therapy as they have inappropriately high osmolalities and low sodium concentrations. A clinical evaluation plan and management strategy for children with moderate to severe diarrhea is outlined in Figure 337-5 and Table 337-7. Oral rehydration should be given to infants and children slowly, especially if they have emesis. It can be given initially by a dropper, teaspoon, or syringe, beginning with as little as 5 mL at a time. The volume is increased as tolerated. Replacement for emesis or stool losses is noted in Table 337-7. Oral rehydration can also be given by a nasogastric tube if needed; this is not the usual route.

Limitations to oral rehydration therapy include shock, an ileus, intussusception, carbohydrate intolerance (rare), severe emesis, and high stool output (>10 mL/kg/hr).

ENTERAL FEEDING AND DIET SELECTION. Continued enteral feeding in diarrhea aids in recovery from the episode and a continued age-appropriate diet after rehydration is the norm. Although intestinal brush border surface and luminal enzymes can be affected in children with prolonged diarrhea, there is evidence that satisfactory carbohydrate, protein, and fat absorption can take place on a variety of diets. Once rehydration is complete, food should be reintroduced while oral rehydration can be continued to replace ongoing losses from emesis or stools and for maintenance. Breast-feeding or nondiluted regular formula should be resumed as soon as possible. Foods with complex carbohydrates (rice, wheat, potatoes, bread, and cereals), lean meats, yogurt, fruits, and vegetables are also tolerated. Fatty foods or foods high in simple sugars (juices, carbonated sodas) should be avoided. The usual energy density of any diet used for the therapy of diarrhea should be around 1 kcal/g, aiming to provide an energy intake of a minimum of 100 kcal/kg/day and a protein intake of between 2 and 3 g/kg/day. In selected circumstances when adequate intake of energy-dense food is problematic, the addition of amylase to the diet through germination techniques can also be helpful.

With the exception of acute lactose intolerance in a small subgroup, most children with diarrhea are able to tolerate milk and lactose-containing diets. Withdrawal of milk and replacement with specialized (and expensive) lactose-free formulations are unnecessary. Although children with persistent diarrhea are not lactose intolerant, administration of a lactose load exceeding 5 g/kg/day may be associated with higher purging rates and treatment failure. Alternative strategies for reducing the lactose load while feeding malnourished children with prolonged diarrhea include addition of milk to cereals as well as replacement of milk with fermented milk products such as yogurt.

Rarely, when dietary intolerance precludes the administration of cow's milk–based formulations or milk it may be necessary to administer specialized milk-free diets such as a comminuted or blenderized chicken-based diet or an elemental formulation. Although effective in some settings, the latter are unaffordable in most developing countries. In addition to rice-lentil formulations, the addition of green banana or pectin to the diet has also been shown to be effective in the treatment of persistent diarrhea. Figure 337-6 indicates a suggestive algorithm for the management of children with prolonged diarrhea in developing countries.

ZINC SUPPLEMENTATION. There is strong evidence that zinc supplementation in children with diarrhea in developing countries leads to reduced duration and severity of diarrhea and could potentially prevent 300,000 deaths. WHO and UNICEF recommend that all children with acute diarrhea in at-risk areas should receive oral zinc in some form for 10–14 days during and after diarrhea (10 mg/day for infants <6 mo of age and 20 mg/day for those >6 mo). In addition to improving diarrhea, administration of zinc in community settings leads to increased use of ORS and reduction in the use of antimicrobials.

ADDITIONAL THERAPIES. The use of probiotic nonpathogenic bacteria for prevention and therapy of diarrhea has been successful in developing countries. There are a variety of organisms (*Lactobacillus, Bifidobacterium*) that have a good safety record; therapy has not been standardized and the most effective (and safe) organism has not been identified.

Antimotility agents (loperamide) are contraindicated in children with dysentery and probably have no role in the management of acute watery diarrhea in otherwise healthy children. Similarly, **antiemetic** agents such as the phenothiazines are of little value and are associated with potentially serious side effects (lethargy, dystonia, malignant hyperpyrexia). Nonetheless, ondansetron is an effective and less toxic antiemetic agent. Because persistent vomiting may limit oral rehydration therapy, a single sublingual dose of an oral dissolvable tablet of ondansetron (2 mg children 8–15 kg; 4 mg children ≥15–30 kg; 8 mg children >30 kg) may be given. However, most children do not require specific antiemetic therapy; careful oral rehydration therapy is usually sufficient (see Chapter 55.1).

Racecadotril, an enkephalinse inhibitor, has been shown to reduce stool output in patients with diarrhea. Experience with this drug in children is limited, and for the average child with acute diarrhea it may be unnecessary.

ANTIBIOTIC THERAPY. Timely antibiotic therapy in select cases of diarrhea may reduce the duration and severity of diarrhea and prevent complications (Table 337-9). While these agents are important to use in specific cases, their widespread and indiscriminate use leads to the development of antimicrobial resistance. **Nitazoxanide**, an anti-infective agent, has been effective in the treatment of a wide variety of pathogens including *Cryptosporidum parvum*, *Giardia lamblia*, *Entamoeba histolytica*, *Blastocystis hominis*, *C. difficile*, and rotavirus.

PREVENTION

In many developed countries, diarrhea due to pathogens such as *Clostridum botulinum*, *E. coli* 0157 : H7, *Salmonella*, *Shigella*, *V. cholerae*, *Cryptosporidium*, and *Cyclospora* is a notifiable disease and, thus, contact tracing and source identification is important in preventing outbreaks.

Many developing countries struggle with huge disease burdens of diarrhea where a wider approach to diarrhea prevention may be required. Preventive strategies may be of relevance to both developed and developing countries.

PROMOTION OF EXCLUSIVE BREAST-FEEDING. Exclusive breast-feeding (administration of no other fluids or foods for the 1st 6 mo of life) is not common. Exclusive breast-feeding protects very young infants from diarrheal disease through the promotion of passive immunity (see Chapters 42 and 94) and through reduction in the intake of potentially contaminated food and water. Breast milk contains all the nutrients needed in early infancy, and when continued during diarrhea, also diminishes the adverse impact on nutritional status.

IMPROVED COMPLEMENTARY FEEDING PRACTICES. There is a strong inverse association between appropriate, safe complemen-

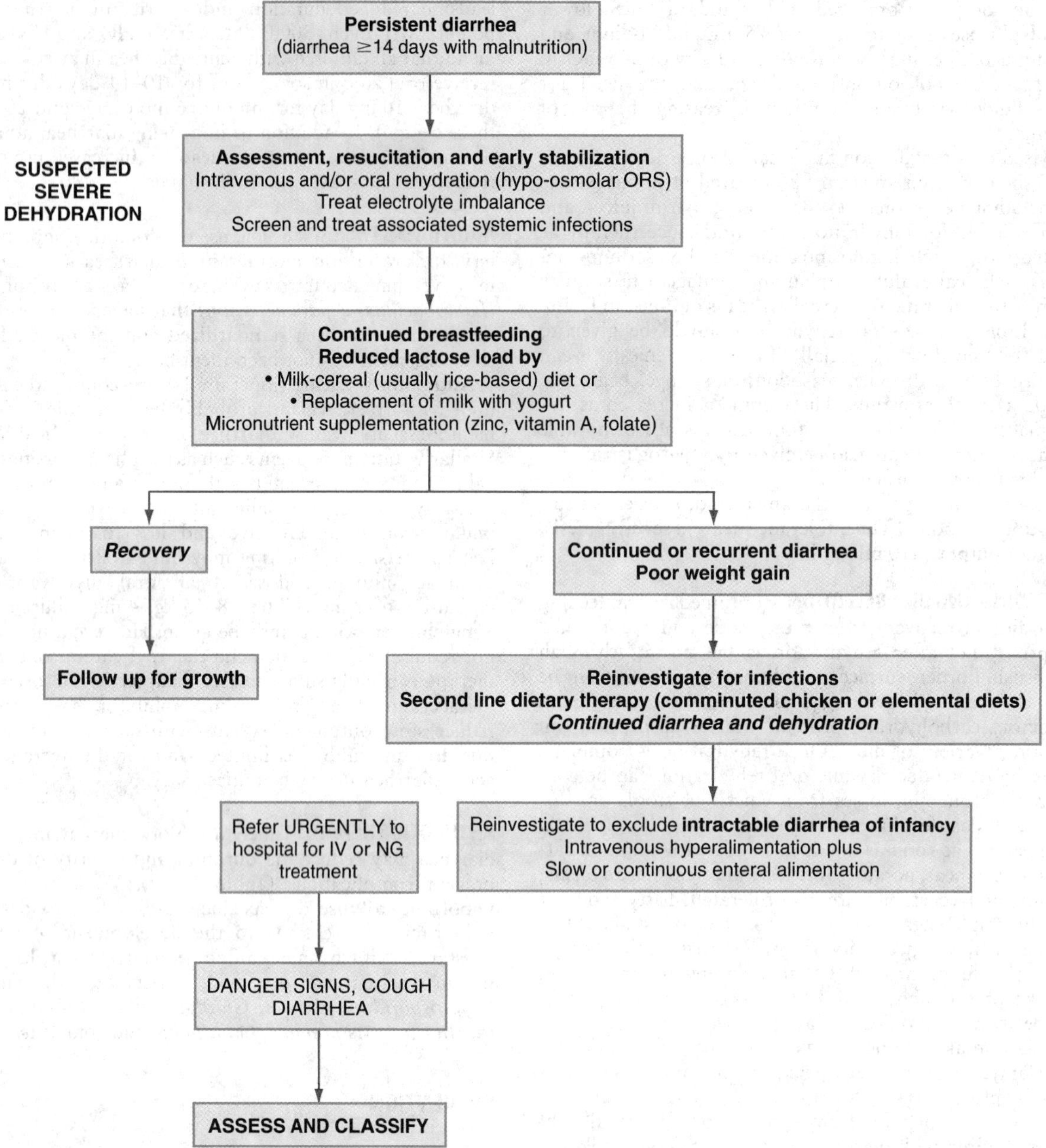

Figure 337-6. Persistent diarrhea. NG, nasogastric tube; ORS, oral rehydration solution.

tary feeding and mortality in children age 6–11 mo; malnutrition is an independent risk for the frequency and severity of diarrheal illness. Complementary foods should be introduced at 6 mo of age while breast-feeding should continue for up to 1 yr (longer period for developing countries). Complementary foods in developing countries are generally poor in quality and frequently heavily contaminated, thus predisposing to diarrhea. Contamination of complementary foods can be potentially reduced through caregivers' education and improving home food storage. Vitamin A supplementation reduces childhood mortality by 34%; improved vitamin A status reduces the frequency of severe diarrhea.

ROTAVIRUS IMMUNIZATION. Most infants acquire rotavirus diarrhea early in life; an effective rotavirus vaccine would have a major effect on reducing diarrhea mortality in developing countries. In 1998, a quadrivalent Rhesus rotavirus–derived vaccine was licensed in the United States but subsequently withdrawn due to an increased risk of intussusception. Newer vaccines are approved for both developed and developing countries and significantly reduce diarrhea mortality (see Chapters 170, 262).

Other vaccines that could potentially reduce the burden of severe diarrhea and mortality in young children are vaccines against *Shigella* and ETEC.

IMPROVED WATER AND SANITARY FACILITIES AND PROMOTION OF PERSONAL AND DOMESTIC HYGIENE. Much of the reduction in diarrhea prevalence in the developed world is the result of improvement in standards of hygiene, sanitation, and water supply. In addition, routine handwashing with plain soap in the home can reduce the incidence of diarrhea in all environments.

TABLE 337-9. Antibiotic Therapy for Infectious Diarrhea

ORGANISM	DRUG OF CHOICE	DOSE AND DURATION OF TREATMENT
Shigella (severe dysentery and EIEC dysentery)	Ciprofloxacin, ampicillin, ceftriaxone, or trimethoprim-sulfamethoxazole (TMP-SMX). Most strains are resistant to many antibiotics.	Ceftriaxone IV, IM 50–100 mg/kg/d qd, bid × 7 d Ciprofloxacin PO 20–30 mg/kg/d bid × 7–10 d 10 mg/kg/d of TMP and 50 mg/kg/d of SMX bid × 5 d Ampicillin PO, IV 50–100 mg/kg/d qid × 7 d
EPEC, ETEC, EIEC	TMP-SMX or ciprofloxacin	10 mg/kg/d of TMP and 50 mg/kg/d of SMX bid × 5 d Ciprofloxacin PO 20–30 mg/kg/d qid for 5–10 d
Salmonella	No antibiotics for uncomplicated gastroenteritis in normal hosts caused by non-typhoidal species. **Treatment** indicated in infants <3 mo, and patients with malignancy, chronic GI disease, severe colitis hemoglobinopathies, or HIV infection, and other immunoincompetent patients. Most strains have become resistant to multiple antibiotics.	See treatment of *Shigella*
Aeromonas/Plesiomonas	TMP-SMX Ciprofloxacin	10 mg/kg/d of TMP and 50 mg/kg/d of SMX bid for 5 d Ciprofloxacin PO 20–30 mg/kg/d divided bid × 7–10 d
Yersinia spp.	Antibiotics are not usually required for diarrhea. Deferoxamine therapy should be withheld for severe infections or associated bacteremia. Treat sepsis as for immunocompromised hosts, using combination therapy with parenteral doxycycline, aminoglycoside, TMP-SMX, or fluoroquinolone.	
Campylobacter jejuni	Erythromycin or azithromycin	Erythromycin PO, 50 mg/kg/d divided tid × 5 d Azithromycin PO, 5–10 mg/kg/d qid × 5 d
Clostridium difficile	Metronidazole (first line) Discontinue initiating antibiotic Vancomycin (2nd line)	PO 30 mg/kg/d divided tid × 5 d PO 40 mg/kg/d qid × 7 d
Entamoeba histolytica	Metronidazole followed by iodoquinol or paromomycin	PO 30–40 mg/kg/d tid × 7–10 d PO 30–40 mg/kg/d tid × 20 d PO 25–35 mg/kg/d tid × 7 d
Giardia lamblia	Furazolidone or metronidazole or albendazole or quinacrine	Furazolidone PO 25 mg/kg/d qid for 5–7 d Metronidazole PO 30–40 mg/kg/d tid × 7 d Albendazole PO 200 mg bid × 10 d
Cryptosporidium spp.	Nitazoxanide PO treatment may not be needed in normal hosts. In immunocompromised, PO immunoglobulin + aggressively treat HIV, etc.	Children 1–3 yr: 100 mg bid × 3 d Children 4–11 yr: 200 mg bid Adults: 500 mg bid
Isospora spp.	TMP-SMX	PO 5 mg/kg/d and 25 mg/kg/d, respectively, bid × 7–10 d
Cyclospora spp.	TMP/SMX	PO 5 mg/kg/d and 25 mg/kg/d respectively, bid × 7 d
Blastocystis hominis	Metronidazole or iodoquinol	Metronidazole PO 30–40 mg/kg/d tid × 7–10 d Iodoquinol PO 40 mg/kg/d tid × 20 d

bid, 2 times a day; EIEC, Enteroinvasive *Escherichia coli*; EPEC, *Enteropathogenic E. coli*; ETEC, *Enterotoxigenic E. coli*; IM, intramuscular; IV, intravenous; PO, oral; qd, daily; qid, 4 times a day, SMX, sulfamethoxazole; tid, 3 times a day; TMP, trimethoprim.

Behavioral change strategies through promotion of handwashing indicate that handwashing promotion and access to soap reduces the burden of diarrhea in developing countries.

IMPROVED CASE MANAGEMENT OF DIARRHEA. Improved management of diarrhea through prompt identification and appropriate therapy significantly reduces diarrhea duration, its nutritional penalty, and risk of death in childhood. Improved management of acute diarrhea is a key factor in reducing the burden of prolonged episodes and persistent diarrhea. The WHO/UNICEF recommendations to use low osmolality ORS and zinc supplementation for the management of diarrhea, coupled with selective and appropriate use of antibiotics, have the potential to reduce the number of diarrheal deaths among children.

337.1 • Traveler's Diarrhea (See Chapter 173) •

Zulfiqar Ahmed Bhutta

Traveler's diarrhea is a common complication of visitors to developing countries and is caused by a variety of pathogens, in part dependent on the season and region visited (Table 337-10). Traveler's diarrhea has a high attack rate among travelers from higher income countries visiting, during the summer, countries in a warmer climate that have a high prevalence of indigenous infectious diarrhea. Traveler's diarrhea may manifest with watery diarrhea or as dysentery.

TREATMENT. Traveler's diarrhea is often self-limiting but requires particular attention to avoid dehydration. For infants and children, rehydration as discussed in Chapter 337 is appropriate, followed by a standard diet. Adolescents and adults should increase their intake of electrolyte-rich fluids. Kaolin-pectin, anticholinergic agents, *Lactobacillus*, and bismuth salicylate have not been effective therapies. Loperamide, an antimotility and antisecretory agent, reduces the number of stools in older children with watery diarrhea, but it should be used with great caution or not at all in febrile or toxic patients with dysentery.

TABLE 337-10. Regional Distribution of the Most Common Pathogens That Cause Traveler's Diarrhea

	Asia	Latin America	Africa
BACTERIAL			
Enterotoxigenic *E. coli*	6–37%	17–70%	8–42%
Other *E. coli*	3–4%	7–22%	2–9%
Campylobacter jejuni	9–39%	1–5%	1–28%
Salmonella spp.	1–33%	1–16%	4–25%
Shigella spp.	0–17%	2–30%	0–9%
Plesiomonas shigelloides	3–13%	0–6%	3–5%
Aeromonas spp.	1–57%	1–5%	0–9%
VIRAL			
Rotavirus	1–8%	0–6%	0–36%
PARASITIC			
Entamoeba histolytica	5–11%	<1%	2–9%
Giardia lambia	1–12%	1–2%	0–1%
Cryptosporidium spp.	1–5%	<1%	2%
Cyclospora cayetanensis	1–5%?	<1%?	<1%?
No pathogen identified	10–56%	24–62%	15–53%

From: Al-Abri SS, Beeching NJ, Nye FJ: Traveller's diarrhoea. *Lancet Infect Dis* 2005;5:349–360.

Antibiotics, with or without loperamide, reduce the number of unformed stools. Short (3 days) duration therapy with fluoroquinolones, trimethoprim-sulfamethoxazole, azithromycin, or rifaximin is effective; the choice of antibiotic depends on the age of the patient, the potential organism, and the organism's local resistance patterns. For up to date information on local pathogens and resistant patterns, see www.cdc.gov/travel.

PREVENTION. Travelers should drink bottled or canned beverages, or boiled water. They should avoid ice, salads, and fruit they did not peel themselves. Food should be eaten hot if possible. Raw or poorly cooked seafood is a risk, as is eating in a restaurant rather than a private home. Swimming pools and other recreational water sites can also be contaminated.

Chemoprophylaxis is not routinely recommended for previously healthy children or adults.

Al-Abri SS, Beeching NJ, Nye FJ: Traveller's diarrhoea. *Lancet Infect Dis* 2005;5:349–360.

American Medical Association, American Nurses Association–American Nurses Foundation, Centers for Disease Control and Prevention, et al: Diagnosis and management of foodborne illnesses: A primer for physicians and other health care professionals. *MMWR Recomm Rep* 2004;53:1–33.

Ashkenazi S: *Shigella* infections in children: New insights. *Semin Pediatr Infect Dis* 2004;15:246–252.

Bhatnagar S, Bahl R, Sharma PK, et al: Zinc with oral rehydration therapy reduces stool output and duration of diarrhea in hospitalized children: A randomized controlled study. *J Pediatr Gastroenterol Nutr* 2004;38:34–40.

Bhutta ZA, Ghishan F, Lindley K, et al: Persistent and chronic diarrhea and malabsorption: Working Group report of the Second World Congress of Pediatric Gastroenterology, Hepatology, and Nutrition. *J Pediatr Gastroenterol Nutr* 2004;39:S711–S716.

Bouckenooghe AR, Jiang ZD, de la Cabada FJ, et al: Enterotoxigenic *Escherichia coli* as cause of diarrhea among Mexican adults and US travelers in Mexico. *J Travel Med* 2002;9:137–140.

Caeiro JP, DuPont HL, Albrecht H, Ericsson CD: Oral rehydration therapy plus loperamide versus loperamide alone in the treatment of traveler's diarrhea. *Clin Infect Dis* 1999;28:1286–1289.

Cartwright RY: Food and waterborne infections associated with package holidays. *J Appl Microbiol* 2003;94:12S–24S.

Centers for Disease Control and Prevention: Ongoing multistate outbreak of *Escherichia coli* serotype 0157 : H7 infections associated with consumption of fresh spinach—United States, September 2006. *MMWR* 2006;55:1045–1046.

Centers for Disease Control and Prevention (CDC): Outbreak of cyclosporiasis associated with snow peas—Pennsylvania, 2004. *MMWR* 2004;53:876–878.

Centers for Disease Control and Prevention: Outbreaks of multidrug-resistant *Shigella sonnei* gastroenteritis associated with day care centers—Kansas, Kentucky, and Missouri, 2005. *MMWR* 2006;55:1068–1070.

Centers for Disease Control and Prevention: Preliminary food net data on the incidence of infection with pathogens transmitted commonly through food—10 states, United States, 2005. *MMWR* 2006;55:392–395.

Chouraqui JP, Van Egroo LD, Fichot MC: Acidified milk formula supplemented with *Bifidobacterium lactis*: Impact on infant diarrhea in residential care settings. *J Pediatr Gastroenterol Nutr* 2004;38:288–292.

De Bruyn G, Hahn S, Borwick A: Antibiotic treatment fot travellers' diarrhoea. *Cochrane Database Syst Rev* 2000;3:CD002242.

Denno DM, Stapp JR, Boster DR, et al: Etiology of diarrhea in pediatric outpatient settings. *Pediatr Infect Dis J* 2005;24:142–148.

Elliott EJ: Acute gastroenteritis in children. *BMJ* 2007;334:35–40.

Finley R, Reid-Smith R, Weese JS: Human health implications of Salmonella-contaminated natural pet treat and raw pet food. *CID* 2006;42:686–691.

Fonseca BK, Holdgate A, Craig JC: Enteral vs intravenous rehydration therapy for children with gastroenteritis. *Arch Pediatr Adolesc Med* 2004;158:483–490.

Freedman SB, Adler M, Seshadri R, Powell EC: Oral ondansetron for gastroenteritis in a pediatric emergency department. *N Engl J Med* 2006;354:1698–1705.

Fullerton KE, Ingram A, Jones TF, et al: Sporadic *Campylobacter* infection in infants: a population-based surveillance case-control study. *Pediatr Infect Dis J* 2007;26:19–24.

Guandalini S, Pensabene L, Zikri MA, et al: *Lactobacillus* GG administered in oral rehydration solution to children with acute diarrhoea: A multicenter European trial. *J Pediatr Gastroenterol Nutr* 2000;30:54–60.

Hahn S, Kim Y, Garner P: Reduced osmolarity oral rehydration solution for treating dehydration due to diarrhoea in children: Systematic review. *Br Med J* 2001;323:s81–s85.

Högenauer C, Langner C, Beubler E, et al: *Klebsiella oxytoca* as a causative organism of antibiotic-associated hemorrhagic colitis. *N Engl J Med* 2006;355:2418–2426.

Huang DB, Awasthi M, Le B, et al: The role of diet in the treatment of traveler's diarrhea: A pilot study. *Clin Infect Dis* 2004;39:468–771.

Jalava K, Hakkinen M, Valkonen M, et al: An outbreak of gastrointestinal illness and erythema nodosum from grated carrots contaminated with *Yersinia pseudotuberculosis. JID* 2006;194:1209–1216.

Jones TF, Angulo FJ: Eating in restaurants: a risk factor for foodbourne disease? *CID* 2006;43:1324–1328.

Kang G, Ramakrishna BS, Daniel J, et al: Epidemiological and laboratory investigations of outbreaks of diarrhoea in rural South India: Implications for control of disease. *Epidemiol Infect* 2001;127:107–112.

King CK, Glass R, Bresee JS, Duggan C; Centers for Disease Control and Prevention: Managing acute gastroenteritis among children: Oral rehydration, maintenance, and nutritional therapy. *MMWR Recomm Rep* 2003;52:1–16.

Kirkwood C: Viral gastroenteritis in Europe: A new norovirus variant? *Lancet* 2004;363:671–672.

Kosek M, Bern C, Guerrant RL: The global burden of diarrhoeal disease, as estimated from studies published between 1992 and 2000. *Bull World Health Organ* 2003;81:197–204.

Luby SP, Agboatwalla M, Painter J, et al: Effect of intensive handwashing promotion on childhood diarrhea in high-risk communities in Pakistan. *JAMA* 2004;291:2547–2554.

Maki DG: Don't eat the spinach—controlling foodborne infectious disease. *N Engl J Med* 2006;355:1952–1955.

Murata T, Katsushima N, Mizuta K, et al: Prolonged norovirus shedding in infants ≤6 months of age with gastroenteritis. *Pediatr Infect Dis J* 2007;26:46–49.

Musher DM, Musher BL: Contagious acute gastrointestinal infections. *N Engl J Med* 2004;351:2417–2427.

O'Ryan M, Diaz J, Mamani N, et al: Impact of rotavirus infections on outpatient clinic visits in Chile. *Pediatr Infect Dis J* 2007;26:41–45.

O'Ryan M, Prado V, Pickering L: A millennium update on pediatric diarrheal illness in the developing world. *Semin Pediatr Infect Dis* 2005;16:125–136.

Rossignol JF, Abu-Zakry M, Hussein A, Santoro MG: Effect of nitazoxanide for treatment of severe rotavirus diarrhoea: randomized double-blind placebo-controlled trial. *Lancet* 2006;368:124–129.

Shavit I, Brant R, Nijsen-Jordan C, et al: A novel imaging technique to measure capillary-refill time: improving diagnostic accuracy for dehydration in young children with gastroenteritis. *Pediatrics* 2006;118:2402–2408.

Spandorfer PR, Alessandrini EA, Joffe MD, et al: Oral versus intravenous rehydration of moderately dehydrated children: A randomized, controlled trial. *Pediatrics* 2005;115:295–301.

Stauffer WM, Konop RJ, Kamat D: Traveling with infants and young children. Part III: Traveler's diarrhea. *J Travel Med* 2002;9:141–150.

Swanson SJ, Snider C, Branden CR, et al: Multidrug-resistant *Salmonella enterica* serotype typhimurium associated with pet rodents. *N Engl J Med* 2007;356:21–28.

Taylor JA: Oral rehydration. *Arch Pediatr Adolesc Med* 2004;158:420–421.

Thapar M, Sanderson IR: Diarrhoea in children: An interface between developing and developed countries. *Lancet* 2004;363:641–653.

Thielman NM, Guerrant RL: Acute infectious diarrhea. *N Engl J Med* 2004; 350:38–47.

Turck D, Bernet JP, Marx J, et al: Incidence and risk factors of oral antibiotic-associated diarrhea in an outpatient pediatric population. *J Pediatr Gastroenterol Nutr* 2003;37:22–26.

Widdowson MA, Cramer EH, Hadley L, et al: Outbreaks of acute gastroenteritis on cruise ships and on land: Identification of a predominant circulating strain of norovirus—United States, 2002. *J Infect Dis* 2004;190: 27–36.

337.2 • Probiotics in Gastrointestinal Disorders • David Branski and Michael Wilschanski

Probiotics are living microorganisms or components of microbial cells that have a beneficial effect on the host. They are mainly lactic acid–producing bacilli, mostly *Lactobacilli* and *Bifidobacteria,* and also the yeast *Saccharomyces boulardii.*

A probiotic agent must fulfill the following criteria: be of human source, nonpathogenic, and safe; resist gastric, bile, and pancreatic digestion; and adhere to and colonize the enterocytes. Moreover, it should produce antimicrobial substances, have favorable immunomodulation properties, and have the ability to influence metabolic activities.

Prebiotics include materials that enhance the proliferation and development of probiotic microorganisms; they include substances such as fructo- and galacto-oligosaccharides, inulin, germinated barley foodstuff, and psyllium. Prebiotics should pass harmlessly through the upper digestive tract and be a substrate for selective probiotic agents in the large bowel.

The combined approach utilizing prebiotics and probiotics to induce synergistic effects so as to produce a more favorable host intestinal environment is termed **synbiotics.**

PHYSIOLOGIC MECHANISMS

The mucosal immune response to commensals (nonpathologic flora) is markedly different from the response to pathogens. This difference is explained by the presence of virulence factors produced by pathogens, which are absent in the commensals. This immunologic "tolerance" toward the commensal microorganisms enables them to successfully colonize and thrive inside the bowel lumen. Moreover, a cross talk is established between the probiotic agents and the host mucosal immune system. In the gut epithelium, Toll-like receptors (TLRs) and nucleotide-binding oligomerization domain isoforms (NODs) identify commensals as such, thereby avoiding the initiation of immune responses that would otherwise eliminate them as they do pathogens.

Probiotics favorably affect the host by local and/or immune modulation pathways. In the gut, the probiotic agents compete with pathogens for nutrients. They produce bacteriocins, which act as local antibiotics against pathogens. In the gut, they also induce the synthesis of antimicrobial peptides such as human β-defensin 2. The probiotic agents are able to decrease enteroaggregative *E. coli* virulence factor by downregulating the expression of the transcriptional regulator aggR, concomitant with increased expression of commensal bacteria.

Some probiotic bacteria produce lactic and acetic acids that can inhibit pathogen growth by lowering luminal pH. Moreover, probiotic agents occupy binding sites on the epithelial mucosa, preventing adherence of pathogenic bacteria to the mucosa. Even inactivated probiotic bacteria or isolated DNA sequence repeats obtained from probiotic bacteria can modify the toxin receptor.

DNA obtained from a mixture of probiotic strains was shown to attenuate colitis in an animal model, an effect that was dependent on TLR-9. DNA obtained from a probiotic combination can inhibit the activation of the transcription factor NF-πB (nuclear factor πB) as well as the secretion of proinflammatory cytokines in human epithelial cells.

Probiotics may improve the integrity of the mucosal barrier function by stimulating mucin production. They inhibit the increased paracellular permeability induced by pathogens. Probiotic agents have the capacity to attenuate the muscular hypercontractility that is seen in postinfectious gut dysmotility.

Certain probiotic bacteria decrease the synthesis of potent proinflammatory cytokines such as tumor necrosis factor–α (TNF-α), interferon-γ (IFN-γ), interleukin 12 (IL-12) and also platelet activating factor (PAF), whereas they enhance the production of antinflammatory cytokines such as IL-10. The increased IL-10 production is accompanied by an increase in transforming growth factor–β (TGF-β) through ligation of certain probiotic antigens to TLRs. Probiotics could skew the Th1/Th2 balance toward Th1, with consequent downregulation of the activity of Th2-mediated allergic response.

THE EFFECTS OF PROBIOTICS IN VARIOUS DISORDERS

ACUTE INFECTIOUS DIARRHEA. Specific probiotic strains can contribute to both the prophylactic and therapeutic management of acute infectious diarrhea in children, decreasing its incidence and duration (see Chapter 337). When children with rotavirus gastroenteritis are treated with probiotics, the diarrhea is briefer and milder. Probiotic-treated children also produce higher levels of immunoglobulin A (IgA) antibodies. The beneficial effect of probiotics has also been demonstrated in infectious diarrhea in adults.

ANTIBIOTIC-ASSOCIATED DIARRHEA. Antibiotic-associated diarrhea is common; it occurs in up to a third of all hospitalized patients who receive antibiotics (see Chapters 209 and 337). It can range from mild diarrhea to colitis to pseudomembranous enterocolitis (PMC), which can be recurrent and may be fatal. The cause of PMC is multifactorial, including toxin produced by *Clostridium difficile,* altered bowel flora due to prior antibiotic treatment, and impaired host immunity. Because one of the proposed mechanisms for antibiotic-associated diarrhea is alteration in the gut flora, probiotic agents might be beneficial, and, indeed, several agents have been demonstrated to display preventive properties. The most studied microorganism in this regard is *Saccharomyces boulardii.*

NEONATAL NECROTIZING ENTEROCOLITIS (NEC). The colonic flora of preterm infants, particularly those in the neonatal intensive care units, is different from that of healthy, term infants. *Bifidobacteria* spp., which is commonly cultured from healthy, breast-fed term neonates, only appears several weeks after birth. Preterm infants are exposed late to maternal microflora; they tend to receive broad-spectrum antibiotics and sterile feeds. Thus, the colon in these infants can harbor potentially harmful, antibiotic-resistant organisms. Prophylactic administration of oral probiotics given to this population reduces the incidence and severity of NEC (see Chapter 102.2).

LACTASE DEFICIENCY. Lactase deficiency is a very frequent phenomenon in children, with digestive complaints related to the consumption of milk and dairy products (see Chapter 335.11). These complaints can include flatulence, diarrhea, and abdominal distention. Probiotic bacteria are capable of digesting lactose that would otherwise remain poorly digested, thereby alleviating the symptoms of lactase deficiency in susceptible subjects. Indeed, in children with lactase deficiency, yogurt, but not milk, containing these probiotic bacteria alleviated the symptoms and also decreased the exhaled hydrogen concentrations.

IRRITABLE BOWEL SYNDROME (IBS). This functional digestive disorder encompasses such entities as chronic nonspecific diarrhea or "toddler diarrhea" and recurrent abdominal pain, which according to the Rome II criteria should be termed *functional abdominal pain* (see Chapter 339). It affects mainly children >5 yr of age and adolescents. In adults suffering from IBS, specific probiotic bacteria improve their symptoms. Moreover, the basal IL-10 : IL-12 ratio that is low prior to the probiotic treatment can become normal after probiotic treatment.

INFLAMMATORY BOWEL DISEASE (IBD). IBD has a complex etiology, with both environmental and genetic involvement (see Chapter 333). These factors may alter the host's immune response to bacterial flora. Rodents with dysfunctional immune systems, which serve as models of IBD, do not develop inflammation when kept under germ-free conditions. This implies that commensal enteric bacteria may have an important role in the development of disease. The accumulating evidence for an important role of luminal flora in the pathogenesis of IBD has led to the proposition that manipulation of the intestinal flora may yield therapeutic benefits.

Administering probiotics to IL-10 deficient mice with bowel inflammation decreased the levels of proinflammatory cytokines TNF-α and IL-12 and reduced intestinal inflammation. Despite promising results with animal models, the efficacy of probiotic use in humans with IBD is unclear. The one disorder associated with IBD in which probiotics have been shown to be efficacious is pouchitis. A probiotic mixture of eight bacterial species is effective in the treatment and prevention of pouchitis following ileoanal pouch creation. Studies using a probiotic mixture in patients with ulcerative colitis (UC) who did not have surgery showed induction of remission in >75% of the patients. The efficacy of probiotics in UC is still controversial, however.

Clinical trials have also been conducted in Crohn disease, comparing mesalazine with probiotics; the latter contribute to a decreased recurrence rate. In children, the most widely used probiotic is *Lactobacillus* GG (LGG). The addition of LGG to prednisone decreased disease activity in a small study of children with Crohn disease. In a larger study of children, however, there was no difference in remission rate observed over 2 yr.

CELIAC DISEASE. Gliadin and respective prolamins contain the "toxic" amino acid sequences that are responsible for the symptoms of gluten-sensitive enteropathy in immunologically susceptible subjects (see Chapter 335). These epitopes, including the 33-mer peptides corresponding to 57–89 of α2-gliadin, are very resistant to digestion. In vitro, the prolyl endopeptidase of probiotic bacteria origin is able to digest these 33-mer peptides. Only a mixture of probiotic strains contains the entire portfolio of peptidases that are able to degrade gliadins.

A modified biotechnology of bread-baking, using long fermentation times with selective probiotic bacilli and added nontoxic flours, decreases the level of gluten intolerance in celiac subjects. Bacterial prolyl endopeptidase promotes digestion of cereal proteins, enabling the attack on T-cell multipotent epitopes, which may consequently detoxify "toxic" sequences.

It remains to be seen to what extent this intraluminal digestion process will detoxify peptides that otherwise contribute to the harmful effects of gliadin on the mucosal layer of the proximal small intestine.

FOOD PROTEIN HYPERSENSITIVITY. The commensal flora stimulates development of the gut-associated lymphoid tissue and is important for the development of oral tolerance to food antigens (see Chapters 144 and 151). It is suggested that intestinal microbes are pivotal in the development of allergic disorders by creating an immune imbalance. The intestinal flora of atopic children is markedly different from that of controls; for example, *Bifidobacteria* spp., which are markers for healthy commensal development, are reduced in such children even before they develop allergy. Certain commensal bacteria induce lymphocytes to produce Th1 secretion such as IL-10, TGF-β, and IFN-γ. Probiotics have been confirmed in vitro as well as in animal models to stimulate Th1 and Th Reg production. This has been observed in clinical trials both in infants with atopic eczema and cow's milk protein hypersensitivity. LGG administered to pregnant women with a strong family history of allergic disorder reduces the frequency of atopic eczema in their infants, which is maintained for a further 4 yr. Probiotics reverse the increased intestinal permeability and enhance specific IgA responses that are frequently defective in children with food allergy.

HELICOBACTER PYLORI. Studies have shown that probiotics can inhibit or kill *Helicobacter pylori* in vitro. A small number of clinical studies have been carried out with encouraging results in adults and children.

OTHER CONDITIONS. The potential role of probiotics in the prevention and treatment of constipation, traveler's diarrhea, and acute pancreatitis and lowering cholesterol levels should be further researched and evaluated.

THE RATIONAL APPROACH TO THE USE OF PROBIOTICS

After having demonstrated the advantageous effects of probiotics on the host, the question arises as to whether they should be recommended as a food additive or even included in infant formulas.

To address this dilemma, the clinician should 1st consider the safety issues. There have been reports documenting mild gastrointestinal complaints such as diarrhea, flatulence, and change of bowel habit with probiotic use. There are also isolated rare anecdotal descriptions of bacteremia or endocarditis among children treated with probiotics, mainly in those who suffered from immune deficiency states or cardiac anomalies, and fungemia, mainly among adults in intensive care units treated with *Saccharomyces cerevisia*. It should be stressed that enteric epithelial cells under metabolic stresses might perceive the host's own commensal "friendly" flora as offensive agents, resulting in increased IL-8 synthesis, decreased enterocyte barrier function, and, subsequently, increased translocation.

Another important consideration is the potential transfer of virulence and/or resistance factors to antibiotic agents from microorganisms in probiotic material to the commensal gut flora. This needs to be borne in mind, particularly if considering supplementing infant formulas with probiotics. Probiotic supplementation of infant formulas may modulate the bowel flora and help in the prevention of allergy. Two strains of *Lactobacilli*, however, caused a higher incidence of mortality in neonatal athymic mice but not athymic adult mice. Thus, probiotics may be unsafe in immunodeficient neonates. It is recommended that currently marketed infant formulas enriched with probiotics should be used only in immunocompetent infants >4–5 mo of age.

Another potential ill effect of probiotics is in regard to dental care. Several *Lactobacilli* may potentially contribute to dental caries, presumably due to their ability to produce organic acids that decalcify the dental matrix.

It is extremely important to define more accurately the particular beneficial strains or optimal combinations of strains of probiotic organisms for any specific target. In one situation, a commensal can contribute to beneficial immunomodulation, whereas in another situation, it can have no effect or cause a general indiscriminate stimulation of the immune response. Moreover, a specific strain can have a beneficial effect when administered alone, whereas when included in a mixture of probiotics, this effect might be eliminated.

Agostoni C, Axelsson I, Braegger C, et al: Probiotic bacteria in dietetic products for infants: A commentary by the ESPGHAN Committee on Nutrition. *J Pediatr Gastroenterol Nutr* 2004;38:365–374.

Bin-Nun A, Bromiker R, Wilschanski M, et al: Oral probiotics prevent necrotizing enterocolitis in very low birth weight neonates. *J Pediatr* 2005;147:192–196.

Di Marzio L, Russo FP, D'Alo S, et al: Apoptotic effects of selected strains of lactic acid bacteria on a human T leukemia cell line are associated with bacterial arginine deiminase and/or sphingomyelinase activities. *Nutr Cancer* 200;40:185–196.

Ezendam J, van Loveren H: Probiotics: Immunomodulation and evaluation of safety and efficacy. *Nutr Rev* 2006;64:1–14.

Gionchetti P, Rizzello F, Helwig U, et al: Prophylaxis of pouchitis onset with probiotic therapy: A double-blind, placebo-controlled trial. *Gastroenterology* 2003;124:1202–1209.

Kalliomaki M, Salminen S, Poussa T, et al: Probiotics and prevention of atopic disease: 4-year follow-up of a randomised placebo-controlled trial. *Lancet* 2003;361:1869–1871.
Rachmilewitz D, Karmeli F, Takabayashi K, et al: Immunostimulatory DNA ameliorates experimental and spontaneous murine colitis. *Gastroenterology* 2002;122:1428–1441.
Sazawal S, Hiremath G, Dhingra U, et al: Efficacy of probiotics in prevention of acute diarrhoea: A meta-analysis of masked, randomised, placebo-controlled trials. *Lancet Infect Dis* 2006;6:374–382.
Szajewska H, Setty M, Mrukowicz J, et al: Probiotics in gastrointestinal diseases in children: Hard and not-so-hard evidence of efficacy. *J Pediatr Gastroenterol Nutr* 2006;42:454–475.
Weizman Z, Asli G, Alsheikh A: Effect of a probiotic infant formula on infections in child care centers: Comparison of two probiotic agents. *Pediatrics* 2005;115:5–9.

Chapter 338 ■ Chronic Diarrhea

Fayez K. Ghishan

(See also Chapters 335 and 337.)

Diarrhea in children accounts for ≈5,000,000 deaths per year in the developing world. In the United States, diarrhea accounts for 10% of all outpatient visits and 14 hospital admissions each year per 1,000 children <1 yr of age (see Chapter 337).

DEFINITION. Diarrhea, defined as increased total daily stool output, is usually associated with increased stool water content (see Chapters 303 and 337). For infants and children, this would result in stool output >10 g/kg/24 hr, or more than the adult limit of 200 g/24 hr. When diarrhea lasts >2 wk, it is considered chronic. Diarrhea results from altered intestinal water and electrolyte transport. The gastrointestinal tract of the infant handles ≈285 mL/kg/24 hr of fluid (intake plus intestinal secretion) with a stool output of 5–10 g/kg/24 hr. The efficient mechanisms responsible for this absorptive capacity are due to the function of several transport proteins located at the brush border membrane of the small and large intestine. The transport of electrolytes across the gastrointestinal tract contributes to the overall absorptive process of the small and large intestine. The stool output in infants and children contains approximately, per liter: 20–25 mEq of sodium, 50–70 mEq of potassium, and 20–25 of mEq of chloride. The normal cellular mechanisms responsible for the transport of nutrients and electrolytes across the gastrointestinal tract are noted in Figure 338-1.

FUNCTIONAL ANATOMY OF THE INTESTINAL MUCOSA. The villus, the functional unit of the small intestine, greatly amplifies the absorptive and digestive surface of the intestinal mucosa. The tip of the villus represents the highly differentiated absorptive cells, whereas the crypt epithelia represent undifferentiated secretory cells. The epithelial cells at the tip of the villus are continually renewed every 4–5 days from the undifferentiated crypt cells. Digestive enzymes and transport proteins responsible for the movements of electrolytes across the intestinal mucosa are located at the brush border membrane of the villus cells. The gastrointestinal epithelia are leaky epithelia that adjust the osmotic load presented to the small intestine. Tight junctions, dynamic structures that occur between the epithelial cells, contribute to overall movement of water and electrolytes. Transport of electrolytes across the intestinal epithelia occurs through several mechanisms, including the glucose-sodium co-transporter. This transport protein requires the presence of a sodium gradient

Normal Transport of Nutrients and Electrolytes Across the Gastrointestinal Tract of an Infant

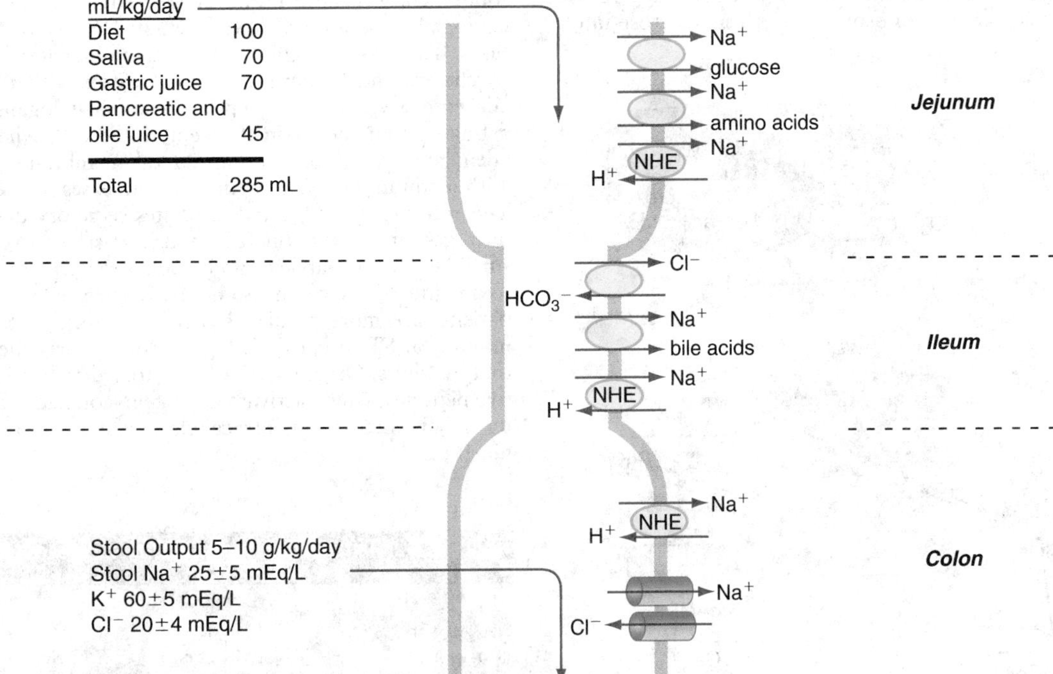

Figure 338-1. The gastrointestinal tract of the infant handles 285 mL/kg/day of dietary and endogenous fluids. The majority of the nutrients and fluids are absorbed via transport protein depicted schematically. NHE-2, NHE-3, and NHE-8 indicate Na^+/H^+ exchanger isoforms 2, 3, and 8. The colon absorbs mainly water and electrolytes via the electroneutral NaCl and the electrogenic Na^+ process.

across the brush border membrane that is maintained by the sodium potassium adenosine triphosphatase (ATPase) pump at the basolateral membranes of the enterocyte. The defect in glucose-galactose malabsorption is a missense mutation in the sodium-glucose co-transporter gene (see Chapter 335.11).

A 2nd mechanism of electrolyte transport across the intestinal epithelia is the electroneutral sodium chloride–coupled pathway that involves the double exchange mechanism by the sodium-hydrogen exchanger and the chloride-bicarbonate exchanger. Three sodium-hydrogen exchangers (NHE-2, -3, and -8) located at the apical membrane appear to be involved in the transport of sodium. Defects of the genes of sodium-hydrogen and chloride-bicarbonate exchangers are candidates for congenital sodium and chloride diarrhea, respectively. Sodium is absorbed in the colon by the electroneutral sodium chloride–coupled pathway and by an electrogenic mechanism, which is regulated by aldosterone. Intestinal secretion occurs primarily from the crypt cells and is stimulated by an increase in the intracellular level of cyclic adenosine monophosphate (cAMP), cyclic gyanosine monophosphate (cGMP), and calcium. These mediators inhibit the neutral sodium chloride entry and permit the entry of chloride into the cells through the basolateral membrane via the sodium-potassium-2 chloride transporter (Na^+-K^+–$2Cl^-$). Chloride is then secreted through the opening of chloride channel (cystic fibrosis transmembrane conductor regulator [CFTR]) at the apical membrane of the crypt cells. Sodium and, thus, water secretion will result in secretory diarrhea. The sodium-glucose co-transporter is not altered by the intracellular mediators, however, and, thus, this concept forms the basis of oral rehydration solutions. Figure 338-2 depicts a model for intestinal secretion induced by enterotoxins.

PATHOPHYSIOLOGY. The pathophysiologic mechanisms of diarrhea include osmotic diarrhea, secretory diarrhea, mutations in apical membrane transport proteins, a reduction in anatomic surface area, alteration in intestinal motility, and inhibition of transport of electrolytes by inflammatory mediators (see Table 303-4).

Osmotic Diarrhea. Osmotic diarrhea is caused by the presence of nonabsorbable solutes in the gastrointestinal tract (Table 338-1). The classic example of osmotic diarrhea is lactose intolerance due to lactose enzyme deficiency in which lactose is not absorbed in the small intestine and reaches the colon intact (see Chapter 335.9). The colonic bacteria ferment the nonabsorbed lactose to short-chain organic acids, generating an osmotic load and causing water to be secreted into the lumen. Other examples include ingestion of excessive amounts of carbonated fluids that exceed the transport capacity, especially in toddlers, and ingestion of magnesium hydroxide and sorbitol, neither of which are absorbed, resulting in an osmotic load. Lactulose, a synthetic therapeutic disaccharide composed of galactose and fructose, is not digested in the small intestine and is fermented by the colonic bacteria to form organic acids, resulting in osmotic diarrhea. Osmotic diarrhea stops with fasting, has a low pH, and is positive for reducing substances. The sum of sodium plus potassium multiplied by two in the stools will be less than the measured stool osmolarity, a finding suggesting the presence of other osmols in the stool. The main diagnostic points that differentiate osmotic from secretory diarrhea are noted in Table 338-2.

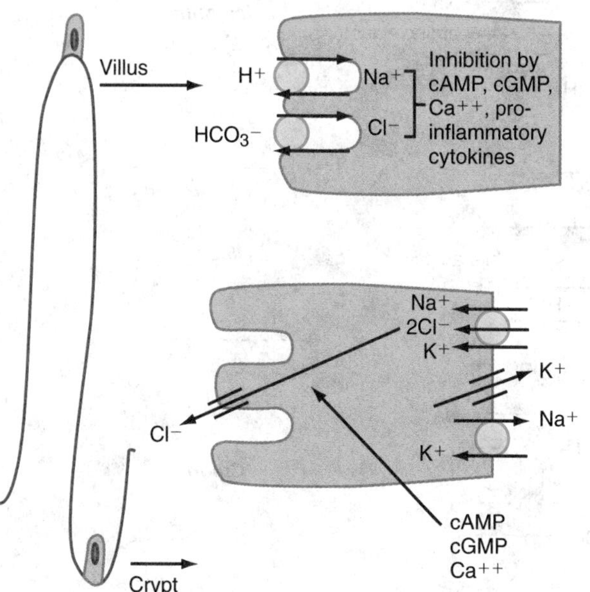

Figure 338-2. Model for intestinal secretion: Enterotoxins increase intracellular mediators (cAMP, cGMP, Ca^{2+}), which open chloride channels in the crypt cells and inhibit the neutral NaCl coupled pathway at the villus cells.

TABLE 338-1. Causes of Osmotic Diarrhea

MALABSORPTION OF WATER-SOLUBLE NUTRIENTS
Glucose-galactose malabsorption
Congenital
Acquired
Disaccharidase deficiencies (lactase and sucrase-isomaltase)
Congenital
Acquired
EXCESSIVE INTAKE OF CARBONATED FLUIDS
EXCESSIVE INTAKE OF NONABSORBABLE SOLUTES
Sorbitol
Lactulose
Magnesium hydroxide

Secretory Diarrhea. The major causes of secretory diarrhea are depicted in Table 338-3. The mechanisms for secretory diarrhea include activation of the intracellular mediators such as cAMP, cGMP, and intracellular calcium, which stimulate active chloride secretion from the crypt cells and inhibit the neutral coupled sodium chloride absorption. These mediators alter the paracellular ion flux because of toxin-mediated injury to the tight junctions. The classic example of secretory diarrhea is that induced by cholera and *Escherichia coli* enterotoxins that bind to a specific enterocyte surface receptor (the monosialoganglioside GM_1); a fragment of the toxin then enters the cell, where it activates adenylate cyclase on the basolateral membrane via interaction with a stimulatory G protein. This increases intracellular cAMP. The enterotoxigenic *E. coli* mediates secretory diarrhea by producing heat-labile toxin (LT) and heat-stable toxin (ST) in the small bowel. The labile toxin is similar in its action to the cholera toxin and binds to the same GM_1 surface receptor. Younger patients are more predisposed to the effects of ST because the number of ST receptors is higher during early life compared to that in adults. Other causes of secretory diarrhea include vasoactive peptides, which activate G protein–coupled receptors, resulting in an increase in intracellular mediators causing secretory diarrhea.

TABLE 338-2. Differential Diagnosis of Osmotic Vs Secretory Diarrhea

	OSMOTIC DIARRHEA	SECRETORY DIARRHEA
Volume of stool	<200 mL/24 hr	>200 mL/24 hr
Response to fasting	Diarrhea stops	Diarrhea continues
Stool Na^+	<70 mEq/L	>70 mEq/L
Reducing substances*	Positive	Negative
Stool pH	<5	>6

*Sucrose is not a reducing agent. Add 5 drops of 0.1 N HCl to a stool sample before adding reducing agent (Clinitest tablet).

TABLE 338-3. Causes of Secretory Diarrhea

ACTIVATION OF CYCLIC ADENOSINE MONOPHOSPHATE
Bacterial toxins: enterotoxins of cholera, *Escherichia coli* (heat-labile), *Shigella, Salmonella, Campylobacter jejuni, Pseudomonas aeruginosa*
Hormones: vasoactive intestinal peptide, gastrin, secretin
Anion surfactants: bile acids, ricinoleic acid
ACTIVATION OF CYCLIC GUANOSINE MONOPHOSPHATE
Bacterial toxins: *E. coli* (heat-stable) enterotoxin, *Yersinia enterocolitica* toxin
CALCIUM-DEPENDENT
Bacterial toxins: *Clostridium difficile* enterotoxin
Neurotransmitters: acetylcholine, serotonin
Paracrine agents: bradykinin

Secretory diarrhea is characterized by high volume; the stools are extremely watery. Stool analysis reveals high sodium and chloride content (>70 mEq/L). Secretory diarrhea continues with fasting.

Mutational Defects in Ion Transport Proteins. Congenital defects of sodium-hydrogen exchange, chloride-bicarbonate exchange, and sodium–bile acid transport proteins result in secretory diarrhea presenting at birth. The defects in chloride-bicarbonate exchange and sodium–bile acid transporters have gene mutations that encode their corresponding transport proteins. The defect in sodium-hydrogen exchange is believed to represent defects in the apical sodium-hydrogen exchangers. Patients with these defects present with secretory diarrhea and failure to thrive during the neonatal period. The defect in chloride-bicarbonate exchange is well characterized, and is more common compared with the defects in sodium-hydrogen exchange and sodium–bile acid transporter (see Chapter 335.11). Patients with chloride diarrhea have hypochloremic metabolic alkalosis with low serum chloride concentration, high stool chloride content coupled with chloride-free urine, low serum potassium, and high serum bicarbonate. Hydramnios is present in the mothers.

Reduction in Anatomic Surface Area. Short bowel syndrome results from resection of the bowel secondary to surgical indications such as necrotizing enterocolitis, midgut volvulus, or intestinal atresia (see Chapter 335.7). Celiac disease results in flattening of the proximal intestinal surface area with marked decrease in the digestive and absorptive function of the villus epithelium (see Chapter 335.2). Diarrhea is characterized by loss of fluids, electrolytes, macronutrients, and micronutrients.

Alteration in Intestinal Motility. The causes of altered intestinal motility include malnutrition, scleroderma, intestinal pseudo-obstruction syndromes, and diabetes mellitus. Malnutrition, in general, results in hypomotility, allowing bacterial overgrowth that leads to deconjugation of bile salts, resulting in an increase in the intracellular mediator cAMP and leading to secretory diarrhea.

ETIOLOGY. A simple classification for the etiology of chronic diarrhea is shown in Table 338-4. The two major factors resulting in diarrhea include intraluminal factors and mucosal factors. Intraluminal factors are involved in the digestion process, whereas mucosal factors are involved in the digestion and transport of nutrients across the mucosa. In many situations, both intraluminal and mucosal factors cause diarrhea. The intraluminal factors involve disorders of the pancreas, liver, and the brush border membrane of the enterocytes. In ≈85% of patients with **cystic fibrosis,** pancreatic insufficiency results in malabsorption of fats and proteins. Short stature, exocrine pancreatic hypoplasia, normal sweat chloride concentrations, and the variable features of neutropenia and skeletal changes characterize **Shwachman syndrome** (see Chapter 346). **Johannson-Blizzard syndrome** is characterized by anal imperforation, agenesis of the nasal cartilage, hair anomalies, mental retardation, deafness, hypothyroidism, and pancreatic insufficiency (see Chapter 346). The isolated pancreatic enzyme defects are congenital, and result in malabsorption of fat or proteins, depending on the defect. These defects include congenital lipase/colipase deficiency and congenital trypsinogen deficiency. Patients with **chronic pancreatitis** can present with pancreatic insufficiency and insulin-dependent diabetes. **Familial pancreatitis,** secondary to a mutation in the trypsinogen gene, can result in chronic pancreatitis and pancreatic insufficiency. **Pearson syndrome** is characterized by refractory sideroblastic anemia with vacuolization of bone marrow precursors, exocrine pancreatic insufficiency, and mitochondrial DNA deletions and duplications. Disorders of the liver, such as cholestasis, result in a decrease in bile acid pool size with malabsorption of fats. Bile acid loss with fat malabsorption can occur with terminal ileum disease, such as Crohn disease, or with terminal ileum resection. **Primary bile acid malabsorption** is a rare disorder secondary to a mutation in the ileal bile acid transporter. Patients present with fat malabsorption and diarrhea. Bacterial overgrowth in the gastrointestinal tract results in deconjugation and dehydroxylation of bile salts, resulting in diarrhea. Long-term use of bile acid sequestrants, such as cholestyramine, can lead to a decrease in bile acid pool size because of the continued loss of bile acids in the stools. Intraluminal osmolarity, resulting from malabsorption of carbohydrates, presents with an osmotic type of diarrhea. The causes of carbohydrate malabsorption include congenital and acquired causes of monosaccharide and disaccharide deficiencies. Excessive carbonated fluid intake that exceeds the transport capacity of the small intestine in younger infants results in nonspecific diarrhea. Excessive intake of nonabsorbable solutes, such as sorbitol, magnesium hydroxide, and lactulose, results in osmotic diarrhea.

The mucosal factors that lead to chronic diarrhea could be secondary to altered mucosal integrity from infections such as bacterial, viral, parasitic, and fungal agents. Parasitic infestations

TABLE 338-4. Etiology of Chronic Diarrhea

INTRALUMINAL FACTORS	MUCOSAL FACTORS
PANCREATIC DISORDERS	**ALTERED INTEGRITY**
Cystic fibrosis	Infections: bacterial, viral, fungal
Shwachman-Diamond syndrome	Infestations: parasitic
Johannson-Blizzard syndrome	Cow's milk and soy protein intolerance
Isolated pancreatic enzyme deficiencies	Inflammatory bowel disease (ulcerative colitis, microscopic colitis, Crohn)
Chronic pancreatitis	
Pearson syndrome	**ALTERED IMMUNE FUNCTION**
BILE ACID DISORDERS	Autoimmune enteropathy
Chronic cholestasis	Eosinophilic gastroenteropathy
Terminal ileum resection	AIDS
Bacterial overgrowth	Combined immunodeficiency syndromes
Chronic use of bile acid sequestrants	Immunoglobulin A and G deficiencies
Primary bile acid malabsorption	**ALTERED FUNCTION**
INTESTINAL DISORDERS	Defects in Cl^-/HCO_3^-, Na^+/H^+, bile acids, acrodermatitis enteropathica, selective folate deficiency, abetalipoproteinemia
Intraluminal osmolarity	
Carbohydrate malabsorption	
Congenital and acquired sucrase, lactase deficiencies	**ALTERED DIGESTIVE FUNCTION**
Congenital and acquired monosaccharide deficiency	Enterokinase deficiency
	Glucoamylase deficiency
Excessive carbonated fluid intake	**ALTERED SURFACE AREA**
Excessive intake of sorbitol, $Mg(OH)_2$, and lactulose	Celiac disease, postgastroenteritis syndrome
	Microvillus inclusion disease
	Short bowel syndrome
	ALTERED SECRETORY FUNCTION
	Enterotoxin-producing bacteria
	Tumors secreting vasoactive peptides
	ALTERED ANATOMIC STRUCTURES
	Hirschsprung disease
	Partial small bowel obstruction
	Malrotation

such as with *Giardia* or cryptosporidia can present with chronic diarrhea. Inflammatory bowel disease such as ulcerative colitis, Crohn disease, and microscopic colitis can lead to alteration in the mucosal integrity, resulting in the decreased absorption of water and electrolytes through the gastrointestinal tract. Cow's milk and soy protein intolerance can present with diarrhea secondary to partial villus atrophy or allergic colitis. Altered immune function, as seen in patients with agammaglobulinemia, isolated immunoglobulin A (IgA) deficiency, and combined immunodeficiency disorders, can result in diarrhea. Patients with AIDS are more predisposed to bacterial, viral, and fungal infections. Similarly, **autoimmune enteropathy** and **eosinophilic gastroenteropathy** are believed to be disorders involving alteration of the mucosal immune function, and can result in diarrhea. Altered mucosa transport function, as seen in congenital disorders involving sodium-hydrogen exchange, chloride-bicarbonate exchange, bile acid transport, and glucose-galactose transport, results in diarrhea early in the neonatal period. Similarly, defects in the absorption of zinc, such as acrodermatitis anteropathica and folate transport, can result in diarrhea.

Abetalipoproteinemia is characterized by fat malabsorption, neurologic lesions, and ocular abnormalities, such as retinitis pigmentosa (see Chapter 86.3). The diagnosis is confirmed by the typical hematologic finding of acanthocytosis and the appearance of the small bowel biopsy in which the enterocyte tips are filled with lipid droplets. Altered mucosal digestive function includes congenital enterokinase deficiency that results in loss of activation of trypsinogen to trypsin with protein malabsorption (see Chapter 335.9). α-Glucoamylase deficiency is rare and results in loss of hydrolysis of glucose polymers.

Altered mucosal surface area is seen in **celiac disease**, partial villus atrophy secondary to postgastroenteritis malabsorption syndrome, tropical sprue, microvillus inclusion disease, Whipple disease, and short bowel syndrome. In these disorders, the height and structure of the villi are altered so that the absorptive capacity of the mucosal surface area is markedly decreased. Celiac disease occurs secondary to gluten sensitivity (see Chapter 335.2). Postgastroenteritis syndrome is a nutritional disorder that occurs after a prolonged episode of gastroenteritis and decreased energy intake. Microvillus inclusion disease is characterized by diarrhea, failure to thrive, and a histologic picture of microvillus inclusions (see Chapter 335.3). The mucosal surface lacks brush border membranes or possesses irregular blunted microvilli. Whipple disease is mainly seen in adults and is secondary to an actinomycete, *Tropheryma whippelii*. Patients present with weight loss, diarrhea, and arthropathy. The diagnosis is established by a small bowel biopsy, and patients respond to prolonged administration of trimethoprim-sulfamethoxazole. Tropical sprue is commonly seen in patients living or returning from trips to developing countries (see Chapter 335.4). Patients present with diarrhea and nutritional deficiencies, especially folate. Alteration in the anatomic structure, as seen in Hirschsprung disease, malrotation, and partial small bowel obstruction, can result in diarrhea secondary to bacterial overgrowth. Altered mucosal secretory function includes enterotoxin-producing bacteria and tumors that secrete vasoactive peptides. Table 338-5 summarizes the most common causes of chronic diarrhea at various age groups.

TABLE 338-5. Common Causes of Chronic Diarrhea

INFANCY
Postgastroenteritis malabsorption syndrome
Cow's milk/soy protein intolerance
Secondary disaccharidase deficiencies
Cystic fibrosis
CHILDHOOD
Chronic nonspecific diarrhea
Secondary disaccharidase deficiencies
Giardiasis
Postgastroenteritis malabsorption syndrome
Celiac disease
Cystic fibrosis
ADOLESCENCE
Irritable bowel syndrome
Inflammatory bowel disease
Giardiasis
Lactose intolerance

EVALUATION OF PATIENTS. The evaluation of patients with chronic diarrhea is depicted in Table 338-6. First, it is important to determine that the patient indeed has diarrhea, as patients with encopresis may be mistakenly considered to have diarrhea secondary to constant fecal soiling. In phase I, the history and physical examination, which include a nutritional assessment, are the initial steps. The clinical history should include the amount and type of fluid ingested per day. If the patient's clinical history suggests excessive carbonated drink or fruit juice intake of >150 mL/kg/24 hr, with normal growth and height parameters, **chronic nonspecific diarrhea** needs to be considered. A decrease in the amount of fluid to no more than 90 mL/kg/24 hr will result in resolution of the diarrhea. If the patient is ingesting nonabsorbable nutrients such as sorbitol in excessive amounts, a dietary adjustment needs to be made before extensively investigating the patient.

The stool examination is an integral step in investigating a patient with chronic diarrhea. The most recently evacuated stool, including its liquid content, is useful for diagnostic purposes. Various collection techniques are helpful, including the placement of a urine collection bag over the anus and everting a disposable diaper to collect the stool. The stool specimen should be stored in a refrigerator until examination is performed. Specimens for bacterial culture should be transported immediately to the bacteriology laboratory for inoculation into growth media. The gross examination of the stool should allow the physician to determine whether the patient has diarrhea and whether blood or mucus is present in the stool, a finding suggesting inflammation of the colon. The color of the stool is rarely helpful unless it is bloody. Occult testing for blood is useful to determine whether the patient has microscopic blood loss. Carbohydrate malabsorption is detected by analysis of the liquid fraction of a fresh specimen. A pH <5 or the presence of moderate reducing substances indicates the presence of reducing carbohydrates (sucrose is not a direct

TABLE 338-6. Evaluation of Patients with Chronic Diarrhea

PHASE I
Clinical history including specific amounts of fluids ingested per day
Physical examination including nutritional assessment
Stool exam (pH, reducing substances, smear for white blood count, fat, ova, and parasites)
Stool cultures
Stool for *Clostridium difficile* toxin
Blood studies (complete blood count, erythrocyte sedimentation rate, electrolytes, blood urea nitrogen, creatinine)
PHASE II
Sweat chloride
72 hr stool collection for fat determination
Stool electrolytes, osmolality
Stool for phenolphthalein, magnesium sulfate, phosphate
Breath H_2 tests
Phase III
Endoscopic studies
Small bowel biopsy
Sigmoidoscopy or colonoscopy with biopsies
Barium studies
Phase IV
Hormonal studies vasoactive intestinal polypeptide, gastrin, secretin, 5-hydroxyindoleacetic assays

reducing substance). The stools should be sent for electrolytes and osmolality testing if secretory diarrhea is considered (see Table 338-2).

Microscopic examination of the stool helps to determine the presence of white blood cells, which signifies colonic inflammation. The stools could be examined for ova and parasites such as *Giardia,* amebae, or cryptosporidia. Trichrome stain or acid-fast stain can be of value in identifying *Cryptosporidium* spp. Stool should be examined for the presence of *Giardia* antigen. Sudan stain can be used either on a plain stool smear or with the addition of acetic acid and heat to determine the presence of triglycerides and split fats.

In the event that phase I investigation has failed to reveal a cause, a phase II work-up is indicated, and includes a sweat chloride test to rule out cystic fibrosis. A 72-hr stool collection for fat determination is the standard to determine whether the patient has fat malabsorption in the setting of a negative sweat chloride test. Stools could also be checked for phenolphthalein, magnesium, sulfate, and phosphate to determine whether the diarrhea is secondary to the ingestion of **laxatives** (factitious diarrhea). Breath hydrogen tests can be used to determine a specific carbohydrate malabsorption. A breath hydrogen test for glucose or lactulose can be used to diagnose bacterial overgrowth.

Phase III investigation includes endoscopic studies for small bowel and colonic biopsies. Barium studies, such as an upper gastrointestinal series or a barium enema, can be used to rule out anatomic lesions in the gastrointestinal tract. If none of these tests are revealing, phase IV evaluation includes hormonal studies and neurohormonal and neurotransmittal studies such as vasoactive intestinal polypeptide, gastrin, secretin, and 5-hydroxyindoleacetic assays.

TREATMENT. Figure 338-3 depicts the general therapeutic approaches to the management of chronic diarrhea. The 1st principle is to maintain adequate nutritional intake to permit normal growth and development. The height, weight, and nutritional status of the patient must be documented. If nutritional parameters, including weight and height, are normal, and the stool examination does not show any fat, the possibility of chronic nonspecific diarrhea needs to be considered. The pathogenesis of this condition includes excessive carbonated fluid intake, nondigestible carbohydrate malabsorption from excessive juice ingestion, and low fat intake.

Chronic nonspecific diarrhea generally presents in well-appearing toddlers between 1 and 3 yr of age (toddler's diarrhea). The diarrhea is often brown and watery, at times containing undigested food particles. If the child's fluid intake is >150 mL/kg/24 hr, fluid intake should be reduced to no more than 90 mL/kg/24 hr. Parents may note that the child is irritable in the 1st 2 days after the fluid restriction; however, persistence in this approach for several more days results in a decrease in the stool frequency and volume. If the dietary history suggests that the child is ingesting significant amounts of fruit juices, then the offending juices should be decreased. Sorbitol, which is a nonabsorbable sugar, is found in apple, pear, and prune juices, and can cause diarrhea in toddlers. Moreover, apple and pear juices contain higher amounts of fructose in excess of glucose concentration, a feature postulated to cause diarrhea in toddlers.

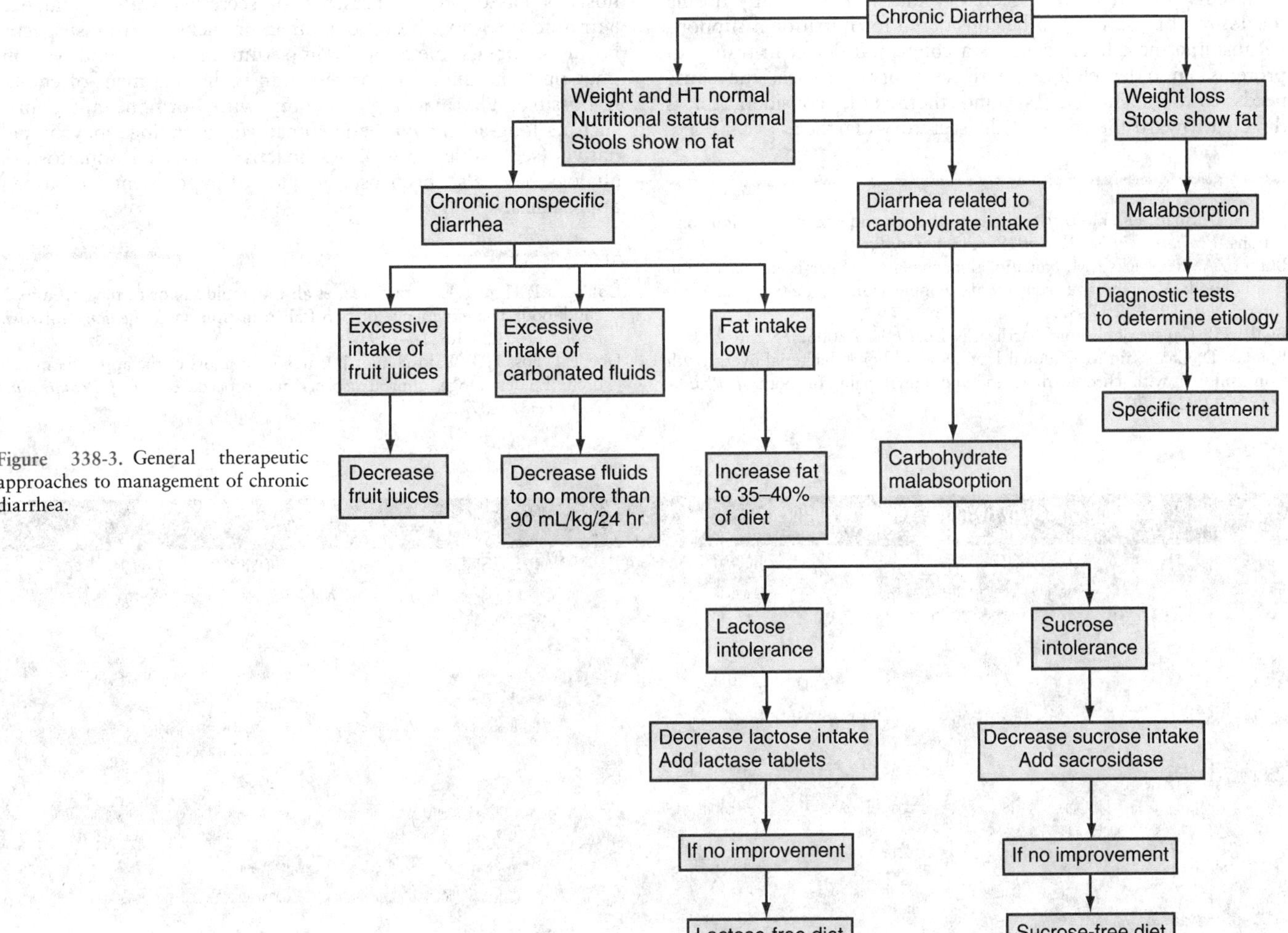

Figure 338-3. General therapeutic approaches to management of chronic diarrhea.

Levels of dietary fat intake may also play a role in chronic diarrhea. If the child's fat intake has been restricted by the parents, then fat intake can be increased to ≈40% of the total calories per day.

If the diarrhea is secondary to carbohydrate intolerance, then a trial period of decreased lactose or sucrose may be initiated. Lactase (LactAid) can be used to aid in the digestion of lactose. If diarrhea persists, a trial of a lactose-free or sucrose-free diet is indicated. Alternatively, breath hydrogen tests can document the presence of lactose or sucrose intolerance. A glucose or lactulose breath hydrogen test can be used for the diagnosis of bacterial overgrowth.

If the patient presents with weight loss and the stool examination shows fat, the possibility of chronic diarrhea secondary to a malabsorption syndrome needs to be considered. The most common cause of chronic diarrhea associated with the malabsorption is postgastroenteritis malabsorption syndrome. These patients respond well to a predigested formula. In the event that the patient shows intolerance to oral feeding with a predigested formula such as Pregestimil or Alimentum, nasogastric drip-feeding with an elemental formula should be considered for a period of 3–4 wk.

A patient presenting with suspected small intestinal bacterial overgrowth should undergo evaluation for surgical, medical, and nutritional support. Surgical treatment is indicated if the patient has malrotation or partial small bowel obstruction. Antibiotic therapy is usually initiated with metronidazole in combination with ampicillin or trimethoprim-sulfamethoxazole. Diarrhea caused by *Giardia lamblia* can be treated with metronidazole or nitazoxanide, whereas *Cryptosporidium parvum* is treated with nitazoxanide.

Patients presenting with secretory diarrhea, especially during the 1st mo of life, need to be considered for nutritional support, because the most likely cause is a congenital defect in transport proteins. In older children with secretory diarrhea, the cause needs to be identified 1st, and therapeutic consideration is directed toward the cause of the secretory diarrhea.

Acra S, Ghishan, FK: Electrolyte fluxes in the gut and oral rehydration solutions. *Pedriatr Clin North Am* 1996;43:433–449.

Bhutta ZA, Hendricks KM: Nutritional management of persistent diarrhea in childhood: A perspective from the developing world. *J Pediatr Gastroenterol Nutr* 1996;22:17–37.

Binder HJ: Causes of chronic diarrhea. *N Engl J Med* 2006;355:236–239.

Boissieu D, Chaussain M, Badoual J, et al: Small-bowel bacterial overgrowth in children with chronic diarrhea, abdominal pain, or both. *J Pediatr* 1996;128:203–207.

Castro-Rodriguez JA, Salazar-Lindo E, Leon-Barua R: Differentiation of osmotic and secretory diarrhea by stool carbohydrate and osmolar gap measurements. *Arch Dis Child* 1997;77:201–205.

Cutz E, Sherman PM, Davidson GP: Enteropathies associated with protracted diarrhea of infancy: Clinicopathological features, cellular and molecular mechanisms. *Pediatr Pathol Lab Med* 1997;17:335–368.

Dellert SF, Cohen MB: Diarrheal disease. *Pediatr Gasterol* 1994;23:637–654.

Donowitz M, Kokke FT, Saidi R: Evaluation of patients with chronic diarrhea. *N Engl J Med* 1995;332:725–729.

Duggan C, Nurko S: Feeding the gut: The scientific basis for continued enteral nutrition during acute diarrhea. *J Pediatr* 1997;131:801–808.

Greene HL, Ghishan FK: Excessive fluid intake as a cause of chronic diarrhea in young children. *J Pediatr* 1983;102:836–840.

Kneepkens CM, Hoekstra JH: Chronic nonspecific diarrhea of childhood: Pathophysiology and management. *Pediatr Clin North Am* 1996;43: 375–390.

338.1 • Diarrhea from Hormone-Secreting Tumors • Joel Shilyansky

Certain hormone-producing tumors cause a marked increase in intestinal secretion, leading to severe chronic watery diarrhea (Table 338-7). The secretory diarrhea persists even if food is withheld. These tumors originate in the neural crest–derived APUD cells (*a*mine content, *p*recursor *u*ptake, amino acid *d*ecarboxylation) of the gastroenteropancreatic endocrine system and in adrenal or extra-adrenal neurogenic sites. Diarrhea is massive and results in fluid and electrolyte imbalance and weight loss. Diagnosis is based on the presence of secretory watery diarrhea, extraintestinal manifestations, measurement of the suspected hormone or its metabolites in serum or urine, and various imaging techniques. Tumor resection is the treatment of choice, if possible. Pharmacologic therapy with hormone antagonists such as long-acting synthetic somatostatin analogs may be palliative (see Table 338-7). Radioactively labeled somatostatin analogs have also been used as part of experimental treatment approaches.

Dall'Igna P, Ferrari A, Luzzatto C, et al: Carcinoid tumor of the appendix in childhood: The experience of two Italian institutions. *J Pediatr Gastroenterol Nutr* 2005;40:216–219.

Doede T, Foss HD, Waldschmidt J: Carcinoid tumors of the appendix in children: Epidemiology, clinical aspects and procedure. *Eur J Pediatr Surg* 2000;10:372–377.

TABLE 338-7. Diarrhea Caused by Hormone-Secreting Tumors

NAME	SITE	HORMONE	MANIFESTATIONS	THERAPY
Carcinoid	Intestinal argentaffin cells Appendix, ileum, colon, jejunum, rectum Bronchial tree	Serotonin	Diarrhea, crampy abdominal pain, flushing, wheezing, cardiac valve damage	Somatostatin analog, resection
Gastrinoma	Pancreas	Gastrin	Peptic ulcer, diarrhea	H_2-blocking agents, omeprazole, tumor resection, (gastrectomy)
Mastocytoma	Cutaneous, intestine, liver, spleen	Histamine, VIP	Pruritus, flushing, apnea, if VIP(+)-diarrhea	H_1- and H_2-blocking agents, cromolyn, steroids, resection if solitary
Medullary carcinoma	Thyroid	Calcitonin, VIP, prostaglandins	Watery diarrhea	Thyroidectomy
Ganglioneuroma, Ganglioneuroblastoma, Neuroblastoma, Pheochromocytoma	Chromaffin cells; abdominal > other sites; extra-adrenal or adrenal	Catecholamines, VIP	Hypertension, tachycardia, sweating, anxiety, watery diarrhea[†]	α-Adrenergic blockade for BP control, β-adrenergic blockade for tachycardia, resection
Somatostatinoma	Pancreas	Somatostatin	Massive diarrhea	Resection
VIPoma	Pancreas	VIP	Watery diarrhea, achlorhydria, hypokalemia	Somatostatin analogs, resection

[†] *Diarrhea has been reported only in adult patients with pheochromocytoma.*

BP, blood pressure; H_1, histamine receptor type 1; H_2, histamine receptor type 2; VIP, vasoactive intestinal polypeptide.

Oberg K: Chemotherapy and biotherapy in the treatment of neuroendocrine tumours. *Ann Oncol* 2001;12:S111–S114.
Soga J: Early-stage carcinoids of the gastrointestinal tract: An analysis of 1914 reported cases. *Cancer* 2005;103:1587–1595.

Chapter 339 ■ Recurrent Abdominal Pain of Childhood

Robert Wyllie

Chronic abdominal pain is classified as either organic or nonorganic, depending on whether a specific cause of the pain is identified. Nonorganic pain or "functional" abdominal pain refers to pain that cannot be explained on a structural, physiologic, or biochemical basis. Recurrent abdominal pain (RAP) in children is defined as episodes of pain occurring at least monthly for 3 consecutive months with a severity that interrupts routine functioning. RAP affects ≈15% of middle and high school students. Approximately 10% of students who experience abdominal pain seek medical evaluation. The likelihood of seeking medical attention is proportional to the severity and frequency of abdominal pain and its impact on school attendance.

Early investigators found an organic cause for RAP in 5–10% of children. With advancement in medical technology, including endoscopy, breath hydrogen testing for carbohydrate malabsorption, intestinal motility, and radiographic analysis, the percentage of patients with unexplained pain is decreasing. For the majority of teenagers with RAP, no specific cause can be found with current diagnostic techniques; many will eventually be diagnosed with irritable bowel syndrome.

Periumbilical abdominal pain is the most common pain location in children with RAP. Epigastric pain is frequently associated with symptoms of early satiety, nausea, bloating, or belching and, in the presence of a negative evaluation and no response to acid-blocking medication, is referred to as *nonulcer dyspepsia.* Pain below the umbilicus is often accompanied by abdominal cramps, bloating, and distention with an altered bowel pattern. This complex of symptoms is consistent with irritable bowel syndrome (IBS) in the adult population. IBS-type symptoms have been documented in ≈35% of the children with RAP. The Rome II diagnostic criteria for IBS-like symptoms in children include: pain or discomfort for 12 wk in the last 12 mo plus two of the following three:

- abdominal pain relieved by defecation
- onset of pain with a change in stool frequency (>3 movements/day or <3 movements/wk)
- onset of pain with change in stool form (lumpy, loose, hard), the presence of mucus, bloating, abnormal passage (straining, urgency, incomplete evacuation)

Gastrointestinal tract symptoms are positively related to both anxiety and depression, particularly in children with IBS-type symptoms. Improvement in symptoms during weekends and school vacations suggests functional pain, but the absence of this pattern does not rule out this diagnosis.

Investigations into the etiology of RAP have focused on the autonomic nervous system and intestinal motility abnormalities. The dorsal horn of the spinal cord regulates conduction of impulses from peripheral nociceptive receptors to the spinal cord and brain, and the pain experience is further influenced by cognitive and emotional centers. Chronic peripheral pain can produce increased neural activity in higher central nervous system centers, leading to perpetuation of pain. Psychosocial stress can affect pain intensity and quality through these mechanisms. Manometric and radionucleotide emptying studies suggest that altered motility in combination with heightened awareness in certain children may cause abdominal pain. Differences in visceral sensation may contribute to differences in perception of pain.

The child's response to pain can be influenced by stress, by personality type, and by the reinforcement of illness behavior within the family. A significantly higher proportion of children with RAP have relatives with somatization disorders, alcoholism, and antisocial behavior problems. Parents and siblings are more likely to have complaints of abdominal pain, nervous breakdown, and migraine headaches. Children with functional abdominal pain are more likely to experience stressors. Sexual abuse as a child may be associated with RAP. This possibility should always be considered, especially in a girl whose abdominal symptoms begin in the pre-teenage or teenage years.

DIAGNOSIS. A wide range of potential organic causes of RAP (see Table 303-4) must be considered before establishing a diagnosis of functional pain. Among the more common causes are chronic constipation, parasitic infection *(Giardia),* gastroesophageal reflux, inflammatory bowel disease, and lactase deficiency. Lactose intolerance is so common that the finding may be coincidental; the clinician must be cautious in attributing chronic abdominal pain to this condition. Pinworms are unlikely to be the cause of abdominal pain.

The characteristic presentation of children with RAP includes onset later than 6 yr of age and midline paroxysmal pain, most often periumbilical but also localized to the epigastric or suprapubic area. The pain interrupts normal activity, but there is usually no relationship with meals. Children with IBS typically have abdominal pain relieved by defecation. They may notice mucus in their stools and looser or more frequent stools at the outset of their pain. Bloating or the sense of incomplete evacuation may also be present.

Symptoms suggestive of an organic etiology include age <6 yr, fever, weight loss, joint symptoms, or abnormal growth. Organic pain is usually localized away from the umbilicus and may wake the patient from sleep. Vomiting, diarrhea, and blood in the stool are suggestive of an organic etiology. Children with RAP have a normal physical examination, whereas those with organic etiology may have abdominal tenderness, rectal fissures, or evidence of occult blood in the stool. Serial growth points should be plotted, if available, because growth deceleration is frequently associated with organic causes of abdominal pain.

EVALUATION. The laboratory, radiologic, or endoscopic evaluation of children with chronic abdominal pain should be individualized, depending on the findings suggested by a detailed history and physical examination. Laboratory studies may be unnecessary if the history and physical examination clearly lead to a diagnosis of functional abdominal pain. A complete blood cell count, sedimentation rate, stool test for parasites (especially *Giardia*), and urinalysis are reasonable screening studies. If inflammatory bowel disease is suspected, the sedimentation rate is often elevated. The finding of an abnormal sedimentation rate or other acute phase reactant should prompt the clinician to look further for an organic etiology of the complaints. Elevated stool calprotectin levels also suggest an organic etiology. If indicated, an ultrasound examination of the abdomen can give information about kidneys, gallbladder, and pancreas; with lower abdominal pain, a pelvic ultrasonogram may be indicated. An upper gastrointestinal tract x-ray series is indicated if one suspects a disorder of the stomach or small intestine. *Helicobacter pylori* infection does not seem to be associated with RAP. In patients with symptoms suggestive of gastritis or ulcer, an *H. pylori* test (serum or fecal) may be performed to document the infection. Esophagogastroduodenoscopy is indicated with symptoms suggestive of persistent upper gastrointestinal pathology. In the absence of this suspicion, esophagogastroduodenoscopy is unlikely to identify an abnormality and is usually not necessary.

TREATMENT. The family and the child with functional RAP may worry about the inability to identify an organic cause and may be resistant to a diagnosis of nonorganic disease. After a thorough history and physical examination, the most important component of the treatment is reassurance of the child and family members. Specifically, they need to be reassured that no evidence of a serious underlying disorder is present. Children of families that do not accept a psychologic cause of the symptoms are more likely to have persistent somatic complaints and school absences. The parents should be instructed to avoid reinforcing the symptom with secondary gain. Furthermore, if children have missed school or have been removed from routine activities because of the pain, it is important that they return to regular activities. Medications are generally unhelpful or, at best, offer transient placebo effect. Gastric acid blockers or visceral muscle relaxants (anticholinergics) can be tried empirically, but they are most often unhelpful in the absence of specific indication. Biofeedback, guided imagery, and relaxation techniques have been useful in some children with functional pain.

If lactose intolerance is suspected, the diagnosis can be documented by breath hydrogen testing. Institution of a lactose-free diet usually results in resolution of the pain. Symptoms of gastroesophageal reflux will generally subside with the use of acid blockers. Recurrent symptoms are usually an indication for formal testing before instituting chronic therapy. Children with symptoms of irritable bowel and loose stools often benefit from fiber supplementation. Anticholinergics or tricyclic antidepressants may be useful in some patients. Adults with IBS have been treated with 5-hydroxytryptamine receptor antagonists (for diarrhea predominant) or agonists (for constipation). $5HT_3$ (alosetron) receptor antagonists are associated with ischemic colitis and are not recommended. If chronic constipation is identified, it should be treated in the standard fashion (see Chapters 22.4 and 329).

Successful management depends on close follow-up. The parents can try new approaches to the child's symptoms without fear that the physician is abandoning them if they know that follow-up by telephone or office visit has been arranged. Often, it is during the follow-up visits that the pediatrician comes to know the child and fully understand the symptoms. It is possible that an organic problem may not have been apparent on the initial visit but, with time, the symptom complex becomes more typical.

These approaches often result in reduction or elimination of the abdominal symptoms. Children with functional abdominal pain are likely to become adults with functional disorders, although the nature of the symptoms may change.

Ball TM, Shapiro DE, Monheim CJ, Weydert JA: A pilot study of the use of guided imagery for the treatment of recurrent abdominal pain in children. *Clin Pediatr (Phila)* 2003;42:527–532.

Ball TM, Weydert JA: Methodological challenges to treatment trials for recurrent abdominal pain in children. *Arch Pediatr Adolesc Med* 2003;157:1121–1127.

Biggs AM, Aziz Q, Tomenson B, Creed F: Effect of childhood adversity on health related quality of life in patients with upper abdominal or chest pain. *Gut* 2004;53:180–186.

Biggs AM, Aziz Q, Tomenson B, Creed F: Do childhood adversity and recent social stress predict health care use in patients presenting with upper abdominal or chest pain? *Psychosom Med* 2003;65:1020–1028.

Chang L, Ameen VZ, Dukes GE, et al: A dose-ranging, phase II study of the efficacy and safety of alosetron in men with diarrhea-predominant IBS. *Am J Gastroenterol* 2005;100:115–123.

Chitkara DK, Camilleri M, Zinsmeister AR, et al: Gastric sensory and motor dysfunction in adolescents with functional dyspepsia. *J Pediatr* 2005;146:500–505.

Crushell E, Rowland M, Doherty M, et al: Importance of parental conceptual model of illness in severe recurrent abdominal pain. *Pediatrics* 2003;112:1368–1372.

El-Matary W, Spray C, Sandhu B: Irritable bowel syndrome: The commonest cause of recurrent abdominal pain in children. *Eur J Pediatr* 2004;163:584–588.

Farthing MJG: Treatment of irritable bowel syndrome. *Br Med J* 2005;330: 429–430.

Faure C, Wieckowska A: Somatic referral of visceral sensations and rectal sensory threshold for pain in children with functional gastrointestinal disorders. *J Pediatr* 2007;150:66–71.

Ghandour RM, Overpeck MD, Huang ZJ, et al: Headache, stomachache, backache, and morning fatigue among adolescent girls in the United States: Associations with behavioral, sociodemographic, and environmental factors. *Arch Pediatr Adolesc Med* 2004;158:797–803.

Gremse DA, Greer AS, Vacik J, DiPalma JA: Abdominal pain associated with lactose ingestion in children with lactose intolerance. *Clin Pediatr (Phila)* 2003;42:341–345.

Haim A, Pillar G, Pecht A, et al: Sleep patterns in children and adolescents with functional recurrent abdominal pain: Objective versus subjective assessment. *Acta Paediatr* 2004;93:677–680.

Lindley KJ, Glaser D, Milla PJ: Consumerism in healthcare can be detrimental to child health: Lessons from children with functional abdominal pain. *Arch Dis Child* 2005;90:335–337.

Tibble JA, Sigthorsson G, Foster R, et al: Use of surrogate markers of inflammation and Rome criteria to distinguish organic from nonorganic intestinal disease. *Gastroenterology* 2002;123:450–460.

Walker LS, Lipani TA, Greene JW, et al: Recurrent abdominal pain: Symptom subtypes based on the Rome II Criteria for pediatric functional gastrointestinal disorders. *J Pediatr Gastroenterol Nutr* 2004;38:187–191.

Weydert JA, Ball TM, Davis MF: Systematic review of treatments for recurrent abdominal pain. *Pediatrics* 2003;111:e1–e11.

Chapter 340 ■ Acute Appendicitis

John J. Aiken and Keith T. Oldham

Acute appendicitis, despite a declining incidence in the United States in the past half-century, remains the most common acute surgical condition in children and a major cause of childhood morbidity. Presently, ≈80,000 children are affected in the United States annually, a rate of 4/1,000 children <14 yr of age. Although in the past decade there has been a trend toward shorter hospital stays, appendicitis accounts for >1 million hospital days utilized per year. A primary focus is improved diagnosis to avoid complications and the significant morbidity associated with perforation. Appendicitis is most common in older children with peak incidence between the ages of 12 and 18 yr; it is rare in children <5 yr of age (<5% of cases) and extremely rare (<1% of cases) in children <3 yr of age. It affects males slightly more often than females and whites more often than blacks in the United States. There is a seasonal peak incidence in autumn and spring. There appears to be a familial predisposition in some cases, particularly in children in whom appendicitis develops before age 6 yr. Despite advances in imaging technology and computer-assisted decision-making models/scoring systems, accurate diagnosis can be difficult and perforation rates are reported to be as high as 20%. Management has changed significantly in the past several decades with the use of antibiotics, improved imaging techniques, initial nonoperative management in selected cases, percutaneous drainage procedures by interventional radiology, and the use of laparoscopy. Mortality is low, but morbidity remains high, mostly in association with perforated appendicitis. There is an increased incidence of perforated appendicitis in children of minority race and children with Medicaid health insurance.

PATHOLOGY

Acute appendicitis is most likely a disease of multiple etiologies, the final common pathway of which involves invasion of the appendiceal wall by bacteria. One pathway to acute appendicitis begins with luminal obstruction; inspissated fecal material, lymphoid hyperplasia, ingested foreign body, parasites, and tumors have all been implicated as causative factors. Obstruction of the appendiceal lumen results in increasing intraluminal pressures from bacterial proliferation and continued secretion of mucus. Elevated intraluminal pressure, in turn, leads to lymphatic and venous congestion and edema followed by impaired arterial perfusion eventually leading to ischemia of the wall of the appendix, bacterial invasion with inflammatory infiltrate of all layers of the appendiceal wall and necrosis. This progression correlates clinically with progression from simple appendicitis to gangrenous appendicitis and, thereafter, appendiceal perforation. Submucosal lymphoid follicles, which can obstruct the appendiceal lumen, are few in number at birth but multiply steadily during childhood, reaching a peak in number during the teen years when acute appendicitis is most common and declining after age 30 yr. Both fecaliths and appendicitis are more frequent in developed countries with refined, low-fiber diets than in developing countries with a high-fiber diet; no causal relationship has been established between lack of dietary fiber and appendicitis. The finding that <50% of specimens from cases of acute appendicitis demonstrate luminal obstruction on histologic examination has lead to investigations of alternative etiologies. Enteric infection likely plays a role in many cases in association with mucosal ulceration and invasion of the appendiceal wall by bacteria. Bacteria such as *Yersinia, Salmonella,* and *Shigella* spp. and viruses such as mumps, coxsackie B, and adenovirus have all been implicated. In addition, case reports demonstrate the occurrence of appendicitis from ingested foreign bodies, in association with carcinoid tumors of the appendix or *Ascaris* and after blunt abdominal trauma. Children with cystic fibrosis have an increased incidence of appendicitis and the cause is believed to be the abnormal thickened mucus characteristic of this disease. Appendicitis in neonates is rare and warrants evaluation for cystic fibrosis as well as Hirschsprung disease.

A primary focus in the management of acute appendicitis is avoidance of sepsis and the infectious complications mostly seen in association with perforation. Bacteria can be cultured from the serosal surface of the appendix before microscopic or gross perforation and bacterial invasion of the mesenteric veins can result in portal vein sepsis (pylephlebitis) and possible liver abscess. Subsequent to perforation, the microbiologic fecal contamination may be localized to the right lower quadrant or pelvis by the omentum and adjacent loops of bowel, resulting in a localized abscess or inflammatory mass (phlegmon), or alternatively, the fecal contamination may spread throughout the peritoneal cavity causing diffuse peritonitis. Young children typically have a poorly developed omentum and are frequently unable to control the infection locally. Perforation and abscess formation with appendicitis can lead to fistula formation in adjacent organs, scrotal cellulitis and abscess through a patent processus vaginalis (congenital indirect inguinal hernia), or small bowel obstruction.

CLINICAL MANIFESTATIONS

There are several predictable "forms" of acute appendicitis; the signs and symptoms can be classic or quite variable, depending on the timing of presentation, the position of the appendix, and individual variability in the evolution of the disease process. Whereas the classic presentation of acute appendicitis is well described, this represents less than half the cases; therefore, most cases have an "atypical" presentation. Despite advances in imaging technology, the hallmark of diagnosing acute appendicitis remains a careful and thorough history and physical examination. A primary focus of the initial assessment is attention to the temporal evolution of illness in relation to specific presenting signs and symptoms.

Classically, acute appendicitis begins as an insidious illness with generalized malaise and anorexia. Abdominal pain is consistently the primary symptom and begins shortly (hours) after the onset of illness. The pain is initially vague, unrelated to activity or position, often colicky, and periumbilical in location as a result of visceral inflammation from a distended appendix. Progression of the inflammatory process in the next 12–24 hr leads to involvement of the adjacent parietal surfaces, resulting in somatic pain localized to the right lower quadrant. The pain becomes steady and more severe and is exacerbated by movement. The child often describes marked discomfort with the "bumpy" car ride to the hospital, moves cautiously, and has difficulty getting on to the examining room stretcher. Nausea and vomiting occur in more than half the patients and almost always follow the onset of abdominal pain by several hours. Anorexia is a classic and consistent finding in acute appendicitis, but occasionally, affected patients are hungry. Diarrhea and urinary symptoms are also common, particularly in cases of perforated appendicitis when there is likely inflammation and possible abscess in the pelvis. Fever is typically low-grade unless perforation has occurred. Most patients demonstrate at least mild tachycardia. The temporal progression of symptoms from vague mild pain, malaise, and anorexia to severe localized pain, fever, and vomiting occurs rapidly, in 24–48 hr in the majority of cases. If the diagnosis is delayed beyond 36–48 hr, the perforation rate exceeds 65%. Many patients experience a period after perforation of lessened abdominal pain and acute symptoms, presumably with the elimination of pressure within the appendix. If the omentum or adjacent intestine is able to "wall off" the infectious process, the evolution of illness is less predictable and delay in presentation is likely. If perforation leads to diffuse peritonitis, the child generally has escalating diffuse abdominal pain and rapid development of toxicity evidenced by dehydration and signs of sepsis including: hypotension, oliguria, acidosis, and high-grade fever. When several days have elapsed in the progression of appendicitis, patients frequently develop signs and symptoms of developing small bowel obstruction. If the appendix is **retrocecal** in location, appendicitis predictably evolves more slowly and patients are likely to relate 4–5 days of illness preceding evaluation. In addition, the pain will be lateral and posterior and may mimic the symptoms associated with septic arthritis of the hip or a psoas muscle abscess.

Physical examination remains primary in accurate diagnosis of acute appendicitis and begins with inspection of the child's demeanor as well as the appearance of the abdomen. Children with early appendicitis typically appear mildly ill and move tentatively, hunched forward and often with a slight limp favoring the right side. Supine, they are frequently lying quietly, on their right side with their knees pulled up to relax the abdominal muscles, and when asked to lie flat or sit up, they move cautiously and may use a hand to protect the right lower quadrant. Early in appendicitis, the abdomen is typically flat; abdominal distention suggests more advanced disease characteristic of perforation or developing small bowel obstruction. Auscultation may reveal normal or hyperactive bowel sounds in early appendicitis, to be replaced by hypoactive bowel sounds as the disease progresses to perforation. **Localized abdominal tenderness is the single most reliable finding in the diagnosis of acute appendicitis.** The judicious use of morphine analgesia to relieve abdominal pain does not change diagnostic accuracy or interfere with surgical decision-making and patients should receive adequate pain control. In 1889, McBurney described the classic point of localized tenderness in acute appendicitis, which is the junction of the lateral and middle thirds of the line joining the right anterior-superior iliac spine and the umbilicus, but the tenderness can also localize to any of the aberrant locations of the appendix. In addition, localized tenderness is a later and less consistent finding when the appendix is retrocecal in position. A gentle touch on the child's arm at the beginning of the examination with the reassurance that the abdominal examination will be similarly gentle may help to establish trust and increase the chance for a reliable and reproducible examination. The examination is best initiated in the left lower abdomen so that the immediate part of the exam is not uncomfortable, and conducted in a counterclockwise direction moving to the left upper abdomen, right upper abdomen, and, lastly, the right lower abdomen. This should alleviate anxiety, allow for relaxation of the abdominal musculature, and enhance trust. The examiner makes several "circles" of the abdomen with sequentially more pressure. A consistent finding in acute appendicitis is rigidity of the overlying rectus muscle. This rigidity may be voluntary to protect the area of tenderness from the examiner's hand or involuntary, secondary to peritonitis causing spasm of the overlying muscle. Physical examination findings must be interpreted relative to the temporal evolution of the illness. Abdominal tenderness may be vague or even absent early in the course of appendicitis and is often diffuse after rupture. Rebound tenderness and referred rebound tenderness (**Rovsing sign**) are also consistent findings in acute appendicitis but not always present. Rebound tenderness is elicited by deep palpation of the abdomen followed by the sudden release of the examining hand. This is often very painful to the child and has demonstrated poor correlation with peritonitis, so it should be avoided. Gentle finger percussion is a better test for peritoneal irritation. Similarly, digital rectal examination is uncomfortable and unlikely to contribute to the evaluation of appendicitis in most cases. Rectal examination may be helpful in selected cases, including when the diagnosis is in doubt, when a pelvic appendix or abscess is suspected, or in adolescent females when ovarian pathology is suspected. Psoas and obturator internus signs are pain with passive stretch of these muscles. The psoas sign is elicited with active right thigh flexion or passive extension of the hip and typically positive in cases of a retrocecal appendix. The obturator sign is demonstrated by adductor pain after internal rotation of the flexed thigh and typically positive in cases of a pelvic appendix. Physical examination may demonstrate a mass in the right lower quadrant representing an inflammatory phlegmon around the appendix or a localized abscess.

LABORATORY FINDINGS

A variety of laboratory tests have been utilized in the evaluation of children with suspected appendicitis. Individually, none are very sensitive or specific for appendicitis but may affect the clinician's decision-making relative to the need for urgent appendectomy, a period of observation and serial examination, or further diagnostic (imaging) studies. Findings should be interpreted with attention to the temporal evolution of the illness. A complete blood count with differential and urinalysis are commonly obtained. The leukocyte count in early appendicitis (<24 hr of illness) may be normal and, typically, is mildly elevated (11,000–16,000/mm^3) as the illness progresses in the 1st 24–48 hr. Whereas a normal white blood cell (WBC) count never completely eliminates appendicitis, a count <8,000/mm^3 in a patient with a history of illness >48 hr should be viewed as highly suspicious for an alternative diagnosis. The leukocyte count may be markedly elevated (>20,000/mm^3) in perforated appendicitis and rarely in nonperforated cases; a markedly elevated WBC count most often raises suspicion of an alternative diagnosis. Urinalysis frequently demonstrates a few white or red blood cells, due to proximity of the inflamed appendix to the ureter or bladder, but should be free of bacteria. Gross hematuria is uncommon and suggests primary renal pathology. The urine is often concentrated and contains ketones from diminished oral intake and vomiting. Electrolytes and liver chemistries are generally normal unless there has been a delay in diagnosis leading to severe dehydration and/or sepsis. Amylase and liver enzymes are only helpful to exclude alternative diagnoses such as pancreatitis and cholecystitis and are not obtained if appendicitis is the strongly suspected diagnosis. C-reactive protein increases in proportion to the degree of appendiceal inflammation but is nonspecific and not widely utilized. Serum amyloid A protein is consistently elevated in patients with acute appendicitis with a sensitivity and specificity of 86% and 83%, respectively. Several reports have described clinical scoring systems and computer-assisted decision-making models incorporating specific elements of the history, physical examination, and laboratory studies designed to improve diagnostic accuracy in acute appendicitis. To date, none has demonstrated improved accuracy over experienced clinical judgment.

RADIOLOGIC STUDIES.

Plain Films. Plain abdominal x-rays may demonstrate several findings in acute appendicitis, including sentinel loops of bowel and localized ileus, scoliosis from psoas muscle spasm, a colonic air-fluid level above the right iliac fossa (colon cutoff sign), or a fecalith (5–10% of cases), but have a low sensitivity for appendicitis and are not generally recommended (Fig. 340-1). Plain films are most helpful in evaluation of complicated cases in which small bowel obstruction or free air is suspected.

Ultrasound. Ultrasound (US) is frequently utilized in the evaluation of acute appendicitis and has demonstrated >90% sensitivity and specificity in pediatric centers experienced in the technique. Graded abdominal compression is used to displace the cecum and ascending colon and identify the appendix, which has a typical target appearance (Fig. 340-2). The ultrasound criteria for appendicitis include wall thickness ≥6 mm, luminal distention, lack of compressibility, a complex mass in the right lower quadrant, or a fecalith. The visualized appendix usually coincides with the site of localized pain and tenderness. Findings suggestive of advanced appendicitis on ultrasound include asymmetric wall thickening, abscess formation, associated free intraperitoneal fluid, surrounding tissue edema, and decreased local tenderness to compression. The main limitation of ultrasound is inability to visualize the appendix, which is reported in up to 20% of cases. A normal appendix must be visualized to exclude

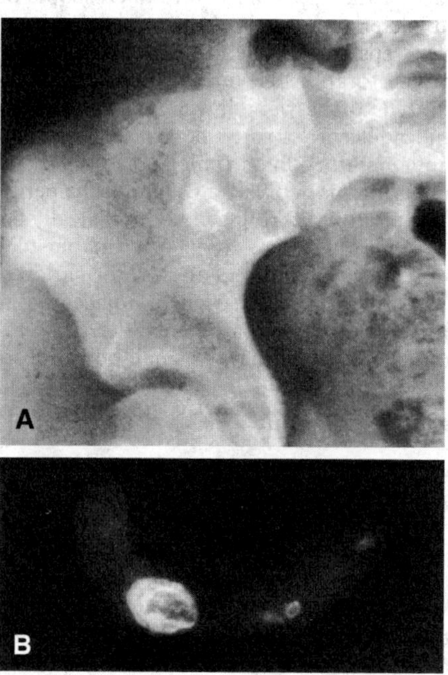

Figure 340-1. Calcified appendicoliths are seen in a coned-down anteroposterior view of the right lower quadrant and in the resected appendix of a 10 yr old girl with acute appendicitis. (From Kuhn JP, Slovis TL, Haller JO: *Caffrey's Pediatric Diagnostic Imaging,* vol 2, 10th ed. Philadelphia, Mosby, 2004, p 1682.)

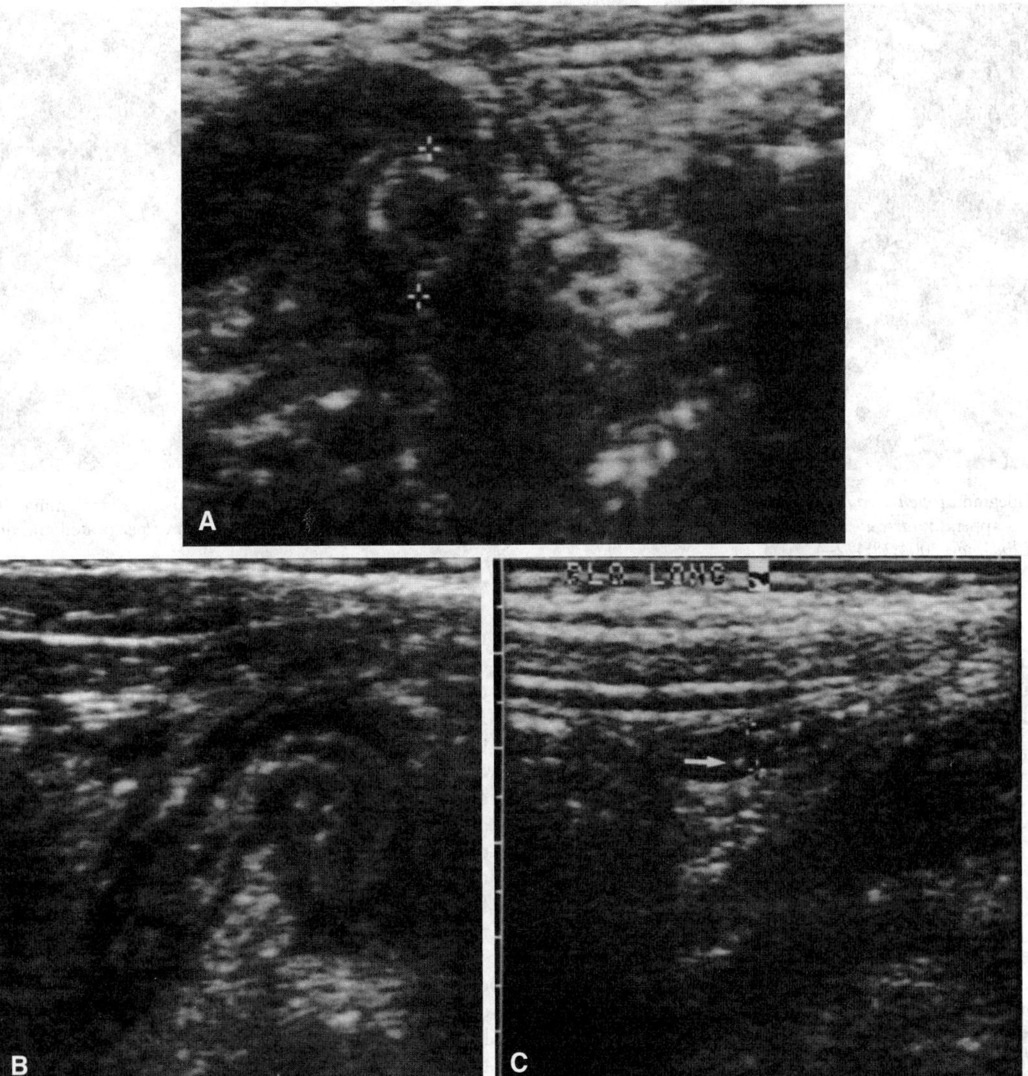

Figure 340-2. Ultrasound examination of patients with appendicitis. *A,* Transverse ultrasound scan of the appendix demonstrates the characteristic "target sign." In this case, the innermost portion is sonolucent, compatible with fluid or pus. *B,* Longitudinal view of another patient demonstrates the alternating hyperechoic and hypoechoic layers with an outermost hypoechoic layer, suggesting periappendiceal fluid. *C,* Longitudinal ultrasound scan of the right lower quadrant demonstrates a dilated, noncompressible appendix. The bright echo within the appendix represents an appendicolith with acoustic shadowing *(arrow).* (From Kuhn JP, Slovis TL, Haller JO: *Caffrey's Pediatric Diagnostic Imaging,* vol 2, 10th ed. Philadelphia, Mosby, 2004, p 1684.)

appendicitis by ultrasound. Certain conditions decrease the sensitivity and reliability of ultrasound for appendicitis, including obesity, bowel distention, and pain. Major advantages of ultrasound include its low cost and freedom from ionizing radiation. Ultrasound can be particularly helpful in adolescent females because of its ability to evaluate for ovarian pathology without ionizing radiation.

CT SCAN. CT is the gold standard imaging study for evaluating children with abdominal pain and suspected appendicitis. Some authors have recommended a CT scan in evaluation of all patients with suspected appendicitis to facilitate decision-making and avoid unnecessary surgery. CT examination can be performed in several ways, including standard CT scan with or without oral and intravenous contrast, examination of both the abdomen and pelvis or pelvis alone, helical appendiceal CT, and helical appendiceal CT with rectal contrast. All of these techniques have demonstrated >95% sensitivity and specificity for acute appendicitis. Findings on CT scan consistent with appendicitis include a distended thick-walled appendix, inflammatory streaking of surrounding fat, or a pericecal phlegmon or abscess (Figs. 340-3 and 340-4). Appendicoliths are more readily demonstrated on CT scan than on plain radiographs. CT scan is also useful in advanced appendicitis to identify and guide percutaneous drainage of fluid collections and identification of an inflammatory mass, which might prompt a plan for initial nonoperative management. Disadvantages of CT scan include: greater cost; radiation exposure; possible need for intravenous, oral, or rectal contrast; and possible need for sedation. Oral contrast is particularly problematic if appendicitis is confirmed, because of the risk for aspiration at induction of anesthesia. Because the finding of fat stranding is a critical component of CT evaluation for appendicitis, CT is less reliable in thin children with minimal body fat. For this reason, rectal contrast may significantly add to diagnostic accuracy in this group. CT imaging is also helpful in demonstrating nonappendiceal causes of abdominal pain.

MRI/WBC SCAN. MRI has been demonstrated to be at least equivalent to CT in diagnostic accuracy for appendicitis and does not involve ionizing radiation. The use of MRI in the evaluation of

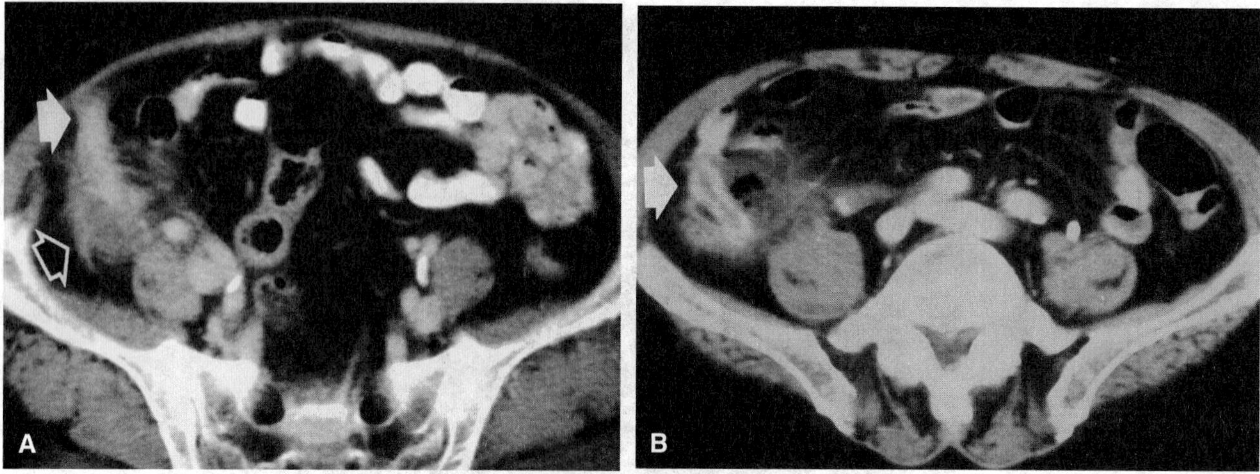

Figure 340-3. *A*, Phlegmon *(open arrow)* is noted around the enlarged appendix *(solid arrow)* in perforated appendicitis. *B*, Extraluminal air is shown adjacent to the wall-enhanced appendix *(arrow)* in perforated appendicitis. (From Yeung KW, Chang MS, Hsiao CP: Evaluation of perforated and nonperforated appendicitis with CT. *J Clin Imag* 2004;28:422–427.)

appendicitis is limited because it is less available, more costly, most often requires sedation, and does not offer equivalent access for percutaneous drainage of fluid collections. Radionuclide-labeled WBC scans have also been used in some centers in evaluating atypical cases of possible appendicitis in children and demonstrated a high sensitivity (97%) but only modest specificity (80%).

DIAGNOSTIC APPROACH

A diagnosis of acute appendicitis is made in only 50–70% of children at the time of initial assessment. Historically, early surgery in equivocal cases was the standard because complications and morbidity rise dramatically in appendicitis after perforation. Negative laparotomy rates of 10–20% were deemed acceptable to keep perforation rates low. In concert with improved imaging technology, there has been a focus to improve diagnostic accuracy in acute appendicitis and, thereby, lower both rates of perforation and unnecessary surgery when the appendix is found to be normal. Current data collected from 36 pediatric centers report a negative appendectomy rate of only 3%. Some clinicians remain steadfast to the primacy of careful history and physical examination and rarely order imaging studies. In uncertain cases, they are likely to proceed with a plan of "active observation." Many clinicians support active observation with serial examination over a period of 12–24 hr in equivocal cases to improve diagnostic accuracy with clinical criteria alone, simplifying the decision to proceed with appendectomy or discharge the patient, and report no correlation between surgical morbidity and timing of surgery. This approach is cost-effective and often avoids radiologic imaging. Fewer than 2% of children's appendixes will perforate while under observation. Other clinicians frequently use radiologic imaging as an adjunct to physical examination and some have even recommended imaging in **all** atypical cases to decrease morbidity and optimize management plans and clinical outcomes. Current data from 36 children's hospitals report some hospitals with negative appendectomy rates as low as 1–2% with the aid of diagnostic imaging. It has also been reported that the likelihood of perforated appendicitis is affected by socioeconomic factors such as access to health care, insurance status, and patient-referral patterns.

It seems likely that if imaging studies are obtained in all patients with equivocal presentations and a brief duration of

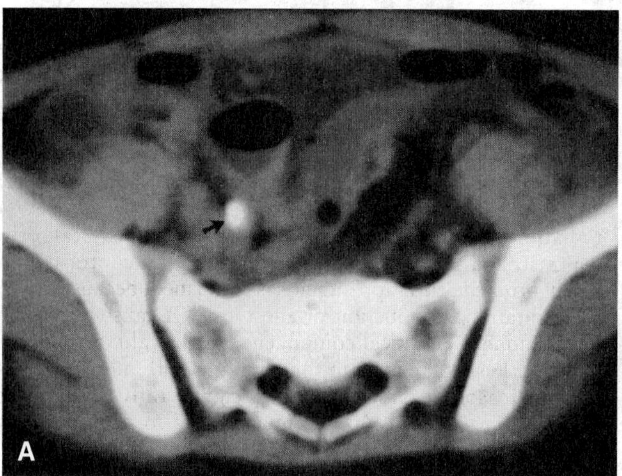

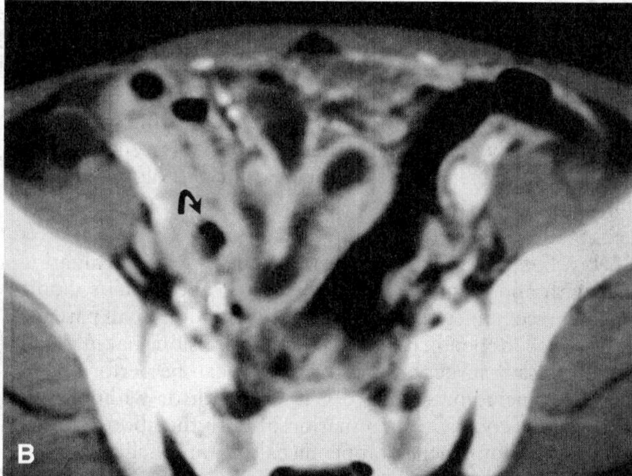

Figure 340-4. *A*, Pre-contrast-enhanced CT reveals an appendicolith *(arrow)* in perforated appendicitis. *B*, Post-contrast-enhanced CT (being 1 cm below the level of *A*) reveals intraluminal air of the appendix *(curved arrow)* associated with ileal wall enhancement in perforated appendicitis. (From Yeung KW, Chang MS, Hsiao CP: Evaluation of perforated and nonperforated appendicitis with CT. *J Clin Imag* 2004;28:422–427.)

illness (<24 hr), the false-negative rate of the imaging studies will increase. Maximum benefit and effectiveness of imaging is obtained when it is used selectively in children for whom the diagnosis is equivocal after careful history and physical examination by an experienced clinician and not too early in the temporal evolution of the illness. A thoughtful approach in equivocal cases of appendicitis is to begin with ultrasound if it is readily available and the hospital has experience with ultrasound for suspected appendicitis. CT scan is used if ultrasound is unavailable or inconclusive, or as the first-line test in obese patients, in the event of probable advanced appendicitis, or when there is gaseous distention of the bowel. This approach has proven both highly accurate and cost-effective.

DIFFERENTIAL DIAGNOSIS

The diagnosis of acute appendicitis can humble even the most experienced clinicians. The list of illnesses that can mimic acute appendicitis is extensive and even limited to common conditions includes: gastroenteritis; mesenteric adenitis; Meckel diverticulitis; inflammatory bowel disease; pneumonia; cholecystitis; pancreatitis; urinary tract infection; infectious enteritis; and in females, ovarian torsion, ectopic pregnancy, ruptured ovarian cysts, and pelvic inflammatory disease (including tubo-ovarian abscess). Intestinal tract lymphoma, tumors of the appendix (carcinoid in children), and ovarian tumors can also masquerade as acute appendicitis. Children <3 yr of age and adolescent females have proven to be at highest risk for an incorrect diagnosis. Most important is differentiation of the patient with gastroenteritis, the most common misdiagnosis, from the one with appendicitis, as significant morbidity and malpractice surround this distinction. The time course of illness (hours, days, or weeks) leading to presentation is a critical component of the history. The classic patient with acute appendicitis describes abdominal pain as the preeminent symptom. Acute appendicitis most often begins insidiously as generalized malaise or anorexia, but there is early onset of abdominal pain and the illness typically escalates rapidly in the 1st 24–48 hr. Whereas most patients with acute appendicitis have one or two episodes of vomiting in the 1st 24–48 hr of illness, multiple episodes of vomiting are unusual during early appendicitis. In contrast, when gastroenteritis is the diagnosis, diarrhea and vomiting may be predominant symptoms early in the illness and abdominal pains may seem associated with the frequent episodes of diarrhea or vomiting. In patients with an acute presentation (<72 hr of illness), vomiting preceding pain, large-volume diarrhea, large amounts of vomiting, and high fever suggest gastroenteritis. In addition, patients with appendicitis typically have normal or hypoactive bowel sounds, whereas gastroenteritis typically produces persistently hyperactive bowel sounds. In the classic child with acute appendicitis who presents within 48 hr of the onset of illness, the WBC count can be low, normal, or elevated but is only rarely elevated above 20,000. WBC counts in this range should prompt consideration of alternative diagnoses and further studies.

Children who present with a history of illness >3–4 days are often more challenging. If the diagnosis is appendicitis, perforation has likely occurred and the child's presentation should evidence signs and symptoms of localized abscess/phlegmon in the right lower quadrant or diffuse peritonitis. At this point in the illness, the WBC count should be elevated (>12,000) with a left shift; whereas a WBC count <7,000 with a lymphocytosis would be distinctly unusual and more typical of gastroenteritis. An abnormal hemogram combined with purpuric skin lesions, arthritis, and nephritis suggests a diagnosis of Henoch-Schönlein purpura or hemolytic-uremic syndrome. Torsion of an undescended testis and epididymitis are common but should be discovered on physical examination. Meckel diverticulitis is an infrequent condition, but the clinical presentation closely mimics appendicitis and the diagnosis is usually made at surgery. Primary spontaneous peritonitis in prepubertal females is frequently mistaken for appendicitis. It should be recognized that "missed" appendicitis is the most common cause of small bowel obstruction in children without history of prior abdominal surgery. Atypical presentations of appendicitis are expected in association with other conditions such as pregnancy, Crohn disease, steroid treatment, or immunosuppressive therapy. Appendicitis in association with Crohn disease often has a protracted presentation with an atypical pattern of recurring but localized abdominal pain.

The diagnosis of appendicitis in adolescent females is especially challenging and some series report negative appendectomy rates as high as 30%. Ovarian cysts are frequently painful as a result of rupture, rapid enlargement, or hemorrhage. Rupture of an ovarian follicle associated with ovulation frequently causes midcycle lateralizing pain (mittelschmerz), but there is no progression of symptoms and systemic illness is absent. Ovarian tumors and torsion can also mimic acute appendicitis, although ovarian torsion is typically characterized by the acute onset of severe pain and associated with more dramatic nausea and vomiting than normally seen in early appendicitis. In pelvic inflammatory disease, the pain is typically suprapubic, bilateral, and of longer duration. The need for accurate urgent diagnosis in females is influenced by concern that perforated appendicitis may predispose the patient to future ectopic pregnancy or tubal infertility, although data has not consistently demonstrated increased incidence of infertility after perforated appendicitis. For these reasons, the majority of adolescent females warrant further diagnostic studies by ultrasonography, CT, or laparoscopy.

TREATMENT

Once the diagnosis of appendicitis is confirmed or highly suspected, the treatment for acute appendicitis is most often prompt appendectomy. Antibiotics and advances in interventional radiology have permitted drainage of fluid collections and initial nonoperative management as an alternative option in late presentations, depending on both the patient's general condition and the state of the appendix. Emergency surgery is rarely indicated and most patients require preoperative supportive measures to ensure the safety of the procedure and improve outcomes. Whereas the traditional surgical approach has been to proceed with surgery as soon as the diagnosis is confirmed, appendectomy should rarely be undertaken in the middle of the night. Frequently unexpected pathology (appendiceal tumors, intestinal lymphoma, congenital renal anomalies, complicated inflammatory bowel disease) may be discovered at operation and intraoperative consultation and frozen section may be needed. There is no correlation between timing of surgery and perforation rates or postoperative morbidity when the operation proceeds within 12–24 hr of diagnosis. In addition, appendectomy can be a challenging operation, with potential for major complications including injury to adjacent intestine, the iliac vessels, or the right ureter. The operation should proceed semi-electively within 12–24 hr of diagnosis. Children with appendicitis are typically at least mildly dehydrated and require preoperative fluid resuscitation to correct hypovolemia and electrolyte abnormalities before anesthesia. Fever, if present, should be treated. Pain management begins even before a definitive diagnosis is made and consultation of a pain service, if available, is appropriate once a decision is made to proceed to surgery. In the majority of cases, preoperative management can often be accomplished during the period of diagnostic evaluation and prompt appendectomy performed.

In patients identified as having perforated appendicitis at the time of diagnosis, the operation is even less urgent and proper preoperative management more critical. When the illness is protracted due to a delay in diagnosis or presentation, patients can demonstrate significant physiologic alterations including severe dehydration, hypotension, acidosis, and renal failure. These patients require a longer period of stabilization with fluid resuscitation and antibiotics, including, in occasional cases, admission to an intensive care unit, before proceeding with more definitive management. Based on patient status, findings on CT scan, and availability of experienced radiologists, the initial plan may be percutaneous drainage of fluid collections by interventional radiology and continued fluid resuscitation and antibiotics. A phlegmon without an identifiable fluid component may respond to nonoperative antibiotic treatment initially. Placement of one or more drainage catheters under imaging (CT or ultrasound) guidance has been successful in >80% of patients. Most patients still require delayed (during the same hospitalization) or interval appendectomy (4–6 wk after the initial presentation).

If diffuse peritonitis exists, most surgeons proceed promptly with appendectomy after a brief period of intravenous fluids and antibiotics. Others continue nonoperative management provided the patient demonstrates clinical improvement by physiologic criteria including hemodynamic stability, urine output, control of fever, and declining leukocyte count. If the patient demonstrates clinical recovery by resolution of fever, sepsis, and return of bowel function, a 2 wk course of antibiotics is completed and a decision is made regarding interval appendectomy in 6–8 wk. A child who fails to improve within 24–72 hr needs appendectomy to control sepsis. Emergency appendectomy should only be performed in the occasional circumstance when physiologic resuscitation requires urgent control of advanced peritoneal sepsis not amenable to interventional drainage or this is not available.

ANTIBIOTICS. Antibiotics lower the incidence of postoperative wound infections and intraperitoneal abscesses in perforated appendicitis, but their role is less well defined in simple appendicitis. The antibiotic regimen should be directed against the typical bacterial flora found in the appendix, including anaerobic organisms (*Bacteroides, Clostridia,* and *Peptostreptococcus* spp.) and gram-negative aerobic bacteria (*Escherchia coli, Pseudomonas aeruginosa, Enterobacter,* and *Klebsiella* spp.). Gram-positive organisms are less commonly found in the colon and the need to provide antibiotic coverage for them (primarily enterococcus) is controversial. Many combinations have demonstrated equivalent efficacy in controlled trials in terms of wound infection rate, resolution of fever, duration of stay, and incidence of complications. For simple nonperforated appendicitis, one preoperative dose of a single broad-spectrum agent (cefoxitin) or equivalent is sufficient, although most surgeons continue coverage for 24 hours. In perforated or gangrenous appendicitis, most surgeons prefer either traditional "triple" antibiotics (ampicillin, gentamycin, and clindamycin or metronidazole) or a combination such as ceftriaxone-metronidazole or ticarcillin-clavulanate plus gentamycin, and antibiotic coverage is continued postoperatively for 3–5 days. Oral antibiotics have proven equally effective as intravenous and, therefore, the patient can be switched to an oral regimen once bowel function returns.

INTERVAL APPENDECTOMY. Appendicitis complicated by an inflammatory mass or abscess can be treated without immediate appendectomy. This strategy is intended to avoid a predictable increased surgical complication rate and is often helpful in children, in whom the overall incidence of perforation approaches 50%. In this group of patients, debate exists over the need for interval appendectomy. The risk of developing recurrent appendicitis if the appendix is not removed is unknown and published reports vary between 10% and 80%. Most cases of recurrent appendicitis develop within 2 yr of the initial illness. Some authors believe interval appendectomy is unnecessary because of the low risk for recurrent appendicitis. Others believe interval appendectomy should be performed to avoid recurrent appendicitis and to confirm the original diagnosis, citing an incidence of unexpected pathology in 30% of interval appendectomy specimens. The vast majority of pediatric surgeons perform interval appendectomy routinely after nonoperative management of perforated appendicitis.

Surgical Technique. Appendectomy is traditionally performed through a right lower quadrant muscle-splitting incision. Laparoscopic appendectomy is also popular among pediatric surgeons for both simple and perforated appendicitis. Studies that have compared the open surgical approach to laparoscopic appendectomy demonstrate differences in both administrative factors (cost, resource utilization, length of stay) and clinical outcome measures (wound infections, intra-abdominal abscess, analgesic requirements, return to full activity) but have failed to establish an evidence-based preference between laparoscopic and open appendectomy in children. In simple appendicitis, laparoscopic appendectomy appears to have lower narcotic analgesic requirements, decreased wound morbidity, and improved cosmesis, but operative times and costs seem slightly higher when compared to the open procedure. Length of hospitalization is similar for both approaches. The role for laparoscopy in perforated appendicitis is less well defined. There is not convincing data to recommend one approach in all patients. Most pediatric surgeons use both approaches selectively. The laparoscopic approach is used most often for obese patients, when alternative diagnoses are suspected, and in adolescent females to better evaluate for ovarian pathology and pelvic inflammatory disease, while avoiding the ionizing radiation associated with CT imaging. Injection of bupivacaine into the wound has been shown to reduce postoperative pain significantly in a randomized controlled trial in children.

COMPLICATIONS. **Morbidity rates** for appendicitis vary widely in large series from 10% to 45%. The principal determinant of complications is the severity of the appendicitis. In simple acute appendicitis, an overall complication rate of 5–10% is expected. With gangrenous or perforated appendicitis, the complication rate rises to 15–30%. The most common complications are wound infections and intra-abdominal abscesses; both are more common after perforation. Perforation rates are consistently >80% in children <5 yr of age. Patients with advanced appendicitis can progress to sepsis and multisystem organ failure, but usually these patients respond promptly to antibiotics, fluids, and other supportive measures. **Mortality** after appendicitis is rare (<0.3%) and seen mostly in neonates and immunocompromised patients. Perforation and abscess formation can also lead to fistula formation in adjacent organs. Other potential complications include postoperative ileus, diffuse peritonitis, portal vein pylephlebitis, and adhesive small bowel obstruction.

POSTOPERATIVE CARE. Most surgeons continue antibiotics for 24 hr and the diet is advanced as tolerated in simple acute appendicitis. The majority of children are discharged from the hospital within 24–48 hr. In perforated appendicitis, there is established infection and intravenous antibiotics are typically continued for 3–5 days postoperatively, followed by a short course of oral antibiotics. Some clinicians use clinical criteria and discontinue the antibiotics when the patient has been afebrile for 24 hr and has a normal WBC count. Oral antibiotics have equivalent efficacy compared to intravenous and patients can therefore complete the antibiotic course at home once there is return of bowel function and the patient meets other discharge criteria.

Applegate, KE, Sivit CJ, Salvator AE, et al: Effect of cross-sectional imaging on negative appendectomy and perforation rates in children. *Radiology* 2001;220:103–107.

Benjamin IS, Patel AG: Managing acute appendicitis. *Br Med J* 2002; 325:505–506.

Brown CV, Abrishami M, Muller M, et al: Appendiceal abscess: Immediate operation or percutaneous drainage? *Am Surg* 2003;69:829–832.

Cappendijk VC, Hazebroek FWJ: The impact of diagnostic delay on the course of acute appendicitis. *Arch Dis Child* 2000;83:64–66.
Chong CF, Wang TL, Chen CC, et al: Preconsultation use of analgesics on adults presenting to the emergency department with acute appendicitis. *Emerg Med* 2004;21:41–43.
Garcia Pena BM, Taylor GA, Fishman SJ, Mandl KD: Costs and effectiveness of ultrasonography and limited computed tomography for diagnosing appendicitis in children. *Pediatrics* 2000;106:672–676.
Guillerman RP, Brody AS, Kraus SJ: Evidence-based guidelines for pediatric imaging: The example of the child with possible appendicitis. *Pediatr Ann* 2002;31:629–640.
Humes DJ, Simpson J: Acute appendicitis. *BMJ* 2006;333:530–534.
Kaiser S, Mesas-Burgos C, Soderman E, et al: Appendicitis in children—Impact of US and CT on the negative appendectomy rate. *Eur J Ped Surg* 2004; 14:260–264.
Kim MK, Strait RT, Sato TT, et al: A randomized clinical trial of analgesia in children with acute abdominal pain. *Acad Emerg Med* 2002;9:281–287.
Kokki H, Lintula H, Vanamo K, et al: Oxycodone vs placebo in children with undifferentiated abdominal pain. *Arch Pediatr Adolesc Med* 2005;159: 320–325.
Kosloske AM, Love CL, Rohrer JE, et al: The diagnosis of appendicitis in children: Outcomes of a strategy based on pediatric surgical evaluation. *Pediatrics* 2004;113:29–34.
Lee JH, Jeong YK, Hwang JC, et al: Graded compression sonography with adjuvant use of posterior manual compression technique in the sonographic diagnosis of acute appendicitis. *AJR Am J Roentgenol* 2002;178:863–868.
Lintula H, Kokki H, Vanamo K: Single-blind randomized clinical trial of laparoscopic versus open appendectomy in children. *Br J Surg* 2001;88: 510–514.
Lycopoulou L, Mamoulakis C, Hantzi E, et al: Serum amyloid A protein levels as a positive aid in the diagnosis of acute appendicitis in children. *Clin Chem Lab Med* 2005;43:49–53.
Martin AE, Vollman D, Adler B, et al: CT scans may not reduce the negative appendectomy rate in children. *J Pediatr Surg* 2004;39:886–890.
Mittal VK, Goliath J, Sabir M, et al: Advantages of focused helical computed tomographic scanning with rectal contrast only vs triple contrast in the diagnosis of clinically uncertain acute appendicitis. *Arch Surg* 2004;139: 495–500.
Morrow SE, Newman KD: Appendicitis. In Ashcraft KW, Holcomb, GW III, Murphy JP: *Pediatric Surgery,* 4th ed. Philadelphia, Elsevier Saunders, 2005, pp 577–585.
Nance ML, Adamson WT, Hedrick HL: Appendicitis in the very young child: A continuing diagnostic challenge. *Pediatr Emerg Care* 2000;16:160–162.
Newman K, Ponsky T, Little K, et al: Appendicitis 2000: Variability in practice, outcomes, and resource utilization at 30 pediatric hospitals. *J Pediatr Surg* 2003;38:372–379.
Ponsky TA, Huang ZJ, Kittle K, et al: Hospital and patient-level characteristics and the risk of appendiceal rupture and negative appendectomy in children. *JAMA* 2004;292:1977–1982.
Prommeger R, Obrist P, Ensinger C, et al: Retrospective evaluation of carcinoid tumors of the appendix in children. *World J Surg* 2002;26:1489–1492.
Sauerland S, Lefering R, Neugebauer EA: Laparoscopic versus open surgery for suspected appendicitis. *Cochrane Database Sys Rev* 2002:CD001546.
Smink DS, Finkelstein JA, Garcia Pena BM, et al: Diagnosis of acute appendicitis in children using a clinical practice guideline. *J Pediatr Surg* 2004;39:458–463.
Taylor, GA: Suspected appendicitis in children: In search of the single best diagnostic test. *Radiology* 2004;231:293–295.
Ziegler, MM: The diagnosis of appendicitis: An evolving paradigm. *Pediatrics* 2004;113:130–132.

Chapter 341 ■ Surgical Conditions of the Anus, Rectum, and Colon

Michael D. Klein and Robert P. Thomas

341.1 • Anorectal Malformations

In understanding the spectrum of anorectal anomalies, it is important to consider the importance of the sphincter complex, a mass of muscle fibers surrounding the anorectum (Fig. 341-1). This complex is the combination of the puborectalis, levator ani, external and internal sphincters, and the superficial external sphincter muscles, all meeting at the rectum. Anorectal malformations are defined by the relationship of the rectum to this complex and include varying degrees of stenosis to complete atresia; the incidence is 1/4,000 live births. Significant long-term concerns focus on bowel control and urinary and sexual functions.

EMBRYOLOGY

The hindgut forms early as that part of the primitive gut tube, which extends into the tail fold in the 2nd week of gestation. At about day 13, it develops a ventral diverticulum, the allantois or primitive bladder. The junction of allantois and hindgut become

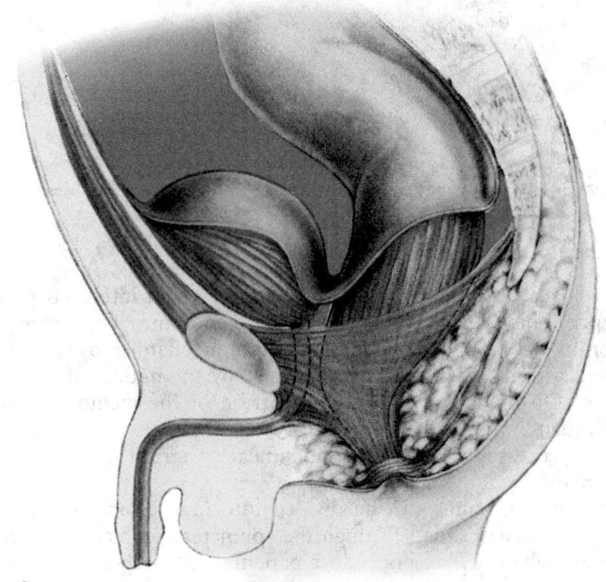

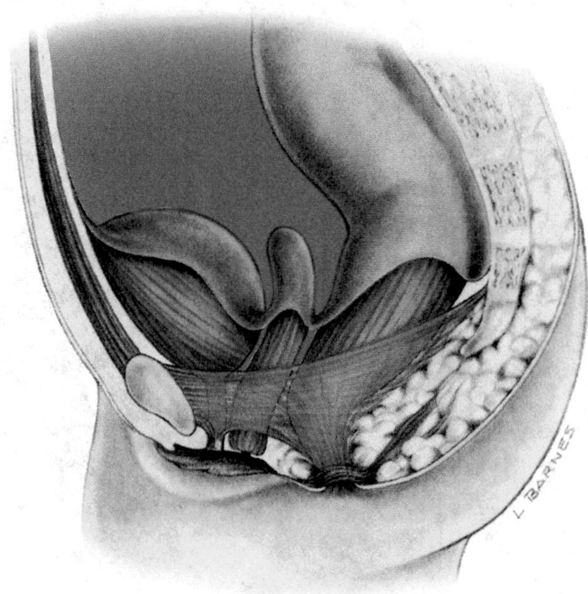

Figure 341-1. Normal anorectal anatomy in relation to pelvic structures. *A*, Male. *B*, Female. (From Peña A: *Atlas of Surgical Management of Anorectal Malformations*. Springer-Verlag, New York, 1989, p 3.)

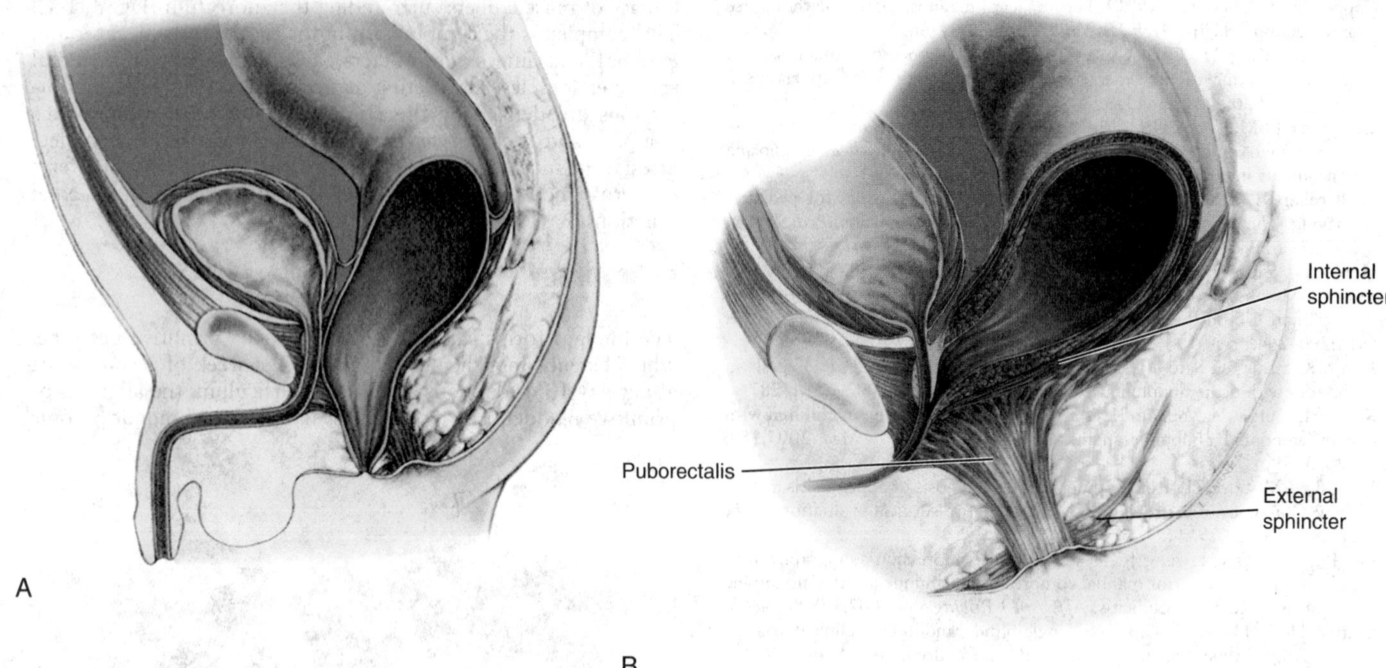

Figure 341-2. Imperforate anus in males. *A*, Low lesions. *B*, High lesions. (From Peña A: *Atlas of Surgical Management of Anorectal Malformations.* Springer-Verlag, New York, 1989, pp 7, 26.)

the cloaca, into which the genital, urinary, and intestinal tubes empty. This is covered by a cloacal membrane. The urorectal septum descends to divide this common channel by forming lateral ridges, which grow in and fuse by the middle of the 7th week. Opening of the posterior portion of the membrane (the anal membrane) occurs in the 8th week. Failures in any part of these processes can lead to the clinical spectrum of anogenital anomalies.

Imperforate anus can be divided into low lesions where the rectum has descended through the sphincter complex, and high lesions where it has not. Most patients with imperforate anus have a fistula. There is a spectrum of malformation in both males and females (Fig. 341-1). In males, low lesions usually present with meconium staining somewhere on the perineum along the median raphe (Fig. 341-2*A*). Girls with low lesions also present as a spectrum, from an anus that is only slightly anterior on the perineal body to a fourchette fistula that opens on the moist mucosa of the introitus distal to the hymen (Fig. 341-3*A*). A high imperforate anus in a male has no apparent cutaneous opening or fistula, but usually has a fistula to the urinary tract, either the urethra or the bladder (Fig. 341-2*B*). Although there is occasionally a rectovaginal fistula, in girls, high lesions are usually

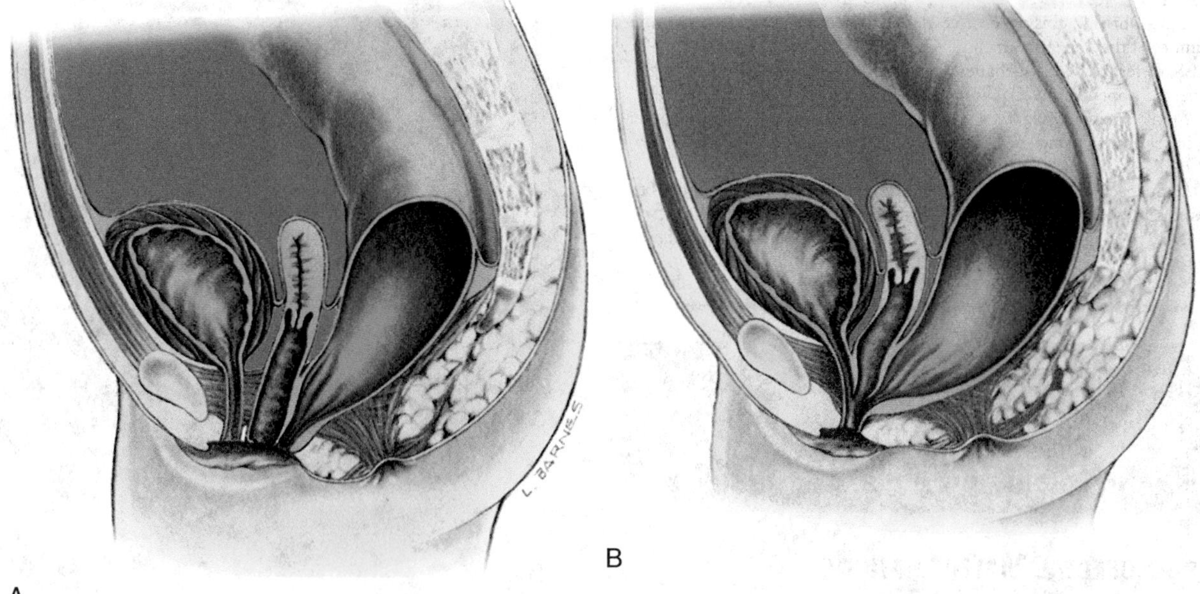

Figure 341-3. Imperforate anus in females. *A*, Vestibular fistula. *B*, Cloaca. (From Peña A: *Atlas of Surgical Management of Anorectal Malformations.* Springer-Verlag, New York, 1989, pp 50, 60.)

TABLE 341-1. Associated Malformations

GENITOURINARY	**CARDIOVASCULAR**
Vesicoureteric reflux	Tetralogy of Fallot
Renal agenesis	Ventricular septal defect
Renal dysplasia	Transposition of the great vessels
Ureteral duplication	Hypoplastic left heart syndrome
Cryptorchidism	**GASTROINTESTINAL**
Hypospadias	Tracheoesophageal fistula
Bicornuate uterus	Duodenal atresia
Vaginal septums	Malrotation
VERTEBRAL	Hirschsprung disease
Spinal dysraphism	
Tethered chord	
Presacral masses	
Meningocele	
Lipoma	
Dermoid	
Teratoma	

cloacal anomalies in which the rectum, vagina, and urethra all empty into a common channel or cloacal stem of varying length (Fig. 341-3*B*). The interesting category of boys with imperforate anus and no fistula occurs mainly in children with trisomy 21.

ASSOCIATED ANOMALIES

There are many anomalies associated with anorectal malformations (Table 341-1). The most common are anomalies of the kidneys and urinary tract in conjunction with abnormalities of the sacrum. This complex is often referred to as the **caudal regression syndrome.** Males with a rectovesical fistula and patients with a persistent cloaca have a 90% risk of urologic defects. Other common associated anomalies are cardiac anomalies and esophageal atresia with or without tracheoesophageal fistula. These can cluster in any combination in a patient. When combined, they are often accompanied by abnormalities of the radial aspect of the upper extremity and are termed the VATERR (*v*ertebral, *a*nal, *t*racheal, *e*sophageal, *r*adial, *r*enal) or VACTERL (*v*ertebral, *a*nal, *c*ardiac, *t*racheal, *e*sophageal, *r*enal, *l*imb) anomalad.

A good correlation exists between the degree of sacral development and future function. Patients with an absent sacrum usually have permanent fecal and urinary incontinence. Spinal abnormalities and different degrees of dysraphism are frequently associated with these defects. Tethered cord occurs in ≈ 25% of patients with anorectal malformations. The diagnosis of spinal defects can be established in the 1st 3 mo of life by spinal ultrasound; in older patients, MRI is needed.

MANIFESTATIONS AND DIAGNOSIS

LOW LESIONS. Examination of a newborn includes the inspection of the perineum. The absence of an anal orifice in the correct position leads to further evaluation. Mild forms of imperforate anus are often called anal stenosis or anterior ectopic anus. These are probably imperforate anus with a perineal fistula. The normal position of the anus on the perineum is approximately halfway (0.5 ratio) between the coccyx and the scrotum or introitus. Although symptoms, primarily constipation, have been attributed to anterior ectopic anus (ratio <0.34 in females: <0.46 in males), many patients have no symptoms.

If no anus or fistula is visible, there may be a low lesion or "covered anus." In these cases, there are well-formed buttocks and often a thickened raphe or "bucket handle" (also called "black ribbon.") After 24 hr, meconium bulging may be seen creating a blue or black appearance. In these cases, an immediate perineal procedure can often be performed followed by a dilation program.

In a male, the perineal (cutaneous) fistula may track anteriorly along the median raphe across the scrotum and even down the penile shaft. This is usually a thin track, with a normal rectum often just a few mm from the skin. Extraintestinal anomalies are seen in <10% of these patients.

In a female, a low lesion enters the vestibule or fourchette (the moist mucosa outside the hymen, but within the introitus). In this case, the rectum has descended through the sphincter complex.

Children with a low lesion can usually be treated initially with perineal manipulation and dilation. Visualizing these low fistulas is so important in the evaluation and treatment that one should avoid passing a nasogastric tube for the 1st 24 hr to allow the abdomen and bowel to distend, pushing meconium down into the distal rectum.

HIGH LESIONS. In a boy with a high imperforate anus, the perineum appears flat. There may be air or meconium passed via the penis (urethra) when the fistula is high, entering the bulbar or prostatic urethra, or even the bladder. In **rectourethral fistulas** (the most common in males), the sphincter mechanism is satisfactory, the sacrum may be underdeveloped, and an anal dimple is present. In **rectoprostatic fistulas,** the sacrum is poorly developed, the scrotum may be bifid, and the anal dimple is near the scrotum. In **retrovesicular fistulas,** the sphincter mechanism is poorly developed and the sacrum is hypoplastic or absent. In boys with trisomy 21, all the features of a high lesion may be present, but there will be no fistula, the sacrum and sphincter mechanisms are usually well developed, and the prognosis is good.

In girls with high imperforate anus, there may be the appearance of a rectovaginal fistula. A true rectovaginal fistula is rare. Most are fistulas to the vestibule outside the hymen orifice. These have a good prognosis with a normal sacrum, an anal dimple, and intact sphincter function.

Persistent Cloaca. This is usually a form of cloaca wherein the rectum, urethra, and vagina communicate with the cloaca. It is important to realize this, as the repair will often require repositioning of the urethra and vagina as well as the rectum. Children of both sexes with a high lesion require a colostomy before repair.

Rectal Atresia. Rectal atresia is a rare defect occurring in only 1% of anorectal anomalies. It has the same characteristics in both sexes. The unique feature of this defect is that affected patients have a normal anal canal and a normal anus. The defect is frequently discovered while rectal temperature is being taken. An obstruction is present about 2 cm above the skin level. These patients need a protective colostomy. The functional prognosis is excellent because they have a normal sphincteric mechanism (and normal sensation), which resides in the anal canal.

APPROACH TO THE PATIENT

Good clinical evaluation and a urinalysis provide enough data in 80–90% of **male** patients to determine the need for a colostomy. If a patient has a perineal or rectourinary fistula, meconium may not be seen at the perineum or in the urine before 16–24 hr after birth. Voluntary sphincteric muscles surround the most distal part of the bowel in cases of perineal and rectourethral fistulas; the intraluminal bowel pressure must be sufficiently high to overcome the tone of those muscles before meconium can be seen in the urine or in the perineum. At birth, the bowel is not distended; therefore, clinical and radiologic evaluations are not reliable during the 1st 16–24 hr of life. A piece of gauze is placed around the tip of the penis; one checks for particles of filtered meconium. The presence of meconium in the urine and a flat bottom are considered indications for the creation of a protective colostomy. Clinical findings consistent with the diagnosis of a perineal fistula represent an indication for an anoplasty without a protective colostomy. Sometimes none of the clinical signs already described becomes evident after 24 hr of observation; a radiologic evaluation is then indicated. A cross-table lateral film with the patient in a prone position taken after 16–24 hr of life is valuable for determining the position of the rectal pouch. When this pouch is separated from the skin by >1 cm, the patient needs a colostomy.

More than 90% of the time, the diagnosis in **females** can be established on perineal inspection. These patients must be observed during the 1st 16–24 hr of life. The presence of a single perineal orifice is a cloaca. A palpable pelvic mass (hydrocolpos) reinforces this diagnosis. A vestibular fistula is diagnosed by careful separation of the labia exposing the vestibule. The rectal orifice is located immediately behind the hymen within the female genitalia and in the vestibule. A perineal fistula is easy to diagnose. The rectal orifice is located somewhere between the female genitalia and the center of the sphincter and is surrounded by skin; the term *anterior anus,* which is sometimes used for this defect, is inadequate because these are abnormal fistula orifices not surrounded by a normal sphincteric mechanism. Fewer than 10% of these patients fail to pass meconium through the genitalia or perineum after 24 hr of observation. Those patients may require a cross-table lateral film.

Evaluation also consists of identifying associated anomalies (see Table 341-1). Careful inspection of the perineum is important to determine the presence or absence of a fistula. If the fistula can be seen there, it is a low lesion. The invertogram or upside-down x-ray is of little value, but a plain x-ray of the entire sacrum, including both iliac wings, is important to identify sacral anomalies and the adequacy of the sacrum. If there are any anomalies or if the sacral ratio is <0.52, the prognosis for true continence is very poor; there are no reports of good bowel control with a ratio of <0.3. An abdominal-pelvic ultrasound and voiding cystourethrogram (VCUG) must be performed. The clinician should also pass a nasogastric tube to identify esophageal atresia, and obtain an echocardiogram. In boys with a high lesion, the VCUG often identifies the rectourinary fistula. In girls with a high lesion, more invasive evaluation, including vaginogram and endoscopy, is often necessary for careful detailing of the cloacal anomaly.

OPERATIVE REPAIR

Sometimes a perineal fistula, if it opens in good position, can be treated by simple dilation. Hegar dilators are employed, starting with a #5 or 6 and letting the baby go home when the mother can use a #8. Twice-daily dilations are done at home, increasing the size every few weeks until a #14 is achieved. By 1 yr of age, the stool is usually well formed and further dilation is not necessary. By the time size 14 is reached, the examiner can usually insert a little finger. If the anal ring is soft and pliable, dilation can be reduced in frequency or discontinued.

Occasionally, there is no visible fistula, but the rectum can be seen to be filled with meconium bulging on the perineum, or a covered anus is otherwise suspected. If confirmed by plain x-ray or ultrasound of the perineum that the rectum is <2 cm from the skin, the clinician can do a minor perineal procedure to perforate the skin and then proceed with dilation or do a simple perineal anoplasty.

When the fistula orifice is very close to the introitus or scrotum, it is often appropriate to move it back surgically. This also requires postoperative dilation to prevent stricture formation. This procedure can be done anytime from the newborn period to 1 yr. It is preferable to wait until dilations have been done for several weeks and the child is bigger. The anorectum is a little easier to dissect at this time. The posterior sagittal approach of Peña is used, making an incision around the fistula and then in the midline to the site of the posterior wall of the new location. The dissection is continued in the midline using a muscle stimulator to be sure there is adequate muscle on both sides. The fistula must be dissected cephalad for several cm to allow posterior positioning without tension. If appropriate, some of the distal fistula is resected before the anastomosis to the perineal skin.

Children with a high lesion have a double-barrel colostomy performed. This effectively separates the fecal stream from the urinary tract. It also allows the performance of an augmented pressure colostogram before repair to identify the exact position of the distal rectum and the fistula. The definitive repair or posterior sagittal anorectoplasty (PSARP) is performed at about 1 yr of age. A midline incision is made, often splitting the coccyx and even the sacrum. Using a nerve and muscle stimulator, the surgeon stays strictly in the midline and divides the sphincter complex and identifies the rectum. The rectum is then opened in the midline and the fistula is identified from within the rectum. This allows a division of the fistula without injury to the urinary tract. The rectum is then dissected proximally until enough length is gained to suture it to an appropriate perineal position. The muscles of the sphincter complex are then sutured around (and especially behind) the rectum.

A similar procedure can be done for female high anomalies with variations to deal with separating the vagina and rectum from within the cloacal stem. When the stem is longer than 3 cm, this is an especially difficult and complex procedure.

Usually, the colostomy can be closed 6 wks or more after the PSARP. Two weeks after any anal procedure, twice-daily dilations are performed by the family. By doing frequent dilations, each one is not so painful and there is less tissue trauma, inflammation, and scarring.

OUTCOME

Patients with low lesions are more likely to achieve true continence. They are also, however, much more prone to constipation, which leads to overflow incontinence. It is very important that all these patients are followed closely, and that the constipation and anal dilation is well managed until toilet training is successful. Tables 341-2 and 341-3 outline the results of continence and constipation in relation to the malformation encountered. Children with high lesions, especially males with rectoprostatic urethral fistulas and females with cloacal anomalies, have a poorer chance of being continent, but they can usually achieve a socially acceptable defecation pattern with a bowel management program (without a colostomy). Frequently, the bowel management program consists of a daily enema to keep the colon empty and the patient clean until the next enema. If this is successful, an antegrade continence enema procedure (ACE or Malone procedure) may improve the patient's quality of life. These procedures provide access to the right colon either by bringing the appendix out the umbilicus in a non-refluxing fashion or by putting a

TABLE 341-2. Results of Surgical Treatment of Anorectal Malformations: Total Continence*

LOW	
Perineal fistula	100%
Rectal atresia/stenosis	88
Vestibular fistula	55
HIGH	
Imperforate with no fistula	52
Bulbar urethral fistula	31
Short cloaca	28
Prostatic fistula	20
Long cloaca	17
Bladder neck fistula	0

*Voluntary bowel movements, no soiling.
Modified from Peña A, Hong A: Advances in the management of anorectal malformations. *Am J Surg* 2000;180:370–376.

TABLE 341-3. Constipation and Type of Anogenital Malformation*

Vestibular fistula	61%
Bulbar urethral fistula	59
Rectal atresia/stenosis	57
Imperforate with no fistula	55
Perineal fistula	50
Long cloaca	48
Prostatic fistula	45
Short cloaca	39
Bladder neck fistula	15

*Modified from Peña A, Hong A: Advances in the management of anorectal malformations. *Am J Surg* 2000;180:370–376.

plastic button in the right lower quadrant to access the cecum. The patient can then sit on the toilet and administer the enema through the ACE, thus flushing out the entire colon. Antegrade regimens can produce successful 24 hr cleanliness rates of up to 95%.

341.2 • Anal Fissure

Anal fissure is a laceration of the anal mucocutaneous junction. It is an acquired lesion of unknown etiology thought to be secondary to the forceful passage of a hard stool, mainly seen in infants <1 yr of age. Fissures may be the consequence and not the cause of constipation.

CLINICAL MANIFESTATIONS. A history of constipation is often noted. A patient may have a painful bowel movement, which may correspond to the fissure formation after passing of hard stool. The patient then voluntarily retains stool to avoid another painful bowel movement. This exacerbates the constipation, and, eventually, the passing of harder stools. Pain on defecation and bright red blood on the surface of the stool may be observed. The diagnosis is established by inspection of the perineal area. The infant's hips are held in acute flexion, the buttocks are separated to expand the folds of the perianal skin, and the fissure becomes evident as a minor laceration. Sometimes, peripheral to the laceration, the patient has a little skin appendage that actually represents epithelialized granulomatous tissue, secondary to the chronic inflammation; this is usually known as a "tag." On rectal examination, there may be hard stool in the ampulla and rectal spasm.

TREATMENT. The parents must understand the origin of the laceration and the mechanism of the cycle of constipation. The goal is to guarantee that the patient has soft stools to avoid overstretching the anus. The healing process can take several days or even several weeks. A single episode of impaction with passing of a hard stool can exacerbate the problem. A stool softener is indicated; the parents must adjust the dose to the response of the patient. The primary cause of the constipation, if identified, must be treated. No scientific basis supports other types of treatments, including stretching of the anus, "internal" anal sphincterotomy, or excision of the fissure.

Chronic anal fissures in older patients have been associated with constipation, prior rectal surgery, Crohn disease, and chronic diarrhea. They are managed initially like fissures in infants, with stool softeners with the addition of sitz baths. Topical 0.2% glyceryl trinitrate reduces anal spasm and heals fissures. In addition, local anesthetics such as 10% lidocaine or EMLA (5% prilocaine, 5% lidocaine) may be effective. Patients who do not respond may be managed with the local injection of botulinum toxin to treat the associated contraction of the sphincter.

341.3 • Perianal Abscess and Fistula

Perianal abscess and fistula are observed in two groups of pediatric patients with different causes, pathogenesis, and treatments. These are (1) infants with no predisposing conditions, and (2) older children with predisposing conditions. This disorder is relatively common in the 1st group, which includes infants, usually boys <2 yr of age. This is usually a benign, self-limited condition that may also involve the surrounding skin; the abscess has a communication with one of the crypts of the pectinate line of the anal canal. The crypt may be the source of contamination. The abscess eventually drains through an orifice in the perianal area, but a fistula remains that communicates with the affected crypt to the perianal external orifice. The fistula becomes chronic but usually disappears spontaneously before 2 yr of age. Because the fistula is located close to the lumen of the anus, it is a benign condition because the sphincter is not affected.

Patients >2 yr of age with a perianal or perirectal abscess have a predisposing illness, including drug-induced or autoimmune neutropenia, leukemia, AIDS, diabetes mellitus, Crohn disease, prior rectal surgery (Hirschsprung disease, imperforate anus), or sequelae from the use of immunosuppressant drugs. The prognosis is intimately related to that of the predisposing disease. The abscess may be deep and may rapidly expand with severe toxic symptoms, particularly when the predisposing illness is associated with immunosuppression or neutropenia. Bacteriologic examination of abscess material reveals mixed aerobic *(Escherichia coli, Klebsiella pneumoniae, Staphylococcus aureus)* and anaerobic (*Bacteroides* spp., *Clostridium, Veillonella*) flora. Ten to 15% yield pure growth of *E. coli, S. aureus,* or *Bacteroides fragilis.* Neutropenic patients may also have bacteremia that inconsistently has the same organism as the abscess.

CLINICAL MANIFESTATIONS. The infants with no predisposing conditions have mild clinical manifestations, sometimes including low-grade fever, mild rectal pain, and an area of perianal cellulitis. Subsequently, a pustule is formed and the abscess drains through that orifice. This alleviates the symptoms. The inflammation disappears and the pustule heals. One or several weeks later, pus drainage reappears and continues in an intermittent, chronic way. This condition usually heals spontaneously before 2 yr of age.

Children with predisposing conditions have a much more serious clinical course. They may or may not have fever depending on their immunologic status. Cellulitis may rapidly expand with warmth, erythema, induration, tenderness, and fluctuation over the ischiorectal fossa. Patients may experience severe toxicity and may become septic. They may have symptoms of the predisposing illness. A biopsy of the abscess wall may show granulomas as evidence of Crohn disease.

TREATMENT. Infants with no predisposing disease and a self-limited condition do not usually require treatment. Conservative management (observation) is accepted because, in most cases, the fistula disappears spontaneously before 2 yr of age. Antibiotics are not useful in these patients. Occasionally, when the patient is extremely uncomfortable, the abscess can be drained under local anesthesia. Examination under anesthesia with sigmoidoscopy can define the anatomy and allow for incision, curettage and/or drainage as indicated. Supralevator abscesses can be confirmed by palpation of the fluctulent mass above the sphincter. Simple draining may not be effective and may injure the sphincter. Instead, a heavy suture is passed up the fistula, retrieved from inside the anus, and tied tightly to divide the sphincter slowly.

Another approach to a chronic fistula is a fistulotomy under general anesthesia. The anal canal and lower part of the rectum are exposed with an adequate retractor, and a lacrimal probe is passed through the external orifice of the fistula, coming out through one of the crypts. The tissue between the fistula and the lumen of the anal canal is divided with cautery. The wound is left open to granulate spontaneously. This treatment usually runs a 20% chance of recurrence.

Older children with predisposing diseases require more aggressive fistula treatment with treatment of the predisposing condition. Antibiotics must be administered, including a combination that covers enteric gram-negative organisms, *S. aureus,* and fecal anaerobic flora. Wide excision and drainage are mandatory in cases of sepsis and expanding cellulitis.

Fistulas in older patients are mainly associated with Crohn disease or with a history of pull-through surgery for the treatment of Hirschsprung disease. Those fistulas are difficult to treat. The treatment is the same as that of the predisposing condition.

341.4 • Hemorrhoids

Dilated hemorrhoid veins in children are usually benign but should always raise the concern of portal hypertension, a rare entity in children. The mass of dilated veins is associated with rectal bleeding, itching, and discomfort. If portal hypertension is excluded, older children and adolescents with acute and excruciating anal pain may have an acute thrombosis of a pre-existing external hemorrhoid. This is best treated with local infiltration of bupivacaine 0.25% with epinephrine 1:200,000, followed by incision of the vein or skin tag and extraction of the clot. This provides immediate relief; recurrence is rare and further follow-up unnecessary. Any associated constipation or fecal impaction must be treated to avoid recurrences. Additional approaches to chronic refractory hemorrhoids may include stapled hemorrhoidopexy, coagulation, or excision.

341.5 • Rectal Prolapse

Rectal prolapse is the exteriorization of the rectal mucosa through the anus. In the unusual occurrence when all of the layers of the rectal wall are included, it is called **procidentia.** Most cases of rectal tissue protruding through the anus are prolapse and not polyps, intussusception, or other tissue.

Most cases of prolapse are idiopathic. The onset is often between age 1 and 5 yr (mean, 3 yr). Prolapse usually presents when the child begins standing and then resolves by ≈3–5 yr of age when the sacrum has taken its more adult shape and the anal lumen is oriented posteriorly. Thus, the entire weight of the abdominal viscera is not pushing down on the rectum as it is earlier in development.

Other predisposing factors include intestinal parasites (particularly in endemic areas), malnutrition, diarrhea, ulcerative colitis, pertussis, Ehlers-Danlos syndrome, meningocele (more frequently associated with procidentia owing to the lack of perineal muscle support), cystic fibrosis, and chronic constipation. Patients treated surgically for imperforate anus can have different degrees of rectomucosal prolapse. This is particularly common in patients with poor sphincteric development.

CLINICAL MANIFESTATIONS. Prolapse of the rectum usually occurs during defecation, especially during toilet training. Afterward, the prolapse is reduced spontaneously or manually by the patient or parent. In severe cases, the prolapsed rectum is chronically exteriorized, becoming congested and edematous, making it more difficult to reduce. Rectal prolapse is usually painless or produces mild discomfort. If the rectum is prolapsed after defecation, it can be traumatized by underwear, with resultant bleeding and wetness. The exposed rectum can become ulcerated. The protruding mass varies from bright red to dark red; it can be as long as 10–12 cm. See Chapter 342 for a distinction from a prolapsed polyp.

TREATMENT. The evaluation should include all the necessary tests to rule out the already stated predisposing conditions, especially cystic fibrosis and sacral root lesions. Reduction of protrusion is aided by pressure with warm compresses. An easy method of reduction is to cover the finger with a piece of toilet paper, introduce it into the lumen of the mass, and gently push it into the patient's rectum. The finger is then immediately withdrawn. The toilet paper adheres to the mucous membrane, permitting release of the finger; the paper, when softened, is later expelled.

General measures should include careful manual reduction of the prolapse after an episode of defecation, attempts to avoid excessive pushing during bowel movements (with patient's feet off the floor), use of laxatives and stool softeners in cases of constipation, avoidance of inflammatory conditions of the rectum, and treatment of intestinal parasitosis when present. If all this fails, surgical treatment may be indicated. None of the existing operations is considered ideal because each has risks and disadvantages. Therefore, medical treatment should always be tried first.

Rectal mucosal prolapse can be treated with linear cauterization. In the operating room, the prolapse is recreated by traction on the mucosa. With a Bovie, linear burns are made through nearly the full thickness of the mucosa. One can usually make eight linear burns on the outside and four on the inside of the prolapsed mucosa. In the immediate postoperative period, prolapse can still occur, but in the next several weeks, the burned areas will contract and keep the mucosa within the anal canal.

341.6 • Pilonidal Sinus and Abscess

There are at least three suggestions as to the etiology of pilonidal disease. One states that trauma such as may occur with prolonged sitting impacts hair into the subcutaneous tissue, which serves as a nidus for infection. Another suggests that, in some individuals, hair follicles exist in the subcutaneous tissues, perhaps due to some embryologic abnormality, and that they again serve as a focal point for infection, especially with secretion of hair oils. A third hypothesis is that motion of the buttocks disturbs a particularly deep midline crease and works bacteria and hair beneath the skin. This theory arises from the apparent improved short-term and long-term results of operations that close the wound off the midline, obliterating the deep natal cleft.

Pilonidal disease usually presents in adolescence or young adults with significant hair over the midline sacral and coccygeal areas but not related to perianal disease. It can present as an acute abscess with a tender, warm, fluctulent, erythematous swelling. It can also present as one or more sinus tracts draining only small amounts of serous, bloody, and/or purulent fluid. This disease does not resolve with nonoperative treatment. An acute abscess should be drained and packed open with appropriate anesthesia. Oral antibiotics are helpful; the patient's family withdraws the packing a few inches each day. When the packing has been totally removed, the area can be kept clean by a bath or shower. The wound usually heals completely in 6 wk. Once healed, elective excision should be scheduled to avoid recurrence. Usually, patients who present with sinus tracts can only be managed with a single elective excision.

Most surgeons carefully identify the extent of each sinus tract and excise all skin and subcutaneous tissue involved to the fascia covering the sacrum and coccyx. Some close the wound in the midline; others leave it open and packed for healing by secondary intention. Some marsupialize the wound by suturing the skin edges down to the exposed fascia covering the sacrum and coccyx. There appears to be improved success with excision and closure in such a way that the suture line is not in the midline.

Recurrence or wound-healing problems are relatively common. Some have treated these with VAC sponge dressings. This is a system that applies continuous suction to a porous dressing. It is usually changed every 3 days and can be done at home with the assistance of a nurse. Recalcitrant cases are treated by a large, full-thickness, gluteal flap.

A simple dimple located in the midline intergluteal cleft, at the level of the coccyx, is seen relatively frequently in normal infants. No evidence indicates that this little sinus provokes any problems for the patient. Malignant degeneration of pilonidal sinus cyst has been reported only in patients with chronic infections and abscesses. An open dermal sinus is a benign condition and is usually asymptomatic.

Ashcraft KW, Garred JL, Holder TM, et al: Rectal prolapse: 17 year experience with the posterior repair and suspension. *J Pediatr Surg* 1990;15:992–994.
Georgeson KE, Inge TH, Albanese CT: Laparoscopically assisted anorectal pull-through for high imperforate anus—A new technique. *J Pediatr Surg* 2000;35:927–930.
Levitt MA, Patel M, Rodriguez G, et al: The tethered spinal cord in patients with anorectal malformations. *J Pediatr Surg* 1997;32:462–468.
Levitt MA, Soffer SZ, Peña A: Continent appendicostomy in the bowel management of fecally incontinent children. *J Pediatr Surg* 1997;32:1630–1633.
Madoff RD, Fleshman JW: AGA technical review on the diagnosis and care of patients with anal fissure. *Gastroenterology* 2003;124:235–245.
Nelson RL: Treatment of anal fissure. *Br Med J* 2003;327:354–355.
Peña A: Anorrectal malformations. *Semin Pediatr Surg* 1995;4:35–47.
Peña A, Guardino K, Tovilla JM, et al: Bowel management for fecal incontinence in patients with anorectal malformations. *J Pediatr Surg* 1998; 33:133–137.
Peña A, Hong AR: Advances in the management of anorectal malformations. *Am J Surg* 2000;180:370–376.
Piazza DJ, Radhakrishnan J: Perianal abscess and fistula-in-ano in children. *Dis Colon Rectum* 1990;33:1014–1016.
Rakhimov S: Treatment of rectal prolapse in children. *Vestn Khir Im II Grek* 1989;142:72–74.
Rosen R, Buonomo C, Andrade R, Nurko S: Incidence of spinal cord lesions in patients with intractable constipation. *J Pediatr* 2004;145:409–411.
Sigalet DL, Laberge JM, Adolph VR, Guttman FM: The anterior sagittal approach for high imperforate anus: A simplification of the mollard approach. *J Pediatr Surg* 1996;31:625–629.
Smyth EF, Baker RP, Wilken BJ, et al: Stapled versus excision haemorrhoidectomy: Long-term follow up of a randomized controlled trial. *Lancet* 2003;361:1437–1438.
Sonmez K, Demirogullari B, Ekingen G, et al: Randomized, placebo-controlled treatment of anal fissures by lidocaine, EMLA and GTN in children. *J Pediatr Surg* 2002;37:1313–1316.
Torres R, Levitt MA, Tovilla JM, et al: Anorectal malformations and Down's syndrome. *J Pediatr Surg* 1998;33:194–197.
Tsakayannis DE, Shamberger RC: Association of imperforate anus with occult spinal dysraphism. *J Pediatr Surg* 1995;30:1010–1012.

Chapter 342 ■ Tumors of the Digestive Tract Joel Shilyansky

FAMILIAL POLYPOSIS SYNDROMES. The familial syndromes associated with intestinal polyps are particularly important because they confer an increased risk for developing cancer (Table 342-1). Children need to be followed regularly and a plan for appropriate intervention formulated in advance. In addition, genetic testing should be offered in order to identify family members at risk.

HAMARTOMATOUS POLYPOSIS SYNDROMES. Juvenile colonic polyps, also known as retention or inflammatory polyps, are the most common childhood bowel tumors, present in 1–3% of people <21 yr of age. Polyps rarely appear before 1 yr of age and most present between 2 and 10 yr of age. Juvenile polyps are uncommon beyond 15 yr of age. The polyps are evenly distributed through the colon. Solitary polyps are common, but two or more juvenile polyps may occur. Most juvenile polyps are erythematous, friable and pedunculated, and range in size from a few mm to 3 cm. Histologic examination demonstrates hamartomatous proliferation of mucus-filled glandular and stromal elements, marked vascularity, and infiltration with lymphocytes, eosinophils, and polymorphonuclear and plasma cells. The polyps have characteristic mucus-filled cystic glands and are covered by a fragile, single layer of epithelium. The typical juvenile polyp with no adenomatous changes has no potential for malignancy. Juvenile polyps with an adenomatous component have rarely been reported.

Clinical manifestations usually include bright red, painless rectal bleeding during or immediately after defecation. Exsanguinating hemorrhage is rare; bleeding often stops spontaneously. Iron-deficiency anemia is present in 30% of children, but it is rarely the initial chief complaint. Lower abdominal pain and cramps are uncommon and are associated with intussusception. Prolapsed polyps appear as dark, beefy red, pedunculated masses, in contrast to the lighter pink mucosal appearance of rectal prolapse. Perianal pruritus and mucous discharge are often associated with prolapse. Spontaneous polyp infarction and self-amputation are common; diarrhea and obstruction are uncommon. The **differential diagnosis** includes other forms of intestinal polyposis, Meckel diverticulum, anal fissure, inflammatory bowel disease, intestinal infections, Henoch-Schönlein purpura (HSP), and coagulation disorders.

The **diagnosis** is usually made by colonoscopy. Polyps appear as smooth, pedunculated lesions. Air-contrast barium enema can demonstrate polyps, but colonoscopy is still required for

TABLE 342-1. General Features of the Inherited Colorectal Cancer Syndromes

SYNDROME	POLYP HISTOLOGY	POLYP DISTRIBUTION	AGE OF ONSET	RISK OF COLON CANCER	GENETIC LESION	CLINICAL MANIFESTATIONS	ASSOCIATED LESIONS
Familial adenomatous polyposis	Adenoma	Large intestine	16 yr (range 8–34 yr)	100%	5q (*APC* gene)	Rectal bleeding, abdominal pain, bowel obstruction	Desmoids, CHRPE
Gardner syndrome	Adenoma	Large and small intestine	16 yr (range 8–34 yr)	100%	5q (*APC* gene)	Rectal bleeding, abdominal pain, bowel obstruction	Desmoids, CHRPE
Peutz-Jeghers syndrome	Hamartoma	Large and small intestine	1st decade	Increased	19p (*STK11*)	Possible rectal bleeding, abdominal pain, intussusception	Orocutaneous melanin pigment spots
Juvenile polyposis	Hamartoma (rarely adenoma)	Large and small intestine	1st decade	≈10–50%	*PTEN, SMAD4, BMPR1*	Possible rectal bleeding, abdominal pain, intussusception	Congenital abnormalities in 20% of the nonfamilial type
Heriditary nonpolyposis colon cancer	Adenoma	Large intestine	40 yr (range 18–65 yr)	30%	Mismatch repair genes*	Rectal bleeding, abdominal pain, bowel obstruction	Other tumors (e.g., ovary, ureter, pancreas, stomach)

*Including *hMSH2, hMSH3, hMSH6, hMLH1, hPMS1*, and *hPMS2*.
CHRPE, congenital hypertrophy of the retinal pigment epithelium.
From Goldman L, Ausiello D: *Cecil Textbook of Medicine*, 22nd ed. Philadelphia, WB Saunders, 2004, p 1213.

treatment. **Treatment** includes the removal of the polyp at colonoscopy by snare cautery or, rarely, by transabdominal polypectomy. Retrieval of polyps for histologic confirmation of the diagnosis should always be performed. Recurrences are occasionally seen.

Juvenile polyposis (JPS) is characterized by multiple juvenile gastrointestinal polyps (>5), occurs in families as an autosomal dominant trait, and may be associated with congenital anomalies (20% of new cases are sporadic). In a subset of families, inactivating mutations were found in the *MADH4 (SMAD4)* and bone morphogenetic protein receptor 1A genes (*BMR1A*), resulting in interruption of intracellular signaling of the transforming growth factor–β (TGF-β). These polyps are identical to solitary polyps; affected individuals are at greatly increased risk for gastrointestinal cancer (10–50%). Children can present with painless bleeding, intussusception or, occasionally, when the entire gastrointestinal tract is involved, with failure to thrive, malabsorption, anemia, hypoalbumenemia, and abdominal pain.

The risk of cancer is low in patients without family history of cancer and two or fewer polyps, whereas patients with three or more polyps are at greatly increased risk for malignancy. Thus, patients with multiple juvenile polyps or family history of juvenile polyposis should undergo esophagogastroduodenoscopy, colonoscopy, and upper gastrointestinal contrast radiography with small bowel follow-through every 2 yr. The frequency of examinations should increase in adult patients. Capsule endoscopy is an attractive novel modality that may be used in the future to screen patients with JPS.

Cowden syndrome (CS) and Bannayan-Riley-Ruvalcaba syndrome (BRRS) are rare autosomal dominant syndromes associated with multiple, distinct anomalies, and hamartomas in skin (99% of patients), breast, thyroid, endometrium, brain, and gastrointestinal tract (60% of patients). Both syndromes are associated with mutations in a tumor suppressor gene *protein tyrosine phosphatase and tensin homologue (PTEN)*. Affected individuals are at increased risk for cancer of the thyroid and breast, whereas the risk of gastrointestinal neoplasm is uncertain.

Peutz-Jeghers syndrome (PJS) is a rare, autosomal dominant inherited syndrome characterized by mucosal pigmentation of the lips and gums and hamartomas of the gastrointestinal tract. The incidence is ≈1/120,000. Deeply pigmented discrete freckles are seen at birth or appear during infancy on the lips and buccal mucosa and even around the mouth (Fig. 342-1). Evidence of intestinal lesions can come from bleeding but more commonly arises from painful intestinal cramps associated with obstruction due to recurrent intussusceptions.

Polyps in PJS are benign hamartomas characterized as "frond-like" cores of stromal tissue and smooth muscle surrounded by normal-appearing intestinal epithelium. Intestinal lesions should be excised if they are causing significant and persistent symptoms. Intestinal involvement is usually too extensive to remove all the polyps, although such treatment has been advocated in some patients.

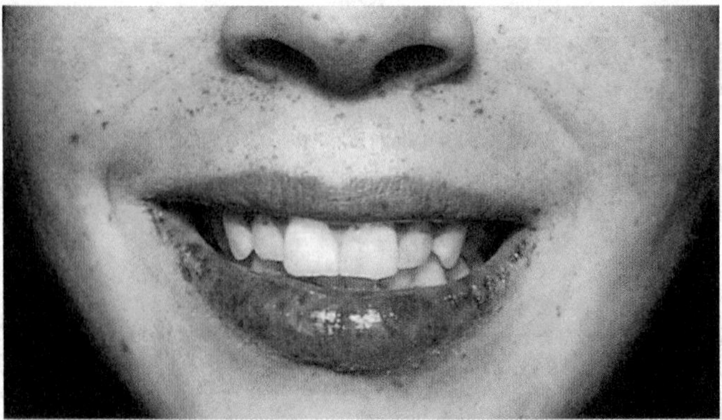

Figure 342-1. Peutz-Jeghers syndrome. Note the pigmentary changes. (From Swartz MH: *Textbook of Physical Diagnosis: History and Examination*, 4th ed. Philadelphia, WB Saunders, 2002, p 295.)

Family studies and genetic counseling may reveal relatives with either partial or complete manifestations of the syndrome. Fifty per cent of patients have no family member with the disorder, a finding suggesting a high rate of new mutation. Inactivating mutations in a gene located on chromosome 19p13.3, *LKB1 (STK11)*, encoding a serine/threonine kinase has been implicated in the pathogenesis of the syndrome. PJS is the 1st cancer-susceptibility syndrome identified that results from inactivating mutations of a protein kinase. Cancer develops in up to 50% of people with PJS, most commonly, middle-aged adults. Colorectal, breast, and gynecologic tumors are seen most frequently. Mammography, gynecologic examination, and colonoscopy starting in the patient's late 20s or early 30s are recommended.

FAMILIAL ADENOMATOUS POLYPOSIS (FAP). Large numbers of adenomatous lesions throughout the colon characterize these autosomal dominant, premalignant conditions. All are caused by germ line mutations in the adenomatous polyposis coli *(APC)* gene, a tumor suppressor gene localized to chromosome 5q21. *APC* gene mutations result in truncation of the cytoplasmic protein, which is responsible for binding and regulating the degradation of β-catenin. Intracellular accumulation of β-catenin may play an important role in colonic epithelial cell proliferation and the formation of adenomas. The incidence of FAP is between 1/5,000 and 1/17,000 persons, with usual onset of polyp development late in the 1st decade of life or during adolescence. **By definition,** more than five adenomatous polyps are present in the colon at the time of diagnosis. Usually, more than 100 (often >1,000) visible adenomas are present when the patient is in the 2nd or 3rd decade. Congenital hypertrophy of retinal pigment epithelial cells is also present from birth in most patients. Variability in the clinical features, including extracolonic manifestations, depends on the location of the mutation in the *APC* gene. Thus mutations of the *APC* gene are also responsible for **Gardner syndrome** (multiple colorectal polyps, periampullary polyps, osteomas [mandibular], lipomas, fibromas, epidermoid cysts, and desmoid tumors) and some, but not all cases of **Turcot syndrome** (primary brain tumor–medulloblastoma and multiple colorectal polyps). The soft tissue lesions (desmoid tumors) and osteomas may appear in childhood, whereas intestinal polyps may not become apparent until adolescence or early adult life. The premalignant polyps can develop anywhere along the digestive tract; however, colonic, gastric, and duodenal (periampullary) lesions predominate. The relative risk of hepatoblastoma, thyroid carcinoma, and cholangiocarcinoma is also increased in FAP patients. Some families who do not meet the criteria for FAP but who have a high frequency of adenomatous polyps and colonic cancer may also have a mutation of the *APC* gene.

In the **clinical presentation,** initially, the polyps are asymptomatic; many often remain so. When symptomatic, adenomatous polyps cause hematochezia, occasionally cramps, or, rarely, diarrhea. The presence of symptoms does not correlate with dysplastic changes. Malignancy arising from pre-existing adenomatous polyps has been reported in children as young as 10 yr, although these lesions more commonly appear in young adults. Most affected individuals will have cancer by age 40 yr.

The **diagnosis** should be suspected from the family history and confirmed by colonoscopy. The polyps are numerous; biopsies demonstrate the adenomatous nature in contrast to the inflammatory and cystic finding of juvenile polyps. *APC* gene mutations are detected in 80–90% of families with FAP, a finding allowing for presymptomatic testing in association with genetic counseling. If a mutation is identified in the index patient, affected family members can be differentiated from unaffected members by gene testing. If the index patient is among the 10–20% of individuals with this disorder in whom the mutation is not defined, genetic testing of family members may identify novel mutations in the *APC* gene. Because a negative result can be misleading, caution should be exercised in counseling families. A child with a diagnosis of FAP or a family history of FAP and a positive gene test should be followed with colonoscopy every 6–12 mo until definitive surgical treatment is undertaken. If genetic testing is negative in a family with an identified mutation, the child is likely not to have FAP. Patients with Gardner syndrome should also undergo regular gastroduodenoscopy to remove gastric and duodenal polyps. Premalignant lesions of the ampulla of Vater occur in adulthood and can be usually treated with local resection, although pancreaticoduodenectomy may be needed.

Definitive **treatment** of FAP requires prophylactic proctocolectomy to prevent cancer. Ileoanal pull-through restores bowel continuity with excellent functional results. Although controversy regarding the timing of surgery exists, the success of reconstruction has allowed earlier resection, thus averting the risk of invasive carcinoma. Nonsteroidal anti-inflammatory drugs such as sulindac and more selective cyclo-oxygenase-2 inhibitors such as celecoxcib may slow polyp development; their efficacy in preventing malignant transformation is unknown and their use remains investigational, especially in light of potential cardiac morbidity.

CARCINOMA. Epithelial tumors of the digestive tract are rare in children, which argues for a measured diagnostic approach to many gastrointestinal symptoms in this age group. Several childhood conditions predispose to development of gastrointestinal adenocarcinoma in early adulthood, for example, familial adenomatous polyposis, hereditary nonpolyposis colon carcinoma (HNPCC), Peutz-Jeghers syndrome, juvenile polyposis, ulcerative colitis, Crohn disease, and disorders associated with chromosomal fragility. The usual site is the colon, but gastric and duodenal lesions are reported. Diagnosis is made based on family history, endoscopic findings, gastrointestinal bleeding, or obstruction. Symptoms are nonspecific: abdominal pain, an abdominal mass, constipation, and, less frequently, bleeding. The tumors are relatively undifferentiated and highly malignant. The **treatment** of colorectal carcinoma is primarily surgical. Prognosis is related to stage of disease. Carcinoma of the colon without any known predisposing factors is rare in children. It is important to obtain a complete family history and provide effective genetic screening and counseling to cancer patients (index cases) and their families to identify at-risk family members. Mutations in the *APC* gene, leading to FAP and DNA mismatch repair genes *(hMSH2, hMSH6, PMS1, PMS2,* and *hMLH1),* leading, in turn, to HNPCC, are most commonly associated with colorectal carcinoma in children and young adults. Diagnosis of HNPCC should be suspected in the presence of family history of early onset colon carcinoma and could be confirmed by genetic analysis. While the great majority of patients with HNPCC do not develop cancers until adulthood, adolescents can be affected. The age to begin endoscopic surveillance remains controversial and should be tailored to the individual patient. In addition, the risk of uterine, ovarian, pancreatic, biliary, and gastric cancer is also increased. Ethical, social, and psychologic impact must be considered when genetic screening is contemplated.

VASCULAR MALFORMATIONS (HEMANGIOMA). These rare benign lesions can cause massive, even fatal hemorrhage. The usual clinical manifestation is painless bleeding beginning in childhood. The blood loss can be subtle and chronic or sudden and massive. Usually, the patient has no additional intestinal symptoms, but intussusception with obstructive symptoms can occur. About 50% of patients have cutaneous hemangiomas or telangiectasias, and some may have a family history of similar lesions. Vascular malformations of the gastrointestinal tract can be associated with blue rubber bleb nevus syndrome (BRBNS) or hereditary hemorrhagic telangiectasia (HHT). About half of these lesions are in the colon, where they can be seen by colonoscopy. During a period of bleeding, selective mesenteric arteriography may be useful in locating a lesion. Surgery can provide definitive treatment of isolated lesions.

LEIOMYOMA. This rare benign tumor occurs most commonly in the stomach, jejunum, and distal ileum. It can remain asymptomatic for long periods. Symptoms can result from intussusception, volvulus, central necrosis, and obstruction. Leiomyoma can be difficult to differentiate from leiomyosarcoma, a malignant tumor that occurs rarely in the gastrointestinal tract in children. Smooth muscle tumors occur at increased frequency in children with AIDS or those requiring immunosuppression after transplantation.

LYMPHOMA. Lymphoma is the most common malignancy of the gastrointestinal tract in children (see Chapter 496). About 30% of children with non-Hodgkin lymphoma present with abdominal tumors. Disorders that predispose to lymphoma include AIDS, ataxia-telangiectasia, Wiskott-Aldrich syndrome, agammaglobulinemia, severe combined immunodeficiency syndrome, bone marrow or solid organ transplantation, and long-standing celiac disease. Lymphoma can arise in the stomach, distal ileum, cecum, or appendix and may present with crampy abdominal pain, vomiting, distention, or a palpable abdominal mass. Perforation is uncommon. Bowel lymphoma should be considered in children >3 yr of age presenting with an acute intussusception. It can be difficult to differentiate symptoms of small bowel lymphoma from Crohn disease.

CARCINOID TUMORS. These tumors of the enterochromaffin cells of the intestine usually occur in the appendix in children and are very low grade malignancies. They may be found incidentally in the appendix at appendectomy. Complete resection with clear surgical margins of a carcinoid tumor of the appendix less than 1 cm in size is usually curative. Carcinoid tumors outside the appendix (rectum, stomach, duodenum, ileojejunum, and colon, in order of frequency) commonly metastasize, and lesions metastatic to the liver can give rise to the carcinoid syndrome, which is the result of hormones produced by the tumor. These hormones produce episodic intestinal hypermotility and diarrhea, vasomotor disturbances (flushing), bronchoconstriction (wheezing), and right heart failure. The most important active agent is serotonin. Finding high urinary levels of the serotonin metabolite, 5-hydroxyindoleacetic acid (5-HIAA), usually suggests the diagnosis. Functional neoplasms are rare in children. Carcinoid can also spread to the small bowel mesentery, inducing severe retroperitoneal and mesenteric fibrosis. Resection is the primary mode of therapy. Treatment with long-acting somatostatin analogs can provide significant palliation.

NODULAR LYMPHOID HYPERPLASIA (NLH). Lymphoid follicles in the lamina propria of the gut normally aggregate in Peyer patches, which are more prominent in the distal ileum. Hyperplastic follicles appear as submucosal nodules on contrast roentgenograms and can be mistaken for an abnormality. NLH can occur in the colon or the small bowel. Diffuse small bowel NLH may be seen in cases of immunoglobulin deficiency, with or without *Giardia lamblia* infestation. Patients may have rectal bleeding, diarrhea, and abdominal cramps, but symptoms are generally mild. In infants with dietary protein hypersensitivity, NLH can occur in association with enterocolitis. NLH has also been noted to occur in inflammatory bowel disease and Castleman disease. The major importance of this entity is the similarity of its manifestations to more serious disorders. NLH usually resolves spontaneously and rarely requires specific treatment. Cyproheptadine or prednisone has been used for extreme bleeding or abdominal pain.

Amos CI, Keitheri-Cheteri MB, Sabripour M, et al: Genotype-phenotype correlations in Peutz-Jeghers syndrome. *J Med Genet* 2004;41:327–333.

Attard TM, Cuffari C, Tajouri T, et al: Multicenter experience with upper gastrointestinal polyps in pediatric patients with familial adenomatous polyposis. *Am J Gastroenterol* 2004;99:681–686.

Bisgaard ML, Ripa RS, Bulow S: Mutation analysis of the adenomatous polyposis coli (*APC*) gene in Danish patients with familial adenomatous polyposis (FAP). *Hum Mutat* 2004;23:522.

Bulow S, Bjork J, Christensen IJ, et al: Duodenal adenomatosis in familial adenomatous polyposis. *Gut* 2004;53:381–386.

Burt R, Neklason DW: Genetic testing for inherited colon cancer. *Gastroenterology* 2005;128:1696–1716.

Corredor J, Wambach J, Barnard J: Gastrointestinal polyps in children: Advances in molecular genetics, diagnosis, and management. *J Pediatr* 2001;138:621–628.

Durno CA, Aronson M, Bapat B, et al: Family history and molecular features of children, adolescents and young adults with colorectal carcinoma. *Gut* 2005;54:1146–1150.

Gupta SK, Fitzgerald JF, Croffie JM, et al: Experience with juvenile polyps in North American children: The need for pancolonoscopy. *Am J Gastroenterol* 2001;96:1695–1697.

Hampel H, Frankel WL, Martin E, et al: Screening for the Lynch syndrome (hereditary nonpolyposis colorectal cancer). *N Engl J Med* 2005; 352:1851–1860.

Howe JR, Sayed MG, Ahmed AF, et al: The prevalence of *MADH4* and *BMPR1A* mutations in juvenile polyposis and absence of *BMPR2*, *BMPR1B*, and *ACVR1* mutations. *J Med Genet* 2004;41:484–491.

Latchford AR, Phillips RK: Duodenal adenoma and cancer in FAP. *Gut* 2005;54:171.

Merg A, Howe JR; Genetic conditions associated with intestinal juvenile polyps. *Am J Med Genet C Semin Med Genet* 2004;129:44–55.

Molle ZL, Moallem H, Desai N, et al: Endoscopic features of smooth muscle tumors in children with AIDS. *Gastrointest Endosc* 2000;52:91–94.

Parc Y, Piquard A, Dozois RR, et al: Long-term outcome of familial adenomatous polyposis patients after restorative coloproctectomy. *Ann Surg* 2004;239:378–382.

Samowitz WS, Curtin K, Lin HH, et al: The colon cancer burden of genetically defined hereditary nonpolyposis colon cancer. *Gastroenterology* 2001;121:830–838.

Schreibman IR, Baker M, Amos C, McGarrity TJ: The hamartomatous polyposis syndromes: A clinical and molecular review. *Am J Gastroenterol* 2005;100:476–490.

Strate LL, Syngal S: Hereditary colorectal cancer syndromes. *Cancer Causes Control* 2005;16:201–213.

Tonelli F, Valanzano R, Monaci I, et al: Restorative proctocolectomy or rectum-preserving surgery in patients with familial adenomatous polyposis: Results of a prospective study. *World J Surg* 1997;21:653–658, discussion 659.

Vasen HFA: Clinical diagnosis and management of hereditary colorectal cancer syndromes. *J Clin Oncol* 2000;18:81–92.

Chapter 343 ■ Inguinal Hernias

John J. Aiken and Keith T. Oldham

Inguinal hernias are one of the most common conditions seen in pediatric practice. The frequency of this condition in concert with its potential morbidity of ischemic injury to the intestine, testis, or ovary makes proper diagnosis and management an important part of daily practice for pediatric practitioners and pediatric surgeons. The overwhelming majority of inguinal hernias in infants and children are congenital indirect hernias (99%) as a consequence of a patent processus vaginalis. Other types of inguinal hernias include direct or acquired (0.5–1.0%) and femoral (<0.5%). Approximately one half of inguinal hernias present clinically in the 1st year of life, most in the 1st 6 mo. Advances in neonatal intensive care have enabled more premature infants to survive with risk factors for development of an inguinal hernia; these infants have an incidence of inguinal hernia approaching 30%. Furthermore, the risk of incarceration and possible strangulation of an inguinal hernia is greatest in the 1st year of life (30–40%) and mandates prompt identification and operative repair to minimize morbidity and complications.

EMBRYOLOGY AND PATHOGENESIS

Most inguinal hernias in infants and children are congenital and result from a persistent patency of the processus vaginalis. The pertinent developmental anatomy of congenital indirect inguinal hernia relates to development of the gonads and descent of the testis through the internal ring and into the scrotum late in gestation. The gonads develop near the kidney as a result of migration of primitive germ cells from the yolk sac to the genital ridge, which is completed by 6 wk gestation. Differentiation into testes or ovary occurs by 7 or 8 wk gestation under hormonal influences. The testes descend from the urogenital ridge in the retroperitoneum to the area of the internal ring by about 28 wk gestation. The processus vaginalis is present in the developing fetus at 12 wk gestation as a peritoneal outpouching that extends through the internal inguinal ring and accompanies the testis as it exits the abdomen and descends into the scrotum. The gubernaculum testis forms from the mesonephros, attaches to the lower pole of the testes, and directs the testis through the internal ring and inguinal canal and into the scrotum. The testis passes through the inguinal canal in a few days but takes about 4 wk to migrate from the external ring to the scrotum. The ovaries also descend into the pelvis from the urogenital ridge but do not exit from the abdominal cavity. The cranial portion of the gubernaculum in girls differentiates into the ovarian ligament, and the inferior aspect of the gubernaculum becomes the round ligament, which passes through the internal ring and attaches to the labia majoris. The processus vaginalis in girls extends into the labia majoris through the inguinal canal and is also known as the canal of Nuck.

Androgenic hormones, adequate end-organ receptors, and mechanical factors such as increased intra-abdominal pressure influence complete descent of the testis through the inguinal canal. The testes and spermatic cord structures (spermatic vessels and vas deferens) are located in the retroperitoneum but affected by increases in intra-abdominal pressure as a consequence of their intimate attachment to the processus vaginalis. The genitofemoral nerve also has an important role; it innervates the cremaster muscle, which develops within the gubernaculum, and experimental division or injury to both nerves in the fetus prevents testicular descent. The cordlike structures of the gubernaculum occasionally pass to ectopic locations (perineum or femoral region), resulting in ectopic testes. In the last few weeks of gestation or shortly after birth, the layers of the processus vaginalis normally fuse together and obliterate the patency from the peritoneal cavity through the inguinal canal to the testis. The processus vaginalis also obliterates just above the testes, with the portion of the processus vaginalis that envelops the testis becoming the tunica vaginalis. In girls, the processus vaginalis obliterates earlier, at about 7 mo of gestation. Failure of closure of the processus vaginalis permits fluid or abdominal viscera to escape the peritoneal cavity and accounts for a variety of inguinal-scrotal abnormalities seen in infancy and childhood (Fig. 343-1).

PATHOLOGY

Patency of the processus vaginalis after birth is a potential hernia, but not all patients with a patent processus vaginalis develop a

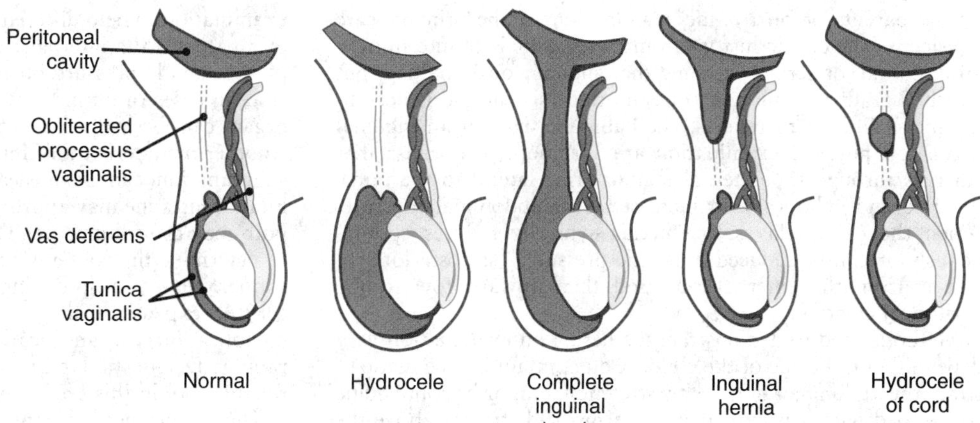

Figure 343-1. Hernia and hydroceles. (Modified from Scherer LR III, Grosfeld JL: Inguinal and umbilical anomalies. *Pediatr Clin North Am* 1993;40: 1121–1131.)

clinical hernia. An inguinal hernia occurs when intra-abdominal contents escape the abdominal cavity and enter the inguinal region through a patent processus vaginalis. Based on their location in the inguinal canal (lateral to the inferior epigastric vessels), they are indirect inguinal hernias but are rarely associated with a muscular weakness or defect as would be typical of an adult hernia. Depending on the extent of patency of the distal processus, the hernia may be confined to the inguinal region or pass down into the scrotum. Complete failure of obliteration of the processus predisposes to a complete inguinal hernia characterized by a protrusion of abdominal contents into the inguinal canal and possibly extending into the scrotum. Obliteration of the processus vaginalis distally (around the testis) with patency proximally results in the classic indirect inguinal hernia with the protrusion in the inguinal canal.

A **hydrocele** is when only fluid enters the patent processus vaginalis and the swelling may exist only in the scrotum (scrotal hydrocele), only along the spermatic cord in the inguinal region (hydrocele of the spermatic cord), or extend from the scrotum through the inguinal canal and even into the abdomen (abdominal-scrotal hydrocele). A hydrocele is termed a *communicating hydrocele* if it demonstrates fluctuation in size, often increasing in size after activity and, at other times, being smaller when the fluid decompresses into the peritoneal cavity. Occasionally, hydroceles in older children follow trauma, inflammation, or tumors affecting the testis. Although reasons for failure of closure of the processus vaginalis are unknown, it is more common in cases of testicular nondescent and prematurity. In addition, persistent patency of the processus vaginalis is twice as common on the right side, presumably related to later descent of the right testis and interference from the developing inferior vena cava and external iliac vein. Risk factors identified as contributing to the development of congenital inguinal hernia relate to conditions that predispose to failure of obliteration of the processus vaginalis and are listed in Table 343-1. Patients with cystic fibrosis have an ≈15% incidence of inguinal hernia believed to be related to an altered embryogenesis of the wolffian duct structures, which leads to an absent vas deferens in males with this condition. There is also an increased incidence of inguinal hernia in patients with testicular feminization syndrome and other forms of ambiguous genitalia. The rate of recurrence after repair of an inguinal hernia in patients with a connective tissue disorder approaches 50% and, frequently, the diagnosis of connective tissue disorders in children results from investigation after development of a recurrent inguinal hernia.

INCIDENCE

The incidence of congenital indirect inguinal hernia in full-term newborn infants is 3.5–5.0%. The incidence of hernia in preterm and low birthweight infants is considerably higher, ranging from 9% to 11%, and approaches 30% in very low birthweight infants (<1,000 g) and preterm infants <28 wk of gestation. Inguinal hernia is much more common in boys than girls, with a male to female ratio of 6 : 1. Sixty per cent of inguinal hernias occur on the right side, 30% are on the left side, and 10% are bilateral. The incidence of bilateral hernias is higher in females and appears to be 20–40%. The increased frequency on the right side is presumably related to the later descent of the right testis and interference with obliteration of the processus vaginalis from the developing inferior vena cava. An increased incidence of congenital inguinal hernia has been documented in twins and in individuals from families of patients with inguinal hernia. There is a history of another inguinal hernia in the family in 11.5% of patients.

CLINICAL PRESENTATION

An inguinal hernia typically appears as a bulge in the inguinal region or extending through the inguinal region into the scrotum. In girls, the mass typically presents in the upper portion of the labia majora. The bulge or mass is most visible at times of irritability or increased intra-abdominal pressure (crying, straining, coughing). It may be present at birth or may not appear until weeks, months, or years later. The bulge is most often 1st noted

TABLE 343-1. Predisposing Factors for Hernias
PREMATURITY
UROGENITAL
Cryptorchidism
Exstrophy of the bladder or cloaca
Ambiguous genitalia
Hypospadius/epispadius
INCREASED PERITONEAL FLUID
Ascites
Ventriculoperitoneal shunt
Peritoneal dialysis catheter
INCREASED INTRA-ABDOMINAL PRESSURE
Repair of abdominal wall defects
Severe ascites (chylous)
Meconium peritonitis
CHRONIC RESPIRATORY DISEASE
Cystic fibrosis
CONNECTIVE TISSUE DISORDERS
Ehlers-Danlos syndrome
Hunter-Hurler syndrome
Marfan syndrome
Mucopolysaccharidosis

by the parents or on routine examination by the primary care physician. The classic history from the parents is of intermittent groin, labial, or scrotal swelling that spontaneously reduces but which is gradually enlarging or is more persistent and is becoming more difficult to reduce. The **hallmark signs** of an inguinal hernia on physical examination are a smooth, firm mass that emerges through the external inguinal ring lateral to the pubic tubercle and enlarges with increased intra-abdominal pressure. When the child relaxes, the hernia typically reduces spontaneously or can be reduced by gentle pressure, 1st posteriorly to free it from the external ring and then upward toward the peritoneal cavity.

Methods used to demonstrate the hernia on examination vary depending on the age of the child. A quiet infant can be made to strain the abdominal muscles by stretching him or her out supine on the bed with legs extended and arms held straight above the head. Most infants struggle to get free, thus increasing the intra-abdominal pressure and pushing out the hernia. Older patients can be asked to perform the Valsalva maneuver by blowing up a balloon or coughing. The older child should be examined while standing and examination after voiding can also be helpful. With increased intra-abdominal pressure, the protruding mass is obvious on inspection of the inguinal region or can be palpated by an examining finger invaginating the scrotum to palpate at the external ring. In the female infant, the ovary and fallopian tube can be contained within the hernia sac, presenting as a firm, discrete, nontender mass in the labia. Another test is the **"silk glove sign,"** which describes the feeling of the layers of the hernia sac (processus vaginalis) as they slide over the spermatic cord structures, with rolling of the spermatic cord beneath the index finger at the pubic tubercle. If the bulge is located below the inguinal canal on the medial aspect of the thigh, a femoral hernia should be suspected. In the absence of a bulge, the finding of increased thickness of the inguinal canal structures on palpation also suggests the diagnosis of an inguinal hernia. It is important on examination to note the position of the testes because retractile testes are common in infants and young children and can mimic an inguinal hernia with a bulge in the region of the external ring. Because in the female patient ≈20–25% of inguinal hernias are sliding hernias (the contents of the hernia sac are adherent within the sac and therefore not reducible), a fallopian tube or ovary can be palpated in the inguinal canal.

EVALUATION OF THE ACUTE INGUINAL-SCROTAL SWELLING

Occasionally, an inguinal-scrotal mass appears suddenly in an infant or child and is associated with discomfort. The **differential diagnosis** includes incarcerated inguinal hernia, acute hydrocele, torsion of an undescended testis, and suppurative inguinal lymphadenitis. Differentiation between the incarcerated inguinal hernia and the acute hydrocele is probably the most difficult. The infant or child with an incarcerated inguinal hernia is likely to have associated findings suggestive of intestinal obstruction such as colicky abdominal pain, abdominal distention, vomiting, and cessation of stool and may appear ill. The infant with an acute hydrocele may have discomfort but is consolable and tolerates feedings without signs or symptoms suggestive of intestinal obstruction. When the diagnosis is incarcerated inguinal hernia, plain radiographs typically demonstrate multiple air-fluid levels. On examination of the child with the acute hydrocele, the clinician may note that the mass is somewhat mobile. In addition, in the area between the suspected hydrocele mass and the internal ring, the cord structures may appear only slightly thickened. With the incarcerated hernia, there is a lack of mobility of the groin mass as well as marked swelling or mass extending from the scrotal mass through the inguinal area and up to and including the internal ring. An experienced clinician can use a bimanual examination to help differentiate groin abnormalities. The examiner palpates the internal ring per rectum, with the other hand placing gentle pressure on the inguinal region over the internal ring. In cases of an indirect inguinal hernia, an intra-abdominal organ can be palpated extending through the internal ring. Another method is **transillumination.** It must be noted that transillumination can be misleading because the thin wall of the infant's intestine may approximate that of the hydrocele wall and both may transilluminate. This is also the reason why aspiration to determine the contents of a groin mass is discouraged. **Ultrasonography** can help distinguish between a hernia and a hydrocele. An expeditious diagnosis is important to avoid the potential complications of an incarcerated hernia, which can develop rapidly. Diagnostic laparoscopy has emerged as an effective and reliable tool in this setting but requires general anesthesia.

The occurrence of suppurative adenopathy in the inguinal region can be confused with an incarcerated inguinal hernia. Examination of the watershed area of the inguinal lymph node may reveal a superficial infected or crusted lesion. In addition, the swelling associated with inguinal lymphadenopathy is typically located more inferior and lateral than the mass of an inguinal hernia and there may be other associated nodes in the area. Torsion of an undescended testis may present as a painful erythematous mass in the groin. The absence of a gonad in the scrotum in the ipsilateral side should clinch this diagnosis.

INCARCERATED HERNIA. This is a hernia in which the contents of the hernia sac cannot be reduced into the abdominal cavity. Contained structures can include small bowel, appendix, omentum, colon, or, rarely, Meckel diverticulum. In females, the ovary, fallopian tube, or both are commonly incarcerated. Rarely, the uterus in infants can also be pulled into the hernia sac. A **strangulated hernia** is one that is tightly constricted in its passage through the inguinal canal and, as a result, the hernia contents have become ischemic or gangrenous. Although incarceration may be tolerated in adults for years, most nonreducible inguinal hernias in children, unless treated, rapidly progress to strangulation with potential infarction of the hernia contents. Initially, pressure on the herniated viscera as they pass through the internal ring, inguinal canal, and external ring leads to impaired lymphatic and venous drainage. This leads, in turn, to swelling of the herniated viscera, which further increases the compression in the inguinal canal, ultimately resulting in total occlusion of the arterial supply to the trapped viscera. Progressive ischemic changes take place, culminating in gangrene and/or perforation of the herniated viscera. The testis is also at risk of ischemia because of compression of the spermatic cord structures by the strangulated hernia. In females, herniation of the ovary places it at risk of strangulation and torsion. The incidence of incarceration of an inguinal hernia is between 12% and 17%. Two thirds of incarcerated hernias occur in the 1st year of life. The greatest risk is in infancy with reported incidences of between 25% and 30% for infants <6 mo of age. The incidence of incarceration is slightly less in premature infants, although the reasons are unclear.

The symptoms of an incarcerated hernia are irritability, pain in the groin and abdomen, abdominal distention, and vomiting. A somewhat tense, nonfluctuant mass is present in the inguinal region and may extend down into the scrotum or labia majora. The mass is well defined, may be tender, and does not reduce. With the onset of ischemic changes, the pain intensifies, and the vomiting becomes bilious or feculent. Blood may be noted in the stools. The mass is typically tender, and there is often edema and erythema of the overlying skin, with fever and signs of intestinal obstruction. The testes may be normal, but also may be swollen and hard on the affected side because of venous congestion resulting from compression of the spermatic veins and lymphatic channels at the inguinal ring by the tightly strangulated hernia mass. Abdominal radiographs demonstrate features of partial or complete intestinal obstruction, and gas within the incarcerated bowel segments may be seen below the inguinal ligament or within the scrotum.

AMBIGUOUS GENITALIA. Infants with intersex problems frequently present with inguinal hernias, often containing a gonad and require special consideration. Female infants with inguinal hernias, particularly if the presentation is bilateral inguinal masses, should be suspected of having **testicular feminization syndrome** because >50% of patients with testicular feminization have an inguinal hernia (see Chapter 584). Conversely, the true incidence of testicular feminization in all female infants with inguinal hernias is difficult to determine but is ≈1%. In phenotypic females, if the diagnosis of testicular feminization is suspected preoperatively, the child should be screened with a buccal smear for Barr bodies and appropriate genetic evaluation before proceeding with the hernia repair. The diagnosis of testicular feminization is occasionally made at the time of operation, by identifying an abnormal gonad (testis) within the hernia sac or absence of the uterus on rectal examination. In the normal female infant, the uterus is easily palpated as a distinct midline structure beneath the symphysis pubis on rectal examination. Preoperative diagnosis of testicular feminization syndrome or other intersex disorders such as mixed gonadal dysgenesis and selected pseudohermaphrodites enables the family to receive counseling, and gonadectomy can be accomplished at the time of the hernia repair.

MANAGEMENT

The presence of an inguinal hernia in the pediatric age group constitutes the indication for operative repair. An inguinal hernia does not resolve spontaneously and early repair eliminates the risk of incarceration and the associated potential complications, particularly in the 1st 6–12 mo of life. The timing of operative repair depends on several factors including age, general condition of the patient, and co-morbid conditions. In infants <1 yr of age diagnosed with an inguinal hernia, repair should proceed promptly because as many as 70% of incarcerated inguinal hernias requiring emergency operation for reduction and repair occur in the 1st year of life. In addition, the incidence of testicular atrophy after incarceration in infants <3 mo of age has been reported as high as 30%. In children >1 yr, the risk of incarceration is less and the repair can be scheduled with less urgency. For the routine reducible hernia, the operation should be carried out electively shortly after diagnosis. Elective inguinal hernia repair can be safely performed in an outpatient setting with an expectation for full recovery within 48 hr. The operation should be performed at a facility with the ability to admit the patient to an inpatient unit as needed. Certain conditions may dictate postponement of repair, such as marked prematurity, intercurrent pneumonia (especially respiratory syncytial virus [RSV]), other infections, or severe congenital heart disease. In cases of marked prematurity (1,800–2,000 g), repair is typically performed before discharge home from the neonatal intensive care unit.

The operation is most often performed under general anesthesia, but can be performed under spinal or caudal anesthesia if avoidance of intubation is preferable due to chronic lung disease or bronchopulmonary dysplasia. Prophylactic antibiotics are not routinely used except for associated conditions such as congenital heart disease or the presence of a venticuloperitoneal shunt. Preterm infants mandate special consideration because of their higher risk for apnea and bradycardia after general anesthesia (see Chapter 76). Infants <44 wk postconceptual age and full-term infants <3 mo of age and with co-morbid conditions should be observed overnight with appropriate apnea and cardiorespiratory monitors.

An incarcerated, irreducible hernia without evidence of strangulation in a clinically stable patient should initially be managed nonoperatively. Reduction by gentle compression of the hernia can be attempted. The attempt should not be continued if the infant is crying and resisting the pressure on the hernia. The use of sedation or analgesia before attempting reduction can be helpful; this reduces intra-abdominal pressure and relieves the pressure on the neck of the hernia sac at the inguinal ring. Care must be taken to avoid respiratory depression, especially in the premature infant. Other techniques advocated to assist in the nonoperative reduction of an incarcerated inguinal hernia include elevation of the lower torso and legs and brief exposure to an ice pack. Many practitioners do not favor the use of an ice pack in infants because of the risk of hypothermia. Manual reduction is performed first with traction caudad and posteriorly to free the mass from the external inguinal ring, and then upward to reduce the contents back into the peritoneal cavity. If reduction is successful but difficult, the patient should be observed to ensure that feedings are tolerated and there is no concern that necrotic intestine was reduced. Elective repair is performed 24–48 hours later, by which time there is less edema, handling of the sac is easier, and the risk of complications is reduced. A common presentation in female patients is the presence of an irreducible ovary in the inguinal hernia in an otherwise asymptomatic patient. The inguinal mass is soft, nontender to gentle exam, and there is no swelling or edema; thus, there are no findings suggestive of strangulation. This represents a "sliding" hernia with the fallopian tube and ovary fused to the posterior-medial wall of the hernia sac. Overzealous attempts to reduce the hernia are unwarranted and potentially harmful to the tube and ovary. The risk that incarceration of the ovary in this setting will lead to strangulation is not known. Most pediatric surgeons recommend elective repair of the hernia within 48–72 hr. For any patient who presents with a prolonged history of incarceration, signs of peritoneal irritation, or small bowel obstruction, surgery and operative reduction and repair of the hernia should be performed.

OPERATIVE MANAGEMENT. When the hernia cannot be reduced or is strangulated, immediate operation is indicated to prevent further damage to the contents of the hernia sac or testis. If there are signs of intestinal obstruction or strangulation, initial management includes nasogastric intubation, intravenous fluids, and administration of broad-spectrum antibiotics. When fluid and electrolyte imbalance has been corrected and the child's condition is satisfactory, exploration is undertaken. The operation consists of reduction of the contents of the hernia sac, separation of the hernia sac from the spermatic cord vessels and vas deferens in the inguinal canal, and high ligation of the hernia sac at the internal ring. Resection of nonviable structures within the hernia sac or of an infarcted testis may be indicated based on the experience and judgment of the surgeon. It is important to note that, although the testis may appear ischemic, most will recover after relief of the incarceration and do no require removal.

The elective operative repair of a congenital indirect inguinal hernia is straightforward and consists of high ligation of the hernia sac (patent processus vaginalis) at the level of the internal ring, thus preventing protrusion of abdominal contents into the inguinal canal. In males, this requires careful separation of the sac from the spermatic cord structures and avoidance of injury to these vital structures. In females, surgical repair is simpler because the hernia sac and round ligament can be ligated without concern for injury to the ovary and its blood supply, which generally remain within the abdomen. The fallopian tube is routinely visualized to rule out testicular feminization syndrome. If the ovary and fallopian tube are within the sac and not reducible, most often the sac is ligated distal to these structures and the internal ring closed after reducing the sac and its contents to the abdominal cavity.

CONTRALATERAL INGUINAL EXPLORATION. Controversy exists regarding when to proceed with contralateral groin exploration in infants and children with a unilateral indirect inguinal hernia. The only purpose of contralateral exploration is to avoid the occurrence of a hernia on that side at a later date. The incidence of a contralateral patent processus vaginalis is ≈60% at 2 mo of age and decreases to 40% at 2 yr of age. A patent processus represents only a potential hernia, and many risk factors influence the likelihood of development of an actual inguinal hernia. The advantages of contralateral exploration include avoidance of (1) parental anxiety and possibly a second anesthesia, (2) the cost of additional surgery, and (3) the risk of contralateral incarceration. The disadvantages include (1) potential injury to the spermatic cord vessels, vas deferens, and testis; (2) increased operative time; and (3) the fact that, in many infants, it is an unnecessary procedure. The relevant issues in the debate revolve around the frequency of occurrence of contralateral hernias after one-sided hernia repair and the relation of this to age, gender, and side of the clinically apparent hernia. Historically, most large series noted a chance of developing a contralateral hernia as 30–40% in children <2 yr of age, leading most pediatric surgeons to recommend routine contralateral exploration in this age group. In females, because of the higher incidence of bilateral inguinal hernias and elimination of concern for injury to the spermatic cord or testis, routine contralateral exploration has been recommended up to age 5 or 6 yr. Infants and children with risk factors for development of an inguinal hernia or with medical conditions that increase the risk of general anesthesia should be approached with a low threshold for routine contralateral exploration. Laparoscopy enables assessment of the contralateral side without risk of injury to the spermatic cord structures or testis. This procedure can be performed through an umbilical incision or by passing a 30-degree or 70-degree oblique scope through the open hernia sac just before ligation of the hernia sac on the involved side. If patency of the contralateral side is demonstrated, the surgeon can proceed with bilateral hernia repair, and if the contralateral side is properly obliterated, exploration and potential complications are avoided (Figs. 343-2 and 343-3).

DIRECT INGUINAL HERNIA

These hernias are rare in children. Direct hernias appear as groin masses that extend toward the femoral vessels with exertion or straining. The etiology is from a muscular defect or weakness in the floor of the inguinal canal medial to the epigastric vessels. As such, direct inguinal hernias in children are generally considered an acquired defect. In one third of cases, the patient has history of a prior indirect hernia repair on the side of the direct hernia, which suggests a possible injury to the floor muscles of the inguinal canal at the time of the first herniorrhaphy. In addition, patients with **connective tissue disorders** such as Ehlers-Danlos syndrome or Marfan syndrome and mucopolysaccharidosis such as Hunter-Hurler syndrome are at increased risk for the development of direct inguinal hernias either independently or after indirect inguinal hernia repair. Operative repair of a direct inguinal hernia involves strengthening of the floor of the inguinal canal and many standard techniques have been described, similar to repair techniques used in adults. The repair can be performed through a single limited incision and, therefore, laparoscopic repair does not offer any significant advantage. Recurrence after repair, in contrast to that in adults, is extraordinarily rare. Prosthetic material for direct hernia repair or other approaches, such as preperitoneal repair, are rarely required in the pediatric age group. The older child with a direct inguinal hernia and a connective tissue disorder may be the exception and a laparoscopic approach and prosthetic material in such a case can be useful for repair.

FEMORAL HERNIA

Femoral hernias are also rare in children. They are more common in girls than boys, with a ratio of 2 : 1. Femoral hernias represent a protrusion through the femoral canal. The bulge of a femoral hernia is located below the inguinal ligament and typi-

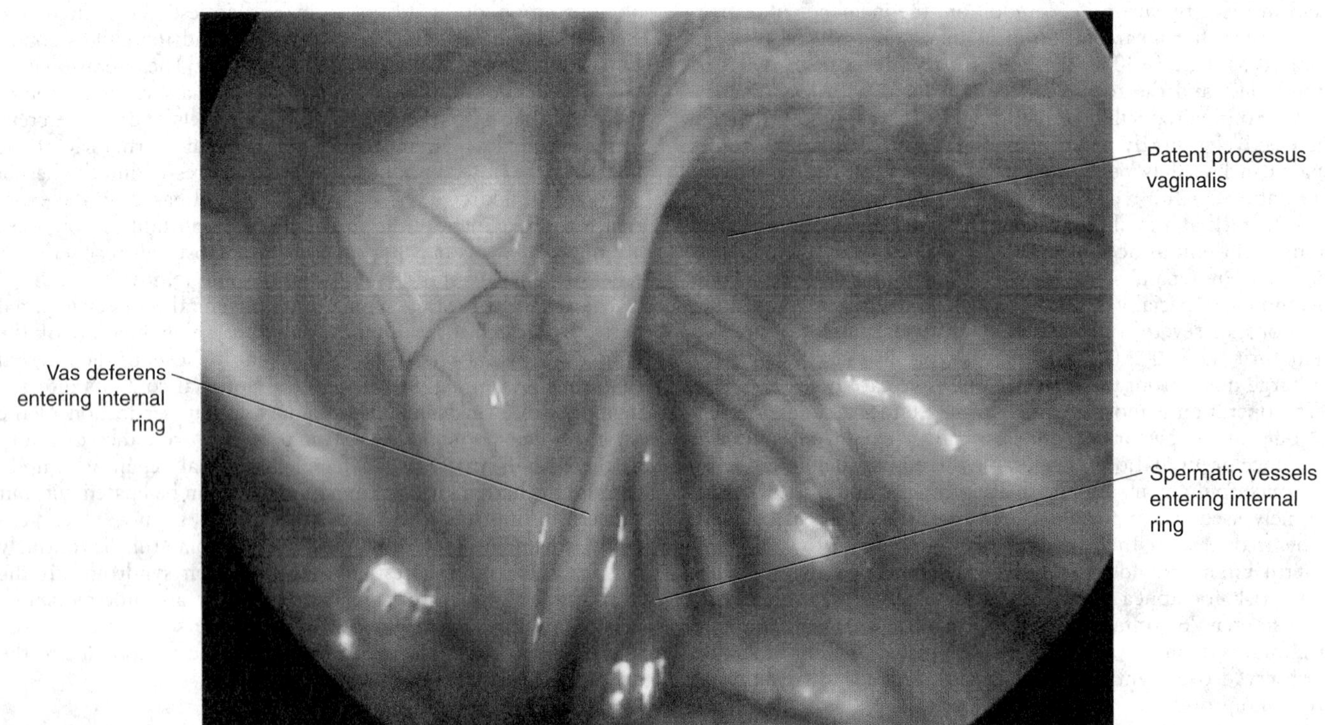

Figure 343-2. Image on laparoscopy of patent processus vaginalis on right side.

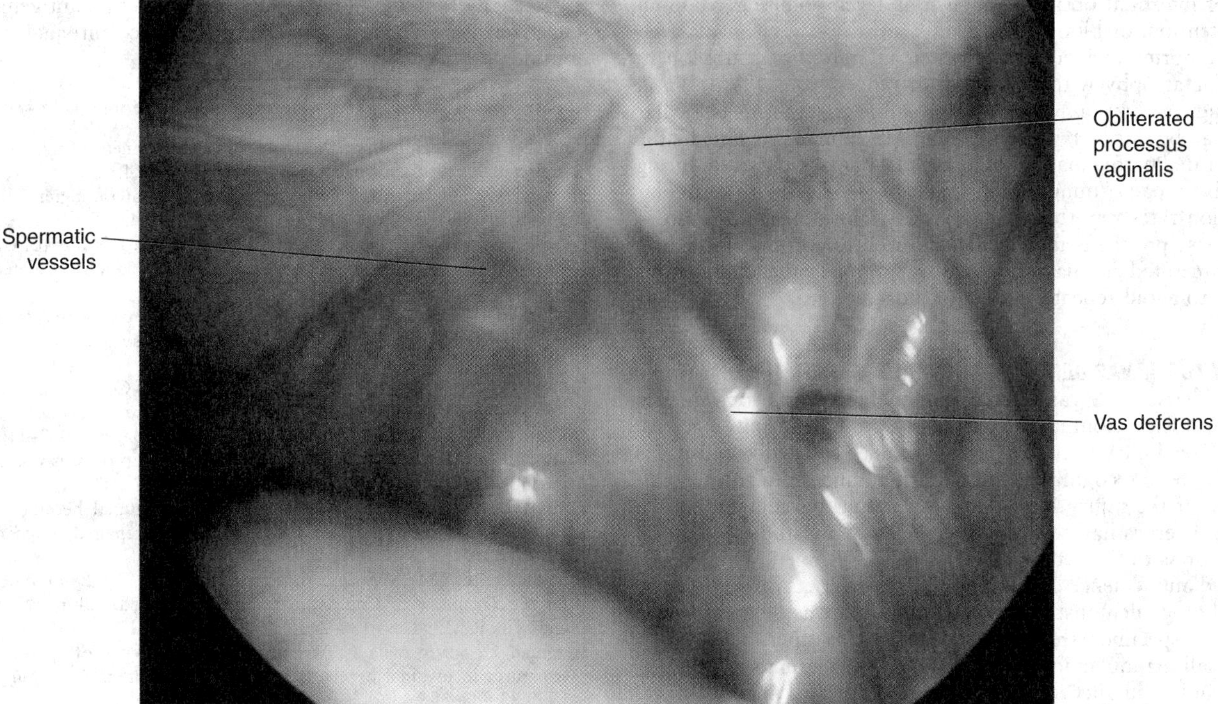

Figure 343-3. Image on diagnostic laparoscopy of obliterated processus vaginalis on left side.

cally projects toward the medial aspect of the thigh. Femoral hernias are more often missed clinically than direct hernias on physical examination or at the time of indirect hernia repair. Repair of a femoral hernia involves closure of the defect at the femoral canal, generally suturing the inguinal ligament to the pectineal ligament and pectineal fascia.

COMPLICATIONS

Complications after elective inguinal hernia repair are uncommon (1.5%) but significantly higher in association with incarceration (10%). Some complications are related to technical factors (recurrence, iatrogenic cryptorchidism), whereas others are related to the underlying process, such as bowel ischemia, gonadal infarction, and testicular atrophy related to an incarcerated hernia. The majority of complications are related to episodes of incarceration or occur after emergency operative reduction and hernia repair.

WOUND INFECTION. Wound infection occurs in <1% of elective inguinal hernia repairs in infants and children, but the incidence increases to 5–7% in association with incarceration and emergent repair. The patient typically develops fever and irritability 3–5 days after the surgery and the wound demonstrates warmth, erythema, and fluctuance. Management consists of opening and draining the wound, a short course of antibiotics, and a daily wound dressing. Most common organisms are gram positive (*Staphylococcus* and *Streptococcus* spp.) and consideration should be given to coverage of methicillin-resistant *Staphlococcus aureus*. The wound generally heals in 1–2 wk with low morbidity and a good cosmetic result.

RECURRENT HERNIA. The recurrence rate of inguinal hernias after elective inguinal hernia repairs is generally reported as 0.5–1.0%, with rates as high as 2% for premature infants. The rate of recurrence after emergency repair of an incarcerated hernia is significantly higher, reported as 3–6% in most large series. The true incidence of recurrence is most certainly even higher, given the problem of accurate long-term follow-up. In the group of patients who develop recurrent inguinal hernia, the recurrence occurs in 50% within 1 yr of the initial repair and in 75% by 2 yr.

Recurrence of an indirect hernia is most likely due to a technical problem in the original procedure such as failure to identify the sac properly, failure to perform high ligation of the sac at the level of the internal ring, or a tear in the sac that leaves a strip of peritoneum along the cord structures. Recurrence as a direct hernia can result from injury to the inguinal floor (transversalis fascia) during the original procedure or failure to identify a direct hernia during the original exploration. Patients with connective tissue disorders (collagen deficiency) or conditions that cause increased intra-abdominal pressure (ventriculoperitoneal shunts, ascites, peritoneal catheter for dialysis) are at increased risk for recurrence.

IATROGENIC CRYPTORCHIDISM. Iatrogenic cryptorchidism describes malposition of the testis after inguinal hernia repair. This complication is usually related to disruption of the testicular attachment or failure to recognize an undescended testis during the original procedure, allowing the testis to retract, typically to the region of the external ring. At the completion of inguinal hernia repair, the testis should be placed in a dependent intrascrotal position. If the testis will not remain in this position, an orchiopexy should be performed at the time of the hernia repair.

INCARCERATION. Incarceration of an inguinal hernia can result in injury to the intestines, the fallopian tube and ovary, or the ipsilateral testis. The incidence of incarceration of a congenital indirect inguinal hernia is reported as between 6% and 18% and as high as 30% for infants <3 mo of age. Intestinal injury requiring bowel resection is uncommon, occurring in 1–2% of incarcerated hernias. In cases of incarceration in which the hernia is reduced nonoperatively, the likelihood of intestinal injury is low, but these patients should be observed closely for persistent signs and symptoms of intestinal obstruction, such as fever, vomiting, abdominal distention, or bloody stools.

The reported incidence of testicular infarction and subsequent testicular atrophy with incarceration ranges from 4% to 12%, with higher rates among the irreducible cases. The testicular insult can be caused by compression of the gonadal vessels by the incarcerated hernia mass or as a result of damage incurred during operative repair. Young infants are at higher risk, with testicular infarction rates reported as high as 30% in infants <2–3 mo of age. These problems underscore the need for prompt reduction of incarcerated hernias and early repair once the diagnosis is known to avoid repeat episodes of incarceration.

INJURY TO THE VAS DEFERENS AND MALE FERTILITY. Similar to the gonadal vessels, the vas deferens can be injured as a consequence of compression from an incarcerated hernia or during operative repair. This injury is almost certainly underreported because it is unlikely to be recognized until adulthood and, even then, possibly only if the injury is bilateral. Although the vulnerability of the vas deferens has been documented in many studies, no good data exist as to the actual incidence of this problem. One review reported an incidence of injury to the vas deferens of 1.6% based on pathology demonstrating segments of the vas deferens in the hernia sac specimen; this may be overstated, as others have shown that small glandular inclusions found in the hernia sac can represent müllerian duct remnants and are of no clinical importance. The relationship between male fertility and previous inguinal hernia repair is also unknown. There appears to be an association between infertile males with testicular atrophy and abnormal sperm count and a previous hernia repair. A relationship has also been reported between infertile males with spermatic autoagglutinating antibodies and previous inguinal hernia repair. The proposed etiology is that operative injury to the vas deferens during inguinal hernia repair may result in obstruction of the vas with diversion of spermatozoa to the testicular lymphatics, and this breach of the blood-testis barrier produces an antigenic challenge resulting in formation of spermatic autoagglutinating antibodies.

Gallagher TM: Regional anesthesia for surgical treatment of inguinal hernia in preterm babies. *Arch Dis Child* 1993;69:623–624.

Holcomb GW: Laparoscopic evaluation for a contralateral inguinal hernia or a nonpalpable testis. *Pediatr Ann* 1993;22:678–684.

Lobe TE, Schropp KP: Inguinal hernias in pediatrics: Initial experience with laparoscopic inguinal exploration of the asymptomatic contralateral side. *J Laparoendosc Surg* 1992;2:135–140.

Owings EF, Georgeson KE: A new technique for laparoscopic exploration to find contralateral patent processus vaginalis. *Surg Endosc* 2000; 14:114–116.

Rescorla FJ: Hernias and umbilicus. In Oldham KT, Colambani PM, Foglia RP, Skinner MA (editors): *Principles and Practice of Pediatric Surgery.* Philadelphia, Lippincott Williams and Wilkins, 2005, pp 1087–1101.

Rowe MI, Copelson LW, Clatworthy HW: The patent processus vaginalis and the inguinal hernia. *J Pediatr Surg* 1969;4:102–107.

Shier F, Montupet P, Esposito C: Laparoscopic inguinal herniorrhaphy in children: A three center experience with 933 repairs. *J Pediatr Surg* 2002;37:395–397.

Skandalakis JE, Gray SW: *Embryology for Surgeons: The Embryologic Basis for the Treatment of Congenital Anomalies,* 2nd ed. Baltimore, Williams and Wilkins, 1994, pp 184–241.

Stergman C, Sotelo-Avila C, Weber TR: The incidence of spermatic cord structures in inguinal hernia sacs from male children. *Am J Surg Pathol* 1999;23:883–885.

Tacket LD, Breuer CK, Luks FI, et al: Incidence of contralateral inguinal hernia: A prospective analysis. *J Pediatr Surg* 1999;34:684–687.

Weber TR, Tracy TF Jr, Keller MS: Groin hernias and hydroceles. In Ashcraft KW, Holcomb GW III, Murphy JP (editors): *Pediatric Surgery*, 4th ed. Philadelphia, WB Saunders, 2005, pp 697–705.

Wiener ES, Touloukian RJ, Rodgers BM, et al: Hernia survey of the Section on Surgery of the American Academy of Pediatrics. *J Pediatr Surg* 1996;31:1166–1169.

Section 5 — Exocrine Pancreas — Steven L. Werlin

Chapter 344 ■ Embryology, Anatomy, and Physiology

The human pancreas develops from evaginations of primitive duodenum beginning at about the 5th wk of gestation. The larger dorsal anlage, which develops into the tail, body, and part of the head of the pancreas, grows directly from the duodenum. The smaller ventral anlage develops as one or two buds from the primitive liver and eventually forms the major portion of the head of the pancreas. At about the 17th wk of gestation, the dorsal and ventral anlagen fuse as the buds develop and the gut rotates. The ventral duct forms the proximal portion of the major pancreatic duct of Wirsung, which opens into the ampulla of Vater. The dorsal duct forms the distal portion of the duct of Wirsung and the accessory duct of Santorini, which empties independently in ≈15% of people. Variations in fusion may account for pancreatic developmental anomalies. Pancreatic agenesis has been associated with a base pair deletion in the *ipf1* HOX gene, *PDX1*. Other genes involved in pancreatic organogenesis include the sonic hedgehog and transforming growth factor (TGF) 1β genes.

The pancreas lies transversely in the upper abdomen between the duodenum and the spleen in the retroperitoneum. The head, which rests on the vena cava and renal vein, is adherent to the C loop of the duodenum and surrounds the distal common bile duct. The tail of the pancreas reaches to the left splenic hilum and passes above the left kidney. The lesser sac separates the tail of the pancreas from the stomach.

By the 13th wk of gestation, exocrine and endocrine cells can be identified. Primitive acini containing immature zymogen granules are found by the 16th wk. Mature zymogen granules containing amylase, trypsinogen, chymotrypsinogen, and lipase are present at the 20th wk. Centroacinar and duct cells, which are responsible for water, electrolyte, and bicarbonate secretion, are also found by the 20th wk. The final three-dimensional structure of the pancreas consists of a complex series of branching ducts surrounded by grapelike clusters of epithelial cells. Cells containing glucagon are present at the 8th wk. Islets of Langerhans appear between the 12th and 16th wks.

344.1 • Anatomic Abnormalities

Complete or partial *pancreatic agenesis* is a rare condition. Complete agenesis is associated with severe neonatal diabetes and usually death at an early age. Partial or dorsal pancreatic agenesis is often asymptomatic but may be associated with diabetes, congenital heart disease, polysplenia, and recurrent pancreatitis. Pancreatic agenesis is also associated with malabsorption.

An *annular pancreas* results from incomplete rotation of the left (ventral) pancreatic anlage. Patients usually present in infancy with symptoms of complete or partial bowel obstruction. There is frequently a history of maternal polyhydramnios. Some children present with chronic vomiting, pancreatitis, or biliary colic. The treatment of choice is duodenojejunostomy. Division of the pancreatic ring is not attempted, because a duodenal diaphragm or duodenal stenosis frequently accompanies annular pancreas. Annular pancreas may be associated with Down syndrome, intestinal atresia, imperforate anus, pancreatitis, and malrotation.

Ectopic pancreatic rests in the stomach or small intestine occur in ≈3% of the population. Most cases (70%) are found in the upper intestinal tract. Recognized on barium contrast studies by their typical umbilicated appearance, they are rarely of clinical importance. On endoscopy, they are irregular, yellow nodules 2–4 mm in diameter. A pancreatic rest may occasionally be the lead point of an intussusception, produce hemorrhage, or cause bowel obstruction.

Pancreas divisum, which occurs in 5–15% of the population, is the most common pancreatic developmental anomaly. As the result of failure of the dorsal and ventral pancreatic anlagen to fuse, the tail, body, and part of the head of the pancreas drain through the small accessory duct of Santorini rather than the main duct of Wirsung. This anomaly may be associated with recurrent pancreatitis when there is relative obstruction of the outflow of the ventral pancreas. The treatment of choice of recurrent pancreatitis associated with pancreas divisum is endoscopic insertion of an endoprosthetic stent. If the episodes stop, surgical sphincterotomy is indicated.

Choledochal cysts are dilatations of the biliary tract and usually cause biliary tract symptoms, such as jaundice, pain, and fever. On occasion, the presentation may be pancreatitis. The diagnosis is usually easily made with ultrasonography, CT scanning, or biliary tract scan. Similarly, a choledochocele, an intraduodenal choledochal cyst, may present with pancreatitis. The diagnosis can be difficult and require magnetic resonance cholangiopancreatography (MRCP) or endoscopic retrograde cholangiopancreatography (ERCP).

A number of rare conditions, such as Ivemark and Johanson-Blizzard syndromes, include pancreatic dysgenesis or dysfunction among their features. Many of these syndromes include renal and hepatic dysgenesis along with the pancreatic anomalies. Absence of islet cells and agenesis of the pancreas produce permanent diabetes mellitus, which begins in the neonatal period (see Chapter 590).

Hill ID, Lebenthal E: Congenital abnormalities of the exocrine pancreas. In Go VLW, et al (editors): *The Exocrine Pancreas: Biology, Pathology, and Diseases,* 2nd ed. New York, Raven Press, 1993, pp 1029–1040.

Klein SD, Affronti JP: Pancreas divisum, an evidence-based review: Part I, pathophysiology. *Gastrointest Endosc* 2004;60:9–25.

Klein SD, Affronti JP: Pancreas divisum, an evidence-based review: Part II, patient selection and treatment. *Gastrointest Endosc* 2004;60:585–589.

344.2 • Physiology

The acinus is the functional unit of the exocrine pancreas. Acinar cells are arrayed in a semicircle around a lumen. Ducts that drain the acini are lined by centroacinar and ductular cells. This arrangement allows the secretions of the various cell types to mix.

The acinar cell synthesizes, stores, and secretes >20 enzymes. These enzymes are stored in zymogen granules, some in inactive forms. The relative concentration of the various enzymes in pancreatic juice is affected and perhaps controlled by the diet, probably by regulating the synthesis of specific messenger RNA. Diets high in fat increase the concentration of lipase; a high-protein diet increases pancreatic content of proteases; and a high-carbohydrate diet leads to increased content of amylase in the pancreatic juice. Amylase splits starch into maltose, isomaltose, maltotriose, and dextrins. Trypsin and chymotrypsin, both endopeptidases, and carboxypeptidase, an exopeptidase, are secreted by the pancreas as the inactive proenzymes trypsinogen and chymotrypsinogen. Trypsinogen is activated in the gut lumen by enterokinase, a brush border enzyme. Trypsin can then activate trypsinogen, chymotrypsinogen, and procarboxypeptidase into their respective active forms.

Pancreatic lipase requires colipase, a coenzyme also found in pancreatic fluid, for activity. Lipase liberates fatty acids from the one and three positions of triglycerides, leaving a monoglyceride. The stimuli for exocrine pancreatic secretion are neural and hormonal. Acetylcholine mediates the cephalic phase; cholecystokinin (CCK) mediates the intestinal phase. CCK is released from the duodenal mucosa by luminal amino acids and fatty acids. Feedback regulation of pancreatic secretion is mediated by pancreatic proteases in the duodenum. Secretion of CCK is inhibited by the digestion of a trypsin-sensitive, CCK-releasing peptide released in the lumen of the small intestine or by a monitor peptide released in pancreatic fluid.

Centroacinar and duct cells secrete water and bicarbonate. Bicarbonate secretion is under feedback control and is regulated by duodenal intraluminal pH. The stimulus for bicarbonate production is secretin in concert with CCK. Secretin cells are abundant in the duodenum.

Although normal pancreatic function is required for digestion, maldigestion occurs only after considerable reduction in pancreatic function; lipase and colipase secretion must be decreased by 90–98% before fat maldigestion occurs.

Although amylase and lipase are present in the pancreas early in gestation, secretion of both amylase and lipase is low in the infant. Adult levels of these enzymes are not reached in the duodenum until late in the 1st yr of life. Digestion of the starch found in many infant formulas depends in part on the low levels of salivary amylase that reach the duodenum. This explains the diarrhea that may be seen in infants who are fed formulas high in glucose polymers or starch. Neonatal secretion of trypsinogen and chymotrypsinogen is at ≈70% of the level found in the 1 yr old infant. The low levels of amylase and lipase in duodenal contents of infants may be partially compensated by salivary amylase and lingual lipase. This explains the relative starch and fat intolerance of premature infants.

Christian M, Edwards C, Weaver LT: Starch digestion in infancy. *J Pediatr Gastroenterol Nutr* 1999;29:116–124.

Werlin SL, Lee PC: Development of the exocrine pancreas. In Polin RA, Fox WW (editors): *Fetal and Neonatal Physiology,* 3rd ed. Philadelphia, WB Saunders, 2003, pp 1142–1151.

Chapter 345 ■ Pancreatic Function Tests

Pancreatic function can be measured by direct and indirect methods. Direct stimulation of the pancreas with a test (**Lundh**) meal of corn oil, skim milk powder, and dextrose or with secretin plus cholecystokinin can be performed. Classically, a triple-lumen tube is used to isolate the pancreatic secretions in the duodenum. Measurement of bicarbonate concentration and enzyme activity (trypsin, chymotrypsin, lipase, and amylase) is performed on the aspirated secretions. The most commonly used direct test today is collection of pancreatic juice after stimulation with secretin and cholecystokinin at endoscopy.

A 72 hr stool collection for quantitative analysis of fat content is the gold standard for the diagnosis of malabsorption. The collection is usually performed at home, and the parent is asked to keep a careful dietary record, from which fat intake is calculated. A pre-weighed, sealable plastic container is used, which the parent keeps in the freezer. Freezing helps preserve the specimen and reduce odor. Infants are dressed in disposable diapers with the plastic side facing the skin so that the complete sample can be transferred to the container. Normal fat absorption is >93% of intake. Pancreatic enzyme activities can be measured in stool. Qualitative examination of the stool for microscopic fat globules may give both false-positive and false-negative results. Fecal elastase, the standard screening test for pancreatic insufficiency, has a sensitivity and specificity >90%. Falsely abnormal results can occur in many enteropathies.

The elevated serum levels of trypsinogen found in neonates with cystic fibrosis form the basis of the newborn screening test being adapted in many states. With advancing pancreatic damage, serum trypsinogen levels eventually fall below normal.

Pancreatic function can also be measured by breath tests. A labeled triglyceride, most commonly ^{14}C-triolein, is ingested and digested by pancreatic lipase in the duodenum, liberating $^{14}CO_2$, which is detected in the expired air. Because of the radioactivity and long half-life of ^{14}C, this test is not appropriate for use in children. Triolein labeled with ^{13}C, a stable, nonradioactive isotope, is safe for pediatric use. It has not gained widespread acceptance because the test is relatively insensitive in detecting mild cases of pancreatic insufficiency and detection of $^{13}CO_2$ requires a mass spectrophotometer that is not generally available.

Beharry S, Ellis L, Corey M, et al: How useful is fecal pancreatic elastase 1 as a marker of exocrine pancreatic disease? *J Pediatr* 2002;141:84–90.

Del Rosario MA, Fitzgerald JF, Gupta SK, et al: Direct pancreatic measurement of pancreatic enzymes after stimulation with secretin versus secretin plus cholecystokinin. *J Pediatr Gastroenterol Nutr* 2000;31:28–32.

Chapter 346 ■ Disorders of the Exocrine Pancreas

DISORDERS ASSOCIATED WITH PANCREATIC INSUFFICIENCY. Other than cystic fibrosis, conditions that cause pancreatic insufficiency are rare in children. They include Shwachman-Diamond syndrome, isolated enzyme deficiencies, enterokinase deficiency (see Chapter 335), chronic pancreatitis, and protein-calorie malnutrition (see Chapter 335).

Cystic Fibrosis (See Chapter 400). Cystic fibrosis is the most common lethal genetic disease and the most common cause of malabsorption among white American or European children. By the end of the 1st yr of life, 85–90% of children with cystic fibrosis (CF) have pancreatic insufficiency, which, if untreated, can lead to malnutrition. Treatment of the associated pancreatic insufficiency leads to improvement in absorption, better growth, and normalized stools. Pancreatic function can be monitored in children with CF with serial measurements of fecal elastase. Certain mutations in the cystic fibrosis gene have been associated with idiopathic chronic pancreatitis.

Shwachman-Diamond Syndrome (SDS) [See Chapter 130]. SDS is an autosomal recessive syndrome (1/20,000 births), consisting of pancreatic insufficiency; neutropenia, which may be cyclic; neutrophil chemotaxis defects; metaphyseal dysostosis; failure to thrive; and short stature. Some patients with SDS have liver or kidney involvement or learning difficulty. Patients typically present in infancy with poor growth and greasy, foul-smelling stools that are characteristic of malabsorption. These children can be readily differentiated from those with cystic fibrosis by their normal sweat chloride levels, lack of the cystic fibrosis gene, characteristic metaphyseal lesions, and fatty pancreas on CT examination. Despite adequate pancreatic replacement therapy, poor growth frequently continues. Pancreatic insufficiency is often transient, and steatorrhea may spontaneously improve with age. Recurrent pyogenic infections (otitis media, pneumonia, osteomyelitis, dermatitis, sepsis) are common and are a frequent cause of death. Thrombocytopenia is found in 70% of patients and anemia in 50%. Development of a *myelodysplastic syndrome* may occur and transformation to *acute myeloid leukemia* has been reported in up to 33% and 24% of patients, respectively. The gene for SDS is found on chromosome 7. Pathologically, the pancreatic acini are replaced by fat with little fibrosis. Islet cells and ducts are normal. The fatty pancreas has a characteristic hypodense appearance on CT and MRI scans.

Pearson Syndrome. This is a sporadic mitochondrial DNA mutation affecting oxidative phosphorylation that manifests in infants with severe macrocytic anemia and variable thrombocytopenia. The bone marrow demonstrates vacuoles in erythroid and myeloid precursors as well as ringed sideroblasts. In addition to its role in severe bone marrow failure, pancreatic insufficiency contributes to growth failure. Other mitochondrial DNA mutations are associated with the development of diabetes mellitus (Kearns-Sayre, chronic progressive external ophthalmoplegia, diabetes with deafness syndromes). Mitochondrial DNA mutations are transmitted through maternal inheritance to both sexes or are sporadic.

Isolated Enzyme Deficiencies. Isolated deficiencies of trypsinogen, enterokinase, lipase, and colipase have been reported. Although enterokinase is a brush border enzyme, deficiency causes pancreatic insufficiency because pancreatic proteases remain inactive. Deficiencies of trypsinogen or enterokinase manifest with failure to thrive, hypoproteinemia, and edema. Isolated amylase deficiency is typically developmental and resolves by age 2–3 yr.

SYNDROMES ASSOCIATED WITH PANCREATIC INSUFFICIENCY. Pancreatic agenesis, the Johanson-Blizzard syndrome (pancreatic insufficiency, deafness, low birthweight, microcephaly, midline ectodermal scalp defects, psychomotor retardation, hypothyroidism, dwarfism, absent permanent teeth, and aplasia of the alae nasae), congenital pancreatic hypoplasia, and congenital rubella are rare causes of pancreatic insufficiency. Some children with both syndromic (Alagille) and nonsyndromic paucity of intrahepatic bile ducts also have pancreatic insufficiency associated with their liver disease. Pancreatic insufficiency has also been reported in duodenal atresia and stenosis and may also be seen in the infant with familial or nonfamilial hyperinsulinemic hypoglycemia (formerly called nesidioblastosis) who requires 95–100% pancreatectomy to control hypoglycemia.

Boocock GR, Morrison JA, Popovic M, et al: Mutations in SBDS are associated with Shwachman-Diamond syndrome. *Nat Genet* 2003;33:97–101.
Toth T, Bokay J, Szonyi L: Detection of mtDNA deletion in Pearson syndrome by two independent PCR assays from Guthrie card. *Clin Genet* 1998;53:210–213.

Chapter 347 ■ Treatment of Pancreatic Insufficiency

Treatment of exocrine pancreatic insufficiency by oral enzyme replacement usually corrects creatorrhea, but steatorrhea is difficult to correct completely. This is due to variability of lipase activity in different commercial preparations, inadequate dosage, incorrect timing of doses, lipase inactivation by gastric acid, and the observation that chymotrypsin in the enzyme preparation digests and thus inactivates lipase. In enzyme supplements, the true lipase activity has been shown to be as much as twice the labeled amount. Pancrease, Creon, Ultrase, and Panceacarb are the preparations most widely used. These products are enteric-coated preparations that resist gastric acid inactivation. Generic enzyme preparations are less effective and should be avoided.

The dosage of pancreatic replacement for children depends on the amount of food eaten and is established by trial and error. Because these products contain excess protease compared with lipase, the dosage is estimated from the lipase requirement of 500–1,500 IU/kg/meal. An adequate dose is one that is followed by the return of the stools to normal fat content, size, color, and odor. Enzyme replacement should be given at the beginning of and with the meal. Tablets should be chewed; powder and granules can be mixed with a small quantity of food. Enzymes must also be given with snacks. Increasing enzyme supplements beyond the recommended dose does not improve absorption, may retard growth, and may cause fibrosing colonopathy.

When adequate fat absorption is not achieved, gastric acid neutralization with an H_2-receptor antagonist or a proton pump inhibitor decreases enzyme inactivation by gastric acid and improves delivery of lipase into the intestine. The coating of enteric-coated preparations also protects lipase from acid inactivation.

Untoward effects secondary to pancreatic enzyme replacement therapy include allergic reactions, increased uric acid levels, and kidney stones. Fibrosing colonopathy, consisting of colonic fibrosis and strictures, occurs 7–12 mo after high-dose pancreatic supplement therapy (ranging from 6,500 to 58,000 IU lipase/kg/meal).

Baker SS, Borowitz D, Duffy D: Pancreatic enzyme therapy and clinical outcomes in cystic fibrosis. *J Pediatr* 2005;146:189–193.
Borowitz D, Baker RD, Stallings V: Census report in nutrition for pediatric patients with cystic fibrosis. *J Pediatr Gastroenterol Nutr* 2002;35:246–259.
Powell CJ: Colonic toxicity from pancreatins: A contemporary safety issue. *Lancet* 1999;353:911–915.

Chapter 348 ■ Pancreatitis

348.1 • Acute Pancreatitis

Acute pancreatitis, the most common pancreatic disorder in children, is increasing in frequency. At least 30–50 cases are now seen in major pediatric centers per year. Blunt abdominal injuries, multisystem disease, biliary stones or microlithiasis (sludging), and drug toxicity are the most common etiologies. Valproic acid is the most common cause of drug-induced pancreatitis in children. Other cases follow organ transplantation, or are due to infections and metabolic disorders. Fewer cases are idiopathic or due to other etiologies (Table 348-1).

PATHOGENESIS. The classic etiologic theory suggests that after an initial insult, such as ductal disruption or obstruction, lysosomal hydrolases co-localize with pancreatic proenzymes within the acinar cell. Pancreastasis (similar in concept to cholestasis) with

TABLE 348-1. Etiology of Acute Pancreatitis in Children

DRUGS AND TOXINS	**OBSTRUCTIVE**
Acetaminophen overdose	Ampullary disease
Alcohol	Ascariasis
5-aminosalicytate	Biliary tract malformations
L-asparaginase	Choledochal cyst
Azathioprine	Choledochocele
Cimetidine	Choleithiasis, microlithiasis, and choledocholithiasis (stones or sludge)
Corticosteroids	Duplication cyst
DDC	Endoscopic retrograde cholangiopancreatography (ERCP) complication
DDI	Pancreas divisum
Enalapril	Pancreatic ductal abnormalities
Erythromycin	Postoperative
Estrogen	Sphincter of Oddi dysfunction
Furosemide	Tumor
Isoniazid	**SYSTEMIC DISEASE**
6-Mercaptopurine	α_1-antitrypsin deficiency
Mesalamine	Bone marrow transplantation
Methyldopa	Brain tumor
Metronidazole	Collagen vascular diseases
Pentamidine	Crohn disease
Sulfonamides	Cystic fibrosis
Sulindac	Diabetes mellitus
Tetracycline	Head trauma
Thiazides	Hemochromatosis
Trimethoprim	Hemolytic uremic syndrome
Valproic acid	Hyperlipidemia: type I, IV, V
Venom (spider, scorpion, Gila monster lizard)	Hyperparathyroidism/Hypercalcemia
Vincristine	Kawasaki disease
HEREDITARY PANCREATITIS	Malnutrition
Cationic trypsinogen gene	Organic academia
Cystic fibrosis gene	Peptic ulcer
SPINK1 gene	Periarteritis nodosa
INFECTIOUS	Renal failure
Ascariasis	Systemic lupus erythematosus
Coxsackie B virus	Transplantation: bone marrow, heart, liver, kidney, pancreas
Epstein-Barr virus	Vasculitis
Hepatitis A, B	**TRAUMATIC**
Influenza A, B	Blunt injury
Leptospirosis	Burns
Malaria	Child abuse
Measles	Hypothermia
Mumps	Surgical trauma
Mycoplasma	Total body cast
Rubella	
Rubeola	
Reye syndrome: varicella, influenza B	
Septic shock	

continued synthesis of enzymes occurs. Trypsinogen is activated to trypsin, which then activates other pancreatic proenzymes, leading to autodigestion, further enzyme activation, and release of active proteases. Lecithin is activated by phospholipase A2 into the toxic lysolecithin. Prophospholipase is unstable and can be activated by minute quantities of trypsin. Another theory suggests that after an insult, release of cytokines and subsequent depletion of antioxidants leads to pancreastasis and the further activation of pancreatic proenzymes.

The healthy pancreas is protected by: (1) pancreatic proteases that are synthesized as inactive proenzymes; (2) digestive enzymes that are segregated into secretory granules at pH 6.2 with low calcium concentration, which minimizes trypsin activity; (3) the presence of protease inhibitors both in the cytoplasm and zymogen granules; and (4) enzymes that are secreted directly into the ducts. Histopathologically, interstitial edema appears early. Later, as the episode of pancreatitis progresses, localized and confluent necrosis, blood vessel disruption leading to hemorrhage, and an inflammatory response in the peritoneum may develop.

CLINICAL MANIFESTATIONS. The patient with acute pancreatitis has severe abdominal pain, persistent vomiting, and fever. The pain is epigastric or in either upper quadrant and steady, often resulting in the child's assuming an antalgic position with hips and knees flexed, sitting upright, or lying on the side. The child is very uncomfortable and irritable and appears acutely ill. The abdomen may be distended and tender. A mass may be palpable. The pain increases in intensity for 24–48 hr, during which time vomiting may increase and the patient may require hospitalization for dehydration and may need fluid and electrolyte therapy. The prognosis for complete recovery in the acute uncomplicated case is excellent.

Severe acute pancreatitis is rare in children. In this life-threatening condition, the patient is acutely ill with severe nausea, vomiting, and abdominal pain. Shock, high fever, jaundice, ascites, hypocalcemia, and pleural effusions can occur. A bluish discoloration may be seen around the umbilicus (***Cullen*** sign) or in the flanks (***Grey Turner*** sign). The pancreas is necrotic and can be transformed into an inflammatory hemorrhagic mass. The mortality rate, which is ≈25%, is related to the systemic inflammatory response syndrome with multiple organ dysfunction (MOD): shock, renal failure, acute respiratory distress syndrome, disseminated intravascular coagulation, massive gastrointestinal bleeding, and systemic or intra-abdominal infection. An elevated APACHE II score, high serum C-reactive protein (CRP) levels, persistent MOD for >1 wk, the percent necrosis seen on CT scan, and failure of pancreatic tissue to enhance on CT scan (suggesting necrosis) may predict severe disease with a poor prognosis.

DIAGNOSIS. Acute pancreatitis is usually diagnosed by measurement of serum amylase and lipase activities. The serum amylase level is typically elevated for up to 4 days. A variety of other conditions can also cause hyperamylasemia without pancreatitis (Table 348-2). Elevation of salivary amylase can mislead the clinician into making the diagnosis of pancreatitis in a child with abdominal pain, but the laboratory can separate amylase isoenzymes into pancreatic and salivary fractions. Initially, serum amylase levels are normal in 10–15% of patients. Serum lipase is more specific than amylase for acute inflammatory pancreatic disease and should be determined when pancreatitis is suspected and the amylase level is normal. The serum lipase rises by 4–8 hr, peaks at 24–48 hr, and remains elevated 8–14 days longer than serum amylase. Serum lipase can also be elevated in nonpancreatic diseases.

Other laboratory abnormalities that may be present in acute pancreatitis include hemoconcentration, coagulopathy, leukocytosis, hyperglycemia, glucosuria, hypocalcemia, elevated γ-glutamyl transpeptidase, and hyperbilirubinemia.

TABLE 348-2. Differential Diagnosis of Hyperamylasemia

PANCREATIC PATHOLOGY
Acute or chronic pancreatitis
Complications of pancreatitis (pseudocyst, ascites, abscess)
Factitious pancreatitis
SALIVARY GLAND PATHOLOGY
Parotitis (mumps, *Staphylococcus aureus,* cytomegalovirus, HIV, Epstein-Barr virus)
Sialadenitis (calculus, radiation)
Eating disorders (anorexia nervosa, bulimia)
INTRA-ABDOMINAL PATHOLOGY
Biliary tract disease (cholelithiasis)
Peptic ulcer perforation
Peritonitis
Intestinal obstruction
Appendicitis
SYSTEMIC DISEASES
Metabolic acidosis (diabetes mellitus, shock)
Renal insufficiency, transplantation
Burns
Pregnancy
Drugs (morphine)
Head injury
Cardiopulmonary bypass

Roentgenography of the chest and abdomen may demonstrate nonspecific findings. The chest roentgenogram may demonstrate platelike atelectasis, basilar infiltrates, elevation of the hemidiaphragm, left- (rarely right-) sided pleural effusions, pericardial effusion, and pulmonary edema. Abdominal roentgenograms may demonstrate a sentinel loop, dilatation of the transverse colon (cutoff sign), ileus, pancreatic calcification (if recurrent), blurring of the left psoas margin, a pseudocyst, diffuse abdominal haziness (ascites), and peripancreatic extraluminal gas bubbles.

Ultrasound and, more specifically, CT scanning have major roles in the diagnosis and follow-up of children with pancreatitis. Findings can include pancreatic enlargement, a hypoechoic, sonolucent edematous pancreas, pancreatic masses, fluid collections, and abscesses (Fig. 348-1); at least 20% of children with acute pancreatitis initially have normal imaging studies. In adults, CT findings are the basis of a widely accepted prognostic system. Endoscopic retrograde cholangiopancreatography (ERCP) or more often ***magnetic resonance cholangiopancreatography (MRCP)*** are essential in the investigation of recurrent pancreatitis, pancreas divisum, sphincter of Oddi dysfunction, and disease associated with gallbladder pathology. Endoscopic ultrasonography also helps visualize the pancreaticobiliary system.

TREATMENT. The aims of medical management are to relieve pain and restore metabolic homeostasis. Analgesia should be given in adequate doses. Fluid, electrolyte, and mineral balance should be restored and maintained. Nasogastric suction is useful in patients who are vomiting. While vomiting, the patient should be maintained with nothing by mouth. Prophylactic antibiotics (imipenem/cilastatin) are controversial but are used in severe cases to prevent infected pancreatic necrosis or to treat infected necrosis. Recovery is usually complete within 4–5 days. Refeeding can commence when vomiting has resolved, the serum amylase is falling, and clinical symptoms are resolving.

The treatment of severe acute pancreatitis can involve antibiotics, gastric acid suppression, and peritoneal lavage to reduce the risk of secondary infection. Endoscopic therapy can be of benefit when pancreatitis is caused by anatomic abnormalities, such as strictures or stones. Enteral alimentation is superior to parenteral nutrition. Enteral alimentation by mouth, nasogastric tube, or nasojejunal tube (in severe cases or for those intolerant of oral or nasogastric feedings), within 2–3 days of onset, reduces

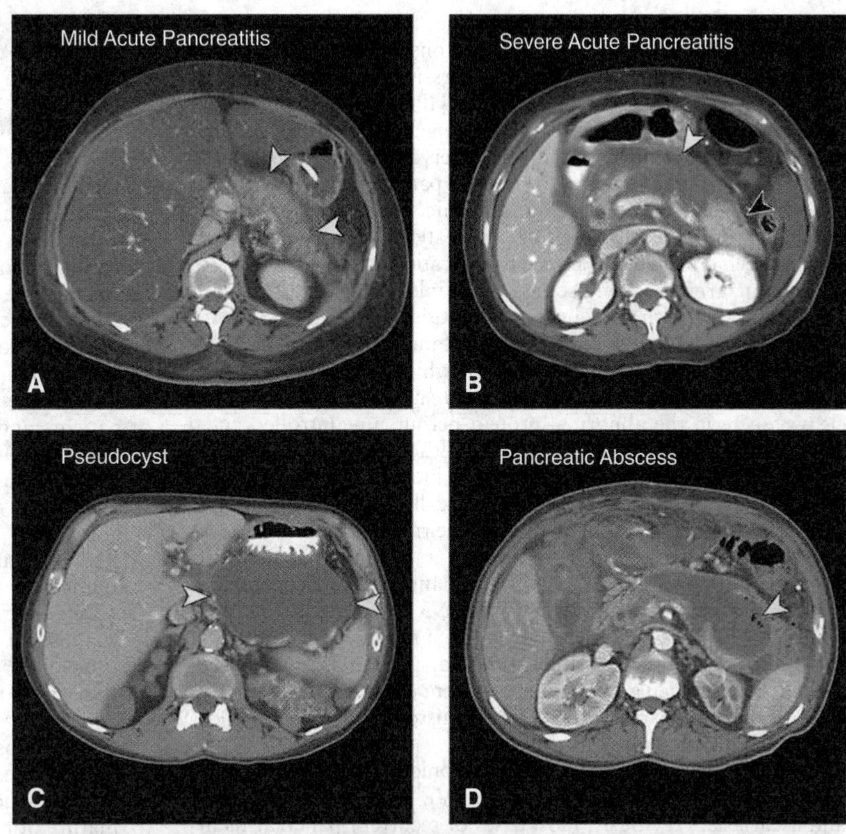

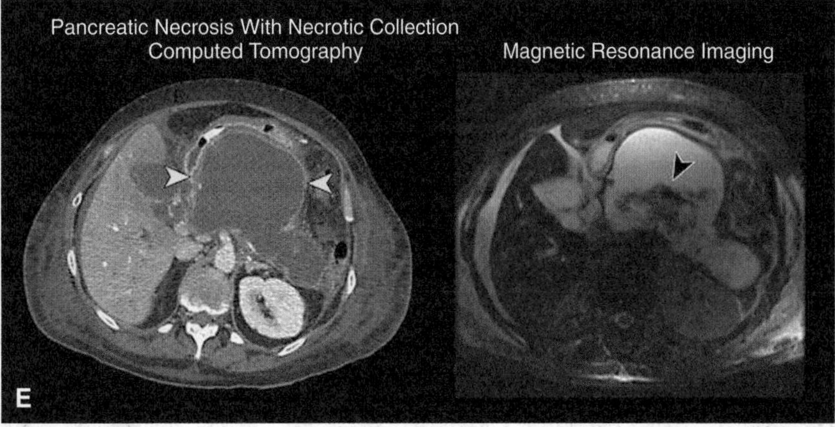

Figure 348-1. Computed tomography (CT) and magnetic resonance imaging (MRI) appearance of pancreatitis. Panels *A* through *E (left)*, CT images; panel *E (right)*, MRI. *A*, Mild acute pancreatitis showing normal enhancement of the body of pancreas *(arrowheads)* after intravenous contrast. *B*, Severe acute pancreatitis showing pancreatic necrosis with areas of the pancreas not enhancing *(arrowhead)* after contrast administration compared with areas that are normally perfused *(black arrowhead)*. *C*, Pseudocyst of the pancreas *(arrowheads)* with clear-appearing fluid within the collection near the pancreas. *D*, Pancreatic abscess with presence of gas *(arrowhead)* inside the cavity. *E*, Pancreatic necrosis (necrotic collection), which appears on CT scan as a clear fluid collection *(yellow arrowheads)*. The same collection on MRI shows areas of necrotic debris *(black arrowhead)* not observed on CT scan, a distinction that has prognostic and therapeutic implications. (From Swaroop VS, Chari ST, Clain JE: Severe acute pancreatitis. *JAMA* 2004;291:2865–2868.)

the need for surgery and the risk of infectious complications as well as the length of hospitalization. Surgical therapy of acute pancreatitis is rarely required, but may include drainage of necrotic material or abscesses.

PROGNOSIS. Children with uncomplicated acute pancreatitis do well and recover within 4–5 days. When pancreatitis is associated with trauma or systemic disease, the prognosis is typically related to the associated medical conditions. A pediatric prognostic system based on admission and 48 hour clinical criteria has recently been proposed but has not yet been validated by other authors.

DeBanto JR, Goday PS, Pedroso MRA, et al: Acute pancreatitis in children. *Am J Gastroenterol* 2002;97:1726–1731.

Johnson CD, Abu-Hilal M: Persistent organ failure during the first week as a marker of fatal outcome in acute pancreatitis. *Gut* 2004;53:1340–1344.

Lopez M: The changing incidence of acute pancreatitis in children: A single-institution perspective. *J Pediatr* 2002;140:622–624.

Makola D, Krenitsky J, Parrish C, et al: Efficacy of enteral nutrition for the treatment of pancreatitis using standard enteral formula. *Am J Gastroenterol* 2006;101:2347–2355.

Marik PE, Zaloga GP: Meta-analysis of parenteral nutrition versus enteral nutrition in patients with acute pancreatitis. *Br Med J* 2004;328:1407.

Mitchell RMS, Byrne MF, Baillie J: Pancreatitis. *Lancet* 2003;361:1447–1455.

Nathens AB, Curtis R, Beale RJ, et al: Management of the critically ill patient with severe acute pancreatitis. *Crit Care Med* 2004;32:2524–2536.

Swaroop VS, Chari ST, Clain JE: Severe acute pancreatitis. *JAMA* 2004; 291:2865–2868.

Werlin SL, Kugathasan S, Frautschy B: Pancreatitis in children. *J Pediatr Gastroenterol Nutr* 2003;37:591–595.

348.2 • Chronic Pancreatitis

Chronic, relapsing pancreatitis in children is frequently hereditary or due to congenital anomalies of the pancreatic or biliary ductal system. Hereditary pancreatitis (HP) is most often transmitted as an autosomal dominant trait with incomplete penetrance but variable expressivity. Symptoms frequently begin in the 1st decade but are usually mild at the onset. Although spontaneous recovery from each attack occurs in 4–7 days, episodes become progressively severe. Clinically, HP may be diagnosed by the presence of the disease in successive generations of a family. An evaluation during symptom-free intervals may be unrewarding until calcifications, pseudocysts, or pancreatic exocrine and endocrine insufficiency develop. Chronic pancreatitis is a risk factor for future development of pancreatic cancer. The gene for HP has been cloned and mapped to the cationic trypsinogen gene on the long arm of chromosome 7. Multiple mutations of the HP gene associated with hereditary pancreatitis have been described. Other alleles may be identified in nonfamilial cases of chronic pancreatitis. Cationic trypsinogen, which autoactivates to trypsin, has a trypsin-sensitive cleavage site. In HP, loss of this cleavage site in the abnormal protein permits uncontrolled activation of trypsinogen to trypsin, which leads to autodigestion of the pancreas. Mutations of other genes, including heterozygosity for the cystic fibrosis gene *(CFTR),* typically in the 5T promoter region, and the *SPINK1* gene (pancreatic trypsin inhibitor), have also been associated with recurrent or chronic pancreatitis. Trypsin inhibitor acts as a fail-safe mechanism to prevent uncontrolled autoactivation of trypsin. In *SPINK1* mutations, this fail-safe mechanism is lost; this gene may be a modifier gene and not the direct etiologic factor. Indications for genetic testing for the cationic trypsinogen gene include recurrent episodes of acute pancreatitis, chronic pancreatitis, a family history of pancreatitis, or unexplained pancreatitis in children.

Other conditions associated with chronic, relapsing pancreatitis are hyperlipidemia (types I, IV, and V), hyperparathyroidism, and ascariasis. Previously, most cases of recurrent pancreatitis in childhood were considered idiopathic; with the discovery of at least three gene families associated with recurrent pancreatitis, this has changed. Congenital anomalies of the ductal systems, such as pancreas divisum, are probably more common than previously recognized.

A thorough diagnostic evaluation of every child with more than one episode of pancreatitis is indicated. Serum lipid, calcium, and phosphorus levels are determined. Stools are evaluated for ascaris, and a sweat test is performed. Plain abdominal films are evaluated for the presence of pancreatic calcifications. Abdominal ultrasound or CT scanning is performed to detect the presence of a pseudocyst. The biliary tract is evaluated for the presence of stones. After genetic counseling evaluation of HP, *SPINK1* and the *CFTR* genotypes can be performed.

MRCP and ERCP are techniques that can be used to define the anatomy of the gland and are mandatory if surgery is considered. One of these studies should be performed as part of the evaluation of any child with idiopathic, nonresolving, or recurrent pancreatitis and in patients with a pseudocyst before surgery. In these cases, MRCP or ERCP may detect a previously undiagnosed anatomic defect that may be amenable to endoscopic or surgical therapy. Endoscopic treatments include sphincterotomy, stone extraction, and insertion of pancreatic or biliary endoprosthetic stents. These treatments allow for successful nonsurgical management of conditions previously requiring surgical intervention.

Kingsnorth A, O'Reilly D: Acute pancreatitis. *BMJ* 2006;332:1072–1076.

Stevens T, Conwell DL, Zuccaro G: Pathogenesis of chronic pancreatitis: An evidence-based review of past theories and recent developments. *Am J Gastroenterol* 2004;99:2256–2270.

Werlin SL, Taylor A: ERCP. In Howard ER, Stringer MD, Colombani PM (editors): *Surgery of the Liver, Bile Ducts and Pancreas in Children,* 2nd ed. London, STM Publishing, 2002, pp 509–520.

Whitcomb DC: Acute pancreatitis. *N Engl J Med* 2006;354:2142–2150.

Witt H, Becker M: Genetics of chronic pancreatitis. *J Pediatr Gastoenterol Nutr* 2002;34:125–136.

Chapter 349 ■ Pseudocyst of the Pancreas

Pancreatic pseudocyst formation is an uncommon sequela to acute or chronic pancreatitis. Pseudocysts are sacs delineated by a fibrous wall in the lesser peritoneal sac. They may enlarge or extend in almost any direction, thus producing a wide variety of symptoms (see Fig. 348-1).

A pancreatic pseudocyst is suggested when an episode of pancreatitis fails to resolve or when a mass develops after an episode of pancreatitis. Clinical features usually include pain, nausea, and vomiting. The most common signs are a palpable mass in 50% of patients and jaundice in 10%. Other findings include ascites and pleural effusions (usually left-sided).

The most useful diagnostic techniques are ultrasonography, CT scanning, endoscopic retrograde cholangiopancreatography (ERCP), and magnetic resonance cholangiopancreatography (MRCP). Because of its ease, availability, and reliability, ultrasonography is the 1st choice. Sequential ultrasonography studies have demonstrated that most small pseudocysts (<6 cm) resolve spontaneously. It is recommended that the patient with acute pancreatitis undergo an ultrasonographic evaluation 2–4 wk after resolution of the acute episode for an evaluation of possible pseudocyst formation.

Percutaneous or endoscopic drainage of pseudocysts has replaced open surgical drainage, except for complicated or recurrent pseudocysts. Whereas a pseudocyst must be allowed to mature for 4–6 wk before surgical drainage is attempted, percutaneous or endoscopic drainage can be attempted earlier. MRCP or ERCP should precede surgical treatment to help the surgeon plan the approach and define anatomic abnormalities.

Baillie J: Pancreatic pseudocysts (part 1). *Gastrointest Endosc* 2004; 59:873–879.

Baillie J: Pancreatic pseudocysts (part 2). *Gastrointest Endosc* 2004; 60:105–113.

Chapter 350 ■ Pancreatic Tumors

NEOPLASIA. Pancreatic tumors can be of either endocrine or nonendocrine origin. Tumors of endocrine origin include insulinomas and gastrinomas. These and other functioning tumors occur in the autosomal dominantly inherited multiple endocrine neoplasia type 1 (MEN-1). Hypoglycemia accompanied by higher than expected insulin levels or refractory gastric ulcers (Zollinger-Ellison syndrome) indicate the possibility of a pancreatic tumor (see Chapter 342). Most gastrinomas arise outside the pancreas. The treatment of choice is surgical removal. If the primary tumor cannot be found or if it has metastasized, cure may not be possible. Treatment with a proton pump inhibitor to inhibit gastric acid secretion is then indicated.

The *watery diarrhea–hypokalemia–acidosis syndrome* is usually produced by the secretion of vasoactive intestinal peptide (VIP) by a non-α-cell tumor (VIPoma) [see Table 342-2]. VIP levels are frequently, but not always, increased in the serum. Treatment is surgical removal of the tumor. When this is not possible, symptoms may be controlled by the use of octreotide acetate (cyclic somatostatin, Sandostatin), a synthetic analog of somatostatin. Pancreatic tumors secreting a variety of hormones, including glucagon, somatostatin, and pancreatic polypeptide, have also been described. The treatment is surgical resection when possible.

Pancreatoblastomas, pancreatic adenocarcinomas, cystadenomas, and rhabdomyosarcomas are rarely encountered. Peculiar to childhood are pancreatoblastomas, which are embryonal tumors that secrete α-fetoprotein and may contain both endocrine and exocrine elements. Their clinical behavior is malignant but not well characterized, owing to their rarity. Presurgical chemotherapy should be considered for lesions not primarily resectable. Resection can be curative; adjuvant chemotherapy has been used, but its effectiveness is not established. Carcinoma of the exocrine pancreas is a major problem in adults, accounting for 2% of diagnoses and 5% of deaths due to cancer. It is very rare in childhood. No definite causes are known. Several genetic syndromes including hereditary pancreatitis and MEN-1 lead to an increased incidence of pancreatic cancer in adult life. The Frantz tumor is a papillary cystic tumor usually found in girls and young women. Typical presenting symptoms are abdominal pain, mass, or jaundice. The treatment of choice is total surgical removal.

Insulinomas and persistent hyperinsulinemic hypoglycemia of infancy (nesidioblastosis) produce symptomatic hypoglycemia. Massive subtotal or total pancreatectomy is the treatment of choice when medical treatment fails (see Chapter 92). These children may then develop pancreatic insufficiency and diabetes as a complication of treatment.

Cysts of the pancreas occur in von Hippel-Lindau disease. Solid and cystic papillary tumors mimic pancreatic ontogeny. Their natural history is still being determined. Metastases have been reported, but adjuvant therapy after surgical excision cannot yet be recommended. The diagnosis is suggested by CT scanning. Surgery is the only known effective therapy.

Prognosis is good for completely resected endocrine tumors but very poor for carcinomas, even with extensive surgery. Children who survive partial or complete pancreatectomy may have decreased pancreatic exocrine and endocrine reserve.

Shorter NA, Glick RD, Klimstra DS, et al: Malignant pancreatic tumors in childhood and adolescence: The Memorial Sloan-Kettering experience, 1967–present. *J Pediatr Surg* 2002;37:887–892.

Tomassetti P, Migliori M, Lalli S, et al: Epidemiology, clinical features and diagnosis of gastroenteropancreatic endocrine tumours. *Ann Oncol* 2001;12:S95–S99.

Section 6 — The Liver and Biliary System

Chapter 351 ■ Morphogenesis of the Liver and Biliary System

Michael D. Bates and William F. Balistreri

The morphogenesis of the liver and biliary system is a complex process; altered development has significant consequences, including disorders featuring cholestasis such as Alagille syndrome and the neonatal presentation of biliary atresia. During the early embryonic process of gastrulation, the three embryonic germ layers (endoderm, mesoderm, ectoderm) are formed. The liver and biliary system arise from cells of the ventral foregut endoderm; their development can be divided into three distinct processes (Fig. 351-1). First, through unknown mechanisms, the ventral foregut endoderm acquires *competence* to receive signals arising from the cardiac mesoderm. These mesodermal signals, in the form of various fibroblast growth factors (FGFs) and bone morphogenetic proteins (BMPs), result in *specification* of cells that will form the liver and activation of liver-specific genes. This specification occurs in animal models just before visible budding of the liver. These newly specified cells then migrate in a cranial ventral direction into the septum transversum in the 4th wk of human gestation to initiate liver *morphogenesis*. The growth and development of the newly budded liver require interactions with endothelial cells. Certain proteins are important for liver development in animal models (Table 351-1).

Within the ventral mesentery, proliferation of migrating cells forms anastomosing hepatic cords, with the network of primitive liver cells, sinusoids, and septal mesenchyme establishing the basic architectural pattern of liver lobule (Fig. 351-2). The solid *cranial* portion of the hepatic diverticulum (pars hepatis) eventually forms the hepatic parenchyma and the intrahepatic bile ducts; the *caudal* portion (pars cystica) becomes the gallbladder, cystic duct, and common bile duct. The hepatic lobules are identifiable in the 6th human gestational wk. The bile canalicular structures that include microvilli and junctional complexes are specialized loci of the liver cell membrane; these appear very early in gestation, and by 6–7 wk, large canaliculi bounded by several hepatocytes are seen. The intrahepatic bile ducts are derived through branching and remodeling of the hepatic duct; formation is complete by the 3rd mo. The cystic duct and the gallbladder are fully recanalized by the 7th–8th wk (see Fig. 351-2C).

In the hepatic excretory (biliary) system, bile canaliculi empty into the smallest bile ductules, which unite to form interlobular bile ducts that follow the terminal branches of the portal vein. At the hilum of the liver, the intrahepatic ducts leave the branches of the portal vein and merge to form the extrahepatic biliary system. The ducts of the right and left lobes form the common hepatic duct. The common bile duct is formed from the merger of the common hepatic duct and cystic duct; it extends along the right edge of the lesser omentum, terminating in the duodenum as the intramural papilla of Vater. Union of the biliary tract with the pancreatic ducts forms the ampulla of Vater, which, with the sphincter of Oddi, regulates the flow of bile into the intestine, prevents entry of bile into the pancreatic duct, and inhibits reflux of intestinal contents into the ducts.

Fetal hepatic blood flow is derived from the hepatic artery and from the portal and umbilical veins, which form the portal sinus. The portal venous inflow is directed mainly to the right lobe of the liver; umbilical flow is primarily to the left. The ductus venosus shunts blood from the portal and umbilical veins to the hepatic vein, bypassing the sinusoidal network. After birth, the ductus venosus becomes obliterated when oral feedings are initi-

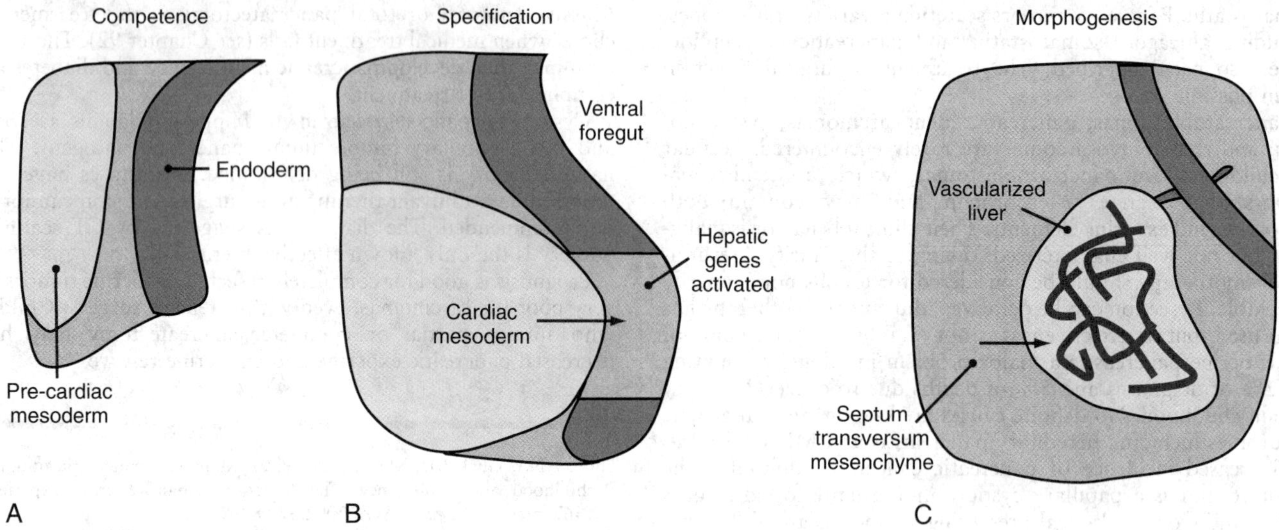

Figure 351-1. Processes involved in early liver development. *A*, The ventral foregut endoderm acquires *competence* to receive signals arising from the cardiac mesoderm. *B*, Specific cells of the ventral foregut endoderm undergo *specification* and activation of liver-specific genes under the influence of mesodermal signals. *C*, Liver *morphogenesis* is initiated as the newly specified cells migrate into the septum transversum under the influence of signaling molecules and extracellular matrix released by septum transversum mesenchymal cells and of primitive endothelial cells. (Reprinted from Zaret KS: Liver specification and early morphogenesis. *Mech Dev* 92:83–88; © 2000, with permission from Elsevier Science.)

ated. The fetal oxygen saturation is lower in portal than in umbilical venous blood; accordingly, the right hepatic lobe has lower oxygenation and greater hematopoietic activity than the left hepatic lobe. The fetal sinusoidal endothelium is the site of large macrophages, which become the Kupffer (reticuloendothelial) cell network.

The transport and metabolic activities of the liver are facilitated by the structural arrangement of liver cell cords, which are formed by rows of hepatocytes, separated by sinusoids that converge toward the tributaries of the hepatic vein (the central vein) located in the center of the lobule (see Fig. 351-2*D*). This establishes the pathways and patterns of flow for substances to and from the liver. In addition to arterial input from the systemic circulation, the liver also receives venous input from the gastroin-

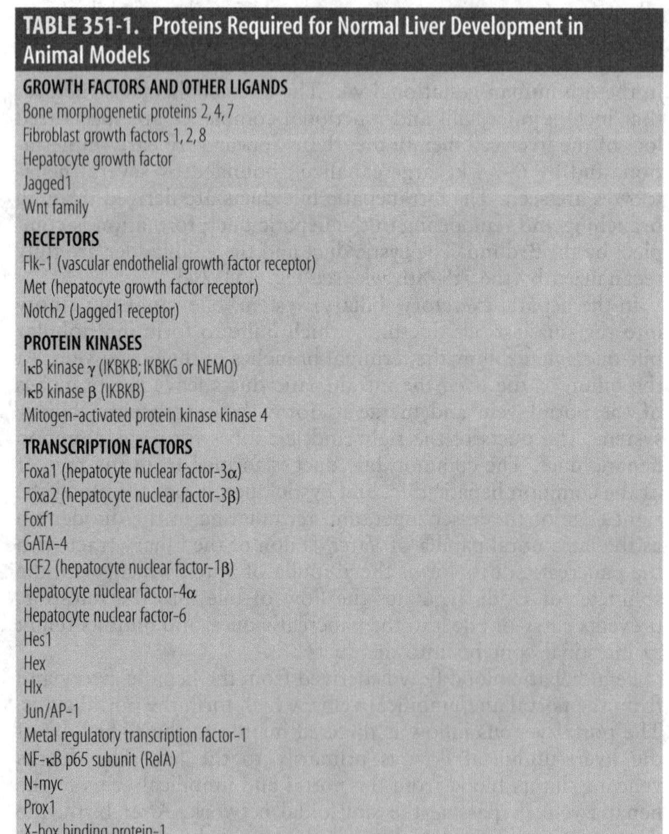

TABLE 351-1. Proteins Required for Normal Liver Development in Animal Models

GROWTH FACTORS AND OTHER LIGANDS
Bone morphogenetic proteins 2, 4, 7
Fibroblast growth factors 1, 2, 8
Hepatocyte growth factor
Jagged1
Wnt family
RECEPTORS
Flk-1 (vascular endothelial growth factor receptor)
Met (hepatocyte growth factor receptor)
Notch2 (Jagged1 receptor)
PROTEIN KINASES
IκB kinase γ (IKBKB; IKBKG or NEMO)
IκB kinase β (IKBKB)
Mitogen-activated protein kinase kinase 4
TRANSCRIPTION FACTORS
Foxa1 (hepatocyte nuclear factor-3α)
Foxa2 (hepatocyte nuclear factor-3β)
Foxf1
GATA-4
TCF2 (hepatocyte nuclear factor-1β)
Hepatocyte nuclear factor-4α
Hepatocyte nuclear factor-6
Hes1
Hex
Hlx
Jun/AP-1
Metal regulatory transcription factor-1
NF-κB p65 subunit (RelA)
N-myc
Prox1
X-box binding protein-1

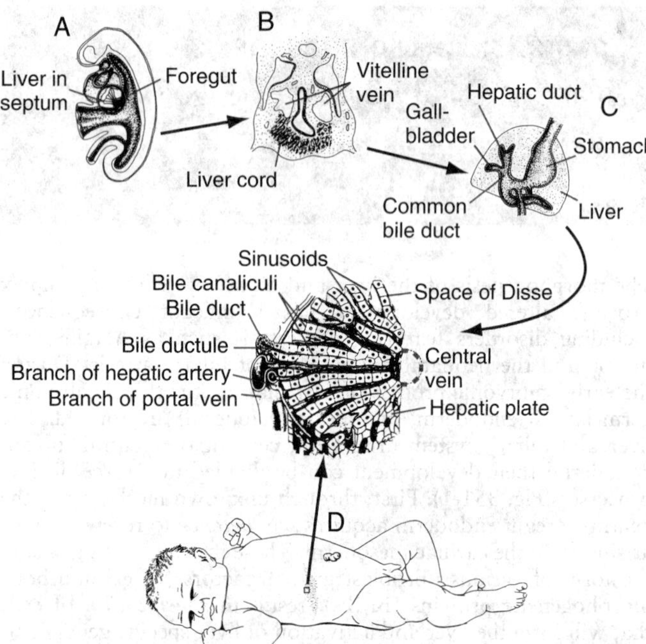

Figure 351-2. Hepatic morphogenesis. *A*, Ventral outgrowth of hepatic diverticulum from foregut endoderm in the 3.5 wk embryo. *B*, Between the two vitrelline veins, the enlarging hepatic diverticulum buds off epithelial (liver) cords that become the liver parenchyma, around which the endothelium of capillaries (sinusoids) align (4 wk embryo). *C*, Hemisection of embryo at 7.5 wk demonstrating recanalization of the biliary tract. *D*, Three-dimensional representation of the hepatic lobule as present in the newborn. (Reprinted from Andres JM, Mathis RK, Walker WA: Liver disease in infants. Part I: Developmental hepatology and mechanisms of liver dysfunction. *J Pediatr* 1977;90:686–697.)

testinal tract via the portal system. The products of the hepatobiliary system are released by two different paths: through the hepatic vein, and through the biliary system back into the intestine. Plasma proteins and other plasma components are secreted by the liver. Absorbed and circulating nutrients arrive through the portal vein or the hepatic artery and pass through the sinusoids and past the hepatocytes to the systemic circulation at the central vein. Biliary components are transported via the series of enlarging channels from the bile canaliculi through the bile ductule to the common bile duct.

Bile secretion is noted at the 12th gestational wk. The major components of bile vary with stage of development. Near term, cholesterol and phospholipid content is relatively low; low concentrations of bile acids, the absence of bacterially derived (secondary) bile acids, and the presence of unusual bile acids reflect low rates of bile flow and immature bile acid synthetic pathways.

The liver reaches a peak relative size at the 9th wk at about 10% of the fetal weight. Early in development, the liver is a primary site of hematopoiesis; in the 7th wk, hematopoietic cells outnumber functioning hepatocytes in the hepatic anlage. These early hepatocytes are smaller than at maturity (≈20 µm vs 30–35 µm) and contain less glycogen. Near term, the hepatocyte mass expands to dominate the organ, as cell size and glycogen content increase. Hematopoiesis is virtually absent by the 2nd postnatal month in full-term infants. As the density of hepatocytes increases with gestational age, the relative volume of the sinusoidal network decreases. The liver constitutes 5% of body weight at birth but only 2% in an adult.

Several metabolic processes are immature in a healthy newborn infant, owing in part to the fetal patterns of activity of various enzymatic processes. Many fetal hepatic functions are carried out by the maternal liver, which provides nutrients and serves as a route of elimination of metabolic end products and toxins. Fetal liver metabolism is devoted primarily to the production of proteins required for growth. Toward term, primary functions become production and storage of essential nutrients, excretion of bile, and establishment of processes of elimination. Extrauterine adaptation requires de novo enzyme synthesis. Modulation of these processes depends on substrate and hormonal input via the placenta and on dietary and hormonal input in the postnatal period.

HEPATIC ULTRASTRUCTURE

Hepatocytes exhibit various ultrastructural features that reflect their biologic functions (Fig. 351-3). First, hepatocytes, like other epithelial cells, are polarized, meaning that their structure and function are directionally oriented. One result of this polarity is that various regions of the hepatocyte plasma membrane exhibit specialized functions. Bidirectional transport occurs at the sinusoidal surface, where materials reaching the liver via the portal system enter and compounds secreted by the liver leave the hepatocyte. Canalicular membranes of adjacent hepatocytes form bile canaliculi, which are bounded by tight junctions preventing transfer of secreted compounds back into the sinusoid. Within hepatocytes, metabolic and synthetic activities are contained within a number of different cell organelles. The oxidation and metabolism of heterogeneous classes of substrates, fatty acid oxidation, key processes in gluconeogenesis, and the storage and release of energy occur in the abundant mitochondria. The endoplasmic reticulum (ER), a continuous network of rough- and smooth-surfaced tubules and cisternae, is the site of various processes, including protein and triglyceride synthesis and drug metabolism. Low fetal activity of ER-bound enzymes accounts for a relative inefficiency of xenobiotic (drug) metabolism. The Golgi apparatus is active in protein packaging and possibly in bile secretion. Hepatocyte peroxisomes are single-membrane-limited cytoplasmic organelles that contain enzymes such as oxidases and catalase and those that have a role in lipid and bile acid metabolism.

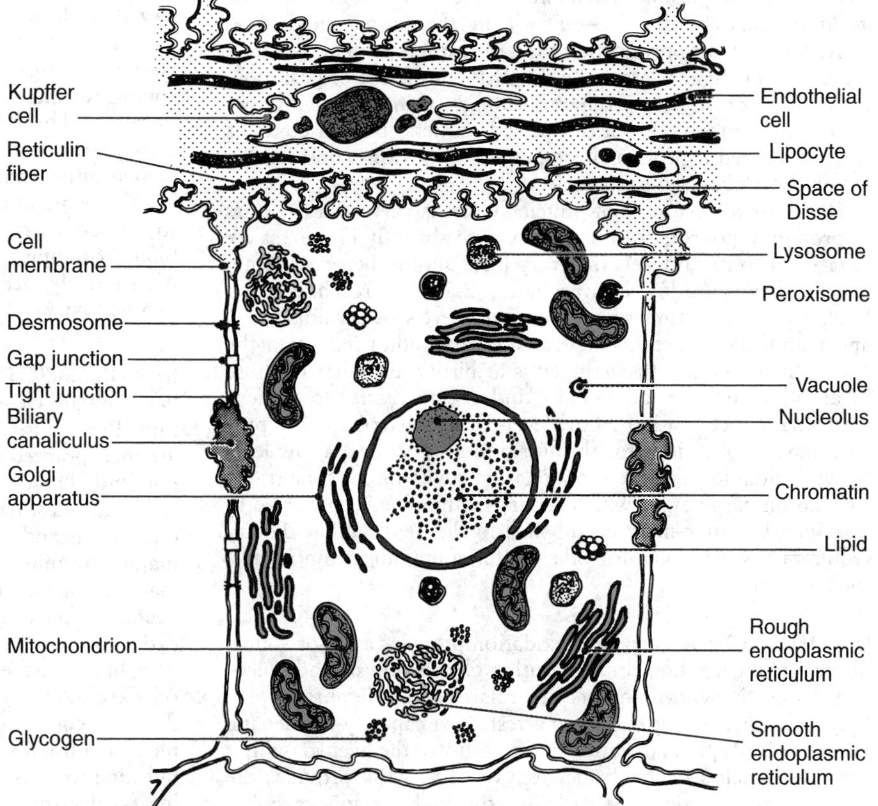

Figure 351-3. Schematic view of the ultrastructure and organelles of hepatocytes. (Reprinted from Sherlock S: Hepatic cell structure. In Sherlock S [editor]: *Diseases of the Liver and Biliary System,* 6th ed. Oxford, Blackwell Scientific, 1981, p 10; with permission from Blackwell Scientific.)

Lysosomes contain numerous hydrolases that have a role in intracellular digestion. The hepatocyte cytoskeleton, composed of actin and other filaments, is distributed throughout the cell and concentrated near the plasma membrane. Microfilaments and microtubules have a role in receptor-mediated endocytosis, in bile secretion, and in maintaining hepatocyte architecture and motility.

METABOLIC FUNCTIONS OF THE LIVER

CARBOHYDRATE METABOLISM. The liver regulates serum glucose levels closely. It stores excess carbohydrate as glycogen, a polymer of glucose readily hydrolyzed to glucose during fasting. To maintain serum glucose levels, hepatocytes produce free glucose by either glycogenolysis or gluconeogenesis. Immediately after birth, an infant is dependent on hepatic glycogenolysis. Gluconeogenic activity is present at a low level in the fetal liver and increases rapidly after birth. Fetal glycogen synthesis begins at about the 9th wk of gestation, with glycogen stores most rapidly accumulated near term, when the liver contains two to three times the amount of glycogen of adult liver. Most of this stored glycogen is used in the immediate postnatal period. Reaccumulation is initiated at about the 2nd wk of postnatal life, and glycogen stores reach adult levels at approximately the 3rd wk in healthy full-term infants. The fluctuations in serum glucose levels in preterm infants are due in part to the fact that efficient regulation of the synthesis, storage, and degradation of glycogen develops only near the end of full-term gestation. Dietary carbohydrates such as galactose are converted to glucose, but there is a substantial dependence on gluconeogenesis for glucose in early life, especially if glycogen stores are limited.

PROTEIN METABOLISM. During the rapid fetal growth phase, specific decarboxylases that are rate limiting in the biosynthesis of physiologically important polyamines have higher activities than in the mature liver. The rate of synthesis of albumin and secretory proteins in the developing liver parallels the quantitative changes in endoplasmic reticulum. Synthesis of albumin appears at approximately the 7th–8th wk in the human fetus and increases in inverse proportion to that of α-fetoprotein, which is the dominant fetal protein. By the 3rd–4th month of gestation, the fetal liver is able to produce fibrinogen, transferrin, and low-density lipoproteins. From this period on, fetal plasma contains each of the major protein classes, at concentrations considerably below those achieved at maturity.

The *postnatal* patterns of protein synthesis vary with the class of protein. Lipoproteins of each class rise abruptly in the 1st wk after birth to reach levels that vary little until puberty. Albumin concentrations are low in a neonate (≈2.5 g/dL), reaching adult levels (≈3.5 g/dL) after several months. Levels of ceruloplasmin and complement factors increase slowly to adult values in the 1st yr. In contrast, transferrin levels at birth are similar to those of an adult, decline for 3–5 mo, and rise thereafter to achieve their final concentrations. Low levels of activity of specific proteins have implications for the nutrition of an infant; a low level of cystathionine γ-lyase (cystathionase) activity impairs the trans-sulfuration pathway by which dietary methionine is converted to cysteine; the latter must be supplied in the diet. Similar dietary requirements may exist for other sulfur-containing amino acids, such as taurine.

LIPID METABOLISM. Fatty acid oxidation provides a major source of energy in early life, complementing glycogenolysis and gluconeogenesis. Newborn infants are relatively intolerant of prolonged fasting, owing in part to a restricted capacity for hepatic ketogenesis. Rapid maturation of the ability of the liver to oxidize fatty acid occurs in the 1st few days of life. Milk provides the major source of calories in early life; this high-fat, low-carbohydrate diet mandates active gluconeogenesis to maintain blood sugar levels. When the glucose supply is limited, ketone body production from endogenous fatty acids may provide energy for hepatic gluconeogenesis and an alternative fuel for brain metabolism. When carbohydrates are in excess, the liver produces triglycerides. Metabolic processes involving lipids and lipoproteins are predominantly hepatic; liver immaturity or disease affects lipid concentrations and lipoproteins.

BIOTRANSFORMATION. Newborn infants have a decreased capacity to metabolize and detoxify certain drugs, owing to underdevelopment of the hepatic microsomal component that is the site of the specific oxidative, reductive, hydrolytic, and conjugation reactions required for these biotransformations. The major components of the mono-oxygenase system, such as cytochrome P450, cytochrome-*c* reductase, and the reduced form of nicotinamide-adenine dinucleotide phosphate (NADPH), are present in low concentrations in fetal microsomal preparations. In full-term infants, hepatic uridine diphosphate (UDP) glucuronosyltransferase and enzymes involved in the oxidation of polycyclic aromatic hydrocarbons have very low activities. Age-related differences in pharmacokinetics vary from compound to compound. The half-life of acetaminophen in a newborn is similar to that of an adult, whereas theophylline has a half-life of ≈100 hr in a premature infant, as compared to 5–6 hr in an adult. These differences in metabolism, as well as factors such as binding to plasma proteins and renal clearance, determine appropriate drug dosage to avoid toxicity. Dramatic examples of the susceptibility of newborn infants to drug toxicity are the responses to chloramphenicol ("gray baby" syndrome) or to benzoyl alcohol and its metabolic products, which involve ineffective glucuronide and glycine conjugation, respectively. The low concentrations of antioxidants (vitamin E, superoxide dismutase, glutathione peroxidase) in the fetal and early newborn liver lead to increased susceptibility to deleterious effects of oxygen toxicity and oxidant injury through lipid peroxidation.

Conjugation reactions, which convert drugs or metabolites into water-soluble forms that can be eliminated in bile, are also catalyzed by hepatic microsomal enzymes. Newborn infants have decreased activity of UDP glucuronosyltransferase, which converts unconjugated bilirubin to the readily excreted glucuronide conjugate and is the rate-limiting enzyme in the excretion of bilirubin. There is rapid postnatal development of transferase activity irrespective of gestational age, which suggests that birth-related rather than age-related factors are of primary importance in the postnatal development of activity of this enzyme. Microsomal activity can be stimulated by administration of phenobarbital, rifampin, or other inducers of cytochrome P450. Alternatively, drugs such as cimetidine may inhibit microsomal P450 activity.

HEPATIC EXCRETORY FUNCTION. Hepatic excretory function and bile flow are closely related to bile acid excretion and recirculation. Bile acids, the major products of cholesterol degradation, are incorporated into mixed micelles with cholesterol and phospholipid. These micelles act as an efficient vehicle for solubilization and intestinal absorption of lipophilic compounds, such as dietary fats and fat-soluble vitamins. Secretion of bile acids is the major determinant of bile flow in the mature animal. Accordingly, maturity of bile acid metabolic processes affects overall hepatic excretory function, including biliary excretion of endogenous and exogenous compounds.

In humans, the two primary bile acids, cholic acid and chenodeoxycholic acid, are synthesized in the liver. Before excretion, they are conjugated with glycine and taurine. In response to a meal, contraction of the gallbladder delivers bile acids to the intestine to assist in fat digestion and absorption. After mediating fat digestion, the bile acids themselves are reabsorbed from

TABLE 351-2. Causes of Impaired Bile Acid Metabolism and Enterohepatic Circulation

DEFECTIVE BILE ACID SYNTHESIS OR TRANSPORT
Inborn errors of bile acid synthesis (reductase deficiency, isomerase deficiency)
Progressive familial intrahepatic cholestasis (PFIC1, 2, 3)
Intrahepatic cholestasis (neonatal hepatitis)
Acquired defects in bile acid synthesis secondary to severe liver disease

ABNORMALITIES OF BILE ACID DELIVERY TO THE BOWEL
Celiac disease (sluggish gallbladder contraction)
Extrahepatic bile duct obstruction (e.g., biliary atresia, gallstones)

LOSS OF ENTEROHEPATIC CIRCULATION OF BILE ACIDS
External bile fistula
Cystic fibrosis
Small bowel bacterial overgrowth syndrome (with bile acid precipitation, increased jejunal absorption, and "short-circuiting")
Drug-induced entrapment of bile acids in intestinal lumen (e.g., cholestyramine)

BILE ACID MALABSORPTION
Primary bile acid malabsorption (absent or inefficient ileal active transport)
Secondary bile acid malabsorption
  Ileal disease or resection
  Cystic fibrosis

DEFECTIVE UPTAKE OR ALTERED INTRACELLULAR METABOLISM
Parenchymal disease (acute hepatitis, cirrhosis)
Regurgitation from cells
Portosystemic shunting
Cholestasis

the terminal ileum through specific active transport processes. They return to the liver via portal blood, are taken up by liver cells, and are re-excreted in bile. In an adult, this enterohepatic circulation involves 90–95% of the circulating bile acid pool. Bile acids that escape ileal reabsorption reach the colon, where the bacterial flora, through dehydroxylation and deconjugation, produce the secondary bile acids, deoxycholate and lithocholate. In an adult, the composition of bile reflects the excretion of the primary and also the secondary bile acids, which are reabsorbed from the distal intestinal tract.

Neonates have inefficient ileal reabsorption of bile acids and a low rate of hepatic clearance of bile acids from portal blood. The latter results in elevated serum concentrations of bile acids in healthy newborns, often to levels that would suggest liver disease in older individuals. The size of the bile acid pool in a neonate is about half that of an adult, and the bile acid concentration in the proximal intestinal lumen is similarly decreased to levels that are frequently below the concentration required for micelle formation (2 mM); accordingly, absorption of dietary fats and fat-soluble vitamins is reduced, albeit not sufficiently to produce malabsorption. Transient phases of "physiologic cholestasis" and "physiologic steatorrhea" have a role in the nutrition of low birthweight infants but are of minor importance to healthy full-term newborns. Beyond the neonatal period, disturbances in bile acid metabolism may be responsible for diverse effects on hepatobiliary and intestinal function (Table 351-2).

Bates MD, Balistreri WF: The gastrointestinal tract: Development of the human digestive system. In Fanaroff AA, Martin RJ (editors): *Neonatal-Perinatal Medicine: Diseases of the Fetus and Infant,* 7th ed. St. Louis, Mosby, 2002, pp 1255–1263.

Beath SV: Hepatic function and physiology in the newborn. *Semin Neonatol* 2003;8:337–346.

Costa RH, Kalinichenko VV, Holterman AL, Wang X: Transcription factors in liver development, differentiation, and regeneration. *Hepatology* 2003;38:1331–1347.

Desmet VJ: Congenital diseases of intrahepatic bile ducts: Variations on the theme "ductal plate malformation." *Hepatology* 1992;16:1069–1083.

Karpen SJ, Suchy FJ: Structural and functional development of the liver. In Suchy FJ, Sokol RJ, Balistreri WF (editors): *Liver Disease in Children,* 2nd ed. Philadelphia, Lippincott Williams and Wilkins, 2001, pp 3–21.

Lemaigre F, Zaret KS: Liver development update: New embryo models, cell lineage control, and morphogenesis. *Curr Opin Genet Dev* 2004;14:582–590.

Meier PJ, Stieger B: Molecular mechanisms of bile formation. *News Physiol Sci* 2000;15:89–93.

Rudolph AM: Hepatic and ductus venosus blood flows during fetal life. *Hepatology* 1983;3:254–258.

Shneider BL: Intestinal bile acid transport: Biology, physiology, and pathophysiology. *J Pediatr Gastroenterol Nutr* 2001;32:407–417.

Zaret KS: Regulatory phases of early liver development: Paradigms of organogenesis. *Nat Rev Genet* 2002;3:499–512.

Chapter 352 ■ Manifestations of Liver Disease

Lynelle Boamah and William F. Balistreri

Liver disease can often be life threatening and difficult to recognize. The clinical presentation varies depending on the etiology and severity of the liver insult. Knowledge of the varied manifestations, a high index of suspicion, and use of clinical diagnostic skills are the 1st steps in identifying pediatric liver disease.

PATHOLOGIC MANIFESTATIONS

Alterations in hepatic structure and function can be acute or chronic, with varying patterns of reaction of the liver to cell injury. Hepatocyte injury can result in inflammatory cell infiltration or cell death (necrosis), which may be followed by a healing process of scar formation (fibrosis) and, potentially, nodule formation (regeneration). Cirrhosis is the end result of any progressive liver disease.

Injury to individual hepatocytes can result from viral infection, drugs or toxins, hypoxia, immunologic disorders, or inborn errors of metabolism. The evolving process leads to repair, continuing injury with chronic changes, or, in rare cases, to massive hepatic damage.

Cholestasis is an alternative or concomitant response to injury caused by extrahepatic or intrahepatic obstruction to bile flow. Accumulation in serum of substances normally excreted in bile, such as conjugated bilirubin, cholesterol, bile acids, and trace elements, occurs. Bile pigment accumulation in liver parenchyma can be seen in liver biopsy. In extrahepatic obstruction, bile pigment may be visible in the intralobular bile ducts or throughout the parenchyma as bile lakes or infarcts. In intrahepatic cholestasis, an injury to hepatocytes or an alteration in hepatic physiology leads to a reduction in the rate of secretion of solute and water. Likely causes include alterations in: enzymatic or canalicular transporter activity, permeability of the bile canalicular apparatus, organelles responsible for bile secretion, or ultrastructure of the cytoskeleton of the hepatocyte. The end result can be clinically indistinguishable from obstructive cholestasis.

Cirrhosis, defined histologically by the presence of bands of fibrous tissue that link central and portal areas and form parenchymal nodules, is a potential end stage of any acute or chronic liver disease. Cirrhosis can be *posthepatitic* (after acute or chronic hepatitis) or *postnecrotic* (after toxic injury), or it can follow chronic biliary obstruction *(biliary cirrhosis).* Cirrhosis can be macronodular, with nodules of various sizes (up to 5 cm) separated by broad septa, or micronodular, with nodules of uniform size (<1 cm) separated by fine septa; mixed forms occur. The progressive scarring of cirrhosis results in altered hepatic blood flow, with further impairment of liver cell function. In addition, the increased intrahepatic resistance to portal blood flow leads to portal hypertension.

Primary tumors of the liver are discussed in Chapter 504. The liver can be secondarily involved in neoplastic (metastatic) and non-neoplastic (storage diseases, fat infiltration) processes as well as a number of systemic conditions and infectious processes. The liver can also be affected by chronic passive congestion or acute hypoxia, with hepatocellular damage.

CLINICAL MANIFESTATIONS

HEPATOMEGALY. Enlargement of the liver can be due to several mechanisms (Table 352-1). Normal liver size estimations are based on age-related clinical indices, such as: the degree of extension of the liver edge below the costal margin; the span of dullness to percussion; or the length of the vertical axis of the liver, as estimated from imaging techniques. In children, the normal liver edge can be felt up to 2 cm below the right costal margin. In a newborn infant, extension of the liver edge >3.5 cm below the costal margin in the right midclavicular line suggests hepatic enlargement. Measurement of liver span is carried out by percussing the upper margin of dullness and by palpating the lower edge in the right midclavicular line; it may be more reliable than an extension of the liver edge alone; the two measurements may correlate poorly.

The liver span increases linearly with body weight and age in both sexes, ranging from ≈4.5–5.0 cm at 1 wk of age to ≈7–8 cm in boys and 6.0–6.5 cm in girls by 12 yr of age. The lower edge of the right lobe of the liver extends downward (Riedel lobe) and is palpable as a broad mass in some normal people. An enlarged left lobe of the liver is palpable in the epigastrium of some patients with cirrhosis. Downward displacement of the liver by the diaphragm (hyperinflation) or thoracic organs can create an erroneous impression of hepatomegaly.

Examination of the liver should note the consistency, contour, tenderness, or the presence of any masses or bruits, as well as assessment of spleen size. Documentation of the presence of ascites and any stigmata of chronic liver disease is important.

Ultrasonography is useful in assessment of liver size and consistency, as well as gallbladder size. Hyperechogenic hepatic parenchyma can be seen with metabolic disease (glycogen storage disease) or fatty liver (obesity, malnutrition, hyperalimentation, corticosteroids).

Gallbladder length normally varies from 1.5–5.5 cm (average, 3.0) in infants to 4–8 cm in adolescents; width ranges from 0.5 to 2.5 cm for all ages. Gallbladder distention may be seen in infants with sepsis. The gallbladder is often absent in infants with biliary atresia.

JAUNDICE (ICTERUS). Yellow discoloration of the sclera, skin, and mucous membranes is a sign of hyperbilirubinemia (see Chapter 102.3). Clinically apparent jaundice in children and adults occurs when the serum concentration of bilirubin reaches 2–3 mg/dL (34–51 μmol/L); the neonate may not appear icteric until the bilirubin level is >5 mg/dL (85 μmol/L). Jaundice may be the earliest and only sign of hepatic dysfunction. Liver disease must be suspected in the infant who appears only mildly jaundiced but has dark urine or acholic (light-colored) stools. Immediate evaluation to establish the cause is required.

Measurement of the total serum bilirubin concentration allows quantitation of jaundice. Bilirubin occurs in plasma in four forms: unconjugated bilirubin tightly bound to albumin; free or unbound bilirubin (the form responsible for kernicterus, because it can cross cell membranes); conjugated bilirubin (the only fraction to appear in urine); and δ fraction (bilirubin covalently bound to albumin), which appears in serum when hepatic excretion of conjugated bilirubin is impaired in patients with hepatobiliary disease. The δ fraction permits conjugated bilirubin to

TABLE 352-1. Mechanisms of Hepatomegaly

INCREASE IN THE NUMBER OR SIZE OF THE CELLS INTRINSIC TO THE LIVER

Storage

Fat: malnutrition, obesity, metabolic liver disease (diseases of fatty acid oxidation and Reye syndrome–like illnesses), lipid infusion (total parenteral nutrition), cystic fibrosis, diabetes mellitus, medication related, pregnancy

Specific lipid storage diseases: Gaucher, Niemann-Pick, Wolman disease

Glycogen: glycogen storage diseases (multiple enzyme defects); total parenteral nutrition; infant of diabetic mother, Beckwith syndrome

Miscellaneous: α1-antitrypsin dificiency, Wilson disease, hypervitaminosis A, neonatal iron storage disease

Inflammation

- Hepatocyte enlargement (hepatitis)
  - Viral: acute and chronic
  - Bacterial: sepsis, abscess, cholangitis
  - Toxic: drugs
  - Autoimmune
- Kupffer cell enlargement
  - Sarcoidosis
  - Systemic lupus erythematosus
  - Mast cell activating syndrome

INFILTRATION OF CELLS

Primary Liver Tumors

- Benign
  - Hepatocellular
    - Focal nodular hyperplasia
    - Nodular regenerative hyperplasia
    - Hepatocellular adenoma
  - Mesodermal
    - Infantile hemangioendothelioma
    - Mesenchymal hamartoma
  - Cystic masses
    - Choledochal cyst
    - Hepatic cyst
    - Hematoma
    - Parasitic cyst
    - Pyogenic or amebic abscess
- Malignant
  - Hepatocellular
    - Hepatoblastoma
    - Hepatocellular carcinoma
  - Mesodermal
    - Angiosarcoma
    - Undifferentiated embryonal sarcoma
  - Secondary or metastatic processes
    - Lymphoma
    - Leukemia
    - Histiocytosis
    - Neuroblastoma
    - Wilms tumor

INCREASED SIZE OF VASCULAR SPACE

- Intrahepatic obstruction to hepatic vein outflow
  - Veno-occlusive disease
  - Hepatic vein thrombosis (Budd-Chiari syndrome)
  - Hepatic vein web
- Suprahepatic
  - Congestive heart failure
  - Pericardial disease
  - Tamponade
- Constrictive pericarditis
- Hematopoietic: sickle cell anemia, thalassemia

INCREASED SIZE OF BILIARY SPACE

Congenital hepatic fibrosis

Caroli disease

Extrahepatic obstruction

IDIOPATHIC (? "BENIGN")

persist in the circulation and delays resolution of jaundice. Although the terms *direct* and *indirect* bilirubin are used equivalently with *conjugated* and *unconjugated* bilirubin, this is not quantitatively correct, because the direct fraction includes both conjugated bilirubin and δ bilirubin. An elevation of serum bile acids is frequently seen in the presence of any form of cholestasis.

Investigation of jaundice in an infant or older child must include determination of the accumulation of both unconjugated and conjugated bilirubin. Unconjugated hyperbilirubinemia may indicate increased production, hemolysis, reduced hepatic removal, or altered metabolism of bilirubin (Table 352-2). Conjugated hyperbilirubinemia reflects decreased excretion by damaged hepatic parenchymal cells or disease of the biliary tract, which may be due to obstruction, sepsis, toxins, inflammation, and genetic or metabolic disease (Table 352-3).

PRURITUS. Intense generalized itching, often with skin excoriation, can occur in patients with cholestasis (conjugated hyperbilirubinemia). Pruritus is unrelated to the degree of hyperbilirubinemia; deeply jaundiced patients can be asymptomatic. Although retained components of bile are likely important, the cause is probably multifactorial, as evidenced by the symptomatic relief of pruritus after administration of various therapeutic agents including bile acid–binding agents (cholestyramine), choleretic agents (ursodeoxycholic acid), opiate antagonists, antihistamines, and antibiotics (rifampin). Surgical diversion of bile (partial external biliary diversion) has provided relief for medically refractory pruritus.

SPIDER ANGIOMAS. Vascular spiders (telangiectasias), characterized by central pulsating arterioles from which small, wiry venules radiate, may be seen in patients with chronic liver disease; these are usually most prominent on the face and chest. They are presumably reflective of altered estrogen metabolism in the presence of hepatic dysfunction.

PALMAR ERYTHEMA. Blotchy erythema, most noticeable over the thenar and hypothenar eminences and on the tips of the fingers, is also noted in patients with chronic liver disease. This may be due to vasodilation and increased blood flow.

XANTHOMAS. The marked elevation of serum cholesterol levels (to >500 mg/dL) associated with chronic cholestasis can cause the deposition of lipid in the dermis and subcutaneous tissue. Brown nodules may develop, 1st over the extensor surfaces of the extremities; rarely, xanthelasma of the eyelids develops.

PORTAL HYPERTENSION. The portal vein drains the splanchnic area (abdominal portion of the gastrointestinal tract, pancreas, and spleen) into the hepatic sinusoids. Normal portal pressure gradient, the pressure difference between the portal vein and the systemic veins (hepatic veins or inferior vena cava), is 3–6 mm Hg. Clinically significant portal hypertension exists when pressure exceeds a threshold of 10 mm Hg. Portal hypertension is the main complication of cirrhosis, directly responsible for two of its most common and potentially lethal complications: ascites and variceal hemorrhage.

ASCITES. The onset of ascites in the child with chronic liver disease means that the two prerequisite conditions for ascites are present: portal hypertension and hepatic insufficiency. Ascites can also be associated with nephrotic syndrome and other urinary tract abnormalities, metabolic diseases (such as lysosomal storage diseases), congenital or acquired heart disease, and hydrops fetalis. Factors favoring the intra-abdominal accumulation of fluid include: decreased plasma colloid osmotic pressure, increased capillary hydrostatic pressure, increased ascitic colloid osmotic fluid pressure, and decreased ascitic fluid hydrostatic pressure. Abnormal renal sodium retention must be considered (see Chapter 367).

VARICEAL HEMORRHAGE. Gastroesophageal varices are the more clinically significant portosystemic collaterals because of their propensity to rupture and cause life-threatening hemorrhage. Variceal hemorrhage results from increased pressure within the

TABLE 352-2. Differential Diagnosis of Unconjugated Hyperbilirubinemia

INCREASED PRODUCTION OF UNCONJUGATED BILIRUBIN FROM HEME
Hemolytic disease (hereditary or acquired)
Isoimmune hemolysis (neonatal; acute or delayed transfusion reaction; autoimmune)
Rh incompatibility
ABO incompatibility
Other blood group incompatibilities
Congenital spherocytosis
Hereditary elliptocytosis
Infantile pyknocytosis
Erythrocyte enzyme defects
Hemoglobinopathy
Sickle cell anemia
Thalassemia
Others
Sepsis
Microangiopathy
Hemolytic-uremic syndrome
Hemangioma
Mechanical trauma (heart valve)
Ineffective erythropoiesis
Drugs
Infection
Enclosed hematoma
Polycythemia
Diabetic mother
Fetal transfusion (recipient)
Delayed cord clamping
DECREASED DELIVERY OF UNCONJUGATED BILIRUBIN (IN PLASMA) TO HEPATOCYTE
Right-sided congestive heart failure
Portacaval shunt
DECREASED BILIRUBIN UPTAKE ACROSS HEPATOCYTE MEMBRANE
Presumed enzyme transporter deficiency
Competitive inhibition
Breast milk jaundice
Lucey-Driscoll syndrome
Drug inhibition (radiocontrast material)
Miscellaneous
Hypothyroidism
Hypoxia
Acidosis
DECREASED STORAGE OF UNCONJUGATED BILIRUBIN IN CYTOSOL (DECREASED Y AND Z PROTEINS)
Competitive inhibition
Fever
DECREASED BIOTRANSFORMATION (CONJUGATION)
Neonatal jaundice (physiologic)
Inhibition (drugs)
Hereditary (Crigler-Najjar)
Type I (complete enzyme deficiency)
Type II (partial deficiency)
Gilbert disease
Hepatocellular dysfunction
ENTEROHEPATIC RECIRCULATION
Breast milk jaundice
Intestinal obstruction
Ileal atresia
Hirschsprung disease
Cystic fibrosis
Pyloric stenosis
Antibiotic administration

TABLE 352-3. Differential Diagnosis of Neonatal and Infantile Cholestasis

INFECTIOUS
Generalized bacterial sepsis
Viral hepatitis
Hepatitis A, B, C (rare)
Cytomegalovirus
Rubella virus
Herpes virus: HSV, HHV 6 and 7
Varicella virus
Coxsackievirus
Echovirus
Reovirus type 3
Parvovirus B19
HIV
Others
Toxoplasmosis
Syphilis
Tuberculosis
Listeriosis
TOXIC
Parenteral nutrition related
Sepsis (urinary tract) with endotoxemia
Drug related
METABOLIC
Disorders of amino acid metabolism
Tyrosinemia
Disorders of lipid metabolism
Wolman disease
Niemann-Pick disease (type C)
Gaucher disease
Disorders of carbohydrate metabolism
Galactosemia
Fructosemia
Glycogenosis IV
Disorders of bile acid biosynthesis
Other metabolic defects
α1-Antitrypsin deficiency
Cystic fibrosis
Idiopathic hypopituitarism
Hypothyroidism
Zellweger (cerebrohepatorenal) syndrome
Neonatal iron storage disease
Indian childhood cirrhosis/infantile copper overload
Congenital disorders of glycosylation
Mitochrondrial hepatopathies
Citrin deficiency
GENETIC/CHROMOSOMAL
Trisomy E
Down syndrome
INTRAHEPATIC CHOLESTASIS SYNDROME
"Idiopathic" neonatal hepatitis
Alagille syndrome (arteriohepatic dysplasia)
Progressive familial intrahepatic cholestasis (PFIC)
Familial benign recurrent cholestasis associated with lymphedema (Aagenaes)
Congenital hepatic fibrosis
Caroli disease (cystic dilatation of intrahepatic ducts)
CD14 endotoxin receptor gene polymorphisms
EXTRAHEPATIC DISEASES
Biliary atresia
Sclerosing cholangitis
Bile duct stenosis
Choledochal-pancreaticoductal junction anomaly
Spontaneous perforation of the bile duct
Choledochal cyst
Mass (neoplasia, stone)
Hemophagocytic lymphohistiocytosis (HLH)
Bile/mucous plug ("inspissated bile")
MISCELLANEOUS
Shock and hypoperfusion
Associated with enteritis
Associated with intestinal obstruction
Neonatal lupus erythematosus
Myeloproliferative disease (trisomy 21)

varix, which leads to changes in the diameter of the varix and increased wall tension. When the variceal wall strength is exceeded, physical rupture of the varix results. Given the high blood flow and pressure in the portosystemic collateral system, coupled with the lack of a natural mechanism to tamponade variceal bleeding, the rate of hemorrhage can be striking.

ENCEPHALOPATHY. Hepatic encephalopathy can involve any neurologic function, and it can be prominent or present in subtle forms such as deterioration of school performance, depression, or emotional outbursts. It can be recurrent and precipitated by intercurrent illness, drugs, bleeding, or electrolyte and acid-base disturbances. The appearance of hepatic encephalopathy depends on the presence of portosystemic shunting, alterations in the blood-brain barrier, and the interactions of toxic metabolites with the central nervous system. Postulated causes include altered ammonia metabolism, synergistic neurotoxins, or false neurotransmitters with plasma amino acid imbalance.

ENDOCRINE ABNORMALITIES. Endocrine abnormalities are more common in adults with hepatic disease than in children. They reflect alterations in hepatic synthetic, storage, and metabolic functions, including those concerned with hormonal metabolism in the liver. Proteins that bind hormones in plasma are synthesized in the liver, and steroid hormones are conjugated in the liver and excreted in the urine; failure of such functions can have clinical consequences. Endocrine abnormalities can also result from malnutrition or specific deficiencies.

RENAL DYSFUNCTION. Systemic disease or toxins can affect the liver and kidneys simultaneously, or parenchymal liver disease can produce secondary impairment of renal function. In hepatobiliary disorders, there may be renal alterations in sodium and water economy, impaired renal concentrating ability, and alterations in potassium metabolism. Ascites in patients with cirrhosis may be related to inappropriate retention of sodium by the kidneys and expansion of plasma volume, or to sodium retention mediated by diminished effective plasma volume. **Hepatorenal syndrome** (**HRS**) is defined as functional renal failure in patients with end-stage liver disease. The pathophysiology of HRS is poorly defined, but the hallmark is intense renal vasoconstriction (mediated by hemodynamic, humoral, or neurogenic mechanisms) with coexistent systemic vasodilation. The diagnosis is supported by the findings of oliguria (<1 mL/kg/day), a characteristic pattern of urine electrolyte abnormalities (urine sodium of <10 mEq/L, fractional excretion of sodium of <1%, urine : plasma creatinine ratio <10, and normal urinary sediment), absence of hypovolemia, and exclusion of other kidney pathology. The best treatment of HRS is timely liver transplantation, as complete renal recovery can be expected.

PULMONARY INVOLVEMENT. **Hepatopulmonary syndrome** is characterized by the typical triad of hypoxemia, intrapulmonary vascular dilations, and liver disease. There is intrapulmonic right-to-left shunting of blood, which results in systemic desaturation. It should be suspected and investigated in the child with chronic liver disease with history of shortness of breath or exercise intolerance and clinical examination findings of cyanosis (particularly of the lips and fingers), digital clubbing, and oxygen saturations <96%, particularly in the upright position. Treatment is timely liver transplantation; successful pulmonary resolution follows.

RECURRENT CHOLANGITIS. Ascending infection of the biliary system is often seen in pediatric cholestatic disease, due most commonly to gram-negative enteric organisms, such as *Escherichia coli*, *Klebsiella*, *Pseudomonas*, and *Enterococcus*. Liver transplantation is the definitive effective treatment for recurrent cholangitis in the child with chronic cholestatic liver disease, especially when medical therapy is not effective.

MISCELLANEOUS MANIFESTATIONS OF LIVER DYSFUNCTION. Nonspecific signs of acute and chronic liver disease include: anorexia, which often affects patients with anicteric hepatitis and with cirrhosis associated with chronic cholestasis; abdominal pain or distention resulting from ascites, spontaneous peritonitis, or visceromegaly; malnutrition and growth failure; and bleeding, which may be due to altered synthesis of coagulation factors (biliary obstruction with vitamin K deficiency or excessive hepatic damage) or to portal hypertension with hypersplenism. In the presence of hypersplenism, there can be decreased synthesis of specific clotting factors, production of qualitatively abnormal proteins, or alterations in platelet number and function. Altered drug metabolism may prolong the biologic half-life of commonly administered medications.

352.1 • Evaluation of Patients with Possible Liver Dysfunction

Adequate evaluation of an infant, child, or adolescent with suspected liver disease involves an appropriate and accurate history, a carefully performed physical examination, and skillful interpretation of signs and symptoms. Further evaluation is aided by judicious selection of diagnostic tests, followed by the use of imaging modalities or a liver biopsy. Most of the so-called liver function tests do not measure specific hepatic functions: a rise in serum aminotransferase levels reflects liver cell injury, an increase in immunoglobulin levels reflects an immunologic response to injury, or an elevation in serum bilirubin levels can reflect any of several disturbances of bilirubin metabolism (see Tables 352-2 and 352-3). Any single biochemical assay provides limited information, which must be placed in the context of the entire clinical picture. The most cost-efficient approach is to become familiar with the rationale, implications, and limitations of a selected group of tests so that specific questions can be answered. Young infants with cholestatic jaundice should be evaluated promptly to identify those patients needing surgical intervention.

For a patient with suspected liver disease, evaluation addresses the following issues in sequence: Is liver disease present? If so, what is its nature? What is its severity? Is specific treatment available? How can we monitor the response to treatment? and What is the prognosis?

BIOCHEMICAL TESTS. Laboratory tests commonly used to screen for or to confirm a suspicion of liver disease include measurements of serum aminotransferase, bilirubin (total and fractionated), and alkaline phosphatase (AP) levels, as well as determinations of prothrombin time (PT) or international normalized ratio (INR) and albumin level. These tests are complementary, provide an estimation of synthetic and excretory functions, and may suggest the nature of the disturbance (inflammation or cholestasis).

Acute liver cell injury (parenchymal disease) in viral hepatitis, drug- or toxin-induced liver disease, shock, hypoxemia, or metabolic disease is best reflected by marked increases in serum aminotransferase levels. Cholestasis (obstructive disease) involves regurgitation of bile components into serum; the serum levels of total and conjugated bilirubin and serum bile acids are elevated. Elevations in serum AP, 5′ nucleotidase (5′NT), and γ-glutamyl transpeptidase (GGT) levels are also sensitive indicators of obstruction or inflammation of the biliary tract.

The severity of the liver disease may be reflected in clinical signs (the occurrence of encephalopathy, variceal hemorrhage, worsening jaundice, apparent shrinkage of liver mass owing to massive necrosis, or onset of ascites) or in biochemical alterations (hypoglycemia, hyperammonemia, electrolyte imbalance, continued hyperbilirubinemia, marked hypoalbuminemia, or a prolonged PT or INR that is unresponsive to parenteral administration of vitamin K).

Fractionation of the total serum bilirubin level into conjugated and unconjugated bilirubin fractions helps to distinguish between elevations caused by hemolysis and those caused by hepatic dysfunction. A predominant elevation in the conjugated bilirubin level provides a relatively sensitive index of hepatocellular disease or hepatic excretory dysfunction, whereas elevation in aminotransferase levels are more highly sensitive indices of hepatocellular damage.

Alanine aminotransferase (ALT, serum glutamate pyruvate transaminase) is liver specific, whereas aspartate aminotransferase (AST, serum glutamic-oxaloacetic transaminase) is derived from other organs in addition to the liver. The most marked rises of both AST and ALT levels may occur with acute hepatocellular injury; a several thousand–fold elevation can result from acute viral hepatitis, toxic injury, hypoxia, or hypoperfusion. After blunt abdominal trauma, parallel elevations in aminotransferase levels may provide an early clue to hepatic injury. A differential rise or fall in AST and ALT levels can sometimes provide useful information. In acute hepatitis, the rise in ALT may be greater than the rise in AST. In alcohol-induced liver injury, fulminant echovirus infection, and various metabolic diseases, more predominant rises in the AST level are reported. In chronic liver disease or in intrahepatic and extrahepatic biliary obstruction, AST and ALT elevations may be less marked. Nonalcoholic steatohepatitis (NASH) and other forms of nonalcoholic fatty liver disease are chronic liver disorders seen in obese children presenting with elevated serum aminotransferase levels. The notable characteristic is the similar histology to alcoholic-induced liver injury in the absence of alcohol abuse.

Hepatic synthetic function is reflected in serum albumin and protein levels and in the PT or INR. Examination of serum globulin concentration and of the relative amounts of the globulin fractions may be helpful. Patients with autoimmune hepatitis often have high gamma-globulin levels and increased titers of anti–smooth muscle, antinuclear, and anti–liver-kidney-microsome antibodies. Antimitochondrial antibodies may also be found in patients with autoimmune hepatitis. A resurgence in α-fetoprotein levels may suggest hepatoma, hepatoblastoma, or hereditary tyrosinemia. Hypoalbuminemia caused by depressed synthesis can complicate severe liver disease and serve as a prognostic factor. Deficiencies of factor V and of the vitamin K–dependent factors (II, VII, IX, and X) can occur in patients with severe liver disease or fulminant hepatic failure. If the PT or INR is prolonged as a result of intestinal malabsorption of vitamin K (resulting from cholestasis) or decreased nutritional intake of vitamin K, then parenteral administration of vitamin K should correct the coagulopathy, leading to normalization within 12–24 hr. Unresponsiveness to vitamin K suggests severe hepatic disease. Persistently low levels of factor VII are evidence of a poor prognosis in fulminant liver disease.

Interpretation of results of biochemical tests of hepatic structure and function must be made in the context of age-related changes. The activity of AP varies considerably with age. Normal growing children have significant elevations of serum AP activity originating from influx into serum of the isoenzyme that originates in bone, particularly in rapidly growing adolescents. Therefore, an isolated increase in AP does not indicate hepatic or biliary disease if other liver function test results are normal. Other enzymes such as 5′NT and GGT are increased in cholestatic conditions, and may be more specific for hepatobiliary disease. 5′NT is not found in bone. GGT exhibits high enzyme activity in early life that declines rapidly with age. Cholesterol concentrations increase throughout life. Cholesterol levels may be markedly elevated in patients with intra- or extrahepatic cholestasis and decreased in severe acute liver disease such as hepatitis.

Interpretation of serum ammonia values must be carried out with caution because of variability in their physiologic determinants and the inherent difficulty in laboratory measurement.

LIVER BIOPSY. Liver biopsy combined with clinical data can suggest a cause in most cases. Specimens of liver tissue can be used: to provide a precise histologic diagnosis in patients with neonatal cholestasis, chronic active hepatitis, metabolic liver disease, suspected Reye syndrome, intrahepatic cholestasis (paucity of bile ducts), congenital hepatic fibrosis, or undefined portal hypertension; for enzyme analysis to detect inborn errors of metabolism; and for analysis of stored material such as iron, copper, or specific metabolites. Liver biopsies can monitor responses to therapy or detect complications of treatment with potentially hepatotoxic agents, such as aspirin, anti-infectives (erythromycin, minocycline, ketoconazole, isoniazid), antimetabolites, antineoplastics, or anticonvulsant agents.

In infants and children, needle biopsy of the liver is easily accomplished percutaneously. The amount of tissue obtained, even in small infants, is usually sufficient for histologic interpretation and for biochemical analyses, if the latter are deemed necessary. Percutaneous liver biopsy can be performed safely in infants as young as 1 wk of age. Patients usually require only conscious sedation and local anesthesia. Contraindications to the percutaneous approach include prolonged PT or INR; thrombocytopenia; suspicion of a vascular, cystic, or infectious lesion in the path of the needle; and severe ascites. If administration of fresh frozen plasma or of platelet transfusions fails to correct a prolonged PT, INR, or thrombocytopenia, a tissue specimen can be obtained via alternative techniques. Considerations include either the open laparotomy (wedge) approach by a general surgeon, or the transjugular approach under ultrasound and fluoroscopic guidance by an experienced pediatric interventional radiologist in an appropriately equipped fluoroscopy suite. The risk of development of a complication such as hemorrhage, hematoma, creation of an arteriovenous fistula, pneumothorax, or bile peritonitis is small.

HEPATIC IMAGING PROCEDURES. Various techniques help define the size, shape, and architecture of the liver and the anatomy of the intrahepatic and extrahepatic biliary trees. Although imaging may not provide a precise histologic and biochemical diagnosis, specific questions can be answered, such as whether hepatomegaly is related to accumulation of fat or glycogen or is due to a tumor or cyst. These studies may direct further evaluation such as percutaneous biopsy and make possible prompt referral of patients with biliary obstruction to a surgeon. Choice of imaging procedure should be part of a carefully formulated diagnostic approach, with avoidance of redundant demonstrations by several techniques.

A plain roentgenographic study may suggest hepatomegaly, but a carefully performed physical examination gives a more reliable assessment of liver size. The liver may appear less dense than normal in patients with fatty infiltration or more dense with deposition of heavy metals such as iron. A hepatic or biliary tract mass may displace an air-filled loop of bowel. Calcifications may be evident in the liver (parasitic or neoplastic disease), in the vasculature (portal vein thrombosis), or in the gallbladder or biliary tree (gallstones). Collections of gas may be seen within the liver (abscess), biliary tract, or portal circulation (necrotizing enterocolitis).

Ultrasonography (US) provides information about the size, composition, and blood flow of the liver. Increased echogenicity is observed with fatty infiltration; mass lesions as small as 1–2 cm may be shown. US has replaced cholangiography in detecting stones in the gallbladder or biliary tree. Even in neonates, US can assess gallbladder size, detect dilatation of the biliary tract, and define a choledochal cyst. In infants with biliary atresia, US findings may include small or absent gallbladder; nonvisualization of the common duct; and presence of the triangular cord sign, a triangular/tubular-shaped echogenic density in the bifurcation of the portal vein, representing fibrous remnants at the porta hepatis. In patients with portal hypertension, Doppler US can evaluate patency of the portal vein, demonstrate collateral circulation, and assess size of spleen and amount of ascites. Relatively small amounts of ascitic fluid can also be detected. The use of Doppler US has been helpful in determining vascular patency after liver transplantation.

CT scanning provides information similar to that obtained by US but is less suitable for use in patients <2 yr of age because of the small size of structures, the paucity of intra-abdominal fat for contrast, and the need for heavy sedation or general anesthesia. MRI is a useful alternative. Magnetic resonance cholangiography can be of value in differentiating biliary tract lesions. CT scan or MRI may be more accurate than US in detecting focal lesions such as tumors, cysts, and abscesses. When enhanced by contrast medium, CT scanning may reveal a neoplastic mass density only slightly different from that of a normal liver. When a hepatic tumor is suspected, CT scanning is the best method to define anatomic extent, solid or cystic nature, and vascularity. CT scanning can also reveal subtle differences in density of liver parenchyma, the average liver attenuation coefficient being reduced with fatty infiltration. Increases in density may occur with diffuse iron deposition or with glycogen storage. In differentiating obstructive from nonobstructive cholestasis, CT scanning or MRI identifies the precise level of obstruction more frequently than US. Either CT scanning or US may be used to guide percutaneously placed fine needles for biopsies, aspiration of specific lesions, or cholangiography.

Radionuclide scanning relies on selective uptake of a radiopharmaceutical agent. Commonly used agents include: technetium 99m-labeled sulfur colloid, which undergoes phagocytosis by Kupffer cells; ^{99m}Tc-iminodiacetic acid agents, which are taken up by hepatocytes and excreted into bile in a fashion similar to bilirubin; and gallium 67, which is concentrated in inflammatory and neoplastic cells. The anatomic resolution possible with hepatic scintiscans is generally less than that obtained with CT scanning, MRI, or US.

The ^{99m}Tc-sulfur colloid scan can detect focal lesions (tumors, cysts, abscesses) >2–3 cm in diameter. This modality can help to evaluate patients with possible cirrhosis and with patchy hepatic uptake and a shift of colloid uptake from liver to bone marrow.

The ^{99m}Tc-substituted iminodiacetic acid dyes may differentiate intrahepatic cholestasis from extrahepatic obstruction in neonates. Imaging results are best when scanning is preceded by a 5–7 day period of treatment with phenobarbital to stimulate bile flow. After intravenous injection, the isotope is normally detected in the bowel within 1–2 hr. In the presence of extrahepatic obstruction, excretion of the isotope is delayed; accordingly, serial scans should be made for up to 24 hr after injection. Early in the course of biliary atresia, hepatocyte function is usually good; uptake (clearance) occurs rapidly, but excretion into the intestine is absent. In contrast, uptake is poor in parenchymal liver disease, such as neonatal hepatitis, but excretion into the bile and intestine eventually ensues.

Cholangiography, direct visualization of the intrahepatic and extrahepatic biliary tree after injection of opaque material, may be required in some patients to evaluate the cause, location, or extent of biliary obstruction. Percutaneous transhepatic cholangiography with a fine needle is the technique of choice in infants and young children. The likelihood of opacifying the biliary tract is excellent in patients in whom CT scanning, MRI, or ultrasonography demonstrates dilated ducts. Percutaneous transhepatic cholangiography has been used to outline the biliary ductal system.

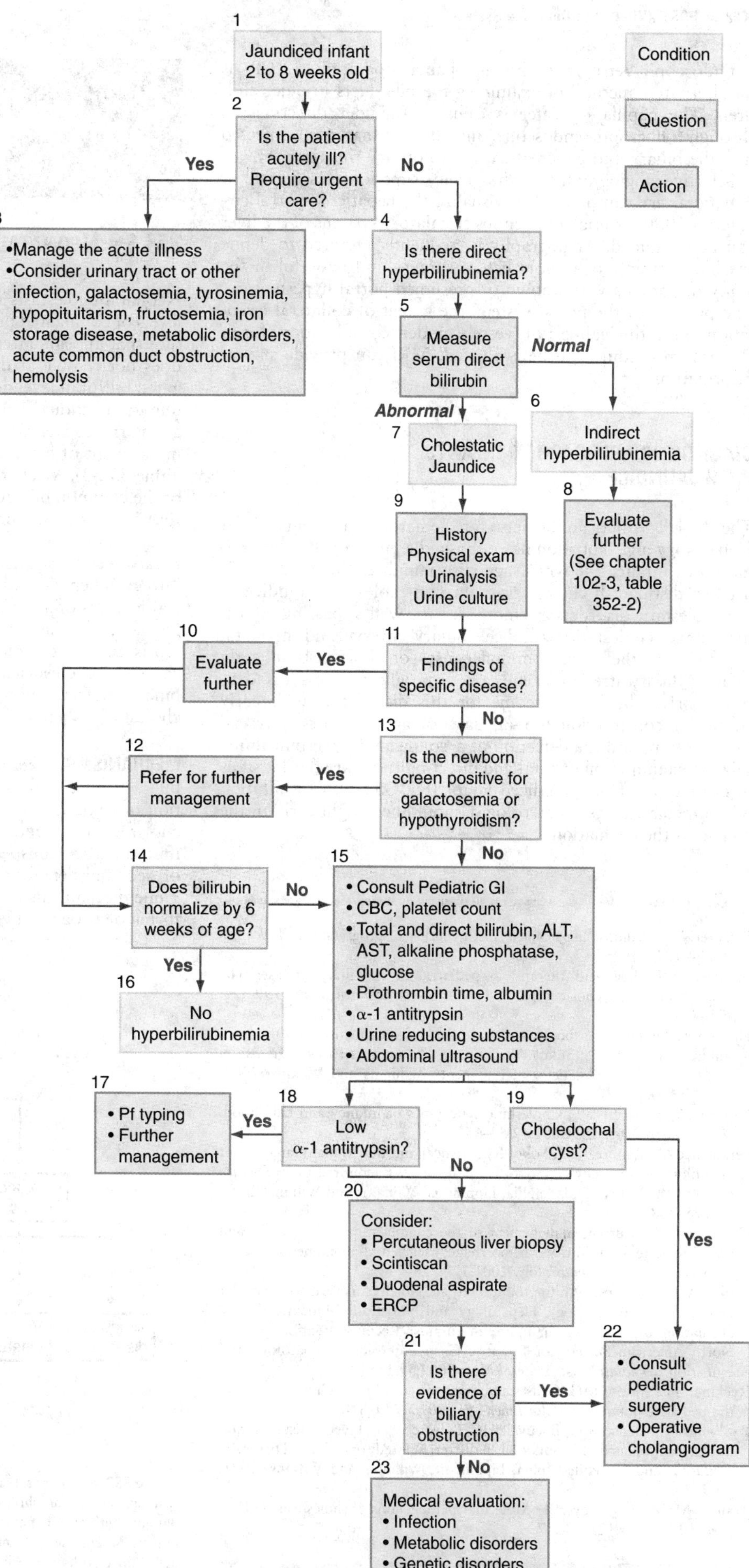

Figure 352-1. Cholestasis clinical practice guideline. Algorithm for a 2–8 wk old. ALT, alanine aminotransferase; AST, aspartate aminotransferase; ERCP, endoscopic retrograde cholangiopancreatography; PT, prothrombin time. (Moyer V, Freese DK, Whitington PF, et al; North American Society for Pediatric Gastroenterology, Hepatology and Nutrition: Guideline for the evaluation of cholestatic jaundice in infants: Recommendations of the North American Society for Pediatric Gastroenterology, Hepatology and Nutrition. *J Pediatr Gastroenterol Nutr* 2004;39:115–128.)

Endoscopic retrograde cholangiopancreatography (ERCP) is an alternative method of examining the bile ducts in older children. The papilla of Vater is cannulated under direct vision through a fiberoptic endoscope, and contrast material is injected into the biliary and pancreatic ducts to outline the anatomy.

Selective angiography of the celiac, superior mesenteric, or hepatic artery can be used to visualize the hepatic or portal circulation. Both arterial and venous circulatory systems of the liver can be examined. Angiography is frequently required to define the blood supply of tumors before surgery and is useful in the study of patients with known or presumed portal hypertension. The patency of the portal system, the extent of collateral circulation, and the caliber of vessels under consideration for a shunting procedure can be evaluated. MRI can provide similar information.

DIAGNOSTIC APPROACH TO INFANTS WITH JAUNDICE

The North American Society for Pediatric Gastroenterology, Hepatology and Nutrition has published a guideline for the evaluation of infants 2–8 wk of age with jaundice. The guideline is used to distinguish cholestatic from non-cholestatic jaundice as the cholestatic disorders are more serious. Well-appearing infants may have cholestatic jaundice. Biliary atresia and neonatal hepatitis are the most common causes of cholestasis in early infancy. Biliary atresia portends a poor prognosis unless it is identified early. The best outcome for this disorder is with early surgical reconstruction (45–60 days of age). History, physical examination, and the detection of a conjugated hyperbilirubinemia via examination of total and direct bilirubin are the 1st steps in evaluation of the jaundiced infant (Fig. 352-1). Consultation with a pediatric gastroenterologist should be sought early in the course of the evaluation.

Balistreri WF: Pediatric hepatology. A half-century of progress. *Clin Liver Dis* 2000;4:191–210.

Balistreri WF: Bile acid therapy in pediatric hepatobiliary disease: The role of ursodeoxycholic acid. *J Pediatr Gastroenterol Nutr* 1997;24:573–589.

Batres LA, Maller ES: Laboratory assessment of liver function and injury in children: In Suchy FS, Sokol RJ, Balistreri WF (editors): *Liver Disease in Children,* 2nd ed. Philadelphia, Lippincott, Williams and Wilkins, 2001, pp 155–170.

Bezerra JA, Balistreri WF: Cholestatic syndromes of infancy and childhood. *Semin Gastrointest Dis* 2001;12:54–65.

Feranchak AP, Ramirez RO, Sokol RJ: Medical and nutritional management of cholestasis: In Suchy FS, Sokol RJ, Balistreri WF (editors): *Liver Disease in Children,* 2nd ed. Philadelphia, Lippincott, Williams and Wilkins, 2001, pp 195–238.

Garcia-Tsao G: Current management of the complications of cirrhosis and portal hypertension: Variceal hemorrhage, ascites and spontaneous bacterial peritonitis. *Gastroenterology* 2001;120:726–748.

Moyer V, Freese DK, Whitington PF, et al; North American Society for Pediatric Gastroenterology, Hepatology and Nutrition: Guideline for the evaluation of cholestatic jaundice in infants: Recommendations of the North American Society for Pediatric Gastroenterology, Hepatology and Nutrition. *J Pediatr Gastroenterol Nutr* 2004;39:115–128.

Ryckman FC, Alonso MH: Causes and management of portal hypertension in the pediatric population. *Clin Liver Dis* 2001;5:789–818.

Ryckman FC, Alonso MH, Bucuvalas JC, Balistreri WF: Liver transplantation in children: In Suchy FS, Sokol RJ, Balistreri WF (editors): *Liver Disease in Children,* 2nd ed. Philadelphia, Lippincott, Williams and Wilkins, 2001, pp 949–974.

Trauner M, Meier PJ, Boyer JL: Molecular pathogenesis of cholestasis. *N Engl J Med* 1998;339:1217–1227.

Chapter 353 ■ Cholestasis

Hassan H. A-Kader and William F. Balistreri

353.1 • Neonatal Cholestasis

Neonatal cholestasis is defined as prolonged elevation of serum levels of conjugated bilirubin beyond the 1st 14 days of life. Jaundice that appears after 2 wk of age, progresses after this time, or does not resolve at this time should be evaluated and a conjugated bilirubin level determined. Cholestasis in a newborn can be due to infectious, genetic, metabolic, or undefined abnormalities giving rise to *mechanical* obstruction of bile flow or to *functional* impairment of hepatic excretory function and bile secretion (see Table 352-3). Mechanical lesions include stricture or obstruction of the common bile duct; biliary atresia is the prototypic obstructive abnormality. Functional impairment of bile secretion can result from congenital defects or damage to liver cells or to the biliary secretory apparatus. Neonatal cholestasis can be divided into extrahepatic and intrahepatic disease (Fig. 353-1). The clinical features of any form of cholestasis are similar. In an affected neonate, the diagnosis of certain entities, such as galactosemia, sepsis, or hypothyroidism, is relatively simple. In most cases, the cause of cholestasis is more obscure. Differentiation among biliary atresia, idiopathic neonatal hepatitis, and intrahepatic cholestasis is particularly difficult.

MECHANISMS. Metabolic liver disease caused by inborn errors of bile acid metabolism or transport is associated with accumulation of toxic primitive bile acids and failure to produce normal choleretic and trophic bile acids. The clinical and histologic manifestations are nonspecific and are similar to those in other forms of neonatal hepatobiliary injury. It is also possible that autoimmune mechanisms may be responsible for some of the enigmatic forms of neonatal liver injury. Overall, the mechanisms are not

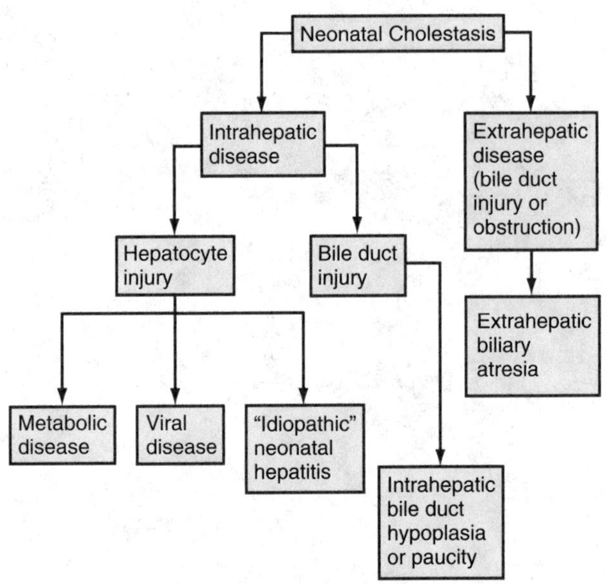

Figure 353-1. Neonatal cholestasis. Conceptual approach to the group of diseases presenting as cholestasis in the neonate. There are areas of overlap—patients with extrahepatic biliary atresia may have some degree of intrahepatic injury. Patients with "idiopathic" neonatal hepatitis may, in the future, be determined to have a primary metabolic or viral disease.

well documented. Some of the histologic manifestations of hepatic injury in early life are not seen in older individuals. Giant cell transformation of hepatocytes occurs frequently in infants with cholestasis and may occur in any form of neonatal liver injury. It is more frequent and more severe, however, in intrahepatic forms of cholestasis. The clinical and histologic findings that exist in patients with neonatal hepatitis and in those with biliary atresia are quite disparate; the basic process is an undefined initiating insult causing inflammation of the liver cells or of the cells within the biliary tract. If bile duct epithelium is the predominant site of disease, cholangitis can result and lead to progressive sclerosis and narrowing of the biliary tree, the ultimate state being complete obliteration (biliary atresia). Injury to liver cells can present the clinical and histologic picture of "neonatal hepatitis." This concept does not account for the precise mechanism, but offers an explanation for well-documented cases of unexpected postnatal evolution of these disease processes; infants initially regarded as having neonatal hepatitis, with a patent biliary system shown on cholangiography, can later develop biliary atresia.

Functional abnormalities in the generation of bile flow may also have a role in neonatal cholestasis. Bile flow is directly dependent on effective hepatic bile acid excretion.

During the phase of relatively inefficient liver cell transport and metabolism of bile acids in early life, minor degrees of hepatic injury can further decrease bile flow and lead to production of abnormal toxic bile acids. Selective impairment of a single step in the series of events involved in hepatic excretion produces the full expression of a cholestatic syndrome. Specific defects in bile acid synthesis are found in infants with intrahepatic cholestasis and in infants with Zellweger syndrome. Severe forms of familial cholestasis have been associated with neonatal hemochromatosis and an aberration in the contractile proteins that compose the cytoskeleton of the hepatocyte. Neonatal hemochromatosis may also be an alloimmune-mediated gestational disease responsive to maternal intravenous immunoglobulin (IVIG). Sepsis is known to cause cholestasis, presumably mediated by an endotoxin produced by *Escherichia coli.*

EVALUATION. The evaluation of the infant with jaundice should follow a logical, cost-effective sequence in a multistep process (Table 353-1). Although cholestasis in the neonate may be the initial manifestation of numerous disorders, the clinical manifestations are usually similar and provide very few clues about etiology. Affected infants have icterus, dark urine, light or acholic stools, and hepatomegaly, all resulting from decreased bile flow due to either hepatocyte injury or bile duct obstruction. Hepatic synthetic dysfunction can lead to hypoprothrombinemia and bleeding. Administration of vitamin K should be the initial treatment of cholestatic infants to prevent hemorrhage.

TABLE 353-1. Value of Specific Tests in the Evaluation of Patients with Suspected Neonatal Cholestasis

TEST	RATIONALE
Serum bilirubin fractionation	Documents cholestasis
Assessment of stool color	Indicates bile flow into intestine
Urine/serum bile acids measurement	Confirms cholestasis; may indicate inborn error of bile acid biosynthesis
Hepatic synthetic function (albumin, coagulation profile)	Indicates severity of hepatic dysfunction
α1-antitrypsin phenotype	Suggests (or excludes) PiZZ
Thyroxine and TSH	Suggests (or excludes) endocrinopathy
Sweat chloride/mutation analysis	Suggests (or excludes) cystic fibrosis
Urine/serum amino acids and urine reducing substances	Suggests (or excludes) metabolic liver disease
Ultrasonography	Suggests (or excludes) choledochal cyst; may detect the triangular cord (TC) sign, suggesting biliary atresia
Hepatobiliary scintigraphy	Documents bile duct patency or obstruction
Liver biopsy	Distinguishes biliary atresia from neonatal hepatitis; suggests alternative diagnosis

PiZZ, protease inhibitor ZZ phenotype; TSH, thyroid stimulating hormone.

TABLE 353-2. Proposed Subtypes of Intrahepatic Cholestasis

A. Disorders of membrane transport and secretion
   1. Disorders of canalicular secretion
      a. Bile acid transport—BSEP deficiency
         i. Persistent, progressive (PFIC type 2)
         ii. Recurrent, benign (BRIC type 2)
      b. Phospholipid transport—MDR3 deficiency (PFIC type 3)
      c. Ion transport—cystic fibrosis (CFTR)
   2. Complex/multi-organ disorders
      a. FIC1 deficiency
         i. Persistent, progressive (PFIC Type 1, Byler disease)
         ii. Recurrent, benign (BRIC type 1)
      b. Neonatal sclerosing cholangitis *(CLDN1)*
      c. Arthrogryposis–renal dysfunction–cholestasis syndrome (*VPS33B*)
B. Disorders of bile acid biosynthesis and conjugation
   1. 3-oxo-4-steroid 5β-reductase deficiency
   2. 3β-hydroxy-5-C27-steroid dehydrogenase/isomerase deficiency
   3. Oxysterol 7α-hydroxylase deficiency
   4. BAAT deficiency (familial hypercholanemia)
C. Disorders of embryogenesis
   1. Alagille syndrome (Jagged1 defect, syndromic bile duct paucity)
   2. Ductal plate malformation (ARPKD, ADPLD, Caroli disease)
D. Unclassified (idiopathic "neonatal hepatitis")-mechanism unknown

Note: FIC1 deficiency, BSEP deficiency, and some of the disorders of bile acid biosynthesis are characterized clinically by low levels of serum GGT despite the presence of cholestasis. In all other disorders listed, the serum GGT level is elevated.
ADPLD, autosomal dominant polycystic liver disease (cysts in liver only); ARPKD, autosomal recessive polycystic kidney disease (cysts in liver and kidney); BAAT, bile acid transporter; BRIC, benign recurrent intrahepatic cholestasis; BSEP, bile salt export pump in; PFIC, progressive familial intrahepatic cholestasis.
From Balistreri WF, Bezerra JA, Jansen P, et al: Intrahepatic cholestasis: Summary of an American Association for the Study of Liver Diseases single-topic conference. *Hepatology* 2005;42:222–235.

In contrast to unconjugated hyperbilirubinemia, which can be physiologic, cholestasis (conjugated bilirubin elevation of any degree) in the neonate is **always pathologic** and prompt differentiation is imperative. The initial step is identification of cholestasis. The next step is to recognize conditions that cause cholestasis and for which specific therapy is available to prevent further damage and avoid long-term complications such as sepsis, an endocrinopathy (hypothyroidism, panhypopituitarism), nutritional hepatotoxicity caused by a specific metabolic illness (galactosemia), or other metabolic diseases (tyrosinemia).

Hepatobiliary disease can be the initial manifestation of homozygous α_1-antitrypsin deficiency or of cystic fibrosis. Neonatal liver disease can also be associated with congenital syphilis and specific viral infections, notably echo virus and herpesviruses including cytomegalovirus (CMV). The hepatitis viruses (A, B, C) rarely cause neonatal cholestasis.

The final and critical step in evaluating neonates with cholestasis is to differentiate extrahepatic biliary atresia from neonatal hepatitis.

INTRAHEPATIC CHOLESTASIS

NEONATAL HEPATITIS. The term *neonatal hepatitis* implies intrahepatic cholestasis (see Fig. 353-1), which has various forms (Tables 353-2 and 353-3).

Idiopathic neonatal hepatitis, which can occur in either a sporadic or a familial form, is a disease of unknown cause. Patients presumably are afflicted with a specific yet undefined metabolic or viral disease. In the past, patients with α_1-antitrypsin deficiency were included in this category; after characterization of this specific metabolic disease, it is possible to define this subgroup of patients precisely.

Infectious hepatitis in a neonate may be shown to be due to a specific virus, such as herpes simplex, enteroviruses, CMV, or,

TABLE 353-3. Molecular Defects Causing Liver Disease

GENE	PROTEIN	FUNCTION, SUBSTRATE	DISORDER
ATP8b1	FIC1	P-type ATPase; aminophospholipid translocase that flips phosphatidylserine and phosphatidylethanolamine from the outer to the inner layer of the canalicular membrane	PFIC1 (Byler disease), BRIC1, GFC
ABCB11	BSEP	Canalicular protein with ATP-binding cassette (ABC family of proteins); works as a pump transporting bile acids through the canalicular domain	PFIC 2, BRIC 2
ABCB4	MDR3	Canalicular protein with ATP-binding cassette (ABC family of proteins); works as a phospholipid flippase in canalicular membrane	PFIC3, ICP, Cholelithiasis
AKR1D1	5β-reductase	3-oxoΔ-4-steroid 5β-reductase gene; regulates bile acid synthesis	BAS: Neonatal cholestasis with giant cell hepatitis
HSD3B7	C27-3β-HSD	3β-hydroxy-5-C27-steroid oxido-reductase (C27-3β-HSD) gene; regulates bile acid synthesis	BAS: Chronic intrahepatic cholestasis
CYP7BI	CYP7BI	Oxysterol 7α-hydroxylase; regulates the acidic pathway of bile acid synthesis	BAS: Neonatal cholestasis with giant cell hepatitis
JAG1	JAG1	Transmembrane, cell-surface proteins that interact with Notch receptors to regulate cell fate during embryogenesis	Alagille syndrome
TJP2	Tight junction protein	Belongs to the family of membrane-associated guanylate kinase homologs that are involved in the organization of epithelial and endothelial intercellular junction; regulates paracellular permeability	FHC
BAAT	BAAT	Enzyme that transfers the bile acid moiety from the acyl coenzyme A thioester to either glycine or taurine	FHC
EPHX1	Epoxide hydrolase	Microsomal epoxide hydrolase regulates the activation and detoxification of exogenous chemicals	FHC
ABCC2	MRP2	Canalicular protein with ATP-binding cassette (ABC family of proteins); regulates canalicular transport of GSH conjugates and arsenic	Dubin-Johnson syndrome
ATP7B	ATP7B	P-type ATPase; function as copper export pump	Wilson disease
CLDN1	Claudin 1	Tight junction protein	NSC
CIRH1A	Cirhin	Cell signaling?	NAICC
CFTR	CFTR	Chloride channel with ATP-binding cassette (ABC family of proteins); regulates chloride transport	Cystic fibrosis
PKHD1	Fibrocystin	Protein involved in ciliary function and tubulogenesis	ARPKD
PRKCSH	Hepatocystin	Assembles with glucosidase II α subunit in endoplasmic reticulum	ADPLD
VPS33B	Vascular Protein sorting 33	Regulates fusion of proteins to cellular membrane	ARC

ADPLD, autosomal dominant polycystic liver disease; ARC, arthrogryposis–renal dysfunction–cholestasis syndrome*; ARPKD, autosomal recessive polycystic kidney disease; BAAT, bile acid transporter; BAS, bile acid synthetic defect; BRIC, benign recurrent intrahepatic cholestasis; BSEP, bile salt export pump; CFTF, cystic fibrosis transmembrane conductance regulator; FHC, familial hypercholanemia; GFC, greenland familial cholestasis; GSH, glutathione; ICP, intrahepatic cholestasis of pregnancy; NAICC, North American Indian childhood cirrhosis; NSC, neonatal sclerosing cholangitis with ichthyosis, leukocyte vacuoles, and alopecia; PFIC, progressive familial intrahepatic cholestasis*.

*, low GGT (PFIC type 1 & 2, BRIC type 1 & 2, ARC)

From Balistreri WF, Bezerra JA, Jansen P, et al: Intrahepatic cholestasis: Summary of an American Association for the Study of Liver Diseases single-topic conference. *Hepatology* 2005; 42:222–235.

rarely, hepatitis B. This accounts for a small percentage of cases of neonatal hepatitis syndrome.

Aagenaes syndrome is a form of idiopathic familial intrahepatic cholestasis associated with lymphedema of the lower extremities. The relationship between the liver disease and lymphedema is not understood and may be attributable to decreased hepatic lymph flow or hepatic lymphatic hypoplasia. Affected patients usually present with episodic cholestasis with elevation of serum aminotransferases, alkaline phosphatase, and bile acids. Between episodes, the patients are usually asymptomatic and biochemical indices improve. The locus for Aagenaes syndrome is mapped to a 6.6 cM interval on chromosome 15q.

Zellweger (cerebrohepatorenal) syndrome is a rare autosomal recessive genetic disorder marked by progressive degeneration of the liver and kidneys (see Chapter 86.2). The incidence is estimated to be 1/100,000 births; the disease is usually fatal in 6–12 mo. Affected infants have severe, generalized hypotonia and markedly impaired neurologic function with psychomotor retardation. Patients have an abnormal head shape and unusual facies, hepatomegaly, renal cortical cysts, stippled calcifications of the patellas and greater trochanter, and ocular abnormalities. Hepatic cells on ultrastructural examination show an absence of peroxisomes.

Neonatal iron storage disease (NISD; neonatal hemochromatosis) is a rapidly progressive disease characterized by increased iron deposition in the liver, heart, and endocrine organs without increased iron stores in the reticuloendothelial system. Patients have multiorgan failure and shortened survival. Familial cases are reported; the disease can be transmitted in an autosomal recessive or codominant pattern. Laboratory findings include hypoglycemia, hyperbilirubinemia, hypoalbuminemia, and profound hypoprothrombinemia. Serum aminotransferase levels may be high initially but normalize with the progression of the disease. The diagnosis is usually confirmed by buccal mucosal biopsy or MRI demonstrating extrahepatic siderosis. The prognosis is poor; liver transplantation can be curative. Despite initially encouraging reports, the use of a combination of antioxidants and prostaglandin infusion with chelation may not uniformly improve outcome in patients with NISD.

NISD in some patients may be due to an alloimmune-mediated mechanism that developed after a previous fetus sensitized the mother to an unknown fetal antigen. Treating the mother with 1gm/kg of IVIG/wk starting at 18 wk gestation improves the outcome of the subsequent pregnancy.

DISORDERS OF TRANSPORT, SECRETION, CONJUGATION, AND BIOSYNTHESIS OF BILE ACIDS. Progressive familial intrahepatic cholestasis type 1 (PFIC 1) or FIC1 disease (formerly known as **Byler disease**) is a severe form of intrahepatic cholestasis. The disease was initially described in the Amish kindred of Jacob Baylor. Affected patients present with steatorrhea, pruritus, vitamin D–deficient rickets, gradually developing cirrhosis, and **low** γ-glutamyl transpeptidase levels. The absence of bile duct paucity and extrahepatic features differentiate this disorder from Alagille syndrome.

PFIC 1 (FIC-1 deficiency) has been mapped to chromosome 18q12 and results from defect in the gene F1C1 (ATP8B1; see Table 353-3). F1C1 is a P-type adenosine triphosphatase (ATPase) that functions as aminophospholipid flippase facilitating the transfer of phosphatidyl serine and phosphatidyl ethanolamine from the outer to inner hemileaflet of cellular membrane. F1C1 may also play a role in intestinal bile acids absorption, as suggested by the high level of expression in the intestine. Defective F1C1 may also result in another form of intrahepatic cholestasis: **benign recurrent intrahepatic cholestasis (BRIC) type I.** The disease is characterized by recurrent bouts of cholestasis, jaundice, and severe pruritus lasting from 2 wk to 6 mo; it can last up to 5 yr. Nonsense, frame shift, and deletional mutation cause PFIC type I; missense and split type mutation result in BRIC type I. Typically, patients with BRIC type I have normal cholesterol and γ-glutamyl transpeptidase levels. Although the disease is supposed to be a benign disorder, some cases can develop severe liver damage.

PFIC type 2 (BSEP deficiency) is mapped to chromosome 2q24 and is similar to PFIC 1 but is present in non-Amish families (Middle Eastern European). The disease results from defects in the canalicular ATP-dependent bile acid transporter BSEP (ABCB11). The progressive liver disease results from accumulation of bile acids secondary to reduction in canalicular bile acid secretion. Mutation in ABC11 is also described in another disorder, BRIC type 2, characterized by recurrent bouts of cholestasis associated with cholelithiasis and watery diarrhea.

In contrast to PFIC 1 and 2, patients with **PFIC type 3** (MDR3 disease) have **high** levels of γ-glutamyl transpeptidase. The disease results from defects in a canalicular phospholipids flippase, MDR3 (ABCB4), which results in deficient translocation of phosphatidylcholine across the canalicular membrane. Mothers who are heterozygous for this gene can develop intrahepatic cholestasis during pregnancy.

Familial hypercholanemia (FHC) is characterized by elevated serum bile acid concentration, pruritus, failure to thrive, and coagulopathy. FHC is a complex genetic trait associated with mutation of bile acid coenzyme A (CoA): amino acid N-acyltransferase (encoded by BAAT) as well as mutations in tight junction protein 2 (encoded by TJP 2, also known as ZO-2). Mutation of BAAT, which is a bile acid conjugating enzyme, abrogates the enzyme activity. Patients who are homozygous for this mutation have only unconjugated bile acids in their bile. Mutation of both BAAT and TJP 2 can disrupt bile acid transport and circulation. Patients with FHC usually respond to the administration of ursodeoxycholic acid.

Defective bile acid biosynthesis has been postulated to be an initiating or perpetuating factor in neonatal cholestatic disorders; the hypothesis is that inborn errors in bile acid biosynthesis lead to absence of normal trophic or choleretic primary bile acids and accumulation of primitive (hepatotoxic) metabolites. Inborn errors of bile acid biosynthesis cause acute and chronic liver disease; early recognition allows institution of targeted bile acid replacement, which reverses the hepatic injury. Several specific defects have been described, as follows.

Deficiency of Δ^4–3-oxosteroid-5β reductase, the 4th step in the pathway of cholesterol degradation to the primary bile acids, manifests with significant cholestasis and liver failure developing shortly after birth, with coagulopathy and metabolic liver injury resembling tyrosinemia. Hepatic histology is characterized by lobular disarray with giant cells, pseudoacinar transformation, and canalicular bile stasis. Mass spectrometry is required to document increased urinary bile acid excretion and the predominance of oxo-hydroxy and oxo-dihydroxy cholenoic acids. **Treatment** with cholic acid and ursodeoxycholic acid is associated with normalization of biochemical, histologic, and clinical features.

Deficiency of 3β-hydroxy C_{27}-steroid dehydrogenase (3β-HSD) isomerase, the 2nd step in bile acid biosynthesis, causes progressive familial intrahepatic cholestasis. Affected patients usually have jaundice with increased aminotransferase levels and hepatomegaly; γ-glutamyl transpeptidase levels and serum cholylglycine levels are **normal.** The histology is variable, ranging from giant cell hepatitis to chronic hepatitis. The diagnosis, suggested by mass spectrometry detection of C^{24} bile acids in urine, which retain the 3β-hydroxy-Δ^5 structure, can be confirmed by determination of 3β-HSD activity in cultured fibroblasts using 7α-hydroxy-Δ^5 cholesterol as a substrate. Primary bile acid therapy, administered orally to downregulate cholesterol 7α-hydroxylase activity, to limit the production of 3β-hydroxy-Δ^5 bile acids, and to facilitate hepatic clearance, has been effective in reversing hepatic injury.

DISORDERS OF EMBRYOGENESIS

Alagille syndrome (arteriohepatic dysplasia) is the most common syndrome with intrahepatic bile duct paucity. Bile duct "paucity" (often erroneously called intrahepatic biliary atresia) designates an absence or marked reduction in the number of interlobular bile ducts in the portal triads, with normal-sized branches of portal vein and hepatic arteriole. Biopsy in early life often reveals an inflammatory process involving the bile ducts; subsequent biopsy specimens then show subsidence of the inflammation with residual reduction in the number and diameter of bile ducts, analogous to the "disappearing bile duct syndrome" noted in adults with immune-mediated disorders. Serial assessment of hepatic histology often suggests progressive destruction of bile ducts. **Clinical manifestations** of Alagille syndrome are expressed in various degrees and can be nonspecific; they include unusual facial characteristics (broad forehead; deep-set, widely spaced eyes; long, straight nose; and an underdeveloped mandible). There may also be ocular abnormalities (posterior embryotoxon), cardiovascular abnormalities (usually peripheral pulmonic stenosis, sometimes tetralogy of Fallot), vertebral arch defects and failure of anterior vertebral arch fusion (butterfly vertebrae), and tubulointerstitial nephropathy. Other findings such as growth retardation and defective spermatogenesis may reflect nutritional deficiency. The prognosis for prolonged survival is good, but patients are likely to have pruritus, xanthomas with markedly elevated serum cholesterol levels, and neurologic complications of vitamin E deficiency if untreated. Mutations in human Jagged1 gene (JAG1), which encodes a ligand for the notch receptor, are linked to Alagille syndrome.

BILIARY ATRESIA

The term *biliary atresia* is imprecise because the anatomy of abnormal bile ducts in affected patients varies markedly. A more appropriate terminology would reflect the pathophysiology—namely, progressive obliterative cholangiopathy. Patients may have distal segmental bile duct obliteration with patent extrahepatic ducts up to the porta hepatis. This is a surgically correctable lesion, but it is uncommon. The most common form of biliary atresia, accounting for ≈85% of the cases, however, is obliteration of the entire extrahepatic biliary tree at or above the porta hepatis. This presents a much more difficult problem in surgical management. Most patients with biliary atresia (85–90%) have a postnatal onset; embryonic fetal onset presents at birth and is associated with other congenital anomalies within the polysplenia spectrum (biliary atresia splenic malformation [BASM]) (Fig. 353-2) [see Chapter 431.11].

INCIDENCE. Biliary atresia has been detected in 1/10,000–15,000 live births, idiopathic neonatal hepatitis in 1/5,000–10,000. Intrahepatic bile duct paucity appears much less commonly, in about 1/50,000–75,000 live births.

DIFFERENTIATION OF IDIOPATHIC NEONATAL HEPATITIS FROM BILIARY ATRESIA. It may be difficult to clearly differentiate infants with biliary atresia, who require surgical correction, from those with intrahepatic disease (neonatal hepatitis) and patent bile ducts. No single biochemical test or imaging procedure is entirely satisfactory. Diagnostic schemas incorporate clinical, historical, biochemical, and radiologic features.

Idiopathic neonatal hepatitis has a familial incidence of ≈20%, whereas biliary atresia is unlikely to recur within the same family. A few infants with fetal onset of biliary atresia have an increased incidence of other abnormalities, such as the polysplenia syndrome with abdominal heterotaxia, malrotation, levocardia, and intra-abdominal vascular anomalies. Neonatal hepatitis appears to be more common in premature or small for gestational age infants. Persistently acholic stools suggest biliary obstruction (biliary atresia), but patients with severe idiopathic neonatal hepatitis may have a transient severe impairment of bile excretion. Consistently pigmented stools rule against biliary atresia. The finding of bile-stained fluid on duodenal intubation also excludes biliary atresia. Palpation of the liver may find an abnormal size or consistency in patients with extrahepatic biliary atresia; this is less common with neonatal hepatitis.

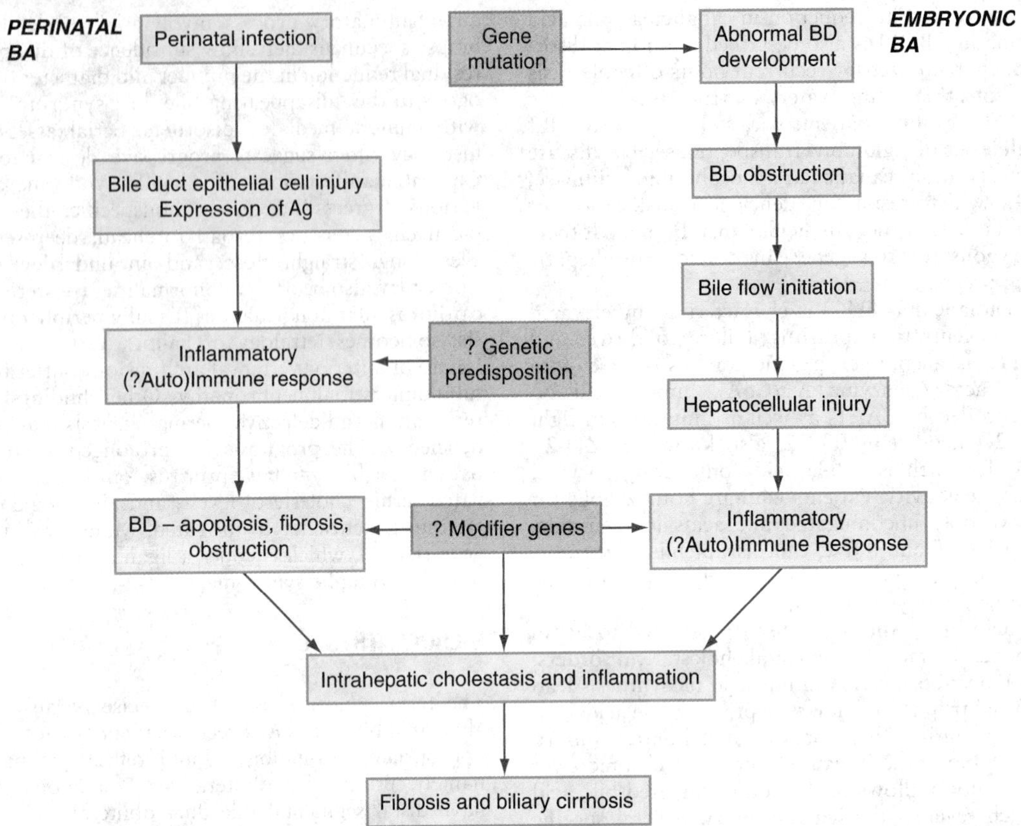

Figure 353-2. Proposed pathways for pathogenesis of 2 forms of biliary atresia (BA). *Perinatal* BA may develop when a perinatal insult, such as a cholangiotropic viral infection, triggers bile duct (BD) epithelial cell injury and exposure of self-antigens or neoantigens that elicit a subsequent immune response. The resulting inflammation induces apoptosis and necrosis of extrahepatic BD epithelium resulting in fibro-obliteration of the lumen and obstruction of the BD. Intrahepatic bile ducts can also be targets in the ongoing TH1 immune (autoimmune?) attack and the cholestatic injury, resulting in progressive portal fibrosis and culminating in biliary cirrhosis. *Embryonic* BA may be the result of mutations in genes controlling normal bile duct formation or differentiation, which secondarily induces an inflammatory/immune response within the common bile duct and liver after the initiation of bile flow at ≈11–13 wk of gestation. Secondary hepatocyte and intrahepatic bile duct injury ensue either as a result of cholestatic injury or as targets for the immune (autoimmune?) response that develops. The end result is intrahepatic cholestasis and portal tract fibrosis, culminating in biliary cirrhosis. Other major factors may be the role played by genetic predisposition to autoimmunity and modifier genes that determine the extent and type of cellular and immune response and the generation of fibrosis. (From Mack CL, Sokol RJ: Unraveling the pathogenesis and etiology of biliary atresia. *Pediatr Res* 2005;57:87R–94R.)

Abdominal ultrasound is a helpful diagnostic tool in the evaluation of neonatal cholestasis because it will identify choledocholithiasis, perforation of the bile duct, or other structural abnormalities of the biliary tree such as a choledochal cyst. In patients with biliary atresia, ultrasound may detect associated anomalies such as abdominal polysplenia and vascular malformations. The gallbladder is either not visualized or a microgallbladder is seen in patients with biliary atresia. Children with intrahepatic cholestasis caused by idiopathic neonatal hepatitis, cystic fibrosis, or total parenteral nutrition may have similar ultrasonographic findings. Ultrasonographic triangular cord (TC) sign, which represents a cone-shaped fibrotic mass cranial to the bifurcation of the portal vein, may be seen in patients with biliary atresia (Figs. 353-3 and 353-4). The echogenic density, which represents the fibrous remnants at the porta hepatis of biliary atresia cases at surgery, may be a helpful diagnostic tool in the evaluation of patients with neonatal cholestasis.

Hepatobiliary scintigraphy with technetium-labeled iminodiacetic acid derivatives is used to differentiate biliary atresia from nonobstructive causes of cholestasis. The hepatic uptake of the agent is normal in patients with biliary atresia, but excretion into the intestine is absent. Although the uptake may be impaired in neonatal hepatitis, excretion into the bowel will eventually occur. Obtaining a follow-up scan after 24 hr is of value to determine the patency of the biliary tree. The administration of phenobarbital (5 mg/kg/day) for 5 days before the scan is recommended because it may enhance biliary excretion of the isotope. Hepatobiliary scintigraphy is a sensitive but not specific test for biliary atresia. It fails to identify other structural abnormalities of the biliary tree or vascular anomalies. The lack of the specificity of the test and the need to wait for 5 days makes this procedure less practical and of limited usefulness in the evaluation of children suspected to have biliary atresia.

Percutaneous liver biopsy is the most valuable procedure in the evaluation of neonatal hepatobiliary diseases and provides the most reliable discriminatory evidence. Biliary atresia is characterized by bile ductular proliferation, the presence of bile plugs, and portal or perilobular edema and fibrosis, with the basic hepatic lobular architecture intact. In neonatal hepatitis, there is severe, diffuse hepatocellular disease, with distortion of lobular architecture, marked infiltration with inflammatory cells, and focal hepatocellular necrosis; the bile ductules show little alteration. Giant cell transformation is found in infants with either condition and has no diagnostic specificity.

The histologic changes seen in patients with idiopathic neonatal hepatitis can occur in other diseases, including α_1-antitrypsin deficiency, galactosemia, and various forms of intrahepatic cholestasis. Although paucity of intrahepatic bile ductules may be detected on liver biopsy even in the 1st few weeks of life, later biopsies in such patients reveal a more characteristic pattern.

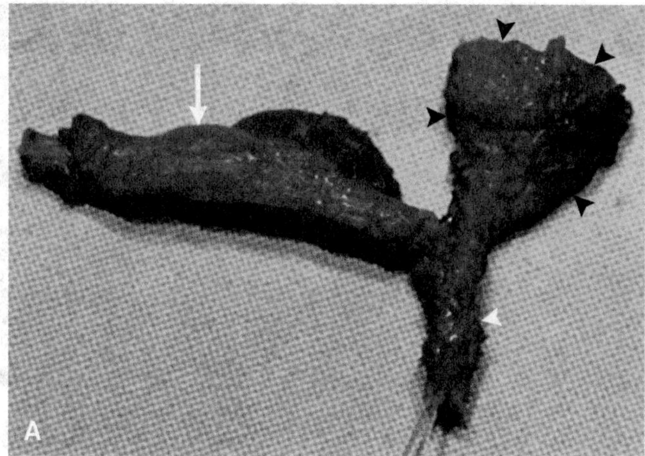

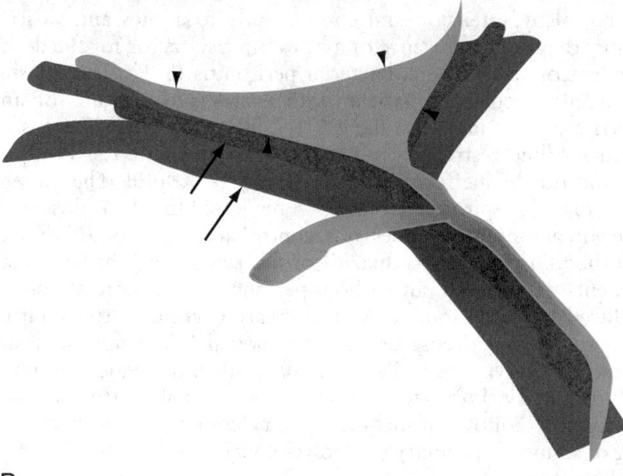

Figure 353-3. Surgical findings of biliary atresia. *A,* Photograph of surgical specimen of obliterated extrahepatic bile ducts shows the fibrous ductal remnant *(black arrowheads)* in the porta hepatis, atretic gallbladder *(arrow),* and fibrous common bile duct *(white arrowhead).* The fibrous ductal remnant is a triangular cone-shaped mass. *B,* Schematic drawing represents the anatomic relationship between the fibrous ductal remnant and blood vessels around the porta hepatis. The triangular, cone-shaped, fibrous ductal remnant *(black arrowheads, green)* is positioned anterior and slightly superior to the portal vein *(long arrow, blue)* and the hepatic artery *(short arrow, red).* (From Lee HJ, Lee SM, Park WH, Choi SO: Objective criteria of triangular cord sign in biliary atresia on US scans. *Radiology* 2003;229:395–400.)

MANAGEMENT OF PATIENTS WITH SUSPECTED BILIARY ATRESIA. All patients suspected of having biliary atresia should undergo exploratory laparotomy and direct cholangiography to determine the presence and site of obstruction. Direct drainage can be accomplished in the few patients with a correctable lesion. When no correctable lesion is found, an examination of frozen sections obtained from the transected porta hepatis can detect the presence of biliary epithelium and determine the size and patency of the residual bile ducts. In some cases, the cholangiogram indicates that the biliary tree is patent but of diminished caliber, suggesting that the cholestasis is not due to biliary tract obliteration but to bile duct paucity or markedly diminished flow in the presence of intrahepatic disease. In these cases, transection of or further dissection into the porta hepatis should be avoided.

For patients in whom no correctable lesion is found, the **hepatoportoenterostomy (Kasai) procedure** should be performed. The rationale for this operation is that minute bile duct remnants, representing residual channels, may be present in the fibrous tissue of the porta hepatis; such channels may be in direct continuity with the intrahepatic ductule system. In such cases, transection of the porta hepatis with anastomosis of bowel to the proximal surface of the transection may allow bile drainage. If flow is not rapidly established in the 1st months of life, progressive obliteration and cirrhosis ensue. If microscopic channels of patency >150 µm in diameter are found, postoperative establishment of bile flow is likely. The success rate for establishing good bile flow after the Kasai operation is much higher (90%) if performed before 8 wk of life. Therefore, the importance of early referral and prompt evaluation of infants with suspected biliary atresia is emphasized.

Some patients with biliary atresia, even of the "non-correctable" type, derive long-term benefits from interventions such as the Kasai procedure. In most, a degree of hepatic dysfunction persists. Patients with biliary atresia usually have persistent inflammation of the intrahepatic biliary tree, which suggests that biliary atresia reflects a dynamic process involving the entire hepatobiliary system. This may account for the ultimate development of complications such as portal hypertension. The short-term benefit of hepatoportoenterostomy is decompression and drainage sufficient to forestall the onset of cirrhosis and sustain growth until a successful liver transplantation can be done (see Chapter 365).

MANAGEMENT OF CHRONIC CHOLESTASIS

With any form of neonatal cholestasis, whether the primary disease is idiopathic neonatal hepatitis, intrahepatic cholestasis, or biliary atresia, affected patients are at increased risk for chronic complications. These reflect various degrees of residual hepatic functional capacity and are due directly or indirectly to diminished bile flow. Any substance normally excreted into bile is retained in the liver, with subsequent accumulation in tissue and in serum. Involved substances include bile acids, bilirubin, cholesterol, and trace elements. Decreased delivery of bile acids to the proximal intestine leads to inadequate digestion and absorption of dietary long-chain triglycerides and fat-soluble vitamins. Impairment of hepatic metabolic function can alter hormonal balance and utilization of nutrients. Progressive liver damage can lead to biliary cirrhosis, portal hypertension, and liver failure.

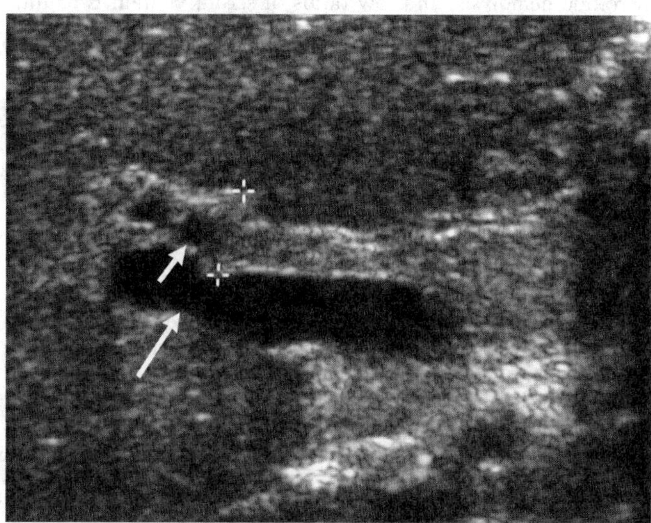

Figure 353-4. Depiction of triangular cord (TC) sign. The echogenic anterior wall of the right portal vein (EARPV) was 5.4 mm thick on this longitudinal US scan, which shows the TC sign *(cursors)* as a thick, tubular, echogenic area along the anterior aspect of the right portal vein *(long arrow).* The right hepatic artery *(short arrow)* is encased within the EARPV. (From Lee HJ, Lee SM, Park WH, Choi SO: Objective criteria of triangular cord sign in biliary atresia on US scans. *Radiology* 2003;229:395–400.)

TABLE 353-4. Suggested Medical Management of Persistent Cholestasis

CLINICAL IMPAIRMENT	MANAGEMENT
Malnutrition resulting from malabsorption of dietary long-chain triglycerides	Replace with dietary formula or supplements containing medium-chain triglycerides
Fat-soluble vitamin malabsorption:	
Vitamin A deficiency (night blindness, thick skin)	Replace with 10,000–15,000 IU/day as Aquasol A
Vitamin E deficiency (neuromuscular degeneration)	Replace with 50–400 IU/day as oral α-tocopherol or TPGS
Vitamin D deficiency (metabolic bone disease)	Replace with 5,000–8,000 IU/day of D_2 or 3–5 μg/kg/day of 25-hydroxycholecalciferol
Vitamin K deficiency (hypoprothrombinemia)	Replace with 2.5–5.0 mg every other day as water-soluble derivative of menadione
Micronutrient deficiency	Calcium, phosphate, or zinc supplementation
Deficiency of water-soluble vitamins	Supplement with twice the recommended daily allowance
Retention of biliary constituents such as cholesterol (itch or xanthomas)	Administer choleretic bile acids and ursodeoxycholic acid, 15–20 mg/kg/day
Progressive liver disease; portal hypertension (variceal bleeding, ascites, hypersplenism)	Interim management (control bleeding; salt restriction; spironolactone)
End-stage liver disease (liver failure)	Transplantation

TPGS, D-tocopherol polyethylene glycol 1000 succinate.

Treatment of such patients is empirical, and is guided by careful monitoring (Table 353-4). No therapy is known to be effective in halting the progression of cholestasis or in preventing further hepatocellular damage and cirrhosis.

Growth failure is a major concern and is related in part to malabsorption and malnutrition resulting from ineffective digestion and absorption of dietary fat. Use of a medium-chain triglyceride–containing formula may improve caloric balance.

With chronic cholestasis and prolonged survival, children with hepatobiliary disease may experience deficiencies of the fat-soluble vitamins (A, D, E, K). Inadequate absorption of fat and fat-soluble vitamins may be exacerbated by administration of the bile acid binder cholestyramine. Metabolic bone disease is common.

Serum vitamin A concentration can usually be maintained at normal levels in patients who have chronic cholestasis and who receive oral supplementation of vitamin A esters. It is essential to monitor the vitamin A status in such patients.

A degenerative neuromuscular syndrome is found with chronic cholestasis, caused by malabsorption and vitamin E deficiency; affected children experience progressive areflexia, cerebellar ataxia, ophthalmoplegia, and decreased vibratory sensation. Specific morphologic lesions have been found in the central nervous system, peripheral nerves, and muscles. These lesions are potentially reversible in young children (<3–4 yr). Affected children have low serum vitamin E concentrations, increased hydrogen peroxide hemolysis, and low ratios of serum vitamin E to total serum lipids (<0.6 mg/g for children <12 yr and <0.8 mg/g for older patients). Vitamin E deficiency may be prevented by oral administration of large doses (up to 1,000 IU/day); patients unable to absorb sufficient quantities may require administration of d-α-tocopheryl polyethylene glycol 1000 succinate orally. Serum levels may be monitored as a guide to efficacy.

Pruritus is a particularly troublesome complication of chronic cholestasis, often with the appearance of xanthomas. Both features seem to be related to the accumulation of cholesterol and bile acids in serum and in tissues. Elimination of these retained compounds is difficult when bile ducts are obstructed, but if there is any degree of bile duct patency, administration of ursodeoxycholic acid may increase bile flow or interrupt the enterohepatic circulation of bile acids and thus decrease the xanthomas and ameliorate the pruritus (see Table 353-4). Ursodeoxycholic acid therapy may also lower serum cholesterol levels. The recommended initial dose is 15 mg/kg/24 hr.

Partial external biliary is efficacious in the management of pruritus refractory to medical therapy and provides a favorable outcome in a select group of patients with chronic cholestasis who have not yet developed cirrhosis. The surgical technique involves resecting a segment of intestine to be used as a biliary conduit. One end of the conduit is attached to the gallbladder and the other end is brought out to the skin, forming a stoma. The main drawback of the procedure is the lifelong need to use an ostomy bag.

Progressive fibrosis and cirrhosis will lead to the development of portal hypertension and consequently to ascites and variceal hemorrhage. The presence of ascites is a risk factor for the development of spontaneous bacterial peritonitis (SBP). The 1st step in the management of patients with ascites is to rule out SBP and restrict sodium intake to 0.5 g (≈1–2 mEq/kg/24 hr). There is no need for fluid restriction in patients with adequate renal output. Should this be ineffective, diuretics may be helpful. The diuretic of choice is spironolactone (3–5 mg/kg/24 hr in 4 doses). If spironolactone alone does not control ascites, the addition of another diuretic such as thiazide or furosemide may be beneficial. Patients with ascites but without peripheral edema are at risk for reduced plasma volume and decreased urine output during diuretic therapy. Tense ascites alters renal blood flow and systemic hemodynamics. Paracentesis and intravenous albumin infusion may improve hemodynamics, renal perfusion, and symptoms. Follow-up includes dietary counseling and monitoring of serum and urinary electrolyte concentrations (see Chapters 361 and 364).

In patients with portal hypertension, variceal hemorrhage and the development of hypersplenism are common. It is important to ascertain the cause of bleeding because episodes of gastrointestinal hemorrhage in patients who have chronic liver disease may be due to gastritis or peptic ulcer disease. Because the management of these various complications differs, differentiation, perhaps via endoscopy, is necessary before treatment is initiated (see Chapter 364). If the patient is volume depleted, blood transfusion should be carefully administered, avoiding overtransfusion, which can precipitate further bleeding. The use of balloon tamponade is not recommended in children because it can be associated with significant complications. Sclerotherapy or endoscopic variceal ligation may be useful palliative measures in the management of bleeding varices and may be superior to surgical alternatives.

For patients with advanced liver disease, hepatic transplantation has a success rate >85% (see Chapter 365). If the operation is technically feasible, it will prolong life and may correct the metabolic error in diseases such as α_1-antitrypsin deficiency, tyrosinemia, and Wilson disease. Success depends on adequate intraoperative, preoperative, and postoperative care and on cautious use of immunosuppressive agents. Scarcity of donors of small livers severely limits the application of liver transplantation for infants and children. The use of reduced-size transplants and living donors increases the ability to treat small children successfully.

PROGNOSIS

For patients with idiopathic neonatal hepatitis, the variable prognosis may reflect the heterogeneity of the disease. In sporadic cases, 60–70% recover with no evidence of hepatic structural or functional impairment. Approximately 5–10% have persistent fibrosis or inflammation, and a smaller percentage have more severe liver disease, such as cirrhosis. Death of infants usually occurs early in the course of the illness, owing to hemorrhage or sepsis. Of infants with idiopathic neonatal hepatitis of the familial variety, only 20–30% recover; 10–15% acquire chronic liver disease with cirrhosis. Liver transplantation may be required.

353.2 • Cholestasis in the Older Child

Most cases of cholestasis with onset after the neonatal period are due to acute viral hepatitis or hepatotoxic drugs. Many of the conditions causing neonatal cholestasis can also cause chronic cholestasis in older patients. Adolescents with conjugated hyperbilirubinemia should be evaluated for acute and chronic hepatitis, α_1-antitrypsin deficiency, Wilson disease, liver disease associated with inflammatory bowel disease, autoimmune hepatitis, and the syndromes of intrahepatic cholestasis. Other causes include obstruction caused by cholelithiasis, abdominal tumors, enlarged lymph nodes, or hepatic inflammation resulting from drug ingestion. Management of cholestasis in the older child is similar to that proposed for neonatal cholestasis (see Table 353-4).

Aagenaes O: Hereditary recurrent cholestasis with lymphedema: Two new families. *Acta Pediatr Scand* 1974;63:465–471.

Alagille D, Estrada A, Hadchovel M, et al: Syndromic paucity of interlobular bile ducts (Alagille syndrome or arteriohepatic dysplasia): Review of 80 cases. *J Pediatr* 1987;110:195–200.

Balistreri WF, Bezerra JA, Jansen P, et al: Intrahepatic cholestasis: Summary of an American Association for the Study of Liver Diseases single-topic conference. *Hepatology* 2005;42:222–235.

Carlton VE, Harris BZ, Puffenberger EG, et al: Complex inheritance of familial hypercholanemia with associated mutations in TJP2 and BAAT. *Nat Genet* 2003;34:91–96.

Chardot C, Carton M, Spire-Bendelac N, et al: Is the Kasai operation still indicated in children older than 3 months diagnosed with biliary atresia? *J Pediatr* 2001;138:224–228.

Chardot C, Serinet MO: Prognosis of biliary atresia: What can be further improved. *J Pediatr* 2006;148:432–435.

Chen J, Raymond K: Nuclear receptors, bile-acid detoxification, and cholestasis. *Lancet* 2006;367:454–456.

Danks DM, Campbell PE, Smith AL, et al: Prognosis of babies with neonatal hepatitis. *Arch Dis Child* 1977;52:368–372.

Davenport M, De Ville de Goyet J, Stringer MD, et al: Seamless management of biliary atresia in England and Wales (1999–2002). *Lancet* 2004; 363:1354–1357.

Davenport M, Tizzard SA, Underhill J, et al: The biliary atresia splenic malformation syndrome: A 28-year single-center retrospective study. *J Pediatr* 2006;149:393–400.

Gissen P, Kelly D: New hope for treatment of neonatal haemochromatosis. *Lancet* 2004;364:1644–1645.

Hinds R, Davenport M, Mieli-Vergani G, et al: Antenatal presentation of the biliary atresia. *J Pediatr* 2004;144:43–46.

Jansen PLM, Muller M: The molecular genetics of familial intrahepatic cholestasis. *Gut* 2000;47:1–5.

Jansen PLM, Sturm E: Paediatric cholestasis: Is villin the villain? *Lancet* 2003;362:1090–1091.

Klomp LW, Vargas JC, van Mil SW, et al: Characterization of mutations in ATP8B1 associated with hereditary cholestasis. *Hepatology* 2004;40:27–38.

Lee HJ, Lee SM, Park WH, Choi SO: Objective criteria of triangular cord sign in biliary atresia on US scans. *Radiology* 2003;229:395–400.

Mack CL, Sokol RJ: Unraveling the pathogenesis and etiology of biliary atresia. *Pediatr Res* 2005;57:87R–94R.

Miga D, Sokol RJ, MacKenzie T, et al: Survival after first esophageal variceal hemorrhage in patients with biliary atresia. *J Pediatr* 2001;139:291–296.

Mowat AP, Psacharopoulos HT, Williams R: Extrahepatic biliary atresia versus neonatal hepatitis: Review of 137 prospectively investigated infants. *Arch Dis Child* 1976;51:763–770.

Nio M, Ohi R, Miyano T, et al: Five- and 10-year survival rates after surgery for biliary atresia: A report from the Japanese biliary atresia registry. *J Pediatr Surg* 2003;38:997–1000.

Oda T, Elkahloun AG, Pike BL, et al: Mutations in the human Jagged1 gene are responsible for Alagille syndrome. *Nat Genet* 1997;16:235–292.

Setchell KD, Schwarz M, O'Connell NC, et al: Identification of a new inborn error in bile acid synthesis: Mutation of the oxysterol 7alpha-hydroxylase gene causes severe neonatal liver disease. *J Clin Invest* 1998; 102:1690–1703.

Shih HH, Lin TM, Chuang JH, et al: Promotor polymorphism of the CD14 endotoxin receptor gene is associated with biliary atresia and idiopathic neonatal cholestasis. *Pediatrics* 2005;116:437–441.

Shneider BL, Brown MB, Haver B, et al: A multicenter study of the outcome of biliary atresia in the United States, 1997 to 2000. *J Pediatr* 2006;148: 467–474.

Sokol RJ, Heubi JE, Butler-Simon N, et al: Treatment of vitamin E deficiency during chronic childhood cholestasis with oral d-alpha-tocopheryl polyethylene glycol-1000 succinate. *Gastroenterology* 1987;93:975–985.

Stringer MD, Dhawan A, Davenport M, et al: Choledochal cysts: Lessons from a 20 year experience. *Arch Dis Child* 1995;73:528–531.

Utterson EC, Shepherd RW, Sokol RJ, et al: Biliary atresia: Clinical profiles, risk factors, and outcomes of 755 patients listed for liver transplantation. *J Pediatr* 2005;147:180–185.

van Mil SW, van der Woerd WL, van der Brugge G, et al: Benign recurrent intrahepatic cholestasis type 2 is caused by mutations in ABCB11. *Gastroenterology* 2004;127:379–384.

Whitington PF, Hibbard JU: High-dose immunoglobulin during pregnancy for recurrent neonatal haemochromatosis. *Lancet* 2004;364:1690–1698.

Yeh JN, Jeng YM, Chen HL, et al: Hepatic steatosis and neonatal intrahepatic choleostasis caused by citrin deficiency (NICCD) in Taiwanese infants. *J Pediatr* 2006;148:642–646.

Yoon PW, Bresee JS, Olney RS, et al: Epidemiology of biliary atresia: A population-based study. *Pediatrics* 1997;99:376–382.

Chapter 354 ■ Metabolic Diseases of the Liver

Rebecca G. Carey and William F. Balistreri

Because the liver has a central role in synthetic, degradative, and regulatory pathways involving carbohydrate, protein, lipid, trace element, and vitamin metabolism, many metabolic abnormalities or specific enzyme deficiencies affect the liver primarily or secondarily (Table 354-1). Many metabolic diseases are detected in expanded newborn metabolic screening programs (see Chapter 84). Liver disease can arise when absence of an enzyme produces a block in a metabolic pathway, when unmetabolized substrate accumulates proximal to a block, when deficiency of an essential substance produced distal to an aberrant chemical reaction develops, or when synthesis of an abnormal metabolite occurs. The spectrum of pathologic changes includes: **hepatocyte injury,** with subsequent failure of other metabolic functions, often eventuating in cirrhosis, liver tumors, or both; **storage** of lipid, glycogen, or other products manifested as hepatomegaly, often with complications specific to deranged metabolism (hypoglycemia with glycogen storage disease); and absence of structural change despite profound **metabolic effects,** as with urea cycle defects. The clinical manifestations of metabolic diseases of the liver mimic infections, intoxications, and hematologic and immunologic diseases (Table 354-2). Further clues are provided by family history of a similar illness or by the observation that the onset of symptoms is closely associated with a change in dietary habits; for example, in patients with hereditary fructose intolerance, symptoms follow ingestion of fructose. Clinical and laboratory evidence often guides the evaluation. Liver biopsy offers

TABLE 354-1. Inborn Errors of Metabolism That Affect the Liver

DISORDERS OF CARBOHYDRATE METABOLISM
Disorders of galactose metabolism
Galactosemia
Disorders of fructose metabolism
Hereditary fructose intolerance (aldolase deficiency)
Fructose-1,6 diphosphatase deficiency
Glycogen storage diseases
Type I
Von Gierke (Ia)
Type 1b
Type III (Cori/Forbes)
Type IV (Andersen)
Type VI (Hers)
Congenital disorders of glycosylation (CGD)
DISORDERS OF AMINO ACID AND PROTEIN METABOLISM
Disorders of tyrosine metabolism
Hereditary tyrosinemia (type I)
Tyrosinemia, type II
Inherited urea cycle enzyme defects
CPS deficiency
OTC deficiency (X-linked dominant)
Citrullinemia
Argininosuccinic aciduria
Argininemia
N-AGS deficiency
DISORDERS OF LIPID METABOLISM
Wolman disease
Cholesteryl ester storage disease
Gaucher disease
Niemann-Pick type C
DISORDERS OF BILE ACID METABOLISM
Isomerase deficiency
Reductase deficiency
Zellweger syndrome (cerebrohepatorenal)
DISORDERS OF METAL METABOLISM
Wilson disease
Hepatic copper overload
Indian childhood cirrhosis
Neonatal iron storage disease (perinatal hemochromatosis)
DISORDERS OF BILIRUBIN METABOLISM
Crigler-Najjar
Type I
Type II
Gilbert disease
Dubin-Johnson syndrome
Rotor syndrome
MISCELLANEOUS
α_1-Antitrypsin deficiency
Cystic fibrosis
Erythropoietic protoporphyria
Citrin deficiency

CPS, Citrin deficiency carbamoyl phosphate synthetase; N-AGS, N-acetylglutamate synthetase; OTC, ornithine transcarbamoylase.

morphologic study and permits enzyme assays, as well as quantitative and qualitative assays of various other constituents. Genetic/molecular diagnosis is also available. Such studies require cooperation of experienced laboratories and careful attention to collection and handling of specimens.

TABLE 354-2. Clinical Manifestations That Suggest the Possibility of Metabolic Disease

Recurrent vomiting, failure to thrive, short stature, dysmorphic features, edema/anasarca
Jaundice, hepatomegaly (± splenomegaly), fulminant hepatic failure
Hypoglycemia, organic acidemia, lactic acidemia, hyperammonemia, bleeding (coagulopathy)
Developmental delay/psychomotor retardation, hypotonia, progressive neuromuscular deterioration, seizures
Cardiac dysfunction/failure, unusual odors, rickets, cataracts

354.1 • Inherited Deficient Conjugation of Bilirubin (Familial Nonhemolytic Unconjugated Hyperbilirubinemia)

Bilirubin is the metabolic end product of heme. Before excretion into bile, it is 1st glucuronidated by the enzyme bilirubin-uridinediphosphoglucuronate glucuronosyltransferase (UDPGT). UDPGT activity is deficient or altered in three genetically and functionally distinct disorders (Crigler-Najjar syndromes type I and II and Gilbert syndrome), producing congenital nonobstructive, nonhemolytic, unconjugated hyperbilirubinemia. UGT1A1 is the primary UDPGT isoform needed for bilirubin glucuronidation, and complete absence of UGT1A1 activity causes CN type I. CN type II is due to decreased UGT1A1 activity; Gilbert syndrome is caused by a polymorphism in the promoter region of UGT1A1 that also decreases normal gene activity but only to ≈30%. Unlike the Crigler-Najjar syndromes, Gilbert syndrome is benign and no treatment is required; however, it is more common, affecting up to 5–10% of the white population.

CRIGLER-NAJJAR SYNDROME TYPE I (GLUCURONYL TRANSFERASE DEFICIENCY). This form is inherited as an autosomal recessive trait and is usually secondary to mutations that cause a premature stop codon or frameshift mutation and thereby abolish UGT1A1 activity. More than 35 mutations have been identified to date. Parents of affected children have partial defects in conjugation as determined by hepatic enzyme assay or by measurement of glucuronide formation; their serum bilirubin concentrations are normal.

Clinical Manifestations. Severe unconjugated hyperbilirubinemia develops in homozygous affected infants in the 1st 3 days of life, and without treatment, serum unconjugated bilirubin concentrations of 25–35 mg/dL are reached in the 1st mo. Kernicterus, an almost universal complication of this disorder, is usually 1st noted in the early neonatal period; some treated infants have survived childhood without clinical sequelae. Stools are pale yellow. Persistence of unconjugated hyperbilirubinemia at levels >20 mg/dL after the 1st wk of life in the absence of hemolysis should suggest the syndrome.

Diagnosis. The diagnosis of Crigler-Najjar type I is based on the early age of onset and the extreme level of bilirubin elevation in the absence of hemolysis. In the bile, bilirubin concentration is <10 mg/dL compared with normal concentrations of 50–100 mg/dL; there is no bilirubin glucuronide. Definitive diagnosis is established by measuring hepatic glucuronyl transferase activity in a liver specimen obtained by a closed biopsy; open biopsy should be avoided because surgery and anesthesia can precipitate kernicterus. DNA diagnosis is also available and may be preferable. Identification of the heterozygous state in parents is also strongly suggestive of the diagnosis. The differential diagnosis of unconjugated hyperbilirubinemia is discussed in Chapter 102.3.

Treatment. The serum unconjugated bilirubin concentration should be kept below 20 mg/dL for at least the 1st 2–4 wk of life; in low birthweight infants, the levels should be kept lower. This usually requires repeated exchange transfusions and phototherapy. Phenobarbital therapy should be considered to determine responsiveness and differentiation between type I and II (see later). The risk of kernicterus persists into adult life, although the serum bilirubin levels required to produce brain injury beyond the neonatal period are considerably higher (usually >35 mg/dL). Therefore, phototherapy is generally continued through the early years of life. In older infants and children, phototherapy is used mainly during sleep so as not to interfere with normal activities. Despite the administration of increasing intensities of light for longer periods, the serum bilirubin decrement response to phototherapy decreases with age. Adjuvant therapy using agents that bind photobilirubin products such as calcium phosphate, cholestyramine, or agar can be used to interfere with the enterohepatic recirculation of bilirubin. Prompt treatment of intercurrent infections, febrile episodes, and other types of illness may help prevent the later development of kernicterus, which may occur at bilirubin levels of 45–55 mg/dL. All patients with type I have eventually experienced severe kernicterus by young adulthood, despite vigorous continuous management that maintained neurologic normality during childhood. Orthotopic hepatic transplantation cures the disease and has been successful in a small number of patients; isolated hepatocyte transplantation has been reported in one patient; however, this patient eventually required orthotopic transplantation. Other therapeutic modalities have included plasmapheresis and limitation of bilirubin production. The latter option, inhibiting bilirubin generation, is possible via inhibition of heme oxygenase using metalloporphyrin therapy. Genetically engineered enzymatic replacement therapy and liver-directed gene therapy remain potential therapeutic options for the future; however, to date, this has only been investigated in animal models.

CRIGLER-NAJJAR SYNDROME TYPE II (PARTIAL GLUCURONYL TRANSFERASE DEFICIENCY). Like Crigler-Najjar type I, type II is an autosomal recessive disease; it is caused by homozygous missense mutations in UGT1A1 resulting in reduced (partial) enzymatic activity. More than 18 mutations have been identified to date. Type II disease can be distinguished from type I by the marked decline in serum bilirubin level that occurs in type II disease after treatment with phenobarbital secondary to an inducible phenobarbital response element on the UGT1A1 promoter.

Clinical Manifestations. When this disorder presents in the neonatal period, unconjugated hyperbilirubinemia usually occurs in the 1st 3 days of life; serum bilirubin concentrations can be in a range compatible with physiologic jaundice or can be at pathologic levels. The concentrations characteristically remain elevated into and after the 3rd wk of life, persisting in a range of 1.5–22 mg/dL; concentrations in the lower part of this range can create uncertainty about whether chronic hyperbilirubinemia is present. The onset of kernicterus is unusual. Stool color is normal, and the infants are without clinical signs or symptoms of disease. There is no evidence of hemolysis.

Diagnosis. Concentration of bilirubin in bile is nearly normal in Crigler-Najjar type II. Jaundiced infants and young children having type II syndrome respond readily to 5 mg/kg/24 hr of oral phenobarbital, with a decrease in serum bilirubin concentration to 2–3 mg/dL in 7–10 days.

Treatment. Long-term reduction in serum bilirubin levels can be achieved with continued administration of phenobarbital at 5 mg/kg/24 hr. The cosmetic and psychosocial benefit should be weighed against the risks of an effective dose of the drug because there is a small long-term risk of kernicterus even in the absence of hemolytic disease.

INHERITED CONJUGATED HYPERBILIRUBINEMIA

Conjugated hyperbilirubinemia can be due to a small number of rare conditions that are autosomal recessive disorders characterized by mild jaundice. The transfer of bilirubin and other organic anions from liver to bile is defective. Chronic mild conjugated hyperbilirubinemia is usually detected during adolescence or early adulthood but can occur as early as the 2nd yr of life. The results of routine liver function tests are normal. Jaundice can be exacerbated by infection, pregnancy, oral contraceptives, alcohol consumption, and surgery. There is usually no morbidity and life expectancy is normal, but these disorders can initially present difficult problems in the differential diagnosis of more serious diseases.

DUBIN-JOHNSON SYNDROME. Dubin-Johnson syndrome is an autosomal recessive inherited defect in hepatocyte secretion of bilirubin glucuronide. The defect in hepatic excretory function is not limited to conjugated bilirubin excretion but also involves several organic anions normally excreted from the liver cell into bile. Absent function of multiple drug-resistant protein (MRP2), an adenosine triphosphate (ATP)–dependent canalicular transporter, is the responsible defect. Approximately 10 different mutations have been identified and affect either localization of MRP2 with resultant increased degradation or impair MRP2 transport activity in the canalicular membrane. Bile acid excretion and serum bile acid levels are normal. Total urinary coproporphyrin excretion is normal in quantity but coproporphrin I excretion increases to ≈80% with a concomittent decrease in coproporphyrin III excretion. Normally, coproporphyrin III is >75% of the total. Cholangiography fails to visualize the biliary tract and roentgenography of the gallbladder is also abnormal. The liver cells contain black pigment similar to melanin.

ROTOR SYNDROME. These patients have an additional deficiency in organic anion uptake. Unlike Dubin-Johnson syndrome, total urinary coproporphyrin excretion is elevated, with a relative increase in the amount of the coproporphyrin I isomer. The gallbladder is normal by roentgenography, and liver cells contain no black pigment. In both Dubin-Johnson and Rotor syndromes, sulfobromophthalein excretion is often abnormal.

354.2 • Wilson Disease

Wilson disease (hepatolenticular degeneration) is an autosomal recessive disorder characterized by degenerative changes in the brain, liver disease, and Kayser-Fleischer rings in the cornea. The incidence is 1/500,000 to 1/100,000 births. It is progressive and fatal if untreated; specific effective treatment is available. Rapid diagnostic investigation of the possibility of Wilson disease in a patient presenting with any form of liver disease, particularly if >5 yr of age, not only facilitates early institution of management of Wilson disease and related genetic counseling but also allows appropriate treatment of non-Wilsonian liver disease once copper toxicosis is ruled out.

PATHOGENESIS. The abnormal gene for Wilson disease is localized to the long arm of chromosome 13 (13q14.3). The Wilson disease gene encodes a copper transporting P-type ATPase, ATP7B. ATP7B is mainly but not exclusively expressed in hepatocytes and is thought to be critical for biliary copper excretion and for copper incorporation into ceruloplasmin. Absence or malfunction of ATP7B results in decreased biliary copper excretion and diffuse accumulation of copper in the cytosol of hepatocytes. When liver cells become overloaded, copper is redistributed to other tissues including the brain and kidneys, to which it is toxic, primarily as a potent inhibitor of enzymatic processes. Ionic copper inhibits pyruvate oxidase in brain and ATPase in membranes, leading to decreased ATP-phosphocreatine and potassium content of tissue.

More than 250 mutations in the gene have been identified, making diagnosis by DNA mutational analysis a difficult task unless a proband mutation is known. Most patients are compound heterozygotes. Mutations that completely knock out gene function are associated with an onset of disease symptoms as early as 2–3 yr of age, when Wilson disease may not typically be considered in the differential diagnosis. Milder mutations can be associated with neurologic symptoms or liver disease as late as 70 yr of age. Cloning of the gene for Wilson disease raises the prospect of precise presymptomatic detection of Wilson disease, timely initiation of therapy, and, ultimately, gene therapy.

CLINICAL MANIFESTATIONS. Forms of Wilsonian hepatic disease include asymptomatic hepatomegaly (with or without splenomegaly), subacute or chronic hepatitis, and fulminant hepatic failure. Cryptogenic cirrhosis, portal hypertension, ascites, edema, variceal bleeding, or other effects of hepatic dysfunction (delayed puberty, amenorrhea, coagulation defect) can be manifestations of Wilson disease.

Disease presentations are variable, with a tendency to familial patterns. The younger the patient, the more likely hepatic involvement will be the predominant manifestation. Females are three times more likely than males to present with fulminant hepatic failure. After 20 yr of age, neurologic symptoms predominate.

Neurologic disorders can develop insidiously or precipitously, with intention tremor, dysarthria, dystonia, lack of motor coordination, deterioration in school performance, or behavioral changes. Kayser-Fleischer rings may be absent in young patients with liver disease but are always present in patients with neurologic symptoms. Psychiatric manifestations include depression, anxiety, or psychosis. Coombs-negative hemolytic anemia may be an initial manifestation, possibly related to the release of large amounts of copper from damaged hepatocytes; this form of Wilson disease is usually fatal without transplantation. During hemolytic episodes, urinary copper excretion and serum copper levels (non-ceruloplasmin-bound) are markedly elevated. Manifestations of renal Fanconi syndrome and progressive renal failure with alterations in tubular transport of amino acids, glucose, and uric acid may be present. Unusual manifestations include arthritis, cardiomyopathy, and endocrinopathies (hypoparathyroidism).

PATHOLOGY. All grades of hepatic injury occur with steatosis, heptocellular ballooning and degeneration, glycogen granules, minimal inflammation, and enlarged Kupffer cells. The lesion may be indistinguishable from that of autoimmune hepatitis. With progressive parenchymal damage, fibrosis and cirrhosis develop. Ultrastructural changes primarily involve the mitochondria and include increased density of the matrix material, inclusions of lipid and granular material, and increased intracristal space with dilatation of the tips of the cristae. Liver copper content is elevated.

DIAGNOSIS. Wilson disease should be considered in children and teenagers with unexplained acute or chronic liver disease, neurologic symptoms of unknown cause, acute hemolysis, psychiatric illnesses, behavioral changes, Fanconi syndrome, or unexplained bone disease. The clinical suspicion is confirmed by study of indices of copper metabolism.

The best screening test is to measure the serum ceruloplasmin level. Most patients with Wilson disease have decreased ceruloplasmin levels. The failure of copper to be incorporated into ceruloplasmin leads to a plasma protein with a shorter half-life and, therefore, a reduced steady state concentration of ceruloplasmin in the circulation. Caution should be used in interpreting serum ceruloplasmin levels, as they may be elevated in acute inflammation and in states of elevated estrogen such as pregnancy, estrogen supplementation, or oral contraceptive use. The serum copper level may be elevated in early Wilson disease, and urinary copper excretion (usually <40 µg/day) is increased to >100 µg/day and often up to 1,000 µg or more per day. In equivocal cases, the response of urinary copper output to chelation may be of diagnostic help. During the 24 hr urine collection patients are given two 500 mg oral doses of D-penicillamine 12 hr apart; affected patients excrete 1,200–2,000 µg/24 hr. Demonstration of Kayser-Fleischer rings, which may not be present in younger children, requires a slit-lamp examination by an ophthalmologist.

Liver biopsy is of value for determining the extent and severity of liver disease, and for measurement of the hepatic copper content (normally <10 µg/g dry weight). In Wilson disease, hepatic copper content exceeds 250 µg/g dry weight. In healthy heterozygotes, levels may be intermediate.

Family members of patients with proven cases require screening for presymptomatic Wilson disease. Such screening should include determination of the serum ceruloplasmin level and urinary copper excretion. If these results are abnormal or equivocal, liver biopsy should be carried out to determine morphology and hepatic copper content. Genetic screening by either linkage analysis or direct DNA mutation analysis is possible, especially if the mutation for the proband case is known or the patient is from an area where a specific mutation is known (in central and eastern Europe, the *H1069Q* mutation is present in 50–80% of patients).

TREATMENT. A major attempt should be made to restrict copper intake to <1 mg/day. Foods such as liver, shellfish, nuts, and chocolate should be avoided. If the copper content of the drinking water exceeds 0.1 mg/L, it may be necessary to demineralize. Administration of copper-chelating agents leads to rapid excretion of excess deposited copper in patients with Wilson disease. Chelation therapy is best managed with oral administration of D-penicillamine (β,β-dimethylcysteine) in a dose of 1 g/day in two doses before meals for adults and 20 mg/kg/day for pediatric patients. In response to penicillamine, urinary copper excretion markedly increases, and with continued administration, urinary copper levels may become normal, with marked improvement in hepatic and neurologic function and the disappearance of Kayser-Fleischer rings. However, 10–50% of patients initially treated with penicillamine for neurologic symptoms have a worsening of their condition. Toxic effects of penicillamine occur in 10–20% and consist of hypersensitivity reactions (Goodpasture syndrome, systemic lupus erythematosus, polymyositis), interaction with collagen and elastin, deficiency of other elements such as zinc, and aplastic anemia and nephrosis. Because penicillamine is an antimetabolite of vitamin B_6, additional amounts of this vitamin are necessary. For those patients who are unable to tolerate penicillamine, triethylene tetramine dihydrochloride (Trien, TETA, trientine) at a dose of 0.5–2.0 g/day for adults and 20 mg/kg/day for children is an acceptable alternative. Ammonium tetrathiomolybdate is another alternate chelating agent under investigation for patients with neurologic disease; initial results suggest that significantly fewer patients experience neurologic deterioration with this drug compared to penicillamine. The initial dose is 120 mg/day (20 mg between meals tid and 20 mg with meals tid). If a nighttime snack is eaten, another 20 mg is given with the snack. Side effects include anemia, leukopenia, thrombocytopenia, and mild elevations of transaminases. Zinc has also been used as adjuvant therapy, maintenance therapy, or primary therapy in presymptomatic patients, owing to its unique ability to impair the gastrointestinal absorption of copper. Zinc acetate is given in adults at a dose of 25–50 mg of elemental zinc three times a day, and 25 mg three times a day in children >5 yr of age.

PROGNOSIS. Untreated patients with Wilson disease die of the hepatic, neurologic, renal, or hematologic complications. The prognosis for patients receiving prompt and continuous penicillamine is variable and depends on the time of initiation of and the individual response to chelation. Liver transplantation should be considered for patients with fulminant liver disease, decompensated cirrhosis, or progressive neurologic disease; the latter indication remains controversial. Liver transplantation is curative with a survival rate of ≈85–90%. In asymptomatic siblings of affected patients, early institution of chelation therapy can prevent expression of the disease.

354.3 • Indian Childhood Cirrhosis

Copper also has a role in non-Wilsonian liver diseases that affect young children with other genetic and, as yet, mostly unknown abnormalities of copper metabolism. Indian childhood cirrhosis (ICC) occurs predominantly in rural areas in India and presents with jaundice, pruritus, lethargy, and hepatosplenomegaly. Histologically, it is characterized by hepatocyte necrosis, Mallory bodies, intralobular fibrosis, and inflammation. There is an increased hepatic copper content, usually >700 µg/g dry weight. ICC has been linked to excess dietary ingestion of copper primarily through the use of contaminated utensils used to feed babies animal milk. This high hepatic copper content cannot be completely explained by the amount ingested and suggests a genetic susceptibility to copper toxicosis. Untreated ICC has a mortality of 45% within 4 wk. Administration of penicillamine early in the course of disease at similar doses used to treat Wilson disease decreases the mortality rate by half. After education about the association between contaminated utensils and ICC, the incidence of ICC decreased as families found alternate feeding utensils. Variants of this syndrome have been named according to the population where it has been described, such as Tyrolean childhood cirrhosis. It has also been reported in the Middle East, West Africa, and North and Central America.

354.4 • Neonatal Iron Storage Disease (NISD)

NISD, also known as **neonatal hemochromatosis,** is a rare form of fulminant liver disease that presents in the 1st few days of life. Evidence of a gestational insult is given by the fact that affected infants may be born prematurely or with intrauterine growth retardation. Several infants with NISD also have renal dysgenesis. Clinically, NISD is a rapidly fatal, progressive illness characterized by hepatomegaly, hypoglycemia, hypoprothrombinemia, hypoalbuminemia, hyperferritinemia, and hyperbilirubinemia. The coagulopathy is refractory to therapy with vitamin K. The diagnosis can be confirmed through documentation of extrahepatic siderosis (biopsy material of buccal mucosal glands is laden with iron) or MRI determination of iron storage in organs such as the pancreas.

NISD has a high rate of recurrence in families, with ≈80% probability that subsequent infants will be affected. NISD may be a gestational alloimmune disease; the proposed target of the maternal alloimmune response is a fetal liver antigen. Recurrences of NISD may be modified with intravenous immunoglobulin (IVIg) administered to the mother once a week from the 18th week of gestation until delivery. The largest experience to date reports 18 women with previous infants with NISD who successfully delivered 22 babies (two sets of twins) after IVIg treatment. All infants survived with medical therapy or no therapy. The majority of babies had biochemical evidence of liver disease with elevated serum α-fetoprotein and ferritin. Liver biopsies were obtained in four patients and showed severe hepatitis with necrosis and iron deposition. Some patients with NISD have been successfully treated with iron chelating agents (deferoxamine) combined with aggressive antioxidant therapy. This may be effective if initiated very early. Liver transplantation should also be an early consideration.

354.5 • Miscellaneous Metabolic Diseases of the Liver

α_1-ANTITRYPSIN DEFICIENCY

A small percentage of individuals homozygous for deficiency of the major serum protease inhibitor α_1-antitrypsin manifest neonatal cholestasis or later onset childhood cirrhosis. α_1-Antitrypsin, a protease inhibitor synthesized by the liver, protects lung alveolar tissues from destruction by neutrophil elastase (see Chapter 389). α_1-Antitrypsin is present in >20 different codominant alleles, only a few of which are associated with defective protease inhibitors. The most common allele of the protease inhibitor (Pi) system is M, and the normal phenotype is PiMM. The Z allele predisposes to clinical deficiency; patients with liver disease are usually PiZZ and have serum α_1-antitrypsin levels <2 mg/mL (≈10–20% of normal). The incidence of the PiZZ genotype in the white population is estimated at 1/2,000–4,000. Compound heterozygotes PiZ-, PiSZ, PiZI have also been associated with liver disease, whereas the null genotype is not associated with liver disease.

Newly formed α_1-antitrypsin peptide normally enters the endoplasmic reticulum, where it undergoes enzymatic modification and folding before transport to the plasma membrane, where it is excreted as a 55kDa glycoprotein. In affected patients with PiZZ, the rate at which the α_1-antitrypsin peptide folds is decreased and this delay allows the formation of polymers that are retained in the endoplasmic reticulum. In liver biopsies from patients, polymerized α_1-antitrypsin peptides can be seen by electron microscopy and histochemically as PAS-positive diastase-resistant globules primarily in periportal hepatocytes but also in Kupffer cells and biliary epithelial cells. How the polymers cause liver damage is unknown. The pattern of neonatal liver injury can be highly variable and liver biopsies may demonstrate heptocellular necrosis, inflammatory cell infiltration, bile duct proliferation, periportal fibrosis, or cirrhosis.

In affected patients, the course of liver disease is also highly variable. Prospective studies in Sweden have shown that only 10% of patients develop clinically significant liver disease by their 4th decade. Genetic traits or environmental factors must influence the development of disease in α_1-antitrypsin deficient individuals. Infants with liver disease are indistinguishable from other infants with "idiopathic" neonatal hepatitis, of whom they constitute ≈5–10%. Jaundice, acholic stools, and hepatomegaly are present in the 1st wk of life, but the jaundice usually clears in the 2nd–4th mo. Complete resolution, persistent liver disease, or the development of cirrhosis may follow. Older children may present with asymptomatic hepatomegaly or manifestations of chronic liver disease or cirrhosis, with evidence of portal hypertension.

Liver transplantation has been curative.

Ala A, Walker AP, Ashkan K, et al: Wilson's disease. *Lancet* 2007;369:397–408.

Bosma PJ: Inherited disorders of bilirubin metabolism. *J Hepatol* 2003;38:107–117.

Bove KE, Daugherty CC, Tyson W, et al: Bile acid synthetic defects and liver disease. *Pediatr Dev Pathol* 2000;3:1–16.

Brewer GJ, Hedera P, Kluin KJ, et al: Treatment of Wilson disease with ammonium tetrathiomolybdate. *Arch Neurol* 2003;60:379–385.

Feranchak AP, Sokol RJ: Cholangiocyte biology and cystic fibrosis liver disease. *Semin Liver Dis* 2001;21:471–488.

Fox IJ, Chowdhury JR: Hepatocyte transplantation. *Am J Transplant* 2004;4:7–13.

Grabhorn E, Richter A, Burdelski M, et al: Neonatal hemochromatosis: Long-term experience with favorable outcome. *Pediatrics* 2006;118:2060–2065.

Grompe M: The pathophysiology and treatment of hereditary tyrosinemia type 1. *Semin Liver Dis* 2001;21:563–571.

Kadakol A, Ghosh SS, Sappal BS, et al: Genetic lesions of bilirubin uridine-diphosphoglucuronate glucuronosyltransferase (UGT1A1) causing Crigler-Najjar and Gilbert syndromes: Correlation of genotype to phenotype. *Hum Mutat* 2000;16:297–306.

Keitel V, Nies AT, Brom M, et al: A common Dubin-Johnson syndrome mutation impairs protein maturation and transport activity of MRP2 (ABCC2). *Am J Physiol Gastrointest Liver Physiol* 2003;284:G165–G174.

Kelley AL, Lunt PW, Rodrigues F, et al: Classification and genetic features of neonatal haemochromatosis: A study of 27 affected pedigrees and molecular analysis of genes implicated in iron metabolism. *J Med Genet* 2001;38:599–610.

Loudinos G, Gitlin JD: Wilson's disease. *Semin Liver Dis* 2000;20:353–364.

Mor-Cohen R, Zivelin A, Rosenberg N, et al: Identification and functional analysis of two novel mutations in the multidrug resistance protein 2 gene in Israeli patients with Dubin-Johnson syndrome. *J Biol Chem* 2001;276:36923–36930.
Perlmutter DH: Alpha-1-antitrypsin deficiency: Diagnosis and treatment. *Clin Liver Dis* 2004;8:839–859.
Primhak RA, Tanner MS: Alpha-1 antitrypsin deficiency. *Arch Dis Child* 2001;85:2–5.
Schilsky ML: Wilson disease: New insights into pathogenesis, diagnosis, and future therapy. *Curr Gastroenterol Rep* 2005;7:26–31.
Taly AB, Meenakshi-Sundaram S, Sinha S, et al: Wilson disease. Description of 282 patients evaluated over 3 decades. *Medicine* 2007;82:112–121.
Tanner MS: Role of copper in Indian childhood cirrhosis. *Am J Clin Nutr* 1998;67:1074S–1081S.
Tao TY, Gitlin JD: Hepatic copper metabolism: Insights from genetic disease. *Hepatology* 2003;37:1241–1247.
Whitington PF, Malladi P: Neonatal hemochromatosis: Is it an alloimmune disease? *J Pediatr Gastroenterol Nutr* 2005;40:544–549.

Chapter 355 ■ Viral Hepatitis

Nada Yazigi and William F. Balistreri

Viral hepatitis is a major health problem in both developing and developed countries. This disorder is caused by at least five pathogenic hepatotropic viruses recognized to date: hepatitis A, B, C, D, and E viruses (Table 355-1). Many other viruses can cause hepatitis, usually as one component of a multisystem disease; these include herpes simplex virus (HSV), cytomegalovirus (CMV), Epstein-Barr virus (EBV), varicella-zoster virus, HIV, rubella, adenoviruses, enteroviruses, parvovirus B19, and arboviruses. Hepatitis G virus (GBV) and transfusion transmissible virus (TTV) often infect the liver as a co-infection with another hepatotropic virus, and may produce acute or chronic viremia but rarely produce hepatocellular injury on their own.

The hepatotropic viruses are a heterogeneous group of infectious agents that cause similar acute clinical illness. In most pediatric-aged patients, the acute phase causes no or mild clinical disease. Morbidity is related to rare cases of **acute liver failure** triggered in susceptible patients and to the chronic disease state and attendant complications that three of these viruses (B, C, D) can cause. As the epidemiology of these forms of viral hepatitis varies widely geographically, so does their medical impact.

ISSUES COMMON TO ALL FORMS OF VIRAL HEPATITIS

DIFFERENTIAL DIAGNOSIS. Often what brings the patient to medical attention is clinical icterus, which, in hepatitis, is a mixed or conjugated (direct) reacting hyperbilirubinemia.

TABLE 355-1. Features of the Hepatotropic Viruses

	HAV	HBV	HCV	HDV	HEV	HGV*	TTV**
Virology	RNA	DNA	RNA	RNA	RNA	RNA	DNA
Incubation (days)	15–19	60–180	14–160	21–42	21–63	?	?
Transmission							
Parenteral	Rare	Yes	Yes	Yes	No	Yes	Yes
Fecal-oral	Yes	No	No	No	Yes	Possible	Possible
Sexual	No	Yes	Yes	Yes	No	Yes	Possible
Perinatal	No	Yes	Rare	Yes	No	Yes	Yes
Chronic infection	No	Yes	Yes	Yes	No	Yes	Yes
Fulminant disease	Rare	Yes	Rare	Yes	Yes	No	No

HAV, hepatitis A virus; ?, unknown
*Also called GBV-C (rarely produces liver disease, often co-infection)
**Transfusion transmissible virus (often co-infection with other hepatitis viruses, alone rarely causes liver disease)

In the **newborn period,** infection is a common cause of direct reacting hyperbilirubinemia; the infectious cause is either a bacterial agent *(Escherichia coli, Listeria)* or one of the non-hepatotropic viruses (HSV, enteroviruses, CMV). Metabolic and anatomic causes (tyrosinemia, biliary atresia, choledochal cysts) should always be excluded (see Chapter 353.1).

In later **childhood,** extrahepatic obstruction (gallstones, primary sclerosing cholangitis, pancreatic pathology), inflammatory conditions (autoimmune hepatitis, juvenile rheumatoid arthritis, Kawasaki disease, immune dysregulation), infiltrative disorders (malignancies), toxins/medications, metabolic disorders (Wilson disease, cystic fibrosis), and infection (EBV, varicella, malaria, leptospirosis, syphilis) should be ruled out.

PATHOGENESIS. The acute response of the liver to hepatotropic viruses involves a direct cytopathic as well as an immune-mediated injury. The entire liver is involved. Necrosis when present, is usually most marked in the centrilobular areas. An acute mixed inflammatory infiltrate predominates in the portal areas but also affects the lobules. The lobular architecture remains intact, although balloon degeneration and necrosis of single or groups of parenchymal cells occur frequently. Fatty change is rare except with HCV infection. Bile duct proliferation but not bile duct damage is common. Diffuse Kupffer cell hyperplasia is noticed in the sinusoids. Neonates often respond to hepatic injury by forming **giant cells.**

In **fulminant hepatitis,** parenchymal collapse occurs on the just described background. With recovery, the liver returns to its morphologic normal within 3 mo of the acute infection. If chronic hepatitis develops, the inflammatory infiltrate settles in the periportal areas and often leads to progressive scarring; both of these hallmarks of chronic hepatitis are seen in cases of HBV and HCV.

COMMON BIOCHEMICAL PROFILES IN THE ACUTE INFECTIOUS PHASE. Acute liver injury caused by the hepatotropic viruses manifests in three main functional liver biochemical profiles. These serve as an important guide to supportive care and monitoring in the acute phase of the infection for all viruses.

1. As a reflection of **cytopathic injury** to the hepatocytes, there is a rise in serum levels of alanine aminotransferase (ALT, formerly serum glutamic-pyruvic transaminase) and aspartate aminotransferase (AST, formerly serum glutamic-oxaloacetic transaminase). The magnitude of enzyme elevation does not correlate with the extent of hepatocellular necrosis and has little prognostic value. There is usually slow improvement in the levels over several weeks, but AST/ALT levels lag behind the serum bilirubin level, which tends to normalize first. Rapidly falling aminotransferase levels may predict a poor outcome, particularly if their decline occurs in conjunction with a rising bilirubin level and a prolonged prothrombin time (PT); this combination of findings usually indicates that massive hepatic injury has occurred.
2. **Cholestasis,** defined by elevated serum conjugated bilirubin levels, results from abnormal biliary flow at the canalicular and cellular level due to hepatocyte damage and inflammatory mediators. Elevation of serum alkaline phosphatase (ALP), 5′-nucleotidase, γ-glutamyl transpeptidase (GGT), and urobilinogen all mark cholestasis. Improvement tends to parallel the acute hepatitis phase. Absence of cholestatic markers does not rule out progression to chronicity in HCV or HBV infections.
3. The most important marker of liver injury is altered **synthetic function.** Monitoring of synthetic function should be the main focus in clinical follow-up to define the acuity of the disease. In the acute phase, the degree of liver synthetic dysfunction guides treatment and helps to establish intervention criteria. Abnormal liver synthetic function is a marker of **liver failure** and is an indication for prompt referral to a transplant center. Serial assessment is necessary because liver dysfunction does not progress linearly. Synthetic dysfunction is reflected by abnormal protein synthesis (prolonged prothrombin time, high INR, low serum albumin levels, hypoglycemia, lactic acidosis, hyperammonemia) or clinical signs, such as poor clearance of medications dependant on liver function and altered sensorium with increased deep tendon reflexes (hepatic encephalopathy; see Chapter 361).

HEPATITIS A

Hepatitis A virus (HAV) is the most prevalent of the five viruses in the United States and worldwide. This virus is also responsible for most forms of acute and benign hepatitis; although fulminant hepatic failure can occur, it is rare and occurs more often in adults than in children.

ETIOLOGY. HAV is an RNA virus, a member of the picornavirus family. It is heat stable and has limited host range—namely, the human and other primates.

EPIDEMIOLOGY. HAV infection occurs throughout the world but is most prevalent in the developing countries. In the United States, 30–40% of the adult population has evidence of previous HAV infection. Hepatitis A is thought to account for ≈50% of all clinically apparent acute viral hepatitis in the United States. As a result of aggressive implementation of a childhood vaccination strategy, the prevalence of symptomatic HAV cases in the United States has declined significantly. However, outbreaks in daycare centers (where the spread from young, non-icteric, infected children can occur easily) as well as multiple food and water-borne outbreaks in recent years have justified the implementation of a universal vaccination program in multiple states.

HAV is highly contagious. Transmission is almost always by person-to-person contact through the fecal-oral route. Parenteral transmission occurs rarely; no other form of transmission is recognized. HAV infection during pregnancy or at the time of delivery does not appear to result in increased complications of pregnancy or clinical disease in the newborn. In the United States, increased risk of infection is found in contacts with infected persons, child-care centers, and household contacts. Infection has also been associated with contact with contaminated food or water and after travel to endemic areas. Common source food-borne and water-borne outbreaks have occurred, including several due to contaminated shellfish, frozen berries, and raw vegetables; no known source is found in about half of the cases. The mean incubation period for HAV is ≈3 wk. Fecal excretion of the virus starts late in the incubation period, reaches its peak just before the onset of symptoms, and resolves by 2 wk after the onset of jaundice in older subjects. The duration of viral excretion is prolonged in infants. The patient is therefore contagious before clinical symptoms are apparent, and remains so until viral shedding stops.

CLINICAL MANIFESTATIONS. HAV is responsible for acute hepatitis only. Often, this is an anicteric illness, with clinical symptoms indistinguishable from other forms of viral gastroenteritis, particularly in young children.

The illness is much more likely to be symptomatic in older adolescents or adults, in patients with underlying liver disorders, and in those who are immunocompromised. It is characteristically an acute febrile illness with an abrupt onset of anorexia, nausea, malaise, vomiting, and jaundice. The typical duration of illness is 7–14 days (Fig. 355-1).

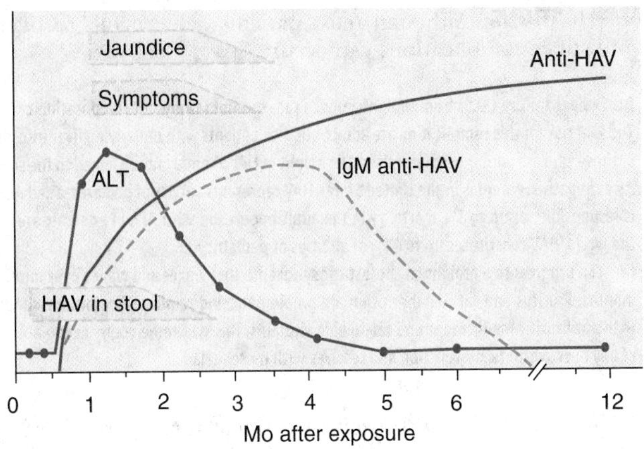

Figure 355-1. The serologic course of acute hepatitis A. ALT, alanine aminotransferase; HAV, hepatitis A virus. (From Goldman L, Ausiello D: *Cecil Textbook of Medicine*, 22nd ed. Philadelphia, Saunders, 2004, p 913.)

Other organ systems can be affected during acute HAV infection. Regional lymph nodes and the spleen may be enlarged. The bone marrow may be moderately hypoplastic, and aplastic anemia has been reported. Small intestinal tissue may show changes in villous structure, and ulceration of the gastrointestinal tract can occur, especially in fatal cases. Acute pancreatitis and myocarditis have been reported, though rarely, and nephritis, arthritis, vasculitis, and cryoglobulinemia can result from circulating immune complexes.

DIAGNOSIS. Acute HAV infection is diagnosed by detecting antibodies to HAV, specifically, anti-HAV (immunoglobulin [Ig] M) by radioimmunoassay or, rarely, by identifying viral particles in stool. A viral polymerase chain reaction (PCR) assay is available for research use (Table 355-2). Anti-HAV is detectable when the symptoms are clinically apparent, and remains positive for 4–6 mo after the acute infection. A neutralizing anti-HAV (IgG) is usually detected within 8 wk of symptoms onset, and is measured as part of a total anti-HAV in the serum, conferring long-term protection.

The virus is excreted in stools from 2 wk before to 1 wk after the onset of illness. Rises in ALT, AST, bilirubin, ALP, 5′-nucleotidase, and GGT are almost universally found and do not help to differentiate the cause of hepatitis.

TABLE 355-2. Diagnostic Blood Tests: Serology and Viral PCRs

	HAV	HBV	HCV	HDV	HEV
Acute Infection	Anti-HAV IgM (+) Blood PCR (+)*	Anti-HBc IgM (+) HBsAg (+) Anti-HBs HBV DNA (+) (PCR)	Anti-HCV (+) HCV RNA (+) (PCR)	Anti-HDV IgM (+) Blood PCR (+) HBsAg (+) Anti-HBs (−)	Anti-HEV IgM (+) Blood PCR (+)
Past infection (recovered)	Anti-HAV IgG (+)	Anti-HBs (+) Anti-HBc IgG (+)	Anti-HCV (−) Blood PCR (−)	Anti-HDV IgG (+) Blood PCR (−)	Anti-HEV IgG (+) Blood PCR (−)
Chronic infection	N/A	Anti-HBc IgG (+) HBsAg (+) Anti-HBs PCR (+) or (−)	Anti-HCV (+) Blood PCR (+)	Anti-HDV IgG (+) Blood PCR (−) HBsAg (+)	N/A
Vaccine response	Anti-HAV IgG (+)	Anti-HBs (+) Anti-HBc (−)	N/A	N/A	N/A

*Research tool.
HAV, hepatitis A virus; HBs, hepatitis B surface; HBsAg, hepatitis B surface antigen; Ig, immunoglobulin; PCR, polymerase chain reaction.

COMPLICATIONS. Although most patients achieve full recovery, two distinct complications can occur:

1. **Acute liver failure (ALF) from HAV infection, a rare but not infrequent complication of HAV. Those at risk for this complication are adults, but also patients with underlying liver disorders or those who are immunocompromised. The height of HAV viremia may be linked to the severity of hepatitis. Whereas in the United States, HAV represents <0.5% of pediatric-aged ALF, it is responsible for up to 3% mortality in the adult population with ALF. In endemic areas of the world, HAV constitutes up to 40% of all cases of pediatric ALF.**
2. **HAV can progress to a prolonged cholestatic syndrome that waxes and wanes over multiple months. Pruritus and fat malabsorption are problematic and require symptomatic support with antipruritic medications and fat-soluble vitamins. This syndrome occurs in the absence of any liver synthetic dysfunction and resolves with no sequelae.**

TREATMENT. There is no specific treatment for hepatitis A. Supportive treatment consists of intravenous hydration as needed and antipruritic agents and fat-soluble vitamins for the prolonged cholestatic form of disease. Serial monitoring for signs of acute liver failure and early referral to a transplantation center can be lifesaving.

PREVENTION. Patients infected with HAV are contagious for 2 wk before and about 7 days after the onset of jaundice and should be excluded from school, child care, or work during this period. Careful handwashing is necessary, particularly after changing diapers and before preparing or serving food. In hospital settings, contact and standard precautions are recommended for 1 wk after onset of symptoms.

Vaccine. The availability of two inactivated, highly immunogenic, and safe HAV vaccines has had a major impact on the prevention of HAV infection. Both vaccines are approved for children >1 yr of age. They are administered intramuscularly in a two-dose schedule, with the 2nd dose given 6–12 mo after the 1st dose. Seroconversion rates in children exceed 90% after an initial dose and approach 100% after the 2nd dose. The immune response in immunocompromised persons may be suboptimal. HAV vaccine can be administered simultaneously with other vaccines at separate sites. For persons >1 yr of age, vaccine is preferable to immunoglobulin for pre-exposure prophylaxis (Table 355-3). Greater consideration is being given, however, to other at-risk groups, including: (1) children >1 yr of age in defined and circumscribed communities with endemic rates or periodic outbreaks of HAV infection (e.g., Native Americans or Alaskan Natives); (2) patients with chronic liver disease; (3) individuals at occupational risk of exposure; and (3) persons with clotting factors and immune disorders. In the U.S. and some other countries, universal vaccination is recommended for all children >1 yr of age.

Mass immunization of school children has been used when epidemics have been school centered. The vaccine is effective in curbing outbreaks of hepatitis A and also when administered postexposure, due to rapid seroconversion and the long incubation period of the disease. Available data are still not sufficient, however, to recommend HAV vaccine alone for postexposure prophylaxis.

Immunoglobulin (Ig). Indications for intramuscular administration of Ig include pre-exposure and postexposure prophylaxis (see Table 355-3). Intravenous Ig is likely to be effective against HAV infection, but appropriate dose, efficacy, and duration of protection have not been defined. Ig is recommended for pre-exposure prophylaxis for all susceptible travelers to countries where HAV is endemic. For children >2 yr of age, HAV immunization is preferred if the interval before departure is >1 mo after dose 1. Ig as prophylaxis in postexposure situations is used for: (1) household and sexual contacts of HAV cases; (2) newborn infants of HAV-infected mothers; (3) child-care center staff, employees, children, and their household contacts during an outbreak; and (4) outbreaks in institutions and hospitals. The use of Ig >2 wk after exposure is not indicated. Ig is not routinely recommended for sporadic nonhousehold exposure (e.g., protection of hospital personnel or schoolmates).

TABLE 355-3. Hepatitis A Virus (HAV) Prophylaxis

AGE	EXPOSURE	DOSE
PRE-EXPOSURE PROPHYLAXIS (TRAVELERS TO ENDEMIC REGIONS)		
<1 yr	Expected <3 mo	Ig 0.02 mL/kg
	Expected 3–5 mo	Ig 0.06 mL/kg
	Expected long term	Ig 0.06 mL/kg at departure and every 5 mo thereafter
≥1 yr	Expected <3 mo	HAV vaccine* or IG 0.02 mL/kg
	Expected 3–5 mo	HAV vaccine* or IG 0.06 mL/kg
	Expected long term	HAV vaccine*
POSTEXPOSURE PROPHYLAXIS		
	≤2 wk since exposure	Ig 0.02 mL/kg and HAV vaccine if >1 yr and future exposure likely
	>2 wk since exposure	No prophylaxis. Consider HAV vaccine if >1 yr and future exposure likely

*Two inactivated vaccines are approved for use in persons ≥1 yr of age.
Ig, immunoglobulin.

PROGNOSIS. The prognosis is excellent, with no long-term sequelae. The only feared complication is ALF. HAV infection remains a cause of major morbidity, however, and has a high socioeconomic impact during epidemics and in endemic areas.

HEPATITIS B

ETIOLOGY. HBV is a member of the Hepadnaviridae family, which includes a hepatotropic group of DNA viruses. HBV has a circular, partially double-stranded DNA genome composed of ≈3,200 nucleotides. Four genes have been identified: the S (surface), C (core), X, and P (polymer) genes. The surface of the virus includes particles designated *hepatitis B surface antigen (HBsAg)*, which is a 22 nm diameter spherical particle and a 22 nm wide tubular particle with a variable length of up to 200 nm. The inner portion of the virion contains hepatitis B core antigen (HBcAg), the nucleocapsid that encodes the viral DNA, and a nonstructural antigen called hepatitis B e antigen (HBeAg), a nonparticulate soluble antigen derived from HBcAg by proteolytic self-cleavage. HBeAg serves as a marker of active viral replication and usually correlates with HBV DNA levels. Replication of HBV occurs predominantly in the liver but also occurs in the lymphocytes, spleen, kidney, and pancreas.

EPIDEMIOLOGY. HBV has a worldwide spread, with an estimated 400 million persons chronically infected. The areas of highest prevalence of HBV infection are sub-Saharan Africa, China, parts of the Middle East, the Amazon basin, and the Pacific Islands. In the United States, the Eskimo population in Alaska had the highest prevalence rate before the implementation of universal vaccination programs. An estimated 1.25 million persons in the United States are chronic HBV carriers, with ≈300,000 new cases of HBV occurring each year, the highest incidence being among adults 20–39 yr of age. One of four chronic HBV carriers will develop serious sequelae in their lifetime. The number of new cases in children reported each year is thought to be low but is difficult to estimate because many infections in children are asymptomatic. In the United States, since 1982 when the 1st vaccine for HBV was introduced, the overall incidence of HBV infection has been reduced by more than half. Since the implementation of universal vaccination programs in the United States, substantial progress has been made toward eliminating HBV infection in children.

HBV is present in high concentrations in blood, serum, and serous exudates and in moderate concentrations in saliva, vaginal fluid, and semen; efficient transmission occurs through blood exposure and sexual contact. Risk factors for HBV infection in children and adolescents include intravenous acquisition by drugs or blood products, acupuncture or tattoos, sexual contact, institutional care, and intimate contact with carriers. No risk factors are identified in ≈40% of cases. HBV is not thought to be transmitted via indirect exposure such as sharing toys. In children, the most important risk factor for acquisition of HBV remains perinatal exposure to an HBsAg-positive mother. The risk of transmission is greatest if the mother is also HBeAg positive; up to 90% of their infants become chronically infected if untreated; intrauterine infection occurs in 2.5% of their infants. In most cases, serologic markers of infection and antigenemia appear 1–3 mo after birth, suggesting that transmission occurred at the time of delivery; virus contained in amniotic fluid or in maternal feces or blood may be the source. Immunoprophylaxis of those infants is very effective in preventing infection and protects >95% of neonates. Of the 22,000 infants born each year to HBsAg-positive mothers in the United States, >98% receive immunoprophylaxis and are thus protected.

HBsAg is inconsistently recovered in human milk of infected mothers. Breast-feeding of nonimmunized infants by infected mothers does not confer a greater risk of hepatitis than does formula feeding.

The risk of developing **chronic HBV** infection, defined as being positive for HBsAg for >6 mo, is inversely related to age of acquisition. In the United States, although <10% of infections occur in children, these infections account for 20–30% of all chronic cases. This risk of chronic infection is 90% in children <1 yr; the risk is 30% for those 1–5 yr and 2% for adults. Chronic infection is associated with the development of chronic liver disease, as well as hepatocellular carcinoma. The carcinoma risk is independent of the presence of cirrhosis and was the most prevalent cancer-related death in young adults in Asia where HBV was endemic.

HBV has eight genotypes (A–H). A is pandemic, B and C are prevalent in Asia, D is seen in Southern Europe, E in Africa, F in the United States, G in the United States and France, and H in Central America. In addition, genetic variants have become resistant to antiviral agents. After infection, the incubation period ranges from 45 to 160 days, with a mean of about 120 days.

PATHOGENESIS. The acute response of the liver to HBV is the same as for all hepatotropic viruses. Persistence of histologic changes in patients with hepatitis B indicates development of chronic liver disease. HBV, unlike the other hepatotropic viruses, is a predominantly non-cytopathogenic virus that causes injury predominantly by immune-mediated processes. The severity of hepatocyte injury reflects the degree of the immune response, with the most complete immune response being associated with the greatest likelihood of viral clearance and the most severe injury to hepatocytes. The 1st step in the process of **acute hepatitis** is infection of hepatocytes by HBV, resulting in expression of viral antigens on the cell surface. The most important of these viral antigens may be the nucleocapsid antigens HBcAg and HBeAg. These antigens, in combination with class I major histocompatibility (MHC) proteins, make the cell a target for cytotoxic T-cell lysis. The mechanism for development of **chronic hepatitis** is less well understood. To permit hepatocytes to continue to be infected, the core protein or MHC class I protein may not be recognized, the cytotoxic lymphocytes may not be activated, or some other, yet unknown mechanism may interfere with destruction of hepatocytes. This **tolerance** phenomenon predominates in the cases acquired perinatally, resulting in a high incidence of chronic carrier state in those children with no or little inflammation in the liver. Although end-stage liver disease rarely develops, the inherent hepatocellular carcinoma risk is very high, possibly related, in part, to uncontrolled viral replication cycles.

Further, **ALF** has been seen in infants of chronic carrier mothers who have anti-HBe or are infected with a precore-mutant strain. This fact led to the postulate that HBeAg exposure in utero in infants of chronic carriers likely induces tolerance to the virus once infection occurs postnatally. In the absence of this tolerance, the liver is massively attacked by T cells and the patient presents with ALF.

Immune-mediated mechanisms are also involved in the **extrahepatic conditions** that can be associated with HBV infections. **Circulating immune complexes** containing HBsAg can occur in patients who develop associated polyarteritis nodosa, membranous or membranoproliferative glomerulonephritis, polymyalgia rheumatica, leukocytoclastic vasculitis, and Guillain-Barré syndrome.

CLINICAL MANIFESTATIONS. Many acute cases of HBV infection in children are asymptomatic, as evidenced by the high carriage rate of serum markers in persons who have no history of acute hepatitis. The usual acute symptomatic episode is similar to that of HAV and HCV infections but may be more severe and is more likely to include involvement of skin and joints (Fig. 355-2). The 1st biochemical evidence of HBV infection is elevation of ALT levels, which begin to rise just before development of lethargy, anorexia, and malaise, which occurs about 6–7 wk after exposure. The illness may be preceded in a few children by a serum sickness–like prodrome marked by arthralgia or skin lesions, including urticarial, purpuric, macular, or maculopapular rashes. Papular acrodermatitis, the Gianotti-Crosti syndrome, may also occur. Other extrahepatic conditions associated with HBV infections in children include polyarteritis, glomerulonephritis, and aplastic anemia. Jaundice, which is present in ≈25% of infected individuals, usually begins ≈8 wk after exposure and lasts for ≈4 wk. In the usual course of resolving HBV infection, symptoms are present for 6–8 wk. The percentage of children in whom clinical evidence of hepatitis develops is higher for HBV than for HAV, and the rate of ALF is also greater. Most patients do recover, but the "chronic carrier state" complicates up to 10% of cases acquired in adulthood. The rate of acquisition of chronic infection depends largely on the mode and age of acquisition, and is up to 90% in the perinatal cases. Chronic hepatitis cirrhosis and hepatocellular carcinoma are seen with chronic infection.

On physical examination, symptomatic infection results in icteric skin and mucous membranes. The liver is usually enlarged and tender to palpation and percussion. Splenomegaly and lymphadenopathy are common. Clinical signs of altered sensorium and hyper-reflexivity should be carefully looked for, as they mark the onset of encephalopathy and ALF (see Chapter 361).

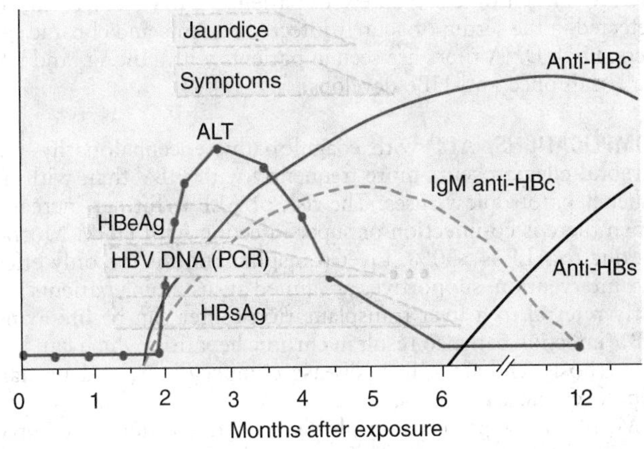

Figure 355-2. The serologic course of acute hepatitis B. HBc, hepatitis B core; HBeAG, hepatitis B e antigen; HBs, hepatitis B surface; HBsAg, hepatitis B surface antigen; HBV, hepatitis B virus; PCR, polymerase chain reaction. (From Goldman L, Ausiello D: *Cecil Textbook of Medicine,* 22nd ed. Philadelphia, Saunders, 2004, p 914.)

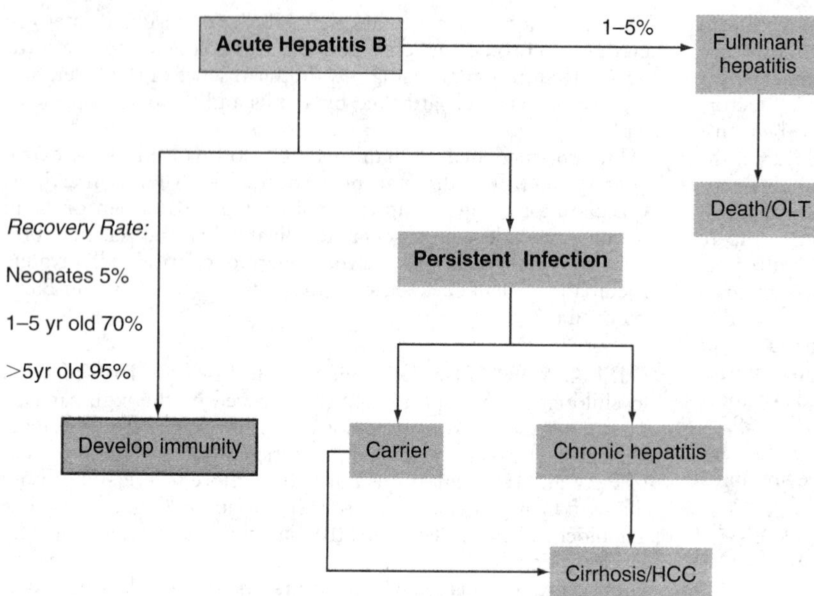

Figure 355-3. Natural history of hepatitis B virus (HBV) infection. HCC, hepatocellular carcinoma; OLT, orthotopic liver transplant.

DIAGNOSIS. The serologic profile of HBV infection is more complex than for HAV infection and differs depending on whether the disease is acute or chronic (Fig. 355-3). Several antigens and antibodies are used to confirm the diagnosis of acute HBV infection (see Table 355-2). Routine screening for HBV infection requires assay of at least three serologic markers (HBsAg, anti-HBc, anti-HBs). HBsAg is the 1st serologic marker of infection to appear and is found in almost all infected persons; its rise closely coincides with the onset of symptoms. Because HBsAg levels fall before symptoms wane, IgM antibody to HBcAg (anti-HBc IgM) helps to identify acute infection, as it rises early after infection and remains positive for many months before being replaced by anti-HBc IgG, which persists for years. Anti-HBc is the most valuable single serologic marker of acute HBV infection because it is present almost as early as HBsAg and continues to be present later in the course of the disease when HBsAg has disappeared. Anti-HBs marks serologic recovery and protection. Only anti-HBs is present in persons immunized with hepatitis B vaccine, whereas both anti-HBs and anti-HBc are detected in persons with resolved infection. HBeAg is present in active acute or chronic infections and is a marker of infectivity. The development of anti-HBe marks improvement and is a goal of therapy in chronically infected patients. HBV DNA can be detected in the serum of acutely infected patients and chronic carriers. High DNA titers are seen in patients with HBeAg, and typically fall once anti-HBe develops.

COMPLICATIONS. ALF with coagulopathy, encephalopathy, and cerebral edema occurs more frequently with HBV than with the other hepatotropic viruses. The risk of ALF is further increased when there is co-infection or super-infection with HDV. Mortality due to ALF is >30%. Liver transplantation is the only effective intervention; supportive care aimed at sustaining patients and early referral to a liver transplantation center can be lifesaving. HBV infection can also result in **chronic hepatitis,** which can lead to cirrhosis, end-stage liver disease complications, and primary **hepatocellular carcinoma.**

Membranous glomerulonephritis with deposition of complement and HBeAg in glomerular capillaries is a rare complication of HBV infection.

TREATMENT. No currently available medical therapy is reliably successful in the majority of persons infected with HBV. Treatment of the acute infection is largely supportive. Interferon-α-2b (IFN-α2b) and lamivudine (synthetic nucleoside analog) are the current therapies approved for treatment of **chronic** hepatitis B in adults >18 yr of age with compensated liver disease and HBV replication. IFN-α2b has also been used in children, with long-term eradication rates similar to the 25% rate reported in adults. Combination therapy in children using both agents did not seem to improve the rates of response. Recombinant interferons have immunomodulatory and antiviral effects whereas lamivudine inhibits the viral enzyme reverse transcriptase. Patients most likely to respond have low serum HBV DNA titers, are HBeAg positive, have active hepatic inflammation (ALT greater than twice the upper limit of normal), and recently acquired disease. Peginterferon-α2 and two new nucleotide/nucleoside analogs (adefovir dipivoxil and entecavir) are approved for use in adults. No data are yet available on their use in children. They seem to have an improved efficacy and less viral resistance than IFN-α2b or lamuvidine in the adult population. There is greater improvement among adults who are HBeAg positive chronic carriers when treated with entecavir than lamivudine. Treatment of chronic HBV infection in children should be individualized and done under the care of a pediatric gastroenterologist experienced in treating liver disease. The goal of treatment is cessation of active replication as manifested by HBeAg seroconversion. HBsAg seroconversion occurs in a minority of untreated patients.

PREVENTION. Hepatitis B vaccine and hepatitis B immunoglobulin (HBIG) are available for prevention of HBV infection. Two recombinant DNA vaccines are available in the United States; both are highly immunogenic in children. The safety profile of HBV vaccine is excellent. The most reported side effects are pain at the injection site (up to 29% of cases) and fever (up to 6% of cases).

Household, sexual, and needle-sharing contacts should be identified and vaccinated if they are susceptible to HBV infection. Patients should be advised about the perinatal and intimate contact risk of transmission of HBV. HBV is not spread by breast-feeding, kissing, hugging, or sharing water or utensils. Children with HBV should not be excluded from school, play, child care, or work, unless they are prone to biting. A support group might help children to cope better with their disease. All individuals positive for HBsAg should be reported to the state or local health department, and chronicity is diagnosed if they remain positive past 6 mo.

Hepatitis B Immunoglobulin. HBIG is indicated only for specific postexposure circumstances and provides only temporary protection (3–6 mo) [Table 355-4].

Universal Vaccination. In 2005, the Centers for Disease Control and Prevention (CDC) Advisory Committee on Immunization Practices revised its recommendations regarding HBV vaccination. These recommendations have been incorporated into the American Academy of Pediatrics Revised Vaccine schedule. A main focus is **universal infant vaccination,** beginning at birth, to provide a "safety net" for prevention of perinatal infection, prevent early childhood infection, facilitate implementation of universal vaccine recommendations, and prevent infection in adolescents and adults. The ultimate goal is to eliminate HBV transmission in the United States and to integrate HBV vaccination in a harmonized childhood vaccination.

Two single antigen vaccines (Recombivax HB and Engerix-B) are approved for children, and are the only preparations approved for infants <6 mo old. Three combination vaccines can be used for subsequent immunization dosing and enable integration of the HBV vaccine into the regular immunization schedule. Seropositivity is >95% with all vaccines, achieved after the 2nd dose in most patients. The 3rd dose serves as a booster and may have an effect on maintaining long-term immunity. In immunosuppressed individuals and infants <2,000 g birthweight, a 4th dose is recommended, as is checking for seroconversion. Despite declines in the anti-HBs titer in time, most vaccinated individuals remain protected against HBV infection.

Current vaccination recommendations are as follows (see Table 355-4):

1. For all medically stable infants weighing >2,000 g at birth and born to HBsAg-*negative* mothers, the 1st dose of HBV vaccine should be administered before hospital discharge; single-dose antigen HBV vaccine should be used for the birth dose. Subsequent doses to complete the series are given at 1–4 mo, and at 6–18 mo of age. Routine postvaccination testing of immunized infants born to HBsAg-negative women or with anti-HBs is not recommended.
2. In rare circumstances (on a case-by-case basis), the 1st dose may be delayed (up to 2 mo) until after hospital discharge. When a decision to delay is made, however, a physician's order to withhold the birth dose, along with a copy of the original laboratory report indicating that the mother was HBsAg *negative,* should be placed on the medical record.
3. Preterm infants weighing <2,000 g at birth and born to HBsAg-*negative* mothers should have their initial dose delayed until 1 mo of age or before hospital discharge.
4. Improve vaccine coverage of children and adolescents not previously vaccinated. To increase coverage, many states have made immunization a requirement for entry into junior high school.
5. Prevent **perinatal transmission** through improved maternal screening and immunoprophylaxis of infants born to HbsAg-**positive** mothers. **Infants born to HBsAg-positive women** should receive vaccine at birth, 1–2 mo, and 6 mo of age (see Table 355-4). The 1st dose should be accompanied by administration of 0.5 mL of HBIG as soon after delivery as possible (within 12 hr) because the effectiveness decreases rapidly with increased time after birth. Postvaccination testing for HBsAg and anti-HBs should be done at 9–18 mo. If the result is positive for anti-HBs, the child is immune to HBV. If the result is positive for HBsAg only, the parent should be counseled and the child evaluated by a pediatric gastroenterologist. If the result is negative for both HBsAg and anti-HBs, a 2nd complete hepatitis B vaccine series should be administered, followed by testing for anti-HBs to determine if subsequent doses are needed. Administration of four doses of vaccine is permissible when combination vaccines are used after the birth dose; this does not increase vaccine reactogenicity.

Postexposure Prophylaxis. Recommendations for postexposure prophylaxis for prevention of hepatitis B infection depend on the conditions under which the person is exposed to HBV (see Table 355-4). Vaccination should never be postponed if written records of the exposed individual's immunization history are not available, but every effort should still be made to obtain those records.

PROGNOSIS. In general, the outcome after acute HBV infection is favorable, despite a risk of ALF. The risk of developing chronic infection brings the risks of liver cirrhosis and hepatocellular carcinoma to the forefront. Perinatal transmission leading to chronicity is responsible for the high incidence of hepatocellular carcinoma in young adults in the endemic areas. Importantly, HBV infection and its complications are effectively controlled with vaccination.

HEPATITIS C

ETIOLOGY. HCV is the cause of most cases previously known as "transfusion-related non-A, non-B hepatitis." HCV is a single-

TABLE 355-4. Indications and Dosing Schedule for Hepatitis B Vaccine and Hepatitis B Immunoglobulin (HBIG)

	VACCINE DOSE		
	RECOMBIVAX HB (μg)	ENGERIX-B (μg)	SCHEDULE
UNIVERSAL PROPHYLAXIS			
Infants of HBsAg-negative women	5	10	Birth, 1–2, 6–18 mo
Children and adolescents (11–19 yr)	5	10	0, 1, and 6 mo
POSTEXPOSURE PROPHYLAXIS IN SUSCEPTIBLE INDIVIDUALS			
Contact with HBsAg-positive source			
Infants of HBsAg (+) women	5	10	Birth* *(+HBIG∫),* 1 and 6 mo
Intimate or identifiable blood exposure			
0–19 yr old	5	10	Exposure *(+HBIG∫),* 1 and 6 mo
>19 yr old	10	20	Exposure *(+HBIG∫),* 1 and 6 mo
Household			
0–19 yr old	5	10	Exposure, 1 and 6 mo
>19 yr old	10	20	Exposure, 1 and 6 mo
Casual	None	None	None
Immunocompromised¶	40	40	Exposure *(+HBIG∫),* 1 and 6 mo
Contact with unknown HBsAg status			
Intimate or identifiable blood exposure			
>19 yr old	10	20	Exposure, 1 and 6 mo
Immunocompromised¶	40	40	Exposure *(+HBIG∫),* 1 and 6 mo

*Both HBIG and vaccine should be administered within 12 hr of infant's birth, and within 24 hr of identifiable blood exposure. HBIG can be given up to 14 days after sexual exposure.
∫HBIG dose: 0.5 μL for newborns of HBsAg-positive mothers, and 0.06 μL/kg for all others when recommended.
¶Immunocompromised patients should have their seroconversion status checked 1–2 months after the last dose of vaccine, and yearly thereafter. Booster doses of vaccine should be administered if the anti-HBs titer is <10 mIU/mL. Nonresponsive patients should be considered at high risk for HBV acquisition and counseled about preventive measures.
HBs, hepatitis B surface; HBsAg, hepatitis B surface antigen; HBV, hepatitis B virus.

stranded RNA virus, classified as a separate genus within the Flaviviridae family, with marked genetic heterogeneity. It has six major genotypes and numerous subtypes and quasi-species, which permit the virus to escape host immune surveillance. Genotype variation may partially explain the differences in clinical course and response to treatment. Genotype 1b is the most common genotype in the United States, and the least responsive to the available medications.

EPIDEMIOLOGY. In the United States, HCV infection is the most common cause of chronic liver disease in adults and causes 8,000–10,000 deaths per year. About 4 million people in the United States and 170 million people worldwide are estimated to be infected with HCV. Approximately 85% of infected adults remain chronically infected. In children, sero-prevalence of HCV is 0.2% in children younger than 11 yr of age and 0.4% in children ≥11 yr of age.

Risk factors for HCV transmission in the United States previously included blood transfusion as the most common route of infection, but, with the current screening practices, the risk of HCV transmission is now about 0.001% per unit transfused. Illegal drug use with exposure to blood or blood products from HCV-infected individuals accounts for more than half of adult cases in the United States. Sexual transmission, especially through multiple sexual partners, is the 2nd most common cause of infection. Other risk factors include imprisonment and occupational exposure; ≈10% of new infections have no known transmission source. In children, perinatal transmission is the most prevalent mode of transmission (see Table 355-1). Vertical transmission occurs in up to 5% of infants born to viremic mothers. HIV co-infection and high viremia titers (HCV RNA positive) in the mother can increase the transmission rate to 20%. The incubation period is 7–9 wk (range of 2–24 wk).

PATHOGENESIS. The pattern of acute hepatic injury is indistinguishable from that of other hepatotropic viruses. In chronic cases, lymphoid aggregates or follicles in portal tracts are found, either alone or as part of a general inflammatory infiltration of the tracts. Steatosis is also often seen in these liver specimens. HCV appears to cause injury primarily by cytopathic mechanisms, but immune-mediated injury may also occur. The cytopathic component appears to be mild, as the acute illness is typically the least severe of all hepatotropic virus infections.

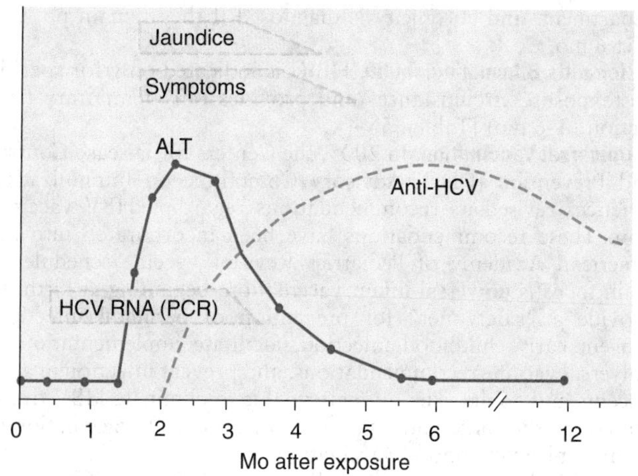

Figure 355-4. The serologic course of acute hepatitis C. HCV, hepatitis C virus; PCR, polymerase chain reaction. (From Goldman L, Ausiello D: *Cecil Textbook of Medicine,* 22nd ed. Philadelphia, Saunders, 2004, p 915.)

CLINICAL MANIFESTATIONS. Acute HCV infection tends to be mild and insidious in onset (Fig. 355-4; see also Table 355-1). Acute liver failure rarely occurs. However, HCV is the most likely hepatotropic virus to cause chronic infection (Fig. 355-5). In affected adults, <15% clear the virus; the rest develop chronic hepatitis. In pediatric studies, 6–19% of children achieved spontaneous sustained clearance of the virus during a 6 yr follow-up, regardless of the mode of acquisition. Chronic hepatitis C is also clinically silent until a complication develops. Serum aminotransferase levels fluctuate and are sometimes normal, but histologic inflammation is universal. Progression of liver fibrosis is slow over several years, unless co-morbid factors are present, which can accelerate fibrosis progression. About 25% of infected patients ultimately progress to cirrhosis, liver failure, and, occasionally, primary hepatocellular carcinoma (HCC) within 20–30 yr of the

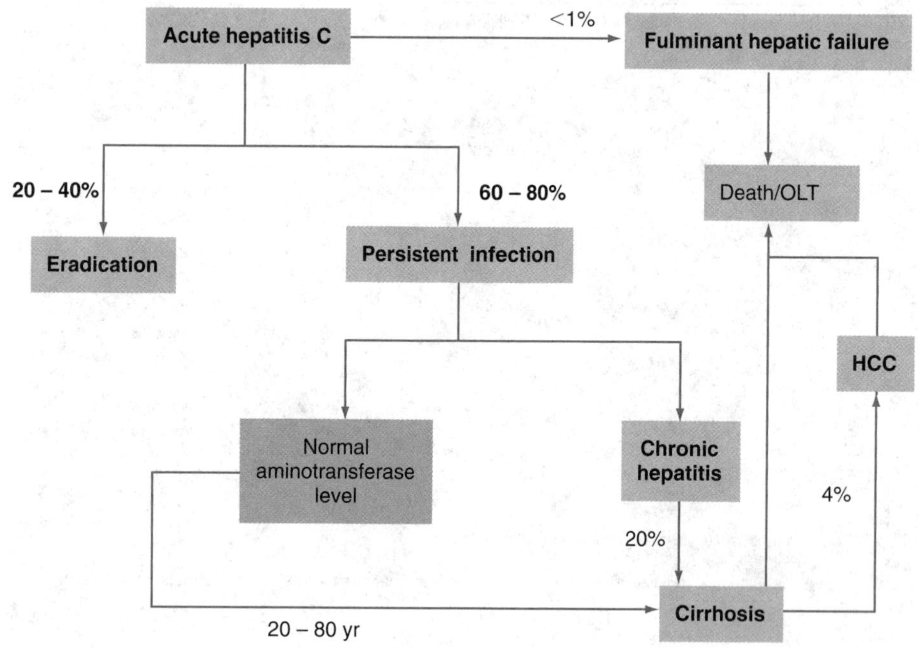

Figure 355-5. Natural history of hepatitis C virus (HCV) infection. HCC, hepatocellular carcinoma; OLT, orthotopic liver transplant. (From Hochman JA, Balistreri WF: Chronic viral hepatitis: Always be current! *Pediatr Rev* 2003;24: 399–410.)

acute infection. Although progression is rare within the pediatric age range, cirrhosis and HCC from HCV have been reported in children. The long-term morbidities constitute the rationale for diagnosis and treatment in children with HCV.

Chronic HCV infection can be associated with **small vessel vasculitis** and is a common cause of essential mixed cryoglobulinemia. Other extrahepatic manifestations predominantly seen in adults include cutaneous vasculitis, peripheral neuropathy, cerebritis, membranoproliferative glomerulonephritis, and nephrotic syndrome. Antibodies to smooth muscle, antinuclear antibodies, and low thyroid levels may also be present.

DIAGNOSIS. The clinically available assays for detection of HCV infection are based on detection of antibodies to HCV antigens or detection of viral RNA (see Table 355-2); neither can predict the severity of liver disease.

The most widely used **serologic test** is the third-generation enzyme immunoassay (EIA) to detect anti-HCV. The predictive value of this assay is greatest in high-risk populations, but the false-positive rate can be as high as 50–60% in low-risk populations. False-negative results also occur because antibodies remain negative for as long as 1–3 mo after clinical onset of illness. Anti-HCV is not a protective antibody and does not confer immunity; it is usually present simultaneously with the virus.

The most commonly used **virologic assay** for HCV is a PCR assay, which permits detection of small amounts of **HCV RNA** in serum and tissue samples within days of infection. The qualitative PCR detection is especially useful in patients with recent or perinatal infection, hypogammaglobulinemia, or immunosuppression and is very sensitive. The quantitative PCR aids in identifying patients who are likely to respond to therapy and in monitoring response to therapy.

Screening for HCV should include all patients with the following risk factors: history of illegal drug use (even if only once), receiving clotting factors made before 1987 (when inactivation procedures were introduced) or blood products before 1992, hemodialysis, idiopathic liver disease, and children born to HCV-infected women (qualitative PCR in infancy and anti-HCV after 12 mo of age). Routine screening of all *pregnant women* is not recommended.

Determining HCV **genotype** is also important, particularly when therapy is considered since the response to the current therapeutic agents varies greatly. Genotype 1 is poorly responsive; genotypes 2 and 3 are more reliably responsive to therapy (as discussed later).

Aminotransferase levels typically fluctuate during HCV infection and do not correlate with the degree of liver fibrosis.

A liver biopsy is the only means to assess the presence and extent of hepatic fibrosis, outside of overt signs of chronic liver disease. A liver biopsy is indicated only before starting any treatment and to rule out other causes of overt liver disease.

COMPLICATIONS. The risk of acute liver failure due to HCV is low, but the risk of **chronic hepatitis** is the highest of all the hepatotropic viruses. In adults, risk factors for progression to hepatic fibrosis include older age, obesity, male sex, and even moderate alcohol ingestion (two 1 oz drinks per day). Progression to cirrhosis or HCC is a major cause of morbidity and the most frequent indication for liver transplantation in adults in the United States.

TREATMENT. In adults, peginterferon (subcutaneous, weekly) combined with oral daily ribavirin is the most effective therapy; this combination is not approved for children at present. Patients most likely to respond have mild hepatitis, shorter duration of infection, and low viral titers. Genotypes 2 and 3 are the most sensitive to treatment; patients with genotype 1 virus respond poorly. The goal of treatment is to achieve a sustained viral response (SVR), as defined by the absence of viremia 6 mo after stopping the medications; SVR is associated with improved histology and decreased risk of morbidities.

The natural history of HCV infection in children is still being defined, but emerging data suggest that children have a higher likelihood of spontaneously clearing the virus as well as a lower risk of advanced or rapidly progressive liver disease. These features justify the current approach of serial monitoring and waiting for new, more effective therapies. There are rare reported cases of cirrhosis and even HCC seen in children. Shorter duration of infection and fewer co-morbid conditions than the adult counterpart would seemingly imply that children may be better candidates for treatment; given the adverse effects of currently available therapy, these authors do not recommend treatment outside of clinical trials.

Only IFN-α2b and ribavirin are approved for use by the Food and Drug Administration (FDA) in children >3 yr of age with HCV hepatitis. Studies of IFN monotherapy in children have shown a higher SVR than in adults, with better compliance and fewer side effects. A single study that evaluated combination therapy, showed a 49% SVR. Factors associated with a higher likelihood of response are age <12 yr, genotypes 2 and 3, and, in patients with genotype 1b, an RNA titer <2 million copies/mL of blood. Side effects of medications lead to discontinuation of treatment in a high proportion of patients; these include anemia, neutropenia, and influenza-like symptoms.

Treatment should be considered for all children infected with genotypes 2 and 3, as they have a high response rate to therapy. If the child has genotype type 1b virus, the treatment choice should be individualized, and offered only to patients with evidence of advanced fibrosis or injury on liver biopsy.

PREVENTION. No vaccine is available to prevent HCV. Immunoglobulin preparations are not beneficial. Immunoglobulin produced in the United States does not contain antibodies to HCV because blood and plasma donors are screened for anti-HCV and excluded from the donor pool. Once HCV infection is identified, patients should be screened yearly with a liver ultrasound and serum α-fetoprotein for HCC, as well as for any clinical evidence of liver disease. Vaccinating the affected patient against HAV and HBV will prevent super-infection with these viruses and the increased risk of developing severe liver failure.

PROGNOSIS. Viral titers should be checked yearly to document spontaneous remission. Most patients develop chronic hepatitis. Progressive liver damage is higher in those with additional co-morbid factors such as alcohol consumption, viral genotypic variations, and underlying genetic predispositions. Referral to a pediatric gastroenterologist is strongly advised to take advantage of up-to-date monitoring regimens and to optimize their enrollment in treatment protocols when available.

HEPATITIS D

ETIOLOGY. HDV, the smallest known animal virus, is considered defective because it cannot produce infection without a concurrent HBV infection. The 36 nm diameter virus is incapable of making its own coat protein; its outer coat is composed of excess HBsAg from HBV. The inner core of the virus is single-stranded circular RNA that expresses the HDV antigen.

EPIDEMIOLOGY. HDV cannot produce infection without HBV as a helper virus. HDV can cause an infection at the same time as the initial HBV infection (**co-infection**), or HDV can infect a person who is already infected with HBV (**super-infection**). Transmission usually occurs by intrafamilial or intimate contact in areas of high prevalence, which are primarily developing countries (see Table 355-1). In areas of low prevalence, such as the United States, the parenteral route is far more common. HDV infections are uncommon in children in the United States but must be considered when acute liver failure occurs. The incubation period for HDV super-infection is about 2–8 wk; with co-infection, the incubation period is similar to that of HBV infection.

PATHOGENESIS. Liver pathology in HDV hepatitis has no distinguishing features except that damage is usually quite severe. In contrast to HBV, HDV causes injury directly by cytopathic mechanisms. Many of the most severe cases of HBV infection appear to be a result of co-infection of HBV and HDV.

CLINICAL MANIFESTATIONS. The symptoms of hepatitis D infection are similar to but usually more severe than those of the other hepatotropic viruses. The clinical outcome for HDV infection depends on the mechanism of infection. In co-infection, acute hepatitis, which is much more severe than for HBV alone, is common, but the risk of developing chronic hepatitis is low. In super-infection, acute illness is rare and chronic hepatitis is common. The risk of ALF is highest in super-infection. Hepatitis D should be considered in any child who experiences acute liver failure.

DIAGNOSIS. HDV has not been isolated and no circulating antigen has been identified. The diagnosis is made by detecting IgM antibody to HDV; the antibodies to HDV develop ≈2–4 wk after co-infection and ≈10 wk after a super-infection. A test for anti-HDV antibody is commercially available. PCR assays for viral RNA are available as research tools (see Table 355-2).

COMPLICATIONS. HDV must be considered in all cases of ALF. Co-infection with HBV can also result in a more severe chronic disease.

TREATMENT. The treatment is based on supportive measures once an infection is identified. There are no specific HDV-targeted treatments to date. The treatment is mostly based on controlling and treating HBV infection, without which HDV cannot induce hepatitis.

PREVENTION. There is no vaccine for hepatitis D. Because HDV replication cannot occur without hepatitis B co-infection immunization against HBV also prevents HDV infection. Hepatitis B vaccines and HBIG are used for the same indications as for hepatitis B alone.

HEPATITIS E

ETIOLOGY. HEV has not been isolated but has been cloned using molecular techniques. This RNA virus has a non-enveloped sphere shape with spikes and is similar in structure to the caliciviruses.

EPIDEMIOLOGY. Hepatitis E is the epidemic form of what was formally called non-A, non-B hepatitis. Transmission is fecal-oral (often water-borne) and is associated with shedding of 27–34 nm particles in the stool (see Table 355-1). The highest prevalence of HEV infection has been reported in the Indian subcontinent, the Middle East, Southeast Asia, and Mexico, especially in areas with poor sanitation. In the United States, the only reported cases have been in persons who have visited or emigrated from endemic areas. The mean incubation period is ≈40 days (range of 15–60 days).

PATHOGENESIS. HEV appears to act as a cytopathic virus. The pathologic findings are similar to those of the other hepatitis viruses.

CLINICAL MANIFESTATIONS. The clinical illness associated with HEV infection is similar to HAV but is often more severe. As with HAV, chronic illness does not occur. In addition to often causing a more severe episode than HAV, HEV tends to affect older patients with a peak age between 15 and 34 yr. HEV is a major pathogen in pregnant women, in whom it causes ALF with a high fatality incidence.

COMPLICATIONS. HEV is associated with a high risk of death in pregnant women. No other complications are recognized in association with this virus.

DIAGNOSIS. Recombinant DNA technology has resulted in development of antibodies to HEV particles, and IgM and IgG assays are available to distinguish between acute and resolved infections (see Table 355-2). IgM antibody to viral antigen becomes positive after ≈1 wk of illness. Viral RNA can be detected in stool and serum by PCR.

PREVENTION. A recombinant hepatitis E vaccine is highly effective in adults. No evidence suggests that immunoglobulin is effective in preventing HEV infections. Immunoglobulin pooled from patients in endemic areas may prove to be effective.

APPROACH TO ACUTE OR CHRONIC HEPATITIS

Although new treatment modalities for chronic viral hepatitis are continuously being developed, and treatment outcomes have improved, the major medical breakthrough in regard to the pediatric population is prevention, with the availability of effective and safe vaccines for the HAV and HBV infections. The availability of more sensitive and reliable diagnostic tools may lead to improved care for affected patients. The primary care physician is at the forefront of the care and control of patients exposed to these viruses. Aggressive perinatal, childhood, and adolescent immunization strategies have already had a major impact in endemic HAV and HBV areas.

Identifying deterioration of the patient with acute hepatitis and the development of acute liver failure is a major contribution of the primary pediatrician (Fig. 355-6). If ALF is identified, the clinician should immediately refer the patient to a transplant center; this can be lifesaving.

Once chronic infection is identified, close follow-up and referral to a pediatric gastroenterologist is recommended to enroll the patient in appropriate treatment trials. Treatment of both chronic HBV and HCV in children should preferably be delivered within controlled trials, as indications, timing, regimen, and outcomes remain to be defined and cannot simply be extrapolated from adult data. All patients with chronic viral hepatitis should avoid, as much as possible, further insult to the liver: HAV vaccine is recommended, avoid alcohol consumption, and exercise care when taking new medications, including over-the-counter drugs and herbal medications.

International adoption and ease of travel continue to change the epidemiology of these viruses. In the United States, chronic HBV and HCV have a high prevalence among international adoptee patients; vigilance is required to establish early diagnosis in order to offer appropriate treatment as well as prophylactic measures to limit viral spread.

Chronic hepatitis can be a stigmatizing disease for children and their families. The pediatrician should offer, with proactive advocacy, appropriate support for them as well as needed education for their social circle. Scientific data and information about support groups are available for families on the websites for the American Liver Foundation (www.liverfoundation-ne.org) and the North American Society for Pediatric Gastroenterology, Hepatology and Nutrition (www.naspghan.org), as well as through pediatric gastroenterology centers.

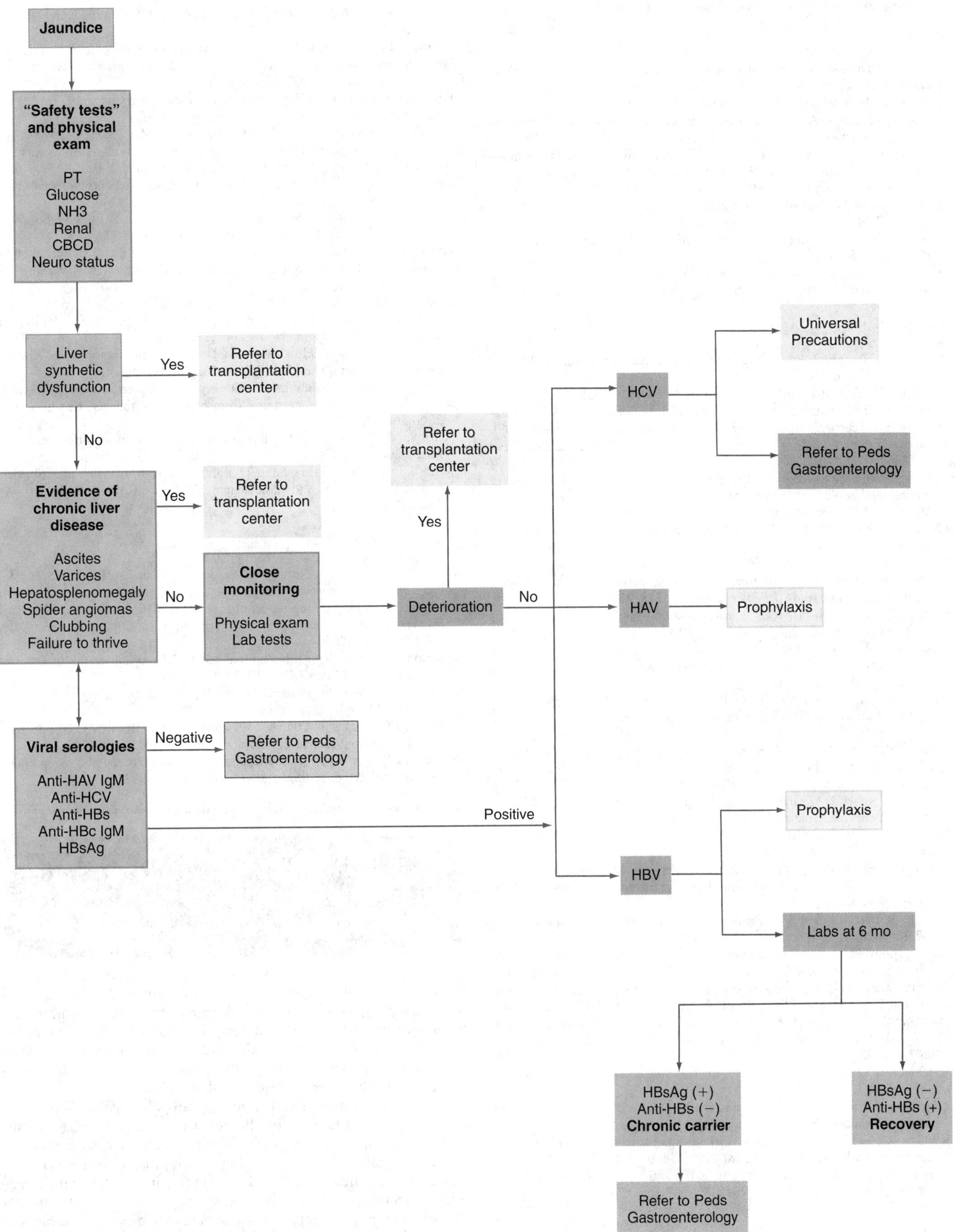

Figure 355-6. Clinical approach to viral hepatitis. CBCD, complete blood count with differential; HAV, hepatitis A virus; HBs, hepatitis B surface; HBsAg, hepatitis B surface antigen; HBV, hepatitis B virus; HCV, hepatitis C virus; IgM, immunoglobulin M; NH_3, ammonia; PT, prothrombin time.

Hepatitis A

Centers for Disease Control and Prevention (CDC): Multistate outbreak of hepatitis A among young adult concert attendees—United States, 2003. *MMWR Morb Mortal Wkly Rep* 2003;52:844–845.

Dagan R, Leventhal A, Anis E, et al: Incidence of hepatitis A in Israel following universal immunization of toddlers. *JAMA* 2005;294:202–210.

Nainan OV, Armstrong GL, Han XH, et al: Hepatitis A molecular epidemiology in the United States, 1996–1997: Sources of infection and implications of vaccination policy. *J Infect Dis* 2005;191:957–963.

Rein DB, Fiore AE, Bell BP: What's next for the hepatitis A vaccine? *Lancet* 2006;367:546–548.

Temte JL: Should all children be immunized against hepatitis A? *Br Med J* 2006;332:715–718.

Wheeler C, Vogt TM, Armstrong GL: An outbreak of hepatitis A associated with green onions. *N Engl J Med* 2005;353:890–897.

Hepatitis B

Aggarwal R, Ranjan P: Preventing and treating hepatitis B infection. *Br Med J* 2004;329:1080–1086.

Beeching NJ: Hepatitis B infections. *Br Med J* 2004;329:1059–1060.

Boxall EH, Sira J, Standish RA, et al: Natural history of hepatitis B in perinatally infected carriers. *Arch Dis Child Fetal Neonatal Ed* 2004;89:F456–F460.

Broderick A, Jonas MM: Management of hepatitis B in children. *Clin Liver Dis* 2004;8:387–401.

Centers for Disease Control and Prevention (CDC): Acute hepatitis B among children and adolescents, United States, 1990–2002. *MMWR Morb Mortal Wkly Rep* 2004;53:1015–1018.

Chang TT, Gish RG, de Man R, et al: A comparison of entecavir and lamivudine for HBeAg-positive chronic hepatitis B. *N Engl J Med* 2006;354:1001–1010.

D'Antiga L, Aw M, Mieli-Vergani G, et al: Combined lamuvidine/interferon alpha treatment in immunotolerant children perinatally infected with hepatitis B: A pilot study. *J Pediatr* 2006;148:228–233.

Ganem D, Prince AM: Hepatitis B virus infection—Natural history and clinical consequences. *N Engl J Med* 2004;350:1118–1129.

Hadziyannis SJ, Tassopoulos NC, Heathcoate EJ, et al: Long-term therapy with adefovir dipivoxil for HBeAg-negative chronic hepatitis B. *N Engl J Med* 2005;352:2673–2681.

Hadziyannis SJ, Tassopoulos NC, Heathcoate EJ, et al: Adefovir dipivoxil for the treatment of hepatitis B e antigen–negative chronic hepatitis B. *N Engl J Med* 2003;348:800–806.

Janssen HLA, van Zonneveld M, Senturk H, et al: Pegylated interferon alfa-2b alone or in combination with lamivudine for HBeAg-positive hepatitis B: A randomised trial. *Lancet* 2005;365:123–128.

Jonas MM, Kelley DA, Mizerski J, et al: Clinical trial of lamivudine in children with chronic hepatitis B. *N Engl J Med* 2002;346:1706–1713.

Kao JH, Chen DS: Hepatitis B vaccination: To boost or not to boost? *Lancet* 2005;366:1337–1338.

Kobak GE, MacKenzie T, Sokol RJ, et al: Interferon treatment for chronic hepatitis B: Enhanced response in children 5 years old or younger. *J Pediatr* 2004;145:340–345.

Lai CL, Ratziu V, Yuen MF, Poynard T: Viral hepatitis B. *Lancet* 2003; 362:2089–2094.

Lai CL, Shouval D, Lok AS, et al: Entecavir versus lamivudine for patients with HBeAg-negative chronic hepatitis B. *N Engl J Med* 2006;354:1011–1020.

Liaw YF, Sung JJY, Cheng Chow W, et al: Lamivudine for patients with chronic hepatitis B and advanced liver disease. *N Engl J Med* 2004;351:1521–1530.

Marcellin P, Chang TT, Gee Lim S, et al: Adefovir dipivoxil for the treatment of hepatitis B e antigen–positive chronic hepatitis B. *N Engl J Med* 2003;348:808–816.

The Medical Letter: Telbivudine *(Tyzeka)* for chronic hepatitis B. *Med Lett* 2007;49:11–12.

Poland GA, Jacobson RM: Clinical practice: Prevention of hepatitis B with the hepatitis B vaccine. *N Engl J Med* 2004;351:2832–2838.

Schildgen O, Sirma H, Funk A, et al: Variant of hepatitis B virus with primary resistance to adefovir. *N Engl J Med* 2006;354:1807–1812.

Yang HI, Lu SN, Liaw YF, et al: Hepatitis B e antigen and the risk of hepatocellular carcinoma. *N Engl J Med* 2002;347:168–174.

Hepatitis C

Bair RM, Baillargeon JG, Kelly PJ, et al: Prevalence and risk factors for hepatitis C virus infection among adolescents in detention. *Arch Pediatr Adolesc Med* 2005;159:1015–1018.

Cagle HH, Jacob J, Homan CE, et al: Results of a general hepatitis C lookback program for persons who received blood transfusions in a neonatal intensive care unit between January 1975 and July 1992. *Arch Pediatr Adolesc Med* 2007;161:125–130.

Carrat F, Bani-Sadr F, Pol S, et al: Pegylated interferon alfa-2b vs standard interferon alfa-2b, plus ribavirin, for chronic hepatitis C in HIV-infected patients. *JAMA* 2004;292:2839–2848.

Elisofon SA, Jonas MM: Hepatitis B and C in children: Current treatment and future strategies. *Clin Liver Dis* 2006;10:133–148.

Flamm SL: Chronic hepatitis C virus infection. *JAMA* 2003;289:2413–2417.

Fried MW, Shiffman ML, Reddy R, et al: Peginterferon alfa-2a plus ribavirin for chronic hepatitis C virus infection. *N Engl J Med* 2002;347:975–982.

Hoofnagle JH, Seeff LB: Peginterferon and ribavirin for chronic hepatitis C. *N Engl J Med* 2006;355:2444–2451.

Iorio R, Giannattasio A, Sepe A, et al: Chronic hepatitis C in childhood: An 18-year experience. *Clin Infect Dis* 2005;41:1431–1437.

Jara P, Resti M, Hierro L, et al: Chronic hepatitis C virus infection in childhood: Clinical patterns and evolution in 224 white children. *Clin Infect Dis* 2003;36:275–280.

Mast EE, Hwang LY, Seto DSY, et al: Risk factors for perinatal transmission of hepatitis C virus (HCV) and the natural history of HCV infection acquired in infancy. *J Infect Dis* 2005;192:1880–1889.

Patel K, Muir AJ, McHutchison JG: Diagnosis and treatment of chronic hepatitis C infection. *Br Med J* 2006;332:1013–1017.

Poynard T, Yuen MF, Ratziu V, Lai CL: Viral hepatitis C. *Lancet* 2003;362:2095–2100.

Schiff ER: Prevention of mortality from hepatitis B and hepatitis C. *Lancet* 2006;368:896–897.

Vento S, Nobili V, Cainelli F: Clinical course of infection with hepatitis C. *Br Med J* 2006;332:374–375.

Wirth S, Pieper-Boustani H, Lang T, et al: Peginterferon alfa-2b plus ribavirin treatment in children and adolescents with chronic hepatitis C. *Hepatology* 2005;41:1013–1018.

Other Viral Agents

Chang MH, Hadzic D, Rouassant AH, et al: Asian Pan-Pacific Society for Pediatric Gastroenterology, Hepatology, and Nutrition: Acute and chronic hepatitis: Working Group report of the Second World Congress of Pediatric Gastroenterology, Hepatology, and Nutrition. *J Pediatr Gastroenterol Nutr* 2004;39:S584–S588.

Emerson SU, Purcell RH: Running like water—The omnipresence of hepatitis E. *N Engl J Med* 2004;351:2367–2368.

Kelly D, Skidmore S: Hepatitis C–Z: Recent advances. *Arch Dis Child* 2002;86:339–343.

Mehrishi JN, Bakács T: HIV and hepatitis G virus/GB virus C co-infection: Beneficial or not? *Lancet* 2005;5:464–466.

Shrestha MP, Scott RM, Joshi DM, et al: Safety and efficacy of a recombinant hepatitis 5 vaccine. *N Engl J Med* 2007;356:895–902.

Chapter 356 ■ Liver Abscess

Stavra A. Xanthakos and William F. Balistreri

Pyogenic liver abscesses are rare in children. In developed countries, liver abscesses most often occur in the setting of immunosuppression (40–45% of cases); by contrast, in developing countries, malnutrition, sepsis, and parasitic infections play a greater role. Pyogenic hepatic abscesses can be caused by bacteria entering the liver via the portal circulation in cases of pylephlebitis, intra-abdominal infection or abscess secondary to appendicitis or inflammatory bowel disease, or generalized sepsis; ascending cholangitis associated with biliary tract obstruction caused by gallstones or sclerosing cholangitis, after a Kasai procedure, or secondary to choledochal cysts; and cryptogenic biliary tract infections. Very rarely, liver abscesses occur after percutaneous liver biopsy. Hepatic abscesses can also occur in infants in association with sepsis, umbilical vein infection, or cannulation. In adults with pyogenic liver abscesses, liver transplantation has emerged as a significant risk factor; it is not known if pediatric liver transplant patients are also at increased risk.

In children with pyogenic liver abscesses, the most common pathogenic organisms include *Staphylococcus aureus, Strepto-*

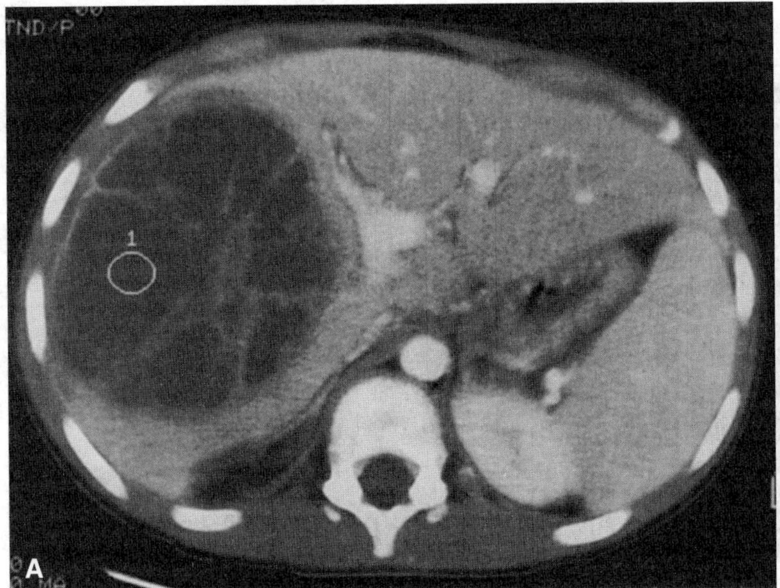

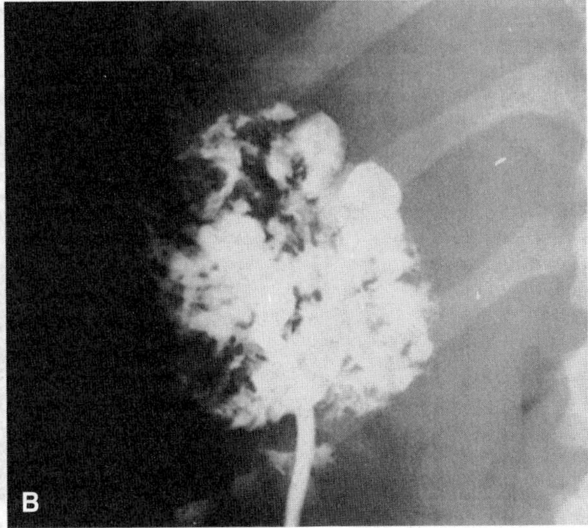

Figure 356-1. Liver abscess. *A,* Contrast-enhanced CT scan demonstrates a multioculated septated mass of decreased attenuation in the right lobe of the liver. There is increased attenuation of the septa. There is also faintly seen edema between the abscess and the enhanced normal liver. *B,* Injection of contrast material after percutaneous drainage of this documented streptococcal abscess demonstrates the multiocular nature of the lesion and its irregularly marginated wall. (From Kuhn JP, Slovis TL, Haller JO: *Caffrey's Pediatric Diagnostic Imaging,* vol 2, 10th ed. Philadelphia, Mosby, 2004, p 1470.)

coccus spp., *Escherichia coli, Salmonella,* and anaerobic organisms; *Entamoeba histolytica* or *Toxocara canis*–associated liver abscesses have also been reported in developing countries or endemic areas. In adult patients, *Klebsiella* spp. have emerged as a significant cause of pyogenic liver abscesses and are also associated with increased risk of metastatic septic endopthalmitis, especially in patients with diabetes mellitus. Microabscesses are most commonly secondary to bacteremia, candidemia, or cat scratch disease. Multiple infectious hepatic (and/or splenic) granulomas can also be seen with cat scratch disease or fungi.

Signs and symptoms are nonspecific and can include fever, chills, night sweats, malaise, fatigue, nausea, abdominal pain with right upper quadrant tenderness, and mild hepatomegaly; jaundice is uncommon. Diagnosis can be challenging and is often delayed; a high index of suspicion is necessary in children with risk factors. Serum aminotransferase and alkaline phosphatase levels may be mildly elevated. The erythrocyte sedimentation rate is high, and leukocytosis may be noted. The results of blood cultures are not always positive. Chest roentgenographs may show elevation of the right hemidiaphragm with decreased mobility or a right pleural effusion. Ultrasound or CT can confirm diagnosis (Figs. 356-1, 356-2, and 356-3). Solitary liver abscesses in the right lobe of the liver are more common than multiple abscesses or solitary left lobe abscesses. **Treatment** requires percutaneous ultrasonogram- or CT-guided needle aspiration and, in some cases, open surgical drainage, particularly if multiple or large

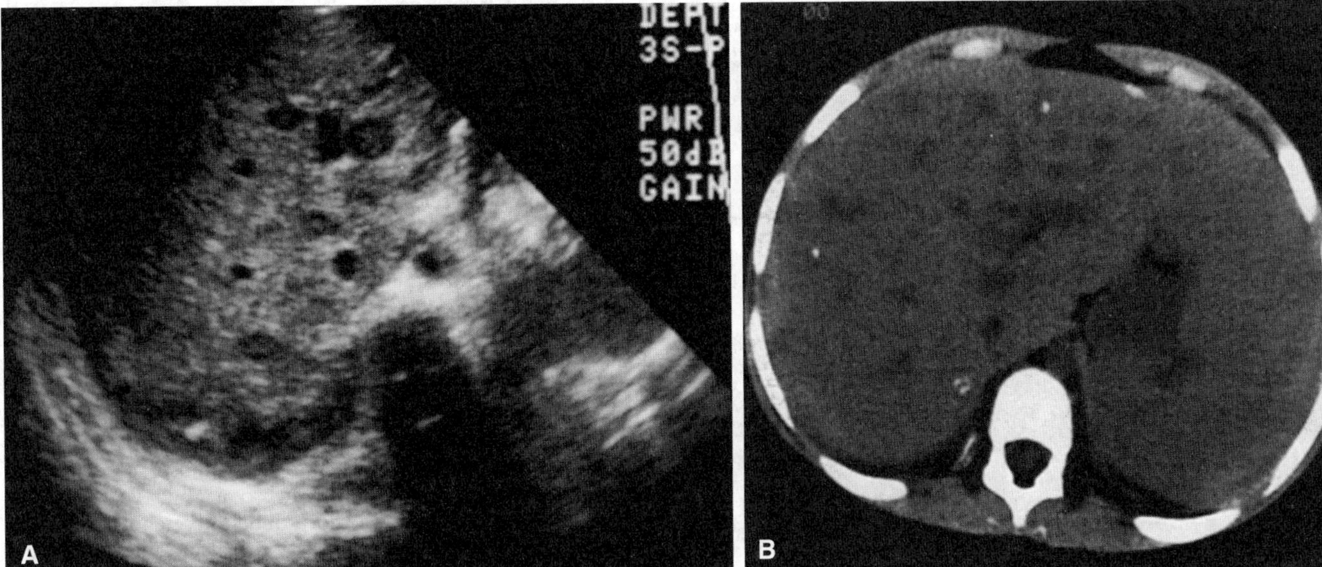

Figure 356-2. Hepatic candidiasis. Transverse sonogram *(A)* and CT scan *(B)* of the upper abdomen demonstrate "bull's-eye" lesions in the right lobe of the liver in an immunocompromised patient. The calcifications seen on the CT scan are presumed to represent sequelae of prior infection. Liver biopsy demonstrated candidiasis. (From Kuhn JP, Slovis TL, Haller JO: *Caffrey's Pediatric Diagnostic Imaging,* vol 2, 10th ed. Philadelphia, Mosby, 2004, p 1472.)

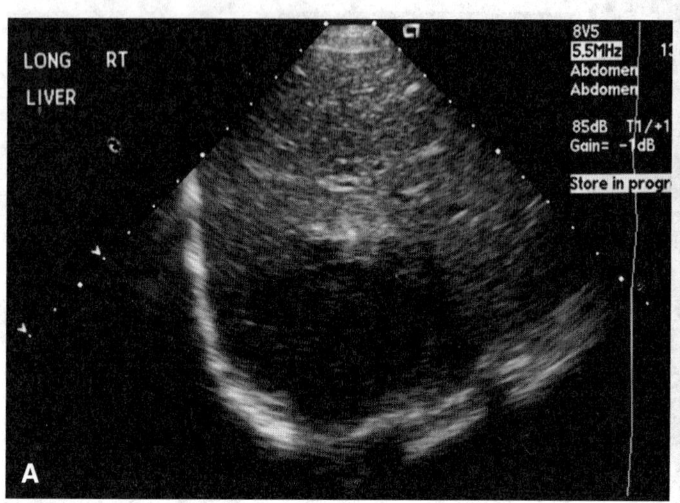

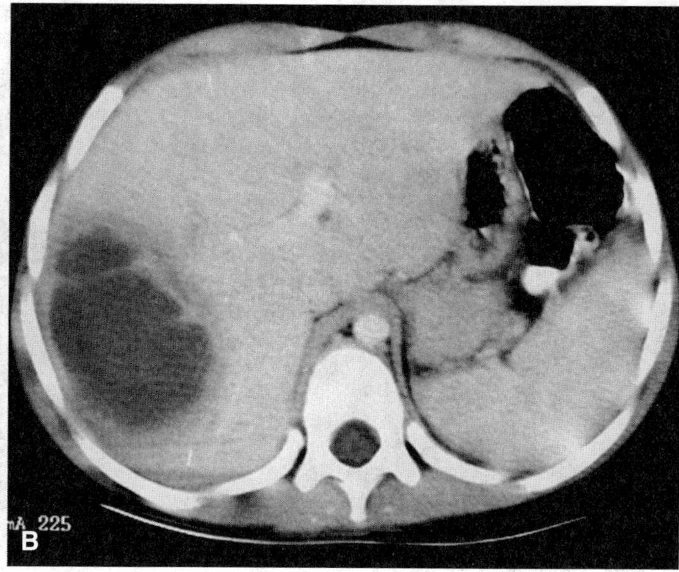

Figure 356-3. Amebic abscess. *A,* Sonogram demonstrates a hypoechogenic mass in the right lobe of the liver with a more hypoechoic surrounding rim. *B,* CT scan demonstrates a low-attenuation mass in the right lobe of the liver with a prominent halo. (From Kuhn JP, Slovis TL, Haller JO: *Caffrey's Pediatric Diagnostic Imaging,* vol 2, 10th ed. Philadelphia, Mosby, 2004, p 1473.)

abscesses are present. Aerobic and anaerobic cultures should be obtained. Antibiotic therapy should initially be broad spectrum but then narrowed, based on the culture results of the abscess fluid. Antibiotic therapy is intravenous and prolonged for at least 4–8 wk, although no evidence-based data exist to guide duration. Mortality has decreased significantly in the past three decades with early diagnosis and initiation of appropriate therapy.

Fung CP, Change SC, Hu BS, et al: A global emerging disease of *Klebsiella pneumoniae* liver abscess: Is serotype K1 an important factor for complicated endopthalmitis? *Gut* 2002;50:420–424.

Kaplan GG, Gregson DB, Laupland KB: Population-based study of the epidemiology of and the risk factors for pyogenic liver abscess. *Clin Gastroenterol Hepatol* 2004;2:1032–1038.

Kumar A, Srinivasan S, Sharma AK: Pyogenic liver abscess in children—South Indian experiences. *J Pediatr Surg* 1998;33:417–421.

Margalit M, Elinav H, Ilan Y, et al: Liver abscess in inflammatory bowel disease: Report of two cases and review of the literature. *J Gastroenterol Hepatol* 2004;19:1338–1342.

Pereira FE, Musso C, Castelo JS: Pathology of pyogenic liver abscess in children. *Pediatr Dev Pathol* 1999;2:537–543.

Pineiro-Carrero VM, Andres JM: Morbidity and mortality in children with pyogenic liver abscess. *Am J Dis Child* 1989;143:1424–1427.

Chapter 357 ■ Liver Disease Associated with Systemic Disorders

Stavra A. Xanthakos and William F. Balistreri

Liver disease is found in a wide variety of systemic illnesses, both as a result of the primary pathologic process and as a secondary complication of the disease or associated therapy.

INFLAMMATORY BOWEL DISEASE (IBD). Ulcerative colitis and Crohn disease (see Chapter 333) are associated with hepatobiliary disease that includes autoimmune and inflammatory processes related to IBD (sclerosing cholangitis, autoimmune hepatitis), drug toxicity (mercaptopurine, methotrexate, 6-thioguanine), malnutrition and disordered physiology (fatty liver, cholelithiasis), bacterial translocation and systemic infections (hepatic abscess, portal vein thrombosis), hypercoagulability (infarction), and long-term complications of these liver diseases, such as ascending cholangitis, cirrhosis, portal hypertension, and biliary carcinoma.

Sclerosing cholangitis is a common hepatobiliary diseases associated with IBD, occurring in 2–8% of adult patients with ulcerative colitis, and less often in Crohn disease. In pediatric patients with IBD, the diagnosis typically occurs in the 2nd decade of life. Sclerosing cholangitis is characterized by progressive inflammation and fibrosis of segments of the intra- and extrahepatic bile ducts, and can progress to complete obliteration. Genetic susceptibility, with associations with several human leukocyte antigens, has been demonstrated. Many patients are asymptomatic and initially diagnosed by routine liver function testing that reveals elevated serum alkaline phosphatase (ALP), 5′-nucleotidase, or γ-glutamyl transpeptidase (GGT) activities. Antinuclear or anti–smooth muscle antibodies may also be present in the serum. Ten to 15% of adult patients present with symptoms including anorexia, weight loss, pruritus, fatigue, right upper quadrant pain, and jaundice; intermittent acute cholangitis accompanied by fever, jaundice, and right upper quadrant pain can also occur. Portal hypertension can develop with progressive disease. These symptoms are less common in children in whom hepatobiliary disease is often recognized by routine screening of liver function tests. Occasionally, children present initially with sclerosing cholangitis, and the associated IBD is discovered only on subsequent endoscopy. Definitive diagnosis of sclerosing cholangitis requires liver biopsy, which typically reveals periductal fibrosis and inflammation, fibro-obliterative cholangitis, and portal fibrosis. Cholangiography may reveal beading and irregularity of the intrahepatic and extrahepatic bile ducts.

There is no definitive medical treatment for sclerosing cholangitis; liver transplantation is the only long-term option for progressive cirrhosis; and autoimmune disease may recur in the allograft. Short-term therapy aims at improving biliary drainage and attempting to slow the obliterative process. Ursodeoxycholic acid, at a dose of 15 mg/kg/24 hr, improves bile flow and laboratory parameters but has not been shown to improve clinical outcome. Oral vancomycin may also improve serum biochemical levels. Dominant extrahepatic biliary strictures may be dilated or endoscopically stented. Immunosuppressive therapy with corticosteroids and/or azathioprine improves biochemical parameters but has been disappointing in halting long-term histologic progression. Symptomatic therapy should be initiated for pruritus (rifampin, ursodeoxycholic acid, diphenhydramine), malnutrition (enteral supplementation), and ascending cholangitis (antibiotics) as indicated. Total colectomy has not been beneficial in preventing or managing hepatobiliary complications in patients with ulcerative colitis.

IBD-associated **autoimmune hepatitis** (AIH) can closely resemble IBD-associated sclerosing cholangitis, a condition often referred to as **overlap syndrome** or autoimmune sclerosing cholangitis (ASC). These patients typically exhibit hyperglobulinemia (marked increase in serum immunoglobulin [Ig] G levels). Some children are initially diagnosed with AIH and later found to have sclerosing cholangitis after cholangiography; in other cases, AIH presents years after diagnosis of IBD-associated sclerosing cholangitis. Liver biopsy in patients with AIH/sclerosing cholangitis overlap syndrome (ASC) shows interface hepatitis, in addition to the bile duct injury associated with sclerosing cholangitis. Immunosuppressive medication (corticosteroids and/or azathioprine) is the mainstay of therapy for ASC; long-term response does not appear to be as favorable as in AIH alone. Long-term survival in children with ASC appears to be similar to those with sclerosing cholangitis, with an overall median (50%) survival free of liver transplantation of 12.7 yr.

Fatty liver disease may also be more prevalent in adult patients with IBD, ranging from 25 to 40% in one large series. Gallstones are more prevalent in those with Crohn disease (11%) than in those with ulcerative colitis (7.5%) and normal subjects (5%). The true prevalence of these IBD-associated liver diseases in pediatric patients is unknown, however.

BACTERIAL SEPSIS (SEE CHAPTERS 109 AND 176). Sepsis can mimic liver disease and should be excluded in any critically ill patient that develops cholestasis in the absence of markedly elevated serum aminotransferase or ALP levels, even when other signs of infection are not evident. Gram-negative organisms are most often isolated from blood cultures, in particular *Escherichia coli, Klebsiella pneumoniae,* and *Pseudomonas aeruginosa.* Lipopolysaccharides and other bacterial endotoxins are thought to interfere with bile secretion by directly altering the structure or function of bile canalicular membrane transport proteins. The serum bilirubin level is elevated, usually predominantly the conjugated fraction. Serum ALP and aminotransferase activities are not necessarily elevated. Liver biopsy shows intrahepatic cholestasis with little or no hepatocyte necrosis. Kupffer cell hyperplasia and an increase in inflammatory cells are also common. Similar findings can occur with urosepsis.

CARDIAC DISEASE. Hepatic injury can occur as a complication of severe acute or chronic congestive heart failure (see Chapter 442), cyanotic congenital heart disease (see Chapters 429 and 430), and acute ischemic shock. In all conditions, both passive congestion and reduced cardiac output can contribute to liver damage. Elevated central venous pressure is transmitted to the hepatic veins, smaller venules, and, ultimately, the surrounding hepatocytes, resulting in hepatocellular atrophy in the centrilobular zone of the liver. Due to decreased cardiac output, there is decreased hepatic arterial blood flow and centrilobular hypoxia results. Hepatic necrosis leads to lactic acidosis, elevated aminotransferase levels, cholestasis, prolonged partial thromboplastin time, and possibly hypoglycemia due to impaired hepatocellular metabolism. Jaundice, tender hepatomegaly, and, in some cases, ascites and splenomegaly can occur.

After acute hypovolemic shock, serum aminotransferase levels may rise dramatically but rapidly return to normal when perfusion and cardiac function improve. Hepatic necrosis or acute liver failure can occur in infants with hypoplastic left heart syndrome and coarctation of the aorta. High systemic venous pressures after Fontan procedures can also lead to hepatic dysfunction, marked by prolonged prothrombin time. The aim of therapy in all causes of cardiac-associated liver disease is to improve cardiac output, reduce systemic venous pressures, and monitor for other signs of hypoperfusion by closely following renal output and mental status.

OBESITY. Nonalcoholic fatty liver disease (NAFLD) is part of the spectrum of liver disease strongly associated with obesity. NAFLD can range from fatty liver alone to a triad of fatty infiltration, inflammation, and fibrosis (nonalcoholic steatohepatitis [NASH]) that resembles alcoholic liver disease but occurs with little or no exposure to ethanol. NAFLD was thought to occur mainly in older obese adults (mainly women) with central obesity, insulin resistance, and type II diabetes mellitus, but it has been increasingly described in children as well. The true prevalence in children is unknown because diagnosis requires liver biopsy. Elevated serum aminotransferase levels are not sensitive or specific markers for NAFLD. Likewise, no current imaging modalities distinguish between steatosis and NASH. The estimated prevalence in adults is thought to be as high as 15–20% for NAFLD overall and 2–4% for NASH. Risk factors in pediatric cohorts include obesity, male gender, white or Hispanic ethnicity, hypertriglyceridemia, and insulin resistance.

Hepatic steatosis alone may be benign, but up to a quarter of individuals with NASH may develop progressive fibrosis with resultant cirrhosis. The long-term prognosis of NASH that has developed in childhood is unknown. Gradual slow weight loss is effective in normalizing serum ALT and improving NAFLD. Vitamin E and metformin are under investigation in children and may be beneficial in improving serum biochemical abnormalities; it is not known whether they improve liver histopathology. Thiazolidenediones improve liver histology in adults with NASH but have not been studied in children.

CHOLESTASIS ASSOCIATED WITH TOTAL PARENTERAL NUTRITION (TPN). TPN can cause a variety of liver diseases including hepatic steatosis, gallbladder and bile duct damage, and cholestasis. Cholestasis is the most severe complication and can lead to progressive fibrosis and cirrhosis, particularly in infants and young children on prolonged TPN. It is the major factor limiting effective long-term use of TPN in both children and adults. Risk factors for TPN-associated cholestasis include prolonged duration of TPN, prematurity, low birthweight, sepsis, necrotizing enterocolitis, and short bowel syndrome. In low birthweight infants, TPN-associated cholestasis develops in nearly half of infants with birthweight <1,000 g, in 20% of those 1,000–1,500 g, and in 5–10% of those 1,500–2,000 g.

The pathogenesis of TPN-associated cholestasis is multifactorial. Sepsis; excess caloric intake; high amounts of protein, fat, or carbohydrate; specific amino acid toxicities; nutrient deficiencies; and toxicities related to components such as manganese, aluminum, and copper can all contribute to hepatic injury. Prolonged enteral fasting compromises mucosal integrity and increases bacterial mucosal translocation. Fasting also decreases release of enteral hormones such as cholecystokinin, which promote bile flow. Sepsis, in particular due to gram-negative bacteria, and associated endotoxins can exacerbate liver damage.

Early histologic findings include macrovesicular steatosis, canalicular cholestasis, and portal triad inflammation. These changes can regress after cessation of short-term TPN. Prolonged duration of TPN is marked by bile duct proliferation, portal fibrosis, and expansion of portal triads and it can progress to cirrhosis and end-stage liver disease.

Clinical onset is typically marked by gradual onset of cholestasis, developing after >2 wk of TPN. In low birthweight infants, the onset of jaundice may overlap the phase of physiologic (unconjugated) hyperbilirubinemia. Any icteric infant who has received TPN for >1 wk should have all bilirubin determinations fractionated. With prolonged duration, hepatic enlargement or splenomegaly may develop. Serum bile acid concentrations may increase. Rises in serum aminotransferase activities may be a late finding. An elevation in serum ALP activity may be due to rickets, a common complication of TPN in low birthweight infants.

In addition to cholestasis, biliary complications of intravenous nutrition include cholelithiasis and the development of biliary sludge, associated with thick, inspissated gallbladder contents. These may be asymptomatic. Hepatic steatosis or elevated serum aminotransferase levels can also occur in the absence of cholestasis, particularly in older children. This is generally mild and resolves after TPN is discontinued. Serum bilirubin and bile acid levels remain within the normal range. Other causes of liver disease should also be considered, especially if evidence of hepatic dysfunction persists despite weaning TPN and initiating enteral feeds. The risk group in which TPN-associated cholestasis most frequently occurs often receives blood products or drugs. Therefore, hepatic disease related to viral or drug-induced liver disease is a consideration. If serum ALP or aminotransferase levels remain elevated, liver biopsy may be necessary for accurate diagnosis.

Treatment of TPN-associated cholestasis is focused on avoiding progressive liver injury by limiting duration whenever possible. Enteral feeding should be initiated as soon as tolerated and prolonged fasting avoided. Even small volumes of nutrients given by intermittent oral feedings or by continuous nasogastric drip promote bile flow, enterohepatic recirculation of bile acids, intestinal motility, and enhance mucosal barrier function, reducing the risk of bacterial translocation. Improved TPN solutions that meet the specific needs of neonates may prevent deficiencies and avoid toxicities. The risk of further hepatic injury should always be considered when weighing the option of continuing TPN indefinitely and all efforts should be made to try to advance enteral feeds whenever possible. Ursodeoxycholic acid therapy may be beneficial in improving jaundice and hepatosplenomegaly. Other therapies, such as administration of antibiotics to reduce intraluminal bacterial overgrowth or oral administration of taurine or cholecystokinin, remain experimental.

CYSTIC FIBROSIS (CF). CF is caused by mutations in the cystic fibrosis transmembrane conductance regulator (CFTR) gene, which impair chloride transport across the apical membranes of epithelial cells in numerous organs (including cholangiocytes) [see Chapter 400]. The reported prevalence of liver disease in CF is as high as 37% but may be increasing with the longer life span of CF patients and growing awareness of CF-associated liver disease.

Liver disease in patients with CF is postulated to result, in part, from impaired secretory function of the bile duct epithelium; bile ducts contain inspissated granular eosinophilic material, which leads to focal biliary cirrhosis. Gradual progression to multilobular cirrhosis may occur and result in portal hypertension and end-stage liver disease. Liver disease tends to occur mainly in patients with pancreatic insufficiency; the association is not well understood. Familial clustering suggests a genetic predisposition; however, no specific genotype-phenotype association with specific CFTR mutations has been found. Mutational analysis is not helpful at this time in predicting which patients with CF will develop liver disease. Clinical risk factors that may be associated with liver disease include older age, pancreatic insufficiency, male gender, and possibly a history of meconium ileus.

Treatment with oral ursodeoxycholic acid (10–15 mg/kg/day) may be beneficial in improving liver function, presumably by improving bile flow; further research is necessary to determine whether a true long-term benefit exists. Because it is difficult to predict which patients will develop liver disease, prophylactic therapy is not possible. Progression of liver disease is generally slow. Patients who develop end-stage liver disease may require liver transplantation for survival.

BONE MARROW TRANSPLANTATION. Liver disease is common in patients who have received hematopoietic stem cell transplantation (SCT), whether the cells are harvested from bone marrow or peripheral blood (see Chapters 134–138). The pathogenesis is varied and includes: infections (viral, bacterial, or fungal); toxicity from drugs, parenteral nutrition, chemotherapy, or radiation; veno-occlusive disease (VOD); graft vs host disease (GVHD); or hemosiderosis secondary to iron overload from frequent blood transfusions. GVHD, drug toxicity, and sepsis are the most common causes of liver dysfunction after allogeneic stem cell transplantation. Diagnosis is often challenging due to the coexistence of multiple risk factors. Clinical course, symptoms and signs, as well as biochemical liver function and viral serologic tests must be considered in making the correct diagnosis. Percutaneous liver biopsy may be necessary; histology may show extensive bile duct injury in GVHD, viral inclusions in cytomegalovirus disease, or the characteristic endothelial lesion in VOD. It is important to diagnose the cause accurately, as treatment for GVHD differs markedly from that of other conditions (i.e., GVHD treatment involves initiating immunosuppression) and may worsen hepatitis secondary to infections.

GVHD of the liver can be acute or chronic but often occurs with the presence of GVHD in other target organs such as the skin and gut (see Chapter 136). Hepatic GVHD is caused by immunologic reaction to bile duct epithelium, leading to a nonsuppurative cholangitis. Histologic features of GVHD include loss of intralobular bile ducts, endothelial injury of hepatic and portal venules, and hepatocellular necrosis.

Onset typically occurs at the time of donor engraftment (days 14–21 after SCT). In acute hepatic GVHD, serum aminotransferase levels may rise markedly in the absence of elevated bilirubin, ALP, and GGT levels, mimicking viral hepatitis. Acute hepatic GVHD can present both early (days 14–21) and late (>day 70) after allogeneic SCT. In chronic hepatic GVHD, serum aminotransferase levels are not as markedly elevated and cholestasis is more prominent with marked rises in serum conjugated bilirubin, GGT, and ALP levels. Other signs and symptoms can include hepatic tenderness, dark urine, acholic stools, itching, and anorexia.

VOD of the liver usually develops in the 1st 3 wk after SCT. The incidence is <10%, with a mortality rate of <4%. Risk factors include trauma, coagulopathies, sickle cell anemia, leukemia, polycythemia vera, hepatic abscesses, irradiation, and GVHD. VOD is caused by fibrous obliteration of the terminal hepatic venules and small lobular veins, with resultant damage to the surrounding hepatocytes and sinusoids. It is not associated with thrombus formation, in contrast with Budd-Chiari syndrome, which involves occlusion of the larger hepatic veins or inferior vena cava by a web, mass, or thrombus. The cause of VOD after bone marrow transplantation is not clear; risk factors for VOD include high-dose conditioning regimens, radiation, leukemia, advanced age, and pre-existing liver disease.

Pathologic changes in patients with VOD are best demonstrated using special (trichrome) stains to highlight the central veins. An early lesion is concentric narrowing of the lumina of small central veins, owing to edema in the subendothelial zone. There is a dense, wavy continuous band of collagen in the central veins and centrilobular hemorrhagic necrosis. The lesions may be patchy. Later in the course, hepatic venules may be completely obliterated.

Symptoms typically include jaundice, painful hepatomegaly, rapid weight gain, and ascites. VOD resolves in the majority of patients but can also lead to multisystem organ failure, hepatic encephalopathy, and fulminant hepatic failure. Less severe forms may be characterized by jaundice and ascites with a slow resolution; in very mild cases, histologic changes may be the sole manifestation. The diagnosis rests on the exclusion of other diseases, such as GVHD, congestive cardiomyopathy, constrictive pericarditis, and Budd-Chiari syndrome.

There is no effective prophylaxis or therapy for VOD. Prophylactic therapeutic agents under investigation include intravenous or low molecular weight heparin, prostaglandin E_1, and ursodeoxycholic acid. Oral ursodeoxycholic acid can decrease the incidence of severe liver disease in patients undergoing SCT, but its direct benefit in preventing VOD is unclear. Supportive management includes maintaining intravenous hydration and renal perfusion. Severe VOD has been treated with difibrotide, an experimental agent with antithrombotic and thrombolytic properties, in high-risk adult patients.

HEMOGLOBINOPATHIES. Patients with sickle cell anemia (see Chapter 462.1) or sickle cell thalassemia (Chapter 462.1) can have hepatic dysfunction due to acute or chronic viral hepatitis, hemosiderosis from frequent transfusion therapy, hepatic crises related to severe intrahepatic cholestasis, sequestration, or ischemic necrosis. In addition, cholelithiasis is common.

Hepatic sickle cell crisis or "sickle hepatopathy" occurs in ≈10% of patients with sickle cell disease. It presents with intense right upper quadrant pain, fever, leukocytosis, right upper quadrant tenderness, and jaundice. Bilirubin levels may be markedly elevated; serum ALP levels may be only moderately elevated. It can be difficult to distinguish sickle hepatopathy from viral hepatitis or acute cholecystitis/choledocholithiasis; therefore, these conditions should be excluded. Generally, hepatic sickle cell crisis is self-limited. **Sickle cell intrahepatic cholestasis** presents as hepatomegaly, abdominal pain, hyperbilirubinemia, and coagulopathy and can progress to acute liver failure, leaving transplantation as the only therapeutic option. Transplantation carries a high risk for graft loss due to vascular complications. Fortunately, intrahepatic cholestasis occurs infrequently.

On occasion, children with sickle cell disease experience bilirubin levels >20 mg/dL but unaccompanied by severe pain or fever. There is no change in hematocrit or reticulocyte count nor any association with a hemolytic crisis. The clinical course is benign.

COLLAGEN VASCULAR DISEASE. Liver enzyme abnormalities are commonly associated with collagen vascular diseases in children, including systemic lupus erythematosus, rheumatoid arthritis, and mixed connective tissue diseases. Hepatic arteritis, nonspecific reactive hepatitis, autoimmune hepatitis, nodular regenerative hyperplasia, steatosis, and hepatic infarction have all been reported. Drug toxicity and viral hepatitis must be excluded. In cases of persistent idiopathic biochemical abnormalities, liver biopsy may be necessary for specific diagnosis.

Ahmad J, Slivka A: Hepatobiliary disease in inflammatory bowel disease. *Gastroenterol Clin North Am* 2002;31:329–345.

Bargiggia S, Maconit G, Elli M, et al: Sonographic prevalence of liver steatosis and biliary tract stones in patients with inflammatory bowel disease: Study of 511 subjects at a single center. *J Clin Gastroenterol* 2003;36:417–420.

Beale E, Nelson R, Bucciarelli R, et al: Intrahepatic cholestasis associated with parenteral nutrition in premature infants. *Pediatrics* 1979;64:342–347.

Buchanan GR, Glader BE: Benign course of extreme hyperbilirubinemia in sickle cell anemia: Analysis of six cases. *J Pediatr* 1977;91:21–24.

Chen CY, Tsao PN, Chen HL, et al: Ursodeoxycholic acid (UDCA) therapy in very-low-birth-weight infants with parenteral nutrition–associated cholestasis. *J Pediatr* 2004;145:317–321.

Colombo C, Battezzati PM, Podda M, et al: Ursodeoxycholic acid for liver disease associated with cystic fibrosis: A double-blind multicenter trial. The Italian Group for the Study of Ursodeoxycholic Acid in Cystic Fibrosis. *Hepatology* 1996;23:1484–1490.

Columbo C, Battezzati PM, Strazzabosco M, et al: Liver and biliary problems in cystic fibrosis. *Semin Liver Dis* 1998;18:227–235.

Debray D, Pariente D, Urvoas E, et al: Sclerosing cholangitis in children. *J Pediatr* 1994;124:49–56.

Feldstein AE, Perrault J, El-Youssif M, et al: Primary sclerosing cholangitis in children: A long-term follow-up study. *Hepatology* 2003;38:210–217.

Fujii N, Takenaka K, Shinagawa K et al: Hepatic graft-versus-host disease presenting as acute hepatitis after allogeneic peripheral blood stem cell transplantation. *Bone Marrow Transplant* 2001;27:1007–1010.

Giallourakis CC, Rosenberg P, Friedman LS: The liver in heart failure. *Clin Liver Dis* 2002;6:947–967.

Gregorio GV, Portmann B, Karani J, et al: Autoimmune hepatitis/sclerosing cholangitis overlap syndrome in childhood: A 16-year prospective study. *Hepatology* 2001;33:544–553.

Hong-Curtis J, Yeh MM, Jain D, et al: Rapid progression of autoimmune hepatitis in the background of primary sclerosing cholangitis. *J Clin Gastroenterol* 2004;38:906–909.

Kaufman SS: Prevention of parenteral nutrition-associated liver disease in children. *Pediatr Transplant* 2002;6:37–42.

Khurshid I, Anderson L, Downie GH, et al: Sickle cell disease, extreme hyperbilirubinemia, and pericardial tamponade: Case report and review of the literature. *Crit Care Med* 2002;30:2363–2367.

Kim BK, Chung KW, Sun HS: Liver disease during the first post-transplant year in bone marrow transplantation recipients: Retrospective study. *Bone Marrow Transplant* 2000;26:193–197.

Kwan V and George J: Liver disease due to parenteral and enteral nutrition. *Clin Liver Dis* 2004;8:893–913.

Lavine JE: Vitamin E treatment of nonalcoholic steatohepatitis in children: A pilot study. *J Pediatr* 2000;136:734–738.

Levine A, Maayan A, Shamir R, et al: Parenteral nutrition–associated cholestasis in preterm neonates: Evaluation of ursodeoxycholic acid treatment. *J Pediatr Endocrinol Metab* 1999;12:549–553.

Margalit M, Elinav H, Ilan Y, et al: Liver abscess in inflammatory bowel disease: Report of two cases and review of the literature. *J Gastroenterol Hepatol* 2004;19:1338–1342.

Matsumoto T, Kobayashi S, Shimizu H, et al: The liver in collagen diseases: Pathologic study of 160 cases with particular reference to hepatic arteritis, primary biliary cirrhosis, autoimmune hepatitis and nodular regenerative hyperplasia of the liver. *Liver* 2000;20:366–373.

Moseley RH: Sepsis and cholestasis. *Clin Liver Dis* 2004;8:83–94.

Narkewicz MR, Sondheimer HM, Ziegler JW, et al: Hepatic dysfunction following the Fontan procedure. *J Pediatr Gastroenterol Nutr* 2003;36: 352–357.

Ribaud P, Gluckman E: Hepatic veno-occlusive disease. *Pediatr Transplant* 1999;3:41–44.

Roberts EA: Nonalcoholic steatohepatitis in children. *Curr Gastroenterol Rep* 2003;5:253–259.

Ruutu T, Eriksson B, Juvonen E, et al: Ursodeoxycholic acid for the prevention of hepatic complications in allogeneic stem cell transplantation. *Blood* 2002;100:1977–1983.

Schubert TT: Hepatobiliary system in sickle cell disease. *Gastroenterology* 1986;90:2013–2021.

Schwimmer JB, Deutsch R, Kahen T, et al: Prevalence of fatty liver in children and adolescents. *Pediatrics* 2006;118:1388–1393.

Schwimmer JB, Deutsch R, Rauch JB, et al: Obesity, insulin resistance and other clinicopathological correlates of pediatric nonalcoholic fatty liver disease. *J Pediatr* 2003;143:500–505.

Strauss RS, Barlow SE, Dietz WH: Prevalence of abnormal serum aminotransferase values in overweight and obese adolescents. *J Pediatr* 2000;136: 727–733.

Wilschanski M, Rivlin J, Cohen S, et al: Clinical and genetic risk factors for cystic fibrosis–related liver disease. *Pediatrics* 1999;103:52–57.

Zakrzewski JL, Ballauff A, Wieland R: Differential diagnosis of cholestasis following allogeneic hematopoietic stem cell transplantation: The contribution of serum bile acid levels in relation to other liver tests. *Pediatr Hematol Oncol* 2004;21:697–705.

Chapter 358 ■ Mitochondrial Hepatopathies

Rebecca G. Carey and William F. Balistreri

Hepatocytes are rich in mitochondria due to the energy required for the process of metabolism and are a target organ for disorders in mitochondrial function. Defects in mitochondrial function can lead to impaired oxidative phosphorylation (OXPHOS), increased generation of reactive oxygen species, impairment of other metabolic pathways, and activation of mechanisms of cellular death. Mitochondrial disorders can be divided into primary, in which the mitochondrial defect is the primary cause of the disorder, and secondary, in which mitochondrial function is affected by exogenous injury or a genetic mutation in a non-mitochondrial gene (see Chapter 87.4). Primary mitochondrial disorders can be caused either by mutations affecting mitochondrial DNA (mtDNA) or by nuclear genes that encode mitochondrial proteins or cofactors (Table 358-1). Secondary mitochondrial disorders include diseases with an uncertain etiology such as Reye syndrome; disorders caused by endogenous or exogenous toxins, drugs, or metals; and other conditions in which mitochondrial oxidative injury may be involved in the pathogenesis of liver injury.

EPIDEMIOLOGY. More than 200 gene mutations that involve mtDNA and nuclear DNA that encodes mitochondrial proteins have been identified. Mitochondrial genetics are unique because mitochondria are able to replicate, transcribe, and translate their DNA independently. The mitochondrial genome encodes 2 ribosomal RNAs, 22 transfer RNAs, and 13 proteins of complex I, III, IV, and V of the respiratory chain. OXPHOS (the process of adenosine triphosphate [ATP] production) occurs in the respiratory chain located in the inner mitochondrial membrane and is divided into five multienzyme complexes: reduced nicotinamide adenine dinucleotide (NADH) coenzyme Q (CoQ) reductase (Complex I), succinate-CoQ reductase (Complex II), reduced CoQ-cytochrome c reductase (Complex III), cytochrome-*c* oxidase (Complex IV), and ATP synthase (Complex V). The polypeptides that form these complexes are transcribed from both mitochondrial and nuclear DNA; mutations in either genome can result in disorders of OXPHOS. Expression of mitochondrial disorders is complex and epidemiologic studies are hampered by technical difficulties collecting and processing tissue specimens needed to make accurate diagnoses, the variability in clinical presentation, and the fact that most disorders display maternal inheritance with variable penetrance (see Chapter 80). Moreover, mtDNA mutates 10 times more frequently than nuclear DNA secondary to a lack of introns, protective histones, and an effective repair system in mitochandria. Mitochondrial genetics also display a threshold effect in that the type and severity of mutation required for clinical expression varies among people and organ systems. Despite this, it has been estimated that mitochondrial diseases have a prevalence of 11.5 cases per 100,000 individuals.

TABLE 358-1. Primary Mitochondrial Hepatopathies

Electron transport (respiratory chain) defects
Neonatal liver failure: Complex I deficiency (NADH: ubiquinone oxidoreductase), complex IV deficiency (cytochrome-*c* oxidase), complex III deficiency (ubiquinol: cytochrome c oxidoreductase), multiple complex deficiencies
Mitochondrial DNA depletion syndrome (deoxyguanosine kinase)
Alpers disease (complex I deficiency, DNA polymerase-γA)
Pearson marrow-pancreas syndrome (mtDNA deletion)
Mitochondrial neurogastrointestinal encephalomyopathy (thymidine phosphorylase, tryptophan tRNA)
Chronic diarrhea (villous atrophy) with hepatic involvement (complex III deficiency)
Navajo neurohepatopathy
Mitochondrial translation defects (elongation factor G1)
Long-chain hydroxyacyl CoA dehydrogenase deficiency
Acute fatty liver of pregnancy (AFLP)
Fatty acid oxidation and transport defects
Carnitine palmitoyltransferase I and II deficiencies
Carnitine-acylcarnitine translocase deficiency
Urea cycle enzyme deficiencies
Electron-transfer flavoprotein (EFT) and EFT-dehydrogenase deficiencies
Phosphoenolpyruvate carboxykinase (PEPCK) deficiency (mitochondrial)
Nonketotic hyperglycinemia (gylcine cleavage enzyme deficiency)

CoA, coenzyme A; mtDNA, mitochondrial DNA; NADH, nicotinamide adenine dinucleotide.

CLINICAL MANIFESTATIONS. Defects in OXPHOS can affect any tissue to a variable degree, with the most energy-dependent organs being the most vulnerable. One should consider the diagnosis of a mitochondrial disorder in a patient of any age that presents with progressive, multisystem involvement that cannot be explained by a specific diagnosis. Gastrointestinal complaints include vomiting, diarrhea, constipation, failure to thrive (FTT), and abdominal pain; certain mitochondrial disorders have characteristic gastrointestinal presentations. Pearson marrow-pancreas syndrome presents with sideroblastic anemia and exocrine pancreatic insufficiency, whereas mitochondrial neurogastrointestinal encephalomyopathy (MNGIE) presents with chronic intestinal pseudo-obstruction and cachexia. Hepatic presentations range from chronic cholestasis, hepatomegaly, or steatosis to fulminant hepatic failure and death.

PRIMARY MITOCHONDRIAL HEPATOPATHIES

A common presentation of respiratory chain defects is severe liver failure in the 1st few months of life, characterized by lactic acidosis, jaundice, hypoglycemia, renal dysfunction, and hyperammonemia. Symptoms are nonspecific and include lethargy and vomiting. Most patients additionally have neurologic involvement manifested as a weak suck, recurrent apnea, or myoclonic epilepsy. Liver biopsy shows predominantly microvesicular steatosis, cholestasis, bile duct proliferation, glycogen depletion, and iron overload. With standard therapy, the prognosis is very poor and most patients die from liver failure or infection in the 1st few months of life. **Cytochrome-*c* oxidase** (Complex IV), a nuclear encoded gene, is the most common deficiency in these infants (see Table 358-1).

Alpers syndrome (Alpers-Huttenlocher syndrome or Alpers hepatopathic poliodystrophy) also presents in infancy with seizures, hypotonia, feeding difficulties, and ataxia. Patients typically develop hepatomegaly and jaundice and have a slower progression to liver failure than those with cytochrome-*c* oxidase deficiency. The disease is inherited in an autosomal recessive fashion and mutations in the catalytic subunit of the nuclear gene mtDNA polymerase-γA have been identified in one family with Alpers syndrome.

MITOCHONDRIAL DNA DEPLETION SYNDROME (MDS). MDS is characterized by a tissue-specific reduction in mtDNA copy number. MDS presents with phenotypic heterogeneity, and multisystem and localized disease forms include myopathic, hepatocerebral, and liver-restricted presentations. Infants with the hepatocerebral form present in the neonatal period with progressive liver failure, neurologic abnormalities, hypoglycemia, and lactic acidosis. Death usually occurs by 1 yr of age. Spontaneous recovery has been reported in one patient with liver-restricted disease. Inheritance is autosomal recessive and mutations in the **deoxyguanosine kinase (dGK)** gene have been identified in many patients with hepatocerebral MDS. No known genetic defect has been identified in liver-restricted MDS. dGK is a nuclear gene whose protein product phosphorylates deoxyguanosine to deoxyguanosine monophosphate, confirming the importance of nucleotide pool homeostasis in mtDNA stability and maintenance. Liver biopsies of patients with MDS show microvesicular steatosis, cholestasis, focal cytoplasmic biliary necrosis, and cytosiderosis in hepatocytes and sinusoidal cells. Ultrastructural changes are characteristic with oncocytic transformation of mitochondria, which is characterized by mitochondria with sparse cristae, granular matrix, and dense or vesicular inclusions. **Diagnosis** is established by demonstration of a low ratio of mtDNA (<10%) to nuclear DNA in affected tissues and/or genetic testing. Importantly, the sequence of the mitochondrial genome is normal.

NAVAJO NEUROHEPATOPATHY (NNH). NNH is an autosomal recessive sensorimotor neuropathy with progressive liver disease found only in Navajo Indians of the southwestern United States. The incidence is 1/1,600 live births. Diagnostic criteria have been defined and include sensory neuropathy; motor neuropathy; corneal anesthesia; liver disease; metabolic or infectious complications including FTT, short stature, delayed puberty or systemic infection; and evidence of central nervous system (CNS) demyelination on radiographic imaging. A definite case requires four of these criteria or three with a sibling previously diagnosed with NNH.

NNH has been divided into three phenotypic variations based on age of presentation and clinical findings. Different presentations have been noted within single families. First, **classical NNH** presents in infancy with severe progressive neurologic deterioration manifesting clinically as weakness, hypotonia, loss of sensation with accompanying acral mutilation and corneal ulcerations, and poor growth. Liver disease, present in the majority of patients, is secondary and variable and includes asymptomatic elevations of liver function tests, Reye syndrome–like episodes, hepatocellular carcinoma, or cirrhosis. γ-Glutamyl transpeptidase (GGT) levels tend to be higher than in other forms of NNH. Liver biopsy may show chronic portal tract inflammation and cirrhosis, but it shows less cholestasis, hepatocyte ballooning, and giant cell transformation than other forms of NNH. **Infantile NNH** presents between the age of 1 and 6 mo with jaundice and failure to thrive and progresses to liver failure and death by 2 yr of age. Patients have hepatomegaly with moderate elevations in SGOT, SGPT, and GGT. Liver biopsy demonstrates pseudo-acinar formation, multinucleate giant cells, portal and lobular inflammation, canalicular cholestasis, and microvesicular steatosis. Progressive neurologic symptoms are not usually noticed at presentation but do develop later. **Childhood NNH** presents from age 1 to 5 yr with the acute onset of fulminant hepatic failure that leads to death within months. Most patients also have evidence of neuropathy at presentation. Liver biopsies are similar to those in infantile NNH, except significant hepatocyte ballooning and necrosis, bile duct proliferation, and cirrhosis are also seen. Nerve biopsy in all types may show reduction of large- and small-caliber myelinated nerve fibers and degeneration and regeneration of unmyelinated nerve fibers. There is no effective treatment for any of the forms of NNH and neurologic symptoms often preclude liver transplantation. The underlying genetic defect is unknown; a mitochondrial cause is strongly suspected, secondary to ultrastructural mitochondrial changes, elevated serum lactate levels, evidence of mitochondrial depletion, and decreased activity of multiple respiratory chain enzymes.

SECONDARY MITOCHONDRIAL HEPATOPATHIES

Secondary mitochondrial hepatopathies are caused by a hepatotoxic metal, drug, toxin, or endogenous metabolite. In the past, the most common secondary mitochondrial hepatopathy was **Reye syndrome,** the prevalence of which peaked in the 1970s and which had a mortality rate of >40%. Even though mortality has not changed, the prevalence has decreased from >500 cases in 1980 to ≈35 cases per yr in the 1990s. It is precipitated in a genetically susceptible individual by the interaction of a viral infection (influenza, varicella) and salicylate use. Clinically, it is characterized by a preceding viral illness that appears to be resolving and the acute onset of vomiting and encephalopathy (Table 358-2). Neurologic symptoms can rapidly progress to seizures, coma, and death. Liver dysfunction is invariably present when vomiting develops, with coagulopathy and elevated SGOT, SGPT, and ammonia. Importantly, patients remain anicteric and serum bilirubin levels are normal. Liver biopsies show microvesicular steatosis without evidence of liver inflammation or necrosis. Death is usually secondary to increased intracranial pressures and herniation. Patients that survive have full recovery of liver function, but should be carefully screened for fatty-acid oxidation and fatty-acid transport defects (Table 358-3).

Acquired abnormalities of mitochondrial function can be caused by several drugs and toxins, including valproic acid, cyanide, amiodarone, chloramphenicol, iron, antimycin A, the emetic toxin of *Bacillus cereus,* and nucleoside analogs. Valproic acid is a branched fatty acid that can be metabolized into the mitochondrial toxin 4-envalproic acid. Children with underlying respiratory chain defects appear more sensitive to the toxic effects of this drug and it has been reported to precipitate liver failure in patients with **Alpers syndrome** and **cytochrome-*c* oxidase deficiency.** Nucleoside analogs directly inhibit mitochondrial respiratory chain complexes. Fialuridine, used to treat hepatitis B infection, can produce fatal lactic acidosis and liver failure. The mechanism of mitochondrial injury involves the direct incorporation of fialuridine into mtDNA, replacing thymidine and thereby directly inhibiting DNA transcription, which leads to acquired mtDNA depletion syndrome. The reverse transcriptase inhibitors zidovudine, didanosine, stavudine, and zalcitabine used to treat HIV-infected patients inhibit DNA polymerase-γ of mitochondria and may block elongation of mtDNA, leading to mtDNA depletion. Other conditions that can lead to mitochondrial oxidative stress include cholestasis, nonalcoholic steatohepatitis, α_1-antitrypsin deficiency and Wilson disease.

There is no effective therapy for most patients with mitochondrial hepatopathies; neurologic involvement often precludes

TABLE 358-2. Clinical Staging of Reye Syndrome

SYMPTOMS AT TIME OF ADMISSION	
I.	Usually quiet, **lethargic** and sleepy, vomiting, laboratory evidence of liver dysfunction
II.	Deep lethargy, **confusion,** delirium, combative, hyperventilation, hyper-reflexic
III.	Obtunded, **light coma** ± seizures, decorticate rigidity, intact pupillary light reaction
IV.	Seizures, deepening coma, **decerebrate rigidity,** loss of oculocephalic reflexes, fixed pupils
V.	Coma, loss of deep tendon reflexes, respiratory arrest, fixed dilated pupils, **flaccidity/decerebrate** (intermittent); isoelectric electroencephalogram

TABLE 358-3. Diseases That Present a Clinical/Pathologic Picture Resembling Reye Syndrome

Metabolic disease
- Organic acidurias
- Disorders of oxidative phosphorylation
- Urea cycle defects (carbamoyl phosphate synthetase, ornithine transcarbamylase)
- Defects in fatty acid oxidation metabolism
- Acyl-CoA dehydrogenase deficiencies
- Systemic carnitine deficiency
- Hepatic carnitine palmitoyltransferase deficiency
- 3-OH, 3-methylglutaryl-CoA lyase deficiency
- Fructosemia

Central nervous system infections or intoxications (meningitis), encephalitis, toxic encephalopathy
Hemorrhagic shock with encephalopathy
Drug or toxin ingestion (salicylate, valproate)

CoA, coenzyme A.

orthotopic liver transplantation. Several drug mixtures that include antioxidants, vitamins, cofactors, and electron acceptors have been proposed, but no randomized controlled trials have been completed to evaluate these drug combinations. Therefore, current treatment strategies are supportive.

Belay E, Bresee JS, Holman RC, et al: Reye's syndrome in the United States from 1981 through 1997. *N Engl J Med* 1999;340:1377–1382.

Bougneres PF, Rocchiccioli F, Koluraa S, et al: Medium-chain acyl-CoA dehydrogenase deficiency in two siblings with a Reye-like syndrome. *J Pediatr* 1985;106:918–921.

Casteels-Van Daele M, Van Geet C, Wounter C, et al: Reyes syndrome revisited: A descriptive term covering a group of heterogeneous disorders. *Eur J Pediatr* 2000;159:641–648.

Ducluzeau PH, Lachaux A, Bouvier R, et al: Progressive reversion of clinical and molecular phenotype in a child with liver mitochondrial DNA depletion. *J Hepatol* 2002:36:698–703.

Gillis LA, Sokol RJ: Gastrointestinal manifestations of mitochondrial disease. *Gastroenterol Clin North Am* 2003;32:789–817.

Holve S, Hu D, Shub M, et al: Liver disease in Navajo neuropathy. *J Pediatr* 1999;135:482–493.

Mancuso M, Filosto M, Tsujino S, et al: Muscle glycogenosis and mitochondrial hepatopathy in an infant with mutations in both the myophosphorylase and deoxyguanosine kinase genes. *Arch Neurol* 2003;60:1445–1447.

Rabinowitz SS, Gelfond D, Chen CK, et al: Hepatocerebral mitochondrial DNA depletion syndrome: Clinical and morphologic features of a nuclear gene mutation. *J Pediatr Gastroenterol Nutr* 2004;38:216–220.

Teitelbaum JE, Berde CB, Nurko C, et al: Diagnosis and management of MNGIE syndrome in children: Case report and review of the literature. *J Pediatr Gastroenterol Nutr* 2002;35:377–383.

Chapter 359 ■ Autoimmune and Chronic Hepatitis

Benjamin L. Shneider and Frederick J. Suchy

Autoimmune hepatitis is a chronic hepatic inflammatory process manifested by elevated serum aminotransaminase concentrations and liver-associated serum autoantibodies and hypergammaglobulinemia. The target of the inflammatory process can include both hepatocytes and bile duct epithelium. Chronicity is determined either by duration of liver disease (typically >3–6 mo) or by evidence of either severe liver disease or physical stigmata of chronic liver disease (clubbing, spider telangiectasia, hepatosplenomegaly). The severity is variable; the affected child may have only biochemical evidence of liver dysfunction, may have stigmata of chronic liver disease, or may present in hepatic failure.

Chronic hepatitis can also be caused by persistent viral infection (see Chapter 355), drugs (see Chapter 360), metabolic diseases (see Chapter 358), or unknown factors (Table 359-1). Approximately 15–20% of cases are associated with hepatitis B infection; unusually severe disease may be caused by superimposed infection with hepatitis D (a defective RNA virus that is dependent on replicating hepatitis B virus [HBV]). More than 90% of hepatitis B infections in the 1st yr of life become chronic, compared with 5–10% among older children and adults. Chronic hepatitis develops in >50% of acute hepatitis C virus infections. Patients receiving blood products or who have had massive transfusions are at increased risk. Hepatitis A or E viruses do not cause chronic hepatitis. **Drugs** commonly used in children that can cause chronic liver injury include isoniazid, methyldopa, pemoline, nitrofurantoin, dantrolene, minocycline, pemoline, and the

TABLE 359-1. Disorders Producing Chronic Hepatitis

CHRONIC VIRAL HEPATITIS
Hepatitis B
Hepatitis C
Hepatitis D
AUTOIMMUNE HEPATITIS
Antiactin antibody positive
Anti–liver-kidney microsomal antibody positive
Antisoluble liver antigen antibody positive
Others (includes antibodies to liver-specific lipoproteins or asialoglycoprotein)
Overlap syndrome with sclerosing cholangitis and autoantibodies
Systemic lupus erythematosus
Celiac disease
DRUG-INDUCED HEPATITIS
METABOLIC DISORDERS ASSOCIATED WITH CHRONIC LIVER DISEASE
Wilson disease
α_1-Antitrypsin deficiency
Tyrosinemia
Niemann-Pick disease type 2
Glycogen storage disease type IV
Cystic fibrosis
Galactosemia
BILE ACID BIOSYNTHETIC ABNORMALITIES

sulfonamides. **Metabolic diseases** can lead to chronic hepatitis including α_1-antitrypsin deficiency, inborn errors of bile acid biosynthesis, and Wilson disease. **Steatohepatitis,** usually associated with obesity and insulin resistance, is another common cause of chronic hepatitis; it is relatively benign and responds to weight reduction and/or vitamin E therapy. Progression to cirrhosis has been described in adults. In most cases, the cause of chronic hepatitis is unknown; in many, an autoimmune mechanism is suggested by the finding of serum antinuclear and anti–smooth muscle antibodies and by multisystem involvement (arthropathy, thyroiditis, rashes, Coombs-positive hemolytic anemia).

Histologic features help characterize chronic hepatitis. Subdivision of chronic hepatitis into a persistent vs active form on the basis of histologic findings is not as useful as once thought. The finding of inflammation contained within the limiting plate of the portal tract (chronic persistent hepatitis) and the absence of fibrosis/cirrhosis suggest a more benign course. The finding of activity on biopsy may be predictive of response to antiviral therapy if hepatitis B infection is present and is a criterion used in the diagnosis of autoimmune hepatitis. Histologic features help identify the etiology; characteristic PAS-positive, diastase-resistant granules are seen in α_1-antitrypsin deficiency, while macrovesicular and microvesicular neutral fat accumulation within hepatocytes is a feature of steatohepatitis. Bile duct injury may suggest an autoimmune cholangiopathy. Ultrastructural analysis may suggest distinct types of storage disorders.

Autoimmune hepatitis is a clinical constellation that suggests an immune-mediated process; it is responsive to immunosuppressive therapy (Table 359-2). Autoimmune hepatitis typically refers to a primarily hepatocyte-specific process, whereas autoimmune cholangiopathy and sclerosing cholangitis are predominated by intra- and extrahepatic bile duct injury. Overlap of the process involving both hepatocyte and bile duct directed injury may be common in children. De novo hepatitis is seen in a subset of liver transplant recipients whose initial disease was not autoimmune.

ETIOLOGY. The cause of autoimmune hepatitis is unknown. It may be the result of an imbalance between CD4 and CD8 T-lymphocyte activity. Genetic predisposition may play an important role in the development of autoimmune hepatitis, although viral infection or drug exposure may initiate the process.

TABLE 359-2. Classification of Autoimmune Hepatitis

VARIABLE	TYPE 1 AUTOIMMUNE HEPATITIS	TYPE 2 AUTOIMMUNE HEPATITIS
Characteristic autoantibodies	Antinuclear antibody* Smooth-muscle antibody* Antiactin antibody† Autoantibodies against soluble liver antigen and liver-pancreas antigen‡ Atypical perinuclear antineutrophil cytoplasmic antibody	Antibody against liver-kidney microsome 1* Antibody against liver cytosol 1*
Geographic variation	Worldwide	Worldwide; rare in North America
Age at presentation	Any age	Predominantly childhood and young adulthood
Sex of patients	Female in approximately 75% of cases	Female in approximately 95% of cases
Association with other autoimmune diseases	Common	Common§
Clinical severity	Broad range	Generally severe
Histopathologic features at presentation	Broad range	Generally advanced
Treatment failure	Infrequent	Frequent
Relapse after drug withdrawal	Variable	Common
Need for long-term maintenance	Variable	Approximately 100%

*The conventional method of detection is immunofluorescence.
†Tests for this antibody are rarely available in commercial laboratories.
‡This antibody is detected by enzyme-linked immunosorbent assay.
§Autoimmune polyendocrinopathy-candidiasis-ectodermal dystrophy is seen only in patients with type 2 disease.
From Krawitt EL: Autoimmune hepatitis. *N Engl J Med* 2006;354:54–66.

PATHOLOGY. The histologic features common to untreated cases include (1) inflammatory infiltrates, consisting of lymphocytes and plasma cells that expand portal areas and often penetrate the lobule; (2) moderate to severe piecemeal necrosis of hepatocytes extending outward from the limiting plate; and (3) variable necrosis, fibrosis, and zones of parenchymal collapse spanning neighboring portal triads or between a portal triad and central vein (bridging necrosis); and (4) variable degrees of bile duct epithelial injury. Distortion of hepatic architecture can be severe; cirrhosis may be present in children at the time of diagnosis. Histologic features in acute liver failure may be obscured by massive necrosis.

CLINICAL MANIFESTATIONS. The clinical features and course of autoimmune hepatitis are extremely variable. Signs and symptoms at the time of presentation include a wide spectrum of disease including a substantial number of asymptomatic patients and some who have an acute, even fulminant, onset. In 25–30% of patients with autoimmune hepatitis, particularly children, the illness mimics acute viral hepatitis. In most, the onset is insidious. Patients can be asymptomatic or have fatigue, malaise, behavioral changes, anorexia, and amenorrhea, sometimes for many months before jaundice or stigmata of chronic liver disease are recognized. Extrahepatic manifestations can include arthritis, vasculitis, nephritis, thyroiditis, Coombs-positive anemia, and rash. Some patients' initial clinical features reflect cirrhosis (ascites, bleeding esophageal varices, or hepatic encephalopathy).

There is usually mild to moderate jaundice. Spider telangiectasias and palmar erythema may be present. The liver is often tender and slightly enlarged but may not be felt in patients with cirrhosis. The spleen is commonly enlarged. Edema and ascites may be present in advanced cases. Evidence of involvement of other organ systems may be found.

LABORATORY FINDINGS. The findings are related to the severity of presentation. In many asymptomatic cases, serum aminotransferase ranges between 100 and 300 IU/L, whereas levels in excess of 1,000 IU/L can be seen in symptomatic young patients. Serum bilirubin concentrations (predominantly the direct-reacting fraction) are commonly 2–10 mg/dL. Serum alkaline phosphatase (ALP) and γ-glutamyl transpeptidase (GGT) activities are normal to slightly increased but may be more significantly elevated in autoimmune cholangiopathy. Serum gamma-globulin levels may show marked polyclonal elevations. Hypoalbuminemia is common. The prothrombin time is prolonged, most often as a result of vitamin K deficiency but also as a reflection of impaired hepatocellular function. A normochromic normocytic anemia, leukopenia, and thrombocytopenia are present and become more severe with the development of portal hypertension and hypersplenism.

Most patients with autoimmune hepatitis have hypergammaglobulinemia. Serum immunoglobulin (Ig) G levels usually exceed 16 g/L. Characteristic patterns of serum **autoantibodies** define several subgroups of autoimmune hepatitis (see Table 359-2). The most common pattern is the formation of non–organ specific antibodies, such as antiactin (smooth muscle), antinuclear, and antimitochondrial antibodies. Approximately 50% of these patients are 10–20 yr of age. High titers of a liver-kidney microsomal (LKM) antibody are detected in another form that usually affects children 2–14 yr of age. A subgroup of primarily young women may demonstrate autoantibodies against a soluble liver antigen but not against nuclear or microsomal proteins. Antineutrophil cytoplasmic antibodies may be seen more commonly in autoimmune cholangiopathy. Autoantibodies are rare in healthy children so that titers as low as 1 : 40 should be considered significant. Up to 20% of patients with apparent autoimmune hepatitis may not have autoantibodies at presentation. Antibodies to a cytochrome P450 component of LKM are commonly found in adult patients with chronic hepatitis C infection. Homologies in antigenic peptide epitopes between the hepatitis C virus and cytochrome P450 may explain this. Other less common autoantibodies include rheumatoid factor, anti–parietal cell antibodies, and antithyroid antibodies. A Coombs-positive hemolytic anemia may be present.

DIAGNOSIS. Autoimmune hepatitis is a clinical diagnosis based on certain diagnostic criteria; no single test will make this diagnosis. Diagnostic criteria with scoring systems have been developed for adults and modified slightly for children. Important positive features include female gender, primary elevation in transaminases and not ALP, elevated gamma-globulin levels, the presence of autoantibodies (most commonly antinuclear, smooth muscle, or liver-kidney microsome), and characteristic histologic findings (Fig. 359-1). Important negative features include the absence of viral markers (hepatitis B, C, D) of infection, absence of a history of drug or blood product exposure, and negligible alcohol consumption.

All other conditions that might lead to chronic hepatitis should be excluded (see Table 359-1). The differential diagnosis includes α_1-antitrypsin deficiency (see Chapter 354) and Wilson disease (see Chapter 354.2). The former disorder must be excluded by performing α_1-antitrypsin phenotyping and the latter by measuring serum ceruloplasmin and 24 hr urinary copper excretion and hepatic copper levels. Chronic active hepatitis may occur in patients with inflammatory bowel disease, but liver dysfunction in such patients is more commonly due to pericholangitis or sclerosing cholangitis. Celiac disease (see Chapter 335.2) is associated with liver disease that is akin to autoimmune hepatitis, and appropriate serologic testing should be performed, including assays for tissue transglutaminase. An ultrasonogram should be done to identify a choledochal cyst or other structural disorders of the biliary system. Magnetic resonance cholangiography may be very useful for screening for evidence of sclerosing cholangitis. Dilated or obliterated veins on ultrasonography suggest the possibility of the Budd-Chiari syndrome.

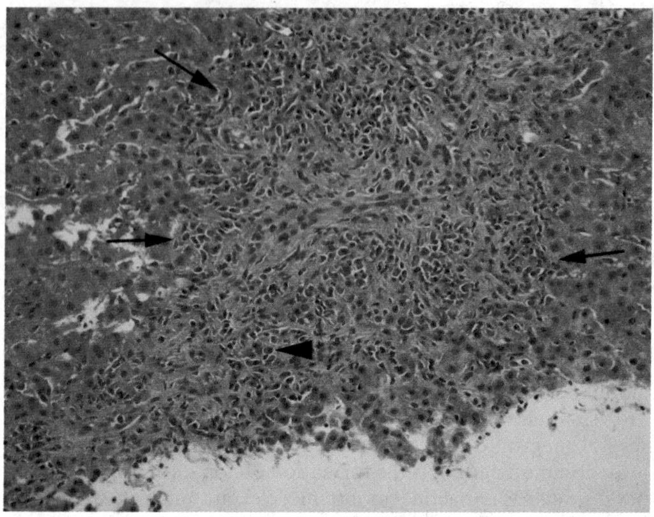

Figure 359-1. Autoimmune hepatitis. Liver biopsy showing fibrous expansion of the portal tracts with moderate portal lymphocytic infiltrates rich in plasma cells *(arrowhead)*. There is extensive interface hepatitis *(arrows)*. Original magnification = 20×. (Courtesy of Margret Magid, Mount Sinai School of Medicine.)

TREATMENT. Prednisone, with or without azathioprine or 6-mercaptopurine, improves the clinical, biochemical, and histologic features in most patients with autoimmune hepatitis and prolongs survival in most patients with severe disease. The choleretic agent ursodeoxycholic acid may be particularly useful in patients with biliary features of their disease.

The goal is to suppress or eliminate hepatic inflammation with minimal side effects. Prednisone at an initial dose of 1–2 mg/kg/24 hr is continued until aminotransferase values return to less than twice the upper limit of normal. The dose should then be lowered in 5 mg decrements over 2–4 mo until a maintenance dose of 0.1–0.3 mg/kg/24 hr is achieved. In patients who respond poorly, who experience severe side effects, or who cannot be maintained on low-dose steroids, azathioprine (1.5–2.0 mg/kg/24 hr, up to 100 mg/24 hr) can be added, with frequent monitoring for bone marrow suppression. Monitoring of metabolites of azathioprine may be useful in tailoring therapy for an individual patient. Single-agent therapy with alternate-day corticosteroids should be used with great caution, although addition of azathioprine to alternate-day steroids can be an effective approach that minimizes corticosteroid related toxicity. In patients with a mild and relatively asymptomatic presentation, some favor a lower starting dose of prednisone (10–20 mg) coupled with the simultaneous early administration of either 6-mercaptopurine (1.0–1.5 mg/kg/ 24 hr) or azathioprine (1.5–2.0 mg/kg/24 hr). Anecdotal reports have shown a potential for cyclosporine, tacrolimus, mycophenylate mofetil, and sirolimus in the management of cases refractory to standard therapy. Use of these agents should be reserved for practitioners with extensive experience in their administration, because the agents have a poor therapeutic to toxic ratio.

Histologic progress does not necessarily need to be assessed by sequential liver biopsies, although biochemical remission does not ensure histologic resolution. Follow-up liver biopsy is, therefore, especially important in those patients for whom consideration is given to discontinuing corticosteroid therapy. In patients with disappearance of symptoms and biochemical abnormalities and resolution of the necroinflammatory process on biopsy, an attempt at gradual discontinuation of medication is justified. There is a high rate of relapse after discontinuation of therapy. Relapse may require reinstitution of high levels of immunosuppression to control disease.

The therapy for chronic viral hepatitis differs from that for autoimmune disease (see also Chapter 355). **Chronic hepatitis B infection** is defined by persistently elevated serum levels of HBV DNA and hepatitis B surface antigen (HBsAg), with or without hepatitis B e antigen (HBeAg). In addition, there is persistent elevated serum aminotransferases and histologic evidence of chronic hepatitis. Therapy with interferon-α (5–10 MU/m^2 body surface area subcutaneously 3 times/wk) for 4–6 mo will induce a seroconversion (defined as conversion from HBeAg to HBeAg positivity) in 25–40% of children. Pegylated interferon-α2b preparations prolong the half-life of interferon, permitting weekly injections, and more constant blood levels are also highly affective. This seroconversion is presumed to be associated with a reduction in the long-term risk of developing cirrhosis and/or hepatocellular carcinoma. Side effects of interferon-α include systemic flu-like episodes, behavioral and cognitive changes, development of autoantibodies, and increased susceptibility to bacterial infection. Lamivudine, an oral nucleoside analog that inhibits viral DNA polymerase, is less toxic and is effective in delaying progression in adults.

Chronic hepatitis C virus is defined by the presence of HCV RNA in blood. Progression to end-stage liver disease has been seen in some children, and thus, chronically elevated aminotransferases and histologic evidence of activity may be an indication for treatment. Therapy includes combination therapy with interferon-α (3 MU/m^2 body surface subcutaneously 3 times/wk) and ribavirin (15/mg/kg divided, twice a day) for 6 (genotypes 2 and 3) to 12 (genotype 1) mo. Long-term clearance of virus is seen in 40–50% of treated children, with sustained viral responses in 80–90% of children with genotypes 2 and 3. The use of pegylated interferon in children is under study.

PROGNOSIS. The initial response to therapy in autoimmune hepatitis is generally prompt, with a >75% rate of remission. Transaminases and bilirubin fall to near-normal levels, often in the 1st 1–3 mo. When present, abnormalities in serum albumin and prothrombin time respond over a longer period (3–9 mo). In patients meeting the criteria for tapering and then withdrawal of treatment (25–40% of children), 50% are weaned from all medication; in the other 50%, relapse occurs after a variable period. Relapse usually responds to retreatment. Many children will not meet the criteria for an attempt at discontinuation of immunosuppression and should be maintained on the smallest dose of prednisone that minimizes biochemical activity of the disease. A careful balance of the risks of continued immunosuppression and ongoing hepatitis must be continually evaluated. This requires continual screening for complications of medical therapy (ophthalmologic examination, bone density measurement, blood pressure monitoring). Intermittent flares of hepatitis can occur and may necessitate recycling of prednisone therapy. Some children have a relatively steroid-resistant form of hepatitis. More extensive evaluations of the etiology of their hepatitis should be undertaken, directed particularly at reassessing for the presence of either sclerosing cholangitis or Wilson disease. Progression to cirrhosis can occur in autoimmune hepatitis despite a good response to drug therapy and prolongation of life. Corticosteroid therapy in fulminant autoimmune disease may be useful, although it should be administered with caution, given the predisposition of these patients to systemic bacterial and fungal infections.

Orthotopic liver transplantation has been successful in patients with end-stage liver disease associated with autoimmune hepatitis (see Chapter 365). Disease may recur after transplantation. Indication for transplantation should include evidence of hepatic decompensation.

Alvarez F, Berg PA, Bianchi FB, et al: International Autoimmune Hepatitis Group Report: Review of criteria for diagnosis of autoimmune hepatitis. *J Hepatol* 1999;31:929–938.

Andries S, Casamayou L, Sempoux C, et al: Posttransplant immune hepatitis in pediatric liver transplant recipients: Incidence and maintenance therapy with azathioprine. *Transplantation* 2001;72:267–272.

Bahar R, Yanni G, Martin M, et al: Orthotopic liver transplantation for autoimmune hepatitis and cryptogenic cirrhosis in children. *Transplantation* 2001;72:829–833.

Carrat F, Bani-Sadr F, Pol S, et al: Pegylated interferon alfa-2b vs standard interferon alfa-2b, plus ribavirin, for chronic hepatitis C in HIV-infected patients. *JAMA* 2004;292:2839–2848.

Czaja AJ, Bianchi FB, Carpenter HA, et al: Treatment challenges and investigational opportunities in autoimmune hepatitis. *Hepatology* 2005;41:207–215.

Ebbeson RL, Schreiber RA: Diagnosing autoimmune hepatitis in children: Is the International Autoimmune Hepatitis Group Scoring System useful? *Clin Gastroenterol Hepatol* 2004;10:935–940.

Gregorio GV, Portmann B, Reid F, et al: Autoimmune sclerosing cholangitis overlap syndrome in childhood: A 16 year prospective study. *Hepatology* 2001;33:544–553.

Janssen HLA, van Zonneveld M, Senturk H, et al: Pegylated interferon alfa-2b alone or in combination with lamivudine for HBeAg-positive chronic hepatitis B: A randomised trial. *Lancet* 2005;365:123–128.

Krawitt EL: Autoimmune hepatitis. *N Engl J Med* 2006;354:54–66.

Oettinger R, Brunnberg A, Gerner P, et al: Clinical features and biochemical data of Caucasian children at diagnosis of autoimmune hepatitis. *J Autoimmun* 2005;24:79–84.

Rumbo C, Emerick KM, Emre S, et al: Azathioprine metabolite measurements in the treatment of autoimmune hepatitis in pediatric patients: A preliminary report. *J Pediatr Gastroenterol Nutr* 2002;35:391–398.

Sokal E, Conjeevaram H, Roberts E, et al: Interferon alfa therapy for chronic hepatitis B in children: A multinational randomized controlled trial. *Gastroenterology* 1998;114:988–995.

Squires RH: Autoimmune hepatitis in children. *Curr Gastroenterol Rep* 2004;6:225–230.

Wen L, Ma Y, Bogdanos DP, et al: Pediatric autoimmune liver diseases: The molecular basis of humoral and cellular immunity. *Curr Mol Med* 2001;3:379–389.

Chapter 360 ■ Drug- and Toxin-Induced Liver Injury

Frederick J. Suchy

The liver is the main site of drug metabolism and is particularly susceptible to structural and functional injury after ingestion, parenteral administration, or inhalation of chemical agents, drugs, plant derivatives (home remedies), or environmental toxins. The possibility of drug use or toxin exposure at home or in the parental workplace should be explored for every child with liver dysfunction. The clinical spectrum of illness can vary from asymptomatic biochemical abnormalities of liver function to fulminant failure. Liver injury may be the only clinical feature of an adverse drug reaction or may be accompanied by systemic manifestations and damage to other organs.

Hepatic metabolism of drugs and toxins is mediated by a sequence of enzymatic reactions that, in large part, transform hydrophobic, less soluble molecules into more nontoxic, hydrophilic compounds that can be readily excreted in urine or bile. Relative liver size, liver blood flow, and extent of protein binding also influence drug metabolism. Phase 1 of the process involves enzymatic activation of the substrate to reactive intermediates containing a carboxyl, phenol, epoxide, or hydroxyl group. Mixed-function mono-oxygenase, cytochrome-*c* reductase, various hydrolases, and the cytochrome P450 (CYP) system are involved in this process. Nonspecific induction of these enzymatic pathways, which can occur during intercurrent viral infection, with starvation, and with administration of certain drugs such as anticonvulsants, can alter drug metabolism and increase the potential for hepatotoxicity. A single agent can be metabolized by more than one biochemical reaction. The reactive intermediates that are potentially damaging to the cell are enzymatically conjugated in phase 2 reactions with glucuronic acid, sulfate, acetate, glycine, or glutathione. Some drugs may be directly metabolized by these conjugating reactions without 1st undergoing phase 1 activation. Phase 3 is the energy-dependent excretion of drug metabolites and their conjugates by an array of membrane transporters such as the multiple drug resistant protein 1 (MDR-1).

Pathways for biotransformation are expressed early in the fetus and infant, but many phase 1 and 2 enzymes are immature, particularly in the 1st yr of life. CYP3A4 is the primary hepatic CYP expressed postnatally, and metabolizes >75 commonly used therapeutic drugs and several environmental pollutants and procarcinogens. Hepatic CYP3A4 activity is poorly expressed in the fetus but increases after birth to reach 30% of adult values by 1 mo, and 50% of adult values between 6 and 12 mo of age. CYP3A4 can be induced by a number of drugs, including phenytoin, phenobarbital, and rifampin. Enhanced production of toxic metabolites can overwhelm the capacity of phase 2 reactions. Conversely, numerous inhibitors of CYP3A4 from several different drug classes, such as erythromycin and cimetidine, can lead to toxic accumulations of CYP3A4 substrates. By contrast, although CYP2D6 is also developmentally regulated (maturation by 10 yr of age), its activity is more dependent on genetic polymorphisms than on sensitivity to inducers and inhibitors since >70 allelic variants of CYP2D6 significantly influence the metabolism of many drugs. UDP-glucuronosyltransferase 1A6, a phase 2 enzyme that glucuronidates acetaminophen, is also absent in the human fetus, increases slightly in the neonate, but does not reach adult levels until sometime after 10 yr of age. Mechanisms for the uptake and excretion of organic ions can also be deficient early in life. Impaired drug metabolism via phrase 1 and 2 reactions present in the 1st few months of life is followed by a period of enhanced metabolism of many drugs in children through 10 yr of age compared with adults.

Genetic polymorphisms in genes encoding enzymes and transporters mediating phase 1, 2, and 3 reactions can also be associated with impaired drug metabolism and an increased risk of hepatotoxicity. Some cases of idiosyncratic hepatotoxicity can occur as a result of aberrations (polymorphisms) in phase 1 drug metabolism, producing intermediates of unusual hepatotoxic potential combined with developmental, acquired, or relative inefficiency of phase 2 conjugating reactions. Children may be more or less susceptible than adults to hepatotoxic reactions; liver injury after the use of the anesthetic halothane is rare in children, and acetaminophen toxicity is unusual in infants compared with adolescents, whereas most cases of fatal hepatotoxicity associated with sodium valproate use have been reported in children. Excess or prolonged therapeutic administration of acetaminophen combined with reductions in caloric or protein intake can produce hepatotoxicity in children. In this setting, acetaminophen metabolism may be impaired by reduced synthesis of sulfated and glucuronated metabolites and reduced stores of glutathione. Immaturity of hepatic drug metabolic pathways may prevent degradation of a toxic agent; under other circumstances, the same immaturity might limit the formation of toxic metabolites.

Chemical hepatotoxicity can be (1) predictable or (2) idiosyncratic. Predictable hepatotoxicity implies a high incidence of hepatic injury in exposed individuals, with dose dependence. It is understandable that only a few drugs in clinical use fall into this category. These agents may damage the hepatocyte directly through alteration of membrane lipids (peroxidation) or through denaturation of proteins; such agents include carbon tetrachloride and trichloroethylene. Indirect injury can occur through interference with metabolic pathways essential for cell integrity or through distortion of cellular constituents by covalent binding of a reactive metabolite; examples include the liver injury produced by acetaminophen or by antimetabolites such as methotrexate or 6-mercaptopurine.

Idiosyncratic hepatotoxicity is infrequent and unpredictable but accounts for the majority of adverse reactions. The likelihood of injury is not dose dependent and may occur at any time during exposure to the agent. Idiosyncratic drug reactions in certain patients may reflect aberrant pathways for drug metabolism, possibly related to genetic polymorphisms, with production of toxic intermediates (isoniazid and sodium valproate may cause liver damage through this mechanism). Duration of drug use before liver injury varies (weeks to ≥1 yr) and the response to re-exposure may be delayed.

An idiosyncratic reaction can also be immunologically mediated as a result of prior sensitization (hypersensitivity); extrahepatic manifestations of hypersensitivity can include fever, rash, arthralgia, and eosinophilia. Duration of exposure before reaction is generally 1–4 wk, with prompt recurrence of injury on re-exposure. Studies indicate that arene oxides, generated through oxidative (cytochrome P450) metabolism of aromatic anticonvulsants (phenytoin, phenobarbital, carbamazepine), may initiate the pathogenesis of some hypersensitivity reactions. Arene oxides, formed in vivo, may bind to cellular macromolecules, thus perturbing cell function and possibly initiating immunologic mechanisms of liver injury.

Activation of liver nonparenchymal Kupffer cells and infiltration by neutrophils perpetuate toxic injury by many drugs by release of reactive oxygen and nitrogen species as well as cytokines. Stellate cells may also be activated, potentially leading to hepatic fibrosis and cirrhosis.

The pathologic spectrum of drug-induced liver disease is extremely wide, is rarely specific, and can mimic other liver diseases (Table 360-1). Predictable hepatotoxins such as acetaminophen produce centrilobular necrosis of hepatocytes. Steatosis is an important feature of tetracycline (microvesicular) and ethanol (macrovesicular) toxicities. A cholestatic hepatitis can be observed, with injury caused by erythromycin estolate and chlorpromazine. Cholestasis without inflammation may be a toxic effect of estrogens and anabolic steroids. Use of oral contraceptives and androgens has also been associated with benign and malignant liver tumors. Some idiosyncratic drug reactions can produce mixed patterns of injury, with diffuse cholestasis and cell necrosis. Several antineoplastic drugs and some herbal remedies have produced hepatic veno-occlusive disease. Chronic hepatitis has been associated with the use of methyldopa and nitrofurantoin. Some herbal supplements are associated with hepatic failure (Table 360-2).

Clinical manifestations can be mild and nonspecific, such as fever and malaise. Fever, rash, and arthralgia may be prominent in cases of hypersensitivity. In ill, hospitalized patients, the signs and symptoms of hepatic drug toxicity may be difficult to separate from the underlying illness. The differential diagnosis should include acute and chronic viral hepatitis, biliary tract disease, septicemia, ischemic and hypoxic liver injury, malignant infiltration, and inherited metabolic liver disease.

TABLE 360-1. Patterns of Hepatic Drug Injury

DISEASE	DRUG
Centrilobular necrosis	Acetaminophen Halothane
Microvesicular steatosis	Valproic acid
Acute hepatitis	Isoniazid
General hypersensitivity	Sulfonamides Phenytoin
Fibrosis	Methotrexate
Cholestasis	Chlorpromazine Erythromycin Estrogens
Veno-occlusive disease	Irradiation plus busulfan Cyclophosphamide
Portal and hepatic vein thrombosis	Estrogens Androgens
Biliary sludge	Ceftriaxone
Hepatic adenoma or hepatocellular carcinoma	Oral contraceptives Anabolic steroids

TABLE 360-2. Potentially Hepatotoxic Herbal or Dietary Supplements

Kava (*Kava kava*, awa, kew)
Chaparral (creosote bush, greasewood, *Larrea tridentata*)
Ma Huang (*Ephedra*)
Comfrey leaves (pyrrolizidine alkaloids)
Germander extracts (*Trucrium chamaedrys*)
Valerian with skullcap
Mushroom (*Amanita phalloides, Galerina*)
LipoKinetix (phenylpropanolamine, sodium usinate, diiodothyronine, yohimbine, caffeine)

The **laboratory features** of drug- or toxin-related liver disease are extremely variable. Hepatocyte damage can lead to elevations of serum aminotransferase activities and serum bilirubin levels and to impaired synthetic function as evidenced by decreased serum coagulation factors and albumin. Hyperammonemia can occur with liver failure or with selective inhibition of the urea cycle (sodium valproate). Toxicologic screening of blood and urine specimens can aid in the detection of drug or toxin exposure. Percutaneous liver biopsy may be necessary to distinguish drug injury from complications of an underlying disorder or from intercurrent infection.

Slight elevation of serum aminotransferase activities (generally <2–3 times normal) may occur during therapy with drugs, particularly anticonvulsants, capable of inducing microsomal pathways for drug metabolism. Liver biopsy reveals proliferation of smooth endoplasmic reticulum but no significant liver injury. Liver test abnormalities often resolve with continued drug therapy.

Treatment of drug- or toxin-related liver injury is mainly supportive. Contact with the offending agent should be avoided. Corticosteroids may have a role in immune-mediated disease. N-acetylcysteine therapy, by stimulating glutathione synthesis, is effective in preventing hepatotoxicity when administered within 16 hr after an acute overdose of acetaminophen and appears to improve survival in patients with severe liver injury even up to 36 hr after ingestion (also see Chapter 758). Orthotopic liver transplantation may be required for treatment of drug- or toxin-induced hepatic failure.

The prognosis of drug- or toxin-induced liver injury depends on its type and severity. Injury is usually completely reversible when the hepatotoxic factor is withdrawn. The mortality of submassive hepatic necrosis with fulminant liver failure may, however, exceed 50%. With continued use of certain drugs, such as methotrexate, effects of hepatoxicity can proceed insidiously to cirrhosis. Neoplasia can follow long-term androgen therapy. Rechallenge with a drug suspected of having caused previous liver injury is rarely justified and can result in fatal hepatic necrosis.

Bessmertny O, Hatton RC, Gonzalez-Peralta RP: Antiepileptic hypersensitivity syndrome in children. *Ann Pharmacother* 2001;35:533–538.

Blake MJ, Castro L, Leeder JS, Kearns GL: Ontogeny of drug metabolizing enzymes in the neonate. *Semin Fetal Neonatal Med* 2005;10:123–138.
Clarkson A, Choonara I: Surveillance for fatal suspected adverse drug reactions in the UK. *Arch Dis Child* 2002;87:462–466.
Estes JD, Stolpman D, Olyaei A, et al: High prevalence of potentially hepatotoxic herbal supplement use in patients with fulminant hepatic failure. *Arch Surg* 2003;138:852–858.
Heubi JE, Barbacci MB, Zimmerman HJ: Therapeutic misadventures with acetaminophen: Hepatotoxicity after multiple doses in children. *J Pediatr* 1998;132:22–27.
James LP, Wells E, Beard RH, Farrar HC: Predictors of outcome after acetaminophen poisoning in children and adolescents. *J Pediatr* 2002;140:522–526.
Kearns GL, Abdel-Rahman SM, Alander SW, et al: Developmental pharmacology—Drug disposition, action, and therapy in infants and children. *N Engl J Med* 2003;349:1157–1167.
Lee WM: Drug-induced hepatotoxicity. *N Engl J Med* 1995;333:1118–1127.
Leeder JS: Pharmacogenetics and pharmacogenomics. *Pediatr Clin North Am* 2001;48:765–781.
Navarro VJ, Senior JR: Drug-related hepatotoxicity. *N Engl J Med* 2006;354: 731–739.
Roberts EA: Drug-induced liver disease in children. In Suchy FJ, Sokol RJ, Balistreri WF (editors): *Liver Disease in Children,* 2nd ed. Philadelphia, Lippincott, William & Wilkins 2001, pp 463–492.
Russo MW, Galanko JA, Shrestha R, et al: Liver transplantation for acute liver failure from drug induced liver injury in the United States. *Liver Transpl* 2004;10:1018–1023.

Chapter 361 ■ Fulminant Hepatic Failure

Frederick J. Suchy

Fulminant hepatic failure is a clinical syndrome resulting from massive necrosis of hepatocytes or from severe functional impairment of hepatocytes. Synthetic, excretory, and detoxifying functions of the liver are all severely impaired. In adults, hepatic encephalopathy has been an essential diagnostic feature. This narrow definition may be problematic because early hepatic encephalopathy can be difficult to detect in infants and children. The currently accepted definition in children includes: (1) biochemical evidence of acute liver injury (usually <8 wk duration); (2) no evidence of chronic liver disease; and (3) hepatic-based coagulopathy defined as a prothrombin time (PT) >15 sec or international normalized ratio (INR) >1.5 not corrected by vitamin K in the presence of clinical hepatic encephalopathy, or a PT >20 sec or INR >2 regardless of the presence of clinical hepatic encephalopathy. Liver failure in the perinatal period can be associated with prenatal liver injury and even cirrhosis. Examples include neonatal iron storage (hemochromatosis) disease, tyrosinemia, and some cases of congenital viral infection. Liver disease may be noticed at birth or after several days of apparent well-being. Fulminant Wilson disease also occurs in older children who were previously asymptomatic but, by definition, have pre-existing liver disease. Moreover, in some cases of liver failure, particularly in the idiopathic form of acute hepatic failure, the onset of encephalopathy occurs later, from 8 to 28 wk after the onset of jaundice.

ETIOLOGY. Fulminant hepatic failure can be a complication of viral hepatitis (A, B, D, E). An unusually high risk of fulminant hepatic failure occurs in young people who have combined infections with the hepatitis B virus (HBV) and hepatitis D. Mutations in the precore and/or promoter region of HBV DNA have been associated with fulminant and severe hepatitis. HBV is also responsible for some cases of fulminant liver failure in the absence of serologic markers of HBV infection but with HBV DNA found in the liver. Hepatitis C and E viruses are uncommon causes of fulminant hepatic failure in the United States. Patients with chronic HCV are at risk if they have superinfection with HAV. Epstein-Barr virus, herpes simplex virus, adenovirus, enterovirus, cytomegalovirus, parvovirus B19, and varicella-zoster infections can produce fulminant hepatitis in children. Fulminant hepatic failure may also be caused by autoimmune hepatitis. An idiopathic form of fulminant hepatic failure accounts for 40–50% of cases in children. The disease occurs sporadically and usually without the risk factors for common causes of viral hepatitis. It is likely that the etiology of these cases is heterogeneous, including unidentified or variant viruses and undiagnosed metabolic disorders.

Various hepatotoxic drugs and chemicals can also cause fulminant hepatic failure. Predictable liver injury may occur after exposure to carbon tetrachloride and *Amanita phalloides* mushroom or after acetaminophen overdose. The latter drug is a common etiology of hepatic failure in children and adolescents. Idiosyncratic damage can follow the use of drugs such as halothane or sodium valproate. Ischemia and hypoxia resulting from hepatic vascular occlusion, congestive heart failure, cyanotic congenital heart disease, or circulatory shock can produce liver failure. Metabolic disorders associated with hepatic failure include Wilson disease, acute fatty liver of pregnancy, galactosemia, hereditary tyrosinemia, hereditary fructose intolerance, neonatal iron storage disease, defects in β-oxidation of fatty acids, and deficiencies of mitochondrial electron transport. Herbal supplements are additional causes of hepatic failure (see Table 360-2).

PATHOLOGY. Liver biopsy usually reveals patchy or confluent massive necrosis of hepatocytes. Multilobular or bridging necrosis can be associated with collapse of the reticulin framework of the liver. There may be little or no regeneration of hepatocytes. A zonal pattern of necrosis may be observed with certain insults (centrilobular damage is associated with acetaminophen hepatotoxicity or with circulatory shock). Evidence of severe hepatocyte dysfunction rather than cell necrosis is occasionally the predominant histologic finding (microvesicular fatty infiltrate of hepatocytes is observed in Reye syndrome, β-oxidation defects, and tetracycline toxicity).

PATHOGENESIS. The mechanisms that lead to fulminant hepatic failure are poorly understood. It is unknown why only about 1–2% of patients with viral hepatitis experience liver failure. Massive destruction of hepatocytes may represent both a direct cytotoxic effect of the virus and an immune response to the viral antigens. One third to one half of patients with HBV-induced liver failure become negative for serum hepatitis B surface antigen within a few days of presentation and often have no detectable HBV antigen or HBV DNA in serum. These findings suggest a hyperimmune response to the virus that underlies the massive liver necrosis. Formation of hepatotoxic metabolites that bind covalently to macromolecular cell constituents is involved in the liver injury produced by drugs such as acetaminophen and isoniazid; fulminant hepatic failure may follow depletion of intracellular substrates involved in detoxification, particularly glutathione. Whatever the initial cause of hepatocyte injury, various factors may contribute to the pathogenesis of liver failure, including impaired hepatocyte regeneration, altered parenchymal perfusion, endotoxemia, and decreased hepatic reticuloendothelial function.

The pathogenesis of hepatic encephalopathy may relate to increased serum levels of ammonia, false neurotransmitters, amines, increased γ-aminobutyric acid (GABA) receptor activity, or increased circulating levels of endogenous benzodiazepine-like compounds. Decreased hepatic clearance of these substances may produce marked central nervous system dysfunction.

CLINICAL MANIFESTATIONS. Fulminant hepatic failure can be the presenting feature of liver disease or it can complicate previously known liver disease. A history of developmental delay and/or neuromuscular dysfunction may indicate an underlying mitochondrial or β-oxidation defect. A child with fulminant hepatic failure has usually been previously healthy and most often has no risk factors for liver disease such as toxin or blood product exposure. Progressive jaundice, fetor hepaticus, fever, anorexia, vomiting, and abdominal pain are common. A rapid decrease in liver size without clinical improvement is an ominous sign. A hemorrhagic diathesis and ascites may develop. Patients should be closely observed for hepatic encephalopathy, which is initially characterized by minor disturbances of consciousness or motor function. Irritability, poor feeding, and a change in sleep rhythm may be the only findings in infants; asterixis may be demonstrable in older children. Patients are often somnolent, confused, or combative on arousal and may eventually become responsive only to painful stimuli. Patients can rapidly progress to deeper stages of coma in which extensor responses and decerebrate and decorticate posturing appear. Respirations are usually increased early, but respiratory failure can occur in stage IV coma (Table 361-1).

LABORATORY FINDINGS. Serum direct and indirect bilirubin levels and serum aminotransferase activities may be markedly elevated. Serum aminotransferase activities do not correlate well with the severity of the illness and may actually decrease as a patient deteriorates. The blood ammonia concentration is usually increased, but hepatic coma can occur in patients with a normal blood ammonia level. PT is always prolonged and often does not improve after parenteral administration of vitamin K. Hypoglycemia can occur, particularly in infants. Hypokalemia, hyponatremia, metabolic acidosis, or respiratory alkalosis may develop.

TREATMENT. Management of fulminant hepatic failure is supportive. No therapy is known to reverse hepatocyte injury or to promote hepatic regeneration. An infant or child with acute hepatic failure should be cared for in an institution able to perform a liver transplantation if necessary and managed in an intensive care unit with continuous monitoring of vital functions. Endotracheal intubation may be required to prevent aspiration, to reduce cerebral edema by hyperventilation, and to facilitate pulmonary toilet. Mechanical ventilation and supplemental oxygen are often necessary in advanced coma. Sedatives should be avoided unless needed in the intubated patient because these agents can aggravate or precipitate encephalopathy. Prophylactic use of antacids, H_2 receptor blockers, or both should be considered because of the high risk of gastrointestinal bleeding. Hypovolemia should be avoided and treated with cautious infusions of fluids and blood products. Renal dysfunction can result from dehydration, acute tubular necrosis, or functional renal failure (hepatorenal syndrome). Electrolyte and glucose solutions should be administered intravenously to maintain urine output, to correct or prevent hypoglycemia, and to maintain normal serum potassium concentrations. Hyponatremia is common but is usually dilutional and not a result of sodium depletion. Parenteral supplementation with calcium, phosphorus, and magnesium may be required. Hypophosphatemia, probably a reflection of liver regeneration, and early phosphorus administration are associated with a better prognosis in acute liver failure, whereas hyperphosphatemia predicts a failure of spontaneous recovery.

Coagulopathy should be treated with parenteral administration of vitamin K and may require infusion of fresh frozen plasma and platelets to treat clinically significant bleeding; disseminated intravascular coagulation may also occur. Plasmapheresis may permit temporary correction of the bleeding diathesis without resulting in volume overload. Recombinant factor VIIa has been used for transient correction of coagulopathy refractory to fresh frozen plasma infusions and may facilitate the performance of invasive procedures such as placement of a central line or an intracranial pressure monitor. Continuous hemofiltration is useful for management of fluid overload and acute renal failure.

Patients should be monitored closely for infection, including sepsis, pneumonia, peritonitis, and urinary tract infections. At least 50% of patients experience serious infection. Gram-positive organisms (*Staphylococcus aureus, S. epidermidis*) are the most common pathogens, but gram-negative and fungal infections are also observed.

Gastrointestinal hemorrhage, infection, constipation, sedatives, electrolyte imbalance, and hypovolemia can precipitate encephalopathy and should be identified and corrected. Protein intake should be initially restricted or eliminated, depending on the degree of encephalopathy. The gut should be purged with several enemas. Lactulose should be given every 2–4 hr orally or by nasogastric tube in doses (10–50 mL) sufficient to cause diarrhea. The dose is then adjusted to produce several acidic, loose bowel movements daily. Lactulose syrup diluted with 1–3 volumes of water can also be given as a retention enema every 6 hr. Lactulose, a nonabsorbable disaccharide, is metabolized to organic acids by colonic bacteria; it probably lowers blood ammonia levels through decreasing microbial ammonia production and through trapping of ammonia in acidic intestinal contents. Oral or rectal administration of a nonabsorbable antibiotic such as neomycin may reduce enteric bacteria responsible for ammonia production. Oral antibiotics may be more effective than lactulose in lowering serum ammonia levels. Flumazenil, a benzodiazepine antagonist, may temporally reverse early hepatic encephalopathy. Cerebral edema is an extremely serious complication of hepatic encephalopathy that responds poorly to measures such as corticosteroid administration and osmotic diuresis. Monitoring intracranial pressure can be useful in preventing severe cerebral edema, in maintaining cerebral perfusion pressure, and in establishing the suitability of a patient for liver transplantation.

Controlled trials have shown a worsened outcome of fulminant hepatic failure in patients treated with corticosteroids. Immunosuppressive therapy may be effective in fulminant autoimmune hepatitis. The antiviral drug pleconaril is the treatment of choice for fulminant enteroviral hepatitis in the neonate.

Temporary liver support continues to be evaluated as a bridge for the patient with liver failure to liver transplantation or regeneration. Nonbiologic systems, essentially a form of liver dialysis

TABLE 361-1. Stages of Hepatic Encephalopathy

	STAGES			
	I	II	III	IV
Symptoms	Periods of lethargy, euphoria; reversal of day-night sleeping; may be alert	Drowsiness, inappropriate behavior, agitation, wide mood swings, disorientation	Stupor but arousable, confused, incoherent speech	Coma IVa responds to noxious stimuli IVb no response
Signs	Trouble drawing figures, performing mental tasks	Asterixis, fetor hepaticus, incontinence	Asterixis, hyperreflexia, extensor reflexes, rigidity	Areflexia, no asterixis, flaccidity
Electroencephalogram	Normal	Generalized slowing, θ waves	Markedly abnormal, triphasic waves	Markedly abnormal bilateral slowing, δ waves, electric-cortical silence

with an albumin-containing dialysate, and biologic liver support devices that involve perfusion of the patient's blood through a cartridge containing liver cell lines or porcine hepatocytes can remove some toxins, improve serum biochemical abnormalities, and, in some cases, improve neurologic function, but there has been little evidence of improved survival and few children have been treated.

Orthotopic liver transplantation (OLT) can be lifesaving in patients who reach advanced stages of hepatic coma. Reduced-size allografts and living donor transplantation have been important advances in the treatment of infants with hepatic failure. Partial auxiliary orthotopic or heterotopic liver transplantation is successful in a small number of children and, in some cases, has allowed regeneration of the native liver and eventual withdrawal of immunosuppression. OLT should not be done in patients with liver failure and neuromuscular dysfunction secondary to a mitochondrial disorder since progressive neurologic deterioration is likely to continue post transplant.

PROGNOSIS. Children with hepatic failure may fare somewhat better than adults, but overall mortality with supportive care alone exceeds 70%. The prognosis varies considerably with the cause of liver failure and stage of hepatic encephalopathy. With intensive medical support, survival rates of 50–60% occur with hepatic failure complicating acetaminophen overdose (may be as high as 90%) and with fulminant HAV or HBV infection. By contrast, spontaneous recovery can be expected in only 10–20% of patients with liver failure caused by the idiopathic form of acute liver failure or an acute onset of Wilson disease. In patients who progress to stage IV coma (see Table 361-1), the prognosis is extremely poor. Brainstem herniation is the most common cause of death. Major complications such as sepsis, severe hemorrhage, or renal failure increase the mortality. The prognosis is particularly poor in patients with liver necrosis and multiorgan failure. Age <1 yr, stage 4 encephalopathy, and the need for dialysis before transplantation have been associated with increased mortality. Pretransplant serum bilirubin concentration and the INR of coagulation are not predictive of post-tranplant survival. Children diagnosed with acute hepatic failure are more likely to die while on the waiting list compared to children with other diagnoses. Moreover, owing to the severity of their illness, the 6 mo post liver transplantation survival of ≈75% is significantly lower than the ≥90% now being achieved in children with chronic liver disease. Patients who recover from fulminant hepatic failure with only supportive care do not usually develop cirrhosis or chronic liver disease. Aplastic anemia occurs in ≈10% of children with the idiopathic form of fulminant hepatic failure and is often fatal.

Als-Nielsen B, Gluud LL, Gluud C: Non-absorbable disaccharides for hepatic encephalopathy: Systematic review of randomized trials. *Br Med J* 2004;328:1046–1050.

Baliga P, Alvarez S, Lindblad A, Zeng L: Posttransplant survival in pediatric fulminant hepatic failure: The SPLIT experience. *Liver Transpl* 2004;10:1364–1371.

Dhawan A, Cheeseman P, Mieli-Vergani G: Approaches to acute liver failure in children. *Pediatr Transplant* 2004;8:584–588.

Dubern B, Broue P, Dubuisson C, et al: Orthotopic liver transplantation for mitochondrial respiratory chain disorders: A study of 5 children. *Transplantation* 2001;71:633–637.

Emre S, Schwartz ME, Shneider B, et al: Living related liver transplantation for acute liver failure in children. *Liver Transpl Surg* 1999;5:161–165.

Gines P, Guevara M, Arroyo V, Rodes J: Hepatorenal syndrome. *Lancet* 2003;362:1819–1826.

Lee WM: Management of acute liver failure. *Semin Liver Dis* 1996;16:369–378.

Shawcross D, Jalan R: Dispelling myths in the treatment of hepatic encephalopathy. *Lancet* 2005;265:431–433.

Shneider BL, Rinaldo P, Emre S, et al: Abnormal concentrations of esterified carnitine in bile: A feature of pediatric acute liver failure with poor prognosis. *Hepatology* 2005;41:717–721.

Singer AL, Olthoff KM, Kim H, et al: Role of plasmapheresis in the management of acute hepatic failure in children. *Ann Surg* 2001;234:418–424.

Squires RH, Shneider BL, Bucuvalus J, et al: Acute liver failure in children: The first 348 patients in the pediatric acute liver failure study group. *J Pediatr* 2006;148:652–658.

Teo EK, Ostapowicz G, Hussain M, et al: Hepatitis B infection in patients with acute liver failure in the United States. *Hepatology* 2001;33:972–976.

van de Kerkhove MP, Hoekstra R, Chamuleau RA, van Gulik TM: Clinical application of bioartificial liver support systems. *Ann Surg* 2004; 240:216–230.

Chapter 362 ■ Cystic Diseases of the Biliary Tract and Liver

Frederick J. Suchy

Cystic lesions of liver may be initially recognized during infancy and childhood. Hepatic fibrosis can also occur as part of an underlying developmental defect. Cystic renal disease is usually associated and often determines the clinical presentation and prognosis. Virtually all proteins encoded by genes mutated in combined cystic diseases of the liver and kidney are at least partially localized to primary cilia in renal tubular cells and cholangiocytes.

CHOLEDOCHAL CYSTS. These are congenital dilatations of the common bile duct that can cause progressive biliary obstruction and biliary cirrhosis. Cylindrical and spherical cysts of the extrahepatic ducts are the most common types. Segmental or diffuse dilatation can be observed. A diverticulum of the common bile duct or dilatation of the intraduodenal portion of the common duct (choledochocele) is a variant. Cystic dilatation of the intrahepatic bile ducts may be associated with a choledochal cyst.

The pathogenesis of choledochal cysts remains uncertain. Some reports have suggested that junction of the common bile duct and the pancreatic duct before their entry into the sphincter of Oddi may allow reflux of pancreatic enzymes into the common bile duct, causing inflammation, localized weakness, and dilatation of the duct. Other possibilities are that choledochal cysts represent malformations of the common duct or that they occur as part of the spectrum of an infectious disease that includes neonatal hepatitis and biliary atresia. Consistent with this theory, reovirus RNA has been detected in liver and biliary tissues of some infants with choledochal cysts.

Approximately 75% of cases appear during childhood. The infant typically presents with cholestatic jaundice; severe liver dysfunction including ascites and coagulopathy can rapidly evolve if biliary obstruction is not relieved. An abdominal mass is rarely palpable. In an older child, the **classic triad** of abdominal pain, jaundice, and mass occurs in <33% of patients. Features of acute cholangitis (fever, right upper quadrant tenderness, jaundice, leukocytosis) may be present. The diagnosis is made by ultrasonography; choledochal cysts have been identified prenatally using this technique. Magnetic resonance cholangiography is useful in the preoperative assessment of choledochal cyst anatomy.

The **treatment of choice** is primary excision of the cyst and a Roux-en-Y choledochojejunostomy. Simple drainage into the small bowel is less satisfactory owing to a risk of development of carcinoma in the residual cystic tissue. The postoperative course can be complicated by recurrent cholangitis or stricture at the anastomotic site.

CYSTIC DILATATION OF THE INTRAHEPATIC BILE DUCTS (CAROLI DISEASE). Congenital saccular dilatation can affect several segments of the intrahepatic bile ducts; the dilated ducts are lined by cuboidal epithelium and are in continuity with the main duct system, which is usually normal. Caroli actually described two variants: Caroli disease, characterized by ectasias of the intrahepatic bile ducts without other abnormalities; and Caroli syndrome, in which congenital ductal dilatation is associated with features of congenital hepatic fibrosis and the renal lesion of autosomal recessive polycystic renal disease. Caroli syndrome is more common, but both varieties can occur in the same family and are inherited in an autosomal recessive fashion. Choledochal cysts have also been associated with Caroli disease. There is a marked predisposition to ascending cholangitis and calculus formation within the abnormal bile ducts.

Affected patients usually experience symptoms of acute cholangitis as children or young adults. Fever, abdominal pain, mild jaundice, and pruritus occur; and a slightly enlarged, tender liver is palpable. Elevated alkaline phosphatase (ALP) activity, direct-reacting bilirubin levels, and leukocytosis may be observed during episodes of acute infection. In patients with Caroli syndrome, clinical features may be due to a combination of recurring bouts of cholangitis reflecting the intrahepatic ductal abnormalities and portal hypertensive bleeding resulting from hepatic fibrosis. Ultrasonography shows the dilated intrahepatic ducts, but definitive diagnosis and extent of disease must be determined by percutaneous transhepatic, endoscopic, or magnetic resonance cholangiography.

Cholangitis and sepsis are treated with appropriate antibiotics. Calculi may require surgery. Partial hepatectomy may be curative in rare cases in which disease is confined to a single lobe. The prognosis is otherwise guarded, largely owing to difficulties in controlling cholangitis and biliary lithiasis and to a significant risk for developing cholangiocarcinoma. Liver transplantation may be required.

CONGENITAL HEPATIC FIBROSIS. This is an autosomal recessive disorder characterized pathologically by diffuse periportal and perilobular fibrosis in broad bands that contain distorted bile duct–like structures and that often compress or incorporate central or sublobular veins. Irregularly shaped islands of liver parenchyma contain normal-appearing hepatocytes. Caroli disease and choledochal cysts have been associated. About 75% of patients have renal disease, mostly autosomal recessive polycystic renal disease and rarely nephronophthisis. Congenital hepatic fibrosis also occurs as part of the COACH syndrome (*c*erebellar vermis hypoplasia, *o*ligophrenia, congenital *a*taxia, *c*oloboma, and *h*epatic fibrosis). Congenital hepatic fibrosis has been described in children with a congenital disorder of glycosylation caused by mutations in the gene encoding phosphomannose isomerase (see Chapter 87.6).

The disorder usually has its clinical onset in childhood, with hepatosplenomegaly or with bleeding secondary to portal hypertension. Cholangitis may occur in patients who have associated abnormalities of bile ducts.

Hepatocellular function is well preserved. Serum aminotransferase activities and bilirubin levels are usually normal; serum ALP activity may be slightly elevated. The serum albumin level and prothrombin time are normal. Liver biopsy is usually required for diagnosis.

Treatment of this disorder should focus on control of bleeding from esophageal varices. Infrequent mild bleeding episodes may be managed by endoscopic sclerotherapy or band ligation of the varices. After more severe hemorrhage, portacaval anastomosis may bring relief of portal hypertension. The prognosis may be greatly improved by a shunting procedure, but survival in some patients may be limited by renal failure.

AUTOSOMAL DOMINANT POLYCYSTIC KIDNEY DISEASE (ADPKD) [SEE CHAPTER 521.3]. ADPKD, a common inherited disease, affects 1/1,000 live births. It is characterized by progressive renal cyst development and cyst enlargement and an array of extrarenal manifestations. There is a high degree of intrafamilial and interfamilial variability in the clinical expression of the disease.

ADPKD is caused by mutation in one of two genes, *PKD1* or *PKD2*, which account for 85–90% and 10–15% of cases, respectively. The proteins encoded by these genes, polycystin-1 and polycystin-2, are expressed in renal tubule cells and in cholangiocytes. Polycystin-1 functions as a mechanosensor in cilia, detecting the movement of fluid through tubules and transmitting the signal through polycystin-2, which acts as a calcium channel.

Multiple hepatic lesions have been associated with ADPKD and include the ductal plate malformation with cystic communicating duct elements, dilated and apparently noncommunicating cysts, and biliary microhamartomas (the so-called von Meyenburg complexes). Segmental dilatation of the intrahepatic ducts (Caroli disease) and congenital hepatic fibrosis have been reported. Approximately 50% of patients with renal failure have demonstrable hepatic cysts that are derived from but not in continuity with the biliary tract. The hepatic cysts increase with age but are extremely uncommon before the age of 16 yr. Hepatic cystogenesis appears to be influenced by estrogens. Although the frequency of cysts is similar in males and females, the development of large hepatic cysts is mainly a complication in females. Hepatic cysts are often asymptomatic but can cause pain and are occasionally complicated by hemorrhage, infection, jaundice from bile duct compression, portal hypertension with variceal bleeding, or hepatic venous outflow obstruction from mechanical compression of hepatic veins, resulting in tender hepatomegaly and exudative ascites. Cholangiocarcinoma can occur. Selected patients with severe symptomatic polycystic liver disease and favorable anatomy benefit from liver resection or fenestration.

Subarachnoid hemorrhage may result from the associated cerebral arterial aneurysms.

AUTOSOMAL DOMINANT POLYCYSTIC LIVER DISEASE (ADPLD). ADPLD is a distinct clinical and genetic identity in which multiple cysts develop and are unassociated with cystic kidney disease. Liver cysts arise from but are not in continuity with the biliary tract. Females are more commonly affected than males, and the cysts often enlarge during pregnancy. Cysts are rarely identified in children. Cyst complications are related to effects of local compression, infection, hemorrhage, or rupture. Genes associated with ADPLD are *PRKCSH* and *SEC63*, which encode hepatocystin and Sec63, respectively. Hepatocystin is a protein kinase c substrate adK-H that is involved in the proper folding and maturation of glycoproteins. It has been localized to the endoplasmic reticulum. *SEC63* encodes a protein SEC63P, which is a component of the protein translocation machinery in the endoplasmic reticulum.

A solitary liver cyst (nonparasitic) rarely occurs in childhood. Abdominal distention and pain may be present, and a poorly defined right upper quadrant mass may be palpable. These benign lesions are best left undisturbed unless they compress adjacent structures or a complication occurs, such as hemorrhage into the cyst.

AUTOSOMAL RECESSIVE POLYCYSTIC KIDNEY DISEASE (ARPKD) [SEE CHAPTER 521.2]. ARPKD presents predominantly in childhood. Bilateral enlargement of the kidneys is caused by a generalized dilatation of the collecting tubules. The disorder is invariably associated with congenital hepatic fibrosis and various degrees of biliary ductal ectasia.

The gene for ARPKD encodes a protein that is called fibrocystin or polyductin. Fibrocystin has been localized to cilia on the apical domain of renal collecting cells and cholangiocytes. The primary defect in ARPKD may be ciliary dysfunction related to the abnormality in this protein. In ARPKD, the cysts arise as ectatic expansions of the collecting tubules and bile ducts that remain in continuity with their structures of origin.

ARPKD normally presents in early life, often shortly after birth, and is generally more severe than ADPKD. Patients with ARPKD may die in the perinatal period owing to renal failure or lung dysgenesis. The kidneys in these patients are usually markedly enlarged and dysfunctional. Respiratory failure can result from compression of the chest by grossly enlarged kidneys, from fluid retention, or from concomitant pulmonary hypoplasia. The clinical pathologic findings within a family tend to breed true, although there has been some variability in the severity of the disease and the time for presentation within the same family.

The liver in patients with ARPKD demonstrates various degrees of periportal fibrosis, bile ductular hyperplasia, and biliary dysgenesis. Liver disease and complications from hepatic fibrosis are most likely to be clinically significant in patients whose kidney disease allows prolonged survival. The most prominent clinical problem in older patients with ARPKD and congenital hepatic fibrosis is portal hypertension. Although portal hypertensive bleeding can occur in the 1st year of life, it more commonly presents in older children with hematemesis or melena. Firm or hard hepatomegaly is usually present. Splenomegaly is a frequent finding accompanied by hypersplenism. Owing to dilatation of the intrahepatic bile ducts, these patients are at increased risk of bacterial cholangitis. Caroli disease or a congenital, segmental, saccular dilatation of the intrahepatic bile ducts may coexist with congenital hepatic fibrosis and ARPKD.

Hemorrhage from esophageal varices can be initially managed by using endoscopic sclerotherapy or banding. Some patients with well-preserved hepatic function may benefit from a selective portacaval shunt. Biliary sepsis should be aggressively treated. Recurrent bouts of bacterial cholangitis can lead to progressive loss of hepatic function. Rare patients have unilateral involvement that can be treated by hepatic resection. Hepatic transplantation may be required for patients with hepatic failure.

Variable abnormalities of bile ducts (irregular dilatation, proliferation, cysts) and portal fibrosis can be associated with Meckel syndrome, trisomy 17–18, tuberous sclerosis, and asphyxiating thoracic dystrophy.

Choledochal Cysts

Miyano T, Yamataka A: Choledochal cysts. *Curr Opin Pediatr* 1997;9:283–288.

Okada T, Sasaki F, Ueki S, et al: Postnatal management for prenatally diagnosed choledochal cysts. *J Pediatr Surg* 2004;39:1055–1058.

Stringer MD, Dhawan A, Davenport M, et al: Choledochal cysts: Lessons from a 20-year experience. *Arch Dis Child* 1995;73:528–531.

Caroli Disease

Asselah T, Ernst O, Sergent G, et al: Caroli's disease: A magnetic resonance cholangiopancreatography diagnosis. *Am J Gastroenterol* 1998;93:109–110.

Desmet VJ: Ludwig symposium on biliary disorders—Part I. Pathogenesis of ductal plate abnormalities. *Mayo Clin Proc* 1998;73:80–89.

Keane F, Hadzic N, Wilkinson ML, et al: Neonatal presentation of Caroli's disease. *Arch Dis Child Fetal Neonatal Ed* 1997;77:F145–F146.

Congenital Hepatic Fibrosis

Desmet VJ: What is congenital hepatic fibrosis? *Histopathology* 1992;20:465–477.

Perisic VN: Long-term studies on congenital hepatic fibrosis in children. *Acta Paediatr* 1995;84:695–696.

Polycystic Diseases of the Liver and Kidney

Davila S, Furu L, Gharavi AG: Mutations in *SEC63* cause autosomal dominant polycystic liver disease. *Nat Genet* 2004;36:575–577.

Everson GT, Taylor MR: Management of polycystic liver disease. *Curr Gastroenterol Rep* 2005;7:19–25.

Guay-Woodford LM, Desmond RA: Autosomal recessive polycystic kidney disease: The clinical experience in North America. *Pediatrics* 2003;111:1072–1080.

Johnson CA, Gissen P, Sergi C: Molecular pathology and genetics of congenital hepatorenal fibrocystic syndromes. *J Med Genet* 2003;40:311–319.

Lina F, Satlinb LM: Polycystic kidney disease: The cilium as a common pathway in cystogenesis. *Curr Opin Pediatr* 2004;16:171–176.

Qian Q, Li A, King BF, et al: Clinical profile of autosomal dominant polycystic liver disease. *Hepatology* 2003;37:164–171.

Wilson PD: Polycystic kidney disease. *N Engl J Med* 2004;350:151–164.

Chapter 363 ■ Diseases of the Gallbladder

Frederick J. Suchy

ANOMALIES. The gallbladder is congenitally absent in about 0.1% of the population. Hypoplasia or absence of the gallbladder can be associated with extrahepatic biliary atresia or cystic fibrosis. Duplication of the gallbladder occurs rarely.

ACUTE HYDROPS (TABLE 363-1). Acute noncalculous, noninflammatory distention of the gallbladder can occur in infants and children. It is defined by the absence of calculi, bacterial infection, or congenital anomalies of the biliary system. The disorder may complicate acute infections, but the cause is often not identified. Hydrops of the gallbladder may also develop in patients receiving long-term parenteral nutrition, presumably as a result of gallbladder stasis during the period of enteral fasting. Hydrops is distinguished from acalculous cholecystitis by the absence of a significant inflammatory process and a generally benign prognosis.

Affected patients usually have right upper quadrant pain with a palpable mass. Fever, vomiting, and jaundice may be present and are usually associated with a systemic illness such as streptococcal infection. Ultrasonography shows a markedly distended, echo-free gallbladder, without dilatation of the biliary tree. Acute hydrops is usually treated conservatively with a focus on supportive care and managing the intercurrent illness; cholecystostomy and drainage are rarely needed. Spontaneous resolution and return of normal gallbladder function usually occur over a period of several weeks. If a laparotomy is required, a large, edematous gallbladder is found to contain white, yellow, or green bile. Obstruction of the cystic duct by mesenteric adenopathy is occasionally observed. Cholecystectomy is required if the gallbladder is gangrenous. Pathologic examination of the gallbladder

TABLE 363-1. Conditions Associated with Hydrops of the Gallbladder

Kawasaki disease	Thalassemia
Streptococcal pharyngitis	Total parenteral nutrition
Staphylococcal infection	Prolonged fasting
Leptospirosis	Viral hepatitis
Ascariasis	Sepsis
Threadworm	Henoch-Schönlein purpura
Sickle cell crisis	Mesenteric adenitis
Typhoid fever	Necrotizing enterocolitis

wall shows edema and mild inflammation. Cultures of bile are usually sterile.

CHOLECYSTITIS AND CHOLELITHIASIS. Acute acalculous cholecystitis is uncommon in children and is usually caused by infection. Pathogens include streptococci (groups A and B), gram-negative organisms, particularly *Salmonella* and *Leptospira interrogans*. Parasitic infestation with ascaris or *Giardia lamblia* may be found. Calculous cholecystitis may rarely follow abdominal trauma or burn injury or is associated with a systemic vasculitis, such as periarteritis nodosa.

Clinical features include right upper quadrant or epigastric pain, nausea, vomiting, fever, and jaundice. Right upper quadrant guarding and tenderness are present. Ultrasonography discloses an enlarged, thick-walled gallbladder, without calculi. Serum alkaline phosphatase (ALP) activity and direct-reacting bilirubin levels are elevated. Leukocytosis is usual.

Patients may recover with treatment of systemic and biliary infection. Since the gallbladder can become gangrenous, daily ultrasonography is useful in monitoring gallbladder distention and wall thickness. Cholecystectomy is required in patients who fail to improve with conservative management. Cholecystostomy drainage is an alternative approach in a critically ill patient.

Cholelithiasis is relatively rare in otherwise healthy children, occurring more commonly in patients with various predisposing disorders (Table 363-2). In children, >70% of gallstones are the pigment type, 15–20% are cholesterol stones, and the remainder are composed of a mixture of cholesterol, organic matrix, and calcium bilirubinate. Black pigment gallstones, composed mostly of calcium bilirubinate and glycoprotein matrix, are a frequent complication of chronic hemolytic anemias. Brown pigment stones form mostly in infants as a result of biliary tract infection. Unconjugated bilirubin is the predominant component, formed by the high β-glucuronidase activity of infected bile. Cholesterol gallstones are composed purely of cholesterol or contain >50% cholesterol along with a mucin glycoprotein matrix and calcium bilirubinate. Calcium carbonate stones have also been described in children.

Patients with hemolytic disease (including sickle cell anemia, the thalassemias, and red blood cell enzymopathies) and Wilson disease are at increased risk for black pigment cholelithiasis. In sickle cell disease, pigment gallstones can develop before age 4 yr and have been reported in 17–33% of patients aged 2 to 18 yr. Genetic variation in the promoter of uridine diphosphate (UDP)-glucuronosyltransferase 1A1 (the [TA]7/[TA]7 and [TA]7/[TA]8 genotypes) underlies Gilbert syndrome, a chronic form of unconjugated hyperbilirubinemia, and is a risk factor for pigment gallstone formation in sickle cell disease.

Cirrhosis and chronic cholestasis also increase the risk for pigment gallstones. Sick premature infants may also have gallstones; their treatment is often complicated by such factors as bowel resection, necrotizing enterocolitis, prolonged parenteral nutrition without enteral feeding, cholestasis, frequent blood transfusions, and use of diuretics. Cholelithiasis in premature infants is often asymptomatic and may resolve spontaneously. Brown pigment stones are found in infants with obstructive jaundice and infected intra- and extrahepatic bile ducts. These stones are usually radiolucent, owing to a lower content of calcium phosphate and carbonate and a higher amount of cholesterol than in black pigment stones. Biliary dyskinesia, a disorder of impaired gallbladder contractility, is an abnormality predisposing to gallstones in late childhood and teenage years.

TABLE 363-2. Conditions Associated with Cholelithiasis
Chronic hemolytic disease (sickle cell anemia, spherocytosis)
Obesity
Ileal resection or disease
Cystic fibrosis
Chronic liver disease
Crohn disease
Prolonged parenteral nutrition
Prematurity with complicated medical or surgical course
Prolonged fasting or rapid weight reduction
Treatment of childhood cancer
Abdominal surgery
Pregnancy

Cholesterol cholelithiasis in children most frequently affects obese adolescent girls. Cholesterol gallstones are also found in children with disturbances of the enterohepatic circulation of bile acids, including patients with ileal disease and bile acid malabsorption, such as those with ileal resection, ileal Crohn disease, and cystic fibrosis. Pigment stones can also occur in these patients.

Cholesterol gallstone formation seems to result from an excess of cholesterol in relation to the cholesterol-carrying capacity of micelles in bile. Supersaturation of bile with cholesterol, leading to crystal and stone formation, could result from decreased bile acid or from an increased cholesterol concentration in bile. Other initiating factors that may be important in stone formation include gallbladder stasis or the presence in bile of abnormal mucoproteins or bile pigments that may serve as a nidus for cholesterol crystallization.

Prolonged use of high-dose ceftriaxone, a third-generation cephalosporin, has been associated with the formation of calcium-ceftriaxone salt precipitates *(biliary pseudolithiasis)* in the gallbladder. Biliary sludge or cholelithiasis can be detected in >40% of children treated with ceftriaxone for at least 10 days. In rare cases, children become jaundiced and develop abdominal pain; precipitates usually resolve spontaneously within several months after discontinuation of the drug.

Acute or chronic cholecystitis is often associated with gallstones. The acute form may be precipitated by impaction of a stone in the cystic duct. Proliferation of bacteria within the obstructed gallbladder lumen can contribute to the process and lead to biliary sepsis. Chronic calculous cholecystitis is more common. It can develop insidiously or follow several attacks of acute cholecystitis. The gallbladder epithelium commonly becomes ulcerated and scarred.

The most important clinical feature of cholelithiasis is recurrent abdominal pain, which is often colicky and localized to the right upper quadrant. An older child may have intolerance for fatty foods. Acute cholecystitis may be the 1st manifestation, with fever, pain in the right upper quadrant, and often a palpable mass. Jaundice occurs more commonly in children than adults. Pain may radiate to an area just below the right scapula. A plain roentgenogram of the abdomen may reveal opaque calculi, but radiolucent (cholesterol) stones are not visualized. Accordingly, ultrasonography is the method of choice for gallstone detection. Hepatobiliary scintography is a valuable adjunct in that failure to visualize the gallbladder provides evidence of cholecystitis.

Cholecystectomy is curative. Laparoscopic cholecystectomy is routinely performed in symptomatic infants and children with cholelithiasis. Common bile duct stones are unusual in children, occurring in 2–6% of cases with cholelithiasis, often in association with obstructive jaundice and pancreatitis. Operative cholangiography should be done at the time of surgery, however, to detect unsuspected common duct calculi. Endoscopic retrograde cholangiography with extraction of common duct stones is an option before laparoscopic cholecystectomy in older children and adolescents.

Asymptomatic patients with cholelithiasis pose a more difficult management problem. Studies in adults indicate a lag time of more than a decade between initial formation of a gallstone and development of symptoms. Spontaneous resolution of cholelithiasis has been reported in infants and children. If surgery is deferred for any patient, however, parents should be counseled about signs and symptoms consistent with cholecystitis or obstruction of the common bile duct by a gallstone. In patients with chronic hemolysis or ileal disease, cholecystectomy can be carried out at the same time as another surgical procedure. Since laparoscopic surgery can safely be performed in children with sickle cell disease, elective cholecystectomy is being done more frequently at the time of gallstone diagnosis, before symptoms or complications develop. In cases associated with liver disease, severe obesity, or cystic fibrosis, the surgical risk of cholecystectomy may be substantial so that the risks and benefits of the operation need to be carefully considered.

Barton LL, Luisiri A, Dawson JE: Hydrops of the gallbladder in childhood infections. *Pediatr Infect Dis J* 1995;14:163–164.

Bor O, Dinleyici EC, Kebapci M, Aydogdu SD: Ceftriaxone-associated biliary sludge and pseudocholelithiasis during childhood: A prospective study. *Pediatr Int* 2004;46:322–324.

Chaar V, Keclard L, Diara JP, et al: Association of UGT1A1 polymorphism with prevalence and age at onset of cholelithiasis in sickle cell anemia. *Haematologica* 2005;90:188–199.

Lobe TE: Cholelithiasis and cholecystitis in children. *Semin Pediatr Surg* 2000;9:170–176.

Rescorla FJ: Cholelithiasis, cholecystitis, and common bile duct stones. *Curr Opin Pediatr* 1997;9:276–282.

Stringer MD, Taylor DR, Soloway RD: Gallstone composition: Are children different? *J Pediatr* 2003;142:435–440.

Suchy FJ: Anatomy, anomalies and pediatric disorders of the biliary tract. In Feldman M, Friedman LS, Sleisenger MH (editors): *Gastrointestinal and Liver Disorders*, 7th ed. Philadelphia, WB Saunders, 2002, pp 1019–1036.

Suell MN, Horton TM, Dishop MK, et al: Outcomes for children with gallbladder abnormalities and sickle cell disease. *J Pediatr* 2004;145:617–621.

Walker TM, Hambleton IR, Serjeant GR: Gallstones in sickle cell disease: Observations from the Jamaican Cohort study. *J Pediatr* 2000;136:80–85.

Chapter 364 ■ Portal Hypertension and Varices

Frederick J. Suchy

Portal hypertension, defined as an elevation of portal pressure >10–12 mm Hg, is a major cause of morbidity and mortality in children with liver disease. The normal portal venous pressure is ≈7 mm Hg. The clinical features of the various forms of portal hypertension may be similar, but the associated complications, management, and prognosis can vary significantly and depend on whether the process is complicated by hepatic insufficiency.

ETIOLOGY. Portal hypertension can result from obstruction to portal blood flow anywhere along the course of the portal venous system. The various disorders associated with portal hypertension are outlined in Table 364-1. Portal hypertension can occur as a result of prehepatic, intrahepatic, or posthepatic obstruction to the flow of portal blood.

Extrahepatic portal vein obstruction is an important cause of portal hypertension in childhood. The obstruction can occur at any level of the portal vein. Umbilical infection (omphalitis) with or without a history of catheterization of the umbilical vein may be causal in neonates. The infection can potentially spread from the umbilical vein to the left branch of the portal vein and eventually to the main portal venous channel. Intra-abdominal infections, including acute appendicitis and primary peritonitis, can be causal in older children. Portal vein thrombosis has also been associated with neonatal dehydration and systemic infection. In older children, inflammatory bowel disease can be associated with a hypercoagulable state and portal venous obstruction.

TABLE 364-1. Causes of Portal Hypertension

EXTRAHEPATIC PORTAL HYPERTENSION
Portal vein agenesis, atresia, stenosis
Portal vein thrombosis or cavernous transformation
Splenic vein thrombosis
Increased portal flow
Arteriovenous fistula
INTRAHEPATIC PORTAL HYPERTENSION
Hepatocellular Disease
Acute and chronic viral hepatitis
Cirrhosis
Congenital hepatic fibrosis
Wilson disease
α_1-Antitrypsin deficiency
Glycogen storage disease type IV
Hepatotoxicity
Methotrexate
Parenteral nutrition
Biliary Tract Disease
Extrahepatic biliary atresia
Cystic fibrosis
Choledochal cyst
Sclerosing cholangitis
Intrahepatic bile duct paucity
Idiopathic Portal Hypertension
Postsinusoidal Obstruction
Budd-Chiari syndrome
Veno-occlusive disease

Thrombosis of the portal vein has also occurred in association with biliary tract infections and primary sclerosing cholangitis. Portal vein thrombosis has also been associated with hypercoagulable states such as deficiencies of factor V Leiden, protein C, or protein S. The portal vein can be replaced by a fibrous remnant or contain an organized thrombus. Rare developmental anomalies producing extrahepatic portal hypertension include agenesis, atresia, or stenosis of the portal vein. Obstruction by a web or diaphragm can also occur. At least half of reported cases have no defined cause.

Uncommonly, presinusoidal hypertension can be caused by increased flow through the portal system as a result of a congenital or acquired arteriovenous fistula.

The intrahepatic causes of portal hypertension are numerous. Obstruction to flow can occur on the basis of a presinusoidal process, including acute and chronic hepatitis, congenital hepatic fibrosis, and schistosomiasis. Portal infiltration with malignant cells or granulomas can also contribute. An idiopathic form of portal hypertension characterized by splenomegaly, hypersplenism, and portal hypertension without occlusion of portal or splenic veins and with no obvious disease in the liver has been described. In some patients, noncirrhotic portal fibrosis has been observed.

Cirrhosis is the predominant cause of portal hypertension and is related to obstruction of bloodflow through the portal vein. The numerous causes of cirrhosis include recognized disorders such as biliary atresia, autoimmune hepatitis, chronic viral hepatitis, and metabolic liver disease such as α_1-antitrypsin deficiency, Wilson disease, glycogen storage disease type IV, hereditary fructose intolerance, and cystic fibrosis.

Postsinusoidal causes of portal hypertension are also observed in childhood. The Budd-Chiari syndrome occurs with obstruction to hepatic veins anywhere between the efferent hepatic veins and the entry of the inferior vena cava into the right atrium. In most cases, no specific cause can be found, but thrombosis can occur from inherited and acquired hypercoagulable states (antithrombin III deficiency, protein C or S deficiency, factor V Leiden or prothrombin mutations, paroxysmal nocturnal hemoglobinemia, pregnancy, oral contraceptives) and can complicate hepatic or metastatic neoplasms, collagen vascular disease, infection, and trauma. Additional causes of the Budd-Chiari syndrome include Behçet syndrome, inflammatory bowel disease, aspergillosis, dacarbazine therapy, and inferior vena cava webs. Veno-occlusive disease is the most frequent cause of hepatic vein obstruction in children. In this disorder, occlusion of the centrilobular venules or sublobular hepatic veins occurs. The disorder occurs after total body irradiation with or without cytotoxic drug therapy that is commonly used before bone marrow transplantation. The disease has also occurred after ingestion of herbal remedies containing the pyrrolizidine alkaloids, which are sometimes taken as medicinal teas.

PATHOPHYSIOLOGY. The primary hemodynamic abnormality in portal hypertension is increased resistance to portal blood flow. This is the case whether the resistance to portal flow has an intrahepatic cause such as cirrhosis or is due to portal vein obstruction. Portosystemic shunting should decompress the portal system and thus significantly lower portal pressures. Despite the development of significant collaterals deviating portal blood into systemic veins, portal hypertension is maintained by an overall increase in portal venous flow and thus maintenance of portal hypertension. A hyperdynamic circulation is achieved by tachycardia, an increase in cardiac output, and decreased systemic vascular resistance. Splanchnic dilatation also occurs. Overall, the increase in portal flow likely contributes to an increase in variceal transmural pressure. The increase in portal blood flow is related to the contribution of hepatic and collateral flow; the actual portal blood flow reaching the liver is reduced. It is also likely that hepatocellular dysfunction and portosystemic shunting lead to the generation of various humoral factors that cause vasodilatation and an increase in plasma volume.

Many of the portal hypertension complications can be accounted for by the development of a remarkable collateral circulation. Collateral vessels may form prominently in areas in which absorptive epithelium joins stratified epithelium, particularly in the esophagus or anorectal region. The superficial submucosal collaterals, especially those in the esophagus and stomach and, to a lesser extent, those in the duodenum, colon, or rectum, are prone to rupture and bleeding under increased pressure. In portal hypertension, the vascularity of the stomach is also abnormal and demonstrates prominent submucosal arteriovenous communications between the muscularis mucosa and dilated precapillaries and veins. The resulting lesion, a vascular ectasia, has been called *congestive gastropathy* and contributes to a significant risk of bleeding from the stomach.

CLINICAL MANIFESTATIONS. Bleeding from esophageal varices is the most common presentation. In patients with underlying hepatic disease, physical examination may show jaundice and stigmata of cirrhosis such as palmar erythema and vascular telangiectasias. Growth retardation can occur in patients with cirrhosis and, to a lesser extent, in children with isolated extrahepatic portal vein obstruction. Ascites may be present in patients with intrahepatic causes of portal hypertension and may transiently occur with portal vein obstruction. Dilated cutaneous collateral vessels carrying blood from the portal to systemic circulation may be apparent in the periumbilical region. In the absence of clinical or biochemical features of liver disease and with a liver of normal size, portal vein obstruction is most likely. Well-compensated cirrhosis cannot be completely ruled out under these conditions. Cholestasis and liver dysfunction with elevated serum bilirubin and aminotransferases may occur uncommonly in portal vein obstruction as a result of external compression of bile ducts by cavernous transformation of the portal vein. An enlarged, hard liver with minimal disturbance of hepatic function suggests the possibility of congenital hepatic fibrosis. Hemorrhage, particularly in children with portal vein obstruction, can be precipitated by minor febrile, intercurrent illness. The mechanism is often unclear; aspirin or other nonsteroidal anti-inflammatory drugs may be a contributing factor by damaging the integrity of a congested gastric mucosa or interfering with platelet function. Coughing during a respiratory illness can also increase intravariceal pressure. The bleeding may become apparent with hematemesis or with melena. Gastrointestinal hemorrhage can also originate from portal hypertensive gastropathy or from gastric, duodenal, peristomal, or rectal varices. Splenomegaly, sometimes with hypersplenism, is the next most common presenting feature in portal vein obstruction and may be discovered 1st on routine physical examination. Because more than half of patients in many series with portal vein obstruction do not experience bleeding until after age 6 yr, the diagnosis should be suggested in a child without hepatocellular disease who had a complicated neonatal course and in whom asymptomatic splenomegaly later developed.

Children with portal hypertension, regardless of the underlying cause, may have recurrent bouts of life-threatening hemorrhage. In patients with portal vein obstruction and normal hepatic function, the bleeding usually stops spontaneously. In patients with intrahepatic disease, the combination of portal hypertension and poor liver synthetic ability (coagulopathy) can make bleeding much more difficult to control. Moreover, esophageal hemorrhage and cirrhosis may have injurious effects on the liver, further impairing hepatic function and sometimes precipitating jaundice, ascites, and encephalopathy.

Another serious complication of portal hypertension is the hepatopulmonary syndrome, which develops in at least 10% of patients with cirrhosis. It is defined as an arterial oxygenation defect induced by intrapulmonary microvascular dilatation, resulting from release of mediators such as nitric oxide into the venous circulation.

DIAGNOSIS. In patients with established chronic liver disease or in those in whom portal vein obstruction is suspected, an experienced ultrasonographer should be able to demonstrate the patency of the portal vein. In addition, the use of Doppler flow ultrasonography can demonstrate the direction of flow within the portal system. The pattern of flow correlates with the severity of cirrhosis and encephalopathy. Reversal of portal vein bloodflow (hepatofugal flow) is more likely to be associated with variceal bleeding. Ultrasonography is also effective in detecting the presence of esophageal varices. Another important feature of extrahepatic portal vein obstruction is so-called cavernous transformation of the portal vein, in which an extensive complex of small collateral vessels form in the paracholedochal and epicholedochal venous system to bypass the obstruction. Other imaging techniques also contribute to further definition of the portal vein anatomy but are required less often; contrast-enhanced CT and magnetic resonance angiography provide similar information to ultrasonography. Selective arteriography of the celiac axis, superior mesenteric artery, and splenic vein may be useful in precise mapping of the extrahepatic vascular anatomy. This is not required to establish a diagnosis but may prove valuable in planning surgical decompression of portal hypertension.

In a patient with hypoxia (hepatopulmonary syndrome), intrapulmonary microvascular dilatation is demonstrated with contrast-enhanced echocardiography that shows delayed appearance in the left heart of microbubbles from a saline bolus injected into a peripheral vein.

Endoscopy is the most reliable method for detecting esophageal varices and for identifying the source of gastrointestinal bleeding. Although bleeding from esophageal or gastric varices is most common in children with portal hypertension, up to one third of patients, particularly those with cirrhosis, may have bleeding from some other source such as portal hypertensive gastropathy or gastric or duodenal ulcerations. There is a strong correlation between variceal size as assessed endoscopically and the probability of hemorrhage. Red spots apparent over varices at the time of endoscopy are a strong predictor of imminent hemorrhage.

TREATMENT. The therapy of portal hypertension can be divided into emergency treatment of potentially life-threatening hemorrhage and prophylaxis directed at prevention of initial or subsequent bleeding. It must be emphasized that many trials of therapy are based on experience with adults with portal hypertension.

Treatment of patients with variceal hemorrhage must focus on fluid resuscitation, initially in the form of crystalloid infusion, followed by the replacement of red blood cells. Correction of coagulopathy by administration of vitamin K or the infusion of platelets or fresh frozen plasma, or both therapies, may be required. A nasogastric tube should be placed to document the presence of blood within the stomach and to monitor for ongoing bleeding. An H_2 receptor blocker such as ranitidine should be given intravenously to reduce the risk of bleeding from gastric erosions. In most patients, particularly those with extrahepatic portal hypertension and with normal hepatic synthetic function, bleeding usually stops spontaneously. Care should be taken in fluid resuscitation of children after bleeding to avoid producing an excessively high venous pressure and an increased risk for further bleeding.

Pharmacologic therapy to decrease portal pressure may be considered in patients with continued bleeding. Vasopressin or one of its analogs has been commonly used and is thought to act by increasing splanchnic vascular tone and thus decreasing portal blood flow. Vasopressin is administered initially with a bolus of 0.33 U/kg over 20 min, followed by a continued infusion of the same dose on an hourly basis or a continuous infusion of 0.2 U/1.73 m^2/min. The drug has a half-life of ≈30 min. Its use may be limited by the side effects of vasoconstriction, which can impair cardiac function and perfusion to the heart, bowel, and kidneys and may also, as a result, exacerbate fluid retention. Nitroglycerin, usually given as a portion of a skin patch, has also been used to decrease portal pressure and, when used in conjunction with vasopressin, may ameliorate some of its untoward effects. The somatostatin analog octreotide decreases splanchnic blood flow with fewer side effects and may be administered by continuous intravenous infusion of 1.0–5.0 μg/kg/hr. Although studies in adults are promising, its use and efficacy in children have not been well evaluated.

After an episode of variceal hemorrhage or in patients in whom bleeding cannot be controlled, endoscopic sclerosis or elastic band ligation of esophageal varices are important options. In endoscopic sclerosis, sclerosants are injected either intravariceally or paravariceally until bleeding has stopped. Although bleeding can be controlled acutely in most cases, further sessions of sclerotherapy are required to achieve temporary obliteration of the varices. Treatments may be associated with further bleeding, bacteremia, esophageal ulceration, and stricture formation. Most centers do not perform endoscopic sclerotherapy of varices prophylactically but use the procedure as a bridge to the time of liver transplantation or until collateral circulation develops in extrahepatic portal vein obstruction. Endoscopic elastic band ligation of varices has been shown in adult and pediatric studies to be more effective and associated with fewer complications than is sclerotherapy.

In patients who continue to bleed despite pharmacologic and endoscopic methods to control hemorrhage, a Sengstaken-Blakemore tube can be placed to stop hemorrhage by mechanically compressing esophageal and gastric varices. The device may be the only option to control life-threatening hemorrhage but carries a significant rate of complications and a high rate of bleeding when the device is removed. It poses a particularly high risk for pulmonary aspiration, and the tube is not well tolerated in children without significant sedation.

Various surgical procedures have been devised to divert portal blood flow and to decrease portal pressure. A portacaval shunt diverts nearly all of the portal blood flow into the subhepatic inferior right vena cava. Although portal pressure is significantly reduced, because of the significant diversion of blood from the liver, patients with parenchymal liver disease have a marked risk for hepatic encephalopathy. More selective shunting procedures, such as mesocaval or distal splenorenal shunt, may effectively decompress the portal system while allowing a greater amount of portal blood flow to the liver. The small size of the vessels makes these operations technically challenging in infants and small children, and there is a significant risk of failure as a result of shunt thrombosis. Portal vein thrombosis has been managed with the REX shunt (mesenterico–left portal vein bypass), which restores physiologic portal blood flow and inflow of hepatotrophic factors.

Orthotopic liver transplantation represents a much better therapy for portal hypertension resulting from intrahepatic disease. A prior portosystemic shunting operation does not preclude a successful liver transplantation but makes the operation technically more difficult. Portosystemic shunting may remain an option in children with extrahepatic portal hypertension, particularly in those patients who are suffering from potentially life-threatening hemorrhage not effectively controlled by other measures and who reside a great distance from emergency medical care. A transjugular intrahepatic portosystemic shunt (TIPS), in which a stent is placed by an interventional radiologist between the right hepatic vein and the right or left branch of the portal vein, can aid in the management of portal hypertension in children, especially in those needing temporary relief before liver transplantation. The TIPS procedure can precipitate hepatic encephalopathy, however, and is prone to thrombosis.

Long-term treatment with nonspecific β blockers such as propranolol has been used extensively in adults with portal hypertension. These agents may act by lowering cardiac output and portal perfusion. Evidence in adult patients shows that β blockers may reduce the incidence of variceal hemorrhage and improve long-term survival. A therapeutic effect is thought to result when the pulse rate is reduced by at least 25%. There is limited published experience with the use of this therapy in children.

PROGNOSIS. Portal hypertension secondary to intrahepatic disease has a poor prognosis. Portal hypertension is usually progressive in these patients and is often associated with deteriorating liver function. Efforts should be directed toward prompt treatment of acute bleeding and prevention of recurrent hemorrhage with available methods. Patients with progressive liver disease and significant esophageal varices ultimately require orthotopic liver transplantation. Liver transplantation is the only effective therapy for hepatopulmonary syndrome and should also be considered for patients with portal hypertension secondary to hepatic vein obstruction or resulting from severe veno-occlusive disease.

In patients with portal vein obstruction, episodes of bleeding may become less frequent and severe with age as a collateral circulation develops. Most patients can be treated conservatively with endoscopic sclerotherapy when necessary. Children may continue to experience significant bleeding during adolescence, however, and may eventually require a portosystemic shunting procedure.

Botha JF, Campos, BD, Grant, WJ, et al: Portosystemic shunts in children: A 15-year experience. *J Am Coll Surg* 2004;199:179–185.

Gauthier-Villars M, Franchi S, Gauthier F, et al: Cholestasis in children with portal vein obstruction. *J Pediatr* 2005;146:568–573.

Gentil-Kocher S, Bernard O, Brunelle F, et al: Budd-Chiari syndrome in children: Report of 22 cases. *J Pediatr* 1988;113:30–38.

Heyman MB, LaBerge JM, Somberg KA, et al: Transjugular intrahepatic portosystemic shunts (TIPS) in children. *J Pediatr* 1997;131:914–919.
Hoeper MM, Krowka MJ, Strassburg CP: Portopulmonary hypertension and hepatopulmonary syndrome. *Lancet* 2004;363:1461–1468.
Lykavieris P, Gauthier F, Hadchouel P, et al: Risk of gastrointestinal bleeding during adolescence and early adulthood in children with portal vein obstruction. *J Pediatr* 2000;136:805–808.
Miga D, Sokol RJ, Mackenzie T, et al: Survival after first esophageal variceal hemorrhage in patients with biliary atresia. *J Pediatr* 2001;139:291–296.
Narayanan Menon KV, Shah V, Kamath PS: The Budd-Chiari syndrome. *N Engl J Med* 2004;350:578–584.
Peter L, Dadhich SK, Yachha SK: Clinical and laboratory differentiation of cirrhosis and extrahepatic portal venous obstruction in children. *J Gastroenterol Hepatol* 2003;18:185–189.
Ryckman FC, Alonso MH: Causes and management of portal hypertension in the pediatric population. *Clin Liver Dis* 2001;5:789–818.
Sarin SK, Agarwal SR: Extrahepatic portal vein obstruction. *Semin Liver Dis* 2002;22:43–58.
Shashidhar H, Langhans N, Grand RJ: Propranolol in prevention of portal hypertensive hemorrhage in children: A pilot study. *J Pediatr Gastroenterol Nutr* 1999;29:12–17.

Chapter 365 ■ Liver Transplantation

Melissa Hurwitz and Kenneth L. Cox

Liver transplantation is standard therapy for children with end-stage liver disease, life-threatening hepatic metabolic disorders, severe drug (acetaminophen) or toxin (mushroom) mediated hepatic failure, and localized cancers of the liver. With current immunosuppression and surgical techniques, 1 and 5 yr survival rates for children after liver transplantation are 87% and 77%, respectively. One third of pediatric liver transplant recipients are <1 yr of age at the time of transplant and have a significantly poorer 1 yr survival rate (85%) as compared with older children (90%). Approximately 500 children in the United States undergo liver transplantation each year, with 6% having more than one organ transplanted simultaneously, which usually includes either a kidney or small intestine (see Chapter 336).

The most frequent indication for liver transplantation is extrahepatic biliary atresia after a failed portoenterostomy (Kasai) procedure. Metabolic liver disease and acute hepatic necrosis are next in frequency (Table 365-1). The decision to perform transplantation in patients with metabolic liver disease includes: Is the disease hepatic in origin, can it be successfully treated medically, and are the extrahepatic manifestations reversible?

Early referral to a transplant center is important so that patients and their families can be evaluated and treated in a timely fashion. Medical and psychological issues are assessed to determine the appropriateness of transplant, optimal management, and urgency. Age (<1 yr), growth failure (defined as height or weight 2 standard deviations below normal), hyperbilirubinemia, hypoalbuminemia, and coagulopathy as indicated by prolonged international normalized ratio (INR) have been predictive of increased morbidity and mortality from liver disease and are used to determine the urgency for liver transplantation. Other variables that also indicate the need for liver transplantation are ascites, encephalopathy, variceal bleeding, and renal failure. Prompt referral of patients with fulminant hepatic failure is critical because a majority quickly die without liver transplantation. Counseling families about the special needs of children with chronic illness improves the psychosocial outcome. Early evaluation allows sufficient time to find a donor and for families to learn about liver transplantation. Pretransplantation management is critical to the success of the procedure and to limiting morbidity from the liver disease (see Chapters 353, 361, and 364). Portoenterostomies should be performed in children with biliary atresia because they often delay and occasionally obviate the need for liver transplantation. Even children with biliary atresia who are >3 mo of age may benefit from this procedure.

TABLE 365-1. Indications for Pediatric Liver Transplantation

INDICATIONS	PER CENT OF TRANSPLANTS (%)
Biliary atresia	39
Metabolic liver disease	13
α_1-Antitrypsin deficiency	5
Tyrosinemia	1
Wilson disease	1
Other*	6
Acute hepatic necrosis	12
Biliary hypoplasia including Alagille syndrome	5
TPN-associated liver disease	5
Idiopathic cirrhosis	4
Autoimmune hepatitis	3
Tumors including hepatoblastoma	3
Neonatal hepatitis	2
Cystic fibrosis	2
Primary sclerosing cholangitis	2
Congenital hepatic fibrosis	1
Other	9

*Includes urea cycle defects.
Data are from the United Network for Organ Sharing Data Base for 8,950 pediatric liver transplants performed on children between January 1, 1988, and October 31, 2004.

Areas of major importance are nutrition and immunizations. Patients with liver disease have malabsorption as well as anorexia, which lead to growth retardation. Formula containing medium-chain triglycerides is helpful because bile salts are not necessary for their absorption. Caloric requirements may be as high as 150 kcal/kg/day. Nocturnal nasogastric tube feedings and intravenous nutrition, especially lipids, may be required because of the anorexia and malabsorption.

Fat-soluble vitamin deficiencies must be prevented by providing vitamin supplements. Vitamin E deficiency (ataxia, peripheral neuropathy, gross motor delay) is best avoided by using a well-absorbed water-soluble preparation containing d-α-tocopherol polyethylene glycol succinate. Vitamin D deficiency–associated bone disease is prevented with oral preparations of 25-hydroxyvitamin D_3. Early changes of vitamin A deficiency appear in the conjunctiva and cornea; they are prevented by using an oral, water-soluble preparation of vitamin A. Vitamin K deficiency is commonly encountered as a prolonged prothrombin time, which may respond to oral supplementation but often requires parenteral vitamin K. Vitamin and fat absorption may be enhanced with oral ursodeoxycholic acid as a choleretic (increases bile flow into the intestine) and an intraluminal bile acid. Prothrombin time and serum levels of vitamins E, D, and A should be monitored. Iron deficiency due to occult blood loss and zinc deficiency associated with chronic diarrhea may occur.

Immunizations should be given for hepatitis A and B to avoid additional hepatic injury caused by these infections; immunizations containing live viruses (measles-mumps-rubella, varicella) should be given on schedule because immunosuppression after transplantation may prevent administration.

Medical management should also be directed toward control of variceal bleeding, ascites, encephalopathy, coagulopathy, and sepsis. While waiting for transplantation, morbidity and mortality from liver failure can be reduced by prompt diagnosis and aggressive treatment of these complications. The success of transplantation has been enhanced by better preservation of the organ (up to 18 hr ex vivo with <2% primary non-function), refinement of surgical techniques, and advances in immunosuppressive therapy. The pediatric donor pool size has been expanded by using a lobe or segment of the liver from a cadaver or living donor and by using ABO blood type mismatches. Living related donation using the right lobe of the liver has also been successful in adolescent and adult recipients. Most frequently, the biliary tract in young children is connected to a Roux-en-Y loop of jejunum and direct vascular connections are made. Donor venous grafts are occasionally used if pretransplant portal vein thrombosis is present.

Steroids and either cyclosporine (Sandimmune or Neoral) or tacrolimus (Prograf, FK506) are standard therapies to prevent rejection. Many children are weaned off steroids within 1 yr of the transplantation. Compared with cyclosporine (Sandimmune), tacrolimus has been associated with lower rates of acute and chronic rejection. The water-soluble microemulsion of cyclosporine (Neoral) has been better absorbed than the bile salt–dependent, fat-soluble form (Sandimmune) and may be more comparable to tacrolimus in the prevention of rejection. Hirsutism and gingival hyperplasia are specific side effects of cyclosporine.

Early complications in the postoperative period include fluid shifts, electrolyte imbalance, renal dysfunction, and hypertension. Primary nonfunction of the graft or vascular complications, such as thrombosis of graft vessels, is an ominous early problem that often results in death unless the graft is replaced within 48 hrs. After this early phase, infection and organ rejection are the most frequent problems. Bacterial infections including cholangitis are most common, followed by viral (cytomegalovirus, adenovirus), fungal, and, rarely, parasitic *(Pneumocystis carinii)* infections. Hospital stays are usually 2–3 wks but may be several months. Late complications may arise (rejection, cyclosporine- or tacrolimus-induced renal dysfunction, Epstein-Barr virus [EBV] –associated post-transplant lymphoproliferative disease). The latter may progress to lymphoma. Rejection in older children is often due to poor compliance.

When rejection has required high doses of cyclosporine or tacrolimus and/or continued use of steroids, azathioprine (Imuran), sirolimus (Rapamune), or mycophenolate mofetil (Cellcept) may control rejection and allow reduction of the doses of these more toxic drugs. Mouse anti–T-cell monoclonal antibodies (OKT3) have been used to treat severe, steroid-resistant rejection. Less toxic, genetically engineered monoclonal anti-interleukin 2 (IL-2)–receptor antibodies can be used instead of OKT3. In addition, thymoglobulin, a polyclonal antilymphocyte preparation, can be used for severe rejection.

Post-transplant lymphoproliferative disease (PTLD) occurs in 4–11% of children, is associated with high-dose immunosuppression and EBV infection, and has resulted in a 10–20% mortality rate. The EBV-naïve, younger age groups are at particularly high risk for developing primary EBV infection in the post-transplant period. The morbidity and mortality from PTLD has been reduced by early diagnoses with frequent monitoring of EBV serology and quantitative blood EBV PCR, the use of intravenous ganciclovir in the post-transplant period for high-risk patients, and lowering or discontinuing immunosuppression as soon as EBV infection is detected.

Blood pressure and creatinine clearance should be monitored because hypertension and renal failure are common long-term complications, especially in children on high doses of cyclosporine or tacrolimus.

The prognosis for survivors is very encouraging. Most children have improvement in growth and development and the stigmata of chronic liver disease resolve. Children and their families resume more normal lives. Close follow-up of medical and psychosocial issues is necessary. Though some children may become tolerant of their graft and not need immunosuppression, many will reject up to 4 yr after immunosuppression has been discontinued. Children are usually left on immunosuppression indefinitely, awaiting the development of methods to identify those who are tolerant.

Bartosh, S, Thomas SE, Sutton MM, et al: Linear growth after pediatric liver transplantation. *J Pediatr* 1999;135:624–631.

Cacciarelli TV, Reyes J, Jaffe R, et al: Primary tacrolimus (FK506) therapy and the long-term risk of post-transplant lymphoproliferative disease in pediatric liver transplant recipients. *Pediatr Transplant* 2001;5:359–364.

Chardot C, Carton M, Spire-Bendelac N, et al: Is the Kasai operation still indicated in children older than 3 months diagnosed with biliary atresia? *J Pediatr* 2001;138:224–228.

Cherqui D, Soubrane O, Husson E, et al: Laparoscopic living donor hepatectomy for liver transplantation in children. *Lancet* 2002;359:392–396.

Cox K, Rodriguez-Baez N, Nasr A, et al: Mortality rate correlated with the number of pediatric liver transplants performed at a center. *Transplant Proc* 2001;33:1512–1513.

Hurwitz M, Desai DM, Cox KL, et al: Complete immunosuppressive drug withdrawal as a uniform approach to post-transplant lymphoproliferative disease in pediatric liver transplantation. *Pediatr Transplant* 2004;8:267–272.

McDiarmid SV: Liver transplantation: The pediatric challenge. *Clin Liver Dis* 2000;4:879–927.

Split Research Group: Studies of Pediatric Liver Transplantation (SPLIT): Year 2000 outcomes. *Transplantation* 2001;72:463–476.

United Network for Organ Sharing (UNOS) Scientific Registry data as of December 31, 2004. Available online at www.unos.org/data

Van Mourik IDM, Beath SV, Brook GA, et al: Long-term nutritional and neurodevelopmental outcomes of liver transplantation in infants aged less than 12 month. *J Pediatr Gastroenterol Nutr* 2000;30:269–275.

Wayman KI, Cox KL, Esquivel CO: Neurodevelopmental outcome of young children with extrahepatic biliary atresia 1 year after liver transplantation. *J Pediatr* 1997;131:894–898.

Section 7 — Peritoneum

Chapter 366 ■ Malformations

Jeffrey S. Hyams

Congenital peritoneal bands may be responsible for intestinal obstruction; numerous other anomalies may occur in the course of the development of the peritoneum but are rarely of clinical importance. Intra-abdominal herniations infrequently occur through ring-like formations produced by anomalous peritoneal bands. Absence of the omentum or its duplication occurs rarely. Omental cysts arise in obstructed lymphatic channels within the omentum. They may be congenital or may result from trauma and are usually asymptomatic. Abdominal pain or partial small bowel obstruction can result from compression or torsion of the small bowel from traction on the omentum.

Chapter 367 ■ Ascites Jeffrey S. Hyams

Ascites is an accumulation of serous fluid within the peritoneal cavity. Multiple causes of ascites have been described (Table 367-1). In children, hepatic, renal, and cardiac disease are the most common causes.

The clinical hallmark of ascites is abdominal distention, but this can also be caused by other conditions, including gaseous distention, fecal retention, tumor masses, peritoneal hemorrhage, extreme bladder distention, pregnancy, and obesity. Considerable intraperitoneal fluid may accumulate before ascites is detectable by the five classic physical signs: bulging flanks, flank dullness, shifting dullness, fluid wave, and the "puddle sign" (decreased auscultation of high-frequency vibrations in central abdomen when flicking side of abdomen, with patient on hands and knees). Umbilical herniation can be associated with tense ascites. Ultrasound examination can detect small amounts of ascites.

The course, prognosis, and treatment of ascites depend entirely on the cause. Patients with any type of ascites are at increased risk for spontaneous bacterial peritonitis.

Sabri M, Saps M, Peters JM: Pathophysiology and management of pediatric ascites. *Curr Gastroenterol Rep* 2003;5:240–246.

367.1 • Chylous Ascites

Chylous ascites can result from an anomaly, injury, or obstruction of the intra-abdominal portion of the thoracic duct. Although uncommon, it can occur at any age. Causes include congenital malformations, peritoneal bands, generalized lymphangiomatosis, chronic inflammatory processes of the bowel, tumors, enlarged lymph nodes, previous abdominal surgery, and trauma. Congenital anomalies of the lymphatic system are associated with Turner, Noonan, yellow nail, and Klippel-Trenaunay-Weber syndromes.

TABLE 367-1. Causes of Ascites

HEPATIC	**GASTROINTESTINAL**
Cirrhosis	Infarcted bowel
Congenital hepatic fibrosis	Perforation
Portal vein obstruction	**NEOPLASTIC**
Fulminant hepatic failure	Lymphoma
Budd-Chiari syndrome	Neuroblastoma
Lysosomal storage disease	**GYNECOLOGIC**
RENAL	Ovarian tumors
Nephrotic syndrome	Ovarian torsion, rupture
Obstructive uropathy	**PANCREATIC**
Perforation of urinary tract	Pancreatitis
Peritoneal dialysis	Ruptured pancreatic duct
CARDIAC	**MISCELLANEOUS**
Heart failure	Systemic lupus erythematosus
Constrictive pericarditis	Ventriculoperitoneal shunt
Inferior vena cava web	Eosinophilic ascites
INFECTIOUS	Chylous ascites
Abscess	Hypothyroidism
Tuberculosis	
Chlamydia	
Schistosomiasis	

In neonates, rapidly progressing abdominal distention is noted, along with poor weight gain and loose stools. Peripheral edema is common. Massive chylous ascites can result in scrotal edema, inguinal and umbilical herniation, and respiratory embarrassment.

Diagnosis of chylous ascites depends on the demonstration of milky ascitic fluid obtained via paracentesis after a fat-containing feeding. Fluid analysis will reveal a high-protein content, elevated triglycerides, and lymphocytosis. If the patient has had nothing by mouth, the fluid will appear serous. Hypoalbuminemia, hypogammaglobulinemia, and lymphopenia are common.

Treatment includes the provision of a high-protein, low-fat diet supplemented with medium-chain triglycerides that are absorbed directly into the portal circulation. Parenteral alimentation may be necessary if nutrition remains impaired on oral feedings and also in order to decrease lymph flow to facilitate sealing at the point of lymph leakage. Octreotide, a somatostatin analog, has been used. Paracentesis should be repeated only if abdominal distention causes respiratory distress. Laparotomy may be indicated to search for the site of the leak if a trial of dietary management has been unsuccessful.

Aalami AO, Allen DB, Organ CH: Chylous ascites: A collective review. *Surgery* 2000;128:761–768.

Caty MG, Hilfiker ML, Azizkhan RG, et al: Successful treatment of congenital chylous ascites with somatostatin analogue. *Pediatr Surg Int* 1996;11:396–397.

Man DW, Spitz L: The management of chylous ascites in children. *J Pediatr Surg* 1985;20:72–75.

Chapter 368 ■ Peritonitis Elias S. Hyams and Jeffrey S. Hyams

Inflammation of the peritoneal lining of the abdominal cavity can result from infectious, autoimmune, neoplastic, and chemical processes. Infectious peritonitis is usually defined as primary (spontaneous) or secondary. In primary peritonitis, the source of infection originates outside the abdomen and seeds the peritoneal cavity via hematogenous, lymphatic, or transmural spread. Secondary peritonitis arises from the abdominal cavity itself through extension from or rupture of an intra-abdominal viscus, or an abscess within an organ. Tertiary peritonitis refers to recurrent diffuse or localized disease, and is associated with poorer outcomes than secondary peritonitis.

Peritonitis in the neonatal period can arise from a transplacental in utero infection; more frequently, it is the result of infection acquired during or shortly after birth. It may be a manifestation of septicemia, a direct extension from an umbilical infection or from perforation of the intestine, necrotizing enterocolitis, or, rarely, the sequela of a ruptured appendix or Meckel diverticulum. Meconium peritonitis is described in Chapters 102.1 and 327.

Evans HL, Raymond DP, Pelletier SJ, et al: Tertiary peritonitis (recurrent diffuse or localized disease) is not an independent predictor of mortality in surgical patients with intra-abdominal infection. *Surg Infect* 2001;2:255–263.

368.1 • Acute Primary Peritonitis

ETIOLOGY AND EPIDEMIOLOGY. Primary peritonitis usually refers to bacterial infection of the peritoneal cavity without a demonstrable intra-abdominal source. Most cases occur in children with ascites resulting from nephrotic syndrome or cirrhosis. Infection can result from translocation of gut bacteria as well as immune dysfunction. Rarely, primary peritonitis occurs in previously healthy children. Pneumococci (most frequent), group A streptococci, enterococci, staphylococci, and gram-negative enteric bacteria, especially *Escherichia coli* and *Klebsiella pneumoniae,* are also commonly found. The genders are affected equally; most cases occur before 6 yr of age. *Mycobacterium tuberculosis* and *M. bovis* are rare causes.

CLINICAL MANIFESTATIONS. Onset may be insidious or rapid and is characterized by fever, abdominal pain, vomiting, diarrhea, and a "toxic appearance." Hypotension and tachycardia are common along with shallow, rapid respirations because of discomfort associated with breathing. Abdominal palpation may demonstrate rebound tenderness and rigidity. Bowel sounds are hypoactive or absent. The prior use of corticosteroids can diminish the clinical expression of peritonitis and delay diagnosis.

DIAGNOSIS AND TREATMENT. Peripheral leukocytosis with a marked predominance of polymorphonuclear cells is common, although the white blood cell (WBC) count can be affected by preexisting hypersplenism in patients with cirrhosis. Subjects with nephrotic syndrome generally have proteinuria, and low serum albumin in these patients is associated with increased risk of peritonitis. Roentgenographic examination of the abdomen reveals dilatation of the large and small intestines, with increased separation of loops secondary to bowel wall thickening. Distinguishing primary peritonitis from appendicitis may be impossible in patients without a history of nephrotic syndrome or cirrhosis; accordingly, the diagnosis of primary peritonitis is made by CT scan, laparoscopy, or laparotomy. In a child with known renal or hepatic disease and ascites, the presence of peritoneal signs should prompt diagnostic paracentesis. Infected fluid usually reveals a WBC count of ≥250 cells/mm^3, with >50% polymorphonuclear cells.

Other peritoneal fluid findings suggestive of primary peritonitis include a pH <7.35, arterial-ascitic fluid pH gradient >0.1, and elevated lactate. Gram stain of the ascitic fluid characteristically reveals a single species of gram-positive or, less often, gram-negative bacteria. The presence of mixed bacterial flora on ascitic fluid examination or free air on abdominal roentgenogram in children with presumed primary peritonitis mandates laparotomy to localize a perforation as a likely intra-abdominal source of the infection. Inoculation of ascitic fluid obtained at paracentesis directly into blood culture bottles will increase the yield of positive cultures. Parenteral antibiotic therapy with cefotaxime and an aminoglycoside should be started promptly, with subsequent changes dependent on sensitivity testing (vancomycin for resistant pneumococci). Therapy should be continued for 10–14 days.

Culture-negative neutrocytic ascites is a variant of primary peritonitis with a WBC count of 500 cells/mm^3, a negative culture, no intra-abdominal source of infection, and no prior treatment with antibiotics. It should be treated in a similar manner as primary peritonitis.

Garcia-Tsao G: Spontaneous bacterial peritonitis: A historical perspective. *J Hepatology* 2004;41:522–527.

Hingorani SR, Weiss NS, Watkins SL: Predictors of peritonitis in children with nephrotic syndrome. *Pediatr Nephrol* 2002;17:678–682.

Runyon BA: Early events in spontaneous bacterial peritonitis. *Gut* 2004;53:782–784.

368.2 • Acute Secondary Peritonitis

This is most often due to the entry of enteric bacteria into the peritoneal cavity through a necrotic defect in the wall of the intestines or other viscus as a result of obstruction or infarction or after rupture of an intra-abdominal visceral abscess. It most commonly follows perforation of the appendix. Other gastrointestinal causes include incarcerated hernias, rupture of a Meckel diverticulum, midgut volvulus, intussusception, hemolytic uremic syndrome, peptic ulceration, inflammatory bowel disease, necrotizing cholecystitis, necrotizing enterocolitis, typhlitis, and traumatic perforation. Peritonitis in the neonatal period most often occurs as a complication of necrotizing enterocolitis but may be associated with meconium ileus or spontaneous (or indomethacin-induced) rupture of the stomach or intestines. In postpubertal females, bacteria from the genital tract *(Neisseria gonorrhoeae, Chlamydia trachomatis)* may gain access to the peritoneal cavity via the fallopian tubes, causing secondary peritonitis. The presence of a foreign body, such as a ventriculoperitoneal catheter or peritoneal dialysis catheter, can predispose to peritonitis, with skin microorganisms, such as *Staphylococcus epidermidis, S. aureus,* and *Candida albicans,* contaminating the shunt. Secondary peritonitis results from direct toxic effects of bacteria as well as local and systemic release of inflammatory mediators in response to organisms and their products (LPS/endotoxin). The development of sepsis depends on various host and disease factors, as well as promptness of antimicrobial and surgical intervention.

CLINICAL MANIFESTATIONS. Similar to primary peritonitis, characteristic symptoms include fever (≥39.5°C), diffuse abdominal pain, nausea, and vomiting. Physical findings of peritoneal inflammation include rebound tenderness, abdominal wall rigidity, a paucity of body motion (lying still), and decreased or absent bowel sounds from a paralytic ileus. Massive exudation of fluid into the peritoneal cavity, along with the systemic release of vasodilatory substances, can lead to the rapid development of shock. A "toxic" appearance, irritability, and restlessness are common. Basilar atelectasis as well as intrapulmonary shunting can develop, with progression to acute respiratory distress syndrome.

Laboratory studies reveal a peripheral WBC count >12,000 cells/mm^3, with a marked predominance of polymorphonuclear forms. Roentgenograms of the abdomen may reveal free air in the peritoneal cavity, evidence of ileus or obstruction, peritoneal fluid, and obliteration of the psoas shadow.

TREATMENT. Aggressive fluid resuscitation and support of cardiovascular function should begin immediately. Stabilization of the patient before surgical intervention is mandatory. Antibiotic therapy must provide coverage for those organisms that predominate at the site of presumed origin of the infection. For perforation of the lower gastrointestinal tract, a regimen of ampicillin, gentamicin, and clindamycin will adequately address infection by *E. coli, Klebsiella,* and *Bacteroides* spp., and enterococci. Alternative therapy could include ticarcillin-clavulanic acid and an aminoglycoside. Surgery to repair a perforated viscus should proceed after the patient is stabilized and antibiotic therapy initiated. Intraoperative peritoneal fluid cultures will indicate whether a change in the antibiotic regimen is warranted. Empiric treatment for peritoneal dialysis (PD) catheter-related peritonitis may include cefazolin plus ceftazidime, imipenem/cilastin, or vancomycin/ciprofloxacin. Serious infection from PD catheters can generally be prevented with good catheter hygiene and prompt removal/replacement with signs of progressive infection.

Anaya DA, Nathens AB: Risk factors for severe sepsis in secondary peritonitis. *Surg Infect (Larchmt)* 2003;4:355–362.
Goffin E, Herbiet L, Pouthier D, et al: Vancomycin and ciprofloxacin: Systemic antibiotic administration for peritoneal dialysis-associated peritonitis. *Perit Dial Int* 2004;24:433–439.
Leung CB, Szeto CC, Chow KM, et al: Cefazolin plus ceftazidime versus imipenem/cilastatin monotherapy for treatment of CAPD peritonitis—A randomized control trial. *Perit Dial Int* 2004;24:440–446.
Malangoni MA: Current concepts in peritonitis. *Curr Gastroenterol Rep* 2003;5:295–301.
Piraino B: New insights on preventing and managing peritonitis. *Pediatr Nephrol* 2004;19:125–127.

368.3 • Acute Secondary Localized Peritonitis (Peritoneal Abscess)

ETIOLOGY. Intra-abdominal abscesses occur less commonly in children and infants than in adults but can develop in visceral intra-abdominal organs (hepatic, splenic, renal, pancreatic, tubo-ovarian abscesses) or in the interintestinal, periappendiceal, subdiaphragmatic, subhepatic, pelvic, or retroperitoneal spaces. Most commonly, periappendiceal and pelvic abscesses arise from a perforation of the appendix. Transmural inflammation with fistula formation can result in intra-abdominal abscess formation in children with Crohn disease.

CLINICAL MANIFESTATIONS. Prolonged fever, anorexia, vomiting, and lassitude are suggestive of the development of an intra-abdominal abscess. The peripheral WBC count is elevated, as is the erythrocyte sedimentation rate. With an appendiceal abscess, there is localized tenderness and a palpable mass in the right lower quadrant.

A pelvic abscess is suggested by abdominal distention, rectal tenesmus with or without the passage of small-volume mucous stools, and bladder irritability. Rectal examination may reveal a tender mass anteriorly. Subphrenic gas collection, basal atelectasis, elevated hemidiaphragm, and pleural effusion may be present with a subdiaphragmatic abscess. Psoas abscess can develop from extension of infection from a retroperitoneal appendicitis, Crohn disease, or a perirenal or intrarenal abscess. Abdominal findings may be minimal, and presentation may include a limp, hip pain, and fever. Both ultrasound examination and CT scanning can be used to localize intra-abdominal abscesses, though CT scanning has superior sensitivity and can assess the retroperitoneal space.

TREATMENT. An abscess should be drained and appropriate antibiotic therapy provided. Drainage can be performed under radiologic control (ultrasonogram or CT guidance) and an indwelling drainage catheter left in place. Initial broad-spectrum antibiotic coverage with ampicillin, gentamicin, and clindamycin should be started and can be modified depending on the results of sensitivity testing. The treatment of appendiceal rupture complicated by abscess formation may be problematic because intestinal phlegmon formation can make surgical resection more difficult. Intensive antibiotic therapy for 4–6 wk followed by an interval appendectomy is often the treatment course followed.

Brook I: Intra-abdominal, retroperitoneal, and visceral abscesses in children. *Eur J Pediatr Surg* 2004;14:265–273.
Wilson-Storey D, Scobie WG: Appendix masses—A 15-year review. *Pediatr Surg Int* 1989;4:168–170.

Chapter 369 ■ Epigastric Hernia

John J. Aiken and Keith T. Oldham

Epigastric hernias are ventral hernias in the midline of the abdominal wall between the xyphoid and the umbilicus. Epigastric hernias result from defects in the decussating fibers of the linea alba and are more likely congenital than acquired. Most epigastric hernias are small and asymptomatic; therefore, the true incidence is unknown, but the reported incidence in childhood varies from <1% to as high as 5%. Epigastric hernias may be single or multiple and are two to three times more common in males than females. The defect typically contains only preperitoneal fat without a peritoneal sac or abdominal viscera. Epigastric (incisional) hernias can occur in a previous incision site or be associated with ventricular-peritoneal shunts.

CLINICAL PRESENTATION. Epigastric hernias typically present in young children as a visible or palpable mass in the midline, between the umbilicus and the xyphoid, noted by the parents or primary care practitioner. The mass is almost always small (<1 cm) and asymptomatic. The mass is typically present at all times but most apparent at times of irritability or straining. Occasionally, the mass is intermittent and the child relates pain localized to the site of the hernia. Physical examination demonstrates a firm mass, directly in the midline, anywhere between the umbilicus and the xyphoid. Epigastric hernias typically contain only preperitoneal fat and are not reducible due to the small size of the fascial defect. Rarely, a fascial defect is noted without a palpable mass. The mass may be intermittent if the fat reduces with relaxation of the abdominal muscles. Herniation of intestines or abdominal viscera in an epigastric hernia would be exceptionally rare. The mass may be tender to examination, but strangulation of the hernia contents is uncommon. Physical examination is almost always diagnostic and imaging studies are unnecessary.

The natural history of epigastric hernias is for gradual enlargement over time as intermittently more preperitoneal fat is extruded through the defect at times of straining or increased intra-abdominal pressure. Left untreated, the defect can enlarge and enable herniation of intra-abdominal viscera within a peritoneal sac. Epigastric hernias do not resolve spontaneously and, therefore, operative repair is the recommended treatment. The site should be carefully marked preoperatively because the mass and defect can be difficult to localize after induction of anesthesia. A limited transverse incision is made over the mass and dissection is performed to delineate the edges of the fascial defect. If herniated fat is present, it is dissected free of the subcutaneous tissues and can be reduced or ligated and excised. The defect is closed using absorbable suture. The skin is closed with an absorbable subcuticular suture. Postoperative complications are rare and the recurrence rate is low.

Coats RD, Helikson MA, Burd RS: Presentation and management of epigastric hernias in children. *J Pediatr Surg* 2000;35:1754–1756.
Richards AT, Quinn TH, Fitzgibbons RJ Jr: Epigastric hernias. In Mulholland MW, Lillemoe KD, Doherty GM, et al (editors): *Greenfield's Surgery: Scientific Principles and Practice,* 4th ed. Philadelphia, Lippincott Williams and Wilkins, 2006, pp 1201–1202.
Skandalakis J, Gray SQW, Rickets R: The anterior abdominal wall. In Skandalakis JG (editor): *Embryology for Surgeons,* 2nd ed. Baltimore, Williams and Wilkins, 1994, pp 540–593.

369.1 • Incisional Hernia

Hernia formation at the site of a previous laparotomy is uncommon in childhood. Factors associated with an increased risk of incisional hernia include increased intra-abdominal pressure, wound infection, and midline incision. Transverse abdominal incisions are favored because of their increased strength and blood supply, which reduce the likelihood of wound infection and incisional hernia. Although most incisional hernias require repair, operation should be deferred until the child is in optimal medical condition. Some incisional hernias resolve, especially those occurring in infants. Some recommend elastic bandaging to discourage enlargement of the hernia and to promote spontaneous healing. Newborns with abdominal wall defects represent the largest group of children with incisional hernias. Initial management should be conservative, with repair deferred until about 1 yr of age. Incarceration is very uncommon but is an indication for prompt repair.

Coats RD, Helikson MA, Burd RS: Presentation and management of epigastric hernias in children. *J Pediatr Surg* 2000;35:1754–1756.

Neblett KW, Holcomb TM: Umbilical and other abdominal wall hernias. In Ashcraft KW, Holder TM (editors): *Pediatric Surgery.* Philadelphia, WB Saunders, 1993, pp 557–561.

Part XVIII ■ Respiratory System

Section 1 — Development and Function

Chapter 370 ■ Respiratory Pathophysiology and Regulation

Ashok P. Sarnaik and
Sabrina M. Heidemann

The age- and growth-dependent changes in physiology and anatomy of the respiratory control mechanism, airway dynamics, and lung parenchymal characteristics have a profound influence on the pathophysiologic manifestations of the disease process. Smaller airways, a more compliant chest wall, and poor hypoxic drive render a younger infant more vulnerable compared to an older child with similar severity of disease. The main function of the respiratory system is to supply sufficient oxygen to meet metabolic demands and remove carbon dioxide. A variety of processes including ventilation, perfusion, and diffusion are involved in tissue oxygenation and carbon dioxide removal. Abnormalities in any one of these mechanisms can lead to respiratory failure. A child may be identified as being in respiratory distress because of the presence of signs such as cyanosis, nasal flaring, grunting, tachypnea, wheezing, chest wall retractions, and stridor. Respiratory failure can be present without respiratory distress; a patient with abnormalities of central nervous system (CNS) or neuromuscular disease may not be able to mount sufficient effort to appear in respiratory distress. A child who appears in respiratory distress may not have a respiratory illness; a patient with primary metabolic acidosis (diabetic ketoacidosis) or central nervous system excitatory states (encephalitis) may present in severe respiratory distress without respiratory disease.

370.1 • Lung Volumes and Capacities in Health and Disease

Lung volumes are traditionally measured with a spirogram (Fig. 370-1). **Tidal volume** (V_T) is the amount of air moved in and out of the lungs during each breath. At rest, it is usually 6–7 mL/kg body weight. **Inspiratory capacity** (**IC**) is the amount of air inspired by maximum inspiratory effort after tidal expiration. **Expiratory reserve volume** (**ERV**) is the amount of air exhaled by maximum expiratory effort after tidal expiration. The volume of gas remaining in the lungs after maximum expiration is **residual volume** (**RV**). **Vital capacity** (**VC**) is defined as the amount of air moved in and out of the lungs with maximum inspiration and expiration. VC, IC, and ERV are decreased in lung pathology but are also effort dependent. **Total lung capacity** (**TLC**) is the volume of gas occupying the lungs after maximum inhalation.

Functional residual capacity (**FRC**) is the amount of air left in the lungs after tidal expiration. FRC has important pathophysiologic implications. Alveolar gas composition changes during inspiration and expiration. **Alveolar** PO_2 (P_AO_2) increases and **alveolar** PCO_2 (P_ACO_2) decreases during inspiration as fresh atmospheric gas enters the lungs. During exhalation, P_AO_2 decreases and P_ACO_2 increases as pulmonary capillary blood continues to remove oxygen from and add CO_2 into the alveoli (Fig. 370-2). FRC acts as a buffer, minimizing the changes in P_AO_2 and P_ACO_2 during inspiration and expiration. FRC represents the environment available for pulmonary capillary blood for gas exchange at all times. A decrease in FRC is often encountered in alveolar interstitial diseases and thoracic deformities. The major pathophysiologic consequence of decreased FRC is **hypoxemia.** Reduced FRC results in a sharp decline in P_AO_2 during exhalation because a limited volume is available for gas exchange. PO_2 of pulmonary capillary blood therefore falls excessively during exhalation, leading to a decline in **arterial PO2** (PaO_2). Any increase in P_AO_2 (and therefore PaO_2) during inspiration cannot compensate for the decreased PaO_2 during expiration. The explanation for this lies in the shape of O_2-hemoglobin dissociation curve, which is sigmoid shaped (Fig. 370-3). Since most of the oxygen in blood is combined with the hemoglobin, it is the percentage of **oxyhemoglobin** (**SO_2**) that gets averaged rather than the PO_2. While an increase in arterial PO_2 cannot increase oxygen-hemoglobin saturation more than 100%, there is a steep desaturation of hemoglobin below a PO_2 of 50 torr; thus, decreased SO_2 during exhalation as a result of low FRC leads to overall arterial desaturation and hypoxemia. The adverse pathophysiologic consequences of decreased FRC are ameliorated by application of **positive end expiratory pressure** (**PEEP**) and increasing the inspiratory time during mechanical ventilation.

The lung pressure-volume relationship is markedly influenced by FRC (Fig. 370-4). Pulmonary compliance is decreased at abnormally low or high FRC.

FRC is abnormally increased in intrathoracic airway obstruction, which results in incomplete exhalation, and abnormally decreased alveolar-interstitial diseases. At excessively low or high FRC, tidal respiration requires higher inflation pressures compared to normal FRC. Abnormalities of FRC result in increased work of breathing with spontaneous respiration and increased barotrauma in mechanical ventilation.

370.2 • Chest Wall

One important area where an infant's respiratory system differs from that of an older child or adult is its chest wall. Although a soft, highly compliant chest wall is beneficial to a baby in its passage through the birth canal and allows future lung growth, it places the young infant in a vulnerable situation under certain pathologic conditions. Chest wall compliance is a major determinant of FRC. Since the chest wall and the lungs recoil in opposite directions at rest, FRC is reached at the point where the outward elastic recoil of the thoracic cage counterbalances the inward lung recoil. This balance is attained at a lower lung volume in a young infant because of the extremely high thoracic compliance compared to older children (Fig. 370-5). The measured FRC in infants is higher than expected because respiratory

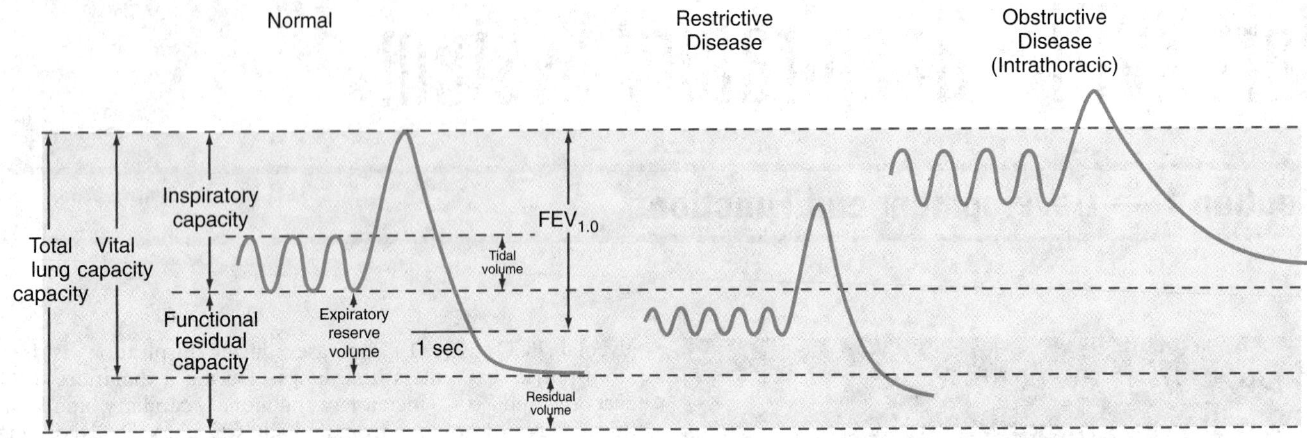

Figure 370-1. Spirogram showing lung volumes and capacities. $FEV_{1.0}$ is the maximum volume exhaled in 1 sec after maximum inspiration. Restrictive diseases are usually associated with decreased lung volumes and capacities. Intrathoracic airway obstruction is associated with air trapping and abnormally high functional residual capacity and residual volume. $FEV_{1.0}$ and vital capacity are decreased in both restrictive and obstructive diseases. The ratio of $FEV_{1.0}$ to vital capacity is normal in restrictive disease but decreased in obstructive disease. FEV, Forced expiratory volume.

muscles of infants maintain the thoracic cage in a slight inspiratory position at all times. Additionally, some amount of air trapping during expiration occurs in young infants.

The increased chest wall compliance is a distinct disadvantage to the young infant under several pathologic conditions. A decrease in muscle tone, as occurs in *rapid eye movement (REM)* sleep or with CNS depression, allows greater chest wall retraction because of less opposition to the lung recoil; the FRC decreases in such states. The respiratory muscles of infants are poorly equipped to sustain large workloads. They are more easily fatigued than those of older children, limiting their ability to maintain adequate ventilation in lung disease. In diseases of poor lung compliance (atelectasis, pulmonary edema), excessive lung recoil results in greater retraction of the soft chest wall and more loss of FRC than occurs in older children and adults with stiffer chest walls. Increased negative intrathoracic pressure required to overcome airway resistance in obstructive lung disease also produces greater chest wall recoil and reduced FRC in young infants. Application of PEEP is beneficial in such states for stabilization of the chest wall and restoration of FRC.

Abnormalities of the chest wall are encountered in certain pathologic conditions. Chest wall instability can result from trauma (fractured ribs, thoracotomy) and neuromuscular diseases that lead to intercostal and diaphragmatic muscle weakness. The increased chest wall compliance makes such children more vulnerable to respiratory decompensation when faced with similar pulmonary pathology compared to older children and adults with stiffer chest walls. Children with rigid, noncompliant chest wall

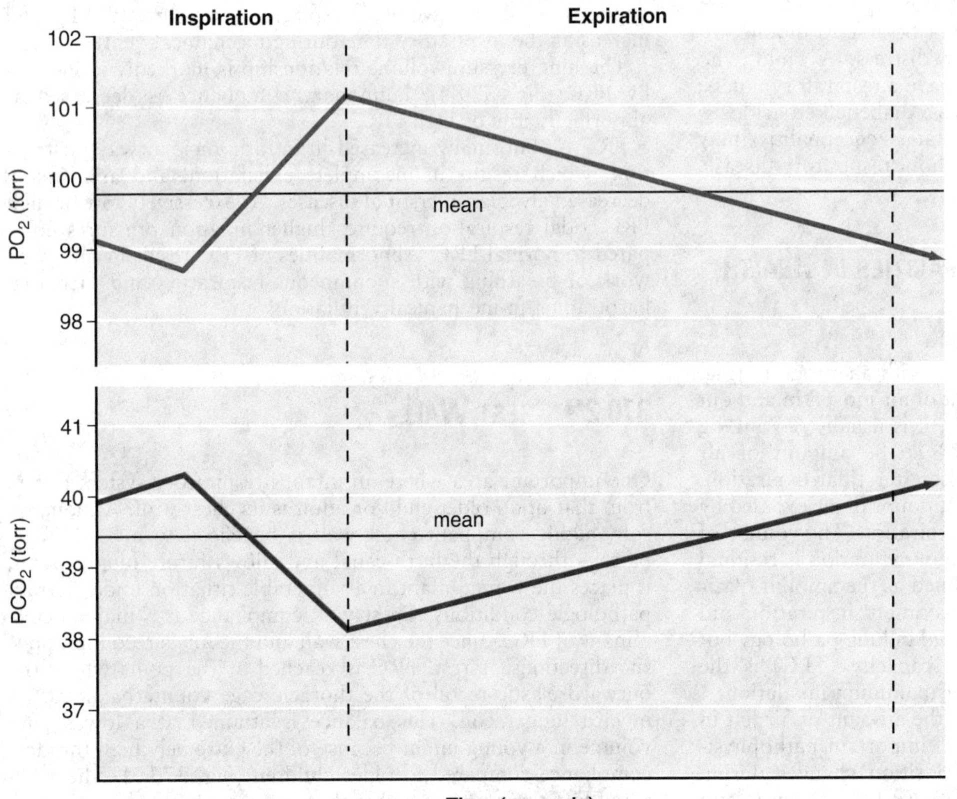

Figure 370-2. Alveolar PO_2 rises and PCO_2 falls during inspiration as fresh atmospheric gas is brought into the lungs. During expiration, the opposite changes occur as pulmonary capillary blood continues to remove O_2 and add CO_2 from the alveoli without atmospheric enrichment. Note that during the early part of inspiration, alveolar PO_2 continues to fall and PCO_2 continues to rise because of inspiration of the dead space that is occupied by the previously exhaled gas. (Modified from Comroe JH: Physiology of Respiration, 2nd ed. Chicago, Year Book Medical Publishers, 1974, p 12.)

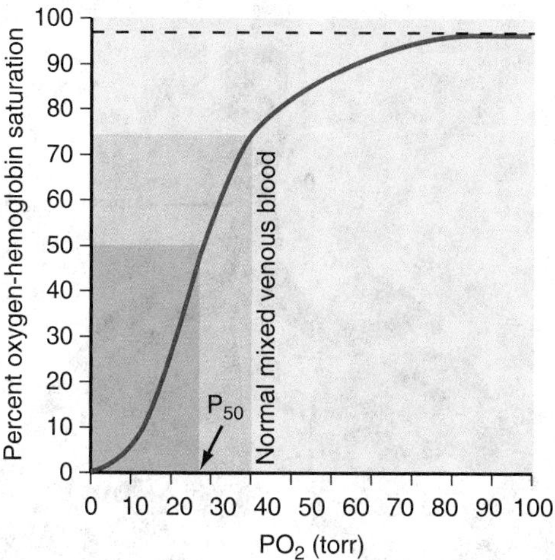

Figure 370-3. Oxygen-hemoglobin dissociation curve. P_{50} of adult blood is around 27 torr. Under basal conditions, mixed venous blood has PO_2 of 40 torr and oxygen-hemoglobin saturation of 75%. In arterial blood, these values are 100 torr and 97.5%, respectively. Note that there is a steep decline in oxygen-hemoglobin saturation at $PaO_2 < 50$ torr, but relatively little increase in saturation is gained at $PO_2 > 70$ torr.

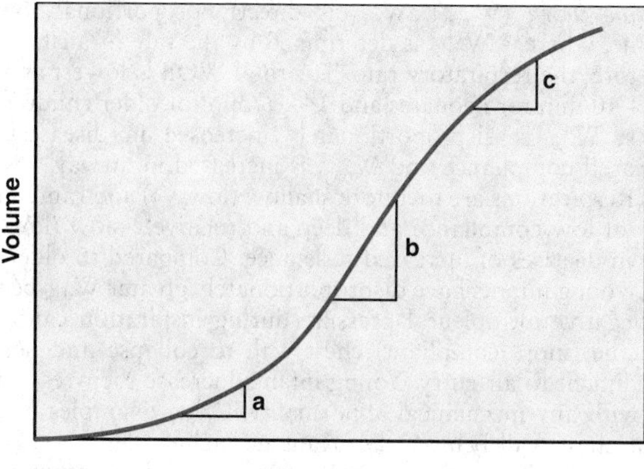

Figure 370-4. Lung compliance is significantly influenced by the functional residual capacity (FRC). The same change in pressure is associated with less change in volume when FRC is abnormally decreased *(a)* or abnormally increased *(c)* compared to the normal state *(b)*.

(asphyxiating thoracic dystrophy of Jeune [see Chapters 416.3 and 698], achondroplasia [see Chapter 416.4]) have markedly diminished lung volumes and capacities.

370.3 • Pulmonary Mechanics and Work of Breathing in Health and Disease

For air to move in and out of the lungs, a sufficient pressure gradient is needed between alveoli and atmosphere during both inspiration and expiration. Part of the pressure gradient is required to overcome the lung and chest wall elastance; another part is needed to overcome airway resistance. **Elastance** refers to the property of a substance to oppose deformation or stretching. It is calculated as a change in pressure (ΔP) ÷ change in volume (ΔV). Elastic recoil is a property of a substance that enables it to return to its original state after it is no longer subjected to pressure. **Compliance** ($\Delta V \div \Delta P$) is the reciprocal of elastance. In the context of the pulmonary parenchyma, airways, and the chest wall, the compliance refers to their distensibilty. **Resistance** is calculated as the amount of pressure required to generate flow of gas across the airways. Resistance to laminar flow is governed by *Poiseuille's law* stated as: $R = 8\, l\eta \div \Pi r^4$ where R is resistance, l length, η viscosity, and r radius. The practical implication of pressure-flow relationship is that airway resistance is inversely proportional to its radius raised to the 4th power. If the airway lumen is decreased in half, the resistance will increase 16-fold. Newborns and young infants with their inherently smaller airways are especially prone to marked increase in airway resistance from inflamed tissues and secretions. In diseases in which airway resistance is increased, flow often becomes turbulent. **Turbulence** depends to a great extent on the *Reynolds number* (Re), a dimensionless entity, which is calculated as $Re = 2rvd \div \eta$ where r is radius, v velocity, d density, and η viscosity. Turbulence in gas flow is most likely to occur when Re exceeds 2000. Resistance to turbulent flow is greatly influenced by density. A low-density gas such as helium-oxygen mixture decreases turbulence in obstructive airway diseases such as viral laryngotracheobronchitis and asthma. Neonates and young infants are predominantly nose breathers and, therefore, even a minimal amount of nasal obstruction is poorly tolerated.

The diaphragm is the major muscle of respiration. When additional *work of breathing* (WOB) is required, intercostal and other accessory muscles of respirations also contribute to the increased work. The tidal volume and respiratory rate are adjusted, both in health and disease, to maintain the required minute volume with the least amount of energy expenditure. The total WOB (necessary to create pressure gradients to move air) is divided into 2 parts. The 1st part is to overcome the lung and chest wall elastance, and is referred to as *elastic work* (W_{elast}). The 2nd part is to overcome airway and tissue resistance, and is referred to as

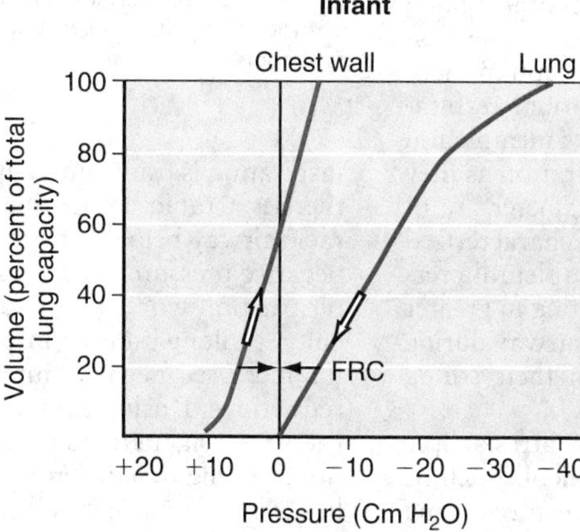

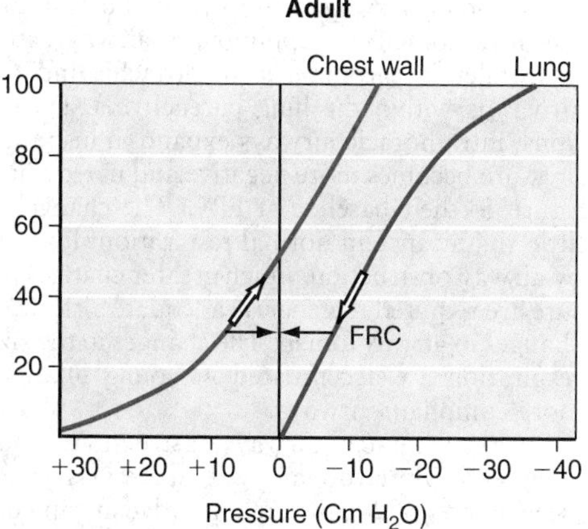

Figure 370-5. Schematic representation of interaction between chest wall and lung recoil in infants compared to adults. The elastic recoil of a relatively more compliant chest wall is balanced by the lung recoil at a lower volume (FRC) in infants compared to adults. FRC, functional residual capacity.

resistive work (W_{resist}). W_{elast} is directly proportional to tidal volume, whereas W_{resist} is determined by the rate of airflow and, therefore, the respiratory rate. The total WOB is lowest at a rate of 35–40/min for neonates and 14–16/min for older children and adults. W_{elast} is disproportionately increased in diseases with decreased compliance and W_{resist} is increased in airway obstruction. Respirations are therefore shallow (low V_T) and rapid in diseases of low compliance and deep and relatively slow (low flow rate) in diseases of increased resistance. Compared to older children, young infants have disproportionately greater W_{elast} because the negative intrapleural pressure during inspiration causes the retractile (more compliant) chest wall to collapse and pose an impediment to air entry. Young infants increase their respiratory rate with any mechanical abnormality. Other examples of compliant chest wall being a disadvantage include flail chest resulting from rib fractures, thoracotomy, and neuromuscular weakness. One of the salutary effects of continuous positive airway pressure in such situations is the stabilization of the chest wall.

Time constant, measured in seconds, is a product of compliance and resistance. It is a reflection of the amount of time required for proximal airway pressure (and, therefore, volume) to equilibrate with alveolar pressure. It takes 3 time constants for 95%, and 5 time constants for 99% of pressure equilibration to occur. Since airways expand during inspiration and narrow during expiration, expiratory time constant is longer than inspiratory time constant. Diseases characterized by decreased compliance (pneumonia, pulmonary edema, atelectasis) are associated with a shorter time constant and therefore require less time for alveolar inflation and deflation. Diseases associated with increased resistance (asthma, bronchiolitis, aspiration syndromes) have prolonged time constant, and therefore require more time for alveolar inflation and deflation. Pathologic alterations in time constants have practical significance during mechanical ventilation. Patients with shorter time constants are best ventilated with relatively smaller tidal volumes and faster rates to minimize peak inflation pressure. In patients with increased airway resistance, a fast respiratory rate (and, therefore, less time) does not allow enough pressure equilibration to occur between the proximal airway and the alveoli. Inadequate inspiratory time results in lower tidal volume, whereas insufficient exhalation time results in inadvertent PEEP, often referred to as auto-PEEP or intrinsic PEEP. Such patients are therefore best ventilated with relatively slower rates and larger tidal volumes.

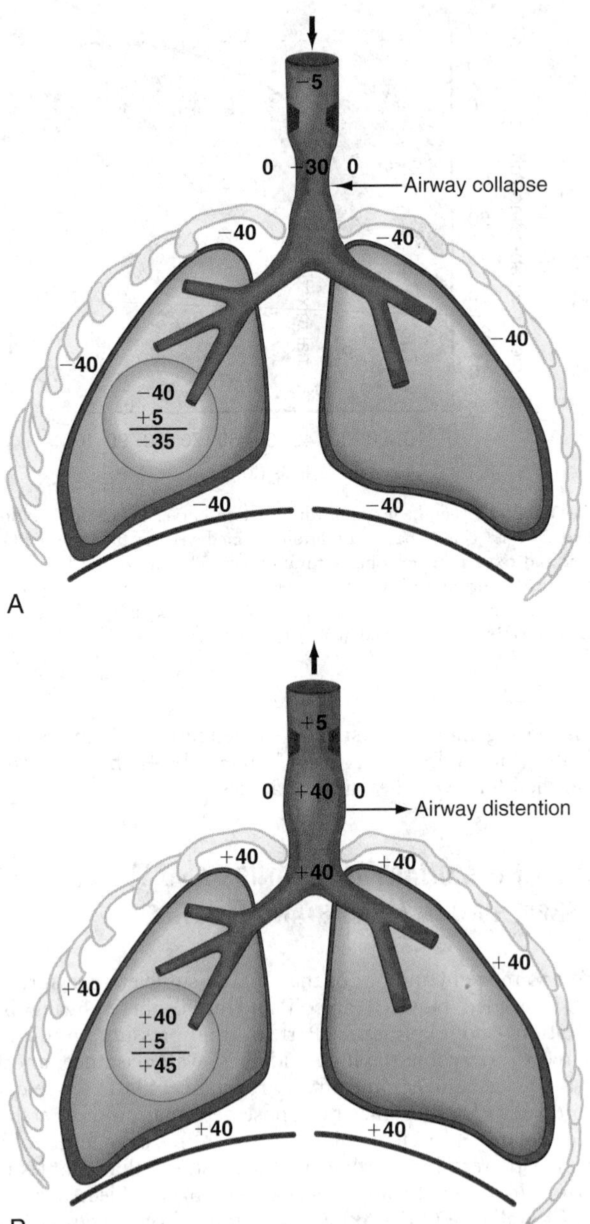

Figure 370-6. *A,* In extrathoracic airway obstruction, the increased negative pressure during inspiration is transmitted up to the site of obstruction. This results in collapse of the extrathoracic airway below the site of obstruction, making the obstruction worse during inspiration. Note that the pressures are compared to the atmospheric pressure which is traditionally represented as 0 cm. Terminal airway pressure is calculated as (intrapleural pressure + lung recoil pressure). Lung recoil pressure is arbitrarily chosen as 5 cm for the sake of simplicity. *B,* During expiration, the positive pressure below the site of obstruction results in distention of extrathoracic airway and amelioration of symptoms.

370.4 • Airway Dynamics in Health and Disease

The trachea and airways of an infant are much more compliant than those of older children and adults, thus changes in intrapleural pressure result in much greater changes in airway diameter. The airway can be divided into 3 anatomic parts: the extrathoracic airway extends from the nose to the thoracic inlet; the intrathoracic-extrapulmonary airway extends from the thoracic inlet to the main stem bronchi; and the intrapulmonary airway is within the lung parenchyma. During normal respirations, intrathoracic airways expand in inspiration as intrapleural pressure becomes more negative and narrow in expiration as they return to their baseline at FRC. The changes in diameter are of little significance in normal respiration. In diseases characterized by airway obstruction, much greater changes in intrapleural pressure are required to generate adequate airflow, resulting in greater changes in airway lumen. The changes in the size of airway during respiration are accentuated in young infants with their softer, more compliant airways.

In extrathoracic airway obstruction (choanal atresia [see Chapter 373], retropharyngeal abscess, laryngotracheobronchitis [see Chapter 382]), the high negative intrapleural pressure during inspiration is transmitted up to the site of obstruction, after which there is a rapid dissipation of pressure. Therefore, the extrathoracic airway below the site of obstruction has markedly increased negative pressure inside, resulting in its collapse, which makes the obstruction worse (Fig. 370-6*A*). This produces inspiratory difficulty, prolongation of inspiration, and inspiratory stridor. Also, the increased negative intrapleural pressure results in chest wall retractions. During expiration, the increased positive intrapleural pressure is again transmitted up the airways to the site of obstruction, leading to a distension of the extrathoracic airway and amelioration of obstruction (Fig. 370-6*B*).

Because of the increased positive intrapleural pressure, the chest wall tends to bulge out, which produces the **classical paradoxical respiration,** in which the chest retracts during inspiration and bulges out during expiration. The younger the child, the softer is the chest wall and the more marked is the paradoxical respiration of extrathoracic airway obstruction. A pattern of seesaw respiration may also be evident in newborns and young infants as the compliant chest wall is sucked in and the abdomen bulges out during inspiration, with the converse happening during expiration.

In obstruction of intrathoracic-extrapulmonary airway (vascular ring [see Chapter 383], mediastinal tumors) and intrapulmonary airway (asthma, bronchiolitis), the increased negative intrapleural pressure results in a distention of intrathoracic airways during inspiration, thus providing some relief from obstruction (Fig. 370-7*A*).

During expiration, the increased positive intrathoracic pressure is transmitted up to the site of obstruction, after which it dissipates rapidly. The intrathoracic airway above the site of obstruction is therefore subjected to much greater intrapleural pressure from outside, which cannot be adequately balanced by enough positive pressure inside, resulting in collapse above the site of obstruction (Fig. 370-7*B*).

The site at which pressures inside and outside the airway during exhalation are equal is referred to as the *equal pressure point* (EPP). With intrathoracic airway obstruction, the EPP is shifted distally toward the alveolus, causing airway collapse above. Marked inspiratory/expiratory changes in a young infant's airway lumen above the EPP is often termed *collapsible trachea.* **Tracheal collapse** is often a sign of airway obstruction, and even contributes to its severity, but is rarely the primary abnormality. With intrapulmonary airway obstruction, an even wider portion of intrathoracic airway is subjected to pressure swings during inspiration and expiration (Fig. 370-8).

Both intrathoracic-extrapulmonary and intrapulmonary airway obstruction result in increasing difficulty during expiration, prolongation of expiration, and expiratory wheezing. Any airway obstruction within the thorax results in expiratory wheezing.

370.5 • Interpretation of Clinical Signs to Localize the Site of Pathology

Appropriate interpretation of clinical findings is the 1st step in establishing the diagnosis of respiratory disease. Respiratory distress can occur without respiratory disease, and severe respiratory failure can be present without significant respiratory distress. Diseases characterized by CNS excitation, such as encephalitis, and neureoexcitatory drugs are associated with central neurogenic hyperventilation. Similarly, diseases that produce metabolic acidosis, such as diabetic ketoacidosis, salicylism, and shock, result in hyperventilation as a compensatory response. Patients in either group could be considered clinically to have respiratory distress; they are distinguished from patients with respiratory disease by their increased tidal volume as well as the respiratory rate. Their blood gas values reflect a low $PaCO_2$ and a normal PaO_2. Patients with neuromuscular diseases, such as Guillain-Barré syndrome or myasthenia gravis, and those with an abnormal respiratory drive may develop severe respiratory failure but are not able to mount sufficient effort to appear in respiratory distress. In these patients, respirations are ineffective or may even appear normal in the presence of respiratory acidosis and hypoxemia.

The rate and depth of respiration and the presence of retractions, stridor, wheezing, and grunting are valuable signs in localizing the site of respiratory pathology (Table 370-1 and Fig. 370-9). Rapid and shallow respirations (**tachypnea**) are characteristic of parenchymal pathology, in which the elastic work of breathing is increased disproportionately to the resistive work of breathing. Chest wall, intercostal, and suprasternal **retractions** are most striking, with increased negative intrathoracic pressure during inspiration. This occurs in extrathoracic airway obstruction as well as diseases of decreased compliance. Inspiratory **stridor** is a hallmark of extrathoracic airway obstruction. Expiratory **wheezing** is characteristic of intrathoracic airway obstruction, either extrapulmonary or intrapulmonary. **Grunting** is produced by expiration against a partially closed glottis and is an

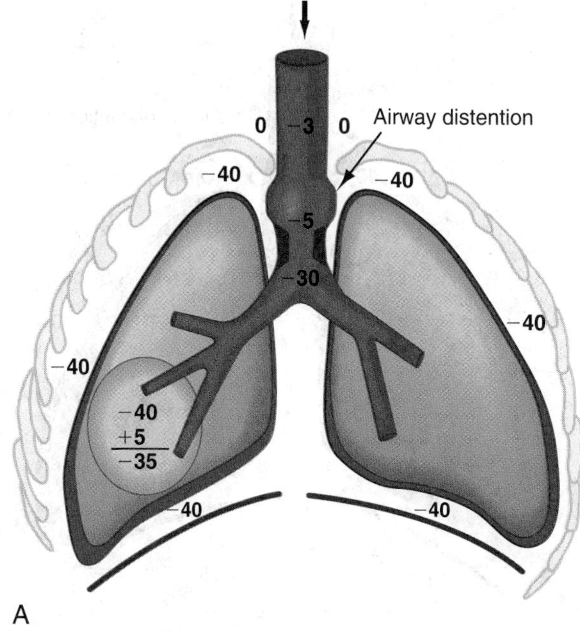

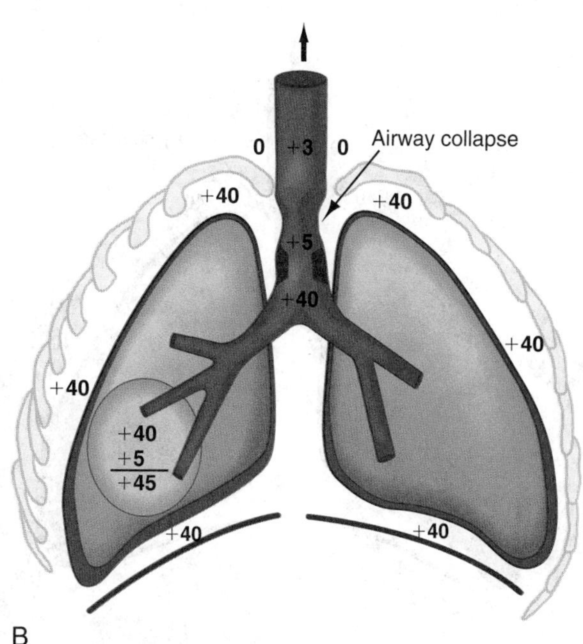

Figure 370-7. *A,* In intrathoracic-extrapulmonary airway obstruction, the increased negative pressure during inspiration is transmitted up to the site of obstruction. This results in the distension of the intrathoracic airway above the lesion since it is surrounded by an even greater negative intrapleural pressure. *B,* During expiration, the increased positive airway pressure rapidly dissipates above the obstruction. Consequently, there is a collapse of the intrathoracic airway above the obstruction as it is subjected to markedly increased positive intrapleural pressure, making the obstruction worse during expiration.

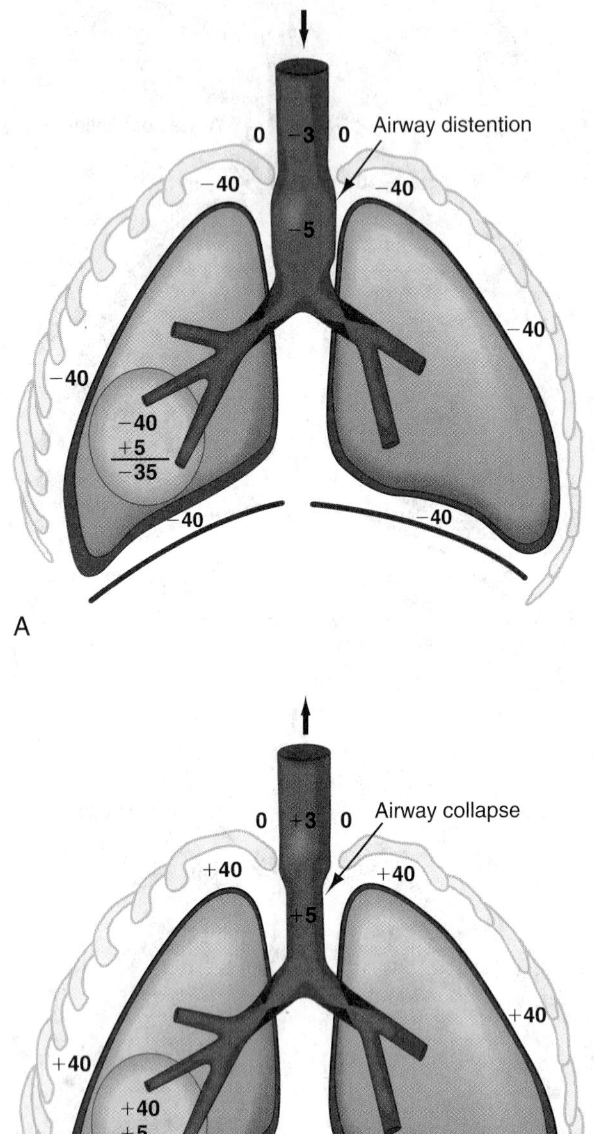

Figure 370-8. *A* and *B*, In intrapulmonary airway obstruction, even a wider segment of intrathoracic airway is subjected to pressure changes compared to those observed in intrathoracic-extrapulmonary airway obstruction. Such lesions are associated with marked increase in airway obstruction during expiration.

attempt to maintain positive airway pressure during expiration for as long as possible. Such prolongation of positive pressure is most beneficial in alveolar diseases that produce widespread loss of FRC, such as in pulmonary edema, hyaline membrane disease, and pneumonia. Grunting is also effective in small airway obstruction (bronchiolitis) to maintain a higher positive pressure in the airway during expiration, decreasing the airway collapse.

370.6 • Ventilation-Perfusion (V/Q) Relationship in Health and Disease

During tidal respiration, alveoli and airways in the nondependent parts (the upper lobes in upright position) of the lung are subjected to greater negative intrapleural pressure, and therefore kept relatively more inflated, compared to the dependent alveoli and airways (the lower lobes in upright position). This is because of the gravitational force pulling the lung away from the nondependent part of the parietal pleura. The nondependent alveoli are less compliant because they are already more inflated. During tidal inspiration, ventilation therefore occurs preferentially in the dependent portions of the lung that are more amenable to expansion. Although perfusion is also greater in the dependent portions of the lung because of greater pulmonary arterial hydrostatic pressure due to gravity, the increase in perfusion is greater than the increase in ventilation in the dependent portions of the lung. Thus, the V/Q ratios favor ventilation in the nondependent portions and perfusion in the dependent portions. Since the airways in the dependent portion of the lung are narrower, they close earlier during expiration. The lung volume at which the dependent airways start to close is referred to as the *closing capacity.* In normal children, *the FRC is greater than the closing capacity.* During tidal respiration, airways remain patent both in the dependent and the nondependent portions of the lung. In newborns, the closing capacity is greater than the FRC, resulting in perfusion of poorly ventilated alveoli during tidal respiration; therefore, normal neonates have a lower PaO_2 compared to older children.

The V/Q relationship is adversely affected in a variety of pathophysiologic states (Fig. 370-10). Air movement in areas that are poorly perfused is referred to as **dead space ventilation.** Examples of dead space ventilation include pulmonary thromboembolism and hypovolemia. Perfusion of poorly ventilated alveoli is referred to as intrapulmonary right-to-left shunting or venous admixture. Examples include pneumonia, asthma, and hyaline membrane disease. In intrapulmonary airway obstruction, the closing capacity is abnormally increased and may exceed the FRC. In such situations, perfusion of poorly ventilated alveoli during tidal respiration results in venous admixture.

370.7 • Gas Exchange in Health and Disease

The main function of the respiratory system is to remove carbon dioxide from and add oxygen to the systemic venous blood brought to the lung. The composition of the inspired gas, venti-

TABLE 370-1. Interpreting the Clinical Signs of Respiratory Disease

SIGN	EXTRATHORACIC AIRWAY OBSTRUCTION	INTRATHORACIC-EXTRAPULMONARY AIRWAY OBSTRUCTION	INTRAPULMONARY AIRWAY OBSTRUCTION	PARENCHYMAL PATHOLOGY
Tachypnea	+	+	++	++++
Retractions	++++	++	++	+++
Stridor	++++	++	−	−
Wheezing	±	+++	++++	±
Grunting	±	±	++	++++

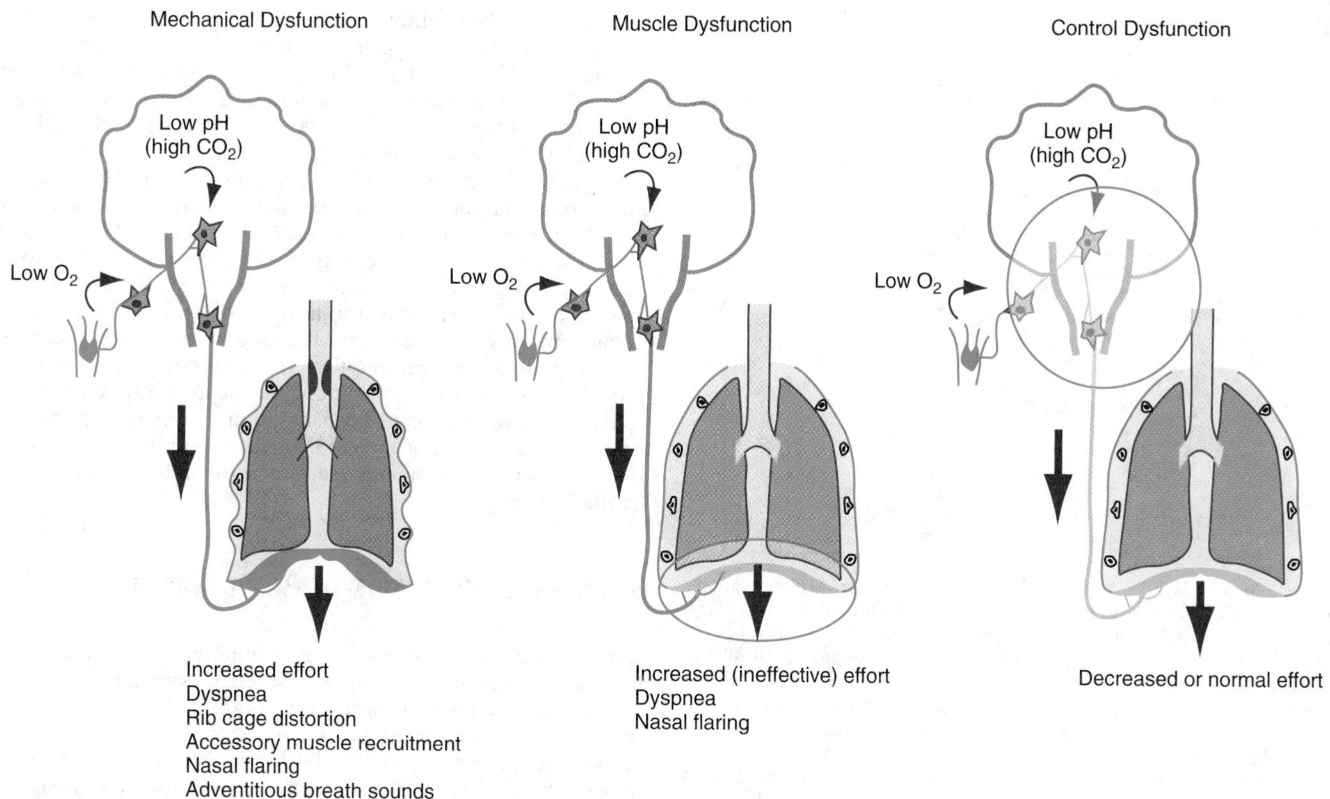

Figure 370-9. Presentation profiles of respiratory failure in childhood. When a mechanical dysfunction is present (by far, the most common circumstance), arterial hypoxemia and hypercapnia (and hence, pH) are sensed by peripheral (carotid bodies) and central (medullary) chemoreceptors. After being integrated with other sensory information from the lungs and chest wall, chemoreceptor activation triggers an increase in the neural output to the respiratory muscles *(vertical arrows)*, which results in the physical signs that characterize respiratory distress. When the problem resides with the respiratory muscles (or their innervation), the same increase in neural output occurs *(arrow)*, but the respiratory muscles cannot increase their effort as demanded; therefore, the physical signs of distress are more subtle. Finally, when the control of breathing is itself affected by disease, the neural response to hypoxemia and hypercapnia is absent or blunted and the gas exchange abnormalities are not accompanied by respiratory distress.

lation, perfusion, diffusion, and tissue metabolism have a significant influence on the arterial blood gases.

The total pressure of the atmosphere at sea level is 760 torr. With increasing altitude, the atmospheric pressure decreases. The total atmospheric pressure is equal to the sum of partial pressures exerted by each of its component gases. Alveolar air is 100% humidified and, therefore, for alveolar gas calculations, the inspired gas is also presumed to be 100% humidified. At a temperature of 37°C and 100% humidity, water vapor exerts pressure of 47 torr, regardless of altitude. In a natural setting, the atmosphere consists of 20.93% oxygen. *Partial pressure of oxygen in inspired gas* (PiO_2) at sea level is therefore $(760 - 47) \times 20.93\% = 149$ torr. When breathing 40% oxygen at sea level, PiO_2 is $(760 - 47) \times 40\% = 285$ torr. At higher altitudes, breathing different concentrations of oxygen, PiO_2 is less than at sea level, depending on the prevalent atmospheric pressures. In Denver (altitude of 5,000 feet and barometric pressure of 632 torr), PiO_2 in room air is $(632 - 47) \times 20.93\% = 122$ torr; and in 40% oxygen, it is $(632 - 47) \times 40\% = 234$ torr.

Minute volume is a product of V_T and respiratory rate. Part of the V_T occupies the conducting airways (anatomic dead space), which does not contribute to gas exchange in the alveoli. **Alveolar ventilation** is the volume of atmospheric air entering the alveoli and is calculated as $(V_T - \text{dead space}) \times$ respiratory rate. Alveolar ventilation is inversely proportional to alveolar PCO_2 (P_ACO_2). When alveolar ventilation is halved, P_ACO_2 is doubled. Conversely, doubling of alveolar ventilation decreases P_ACO_2 by 50%. *Alveolar PO_2* (P_AO_2) is calculated by the **alveolar air equation** as follows: $P_AO_2 = PiO_2 - (P_ACO_2 \div R)$; where R is the respiratory quotient. For practical purposes, P_ACO_2 is substituted by *arterial PCO_2* ($PaCO_2$) and R is assumed to be 0.8. According to the alveolar air equation, for a given PiO_2, a rise in $PaCO_2$ of 10 torr results in a decrease in P_AO_2 by $10 \div 0.8$ or 10×1.25 or 12.5 torr. Thus, proportionately inverse changes in P_AO_2 occur to the extent of 1.25× the changes in P_ACO_2 (or $PaCO_2$).

After the alveolar gas composition is determined by the inspired gas conditions and process of ventilation, gas exchange occurs by the process of diffusion and equilibration of alveolar gas with pulmonary capillary blood. Diffusion depends on the alveolar capillary barrier and amount of available time for equilibration. In health, the equilibration of alveolar gas and pulmonary capillary blood is complete for both oxygen and carbon dioxide. In diseases in which alveolar capillary barrier is abnormally increased (alveolar interstitial diseases) and/or when the time available for equilibration is decreased (increased blood flow velocity), diffusion is incomplete. Because of its greater solubility in liquid medium, carbon dioxide is 20 times more diffusible than oxygen. Therefore, diseases with diffusion defects are characterized by marked *alveolar-arterial oxygen* ($A - aO_2$) gradient and hypoxemia. Significant elevation of CO_2 does not occur as a result of a diffusion defect unless there is coexistent hypoventilation.

Venous blood brought to the lungs is "arterialized" after diffusion is complete. After complete arterialization, the pulmonary capillary blood should have the same PO_2 and PCO_2 as in the alveoli. The arterial blood gas composition, however, is different from that in the alveoli, even in normal conditions. This is because there is a certain amount of dead space ventilation as well as venous admixture in a normal lung. Dead space ventila-

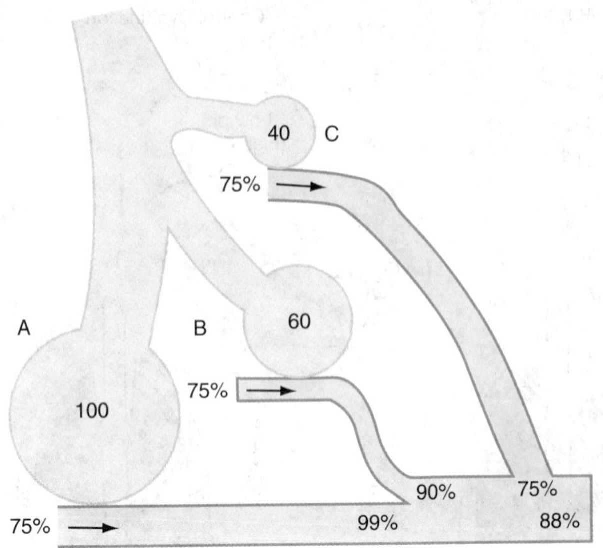

Figure 370-10. Diagram demonstrating the effects of decreased ventilation-perfusion ratios on arterial oxygenation in the lungs. Three alveolar-capillary units are illustrated. Unit A has normal ventilation and an alveolar PO_2 of 100 mm mL/min Hg (shown by the number in the middle of the space). The blood that circulates through this unit raises its oxygen saturation from 75% (the saturation of mixed venous blood) to 99%. Unit B has a lower ventilation-perfusion ratio and a lower alveolar PO_2 of 60 mm Hg. The blood that circulates through this unit reaches a saturation of only 90%. Finally, unit C is not ventilated at all. Its alveolar PO_2 is equivalent to that of the venous blood, which travels through the unit unaltered. The oxygen saturation of the arterial blood reflects the weighted contributions of these 3 units. If it is assumed that each unit has the same blood flow, the arterial blood would have a saturation of only 88%. Ventilation-perfusion mismatch is the most common mechanism of arterial hypoxemia in lung disease. Supplemental oxygen increases the arterial PO_2 by raising the alveolar PO_2 in lung units that, like B, have a ventilation-perfusion ratio greater than zero.

tion results in a higher $PaCO_2$ than P_ACO_2, whereas venous admixture or right-to-left shunting results in a lower PaO_2 compared to the alveolar gas composition (see Fig. 370-10). PaO_2 is a reflection of the amount of oxygen dissolved in blood, which is a relatively minor component of total blood oxygen content. For every 100 torr PO_2, there is 0.3 mL of dissolved O_2 in 100 mL of blood. The total blood oxygen content is composed of the dissolved oxygen and the oxygen bound to hemoglobin. Each gram of hemoglobin carries 1.34 mL of O_2 when 100% saturated with oxygen. Thus, 15 g of hemoglobin carries 20.1 mL of oxygen. *Arterial oxygen content* (CaO_2), expressed as mL O_2/dL blood, can be calculated as ($PaO_2 \times 0.003$) + (Hb $\times$ 1.34 $\times$ SO_2), where Hb is grams of hemoglobin per dL blood and SO_2 is percent of oxyhemoglobin saturation. The relationship of PO_2 and the amount of oxygen carried by the hemoglobin is the basis of the oxygen-hemoglobin (O_2-Hb) dissociation curve (see Fig. 370-3). The PO_2 at which hemoglobin is 50% saturated is referred to as P_{50}. At a normal pH, hemoglobin is 94% saturated at PO_2 of 70, and little further gain in saturation is accomplished at a higher PO_2. At PO_2 below 50, there is a steep decline in saturation and, therefore, the oxygen content.

Oxygen delivery to the tissues is a product of oxygen content and cardiac output. When hemoglobin is near 100% saturated, the blood contains ≈20 mL oxygen per 100 mL or 200 mL/L. In a healthy adult, the cardiac output is ≈5 L/min, oxygen delivery 1,000 mL/min, and oxygen consumption 250 mL/min. Mixed venous blood returning to the heart has PO_2 of 40 torr and is 75% saturated with oxygen. Blood oxygen content, cardiac output, and oxygen consumption are important determinants of mixed venous oxygen saturation. Given a steady state blood oxygen content and oxygen consumption, the mixed venous saturation is an important indicator of cardiac output. A declining mixed venous saturation in such a state indicates decreasing cardiac output.

370.8 • Interpretation of Blood Gases

Interpretation of blood gas values is important in localizing the site of the lesion and estimating its severity, especially when considered with clinical observations (Table 370-2). In airway obstruction above the carina (subglottic stenosis, vascular ring), blood gases reflect overall alveolar hypoventilation. This is manifested by an elevated P_ACO_2 and a proportionate decrease in P_AO_2 as determined by the alveolar air equation. A rise in P_ACO_2 of 20 torr will decrease P_AO_2 by 20×1.25 or 25 torr. In the absence of a significant parenchymal disease and intrapulmonary shunting, such lesions respond very well to supplemental oxygen in reversing hypoxemia. Similar blood gas values, demonstrating alveolar hypoventilation and response to supplemental oxygen, are observed in patients with a depressed respiratory center and ineffective neuromuscular function, resulting in respiratory insufficiency (see Fig. 370-9). Such patients can be easily distinguished from those with airway obstruction by their poor respiratory effort.

In intrapulmonary airway obstruction (asthma, bronchiolitis), blood gases reflect ventilation perfusion imbalance and venous admixture. In these diseases, the obstruction is not uniform throughout the lungs, resulting in areas that are hyperventilated and others that are hypoventilated. Pulmonary capillary blood coming from hyperventilated areas has a higher PO_2 and lower PCO_2, whereas that coming from hypoventilated regions has a lower PO_2 and higher PCO_2. A lower blood PCO_2 can compensate for the higher PCO_2 since the hemoglobin-CO_2 dissociation curve is relatively linear. In mild disease, the hyperventilated areas predominate, resulting in hypocarbia. An elevated PaO_2 in hyperventilated areas cannot compensate for the decreased PaO_2 in

TABLE 370-2. Interpretation of Arterial Blood Gas (ABG) Values

LESION	EFFECT	TYPICAL ABG
Central (above the carina) airway obstruction, or Depressed respiratory center, or Ineffective neuromuscular function	Uniform alveolar hypoventilation	* Early increase in PCO_2 * Proportionate decrease in PO_2 depending on alveolar air equation * Response to supplemental oxygen: Excellent
Intrapulmonary airway obstruction	Venous admixture V/Q mismatch	* Mild: ↓ PCO_2, ↓ PO_2 * Moderate: "Normal" PCO_2, ↓↓ PO_2 * Severe: ↑↑ PCO_2, ↓↓↓ PO_2 * Response to supplemental oxygen: Good
Alveolar-interstitial pathology	Diffusion defect R → L shunt	* Early decrease in PO_2 depending on severity * Normal or low PCO_2, ↑ PCO_2 if fatigue develops * Response to supplemental oxygen: Fair to poor

V/Q, ventilation-perfusion.

hypoventilated areas because of the shape of the O_2-Hb dissociation curve. This results in venous admixture, arterial desaturation, and decreased PaO_2 (see Fig. 370-10). With increasing disease severity, more areas become hypoventilated, resulting in normalization of $PaCO_2$ with a further decrease in PaO_2. A normal or slightly elevated $PaCO_2$ in asthma should be viewed with concern as a potential indicator of impending respiratory failure. In severe intrapulmonary airway obstruction, hypoventilated areas predominate, leading to hypercarbia, respiratory acidosis, and hypoxemia. The degree to which supplemental oxygenation raises PaO_2 depends on the severity of the illness and the degree of venous admixture.

In alveolar and interstitial diseases, blood gas values reflect both intrapulmonary right-to-left shunting and a diffusion barrier. Hypoxemia is a hallmark of such conditions occurring early in the disease process. $PaCO_2$ is either normal or decreased. An increase in $PaCO_2$ is observed only later in the course, as muscle fatigue and exhaustion result in hypoventilation. Response to supplemental oxygen is relatively poor with shunting and diffusion disorders compared to other lesions.

Most clinical entities present with mixed lesions. A child with a vascular ring may also have an area of atelectasis; the arterial blood gas reflects both processes. The blood gas values reflect the more dominant lesion.

370.9 • Pulmonary Vasculature in Health and Disease

During intrauterine fetal development, the tunica media of pulmonary arteries become more muscular in the last trimester of pregnancy (see Chapter 101.1). Up to 90% of the systemic venous return is shunted away from the pulmonary arterial circulation to the systemic arterial circulation through the foramen ovale and the ductus arteriosus. After birth, with functional closure of the foramen ovale and the ductus arteriosus, and dilatation of the pulmonary arterial circulation with consequent decrease in **pulmonary vascular resistance** (PVR), all of the right ventricular output passes through the lung. The PVR is ≈50% of the systemic arterial resistance 3 days after birth. In the next several wk after birth, there is a further decline in PVR and, therefore, the pulmonary artery pressure, as pulmonary arterial musculature in the tunica media involutes. Two to 3 mo after birth, the PVR and the pulmonary artery pressure are ≈15% of the systemic values, a relationship that exists through childhood and adolescence. Pulmonary vasculature constricts in response to hypoxemia, acidosis, and hypercarbia, and dilates with increased alveolar and arterial PO_2, alkalosis, and hypocarbia. Younger infants, with their relatively muscular pulmonary arteries, are especially susceptible to pulmonary vasoconstrictive stimuli.

Failure of the pulmonary arterial circulation to dilate after birth results in **persistent pulmonary hypertension of the newborn** (**PPHN**; see Chapter 101.8). Because of the persistently high PVR, the systemic venous blood returning to the right side of the heart continues to be shunted across the foramen ovale and the ductus arteriosus to the systemic arterial circulation, leading to a vicious cycle of hypoxemia, acidosis, and further pulmonary vasoconstriction.

The relatively high PVR opposes excessive left-to-right shunting in full-term neonates with ventricular septal defect and patent ductus arteriosus (see Chapter 426). Such infants do not usually manifest heart failure until 2–3 mo after birth, when PVR has sufficiently declined. Premature infants, with lesions capable of left-to-right shunting, are susceptible to developing heart failure earlier in life because of less musculature in pulmonary artery tunica media and, therefore, a lower PVR. Persistent and long-term left-to-right shunting carries the risk of development of secondary pulmonary vascular disease characterized by the postnatal development of medial muscular hypertrophy followed by intimal proliferation and increased PVR. Early changes in pulmonary vasculature are reversible with correction of the congenital heart defect responsible for left-to-right shunting. Advanced pulmonary vascular disease is characterized by irreversible intimal and medial changes. When PVR is increased to suprasystemic levels, right-to-left shunting occurs and is characterized by a cyanotic state (Eisenmenger syndrome), making the heart defect inoperable in the absence of an accompanying lung transplantation (see Chapter 433.2).

Pulmonary hypertension can develop without a well-defined etiology (primary pulmonary hypertension) or as a consequence of an underlying disease (secondary pulmonary hypertension) (see Chapter 433). Adverse effects of pulmonary hypertension are related to an increased right ventricular afterload, decreased cardiac output, and heart failure characterized by increased systemic venous pressure, hepatomegaly, and edema. In an acute situation, right ventricular failure and decreased cardiac output can worsen oxygen delivery and hypoxemia. Right ventricular failure secondary to pulmonary pathology is referred to as **cor pulmonale.** Secondary pulmonary hypertension is a common occurrence in end-stage chronic obstructive pulmonary disease such as cystic fibrosis and bronchopulmonary dysplasia. Pulmonary arterial involvement is sometimes encountered in collagen vascular diseases such as scleroderma (see Chapter 159) and dermatomyositis (see Chapter 158). Functional or structural upper airway obstruction may also produce right ventricular failure. Children with marked obesity are also susceptible to chronic alveolar hypoventilation and right heart failure, termed **Pickwickian syndrome.** Treatment of the underlying cause is the 1st priority in patients with secondary pulmonary hypertension (see Chapter 433).

370.10 • Immune Response of the Lung to Injury

Various disease entities, local or systemic, can potentially induce an inflammatory response in the lung. Local diseases of the lung capable of inducing the inflammatory response include infectious processes, aspiration, asphyxia, pulmonary contusion, and inhalation of chemical irritants; systemic diseases include sepsis, shock, trauma, and cardiopulmonary bypass. This inflammatory response is mediated through the release of cytokines and other mediators. In the lung, alveolar macrophages are the chief architects of the early cytokine response, producing *tumor necrosis factor-α* (TNF-α) and *interleukin 1β* (IL-1β). These cytokines are involved in initiating the inflammatory cascade resulting in the production of other cytokines, prostaglandins, reactive oxygen species, and upregulating cell adhesion molecules, which, in turn, leads to white cell migration into the lung tissue. The pathophysiologic consequences of the inflammatory response include injury to pulmonary capillary endothelium and the alveolar epithelial cells. Various cytokines and eicosanoids produce pulmonary vasoconstriction, resulting in pulmonary hypertension and increased right ventricular afterload. Injury to the capillary endothelium results in increased permeability and exudation of protein-rich fluid into the pulmonary interstitium and alveoli. Cellular debris and fibrin form the characteristic eosinophilic hyaline membranes along the walls of the alveolar duct. There is sloughing of type 1 pneumocytes. Interstitial and alveolar edema results in decreased FRC, diffusion barrier, intrapulmonary right-to-left shunting across poorly ventilating alveoli and increase in the alveolar–arterial (A-aO_2) gradient. Clinically, A-aO_2 gradient >200 is characterized as *acute lung injury* and a gradient >300 is termed acute **respiratory distress syndrome (ARDS)** [see Chapter 69].

The clinician must consider the potential adverse effects of therapeutic interventions such as oxygen, endotracheal intubation, and mechanical ventilation as part of the pathophysiologic consequences of ARDS. High concentrations of inspired oxygen have a risk of pulmonary capillary and epithelial cell injury; the concentration of oxygen below which it can be considered safe has not been established. In addition to the potential for nosocomial pneumonia, mechanical ventilation carries the risk of ventilator-induced lung injury due to physical stress applied to terminal airways, alveolar epithelium, and pulmonary capillaries. Excessive tidal volume can, in and of itself, result in mechanical disruption capable of perpetuating the inflammatory response. If alveoli are allowed to deflate excessively during exhalation, they are subjected to greater stress injury from alveolar recruitment and derecruitment. The mechanical ventilation strategy aimed at minimizing ventilator-induced lung injury in ARDS includes alveolar recruitment and maintenance of adequate FRC throughout the respiratory cycle with an optimum PEEP, and ventilation with relatively low (6–8 mL/kg) tidal volume.

370.11 • Regulation of Respiration

The main function of respiration is to maintain normal blood gas homeostasis to match the metabolic needs of the body with the least amount of energy expenditure. Respiratory rate and tidal volume are regulated by a complex interaction of *controllers, sensors,* and *effectors.* The central respiratory controller consists of a group of neurons in the CNS that receive and integrate the afferent information from sensors, and send motor impulses to effectors to initiate and maintain respiration. Sensors are a variety of receptors located throughout the body. They gather chemical and physical information that is sent to the controller either to stimulate or to inhibit its activity. Effectors are the various muscles of respiration that, under the influence of the controller, move air in and out of the lung at a given tidal volume and rate. The respiratory regulatory mechanism itself undergoes a significant maturation process from the neonatal period throughout infancy and early childhood. **Sleep states** have the potential for profound influences on the control of respiration.

CENTRAL RESPIRATORY CONTROLLER. The respiratory controller mechanism comprises 2 functionally and anatomically distinct groups of neurons located in the CNS: 1 for voluntary and the other for automatic control. These areas of respiratory control can function independently but are also capable of interacting with each other.

Voluntary control of respiration resides in the cerebral motor cortex and limbic forebrain structure. Information is received from sensory neurons such as pain, touch, temperature, smell, vision, and emotions, and impulses are sent directly to the respiratory muscles through corticobulbar and corticospinal tracts. Voluntary control of respiration is important for protection from aspiration and inhalation of noxious gases. A certain level of consciousness is necessary to exercise voluntary control of respiration. Patients with CNS injury and toxic/metabolic encephalopathies lose voluntary control of respirations to varying degrees, depending on the extent of CNS dysfunction.

Automatic control of respiration resides in the brainstem. A group of 150–200 neurons, designated as the *pre-Botzinger complex* (preBotC), are located in the medullary region. PreBotC is responsible for maintaining respiratory rhythmicity and it can be considered the pacemaker for the automatic respiratory activity. PreBotC neurons are responsible for various patterns of respiration, including eupneic gasping and sighing, depending on the afferent input. These neurons have specific receptors for neurotransmitters, which may stimulate, inhibit, or modify their activity; such receptors include those for substance P (neurokinin), acetylcholine (nicotinic), glutamate, and opioid μ receptors. Several genes such as Hox paralogs and Hox-regulating genes kreisler/mafB and Krox20 regulate the embryonic generation of brainstem neurons and their intrinsic connections. A group of neurons located in the lower pons is collectively termed the *apneustic center,* which stimulates preBotC, resulting in prolonged inspiratory gasps (apneuses) interrupted by transient expiratory efforts. Another group of neurons in the upper pons, called the *pneumotaxic center,* is involved in inhibiting the activity of preBotC. The role of apneustic and pneumotaxic centers is to "fine-tune" the rhythmic respiratory activity generated by preBotC neurons.

Abnormalities of respirations are commonly encountered in CNS dysfunction. Global CNS depression may manifest as slow and shallow respirations with resultant hypoventilation and respiratory acidosis. Bihemispheric and diancephalic pathology can lead to **Cheyne-Stokes respirations,** characterized by periods of apnea interspersed with hyperventilation. Injuries within the rostral brainstem or tegmentum can lead to central neurogenic hyperventilation and respiratory alkalosis. Mid to caudal pontine lesion can result in an apneustic breathing pattern characterized by a prolonged inspiratory pause. Medullary lesions result in ataxic, irregular breathing or apnea.

SENSORS. Various receptors throughout the body are responsible for sensing afferent information that modulates the activity of the central respiratory controller. These receptors are sensory nerve endings that respond to changes in their environment. They are termed either *chemoreceptors* or *mechanoreceptors,* depending on the type of stimulus that is sensed. Chemoreceptors are classified as central or peripheral, depending on their location.

Central chemoreceptors are so termed because of their location within the CNS. Chemoreceptors sense a change in the chemical composition of body fluid to which they are exposed. Central chemoreceptors reside over a wide area that includes the posterior hypothalamus, cerebellum, locus ceruleus, raphe, and multiple nuclei within the brainstem. Central chemoreceptors bathe in the extracellular fluid of the brain and respond to the changes in the H^+ concentration. Information sensing an increase in H^+ concentration stimulates ventilatory response of the controller, whereas a decrease inhibits it. The brain's extracellular fluid, represented by the cerebrospinal fluid (CSF), is separated from the blood by the blood-brain barrier, which is relatively impermeable to H^+ and $HCO_3{-}$ ions, but readily permeable to CO_2. A rise in $PaCO_2$ is quickly reflected in a similar rise in the CSF. The consequent fall in CSF pH is sensed by the central chemoreceptors, causing stimulation of the controller and increase in ventilation. Changes in $PaCO_2$ result in stimulation or inhibition of ventilation by changes in CSF pH. CSF pH in normal conditions is ≈7.32. Compared to blood, CSF has much less CO_2 buffering capacity because of a much lower protein concentration. Consequently, the change in CSF pH is more pronounced than that in the blood for the same change in $PaCO_2$. With a persistent elevation in $PaCO_2$, the CSF pH eventually tends to normalize as HCO_3^- equilibrates across the blood-brain barrier. Patients with chronic obstructive lung disease therefore have a relatively normal CSF pH, and they do not show the ventilatory response that is observed with an acute rise in $PaCO_2$.

Hypoxia can depress global CNS function; nonetheless, multiple regions in the brain show an excitatory response to hypoxia, which contributes to the increase in ventilation.

Peripheral chemoreceptors are located in carotid bodies just above the bifurcation of the common carotid arteries, and in the aortic bodies above and below the aortic arch; the carotid bodies are the most important in humans. The most important variable in determining the activity of the carotid bodies is changes in PaO_2. Although the carotid bodies have a relatively high metabolic rate, they receive a very high flow for their rather small size. As long as a normal blood flow is maintained, the dissolved oxygen reflected by PaO_2 is sufficient for their metabolism. Stimulation of carotid bodies resulting in increased ventilation occurs

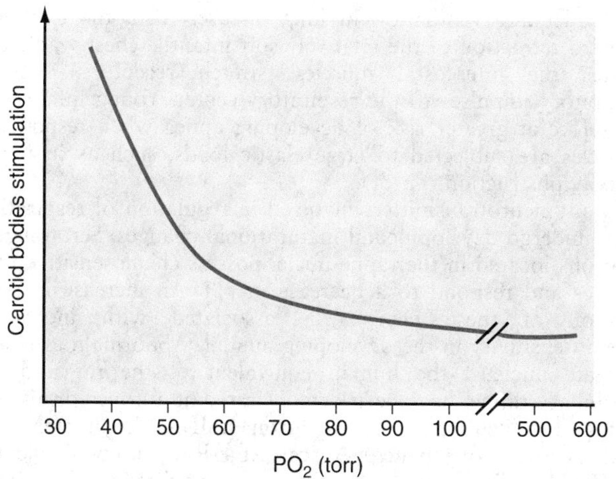

Figure 370-11. Significant stimulation of carotid bodies occurs with PaO_2 level <100 torr. A subjective feeling of dyspnea does not occur, however, until PaO_2 is <50 torr, at which point, stimulation of the carotid bodies increases exponentially.

when their oxygen supply is decreased below their metabolic requirements. This occurs when there is (1) decreased PaO_2, (2) decreased blood flow (low cardiac output), and (3) impaired oxygen utilization (cyanide poisoning). In anemia, carbon monoxide poisoning, and methemoglobinemia, carotid bodies are not stimulated as long as the PaO_2 and the cardiac output are not compromised. The relationship of PaO_2 and the stimulation of carotid bodies is nonlinear (Fig. 370-11).

Carotid bodies are activated at a PaO_2 of <500 torr. This is substantiated by the observation that there is a small but distinct decrease in ventilation when 100% oxygen is breathed by normal individuals when PaO_2 exceeds 500 torr. A relatively small increase in ventilation occurs until the PaO_2 reaches 100 torr. Where the PaO_2 is <100 torr the carotid body stimulation increases significantly. The carotid body receptor response rate is fast enough to alter their discharge rate during the respiratory cycle as a result of small cyclic changes in PaO_2 during inspiration and expiration. At PaO_2 levels <50 torr, carotid body stimulation increases exponentially. The most important effect of carotid body stimulation is an increase in respiratory rate and tidal volume. Additional effects include vasoconstriction, bradycardia, systemic hypertension, release of antidiuretic hormone, and stimulation of the adrenal medulla and adrenal cortex. The bradycardic effect of carotid body stimulation is overshadowed by the pulmonary reflex, which is induced by lung inflation and results in tachycardia. Patients in whom lung inflation is prevented are more likely to develop bradycardia after hypoxic stimulation of carotid bodies. Examples of such situations are: fetal hypoxia, CNS depression, neuromuscular blockade, myopathy, neuropathy, and controlled ventilation. The peripheral chemoreceptors are responsible for almost all the increase in ventilation that occurs in response to hypoxemia.

Peripheral chemoreceptors are also stimulated by an increase in $PaCO_2$; this response requires a relatively large change in $PaCO_2$ and results in a smaller rise in minute ventilation compared to the effect of CO_2 on central chemoreceptors. The peripheral chemoreceptors respond much more quickly (within 1 sec), however, whereas the central chemoreceptors may take minutes to respond. Thus peripheral chemoreceptors are important in the immediate rise in ventilation in response to a large and abrupt increase in $PaCO_2$. Decreased pH also stimulates the peripheral chemoreceptors. The effect of pH is regardless of whether the acidosis is due to respiratory or metabolic causes. Decreased PaO_2, increased $PaCO_2$, and decreased pH act synergistically on carotid bodies. The combined effect is greater than the sum of their individual actions.

In contrast to the central chemoreceptors, the peripheral chemoreceptors are not easily depressed, such as by anesthesia or opiates. They also do not adapt easily to a persistent stimulus such as hypoxia, as do the central chemoreceptors to hypercarbia. The central chemoreceptors in hypoxic patients are relatively unresponsive to CO_2 at a time when respirations are predominantly stimulated by effects of hypoxia on peripheral chemoreceptors.

LUNG RECEPTORS. *Stretch receptors* are located within the airway smooth muscle. They are stimulated by lung inflation and the impulse is conducted via the vagus nerve. The main effect of these receptors is to decrease the respiratory rate due to an inhibition of inspiratory muscle activity and an increase in exhalation time. This reflex is termed Hering-Breuer inflation reflex. Hering-Breuer deflation reflex stimulates inspiratory muscle activity in response to deflation of the lung. These reflexes are not operative during normal breathing in adults but may be important in newborns. Stretch receptors play an important role in minimizing the energy required for the work of breathing in respiratory disease. In diseases in which airway resistance is increased (asthma), more energy is needed to overcome airway resistance. Slow and deep breathing is most economical in such a situation because of relatively lower flow rate, and greater alveolar inflation is possible without stretching of the airway smooth muscle earlier during inspiration. In diseases of compliance, (pulmonary edema), rapid and shallow breathing is most economical to keep the elastic work at minimum. Because of the stiffer alveoli in such situations, the transpulmonary pressure is transmitted to the airway smooth muscle earlier during inspiration, stimulating the stretch receptors and turning off inspiration.

Irritant receptors are present in between the epithelial cells in the airway mucous membrane. They are stimulated by particulate matter, noxious gases, and chemical fumes in the inspired gas, and also by cold air. The vagus nerve is responsible for conducting the impulse. Stimulation of irritant receptors results in bronchoconstriction and hyperpnea.

J receptors derive their name because of their "juxta-capillary" location. They lie in the alveolar walls close to the pulmonary capillaries. Pulmonary capillary engorgement and interstitial and alveolar wall edema provide stimuli for activation of the J receptors, resulting in shallow and rapid respirations and dyspnea. This is seen in left heart failure, ARDS, and interstitial diseases.

Muscle receptors important for regulation of respirations are those in the diaphragm and the intercostals. Stretch of the muscle sensed by the muscle spindle is used to control the strength of contraction. Excessive distortion of the diaphragm and the intercostals inhibits inspiratory activity when large negative intrathoracic pressure is required to move air, such as in airway obstruction. The soft chest walls of newborns and young infants are more susceptible to distortion; such children may respond to upper airway obstruction by premature cessation of inspiration and apnea rather than by the prolongation of inspiration required to move sufficient air past the obstruction.

Arterial baroreceptors located in aortic arch and carotid sinuses can influence respiration depending on arterial blood pressure. A decrease in blood pressure results in hyperventilation and an increased blood pressure causes hypoventilation.

Pain and temperature receptors also influence respirations and they are especially pronounced in the neonates and young infants. A painful stimulus causes breath holding followed by hyperventilation. Increased skin temperature causes hyperventilation and hypothermia results in hypoventilation. In the context of cold stimulus, the facial area is most important in causing apnea.

EFFECTORS. The most important effectors of respiration are the diaphragm, intercostals, and abdominal muscles. They receive impulses from the controller and effect ventilation. Accessory effectors such as sternocleidomastoids and paraspinal muscles may be called on to make additional contribution to the respiratory efforts in times of need. The effectors can be seriously impaired in malnutrition, spinal injury, and neuromuscular disease.

SLEEP STATES. Respiratory regulation is considerably affected by sleep. Sleep, in general, decreases central chemosensitivity to CO_2. $PaCO_2$ is increased by a few torr compared to that in the wakeful state. Two broad categories of sleep states exist: *nonrapid eye movement* (NREM) and *rapid eye movement* (REM) sleep (see Chapter 18). NREM sleep is characterized by high-voltage, slow waves on electroencephalogram (EEG), and is associated with fragmented mental activity. Muscle tone and movements are relatively unaffected. NREM sleep is likened to a "relatively inactive brain in a movable body." REM sleep is so termed because of the presence of episodic bursts of rapid eye movements. The most clinically significant aspect of REM sleep is marked suppression of postural muscle tone and lack of spontaneous movements. REM sleep is likened to "a highly activated brain in a paralyzed body." Descending axons from the dorsal pontine tegmentum region are responsible for the REM sleep-specific characteristic atonia and paralysis. The predominant sleep pattern in premature babies is REM sleep. A full-term newborn has 50% REM sleep. Most of the sleep maturation occurs in the 1st 6 mo of life. Older children and adults spend ≈20% of their sleep in the REM state. Sleep-related respiratory abnormalities are encountered predominantly in REM sleep. Depression of muscle tone during REM sleep has 2 major effects. The relaxed and therefore increasingly compliant chest wall retracts inward much more during inspiration than a less compliant chest wall would, resulting in an impediment to air inflow and s paradoxical (seesaw) pattern of breathing, in which the abdomen and the chest wall move asynchronously. The 2nd effect is that of relaxation of the genioglossus, palatal, and other upper airway muscles, causing airway obstruction. REM sleep-related respiratory abnormalities are commonly encountered in premature infants and those children with coexistent anatomic upper airway obstruction, obesity, and neuromuscular dysfunction.

REGULATION OF RESPIRATION IN SPECIAL SITUATIONS.

Fetus, Newborns, and Young Infants. At various stages of development, the response to chemoreceptor and mechanoreceptor stimulation and the efficiency of effectors are markedly different. Unlike adults who show an immediate and sustained response to hypoxemia characterized by hyperventilation, the newborn exhibits a biphasic response. After an initial brief period (1–2 min) of hyperventilation, the neonate and young infant develop hypoventilation and apnea when hypoxemia is sustained. This explains why such infants are much more prone to develop respiratory arrest in hypoxic states than are older children and adults. Lower gestational age of the infant is associated with a more pronounced and earlier apneic response to hypoxemia. Fetal respiratory activity, for example, is switched off when faced with oxygen deprivation. Maturation of carotid chemoreceptors may be an explanation for the differences in hypoxic response at various stages of development. Sensitivity of CO_2 sensors also undergoes maturation. Compared to adults and older children, neonates and young infants have decreased CO_2 responsiveness, as measured by an increase in minute alveolar ventilation for a given increase in $PaCO_2$. Theophylline and caffeine have been shown to increase the central chemoreceptor ventilatory response to CO_2 and decrease the number of apneic spells in premature babies.

The neonatal respiratory muscles are poorly equipped to sustain large workloads; they are more easily fatigued than in older children, and this significantly limits their ability to maintain adequate ventilation in lung disease. Also, the excessive inward retraction of the relatively soft infantile chest wall stimulates the intercostal muscles' stretch receptors, sending inhibitory impulses to the respiratory center. Young infants are therefore at greater risk of developing apnea when respiratory muscles are subjected to large elastic loads, such as in upper airway obstruction.

Many neurotransmitters involved in regulation of respiration also undergo developmental maturational changes. Serotonergic neurons located in the raphe nuclei possess chemosensitive properties and respond to a decrease in pH. An increase in population of these neurons is associated with increasing chemosensitivity in the developing animal. Abnormalities of the arcuate nucleus, the human equivalent of the rat and cat medullary raphe, have been demonstrated at autopsy on infants dying of sudden infant death syndrome (SIDS; see Chapter 372). Cohort studies of Japanese, African-American, and white victims of SIDS have implicated a homozygous gene that encodes for the long allele of the serotonin transporter promoter. SIDS victims are more likely to express the long allele of the serotonin transporter promoter and miss the short allele compared to controls. The delay in development of serotonergic neurons or overexpression of the long allele for serotonin transporter promoter may explain the abnormal respiratory response to adverse conditions, which results in SIDS. Central chemoreception is also severely impaired in congenital central hypoventilation syndrome.

Chronic Hypoxia and Hypercarbia. The respiratory control mechanism is altered when exposed to chronic conditions. In patients with chronic pulmonary insufficiency with elevated $PaCO_2$, the CSF pH has been normalized and the central chemoreceptors become unresponsive to CO_2. Furthermore, renal compensation results in bicarbonate retention and relative normalization of blood pH. Arterial hypoxemia remains the chief stimulus for ventilation, which is predominantly dependent on peripheral chemoreceptor stimulation by a low PaO_2. Administration of a high amount of oxygen in such patients carries a risk of sudden removal of the hypoxic stimulus, cessation of breathing, exacerbation of hypercarbia and CO_2 narcosis, and coma. Patients with chronic obstructive lung disease and neuromuscular disease are especially susceptible to this complication. Children with bronchopulmonary dysplasia or with muscular dystrophy who have had a high $PaCO_2$, with or without supplemental oxygen, may develop serious hypoventilation and respiratory acidosis when their PaO_2 is increased more than their baseline with administration of a higher amount of oxygen.

Chronically hypoxic patients such as those living at high altitude and those with cyanotic heart disease and interstitial lung disease have a blunted chemoreceptor function and poor response to further hypoxemia. It is of interest to the clinician that children with poorly controlled asthma also show a blunted hypoxic response and may appear to be breathing relatively comfortably in spite of dangerously low PaO_2. Such children and their caretakers are at risk of failing to appreciate the severity of their disease, which can result in delay in the institution of appropriate therapy.

Abu-Shaweesh JM: Maturation of respiratory responses in the fetus and neonate. *Semin Neonatol* 2004;9:169–180.

Carskadon MA, Dement WC: Normal human sleep: An overview. In Kryger MH, Roth T, Dement WC (editors): *Principles and Practice of Sleep Medicine*. Philadelphia, W B Saunders, 2000, 3rd ed, pp 15–25.

Chokroverty S: Physiology of sleep. In Chokroverty S, Daroff RB (editors): *Sleep Disorders Medicine: Basic Science, Technical Considerations, and Clinical Aspects*. Boston, Butterworth-Heinemann, 2nd ed, 1999, pp 95–126.

Feldman JL, Mitchell GS, Nattie EE: Breathing: Rhythmicity, plasticity, chemosensitivity. *Annu Rev Neurosci* 2003;26:239–266.

Gozal D: New concepts in abnormalities of respiratory control in children. *Curr Opin Pediatr* 2004;19:305–308.

Polgar G, Weng T: The functional development of the respiratory system from the period of gestation to adulthood. *Am Rev Respir Dis* 1979;120:625–695.
Smith JC, Ellenberger HH, Ballanyi K, et al: Pre-Botzinger complex: A brain stem region that may generate respiratory rhythm in mammals. *Science* 1991;254:726–729.
West JB: *Respiratory Physiology: The Essentials,* 7th ed. Baltimore, Lippincott Williams and Wilkins, 2005.

Chapter 371 ■ Diagnostic Approach to Respiratory Disease Gabriel G. Haddad and Thomas P. Green

The appropriate diagnosis of a child presenting with respiratory signs and symptoms depends most heavily on a careful history and physical examination. In some patients, complementary diagnostic tests and modalities are required.

HISTORY

The history should include questions about respiratory symptoms (dyspnea, cough, pain, wheezing, snoring, apnea, cyanosis), chronicity, timing during day or night, and associations with activities such as exercise or food intake. The respiratory system interacts with a number of other systems, and questions related to cardiac, gastrointestinal, central nervous, hematologic, and immune systems may be relevant. Questions related to gastrointestinal reflux or immune status may be important in a patient with repeated pneumonias. The family history is essential and should include inquiries about siblings and other close relatives with similar symptoms or any chronic disease with respiratory components.

PHYSICAL EXAMINATION

Respiratory dysfunction usually produces detectable alterations in the pattern of breathing. Values for normal respiratory rates are presented in Table 66-3 and depend on many factors, most importantly, age. Repeated respiratory rate measurements are necessary because respiratory rates, especially in the young, are exquisitely sensitive to extraneous stimuli. Sleeping respiratory rates are more reproducible in infants than those obtained during feeding or activity. These rates vary among infants but average 40–50 breaths/min in the 1st weeks of life and usually <60 breaths/min in the 1st few days of life. Respiratory control abnormalities may cause the child to breathe at a low rate or periodically. Mechanical abnormalities produce compensatory changes that are generally directed at maintaining or increasing alveolar ventilation. Decreases in lung compliance require increases in muscular force and breathing rate leading to variable increases in chest wall retractions and nasal flaring. The respiratory excursions of children with restrictive disease are shallow. An expiratory grunt is common as the child attempts to raise the *functional residual capacity* (FRC) by closing the glottis at the end of expiration.

Children with obstructive disease take slower, deeper breaths (see Chapter 370). When the obstruction is **extrathoracic** (from the nose to the mid-trachea), inspiration is more prolonged than is expiration, and an inspiratory stridor can usually be heard. When the obstruction is **intrathoracic,** expiration is more prolonged than is inspiration, and the patient often has to make use of accessory expiratory muscles.

TABLE 371-1. Lung Sound Nomenclature

	SOUND
DISCONTINUOUS	
Fine (high pitched, low amplitude, short duration)	Fine crackles
Coarse (low pitched, high amplitude, long duration)	Coarse crackles
CONTINUOUS	
High pitched	Wheezes
Low pitched	Rhonchus

Recommendation from the 1985 International Symposium on Lung Sounds in Tokyo for a unified nomenclature of adventitious sounds. (From Cugell DW: Lung sound nomenclature. *Am Rev Respir Dis* 1987;136:1016, with permission.)
From Chernick V, Boat TF: *Kendig's Disorders of the Respiratory Tract in Children,* 6th ed. Philadelphia, WB Saunders, 1998, p 97.

Lung percussion has limited value in small infants because it cannot discriminate between noises originating from tissues that are close to each other. In adolescents and adults, percussion is usually dull in restrictive lung disease and with a pleural effusion, pneumonia, and atelectasis, and tympanitic in obstructive disease (asthma, pneumothorax).

Auscultation confirms the presence of inspiratory or expiratory prolongation and provides information about the symmetry and quality of air movement. In addition, it often detects abnormal or adventitious sounds such as **stridor** (a predominant inspiratory monophonic noise), **crackles** (high pitch, interrupted sounds found during inspiration and more rarely during early expiration, which denote opening of previously closed air spaces), or **wheezes** (musical, continuous sounds usually caused by the development of turbulent flow in narrow airways) [Table 371-1]. **Digital clubbing** is a sign of chronic hypoxia (Fig. 371-1) but may be due to nonpulmonary etiologies (Table 371-2).

BLOOD GAS ANALYSIS

An arterial blood gas analysis is probably the single most useful rapid test of pulmonary function. Although this analysis does not

TABLE 371-2. Nonpulmonary Diseases Associated with Clubbing

CARDIAC
Cyanotic congenital heart disease
Subacute bacterial endocarditis
Chronic congestive heart failure
HEMATOLOGIC
Thalassemia
Congenital methemoglobinemia (rare)
GASTROINTESTINAL
Crohn disease
Ulcerative colitis
Chronic dysentery, sprue
Polyposis coli
Severe gastrointestinal hemorrhage
Small bowel lymphoma
Liver cirrhosis (including α_1-antitrypsin deficiency)
OTHER
Thyroid deficiency (thyroid acropachy)
Chronic pyelonephritis (rare)
Toxic (e.g., arsenic, mercury, beryllium)
Lymphomatoid granulomatosis
Fabry disease
Raynaud disease, scleroderma
UNILATERAL CLUBBING
Vascular disorders (e.g., subclavian arterial aneurysm, brachial arteriovenous fistula)
Subluxation of shoulder
Median nerve injury
Local trauma

From Chernick V, Boat TF: *Kendig's Disorders of the Respiratory Tract in Children,* 6th ed. Philadelphia, WB Saunders, 1998, p 102.

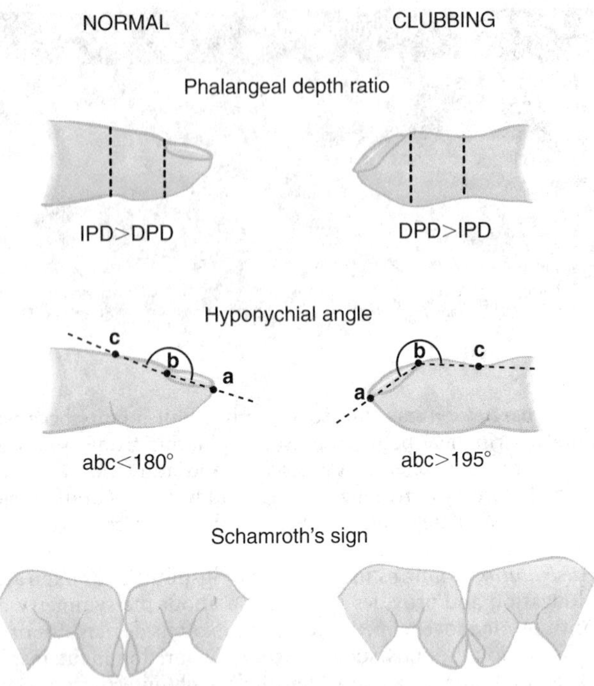

Figure 371-1. Finger clubbing can be measured in different ways. The ratio of the distal phalangeal diameter (DPD) over the interphalangeal diameter (IPD), or the phalangeal depth ratio, is <1 in normal subjects but increases to >1 with finger clubbing. The DPD/IPD can be measured with calipers or, more accurately, with finger casts. The hyponychial angle can be measured from lateral projections of the finger contour on a magnifying screen and is usually <180 degrees in normal subjects but >195 degrees in patients with finger clubbing. For bedside clinical assessment, the Schamroth sign is useful. The dorsal surfaces of the terminal phalanges of similar fingers are placed together. With clubbing, the normal diamond-shaped aperture or "window" at the bases of the nail beds disappears, and a prominent distal angle forms between the ends of the nails. In normal subjects, this angle is minimal or nonexistent. (From Chernick V, Boat TF: *Kendig's Disorders of the Respiratory Tract in Children,* 6th ed. Philadelphia, WB Saunders, 1998.)

specify the cause of the condition or the specific nature of the disease process, it can give an overall assessment of the functional state of the respiratory system and clues about the pathogenesis of the disease. Because the detection of cyanosis is influenced by skin color, perfusion, and blood hemoglobin concentration, the clinical detection by inspections is an unreliable sign of hypoxemia. Arterial hypertension, tachycardia, and diaphoresis are late, and not exclusive, signs of hypoventilation.

Blood gas exchange is evaluated most accurately by the direct measurement of arterial PO_2, PCO_2, and pH (see Chapters 64, 101.4, and 370). The blood specimen is best collected anaerobically in a heparinized syringe containing only enough heparin solution to displace the air from the syringe. The syringe should be sealed, placed in ice, and carried to the laboratory for immediate analysis. Although these measurements have no substitute in many conditions, they require arterial puncture and have been replaced to a great extent by noninvasive monitoring.

The age and clinical condition of the patient need to be taken into account when interpreting blood gas tensions. With the exception of neonates, values of arterial $PO_2 < 85$ mm Hg are usually abnormal for a child breathing room air at sea level. Calculation of the alveolar-arterial oxygen gradient is useful in the analysis of arterial oxygenation, particularly when the patient is not breathing room air or in the presence of hypercarbia. Values of arterial $PCO_2 > 45$ mm Hg usually indicate hypoventilation or a severe ventilation-perfusion mismatch, unless they reflect respiratory compensation for metabolic alkalosis (see Chapter 52).

TRANSILLUMINATION OF THE CHEST

In infants up to at least 6 mo of age, a pneumothorax can often be diagnosed by transillumination of the chest wall using a fiberoptic light probe. Free air in the pleural space often results in an unusually large halo of light in the skin surrounding the probe. Comparison with the contralateral chest is often very helpful in interpreting findings. This test is unreliable in older patients or in those with subcutaneous emphysema or atelectasis.

RADIOGRAPHIC TECHNIQUES

CHEST ROENTGENOGRAMS. Whenever possible, a posteroanterior and a lateral view (upright and in full inspiration) should be obtained. Portable films, although useful, can give a somewhat distorted image. Expiratory films can be misinterpreted, although a comparison of expiratory and inspiratory films may be useful in the evaluation of a child with suspected foreign body (localized failure of the lung to empty reflects bronchial obstruction). If pleural fluid is suspected, decubitus films are indicated. Films taken in a recumbent position are difficult to interpret if there is fluid within the pleural space or a cavity.

UPPER AIRWAY FILM. A lateral view of the neck can yield invaluable information about upper airway obstruction and particularly about the condition of the retropharyngeal, supraglottic, and subglottic spaces (which should also be viewed in an anteroposterior projection). Knowing the phase of respiration during which the film was taken is often essential for accurate interpretation. Magnified airway films are often helpful in delineating the upper airways. Patients with suggested obstruction should not be sent unattended to the radiology department.

SINUS AND NASAL FILMS. The utility of roentgenographic examination of the sinuses is uncertain. Imaging studies are not necessary to confirm the diagnosis of sinusitis in children <6 yr. CT scans are indicated if surgery is required, in cases of complications due to sinus infection, in immunodeficient patients, and for recurrent infections that are not responsive to medical management.

CHEST CT AND MRI. CT delineates the internal structure of the thorax in much greater detail than is possible with plain roentgenograms. Technical advances have greatly enhanced the utility of this diagnostic modality (three-dimensional reconstruction is often feasible), and have potentially decreased radiation exposure. CT scans are of particular importance in the evaluation of mediastinal and pleural lesions, solid or cystic parenchymal lesions, pulmonary embolisms, and bronchiectasis. Intravenous contrast material can be infused during the scan to enhance vascular structures, thereby allowing distinction of vessels from other soft tissue densities. MRI can be useful for the same disease entities as CT. MRI is an excellent procedure to delineate hilar and vascular anatomy associated with vascular rings or slings.

FLUOROSCOPY. Fluoroscopy is especially useful for evaluating stridor and abnormal movement of the diaphragm or mediastinum. Many procedures, such as needle aspiration or biopsy of a peripheral lesion, are also best accomplished with the aid of fluoroscopy, CT, or ultrasonography. Videotape recording, which does not increase radiation exposure, may allow detailed study through "replay" capability during a brief exposure to fluoroscopy.

BARIUM SWALLOW. This study, performed with fluoroscopy and spot films, is indicated in the evaluation of patients with recurrent pneumonia, persistent cough of undetermined cause, stridor, or persistent wheezing. The technique can be modified by using barium of different textures and thicknesses, ranging from thin liquid to solids, to evaluate swallowing mechanics, the presence of vascular rings, and tracheoesophageal fistulas, especially when aspiration is suspected. A contrast esophagram has been used in the evaluation of newborns with suggested esophageal atresia, but this procedure entails a high risk of pulmonary aspiration and is not usually recommended. Barium swallows are useful in the evaluation of suggested gastroesophageal reflux, but because of the high incidence of asymptomatic reflux in infants, the applicability of the findings to the clinical problem may be complicated.

BRONCHOGRAPHY. The details of smaller bronchi that cannot be easily evaluated by plain films or even bronchoscopy can be delineated by instilling contrast material directly into the airway. This technique has been used in the past to diagnose suspected bronchiectasis or airway anomalies that may need surgery; CT and MRI have largely replaced bronchography, which requires sedation and topical or general anesthesia.

PULMONARY ARTERIOGRAPHY AND AORTOGRAMS. Pulmonary arteriography has been used to allow detailed evaluation of the pulmonary vasculature; has been helpful in assessing pulmonary blood flow and in diagnosing congenital anomalies, such as lobar agenesis, unilateral hyperlucent lung, vascular rings, and arteriovenous malformations; and is sometimes useful in evaluating solid or cystic lesions. Thoracic aortograms demonstrate the aortic arch, its major vessels, and the systemic (bronchial) pulmonary circulation. They are useful in evaluating vascular rings and suspected pulmonary sequestration. Although most hemoptysis is from the bronchial arteries, bronchial arteriography is seldom helpful in diagnosing or treating intrapulmonary bleeding in children. Real-time and Doppler echocardiography and thoracic CT with contrast are noninvasive methods that often reveal similar information and should be performed before arteriography is considered.

RADIONUCLIDE LUNG SCANS. The usual scan uses intravenous injection of material (macroaggregated human serum albumin labeled with ^{99m}Tc) that will be trapped in the pulmonary capillary bed. The distribution of radioactivity, proportional to pulmonary capillary blood flow, is useful in evaluating pulmonary embolism and congenital cardiovascular and pulmonary defects. Acute changes in the distribution of pulmonary perfusion may reflect alterations of pulmonary ventilation.

The distribution of pulmonary ventilation can also be determined by scanning after the patient inhales a radioactive gas such as xenon-133. After the intravenous injection of xenon-133 dissolved in saline, both pulmonary perfusion and ventilation can be evaluated by continuous recording of the rate of appearance and disappearance of the xenon over the lung. Appearance of xenon early after injection is a measure of perfusion, whereas the rate of washout during breathing is a measure of ventilation in the pediatric population. The most important indication for this test is to demonstrate defects in the pulmonary arterial distribution that can occur with congenital malformations or pulmonary embolism. **Spiral reconstruction** CT with contrast medium enhancement is being increasingly used in the evaluation of pulmonary thrombi and emboli. Abnormalities in regional ventilation are also easily demonstrable in congenital lobar emphysema, cystic fibrosis, and asthma.

PULMONARY FUNCTION TESTING

The measurement of respiratory function in infants and young children can be difficult because of the lack of cooperation. Attempts have been made to overcome this limitation by creating standard tests that do not require the patient's active participation. Respiratory function tests still provide only a partial insight into the mechanisms of respiratory disease at early ages.

Whether restrictive or obstructive, most forms of respiratory disease cause alterations in lung volume and its subdivisions (see Chapter 370). Restrictive diseases typically decrease **total lung capacity** (TLC). TLC includes residual volume, which is not accessible to direct determinations. It must therefore be measured indirectly by gas dilution methods or, preferably, by **plethysmography.** Restrictive disease also decreases **vital capacity** (VC). VC can be measured by **spirometry** (see Fig. 370-1) and is commonly used at the bedside to assess the progression of neuromuscular disorders. Obstructive diseases produce gas trapping and thus increase residual volume and FRC, particularly when these measurements are considered with respect to TLC.

Airway obstruction is most frequently evaluated from determinations of gas flow in the course of a forced expiratory maneuver. The **peak expiratory flow** is reduced in advanced obstructive disease. The wide availability of simple devices that perform this measurement at the bedside makes it useful for assessing children with airway obstruction. Evaluation of peak flows requires a voluntary effort, and peak flows may not be altered when the obstruction is moderate or mild. Other gas flow measurements require that the child inhale to TLC and then exhale as far and as fast as possible for several seconds. Cooperation and good muscle strength are therefore necessary for the measurements to be reproducible. The **forced expiratory volume in 1 sec** (FEV_1) correlates well with the severity of obstructive diseases. The **maximal midexpiratory flow rate,** the average flow during the middle 50% of the forced vital capacity, is a more reliable indicator of mild airway obstruction. Its sensitivity to changes in residual volume and vital capacity, however, limits its use in children with more severe disease. The construction of flow-volume relationships during the forced vital capacity maneuvers overcomes some of these limitations by expressing the expiratory flows as a function of lung volume (see Chapter 370).

A spirometer is used to measure VC and its subdivisions and expiratory (or inspiratory) flow rates (see Fig. 370-1). A simple manometer can measure the maximal inspiratory and expiratory force a subject generates, normally at least 30 cm H_2O, which is useful in evaluating the neuromuscular component of ventilation. Expected normal values for VC, FRC, TLC, and residual volume are obtained from prediction equations based on body height.

Flow rates measured by spirometry usually include the FEV_1 and the **maximal midexpiratory flow rate.** More information results from a maximal expiratory flow-volume curve, in which expiratory flow rate is plotted against expired lung volume (expressed in terms of either VC or TLC). Flow rates at lung volumes less than about 75% VC are relatively independent of effort. Expiratory flow rates at low lung volumes (<50% VC) are influenced much more by small airways than are flow rates at high lung volumes (FEV_1). The flow rate at 25% VC (V_{25}) is a useful index of small airway function. Low flow rates at high lung volumes associated with normal flow at low lung volumes suggest upper airway obstruction (see Chapter 370).

Airway resistance (R_{AW}) is measured in a plethysmograph, or, alternatively, the reciprocal of R_{AW}, **airway conductance** (G_{AW}), may be used. Because airway resistance measurements vary with the lung volume at which they are taken, it is convenient to use **specific airway resistance,** SR_{AW} ($SR_{AW} = R_{AW}$/lung volume), which is nearly constant in subjects older than 6 yr (normally <7 sec/cm H_2O).

The **diffusing capacity for carbon monoxide** (DLCO) is related to oxygen diffusion and is measured by rebreathing from a container having a known initial concentration of carbon monoxide or by using a single breath technique. Decreases in diffusing capacity for carbon monoxide reflect decreases in effective alveolar capillary surface area or decreases in diffusibility of the gas across the alveolar-capillary membrane. Primary diffusion abnormalities are unusual in children; therefore, this test is most frequently employed in children exposed to toxic drugs to the lungs (e.g., oncology patients) or chest wall radiation. Regional gas exchange can be conveniently estimated with the perfusion-ventilation xenon scan. Determining arterial blood gas levels also discloses the effectiveness of alveolar gas exchange.

Pulmonary function testing, although rarely resulting in a diagnosis, is helpful in defining the type of process (obstruction, restriction) and the degree of functional impairment, in following the course and treatment of disease, and in estimating the prognosis. It is also useful in preoperative evaluation and in confirmation of functional impairment in patients having subjective complaints but a normal physical examination. In most patients with obstructive disease, a repeat test after administering a bronchodilator is warranted.

Most tests require some cooperation and understanding by the patient, and interpretation is greatly facilitated if the test conditions and the patient's behavior during the test are known. Infants and young children who cannot or will not cooperate with test procedures can be studied in a limited number of ways, which often require sedation. Flow rates and pressures during tidal breathing, with or without transient interruption of the flow, may be useful to assess some aspects of airway resistance or obstruction and to measure compliance of the lungs and thorax. Expiratory flow rates can be studied in sedated infants with passive compression of the chest and abdomen with a rapidly inflatable jacket. Gas dilution or plethysmographic methods can also be used in sedated infants to measure FRC and R_{AW}.

MICROBIOLOGY: EXAMINATION OF LUNG SECRETIONS

The specific diagnosis of infection in the lower respiratory tract depends on the proper handling of an adequate specimen obtained in an appropriate fashion. Nasopharyngeal or throat cultures are often used but may not correlate with cultures obtained by more direct techniques from the lower airways. Sputum specimens are preferred and are often obtained from patients who do not expectorate by deep throat swab immediately after coughing or by saline nebulization. Specimens can also be obtained directly from the tracheobronchial tree by nasotracheal aspiration (usually heavily contaminated), by transtracheal aspiration through the cricothyroid membrane (useful in adults and adolescents but hazardous in children), and in infants and children by a sterile catheter inserted into the trachea either during direct laryngoscopy or through an endotracheal tube. A specimen can also be obtained at bronchoscopy. A percutaneous lung tap or an open biopsy is the only way to obtain a specimen absolutely free of oral flora.

A specimen obtained by direct expectoration is usually assumed to be of tracheobronchial origin, but often, especially in children, it is not from this source. The presence of alveolar macrophages (large, mononuclear cells) is the hallmark of tracheobronchial secretions. Both nasopharyngeal and tracheobronchial secretions may contain ciliated epithelial cells, which are more commonly found in sputum. Nasopharyngeal and oral secretions often contain large numbers of squamous epithelial cells. Sputum may contain both ciliated and squamous epithelial cells.

During sleep, mucociliary transport continually brings tracheobronchial secretions to the pharynx, where they are swallowed. An early morning fasting gastric aspirate often contains material from the tracheobronchial tract that is suitable for culture for acid-fast bacilli.

The absence of polymorphonuclear leukocytes in a Wright-stained smear of sputum or **bronchoalveolar lavage** (BAL) fluid containing adequate numbers of macrophages may be significant evidence against a bacterial infectious process in the lower respiratory tract, assuming that the patient has normal neutrophil counts and function. Eosinophils suggest allergic disease. Iron stains may reveal hemosiderin granules within macrophages, suggesting pulmonary hemosiderosis. Specimens should also be examined by Gram stain. Bacteria within or near macrophages and neutrophils can be significant. Viral pneumonia may be accompanied by intranuclear or cytoplasmic inclusion bodies visible on Wright-stained smears, and fungal forms may be identifiable on Gram or silver stains.

EXERCISE TESTING

Exercise testing (see Chapter 423.5) is a more direct approach for detecting diffusion impairment as well as other forms of respiratory disease. Measurements of heart and respiratory rate, minute ventilation, oxygen consumption, carbon dioxide production, and arterial blood gases during incremental exercise loads often provide invaluable information about the functional nature of the disease. Often a simple assessment of the patient's exercise tolerance in conjunction with other, more static forms of respiratory function testing can allow a distinction between respiratory and nonrespiratory disease in children.

SLEEP STUDIES

The sleep state has an important influence on respiratory function, particularly in the newborn and young infant (see Chapter 18). Polysomnographic studies are often helpful when abnormalities of central respiratory control, muscular disorders, or respiratory complications from **gastroesophageal reflux** (GER) are suspected. Polysomnography is now considered to be the gold standard test for obstructive sleep apnea or hypoventilation during sleep. pH probe studies are indicated and are added to such sleep studies when GER is suspected. In these studies, a pH probe is placed in the esophagus and prolonged (usually over several hours) monitoring is undertaken (see Chapter 320). These studies, which usually include the simultaneous assessment of ventilatory effort, airway gas flow, gas exchange, and sleep state, are also useful in the diagnosis and management of disorders of respiratory control and nocturnal hypoxemia and hypercapnia in children with chronic respiratory disease (see Chapter 370).

LUNG VISUALIZATION AND LUNG SPECIMEN–BASED DIAGNOSTIC TESTS

LARYNGOSCOPY. The evaluation of stridor, problems with vocalization, and other upper airway abnormalities usually require direct inspection. Although indirect (mirror) laryngoscopy may be reasonable in older children and adults, it is rarely feasible in infants and small children. Direct laryngoscopy can be performed with either a rigid or a flexible instrument. The safe use of the rigid scope for examination of the upper airway requires topical anesthesia and either sedation or general anesthesia, whereas the flexible laryngoscope can often be used in the office setting with or without sedation. Further advantages to the flexible scope include the ability to assess the airway without the distortion that may be introduced by the use of the rigid scope and the ability to assess airway dynamics more accurately. Because there is a relatively high incidence of concomitant lesions in the upper and lower airways, it is often prudent to examine the airways above and below the glottis, even when the primary indication is in the upper airway (stridor).

BRONCHOSCOPY AND BRONCHEOALVEOLAR LAVAGE (BAL). Bronchoscopy is the inspection of the airways. BAL is a method used to obtain a representative specimen of fluid and secretions from the lower respiratory tract, which is useful for the cytologic and microbiologic diagnosis of lung diseases, especially in those who are unable to expectorate sputum. BAL is performed after the general inspection of the airways and before tissue sampling with a brush or biopsy forceps. BAL is accomplished by gently wedging the scope into a lobar, segmental, or subsegmental bronchus and sequentially instilling and withdrawing sterile nonbacteriostatic saline in a volume sufficient to ensure that some of the aspirated fluid contains material that originated from the alveolar space. Nonbronchoscopic BAL can be performed, although with less accuracy and, therefore, less reliable results, in intubated patients by instilling and withdrawing saline through a catheter passed though the artificial airway and blindly wedged into a distal airway. In either case, the presence of alveolar macrophages documents that an alveolar sample has been obtained. Because the methods used to perform BAL involve passage of the equipment through the upper airway, there is a risk of contamination of the specimen by upper airway secretions. Careful cytologic examination and quantitative microbiologic cultures are important for correct interpretation of the data. BAL can often obviate the need for more invasive procedures such as open lung biopsy, especially in immunocompromised individuals.

Indications for diagnostic bronchoscopy and BAL include recurrent or persistent pneumonia or atelectasis, unexplained or localized and persistent wheeze, the suspected presence of a foreign body, hemoptysis, suspected congenital anomalies, mass lesions, interstitial disease, and pneumonia in the immunocompromised host. Indications for therapeutic bronchoscopy and BAL include bronchial obstruction by mass lesions, foreign bodies or mucous plugs, and general bronchial toilet and bronchopulmonary lavage. The individual undergoing bronchoscopy ventilates around the flexible scope, whereas, with the rigid scope, ventilation is accomplished through the scope. Rigid bronchoscopy is preferentially indicated for the extraction of foreign bodies, for the removal of tissue masses, and in patients with massive hemoptysis. In other cases, the flexible scope offers the advantages that it can be passed through endotracheal or tracheostomy tubes, can be introduced into bronchi that come off the airway at acute angles, and can be safely and effectively inserted with topical anesthesia and conscious sedation.

Regardless of the instrument used, the procedure performed, or its indications, the most common complications are related to sedation. The relatively more common complications include transient hypoxemia, laryngospasm, bronchospasm, and cardiac arrhythmias. Iatrogenic infection, bleeding, pneumothorax, and pneumomediastinum are rare but reported complications of bronchoscopy or BAL. Bronchoscopy in the setting of possible pulmonary abcess or hemoptysis must be undertaken with advance preparations for definitive airway control, mindful of the possibility that pus or blood might flood the airway. Subglottic edema is a more common complication of rigid bronchoscopy than of flexible procedures, in which the scopes are smaller and less likely to traumatize the mucosa. Postbronchoscopy croup is treated with oxygen, mist, vasoconstrictor aerosols, and corticosteroids as necessary.

THORACOSCOPY. The pleural cavity can be examined through a thoracoscope, which is similar to a rigid bronchoscope. The thoracoscope is inserted through an intercostal space and the lung is partially deflated, thus allowing the operator to view the surface of the lung, the pleural surface of the mediastinum and diaphragm, and the parietal pleura. Multiple thoracoscopic instruments can be inserted, allowing endoscopic lung or pleural biopsy, bleb resection, pleural abrasion, and ligation of vascular rings.

THORACENTESIS. For diagnostic or therapeutic purposes, fluid can be removed from the pleural space by needle. Generally, as much fluid as possible should be withdrawn, and an upright chest roentgenogram should be obtained after the procedure. Complications of thoracentesis include infection, pneumothorax, and bleeding. Thoracentesis on the right may be complicated by puncture or laceration of the capsule of the liver and, on the left, by puncture or laceration of the capsule of the spleen. Specimens obtained should always be cultured, examined microscopically for evidence of bacterial infection, and evaluated for total protein and total differential cell counts. Lactic acid dehydrogenase, glucose, cholesterol, triglyceride (chylous), and amylase determinations may also be useful. If malignancy is suspected, cytologic examination is imperative.

Transudates result from mechanical factors influencing the rate of formation or reabsorption of pleural fluid and generally require no further diagnostic evaluation. Exudates result from inflammation or other disease of the pleural surface and underlying lung and require a more complete diagnostic evaluation. In general, transudates have a total protein of <3 g/dL or a ratio of pleural protein to serum protein <0.5, a total leukocyte count of fewer than $2,000/mm^3$ with a predominance of mononuclear cells, and low lactate dehydrogenase levels. Exudates have high protein levels and a predominance of polymorphonuclear cells (although malignant or tuberculous effusions may have a higher percentage of mononuclear cells). Complicated exudates often require continuous chest tube drainage and have a $pH < 7.2$. Tuberculous effusions may have low glucose and high cholesterol content.

LUNG TAP. Using a technique similar to that used for thoracentesis, a percutaneous lung tap is the most direct method of obtaining bacteriologic specimens from the pulmonary parenchyma and is the only technique other than open lung biopsy not associated with at least some risk of contamination by oral flora. After local anesthesia, a needle attached to a syringe containing nonbacteriostatic sterile saline is inserted using aseptic technique through the inferior aspect of an intercostal space in the area of interest. The needle is rapidly advanced into the lung; the saline is injected and reaspirated, and the needle is withdrawn. These actions are performed as quickly as possible. This procedure usually yields a few drops of fluid from the lung, which should be cultured and examined microscopically.

Major indications for a lung tap are roentgenographic infiltrates of undetermined cause, especially those unresponsive to therapy in immunosuppressed patients who are susceptible to unusual organisms. Complications are the same as for thoracentesis, but the incidence of pneumothorax is higher and somewhat dependent on the nature of the underlying disease process. In patients with poor pulmonary compliance, such as children with *Pneumocystis* pneumonia, the rate may approach 30%, with 5% requiring chest tubes. Bronchopulmonary lavage has replaced lung taps for most purposes.

LUNG BIOPSY. Lung biopsy may be the only way to establish a diagnosis, especially in protracted, noninfectious disease. In infants and small children, thoracoscopic or open surgical biopsies are the procedures of choice, and in expert hands, there is low morbidity. Biopsy through the 3.5 mm diameter pediatric bronchoscopes limits the sample size and diagnostic abilities. As well as ensuring that an adequate specimen is obtained, the surgeon can inspect the lung surface and choose the site of biopsy. In older children, transbronchial biopsies can be performed using flexible forceps through a bronchoscope, an endotracheal tube, a rigid bronchoscope, or an endotracheal tube, usually with fluoroscopic guidance. This technique is most appropriately used when the disease is diffuse, as in the case of *Pneumocystis* pneumonia, or after rejection of a transplanted lung. The diagnostic limitations related to the small size of the biopsy specimens can be mitigated by the ability to obtain several samples. The risk of pneumothorax related to bronchoscopy is increased when transbronchial biopsies are part of the procedure; however, the ability to obtain biopsy specimens in a procedure performed with topical anesthesia and conscious sedation offers advantages to the select population for whom this procedure offers a reasonable diagnostic yield.

SWEAT TESTING. See Chapter 400.

American Academy of Pediatrics, Subcommittee on Management of Sinusitis and Committee on Quality Improvement: Clinical practice guideline: Management of sinusitis. *Pediatrics* 2001;108:798–808.

Baughman RP (editor): *Bronchoalveolar Lavage*. St. Louis, Mosby–Year Book, 1992.

Goodman TR, McHugh K: The role of radiology in the evaluation of stridor. *Arch Dis Child* 1999;81:456–459.

Margolis P, Ferkol T, Marsocci S, et al: Accuracy of the clinical examination in detecting hypoxemia in infants with respiratory illness. *J Pediatr* 1994;124:552–560.

Saccomanno G: *Diagnostic Pulmonary Cytology*. Chicago, American Society of Clinical Pathologists Press, 1986.

Schechter MS: Snoring: Investigations guidelines. *Pediatr Pulmonol Suppl* 2004;26:172–174.

Schechter, MS; Section on Pediatric Pulmonology, Subcommittee on Obstructive Sleep Apnea Syndrome: Technical report: Diagnosis and management of childhood obstructive sleep apnea syndrome. *Pediatrics* 2002;109:e69.

Welsby PD, Earis JE: Some high pitched thoughts on chest examination. *Postgrad Med J* 2001;77:617–620.

Chapter 372 ■ Sudden Infant Death Syndrome

Carl E. Hunt and Fern R. Hauck

Sudden infant death syndrome (SIDS) is defined as the sudden death of an infant that is unexpected by history and unexplained by a thorough postmortem examination, which includes a complete autopsy, investigation of the scene of death, and review of the medical history. An autopsy is essential to identify natural causes of sudden, unexpected death such as congenital anomalies or infection and to diagnosis traumatic child abuse (Tables 372-1, 372-2, 372-3). The autopsy cannot reliably distinguish between SIDS and intentional suffocation, but the scene investigation and medical history may be of help if inconsistencies are evident.

EPIDEMIOLOGY. SIDS is the 3rd leading cause of infant mortality in the United States, accounting for 8% of all infant deaths. It is the most common cause of postneonatal infant mortality, accounting for 40–50% of all deaths between 1 mo and 1 yr of age. The annual rate of SIDS in the United States was stable at 1.3–1.4/1,000 live births (about 7,000 infants/yr) before 1992, the year in which the American Academy of Pediatrics recommended that infants sleep non-prone as a way to reduce risk for SIDS. Since then, particularly after initiation of the national Back to Sleep campaign in 1994, the rate of SIDS progressively declined and then leveled off in 2002 at 0.57/1,000 live births (2,295 infants). The decline in the number of SIDS deaths in the United States and other countries around the world has been attributed to the increasing use of the supine position for sleep. Several other countries have decreased prone sleeping prevalence to ≤2%, but in the United States in 2004, 13% of infants were still being placed prone for sleeping.

PATHOLOGY. There are no autopsy findings pathognomonic of SIDS and no findings required for the diagnosis, although there are some common findings. Petechial hemorrhages are found in 68–95% of cases and are more extensive than in explained causes of infant mortality. Pulmonary edema is often present and may be substantial. The reasons for these findings are unknown.

SIDS victims have several identifiable changes in the lungs and other organs and in brainstem structure and function. Nearly ⅔ of SIDS victims have structural evidence of pre-existing, chronic low-grade asphyxia, while other studies have identified biochemical markers of asphyxia. SIDS victims have higher expression of vascular endothelial growth factor (VEGF) in the cerebrospinal fluid (CSF), which is upregulated by hypoxia, providing independent evidence of recent single or multiple hypoxemic events. Brainstem findings in SIDS victims include a persistent increase of dendritic spines and delayed maturation of synapses in the medullary respiratory centers, and decreased tyrosine hydroxylase immunoreactivity and catecholaminergic neurons. Decreases in 5-hydroxytryptamine (5-HT) 1A and 5-HT 2A receptor immunoreactivity have been observed in the dorsal nucleus of the vagus, solitary nucleus, and ventrolateral medulla, whereas increases are present in periaqueductal gray matter of the midbrain. The decreased immunoreactivity of receptors is accompanied by brainstem gliosis and it is therefore unclear whether the decreases are secondary to hypoxia or ischemia, or whether they reflect primary alterations in 5-HT metabolism or transport (see later discussion of 5-HT polymorphisms).

The arcuate nucleus in the ventral medulla has been a particular focus for studies in SIDS victims. It is an integrative site for vital autonomic functions including breathing and arousal and is integrated with other regions that regulate arousal and autonomic chemosensory function. Quantitative 3-dimensional anatomic studies indicate that some SIDS victims have hypoplasia of the

TABLE 372-1. Differential Diagnosis of Sudden Unexpected Death in Infancy

CAUSE OF DEATH	PRIMARY DIAGNOSTIC CRITERIA	CONFOUNDING FACTOR(S)	FREQUENCY DISTRIBUTION
EXPLAINED AT AUTOPSY			
Natural			18–20%*
Infections	History, autopsy, and cultures	If minimal findings: SIDS	35–46%†
Congenital anomaly	History and autopsy	If minimal findings: SIDS or intentional suffocation	14–24%†
Unintentional injury	History, scene investigation, autopsy	Traumatic child abuse	15%*
Traumatic child abuse	Autopsy and scene investigation	Unintentional injury	13–24%*
Other natural causes	History and autopsy	If minimal findings: SIDS or intentional suffocation	12–17%*
UNEXPLAINED AT AUTOPSY			
Sudden infant death syndrome (SIDS)	History, scene investigation, absence of explainable cause at autopsy	Intentional suffocation	80–82%
Intentional suffocation (filicide)	Perpetrator confession, absence of explainable cause at autopsy	SIDS	Unknown

*As a percentage of all sudden unexpected infant deaths explained at autopsy.
†As a percentage of all natural causes of sudden unexpected infant deaths explained at autopsy.
Adapted from Hunt CE: Sudden infant death syndrome and other causes of infant mortality: Diagnosis, mechanisms and risk for recurrence in siblings. *Am J Respir Crit Care Med* 2001;164:346–357.

TABLE 372-2. Condition That May Cause Apparent Life-threatening Events or Sudden Death

CAUSE	COMMENT
CNS	Arteriovenous malformation, seizures, congenital central hypoventilation, neuromuscular disorders (Werdnig-Hoffmann disease), Arnold-Chiari crisis, Leigh syndrome
Cardiac	Subendocardial fibroelastosis, aortic stenosis, anomalous coronary artery, myocarditis, cardiomyopathy, arrhythmias (prolonged Q-T syndrome, Wolff-Parkinson-White syndrome, congenital heart block)
Pulmonary	Pulmonary hypertension, vocal cord paralysis, aspiration, laryngotrachael disease
Gastrointestinal	Pancreatitis, diarrhea and/or dehydration, gastroesophageal reflux, volvulus
Endocrine-metabolic	Congenital adrenal hyperplasia, malignant hyperpyrexia, long- or medium-chain acyl coenzyme A deficiency, hyperammonemias (urea cycle enzyme deficiencies), glutaricaciduria, carnitine deficiency (systemic or secondary), glycogen storage disease type I, maple syrup urine disease, congenital lactic acidosis, biotinidase deficiency
Infection	Sepsis, meningitis, encephalitis, brain abscess, hepatitis, pyelonephritis, bronchiolitis (RSV), infant botulism, pertussis
Trauma	Child abuse, suffocation, physical trauma, Munchausen syndrome by proxy
Poisoning	Boric acid, carbon monoxide, salicylates, barbiturates, ipecac, cocaine, insulin

CNS, central nervous system; RSV, respiratory syncytial virus.
From Kliegman RM, Greenbaum LA, Lye PS: *Practical Strategies in Pediatric Diagnosis and Therapy*, 2nd ed. Philadelphia, Elsevier Saunders, 2004, p 98.

arcuate nucleus and up to 60% of SIDS victims have histopathologic evidence of less extensive bilateral or unilateral hypoplasia. Considering the apparent overlap between putative mechanisms for SIDS and for unexpected late fetal deaths, it is of interest that ≈30% of late unexpected and unexplained stillbirths also have hypoplasia of the arcuate nucleus.

Neurotransmitter studies of the arcuate nucleus have also identified receptor abnormalities in some SIDS victims that involve several receptor types relevant to state-dependent autonomic control overall and to ventilatory and arousal responsiveness in particular. These deficits include significant decreases in binding to kainate, muscarinic cholinergic, and serotonergic (5-HT) receptors. High neuronal levels of interleukin 1β (IL-1β) are present in the arcuate and dorsal vagal nuclei in SIDS victims compared to controls, perhaps contributing to molecular interactions affecting cardiorespiratory and arousal responses.

The postmortem data summarized here do not establish any genetic risk factors for sudden unexpected deaths in infants (SUDI) to the exclusion of environmental risk factors. Recent genetic studies in SIDS victims, however, have identified several ways in which infants dying from SIDS differ genetically from both healthy infants and infants dying of other causes (see the "Genetic Risk Factors" section and Table 372-4).

ENVIRONMENTAL RISK FACTORS. Declines of 50% or more in rates of SIDS in the United States and around the world have occurred in the past decade, at least in part as a result of national education campaigns directed at reducing risk factors associated with SIDS. The reductions in risk appear to be related primarily to decreases in placing infants prone for sleep and increases in placing them supine. A number of other risk factors also have significant associations with SIDS (Table 372-5); although many are nonmodifiable and most of the modifiable factors have not changed appreciably, self-reported maternal smoking prevalence during pregnancy has decreased by 25% in the past decade.

TABLE 372-3. Differential Diagnosis of Recurrent Sudden Infant Death in a Sibship

Idiopathic	Recurrent true sudden infant death syndrome
CNS	Congenital central hypoventilation, neuromuscular disorders, Leigh syndrome
Cardiac	Endocardial fibroelastosis, Wolff-Parkinson-White syndrome, prolonged Q-T syndrome, congenital heart block
Pulmonary	Pulmonary hypertension
Endocrine-metabolic	See Table 372-2
Infection	Disorders of immune host defense
Child abuse	Filicide, infanticide, Munchausen syndrome by proxy

CNS, central nervous system.
From Kliegman RM, Greenbaum LA, Lye PS: *Practical Strategies in Pediatric Diagnosis and Therapy*, 2nd ed. Philadelphia, Elsevier Saunders, 2004, p 101.

TABLE 372-4. Identified Genes for Which the Distribution of Polymorphisms Differs in SIDS Victims Compared to Control Infants

Sodium and potassium cardiac ion channel genes *(SCN5A)*
Serotonin (5-hydroxytrypamine) transporter protein promoter region (5-HTT)
Genes pertinent to development of autonomic nervous system
- Paired-like homeobox 2a *(PHOX2a)*
- Rearranged during transfection factor *(RET)*
- Endothelin converting enzyme-1 *(ECE1)*
- T-cell leukemia homeobox *(TLX3)*
- Engrailed-1 *(EN1)*
- Testis-specific Y-like *(TSPYL)* gene
- Complement C4A and C4B genes
- Interleukin 10 gene polymorphisms

SIDS, sudden infant death syndrome.
Adapted from Hunt CE: Gene-environment interations: Implications for sudden unexpected deaths in infancy. *Arch Dis Child* 2005;90:48–53.

TABLE 372.5. Environmental Factors Associated with Increased Risk for SIDS

MATERNAL AND ANTENATAL RISK FACTORS
- Elevated 2nd trimester serum α-fetoprotein
- Smoking
- Alcohol use
- Drug use (cocaine, heroin)
- Nutritional deficiency
- Inadequate prenatal care
- Low socioeconomic status
- Younger age
- Lower education
- Single marital status
- Shorter interpregnancy interval
- Intrauterine hypoxia
- Fetal growth restriction

INFANT RISK FACTORS:
- Age (peak 2–4 mo, but may be decreasing)
- Male gender
- Race/ethnicity (African-American and Native American)
- Growth failure
- No pacifier (dummy)
- Prematurity
- Prone and side sleep position
- Recent febrile illness
- Smoking exposure (prenatal and postnatal)
- Soft sleeping surface, soft bedding
- Infant-mother or -parent bed sharing
- Thermal stress/overheating
- Colder season, no central heating

SIDS, sudden infant death syndrome.

NONMODIFIABLE RISK FACTORS. Although SIDS affects infants from all social strata, lower socioeconomic status is consistently associated with higher risk. In the United States, African-American, Native American, and Alaskan Native infants are 2 to 3 times more likely than white infants to die of SIDS, whereas Asian, Pacific Islander, and Hispanic infants have the lowest incidence. Some of this disparity may be related to the higher concentration of poverty and other adverse environmental factors found within the higher incidence communities.

Infants are at greatest risk of SIDS at 2–4 mo of age, with most deaths having occurred by 6 mo. This characteristic age has decreased in some countries as the SIDS incidence has declined, with deaths occurring at earlier ages and with a flattening of the peak incidence. Similarly, the commonly found winter seasonal predominance of SIDS has declined or disappeared in some countries as prone prevalence has decreased, supporting prior findings of an interaction between sleep position and factors more common in colder months (overheating, infection). Male infants are 30–50% more likely to be affected than females.

MODIFIABLE RISK FACTORS.

Pregnancy-Related Factors. An increased SIDS risk is associated with numerous obstetric factors, suggesting that the in utero environment of future SIDS victims is suboptimal. SIDS infants are more commonly of higher birth order, independent of maternal age, and of gestations after shorter interpregnancy intervals. Mothers of SIDS infants generally receive less prenatal care and initiate care later in pregnancy. Additionally, low birthweight, preterm birth, and slower intrauterine and postnatal growth rates are risk factors.

Cigarette Smoking. There is a major association between intrauterine exposure to cigarette smoking and risk for SIDS. The incidence of SIDS is about 3 times greater among infants of mothers who smoke in studies conducted before SIDS risk reduction campaigns and 5 times higher after implementation of risk reduction campaigns. The risk of death is progressively greater as daily cigarette use increases. The effects of smoking by the father and other household members are more difficult to interpret because they are highly correlated with maternal smoking. There appears to be a small independent effect of paternal smoking, but data on other household members have been inconsistent.

It is very difficult to assess the independent effect of infant exposure to environmental tobacco smoke (ETS) because parental smoking behaviors during and after pregnancy are also highly correlated. An increased risk of SIDS is also found for infants exposed to only postnatal maternal ETS. There is a dose response for the number of household smokers, number of people smoking in the same room as the infant, and the number of cigarettes smoked. Maternal smoking is currently the most important risk factor for SIDS.

Drug and Alcohol Use. Overall, most studies do link maternal prenatal drug use with an increased risk of SIDS. Most studies have not found an association between maternal alcohol use prenatally or postnatally and SIDS. In one study of Northern Plains Indians, periconceptional alcohol use and binge drinking in the 1st trimester were associated with a sixfold and an eightfold increased risk of SIDS, respectively. Siblings of infants with fetal alcohol syndrome have a tenfold increased risk of SIDS compared to controls.

Infant Sleep Environment. Sleeping prone has consistently been shown to increase the risk of SIDS. As rates of prone positioning have decreased in the general population, the odds ratios for SIDS in infants still sleeping prone have increased. The highest risk of SIDS may occur in infants who are usually placed non-prone but placed prone for last sleep ("unaccustomed prone") or found prone ("secondary prone"). The "unaccustomed prone" position is more likely to occur in daycare or other settings outside the home and highlights the need for all infant caretakers to be educated about appropriate sleep positioning.

The initial SIDS risk reduction campaign recommendations considered side sleeping to be nearly equivalent to the supine position in reducing the risk of SIDS. Subsequent studies have indicated that, although safer than the prone position, side-sleeping infants are twice as likely to die of SIDS as infants sleeping supine. This increased risk may relate to the relative instability of the position, with some infants placed on the side rolling to the prone position. The **current recommendations** call for **supine position** for sleeping for all infants except those few with specific medical conditions for which recommending a different position may be justified. Many parents and health care providers were initially concerned that supine sleeping would be associated with an increase in adverse consequences, such as difficulty sleeping, vomiting, or aspiration. Evidence suggests that the risk of regurgitation and choking are highest for prone-sleeping infants. Some newborn nursery staff still tend to favor side positioning, which models inappropriate infant care practice to parents. Infants sleeping on their backs do not have more episodes of cyanosis or apnea; reports of apparent life-threatening events decreased in Scandinavia after increased use of the supine position. Among infants in the United States who maintained the same sleep position at 1, 3, and 6 mo of age, no clinical symptoms or reasons for outpatient visits (including fever, cough, wheezing, trouble breathing or sleeping, vomiting, diarrhea, or respiratory illness) are more common in infants sleeping supine or on their side compared with infants sleeping prone. Three symptoms are actually less common in infants sleeping supine or on their side: fever at 1 mo, stuffy nose at 6 mo, and trouble sleeping at 6 mo. Outpatient visits for ear infection are less common at 3 and 6 mo for infants sleeping supine and also less common at 3 mo for infants sleeping on their side. These results provide reassurance for parents and health care providers and will lead, it is hoped, to universal acceptance of supine as the safest and optimal sleep position for infants.

Soft sleep surfaces or bedding, such as comforters, pillows, sheepskins, polystyrene bean pillows, and older or softer mattresses are associated with increased risk of SIDS. Head and face covering by loose bedding, particularly heavy comforters, is also associated with increased risk. Overheating has been associated with increased risk for SIDS based on indicators such as higher room temperature, high body temperature, sweating, and excessive clothing or bedding. Some studies have identified an interaction between overheating and prone sleeping, with overheating increasing the risk of SIDS only when infants were sleeping prone. Higher external environmental temperatures have not been associated with increased SIDS incidence in the United States.

Several studies have implicated bed sharing as a risk factor for SIDS. Bed sharing is associated with increased risk of SIDS among infants up to 3 mo of age even if their mothers did not smoke. Bed sharing is particularly hazardous when other children are in the same bed, when the parent is sleeping with an infant on a couch or other soft or confining sleeping surface, and for infants <4 mo of age. Risk is also increased with longer duration of bed sharing during the night; returning the infant to his or her own crib is not associated with increased risk. There is increasing evidence that room sharing without bed sharing is associated with lower SIDS rates; the safest place for infants to sleep may be in their own crib in the parents' room.

Infant Feeding Care Practices and Exposures. A number of studies have demonstrated a protective effect of breast-feeding that is not present after adjusting for potentially confounding factors. This suggests that breast-feeding is a marker for lifestyle or socioeconomic status rather than an independent factor. Although the benefits of breast-feeding are many, data are inadequate to recommend it as a strategy to reduce risk for SIDS.

Pacifier (dummy) use lowers the risk of SIDS in the majority of studies when used for last/reference sleep. A meta-analysis found this reduced risk to be equal to an adjusted summary odds ratio of 0.39 (95% confidence intervals 0.31–0.50). Although it is not known if this is a direct effect of the pacifier itself or from associated infant or parental behaviors, there is increasing evidence that pacifier use and dislodgment may increase the arousability of infants during sleep. Concerns have been expressed about recommending pacifiers as a means of reducing the risk of SIDS for fear of creating adverse consequences, particularly interference with breast-feeding. In well-designed studies, however, no association between pacifiers and breast-feeding duration has been found. A small increased incidence of otitis media and of respiratory and gastrointestinal illness has been reported for pacifier users compared with non-users. The Netherlands (for bottle-fed babies) and Germany have recommended pacifier use as a potential way to reduce the risk of SIDS. The most recent American Academy of Pediatrics guidelines recommend pacifier use once breast-feeding has been established.

Upper respiratory tract infections have generally not been found to be an independent risk factor for SIDS. These and other minor infections, however, may play a role in the pathogenesis of SIDS. Risk for SIDS has been found to be increased after illness among prone sleepers, those who were heavily wrapped, and those whose heads were covered during sleep.

No association between immunizations and SIDS has been found. SIDS infants are less likely to be immunized than control infants, and in immunized infants, no temporal relationship between vaccine administration and death has been identified. Parents should be reassured that immunizations do not present a risk for SIDS.

SIDS rates remain higher among Native Americans, Alaskan Natives, and African-Americans. This may be due, in part, to group differences in adopting supine sleeping or other risk-reduction behaviors. Greater efforts are needed to address this persistent disparity and to ensure that SIDS risk-reduction education reaches all parents. The messages must reach all care providers, including grandparents, other relatives, and personnel at daycare centers.

GENETIC RISK FACTORS. Genetic studies have identified multiple ways in which SIDS victims differ from healthy infants and infants dying from other causes (see Table 372-4). Differences include sodium and potassium ion channel gene defects, serotonin (5-HT) transporter (5-HTT) gene, autonomic nervous system (ANS) development genes, complement C4, and IL-10. Long Q-T syndrome (LQTS) is associated with sodium channel gene *(SCN5A)* defects. SCN5A has emerged as the leading candidate ion channel gene having relevance for SIDS, with 2% of 93 SIDS cases in one study having a distinct *SCN5A* channel defect. These findings suggest that mutations in cardiac ion channels may provide a lethal arrhythmogenic substrate in some infants at risk for SIDS (Fig. 372-1).

Polymorphisms in the 5-HTT gene are illustrative of the way in which alterations in individual genes could influence risk for SIDS. 5-HT is a widespread neurotransmitter affecting breathing, cardiovascular control, temperature, and mood. It modulates activity of the circadian clock and is the major neurotransmitter of nonrapid eye movement (NREM or quiet) sleep. Many genes are involved in the control of 5-HT synthesis, storage, membrane uptake, and metabolism. Several polymorphisms have been identified in the promoter region of the *5-HTT* gene, which is located on chromosome 17. Variations in the promoter region of the *5-HTT* gene appear to have a role in 5-HT membrane uptake and regulation. White, African-American, and Japanese SIDS victims are more likely than matched controls to have the "L" (long) allele. There is also a negative association between SIDS and the S/S genotype. An association has also been observed between SIDS and a *5-HTT* intron 2 polymorphism that differentially regulates *5-HTT* expression. These transporter polymorphisms would lead to reduced serotonin concentrations at nerve endings with the "L" allele in comparison to the short "S" allele. The L/L genotype is associated with increased serotonin transporters on neuroimaging and postmortem binding studies.

Molecular genetic studies in SIDS victims have identified mutations pertinent to early embryologic development of the ANS. The relevant genes include mammalian achaete-scute homolog-1 *(MASH1)*, bone morphogenic protein-2 *(BMP2)*, paired-like homeobox 2a *(PHOX2a)*, *PHOX2b*, rearranged during transfection factor (RET), endothelin converting enzyme-1 (ECE1), endothelin-1 (EDN1), T-cell leukemia homeobox (TLX3), and engrailed-1 (EN1).

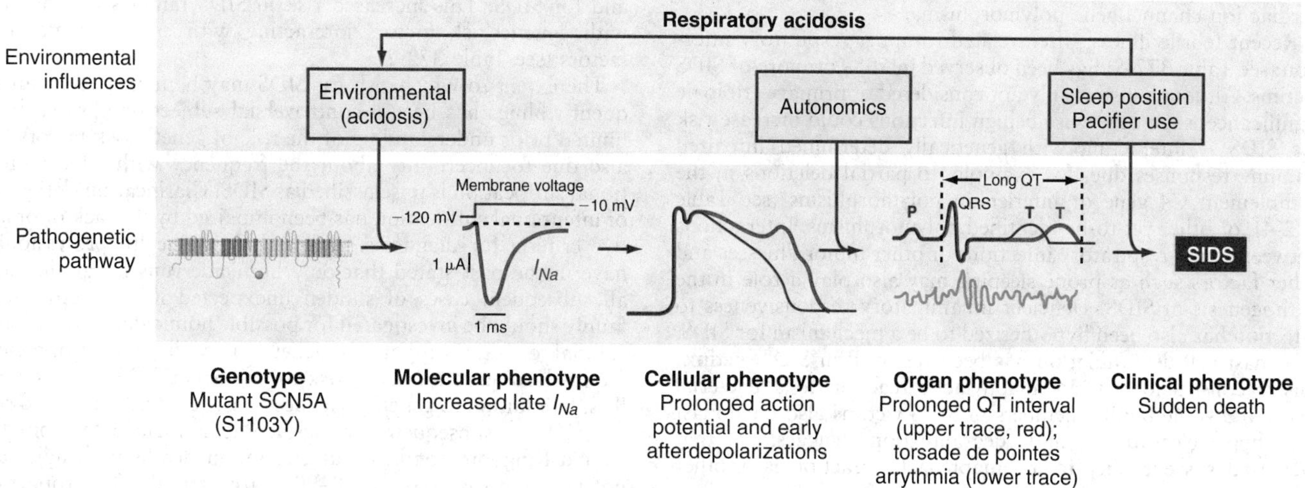

Figure 372-1. An arrhythmogenic pathogenetic pathway for sudden infant death syndrome (SIDS) from patient genotype to clinical phenotype, with environmental influences noted. The genetic abnormality, in this instance, a polymorphism in the cardiac Na^+ channel SCN5A, causes a molecular phenotype of increased late Na^+ current (I_{Na}) under the influence of environmental factors such as acidosis. Interacting with other ion currents that may themselves be altered by genetic and environmental factors, the late Na^+ current causes a cellular phenotype of prolonged action potential duration as well as early afterdepolarizations. Prolonged action potential in the cells of the ventricular myocardium and further interaction with environmental factors such as autonomic innervation, which, in turn, may be affected by genetic factors, produce a tissue/organ phenotype of a prolonged Q-T interval on the electrocardiogam (ECG) and torsades de pointes arrhythmia in the whole heart. If this is sustained or degenerates to ventricular fibrillation, the clinical phenotype of SIDS results. Environmental and multiple genetic factors may interact at many different levels to produce the characteristic phenotypes at the molecular, cellular, tissue, organ, and clinical levels. (From Makielski JC: SIDS: Genetic and environmental influences may cause arrhythmia in this silent killer. *J Clin Invest* 2006;116:297–299.)

Genetic differences among SIDS infants have also been reported for the complement C4 gene, with SIDS victims who had mild upper respiratory infection before death more likely to have deletion of either the C4A or the C4B gene compared to SIDS victims without infection or to living controls. These data suggest that partial deletions of the C4 gene in combination with a mild upper respiratory infection place infants at increased risk for SIDS.

SIDS victims have also been reported to have polymorphisms in the gene promoter region for IL-10, an anti-inflammatory cytokine. Sudden infant death was strongly associated with IL-10 genotype, both with the ATA haplotype and with presence of the –592*A and –592*C alleles. These IL-10 polymorphisms are associated with decreased IL-10 levels and hence could contribute to SIDS by delaying initiation of protective antibody production or reduced capacity to inhibit inflammatory cytokine production.

An uncommon cause of SIDS is due to mutations in the testis-specific Y-like gene *(TSPYL),* which also demonstrates testicular dysgenesis.

GENE-ENVIRONMENT INTERACTIONS. The actual risk for SIDS in individual infants is determined by complex interactions between genetic and environmental risk factors (see Fig. 372-1). There appears, for example, to be an interaction between prone sleep position and impaired ventilatory and arousal responsiveness. Facedown or nearly facedown sleeping does occasionally occur in prone-sleeping infants and can result in episodes of airway obstruction and asphyxia in healthy full-term infants. Healthy infants arouse before such episodes become life-threatening, but infants with insufficient arousal responsiveness to asphyxia may be at risk for sudden death. There may also be links between modifiable risk factors such as soft bedding, prone sleep position, and thermal stress, and links between genetic risk factors such as ventilatory and arousal abnormalities and temperature or metabolic regulation deficits. Cardiorespiratory control deficits could be related to 5-HTT polymorphisms, for example, or to polymorphisms in genes pertinent to ANS development. Affected infants could be at increased risk for sleep-related hypoxemia and, hence, more susceptible to adverse effects associated with unsafe sleep position or bedding. Infants at increased risk for sleep-related hypoxemia could also be at greater risk for fatal arrhythmias in the presence of a sodium or potassium cardiac ion channel gene polymorphism.

Recent febrile illness, often related to upper respiratory infection (see Table 372-5) has been observed in 50% or more of SIDS victims. Although historically not considered of primary etiologic significance, such otherwise benign infections could increase risk for SIDS if interacting with genetically determined impaired immune responses due, for example, to partial deletions in the complement C4 gene or interleukin polymorphisms (see Table 372-4), or other yet-to-be-identified polymorphisms. Interactions between upper respiratory infections or other minor illnesses and other factors such as prone sleeping may also play a role in the pathogenesis of SIDS. Deficient inflammatory responsiveness to infection has also been hypothesized to be a mechanism for SIDS, and mast cell degranulation has been reported in SIDS victims; this is consistent with an anaphylactic reaction to a bacterial toxin and some family members of SIDS victims also have mast cell hyperreleasability and degranulation, suggesting that increased susceptibility to an anaphylactic reaction is another genetic factor influencing fatal outcomes to otherwise minor infections in infants.

The increased risk for SIDS associated with fetal and postnatal exposure to cigarette smoke also appears, at least in part, to depend on genetic factors affecting brainstem autonomic control. Maternal smoking can potentiate hyperplasia of pulmonary neuroendocrine cells and dysfunction of these cells may contribute to the pathophysiology of SIDS. Both animal and clinical studies indicate decreased ventilatory and arousal responsiveness to hypoxia after fetal exposure, including impaired autoresuscitation after apnea in association with postnatal nicotine exposure. Decreased brainstem immunoreactivity to selected protein kinase C and neuronal nitric oxide synthase isoforms has been observed in rats exposed to cigarette smoke prenatally, which could be associated with impaired ventilatory and arousal responsiveness to hypoxia. Hence, the age-specific attenuation of hypoxic defenses after nicotine exposure appears related, at least in part, to impaired brain catecholamine metabolism, but no genetic polymorphisms contributing to these smoking-related metabolic changes have yet been identified. In vitro studies also suggest that smoking increases risk for SIDS, due to greater susceptibility to viral and bacterial infections and enhanced bacterial binding after passive coating of mucosal surfaces with smoke components, hence suggesting interactions between smoking, cardiorespiratory control, and immune status.

INFANT GROUPS AT INCREASED RISK FOR SIDS

UNEXPLAINED APPARENT LIFE-THREATENING EVENTS. Infants with an unexplained apparent life-threatening event (ALTE) are at increased risk for SIDS. A history of an unexplained ALTE has been reported in 5–9% of SIDS victims, and the risk of SIDS appears to be higher with 2 or more unexplained events, but no definitive incidence rates are available. Compared with healthy control infants, the risk for SIDS may be as much as 3 to 5 times greater in infants having experienced an ALTE. Although most studies of ALTE have not specified gestational age, 30% of ALTE infants in the Collaborative Home Infant Monitoring Evaluation were ≤37 wk at birth.

SUBSEQUENT SIBLINGS OF A SIDS VICTIM. The next-born siblings of first-born infants dying of any noninfectious natural cause are at significantly increased risk for infant death from the same cause, including SIDS. The relative risk is 9.1 for the same cause of recurrent death vs 1.6 for a different cause of death. The relative risk for recurrence of SIDS (range 5.4–5.8) is similar to the relative risk for non-SIDS causes of recurrent death (range 4.6–12.5). The risk for recurrent infant mortality from the same cause as in the index sibling thus appears to be increased to a similar degree in subsequent siblings for both explained causes and for SIDS. This increased risk in SIDS families is consistent with genetic risk factors interacting with environmental risk factors (see Table 372-2).

The extent to which risk for SIDS may be increased in subsequent siblings has been a controversial subject due primarily to limited prior understanding of the role of genetic risk factors but also due to uncertainty about the frequency with which intentional suffocation is misclassified as SIDS. Clarification of the role of intentional suffocation has been impaired by the lack of objective criteria for diagnosis. Although some health professionals have in the past stated that only homicide runs in families and all subsequent cases of sudden unexpected infant deaths in a family should be investigated for possible homicide, there are substantial data in support of genetic as well as environmental factors leading to increased risk for recurrent SIDS in some families. In addition to genetic evidence consistent with increased risk for SIDS in subsequent siblings, epidemiologic data from the United Kingdom confirm that 2nd infant deaths in families are not rare and that at least 80–90% are natural. The proportion of recurrent infant death from SIDS in subsequent siblings was 5.9 times greater than the proportion of probable homicides.

PREMATURITY. Many studies have identified an inverse relationship between risk for SIDS and birthweight/gestational age. The environmental risk factors associated with SIDS in preterm infants are not substantially different from those observed in full-term infants, including prone and side sleeping. The postnatal age of preterm infants dying of SIDS is 5–7 wk older than that of full-term infants, and the postconceptional age is 4–6 wk younger than that of full-term infants. Compared with infants with birthweight >2,500 g, infants with birthweights of 1,000–1,499 g and 1,500–2,499 g are approximately 4 and 3 times more likely to die of SIDS, respectively.

PHYSIOLOGIC STUDIES. Physiologic studies have been performed on healthy infants in early infancy, a few of whom later died of SIDS. Physiologic studies have also been performed on infant groups at increased risk for SIDS, especially infants having experienced an unexplained ALTE and subsequent siblings of SIDS victims. In the aggregate, these studies are indicative of a brainstem abnormality related to neuroregulation of cardiorespiratory control or other autonomic functions and are consistent with the autopsy findings including genetic studies in SIDS victims (see the "Pathology" and "Genetic Risk Factors" sections). The observed physiologic abnormalities affect respiratory patterns, chemoreceptor sensitivity, control of heart and respiratory rate or variability, and asphyxic arousal responsiveness. A deficit in arousal responsiveness may be a necessary prerequisite for SIDS to occur but may be insufficient to cause SIDS in the absence of other genetic or environmental risk factors. Autoresuscitation (gasping) is a critical component of the asphyxic arousal response, and a failure of autoresuscitation in victims of SIDS may be the final and most devastating physiologic failure. Most full-term infants <9 wk of age arouse in response to mild hypoxia, but only 10–15% of normal infants >9 wk of age arouse. These data thus suggest that as infants mature, their ability to arouse to mild-moderate hypoxic stimuli diminishes as they reach the age range of greatest risk for SIDS.

The ability to shorten the Q-T interval as heart rate increases appears to be impaired in some SIDS victims, suggesting that such infants may be predisposed to ventricular arrhythmia. This is consistent with the observations of cardiac ion channel gene polymorphisms in other SIDS victims (see Table 372-4), but there are no ante mortem Q-T interval data in the SIDS infants having postmortem genetic data. Infants studied physiologically and later dying of SIDS have higher heart rates in all sleep-waking states, diminished heart rate variability during wakefulness, and significantly lower heart rate variability at the respiratory frequency across all sleep-waking cycles.

Part of the decreased heart rate variability and increased heart rate observed in infants who later die of SIDS may be related to decreased vagal tone. This decreased tone appears, at least in part, to be related to vagal neuropathy or to brainstem damage in areas responsible for parasympathetic cardiac control. In a comparison of heart rate power spectra before and after obstructive apneas in infants, future SIDS victims do not have the decreases in low-frequency to high-frequency power ratios observed in control infants. Some future SIDS victims thus have different autonomic responsiveness to obstructive apnea, perhaps indicating impaired ANS control associated with higher vulnerability to external or endogenous stress factors and hence to reduced electrical stability of the heart.

Sweating during sleep has been observed in some infants who have had an idiopathic ALTE or have died of SIDS. Although overheating may be the cause of this sweating, it may also be caused by alveolar hypoventilation and secondary asphyxia or by autonomic dysfunction as part of a more generalized deficiency in brainstem function.

Although home cardiorespiratory monitors with memory capability have recorded the terminal events in some SIDS victims, these recordings have not included pulse oximetry and do not permit identification of obstructed breaths due to reliance on transthoracic impedance for breath detection. In most instances, there has been sudden and rapid progression of severe bradycardia that is either unassociated with central apnea or appears to occur too soon to be explained by the central apnea. These observations are consistent with an abnormality in autonomic control of heart rate variability, or with obstructed breaths and associated bradycardia or hypoxemia.

CLINICAL STRATEGIES

MONITORING. SIDS cannot currently be prevented in individual infants because it is not, at this time, possible to identify prospective SIDS victims and no effective intervention has been established even if victims could be prospectively identified. Studies of cardiorespiratory pattern or other autonomic abnormalities do not have sufficient sensitivity and specificity to be clinically useful as a screening test. Home electronic surveillance using existing technology has not been shown to reduce the risk of SIDS. Although prolonged Q-T interval in an infant may be treated if diagnosed, neither the role of routine postnatal electrocardiographic (ECG) screening nor the safety of treatment has been established (see Chapter 435.5). Parental ECG screening is not likely to be helpful because spontaneous mutations are common.

REDUCING THE RISK OF SIDS. The American Academy of Pediatrics guidelines to reduce the risk of SIDS in individual infants are appropriate for most infants, but physicians and other health care providers may, on occasion, need to consider alternative approaches. The major components are as follows:

1. **Full-term and premature infants should be placed for sleep in the supine position. There are no adverse health outcomes from supine sleeping. Side sleeping is not recommended.**
2. **It is recommended that infants sleep in the same room as their parents, but in their own crib or bassinette that conforms to the safety standards of the Consumer Product Safety Commission. Placing the crib or bassinette near the mother's bed facilitates nursing and contact.**
3. **Infants should be put to sleep on a firm mattress. Waterbeds, sofas, soft mattresses, or other soft surfaces should not be used.**
4. **Soft materials in the infant's sleep environment—over, under, or near the infant—should be avoided. These include pillows, comforters, quilts, sheepskins, cushion-like bumper pads, and stuffed toys. Because loose bedding may be hazardous, blankets, if used, should be tucked in around the crib mattress. Sleeping clothing, such as a sleep sack, can be used in place of blankets.**
5. **Avoid overheating and overbundling. The infant should be lightly clothed for sleep and the thermostat set at a comfortable temperature.**
6. **Infants should have some time in the prone position (tummy time) while awake and observed. Alternating the placement of the infant's head as well as his or her orientation in the crib can also minimize the risk of head flattening from supine sleeping (positional plagiocephaly).**
7. **Devices advertised to maintain sleep position, "protect" a bed-sharing infant, or reduce the risk of rebreathing are not recommended.**
8. **Home respiratory, cardiac, and O_2 saturation monitoring may be of value for selected infants who have extreme instability, but there is no evidence that monitoring decreases the incidence of SIDS and it is, therefore, not recommended for this purpose.**
9. **Consider offering a pacifier at bedtime and naptime. The pacifier should be used when placing the infant down for sleep and not be reinserted once it falls out. For breast-fed infants, delay introduction of the pacifier until breast-feeding is well established.**
10. **Mothers should not smoke during pregnancy and infants should not be exposed to second-hand smoke.**
11. **The national Back to Sleep campaign should continue and be expanded to emphasize the multiple characteristics of a safe sleeping environment and to focus on the groups who continue to have higher rates of SIDS. Educational strategies must be tailored to each racial-ethnic group to ensure acceptance within that cultural context. Secondary care providers need to be targeted to receive these educational messages, including daycare providers, grandparents, foster parents, and babysitters. Health care professionals in intensive care and normal newborn nurseries should implement these recommendations well before anticipated discharge.**

Ackerman MJ, Siu BL, Sturner WQ, et al: Postmortem molecular analysis of SCN5A defects in SIDS. *JAMA* 2001;286:2264–2269.

American Academy of Pediatrics Task Force on Infant Sleep Position and Sudden Infant Death Syndrome: The changing concept of sudden infant death syndrome: Diagnostic coding shifts, controversies regarding the sleeping environment, and new variables to consider in reducing risk. *Pediatrics* 2005;116:1245–1255.
Blair PS, Sidebotham P, Berry PJ, et al: Major epidemiological changes in sudden infant death syndrome: A 20-year population-based study in the UK. *Lancet* 2006;367:314–319.
Carpenter RG, Irgens LM, Blair PS, et al: Sudden unexplained infant death in 20 regions in Europe: Case control study. *Lancet* 2004;363:185–190.
Carpenter RG, Waite A, Coombs RC, et al: Repeat sudden unexpected and unexplained infant deaths: Natural or unnatural? *Lancet* 2005;365:29–35.
Centers for Disease Control and Prevention: Release of sudden, unexplained infant death investigation reporting form. *MMWR* 2006;55:212–213.
Corwin MJ, Lesko SM, Heeren T, et al: Secular changes in sleep position during infancy: 1995–1998. *Pediatrics* 2003;111:52–60.
Gaultier C: Functional brain deficits in congenital central hypoventilation syndrome. *Pediatr Res* 2005;57:471–472.
Gordon AE, El Ahmer OR, Chan R, et al: Why is smoking a risk factor for sudden infant death syndrome? *Child Care Health Dev* 2002;28:23–25.
Hauck FR, Omojokun OO, Siadaty MS: Do pacifiers reduce the risk of sudden infant death syndrome? A meta-analysis. *Pediatrics* 2005;116:e716–e723.
Horn MH, Kinnamon DD, Ferraro N, Curley MAQ: Smaller mandibular size in infants with a history of an apparent life-threatening event. *J Pediatr* 2006;149:499–504.
Hunt CE: Gene-environment interactions: Implications for sudden unexpected deaths in infancy. *Arch Dis Child* 2005;90:48–53.
Hunt CE, Lesko SM, Vezina RM, et al: Infant sleep position and associated health outcomes. *Arch Pediatr Adolesc Med* 2003;157:469–474.
Immunization Safety Review Committee. Stratton K, Almario DA,Wizemann TM, McCormick MC (eds): Immunization safety review. Vaccinations and sudden unexpected death in infancy. Washington DC, National Academies Press, 2003. National Infant Sleep Position website (http://dccwww.bumc.bu.edu/ChimeNisp/Main_Nisp.asp), accessed April 8, 2005.
Iyasu S, Randall LL, Welty TK, et al: Risk factors for sudden infant death syndrome among northern plains Indians. *JAMA* 2002;288:2717–2723.
Jones KL, Krous HF, Nadeau J, et al: Vascular endothelial growth factor in the cerebrospinal fluid of infants who died of sudden infant death syndrome: Evidence for antecedent hypoxia. *Pediatrics* 2003;111:358–363.
Kadhim H, Kahn A, Sébire G: Distinct cytokine profile in SIDS brain: A common denominator in a multifactorial syndrome. *Neurology* 2003;61:1256–1259.
Kinney HC, Randall LL, Sleeper LA, et al: Serotonergic brainstem abnormalities in northern plains Indians with the sudden infant death syndrome. *J Neuropathol Exp Neurol* 2003;62:1178–1191.
Korachi M, Pravica V, Barson AJ, et al: Interleukin 10 genotype as a risk factor for sudden infant death syndrome: Determination of IL-10 genotype from wax-embedded postmortem samples. *FEMS Immunol Med Microbiol* 2004;42:125–129.
Li DK, Willinger M, Petitti DB, et al: Use of a dummy (pacifier) during sleep and risk of sudden infant death syndrome (SIDS): Population based case-control study. *Br Med J* 2006;332:18–21.
Makielski JC: SIDS: Genetic and environmental influences may cause arrhythmia in this silent killer. *J Clin Invest* 2006;116:297–299.
Matthews T: Sudden unexpected infant death: Infanticide or SIDS? *Lancet* 2005;365:3–4.
Matturri L, Biondo B, Suarez-Mier MP, et al: Brain stem lesions in the sudden infant death syndrome: Variability in the hypoplasia of the arcuate nucleus. *Acta Neuropathol (Berl)* 2002;104:12–20.
McGovern MC, Smith MBH: Causes of apparent life threatening events in infants: A systematic review. *Arch Dis Child* 2004;89:1043–1048.
Opdal SH, Rognum TO: New insight into sudden infant death syndrome. *Lancet* 2004;364:825–826.
Opdal SH, Rognum TO: The sudden infant death syndrome gene: Does it exist? *Pediatrics* 2004;114:e506–e512.
Ramanathan R, Corwin MJ, Hunt CE, et al: Collaborative Home Infant Monitoring Evaluation (CHIME) Study Group: Cardiorespiratory events recorded on home monitors: Comparison of healthy infants with those at increased risk for SIDS. *JAMA* 2001;285:2199–2207.
Skinner JR, Chung SK, Montgomery D, et al: Near-miss SIDS due to Brugada syndrome. *Arch Dis Child* 2005;90:528–529.
Smith GCS, Wood AM, Pell JP, et al: Second-trimester maternal serum levels of alpha-fetoprotein and the subsequent risk of sudden infant death syndrome. *N Engl J Med* 2004;351:978–986.
Van Wouwe J, HiraSing RA: Prevention of sudden unexpected infant death. *Lancet* 2006;367:277–278.
Weese-Mayer DE, Berry-Kravis EM, Zhou L, et al: Sudden infant death syndrome: Case-control frequency differences at genes pertinent to early autonomic nervous system embryologic development. *Pediatr Res* 2004;56:391–396.
Weese-Mayer DE, Zhou L, Berry-Kravis, et al: Association of the serotonin transporter gene with sudden infant death syndrome: A haplotype analysis. *Am J Med Genet A* 2003;122:238–245.
Willinger M, Ko C-W, Hoffman HJ, et al: Factors associated with caregivers' choice of infant sleep position, 1994–1998. The National Infant Sleep Position Study. *JAMA* 2000;283:2135–2142.

Section 2 — Disorders of the Respiratory Tract

Chapter 373 ■ Congenital Disorders of the Nose

Joseph Haddad Jr.

NORMAL NEWBORN NOSE. Although children and adults preferentially breathe through their nose unless nasal obstruction interferes, most newborn infants are obligate nasal breathers and significant nasal obstruction presenting at birth, such as choanal atresia, may be a life-threatening situation for the infant unless an alternative to the nasal airway is established. Nasal congestion with obstruction is common in the 1st year of life and can affect the quality of breathing during sleep; it may be associated with a narrow nasal airway, viral or bacterial infection, enlarged adenoids, or maternal estrogenic stimuli similar to rhinitis of pregnancy. The internal nasal airway doubles in size in the 1st 6 mo of life, leading to resolution of symptoms in many infants. Supportive care with a bulb syringe and saline nose drops, topical nasal decongestants, and antibiotics, when indicated, improve symptoms in affected infants.

PHYSIOLOGY. The nose is responsible for olfaction and initial warming and humidification of inspired air. In the anterior nasal cavity, turbulent airflow and coarse hairs enhance the deposition of large particulate matter; the remaining nasal airways filter out particles as small as 6 μm in diameter. In the turbinate region, the airflow becomes laminar and the airstream is narrowed and directed superiorly, enhancing particle deposition, warming, and humidification. Nasal passages contribute as much as 50% of the total resistance of normal breathing. Nasal flaring, a sign of respiratory distress, reduces the resistance to inspiratory airflow through the nose and may improve ventilation.

Although the nasal mucosa is more vascular, especially in the turbinate region than in the lower airways, the surface epithelium is similar, with ciliated cells, goblet cells, submucosal glands, and a covering blanket of mucus. The nasal secretions contain lysozyme and secretory immunoglobulin A (IgA), both of which have antimicrobial activity, and IgG, IgE, albumin, histamine, bacteria, lactoferrin, and cellular debris, as well as mucous glycoproteins, which provide viscoelastic properties. Aided by the ciliated cells, mucus flows toward the nasopharynx, where the airstream widens, the epithelium becomes squamous, and secretions are wiped away by swallowing. Replacement of the mucous layers occurs about every 10–20 min. Estimates of daily mucus production vary from 0.1–0.3 mg/kg/24 hr, with most of the mucus being produced by the submucosal glands.

CONGENITAL DISORDERS. Congenital *structural nasal malformations* are uncommon compared with acquired abnormalities. The nasal bones can be congenitally absent so that the bridge of the nose fails to develop, resulting in *nasal hypoplasia.* Congenital absence of the nose *(arhinia),* complete or partial duplication, or a single centrally placed nostril can occur in isolation but is usually part of a malformation syndrome. Rarely, *supernumerary teeth* are found in the nose, or teeth grow into it from the maxilla.

Nasal bones can be sufficiently malformed to produce severe narrowing of the nasal passages. Often, such narrowing is associated with a high and narrow hard palate. Children with these defects may have significant obstruction to airflow during infections of the upper airways and are more susceptible to the development of chronic or recurrent hypoventilation (see Chapter 18). Rarely, the alae nasi are sufficiently thin and poorly supported to result in inspiratory obstruction, or there may be congenital nasolacrimal duct obstruction with cystic extension into the nasopharynx, causing respiratory distress.

CHOANAL ATRESIA. This is the most common congenital anomaly of the nose and has a frequency of ≈1/7,000 live births. It consists of a unilateral or bilateral bony (90%) or membranous (10%) septum between the nose and the pharynx; most cases are a combination of bony and membranous atresia. Nearly 50% of affected infants have other congenital anomalies, with the anomalies occurring more frequently in bilateral cases. The **CHARGE syndrome** (*c*oloboma, *h*eart disease, *a*tresia choanae, *r*etarded growth and development or CNS anomalies or both, *g*enital anomalies or hypogonadism or both, and *e*ar anomalies or deafness or both) is one of the more common anomalies associated with choanal atresia. Most patients with CHARGE syndrome have mutations in the *CHD7* gene, which is involved in chromatin organization.

Clinical Manifestations. Newborn infants have a variable ability to breathe through their mouths, so nasal obstruction does not produce the same symptoms in every infant. When the obstruction is unilateral, the infant may be asymptomatic for a prolonged period, often until the 1st respiratory infection, when unilateral nasal discharge or persistent nasal obstruction may suggest the diagnosis. Infants with bilateral choanal atresia who have difficulty with mouth breathing make vigorous attempts to inspire, often suck in their lips, and develop cyanosis. Distressed children then cry (which relieves the cyanosis) and become calmer, with normal skin color, only to repeat the cycle after closing their mouths. Those who are able to breathe through their mouths at once experience difficulty when sucking and swallowing, becoming cyanotic when they attempt to feed.

Diagnosis. This is established by the inability to pass a firm catheter through each nostril 3–4 cm into the nasopharynx. The atretic plate may be seen directly with fiberoptic rhinoscopy. The anatomy is best evaluated by using high-resolution CT (Fig. 373-1)

Treatment. Initial treatment consists of prompt placement of an oral airway, maintaining the mouth in an open position, or intubation. A standard oral airway (such as that used in anesthesia) can be used, or a feeding nipple can be fashioned with large holes at the tip to facilitate air passage. Once an oral airway is established, the infant can be fed by gavage until breathing and eating without the assisted airway is possible. In bilateral cases, intubation or, less often, tracheotomy may be indicated. If the child is free of other serious medical problems, operative intervention is considered in the neonate; transnasal repair is the treatment of choice with the introduction of small magnifying endoscopes and smaller surgical instruments and drills. Stents are usually left in place for weeks after the repair to prevent closure or stenosis. Tracheotomy should be considered in cases of bilateral atresia in which the child has other potentially life-threatening problems and in whom early surgical repair of the choanal atresia may not be appropriate or feasible. Operative correction of unilateral obstruction may be deferred for several yr. In both unilateral and bilateral cases, restenosis necessitating dilation or reoperation, or both, is common. Mitomycin C has been used to help prevent the development of granulation tissue and stenosis.

CONGENITAL DEFECTS OF THE NASAL SEPTUM. Perforation of the septum is most commonly acquired after birth secondary to infection, such as syphilis, tuberculosis, or trauma; rarely, it is developmental. Continuous positive airway pressure cannulas are a cause of iatrogenic perforation. Trauma from delivery is the most common cause of septal deviation noted at birth. When recognized early, it can be corrected with immediate realignment using blunt probes, cotton applicators, and topical anesthesia. Formal surgical correction, when required, is usually postponed to avoid disturbance of midface growth.

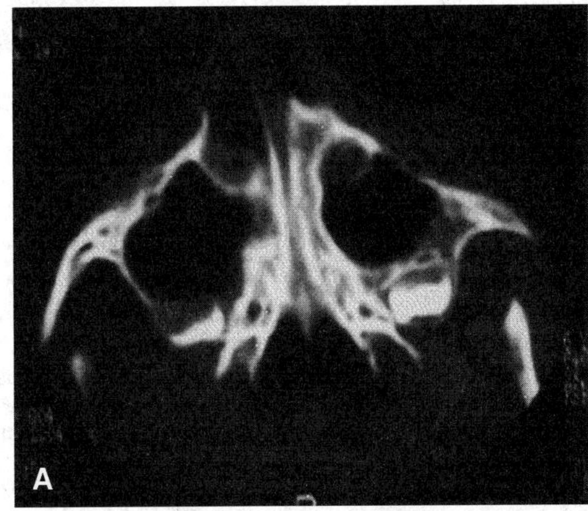

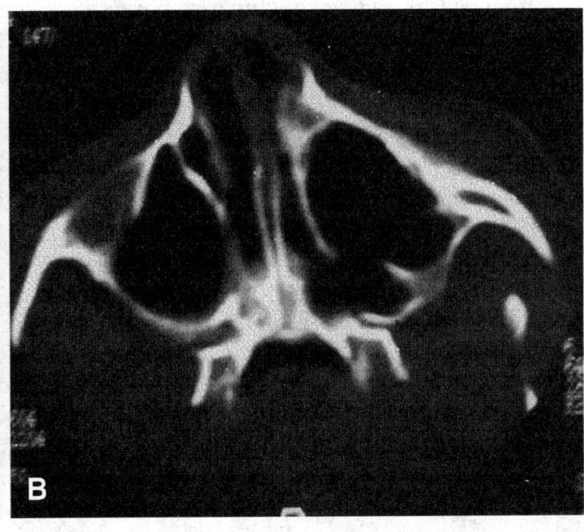

Figure 373-1. CT scan showing (a) hypoplastic nasal cavities, and (b) bony and mucosal choanal atresia. (From Altuntas A, Yilmaz MD, Kahveci OK, et al: Coexistence of choanal atresia and Tessier's facial cleft number 2. *Int J Pediatr Otorhinolaryngol* 2004;68:1083.)

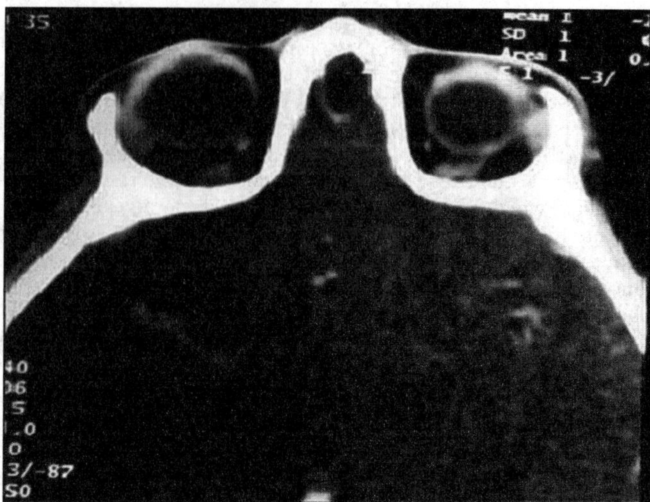

Figure 373-2. CT axial view showing nasal dermoid extension into the anterior cranial fossa through a defect in the cribriform plate. (From Meher R, Singh I, Aggarwal S: Nasal dermoid with intracranial extension. *J Postgrad Med* 2005;51:39.)

Mild septal deviations are common and usually asymptomatic; abnormal formation of the septum is infrequent unless other malformations are present, such as cleft lip or palate.

PYRIFORM APERTURE STENOSIS. Infants with this bony abnormality of the anterior nasal aperture present with severe nasal obstruction at birth or shortly thereafter. Diagnosis is made by CT of the nose; surgical repair by means of an anterior, sublabial approach may be needed if the child cannot feed or breathe without difficulty.

CONGENITAL MIDLINE NASAL MASSES. *Dermoids, gliomas,* and *encephaloceles* (in descending order of frequency) present intranasally or extranasally and may have intracranial connections. Nasal dermoids often have a dimple or pit on the nasal dorsum, sometimes with hair being present, and can predispose to intracranial infections if an intracranial fistula or sinus is present. Recurrent infection of the dermoid itself is more common. Gliomas or heterotopic brain tissue are firm, whereas encephaloceles are soft and enlarge with crying or the Valsalva maneuver. Diagnosis is based on physical examination findings and results from imaging studies. CT provides the best bony detail, but MRI allows sagittal views, which may be needed to further define intracranial extension (Fig. 373-2) Surgical excision of these masses is generally required, with the extent and surgical approach based on the type and size of the mass.

Other nasal masses include *hemangiomas, congenital nasolacrimal duct obstruction* (which may present as an intranasal mass), nasal polyps, and tumors such as rhabdomyosarcoma (see Chapter 500). Nasal polyps are rarely present at birth, but the other masses often present at birth or in early infancy (see Chapter 375).

Poor development of the paranasal sinuses and a narrow nasal airway are associated with recurrent or chronic upper airway infection in Down syndrome (see Chapter 81).

DIAGNOSIS AND TREATMENT. In children with congenital nasal disorders, supportive care of the airway is given until the diagnosis is established. Diagnosis is made through a combination of flexible scoping and imaging studies, primarily CT scan. In the case of surgically correctable congenital problems such as choanal atresia, surgery is performed once the child is deemed healthy and free of life-threatening problems such as congenital heart disease.

Aramaki M, Udaka T, Kosaki R, et al: Phenotypic spectrum of CHARGE syndrome with *CHD7* mutations. *J Pediatr* 2006;148:410–414.

Brown OE, Myer CM, Manning SC: Congenital nasal pyriform aperture stenosis. *Laryngoscope* 1989;99:86–91.

Giffon SD, Goncalves VM, Zanardi VA, gil-da-Silva Lopes VL: Cerebellar involvement in midline facial defects with ocular hypertelorism. *Cleft Palate Craniofac J* 2006;43:466–470.

Harley EH: Pediatric congenital nasal masses. *Ear Nose Throat J* 1991; 70:28–32.

Jongmans MCJ, Admiraal RJ, vander Donk KP, et al: CHARGE syndrome: the phenotypic spectrum of mutations in the *CHD7* gene. *J Med Genet* 2006;43:306–314.

Khafagy YW: Endoscopic repair of bilateral congenital choanal atresia. *Laryngoscope* 2002;112:316–319.

Lusk RP, Lee PC: Magnetic resonance imaging of congenital midline nasal masses. *Otolaryngol Head Neck Surg* 1986;95:303–306.

Rahbar R, Jones DT, Nuss RC, et al: The role of mitomycin in the prevention and treatment of scar formation in the pediatric aerodigestive tract: Friend or foe? *Arch Otolaryngol Head Neck Surg* 2002;128:401–406.

Rohrich RJ, Lowe JB, Schwartz MR: The role of open rhinoplasty in the management of nasal dermoid cysts. *Plast Reconstr Surg* 1999;10:2163–2170.

Samadi DS, Shah UK, Handler SD, et al: Choanal atresia: A twenty-year review of medical comorbidities and surgical outcomes. *Laryngoscope* 2003;113:254–258.

Sanlaville D, Etehevers HC, Gonzales M, et al: Phenotypic spectrum of CHARGE syndrome in fetuses with *CHD7* truncating mutations correlates with expression during human development. *J Med Genet* 2006;43: 211–217.

Van Den Abbeele T, Triglia JM, Francois M, Narcy P: Congenital nasal pyriform aperture stenosis: Diagnosis and management of 20 cases. *Ann Otol Rhinol Laryngol* 2001;110:70–75.

Veruloed MPJ, Hoevenadrs-van den Boom MAA, Knoors H, et al: CHARGE syndrome: Relations between behavioral characteristics and medical conditions. *Am J Med Genet* 2006;140A:851–862.

Chapter 374 ■ Acquired Disorders of the Nose

Joseph Haddad Jr.

GENERAL. Many acquired abnormalities of the nose and paranasal sinuses, such as tumors and septal perforations, present as epistaxis. Midface trauma with a nasal or facial fracture may be accompanied by epistaxis. Trauma to the nose can cause a *septal hematoma;* if treatment is delayed, this can lead to necrosis of septal cartilage and a resultant *saddle-nose deformity.* Other abnormalities that can cause a change in the shape of the nose and paranasal bones, with obstruction but few other symptoms, include *fibro-osseus lesions* (ossifying fibroma, fibrous dysplasia, cementifying fibroma) and *mucoceles of the paranasal sinuses.* These conditions may be suspected on physical examination and confirmed by CT scan and biopsy. Although these are considered benign lesions, they can all greatly change the anatomy of surrounding bony structures and often require surgical intervention for management.

374.1 • Foreign Body

ETIOLOGY. Food, crayons, small toys, erasers, paper wads, beads, beans, stones, pieces of sponge, and other foreign bodies are frequently introduced into the nose by young or developmentally delayed children. Initial symptoms are unilateral obstruction, sneezing, relatively mild discomfort, and, rarely, pain. In one retrospective study, presenting clinical symptoms included history of insertion of foreign bodies (86%), mucopurulent nasal discharge

(24%), foul nasal odor (9%), epistaxis (6%), nasal obstruction (3%), and mouth breathing (2%). Irritation results in mucosal swelling because some foreign bodies are hygroscopic and increase in size as water is absorbed; signs of local obstruction and discomfort may increase with time. The patient may also present with a generalized body odor known as *bromhidrosis*.

DIAGNOSIS. Unilateral nasal discharge and obstruction should suggest the presence of a foreign body, which can often be seen on examination with a nasal speculum or wide otoscope placed in the nose. Often, purulent secretions must be removed so that the foreign object can actually be seen; a headlight, suction, and topical decongestants are often needed. The object is usually situated anteriorly at first, but through unskilled attempts at removal it can be forced deeper into the nose. When of long standing, a foreign body can become embedded in granulation tissue or mucosa and appear as a nasal mass. A lateral skull radiograph assists in diagnosis if the foreign body is metallic or radiopaque.

COMPLICATIONS. Infection often follows and gives rise to a purulent, malodorous, or bloody discharge Local tissue damage from long-standing foreign body, or alkaline injury from a disk battery, can lead to local tissue loss and cartilage destruction. A synechia or scar band can then form, causing nasal obstruction. Loss of septal mucosa and cartilage can cause a septal perforation. Disk batteries are dangerous when placed in the nose; they leach base, which causes pain and local tissue destruction in a matter of hours.

TREATMENT. A quick examination of the nose is made to determine if a foreign body is present, and whether it needs to be removed emergently. Planning is then made for office or operating room extrication of the foreign body. Prompt removal minimizes the danger of aspiration and local tissue necrosis. This can usually be performed with topical anesthesia, using either forceps or nasal suction. If there is marked swelling, bleeding, or tissue overgrowth, general anesthesia may be needed to remove the object. Infection usually clears promptly after the removal of the object and, generally, no further therapy is necessary.

COMPLICATIONS. Tetanus is a rare complication of long-standing nasal foreign bodies in nonimmunized children. Toxic shock syndrome is also rare but when it does occur in this setting, it most commonly occurs from nasal surgical packing (see Chapter 180.2).

PREVENTION. Tempting objects such as round, shiny beads should only be used under adult supervision. Disk batteries should be stored away from the reach of small children.

Figueiredo RR, Azevedo AA, Kos AO, Tomita S: Nasal foreign bodies: description of types and complications in 420 cases. *Rev Bras Otorrinolaringol* 2006;72:18–23.

Haddad J Jr: Foreign bodies of the ear, nose and pharynx. In Burg FD, Gershon A, Indelfinger JR, Polin RA (eds): *Current Pediatric Therapy,* 17th ed. Philadelphia, WB Saunders, 2002, p 23.

Lin VY, Daniel SJ, Papsin BC: Button batteries in the ear, nose and upper aerodigestive tract. *Int J Pediatr Otorhinolaryngol* 2004;68:473–479.

Ogunleye AO, Sogebi OA: Nasal foreign bodies in the African children. *Afr J Med Sci* 2004;33:225–228.

374.2 • Epistaxis

Nosebleeds are rare in infancy and common in childhood; their incidence decreases after puberty. Diagnosis and treatment depend on the location and cause of the bleeding.

ANATOMY. The most common site of bleeding is the Kiesselbach plexus, an area in the anterior septum where vessels from both the internal carotid (anterior and posterior ethmoid arteries) and external carotid (sphenopalatine and terminal branches of the internal maxillary arteries) converge. The thin mucosa in this area, as well as the anterior location, makes it prone to exposure to dry air and trauma.

ETIOLOGY. Common causes of nosebleeds from the anterior septum include digital trauma, foreign bodies, dry air, and inflammation, including upper respiratory tract infections, sinusitis, and allergic rhinitis. Nasal steroid sprays are commonly used in children, and their chronic use may be associated with bleeding. Young infants with significant gastroesophageal reflux into the nose may occasionally present with epistaxis secondary to mucosal inflammation. There is frequently a family history of childhood epistaxis. Susceptibility is increased during respiratory infections and in the winter when dry air irritates the nasal mucosa, resulting in formation of fissures and crusting. Severe bleeding may be encountered with congenital vascular abnormalities, such as *hereditary hemorrhagic telangiectasia* (see Chapter 432.3), varicosities, hemangiomas, and, in children with thrombocytopenia, deficiency of clotting factors, particularly von Willebrand disease, hypertension, renal failure, or venous congestion. Nasal polyps or other intranasal growths may be associated with epistaxis. Recurrent, and frequently severe, nosebleeds may be the initial presenting symptom in **juvenile nasal angiofibromas,** which occur in adolescent males. The incidence of Kiesselbach plexus bleeding decreases in adolescence.

CLINICAL MANIFESTATIONS. Epistaxis usually occurs without warning, with blood flowing slowly but freely from one nostril or occasionally from both. In children with nasal lesions, bleeding may follow physical exercise. When bleeding occurs at night, the blood may be swallowed and become apparent only when the child vomits or passes blood in the stools. Posterior epistaxis can manifest as anterior nasal bleeding or, if copious, the patient may vomit blood as the initial symptom.

TREATMENT. Most nosebleeds stop spontaneously in a few min. The nares should be compressed and the child kept as quiet as possible, in an upright position with the head tilted forward to avoid blood trickling back into the throat. Cold compresses applied to the nose can also help. If these measures do not stop the bleeding, local application of a solution of oxymetazoline (Afrin) or Neo-Synephrine (0.25–1%) may be useful. If bleeding persists, an anterior nasal pack may need to be inserted; if bleeding originates in the posterior nasal cavity, combined anterior and posterior packing is necessary. After bleeding has been controlled, and if a bleeding site is identified, its obliteration by cautery with silver nitrate may prevent further difficulties. Because the septal cartilage derives its nutrition from the overlying mucoperichondrium, only 1 side of the septum should be cauterized at a time to reduce the chance of a septal perforation. During the winter, or in a dry environment, a room humidifier, saline drops, and petrolatum (Vaseline) applied to the septum may help to prevent epistaxis. Three studies examining treatment options (antiseptic cream vs no treatment, petroleum jelly [Vaseline] vs no treatment, and antiseptic cream vs silver nitrate cautery) found no differences between the compared treatments.

In patients with severe or repeated epistaxis, blood transfusions may be necessary. Otolaryngologic evaluation is indicated for these children and for those with bilateral bleeding or with hemorrhage that does not arise from the Kiesselbach plexus. Hematologic evaluation (for coagulopathy and anemia), along with nasal endoscopy and diagnostic imaging, may be needed to make a definitive diagnosis in cases of severe recurrent epistaxis. Replacement of deficient clotting factors may be required for patients who have an underlying hematologic disorder (see Chapter 476). Profuse unilateral epistaxis associated with a nasal mass in an adolescent boy near puberty may signal a **juvenile nasopharyngeal angiofibroma.** This unusual tumor has also been reported in a 2 yr old and in 30–40 yr olds, but the incidence peaks in adolescent and preadolescent boys. CT with contrast medium enhancement and MRI are part of the initial evaluation; arteriography, embolization, and extensive surgery may be needed.

Surgical intervention may also be needed for bleeding from the internal maxillary artery or other vessels that can cause bleeding in the posterior nasal cavity.

PREVENTION. The discouragement of nose picking, and attention to proper humidification of the bedroom during dry winter months helps to prevent many nosebleeds. Prompt attention to nasal infections and allergies is beneficial to nasal hygiene. Prompt cessation of nasal steroid sprays prevents ongoing bleeding.

Burton MJ, Doree CJ: Interventions for recurrent idiopathic epistaxis (nosebleeds) in children. *Cochrane Database Syst Rev* 2004;CD004461.

Makura ZG, Porter GC, McCormick MS: Paediatric epistaxis: Alder Hey experience. *J Laryngol Otol* 2002;116:903–906.

Wurman LH: Epistaxis. In Gates GA (ed): *Current Therapy in Otolaryngology—Head and Neck Surgery,* 5th ed. St Louis, Mosby, 1994, p 354.

Chapter 375 ■ Nasal Polyps

Joseph Haddad Jr.

ETIOLOGY. Nasal polyps are benign pedunculated tumors formed from edematous, usually chronically inflamed nasal mucosa. They commonly arise from the ethmoidal sinus and present in the middle meatus. Occasionally, they appear within the maxillary antrum and can extend to the nasopharynx (antrochoanal polyp) [Fig. 375-1]. Whereas antrochoanal polyps represent only 4–6% of all nasal polyps in the general population, they represent about 33% of polyps in the pediatric population. Large or multiple polyps can completely obstruct the nasal passage. The polyps originating from the ethmoidal sinus are usually smaller and multiple, as compared with the large and usually single antrochoanal polyp.

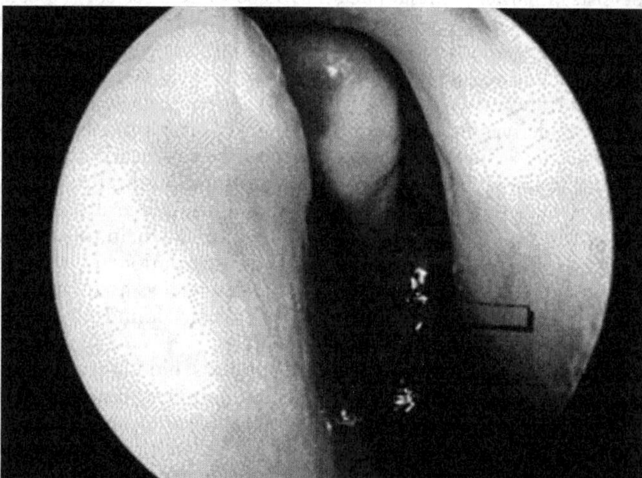

Figure 375-1. Antrochoanal polyp viewed endoscopically *(arrow)*. (From Basak S, Karaman CZ, Akdilli A, Metin KK: Surgical approaches to antrochoanal polyps in children. *Int J Pediatr Otorhinolaryngol* 1998;46:197–205.)

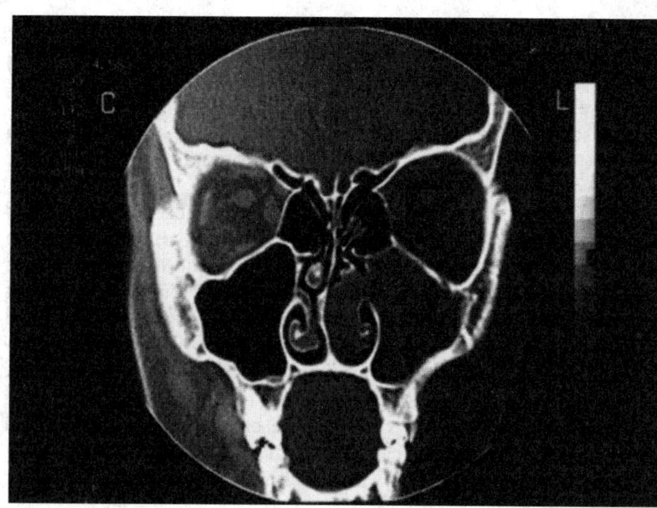

Figure 375-2. A typical CT image of an isolated antrochoanal polyp on the left side. (From Basak S, Karaman CZ, Akdilli A, Metin KK: Surgical approaches to antrochoanal polyps in children. *Int J Pediatr Otorhinolaryngol* 1998;46:197–205.)

Cystic fibrosis is the most common childhood cause of nasal polyposis and should be suspected in any child <12 yr old with nasal polyps, even in the absence of typical respiratory and digestive symptoms; as many as 30% of children with cystic fibrosis acquire nasal polyps. Nasal polyposis is also associated with chronic sinusitis and allergic rhinitis. In the uncommon Samter triad, nasal polyps are associated with aspirin sensitivity and asthma.

CLINICAL MANIFESTATIONS. Obstruction of nasal passages is prominent, with associated hyponasal speech and mouth breathing. Profuse unilateral mucoid or mucopurulent rhinorrhea may also be present. An examination of the nasal passages shows glistening, gray, grapelike masses squeezed between the nasal turbinates and the septum.

DIAGNOSIS AND DIFFERENTIAL DIAGNOSIS. Examination of the external nose and rhinoscopy is performed. Ethmoidal polyps can be readily distinguished from the well-vascularized turbinate tissue, which is pink or red; antrochoanal polyps may have a more fleshy appearance. Antrochoanal polyps may prolapse into the nasopharynx; flexible nasopharyngoscopy can assist in making this diagnosis. Prolonged presence of ethmoidal polyps in a child can widen the bridge of the nose and erode adjacent osseous structures. Tumors of the nose cause more local destruction and distortion of the anatomy. CT scan of the midface is key to diagnosis and planning for surgical treatment (Fig. 375-2).

TREATMENT. Local or systemic decongestants are not usually effective in shrinking the polyps, although they may provide symptomatic relief from the associated mucosal edema. Intranasal steroid sprays, and sometimes systemic steroids, may provide some shrinkage of nasal polyps with symptomatic relief and have proved useful in children with cystic fibrosis and adults with nasal polyps. Polyps should be removed surgically if complete obstruction, uncontrolled rhinorrhea, or deformity of the nose appears. If the underlying pathogenic mechanism cannot be eliminated (cystic fibrosis), the polyps may soon return. Functional endoscopic sinus surgery provides more complete polyp removal and treatment of other associated nasal disease; in some cases, this has reduced the need for frequent surgeries. Nasal steroid sprays should also be started preventively, once postsurgical healing occurs.

Antrochoanal polyps do not respond to medical measures and must be removed surgically. Because these types of polyps are not generally associated with any other underlying disease process, the recurrence rate is much less than for other types of polyps.

Basik S, Karaman CZ, Akdilli A, Metin KK: Surgical approaches to antrochoanal polyps in children. *Int J Pediatr Otorhinolaryngol* 1998; 46:197–205.

Magit AE: Tumors of the nose, paranasal sinuses, and nasopharynx. In Bluestone CD, Stool SE, Kenna MA (eds): *Pediatric Otolaryngology,* 3rd ed. Philadelphia, WB Saunders, 1996, pp 893–904.

Orvidas LJ, Beatty CW, Weaver AL: Antrochoanal polyps in children. *Am J Rhinol* 2001;15:321–325.

Stjärne P, Mösges R, Jorissen M, et al: A randomized controlled trial of mometasonc furoate nasal spray for the treatment of nasal polyposis. *Arch Otolaryngol Head Neck Surg* 2006;132:179–185.

Chapter 376 ■ The Common Cold

Ronald B. Turner and Gregory F. Hayden

The common cold is a viral illness in which the symptoms of rhinorrhea and nasal obstruction are prominent; systemic symptoms and signs such as myalgia and fever are absent or mild. It is often termed *rhinitis* but includes self-limited involvement of the sinus mucosa and is more correctly termed *rhinosinusitis.*

ETIOLOGY. The most common pathogens associated with the common cold are the rhinoviruses (see Chapter 260), but the syndrome can be caused by many different viruses (Table 376-1).

EPIDEMIOLOGY. Colds occur year-round, but the incidence is greatest from the early fall until the late spring, reflecting the seasonal prevalence of the viral pathogens associated with cold symptoms. The highest incidence of rhinovirus infection occurs in the early fall (August–October) and in the late spring (April–May). The seasonal incidence for parainfluenza viruses (see Chapter 256) usually peaks in the late fall, and is highest between December and April for respiratory syncytial virus (RSV; see Chapter 257) and influenza viruses (see Chapter 255).

Young children have an average of 6–8 colds per year but 10–15% of children have at least 12 infections per year. The incidence of illness decreases with age, with 2 to 3 illnesses per year by adulthood. Children in out-of-home daycare centers during the 1st year of life have 50% more colds than children cared for only at home. The difference in the incidence of illness between these groups of children decreases as the length of time spent in daycare increases, although the incidence of illness remains higher in the daycare group through at least the 1st 3 yr of life.

TABLE 376-1. Pathogens Associated with the Common Cold

ASSOCIATION	PATHOGEN	RELATIVE FREQUENCY*
Agents primarily associated with colds	Rhinoviruses	Frequent
	Coronaviruses	Occasional
Agents primarily associated with other clinical syndromes that also cause common cold symptoms	Respiratory syncytial viruses	Occasional
	Human metapneumovirus	Occasional
	Influenza viruses	Uncommon
	Parainfluenza viruses	Uncommon
	Adenoviruses	Uncommon
	Enteroviruses	Uncommon
	Bocavirus	Uncommon

*Relative frequency of colds caused by the agent.

PATHOGENESIS. Viruses that cause the common cold are spread by small-particle aerosols, large-particle aerosols, and direct contact. Although the different common cold pathogens can presumably be spread by any of these mechanisms, some routes of transmission appear to be more efficient than others for particular viruses. Studies of rhinoviruses and RSV suggest that direct contact is an efficient mechanism of transmission of these viruses, although transmission by large-particle aerosols may also occur. In contrast to rhinoviruses and RSV, influenza viruses appear to be most efficiently spread by small-particle aerosols.

The respiratory viruses have evolved different mechanisms to avoid host defenses. Infections with rhinoviruses and adenoviruses result in the development of serotype-specific protective immunity. Repeated infections with these pathogens occur because there are a large number of distinct serotypes of each virus. Influenza viruses have the ability to change the antigens presented on the surface of the virus and thus behave as though there were multiple viral serotypes. The interaction of coronaviruses (see Chapter 261) with host immunity is not well defined, but it appears that multiple distinct strains of coronaviruses are capable of inducing at least short-term protective immunity. The parainfluenza viruses and RSV each have a small number of distinct serotypes. Reinfection with these viruses occurs because protective immunity to these pathogens does not develop after an infection. Although reinfection is not prevented by the adaptive host response to these viruses, the severity of subsequent illness is moderated by pre-existing immunity.

Viral infection of the nasal epithelium can be associated with destruction of the epithelial lining, as with influenza viruses and adenoviruses, or there can be no apparent histologic damage, as with rhinoviruses, RSV, and coronaviruses. Regardless of the histopathologic findings, infection of the nasal epithelium is associated with an acute inflammatory response characterized by release of a variety of inflammatory cytokines and infiltration of the mucosa by inflammatory cells. This acute inflammatory response appears to be responsible, at least in part, for many of the symptoms associated with the common cold. Inflammation can obstruct the sinus ostium or eustachian tube and predispose to bacterial sinusitis or otitis media.

CLINICAL MANIFESTATIONS. The onset of common cold symptoms typically occurs 1–3 days after viral infection. The 1st symptom noted is frequently sore or "scratchy" throat, followed closely by nasal obstruction and rhinorrhea. The sore throat usually resolves quickly and, by the 2nd and 3rd day of illness, nasal symptoms predominate. Cough is associated with ≈30% of colds and usually begins after the onset of nasal symptoms. Influenza viruses, RSV, and adenoviruses are more likely than rhinoviruses or coronaviruses to be associated with fever and other constitutional symptoms. The usual cold persists for about 1 wk, although 10% last for 2 wk.

The physical findings of the common cold are limited to the upper respiratory tract. Increased nasal secretion is frequently obvious to the examiner. A change in the color or consistency of the secretions is common during the course of the illness and is not indicative of sinusitis or bacterial superinfection. Examination of the nasal cavity may reveal swollen, erythematous nasal turbinates, although this finding is nonspecific and of limited diagnostic value.

DIAGNOSIS. The most important task of the physician caring for a patient with a cold is to exclude other conditions that are poten-

TABLE 376-2. Conditions That Can Mimic the Common Cold

CONDITION	DIFFERENTIATING FEATURES
Allergic rhinitis	Prominent itching and sneezing Nasal eosinophils
Foreign body	Unilateral, foul-smelling secretions Bloody nasal secretions
Sinusitis	Presence of fever, headache or facial pain, or periorbital edema or persistence of rhinorrhea or cough for >14 days
Streptococcosis	Nasal discharge that excoriates the nares
Pertussis	Onset of persistent or severe cough
Congenital syphilis	Persistent rhinorrhea with onset in the 1st 3 mo of life

tially more serious or treatable. The differential diagnosis of the common cold includes noninfectious disorders as well as other upper respiratory tract infections (Table 376-2).

LABORATORY FINDINGS. Routine laboratory studies are not helpful for the diagnosis and management of the common cold. A nasal smear for eosinophils may be useful if allergic rhinitis is suspected (see Chapter 142). A predominance of polymorphonuclear leukocytes in the nasal secretions is characteristic of uncomplicated colds and does not indicate bacterial superinfection.

The viral pathogens associated with the common cold can be detected by culture, antigen detection, polymerase chain reaction (PCR), or serologic methods. These studies are generally not indicated in patients with colds because a specific etiologic diagnosis is useful only when treatment with an antiviral agent is contemplated. Bacterial cultures or antigen detection are useful only when group A streptococcus (see Chapter 182), *Bordetella pertussis* (see Chapter 194), or nasal diphtheria (see Chapter 186) is suspected. The isolation of other bacterial pathogens is not an indication of bacterial nasal infection and is not a specific predictor of the etiologic agent in sinusitis.

TREATMENT. The management of the common cold consists primarily of symptomatic treatment.

Antiviral Treatment. Specific antiviral therapy is not currently available for rhinovirus infections. Ribavirin, which is approved for treatment of RSV infections, has no role in the treatment of the common cold. The neuraminidase inhibitors oseltamivir and zanamivir have a modest effect on the duration of symptoms associated with influenza viral infections in children. Oseltamivir also reduces the frequency of influenza-associated otitis media. The difficulty of distinguishing influenza from other common cold pathogens and the necessity that therapy be started early in the illness (within 48 hr of onset of symptoms) to be beneficial are practical limitations to the use of these agents for mild upper respiratory tract infections. Other antiviral agents such as pleconaril for treatment of rhinovirus infections are being developed, although the role, if any, of these agents in routine treatment of the common cold remains to be determined. Antibacterial therapy is of no benefit in the treatment of the common cold.

Symptomatic Treatment. The use of symptomatic therapies in children is controversial; although some of these medications are effective in adults, no studies have demonstrated a significant effect in children. Young children cannot assist in these measurements, so studies of these treatments in children have generally been based on observations by parents or other observers. The use of symptomatic therapies in children can only be based on an assumption that the effects of symptomatic treatments may be similar in adults and children. A decision to use these medications in children must be balanced against the potential adverse effects of each drug. The prominent or most bothersome symptoms of colds vary in the course of the illness and, therefore, if symptomatic treatments are used, it is reasonable to target therapy to specific bothersome symptoms. If symptomatic treatments are recommended, care should be taken to ensure that caregivers understand the intended effect and can determine the proper dosage of the medications.

FEVER. Fever is infrequently associated with an uncomplicated common cold and antipyretic treatment is generally not indicated.

NASAL OBSTRUCTION. Either topical or oral adrenergic agents can be used as nasal decongestants. Effective topical adrenergic agents such as xylometazoline, oxymetazoline, or phenylephrine are available as either intranasal drops or nasal sprays. Reduced-strength formulations of these medications are available for use in younger children, although they are not approved for use in children <2 yr old. Systemic absorption of the imidazolines (oxymetazoline, xylometazoline) has very rarely been associated with bradycardia, hypotension, and coma. Prolonged use of the topical adrenergic agents should be avoided to prevent the development of **rhinitis medicamentosa,** an apparent rebound effect that causes the sensation of nasal obstruction when the drug is discontinued. The oral adrenergic agents are less effective than the topical preparations and are occasionally associated with systemic effects such as central nervous system stimulation, hypertension, and palpitations.

RHINORRHEA. The first-generation antihistamines reduce rhinorrhea by 25–30%. The effect of the antihistamines on rhinorrhea appears to be related to the anticholinergic rather than the antihistaminic properties of these drugs and therefore the second-generation or "nonsedating" antihistamines have no effect on common cold symptoms. The major adverse effect associated with the use of the antihistamines is sedation, although there is some evidence that this adverse effect is less bothersome in children than in adults. Rhinorrhea can also be treated with ipratropium bromide, a topical anticholinergic agent. This drug produces an effect comparable to the antihistamines but is not associated with sedation. The most common side effects of ipratropium are nasal irritation and bleeding.

SORE THROAT. The sore throat associated with colds is generally not severe, but treatment with mild analgesics is occasionally indicated, particularly if there is associated myalgia or headache. The use of acetaminophen during rhinovirus infection has been associated with suppression of neutralizing antibody responses, but this observation has no apparent clinical significance. Aspirin should not be given to children with respiratory infections because of the risk of Reye syndrome in children with influenza (see Chapter 598).

COUGH. Cough suppression is generally not necessary in patients with colds. Cough in some patients appears to be due to upper respiratory tract irritation associated with postnasal drip. Cough in these patients is most prominent during the time of greatest nasal symptoms, and treatment with a first-generation antihistamine may be helpful. Sugar-containing cough drops or lozenges may be temporarily effective. In other patients, cough can be a result of virus-induced **reactive airway disease.** These patients may have cough that persists for days to weeks after the acute illness and may benefit from inhaled steroids and bronchodilator therapy. Codeine or dextromethorphan hydrobromide has no effect on cough from colds. Expectorants such as guaifenesin are not effective antitussive agents.

Ineffective Treatments. Vitamin C, guaifenesin, and inhalation of warm, humidified air are no more effective than placebo for the symptomatic treatment of colds.

Zinc, given as oral lozenges, has been evaluated in several studies as a treatment for common cold symptoms. The function of the rhinovirus 3C protease, an essential enzyme for rhinovirus replication, is inhibited by zinc, but there has been no evidence of an antiviral effect of zinc in vivo. The effect of zinc on symptoms has been inconsistent, with some studies reporting dramatic treatment effects (in adults), whereas other studies find no benefit. A synthesis of these disparate results is difficult, but it appears unlikely that zinc has a clinically significant impact on common cold symptoms in children.

Echinacea is a popular herbal treatment for the common cold. Although echinacea extracts have been shown to have biologic effects, echinacea is not effective as a common cold treatment in children. The lack of standardization of commercial products containing echinacea also presents a formidable obstacle to the rational evaluation or use of this therapy.

COMPLICATIONS. The most common complication of a cold is **otitis media** (see Chapter 639), which is reported in 5–30% of children who have a cold, with the higher incidence occurring in children cared for in a group daycare setting. Symptomatic treatment has no effect on the development of acute otitis media, but treatment with oseltamivir may reduce the incidence of otitis media in patients with influenza.

Sinusitis is another complication of the common cold (see Chapter 377). Self-limited sinus inflammation is a part of the pathophysiology of the common cold, but 0.5–2% of viral upper respiratory tract infections in adults, and 5–13% in children, are complicated by acute bacterial sinusitis. The differentiation of common cold symptoms from bacterial sinusitis may be difficult. The diagnosis of bacterial sinusitis should be considered if rhinorrhea or daytime cough persists without improvement for at least 10–14 days or if signs of more severe sinus involvement such as fever, facial pain, or facial swelling develop. There is no evidence that symptomatic treatment of the common cold alters the frequency of development of bacterial sinusitis.

Exacerbation of **asthma** is a relatively uncommon but potentially serious complication of colds. The majority of asthma exacerbations in children are associated with the common cold. There is no evidence that treatment of common cold symptoms prevents this complication.

Although not a complication, another important consequence of the common cold is the inappropriate use of antibiotics for these illnesses and the associated contribution to the problem of increasing antibiotic resistance of pathogenic respiratory bacteria. In 1998 in the United States, there were an estimated 25 million primary care office visits for the common cold, with 30% of these visits resulting in an inappropriate prescription for antibiotics.

PREVENTION. Chemoprophylaxis or immunoprophylaxis is generally not available for the common cold. Immunization or chemoprophylaxis against influenza may be useful for prevention of colds caused by this pathogen; however, influenza is responsible for only a small proportion of all colds. Vitamin C and echinacea do not prevent the common cold.

Interrupting the chain involved in the spread of virus by direct contact may prevent colds. In the hospital setting, prevention of transmission of respiratory viruses has been achieved by personnel wearing protective face shields to prevent hand-to-eye or hand-to-nose contact. Prevention of the spread of viruses by direct contact can be most readily accomplished by good handwashing by the infected individual and/or the susceptible contact.

Arnold JC, Singh KK, Spector SA, Sawyer MA: Human bocavirus: prevalence and clinical spectrum at a children's hospital. *CID* 2006;43:283–288.
Butler CC, Kinnersley P, Hood K, et al: Clinical course of acute infection of the upper respiratory tract in children: Cohort study. *Br Med J* 2003; 327:1088–1089.
Eccles R: Efficacy and safety of over-the-counter analgesics in the treatment of common cold and flu. *J Clin Pharm Ther* 2006;31:309–319.
Gonzales R, Malone DC, Maselli JH, et al: Excessive antibiotic use for acute respiratory infections in the United States. *Clin Infect Dis* 2001;33:757–762.
Hampton T: New guidelines released for managing cough. *JAMA* 2006;295:746–747.
Hedrick JA, Barzilai A, Behre U, et al: Zanamivir for treatment of symptomatic influenza A and B infection in children five to twelve years of age: A randomized controlled trial. *Pediatr Infect Dis J* 2000;19:410–417.
Hrastinger A, Dietz B, Bauer R, et al: Is there clinical evidence supporting the use of botanical dietary supplements in children? *J Pediatr* 2005:146: 311–317.
Jackson JL, Peterson C, Lesho E: A meta-analysis of zinc salts lozenges and the common cold. *Arch Intern Med* 1997;157:2373–2376.
Kusel MMH, de Klerk NH, Holt PG, et al: Role of respiratory viruses in acute upper and lower respiratory tract illness in the first year of life. *Pediatr Infect Dis J* 2006;25:680–686.
Simon HK, Weinkle DA: Over-the-counter medications. Do parents give what they intend to give? *Arch Pediatr Adolesc Med* 1997;151:654–656.
Taylor JA, Weber W, Standish L, et al: Efficacy and safety of Echinacea in treating upper respiratory tract infections in children: A randomized controlled trial. *JAMA* 2003;290:2824–2830.
Turner RB: The treatment of rhinovirus infections: Progress and potential. *Antiviral Res* 2001;49:1–14.

Chapter 377 ■ Sinusitis

Diane E. Pappas and J. Owen Hendley

Sinusitis is a common illness of childhood and adolescence with significant acute and chronic morbidity as well as the potential for serious complications. There are 2 types of acute sinusitis: viral and bacterial. The common cold produces a viral, self-limited rhinosinusitis (see Chapter 376). Approximately 0.5–2% of viral upper respiratory tract infections in children and adolescents are complicated by acute bacterial sinusitis. Some children with underlying predisposing conditions have chronic sinus disease that does not appear to be infectious. The means for appropriate diagnosis and optimal treatment of sinusitis remain controversial.

Both the **ethmoidal** and **maxillary** sinuses are present at birth, but only the ethmoidal sinuses are pneumatized (Fig. 377-1). The maxillary sinuses are not pneumatized until 4 yr of age. The **sphenoidal** sinuses are present by 5 yr of age, whereas the **frontal sinuses** begin development at age 7–8 yr and are not completely developed until adolescence. The ostia draining the sinuses are narrow (1–3 mm) and drain into the ostiomeatal complex in the middle meatus. The **paranasal sinuses** are normally sterile, maintained by the mucociliary clearance system.

ETIOLOGY. The bacterial pathogens causing acute bacterial sinusitis in children and adolescents include *Streptococcus pneumoniae*

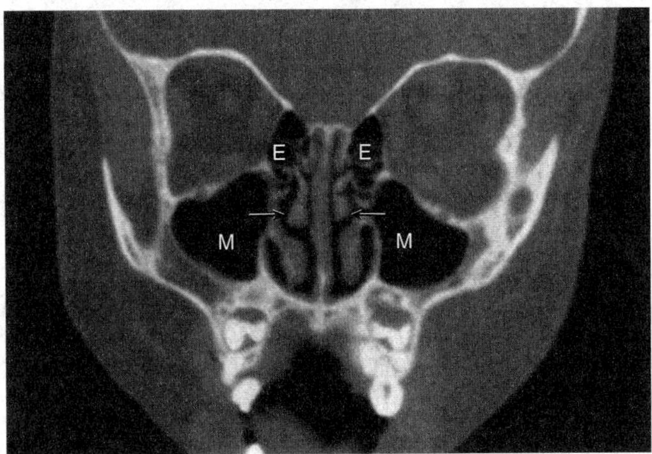

Figure 377-1. Coronal CT scan of normal 3 yr old child. *Arrows* point to middle meatus. E, ethmoid sinuses; M, maxillary sinuses. (From Isaacson G: Sinusitis in childhood. *Pediatr Clin North Am* 1996;43:1297–1317.)

(≈30%), nontypable *Haemophilus influenzae* (≈20%), and *Moraxella catarrhalis* (≈20%). Approximately 50% of *H. influenzae* and 100% of *M. catarrhalis* are β-lactamase positive. About 25% of *S. pneumoniae* may be penicillin resistant. *Staphylococcus aureus,* other streptococci, and anaerobes are uncommon causes of acute bacterial sinusitis in children. *H. influenzae,* α- and β-hemolytic streptococci, *M. catarrhalis, S. pneumoniae,* and coagulase-negative staphylococci are commonly recovered from children with **chronic sinus disease.**

EPIDEMIOLOGY. Acute bacterial sinusitis can occur at any age. Predisposing conditions include viral upper respiratory tract infections (associated with out-of-home daycare or a school-aged sibling), allergic rhinitis, and cigarette smoke exposure. Children with immune deficiencies particularly of antibody production (immunoglobulin G [IgG], IgG subclasses, IgA) [see Chapter 123], cystic fibrosis (see Chapter 400), ciliary dysfunction (see Chapter 401), abnormalities of phagocyte function, gastroesophageal reflux, anatomic defects (cleft palate), nasal polyps, and nasal foreign bodies (including nasogastric tubes) can develop chronic sinus disease. Immunosuppression for bone marrow transplantation or malignancy with profound neutropenia and lymphopenia predisposes to severe fungal (aspergillus, mucor) sinusitis, often with intracranial extension. Patients with nasotracheal intubation or nasogastric tubes may have obstruction of the sinus ostia and develop sinusitis with the multiple-drug resistant organisms of the intensive care unit (ICU).

PATHOGENESIS. Acute bacterial sinusitis typically follows a viral upper respiratory tract infection. Initially, the viral infection produces a viral rhinosinusitis; MRI evaluation of the paranasal sinuses demonstrates major abnormalities (mucosal thickening, edema, inflammation) of the paranasal sinuses in 68% of healthy children in the normal course of the common cold. Nose blowing has been demonstrated to generate sufficient force to propel nasal secretions into the sinus cavities. Bacteria from the nasopharynx that enter the sinuses are normally cleared readily, but during viral rhinosinusitis inflammation and edema may block sinus drainage and impair mucociliary clearance of bacteria. The growth conditions are favorable and high titers of bacteria are produced.

CLINICAL MANIFESTATIONS. Children and adolescents with sinusitis may present with nonspecific complaints, including nasal congestion, purulent nasal discharge (unilateral or bilateral), fever, and cough. Less common symptoms include bad breath (halitosis), a decreased sense of smell, and periorbital edema. Complaints of headache and facial pain are rare in children. Additional symptoms include maxillary tooth discomfort, pain or pressure exacerbated by bending forward, and hyposmia. Physical examination may reveal erythema and swelling of the nasal mucosa with purulent nasal discharge. Sinus tenderness may be detectable in adolescents and adults. Transillumination reveals an opaque sinus that transmits light poorly.

DIAGNOSIS. The clinical diagnosis of acute bacterial sinusitis is based solely on history. Persistent symptoms of upper respiratory tract infection, including nasal discharge and cough, for >10–14 days without improvement, or severe respiratory symptoms, including temperature of at least 102°F (39°C) and purulent nasal discharge for 3–4 consecutive days, are suggestive of a complicating acute bacterial sinusitis. Bacteria are recovered from maxillary sinus aspirates in 70% of children with such persistent or severe symptoms studied. Children with chronic sinusitis have a history of persistent respiratory symptoms, including cough, nasal discharge, or nasal congestion, lasting >90 days.

Sinus aspirate culture is the only accurate method of diagnosis but is not practical for routine use for immunocompetent patients. It may be a necessary procedure for immunosuppressed patients with suspected fungal sinusitis. In adults, *rigid nasal endoscopy* is a less invasive method for obtaining culture material from the sinus but detects a great excess of positive cultures compared to aspirates. *Transillumination* of the sinus cavities may demonstrate the presence of fluid but cannot reveal whether it is viral or bacterial in origin. In children, transillumination is difficult to perform and is unreliable. Findings on radiographic studies (sinus plain films, CT scans) including opacification, mucosal thickening, or presence of an air-fluid level are not totally diagnostic (Fig. 377-2). Such findings can confirm the presence of sinus inflammation but cannot be used to differentiate between viral, bacterial, or allergic causes of inflammation.

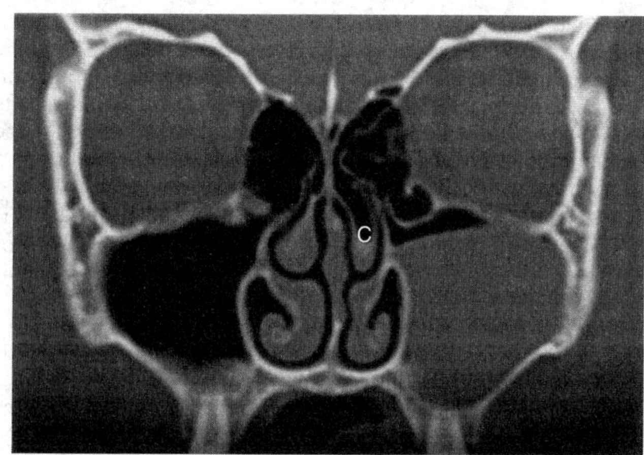

Figure 377-2. Acute left maxillary sinusitis with an air-fluid level. Note concha bullosa *(C)*. (From Isaacson G: Sinusitis in childhood. *Pediatr Clin North Am* 1996;43:1297–1317.)

Given the nonspecific clinical picture, differential diagnostic considerations include viral upper respiratory tract infection, allergic rhinitis, nonallergic rhinitis, and nasal foreign body. Viral upper respiratory tract infections are characterized by clear and usually nonpurulent nasal discharge, cough, and initial fever; symptoms do not usually persist beyond 10–14 days, although a few children (10%) have persistent symptoms even at 14 days. Allergic rhinitis can be seasonal; evaluation of nasal secretions should reveal significant eosinophilia.

TREATMENT. It is unclear whether antimicrobial treatment of clinically diagnosed acute bacterial sinusitis offers any substantial benefit. A randomized, placebo-controlled trial comparing 14 day treatment of children with clinically diagnosed sinusitis with amoxicillin, amoxicillin-clavulanate, or placebo found that antimicrobial therapy did not affect symptom resolution, duration of symptoms, or days missed from school. Guidelines from the American Academy of Pediatrics recommend antimicrobial treatment for acute bacterial sinusitis to promote resolution of symptoms and prevent suppurative complications, although 50–60% of children with acute bacterial sinusitis recover without antimicrobial therapy. Initial therapy with amoxicillin (45 mg/kg/day) is adequate for the majority of children with uncomplicated acute bacterial sinusitis. Alternative treatments for the penicillin-allergic patient include trimethoprim-sulfamethoxazole, cefuroxime axetil, cefpodoxime, clarithromycin, or azithromycin. For children with risk factors (antibiotic treatment in the preceding 1–3 mo, daycare attendance, or age <2 yr) for the presence of resistant bacterial species, and for children who fail to respond to initial therapy with amoxicillin within 72 hr, treatment with "high dose" amoxicillin-clavulanate (80–90 mg/kg/day of amoxicillin and 6.4 mg/ kg/day of clavulanate) should be initiated. Azithromycin (or in older children, levofloxacin) is an alternative antibiotic. Failure to respond to this regimen necessitates referral to an otolaryngologist for further evaluation because maxillary sinus aspiration for culture and susceptibility testing may be necessary. The appropriate duration of therapy for sinusitis has yet to be determined; individualization of therapy is a reasonable approach, with treatment recommended for 7 days after resolution of symptoms.

Frontal sinusitis can rapidly progress to serious intracranial complications and necessitates initiation of parenteral ceftriaxone until substantial clinical improvement is achieved (Figs. 377-3 and 377-4). Treatment is then completed with oral antibiotic therapy.

The use of decongestants, antihistamines, mucolytics, and intranasal corticosteroids has not been adequately studied in children and is not recommended for the treatment of acute uncomplicated bacterial sinusitis. Likewise, saline nasal washes or nasal sprays may help to liquefy secretions and act as a mild vasoconstrictor, but the effects have not been systematically evaluated in children.

COMPLICATIONS. Because of the close proximity of the paranasal sinuses to the brain and eyes, serious orbital and/or intracranial complications can result from acute bacterial sinusitis and progress rapidly. Orbital complications, including *periorbital cellulitis* and *orbital cellulitis* (see Chapter 633), are most often secondary to acute bacterial ethmoiditis. Infection can spread directly through the lamina papyracea, the thin bone that forms the lateral wall of the ethmoidal sinus. Periorbital cellulitis produces erythema and swelling of the tissues surrounding the globe, whereas orbital cellulitis involves the intraorbital structures and produces proptosis, chemosis, decreased visual acuity, double vision and impaired extraocular movements, and eye pain. Evaluation should include CT scan of the orbits and sinuses with ophthalmology and otolaryngology consultations. Treatment with intravenous antibiotics should be initiated. Orbital cellulitis may require surgical drainage of the ethmoidal sinuses.

Intracranial complications can include epidural abscess, meningitis, cavernous sinus thrombosis, subdural empyema, and brain abscess (see Chapter 602). Children with altered mental status, nuchal rigidity, or signs of increased intracranial pressure (headache, vomiting) require immediate CT scan of the brain, orbits, and sinuses to evaluate for the presence of intracranial complications of acute bacterial sinusitis. Treatment with broad-spectrum intravenous antibiotics (usually cefotaxime or ceftriaxone combined with vancomycin) should be initiated immediately, pending culture and susceptibility results. In 50% the abscess is a polymicrobial infection. Abscesses may require surgical drainage. Other complications include osteomyelitis of the frontal bone (**Pott puffy tumor**), which is characterized by edema and swelling of the forehead (see Fig. 377-3), and **mucoceles,** which are chronic inflammatory lesions commonly located in the frontal sinuses that can expand, causing displacement of the eye with resultant diplopia. Surgical drainage is usually required.

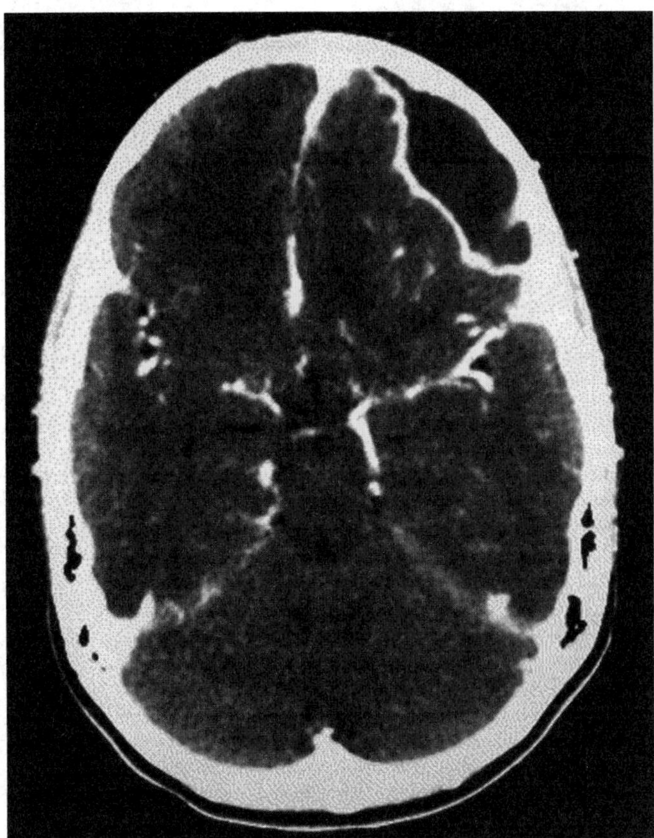

Figure 377-4. Axial plane contrast-enhanced CT scan of an 11 yr old obtunded female with a subfrontal lobe abscess secondary to frontal sinusitis. The CT scan demonstrates an eliptiform ring-enhancing fluid-filled cavity adjacent to the frontal lobe with contralateral shift of the midline. (From Parikh SR, Brown SM: Image-guided frontal sinus surgery in children. *Operative Tech Otolaryngol Head Neck Surg* 2004;15:37–41.)

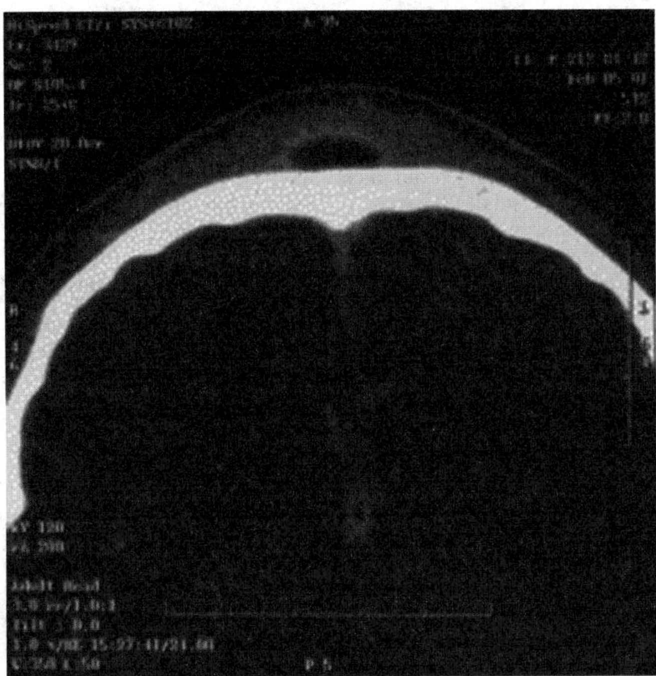

Figure 377-3. Axial plane contrast-enhanced CT scan of an 11 yr old male with a frontal subperiosteal abscess secondary to acute frontal sinusitis. The CT scan demonstrates a ring-enhancing midline fluid density over the frontal bone. (From Parikh SR, Brown SM: Image-guided frontal sinus surgery in children. *Operative Tech Otolaryngol Head Neck Surg* 2004;15:37–41.)

PREVENTION. Prevention is best accomplished by frequent handwashing and avoiding persons with colds. Because acute bacterial sinusitis can complicate influenza infection, prevention of influenza infection by yearly influenza vaccine will prevent some cases of complicating sinusitis. Immunization or chemoprophylaxis against influenza with oseltamivir or zanamivir may be useful for prevention of colds caused by this pathogen and the associated complications; influenza is responsible for only a small proportion of all colds.

American Academy of Pediatrics, Subcommittee on Management of Sinusitis and Committee on Quality Improvement: Clinical practice guideline: Management of sinusitis. *Pediatrics* 2001;108:798–808.

Arroll B, Kenealy T: Are antibiotics effective for acute purulent rhinitis? Systematic review and meta-analysis of placebo controlled randomised trials. *BMJ* 2006;333:279–280.

Brook I, Gooch WM III, Jenkins SG, et al: Medical management of acute bacterial sinusitis: Recommendations of a clinical advisory committee on pediatric and adult sinusitis. *Ann Otol Rhinol Laryngol* 2000;109:1–20.

Butler C, Kinnersley P, Hood K, et al: Clinical course of acute infection of the upper respiratory tract in children: Cohort study. Br Med J 2003;327:1088–1089.

Chan KH, Abzug MJ, Coffinet L, et al: Chronic rhinosinusitis in young children differs from adults: A histopathology study. *J Pediatr* 2004;144:206–212.

Don DM, Yellon RF, Casselbrant ML, et al: Efficacy of a stepwise protocol that includes intravenous antibiotic therapy for the management of chronic sinusitis in children and adolescents. *Arch Otolaryngol Head Neck Surg* 2001;127:1093–1098.

Garbutt JM, Goldstein M, Gellman E, et al: A randomized, placebo-controlled trial of antimicrobial treatment for children with clinically diagnosed acute sinusitis. *Pediatrics* 2001;107:619–24.

Germiller JA, Monin DL, Sparano AM, et al: Intracranial complications of sinusitis in children and adolescents and their outcomes. *Arch Otolaryngol Head Neck Surg* 2006;132:969–976.

Goldsmith AJ, Rosenfeld RM: Treatment of pediatric sinusitis. *Pediatr Clin North Am* 2003;50:413–426.

Isaacson G: Sinusitis in childhood. *Pediatr Clin North Am* 1996;43:1297–1317.

Kristo A, Uhari M, Luotonen J, et al: Paranasal sinus findings in children during respiratory infection evaluated with magnetic resonance imaging. *Pediatrics* 2003;111:e586–e589.

[No authors listed]: Antimicrobial treatment guidelines for acute bacterial rhinosinusitis. Sinus and Allergy Health Partnership. *Otolaryngol Head Neck Surg* 2000;123:5–31.

Parikh SR, Brown SM: Image-guided frontal sinus surgery in children. *Operative Tech Otolaryngol Head Neck Surg* 2004;15:37–41.

Phipps CD, Wood WE, Gibson WS, et al: Gastroesophageal reflux contributing to chronic sinus disease in children: A prospective analysis. *Arch Otolaryngol Head Neck Surg* 2000;126:831–836.

Piccirillo JF: Acute bacterial sinusitis. *N Engl J Med* 2004;351:902–910.

Slavin RG, Spector RL, Bernstein IL: The diagnosis and management of sinusitis: A practice parameter update. *J Allergy Clin Immunol* 2005;116: S13–S47.

Steele RW: Rhinosinusitis in children. *Curr Allergy Asthma Rep* 2006;6: 508–512.

Talbot G, Kennedy D, Scheld W, et al: Rigid nasal endoscopy versus sinus puncture and aspiration for microbiologic documentation of acute bacterial maxillary sinusitis. *Clin Infect Dis* 2001;33:1668–1675.

Chapter 378 ■ Acute Pharyngitis

Gregory F. Hayden and Ronald B. Turner

Upper respiratory tract infections account for a substantial portion of visits to pediatricians. Approximately ⅓ of such illnesses feature a sore throat as the primary symptom.

ETIOLOGY. The most important agents causing pharyngitis are viruses, (adenoviruses, coronaviruses, enteroviruses, rhinoviruses, respiratory syncytial virus [RSV], Epstein-Barr virus [EBV], herpes simplex virus [HSV], metapneumovirus) and group A β-hemolytic streptococcus (GABHS). Other organisms sometimes associated with pharyngitis include group C streptococcus, *Arcanobacterium haemolyticum, Francisella tularensis, Mycoplasma pneumoniae, Neisseria gonorrhoeae,* and *Corynebacterium diphtheriae.* Other bacteria, such as *Haemophilus influenzae* and *Streptococcus pneumoniae,* may be cultured from the throats of children with pharyngitis, but their role in causing pharyngitis has not been established.

EPIDEMIOLOGY. Viral upper respiratory tract infections are spread by close contact and occur most commonly in fall, winter, and spring. Streptococcal pharyngitis is uncommon before 2–3 yr of age, has a peak incidence in the early school years, and declines in late adolescence and adulthood. Illness occurs most often in winter and spring and spreads among siblings and classmates. Pharyngitis from group C streptococcus and *A. haemolyticum* occurs most frequently among adolescents and adults. Primary infection with HIV also manifests with pharyngitis and a mononucleosis-like syndrome.

PATHOGENESIS. Colonization of the pharynx by GABHS can result in either asymptomatic carriage or acute infection. The M protein is the major virulence factor of GABHS and facilitates resistance to phagocytosis by polymorphonuclear neutrophils. Type-specific immunity develops during infection and provides protective immunity to subsequent infection with that particular M serotype.

Scarlet fever is caused by GABHS that produces 1 of 3 streptococcal erythrogenic exotoxins (A, B, and C) that can induce a fine papular rash (see Chapter 182). Exotoxin A appears to be most strongly associated with scarlet fever. Exposure to each exotoxin confers specific immunity only to that toxin and, therefore, scarlet fever can occur up to 3 times.

CLINICAL MANIFESTATIONS. The onset of streptococcal pharyngitis is often rapid with prominent sore throat, absence of cough, and fever. Headache and gastrointestinal symptoms (abdominal pain, vomiting) are frequent. The pharynx is red, and the tonsils are enlarged and classically covered with a yellow, blood-tinged exudate. There may be petechiae or "doughnut" lesions on the soft palate and posterior pharynx, and the uvula may be red, stippled, and swollen. The anterior cervical lymph nodes are enlarged and tender. The incubation period is 2–5 days. Some patients demonstrate the additional stigmata of scarlet fever: circumoral pallor, strawberry tongue, and a red, finely papular rash that feels like sandpaper and resembles sunburn with goose pimples (see Chapter 182).

The onset of viral pharyngitis may be more gradual, and symptoms more often include rhinorrhea, cough, and diarrhea. A viral etiology is suggested by the presence of conjunctivitis, coryza, hoarseness, and cough. Adenovirus pharyngitis may feature concurrent conjunctivitis and fever (pharyngoconjunctival fever). Coxsackievirus pharyngitis may produce small (1–2 mm) grayish vesicles and punched-out ulcers in the posterior pharynx (herpangina), or small (3–6 mm) yellowish-white nodules in the posterior pharynx (acute lymphonodular pharyngitis). In EBV pharyngitis, there may be prominent tonsillar enlargement with exudate, cervical lymphadenitis, hepatosplenomegaly, rash, and generalized fatigue as part of the infectious mononucleosis syndrome (see Chapter 251). Primary HSV infections in young children often present as high fever and gingivostomatitis, but pharyngitis may be present (see Chapter 249).

The illnesses attributed to group C streptococcus and *A. haemolyticum* are generally similar to those caused by GABHS. Infections with *A. haemolyticum* are sometimes accompanied by a blanching, erythematous, maculopapular rash. Gonococcal pharyngeal infections are usually asymptomatic but can cause acute pharyngitis with fever and cervical lymphadenitis.

DIAGNOSIS. The goal of specific diagnosis is to identify GABHS infection. The clinical presentations of streptococcal and viral pharyngitis show considerable overlap. Physicians using clinical judgment often overestimate the likelihood of a streptococcal etiology, so laboratory testing is useful in identifying children who are most likely to benefit from antibiotic therapy. Throat culture remains an imperfect gold standard for diagnosing streptococcal pharyngitis. False-positive cultures can occur if other organisms are misidentified as GABHS, and children who are streptococcal carriers can also have positive cultures. False-negative cultures are attributed to a variety of causes, including inadequate throat swab specimens and patients' surreptitious use of antibiotics. The specificity of rapid tests to detect group A streptococcal antigen is high, so if a rapid test is positive, throat culture is unnecessary and appropriate treatment is indicated. Because rapid tests are generally less sensitive than culture, confirming a negative rapid test with a throat culture is recommended, especially if the clinical suspicion of GABHS is high. Special culture media and a prolonged incubation are required to detect *A. haemolyticum*. Viral cultures are often unavailable and are generally too expensive and slow to be clinically useful. Viral polymerase chain reaction (PCR) is more rapid and may be useful but is not always necessary. A complete blood cell (CBC) count showing many atypical lymphocytes and a positive slide agglutination (or "spot") test can help to confirm a clinical diagnosis of EBV infectious mononucleosis.

TREATMENT. Most untreated episodes of streptococcal pharyngitis resolve uneventfully in a few days, but early antibiotic therapy hastens clinical recovery by 12–24 hr. The primary benefit of treatment is the prevention of acute rheumatic fever, which is almost completely successful if antibiotic treatment is instituted within 9 days of illness. Antibiotic therapy should be started immediately without culture for children with symptomatic pharyngitis and a positive rapid streptococcal antigen test, clinical diagnosis of scarlet fever, a household contact with documented streptococcal pharyngitis, a past history of acute rheumatic fever, or a recent history of acute rheumatic fever in a family member.

A variety of antimicrobial agents are effective. GABHS remains universally susceptible to penicillin, which has a narrow spectrum and few adverse effects. Penicillin V is inexpensive and is given bid or tid for 10 days: 250 mg/dose for children and 500 mg/dose for adolescents and adults. Oral amoxicillin is often preferred for children because of taste and availability as chewable tablets. A once-daily 750 mg dose of amoxicillin given orally for 10 days may be as effective as 250 mg of penicillin given tid for 10 days. A shorter, 6 day course of oral amoxicillin (50 mg/kg/day divided bid: adult dose 1 gm bid) may be as effective as a 10 day course of penicillin V given tid. If the efficacy of these regimens is confirmed, the advantages will make amoxicillin a popular option. A single intramuscular dose of benzathine penicillin (600,000 U for children <27 kg [60 lb]; 1.2 million U for larger children and adults) or a benzathine-procaine penicillin G combination is painful but ensures compliance and provides adequate blood levels for more than 10 days. Reports that a high proportion of patients treated with oral or intramuscular penicillin remain culture positive after treatment deserve further evaluation. Erythromycin (erythromycin ethyl succinate 40 mg/kg/day divided bid, tid, or qid orally for 10 days; or erythromycin estolate 20–40 mg/kg/day divided bid, tid, or qid orally for 10 days; maximum dose for either drug 1 gm per 24 hr) is recommended for patients allergic to β-lactam antibiotics. Azithromycin offers the convenience of once-daily administration and a shorter length of therapy, which may improve compliance, but this drug is more expensive and the increased use of macrolide antibiotics has been correlated with increased rates of resistance to erythromycin among group A streptococci. Based on the proportion of cultures that remain positive for GABHS after therapy, cephalosporins appear to be as good as, or better than, penicillin, perhaps because these drugs are more effective in eradicating streptococcal carriage. Evidence is not sufficient to recommend shorter courses of cephalosporins for routine therapy at this time.

Follow-up cultures are unnecessary unless symptoms recur. Some treated patients continue to harbor GABHS in their pharynx and become streptococcal carriers. Carriage generally poses little risk to patients and their contacts, but it may confound the test results used to determine the etiology of subsequent episodes of sore throat. The treatment regimen most effective for eradicating streptococcal carriage is clindamycin, 20 mg/kg/day divided in 3 doses (adult dose: 150–450 mg tid or qid; maximum dose 1.8 gm/day) orally for 10 days.

Specific therapy is unavailable for most viral pharyngitis. On the basis of in vitro susceptibility data, oral penicillin is often suggested for patients with group C streptococcal isolates and oral erythromycin is recommended for patients with *A. haemolyticum*, but the clinical benefit of such treatment is uncertain.

Nonspecific, symptomatic therapy can be an important part of the overall treatment plan. An oral antipyretic/analgesic agent (acetaminophen or ibuprofen) may relieve fever and sore throat pain. Gargling with warm salt water is often comforting, and anesthetic sprays and lozenges (often containing benzocaine, phenol, or menthol) may provide local relief.

RECURRENT PHARYNGITIS. Recurrent streptococcal pharyngitis may represent relapse with an identical strain. If antibiotic compliance has been poor, intramuscular benzathine penicillin is suggested. The possibility of resistance should be considered if a nonpenicillin treatment such as erythromycin was given. Recurrences can also be caused by a different strain resulting from new exposures or may represent pharyngitis of another cause accompanied by streptococcal carriage. This last possibility is likely if the illnesses are mild and otherwise atypical for streptococcal pharyngitis. If GABHS is detected by repeat culture a few days after completing treatment, therapy to eliminate carriage is recommended. Prolonged pharyngitis (>1–2 wk) suggests another disorder such as neutropenia or recurrent fever syndromes.

Tonsillectomy lowers the incidence of pharyngitis for 1–2 yr among children with recurrent, culture-positive GABHS pharyngitis that has been severe and frequent (more than 7 episodes in the previous year, or more than 5 in each of the preceding 2 yr). Most children spontaneously have fewer episodes over time, however, so the anticipated clinical benefit must be balanced against the risks of anesthesia and surgery. Undocumented histories of recurrent pharyngitis are an inadequate basis for recommending tonsillectomy.

Complications and Prognosis. Viral respiratory tract infections may predispose to bacterial middle ear infections. The complications of streptococcal pharyngitis include local suppurative complications, such as parapharyngeal abscess, and later nonsuppurative illnesses, such as acute rheumatic fever (see Chapter 182.1) and acute postinfectious glomerulonephritis (see Chapter 511.1).

Prevention. Multivalent streptococcal vaccines based on M protein peptides are under development. Antimicrobial prophylaxis with daily oral penicillin prevents recurrent GABHS infections but is recommended only to prevent recurrences of acute rheumatic fever (see Chapter 182.1).

Bisno AL: Are cephalosporins superior to penicillin for treatment of acute streptococcal pharyngitis? *Clin Infect Dis* 2004;38:1535–1537.

Bisno AL: Acute pharyngitis. *N Engl J Med* 2001;344:205–211.

Bisno AL, Gerber MA, Gwaltney JM Jr, et al: Practice guidelines for the diagnosis and management of group A streptococcal pharyngitis. *Clin Infect Dis* 2002;35:113–125.

Bisno AL, Robin FA, Cleary PP, Dale JB: Prospects for a group A streptococcal vaccine: rationale, feasibility, and obstacles—report of a NIAID workshop. *Clin Infect Dis* 2005;41:1150–1156.

Casey JR, Pichichero ME: Meta-analysis of cephalosporin versus penicillin treatment of group A streptococcal tonsillopharyngitis in children. *Pediatrics* 2004;113:866–882.

Clegg HW, Ryan AG, Dallas SD, et al: Treatment of streptococcal pharyngitis with once daily compared with twice daily amoxicillin: a mono-inferiority trial. *Pediatr Infect Dis J* 2006;25:761–767.

Gerber MA: Diagnosis and treatment of pharyngitis in children. *Pediatr Clin N Amer* 2005;52:729–747.
Gerber MA, Shulman ST: Rapid diagnosis of pharyngitis caused by group A streptococci. *Clin Microbiol Rev* 2004;17:571–580.
Jaggi P, Shulman ST: Group A streptococcal infections. *Pediatr Rev* 2006;27:99–105.
Martin JM, Green M: Group A streptococcus. *Semin Pediatr Infect Dis* 2006;3:140–148.
McIsaac WJ, Kellner JD, Aufricht P, et al: Empirical validation of guidelines for the management of pharyngitis in children and adults. *JAMA* 2004;291:1587–1595.
Shulman ST, Gerber MA: So what's wrong with penicillin for strep throat? *Pediatrics* 2004;113:1816–1819.

Chapter 379 ■ Retropharyngeal Abscess, Lateral Pharyngeal (Parapharyngeal) Abscess, and Peritonsillar Cellulitis/Abscess

Diane E. Pappas and J. Owen Hendley

The neck contains deeply located lymph nodes including *retropharyngeal nodes* and *lateral pharyngeal nodes* that drain the mucosal surfaces of the upper airway and digestive tracts. These nodes lie within the *retropharyngeal space* (located between the pharynx and the cervical vertebrae and extending down into the superior mediastinum) and the *lateral pharyngeal space* (bounded by the pharynx medially, the carotid sheath posteriorly, and the muscles of the styloid process laterally), which are interconnected. The lymph nodes in these deep neck spaces communicate with each other, allowing bacteria from either cellulitis or node abscess to spread to other nodes. Infection of the nodes usually occurs as a result of extension from a localized infection of the oropharynx. Retropharyngeal abscess can result from penetrating trauma to the oropharynx, dental infection, and vertebral osteomyelitis. Once infected, the nodes may progress through three stages: *cellulitis, phlegmon,* and *abscess.* Infection in the retropharyngeal and lateral pharyngeal spaces may result in airway compromise or posterior mediastinitis, making timely diagnosis important.

RETROPHARYNGEAL AND LATERAL PHARYNGEAL ABSCESS. Retropharyngeal abscess occurs most commonly in children <3–4 yr of age, with boys affected more often than girls. Up to 67% of patients have a history of recent ear, nose, or throat infection. The retropharyngeal nodes involute after 5 yr of age and, therefore, infection in older children and adults is much less common.

Clinical manifestations of retropharyngeal abscess are nonspecific and include fever, irritability, decreased oral intake, and drooling. Neck stiffness, torticollis, and refusal to move the neck may also be present. The verbal child may complain of sore throat and neck pain. Other signs may include muffled voice, stridor, and respiratory distress. Physical examination may reveal bulging of the posterior pharyngeal wall, although this is present in <50% of infants with retropharyngeal abscess. Cervical lymphadenopathy may also be present. Lateral pharyngeal abscess commonly presents as fever, dysphagia, and a prominent bulge of the lateral pharyngeal wall, sometimes with medial displacement of the tonsil.

The *differential diagnosis* includes acute epiglottitis and foreign body aspiration. In the young child with limited neck mobility, meningitis must also be considered. Other possibilities include lymphoma, hematoma, and vertebral osteomyelitis.

Incision for drainage and culture of an abscessed node provides the definitive diagnosis, but CT can be useful in identifying the presence of a retropharyngeal or lateral pharyngeal abscess (Fig. 379-1). With CT scans, deep neck infections can be accurately identified and localized, but CT accurately identifies abscess formation in only 63% of patients. Soft tissue neck films taken during inspiration with the neck extended may show increased width or an air-fluid level in the retropharyngeal space. CT with contrast medium enhancement may reveal central lucency, ring enhancement, or scalloping of the walls of a lymph node. Scalloping of the abscess wall is thought to be a late finding and is predictive of abscess formation.

Retropharyngeal and lateral pharyngeal infections are most often polymicrobial; the usual pathogens include group A streptococcus (see Chapter 182), oropharyngeal anaerobic bacteria (see Chapter 210), and *Staphylococcus aureus* (see Chapter 180.1). Studies have documented an increased incidence of group A streptococcus recovered from such abscesses. Other pathogens may include *Haemophilus influenzae, Klebsiella,* and *Mycobacterium avium-intracellulare.*

Treatment options include intravenous antibiotics with or without surgical drainage. A 3rd-generation cephalosporin combined with ampicillin-sulbactam or clindamycin to provide anaerobic coverage is effective. Studies have shown that >50% of children with retropharyngeal or lateral pharyngeal abscess as identified by CT can be successfully treated without surgical drainage. Drainage is necessary, however, in the patient with respiratory distress or failure to improve with intravenous antibiotic treatment. The optimal duration of treatment is unknown, but therapy for several days with intravenous antibiotics until the patient has begun to improve followed by a course of oral antibiotic is typically utilized.

Complications of retropharyngeal or lateral pharyngeal abscess include significant upper airway obstruction, rupture leading to aspiration pneumonia, and extension to the mediastinum. Thrombophlebitis of the internal jugular vein and erosion of the carotid artery sheath may also occur.

An uncommon but characteristic infection of the parapharyngeal space is **Lemierre disease,** in which infection from the oropharynx extends to cause septic thrombophlebitis of the internal jugular vein and metastatic abscesses in the lungs (Fig. 379-2). The causative pathogen is *Fusobacterium necrophorum,* an anaerobic bacterial constituent of the oropharyngeal flora. The typical presentation is that of a previously healthy adolescent or young adult with a history of recent pharyngotonsillar disease who becomes acutely ill with fever and pulmonary symptoms. Chest radiography demonstrates multiple cavitary nodules, often bilateral, and often accompanied by pleural effusion. Blood culture may be positive. Treatment involves prolonged intravenous antibiotic therapy with penicillin or cefoxitin; surgical drainage of extrapulmonary metastatic abscesses may be necessary.

PERITONSILLAR CELLULITIS/ABSCESS. Peritonsillar cellulitis/abscess, which is relatively common compared to the deep neck infections, is caused by bacterial invasion through the capsule of the tonsil, leading to cellulitis and/or abscess formation in the surrounding tissues. The typical patient with a peritonsillar abscess is an adolescent with a recent history of acute pharyngotonsillitis. *Clinical manifestations* include sore throat, fever, trismus, and dysphagia. *Physical examination* reveals an asymmetric tonsillar bulge with displacement of the uvula. An asymmetric tonsillar bulge is diagnostic, but it may be poorly visualized because of trismus. CT is helpful for revealing the abscess. Group A streptococci and mixed oropharyngeal anaerobes are the most common pathogens, with more than 4 bacterial isolates per abscess typically recovered by needle aspiration.

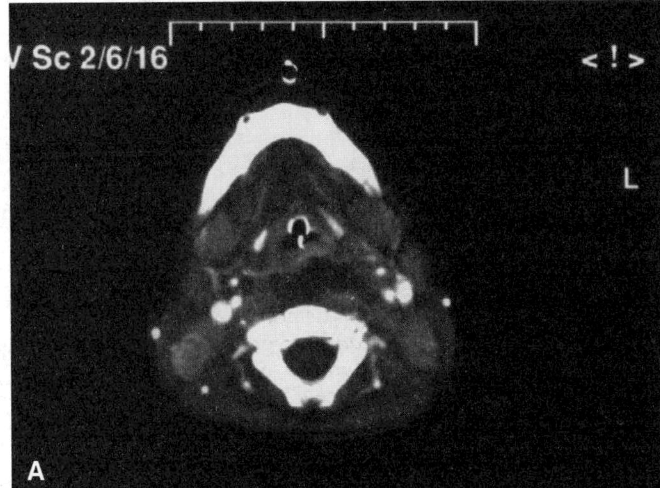

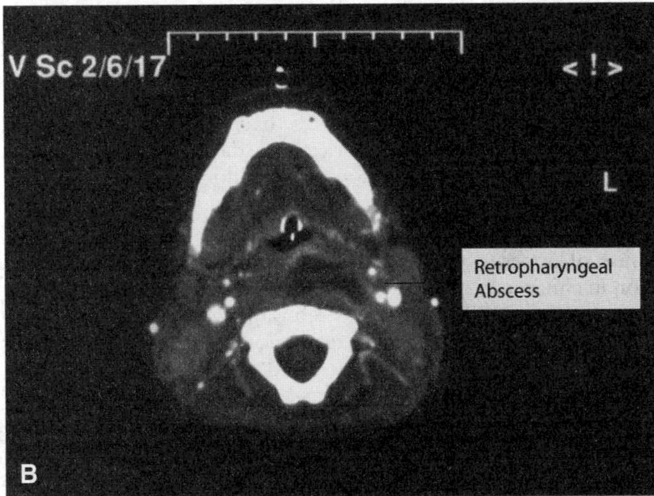

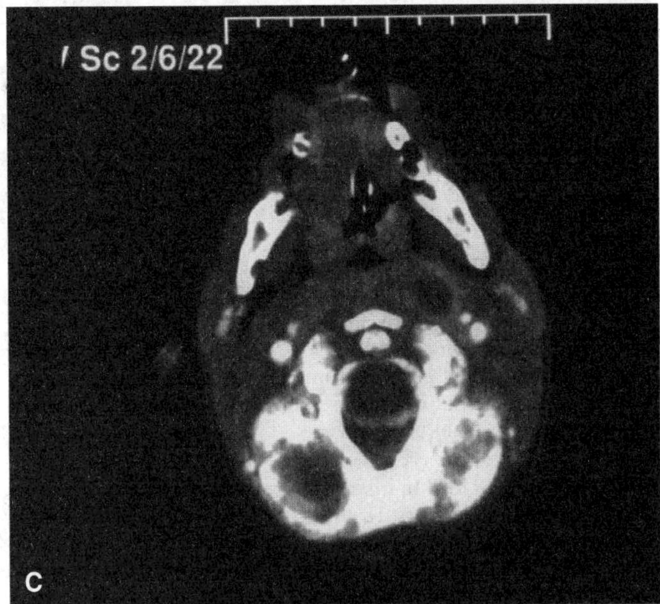

Figure 379-1. CT of retropharyngeal abscess. *A*, CT image at level of epiglottis. *B*, Sequential CT slice exhibiting ring-enhancing lesion. *C*, Further sequential CT slice demonstrating inferior extent of lesion. (From Philpott CM, Selvadurai D, Banerjee AR: Paediatric retropharyngeal abscess. *J Laryngol Otol* 2004;118:925.)

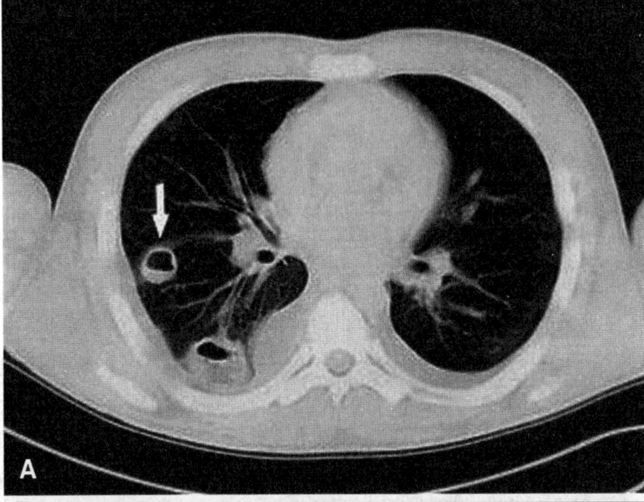

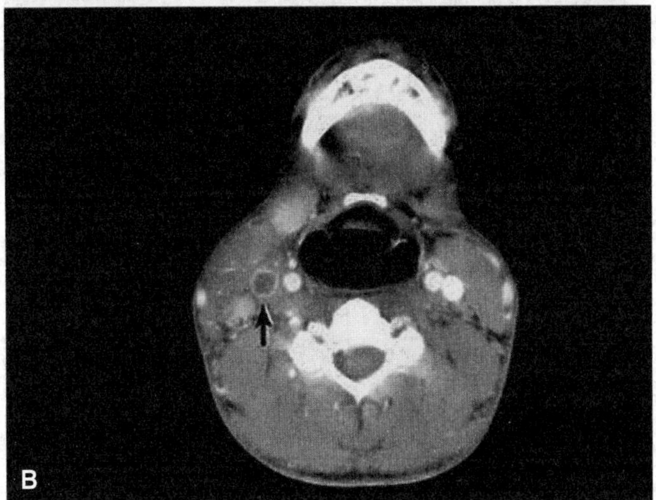

Figure 379-2. CT of Lemierre disease. *A*, CT demonstrating nodular appearance of pulmonary infiltrates *(arrow)*. *B*, CT of neck demonstrating thrombosis of right internal jugular vein *(arrow)*. (From Plymyer MR, Zoccola DC, Tallarita G: An 18 year old man presenting with sepsis following a recent pharyngeal infection. *Arch Pathol Lab Med* 2004;128:813. Reprinted with permission from Archives of Pathology & Laboratory Medicine. Copyright 2004. College of American Pathologists.)

Treatment includes surgical drainage and antibiotic therapy effective against group A streptococci and anaerobes. Surgical drainage may be accomplished through needle aspiration, incision and drainage, or tonsillectomy. Needle aspiration may involve aspiration of the superior, middle, and inferior aspects of the tonsil to locate the abscess. General anesthesia may be required for the uncooperative patient. Approximately 95% of peritonsillar abscesses resolve after needle aspiration and antibiotic therapy. A small percentage of these patients require a repeat needle aspiration. The 5% who fail to resolve after needle aspiration require incision and drainage. Tonsillectomy should be considered if there is failure to improve within 24 hours of antibiotic therapy and needle aspiration, history of recurrent peritonsillar abscess or recurrent tonsillitis, or complications from peritonsillar abscess. The feared, albeit rare, complication is rupture of the abscess, with resultant aspiration pneumonitis. There is a 10% recurrence risk for peritonsillar abscess.

Azimi PH, Grossman M: Irritability and neck stiffness in a five-month-old infant. *Pediatr Infect Dis J* 2001;20:724, 728–729.

Blotter JW, Yin L, Glyn M, et al: Otolaryngology consultation for peritonsillar abscess in the pediatric population. *Laryngoscope* 2000;110:1698–1701.

Conway JH, Nyquist AC, Goldson E: Posterior mediastinal abscess caused by invasive group A Streptococcus infection. *Pediatr Infect Dis J* 1996;15:547–549.

Coticchia JM, Getnick GS, Yun RD, et al: Age-, site-, and time-specific differences in pediatric deep neck abscesses. *Arch Otolaryngol Head Neck Surg* 2004;130:201–207.

Friedman NR, Mitchell RB, Pereira KD, et al: Peritonsillar abscess in early childhood: Presentation and management. *Arch Otolaryngol Head Neck Surg* 1997;123:630–632.

Herzon FS: Peritonsillar abscess: Incidence, current management practices, and a proposal for treatment guidelines. *Laryngoscope* 1995;105:1–17.

Jousimies-Somer H, Savolainen S, Mäkitie A, et al: Bacteriologic findings in peritonsillar abscesses in young adults. *Clin Infect Dis* 1993;16:S292–S298.

Kirse DJ, Roberson DW: Surgical management of retropharyngeal space infections in children. *Laryngoscope* 2001;111:1413–1422.

Lee SS, Schwartz RH, Bahadori RS: Retropharyngeal abscess: Epiglottitis of the new millennium. *J Pediatr* 2001;138:435–437.

Moreno S, Garcia Altozano J, Pinilla JC, et al: Lemierre's disease: Postanginal bacteremia and pulmonary involvement caused by Fusobacterium necrophorum. *Rev Infect Dis* 1989;11:319–324.

Philpott CM, Selvadurai D, Banerjee AR: Paediatric retropharyngeal abscess. *J Laryngol Otol* 2004;118:919–926.

Plymyer MR, Zoccola DC, Tallarita G: An 18 year old man presenting with sepsis following a recent pharyngeal infection. *Arch Pathol Lab Med* 2004;128:813–814.

Vural C, Gungor A, Comerci S: Accuracy of computerized tomography in deep neck infections in the pediatric population. *Am J Otolaryngol* 2003;24:143–148.

Weinberg E, Brodsky L, Stanievich J, et al: Needle aspiration of peritonsillar abscess in children. *Arch Otolaryngol Head Neck Surg* 1993;119:169–172.

Chapter 380 ■ Tonsils and Adenoids

Ralph F. Wetmore

ANATOMY. *Waldeyer ring* consists of lymphoid tissue that surrounds the opening of the oral and nasal cavities into the pharynx and includes the palatine tonsils, the pharyngeal tonsil or adenoid, lymphoid tissue surrounding the eustachian tube orifice in the lateral walls of the nasopharynx, the lingual tonsil at the base of the tongue, and scattered lymphoid tissue throughout the remainder of the pharynx but especially behind the posterior pharyngeal pillars and along the posterior pharyngeal wall. Lymphoid tissue located between the palatoglossal fold (anterior tonsillar pillar) and the palatopharyngeal fold (posterior tonsillar pillar) forms the *palatine tonsil.* This lymphoid tissue is separated from the surrounding pharyngeal musculature by a thick fibrous capsule. The *adenoid* is a single aggregation of lymphoid tissue that occupies the space between the nasal septum and the posterior pharyngeal wall. A thin fibrous capsule separates it from the underlying structures; the adenoid does not contain the complex crypts that are found in the palatine tonsils but rather more simple crypts. Lymphoid tissue at the base of the tongue forms the *lingual tonsil* that also contains simple tonsillar crypts.

NORMAL FUNCTION. Approximately 65% of the lymphocytes that make up the lymphoid tissue of Waldeyer ring are B lymphocytes, the remainder being either T lymphocytes or plasma cells (see Chapter 122). The immunologic role of the tonsils and adenoid is to induce secretory immunity and to regulate the production of the secretory immunoglobulins. Situated at the opening of the pharynx to the external environment, the tonsils and adenoid are in a position to provide primary defense against foreign matter. Deep crevices within tonsillar tissue form tonsillar crypts that are lined with squamous epithelium but have a concentration of lymphocytes at their bases. Lymphoid tissue of Waldeyer ring is most immunologically active between 4 and 10 yr of age, with a decrease after puberty. No major immunologic deficiency has been demonstrated after removal of either or both of the tonsils and adenoid.

PATHOLOGY

ACUTE INFECTION. Most episodes of acute pharyngotonsillitis are caused by viruses (see Chapter 378). Group A β-hemolytic streptococcus (GABHS) is the most common cause of bacterial infection in the pharynx (see Chapter 182). Additional bacterial organisms can include other β-hemolytic streptococcal species (group C), *Staphylococcus aureus,* gram-negative organisms, *Mycoplasma pneumoniae,* and, rarely, *Neisseria gonorrhoeae* and *Corynebacterium diphtheriae* (see Chapter 186). Oral candidiasis can occur in immunocompromised patients or children who have been treated chronically with antibiotics or inhaled steroids.

CHRONIC INFECTION. The tonsils and adenoid can be chronically infected by multiple microbes, which may include a high incidence of β-lactamase–producing organisms. Both aerobic species, such as streptococci and *Haemophilus influenzae,* and anaerobic species, such as *Peptostreptococcus, Prevotella,* and *Fusobacterium,* predominate. The tonsillar crypts can accumulate desquamated epithelial cells, lymphocytes, bacteria, and other debris, causing cryptic tonsillitis. With time, these cryptic plugs can calcify into tonsillar concretions or tonsillolith.

AIRWAY OBSTRUCTION. Both the tonsils and adenoid are a major cause of upper airway obstruction in children. Airway obstruction in children is typically manifested in sleep-disordered breathing, including obstructive sleep apnea, obstructive sleep hypopnea, and upper airway resistance syndrome (see Chapter 18).

TONSILLAR NEOPLASM. Rapid enlargement of one tonsil is highly suggestive of a tonsillar malignancy, typically lymphoma in children.

CLINICAL MANIFESTATIONS

ACUTE INFECTION. Symptoms of GABHS infection include odynophagia, dry throat, malaise, fever and chills, dysphagia, referred otalgia, headache, muscular aches, and enlarged cervical nodes. Signs include dry tongue, erythematous enlarged tonsils, tonsillar or pharyngeal exudate, palatine petechiae, and enlargement and tenderness of the jugulodigastric lymph nodes (Fig. 380-1; see also Chapters 182 and 378).

CHRONIC INFECTION. Children with chronic or cryptic tonsillitis frequently present with halitosis, chronic sore throats, foreign body sensation, or a history of expelling foul-tasting and smelling cheesy lumps. Examination may reveal tonsils of almost any size and, frequently, they contain copious debris within the crypts. Because the offending organism is not usually GABHS, streptococcal culture is usually negative.

AIRWAY OBSTRUCTION. In many children, the diagnosis of airway obstruction (see Chapters 18 and 370) can be made by history and physical examination. Daytime symptoms of airway obstruction, secondary to adenotonsillar hypertrophy, include chronic mouth breathing, nasal obstruction, hyponasal speech, hyposmia, decreased appetite, poor school performance, and, rarely, symptoms of right-sided heart failure. Nighttime symptoms consist of loud snoring, choking, gasping, frank apneas, restless sleep, abnormal sleep positions, somnambulism, night terrors, diaphoresis, enuresis, and sleep talking. Large tonsils are typically

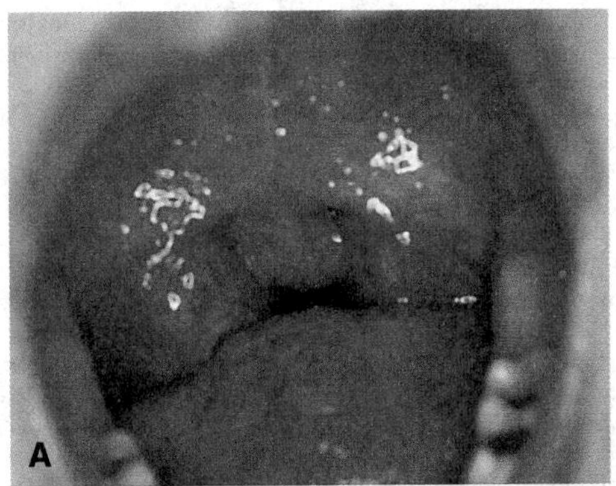

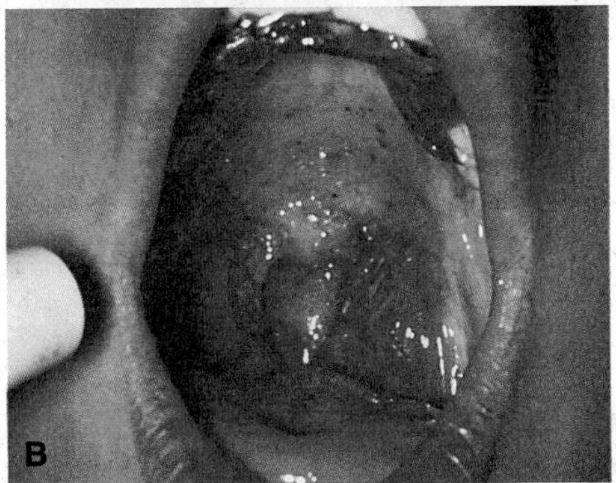

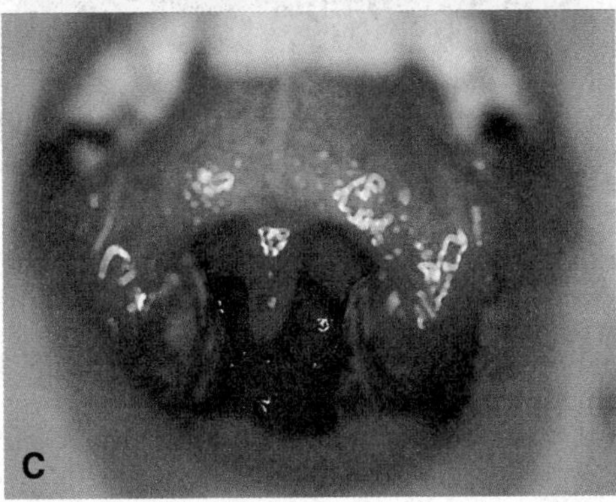

Figure 380-1. Pharyngotonsillitis. This common syndrome has a number of causative pathogens and a wide spectrum of severity. *A,* The diffuse tonsillar and pharyngeal erythema seen here is a nonspecific finding that can be produced by a variety of pathogens. *B,* This intense erythema, seen in association with acute tonsillar enlargement and palatal petechiae, is highly suggestive of group A β-streptococcal infection, though other pathogens can produce these findings. *C,* This picture of exudative tonsillitis is most commonly seen with either group A streptococcal or Epstein-Barr virus infection. (*B,* Courtesy of Michael Sherlock, MD, Lutherville, MD.) (From Yellon RF, McBride TP, Davis HW: Otolaryngology. In Zitelli BJ, Davis HW [editors]: *Atlas of Pediatric Physical Diagnosis,* 4th ed. Philadelphia, Mosby, 2002, p 852.)

seen on examination, although the absolute size may not be indicative of the degree of obstruction. The size of the adenoid tissue can be demonstrated on a lateral neck radiograph or with flexible endoscopy. Other signs that can contribute to airway obstruction include the presence of a craniofacial syndrome or hypotonia.

TONSILLAR NEOPLASM. The rapid unilateral enlargement of a tonsil, especially if accompanied by systemic signs of night sweats, fever, weight loss, and lymphadenopathy, is highly suggestive of a tonsillar malignancy. The diagnosis of a tonsillar malignancy should also be entertained if the tonsil appears grossly abnormal.

TREATMENT

MEDICAL MANAGEMENT. The treatment of acute pharyngotonsillitis is discussed in Chapter 378 and antibiotic treatment of GABHS in Chapter 182. Because co-pathogens such as staphylococci or anaerobes can produce β-lactamase that can inactivate penicillin, the use of cephalosporins or clindamycin may be more efficacious in the treatment of chronic throat infections. Children with cryptic tonsillitis may be able to express tonsillolith or debris manually with either a cotton-tipped applicator or a water jet. Chronically infected tonsillar crypts can be cauterized using silver nitrate.

TONSILLECTOMY. Tonsillectomy alone is usually performed for recurrent or chronic pharyngotonsillitis. Indications for surgery remain uncertain; there are large variations in surgical rates across countries: 115/10,000 children in the Netherlands; 65/10,000 in England; and 50/10,000 in the United States. One criteria is 7 or more throat infections treated with antibiotics in the preceding yr, 5 or more throat infections treated in each of the preceding 2 yr, or 3 or more throat infections treated with antibiotics in each of the preceding 3 yr. The American Academy of Otolaryngology–Head and Neck Surgery offers guidelines of 3 or more infections of tonsils and/or adenoids per yr despite adequate medical therapy while the Scottish Intercollegiate Tonsillectomy recommends 5 or more episodes per yr of tonsillitis with disabling symptoms and lasting for longer than a yr. Tonsillectomy has been shown to be effective in reducing the number of infections and the symptoms of chronic tonsillitis such as halitosis, persistent or recurrent sore throats, and recurrent cervical adenitis. In resistant cases of cryptic tonsillitis, tonsillectomy may be curative. Rarely in children, tonsillectomy may be indicated for biopsy of a unilaterally enlarged tonsil to exclude a neoplasm or to treat recurrent hemorrhage from superficial tonsillar blood vessels. Tonsillectomy has not been shown to offer clinical benefit over conservative treatment in children with mild symptoms.

ADENOIDECTOMY. Adenoidectomy alone may be indicated for the treatment of chronic nasal infection (chronic adenoiditis), chronic sinus infections that have failed medical management, and recurrent bouts of acute otitis media, including those in children with tympanostomy tubes who suffer from recurrent otorrhea. In addition, adenoidectomy may be helpful in children with chronic or recurrent otitis media with effusion. Adenoidectomy alone may be curative in the management of patients with nasal obstruction, chronic mouth breathing, and loud snoring suggestive of sleep-disordered breathing. Adenoidectomy may also be indicated for children in whom upper airway obstruction is suspected of causing craniofacial or occlusive developmental abnormalities.

TONSILLECTOMY AND ADENOIDECTOMY. The criteria for both tonsillectomy and adenoidectomy for recurrent infection are the same as those for tonsillectomy alone. The other major indication for performing both procedures together is upper airway obstruction secondary to adenotonsillar hypertrophy that results in sleep-disordered breathing, failure to thrive, craniofacial or occlusive developmental abnormalities, speech abnormalities, or, rarely, cor pulmonale.

COMPLICATIONS

ACUTE PHARYNGOTONSILLITIS. The 2 major complications of untreated GABHS infection are post-streptococcal glomerulonephritis and acute rheumatic fever (see Chapters 511 and 182).

PERITONSILLAR INFECTION. Peritonsillar infection can occur as either cellulitis or a frank abscess in the region superior and lateral to the tonsillar capsule (see Chapter 379). These infections usually occur in children with a history of recurrent tonsillar infection and are polymicrobial, including both aerobes and anaerobes. Unilateral throat pain, referred otalgia, drooling, and trismus are presenting symptoms. The affected tonsil is displaced down and medial by swelling of the anterior tonsillar pillar and palate. The diagnosis of an abscess can be confirmed by CT or by needle aspiration, the contents of which should be sent for culture. See Chapter 379 for treatment.

RETROPHARYNGEAL SPACE INFECTION. Infections in the retropharyngeal space develop in the lymph nodes that drain the oropharynx, nose, and nasopharynx. See Chapter 379.

PARAPHARYNGEAL SPACE INFECTION. Tonsillar infection can extend into the parapharyngeal space, causing symptoms of fever, neck pain and stiffness, and signs of swelling of the lateral pharyngeal wall and neck on the affected side. The diagnosis is confirmed by contrast medium enhanced CT, and treatment includes intravenous antibiotics and external incision and drainage if an abscess is demonstrated on CT (see Chapter 379). Septic thrombophlebitis of the jugular vein, **Lemierre syndrome,** presents with fever, toxicity, neck pain and stiffness, and respiratory distress due to multiple septic pulmonary emboli and is a complication of a parapharyngeal space or odontogenic infection from *Fusobacterium necrophorum.* Concurrent Epstein-Barr virus mononucleosis can be a predisposing event before the sudden onset of fever, chills, and respiratory distress in an adolescent patient. Treatment includes high-dose intravenous antibiotics (ampicillin-sulbactam, clindamycin, penicillin, or ciprofloxacin) and heparinization.

RECURRENT OR CHRONIC PHARYNGOTONSILLITIS. See Chapter 378.

CHRONIC AIRWAY OBSTRUCTION (SEE ALSO CHAPTER 18). Although rare, children with chronic airway obstruction from enlarged tonsils and adenoids can present with cor pulmonale.

The effects of chronic airway obstruction and mouth breathing on facial growth remain a subject of controversy. Studies of chronic mouth breathing, both in humans and animals, have shown changes in facial development, including prolongation of the total anterior facial height and a tendency toward a retrognathic mandible, the so-called adenoid facies. Adenotonsillectomy may reverse some of these abnormalities. Other studies have disputed these findings.

TONSILLECTOMY AND ADENOIDECTOMY. Bleeding may occur in the immediate postoperative period or be delayed after separation of the eschar. Swelling of the tongue and soft palate may lead to acute airway obstruction in the 1st few hours after surgery. Children with underlying hypotonia or craniofacial anomalies are at greater risk of suffering this complication. Dehydration from odynophagia is not uncommon in the 1st postoperative week. Rare complications include velopharyngeal insufficiency, nasopharyngeal or oropharyngeal stenosis, and psychologic problems.

American Academy of Otolaryngology–Head and Neck Surgery. (2000.) Clinical indicators: Tonsillectomy, adenoidectomy, adenotonsillectomy. Available at www.entlink.net/practice/products/indicators/tonsillectomy.html.

Brook I, Shah K: Bacteriology of adenoids and tonsils in children with recurrent adenotonsillitis. *Ann Otol Rhinol Laryngol* 2001;110:844–848.

de Serres LM, Derkay C, Sie K, et al: Impact of adenotonsillectomy on quality of life in children with obstructive sleep disorders. *Arch Otolaryngol Head Neck Surg* 2002;128:489–496.

Ebert CS, Drake AF: The impact of sleep-disordered breathing on cognition and behavior in children: A review and meta-synthesis of the literature. *Otolaryngol Head Neck Surg* 2004;131:814–1826.

Gozal D: Sleep-disordered breathing and school performance in children. *Pediatrics* 1998;102:616–620.

Johnson RF, Stewart MG, Wright CC: An evidence-based review of the treatment of peritonsillar abscess. *Otolaryngol Head Neck Surg* 2003:128:332–343.

Paradise JL, Bluestone CD, Colborn DK, et al: Tonsillectomy and adenotonsillectomy for recurrent throat infection in moderately affected children. *Pediatrics* 2002;110:7–15.

Ramirez S, Hild TG, Rudolph CN, et al: Increased diagnosis of Lemierre syndrome and other *Fusobacterium necrophorum* infections at a children's hospital. *Pediatrics* 2003;112:e380–e385.

Scottish Intercollegiate Guidelines Network. (1999.) Management of sore throat and indications for tonsillectomy. Available at www.sign.ac.uk/guidelines.

van Staaij BK, van den Akker EH, Rovers MM, et al: Effectiveness of adenotonsillectomy in children with mild symptoms of throat infections or adenotonsillar hypertrophy: Open, randomised controlled trial. *Br Med J* 2004;329:651.

Chapter 381 ■ Chronic or Recurrent Respiratory Symptoms

Thomas F. Boat and Thomas P. Green

Respiratory tract symptoms such as cough, wheeze, and stridor occur frequently or persist for long periods in a substantial number of children; others have persistent or recurring lung infiltrates with or without symptoms. Determining the cause of these chronic findings can be difficult because symptoms can be caused by a close succession of unrelated acute respiratory tract infections or by a single pathophysiologic process; there is a paucity of easily performed, specific diagnostic tests for many acute and chronic respiratory conditions. Pressure from the affected child's family for a quick remedy because of concern over symptoms related to breathing may complicate diagnostic and therapeutic efforts.

A systematic approach to the diagnosis and treatment of these children consists of assessing whether the symptoms are the manifestation of a minor problem or a life-threatening process; determining the most likely underlying pathogenic mechanism; selecting the simplest effective therapy for the underlying process, which may often be only symptomatic therapy; and carefully evaluating the effect of therapy. Failure of this approach to identify the process responsible or to effect improvement signals the need for more extensive and perhaps invasive diagnostic efforts, including bronchoscopy.

JUDGING THE SERIOUSNESS OF CHRONIC RESPIRATORY COMPLAINTS

Clinical manifestations suggesting that a respiratory tract illness may be life-threatening or associated with the potential for chronic disability are listed in Table 381-1. If none of these findings is detected, the chronic respiratory process is more likely to be benign. Active, well-nourished, and appropriately growing infants who present with intermittent noisy breathing but no other physical or laboratory abnormalities require only symptomatic treatment and parental reassurance. Benign-appearing but persistent symptoms are occasionally the harbinger of a serious lower respiratory tract problem and, conversely, a few children (those with infection-related asthma) have recurrent life-threat-

TABLE 381-1. Indicators of Serious Chronic Lower Respiratory Tract Disease in Children
Persistent fever
Ongoing limitation of activity
Failure to grow
Failure to gain weight appropriately
Clubbing of the digits
Persistent tachypnea and labored ventilation
Chronic purulent sputum
Persistent hyperinflation
Substantial and sustained hypoxemia
Refractory infiltrates on chest x-ray
Persistent pulmonary function abnormalities
Family history of heritable lung disease
Cyanosis and hypercarbia

ening episodes but few or no symptoms in the intervals. Repeated examinations over an extended period, both when the child appears healthy and when the child is symptomatic, are often helpful in sorting out the severity and chronicity of lung disease.

RECURRENT OR PERSISTENT COUGH

Cough is a reflex response of the lower respiratory tract to stimulation of irritant or cough receptors in the airways' mucosa. The most common cause in children is reactive airways (asthma). Because cough receptors also reside in the pharynx, paranasal sinuses, stomach, and external auditory canal, the source of a persistent cough may need to be sought beyond the lungs. Specific lower respiratory stimuli include excessive secretions, aspirated foreign material, inhaled dust particles or noxious gases, and an inflammatory response to infectious agents or allergic processes. Some of the conditions responsible for chronic cough are listed in Table 381-2.

Characteristics of cough that may aid in distinguishing its origin are presented in Table 381-3. Additional useful information may include a history of atopic conditions (asthma, eczema, urticaria, allergic rhinitis), a seasonal or environmental variation in frequency or intensity of cough, and a strong family history of atopic conditions, all suggesting an allergic cause; symptoms of malabsorption or family history indicative of cystic fibrosis; symptoms related to feeding, suggesting aspiration; a choking episode, suggesting foreign body aspiration; headache or facial edema associated with sinusitis; and a smoking history in older children and adolescents or the presence of a smoker in the house (Table 381-4).

Considerable information pertaining to the cause of chronic cough can be obtained during the physical examination. Posterior pharyngeal drainage combined with a nighttime cough suggests chronic upper airway disease such as sinusitis. An overinflated chest suggests chronic airway obstruction, as in asthma or cystic fibrosis. An expiratory wheeze, with or without diminished intensity of breath sounds, strongly suggests asthma or asthmatic bronchitis but may also be consistent with a diagnosis of cystic fibrosis, vascular ring, aspiration of foreign material, or pulmonary hemosiderosis. Careful auscultation during forced expiration may reveal expiratory wheezes that are otherwise undetectable and that are the only indication of underlying reactive airways. Coarse crackles suggest bronchiectasis, includ-

TABLE 381-2. Differential Diagnosis of Recurrent and Persistent Cough in Children
RECURRENT COUGH
Bronchial reactivity, including allergic asthma
Drainage from upper airways
Aspiration syndromes
Frequently recurring respiratory tract infections in immunocompetent or immunodeficient patients
Idiopathic pulmonary hemosiderosis
PERSISTENT COUGH
Hypersensitivity of cough receptors after infection
Reactive airways disease (asthma)
Chronic sinusitis
Bronchitis, tracheitis due to chronic infection, active or passive smoking
Bronchiectasis, including cystic fibrosis, primary ciliary dyskinesia, immunodeficiency
Foreign body aspiration
Recurrent aspiration owing to pharyngeal incompetence, tracheolaryngoesophageal cleft, tracheoesophageal fistula
Gastroesophageal reflux, with or without aspiration
Pertussis syndrome
Extrinsic compression of the tracheobronchial tract (vascular ring, neoplasm, lymph node, lung cyst)
Tracheomalacia, bronchomalacia
Endobronchial or endotracheal tumors
Endobronchial tuberculosis
Habit cough
Hypersensitivity pneumonitis
Fungal infections
Inhaled irritants, including tobacco smoke
Irritation of external auditory canal

TABLE 381-3. Characteristics of a Chronic Cough and Their Etiologic Significance

TYPE OF COUGH	LIKELY RESPONSIBLE CONDITION
Loose (discontinuous), productive	Bronchitis, asthmatic bronchitis, cystic fibrosis, bronchiectasis
Brassy	Tracheitis, habit cough
With stridor	Laryngeal obstruction, pertussis
Paroxysmal (with or without gagging)	Cystic fibrosis, pertussis syndrome, and foreign body
Staccato	Chlamydial pneumonitis
Nocturnal	Upper or lower respiratory tract allergic reaction, or both, sinusitis
Most severe on awaking in morning	Cystic fibrosis, bronchiectasis, chronic bronchitis
With vigorous exercise	Exercise-induced asthma, cystic fibrosis, bronchiectasis
Disappears with sleep	Habit cough, mild hypersecretory states such as in cystic fibrosis and asthma
Tight (wheezy)	Reactive airways

TABLE 381-4. Clinical Clues About Cough

CHARACTERISTIC	THINK OF
Staccato, paroxysmal	Pertussis, cystic fibrosis, foreign body, *Chlamydia* spp., *Mycoplasma* spp.
Followed by "whoop"	Pertussis
All day, never during sleep	Psychogenic, habit
Barking, brassy	Croup, psychogenic, tracheomalacia, tracheitis, epiglottitis
Hoarseness	Laryngeal involvement (croup, recurrent laryngeal nerve involvement)
Abrupt onset	Foreign body, pulmonary embolism
Follows exercise	Reactive airways disease
Accompanies eating, drinking	Aspiration, gastroesophageal reflux, tracheoesophageal fistula
Throat clearing	Postnasal drip
Productive (sputum)	Infection
Night cough	Sinusitis, reactive airways disease
Seasonal	Allergic rhinitis, reactive airways disease
Immunosuppressed patient	Bacterial pneumonia, *Pneumocystis carinii, Mycobacterium tuberculosis, Mycobacterium avium–intracellulare*, cytomegalovirus
Dyspnea	Hypoxia, hypercarbia
Animal exposure	*Chlamydia psittaci* (birds), *Yersinia pestis* (rodents), *Francisella tularensis* (rabbits), Q fever (sheep, cattle), hantavirus (rodents), histoplasmosis (pigeons)
Geographic	Histoplasmosis (Mississippi, Missouri, Ohio River Valley), coccidioidomycosis (southwest), blastomycosis (north and midwest)
Workdays with clearing on days off	Occupational exposure

From Kliegman RM, Greenbaum LA, Lyle PS: *Practical Strategies in Pediatric Diagnosis and Therapy*, 2nd ed. Philadelphia, Elsevier Saunders, 2004, p 19.

ing cystic fibrosis, but can also occur with an acute or subacute exacerbation of asthma. Clubbing of the digits is seen in most patients with bronchiectasis but in only a few other respiratory conditions with chronic cough (see Fig. 371-1 and Table 371-2). Tracheal deviation suggests foreign body aspiration or a mediastinal mass.

It is essential to allow sufficient examination time to detect a spontaneous cough. If not spontaneous, most children can cough on request by 4–5 yr of age. Asking the child to take a maximal breath and forcefully exhale repeatedly usually induces a cough reflex. Children who cough as often as several times a min with regularity are likely to have a habit (tic) cough. If the cough is loose, every effort should be made to obtain sputum; many older children can comply. It is sometimes possible to pick up small bits of sputum with a throat swab quickly inserted into the lower pharynx while the child coughs with the tongue protruding. Clear mucoid sputum is most often associated with an allergic reaction or asthmatic bronchitis. Cloudy (purulent) sputum suggests a respiratory tract infection but can also reflect increased cellularity (eosinophilia) due to an asthmatic process. Very purulent sputum is characteristic of bronchiectasis. Malodorous expectorations suggest anaerobic infection of the lungs. In cystic fibrosis, the sputum, even when purulent, is rarely foul smelling.

Laboratory tests may help in the evaluation of a chronic cough. Only sputum specimens containing alveolar macrophages should be interpreted as reflecting lower respiratory tract processes. Sputum eosinophilia suggests asthma, asthmatic bronchitis, or hypersensitivity reactions of the lung, but a polymorphonuclear cell response suggests infection; if sputum is unavailable, the presence of eosinophilia in nasal secretions also suggests atopic disease. If most of the cells in sputum are macrophages, postinfectious hypersensitivity of cough receptors should be suspected. Sputum macrophages can be stained for hemosiderin content, which is diagnostic of pulmonary hemosiderosis, or for lipid content, which in large amounts suggests, but is not specific for, repeated aspiration. Children whose coughs persist >6 wk should be tested for cystic fibrosis. Sputum culture is helpful for diagnosis of cystic fibrosis but less so for other conditions because throat flora may contaminate the sample.

Hematologic assessment may reveal anemia that is the result of pulmonary hemosiderosis or eosinophilia that accompanies asthma and other hypersensitivity reactions of the lung. Infiltrates on the chest radiograph suggest cystic fibrosis, bronchiectasis, foreign body, hypersensitivity pneumonitis, or tuberculosis. When asthma-equivalent cough is suggested, a trial of bronchodilator therapy may be diagnostic. If the cough does not respond to initial therapeutic efforts, more specific diagnostic procedures may be indicated, including an immunologic or allergic evaluation, chest and paranasal sinus imaging, esophagograms, tests for gastroesophageal reflux, special microbiologic studies including rapid viral testing, evaluation of ciliary morphologic features, and bronchoscopy.

Habit cough ("psychogenic cough" or "cough tic") must be considered in any child with a cough that has lasted for weeks or months, that has been refractory to treatment, and that disappears with sleep or with distraction. Typically the cough is abrupt and loud, and has a harsh, honking, "barking" quality. A disassociation between the intensity of the cough and the child's affect is typically striking. This cough may be absent if the physician listens outside the examination room, but it will reliably appear immediately on direct attention to the child and the symptom. It typically begins with an upper respiratory infection but then lingers. The child misses many days of school because the cough disrupts the classroom. This disorder accounts for many unnecessary medical procedures and courses of medication. It is treatable with assurance that a pathologic lung condition is absent and that the child should resume full activity, including school. This assurance, together with speech therapy techniques that allow the child to reduce musculoskeletal tension in the neck and chest and that increase the child's awareness of the initial sensations that trigger cough, has been very successful. This approach does not depend on deception, unlike one technique that involves wrapping the *highly suggestive* child's chest with a bedsheet to "strengthen weakened muscles" until the coughing stops. Self-hypnosis is another successful therapy, often effective with 1 session. The designation "habit cough" is preferable to "psychogenic cough" because it carries no stigma and because most of these children do not have significant emotional problems. When the cough disappears, it does not re-emerge as another symptom. Nonetheless, other symptoms such as irritable bowel syndrome may be present in the patient or family.

FREQUENTLY RECURRING OR PERSISTENT STRIDOR

Stridor, a harsh, medium-pitched, inspiratory sound associated with obstruction of the laryngeal area or the extrathoracic trachea, is often accompanied by a croupy cough and hoarse voice. Stridor is most commonly observed in children with croup; foreign bodies and trauma can also cause acute stridor. A small number of children, however, acquire recurrent stridor or have persistent stridor from the 1st days or weeks of life (Table 381-5). Most congenital anomalies of large airways that produce stridor become symptomatic soon after birth. Increase of stridor when a child is supine suggests laryngomalacia or tracheomalacia. An accompanying history of hoarseness or aphonia suggests involvement of the vocal cords.

Physical examination for recurrent or persistent stridor is usually unrewarding, although changes in its severity and intensity due to changes of body position should be assessed. Anteroposterior and lateral roentgenograms, contrast esophagography, fluoroscopy, CT, and MRI are potentially useful diagnostic tools.

TABLE 381-5. Causes of Recurrent or Persistent Stridor in Children
RECURRENT
Allergic (spasmodic) croup
Respiratory infections in a child with otherwise asymptomatic anatomic narrowing of the large airways
Laryngomalacia
PERSISTENT
Laryngeal obstruction
Laryngomalacia
Papillomas, other tumors
Cysts and laryngoceles
Laryngeal webs
Bilateral abductor paralysis of the cords
Foreign body
Tracheobronchial disease
Tracheomalacia
Subglottic tracheal webs
Endotracheal, endobronchial tumors
Subglottic tracheal stenosis
Congenital
Acquired
Extrinsic masses
Mediastinal masses
Vascular ring
Lobar emphysema
Bronchogenic cysts
Thyroid enlargement
Esophageal foreign body
Tracheoesophageal fistulas
OTHER
Gastroesophageal reflux
Macroglossia, Pierre Robin syndrome
Cri-du-chat syndrome
Hysterical stridor
Hypocalcemia
Vocal cord paralysis
Chiari crisis

In most cases, direct observation by laryngoscopy is necessary for diagnosis. Undistorted views of the larynx are best obtained with fiberoptic laryngoscopy.

RECURRENT OR PERSISTENT WHEEZE

Parents frequently complain that their child "wheezes," when, in fact, they are reporting respiratory sounds that are audible without a stethoscope, produce palpable resonance throughout the chest, and occur most prominently in inspiration. Some of these children have stridor, although many have audible sounds when the supraglottic airway is incompletely cleared of feedings or secretions.

By contrast, true **wheezing** is a relatively frequent and particularly troublesome manifestation of obstructive *lower* respiratory tract disease in children. The site of obstruction may be anywhere from the intrathoracic trachea to the small bronchi or large bronchioles, but the sound is generated by turbulence in larger airways that collapse with forced expiration. Children <2–3 yr of age are especially prone to wheezing, because bronchospasm, mucosal edema, and accumulation of excessive secretions have a relatively greater obstructive effect on their smaller airways. In addition, the compliant airways in young children collapse more readily with active expiration. Isolated episodes of acute wheezing, such as may occur with bronchiolitis, are not uncommon, but wheezing that recurs or persists for >4 wk suggests other diagnoses (see Table 388-2). Most recurrent or persistent wheezing in children is the result of reactive airways disease. Nonspecific environmental factors such as cigarette smoke may be important contributors.

Frequently recurring or persistent wheezing starting at or soon after birth suggests a variety of other diagnoses, including congenital structural abnormalities involving the lower respiratory tract or tracheobronchomalacia. Wheezing that attends cystic fibrosis is most common in the 1st year of life. Sudden onset of severe wheezing in a previously healthy child should suggest foreign body aspiration.

Repeated examination may be required to verify a history of wheezing in a child with episodic symptoms and should be directed toward assessing air movement, ventilatory adequacy, and evidence of chronic lung disease, such as fixed overinflation of the chest, growth failure, and digital clubbing. Clubbing suggests chronic lung infection and is rarely prominent in uncomplicated asthma. Tracheal deviation from foreign body aspiration should be sought. It is essential to rule out wheezing secondary to congestive heart failure. Allergic rhinitis, urticaria, eczema, or evidence of ichthyosis vulgaris suggests asthma or asthmatic bronchitis. The nose should be examined for polyps, which may exist with allergic conditions or cystic fibrosis.

Sputum eosinophilia and elevated serum immunoglobulin E (IgE) levels suggest allergic reactions. An FEV_1 (forced expiratory volume in 1 sec) increase of 15% in response to bronchodilators is confirmatory of reactive airways. Specific microbiologic studies, special imaging studies of the airways and cardiovascular structures, diagnostic studies for cystic fibrosis, and bronchoscopy should be considered if the response is unsatisfactory.

RECURRENT AND PERSISTENT LUNG INFILTRATES

Radiographic lung infiltrates resulting from acute pneumonia usually resolve within 1–3 wk, but a substantial number of children, particularly infants, fail to completely clear infiltrates within a 4 wk period. These children may be febrile or afebrile and may display a wide range of respiratory symptoms and signs. Persistent or recurring infiltrates present a diagnostic challenge (Table 381-6).

Symptoms associated with chronic lung infiltrates in the 1st several weeks of life (but not related to neonatal respiratory distress syndrome) suggest infection acquired in utero or during descent through the birth canal. Early appearance of chronic infiltrates can also be associated with cystic fibrosis or congenital anomalies that result in aspiration or airway obstruction. A history of recurrent infiltrates, wheezing, and cough may reflect asthma, even in the 1st year of life.

TABLE 381-6. Diseases Associated with Recurrent, Persistent, or Migrating Lung Infiltrates Beyond the Neonatal Period
Asthma
Repeated aspiration
Hypersensitivity pneumonitis
Pulmonary hemosiderosis
Foreign body
Sickle cell disease
Cystic fibrosis
Congenital infection
Cytomegalovirus
Rubella
Syphilis
Acquired infection
Cytomegalovirus
Tuberculosis
HIV
Other viruses
Chlamydia
Mycoplasma, Ureaplasma
Pertussis
Fungal organisms
Pneumocystis carinii
Inadequately treated bacterial infection
Congenital anomalies
Lung cysts
Pulmonary sequestration
Bronchial stenosis
Vascular ring
Congenital heart disease with large left-to-right shunt
Aspiration
Pharyngeal incompetence (e.g., cleft palate)
Laryngotracheoesophageal cleft
Tracheoesophageal fistula
Gastroesophageal reflux
Foreign body
Lipid aspiration
Immunodeficiency, phagocytic deficiency
Humoral, cellular, combined immunodeficiency states
Chronic granulomatous disease and related phagocytic defects
Complement deficiency states
Allergy-hypersensitivity
Pulmonary hemosiderosis (cow's milk–related, other)
Asthma
Hypersensitivity pneumonitis (allergic alveolitis)
Cystic fibrosis
Primary ciliary dyskinesia (Kartagener syndrome)
Other bronchiectases
Sarcoidosis
Neoplasms (primary, metastatic)
Interstitial pneumonitis and fibrosis
Usual
Lymphoid (AIDS)
Genetic disorders of surfactant synthesis, secretion
Desquamative
Acute (Hamman-Rich)
Alveolar proteinosis
Pulmonary lymphangiectasia
α1-Antitrypsin deficiency
Drug-induced, radiation-induced inflammation and fibrosis
Collagen-vascular diseases
Eosinophilic pneumonias
Visceral larva migrans
Histiocytosis
Leukemia

One uncommon but characteristic syndrome appearing in the 1st year of life with recurrent lung infiltrates is pulmonary hemosiderosis related to cow's milk hypersensitivity or unknown causes. Children with a history of bronchopulmonary dysplasia frequently have episodes of respiratory distress attended by wheezing and new lung infiltrates. Recurrent pneumonia in a child with frequent otitis media, nasopharyngitis, adenitis, or dermatologic manifestations suggests an immunodeficiency state, complement deficiency, or phagocytic defect (see Chapters 123–126). Particular attention must be directed to the possibility that the infiltrates represent lymphocytic interstitial pneumonitis or opportunistic infection associated with HIV infection (see Chapter 273). A history of paroxysmal coughing in an infant suggests pertussis syndrome or cystic fibrosis. Persistent infiltrates, especially with loss of volume, in a toddler should suggest foreign body aspiration.

Overinflation and infiltrates suggest cystic fibrosis or chronic asthma. A "silent chest" with infiltrates should arouse suspicion of alveolar proteinosis, *Pneumocystis carinii* infection, genetic disorders of surfactant synthesis and secretion causing interstitial pneumonitis, or tumors. Growth should be carefully assessed to determine whether the lung process has had systemic effects, indicating substantial severity and chronicity as in cystic fibrosis or alveolar proteinosis. Cataracts, retinopathy, or microcephaly suggest in utero infection. Chronic rhinorrhea can be associated with atopic disease, cow's milk intolerance, cystic fibrosis, or congenital syphilis. The absence of tonsils and cervical lymph nodes suggests an immunodeficiency state.

Diagnostic studies should be performed selectively, based on information obtained from history and physical examination and on a thorough understanding of the conditions listed in Table 381-6. Cytologic evaluation of sputum, if available, may be helpful. Chest CT often provides more precise anatomic detail concerning the infiltrate. Bronchoscopy is indicated for detecting foreign bodies, congenital or acquired anomalies of the tracheobronchial tract, and obstruction by endobronchial or extrinsic masses. Bronchoscopy provides access to secretions that can be studied cytologically and microbiologically. Alveolar lavage fluid is diagnostic for alveolar proteinosis and persistent pulmonary hemosiderosis and may suggest aspiration syndromes. If all appropriate studies have been completed and the condition remains undiagnosed, lung biopsy may yield a definitive diagnosis.

Optimal medical or surgical treatment of chronic lung infiltrates frequently depends on a specific diagnosis, but chronic conditions may be self-limiting (severe and prolonged viral infections in infants); in these cases, symptomatic therapy may maintain adequate lung function until spontaneous improvement occurs. Helpful measures include inhalation and physical therapy for excessive secretions, antibiotics for bacterial infections, supplementary oxygen for hypoxemia, and maintenance of adequate nutrition. Because the lung of a young child has remarkable recuperative potential, normal lung function may ultimately be achieved with treatment despite the severity of pulmonary insult occurring in infancy or early childhood.

Anbar RD, Hall HR: Childhood habit cough treated with self-hypnosis. *J Pediatr* 2004;144:213–217.

Blager F, Gay M, Wood R: Voice therapy techniques adapted to treatment of habit cough: A pilot study. *J Commun Disord* 1988;21:393–400.

Chang AB, Newman RG, Carlin JB, et al: Subjective scoring of cough in children: Parent-completed vs child-completed diary cards vs an objective method. *Eur Respir J* 1998;11:462–466.

De Jongste JC, Shields MD: Cough 2: Chronic cough in children. *Thorax* 2003;58:998–1003.

del Rosario JF, Orenstein SR: Evaluation and management of gastroesophageal reflux and pulmonary disease. *Curr Opin Pediatr* 1996;8:209–215.

Hay AD, Schroeder K, Fahey T: Acute cough in children. *Br Med J* 2004;328:1062–1063.

Irwin RS, Madison JM: The diagnosis and treatment of cough. *N Engl J Med* 2000;343:1715–1721.

Mamlock R: A cost-effective approach to the diagnosis and treatment of the wheezing infant. *Allergy Asthma Proc* 1997;18:149–152.

Mancuso RF: Stridor in neonates. *Pediatr Clin North Am* 1996;43:1339–1356.

Martinez FD, Wright AL, Taussig LM, et al: Asthma and wheezing in the first six years of life. *N Engl J Med* 1995;332:133–138.

Morgan WJ, Taussig LM: The child with persistent cough. *Pediatr Rev* 1987;8:249–253.

Nogee LM: Alterations of SP-B and SP-C expression in neonatal lung disease. *Ann Rev Physiol* 2004;66:601–623.

Chapter 382 ■ Acute Inflammatory Upper Airway Obstruction (Croup, Epiglottitis, Laryngitis, and Bacterial Tracheitis)

Genie E. Roosevelt

GENERAL CONSIDERATIONS. Because airway resistance is inversely proportional to the 4th power of the radius, minor reductions in cross-sectional area due to mucosal edema or other inflammatory processes cause an exponential increase in airway resistance and a significant increase in the work of breathing. The larynx is composed of 4 major cartilages (epiglottic, arytenoid, thyroid, and cricoid cartilages, ordered from superior to inferior) and the soft tissues that surround them. The cricoid cartilage encircles the airway just below the vocal cords and defines the narrowest portion of the upper airway in children <10 yr of age.

Inflammation involving the vocal cords and structures inferior to the cords is called *laryngitis, laryngotracheitis,* or *laryngotracheobronchitis,* and inflammation of the structures superior to the cords (i.e., arytenoids, aryepiglottic folds ["false cords"], epiglottis) is called *supraglottitis.* The term **croup** refers to a heterogeneous group of mainly acute and infectious processes that are characterized by a barklike or brassy cough and may be associated with hoarseness, inspiratory stridor, and respiratory distress. **Stridor** is a harsh, high-pitched respiratory sound, which is usually inspiratory but it can be biphasic and is produced by turbulent airflow; it is not a diagnosis but a sign of upper airway obstruction (see Chapter 371). Croup typically affects the larynx, trachea, and bronchi. When the involvement of the larynx is sufficient to produce symptoms, they dominate the clinical picture over the tracheal and bronchial signs. Traditionally, a distinction has been made between spasmodic or recurrent croup and laryngotracheobronchitis. Some clinicians believe that spasmodic croup may have an allergic component and improves rapidly without treatment, whereas laryngotracheobronchitis is always associated with a viral infection of the respiratory tract. Others believe that the signs and symptoms are similar enough to consider them within the spectrum of a single disease.

382.1 • Infectious Upper Airway Obstruction

ETIOLOGY AND EPIDEMIOLOGY. Viral agents account for most acute infectious upper airway obstructions. The exceptions are diphtheria, bacterial tracheitis, and epiglottitis. The parainfluenza viruses (types 1, 2, and 3; see Chapter 256) account for ≈75% of cases; other viruses associated with this disease include influenza A and B, adenovirus, respiratory syncytial virus (RSV), and measles. Influenza A has been associated with severe laryngotracheobronchitis. *Mycoplasma pneumoniae* has rarely been isolated from children with croup and causes mild disease (see Chapter 220). Most patients with croup are between the ages of 3 mo and 5 yr, with the peak in the 2nd yr of life. The incidence of croup is higher in males; it occurs most commonly in the late fall and winter but may occur throughout the year. Recurrences are frequent from 3–6 yr of age and decrease with growth of the airway. Approximately 15% of patients have a strong family history of croup.

In the past, *Haemophilus influenzae* type b was the most commonly identified etiology of acute epiglottitis. Since the widespread use of the HiB vaccine, invasive disease due to *H. influenzae* type b in pediatric patients has been reduced by 80–90% (see Chapter 192). Therefore, other agents, such as *Streptococcus pyogenes, Streptococcus pneumoniae,* and *Staphylococcus aureus,* now represent a larger portion of pediatric cases of epiglottitis in vaccinated children. In the prevaccine era, the typical patient with epiglottitis due to *H. influenza* type b was 2–4 yr of age, although cases were seen in the 1st year of life and in patients as old as 7 yr of age. The typical patient with epiglottitis is an adult with a sore throat, although cases still do occur in underimmunized children; vaccine failures have been reported.

CLINICAL MANIFESTATIONS.

Croup (Laryngotracheobronchitis). Viruses most commonly cause croup, the most common form of acute upper respiratory obstruction. The term *laryngotracheobronchitis* refers to viral infection of the glottic and subglottic regions. Some clinicians use the term *laryngotracheitis* for the most common and most typical form of croup and reserve the term *laryngotracheobronchitis* for the more severe form that is considered an extension of laryngotracheitis associated with bacterial superinfection that occurs 5–7 days into the clinical course.

Most patients have an upper respiratory tract infection with some combination of rhinorrhea, pharyngitis, mild cough, and low-grade fever for 1–3 days before the signs and symptoms of upper airway obstruction become apparent. The child then develops the characteristic "barking" cough, hoarseness, and inspiratory stridor. The low-grade fever may persist, although temperatures may reach 39–40°C (102.2–104°F); some children are afebrile. Symptoms are characteristically worse at night and often recur with decreasing intensity for several days and resolve completely within a wk. Agitation and crying greatly aggravate the symptoms and signs. The child may prefer to sit up in bed or be held upright. Older children usually are not seriously ill. Other family members may have mild respiratory illnesses with laryngitis. Most young patients with croup progress only as far as stridor and slight dyspnea before they start to recover.

Physical examination may reveal a hoarse voice, coryza, normal to moderately inflamed pharynx, and a slightly increased respiratory rate. Patients vary substantially in their degree of respiratory distress. Rarely, the upper airway obstruction progresses and is accompanied by an increasing respiratory rate; nasal flaring; suprasternal, infrasternal, and intercostal retractions; and continuous stridor. Croup is a disease of the upper airway, and alveolar gas exchange is usually normal. Hypoxia and low oxygen saturation are seen only when complete airway obstruction is imminent. The child who is hypoxic, cyanotic, pale, or obtunded needs immediate airway management. Occasionally, the pattern of severe laryngotracheobronchitis is difficult to differentiate from epiglottitis, despite the usually more acute onset and rapid course of the latter.

Croup is a clinical diagnosis and does not require a radiograph of the neck. Radiographs of the neck may show the typical subglottic narrowing or "steeple sign" of croup on the posteroanterior view (Fig. 382-1). However, the "steeple sign" may be absent in patients with croup, may be present in patients without croup as a normal variant, and may occasionally be present in patients with epiglottitis. The radiographs do not correlate well with disease severity. Radiographs should be considered only after airway stabilization in children who have an atypical presentation or clinical course. Radiographs may be helpful in distinguishing between severe laryngotracheobronchitis and epiglottitis, but airway management should always take priority.

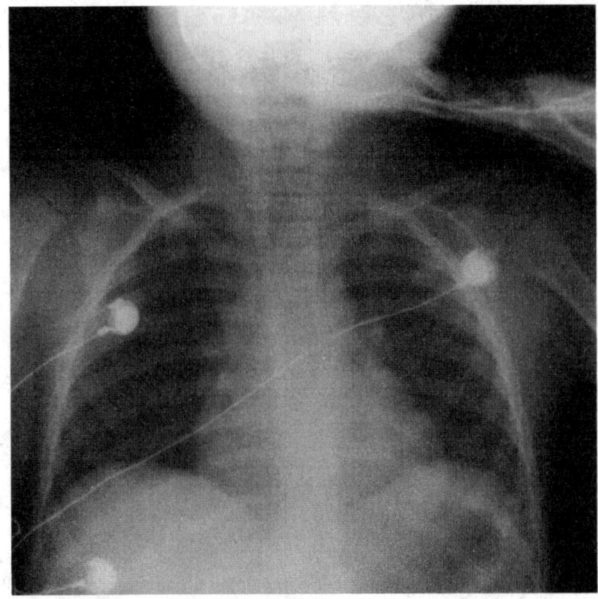

Figure 382-1. Radiograph of an airway of a patient with croup, showing typical subglottic narrowing ("steeple sign").

Acute Epiglottitis (Supraglottitis). This dramatic, potentially lethal condition is characterized by an acute potentially fulminating course of high fever, sore throat, dyspnea, and rapidly progressing respiratory obstruction. The degree of respiratory distress at presentation is variable. The initial lack of respiratory distress can deceive the unwary clinician; respiratory distress can also be the 1st manifestation, however. Often, the otherwise healthy child suddenly develops a sore throat and fever. Within a matter of hours, the patient appears toxic, swallowing is difficult, and breathing is labored. Drooling is usually present and the neck is hyperextended in an attempt to maintain the airway. The child may assume the tripod position, sitting upright and leaning forward with the chin up and mouth open while bracing on the arms. A brief period of air hunger with restlessness may be followed by rapidly increasing cyanosis and coma. Stridor is a late finding and suggests near-complete airway obstruction. Complete obstruction of the airway and death can ensue unless adequate treatment is provided. The barking cough typical of croup is rare. Usually, no other family members are ill with acute respiratory symptoms.

The diagnosis requires visualization of a large, "cherry red" swollen epiglottis by laryngoscopy. Occasionally, the other supraglottic structures, especially the aryepiglottic folds, are more involved than the epiglottis itself. In a patient in whom the diagnosis is certain or probable based on clinical grounds, laryngoscopy should be performed expeditiously in a controlled environment such as an operating room or intensive care unit. Anxiety-provoking interventions such as phlebotomy, intravenous line placement, placing the child supine, or direct inspection of the oral cavity should be avoided until the airway is secure. If epiglottitis is thought to be possible but not certain in a patient with acute upper airway obstruction, the patient can undergo lateral radiographs of the upper airway first. Classic radiographs of a child who has epiglottitis show the "thumb sign" (Fig. 382-2). Proper positioning of the patient for the lateral neck radiograph is crucial in order to avoid some of the pitfalls associated with interpretation of the film. Adequate hyperexten-

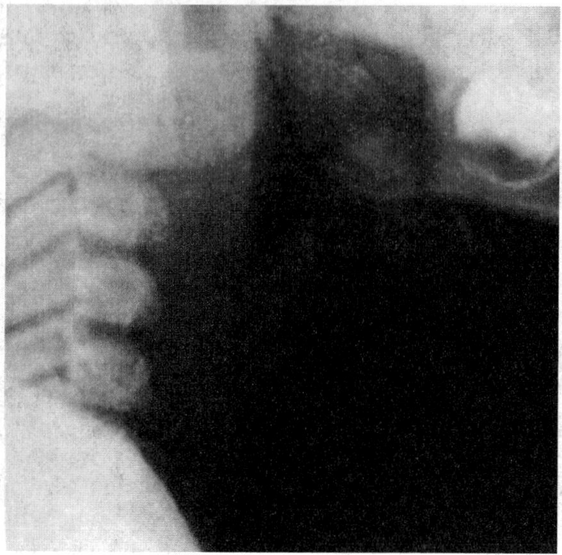

Figure 382-2. Lateral roentgenogram of the upper airway reveals the swollen epiglottis ("thumb sign").

sion of the head and neck is necessary. In addition, the epiglottis can appear to be round if the lateral neck is taken at an oblique angle. If the concern for epiglottitis still exists after the radiographs, direct visualization should be performed. A physician skilled in airway management and use of intubation equipment should accompany patients with suspected epiglottitis at all times. An older cooperative child may voluntarily open the mouth wide enough for a direct view of the inflamed epiglottis.

Establishing an airway by nasotracheal intubation or, less often, by tracheostomy is indicated in patients with epiglottitis, regardless of the degree of apparent respiratory distress, because as many as 6% of children with epiglottitis without an artificial airway die, compared with <1% of those with an artificial airway. No clinical features have been recognized that predict mortality. Pulmonary edema can be associated with acute airway obstruction. The duration of intubation depends on the clinical course of the patient and the duration of epiglottic swelling, as determined by frequent examination using direct laryngoscopy or flexible fiberoptic laryngoscopy. In general, children with acute epiglottitis are intubated for 2–3 days, because the response to antibiotics is usually rapid (see later). Most patients have concomitant bacteremia; occasionally, other infections are present, such as pneumonia, cervical adenopathy, or otitis media. Meningitis, arthritis, and other invasive infections with *H. influenzae* type b are rarely found in conjunction with epiglottitis.

Acute Infectious Laryngitis. Laryngitis is a common illness. Viruses cause most cases; diphtheria is an exception but is extremely rare in developed countries (see Chapter 186). The onset is usually characterized by an upper respiratory tract infection during which sore throat, cough, and hoarseness appear. The illness is generally mild; respiratory distress is unusual except in the young infant. Hoarseness and loss of voice may be out of proportion to systemic signs and symptoms. The physical examination is usually not remarkable except for evidence of pharyngeal inflammation. Inflammatory edema of the vocal cords and subglottic tissue may be demonstrated laryngoscopically. The principal site of obstruction is usually the subglottic area.

Spasmodic Croup. Spasmodic croup occurs most often in children 1–3 yr of age and is clinically similar to acute laryngotracheobronchitis, except that the history of a viral prodrome and fever in the patient and family are frequently absent. The cause is viral in some cases, but allergic and psychologic factors may be important in others. Laryngoscopy reveals pale, watery edema with preservation of the epithelium (unlike the erythematous edema and destruction of the epithelium of acute infectious laryngotracheobronchitis).

Occurring most frequently in the evening or nighttime, spasmodic croup begins with a sudden onset that may be preceded by mild to moderate coryza and hoarseness. The child awakens with a characteristic barking, metallic cough, noisy inspiration, and respiratory distress and appears anxious and frightened. The patient is usually afebrile. Usually, the severity of the symptoms diminishes within several hr, and the following day, the patient often appears well except for slight hoarseness and cough. Similar, but usually less severe, attacks without extreme respiratory distress may occur for another night or 2. Such episodes often recur several times. Spasmodic croup may represent more of an allergic reaction to viral antigens than direct infection, although the pathogenesis is unknown.

DIFFERENTIAL DIAGNOSIS. These 4 syndromes must be differentiated from one another and from a variety of other entities that can present as upper airway obstruction. **Bacterial tracheitis** is the most important differential diagnostic consideration. Diphtheritic croup is extremely rare in North America, although a major epidemic of diphtheria occurred in countries of the former Soviet Union beginning in 1990 from the lack of routine immunization of adults (see Chapter 186). Early symptoms of diphtheria include malaise, sore throat, anorexia, and low-grade fever. Within 2–3 days, pharyngeal examination reveals the typical gray-white membrane, which may vary in size from covering a small patch on the tonsils to covering most of the soft palate. The membrane is adherent to the tissue, and forcible attempts to remove it cause bleeding. The course is usually insidious, but respiratory obstruction can occur suddenly. Measles croup almost always coincides with the full manifestations of systemic disease and the course may be fulminant (see Chapter 243).

Sudden onset of respiratory obstruction can be caused by aspiration of a **foreign body** (see Chapter 384). The child is usually 6 mo–3 yr of age. Choking and coughing occur suddenly, usually without prodromal signs of infection, although children with a viral infection can also aspirate a foreign body. A **retropharyngeal** or **peritonsillar abscess** can mimic respiratory obstruction (see Chapter 379). CT scans of the upper airway are essential in evaluating these possibilities. Other possible causes of upper airway obstruction include extrinsic compression of the airway (laryngeal web, vascular ring) and intraluminal obstruction from masses (laryngeal papilloma, subglottic hemangioma); these tend to have chronic or recurrent symptoms.

Upper airway obstruction is occasionally associated with **angioedema** of the subglottic areas as part of anaphylaxis and generalized allergic reactions, edema after endotracheal intubation for general anesthesia or respiratory failure, hypocalcemic tetany, infectious mononucleosis, trauma, and tumors or malformations of the larynx. A croupy cough may be an early sign of asthma. Vocal cord dysfunction can also occur. Epiglottitis, with the characteristic manifestations of drooling or dysphagia and stridor, can also result from the accidental ingestion of very hot liquid.

COMPLICATIONS. Complications occur in ≈15% of patients with viral croup. The most common is extension of the infectious process to involve other regions of the respiratory tract, such as the middle ear, the terminal bronchioles, or the pulmonary parenchyma. Bacterial tracheitis may be a complication of viral croup rather than a distinct disease. If associated with *S. aureus,* toxic shock syndrome may develop. Pneumonia, cervical lymphadenitis, otitis media, or, rarely, meningitis or septic arthritis can occur in the course of epiglottitis. Mediastinal emphysema and pneumothorax are the most common complications of tracheotomy.

TREATMENT. The mainstay of treatment for children with **croup** is airway management. Treatment of the respiratory distress should take priority over any testing. Most children with either acute spasmodic croup or infectious croup can be managed safely at home. Mist has been traditionally used to treat croup. Given the risk of burns and the observation that cold night air is also beneficial led to the use of cool mist. There is no evidence to support the effectiveness of mist therapy. Children with both wheezing and croup may experience worsening of their bronchospasm with cool mist.

Nebulized racemic epinephrine is an accepted treatment for moderate or severe croup. The mechanism of action is believed to be constriction of the precapillary arterioles through the β-adrenergic receptors, causing fluid resorption from the interstitial space and a decrease in the laryngeal mucosal edema. Traditionally, racemic epinephrine, a 1 : 1 mixture of the d- and l-isomers of epinephrine, has been administered. A dose of 0.25–0.75 mL of 2.25% racemic epinephrine in 3 mL of normal saline can be used as often as every 20 min. Racemic epinephrine was initially chosen over the more active and more readily available l-epinephrine to minimize anticipated cardiovascular side effects such as tachycardia and hypertension. There is evidence that l-epinephrine (5 mL of 1 : 1,000 solution) is equally effective as racemic epinephrine and does not carry the risk of additional adverse effects. This information is both practical and important, because racemic epinephrine is not available outside the United States.

The indications for the administration of nebulized epinephrine include moderate to severe **stridor at rest,** the possible need for intubation, respiratory distress, and hypoxia. The duration of activity of racemic epinephrine is <2 hr. Therefore, observation is mandated. The symptoms of croup may reappear, but racemic epinephrine does not cause rebound worsening of the obstruction. Patients can be safely discharged home after a 2–3 hr period of observation provided they have no stridor at rest; have normal air entry, normal color, and normal level of consciousness; and have received steroids (see later). Nebulized epinephrine should still be used cautiously in patients with tachycardia, heart conditions such as tetralogy of Fallot, or ventricular outlet obstruction because of possible side effects.

The effectiveness of oral corticosteroids in viral croup is well established. Corticosteroids decrease the edema in the laryngeal mucosa through their anti-inflammatory action. Oral steroids are beneficial, even in mild croup, as measured by reduced hospitalization, shorter duration of hospitalization, and reduced need for subsequent interventions such as epinephrine administration. Most studies that demonstrated the efficacy of oral dexamethasone used a *single dose of 0.6 mg/kg*; a dose as low as 0.15 mg/kg may be just as effective. Intramuscular dexamethasone and nebulized budesonide have an equivalent clinical effect; oral dosing of dexamethasone is as effective as intramuscular administration. The only adverse effect described in the treatment of croup with corticosteroids was the development of *Candida albicans* laryngotracheitis in a patient who received dexamethasone, 1 mg/kg/24 hr, for 8 days. Corticosteroids should not be administered to children with varicella or tuberculosis (unless the patient is receiving appropriate antituberculosis therapy) because they worsen the clinical course.

Antibiotics are not indicated in croup. A helium-oxygen mixture (Heliox) may be effective in children with severe croup who may need intubation. Children with croup should be hospitalized for any of the following: progressive stridor, severe stridor at rest, respiratory distress, hypoxia, cyanosis, depressed mental status, poor oral intake, or the need for reliable observation.

Epiglottitis is a medical emergency and warrants immediate treatment with an **artificial airway** placed under controlled conditions, either in an operating room or intensive care unit. All patients should receive oxygen en route unless the mask causes excessive agitation. Racemic epinephrine and corticosteroids are ineffective. Cultures of blood, epiglottic surface, and, in selected cases, cerebrospinal fluid should be collected after airway stabilization. *Ceftriaxone, cefotaxime, or a combination of ampicillin and sulbactam* should be given parenterally, pending culture and susceptibility reports, because from 10–40% of *H. influenzae* type b cases are resistant to ampicillin. After insertion of the artificial airway, the patient should improve immediately, and respiratory distress and cyanosis should disappear. Epiglottitis resolves after a few days of antibiotics, and the patient may be extubated; antibiotics should be continued for 7–10 days. Chemoprophylaxis is not routinely recommended for household, child-care, or nursery contacts of patients with invasive *H. influenzae* type b infections, but careful observation is mandatory with prompt medical evaluation when exposed children develop a febrile illness. *Indications for rifampin prophylaxis* (20 mg/kg orally once a day for 4 days; maximum dose, 600 mg) for all household members are: (1) any contact <48 mo of age who is incompletely immunized; (2) any contact <12 mo who has not received the primary vaccination series; or (3) an immunocompromised child in the household.

Acute laryngeal swelling on an allergic basis responds to epinephrine (1 : 1,000 dilution in dosage of 0.01 mL/kg to a maximum of 0.5 mL/dose) administered subcutaneously or racemic epinephrine (dose of 0.25–0.75 mL of 2.25% racemic epinephrine in 3 mL of normal saline) [see Chapter 148]. Corticosteroids are frequently required (2–4 mg/kg/24 hr of prednisone). After recovery, the patient and parents should be discharged with a preloaded syringe of epinephrine to be used in emergencies. Reactive mucosal swelling, severe stridor, and respiratory distress unresponsive to mist therapy may follow endotracheal intubation for general anesthesia in children. Racemic epinephrine and corticosteroids are helpful.

Tracheotomy and Endotracheal Intubation. With the introduction of routine nasotracheal intubation or, less often, tracheotomy for epiglottitis, the mortality rate for epiglottis has dropped to almost zero. Both procedures should always be performed in an operating room or intensive care unit if time permits; prior intubation and general anesthesia greatly facilitate performing a tracheotomy without complications. The use of a nasotracheal tube that is 0.5–1.0 mm smaller than estimated by age is recommended to facilitate intubation and reduce long-term sequelae. The choice of procedure should be based on the local expertise and experience with the procedure and the postoperative care involved with each.

Endotracheal intubation or tracheotomy is required for most patients with bacterial tracheitis and all young patients with epiglottitis. It is rarely required for patients with laryngotracheobronchitis, spasmodic croup, or laryngitis. Severe forms of laryngotracheobronchitis that require intubation in a high proportion of patients have been reported during severe measles and influenza A virus epidemics. Assessing the need for these procedures requires experience and judgment because they should not be delayed until cyanosis and extreme restlessness have developed (see Chapters 64 and 69).

The endotracheal tube or tracheostomy must remain in place until edema and spasm have subsided and the patient is able to handle secretions satisfactorily. It should be removed as soon as possible, usually within a few days. Adequate resolution of epiglottic inflammation that has been accurately confirmed by fiberoptic laryngoscopy, permitting much more rapid extubation, often occurs within 24 hr. Racemic epinephrine and dexamethasone (0.5 mg/kg/dose every 6 hr as needed) may be useful in the treatment of croup associated with extubation.

PROGNOSIS. In general, the length of hospitalization and the mortality rate for cases of acute infectious upper airway obstruction increase as the infection extends to involve a greater portion of the respiratory tract, except in epiglottitis, in which the localized infection itself may prove to be fatal. Most deaths from croup are caused by a laryngeal obstruction or by the complications of tracheotomy. Rarely, fatal out-of-hospital arrests due to viral laryngotracheobronchitis have been reported, particularly in infants and those patients whose course has been complicated by bacterial tracheitis. Untreated epiglottitis has a mortality rate of 6% in some series, but if the diagnosis is made and appropriate treatment is initiated before the patient is moribund, the prognosis is excellent. The outcome of acute laryngotracheobronchitis, laryngitis, and spasmodic croup is also excellent. As a group, children who need to be hospitalized for croup have somewhat increased bronchial reactivity compared with normal children when tested several yr later, but the significance is uncertain.

Laryngotracheobronchitis

Bjornson CL, Klassen TP, Williamson J, et al: A randomized trial of a single dose of oral dexamethasone for mild croup. *N Engl J Med* 2004;351:1306–1313.

Fogel JM, Berg IJ, Gerber MA, et al: Racemic epinephrine in the treatment of croup: Nebulization alone versus nebulization with intermittent positive pressure breathing. *J Pediatr* 1982;101:1028–1031.

Geelhoed GC, Turner J, MacDonald WB: Efficacy of a small single dose of oral dexamethasone for outpatient croup: A double blind placebo controlled trial. *Br Med J* 1996;313:140–142.

Kristjansson S, Berg-Kelly K, Winso E: Inhalation of racemic adrenaline in the treatment of mild and moderately severe croup: Clinical symptom score and oxygen saturation measurements for evaluation of treatment effects. *Acta Pediatr* 1994;83:1156–1160.

Ledwith CA, Shea LM, Mauro RD: Safety and efficacy of nebulized racemic epinephrine in conjunction with oral dexamethasone and mist in the outpatient treatment of croup. *Ann Emerg Med* 1995;25:331–337.

Luria JW, Gonzalez-del-Rey JA, DiBiulio GA, et al: Effectiveness of oral or nebulized dexamethasone for children with mild croup. *Pediatr Adolesc Med* 2001;155:1340–1345.

Rittichier KK, Ledwith CA: Outpatient treatment of moderate croup with dexamethasone: Intramuscular versus oral dosing. *Pediatrics* 2000;106:1344–1348.

Scolnik D, Coates AL, Stephens D, et al: Controlled delivery of high vs low humidity vs mist therapy for croup in emergency departments. *JAMA* 2006;295:1274–1280.

Waisman Y, Klein BL, Boenning DA, et al: Prospective randomized double-blind study comparing L-epinephrine and racemic epinephrine aerosols in the treatment of laryngotracheitis. *Pediatrics* 1992;89:302–306.

Walner DL, Ouanounou S, Donnelly LF, et al: Utility of radiographs in the evaluation of pediatric upper airway obstruction. *Ann Otol Rhinol Laryngol* 1999;108:378–383.

Weber JE, Chudnofsky CR, Younger JG, et al: A randomized comparison of helium-oxygen mixture (Heliox) and racemic epinephrine for the treatment of moderate to severe croup. *Pediatrics* 2001;107:E96.

Epiglottitis

Adams WG, Deaver KA, Cochi SL, et al: Decline in childhood Haemophilus influenzae type b (HiB) in the HiB vaccine era. *JAMA* 1993; 269:221–226.

Frantz TD, Rasgon BM: Acute epiglottitis: Changing epidemiologic patterns. *Otolaryngol Head Neck Surg* 1993;109:457–460.

Gorelick MH, Baker MD: Epiglottitis in children, 1979 through 1992: Effects of *Haemophilus influenzae* type b immunization. *Arch Pediatr Adolesc Med* 1994;148:47–50.

Hickerson SL, Kirby RS, Wheeler JG, et al: Epiglottitis: A 9-year case review. *South Med J* 1996;89:487–490.

Kulick RM, Selbst SM, Baker MD, et al: Thermal epiglottitis after swallowing hot beverages. *Pediatrics* 1988;81:441–444.

Murrage KJ, Janzen VD, Ruby RR: Epiglottitis: Adult and pediatric comparisons. *J Otolaryngol* 1988;17:194–198.

Senior BA, Radkowski D, MacArthur C, et al: Changing patterns in pediatric epiglottis: A multi-institutional review, 1980 to 1992. *Laryngoscope* 1994;104:1314–1322.

382.2 • Bacterial Tracheitis

Bacterial tracheitis, an acute bacterial infection of the upper airway, does not involve the epiglottitis but, like epiglottitis and croup, is capable of causing life-threatening airway obstruction. *Staphylococcus aureus* is the most commonly isolated pathogen. *Moraxella catarrhalis*, non-typable *H. influenzae*, and anaerobic organisms have also been implicated. Historically, most patients were <3 yr of age, but in more recent cases series, the mean age has been between 5 and 7 yr. Incidence and severity do not differ by gender. Bacterial tracheitis often follows a viral respiratory infection (especially laryngotracheitis), so it may be considered a bacterial complication of a viral disease, rather than a primary bacterial illness. This life-threatening entity is more common than epiglottitis in vaccinated populations.

CLINICAL MANIFESTATIONS. Typically, the child has a brassy cough, apparently as part of a viral laryngotracheobronchitis. High fever and "toxicity" with respiratory distress may occur immediately or after a few days of apparent improvement. The patient can lie flat, does not drool, and does not have the dysphagia associated with epiglottitis. The usual treatment for croup (racemic epinephrine) is ineffective. Intubation or tracheostomy may be necessary, but in more recent case series, only 50–60% of patients required intubation for management; younger patients are more likely to need intubation. The major pathologic feature appears to be mucosal swelling at the level of the cricoid cartilage, complicated by copious thick, purulent secretions, sometimes causing pseudomembranes. Suctioning these secretions, although occasionally affording temporary relief, usually does not sufficiently obviate the need for an artificial airway.

DIAGNOSIS. The diagnosis is based on evidence of bacterial upper airway disease, which includes high fever, purulent airway secretions, and an absence of the classic findings of epiglottitis. X-rays are not needed but may show the classic findings (Fig. 382-3); purulent material is noted below the cords during endotracheal intubation (Fig. 382-4).

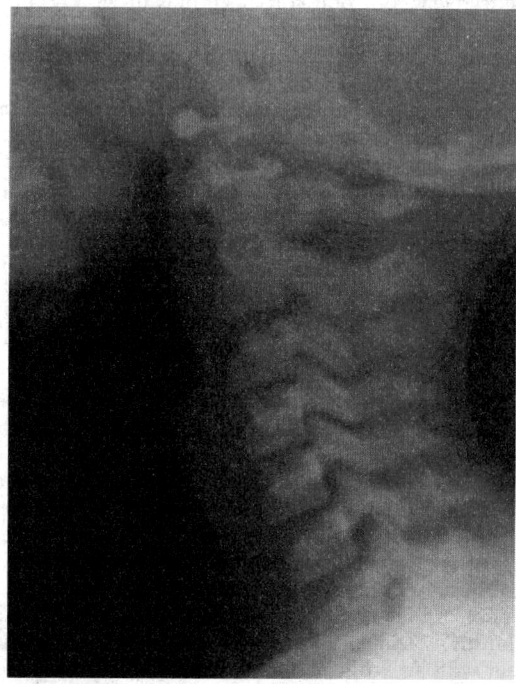

Figure 382-3. Lateral radiograph of the neck of a patient with bacterial tracheitis, showing pseudomembrane detachment in the trachea. (From Stroud RH, Friedman NR: An update on inflammatory disorders of the pediatric airway: Epiglottitis, croup, and tracheitis. *Am J Otolaryngol* 2001; 22:268–275. Photo courtesy of the Department of Radiology, University of Texas Medical Branch at Galveston.)

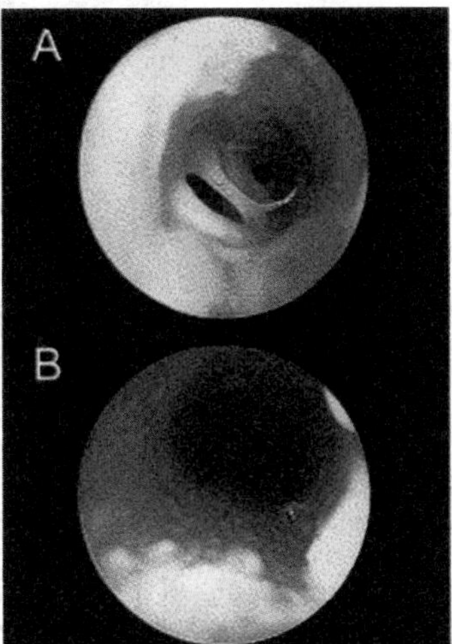

Figure 382-4. Thick tracheal membranes seen on rigid bronchoscopy. The supraglottis was normal. *A,* Thick adherent membranous secretions. *B,* The distal tracheobronchial tree is unremarkable. In contrast to croup, tenacious secretions are seen throughout the trachea, and in contrast to bronchitis, the bronchi are not affected. (From Salamone FN, Bobbitt DB, Myer CM, et al: Bacterial tracheitis reexamined: Is there a less severe manifestation? *Otolaryngol Head Neck Surg* 2004;131:871–876. © 2004 American Academy of Otolaryngology—Head and Neck Surgery Foundation, Inc.)

TREATMENT. Appropriate antimicrobial therapy, which usually includes antistaphylococcal agents, should be instituted in any patient whose course suggests bacterial tracheitis. When bacterial tracheitis is diagnosed by direct laryngoscopy or is strongly suspected on clinical grounds, an artificial airway should be strongly considered. Supplemental oxygen may be necessary.

COMPLICATIONS. Chest radiographs often show patchy infiltrates and may show focal densities. Subglottic narrowing and a rough and ragged tracheal air column can often be demonstrated radiographically. If airway management is not optimal, cardiorespiratory arrest can occur. Toxic shock syndrome has been associated with staphylococcal tracheitis (see Chapter 180.2).

PROGNOSIS. The prognosis for most patients is excellent. Patients usually become afebrile within 2–3 days of the institution of appropriate antimicrobial therapy, but prolonged hospitalization may be necessary. In recent years, there appears to be a trend toward a less morbid condition. With a decrease in mucosal edema and purulent secretions, extubation can be accomplished safely, and the patient should be observed carefully while antibiotics and oxygen therapy are continued.

Berstein T, Brilli R, Jacobs B: Is bacterial tracheitis changing? A 14-month experience in a pediatric intensive care unit. *Clin Infect Dis* 1998;27:458–462.

Brook I: Aerobic and anerobic microbiology of bacterial tracheitis in children. *Pediatr Emerg Care* 1997;13:16–18.

Donnelly LF: *Diagnostic Imaging Pediatrics.* Salt Lake City, Amirys, 2005, p 17.

Eckel HE, Widemann B, Damm M, et al: Airway endoscopy in the diagnosis and treatment of bacterial tracheitis in children. *Int J Pediatr Otorhinolaryngol* 1993;27:147–157.

Faden H: The dramatic change in the epidemiology of pediatric epiglottitis. *Pediatr Emerg Care* 2006;22:443–444.

Salamone FN, Bobbitt DB, Myer CM, et al: Bacterial tracheitis reexamined: Is there a less severe manifestation? *Otolaryngol Head Neck Surg* 2004;131:871–876.

Chapter 383 ■ Congenital Anomalies of the Larynx, Trachea, and Bronchi

Lauren D. Holinger

The larynx functions as a breathing passage, a valve to protect the lungs, and the primary organ of communication. Symptoms of laryngeal anomalies are those of airway obstruction, difficulty feeding, and abnormalities of phonation. With airway obstruction, the severity of the obstructing lesion determines the necessity for diagnostic procedures and surgical intervention. Obstructive symptoms vary from mild stridor to severe obstruction with episodes of apnea, cyanosis, suprasternal (tracheal tugging) and subcostal retractions, dyspnea, and tachypnea. Chronic obstruction may cause failure to thrive.

Congenital anomalies of the trachea and bronchi can create serious respiratory difficulties from the 1st minutes of life. These **intrathoracic** lesions typically cause expiratory wheezing or stridor, frequently masquerading as asthma. The expiratory wheezing contrasts to the inspiratory stridor caused by the **extrathoracic** lesions of congenital laryngeal anomalies, specifically laryngomalacia and bilateral vocal cord paralysis.

383.1 • Laryngomalacia

CLINICAL MANIFESTATIONS. Of congenital laryngeal anomalies in children with stridor, 60% are caused by laryngomalacia, the most common congenital laryngeal anomaly and the most frequent cause of stridor in infants and children. Typically, stridor is inspiratory, low pitched, and exacerbated by any exertion (crying, agitation, feeding), supine position, and viral infections of the upper airway. Stridor results from the collapse of supraglottic structures inward during inspiration. Symptoms usually appear in the first 2 wk of life and increase in severity for up to 6 mo, although gradual improvement can begin at any time. Laryngopharyngeal reflux is commonly associated with laryngomalacia.

DIAGNOSIS. The diagnosis is confirmed by flexible laryngoscopy in the office. When the work of breathing is moderate to severe, airway films and chest radiographs are indicated. With associated dysphagia, a contrast swallow study and esophagogram may be indicated. Because 15–60% of infants with laryngomalacia have synchronous airway anomalies, complete bronchoscopy is undertaken for patients with moderate to severe obstruction.

TREATMENT. Expectant observation is suitable for most infants because most symptoms resolve spontaneously. Laryngopharyngeal reflux is managed aggressively. For those few patients who have such severe obstruction that surgical intervention is unavoidable (patients with apparent life-threatening events, cor pulmonale, cyanosis, failure to thrive), endoscopic supraglottoplasty can be used to avoid tracheotomy.

383.2 • Congenital Subglottic Stenosis

Congenital subglottic stenosis is the 2nd most common cause of stridor. Stridor is biphasic or primarily inspiratory. Recurrent or persistent croup is typical. First symptoms often occur with a respiratory tract infection as edema and thickened secretions of a common cold narrow an already compromised airway (see Chapter 385.1).

383.3 • Vocal Cord Paralysis

Vocal cord paralysis is the 3rd most common congenital laryngeal anomaly producing stridor in infants and children. Congenital central lesions such as myelomeningocele, Arnold-Chiari malformation, and hydrocephalus are often associated. Paralysis can occur as a result of surgical correction of congenital cardiac anomalies or tracheoesophageal fistula.

Bilateral vocal cord paralysis typically produces airway obstruction manifested by high-pitched inspiratory stridor: a phonatory sound or inspiratory cry. Unilateral paralysis causes aspiration, coughing, and choking. The cry is weak and breathy, but stridor and other symptoms of airway obstruction are less common.

The diagnosis of vocal cord paralysis is made by awake flexible laryngoscopy. A thorough investigation for the underlying cause is indicated. Because of the association with other congenital lesions, evaluation includes neurology and cardiology consultations as well as diagnostic endoscopy of the larynx, trachea, and bronchi.

Vocal cord paralysis in infants usually resolves spontaneously within 6–12 mo. Bilateral paralysis may require temporary tracheotomy. For unilateral vocal cord paralysis with aspiration, the paralyzed vocal cord is injected laterally so that it touches the non-paralyzed cord medially, reducing aspiration and related complications.

383.4 • Congenital Laryngeal Webs and Atresia

Most congenital laryngeal webs are glottic with subglottic extension and associated subglottic stenosis (Fig. 383-1). The cry may be high pitched. Airway obstruction is not always present and may be related to the subglottic stenosis. Thick webs may be suspected in lateral radiographs of the airway. Diagnosis is made by direct laryngoscopy. Treatment may require only incision or dilation. Webs with associated subglottic stenosis are likely to require cartilage augmentation of the cricoid (laryngotracheal reconstruction).

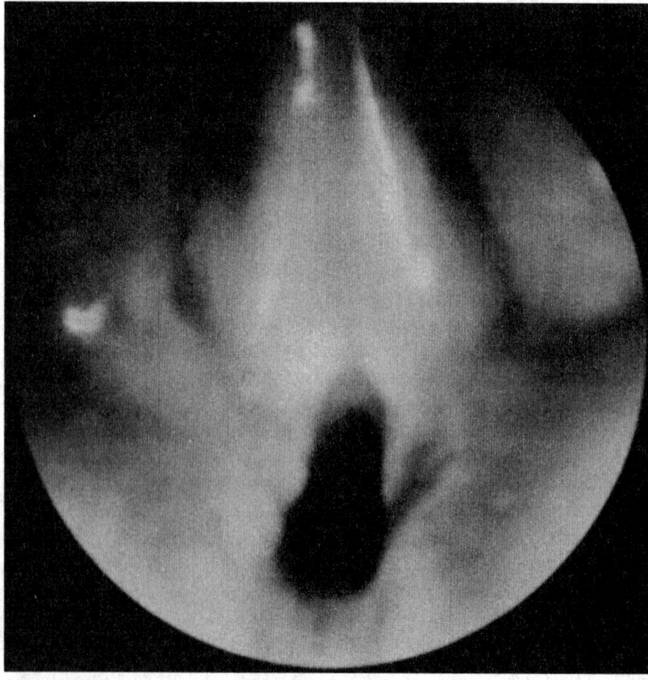

Figure 383-1. Anterior glottic web. Most of the membranous true vocal cords are involved. (From Milczuk HA, Smith JD, Everts EC: Congenital laryngeal webs: Surgical management and clinical embryology. *Int J Pediatr Otorhinolaryngol* 2000;52:4.)

Laryngeal atresia occurs as a complete glottic web and is commonly associated with tracheal agenesis and tracheoesophageal fistula. It is not compatible with long-term survival.

383.5 • Congenital Subglottic Hemangioma

Symptoms of airway obstruction typically occur in the 1st 2 mo of life. Stridor is biphasic but usually more prominent during inspiration. A barking cough, hoarseness, and symptoms of recurrent or persistent croup are typical. Chest and neck radiographs may show the characteristic asymmetric narrowing of the subglottic larynx. Treatment is discussed in Chapter 387.3.

383.6 • Laryngoceles and Saccular Cysts

A laryngocele is an abnormal air-filled dilation of the laryngeal saccule. It communicates with the laryngeal lumen, and when intermittently filled with air, causes hoarseness and dyspnea. A saccular cyst (congenital cyst of the larynx) is distinguished from the laryngocele in that its lumen is isolated from the interior of the larynx and it contains mucus, not air. A saccular cyst may be visible on radiography, but the diagnosis is made by laryngoscopy. Needle aspiration of the cyst confirms the diagnosis but rarely provides a cure. Endoscopic CO_2 laser excision may suffice, but external excision is often necessary.

383.7 • Posterior Laryngeal Cleft (PLC) and Laryngotracheoesophageal Cleft (LTEC)

The rare posterior laryngeal cleft (PLC) is characterized by deficiency in the midline of the posterior larynx. In severe cases, the cleft extends inferiorly into the cervical or thoracic trachea so there is no separation between the trachea and esophagus-laryngotracheoesophageal cleft (LTEC). Laryngeal clefts can occur in families and are likely to be associated with tracheal agenesis, tracheoesophageal fistula, and multiple congenital anomalies, as with G syndrome, Opitz-Frias syndrome, and Pallister-Hall syndrome.

Initial symptoms are those of aspiration and respiratory difficulties. The cry may be weak or absent. An esophagogram is done with extreme caution. Confirmation of the diagnosis is made by direct laryngoscopy and bronchoscopy. Stabilization of the airway is the 1st priority. Gastroesophageal reflux must be controlled, and a careful assessment for other congenital anomalies should be undertaken.

383.8 • Vascular and Cardiac Anomalies

The aberrant innominate artery is the most common cause of secondary tracheomalacia. Expiratory wheezing and cough occur and, rarely, reflex apnea or "dying spells." Surgical intervention is rarely necessary. Infants are treated expectantly because the problem is self-limited.

The term *vascular ring* is used to describe vascular anomalies that result from abnormal development of the aortic arch complex (see Chapter 432). The double aortic arch is the most common complete vascular ring, encircling both the trachea and esophagus, compressing both. With rare exception, these patients are symptomatic by 3 mo of age. Respiratory symptoms predominate, but dysphagia may be present. The diagnosis is established by barium esophagram, which shows a posterior indentation of the esophagus by the vascular ring. CT scan with contrast or MRI provides the surgeon the information needed (see Chapter 432).

Other vascular anomalies include the pulmonary artery sling, which also requires surgical correction. The most common open (incomplete) vascular ring is the aberrant right subclavian artery. Although common, it is usually asymptomatic and of academic interest only.

Congenital cardiac defects are likely to compress the left main bronchus or left lower trachea. Any condition that produces significant pulmonary hypertension increases the size of the pulmonary arteries, which, in turn, causes compression of the left main bronchus. Correction of the underlying pathology to relieve pulmonary hypertension relieves the airway compression.

383.9 • Tracheal Stenoses, Webs, and Atresia

Congenital soft tissue stenoses and thin webs are rare. Dilation may be all that is required. Long-segment congenital tracheal stenosis with complete tracheal rings typically presents in the 1st year of life, usually after a crisis has been precipitated by an acute respiratory illness. The diagnosis may be suggested by plain radiographs. CT with contrast delineates associated intrathoracic anomalies such as the pulmonary artery sling, which occurs in ⅓ of patients; ¼ have associated cardiac anomalies. Bronchoscopy is the best method to define the degree and extent of the stenosis.

With an adequate airway, surgical intervention is not necessary. When the severity of obstruction dictates surgical intervention, resection of the narrowed segment and re-anastomosis suffices for short segments. For long-segment congenital tracheal stenosis with complete tracheal rings, slide tracheoplasty or free tracheal autograft is undertaken with cardiopulmonary bypass.

Tracheal agenesis and atresia are rare anomalies that are incompatible with life. They are often associated with other congenital anomalies, particularly laryngeal conditions and tracheoesophageal fistula. The diagnosis is made by bronchoscopy in the newborn with severe respiratory distress.

383.10 • Foregut Cysts

The bronchogenic cyst, intramural esophageal cyst (esophageal duplication), and enteric cyst can all produce symptoms of respiratory obstruction and dysphagia. The diagnosis is suspected when chest radiographs or CT scan delineate the mass and, in the case of an enteric cyst, the associated vertebral anomaly. The treatment of all foregut cysts is surgical excision.

383.11 • Tracheomalacia and Bronchomalacia

See Chapter 386.

Backer CM, Mavroudis, C, Dunham ME, et al: Free tracheal autograft for long segment congenital tracheal stenosis. *J Pediatr Surg* 2000;35:813–819.

Civantos FJ, Holinger LD: Laryngoceles and saccular cysts in infants and children. *Arch Otolaryngol Head Neck Surg* 1992;118:296–300.

Holinger LD: Histopathology of congenital subglottic stenosis. *Ann Otol Rhinol Laryngol* 1999;108:101–111.

Hughes CA, Rezaee A, Ludemann JP, et al: Management of congenital subglottic hemangioma. *J Otolaryngol* 1999;28:223–228.

Mavroudis C, Backer CL: Vascular rings and pulmonary artery sling. In Mavroudis C, Backer CL (eds): *Pediatric Cardiac Surgery.* Chicago, Mosby, 1994, p 147.

Men S, Ikiz AO, Topcu I, et al: CT and virtual endoscopy findings in congenital laryngeal web. *Int J Pediatr Otorhinolaryngol* 2006;70(6): 1125–1127.

Milczuk HA, Smith JD, Everts EC: Congenital laryngeal webs: Surgical management and clinical embryology. *Int J Pediatr Otorhinolaryngol* 2000;52:1–9.

Moungthong G, Holinger LD: Laryngotracheoesophageal clefts. *Ann Otol Rhinol Laryngol* 1997;106:1002–1011.

Myer CM III, O'Connor DM, Cotton RT: Proposed grading system for subglottic stenosis based on endotracheal tube sizes. *Ann Otol Rhinol Laryngol* 1994;103:319–323.

Chapter 384 ■ Foreign Bodies of the Airway

Lauren D. Holinger

EPIDEMIOLOGY AND ETIOLOGY

Infants and toddlers use their mouths to explore their surroundings. Although there has been a decrease in childhood deaths from asphyxiation by ingested objects, the incidence of foreign body aspiration has not changed significantly. Most victims of foreign body aspiration are older infants and toddlers. Children <3 yr of age account for 73% of cases. Preambulatory toddlers may aspirate objects given to them by older siblings. One third of aspirated objects are nuts, particularly peanuts. Fragments of raw carrot, apple, dried beans, popcorn, and sunflower or watermelon seeds are also common, as are small toys or toy parts.

The most serious complication of foreign body aspiration is complete obstruction of the airway. Globular or round food objects such as hotdogs, grapes, nuts, and candies are the most frequent offenders. Hotdogs are rarely seen as airway foreign bodies since toddlers who choke on hotdogs asphyxiate on the spot unless treated immediately. Complete airway obstruction is recognized in the conscious child as sudden respiratory distress followed by inability to speak or cough.

CLINICAL MANIFESTATIONS

Three stages of symptoms may result from aspiration of an object into the airway:

1. **Initial event**—violent paroxysms of coughing, choking, gagging, and possibly airway obstruction occur immediately when the foreign body is aspirated.
2. **Asymptomatic interval**—the foreign body becomes lodged, reflexes fatigue, and the immediate irritating symptoms subside. This stage is most treacherous and accounts for a large percentage of delayed diagnoses and overlooked foreign bodies. It is during this 2nd stage that the physician may minimize the possibility of a foreign body accident, being reassured by the absence of symptoms that no foreign body is present.
3. **Complications**—obstruction, erosion, or infection develops to direct attention again to the presence of a foreign body. In this 3rd stage, complications include fever, cough, hemoptysis, pneumonia, and atelectasis.

A positive history must never be ignored. A negative history may be misleading. Choking or coughing episodes accompanied by wheezing are highly suggestive of an airway foreign body. Since nuts are the most common bronchial foreign body, the physician specifically questions the toddler's parents about nuts. If there is any history of eating nuts, bronchoscopy is carried out promptly.

Most airway foreign bodies lodge in a bronchus (right bronchus in ≈58% of cases); laryngeal or tracheal locations occur in ≈10% of cases. An esophageal foreign body can compress the

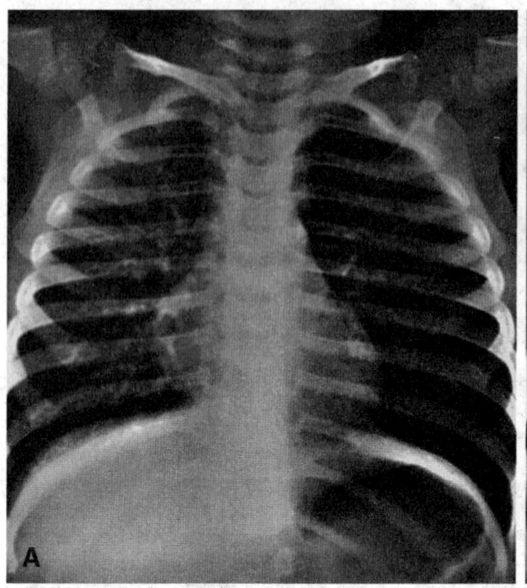

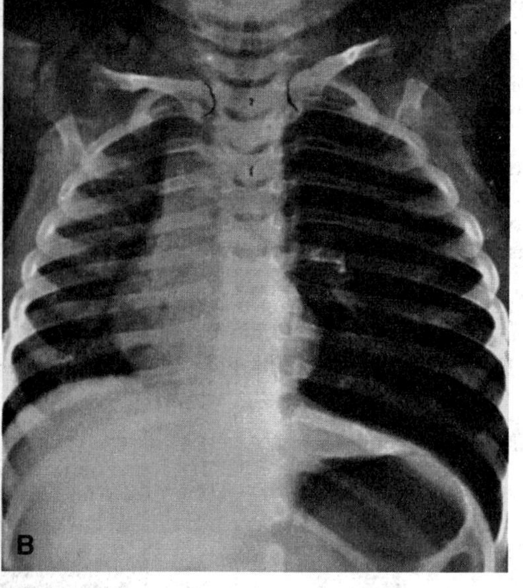

Figure 384-1. *A,* Normal inspiratory chest radiograph in a toddler with a peanut fragment in the left main bronchus. *B,* Expiratory radiograph of the same child showing the classic obstructive emphysema (air trapping) on the involved (left) side. Air leaves the normal right side, allowing the lung to deflate. The mediastinum shifts toward the unobstructed side.

trachea and be mistaken for an airway foreign body. The patient is asymptomatic and the x-ray normal in 15–30% of cases. Opaque foreign bodies occur in only 10–25% of cases. CT or MRI may help define radiolucent foreign bodies. If there is a high index of suspicion, bronchoscopy should be performed despite negative imaging studies.

TREATMENT

The treatment of choice for airway foreign bodies is prompt endoscopic removal with rigid instruments. Bronchoscopy is deferred only until preoperative studies have been obtained and the patient has been prepared by adequate hydration and emptying of the stomach. Airway foreign bodies are usually removed the same day the diagnosis is 1st considered.

384.1 • Laryngeal Foreign Bodies

Complete obstruction rapidly asphyxiates the child unless promptly relieved with the Heimlich maneuver. Objects that are partially obstructive are usually flat and thin. They lodge between the vocal cords in the sagittal plane, causing symptoms of croup, hoarseness, cough, stridor, and dyspnea.

384.2 • Tracheal Foreign Bodies

Choking and aspiration occurs in 90% of patients with tracheal foreign bodies, stridor in 60%, and wheezing in 50%. Posteroanterior and lateral soft tissue neck radiographs (airway films) are abnormal in 92% of children, whereas chest radiographs are abnormal in only 58%.

384.3 • Bronchial Foreign Bodies

Posteroanterior and lateral chest radiographs are standard in the assessment of infants and children suspected of having aspirated a foreign object. The abdomen is included. A good expiratory posteroanterior chest film is most helpful. During expiration, the bronchial foreign body obstructs the exit of air from the obstructed lung, producing obstructive emphysema (air trapping) with persistent inflation of the obstructed lung and shift of the mediastinum toward the opposite side (Fig. 384-1). Air trapping is an immediate complication in contrast to atelectasis, which is a late finding. Lateral decubitus chest films or fluoroscopy may provide the same information but are unnecessary. History and physical examination, not radiographs, determine the indication for bronchoscopy, which is both diagnostic and therapeutic.

Babin E, Sigston E, Bigeon JY, et al: How we do it: Management of tracheobronchial foreign bodies in children. *Clin Otolaryngol Allied Sci* 2004;29:750–753.

Nova A, Muntz H, Clary R: Utility of conventional radiography in pediatric airway foreign bodies. *Ann Otol Rhinol Laryngol* 1998;107:834–838.

White DR, Zdanski CJ, Drake AF: Comparison of pediatric airway foreign bodies over fifty years. *South Med J* 2004;97:434–436.

Williams H: Inhaled foreign bodies. *Arch Dis Child Educ Pract Ed* 2005;90:ep31–ep33.

Chapter 385 ■ Laryngotracheal Stenosis, Subglottic Stenosis

Lauren D. Holinger

Laryngotracheal stenosis is the most frequent cause of airway obstruction requiring tracheostomy in infants. The glottis (vocal cords) and the upper trachea are also compromised in most laryngeal stenoses, particularly those due to endotracheal intubation. Subglottic stenosis is considered to be congenital when there is no other apparent cause, such as a history of laryngeal trauma or intubation.

385.1 • Congenital Subglottic Stenosis (See Chapter 383.2)

CLINICAL MANIFESTATIONS. Stridor, biphasic or primarily inspiratory, is the typical presenting symptom for congenital subglottic stenosis. Recurrent or persistent croup occurs in these children at 6 mo of age or younger. The small amount of edema associated with an upper respiratory tract infection or laryngopharyngeal gastroesophageal reflux events compromises the already narrowed airway. The diagnosis is suggested by airway radiographs and confirmed by direct laryngoscopy. Treatment is dictated by the severity of the obstruction and is the same as for acquired subglottic stenosis. Because most cases of congenital stenosis are cartilaginous, dilatation or laser surgery are not uniformly effective. Anterior laryngotracheal decompression (**cricoid split**) or reconstruction with cartilage grafting usually avoids tracheostomy.

385.2 • Acquired Laryngotracheal Stenosis

Ninety per cent of acquired stenoses are related to endotracheal intubation. When the pressure of the endotracheal tube against the mucosa is greater than the capillary pressure, ischemia occurs, followed by necrosis and ulceration. Secondary infection and perichondritis develop with exposure of cartilage. Granulation tissue forms around the ulcerations. These changes and edema throughout the larynx usually resolve spontaneously after extubation. Chronic edema and fibrous stenosis develop in a small percentage of cases.

Factors that predispose to the development of laryngeal stenosis include: (1) Laryngopharyngeal reflux of acid and pepsin from the stomach exacerbates endotracheal tube trauma. More damage is caused in areas left unprotected, owing to loss of mucosa. (2) Congenital subglottic stenosis narrows the larynx and is more likely to be traumatized by an endotracheal tube of age-appropriate size. (3) Other patient factors include sepsis and infection, dehydration, malnutrition, chronic inflammatory disorders, and immunosuppression. (4) An oversized endotracheal tube is the most common cause of laryngeal injury. A tube that allows a small air leak at the end of the inspiratory cycle minimizes potential trauma. (5) Other extrinsic factors—traumatic intubation, multiple reintubations, movement of the endotracheal tube, and duration of intubation—may contribute to varying degrees in individual patients.

Clinical manifestations of acquired and congenital stenosis (see Chapter 383.2) are similar. Spasmodic croup, the sudden onset of severe croup in the early morning hours, is usually due to an episode of laryngopharyngeal reflux with transient laryngospasm and subsequent laryngeal edema. These frightening episodes resolve rapidly, often before the family and child reach the emergency department.

DIAGNOSIS. The diagnosis is confirmed by direct laryngoscopy and bronchoscopy. High-resolution CT imaging is of limited value.

TREATMENT. The severity, location, and type (cartilaginous or soft tissue) of the stenosis determines the treatment. Mild cases can be managed without operative intervention since the airway will improve as the child grows. Moderate soft tissue stenosis is treated by endoscopy using gentle dilations or CO_2 laser. Severe laryngotracheal stenosis is likely to require laryngotracheal expansion surgery or resection of the narrowed portion of the laryngeal and tracheal airway (cricotracheal resection). Every effort is made to avoid tracheotomy using endoscopic techniques or open surgical procedures such as the anterior laryngotracheal decompression (cricoid split).

Benjamin B: Prolonged intubation injuries of the larynx: Endoscopic diagnosis, classification, and treatment. *Ann Otol Rhinol Laryngol Suppl* 1993;160:1–15.

Cotton RT, Gray SD, Miller RP, et al: Update of the Cincinnati experience in pediatric laryngotracheal reconstruction. *Laryngoscope* 1989;99:1111–1116.

Gerber M, Stern Y, Walner D, et al: Role of laryngoscopy, dual pH probe monitoring, and laryngeal mucosa biopsy in the diagnosis of pharyngoesophageal reflux. *Ann Otol Rhinol Laryngol* 2001;110:299–304.

Liu H, Chen J, Holinger L, et al: Histopathologic fundamentals of acquired laryngeal stenosis. *Pediatr Pathol Lab Med* 1995;15:655–677.

Chapter 386 ■ Bronchomalacia and Tracheomalacia

Jonathan D. Finder

Chondromalacia of the trachea or of a main bronchus is a common cause of persistent wheezing in infancy. In these disorders, there is insufficient cartilage to maintain the airway patency throughout the respiratory cycle. Tracheomalacia and bronchomalacia can be either primary or secondary (Table 386-1). Although primary tracheomalacia and bronchomalacia are seen frequently in premature infants, most affected patients are born at term. Secondary tracheomalacia and bronchomalacia refers to the situation in which the central airway is compressed by adjacent structure (e.g., vascular ring) or deficient in cartilage due to tracheoesophageal fistula. Laryngomalacia may accompany primary bronchomalacia or tracheomalacia (see also Chapter 383.1). Involvement of the entire central airway (laryngotracheobronchomalacia) is also seen.

CLINICAL MANIFESTATIONS. Primary tracheomalacia and bronchomalacia are principally disorders of infants, with a male: female ratio of 2 : 1. The dominant finding, low-pitched monophonic wheezing, is most prominent over the central airways. Parents often describe persistent respiratory congestion even in the absence of a viral respiratory infection. When the lesion involves only one main bronchus (more commonly the left), the wheezing is louder on that side. In cases of tracheomalacia, the wheeze is loudest over the trachea. Hyperinflation and/or subcostal retractions do not occur unless the patient also has asthma or another cause of small airways obstruction. In the absence of asthma, patients with tracheomalacia and bronchomalacia are not helped by administration of a bronchodilator. Acquired tracheomalacia and bronchomalacia are seen in association with vascular rings (and may persist after surgical correction), tracheoesophageal fistula, and cardiomegaly, and after lung transplantation.

DIAGNOSIS. The definitive diagnosis of tracheomalacia and bronchomalacia is established by flexible or rigid bronchoscopy. The lesion is difficult to detect on plain radiographs, but fluoroscopy may demonstrate dynamic collapse and can avoid the need for invasive diagnostic techniques. Pulmonary function testing may show a pattern of decreased peak flow and flattening of the flow-

TABLE 386-1. Classification of Tracheomalacia
PRIMARY TRACHEOMALACIA
Congenital absence of tracheal-supporting cartilages
SECONDARY TRACHEOMALACIA
Esophageal atresia/tracheo-esophgeal fistula
Vascular rings (double aortic arch)
Tracheal compression from an aberrant innominate artery
Tracheal compression from mediastinal masses
Abnormally soft tracheal cartilages associated with connective tissue disorders
Prolonged mechanical ventilation/chronic lung disease

From McNamara VM, Crabbe DC: Tracheomalacia. *Paediatr Respir Rev* 2004;5:147–154.

volume loop. Other important diagnostic modalities include MRI and CT scanning. MRI is especially useful when there is a possibility of vascular ring and should be performed when a right aortic arch is seen on plain film radiography.

TREATMENT. Postural drainage may help with clearance of secretions. β-Adrenergic agents should be avoided in the absence of asthma. Nebulized ipratropium bromide may be useful. Endobronchial stents have been used in severely affected patients but have a high incidence of complications, ranging from airway obstruction from granulation tissue to erosion into adjacent vascular structures. Constant positive airway pressure (CPAP) via tracheostomy may be indicated for severe cases. Surgical approach (aorticopexy and bronchopexy) is rarely required and only for patients who have life-threatening apnea, cyanosis, and bradycardia ("cyanotic spells") from airway obstruction.

PROGNOSIS. Primary bronchomalacia and tracheomalacia have excellent prognoses, because airflow improves as the airways grow. Wheezing at rest is usually gone by age 3 yr. Prognosis in secondary and acquired forms varies with cause. Patients with concurrent asthma need considerable supportive treatment.

Boogaard R, Huijsmans SH, Pijnenburg MW, et al: Tracheomalacia and bronchomalacia in children: incidence and patient characteristics. *Chest* 2005;128:3391–3397.

Carden KA, Boiselle PM, Waltz DA, et al: Tracheomalacia and tracheobronchomalacia in children and adults: An in-depth review. *Chest* 2005;127:984–1005.

Filler RM, Forte V, Chait P: Tracheobronchial stenting for the treatment of airway obstruction. *J Pediatr Surg* 1998;33:304–311.

Finder JD: Primary bronchomalacia in infants and children. *J Pediatr* 1997;130:59–66.

Masters IB, Chang AB, Patterson L, et al: Series of laryngomalacia, tracheomalacia, and bronchomalacia disorders and their associations with other conditions in children. *Pediatr Pulmonol* 2002;34:189–195.

McNamara VM, Crabbe DC: Tracheomalacia. *Paediatr Respir Rev* 2004;5:147–154.

Panitch HB, Keklikian EN, Motley RA, et al: Effect of altering smooth muscle tone on maximal expiratory flows in patients with tracheomalacia. *Pediatr Pulmonol* 1990;9:170–176.

Yalcin E, Dogru D, Ozcelik U, et al: Tracheomalacia and bronchomalacia in 34 children: clinical and radiologic profiles and associations with other diseases. *Clin Pediatr* 2005;44:777–781.

Chapter 387 ■ Neoplasms of the Larynx, Trachea, and Bronchi

Lauren D. Holinger

387.1 • Vocal Nodules

Although vocal nodules are not true neoplasms, they are the most common cause of chronic hoarseness in children. Chronic vocal abuse or misuse produces nodules at the junction of the anterior and middle thirds of the phonating edge of the vocal cords. These symmetric, bilateral swellings interfere with voice production and cause children to strain the voice. Vocal nodules can occur in infants and are exacerbated by laryngopharyngeal reflux.

Voice therapy may be effective in the cooperative child, but for most toddlers and older children, behavioral therapy is necessary. Nodules usually resolve by early teenage years as the child matures and vocal abuse is moderated. Surgical excision is rarely indicated but may be necessary if the child is unable to communicate adequately, becomes aphonic, or tension and straining are necessary to make any utterances whatsoever.

Laryngopharyngeal reflux commonly exacerbates vocal abuse, adding to swelling of the vocal cords. When vocal abuse is the main factor, the voice is worse in the evenings; with laryngopharyngeal reflux, hoarseness is worse in the morning. An anti-reflux regimen is indicated (see Chapter 320.1).

387.2 • Recurrent Respiratory Papillomatosis (RRP)

EPIDEMIOLOGY AND ETIOLOGY. Papillomas are the most common respiratory tract neoplasms in children, occurring in 4.3/100,000. They are simply warts, benign tumors, due to the human papillomavirus (HPV) (see Chapter 263); the same pathology is found in condylomata acuminata (vaginal warts). HPV types 6 and 11 are most commonly associated with laryngeal disease. Fifty per cent occur in children <5 yr but the diagnosis can be made at any age. Sixty-seven per cent of children with RRP are born to mothers who had condylomata during pregnancy or parturition. The risk for transmission is ≈1/500 vaginal births in mothers with active condylomata. Many neonates have been reported to have RRP, suggesting intrauterine transmission of HPV.

CLINICAL MANIFESTATIONS. These benign squamous lesions can produce chronic hoarseness in the infant. Most are solitary and occur in the larynx, specifically on the vocal cords, but in 31%, these lesions occur in other areas of the respiratory tract: nose, pharynx (especially the uvula and posterior soft palate), trachea, bronchi, and lungs. As growth on the vocal cords progresses, hoarseness increases and communication becomes difficult. Respiratory distress may develop. Surgical excision is a quality of life issue warranting removal to improve the voice. Intervention becomes a medical necessity when airway obstruction progresses. Symptoms often occur 1st during sleep, with symptoms typical of obstructive sleep apnea. Progressive respiratory distress with sleep, exertion, daily activities, and, finally, at rest indicates the need for surgical intervention.

TREATMENT. The treatment of RRP is endoscopic surgical removal. Most surgeons in North America prefer the microdebrider or, less commonly, the CO_2 laser. Tracheostomy is rarely required; medical management including injection of cidofovir may have some benefit for severe and recurrent lesions. Laryngopharyngeal reflux may require treatment when reflux laryngitis is a factor.

HPV vaccination may decrease maternal infection and its perinatal transmission to the infant.

387.3 • Congenital Subglottic Hemangioma

Hemangiomas are symptomatic within the 1st 2 mo of life, almost all presenting before 6 mo of age. Stridor is biphasic but usually more prominent during inspiration. The infant may be hoarse, have a barking cough, and present with croup. Fifty per cent of congenital subglottic hemangiomas are associated with cutaneous lesions often in the facial beard distribution. Radiographs classically delineate an asymmetric subglottic narrowing. The diagnosis is made by direct laryngoscopy.

Medical management includes systemic steroids. Prednisone (2–4 mg/kg/day) is given orally for 4–6 wk, or less if the lesions stabilize sooner. The dosage is then tapered. If there is no response, the drug is discontinued. Interferon-α2a has also been used for the treatment of life-threatening corticosteroid-resistant hemangiomas that involve the airway and massively endanger vital structures (see Chapter 649).

Although tracheostomy establishes a safe airway, every effort should be made to find an alternative. Corticosteroids can be injected directly into the lesion. Endoscopic excision with the CO_2 laser is effective. Combining several modalities increases the possibility of avoiding tracheotomy. External surgical excision is suitable for rare lesions.

387.4 • Vascular Anomalies

Vascular malformations are not true neoplastic lesions. They have a normal rate of endothelial turnover and various channel abnormalities. They are categorized by their predominant type (capillary, venous, arterial, lymphatic, or a combination thereof). Slow-flow malformations have capillary, lymphatic, or venous components. In the past, these have been incorrectly called capillary hemangiomas, cystic hygromas or lymphangiomas, and cavernous hemangiomas, respectively.

Lymphatic malformations (cystic hygromas) rarely occur in the larynx. When they do, they are invariably an extension of disease from elsewhere in the head and neck. Airway obstruction may necessitate tracheostomy. The lesion can be debulked with the CO_2 laser.

387.5 • Other Laryngeal Neoplasms

Neurofibromatosis (see Chapter 596.1) rarely involves the larynx. When children are affected, limited local resection is undertaken to maintain an airway and optimize the voice. Complete surgical extirpation is virtually impossible without debilitating resection of vital laryngeal structures. Most surgeons select the option of less aggressive symptomatic surgery because of the poorly circumscribed and infiltrative nature of these fibromas. *Rhabdomyosarcoma* (see Chapter 500) and other malignant tumors of the larynx are rare. Symptoms of hoarseness and progressive airway obstruction prompt initial evaluation by flexible laryngoscopy in the office.

387.6 • Tracheal Neoplasms

The majority of tracheal tumors are benign; the 2 most common are *inflammatory pseudotumor* and *hamartoma.* The inflammatory pseudotumor is probably a reaction to a previous bronchial infection or traumatic insult. Growth is slow and the tumor may be locally invasive. Hamartomas are tumors of primary tissue elements that are abnormal in proportion and arrangement.

Tracheal neoplasms present with stridor, wheezing, cough, or pneumonia and are rarely diagnosed until 75% of the lumen has been obstructed. Symptoms mimic asthma and are frequently misdiagnosed as such. Chest radiographs or airway films may identify the obstruction. Pulmonary function studies demonstrate an abnormal flow-volume loop. A mild response to bronchodilator therapy may be misleading.

387.7 • Bronchial Tumors

Bronchial tumors are rare. Two thirds are malignant. Bronchial "adenomas" are the most common, representing 30% of all lung tumors. Bronchogenic carcinoma is the 2nd most common and occurs in ≈20% of cases. The diagnosis is confirmed at bronchoscopy and biopsy; treatment depends on the histopathology.

Derkay CS: Recurrent respiratory papillomatosis. *Laryngoscope* 2001;111:57–67.

Desai DP, Maddalozzo J, Holinger LD: Granular cell tumor of the trachea. *Otolaryngol Head Neck Surg* 1999;120:595–598.

Desai DP, Mahoney EM, Miller RP, et al: Case report: Mucoepidermoid carcinoma of the trachea in a child. *Int J Pediatr Otorhinolaryngol* 1998;45:259–263.

Hughes CA, Rezaee A, Ludemann JP, et al: Management of congenital subglottic hemangioma. *J Otolaryngol* 1999;28:223–228.

Newhouse MT, Martin L, Kay JM, Miller JD: Laser resection of a pedunculated tracheal adenoma. *Chest* 2000;118:262–265.

Reeves WC, Ruparelia SS, Swanson KI, et al: National registry for juvenile-onset recurrent respiratory papillomatosis. *Arch Otolaryngol Head Neck Surg* 2003;129:976–982.

Ruparelia S, Unger ER, Nisenbaum R, et al: Predictors of remission in juvenile-onset recurrent respiratory papillomatosis. *Arch Otolaryngol Head Neck Surg* 2003;129:1275–1278.

Schraff S, Derkay CS, Burke B, Lawson L: American Society of Pediatric Otolaryngology members' experience with recurrent respiratory papillomatosis and the use of adjuvant therapy. *Arch Otolaryngol Head Neck Surg* 2004;130:1039–1042.

Tasca RA, Clarke RW: Recurrent respiratory papillomatosis. *Arch Dis Child* 2006;91:689–691.

Vijavasekaram S, White DR, Hartley BB, et al: Open excision of subglottic hemangiomas to avoid tracheostomy. *Arch Otolaryngol Head Neck Surg* 2006;132:159–163.

Zacharisen MC, Conley SF: Recurrent respiratory papillomatosis in children: masquerader of common respiratory diseases. *Pediatrics* 2006;118:1925–1931.

Chapter 388 ■ Wheezing, Bronchiolitis, and Bronchitis

388.1 • Wheezing in Infants: Bronchiolitis •

Kimberly Danieli Watts and
Denise M. Goodman

DEFINITIONS AND GENERAL PATHOPHYSIOLOGY

A **wheeze** is a musical and continuous sound that originates from oscillations in narrowed airways. Wheezing is heard mostly on expiration as a result of critical airway obstruction. Wheezing is **polyphonic** when there is widespread narrowing of the airways causing various pitches or levels of obstruction to airflow as seen in asthma. **Monophonic** wheezing refers to a single-pitch sound that is produced in the larger airways during expiration as in distal tracheomalacia or bronchomalacia. When obstruction occurs in the extrathoracic airways during inspiration, the noise is referred to as **stridor.**

Infants are prone to wheeze due to a differing set of lung mechanics in comparison to older children and adults. The obstruction to flow is affected by the airway caliber and compliance of the infant lung. Resistance to airflow through a tube is inversely related to the radius of the tube to the 4th power. In children <5 yr old, small caliber peripheral airways can contribute up to 50% of the total airway resistance. Marginal additional narrowing can cause further flow limitation and a subsequent wheeze.

With the very compliant newborn chest wall, the inward pressure produced in expiration subjects the intrathoracic airways to collapse. Flow limitation is further affected in infants by the differences in tracheal cartilage composition and airway smooth muscle tone causing further increase in airway compliance in comparison to older children. All of these mechanisms combine to make the infant more susceptible to airway collapse, increased resistance, and subsequent wheezing. Many of these conditions are outgrown in the 1st year of life.

Immunologic and molecular influences can contribute to the infant's propensity to wheeze. In comparison to older children and adults, infants tend to have higher levels of lymphocytes and neutrophils, rather than mast cells and eosinophils, in bronchoalveolar lavage fluid. A variety of inflammatory mediators have also been implicated in the wheezing infant such as histamine, leukotrienes, and interleukins. Fetal and/or early postnatal "programming" in which the structure and function of the lung are affected by factors including fetal nutrition and fetal and neonatal exposure to maternal smoking may also occur.

ETIOLOGY

Most wheezing in infants is caused by inflammation (generally bronchiolitis), but many other entities can present with wheezing (Table 388-1).

ACUTE BRONCHIOLITIS AND INFLAMMATION OF THE AIRWAY. Infection can cause obstruction to flow by internal narrowing of the airways.

Acute bronchiolitis is predominantly a viral disease. Respiratory syncytial virus (RSV) is responsible for >50% of cases (see Chapter 257). Other agents include parainfluenza (see Chapter 256), adenovirus, *Mycoplasma,* and, occasionally, other viruses. Human metapneumovirus (see Chapter 258) is an important primary cause of viral respiratory infection or it can occur as a co-infection with RSV. There is no evidence of a bacterial cause for bronchiolitis, although bacterial pneumonia is sometimes confused clinically with bronchiolitis and bronchiolitis is rarely followed by bacterial superinfection.

Approximately 50,000–80,000 of hospitalizations annually among children <1 yr old are attributable to RSV infection, with 200–500 deaths per yr in the United States. Increasing rates of hospitalization may reflect increased attendance of infants in daycare centers, changes in criteria for hospital admission, and/or improved survival of premature infants and others at risk for severe RSV-associated disease.

Bronchiolitis is more common in males, in those who have not been breast-fed, and in those who live in crowded conditions. Older family members are a common source of infection; they may only experience minor respiratory symptoms. The clinical manifestations of lower respiratory tract illness (LRTI) seen in young infants may be minimal in older patients, in whom bronchiolar edema is better tolerated.

Not all infected infants develop LRTI. Host anatomic and immunologic factors seem to play a significant role in the severity of the clinical syndrome. Infants with pre-existent smaller airways and diminished lung function have a more severe course. In addition, RSV infection incites a complex immune response. Eosinophils degranulate and release eosinophil cationic protein, which is cytotoxic to airway epithelium. Immunoglobulin E (IgE) antibody release may also be related to wheezing. Other mediators invoked in the pathogenesis of airway inflammation include chemokines such as interleukin 8 (IL-8), macrophage inflammatory protein (MIP) 1α, and RANTES (*r*egulated on *a*ctivation, *n*ormal *T* cell *e*xpressed and *s*ecreted). RSV-infected infants who wheeze express higher levels of interferon-γ in the airway as well as leukotrienes. RSV co-infection with metapneumovirus can be more severe than monoinfection.

Acute bronchiolitis is characterized by bronchiolar obstruction with edema, mucus, and cellular debris. Even minor bronchiolar wall thickening significantly affects airflow because resistance is inversely proportional to the 4th power of the radius of the bronchiolar passage. Resistance in the small air passages is increased during both inspiration and exhalation, but because the radius of an airway is smaller during expiration, the resultant respiratory obstruction leads to early air trapping and overinflation. If obstruction becomes complete, there will be resorption of trapped distal air, and the child will develop atelectasis.

Hypoxemia is a consequence of ventilation-perfusion mismatch early in the course. With severe obstructive disease and tiring of respiratory effort, hypercapnia may develop.

TABLE 388-1. Differential Diagnosis of Wheezing in Infancy
INFECTION
Viral
Respiratory syncytial virus (RSV)
Human metapneumovirus
Parainfluenza
Adenovirus
Influenza
Rhinovirus
Other
Chlamydia trachomatis
Tuberculosis
Histoplasmosis
Papillomatosis
ASTHMA
Transient wheezer
Initial risk factor is primarily diminished lung size
Persistent wheezers
Initial risk factors include passive smoke exposure, maternal asthma history, and an elevated immunoglobulin E (IgE) level in the 1st year of life
At increased risk of developing clinical asthma
Late-onset wheezer
ANATOMIC ABNORMALITIES
Central airway abnormalities
Malacia of the larynx, trachea, and/or bronchi
Tracheoesophageal fistula (specifically H-type fistula)
Laryngeal cleft (resulting in aspiration)
Extrinsic airway anomalies resulting in airway compression
Vascular ring or sling
Mediastinal lymphadenopathy from infection or tumor
Mediastinal mass/tumor
Esophageal foreign body
Intrinsic airway anomalies
Airway hemangioma, other tumor
Cystic adenomatoid malformation
Bronchial/lung cyst
Congenital lobar emphysema
Aberrant tracheal bronchus
Sequestration
Congenital heart disease with left-to-right shunt (increased pulmonary edema)
Foreign body
IMMUNODEFICIENCY STATES
IgA deficiency
B-cell deficiencies
Primary ciliary dyskinesia
AIDS
Bronchiectasis
MUCOCILIARY CLEARANCE DISORDERS
Cystic fibrosis
Primary ciliary dyskinesias
Bronchiectasis
BRONCHOPULMONARY DYSPLASIA
ASPIRATION SYNDROMES
Gastroesophageal reflux disease
Pharyngeal/swallow dysfunction
INTERSTITIAL LUNG DISEASE, INCLUDING BRONCHIOLITIS OBLITERANS
HEART FAILURE
ANAPHYLAXIS
INHALATION INJURY—BURNS

Chronic infectious causes of wheezing should be considered in those infants who seem to fall out of the range of a normal clinical course. Cystic fibrosis is one such entity; suspicion increases in a patient with persistent respiratory symptoms, digital clubbing, malabsorption, failure to thrive, electrolyte abnormalities, or a resistance to bronchodilator treatment (see Chapter 400).

Allergy and asthma are important causes of wheezing and probably generate the most questions by the parents of a wheezing infant. Asthma is characterized by airway inflammation, bronchial hyperreactivity, and reversibility of obstruction (see Chapter 143). Three identified patterns of infant wheezing are: the transient early wheezer, 19.9% of the general population, had wheezing at least once with a lower respiratory infection before the age of 3 yr but never wheezed again; the persistent wheezer, 13.7% of the general population, had wheezing episodes before 3 yr and was still wheezing at 6 yr of age; and the late onset wheezer, 15% of the general population, had no wheezing by 3 yr but was wheezing by 6 yr. The other ½ of the children had never wheezed by 6 yr. Of all the infants who wheezed before 3 yr old, almost 60% stopped wheezing by 6 yr. Risk factors for persistent wheezing included maternal asthma, maternal smoking, persistent rhinitis (apart from acute upper respiratory tract infections), and eczema at <1 yr of age.

OTHER CAUSES. **Congenital malformations** of the respiratory tract cause wheezing in early infancy. These findings can be diffuse or focal and can be from an external compression or an intrinsic abnormality. *External vascular compression* includes a vascular ring, in which the trachea and esophagus are surrounded completely by vascular structures, or a vascular sling, in which the trachea and esophagus are not completely encircled (see Chapter 432). *Cardiovascular causes* of wheezing include dilated chambers of the heart including massive cardiomegaly, left atrial enlargement, and dilated pulmonary arteries. Pulmonary edema caused by heart failure can also cause wheezing by lymphatic and bronchial vessel engorgement that leads to obstruction and edema of the bronchioles and further obstruction (see Chapter 442).

Foreign body aspiration (see Chapter 384) can cause acute or chronic wheezing. It is estimated that 78% of those who die from foreign body aspiration are between 2 mo and 4 yr old. Even in young infants, a foreign body can be ingested if given to the infant by another person such as an older sibling. Infants who have atypical histories or misleading clinical and radiologic findings may be misdiagnosed with asthma or another obstructive disorder as inflammation and granulation develop around the foreign body. Esophageal foreign body can transmit pressure to the membranous trachea, causing compromise of the airway lumen.

Gastroesophageal reflux (see Chapter 320.1) can cause wheezing with or without direct aspiration into the tracheobronchial tree. Without aspiration, the reflux is thought to trigger a vagal or neural reflex, causing increased airway resistance and airway reactivity. Aspiration from gastroesophageal reflux or from the direct aspiration from oral liquids can also cause wheezing.

Trauma and tumors are much more rare causes of wheezing in infants. Trauma of any type to the tracheobronchial tree can cause an obstruction to airflow. Accidental or nonaccidental aspirations, burns, or scalds of the tracheobronchial tree can cause inflammation of the airways and subsequent wheezing. Any space-occupying lesion either in the lung itself or extrinsic to the lung can cause tracheobronchial compression and obstruction to airflow.

CLINICAL MANIFESTATIONS

HISTORY AND PHYSICAL EXAMINATION. Initial history of a wheezing infant should include accounts of the recent event including onset, duration, and associated factors (Table 388-2). *Birth history* includes weeks of gestation, neonatal intensive care unit admission, history of intubation or oxygen requirement, maternal complications including infection, herpes simplex virus (HSV) status, HIV status, and prenatal smoke exposure. Past medical history includes any co-morbid conditions including syndromes or associations. *Family history* of cystic fibrosis, immunodeficiencies, asthma in a 1st-degree relative, or any other recurrent respiratory conditions in children should be obtained. *Social history* should include an environmental history including any smokers at home, inside or out, daycare exposure, number of siblings, occupation of inhabitants of the home, pets, tuberculosis exposure, and concerns regarding home environment (i.e. dust mites, construction dust, heating and cooling techniques, mold, cockroaches).

TABLE 388-2. Pertinent Medical History in the Wheezing Infant

Did the onset of symptoms begin at birth or thereafter?
Is the infant a noisy breather and when is it most prominent?
Is there a history of cough apart from wheezing?
Was there an earlier lower respiratory tract infection?
Have there been any emergency department visits, hospitalizations, or intensive care unit admissions for respiratory distress?
Is there a history of eczema?
Does the infant cough after crying or cough at night?
How is the infant growing and developing?
Is there associated failure to thrive?
Is there failure to thrive without feeding difficulties?
Is there a history of electrolyte abnormalities?
Are there signs of intestinal malabsorption including frequent, greasy, or oily stools?
Is there a maternal history of genital herpes simplex virus (HSV) infection?
What was the gestational age at delivery?
Was the patient intubated as a neonate?
Does the infant bottle-feed in the bed or the crib, especially in a propped position?
Are there any feeding difficulties including choking, gagging, arching, or vomiting with feeds?
Any new food exposure?
Is there a toddler in the home or lapse in supervision in which foreign body aspiration could have occurred?
Change in caregivers or chance of nonaccidental trauma?

On **physical examination,** evaluation of the patient's vital signs with special attention to the respiratory rate and the pulse oximetry reading for oxygen saturation is an important initial step. There should also be a thorough review of the patient's growth chart for signs of failure to thrive. Wheezing produces an expiratory whistling sound that can be polyphonic or monophonic in nature. Prolonged expiratory time may be present. Biphasic wheezing can occur if there is a central, large airway obstruction. The lack of audible wheezing is not reassuring if the infant shows other signs of respiratory distress because complete obstruction to airflow can eliminate the turbulence, which causes the sound to resonate. Aeration should be noted and a trial of a bronchodilator may be warranted to evaluate for any change in wheezing after treatment. Listening to breath sounds over the neck will help differentiate upper airway from lower airway sounds. The absence or presence of stridor should be noted and appreciated on inspiration. Signs of respiratory distress include tachypnea, increased respiratory effort, nasal flaring, tracheal tugging, subcostal and intercostal retractions, and excess use of accessory muscles. In the upper airway, signs of atopy, including boggy turbinates and posterior oropharynx cobblestoning, can be evaluated in older infants. It is also useful to evaluate the skin of the patient for eczema and any significant hemangiomas; midline lesions may be associated with an intrathoracic lesion. Digital clubbing should be noted (see Chapter 371).

Acute bronchiolitis is usually preceded by exposure to an older contact with a minor respiratory syndrome within the previous wk. The infant 1st develops a mild upper respiratory tract infection with sneezing and clear rhinorrhea. This may be accompanied by diminished appetite and fever of 38.5–39°C (101–102°F), although the temperature may range from subnormal to markedly elevated. Gradually, respiratory distress ensues, with paroxysmal wheezy cough, dyspnea, and irritability. The infant is often tachypneic, which may interfere with feeding. The child does not usually have other systemic complaints, such as diarrhea or vomiting. Apnea may be more prominent than wheezing early in the course of the disease, particularly with very young infants (<2 mo old) or former premature infants.

The **physical examination** is characterized most prominently by wheezing. The degree of tachypnea does not always correlate with the degree of hypoxemia or hypercarbia, so the use of pulse oximetry and noninvasive carbon dioxide determination is essential. Work of breathing may be markedly increased, with nasal flaring and retractions. Auscultation may reveal fine crackles or overt wheezes, with prolongation of the expiratory phase of breathing. Barely audible breath sounds suggest very severe disease with nearly complete bronchiolar obstruction. Hyperinflation of the lungs may permit palpation of the liver and spleen.

DIAGNOSTIC EVALUATION. Initial evaluation is dependent on likely etiology; a baseline chest radiograph, including posteroanterior and lateral films, is warranted in many cases and for any infant in acute respiratory distress. Focal infiltrates are most often found in wheezing infants who have a pulse oximetry reading <93%, grunting, decreased breath sounds, prolonged inspiratory to expiratory ratio, and crackles. The chest radiograph may also be useful for evaluation of hyperinflation (common in bronchiolitis and viral pneumonia), signs of chronic disease such as bronchiectasis, or a space-occupying lesion causing airway compression. A trial of bronchodilator may be diagnostic as well as therapeutic because these medications can reverse conditions such as bronchiolitis (occasionally) and asthma but will not affect a fixed obstruction. Bronchodilators may potentially worsen a case of wheezing caused by tracheal or bronchial malacia. A sweat test to evaluate for cystic fibrosis and evaluation of baseline immune status are reasonable in infants with recurrent wheezing or complicated courses. Further evaluation such as upper gastrointestinal (GI) contrast x-rays, chest CT, bronchoscopy, infant pulmonary function testing, video swallow study, and pH probe can be considered second-tier diagnostic procedures in complicated patients.

In **acute bronchiolitis,** chest radiography reveals hyperinflated lungs with patchy atelectasis. The white blood cell and differential counts are usually normal. Viral testing (usually rapid immunofluorescence, polymerase chain reaction, or viral culture) is helpful if the diagnosis is uncertain or for epidemiologic purposes. The diagnosis is clinical, particularly in a previously healthy infant presenting with a first-time wheezing episode during a community outbreak. Because concurrent bacterial infection (sepsis, pneumonia, meningitis) is highly unlikely, confirmation of viral bronchiolitis may obviate the need for a sepsis evaluation in a febrile infant and assist with respiratory precautions and isolation if the patient requires hospitalization.

TREATMENT

Treatment of an infant with wheezing depends on the underlying etiology. Response to bronchodilators is unpredictable, regardless of cause, but suggests a component of bronchial hyperreactivity. It is appropriate to administer albuterol aerosol and objectively observe the response. For infants <3 yr of age, it is acceptable to continue to administer inhaled medications through an MDI with mask and spacer if a therapeutic benefit is demonstrated. Therapy should be continued in all patients with asthma exacerbations from a viral illness.

The use of ipratropium bromide in this population is controversial, but it appears to be somewhat effective as an adjunct therapy. It is also useful in infants with significant tracheal and bronchial malacia who may be made worse by β-2 agonists such as albuterol because of the subsequent decrease in smooth muscle tone.

A trial of inhaled steroids may be warranted in a patient who has responded to multiple courses of oral steroids, has moderate to severe wheezing, or a significant history of atopy including food allergy or eczema. Inhaled steroids are appropriate for maintenance therapy in patients with known reactive airways but are controversial when used for episodic or acute illnesses.

Oral steroids are generally reserved for atopic wheezing infants thought to have asthma that is refractory to other medications. Their use in first-time wheezing infants or those infants that do not warrant hospitalization is controversial.

Infants with **acute bronchiolitis** who are experiencing respiratory distress should be hospitalized; the mainstay of treatment is supportive. If hypoxemic, the child should receive cool humidified oxygen. Sedatives are to be avoided because they may depress respiratory drive. The infant is sometimes more comfortable if sitting with head and chest elevated at a 30-degree angle with neck extended. The risk of aspiration of oral feedings may be high in infants with bronchiolitis, owing to tachypnea and the increased work of breathing. The infant may be fed through a nasogastric tube. If there is any risk for further respiratory decompensation potentially necessitating tracheal intubation, however, the infant should not be fed orally but be maintained with parenteral fluids. Frequent suctioning of nasal and oral secretions often provides relief of distress or cyanosis. Oxygen is indicated in all infants with hypoxia.

A number of agents have been proposed as adjunctive therapies for bronchiolitis. Bronchodilators produce modest short-term improvement in clinical features, but the statistical improvement in clinical scoring systems seen with them is not always clinically significant. Several studies have included both infants with 1st-time wheezing and those with recurrent wheezing, complicating interpretation of the data. Nebulized epinephrine may be more effective than β-agonists. A trial dose of inhaled bronchodilator may be reasonable, with further therapy predicated on response in the individual patient. Corticosteroids, whether parenteral, oral, or inhaled, have been used for bronchiolitis despite conflicting and often negative studies. Differences of diagnostic criteria, measures of effect, timing and route of administration, and severity of illness complicate these studies. Corticosteroids are not recommended in previously healthy infants with RSV. Ribavirin, an antiviral agent administered by aerosol, has been used for infants with congenital heart disease or chronic lung disease. There is no convincing evidence of a positive impact on clinically important outcomes such as mortality and duration of hospitalization. Antibiotics have no value unless there is secondary bacterial pneumonia. Likewise, there is no support for RSV immunoglobulin administration during acute episodes of RSV bronchiolitis.

PROGNOSIS

Infants with **acute bronchiolitis** are at highest risk for further respiratory compromise in the 1st 48–72 hr after onset of cough and dyspnea; the child may be desperately ill with air hunger, apnea, and respiratory acidosis. The case fatality rate is <1%, with death attributable to apnea, uncompensated respiratory acidosis, or severe dehydration. After this critical period, symptoms may persist. The median duration of symptoms in ambulatory patients is ≈12 days. Infants with conditions such as congenital heart disease, bronchopulmonary dysplasia, and immunodeficiency often have more severe disease, with higher morbidity and mortality. There is a higher incidence of wheezing and asthma in children with a history of bronchiolitis unexplained by family history or other atopic syndromes. It is unclear whether bronchiolitis incites an immune response that manifests as asthma later or whether those infants have an inherent predilection for asthma that is merely unmasked by their episode of RSV. Approximately 60% of infants who wheeze will stop wheezing.

PREVENTION

Reduction in the severity and incidence of **acute bronchiolitis** due to RSV is possible through the administration of pooled hyperimmune RSV intravenous immunoglobulin (RSV-IVIG, RespiGam) and palivizumab (Synagis), an intramuscular monoclonal antibody to the RSV F protein, before and during RSV season. Palivizumab is recommended for infants <2 yr of age with chronic lung disease (bronchopulmonary dysplasia) or prematurity. Meticulous handwashing is the best measure to prevent nosocomial transmission.

388.2 • Bronchitis • Denise M. Goodman

Bronchitis refers to nonspecific bronchial inflammation and is associated with a number of childhood conditions. *Acute bronchitis* is a syndrome, usually viral in origin, with cough as a prominent feature.

Acute tracheobronchitis is a term used when the trachea is prominently involved. Nasopharyngitis may also be present, and a variety of viral and bacterial agents, such as those causing influenza, pertussis, and diphtheria, may be responsible. Isolation of common bacteria such as pneumococcus, *Staphylococcus aureus*, and *Streptococcus pneumoniae* from the sputum may not imply a bacterial cause requiring antibiotic therapy.

ACUTE BRONCHITIS

CLINICAL MANIFESTATIONS. Acute bronchitis is commonly preceded by a viral upper respiratory tract infection. It is more common in the winter when respiratory viral syndromes predominate. The tracheobronchial epithelium is invaded by the infectious agent, leading to activation of inflammatory cells and release of cytokines. Constitutional symptoms, such as fever and malaise, follow. The tracheobronchial epithelium may become significantly damaged or hypersensitized, leading to a protracted cough lasting 1–3 wk.

The child 1st presents with nonspecific upper respiratory infectious symptoms, such as rhinitis. Three to 4 days later, a frequent, dry, hacking cough develops, which may or may not be productive. After several days, the sputum may become purulent, indicating leukocyte migration but not necessarily bacterial infection. Many children swallow their sputum, and this may produce emesis. Chest pain may be a prominent complaint in older children, exacerbated by coughing. The mucus gradually thins, usually within 5–10 days, and then the cough gradually abates. The entire episode usually lasts about 2 wk and seldom longer than 3 wk.

Findings on physical examination vary with age of the patient and stage of the disease. Early findings are absent or are low-grade fever and upper respiratory signs such as nasopharyngitis, conjunctivitis, and rhinitis. Auscultation of the chest may be unremarkable at this early phase. As the syndrome progresses and cough worsens, breath sounds become coarse, with coarse and fine crackles and scattered high-pitched wheezing. Chest radiographs are normal or may have increased bronchial markings.

The principal objective of the clinician is to exclude pneumonia, which is more likely caused by bacterial agents requiring antibiotic therapy. In adults, absence of abnormality of vital signs (tachycardia, tachypnea, fever) and a normal physical examination of the chest reduce the likelihood of pneumonia.

DIFFERENTIAL DIAGNOSIS. Persistent or recurrent symptoms should lead the clinician to consider entities other than acute bronchitis. Many entities manifest with cough as a prominent symptom (Table 388-3).

TABLE 388-3. Disorders with Cough as a Prominent Finding

CATEGORY	DIAGNOSES
Inflammatory	Asthma
Chronic pulmonary processes	Bronchopulmonary dysplasia/chronic lung disease
	Postinfectious bronchiectasis
	Cystic fibrosis
	Tracheo- or bronchomalacia
	Ciliary abnormalities
Other chronic disease/congenital disorders	Laryngeal cleft
	Swallowing disorders
	Gastroesophageal reflux
	Airway compression (such as a vascular ring or hemangioma)
	Congenital heart disease
Infectious/immune disorders	Immunodeficiency
	Tuberculosis
	Allergy
	Sinusitis
	Tonsillitis or adenoiditis
	Chlamydia, Ureaplasma (infants)
	Bordetella pertussis
	Mycoplasma pneumoniae
Acquired	Foreign body aspiration, tracheal or esophageal

TREATMENT. There is no specific therapy for acute bronchitis. The disease is self-limited, and antibiotics, although frequently prescribed, do not hasten improvement. Frequent shifts in position may facilitate pulmonary drainage in infants. Older children are sometimes more comfortable with humidity, but this does not shorten the disease course. Cough suppressants may produce symptomatic relief but may also increase the risk of suppuration and inspissated secretions and, therefore, should be used judiciously. Antihistamines dry secretions and are not helpful; expectorants are likewise not indicated.

CHRONIC BRONCHITIS

Chronic bronchitis is well recognized in adults, formally defined as ≥3 mo of productive cough each year for ≥2 yr. The disease may develop insidiously, with episodes of acute obstruction alternating with quiescent periods. A number of predisposing conditions can lead to progression of airflow obstruction or chronic obstructive pulmonary disease (COPD), with smoking as the major factor (up to 80% of patients have a smoking history). Other conditions include air pollution, occupational exposures, and repeated infections. In children, cystic fibrosis, bronchopulmonary dysplasia, and bronchiectasis must be ruled out.

The applicability of this definition to children is unclear. The existence of chronic bronchitis as a distinct entity in children is controversial. Like adults, however, children with chronic inflammatory diseases or those with toxic exposures can develop damaged pulmonary epithelium. Thus, chronic or recurring cough in children should lead the clinician to search for underlying pulmonary or systemic disorders (see Table 388-3).

CIGARETTE SMOKING AND AIR POLLUTION

Exposure to environmental irritants, such as tobacco smoke and air pollution, can incite or aggravate cough. There is a well-established association between tobacco exposure and pulmonary disease, including bronchitis and wheezing. This can occur through cigarette smoking or by exposure to passive smoke. Marijuana smoke is another irritant sometimes overlooked when eliciting a history. There is some evidence that women may be particularly susceptible to long-term pulmonary disease as a consequence of childhood smoking.

A number of pollutants compromise lung development and likely precipitate lung disease, including particulate matter, ozone, acid vapor, and nitrogen dioxide. Because these substances coexist in the atmosphere, the relative contribution of any 1 to pulmonary symptoms is difficult to discern. Proximity to motor vehicle traffic is an important source of these pollutants.

Wheezing and Bronchiolitis

Bush A: Treatment options of asthma in infancy. *Pediatr Pulmonol Suppl* 2004;26:20–22.

Castro-Rodriguez JA, Rodrigo GJ: Beta agonists through metered-dose inhaler with valved holding chamber versus nebulizer for acute exacerbation of wheezing or asthma in children under five years of age: A systematic review with meta-analysis. *J Pediatr* 2004;172–177.

Covar RA, Spahn JD: Treating the wheezing infant. *Pediatr Clin North Am* 2003;50:631–654.

Frey U, Makkonen K, Wellman T, et al: Alterations in airway wall properties in infants with a history of wheezing disorders. *Am J Respir Crit Care Med* 2000;161:1825–1829.

Hartling L, Wiebe N, Russell K, et al: A meta-analysis of randomized controlled trials evaluating the efficacy of epinephrine for the treatment of acute viral bronchiolitis. *Arch Pediatr Adolesc Med* 2003;157:957–964.

Hofhuis W, van der Wiel EC, et al: Bronchodilation in infants with malacia or recurrent wheeze. *Arch Dis Child* 2003;88:246–249.

Joseph L, Goldberg S, Picard E: A randomized trial of home oxygen therapy from the emergency department for acute bronchiolitis. *Pediatrics* 2006; 118:1319–1320.

King VJ, Viswanathan M, Bordley WC, et al: Review: Commonly used pharmacological treatments for bronchiolitis in children do not seem to be effective. *Arch Pediatr Adolesc Med* 2004;158:127–137.

Klinnert MD, Liu AH, Pearson MR, et al: Short-term impact of a randomized multifaceted intervention for wheezing infants in low-income families. *Arch Pediatr Adolesc Med* 2005;159:75–82.

Klinnert MD, Price MR, Liu AH, Robinson JL: Morbidity patterns among low-income wheezing infants. *Pediatrics* 2003;112:49–57.

Kussman BD, Geva T, McGowan FX: Cardiovascular causes of airway compression. *Paediatr Anaesth* 2004;14:60–74.

Martinez FD, Wright AL, Taussig LM, et al: Asthma and wheezing in the first six years of life. *N Engl J Med* 1995;332:133–138.

Meates-Dennis M: Bronchiolitis. *Arch Dis Child* 2005;90:ep81–ep86.

Morton RL, Sheikh S, Corbett ML, Eid NS: Evaluation of the wheezy infant. *Ann Allergy Asthma Immunol* 2001;86:251–256.

Principi N, Esposito S: Emerging role of *Mycoplasma pneumoniae* and *Chlamydia pneumoniae* in paediatric respiratory tract infection. *Lancet* 2001;1:334–344.

Semple MG, Cowell A, Dove W, et al: Dual infection of infants by human metapneumovirus and human respiratory syncytial virus is strongly associated with severe bronchiolitis. *J Infect Dis* 2005;191:382–386.

Silvestri M, Sabatini F, Defilippi AC, Rossi GA: The wheezy infant—immunological and molecular considerations. *Paediatr Respir Rev* 2004;5:S81–S87.

Smyth RL, Openshaw PJM: Bronchiolitis. *Lancet* 2006;368:312–322.

Subcommittee on Diagnosis and Management of Bronchitis: Diagnosis and management of bronchitis. *Pediatrics* 2006;118:1774–1793.

Tokar B, Ozkan R, Ilhan H: Tracheobronchial foreign bodies in children: Importance of accurate history and plain chest radiography in delayed presentation. *Clin Radiol* 2004;59:609–615.

Weinberger M: Corticosteroids for first-time young wheezers: Current status of the controversy. *J Pediatr* 2003;143:700–702.

Williams JV, Harris PA, Tollefson SJ, et al: Human metapneumovirus and lower respiratory tract disease in otherwise healthy infants and children. *N Engl J Med* 2004;350:443–450.

Bronchitis

Arnold JC, Singh KK, Spector SA, et al: Human bocavirus: Prevalence and clinical spectrum at a children's hospital. *CID* 2006;43:283–288.

Arroll B, Kenealy T: Antibiotics for acute bronchitis. *Br Med J* 2001;322:939–940.

Gauderman WJ, Avol E, Gilliland F, et al: The effect of air pollution on lung development from 10 to 18 years of age. *N Engl J Med* 2004;351: 1057–1067.

Gergen PJ, Fowler JA, Maurer KR, et al: The burden of environmental tobacco smoke exposure on the respiratory health of children 2 months through 5 years of age in the United States: Third National Health and Nutrition Examination Survey, 1988 to 1994. *Pediatrics* 1998;101:e8.

Gonzales R, Sande MA: Uncomplicated acute bronchitis. *Ann Intern Med* 2000;133:981–991.

Irwin RS, Madison JM: The diagnosis and treatment of cough. *N Engl J Med* 2000;343:1715–1721.

Kim JJ, Smorodinsky S, Lipsett M, et al: Traffic-related air pollution near busy roads: The East Bay Children's Respiratory Health Study. *Am J Respir Crit Care Med* 2004;170:520–526.

Morice AH, et al: The diagnosis and management of chronic cough. *Eur Respir J* 2004;24:481–492.

Patel BD, Luben RN, Welch AA, et al: Childhood smoking is an independent risk factor for obstructive airways disease in women. *Thorax* 2004;59:682–686.

Peters JM, Avol E, Navidi W, et al: A study of twelve Southern California communities with differing levels and types of air pollution: I. Prevalence of respiratory morbidity. *Am J Respir Crit Care Med* 1999;159:760–767.

Peters JM, Avol E, Gauderman WJ, et al: A study of twelve Southern California communities with differing levels and types of air pollution: II. Effects on pulmonary function. *Am J Respir Crit Care Med* 1999;159:768–775.

Snow V, Mottur-Pilson C, Gonzales R, et al: Principles of appropriate antibiotic use for treatment of acute bronchitis in adults. *Ann Intern Med* 2001;134:518–520.

Chapter 389 ■ Emphysema and Overinflation

Steven Boas and Glenna B. Winnie

Pulmonary emphysema is distention of air spaces with irreversible disruption of the alveolar septa. It can be generalized or localized, involving part or all of a lung. Overinflation is distention with or without alveolar rupture and is often reversible.

Compensatory overinflation can be acute or chronic and occurs in normally functioning pulmonary tissue when, for any reason, a sizable portion of the lung is removed or becomes partially or completely airless, which can occur with pneumonia, atelectasis, empyema, and pneumothorax.

Obstructive overinflation results from partial obstruction of a bronchus or bronchiole, when it becomes more difficult for air to leave the alveoli than to enter; there is a gradual accumulation of air distal to the obstruction, the so-called bypass, ball valve, or check valve type of obstruction (see Chapter 384).

LOCALIZED OBSTRUCTIVE OVERINFLATION

When a ball-valve type of obstruction partially occludes the main stem bronchus, the entire lung becomes overinflated; individual lobes are affected when the obstruction is in lobar bronchi. Segments or subsegments are affected when their individual bronchi are blocked. Localized obstructions that can be responsible for overinflation include foreign bodies and the inflammatory reaction to them, abnormally thick mucus (cystic fibrosis, see Chapter 400), endobronchial tuberculosis or tuberculosis of the tracheobronchial lymph nodes (see Chapter 212), and endobronchial or mediastinal tumors. When most or all of a lobe is involved, the percussion note is hyperresonant over the area, and the breath sounds are decreased in intensity. The distended lung may extend across the mediastinum into the opposite hemithorax. Under fluoroscopic scrutiny during exhalation, the overinflated area does not decrease in size, and the heart and the mediastinum shift to the opposite side because the unobstructed lung empties normally.

Unilateral hyperlucent lung can be associated with a variety of cardiac and pulmonary diseases of children, but in some patients, it occurs without demonstrable underlying active disease. More than half the cases follow 1 or more episodes of pneumonia; a rising titer to adenovirus (see Chapter 259) has been documented in several children. This condition may follow bronchiolitis obliterans and may include obliterative vasculitis as well, accounting for the greatly diminished perfusion and vascular marking on the affected side.

Patients with unilateral hyperlucent lung may present with **clinical manifestations** of pneumonia, but some patients are discovered only when a chest radiograph is obtained for an unrelated reason. A few patients have hemoptysis. Physical findings may include hyperresonance and a small lung with the mediastinum shifted toward the more abnormal lung. This condition has been labeled **Swyer-James** or **Macleod syndrome.** Some patients show a mediastinal shift away from the lesion with exhalation. CT scanning or bronchography may demonstrate bronchiectasis. In some patients, previous chest radiographs have been normal or have shown only an acute pneumonia, suggesting that a hyperlucent lung is an acquired lesion. No specific treatment is known; it may become less symptomatic with time.

Congenital lobar emphysema (CLE) can result in severe respiratory distress in early infancy and can be caused by localized obstruction. Familial occurrence has been reported. In 50% of cases, a cause of CLE can be identified. Congenital deficiency of the bronchial cartilage, external compression by aberrant vessels, bronchial stenosis, redundant bronchial mucosal flaps, and kinking of the bronchus caused by herniation into the mediastinum have been described as leading to bronchial obstruction and subsequent CLE.

Clinical manifestations usually become apparent in the neonatal period but are delayed for as long as 5–6 mo in 5% of patients. Many are diagnosed by antenatal ultrasonography. Prenatally diagnosed cases are not always symptomatic at birth. Some patients remain undiagnosed until school age or beyond. Signs range from mild tachypnea and wheeze to severe dyspnea with cyanosis. CLE affects the upper and middle lobes, with the left upper lobe the most common site. The affected lobe is essentially nonfunctional because of the overdistention, and atelectasis of the ipsilateral normal lung may ensue. With further distention, the mediastinum is shifted to the contralateral side with impaired function seen as well (Fig. 389-1). A radiolucent lobe and a mediastinal shift are often revealed by radiographic examination. A CT scan may demonstrate the aberrant anatomy of the lesion, and MRI/MRA will demonstrate any vascular lesions, which might be causing extraluminal compression. Nuclear imaging studies are useful to demonstrate perfusion defects in the affected lobe. Figure 389-2 outlines evaluation of an infant presenting

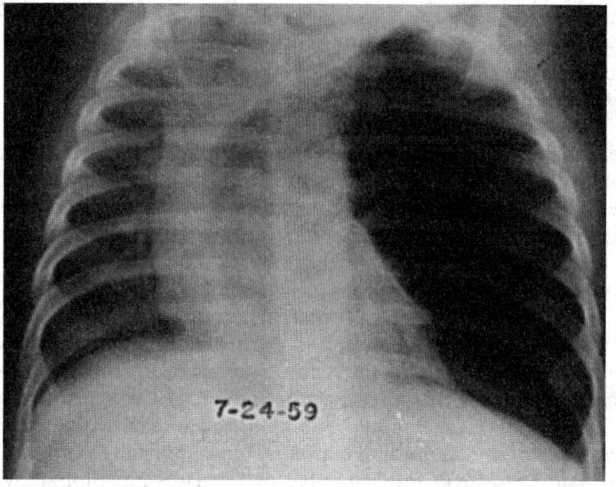

Figure 389-1. Congenital left upper lobe emphysema. Note the extension of the emphysematous lobe into the left lower lobe and its displacement of the mediastinum toward the right.

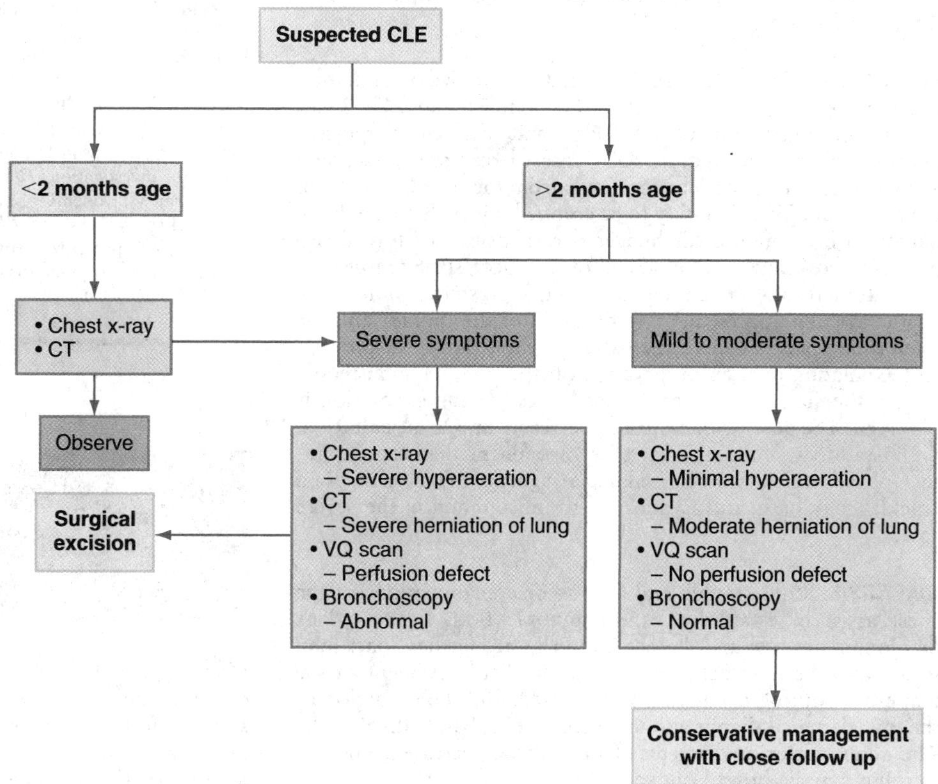

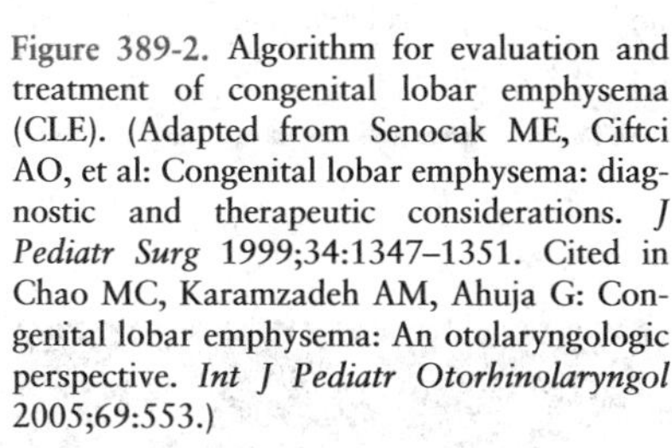
Figure 389-2. Algorithm for evaluation and treatment of congenital lobar emphysema (CLE). (Adapted from Senocak ME, Ciftci AO, et al: Congenital lobar emphysema: diagnostic and therapeutic considerations. *J Pediatr Surg* 1999;34:1347–1351. Cited in Chao MC, Karamzadeh AM, Ahuja G: Congenital lobar emphysema: An otolaryngologic perspective. *Int J Pediatr Otorhinolaryngol* 2005;69:553.)

with suspected CLE. The differential diagnosis includes pneumonia with or without an effusion and cystic adenomatoid malformation.

Treatment by immediate surgery and excision of the lobe may be lifesaving when cyanosis and severe respiratory distress are present, but some patients respond to medical treatment. Selective intubation of the unaffected lung may be of value. Some children with apparent congenital lobar emphysema have reversible overinflation, without the classic alveolar septal rupture implied in the term *emphysema*. Bronchoscopy may reveal an endobronchial lesion.

Overinflation of all three lobes of the right lung has been produced by anomalous location of the left pulmonary artery, which impinges on the right main stem bronchus. Hyperinflation also occurs in patients with the absent pulmonary valve type of tetralogy of Fallot (see Chapter 430.1) and secondary aneurysmal dilatation of the pulmonary artery, which partially compresses the main stem bronchi. A number of neonates have lobar overinflation while being treated for hyaline membrane disease with assisted ventilation, suggesting an acquired cause. Medical management with selective intubation of the unaffected bronchus or high-frequency ventilation has occasionally been successful and lobectomy avoided.

GENERALIZED OBSTRUCTIVE OVERINFLATION

Acute generalized overinflation of the lung results from widespread involvement of the bronchioles and is usually reversible. It occurs more commonly in infants than in children and may be secondary to a number of clinical conditions, including asthma, cystic fibrosis, acute bronchiolitis, interstitial pneumonitis, atypical forms of acute laryngotracheobronchitis, aspiration of zinc stearate powder, chronic passive congestion secondary to a congenital cardiac lesion, and miliary tuberculosis.

PATHOLOGY. In chronic overinflation, many of the alveoli are ruptured and communicate with one another, producing distended saccules. Air may also enter the interstitial tissue (i.e., interstitial emphysema), resulting in pneumomediastinum and pneumothorax (see Chapters 410 and 411).

CLINICAL MANIFESTATIONS. Generalized obstructive overinflation is characterized by dyspnea, with difficulty in exhaling. The lungs become increasingly overdistended, and the chest remains expanded during exhalation. An increased respiratory rate and decreased respiratory excursion result from the overdistention of the alveoli and their inability to be emptied normally through the narrowed bronchioles. Air hunger is responsible for forced respiratory movements. Overaction of the accessory muscles of respiration results in retractions at the suprasternal notch, the supraclavicular spaces, the lower margin of the thorax, and the intercostal spaces. Unlike the flattened chest during inspiration and exhalation in cases of laryngeal obstruction, minimal reduction in the size of the overdistended chest during exhalation is observed. The percussion note is hyperresonant. On auscultation, the inspiratory phase is usually less prominent than the expiratory phase, which is prolonged and roughened. Fine or medium crackles may be heard. Cyanosis is more common in the severe cases.

DIAGNOSIS. Radiographic and fluoroscopic examinations of the chest assist in establishing the diagnosis. Both leaves of the diaphragm are low and flattened, the ribs are farther apart than usual, and the lung fields are less dense. The movement of the diaphragm during exhalation is decreased, and the excursion of the low, flattened diaphragm in severe cases is barely discernible. The anteroposterior diameter of the chest is increased, and the sternum may be bowed outward.

Bullous Emphysema. Bullous emphysematous blebs or cysts (pneumatoceles) result from overdistention and rupture of alveoli during birth or shortly thereafter, or they may be sequelae of pneumonia and other infections. They have been observed in tuberculosis lesions during specific antibacterial therapy. These emphysematous areas presumably result from rupture of distended alveoli, forming a single or multiloculated cavity. The cysts may become large and may contain some fluid; an air-fluid level may be demonstrated on the radiograph. The cysts should be differentiated from pulmonary abscesses. In most cases, the cysts disappear spontaneously within a few mo, although they may persist for a yr or more. Aspiration or surgery is not indicated except in cases of severe respiratory and cardiac compromise.

Subcutaneous Emphysema. Subcutaneous emphysema results from any process that allows free air to enter into the subcutaneous tissue. The most common causes include pneumomediastinum or pneumothorax (see Chapters 410 and 411). Additionally, it can be a complication of fracture of the orbit, which permits free air to escape from the nasal sinuses. In the neck and thorax, subcutaneous emphysema can follow tracheotomy, deep ulceration in the pharyngeal region, esophageal wounds, or any perforating lesion of the larynx or trachea. It is occasionally a complication of thoracentesis, asthma, or abdominal surgery. Rarely, air is formed in the subcutaneous tissues by gas-producing bacteria.

Tenderness over the site of emphysema and a "crepitant" quality on palpation of the skin are classic manifestations. Subcutaneous emphysema is usually a self-limited process and requires no specific treatment. Minimization of activities that may increase airway pressure (cough, performance of high-pressure pulmonary function testing maneuvers) is recommended. Resolution occurs by resorption of subcutaneous air after elimination of its source. Rarely, dangerous compression of the trachea by air in the surrounding soft tissue requires surgical intervention.

Chao MC, Karamzadeh AM, Ahuja G: Congenital lobar emphysema: An otolaryngologic perspective. *Int J Pediatr Otorhinolaryngol* 2005;69:549–554.

Cumming GR, Macpherson RI, Chernick V: Unilateral hyperlucent lung syndrome in children. *J Pediatr* 1971;78:250–260.

Horak E, Bodner J, Gassner I, et al: Congenital cystic lung disease: Diagnostic and therapeutic considerations. *Clin Pediatr* 2003;42:251–261.

Karnak I, Senocak ME, Ciftci AO, et al: Congenital lobar emphysema: Diagnostic and therapeutic considerations. *J Pediatr Surg* 1999;34:1347–1351.

McKenzie SA, Allison DJ, Singh MP, et al: Unilateral hyperlucent lung: The case for investigation. *Thorax* 1980;35:745–750.

Mei-Zahar M, Konen O, Manson D, Langer JC: Is congenital lobar emphysema a surgical disease? *J Pediatr Surg* 2006;41:1058–1061.

Mura M, Zompatori M, Mussoni A, et al: Bullous emphysema versus diffuse emphysema: A functional and radiologic comparison. *Respir Med* 2005;99:171–178.

Chapter 390 ■ α_1-Antitrypsin Deficiency and Emphysema

Glenna B. Winnie and Steven Boas

Homozygous deficiency of α_1-antitrypsin (α-AT) is an important cause of the early onset of severe panacinar pulmonary emphysema in adults in the 3rd and 4th decades of life and an important cause of liver disease in children; it rarely causes lung disease in children (see Chapter 354.5).

PATHOGENESIS. The type and concentration of α_1-antitrypsin are inherited as a series of codominant alleles on chromosomal segment 14q32.1. See Chapter 354.5 for discussion of genotypes and liver disease. The autosomal recessive deficiency affects 1/1,600–1,800 individuals, or ≈100,000 people in the United States. It occurs most commonly in whites of European ancestry. The normal α_1-antitrypsin PiM protein is secreted by the liver into the circulation at a rate of ≈34 mg/kg/day. Mutant protein is not produced (null), or is misfolded (PiZ and others); it may polymerize in the endoplasmic reticulum or be degraded, with subsequent low serum levels. Early adult-onset emphysema associated with α_1-antitrypsin deficiency occurs most frequently with PiZZ (mutation in *SERPINA1* gene), although Pi (null) (null) and, to a lesser extent, other mutant Pi types such as SZ have been associated with emphysema.

α_1-Antitrypsin and other serum antiproteases are important in the inactivation of proteolytic enzymes released from dead bacteria or leukocytes in the lung. Deficiency of these antiproteases leads to an accumulation of proteolytic enzymes in the lung, resulting in destruction of pulmonary tissue with subsequent development of emphysema. Furthermore, polymerized mutant protein in the lungs may be proinflammatory. The concentration of proteases (elastase) in the patients' leukocytes may also be an important factor in determining the severity of clinical pulmonary disease with a given level of α_1-antitrypsin.

CLINICAL MANIFESTATIONS. Most patients who have the PiZZ defect have little or no detectable pulmonary disease during childhood. A few have early onset of chronic pulmonary symptoms, including dyspnea, wheezing, and cough, and panacinar emphysema has been documented by lung biopsy; it is probable that these findings occur secondarily to infection, causing inflammation with consequent early disease. Smoking greatly increases the risk of emphysema developing in mutant Pi types. Although newborn screening to identify children with PiZZ phenotype does not affect parental smoking habits, it does decrease smoking rates among affected adolescents.

Physical examination in childhood is usually normal. It very rarely reveals growth failure, an increased anteroposterior diameter of the chest with a hyperresonant percussion note, crackles if there is active infection, and clubbing. Severe emphysema can depress the diaphragm, making the liver and spleen more easily palpable.

LABORATORY FINDINGS. Serum immunoassay measures low levels of α_1-antitrypsin; normal serum levels are 180–280 mg/dL. Serum electrophoresis reveals the phenotype, and genotype is determined by polymerase chain reaction. In the rare patient with lung disease in adolescence, chest radiograph reveals overinflation with depressed diaphragms, and chest CT may show more hyperexpansion in the lower lung zones, with occasional bronchiectasis.

TREATMENT. Therapy for α_1-antitrypsin deficiency is replacement with enzyme derived from pooled human plasma. A level of 80 mg/dL is protective for emphysema, and this target level for augmentation therapy results in the appearance of the transfused antiprotease in pulmonary lavage fluid. It is usually achieved with doses of 60 mg/kg IV weekly. The Food and Drug Administration has approved the use of purified blood-derived human enzyme for ZZ and null-null patients. The benefit of this therapy has not yet been clearly established. Replacement therapy appears most beneficial for those with moderately severe obstructive lung disease (forced expiratory volume in 1 sec [FEV_1] is 30–65% of predicted) or those with mild lung disease experiencing a rapid decline in lung function. Recombinant sources of α_1-antitrypsin are under development and may be useful for inhalation therapy, although current products are rapidly cleared from the circulation when given intravenously.

Standard supportive therapy for chronic lung disease includes aggressive treatment of pulmonary infection, routine use of pneumococcal and influenza vaccines, bronchodilators, and advice about the serious risks of smoking. Such treatment is also indicated for other members of the family found to have PiZZ phenotypes or null-null, even if they are asymptomatic. Persons with the MZ Pi type do not have an increased risk for the development of pulmonary disease. The clinical significance of the SZ Pi type is unknown, but nonspecific treatment is reasonable. All persons with low levels of serum antiprotease should be warned that the eventual development of emphysema is partially related to environmental factors, including exposure to industrial fumes, respiratory tract infections, and particularly cigarette smoking. Although identification of affected individuals could help prevent development of obstructive lung disease, screening programs are currently suspended, due to concerns about employment and health care insurance discrimination.

Abboud RT, Ford GT, Chapman KR: Standards Committee of the Canadian Thoracic Society: Alpha1-antitrypsin deficiency: A position statement of the Canadian Thoracic Society. *Can Respir J* 2001;8:81–88.

Primhak RA, Tanner MS: Alpha 1-antitrypsin deficiency. *Arch Dis Child* 2001;85:2–5.

Sandhaus RA: Alpha1-antitrypsin deficiency: New and emerging treatments for alpha1-antitrypsin deficiency. *Thorax* 2004;59:904–909.

Stoller JK, Aboussouan LS: Alpha1-antitrypsin deficiency. *Lancet* 2005; 365:2225–2236.

Strange C, Moseley MA, Jones Y, et al: Genetic testing of minors for alpha 1-antitrypsin deficiency. *Arch Pediatr Adolesc Med* 2006;160:531–534.

von Ehrenstein OS, Maier EM, Weiland SK, et al: Alpha1 antitrypsin and the prevalence and severity of asthma. *Arch Dis Child* 2004;89:230–231.

Chapter 391 ■ Other Distal Airway Diseases

Steven Boas

391.1 • Bronchiolitis Obliterans

EPIDEMIOLOGY. Bronchiolitis obliterans (BO) is a rare, chronic lung disease of the bronchioles and smaller airways. BO most commonly occurs in the pediatric population after respiratory infections (adenovirus, *Mycoplasma,* measles, legionella, influenza, pertussis). Other causes include inflammatory diseases (juvenile rheumatoid arthritis, systemic lupus erythematosus, scleroderma, Stevens-Johnson syndrome), toxin fume inhalation (NO_2, NH_3), as well as a manifestation after lung and bone marrow transplantation. BO occurs in all age groups, and the prevalence in 1 pediatric autopsy series was 2/1,000.

PATHOGENESIS. After the initial insult, inflammation affecting terminal bronchioles, respiratory bronchioles, and alveolar ducts may result in the obliteration of the airway lumen. Epithelial damage resulting in abnormal repair is characteristic of BO. Complete or partial obstruction of the airway lumen may result in air trapping or atelectasis. Bronchiolitis obliterans organizing pneumonia (BOOP) is a fibrosing lung disease that includes the histologic features of BO with extension of the inflammatory process from distal alveolar ducts into alveoli and proliferation of fibroblasts. Bronchiolitis obliterans syndrome (BOS) is a clinical entity that relates to graft deterioration after transplantation due to progressive airway disease that appears histologically similar to BO. The etiology of BOS is unclear, however, and may be unrelated to the mechanisms responsible for BO in nontransplant patients.

CLINICAL MANIFESTATIONS/DIAGNOSIS. Cough, fever, cyanosis, dyspnea, chest pain, and respiratory distress followed by initial improvement may be the initial signs of BO. In this phase, BO is easily confused with pneumonia, bronchitis, or bronchiolitis. Progression of the disease may ensue, with increasing dyspnea, chronic cough, sputum production, and wheezing. Physical examination findings are usually nonspecific and may include wheezing and crackles. Chest radiographs may be relatively normal compared with the extent of physical findings but may demonstrate hyperlucency and patchy infiltrates. Occasionally, a Swyer-James syndrome (unilateral hyperlucent lung; see Chapter 389) develops. Pulmonary function tests demonstrate variable findings but typically show signs of airway obstruction. Ventilation-perfusion scans reveal a typical moth-eaten appearance of multiple matched defects in ventilation and perfusion. Chest CT often demonstrates patchy areas of hyperlucency and bronchiectasis. Open lung biopsy or transbronchial biopsy remains the best means of establishing the diagnosis of BO or BOOP.

TREATMENT. No definitive therapy exists for BO. Administration of corticosteroids may be beneficial. Immunomodulatory agents such as sirolimus, tacrolimus, aerosolized cyclosporine, and macrolide antibiotics have been utilized in post–lung transplant recipients with BO with variable success. Infliximab, a monoclonal antibody that binds tumor necrosis factor-α (TNF-α), has been successful in 1 patient with BO after a bone marrow transplant. For BOOP, use of oral corticosteroids for up to 1 yr has been advocated as first-line therapy for symptomatic and progressive disease. Patients with asymptomatic or nonprogressive BOOP can be observed.

PROGNOSIS. Some patients with BO experience rapid deterioration in their condition and die within wk of the initial symptoms; most nontransplant patients survive with chronic disability. Unlike in BO, total recovery is seen in 60–80% of patients with BOOP, although this depends on the underlying systemic disease. Relapse of BOOP can occur, especially if treatment is <1 yr and is amenable to repeat courses of oral corticosteroids. Unlike the more common idiopathic BOOP, progressive BOOP characterized by acute respiratory distress syndrome (ARDS) is rare but is aggressive in its clinical course leading to death.

Epler GR: Bronchiolitis obliterans organizing pneumonia. *Arch Intern Med* 2001;161;158–164.

Fullmer JJ, Fan LL, Dishop MK, et al: Successful treatment of bronchiolitis obliterans in a bone marrow transplant patient with tumor necrosis factor-a blockade. *Pediatrics* 2005;116:767–770.

Hardy KA, Schidlow DV, Zaeri N: Obliterative bronchiolitis in children. *Chest* 1988;93:460–466.

Kurland G, Michelson P: Bronchiolitis obliterans in children. *Pediatr Pulmonol* 2005;39:193–208.

Zhang L, Irion K, Kozakewich H, et al: Clinical course of postinfectious bronchiolitis obliterans. *Pediatr Pulmonol* 2000;29:341–350.

391.2 • Follicular Bronchitis

Follicular bronchitis (FB) is a lymphoproliferative lung disorder characterized by the presence of lymphoid follicles coursing alongside the airways (bronchi or bronchioles). FB is rare in children. Although the cause is unknown, an infectious etiology (viral) has been proposed. Onset of symptoms generally occurs by 6 wk of age and peaks between 6 and 18 mo. Cough, moderate respiratory distress, fever, and fine crackles are common clinical findings. Fine crackles generally persist over time, and recurrence of symptoms is common. Chest radiographs may be relatively benign initially (air trapping, peribronchial thickening) but evolve into the typical interstitial pattern. Chest CT may show a fine reticular pattern. Definitive diagnosis is made by open lung biopsy. Some individuals with FB may respond to therapy with corticosteroids. Prognosis is variable, with some individuals having significant progression of pulmonary disease and others developing only mild obstructive airway disease. The differential diagnosis includes the pulmonary complications of HIV infection.

Bramson RT, Cleveland R, Blickman JG, et al: Radiographic assessment of follicular bronchitis in children. *AJR Am J Roentgenol* 1996;166:1447–1450.

Kinane BT, Mansell AL, Zwerdling RG, et al: Follicular bronchitis in the pediatric population. *Chest* 1993;104:1183–1186.

Yousem SA, Colby TV, Carrington CB: Follicular bronchitis/bronchiolitis. *Hum Pathol* 1985;16:700–706.

391.3 • Pulmonary Alveolar Microlithiasis

Approximately 400 cases of this unusual disorder have been reported. Although the underlying cause of pulmonary alveolar microlithiasis (PAM) is unknown, the disease is characterized by the formation of lamellar concretions of calcium phosphate or "microliths" within the alveoli, creating a classic pattern on the radiograph (Fig. 391-1).

EPIDEMIOLOGY AND ETIOLOGY. Although the mean age at time of diagnosis is in the mid 30s, the onset of the disease can occur in childhood. A strong familial association is seen in ½ of the

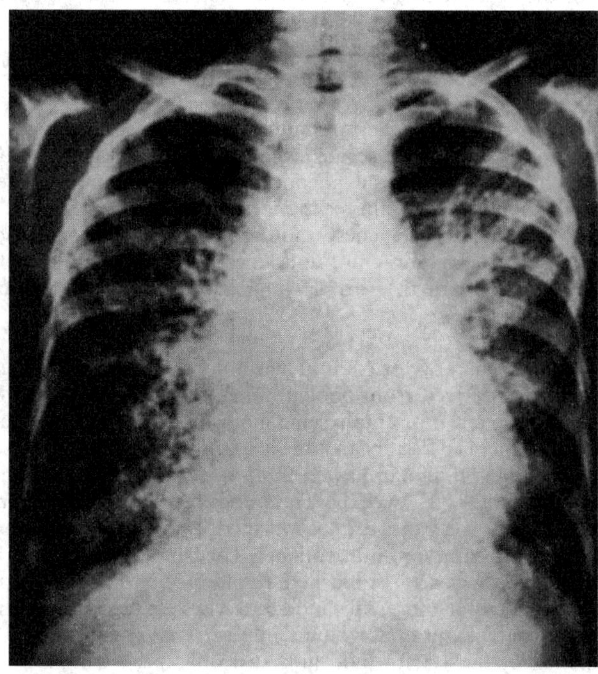

Figure 391-1. Radiograph of the chest of a 7 yr old boy with pulmonary alveolar microlithiasis. (From Clark RB III, Johnson FC: Idiopathic pulmonary alveolar microlithiasis: A case report and brief review of the literature. *Pediatrics* 1961;28:650.)

reported cases, with a probable autosomal recessive pattern of inheritance. In some families, a rapid progression of disease occurs. An equal male and female frequency is noted. A relatively large proportion of patients with PAM have Turkish ancestry. The nonfamilial or sporadic form appears to be associated with other medical conditions including mitral stenosis, nephrolithiasis, pulmonary fibrosis, milk alkalai syndrome, or environmental factors (sand).

CLINICAL MANIFESTATIONS. When symptomatic, individuals with PAM usually complain of dyspnea on exertion and nonproductive cough. Physical examination of the lungs may reveal fine inspiratory crackles and diminished breath sounds. Clubbing occurs, although this is usually a more advanced sign. Discordance between the clinical and radiographic manifestations is common. Children are often asymptomatic on initial presentation. Complications of pneumothorax, pleural adhesions and calcifications, pleural fibrosis, apical bulla, and extrapulmonary sites of microliths have been reported (kidneys, prostate, sympathetic chain, and testes).

DIAGNOSIS. Chest radiography typically reveals bilateral infiltrates with a fine sandlike micronodular appearance or "sandstorm" appearance with greater density in the lower and middle lung fields (see Fig. 391-1). CT of the chest shows diffuse micronodular calcified densities with thickening of the microliths along the septa and around distal bronchioles, especially in the inferior and posterior regions. Diffuse uptake of technetium-99 methylene diphosphonate (^{99m}Tc) by nuclear scan has been reported. Open lung and transbronchial lung biopsy reveal 0.1–0.3 mm laminated calcific concretions within the alveoli. Although the alveoli are often normal initially, progression to pulmonary fibrosis with advancing disease usually ensues. Sputum expectoration may reveal small microliths, although this finding is not diagnostic for PAM and is not typically seen in children. Pulmonary function testing reveals restrictive lung disease with impaired diffusing capacity as the disease progresses, whereas exercise testing demonstrates arterial oxygen desaturation. The differential diagnosis includes sarcoidosis, miliary tuberculosis, hemosiderosis, healed disseminated histoplasmosis, pulmonary calcinosis, and metastatic pulmonary calcifications.

TREATMENT. No specific treatment is effective, although some clinicians have used glucocorticosteroids, etidronate disodium, and bronchopulmonary lavage with limited success. Lung transplantation has been performed for this condition, although it is unknown whether the disease recurs after transplantation.

PROGNOSIS. Progressive cardiopulmonary disease may ensue, leading to cor pulmonale, superimposed infections, and subsequent death in mid-adulthood. Because of the familial nature of this disease, counseling and chest radiographs of family members are indicated.

Edelman, JD, Bavaria J, Kaiser LR, et al: Bilateral sequential lung transplantation for pulmonary alveolar microlithiasis. *Chest* 1997;112:1140–1144.

Erelel M, Kiyan E, Cuhadaroglu C, et al: Pulmonary alveolar lithiasis in two siblings. *Respiration* 2001;68:327–330.

Mariotta S, Ricci A, Papale M, et al: Pulmonary alveolar microlithiasis: report on 576 cases published in the literature. *Sarcoidosis Vase Diffuse Lung Dis* 2004;21(3):173–181.

Schmidt H, Lorcher U, Kitz R, et al: Pulmonary alveolar microlithiasis in children. *Pediatr Radiol* 1996;26:33–36.

Wallis C, Whitehead B, Malone M, et al: Pulmonary alveolar microlithiasis in childhood: Diagnosis by transbronchial biopsy. *Pediatr Pulmonol* 1996;21:62–64.

Chapter 392 ■ Congenital Disorders of the Lung

Jonathan D. Finder and Peter H. Michelson

392.1 • Pulmonary Agenesis and Aplasia

ETIOLOGY AND PATHOLOGY. Pulmonary agenesis differs from hypoplasia in that it entails the complete absence of a lung; it differs from aplasia in the absence of a bronchial stump or carina with agenesis. Bilateral pulmonary agenesis is incompatible with life, presenting as severe respiratory distress and failure. Based on reports of patients with parental consanguinity, pulmonary agenesis is thought to be an autosomal recessive trait.

CLINICAL MANIFESTATIONS AND PROGNOSIS. Unilateral agenesis or hypoplasia may have few symptoms and nonspecific findings, resulting in only ⅓ of the cases being diagnosed while the patient is living. Symptoms tend to be related to central airway complications of stenosis and/or tracheobronchomalacia. In patients in whom the right lung is absent, the aorta can compress the trachea and lead to symptoms of central airway compression; right lung agenesis has a higher morbidity and mortality than left lung agenesis. Pulmonary agenesis is often seen in association with other congenital anomalies, such as the VACTERL sequence (vertebral anomalies, anal atresia, congenital heart disease, tracheoesophageal fistula, renal anomalies, and limb anomalies), ipsilateral facial and skeletal malformations, and central nervous system and cardiac malformations. Compensatory growth of the remaining lung allows for improved gas exchange, but the mediastinal shift can lead to scoliosis and airway compression.

DIAGNOSIS AND TREATMENT. Chest radiographic findings of unilateral lung or lobar collapse with a shift of mediastinal structures toward the affected side may prompt referral for suspected foreign body aspiration, mucous plug occlusion or other bronchial mass lesions. The diagnosis requires a high index of suspicion to avoid the unnecessary risks of bronchoscopy including potential perforation of the rudimentary bronchus. CT of the chest is diagnostic, although the diagnosis may be suggested by chronic changes in the contralateral aspect of the chest wall and lung expansion on chest radiographs. Conservative treatment is usually recommended, although surgery has offered benefit in selected cases.

392.2 • Pulmonary Hypoplasia

ETIOLOGY AND PATHOLOGY. Pulmonary hypoplasia is usually secondary to other intrauterine disorders that produce an impairment of normal lung development (see Chapter 101). Conditions such as deformities of the thoracic spine and rib cage (thoracic dystrophy), pleural effusions with fetal hydrops, cystic adenomatoid malformation, and congenital diaphragmatic hernia physically constrain the developing lung. Any condition that produces oligohydramnios (fetal renal insufficiency or prolonged premature rupture of membranes) can also lead to diminished lung growth. In these conditions, airway and arterial branching are inhibited, thereby limiting the capacity for capillary and gas exchange surface area. Pulmonary hypoplasia involves a decrease in both the number of alveoli and the number of airway generations. The hypoplasia may be bilateral because of the presence of bilateral lung constraint, as occurs in oligohydramnios or thoracic dystrophy. Large, unilateral lesions, such as congenital diaphragmatic hernia and cystic adenomatoid malformation, can displace the mediastinum and thereby produce a contralateral hypoplasia, although usually not as severe as that seen on the ipsilateral side.

CLINICAL MANIFESTATIONS. Pulmonary hypoplasia is usually recognized in the newborn period due to either the respiratory insufficiency or the presentation of persistent pulmonary hypertension. Later presentation (tachypnea) with stress or respiratory viral infection can be seen in infants with mild pulmonary hypoplasia.

TREATMENT. Mechanical ventilation and oxygen may be required to support gas exchange. Specific therapy to control associated pulmonary hypertension, such as inhaled nitric oxide, may be useful. In cases of severe hypoplasia, the limited capacity of the lung for gas exchange may be inadequate to sustain life. Extracorporeal membrane oxygenation may provide gas exchange for a critical period of time and permit survival. Rib expanding devices may improve the survival of patients with thoracic dystrophies (see Chapter 678 and 692).

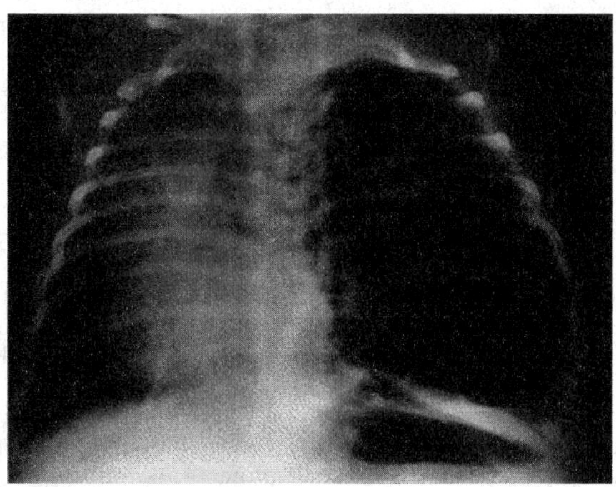

Figure 392-1. Neonatal chest x-ray showing large multicystic mass in the left hemithorax with mediastinal shift due to congenital cystic adenomatoid malformation (CCAM). (From Williams HJ, Johnson KJ: Imaging of congenital cystic lung lesions. *Paediatr Resp Rev* 2002;3:120–127.)

392.3 • Cystic Adenomatoid Malformation

PATHOLOGY. Congenital cystic adenomatoid malformation (CCAM) is a common (1–4/100,000 births) pulmonary congenital anomaly and consists of hamartomatous or dysplastic lung tissue mixed with more normal lung; it is usually confined to one lobe. Three histologic patterns have been described, although the relationship between the histologic appearance and outcome is controversial. **Type 1** (50%) is macrocystic and consists of a single or several large (>2 cm in diameter) cysts lined with ciliated pseudostratified epithelium. The wall of the cyst contains smooth muscle cells and elastic tissue. One third of cases have mucus-secreting cells. Cartilage is rarely seen in the wall of the cyst. This type has a good prognosis for survival. **Type 2** (40%) is microcystic and consists of multiple small cysts with similar histology to that of the type 1 lesion. Type 2 is associated with other congenital anomalies and carries a poor prognosis. In **type 3** (<10%), the lesion is solid with bronchiole-like structures lined with cuboidal ciliated epithelium and separated by areas of nonciliated cuboidal epithelium. This lesion carries the poorest prognosis and can be fatal.

ETIOLOGY. The lesion probably results from an embryologic insult, before the 35th day of gestation, with maldevelopment of terminal bronchiolar structures. Histologic examination reveals little normal lung and many glandular elements. Cysts are very common; cartilage is rare. The presence of cartilage may indicate a somewhat later embryologic insult, perhaps extending into the 10th–24th wk. Although growth factor interactions and signaling mechanisms have been implicated in altered lung branching morphogenesis, the exact roles in the maldevelopment seen here remain obscure.

DIAGNOSIS. Cystic adenomatoid malformations can be diagnosed in utero by ultrasonography. In one series of 67 fetuses with a cystic lung abnormality diagnosed, including 40% with cystic adenomatoid malformations, 14% with pulmonary sequestration (see Chapter 392.4) and 26% with both, the median age at diagnosis was 21 wk gestation. In this series, 7% had severe signs of fetal distress including hydrops ($n = 4$), pleural effusion ($n = 2$), polyhydramnios ($n = 1$), ascites ($n = 1$), and severe facial edema ($n = 1$); 96% of the fetuses were born alive, 2 of whom died in the neonatal period. Antenatal ultrasound scan features and macroscopic or histologic appearance are poor prognostic indicators. Lesions causing fetal hydrops have a poor prognosis. Large lesions, by compressing adjacent lung, may produce pulmonary hypoplasia in nonaffected lobes (see Chapter 392.2). Even lesions that appear large in early gestation may regress considerably or decrease in relative size and be associated with good pulmonary function in childhood. CT allows for accurate sizing of the lesion.

CLINICAL MANIFESTATIONS. Patients who present in the newborn period or early infancy have respiratory distress, recurrent respiratory infection, and pneumothorax. The lesion may be confused with a diaphragmatic hernia. Patients with smaller lesions are asymptomatic until mid-childhood, when brief episodes of recurrent or persistent pulmonary infection or relatively acute chest pain occur. Breath sounds may be diminished, with mediastinal shift away from the lesion on physical examination. Chest radiographs reveal a cystic mass, sometimes with mediastinal shift (Fig. 392-1). Occasionally, an air-fluid level suggests a lung abscess.

TREATMENT. Antenatal intervention in affected infants is controversial but may include excision of the affected lobe for microcystic lesions, aspiration of macrocystic lesions, and open fetal surgery. In the postnatal period, surgery is indicated for all symptomatic patients. Although surgery may be delayed for asymptomatic infants because postnatal resolution has been reported, true resolution appears to be very rare with abnormalities detectable on CT or MRI. Sarcomatous and carcinomatous differentiation has been described in patients with CCAM so surgical resection by 1 yr of age is recommended to limit malignant potential. The mortality rate is <10%.

392.4 • Pulmonary Sequestration

Pulmonary sequestration, a congenital anomaly of lung development, is defined as intrapulmonary or extrapulmonary, depending on the location within the visceral pleura. The majority of sequestrations are intrapulmonary.

PATHOPHYSIOLOGY. The lung tissue in a sequestration does not connect to a bronchus and receives its arterial supply from the systemic arteries (commonly off the aorta) and returns its venous blood to the right side of the heart through the inferior vena cava (extralobar) or pulmonary veins (intralobar). The sequestration functions as a space-occupying lesion within the chest; it does not function in gas exchange and does not contribute to a left-to-right shunt or the dead space. Communication with the airway can occur as the result of rupture of infected material into an adjacent airway. In addition, collateral ventilation within intrapulmonary lesions via pores of Kohn may occur. Pulmonary sequestrations may arise through the same pathoembryologic mechanism as a remnant of a diverticular outgrowth of the esophagus. Some propose that intrapulmonary sequestration is an acquired lesion primarily caused by infection and inflammation; inflammation leads to cystic changes and hypertrophy of a feeding systemic artery. This is consistent with the rarity of this lesion in autopsy series of newborns. Gastric or pancreatic tissue may be found within the sequestration. Cysts may also be present. Other congenital anomalies, including CCAM, diaphragmatic hernia, and esophageal cysts, are not uncommon. Some believe that intrapulmonary sequestration is often a manifestation of cystic adenomatoid malformation and have questioned the existence of intrapulmonary sequestration as a separate entity.

CLINICAL MANIFESTATIONS AND DIAGNOSIS. Physical findings in patients with sequestration include an area of dullness to percussion and decreased breath sounds over the lesion. During infection, crackles may also be present. A continuous or purely systolic murmur may be heard over the back. If findings on routine chest radiographs are consistent with the diagnosis, further delineation is indicated before surgical intervention (Fig. 392-2). CT with contrast can demonstrate both the extent of the lesion and its vascular supply. Magnetic resonance angiography (MRA) is also useful. Ultrasonography can help rule out a diaphragmatic hernia and demonstrate the systemic artery. Surgical removal is recommended. Identifying the blood supply before surgery avoids inadvertently severing its systemic artery.

Intrapulmonary sequestration is generally found in a lower lobe and does not have its own pleura. Patients usually present with infection. In older patients, hemoptysis is common. A chest radiograph during a period when there is no active infection reveals a mass lesion; an air-fluid level may be present. During infection, the margins of the lesion may be blurred. There is no difference in the incidence of this lesion in each lung.

Extrapulmonary sequestration is much more common in males and almost always involves the left lung. This lesion is enveloped by a pleural covering and is associated with diaphragmatic hernia and other abnormalities such as colonic duplication, vertebral abnormalities, and pulmonary hypoplasia. Many of these patients are asymptomatic when the mass is discovered by routine chest radiography. Other patients present with respiratory symptoms or heart failure. Subdiaphragmatic extrapulmonary sequestration may present as an abdominal mass on prenatal ultrasonography. The advent of prenatal ultrasonography has also enabled evidence that fetal pulmonary sequestrations can spontaneously regress.

TREATMENT. Treatment of intrapulmonary sequestration is surgical removal of the lesion, a procedure that usually requires excision of the entire involved lobe. Segmental resection occasionally suffices. Surgical resection of the involved area is recommended for extrapulmonary sequestration.

392.5 • Bronchogenic Cysts

ETIOLOGY AND PATHOLOGY. Bronchogenic cysts arise from abnormal budding of the tracheal diverticulum of the foregut before the 16th wk of gestation and are originally lined with ciliated epithelium. They are more commonly found on the right and near a midline structure (trachea, esophagus, carina), but peripheral lower lobe and perihilar intrapulmonary cysts are not infrequent. Diagnosis may be precipitated by enlargement of the cyst, which causes symptoms by pressure on an adjacent airway. When the diagnosis is delayed until an infection occurs, the ciliated epithelium may be lost, and accurate pathologic diagnosis is then impossible. Cysts are rarely demonstrable at birth. Later, some cysts become symptomatic by becoming infected or by enlarging in size and compromising the function of an adjacent airway.

CLINICAL MANIFESTATIONS AND TREATMENT. Fever, chest pain, and productive cough are the most common presenting symp-

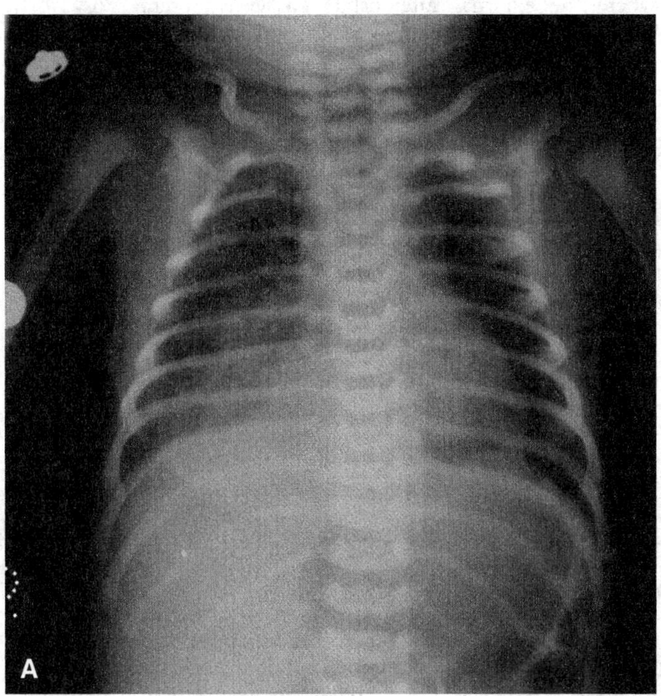

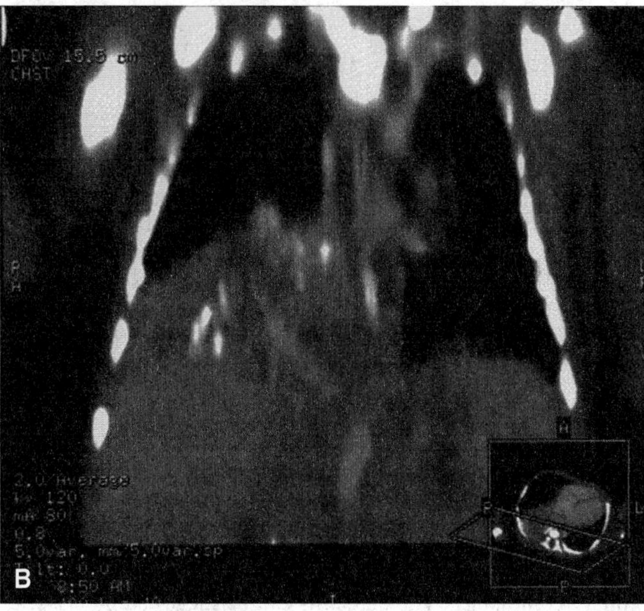

Figure 392-2. *A*, Plain chest x-ray showing changes in the region of the right lower/middle lobe of the lung. *B*, CT showing parenchymal changes in the right lower lobe of the lung in keeping with a sequestration. (From Corbett HJ, Humphrey GME: Pulmonary sequestration. *Paediatr Resp Rev* 2004;5:59–68.)

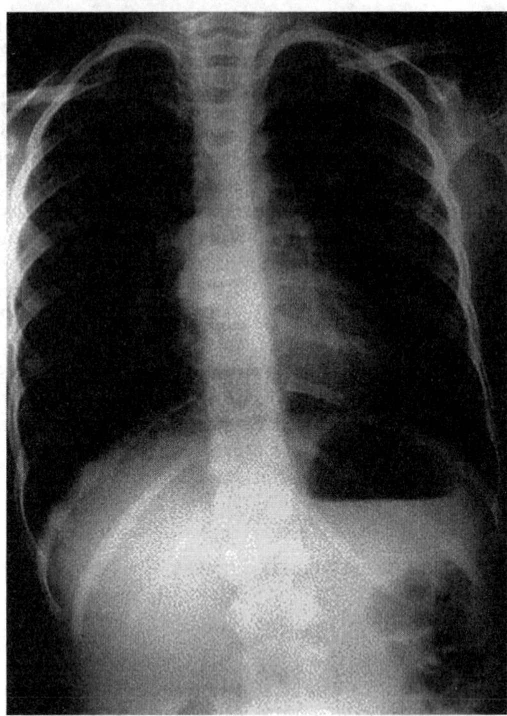

Figure 392-3. Chest x-ray showing an ovoid, well-defined, soft-tissue density causing splaying of the carina due to bronchogenic cyst. (From Williams HJ, Johnson KJ: Imaging of congenital cystic lung lesions. *Paediatr Resp Rev* 2002;3:120–127.)

toms. Dysphagia may be present; some bronchogenic cysts are asymptomatic. A chest radiograph reveals the cyst, which may contain an air-fluid level (Fig. 392-3). CT scan or MRI is obtained in most cases to better demonstrate anatomy and extent of lesion before surgical resection. Treatment of symptomatic cysts is surgical excision after appropriate antibiotic management. Asymptomatic cysts are generally excised in view of the high rate of infection.

392.6 • Congenital Pulmonary Lymphangiectasia

ETIOLOGY AND PATHOLOGY. This disease, characterized by greatly dilated lymphatic ducts throughout the lung, can occur in 3 pathologic circumstances: (1) pulmonary venous obstruction produces an elevated transvascular pressure and engorges the pulmonary lymphatics; (2) generalized lymphangiectasia is a generalized disease of several organ systems, including lungs and the intestines, and is associated with Noonan syndrome; and (3) lymphangiectasia may be limited to the lung.

CLINICAL MANIFESTATIONS AND TREATMENT. Children with pulmonary venous obstruction or severe pulmonary lymphangiectasia present with dyspnea and cyanosis in the newborn period. Chest radiographs reveal diffuse, dense, reticular densities with prominence of Kerley B lines. If the lung is not completely involved, the spared areas appear hyperlucent. Respiration is compromised because of impaired diffusion and decreased pulmonary compliance. The diagnosis can be suggested by CT scan and cardiac catheterization; definitive diagnosis requires lung biopsy (either thoracoscopic or open). Treatment is supportive and includes administration of oxygen, mechanical ventilation, nutritional support (including gastrostomy placement), and careful fluid management with diuretics. Primary pulmonary lymphangiectasia can produce severe pulmonary dysfunction that may require long-term mechanical ventilation; long-term survival is possible even in severe cases. Occasionally, the pulmonary venous obstruction is secondary to left-sided cardiac lesions, and relief of the latter can produce improvement in pulmonary dysfunction. Generalized lymphangiectasia generally produces milder pulmonary dysfunction, and survival to mid-childhood and beyond is not unusual.

392.7 • Lung Hernia

ETIOLOGY AND PATHOLOGY. A lung hernia is a protrusion of the lung beyond its normal thoracic boundaries. About 20% are congenital; the balance of cases are noted after chest trauma or thoracic surgery or in patients with pulmonary diseases such as cystic fibrosis or asthma, which cause frequent cough and generate high intrathoracic pressure. A congenital weakness of the suprapleural membranes or musculature of the neck may play a role in the appearance of a lung hernia. More than half of congenital lung hernias and almost all acquired hernias are **cervical.** Congenital cervical hernias usually occur anteriorly through a gap between the scalenus anterior and sternocleidomastoid muscles. Cervical herniation is usually prevented by the trapezius muscle (posteriorly, at the thoracic inlet) and by the three scalene muscles (laterally).

CLINICAL MANIFESTATIONS AND TREATMENT. The presenting sign of a cervical hernia ("Sibson hernia") is usually a neck mass noticed while straining or coughing. Some lesions are asymptomatic and detected only when a chest film is taken for another reason. Findings on physical examination are normal except during Valsalva maneuver, when a soft bulge may be noticed in the neck. In most cases, no treatment is necessary. These hernias may cause problems, however, during attempts to place a central venous catheter through the jugular or subclavian veins. Spontaneous resolution can occur.

Paravertebral or parasternal hernias are usually associated with rib anomalies. Intercostal hernias usually occur parasternally, where the external intercostal muscle is absent. Posteriorly, despite the seemingly inadequate internal intercostal muscle, the paraspinal muscles usually prevent herniation. Straining, coughing, or playing a musical instrument may have a role in causing intercostal hernias, but in most cases, there is probably a preexisting defect in the thoracic wall.

Surgical treatment for lung hernia is occasionally justified for cosmetic reasons. In patients with severe chronic pulmonary disease and chronic cough and for whom cough suppression is contraindicated, permanent correction may not be achieved.

392.8 • Other Congenital Malformations of the Lung

CONGENITAL LOBAR EMPHYSEMA AND PULMONARY CYSTS. See Chapter 389.

PULMONARY ARTERIOVENOUS MALFORMATION. See Chapters 432 and 444.

BRONCHOBILIARY FISTULA. This rare anomaly usually presents life-threatening problems in early infancy, but diagnosis has occasionally been delayed until adulthood. Females are more commonly affected. The bronchobiliary fistula consists of a fistulous connection between the right middle lobe bronchus and the left hepatic ductal system. All patients have recurrent severe bronchopulmonary infection starting in early infancy. *Definitive diagnosis* requires endoscopy and bronchography or exploratory surgery. *Treatment* includes surgical excision of the entire intrathoracic portion of the fistula. If the hepatic portion of the fistula does not communicate with the biliary system or duodenum, the involved segment may also have to be resected. Bronchobiliary communications also occur as acquired lesions resulting from hepatic disease complicated by infection.

Bentsianov BL, Goldstein NA, Giuste R, Har-El G: Unilateral pulmonary agenesis presenting as an airway lesion. *Arch Otolaryngol Head Neck Surg* 2000;126:1386–1389.

Calvert JK, Boyd PA, Chamberlain PC, et al: Outcome of antenatally suspected congenital cystic adenomatoid malformation of the lung: 10 years' experience 1991–2001. *Arch Dis Child* 2006;91:F26–F28.

Carpentieri DF, Guttenberg M, Quinn TM, Adzick NS: Subdiaphragmatic pulmonary sequestration: A case report with review of the literature. *J Perinatol* 2000;20:60–62.

Chung CJ, Fordham LA, Barker P, Cooper LL: Children with congenital pulmonary lymphangiectasia: After infancy. *AJR Am J Roentgenol* 1999;173:1583–1588.

Davenport M, Warne SA, Cacciaguerra S, et al: Current outcome of antenally diagnosed cystic lung disease. *J Pediatr Surg* 2004;39:549–556.

Garcia-Pena P, Lucaya J, Hendry GM, et al: Spontaneous involution of pulmonary sequestration in children: A report of two cases and review of the literature. *Pediatr Radiol* 1998;28:266–270.

Glenn C, Bonekat W, Cua A, et al: Lung hernia. *Am J Emerg Med* 1997;15:260–262.

Granata C, Gambini C, Balducci T, et al: Bronchioloalveolar carcinoma arising in congenital cystic adenomatoid malformation in a child: A case report and review on malignancies originating in congenital cystic adenomatoid malformation. *Pediatr Pulmonol* 1998; 25:62–66.

Krivchenya DU, Dubrovin AG, Krivchenya TD, et al: Aplasia of the right lung in a 4-year-old child: Surgical stabilization of the mediastinum by diaphragm translocation leading to complete recovery from respiratory distress syndrome. *J Pediatr Surg* 2000;35:1499–1502.

Nicolette LA, Kosloske AM, Bartow SA, Murphy S: Intralobar pulmonary sequestration: A clinical and pathological spectrum. *J Pediatr Surg* 1993;28:802–805.

Riedlinger WF, Vargas SO, Jennings RW, et al: Bronchial atresia is common to extralobar sequestration, intralobar sequestration, congenital cystic adenomatoid malformation, and lobar emphysema. *Pediatr Dev Pathol* 2006;9:361–373.

Sauvat F, Michel JL, Benachi A, et al: Management of asymptomatic neonatal cystic adenomatoid malformations. *J Pediatr Surg* 2003; 38:548–552.

Schmittenbecher P: Congenital cystic adenomatoid malformation of the lung: Indications and timing of surgery. *J Pediatr Surg* 2005;40:891–892.

Schwartz D, Reyes-Mugica M, Keller M: Imaging of surgical diseases of the newborn chest. *Radiol Clin North Am* 1999;37:1067–1078.

Zach MS: Adult outcome of congenital lower respiratory tract malformations. *Thorax* 2001;56:65–72.

Chapter 393 ■ Pulmonary Edema

Thomas Bahk, Robert Mazor, and Thomas P. Green

Pulmonary edema is an excessive accumulation of fluid in the interstitium and air spaces of the lung, resulting in oxygen desaturation and respiratory distress. It is a common problem in the acutely ill child and a sequela of several different pathologic processes.

PATHOPHYSIOLOGY. Although pulmonary edema is traditionally separated into two categories according to cause (*cardiogenic* and *noncardiogenic*), the end result of both processes is a net fluid accumulation within the interstitial and alveolar spaces. Noncardiogenic pulmonary edema, in its most severe state, is also known as **acute respiratory distress syndrome (ARDS)** [see Chapter 69].

The pressure and osmolarity on either side of a pulmonary capillary and capillary permeability are the physical factors that determine fluid movement through the capillary wall. Baseline conditions lead to a net filtration of fluid from the intravascular space into the interstitium. This "extra" interstitial fluid is usually rapidly reabsorbed by pulmonary lymphatics. Conditions that lead to altered capillary permeability, increased pulmonary capillary pressure, or decreased intravascular oncotic pressure increase the net flow of fluid out of the capillary (Table 393-1) and thereby lead to water accumulation in the lung.

To understand the sequence of lung water accumulation, it is helpful to consider its distribution among 4 distinct compartments.

1. **Vascular compartment:** This compartment consists of all blood vessels that participate in fluid exchange with the interstitium. The vascular compartment is separated from the interstitium by capillary endothelial cells. Several endogenous inflammatory mediators, as well as exogenous toxins, are implicated in the pathogenesis of pulmonary capillary endothelial damage, leading to the "leakiness" seen in several systemic processes.
2. **Interstitial compartment:** The importance of this space lies in its interposition between the alveolar and vascular compartments. As fluid leaves the vascular compartment, it collects in the interstitium before overflowing into the air spaces of the alveolar compartment.
3. **Alveolar compartment:** This compartment is lined with type 1 and type 2 epithelial cells. These epithelial cells have a role in active fluid transport from the alveolar space.
4. **Pulmonary lymphatic compartment:** There is an extensive network of pulmonary lymphatics. Excess fluid present in the alveolar and interstitial compartments is drained via the lymphatic system. When the capacity for drainage of the lymphatics is surpassed, fluid accumulation occurs.

ETIOLOGY. The specific clinical findings vary according to the underlying mechanism (see Table 393-1).

TABLE 393-1. Etiology of Pulmonary Edema

INCREASED PULMONARY CAPILLARY PRESSURE
Cardiogenic, such as left ventricular failure
Noncardiogenic, as in pulmonary veno-occlusive disease, pulmonary venous fibrosis, mediastinal tumors
INCREASED CAPILLARY PERMEABILITY
Bacterial and viral pneumonia
Acute respiratory distress syndrome (ARDS)
Inhaled toxic agents
Circulating toxins
Vasoactive substances such as histamine, leukotrienes, thromboxanes
Diffuse capillary leak syndrome, as in sepsis
Immunologic reactions, such as transfusion reactions
Smoke inhalation
Aspiration pneumonia/pneumonitis
Drowning and near drowning
Radiation pneumonia
Uremia
LYMPHATIC INSUFFICIENCY
Congenital and acquired
DECREASED ONCOTIC PRESSURE
Hypoalbuminemia, as in renal and hepatic diseases, protein-losing states, and malnutrition
INCREASED NEGATIVE INTERSTITIAL PRESSURE
Upper airway obstructive lesions, such as croup and epiglottitis
Re-expansion pulmonary edema
MIXED OR UNKNOWN CAUSES
Neurogenic pulmonary edema
High-altitude pulmonary edema
Eclampsia
Pancreatitis
Pulmonary embolism
Heroin (narcotic) pulmonary edema

Modified from Robin E, Carroll C, Zelis R: Pulmonary edema. *N Engl J Med* 1973;288:239, 292; and Desphande J, Wetzel R, Rogers M: In Rogers M (editor): *Textbook of Pediatric Intensive Care*, 3rd ed. Baltimore, Williams & Wilkins, 1996, pp 432–442.

Increases in pulmonary vascular pressure *(capillary hydrostatic pressure)* lead to increased flow of fluid from the vessel. *Cardiac processes* that lead to failure of left-sided forward flow (myocarditis) or to an increase left-sided back flow (mitral valve regurgitation) increase pulmonary capillary pressure. In addition, there are noncardiac causes involving abnormalities of the pulmonary veins that obstruct venous drainage, leading to an *increase in capillary pressure.*

Increased capillary permeability is usually secondary to damage to the endothelium. This can occur secondary to direct injury to the alveolar epithelium, or indirectly through systemic processes that deliver circulating inflammatory mediators or toxins to the lungs. Because of the large amount of pulmonary blood flow, the lung is especially susceptible to circulating toxins. Inflammatory mediators (tumor necrosis factor, leukotrienes, thromboxanes) and vasoactive agents (nitric oxide, histamine) formed during pulmonary and systemic processes play a role in the endothelial damage and the altered capillary permeability that occurs in many disease processes, with sepsis being a common cause.

Fluid homeostasis in the lung is largely dependent on drainage via the lymphatics. Experimentally, pulmonary edema occurs with obstruction of the lymphatic system. Increased lymph flow and dilation of lymphatic vessels occur in chronic edematous states.

By decreasing the forces promoting fluid re-entry into the vascular space, decreases in intravascular oncotic pressure lead to pulmonary edema. This occurs in dilutional disorders such as fluid overload with hypotonic solutions and in protein-losing states such as nephrotic syndrome and malnutrition.

Increased negative interstitial pressure is invoked in disorders in which upper airway obstruction exists, such as croup. Other mechanisms may also be involved. Theories implicate an increase in CO_2 tension, decreased O_2 tension, and extreme increases in cardiac afterload, leading to transient cardiac insufficiency.

The mechanism causing neurogenic pulmonary edema is not clear. A massive sympathetic discharge secondary to a cerebral injury may produce increased pulmonary and systemic vasoconstriction, resulting in a shift of blood to the pulmonary vasculature, an increase in capillary pressure, and edema formation. The mechanism causing high-altitude pulmonary edema is unclear, but it may also be related to sympathetic outflow, increased pulmonary vascular pressures, and hypoxia-induced increases in capillary permeability.

CLINICAL MANIFESTATIONS. The clinical features that arise depend on the mechanism of edema formation. In general, the interstitial and alveolar edema prevent the inflation of alveoli, leading to atelectasis and decreased surfactant production, resulting in decreased pulmonary compliance and decreased tidal volumes. Increased respiratory effort is required to preserve tidal volume and/or increase respiratory rate. The earliest clinical signs include increased work of breathing in the form of tachypnea and dyspnea. With the accumulation of fluid in the alveolar space, auscultation reveals fine crackles and wheezing, especially in dependent lung fields. In cardiogenic pulmonary edema, a gallop may be present as well as peripheral edema and jugular venous distension.

Chest radiographs can provide useful ancillary data, although initial radiographs may be normal. Early radiographic signs include peribronchial and perivascular cuffing, representing accumulation of interstitial edema. Diffuse streakiness reflects interlobular edema and distended pulmonary lymphatics. Diffuse, patchy densities secondary to alveolar filling are a late sign, including the classic description of the "butterfly" appearance, representing bilateral interstitial or alveolar infiltrates. Cardiomegaly and increased pulmonary vascular markings are seen with causes involving left ventricular dysfunction. Heart size is usually normal in noncardiogenic pulmonary edema (see Table 393-2). Chest tomography demonstrates that edema accumulates in the dependent areas of the lung. Therefore, changing the patient position can alter regional differences in lung compliance and alveolar ventilation.

TABLE 393-2. Radiographic Features That May Help to Differentiate Cardiogenic from Noncardiogenic Pulmonary Edema

RADIOGRAPHIC FEATURE	CARDIOGENIC EDEMA	NONCARDIOGENIC EDEMA
Heart size	Normal or greater than normal	Usually normal
Width of the vascular pedicle*	Normal or greater than normal	Usually normal or less than normal
Vascular distribution	Balanced or inverted	Normal or balanced
Distribution of edema	Even or central	Patchy or peripheral
Pleural effusions	Present	Not usually present
Peribronchial cuffing	Present	Not usually present
Septal lines	Present	Not usually present
Air bronchograms	Not usually present	Usually present

*The width of the vascular pedicle in adults is determined by dropping a perpendicular line from the point at which the left subclavian artery exits the aortic arch and measuring across to the point at which the superior vena cava crosses the right mainstem bronchus. A vascular-pedicle width >70 mm on a portable digital anteroposterior radiograph of the chest when the patient is supine is optimal for differentiating high from normal-to-low intravascular volume.

From Ware LB, Matthay MA: Acute pulmonary edema. *N Engl J Med* 2005;353:2788–2796.

Measurement of brain natriuretic peptide (BNP), which is elevated in heart disease, can help differentiate cardiac from pulmonary causes of pulmonary edema. A BNP level >500 pg/mL suggests heart disease; <100 pg/mL suggests lung disease.

TREATMENT. The treatment of a patient with noncardiogenic pulmonary edema is largely supportive, with the primary goals to ensure adequate ventilation and oxygenation. Additional therapy is directed toward the underlying cause. Patients should receive supplemental oxygen in an effort to increase alveolar oxygen tension and decrease pulmonary vasoconstriction. Patients with cardiogenic causes should be managed with inotropic agents and systemic vasodilators to produce afterload reduction (see Chapter 442). Judicious use of diuretics is valuable in the treatment of pulmonary edema associated with total body fluid overload (sepsis, renal insufficiency). Morphine is often helpful as a vasodilator and a mild sedative.

Positive airway pressure effectively improves gas exchange in patients with pulmonary edema. Positive airway pressure can be provided as **positive end-expiratory pressure (PEEP)** in tracheally intubated patients or in noninvasive forms by continuous positive airway pressure (CPAP) with a mask or nasal prong. The mechanism by which positive airway pressure improves pulmonary edema is not entirely clear but is not associated with decreasing lung water. CPAP prevents closure of alveoli and may reopen collapsed alveolar units. This leads to increased functional residual capacity (FRC) and improved pulmonary compliance, improved surfactant function, and decreased pulmonary vascular resistance. The net effect is to decrease the work of breathing, improve oxygenation, and decrease cardiac afterload.

When mechanical ventilation becomes necessary, especially in noncardiogenic pulmonary edema, care must be taken to minimize the risk of developing complications from barotrauma, including pneumothorax, pneumomediastinum, and primary alveolar damage (see Chapter 70). Lung protective strategies include setting low tidal volumes, relatively high PEEPs, and allowing for permissive hypercapnia.

High altitude pulmonary edema (HAPE) should be managed with descent and supplemental oxygen. Portable CPAP or a portable hyperbaric chamber is also helpful. Nifedipine (10 mg initially, then 20–30 mg slow release every 12–24 hr) in adults is also helpful. If there is a history of HAPE, nifedipine and β-adrenergic agonists (inhaled) may prevent recurrence.

Basnyat B, Murdoch DR: High-altitude illness. *Lancet* 2003;361:1967–1974.

Cotter G, Kaluski E, Moshkoviz Y, et al: Pulmonary edema: New insight on pathogenesis and treatment. *Curr Opin Cardiol* 2001;16:159–163.

Mahfood S, Hix WR, Aaron BL, et al: Reexpansion pulmonary edema. *Ann Thorac Surg* 1988;45:340–345.
Masip J, Roque M, Sanchez B, et al: Noninvasive ventilation in acute cardiogenic pulmonary edema. *JAMA* 2005;294:3124–3130.
Perina DG: Noncardiogenic pulmonary edema. *Emerg Med Clin North Am* 2003;21:385–393.
Peter JV, Moran JL, Phillips-Hughes J, et al: Effect of non-invasive positive pressure ventilation (NIPPV) on mortality in patients with acute cardiogenic pulmonary oedema: a meta-analysis. *Lancet* 2006;367:1155–1162.
Piantadosi C, Schwartz D: The acute respiratory distress syndrome. *Ann Intern Med* 2004;141:460–470.
Ware LB, Matthay MA: Acute pulmonary edema. *N Engl J Med* 2005;353:2788–2796.

Chapter 394 ■ Aspiration Syndromes

John L. Colombo

The spectrum of aspiration spans from an asymptomatic condition to acute life-threatening events, such as occurs with massive aspiration of gastric contents or hydrocarbon products. Other chapters discuss mechanical obstruction of large or intermediate-sized airways (as occurs with foreign bodies; see Chapter 384) and infectious complications of aspiration and recurrent microaspiration (see Chapter 395), such as may occur with gastroesophageal reflux (see Chapter 320.1) or dysphagia (see Chapter 303). Occult aspiration of nasopharyngeal secretions into the lower respiratory tract is a normal event in healthy people, usually without apparent clinical significance.

GASTRIC CONTENTS. Large volume aspiration of gastric contents usually occurs after vomiting; it is an infrequent complication of general anesthesia, gastroenteritis, and an altered level of consciousness. Pathophysiologic consequences can vary, depending primarily on the pH and volume of the aspirate and the amount of particulate material. Increased clinical severity is noted with volumes greater than approximately 0.8 mL/kg and/or pH < 2.5. Hypoxemia, hemorrhagic pneumonitis, atelectasis, intravascular fluid shifts, and pulmonary edema all occur rapidly after massive aspiration. These occur earlier, become more severe, and last longer with acid aspiration. Most clinical changes are present within minutes to 1–2 hr after the aspiration event. In the next 24–48 hr, there is a marked increase in lung parenchymal neutrophil infiltrations, mucosal sloughing and alveolar consolidation that often correlates with increasing infiltrates on chest radiographs. These changes tend to occur significantly later and are more prolonged after aspiration of particulate material. Infection usually does not have a role in initial lung injury after aspiration of gastric contents; aspiration may impair pulmonary defenses, predisposing the patient to secondary bacterial pneumonia. In the patient who has shown clinical improvement but then develops clinical worsening, especially with fever and leukocytes, secondary bacterial pneumonia should be suspected.

Treatment. If a patient has had large volume or highly toxic substance aspiration and already has an artificial airway in place, it is important to perform immediate suctioning of the airway. When immediate suctioning cannot be performed, later suctioning or bronchoscopy is usually of limited therapeutic value. An exception to this is if significant particulate aspiration is suspected. Attempts at acid neutralization are not warranted because acid is rapidly neutralized by the respiratory epithelium. Patients suspected of large volume or toxic aspiration should be observed, have oxygenation measured by oximetry or blood gas analysis, and have a chest radiograph taken, even if asymptomatic. If the chest radiograph and oxygen saturation are normal, and the patient remains asymptomatic, home observation, after a period of observation in the hospital or office, is adequate. No treatment is indicated at that time, but the caregivers should be instructed to bring the child back in for medical attention should respiratory symptoms or fever develop. For those patients who present with or develop abnormal findings during observation, oxygen therapy is given to correct hypoxemia. Endotracheal intubation and mechanical ventilation are often necessary for more severe cases. Bronchodilators may be tried, although they are usually of limited benefit. Animal studies indicate that treatment with corticosteroids does not appear to have any benefit, unless given nearly simultaneously with the aspiration event; their use may increase the risk of secondary infection. Prophylactic antibiotics are not indicated, although in the patient with very limited reserve, early antibiotic coverage may be appropriate. If used, antibiotics should be used that cover for anaerobic microbes. If the aspiration event occurs in a hospitalized or chronically ill patient, coverage of *Pseudomonas* and enteric gram-negative organisms should also be considered. A mortality rate of ≤5% is seen if 3 or fewer lobes are involved. Unless complications develop, such as infection or barotrauma, most patients will recover in 2–3 wk, although prolonged lung damage may persist, with scarring and bronchiolitis obliterans.

Prevention. Prevention of aspiration should always be the goal when airway manipulation is necessary for intubation or other invasive procedures. Feeding with enteral tubes passed beyond the pylorus and elevating the head of the bed in mechanically ventilated patients have been shown to reduce the incidence of aspiration complications in the intensive care unit.

HYDROCARBON ASPIRATION. The most dangerous consequence of acute hydrocarbon ingestion is usually aspiration and resulting pneumonitis (see Chapter 58). Although significant pneumonitis occurs in <2% of all hydrocarbon ingestions, there are an estimated 20 deaths annually from hydrocarbon aspiration in both children and adults. Some of these deaths represent suicides. Hydrocarbons with lower surface tensions (gasoline, turpentine, naphthalene) have more potential for aspiration toxicity than heavier mineral or fuel oils. Ingestion of >30 mL (approximate volume of an adult swallow) of hydrocarbon is associated with an increased risk of severe pneumonitis. Clinical findings of chest retractions, grunting, cough, and fever may occur as soon as 30 min after aspiration, or may be delayed for several hr. Lung radiograph changes usually occur within 2–8 hr, peaking in 48–72 hr. Pneumatoceles and pleural effusions may occur. Patients presenting with cough, shortness of breath, or hypoxemia are at high risk for pneumonitis. Persistent pulmonary function abnormalities can be present many years after hydrocarbon aspiration. Other organ systems, especially the liver, central nervous system, and heart, may suffer serious injury. Cardiac dysrhythmias may occur and be exacerbated by hypoxia and acid-base or electrolyte disturbances.

Treatment. Gastric emptying is nearly always contraindicated because the risk of aspiration is greater than any systemic toxicity. Treatment is generally supportive with oxygen, fluids, and ventilatory support as necessary. The child who has no symptoms and a normal chest radiograph should be observed for 6–8 hr to ensure safe discharge. Certain hydrocarbons have more inherent systemic toxicity. The pneumonic **CHAMP** refers collectively to these: **c**amphor, **h**alogenated carbons, **a**romatic hydrocarbons, and those associated with **m**etals and **p**esticides. Patients who ingest these compounds in volumes >30 mL, such as might occur with intentional overdose, may benefit from gastric emptying. This is still a high-risk procedure that can result in further aspiration. If a cuffed endotracheal tube can be placed without inducing vomiting, this should be considered, especially in the presence of altered mental status. Treatment of each case should be considered individually, with guidance from a poison control center.

Other substances that are particularly toxic and cause significant lung injury when aspirated or inhaled include baby powder, chlorine, shellac, beryllium, and mercury vapors. Repeated exposure to low concentration of these agents can lead to chronic lung disease, such as intersitial pneumonitis and granuloma formation. Corticosteroids may help reduce fibrosis development and improve pulmonary function, although the evidence is limited.

Bynum L, Pierce A: Pulmonary aspiration of gastric contents. *Am Rev Respir Dis* 1976;114:1129–1136.

Colombo JL, Sammut PH: Aspiration syndromes: In Taussig LM, Landau LI (eds): *Pediatric Respiratory Medicine*. St. Louis, Mosby, 1999, pp 439–441.

DeLegge MH: Aspiration pneumonia: Incidence, mortality, and at-risk populations. *JPEN J Parenter Enteral Nutr* 2002;26:S19–S25.

Gleeson K, Eggli D, Maxwell S: Quantitative aspiration during sleep in normal subjects. *Chest* 1997;111:1266–1272.

Marik PE: Aspiration pneumonitis and aspiration pneumonia. *N Engl J Med* 2001;344:665–671.

Mickiewicz M, Gomez HF: Hydrocarbon toxicity: General review and management guidelines. *Air Med J* 2001;20:8–11.

Vale J, Kulig K: American Academy of Clinical Toxicology; European Association of Poisons Centres and Clinical Toxicologists: Position paper: Gastric lavage. *J Toxicol Clin Toxicol* 2004;42:933–943.

Warner MA, Warner ME, Warner DO, et al: Perioperative pulmonary aspiration in infants and children. *Anesthesiology* 1999;90:66–71.

Chapter 395 ■ Chronic Recurrent Aspiration

John L. Colombo

ETIOLOGY. The recurrent aspiration of small quantities of gastric, nasal, or oral contents can lead to several clinical presentations. These include recurrent bronchitis or bronchiolitis, recurrent pneumonia, atelectasis, wheezing, cough, apnea, and laryngospasm. Pathologic outcomes may include granulomatis inflammation, interstitial inflammation, fibrosis, lipoid pneumonia, and bronchiolitis obliterans. Most cases, although associated with significant morbidity, do not come to pathologic inspection, but clinically manifest as airway inflammation. Table 395-1 lists the underlying disorders frequently associated with recurrent aspiration. Oropharyngeal incoordination is reportedly the most common underlying problem associated with recurrent pneumonias of hospitalized children. In one series of hospitalized children with recurrent pneumonia, 48% were found to have dysphagia as their underlying problem. Lipoid pneumonia may occur after the use of home/folk remedies involving oral or nasal administration of animal or vegetable oils to treat various childhood illnesses. Lipoid pneumonia has been reported as a complication of these practices in the Middle East, Asia, India, Brazil, and Mexico. The initial underlying disease, language barriers, and a belief that these are not "medications" may delay the diagnosis.

Gastroesophageal reflux (see Chapter 320.1) is also a common underlying finding that may predispose to recurrent respiratory disease, but it is less frequently associated with recurrent pneumonia. Aspiration has also been observed in infants with respiratory symptoms but no other apparent abnormalities. Recurrent microaspiration has been reported in otherwise apparently normal newborns, especially premature infants. Aspiration is also a risk in patients suffering from acute respiratory illness from other causes, especially respiratory syncytial virus infection (see Chapter 257). These patients, when studied with modified barium swallow and videofluoroscopy, have been seen to have silent aspiration. This emphasizes the need for a high degree of clinical suspicion of ongoing aspiration in a child with an acute respiratory illness who is being fed enterally and who deteriorates unexpectedly.

TABLE 395-1. Conditions Predisposing to Aspiration Lung Injury in Children

ANATOMICAL AND MECHANICAL
Tracheoesophageal fistula
Laryngeal cleft
Vascular ring
Cleft palate
Micrognathia
Macroglossia
Achalasia
Esophageal foreign body
Tracheostomy
Endotracheal tube
Nasoenteric tube
Collagen vascular disease (scleroderma, dermatomyositises)
Gastroesophageal reflux disease
Obesity
NEUROMUSCULAR
Altered consciousness
Immaturity of swallowing/prematurity
Dysautonomia
Increased intracranial pressure
Hydrocephalus
Vocal cord paralysis
Cerebral palsy
Muscular dystrophy
Myasthenia gravis
Guillain-Barré syndrome
Werdnig-Hoffmann disease
Ataxia-telangiectasia
Cerebral vascular accident
MISCELLANEOUS
Poor oral hygiene
Gingivitis
Prolonged hospitalization
Gastric outlet or intestinal obstruction
Poor feeding techniques (bottle propping, overfeeding, inappropriate foods for toddlers)
Bronchopulmonary dysplasia
Viral infection

DIAGNOSIS. Underlying predisposing factors (see Table 395-1) are frequently clinically apparent but may require specific further evaluation. The caregiver should be asked about spitting, vomiting, arching, or epigastric discomfort in an older child; and the timing of symptoms in relation to feedings, positional changes, and nocturnal symptoms such as coughing or wheezing. It is important to remember that coughing or gagging may be minimal or absent in a child with a depressed cough or gag reflex. Observation of a feeding is an essential part of the examination when considering a diagnosis of recurrent aspiration. Particular attention should be given to nasopharyngeal reflux, difficulty with sucking or swallowing, and associated coughing and choking. The oral cavity should be inspected for gross abnormalities and stimulated to assess the gag reflex. Drooling or excessive accumulation of secretions in the mouth suggests dysphagia. Lung auscultation may reveal transient crackles or wheezes after feeding, particularly in the dependent lung segments.

The diagnosis of recurrent microaspiration is challenging because of the lack of highly specific and sensitive tests. A plain chest radiograph is the usual initial study for a child suspected of recurrent aspiration. The classic findings of segmental or lobar infiltrates localized to dependent areas may be apparent (Fig. 395-1), but there are a wide variety of radiographic findings, including diffuse infiltrates, lobar infiltrates, bronchial wall thickening, hyperinflation, and even normal-appearing chest x-rays. Radiologic findings consistent with aspiration may be incidental findings when such imaging is done for other reasons.

A carefully performed barium esophagram is useful in looking for anatomic abnormalities such as vascular ring, stricture, hiatal hernia, or tracheoesophageal fistula. It also yields qualitative information about esophageal motility and, when extended, of gastric emptying. The esophagram is insensitive and nonspecific for aspiration or gastroesophageal reflux.

A modified barium swallow with videofluoroscopy is generally considered the gold standard for evaluating the swallowing mechanism. This study is preferably done with the assistance of a pediatric feeding specialist and a caregiver to try to simulate the usual feeding technique of the child. The modified barium swallow occasionally detects aspiration in patients without apparent respiratory abnormalities.

A gastroesophageal "milk" scintiscan offers theoretical advantages over a barium swallow in being more physiologic and providing a longer window of viewing than the barium esophagram for detecting aspiration and gastroesophageal reflux. This procedure has been a relatively insensitive test for detecting aspiration. The "salivagram," another radionuclide study, may be useful in assessing aspiration of esophageal contents, although its sensitivity has not been well studied. Fiberoptic endoscopic evaluation of swallowing, used effectively in adults, has been reported to be useful in pediatric patients. With this technique, the swallowing is observed directly, without radiation exposure. A child's reaction to placement of the endoscope may alter the assessment of function, depending on level of comfort and cooperation.

Incidental findings on CT scans (generally not indicated to establish a diagnosis of aspiration) may show infiltrates with decreased attenuation suggestive of lipoid pneumonia (Fig. 395-2).

Tracheobronchial aspirates can be examined to evaluate for aspiration. For patients with artificial airways, the use of an oral dye and visual examination of tracheal secretions is useful. This test should not be done on a chronic basis due to possible dye toxicity. It is important to use an adequate volume of dye, but even this may be relatively insensitive compared to measuring lactose or glucose in airway secretions. Quantitation of lipid-laden alveolar macrophages from bronchial aspirates has been shown to be a sensitive test for aspiration in children, but false-positive tests occur, especially with endobronchial obstruction, use of intravenous lipids, sepsis, and pulmonary bleeding. Bronchial washings may also be examined for various food substances, including lactose, glucose, food fibers, and milk antigens.

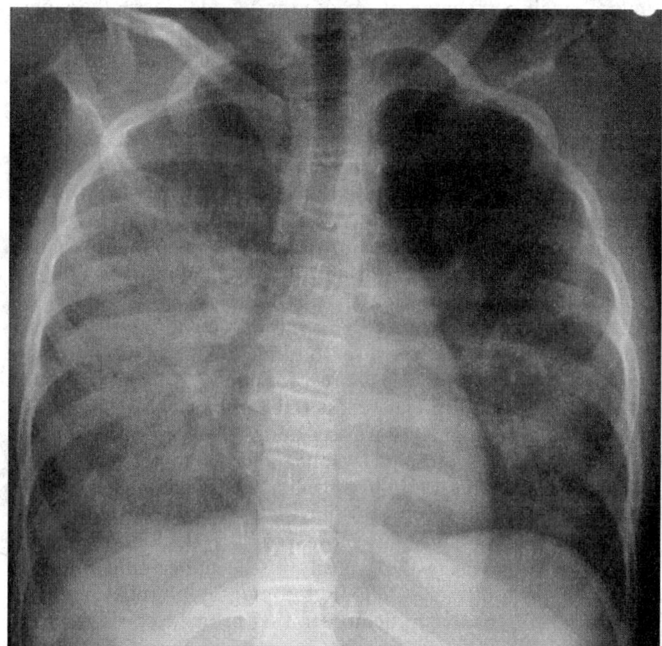

Figure 395-1. Chest radiograph of a developmentally delayed 15 yr old with chronic aspiration of oral formula. Note posterior (dependent areas) distribution with sparing of heart borders.

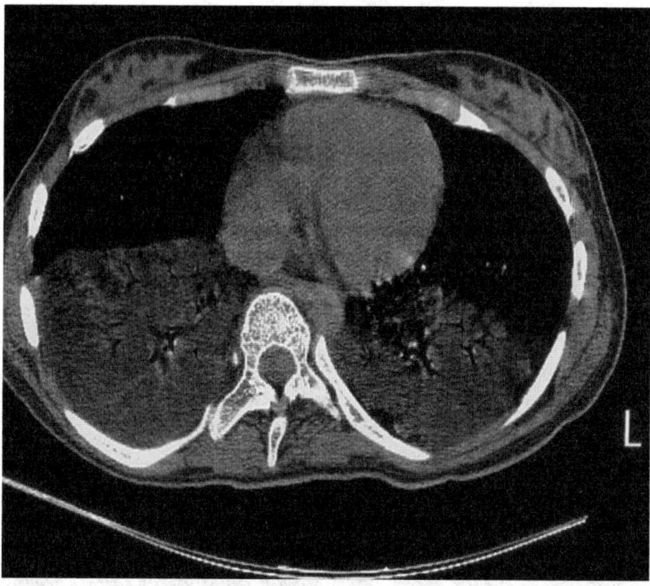

Figure 395-2. Chest CT scan of same patient as in Figure 395-1. Note lung consolidation in dependent region is of similar density to subcutaneous fat.

TREATMENT. If chronic aspiration is associated with another underlying medical condition, treatment should be directed toward that problem. The level of morbidity from respiratory problems should determine the level of intervention. Often, milder dysphagia can be treated with alteration of feeding position, limiting texture of foods to those best tolerated on modified barium esophagram (usually thicker foods), or limiting quantity per feeding. Nasogastric tube feedings can be utilized temporarily during periods of transient vocal cord dysfunction or other dysphagia. Post-pyloric feedings may also be helpful, especially if gastroesophageal reflux is present. Several surgical procedures may be considered. Tracheostomy, although sometimes predisposing to aspiration, may provide overall benefit from improved bronchial hygiene and the ability to suction aspirated material. Fundoplication with gastrostomy or jejunostomy feeding tube will reduce the probability of gastroesophageal reflux–induced aspiration, but recurrent pneumonias often persist because of dysphagia and presumed aspiration of upper airway secretions. Medical treatment with anticholinergics, such as glycopyrrolate or scopolamine, or botulism toxin may significantly reduce morbidity from salivary aspiration but often has side effects. Aggressive surgical intervention with salivary gland excision, ductal ligation, laryngotracheal separation, or esophagogastric disconnection can be considered in severe, unresponsive cases.

Celedon JC, Litonjua A, Ryan L, et al: Bottle feeding in the bed or crib before sleep time and wheezing in early childhood. *Pediatrics* 2002;110:e77.

Colombo JL, Hallberg TK: Pulmonary aspiration and lipid-laden macrophages: In search of gold (standards). *Pediatr Pulmonol* 1999;28:79–82.

Heuschkel RB, Fletcher K, Hill A, et al: Isolated neonatal swallowing dysfunction: A case series and review of the literature. *Dig Dis Sci* 2003;48:30–35.

Hoffman LR, Yen EH, Kanne JP, et al: Lipoid pneumonia due to Mexican folk remedies. *Arch Pediatr Adolesc Med* 2005;159:1043–1048.

Khoshoo V, Ross G, Kelly B, et al: Benefits of thickened feeds in previously healthy infants with respiratory syncytial viral bronchiolitis. *Pediatr Pulmonol* 2001;31:301–302.
Link DT, Willging JP, Miller CK, et al: Pediatric laryngopharyngeal sensory testing during flexible endoscopic evaluation of swallowing: Feasible and correlative. *Ann Otol Rhinol Laryngol* 2000;109:899–905.
Mercado-Deane MG, Burton EM, Harlow SA, et al: Swallowing dysfunction in infants less than 1 year of age. *Pediatr Radiol* 2001;31:423–428.
Newman LA, Keckley C, Petersen MC, et al: Swallow function and medical diagnoses in infants suspected of dysphagia. *Pediatrics* 2001;108:E106.
Owayaed AF, Campbell DM, Wange GG: Underlying causes of recurrent pneumonia in children. *Arch Pediatr Adolesc Med* 2000;154:190–194.
Sheikh S, Allen E, Shell R, et al: Chronic aspiration without gastroesophageal reflux as a cause of chronic respiratory symptoms in neurologically normal infants. *Chest* 2001;120:1190–1195.
Takamizawa S, Tsugawa C, Nishijima E, et al: Laryngotracheal separation for intractable aspiration pneumonia in neurologically impaired children: Experience with 11 cases. *J Pediatr Surg* 2003;38:975–977.

Chapter 396 ■ Parenchymal Disease with Prominent Hypersensitivity, Eosinophilic Infiltration, or Toxin-Mediated Injury

Oren Lakser

396.1 • Hypersensitivity to Inhaled Materials

Hypersensitivity pneumonitis (HP) or **extrinsic allergic alveolitis** is an immunologically mediated diffuse inflammatory disease of the pulmonary interstitium caused by inhalation of a variety of organic antigens. Usually these antigens are of animal or vegetable origin and are typically 1–5 μm in size and therefore deposit in the alveoli. Reactive antigens, such as a variety of drugs, can occasionally cause HP.

ETIOLOGY. Although typically an adult disease, HP has been reported in children and even infants. There are many types of HP, each related to the offending antigen. The most common forms in the United States include **farmer's lung** (from moldy hay; antigen is thermophilic actinomycetes), **bird fancier** or **breeder lung** (from the feces or urine of a wide variety of bird and animal species), and ventilation or **humidifier HP** (from contaminated humidifiers or air conditioners; also caused by thermophilic actinomycetes). Exposure to pigeons (**pigeon breeder disease**) is the most common form in Turkey and Mexico, among other countries. Most case reports of HP in children have been the result of antigens inhaled during avian exposure or exposure to molds. There has been 1 report of HP after exposure to cat hair antigen.

PATHOLOGY AND PATHOGENESIS. HP can present as an acute, subacute, or chronic illness. These forms can be distinguished based on the morphologic features of the pulmonary involvement. In the acute stage, alveolar walls are infiltrated by neutrophils, lymphocytes, plasma cells, and macrophages (Fig. 396-1). The alveolar lumen may contain a proteinaceous exudate mixed with inflammatory cells. Repeated or continuous exposure may result in a subacute presentation characterized by the classic noncaseating granuloma associated with HP. Often, there is an associated terminal and respiratory bronchiolitis; alveoli may have pale foamy macrophages. The chronic form demonstrates further progression of the granulomatous alveolitis, resulting in interstitial fibrosis and honeycombing, primarily affecting the upper lobes.

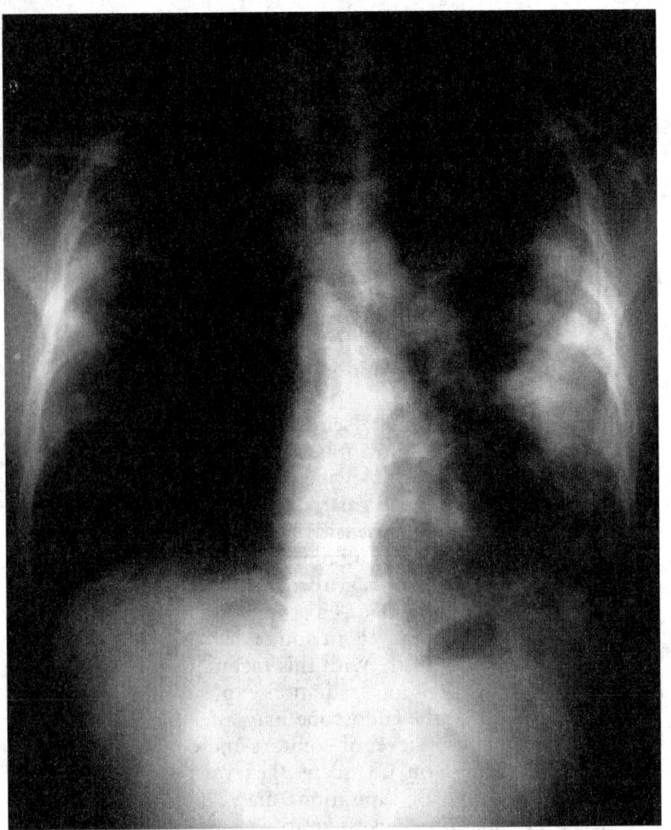

Figure 396-1. Chest radiograph shows bilateral patchy alveolar infiltrate with peripheral consolidation. (From Wubbel C, Fulmer D, Sherman J: Chronic eosinophilic pneumonia: A case report and national survey. *Chest* 2003;123:1763–1766.)

The immune mechanisms involved with inducing these morphologic changes may include immune complex (type III) hypersensitivity (particularly in the acute presentation), delayed cellular (type IV) hypersensitivity, and the alternate complement pathway. Only a small percentage of exposed individuals actually experience clinical symptoms, suggesting an interaction between the nature of the offending antigen, the intensity and duration of exposure, and genetic factors in determining the host response.

CLINICAL MANIFESTATIONS. Acute attacks generally occur 4–8 hr after an exposure. Typical symptoms include fever, chills, cough, dyspnea, myalgia, and malaise that can persist for up to 48 hr. Physical examination usually reveals an ill-appearing, dyspneic child with bibasilar crackles or normal lung examination. Chest radiographs may also be normal or may demonstrate bilateral ground-glass haziness, often sparing the lung apices and bases, with fine nodulations. These patients may progress to the subacute presentation if exposure continues or recurs. The cough worsens, dyspnea becomes more prominent, and anorexia and weight loss may occur. The chest radiograph at this stage has a more reticulonodular appearance. Long-term exposure can lead to the chronic presentation. Dyspnea and cough are severe, with weight loss, weakness, and hypoxemia. These patients eventually develop chronic alveolitis and fibrosis that can lead to cor pulmonale. Chest radiographs show coarse reticulonodular infiltrates and bronchiectasis primarily in the upper- and mid-lung zones. High-resolution computed tomography (HRCT) scans may be more sensitive in demonstrating bronchiectasis.

DIAGNOSIS. The diagnosis of HP is based primarily on the clinical presentation in association with a suspicious exposure. Because the clinical presentation is nonspecific, a high index of suspicion is crucial. Children with HP will meet most of the basic diagnostic criteria that have been proposed for adults. Major criteria include symptoms compatible with HP, evidence of exposure (antibody studies), compatible chest x-ray or HRCT findings, bronchoalveolar lavage (BAL) lymphocytosis, histologic changes compatible with HP, and a positive antigen provocation challenge. Minor criteria include bibasilar crackles, decreased diffusion capacity, and hypoxemia. The presence of 4 major and 2 minor criteria are very suggestive of HP, especially when other diseases with similar presentations have been excluded. A number of laboratory tests may also be helpful in confirming a strong clinical suspicion. HP patients often demonstrate a modest leukocytosis with neutrophilia with a left shift, and modest elevation of the erythrocyte sedimentation rate. Serum levels of immunoglobulins (IgG, IgM, and IgA) are often elevated. Skin testing to particular antigens lacks sensitivity and specificity, as do serum precipitins to specific antigens. Both these tests may indicate exposure but are often positive in individuals without the clinical disease. In adults, BAL fluid typically demonstrates a marked lymphocytosis (often up to 70%) particularly of the $CD8^+$ suppressor T cells, although in children the CD4 : CD8 ratio is not increased. BAL fluid may also contain higher levels of immunoglobulins. Pulmonary function tests classically demonstrate a **restrictive pattern** with impaired gas exchange (diffusion capacity). The presence of a mild obstructive pattern during the acute stage is a poor prognostic indicator. Some have advocated an inhalational challenge either in the laboratory or by re-exposure to the environment. Challenge testing can be dangerous and therefore should be undertaken only in appropriately equipped diagnostic centers.

TREATMENT. The most effective therapeutic approach is complete avoidance of the suspected antigen. Prednisone (1–2 mg/kg/24 hr) is of some benefit, but an extended course, perhaps up to 6 mo, is required. In general, prognosis is quite good, but if exposure persists, pulmonary fibrosis may occur and patients may not completely recover their baseline lung function.

Ceviz N, Kaynar H, Olgun H, et al: Pigeon breeder's lung in childhood: is family screening necessary? *Pediatr Pulmonol* 2006;41:279–282.

Fan LF: Hypersensitivity pneumonitis in children. *Curr Opin Pediatr* 2002;14:323–326.

Knutsen AP, Sotelo-Avila C, Albers GM: Hypersensitivity pneumonitis in children. *Pediatr Asthma Allergy Immunol* 2003;16:247–264.

Lacasse Y, Selman M, Costabel U, et al: Clinical diagnosis of hypersensitivity pneumonitis. *Am J Respir Crit Care Med* 2003;168:952–958.

Martinez-Cordero E, Aguilar Leon DE, Retana VN: IgM antiavian antibodies in sera from patients with pigeon breeder's disease. *J Clin Lab Anal* 2000;14:201–207.

Morell F, Roger A, Cruz MJ: Usefulness of specific skin tests in the diagnosis of hypersensitivity pneumonitis. *J Allergy Clin Immunol* 2002;110:939.

Nacar N, Kiper N, Yalcin E, et al: Hypersensitivity pneumonitis in children: Pigeon breeder's disease. *Ann Trop Paediatr* 2004;24:349–355.

Patel AM, Ryu JH, Reed CE: Hypersensitivity pneumonitis: Current concepts and future questions. *J Allergy Clin Immunol* 2001;108:661–670.

Ratjen F, Costabel U, Griese M, et al: Bronchoalveolar lavage fluid findings in children with hypersensitivity pneumonitis. *Eur Respir J* 2003;21:144–148.

Selman M: Hypersensitivity pneumonitis: A multifaceted deceiving disorder. *Clin Chest Med* 2004;25:531–547.

Stauffer Ettlin M, Pache JC, Renevey F, et al: Bird breeder's disease: A rare diagnosis in young children. *Eur J Pediatr* 2006;165:55–61. Epub 2005, Nov 4.

396.2 • Silo Filler Disease

Silo filler disease, also known as **silage gas poisoning** or **silo filler pneumoconiosis,** is typically caused by nitrogen dioxide toxicity. Nitrogen dioxide is produced in silos (particularly corn silos) within a few hr of filling and reaches a maximum concentration within about 2 days. Dangerous concentrations of gas can remain in a closed silo for as long as 2 wk. After entering a silo within this time frame without proper protection, a person may experience various degrees of silo filler disease.

PATHOGENESIS. The degree of lung injury depends on the duration of exposure and the concentration of nitrogen dioxide. Shortly after inhalation, nitrogen dioxide is hydrolyzed to nitrous and nitric acid, causing chemical pneumonitis and pulmonary edema, primarily affecting type I pneumocytes and ciliated cells lining the airways. Biopsy or autopsy findings include diffuse pulmonary edema, hyperplastic airway epithelium, widened intralobular septa, and bronchiolitis obliterans. With severe exposures, methemoglobinemia can occur. Alteration of macrophage activity and immune function can also occur, resulting in increased risk of infection.

CLINICAL MANIFESTATIONS AND DIAGNOSIS. Most exposures result in mild symptoms that are self-limited. Cough and dyspnea typically occur immediately on entering the silo and are often associated with wheezing, nausea, a choking sensation, ocular irritation, and fatigue. Rarely, symptoms are delayed days or even weeks after exposure. Radiologic manifestations include pulmonary edema in the perihilar areas and bases. Some patients recover and the pulmonary edema clears rapidly. Often, however, this initial phase is followed by a period of remission for 2–3 wk. This quiescent period gives way to a 2nd phase characterized by fever, progressive dyspnea, cyanosis, and cough associated with widespread, scattered miliary opacities that can become confluent and take on a more patchy and nodular appearance. These patients may suffer from methemoglobinemia. Complications include secondary infection and bronchiolitis obliterans. Diagnosis necessitates a careful medical and occupational history, as specific laboratory confirmation of silo filler disease is unavailable.

TREATMENT. Prevention of silo filler disease by minimizing exposure during the initial 2 wk after filling is key. Although no controlled trial has been conducted, high-dose prednisone (up to 30 mg/kg/day) is of some benefit in reducing the severity and duration of the symptoms. Bronchodilators may also be of some limited benefit. Methemoglobinemia is treated with methylene blue in severe cases. Counterintuitively, nitric oxide therapy has been reported to improve oxygenation in patients with silo filler disease. Silo filler disease can be fatal, result in complete recovery, or leave patients with chronic lung disease associated with fibrosis and emphysema.

Dambro MR: Silo filler disease. In Griffith JA: *5 Minute Clinical Consult.* Philadelphia, Lippincott Williams and Wilkins, 2001.

Frampton MW, Boscia J, Roberts NJ Jr, et al: Nitrogen dioxide exposure: Effects on airway and blood cells. *Am J Physiol Lung Cell Mol Physiol* 2002;282:L155–L165.

Leavey JF, Dubin RL, Singh N, et al: Silo-filler's disease, the acute respiratory distress syndrome, and oxides of nitrogen. *Ann Intern Med* 2004; 141:410–411.

Rasmussen MD, Bascom R: Silo filler's disease. Available at emedicine website (www.emedicine.com).

396.3 • Paraquat Lung

Paraquat is the most toxic dipyridilium herbicide. Concentrated solutions (12–20%) tend to be more dangerous than dilute solutions. Its toxic effects result from the production of superoxides and other highly reactive free radicals that cause the peroxidation of cell membranes and selective mitochondrial damage, resulting in cell death. Paraquat selectively concentrates in the lungs because of an amine uptake process that exists in alveolar epithelial cells. Additionally, paraquat-induced injury is significantly increased in the presence of high concentrations of oxygen. Although its use is banned or restricted in some countries, paraquat is still used extensively, particularly in many developing countries.

Pathophysiologically, there is direct injury to the alveolar-capillary membrane and surfactant loss, acute respiratory distress syndrome, progressive intra-alveolar pulmonary fibrosis, and respiratory failure.

CLINICAL MANIFESTATIONS. There are 3 degrees of paraquat intoxication that are dose related. Patients with mild poisoning after ingestion of <20 mg of paraquat ion/kg body weight are usually asymptomatic or may develop vomiting, diarrhea, and mild impairment of gas exchange. Moderate to severe poisoning follows ingestion of 20–40 mg of paraquat ion/kg. These patients typically suffer from vomiting, diarrhea, and caustic injury to the oral or esophageal mucosa and may develop renal failure, hepatic dysfunction, and progressive pulmonary fibrosis, resulting in respiratory failure and death. Acute fulminant poisoning follows ingestion of >40 mg of paraquat ion/kg. Marked ulceration of the oropharynx and esophagus occurs, with multiorgan failure and 100% mortality within hours of ingestion. Measuring the plasma paraquat concentration may be the best marker of exposure and severity (paraquat nomograms) and for predicting prognosis.

TREATMENT. Treatment is generally supportive because no antidote exists. Gastric lavage, activated charcoal, hemoperfusion, and hemodialysis are of limited value in significant poisoning. There have been rare individual case reports of successful treatment of paraquat poisoning with antioxidant therapy consisting of deferoxamine infusion and acetylcysteine. Others have reported some success with combination immunosuppressive therapy consisting of intravenous corticosteroids and cyclophosphamide or prolonged repeated pulse corticosteroid therapy. Results after lung transplantation are poor, likely related to long-term storage of paraquat in muscle and eventual reaccumulation in the transplanted lungs. One patient survived with lung transplantation when the transplant was delayed for >40 days after the ingestion.

Overall prognosis is poor. Survivors generally suffer from a persistent restrictive defect with impaired diffusion capacity on tests of pulmonary function.

Chen G, Lin J, Huang Y: Combined methylprednisolone and dexamethasone therapy for paraquat poisoning. *Crit Care Med* 2002;30:2584–2587.

Dalvie MA, White N, Raine R: Long-term respiratory health effects of the herbicide, paraquat, among workers in the Western Cape. *Occup Environ Med* 1999;56:391–396.

Eddleston M, Wilks MF, Buckley NA: Prospects for treatment of paraquat-induced lung fibrosis with immunosuppressive drugs and the need for better prediction of outcome: A systematic review. *Q J Med* 2003;96:809–824.

Ellenhorn MJ, Schonwald S, Ordog J, et al: Pesticides. In Ellenhorn MJ (ed): *Medical Toxicology: Diagnosis and Treatment of Human Poisoning*, 2nd ed. Baltimore, Williams and Wilkins, 1997.

Lo Sasso AA, Osterhoudt K, Meier FA, et al: A 16-year-old boy with rapidly progressing pulmonary fibrosis. *J Pediatr* 2002;140:270–275.

Schenker MB: Pulmonary function and exercise-associated changes with chronic low-level paraquat exposure. *Am J Respir Crit Care Med* 2004;170:773–779.

396.4 • Eosinophilic Lung Disease (Formerly Löffler Syndrome)

Eosinophilic lung diseases are a heterogeneous group of disorders linked by the common findings of pulmonary infiltrates and circulating or tissue eosinophilia. Many clinicians have adopted the term **pulmonary infiltrates with eosinophilia** (PIE) as a more accurate label for these disorders. There are numerous classification schemes for these types of lung disease. PIE syndromes can be divided into simple pulmonary eosinophilia (Löffler syndrome), prolonged pulmonary eosinophilia, tropical pulmonary eosinophilia, pulmonary eosinophilia with asthma, polyarteritis nodosa, chronic eosinophilic pneumonia, and acute eosinophilic pneumonia. Others have included **Churg-Strauss syndrome, allergic bronchopulmonary aspergillosis** (ABPA), and **idiopathic hypereosinophilia syndrome.** Additional lung diseases such as idiopathic pulmonary fibrosis, Langerhans cell granuloma, and other interstitial lung diseases may have associated eosinophilia but are better classified elsewhere.

Löffler syndrome, the most common PIE syndrome reported in children, is characterized by migrating pulmonary infiltrates accompanied by peripheral blood eosinophilia but minimal respiratory symptoms. This term is rarely used today, and it is likely that most patients with this diagnosis have allergic bronchopulmonary helminthiasis (parasites), medication reactions, or ABPA.

EPIDEMIOLOGY. PIE syndromes appear to be much less common in the pediatric population than in adults. In one series, only 6% of cases occurred in persons <20 yr of age. There have been scattered case reports of acute eosinophilic pneumonia and chronic eosinophilic pneumonia in children. Children previously classified as having Löffler syndrome make up the majority of pediatric cases. Most pediatric case reports suggest an equal number of males and females being affected; there may be geographic differences because 1 group reports a female preponderance in children, similar to adult patients with PIE syndromes. Age at presentation ranges from infancy to adolescence.

PATHOLOGY AND PATHOGENESIS. In the pediatric population, the most common etiology of PIE syndromes includes parasite infections and drug reactions. The prevalence of individual parasite infections varies geographically. The most common parasite causing PIE syndromes in the United States is *Ascaris lumbricoides.* The eggs are ingested. After the larvae hatch, they pass through the intestinal wall and migrate to the lungs, causing an intense inflammatory reaction. Alveolar macrophages, lymphocytes, neutrophils, and eosinophils are the most striking inflammatory cells. Other common parasites include *Strongyloides* species, *Toxocara canis* (dog roundworm, visceral larva migrans), and *Ancylostoma braziliense* ("creeping eruption"). In Africa, South America, and Southeast Asia, the filarial worms *Wuchereria bancrofti* and *Brugia malayi* cause tropical pulmonary eosinophilia.

Several drugs have also been reported to cause PIE syndromes. Sulfasalazine, penicillin, ampicillin, ibuprofen, and cromolyn are a few of these drugs that are of common use in pediatric patients. Immunologic mechanisms may be the means by which these drugs result in an intense pulmonary inflammatory reaction.

CLINICAL MANIFESTATIONS. Patients with PIE syndromes caused by parasites or drugs present with malaise, chronic cough, intermittent fevers, dyspnea, wheezing, and, occasionally, abdominal pain, rash, and weight loss. Symptom duration varies. In acute eosinophilic pneumonia, symptoms are usually present for less than a month and typically do not recur once treated. In chronic eosinophilic pneumonia, symptoms are present for more than 6 mo and often recur despite successful treatment. Results of physical examination vary but often show tachypnea, crackles, and wheezing.

DIAGNOSIS. The diagnosis of a PIE syndrome is made by clinical manifestations with associated blood eosinophilia and chest radiographic findings. Radiologically, these patients present with nonspecific interstitial, alveolar, or mixed infiltrates. The infiltrates tend to be bilateral and diffuse. Patients with chronic eosinophilic pneumonia demonstrate peripheral infiltrates with central sparing ("photographic negative of pulmonary edema"). In addition, eosinophilic lung diseases can be diagnosed by the presence of pulmonary infiltrates and eosinophilia on bronchoalveolar lavage or the presence of parasitic larvae in bronchoscopic or gastric lavage. Lung biopsy can be used to make the diagnosis.

TREATMENT. Therapy varies with the type of PIE syndrome. Parasite and drug-induced PIE syndromes have a good prognosis and resolve spontaneously with supportive care and removal of exposure. Rarely, medications to eradicate the parasites may be warranted. Patients with other forms of eosinophilic lung diseases including acute eosinophilic pneumonia and chronic eosinophilic pneumonia may require a course of corticosteroids. Prognosis for patients with most forms of eosinophilic lung disease is good. Acute eosinophilic pneumonia, however, can be life-threatening.

Allen JN, Magro CM, King MA: The eosinophilic pneumonias. *Semin Respir Crit Care Med* 2002;23:127–143.

O'Connor DL: Recognizing eosinophilic lung syndromes. *Resp Rev* 2001;6:6.

Oermann CM, Panesar KS, Langston C, et al: Pulmonary infiltrates with eosinophilia syndromes in children. *J Pediatr* 2000;136:351–358.

Savani DM, Sharma OP: Eosinophilic lung disease in the tropics. *Clin Chest Med* 2002;23:377–396.

Talmaciu I: Loffler syndrome. Available at emedicine website (www.emedicine.com).

Wubbel C, Fulmer D, Sherman J: Chronic eosinophilic pneumonia: A case report and national survey. *Chest* 2003;123:1763–1766.

Chapter 397 ■ Pneumonia

Theodore C. Sectish and Charles G. Prober

Pneumonia is an inflammation of the parenchyma of the lungs. Although most cases of pneumonia are caused by microorganisms, noninfectious causes include aspiration of food or gastric acid, foreign bodies, hydrocarbons, and lipoid substances, hypersensitivity reactions, and drug- or radiation-induced pneumonitis. The causes of lung infection in neonates (see Chapter 109) and immunocompromised hosts (see Chapter 177) are distinct from those affecting otherwise normal infants and children.

EPIDEMIOLOGY. Pneumonia is a substantial cause of morbidity and mortality in childhood (particularly among children <5 yr of age) throughout the world, rivaling diarrhea as a cause of death in developing countries. With an estimated 146–159 million new episodes per yr in developing countries, pneumonia is estimated to cause approximately 4 million deaths among children worldwide. Currently, the incidence of community-acquired pneumonia in developed countries is estimated to be 0.026 episodes per child-year compared to 0.280 episodes per child-year in developing countries.

In the United States from 1939–1996, mortality caused by pneumonia in children declined by 97%. It is hypothesized that this decline is attributable to the introduction of antibiotics, vaccines, and the expansion of medical insurance coverage for children. *Haemophilus influenzae* type b (see Chapter 192) was an important cause of bacterial pneumonia in young children but has become uncommon with the routine use of effective vaccines. The introduction of heptavalent pneumococcal conjugate vaccine and its impact on pneumococcal disease (see Chapter 181) has reduced the overall incidence of pneumonia in infants and children in the United States by ≈30% in the 1st yr of life, ≈20% in the 2nd yr of life, and ≈10% in children >2 yr of age.

ETIOLOGY. The cause of pneumonia in an individual patient is often difficult to determine because direct culture of lung tissue is invasive and rarely performed. Cultures performed on specimens obtained from the upper respiratory tract or "sputum" generally do not accurately reflect the cause of lower respiratory tract infection. Using "state-of-the-art" diagnostic testing, a bacterial or viral cause of pneumonia can be identified in 40–80% of children with community-acquired pneumonia. *Streptococcus pneumoniae* (pneumococcus) is the most common bacterial pathogen, followed by *Chlamydia pneumoniae* and *Mycoplasma pneumoniae*. In addition to pneumococcus, other bacterial causes of pneumonia in previously healthy children in the United States include group A streptococcus (*Streptococcus pyogenes;* see Chapter 182) and *Staphylococcus aureus* (see Chapter 180.1) [Table 397-1].

Streptococcus pneumoniae, Haemophilus influenzae, and *Staphylococcus aureus* are the major causes of hospitalization and death from pneumonia among children in developing countries, although in children with HIV infection, *Mycobacterium tuberculosis* (see Chapter 212), atypical mycobacterium, *Salmonella* (see Chapter 195), *Escherichia coli* (see Chapter 197), and *Pneumocystis jirovecii* (see Chapter 241) must be considered.

Viral pathogens are a prominent cause of lower respiratory tract infections in infants and children <5 yr of age. Viruses are responsible for 45% of the episodes of pneumonia identified in hospitalized children in Dallas. Unlike bronchiolitis, for which the peak incidence is in the 1st yr of life, the highest frequency of viral pneumonia occurs between the ages of 2 and 3 yr, decreasing slowly thereafter. Of the respiratory viruses, influenza virus (Chapter 255) and respiratory syncytial virus (RSV) (Chapter 257) are the major pathogens, especially in children <3 yr of age. Other common viruses causing pneumonia include parainfluenza viruses, adenoviruses, rhinoviruses, and metapneumovirus. The age of the patient may help identify possible pathogens (Table 397-2).

Lower respiratory tract viral infections in the United States are much more common in the fall and winter, related to the seasonal epidemics of respiratory viral infection that occur each yr. The typical pattern of these epidemics usually begins in the fall when parainfluenza infections appear and most often manifest as croup. Later in winter, RSV, metapneumovirus, and influenza viruses cause widespread infection, including upper respiratory tract infections, bronchiolitis, and pneumonia. RSV attacks infants and young children, whereas influenza virus causes disease and excess hospitalization for acute respiratory illness in all age groups. The knowledge of the prevailing viral epidemic may lead to a presumptive initial diagnosis.

Immunization status is relevant because children fully immunized against *H. influenzae* type b and *S. pneumoniae* are less likely to be infected with these pathogens. Children who are immunosuppressed or who have an underlying illness may be at risk for specific pathogens, such as *Pseudomonas* spp. in patients with cystic fibrosis.

PATHOGENESIS. The lower respiratory tract is normally kept sterile by physiologic defense mechanisms, including the mucocil-

TABLE 397-1. Causes of Infectious Pneumonia

Bacterial	
Common	
Streptococcus pneumoniae	
Group B streptococci	Neonates
Group A streptococci	
*Mycoplasma pneumoniae**	Adolescents; summer-fall epidemics
*Chlamydia pneumoniae**	Adolescents
Chlamydia trachomatis	Infants
Mixed anaerobes	Aspiration pneumonia
Gram-negative enteric	Nosocomial pneumonia
Uncommon	
Haemophilus influenzae type B	Unimmunized
Staphylococcus aureus	Pneumatoceles; infants
Moraxella catarrhalis	
Neisseria meningitides	
Francisella tularensis	Animal, tick, fly contact
Nocardia species	Immunosuppressed persons
*Chlamydia psittaci**	Bird contact
Yersinia pestis	Plague
Legionella species*	Exposure to contaminated water; nosocomial
Viral	
Common	
Respiratory synctial virus	Bronchiolitis
Parainfluenza types 1–3	Croup
Influenza A, B	High fever; winter months
Adenovirus	Can be severe; often occurs between January and April
Metapneumovirus	Similar to RSV
Uncommon	
Rhinovirus	Rhinorrhea
Enterovirus	Neonates
Herpes simplex	Neonates
Cytomegalovirus	Infants, immunosuppressed persons
Measles	Rash, coryza, conjunctivitis
Varicella	Adolescents
Hantavirus	Southwestern United States, rodents
SARS agent	Asia
Fungal	
Histoplasma capsulatum	Geographic region; bird, bat contact
Cryptococcus neoformans	Bird contact
Aspergillus species	Immunosuppressed
Mucormycosis	Immunosuppressed
Coccidioides immitis	Geographic region
Blastomyces dermatitides	Geographic region
Rickettsial	
*Coxiella burnetii**	Q fever, animal (goat, sheep, cattle) exposure
Rickettsia rickettsiae	Tick bite
Mycobacterial	
Mycobacterium tuberculosis	Developing countries
Mycobacterium avium-intracellulare	Immunosuppressed persons
Parasitic	
Pneumocystis carinii	Immunosuppressed, steroids
Eosinophilic	Various parasites (e.g., Ascaris *Strongyloides* species)

*Atypical pneumonia syndrome; atypical in terms of extrapulmonary manifestations, low-grade fever, patchy diffuse infiltrates, poor response to penicillin-type antibiotics, and negative sputum Gram stain.
SARS, severe acute respiratory syndrome.
From Kliegman RM, Greenbaum LA, Lye PS: *Practical Strategies in Pediatric Diagnosis & Therapy,* 2nd ed, Philadelphia, Elsevier, 2004, p. 29.

TABLE 397-2. Etiologic Agents Grouped by Age of the Patient

AGE GROUP	FREQUENT PATHOGENS (IN ORDER OF FREQUENCY)
Neonates (<1 mo)	Group B streptococcus, *Escherichia coli,* other gram-negative bacilli, *Streptococcus pneumoniae, Haemophilus influenzae* (type b,* nontypable)
1–3 mo	
Febrile pneumonia	Respiratory syncytial virus, other respiratory viruses (parainfluenza viruses, influenza viruses, adenoviruses), *S. pneumoniae, H. influenzae* (type b,* nontypable)
Afebrile pneumonia	*Chlamydia trachomatis, Mycoplasma hominis, Ureaplasma urealyticum,* cytomegalovirus
3–12 mo	Respiratory syncytial virus, other respiratory viruses (parainfluenza viruses, influenza viruses, adenoviruses), *S. pneumoniae, H. influenzae* (type b,* nontypable), *C. trachomatis, Mycoplasma pneumoniae,* group A streptococcus
2–5 yr	Respiratory viruses (parainfluenza viruses, influenza viruses, adenoviruses), *S. pneumoniae, H. influenzae* (type b,* nontypable), *M. pneumoniae, Chlamydophila pneumoniae, S. aureus,* group A streptococcus
5–18 yr	*M. pneumoniae, S. pneumoniae, C. pneumoniae, H. influenzae* (type b,* nontypable), *influenza* viruses, adenoviruses, other respiratory viruses
≥18 yr	*M. pneumoniae, S. pneumoniae, C. pneumoniae, H. influenzae* (type b,* nontypable), *influenza* viruses, adenoviruses, *Legionella pneumophila*

**H. influenzae* type b is uncommon with universal *H. influenza* type b immunization.
From Kliegman RM, Marcdante KJ, Jenson HJ, Behrman RE: *Nelson Essentials of Pediatrics,* 5th ed Philadelphia, Elsevier, 2006, p. 504.

iary clearance, the properties of normal secretions such as secretory immunoglobulin A (IgA), and clearing of the airway by coughing. Immunologic defense mechanisms of the lung that limit invasion by pathogenic organisms include macrophages that are present in alveoli and bronchioles, secretory IgA, and other immunoglobulins.

Viral pneumonia usually results from spread of infection along the airways, accompanied by direct injury of the respiratory epithelium, resulting in airway obstruction from swelling, abnormal secretions, and cellular debris. The small caliber of airways in young infants makes them particularly susceptible to severe infection. Atelectasis, interstitial edema, and ventilation-perfusion mismatch causing significant hypoxemia often accompany airway obstruction. Viral infection of the respiratory tract can also predispose to secondary bacterial infection by disturbing normal host defense mechanisms, altering secretions, and modifying the bacterial flora.

When bacterial infection is established in the lung parenchyma, the pathologic process varies according to the invading organism. *M. pneumoniae* attaches to the respiratory epithelium, inhibits ciliary action, and leads to cellular destruction and an inflammatory response in the submucosa. As the infection progresses, sloughed cellular debris, inflammatory cells, and mucus cause airway obstruction, with spread of infection occurring along the bronchial tree, as it does in viral pneumonia.

S. pneumoniae produces local edema that aids in the proliferation of organisms and their spread into adjacent portions of lung, often resulting in the characteristic focal lobar involvement.

Group A streptococcus infection of the lower respiratory tract results in more diffuse infection with interstitial pneumonia. The pathology includes necrosis of tracheobronchial mucosa; formation of large amounts of exudate, edema, and local hemorrhage, with extension into the interalveolar septa; and involvement of lymphatic vessels and the increased likelihood of pleural involvement.

S. aureus pneumonia manifests in confluent bronchopneumonia, which is often unilateral and characterized by the presence of extensive areas of hemorrhagic necrosis and irregular areas of cavitation of the lung parenchyma, resulting in pneumatoceles, empyema, or, at times, bronchopulmonary fistulas.

Recurrent pneumonia is defined **as 2 or more** episodes in a single yr **or 3 or more** episodes ever, with radiographic clearing between occurrences. An underlying disorder should be considered if a child experiences recurrent bacterial pneumonia (Table 397-3). Additional factors that promote pulmonary infection include trauma, anesthesia, and aspiration.

Slowly resolving pneumonia refers to the persistence of symptoms or radiographic abnormalities beyond the expected time course. The time course varies, depending on the organism involved, the extent of disease, and the presence of associated complicating conditions.

CLINICAL MANIFESTATIONS. Viral and bacterial pneumonias are often preceded by several days of symptoms of an upper respiratory tract infection, typically rhinitis and cough. In viral pneu-

TABLE 397-3. Differential Diagnosis of Recurrent Pneumonia

Hereditary Disorders
Cystic fibrosis
Sickle cell disease
Disorders of Immunity
AIDS
Bruton agammaglobulinemia
Selective IgG subclass deficiencies
Common variable immunodeficiency syndrome
Severe combined immunodeficiency syndrome
Disorders of Leukocytes
Chronic granulomatous disease
Hyperimmunoglobulin E syndrome (Job syndrome)
Leukocyte adhesion defect
Disorders of Cilia
Immotile cilia syndrome
Kartagener syndrome
Anatomic Disorders
Sequestration
Lobar emphysema
Esophageal reflux
Foreign body
Tracheoesophageal fistula (H type)
Gastroesophageal reflux
Bronchietasis
Aspiration (oropharyngeal incoordination)

From Kliegman RM, Marcdante KJ, Jenson HJ, Behrman RE: *Nelson Essentials of Pediatrics*, 5th ed, Philadelphia, Elsevier, 2006, p. 507.

monia, fever is usually present; temperatures are generally lower than in bacterial pneumonia. Tachypnea is the most consistent clinical manifestation of pneumonia. Increased work of breathing accompanied by intercostal, subcostal, and suprasternal retractions, nasal flaring, and use of accessory muscles is common. Severe infection may be accompanied by cyanosis and respiratory fatigue, especially in infants. Auscultation of the chest may reveal crackles and wheezing, but it is often difficult to localize the source of these adventitious sounds in very young children with hyperresonant chests. It is often not possible to distinguish viral pneumonia clinically from disease caused by *Mycoplasma* and other bacterial pathogens.

Bacterial pneumonia in adults and older children typically begins suddenly with a shaking chill followed by a high fever, cough, and chest pain. In older children and adolescents, a brief upper respiratory tract illness is followed by the abrupt onset of shaking chills and high fever accompanied by drowsiness with intermittent periods of restlessness; rapid respirations; a dry, hacking, unproductive cough; anxiety; and, occasionally, delirium. Circumoral cyanosis may be observed. Many children are noted to be splinting on the affected side to minimize pleuritic pain and improve ventilation; they may lie on their side with their knees drawn up to their chest.

Physical findings depend on the stage of pneumonia. Early in the course of illness, diminished breath sounds, scattered crackles, and rhonchi are commonly heard over the affected lung field. With the development of increasing consolidation or complications of pneumonia such as effusion, empyema, or pyopneumothorax, dullness on percussion is noted and breath sounds may be diminished. A lag in respiratory excursion often occurs on the affected side. Abdominal distention may be prominent because of gastric dilation from swallowed air or ileus. Abdominal pain is common in lower lobe pneumonia. The liver may seem enlarged because of downward displacement of the diaphragm secondary to hyperinflation of the lungs or superimposed congestive heart failure. Nuchal rigidity, in the absence of meningitis, may also be prominent, especially with involvement of the right upper lobe.

Symptoms described in adults with pneumococcal pneumonia may be noted in older children but are rarely observed in infants and young children, in whom the clinical pattern is considerably more variable. In infants, there may be a prodrome of upper respiratory tract infection and diminished appetite, leading to the abrupt onset of fever, restlessness, apprehension, and respiratory distress. These infants appear ill with respiratory distress manifested by grunting; nasal flaring; retractions of the supraclavicular, intercostal, and subcostal areas; tachypnea; tachycardia; air hunger; and often cyanosis. Results of physical examination may be misleading, particularly in young infants, with meager findings disproportionate to the degree of tachypnea. Some infants with bacterial pneumonia may have associated gastrointestinal disturbances characterized by vomiting, anorexia, diarrhea, and abdominal distention secondary to a paralytic ileus. Rapid progression of symptoms is characteristic in the most severe cases of bacterial pneumonia.

DIAGNOSIS. The chest radiograph confirms the diagnosis of pneumonia and may indicate a complication such as a pleural effusion or empyema. Viral pneumonia is usually characterized by hyperinflation with bilateral interstitial infiltrates and peribronchial cuffing (Fig. 397-1). Confluent lobar consolidation is typically seen with pneumococcal pneumonia (Fig. 397-2). The radiographic appearance alone is not diagnostic and other clinical features must be considered. Repeat chest x-rays are not required for proof of cure for patients with uncomplicated pneumonia.

The peripheral white blood cell (WBC) count can be useful in differentiating viral from bacterial pneumonia. In viral pneumonia, the WBC count can be normal or elevated but is usually not higher than 20,000/mm^3, with a lymphocyte predominance. Bacterial pneumonia (occasionally, adenovirus pneumonia) is often associated with an elevated WBC count in the range of 15,000–40,000/mm^3 and a predominance of granulocytes. A large pleural effusion, lobar consolidation, and a high fever at the onset of the illness are also suggestive of a bacterial etiology.

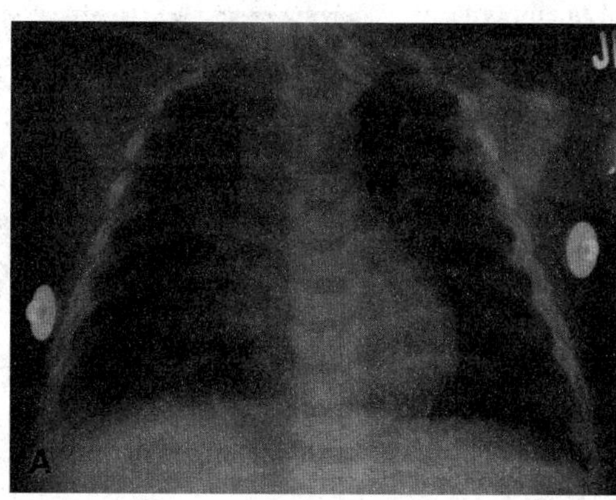

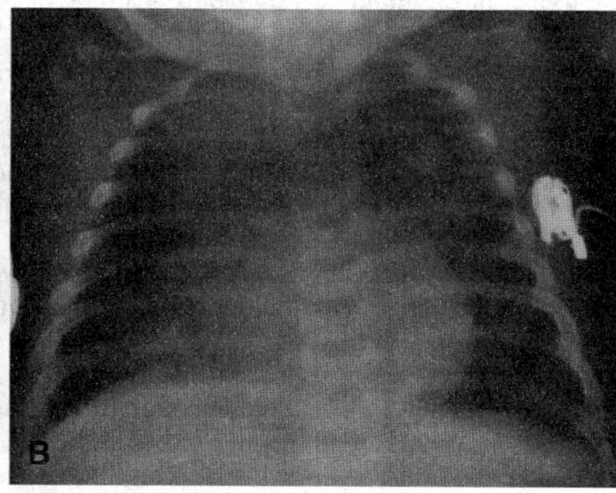

Figure 397-1. *A*, Radiographic findings characteristic of respiratory syncytial virus (RSV) pneumonia in a 6 mo old infant with rapid respirations and fever. Anteroposterior (AP) radiograph of the chest shows hyperexpansion of the lungs with bilateral fine air space disease and streaks of density, indicating the presence of both pneumonia and atelectasis. An endotracheal tube is in place. *B*, One day later, the AP radiograph of the chest shows increased bilateral pneumonia.

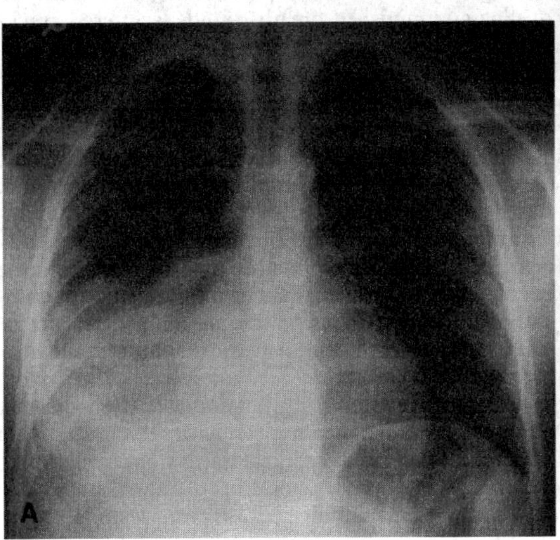

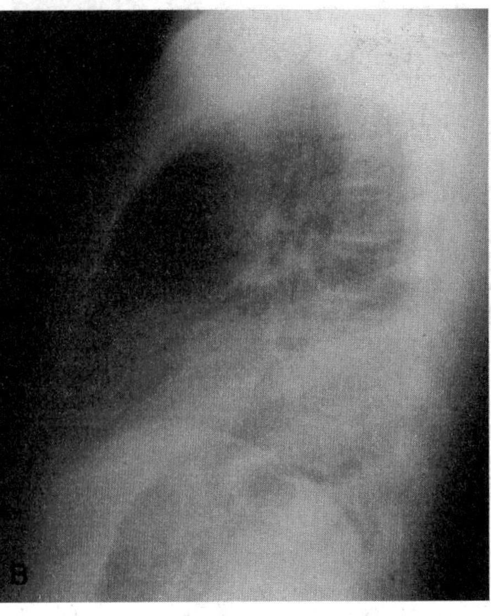

Figure 397-2. Radiographic findings characteristic of pneumococcal pneumonia in a 14 yr old boy with cough and fever. Posteroanterior *(A)* and lateral *(B)* chest radiographs reveal consolidation in the right lower lobe, strongly suggesting bacterial pneumonia.

Atypical pneumonia due to *C. pneumoniae* or *M. pneumoniae* is difficult to distinguish from pneumococcal pneumonia by x-ray and other labs, and although pneumococcal pneumonia is associated with a higher WBC count, erythrocyte sedimentation rate (ESR), and C-reactive protein (CRP), there is considerable overlap.

The definitive diagnosis of a viral infection rests on the isolation of a virus or detection of the viral genome or antigen in respiratory tract secretions. Growth of respiratory viruses in tissue culture usually requires 5–10 days. Reliable DNA or RNA tests for the rapid detection of RSV, parainfluenza, influenza, and adenoviruses are available and accurate. Serologic techniques can also be used to diagnose a recent respiratory viral infection but generally require testing of acute and convalescent serum samples for a rise in antibodies to a specific viral agent. This diagnostic technique is laborious, slow, and not generally clinically useful because the infection usually resolves by the time it is confirmed serologically. Serologic testing may be valuable as an epidemiologic tool to define the incidence and prevalence of the various respiratory viral pathogens.

The definitive diagnosis of a bacterial infection requires isolation of an organism from the blood, pleural fluid, or lung. Culture of sputum is of little value in the diagnosis of pneumonia in young children. Blood cultures are positive in only 10% of children with pneumococcal pneumonia. In *M. pneumoniae* infections, cold agglutinins at titers >1 : 64 are found in the blood in ≈50% of patients. Cold agglutinins are nonspecific, however, because other pathogens such as influenza viruses may also cause increases. Acute infection caused by *M. pneumoniae* can be diagnosed on the basis of a positive PCR test or seroconversion in an IgG assay. Serologic evidence such as the anti-streptolysin O (ASO) titer may be useful in the diagnosis of group A streptococcal pneumonia.

TREATMENT. Treatment of suspected bacterial pneumonia is based on the presumptive cause and the clinical appearance of the child (see Tables 397-1 and 397-2). For mildly ill children who do not require hospitalization, amoxicillin is recommended. In communities with a high percentage of penicillin-resistant pneumococci, high doses of amoxicillin (80–90 mg/kg/24 hr) should be prescribed. Therapeutic alternatives include cefuroxime axetil or amoxicillin/clavulanate. For school-aged children and in those in whom infection with *M. pneumoniae* or *C. pneumoniae* (atypical pneumonias) is suggested, a macrolide antibiotic such as azithromycin is an appropriate choice. In adolescents, a respiratory fluoroquinolone (levofloxacin, gatifloxacin, moxifloxacin, gemifloxacin) may be considered for atypical pneumonias.

The empirical treatment of suspected bacterial pneumonia in a hospitalized child requires an approach based on the clinical manifestations at the time of presentation. Parenteral cefuroxime (150 mg/kg/24 hr), cefotaxime, or ceftriaxone is the mainstay of therapy when bacterial pneumonia is suggested. If clinical features suggest staphylococcal pneumonia (pneumatoceles, empyema), initial antimicrobial therapy should also include vancomycin or clindamycin.

If viral pneumonia is suspected, it is reasonable to withhold antibiotic therapy, especially for those patients who are mildly ill, have clinical evidence suggesting viral infection, and are in no respiratory distress. Up to 30% of patients with known viral infection may have coexisting bacterial pathogens. Therefore, if the decision is made to withhold antibiotic therapy based on presumptive diagnosis of a viral infection, deterioration in clinical status should signal the possibility of superimposed bacterial infection and antibiotic therapy should be initiated.

Indications for admission to a hospital are noted in Table 397-4. In developing countries, oral zinc (20 mg/day) helps accelerate recovery from severe pneumonia.

RESPONSE TO TREATMENT. Typically, patients with uncomplicated community-acquired bacterial pneumonia respond to therapy with improvement in clinical symptoms (fever, cough, tachypnea, chest pain) within 48–96 hr of initiation of antibiotics. Radiographic evidence of improvement substantially lags behind clinical improvement. A number of factors must be considered when a patient does not improve on appropriate antibiotic therapy (**slowly resolving pneumonia**): (1) complications, such as

TABLE 397-4. Factors Suggesting Need for Hospitalization of Children with Pneumonia

Age <6 mo
Sickle cell anemia with acute chest syndrome
Multiple lobe involvement
Immunocompromised state
Toxic appearance
Severe respiratory distress
Requirement for supplemental oxygen
Dehydration
Vomiting
No response to appropriate oral antibiotic therapy
Noncompliant parents

Adapted from Baltimore RS: Pneumonia. In Jenson HB, Baltimore RS (editors): *Pediatric Infectious Diseases: Principles and Practice.* Philadelphia, WB Saunders, 2002, p. 801.

TABLE 397-5. Differentiation of Pleural Fluid

	TRANSUDATE	EXUDATE	COMPLICATED EMPYEMA
Appearance	Clear	Cloudy	Purulent
Cell count	<1000	>1000	>5000
Cell type	Lymphocytes, monocytes	PMNs	PMNs
LDH	<200 U/L	>200 U/L	>1000 U/L
Pleural/serum LDH ration	<0.6	>0.6	>0.6
Protein >3 g	Unusual	Common	Common
Pleural/serum protein ratio	<0.5	>0.5	>0.5
Glucose*	Normal	Low	Very low*(<40 mg/dL)
pH*	Normal (7.40–7.60)	7.20–7.40	<7.20, chest tube placement required
Gram stain	Negative	Usually positive	>85% positive unless patient received prior antibiotics

*Low glucose or pH may be seen in malignant effusion, tuberculosis, esophageal rupture, pancreatitis (positive pleural amylase), and rheumatologic diseases (e.g., systemic lupus erythematosus).
LDH, lactate dehydrogenase; PMNs, polymorphonuclear neutrophils.
From Kliegman RM, Greenbaum LA, Lye PS: *Practical Strategies in Pediatric Diagnosis & Therapy*, 2nd ed Philadelphia, Elsevier, 2004, p. 30.

empyema; (2) bacterial resistance; (3) nonbacterial etiologies such as viruses and aspiration of foreign bodies or food; (4) bronchial obstruction from endobronchial lesions, foreign body, or mucous plugs; (5) pre-existing diseases such as immunodeficiencies, ciliary dyskinesia, cystic fibrosis, pulmonary sequestration, or cystic adenomatoid malformation; and (6) other noninfectious causes (including bronchiolitis obliterans, hypersensitivity pneumonitis, eosinophilic pneumonia, aspiration, and Wegener granulomatosis). A repeat chest x-ray is the 1st step in determining the reason for delay in response to treatment.

COMPLICATIONS. Complications of pneumonia are usually the result of direct spread of bacterial infection within the thoracic cavity (pleural effusion, empyema, pericarditis) or bacteremia and hematologic spread (Fig. 397-3). Meningitis, suppurative arthritis, and osteomyelitis are rare complications of hematologic spread of pneumococcal or *H. influenzae* type b infection.

S. aureus, S. pneumoniae, and *S. pyogenes* are the most common causes of parapneumonic effusions and of empyema (Table 397-5). The treatment of empyema is based on the stage (exudative, fibrinopurulent, organizing). Imaging studies including ultrasonography and CT are helpful in determining the stage of empyema. The mainstays of therapy include antibiotic therapy and drainage with tube thoracostomy. Additional approaches include the use of fibrinolytic therapy (urokinase, streptokinase, alteplase) and selected video-assisted thoracoscopy (VATS) to debride, lyse adhesions, and drain loculated areas of pus. Early diagnosis and intervention, particularly with VATS, may obviate the need for thoracotomy and open debridement.

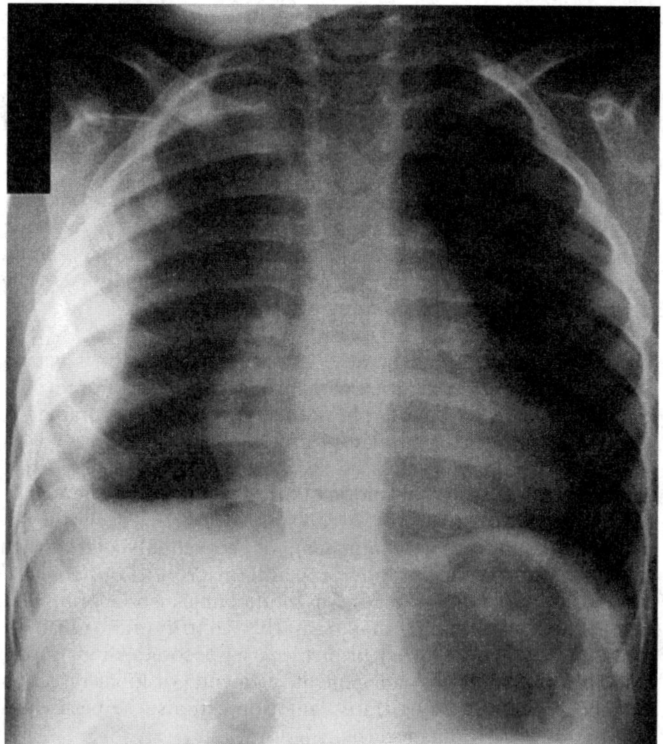

Figure 397-3. Pneumococcal empyema in a 3 yr old child with cold and fever for 3 days. A pleural or extrapleural fluid collection is seen on the right side. The patient had a positive pleural tap and blood culture for pneumococci. The child recovered completely within 3 wk. (From Kuhn JP, Slovis TL, Haller JO: *Caffrey's Pediatric Diagnostic Imaging,* vol 1, 10th ed. Philadelphia, Mosby/Elsevier, 2004, p 1002.)

Addo-Yoba E, Chisaka N, Hassan M, et al: Oral amoxicillin versus injectable penicillin for severe pneumonia in children aged 3 to 59 month: A randomized multicentre equivalency study. *Lancet* 2004;364:1141–1148.

Avansino JR, Goldman B, Sawin RS, Flum DR: Primary operative versus nonoperative therapy for pediatric empyema: A meta-analysis. *Pediatrics* 2005;115:1652–1659.

Baumer JH: Parapneumonic effusion and empyema. *Arch Dis Child* 2005;90:ep21–ep24.

Bhutta ZA: Childhood pneumonia in developing counries. *BMJ* 2006;333:612–613.

Black SB, Shinefeld HR, Ling S, et al: Effectiveness of heptavalent pneumococcal conjugate vaccine in children younger than five years of age for prevention of pneumonia. *Pediatr Infect Dis J* 2002;21:810–815.

Bouros D, Antoniou KM, Light RW: Intrapleural streptokinase for pleural infection. *Br Med J* 2006;332:133–134.

Brooks WA, Yunus M, Santosham M, et al: Zinc for severe pneumonia in very young children: Double-blind placebo-controlled trial. *Lancet* 2004;363:1683–1688.

Duke T: Neonatal pneumonia in developing countries. *Arch Dis Child Fetal Neonatal Ed* 2005;90:F211–F219.

Esposito S, Bosis S, Cavagna R, et al: Characteristics *of Streptococcus pneumoniae* and atypical bacterial infections in children 2–5 years of age with community-acquired pneumonia. *Clin Infect Dis* 2002;35:1345–1352.

File TM Jr: Community-acquired pneumonia. *Lancet* 2003;362:1991–2001.

Kusel MMH, de Klerk NH, Holt PG, et al: Role of respiratory viruses in acute upper and lower respiratory tract illness in the first year of life: a birth cohort study. *Pediatr Infect Dis J* 2006;25:680–686.

Lakhanpaul M, Atkinson M, Stephenson T: Community acquired pneumonia in children: A clinical update. *Arch Dis Child* 2004;89:ep29–ep34.

McCracken GH Jr: Diagnosis and management of pneumonia. *Pediatr Infect Dis J* 2000;19:924–928.

McIntosh K: Community-acquired pneumonia in children. *N Engl J Med* 2002;346:429–437.

Michelow IC, Olsen K, Lozana J, et al: Epidemiology and clinical characteristics of community-acquired pneumonia in hospitalized children. *Pediatrics* 2004;113:701–707.

Nelson JD: Community-acquired pneumonia in children: Guidelines for treatment. *Pediatr Infect Dis J* 2000;19:251–253.

Panitch HB: Evaluation of recurrent pneumonia. *Pediatr Infect Dis J* 2005;24:265–266.

Rudan I, Tomaskovic L, Boschi-Pinto C, Campbell H: WHO Child Health Epidemiology Reference Group: Global estimate of the incidence of clinical pneumonia among children under five years of age. *Bull World Health Organ* 2004;82:895–903.

Schultz KD, Fan LL, Oinsky J, et al: The changing face of pleural empyemas in children: Epidemiology and management. *Pediatrics* 2004;113: 1735–1740.

Tsolia MN, Psarras S, Bossios A, et al: Etiology of community-acquired pneumonia in hospitalized school-age children: Evidence for high prevalence of viral infections. *Clin Infect Dis* 2004;39:686–686.

Ulloa-Guiterrez R, Skippen P, Synnes A, et al: Life-threatening human metapneumovirus pneumonia requiring extracorporal membrane oxygenation in a preterm infant. *Pediatrics* 2004;114:e517–e519.

Wacogne I, Negrine RJS: Are follow up chest x ray examinations helpful in the management of children recovering from pneumonia? *Arch Dis Child* 2003;88:457–458.

Wardlaw T, Salama P, White Johansson E: Pneumonia: the leading killer of children. *Lancet* 2006;368:1048–1050.

Weinstein M, Restrepo R, Chait PG, et al: Effectiveness and safety of tissue plasminogen activator in the management of complicated parapneumonic effusions. *Pediatrics* 2004;113:e182–e185.

Zar HJ: Pneumonia in HIV-infected and HIV-uninfected children in developing countries: Epidemiology, clinical features, and management. *Curr Opin Pulm Med* 2004;10:176–182.

Chapter 398 ■ Bronchiectasis

Oren Lakser

Bronchiectasis is a disease characterized by irreversible abnormal dilatation of the bronchial tree and likely represents a common end stage of a number of nonspecific and unrelated antecedent events. Its incidence has been decreasing overall in developed countries, but it persists as a problem in developing countries. In at least 1 series of children with bronchiectasis (not due to cystic fibrosis), the male to female ratio was 2 : 1.

PATHOPHYSIOLOGY AND PATHOGENESIS. In the developed world, cystic fibrosis (see Chapter 400) is the most common cause of clinically significant bronchiectasis. Other conditions associated with bronchiectasis include ciliary dyskinesia, immune deficiency syndromes, and infection, especially pertussis, measles, and tuberculosis. Bronchiectasis can also be congenital, as in *Williams-Campbell syndrome,* in which there is an absence of annular bronchial cartilage, and *Marnier-Kuhn syndrome* (congenital tracheobronchomegaly), in which there is a connective tissue disorder. Other disease entities associated with bronchiectasis include *right middle lobe syndrome* (chronic extrinsic compression of right middle lobe bronchus by hilar lymph nodes) and *yellow nail syndrome* (pleural effusion, lymphedema, discolored nails).

Three basic mechanisms are involved in the pathogenesis of bronchiectasis. Obstruction can occur because of tumor, foreign body, impacted mucus caused by poor mucociliary clearance, external compression, bronchial webs, and atresia. Infections due to *Bordetella pertussis*, measles, rubella, togavirus, respiratory syncytial virus, and *Mycobacterium tuberculosis* induce chronic inflammation, progressive bronchial wall damage, and dilatation. Chronic inflammation similarly contributes to the mechanism by which obstruction leads to bronchiectasis. The mechanism by which bronchiectasis occurs in congenital forms is likely related to abnormal cartilage formation. The common thread in the pathogenesis of bronchiectasis is difficulty clearing secretions and recurrent infections with a "vicious cycle" of infection and inflammation resulting in airway injury and remodeling.

Bronchiectasis can present in any combination of three pathologic forms, best defined by high-resolution CT (HRCT) scan. In cylindrical bronchiectasis, the bronchial outlines are regular, but there is diffuse dilatation of the bronchial unit. The bronchial lumen ends abruptly because of mucous plugging. In varicose bronchiectasis, the degree of dilatation is greater and local constrictions cause an irregularity of outline resembling varicose veins. There may also be small sacculations. In saccular (cystic) bronchiectasis, bronchial dilatation progresses and results in ballooning of bronchi that end in fluid- or mucus-filled sacs. This is the most severe form of bronchiectasis. Bronchiectasis lies within a disease spectrum of chronic pediatric suppurative lung disease. The following definitions have been proposed: *prebronchiectasis* (chronic or recurrent endobronchial infection with nonspecific HRCT changes); *HRCT bronchiectasis* (clinical symptoms with HRCT evidence of bronchial dilation—may persist, progress, or improve and resolve); *established bronchiectasis* (like the previous but with no resolution within 2 yr).

CLINICAL MANIFESTATIONS. The most common complaints in patients with bronchiectasis are cough and copious purulent sputum production. Younger children may swallow the sputum. Hemoptysis is seen with some frequency. Fever can occur with infectious exacerbations. Anorexia and poor weight gain may occur as time passes. Physical examination typically reveals crackles localized to the affected area, but wheezing as well as digital clubbing may also occur. In severe cases, dyspnea and hypoxemia can occur. Pulmonary function studies may demonstrate an obstructive, restrictive, or mixed pattern. Typically, impaired diffusion capacity is a late finding.

DIAGNOSIS. Chest radiographs of patients with bronchiectasis tend to be nonspecific. Typical findings can include increase in size and loss of definition of bronchovascular markings, crowding of bronchi, and loss of lung volume. In more severe forms, cystic spaces, occasionally with air-fluid levels and honeycombing, may occur. Compensatory overinflation of unaffected lung may be seen. Thin-section HRCT scanning is the gold standard, because it has excellent sensitivity and specificity. CT provides further information on disease location, presence of mediastinal lesions, and the extent of segmental involvement. The addition of radiolabeled aerosol inhalation to CT scanning can provide further information. The CT findings in patients with bronchiectasis typically include cylindrical ("tram lines," "signet ring appearance"), varicose (bronchi with "beaded contour"), cystic (cysts in "strings and clusters"), or mixed forms (Fig. 398-1). The lower lobes are most commonly affected.

TREATMENT. The initial therapy for patients with bronchiectasis is medical and aims at decreasing airway obstruction and controlling infection. Chest physiotherapy (postural drainage), antibiotics, and bronchodilators are essential. Two to 4 wk of parenteral antibiotics are often necessary to manage acute exacerbations adequately. Antibiotic choice is dictated by the identification and sensitivity of organisms found on deep throat, sputum (induced or spontaneous), or bronchoalveolar lavage fluid cultures. Chronic prophylactic oral (macrolide) or nebulized antibiotics may be beneficial. Any underlying disorder (immunodeficiency, aspiration) that may be contributing must be addressed. When localized bronchiectasis becomes more severe or resistant to medical management, segmental or lobar resection may be warranted. Lung transplantation can also be performed in patients with bronchiectasis.

PROGNOSIS. Overall, the prognosis for patients with bronchiectasis has improved considerably in the past few decades. Earlier recognition or prevention of predisposing conditions, more powerful and wide-spectrum antibiotics, and improved surgical outcomes are likely reasons.

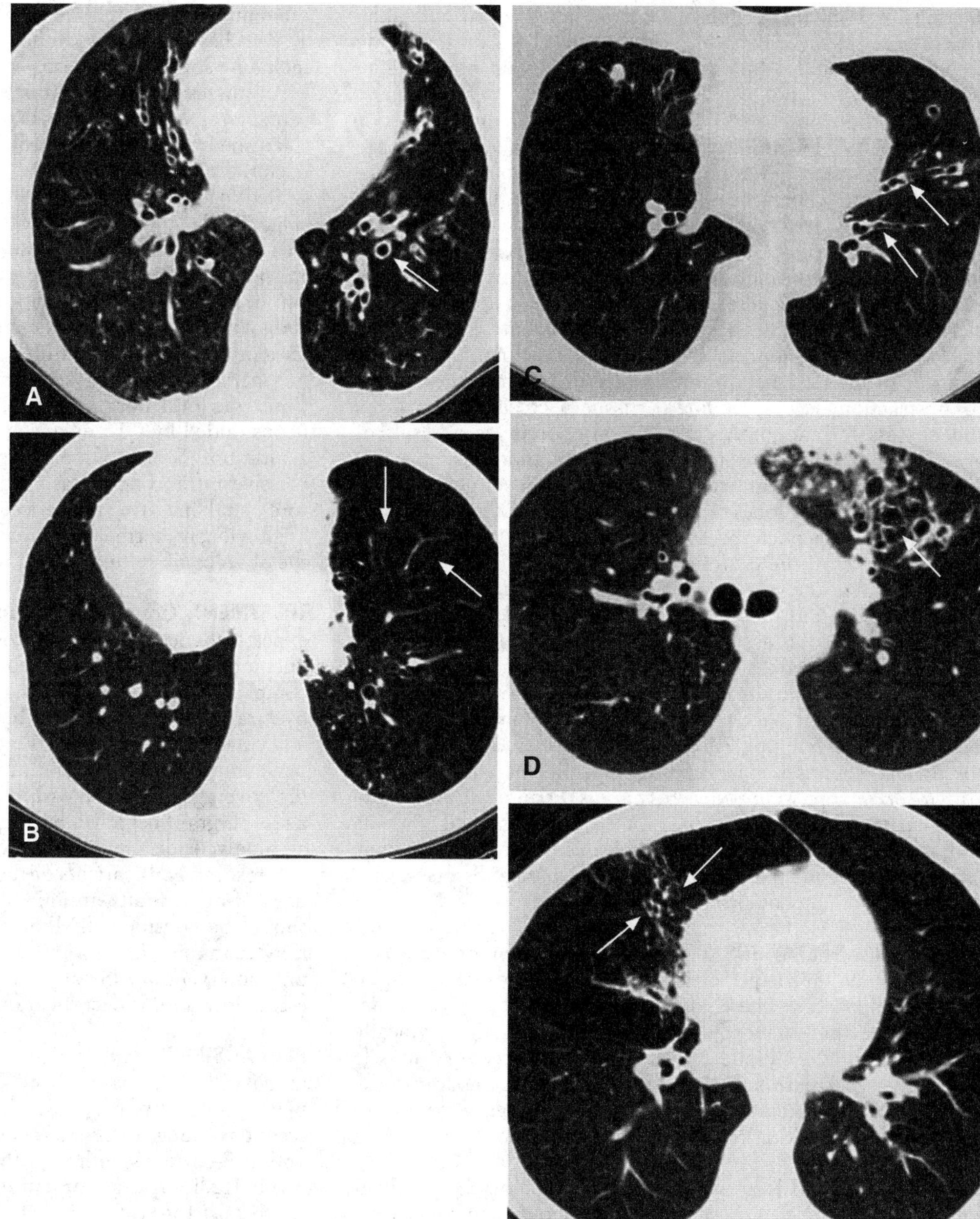

Figure 398-1. High-resolution CT images of lungs with bronchiectasis. Panel *A* shows dilated and thickened airways *(arrow)*. Panel *B* shows airways that do not taper *(arrows)* toward the periphery in a patient with Kartagener syndrome. Panel C shows varicose changes (dilated and beaded airways *[arrows]*). Panel *D* shows clustered cysts or saccules *(arrow)* as well as a peripheral infiltrate. Panel *E* shows middle lobe bronchiectasis *(arrows)* in a patient with *Mycobacterium avium* complex infection. (From Barker AF: Bronchiectasis. *N Engl J Med* 2002;346:1383.)

Barker AF: Bronchiectasis. *N Engl J Med* 2002;346:1383–1393.

Callahan CW, Redding GJ: Bronchiectasis in children: Orphan disease or persistent problem? *Pediatr Pulmonol* 2002;33:492–496.

Chang AB, Grimwood K, Mulholland EK, et al: Bronchiectasis in indigenous children in remote Australian communities. *Med J Aust* 2002;177:200–204.

Eastham KM, Fall AJ, Mitchell L, et al: The need to redefine non-cystic fibrosis bronchiectasis in childhood. *Thorax* 2004;59:324–327.

Evans DJ, Greenstone M: Long-term antibiotics in the management of non-CF bronchiectasis—do they improve outcome? *Respir Med* 2003;97:851–858.

Galvin JR, D'Alessandro MP: Electric diffuse lung: The diagnosis of diffuse lung disease, bronchiectasis. Available at University of Iowa Virtual Hospital website (www.vh.org).

Haciibrahimoglu G, Fazlioglu M, Olcmen A, et al: Surgical management of childhood bronchiectasis due to infectious disease. *J Thorac Cardiovasc Surg* 2004;127:1361–1365.

Karakoc GB, Yilmaz M, Altintas DU, et al: Bronchiectasis: Still a problem. *Pediatr Pulmonol* 2001;32:175–178.

Morrissey BM, Evans SJ: Severe bronchiectasis. *Clin Rev Allergy Immunol* 2003:25:233–248.

Rama M, Yousef E: Bronchiectasis and chronic asthma: How common in pediatrics? *Allergy Asthma Proc* 2006;27:354–358.

Santamaria F, Montella S, Camera L, et al: Lung structure abnormalities, but normal lung function in pediatric bronchiectasis. *Chest* 2006;130:480–486.

Chapter 399 ■ Pulmonary Abscess

Oren Lakser

Pulmonary abscesses are localized areas composed of thick-walled purulent material formed as a result of lung infection that lead to destruction of lung parenchyma, cavitation, and central necrosis. Lung abscesses are much less common in children than in adults. A primary lung abscess occurs in a previously healthy patient with no underlying medical disorders. A secondary lung abscess occurs in a patient with underlying or predisposing conditions.

PATHOLOGY AND PATHOGENESIS. A number of conditions predispose children to the development of pulmonary abscesses, including aspiration, pneumonia, cystic fibrosis (see Chapter 400), gastroesophageal reflux (see Chapter 320.1), tracheoesophageal fistula (see Chapter 316), immunodeficiencies, postoperative complications of tonsillectomy and adenoidectomy, seizures, and a variety of neurologic diseases. In children, aspiration of infected materials or a foreign body is the predominant source of the organisms causing abscesses. Initially, a pneumonitis impairs drainage of fluid or the aspirated material. Inflammatory vascular obstruction occurs, leading to tissue necrosis, liquefaction, and abscess formation. Abscess can also occur as a result of pneumonia and hematogenous seeding from another site.

If the aspiration event occurred in the recumbent position, the right and left upper lobes and apical segment of the right lower lobes are the dependent areas most likely to be affected. If the child was upright, the posterior segments of the upper lobes are dependent and therefore most likely to be affected. Primary abscesses are found most often on the right side, whereas secondary lung abscesses, particularly in immunocompromised patients, have a predilection for the left side.

Both anaerobic and aerobic organisms can cause lung abscesses. Common anaerobic bacteria that can cause a pulmonary abscess include *Bacteroides* spp., *Fusobacterium* spp., and *Peptostreptococcus* spp. Abscesses can be caused by aerobic organisms such as *Streptococcus* spp., *Staphylococcus aureus, Escherichia coli, Klebsiella pneumoniae,* and *Pseudomonas aeruginosa.* All patients with a lung abscess should have aerobic and anaerobic cultures as part of their work-up. Fungi can also cause lung abscesses, particularly in immunocompromised patients.

CLINICAL MANIFESTATIONS. The most common symptoms of pulmonary abscess in the pediatric population include cough, fever, tachypnea, dyspnea, chest pain, vomiting, sputum production, weight loss, and hemoptysis. Physical examination typically reveals tachypnea, dyspnea, retractions with accessory muscle use, decreased breath sounds, and dullness to percussion in the affected area. Crackles and, occasionally, a prolonged expiratory phase may be heard on lung examination.

DIAGNOSIS. Diagnosis is most commonly made on chest radiography. Classically, the chest radiograph shows a parenchymal inflammation with a cavity containing an air-fluid level (Fig. 399-1). A chest CT scan can provide better anatomic definition, including location and size.

An abscess is usually a thick-walled lesion with a low-density center progressing to an air-fluid level. Abscesses should be distinguished from pneumatoceles, which often complicate severe bacterial pneumonias and are characterized by thin- and smooth-walled localized air collections with or without an air-fluid level (Fig. 399-2). Pneumatoceles often resolve spontaneously with the treatment of the specific cause of the pneumonia.

The determination of the etiologic bacteria in a lung abscess can be very helpful in guiding antibiotic choice. Although Gram stain of sputum can provide an early clue as to the class of bacteria involved, sputum cultures typically yield mixed bacteria and are therefore not always reliable. Attempts to avoid contamination from oral flora include direct lung puncture and percutaneous (aided by CT guidance), bronchoscopic, and transtracheal aspiration. Bronchoscopic aspiration can be complicated by massive intrabronchial aspiration, and great care should therefore be taken during the procedure. To avoid invasive procedures in previously normal hosts, empiric therapy can be initiated in the absence of culturable material.

TREATMENT. Conservative management is recommended. Most experts advocate a 2–3 wk course of parenteral antibiotics for uncomplicated cases, followed by a course of oral antibiotics to complete a total of 4–6 wk. Antibiotic choice should be guided by Gram stain and culture but initially should include aerobic and anaerobic coverage. Treatment regimens should include a penicillinase-resistant agent active against *S. aureus* and anaerobic coverage, typically with clindamycin or ticarcillin/clavulinic acid. If gram-negative bacteria are suspected or isolated, an aminoglycoside should be added.

For severely ill patients or those who fail to improve after 7–10 days of appropriate antimicrobial therapy, surgical intervention should be considered. Minimally invasive percutaneous aspiration techniques, often with CT guidance, are the initial and, often, only intervention. In rare complicated cases, thoracotomy with lobectomy and/or decortication may be necessary.

PROGNOSIS. Overall, prognosis for children with primary pulmonary abscesses is excellent. The presence of aerobic organisms may be a negative prognostic indicator, particularly in those with secondary lung abscesses. Most children become asymptomatic within 7–10 days, although the fever can persist for as long as 3 wk. Radiologic abnormalities usually resolve in 1–3 mo but can persist for years.

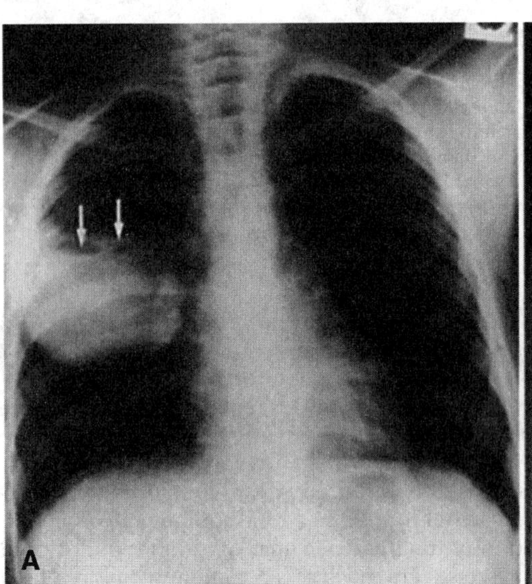

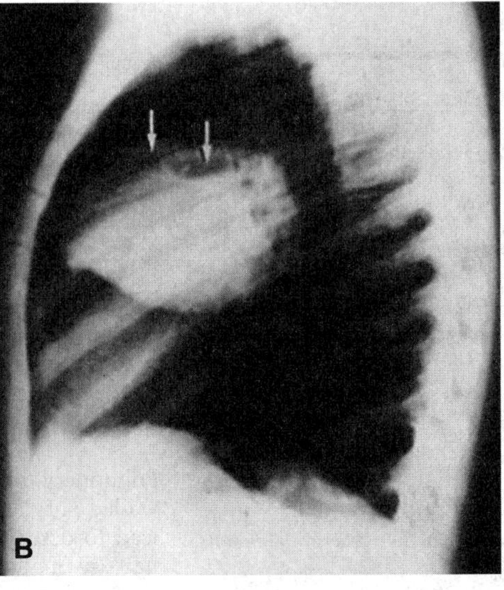

Figure 399-1. Multioculated lung abscess *(arrows).* (From Brook I: Lung abscess and pulmonary infections due to anaerobic bacteria. In Chernick V, Boat TF, Wilmott RW, Bush A [editors]: *Kendig's Disorders of the Respiratory Tract in Children,* 7th ed. Philadelphia, Saunders, 2006, p 482.)

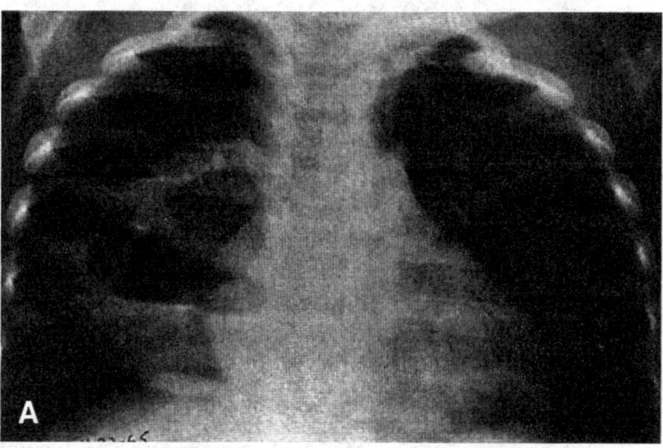
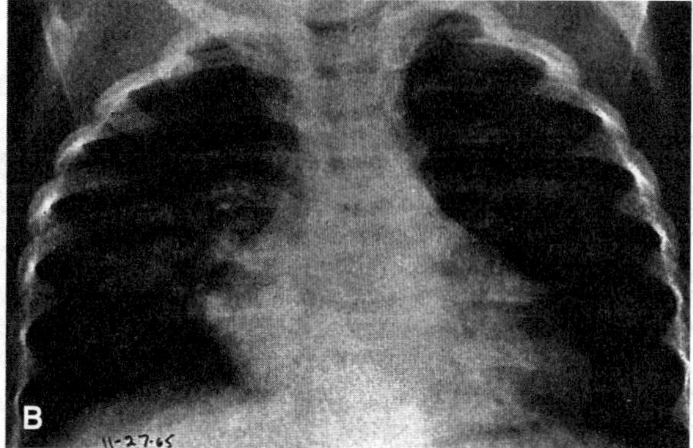

Figure 399-2. Appearance over a period of 5 days of a large multioculated pneumonocele in a segment of alveolar consolidation. *A,* There is a large cavity with two air-fluid levels in a segment of alveolar pneumonia in the right upper lobe. *B,* Five days later, the cavity and most of the pneumonic consolidation have disappeared. (From Silverman FN, Kuhn JP: *Essentials of Caffrey's Pediatric X-Ray Diagnosis.* Chicago, Year Book Medical Publishers, 1990, p 303.)

Brook I: Anaerobic pulmonary infections in children. *Pediatr Emerg Care* 2004;20:636–640.

Chan PC, Huang LM, Wu PS, et al: Clinical management and outcome of childhood lung abscess: a 16-year experience. *J Microbiol Immunol Infect* 2005;38:183–188.

De A, Varaiya A, Mathur M: Anaerobes in pleuropulmonary infections. *Indian J Med Microbiol* 2002;20:150–152.

Mansharamani NG, Koziel H: Chronic lung sepsis: Lung abscess, bronchiectasis, and empyema. *Curr Opin Pulm Med* 2003;9:181–185.

Mueller PR, Berlin L: Complications of lung abscess aspiration and drainage. *AJR Am J Roentgenol* 2002;178:1083–1886.

Tseng YL, Wu MH, Lin MY, et al: Surgery for lung abscess in immunocompetent and immunocompromised children. *J Pediatr Surg* 2001;36:470–473.

Yen C, Tang R, Chen S, et al: Pediatric lung abscess: A retrospective review of 23 cases. *J Microbiol Immunol Infect* 2004;37:45–49.

Young CS: Cough, fever, a lung mass, and a complex history. *JAAPA* 2004;17:31–32, 37–39.

Chapter 400 ■ Cystic Fibrosis

Thomas F. Boat and James D. Acton

Cystic fibrosis (CF) is an inherited multisystem disorder of children and adults, characterized chiefly by obstruction and infection of airways and by maldigestion and its consequences. It is the most common life-limiting recessive genetic trait among whites. A dysfunction of epithelialized surfaces is the predominant pathogenetic feature and is responsible for a broad, variable, and sometimes confusing array of presenting manifestations and complications.

CF is the major cause of severe chronic lung disease in children and is responsible for most exocrine pancreatic insufficiency in early life. It is also responsible for many cases of salt depletion, nasal polyposis, pansinusitis, rectal prolapse, pancreatitis, cholelithiasis, and insulin-dependent hyperglycemia. CF may present as failure to thrive and, occasionally, as cirrhosis or other forms of hepatic dysfunction. Therefore, this disorder enters into the differential diagnosis of many pediatric conditions (Table 400-1).

GENETICS. CF occurs most frequently in white populations of northern Europe, North America, and Australia/New Zealand. The prevalence varies by report but, in general, approximates 1/3,500 live births. Although less frequent in African, Middle Eastern, South Asian, and eastern Asian populations, with improving ascertainment, the prevalence in these groups is considerably higher than previously estimated. The prevalence of CF in 0–14 yr old children in Toronto is only moderately

TABLE 400-1. Complications of Cystic Fibrosis

RESPIRATORY
Bronchiectasis, bronchitis, bronchiolitis, pneumonia
Atelectasis
Hemoptysis
Pneumothorax
Nasal polyps
Sinusitis
Reactive airway disease
Cor pulmonale
Respiratory failure
Mucoid impaction of the bronchi
Allergic bronchopulmonary aspergillosis
GASTROINTESTINAL
Meconium ileus, meconium plug (neonate)
Meconium peritonitis (neonate)
Distal intestinal obstruction syndrome (non-neonatal obstruction)
Rectal prolapse
Intussusception
Volvulus
Fibrosing colonopathy (strictures)
Appendicitis
Intestinal atresia
Pancreatitis
Biliary cirrhosis (portal hypertension: esophageal varices, hypersplenism)
Neonatal obstructive jaundice
Hepatic steatosis
Gastroesophageal reflux
Cholelithiasis
Inguinal hernia
Growth failure (malabsorption)
Vitamin deficiency states (vitamins A, K, E, D)
Insulin deficiency, symptomatic hyperglycemia, diabetes
Malignancy (rare)
OTHER
Infertility
Delayed puberty
Edema-hypoproteinemia
Dehydration-heat exhaustion
Hypertrophic osteoarthropathy-arthritis
Clubbing
Amyloidosis
Diabetes mellitus

Silverman FN, Kuhn JP: *Essentials of Caffrey's Pediatric X-Ray Diagnosis.* Chicago, Year Book Medical Publishers, 1990, p 649.

less for South Asian immigrants than for the general population (1/9,200 vs 1/6,600).

CF is inherited as an autosomal recessive trait. The CF gene codes for a protein of 1,480 amino acids called the *CF transmembrane regulator (CFTR)*. CFTR is expressed largely in epithelial cells of airways, the gastrointestinal tract (including the pancreas and biliary system), the sweat glands, and the genitourinary system. CFTR has ion channel and regulatory functions that are perturbed variably by the different mutations. More than 1,500 CFTR polymorphisms are associated with the CF syndrome. The most prevalent mutation of CFTR is the deletion of a single phenylalanine residue at amino acid 508 (ΔF508). This mutation is responsible for the high incidence of CF in northern European populations and is considerably less frequent in other populations, such as those of southern Europe and Israel. Approximately 50% of individuals with CF who are of northern European ancestry are homozygous for ΔF508, and >70% carry at least one ΔF508 gene. The remainder of patients has an extensive array of mutations, none of which has a prevalence of more than several percent, except in circumscribed populations; the W1282X mutation occurs in 60% of Ashkenazi Jews with CF. The relationship between CFTR genotype and clinical phenotype is highly complex and not predictable for individual patients. Mutations categorized as "severe" (ΔF508) are associated almost uniformly with pancreatic insufficiency but only in general with more rapid progression of lung disease. Modifier gene polymorphisms appear to be responsible for much of the variation in the progression of lung disease. The most compelling association with more severe disease is with a single nucleotide change in the TGF- β1 gene. Variant alleles of the mannose-binding lectin, a key factor in systemic innate immunity, are associated with more serious lung infections and reduced survival. Several mutations (3849 + 10 kb C > T) are found in patients with normal sweat chloride concentrations. Some individuals with polymorphisms of both CFTR genes have few or no CF manifestations until adolescence or adulthood, when they present with pancreatitis, sinusitis, diffuse bronchiectasis, or male infertility. Whereas CFTR mutations are a sine qua non for CF, two mutations of CFTR can cause disorders that do not meet diagnostic criteria for CF and, occasionally, do not cause discernible clinic problems.

Occurrence of liver disease cannot be predicted by CFTR genotype. This suggests a major environmental (acquired) component of organ system dysfunction and the presence of other genes that modify the CF phenotype.

Using probes for 30 of the most frequent mutations, the genotype of 80–90% of Americans with CF can be ascertained, and increasing the number of probes to ≥70 improves mutation ascertainment by only a few percent. Some labs have established protocols for comprehensive screening for all known CFTR mutations. In special cases, sequencing the CFTR gene is necessary to establish the genotype.

The high frequency of CFTR mutations has been hypothetically ascribed to resistance to the morbidity and mortality associated with cholera through the ages. Cultured CF intestinal epithelial cells homozygous for the ΔF508 mutation are unresponsive to the secretory effects of cholera toxin.

PATHOGENESIS. Four long-standing observations are of fundamental pathophysiologic importance: failure to clear mucous secretions, a paucity of water in mucous secretions, an elevated salt content of sweat and other serous secretions, and chronic infection limited to the respiratory tract. In addition, there is a greater negative potential difference across the respiratory epithelia of CF patients than across the respiratory epithelia of control subjects. Aberrant electrical properties were also demonstrated for CF sweat gland duct epithelium. The membranes of CF epithelial cells are unable to secrete chloride ions in response to cyclic adenosine monophosphate (cAMP)–mediated signals and, at least in the respiratory tract, excessive amounts of sodium are absorbed through these membranes (Fig. 400-1). These defects can be traced to a dysfunction of CFTR (Figs. 400-2 and 400-3).

Cyclic AMP-stimulated chloride conductance is a function of CFTR itself; this function is absent in epithelial cells with many different mutations of the CFTR gene. CFTR mutations fall into

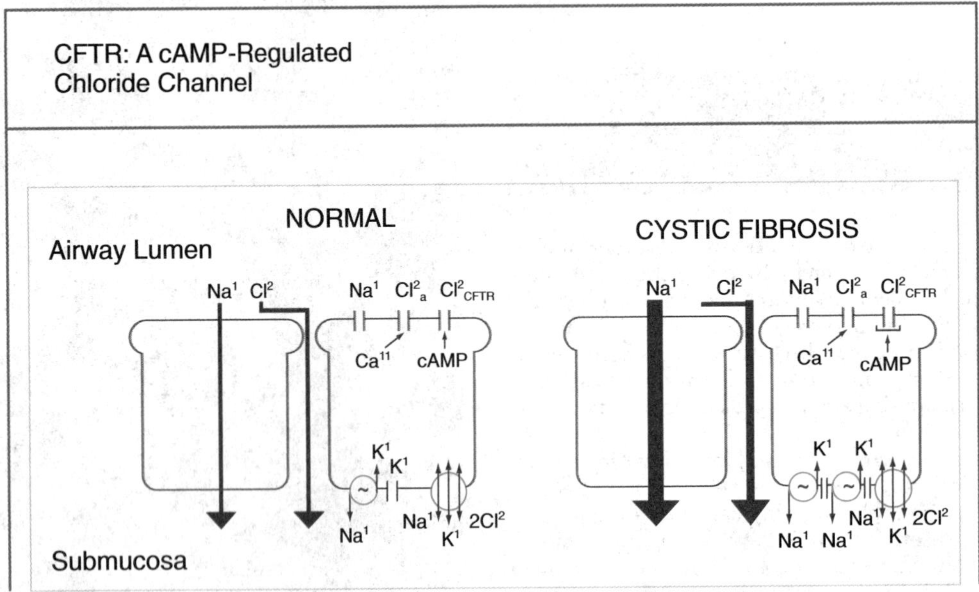

Figure 400-1. The net ion flow across normal and cystic fibrosis (CF) airway epithelia under basal conditions *(large arrows)*. Because water follows salt movement, the predicted net flux of water would be from the airway lumen to the submucosa and would be greater across CF epithelia. The increased Na^+ absorption by CF cells is associated with an increased amiloride-sensitive Na^+ conductance across the apical (luminal) membrane and increased Na^+,K^+-ATPase sites at the basolateral membrane. The cAMP-mediated apical membrane conductance of Cl^- associated with the CF transmembrane regulator (CFTR) does not function in CF epithelia, but an alternative, calcium-activated Cl^- conductance is present in normal and CF cells. It is postulated that CF cells have a limited ability to secrete Cl^- and absorb Na^+ in excessive amounts, limiting the water available to hydrate secretions and allow them to be cleared from the airways lumen. ATP, adenosine triphosphate; cAMP, cyclic adenosine monophosphate. (From Knowles MR: Contemporary perspectives on the pathogenesis of cystic fibrosis. *New Insights Cystic Fibrosis* 1993;1:1.)

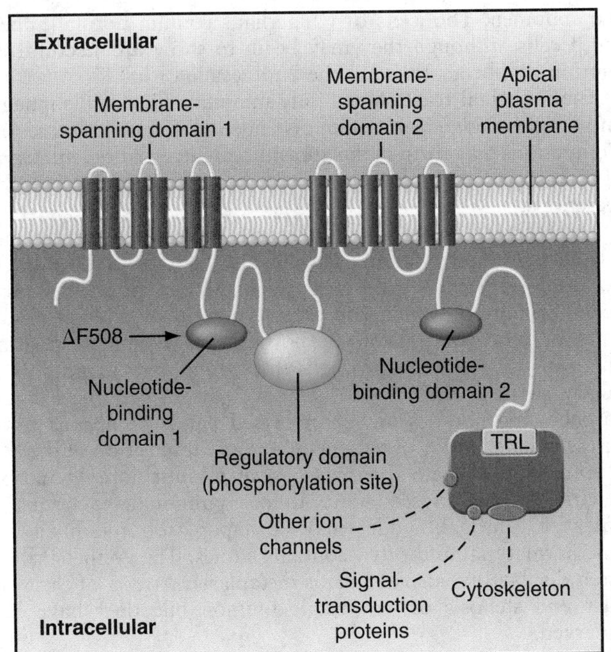

Figure 400-2. Hypothesized structure of cystic fibrosis transmembrane regulator (CFTR). The protein contains 1,480 amino acids and a number of discrete globular and transmembrane domains. Activation of CFTR relies on phosphorylation, particularly through protein kinase A but probably involving other kinases as well. Channel activity is governed by the 2 nucleotide-binding domains, which regulate channel gating. The carboxyl terminal (consisting of threonine, arginine, and leucine [TRL]) of CFTR is anchored through a PDZ-type–binding interaction with the cytoskeleton and is kept in close approximation *(dashed arrows)* to a number of important proteins. These associated proteins influence CFTR functions, including conductance, regulation of other channels, signal transduction, and localization at the apical plasma membrane. Each membrane-spanning domain contains 6 membrane-spanning α helixes, portions of which form a chloride-conductance pore. The regulatory domain is a site of protein kinase A phosphorylation. The common F508 mutation occurs on the surface of nucleotide-binding domain 1. (From Rowe SM, Miller S, Sorscher EJ: Cystic fibrosis. *N Engl J Med* 2005; 352:1992–2001.)

6 classes, albeit with some overlap (see Fig. 400-3). Individuals with class I, II, and III mutations, on average, have shortened survival compared with those who have "mild" genotypes (class IV or V). The clinical importance of these functional categories is limited because they do not uniformly correlate with specific clinical features or their severity. Rather, clinical features correlate with the residual CFTR activity. Individuals with only 1% of normal CFTR activity have lung disease and pancreatic insufficiency; pancreatic function is retained with 5% activity, and 10% results in isolated congenital bilateral absence of the vas deferens or idiopathic chronic pancreatitis. These numbers should be viewed as relative and debate continues as to the absolute level of CFTR activity required to preserve organ system function.

The postulated epithelial pathophysiology in airways involves an inability to secrete salt and secondarily to secrete water in the presence of excessive reabsorption of salt and water. The proposed outcome is insufficient water on the airway surface to hydrate secretions. Desiccated secretions become more viscous and elastic (rubbery) and are harder to clear by mucociliary and other mechanisms. Altered mucus rheology can be aggravated by low HCO_{3^-} and a more acidic pH. These secretions are retained and obstruct airways, starting with those of the smallest caliber, the bronchioles. Airflow obstruction at the level of small airways is the earliest observable physiologic abnormality of the respiratory system.

It is plausible that similar pathophysiologic events take place in the pancreatic and biliary ducts (and in the vas deferens), leading to desiccation of proteinaceous secretions and obstruction. Because the function of sweat gland duct cells is to absorb rather than secrete chloride, salt is not retrieved from the isotonic primary sweat as it is transported to the skin surface; chloride and sodium levels are consequently elevated.

Chronic infection in CF is limited to the airways. The most likely explanation for infection is a sequence of events starting with failure to clear inhaled bacteria promptly and then proceeding to persistent colonization and an inflammatory response in airway walls. An alternative hypothesis is that abnormal CFTR creates a proinflammatory state or amplifies the inflammatory response to initial viral infections. Inflammatory events occur 1st in small airways, perhaps because clearance of altered secretions and microorganisms is more difficult from these regions. Chronic bronchiolitis and bronchitis are the initial lung manifestations, but after months to years, structural changes in airway walls produce bronchiolectasis and bronchiectasis.

The agents of airway injury include neutrophil products, such as oxidative radicals and proteases, and immune reaction products. With advanced lung disease, infection may extend to peribronchial lung parenchyma. Several inflammatory products, including proteases, contribute to the mucus hypersecretion that is characteristic of chronic airway disease.

A finding that is not readily explained is the high prevalence of airway colonization with *Staphylococcus aureus* (see Chapter 180.1), *Pseudomonas aeruginosa* (see Chapter 202), and *Burkholderia cepacia* (see Chapter 202), organisms that rarely infect

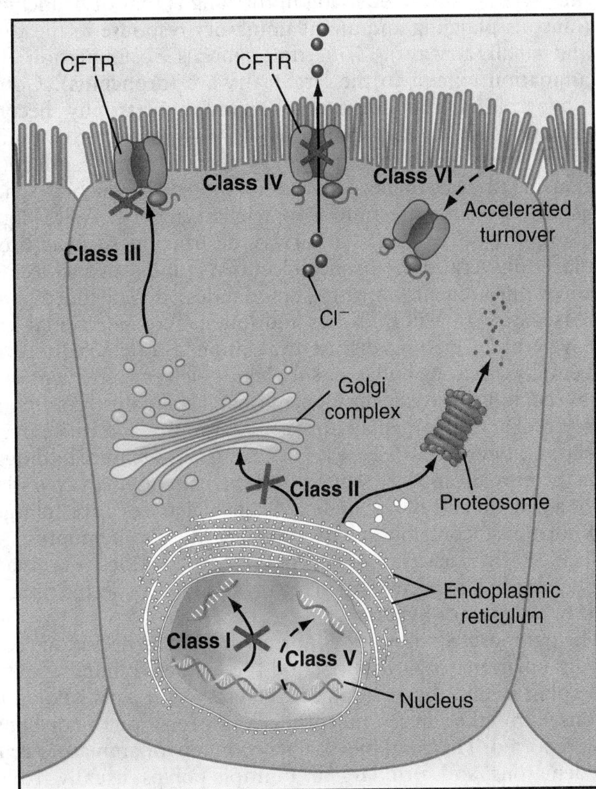

Figure 400-3. Categories of *CFTR* Mutations. Classes of defects in the *CFTR* gene include the absence of synthesis (class I); defective protein maturation and premature degradation (class II); disordered regulation, such as diminished ATP binding and hydrolysis (class III); defective chloride conductance or channel gating (class IV); a reduced number of CFTR transcripts due to a promoter or splicing abnormality (class V); and accelerated turnover from the cell surface (class VI). CFTR, cystic fibrosis transmembrane regulator; ATP, adenosine triphosphate. (From Rowe SM, Miller S, Sorscher EJ: Cystic fibrosis. *N Engl J Med* 2005;352:1992–2001.)

the lungs of other individuals. The CF airway epithelial cells or surface liquids may provide a favorable environment for harboring these organisms. CF airway epithelium may be compromised in its innate defenses against these organisms, through either acquired or genetic alterations. Antimicrobial activity is diminished in CF secretions; this is more likely related to hyperacidified surface liquids or other effects on innate immunity. Another puzzle is the propensity for *P. aeruginosa* to undergo mucoid transformation in the CF airways. The complex polysaccharide produced by these organisms generates a biofilm that provides a hypoxic environment and thereby protects *Pseudomonas* against antimicrobial agents.

Although functional deficits may occur in cellular immunity, mucosal immune function, and the alternate pathway for complement as lung infection progresses to an advanced stage, the immune system in CF appears to be fundamentally intact. Nutritional deficits, including fatty acid deficiency, have been implicated as predisposing factors for respiratory tract infection. More specifically, concentrations of lipoxins, molecules that suppress neutrophilic inflammation, are suppressed in CF airways. The 10–15% of individuals who retain substantial exocrine pancreatic function have statistically lower sweat chloride values, delayed onset of colonization with *P. aeruginosa,* and slower deterioration of lung function. It appears that nutritional factors are only contributory because preservation of pancreatic function does not preclude development of typical lung disease.

PATHOLOGY. Eccrine sweat glands and parotid salivary glands, including ducts, are not involved pathologically, despite abnormalities in the electrolyte content of their secretory product.

The earliest pathologic lesion in the lung is that of **bronchiolitis** (mucous plugging and an inflammatory response in the walls of the small airways). With time, mucus accumulation and inflammation extend to the larger airways (**bronchitis**). Goblet cell hyperplasia and submucosal gland hypertrophy become prominent pathologic expressions of a hypersecretory state, which is most likely a response to chronic airway infection. Organisms appear to be confined to the endobronchial space; invasive bacterial infection is not characteristic. With long-standing disease, evidence of airway destruction such as **bronchiolar obliteration, bronchiolectasis,** and **bronchiectasis** becomes prominent. Imaging modalities demonstrate both increased airway wall thickness and luminal cross-sectional area relatively early in lung disease evaluation. Bronchiectatic cysts and emphysematous bullae or subpleural blebs are frequent with advanced lung disease, the upper lobes being most commonly involved. These enlarged air spaces may rupture and cause pneumothorax. Interstitial disease is not a prominent feature, although areas of fibrosis appear eventually. True emphysema occurs but is not a general pathologic finding. Bronchial arteries are enlarged and tortuous, contributing to a propensity for **hemoptysis** in bronchiectatic airways. Small pulmonary arteries eventually display medial hypertrophy, which would be expected in secondary pulmonary hypertension.

The **paranasal sinuses** are uniformly filled with secretions containing inflammatory products, and the epithelial lining displays hyperplastic and hypertrophied secretory elements. Polypoid lesions within the sinuses, mucopyocele, and erosion of bone have been reported. The nasal mucosa may contain inflammatory cells, be edematous, and form large or multiple polyps, usually from a base surrounding the ostia of the maxillary and ethmoidal sinuses.

The **pancreas** is usually small, occasionally cystic, and often difficult to find at postmortem examination. The extent of involvement varies at birth. In infants, the acini and ducts are often distended and filled with eosinophilic material. In 85–90% of patients, the lesion progresses to complete or almost complete disruption of acini and replacement with fibrous tissue and fat. Infrequently, foci of calcification may be seen on radiographs of the abdomen. The islets of Langerhans contain normal appearing β cells, although they may begin to show architectural disruption by fibrous tissue in the 2nd decade of life.

The **intestinal tract** shows only minimal changes. Esophageal and duodenal glands are often distended with mucous secretions. Concretions may form in the appendiceal lumen or cecum. Crypts of the appendix and rectum may be dilated and filled with secretions.

Focal biliary cirrhosis secondary to blockage of intrahepatic bile ducts is uncommon in early life, although it is responsible for occasional cases of prolonged neonatal jaundice. This lesion becomes more prevalent and extensive with age and is found in 25% or more of patients at postmortem examination. Infrequently, this process proceeds to symptomatic multilobular biliary cirrhosis that has a distinctive pattern of large irregular parenchymal nodules and interspersed bands of fibrous tissue. Approximately 30% of patients have fatty infiltration of the liver, in some cases despite apparently adequate nutrition. At autopsy, hepatic congestion secondary to cor pulmonale is frequently observed. The gallbladder may be hypoplastic and filled with mucoid material and often contains stones. The epithelial lining often displays extensive mucous metaplasia. Atresia of the cystic duct and stenosis of the distal common bile duct have been observed.

Mucus-secreting salivary glands are usually enlarged and display focal plugging and dilatation of ducts.

Glands of the **uterine cervix** are distended with mucus, copious amounts of which collect in the cervical canal. Endocervicitis may be prevalent in teenagers and young women. In >95% of males, the body and tail of the epididymis, the vas deferens, and the seminal vesicles are obliterated or atretic.

Generalized amyloidosis has been reported rarely (see Chapter 163).

CLINICAL MANIFESTATIONS. Mutational heterogeneity and environmental factors appear responsible for highly variable involvement of the lungs, pancreas, and other organs. A list of presenting manifestations is lengthy, although pulmonary and gastrointestinal presentations predominate (Table 400-2).

Respiratory Tract. Cough is the most constant symptom of pulmonary involvement. At first, the cough may be dry and hacking, but eventually it becomes loose and productive. In older patients, the cough is most prominent on arising in the morning or after activity. Expectorated mucus is usually purulent. Some patients remain asymptomatic for long periods or seem to have prolonged but intermittent acute respiratory infections. Others acquire a chronic cough in the 1st weeks of life, or they have pneumonia repeatedly. Extensive bronchiolitis is attended by wheezing, which is a frequent symptom during the 1st years of life. As lung disease slowly progresses, exercise intolerance, shortness of

TABLE 400-2. Presenting Features of More Than 20,000 Cystic Fibrosis Patients in the United States

FEATURE	%
Acute or persistent respiratory symptoms	50.5
Failure to thrive, malnutrition	42.9
Abnormal stools	35.0
Meconium ileus, intestinal obstruction	18.8
Family history	16.8
Electrolyte, acid-base abnormality	5.4
Rectal prolapse	3.4
Nasal polyps, sinus disease	2.0
Hepatobiliary disease	0.9
Other*	1.0–2.0

*Includes pseudotumor cerebri, azoospermia, acrodermatitis-like rash, vitamin deficiency states, hypoproteinemic edema, hypoprothrombinemia with bleeding, meconium plug syndrome.
Data from the Patient Registry, Cystic Fibrosis Foundation, Bethesda, MD.

breath, and failure to gain weight or grow are noted. Exacerbations of lung symptoms, presumably owing to more active airways infection, eventually require repeated hospitalizations for effective treatment. Cor pulmonale, respiratory failure, and death eventually supervene unless lung transplantation is accomplished. Colonization with *Burkholderia cepacia* and other multidrug-resistant organisms may be associated with particularly rapid pulmonary deterioration and death.

The rate of progression of lung disease is the chief determinant of morbidity and mortality. The course of lung disease, however, is largely independent of genotype. Severe mutations tend to be associated with more rapid progression. A few mutations (R117H) may substantially or even fully spare the lungs. Male gender and exocrine pancreatic sufficiency are also associated with a slower rate of pulmonary function decline. Early insults to the lungs (severe viral infections) are likely to be a major determinant of pulmonary outcome.

Early **physical findings** include increased anteroposterior diameter of the chest, generalized hyperresonance, scattered or localized coarse crackles, and digital clubbing. Expiratory wheezes may be heard, especially in young children. Cyanosis is a late sign. Common pulmonary complications include atelectasis, hemoptysis, pneumothorax, and cor pulmonale; these usually appear beyond the 1st decade of life.

Even though the paranasal sinuses are virtually always opacified radiographically, acute sinusitis is infrequent. Nasal obstruction and rhinorrhea are common, caused by inflamed, swollen mucous membranes or, in some cases, nasal polyposis. **Nasal polyps** are most troublesome between 5 and 20 yr of age.

Intestinal Tract. In 15–20% of newborn infants with CF, the ileum is completely obstructed by meconium (**meconium ileus**). The frequency is greater (≈30%) among siblings born subsequent to a child with meconium ileus and particularly striking in monozygotic twins, reflecting a genetic contribution from 1 or more modifying genes. Abdominal distention, emesis, and failure to pass meconium appear in the 1st 24–48 hr of life (see Chapter 102.1). Abdominal radiographs (Fig. 400-4) show dilated loops of bowel with air-fluid levels and, frequently, a collection of granular, "ground-glass" material in the lower central abdomen. Rarely, **meconium peritonitis** results from intrauterine rupture of the bowel wall and can be detected radiographically by the presence of peritoneal or scrotal calcifications. **Meconium plug syndrome** occurs with increased frequency in infants with CF but is less specific than meconium ileus. Ileal obstruction with fecal material (distal intestinal obstruction syndrome or meconium ileus equivalent) occurs in older patients, causing cramping abdominal pain and abdominal distention.

More than 85% of affected children show evidence of maldigestion from exocrine pancreatic insufficiency. Symptoms include frequent, bulky, greasy stools and failure to gain weight even when food intake appears to be large. Nearly 40% of patients display nutritional failure by the criterion of weight/height less than the 10th percentile. Characteristically, stools contain readily visible droplets of fat. A protuberant abdomen, decreased muscle mass, poor growth, and delayed maturation are typical physical signs. Excessive flatus may be a problem. A number of mutations are associated with preservation of some exocrine pancreatic function, including R117H and 3849 + 10 kb C > T. Virtually all individuals homozygous for ΔF508 have pancreatic insufficiency.

Less common gastrointestinal manifestations include intussusception, fecal impaction of the cecum with an asymptomatic right lower quadrant mass, and epigastric pain owing to duodenal inflammation. Acid or bile reflux with esophagitis symptoms is common in older children and adults. Subacute appendicitis and periappendiceal abscess have been encountered. Historically a relatively common event, rectal prolapse occurs much less frequently as the result of earlier diagnosis and initiation of pancreatic enzyme replacement therapy. Occasionally, hypoproteinemia with anasarca appears in malnourished infants, especially if children are fed soy-based preparations. Neurologic dysfunction (dementia, peripheral neuropathy) and hemolytic anemia may occur because of **vitamin E deficiency.** Deficiency of other fat-soluble vitamins is occasionally symptomatic. **Hypoprothrombinemia** owing to vitamin K deficiency may result in a bleeding diathesis. Clinical manifestations of other fat-soluble vitamin deficiencies, such as decreased bone density and night blindness, have been noted. Rickets is rare.

Biliary Tract. Evidence for liver dysfunction is most often detected in the 1st 15 yr of life and can be found in up to 30% of individuals. Biliary cirrhosis becomes symptomatic in only 2–3% of patients. Manifestations can include icterus, ascites, hematemesis from esophageal varices, and evidence of hypersplenism. A neonatal hepatitis-like picture and massive hepatomegaly owing to steatosis have been reported. Biliary colic secondary to cholelithiasis may occur in the 2nd decade or later.

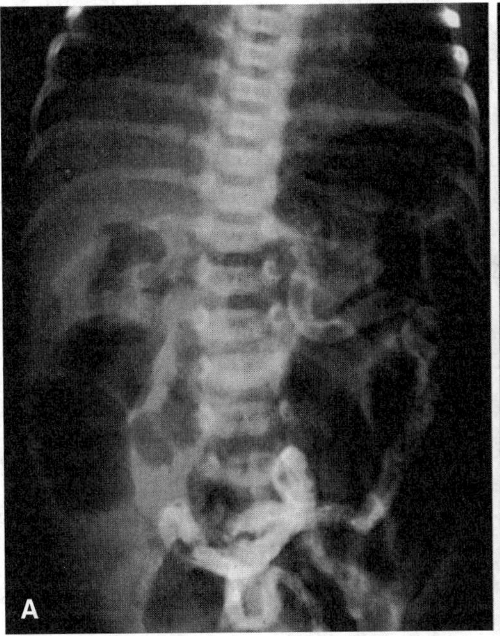

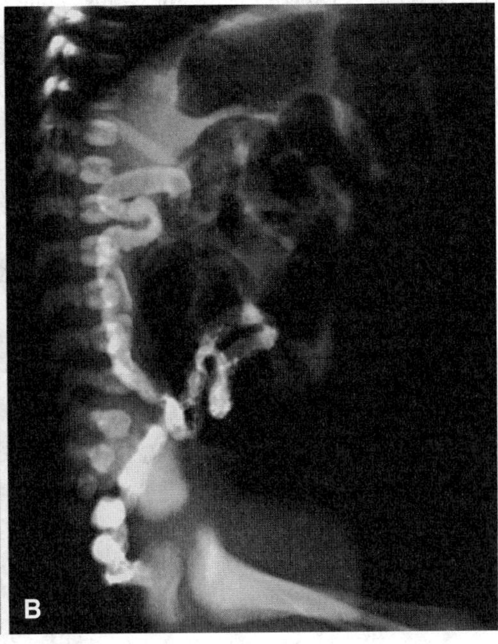

Figure 400-4. *A* and *B*, Contrast enema in a newborn infant with abdominal distention and failure to pass meconium. Notice the small diameter of the sigmoid and ascending colon and dilated, air-filled loops of small intestine. Several air-fluid levels in the small bowel are seen on the upright lateral view.

Liver disease occurs independent of genotype but is associated with meconium ileus and pancreatic insufficiency.

Pancreas. In addition to exocrine pancreatic insufficiency, evidence for hyperglycemia and glycosuria including polyuria and weight loss may appear, especially in the 2nd decade of life. Eight percent of 11–17 yr old patients and 18% of 18–24 yr olds have insulin-dependent diabetes. Ketoacidosis usually does not occur, but eye, kidney, and other vascular complications have been noted in patients living ≥10 yr after the onset of hyperglycemia. Recurrent, acute pancreatitis occurs occasionally in individuals who have residual exocrine pancreatic function and may be the sole manifestation of two CFTR mutations.

Genitourinary Tract. Sexual development is often delayed but only by an average of 2 yr. More than 95% of males are azoospermic because of failure of development of Wolffian duct structures, but sexual function is generally unimpaired. The incidence of inguinal hernia, hydrocele, and undescended testis is higher than expected. Adolescent females may experience secondary amenorrhea, especially with exacerbations of pulmonary disease. Cervicitis and accumulation of tenacious mucus in the cervical canal have been noted. The female fertility rate is diminished. Pregnancy is generally tolerated well by women with good pulmonary function but may accelerate pulmonary progression in those with moderate or advanced lung problems.

Sweat Glands. Excessive loss of salt in the sweat predisposes young children to salt depletion episodes, especially during episodes of gastroenteritis and during warm weather. These children present with **hypochloremic alkalosis.** Frequently, parents notice salt "frosting" of the skin or a salty taste when they kiss the child. A few genotypes (3849 + 10 kb C > T) are associated with normal sweat chloride values.

DIAGNOSIS AND ASSESSMENT. The diagnosis of CF has been based on a positive quantitative sweat test ($Cl^- \geq 60$ mEq/L) in conjunction with 1 or more of the following: typical chronic obstructive pulmonary disease, documented exocrine pancreatic insufficiency, or a positive family history. Diagnostic criteria have been recommended to include additional testing procedures (Table 400-3).

Sweat Testing. The sweat test, using pilocarpine iontophoresis to collect sweat and chemical analysis of its chloride content, is the standard approach to diagnosis. The procedure requires care and accuracy. A 3 mA electric current is used to carry pilocarpine into the skin of the forearm and locally stimulate the sweat glands. After washing the arm with distilled water, sweat is collected on filter paper or gauze (or with a capillary tube) that has been placed on the stimulated skin and covered to prevent evaporation. After 30 min, the filter paper is removed, weighed, and eluted in distilled water. A chloridometer is recommended for the analysis of chloride in these samples. The amount of sweat collected should be measured and reported. For reliable results, at least 75 mg and preferably 100 mg of sweat should be collected. Testing may be difficult in the 1st 2 wk of life because of low sweat rates but is recommended any time after the 1st 48 hrs of life. Positive results should be confirmed; a negative result should be repeated if suspicion of the diagnosis remains.

More than 60 mEq/L of chloride in sweat is diagnostic of CF when 1 or more other criteria are present. Threshold levels of 40 mEq/L for infants have been suggested. Values between 40 and 60 mEq/L have been reported at all ages in cases with typical involvement. In healthy adults, the sweat chloride values increase slightly, but a value of 60 mEq/L still adequately differentiates CF from other conditions. Chloride concentrations in sweat are somewhat lower in individuals who retain exocrine pancreatic function but remain within the diagnostic range. False-negative test results may be encountered in children with hypoproteinemic edema; false-positive results can occur when testing is performed on skin affected by eczema or contaminated with skin creams or lotions.

Non-CF conditions associated with elevated concentrations of sweat electrolytes include untreated adrenal insufficiency, ectodermal dysplasia, hereditary nephrogenic diabetes insipidus, glucose-6-phosphatase deficiency, hypothyroidism, hypoparathyroidism, familial cholestasis, pancreatitis, mucopolysaccharidoses, fucosidosis, and malnutrition. Most of these conditions can be easily distinguished from CF by clinical criteria.

DNA Testing. Several commercial laboratories test for 30–80 of the most common CFTR mutations. This testing identifies ≥90% individuals who carry 2 CF mutations. Some children with typical CF manifestations have 1 or no detectable mutations by this methodology. Some laboratories perform comprehensive mutation analysis, screening for all of the >1,500 identified mutations.

Other Diagnostic Tests. The finding of increased potential differences across nasal epithelium, the loss of this difference with topical amiloride application, and the absence of a voltage response to a β-adrenergic agonist have been used to confirm the diagnosis in patients with equivocal or frankly normal sweat chloride values. Failure to sweat when a combination of isoproterenol and atropine is injected into the skin has also been used to characterize CF variants.

Pancreatic Function. Exocrine pancreatic dysfunction is clinically apparent in many patients. Documentation is desirable if there are questions about the functional status of the pancreas. Measurement of fat balances with a 3 day stool collection or direct documentation of enzyme secretion after duodenal intubation and pancreozymin-secretin stimulation provides a reliable measure, but these methods are cumbersome or invasive for children and are not routinely used. Quantitation of elastase-1 activity in a fresh stool sample is a useful screening test. Measurement of immunoreactive trypsinogen in serum, used for newborn screening, also reliably distinguishes patients with CF, with and without pancreatic insufficiency. Other indirect measures of pancreatic enzyme secretion are available but have limited or unproven clinical value. Endocrine pancreatic dysfunction may be more prevalent than previously recognized. Many advocate yearly monitoring with a modified 2 hr oral glucose tolerance test (OGTT) after 10 yr of age. This approach is more sensitive than spot checks of blood and urine glucose levels and glycosylated hemoglobin levels.

Radiology. Pulmonary radiologic findings suggest the diagnosis but are not specific. Hyperinflation of lungs occurs early and may be overlooked in the absence of infiltrates or streaky densities. Bronchial thickening and plugging and ring shadows suggesting bronchiectasis usually appear 1st in the upper lobes. Nodular densities, patchy atelectasis, and confluent infiltrate follow. Hilar lymph nodes may be prominent. With advanced disease, impressive hyperinflation with markedly depressed diaphragms, anterior bowing of the sternum, and a narrow cardiac shadow are noted. Cyst formation, extensive bronchiectasis, dilated pulmonary artery segments, and segmental or lobar atelectasis are often apparent with advanced disease. Typical progression of lung disease is seen in Figure 400-5. Most CF centers obtain chest x-

TABLE 400-3. Diagnostic Criteria for Cystic Fibrosis (CF)
Presence of typical clinical features (respiratory, gastrointestinal, or genitourinary)
OR
A history of CF in a sibling
OR
A positive newborn screening test
PLUS
Laboratory evidence for CFTR dysfunction:
Two elevated sweat chloride concentrations obtained on separate days
OR
Identification of two CF mutations
OR
An abnormal nasal potential difference measurement
CFTR, CF transmembrane regulator.

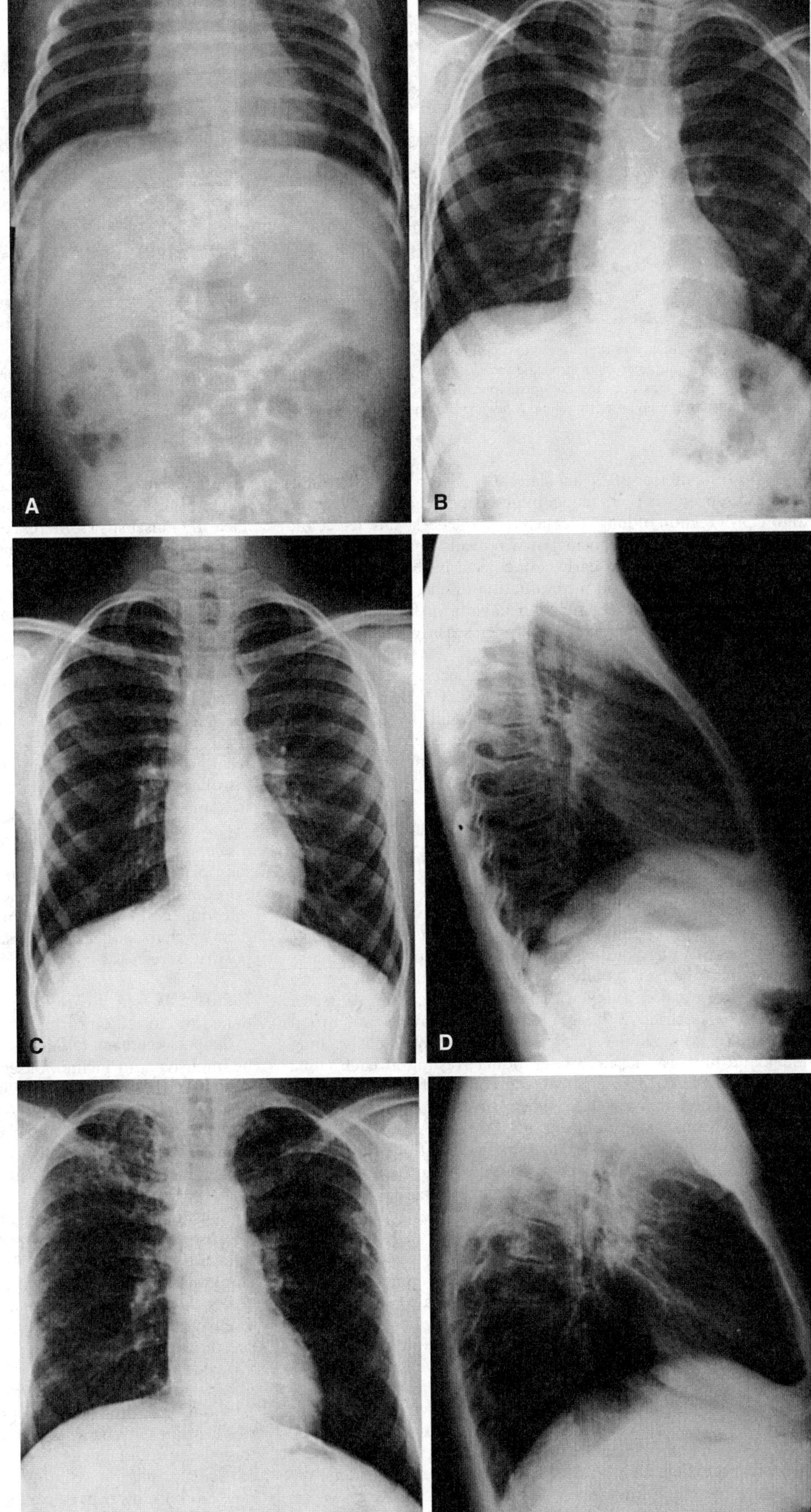

Figure 400-5. Roentgenographic progression of cystic fibrosis lung disease from the diagnosis in infancy to 18 yr of age. *A*, Admitted with cough and wheezing at 2 mo of age. Notice the mild increase in bronchovascular markings, especially in the upper lobe areas. *B*, At age 4 yr, cough was minimal. Bronchovascular markings were mildly increased, and there was some improvement in the upper lobes. The wheeze never recurred. *C* and *D*, At age 13 yr, there was minimal cough and occasional sputum production. The bronchovascular markings were generally further increased, with early bronchiectatic changes in the right upper lobe. The lateral view does not suggest overinflation. *E* and *F*, Age 18 yr. During adolescence, cough and sputum production increased even though outpatient antibiotic therapy was intensified. Small-volume hemoptysis, occasional paroxysms of cough, and weight loss as well as increased nodular infiltrates (especially in the right upper lobe) and hyperinflation (as seen on the lateral view) led to the 1st hospitalization since infancy. Height and weight were maintained in the 25th–50th percentile.

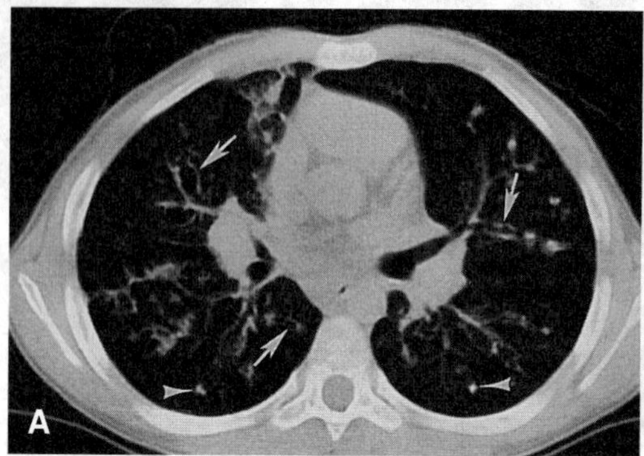

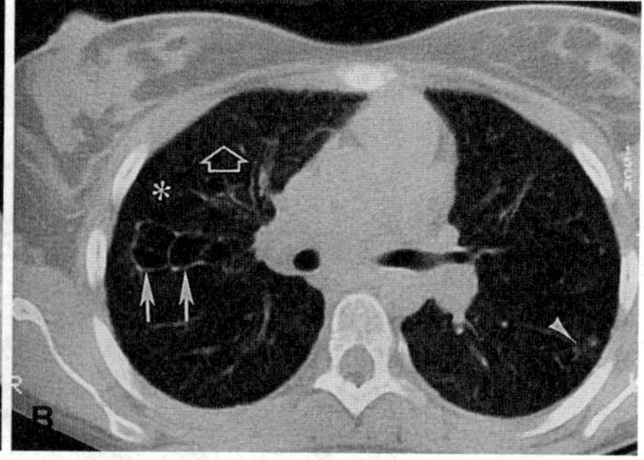

Figure 400-6. CT images of the chest in cystic fibrosis. *A,* A 12 yr old boy with moderate lung disease. Airway and parenchymal changes are present throughout both lungs. Multiple areas of bronchiectasis *(arrows)* and mucous plugging *(arrowheads)* are seen. *B,* A 19 yr old girl has mostly normal lung with 1 area of saccular bronchiectasis in the right upper lobe *(arrows)* and a focal area of peripheral mucous plugging in the right lower lobe *(arrowhead).* Lung density is heterogeneous with areas of normal lung *(open arrow)* and areas of low attenuation reflecting segmental and subsegmental air trapping *(asterisk).*

rays (posteroanterior [PA] and lateral) at least annually. Standardized scoring of roentgenographic changes has been used to follow progression of lung disease. CT of the chest can detect and localize thickening of bronchial airway walls, mucous plugging, focal hyperinflation, and early bronchiectasis (Fig. 400-6); it is generally not used for routine evaluation of chest disease. Many children with normal lung function have bronchiectasis by CT, indicating that this imaging modality is sensitive to early lung changes.

Radiographs of paranasal sinuses reveal panopacification and often failure of frontal sinus development. CT provides better resolution of sinus changes if this information is required clinically. Fetal ultrasonography may suggest ileal obstruction with meconium early in the 2nd trimester, but this finding is not predictive of meconium ileus at birth.

Pulmonary Function. Standard pulmonary function studies are not obtained until 4–6 yr of age, by which time many patients show the typical pattern of obstructive pulmonary involvement (see Chapter 381). Decrease in the midmaximal flow rate is an early functional change, reflecting small airway obstruction. This lesion also affects the distribution of ventilation and increases the alveolar-arterial oxygen difference. The findings of obstructive airway disease and modest responses to a bronchodilator are consistent with the diagnosis of CF at all ages. Residual volume and functional residual capacity are increased early in the course of lung disease. Restrictive changes, characterized by declining total lung capacity and vital capacity, correlate with extensive lung injury and fibrosis and are a late finding. Testing at each clinic visit is recommended to evaluate the course of the pulmonary involvement and intervene early when substantial decrements are documented. Increasing numbers of CF centers are equipped to measure airflow patterns of sedated infants, but this procedure is usually done in the context of research studies. Some patients reach adolescent or adult life with normal pulmonary function and without evidence of overinflation.

Microbiologic Studies. The finding of *S. aureus* or *P. aeruginosa* on culture of the lower airways (sputum) strongly suggests a diagnosis of CF. In particular, mucoid forms of *P. aeruginosa* are often recovered from CF lungs. *B. cepacia* recovery also suggests CF. A wide range of other organisms are frequently recovered, particularly in advanced lung disease, and include a variety of gram-negative rods, fungi, and nontuberculous mycobacterial species. Failure of respiratory symptom flares to respond to usual antibiotics triggers testing for mycoplasma and viruses. Fiberoptic bronchoscopy is used to gather lower respiratory tract secretions of infants and young children who do not expectorate.

Heterozygote Detection and Prenatal Diagnosis. Mutation analysis should be fully informative when testing potential carriers or a fetus, provided that mutations within the family have been previously identified. Testing a spouse of a carrier with a standard panel of probes is ≈90% sensitive. A 1977 National Institutes of Health Consensus Conference recommendation to offer prenatal testing to all couples planning to have children in addition to individuals with a family history of CF and partners of CF women has been reconsidered. Termination of pregnancy is a less popular option because the clinical course is not predictable and expected longevity now approaches 4 decades on average.

Newborn Screening. Most newborns with CF can be identified by determination of immunoreactive trypsinogen and limited DNA testing on blood spots, coupled with confirmatory sweat analysis. This screening test is ≈95% sensitive. Newborn diagnoses can prevent early nutritional deficiencies and improve long-term growth, and may spare cognitive function. Early diagnosis also has the advantage of genetic counseling for the family and, in some cases, avoids protracted diagnostic efforts. *There is as yet no compelling evidence that early diagnosis improves pulmonary outcome and, therefore, survival.* Newborn screening may place infants with CF at increased risk for earlier acquisition of *P. aeruginosa* and other troublesome airway infections if infection control is not vigorously practiced. Parental anxiety dictates that confirmatory testing is arranged promptly when a positive screen is reported.

TREATMENT. The treatment plan should be comprehensive and linked to close monitoring and early, aggressive intervention.

General Approach to Care. Initial efforts after diagnosis should be intensive and include baseline assessment, initiation of treatment, clearing of pulmonary involvement, and education of the patient and parents. Follow-up evaluations are scheduled every 2–3 mo because many aspects of the condition require careful monitoring. An interval history and physical examination should be obtained at each visit. A sputum sample or, if that is not available, a lower pharyngeal swab taken during or after a forced cough is obtained for culture and antibiotic susceptibility studies. Because irreversible loss of pulmonary function from low-grade infection can occur gradually and without acute symptoms, emphasis is placed on a thorough pulmonary history. Table 400-4 lists symptoms and signs that suggest the need for more intensive antibiotic and physical therapy. Immunoprophylaxis specifically against rubeola, pertussis, and influenza is essential. Protection against exposure to methicillin-resistant *S. aureus, P. aeruginosa, B. cepacia,* and other resistant gram-negatives is essential, including isolation procedures and careful attention to sterilization of inhalation therapy equipment. A nurse, respiratory therapist, social worker, dietitian, and psychologist should participate in the care program as needed. Considerable education and empowerment for families and older children to take responsibility for care is likely to result in the best adherence to

TABLE 400-4. Symptoms and Signs Associated with Exacerbation of Pulmonary Infection in Patients with Cystic Fibrosis

SYMPTOMS
Increased frequency and duration of cough
Increased sputum production
Change in appearance of sputum
Increased shortness of breath
Decreased exercise tolerance
Decreased appetite
Feeling of increased congestion in the chest
SIGNS
Increased respiratory rate
Use of accessory muscles for breathing
Intercostal retractions
Change in results of auscultatory examination of chest
Decline in measures of pulmonary function consistent with the presence of obstructive airway disease
Fever and leukocytosis
Weight loss
New infiltrate on chest radiograph

From Ramsey B: Management of pulmonary disease in patients with cystic fibrosis. *N Engl J Med* 1996;335:179.

daily care programs. Standardization of practice, on the part of both caregivers and families, as well as close monitoring and early intervention for new or increasing symptoms appear to result in the best long-term outcomes.

Because secretions of CF patients are not adequately hydrated, attention in early childhood to oral hydration, especially during warm weather or with acute gastroenteritis, may minimize complications associated with impaired mucus clearance. For the same reason, intravenous therapy for dehydration should be initiated early.

The goal of therapy is to maintain a stable condition for prolonged periods. This can be accomplished for most patients by interval evaluation and adjustments of the home treatment program. Some children have episodic acute or low-grade chronic lung infection that progresses. For these patients, ≥2 wk of intensive inhalation and physical therapy and intravenous antibiotics are indicated. Improvement is most reliably accomplished in a hospital setting; selected patients have demonstrated successful outcomes while completing these treatments at home. Intravenous antibiotics may be required infrequently or as often as every 2–3 mo. The goal of treatment is to return patients to their previous pulmonary and functional status.

The basic daily care program varies depending on the age of the child, the degree of pulmonary involvement, other system involvement, and the time available for therapy. The major components of this care are pulmonary and nutritional therapy. Because therapy is medication-intensive, iatrogenic problems frequently arise. Monitoring for these complications is also an important part of management (Table 400-5).

TABLE 400-5. Complications of Therapy for Cystic Fibrosis

COMPLICATION	AGENT
Gastrointestinal bleeding	Ibuprofen
Hyperglycemia	Corticosteroids (systemic)
Growth retardation	Corticosteroids (systemic, inhaled)
Renal dysfunction	
Tubular	Aminoglycosides
Interstitial nephritis	Semisynthetic penicillins, NSAIDs
Hearing loss, vestibular dysfunction	Aminoglycosides
Peripheral neuropathy or optic atrophy	Chloramphenicol (prolonged course)
Hypomagnesemia	Aminoglycosides
Hyperuricemia, colonic stricture	Pancreatic extracts (very large doses)
Goiter	Iodine-containing expectorants
Gynecomastia	Spironolactone
Enamel hypoplasia or staining	Tetracyclines (used in 1st 8 yr of life)

Note: Common hypersensitivity reactions to drugs are not included.
NSAIDs, nonsteroidal anti-inflammatory drugs.

Pulmonary Therapy. The object is to clear secretions from airways and to control infection. The effectiveness of the overall approach, including continuity of care, frequent evaluations, aggressive intervention, and an optimistic outlook, is more important than variations in the use of individual measures. When a child is not doing well, every potentially useful aspect of therapy should be considered.

Inhalation Therapy. Aerosol therapy is used to deliver medications and hydrate the lower respiratory tract. Metered-dose inhalers can deliver some agents such as bronchodilators and corticosteroids, with a spacer for younger children. The mainstay is intermittent delivery using a compressor that drives a hand-held nebulizer. The basic aerosol solution is 0.9% saline. In patients with reactive airways, albuterol or other β agonists are added. β Agonists may decrease PaO_2 acutely by increasing ventilation-perfusion mismatch, a concern if the PaO_2 is marginal.

When the airway pathogens are resistant to oral antibiotics or when the infection is difficult to control at home, aerosolized antibiotics may reduce symptoms, improve pulmonary function, and alleviate the need for hospitalization (see Aerosolized Antibiotic Therapy).

Human recombinant DNase (2.5 mg), given as a single daily aerosol dose, improves pulmonary function, decreases numbers of pulmonary exacerbations, and promotes a sense of well-being in patients who have moderate disease and purulent secretions. Benefit for those with normal forced expiratory volume in 1 sec (FEV_1) values or advanced lung disease has also been documented. Improvement is sustained for ≥12 mo on continuous therapy. Variation in response suggests that an individual trial be conducted to document benefit before embarking on long-term therapy at considerable cost. Another mucolytic agent, *N*-acetylcysteine, is toxic to ciliated epithelium, and repeated administration should be avoided.

Hypertonic saline aerosols are reported to increase mucus clearance and improve pulmonary function. Benefit is quite variable and inferior, on average, to that achieved with DNase.

Airway Clearance Therapy. This treatment usually consists of chest percussion combined with postural drainage and derives its rationale from the idea that cough clears mucus from large airways, but chest vibrations are required to move secretions from small airways where expiratory flow rates are low. **Chest physical therapy (PT)** can be particularly useful for patients with CF because they accumulate secretions in small airways first, even before the onset of symptoms. Although immediate improvement of pulmonary function generally cannot be demonstrated after PT, cessation of chest PT in children with mild to moderate airflow limitation results in deterioration of lung function within 3 wk, and prompt improvement of function occurs when therapy is resumed. Chest PT is recommended 1–4 times a day, depending on the severity of lung dysfunction. Cough, huffing, or forced expirations are encouraged after each lung segment is "drained." Vest-type mechanical percussors may be useful for older patients. Voluntary coughing, repeated forced expiratory maneuvers with and without positive expiratory pressure, patterned breathing, and use of a hand-held flutter device are additional aids to clearance of mucus. Routine aerobic exercise appears to slow the rate of decline of pulmonary function, and benefit has also been documented with weight training.

Antibiotic Therapy. Antibiotics are the mainstay of therapy designed to control progression of lung infection. The goal is to reduce the intensity of endobronchial infection and to delay progressive lung damage. The usual guidelines for acute chest infections, such as fever, tachypnea, or chest pain, are often absent. Consequently, all aspects of the patient's history and examination, including anorexia, weight loss, and diminished activity, must be used to guide the frequency and duration of therapy. Antibiotic treatment varies from intermittent short courses of 1 antibiotic to nearly continuous treatment with 1 or more antibiotics. Dosages for some antibiotics are often 2 to 3 times the amount recommended for minor infections because patients with CF have proportionately more lean body mass and higher clearance rates for many antibiotics than do other individuals. In addition, it is difficult to achieve effective drug levels of many antimicrobials in respiratory tract secretions.

ORAL ANTIBIOTIC THERAPY. Indications include the presence of respiratory tract symptoms and identification of pathogenic organisms in respiratory tract cultures. Whenever possible, the choice of antibiotics should be guided by in vitro sensitivity testing. Common organisms including *S. aureus,* nontypable *Haemophilus influenzae,* and *P. aeruginosa. B. cepacia,* and other gram-negative rods are encountered with increasing frequency. The first 2 can be eradicated from the respiratory tract in CF, but *Pseudomonas* is more difficult to treat. The usual course of therapy is ≥2 wk, and maximal doses are recommended. Useful oral antibiotics are listed in Table 400-6. Tetracycline should be avoided in children <9 yr of age. The quinolones are the only broadly effective oral antibiotics for *Pseudomonas* infection, but resistance emerges rapidly. Infection with mycoplasmal or chlamydial organisms has been documented, providing a rationale for the use of macrolides on an empirical basis for flare of symptoms. Macrolides may reduce the virulence properties of *P. aeruginosa* such as biofilm production and contribute anti-inflammatory effects. Long-term therapy with azithromycin times a week has been shown to improve lung function in patients with chronic *P. aeruginosa* infection.

AEROSOLIZED ANTIBIOTIC THERAPY. *P. aeruginosa* and other gram-negative organisms are frequently resistant to all oral antibiotics. Aerosol delivery of antibiotics offers an option for home delivery of additional agents. Inhaled tobramycin has been studied the most extensively. When given at a dose of 300 mg twice daily on alternate months for 6 mo, *Pseudomonas* density in sputum decreases, fewer hospitalizations are required, and pulmonary function can improve by ≥10%. Toxicity is negligible. This therapy can be recommended for increasing symptoms or to improve long-term function in patients with moderate to severe disease. Other antimicrobials such as colistin (75–150 mg) have been aerosolized 2 to 4 times a day. Sensitization or resistance to inhaled antibiotics can occur, but both are surprisingly infrequent. Bronchospasm may complicate aerosolized colistin therapy. Another indication for aerosolized antibiotic therapy is the emergence of *Pseudomonas* colonization in the airways. Early infection may be eliminated for mo to several yr by oral ciprofloxacin with aerosolized colistin or tobramycin. Established infection is rarely eradicated. Consensus is building that ongoing surveillance for *P. aeruginosa* and prompt intensive therapy are indicated.

INTRAVENOUS ANTIBIOTIC THERAPY. For the patient who has progressive or unrelenting symptoms and signs despite intensive home measures, intravenous antibiotic therapy is indicated. This therapy is usually initiated in the hospital but may be completed on an ambulatory basis. Although many patients improve within 7 days, it is usually advisable to extend the period of treatment to at least 14 days. Permanent intravenous access can be provided for long-term or frequent courses of therapy in the hospital or at home.

Several studies have found a surprisingly high occurrence of thrombophilia, both genetic and acquired. Thrombophilia screening should be considered before using totally implantable intravenous devices or for recurring problems with venous catheters.

Commonly used intravenous antibiotics are listed in Table 400-6. In general, treatment of *Pseudomonas* infection requires 2-drug therapy. A 3rd agent may be required for optimal coverage of *S. aureus* or other organisms. Simultaneous administration of aerosolized antimicrobial agents can increase endobronchial concentrations. The aminoglycosides have a relatively short half-life in many patients with CF. The initial parenteral dose, noted in Table 400-6, is generally given every 8 hr. After blood levels have

TABLE 400-6. Antimicrobial Agents for Cystic Fibrosis Lung Infection

ROUTE	ORGANISMS	AGENTS	DOSAGE (mg/kg/24 hr)	DOSES/24 hr
Oral	*Staphylococcus aureus*	Dicloxacillin	25–50	4
		Linezolid	20	2
		Cephalexin	50	4
		Clindamycin	25–40	3–4
		Amoxicillin-clavulanate	25–45	2–3
	Haemophilus influenzae	Amoxicillin	50–100	2–3
	Pseudomonas aeruginosa	Ciprofloxacin	15–30	2–3
	Burkholderia cepacia	Trimethoprim-sulfamethoxazole	20*	2–4
	Empirical	Azithromycin	10, day 1; 5, days 2–5	1
		Erythromycin	30–50	3–4
Intravenous	*S. aureus*	Nafcillin	100-200	4–6
		Vancomycin	40	3–4
	P. aeruginosa	Tobramycin	8–20	1–3
		Amikacin	15–30	2–3
		Netilmicin	6–12	2–3
		Carbenicillin	400	4
		Ticarcillin	400	4
		Piperacillin	300–400	4
		Ticarcillin-clavulanate	400†	4
		Piperacillin-Tazobactam	240–400††	3
		Meropenem	60–120	3
		Cefipime	150	3
		Imipenem-cilastatin	45–100	3–4
		Ceftazidime	150	3
		Aztreonam	150–200	4
	B. cepacia	Chloramphenicol	50–100	4
		Meropenem	60–120	3
Aerosol		Tobramycin (inhaled)	300‡	2

*Quantity of trimethoprim.
†Quantity of ticarcillin.
††Quantity of piperacillin.
‡In mg per dose.

been determined, the total daily dose should be adjusted. Peak levels of 10–15 mg/L are desirable, and trough levels should be kept at <2 mg/L to minimize the risk of ototoxicity and nephrotoxicity. Once- or twice-daily aminoglycoside dosing may have advantages over dosing every 8 hr. Changes in therapy should be guided by culture results and by lack of improvement. If patients do not improve, complications such as heart failure and reactive airways or infection with viruses, *Aspergillus fumigatus* (see Chapter 234), nontuberculous mycobacteria (see Chapter 214), or other unusual organisms should be considered. *B. cepacia* is the most frequent of a growing list of gram-negative rods that may be particularly refractory to antimicrobial therapy.

Bronchodilator Therapy. Reversible airway obstruction occurs in many children with CF, sometimes in conjunction with frank asthma or acute bronchopulmonary aspergillosis (see Chapter 234). Reversible obstruction is defined as improvement of ≥15% in flow rates after inhalation of a bronchodilator. Many CF patients may improve by only 5–10%, however. Nevertheless, subjective benefit is claimed by many following a β-adrenergic agonist aerosol. Cromolyn sodium or ipratropium hydrochlorides are alternative agents, but their efficacy has not been studied systematically.

Anti-Inflammatory Agents. Corticosteroids are useful for the treatment of allergic bronchopulmonary aspergillosis and severe reactive airway disease occasionally encountered in children with CF. Prolonged treatment of standard CF lung disease using an alternate-day regimen initially appeared to improve pulmonary function and diminish hospitalization rates. However, a 4 yr double-blind, multicenter study of this regimen for patients with mild to moderate lung disease found only modest efficacy and prohibitive side effects, including growth retardation, cataracts, and abnormalities of glucose tolerance at a dose of 2 mg/kg and growth retardation at 1 mg/kg. Inhaled corticosteroids have theoretical appeal, but there are few data documenting their efficacy and safety. Ibuprofen, given chronically (dose adjusted to achieve a peak serum concentration of 50–100 µg/mL) for 4 yr, is associated with an impressive slowing of disease progression, particularly in younger patients with mild lung disease. Side effects of nonsteroidal anti-inflammatory drugs have been encountered (see Table 400-5) and this therapy has not gained broad acceptance.

Endoscopy and Lavage. Treatment of obstructed airways sometimes includes tracheobronchial suctioning or lavage, especially if atelectasis or mucoid impaction is present. Bronchopulmonary lavage can be performed by the instillation of saline or a mucolytic agent through a fiberoptic bronchoscope. Antibiotics (usually gentamicin or tobramycin) can also be instilled directly at lavage, transiently achieving a much higher endobronchial concentration than can be obtained by using intravenous therapy. There is no evidence for sustained benefit from repeated endoscopic or lavage procedures.

Other Therapies. Expectorants such as iodides and guaifeusin do not effectively assist with the removal of secretions from the respiratory tract. Inspiratory muscle training can enhance maximum oxygen consumption during exercise as well as FEV_1.

TREATMENT OF PULMONARY COMPLICATIONS. A number of pulmonary complications require extra attention or special measures.

Atelectasis. Lobar atelectasis occurs relatively infrequently; it may be asymptomatic and noted only at the time of a routine chest radiograph. Aggressive intravenous therapy with antibiotics and increased chest PT directed at the affected lobe may be effective. If there is no improvement in 5–7 days, bronchoscopic examination of the airways may be indicated. If the atelectasis does not resolve, continued intensive home therapy is indicated, because atelectasis may resolve during a period of weeks or months. Persistent atelectasis may be asymptomatic. Lobectomy should be considered only if expansion is not achieved and the patient has progressive difficulty from fever, anorexia, and unrelenting cough (see Chapter 407).

Hemoptysis. Endobronchial bleeding usually reflects airway wall erosion secondary to infection. With increasing numbers of older patients, hemoptysis has become a relatively frequent complication. Blood streaking of sputum is particularly common. Small volume hemoptysis (<20 mL) should not trigger panic and is usually viewed as a need for intensified antimicrobial therapy and chest PT. When the hemoptysis is persistent or increases in severity, hospital admission is indicated. **Massive hemoptysis,** defined as total blood loss of ≥250 mL in a 24 hr period, is rare in the 1st decade and occurs in <1% of adolescents, but it requires close monitoring and the capability to replace blood losses rapidly. Chest PT is often discontinued until 12–24 hr after the last brisk bleeding episode and is then gradually reinstituted. Patients should receive vitamin K for an abnormal prothrombin time. During brisk hemoptysis, the child and parents require a great deal of reassurance that the bleeding will stop. Blood transfusion is not indicated unless there is hypotension or the hematocrit is significantly reduced. Ticarcillin, salicylates, or nonsteroidal anti-inflammatory drugs interfere with platelet function and may aggravate hemoptysis. Bronchoscopy rarely reveals the site of bleeding. Lobectomy is to be avoided, if possible, because functioning lung should be preserved. Bronchial artery embolization can be useful to control persistent, significant hemoptysis.

Pneumothorax. Pneumothorax (see Chapter 410) is encountered in <1% of children and teenagers with CF, but it is more frequently encountered in older patients and may be life-threatening. The episode may be asymptomatic but is often attended by chest and shoulder pain, shortness of breath, or hemoptysis. A small air collection that does not grow can be observed closely. Chest tube placement with or without pleurodesis is often the initial therapy. An open thoracotomy or video-assisted thoracoscopy (VATS) with plication of blebs, apical pleural stripping, and basal pleural abrasion should be considered if the air leak persists. Surgical intervention is usually well tolerated even in cases of advanced lung disease. Intravenous antibiotics are also begun on admission. The thoracotomy tube is removed as soon as possible, usually on the 2nd or 3rd postoperative day. The patient can then be mobilized and full postural drainage therapy resumed. Rarely, bilateral simultaneous pneumothorax is encountered; in this case, control of the air leak must be achieved immediately, at least on one side. Previous pneumothorax with or without pleurodesis is not a contraindication for subsequent lung transplantation.

Allergic Aspergillosis. This complication occurs in 5–10% of patients and may present as wheezing, increased cough, shortness of breath, and marked hyperinflation (see Chapters 234 and 396). In some patients, there are new, focal infiltrates on the chest radiograph. The presence of rust-colored sputum, the recovery of *Aspergillus* organisms from the sputum, the demonstration of serum precipitating and specific immunoglobulin E (IgE) and IgG antibodies against *A. fumigatus,* or the presence of eosinophils in a fresh sputum sample support the diagnosis. The serum IgE level is usually high. Treatment is directed at controlling the inflammatory reaction with oral corticosteroids and preventing central bronchiectasis. For refractory cases, oral itraconazole may be required.

Nontuberculous Mycobacteria (NTM) Infection (See Chapter 214). Injured airways with poor clearance may be colonized by *Mycobacterium avium-complex,* but also *M. abscessus* and *M. kansasii.* Distinguishing endobronchial colonization (frequent) from invasive infection (infrequent) is challenging. Persistent fevers and new infiltrates or cystic lesions coupled with acid-fast organisms on sputum smear suggest infection. Treatment is prolonged and requires multiple antimicrobial agents. Symptoms may improve, but NTM is not usually cleared from the lungs.

Bone and Joint Complications. Hypertrophic osteoarthropathy causes elevation of the periosteum over the distal portions of long bones and bone pain, overlying edema, and joint effusions. Acetaminophen or ibuprofen may provide relief. Control of lung infection usually reduces symptoms. Intermittent arthropathy unrelated to other rheumatologic disorders occurs occasionally, has no recognized pathogenesis, and usually responds to nonsteroidal anti-inflammatory agents. Back pain or rib fractures from vigorous coughing may require pain management to permit adequate airway clearance. These and other fractures may stem from diminished bone mineralization, the result of reduced vitamin D absorption, corticosteroid therapy, diminished weight bearing exercises, and, perhaps, other factors.

Sleep-Disordered Breathing. Particularly with advanced pulmonary disease and during chest exacerbations, individuals with CF may experience more sleep arousals, less time in rapid eye movement (REM) sleep, nocturnal hypoxemia, hypercapnia, and associated neurobehavioral impairment. Nocturnal hypoxemia may hasten onset of pulmonary hypertension and right-sided heart failure. Efficacy of specific interventions has not been systematically assessed. Prompt treatment of airway symptoms and nocturnal oxygen supplementation or bilevel positive airway pressure (BiPAP) support in selected cases should be considered.

Acute Respiratory Failure. Acute respiratory failure (see Chapters 69 and 370) in patients with mild to moderate lung disease rarely occurs and is usually the result of a severe viral or other infectious illness. Because patients with this complication can regain their previous status, intensive therapy is indicated. In addition to aerosol, postural drainage, and intravenous antibiotic treatment, oxygen is required to raise the arterial PaO_2. An increasing PCO_2 may require ventilatory assistance. Endotracheal or bronchoscopic suction may be necessary to clear airway inspissated secretions and can be repeated daily. Right-sided heart failure should be treated vigorously. Recovery is often slow. Intensive intravenous antibiotic therapy and postural drainage should be continued for 1–2 wk after the patient has regained baseline status.

Chronic Respiratory Failure. Patients acquire chronic respiratory failure after prolonged deterioration of lung function. Although this can occur at any age, it is seen most frequently in adult patients. Because a long-standing $PaO_2 < 50$ mm Hg promotes the development of right-sided heart failure, patients usually benefit from low-flow oxygen to raise arterial PO_2 to ≥55 mm Hg. Increasing hypercapnia may prevent the use of optimal FIO_2. Most patients improve somewhat with intensive antibiotic and pulmonary therapy measures and can be discharged from the hospital. Low-flow oxygen therapy is needed at home, especially with sleep. Noninvasive ventilatory support can improve gas exchange and quality of life enhancement has been documented. Ventilatory support may be particularly useful for patients awaiting lung transplantation. These patients usually display cor pulmonale and should be maintained on reduced salt intake and given diuretics. Caution should be exercised to avoid ventilation-suppressing metabolic alkalosis that results from CF-related chloride depletion and, in many cases, from diuretic-induced bicarbonate retention. Chronic pain (headache, chest pain, abdominal pain, and limb pain) is frequent at the end of life and responds to judicious use of analgesics, including opioids. Dyspnea has been ameliorated with nebulized fentanyl.

Lung transplantation is an option for end-stage lung disease (see Chapter 443). Criteria for referral continue to be a subject of investigation, and ideally include estimates of longevity with and without transplant based on lung function and exercise tolerance data. Chest infection with *B. cepacia* and arthropathy are negative predictors of outcome. Quality of life generally improves post transplant. Because of bronchiolitis obliterans and other complications, transplanted lungs cannot be expected to function for the lifetime of a recipient and repeat transplant is increasingly frequent. The demand for donor lungs exceeds the supply and waiting lists as well as duration of waits continue to grow. The protocol for matching donor organs with lung transplant recipients has been revised to account for the severity of the patients' lung disease.

Heart Failure. Some patients experience reversible right-sided heart failure (see Chapters 370 and 442) as the result of an acute event such as a viral infection or pneumothorax. Individuals with long-standing, advanced pulmonary disease, especially those with severe hypoxemia ($PaO_2 < 50$ mm Hg), often acquire chronic right-sided heart failure. The mechanisms include hypoxemic pulmonary arterial constriction and loss of the pulmonary vascular bed. Pulmonary arterial wall changes contribute to increased vascular resistance with time. Evidence for concomitant left ventricular dysfunction is often found. Cyanosis, increased shortness of breath, increased liver size with a tender margin, ankle edema, jugular venous distention, an unusual weight gain, increased heart size seen on chest radiograph, or evidence for right-sided heart enlargement seen on electrocardiogram or echocardiogram help to confirm the diagnosis. Furosemide (1 mg/kg administered intravenously) induced diuresis confirms the suspicion of fluid retention. Repeated doses are often required at 24–48 hr intervals to reduce fluid accumulation and accompanying symptoms. Concomitant use of spironolactone may protect against potassium depletion and facilitate long-term diuresis. Hypochloremic alkalosis complicates the chronic use of loop diuretics. Digitalis is not effective in pure right-sided failure, but may be useful when there is an associated left-sided dysfunction. The arterial PO_2 should be maintained at >50 mm Hg if possible. Intensive pulmonary therapy including intravenous antibiotics is most important. Initially, the salt intake should be limited. Volume overload and antibiotics with high sodium content should be avoided. No clear-cut long-term benefit from pulmonary vasodilators has been demonstrated. The prognosis for heart failure is poor, but a number of patients survive for ≥5 yr after the appearance of heart failure. Lung or heart-lung transplantation is the best option for reversal with advanced lung disease (see Chapter 443).

NUTRITIONAL THERAPY. Up to 90% of patients have loss of exocrine pancreatic function and inadequate digestion and absorption of fats and proteins. They require dietary adjustment, pancreatic enzyme replacement, and supplementary vitamins. In general, children with CF need to exceed the usual required daily caloric intake to grow. The target has been set at 130 Kcal/kg of body weight. Daily supplements of the fat-soluble vitamins are required.

Diet. Many infants at the time of diagnosis have nutritional deficits. Young infants who present with wheezy breathing and are fed soy-protein formulas do not use this protein well and may acquire hypoproteinemia with anasarca. Infants do not routinely need formulas containing predigested protein and medium-chain triglycerides. A low-fat, high-protein, high-calorie diet was generally recommended in the past for older children. Some children on this diet are deficient in essential fatty acids. With the advent of improved pancreatic enzyme products, normal to increased amounts of fat in the diet are usually tolerated and preferred. Fat intake can be adjusted if stools frequently contain undigested oil. Not infrequently, parent-child interactions at feeding time are maladaptive, and behavioral interventions can improve caloric intake.

Most individuals have a higher than normal caloric need because of increased work of breathing and perhaps because of increased metabolic activity related to the basic defect. When anorexia of chronic infection supervenes, weight loss occurs. Encouragement to eat high-calorie foods is important, but weight gain is not generally realized unless lung infection is controlled. With advanced lung disease, weight stabilization or gain sometimes requires nocturnal feeding via nasogastric tube or percutaneous enterostomy or by short-term intravenous hyperalimentation. Long-term benefits of these interventions include improved quality of life and psychologic well-being. Improvement of lung function has not been clearly documented.

Three times a week human recombinant growth hormone therapy has improved nutritional outcomes, including positive effects on nitrogen balance and improved height and weight velocities.

Pancreatic Enzyme Replacement. Extracts of animal pancreas given with ingested food reduce but do not fully correct stool fat and nitrogen losses. Enzyme dosage and product should be individualized for each patient. Enteric-coated, pH-sensitive enzyme microspheres are most often prescribed. Several strengths up to 20,000 IU of lipase/capsule are available. Administration of excessive doses has been linked to **colonic strictures** requiring surgery. Consequently, enzyme replacement should not exceed 2,500 lipase units/kg/meal in most circumstances. One to 3 capsules/meal is sufficient for most patients; infants need 2,000–4,000 lipase units per feeding, which is most easily given mixed with applesauce. Snacks should also be covered. The microsphere preparations usually are sufficiently effective to permit a liberal diet, which should include homogenized milk with vitamin D. Although children with CF display bile salt malabsorption, enzyme preparations containing bile salts are infrequently needed. The dose of enzymes required usually increases with age, but some teenagers and young adults may later have a decrease in their requirement.

Vitamin and Mineral Supplements. Because pancreatic insufficiency results in malabsorption of fat-soluble vitamins (A, D, E, K), vitamin supplementation is recommended. Several vitamin preparations containing all 4 vitamins for CF patients are available. They should be taken daily. Replacement doses may be required when low serum levels are documented or the patient is symptomatic. Infants with zinc deficiency and an acrodermatitis enteropathica–like rash have been reported. In addition, attention should be paid to iron status; in one study, almost ⅓ of children with CF had a low serum ferritin concentration.

TREATMENT OF INTESTINAL COMPLICATIONS.

Meconium Ileus. When meconium ileus (see Chapter 102.1) is suspected, a nasogastric tube is placed for suction and the newborn is hydrated. In many cases, diatrizoate (Gastrografin) enemas with reflux of contrast material into the ileum not only confirm the diagnosis, but have also resulted in the passage of a meconium plug and clearing of the obstruction. Use of this hypertonic solution requires careful correction of water losses into the bowel. Children in whom this procedure fails require operative intervention. Children who are successfully treated generally have a prognosis similar to that of other patients with severe CF mutations. Infants with meconium ileus should be treated as having CF until adequate diagnostic testing can be carried out.

Distal Intestinal Obstruction Syndrome (DIOS, Meconium Ileus Equivalent) and Other Causes of Abdominal Symptoms. Despite appropriate pancreatic enzyme replacement, 2–5% of patients accumulate fecal material in the terminal portion of the ileum and in the cecum, which may result in partial or complete obstruction. For intermittent symptoms, pancreatic enzyme replacement should be continued or even increased and stool softeners (polyethylene glycol [Miralax] or docusate sodium [Colace]) given. Increased fluid intake is also recommended. Failure to relieve symptoms signals the need for large-volume bowel lavage with a balanced salt solution containing polyethylene glycol taken by mouth or by nasogastric tube. When there is complete obstruction, a diatrizoate enema, accompanied by large amounts of intravenous fluids, can be therapeutic. Intussusception (see Chapter 330.3) and volvulus (see Chapter 326.4) must also be considered in the differential diagnosis. Intussusception, usually ileocolic, occurs at any age and often follows a 1–2 day history of "constipation." It can often be diagnosed and reduced by a diatrizoate enema. If a nonreducible intussusception or a volvulus is present, laparotomy is required. Repeated episodes of intussusception may be an indication for cecectomy.

Chronic appendicitis with or without periappendiceal abscess may present with recurrent or persistent abdominal pain, raising the question of need for a laparotomy. A lack of acid buffering in the duodenum appears to promote duodenitis and ulcer formation in some children. Bile reflux is seen in older patients (see following section). Other reasons for surgical procedures include carcinoma of the colon or biliary tract and sclerosing colonopathy.

Gastroesophageal Reflux (see Chapter 320). Because several factors raise intra-abdominal pressure, including cough and obstructed airways, pathologic gastroesophageal reflux is not uncommon and may exacerbate lung disease secondary to reflex wheezing and repeated aspiration. Dietary, positional, and medication therapy should be considered. Cholinergic agonists are contraindicated because they trigger mucus secretion and progressive respiratory difficulty. Reduction of stomach acid secretion can help, with proton pump inhibitors being the most effective agents. Fundoplication is a procedure of last resort.

Rectal Prolapse (see Chapter 341.5). Though uncommon, this occurs most often in infants with CF and less commonly in older children. It is usually related to steatorrhea, malnutrition, and repetitive cough. The prolapsed rectum can usually be replaced manually by continuous gentle pressure with the patient in the knee-chest position. Sedation may be helpful. To prevent an immediate recurrence, the buttocks can be taped closed. Adequate pancreatic enzyme replacement, decreased fat and roughage in the diet, stool softener, and control of pulmonary infection result in improvement. Occasionally, a patient may continue to have rectal prolapse and require sclerotherapy or surgery.

Heptobiliary Disease. Liver function abnormalities associated with biliary cirrhosis can be improved by treatment with ursodeoxycholic acid. The ability of bile acids to prevent progression of cirrhosis has not been clearly documented. Portal hypertension with esophageal varices, hypersplenism, or ascites occurs in ≤2% of children with CF (see Chapter 364). The acute management of bleeding esophageal varices includes nasogastric suction and cold saline lavage. Sclerotherapy is recommended after an initial hemorrhage. In the past, significant bleeding has also been treated successfully with portosystemic shunting. Splenorenal anastomosis has been the most effective. Pronounced hypersplenism may require splenectomy. Cholelithiasis should prompt surgical consultation. The management of ascites is discussed in Chapter 367.

Obstructive jaundice in newborns with CF requires no specific therapy. Hepatomegaly with steatosis requires careful attention to nutrition and may respond to carnitine repletion. Rarely, biliary cirrhosis proceeds to hepatocellular failure, which should be treated as in other patients with hepatic failure (see Chapters 361 and 364). End-stage liver disease is an indication for liver transplantation in children with CF, especially if pulmonary function is good. Outcomes have been encouraging.

Pancreatitis. Pancreatitis can be precipitated by fatty meals, alcohol ingestion, or tetracycline therapy. Serum amylase and lipase levels may remain elevated for long periods. Treatment is discussed in Chapter 348.

Hyperglycemia. Onset occurs most frequently after the 1st decade. Approximately 20% of young adults are treated for hyperglycemia, although the incidence of CF-related diabetes (CFRD) may be higher. Prevalence is greater in females and in ΔF508 homozygotes. Ketoacidosis is rarely encountered. The pathogenesis includes both impaired insulin secretion and insulin resistance. Routine screening consists of a modified 2 hr oral glucose tolerance test performed annually after age 8–10 yrs old. Glucose intolerance without urine glucose losses is usually not treated; glycosylated hemoglobin levels should be followed at least annually. With persistent glycosuria and symptoms, insulin treatment should be instituted. Oral hypoglycemic agents, with or without drugs that reduce insulin resistance, may also be effective. Exocrine pancreatic insufficiency and malabsorption make strict dietary control of hyperglycemia difficult. Corticosteroid therapy should be avoided. The development of significant hyperglycemia favors acquisition of *P. aeruginosa* and *B. cepacia* in the airways and may adversely affect pulmonary function. Thus, careful control of blood sugar is an important goal. Long-term vascular complications of diabetes can occur, providing an additional rationale for good control of blood sugar levels.

OTHER THERAPY

Nasal Polyps. Nasal polyps (see Chapter 375) occur in 15–20% of patients with CF and are most prevalent in the 2nd decade of life. Local corticosteroids and nasal decongestants occasionally provide some relief. When the polyps completely obstruct the nasal airway, rhinorrhea becomes constant, or widening of the nasal bridge is noticed, surgical removal is indicated; polyps may recur promptly or after a symptom-free interval of mo to yr. Polyps inexplicably stop developing in many adults.

Rhinosinusitis. Opacification of paranasal sinuses is not an indication for intervention. Acute or chronic sinus-related symptoms are treated initially with antimicrobials, with or without maxillary sinus aspiration for cultures. Functional endoscopic sinus surgery has anecdotally provided benefit.

Salt Depletion. Sweat salt losses can be high, especially in warm arid climates. Children should have free access to salt, and precautions against overdressing infants should be observed. Regimented salt supplements are no longer prescribed except in hot weather climates. Hypochloremic alkalosis should be suspected in any infant who has had symptoms of gastroenteritis, and prompt fluid and electrolyte therapy should be instituted as needed.

Growth and Maturation. Delayed growth should be vigorously addressed by enhancing nutrition, treating lung disease more vigorously, and, in selected instances, endocrine evaluation and, possibly, growth hormone therapy. The risk-benefit ratio of anabolic steroids does not support their use for undersized children with CF. Delayed sexual maturation, often associated with short stature, occurs fairly frequently. Although many patients have severe pulmonary infection or poor nutrition, delayed puberty also occurs in those with otherwise mild disease and is not well explained. Adolescents with CF should receive specific counseling through their developing years concerning sexual maturation and reproductive potential.

Surgery. Minor surgical procedures, including dental work, should be performed under local anesthesia if possible. Patients with good or excellent pulmonary status can tolerate general anesthesia without any intensive pulmonary measures before the surgery. Those with moderate or severe pulmonary infection usually do better with a 1–2 wk course of intensive antibiotic treatment and increased airway clearance before surgery. If this is impossible, prompt intravenous antibiotic therapy is indicated once it is recognized that major surgery is required. The total time of anesthesia should be kept to a minimum. After induction, tracheal suctioning is useful and should be repeated at least at the end of the operation. Patients with severe disease require monitoring of their blood gases and may require ventilatory assistance in the immediate postoperative period.

After major surgery, cough should be encouraged and airway clearance treatments should be reinstituted as soon as possible, usually within 24 hr. Adequate analgesia is important if early effective therapy is to be achieved. For those with significant pulmonary involvement, intravenous antibiotics are continued for 7–14 postoperative days. Early ambulation and intermittent deep breathing are important; an incentive spirometer can also be helpful. After open thoracotomy for treatment of pneumothorax or lobectomy, the chest tube is the greatest single obstacle to effective pulmonary therapy and should be removed as soon as possible so that full postural drainage therapy can resume.

PROGNOSIS. CF remains a life-limiting disorder, although survival has improved dramatically in the past 30–40 yr. Infants with severe lung disease occasionally succumb, but most children survive this difficult period and are relatively healthy into adolescence or adulthood. The slow progression of lung disease eventually reaches disabling proportions, however. Life table data now indicate a median cumulative survival exceeding 35 yr. Male survival is somewhat better than female survival for reasons that are not readily apparent. Children in socioeconomically disadvantaged families have, on average, a poorer prognosis.

Children with CF usually have good school attendance records and should not be restricted in their activities. A high percentage eventually attends and graduates from college. Most find satisfactory employment, and an increasing number marry. Transitioning care from pediatric to adult care centers by 21 yr of age is an important objective and requires a thoughtful, supportive approach involving both the pediatric and internal medicine specialists.

With increasing life span, a new set of psychosocial considerations has emerged, including dependence-independence issues, self-care, peer relationships, sexuality, reproduction, substance abuse, educational and vocational planning, medical care costs and other financial burdens, and anxiety concerning health and prognosis. Many of these issues are best addressed in an anticipatory fashion, before the onset of psychosocial dysfunction. With appropriate medical and psychosocial support, children and adolescents with CF generally cope well. Achievement of an independent and productive adulthood is a realistic goal for many.

Aaron SD, Vandemheen KL, Ferris W, et al: Combination antibiotic susceptibility testing to treat exacerbations of cystic fibrosis associated with multiresistant bacteria: A randomized, double-blind, controlled clinical trial. *Lancet* 2005;366:463–471.

Colombo C, Battezzati A: Growth failure in cystic fibrosis: A true need for anabolic agents? *J Pediatr* 2005;146:303–305.

Corey M, Edwards L, Levison H, et al: Longitudinal analysis of pulmonary function decline in patients with cystic fibrosis. *J Pediatr* 1997; 131:809–814.

Donaldson SH, Bennett WD, Zeman KL, et al: Mucus clearance and lung function in cystic fibrosis with hypertonic saline. *N Engl J Med* 2006;354: 241–250.

Drumm ML, Konstan MW, Schluchter MD, et al: Genetic modifiers of lung disease in cystic fibrosis. *N Engl J Med* 2005;353:1443–1453.

Elkins MR, Robinson M, Rose BR, et al: A controlled trial of long-term inhaled hypertonic saline on patients with cystic fibrosis. *N Engl J Med* 2006;354:229–240.

Emerson J, Rosenfeld M, McNamara S, et al: *Pseudomonas aeruginosa* and other predictors of mortality and morbidity in young children with cystic fibrosis. *Pediatr Pulmonol* 2002;34:91–100.

Eubanks V, Koppersmith N, Wooldridge N, et al: Effects of megestrol acetate on weight gain, body composition, and pulmonary function in patients with cystic fibrosis. *J Pediatr* 2002;140:439–444.

Ferkol T, Rosenfeld M, Milla CE: Cystic fibrosis pulmonary exacerbations. *J Pediatr* 2006;148:259–264.

FitzSimmons SC, Burkhart GA, Borowitz D, et al: High-dose pancreatic-enzyme supplements and fibrosing colonopathy in children with cystic fibrosis. *N Engl J Med* 1997;336:1283–1289.

Fuchs HJ, Borowitz DS, Christiansen DH, et al: Effect of aerosolized recombinant human DNase on exacerbations of respiratory symptoms and on pulmonary function in patients with cystic fibrosis. The Pulmozyme Study Group. *N Engl J Med* 1994;331:637–642.

Groman JD, Karczeki B, Sheridan M, et al: Phenotypic and genetic characterization of patients with features of nonclassic forms of cystic fibrosis. *J Pediatr* 2005;146:675–680.

Grosse SD, Rosenfeld M, Devine OJ, et al: Potential impact of newborn screening for cystic fibrosis on child survival: A systematic review and analysis. *J Pediatr* 2006;149:362–366.

Hardin DS, Rice J, Ahn C, et al: Growth hormone treatment enhances nutrition and growth in children with cystic fibrosis receiving enteral nutrition. *J Pediatr* 2005;146:324–328.

Kappler M, Griese M: Nutritional supplements in cystic fibrosis. *BMJ* 2006; 332:618–619.

Lenaerts C, Lapierre C, Patriqui H, et al: Surveillance for cystic fibrosis-associated hepatobiliary disease: Early ultrasound changes and predisposing factors. *J Pediatr* 2003;143:343–350.
Li Z, Kosorok MR, Farrell PM, et al: Longitudinal development of mucoid *Pseudomonas aeruginosa* infection and lung disease progression in children with cystic fibrosis. *JAMA* 2005;293:581–588.
Lion RG, Adler FR, Cahill BC, et al: Survival effect of lung transplantation among patients with cystic fibrosis. *JAMA* 2001;286:2683–2689.
McColley SA: Cystic fibrosis lung disease: When does it start, and how can it be prevented? J *Pediatr* 2004;145:6–7.
Moran A, Hardin D, Rodman D, et al: Diagnosis, screening and management of cystic fibrosis related diabetes mellitus: A consensus conference report. *Diabetes Res Clin Pract* 1999;45:61–73.
Poustie VJ, Russell JE, Watling, et al: Oral protein energy supplements for children with cystic fibrosis: CALICO multicentre randomized controlled trial. *BMJ* 2006;332:632–635.
Rajan S, Saiman L: Pulmonary infections in patients with cystic fibrosis. *Semin Respir Infect* 2002;17:47–56.
Rao S, Grigg J: New insights into pulmonary inflammation in cystic fibrosis. *Arch Dis Child* 2006;91:786–788.
Rowe SM, Miller S, Sorscher EJ: Cystic fibrosis. *N Engl J Med* 2005; 352:1992–2001.
Saiman L, Marshall BC, Mayer-Hamblett N, et al: Azithromycin in patients with cystic fibrosis chronically infected with *Pseudomonas aeruginosa:* A randomized controlled trial. *JAMA* 2003;290:1749–1756.
Sims EJ, McCormick J, Mehta G, Mehta A: Newborn screening for cystic fibrosis is associated with reduced treatment intensity. *J Pediatr* 2005; 147:306–311.
Smyth A, Tan KHV, Hyman-Taylor P, et al: Once versus three-times daily regimens of tobramycin treatment for pulmonary exacerbations of cystic fibrosis—the TOPIC study: A randomized controlled trial. *Lancet* 2005;365:573–578.
Smyth RL: Daily activity and disease status in cystic fibrosis: An important area for research. *J Pediatr* 2005;147:281–283.
Smyth RL: Diagnosis and management of cystic fibrosis. *Arch Dis Child* 2005;90:ep1–ep6.
Sun L, Jiang RZ, Steinbach S, et al: The emergence of a highly transmissible lineage of cbl+ *Pseudomonas (Burkholderia)* cepacia causing CF centre epidemics in North America and Britain. *Nat Med* 1995;1:661–666.
Texereau J, Marullo S, Hubert D, et al: Nitric oxide synthase 1 as a potential modifier gene of decline in lung function in patients with cystic fibrosis. *Thorax* 2004;59:156–158.
Vandenbussche HL, Klepser ME: Single daily tobramycin dosing in cystic fibrosis: Is it better for the patients or the bugs? *Lancet* 2005;365:547–548.
Wilschanski M, Yahav Y, Yaacov Y, et al: Gentamicin-induced correction of CFTR function in patients with cystic fibrosis and CFTR stop mutations. *N Engl J Med* 2003;349:1433–1441.
Zeitlin P: Can curcumin cure cystic fibrosis? *N Engl J Med* 2004;351:606–608.

Chapter 401 ■ Primary Ciliary Dyskinesia (Immotile Cilia Syndrome)

Gabriel G. Haddad and Michael Kashgarian

Primary ciliary dyskinesia (PCD) comprises those respiratory disorders having in common the malfunction of airway cilia. The abnormality results from various inherited primary structural defects in the cilia that lead to repeated and chronic lung and sinus infections. The ciliary malfunction in PCD is not a result of acquired repeated pulmonary infections, conditions in which the ciliary abnormalities revert to normal, unlike in PCD. About 50% of patients with PCD have **Kartagener syndrome:** situs inversus, chronic sinusitis and otitis, and airway disease leading to bronchiectasis. Approximately 25% of patients with situs inversus have PCD; the presence of situs inversus does not establish the presence of PCD.

LOCATION AND STRUCTURE. Cilia are finger-like structures that extend from the surface of cells into the lumen of airways. They have a diameter of 0.25 microns and a length of 306 microns. Each cell typically has about 200 cilia on its surface. Each cilia has a *trunk;* a *basal body,* where the cilia attach to the cell; and a *crown,* which is a specialized structure presumed to be important in cilia attachment to mucus. The trunk is made of an outer cell membrane and axonemes or cytoskeletal protein structures. The latter form a circular array of 9 microtubules in pairs with an additional central pair (9 + 2 structure). Each peripheral pair can attach to the other via bridges or dynein arms. Spokes are also cytoskeletal proteins that join peripheral and central microtubules.

Airway cilia are located on epithelial surfaces in the nose, sinuses, ears, and airways. The density of cilia varies, with the majority of cells (50–80%) in the large airways having cilia, far fewer cells in the lower airways having cilia, and no cells in air sacs and alveoli having cilia. The frequency of ciliary beating, or **beatquency,** is 1–20 Hz, with the higher beatquency occurring in the larger airways, correlating with the mucous velocity in various parts of the tracheobronchial tree.

In humans, there are at least 6 types of cilia: *airway, ventricular, embryonic, olfactory,* and *photoreceptor* cilia, and *sperm flagellum.* Whereas the embryonic and photoreceptor cilia contain 9 microtubular doublets and no central singlets (9 + 0 structure), the other types of cilia share the peripheral structures (9 microtubular doublets) but have in addition 2 central singlets (9 + 2 structure). Airway cilia propel mucus in the airways; ventricular cilia are located on the ependymal lining of the brain ventricles and propel cerebrospinal fluid (CSF). An association between ciliary dyskinesia, hydrocephalus, and mental retardation in 4 male siblings in a Jordanian family has been reported and might be caused by a mutation that affects pulmonary toilet and fluid movement in the lung and CSF. Embryonic cilia are located in the embryonic node and presumed to propel morphogens and establish, at this early stage, a morphogenic gradient that is crucial for the development of embryonic sidedness. Indeed, abnormal nodal cilia result in situs inversus.

FUNCTION. Cilia beat and move by a sliding motion of microtubules. At the outset of the beating cycle, they bend at the base and move backward, perpendicular to the surface. Subsequently, they extend ("slide") while rotating in a forward motion. These bending and rotating movements, which are clockwise 3-dimensional rotations, are made possible by adenosine triphosphate (ATP) hydrolysis and the dynein arms, which are ATPases. When visualized under microscopy, airway cilia are seen to coordinate their activity regionally, and *waves of ciliary movements* (many cilia together) occur.

The main function of airway cilia is to transport, through its beating movements, mucus toward the mouth. The effectiveness of this function depends on the beatquency, the composition and thickness of the periciliary fluid and mucous layer above it, and the coordination of ciliary movements. There are a number of neurochemicals that modulate ciliary beating by increasing beatquency, such as β-adrenergic compounds, acetylcholine, bradykinins, and serotonin. Alternatively, lowering airway humidity significantly lowers the frequency of ciliary beating. In addition, increasing bacterial loads decreases its beatquency.

PATHOLOGY. It is estimated that there are >250 polypeptides in the ciliary structure, and primary ciliary dyskinesia is most likely based on the absence of 1 or several ciliary cytoskeletal proteins. There is also some variability in the structural proteins from 1 cilium type to another. The structural abnormalities of these disorders can be seen with electron microscopy.

Ciliary ultrastructual changes of ciliary dyskinesia include the lack of dynein arms, microtubular transposition, compound cilia,

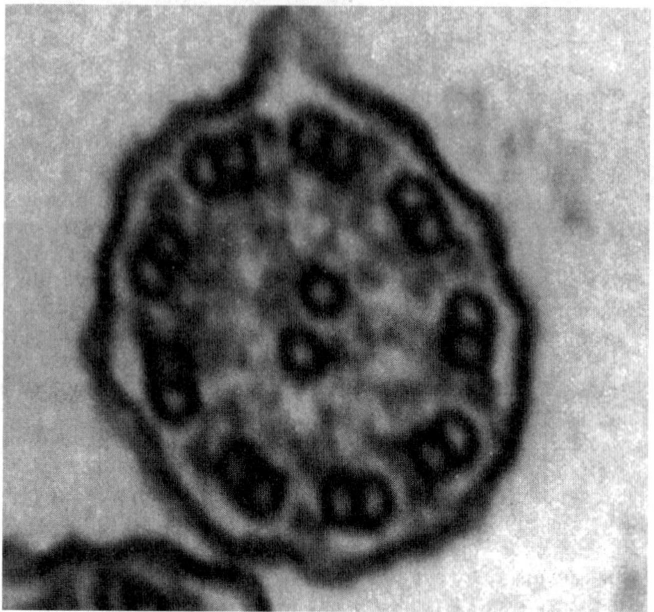

Figure 401-1. Electron micrograph of a normal cilium. Electron micrograph demonstrates the normal 9 + 2 configuration of the axoneme. Both inner and outer dynein arms can be identified but not always on the same microtubule doublet. The outer arms are generally more easily visualized and the spokes are not clearly identified.

random ciliary orientation, abnormal length of cilia, radial spoke and nexin link defects, and absence of cilia with brush border metaplasia. It is important to differentiate those instances that cause transient ciliary defects involving only a subset of cilia (such as acute and chronic respiratory inflammation) from true congenital defects. In classical PCD, there is an *absence of both inner and outer dynein arms,* resulting in a complete dynein arm defect (Figs. 401-1 and 401-2). *Partial dynein arm defects* (in which either inner or outer arms are not visualized) or *defects in central doublets* are generally not associated with situs inversus (see Chapter 431.11) and appear to occur as isolated genetic abnormalities. *Radial spoke defects* are much more difficult to visualize but are generally considered to be a legitimate entity in this spectrum of ciliary abnormalities. *Ciliary aplasia* or *brush border metaplasia* with an absence of cilia in the epithelium may actually be the result of chronic inflammatory changes in an individual with a previous ciliary abnormality. *Random ciliary orientation* is when the sole ultrastructural defect is that the central doublets are arranged in a random orientation rather than a uniform parallel orientation.

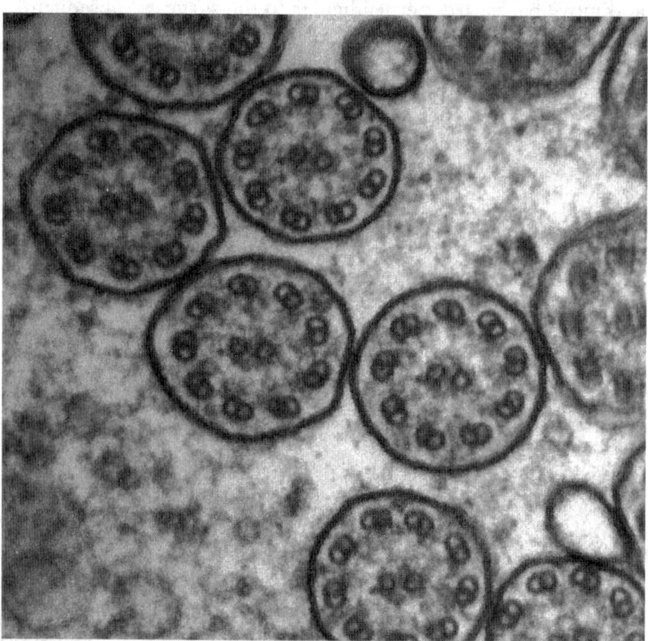

Figure 401-2. Cilia from a patient with Kartagener syndrome. Although the axoneme contains the normal component of 9 + 2 tubule doublets, both inner and outer dynein arms are absent in all the cilia.

Ciliary motility studies may not directly correlate with the ultrastructural findings. Cilia from patients with Kartagener syndrome are immotile. By contrast, single arm defects may show coordinated movement, although ciliary beatquency will be slower than normal. Random axis orientation of cilia results in incoordinate random movement. All these structural defects result in ciliary malfunction characterized by either abnormal beating or immotility of cilia and, therefore, defective mucociliary clearance of airway secretions. The most likely pathogenic sequence is airway mucus retention and failure to clear pathogenic organisms, followed by chronic or frequently recurring respiratory tract infections and, ultimately, injury to airway walls.

GENETICS. Estimates of PCD prevalence range from 1/15,000 to 1/60,000 live births. It is probably the 3rd most common form of inherited chronic airway disease of caucasian children, after cystic fibrosis (CF) and genetic immunodeficiency states. Cases have been reported from multiple ethnic and racial groups including populations from Japan, China, and northern Africa. The inheritance pattern of most PCD cases is autosomal recessive, although there are reported cases of autosomal dominant or even X-linked modalities.

A number of genes have been hypothesized to be at the basis of PCD. *DNAH5* is an axonemal dynein heavy chain gene localized on chromosome 5p (5p14–5p15). This gene is very long (79 exons) and codes for a protein of 4,624 amino acids. It is expressed in lung and kidney and, to a lesser extent, in brain and testis. Several homozygous and heterozygous mutations were found in PCD families. A number of individuals in these families also had situs inversus.

DNAI1, another gene on chromosome 9 (9p13–21), is highly expressed in trachea and testis and is a long gene, with 20 exons. It encodes for an intermediate chain found in the outer dynein arms. Several other mutations in other PCD families have also been found, such as substitution of conserved bases and deletion of base pairs in exons. A 3rd gene *(DNAH11),* which also encodes a heavy chain dynein in the outer arm, maps to the 7th chromosome (7p21) and has been associated with PCD.

CLINICAL MANIFESTATIONS. The course is variable. Individuals with PCD may have unexplained respiratory distress during the newborn period or may survive to adulthood without overt chronic sinusitis and airway disease symptoms. In one study of PCD, 100% of children had productive cough, sinusitis, and otitis. Many present as neonates with nasal congestion, rhinitis, and cough. A feature that is helpful in differentiating PCD from CF is repeated bouts of acute otitis media or chronic serous otitis. Children diagnosed after several years of life have often been treated with tympanostomy tubes; conductive hearing loss is common. Prolonged otorrhea often follows tympanostomy tube placement. Nasal polyps or clubbing is present in ≈20% of patients. Many children with PCD experience frequent wheezing and have an initial diagnosis of asthma. The hallmark symptom is a chronic, often loose or productive cough. Pneumonia may supervene, and lower respiratory tract disease can progress to weight loss, diminished exercise tolerance, and bronchiectasis. Respiratory failure in childhood is uncommon, as are lung complications such as pneumothorax and hemoptysis. Lobar atelectasis occurs frequently. Males are frequently infertile and display absent or poor sperm motility; females are at increased risk for ectopic pregnancy.

DIAGNOSIS. PCD should be suspected in children with chronic or recurring upper and lower respiratory tract symptoms, especially in the presence of substantial middle-ear disease. Presentation often begins as neonates. Radiographic or CT imaging shows involvement of the paranasal sinuses. Chest radiographs may demonstrate overinflation, bronchial wall thickening, and peribronchial infiltrates. Atelectasis and consolidation are often present. **Bronchiectasis** is best detected by CT scanning (see Chapter 398). The presence of a right-sided heart in a child with chronic respiratory tract symptoms is virtually diagnostic, but this configuration occurs in only 50% of these patients. Pulmonary function testing of older children yields a typical obstructive pattern (see Chapter 371).

Mucociliary clearance can be assessed in cooperative children by ascertaining the time to taste perception of a saccharin particle placed on the inferior nasal turbinate (normal is <30 min). Scrapings or brushings of nasal mucosa can be examined directly by light or, preferably, by phase-contrast microscopy for evidence of motility. In most PCD tissue specimens, little or no ciliary motion is seen. Because substantial motility has been documented in scrapings of several individuals with absent dynein arms, light microscopic examination of living tissue can be used as a screening tool only. **The gold standard** is quantitative documentation of abnormal structural elements, such as missing dynein arms or random orientation of cilia in nasal or bronchial biopsies or scrapings on electron microscopic examination. Concordance of ultrastructural abnormalities in cilia and sperm is not complete. To avoid acquired ciliary changes, mucosal specimens should not be obtained until 2 wk after an acute respiratory tract infection. Ultrastructural evaluation should be reserved for highly suspicious cases. Some structural abnormalities are also observed after injury to ciliated epithelial cells by viral infection or sulfur dioxide exposure. Definitive evidence that any structural alteration represents a discrete form of PCD awaits the identification of specific gene mutations.

Exhaled nitric oxide (NO) is markedly decreased in patients with PCD as compared with patients who do not have PCD, particularly those with cystic fibrosis, idiopathic bronchiectasis, sinusitis alone, and normal controls. A low NO measurement may not be diagnostic, but a high level suggests a disease other than PCD.

TREATMENT. Therapy is symptomatic. Cough should be encouraged. Chest physiotherapy assists the clearance of mucus. Antibiotics should be prescribed for evidence of infection of sinuses or lower airways. The choice of antibiotics is best dictated by identification and sensitivity testing of pathogenic organisms, often pneumococcus (see Chapter 181) or untypable *Haemophilus influenzae* (see Chapter 192). Oral antibiotic administration is usually effective. Bronchodilators can be used for symptomatic wheezing or documentation of reversible airway obstruction. Children should be examined several times each yr and followed by periodic chest radiographs and serial pulmonary function testing. Sinus and middle-ear symptoms refractory to medical therapy deserve consultation with an otolaryngologist. Surgical intervention may be helpful in selected cases. Prevention of lung infection by measles, pertussis, influenza, and, possibly, pneumococcal vaccines is highly desirable. Additional preventive measures include avoidance of cigarette smoke and other airway irritants.

PROGNOSIS. Progression of lung disease appears to be much slower for patients with PCD than for those with CF. With proper treatment, disabling lung disease can often be avoided for long periods. A normal life span is possible.

Afzelius BA: Cilia-related diseases. *J Pathol* 2004;204:470–477.

Al-Shroof M, Karnik AM, Karnik AA, et al: Ciliary dyskinesia associated with hydrocephalus and mental retardation in a Jordanian family. *Mayo Clin Proc* 2001;76:1219–1224.

Brueckner M: Cilia propel the embryo in the right direction. *Am J Med Genet* 2001;101:339–344.

Bush A, O'Callaghan C: Primary ciliary dyskinesia. *Arch Dis Child* 2002;87:363–365.

Bush A, Payne D, Pike S, et al: Mucus properties in children with primary ciliary dyskinesia: comparison with cystic fibrosis. *Chest* 2006;129(1):118–123.

Chodhari R, Mitchison HM, Meeks M: Cilia, primary ciliary dyskinesia and molecular genetics. *Pediatr Respir Rev* 2004;5:69–76.

Noone PG, Leigh MW, Sannuti A, et al: Primary ciliary dyskinesia: Diagnostic and phenotypic features. *Am J Respir Crit Care Med* 2004;169:459–467.

Olbrich H, Haffner K, Kispert A, et al: Mutations in DNAH5 cause primary ciliary dyskinesia and randomization of left-right asymmetry. *Nat Genet* 2002;30:143–144.

Rutland J, de Iongh RU: Random ciliary orientation: A cause of respiratory tract disease. *N Engl J Med* 1990;323:1681–1684.

Wodehouse T, Kharitonov SA, Mackay IS, et al: Nasal nitric oxide measurements for the screening of primary ciliary dyskinesia. *Eur Respir J* 2003;21:43–47.

Chapter 402 ■ Interstitial Lung Diseases

Michelle S. Howenstine

The interstitial lung diseases (ILD) in infants and children include a group of uncommon, heterogeneous, familial, or sporadic diseases that cause disruption of alveolar gas exchange and symptoms of restrictive lung disease. Knowledge regarding pediatric ILD is limited because of its rare occurrence, varied spectrum of disease, and lack of controlled clinical trials investigating the disease process and treatment measures. The pathophysiology is believed to be more complex than adult disease because the injury occurs during the process of lung growth and differentiation. In ILD, the initial injury causes damage to the alveolar epithelium and capillary endothelium. Abnormal healing of injured tissue may be more prominent than inflammation in the initial steps of the development of chronic ILD. Some familial cases, inherited as an autosomal dominant trait, may be due to mutations in surfactant protein genes, specifically surfactant protein C (SP-C). Some sporadic cases may also have similar SP-C gene mutations.

CLASSIFICATION AND PATHOLOGY. The classification of ILD in children is not standardized, but it is helpful to separate diseases into those of known and unknown etiology (Table 402-1). Respiratory infections caused by adenoviruses (see Chapter 259), influenza viruses (see Chapter 255), *Chlamydia* (see Chapter 222), and *Mycoplasma pneumoniae* (see Chapter 220) are usually self-limited illnesses but have been associated with prolonged and progressive lung damage, often in the form of bronchiolitis obliterans. **Aspiration** is a frequent cause of chronic lung disease in childhood. Children with developmental delay or neuromuscular weakness are at an increased risk for aspiration of food, saliva, or foreign matter secondary to swallowing dysfunction and/or gastroesophageal reflux. An undiagnosed tracheoesophageal fistula can also result in pulmonary complications related to aspiration of gastric contents and interstitial pneumonia. Children experiencing an exaggerated immunologic response to organic dust, molds, or bird antigens may develop **hypersensitivity pneumonitis.** Children with malignancies may develop ILD related to the primary malignancy, an opportunistic infection, or secondary

TABLE 402-1. Pediatric Interstitial Lung Diseases

INTERSTITIAL LUNG DISEASES OF KNOWN ETIOLOGY
Aspiration syndromes
Chronic infection (viral, bacterial, fungal, parasitic)
Immunocompetent host
Immunocompromised host
Bronchopulmonary dysplasia
Hypersensitivity pneumonitis (drugs, environment or occupation associated)*
Lymphangioleiomyomatosis
Surfactant protein B or C deficiency
INTERSTITIAL LUNG DISEASES OF UNKNOWN ETIOLOGY
Usual interstitial pneumonitis (UIP)
Desquamative pneumonitis (DIP)
Lymphocytic interstitial pneumonitis (LIP) and related disorders
Nonspecific interstitial pneumonitis
Pulmonary hemosiderosis
Goodpasture disease
Pulmonary infiltrates with eosinophilia
Pulmonary interstitial glycogenosis (PIG)
Neuroendocrine cell hyperplasia of infancy (NEHI)
Bronchiolitis obliterans
Bronchiolitis obliterans with organizing pneumonia (BOOP)
Alveolar proteinosis
Pulmonary vascular disorders (proliferative and congenital)
Pulmonary lymphatic disorders
Pulmonary microlithiasis
OTHER DISORDERS WITH PULMONARY INVOLVEMENT
Connective tissue disorders (Rheumatoid arthritis, SLE, Dermatomyositis)
Malignancies
Langerhans cell histiocytosis
Churg-Strauss syndrome
Sarcoidosis
Wegener granulomatosis
Neurocutaneous syndromes (neurofibromatosis, tuberous sclerosis)
Storage diseases (Gaucher disease, Niemann-Pick disease)
Hermansky-Pudlak syndrome

*Drugs include antibiotics (penicillin, nitrofurantoin, cephalosporins, isoniazid sulfonamides), anticancer therapies, drugs of abuse, oxygen, radiation, and dietary supplements. Environmental or occupation exposure includes inorganic and organic dusts, farmer's lung, bird breeder's lung, bagassosis, gases (fumes, vapors), hydrocarbons, resins, and nitrogen oxides.

Modified from Fan LL: Pediatric interstitial lung disease. In Schwartz MI, King TE (editors): *Interstitial Lung Disease,* 3rd ed. Toronto, BC Decker, 1998, p 103.

to chemotherapy or radiation treatment. Unique forms of ILD have been described in infants presenting with chronic tachypnea, retractions, crackles, and hypoxemia (Table 402-2). Defects in surfactant proteins may be associated with forms of familial and sporadic chronic lung disease. The prognosis in these diseases is variable.

Usual interstitial pneumonitis (UIP) is the most common form of ILD in affected adults but is rare in children. The pulmonary lesion is characterized by a mixed distribution of ongoing inflammation and progressive end-stage fibrosis that is patchy and heterogenous. The diagnosis is made by biopsy; there is no definitive clinical or radiologic feature. The diagnosis of *desquamative interstitial pneumonitis (DIP)* depends on biopsy that demonstrates a uniform, homogeneous process characterized by hyperplasia of alveolar epithelial cells with an accumulation of large macrophages within the air spaces. Fibrosis is usually not

TABLE 402-2. Unique Forms of Interstitial Lung Disease in Infancy

Persistent tachypnea of infancy (PTI)
Follicular bronchitis/bronchiolitis
Infantile pulmonary hemosiderosis
Chronic pneumonitis of infancy
Disorders of surfactant protein deficiency
Familial desquamative interstitial pneumonitis (DIP)
Idiopathic pulmonary fibrosis of infancy

From Fan LL: Pediatric interstitial lung disease. In Schwarz MI, King TE (editors): *Interstitial Lung Disease,* 3rd ed. Toronto, BC Decker, 1998, p 104.

seen. Some infants with histology similar to DIP have been diagnosed with surfactant B deficiency. A familial form has been described in infants, which is unusually severe and often fatal.

Lymphocytic interstitial pneumonitis (LIP), the most common form of ILD in children, is a form of pulmonary lymphoproliferative disease. LIP usually develops in association with conditions of impaired immunity, such as an autoimmune disease or immunodeficiency (HIV infection). The pulmonary interstitium is invaded by a diffuse infiltrate of mature lymphocytes. Fibrosis is rare. Infection with a virus such as Epstein-Barr virus (see Chapter 251) is often a contributing factor in the development of pediatric LIP.

Acute interstitial pneumonitis, also known as rapidly progressive interstitial pneumonitis or Hamman-Rich syndrome, is a distinct, rapidly progressive form of ILD. The alveolar damage progresses from an acute exudative process to severe fibrosis. An antecedent injury is often not identified; the fatality rate is >50%.

CLINICAL MANIFESTATIONS. A detailed history is needed to assess the severity of symptoms and the possibility of an underlying systemic disease. Identification of precipitating factors such as exposure to molds or birds or a severe lower respiratory infection is important in establishing the diagnosis and instituting avoidance measures. A positive family history, especially in an affected infant, is suggestive of a genetic or familial disease, such as a surfactant protein B or C deficiency (see Chapters 403 and 404). Tachypnea, cough, dyspnea, and exercise intolerance are present in >65% of patients. The majority have a reduced arterial saturation. Hypercarbia is a late complication. Symptoms are usually insidious and occur in a continuous, not episodic pattern. Tachypnea and basilar crackles are present in >50% of the patients. Retractions, failure to thrive, clubbing, and wheezing are common complaints. Cyanosis and a prominent 2nd heart sound are suggestive of severe disease. Anemia or hemoptysis suggests a pulmonary vascular disease or pulmonary hemosiderosis. Rashes or joint complaints are consistent with an underlying connective tissue disease.

DIAGNOSIS. Noninvasive tests are initially used to determine the extent and severity of the disease. Chest radiographic abnormalities can be classified as interstitial, reticular, nodular, reticulonodular, or honeycombed. The chest film may also be normal, despite significant clinical impairment, and may correlate poorly with the extent of disease. High-resolution CT (HRCT) of the chest better defines the extent and distribution of disease and can provide specific information for selection of a biopsy site. Faster modalities such as helical, spiral, or ultra-fast CT may provide precise resolution of disease patterns in tachypneic infants. Serial HRCT images may be of benefit in monitoring disease progression and severity.

Pulmonary function tests are important in defining the degree of **restrictive lung disease** and in following the response to treatment. In ILD, pulmonary function abnormalities demonstrate a restrictive ventilatory deficit with decreased lung volumes. Functional residual capacity (FRC) is reduced but usually less than vital capacity (VC) and total lung capacity (TLC). The residual volume (RV) is usually maintained; therefore, ratios of FRC : TLC and RV : TLC are often increased. Diffusion of carbon monoxide (DLCO) is usually normal when corrected for the decreased alveolar volume. An impaired DLCO may suggest vascular disease. Bronchoalveolar lavage (BAL) may provide helpful information regarding secondary infection, bleeding, or aspiration but will not usually determine the exact diagnosis. BAL is diagnostic for **pulmonary alveolar proteinosis.** Transthoracic lung biopsy for histopathology is usually the final step and is necessary for a conclusive diagnosis. Conventional thoracotomy or video-assisted thoracoscopy is used to obtain tissue from children with suspected ILD. Evaluation for possible systemic disease may also be necessary.

TREATMENT. Supportive care is essential and includes supplemental oxygen for hypoxia and adequate nutrition for growth failure. Antimicrobial treatment may be necessary for intercurrent infections. Some patients may be responsive to bronchodilators. Anti-inflammatory treatment with corticosteroids remains the initial treatment of choice. Controlled trials in children are lacking, and the clinical responses reported in case studies are variable. The usual dose of prednisone is 1–2 mg/kg/24 hr for 6–8 wk with tapering dictated by clinical response. Alternative, but not adequately evaluated, therapy includes hydroxychloroquine, azathioprine, cyclophosphamide, cyclosporine, methotrexate, intravenous immunoglobulin, and pulsed high-dose steroids. Hydroxychloroquine treatment is successful in some children with classic ILD, particularly those with histopathologic changes of DIP. Lung transplantation for progressive or end-stage ILD is successful in some infants and children. Appropriate treatment for underlying systemic disease is indicated. Preventive measures include avoidance of all inhalation irritants such as tobacco smoke and, when appropriate, molds and bird antigens. Supervised pulmonary rehabilitation programs may be helpful.

PROGNOSIS. The overall mortality of ILD is dependent on specific diagnosis and is as high as 20% in infants and children. Prognosis is variable and poor in children with pulmonary hypertension, failure to thrive, and severe fibrosis.

GENETIC COUNSELING. A high incidence of interstitial lung disease in some families suggests a genetic predisposition to either development of the disease or severity of the disorder. Genetic counseling may be beneficial if a familial history is obtained.

Atival A, Godrey S, Maayan C, et al: Chloroquine treatment of interstitial lung disease in children. *Pediatr Pulmonol* 1994;18:356–360.

Cameron HS, Somaschini M, Carrera P, et al: A common mutation in the surfactant protein C gene associated with lung disease. *J Pediatr* 2005;146:370–375.

Clement A, ERS Task Force: Task force on chronic interstitial lung disease in immunocompetent children. *Eur Respir J* 2004;24:686–697.

Fan LL, Kozinetz CA, Wojtczak HA, et al: The diagnostic value of transbronchial, thoracoscopic and open lung biopsy in immunocompetent children with chronic interstitial lung disease. *J Pediatr* 1997;131:565–569.

Fan LL, Langston C: Chronic interstitial lung disease in children. *Pediatr Pulmonol* 1993;16:184–196.

Nogee LM: Genetics of pediatric interstitial lung disease. *Curr Opin Pediatr* 2006;18:287–292.

Shulenin S, Nogee LM, Annilo T, et at: ABCA3 gene mutations in newborns with fatal surfactant deficiency. *N Engl J Med* 2004;350:1296–1303.

Sondheimer HM, Lum Lung MC, Brugman SM, et al: Pulmonary vascular disorders masquerading as interstitial lung disease. *Pediatr Pulmonol* 1995;20:284–288.

Teirstein AS: The elusive goal of therapy for usual interstitial pneumonia. *N Engl J Med* 2004;350:181–183.

Chapter 403 ■ Pulmonary Alveolar Proteinosis

Aaron Hamvas, Lawrence M. Nogee, Stuart C. Sweet, and F. Sessions Cole

Pulmonary alveolar proteinosis (PAP) is a disorder characterized by the intra-alveolar accumulation of pulmonary surfactant lipoproteins. On histopathologic examination, distal air spaces are filled with a granular, eosinophilic material that stains positively with periodic acid-Schiff reagent and is diastase resistant. Two clinically distinct forms of PAP have been described in children: a fulminant, often fatal form presenting shortly after birth (termed **congenital PAP**); and a gradually progressive type presenting in older infants and children that is similar to PAP observed in adults. PAP in older individuals is often classified as either primary or idiopathic (acquired) or secondary to a number of recognized conditions (malignancy, immunosuppression, inorganic dusts, toxic fumes, infections).

ETIOLOGY AND PATHOPHYSIOLOGY. The early onset of the neonatal form of PAP, its relentless progression toward death, and the observations of familial cases suggest a genetic basis. Single gene disorders that result in the neonatal form of PAP include mutations in the surfactant protein B (SP-B), surfactant protein C (SP-C), the β chain of the granulocyte-macrophage colony–stimulating factor (GM-CSF) receptor, and the adenosine triphosphate (ATP)–binding cassette transporter (ABCA3) genes (see Chapter 404). Alveolar proteinosis has also been reported in children, including young infants, with lysinuric protein intolerance (LPI), a rare autosomal recessive disorder caused by mutations in the cationic amino acid transporter SLC7A7. These children generally present with vomiting, hyperammonemia, and failure to thrive, although their pulmonary disease may prove fatal. The relationship between the basic defect and the development of PAP is unclear, although a case of recurrence of the disease after lung transplantation suggests that alveolar macrophage dysfunction is likely important in the pathogenesis of PAP associated with LPI.

Primary (idiopathic) PAP in adults is an autoimmune disease mediated by autoantibodies against GM-CSF. GM-CSF is essential in regulating macrophage function and clearance of surfactant. High titer, neutralizing immunoglobulin (Ig) G1 and IgG2 autoantibodies directed against GM-CSF can be detected in serum and bronchoalveolar lavage (BAL) fluid in adults with primary PAP. These autoantibodies block GM-CSF binding to its receptor, thereby inhibiting alveolar macrophage function and surfactant clearance. Such antibodies have been found in older children with apparent primary PAP but have not been identified in the congenital forms of alveolar proteinosis.

Secondary alveolar proteinosis can occur in association with infection, particularly in immunocompromised individuals. Environmental exposures to dust, silica, and chemicals have also been associated with the development of secondary alveolar proteinosis.

CLINICAL MANIFESTATIONS. Infants with the congenital form of PAP present in the immediate newborn period and rapidly develop respiratory failure. There is no gender difference in frequency. Congenital PAP is clinically and radiographically indistinguishable from more common disorders of the newborn that lead to respiratory failure, including pneumonia, generalized bacterial infection, respiratory distress syndrome, and total anomalous pulmonary venous return with obstruction. The differential diagnosis also includes primary pulmonary hypertension of the neonate, meconium aspiration, and alveolar capillary dysplasia, although the radiologic findings of these disorders usually differ. The incidence of congenital PAP is unknown; it was listed on death certificates of 37 infants who died in the 1st year of life in a cohort of 1,052,554 births in Missouri between 1979 and 1992.

Idiopathic (acquired) alveolar proteinosis in older infants and children is also rare. Males are affected 3 times as often as females. Usually, there is no identifiable etiologic factor (primary), or it can occur in association with malignancy or infection, particularly in the setting of systemic immunosuppression or congenital immunodeficiency, or after exposure to several inciting agents, including dust or chemicals (secondary). Older infants and children with PAP present with dyspnea, fatigue, cough, weight loss, chest pain, or hemoptysis. In the later stages, cyanosis and digital clubbing may be seen. Pulmonary function changes include decreased diffusing capacity of carbon monoxide (D_LCO), lung volumes with a restrictive abnormality, and arterial blood gases with marked hypoxemia and/or chronic respiratory acidosis.

DIAGNOSIS. Histopathologic examination of lung biopsy specimens is the gold standard for diagnosis in children. In patients with alveolar proteinosis caused by mechanisms other than SP-B deficiency, immunohistochemical staining reveals abundant quantities of alveolar and intracellular surfactant proteins A and B. Latex agglutination tests for the presence of anti–GM-CSF antibodies in BAL fluid or blood are highly sensitive and specific for the acquired forms of alveolar proteinosis. The examination of sputum or BAL fluid for surfactant components has been used diagnostically in adults, but these methods have not been validated in children. Examination of peripheral blood and/or bone marrow for clonogenic stimulation of monocyte-macrophage precursors, GM-CSF receptor and ligand expression, and GM-CSF binding are available through research protocols.

TREATMENT. Alveolar proteinosis in newborns resulting from SP-B deficiency is rapidly fatal and no successful medical therapy has been developed. The natural history of other forms of PAP is significantly more variable, making prognostic and therapeutic decisions difficult. Total lung lavage has been associated with prolonged remissions of PAP in adults and remains a therapeutic option for patients with the later-onset form of PAP. It is ineffective in the congenital form of the disease due to inborn errors of surfactant metabolism. The role of repeated bronchoalveolar lavage in children has not been well studied. It may provide a temporizing measure in some circumstances and benefit in patients with autoimmune or secondary PAP. Subcutaneous or inhaled administration of recombinant GM-CSF may improve pulmonary function in some adults with idiopathic primary (autoimmune) alveolar proteinosis. Anti–GM-CSF antibody titers may decrease during GM-CSF treatment, suggesting that this therapy may desensitize the patient. These interventions have been unsuccessful for the long-term management of newborn infants. Lung transplantation is a therapeutic option, but its use is limited by concerns about disease recurrence in the absence of a defined primary mechanism of lung injury.

Borsani G, Bassi MT, Sperandeo MP, et al: SLC7A7, encoding a putative permease-related protein, is mutated in patients with lysinuric protein intolerance. *Nat Genet* 1999;21:297–301.

de Blic J: Pulmonary alveolar proteinosis in children. *Paediatr Resp Rev* 2004;5:316–322.

Kitamura T, Uchida K, Tanaka N, et al: Serological diagnosis of idiopathic pulmonary alveolar proteinosis. *Am J Respir Crit Care Med* 2000; 162:658–662.

Mahut B, Delacourt C, Scheinmann P, et al: Pulmonary alveolar proteinosis: Experience with eight pediatric cases and a review. *Pediatrics* 1996; 97:117–122.

Seymour JF, Presneill JJ, Schoch OD, et al: Therapeutic efficacy of granulocyte-macrophage colony-stimulating factor in patients with idiopathic acquired alveolar proteinosis. *Am J Respir Crit Care Med* 2001; 163:524–531.

Trapnell BC, Whitsett JA, Nakata K: Pulmonary alveolar proteinosis. *N Engl J Med* 2003;329:2527–2539.

Uchida K, Nakata K, Trapnell BC, et al: High-affinity autoantibodies specifically eliminate granulocyte-macrophage colony-stimulating factor activity in the lungs of patients with idiopathic pulmonary alveolar proteinosis. *Blood* 2004;103:1089–1098.

Chapter 404 ■ Inherited Disorders of Surfactant Metabolism

Aaron Hamvas, Lawrence M. Nogee, and F. Sessions Cole

Pulmonary surfactant is a mixture of phospholipids and proteins synthesized, packaged, and secreted by type II pneumocytes. This mixture forms a monolayer at the air-liquid interface that lowers surface tension at end-expiration of the respiratory cycle and thereby prevents atelectasis and ventilation-perfusion mismatch. Four surfactant-associated proteins have been described: surfactant proteins A and D (SP-A, SP-D) participate in host defense in the lung, whereas surfactant proteins B and C (SP-B, SP-C) contribute to the surface tension-lowering activity of the pulmonary surfactant. Two genes for SP-A *(SFTPA1, SFTPA2)* and one gene for SP-D *(SFTPD)* are located on human chromosome 10, whereas single genes encode SP-B *(SFTPB)* and SP-C *(SFTPC)* located on human chromosomes 2 and 8, respectively. Although inherited deficiencies of SP-A or SP-D have not been identified in humans, genetically engineered mice deficient in these proteins are susceptible to viral and bacterial infections, and lineages deficient in SP-D accumulate lipids and foamy macrophages in their lungs and develop emphysema as they age. Inherited disorders of SP-B and SP-C have been identified in humans. The ATP-binding cassette protein member A3, ABCA3, is a transporter located on the limiting membrane of lamellar bodies, the storage organelle for surfactant within alveolar Type II cells. Encoded on human chromosome 16, recessive mutations in the ABCA3 gene *(ABCA3)* have been associated with lethal surfactant deficiency.

DEFICIENCY OF SURFACTANT PROTEIN B

GENETICS. More than 30 loss-of-function mutations in *SFTPB* have been identified. The most common is a net 2 base-pair insertion in codon 121 (termed *121ins2*) that results in a frameshift, an unstable SP-B transcript and absence of SP-B protein production. The insertion generates a restriction fragment polymorphism (RFLP) that is useful for diagnosis. This mutation has accounted for 60–70% of the alleles found to date in patients identified with SP-B deficiency. Most other mutations have been family specific.

PATHOLOGY. Although SP-B deficiency was 1st described in a patient with newborn-onset alveolar proteinosis, this histology is neither specific for SP-B deficiency nor universally present in lungs of affected infants. Several SP-B deficient patients homozygous for the 121ins2 mutation have had histologic features more typical of **desquamative interstitial pneumonitis** (see Chapter 402) with accumulation of macrophages and little detectable alveolar proteinosis at the time of lung transplantation. Other findings are nonspecific and include variable degrees of interstitial fibrosis and alveolar cell hyperplasia. Ultrastructural findings include a lack of tubular myelin, disorganized lamellar bodies, and an accumulation of abnormal-appearing multivesicular bodies, suggesting abnormal lipid packaging and secretion.

CLINICAL MANIFESTATIONS. Infants with an inherited deficiency of SP-B present in the immediate neonatal period with respiratory failure. This autosomal recessive disorder is clinically and radiographically similar to the respiratory distress syndrome (RDS) of premature infants (see Chapter 101.4) but typically affects full-term infants. The initial degree of respiratory distress is variable, but the disease is progressive and is refractory to mechanical ventilation, surfactant replacement therapy, glucocorticoid administration, and extracorporeal membrane oxygenation. SP-B deficiency has been recognized in diverse racial and ethnic groups. Almost all patients have died unless they had lung transplantation; prolonged survival is possible in cases with a partial deficiency of SP-B. Humans heterozygous for loss-of-function mutations in the SP-B gene are clinically normal as adults and have normal pulmonary function.

DIAGNOSIS. A rapid, definitive diagnosis can be established with analyses of DNA for known mutations in *SFTPB*, particularly the 121ins2 mutation (using RFLP analysis of polymerase chain reaction–amplified genomic DNA). The sensitivity of genetic diagnosis is limited, as disease may result from yet unidentified mutations. In families in which a mutation has been previously identified, antenatal diagnosis can be established by molecular assays of DNA from chorionic villus biopsy or aminocytes. Other laboratory tests remain investigational and include analysis of tracheal effluent by enzyme-linked immunosorbent assay or Western blotting for the presence or absence of SP-B protein and for aberrantly processed precursor proSP-C peptides that have been found in SP-B deficient human infants and animals. Immunostaining of lung biopsy tissue for the surfactant proteins can also support the diagnosis, although, currently, immunohistochemical assays for SP-B and SP-C are only available on a research basis. Generally, staining for SP-B is absent, but robust extracellular staining for proSP-C due to aberrantly processed proSP-C peptides is observed and diagnostic for SP-B deficiency. Such studies require a lung biopsy in a critically ill child, but can also be performed on lung blocks acquired at the time of autopsy, allowing for retrospective diagnosis.

TREATMENT. Virtually all patients with SP-B deficiency die within the 1st year of life. Conventional neonatal intensive care interventions can maintain extrapulmonary organ function for a limited time (weeks to months). Replacement therapy with commercially available surfactants is ineffective. Lung transplantation has been successful, but the pretransplant, transplant, and post-transplant medical and surgical care is highly specialized and only available at pediatric pulmonary transplant centers. Thus, prompt recognition is critical if patients are to be considered for lung transplantation. The oldest living SP-B deficient survivor after lung transplantation was born in 1994. Five year survival following lung transplantation is ≈50% and is no different than that for other causes of infant lung transplantation. Anti SP-B antibodies may develop but have not had an effect on the transplant. Genetic counseling is also important to convey the risks for future pregnancies and the availability of antenatal diagnosis and therapeutic options. Palliative care consultation is also helpful.

SURFACTANT PROTEIN C GENE ABNORMALITIES

SP-C is a very low molecular weight, extremely hydrophobic protein, which, along with SP-B, enhances the surface tension-lowering properties of surfactant phospholipids. It is derived from proteolytic processing of a larger precursor protein (proSP-C).

GENETICS. More than 35 dominantly expressed mutations in *SFTPC* have been identified in association with acute and chronic lung disease in patients ranging in age from newborn to adult. Approximately 55% of these mutations arise spontaneously, resulting in sporadic disease; the remainder are inherited. A threonine substitution for isoleucine in codon 73 (termed *I73T*) has accounted for 25% of the cases identified to date. Mutations in *SFTPC* are thought to result in production of misfolded proSP-C that accumulates within the alveolar type II cell and causes cellular injury. The frequency of mutations and of disease due to mutations in *SFTPC* are unknown. Mutations have been identified in diverse racial and ethnic groups.

PATHOLOGY. The histopathology of lung tissue from patients with mutations in *SFTPC* falls into the category of **interstitial pneumonitis,** with a variety of diagnoses based largely on adult classifications of interstitial lung disease. These include nonspecific interstitial pneumonia, desquamative interstitial pneumonitis, idiopathic pulmonary fibrosis, pulmonary alveolar proteinosis, and chronic pneumonitis of infancy.

CLINICAL MANIFESTATIONS. The clinical presentation of patients with *SFTPC* mutations is quite variable. Some patients present at birth with symptoms, signs, and radiographic findings typical of RDS. Others present later in life, ranging from early infancy until well into adulthood, with gradual onset of respiratory insufficiency, hypoxemia, failure to thrive, and interstitial lung disease on chest radiographs. The age and severity of disease varies even within families with the same mutation. The natural history is also quite variable, with some patients improving either spontaneously or due to therapy, some with persistent respiratory insufficiency, and some progressing to the point of requiring lung transplantation. This variability in severity and course of the disease does not appear to correlate with the specific mutation and also hinders accurate assessment of prognosis.

DIAGNOSIS. In contrast to SP-B deficiency, no biochemical markers are available to permit rapid diagnosis. Sequencing of *SFTPC* gene is the only definitive diagnostic test and is available in some clinical and research laboratories. The relatively small size of the gene facilitates such analyses, which are quite sensitive, but since most *SFTPC* mutations are missense mutations, distinguishing true disease causing mutations from rare, yet benign sequence variants may be difficult.

TREATMENT. No specific treatment is available for patients with lung disease due to mutations in the SP-C gene. Therapeutic approaches used for interstitial lung diseases, such as quinolones or corticosteroids, have been used but not been systematically evaluated. Lung transplantation is reserved for patients with progressive and refractory respiratory failure who would otherwise qualify for transplantation irrespective of their diagnosis. Genetic counseling is important to define the risks for future pregnancies.

DISEASE DUE TO MUTATIONS IN ABCA3

GENETICS. Recessive mutations in *ABCA3* were 1st described in a series of 20 infants who presented with lethal respiratory distress. There is considerable allelic heterogeneity; >20 mutations scattered throughout the gene have been identified, most of which are family specific. No common mutation has been yet identified. The frequency of mutations and disease is unknown, but *ABCA3* mutations may contribute to a substantial proportion of unexplained fatal lung disease in term infants. *ABCA3* mutations have been identified in diverse racial and ethnic groups.

PATHOLOGY. The lung pathology of infants with *ABCA3* mutations is similar to that of infants with *SFTPB* mutations and includes changes of desquamative interstitial pneumonitis and/or alveolar proteinosis. On ultrastructural examination, the lamellar bodies appear small and contain eccentrically placed electron dense inclusions, a finding that may be characteristic for mutations in *ABCA3* and one that indicates that *ABCA3* function is necessary for lamellar body biogenesis.

CLINICAL MANIFESTATIONS. Infants with *ABCA3* mutations typically presented in the neonatal period with severe respiratory failure that was clinically and radiographically similar to that of SP-B deficient infants or premature infants with RDS, and was refractory to standard intensive care interventions. Experience with the disorder is limited, however, and the initial group of infants studied was deliberately selected for the severe nature of their lung disease. The extent of phenotypic variability associated with *ABCA3* mutations is unknown.

DIAGNOSIS. Clinical suspicion is the key to diagnosis. Currently, no biochemical or histopathologic markers definitively establish the diagnosis, though the presence of the dense lamellar body inclusions on electron microscopy of lung tissue is consistent with the diagnosis. The size of the *ABCA3* gene (80 kb with 30 coding exons) and the degree of allelic heterogeneity limit molecular diagnosis, which is currently available on a research basis.

TREATMENT. Specific treatment for patients with *ABCA3* mutations is not available. Infants with progressive respiratory failure may be candidates for lung transplantation. Genetic counseling is important to define the risks for future pregnancies.

Cameron HS, Somaschini M, Carrera P, et al: A common mutation in the surfactant protein C gene associated with lung disease. *J Pediatr* 2005;146:370–375.

Cole FS, Hamvas A, Nogee LM: Genetic disorders of neonatal respiratory function. *Pediatr Res* 2001;50:157–162.

Dunbar AE, Wert SE, Hamvas A, et al: Prolonged survival in hereditary surfactant protein B (SP-B) deficiency associated with a novel splicing mutation. *Pediatr Res* 2000;48:275–282.

Hamvas A: Surfactant protein B deficiency: Insights into inherited disorders of lung cell metabolism. *Curr Prob Pediatr* 1997;27:325–345.

Nogee LM, deMello DE, Dehner LP, et al: Pulmonary surfactant protein B deficiency in congenital pulmonary alveolar proteinosis. *N Engl J Med* 1993;328:406–410.

Nogee LM, Dunbar AE III, Wert SE, et al: A mutation in the surfactant protein C gene associated with familial interstitial lung disease. *N Engl J Med* 2001;344:573–579.

Nogee LM, Garnier G, Singer L, et al: A mutation in the surfactant protein B gene responsible for fatal neonatal respiratory disease in multiple kindreds. *J Clin Invest* 1994;93:1860–1863.

Nogee LM, Wert SE, Proffit SA, et al: Allelic heterogeneity in hereditary surfactant protein B (SP-B) deficiency. *Am J Respir Crit Care Med* 2000;161:973–981.

Palomar LM, Nogee LM, Sweet SC, et al: Long-term outcomes after infant lung transplantation for surfactant protein B deficiency related to other causes of respiratory failure. *J Pediatr* 2006;149:548–553.

Shulenin S, Nogee LM, Annilo T, et al: *ABCA3* gene mutations in newborns with fatal surfactant deficiency. *N Engl J Med* 2004;350:1296–1303.

Thomas AQ, Lane K, Phillips J, et al: Heterozygosity for a surfactant protein C gene mutation associated with usual interstitial pneumonitis and cellular nonspecific interstitial pneumonitis in one kindred. *Am J Respir Crit Care Med* 2002;165:1322–1328.

Chapter 405 ■ Pulmonary Hemosiderosis

Mary A. Nevin

Pulmonary hemorrhage is infrequently encountered in pediatrics; when present, it is often focal and self-limited in nature. Rarely, bleeding reflects **diffuse alveolar hemorrhage (DAH)**. The diagnosis of pulmonary hemosiderosis refers to this more chronic and diffuse alveolar process. Pulmonary hemosiderosis has classically been characterized by the triad of iron-deficiency anemia, hemoptysis, and the alveolar infiltrates on chest radiographs. A high level of clinical suspicion may be required because any or all of these features of the disease can be absent at any point in time. Pulmonary hemosiderosis can exist in isolation, but more commonly, it occurs in association with an underlying condition. A precise etiology for hemorrhage is not always found. When alveolar hemorrhage occurs in isolation and an exhaustive evaluation for underlying disease is found to be negative, the patient is said to have **idiopathic pulmonary hemosiderosis (IPH)**.

ETIOLOGY. Some of the conditions that can be associated with diffuse hemorrhage are noted in Table 406-3. Most cases of DAH are associated with an underlying immunologic, rheumatologic, or vasculitic disorder, but other diagnoses may present with recurrent or chronic pulmonary bleeding.

Pulmonary hemosiderosis can be classified as primary or secondary. **Primary pulmonary hemosiderosis (PPH)** is described as encompassing the diagnoses of IPH, **Goodpasture syndrome** (see Chapter 517), and **Heiner syndrome** (cow's milk hyperreactivity). Among these etiologies, Goodpasture syndrome (or anti–basement membrane antibody disease) appears to be the most common cause of pulmonary hemorrhage.

Secondary pulmonary hemosiderosis refers to the remaining, diverse group of potential etiologies. Among these are cardiac causes of pulmonary hemosiderosis such as congestive heart failure, pulmonary hypertension, and mitral valve stenosis. Vasculitic and collagen vascular diseases such as systemic lupus erythematosus (SLE; see Chapter 157), rheumatoid arthritis, Wegener granulomatosis (see Chapter 166.4), and Henoch-Schönlein purpura (HSP; see Chapter 166.1) are another important group to consider in the differential diagnosis. Coagulopathies are encountered and may be either inherited or acquired. Prematurity is also a recognized risk factor for hemorrhage. Pulmonary hemosiderosis has been well described in association with celiac disease. Postinfectious processes such as hemolytic-uremic syndrome (see Chapter 484.4) and immunodeficiency syndromes, including chronic granulomatous disease (CGD; see Chapter 129) have also been implicated. Finally, numerous medications, environmental exposures, chemicals, and food allergens have been reported as potential etiologies.

EPIDEMIOLOGY. The frequency with which DAH occurs is difficult to quantify. This is largely because of the variety of disorders that can present with a component of alveolar hemorrhage. Similarly, the prevalence of IPH is largely unknown. In fact, many children and young adults who were diagnosed with IPH in the past might have a discoverable etiology for their hemorrhage if they were studied today with the advantage of newer and more advanced diagnostics. Estimates of prevalence obtained from Swedish and Japanese retrospective case analyses vary from 0.24–1.23 cases per million. In general, the manifestations of IPH are seen before the age of 10 yr. Nearly 80% of cases occur in this early age group. The remaining 20% of adult patients are typically diagnosed before the age of 30 yr. The ratio of affected males to females is equal in the childhood diagnosis group, and males are only slightly more affected in the group diagnosed as adults.

PATHOLOGY. With repeated episodes of pulmonary hemorrhage, lung tissue appears brown secondary to the presence of **hemosiderin.** The finding of blood in the airways or alveoli is representative of a recent hemorrhage. Hemosiderin-laden macrophages are seen with recovering, recurrent, or chronic pulmonary hemorrhage. It takes 48–72 hr for the alveolar macrophages to convert iron from erythrocytes into hemosiderin. Hemosiderin-laden macrophages may be detectable for weeks after a hemorrhagic event. Other nonspecific pathologic findings can include thickening of alveolar septae and hypertrophy of type II pneumocytes. Fibrosis may be seen with chronic disease (see also Chapter 413).

PATHOPHYSIOLOGY. In Goodpasture syndrome, anti–basement membrane antibody (ABMA) binds to the basement membrane of both the alveolus and the glomerulus. At the alveolar level, immunoglobulin G (IgG), IgM, and complement are deposited at alveolar septae. Electron microscopy shows disruption of basement membranes and vascular integrity, thereby allowing blood to escape into alveolar spaces.

Pulmonary hemosiderosis in association with **cow's milk hypersensitivity** was first reported by Heiner in 1962. This condition is characterized by variable symptoms of milk intolerance. Symptoms can include grossly bloody or heme-positive stools, vomiting, failure to thrive, symptoms of gastroesophageal reflux, and/or upper airway congestion. Pathologic findings have included elevations of IgE and peripheral eosinophilia as well as alveolar deposits of IgG, IgA, and C3. High titers to cow's milk protein are also typically found in cow milk hypersensitivity.

Alveolar hemorrhage, seen rarely in association with **SLE**, is often severe and potentially life-threatening. Pathologic vasculitic features may be absent. Some immuoflorescent studies have revealed IgG and C3 deposits at the alveolar septae. A clear link between immune complex formation and alveolar hemorrhage has not been established, however.

In **HSP**, pulmonary hemorrhage is a rare but recognized complication. Pathologic findings have included transmural neutrophilic infiltration of small vessels, alveolar septal inflammation, and intra-alveolar hemorrhage. Vasculitis is the proposed mechanism for hemorrhage.

Wegener granulomatosis is a rare etiology for hemorrhage in children. Pulmonary granuloma formation (with or without cavitation) and a necrotizing vasculitis may be appreciated. In children, presentations attributable to the upper airway, including subglottic stenosis, may suggest the diagnosis. Testing for antineutrophil cytoplasmic antibody (ANCA) is generally positive.

A premature infant's neonatal course can frequently be complicated by pulmonary hemorrhage. The alveolar and vascular networks are immature and particularly prone to inflammation and damage by ventilator mechanics, oxidative stress, and infection. Pulmonary hemorrhage may be unrecognized if the volume of blood is insufficient to reach the proximal airways. The chest radiograph findings of pulmonary hemorrhage may be appreciated instead as a worsening picture of respiratory distress syndrome, edema, or infection.

A number of additional associated conditions and exposures exist, as outlined previously. These occur infrequently in the pediatric population and suggested mechanisms for hemorrhage are variable. The diagnosis of IPH is made when there is evidence of chronic or recurrent diffuse alveolar hemorrhage and when exhaustive evaluations for primary or secondary etiologies are negative. A biopsy specimen should not reveal any evidence of granulomatous disease, vasculitis, infection, infarction, immune complex deposition, malignancy, or any other features of associated primary or secondary conditions.

CLINICAL MANIFESTATIONS. The clinical presentation of pulmonary hemosiderosis is highly variable. Symptoms may be reflective of an underlying and associated disease process rather than specifically related to pulmonary hemorrhage. Presentations can vary widely from a relative lack of symptoms to shock or sudden death. Hemorrhage may be significant without remarkable symptomatology. Hemoptysis may not occur. Bleeding may occasionally be recognized by the presence of alveolar infiltrates on a chest radiograph. It should be noted that the absence of an infiltrate does not rule out an ongoing hemorrhagic process.

Because the presence of blood in the lung is typically a source of significant irritation and inflammation, the patient may present after an episode of hemorrhage with wheezing, cough, dyspnea, and alterations in gas exchange, reflecting bronchospasm, edema, mucous plugging, and inflammation. On physical examination, the patient may be pale with tachycardia and tachypnea. During an acute exacerbation, children are frequently febrile. Examination of the chest may reveal retractions and differential or decreased aeration, with crackles or wheezes. The patient may present in shock with respiratory failure from massive hemoptysis. Children in particular may present with symptoms of chronic anemia, such as failure to thrive.

LABORATORY FINDINGS AND DIAGNOSIS. Pulmonary hemorrhage is associated with a decrease in hemoglobin and hematocrit. The classic finding is a microcytic, hypochromic anemia. The reticulocyte count is elevated. The anemia of IPH can mimic a hemolytic anemia. Elevations of plasma bilirubin are caused by absorption and breakdown of hemoglobin in the alveoli. Serum iron is reduced. Iron-binding capacity is generally elevated. Any or all hematologic manifestations may be absent in the face of recent hemorrhage.

White blood count and differential should be evaluated for evidence of infection and eosinophilia. A stool specimen can be heme-positive secondary to swallowed blood. Renal and liver function should be reviewed. A urinalysis should be obtained to assess for evidence of nephritis. A coagulation profile, quantitative immunoglobulins (including IgE), and complement studies are recommended.

Testing for ANCA, antinuclear antibody (ANA), anti–double stranded DNA, rheumatoid factor, antiphospholipid antibody, and anti–glomerular basement membrane antibody (antiGBM) evaluates for a number of primary and secondary etiologies of DAH. An elevated erythrocyte sedimentation rate (ESR) is a nonspecific finding.

Sputum or pulmonary secretions should be analyzed for significant evidence of blood or hemosiderin-laden macrophages (HLM). Gastric secretions may also reveal HLM. Flexible bronchoscopy provides visualization of any areas of active bleeding. With bronchoalveolar lavage, pulmonary secretions may be sent for pathologic review and culture analysis. The ability to perform flexible bronchoscopy will be limited if there are large amounts of blood or clots in the airway. A patient with respiratory failure can be ventilated more effectively through a rigid bronchoscope.

Lung biopsy is warranted when DAH occurs without discernible etiology, extrapulmonary disease, or circulating ABMA. Pulmonary tissue when obtained should be evaluated for evidence of vasculitis, immune complex deposition, and granulomatous disease.

A chest radiograph may reveal evidence of acute or chronic disease. Hyperaeration is frequently seen, especially during an acute hemorrhage. Infiltrates are typically symmetric and may spare the apices of the lung. Atelectasis may also be appreciated. With chronic disease, fibrosis lymphadenopathy and nodularity may be seen. Findings on CT imaging may reveal a subclinical and contributory disease process.

Pulmonary function testing will likely reveal primarily obstructive disease in the acute period. With more chronic disease, fibrosis and restrictive disease tend to predominate. Oxygen saturations may be decreased. Lung volumes may reveal air trapping acutely and decreases in total lung capacity chronically. The diffusing capacity of carbon monoxide (D_LCO) may be low or normal in the chronic phase but is likely to be elevated in the setting of an acute hemorrhage. This is because carbon monoxide binds to the hemoglobin in extravasated red blood cells.

TREATMENT. Supportive therapy including volume resuscitation, ventilatory support, supplemental oxygen, and transfusion of blood products may be warranted. If an associated treatable condition exists, surgical or medical therapy should be directed at that underlying condition. In IPH, early treatment with systemic corticosteroids is the treatment of choice. Therapy is generally initiated at 2–5 mg/kg/day and decreased to 1 mg/kg every other day after resolution of acute symptoms. Early treatment with corticosteroids appears to decrease episodes of hemorrhage. This therapy may also modulate the neutrophil influx and inflammation associated with hemorrhage, thereby decreasing progression toward fibrotic disease.

The goal of gradually tapering systemic steroids may not be tolerated. In addition, a subgroup of patients may not respond optimally to corticosteroid therapy alone. In these cases, immunosuppressive agents such as cyclophosphamide, azathioprine, and chloroquine have been utilized. The indications for and effectiveness of long-term immunosuppressive therapies remain unclear. The numerous potential long-term side effects of corticosteroids and other immunosuppressive agents may limit therapy.

In chronic disease, progression to debilitating pulmonary fibrosis has been described. Lung transplant has been performed in patients with IPH who are refractory to immunosuppressive therapy. In one reported case study, IPH recurred in the transplanted lung.

PROGNOSIS. The outcome of patients suffering from DAH is highly dependent on the underlying disease process. Some conditions, such as cow's milk hypersensitivity, respond well to removal of the offending agent. Other syndromes, especially those with an immunologic mechanism, tend to carry a poor prognosis. In IPH, mortality is often related to massive hemorrhage or, alternatively, to progressive fibrosis, respiratory insufficiency, and right-sided heart failure.

Long-term prognosis in IPH varies among studies. Initial case study reviews suggested an average survival after symptom onset of only 2.5 yr. In this early review, a minority of patients were treated with steroids. A more recent review reported a 5 yr survival rate of 86%. Whether this improvement in survival is primarily related to overall advances in care or long-term immunosuppressive therapy is not established at this time. Spontaneous remissions have been documented.

Boat TF: Pulmonary hemorrhage and hemoptysis. In Chernick V, Boat TF (editors): *Kendig's Disorders of the Respiratory Tract in Children.* Philadelphia, WB Saunders, 1998, pp 623–633.

Calabrese F, Giacometti C, Rea F, et al: Recurrence of idiopathic pulmonary hemosiderosis in a young adult patient after bilateral single-lung transplantation. *Transplantation* 2002;74:1643–1645.

Cohen S: Idiopathic pulmonary hemosiderosis. *Am J Med Sci* 1999; 317:67–74.

Dearborn DG: Pulmonary hemorrhage in infants and children. *Curr Opin Pediatr* 1997;9:219–224.

Godfrey S: Pulmonary hemorrhage/hemoptysis in children. *Pediatr Pulmonol* 2004;37:476–484.

Ioachimescu OC, Sieber S, Kotch A: Idiopathic pulmonary hemosiderosis revisited. *Eur Respir J* 2004;24:162–170.

Le Clainche L, Le Bourgeois M, Fauroux B, et al: Long-term outcome of idiopathic pulmonary hemosiderosis in children. *Medicine* 2000;79: 318–326.

McCoy KS: Hemosiderosis. In Taussig LM, Landau LI (eds): *Pediatric Respiratory Medicine.* St. Louis, Mosby, 1999, pp 835–841.

Moissidi SI, Chaidaroon D, Vichyanond P, Bahna SL: Milk-induced pulmonary disease in infants (Heiner Syndrome). *Pediatr Allergy Immunol* 2005;16(6):545–562.

Saeed MM, Woo MS, MacLaughlin EF, et al: Prognosis in pediatric idiopathic pulmonary hemosiderosis. *Chest* 1999;116:721–725.

Yao TC, Hung IJ, Jaing TH, et al: Pitfalls in the diagnosis of idiopathic pulmonary haemosiderosis. *Arch Dis Child* 2002;86:436–438.

Chapter 406 ■ Pulmonary Embolism, Infarction, and Hemorrhage

Mary A. Nevin

406.1 • Pulmonary Embolus and Infarction

Although children are viewed as less at risk than adults for the development of venous thromboembolic disease (VTE), embolic disease does occur and is well described in children and adolescents with or without risk factors (Table 406-1). Embolic disease in children can be a significant source of morbidity and mortality. Improvements in therapeutics for childhood illnesses and increased survival with chronic illness may contribute to the increased number of children presenting with thromboembolic events.

ETIOLOGY. Commonly appreciated risk factors for thromboembolic disease in adults include immobility, malignancy, pregnancy,

TABLE 406-1. Risk Factors for Pulmonary Embolism (PE)
ENVIRONMENTAL
Long-haul air travel
Obesity
Cigarette smoking
Hypertension
Immobility
WOMEN'S HEALTH
Oral contraceptives, including progesterone-only and, especially, third-generation pills
Pregnancy
Hormone replacement therapy
MEDICAL ILLNESS
Previous PE or deep venous thrombosis (DVT)
Cancer
Congestive heart failure
Chronic obstructive pulmonary disease
Diabetes mellitus
Inflammatory bowel disease
Antipsychotic drug use
Chronic indwelling central venous catheter
Permanent pacemaker
Internal cardiac defibrillator
Stroke with limb paresis
Nursing-home confinement or current or repeated hospital admission
SURGICAL
Trauma
Orthopedic surgery
General surgery
Neurosurgery, especially craniotomy for brain tumor
THROMBOPHILIA
Factor V Leiden mutation
Prothrombin gene mutation
Hyperhomocysteinaemia (including mutation in methylenetetrahydrofolate reductase)
Antiphospholipid antibody syndrome
Deficiency of antithrombin III, protein C, or protein S
High concentrations of factor VIII or XI
Increased lipoprotein a
NONTHROMBOTIC
Air
Foreign particles (e.g., hair, talc, as a consequence of intravenous drug misuse)
Amniotic fluid
Bone fragments, bone marrow
Fat
Tumors (Wilms tumor)

Modified from Goldhaber SZ: Pulmonary embolism. *Lancet* 2004;363:1295–1305.

infection, and hypercoagulability (see Table 406-1). Adults may also have thromboembolic disease without identifiable risk factors. Idiopathic disease has been described in up to 20% of adults with this condition. Children with deep venous thrombosis (DVT) and pulmonary embolism (PE) are much more likely to have 1 or more identifiable conditions or circumstances placing them at risk. In a large Canadian registry, 96% of pediatric patients were found to have 1 risk factor and 90% had 2 or more risk factors.

Embolic disease has variable etiologies in children. An embolus can contain thrombus, air, amniotic fluid, septic material, or metastatic neoplastic tissue; however, thromboemboli are most commonly encountered. A commonly encountered risk factor for DVT and PE in the pediatric population is the presence of a central venous catheter. The presence of a catheter in a vessel lumen as well as instilled medications can induce endothelial damage and favor thrombus formation.

Children with malignancies are also at considerable risk. The risk of PE is more significant in children with solid, rather than with hematologic, malignancies. PE has been described in children with Wilms tumor as well as leukemia. A child with malignancy may have numerous risk factors related to the primary disease process and the therapeutic interventions. Infection from chronic immunosuppression may interact with hypercoagulability of malignancy and chemotherapeutic effects on the endothelium.

In the neonatal period, thromboembolic disease and PE are often related to indwelling catheters used for parenteral nutrition and medication delivery. Emboli in this age group may occasionally reflect maternal risk factors, such as diabetes or toxemia of pregnancy. Infants with congenitally acquired homozygous deficiencies of antithrombin, protein C, and protein S are also likely to present in the neonatal period.

Prothrombotic disease can also present in older infants and children. Disease can be congenital or acquired; DVT/PE may be the initial presentation. *Factor V Leiden mutation* (see Chapter 478), *hyperhomocysteinemia* (see Chapter 85.3), *prothrombin 20210A mutation* (see Chapter 478), *anticardiolipin antibody,* and elevated levels of *lipoprotein A* have all been linked to thromboembolic disease. Children with sickle cell disease are also at high risk for pulmonary embolus and infarction. Acquired prothrombotic disease is represented by *nephrotic syndrome* (see Chapter 527) and *antiphospholipid antibody syndrome.* From 21% to 57% of children with *systemic lupus erythematosus* (see Chapter 157) have thromboembolic disease.

Other risk factors include infection, cardiac disease, recent surgery, and trauma. Surgical risk is thought to be more significant when immobility will be a prominent feature of the recovery. Use of oral contraceptives confers additional risk, although the level of risk in patients taking these medications appears to be decreasing, perhaps resulting from a lower amount of estrogen in current formulations.

Septic emboli are rare in children but may be caused by osteomyelitis, cellulitis, urinary tract infection, jugular vein or umbilical thrombophlebitis, and right-sided endocarditis.

EPIDEMIOLOGY. Younger age appears to be somewhat protective in thromboembolic disease. The DVT incidence in 1 study of hospitalized children was 5.3/10,000 admissions. In a study that analyzed data from 1979 through 2001, there were 0.9 PE/100,000 children/yr, 4.2 DVT/100,000 children/yr, and 4.9 VTE/100,000 children/yr (Table 406-2).

TABLE 406-2. Thromboembolic Disease in Children: 1979–2001

	AGE GROUP	RATE OF DIAGNOSIS/100,000 CHILDREN/YR		
		All	Boys	Girls
PE	0–1	2.2*	—‡	—
	2–14	0.4	—	—
	15–17	2.0*	—	—
	All	0.9	—	—
DVT	0–1	8.7†	9.3	8.0
	2–14	2.1	2.0	2.2
	15–17	9.9†	6.5	13.5
	All	4.2	3.6	4.8
VTE	0–1	10.5†	11.3	9.7
	2–14	2.4	2.3	2.6
	15–17	11.4†	8.1	14.9
	All	4.9	4.3	5.5

*$P < .05$ age 0–1 vs age 2–14, and 15–17 vs age 2–14.
†$P < .001$ age 0–1 vs age 2–14, and age 15–17 vs age 2–14.
‡Insufficient data for interpretation according to age and sex.
DVT, deep venous thrombosis; PE, pulmonary embolism; VTE, venous thromboembolic disease.
From Stein P, Kayali F, Olson R: Incidence of venous thromboembolism in infants and children: Data from the National Hospital Discharge Survey. *J Pediatr* 2004;145:564.

Pediatric autopsy reviews have estimated the incidence between 1% and 4%. Not all of these embolic findings were clinically significant. Thromboembolic pulmonary disease is often unrecognized and ante-mortem studies may underestimate the true incidence. Pediatric deaths from isolated pulmonary emboli are rare. Most thromboemboli are related to central venous catheters. The source of the emboli may be lower or upper extremity veins as well as the pelvis and right heart. The most common location for an embolus unassociated with the presence of an indwelling venous catheter is the lower extremity.

PATHOPHYSIOLOGY. Favorable conditions for thrombus formation include injury to the vessel endothelium, hemostasis, and hypercoagulability. Once an embolus develops and travels to the pulmonary circulation, symptoms of presentation are largely attributable to unequal ventilation and perfusion. The occlusion of the involved vessel prevents perfusion of distal alveolar units, thereby creating an increase in dead space and hypoxia with an elevated a-A O_2 gradient. Most patients are hypocarbic secondary to hyperventilation, which often persists even when oxygenation is optimized. Abnormalities of oxygenation and ventilation are likely to be less significant in the pediatric population, possibly owing to less underlying cardiopulmonary disease and greater reserve. The vascular supply to lung tissue is abundant and pulmonary infarction is unusual with pulmonary embolus but may result from distal arterial occlusion and alveolar hemorrhage. In rare instances of death from massive pulmonary embolus, marked increases in pulmonary vascular resistance and heart failure are usually present. Most of these severe outcomes are expectedly found in those with pre-existing cardiopulmonary disease.

CLINICAL MANIFESTATIONS. Presentation is variable and many pulmonary emboli are silent. Rarely, PE presents with cardiopulmonary failure. Children are more likely to have underlying disease processes or risk factors but might still present asymptomatically with small emboli. Common symptoms and signs of PE include hypoxia (cyanosis), tachypnea, dyspnea, cough, diaphoresis, and chest pain. Localized crackles may occasionally be appreciated on examination. These are nonspecific complaints and may be attributed to an underlying disease process or an unrelated/incorrect diagnosis in many cases. A high level of clinical suspicion is required as the diagnosis of pulmonary embolus is infrequently considered in children. A large number of diagnoses can present with similar symptoms. Therefore, confirmatory testing should follow a clinical diagnosis of PE.

LABORATORY FINDINGS AND DIAGNOSIS. Radiographic images of the chest are often normal. Any abnormalities found on chest radiograph are likely to be nonspecific. Patients with septic emboli may have multiple areas of nodularity and cavitation, which are typically located peripherally in both lung fields. Many patients with PE have hypoxemia. The alveolar-arterial oxygen tension difference or a-A gradient is more sensitive in detecting gas exchange derangements. A review of complete blood count (CBC), urinalysis, and coagulation profile is warranted. Prothrombotic diseases should be highly suspected on the basis of past medical or family history; therefore, additional laboratory evaluations include fibrinogen assays, protein C, protein S, and antithrombin III studies and analysis for factor V Leiden mutation as well as evaluation for lupus anticoagulant and anticardiolipin antibodies.

Electrocardiographs may reveal ST segment changes or evidence of pulmonary hypertension with right ventricular failure (cor pulmonale). These changes are nonspecific and nondiagnostic. Echocardiograms may be warranted to assess ventricular size and function. A transthoracic echocardiogram is required if there is any suspicion of intracardiac thrombi or endocarditis.

Noninvasive venous ultrasound with Doppler flow can be used to confirm DVT in the lower extremities; ultrasound may not detect thrombi in the upper extremities or pelvis. In patients with significant venous thrombosis, D-dimers are usually elevated. When a high level of suspicion exists, confirmatory testing with venography should be pursued. DVT can be recurrent and multifocal and may lead to repeated episodes of pulmonary embolism.

Although a ventilation-perfusion (V-Q) radionuclide scan is a noninvasive and potentially sensitive method of pulmonary embolus detection, the interpretation of V-Q scans is potentially problematic. Helical or spiral CT with intravenous contrast is valuable and the diagnostic test of choice to detect a PE. Specificity exceeds 90%. CT studies detect emboli in lobar and segmental vessels with acceptable sensitivities. Poorer sensitivities may be encountered when evaluating the subsegmental pulmonary vasculature. Pulmonary angiography is the gold standard for diagnosis of PE, but with multidetector spiral CT angiography, it is not necessary except in unusual cases.

TREATMENT. Initial treatment should always be directed toward stabilization of the patient. Careful approaches to ventilation, fluid resuscitation, and inotropic support are always indicated, as improvement in 1 area of decompensation can often exacerbate coexisting pathology.

After the patient with a PE has been stabilized, the next therapeutic approach is anticoagulation. Evaluations for prothrombotic disease must precede anticoagulation. Treatment is generally initiated with heparin. Anticoagulation is usually achieved when the activated partial thromboplastin time (PTT) is 1.5–2 times the control. Long-term therapy with heparin should be avoided whenever possible. Complications of heparin include bleeding and acquired thrombocytopenia.

Heparin therapy continues for several days before beginning oral therapy with warfarin. Anticoagulation may be required for 3–6 mo in the setting of acute thromboembolic disease. Longer treatment is indicated in those patients with ongoing thrombotic disease. Coagulation profiles are obtained regularly to guide warfarin and heparin therapies.

In adults, low molecular weight (LMW) heparin is considered equivalent to therapy with heparin. A longer half-life allows discontinuous dosing and effectiveness appears comparable. Minimal monitoring is involved with drug administration. Other advantages may include decreased risks of both osteoporosis and thrombocytopenia. At this time, LMW heparin is being used in many pediatric patients.

Thrombolytic therapy can be combined with anticoagulants in the early stages of treatment. Thrombolytic agents include urokinase, streptokinase, and recombinant tissue plasminogen activator. Combined therapy may reduce the incidences of progressive thromboembolism, pulmonary embolus, and postphlebitic syndrome. Although mortality rate appears to be unaffected by additional therapies, the additional risk of hemorrhage limits the use of combination therapy in all but the most compromised patients. The use of thrombolytic agents in patients with active bleeding, recent cerebrovascular accidents, or trauma is contraindicated.

Surgical embolectomy is invasive and associated with significant mortality. Its application should be limited to those with persistent hemodynamic compromise refractory to standard therapy.

PROGNOSIS. Mortality in pediatric patients with PE is likely to be attributable to an underlying disease process rather than to the embolus itself. Conditions with a poorer prognosis include malignancy, infection, and cardiac disease. The mortality rate in children from PE is 2.2%. Recurrent thromboembolic disease may complicate recovery. The practitioner must conduct an extensive evaluation for underlying pathology so as to prevent progressive disease. Postphlebitic syndrome is another recognized complication of pediatric thrombotic disease. Venous valvular damage can be initiated by the presence of DVT and lead to persistent venous hypertension with ambulation and valvular reflux. Symptoms include edema, pain, increases in pigmentation, and ulcerations. Affected pediatric patients may suffer lifelong disability.

Andrew M, David M, Adams M, et al: Venous thromboembolic complications (VTE) in children: First analysis of the Canadian registry of VTE. *Blood* 1994;83:1251–1257.

Bonduel M, Hepner M, Sciuccati G, et al: Prothrombotic abnormalities in children with venous thromboembolism. *J Pediatr Hematol Oncol* 2000;22:66–72.

Chan AK, Deveber G, Monagle P, et al: Venous thrombosis in children. *J Thromb Haemost* 2003;1:1443–1455.

Goldhaber SZ: Pulmonary embolism. *Lancet* 2004;363:1295–1305.

Holzer R, Peart I, Ciotti G, et al: Successful treatment with rTPA. *Pediatr Cardiol* 2002;23:548–552.

Hull RD: Diagnosing pulmonary embolism with improved certainty and simplicity. *JAMA* 2006;295:213–215.

Johnson AS, Bolte RG: Pulmonary embolism in the pediatric patient. *Pediatr Emerg Care* 2004;20:555–560.

Manco-Johnson MJ, Nuss R, Hays T, et al: Combined thrombolytic and anticoagulant therapy for venous thrombosis in children. *J Pediatr* 2000;136:446–453.

Perrier A, Roy PM, Sanchez O, et al: Multidetector-row computed tomography in suspected pulmonary embolism. *N Engl J Med* 2005;352:1760–1768.

Robinson GV: Pulmonary embolism in hospital practice. *Br Med J* 2006;332:156–160.

Roy PM, Colombet I, Durieux P, et al: Systemic review and meta-analysis of strategies for the diagnosis of suspected pulmonary embolism. *Br Med J* 2005;331:259–263.

Stein PD, Fowler SE, Goodman LR: Multidetector computed tomography for acute pulmonary embolism. *N Engl J Med* 2006;354:2317–2326.

Stein P, Kayali F, Olson R: Incidence of venous thromboembolism in infants and children: Data from the National Hospital Discharge Survey. *J Pediatr* 2004;145:563–565.

van Belle A, Buller HR, Huisman MV, et al: Christopher Study Investigators: Effectiveness of managing suspected pulmonary embolism using an algorithm combining clinical probability, D-Dimer testing, and computed tomography. *JAMA* 2006;295:172–179.

Wells PS, Anderson DR, Rodger M, et al: Evaluation of d-dimer in the diagnosis of suspected deep-vein thrombosis. *N Engl J Med* 2003;349:1227–1234.

Wong KS, Lin TY, Huang YC, et al: Clinical and radiographic spectrum of septic pulmonary embolism. *Arch Dis Child* 2002;87:312–315.

406.2 • Pulmonary Hemorrhage and Hemoptysis

Pulmonary hemorrhage is a relatively uncommon but potentially fatal occurrence in pediatric practice. Its incidence may be significantly underestimated because many children and young

TABLE 406-3. Etiology of Pulmonary Hemorrhage (Hemoptysis)

FOCAL HEMORRHAGE
- Bronchitis and Bronchiectasis (especially CF related)
- Infection (acute or chronic)
- Tuberculosis
- Trauma
- Pulmonary arteriovenous malformation
- Foreign body (chronic)
- Neoplasm including hemangioma
- Pulmonary embolus with or without infarction

DIFFUSE HEMORRHAGE
- Idiopathic of infancy
- Congenital heart disease (including pulmonary hypertension, veno-occlusive disease, CHF)
- Prematurity
- Cow's milk hyperreactivity (Heiner syndrome)
- Goodpasture syndrome
- Collagen vascular diseases (SLE, rheumatoid arthritis)
- Henoch-Schönlein purpura and vasculitic disorders
- Granulomatous disease (Wegener)
- Celiac disease
- Coagulopathy (congenital or acquired)
- Malignancy
- Immunodeficiency
- Exogenous toxins
- Idiopathic pulmonary hemosiderosis
- Tuberous sclerosis
- Lymphangiomyomatosis or lymphangioleiomyomatosis
- Physical injury or abuse

CF, cystic fibrosis; CHF, coronary heart failure; SLE, systemic lupus erythematosus.

adults swallow rather than expectorate mucus, which may prevent recognition of hemoptysis, the primary presenting symptom of the disorder. Further, diffuse, slow bleeding in the lower airways may become severe and present with anemia, fatigue, or respiratory compromise without the patient ever experiencing episodes of hemoptysis. Hemoptysis must always be separated from episodes of hemetemesis or epistaxis, as all can present similarly in the young patient.

ETIOLOGY. Conditions that can present with pulmonary hemorrhage or hemoptysis in children are found in Table 406-3. The chronic presence (opposed to an acute presence) of a foreign body can lead to inflammation and/or infection, thereby inducing hemorrhage. Although acute infections such as bronchitis or bronchopneumonia can cause hemorrhage, more commonly, hemorrhage is a reflection of chronic inflammation and infection as seen in cystic fibrosis with bronchiectasis or in tuberculosis with cavitary disease. Other relatively common etiologies include congenital heart disease and trauma. Traumatic irritation or damage of the airway is often accidental in nature. Bleeding can also be related to instrumentation of the airway as is commonly seen in a child with a tracheostomy. It is important to note, however, that children who have been victims of nonaccidental trauma or deliberate suffocation can also be found to have blood in the mouth or airway. Less commonly, syndromes associated with vasculitic, autoimmune, and idiopathic disorders can be associated with diffuse alveolar hemorrhage (DAH). The mechanisms of DAH are multiple and are discussed further in Chapter 405.

Acute idiopathic pulmonary hemorrhage (AIPH) occurs in young infants as a distinct entity, but the disorders in Table 406-3 must also be considered.

EPIDEMIOLOGY. The frequency with which pulmonary hemorrhage occurs in the pediatric population is difficult to define. This difficulty is largely related to the variability in disease presentation. Chronic bronchiectases as seen in cystic fibrosis or ciliary dyskinesia can cause hemoptysis but usually in children >10 yr of age. AIPH is defined as evidence of blood in the airway, age ≤ 1 yr, no medical conditions predisposing to pulmonary hemorrhage, and severe respiratory distress leading to respiratory failure. This entity may be more common than previously thought. Most cases are idiopathic, but some have been associated with von Willebrand disease. There is no association between the disorder and house contamination with molds.

PATHOPHYSIOLOGY. Pulmonary hemorrhage can be localized or diffuse. Focal hemorrhage from an isolated bronchial lesion is often secondary to infection or chronic inflammation. Erosion through a chronically inflamed airway into the adjacent bronchial artery is a mechanism for potentially massive hemorrhage. Bleeding from such a lesion is more likely to be bright red, brisk, and secondary to enlarged bronchial arteries and systemic arterial pressures. The severity of more diffuse hemorrhage can be difficult to ascertain. The rate of blood loss may be insufficient to reach the proximal airways. As such, the patient may present without hemoptysis. The diagnosis of pulmonary hemorrhage is generally achieved by finding evidence of blood or hemosiderin in the lung. Within 48–72 hr of an episode of bleeding, alveolar macrophages convert the iron from erythrocytes into hemosiderin. It may take weeks to clear these hemosiderin-laden macrophages completely from the alveolar spaces. This fact may allow differentiation between acute and chronic hemorrhage. Hemorrhage is often followed by the influx of neutrophils and other proinflammatory mediators. With repeated or chronic hemorrhage, pulmonary fibrosis can become a prominent pathologic finding.

CLINICAL MANIFESTATIONS. The severity of patients presenting with hemoptysis and pulmonary hemorrhage is highly variable. Older children and young adults with a focal hemorrhage may complain of warmth or a "bubbling" sensation in the chest wall. This can occasionally aid the clinician in locating the area involved. Rapid and large volume blood loss presents with symptoms of cyanosis, respiratory distress, and shock. Chronic, subclinical blood loss may present with anemia, fatigue, dyspnea, or altered activity tolerance. Less commonly, patients present with persistent infiltrates on chest radiograph or symptoms of chronic illness such as failure to thrive.

LABORATORY FINDINGS AND DIAGNOSIS. Every patient with suspected hemorrhage should have a laboratory evaluation with CBC and coagulation studies. The CBC finding may demonstrate a microcytic, hypochromic anemia. Other laboratory findings are highly dependent on the underlying diagnosis. A urinalysis may show evidence of nephritis in patients with concomitant pulmonary and renal disease. The classic finding, which defines pulmonary hemorrhage, is that of hemosiderin-laden macrophages in pulmonary secretions. These can be obtained by sputum analysis with Prussian blue staining. Chest x-rays may demonstrate fluffy bilateral densities, as seen in AIPH of infancy (Fig. 406-1). Alveolar infiltrates on chest radiograph may be seen as a representation of recent bleeding, but the absence of such an infiltrate does not rule out a hemorrhage. Infiltrates, when present, are often symmetric and diffuse. CT may be indicated to assess for underlying disease processes.

Flexible bronchoscopy with bronchoalveolar lavage is frequently utilized to obtain pulmonary secretions in a child or young adult who is not able to expectorate secretions. Lung biopsy is rarely necessary unless bleeding is chronic or an etiology is unavailable by other methods. Pulmonary function testing, including a determination of gas exchange, is important to assess the severity of the ventilatory defect. In older children, spirometry may demonstrate evidence of predominantly obstructive disease in the acute period. Restrictive disease secondary to fibrosis is typically seen with more chronic disease.

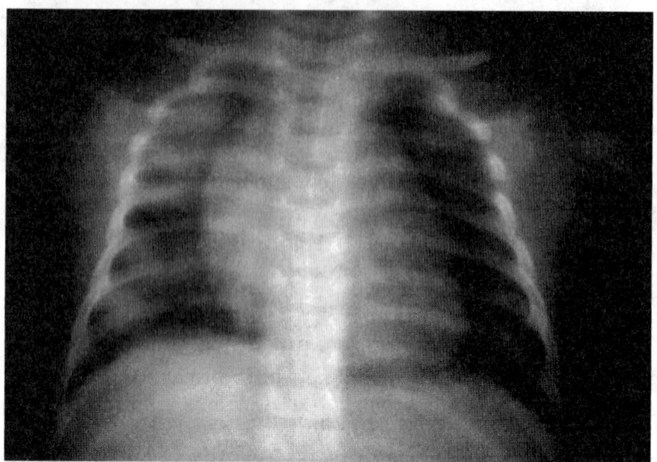

Figure 406-1. Radiographic appearance of acute idiopathic pulmonary hemorrhage in infancy. (From Brown CM, Redd SC, Damon SA; Centers for Disease Control and Prevention (CDC): Acute idiopathic pulmonary hemorrhage among infants: Recommendations from the Working Group for Investigation and Surveillance. *MMWR Recomm Rep* 2004;53:1–12.)

TREATMENT. In the setting of massive blood loss, volume resuscitation and transfusion of blood products are necessary. Maintenance of adequate ventilation and circulatory function are crucial. Rigid bronchoscopy may be utilized for removal of debris or the application of topical vasoconstrictive agents. Ideally, treatment is directed at the specific pathologic process responsible for the hemorrhage. When bronchiectasis is a known entity and a damaged artery can be localized, bronchial artery embolization is often the therapy of choice. If embolization fails, total or partial lobectomy may be required. In circumstances of diffuse hemorrhage, corticosteroids and other immunosuppressive agents have been shown to be of benefit. Prognosis depends largely on the underlying disease process.

Brown CM, Redd SC, Damon SA: Centers for Disease Control and Prevention (CDC): Acute idiopathic pulmonary hemorrhage among infants: Recommendations from the Working Group for Investigation and Surveillance. *MMWR Recomm Rep* 2004;53:1–12.

Centers for Disease Control and Prevention (CDC): Investigation of acute idiopathic pulmonary hemorrhage among infants—Massachusetts, December 2002–June 2003. *MMWR Morb Mortal Wkly Rep* 2004;53:817–820.

Coss-Bu JA, Sachdeva RC, Bricker JT, et al: Hemoptysis: A 10-year retrospective study. *Pediatrics* 1997;100:E7.

Cottin V, Chinet T, Lavolé A, et al: Pulmonary arteriovenous malformations in hereditary hemorrhagic telagiectasia. A series of 126 patients. *Medicine* 2007;86:1–17.

Godfrey S: Pulmonary hemorrhage/hemoptysis in children. *Pediatr Pulmonol* 2004;37;476–484.

Chapter 407 ■ Atelectasis

Ranna A. Rozenfeld

Atelectasis, the incomplete expansion or complete collapse of air-bearing tissue, is common in infants and children. Atelectasis results from obstruction of air intake into the alveolar sacs. Segmental, lobar, or whole lung collapse is associated with the absorption of air contained in the alveoli, which are no longer ventilated.

PATHOPHYSIOLOGY. The causes of atelectasis can be divided into five groups (Table 407-1). Viral infections in young children, specifically respiratory syncytial virus (see Chapter 257), can cause multiple areas of atelectasis. Mucous plugs from whatever etiology are a common predisposing factor to atelectasis. Massive collapse of one or both lungs is most often a postoperative complication but occasionally results from other causes, such as trauma, asthma, pneumonia, tension pneumothorax (see Chapter 410), aspiration of foreign material (see Chapters 384 and 394), paralysis, or after extubation. Massive atelectasis is usually produced by a combination of factors, including immobilization or decreased use of the diaphragm and the respiratory muscles, obstruction of the bronchial tree, and abolition of the cough reflex.

CLINICAL MANIFESTATIONS. Symptoms vary with the cause and extent of the atelectasis. A small area is likely to be asymptomatic. When a large area of previously normal lung becomes atelectatic, especially when it does so suddenly, dyspnea accompanied by rapid shallow respirations, tachycardia, cough, and often cyanosis occurs. If the obstruction is removed, the symptoms disappear rapidly. Although it was once believed that atelectasis alone can cause fever, studies have shown no association between atelectasis and fever. Physical findings include limitation of chest excursion, decreased breath sound intensity, and coarse crackles. Breath sounds are decreased or absent over extensive atelectatic areas.

Massive pulmonary atelectasis usually presents with dyspnea, cyanosis, and tachycardia. An affected child is extremely anxious and, if old enough, complains of chest pain. The chest appears flat on the affected side, where decreased respiratory excursion, dullness to percussion, and feeble or absent breath sounds are also noted. Postoperatively, atelectasis usually presents within 24 hr after operation but may not occur for several days.

Acute lobar collapse is a frequent occurrence in patients receiving intensive care. If undetected, it can lead to impaired gas exchange, secondary infection, and subsequent pulmonary fibrosis. Initially, hypoxemia may result from ventilation-perfusion mismatch. In contrast to adult patients in whom the lower lobes and, in particular, the left lower lobe are most often involved, 90% of cases in children involve the upper lobes and 63% involve the right upper lobe. There is also a high incidence of upper lobe atelectasis and especially right upper lobe collapse in neonatal

TABLE 407-1. Anatomic Causes of Atelectasis

CAUSE	CLINICAL EXAMPLES
External compression on the pulmonary parenchyma	Pleural effusion, pneumothorax, intrathoracic tumors, diaphragmatic hernia
Endobronchial obstruction completely obstructing the ingress of air	Enlarged lymph node, tumor, cardiac enlargement, foreign body, mucoid plug, broncholithiasis
Intraluminal obstruction of a bronchus	Foreign body, granulomatous tissue, tumor, secretions, including mucous plugs, bronchiectasis, pulmonary abscess, asthma, chronic bronchitis, acute laryngotracheobronchitis
Intrabronchiolar obstruction	Bronchiolitis, interstitial pneumonitis, asthma
Respiratory compromise or paralysis	Neuromuscular abnormalities, osseous deformities, overly restrictive casts and surgical dressings, defective movement of the diaphragm, or restriction of respiratory effort

intensive care units. This may be due to the endotracheal tube moving into the right main stem bronchus and obstructing or causing inflammation of the bronchus to the right upper lobe.

DIAGNOSIS. The diagnosis of atelectasis can usually be established by chest radiographic examination. Typical findings include volume loss and displacement of fissures. Atypical presentations include atelectasis presenting as a masslike opacity and atelectasis in an unusual location. Lobar atelectasis may be associated with pneumothorax.

In asthmatic children, chest radiography demonstrates an abnormality rate of 44%, compared with a thorax high-resolution CT (HRCT) scan abnormality rate of 75%. Children with asthma and atelectasis have an increased incidence of right middle lobe syndrome, acute asthma exacerbations, pneumonia, and upper airway infections.

In foreign body aspiration, atelectasis is one of the most common radiographic findings. The site of atelectasis usually indicates the site of the foreign body (see Chapter 374.1). Atelectasis is more common when patients have a delay in diagnosis of >2 wk duration.

Bronchoscopic examination reveals a collapsed main bronchus when the obstruction is at the tracheobronchial junction and may also disclose the nature of the obstruction.

Massive pulmonary atelectasis is generally diagnosed by chest radiograph. Typical findings include elevation of the diaphragm, narrowing of the intercostal spaces, and displacement of the mediastinal structures and heart toward the affected side (Fig. 407-1).

TREATMENT. Treatment depends on the cause of the collapse. If effusion or pneumothorax is responsible, the external compression must first be removed. Often vigorous efforts at cough, deep breathing, and percussion will facilitate expansion. Aspiration with sterile tracheal catheters may facilitate removal of mucous plugs. Continuous positive airway pressure (CPAP) may improve atelectasis.

Bronchoscopic examination is immediately indicated if atelectasis is the result of a foreign body or any other bronchial obstruction that can be relieved. For bilateral atelectasis, bronchoscopic aspiration should also be performed immediately. It is also indicated when an isolated area of atelectasis persists for several weeks. If no anatomic basis for atelectasis is found and no material can be obtained by suctioning, the introduction of a small amount of saline followed by suctioning allows recovery of bronchial secretions for culture and, possibly, for cytologic examination. Frequent changes in the child's position, deep breathing, and chest physiotherapy may be beneficial. Oxygen therapy is indicated when there is dyspnea or desaturation. Intermittent positive pressure breathing and incentive spirometry are recommended when atelectasis does not improve after chest physiotherapy.

In some conditions, such as asthma, bronchodilator and corticosteroid treatment may accelerate atelectasis clearance. Recombinant human DNase (rhDNase), which is approved only for the treatment of cystic fibrosis, has been used off label for patients without cystic fibrosis who have persistent atelectasis. This product reduces the viscosity of purulent bronchial debris. In patients with acute severe asthma, diffuse airway plugging with thick viscous secretions frequently occurs, with the resulting atelectasis often refractory to conventional therapy. rhDNase has been used in both nebulized form for nonintubated patients with acute asthma as well as intratracheally for atelectasis in intubated asthmatics, with resolution of atelectasis unresponsive to conventional asthma therapies.

Lobar atelectasis in cystic fibrosis is discussed in Chapter 400.

Atelectasis can occur in patients with neuromuscular diseases. These patients tend to have ineffective cough and difficulty expelling respiratory tract secretions, which leads to pneumonia and atelectasis. Several devices are available to assist these patients, including intermittent positive pressure breathing, In-Exsufflator, and noninvasive bilevel positive pressure ventilation via nasal mask or full-face mask. Patients with neuromuscular disease who have undergone surgery are at substantial risk of postoperative atelectasis and subsequent pneumonia. **Migrating atelectasis** in the newborn infant is a rare and unique presentation and may be secondary to neuromuscular disease.

There is an association between the development of lobar collapse and the requirement for mechanical ventilation. Although lobar collapse is rarely a cause of long-term morbidity, its occurrence may necessitate the prolongation of mechanical ventilation or reintubation. In patients who are ventilated, positive end-expiratory pressure (PEEP) or CPAP is generally indicated.

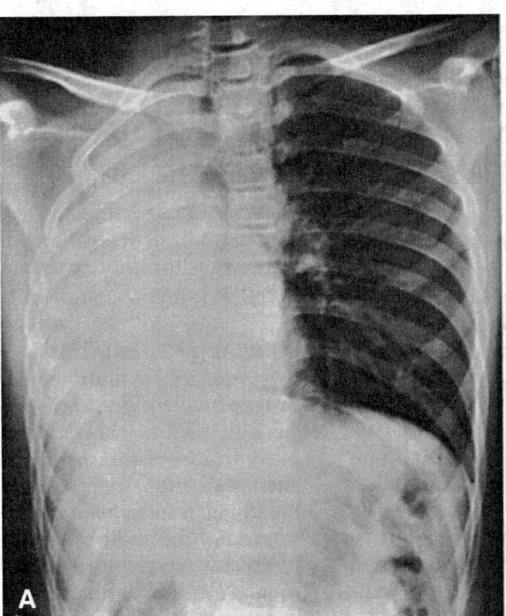

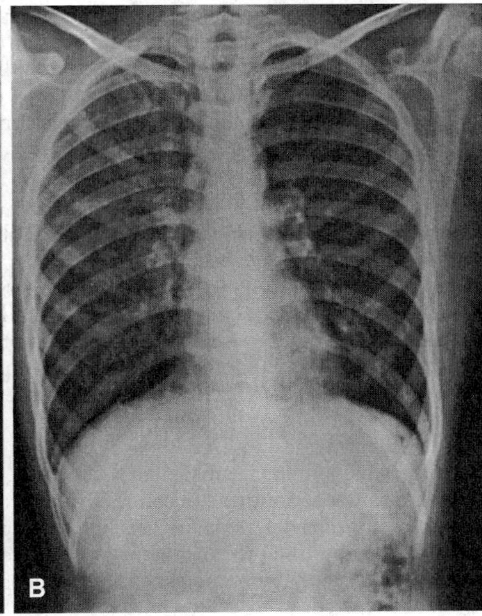

Figure 407-1. *A,* Massive atelectasis of the right lung. The patient has asthma. The heart and other mediastinal structures shift to the right during the atelectatic phase. *B,* Comparison study after re-aeration subsequent to bronchoscopic removal of a mucous plug from the right main stem bronchus.

Ashizawa K, Hayashi K, Aso N, et al: Lobar atelectasis: Diagnostic pitfalls on chest radiography. *Br J Radiol* 2001;74:89–97.

Birnkrant DJ: The assessment and management of the respiratory complications of pediatric neuromuscular diseases. *Clin Pediatr* 2002;41:301–308.

Durward A, Forte V, Shemie SD: Resolution of mucus plugging and atelectasis after intratracheal rhDNase therapy in a mechanically ventilated child with refractory status asthmaticus. *Crit Care Med* 2000;28:560–562.

Engoren M: Lack of association between atelectasis and fever. *Chest* 1995;107:81–84.

Girardi G, Contador AM, Castro-Rodriguez JA: Two new radiological findings to improve the diagnosis of bronchial foreign-body aspiration in children. *Pediatr Pulmonol* 2004;38:261–264.

Miske LJ, Hickey EM, Kolb SM, et al: Use of the mechanical In-Exsufflator in pediatric patients with neuromuscular disease and impaired cough. *Chest* 2004;125:1406–1412.

Nuhoglu Y, Bahceciler N, Yuksel M, et al: Thorax high resolution computerized tomography findings in asthmatic children with unusual clinical manifestations. *Ann Allergy Asthma Immunol* 1999;82:311–314.

Scolieri P, Adappa ND, Coticchia JM: Value of rigid bronchoscopy in the management of critically ill children with acute lung collapse. *Pediatr Emerg Care* 2004;20:384–386.

Thomas K, Habibi P, Britto J, et al: Distribution and pathophysiology of acute lobar collapse in the pediatric intensive care unit. *Crit Care Med* 1999;27:1594–1597.

Tokar B, Ozkan R, Ilhan H: Tracheobronchial foreign bodies in children: Importance of accurate history and plain chest radiography in delayed presentation. *Clin Radiol* 2004;59:609–615.

Tsai SL, Crain EF, Silver EJ, et al: What can we learn from chest radiographs in hypoxemic asthmatics? *Pediatr Radiol* 2002;32:498–504.

Chapter 408 ■ Pulmonary Tumors

Susanna A. McColley

ETIOLOGY. Primary tumors of the lung are rare in children and adolescents. An accurate estimate of frequency is difficult because the literature is limited primarily to case reports and case series. A high incidence of "inflammatory pseudotumors" further clouds the statistics. **Bronchial adenoma** and **carcinoid** are the most common primary tumors. Metastatic lesions are the most common forms of pulmonary malignancy in children; primary processes include Wilms tumor, osteogenic sarcoma, and hepatoblastoma (see Part XXI). Adenocarcinoma and undifferentiated histology are the most common pathologic findings in primary lung cancer; pulmonary blastoma is rarer and frequently occurs in the setting of cystic lung disease. Mediastinal involvement with lymphoma is more common than primary pulmonary malignancies.

CLINICAL MANIFESTATIONS AND EVALUATION. Pulmonary tumors may present with fever, hemoptysis, wheezing, cough, pleural effusion, chest pain, dyspnea, or recurrent or persistent pneumonia or atelectasis. Tumors may be suspected on plain chest x-ray; CT scanning of the chest is necessary for precise anatomic definition. Bronchial tumors are occasionally diagnosed during fiberoptic bronchoscopy performed for persistent or recurrent pulmonary infiltrates or for hemoptysis.

Patients with symptoms or with x-ray or other laboratory findings suggesting pulmonary malignancy should be evaluated carefully for a tumor at another site before surgical excision is carried out. Isolated primary lesions and isolated metastatic lesions discovered long after the primary tumor has been removed are best treated by excision. The prognosis varies and depends on the type of tumor involved.

Eggli KD, Newman B: Nodules, masses, and pseudomasses in the pediatric lung. *Radiol Clin North Am* 1993; 31:651–666.

Epstein DM, Aronchick JM: Lung cancer in childhood. *Med Pediatr Oncol* 1989;17:510–513.

Hancock BJ, Di Lorenzo M, Youssef S, et al: Childhood primary pulmonary neoplasms. *J Pediatr Surg* 1993;28:1133–1136.

Keita O, Lagrange JL, Michiels JF, et al: Primary bronchogenic squamous cell carcinoma in children: Report of a case and review of the literature. *Med Pediatr Oncol* 1995;24:50–52.

McCahon E: Lung tumours in children. *Pediatr Respir Rev* 2006;7(3): 191–196. E-pub 2006; Aug 4.

Roviaro Gc, Varoli F, Zannini P, et al: Lung cancer in the young. *Chest* 1985;87:456–459.

Tian DL, Liu HX, Zhang L, et al: Surgery for young patients with lung cancer. *Lung Cancer* 2003;42:215–220.

Chapter 409 ■ Pleurisy, Pleural Effusions, and Empyema

Glenna B. Winnie

Pleurisy or inflammation of the pleura is often accompanied by an effusion. The most common cause of pleural effusion in children is bacterial pneumonia (see Chapter 397); heart failure (see Chapter 442), rheumatologic causes, and metastatic intrathoracic malignancy are the next most common causes. A variety of other diseases account for the remaining cases, including tuberculosis (see Chapter 212), lupus erythematosus (see Chapter 157), aspiration pneumonitis (see Chapter 394), uremia, pancreatitis, subdiaphragmatic abscess, and rheumatoid arthritis. Males and females are affected equally.

Inflammatory processes in the pleura are usually divided into 3 types: dry or plastic, serofibrinous or serosanguineous, and purulent pleurisy or empyema.

409.1 • Dry or Plastic Pleurisy

ETIOLOGY. Plastic pleurisy may be associated with acute bacterial or viral pulmonary infections or may develop during the course of an acute upper respiratory tract illness. The condition is also associated with tuberculosis and connective tissue diseases such as rheumatic fever.

PATHOLOGY AND PATHOGENESIS. The process is usually limited to the visceral pleura, with small amounts of yellow serous fluid and adhesions between the pleural surfaces. In tuberculosis, the adhesions develop rapidly and the pleura are often thickened. Occasionally, fibrin deposition and adhesions are severe enough to produce a fibrothorax that markedly inhibits the excursions of the lung.

CLINICAL MANIFESTATIONS. The primary disease often overshadows signs and symptoms. Pain is the principal symptom, and is *exaggerated by deep breathing, coughing, and straining.* Occasionally, pleural pain is described as a dull ache, which is less likely to vary with breathing. The pain is often localized over the chest wall and is referred to the shoulder or the back. Pain with breathing is responsible for grunting and guarding of respirations, and the child often lies on the affected side in an attempt to decrease respiratory excursions. Early in the illness, a leathery, rough, inspiratory and expiratory friction rub may be audible, but this usually disappears rapidly. Occasionally, increased dullness on percussion and decreased breath sounds are heard if the layer of exudate is thick. Pleurisy may be asymptomatic. Chronic pleurisy is occasionally encountered with conditions such as atelectasis, pulmonary abscess, connective tissue diseases, and tuberculosis.

LABORATORY FINDINGS. Plastic pleurisy may be detected on radiographs as a diffuse haziness at the pleural surface or a dense, sharply demarcated shadow. The latter finding may be indistinguishable from small amounts of pleural exudate. Chest radiograph may be normal, but ultrasonography or CT will be positive.

DIFFERENTIAL DIAGNOSIS. Plastic pleurisy must be distinguished from other diseases, such as epidemic pleurodynia, trauma to the rib cage (rib fracture), lesions of the dorsal root ganglia, tumors of the spinal cord, herpes zoster, gallbladder disease, and trichinosis. Even if evidence of pleural fluid is not found on physical or radiographic examination, a CT or ultrasound guided pleural tap in suspected cases often results in the recovery of a small amount of exudate, which, when cultured, may reveal the underlying bacterial cause in patients with an acute pneumonia. Patients with pleurisy and pneumonia should always be screened for tuberculosis.

TREATMENT. Therapy should be aimed at the underlying disease. When pneumonia is present, neither immobilization of the chest with adhesive plaster nor therapy with drugs capable of suppressing the cough reflex is indicated. If pneumonia is not present or is under good therapeutic control, strapping of the chest to restrict expansion may afford relief from pain. Analgesia with nonsteroidal anti-inflammatory agents may be helpful.

409.2 • Serofibrinous or Serosanguineous Pleurisy

ETIOLOGY. Serofibrinous pleurisy is defined by a fibrinous exudate on the pleural surface and an exudative effusion of serous fluid into the pleural cavity. It is most frequently associated with infections of the lung or with inflammatory conditions of the abdomen or mediastinum. Less commonly, it is found with connective tissue diseases such as lupus erythematosus, periarteritis, or rheumatoid arthritis. On occasion, it is seen with primary or metastatic neoplasms of the lung, pleura, or mediastinum; tumors are commonly associated with a hemorrhagic pleurisy.

PATHOGENESIS. In health, pleural fluid originates from the capillaries of the parietal pleura and is absorbed from the pleural space via pleural stomas and the lymphatics of the parietal pleura. The rate of fluid formation is dictated by the Starling law, by which fluid movement is determined by the balance of hydrostatic and pressures in the pleural space and pulmonary capillary bed, and the permeability of the pleural membrane. Normally, only 4–12 mL of fluid is present in the pleural space, but if formation exceeds clearance, fluid accumulates. Pleural inflammation increases the permeability of the plural surface, with increased proteinaceous fluid formation; there may also be some obstruction to lymphatic absorption.

CLINICAL MANIFESTATIONS. Because serofibrinous pleurisy is often preceded by the plastic type, early signs and symptoms may be those of plastic pleurisy. As fluid accumulates, pleuritic pain may disappear and the patient may become asymptomatic if the effusion remains small, or there may be only signs and symptoms of the underlying disease. Large fluid collections may produce cough, dyspnea, retractions, tachypnea, orthopnea, or cyanosis. Physical findings depend to some degree on the amount of effusion. Dullness to flatness may be found on percussion. There are decreased or absent breath sounds, a diminution in tactile fremitus, a shift of the mediastinum away from the affected side, and, occasionally, fullness of the intercostal spaces. If the fluid is not loculated, these signs may shift with changes in position. In infants, physical signs are less definite. Instead of decreased or absent breath sounds, bronchial breathing may be heard. If extensive pneumonia is present, crackles and rhonchi may also be audible. Friction rubs are usually detected only during the early or late plastic stage. The process is usually unilateral.

LABORATORY FINDINGS. Radiographic examination shows a generally homogeneous density obliterating the normal markings of the underlying lung. Small effusions may cause obliteration of only the costophrenic or cardiophrenic angles or a widening of the interlobar septa. Examinations should be performed with the patient both supine and upright, to demonstrate a shift of the effusion with a change in position; the decubitus position may be helpful. Ultrasonographic examinations are useful, and may guide thoracentesis if the effusion is loculated. Examination of fluid is essential to differentiate exudates from transudates, and to determine the type of exudate (see Chapter 397). Depending on the clinical scenario, pleural fluid is sent for culture for bacterial, fungal, and mycobacterial cultures; antigen testing; Gram stain; and chemistries including protein, lactic dehydrogenase and glucose, amylase, specific gravity, total cell count and differential, cytologic examination, and pH. **Exudates** usually have at least one of the following: protein level >3.0 g/dL, with pleural fluid/serum protein ratio >0.5; pleural fluid lactic dehydrogenase values >200 IU/L; or fluid to serum lactic dehydrogenase ratio >0.6. A pH < 7.20 suggests an exudate. Glucose is usually <60 mg/dL in malignancy, rheumatoid disease, and tuberculosis; many small lymphocytes and pH < 7.20 suggest tuberculosis. The fluid of serofibrinous pleurisy is clear or slightly cloudy and contains relatively few leukocytes and, occasionally, some erythrocytes. Gram stain may occasionally show bacteria; however, acid-fast stain rarely demonstrates tubercle bacilli.

DIAGNOSIS AND DIFFERENTIAL DIAGNOSIS. Thoracentesis should be performed when pleural fluid is present or is suggested, unless the effusion is small and the patient has a classic appearing lobar pneumococcal pneumonia. Thoracentesis can differentiate serofibrinous pleurisy, empyema, hydrothorax, hemothorax, and chylothorax. Exudates are usually associated with an infectious process. In hydrothorax, the fluid has a specific gravity <1.015, and evaluation reveals only a few mesothelial cells rather than leukocytes. Chylothorax and hemothorax usually have fluid with a distinctive appearance, but differentiating serofibrinous from purulent pleurisy is impossible without microscopic examination of the fluid. Cytologic examination may reveal malignant cells. Serofibrinous fluid may rapidly become purulent.

COMPLICATIONS. Unless the fluid becomes purulent, it usually disappears relatively rapidly, particularly with appropriate treatment of bacterial pneumonia. It persists somewhat longer with tuberculosis and connective tissue diseases and may recur or remain for a long time with neoplasms. As the effusion is absorbed, adhesions often develop between the 2 layers of the pleura, but usually little or no functional impairment results. Pleural thickening may develop and is occasionally mistaken for small quantities of fluid or for persistent pulmonary infiltrates. Pleural thickening may persist for months, but the process usually disappears, leaving no residua.

TREATMENT. Therapy should address the underlying disease, although with large effusions, draining the fluid makes the patient more comfortable. When a diagnostic thoracentesis is performed, as much fluid as possible should be removed for therapeutic purposes. Rapid removal of ≥1 L of pleural fluid may be associated with the development of re-expansion pulmonary edema (see Chapter 393). If the underlying disease is adequately treated, further drainage is usually unnecessary, but if sufficient fluid reaccumulates to cause respiratory embarrassment, chest tube drainage should be performed. In older children with suspected parapneumonic effusion, tube thoracostomy is considered necessary if the pleural fluid pH is <7.20 or the pleural fluid glucose level is <50 mg/dL. If the fluid is clearly purulent, tube drainage is indicated. Systemic acidosis reduces the usefulness of pleural fluid pH measurements. Patients with pleural effusions may need analgesia, particularly after thoracentesis or insertion of a chest tube. Those with acute pneumonia may need supplemental oxygen in addition to specific antibiotic treatment.

409.3 • Purulent Pleurisy or Empyema

ETIOLOGY. Empyema is an accumulation of pus in the pleural space. It is most often associated with pneumonia due to *Streptococcus pneumoniae,* although *Staphylococcus aureus* is most common in developing nations and in post-traumatic empyema (see Chapter 397). The relative incidence of *Haemophilus influenzae* empyema has decreased since the introduction of Hib vaccination. Group A streptococcus, gram-negative organisms, tuberculosis, fungi, and malignancy are less common causes. The disease can also be produced by rupture of a lung abscess into the pleural space, by contamination introduced from trauma or thoracic surgery, or, rarely, by mediastinitis or the extension of intra-abdominal abscesses.

EPIDEMIOLOGY. Empyema is most frequently encountered in infants and preschool children. It occurs in 5–10% of children with bacterial pneumonia.

PATHOLOGY. Empyema has 3 stages: exudative, fibrinopurulent, and organizational. During the *exudative stage,* fibrinous exudate forms on the pleural surfaces. In the *fibrinopurulent stage,* fibrinous septae form, causing loculation of the fluid, with thickening of the parietal pleura. If the pus is not drained, it may dissect through the pleura into lung parenchyma, producing bronchopleural fistulas and pyopneumothorax, or into the abdominal cavity. Rarely, the pus dissects through the chest wall (i.e., empyema necessitatis). During the *organizational stage,* there is fibroblast proliferation, and pockets of loculated pus may develop into thick-walled abscess cavities or the lung may collapse and become surrounded by a thick, inelastic envelope (peel).

CLINICAL MANIFESTATIONS. The initial signs and symptoms are primarily those of bacterial pneumonia. Children treated inadequately or with inappropriate antibiotic agents may have an interval of a few days between the clinical pneumonia phase and the evidence of empyema. Most patients are febrile. In infants, there may be a moderate exacerbation of respiratory distress. The older child is likely to appear more ill and have greater respiratory difficulty. Physical findings are identical to those described for serofibrinous pleurisy, and the 2 conditions are differentiated only by thoracentesis, which should always be performed when empyema is suspected.

LABORATORY FINDINGS. Radiographically, all pleural effusions appear similar, but no shift of fluid with a change of position indicates a loculated empyema; this may be confirmed by ultrasonography or CT scan. The maximal amount of fluid obtainable should be withdrawn by thoracentesis and studied as described in Chapter 409.2. The effusion is empyema if bacteria are present on Gram stain, the pH is <7.20, and there are >100,000 neutrophils/μL. The appearance of pus produced by different organisms is not distinctive; cultures must always be obtained. In pneumococcal empyema the culture is positive in 58% of patients. In patients with negative culture for pneumococcus, the pneumococcal PCR is most helpful in making a diagnosis. Blood cultures have a high yield that might be higher than that of the pleural fluid. Leukocytosis and an elevated sedimentation rate may be found.

COMPLICATIONS. With staphylococcal infections, bronchopleural fistulas and pyopneumothorax commonly develop. Other local complications include purulent pericarditis, pulmonary abscesses, peritonitis secondary to rupture through the diaphragm, and osteomyelitis of the ribs. Septic complications such as meningitis, arthritis, and osteomyelitis may also occur. Septicemia is often encountered in *H. influenzae* and pneumococcal infections. The effusion may organize into a thick "peel," which may restrict lung expansion and be associated with persistent fever.

TREATMENT. Treatment options include antibiotics, thoracentesis, chest tube drainage with or without a fibrinolytic agent, video-assisted thoracoscopic surgery (VATS), or open decortication (see Chapter 397). If empyema is diagnosed early, thoracentesis and antibiotic treatment achieve a complete cure. When pus is obtained by thoracentesis, closed chest tube drainage should be instituted immediately and controlled by an underwater seal or continuous suction. A catheter with the largest possible internal diameter should be inserted; sometimes more than 1 tube is required to drain loculated areas. Closed drainage is usually continued for about 1 wk; chest tubes that are no longer draining should be removed. Multiple aspirations of the pleural cavity rather than closed continuous drainage should not be attempted.

Systemic antibiotic therapy is also required; the selection of the antibiotic should be based on the in vitro sensitivities of the responsible organism. See Chapters 180, 181, and 192 for treatment of infections by *Staphylococcus, Streptococcus pneumoniae,* and *H. influenzae,* respectively. With staphylococcal infections, resolution of the process is very slow, and systemic antibiotic therapy is required for 3–4 wk. Clinical response in nonstaphylococcal empyema is also slow, even with optimal treatment; there may be little improvement for as long as 2 wk. Instillation of antibiotics into the pleural cavity does not improve results obtained with systemic antibiotic therapy alone and is associated with local reactions.

Instillation of fibrinolytic agents into the pleural cavity may promote drainage, decrease fever, lessen need for surgical intervention, and shorten hospitalization; the optimal drug and dosage have not been determined. Streptokinase 15,000 U/kg in 50 mL of 0.9% saline daily for 3–5 days, and urokinase 40,000 U in 40 mL saline every 12 hr for 6 doses have been examined in randomized trials in children. There is a risk of anaphylaxis with streptokinase; both drugs can be associated with hemorrhage and other complications.

Extensive fibrinous changes may take place over the surface of the collapsed lungs, but surgical decortication procedures are rarely indicated. In the child who remains febrile and dyspneic >72 hr after initiation of therapy with intravenous antibiotics and thoracostomy tube drainage, surgical decortication via VATS or, less often, open thoracotomy may speed recovery. If pneumatoceles form, no attempt should be made to treat them surgically or by aspiration, unless they reach sufficient size to cause respiratory embarrassment or become secondarily infected. Pneumatoceles usually resolve spontaneously in time. The long-term clinical prognosis for adequately treated empyema is excellent, and follow-up pulmonary function studies suggest that residual restrictive disease is uncommon, with or without surgical intervention.

Jaffe A, Cohen G: Thoracic empyema: A role for primary video assisted thoracoscopic surgery? *Arch Dis Child* 2003;88:839–841.

Kohn GL, Walston C, Feldstein J, et al: Persistent abnormal lung function after childhood empyema. *Am J Respir Med* 2002;1:441–445.

Kurt BA, Winterhalter KM, Connors RH, et al: Therapy of parapneumonic effusions in children: video-assisted thoracoscopic surgery versus conventional thoracostomy drainage. *Pediatrics* 2006;118:e547–e553.

Le Monnier A, Carbonelle E, Zahar JR, et al: Microbiological diagnosis of empyma in children: comparative evaluations by culture, polymerase chain reaction, and pneumococcal antigen detection in pleural fluids. *CID* 2006;42:1135–1140.

Light RW: A new classification of parapneumonic effusions and empyema. *Chest* 1995;108:299–301.

Noppen M, DeWaele M, Li R, et al: Volume and cellular content of normal pleural fluid in humans examined by pleural lavage. *Am J Resp Crit Care Med* 2000;162:1023–1026.

Paganini H, Guinazu JR, Hernandez C, et al: Comparative analysis of outcome and clinical features in children with pleural empyema caused by penicillin-nonsusceptible and penicillin-susceptible Streptococcus pneumoniae. *Int J Infect Dis* 2001;5:86–88.

Redding GJ, Walund L, Walund D, et al: Lung function in children following empyema. *Am J Dis Child* 1990;144:1337–1342.

Singh M, Mathew JL, Chandra S, et al: Randomized controlled trial of intrapleural streptokinase in empyema thoracis in children. *Acta Paediatr* 2004;93:1443–1445.

Thompson AH, Hull J, Kumar MR, et al: Randomised trial of intrapleural urokinase in the treatment of childhood empyema. *Thorax* 2002; 57:343–347.

Yao CT, Wu JM, Liu CC, et al: Treatment of complicated parapneumonic pleural effusion with intrapleural streptokinase in children. *Chest* 2004;125:566–571.

Chapter 410 ■ Pneumothorax

Glenna B. Winnie

Pneumothorax is the accumulation of extrapulmonary air within the chest. It is uncommon during childhood. Most often, pneumothorax results from leakage of air from within the lung. Air leaks can be primary or secondary and can be spontaneous, traumatic, iatrogenic, or catamenial (Table 410-1). Pneumothorax in the neonatal period is also discussed in Chapter 101.13.

ETIOLOGY AND EPIDEMIOLOGY. A **primary spontaneous pneumothorax** occurs in someone without trauma or underlying lung disease. Spontaneous pneumothorax with or without exertion (Valsalva) occurs occasionally in teenagers and young adults, most frequently in males who are tall, thin, and thought to have subpleural blebs. Families in which many members have had spontaneous pneumothoraces, with the onset ranging from birth to adulthood, have been described. Patients with collagen synthesis defects such as Ehlers-Danlos disease (see Chapter 658) and Marfan syndrome (see Chapter 700) are unusually prone to the development of pneumothorax.

A pneumothorax arising as a complication of an underlying lung disorder but without trauma is a **secondary spontaneous pneumothorax.** Pneumothorax can occur in pneumonia, usually with empyema; it can also be secondary to pulmonary abscess, gangrene, infarct, rupture of a cyst or an emphysematous bleb (in asthma), or foreign bodies in the lung. In infant staphylococcal pneumonia, the incidence of pneumothorax is relatively high. It is found in ≈5% of hospitalized asthmatic children and usually resolves without treatment. Pneumothorax is a serious complication in cystic fibrosis (CF; see Chapter 400). Pneumothorax also

TABLE 410-1. Causes of Pneumothorax in Children

SPONTANEOUS
Primary idiopathic—usually resulting from ruptured subpleural
Secondary blebs
Congenital lung disease
Congenital cystic adenomatoid malformation
Bronchogenic cysts
Pulmonary hypoplasia
Conditions associated with increased intrathoracic pressure
Asthma
Bronchiolitis
Air-block syndrome in neonates
Cystic fibrosis
Airway foreign body
Infection
Pneumatocele
Lung abscess
Bronchopleural fistula
Diffuse lung disease
Langerhans cell histiocytosis
Tuberous sclerosis
Marfan syndrome
Ehlers-Danlos syndrome
Metastatic neoplasm—usually osteosarcoma (rare)
TRAUMATIC
Noniatrogenic
Penetrating trauma
Blunt trauma
Loud music (air pressure)
Iatrogenic
Thoracotomy
Thoracoscopy, thoracentesis
Tracheostomy
Tube or needle puncture
Mechanical ventilation

*Renal agenesis, diaphragmatic hernia, amniotic fluid leaks.
From Kuhn JP, Slovis TL, Haller JO: *Caffey's Pediatric Diagnostic Imaging*, vol 1, 10th ed. Philadelphia, Mosby, 2004, p 885.

occurs in patients with lymphoma or other malignancies, and in graft vs host disease with bronchiolitis obliterans.

External chest or abdominal blunt or penetrating trauma can tear a bronchus or abdominal viscus, with leakage of air into the pleural space. Ecstasy (methylenedioxymethamphetamine) abuse has been associated with pneumothorax.

Iatrogenic pneumothorax can complicate tracheotomy, subclavian line placement, thoracentesis, transbronchial biopsy, or other diagnostic or therapeutic procedures. Pneumothorax may also occur after acupuncture treatment.

Catamenial pneumothorax, an unusual condition that is, by definition, associated with menses, results from passage of intra-abdominal air through diaphragmatic defects.

Pneumothorax can be associated with a serous effusion (hydropneumothorax) or a purulent effusion (pyopneumothorax). Bilateral pneumothorax is rare beyond the neonatal period but has been reported after lung transplantation and with *Mycoplasma pneumoniae* infection and tuberculosis.

PATHOPHYSIOLOGY. The tendency of the lung to collapse, or elastic recoil, is balanced in the normal resting state by the inherent tendency of the chest wall to expand outward; this creates a negative pressure in the intrapleural space. When air enters the pleural space, the lung collapses. Hypoxemia occurs due to alveolar hypoventilation, ventilation-perfusion mismatch, and intrapulmonary shunt. In simple pneumothorax, intrapleural pressure is atmospheric, and the lung collapses up to 30%. In complicated, or tension, pneumothorax, continuing leak causes increasing positive pressure in the pleural space, with further compression of lung, shift of mediastinal structures toward the contralateral side, decreased venous return, and decreased cardiac output.

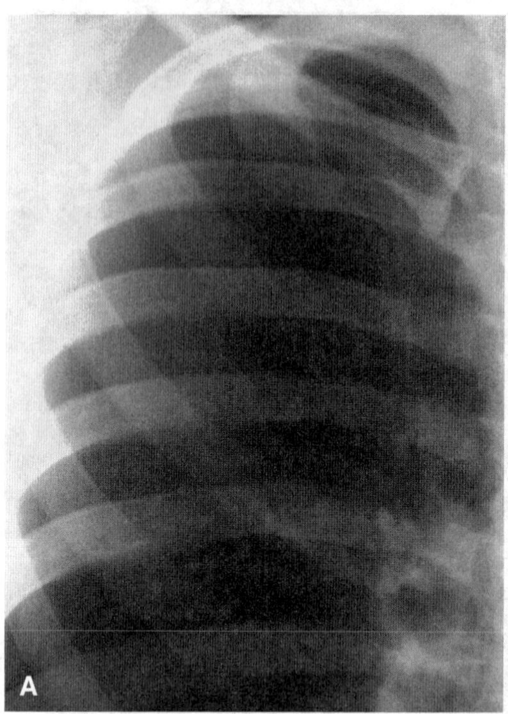

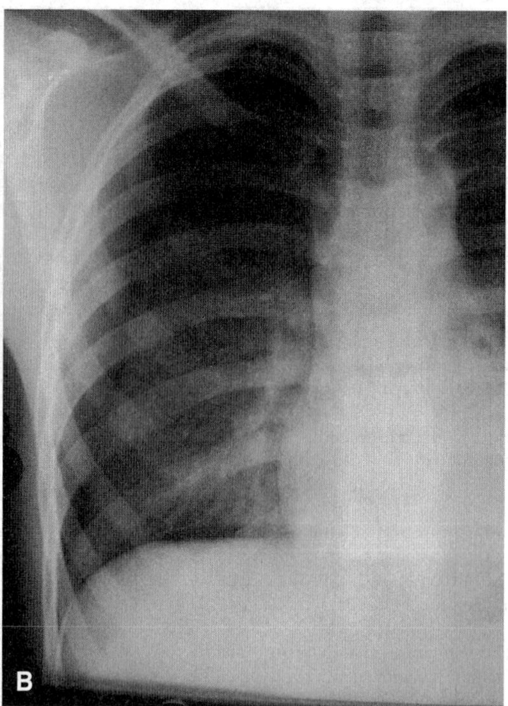

Figure 410-1. Utility of an expiratory film in detection of pneumothorax. *A*, Teenage boy with chest pain and subtle radiolucency laterally in the right upper lobe. The margin of the visceral pleura is very faintly visible. *B*, On expiratory film, the pneumothorax has become obvious as the right lung has deflated and become more opaque, providing better contrast with the air in the pleural space. (From Kuhn JP, Slovis TL, Haller JO: *Caffrey's Pediatric Diagnostic Imaging*, vol 1, 10th ed. Philadelphia, Mosby, 2004, p 885.)

CLINICAL MANIFESTATIONS. The onset is usually abrupt, and the severity of symptoms depends on the extent of the lung collapse and on the amount of pre-existing lung disease. Pneumothorax may cause pain, dyspnea, and cyanosis. In infancy, symptoms and physical signs may be difficult to recognize. Moderate pneumothorax may cause little displacement of the intrathoracic organs and few or no symptoms. The severity of pain usually does not directly reflect the extent of the collapse.

Usually, there is respiratory distress, retractions, and markedly decreased breath sounds over the involved lung. The percussion note over the involved area is tympanitic. The larynx, trachea, and heart may be shifted toward the unaffected side. When fluid is present, there is usually a sharply limited area of tympany above a level of flatness to percussion. The presence of amphoric breathing or, when fluid is present in the pleural cavity, of gurgling sounds synchronous with respirations suggests an open fistula connecting with air-containing tissues.

DIAGNOSIS AND DIFFERENTIAL DIAGNOSIS. The diagnosis is usually established by radiographic examination (Figs. 410-1, 410-2, 410-3). The amount of air outside the lung varies with time. A radiograph that is taken early shows less lung collapse than one taken later if the leak continues. Expiratory views accentuate the contrast between lung markings and the clear area of the pneumothorax (see Fig. 410-1). When considering the possibility of diaphragmatic hernia, a small amount of barium may be necessary to demonstrate that it is not free air but is a portion of the gastrointestinal tract that is in the thoracic cavity. Ultrasound can also be used to establish the diagnosis.

It may be difficult to determine if a pneumothorax is under tension. **Evidence of tension** includes shift of mediastinal structures away from the side of air leak. A shift may be absent in situations in which the other hemithorax resists the shift, such as in the case of bilateral pneumothorax. When the lungs are both stiff, such as in CF or respiratory distress syndrome (RDS), the unaffected lung may not collapse easily and shift may not occur (see Fig. 410-3). On occasion, the diagnosis of tension pneumothorax is made only on the basis of evidence of circulatory compromise or on hearing a "hiss" of rapid exit of air under tension with the insertion of the thoracostomy tube.

Pneumothorax must be differentiated from localized or generalized emphysema, an extensive emphysematous bleb, large pulmonary cavities or other cystic formations, diaphragmatic hernia, compensatory overexpansion with contralateral atelectasis, and gaseous distention of the stomach. In most cases, a chest radiograph or CT differentiates among these conditions.

TREATMENT. Therapy varies with the extent of the collapse and the nature and severity of the underlying disease. A tension pneu-

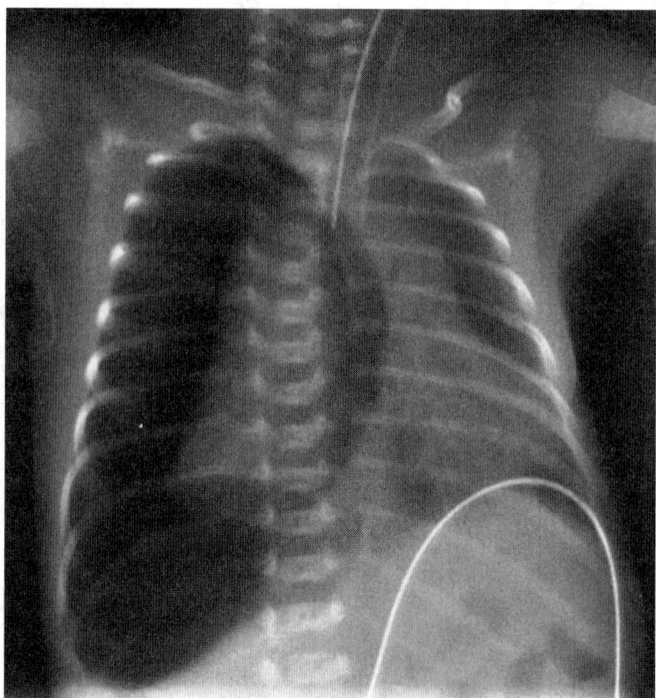

Figure 410-2. Right pneumothorax, compliant lung collapsed. (From Clark DA: *Atlas of Neonatology*, 7th ed. Philadelphia, WB Saunders, 2000, p 91.)

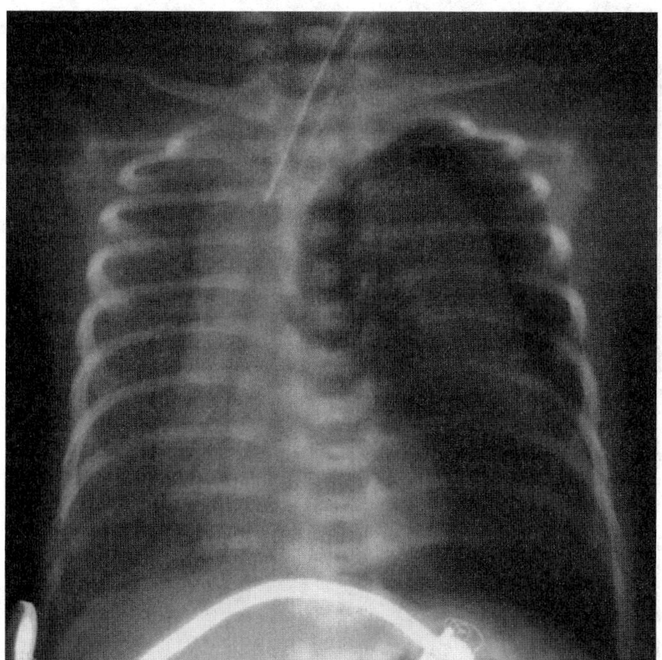

Figure 410-3. Left pneumothorax, lung poorly compliant. (From Clark DA: *Atlas of Neonatology,* 7th ed. Philadelphia, WB Saunders, 2000, p 91.)

mothorax may emergently require drainage by needle thoracostomy. A small or even moderate-sized pneumothorax in an otherwise normal child may resolve without specific treatment, usually within about 1 wk. A small (<5%) pneumothorax complicating asthma may also resolve spontaneously. Administering 100% oxygen may hasten resolution. Patients with chronic hypoxemia should be monitored closely during the administration of supplemental oxygen. Pleural pain deserves analgesic treatment. If there is >5% collapse or if the pneumothorax is recurrent or under tension, chest tube drainage is necessary. Pneumothoraces complicating CF frequently recur, and definitive treatment may be justified with the 1st episode, even with <5% collapse (see Chapter 400). Similarly, if pneumothorax complicating malignancy and its treatment does not improve rapidly with observation, chemical pleurodesis or open thoracotomy is often necessary.

Closed thoracotomy (simple insertion of a chest tube) and drainage of the trapped air through a catheter, the external opening of which is kept in a dependent position under water, is adequate to re-expand the lung in most patients; pigtail catheters are frequently used. When there have been previous pneumothoraces, it may be indicated to induce the formation of strong adhesions between the lung and chest wall by a sclerosing procedure to prevent recurrence. This can be carried out by the introduction of doxycycline or talc into the pleural space (**chemical pleurodesis**). Open thoracotomy through a limited incision, with plication of blebs, closure of fistula, stripping of the pleura (usually in the apical lung where the surgeon has direct vision), and basilar pleural abrasion is also an effective treatment for recurring pneumothorax. Stripping and abrading the pleura leaves raw, inflamed surfaces that heal with sealing adhesions. Postoperative pain is comparable to chemical pleurodesis, but the chest tube can usually be removed in 24–48 hr, compared with the usual 72 hr minimum for closed thoracotomy and pleurodesis. **Video-assisted thoracoscopic surgery** is a preferred therapy for blebectomy, pleural stripping, pleural brushing, and instillation of sclerosing agents, with somewhat less morbidity than occurs with traditional open thoracotomy.

Extensive pleural adhesions help to prevent recurrent pneumothorax, but they also make thoracic surgery difficult. For conditions in which lung transplantation may be a future consideration (e.g., CF), a stepwise approach to treatment of pneumothorax has been proposed. If the patient is comfortable and the pneumothorax is small, no intervention is warranted. For a larger leak or one that does not resolve, simple thoracostomy tube drainage can be attempted. For continuing leak, or recurrence, the next step could be thoracoscopic blebectomy without pleural abrasion. Only after these steps have failed should the full aggressive pleural stripping and abrasion be undertaken. At any step during this approach, the patient and family should be given the option of the definitive procedure if they understand this may make lung transplantation difficult or impossible. It should also be kept in mind that the longer a chest tube is in place, the greater the chance of pulmonary deterioration, particularly in a patient with CF, in whom strong coughing, deep breathing, and postural drainage are important. These are all difficult to accomplish with a chest tube in place.

Treatment of the underlying pulmonary disease should begin on admission and should be continued throughout the course of treatment directed at the air leak.

Liu CM, Hang LW, Chen WK, et al: Pigtail tube drainage in the treatment of spontaneous pneumothorax. *Am J Emerg Med* 2003;21:241–244.

Liu DM, Forkheim K, Rowan K, et al: Utilization of ultrasound for the detection of pneumothorax in the neonatal special-care nursery. *Pediatr Radiol* 2003;33:880–883.

Mathur NN, Kumar S, Bothra R, et al: Multi-lobulated cervical pneumatocoele communicating with pyopneumothorax and bronchopleural fistula. *Int J Pediatr Otorhinolaryngol* 2004;68:1525–1527.

Noppen M, Verbanck S, Harvey J, et al: Music: A new cause of primary spontaneous pneumothorax. *Thorax* 2004;59:722–724.

O'Connor AR, Morgan WE: Radiological review of pneumothorax. *Br Med J* 2005;330:1493–1497.

Ozcan C, McGahren ED, Rodgers BM: Thoracoscopic treatment of spontaneous pneumothorax in children. *J Pediatr Surg* 2003;38:1459–1464.

Ruddy RM: Trauma and the paediatric lung. *Paediatr Resp Rev* 2005;6:61–67.

Shaw KS, Prasil P, Nguyen LT, et al: Pediatric spontaneous pneumothorax. *Semin Pediatr Surg* 2003;12:55–61.

Wammanda RD, Ameh EA, Ali FU: Bilateral pneumothorax complicating miliary tuberculosis in children: Case report and review of the literature. *Ann Trop Paediatr* 2003;23:149–152.

Chapter 411 ■ Pneumomediastinum

Glenna B. Winnie

Pneumomediastinum is the presence or air or gas in the mediastinum.

ETIOLOGY. Pneumomediastinum is usually caused by alveolar rupture during acute or chronic pulmonary disease. A diverse group of nonrespiratory entities can also cause it, and the lung is not always the source of the air. Pneumomediastinum has been reported after dental extractions, normal menses, obstetric delivery, diabetes mellitus with ketoacidosis, acupuncture, and acute gastroenteritis. It can also result from esophageal perforation, penetrating chest trauma, or inhaled foreign body. Occasionally, no underlying cause is found. Acute asthma is the most common cause of pneumomediastinum in older children and teenagers. Simultaneous pneumothorax is unusual in these patients.

PATHOGENESIS. After intrapulmonary alveolar rupture, air dissects through the perivascular sheaths and other soft tissue planes toward the hilum and enters the mediastinum.

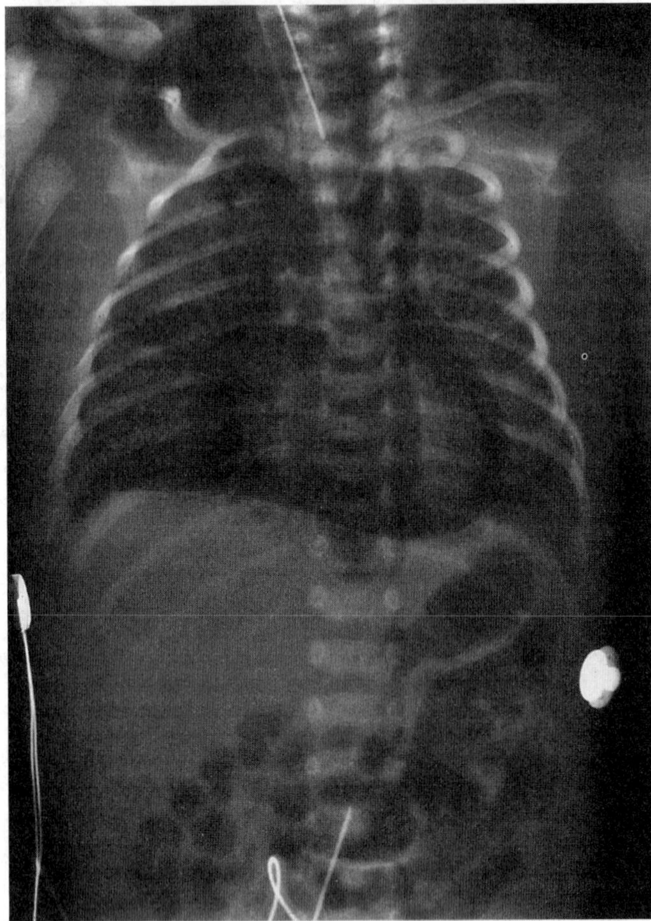

Figure 411-1. Large pneumomediastinum surrounding the heart and dissecting into the neck. (From Clark DA: *Atlas of Neonatology,* 7th ed. Philadelphia, WB Saunders, 2000, p 94.)

CLINICAL MANIFESTATIONS. Transient stabbing chest pain that may radiate to the neck is the principal feature of pneumomediastinum. Isolated abdominal pain and sore throat also occur. The patient may have dyspnea and cough. Pneumomediastinum is difficult to detect by physical examination alone. Subcutaneous emphysema, if present, is diagnostic. Cardiac dullness to percussion may be decreased, but many of these patients' chests are chronically overinflated, and it is unlikely that the clinician can be sure of this finding. A mediastinal "crunch" (Hamman sign) is occasionally heard but is easily confused with a friction rub.

LABORATORY FINDINGS. Chest radiography reveals mediastinal air, with a more distinct cardiac border than normal (Figs. 411-1, 411-2, and 411-3). On the lateral projection, the posterior mediastinal structures are clearly defined, there may be a lucent ring around the right pulmonary artery, and retrosternal air can usually be seen (see Fig. 411-2). Vertical streaks of air in the mediastinum and subcutaneous air are often observed (see Fig. 411-1).

COMPLICATIONS. Pneumomediastinum is rarely a major problem in older children because the mediastinum can be depressurized by escape of air into the neck or abdomen. In the newborn, however, the rate at which air can leave the mediastinum is limited, and pneumomediastinum can lead to dangerous cardiovascular compromise or pneumothorax (see Chapters 101.13 and 410).

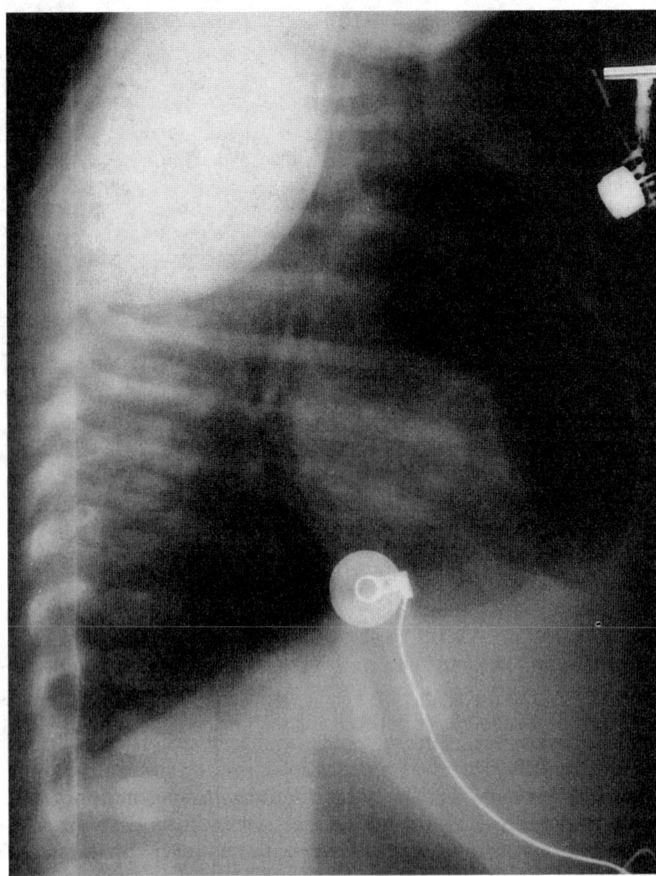

Figure 411-2. Lateral radiograph: upper mediastinal air. (From Clark DA: *Atlas of Neonatology,* 7th ed. Philadelphia, WB Saunders, 2000, p 94.)

TREATMENT. This is directed primarily at the underlying obstructive pulmonary disease or other precipitating condition. Analgesics are occasionally needed for chest pain. Rarely, subcutaneous emphysema can cause sufficient tracheal compression to justify tracheotomy; the tracheotomy also decompresses

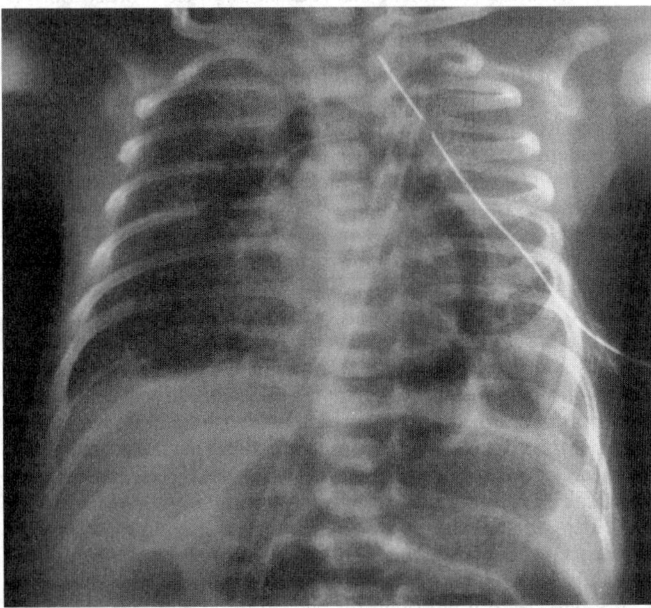

Figure 411-3. Sail sign–thymic elevation. (From Clark DA: *Atlas of Neonatology,* 7th ed. Philadelphia, WB Saunders, 2000, p 94.)

the mediastinum. Collar mediastinotomy and percutaneous drainage catheter placement are other treatment modalities.

Chalumeau M, Le Clainche L, Sayeg N, et al: Spontaneous pneumomediastinum in children. *Pediatr Pulmonol* 2001;31:67–75.
Chapdelaine J, Beaunoyer M, Daigneault P, et al: Spontaneous pneumomediastinum: Are we overinvestigating? *J Pediatr Surg* 2004;39:681–684.
Chau HH, Kwok PC, Lai AK, et al: Percutaneous relief of tension pneumomediastinum in a child. *Cardiovasc Intervent Radiol* 2003;26:561–563.
Damore DT, Dayan PS: Medical causes of pneumomediastinum in children. *Clin Pediatr* 2001;40:87–91.
Nounla J, Trobs R, Bennek J, et al: Idiopathic spontaneous pneumomediastinum: An uncommon emergency in children. *J Pediatr Surg* 2004; 39:E23–E24.

Chapter 412 ■ Hydrothorax

Glenna B. Winnie

Hydrothorax is a transudative pleural effusion usually caused by abnormal pressure gradients in the lung.

ETIOLOGY. Hydrothorax is most often associated with cardiac, renal, or hepatic disease. It can also be a manifestation of severe nutritional edema. Rarely, it results from venous obstruction by neoplasms, enlarged lymph nodes, or adhesions. It may occur from a ventriculoperitoneal shunt.

CLINICAL MANIFESTATIONS. Hydrothorax is usually bilateral, but in cardiac disease it can be bilateral, limited to the right side, or greater on the right than on the left side. The physical signs are the same as those described for serofibrinous pleurisy (see Chapter 409.2), but in hydrothorax, there is more rapid shifting of the level of dullness with changes of position. It is usually associated with an accumulation of fluid in other parts of the body.

LABORATORY FINDINGS. The fluid is noninflammatory, has few cells, and has a lower specific gravity (<1.015) than that of a serofibrinous exudate. The ratio of pleural fluid to serum total protein is <0.5, the ratio of pleural fluid to serum lactic dehydrogenase is <0.6, and the pleural fluid lactic dehydrogenase is less than ⅔ the upper limit of the normal serum lactic dehydrogenase.

TREATMENT. Therapy is directed at the underlying disorder; aspiration may be necessary when pressure symptoms are notable.

Akyuz M, Ucar T, Goksu E: A thoracic complication of ventriculoperitoneal shunt: Symptomatic hydrothorax from intrathoracic migration of a ventriculoperitoneal shunt catheter. *Br J Neurosurg* 2004;18:171–173.
Cho HY, Lee BS, Kang CH, et al: Hydrothorax in a patient with Denys-Drash syndrome associated with a diaphragmatic defect. *Pediatr Nephrol* 2006; Aug 25 (e pub ahead of print).
Karakaya D, Baris S, Ustun E: Hydrothorax: A life threatening complication during thoracotomy. *Paediatr Anaesth* 2002;12:809–810.
Ortiz L, Hazley D, Seikaly MG: Thoracocentesis helps diagnose diaphragmatic defects in peritoneal dialysis patients. *Pediatr Nephrol* 2001;16:105–106.

Chapter 413 ■ Hemothorax

Glenna B. Winnie

Hemothorax is an accumulation of blood in the pleural cavity. It is rare in children.

ETIOLOGY. Bleeding into the chest cavity most commonly occurs after chest trauma, either blunt or penetrating. It can be the result of iatrogenic trauma, including surgical procedures or venous line insertion. Hemothorax can also result from erosion of a blood vessel in association with inflammatory processes such as tuberculosis and empyema. It may complicate a variety of congenital anomalies, including sequestration, patent ductus arteriosus, and pulmonary arteriovenous malformation. It is also an occasional manifestation of intrathoracic neoplasms, blood dyscrasias, bleeding diatheses, or thrombolytic therapy. Rupture of an aneurysm is unlikely during childhood. Hemothorax may occur spontaneously in neonates and older children. A pleural hemorrhage associated with a pneumothorax is a hemopneumothorax.

CLINICAL MANIFESTATIONS. In addition to the symptoms and signs of pleural effusion (see Chapter 409.2), hemothorax is associated with hemodynamic compromise related to the amount and rapidity of bleeding.

DIAGNOSIS. The diagnosis of a hemothorax can be made only by thoracentesis. In every case, an effort must be made to determine and treat the cause.

TREATMENT. Initial therapy is tube thoracostomy. Surgical intervention may be required to control active bleeding, and transfusion may be indicated. Inadequate removal of blood in extensive hemothorax may lead to substantial restrictive disease secondary to organization of fibrin; fibrinolytic therapy or a decortication procedure may then be necessary.

Ambrogi MC, Lucchi M, Dini P, et al: Videothoracoscopy for evaluation and treatment of hemothorax. *J Cardiovasc Surg* 2002;43:109–112.
Bagwell CE, Salzberg AM, Sonnino RE, et al: Potentially lethal complications of central venous catheter placement. *J Pediatr Surg* 2000;35:709–713.
Light RW, Broaddus VC: Pneumothorax, chylothorax, hemothorax and fibrothorax. In Murray RF, Nadel JA: *Textbook of Respiratory Medicine*, 3rd ed. Philadelphia, Elsevier Science, 2000, pp 2043–2055.
Shehata SM, Shabaan BS: Diaphragmatic injuries in children after blunt abdominal trauma. *J Pediatr Surg* 2006;41(10):1727–1731.

Chapter 414 ■ Chylothorax

Glenna B. Winnie

Chylothorax is a pleural collection of fluid formed by the escape of chyle from the thoracic duct or lymphatics into the thoracic cavity.

ETIOLOGY. Chylothorax in children occurs most frequently due to thoracic duct injury as a complication of cardiothoracic surgery. Other cases are associated with chest injury or with primary or metastatic intrathoracic malignancy, particularly lymphoma. In newborns, rapidly increased venous pressure during delivery may lead to thoracic duct rupture. Less common causes include lymphangiomatosis; restrictive pulmonary diseases; thrombosis of the duct, superior vena cava, or subclavian vein; and congenital anomalies of the lymphatic system. Chylothorax can occur in child abuse (see Chapter 36). It is important to establish the etiology, as treatment varies with the cause. In some patients, no specific cause is identified.

CLINICAL MANIFESTATIONS. The signs and symptoms are the same as those due to pleural effusion of similar size. Chyle is not irritating, so pleuritic pain is uncommon. Onset is often gradual; however, after trauma to the thoracic duct, chyle may accumulate in the posterior mediastinum for days and then rupture into the pleural space with sudden onset of dyspnea, hypotension, and hypoxemia. About 50% of newborns with chylothorax present with respiratory distress in the 1st day of life. Chylothorax is rarely bilateral and usually occurs on the right side.

LABORATORY FINDINGS. Thoracentesis demonstrates a chylous effusion, a milky fluid containing fat, protein, lymphocytes, and other constituents of chyle; fluid may be yellow or bloody. In newborn infants who have not yet been fed, the fluid may be clear. A pseudochylous milky fluid may be present in chronic serous effusion, where fatty material arises from degenerative changes in the fluid and not from lymph. In chylothorax, the fluid triglyceride level is >110 mg/dL, pleural fluid to serum triglyceride ratio is >1.0, and pleural fluid to serum cholesterol ratio is <1.0; lipoprotein analysis reveals chylomicrons. The cells are primarily T lymphocytes. Chest radiograph shows an effusion; CT scan shows normal pleural thickness and may reveal a lymphoma as the etiology of the chylothorax. A lymphangiogram may localize the site of the leak in refractory cases when surgical ligation is contemplated.

COMPLICATIONS. Repeated aspirations may be required to relieve the symptoms of pressure. Chyle reaccumulates quickly, and repeated thoracenteses may cause malnutrition with significant loss of calories, protein, and electrolytes. Immunodeficiencies, including hypogammaglobulinemia and abnormal cell-mediated immune responses, have been associated with repeated and chronic thoracenteses for chylothorax. The loss of T lymphocytes is associated with increased risk of infection in neonates; otherwise, infection is uncommon, but patients should not receive live virus vaccines. Lack of resolution of chylothorax can lead to inanition, infection, and death.

TREATMENT. Spontaneous recovery occurs in >50% of cases of neonatal chylothorax. Initial therapy includes enteral feedings with a low-fat or medium-chain triglyceride high-protein diet, or parenteral nutrition. Repeated thoracentesis is done as needed to relieve pressure symptoms; tube thoracostomy is often performed. If there is no resolution in 1–2 wk, total parenteral nutrition is instituted and, if unsuccessful, a pleuroperitoneal shunt or ligation of the thoracic duct is considered. Ligation is done either via open thoracotomy or video-assisted thoracoscopic surgery. Parenteral octreotide has been used successfully in surgical failures. Other therapeutic approaches include pressure control ventilation with positive end-expiratory pressure, talc pleurodesis, and inhalation of nitric oxide. Treatment is similar in traumatic chylothorax. Chemical pleurodesis or radiation is used in malignant chylothorax.

Beghetti M, La Scala G, Belli D, et al: Etiology and management of pediatric chylothorax. *J Pediatr* 2000;136:653–658.

Cormack BE, Wilson NJ, Finucane K, et al: Use of Monogen for pediatric postoperative chylothorax. *Ann Thoracic Surg* 2004;77:301–305.

Coulter DM: Successful treatment with octreotide of spontaneous chylothorax in a premature infant. *J Perinatol* 2004;24:194–195.

Platis IE, Nwogu CE: Chylotherax. *Thorac Surg Clin* 2006;16(3):209–214.

Wasmuth-Pietzuch A, Hansmann M, Bartmann P, et al: Congenital chylothorax: Lymphopenia and high risk of neonatal infections. *Acta Paediatr* 2004;93:220–224.

Chapter 415 ■ Bronchopulmonary Dysplasia Steven Lestrud

Bronchopulmonary dysplasia (BPD) or chronic lung disease during the neonatal period is discussed in detail in Chapter 101.4.

EPIDEMIOLOGY. BPD traditionally occurred in preterm infants with severe respiratory distress syndrome who had been treated with high-inspired oxygen concentrations and prolonged mechanical ventilation with high positive airway pressures. With the increased survival of extremely premature infants (24–26 wk gestation, birth weight <1,000 g), the at-risk group has changed despite the availability of surfactant therapy; the percent of premature infants with **severe** BPD was 9.7% in 1994 and 3.7% in 2002. Milder forms of BPD are frequently seen in very low birthweight infants with mild or no initial respiratory distress syndrome.

CLINICAL MANIFESTATIONS. Physical findings are variable, based on severity of disease. Tachypnea is a common finding. The chest examination demonstrates an increased anteroposterior diameter that suggests air trapping. Intercostal retractions are frequently present. Although breath sounds are frequently clear when the patient is well and only abnormal during an acute exacerbation, many patients will have baseline wheeze or coarse crackles. Fine crackles may be present in patients prone to fluid overload.

The most severely effected patients require prolonged mechanical ventilation to achieve acceptable gas exchange. Infants with significant lung disease will exhibit growth failure due to elevated energy expenditure essential to maintain increased metabolic demands. Many have baseline inspired oxygen requirements to maintain oxygen saturations above 90%. Chronic respiratory insufficiency may be evident by elevated bicarbonate or partial pressure of CO_2 on blood gas analysis.

A **pulmonary exacerbation** is typically triggered during viral upper respiratory infections. Other frequent triggers include sinusitis, otitis media, weather changes, exposure to cigarette smoke, and exacerbations of gastroesophageal reflux. During an exacerbation, the infant will exhibit increased work of breathing, with tachypnea and retractions becoming more prominent. Chest wall configuration may change, with an increased anteroposterior diameter. If wheezing is a prominent baseline finding, poor air entry during an exacerbation may result in less wheezing.

Patients must be monitored for the development of cor pulmonale, especially if they require supplemental oxygen and have chronic respiratory failure. Other complicating conditions may include gastroesophageal reflux disease (GERD) and pulmonary aspiration, particularly during an exacerbation when the infants are most tachypneic and when pulmonary mechanics increase risk of GERD. For severely affected patients and those with disease out of proportion to the risk for development of chronic lung disease, other pulmonary disease may be suspected, such as asthma, cystic fibrosis, and chronic aspiration pneumonitis. Recurrent episodes of respiratory distress may represent anatomic airway abnormalities such as subglottic stenosis and airway malacia.

TREATMENT. Treatment is aimed at decreasing the work of breathing and normalizing gas exchange, to allow for optimal growth and neurodevelopment. Infants requiring supplemental oxygen past 35 wk of postconceptional age have a higher incidence of lower airway obstruction and bronchodilator responsiveness and are more likely to be hospitalized during the toddler years. The etiology of wheezing in BPD may be lower airway inflammation, bronchial smooth muscle irritation, bronchial smooth muscle hypertrophy, and airway malacia. The administration of an inhaled bronchodilator is frequently undertaken to evaluate an individual's response. Inhaled β agonists most commonly initially increase air movement and improve comfort of breathing. For patients who respond, the medication should be continued, especially during high-risk periods when triggers are present, such as an upper respiratory infection or hot humid days. β Agonists may worsen the air exchange, particularly in infants with BPD and concomitant airway malacia. Bronchial smooth muscle may maintain airway caliber in the malacic airway; smooth muscle relaxation after administration of a β agonist results in increased small airway collapse. These patients may benefit from alternative bronchodilators such as inhaled ipratropium or oral methylxanthines. The administration of preventative anti-inflammatory medications such as inhaled glucocorticoids and leukotriene-modifying agents may be considered in patients with frequent inflammatory triggers.

Adequate caloric intake can be difficult for many reasons, including oral aversion, discoordinate suck and swallow, GERD, aspiration, and aspiration with GERD. In addition, tachypnea, episodic respiratory distress, increased work of breathing, and requirement for supplement oxygen place the infant at risk for growth failure. A high caloric intake is necessary, with ranges of 120–160 kcal/kg/day required, frequently combined with fluid restriction. To provide such high caloric intake in the compromised infant, supplemental feedings may be considered through a nasogastric or gastrostomy tube. Careful attention is necessary to maintain fluid balance.

Gastroesophageal reflux is common and must be suspected in patients not responding to therapy and in patients with frequent exacerbations, especially without clear triggers. Definitive diagnosis is necessary because these patients will be subject to prolonged promotility and antacid medications (see Chapter 320). Appropriate antireflux therapy in infants with GERD decreases respiratory complications. Gastroesophageal reflux with pulmonary aspiration or aspiration alone may present as chronic chest congestion, wheezing, and episodic hypoxic spells. Fundoplication with a gastrostomy tube is performed in patients unresponsive to medical therapy. Evaluation and treatment by a speech therapist, pediatric pulmonologist, or otolaryngologist may decrease the risk of developing chronic lung disease associated with aspiration.

Prevention of respiratory viral illness is important; frequent handwashing, especially before handling the baby, and avoidance of contact with children and adults with current respiratory symptoms are important. Respiratory syncytial virus (RSV) immunoprophylaxis should be considered based on the severity of lung disease, gestational age, and current age.

The prognosis for infants with BPD is generally good. Through school age, the family can expect frequent medical interactions for episodes of respiratory distress, frequently triggered by simple upper respiratory tract infections and weather changes. Pulmonary function for severely affected patients will remain decreased, and exercise limitation may be present due to dyspnea. The most severely affected patients will benefit from a multidisciplinary team of caregivers, including the pediatrician, pulmonologist, speech therapist, nutritionist, and developmental specialists.

Ballard RA, Truog WE, Cnaan A, et al: Inhaled nitric oxide in preterm infants undergoing mechanical ventilation. *N Engl J Med* 2006;355:343–352.

Bott L, Béghin L, Devos P, et al: Nutritional status at 2 years in former infants with bronchopulmonary dysplasia influences nutrition and pulmonary outcomes during childhood. *Pediatr Res* 2006;60:340–344.

Clark RH, Gerstmann DR, Jobe AH, Moffitt ST: Lung injury in neonates: Causes, strategies for prevention, and long-term consequences. *J Pediatr* 2001;139:478–486.

Eber E, Zach MS: Long-term sequelae of bronchopulmonary dysplasia (chronic lung disease of infancy). *Thorax* 2001;56:317–323.

Halvorsen T, Skadberg BT, Eide GE, et al: Better care of immature infants; has it influenced long-term pulmonary outcome? *Acta Paediatr* 2006;95:547–554.

Kazzi SNJ, Quasney MW: Deletion allele of angiotensin-converting enzyme is associated with increased risk and severity of bronchopulmonary dysplasia. *J Pediatr* 2005;147:818–822.

Kinsella JP, Cutter GR, Walsh WF, et al: Early inhaled nitric oxide therapy in premature newborns with respiratory failure. *N Engl J Med* 2006;355:354–364.

Kinsella JP, Greenough A, Abman SH: Bronchopulmonary dysplasia. *Lancet* 2006;367:1421–1430.

Robin B, Kim YJ, Huth J, et al: Pulmonary function in bronchopulmonary dysplasia. *Pediatr Pulmonol* 2004;37:236–242.

Smith V, Zupancic J, McCormick M, et al: Trends in severe bronchopulmonary dysplasia rates between 1994 and 2002. *J Pediatr* 2005;146:469–473.

Chapter 416 ■ Skeletal Diseases Influencing Pulmonary Function

Steven R. Boas

Chest wall abnormalities can lead to restrictive or obstructive pulmonary disease, impaired respiratory muscle strength, and decreased ventilatory performance in response to physical stress. The congenital chest wall deformities include pectus excavatum, pectus carinatum, sternal clefts, Poland syndrome, and skeletal and cartilage dysplasias. Additionally, vertebral anomalies such as kyphoscoliosis can alter pulmonary function in children and adolescents.

416.1 • Pectus Excavatum (Funnel Chest)

EPIDEMIOLOGY. Pectus excavatum accounts for >90% of congenital chest wall anomalies. The incidence is ≈1/300 births with a 9 : 1 male preponderance.

ETIOLOGY. Midline narrowing of the thoracic cavity is usually an isolated skeletal abnormality. The cause is unknown. Pectus excavatum can occur in isolation or it may be associated with a connective tissue disorder (Marfan [see Chapter 700] or Ehlers-Danlos syndrome [see Chapter 658]). Additionally, it may be acquired secondarily to chronic lung disease, neuromuscular disease, or trauma.

CLINICAL MANIFESTATIONS. The deformity is present at or shortly after birth but is usually not associated with any symptoms at that time. In time, decreased exercise tolerance, fatigue, chest pain, palpitations, recurrent respiratory infections, wheezing, stridor, and cough may be present. Because of the cosmetic nature of this deformity, children may experience significant psychologic stress. Physical examination may reveal sternal depression, protracted shoulders, kyphoscoliosis, inferior rib flares, rib cage rigidity, forward head tilt, scapular winging, and loss of vertebral contours (Fig. 416-1). Patients exhibit paroxysmal sternal motion

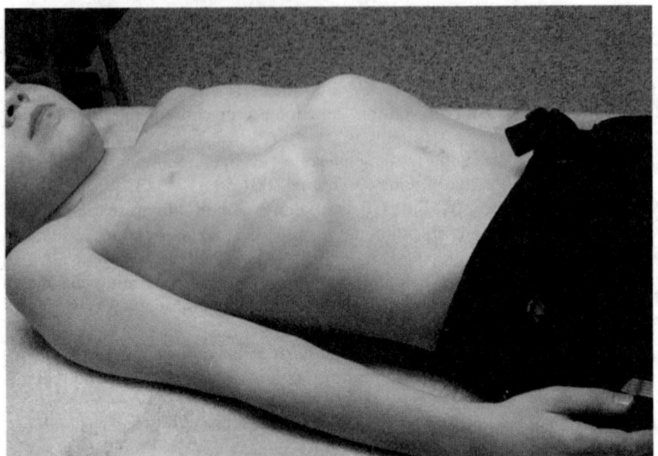

Figure 416-1. Pectus excavatum.

and a shift of point of maximal impulse to the left. Innocent systolic murmurs may be heard.

LABORATORY FINDINGS. Lateral chest radiograms demonstrate the sternal depression. Use of the Haller index on chest CT (maximal internal transverse diameter of the chest divided by the minimal anteroposterior diameter at the same level) compared to age- and gender-appropriate normative values for determining the extent of depression of the chest wall anomaly has become useful in determining the extent of the anatomic abnormality. An electrocardiogram may show a right-axis deviation or Wolff-Parkinson-White syndrome; an echocardiogram may demonstrate mitral valve prolapse and ventricular compression. Results of static pulmonary function tests may be normal but commonly show an obstructive defect in the lower airways and, less commonly, a restrictive defect due to abnormal chest wall mechanics. Exercise testing may demonstrate either normal tolerance or limitations from underlying cardiopulmonary dysfunction that appear associated with the severity of the defect. Ventilatory limitations are commonly seen in younger children and adolescents, whereas cardiac limitations secondary to stroke volume impairments are more commonly seen in older adolescents and young adults.

TREATMENT. Treatment is based on the severity of the deformity and the extent of physiologic compromise. Therapeutic options include careful observation, use of physical therapy to address musculoskeletal compromise, and corrective surgery. For those with significant physiologic compromise, surgical correction may improve the cosmetic deformity and may help minimize or even improve the cardiopulmonary compromise. The 2 main surgical interventions include the Ravitch and Nuss procedures, although superiority of 1 approach has not been established. For teenagers with exercise limitations, surgical repair may result in improved exercise tolerance. Normalization of lung perfusion scans and maximal voluntary ventilation have also been observed after surgery. Ongoing treatment to address the secondary musculoskeletal findings is commonly employed pre- and postoperatively.

Borowitz D, Cerny F, Zallen G, et al: Pulmonary function and exercise response in patients with pectus excavatum after Nuss repair. *J Pediatr Surg* 2003;38:544–547.

Daunt SW, Cohen JH, Miller SF: Age-related normal ranges for the Haller index in children. *Pediatr Radiol* 2004;34:326–330.

Haller JA Jr, Loughlin GM: Cardiorespiratory function is significantly improved following corrective surgery for severe pectus excavatum: Proposed treatment guidelines. *J Cardiovasc Surg* 2000; 41:125–130.

Koumbourlis AC, Stolar CJ: Lung growth and function in children and adolescents with idiopathic pectus excavatum. *Pediatr Pulmonol* 2004;38:339–343.

Malek MH, Fonkalsrud EW, Cooper CB: Ventilatory and cardiovascular responses to exercise in patients with pectus excavatum. *Chest* 2003;124:870–882.

Ohno K, Morotomi Y, Nakahira M, et al: Indications for surgical repair of funnel chest based on indices of chest wall deformity and psychologic state. *Surg Today* 2003;33:662–665.

Rowland T, Moriarty K, Banever G: Effect of pectus excavatum deformity on cardiorespiratory fitness in adolescent boys. *Arch Pediatr Adolesc Med* 2005;159:1069–1073.

Shamberger RC, Welch KJ, Sanders SP: Mitral valve prolapse associated with pectus excavatum. *J Pediatr* 1987;111:404–407.

Zhao L, Feinberg MS, Gaides M, et al: Why is exercise capacity reduced in subjects with pectus excavatum? *J Pediatr* 2000;136:163–167.

416.2 • Pectus Carinatum and Sternal Clefts

PECTUS CARINATUM

ETIOLOGY/EPIDEMIOLOGY. Pectus carinatum (pigeon breast) is an uncommon sternal deformity accounting for 5–15% of congenital chest wall anomalies. Anterior displacement of the mid and lower sternum and adjacent costal cartilages are the most common types with protrusion of the upper sternum, with occasional depression of the lower sternum occurring in only 15% of patients. Asymmetry of the sternum is common, with localized depression of the lower anterolateral chest often observed. Males are affected 4 times more often than females. There is a high familial occurrence and a common association of mild to moderate scoliosis. Mitral valve disease and coarctation of the aorta are associated with this anomaly.

CLINICAL MANIFESTATIONS. In early childhood, symptoms appear minimal. School-age children and adolescents, however, commonly complain of dyspnea with mild exertion, decreased endurance with exercise, and exercise-induced wheezing. The incidence of increased respiratory infections and use of asthma medication is higher than in nonaffected subjects. On physical examination, a marked increase in the anteroposterior chest diameter is seen, with resultant reduction in chest excursion and expansion. The increased residual volume results in tachypnea and diaphragmatic respirations. Chest radiographs show an increased anteroposterior diameter of the chest wall, emphysematous-appearing lungs, and a narrow cardiac shadow. A pectus severity score (analogous to the Haller index) is reduced.

TREATMENT. For symptomatic patients, newer, less invasive surgical correction results in improvement of the clinical symptoms. Surgery is often performed for cosmetic and psychologic reasons.

STERNAL CLEFTS

These are rare congenital malformations that result from the failure of the fusion of the sternum. Partial sternal clefts are more common and may involve the superior sternum in association with other lesions such as vascular dysplasias and supraumbilical raphe, or the inferior sternal clefts, which are often associated with other midline defects (pentalogy of Cantrell). Complete sternal clefts with complete failure of sternal fusion are rare. These disorders may also occur in isolation. The paradoxical movement of thoracic organs with respiration may alter pulmonary mechanics. Rarely, respiratory infections and even significant compromise result. Surgery is required early in life before fixation and immobility take place.

Fonkalsrud EW, Anselmo DM: Less extensive techniques for repair of pectus carinatum: The undertreated chest deformity. *J Am Coll Surg* 2004;198:898–905.

Goretsky MJ, Kelly RE, Croitoru D, Nuss D: Chest wall anomalies: Pectus excavatum amd pectus carinatum. *Adolesc Med Clin* 2004;15:455–471.

Ohye RG, Rutherford JA, Bove EL: Congenital sternal clefts. *Pediatr Cardiol* 2002;23:472–473.

Waters P, Welch K, Micheli LJ, et al: Scoliosis in children with pectus excavatum and pectus carinatum. *J Pediatr Orthop* 1989;9:551–556.

Williams AM, Crabbe DC: Pectus deformities of the anterior chest wall. *Paediatr Resp Rev* 2003;4:237–242.

416.3 • Asphyxiating Thoracic Dystrophy (Thoracic-Pelvic-Phalangeal Dystrophy)

PATHOGENESIS. Also known as Jeune syndrome, this condition is an autosomal recessive disorder that results in a constricted and narrow rib cage with generalized chondrodystrophy. Other systems can be involved, including pelvic, phalangeal, and neurologic anomalies along with renal and hepatic disorders.

CLINICAL MANIFESTATIONS. Most patients with this disorder die shortly after birth from respiratory failure, although less aggressive forms have been reported in older children. For those who survive the neonatal period, progressive respiratory failure often ensues, owing to impaired lung growth, recurrent pneumonia, and atelectasis originating from the rigid chest wall.

DIAGNOSIS. Physical examination reveals a narrowed thorax that, at birth, is much smaller than the head circumference. The ribs are horizontal, and these children have short extremities. Chest radiographs demonstrate a bell-shaped chest cage with short, horizontal, flaring ribs and high clavicles.

TREATMENT. No specific treatment exists, although thoracoplasty to enlarge the chest wall and long-term mechanical ventilation has been tried. Rib-expanding procedures have resulted in improved survival (see Chapters 693–698).

PROGNOSIS. For some children, improvement in the bony abnormalities occurs with age. However, children <1 yr old often succumb to respiratory infection and failure. Progressive renal disease often occurs with older children. Use of vaccines for influenza and other respiratory pathogens is warranted, as is aggressive use of antibiotics for respiratory infections.

Davis JT, Long FR, Adler BH, et al: Lateral thoracic expansion for Jeune syndrome: Evidence of rib healing and new bone formation. *Ann Thorac Surg* 2004;77:445–448.

Kajantic E, Anderson S, Kaitila I: Familial asphyxiating thoracic dysplasia: Clinical variability and impact of improved neonatal intensive care. *J Pediatr* 2001;139:130–133.

Sharoni E, Erez E, Chorev G, et al: Chest reconstruction in asphyxiating thoracic dystrophy. *J Pediatr Surg* 1998;33:1578–1581.

Tahernia AC, Stamps P: "Jeune syndrome" (asphyxiating thoracic dystrophy): Report of a case, a review of the literature, and an editor's commentary. *Clin Pediatr* 1977;16:903–908.

Wiebicke W, Pasterkamp H: Long-term continuous positive pressure in a child with asphyxiating thoracic dystrophy. *Pediatr Pulmonol* 1988;4:54–58.

416.4 • Achondroplasia

This condition is inherited as an autosomal dominant disorder that results in disordered growth (see Chapter 694). The pathogenesis is unknown.

CLINICAL MANIFESTATIONS. Recurrent infections, cor pulmonale, and dyspnea are commonly associated with achondroplasia. There is an increased risk of obstructive sleep apnea, although most patients are not affected. Hypoxemia during sleep is a common feature. Onset of restrictive lung disease can begin at a very young age. On examination, the breathing pattern is rapid and shallow, with associated abdominal breathing. The anteroposterior diameter of the thorax is reduced. Special growth curves for chest circumference of patients with achondroplasia from birth to 7 yr are available. **Three distinct phenotypes** exist, with group 1 possessing relative adenotonsillar hypertrophy, group 2 with muscular upper airway obstruction and progressive hydrocephalus, and group 3 with upper airway obstruction without hydrocephalus. Kyphoscoliosis may develop during infancy.

DIAGNOSIS. Pulmonary function tests reveal a reduced vital capacity that is more pronounced in males. The lungs are small but functionally normal. Chest radiographs demonstrate the decreased anteroposterior diameter along with anterior cupping of the ribs. The degree of foramen magnum involvement correlates with the degree of respiratory dysfunction.

TREATMENT. Treatment of sleep apnea, if present, is supportive (see Chapter 18). Physiotherapy and bracing may minimize the complications of kyphosis and of severe lordosis. Aggressive treatment of respiratory infections and scoliosis is warranted.

PROGNOSIS. The life span is normal for most children with this condition, except for the phenotypic group with hydrocephalus or with severe cervical or lumbar spinal compression.

Hunter AG, Reid CS, Pauli RM, et al: Standard curves of chest circumference in achondroplasia and the relationship of chest circumference to respiratory problems. *Am J Med Genet* 1996;62:91–97.

Mogayzel PJ Jr, Carroll JL, Loughlin GM, et al: Sleep-disordered breathing in children with achondroplasia. *J Pediatr* 1998;132:667–671.

Stokes DC, Phillips JA, Leonard CO, et al: Respiratory complications of achondroplasia. *J Pediatr* 1983;102:534–541.

Stokes DC, Wohl ME, Wise RA, et al: The lungs and airways in achondroplasia: Do little people have little lungs? *Chest* 1990;98:145–152.

Tasker RC, Dundas I, Laverty A, et al: Distinct patterns of respiratory difficulty in young children with achondroplasia: A clinical, sleep, and lung function study. *Arch Dis Child* 1998;79:99–108.

416.5 • Kyphoscoliosis: Adolescent Idiopathic Scoliosis and Congenital Scoliosis

PATHOGENESIS. Adolescent idiopathic scoliosis (AIS) is characterized by lateral bending of the spine (see Chapter 678). It commonly affects children during their teen years and periods of rapid growth. The cause is unknown. Congenital scoliosis is uncommon, affecting girls more than boys, and is apparent in the 1st year of life.

CLINICAL MANIFESTATIONS. The pulmonary manifestations of scoliosis may include chest wall restriction leading to a reduction in total lung capacity. The angle of scoliosis deformity has been correlated with the degree of lung impairment only for those with thoracic curves. Vital capacity, forced expiratory volume in 1 sec (FEV_1), work capacity, diffusion capacity, chest wall compliance, and PaO_2 decrease as the severity of thoracic curve increases. These findings can be seen in even mild to moderate AIS (Cobb angle <30 degrees) but do not occur in other nonthoracic curves. Reduction in peripheral muscle function has been associated with AIS through either intrinsic mechanisms or deconditioning. Severe impairment can lead to cor pulmonale or respiratory failure and can occur before age 20 yr. Children with severe scoliosis, especially boys, may have abnormalities of breathing during sleep, and the resultant periods of hypoxemia may contribute to the eventual development of pulmonary hypertension.

DIAGNOSIS. Physical examination and an upright, posteroanterior radiograph with subsequent measurement of the angle of curvature (Cobb technique) remain the gold standard for assessment. Curves >10 degrees define the presence of scoliosis.

TREATMENT. Depending on the extent of the curve and the degree of skeletal maturation, treatment options include reassurance, observation, bracing, and surgery (spinal fusion). Influenza vaccine should be administered, given the degree of pulmonary compromise that may coexist. Because vital capacity is a strong predictor for the development of respiratory failure in untreated AIS, surgical goals are to diminish the scoliotic curve, maintain the correction, and prevent deterioration in pulmonary function. Abnormal vital capacity and total lung capacity, exercise intolerance, and the rate of change of these variables over time should be taken into consideration for the timing of surgical correction. Preoperative assessment of lung function may assist in predicting postsurgical pulmonary difficulties. Many patients undergoing surgical correction may be managed postoperatively without mechanical ventilation. Even patients with mild scoliosis may have pulmonary compromise immediately after spinal fusion secondary to pain and a body cast that may restrict breathing and interfere with coughing. Rib-expanding procedures have been successful in severe cases of congenital scoliosis (see Chapter 416.5)

Chen S, Huang T, Lee Y, Hsu RW: Pulmonary function after thoracoplasty in adolescent idiopathic scoliosis. *Clin Orthop Related Res* 2002;399:152–161.

Hedequist D, Emans J: Congenital scoliosis. *J Am Acad Orthop Surg* 2004;12:266–275.

Kearon C, Viviani GR, Killian KJ: Factors influencing work capacity in adolescent idiopathic thoracic scoliosis. *Am Rev Respir Dis* 1993;148:295–303.

Leech JA, Ernst P, Rogala EJ, et al: Cardiorespiratory status in relation to mild deformity in adolescent idiopathic scoliosis. *J Pediatr* 1985;106:143–149.

Mezon BL, West P, Israels J, et al: Sleep breathing abnormalities in kyphoscoliosis. *Am Rev Respir Dis* 1980;122:617–621.

416.6 • Congenital Rib Anomalies

CLINICAL MANIFESTATIONS. Isolated defects of the highest and lowest ribs have minimal clinical pulmonary consequences. Missing midthoracic ribs are associated with the absence of the pectoralis muscle, and lung function can become compromised. Associated kyphoscoliosis and hemivertebrae may accompany this defect. If the rib defect is small, no significant sequelae ensue. When the 2nd to 5th ribs are absent anteriorly, lung herniation and significant abnormal respiration ensue. The lung is soft and nontender and may be easily reducible on examination. Complicating sequelae include severe lung restriction (secondary to scoliosis), cor pulmonale, and congestive heart failure. Symptoms are often minimal but can cause dyspnea. Respiratory distress is rare in infancy.

DIAGNOSIS. Chest radiographs demonstrate the deformed and absent ribs with secondary scoliosis. Most rib abnormalities are discovered as incidental findings on a chest film.

TREATMENT. If symptoms are severe enough to cause clinical compromise or significant lung herniation, then homologous rib grafting can be performed. Rib-expanding procedures are also of great value. Adolescent girls may require cosmetic breast surgery.

Bronsther B, Coryllos E, Epstein B, et al: Lung hernias in children. *J Pediatr Surg* 1968;3:544–550.

Mehta MH, Patel RV, Mehta LV, et al: Congenital absence of ribs. *Indian Pediatr* 1992;29:1149–1152.

Rickham PP: Lung hernia secondary to congenital absence of ribs. *Arch Dis Child* 1959;34:14–17.

Chapter 417 ■ Neuromuscular Diseases with Respiratory Dysfunction

David Gozal and Leila Kheirandish

Decreased muscle strength and endurance resulting from neuromuscular disorders can affect any skeletal muscle including those involved in respiratory functions. Of particular concern are those muscles mediating upper airway patency, generation of cough, and lung inflation. Acute respiratory insufficiency is often the most prominent clinical presentation of several acute neuromuscular disorders such as high level spinal cord injury, poliomyelitis, Guillain-Barré syndrome (see Chapter 615), and botulism (see Chapter 207). Although much more insidious in its clinical course, development of respiratory dysfunction constitutes the leading cause of morbidity and mortality in progressive neuromuscular disorders (e.g., Duchenne muscular dystrophy [see Chapter 608], spinal muscular atrophy, congenital myotonic dystrophy, myasthenia gravis [see Chapter 611], Charcot-Marie-Tooth disease [see Chapter 612]).

CLINICAL MANIFESTATIONS. Acute respiratory distress with dyspnea, agitation, diaphoresis, and cyanosis is easily recognizable and these signs should prompt immediate evaluation and therapy. The presence of hypoxemia is documented and monitored by pulse oximetry, and the severity of alveolar hypoventilation can be determined by drawing arterial or capillary blood gases. Radiographic assessment may reveal the presence of segmental or lobar atelectasis, which may be difficult to differentiate from and will often coincide with a pneumonic infiltrate. In children with progressive neuromuscular disorders, decreases in total lung capacity and vital capacity are usually closely linked to the degree of muscular impairment, and the restrictive lung disease is further accentuated by the onset and progression of kyphoscoliosis. The increased work of breathing is further compounded by the decreased chest wall and lung compliance that result from fibrotic changes of the dystrophic chest wall muscles, shortening and stiffening of the unstretched tissues, and widespread microatelectatic changes. Despite the reduction in lung volumes, an increase in residual volume is frequently observed in patients with neuromuscular disorders, and most likely reflects the disproportionate weakness of expiratory muscles. Such preferential weakness of expiratory muscles precludes, in turn, an effective expiration at lung volumes below functional residual capacity, with concomitant reduction of cough and mucociliary clearance efficiency. Since muscle weakness reduces maximal expiratory flows, true airflow obstruction may be concealed during standard spirometric maneuvers, and will require more sophisticated testing, such as the use of the forced oscillation technique, for its detection. Measurement of respiratory muscle strength is an important component of the clinical evaluation of neuromuscular patients, and both maximal inspiratory and expiratory pressures are reduced, albeit to varying degrees. The major implication of this reduction in respiratory force involves the ineffective capacity to develop effective clearance of secretions during cough. In the absence of competent mucociliary clearance, mucous plugs will form and further compromise pulmonary function, in particular, after the onset of an otherwise benign upper respiratory tract infection. Recurrent or chronic infection and fibrosis further accelerate the loss of functional lung parenchyma, leading to hypoxemia, pulmonary hypertension, and, eventually, cor pulmonale.

During sleep (particularly rapid eye movement sleep), normally occurring decreases in central neural ventilatory output may lead to substantial aggravation of alveolar hypoventilation and hypoxemia. Decreased upper airway motor tone further promotes the occurrence of upper airway obstruction. Patients may present with daytime sleepiness, fatigue, exertional dyspnea, morning headache and drowsiness, vomiting, difficulty tolerating the supine posture, and frequent need to be repositioned during the night. Increased clinical awareness of sleep-related disturbances is needed or these symptoms may be misconstrued as related to the neuromuscular disorder.

TREATMENT. Even though gene-targeted therapies are being developed for some neuromuscular disorders, current interventions are primarily directed to provide supportive therapy rather than cure the underlying abnormalities leading to the particular neuromuscular disease. Close surveillance through periodic history intake and physical examination is critical and will guide the need for further laboratory testing. The development of personality changes, such as irritability, decreased attention span, fatigue, or somnolence, may point to the presence of sleep-associated gas exchange abnormalities and sleep fragmentation. Changes in speech and voice characteristics, and the use of alae nasi and other accessory muscles during quiet breathing at rest, may provide sensitive indicators of progressive muscle dysfunction and respiratory compromise. Although the frequency of periodic re-evaluation needs to be individually tailored, tentative guidelines have been recently developed for patients with Duchenne muscular dystrophy; an abbreviated summary of such recommendations, applicable to all children with neuromuscular disorders, is provided in Table 417-1.

Regular administration of physical therapy, postural drainage, and a variety of manually and mechanically assisted cough maneuvers have demonstrated efficacy in the management of both acute pulmonary exacerbations and long-term maintenance therapy. Parents should become proficient in the administration of such interventions. Effective airway clearance is critical for patients with muscular weakness to prevent atelectasis and pneumonia. Ineffective airway clearance can hasten the onset of respiratory failure and death, whereas early intervention to improve airway clearance can prevent hospitalization and reduce the incidence of pneumonia. The role of mucolytic agents such as N-acetylcysteine or inhaled DNAse remains unclear. Respiratory muscle training can improve or at least preserve muscle strength in these children, and should be encouraged. Oral or intravenous antibiotic therapy should be implemented early in the course of respiratory infections, and inhaled bronchodilators may further alleviate any underlying bronchoconstriction. Annual administration of influenza vaccine is generally recommended and pneumococcal vaccine should be strongly considered in younger patients. The roles of theophylline, creatine supplementation, or corticosteroid therapy remain unknown.

When respiratory insufficiency develops in the setting of neuromuscular disease, as evidenced by abnormal respiratory patterns during sleep or wakefulness, mechanical ventilatory support is needed. Tracheotomy should be avoided for as long as possible, since noninvasive mechanical ventilatory support using nasal, oral, or face masks has now clearly supplanted this earlier approach and has become the 1st line of treatment in both the acute and chronic respiratory insufficiency settings. The beneficial effects of mask ventilation on lung volumes, sleep architecture, mucociliary clearance, and overall quality of life have been clearly demonstrated in patients with neuromuscular disease. Supplemental oxygen may be required to alleviate hypoxemia during acute or chronic pulmonary insufficiency, and tracheotomy may ultimately become necessary if patients need frequent suctioning of bronchial secretions, or more particularly, when patients require more than 18 hr of ventilatory support a day on a long-term basis. Despite such supportive measures, most chronic neuromuscular disorders continue to follow their progressive and irreversible course, and social and psychologic assistance should be incorporated into the multidisciplinary management of the patients and their families.

TABLE 417-1. Proposed Guidelines for Initial Evaluation and Follow-up of Patients with Neuromuscular Disease

INITIAL EVALUATION	BASIC INTERVENTION/TRAINING
History/physical/anthropometrics	Nutritional consult and guidance
Lung function and maximal respiratory pressures (PFT)	Regular chest physiotherapy
Arterial blood gases	Use of percussive devices
Polysomnography	Respiratory muscle training
Exercise testing (in selected cases)	Annual influenza vaccine
If vital capacity >60% predicted or maximal respiratory pressures >60 cm H_2O	Evaluate PFT every 6 mo CXR and polysomnography every year
If vital capacity <60% predicted or maximal respiratory pressures <60 cm H_2O	Evaluate PFT every 3–4 mo CXR, MIP/MEP every 6 mo Polysomnography every 6 mo to every year

Please note that if polysomnography is not readily available, multichannel recordings including oronasal airflow, nocturnal oximetry, and end-tidal carbon dioxide levels may provide an adequate alternative.
CXR, chest x-ray; MEP, maximal expiratory pressure; MIP, maximal inspiratory pressure.

Bach JR, Ishikawa Y, Kim H: Prevention of pulmonary morbidity for patients with Duchenne muscular dystrophy. *Chest* 1997;112:1024–1028.

Finder JD, Birnkrant D, Carl J, et al: American Thoracic Society: Respiratory care of the patient with Duchenne muscular dystrophy: ATS consensus statement. *Am J Respir Crit Care Med* 2004;170:456–465.

Gozal D: Pulmonary manifestations of neuromuscular disease: Focus on Duchenne muscular dystrophy and spinal muscular atrophy. *Pediatr Pulmonol* 2000;29:141–150.

Hukins CA, Hillman DR: Daytime predictors of sleep hypoventilation in Duchenne muscular dystrophy. *Am J Respir Crit Care Med* 2000; 161:166–170.

Simonds AK, Ward S, Heather S, et al: Outcome of paediatric domiciliary mask ventilation in neuromuscular and skeletal disease. *Eur Resp J* 2000;16:476–481.

Chapter 418 ■ Extrapulmonary Diseases with Pulmonary Manifestations

Susanna A. McColley

There are a number of respiratory symptoms that originate from extrapulmonary processes. The respiratory system adapts to metabolic demands and is exquisitely responsive to cortical input; therefore, **tachypnea** is common in the presence of metabolic stress such as fever, whereas dyspnea may be related to anxiety. **Cough** most commonly arises from upper or lower respiratory tract disorders, but it can originate from the central nervous system, as with cough tic or psychogenic cough, and it can be a prominent symptom in children with gastroesophageal reflux disease. **Chest pain** does not commonly arise from pulmonary processes in otherwise healthy children but more often has a neuromuscular or inflammatory etiology. **Cyanosis** can be caused by cardiac or hematologic disorders, and **dyspnea** and **exercise intolerance** can have a number of extrapulmonary causes. These disorders may be suspected on the basis of the history and physical examination, or they may be considered in children who have atypical findings on diagnostic studies or poor response to usual therapy. More common causes of such symptoms are listed in Table 418-1.

EVALUATION. In evaluating a child or adolescent with respiratory symptoms, it is important to obtain a detailed past medical history, family history, and review of systems to evaluate the possibility of extrapulmonary origin. A comprehensive physical examination is also essential in obtaining clues to extrapulmonary disease.

Disorders of other organ systems, and many systemic diseases, can have significant respiratory system involvement. Although it is most common to encounter these complications in patients with known diagnoses, respiratory system disease is sometimes the sole or most prominent symptom at the time of presentation. Acute aspiration during feeding can be the presentation of neuromuscular disease in an infant who initially appears to have normal muscle tone and development. Complications can be life-threatening, particularly in immunocompromised patients. The onset of respiratory findings may be insidious; for example, pulmonary vascular involvement in patients with systemic vasculitis may appear as an abnormality in diffusing capacity of the lung for carbon monoxide (DLco) before the onset of symptoms. Disorders that commonly have respiratory complications are listed in Table 418-2.

TABLE 418-1. Respiratory Signs and Symptoms Originating from Outside the Respiratory Tract

SIGN SYMPTOM	NONRESPIRATORY CAUSES	PATHOPHYSIOLOGY	CLUES TO DIAGNOSIS
Chest pain	Cardiac disease	Inflammation (pericarditis), ischemia (anomalous coronary artery, vascular disease)	Precordial pain, friction rub on examination; exertional pain, radiation to arm or neck
Chest pain	Gastroesophageal reflux disease	Esophageal inflammation and/or spasm	Heartburn, abdominal pain
Cyanosis	Congenital heart disease	Right-to-left shunt	Neonatal onset, lack of response to oxygen
Cyanosis	Methemoglobinemia	Increased levels of metHgb interfere with delivery of oxygen to tissues	Drug or toxin exposure, lack of response to oxygen
Dyspnea	Toxin exposure, drug side effect, or overdose	Variable, but often metabolic acidosis	Drug or toxin exposure confirmed by history or toxicology screen, normal Spo_2
Dyspnea	Anxiety, panic disorder	Increased respiratory drive and increased perception of respiratory efforts	Occurs during stressful situation, other symptoms of anxiety or depression
Exercise intolerance	Anemia	Inadequate oxygen deliver to tissues	Pallor, tachycardia, history of bleeding, history of inadequate diet
Exercise intolerance	Deconditioning	Self-explanatory	History of inactivity, obesity
Hemoptysis	Nasal bleeding	Posterior flow of bleeding causes appearance of pulmonary origin	History and physical examination suggest nasal source, normal chest examination, and chest radiography
Hemoptysis	Upper gastrointestinal tract bleeding	Hematemesis mimics hemoptysis	History and physical examination suggest gastrointestinal source, normal chest examination and chest radiography
Wheezing, cough, dyspnea	Congenital or acquired cardiac disease	Pulmonary overcirculation (ASD, VSD, PDA), left ventricular dysfunction	Murmur Refractory to bronchodilators Radiographic changes (prominent pulmonary vasculature, pulmonary edema)
Wheezing, cough	Gastroesophagel reflux disease	Laryngeal and bronchial response to stomach contents ?Vagally mediated bronchoconstriction	Emesis, pain, heartburn Refractory to bronchodilators

ASD, atrial septal defect; PDA, patent ductus arteriosus; VSD, verticular septal defect.

TABLE 418-2. Disorders with Frequent Respiratory Tract Complications

UNDERLYING DISORDER	RESPIRATORY COMPLICATIONS	DIAGNOSTIC TESTS
Autoimmune disorders	Pulmonary vascular disease, restrictive lung disease, pleural effusion (especially lupus), upper airway disease (Wegener granulomatosis)	Spirometry, lung volume determination, oximetry, DL_{CO}, chest radiography, upper airway endoscopy, and/or CT scan
Central nervous system disease (static or progressive)	Aspiration of oral or gastric contents	Chest radiography, videofluoroscopic swallowing study, esophageal pH probe, fiberoptic bronchoscopy
Immunodeficiency	Infection, bronchiectasis	Chest radiography, fiberoptic bronchoscopy, chest CT
Liver disease	Pleural effusion, hepatopulmonary syndrome	Chest radiography, assessment of orthodeoxia
Malignancy and its therapies	Infiltration, metastasis, malignant or infectious effusion, parenchymal infection, graft vs host disease (bone marrow transplant)	Chest radiography, chest CT, fiberoptic bronchoscopy, lung biopsy
Neuromuscular disease	Hypoventilation, atelectasis, pneumonia	Spirometry, lung volume determination, respiratory muscle force measurements
Obesity	Restrictive lung disease, obstructive sleep apnea syndrome	Spirometry, lung volume determination, nocturnal polysomnography

DL_{CO}, diffusing capacity of the lung for carbon monoxide.

Bowman CM: Hemoptysis. In Loughlin GM, Eigen H (editors): *Respiratory Disease in Children: Diagnosis and Management.* Baltimore, Williams and Wilkins, 1994, pp 201–205.
Loughlin GM: Chest pain. In Loughlin GM, Eigen H (editors): *Respiratory Disease in Children: Diagnosis and Management.* Baltimore, Williams and Wilkins, 1994, pp 207–214.
Methemoglobinemia. eMedicine Journal: Medicine, 2002.

Chapter 419 ■ Chronic Severe Respiratory Insufficiency

Zehava Noah and Cynthia Budek

Infants, children, and adolescents with disorders of central control of breathing, disease of the airways, residual lung disease after severe respiratory illness, and neuromuscular disorders may develop hypercarbic and/or hypoxemic chronic respiratory failure (see Chapter 370). Although it is generally possible to identify a primary cause for the respiratory failure, many children have multiple causative factors. Less than 1% of patients admitted to pediatric intensive care units require long-term noninvasive or invasive ventilatory assistance.

ETIOLOGIES

Central Apnea and Central Hypoventilation Syndromes. Common conditions include congenital central hypoventilation syndrome (CCHS, Ondine curse); a small percentage of children with myelomeningocele, hydrocephalus, and Arnold-Chiari malformation; and survivors of brainstem tumors. Children with these disorders do not sense hypercapnia, and some of them do not sense hypoxia. Although some children may be severely bradypneic or apneic during some sleep states, the classic finding in CCHS is hypoventilation in the absence of apnea or bradypnea (see Chapter 370). Polysomnography confirms the diagnosis by documenting episodes of poor or absent respiratory effort and poor or absent airflow during sleep.

Obstructive Sleep Apnea. See Chapter 18.

Lung Disease. Common conditions include bronchopulmonary dysplasia (BPD) and children recuperating from acute respiratory distress syndrome (ARDS). Former premature infants recuperating from respiratory distress syndrome may develop BPD (see Chapters 101.4 and 415). When extreme, BPD may progress to respiratory failure.

Severe Tracheo- and/or Bronchomalacia (Airway Malacia). Conditions associated with airway malacia include tracheoesophageal fistula, innominate artery compression, or pulmonary artery sling after surgical repair (see Chapter 386).

Neuromuscular Weakness. Disease states resulting in neuromuscular weakness include spinal muscular atrophy (see Chapter 611.2), neurodegenerative diseases, myasthenia gravis, spinal cord injuries, and postinfectious neurologic diseases such as Guillain-Barré syndrome (see Chapter 615). Children recuperating from severe illness in the intensive care unit often have neuromuscular weakness from suboptimal nutrition. This neuromuscular weakness can be devastating when coupled with the catabolic effects of severe illness and residual effects of sedatives, analgesics, and muscle relaxants, particularly if steroids were administered. Children with neuromuscular disease have limited ability to increase ventilation and usually do so by increasing respiratory rate. Because of weakness, retractions may not be observed. In severe illness, some of these children respond to increased respiratory load by becoming apneic. A look of panic, changes in vital signs such as significant tachycardia or bradycardia, and cyanosis may be the only signs of respiratory failure.

EVALUATION. Children with chronic respiratory insufficiency require a thorough evaluation to determine the characteristics and severity of the condition and its effect on physical function (see Chapter 370). The evaluation should include a complete history, physical examination, radiologic studies, pulmonary tests, nutritional evaluation, developmental assessment, and analysis of family dynamics. Most children with severe chronic respiratory insufficiency have a combination of factors contributing to their overall clinical status.

LONG-TERM MECHANICAL VENTILATION

Some children with chronic severe respiratory insufficiency benefit from chronic ventilatory support. The goal of such support is to maintain normal oxygenation and ventilation and minimize work of breathing. Long-term ventilation in the home is a complex, physically demanding, emotionally taxing, and expensive process for the family and for society. It changes the family's way of life, priorities, and relationships. It may adversely affect intra- and extra-family relationships.

The prognosis of the disease is a critical factor in deciding whether long-term ventilation should be initiated. The discharge process on ventilatory support should start as soon as the child is medically stable on equipment that can be maintained in the home. Children with degenerative neuromuscular disease, such as type I spinal muscular atrophy (SMA), suffer from respiratory failure very early in life, often triggered by the 1st respiratory illness. Although some parents decide to provide only palliative end-of-life care (see Chapter 40) for the child with SMA, others choose long-term invasive or noninvasive ventilatory support. Young children with chronic lung disease and airway malacia have the potential to improve their pulmonary function and wean successfully off ventilator support, if provided with adequate ventilation, good nutrition, and measures to promote development and prevent further lung injury.

Successful home discharge of a patient receiving mechanical ventilation depends on adequate resources in the community to support the family. Some hospital programs that transition children home on ventilators utilize professional nurses in the home to assist with round-the-clock care. This depends on funding as well as availability of nursing agencies in the community. Housing can be a significant barrier to home discharge because there must be adequate space for the child and caretakers; equipment and supplies; environmental safety, including compliance with building and electrical codes; and home modifications for mobility, including ramping and lifts.

Funding for home care is usually a difficult issue for this population of children. Even if they have private insurance, coverage for home care benefits is frequently limited. In the United States, for children eligible for public aid, most states have funds available to meet the special needs of children who are ventilator dependent, although the extent of coverage varies considerably between geographic areas.

RESPIRATORY EQUIPMENT FOR HOME CARE

Modes of mechanical ventilation support are outlined in Chapters 70 and 70.1.

NONINVASIVE. Supplemental oxygen and positive pressure can be administered by nasal cannula. This system delivers heated, supersaturated, high-flow gases. A number of machines are available for the delivery of continuous and bi-level positive airway pressure. These machines attach to nasal and full-face masks or to nasal pillows, and are best suited for the treatment of obstructive sleep apnea. Long-term use of these devices in small children may result in midface dysplasia. They can occasionally be used for the delivery of positive pressure through a tracheostomy for infants with tracheobronchomalacia. This type of ventilation has also been used in less severely affected patients with recurrent atelectasis, nighttime hypoventilation, or both.

ROCKER BED. A rocker bed moves in a longitudinal seesaw motion at a set rate. The child is secured to the bed with a strap. Movement of the bed promotes diaphragm movement. The bed may be an option for children with mild neuromuscular weakness, for instance, when recuperating from Guillain-Barré syndrome. This device should not be placed in a home with toddlers or young children because they may get trapped in its mechanism.

CUIRASSE. This is a negative pressure device that resembles a turtle shell. It is designed to fit over the anterior chest and provide a tight seal. Cycled negative pressure is applied to the child's chest through a hole in the cuirasse. These devices are suitable only for infants and children with mild neuromuscular weakness. A plastic bag–like device that fits snugly around the chest applies the same principle.

IRON LUNG. The iron lung is a cumbersome device that applies negative pressure to the child's body. The child is placed in the iron lung cylinder with the head extending outside the device. A cuff is placed around the neck to minimize air leaks. Negative pressure is cycled within the iron lung, facilitating chest wall movement. Ventilation is disrupted when the device is opened to deliver care. This device is suitable for children with muscular weakness who require ventilation for part of the day. Its main advantage is that it does not require a tracheostomy; however, upper airway obstruction may occur, and this risk requires ongoing evaluation. A lighter version of this device is available for travel.

DIAPHRAGMATIC PACING. Diaphragmatic pacers may be considered for children with central hypoventilation and those with high spinal cord injury. Electrodes are surgically placed over the phrenic nerves and a receiver is placed in the subcutaneous tissue. The external pacing device is small and light, with antennae secured externally over the receiver. A tracheostomy may be required if there is no coordination between the pacing of the device and the opening of the glottis. Any failure in the electrode pacing wires or the receiver requires surgical intervention.

POSITIVE PRESSURE VENTILATION. Ideally, a ventilator intended for home use should be lightweight and small, be able to entrain room air, preferably have continuous flow, and have a wide range of settings (pressure, volume, pressure support, and rate) that would allow ventilation from infancy to adulthood. Battery support for the ventilator, both internal and external, should be sufficient to permit unrestricted portability in the home and community. The equipment must also be impervious to electromagnetic interference and be relatively easy to understand and troubleshoot. A variety of ventilators that can be used in the home are available, and familiarity with these devices is necessary to choose the best option for the child. Other tools that may be helpful to patients with profound weakness are devices that facilitate mobilization of secretions such as the percussion vest and devices that enhance the patient's cough such as the In-Exsufflator.

DISCHARGE PROCESS

The initial discharge process for a child going home on a ventilator is complex. A multidisciplinary, coordinated team approach is needed to develop a comprehensive plan that addresses medical, psychosocial, developmental, educational, and safety issues. The ventilated child must demonstrate medical stability that can be safely managed at home; interventions to maintain stability should be minimal before discharge. The child should be transitioned to a ventilator suitable for home use that allows portability as well as adequate ventilation. Medical management should also focus on weaning oxygen and ventilator parameters to settings appropriate for home care. Depending on the type of ventilation employed, a tracheostomy may be placed to promote comfort and a stable airway as soon as the decision to ventilate chronically is made.

Nutrition should be optimized to promote growth yet minimize excessive weight gain and carbon dioxide production. The nutritional requirements of a ventilated child are frequently decreased owing to the supported work of breathing. The ventilated child often has problems with swallowing from dyscoordination and oral aversion secondary to intubation. Speech therapy should be introduced early to begin oromotor therapy and return of swallow. Many children require gastrostomy tube placement to replace or supplement oral intake. Evaluation and management of reflux and the risk of aspiration should also be considered because these are common problems in ventilated children. Communication devices to augment speech should be part of the planning.

Training of caregivers should be initiated early in the discharge process and be provided by nurses, respiratory care practitioners, and physical, occupational, and speech therapists. Caregivers must be trained in all aspects of the child's care, including tracheostomy care, ventilator management, and cardiopulmonary resuscitation. Their independence in delivery of care at the bedside and while transporting the child should be emphasized. Special focus should be placed on safety and appropriate response in the event of an emergency. An emergency bag containing critical supplies is developed to accompany the patient at all times. Caregivers must demonstrate their proficiency before the child is discharged.

Community agencies should be identified for provision of home support services. This may include a nursing agency to provide private duty nursing services. It is ideal to train home care nurses about the ventilator and the child's care before home discharge. An equipment vendor who can provide the ventilator equipment, supplies, and service should be selected. A care conference including the hospital team, funding agency, home nursing agency, equipment vendor, and family caregivers should take place before discharge. The conference is important for coordination of last-minute details and, thus, facilitation of a smooth transition to home.

Providing continued support to the child and family after discharge is very important. The pediatrician in the community has a central role in providing coordination of care, well child care, and all other medical needs, with the possible exception of ventilatory care. Equally important is the establishment of lines of communication to the medical center and the provision of timely access for advice and troubleshooting during the intervals between multidisciplinary clinic visits.

Corrado A, Gorini M: Long-term negative pressure ventilation. *Respir Care Clin N Am* 2002;8:545–557.

Gilgoff RL, Gilgoff IS: Long-term follow-up of home mechanical ventilation in young children with spinal-cord injury and neuromuscular conditions. *J Pediatr* 2003;142:476–480.

Miske LJ, Hickey EM, Kolb SM, et al: Use of the mechanical in-exsufflator in pediatric patients with neuromuscular disease and impaired cough. *Chest* 2004;125:1406–1412.

Palfrey JS, Sofis LA, Davidson EJ, et al: The pediatric alliance for coordinated care: Evaluation of a medical home model. *Pediatrics* 2004;113:1507–1516.

Suchada S, Kun SS, Keens TG, et al: Initiation of home mechanical ventilation in children with neuromuscular diseases. *J Pediatr* 2003;142:481–485.

Talmaciu I: Pulmonary function in technology-dependent children two years and older with bronchopulmonary dysplasia. *Pediatr Pulmonol* 2002; 33:181–188.

Trang H, Dehan M, Beaufils F, et al: French CCHS Working Group: The French Congenital Central Hypoventilation Syndrome Registry: General data, phenotype and genotype. *Chest* 2005;127:72–79.

Tzeng AC, Bach JR: Prevention of pulmonary morbidity for patients with neuromuscular disease. *Chest* 2000;118:1390–1396.

Waugh JB: An evaluation of two new devices for nasal high-flow gas therapy. *Respir Care* 2004;49:902–906.

Wright SE, VanDahm K: Long-term care of the tracheostomy patient. *Clin Chest Med* 2003;24:473–487.

Part XIX ▪ The Cardiovascular System

Section 1 — Developmental Biology of the Cardiovascular System — Daniel Bernstein

Chapter 420 ▪ Cardiac Development

Knowledge of the cellular and molecular mechanisms of cardiac development is necessary in understanding congenital heart defects and developing strategies for prevention. Cardiac defects have traditionally been grouped by common morphologic patterns: abnormalities of the outflow tracts (conotruncal lesions such as tetralogy of Fallot and truncus arteriosus) and abnormalities of atrioventricular septation (primum atrial septal defect, complete atrioventricular canal defect). These morphologic categories may not, however, provide an understanding of the mechanisms of genetic alterations that lead to congenital heart disease.

420.1 • Early Cardiac Morphogenesis

In the early presomite embryo, the 1st identifiable cardiac precursors are angiogenetic cell clusters arranged on both sides of the embryo's central axis; these clusters form paired cardiac tubes by 18 days of gestation. The paired tubes fuse in the midline on the ventral surface of the embryo to form the primitive heart tube by 22 days. Premyocardial cells, including epicardial cells and cells derived from the neural crest, continue their migration into the region of the heart tube. Regulation of this early phase of cardiac morphogenesis is controlled in part by the interaction of specific signaling molecules or ligands, usually expressed by one cell type, with specific receptors, usually expressed by another cell type. Positional information is conveyed to the developing cardiac mesoderm by factors such as retinoids (isoforms of vitamin A), which bind to specific nuclear receptors and regulate gene transcription. Migration of epithelial cells into the developing heart tube is directed by extracellular matrix proteins (fibronectin) interacting with cell surface receptors (the integrins). The importance of these ligands is noted by the spectrum of **cardiac teratogenic** effects caused by the retinoid-like drug isotretinoin.

As early as 20–22 days, before cardiac looping, the embryonic heart begins to contract and exhibit phases of the cardiac cycle that are surprisingly similar to those in a mature heart. Morphologists have identified segments of the heart tube that were believed to correspond to structures in a mature heart (Fig. 420-1): the sinus venosus and atrium (right and left atria), the primitive ventricle (left ventricle), the bulbus cordis (right ventricle), and the truncus arteriosus (aorta and pulmonary artery). This model is oversimplified. Only the trabecular (most heavily muscularized) portions of the left ventricular myocardium are present in the early cardiac tube; the cells that will become the inlet portion of the left ventricle migrate into the cardiac tube at a later stage (after looping is initiated). Even later to appear are the primordial cells that give rise to the great arteries (truncus arteriosus), including cells derived from the neural crest, which are not present until after cardiac looping is complete. Chamber-specific transcription factors participate in the differentiation of the right and left ventricles. The basic helix-loop-helix transcription factor dHAND is expressed in the developing right ventricle; disruption of this gene or of other transcriptional factors such as myocyte enhancer factors 2C (MEF2C) in mice leads to hypoplasia of the right ventricle. The transcription factor eHAND is expressed in the developing left ventricle and conotruncus and is also critical to their development.

420.2 • Cardiac Looping

At ≈22–24 days, the heart tube begins to bend ventrally and toward the right (see Fig. 420-1) through as yet unknown biomechanical forces. Looping brings the future left ventricle leftward and in continuity with the sinus venosus (future left and right atria), whereas the future right ventricle is shifted rightward and in continuity with the truncus arteriosus (future aorta and pulmonary artery). This pattern of development explains the relatively common occurrence of the cardiac anomalies double-outlet right ventricle and double-inlet left ventricle and the extreme rarity of double-outlet left ventricle and double-inlet right ventricle (see Chapter 430.5). Cardiac looping, one of the 1st manifestations of right-left asymmetry in the developing embryo, is critical for the successful completion of cardiac morphogenesis. When cardiac looping is abnormal, the incidence of serious cardiac malformations is high.

Potential mechanisms of cardiac looping include differential growth rates for myocytes on the convex vs the concave surface of the curve, differential rates of programmed cell death (apoptosis), and mechanical forces generated within myocardial cells via their actin cytoskeleton. The signal for this directionality may be contained in a concentration gradient between the right and left sides of the embryo by the expression of critical signaling molecules (tumor growth factor-β family of peptide growth factors and signaling peptides such as Sonic hedgehog). In murine models of abnormal looping, one such defect resides in the dynein gene.

420.3 • Cardiac Septation

When looping is complete, the external appearance of the heart is similar to that of a mature heart; internally, the structure resembles a single tube, although it now has several bulges resulting in the appearance of primitive chambers. The common atrium (comprising both the right and left atria) is connected to the primitive ventricle (future left ventricle) via the atrioventricular canal. The primitive ventricle is connected to the bulbus cordis (future right ventricle) via the bulboventricular foramen. The distal portion of the bulbus cordis is connected to the truncus arteriosus via an outlet segment (the conus).

The heart tube now consists of several layers of myocardium and a single layer of endocardium separated by cardiac jelly, an

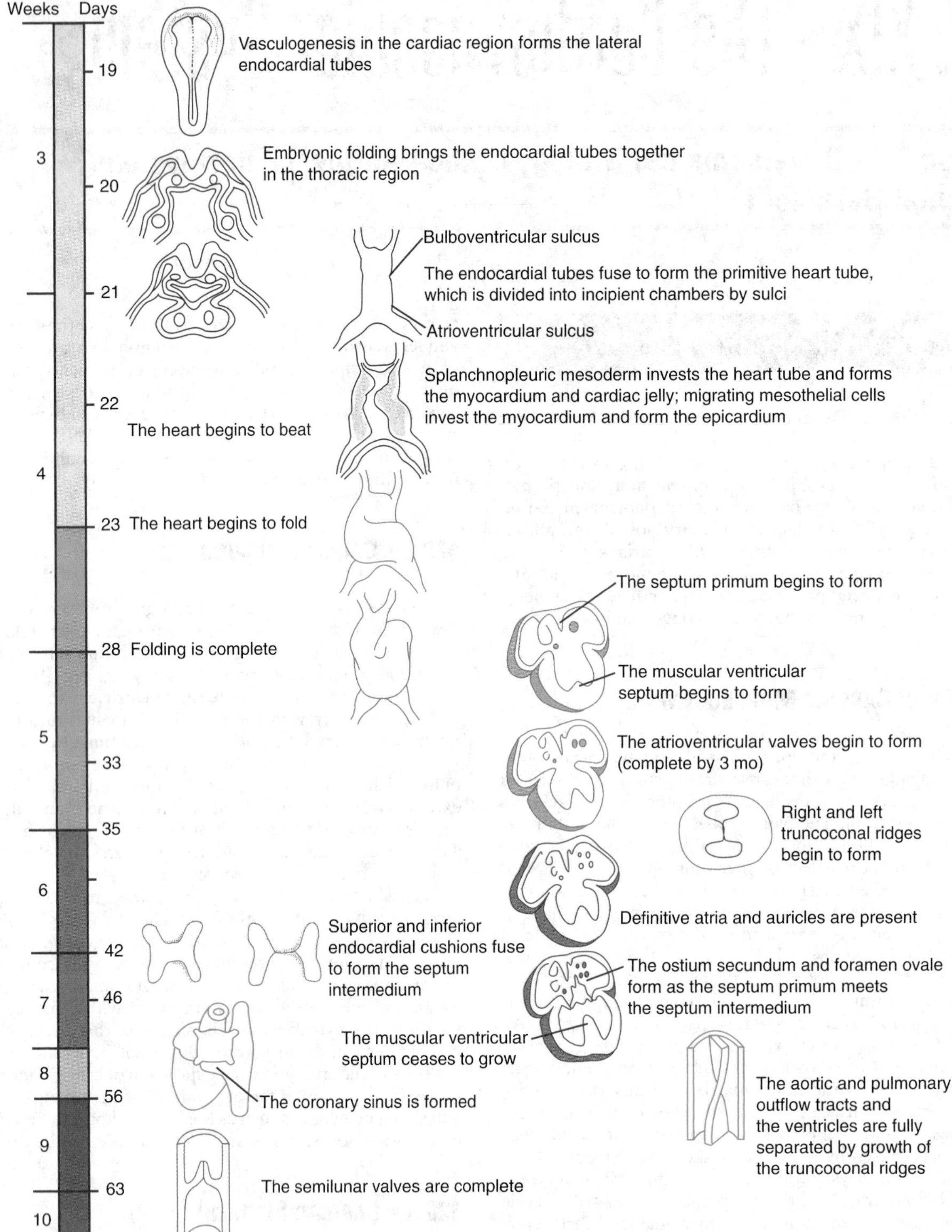

Weeks
Days
3
4
5
6
7
8
9
10
19
20
21
22
23
28
33
35
42
46
56
63
Vasculogenesis in the cardiac region forms the lateral endocardial tubes
Embryonic folding brings the endocardial tubes together in the thoracic region
Bulboventricular sulcus
The endocardial tubes fuse to form the primitive heart tube, which is divided into incipient chambers by sulci
Atrioventricular sulcus
Splanchnopleuric mesoderm invests the heart tube and forms the myocardium and cardiac jelly; migrating mesothelial cells invest the myocardium and form the epicardium
The heart begins to beat
The heart begins to fold
Folding is complete
The septum primum begins to form
The muscular ventricular septum begins to form
The atrioventricular valves begin to form (complete by 3 mo)
Right and left truncoconal ridges begin to form
Definitive atria and auricles are present
Superior and inferior endocardial cushions fuse to form the septum intermedium
The ostium secundum and foramen ovale form as the septum primum meets the septum intermedium
The muscular ventricular septum ceases to grow
The coronary sinus is formed
The aortic and pulmonary outflow tracts and the ventricles are fully separated by growth of the truncoconal ridges
The semilunar valves are complete
TIMELINE. FORMATION OF THE HEART.

Figure 420-1. Timeline of cardiac morphogenesis. (From Larsen WJ: *Essentials of Human Embryology.* New York, Churchill Livingstone, 1998.)

acellular extracellular matrix secreted by the myocardium. Septation of the heart begins at approximately day 26 with the ingrowth of large tissue masses, the endocardial cushions, at both the atrioventricular and conotruncal junctions (see Fig. 420-1). These cushions consist of protrusions of cardiac jelly, which, in addition to their role in development, also serve a physiologic function as primitive heart valves. Endocardial cells dedifferentiate and migrate into the cardiac jelly in the region of the endocardial cushions, eventually becoming mesenchymal cells that will form part of the atrioventricular valves.

Complete septation of the atrioventricular canal occurs with fusion of the endocardial cushions. Most of the atrioventricular valve tissue is derived from the ventricular myocardium in a process involving undermining of the ventricular walls. Because this process occurs asymmetrically, the tricuspid valve annulus sits closer to the apex of the heart than the mitral valve annulus does. Physical separation of these two valves produces the atrioventricular septum, the absence of which is the primary common defect in patients with **atrioventricular canal defects** (see Chapter 426.5). If the process of undermining is incomplete, one of the atrioventricular valves may not separate normally from the ventricular myocardium, a possible cause of **Ebstein anomaly** (see Chapter 430.7).

Septation of the atria begins at ≈30 days with growth of the septum primum downward toward the endocardial cushions (see Fig. 420-1). The orifice that remains is the ostium primum. The endocardial cushions then fuse and, together with the completed septum primum, divide the atrioventricular canal into right and left segments. A 2nd opening appears in the posterior portion of the septum primum, the ostium secundum, and it allows a portion of the fetal venous return to the right atrium to pass across to the left atrium. Finally, the septum secundum grows downward, just to the right of the septum primum. Together with a flap of the septum primum, the ostium secundum forms the foramen ovale, through which fetal blood passes from the inferior vena cava to the left atrium (see Chapter 421).

Septation of the ventricles begins at about embryonic day 25 with protrusions of endocardium in both the inlet (primitive ventricle) and outlet (bulbus cordis) segments of the heart. The inlet protrusions fuse into the bulboventricular septum and extend posteriorly toward the inferior endocardial cushion, where they give rise to the inlet and trabecular portions of the interventricular septum. Ventricular septal defects can occur in any portion of the developing interventricular septum (see Chapter 426.6). The outlet or conotruncal septum develops from ridges of cardiac jelly, similar to the atrioventricular cushions. These ridges fuse to form a spiral septum that brings the future pulmonary artery into communication with the anterior and rightward right ventricle and the future aorta into communication with the posterior and leftward left ventricle. Differences in cell growth of the outlet septum lead to lengthening of the segment of smooth muscle beneath the pulmonary valve (conus), a process that separates the tricuspid and pulmonary valves. In contrast, disappearance of the segment beneath the aortic valve leads to fibrous continuity of the mitral and aortic valves. Defects in these processes are responsible for **conotruncal** and **aortic arch defects** (truncus arteriosus, tetralogy of Fallot, pulmonary atresia, double-outlet right ventricle, interrupted aortic arch), a group of cardiac anomalies often associated with deletions of the DiGeorge critical region of chromosome 22q11 (see Chapters 423 and 424). The transcription factor Tbx1 has been implicated as a candidate gene, which may be responsible for DiGeorge syndrome.

420.4 • Aortic Arch Development

The aortic arch, head and neck vessels, proximal pulmonary arteries, and ductus arteriosus develop from the aortic sac, arterial arches, and dorsal aortae. When the straight heart tube develops, the distal outflow portion bifurcates into the right and left 1st aortic arches, which join the paired dorsal aortae (Fig. 420-2). The dorsal aortae will fuse to form the descending aorta. The proximal aorta from the aortic valve to the left carotid artery arises from the aortic sac. The 1st and 2nd arches largely regress by about 22 days, with the 1st aortic arch giving rise to the maxillary artery and the 2nd to the stapedial and hyoid arteries. The 3rd arches participate in the formation of the innominate artery and the common and internal carotid arteries. The right 4th arch gives rise to the innominate and right subclavian arteries, and the left 4th arch participates in formation of the segment of the aortic arch between the left carotid artery and the ductus arteriosus. The 5th arch does not persist as a major structure in the mature circulation. The 6th arches join the more distal pulmonary arteries, with the right 6th arch giving rise to a portion of the proximal right pulmonary artery and the left 6th arch giving rise to the ductus arteriosus. The aortic arch between the ductus arteriosus and the left subclavian artery is derived from the left-sided dorsal aorta, whereas the aortic arch distal to the left subclavian artery is derived from the fused right and left dorsal aortae. Abnormalities in development of the paired aortic arches are responsible for **right aortic arch, double aortic arch,** and **vascular rings** (see Chapter 432.1).

420.5 • Cardiac Differentiation

The process by which the totipotential cells of the early embryo become committed to specific cell lineages is differentiation. Precardiac mesodermal cells differentiate into mature cardiac muscle cells with an appropriate complement of cardiac-specific contractile elements, regulatory proteins, receptors, and ion channels. Expression of the contractile protein myosin occurs at an early stage of cardiac development, even before fusion of the bilateral heart primordia. Differentiation in these early mesodermal cells is regulated by signals from the anterior endoderm, a process known as induction. Several putative early signaling molecules include fibroblast growth factor, activin, and insulin. Signaling molecules interact with receptors on the cell surface; these receptors activate 2nd messengers, which, in turn, activate specific nuclear transcription factors (GATA-4, MEF2, Nkx, bHLH, and the retinoic acid receptor family) that induce the expression of specific gene products to regulate cardiac differentiation. Some of the primary disorders of cardiac muscle, the **cardiomyopathies,** may be related to defects in some of these signaling molecules (see Chapter 439).

Developmental processes are chamber specific. Early in development, ventricular myocytes express both ventricular and atrial isoforms of several proteins, such as atrial natriuretic peptide (ANP) and myosin light chain (MLC). Mature ventricular myocytes do not express ANP and express only a ventricular-specific MLC 2v isoform, whereas mature atrial myocytes express ANP and an atrial-specific MLC 2a isoform. Heart failure (see Chapter 442), volume overload (see Chapters 426 and 428), and pressure overload hypertrophy (see Chapter 427) are associated with a recapitulation of fetal cell phenotypes in which mature myocytes re-express fetal proteins. Because different isoforms have different contractile behavior (fast vs slow activation, high vs low adenosine triphosphatase activity), expression of different isoforms may have important functional consequences.

The extent to which stem cells can be made to differentiate into cardiac muscle cells is the focus of investigation in the field of regenerative cardiology. Some investigators believe that cardiac precursor cells known as cardiomyoblasts can replace damaged myocytes and, if stimulated with the proper regulatory factors, could be induced to regenerate cardiac muscle. Others believe

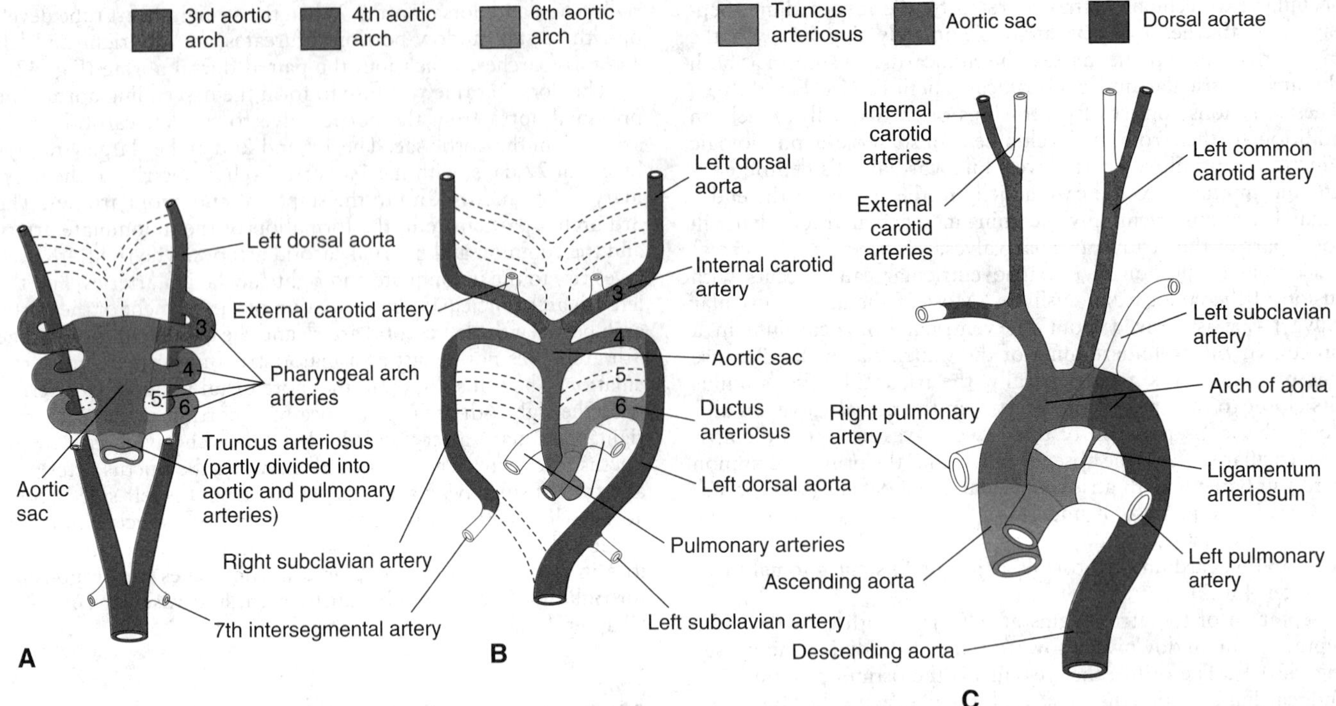

Figure 420-2. Schematic drawings illustrating the changes that result during transformation of the truncus arteriosus, aortic sac, aortic arches, and dorsal aortae into the adult arterial pattern. The vessels that are not shaded or colored are not derived from these structures. *A*, Aortic arches at 6 wk; by this stage the 1st two pairs of aortic arches have largely disappeared. *B*, Aortic arches at 7 wk; the parts of the dorsal aortae and aortic arches that normally disappear are indicated by *broken lines*. *C*, Arterial vessels of a 6 mo old infant. (From Moore KL, Persaud TVN, Torchia M: *The Developing Human*. Philadelphia, Elsevier, 2007.)

that circulating stem cells or bone marrow–derived cells may support cardiac regeneration.

420.6 • Developmental Changes in Cardiac Function

During development, the composition of the myocardium undergoes profound changes that result in an increase in the number and size of myocytes. During prenatal life, this process involves myocyte division (hyperplasia), whereas after the 1st few postnatal weeks, subsequent cardiac growth occurs by an increase in myocyte size (hypertrophy). The myocytes themselves change shape from round to cylindrical, the proportion of myofibrils (which contain the contractile apparatus) increases, and the myofibrils become more regular in their orientation.

The plasma membrane (known as the sarcolemma in myocytes) is the location of the ion channels and transmembrane receptors that regulate the exchange of chemical information from the cell surface to the cell interior. Ion fluxes through these channels control the processes of depolarization and repolarization. Developmental changes have been described for the sodium-potassium pump, the sodium-hydrogen exchanger, and voltage-dependent calcium channels. As the myocyte matures, extensions of the sarcolemma develop toward the interior of the cell (the t-tubule system), which dramatically increases its surface area and enhances rapid activation of the myocyte. Regulation of the membrane's α- and β-adrenergic receptors with development enhances the ability of the sympathetic nervous system to control cardiac function as the heart matures.

The sarcoplasmic reticulum (SR), a series of tubules surrounding the myofibrils, controls the intracellular calcium concentration. A series of pumps regulate calcium release to the myofibrils for initiation of contraction (ryanodine-sensitive calcium channel) and calcium uptake for initiation of relaxation (adenosine triphosphate–dependent SR calcium pump). In immature hearts, this SR calcium transport system is less well developed, and such hearts consequently have an increased dependence on transport of calcium from outside the cell for contraction. In a mature heart, the majority of the calcium to activate contraction comes from the SR. This developmental phenomenon may explain the sensitivity of the infant heart to sarcolemmal calcium channel blockers such as verapamil, which often results in a marked depression in contractility and cardiac arrest (see Chapter 435).

The major contractile proteins (myosin, actin, tropomyosin, and troponin) are organized into the functional unit of cardiac contraction, the sarcomere. Each has several isoforms that are expressed differentially by location (atrium vs ventricle) and by developmental stage (embryo, fetus, newborn, adult).

Changes in myocardial structure and myocyte biochemistry result in easily quantifiable differences in cardiac function with development. Fetal cardiac function is poorly responsive to changes in both preload (filling volume) and afterload (systemic resistance). The most effective means of increasing ventricular function in a fetus is through increasing the heart rate. After birth and with further maturation, preload and afterload play an increasing role in regulating cardiac function. The rate of cardiac relaxation is also developmentally regulated. The decreased ability of the immature SR calcium pump to remove calcium from the contractile apparatus is manifested as a decreased ability of the fetal heart to enhance relaxation in response to sympathetic stimulation. This inability of the immature myocardium to use preload effectively may partly explain the difficulty that most premature infants have in compensating for the left-to-right shunt through a patent ductus arteriosus (see Chapters 101.4 and 426.8).

Baldini A: DiGeorge syndrome: An update. *Curr Opin Cardiol* 2004;19:201–204.

Brand T: Heart development: Molecular insights into cardiac specification and early morphogenesis. *Dev Biol* 2003;258:1–19.

Chen JN, Fishman MC: Genetics of heart development. *Trends Genet* 2000;16:383–388.

Dimmeler S, Zeiher AM, Schneider MD: Unchain my heart: The scientific foundations of cardiac repair. *J Clin Invest* 2005;115:572–583.

Epstein JA, Buck CA: Transcriptional regulation of cardiac development: Implications for congenital heart disease and DiGeorge syndrome. *Pediatr Res* 2000;48:717–724.

Gittenberger-De Groot AC, Bartelings MM, Deruiter MC, et al: Basics of cardiac development for the understanding of congenital heart malformations. *Pediatr Res* 2005;57:169–176.

Kathiriya IS, Srivastava D: Left-right asymmetry and cardiac looping: Implications for cardiac development and congenital heart disease. *Am J Med Genet* 2000;97:271–279.

Person AD, Klewer SE, Runyan RB: Cell biology of cardiac cushion development. *Int Rev Cytol* 2005;243:287–335.

Srivastava D: HAND proteins: Molecular mediators of cardiac development and congenital heart disease. *Trends Cardiovasc Med* 1999;9:11–18.

Towbin JA, Belmont J: Molecular determinants of left and right outflow tract obstruction. *Am J Med Genet* 2000;97:297–303.

Chapter 421 ■ The Fetal to Neonatal Circulatory Transition

421.1 • The Fetal Circulation

The human fetal circulation and its adjustments after birth are similar to those of other large mammals, although rates of maturation differ. In the fetal circulation, the right and left ventricles exist in a parallel circuit, as opposed to the series circuit of a newborn or adult (Fig. 421-1*A*). In the fetus, the placenta provides for gas and metabolite exchange. The lungs do not provide gas exchange, and vessels in the pulmonary circulation are vasoconstricted. Three cardiovascular structures unique to the fetus are important for maintaining this parallel circulation: the ductus venosus, foramen ovale, and ductus arteriosus.

Oxygenated blood returning from the placenta flows to the fetus through the umbilical vein with a PO_2 of about 30–35 mm Hg. Approximately 50% of the umbilical venous blood enters the hepatic circulation, whereas the rest bypasses the liver and joins the inferior vena cava via the ductus venosus, where it partially mixes with poorly oxygenated inferior vena cava blood derived from the lower part of the fetal body. This combined lower body plus umbilical venous blood flow (PO_2 of ≈26–28 mm Hg) enters the right atrium and is preferentially directed across the foramen ovale to the left atrium (see Fig. 421-1*B*). The blood then flows into the left ventricle and is ejected into the ascending aorta. Fetal superior vena cava blood, which is considerably less oxygenated (PO_2 of 12–14 mm Hg), enters the right atrium and preferentially traverses the tricuspid valve, rather than the foramen ovale, and flows primarily to the right ventricle.

From the right ventricle, the blood is ejected into the pulmonary artery. Because the pulmonary arterial circulation is vasoconstricted, only about 10% of right ventricular outflow enters the lungs. The major portion of this blood (which has a PO_2 of ≈18–22 mm Hg) bypasses the lungs and flows through the ductus arteriosus into the descending aorta to perfuse the lower part of the fetal body, after which it returns to the placenta via the two

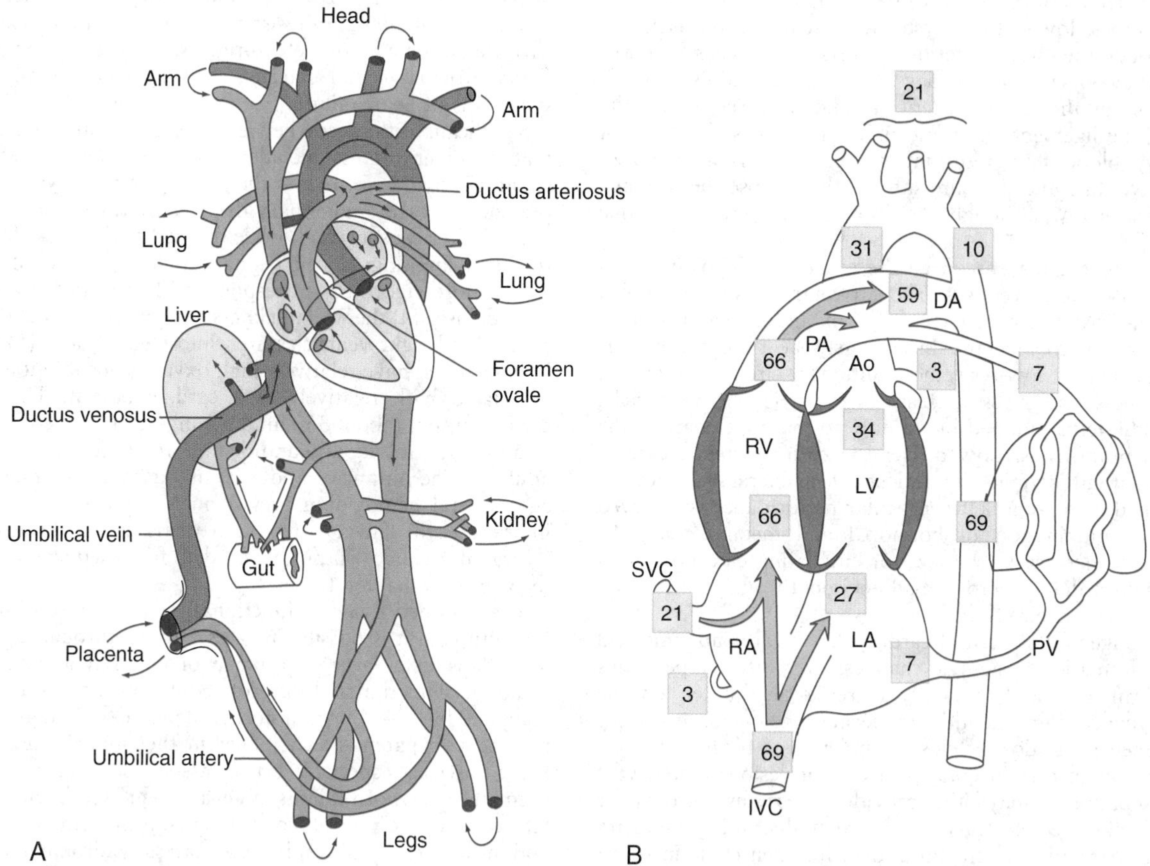

Figure 421-1. *A*, The human circulation before birth (partly after Dawes). *Red* indicates more oxygenated blood, and *arrows* indicate the direction of flow. Highly oxygenated blood from the placenta passes through the foromen ovale from the right to the left atrium, thus bypassing the lungs. *B*, Percentages of combined ventricular output that return to the fetal heart, that are ejected by each ventricle, and that flow through the main vascular channels. Figures are those obtained from study of late-gestation lambs. Ao, aorta; DA, ductus arteriosus; IVC, inferior vena cava; LA, left atrium; LV, left ventricle; PA, pulmonary artery; PV, pulmonary veins; RA, right atrium; RV, right ventricle; SVC, superior vena cava. (From Rudolph AM: *Congenital Diseases of the Heart*. Chicago, Year Book, 1974.)

umbilical arteries. Thus, the upper part of the fetal body (including the coronary and cerebral arteries and those to the upper extremities) is perfused exclusively from the left ventricle with blood that has a slightly higher PO_2 than the blood perfusing the lower part of the fetal body, which is derived mostly from the right ventricle. Only a small volume of blood from the ascending aorta (10% of fetal cardiac output) flows across the aortic isthmus to the descending aorta.

The **total fetal cardiac output**—the combined output of both the left and right ventricles—is ≈450 mL/kg/min. Approximately 65% of descending aortic blood flow returns to the placenta; the remaining 35% perfuses the fetal organs and tissues. In the sheep fetus, right ventricular output is approximately two times that of the left ventricle. In the human fetus, which has a larger percentage of blood flow going to the brain, right ventricular output is probably closer to 1.3 times left ventricular flow. Thus, during fetal life the right ventricle is not only pumping against systemic blood pressure but is also performing a greater volume of work than the left ventricle.

421.2 • The Transitional Circulation

At birth, mechanical expansion of the lungs and an increase in arterial PO_2 result in a rapid decrease in pulmonary vascular resistance. Concomitantly, removal of the low-resistance placental circulation leads to an increase in systemic vascular resistance. The output from the right ventricle now flows entirely into the pulmonary circulation, and because pulmonary vascular resistance becomes lower than systemic vascular resistance, the shunt through the ductus arteriosus reverses and becomes left to right. In the course of several days, the high arterial PO_2 signals constriction of the ductus arteriosus and it closes, eventually becoming the ligamentum arteriosum. The increased volume of pulmonary blood flow returning to the left atrium increases left atrial volume and pressure sufficiently to close the foramen ovale functionally, although the foramen may remain probe patent.

Removal of the placenta from the circulation also results in closure of the ductus venosus. The left ventricle is now coupled to the high-resistance systemic circulation, and its wall thickness and mass begin to increase. In contrast, the right ventricle is now coupled to the low-resistance pulmonary circulation, and its wall thickness and mass decrease slightly. The left ventricle, which in the fetus pumped blood only to the upper part of the body and brain, must now deliver the entire systemic cardiac output (≈350 mL/kg/min), an almost 200% increase in output. This marked increase in left ventricular performance is achieved through a combination of hormonal and metabolic signals, including an increase in the level of circulating catecholamines and the myocardial receptors (β-adrenergic) through which catecholamines have their effect.

When congenital structural cardiac defects are superimposed on these dramatic physiologic changes, they often impede this smooth transition and markedly increase the burden on the newborn myocardium. In addition, because the ductus arteriosus and foramen ovale do not close completely at birth, they may remain patent in certain congenital cardiac lesions. Patency of these fetal pathways may either provide a lifesaving pathway for blood to bypass a congenital defect (a patent ductus in pulmonary atresia or coarctation of the aorta or a foramen ovale in transposition of the great vessels) or present an additional stress to the circulation (patent ductus arteriosus in a premature infant, pathway for right-to-left shunting in infants with pulmonary hypertension). Therapeutic agents may either maintain these fetal pathways (prostaglandin E_1) or hasten their closure (indomethacin).

421.3 • The Neonatal Circulation

At birth, the fetal circulation must immediately adapt to extrauterine life as gas exchange is transferred from the placenta to the lung (see Chapter 101.1). Some of these changes are virtually instantaneous with the 1st breath, whereas others develop over a period of hours or days. After an initial slight fall in systemic blood pressure, a progressive rise occurs with increasing age. The heart rate slows as a result of a baroreceptor response to an increase in systemic vascular resistance when the placental circulation is eliminated. The average central aortic pressure in a term neonate is 75/50 mm Hg.

With the onset of ventilation, pulmonary vascular resistance is markedly decreased as a consequence of both active (PO_2 related) and passive (mechanical related) pulmonary vasodilation. In a normal neonate, closure of the ductus arteriosus and the fall in pulmonary vascular resistance result in a decrease in pulmonary arterial and right ventricular pressures. The major decline in pulmonary resistance from the high fetal levels to the low "adult" levels in the human infant at sea level usually occurs within the 1st 2–3 days but may be prolonged for 7 days or more. Over the 1st several weeks of life, pulmonary vascular resistance decreases even further, secondary to remodeling of the pulmonary vasculature, including thinning of the vascular smooth muscle and recruitment of new vessels. This decrease in pulmonary vascular resistance significantly influences the timing of the clinical appearance of many congenital heart lesions that are dependent on the relative systemic and pulmonary vascular resistance. The left-to-right shunt through a ventricular septal defect may be minimal in the 1st wk after birth when pulmonary vascular resistance is still high. As pulmonary resistance decreases in the next week or two, the volume of the left-to-right shunt through an unrestrictive ventricular septal defect increases and eventually leads to symptoms of heart failure.

Significant differences between the neonatal circulation and that of older infants include: (1) right-to-left or left-to-right shunting may persist across the patent foramen ovale; (2) in the presence of cardiopulmonary disease, continued patency of the ductus arteriosus may allow left-to-right, right-to-left, or bidirectional shunting; (3) the neonatal pulmonary vasculature constricts more vigorously in response to hypoxemia, hypercapnia, and acidosis; (4) the wall thickness and muscle mass of the neonatal left and right ventricles are almost equal; and (5) newborn infants at rest have relatively high oxygen consumption, which is associated with relatively high cardiac output. The newborn cardiac output (about 350 mL/kg/min) falls in the 1st 2 mo of life to about 150 mL/kg/min and then more gradually to the normal adult cardiac output of about 75 mL/kg/min. The high percentage of fetal hemoglobin present in the newborn may actually interfere with delivery of oxygen to tissues in the neonate, so increased cardiac output is needed for adequate delivery of oxygen (see Chapter 101.1).

The foramen ovale is functionally closed by the 3rd mo of life, although it is possible to pass a probe through the overlapping flaps in a large percentage of children and in 15–25% of adults. Functional closure of the ductus arteriosus is usually complete by 10–15 hr in a normal neonate, although the ductus may remain patent much longer in the presence of congenital heart disease, especially when associated with cyanosis. In premature newborn infants, an evanescent systolic murmur with late accentuation or a continuous murmur may be audible, and in the context of respiratory distress syndrome, the presence of a patent ductus arteriosus should be suspected (see Chapter 101.4).

The normal ductus arteriosus differs morphologically from the adjoining aorta and pulmonary artery in that the ductus has a significant amount of circularly arranged smooth muscle in its medial layer. During fetal life, patency of the ductus arteriosus appears to be maintained by the combined relaxant effects of low oxygen tension and endogenously produced prostaglandins, specifically prostaglandin E_2. In a full-term neonate, oxygen is the most important factor controlling ductal closure. When the PO_2 of the blood passing through the ductus reaches about 50 mm Hg, the ductal wall constricts. The effects of oxygen on ductal smooth muscle may be direct or mediated by its effects on prostaglandin synthesis. Gestational age also appears to play an important role; the ductus of a premature infant is less responsive to oxygen, even though its musculature is developed.

421.4 • Persistent Pulmonary Hypertension of the Neonate (Persistence of Fetal Circulatory Pathways)

See Chapter 101.8.

421.5 • The Influence of Fetal Environmental Factors on Adult Cardiovascular and Metabolic Disease

The "fetal origins of adult disease" hypothesis suggests that in utero environmental factors, particularly abnormalities of nutrition, could "program" the fetus to be susceptible to adult diseases such as hypertension and metabolic syndrome (insulin resistance, Type 2 diabetes, obesity). This hypothesis has been supported by epidemiologic studies as well as by experimental studies in animals, examining molecular, metabolic and endocrine adaptations to fetal nutrient deprivation. Fetus with low birth-weight status may "program" their cell development to adapt to a poor in utero nutritional environment by becoming "thrifty." After birth, with ample access to nutrients, the metabolic syndrome may then develop, with complications appearing in adulthood. There is still debate over the exact contribution of fetal "epigenetic" vs traditional genetic factors and their interplay with the postnatal environment.

Abman SH: Abnormal vasoreactivity in the pathophysiology of persistent pulmonary hypertension of the newborn. *Pediatr Rev* 1999;20:e103–e109.

Freed MD, Heymann MA, Lewis AB, et al: Prostaglandin E1 infants with ductus arteriosus-dependent congenital heart disease. *Circulation* 1981;64:899–905.

Gersony WM, Peckham GH, Ellison RC, et al: Effects of indomethacin in premature infants with patent ductus arteriosus: Results of a national collaborative study. *J Pediatr* 1983;102:895–906.

Konduri GG: New approaches for persistent pulmonary hypertension of newborn. *Clin Perinatol* 2004;31:591–611.

McMillen IC, Robinson JS: Developmental origins of the metabolic syndrome: Prediction, plasticity, and programming. *Physiol Rev* 2005;85:571–633.

Ozanne SE, Fernandez-Twinn D, Hales CN: Fetal growth and adult diseases. *Semin Perinatol* 2004;28:81–87.

Rudolph AM: *Congenital Diseases of the Heart: Clinical-Physiological Considerations,* 2nd ed. New York, Futura, 2001.

Trines J, Hornberger LK: Evolution of heart disease in utero. *Pediatr Cardiol* 2004;25:287–298.

Walsh MC, Stork EK: Persistent pulmonary hypertension of the newborn. Rational therapy based on pathophysiology. *Clin Perinatol* 2001;28:609–627.

Section 2 — Evaluation of the Cardiovascular System — Daniel Bernstein

Chapter 422 ■ History and Physical Examination

The importance of the history and physical examination cannot be overemphasized in the evaluation of infants and children with suspected cardiovascular disorders. Patients may require further laboratory evaluation and eventual treatment, or the family may be reassured that no significant problem exists. Although the ready availability of echocardiography may entice the clinician to skip these preliminary steps, an initial evaluation by a skilled cardiologist is preferred for several reasons: (1) a cardiac examination allows the cardiologist to guide the echocardiographic evaluation toward confirming or eliminating specific diagnoses, thereby increasing its accuracy; (2) because most childhood murmurs are innocent, evaluation by a pediatric cardiologist can eliminate unnecessary and expensive laboratory tests; and (3) the cardiologist's knowledge and experience are important in reassuring the patient's family and preventing unnecessary restrictions on healthy physical activity.

HISTORY. A comprehensive cardiac history starts with details of the perinatal period including the presence of cyanosis, respiratory distress, or prematurity. Maternal complications such as gestational diabetes, medications, systemic lupus erythematosus, or substance abuse can be associated with cardiac problems. If cardiac symptoms began during infancy, the timing of the initial symptoms should be noted to provide important clues about the specific cardiac condition.

Many of the symptoms of **heart failure** in infants and children are age specific. In infants, feeding difficulties are common. Inquiry should be made about the frequency of feeding and either the volume of each feeding or the time spent on each breast. An infant with heart failure often takes less volume per feeding and becomes dyspneic or diaphoretic while sucking. After falling asleep exhausted, the baby, inadequately fed, will awaken for the next feeding after a brief time. This cycle continues around the clock and must be carefully differentiated from colic or other feeding disorders. Additional symptoms and signs include those of respiratory distress: rapid breathing, nasal flaring, cyanosis, and chest retractions. In older children, heart failure may be manifested as exercise intolerance, difficulty keeping up with peers during sports or need for a nap after coming home from school, and poor growth. Eliciting a history of fatigue in an older child requires questions about age-specific activities, including stair climbing, walking, bicycle riding, physical education class, and competitive sports; information should be obtained regarding more severe manifestations such as orthopnea and nocturnal dyspnea.

Cyanosis at rest is often overlooked by parents; it may be mistaken for a normal individual variation in color. Cyanosis during crying or exercise, however, is more often noted as abnormal by observant parents. Many infants and toddlers turn "blue around the lips" when crying vigorously or during breath-holding spells; this condition must be carefully differentiated from cyanotic heart disease by inquiring about inciting factors, the length of episodes, and whether the tongue and mucous membranes also appear cyanotic. Newborns have cyanotic extremities (acrocyanosis) when undressed and cold; this response to cold must be carefully differentiated from true cyanosis.

Chest pain is an unusual manifestation of cardiac disease in pediatric patients, although it is a frequent cause for referral to a pediatric cardiologist, especially in adolescents. Nonetheless, a careful history, physical examination, and, if indicated, laboratory or imaging tests will assist in identifying the cause of chest pain (Table 422-1).

TABLE 422-1. Differential Diagnosis of Chest Pain in Pediatric Patients

MUSCULOSKELETAL (COMMON)
Trauma (accidental, abuse)
Exercise, overuse injury (strain, bursitis)
Costochondritis (Tietze syndrome)
Herpes zoster (cutaneous)
Pleurodynia
Fibrositis
Slipping rib
Sickle cell anemia vaso-occlusive crisis
Osteomyelitis (rare)
Primary or metastatic tumor (rare)
PULMONARY (COMMON)
Pneumonia
Pleurisy
Asthma
Chronic cough
Pneumothorax
Infarction (sickle cell anemia)
Foreign body
Embolism (rare)
Pulmonary hypertension (rare)
Tumor (rare)
Bronchiectasis
GASTROINTESTINAL (LESS COMMON)
Esophagitis (gastroesophageal reflux, infectious, pill)
Esophageal foreign body
Esophageal spasm
Cholecystitis
Subdiaphragmatic abscess
Perihepatitis (Fitz-Hugh-Curtis syndrome)
Peptic ulcer disease
CARDIAC (LESS COMMON)
Pericarditis
Postpericardiotomy syndrome
Endocarditis
Cardiomyopathy
Mitral valve prolapse
Aortic or subaortic stenosis
Arrhythmias
Marfan syndrome (dissecting aortic aneurysm)
Kawasaki disease
Cocaine, sympathomimetic ingestion
Angina (familial hypercholesterolemia, anomalous coronary artery)
IDIOPATHIC (COMMON)
Anxiety, hyperventilation
Panic disorder
OTHER (LESS COMMON)
Spinal cord or nerve root compression
Breast-related pathologic condition
Castleman disease (lymph node neoplasm)

Cardiac disease may be a manifestation of a known congenital malformation syndrome with typical physical findings (Table 422-2) or a manifestation of a generalized disorder affecting the heart and other organ systems (Table 422-3). Extracardiac malformations may be noted in 20–45% of infants with congenital heart disease. Between 5 and 10% of patients have a known chromosomal abnormality; the importance of genetics will increase as our knowledge of specific gene defects linked to congenital heart disease increases. A careful family history may also reveal early coronary artery disease or stroke (familial hypercholesterolemia or thrombophilia), generalized muscle disease (muscular dystrophy, dermatomyositis, familial or metabolic cardiomyopathy), or relatives with congenital heart disease.

GENERAL PHYSICAL EXAMINATION. After general assessment of the patient, specific attention is directed toward the presence of cyanosis, abnormalities in growth, and any evidence of respiratory distress. Evaluation of a murmur must always be performed in the context of other physical findings. Frequently, associated findings, such as the quality of the pulses or the presence of a ventricular heave, provide important clues to a specific cardiac diagnosis.

Accurate measurement of height and weight and plotting on a standard growth chart are important because both cardiac failure and chronic cyanosis result in **failure to thrive.** Growth failure is usually manifested predominantly by poor weight gain; if length or head circumference is also affected, additional congenital malformations or metabolic disorders may be present.

Mild cyanosis may be too subtle for early detection, and clubbing of the fingers and toes is not usually manifested until late in the 1st yr of life, even in the presence of severe arterial oxygen desaturation. **Cyanosis** is best observed over the nail beds, lips, tongue, and mucous membranes. Differential cyanosis, manifested as blue lower extremities and pink upper extremities (usually the right arm), is seen with right-to-left shunting across a ductus arteriosus in the presence of coarctation or an interrupted aortic arch. Circumoral cyanosis or blueness around the forehead may be the result of prominent venous plexuses in these areas, rather than decreased arterial oxygen saturation. The extremities of infants often turn blue when the infant is unwrapped and cold (acrocyanosis), and this condition can be distinguished from central cyanosis by examination of the tongue and mucous membranes.

Heart failure in infants and children results in some degree of hepatomegaly and occasionally splenomegaly. The sites of **peripheral** edema are age dependent. In infants, edema is usually seen around the eyes and over the flanks, especially on 1st waking in the morning. Older children and teenagers manifest both periorbital edema and pedal edema. A frequent initial complaint in these older patients is that their clothes no longer fit.

The heart rate of newborn infants is rapid and subject to wide fluctuations (Table 422-4). The average rate ranges from 120 to 140 beats/min and may increase to 170+ beats/min during crying and activity or drop to 70–90 beats/min during sleep. As the child grows older, the average pulse rate decreases and may be as low as 40 beats/min in athletic adolescents. Persistent tachycardia (>200 beats/min in neonates, 150 beats/min in infants, or 120 beats/min in older children), bradycardia, or an irregular heartbeat other than sinus arrhythmia requires investigation to exclude pathologic arrhythmias (see Chapter 435).

Careful evaluation of the character of the **pulses** is an important early step in the physical diagnosis of congenital heart disease. A wide pulse pressure with bounding pulses may suggest an aortic runoff lesion such as patent ductus arteriosus, aortic insufficiency, an arterial-venous communication, or increased cardiac output secondary to anemia, anxiety, or conditions associated with increased catecholamine or thyroid hormone secretion. The presence of diminished pulses in all extremities is associated with pericardial tamponade, left ventricular outflow

TABLE 422-2. Congenital Malformation Syndromes Associated with Congenital Heart Disease

SYNDROME	FEATURES
CHROMOSOMAL DISORDERS	
Trisomy 21 (Down syndrome)	Endocardial cushion defect, VSD, ASD
Trisomy 21p (cat eye syndrome)	Miscellaneous, total anomalous pulmonary venous return
Trisomy 18	VSD, ASD, PDA, coarctation of aorta, bicuspid aortic or pulmonary valve
Trisomy 13	VSD, ASD, PDA, coarctation of aorta, bicuspid aortic or pulmonary valve
Trisomy 9	Miscellaneous
XXXXY	PDA, ASD
Penta X	PDA, VSD
Triploidy	VSD, ASD, PDA
XO (Turner syndrome)	Bicuspid aortic valve, coarctation of aorta
Fragile X	Mitral valve prolapse, aortic root dilatation
Duplication 3q2	Miscellaneous
Deletion 4p	VSD, PDA, aortic stenosis
Deletion 9p	Miscellaneous
Deletion 5p (cri du chat syndrome)	VSD, PDA, ASD
Deletion 10q	VSD, TOF, conotruncal lesions*
Deletion 13q	VSD
Deletion 18q	VSD
SYNDROME COMPLEXES	
CHARGE association (*c*oloboma, *h*eart, *a*tresia choanae, *r*etardation, *g*enital and *e*ar anomalies)	VSD, ASD, PDA, TOF, endocardial cushion defect
DiGeorge sequence, CATCH 22 (*c*ardiac defects, *a*bnormal facies, *t*hymic aplasia, *c*left palate, and *h*ypocalcemia)	Aortic arch anomalies, conotruncal anomalies
Alagille syndrome (arteriohepatic dysplasia)	Peripheral pulmonic stenosis
VATER association (*v*ertebral, *a*nal, *t*racheo *e*sophageal, *r*adial, and *r*enal anomalies)	VSD, TOF, ASD, PDA
FAVS (*f*acio-*a*uriculo-*v*ertebral *s*pectrum)	TOF, VSD
CHILD (*c*ongenital *h*emidysplasia with *i*chthyosiform erythroderma, *l*imb *d*efects)	Miscellaneous
Mulibrey nanism (*mu*scle, *li*ver, *br*ain, *ey*e)	Pericardial thickening, constrictive pericarditis
Asplenia syndrome	Complex cyanotic heart lesions with decreased pulmonary blood flow, transposition of great arteries, anomalous pulmonary venous return, dextrocardia, single ventricle, single atrioventricular valve
Polysplenia syndrome	Acyanotic lesions with increased pulmonary blood flow, azygos continuation of inferior vena cava, partial anomalous pulmonary venous return, dextrocardia, single ventricle, common atrioventricular valve
PHACE syndrome (*p*osterior brain fossa anomalies, facial *h*emangiomas, *a*rterial anomalies, cardiac anomalies and aortic coarctation, *e*ye anomalies)	VSD, PDA, coarctation of aorta, arterial aneurysms
TERATOGENIC AGENTS	
Congenital rubella	PDA, peripheral pulmonic stenosis
Fetal hydantoin syndrome	VSD, ASD, coarctation of aorta, PDA
Fetal alcohol syndrome	ASD, VSD
Fetal valproate effects	Coarctation of aorta, hypoplastic left side of heart, aortic stenosis, pulmonary atresia, VSD
Maternal phenylketonuria	VSD, ASD, PDA, coarctation of aorta
Retinoic acid embryopathy	Conotruncal anomalies
OTHERS	
Apert syndrome	VSD
Autosomal dominant polycystic kidney disease	Mitral valve prolapse
Carpenter syndrome	PDA
Conradi syndrome	VSD, PDA
Crouzon disease	PDA, coarctation of aorta
Cutis laxa	Pulmonary hypertension, pulmonic stenosis
de Lange syndrome	VSD
Ellis-van Creveld syndrome	Single atrium, VSD
Holt-Oram syndrome	ASD, VSD, 1st-degree heart block
Infant of diabetic mother	Hypertrophic cardiomyopathy, VSD, conotruncal anomalies
Kartagener syndrome	Dextrocardia
Meckel-Gruber syndrome	ASD, VSD
Noonan syndrome	Pulmonic stenosis, ASD, cardiomyopathy
Pallister-Hall syndrome	Endocardial cushion defect
Rubinstein-Taybi syndrome	VSD
Scimitar syndrome	Hypoplasia of right lung, anomalous pulmonary venous return to inferior vena cava
Smith-Lemli-Opitz syndrome	VSD, PDA
TAR syndrome (*t*hrombocytopenia and *a*bsent *r*adius)	ASD, TOF
Treacher Collins syndrome	VSD, ASD, PDA
Williams syndrome	Supravalvular aortic stenosis, peripheral pulmonic stenosis

*Conotruncal = TOF, pulmonary atresia, truncus arteriosus, transposition of great arteries.
ASD, atrial septal defect; PDA, patent ductus arteriosus; TOF, tetralogy of Fallot; VSD, ventricular septal defect.

TABLE 422-3. Cardiac Manifestations of Systemic Diseases

SYSTEMIC DISEASE	CARDIAC COMPLICATIONS
INFLAMMATORY DISORDERS	
Sepsis	Hypotension, myocardial dysfunction, pericardial effusion, pulmonary hypertension
Juvenile rheumatoid arthritis	Pericarditis, rarely myocarditis
Systemic lupus erythematosus	Pericarditis, Libman-Sacks endocarditis, coronary arteritis, coronary atherosclerosis (with steroids), congenital heart block
Scleroderma	Pulmonary hypertension, myocardial fibrosis, cardiomyopathy
Dermatomyositis	Cardiomyopathy, arrhythmias, heart block
Kawasaki disease	Coronary artery aneurysm and thrombosis, myocardial infarction, myocarditis, valvular insufficiency
Sarcoidosis	Granuloma, fibrosis, amyloidosis, biventricular hypertrophy, arrhythmias
Lyme disease	Arrhythmias, myocarditis
Löffler hypereosinophilic syndrome	Endomyocardial disease
INBORN ERRORS OF METABOLISM	
Refsum disease	Arrhythmia, sudden death
Hunter-Hurler syndrome	Valvular insufficiency, heart failure, hypertension
Fabry disease	Mitral insufficiency, coronary artery disease with myocardial infarction
Glycogen storage disease IIa (Pompe disease)	Short PR interval, cardiomegaly, heart failure, arrhythmias
Carnitine deficiency	Heart failure, cardiomyopathy
Gaucher disease	Pericarditis
Homocystinuria	Coronary thrombosis
Alkaptonuria	Atherosclerosis, valvular disease
Morquio-Ullrich syndrome	Aortic incompetence
Scheie syndrome	Aortic incompetence
CONNECTIVE TISSUE DISORDERS	
Arterial calcification of infancy	Calcinosis of coronary arteries, aorta
Marfan syndrome	Aortic and mitral insufficiency, dissecting aortic aneurysm, mitral valve prolapse
Congenital contractural arachnodactyly	Mitral insufficiency or prolapse
Ehlers-Danlos syndrome	Mitral valve prolapse, dilatated aortic root
Osteogenesis imperfecta	Aortic incompetence
Pseudoxanthoma elasticum	Peripheral arterial disease
NEUROMUSCULAR DISORDERS	
Friedreich ataxia	Cardiomyopathy
Duchenne dystrophy	Cardiomyopathy, heart failure
Tuberous sclerosis	Cardiac rhabdomyoma
Familial deafness	Occasionally arrhythmia, sudden death
Neurofibromatosis	Pulmonic stenosis, pheochromocytoma, coarctation of aorta
Riley-Day syndrome	Episodic hypertension, postural hypotension
Von Hippel-Lindau disease	Hemangiomas, pheochromocytomas
ENDOCRINE-METABOLIC DISORDERS	
Graves disease	Tachycardia, arrhythmias, heart failure
Hypothyroidism	Bradycardia, pericardial effusion, cardiomyopathy, low-voltage electrocardiogram
Pheochromocytoma	Hypertension, myocardial ischemia, myocardial fibrosis, cardiomyopathy
Carcinoid	Right-sided endocardial fibrosis
HEMATOLOGIC DISORDERS	
Sickle cell anemia	High-output heart failure, cardiomyopathy, pulmonary hypertension
Thalassemia major	High-output heart failure, hemochromatosis
Hemochromatosis (1° or 2°)	Cardiomyopathy
OTHERS	
Appetite suppressants (fenfluramine and dexfenfluramine)	Cardiac valvulopathy, pulmonary hypertension
Cockayne syndrome	Atherosclerosis
Familial dwarfism and nevi	Cardiomyopathy
Jervell and Lange-Nielsen syndrome	Prolonged QT interval, sudden death
Kearns-Sayre syndrome	Heart block
LEOPARD syndrome (lentiginosis)	Pulmonic stenosis, prolonged QT interval
Progeria	Accelerated atherosclerosis
Rendu-Osler-Weber syndrome	Arteriovenous fistula (lung, liver, mucous membrane)
Romano-Ward syndrome	Prolonged QT interval, sudden death
Weill-Marchesani syndrome	Patent ductus arteriosus
Werner syndrome	Vascular sclerosis, cardiomyopathy

LEOPARD, multiple lentigines, electrocardiographic conduction abnormalities, ocular hypertelorism, pulmonary stenosis, abnormal genitals, retardation of growth, sensorineural deafness.

TABLE 422-4. Pulse Rates at Rest

AGE	LOWER LIMITS OF NORMAL		AVERAGE		UPPER LIMITS OF NORMAL	
Newborn	70/min		125/min		190/min	
1–11 mo	80		120		160	
2 yr	80		110		130	
4 yr	80		100		120	
6 yr	75		100		115	
8 yr	70		90		110	
10 yr	70		90		110	
	GIRLS	BOYS	GIRLS	BOYS	GIRLS	BOYS
12 yr	70	65	90	85	110	105
14 yr	65	60	85	80	105	100
16 yr	60	55	80	75	100	95
18 yr	55	50	75	70	95	90

obstruction, or cardiomyopathy. The radial and femoral pulses should always be palpated simultaneously. Normally, the femoral pulse should be appreciated immediately before the radial pulse. In older children with coarctation of the aorta, blood flow to the descending aorta may channel through collateral vessels and result in the femoral pulse being delayed until after the radial pulse (**radial-femoral delay**).

Blood pressure should be measured in the arms as well as in the legs, the latter on at least one occasion to be certain that coarctation of the aorta is not overlooked. Palpation of the femoral or dorsalis pedis pulse, or both, is not reliable alone to exclude coarctation. In older children, a mercury sphygmomanometer with a cuff that covers approximately two thirds of the upper part of the arm or leg may be used for blood pressure measurement. A cuff that is too small results in falsely high readings, whereas a cuff that is too large records slightly decreased pressure. Pediatric clinical facilities should be equipped with 3, 5, 7, 12, and 18 cm cuffs to accommodate the large spectrum of pediatric patient sizes. The 1st Korotkoff sounds indicate systolic pressure. As cuff pressure is slowly decreased, the sounds usually become muffled before they disappear. Diastolic pressure may be recorded when the sounds become muffled (preferred) or when they disappear altogether; the former is usually slightly higher and the latter slightly lower than true diastolic pressure. For lower extremity blood pressure determination, the stethoscope is placed over the popliteal artery. Ordinarily, the pressure recorded in the legs with the cuff technique is about 10 mm Hg higher than that in the arms.

In infants, blood pressure can be determined by auscultation, palpation, or an oscillometric (Dinamap) device that, when properly used, provides accurate measurements in infants as well as older children.

Blood pressure varies with the age of the child and is closely related to height and weight. Significant increases occur during adolescence, and many temporary variations take place before the more stable levels of adult life are attained. Exercise, excitement, coughing, crying, and struggling may raise the systolic pressure of infants and children as much as 40–50 mm Hg greater than their usual levels. Variability in blood pressure in children of approximately the same age and body build should be expected, and serial measurements should always be obtained when evaluating a patient with hypertension (Figs. 422-1 and 422-2).

Though of little use in infants, in cooperative older children, inspection of the **jugular venous pulse** wave provides information about central venous and right atrial pressure. The neck veins should be inspected with the patient sitting at a 90-degree angle. The external jugular vein should not be visible above the clavicles unless central venous pressure is elevated. Increased venous pressure transmitted to the internal jugular vein may appear as

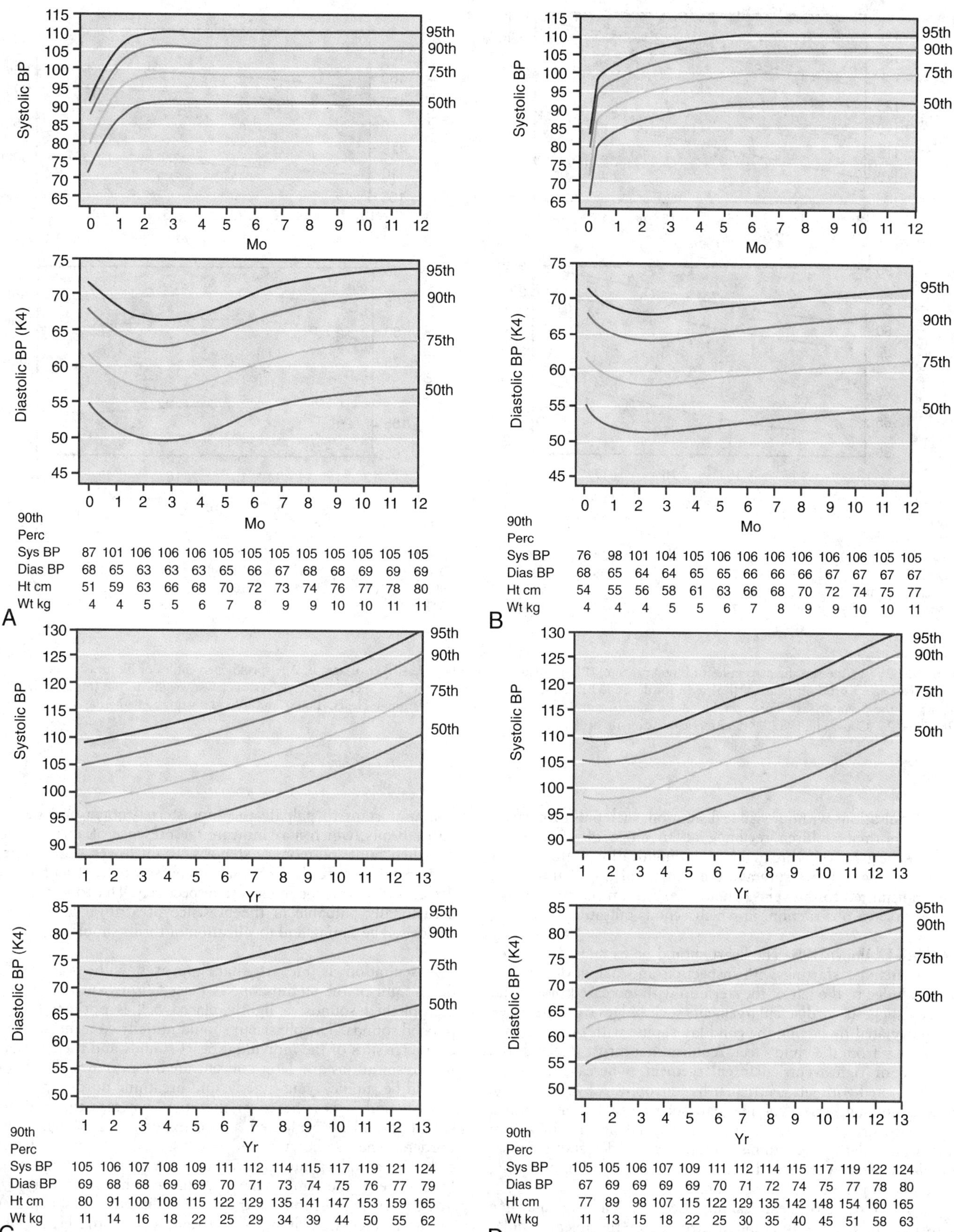

Figure 422-1. *A*, Age-specific percentiles of blood pressure (BP) measurements in boys from birth to 12 mo of age. *B*, Age-specific percentiles of BP measurements in girls from birth to 12 mo of age. *C*, Age-specific percentiles of BP measurements in boys 1–13 yr of age. *D*, Age-specific percentiles of BP measurements in girls 1–13 yr of age; Korotkoff phase IV (K4) used for diastolic BP. Dias, diastolic; Ht, height; Perc, percentile; Sys, systolic; Wt, weight. (From [no authors listed]: Report of the Second Task Force on Blood Pressure Control in Children—1987. National Heart, Lung, and Blood Institute, Bethesda, MD. *Pediatrics* 1987;79:1–25. Copyright 1987 by the American Academy of Pediatrics.)

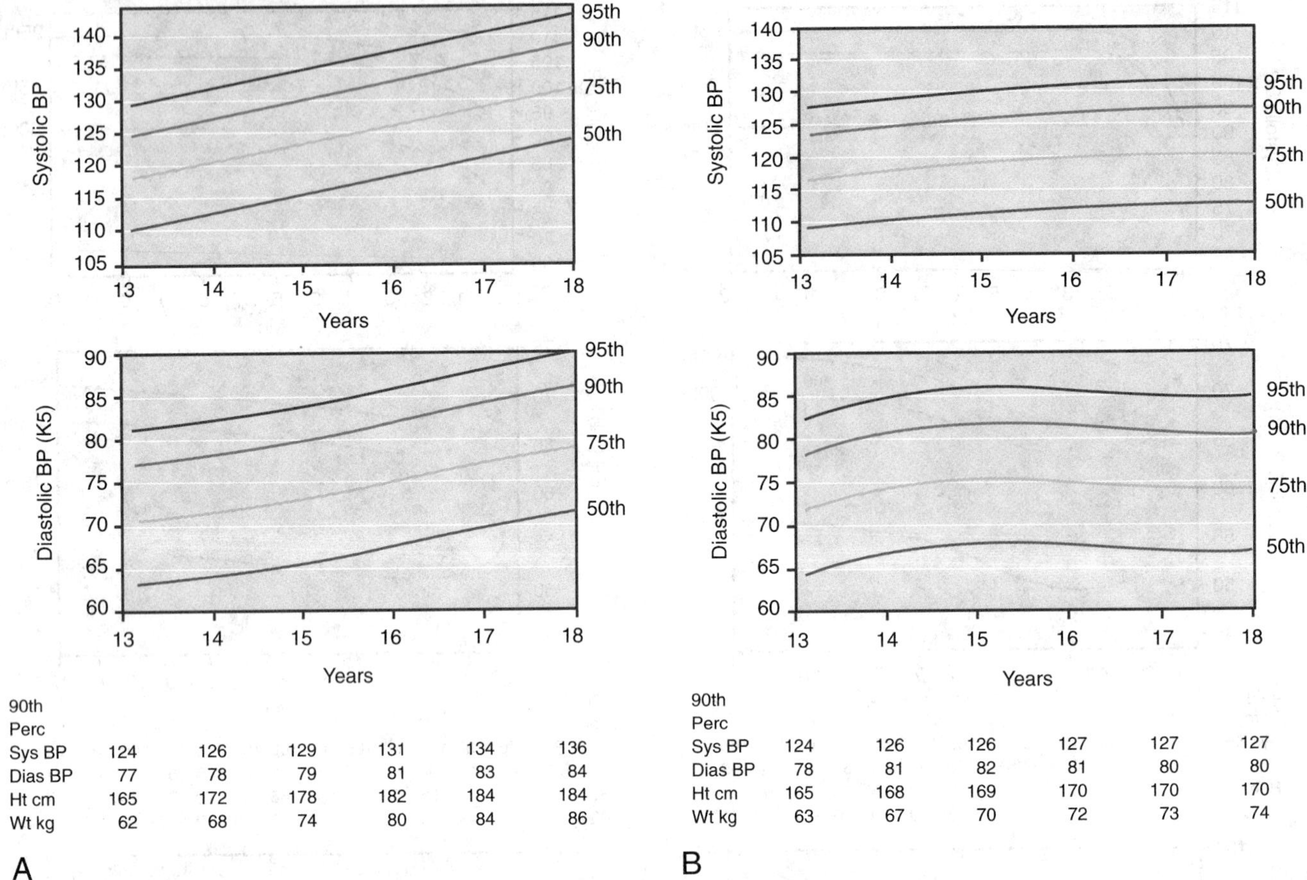

A

90th Perc						
Sys BP	124	126	129	131	134	136
Dias BP	77	78	79	81	83	84
Ht cm	165	172	178	182	184	184
Wt kg	62	68	74	80	84	86

B

90th Perc						
Sys BP	124	126	126	127	127	127
Dias BP	78	81	82	81	80	80
Ht cm	165	168	169	170	170	170
Wt kg	63	67	70	72	73	74

Figure 422-2. *A,* Age-specific percentiles of blood pressure (BP) measurements in boys 13–18 yr of age. *B,* Age-specific percentiles of BP measurements in girls 13–18 yr of age; Korotkoff phase V (K5) used for diastolic BP. Dias, diastolic; Ht, height; Perc, percentile; Sys, systolic; Wt, weight. (From [no authors listed]: Report of the Second Task Force on Blood Pressure Control in Children—1987. National Heart, Lung, and Blood Institute, Bethesda, MD. *Pediatrics* 1987;79:1–25. Copyright 1987 by the American Academy of Pediatrics.)

venous pulsations without visible distention; such pulsation is not seen in normal children reclining at an angle of 45 degrees. Because the great veins are in direct communication with the right atrium, changes in pressure and the volume of this chamber are also transmitted to the veins. The one exception occurs in superior vena cava obstruction, in which venous pulsatility is lost.

CARDIAC EXAMINATION. The heart should be examined in a systematic manner starting with inspection and palpation. A **precordial bulge** to the left of the sternum with increased precordial activity suggests cardiac enlargement; such bulges can often best be appreciated by having the child lay supine with the examiner looking up from the child's feet. A **substernal thrust** indicates the presence of right ventricular enlargement, whereas an apical heave is noted with left ventricular hypertrophy. A hyperdynamic precordium suggests a volume load such as that found with a large left-to-right shunt, although it may be normal in a thin patient. A silent precordium with a barely detectable apical impulse suggests pericardial effusion or severe cardiomyopathy; it may be normal in an obese patient.

The relationship of the **apical impulse** to the midclavicular line is also helpful in the estimation of cardiac size: the apical impulse moves laterally and inferiorly with enlargement of the left ventricle. Right-sided apical impulses signify dextrocardia, tension pneumothorax, or left-sided thoracic space-occupying lesions (e.g., diaphragmatic hernia).

Thrills are the palpable equivalent of murmurs and correlate with the area of maximal auscultatory intensity of the murmur. It is important to palpate the suprasternal notch and neck for aortic bruits, which may indicate the presence of aortic stenosis or, when faint, pulmonary stenosis. Right lower sternal border and apical systolic thrills are characteristic of ventricular septal defect and mitral insufficiency, respectively. Diastolic thrills are occasionally palpable in the presence of atrioventricular valve stenosis. The timing and localization of thrills should be carefully noted.

Auscultation is an art that improves with practice. The diaphragm of the stethoscope is placed firmly on the chest for high-pitched sounds; a lightly placed bell is optimal for low-pitched sounds. The physician should initially concentrate on the characteristics of the individual heart sounds and their variation with respirations and later concentrate on murmurs. The patient should be supine, lying quietly, and breathing normally. The **1st heart sound** is best heard at the apex, whereas the **2nd heart sound** should be evaluated at the upper left and right sternal borders. The 1st heart sound is caused by closure of the atrioventricular valves (mitral and tricuspid); the 2nd sound is caused by closure of the semilunar valves (aortic and pulmonary) [Fig. 422-3]. During inspiration, the decrease in intrathoracic pressure results in increased filling of the right side of the heart, which leads to an increased right ventricular ejection time and thus delayed closure of the pulmonary valve; consequently, **splitting of the 2nd heart** sound increases during inspiration and decreases during expiration.

Often, the 2nd heart sound seems to be single during expiration. The presence of a normally split 2nd sound is strong evi-

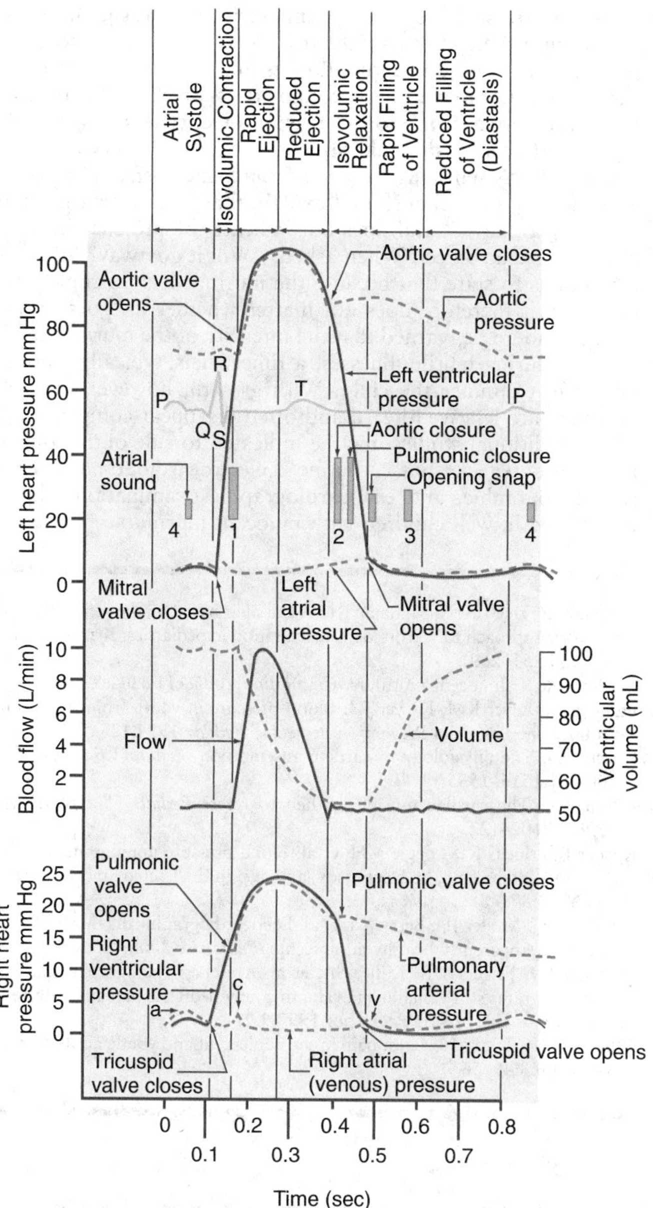

Figure 422-3. Idealized diagram of the temporal events of a cardiac cycle.

dence against the diagnosis of atrial septal defect, defects associated with pulmonary arterial hypertension, severe pulmonary valve stenosis, aortic and pulmonary atresia, and truncus arteriosus. Wide splitting is noted in atrial septal defect, pulmonary stenosis, Ebstein anomaly, total anomalous pulmonary venous return, and right bundle branch block. An accentuated pulmonic component of the 2nd sound with narrow splitting is a sign of pulmonary hypertension. A single 2nd sound occurs in pulmonary or aortic atresia or severe stenosis, truncus arteriosus, and, often, transposition of the great arteries.

A **3rd heart sound** is best heard with the bell at the apex in mid-diastole. A **4th sound** occurring in conjunction with atrial contraction may be heard just before the 1st heart sound in late diastole. The 3rd sound may be normal in an adolescent with a relatively slow heart rate, but in a patient with the clinical signs of heart failure and tachycardia, it may be heard as a gallop rhythm and may merge with a 4th heart sound, a finding known as a summation gallop. A gallop rhythm is attributed to poor compliance of the ventricle, and exaggeration of the normal 3rd sound is associated with ventricular filling.

Ejection clicks, which are heard in early systole, may be related to dilatation of the aorta or pulmonary artery or to a mildly to moderately stenotic semilunar valve. They are heard so close to the 1st heart sound that they may be mistaken for a split 1st sound. Aortic ejection clicks are best heard at the left middle to right upper sternal border and are constant in intensity. They occur in conditions in which the aortic valve is stenotic or the aorta is dilated (tetralogy of Fallot, truncus arteriosus). Pulmonary ejection clicks, which are associated with mild to moderate pulmonary stenosis, are best heard at the left middle to upper sternal border and vary with respirations, often disappearing with inspiration. Split 1st heart sounds are usually heard best at the lower left sternal border. A midsystolic click heard at the apex, often preceding a late systolic murmur, suggests mitral valve prolapse.

Murmurs should be described according to their intensity, pitch, timing (systolic or diastolic), variation in intensity, time to peak intensity, area of maximal intensity, and radiation to other areas. Auscultation for murmurs should be carried out across the upper precordium, down the left or right sternal border, and out to the apex and left axilla. Auscultation should also always be performed in the right axilla and over the back. Systolic murmurs are classified as ejection, pansystolic, or late systolic according to the timing of the murmur in relation to the 1st and 2nd heart sounds. The intensity of systolic murmurs is graded from I to VI: I, barely audible; II, medium intensity; III, loud but no thrill; IV, loud with a thrill; V, very loud but still requiring positioning of the stethoscope at least partly on the chest; and VI, so loud that the murmur can be heard with the stethoscope off the chest.

Systolic ejection murmurs start a short time after a well-heard 1st heart sound, increase in intensity, peak, and then decrease in intensity; they usually end before the 2nd sound. In patients with severe aortic or pulmonary stenosis, however, the murmur may extend beyond the 1st component of the 2nd sound, thus obscuring it. **Pansystolic or holosystolic murmurs** begin almost simultaneously with the 1st heart sound and continue throughout systole, on occasion becoming gradually decrescendo. It is helpful to remember that after closure of the atrioventricular valves (the 1st heart sound), a brief period occurs during which ventricular pressure increases but the semilunar valves remain closed (isovolumic contraction; see Fig. 422-3). Thus, pansystolic murmurs (heard during both isovolumic contraction and the ejection phases of systole) cannot be caused by flow across the semilunar valves because these valves are closed during isovolumic contraction. Pansystolic murmurs are therefore related to blood exiting the contracting ventricle via either an abnormal opening (a ventricular septal defect) or atrioventricular (mitral or tricuspid) valve insufficiency. Systolic ejection murmurs usually imply increased flow or stenosis across one of the ventricular outflow tracts (aortic or pulmonic). In infants with rapid heart rates, it is often difficult to distinguish between ejection and pansystolic murmurs. If a clear and distinct 1st heart sound can be appreciated, the murmur is most likely ejection in nature.

A **continuous murmur** is a systolic murmur that continues or "spills" into diastole and indicates continuous flow, such as in the presence of a patent ductus arteriosus or other aortopulmonary communication. This murmur should be differentiated from a to-and-fro murmur, which indicates that the systolic component of the murmur ends at or before the 2nd sound and the diastolic murmur begins after semilunar valve closure (aortic or pulmonary stenosis combined with insufficiency). A late systolic murmur begins well beyond the 1st heart sound and continues until the end of systole. Such murmurs may be heard after a midsystolic click in patients with mitral valve prolapse and insufficiency.

Several types of **diastolic murmurs** (graded I–IV) can be identified. A decrescendo diastolic murmur is a blowing murmur along the left sternal border that begins with S_2 and diminishes toward mid-diastole. When high-pitched, this murmur is associated with aortic valve insufficiency or pulmonary insufficiency related to pulmonary hypertension. When low-pitched, this murmur is associated with pulmonary valve insufficiency in the absence of pulmonary hypertension. A low-pitched decrescendo diastolic murmur is typically noted after surgical repair of the pulmonary outflow tract in defects such as tetralogy of Fallot or in patients with absent pulmonary valves. A rumbling mid-diastolic murmur at the left middle and lower sternal border may be due to increased blood flow across the tricuspid valve, such as occurs with an atrial septal defect or, less often, because of actual stenosis of this valve. When this murmur is heard at the apex, it is caused by increased flow across the mitral valve, such as occurs with large left-to-right shunts at the ventricular level (ventricular septal defects), at the great vessel level (patent ductus arteriosus, aortopulmonary shunts), or with increased flow because of mitral insufficiency. When an apical diastolic rumbling murmur is longer and is accentuated at the end of diastole (presystolic), it usually indicates anatomic mitral valve stenosis.

The absence of a precordial murmur does not rule out significant congenital or acquired heart disease. Congenital heart defects, some of which are ductal dependent, may not demonstrate a murmur if the ductus arteriosus closes. These lesions include pulmonary or tricuspid valve atresia and transposition of the great arteries. Murmurs may seem insignificant in patients with severe aortic stenosis, atrial septal defects, anomalous pulmonary venous return, atrioventricular septal defects, coarctation of the aorta, or anomalous insertion of a coronary artery. Careful attention to other components of the physical examination (growth failure, cyanosis, peripheral pulses, precordial impulse, heart sounds) increases the index of suspicion of congenital heart defects in these cases. In contrast, loud murmurs may be present in the absence of structural heart disease, for example, in patients with a large noncardiac arteriovenous malformation, myocarditis, severe anemia, or hypertension.

Many murmurs are not associated with significant hemodynamic abnormalities. These murmurs are referred to as functional, normal, insignificant, or innocent (the preferred term). During routine random auscultation, more than 30% of children may have an innocent murmur at one time in their lives; this percentage increases when auscultation is carried out under nonbasal circumstances (high cardiac output because of fever, infection, anxiety). The most **common innocent murmur** is a medium-pitched, vibratory or "musical," relatively short systolic ejection murmur, which is heard best along the left lower and midsternal border and has no significant radiation to the apex, base, or back. It is heard most frequently in children between 3 and 7 yr of age. The intensity of the murmur often changes with respiration and position and may be attenuated in the sitting or prone position. Innocent pulmonic murmurs are also common in children and adolescents and originate from normal turbulence during ejection into the pulmonary artery. They are higher pitched, blowing, brief early systolic murmurs of grade I–II in intensity and are best detected in the 2nd left parasternal space with the patient in the supine position. Features suggestive of heart disease include murmurs that are pansystolic, grade III or higher, harsh, located at the left upper sternal border, and associated with an early or midsystolic click or an abnormal 2nd heart sound.

A **venous hum** is another example of a common innocent murmur heard during childhood. Such hums are produced by turbulence of blood in the jugular venous system; they have no pathologic significance and may be heard in the neck or anterior portion of the upper part of the chest. A venous hum consists of a soft humming sound heard in both systole and diastole; it can be exaggerated or made to disappear by varying the position of the head, or it can be decreased by lightly compressing the jugular venous system in the neck. These simple maneuvers are sufficient to differentiate a venous hum from the murmurs produced by organic cardiovascular disease, particularly a patent ductus arteriosus.

The lack of significance of an innocent murmur should be discussed with the child's parents. It is important to offer complete reassurance because lingering doubts about the importance of a cardiac murmur may have profound effects on child-rearing practices, most often in the form of overprotectiveness. An underlying fear that a cardiac abnormality is present may negatively affect a child's self-image and subtly influence personality development. The physician should explain that an innocent murmur is simply a "noise" and does not indicate the presence of a significant cardiac defect. When asked, "Will it go away?" the best response is to state that because the murmur has no clinical significance, it therefore does not matter whether it "goes away." Parents should be warned that the intensity of the murmur might increase during febrile illnesses, a time when, typically, another physician examines the child. With growth, however, innocent murmurs are less well heard and often disappear completely. At times, additional studies may be indicated to rule out a congenital heart defect, but "routine" electrocardiographic, chest roentgenographic, and echocardiographic examinations should be avoided in well children with innocent murmurs.

Bhatikar SR, DeGroff C, Mahajan RL: A classifier based on the artificial neural network approach for cardiologic auscultation in pediatrics. *Artif Intell Med* 2005;33:251–260.

Biancaniello T: Innocent murmurs. *Circulation* 2005;111:e20–e22.

Hohn AR, Dwyer KM, Dwyer JH: Blood pressure in youth from four ethnic groups: The Pasadena Prevention Project. *J Pediatr* 1994;125:368–373.

Pelech AN: The physiology of cardiac auscultation. *Pediatr Clin North Am* 2004;51:1515–1535.

Pelech AN: The cardiac murmur. When to refer? *Pediatr Clin North Am* 1998;45:107–122.

Rosner B, Prineas RJ, Loggie MH, et al: Blood pressure nomograms for children and adolescents, by height, sex, and age, in the United States. *J Pediatr* 1993;123:871–886.

Steinberger J, Moller JH, Berry JM, et al: Echocardiographic diagnosis of heart disease in apparently healthy adolescents. *Pediatrics* 2000;105:815–818.

Swenson JM, Fischer DR, Miller SA, et al: Are chest radiographs and electrocardiograms still valuable in evaluating new pediatric patients with heart murmurs or chest pain? *Pediatrics* 1997;99:1–3.

Talner NS, Carboni MP: Chest pain in the adolescent and young adult. *Cardiol Rev* 2000;8:49–56.

Chapter 423 ■ Laboratory Evaluation

423.1 • Radiologic Assessment

The chest x-ray may provide information about cardiac size and shape, pulmonary blood flow (vascularity), pulmonary edema, and associated lung and thoracic anomalies that may be associated with congenital syndromes (skeletal dysplasias, extra or deficient number of ribs, abnormal vertebrae, previous cardiac surgery). Variations are due to differences in body build, the phase of respiration or the cardiac cycle, abnormalities of the thoracic cage, position of the diaphragm, or pulmonary disease.

The most frequently used measurement of cardiac size is the maximal width of the cardiac shadow in a posteroanterior chest film taken mid-inspiration. A vertical line is drawn down the middle of the sternal shadow, and perpendicular lines are drawn from the sternal line to the extreme right and left borders of the heart; the sum of the lengths of these lines is the maximal cardiac width. The maximal chest width is obtained by drawing a horizontal line between the right and left inner borders of the rib cage at the level of the top of the right diaphragm. When the maximal cardiac width is more than half the maximal chest width (cardiothoracic ratio >50%), the heart is usually enlarged. Cardiac size should be evaluated only when the film is taken during inspiration with the patient in an upright position. A diagnosis of "cardiac enlargement" on expiratory or prone films is a common cause of unnecessary referrals and laboratory studies.

The cardiothoracic ratio is a less useful index of cardiac enlargement in infants than in older children because the horizontal position of the heart may increase the ratio to >50% in the absence of true enlargement. Furthermore, the thymus may overlap not only the base of the heart but also virtually the entire mediastinum, thus obscuring the true cardiac silhouette.

A lateral chest roentgenogram may be helpful in infants as well as in older children with pectus excavatum or other conditions that result in a narrow anteroposterior chest dimension. In these situations, the heart may appear small in the lateral view and suggest that the apparent enlargement in the posteroanterior projection was due to either the thymic image (anterior mediastinum only) or flattening of the cardiac chambers as a result of a structural chest abnormality.

In the posteroanterior view, the left border of the cardiac shadow consists of three convex shadows produced, from above downward, by the aortic knob, the main and left pulmonary arteries, and the left ventricle (Fig. 423-1). In cases of moderate to marked left atrial enlargement, the atrium may project between the pulmonary artery and the left ventricle. The outflow tract of the right ventricle does not contribute to the shadows formed by the left border of the heart. The aortic knob is not as easily seen in infants and children as in adults. The side of the aortic arch (left or right) can often be inferred as being opposite the side of the midline from which the air-filled trachea is visualized. This observation is important because a right-sided aortic arch is often present in cyanotic congenital heart disease, particularly the tetralogy of Fallot. Three structures contribute to the right border of the cardiac silhouette: From above downward, they are the superior vena cava, the ascending aorta, and the right atrium.

Enlargement of cardiac chambers or major arteries and veins results in prominence of the areas in which these structures are normally outlined on the chest x-ray. In contrast, the electrocardiogram (ECG) is a more sensitive and accurate index of **ventricular hypertrophy.**

It is also important to assess the degree of pulmonary vascularity. Angiocardiographic studies have shown that the hilar shadows are mainly vascular. Pulmonary overcirculation is usually associated with left-to-right shunt lesions, whereas pulmonary undercirculation is associated with obstruction of the outflow tract of the right ventricle.

The esophagus is closely related to the great vessels, and a barium esophagogram can help delineate these structures in the initial evaluation of suspected vascular rings. Echocardiographic examination best defines the morphologic features of intracardiac chambers; CT and MRI best define extracardiac vascular morphology.

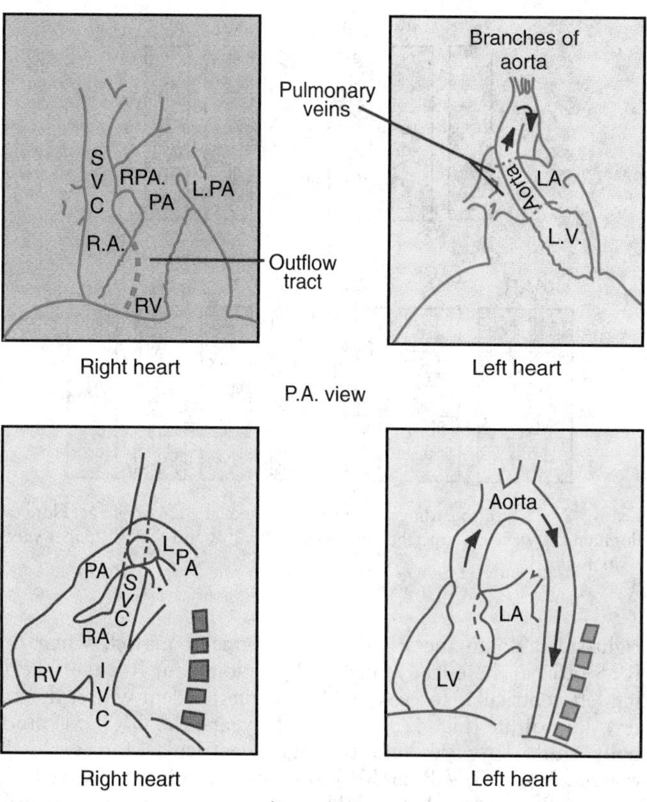

Figure 423-1. Idealized diagrams showing normal position of the cardiac chambers and great blood vessels. IVC, inferior vena cava; LA, left atrium; LPA, left pulmonary artery; LV, left ventricle; PA, pulmonary artery; RA, right atrium; RPA, right pulmonary artery; RV, right ventricle; SVC, superior vena cava. (Adapted and redrawn from Dotter, Steinberg: *Radiology* 1949;53:513.)

423.2 • Electrocardiography

DEVELOPMENTAL CHANGES

The marked changes that occur in cardiac physiology and chamber dominance during the perinatal transition (see Chapter 421) are reflected in the evolution of the ECG during the neonatal period. Because vascular resistance in the pulmonary and systemic circulations is nearly equal in a term fetus, the intrauterine work of the heart results in an equal mass of both the right and left ventricles. After birth, systemic vascular resistance rises when the placental circulation is eliminated, and pulmonary vascular resistance falls when the lungs expand. These changes are reflected in the ECG as the right ventricular wall begins to thin.

The ECG demonstrates these anatomic and hemodynamic features principally by changes in QRS and T-wave morphologic features. It is recommended that a 13-lead ECG be performed in pediatric patients, including either lead V_3R or V_4R, which are important in the evaluation of right ventricular hypertrophy. On occasion, lead V_1 is positioned too far leftward to reflect right ventricular forces accurately. This problem is present particularly in premature infants, in whom the electrocardiographic electrode gel may produce contact among all the precordial leads.

During the 1st days of life, right axis deviation, large R waves, and upright T waves in the right precordial leads (V_3R or V_4R and V_1) are the norm (Fig. 423-2). As pulmonary vascular resistance decreases in the 1st few days after birth, the right precordial T waves become negative. In the great majority of instances, this change occurs within the 1st 48 hr of life. Upright T waves that persist in leads V_3R, V_4R, or V_1 beyond 1 wk of life are an abnormal finding indicating right ventricular hypertrophy or strain, even in the absence of QRS voltage criteria. The T wave in V_1 should never be positive before 6 yr of age and may remain negative into adolescence. This finding represents one of the most important, yet subtle differences between pediatric and adult ECGs and is a common source of error when adult cardiologists interpret pediatric ECGs.

In a newborn, the mean **QRS frontal-plane axis** normally lies in the range of +110 to +180 degrees. The right-sided chest leads reveal a larger positive (R) than negative (S) wave and may do so for months or years because the right ventricle remains relatively thick throughout infancy. Left-sided leads (V_5 and V_6) also reflect

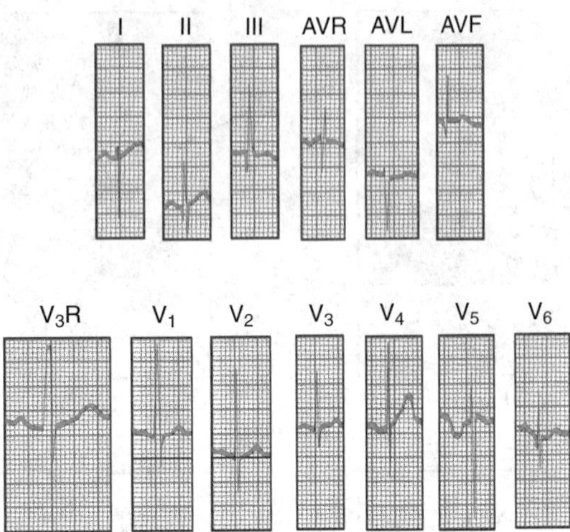

Figure 423-2. Electrocardiogram in a normal neonate <24 hr of age. Note the dominant R wave and upright T waves in leads V_3R and V_1 (V_3R paper speed = 50 mm/sec).

right-sided dominance in the early neonatal period, when the R : S ratio in these leads may be <1. A dominant R wave reflecting left ventricular forces quickly becomes evident within the 1st few days of life (Fig. 423-3). Over the years, the QRS axis gradually shifts leftward, and the right ventricular forces slowly regress. Leads V_1, V_3R, and V_4R display a prominent R wave until 6 mo to 8 yr of age. Most children have an R : S ratio >1 in lead V_4R until they are 4 yr of age. The T waves are inverted in leads V_4R, V_1, V_2, and V_3 during infancy and may remain so into the middle of the 2nd decade of life and beyond. The processes of right ventricular thinning and left ventricular growth are best reflected in the QRS-T pattern over the right precordial leads. The diagnosis of right or left ventricular hypertrophy in a pediatric patient can be made only with an understanding of the normal developmental physiology of these chambers at various ages until adulthood is reached. As the left ventricle becomes dominant, the ECG evolves to the characteristic pattern of older children (Fig. 423-4) and adults (Fig. 423-5).

Ventricular hypertrophy may result in increased voltage in the R and S waves in the chest leads. The height of these deflections is governed by the proximity of the specific electrode to the surface of the heart; by the sequence of electrical activation through the ventricles, which can result in variable degrees of cancellation of forces; and by hypertrophy of the myocardium. Because the chest wall in infants and children, as well as in adolescents, may be relatively thin, the diagnosis of ventricular hypertrophy should not be based on voltage changes alone.

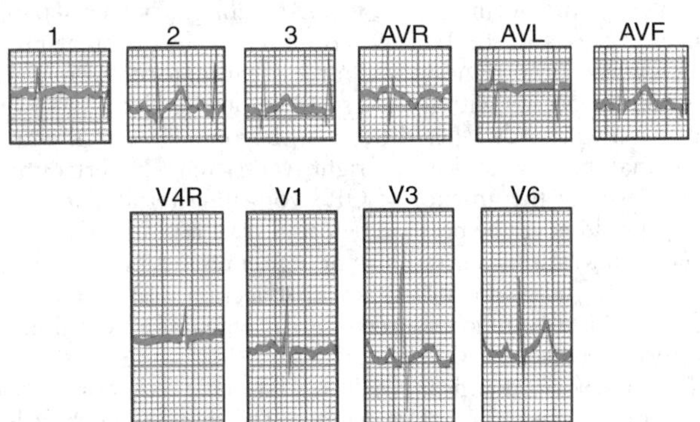

Figure 423-3. Electrocardiogram of a normal infant. Note the tall R and small S waves in V_4R and V_1 and the inverted T wave in these leads. A dominant R wave is also present in V_6.

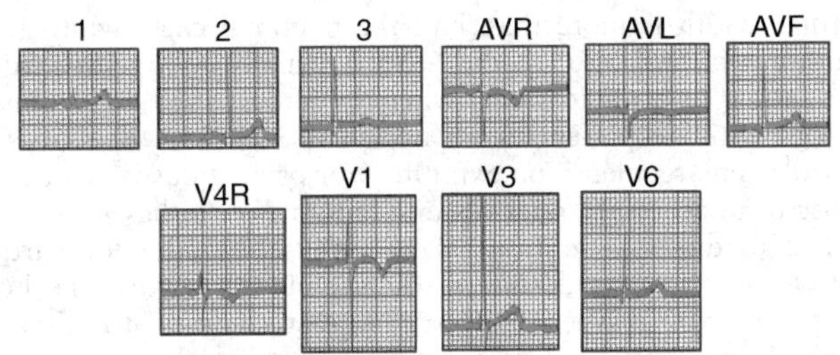

Figure 423-4. Electrocardiogram of a normal child. Note the relatively tall R waves and inversion of the T waves in V_4R and V_1.

The diagnosis of pathologic right ventricular hypertrophy is difficult in the 1st wk of life because physiologic right ventricular hypertrophy is a normal finding. Serial tracings are often necessary to determine whether marked right axis deviation and potentially abnormal right precordial forces or T waves, or both, will persist beyond the neonatal period (Fig. 423-6). In contrast, an adult electrocardiographic pattern (see Fig. 423-5) seen in a neonate suggests left ventricular enlargement. The exception is a premature infant, who may display a more "mature" ECG than a full-term infant (Fig. 423-7) as a result of lower pulmonary vascular resistance secondary to underdevelopment of the medial muscular layer of the pulmonary arterioles. Some premature infants display a pattern of generalized low voltage across the precordium.

The ECG should always be evaluated systematically to avoid the possibility of overlooking a minor, but important abnormality. One approach is to begin with an assessment of rate and rhythm, followed by a calculation of the mean frontal-plane QRS axis, measurements of segment intervals, assessment of voltages, and, finally, assessment of ST and T-wave abnormalities.

RATE AND RHYTHM

A brief rhythm strip should be examined to assess whether a P wave always precedes each QRS complex. The P-wave axis should then be estimated as an indication of whether the rhythm is originating from the sinus node. If the atria are situated normally in the chest, the P wave should be upright in leads I and

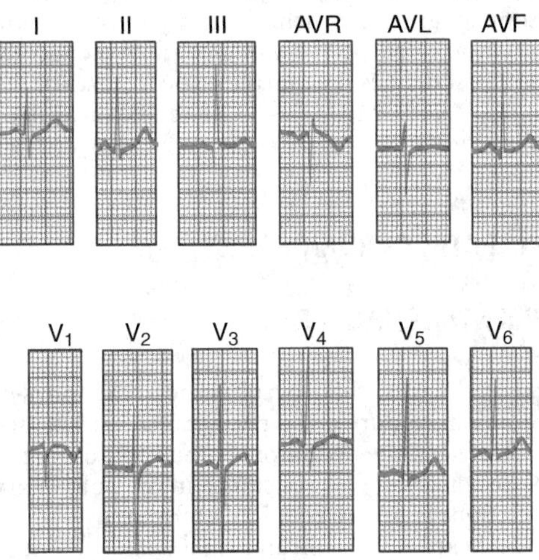

Figure 423-5. Normal adult electrocardiogram. Note the dominant S wave in lead V_1. This pattern in an infant would indicate the presence of left ventricular hypertrophy.

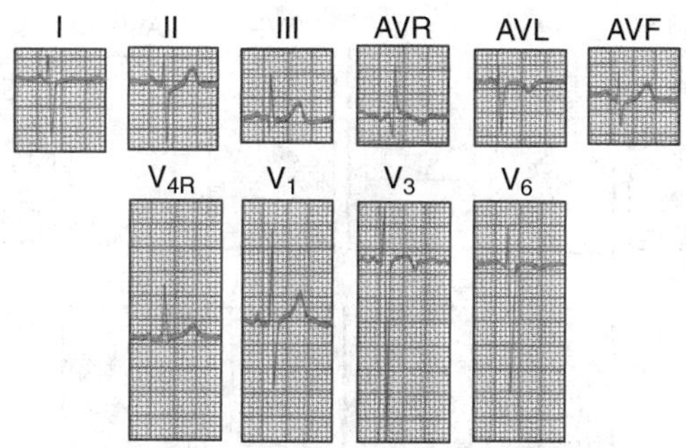

Figure 423-6. Electrocardiogram of an infant with right ventricular hypertrophy (tetralogy of Fallot). Note the tall R waves in the right precordium and deep S waves in V_6. The positive T waves in V_4R and V_1 are also characteristic of right ventricular hypertrophy.

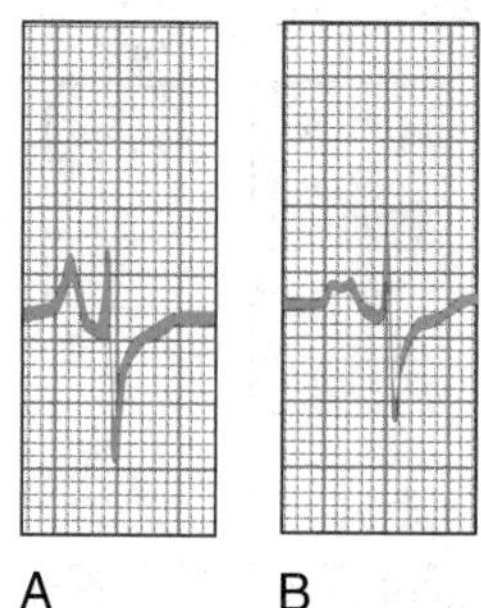

Figure 423-8. Atrial enlargement. *A*, Peaked narrow P waves characteristic of right atrial enlargement. *B*, Wide bifid M-shaped P waves typical of left atrial enlargement.

aVF and inverted in lead aVR. With atrial inversion (situs inversus), the P wave may be inverted in lead I. Inverted P waves in leads II and aVF are seen in nodal or junctional rhythms regardless of atrial position. The absence of P waves indicates a rhythm originating more distally in the conduction system. In this case, the morphologic features of the QRS complexes are important in differentiating a junctional (usually a narrow QRS complex) from a ventricular (usually a wide QRS complex) rhythm.

P WAVES

Tall (>2.5 mm), narrow, and spiked P waves are indicative of **right atrial enlargement** and are seen in congenital pulmonary stenosis, Ebstein anomaly of the tricuspid valve, tricuspid atresia, and sometimes cor pulmonale. These abnormal waves are most obvious in leads II, V_3R, and V_1 (Fig. 423-8*A*). Similar waves are sometimes seen in thyrotoxicosis. **Broad P waves,** commonly **bifid** and sometimes **biphasic,** are indicative of left atrial enlargement (Fig. 423-8*B*). They are seen in some patients with large left-to-right shunts (ventricular septal defect [VSD], patent ductus arteriosus [PDA]) and with severe mitral stenosis or regurgitation. Flat P waves may be encountered in hyperkalemia.

QRS COMPLEX

Right Ventricular Hypertrophy. For the most accurate assessment of ventricular hypertrophy, pediatric ECGs should include the right precordial lead V_3R or V_4R, or both. The diagnosis of right ventricular hypertrophy depends on demonstration of the following changes (see Fig. 423-6): (1) a qR pattern in the right ventricular surface leads; (2) a positive T wave in leads V_3R-V_4R and V_1-V_3 between the ages of 6 days and 6 yr; (3) a monophasic R wave in V_3R, V_4R, or V_1; (4) an rsR′ pattern in the right precordial leads with the 2nd R wave taller than the initial one; (5) age-corrected increased voltage of the R wave in leads V_3R-V_4R or the S wave in leads V_6-V_7, or both; (6) marked right axis deviation (>120 degrees in patients beyond the newborn period); (7) complete reversal of the normal adult precordial RS pattern; and (8) right atrial enlargement. At least two of these changes should be present to support a diagnosis of right ventricular hypertrophy.

Abnormal ventricular loading can be characterized as either systolic (as a result of obstruction of the right ventricular outflow tract, as in pulmonic stenosis) or diastolic (as a result of increased volume load, as in atrial septal defects [ASDs]). These two types of abnormal loads result in distinct electrocardiographic patterns. The **systolic overload pattern** is characterized by tall, pure R waves in the right precordial leads. In older children, the T waves in these leads are initially upright and later become inverted. In infants and children <6 yr, the T waves in V_3R-V_4R and V_1 are abnormally upright. The **diastolic overload pattern** (typically seen in patients with ASDs) is characterized by an rsR′ pattern (Fig. 423-9) and a slightly increased QRS duration (minor right ventricular conduction delay). Patients with mild to moderate pulmonary stenosis may also exhibit an rsR pattern in the right precordial leads.

Left Ventricular Hypertrophy. The following features indicate the presence of left ventricular hypertrophy (Fig. 423-10): (1) depression of the ST segments and inversion of the T waves in the left

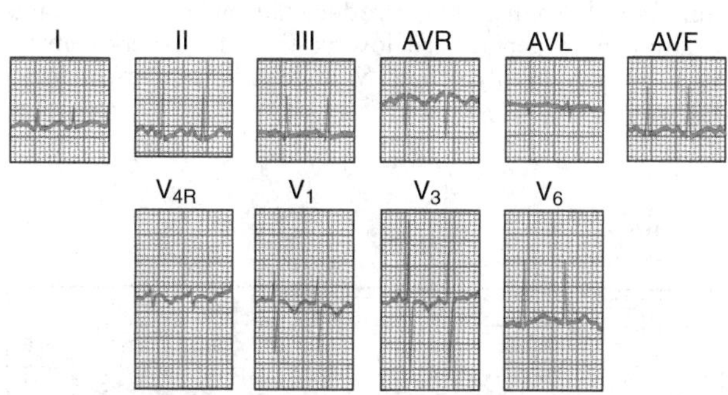

Figure 423-7. Electrocardiogram of a premature infant (weight 2 kg and age 5 wk at the time of the tracing). The cardiovascular system was clinically normal. Left ventricular dominance is manifested by R-wave progression across the chest, similar to tracings obtained from older children. Compare with the tracing from a normal full-term infant (see Fig. 423-3).

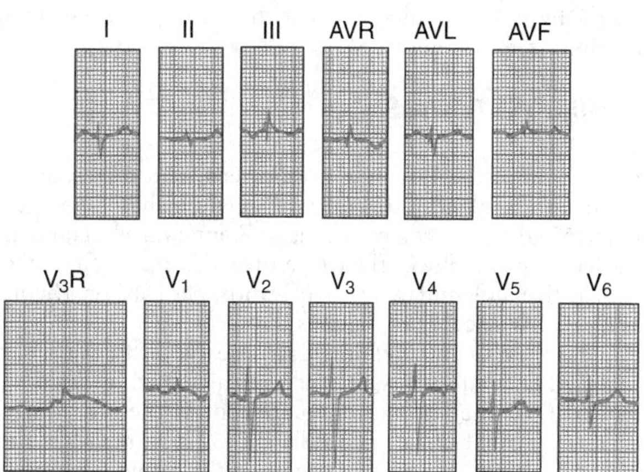

Figure 423-9. Electrocardiogram showing right ventricular conduction delay characterized by an rsR′ pattern in V_1 and a deep S wave in V_6 (V_3R paper speed = 50 mm/sec).

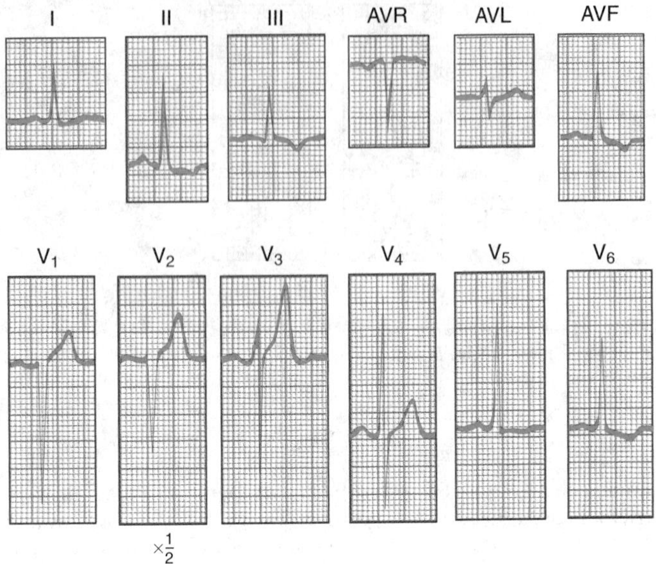

Figure 423-10. Electrocardiogram showing left ventricular hypertrophy in a 12 yr old child with aortic stenosis. Note the deep S wave in V_1-V_3 and tall R in V_5. In addition, T-wave inversion is present in leads II, III, aVF, and V_6.

precordial leads (V_5, V_6, and V_7), known as a left ventricular strain pattern—these findings suggest the presence of a severe lesion; (2) a deep Q wave in the left precordial leads; and (3) increased voltage of the S wave in V_3R and V_1 or the R wave in V_6-V_7, or both. It is important to emphasize that evaluation of left ventricular hypertrophy should not be based on voltage criteria alone. The concepts of systolic and diastolic overload, though not always consistent, are also useful in evaluating left ventricular enlargement. Severe systolic overload of the left ventricle is suggested by straightening of the ST segments and inverted T waves over the left precordial leads; diastolic overload may result in tall R waves, a large Q wave, and normal T waves over the left precordium. Finally, an infant with an ECG that would be considered "normal" for an older child may, in fact, have left ventricular hypertrophy.

Bundle Branch Block. A complete right bundle branch block may be congenital or may be acquired after surgery for congenital heart disease, especially when a right ventriculotomy has been performed, as in repair of the tetralogy of Fallot. Congenital left bundle branch block is rare; this pattern is occasionally seen with cardiomyopathy. A bundle branch block pattern may be indicative of a bypass tract associated with one of the pre-excitation syndromes (see Chapter 435).

P-R AND Q-T INTERVALS

The duration of the P-R interval shortens with increasing heart rate; thus, assessment of this interval should be based on age- and rate-corrected nomograms. A long P-R interval is diagnostic of a **1st-degree heart block,** the cause of which may be congenital, postoperative, inflammatory (myocarditis, pericarditis, rheumatic fever), or pharmacologic (digitalis).

The duration of the Q-T interval varies with the cardiac rate; a corrected Q-T interval (Q-Tc) can be calculated by dividing the measured Q-T interval by the square root of the preceding R-R interval. A normal Q-Tc should be <0.45. It is often lengthened with hypokalemia and hypocalcemia; in the former instance, a U wave may be noted at the end of the T wave (Fig. 423-11). A congenitally prolonged Q-T interval (Fig. 423-12) may also be seen in children with one of the long Q-T syndromes. These

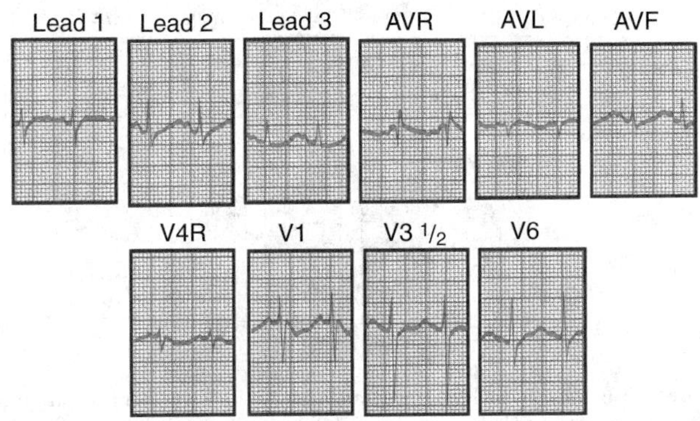

Figure 423-11. Electrocardiogram in hypokalemia (serum potassium, 2.7 mEq/L; serum calcium, 4.8 mEq/L at the time of the tracing). Note the prolongation of electrical systole as evidenced by a widened TU wave, as well as depression of the ST segment in V_4R, V_1, and V_6.

patients are at high risk for ventricular arrhythmias, including a form of ventricular tachycardia known as torsades de pointes, and sudden death (see Chapter 435.5).

ST SEGMENT AND T-WAVE ABNORMALITIES

A slight elevation of the ST segment may occur in normal teenagers and is attributed to early repolarization of the heart. In pericarditis, irritation of the epicardium may cause elevation of the ST segment followed by abnormal T-wave inversion as healing progresses. Administration of digitalis is sometimes associated with sagging of the ST segment and abnormal inversion of the T wave.

Depression of the ST segment may also occur in any condition that produces myocardial damage or ischemia, including severe anemia, carbon monoxide poisoning, aberrant origin of the left coronary artery from the pulmonary artery, glycogen storage disease of the heart, myocardial tumors, and mucopolysaccharidoses. An aberrant origin of the left coronary artery from the pulmonary artery may lead to changes indistinguishable from those of acute myocardial infarction in adults. Similar changes may occur in patients with other rare abnormalities of the coronary arteries and in those with cardiomyopathy, even in the presence of normal coronary arteries. These patterns are often misread in young infants because of the unfamiliarity of pediatricians with this "infarct" pattern, and thus a high index of suspicion must be maintained in infants with symptoms compatible with coronary ischemia.

T-wave inversion may occur in myocarditis and pericarditis, or it may be a sign of either right or left ventricular hypertrophy and strain. Hypothyroidism may produce flat or inverted T waves in association with generalized low voltage. In hyperkalemia, the T waves are commonly of high voltage and are tent-shaped (Fig. 423-13).

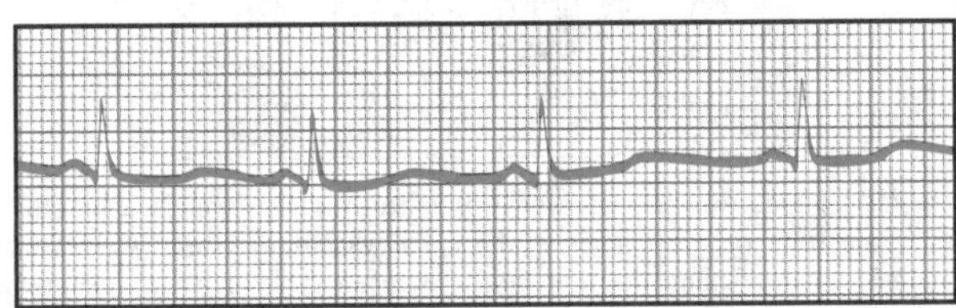

Figure 423-12. Prolonged Q-T interval in a patient with long Q-T syndrome.

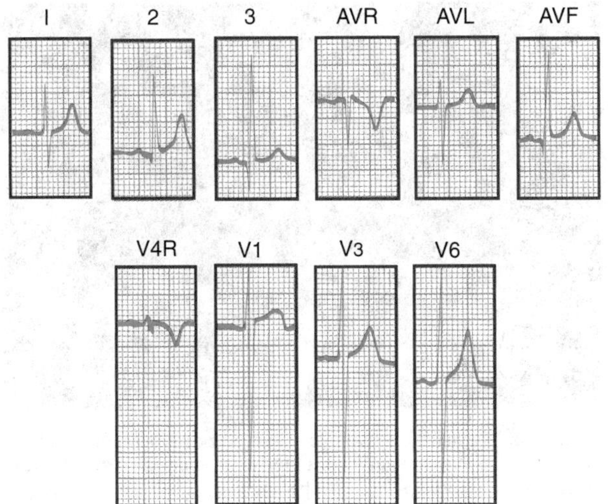

Figure 423-13. Electrocardiogram in hyperkalemia (serum potassium, 6.5 mEq/L; serum calcium, 5.1 mEq/L). Note the tall, tent-shaped T waves, especially in leads I, II, and V_6.

423.3 • Hematologic Data

In acyanotic infants with large left-to-right shunts, the onset of heart failure often coincides with the nadir of the normal physiologic anemia of infancy. Increasing the hematocrit in these patients to >40% may decrease shunt volume and result in an improvement in symptoms; this form of treatment is reserved for infants who are not otherwise surgical candidates (extremely premature infants or those with exceedingly complex congenital heart disease for whom only palliative surgery is possible). In these select infants, regular evaluation of the hematocrit and booster transfusions when appropriate may be helpful in improving growth. In some patients, particularly those who are anemic but stable hemodynamically, erythropoietin (Epogen) can be used to more gradually increase hemoglobin and thus oxygen-carrying capacity.

Polycythemia is frequently noted in cyanotic patients with right-to-left shunts. Patients with severe polycythemia are in a delicate balance between the risks of intravascular thrombosis and a bleeding diathesis. The most frequent abnormalities include accelerated fibrinolysis, thrombocytopenia, abnormal clot retraction, hypofibrinogenemia, prolonged prothrombin time, and prolonged partial thromboplastin time. The preparation of cyanotic, polycythemic patients for elective surgery, such as dental extraction, includes evaluation and treatment of abnormal coagulation.

Because of the high viscosity of polycythemic blood (hematocrit >65%), patients with cyanotic congenital heart disease are at risk for the development of vascular thromboses, especially of cerebral veins. Dehydration increases the risk of thrombosis, and thus adequate fluid intake must be maintained during hot weather or intercurrent gastrointestinal illnesses. Diuretics should be used with caution in these patients and may need to be decreased if fluid intake is a concern. Polycythemic infants with concomitant **iron deficiency** are at even greater risk for cerebrovascular accidents, probably because of the decreased deformability of microcytic red blood cells. Iron therapy produces improvement, but surgical treatment of the cardiac anomaly is the best therapy.

Severely cyanotic patients should have periodic determinations of hemoglobin and hematocrit. Increasing polycythemia, often associated with headache, fatigue, dyspnea, or a combination of these conditions, is one indication for palliative or corrective surgical intervention. In cyanotic patients with inoperable conditions, phlebotomy may be required to treat individuals whose hematocrit has risen to the 65–70% level, usually when the polycythemia is associated with symptoms such as headache. This procedure is not without risk, especially in patients with an extreme elevation in pulmonary vascular resistance. Because these patients do not tolerate wide fluctuations in circulating blood volume, blood should be replaced with fresh frozen plasma or albumin. Whether routine phlebotomy should be performed in polycythemic patients who are asymptomatic is controversial.

423.4 • Echocardiography

Echocardiography dramatically reduces the requirement for invasive studies such as cardiac catheterization. The echocardiographic examination can be used to evaluate cardiac structure in congenital heart lesions, estimate intracardiac pressures and gradients across stenotic valves and vessels, quantitate cardiac contractile function (both systolic and diastolic), determine the direction of flow across a defect, examine the integrity of the coronary arteries, and detect the presence of vegetations from endocarditis, as well as the presence of pericardial fluid, cardiac tumors, and chamber thrombi. Echocardiography may also be used to assist in the performance of pericardiocentesis, balloon atrial septostomy (see Chapter 431.2), and endocardial biopsy and in the placement of flow-directed pulmonary artery (Swan-Ganz) monitoring catheters. **Transesophageal echocardiography** is used to monitor ventricular function in patients during difficult surgical procedures and can provide an immediate assessment of the results of surgical repair of congenital heart lesions. **Fetal echocardiography** can detect the presence of many congenital heart lesions, often as early as 17–19 wk of gestation, and is especially valuable in evaluating fetal cardiac arrhythmias. A complete echocardiographic examination usually entails a combination of M-mode and two-dimensional imaging, as well as pulsed, continuous, and color Doppler flow studies. Three-dimensional echocardiography provides valuable additional information regarding cardiac morphology.

M-Mode Echocardiography

M-mode echocardiography displays a one-dimensional slice of cardiac structure varying over time (Fig. 423-14). It is used mostly for the measurement of cardiac dimensions (wall thickness and chamber size) and cardiac function (fractional shortening, wall thickening). M-mode echocardiography is also useful for assessing the motion of intracardiac structures (opening and closing of valves, movement of free walls and septa) and the anatomy of valves (Fig. 423-15). The most frequently used index of cardiac function in children is percent fractional shortening (%FS), which is calculated as (LVED − LVES)/LVED, where LVED is left ventricular (LV) dimension at end-diastole and LVES is LV dimension at end-systole. Normal fractional shortening is 28–40%. Other M-mode indices of cardiac function include the mean velocity of fiber shortening (mean V_{CF}), systolic time intervals (LVPEP = LV pre-ejection period, LVET = LV ejection time), and isovolemic contraction time. More sophisticated indices of cardiac function can be derived noninvasively with the assistance of echocardiography (pressure-volume relationship, end-systolic wall stress-strain relationship); accuracy is limited when compared with similar measurements in the catheterization laboratory.

Two-Dimensional Echocardiography

Two-dimensional echocardiography provides a real-time image of cardiac structures. With two-dimensional echocardiography, the contracting heart is imaged in real-time using several standard

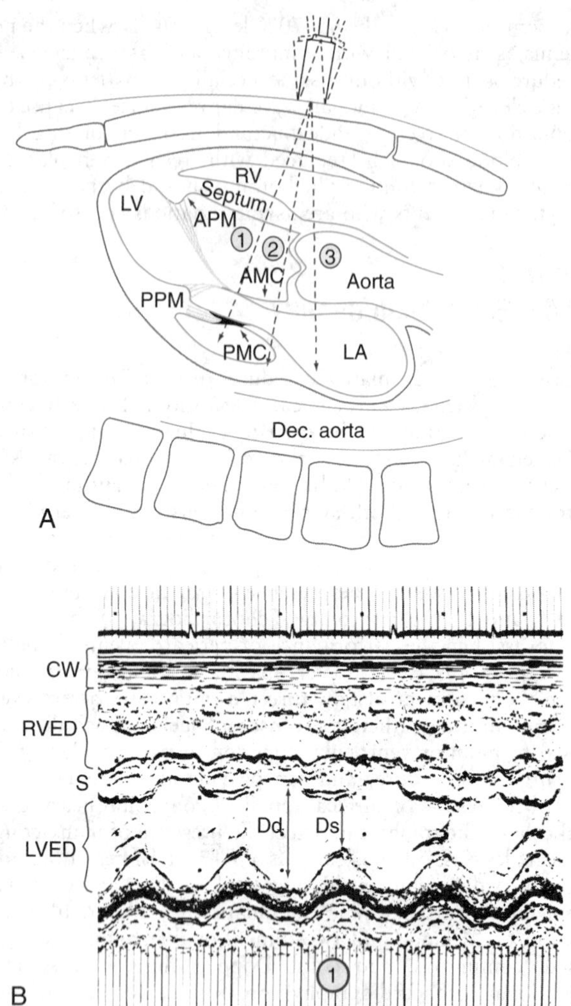

Figure 423-14. M-mode echocardiogram. *A*, Diagram of a sagittal section of a heart showing the structures traversed by the echo beam as it is moved superiorly to positions (1), (2), and (3). AMC, anterior mitral cusp; APM, anterior papillary muscle; Dec. aorta, descending aorta; LA, left atrium; LV, left ventricle; PMC, posterior mitral cusp; PPM, posterior papillary muscle; RV, right ventricle. *B*, Echocardiogram from transducer position (1); this view is the best one for measuring cardiac dimensions and fractional shortening. Fractional shortening is calculated as (LVED – LVES)/LVED; CW, chest wall; Ds, LV dimension in systole; LVED, LV dimension at end-diastole (Dd); RVED, RV dimension at end-diastole.

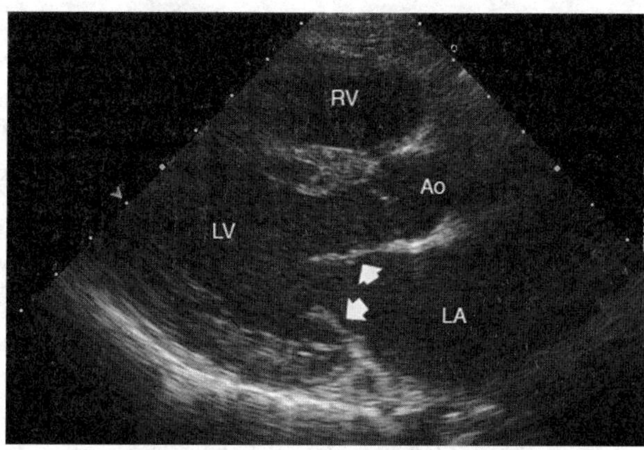

Figure 423-16. Normal parasternal long axis echocardiographic window. The transducer is angulated slightly posteriorly, imaging the left-sided cardiac structures. If the transducer were to be angulated more anteriorly, the right ventricular structures would be imaged. The mitral valve leaflets can be seen in partially open position in early diastole *(arrowheads)*. The closed aortic valve leaflets can be seen just below the label *Ao*. Ao, aorta; LA, left atrium; LV, left ventricle; RV, right ventricle.

views, including parasternal long axis (Fig 423-16), parasternal short axis (Fig. 423-17), apical four chamber (Fig. 423-18), subcostal (Fig. 423-19), and suprasternal (Fig. 423-20) windows, each of which emphasizes specific structures. Two-dimensional echocardiography has replaced cardiac angiography for the preoperative diagnosis of most, but not all congenital heart lesions; it exceeds angiography in imaging the atrioventricular valves and their chordal attachments. When information from the cardiac examination is not consistent with the echocardiogram, cardiac catheterization is an important tool to confirm the anatomic diagnosis and evaluate the degree of physiologic derangement.

DOPPLER ECHOCARDIOGRAPHY

Doppler echocardiography displays blood flow in cardiac chambers and vascular channels based on the change in frequency imparted to a sound wave by the movement of erythrocytes. In pulsed Doppler and continuous wave Doppler, the speed and direction of blood flow in the line of the echo beam change the transducer's reference frequency. This frequency change can be translated into volumetric flow (L/min) data for estimating systemic or pulmonary blood flow and into pressure (mm Hg) data

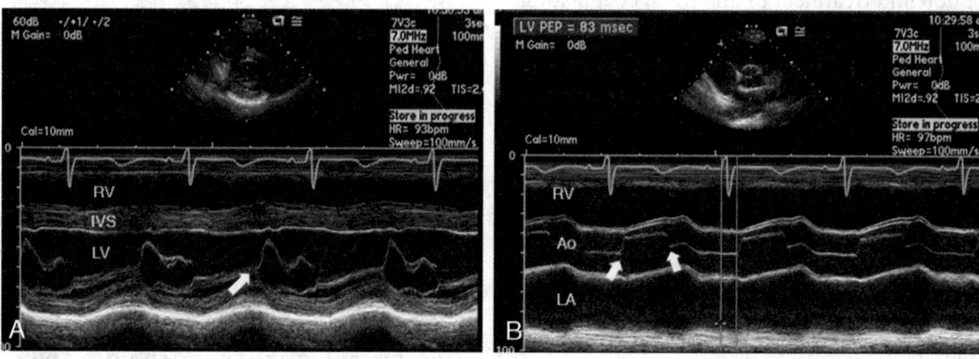

Figure 423-15. M-mode echocardiograms. The small figure at the top of each panel shows the two-dimensional parasternal short axis echo image from which the M-modes are derived. The cursor can be seen midway through the image, indicating the one-dimensional line through which the M-mode is being sampled. *A*, M-mode echocardiogram of a normal mitral valve. *Arrow* shows the opening of the anterior leaflet in early diastole (see ECG tracing above for reference). *B*, M-mode echocardiogram of a normal aortic valve. The opening and closing of the aortic leaflets in systole are outlined by the two *arrows*. Ao, aorta; IVS, interventricular septum; LV, left ventricle; RV, right ventricle.

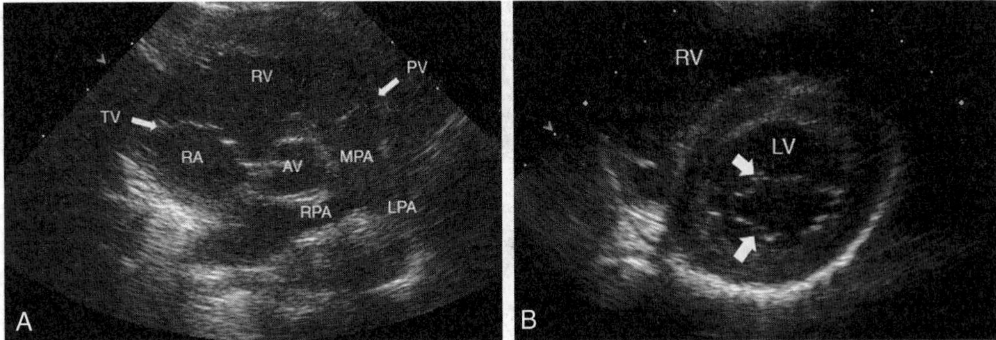

Figure 423-17. Normal parasternal short axis echocardiographic windows. *A,* With the transducer angled superiorly and rightwards, the aortic valve (AV) is imaged, surrounded by both inflow and outflow portions of the right ventricle (RV). LPA, left pulmonary artery; MPA, main pulmonary artery; PV, pulmonary valve; RA, right atrium; RPA, right pulmonary artery; TV, tricuspid valve. *B,* With the transducer angled inferiorly and leftwards, the left ventricular chamber is imaged along with cross-sectional view of the mitral valve *(arrows).* LV, left ventricle; RV, right ventricle.

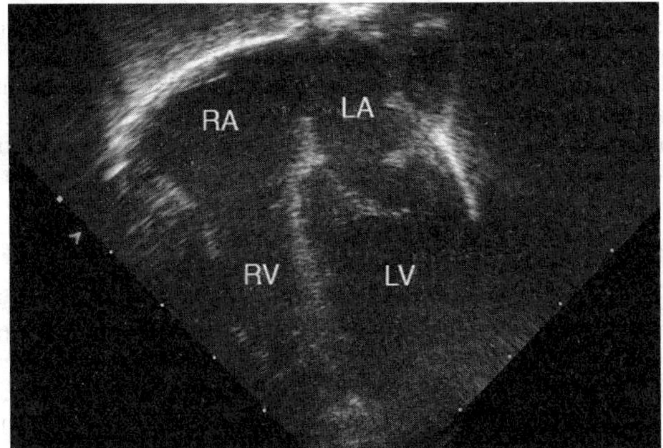

Figure 423-18. Normal apical four chamber echocardiographic window showing all four cardiac chambers and both atrioventricular valves opened in diastole. LA, left atrium; LV, left ventricle; RA, right atrium; RV, right ventricle.

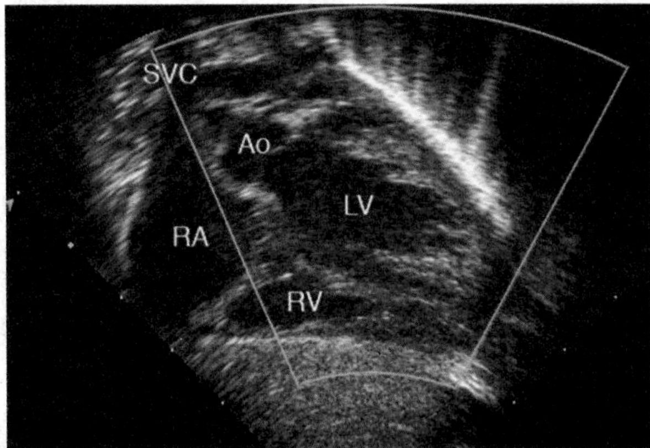

Figure 423-19. Normal subcostal echocardiographic window showing the left ventricular outflow tract. The right-sided structures are not fully imaged in this view. Ao, ascending aorta; LV, left ventricle; RA, right atrium; RV, right ventricle; SVC, superior vena cava.

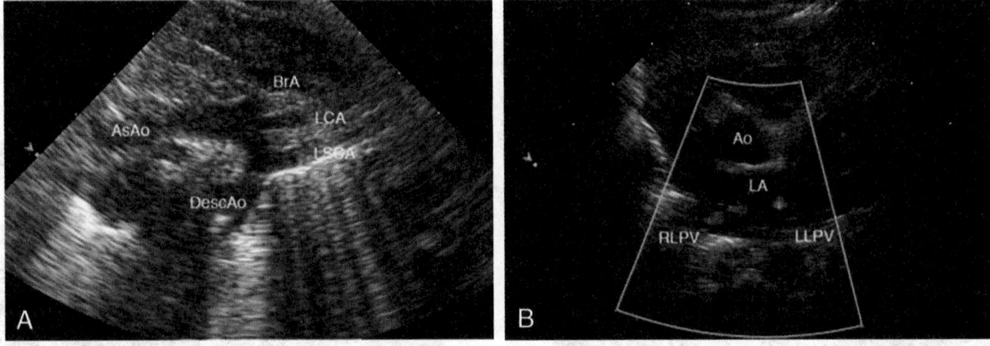

Figure 423-20. *A,* Normal suprasternal echocardiographic window showing the aortic arch and its major branches. AsAo, ascending aorta; BrA, brachiocephalic artery; DescAo, descending aorta; LCA, left carotid artery; LSCA, left subclavian artery. *B,* Normal high parasternal window showing color Doppler imaging of normal pulmonary venous return to the left atrium (LA) of both right (RLPV) and left (LLPV) lower pulmonary veins.

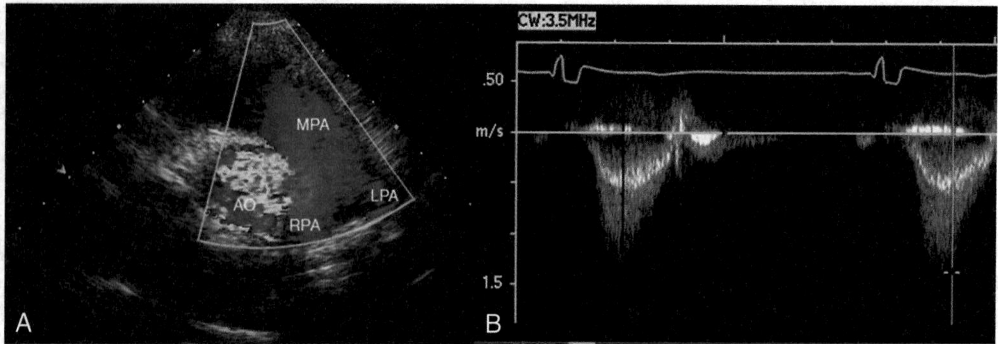

Figure 423-21. Color and pulsed Doppler evaluation of pulmonary arterial flow. *A*, Color Doppler evaluation of a parasternal short axis view showing normal flow through the pulmonary valve to the main and branch pulmonary arteries. The color of the Doppler flow is blue, indicating that the flow is moving away from the transducer (which is located at the top of the figure, at the apex of the triangular ultrasound window). Note that the color assigned to the Doppler signal does not indicate the oxygen saturation of the blood. Ao, aorta; LPA, left pulmonary artery; MPA, main pulmonary artery; RPA, right pulmonary artery. *B*, Pulsed wave Doppler flow pattern through the pulmonary valve showing a low velocity of flow (<1.5 m/sec), indicating the absence of a pressure gradient across the valve. The envelope of the flow signal is below the line, indicating that the flow is moving away from the transducer.

for estimating gradients across the semilunar or atrioventricular valves or across septal defects or vascular communications such as shunts. Color Doppler permits highly accurate assessment of the presence and direction of intracardiac shunts and allows identification of small or multiple left-to-right or right-to-left shunts (Fig. 423-21). The severity of valvular insufficiency can be evaluated with both pulsed and color Doppler (Fig. 423-22).

Sophisticated M-mode, two-dimensional, and Doppler echocardiographic methods of assessing left ventricular systolic and diastolic function (e.g., end-systolic wall stress, dobutamine stress echocardiography, and Doppler tissue imaging) have proved useful in the serial assessment of patients at risk for the development of both systolic and diastolic ventricular dysfunction. Such patients include those receiving anthracycline drugs for cancer chemotherapy, those at risk for iron overload, and those being monitored for rejection or coronary artery disease after heart transplantation.

THREE-DIMENSIONAL ECHOCARDIOGRAPHY

Real-time three-dimensional echocardiographic reconstruction is valuable for the assessment of cardiac morphology (Fig. 423-23). Details of valve structure, the size and location of septal defects, abnormalities of the ventricular myocardium, and details of the great vessels can often be appreciated on 3-D echo, which may not be as readily apparent using 2-D imaging. Reconstruction of the view that the surgeon will encounter in the operating room makes this technique a valuable adjunct for preoperative imaging.

TRANSESOPHAGEAL ECHOCARDIOGRAPHY

Transesophageal echocardiography is an extremely sensitive imaging technique that produces a clearer view of smaller lesions such as vegetations in endocarditis. It is useful in visualizing posteriorly located structures such as the atria, aortic root, and atrioventricular valves. Transesophageal echocardiography is extremely useful as an intraoperative technique for monitoring cardiac function during both cardiac and noncardiac surgery and for screening for residual cardiac defects after cardiopulmonary bypass. This technique has been especially helpful in evaluating the degree of residual regurgitation after repair of atrioventricular septal defects and in searching for small muscular VSDs that may have been missed during the closure of larger defects.

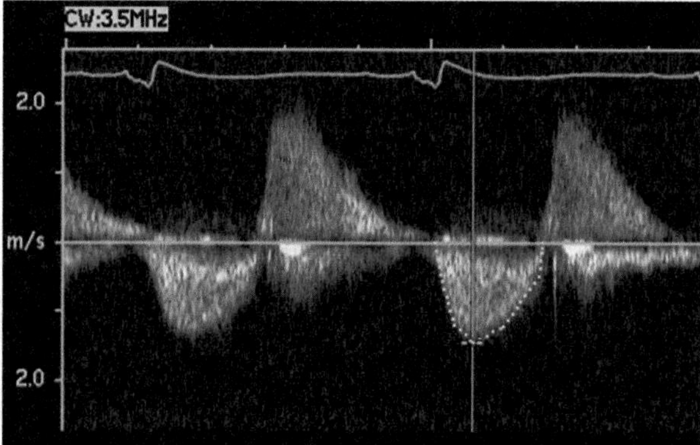

Figure 423-22. Doppler evaluation of a patient who had previously undergone repair of tetralogy of Fallot and who has mild pulmonary stenosis and moderate pulmonary regurgitation. The tracing shows the to-and-fro flow across the pulmonary valve with the signal below the line representing forward flow in systole (see ECG tracing for reference) and the signal above the line representing regurgitation during diastole.

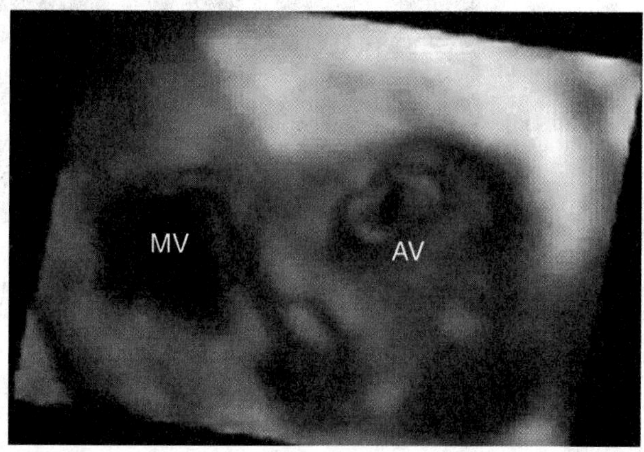

Figure 423-23. 3-D echocardiogram showing a short axis view of the left ventricle. AV, aortic valve; MV, mitral valve. (Courtesy of Dr. Norman Silverman, Stanford University, Stanford, CA.)

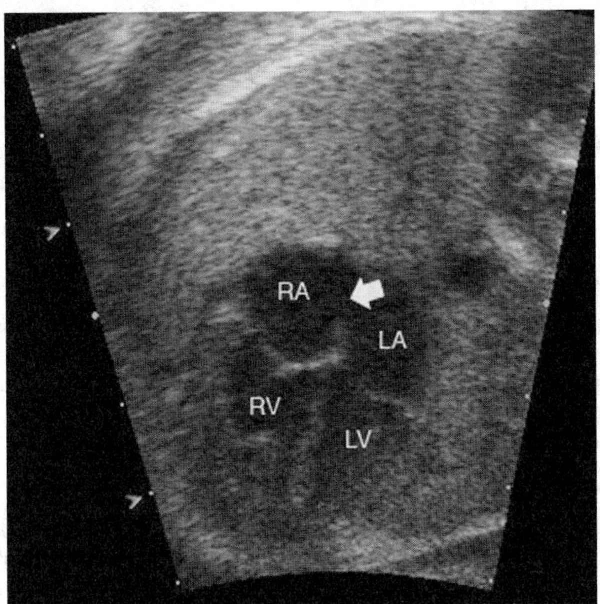

Figure 423-24. Normal four chamber view echocardiogram on a fetus at 20 wk of gestation. The foramen ovale *(arrow)* can be seen between the right and left atria. LA, left atrium; LV, left ventricle; RA, right atrium; RV, right ventricle.

FETAL ECHOCARDIOGRAPHY

Fetal echocardiography can be used to evaluate cardiac structures or disturbances in cardiac rhythm (Fig. 423-24). Perinatologists often detect gross abnormalities in cardiac structure on routine obstetric ultrasonography or may refer the patient because of unexplained hydrops fetalis. Fetal echocardiography is capable of diagnosing many congenital heart lesions as early as 17–19 wk of gestation; however, accuracy at this early stage is still limited and families should understand that these studies cannot totally eliminate the possibility of congenital heart disease. Serial fetal echocardiograms have also demonstrated the importance of flow disturbance in the pathogenesis of congenital heart disease; such studies can show the intrauterine progression of a moderate lesion, such as aortic stenosis, into a more severe lesion, such as hypoplastic left heart syndrome. M-mode echocardiography can diagnose rhythm disturbances in the fetus and can determine the success of antiarrhythmic therapy administered to the mother. A screening fetal echocardiogram is recommended for patients with a previous child or 1st-degree relative with congenital heart disease, for patients who are at higher risk of having a child with cardiac disease (insulin-dependent diabetics, patients with exposure to teratogenic drugs during early pregnancy), and in any fetus in which a chromosomal abnormality is suspected or confirmed.

423.5 • Exercise Testing

The normal cardiorespiratory system adapts to the extensive demands of exercise with a several-fold increase in oxygen consumption and cardiac output. Because of the large reserve capacity for exercise, significant abnormalities in cardiovascular performance may be present without symptoms at rest or during ordinary activities. When patients are evaluated in a resting state, significant abnormalities in cardiac function may not be appreciated, or if detected, their implications for quality of life may not be recognized. Permission for children with cardiovascular disease to participate in various forms of physical activity is frequently based on totally subjective criteria. Exercise testing plays an important role in evaluating symptoms, quantitating the severity of cardiac abnormalities, and assisting in the management of these patients, including prescribing a rational physical activity schedule.

In older children, exercise studies are generally performed on a graded treadmill apparatus with timed intervals of increasing grade and speed. In younger children, exercise studies are performed on a bicycle ergometer. Many laboratories now have the capacity to measure cardiac output and pulmonary function noninvasively during exercise.

As a child grows, the capacity for work is enhanced with increased body size and skeletal muscle mass. All indices of cardiopulmonary function do not increase in a uniform manner. A major response to exercise is an increase in cardiac output, principally achieved through an increase in heart rate, but stroke volume, systemic venous return, and pulse pressure is also increased. Systemic vascular resistance is greatly decreased as the blood vessels in working muscle dilate in response to increasing metabolic demands. As the child becomes older and larger, the response of the heart rate to exercise remains prominent, but cardiac output increases because of growing cardiac volume capacity and, hence, stroke volume. Responses to dynamic exercise are not dependent solely on age. For any given body surface area, boys have a larger stroke volume than size-matched girls. This increase is also mediated by posture. Augmentation of stroke volume with upright, dynamic exercise is facilitated by the pumping action of working muscles, which overcomes the static effect of gravity and increases systemic venous return.

Dynamic exercise testing defines not only endurance and exercise capacity but also the effect of such exercise on myocardial blood flow and cardiac rhythm. Significant ST segment depression reflects abnormalities in myocardial perfusion, for example, the subendocardial ischemia that commonly occurs during exercise in children with hypertrophied left ventricles. The **exercise ECG** is considered abnormal if the ST segment depression is >2 mm and extends for at least 0.06 sec after the J point (onset of the ST segment) in conjunction with a horizontal-, upward-, or downward-sloping ST segment. Provocation of rhythm disturbances during an exercise study is an important method of evaluating selected patients with known or suspected rhythm disorders. The effect of pharmacologic management can also be tested in this manner.

423.6 • MRI, MRA, CT, and Radionuclide Studies

Magnetic resonance imaging (MRI) and **magnetic resonance angiography** (MRA) are extremely helpful in the diagnosis and management of patients with congenital heart disease. These techniques produce tomographic images of the heart in any projection (Fig. 423-25), with excellent contrast resolution of fat, myocardium, and lung, as well as moving blood from blood vessel walls. MRI has been particularly useful in evaluating areas that are less well visualized by echocardiography, such as distal branch pulmonary artery anatomy and anomalies in systemic and pulmonary venous return.

MRA allows the acquisition of images in several tomographic planes. Within each plane, images are obtained at different phases of the cardiac cycle. Thus, when displayed in a dynamic "cine" format, changes in wall thickening, chamber volume, and valve function can be displayed and analyzed. Blood flow velocity and blood flow volume can be calculated. MRA is an excellent technique for following patients serially after repair of complex congenital heart disease, such as tetralogy of Fallot. In these patients, MRA can be used to assess right ventricular volume and mass as well as quantify the amount of regurgitation through either the

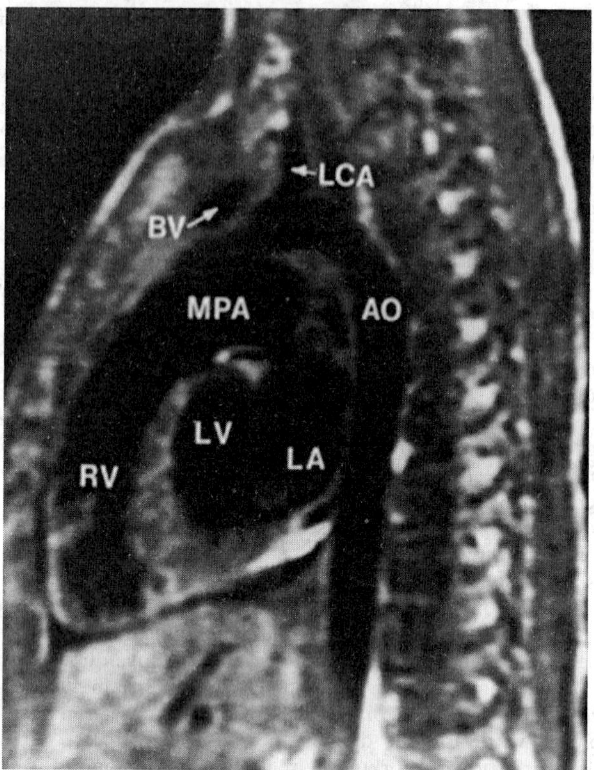

Figure 423-25. Sagittal normal MRI. Ao, aorta; BV, brachiocephalic vein; LA, left atrium; LCA, left coronary artery; LV, left ventricle; MPA, main pulmonary artery; RV, right ventricle. (From Bisset GS III: Cardiac and great vessel anatomy. In El-Khoury GY, Bergman RA, Montgomery WJ [editors]: *Sectional Anatomy by MRI/CT.* New York, Churchill Livingstone, 1990.)

pulmonary or tricuspid valve. **Magnetic resonance spectroscopy (MRS)**, predominantly a research tool at present, provides a means of demonstrating relative concentrations of high-energy metabolites (adenosine triphosphate, adenosine diphosphate, inorganic phosphate, and phosphocreatine) within regions of the working myocardium.

Computer processing of MRA images allows the noninvasive visualization of the cardiovascular system from inside of the heart or vessels, a technique known as fly-through imaging. These images allow the cardiologist to image the interiors of various cardiovascular structures (Fig. 423-26). These imaging techniques are especially helpful in imaging complex peripheral arterial stenoses, especially after attempted balloon angioplasty.

Electron Beam CT (EBCT) scanning is used to perform rapid, respiration-gated cardiac imaging in children with resolutions down to 0.5 mm. Three-dimensional reconstruction of EBCT images (Fig. 423-27) is especially useful in evaluating branch pulmonary arteries, anomalies in systemic and pulmonary venous return, and great vessel anomalies such as coarctation of the aorta.

Radionuclide angiography may be used to detect and quantify shunts and to analyze the distribution of blood flow to each lung. This technique is particularly useful in quantifying the volume of blood flow distribution between the two lungs in patients with abnormalities of the pulmonary vascular tree or after a shunt operation (Blalock-Taussig or Glenn), or to quantify the success of balloon angioplasty and intravascular stenting procedures. Gated blood pool scanning can be used to calculate hemodynamic measurements, quantify valvular regurgitation, and detect regional wall motion abnormalities. Thallium imaging can be performed to evaluate cardiac muscle perfusion. These methods can be used at the bedside of seriously ill children and can be performed serially, with minimal discomfort and low radiation exposure.

423.7 • Diagnostic and Interventional Cardiac Catheterization

As echocardiography, MRI, and CT have become the standards for the diagnosis of most forms of congenital heart disease, the catheterization laboratory has become the site of high-technology interventional procedures, allowing for the minimally invasive repair or palliation of heart defects that once required open heart surgery.

DIAGNOSTIC CARDIAC CATHETERIZAION

Diagnostic catheterization is still performed: (1) to assist in the initial diagnosis of some complex congenital heart lesions (tetralogy of Fallot with pulmonary atresia and major aortopulmonary collateral arteries [MAPCAs], pulmonary atresia with intact ventricular septum and coronary sinusoids); (2) in cases in which other imaging studies are equivocal; (3) in patients for whom hemodynamic assessment is critical (to determine the size of a left-to-right shunt in borderline cases, or to determine the presence or absence of pulmonary vascular disease in a patient with a left-to-right shunt); (4) between stages of repair of complex congenital heart disease (hypoplastic left heart syndrome); (5) for myocardial biopsy in the diagnosis of cardiomyopathy or in screening for cardiac rejection after cardiac transplantation; and (6) for electrophysiologic study in the evaluation of cardiac arrhythmias (see Chapter 435).

Cardiac catheterization should be performed with the patient in as close to a basal state as possible. Conscious sedation is routine; however, if general anesthesia is required, careful choice of an anesthetic agent is warranted to avoid depression of cardiovascular function and subsequent distortion of the calculations of cardiac output, pulmonary and systemic vascular resistance, and shunt ratios.

Cardiac catheterization in critically ill infants with congenital heart disease should be performed in a center where a pediatric cardiovascular surgical team is available in the event that an operation is required immediately afterward. The complication rate of cardiac catheterization and angiography is greatest in critically ill infants; they must be studied in a thermally neutral environment and treated quickly for hypothermia, hypoglycemia, acidosis, or excessive blood loss.

Catheterization may be limited to the right-sided cardiac structures, the left-sided structures, or both the right and left sides of the heart. The catheter is passed into the heart under fluoroscopic guidance through a percutaneous entry point in a femoral or jugular vein. In infants and in a number of older children, the left side of the heart can be accessed by passing the catheter across a patent foramen ovale to the left atrium and left ventricle. If the foramen is closed, the left side of the heart can be catheterized by passing the catheter retrograde via a percutaneous entry site in the femoral artery. The catheter can be manipulated through abnormal intracardiac defects (ASDs, VSDs). Blood samples are obtained for measuring oxygen saturation and calculating shunt volumes, pressures are measured for calculating gradients and valve areas, and radio-opaque contrast is injected to delineate cardiac and vascular structures. A catheter with a thermosensor tip can be utilized for measurement of cardiac output by thermodilution. Specialized catheters can be utilized to measure more sophisticated indices of cardiac function: Those with pressure-transducer tips can be utilized to measure the first derivative of left ventricular pressure (dP/dt); and conductance catheters can be used to produce pressure-volume loops, from which indices of

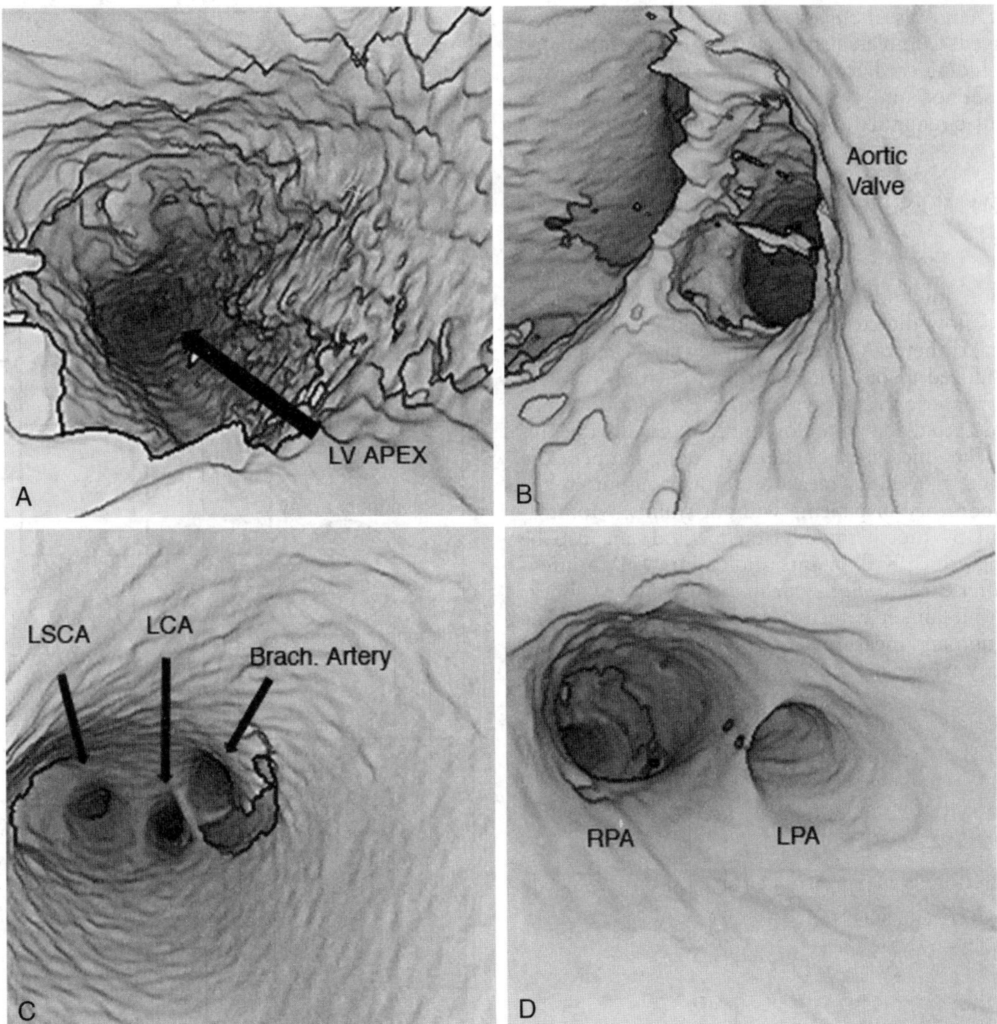

Figure 423-26. Fly-through imaging in a patient with an aortopulmonary window. This series of still frames shows the progression from the left ventricular (LV) chamber *(A)*, through the aortic valve *(B)*, out to the ascending aorta *(C)*, and then through the defect to the branch pulmonary arteries *(D)*. Brach., brachiocephalic artery; LCA, left carotid artery; LPA, left pulmonary artery; LSCA, left subclavian artery; RPA, right pulmonary artery.

Figure 423-27. Three-dimensional reconstruction of electron beam CT images from a neonate with severe coarctation of the aorta. The patent ductus arteriosus can be seen toward the left leading from the main pulmonary artery to the descending aorta. The tortuous and narrow coarctated segment is just to the right of the ductus. The transverse aorta is hypoplastic as well. AAo, ascending aorta; DAo, descending aorta; LA, left atrium; MPA, main pulmonary artery; RAA, right atrial appendage; RPA, right pulmonary artery. (Image courtesy of Dr. Paul Pitlick, Stanford University, Stanford, CA.)

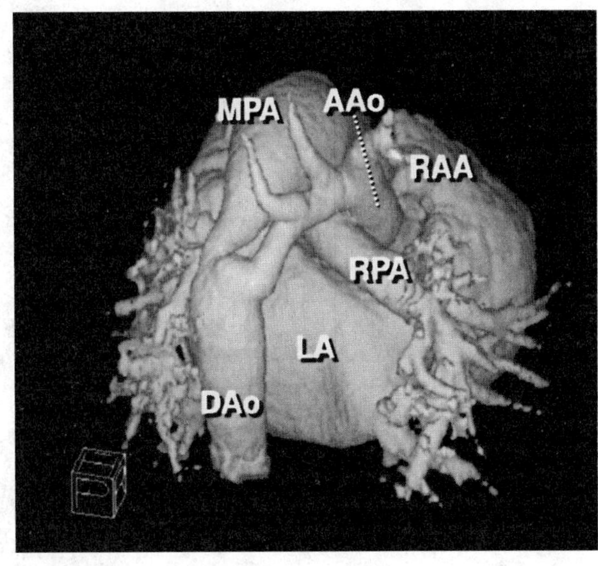

both contractility (end-systolic elastance) and lusitropy (relaxation) can be derived. Complete hemodynamics can be calculated (Table 423-1), including cardiac output, intracardiac left-to-right and right-to-left shunts, and systemic and pulmonary vascular resistance. Normal circulatory dynamics are depicted in Figure 423-28.

THERMODILUTION MEASUREMENT OF CARDIAC OUTPUT

The thermodilution method for measuring cardiac output is performed with a flow-directed, thermistor-tipped, pulmonary artery (Swan-Ganz) catheter. A known change in the heat content of the blood is induced at one point in the circulation (usually the right atrium or inferior vena cava), and the resultant change in temperature is detected at a point downstream (usually the pulmonary artery). The injectate is generally room temperature saline. This method is used to measure cardiac output in the catheterization laboratory in patients without shunts. Monitoring cardiac output by the thermodilution method can also be useful in managing critically ill infants and children in an intensive care setting after cardiac surgery or in the presence of shock. In this case, a triple-lumen catheter is used for both cardiac output determination and measurement of pulmonary artery and pulmonary capillary wedge pressure.

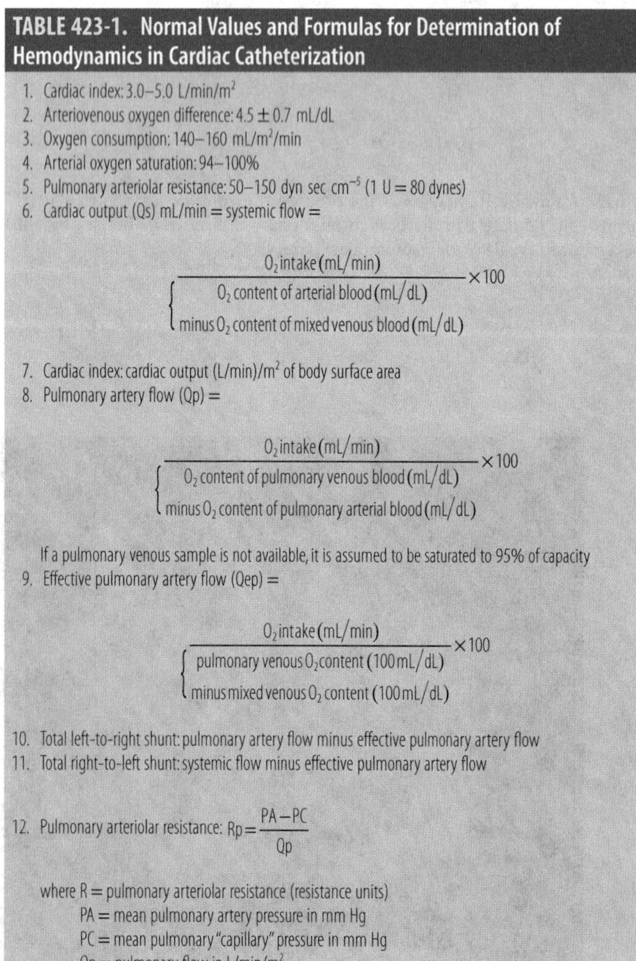

TABLE 423-1. Normal Values and Formulas for Determination of Hemodynamics in Cardiac Catheterization

1. Cardiac index: 3.0–5.0 L/min/m^2
2. Arteriovenous oxygen difference: 4.5 ± 0.7 mL/dL
3. Oxygen consumption: 140–160 mL/m^2/min
4. Arterial oxygen saturation: 94–100%
5. Pulmonary arteriolar resistance: 50–150 dyn sec cm^{-5} (1 U = 80 dynes)
6. Cardiac output (Qs) mL/min = systemic flow =

$$\frac{O_2\,\text{intake}\,(\text{mL/min})}{\left\{\begin{array}{l}O_2\text{ content of arterial blood (mL/dL)}\\ \text{minus } O_2\text{ content of mixed venous blood (mL/dL)}\end{array}\right.}\times 100$$

7. Cardiac index: cardiac output (L/min)/m^2 of body surface area
8. Pulmonary artery flow (Qp) =

$$\frac{O_2\,\text{intake}\,(\text{mL/min})}{\left\{\begin{array}{l}O_2\text{ content of pulmonary venous blood (mL/dL)}\\ \text{minus } O_2\text{ content of pulmonary arterial blood (mL/dL)}\end{array}\right.}\times 100$$

If a pulmonary venous sample is not available, it is assumed to be saturated to 95% of capacity

9. Effective pulmonary artery flow (Qep) =

$$\frac{O_2\,\text{intake}\,(\text{mL/min})}{\left\{\begin{array}{l}\text{pulmonary venous } O_2\text{ content (100 mL/dL)}\\ \text{minus mixed venous } O_2\text{ content (100 mL/dL)}\end{array}\right.}\times 100$$

10. Total left-to-right shunt: pulmonary artery flow minus effective pulmonary artery flow
11. Total right-to-left shunt: systemic flow minus effective pulmonary artery flow
12. Pulmonary arteriolar resistance: $Rp = \frac{PA - PC}{Qp}$

where R = pulmonary arteriolar resistance (resistance units)
PA = mean pulmonary artery pressure in mm Hg
PC = mean pulmonary "capillary" pressure in mm Hg
Qp = pulmonary flow in L/min/m^2

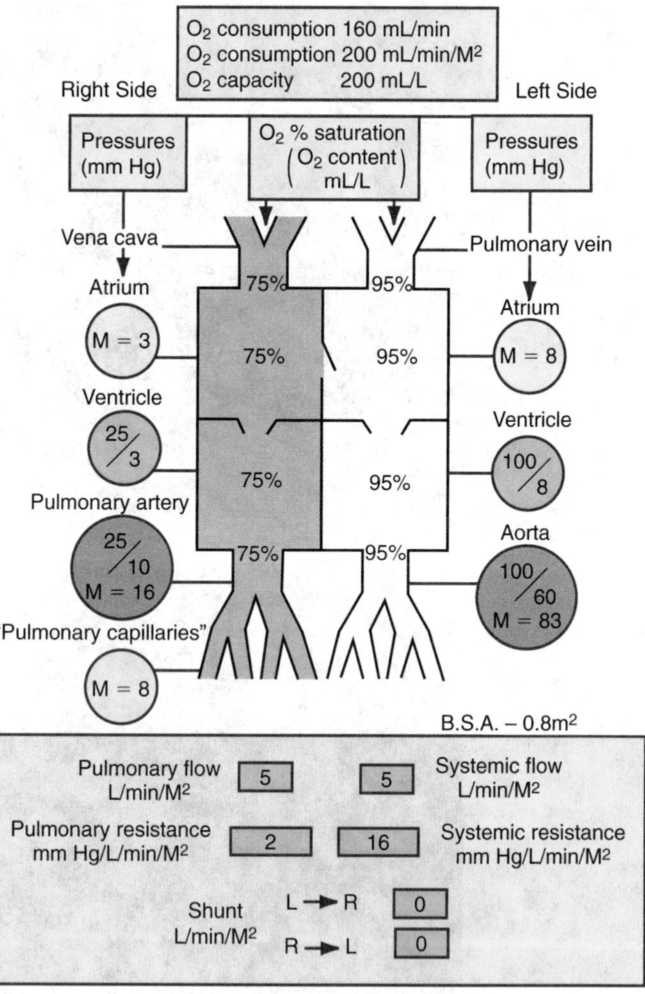

Figure 423-28. Diagram of normal circulatory dynamics with pressure readings, oxygen content, and percent saturation. B.S.A., body surface area. (Modified from Nadas AS, Fyler DC: *Pediatric Cardiology,* 3rd ed. Philadelphia, WB Saunders, 1972.)

ANGIOCARDIOGRAPHY

The major blood vessels and individual cardiac chambers may be visualized by selective angiocardiography, or the injection of contrast material into specific chambers or great vessels. This method allows identification of structural abnormalities without interference from the superimposed shadows of normal chambers. Fluoroscopy is used to visualize the catheter as it passes through the various heart chambers. After the cardiac catheter is properly placed in the chamber to be studied, a small amount of contrast medium is injected with a power injector, and cineangiograms are exposed at rates ranging from 15 to 60 frames/sec. Biplane cineangiocardiography allows detailed evaluation of specific cardiac chambers and blood vessels in two planes simultaneously with the injection of a single bolus of contrast material. This technique is standard in pediatric cardiac catheterization laboratories and allows one to minimize the volume of contrast material used, which is safer for the patient. Various angled views (left anterior oblique, cranial angulation) are used to display specific anatomic features best in individual lesions. Digital imaging has replaced standard roentgenographic film for both diagnostic and archival purposes.

Rapid injection of contrast medium under pressure into the circulation is not without risk, and each injection should be carefully planned. Contrast agents consist of hypertonic solutions, with some containing organic iodides, which can cause complications, including nausea, a generalized burning sensation, central nervous system symptoms, renal insufficiency, and allergic reactions. Intramyocardial injection is generally avoided by careful placement of the catheter before injection. Hypertonicity of the contrast medium may result in transient myocardial depression and a drop in blood pressure, followed soon afterward by tachycardia, an increase in cardiac output, and a shift of interstitial fluid into the circulation. This shift can transiently increase the symptoms of heart failure in critically ill patients.

INTERVENTIONAL CARDIAC CATHETERIZATION

The miniaturization of catheter delivery systems has allowed for the safe application of many of these interventional catheterization techniques, even in neonates and premature infants. Catheter treatment is now the standard of practice for most cases of isolated pulmonary or aortic valve stenosis (see Fig. 427-4) as well as for re-coarctation of the aorta. A special catheter with a sausage-shaped balloon at the distal end is passed through the obstructed valve. Rapid filling of the balloon with a mixture of contrast material and saline solution results in tearing of the stenotic valve tissue, usually at the site of inappropriately fused raphe. Valvular pulmonary stenosis can be treated successfully by balloon angioplasty; in most patients, angioplasty has replaced surgical repair as the initial procedure of choice. The clinical results of this procedure are similar to those obtained by open heart surgery, but without the need for sternotomy or prolonged hospitalization. Balloon valvuloplasty for aortic stenosis has also yielded excellent results, although, as with surgery, aortic stenosis often recurs as the child grows and multiple procedures may thus be required. One complication of both valvuloplasty and surgery is the creation of valvular insufficiency. This complication has more serious implications when it occurs on the aortic vs the pulmonary side of the circulation because regurgitation is less well tolerated at systemic arterial pressures. Balloon angioplasty is the procedure of choice for patients with re-stenosis of coarctation of the aorta after earlier surgery. It is controversial whether angioplasty is the best procedure for native (unoperated) coarctation of the aorta because of reports of later aneurysm formation. Other applications of the balloon angioplasty technique include amelioration of mitral stenosis, dilatation of surgical conduits (Mustard or Senning atrial baffles), relief of branch pulmonary artery narrowing, dilatation of venous obstructions, and the long-used balloon atrial septostomy (Rashkind procedure) for transposition of the great arteries (see Chapter 431.2).

Interventional catheterization techniques are being adapted for use in the **fetus** with lesions such as arotic stenosis in an attempt to prevent their progression to more complex lesions such as hypoplastic left heart syndrome. In these procedures, after administration of appropriate anesthesia, a needle is passed through the maternal abdominal wall, the uterine wall, and the fetal chest wall and directly into the fetal left ventricle (Fig. 431-13). A coronary angioplasty balloon catheter is passed through the needle and across the stenotic aortic valve, which is then dilated. With the restoration of normal left ventricular blood flow, it is to be hoped that normal left ventricular growth potential is restored. Early results with this technique in a limited number of patients are encouraging.

In patients with branch pulmonary artery stenoses, the previously mixed results with balloon angioplasty alone have been enhanced with the use of **intravascular stents** (Fig. 423-29) delivered over a balloon catheter and expanded within the vessel lumen. Once placed, they can often be dilated to successively greater sizes as the patient grows. Placement of stents in small infants and children remains problematic because of subsequent growth. Stents are also being utilized in adolescents and young adults with coarctation of the aorta.

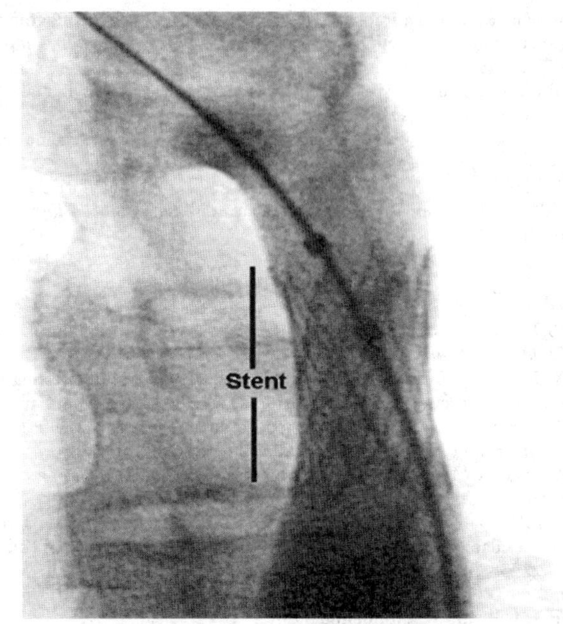

Figure 423-29. Intravascular stent placed in the descending aorta for treatment of recurrent coarctation of the aorta.

Closure of a small patent ductus arteriosus (PDA) is now routinely achieved with catheter-delivered coils (see Fig. 426-11), whereas a larger PDA can be closed with a variety of sandwich-type devices. Closure of anomalous vascular connections (coronary fistulas, veno-venous collaterals in cyanotic heart lesions) can also be achieved using coils. Secundum atrial septal defect (ASD) is now routinely closed with one of several available double disc occluder devices (see Fig. 426-3). Versions of these devices are currently in clinical trials for closure of surgically hard-to-reach muscular VSDs and even for the more common perimembranous VSD. Catheter-delivered devices may also be used as an adjunct to complex surgical repairs (dilation or stenting of branch pulmonary artery or pulmonary vein stenosis or closure of a muscular VSD associated with left-sided obstructive lesions). High-risk patients undergoing the Fontan operation (see Chapter 430.4) often have a small fenestration created between the right and left sides of the circulation to serve as a "popoff valve" for high right-sided pressure in the early surgical period. Patients with these "fenestrated Fontans" are ideal candidates for subsequent closure with a catheter-delivered device.

Electrocardiography

Garson A: *The Electrocardiogram in Infants and Children: A Systematic Approach.* Philadelphia, Lea & Febiger, 1983.

Lipman BF, Massey EF: *Clinical Scalar Electrocardiography.* Chicago, Year Book, 1984.

Marriott H: *Rhythm Quizlets: Self Assessment.* Philadelphia, Lea & Febiger, 1987.

Schwartz PJ, Moss AJ, Vincent GM, et al: Diagnostic criteria for the long QT syndrome: An update. *Circulation* 1993;88:782–784.

Echocardiography

Alagarsamy S, Chhabra M, Gudavalli M, et al: Comparison of clinical criteria with echocardiographic findings in diagnosing PDA in preterm infants. *J Perinat Med* 2005;33:161–164.

Frommelt MA, Frommelt PC: Advances in echocardiographic diagnostic modalities for the pediatrician. *Pediatr Clin North Am* 1999;46:427–439.

Sahn DJ, Vick GW III: Review of new techniques in echocardiography and magnetic resonance imaging as applied to patients with congenital heart disease. *Heart* 2001;86(Suppl 2):II41–II53.

Stevenson JG: Role of intraoperative transesophageal echocardiography during repair of congenital cardiac defects. *Acta Paediatr Suppl* 1995;410:23–33.

Sullivan ID: Prenatal diagnosis of structural heart disease: Does it make a difference to survival? *Heart* 2002;87:405–406.

Todros T: Prenatal diagnosis and management of fetal cardiovascular malformations. *Curr Opin Obstet Gynecol* 2000;12:105–109.

Van Der Velde ME, Perry SB: Transesophageal echocardiography during interventional catheterization in congenital heart disease. *Echocardiography* 1997;14:513–528.

Exercise Testing

Braden DS, Strong WF: Cardiovascular responses to exercise in childhood. *Am J Dis Child* 1990;144:1255–1260.

James FW, Blomqvist CG, Freed MD, et al: Standards for exercise testing in the pediatric age group: American Heart Association Council on Cardiovascular Disease in the Young. Ad hoc committee on exercise testing. *Circulation* 1982;66:1377A–1397A.

Nixon PA, Joswiak ML, Fricker FJ: A six-minute walk test for assessing exercise tolerance in severely ill children. *J Pediatr* 1996;129:362–366.

Washington RL, van Gundy JC, Cohen C, et al: Normal aerobic and anaerobic exercise data for North American school-age children. J Pediatr 1988;112:223–233.

MRI, MRA, CT, and Radionuclide Studies

Nienaber CA, Rehders TC, Fratz S: Detection and assessment of congenital heart disease with magnetic resonance techniques. *J Cardiovasc Magn Reson* 1999;1:169–184.

Strife JL, Sze RW: Radiographic evaluation of the neonate with congenital heart disease. *Radiol Clin North Am* 1999;37:1093–1107.

Wolfson BJ: Radiologic interpretation of congenital heart disease. *Clin Perinatol* 2001;28:71–89.

Diagnostic and Interventional Cardiac Catheterization

Andrews RE, Tulloh RMR: Interventional cardiac catheterization in congenital heart disease. *Arch Dis Child* 2004;89:1168–1173.

Giardini A, Moore P, Brook M, et al: Effect of transcatheter atrial septal defect closure in children on left ventricular diastolic function. *Am J Cardiol* 2005;95:1255–1257.

Holzer R, Balzer D, Cao QL, et al: Device closure of muscular ventricular septal defects using the Amplatzer muscular ventricular septal defect occluder: Immediate and mid-term results of a U.S. registry. *J Am Coll Cardiol* 2004;43:1257–1263.

Knauth AL, Lock JE, Perry SB, et al: Transcatheter device closure of congenital and postoperative residual ventricular septal defects. *Circulation* 2004;110:501–507.

Kreutzer J: Transcatheter intervention in the neonate with congenital heart disease. *Clin Perinatol* 2001;28:137–157.

Masura J, Gavora P, Podnar T: Long-term outcome of transcatheter secundum-type atrial septal defect closure using Amplatzer septal occluders. *J Am Coll Cardiol* 2005;45:505–507.

Simpson JM, Moore P, Teitel DF: Cardiac catheterization of low birth weight infants. *Am J Cardiol* 2001;87:1372–1377.

Tworetzky W, Marshall AC: Fetal interventions for cardiac defects. *Pediatr Clin North Am* 2004;51:1503–1513.

Walsh KP: Interventional paediatric cardiology. *Br Med J* 2003;327:385–388.

Yew G, Wilson NJ: Transcatheter atrial septal defect closure with the Amplatzer septal occluder: Five-year follow-up. *Catheter Cardiovasc Interv* 2005;64:193–196.

Section 3 — Congenital Heart Disease — Daniel Bernstein

Chapter 424 ■ Epidemiology and Genetic Basis of Congenital Heart Disease

PREVALENCE. Congenital heart disease occurs in 0.5–0.8% of live births. The incidence is higher in stillborns (3–4%), spontaneous abortuses (10–25%), and premature infants (about 2% excluding patent ductus arteriosus [PDA]). This overall incidence does not include mitral valve prolapse, PDA of preterm infants, and bicuspid aortic valves (present in 1–2% of adults). Congenital cardiac defects have a wide spectrum of severity in infants: about 2–3 in 1,000 newborn infants will be symptomatic with heart disease in the 1st yr of life. The diagnosis is established by 1 wk of age in 40–50% of patients with congenital heart disease and by 1 mo of age in 50–60% of patients. With advances in both palliative and corrective surgery, the number of children with congenital heart disease surviving to adulthood has increased dramatically. Despite these advances, congenital heart disease remains the leading cause of death in children with congenital malformations. Table 424-1 summarizes the relative frequency of the most common congenital cardiac lesions.

Most congenital defects are well tolerated in the fetus because of the parallel nature of the fetal circulation. Even the most severe cardiac defects (hypoplastic left heart syndrome) can usually be well compensated for by the fetal circulation. In this example, the entire fetal cardiac output would be ejected by the right ventricle via the ductus arteriosus into both the descending and ascending aortae (the latter filling in a retrograde fashion). It is only after birth when the fetal pathways (ductus arteriosus and foramen ovale) are closed that the full hemodynamic impact of an anatomic abnormality becomes apparent. One notable exception is the case of severe regurgitant lesions, most commonly of the tricuspid valve. In these lesions (Ebstein anomaly [see Chapter 430.7]), the parallel fetal circulation cannot compensate for the volume load imposed on the right side of the heart. In utero heart failure, often with fetal pleural and pericardial effusions, and generalized ascites (nonimmune hydrops fetalis) may occur.

Although the most significant transitions in circulation occur in the immediate perinatal period, the circulation continues to undergo changes after birth, and these later changes may also have a hemodynamic impact on cardiac lesions and their apparent incidence. As pulmonary vascular resistance falls in the 1st several weeks of life, left-to-right shunting through intracardiac defects increases and symptoms become more apparent. Thus, in patients with a ventricular septal defect (VSD), heart failure is often manifested between 1 and 3 mo of age (see Chapter 426.6). The severity of various defects can also change dramatically with growth; some VSDs may become smaller and even close as the child ages. Alternatively, stenosis of the aortic or pulmonary valve, which may be mild in the newborn period, may become worse if valve orifice growth does not keep pace with patient growth (see Chapter 427.5). The physician should always be alert for associated congenital malformations, which can adversely affect the patient's prognosis (see Table 422-2).

TABLE 424-1. Relative Frequency of Major Congenital Heart Lesions*

LESION	% OF ALL LESIONS
Ventricular septal defect	35–30
Atrial septal defect (secundum)	6–8
Patent ductus arteriosus	6–8
Coarctation of aorta	5–7
Tetralogy of Fallot	5–7
Pulmonary valve stenosis	5–7
Aortic valve stenosis	4–7
d-Transposition of great arteries	3–5
Hypoplastic left ventricle	1–3
Hypoplastic right ventricle	1–3
Truncus arteriosus	1–2
Total anomalous pulmonary venous return	1–2
Tricuspid atresia	1–2
Single ventricle	1–2
Double-outlet right ventricle	1–2
Others	5–10

*Excluding patent ductus arteriosus in preterm neonates, bicuspid aortic valve, physiologic peripheral pulmonic stenosis, and mitral valve prolapse.

ETIOLOGY. The cause of most congenital heart defects is unknown. Most cases of congenital heart disease were thought to be multifactorial and result from a combination of genetic predisposition and environmental stimulus. A small percentage of congenital heart lesions are related to chromosomal abnormalities, in particular, trisomy 21, 13, and 18 and Turner syndrome; heart disease is found in more than 90% of patients with trisomy 18, 50% of patients with trisomy 21, and 40% of those with Turner syndrome. Other genetic factors may have a role in congenital heart disease; certain types of VSDs (supracristal) are more common in Asian children. The risk of recurrence of congenital heart disease increases if a 1st-degree relative (parent or sibling) is affected.

A growing list of congenital heart lesions has been associated with specific chromosomal abnormalities, and several have even been linked to specific gene defects. Fluorescent in situ hybridization analysis allows clinicians rapid screening of suspected cases once a specific chromosomal abnormality has been identified.

A well-characterized genetic cause of congenital heart disease is the deletion of a large region (1.5–3 Mb) of chromosome 22q11.2, known as the **DiGeorge critical region.** At least 30 genes have been mapped to the deleted region; *Tbx1,* a transcription factor involved in early outflow tract development is implicated as a cause of DiGeorge syndrome. The estimated prevalence of 22q11.2 deletions is 1/4,000 live births. Cardiac lesions associated with 22q11.2 deletions are most often seen in association with either the DiGeorge syndrome or the **Shprintzen (velocardiofacial) syndrome.** The acronym *CATCH 22* has been used to summarize the major components of these syndromes (cardiac defects, abnormal facies, thymic aplasia, cleft palate, and hypocalcemia). The specific cardiac anomalies are conotruncal defects (tetralogy of Fallot, truncus arteriosus, double-outlet right ventricle, subarterial VSD) and branchial arch defects (coarctation of the aorta, interrupted aortic arch, right aortic arch). Congenital airway anomalies such as tracheomalacia and bronchomalacia are sometimes present. Although the risk of recurrence is extremely low in the absence of a parental 22q11.2 deletion, it is 50% if one of the parents carries the deletion. More than 90% of patients with DiGeorge syndrome have a microdeletion at 22q11.2. A second genetic locus on the short arm of chromosome 10 (10p13p14) has also been identified, the deletion of which shares some but not all phenotypic characteristics with the 22q11.2 deletion; patients with del(10p) have an increased incidence of sensorineural hearing loss.

Other structural heart lesions that have been associated with specific chromosomal abnormalities include **familial secundum atrial septal defect** associated with **heart block** (the transcription factor NKX2.5 on chromosome 5q35), familial atrial septal defect without heart block (the transcription factor GATA4), Alagille syndrome (Jagged1 on chromosome 20p12), and Williams syndrome (elastin on chromosome 7q11). Of interest, patients with ventricular septal defects (VSDs) and atrioventricular septal defects (AVSDs) have been found to have multiple NKX2.5 mutations in cells isolated from diseased heart tissues, but not from normal heart tissues or from circulating lymphocytes, indicating a potential role for somatic mutations leading to mosaicism in the pathogenesis of congenital heart defects. A compilation of known genetic causes of congenital heart disease is presented in Table 424-2.

Great progress in identifying the genetic origin of cardiovascular disease has been made in **hypertrophic cardiomyopathy.** Mutations in 10 genes have been implicated, all of which encode protein components of the cardiac sarcomere, either components of the thick or thin fibers or associated regulatory subunits. Mutations of the cardiac β-myosin heavy-chain gene (chromosome 14q1) and the myosin-binding protein C gene (chromosome 11q11) are the most common (see Tables 424-2 and 439-2), with less common mutations including the cardiac troponin T and I genes, α-tropomyosin, regulatory and essential myosin light chains, titin, and the α-myosin heavy chain. Over 200 mutations have been identified in the 10 most common genes, and some patients may carry mutations in more than one gene.

Progress has also been made in identifying the genetic basis of **dilated cardiomyopathy,** which is familial in 20–50% of cases. Autosomal dominant inheritance is most commonly encountered and, to date, 16 genes have been identified (see Table 424-2). X-linked inheritance accounts for 5–10% of cases of familial dilated cardiomyopathy. Mutations in the dystrophin gene (chromosome Xp21) are the most common in this group. Mutations in the gene encoding *tafazzin* are associated with Barth syndrome and some cases of isolated non-compaction of the left ventricle. Autosomal recessive inheritance has been associated with a mutation in cardiac troponin I. Mitochondrial myopathies may be due to mutations of enzymes of the electron transport chain encoded by nuclear DNA (in which inheritance will follow mendelian genetic patterns) or enzymes of fatty acid oxidation encoded by mitochondrial DNA (which is inherited solely from the mother).

The genetic basis of **heritable arrhythmias,** most notably the **long Q-T syndromes,** has been linked to mutations of genes coding for subunits of cardiac potassium and sodium channels (see Table 424-2).

Two to 4% of cases of congenital heart disease are associated with known environmental or adverse maternal conditions and teratogenic influences, including maternal diabetes mellitus, phenylketonuria, or systemic lupus erythematosus; congenital rubella syndrome; and maternal ingestion of drugs (lithium, ethanol, warfarin, thalidomide, antimetabolites, vitamin A derivatives, anticonvulsant agents) [see Table 422-2]. Associated noncardiac malformations noted in identifiable syndromes may be seen in as many as 25% of patients with congenital heart disease (see Table 422-1).

Gender differences in the occurrence of specific cardiac lesions have been identified. Transposition of the great arteries and left-sided obstructive lesions are slightly more common in boys (≈65%), whereas atrial septal defect, VSD, PDA, and pulmonic stenosis are more common in girls. No racial differences in the occurrence of congenital heart lesions as a whole have been noted; for specific lesions such as transposition of the great arteries, a higher occurrence is seen in white infants.

GENETIC COUNSELING. Parents who have a child with congenital heart disease require genetic counseling regarding the probability of a cardiac malformation occurring in subsequent children (see

TABLE 424-2. Genetics of Congenital Heart Disease

CARDIOVASCULAR DISEASE	CHROMOSOMAL LOCATION	GENE*
Structural Heart Defects		
CATCH 22 (DiGeorge syndrome, velocardiofacial syndrome)	22q11.2	Tbx1
	11p13p14	Not known
Familial ASD with heart block	5q35	Nkx2.5
Familial ASD without heart block	8p22-23	GATA4
Alagille syndrome (bile duct hypoplasia, right-sided cardiac lesions)	20p12	Jagged1
Holt-Oram syndrome (limb defects, ASD)	12q2	TBX5
Trisomy 21 (AV septal defect)	21q22	Not known
Isolated familial AV septal defect (without Trisomy 21)	1p31-p21	Not known
	3p25	CRELD1
Familial TAPVR	4p12-q12	Not known
Noonan syndrome (PS, ASD, hypertrophic cardiomyopathy)	12q24	PTPN11
Ellis-van Creveld syndrome (polydactyly, ASD)	4p16	EVC
Char syndrome (craniofacial, limb defects, PDA)	6p12-21.1	TFAP2B
Williams syndrome (supravalvular AS, branch PS, hypercalcemia)	7q11	Elastin
Marfan syndrome (connective tissue weakness, aortic root dilatation)	15q21	Fibrillin
Familial laterality abnormalities (situs inversus, complex congenital heart disease)	Xq24-2q7	ZIC3
	1q42	Not known
	9p13-21	DNAI1
Cardiomyopathies		
Hypertrophic cardiomyopathy	14q1	β-Myosin heavy chain
	15q2	α-Tropomyosin
	1q31	Troponin T
	19p13.2-19q13.2	Troponin I
	11p13-q13	Myosin-binding protein C
	12q23	Cardiac slow myosin regulatory light chain
	13p21	Ventricular slow myosin essential light chain
	2q31	Titin
Hypertrophic cardiomyopathy with Wolf-Parkinson-White syndrome	7q3	Not known
Dilated cardiomyopathy	Xp21	Dystrophin
X-linked	Xp28	G4.5
Autosomal recessive	19p13.2-19q13.2	Troponin I
Autosomal dominant: genes encoding multiple proteins have been identified, including cardiac actin, desmin, δ-sarcoglycan, β-myosin heavy chain, cardiac troponin C and T, α-tropomyosin, titin, metavinculin, myosin-binding protein C, muscle LIM protein, α-actinin-2, phospholamban, Cypher/LIM binding domain 3, α-myosin heavy chain, SUR2A (regulatory subunit of K_{ATP} channel), and lamin A/C.		
Arrhythmias		
Complete heart block	19q13	Not known
Long Q-T syndrome		
LQT1 (autosomal dominant)	11p15.5	KVLQT1 (K^+ channel)
LQT2 (autosomal dominant)	7q35	HERG (K^+ channel)
LQT3 (autosomal dominant)	3p21	SCN5A (Na^+ channel)
LQT4 (autosomal dominant)	4q25-27	Not known
LQT5 (autosomal dominant)	21q22-q22	KCNE1 (K^+ channel)
LQT6	21q22.1	KCNE2 (K^+ channel)
Jervell and Lange-Nielsen syndrome (autosomal recessive, congenital deafness)	11p15.5	KVLQT1 (K^+ channel)
Arrhythmogenic RV dysplasia		
ARVD1	14q24.3	TGF-β3
ARVD2	1q42-q43	RyR2 (Ryanodine receptor)
ARVD3	14q	Not known
ARVD4	2q32.1-q32.3	Not known
ARVD5	3p22-p25	SCN51 (Sodium channel)
ARVD8	6p24	Desmoplakin
Familial atrial fibrillation (autosomal dominant)	10q22-q24	Not known
	11p15.5	KVLQT1 (K^+ channel)
	6q14-16	Not known
Brugada syndrome (familial unexpected nocturnal death syndrome)	3p21-p24	SCN5A

*In many cases, mutation of a single gene has been closely linked to a specific cardiovascular disease, e.g., by finding a high incidence of mutations or deletions of that gene in a large group of patients. These findings are often confirmed by studies in mice in which deletion or alteration of the gene induces a similar cardiac phenotype to the human disease. In others, mutation of a gene may increase the risk of cardiovascular disease, but with decreased penetrance, suggesting that modifier genes or environmental factors play a role. Finally, in some cases, gene mutations have only been identified in a small number of pedigrees and confirmation awaits screening of larger numbers of patients.

AS, aortic stenosis; ASD, atrial septal defect; AV, atrioventricular; PDA, patent ductus arteriosus; PS, pulmonic stenosis; RV, right ventricular; TAPVR, total anomalous pulmonary venous return.

Chapter 83). With the exception of syndromes known to be due to mutation of a single gene, most congenital heart disease is relegated to a multifactorial inheritance pattern, which should result in a low risk of recurrence. As more genetic etiologies are identified, however, these risks will need constant updating. The incidence of congenital heart disease in the normal population is ≈0.8%, and this incidence increases to 2–6% for a 2nd pregnancy after the birth of a child with congenital heart disease or if a parent is affected. This recurrence risk is highly dependent on the type of lesion in the 1st child. When two 1st-degree relatives have congenital heart disease, the risk for a subsequent child may reach 20–30%. When a 2nd child is found to have congenital heart disease, it will tend to be of a similar class as the lesion in their 1st-degree relative (conotruncal lesions, left-sided obstructive lesions, atrioventricular septation defects). The degree of severity may be variable, as is the presence of associated defects. Careful echocardiographic screening of 1st-degree relatives will often uncover mild forms of congenital heart disease that were clinically silent. The incidence of bicuspid aortic valve is more than double (5% vs 2% in the general population) in the relatives of children with left ventricular outflow obstructions (aortic stenosis, coarctation of the aorta, or hypoplastic left heart syndrome). Consultation with a knowledgeable genetic counselor is the most reliable way of providing the family with up-to-date information regarding the risk of recurrence.

Fetal echocardiography improves the rate of detection of congenital heart lesions in high-risk patients (see Chapter 96). The resolution and accuracy of fetal echocardiography are excellent, but not perfect; families should be counseled that a normal fetal echocardiogram does not guarantee the absence of congenital heart disease. Congenital heart lesions may evolve in the course of the pregnancy; moderate aortic stenosis with a normal-sized left ventricle at 18 wk of gestation may evolve into aortic atresia with a hypoplastic left ventricle by 34 wk because of decreased flow through the atria, ventricle, and aorta in the latter half of gestation. This progression has prompted initial clinical trials of interventional treatment, such as fetal aortic balloon valvuloplasty, for the prevention of hypoplastic left heart syndrome (see Chap. 423.7).

The major factor in determining whether a **woman with congenital heart disease,** either unoperated or operated, will be able to carry a fetus to term is the mother's cardiovascular status. In the presence of a mild congenital heart defect or after successful repair of a more severe lesion, normal childbearing is likely. In a woman with poor cardiac function, however, the increased hemodynamic burden imposed by pregnancy may result in a significantly increased risk to both the mother and fetus. The incidence of spontaneous abortion in the presence of severe congenital heart disease is high, especially when the mother is cyanotic. The maternal risk in these situations is also high, and these pregnancies should be managed by an experienced perinatologist in conjunction with a cardiologist with expertise in adult congenital heart disease (see Chap. 434.1). It is important to discuss various methods of birth control with young women who have repaired or palliated congenital heart lesions. Antibiotic prophylaxis against endocarditis is also indicated at the time of delivery.

Berend SA, Spikes AS, Kashork CD, et al: Dual-probe fluorescence in situ hybridization assay for detecting deletions associated with VCFS/DiGeorge syndrome I and DiGeorge syndrome II loci. *Am J Med Genet* 2000;91:313–317.

Boneva RS, Botto LD, Moore CA, et al: Mortality associated with congenital heart defects in the United States: Trends and racial disparities, 1979–1997. *Circulation* 2001;103:2376–2381.

Donnai D, Karmiloff-Smith A: Williams syndrome: From genotype through to the cognitive phenotype. *Am J Med Genet* 2000;97:164–171.

Epstein JA, Buck CA: Transcriptional regulation of cardiac development: Implications for congenital heart disease and DiGeorge syndrome. *Pediatr Res* 2000;48:717–724.

Ferencz C, Rubin JD, McCarter RJ, et al: Congenital heart disease: Prevalence at livebirth. The Baltimore-Washington Infant Study. *Am J Epidemiol* 1985;121:31–36.

Gill HK, Splitt M, Sharland G, et al: Patterns of recurrence of congenital heart disease: An analysis of 6,640 consecutive pregnancies evaluated by detailed fetal echocardiography. *J Am Coll Cardiol* 2003;42:923–929.

Goldmuntz E: The genetic contribution to congenital heart disease. *Pediatr Clin North Am* 2004;51:1721–1737.

Maslen CL: Molecular genetics of atrioventricular septal defects. *Curr Opin Cardiol* 2004;19:205–210.

Reamon-Buettner SM, Hecker H, Spanel-Borowski, et al. Novel NKX2-5 mutations in diseased heart tissues of patients with cardiac malformations. *Am J Pathol* 2004;164:2117–2125.

Schott JJ, Benson DW, Basson CT, et al: Congenital heart disease caused by mutations in the transcription factor NKX2-5. *Science* 1998;281:108–111.

Chapter 425 ■ Evaluation of the Infant or Child with Congenital Heart Disease

The initial evaluation for suspected congenital heart disease involves a systematic approach with three major components. First, congenital cardiac defects can be divided into two major groups based on the presence or absence of cyanosis, which can be determined by physical examination aided by pulse oximetry. Second, these two groups can be further subdivided according to whether the chest radiograph shows evidence of increased, normal, or decreased pulmonary vascular markings. Finally, the electrocardiogram can be used to determine whether right, left, or biventricular hypertrophy exists. The character of the heart sounds and the presence and character of any murmurs further narrow the differential diagnosis. The final diagnosis is then confirmed by echocardiography, CT or MRI, or cardiac catheterization.

ACYANOTIC CONGENITAL HEART LESIONS

Acyanotic congenital heart lesions can be classified according to the predominant physiologic load that they place on the heart. Although many congenital heart lesions induce more than one physiologic disturbance, it is helpful to focus on the primary load abnormality for purposes of classification. The most common lesions are those that produce a volume load, and the most common of these are left-to-right shunt lesions. Atrioventricular (AV) valve regurgitation and some of the cardiomyopathies are other causes of increased volume load. The second major class of lesions causes an increase in pressure load, most commonly secondary to ventricular outflow obstruction (pulmonic or aortic valve stenosis) or narrowing of one of the great vessels (coarctation of the aorta). The chest radiograph and electrocardiogram are useful tools for differentiating between these major classes of volume and pressure overload lesions.

LESIONS RESULTING IN INCREASED VOLUME LOAD. The most common lesions in this group are those that cause left-to-right shunting (see Chapter 426): atrial septal defect, ventricular septal defect (VSD), AV septal defects (AV canal), and patent ductus arteriosus. The pathophysiologic common denominator in this group is communication between the systemic and pulmonary sides of the circulation, which results in shunting of fully oxygenated blood back into the lungs. This shunt can be quantitated by calculating the ratio of pulmonary to systemic blood flow, or Qp : Qs. Thus, a 2:1 shunt implies twice the normal pulmonary blood flow.

The direction and magnitude of the shunt across such a communication depend on the size of the defect and the relative pulmonary and systemic pressure and vascular resistance. These factors are dynamic and may change dramatically with age: Intracardiac defects may grow smaller with time; pulmonary vascular resistance, which is high in the immediate newborn period, decreases to normal adult levels by several weeks of life; and chronic exposure of the pulmonary circulation to high pressure and blood flow results in a gradual increase in pulmonary vascular resistance (Eisenmenger physiology, see Chapter 433.2). Thus, a lesion such as a large VSD may be associated with little shunting and few symptoms during the initial weeks of life. When pulmonary vascular resistance declines in the next several weeks, the volume of the left-to-right shunt increases, and symptoms begin to appear.

The increased volume of blood in the lungs decreases pulmonary compliance and increases the work of breathing. Fluid leaks into the interstitial space and alveoli and causes pulmonary edema. The infant acquires the symptoms we refer to as **heart failure,** such as tachypnea, chest retractions, nasal flaring, and wheezing. The term *heart failure* is a misnomer, however; total left ventricular output is actually several times greater than normal, although much of this output is ineffective because it returns directly to the lungs. To maintain this high level of left ventricular output, heart rate and stroke volume are increased, mediated by an increase in sympathetic nervous system activity. The increase in circulating catecholamines, combined with the increased work of breathing, results in an elevation in total body oxygen consumption, often beyond the oxygen transport ability of the circulation. Such oxygen consumption leads to the additional symptoms of sweating, irritability, and failure to thrive. Remodeling of the heart occurs, with predominantly dilatation and a lesser degree of hypertrophy. If left untreated, pulmonary vascular resistance eventually begins to rise and, by several years of age, the shunt volume will decrease and eventually reverse to right to left (Eisenmenger physiology, Chapter 433.2).

Additional lesions that impose a volume load on the heart include regurgitant lesions (see Chapter 428) and the cardiomyopathies (see Chapter 439). Regurgitation through the AV valves is most commonly encountered in patients with partial or complete AV septal defects (atrioseptal defects, AV canal). In these lesions, the combination of a left-to-right shunt with AV valve regurgitation increases the volume load on the heart and leads to more severe symptoms. Isolated regurgitation through the tricuspid valve is seen in Ebstein anomaly (see Chapter 430.7). Regurgitation involving one of the semilunar valves is usually also associated with some degree of stenosis; however, aortic regurgitation may be encountered in patients with a VSD directly under the aortic valve (supracristal VSD) and in patients with membranous subaortic stenosis.

In contrast to left-to-right shunts, in which intrinsic cardiac muscle function is generally either normal or increased, heart muscle function is decreased in the cardiomyopathies. **Cardiomyopathies** may affect systolic contractility or diastolic relaxation, or both. Decreased cardiac function results in increased atrial and ventricular filling pressure, and pulmonary edema occurs secondary to increased capillary pressure. The major causes of cardiomyopathy in infants and children include viral myocarditis, metabolic disorders, and genetic defects (see Chapter 439).

LESIONS RESULTING IN INCREASED PRESSURE LOAD. The pathophysiologic common denominator of these lesions is an obstruction to normal blood flow. The most frequent are obstructions to ventricular outflow: valvular pulmonic stenosis, valvular aortic stenosis, and coarctation of the aorta (see Chapter 427). Less common are obstruction to ventricular inflow: tricuspid or mitral stenosis and cor triatriatum. Ventricular outflow obstruction can occur at the valve, below the valve (double-chambered right ventricle, subaortic membrane), or above it (branch pulmonary stenosis or supravalvular aortic stenosis). Unless the obstruction is severe, cardiac output will be maintained and the clinical symptoms of heart failure will be either subtle or absent. This compensation predominantly involves an increase in cardiac wall thickness (hypertrophy), but in later stages it also involves dilatation.

The clinical picture is different when obstruction to outflow is severe, which is usually encountered in the immediate newborn period. The infant may become critically ill within several hours of birth. Severe pulmonic stenosis in the newborn period (critical pulmonic stenosis) results in signs of right-sided heart failure (hepatomegaly, peripheral edema), as well as cyanosis from right-to-left shunting across the foramen ovale. Severe aortic stenosis in the newborn period (critical aortic stenosis) is characterized by signs of left-sided heart failure (pulmonary edema, poor perfusion) and right-sided failure (hepatomegaly, peripheral edema), and it may progress rapidly to total circulatory collapse. In older children, severe pulmonic stenosis leads to symptoms of right-sided heart failure, but not to cyanosis unless a pathway persists for right-to-left shunting (e.g., patency of the foramen ovale).

Coarctation of the aorta in older children and adolescents is usually manifested as upper body hypertension and diminished pulses in the lower extremities. In the immediate newborn period, however, the occurrence of coarctation may be delayed because of the presence of a patent ductus arteriosus. In these patients, the open aortic end of the ductus may serve as a conduit for blood flow to partially bypass the obstruction. These infants then become symptomatic, often dramatically, when the ductus finally closes.

CYANOTIC CONGENITAL HEART LESIONS

This group of congenital heart lesions can also be further divided according to pathophysiology: whether pulmonary blood flow is decreased (tetralogy of Fallot, pulmonary atresia with an intact septum, tricuspid atresia, total anomalous pulmonary venous return with obstruction) or increased (transposition of the great vessels, single ventricle, truncus arteriosus, total anomalous pulmonary venous return without obstruction). The chest radiograph is a valuable tool for initial differentiation between these two categories.

CYANOTIC LESIONS WITH DECREASED PULMONARY BLOOD FLOW. These lesions must include both an obstruction to pulmonary blood flow (at the tricuspid valve or right ventricular or pulmonary valve level) and a pathway by which systemic venous blood can shunt from right to left and enter the systemic circulation (via a patent foramen ovale, atrial septal defect, or VSD). Common lesions in this group include tricuspid atresia, tetralogy of Fallot, and various forms of single ventricle with pulmonary stenosis (see Chapter 430). In these lesions, the degree of cyanosis depends on the degree of obstruction to pulmonary blood flow. If the obstruction is mild, cyanosis may be absent at rest. These patients may have hypercyanotic ("tet") spells during conditions of stress. In contrast, if the obstruction is severe, pulmonary blood flow may be dependent on patency of the ductus arteriosus. When the ductus closes in the 1st few days of life, the neonate experiences profound hypoxemia and shock.

CYANOTIC LESIONS WITH INCREASED PULMONARY BLOOD FLOW. This group of lesions is not associated with obstruction to pulmonary blood flow. Cyanosis is caused by either abnormal ventricular-arterial connections or total mixing of systemic venous and pulmonary venous blood within the heart (see

Chapter 431). Transposition of the great vessels is the most common of the former group of lesions. In this condition, the aorta arises from the right ventricle and the pulmonary artery arises from the left ventricle. Systemic venous blood returning to the right atrium is pumped directly back to the body, and oxygenated blood returning from the lungs to the left atrium is pumped back into the lungs. The persistence of fetal pathways (foramen ovale and ductus arteriosus) allows for a small degree of mixing in the immediate newborn period; when the ductus begins to close, these infants become extremely cyanotic.

Total mixing lesions include cardiac defects with a common atrium or ventricle, total anomalous pulmonary venous return, and truncus arteriosus (see Chapter 431). In this group, deoxygenated systemic venous blood and oxygenated pulmonary venous blood mix completely in the heart and, as a result, oxygen saturation is equal in the pulmonary artery and aorta. If pulmonary blood flow is not obstructed, these infants have a combination of cyanosis and heart failure. In contrast, if pulmonary stenosis is present, these infants have cyanosis alone, similar to patients with the tetralogy of Fallot.

Lister G, Moreau G, Moss M, et al: Effects of alterations of oxygen transport on the neonate. *Semin Perinatol* 1984;8:192–204.

Lister G, Pitt BR: Cardiopulmonary interactions in the infant with congenital heart disease. *Clin Chest Med* 1983;4:219–232.

Mair DD, Ritter DG: Factors influencing systemic oxygen saturation in complete transposition of the great arteries. *Am J Cardiol* 1973;31:742–748.

Weeks B, Friedman AH: Training pediatric residents to evaluate congenital heart disease in the current era. *Pediatr Clin North Am* 2004;51: 1641–1651.

Chapter 426 ■ Acyanotic Congenital Heart Disease: The Left-to-Right Shunt Lesions

426.1 • Atrial Septal Defect

Atrial septal defects (ASDs) can occur in any portion of the atrial septum (secundum, primum, or sinus venosus), depending on which embryonic septal structure has failed to develop normally (see Chapter 420). Less commonly, the atrial septum may be nearly absent, with the creation of a functional single atrium. Isolated secundum ASDs account for ≈7% of congenital heart defects. The majority of cases of ASD are sporadic; autosomal dominant inheritance does occur as part of the Holt-Oram syndrome (hypoplastic or absent radii, 1st-degree heart block, ASD) or in families with secundum ASD and heart block.

An isolated valve-incompetent patent foramen ovale (PFO) is a common echocardiographic finding during infancy. It is usually of no hemodynamic significance and is not considered an ASD; a PFO may play an important role if other structural heart defects are present. If another cardiac anomaly is causing increased right atrial pressure (pulmonary stenosis or atresia, tricuspid valve abnormalities, right ventricular dysfunction), venous blood may shunt across the PFO into the left atrium with resultant cyanosis. Because of the anatomic structure of the PFO, left-to-right shunting is unusual outside the immediate newborn period. In the presence of a large volume load or a hypertensive left atrium (secondary to mitral stenosis), the foramen ovale may be sufficiently dilated to result in a significant atrial left-to-right shunt. A valve-competent but probe-patent foramen ovale may be present in 15–30% of adults. An isolated PFO does not require surgical treatment, although it may be a risk for paradoxical (right to left) systemic embolization. Device closure of these defects is considered in adults with a history of thromboembolic stroke.

426.2 • Ostium Secundum Defect

An ostium secundum defect in the region of the fossa ovalis is the most common form of ASD and is associated with structurally normal atrioventricular (AV) valves. Mitral valve prolapse has been described in association with this defect but is rarely an important clinical consideration. Secundum ASDs may be single or multiple (fenestrated atrial septum), and openings ≥2 cm in diameter are common in symptomatic older children. Large defects may extend inferiorly toward the inferior vena cava and ostium of the coronary sinus, superiorly toward the superior vena cava, or posteriorly. Females outnumber males 3 : 1 in incidence. Partial anomalous pulmonary venous return, most commonly of the right upper pulmonary vein, may be an associated lesion.

PATHOPHYSIOLOGY. The degree of left-to-right shunting is dependent on the size of the defect, the relative compliance of the right and left ventricles, and the relative vascular resistance in the pulmonary and systemic circulations. In large defects, a considerable shunt of oxygenated blood flows from the left to the right atrium (Fig. 426-1). This blood is added to the usual venous return to the right atrium and is pumped by the right ventricle to the lungs. With large defects, the ratio of pulmonary to systemic blood flow (Qp : Qs) is usually between 2 : 1 and 4 : 1. The paucity of symp-

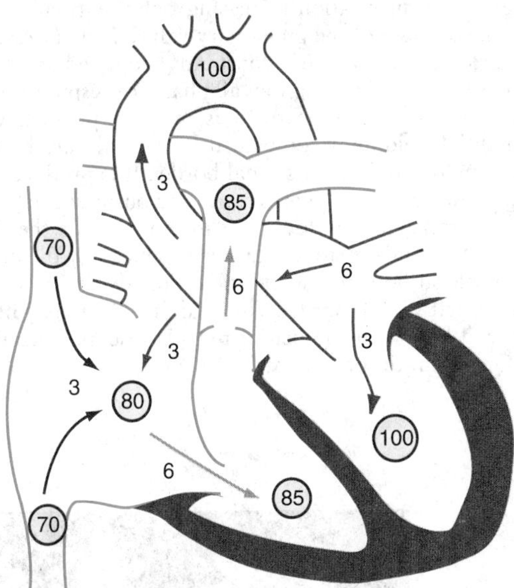

Figure 426-1. Physiology of atrial septal defect (ASD). *Circled numbers* represent oxygen saturation values. The *numbers next to the arrows* represent volumes of blood flow (in L/min/m²). This illustration shows a hypothetical patient with a pulmonary-to-systemic blood flow ratio (Qp : Qs) of 2 : 1. Desaturated blood enters the right atrium from the vena cavae at a volume of 3 L/min/m² and mixes with an additional 3 L of fully saturated blood shunting left to right across the ASD; the result is an increase in oxygen saturation in the right atrium. Six liters of blood flows through the tricuspid valve and causes a mid-diastolic flow rumble. Oxygen saturation may be slightly higher in the right ventricle because of incomplete mixing at the atrial level. The full 6 L flows across the right ventricular outflow tract and causes a systolic ejection flow murmur. Six liters returns to the left atrium, with 3 L shunting left to right across the defect and 3 L crossing the mitral valve to be ejected by the left ventricle into the ascending aorta (normal cardiac output).

toms in infants with ASDs is related to the structure of the right ventricle in early life when its muscular wall is thick and less compliant, thus limiting the left-to-right shunt. As the infant becomes older and pulmonary vascular resistance drops, the right ventricular wall becomes thinner and the left-to-right shunt across the ASD increases. The large blood flow through the right side of the heart results in enlargement of the right atrium and ventricle and dilatation of the pulmonary artery. The left atrium may be enlarged, the left ventricle and aorta normal in size. Despite the large pulmonary blood flow, pulmonary arterial pressure is usually normal because of the absence of a high-pressure communication between the pulmonary and systemic circulations. Pulmonary vascular resistance remains low throughout childhood, although it may begin to increase in adulthood and may eventually result in reversal of the shunt and clinical cyanosis.

CLINICAL MANIFESTATIONS. A child with an ostium secundum ASD is most often asymptomatic; the lesion may be discovered inadvertently during physical examination. Even an extremely large secundum ASD rarely produces clinically evident heart failure in childhood. In younger children, subtle failure to thrive may be present; in older children, varying degrees of exercise intolerance may be noted. Often, the degree of limitation may go unnoticed by the family until after surgical repair, when the child's growth or activity level increases markedly.

The physical findings of an ASD are usually characteristic but fairly subtle and require careful examination of the heart, with special attention to the heart sounds. Examination of the chest may reveal a mild left precordial bulge. A right ventricular systolic lift is generally palpable at the left sternal border. A loud 1st heart sound and sometimes a pulmonic ejection click can be heard. In most patients, the 2nd heart sound is characteristically **widely split and fixed in its splitting** in all phases of respiration. Normally, the duration of right ventricular ejection varies with respiration, with inspiration increasing right ventricular volume and delaying closure of the pulmonary valve. With an ASD, right ventricular diastolic volume is constantly increased and the ejection time is prolonged throughout all phases of respiration. A systolic ejection murmur is heard; it is medium pitched, without harsh qualities, seldom accompanied by a thrill, and best heard at the left middle and upper sternal border. It is produced by the increased flow across the right ventricular outflow tract into the pulmonary artery, not by low-pressure flow across the ASD. A short, rumbling mid-diastolic murmur produced by the increased volume of blood flow across the tricuspid valve is often audible at the lower left sternal border. This finding, which may be subtle and is heard best with the bell of the stethoscope, usually indicates a Qp : Qs ratio of at least 2 : 1.

DIAGNOSIS. The chest roentgenogram shows varying degrees of enlargement of the right ventricle and atrium, depending on the size of the shunt. The pulmonary artery is large, and pulmonary vascularity is increased. These signs vary and may not be conspicuous in mild cases. Cardiac enlargement is often best appreciated on the lateral view because the right ventricle protrudes anteriorly as its volume increases. The electrocardiogram shows volume overload of the right ventricle; the QRS axis may be normal or exhibit right axis deviation, and a minor right ventricular conduction delay (rsR pattern in the right precordial leads) may be present.

The echocardiogram shows findings characteristic of right ventricular volume overload, including an increased right ventricular end-diastolic dimension and flattening and abnormal motion of the ventricular septum (Fig. 426-2). A normal septum moves posteriorly during systole and anteriorly during diastole. With right ventricular overload and normal pulmonary vascular resistance, septal motion is reversed—that is, anterior movement in systole—or the motion may be intermediate so that the septum remains straight. The location and size of the atrial defect are readily appreciated by two-dimensional scanning, with a characteristic brightening of the echo image seen at the edge of the defect (T-artifact). The shunt is confirmed by pulsed and color flow Doppler. Patients with the classic features of a hemodynamically significant ASD on physical examination and chest radiography, in whom echocardiographic identification of an isolated secundum ASD is made, need not be catheterized before surgical closure, with the exception of an older patient, in whom pulmonary vascular resistance may be a concern. If pulmonary vascular disease is suspected, cardiac catheterization confirms the presence of the defect and allows measurement of the shunt ratio and pulmonary pressure.

At catheterization, the oxygen content of blood from the right atrium will be much higher than that from the superior vena cava. This feature is not specifically diagnostic because it may occur with partial anomalous pulmonary venous return to the right atrium, with a ventricular septal defect (VSD) in the presence of tricuspid insufficiency, with AV septal defects associated with left ventricular to right atrial shunts, and with aorta to right atrial communications (ruptured sinus of Valsalva aneurysm). Pressure in the right side of the heart is usually normal, but small to moderate pressure gradients (<25 mm Hg) may be measured across the right ventricular outflow tract because of functional stenosis related to excessive blood flow. In children and adolescents, the pulmonary vascular resistance is almost always normal. The shunt is variable and depends on the size of the defect, but it may be of considerable volume (as high as 20 L/min/m^2). Cineangiography, performed with the catheter through the defect and in the

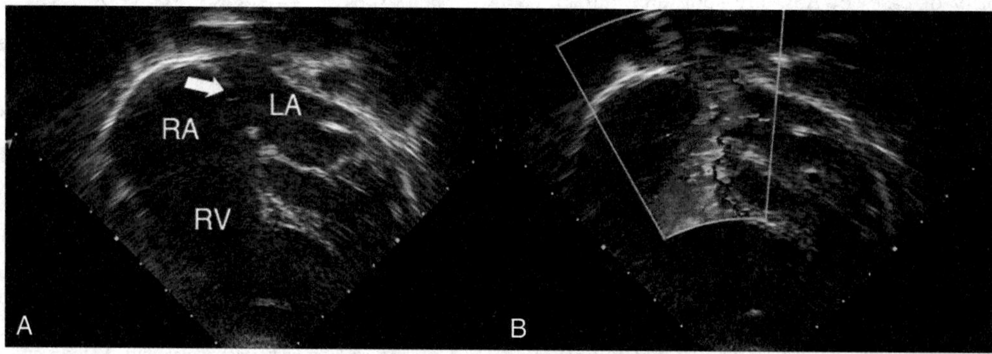

Figure 426-2. Echocardiographic findings in a secundum atrial septal defect (ASD). *A,* 2-D echocardiogram (apical four-chamber view) shows a moderate-sized secundum ASD *(arrow)*. *B,* Color flow Doppler imaging shows left-to-right shunting (the red color represents blood moving toward the ultrasound transducer and does not indicate the level of oxygenation of the blood). LA, left atrium; RA, right atrium; RV, right ventricle.

right upper pulmonary vein, demonstrates the defect and the location of the right upper pulmonary venous drainage. Alternatively, pulmonary angiography demonstrates the defect on the levophase (return of contrast to the left side of the heart after passing through the lungs).

COMPLICATIONS. Secundum ASDs are usually isolated, although they may be associated with partial anomalous pulmonary venous return, pulmonary valvular stenosis, VSD, pulmonary artery branch stenosis, and persistent left superior vena cava, as well as mitral valve prolapse and insufficiency. Secundum ASDs are associated with the autosomal dominant Holt-Oram syndrome. The gene responsible for this syndrome, situated in the region 12q21-q22 of chromosome 12, is TBX5, a member of the T-box transcriptional family. A familial form of secundum ASD associated with AV conduction delay has been linked to mutations in another transcription factor, Nkx2.5. Patients with familial ASD without heart block may carry a mutation in the transcription factor GATA4, located on chromosome 8p22-23.

TREATMENT. Surgical or transcatheter device closure is advised for all symptomatic patients and also for asymptomatic patients with a Qp : Qs ratio of at least 2 : 1. The timing for elective closure is usually after the 1st yr and before entry into school. Closure carried out at open heart surgery is associated with a mortality rate of <1%. Repair is preferred during early childhood because surgical mortality and morbidity are significantly greater in adulthood; the long-term risk of arrhythmia is also greater after ASD repair in adults. Atrial septal occlusion devices are implanted transvenously in the cardiac catheterization laboratory (Fig. 426-3). The results are excellent and patients are discharged the following day. With the latest generation of devices, the incidence of serious complications such as device erosion is 0.1% and can be decreased by identifying high-risk patients such as those with a deficient rim of septum around the device. In patients with small secundum ASDs and minimal left-to-right shunts, the consensus is that closure is not required. It is unclear at present whether the persistence of a small ASD into adulthood increases the risk for stroke enough to warrant prophylactic closure of all these defects.

PROGNOSIS. ASDs detected in term infants may close spontaneously. Secundum ASDs are well tolerated during childhood, and symptoms do not usually appear until the 3rd decade or later. Pulmonary hypertension, atrial dysrhythmias, tricuspid or mitral insufficiency, and heart failure are late manifestations; these symptoms may initially appear during the increased volume load of pregnancy. Infective endocarditis is extremely rare, and antibiotic prophylaxis for isolated secundum ASDs is not recommended.

The results after surgical or device closure in children with moderate to large shunts are excellent. Symptoms disappear rapidly, and growth is frequently enhanced. Heart size decreases to normal, and the electrocardiogram shows decreased right ventricular forces. Late right heart failure and arrhythmias are less frequent in patients who have had early surgical repair, becoming more common in patients who undergo surgery after 20 yr of age. Although early and midterm results with device closure are excellent, the long-term effects are not yet known. Reports of resolution of migraine headaches in patients after device closure of ASD or PFO are intriguing, suggesting a possible thromboembolic etiology; however, there are also paradoxical reports of patients whose migraines began or worsened after placement of one of these devices.

426.3 • Sinus Venosus Atrial Septal Defect

A sinus venosus ASD is situated in the upper part of the atrial septum in close relation to the entry of the superior vena cava. Often, one or more pulmonary veins (usually from the right lung) drain anomalously into the superior vena cava. The superior vena cava sometimes straddles the defect; in this case, some systemic venous blood enters the left atrium, but only rarely does it cause clinically evident cyanosis. The hemodynamic disturbance, clinical picture, electrocardiogram, and roentgenogram are similar to those seen in secundum ASD. The diagnosis can usually be made by two-dimensional echocardiography. If cardiac catheterization is carried out to better define venous drainage, the catheter may enter a right pulmonary vein directly from the superior vena cava. Anatomic correction generally requires the insertion of a patch to close the defect while incorporating the entry of anomalous veins into the left atrium. If the anomalous vein drains high in the superior vena cava, the vein can be left intact and the ASD closed to incorporate the mouth of the cava into the left atrium. The superior vena cava proximal to the venous entrance is then detached and anastomosed directly to the right atrium. Surgical results are generally excellent. Rarely, sinus venosus defects involve the inferior vena cava.

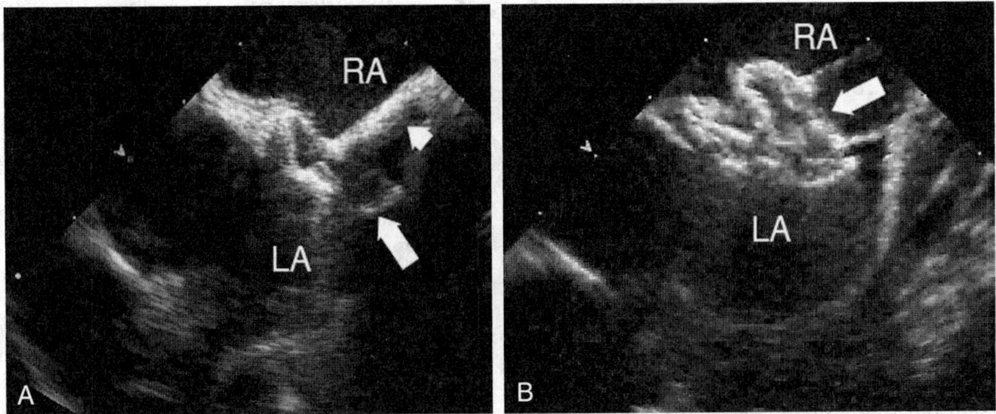

Figure 426-3. Intravascular ultrasound imaging of transcatheter occlusion of an atrial septal defect. *A,* A catheter *(small arrow)* has been advanced across the atrial defect and the left-sided disk of the device *(large arrow)* has been extruded from the sheath into the left atrium (LA). *B,* The right atrial disk *(arrow)* has now been extruded into the right atrium (RA). The two halves of the device are then locked together and the catheter detached from the occluder device and removed.

426.4 • Partial Anomalous Pulmonary Venous Return

One or several pulmonary veins may return anomalously to the superior or inferior vena cava, the right atrium, or the coronary sinus and produce a left-to-right shunt of oxygenated blood. Partial anomalous pulmonary venous return usually involves some or all of the veins from only one lung, more often the right one. When an associated ASD is present, it is generally of the sinus venosus type (see Chapter 426.3). When a sinus venosus ASD is detected by echocardiography, one must search for associated partial anomalous pulmonary venous return. The history, physical signs, and electrocardiographic and roentgenographic findings are indistinguishable from those of an isolated ostium secundum ASD. Occasionally, an anomalous vein draining into the inferior vena cava is visible on chest radiography as a crescentic shadow of vascular density along the right border of the cardiac silhouette (**scimitar syndrome**); in these cases, an ASD is not usually present, but **pulmonary sequestration** and anomalous arterial supply to that lobe are common findings. Total anomalous pulmonary venous return is a cyanotic lesion and is discussed in Chapter 431.7. Echocardiography generally confirms the diagnosis. MRI and CT are also useful for defining pulmonary venous drainage. If cardiac catheterization is performed, the presence of anomalous pulmonary veins is demonstrated by selective pulmonary arteriography.

The prognosis is excellent, similar to that for ostium secundum ASDs. When a large left-to-right shunt is present, surgical repair is performed. The associated ASD should be closed in such a way that pulmonary venous return is directed to the left atrium. A single anomalous pulmonary vein without an atrial communication may be difficult to redirect to the left atrium; if the shunt is small, it may be left unoperated.

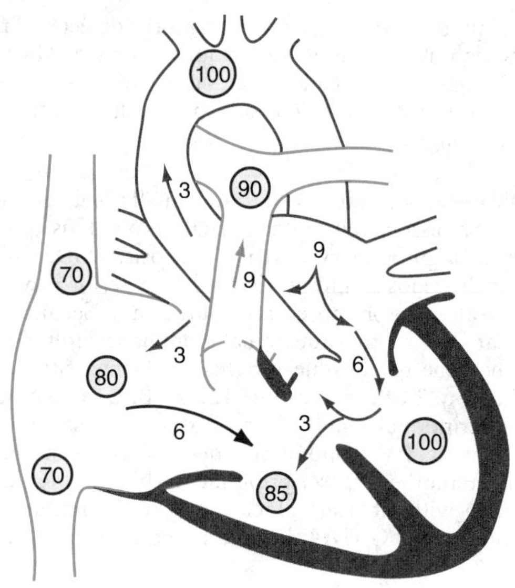

Figure 426-4. Physiology of atrioventricular septal defect (AVSD). *Circled numbers* represent oxygen saturation values. The *numbers next to the arrows* represent volumes of blood flow (in L/min/m²). This illustration shows a hypothetical patient with a pulmonary-to-systemic blood flow ratio (Qp : Qs) of 3 : 1. Desaturated blood enters the right atrium from the vena cavae at a volume of 3 L/min/m² and mixes with 3 L of fully saturated blood shunting left to right across the atrial septal defect; the result is an increase in oxygen saturation in the right atrium. Six liters of blood flows through the right side of the common AV valve, joined by an additional 3 L of saturated blood shunting left to right at the ventricular level, further increasing oxygen saturation in the right ventricle. The full 9 L flows across the right ventricular outflow tract into the lungs. Nine liters returns to the left atrium, with 3 L shunting left to right across the defect and 6 L crossing the left side of the common AV valve and causing a mid-diastolic flow rumble. Three liters of this volume shunts left to right across the VSD, and 3 L is ejected into the ascending aorta (normal cardiac output).

426.5 • Atrioventricular Septal Defects (Ostium Primum and Atrioventricular Canal or Endocardial Cushion Defects)

The abnormalities encompassed by AV septal defects are grouped together because they represent a spectrum of a basic embryologic abnormality, a deficiency of the AV septum. An **ostium primum** defect is situated in the lower portion of the atrial septum and overlies the mitral and tricuspid valves. In most instances, a **cleft** in the **anterior leaflet** of the **mitral valve** is also noted. The tricuspid valve is usually functionally normal, although some anatomic abnormality of the septal leaflet is generally present. The ventricular septum is intact.

An **AV septal defect,** also known as an **AV canal** defect or an endocardial cushion defect, consists of contiguous atrial and ventricular septal defects with markedly abnormal AV valves. The severity of the valve abnormalities varies considerably; in the complete form of AV septal defect, a single AV valve is common to both ventricles and consists of an anterior and a posterior bridging leaflet related to the ventricular septum, with a lateral leaflet in each ventricle. The lesion is common in children with **Down syndrome** and may occasionally occur with pulmonary stenosis.

Transitional varieties of these defects also occur and include ostium primum defects with clefts in the anterior mitral and septal tricuspid valve leaflets, minor ventricular septal deficiencies, and, less commonly, ostium primum defects with normal AV valves. In some patients, the atrial septum is intact, but the inlet VSD simulates that found in the full AV septal defect. These defects are also commonly associated with deformities of the AV valves. Sometimes AV septal defects are associated with varying degrees of hypoplasia of one of the ventricles, known as either left- or right-dominant AVSD. If the affected ventricular chamber is too small, then surgical palliation, aiming for an eventual Fontan procedure, is similar to that for hypoplastic left or right heart syndromes (see Chapters 430.4 and 431.10).

PATHOPHYSIOLOGY. The basic abnormality in patients with ostium primum defects is the combination of a left-to-right shunt across the atrial defect and mitral (or occasionally tricuspid) insufficiency. The shunt is usually moderate to large, the degree of mitral insufficiency is generally mild to moderate, and pulmonary arterial pressure is typically normal or only mildly increased. The physiology of this lesion is therefore similar to that of an ostium secundum ASD.

In AV septal defects, the left-to-right shunt occurs at both the atrial and ventricular levels (Fig. 426-4). Additional shunting may occur directly from the left ventricle to the right atrium because of absence of the AV septum. Pulmonary hypertension and an early tendency to increase pulmonary vascular resistance are common. AV valvular insufficiency increases the volume load on one or both ventricles. Some right-to-left shunting may also occur at both the atrial and ventricular levels and lead to mild but significant arterial desaturation. With time, progressive pulmonary vascular disease increases the right-to-left shunt so that clinical cyanosis develops (Eisenmenger physiology, see Chapter 433.2).

CLINICAL MANIFESTATIONS. Many children with ostium primum defects are asymptomatic, and the anomaly is discovered during a general physical examination. In patients with moderate shunts and mild mitral insufficiency, the physical signs are similar to those of the secundum ASD, but with an additional apical murmur caused by mitral insufficiency.

A history of exercise intolerance, easy fatigability, and recurrent pneumonia may be obtained, especially in infants with large left-to-right shunts and severe mitral insufficiency. In these patients, cardiac enlargement is moderate or marked, and the precordium is hyperdynamic. Auscultatory signs produced by the left-to-right shunt include a normal or accentuated 1st sound; wide, fixed splitting of the 2nd sound; a pulmonary systolic ejection murmur sometimes preceded by a click; and a low-pitched, mid-diastolic rumbling murmur at the lower left sternal edge or apex, or both, as a result of increased flow through the AV valves. Mitral insufficiency may be manifested by a harsh (occasionally very high pitched) apical holosystolic murmur that radiates to the left axilla.

With complete AV septal defects, heart failure and intercurrent pulmonary infection usually appear in infancy. During these episodes, minimal cyanosis may be evident. The liver is enlarged and the infant shows signs of failure to thrive. Cardiac enlargement is moderate to marked, and a systolic thrill is frequently palpable at the lower left sternal border. A precordial bulge and lift may be present as well. The 1st heart sound is normal or accentuated. The 2nd heart sound is widely split if the pulmonary flow is massive. A low-pitched, mid-diastolic rumbling murmur is audible at the lower left sternal border, and a pulmonary systolic ejection murmur is produced by the large pulmonary flow. The harsh apical holosystolic murmur of mitral insufficiency may also be present.

DIAGNOSIS. Chest radiographs of children with complete AV septal defects often show moderate to severe cardiac enlargement caused by the prominence of both ventricles and atria. The pulmonary artery is large, and pulmonary vascularity is increased.

The electrocardiogram in patients with a complete AV septal defect is distinctive. The principal abnormalities are (1) superior orientation of the mean frontal QRS axis with left axis deviation to the left upper or right upper quadrant, (2) counterclockwise inscription of the superiorly oriented QRS vector loop, (3) signs of biventricular hypertrophy or isolated right ventricular hypertrophy, (4) right ventricular conduction delay (RSR′ pattern in leads V_3R and V_1), (5) normal or tall P waves, and (6) occasional prolongation of the P-R interval (Fig. 426-5).

The echocardiogram (Fig. 426-6) is characteristic and shows signs of right ventricular enlargement with encroachment of the mitral valve echo on the left ventricular outflow tract; the abnormally low position of the AV valves results in a "gooseneck" deformity of the left ventricular outflow tract on both echocardiography and angiography. In normal hearts, the tricuspid valve inserts slightly more toward the apex than the mitral valve does.

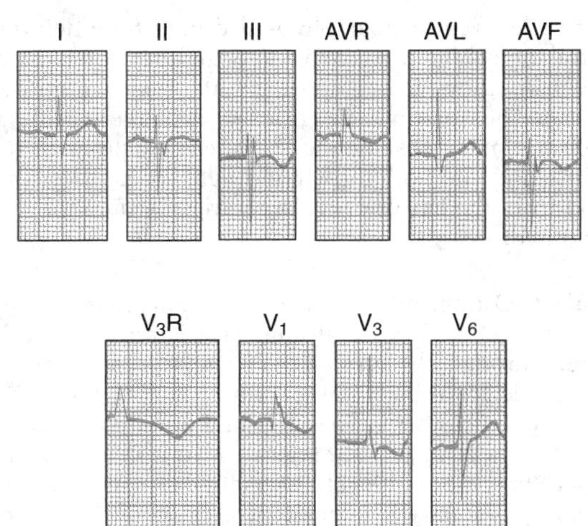

Figure 426-5. Electrocardiogram from a child with an atrioventricular septal defect. Note the QRS axis of −60 degrees and the right ventricular conduction delay with an RSR′ pattern in V1 and V3R (V3R paper speed = 50 mm/sec).

In AV septal defects, both valves insert at the same level because of absence of the AV septum. In complete AV septal defects, the ventricular septal echo is also deficient and the common AV valve is readily appreciated. Pulsed and color flow Doppler echocardiography will demonstrate left-to-right shunting at the atrial, ventricular, or ventricular to atrial levels and semiquantitate the degree of AV valve insufficiency. Echocardiography is useful for determining the insertion points of the chordae of the common AV valve and for evaluating the presence of associated lesions such as patent ductus arteriosus (PDA) or coarctation of the aorta.

Cardiac catheterization and angiocardiography is rarely required in the modern era to confirm the diagnosis unless pulmonary vascular disease is suspected, such as in a patient in whom diagnosis has been delayed beyond infancy. Catheterization demonstrates the magnitude of the left-to-right shunt, the degree of elevation of pulmonary vascular resistance, and the severity of insufficiency of the common AV valve. By oximetry, the shunt is usually demonstrable at both the atrial and ventricular levels. Arterial oxygen saturation is normal or only mildly reduced unless severe pulmonary vascular disease is present. Children with ostium primum defects generally have normal or only moderately elevated pulmonary arterial pressure. Conversely, complete AV septal defects are associated with right ventricular and pulmonary hypertension and, in older patients, with increased pulmonary vascular resistance (see Chapter 433.2).

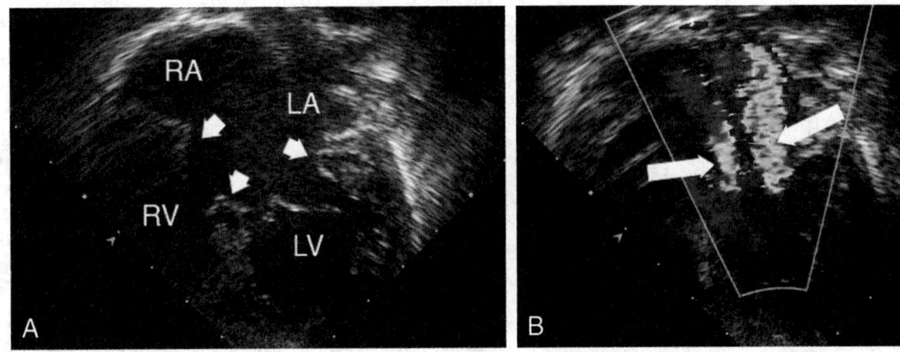

Figure 426-6. Echocardiogram of an atrioventricular septal defect. *A,* Subcostal four-chamber view demonstrating the common atrioventricular valve *(arrows)* spanning the atrial and ventricular septal defects. *B,* Doppler imaging shows two jets of regurgitation through the left side of the common atrioventricular valve *(arrows)*. LA, left atrium; LV, left ventricle; RA, right atrium; RV, right ventricle.

Selective left ventriculography will demonstrate deformity of the mitral or common AV valve and the distortion of the left ventricular outflow tract caused by this valve ("gooseneck" deformity). The abnormal anterior leaflet of the mitral valve is serrated, and mitral insufficiency is noted, usually with regurgitation of blood into both the left and right atria. Direct shunting of blood from the left ventricle to the right atrium may also be demonstrated.

TREATMENT. Ostium primum defects are approached surgically from an incision in the right atrium. The cleft in the mitral valve is located through the atrial defect and is repaired by direct suture. The defect in the atrial septum is usually closed by insertion of a patch prosthesis. The surgical mortality rate for ostium primum defects is very low. Surgical treatment of complete AV septal defects is more difficult, especially in infants with cardiac failure and pulmonary hypertension. Because of the risk of **pulmonary vascular disease** developing as early as 6–12 mo of age, surgical intervention must be performed during infancy. Correction of these defects can be accomplished in infancy, and palliation with pulmonary arterial banding is reserved for the subset of patients who have other associated lesions that make early corrective surgery too risky. The atrial and ventricular defects are patched and the AV valves reconstructed. Complications include surgically induced heart block requiring placement of a permanent pacemaker, excessive narrowing of the left ventricular outflow tract requiring surgical revision, and eventual worsening of mitral regurgitation requiring replacement with a prosthetic valve.

PROGNOSIS. The prognosis for unrepaired complete AV septal defects depends on the magnitude of the left-to-right shunt, the degree of elevation of pulmonary vascular resistance, and the severity of AV valve insufficiency. Death from cardiac failure during infancy used to be frequent before the advent of early corrective surgery. In patients who survived without surgery, pulmonary vascular obstructive disease or, more rarely, pulmonic stenosis usually developed. Most patients with ostium primum defects and minimal AV valve involvement are asymptomatic or have only minor, nonprogressive symptoms until they reach the 3rd–4th decade of life, similar to the course of patients with secundum ASDs. Late postoperative complications include atrial arrhythmias and heart block, progressive narrowing of the left ventricular outflow tract requiring surgical revision, and eventual worsening of atrioventricular valve regurgitation (usually on the left side) requiring replacement with a prosthetic valve.

426.6 • Ventricular Septal Defect

VSD is the most common cardiac malformation and accounts for 25% of congenital heart disease. Defects may occur in any portion of the ventricular septum, but most are of the membranous type. These defects are in a posteroinferior position, anterior to the septal leaflet of the tricuspid valve. VSDs between the crista supraventricularis and the papillary muscle of the conus may be associated with pulmonary stenosis and other manifestations of the tetralogy of Fallot (see Chapter 430.1). VSDs superior to the crista supraventricularis (supracristal) are less common; they are found just beneath the pulmonary valve and may impinge on an aortic sinus and cause aortic insufficiency. VSDs in the midportion or apical region of the ventricular septum are muscular in type and may be single or multiple (Swiss cheese septum).

PATHOPHYSIOLOGY. The physical size of the VSD is a major, but not the only determinant of the size of the left-to-right shunt. The level of pulmonary vascular resistance in relation to systemic vascular resistance also determines the shunt's magnitude. When a small communication is present (usually <0.5 cm^2), the VSD is called **restrictive** and right ventricular pressure is normal. The higher pressure in the left ventricle drives the shunt left to right; the size of the defect limits the magnitude of the shunt. In large **nonrestrictive VSDs** (usually >1.0 cm^2), right and left ventricular pressure is equalized. In these defects, the direction of shunting and shunt magnitude are determined by the ratio of pulmonary to systemic vascular resistance (Fig. 426-7).

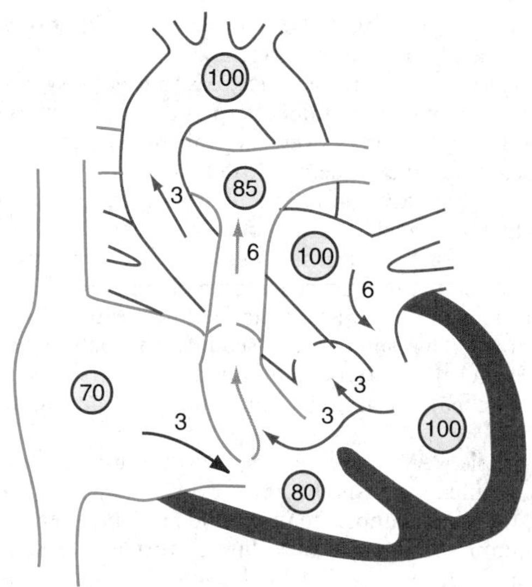

Figure 426-7. Physiology of a large ventricular septal defect (VSD). *Circled numbers* represent oxygen saturation values. The *numbers next to the arrows* represent volumes of blood flow (in L/min/m^2). This illustration shows a hypothetical patient with a pulmonary-to-systemic blood flow ratio (Qp : Qs) of 2 : 1. Desaturated blood enters the right atrium from the vena cava at a volume of 3 L/min/m^2 and flows across the tricuspid valve. An additional 3 L of blood shunts left to right across the VSD, the result being an increase in oxygen saturation in the right ventricle. Six liters of blood is ejected into the lungs. Pulmonary arterial saturation may be further increased because of incomplete mixing at right ventricular level. Six liters returns to the left atrium, crosses the mitral valve, and causes a mid-diastolic flow rumble. Three liters of this volume shunts left to right across the VSD, and 3 L is ejected into the ascending aorta (normal cardiac output).

After birth in patients with a large VSD, pulmonary vascular resistance may remain higher than normal, and thus the size of the left-to-right shunt may initially be limited. As pulmonary vascular resistance continues to fall in the 1st few weeks after birth because of normal involution of the media of small pulmonary arterioles, the size of the left-to-right shunt increases. Eventually, a large left-to-right shunt develops, and clinical symptoms become apparent. In most cases during early infancy, pulmonary vascular resistance is only slightly elevated, and the major contribution to pulmonary hypertension is the extremely large pulmonary blood flow. In some infants with a large VSD pulmonary arteriolar medial thickness never decreases. With continued exposure of the pulmonary vascular bed to high systolic pressure and high flow, pulmonary vascular obstructive disease develops. When the ratio of pulmonary to systemic resistance approaches 1 : 1, the shunt becomes bidirectional, the signs of heart failure abate, and the patient becomes cyanotic (Eisenmenger physiology, see Chapter 433.2).

The magnitude of intracardiac shunts is usually described by the Qp : Qs ratio. If the left-to-right shunt is small (Qp : Qs <1.75 : 1), the cardiac chambers are not appreciably enlarged and the pulmonary vascular bed is probably normal. If the shunt is large (Qp : Qs >2 : 1), left atrial and ventricular volume overload

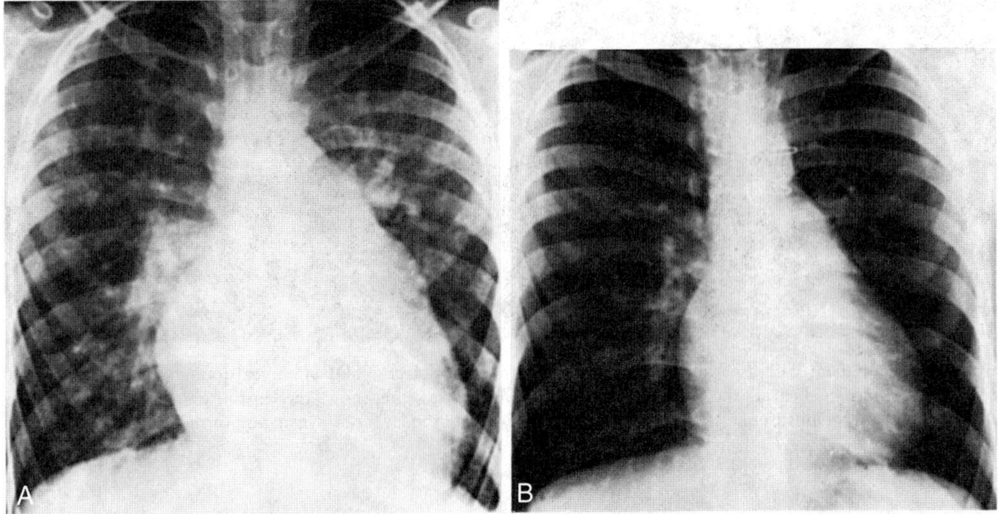

Figure 426-8. *A,* Preoperative roentgenogram in a patient with a ventricular septal defect with a large left-to-right shunt and pulmonary hypertension. Significant cardiomegaly, prominence of the pulmonary arterial trunk, and pulmonary overcirculation are evident. *B,* Three years after surgical closure of the defect, heart size is markedly decreased, and the pulmonary vasculature is normal.

occurs, as does right ventricular and pulmonary arterial hypertension. The main pulmonary artery, left atrium, and left ventricle are enlarged.

CLINICAL MANIFESTATIONS. The clinical findings of patients with a VSD vary according to the size of the defect and pulmonary blood flow and pressure. Small VSDs with trivial left-to-right shunts and normal pulmonary arterial pressure are the most common. These patients are asymptomatic, and the cardiac lesion is usually found during routine physical examination. Characteristically, a loud, harsh, or blowing holosystolic murmur is present and heard best over the lower left sternal border, and it is frequently accompanied by a thrill. In a few instances, the murmur ends before the 2nd sound, presumably because of closure of the defect during late systole. A short, harsh systolic murmur localized to the apex in a neonate is often a sign of a tiny muscular VSD. In the immediate neonatal period, the left-to-right shunt may be minimal because of higher right-sided pressure, and therefore the systolic murmur may not be audible during the 1st few days of life. In premature infants, the murmur may be heard early because pulmonary vascular resistance decreases more rapidly.

Large VSDs with excessive pulmonary blood flow and pulmonary hypertension are responsible for dyspnea, feeding difficulties, poor growth, profuse perspiration, recurrent pulmonary infections, and cardiac failure in early infancy. Cyanosis is usually absent, but duskiness is sometimes noted during infections or crying. Prominence of the left precordium is common, as are a palpable parasternal lift, a laterally displaced apical impulse and apical thrust, and a systolic thrill. The holosystolic murmur of a large VSD is generally less harsh than that of a small VSD and more blowing in nature because of the absence of a significant pressure gradient across the defect. It is even less likely to be audible in the newborn period. The pulmonic component of the 2nd heart sound may be increased as a result of pulmonary hypertension. The presence of a mid-diastolic, low-pitched rumble at the apex is caused by increased blood flow across the mitral valve and indicates a Qp : Qs ratio of ≥2 : 1. This murmur is best appreciated with the bell of the stethoscope.

DIAGNOSIS. In patients with small VSDs, the chest radiograph is usually normal, although minimal cardiomegaly and a borderline increase in pulmonary vasculature may be observed. The electrocardiogram is generally normal but may suggest left ventricular hypertrophy. The presence of right ventricular hypertrophy is a warning that the defect is not small and that the patient has pulmonary hypertension or an associated lesion such as pulmonic stenosis. In large VSDs, the chest radiograph shows gross cardiomegaly with prominence of both ventricles, the left atrium, and the pulmonary artery (Fig. 426-8). Pulmonary vascular markings are increased, and frank pulmonary edema, including pleural effusions, may be present. The electrocardiogram shows biventricular hypertrophy; P waves may be notched or peaked.

The two-dimensional echocardiogram (Fig. 426-9) shows the position and size of the VSD. In small defects, especially those of the muscular septum, the defect itself may be difficult to image and is visualized only by color Doppler examination. In defects of the **membranous septum,** a thin membrane (called a **ventricular septal aneurysm** but consisting of tricuspid valve tissue) can partially cover the defect and limit the volume of the left-to-right shunt. Echocardiography is also useful for estimating shunt size by examining the degree of volume overload of the left atrium and left ventricle; in the absence of associated lesions, the extent of their increased dimensions is a good reflection of the size of the left-to-right shunt. Pulsed Doppler examination shows whether the VSD is pressure restrictive by calculating the pressure gradient across the defect. Such calculation allows an estimation of right ventricular pressure and helps determine whether the patient is at risk for the development of early pulmonary vascular disease. The echocardiogram can also be useful to determine the presence of aortic valve insufficiency or leaflet prolapse in the case of supracristal VSDs.

The hemodynamics of a VSD can also be demonstrated by cardiac catheterization although catheterization is today performed only when the size of the shunt is uncertain after a comprehensive clinical evaluation, when laboratory data do not fit well with the clinical findings, or when pulmonary vascular disease is suspected. Oximetry demonstrates increased oxygen content in the right ventricle; because some defects eject blood almost directly into the pulmonary artery (streaming), this increase is occasionally apparent only when pulmonary arterial blood is sampled. Small, restrictive VSDs are associated with normal right-sided heart pressure and pulmonary vascular resistance. Large, nonrestrictive VSDs are associated with equal or nearly equal pulmonary and systemic systolic pressure. Pul-

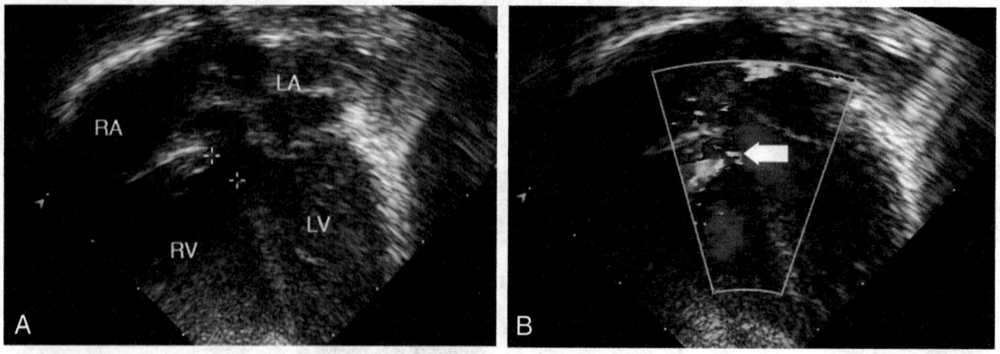

Figure 426-9. Echocardiogram in a patient with a perimembranous ventricular septal defect (VSD). *A,* Apical four-chamber view showing the location of the defect (outlined between two *crosshatches*) beneath the aortic valve. *B,* Color Doppler imaging shows the left-to-right shunt *(arrow)* through the defect (the red color represents blood moving toward the ultrasound transducer and does not indicate the level of oxygenation of the blood). LA, left atrium; LV, left ventricle; RA, right atrium; RV, right ventricle.

monary blood flow may be two to four times systemic blood flow. In patients with such "**hyperdynamic pulmonary hypertension,**" pulmonary vascular resistance is only minimally elevated because resistance is equal to pressure divided by flow. If Eisenmenger syndrome is present, pulmonary artery systolic and diastolic pressure is elevated, the degree of left-to-right shunting is minimal, and desaturation of blood in the left ventricle is encountered. The size, location, and number of ventricular defects are demonstrated by left ventriculography. Contrast medium passes across the defect or defects to opacify the right ventricle and pulmonary artery.

TREATMENT. The natural course of a VSD depends to a large degree on the size of the defect. A significant number (30–50%) of small defects close spontaneously, most frequently during the 1st 2 yr of life. Small muscular VSDs are more likely to close (up to 80%) than membranous VSDs are (up to 35%). The vast majority of defects that close do so before the age of 4 yr, although spontaneous closure has been reported in adults. VSDs that close often have ventricular septal aneurysm tissue limiting the magnitude of the shunt. Most children with small defects remain asymptomatic, without evidence of an increase in heart size, pulmonary arterial pressure, or resistance. A long-term risk is infective endocarditis. Some long-term studies of adults with unoperated small VSDs show an increased incidence of arrhythmia, subaortic stenosis, and exercise intolerance. The Council on Cardiovascular Disease in the Young of the American Heart Association states that an isolated, small, hemodynamically insignificant VSD is not an indication for surgery. The declining risk of open heart surgery has led others to suggest that all VSDs be closed electively by mid-childhood.

It is less common for moderate or large VSDs to close spontaneously, although even defects large enough to result in heart failure may become smaller and up to 8% may close completely. More commonly, infants with large defects have repeated episodes of respiratory infection and heart failure despite optimal medical management. Heart failure may be manifested in many of these infants primarily as failure to thrive. Pulmonary hypertension occurs as a result of high pulmonary blood flow. These patients are at risk for pulmonary vascular disease with time if the defect is not repaired.

Patients with VSD are also at risk for the development of aortic valve regurgitation, the greatest risk occurring in patients with supracristal VSD (see Chapter 426.7). A small number of patients with VSD have **acquired infundibular pulmonary stenosis,** which then protects the pulmonary circulation from the short-term effects of pulmonary overcirculation and the long-term effects of pulmonary vascular disease. In these patients, the clinical picture changes from that of a VSD with a large left-to-right shunt to a VSD with pulmonary stenosis. The shunt may diminish in size, become balanced, or even become a net right-to-left shunt. These patients must be distinguished from those in whom an Eisenmenger physiology develops (see Chapter 433.2).

In patients with small VSDs, parents should be reassured of the relatively benign nature of the lesion, and the child should be encouraged to live a normal life, with no restrictions on physical activity. Surgical repair is currently not recommended. As protection against infective endocarditis, the integrity of primary and permanent teeth should be carefully maintained; antibiotic prophylaxis should be provided for dental visits (including cleanings), tonsillectomy, adenoidectomy, and other oropharyngeal surgical procedures, as well as for instrumentation of the genitourinary and lower intestinal tracts (see Chapter 437). These patients can be monitored by a combination of clinical examination and noninvasive laboratory tests until the VSD has closed spontaneously. The electrocardiogram can be used for screening these patients for possible pulmonary hypertension or pulmonic stenosis as indicated by right ventricular hypertrophy. Echocardiography is used to screen for the development of left ventricular outflow tract pathology (subaortic membrane or aortic regurgitation) and to confirm spontaneous closure.

In infants with a large VSD, medical management has two aims: to control heart failure and prevent the development of pulmonary vascular disease. Therapeutic measures are aimed at control of the heart failure symptoms and maintenance of normal growth (see Chapter 442). If early treatment is successful, the shunt may diminish in size with spontaneous improvement, especially during the 1st yr of life. The clinician must be alert not to confuse clinical improvement caused by a decrease in defect size with clinical changes caused by the development of Eisenmenger physiology. Because surgical closure can be carried out at low risk in most infants, medical management should not be pursued in symptomatic infants after an initial unsuccessful trial. Pulmonary vascular disease can be prevented when surgery is performed within the 1st yr of life.

Indications for surgical closure of a VSD include patients at any age with large defects in whom clinical symptoms and failure to thrive cannot be controlled medically; infants between 6 and 12 mo of age with large defects associated with pulmonary hypertension, even if the symptoms are controlled by medication; and patients older than 24 mo with a Qp : Qs ratio greater than 2 : 1. Patients with supracristal VSD of any size are usually referred for surgery because of the high risk for aortic valve regurgitation (see Chapter 426.7). Severe pulmonary vascular disease is a contraindication to closure of a VSD.

PROGNOSIS. The results of primary surgical repair are excellent, and complications leading to long-term problems (residual ventricular shunts requiring reoperation or heart block requiring a pacemaker) are rare. Pulmonary arterial palliative banding with repair in later childhood is reserved for complicated cases or very premature infants. Surgical risks are higher for defects in the muscular septum, particularly apical defects and multiple (Swiss cheese type) VSDs. These patients may require pulmonary arterial banding if symptomatic, with subsequent debanding and repair of multiple VSDs at an older age. **Catheter occlusion devices** are being tested as a means of closing apical muscular VSDs and other devices are being tested for closing the more common perimembranous defects.

After surgical obliteration of the left-to-right shunt, the hyperdynamic heart becomes quiet, cardiac size decreases toward normal (see Fig. 426-8), thrills and murmurs are abolished, and pulmonary artery hypertension regresses. The patient's clinical status improves markedly. Most infants begin to thrive, and cardiac medications are no longer required. Catch-up growth occurs in most patients within the next 1–2 yr. In some instances after successful surgery, systolic ejection murmurs of low intensity persist for months. The long-term prognosis after surgery is excellent. Patients with a small VSD and those who have undergone surgical closure without residua are considered to be at standard risk for health and life insurance.

426.7 • Supracristal Ventricular Septal Defect with Aortic Insufficiency

A supracristal VSD is complicated by prolapse of the aortic valve into the defect and aortic insufficiency, which may eventually occur in 50–90% of patients. Although it accounts for ≈5% of all patients with VSD, the incidence is highest in Asian children. The VSD, which may be small or moderate in size, is located anterior to and directly below the pulmonary valve in the outlet septum, superior to the crista supraventricularis. Aortic insufficiency is occasionally associated with VSDs located in the membranous septum. The right or, less often, the noncoronary aortic cusp prolapses into the defect and may partially or even completely occlude it. Such occlusion may limit the amount of left-to-right shunting and give the false impression that the defect is not large. Aortic insufficiency is most often not recognized until late in the 1st decade of life or beyond.

Early heart failure secondary to a large left-to-right shunt rarely occurs, but without surgery, severe aortic insufficiency and left ventricular failure may ensue. The murmur of a supracristal VSD is usually heard at the middle to upper left sternal border, as opposed to the lower left sternal border, and it is sometimes confused with that of pulmonic stenosis. The physical signs of aortic insufficiency (diastolic murmur and wide pulse pressure), when present, are added to those of the VSD. These clinical findings must be distinguished from PDA or other defects associated with aortic runoff.

The clinical manifestations vary widely from trivial aortic regurgitation and small left-to-right shunts in asymptomatic children to florid aortic incompetence and massive cardiomegaly in symptomatic adolescents. Closure of all supracristal ventricular VSDs at the time of diagnosis is commonly recommended to prevent the development of aortic regurgitation, even in an asymptomatic child. Patients who already have significant aortic incompetence require surgical intervention to prevent irreversible left ventricular dysfunction. Surgical options depend on the degree of damage to the valve and include valvuloplasty for mild involvement and replacement with a prosthesis or homograft or aortopulmonary translocation (see Chapter 427.5) for severe involvement.

426.8 • Patent Ductus Arteriosus

During fetal life, most of the pulmonary arterial blood is shunted through the ductus arteriosus into the aorta (see Chapter 421). Functional closure of the ductus normally occurs soon after birth, but if the ductus remains patent when pulmonary vascular resistance falls, aortic blood is shunted into the pulmonary artery. The aortic end of the ductus is just distal to the origin of the left subclavian artery, and the ductus enters the pulmonary artery at its bifurcation. Female patients with PDA outnumber males 2 : 1. PDA is also associated with maternal rubella infection during early pregnancy. It is a common problem in premature infants, where it can cause severe hemodynamic derangements and several major sequelae (see Chapter 101.4).

When a term infant is found to have a PDA, the wall of the ductus is deficient in both the mucoid endothelial layer and the muscular media. In a premature infant, the PDA usually has a normal structure; patency is the result of hypoxia and immaturity. Thus, a PDA persisting beyond the 1st few weeks of life in a term infant rarely closes spontaneously or with pharmacologic intervention, whereas if early pharmacologic or surgical intervention is not required in a premature infant, spontaneous closure occurs in most instances. A PDA is seen in 10% of patients with other congenital heart lesions and often plays a critical role in providing pulmonary blood flow when the right ventricular outflow tract is stenotic or atretic (see Chapter 427.6) or in providing systemic blood flow in the presence of aortic coarctation or interruption (see Chapter 427.8).

PATHOPHYSIOLOGY. As a result of the higher aortic pressure, blood shunts left to right through the ductus, from the aorta to the pulmonary artery. The extent of the shunt depends on the size of the ductus and on the ratio of pulmonary to systemic vascular resistance. In extreme cases, 70% of the left ventricular output may be shunted through the ductus to the pulmonary circulation. If the PDA is small, pressure within the pulmonary artery, the right ventricle, and the right atrium is normal. If the PDA is large pulmonary artery pressure may be elevated to systemic levels during both systole and diastole. Patients with a large PDA are at extremely high risk for the development of pulmonary vascular disease if left unoperated. Pulse pressure is wide because of runoff of blood into the pulmonary artery during diastole.

CLINICAL MANIFESTATIONS. A small patent ductus does not usually have any symptoms associated with it. A large PDA will result in heart failure similar to that encountered in infants with a large VSD. Retardation of physical growth may be a major manifestation in infants with large shunts.

A large PDA will result in striking physical signs attributable to the wide pulse pressure, most prominently, bounding peripheral arterial pulses. The heart is normal in size when the ductus is small, but moderately or grossly enlarged in cases with a large communication. The apical impulse is prominent and, with cardiac enlargement, is heaving. A thrill, maximal in the 2nd left interspace, is often present and may radiate toward the left clavicle, down the left sternal border, or toward the apex. It is usually systolic but may also be palpated throughout the cardiac cycle. The classic continuous murmur is described as being like machinery or rolling thunder in quality. It begins soon after onset of the 1st sound, reaches maximal intensity at the end of systole, and wanes in late diastole. It may be localized to the 2nd left intercostal space or radiate down the left sternal border or to the left clavicle. When pulmonary vascular resistance is increased, the diastolic component of the murmur may be less prominent or absent. In patients with a large left-to-right shunt, a low-pitched mitral mid-diastolic murmur may be audible at the apex as a result of the increased volume of blood flow across the mitral valve.

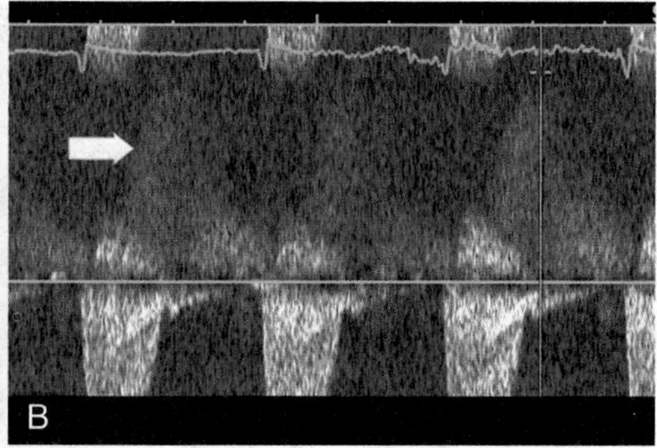

Figure 426-10. Echocardiogram in a newborn with a small- to moderate-sized patent ductus arteriosus (PDA). *A*, Color Doppler performed in a parasternal short axis view shows flow *(arrow)* from the aorta into the main pulmonary artery. *B*, Doppler evaluation demonstrates retrograde diastolic flow into the pulmonary artery. AV, aortic valve; DescAo, descending aorta; LA, left atrium; MPA, main pulmonary artery; RA, right atrium; RV, right ventricle.

DIAGNOSIS. If the left-to-right shunt is small, the electrocardiogram is normal; if the ductus is large, left ventricular or biventricular hypertrophy is present. The diagnosis of an isolated, uncomplicated PDA is untenable when right ventricular hypertrophy is noted.

Radiographic studies in patients with a large PDA show a prominent pulmonary artery with increased intrapulmonary vascular markings. Cardiac size depends on the degree of left-to-right shunting; it may be normal or moderately to markedly enlarged. The chambers involved are the left atrium and ventricle. The aortic knob is normal or prominent.

The echocardiographic view of the cardiac chambers is normal if the ductus is small. With large shunts, left atrial and left ventricular dimensions are increased. The size of the left atrium is usually quantitated by comparison to the size of the aortic root, known as the LA : Ao ratio. Scanning from the suprasternal notch allows direct visualization of the ductus. Color and pulsed Doppler examinations demonstrate systolic or diastolic (or both) retrograde turbulent flow in the pulmonary artery and aortic retrograde flow in diastole (Fig. 426-10).

The clinical pattern is sufficiently distinctive to allow an accurate diagnosis by noninvasive methods in most patients. In patients with atypical findings or when associated cardiac lesions are suspected, cardiac catheterization may be indicated. Cardiac catheterization demonstrates normal or increased pressure in the right ventricle and pulmonary artery, depending on the size of the ductus. The presence of oxygenated blood shunting into the pulmonary artery confirms a left-to-right shunt. The catheter may pass from the pulmonary artery through the ductus into the descending aorta. Injection of contrast medium into the ascending aorta shows opacification of the pulmonary artery from the aorta and identifies the ductus.

Other conditions can produce systolic and diastolic murmurs in the pulmonic area in the absence of cyanosis and must be differentiated. The characteristics of a venous hum are described in Chapter 422. An **aorticopulmonary window** defect may rarely be clinically indistinguishable from a patent ductus, although, in most cases, the murmur is only systolic and is loudest at the right rather than the left upper sternal border. A sinus of Valsalva aneurysm that has ruptured into the right side of the heart or pulmonary artery, coronary arteriovenous fistulas, and an aberrant left coronary artery with massive collaterals from the right coronary display dynamics similar to that of a PDA with a continuous murmur and a wide pulse pressure. Truncus arteriosus with torrential pulmonary flow also has an "aortic runoff" physiology. Pulmonary branch stenosis can be associated with systolic and diastolic murmurs, but the pulse pressure will be normal. A peripheral arteriovenous fistula also results in a wide pulse pressure, but the distinctive murmur of a PDA is not present. VSD with aortic insufficiency and combined rheumatic aortic and mitral insufficiency may be confused with a PDA, but the murmurs should be differentiated by their to-and-fro rather than continuous nature. The combination of a large VSD and a PDA results in findings more like those of an isolated VSD. Echocardiography should be able to eliminate these other diagnostic possibilities. If a PDA is suspected clinically but not visualized on echocardiography, cardiac catheterization is usually indicated.

PROGNOSIS AND COMPLICATIONS. Patients with a small PDA may live a normal span with few or no cardiac symptoms, but late manifestations may occur. Spontaneous closure of the ductus after infancy is extremely rare. Cardiac failure most often occurs in early infancy in the presence of a large ductus but may occur late in life even with a moderate-sized communication. The chronic left ventricular volume load is less well tolerated with aging.

Infective endarteritis may be seen at any age. Pulmonary or systemic emboli may occur. Rare complications include aneurysmal dilatation of the pulmonary artery or the ductus, calcification of the ductus, noninfective thrombosis of the ductus with embolization, and paradoxical emboli. Pulmonary hypertension (Eisenmenger syndrome) usually develops in patients with a large PDA who do not undergo surgical treatment (see Chapter 433.2).

TREATMENT. Irrespective of age, patients with PDA require surgical or catheter closure. In patients with a small PDA, the rationale for closure is prevention of bacterial endarteritis or other late complications. In patients with a moderate to large PDA, closure is accomplished to treat heart failure or prevent the development of pulmonary vascular disease, or both. Once the diagnosis of a moderate to large PDA is made, treatment should not be unduly postponed after adequate medical therapy for cardiac failure has been instituted.

Transcatheter PDA closure is routinely performed in the cardiac catheterization laboratory (Fig. 426-11). Small PDAs are generally closed with intravascular coils. Moderate to large PDAs may be closed with a catheter-introduced sac into which several coils are released or with an umbrella-like device. Surgical closure of PDA can be accomplished by a standard left thoracotomy or using thoracoscopic techniques. Because the case fatality rate with interventional or surgical treatment is considerably less than 1% and the risk without it is greater, closure of the ductus is indicated in asymptomatic patients, preferably before 1 yr of age. Pulmonary hypertension is not a contraindication to surgery at any age if it can be demonstrated at cardiac catheterization that the

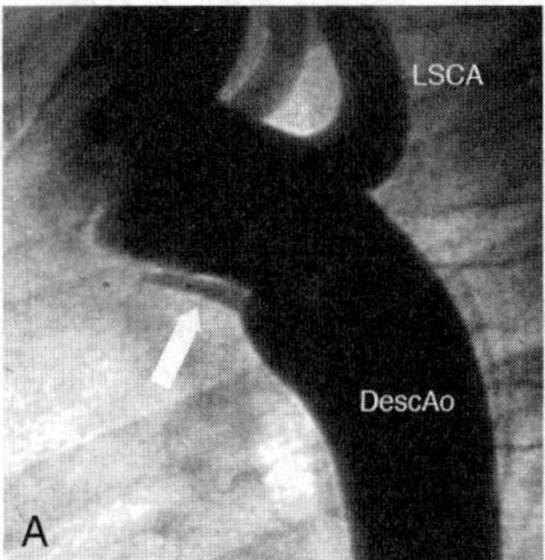

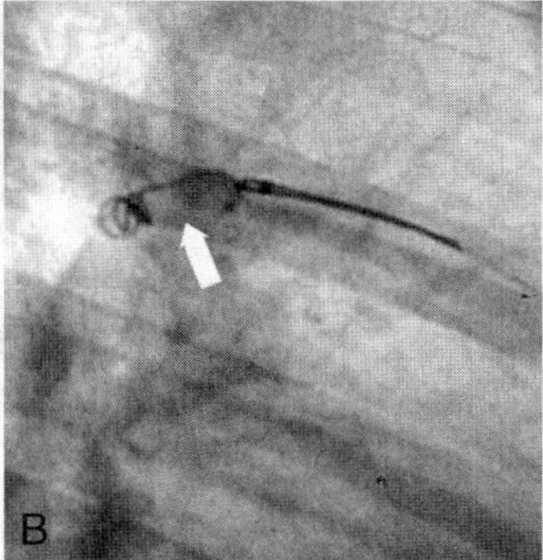

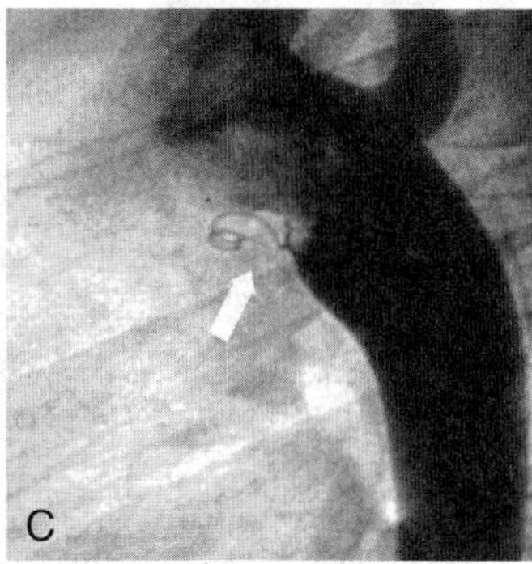

Figure 426-11. Transcatheter closure of a small patent ductus arteriosus using a coil. *A,* Angiogram of transverse and descending aorta shows small PDA *(arrow).* *B,* Coil *(arrow)* has been extruded from sheath and is being positioned in ductal lumen. *C,* Angiogram demonstrating total occlusion of PDA by coil *(arrow).* DescAo, descending aorta; LSCA, left subclavian artery.

shunt flow is still predominantly left to right and that severe pulmonary vascular disease is not present. After closure, symptoms of frank or incipient cardiac failure rapidly disappear. Infants who had failed to thrive usually have immediate improvement in physical development. The pulse and blood pressure return to normal, and the machinery-like murmur disappears. A functional systolic murmur over the pulmonary area may persist; it may represent turbulence in a persistently dilated pulmonary artery. The radiographic signs of cardiac enlargement and pulmonary overcirculation disappear over a period of several months, and the electrocardiogram becomes normal.

Patent Ductus Arteriosus in Low Birthweight Infants. See Chapter 101.4.

426.9 • Aorticopulmonary Window Defect

An aorticopulmonary window defect consists of a communication between the ascending aorta and the main pulmonary artery. The presence of pulmonary and aortic valves and an intact ventricular septum distinguishes this anomaly from truncus arteriosus (see Chapter 431.8). Symptoms of heart failure appear during early infancy; occasionally, minimal cyanosis is present. The defect is usually large, and the cardiac murmur is systolic with a mid-diastolic rumble as a result of the increased blood flow across the mitral valve. In the rare instance when the communication is somewhat smaller and pulmonary hypertension is absent, the findings on examination can mimic those of a PDA (wide pulse pressure and a continuous murmur at the upper sternal borders). The electrocardiogram shows either left ventricular or biventricular hypertrophy. Radiographic studies demonstrate cardiac enlargement and prominence of the pulmonary artery and intrapulmonary vasculature. The echocardiogram shows enlarged left-sided heart chambers; the window defect can best be delineated with color flow Doppler. Magnetic resonance angiography (MRA) can also be utilized to visualize the defect (see Fig 423-20).

Cardiac catheterization reveals a left-to-right shunt at the level of the pulmonary artery, as well as hyperkinetic pulmonary hypertension, because the defect is almost always large. Selective aortography with injection of contrast medium into the ascending aorta demonstrates the lesion, and manipulation of the catheter from the main pulmonary artery directly to the ascending aorta is also diagnostic.

An aorticopulmonary window defect is surgically corrected during infancy with cardiopulmonary bypass. If surgery is not carried out in infancy, survivors carry the risk of progressive pulmonary vascular obstructive disease, similar to that of other patients who have large intracardiac or great vessel communications.

426.10 • Coronary-Arteriovenous Fistula (Coronary-Cameral Fistula)

A congenital fistula may exist between a coronary artery and an atrium, ventricle (especially the right), or pulmonary artery. Sometimes, multiple fistulas exist. Regardless of the recipient chamber, the clinical signs are similar to those of PDA, although the machinery-like murmur may be more diffuse. If the flow is substantial, the involved coronary artery may be dilated or aneurysmal. The anatomic abnormality is usually demonstrable by color flow Doppler echocardiography and, during catheterization, by injection of contrast medium into the ascending aorta. Small fistulas may be hemodynamically insignificant and may even close spontaneously. If the shunt is large, treatment consists of either transcatheter coil embolization or, for lesions not amenable to catheter intervention, surgical closure of the fistula.

426.11 • Ruptured Sinus of Valsalva Aneurysm

When one of the sinuses of Valsalva of the aorta is weakened by congenital or acquired disease, an aneurysm may form and eventually rupture, usually into the right atrium or ventricle. This condition is extremely rare in childhood. The onset is usually sudden. The diagnosis should be suspected in a patient in whom symptoms of acute heart failure develop in association with a new loud to-and-fro murmur. Color Doppler echocardiography and cardiac catheterization demonstrate the left-to-right shunt at the atrial or ventricular level. Urgent surgical repair is generally required. This condition is often associated with infective endocarditis of the aortic valve.

Atrial Septal Defect

Amin Z, Hijazi ZM, Bass JL, et al: Erosion of Amplatzer septal occluder device after closure of secundum atrial septal defects: Review of registry of complications and recommendations to minimize future risk. *Catheter Cardiovasc Interv* 2004;63:496–502.

Beda RD, Gill EA Jr: Patent foramen ovale: Does it play a role in the pathophysiology of migraine headache? *Cardiol Clin* 2005;23:91–96.

Benson DW, Silberbach GM, Kavanaugh-McHugh A, et al: Mutations in the cardiac transcription factor NKX2.5 affect diverse cardiac developmental pathways. *J Clin Invest* 1999;104:1567–1573.

Masura J, Gavora P, Podnar T: Long-term outcome of transcatheter secundum-type atrial septal defect closure using Amplatzer septal occluders. *J Am Coll Cardiol* 2005;45:505–507.

Radzik D, Davignon A, van Doesburg N, et al: Predictive factors for spontaneous closure of atrial septal defects diagnosed in the first 3 months of life. *J Am Coll Cardiol* 1993;22:851–853.

Riggs T, Sharp SE, Batton D, et al: Spontaneous closure of atrial septal defects in premature vs full term neonates. *Pediatr Cardiol* 2000;21:129–134.

Swartz EN: Is transcatheter device occlusion as good as open heart surgery for closure of atrial septal defects? *Arch Dis Child* 2004;89:687–688.

Yew G, Wilson NJ: Transcatheter atrial septal defect closure with the Amplatzer septal occluder: Five-year follow-up. *Catheter Cardiovasc Interv* 2005;64:193–196.

Atrioventricular Septal Defects

Clapp SK, Perry BL, Farooki ZQ, et al: Surgical and medical results of complete atrioventricular canal: A ten-year review. *Am J Cardiol* 1987;59:454–458.

Drinkwater DC Jr, Laks H: Unbalanced atrioventricular septal defects. *Semin Thorac Cardiovasc Surg* 1997;9:21–25.

Marino B, Vairo U, Corno A, et al: Atrioventricular canal in Down syndrome. *Am J Dis Child* 1990;144:1120.

Murphy DJ Jr: Atrioventricular canal defects. *Curr Treat Options Cardiovasc Med* 1999;1:323–334.

Sigfusson G, Ettedgui JA, Silverman NH, et al: Is a cleft in the anterior leaflet of an otherwise normal mitral valve an atrioventricular canal malformation? *J Am Coll Cardiol* 1995;26:508–515.

Ventricular Septal Defect

Glen S, Burns J, Bloomfield P: Prevalence and development of additional cardiac abnormalities in 1448 patients with congenital ventricular septal defects. *Heart* 2004;90:1321–1325.

Holzer R, Balzer D, Cao QL, et al: Device closure of muscular ventricular septal defects using the Amplatzer muscular ventricular septal defect occluder: Immediate and mid-term results of a U.S. registry. *J Am Coll Cardiol* 2004;43:1257–1263.

Hornberger LK, Sahn DJ, Krabill KA, et al: Elucidation of the natural history of ventricular septal defects by serial Doppler color flow mapping studies. *J Am Coll Cardiol* 1989;13:1111–1118.

Knauth AL, Lock JE, Perry SB, et al: Transcatheter device closure of congenital and postoperative residual ventricular septal defects. *Circulation* 2004;110:501–507.

Ramaciotti C, Keren A, Silverman NH: Importance of pseudoaneurysms of the ventricular septum in the natural history of isolated perimembranous ventricular septal defects. *Am J Cardiol* 1986;57:268–272.

Roos-Hesselink JW, Meijboom FJ, Spitaels SE, et al. Outcome of patients after surgical closure of ventricular septal defect at young age: Longitudinal follow-up of 22–34 years. *Eur Heart J* 2004;25:1057–1062.

Patent Ductus Arteriosus

Alagarsamy S, Chhabra M, Gudavalli M, et al: Comparison of clinical criteria with echocardiographic findings in diagnosing PDA in preterm infants. *J Perinat Med* 2005;33:161–164.

Bergwerff M, DeRuiter MC, Gittenberger-de Groot AC: Comparative anatomy and ontogeny of the ductus arteriosus, a vascular outsider. *Anat Embryol (Berl)* 1999;200:559–571.

Gittenberger-de Groot AC, Van Ertbruggen I, Moulaert A, et al: The ductus arteriosus in the preterm infant: Histologic and clinical observations. *J Pediatr* 1980;96:88–93.

Rothman A, Lucas VW, Sklansky MS, et al: Percutaneous coil occlusion of patent ductus arteriosus. *J Pediatr* 1997;130:447–454.

Coronary-Arteriovenous Fistula

Velvis H, Schmidt KG, Silverman NH, et al: Diagnosis of coronary artery fistula by two-dimensional echocardiography, pulsed Doppler ultrasound, and color flow imaging. *J Am Coll Cardiol* 1989;14:968–976.

Chapter 427 ■ Acyanotic Congenital Heart Disease: The Obstructive Lesions

427.1 • Pulmonary Valve Stenosis with Intact Ventricular Septum

Of the various forms of right ventricular outflow obstruction with an intact ventricular septum, the most common is isolated valvular pulmonary stenosis, which accounts for 7–10% of all congenital heart defects. The valve cusps are deformed to various degrees and, as a result, the valve opens incompletely during systole. The valve may be bicuspid or tricuspid and the leaflets partially fused together with an eccentric outlet. This fusion may be so severe that only a pinhole central opening remains. If the valve is not severely thickened, it produces a dome-like obstruction to right ventricular outflow during systole. Isolated infundibular stenosis, supravalvular pulmonary stenosis, and branch pulmonary artery stenosis are less commonly encountered. In cases where pulmonary valve stenosis is associated with a ventricular septal defect (VSD) but without anterior deviation of the infundibular septum, this condition is better classified as pulmonary stenosis with VSD rather than as tetralogy of Fallot (see Chapter 430.1). Pulmonary stenosis and an atrial septal defect (ASD) are also occasionally seen as associated defects. The clinical and laboratory findings reflect the dominant lesion, but it is important to rule out these associated anomalies. Pulmonary stenosis as a result of valve dysplasia is the most common cardiac abnormality in **Noonan syndrome** (see Chapter 81), and is associated in about 50% of cases with a mutation in the gene *PTPN11,* encoding the protein tyrosine phosphotase SHP-2 on chromosome 12. The mechanism for pulmonic stenosis is unknown, although maldevelopment of the distal portion of the bulbus cordis and the sequelae of fetal endocarditis have been suggested. Pulmonary stenosis, either of the valve or the branch pulmonary arteries, is a common finding in patients with arteriohepatic dysplasia, also known as **Alagille syndrome.** In this syndrome and in some patients with isolated pulmonic stenosis, a mutation is present in the *Jagged1* gene.

PATHOPHYSIOLOGY. The obstruction to outflow from the right ventricle to the pulmonary artery results in increased systolic pressure and wall stress, which eventually leads to hypertrophy of the right ventricle (Fig. 427-1). The severity of these abnormalities depends on the size of the restricted valve opening. In severe cases, right ventricular pressure may be higher than systemic arterial systolic pressure, whereas with milder obstruction, right ventricular pressure is only mildly or moderately elevated. Pulmonary artery pressure is normal or decreased. Arterial oxygen saturation will be normal even in cases of severe stenosis, unless an intracardiac communication such as a VSD or ASD is allowing blood to shunt from right to left. When severe pulmonic stenosis occurs in a neonate, markedly decreased right ventricular compliance may lead to cyanosis due to right-to-left shunting through a patent foramen ovale, a condition termed critical pulmonic stenosis.

CLINICAL MANIFESTATIONS AND LABORATORY FINDINGS. Patients with mild or moderate stenosis usually do not have any symptoms. Growth and development are most often normal; older infants and children appear to be well developed and healthy. If the stenosis is severe, signs of right ventricular failure such as hepatomegaly, peripheral edema, and exercise intolerance may be present. In a neonate or young infant with critical pulmonic stenosis, signs of right ventricular failure may be more prominent, and cyanosis is often present because of shunting at the foramen ovale.

With **mild pulmonary stenosis,** venous pressure and pulse are normal. The heart is not enlarged, the apical impulse is normal, and the right ventricular impulse is not palpable. A sharp pulmonic ejection click immediately after the 1st heart sound is heard at the left upper sternal border during expiration. The 2nd heart sound is split, with a pulmonary component of normal intensity that may be slightly delayed. A relatively short, low- or medium-pitched systolic ejection murmur is maximally audible over the pulmonic area and radiates minimally to the lung fields bilaterally. The electrocardiogram is normal or characteristic of mild right ventricular hypertrophy; inversion of the T waves in the right precordial leads may be seen. (Remember that the T wave in lead V_1 should normally be inverted until at least 6–8 y of age. Therefore, a positive T wave in V_1 in a young child is a sign of right ventricular hypertrophy.) The only abnormality demonstrable radiographically is usually poststenotic dilatation of the pulmonary artery. Two-dimensional echocardiography shows right ventricular hypertrophy and a slightly thickened pulmonic valve, which domes in systole; Doppler studies demonstrate a right ventricle to pulmonary artery gradient of ≤30 mm Hg.

In **moderate pulmonic stenosis,** venous pressure may be slightly elevated; in older children, a prominent *a* wave may be noted in the jugular pulse. A right ventricular lift may be palpable at the lower left sternal border. The 2nd heart sound is split, with a delayed and soft pulmonary component. As valve motion becomes more limited with more severe degrees of stenosis, both the pulmonic ejection click and the pulmonic 2nd sound may become inaudible. With increasing degrees of stenosis, the peak of the systolic ejection murmur is prolonged later into systole, and its quality becomes louder and harsher (higher frequency). The murmur radiates more prominently to both lung fields.

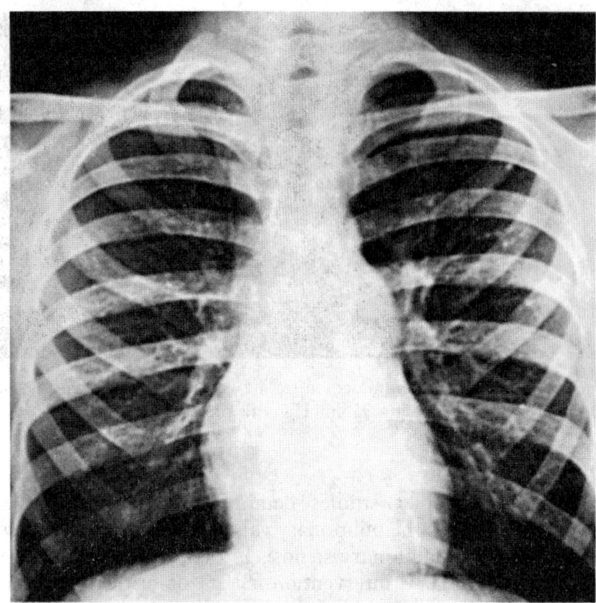
Figure 427-2. Roentgenogram in a patient with valvular pulmonary stenosis and a normal aortic root. The heart size is within normal limits, but poststenotic dilatation of the pulmonary artery is present.

The electrocardiogram reveals varying degrees of right ventricular hypertrophy, sometimes with a prominent spiked P wave. Radiographically, the heart can vary from normal size to mildly enlarged with uptilting of the apex due to prominence of the right ventricle; intrapulmonary vascularity may be normal or slightly decreased. The echocardiogram shows a thickened pulmonic valve with restricted systolic motion. Doppler examination demonstrates a right ventricle to pulmonary artery pressure gradient in the 30–60 mm Hg range. Mild tricuspid regurgitation may be present and allows Doppler confirmation of right ventricular systolic pressure.

In **severe stenosis,** mild to moderate cyanosis may be noted in patients with an interatrial communication (atrial septal defect or patent foramen ovale). If hepatic enlargement and peripheral edema are present, they are an indication of right ventricular failure. Elevation of venous pressure is common and is caused by a large presystolic jugular *a* wave. The heart is moderately or greatly enlarged, and a conspicuous parasternal right ventricular lift is present and frequently extends to the left midclavicular line. The pulmonary component of the 2nd sound is usually inaudible. A loud, long, and harsh systolic ejection murmur, usually accompanied by a thrill, is maximally audible in the pulmonic area and may radiate over the entire precordium, to both lung fields, into the neck, and to the back. The peak of the murmur occurs later in systole as valve opening becomes more restricted. The murmur frequently encompasses the aortic component of the 2nd sound but is not preceded by an ejection click.

The electrocardiogram shows gross right ventricular hypertrophy, frequently accompanied by a tall, spiked P wave. Radiographic studies confirm the presence of cardiac enlargement with prominence of the right ventricle and right atrium. Prominence of the main pulmonary artery segment may be seen due to poststenotic dilatation (Fig. 427-2). Intrapulmonary vascularity is decreased. The two-dimensional echocardiogram shows severe deformity of the pulmonary valve and right ventricular hypertrophy (Fig. 427-3). In the late stages of the disease, systolic dysfunction of the right ventricle may be seen, and in these cases the ventricle may become dilated, with prominent tricuspid

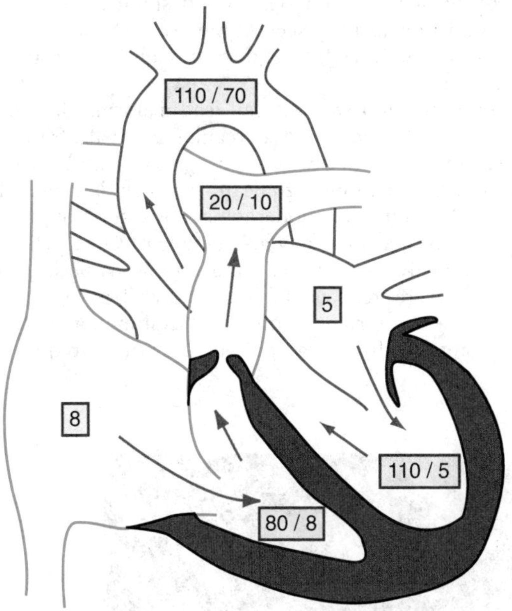

Figure 427-1. Physiology of valvular pulmonary stenosis. Boxed numbers represent pressure in mm Hg. Because of the absence of right-to-left or left-to-right shunting, blood flow through all cardiac chambers is normal at 3 L/min/m². The pulmonary-to-systemic blood flow ratio (Qp : Qs) is 1 : 1. Right atrial pressure is increased slightly as a result of decreased right ventricular compliance. The right ventricle is hypertrophied, and systolic and diastolic pressure is increased. The pressure gradient across the thickened pulmonary valve is 60 mm Hg. The main pulmonary artery pressure is slightly low, and poststenotic dilatation is present. Left heart pressure is normal. Unless right-to-left shunting is occurring through a foramen ovale, the patient's systemic oxygen saturation will be normal.

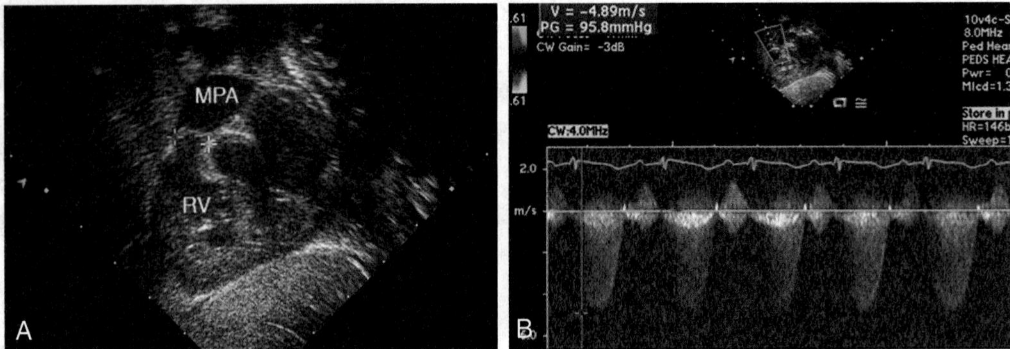

Figure 427-3. Echocardiogram demonstrating valvar pulmonic stenosis. *A,* Subcostal view showing thickened pulmonary valve leaflets (between *crosshatches*). *B,* Doppler study indicating a 95 mm Hg peak pressure gradient across the stenotic valve. MPA, main pulmonary artery; RV, right ventricle.

regurgitation. Doppler studies demonstrate a large gradient (>60 mm Hg) across the pulmonary valve. Fortunately, the classic findings of severe pulmonary stenosis in older children are rarely seen because of early intervention. Signs of critical pulmonic stenosis, with all of the features of severe pulmonic stenosis plus cyanosis, are usually encountered in the neonatal period.

Cardiac catheterization is not generally required for diagnostic purposes but is undertaken as part of a **balloon valvuloplasty** procedure. Catheterization demonstrates an abrupt pressure gradient across the pulmonary valve. Pulmonary artery pressure is either normal or low. The severity of the stenosis is graded based on the ratio of right ventricular systolic pressure to systemic systolic pressure or the right ventricle to pulmonary artery pressure gradient: a gradient of 10–30 mm Hg in mild cases, 30–60 mm Hg in moderate cases, and >60 mm Hg or with right ventricular pressure greater than systemic pressure in severe cases. If cardiac output is low or a significant right-to-left shunt exists across the atrial septum, the pressure gradient may underestimate the degree of valve stenosis. Selective right ventriculography demonstrates the thickened, poorly mobile valve. In mild to moderate stenosis, doming of the valve in systole is readily seen. Flow of contrast medium through the stenotic valve in ventricular systole produces a narrow jet of dye that fills the dilated main pulmonary artery. Subvalvular hypertrophy that may intensify the obstruction may occasionally be present. The angiogram also indicates whether the ventricular septum is intact.

TREATMENT. Patients with moderate or severe isolated pulmonary stenosis require relief of the obstruction. Balloon valvuloplasty is the initial treatment of choice for the majority of patients (Fig. 427-4). Patients with severely thickened pulmonic valves, especially common in those with Noonan syndrome, may require surgical intervention. In a neonate with critical pulmonic stenosis, urgent treatment by either balloon valvuloplasty or surgical valvotomy is warranted.

Excellent results are obtained in most instances. The gradient across the pulmonary valve is markedly reduced or abolished. In the early period after balloon valvuloplasty, a small to moderate residual gradient may remain because of muscular infundibular narrowing; it nearly always resolves with time. A short, early decrescendo diastolic murmur may be heard at the mid to upper left sternal border as a result of pulmonary valvular insufficiency. The degree of insufficiency is not usually clinically significant. No difference in patient status after valvuloplasty or surgery is noted at late follow-up; recurrence is unusual after successful treatment.

PROGNOSIS AND COMPLICATIONS. Heart failure occurs only in severe cases and most often during the 1st mo of life. The development of cyanosis from a right-to-left shunt across a foramen ovale is almost exclusively seen in the neonatal period when the stenosis is severe. Infective endocarditis is a risk but is not common in childhood.

Children with mild stenosis can lead a normal life, but their progress should be evaluated at regular intervals. Patients who have small gradients rarely show progression and do not need intervention, but a more significant gradient is more likely to develop in children with moderate stenosis as they grow older. Worsening of obstruction may also be due to the development of secondary subvalvular muscular and fibrous tissue hypertrophy. In untreated severe stenosis, the course may abruptly worsen with the development of right ventricular dysfunction and cardiac failure. Infants with critical pulmonic stenosis require urgent

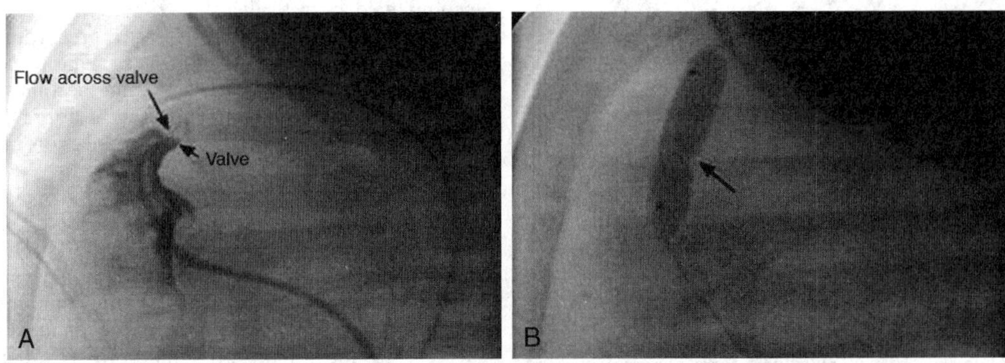

Figure 427-4. Valvar pulmonary stenosis and balloon valvuloplasty. *A,* Right ventricular angiogram showing severely stenotic pulmonary valve with narrow jet of blood flowing across. *B,* Inflation of the balloon catheter showing the indentation *(arrow)* made on the balloon from the stenotic valve. (Photos courtesy of Dr. Jeffrey Feinstein, Stanford University, Stanford, CA.)

catheter balloon valvuloplasty or surgical valvotomy. Development of right ventricular failure many years after pulmonary balloon valvuloplasty is uncommon. Nonetheless, patients should be followed serially for worsening pulmonary insufficiency and right ventricular dilation.

427.2 • Infundibular Pulmonary Stenosis and Double-Chamber Right Ventricle

Infundibular pulmonary stenosis is caused by muscular or fibrous obstruction in the outflow tract of the right ventricle. The site of obstruction may be close to the pulmonary valve or well below it; an infundibular chamber may be present between the right ventricular cavity and the pulmonary valve. In many cases, a VSD may have been present initially and later closed spontaneously. When the pulmonary valve is also stenotic, the combined defect is primarily classified as valvular stenosis with secondary infundibular hypertrophy. The hemodynamics and clinical manifestations of patients with isolated infundibular pulmonary stenosis are similar, for the most part, to those described in the discussion of isolated valvular pulmonary stenosis (see Chapter 427.1).

A common variation in right ventricular outflow obstruction below the pulmonary valve is that of a double-chambered right ventricle. In this condition, a muscular band is present in the mid-right ventricular region; the band divides the chamber into two parts and creates obstruction between the inlet and outlet portions. An associated VSD that may close spontaneously is often noted. Obstruction is not usually seen early in life but may progress rapidly in a similar manner to the progressive infundibular obstruction observed with the tetralogy of Fallot (see Chapter 430.1).

The diagnosis of isolated right ventricular infundibular stenosis or double-chambered right ventricle can be made by echocardiography or cardiac catheterization and angiography, or by both. The ventricular septum must be evaluated carefully to determine whether an associated VSD is present. The prognosis for untreated cases of severe right ventricular outflow obstruction is similar to that for valvular pulmonary stenosis. When the obstruction is moderate to severe, surgery is indicated. After surgery, the pressure gradient is abolished or markedly reduced and the long-term outlook is excellent.

427.3 • Pulmonary Stenosis in Combination with an Intracardiac Shunt

Valvular or infundibular pulmonary stenosis, or both, may be associated with either an ASD or a VSD. In these patients, the clinical features depend on the degree of pulmonary stenosis, which determines whether the net shunt is from left to right or from right to left.

The presence of a large left-to-right shunt at the atrial or ventricular level is evidence that the pulmonary stenosis is mild. These patients have symptoms similar to those of patients with an isolated ASD or VSD. With increasing age, worsening of the obstruction may limit the shunt and result in a gradual improvement in symptoms. Eventually, particularly in patients with pulmonary stenosis and VSD, a further increase in obstruction may lead to right-to-left shunting and cyanosis. When a patient with a VSD has evidence of decreasing heart failure and increased right ventricular forces on the electrocardiogram, one must differentiate between the development of increasing pulmonary stenosis versus the onset of pulmonary vascular disease (Eisenmenger syndrome, see Chapter 433.2).

These anomalies are readily repaired surgically. Defects in the atrial or ventricular septum are closed, and the pulmonary stenosis is relieved by resection of infundibular muscle or pulmonary valvotomy, or both, as indicated. Patients with a predominant right-to-left shunt have symptoms similar to those of patients with the **tetralogy of Fallot** (see Chapter 430.1).

427.4 • Peripheral Pulmonary Stenosis

Single or multiple constrictions may occur anywhere along the major branches of the pulmonary arteries and may range from mild to severe and from localized to extensive. Frequently, these defects are associated with other types of congenital heart disease, including valvular pulmonic stenosis, tetralogy of Fallot, patent ductus arteriosus (PDA), VSD, ASD, and supravalvular aortic stenosis. A familial tendency has been recognized in some patients with peripheral pulmonic stenosis. A high incidence is found in infants with congenital rubella syndrome. The combination of supravalvular aortic stenosis with pulmonary arterial branch stenosis, idiopathic hypercalcemia of infancy, elfin facies, and mental retardation is known as **Williams syndrome,** a condition associated with deletion of the elastin gene in region 7q11.23 on chromosome 7. Peripheral pulmonary stenosis may also be associated with the **Alagille syndrome,** which may be associated with a mutation in the *Jagged1* gene.

A mild constriction has little effect on the pulmonary circulation. With multiple severe constrictions, pressure is increased in the right ventricle and in the pulmonary artery proximal to the site of obstruction. When the anomaly is isolated, the diagnosis is suspected by the presence of murmurs in widespread locations over the chest, either anteriorly or posteriorly. These murmurs are usually systolic ejection in quality but may be continuous. Most often, the physical signs are dominated by the associated anomaly, such as the tetralogy of Fallot (see Chapter 430.1).

In the immediate newborn period, a mild and transient form of peripheral pulmonic stenosis may be present. Physical findings are generally limited to a soft systolic ejection murmur, which can be heard over either or both lung fields. It is the absence of other physical findings of valvular pulmonic stenosis (right ventricular lift, soft pulmonic 2nd sound, systolic ejection click, murmur loudest at the upper left sternal border) that supports this diagnosis. This murmur usually disappears by 1–2 mo.

If the stenosis is severe, the electrocardiogram shows evidence of right ventricular and right atrial hypertrophy, and the chest radiograph shows cardiomegaly and prominence of the main pulmonary artery. The pulmonary vasculature is usually normal; in some cases, however, small intrapulmonary vascular shadows are seen that represent areas of poststenotic dilatation. Echocardiography is limited in its ability to visualize the distal branch pulmonary arteries. Doppler examination demonstrates the acceleration of blood flow through the stenoses and, if tricuspid regurgitation is present, allows an estimation of right ventricular systolic pressure. MRI and CT are extremely helpful in delineating distal obstructions; if moderate to severe disease is suspected, the diagnosis is usually confirmed by cardiac catheterization.

Severe obstruction of the main pulmonary artery and its primary branches can be relieved during corrective surgery for associated lesions such as the tetralogy of Fallot or valvular pulmonary stenosis. If peripheral pulmonic stenosis is isolated, it may be treated by catheter balloon dilatation. When peripheral obstruction occurs distally in the intrapulmonary vessels, it is not usually amenable to surgical repair. These obstructions are often multiple and are best treated with repeat balloon angioplasty, although the rate of recurrence is high. The introduction of expandable intravascular stents, placed by catheter in the distal pulmonary arteries and then dilated with a balloon to the appropriate size, can prevent re-stenosis (see Fig. 423-29).

427.5 • Aortic Stenosis

PATHOPHYSIOLOGY. Congenital aortic stenosis accounts for ≈5% of cardiac malformations recognized in childhood; a bicuspid aortic valve, one of the most common congenital heart lesions overall, is identified in up to 2% of adults and is usually asymptomatic in childhood. Aortic stenosis is more frequent in males (3 : 1). In the most common form, valvular aortic stenosis, the leaflets are thickened and the commissures are fused to varying degrees. Left ventricular systolic pressure is increased as a result of the obstruction to outflow. The left ventricular wall hypertrophies in compensation; as its compliance decreases, end-diastolic pressure increases as well.

Subvalvular (subaortic) stenosis with a discrete fibromuscular shelf below the aortic valve is also an important form of left ventricular outflow tract obstruction. This lesion is frequently associated with other forms of congenital heart disease and may progress rapidly in severity. It is less commonly diagnosed during early infancy and may develop despite previous documentation of no left ventricular outflow tract obstruction. Subvalvular aortic stenosis may become apparent after successful surgery for other congenital heart defects (coarctation of the aorta, PDA, VSD), may develop in association with mild lesions that have not been surgically repaired, or may occur as an isolated abnormality. Subvalvular aortic stenosis may also be due to a markedly hypertrophied ventricular septum in association with hypertrophic cardiomyopathy (see Chapter 439.2).

Supravalvular aortic stenosis, the least common type, may be sporadic, familial, or associated with **Williams syndrome,** which includes mental retardation, elfin facies (full face, broad forehead, flattened bridge of the nose, long upper lip, and rounded cheeks), and idiopathic hypercalcemia of infancy (see Chapter 81). Narrowing of the coronary artery ostia can occur in patients with supravalvar aortic stenosis. Stenosis of other arteries, in particular, the branch pulmonary arteries, may also be present. Williams syndrome has been shown to be due to a deletion involving the elastin gene on chromosome 7q11.23.

CLINICAL MANIFESTATIONS. Symptoms in patients with aortic stenosis depend on the severity of the obstruction. Severe aortic stenosis that occurs in early infancy is termed **critical aortic stenosis** and is associated with left ventricular failure and signs of low cardiac output. Heart failure, cardiomegaly, and pulmonary edema are severe, the pulses are weak in all extremities, and the skin may be pale or grayish. Urine output may be diminished. If cardiac output is significantly decreased, the intensity of the murmur at the right upper sternal border may be minimal. Most children with less severe forms of aortic stenosis remain asymptomatic and display normal growth and development. The murmur is usually discovered during routine physical examination. Rarely, fatigue, angina, dizziness, or syncope may develop in an older child with previously undiagnosed severe obstruction to left ventricular outflow. Sudden death has been reported with aortic stenosis but usually occurs in patients with severe left ventricular outflow obstruction in whom surgical relief has been delayed.

The physical findings are dependent on the degree of obstruction to left ventricular outflow. In mild stenosis, the pulses, heart size, and apical impulse are all normal. With increasing degrees of severity, the pulses become diminished in intensity and the heart may be enlarged, with a left ventricular apical thrust. Mild to moderate valvular aortic stenosis is usually associated with an early systolic ejection click, best heard at the apex and left sternal edge. Unlike the click in pulmonic stenosis, its intensity does not vary with respiration. Clicks are unusual in more severe aortic stenosis or in discrete subaortic stenosis. If the stenosis is severe, the 1st heart sound may be diminished because of decreased compliance of the thickened left ventricle. Normal splitting of the 2nd heart sound is present in mild to moderate obstruction. In patients with severe obstruction, the intensity of aortic valve closure is diminished, and, rarely in children, the 2nd sound may be split paradoxically (becoming wider in expiration). A 4th heart sound may be audible when the obstruction is severe.

The intensity, pitch, and duration of the systolic ejection murmur are other indications of severity. The louder, harsher (higher pitch), and longer the murmur, the greater the degree of obstruction is. The typical murmur is audible maximally at the right upper sternal border and radiates to the neck and the left midsternal border. It is usually accompanied by a thrill in the suprasternal notch. In patients with subvalvular aortic stenosis, the murmur may be maximal along the left sternal border or even at the apex. A soft decrescendo diastolic murmur indicative of aortic insufficiency is often present when the obstruction is subvalvular or in patients with a bicuspid aortic valve. Occasionally, an apical short mid-diastolic rumbling murmur is audible, even in the presence of a normal mitral valve; this murmur should always raise suspicion of associated mitral valve stenosis.

LABORATORY FINDINGS AND DIAGNOSIS. The diagnosis can usually be made on the basis of the physical examination and the severity of obstruction confirmed by laboratory tests. If the pressure gradient across the aortic valve is mild, the electrocardiogram is likely to be normal. The electrocardiogram may occasionally be normal even with more severe obstruction, but evidence of left ventricular hypertrophy and strain (inverted T waves in the left precordial leads) is generally present if severe stenosis is long-standing. The chest radiograph frequently shows a prominent ascending aorta, but the aortic knob is normal. Heart size is typically normal. Valvular calcification has been noted only in older children and adults. Echocardiography identifies both the site and the severity of the obstruction. Two-dimensional imaging shows left ventricular hypertrophy and the thickened and domed aortic valve (Fig. 427-5). The echo will also demonstrate the number of valve leaflets and their morphology, and a subaortic membrane or supravalvar stenosis, if present. Associated anomalies of the mitral valve or aortic arch or a VSD or PDA is present in up to 20% of cases. In the absence of left ventricular failure, the shortening fraction of the left ventricle may be increased because the ventricle is hypercontractile. In infants with critical aortic stenosis, the left ventricular shortening fraction is usually decreased and the endocardium may be bright, indicative of the development of endocardial fibrous scarring, known as **endocardial fibroelastosis.** Doppler studies show the specific site of obstruction and determine the peak and mean systolic left ventricular outflow tract gradients. When severe aortic obstruction is associated with left ventricular dysfunction, the Doppler-derived valve gradient may markedly underestimate the severity of the obstruction because of the low cardiac output.

Graded exercise testing is useful in evaluating the severity of left ventricular outflow tract obstruction in older children. As the severity of the gradient increases, working capacity decreases, systolic blood pressure fails to rise adequately, diastolic blood pressure may increase, and ST segment depression can occur. Because patients with severe aortic stenosis may deny symptoms and have normal electrocardiograms and chest roentgenograms, serial echocardiograms and graded exercise tests may be valuable in determining the timing of cardiac catheterization and surgical or balloon catheter valvuloplasty.

Left heart catheterization demonstrates the magnitude of the pressure gradient from the left ventricle to the aorta. The aortic pressure curve is abnormal if the obstruction is severe. In patients with severe obstruction and decreased left ventricular compliance, left atrial pressure is increased and pulmonary hypertension may be present. The site of obstruction is best identified by selective left ventriculography. Most infants with critical aortic stenosis do not require cardiac catheterization for diagnosis but usually undergo the procedure for balloon valvuloplasty. When a criti-

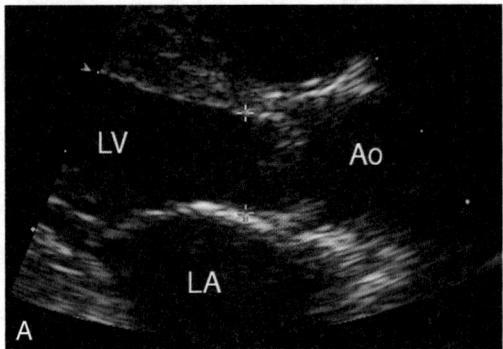

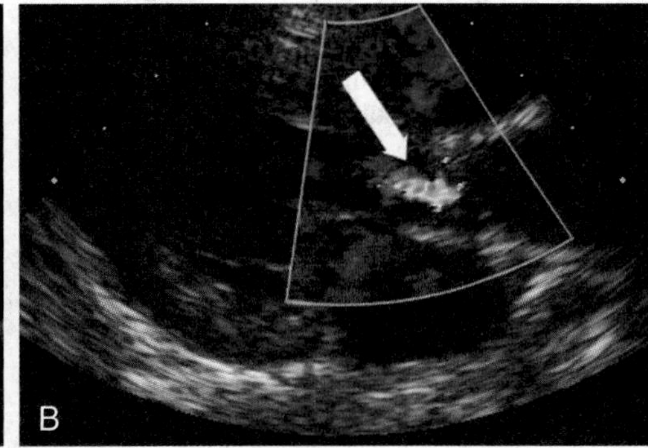

Figure 427-5. Echocardiogram showing valvar aortic stenosis with regurgitation. *A,* In this parasternal long axis view, the stenotic aortic valve can be seen doming in systole. The *crosshatch* marks delineate the aortic annulus. *B,* Doppler study shows the presence of aortic regurgitation *(arrow).* Ao, aorta; LA, left atrium; LV, left ventricle.

cally ill infant with left ventricular outflow tract obstruction undergoes cardiac catheterization, left ventricular function is often markedly decreased. As with the echocardiogram, the gradient measured across the stenotic aortic valve may underestimate the degree of obstruction because of low cardiac output. Actual measurement of cardiac output by thermodilution and calculation of the aortic valve area may be helpful.

TREATMENT. Balloon valvuloplasty is indicated for children with moderate to severe valvular aortic stenosis to prevent progressive left ventricular dysfunction and the risk of syncope and sudden death. It is generally agreed that valvuloplasty should be advised when the peak-to-peak systolic gradient between the left ventricle and aorta exceeds 60–70 mm Hg at rest, assuming normal cardiac output, or for lesser gradients when symptoms or electrocardiographic changes are present. For more rapidly progressive subaortic obstructive lesions, a gradient of 40–50 mm Hg or the presence of aortic insufficieny is considered an indication for surgery. With the development of low-profile balloons and smaller catheters that cause less injury to peripheral arteries, balloon valvuloplasty has become the procedure of choice even in the neonatal period. Surgical treatment is usually reserved for stenotic aortic valves that are not amenable to balloon therapy, generally those that are extremely thickened, or in patients who also have subvalvar or supravalvar stenosis.

Discrete subaortic stenosis can be resected without damage to the aortic valve, the anterior leaflet of the mitral valve, or the conduction system. This type of obstruction is not usually amenable to catheter treatment. Relief of supravalvular stenosis is also achieved surgically, and the results are excellent if the area of obstruction is discrete and not associated with a hypoplastic aorta. In association with supravalvular aortic stenosis, one or both coronary arteries may be stenotic at their origins because of a thick supra-aortic fibrous ridge. For patients who have aortic stenosis in association with severe tunnel-like subaortic obstruction, the left ventricular outflow tract can be enlarged by "borrowing" space anteriorly from the right ventricular outflow tract (the Konno procedure).

Regardless of whether surgical or catheter treatment has been carried out, aortic insufficiency or calcification with re-stenosis is likely to occur years or even decades later and eventually require reoperation and often aortic valve replacement. When recurrence develops, it may not be associated with early symptoms. Signs of recurrent stenosis include electrocardiographic signs of left ventricular hypertrophy, an increase in the Doppler echocardiographic gradient, deterioration in echocardiographic indices of left ventricular function, and recurrence of signs or symptoms during graded treadmill exercise. Evidence of significant aortic regurgitation includes symptoms of heart failure, cardiac enlargement on roentgenogram, and left ventricular dilatation on echocardiogram. The choice of reparative procedure depends on the relative degree of stenosis and regurgitation.

When **aortic valve replacement** is necessary, the choice of procedure often depends on the age of the patient. Homograft valves tend to calcify more rapidly in younger children, but they do not require chronic anticoagulation. Mechanical prosthetic valves are much longer lasting, yet they require anticoagulation, which can be difficult to manage in young children. In adolescent girls who are nearing childbearing age, consideration of the teratogenic effects of warfarin may warrant the use of a homograft valve. None of these options are perfect for a younger child who requires valve replacement because neither homograft nor mechanical valves grow with the patient. An alternative operation is **aortopulmonary translocation (Ross procedure)**; it involves removing the patient's own pulmonary valve and using it to replace the abnormal aortic valve. A homograft is then placed in the pulmonary position. The potential advantage of this procedure is the possibility for growth of the translocated living "neoaortic" valve and the longer longevity of the homograft valve when placed in the lower pressure pulmonary circulation. The long-term success of this operation, especially in young children, is still being investigated. Stent valves, which are tissue valves sewn into the inside of an expandable metal stent, are currently in clinical trials. These can be implanted in the cardiac catheterization laboratory using a percutaneous approach. Tissue-engineered replacement valves grown in the laboratory from the patient's own arterial endothelial cells are the best hope for long-term palliation and are currently under development in animal models.

PROGNOSIS. Neonates with critical aortic stenosis may have severe heart failure and deteriorate rapidly to a low-output shock state. Emergency surgery or balloon valvuloplasty is lifesaving, but the mortality risk is not trivial. Neonates who die of critical aortic stenosis frequently have significant left ventricular endocardial fibroelastosis. Those who survive may develop signs of left ventricular diastolic muscle dysfunction (restrictive cardiomyopathy) later in life (see Chapter 439.3).

In older infants and children with mild to moderate aortic stenosis, the prognosis is reasonably good, although disease progression over a period of 5–10 yr is common. Patients with aortic valve gradients <40–50 mm Hg are considered to have mild disease; those with gradients of 40–70 mm Hg have moderate disease. These patients usually respond well to treatment (either surgery or valvuloplasty), although reoperations on the aortic valve are often required later in childhood or in adult life, and many patients eventually require valve replacement. In unoperated patients with severe obstruction, sudden death is a significant risk and often occurs during or immediately after exercise. Aortic stenosis is one of the causes of sudden cardiac death in the pediatric age group.

Patients with moderate to severe degrees of aortic stenosis should not participate in active competitive sports. In those with milder disease, sports participation is less severely restricted; however, patients should be encouraged to pursue less physically demanding activities. The status of each patient should be reviewed at least annually and intervention advised if progression of signs or symptoms occurs. Lifetime prophylaxis against infective endocarditis is required.

427.6 • Coarctation of the Aorta

Constrictions of the aorta of varying degrees may occur at any point from the transverse arch to the iliac bifurcation, but 98% occur just below the origin of the left subclavian artery at the origin of the ductus arteriosus (juxtaductal coarctation). The anomaly occurs twice as often in males as in females. Coarctation of the aorta may be a feature of **Turner syndrome** (see Chapters 81 and 587.1) and is associated with a bicuspid aortic valve in more than 70% of patients. Mitral valve abnormalities (a supravalvular mitral ring or parachute mitral valve) and subaortic stenosis are potential associated lesions. When this group of left-sided obstructive lesions occurs together, they are referred to as the **Shone complex.**

PATHOPHYSIOLOGY. Coarctation of the aorta can occur as a discrete juxtaductal obstruction or as tubular hypoplasia of the transverse aorta starting at one of the head or neck vessels and extending to the ductal area (previously referred to as preductal or infantile-type coarctation; Fig. 427-6). Often, both components are present. It is postulated that coarctation may be initiated in fetal life by the presence of a cardiac abnormality that results in decreased blood flow anterograde through the aortic valve (e.g., bicuspid aortic valve, VSD). Alternatively, coarctation may be due to abnormal extension of contractile ductal tissue into the aortic wall.

In patients with discrete juxtaductal coarctation, ascending aortic blood flows through the narrowed segment to reach the descending aorta, although left ventricular hypertension and hypertrophy result. In the 1st few days of life, the PDA may serve to widen the juxtaductal area of the aorta and provide temporary relief from the obstruction. Net left-to-right ductal shunting occurs in these acyanotic infants. With more severe juxtaductal coarctation or in the presence of transverse arch hypoplasia, right ventricular blood is ejected through the ductus to supply the descending aorta. Perfusion of the lower part of the body is then dependent on right ventricular output (see Fig. 427-6). In this situation, the femoral pulses are palpable, and differential blood pressures may not be helpful in making the diagnosis. The ductal right-to-left shunting is manifested as differential cyanosis, with the upper extremities being pink and the lower extremities blue.

Such infants may have severe pulmonary hypertension and high pulmonary vascular resistance. Signs of heart failure are prominent. Occasionally, severely hypoplastic segments of the aortic isthmus may become completely atretic and result in an interrupted aortic arch, with the left subclavian artery arising either proximal or distal to the interruption. Coarctation associated with arch hypoplasia was once referred to as infantile type because its severity usually led to recognition of the condition in early infancy. Adult type referred to isolated juxtaductal coarctation, which if mild, was not usually recognized until later childhood. These terms have been replaced with the more accurate anatomic terms describing the location and severity of the defect.

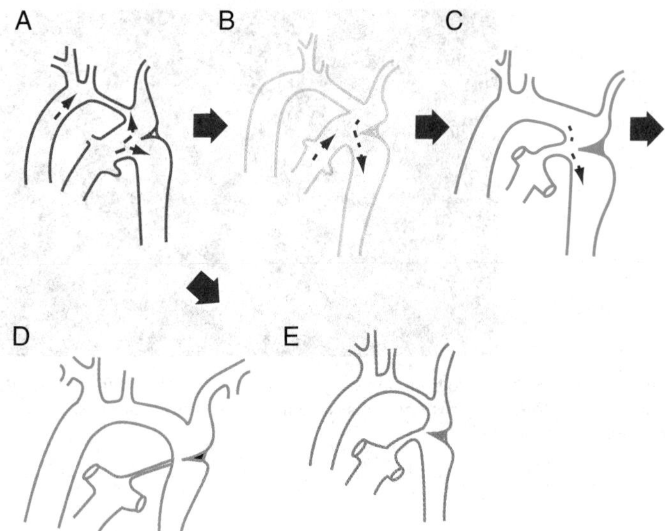

Figure 427-6. Metamorphosis of coarctation. *A*, Fetal prototype with no flow obstruction. *B*, Late gestation. The aortic ventricle increases its output and dilates the hypoplastic segment. Antegrade aortic flow bypasses the shelf via the ductal orifice. *C*, Neonate. Ductal constriction initiates the obstruction by removing the bypass and increasing antegrade arch flow. *D*, Mature juxtaductal stenosis. The bypass is completely obliterated, and intimal hypoplasia on the edge of the shelf is aggravating the stenosis. Collaterals develop. *E*, Persistence of the infantile-type fetal prototype. An intracardiac left-sided heart obstruction precludes an increase in antegrade aortic flow before or after birth. Both isthmus hypoplasia and a contraductal shelf are present. Lower body flow often depends on patency of the ductus. (From Gersony WM: Coarctation of the aorta. In Adams FH, Emmanouilides GC, Riemenshneider T [editors]: *Moss Heart Disease in Infants, Children, and Adolescents,* 4th ed. Baltimore, Williams & Wilkins, 1989.)

Blood pressure is elevated in the vessels that arise proximal to the coarctation; blood pressure as well as pulse pressure is lower below the constriction. The hypertension is not due to the mechanical obstruction alone but also involves neurohumoral mechanisms. Unless operated on in infancy, coarctation of the aorta usually results in the development of an extensive collateral circulation, chiefly from branches of the subclavian, superior intercostal, and internal mammary arteries, to create channels for arterial blood to bypass the area of coarctation. The vessels contributing to the collateral circulation may become markedly enlarged and tortuous by early adulthood.

CLINICAL MANIFESTATIONS. Coarctation of the aorta recognized after infancy is not usually associated with significant symptoms. Some children or adolescents complain about weakness or pain (or both) in the legs after exercise, but in many instances, even patients with severe coarctation are asymptomatic. Older children are frequently brought to the cardiologist's attention when they are found to be hypertensive on routine physical examination.

The classic sign of coarctation of the aorta is a disparity in pulsation and blood pressure in the arms and legs. The femoral, popliteal, posterior tibial, and dorsalis pedis pulses are weak (or absent in up to 40% of patients), in contrast to the bounding pulses of the arms and carotid vessels. The radial and femoral pulses should always be palpated simultaneously for the presence of a radial-femoral delay. Normally, the femoral pulse occurs slightly before the radial pulse. A radial-femoral delay occurs when blood flow to the descending aorta is dependent on collaterals, in which case the femoral pulse is felt after the radial pulse. In normal persons (except neonates), systolic blood pressure in the legs obtained by the cuff method is 10–20 mm Hg higher than

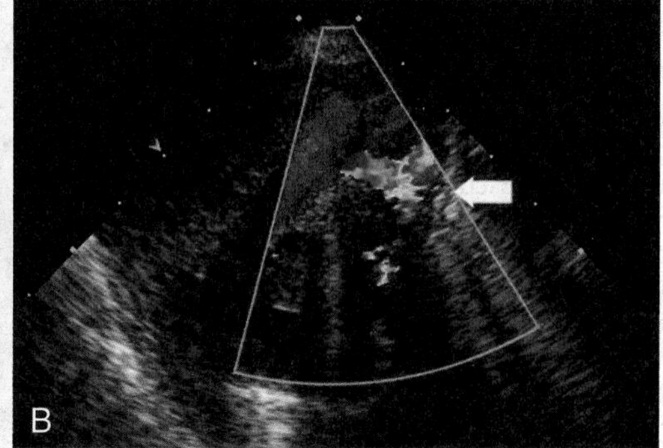

Figure 427-7. Echocardiogram demonstrating coarctation of the aorta with hypoplastic transverse arch. *A*, Suprasternal notch two-dimensional echocardiogram showing marked narrowing beginning just distal to the brachiocephalic artery. *B*, Color Doppler demonstrates turbulent flow in the juxtductal area *(arrow)*. AscAo, ascending aorta; BR, brachiocephalic artery; LCA, left carotid artery; LSCA, left subclavian artery.

that in the arms. In coarctation of the aorta, blood pressure in the legs is lower than that in the arms; frequently, it is difficult to obtain. This differential in blood pressures is common in patients with coarctation who are older than 1 yr, about 90% of whom have systolic hypertension in an upper extremity greater than the 95th percentile for age. It is important to determine the blood pressure in each arm; a pressure higher in the right than the left arm suggests involvement of the left subclavian artery in the area of coarctation. Occasionally, the right subclavian may arise anomalously from below the area of coarctation and result in a left arm pressure that is higher than the right. With exercise, a more prominent rise in systemic blood pressure occurs, and the upper-to-lower extremity pressure gradient will increase.

The precordial impulse and heart sounds are usually normal; the presence of a systolic ejection click or thrill in the suprasternal notch suggests a bicuspid aortic valve (present in 70% of cases). A short systolic murmur is often heard along the left sternal border at the 3rd and 4th intercostal spaces. The murmur is well transmitted to the left infrascapular area and occasionally to the neck. Often, the typical murmur of mild aortic stenosis can be heard in the 3rd right intercostal space. Occasionally, more significant degrees of obstruction are noted across the aortic valve. The presence of a low-pitched mid-diastolic murmur at the apex suggests mitral valve stenosis. In older patients with well-developed collateral blood flow, systolic or continuous murmurs may be heard over the left and right sides of the chest laterally and posteriorly. In these patients, a palpable thrill can occasionally be appreciated in the intercostal spaces on the back.

Neonates or infants with more severe coarctation, usually including some degree of transverse arch hypoplasia, initially have signs of lower body hypoperfusion, acidosis, and severe heart failure. These signs may be delayed days or weeks until after closure of the ductus arteriosus. If detected before ductal closure, patients may exhibit differential cyanosis, best demonstrated by simultaneous oximetry of the upper and lower extremities. On physical examination, the heart is large, and a systolic murmur is heard along the left sternal border with a loud 2nd heart sound.

DIAGNOSIS. Findings on roentgenographic examination depend on the age of the patient and on the effects of hypertension and the collateral circulation. Cardiac enlargement and pulmonary congestion are noted in infants with severe coarctation. During childhood, the findings are not striking until after the 1st decade, when the heart tends to be mildly or moderately enlarged because of left ventricular prominence. The enlarged left subclavian artery commonly produces a prominent shadow in the left superior mediastinum. **Notching** of the **inferior border of the ribs** from pressure erosion by enlarged collateral vessels is common by late childhood. In most instances, the descending aorta has an area of poststenotic dilatation.

The electrocardiogram is usually normal in young children but reveals evidence of left ventricular hypertrophy in older patients. Neonates and young infants display right or biventricular hypertrophy. The segment of coarctation can generally be visualized by two-dimensional echocardiography (Fig. 427-7); associated anomalies of the mitral and aortic valve can also be demonstrated. The descending aorta is hypopulsatile. Color Doppler is useful for demonstrating the specific site of the obstruction. Pulsed and continuous wave Doppler studies determine the pressure gradient directly at the area of coarctation; in the presence of a PDA, however, the severity of the narrowing may be underestimated. CT and MRI are valuable noninvasive tools for evaluation of coarctation when the echocardiogram is equivocal. Cardiac catheterization with selective left ventriculography and aortography is useful in occasional patients with additional anomalies and as a means of visualizing collateral blood flow. In cases that are well defined by echocardiography, CT, or MRI, diagnostic catheterization is not usually required before surgery.

TREATMENT. In neonates with severe coarctation of the aorta, closure of the ductus often results in hypoperfusion, acidosis, and rapid deterioration. These patients should be given an infusion of **prostaglandin E_1** to reopen the ductus and re-establish adequate lower extremity blood flow. Once a diagnosis has been confirmed and the patient stabilized, surgical repair should be performed. Older infants with heart failure but good perfusion should be managed with anticongestive measures to improve their clinical status before surgical intervention. There is usually no reason to delay surgical repair waiting for patient growth; successful repairs have been performed in small premature infants.

Older children with significant coarctation of the aorta should be treated relatively soon after diagnosis. Delay is unwarranted, especially after the 2nd decade of life, when the operation may be less successful because of decreased left ventricular function and degenerative changes in the aortic wall. Nevertheless, if cardiac reserve is sufficient, satisfactory repair is possible well into mid-adult life.

The procedure of choice for isolated juxtaductal coarctation of the aorta is controversial. Surgery remains the treatment of choice at most centers, and several surgical techniques are used. The area of coarctation can be excised and a primary re-anastomosis performed. Often, the transverse aorta is splayed open and an "extended end-to-end" anastomosis performed to increase the effective cross-sectional area of the repair. The subclavian flap procedure, which involves division of the left subclavian artery and incorporation of it into the wall of the repaired coarctation, is used by some, although has grown out of favor due to a higher degree of residual stenosis. Others favor a patch aortoplasty, in which the area of coarctation is enlarged with a roof of prosthetic material. The use of primary angioplasty for native coarctation remains controversial, although is useful in conditions where surgical intervention may be associated with increased risk in patients with severe left ventricular dysfunction.

After surgery, a striking increase in the amplitude of pulsations in the lower extremities is noted. In the immediate postoperative course, **"rebound" hypertension** is common and requires medical management. This exaggerated acute hypertension gradually subsides and, in most patients, antihypertensive medications can be discontinued. Residual murmurs are common and may be due to associated cardiac anomalies, to a residual flow disturbance across the repaired area, or to collateral blood flow. Rare operative problems include spinal cord injury from aortic cross-clamping if the collaterals are poorly developed, chylothorax, diaphragm injury, and laryngeal nerve injury. If a left subclavian flap is used, the radial pulse and blood pressure in the left arm are diminished or absent.

POSTCOARCTECTOMY SYNDROME. Postoperative **mesenteric arteritis** may be associated with acute hypertension and abdominal pain in the immediate postoperative period. The pain varies in severity and may occur in conjunction with anorexia, nausea, vomiting, leukocytosis, intestinal hemorrhage, bowel necrosis, and small bowel obstruction. Relief is usually obtained with antihypertensive drugs (nitroprusside, esmolol, captopril) and intestinal decompression; surgical exploration is rarely required for bowel obstruction or infarction.

PROGNOSIS. Although re-stenosis in older patients after coarctectomy is rare, a significant number of infants operated on before 1 yr of age require revision later in childhood. All patients should be monitored carefully for the development of recoarctation and aortic aneurysm. Should recoarctation occur, **balloon angioplasty** is the procedure of choice. In these patients, scar tissue from previous surgery may make reoperation more difficult yet makes balloon angioplasty safer because of the lower incidence of aneurysm formation. Relief of obstruction with this technique is usually excellent. **Intravascular stents** are commonly used, especially in adolescents and young adults, with generally excellent results.

Repair of coarctation in the 2nd decade of life or beyond may be associated with a higher incidence of premature cardiovascular disease, even in the absence of residual cardiac abnormalities. Early onset of adult chronic hypertension may occur, even in patients with adequately resected coarctation.

Abnormalities of the aortic valve are present in most patients. Bicuspid aortic valves are common but do not generally produce clinical signs unless the stenosis is significant. The association of a PDA and coarctation of the aorta is also common. VSDs and ASDs may be suspected by signs of a left-to-right shunt; they are exacerbated by the increased resistance to flow through the left side of the heart. Mitral valve abnormalities are also occasionally seen, as is subvalvular aortic stenosis.

Severe neurologic damage or even death may rarely occur from associated cerebrovascular disease. Subarachnoid or intracerebral hemorrhage may result from rupture of congenital aneurysms in the circle of Willis, rupture of other vessels with defective elastic and medial tissue, or rupture of normal vessels; these accidents are secondary to hypertension. Children with **PHACE syndrome** (posterior brain fossa anomalies, facial hemangiomas, arterial anomalies, cardiac anomalies and aortic coarctation, eye anomalies) may have strokes (see Table 422-1). Abnormalities of the subclavian arteries may include involvement of the left subclavian artery in the area of coarctation, stenosis of the orifice of the left subclavian artery, and anomalous origin of the right subclavian artery.

Untreated, the great majority of older patients with coarctation of the aorta would succumb between the ages of 20 and 40 yr; some live well into middle life without serious disability. The common serious complications are related to systemic hypertension, which may result in premature coronary artery disease, heart failure, hypertensive encephalopathy, or intracranial hemorrhage. Heart failure may be worsened by associated anomalies. Infective endocarditis or endarteritis is a significant complication in adults. Aneurysms of the descending aorta or the enlarged collateral vessels may develop.

427.7 • Coarctation with Ventricular Septal Defect

Coarctation in the presence of VSD results in both increased preload and afterload on the left ventricle, and patients with this combination of defects will be recognized either at birth or in the 1st mo of life and often have intractable cardiac failure. The magnitude of a left-to-right shunt through a VSD is dependent on the ratio of pulmonary to systemic vascular resistance. In the presence of coarctation, resistance to systemic outflow is enhanced by the obstruction, and the volume of the shunt is markedly increased. The clinical picture is that of a seriously ill infant with tachypnea, failure to thrive, and typical findings of heart failure. Often, the difference in blood pressure between the upper and lower extremities is not very marked because cardiac output may be low. Medical management should be used to stabilize the patient initially; however, it should not be used to delay corrective surgery inordinately.

In most cases, coarctation is the major anomaly causing the severe symptoms, and resection of the coarctated segment results in striking improvement. Many centers routinely repair both the VSD and coarctation at the same operation through a midline sternotomy using cardiopulmonary bypass. Some centers repair the coarctation through a left lateral thoracotomy and, at the same time, place a pulmonary artery band to decrease the ventricular-level shunt. Others do not band the pulmonary artery initially because a number of patients improve sufficiently so that further surgery is not required during early infancy. If heart failure makes it difficult to manage these infants after surgery, open repair of the VSD is then performed soon thereafter. When it is determined that a complicated VSD is present (multiple VSDs, apical muscular VSD), pulmonary arterial banding may be performed at the time of coarctation repair to avoid open heart surgery during infancy for these complex ventricular septal abnormalities.

427.8 • Coarctation with Other Cardiac Anomalies and Interrupted Aortic Arch

Coarctation often occurs in infancy in association with other major cardiovascular anomalies, including hypoplastic left heart, severe mitral or aortic valve disease, transposition of the great arteries, and variations of double-outlet or single ventricle. Severe coarctation may also be associated with endocardial fibroelastosis. The clinical manifestations depend on the effects of the associated malformations, as well as on the coarctation itself.

Coarctation of the aorta associated with severe mitral and aortic valve disease may have to be treated within the context of the hypoplastic left heart syndrome (see Chapter 431.10), even if the left ventricular chamber is not severely hypoplastic. Such patients usually have a long segment of narrow transverse aortic arch with or without an isolated coarctation at the site of the ductus arteriosus. Coarctation of the aorta with transposition of the great arteries or single ventricle may be repaired alone or in combination with other palliative measures.

Complete interruption of the aortic arch is the most severe form of coarctation and is usually associated with other intracardiac pathology. Interruption may occur at any level, although it is most commonly seen between the left subclavian artery and the insertion of the ductus arteriosus (type A), followed in frequency by those between the left subclavian and left carotid arteries (type B). In newborns with an interrupted aortic arch, the ductus arteriosus provides the sole source of blood flow to the descending aorta, and differential oxygen saturation between the right arm (normal saturation) and the legs (decreased) can be noted. When the ductus begins to close, severe congestive heart failure, lower extremity hypoperfusion, anuria, and shock can develop in these infants. Patients with an interrupted aortic arch can be supported with prostaglandin to keep the ductus patent before surgical repair. As one of the conotruncal malformations, an interrupted aortic arch can be associated with the spectrum of lesions known as **CATCH 22** (cardiac defects, abnormal facies, thymic hypoplasia, cleft palate, hypocalcemia). CATCH 22 includes patients with clinical features of the DiGeorge syndrome (hypocalcemia, thymic hypoplasia, mild facial anomalies) and the Shprintzen velocardiofacial syndrome (abnormal facies, cleft palate). Cytogenetic analysis using fluorescence in situ hybridization demonstrates deletion of a segment of chromosome 22q11 known as the DiGeorge critical region, containing the gene *Tbx1,* a transcription factor, which has been implicated in the syndrome.

427.9 • Congenital Mitral Stenosis

Congenital mitral stenosis is a rare anomaly that can be isolated or associated with other defects, the most common being aortic stenosis and coarctation of the aorta (**Shone complex**). The mitral valve may be funnel-shaped, with thickened leaflets and chordae tendineae that are shortened and deformed. Other mitral valve anomalies associated with stenosis include parachute mitral valve, caused by a single papillary muscle, and double-orifice mitral valve.

Symptoms usually appear within the 1st 2 yr of life. These infants are underdeveloped and generally have obvious dyspnea secondary to heart failure; cyanosis and pallor are common. In some patients whose symptoms are mainly wheezing, reactive airway disease may have been diagnosed. Heart enlargement as a result of dilatation and hypertrophy of the right ventricle and left atrium is common. Most patients have rumbling apical diastolic murmurs followed by a loud 1st sound, but the auscultatory findings may be relatively obscure. The 2nd sound is loud and split. An opening snap of the mitral valve may be present. The electrocardiogram reveals right ventricular hypertrophy with normal, bifid, or spiked P waves indicative of left atrial enlargement. Roentgenograms usually show left atrial and right ventricular enlargement and pulmonary congestion. The echocardiogram is characteristic and shows thickened mitral valve leaflets, a diminished E-F slope on the M-mode mitral echocardiogram, and an enlarged left atrium with a normal or small left ventricle. Two-dimensional echocardiographic examination shows a significant reduction of the mitral valve orifice in diastole. Doppler studies demonstrate a mean pressure gradient across the mitral orifice. At cardiac catheterization, an increase in right ventricular, pulmonary arterial, and pulmonary capillary wedge pressure can be noted. Associated anomalies such as aortic stenosis and coarctation are demonstrated. Angiocardiography shows delayed emptying of the left atrium and the small mitral orifice.

The prognosis for untreated patients is poor. The results of surgical treatment have been mixed; a mitral valve prosthesis is usually required, but it must be replaced as the child grows. These patients must be managed by anticoagulation with warfarin, and complications of excessive and insufficient anticoagulation are fairly common in infancy. Transcatheter balloon valvuloplasty has been used by several centers as a palliative procedure with mixed results, depending on the anatomy of the valve and the papillary muscles.

427.10 • Pulmonary Venous Hypertension

A variety of lesions may give rise to chronic pulmonary venous hypertension, which when extreme may result in pulmonary arterial hypertension and right-sided heart failure. These lesions include congenital mitral stenosis, mitral insufficiency, total anomalous pulmonary venous return with obstruction, left atrial myxomas, cor triatriatum (stenosis of a common pulmonary vein), individual pulmonary vein stenosis, and supravalvular mitral rings or webs. Early symptoms can be confused with chronic pulmonary disease such as asthma because of a lack of specific cardiac findings on physical examination. Subtle signs of pulmonary hypertension may be present. The electrocardiogram shows right ventricular hypertrophy with spiked P waves. Roentgenographic studies reveal cardiac enlargement and prominence of the pulmonary veins in the hilar region, the right ventricle and atrium, and the main pulmonary artery; the left atrium is normal in size or only slightly enlarged.

The echocardiogram may demonstrate left atrial myxoma, cor triatriatum, stenosis of one or more pulmonary veins, or a mitral valve abnormality. Cardiac catheterization excludes the presence of a shunt and demonstrates pulmonary hypertension with elevated pulmonary arterial wedge pressure. Left atrial pressure is normal if the lesion is at the level of the pulmonary veins, but it is elevated if the lesion is at the level of the mitral valve. Selective pulmonary arteriography usually delineates the anatomic lesion. Cor triatriatum, left atrial myxoma, and supravalvular mitral webs can all be successfully managed surgically.

The **differential diagnosis** includes pulmonary veno-occlusive disease, an idiopathic process that produces obstructive lesions in the pulmonary veins of children and young adults. The cause is uncertain. Although it is usually encountered in patients after repair of obstructed total anomalous pulmonary venous return (see Chapter 431.7), it can occur in the absence of congenital heart disease. The patient initially presents with left-sided heart failure on the basis of congested lungs with apparent pulmonary edema. Dyspnea, fatigue, and pleural effusions are common; cyanosis, digital clubbing, syncope, and hemoptysis are variable findings. Left atrial pressure is normal, but pulmonary arterial wedge pressure is usually elevated. A normal wedge pressure may be encountered if collaterals have formed or the wedge recording is performed in an uninvolved segment. Angiographically, the pulmonary veins return normally to the left atrium, but one or more pulmonary veins are narrowed, either focally or diffusely.

Lung biopsy demonstrates pulmonary venous and, occasionally, arterial involvement. Pulmonary veins and venules demonstrate fibrous narrowing or occlusion, and pulmonary artery thrombi may be present. Therapy is disappointing, and survival ranges from weeks to months in infants and from months to years in adults. Attempts at surgical repair, balloon dilatation, and transcatheter stenting have not significantly improved the prognosis of these patients. Clinical trials of antiproliferative chemotherapy are currently in progress. Combined heart-lung transplantation (see Chapter 443.2) remains the only moderately successful therapeutic option.

Pulmonary Stenosis

Crosnier C, Lykavieris P, Meunier-Rotival M, et al: Alagille syndrome. The widening spectrum of arteriohepatic dysplasia. *Clin Liver Dis* 2000; 4:765–778.

Krantz ID, Smith R, Colliton RP, et al: Jagged 1 mutations in patients ascertained with isolated congenital heart defects. *Am J Med Genet* 1999; 84:56–60.

Moller JH: Exercise responses in pulmonary stenosis. *Prog Pediatr Cardiol* 1993;2:8–13.

Phoon CK: Estimation of pressure gradients by auscultation: An innovative and accurate physical examination technique. *Am Heart J* 2001;141: 500–506.

Rosales AM, Lock JE, Perry SB, et al: Interventional catheterization management of perioperative peripheral pulmonary stenosis: Balloon angioplasty or endovascular stenting. *Catheter Cardiovasc Interv* 2002;56:272–277.

Yoshida R, Hasegawa T, Hasegawa Y, et al: Protein-tyrosine phosphatase, nonreceptor type 11 mutation analysis and clinical assessment in 45 patients with Noonan syndrome. *J Clin Endocrinol Metab* 2004;89:3359–3364.

Aortic Stenosis

Doyle EF, Arumugham P, Lara E, et al: Sudden death in young patients with congenital aortic stenosis. *Pediatrics* 1974;53:481–489.

Freed MD: Recreational and sports recommendations for the child with heart disease. *Pediatr Clin North Am* 1984;31:1307–1320.

Jahangiri M, Nicholson IA, del Nido PJ, et al: Surgical management of complex and tunnel-like subaortic stenosis. *Eur J Cardiothorac Surg* 2000;17:637–642.

Laudito A, Brook MM, Suleman S, et al: The Ross procedure in children and young adults: A word of caution. *J Thorac Cardiovasc Surg* 2001;122: 147–153.

Leichter DA, Sullivan I, Gersony WM: "Acquired" discrete subvalvular aortic stenosis: Natural history and hemodynamics. *J Am Coll Cardiol* 1989;14: 1539–1544.

Marino BS, Bridges ND, Paridon SM: Aortic insufficiency: Indications for surgery in children. *Semin Thorac Cardiovasc Surg Pediatr Card Surg Annu* 1998;1:147–156.

Ohye RG, Gomez CA, Ohye BJ, et al: The Ross/Konno procedure in neonates and infants: Intermediate-term survival and autograft function. *Ann Thorac Surg* 2001;72:823–830.

Pessotto R, Wells WJ, Baker CJ, et al: Midterm results of the Ross procedure. *Ann Thorac Surg* 2001;71(5 Suppl):S336–S339.

Rocchini A, Beekman RH, Ben Shachar G, et al: Balloon aortic valvuloplasty: Results of the valvuloplasty and angioplasty of congenital anomalies registry. *Am J Cardiol* 1990;65:784–789.

Tweddell JS, Pelech AN, Frommelt PC, et al: Complex aortic valve repair as a durable and effective alternative to valve replacement in children with aortic valve disease. *J Thorac Cardiovasc Surg* 2005;129:551–558.

Coarctation of the Aorta

Daniels SR: Repair of coarctation of the aorta and hypertension: Does age matter? *Lancet* 2001;358:89.

Hamdan MA, Maheshwari S, Fahey JT: Endovascular stents for coarctation of the aorta: Initial results and intermediate-term follow-up. *J Am Coll Cardiol* 2001;38:1518–1523.

Ing FF, Starc TJ, Griffiths SP, et al: Early diagnosis of coarctation of the aorta in children: A continuing dilemma. *Pediatrics* 1996;98:378–382.

Markham LW, Knecht SK, Daniels SR, et al: Development of exercise-induced arm-leg blood pressure gradient and abnormal arterial compliance in patients with repaired coarctation of the aorta. *Am J Cardiol* 2004;94:1200–1202.

Metry DW, Dowd CF, Barkovich J, et al: The many faces of PHACE syndrome. *J Pediatr* 2001;139:117–123.

O'Sullivan JJ, Derrick G, Darnell R: Prevalence of hypertension in children after early repair of coarctation of the aorta: A cohort study using casual and 24 hour blood pressure measurement. *Heart* 2002;88:163–166.

Shone JD, Sellers RD, Anderson RC, et al: The developmental complex of "parachute mitral valve," supravalvar ring of left atrium, subaortic stenosis, and coarctation of the aorta. *Am J Cardiol* 1963;11:714–725.

Mitral Stenosis

Moore P, Adatia I, Spevak PJ, et al: Severe congenital mitral stenosis in infants. *Circulation* 1994;89:2099–2106.

Spevak PJ, Bass JL, Ben-Shachar G, et al: Balloon angioplasty for congenital mitral stenosis. *Am J Cardiol* 1990;66:472–476.

Chapter 428 ■ Acyanotic Congenital Heart Disease: Regurgitant Lesions

428.1 • Pulmonary Valvular Insufficiency and Congenital Absence of the Pulmonary Valve

Pulmonary valvular insufficiency most often accompanies other cardiovascular diseases or may be secondary to severe pulmonary hypertension. Incompetence of the valve is an expected result after surgery for right ventricular outflow tract obstruction, for example, pulmonary valvotomy in patients with valvular pulmonic stenosis or valvotomy with infundibular resection in patients with the tetralogy of Fallot. Isolated congenital insufficiency of the pulmonary valve is rare. These patients are usually asymptomatic because the insufficiency is generally mild.

The prominent physical sign is a decrescendo diastolic murmur at the upper and midleft sternal border, which has a lower pitch than the murmur of aortic insufficiency because of the lower pressure involved. Roentgenograms of the chest show prominence of the main pulmonary artery and, if the insufficiency is severe, right ventricular enlargement. The electrocardiogram is normal or shows minimal right ventricular hypertrophy. Pulsed and color Doppler studies demonstrate retrograde flow from the pulmonary artery to the right ventricle during diastole. The diagnosis can be made at cardiac catheterization if necessary. Pulmonary arterial diastolic pressure is low. Selective pulmonary arteriography shows the incompetent valve, but it is difficult to evaluate in mild cases because the catheter crossing the valve usually results in some iatrogenic insufficiency during the injection. Cardiac magnetic resonance angiography (MRA) is useful for quantifying both right ventricular volume and the regurgitant fraction. Isolated pulmonary valvular insufficiency is generally well tolerated and does not require surgical treatment. When pulmonary insufficiency is severe, especially if significant tricuspid insufficiency is also present, replacement with a homograft valve may become necessary to preserve right ventricular function.

Congenital absence of the pulmonary valve is usually associated with a ventricular septal defect, often in the context of the tetralogy of Fallot (see Chapter 430.1). In many of these neonates, the pulmonary arteries become widely dilated and compress the bronchi, with subsequent recurrent episodes of wheezing, pulmonary collapse, and pneumonitis. The presence and degree of cyanosis are variable. Florid pulmonary valvular incompetence may not be well tolerated, and death may occur from a combination of bronchial compression, hypoxemia, and heart failure. Correction involves plication of the massively dilated pulmonary arteries, closure of the ventricular septal defect, and placement of a homograft across the right ventricular outflow tract.

428.2 • Congenital Mitral Insufficiency

Congenital mitral insufficiency may be isolated but is more often associated with other anomalies, including patent ductus arteriosus, coarctation of the aorta, ventricular septal defect, corrected transposition of the great vessels, anomalous origin of the left coronary artery from the pulmonary artery, or Marfan syndrome. Mitral insufficiency is common in patients with atrioventricular septal defects (see Chapter 426.5). Mitral insufficiency can also be seen in patients with dilated cardiomyopathy (see Chapter 439.1) secondary to dilatation of the valve ring.

In isolated mitral insufficiency, the mitral valve annulus is usually dilated, the chordae tendineae are short and may insert anomalously, and the valve leaflets are deformed. When mitral insufficiency is severe enough to cause clinical symptoms, the left atrium enlarges as a result of the regurgitant flow, and the left ventricle becomes hypertrophied and dilated. Pulmonary venous pressure is increased, and the increased pressure ultimately results in pulmonary hypertension and right ventricular hypertrophy and dilatation. Mild lesions produce no symptoms; the only abnormal sign is the holosystolic murmur of mitral incompetence. Severe regurgitation results in symptoms that can appear at any age, including poor physical development, frequent respiratory infections, fatigue on exertion, and episodes of pulmonary edema or congestive heart failure. Often, a diagnosis of reactive airway disease will have been made because of the similarity in pulmonary symptoms.

The typical murmur of mitral insufficiency is a high-pitched, apical holosystolic murmur. If the insufficiency is moderate to severe, it is usually associated with a low-pitched, apical mid-diastolic rumbling murmur indicative of increased diastolic flow across the mitral valve. The pulmonary component of the 2nd heart sound will be accentuated in the presence of pulmonary hypertension. The electrocardiogram usually shows bifid P waves, signs of left ventricular hypertrophy, and sometimes signs of right ventricular hypertrophy. Roentgenographic examination shows enlargement of the left atrium, which at times is massive. The left ventricle is prominent, and pulmonary vascularity is normal or prominent. The echocardiogram demonstrates the enlarged left atrium and ventricle. Color Doppler demonstrates the extent of insufficiency, and pulsed Doppler of the pulmonary veins detects retrograde flow when mitral insufficiency is severe. Cardiac catheterization shows elevated left atrial pressure. Pulmonary artery hypertension of varying severity may be present. Selective left ventriculography reveals the severity of mitral regurgitation.

Mitral valvuloplasty can result in striking improvement in symptoms and heart size, but in some patients, installation of a prosthetic mechanical mitral valve may be necessary. Before surgery, associated anomalies must be identified. In children older than 3–4 yr, it may be difficult to exclude rheumatic fever as the cause of mitral insufficiency.

428.3 • Mitral Valve Prolapse

Mitral valve prolapse results from an abnormal mitral valve mechanism that causes billowing of one or both mitral leaflets, especially the posterior cusp, into the left atrium toward the end of systole. The abnormality is predominantly congenital but may not be recognized until adolescence or adulthood. Mitral valve prolapse is usually sporadic, is more common in girls, and may be inherited as an autosomal dominant trait with variable expression. It is common in patients with Marfan syndrome, straight back syndrome, pectus excavatum, scoliosis, Ehlers-Danlos syndrome, osteogenesis imperfecta, and pseudoxanthoma elasticum. The dominant abnormal signs are auscultatory, although occasional patients may have chest pain or palpitations. The apical murmur is late systolic and may be preceded by a click, but these signs may vary in the same patient and, at times, only the click is audible. In the standing or sitting position, the click may occur earlier in systole, and the murmur may be more prominent in late systole. Arrhythmias may occur and are primarily unifocal or multifocal premature ventricular contractions.

The electrocardiogram is usually normal but may show biphasic T waves, especially in leads II, III, aVF, and V_6; the T-wave abnormalities may vary at different times in the same patient. The chest roentgenogram is normal. The echocardiogram shows a characteristic posterior movement of the posterior mitral leaflet during mid or late systole or demonstrates pansystolic prolapse of both the anterior and posterior mitral leaflets. These M-mode echocardiographic findings must be interpreted cautiously because the appearance of minimal mitral prolapse may be a normal variant. Prolapse is more precisely defined by single or bileaflet prolapse of >2 mm beyond the long axis annular plane with or without leaflet thickening. Prolapse with valve thickening >5 mm is "classic," a lesser degree is "non-classic." Two-dimensional real-time echocardiography shows that both the free edge and the body of the mitral leaflets move posteriorly in systole toward the left atrium. Doppler can assess the presence and severity of mitral regurgitation.

This lesion is not progressive in childhood, and specific therapy is not indicated. The patient may be at risk for the development of infective endocarditis. Antibiotic prophylaxis is recommended during surgery and dental procedures (see Chapter 437).

Adults (men more often than women) with mitral valve prolapse are at increased risk for cardiovascular complications (sudden death, arrhythmia, cerebrovascular accidents, progressive valve dilatation, heart failure, and endocarditis) in the presence of **thickened** (>5 mm) and **redundant** mitral valve leaflets. Risk factors for morbidity also include poor left ventricular function, moderate to severe mitral regurgitation, and left atrial enlargement.

Often, confusion exists concerning the diagnosis of mitral valve prolapse. The high frequency of mild prolapse on the echocardiogram in the absence of clinical findings suggests that, in these cases, true mitral valve prolapse syndrome is not present. These patients and their parents should be reassured of this fact, and no special recommendations should be made regarding management or frequent laboratory studies. Endocarditis prophylaxis is indicated only in substantiated cases, usually those with mitral insufficiency.

428.4 • Tricuspid Regurgitation

Isolated tricuspid regurgitation is generally associated with **Ebstein anomaly** of the tricuspid valve. Ebstein anomaly may occur either without cyanosis or with varying degrees of cyanosis, depending on the severity of the tricuspid regurgitation and the presence of an atrial-level communication (patent foramen ovale or atrial septal defect). Older children tend to have the acyanotic form, whereas, if detected in the newborn period, Ebstein anomaly is usually associated with severe cyanosis (see Chapter 430.7).

Tricuspid regurgitation often accompanies **right ventricular dysfunction.** When the right ventricle becomes dilated because of volume overload or intrinsic myocardial disease, or both, the tricuspid annulus also enlarges, with resultant valve insufficiency. This form of regurgitation may improve if the cause of the right ventricular dilatation is corrected, or it may require surgical plication of the valve annulus. Tricuspid regurgitation is also encountered in newborns with **perinatal asphyxia.** The cause may be related to an increased susceptibility of the papillary muscles to ischemic damage and subsequent transient papillary muscle dysfunction.

Absent Pulmonary Valve

McDonnell BE, Raff GW, Gaynor JW, et al: Outcome after repair of tetralogy of Fallot with absent pulmonary valve. *Ann Thorac Surg* 1999;67:1391–1395.

Pinsky WW: Absent pulmonary valve syndrome. In Garson A, Bricker JT, Fisher DJ, Neish SR (editors): *The Science and Practice of Pediatric Cardiology.* Baltimore, Williams & Wilkins, 1998, pp 1413–1419.

Mitral Valve Anomalies

American Academy of Pediatrics Committee on Sports Medicine and Fitness: Mitral valve prolapse and athletic participation in children and adolescents. *Pediatrics* 1995;95:789–790.
Bouknight DP, O'Rourke RA: Current management of mitral valve prolapse. *Am Fam Physician* 2000;61:3343–3350, 3353–3354.
Hayek E, Gring CN, Griffin BP: Mitral valve prolapse. *Lancet* 2005;365:507–518.
Jacobs W, Chamoun A, Stouffer GA: Mitral valve prolapse: A review of the literature. *Am J Med Sci* 2001;321:401–410.
Maron BJ, Ackerman MJ, Nishimura RA, et al: Task Force 4: HCM and other cardiomyopathies, mitral valve prolapse, myocarditis, and Marfan syndrome. *J Am Coll Cardiol* 2005;45:1340–1345.

Chapter 429 ■ Cyanotic Congenital Heart Disease: Evaluation of the Critically Ill Neonate with Cyanosis and Respiratory Distress

See also Chapter 101.

A severely ill neonate with cardiorespiratory distress and cyanosis is a diagnostic challenge. The clinician must perform a rapid evaluation to determine whether congenital heart disease is a cause so that potentially lifesaving measures can be instituted. The differential diagnosis of neonatal cyanosis is presented in Table 101-1.

CARDIAC DISEASE. Congenital heart disease produces cyanosis when obstruction to right ventricular outflow causes intracardiac right-to-left shunting or when complex anatomic defects, unassociated with pulmonary stenosis, cause an admixture of pulmonary and systemic venous return in the heart. Cyanosis from pulmonary edema may also develop in patients with heart failure caused by left-to-right shunts, although the degree is usually less severe. Cyanosis may be caused by persistence of fetal pathways, for example, right-to-left shunting across the foramen ovale and ductus arteriosus in the presence of pulmonary outflow tract obstruction or persistent pulmonary hypertension of the newborn (PPHN) (see Chapter 101.8).

DIFFERENTIAL DIAGNOSIS. The initial evaluation of a cyanotic infant begins with observation of the breathing pattern. Weak or irregular respiration is often associated with a weak sucking reflex and a central nervous system (CNS) problem. Convulsions and general depression strongly suggest a CNS cause. An infant with primary cardiac or pulmonary disease, in contrast, displays vigorous or labored respirations with tachypnea.

The **hyperoxia test** is one method of distinguishing cyanotic congenital heart disease from pulmonary disease. Neonates with cyanotic congenital heart disease do not usually have significantly raised arterial PaO_2 during administration of 100% oxygen. If the PaO_2 rises above 150 mm Hg during 100% oxygen administration, an intracardiac shunt can usually be excluded, although the PaO_2 of some patients with cyanotic congenital heart lesions may be transiently increased to >150 mm Hg because of intracardiac streaming patterns. The PaO_2 in patients with pulmonary disease generally increases significantly as ventilation-perfusion inequalities are overcome by oxygen administration. In infants with a CNS disorder, the PaO_2 normalizes completely during artificial ventilation. Hypoxia in many heart lesions is profound and constant, whereas in respiratory disorders and in persistent pulmonary hypertension of the neonate (PPHN), arterial oxygen tension is not as low and often varies with time or changes in ventilator management. Hyperventilation may improve the hypoxia in neonates with PPHN and only occasionally in those with cyanotic heart disease.

Although a significant heart murmur usually suggests a cardiac basis for the cyanosis, several of the more severe cardiac defects (transposition of the great vessels) may not initially be associated with a murmur. The chest roentgenogram may be helpful in the differentiation of pulmonary and cardiac disease; in the latter, it indicates whether pulmonary blood flow is increased, normal, or decreased.

Two-dimensional echocardiography is the definitive noninvasive test to determine the presence of congenital heart disease. Cardiac catheterization is usually performed to examine structures that are not easily visible by echo; distal branch pulmonary arteries or aortopulmonary collateral arteries in patients with tetralogy of Fallot with pulmonary atresia (see Chapter 430.2); coronary arteries and right ventricular sinusoids in patients with pulmonary atresia and intact ventricular septum (see Chapter 430.3). If echocardiography is not immediately available, the clinician caring for a newborn with possible cyanotic heart disease should not hesitate to start a prostaglandin infusion (for a possible ductal-dependent lesion). Because of the risk of hypoventilation associated with prostaglandins, a practitioner skilled in neonatal endotracheal intubation must be available.

Chapter 430 ■ Cyanotic Congenital Heart Lesions: Lesions Associated with Decreased Pulmonary Blood Flow

430.1 • Tetralogy of Fallot

Tetralogy of Fallot is one of the conotruncal family of heart lesions in which the primary defect is an anterior deviation of the infundibular septum (the muscular septum that separates the aortic and pulmonary outflows). The consequences of this deviation are (1) obstruction to right ventricular outflow (pulmonary stenosis), (2) ventricular septal defect (VSD), (3) dextroposition of the aorta with override of the ventricular septum, and (4) right ventricular hypertrophy (Fig. 430-1). Obstruction to pulmonary arterial blood flow is usually at both the right ventricular infundibulum (subpulmonic area) and the pulmonary valve. The main pulmonary artery is often small, and various degrees of branch pulmonary artery stenosis may be present. Complete obstruction of right ventricular outflow (pulmonary atresia with VSD) is classified as an extreme form of tetralogy of Fallot (see Chapter 430.2). The degree of pulmonary outflow obstruction varies, with the severity of the obstruction determining the degree of the patient's cyanosis.

PATHOPHYSIOLOGY. The pulmonary valve annulus may be of nearly normal size or quite small. The valve itself is often bicuspid and, occasionally, is the only site of stenosis. More commonly, the subpulmonic or infundibular muscle, the crista supraventricularis, is hypertrophic, which contributes to the subvalvar stenosis and results in an infundibular chamber of variable size and contour. When the right ventricular outflow tract is completely

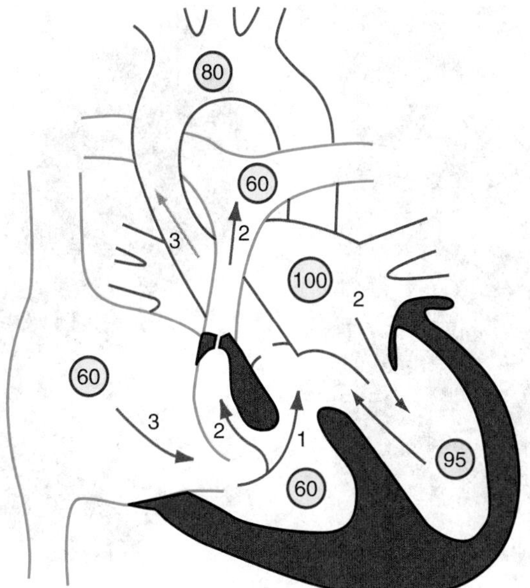

Figure 430-1. Physiology of the tetralogy of Fallot. Circled numbers represent oxygen saturation values. The numbers next to the *arrows* represent volumes of blood flow (in L/min/m^2). Atrial (mixed venous) oxygen saturation is decreased because of the systemic hypoxemia. A volume of 3 L/min/m^2 of desaturated blood enters the right atrium and traverses the tricuspid valve. Two liters flows through the right ventricular outflow tract into the lungs, whereas 1 L shunts right to left through the ventricular septal defect (VSD) into the ascending aorta. Thus, pulmonary blood flow is two thirds normal (Qp : Qs [pulmonary-to-systemic blood flow ratio] of 0.7 : 1). Blood returning to the left atrium is fully saturated. Only 2 L of blood flows across the mitral valve. Oxygen saturation in the left ventricle may be slightly decreased because of right-to-left shunting across the VSD. Two liters of saturated left ventricular blood mixing with 1 L of desaturated right ventricular blood is ejected into the ascending aorta. Aortic saturation is decreased, and cardiac output is normal.

obstructed (**pulmonary atresia**), the anatomy of the branch pulmonary arteries is extremely variable; a main pulmonary artery segment may be in continuity with right ventricular outflow, separated by a fibrous but imperforate pulmonary valve, or the entire main pulmonary artery segment may be absent. Occasionally, the branch pulmonary arteries may be discontinuous. In these more severe cases, pulmonary blood flow may be supplied by a patent ductus arteriosus (PDA) and by multiple **major aortopulmonary collateral arteries (MAPCAs)** arising from the ascending and descending aorta.

The VSD is usually nonrestrictive and large, is located just below the aortic valve, and is related to the posterior and right aortic cusps. Rarely, the VSD may be in the inlet portion of the ventricular septum (atrioventricular septal defect). The normal fibrous continuity of the mitral and aortic valves is usually maintained. The aortic arch is right sided in 20% of cases, and the aortic root is usually large and overrides the VSD to a varying degree. When the aorta overrides the VSD by more than 50% and if there is muscle separating the aortic valve and the mitral annulus (subaortic conus), this defect is usually classified as a form of double-outlet right ventricle; however, the pathophysiology is the same as that of tetralogy of Fallot.

Systemic venous return to the right atrium and right ventricle is normal. When the right ventricle contracts in the presence of marked pulmonary stenosis, blood is shunted across the VSD into the aorta. Persistent arterial desaturation and cyanosis result. Pulmonary blood flow, when severely restricted by the obstruction to right ventricular outflow, may be supplemented by the bronchial collateral circulation (MAPCAs) and, in the newborn, by a PDA. Peak systolic and diastolic pressures in each ventricle are similar and at systemic level. A large pressure gradient occurs across the obstructed right ventricular outflow tract, and pulmonary arterial pressure is normal or lower than normal. The degree of right ventricular outflow obstruction determines the timing of the onset of symptoms, the severity of cyanosis, and the degree of right ventricular hypertrophy. When obstruction to right ventricular outflow is mild to moderate and a balanced shunt is present across the VSD, the patient may not be visibly cyanotic (**acyanotic** or **"pink"** tetralogy of Fallot). When obstruction is severe, cyanosis will be present from birth and worsen when the ductus begins to close.

CLINICAL MANIFESTATIONS. Infants with mild degrees of right ventricular outflow obstruction may initially be seen with heart failure caused by a ventricular-level left-to-right shunt. Often, cyanosis is not present at birth, but with increasing hypertrophy of the right ventricular infundibulum and patient growth, cyanosis occurs later in the 1st yr of life. It is most prominent in the mucous membranes of the lips and mouth and in the fingernails and toenails. In infants with severe degrees of right ventricular outflow obstruction, neonatal cyanosis is noted immediately. In these infants, pulmonary blood flow may be dependent on flow through the ductus arteriosus. When the ductus begins to close in the 1st few hours or days of life, severe cyanosis and circulatory collapse may occur. Older children with long-standing cyanosis who have not undergone surgery may have dusky blue skin, gray sclerae with engorged blood vessels, and marked clubbing of the fingers and toes. Extracardiac manifestations of long-standing cyanotic congenital heart disease are described in Chapter 434.

Dyspnea occurs on exertion. Infants and toddlers play actively for a short time and then sit or lie down. Older children may be able to walk a block or so before stopping to rest. Characteristically, children assume a squatting position for the relief of dyspnea caused by physical effort; the child is usually able to resume physical activity within a few minutes. These findings occur most often in patients with significant cyanosis at rest.

Paroxysmal hypercyanotic attacks (hypoxic, **"blue,"** or **"tet" spells**) are a particular problem during the 1st 2 yr of life. The infant becomes hyperpneic and restless, cyanosis increases, gasping respirations ensue, and syncope may follow. The spells occur most frequently in the morning on initially awakening or after episodes of vigorous crying. Temporary disappearance or a decrease in intensity of the systolic murmur is usual as flow across the right ventricular outflow tract diminishes. The spells may last from a few minutes to a few hours but are rarely fatal. Short episodes are followed by generalized weakness and sleep. Severe spells may progress to unconsciousness and, occasionally, to convulsions or hemiparesis. The onset is usually spontaneous and unpredictable. Spells are associated with reduction of an already compromised pulmonary blood flow, which, when prolonged, results in severe systemic hypoxia and metabolic acidosis. Infants who are only mildly cyanotic at rest are often more prone to the development of hypoxic spells because they have not acquired the homeostatic mechanisms to tolerate rapid lowering of arterial oxygen saturation, such as polycythemia.

Depending on the frequency and severity of hypercyanotic attacks, one or more of the following procedures should be instituted in sequence: (1) placement of the infant on the abdomen in the knee-chest position while making certain that the infant's clothing is not constrictive, (2) administration of oxygen (although increasing inspired oxygen will not reverse cyanosis caused by intracardiac shunting), and (3) injection of morphine subcutaneously in a dose not in excess of 0.2 mg/kg. Calming and holding the infant in a knee-chest position may abort progression of an early spell. Premature attempts to obtain blood samples may cause further agitation and be counterproductive.

Because metabolic acidosis develops when arterial PO_2 is <40 mm Hg, rapid correction (within several minutes) with intravenous administration of sodium bicarbonate is necessary if the spell is unusually severe and the child shows a lack of response to the foregoing therapy. Recovery from the spell is usually rapid once the pH has returned to normal. Repeated blood pH measurements may be necessary because rapid recurrence of acidosis may ensue. For spells that are resistant to this therapy, drugs that increase systemic vascular resistance, such as intravenous phenylephrine, can improve right ventricular outflow, decrease the right-to-left shunt, and improve the symptoms. β-Adrenergic blockade by the intravenous administration of propranolol (0.1 mg/kg given slowly to a maximum of 0.2 mg/kg) is also useful.

Growth and development may be delayed in patients with severe untreated tetralogy of Fallot, particularly when oxygen saturation is chronically <70%. Puberty may also be delayed in patients who do not undergo surgery.

The pulse is usually normal, as is venous and arterial pressure. The left anterior hemithorax may bulge anteriorly because of right ventricular hypertrophy. The heart is generally normal in size, and a substernal right ventricular impulse can be detected. In about half the cases, a systolic thrill is felt along the left sternal border in the 3rd and 4th parasternal spaces. The systolic murmur is usually loud and harsh; it may be transmitted widely, especially to the lungs, but is most intense at the left sternal border. The murmur is generally ejection in quality at the upper sternal border, but it may sound more holosystolic toward the lower sternal border. It may be preceded by a click. The murmur is caused by turbulence through the right ventricular outflow tract. It tends to become louder, longer, and harsher as the severity of pulmonary stenosis increases from mild to moderate; however, it can actually become less prominent with severe obstruction, especially during a hypercyanotic spell. Either the 2nd heart sound is single, or the pulmonic component is soft. Infrequently, a continuous murmur may be audible, especially if prominent collaterals are present.

DIAGNOSIS. Roentgenographically, the typical configuration as seen in the anteroposterior view consists of a narrow base, concavity of the left heart border in the area usually occupied by the pulmonary artery, and normal heart size. The hypertrophied right ventricle causes the rounded apical shadow to be uptilted so that it is situated higher above the diaphragm than normal. The cardiac silhouette has been likened to that of a boot or wooden shoe ("coeur en sabot") (Fig. 430-2). The hilar areas and lung fields are relatively clear because of diminished pulmonary blood flow or the small size of the pulmonary arteries, or both. The aorta is usually large, and in about 20% of patients it arches to the right, which results in an indentation of the leftward-positioned air-filled tracheobronchial shadow in the anteroposterior view.

The electrocardiogram demonstrates right axis deviation and evidence of right ventricular hypertrophy. A dominant R wave appears in the right precordial chest leads (Rs, R, qR, qRs) or an RSR′ pattern. In some cases, the only sign of right ventricular hypertrophy may initially be a positive T wave in leads V_3R and V_1. The P wave is tall and peaked or sometimes bifid (see Fig. 423-8).

Two-dimensional echocardiography establishes the diagnosis (Fig. 430-3) and provides information about the extent of aortic override of the septum, the location and degree of the right ventricular outflow tract obstruction, the size of the proximal branch pulmonary arteries, and the side of the aortic arch. The echocardiogram is also useful in determining whether a PDA is supplying a portion of the pulmonary blood flow. In a patient without pulmonary atresia, echocardiography usually obviates the need for catheterization before surgical repair.

Cardiac catheterization demonstrates a systolic pressure in the right ventricle equal to systemic pressure. If the pulmonary artery is entered, the pressure is markedly decreased, although crossing the right ventricular outflow tract, especially in severe cases, may precipitate a tet spell. Pulmonary arterial pressure is usually lower than normal, in the range of 5–10 mm Hg. The level of arterial oxygen saturation depends on the magnitude of the right-to-left shunt; in "pink tets," systemic saturation may be normal, whereas in a moderately cyanotic patient at rest, it is usually 75–85%.

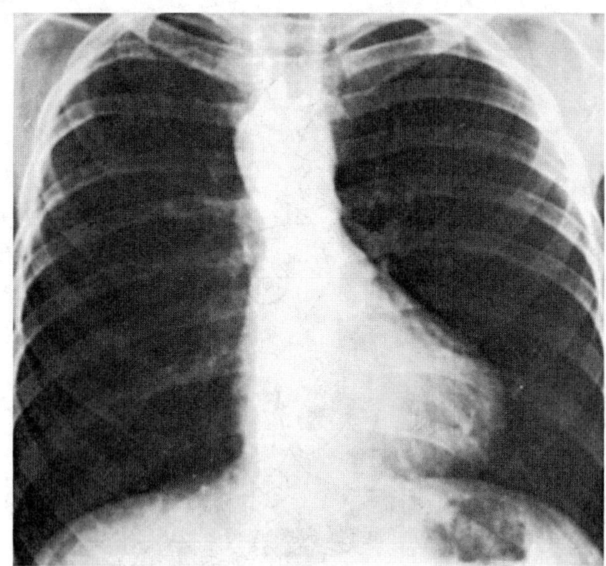

Figure 430-2. Chest x-ray of an 8 yr old boy with the tetralogy of Fallot. Note the normal heart size, some elevation of the cardiac apex, concavity in the region of the main pulmonary artery, right-sided aortic arch, and diminished pulmonary vascularity.

Selective right ventriculography best demonstrates the anatomy of the tetralogy of Fallot. Contrast medium outlines the heavily trabeculated right ventricle. The infundibular stenosis varies in length, width, contour, and distensibility (Fig. 430-4). The pulmonary valve is usually thickened, and the annulus may be small. In patients with pulmonary atresia and VSD, the anatomy of the pulmonary vessels may be extremely complex; for example, there may be discontinuity between the right and left pulmonary arteries. Complete and accurate information regarding the anatomy of the pulmonary arteries and any collateral vessels (MAPCAs) is important when evaluating these children as surgical candidates.

Left ventriculography demonstrates the size of the left ventricle, the position of the VSD, and the overriding aorta; it also

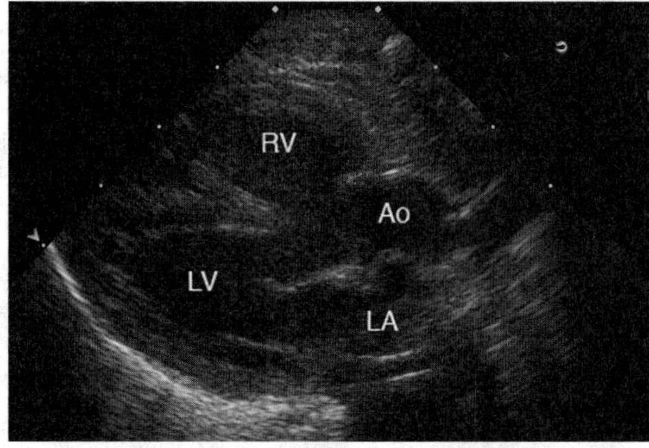

Figure 430-3. Echocardiogram in a patient with the tetralogy of Fallot. This parasternal long-axis two-dimensional view demonstrates anterior displacement of the outflow ventricular septum that resulted in stenosis of the subpulmonic right ventricular outflow tract, overriding of the aorta, and an associated ventricular septal defect. Ao, overriding aorta; LA, left atrium; LV, left ventricle; RV, right ventricle.

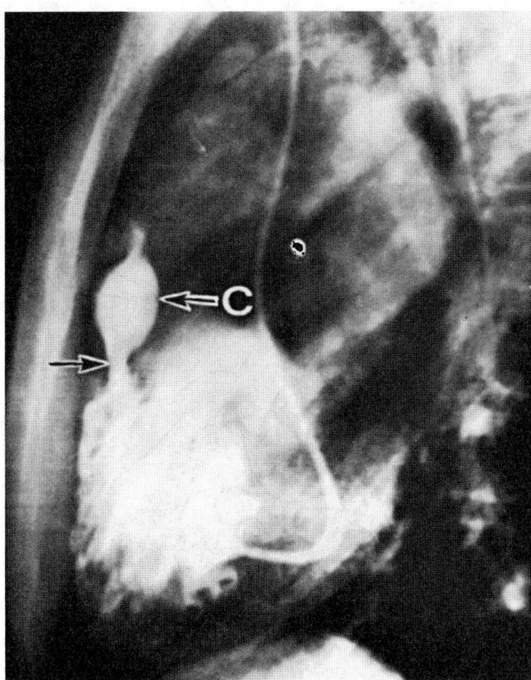

Figure 430-4. Lateral view of a selective right ventriculogram in a patient with the tetralogy of Fallot. The *arrow* points to an infundibular stenosis that is below the infundibular chamber (C). The narrowed pulmonary valve orifice is seen at the distal end of the infundibular chamber.

confirms mitral-aortic continuity, thereby ruling out a double-outlet right ventricle. Aortography or coronary arteriography outlines the course of the coronary arteries. In 5–10% of patients with the tetralogy of Fallot, an aberrant major coronary artery crosses over the right ventricular outflow tract; this artery must not be cut during surgical repair. Verification of normal coronary arteries is important when considering surgery in young infants who may need a patch across the pulmonary valve annulus. Echocardiography can usually delineate the coronary artery anatomy; angiography is reserved for cases in which questions remain.

COMPLICATIONS. Before correction, patients with the tetralogy of Fallot are susceptible to several serious complications. Fortunately, most children undergo palliation or, more often, complete repair in infancy, and these complications are rare. **Cerebral thromboses,** usually occurring in the cerebral veins or dural sinuses and occasionally in the cerebral arteries, are common in the presence of extreme polycythemia and dehydration. Thromboses occur most often in patients younger than 2 yr. These patients may have iron deficiency anemia, frequently with hemoglobin and hematocrit levels in the normal range (but too low for cyanotic heart disease). Therapy consists of adequate hydration and supportive measures. Phlebotomy and volume replacement with albumin or saline are indicated in extremely **polycythemic** patients who are symptomatic.

Brain abscess is less common than cerebral vascular events and extremely rare when most patients are repaired at young ages. Patients with a brain abscess are usually older than 2 yr. The onset of the illness is often insidious and consists of low-grade fever or a gradual change in behavior, or both. Some patients have an acute onset of symptoms that may develop after a recent history of headache, nausea, and vomiting. Seizures may occur; localized neurologic signs depend on the site and size of the abscess and the presence of increased intracranial pressure. CT or MRI confirms the diagnosis. Antibiotic therapy may help keep the infection localized, but surgical drainage of the abscess is usually necessary (see Chapter 603).

Bacterial endocarditis may occur in the right ventricular infundibulum or on the pulmonic, aortic, or, rarely, tricuspid valves. Endocarditis may complicate palliative shunts or, in patients with corrective surgery, any residual pulmonic stenosis or VSD. Antibiotic prophylaxis is essential before and after dental and certain surgical procedures associated with a high incidence of bacteremia (see Chapter 437).

Heart failure is not a usual feature in patients with the tetralogy of Fallot. It may occur in a young infant with "pink" or acyanotic tetralogy of Fallot. As the degree of pulmonary obstruction worsens with age, the symptoms of heart failure resolve and eventually the patient experiences cyanosis, often by 6–12 mo of age. These patients are at increased risk for hypercyanotic spells at this time.

ASSOCIATED ANOMALIES. An associated PDA may be present, and defects in the atrial septum are occasionally seen. A right aortic arch occurs in ≈20% of patients with the tetralogy of Fallot, and other anomalies of the pulmonary arteries and aortic arch may also be seen. Persistence of a left superior vena cava draining into the coronary sinus may be noted. Multiple VSDs are occasionally present and must be diagnosed before corrective surgery. Tetralogy of Fallot may also occur with an atrioventricular septal defect, often associated with Down syndrome.

Congenital absence of the pulmonary valve produces a distinct syndrome that is usually marked by signs of upper airway obstruction (see Chapter 428.1). Cyanosis may be absent, mild, or moderate; the heart is large and hyperdynamic; and a loud to-and-fro murmur is present. Marked aneurysmal dilatation of the main and branch pulmonary arteries results in compression of the bronchi and produces stridulous or wheezing respirations and recurrent pneumonia. If the airway obstruction is severe, reconstruction of the trachea at the time of corrective cardiac surgery may be required to alleviate the symptoms.

Absence of a branch pulmonary artery, most often the left, should be suspected if the roentgenographic appearance of the pulmonary vasculature differs on the two sides; absence of a pulmonary artery is often associated with hypoplasia of the affected lung. It is important to recognize the absence of a pulmonary artery because occlusion of the remaining pulmonary artery during surgery seriously compromises the already reduced pulmonary blood flow.

As one of the conotruncal malformations, the tetralogy of Fallot can be associated with the spectrum of lesions known as **CATCH 22** (cardiac defects, abnormal facies, thymic hypoplasia, cleft palate, hypocalcemia). CATCH 22 includes patients with clinical features of the DiGeorge syndrome (hypocalcemia, thymic hypoplasia, mild facial anomalies) or the **Shprintzen velocardiofacial syndrome** (abnormal facies, cleft palate). Cytogenetic analysis using fluorescence in situ hybridization demonstrates deletions of a large segment of chromosome 22q11 known as the DiGeorge critical region. Deletion or mutation of the gene encoding the transcription factor *Tbx1* has been implicated as a possible cause of DiGeorge syndrome.

TREATMENT. Treatment of the tetralogy of Fallot depends on the severity of the right ventricular outflow tract obstruction. Infants with severe tetralogy require medical treatment and surgical intervention in the neonatal period. Therapy is aimed at providing an immediate increase in pulmonary blood flow to prevent the sequelae of severe hypoxia. The infant should be transported to a medical center adequately equipped to evaluate and treat neonates with congenital heart disease under optimal conditions. It is critical that oxygenation and normal body temperature be maintained during the transfer. Prolonged, severe hypoxia may lead to shock, respiratory failure, and intractable acidosis and will significantly reduce the chance of survival, even when surgically amenable lesions are present. Cold increases oxygen consumption, which places additional stress on a cyanotic infant, whose oxygen delivery is already limited. Blood glucose levels should be monitored because hypoglycemia is more likely to develop in infants with cyanotic heart disease.

Neonates with marked right ventricular outflow tract obstruction may deteriorate rapidly because, as the ductus arteriosus begins to close, pulmonary blood flow is further compromised. The intravenous administration of prostaglandin E_1 (0.01–0.20 μg/kg/min), a potent and specific relaxant of ductal smooth muscle, causes dilatation of the ductus arteriosus and usually provides adequate pulmonary blood flow until a surgical procedure can be performed. This agent should be administered intravenously as soon as cyanotic congenital heart disease is clinically suspected and continued through the preoperative period and during cardiac catheterization.

Infants with less severe right ventricular outflow tract obstruction who are stable and awaiting surgical intervention require careful observation. Prevention or prompt treatment of dehydration is important to avoid hemoconcentration and possible thrombotic episodes. Paroxysmal dyspneic attacks in infancy or early childhood may be precipitated by a relative iron deficiency; iron therapy may decrease their frequency and also improve exercise tolerance and general well-being. Red blood cell indices should be maintained in the normocytic range. Oral propranolol (0.5–1 mg/kg every 6 hr) had been used more commonly in the past to decrease the frequency and severity of hypercyanotic spells, but with the excellent surgery available, surgical treatment is now indicated as soon as spells begin.

Infants with symptoms and severe cyanosis in the 1st mo of life have marked obstruction of the right ventricular outflow tract or pulmonary atresia. Two options are available in these infants. The first, more common in previous years, is a palliative systemic-to-pulmonary artery shunt performed to augment pulmonary artery blood flow. The rationale for this surgery, previously the only option for these patients, is to decrease the amount of hypoxia and improve linear growth, as well as augment growth of the branch pulmonary arteries. The second option is corrective open heart surgery performed in early infancy and even in the newborn period in critically ill infants. This approach has widespread acceptance with excellent short- and long-term results and carries the theoretical advantage in that early physiologic correction allows for improved growth of the branch pulmonary arteries. In infants with less severe cyanosis who can be maintained with good growth and absence of hypercyanotic spells, primary repair is performed electively at between 4 and 6 mo of age.

The modified Blalock-Taussig shunt is currently the most common aortopulmonary shunt procedure and consists of a Gore-Tex conduit anastomosed side to side from the subclavian artery to the homolateral branch of the pulmonary artery (Fig. 430-5). Sometimes the shunt is brought directly from the ascending aorta to the main pulmonary artery and in this case is called a central shunt. The Blalock-Taussig operation can be successfully performed in the newborn period with shunts 3–4 mm in diameter and has also been used successfully in premature infants.

Postoperative complications after a Blalock-Taussig shunt include chylothorax, diaphragmatic paralysis, and Horner syndrome. Chylothorax may require repeated thoracocentesis and, on occasion, reoperation to ligate the thoracic duct. Diaphragmatic paralysis from injury to the phrenic nerve may result in a more difficult postoperative course. Prolonged ventilator support and vigorous physical therapy may be required, but diaphragmatic function usually returns in 1–2 mo unless the nerve was completely divided. Surgical plication of the diaphragm may be indicated. Horner syndrome is usually temporary and does not require treatment. Postoperative cardiac failure may be caused by a large shunt; its treatment is described in Chapter 442. Vascular problems other than a diminished radial pulse and occasional long-term arm length discrepancy are rarely seen in the upper extremity supplied by the subclavian artery used for the anastomosis.

After a successful shunt procedure, cyanosis diminishes. The development of a continuous murmur over the lung fields after the operation indicates a functioning anastomosis. A good continuous shunt murmur may not be heard until several days after surgery. The duration of symptomatic relief is variable. As the child grows, more pulmonary blood flow is needed and the shunt eventually becomes inadequate. When increasing cyanosis develops, a corrective operation should be performed if the anatomy is favorable. If not possible (because of hypoplastic branch pulmonary arteries) or if the 1st shunt lasts only a brief period in a small infant, a second aortopulmonary anastomosis may be required on the opposite side.

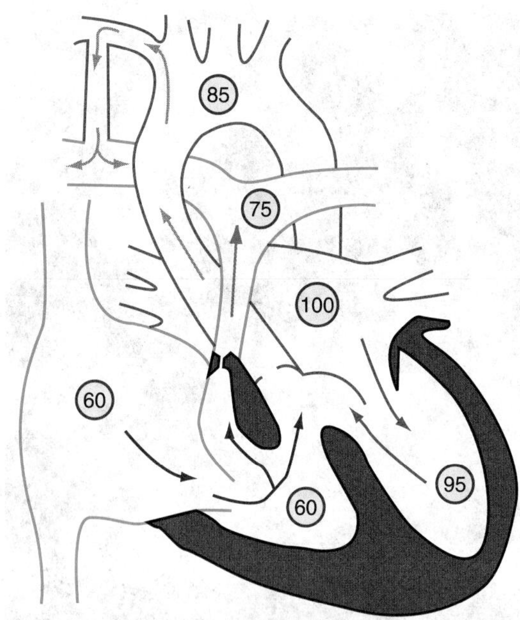

Figure 430-5. Physiology of a Blalock-Taussig shunt in a patient with the tetralogy of Fallot. *Circled numbers* represent oxygen saturation values. The intracardiac shunting pattern is as described for Figure 430-1. Blood shunting left to right across the shunt from the right subclavian artery to the right pulmonary artery increases total pulmonary blood flow and results in a higher oxygen saturation than would exist without the shunt (see Fig. 430-1).

Corrective surgical therapy consists of relief of the right ventricular outflow tract obstruction by removing obstructive muscle bundles and by patch closure of the VSD. If the pulmonary valve is stenotic, a valvotomy is performed. If the pulmonary valve annulus is small or the valve is extremely thickened, a valvectomy may be performed, the pulmonary valve annulus split open, and a transannular patch placed across the pulmonary valve ring. Any previously established systemic-to-pulmonary shunt must be ligated and divided before full repair. The surgical risk of total correction in major centers is <5%. A right ventriculotomy was once the standard approach; however, a **transatrial-transpulmonary** approach is routinely performed to reduce the long-term risks of a right ventriculotomy. Increased bleeding in the immediate postoperative period may be a complicating factor in extremely polycythemic patients.

PROGNOSIS. After successful total correction, patients are generally asymptomatic and are able to lead unrestricted lives. Uncommon immediate postoperative problems include right ventricular failure, transient heart block, residual VSD with left-to-right shunting, and myocardial infarction from interruption of an aberrant coronary artery. Postoperative heart failure (particularly in patients with a transannular outflow patch) may require diuretics and a positive inotropic agent such as digoxin. The long-term effects of isolated, surgically induced pulmonary valvular insufficiency are unknown, but insufficiency is generally well tolerated. The majority of patients after tetralogy repair and all of those with transannular patch repairs have a to-and-fro murmur at the left sternal border, usually indicative of mild outflow obstruction and mild to moderate pulmonary insufficiency. Patients with more marked pulmonary valve insufficiency also have moderate to marked heart enlargement. Patients with a severe residual gradient across the right ventricular outflow tract may require reoperation, but mild to moderate obstruction is usually present and does not require reintervention.

Follow-up of patients 5–20 yr after surgery indicates that the marked improvement in symptoms is generally maintained. Asymptomatic patients nonetheless have lower than normal exercise capacity, maximal heart rate, and cardiac output. These abnormal findings are more common in patients who underwent placement of a transannular outflow tract patch and may be less frequent when surgery is performed at an early age. As these children move into adolescence and adulthood, some (more commonly those with transannular patches) will develop right ventricular dilation due to severe pulmonary regurgitation. Careful lifelong follow-up by a specialist in adult congenital heart disease is important. Serial echocardiography and magnetic resonance angiography (MRA) are valuable tools for assessing the degree of right ventricular dilation, the presence of right ventricular dysfunction, and the regurgitant fraction. Valve replacement is indicated for those patients with increasing right ventricular pathology.

Conduction disturbances can occur after surgery. The atrioventricular node and the bundle of His and its divisions are in close proximity to the VSD and may be injured during surgery. Permanent complete heart block after surgery is rare. When present, it should be treated by placement of a permanently implanted pacemaker. Even transient complete heart block in the immediate postoperative period is rare; it may be associated with an increased incidence of late-onset complete heart block and sudden death. Right bundle branch block after right ventriculotomy is quite common on the postoperative electrocardiogram. The duration of the QRS interval has been shown to predict both the presence of residual hemodynamic derangement and the long-term risk of sudden death. Research is ongoing to determine the effectiveness of biventricular pacing (in which a pacemaker is used to resynchronize the activation of the right and left ventricles) in improving hemodynamics in those patients with long ventricular conduction delays.

A number of children have premature ventricular beats after repair of the tetralogy of Fallot. These beats are of concern in patients with residual hemodynamic abnormalities; 24-hr electrocardiographic (Holter) monitoring studies should be performed to be certain that occult short episodes of ventricular tachycardia are not occurring. Exercise studies may be useful in provoking cardiac arrhythmias that are not apparent at rest. In the presence of complex ventricular arrhythmias or severe residual hemodynamic abnormalities, prophylactic antiarrhythmic therapy is warranted. Re-repair is indicated if significant residual right ventricular outflow obstruction or severe pulmonary insufficiency is present.

430.2 • Tetralogy of Fallot with Pulmonary Atresia

PATHOPHYSIOLOGY. Tetralogy of a Fallot with pulmonary atresia is the most extreme form of the tetralogy of Fallot. The pulmonary valve is atretic, rudimentary, or absent, and the pulmonary trunk is atretic or hypoplastic. The entire right ventricular output is ejected into the aorta. Pulmonary blood flow is then dependent on a PDA or on collateral vessels (MAPCAs). The ultimate prognosis depends on the degree of development of the branch pulmonary arteries, which needs to be assessed by cardiac catheterization. If the pulmonary arteries are severely hypoplastic and fail to grow after palliative shunt procedures, heart-lung transplantation may be the only therapy (see Chapter 443.2). Pulmonary atresia with VSD is also associated with the CATCH 22 deletion and DiGeorge syndrome. The association of severe **tracheomalacia** or **bronchomalacia** with these severe forms of tetralogy/pulmonary atresia may complicate postoperative recovery.

CLINICAL MANIFESTATIONS. Patients with pulmonary atresia and VSD have findings similar to those in patients with severe tetralogy of Fallot. Cyanosis usually appears within the 1st few hours or days after birth, the prominent systolic murmur associated with the tetralogy is usually absent, the 1st heart sound is frequently followed by an ejection click caused by the enlarged aortic root, the 2nd sound is moderately loud and single, and continuous murmurs of a PDA or bronchial collateral flow may be heard over the entire precordium, both anteriorly and posteriorly. Most patients are moderately cyanotic and are initially stabilized with a prostaglandin E_1 infusion pending cardiac catheterization. Patients with several large MAPCAs may be less cyanotic and, once the diagnosis is confirmed, can be taken off prostaglandin while awaiting palliative surgical intervention. Some patients even have heart failure caused by increased pulmonary blood flow via these collateral vessels.

DIAGNOSIS. The chest roentgenogram demonstrates a small or enlarged heart (depending on the degree of pulmonary blood flow), a concavity at the position of the pulmonary arterial segment, and often the reticular pattern of bronchial collateral flow. The electrocardiogram shows right ventricular hypertrophy. The echocardiogram identifies aortic override, a thick right ventricular wall, and atresia of the pulmonary valve. Pulsed and color Doppler echocardiographic studies show an absence of forward flow through the pulmonary valve, with pulmonary blood flow being supplied by the ductus arteriosus or by MAPCAs. At cardiac catheterization, right ventriculography reveals a large aorta, opacified immediately by passage of contrast medium through the VSD, but with no dye entering the lungs through the right ventricular outflow tract. The pathway of pulmonary blood flow from the aorta to the lungs (ductus or collaterals) is demonstrated. Careful delineation of both native pulmonary arteries to determine whether they are continuous or discontinuous and the location and arborization of all MAPCAs by selective contrast injection is required to plan surgical correction.

TREATMENT. The surgical procedure of choice depends on whether the main pulmonary artery segment is adequate and on the size of the branch pulmonary arteries. If these arteries are well developed, a one-stage surgical repair with a homograft conduit between the right ventricle and pulmonary arteries and closure of the VSD is feasible. If the pulmonary arteries are hypoplastic, the prognosis is more guarded, and extensive reconstruction may be required. This usually involved several staged surgical procedures, beginning in early infancy, in which a connection is made between the aorta and the hypoplastic main pulmonary arteries (using either an aortopulmonary window or a central Blalock-Taussig type shunt) to induce growth. The multiple MAPCAs are gathered together (unifocalization procedure) and eventually incorporated into the final repair along with the native pulmonary arteries.

To be a candidate for full repair, the pulmonary arteries must be of adequate size to accept the full volume of right ventricular output. Complete repair includes closure of the VSD and placement of a homograft conduit from the right ventricle to the pulmonary artery. At the time of reparative surgery, previous shunts are taken down. Because of patient growth as well as homograft narrowing due to proliferation of intimal tissue and calcification, replacement of the homograft conduit replacement is usually required in later life, and multiple replacements may be needed. Patients often have malformations of the distal branches of the pulmonary arteries. These vessels are difficult to reconstruct surgically and are addressed by repeated transcatheter balloon dilatation and eventual stenting of the multiple branch pulmonary arterial stenoses.

Acquired total atresia of the right ventricular outflow tract may occur after an aortopulmonary shunt anastomosis for the tetralogy of Fallot. The systolic murmur resulting from pulmonary stenosis becomes attenuated and then disappears. The completeness of obstruction can be confirmed by echocardiography or by right ventriculography. Corrective surgery of the right ventricular outflow tract can be performed in a manner similar to that used for congenital pulmonary atresia.

430.3 • Pulmonary Atresia with Intact Ventricular Septum

PATHOPHYSIOLOGY. In pulmonary atresia with an intact ventricular septum, the pulmonary valve leaflets are completely fused to form a membrane and the right ventricular outflow tract is atretic. Because no VSD is present, no egress of blood from the right ventricle occurs. Right atrial pressure increases, and blood shunts via the foramen ovale into the left atrium, where it mixes with pulmonary venous blood and enters the left ventricle (Fig. 430-6). The combined left and right ventricular output is pumped solely by the left ventricle into the aorta. In a newborn with pulmonary atresia, the only source of pulmonary blood flow occurs via a **PDA.** The right ventricle is usually hypoplastic, although the degree of hypoplasia varies considerably. Patients who have

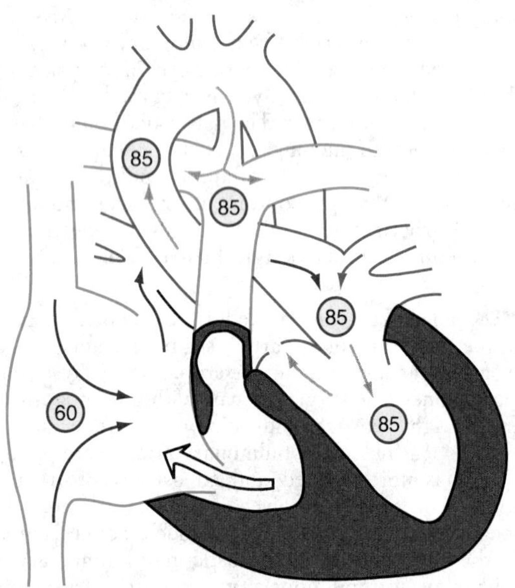

Figure 430-6. Physiology of pulmonary atresia with an intact ventricular septum. *Circled numbers* represent oxygen saturation values. Right atrial (mixed venous) oxygen saturation is decreased secondary to systemic hypoxemia. A small amount of the blood entering the right atrium may cross the tricuspid valve, which is often stenotic as well. The right ventricular cavity is hypertrophied and may be hypoplastic. No outlet from the right ventricle exists because of the atretic pulmonary valve; thus, any blood entering the right ventricle returns to the right atrium via tricuspid regurgitation. Most of the desaturated blood shunts right to left via the foramen ovale into the left atrium, where it mixes with fully saturated blood returning from the lungs. The only source of pulmonary blood flow is via the patent ductus arteriosus. Aortic and pulmonary arterial oxygen saturation will be identical (definition of a total mixing lesion).

a small right ventricular cavity also have a small tricuspid valve annulus, which limits right ventricular inflow. These patients may have **coronary sinusoidal channels** within the right ventricular wall that communicate directly with the coronary arterial circulation. The high right ventricular pressure results in desaturated blood flowing retrograde via collaterals into the coronary arteries and to the aorta. The prognosis in patients with these sinusoids is guarded, especially if they also have proximal stenosis of the coronary arteries. Patients with intermediate-sized or large ventricular cavities may have tricuspid insufficiency, which serves to decompress the right ventricle.

CLINICAL MANIFESTATIONS. As the ductus arteriosus closes in the 1st hours/days of life, infants with pulmonary atresia and an intact ventricular septum become markedly cyanotic. Untreated, most patients die within the 1st wk of life. Physical examination reveals severe cyanosis and respiratory distress. The 2nd heart sound is single and loud. Often, no murmurs are audible, but sometimes a systolic or continuous murmur can be heard secondary to ductal blood flow.

DIAGNOSIS. The electrocardiogram shows a frontal QRS axis between 0 and +90 degrees, the amount of leftward shift reflecting the degree of hypoplasia of the right ventricle. Tall, spiked P waves indicate right atrial enlargement. QRS voltages are consistent with left ventricular dominance or hypertrophy; right ventricular forces are decreased in proportion to the decreased size of the right ventricular cavity. Most patients with small right ventricles have decreased right ventricular forces, but, occasionally, patients with larger, thickened right ventricular cavities may have evidence of right ventricular hypertrophy. The chest roentgenogram shows decreased pulmonary vascularity, the degree depending on the size of the branch pulmonary arteries and the patency of the ductus or the size of any bronchial collaterals (which are much less common than in pulmonary atresia with VSD). The heart may be variable in size. The two-dimensional echocardiogram is useful in estimating right ventricular dimensions and the size of the tricuspid valve annulus, which have been shown to be of prognostic value. Echocardiography can often suggest the presence of sinusoidal channels if they are large. Cardiac catheterization is necessary for complete evaluation and reveals right atrial and right ventricular hypertension. Ventriculography demonstrates the size of the right ventricular cavity, the atretic right ventricular outflow tract, the degree of tricuspid regurgitation, and the presence or absence of intramyocardial sinusoids filling the coronary vessels. Aortography shows filling of the pulmonary arteries via the PDA and is helpful in determining the size and branching patterns of the pulmonary arterial bed. The aortogram is valuable in evaluating for the presence of proximal coronary artery stenosis (right ventricular dependent coronary circulation); the presence of these lesions negatively affects the prognosis.

TREATMENT. Infusion of prostaglandin E_1 (0.01–0.20 μg/kg/min) is usually effective in keeping the ductus arteriosus open before intervention, thus reducing hypoxemia and acidemia before surgery. A surgical pulmonary valvotomy is carried out to relieve outflow obstruction whenever possible. To preserve adequate pulmonary blood flow, an aortopulmonary shunt is often performed during the same procedure. Often, the right ventricular outflow tract is widened with a patch. An alternative approach utilizes interventional catheterization, in which the imperforate pulmonary valve is first punctured either with a wire or a radiofrequency ablation catheter, followed by a balloon valvuloplasty. If this course is taken, it may take days to weeks before the right ventricular muscle regresses enough for the patient to be weaned from prostaglandin, and some of these patients will require surgical intervention. The aim of surgery or interventional catheter-

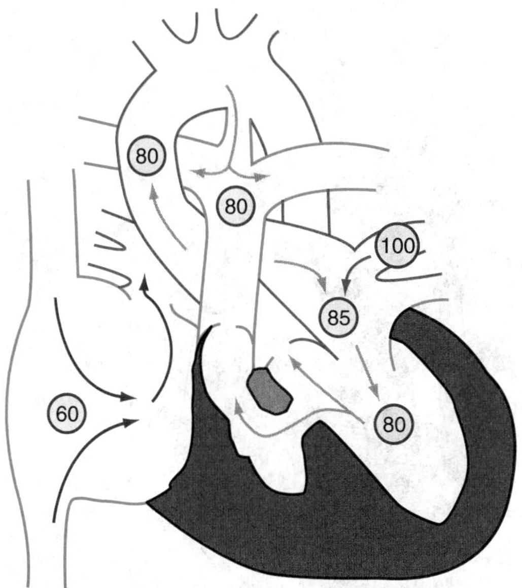

Figure 430-7. Physiology of tricuspid atresia with normally related great vessels. *Circled numbers* represent oxygen saturation values. Right atrial (mixed venous) oxygen saturation is decreased secondary to systemic hypoxemia. The tricuspid valve is nonpatent, and the right ventricle may manifest varying degrees of hypoplasia. The only outlet from the right atrium involves shunting right to left across an atrial septal defect or patent foramen ovale to the left atrium. There, desaturated blood mixes with saturated pulmonary venous return. Blood enters the left ventricle and is ejected either through the aorta or via a ventricular septal defect (VSD) into the right ventricle. In this example, some pulmonary blood flow is derived from the right ventricle, the rest from a patent ductus arteriosus (PDA). In patients with tricuspid atresia, the PDA may close or the VSD may grow smaller and result in a marked decrease in systemic oxygen saturation.

ization is to encourage growth of the right ventricular chamber by allowing some forward flow through the pulmonary valve while using the shunt to ensure adequate pulmonary blood flow. Later, if the tricuspid valve annulus and right ventricular chamber are of adequate size, the shunt is taken down and any remaining atrial level shunt is closed. If the right ventricular chamber remains hypoplastic, a modified **Fontan procedure** (see Chapter 430.4) allows blood to bypass the hypoplastic right ventricle by flowing to the pulmonary arteries directly from the venae cavae. When coronary artery stenoses are present and retrograde coronary perfusion occurs from the right ventricle via myocardial sinusoids, the prognosis may be grave because arrhythmias, coronary ischemia, and sudden death are common. Some of these infants benefit from heart transplantation.

430.4 • Tricuspid Atresia

PATHOPHYSIOLOGY. In tricuspid atresia, no outlet from the right atrium to the right ventricle is present; the entire systemic venous return enters the left side of the heart by means of the foramen ovale or an associated atrial septal defect (Fig. 430-7). Left ventricular blood usually flows into the right ventricle via a VSD. Pulmonary blood flow (and thus the degree of cyanosis) depends on the size of the VSD and the presence and severity of pulmonic stenosis. Pulmonary blood flow may be augmented by or be totally dependent on a PDA. The inflow portion of the right ventricle is always missing in these patients, but the outflow portion is of variable size. If the ventricular septum is intact, the right ventricle is completely hypoplastic and pulmonary atresia is present (see Chapter 430.3). Most patients with tricuspid atresia are recognized in the early months of life by decreased pulmonary blood flow and cyanosis. Alternatively, a large VSD in the absence of right ventricular outflow obstruction can lead to high pulmonary flow; these patients have mild cyanosis, signs of pulmonary overcirculation and heart failure. One variant of tricuspid atresia is associated with **transposition of the great arteries.** In this case, left ventricular blood flows directly into the pulmonary artery, whereas systemic blood must traverse the VSD and right ventricle to reach the aorta. In these patients, pulmonary blood flow is usually massively increased and heart failure develops early. If the VSD is restrictive, aortic blood flow may be compromised.

CLINICAL MANIFESTATIONS. Cyanosis is usually evident at birth, with the extent depending on the degree of limitation to pulmonary blood flow. An increased left ventricular impulse may be noted, in contrast to most other causes of cyanotic heart disease, in which an increased right ventricular impulse is usually present. The majority of patients have holosystolic murmurs audible along the left sternal border; the 2nd heart sound is usually single. The diagnosis is suspected in 85% of patients before 2 mo of age. In older patients, cyanosis, polycythemia, easy fatigability, exertional dyspnea, and occasional hypoxic episodes occur as a result of compromised pulmonary blood flow. Patients with tricuspid atresia are at risk for spontaneous closure of the VSD, which can occur rapidly and lead to a marked increase in cyanosis.

DIAGNOSIS. Roentgenographic studies show either pulmonary undercirculation (usually in patients with normally related great vessels) or overcirculation (usually in patients with transposed great vessels). Left axis deviation and left ventricular hypertrophy are generally noted on the electrocardiogram (except in those with transposition of the great arteries), and these features distinguish tricuspid atresia from most other cyanotic heart lesions. The combination of cyanosis and left axis deviation is highly suggestive of tricuspid atresia. In the right precordial leads, the normally prominent R wave is replaced by an rS complex. The left precordial leads show a qR complex, followed by a normal, flat, biphasic or inverted T wave. RV_6 is normal or tall, and SV_1 is generally deep. The P waves are usually biphasic, with the initial component tall and spiked in lead II. Two-dimensional echocardiography reveals the presence of a fibromuscular membrane in place of a tricuspid valve, the variably small right ventricle, VSD, and the large left ventricle and aorta (Fig. 430-8). The degree of

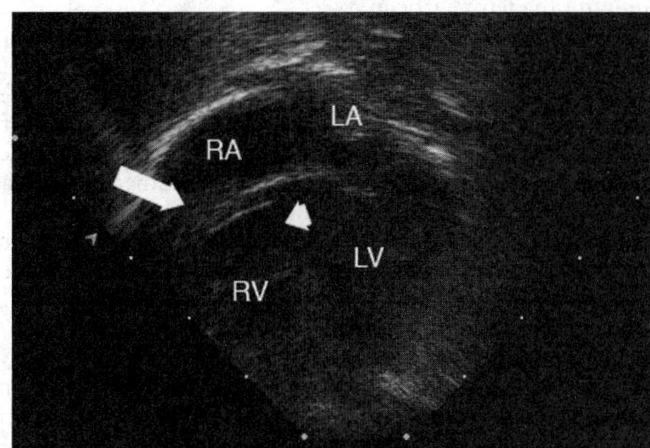

Figure 430-8. Echocardiogram demonstrating tricuspid atresia. The floor of the right atrium consists of a fibromuscular membrane *(large arrow)* instead of the normal tricuspid valve apparatus. The large secundum atrial septal defect can be seen between the right and left atria. The *arrowhead* shows the ventricular septal defect. LA, left atrium; LV, left ventricle; RA, right atrium; RV, right ventricle.

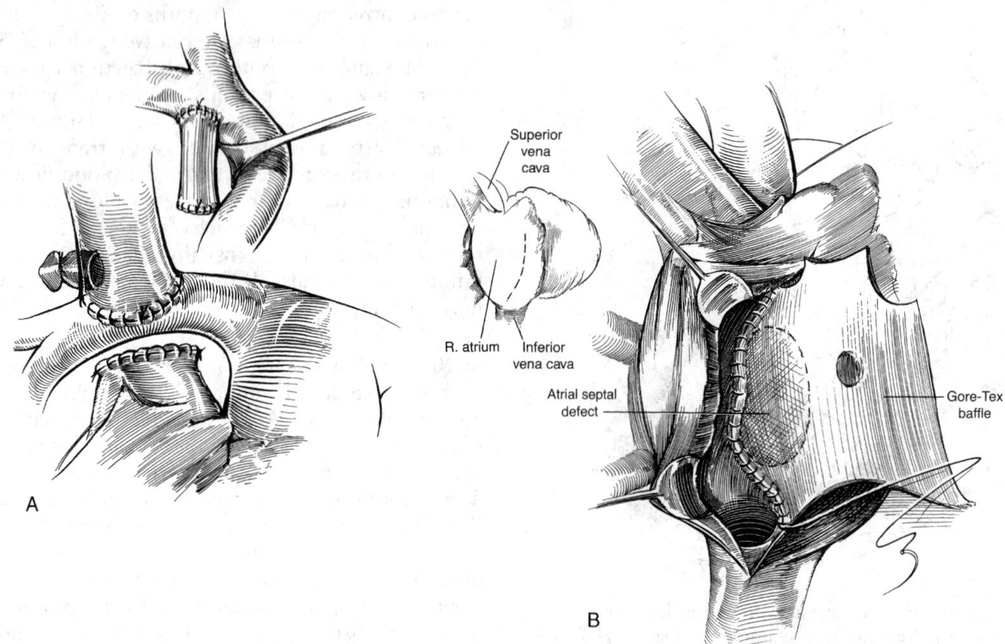

Figure 430-9. *A*, Bidirectional Glenn shunt showing the superior vena cava–right pulmonary anastomosis. *B*, A modified Fontan procedure (cavopulmonary isolation) is completed with placement of a baffle to convey inferior vena cava blood along the lateral wall of the right atrium to the superior vena cava orifice. A 4 mm fenestration is sometimes made on the medial aspect of the polytetrafluoroethylene baffle. (From Castañeda AR, Jonas RA, Mayer JE Jr, Hanley FL: Single-ventricle tricuspid atresia. In *Cardiac Surgery of the Neonate and Infant*. Philadelphia, WB Saunders, 1994.)

obstruction at the level of the VSD or right ventricular outflow tract can be determined by direct measurement and by Doppler examination. The relationship of the great vessels (normal or transposed) can be determined. Blood flow through a patent ductus can be evaluated by color flow and pulsed Doppler examination.

Cardiac catheterization, indicated usually only if questions remain after echocardiography, shows normal or slightly elevated right atrial pressure with a prominent *a* wave. If the right ventricle is entered through the VSD, the pressure may be lower than on the left because of the restrictive nature of the VSD. Right atrial angiography shows immediate opacification of the left atrium from the right atrium followed by left ventricular filling and visualization of the aorta. Absence of direct flow to the right ventricle results in an angiographic filling defect between the right atrium and the left ventricle.

TREATMENT. Management of patients with tricuspid atresia depends on the adequacy of pulmonary blood flow. Severely cyanotic neonates should be maintained on an intravenous infusion of prostaglandin E_1 (0.01–0.20 μg/kg/min) until a surgical aortopulmonary shunt procedure can be performed to increase pulmonary blood flow. The Blalock-Taussig procedure (see Chapter 430.1) or a variation is the preferred anastomosis. Some patients with restrictive atrial-level communications also benefit from a Rashkind balloon atrial septostomy (see Chapter 431.2) or surgical septectomy.

Infants with increased pulmonary blood flow because of an unobstructed pulmonary outflow tract (most often patients with aortopulmonary transposition) require pulmonary arterial banding to decrease the symptoms of heart failure and protect the pulmonary bed from the development of pulmonary vascular disease. Infants with just adequate pulmonary blood flow who are well balanced between cyanosis and pulmonary overcirculation can be watched closely for the development of increasing cyanosis, which may occur as the VSD begins to get smaller and is an indication for surgery.

The next stage of palliation for patients with tricuspid atresia involves the creation of an anastomosis between the superior vena cava and the pulmonary arteries (**bidirectional Glenn shunt;** Fig. 430-9*A*). This procedure is performed after the patient has shown signs of outgrowing a previous aortopulmonary shunt, usually between 4 and 8 mo of age. The benefit of the Glenn shunt is that it reduces the volume load on the left ventricle and may lessen the chance of left ventricular dysfunction developing later in life. Some centers advocate performing the Glenn anastomosis at an even earlier age (2–4 mo) to reduce the volume load on the left ventricle; the long-term benefit of this approach has not yet been confirmed.

The **modified Fontan operation** is the preferred approach to later surgical management. It is often performed between 1.5 and 3 yr of age, usually after the patient is ambulatory. Initially, this procedure was performed by anastomosing the right atrium or atrial appendage directly to the pulmonary artery. A modification of the Fontan procedure, known as a cavopulmonary isolation procedure, involves anastomosing the inferior vena cava to the pulmonary arteries, either via a baffle that runs along the lateral wall of the right atrium (see Fig. 430-9*B*) or via a homograft or Gore-Tex tube running outside the heart. The advantage of this approach is that blood flows by a more direct route into the pulmonary arteries, thereby decreasing the possibility of right atrial dilatation and markedly reducing the incidence of postoperative pleural effusions, which were common with the earlier method. In this completed repair, desaturated blood flows from both venae cavae directly into the pulmonary arteries. Oxygenated blood returns to the left atrium, enters the left ventricle, and is ejected into the systemic circulation. The volume load is completely removed from the left ventricle, and the right-to-left shunt is abolished. Because of the reliance on passive filling of the pulmonary circulation, the Fontan procedure is contraindicated in patients with elevated pulmonary vascular resistance, in those with pulmonary artery hypoplasia, and in patients with left ventricular dysfunction. The patient must be in sinus rhythm and not have significant mitral insufficiency.

Postoperative problems after the Fontan procedure include marked elevation of systemic venous pressure, fluid retention, and pleural or pericardial effusions. In the past, pleural effusions were a problem in 30–40% of patients using the standard Fontan procedure, but the cavopulmonary isolation procedure now in use reduces this risk to about 5%. Late complications include baffle obstruction causing superior or inferior vena cava syndrome, vena cava or pulmonary artery thromboembolism, protein-losing enteropathy, and supraventricular arrhythmias (atrial flutter, paroxysmal atrial tachycardia), occasionally associated with sudden death. Left ventricular dysfunction may be a late occurrence, often in adolescents or young adults. Heart transplantation is a successful treatment option for pediatric patients with "failed" Fontan circuits.

430.5 • Double-Outlet Right Ventricle with Pulmonary Stenosis

Both the aorta and pulmonary artery arising from the right ventricle characterize double-outlet right ventricle with pulmonary stenosis; the outlet from the left ventricle is a VSD into the right ventricle. The aortic and mitral valves are separated by a smooth muscular conus, similar to that seen under the normal pulmonary valve. The aorta may override the VSD by a variable amount but is at least 50% committed to the right ventricle. This defect may be viewed as part of a continuum with the tetralogy of Fallot, depending on the degree of aortic override. The physiology as well as the history, physical examination, electrocardiogram, and roentgenograms are similar to those of the tetralogy of Fallot (see Chapter 430.1). The two-dimensional echocardiogram demonstrates both great vessels arising from the right ventricle and mitral-aortic valve discontinuity. At cardiac catheterization, angiography shows that the aortic and pulmonary valves lie in the same horizontal plane and that the anteriorly displaced aorta arises predominantly or exclusively from the right ventricle. Surgical correction consists of creating an intraventricular tunnel so that the left ventricle ejects blood through the VSD, through the tunnel, and into the aorta. The pulmonary obstruction is relieved either with an outflow patch or with a right ventricular to pulmonary artery homograft conduit (**Rastelli operation**). In small infants, palliation with an aortopulmonary shunt provides symptomatic improvement and allows for adequate growth before corrective surgery is performed.

430.6 • Transposition of the Great Arteries with Ventricular Septal Defect and Pulmonary Stenosis

This combination of anomalies may mimic tetralogy of Fallot in its clinical features (see Chapter 430.1). Because of the transposed great vessels, the site of obstruction is in the left as opposed to the right ventricle. The obstruction can be either valvular or subvalvular; the latter type may be dynamic, related to the interventricular septum or atrioventricular valve tissue, or acquired, as in patients with transposition and VSD after pulmonary arterial banding.

The age at which clinical manifestations initially appear varies from soon after birth to later infancy, depending on the degree of pulmonic stenosis. Clinical findings include cyanosis, decreased exercise tolerance, and poor physical development, similar to those described for the tetralogy of Fallot; however, the heart may be more enlarged. The pulmonary vasculature as seen on the roentgenogram is dependent on the degree of pulmonary obstruction, but it is often normal. The electrocardiogram usually shows right axis deviation, right and left ventricular hypertrophy, and sometimes tall, spiked P waves. Echocardiography confirms the diagnosis and is useful in sequential evaluation of the degree and progression of the left ventricular outflow tract obstruction. Cardiac catheterization, if necessary, shows that pulmonary arterial pressure is low and that oxygen saturation in the pulmonary artery exceeds that in the aorta. Selective right and left ventriculography demonstrates the origin of the aorta from the right ventricle, the origin of the pulmonary artery from the left ventricle, the VSD, and the site and severity of the pulmonary stenosis.

An infusion of prostaglandin E_1 (0.01–0.20 µg/kg/min) should be started in neonates with cyanosis. The preferred surgical treatment in hypoxemic infants is an aortopulmonary shunt (see Chapter 430.1). When necessary, balloon atrial septostomy is performed to improve atrial-level mixing and to decompress the left atrium (see Chapter 431.2). The patient can then be monitored clinically until older, when a Rastelli operation is the preferred corrective procedure. The Rastelli procedure achieves physiologic and anatomic correction by (1) patch closure of the VSD, with left ventricular flow directed to the aorta; and (2) connection of the right ventricle to the pulmonary artery by ligating the proximal pulmonary artery and placing an extracardiac homograft conduit between the right ventricle and the distal pulmonary artery (Fig. 430-10). The conduit may eventually become stenotic or functionally restrictive with growth of the patient and require revision. Surgical correction by the Mustard operation (see Chapter 431.2) with simultaneous closure of the VSD and relief of left ventricular outflow obstruction may be an alternative when the position of the VSD is not suitable for a Rastelli operation. Patients with milder degrees of pulmonary stenosis amenable to simple valvotomy may be able to undergo complete correction with an arterial switch procedure (see Chapter 431.2).

430.7 • Ebstein Anomaly of the Tricuspid Valve

PATHOPHYSIOLOGY. Ebstein anomaly consists of downward displacement of an abnormal tricuspid valve into the right ventricle. The defect may arise from failure of the normal process by which the tricuspid valve is separated from the right ventricular myocardium (see Chapter 420). The anterior cusp of the valve retains some attachment to the valve ring, but the other leaflets are adherent to the wall of the right ventricle. The right ventricle is thus divided into two parts by the abnormal tricuspid valve: the 1st, a thin-walled "atrialized" portion, is continuous with the cavity of the right atrium; the 2nd, often smaller portion consists of normal ventricular myocardium. The right atrium is huge, and the tricuspid valve is generally regurgitant, although the degree is extremely variable. The effective output from the right side of the heart is decreased because of the poorly functioning small right ventricle, tricuspid valve regurgitation, and variable degrees of obstruction of the right ventricular outflow tract produced by the large, sail-like, anterior tricuspid valve leaflet. At times, right ventricular function is so compromised that it is unable to generate enough force to open the pulmonary valve in systole, thus producing "functional" pulmonary atresia. Some infants have true anatomic pulmonary atresia. The increased volume of right atrial blood shunts through the foramen ovale to the left atrium and produces cyanosis (Fig. 430-11).

CLINICAL MANIFESTATIONS. The severity of symptoms and the degree of cyanosis are highly variable and depend on the extent of displacement of the tricuspid valve and the severity of right ventricular outflow tract obstruction. In many patients, symptoms are mild and do not occur until the teenage years or young adult life; the patient may initially have fatigue or palpitations as

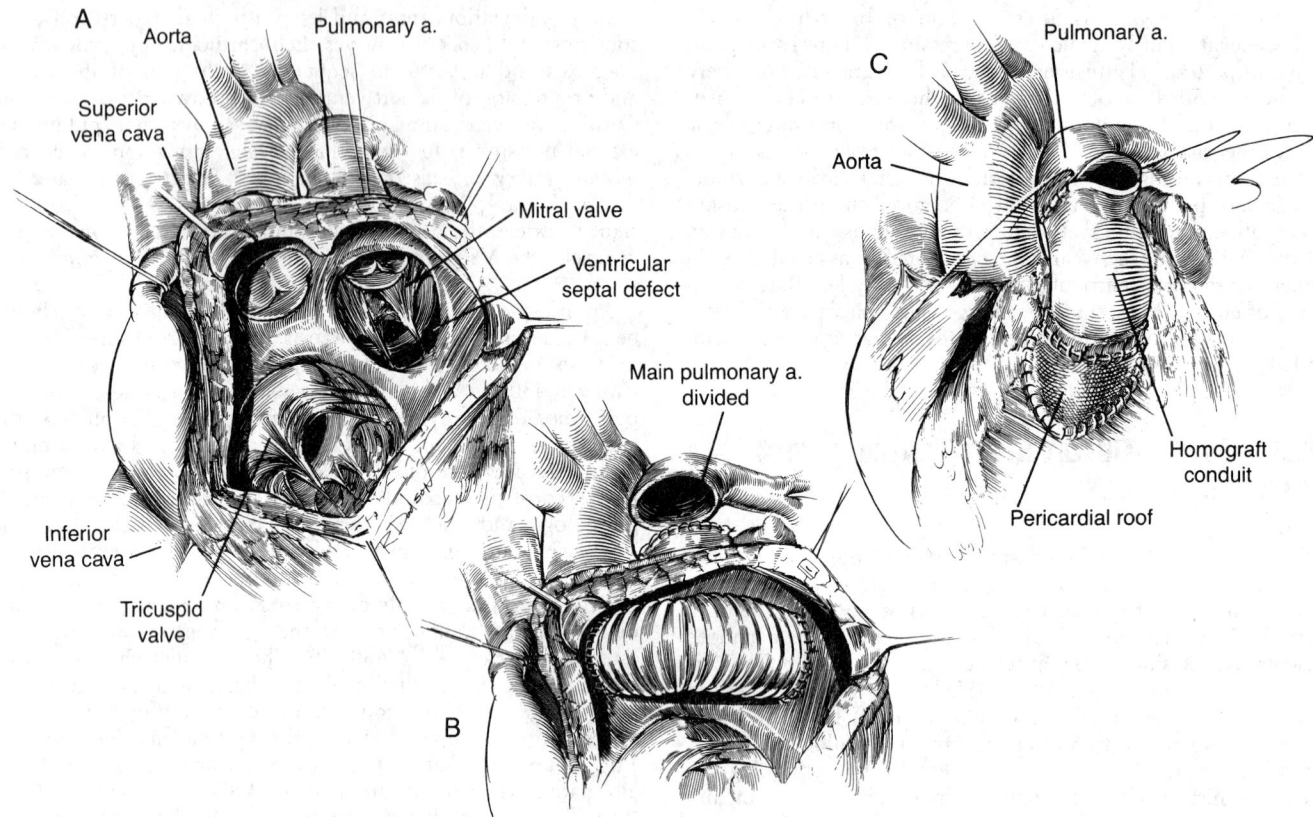

Figure 430-10. *A,* Taussig-Bing type of double-outlet right ventricle with subpulmonary stenosis necessitating repair by the Rastelli technique. *B,* The main pulmonary artery is divided and oversewn proximally. The pulmonary valve lies within the baffle pathway. *C,* Completion of the Rastelli repair with a right ventricle-pulmonary artery allograft conduit. (From Castañeda AR, Jonas RA, Mayer JE Jr, Hanley FL: Single-ventricle tricuspid atresia. In *Cardiac Surgery of the Neonate and Infant.* Philadelphia, WB Saunders, 1994.)

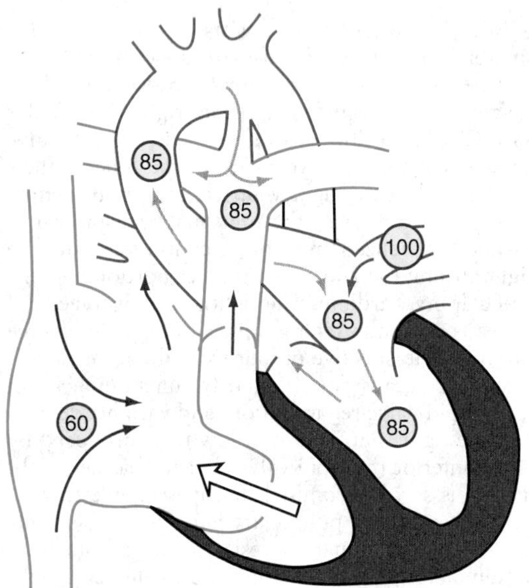

Figure 430-11. Physiology of Ebstein anomaly of the tricuspid valve. *Circled numbers* represent oxygen saturation values. Inferior displacement of the tricuspid valve leaflets into the right ventricle has resulted in a thin-walled, low-pressure "atrialized" segment of right ventricle. The tricuspid valve is grossly insufficient *(clear arrow).* Right atrial blood flow is shunted right to left across an atrial septal defect or patent foramen ovale into the left atrium. Some blood may cross the right ventricular outflow tract and enter the pulmonary artery; however, in severe cases, the right ventricle may generate insufficient force to open the pulmonary valve, and "functional pulmonary atresia" results. In the left atrium, desaturated blood mixes with saturated pulmonary venous return. Blood enters the left ventricle and is ejected via the aorta. In this example, some pulmonary blood flow is derived from the right ventricle, the rest from a patent ductus arteriosus (PDA). Severe cyanosis will develop in neonates with a severe Ebstein anomaly when the PDA closes.

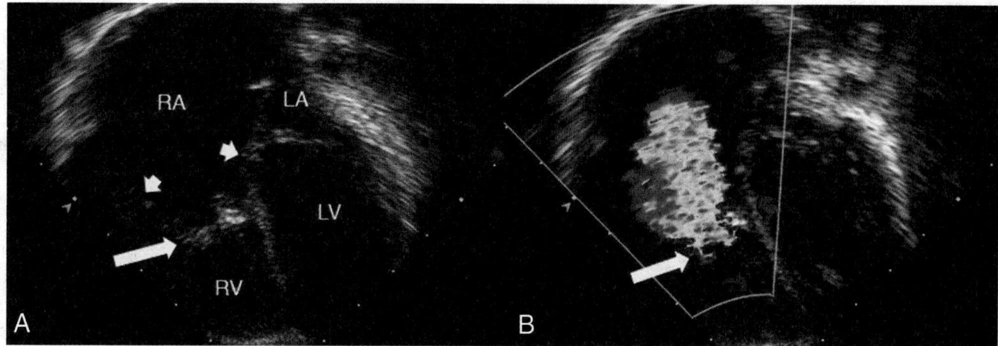

Figure 430-12. Echocardiographic demonstration of Ebstein anomaly of the tricuspid valve. *A,* Subcostal four-chamber two-dimensional view showing severe displacement of the tricuspid valve leaflets *(large arrow)* inferiorly into the right ventricle. The location of the tricuspid valve annulus is outlined by the two *arrowheads.* The portion of the right ventricle between the valve annulus and the valve leaflets is the "atrialized" component. *B,* Color Doppler examination showing severe regurgitation of the dysplastic tricuspid valve. Note that the regurgitant turbulent flow *(arrow)* begins halfway into the right ventricular chamber, at the location of the displaced valve leaflets. LA, left atrium; LV, left ventricle; RA, right atrium; RV, right ventricle.

a result of cardiac dysrhythmias. A right-to-left shunt through the foramen ovale is responsible for cyanosis and polycythemia. Central venous pressure may be normal or increased in those with tricuspid insufficiency. On palpation, the precordium is quiet. A holosystolic murmur caused by tricuspid regurgitation is audible over most of the anterior left side of the chest. A gallop rhythm is common and often associated with multiple clicks at the lower left sternal border. A scratchy diastolic murmur may also be heard at the left sternal border. This murmur is superficial and may mimic a pericardial friction rub.

Newborn infants with severe forms of Ebstein anomaly have marked cyanosis, massive cardiomegaly, and long systolic murmurs. Death may result from cardiac failure and hypoxemia. Spontaneous improvement may occur in some neonates as pulmonary vascular resistance falls normally and improves the ability of the right ventricle to provide pulmonary blood flow. The majority are dependent on a PDA, and thus on a prostaglandin infusion, for pulmonary blood flow.

DIAGNOSIS. The electrocardiogram usually shows a right bundle branch block without increased right precordial voltage, normal or tall and broad P waves, and a normal or prolonged P-R interval. **Wolff-Parkinson-White syndrome** (see Chapter 435) may be present; patients may have episodes of supraventricular tachycardia. On roentgenographic examination, heart size varies from normal to massive, box-shaped cardiomegaly caused by enlargement of the right atrium and ventricle. The pulmonary vasculature can be normal or decreased. Echocardiography shows the degree of displacement of the tricuspid valve leaflets, a dilated right atrium, and any right ventricular outflow tract obstruction (Fig. 430-12). Pulsed and color Doppler examination demonstrates the degree of tricuspid regurgitation. In severe cases, the pulmonary valve may appear immobile and pulmonary blood flow may come solely from the ductus arteriosus. It may be difficult to distinguish true from functional pulmonary valve atresia. Cardiac catheterization, which is not always necessary, confirms the presence of a large right atrium, an abnormal tricuspid valve, and any right-to-left shunt at the atrial level. The risk of arrhythmia is significant during catheterization and angiographic studies.

PROGNOSIS AND COMPLICATIONS. The prognosis in Ebstein anomaly is extremely variable and depends on the spectrum of severity seen. The prognosis is usually poor for neonates or infants with intractable symptoms and cyanosis. Patients with milder degrees of Ebstein anomaly usually survive well into adult life. There is an association of a left ventricular cardiomyopathy (isolated non-compaction) in 18% of patients with Ebstein anomaly.

TREATMENT. Neonates with severe hypoxia who are prostaglandin dependent have been treated with an aortopulmonary shunt alone, by repair of the tricuspid valve, or by surgical patch closure of the tricuspid valve, atrial septectomy, and placement of an aortopulmonary shunt (**Starnes procedure**). Many infants with Ebstein anomaly who have undergone valve repair will still have enough regurgitation that a Glenn shunt is later performed to reduce the volume load on the right ventricle (see Chapter 430.4). In older children with mild or moderate disease, control of supraventricular dysrhythmias is of primary importance; surgical treatment may not be necessary until adolescence or young adulthood. In patients with severe tricuspid regurgitation, repair or replacement of the abnormal tricuspid valve along with closure of the atrial septal defect is then carried out. In some older patients, a bidirectional Glenn shunt is also performed, with the superior vena cava anastomosed to the pulmonary arteries. This procedure reduces the volume of blood that the dysfunctional right side of the heart has to pump, thus creating a "one-and-one-half" ventricle repair.

Tetralogy of Fallot

Boudjemline Y, Fermont L, Le Bidois J, et al: Prevalence of 22q11 deletion in fetuses with conotruncal cardiac defects: A 6-year prospective study. *J Pediatr* 2001;138:520–524.

Dubin AM, Feinstein JA, Reddy VM, et al: Electrical resynchronization: A novel therapy for the failing right ventricle. *Circulation* 2003;107:2287–2289.

Hanley FL: Management of the congenitally abnormal right ventricular outflow tract—what is the right approach? *J Thorac Cardiovasc Surg* 2000;119:1–3.

McCaughan BC, Danielson GK, Driscoll DJ, et al: Tetralogy of Fallot with absent pulmonary valve: Early and late results of surgical treatment. *J Thorac Cardiovasc Surg* 1985;89:280–287.

Pacifico AO, Saro ME, Bargeron LM Jr, et al: Transatrial-transpulmonary repair of tetralogy of Fallot. *J Thorac Cardiovasc Surg* 1987;74:382–395.

Parry AJ, McElhinney DB, Kung GC, et al: Elective primary repair of acyanotic tetralogy of Fallot in early infancy: Overall outcome and impact on the pulmonary valve. *J Am Coll Cardiol* 2000;36:2279–2283.

Reddy VM, McElhinney DB, Amin Z, et al: Early and intermediate outcomes after repair of pulmonary atresia with ventricular septal defect and major aortopulmonary collateral arteries: Experience with 85 patients. *Circulation* 2000;101:1826–1832.

Schultz AH, Wernovsky G: Late outcomes in patients with surgically treated congenital heart disease. *Semin Thorac Cardiovasc Surg Pediatr Card Surg Annu* 2005;8:145–156.

Pulmonary Atresia with Intact Ventricular Septum

Hanley FL, Sade RM, Blackstone EH, et al: Outcomes in neonatal pulmonary atresia with intact ventricular septum. A multiinstitutional study. *J Thorac Cardiovasc Surg* 1993;105:406–423.

Latson LA: Nonsurgical treatment of a neonate with pulmonary atresia and intact ventricular septum by transcatheter puncture and balloon dilatation of the atretic valve membrane. *Am J Cardiol* 1991;68:277–279.

L'Ecuyer TJ, Poulik JM, Vincent JA: Myocardial infarction due to coronary abnormalities in pulmonary atresia with intact ventricular septum. *Pediatr Cardiol* 2001;22:68–70.

Tricuspid Atresia

Anderson RH, Cook AC: Morphology of the functionally univentricular heart. *Cardiol Young* 2004;14(Suppl 1):3–12.

Donnelly JP, Rosenthal A, Castle VP, et al: Reversal of protein-losing enteropathy with heparin therapy in three patients with univentricular hearts and Fontan palliation. *J Pediatr* 1997;130:474–478.

Freedom RM, Hamilton R, Yoo SJ, et al: The Fontan procedure: Analysis of cohorts and late complications. *Cardiol Young* 2000;10:307–331.

Gelatt M, Hamilton R, McCrindle W, et al: Risk factors for atrial tachyarrhythmias after the Fontan operation. *J Am Coll Cardiol* 1994;24:1735–1741.

Hess J: Long-term problems after cavopulmonary anastomosis: Diagnosis and management. *Thorac Cardiovasc Surg* 2001;49:98–100.

Mair DD, Puga FJ, Danielson GK: The Fontan procedure for tricuspid atresia: Early and late results of a 25-year experience with 216 patients. *J Am Coll Cardiol* 2001;37:933–939.

Petrossian E, Reddy VM, McElhinney DB, et al: Early results of the extracardiac conduit Fontan operation. *J Thorac Cardiovasc Surg* 1999;117:688–696.

Shirai LK, Rosenthal DN, Reitz BA, et al: Arrhythmias and thromboembolic complications after the extracardiac Fontan operation. *J Thorac Cardiovasc Surg* 1998;115:499–505.

van den Bosch AE, Roos-Hesselink JW, Van Domburg R, et al: Long-term outcome and quality of life in adult patients after the Fontan operation. *Am J Cardiol* 2004;93:1141–1145.

Ebstein Anomaly of the Tricuspid Valve

Kiziltan HT, Theodoro DA, Warnes CA, et al: Late results of bioprosthetic tricuspid valve replacement in Ebstein's anomaly. *Ann Thorac Surg* 1998;66:1539–1545.

Marianeschi SM, McElhinney DB, Reddy VM, et al: Alternative approach to the repair of Ebstein's malformation: Intracardiac repair with ventricular unloading. *Ann Thorac Surg* 1998;66:1546–1550.

Schreiber C, Cook A, Ho SY, et al: Morphologic spectrum of Ebstein's malformation: Revisitation relative to surgical repair. *J Thorac Cardiovasc Surg* 1999;117:148–155.

Starnes VA, Pitlick PT, Bernstein D, et al: Ebstein's anomaly appearing in the neonate. *J Thorac Cardiovasc Surg* 1991;101:1082–1087.

Chapter 431 ■ Cyanotic Congenital Heart Disease: Lesions Associated with Increased Pulmonary Blood Flow

431.1 • D-Transposition of the Great Arteries

Transposition of the great vessels, a common cyanotic congenital anomaly, accounts for ≈5% of all congenital heart disease. In this anomaly, the systemic veins return normally to the right atrium and the pulmonary veins return to the left atrium. The connections between the atria and ventricles are also normal (atrioventricular concordance). The aorta arises from the right ventricle and the pulmonary artery from the left ventricle (Fig. 431-1). In normally related great vessels, the aorta is posterior and to the right of the pulmonary artery; in d-transposition of the great arteries (d-TGA), the aorta is anterior and to the right of the pulmonary artery (the *d* indicates a dextropositioned aorta). Desaturated blood returning from the body to the right side of the heart goes inappropriately right out the aorta and back to the body again, whereas oxygenated pulmonary venous blood returning to the left side of the heart is returned directly to the lungs. The systemic and pulmonary circulations consist of two parallel circuits. Survival in these newborns is provided by the foramen ovale and the ductus arteriosus, which permit some mixture of oxygenated and deoxygenated blood. About 50% of patients with TGA also have a ventricular septal defect (VSD), which provides for better mixing. The clinical findings and hemodynamics vary in relation to the presence or absence of associated defects. TGA is more common in infants of diabetic mothers and in males (3 : 1). TGA, especially when accompanied by other cardiac defects such as pulmonic stenosis or right aortic arch, can be associated with deletion of chromosome 22q11 (**CATCH 22** [cardiac defects, abnormal facies, thymic aplasia, cleft palate, hypoplasia], DiGeorge syndrome). Before the modern era of corrective or palliative surgery, mortality was >90% in the 1st yr of life.

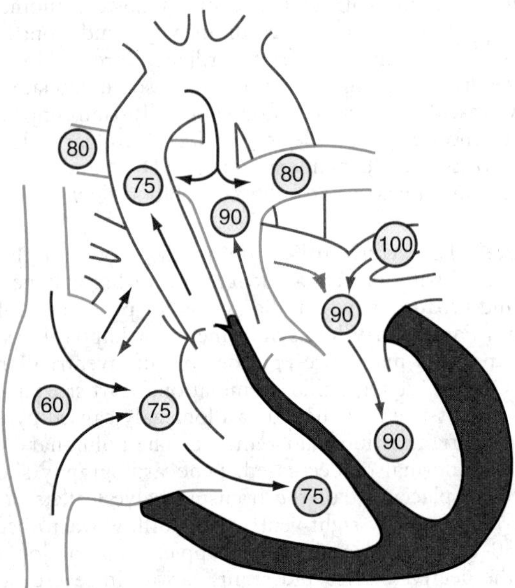

Figure 431-1. Physiology of d-transposition of the great arteries (d-TGA). *Circled numbers* represent oxygen saturation values. Right atrial (mixed venous) oxygen saturation is decreased secondary to systemic hypoxemia. Desaturated blood enters the right atrium, flows through the tricuspid valve into the right ventricle, and is ejected into the transposed aorta with resultant severe aortic desaturation. Fully saturated pulmonary venous blood flows into the left atrium, across the mitral valve into the left ventricle, and across the transposed pulmonary artery into the lungs. Pulmonary arterial oxygen saturation is thus increased. This lesion would not be compatible with life were it not for the ability of blood to shunt via two fetal pathways: the patent foramen ovale (PFO) and patent ductus arteriosus (PDA). Blood may shunt left to right or bidirectionally at the PFO. Because systemic vascular resistance tends to be higher than pulmonary vascular resistance, blood tends to shunt across the PDA mostly from the aorta to the pulmonary artery. As pulmonary resistance drops in the 1st few weeks of life, pulmonary blood flow will gradually increase in patients with d-TGA.

431.2 • D-Transposition of the Great Arteries with Intact Ventricular Septum

D-TGA with an intact ventricular septum is also referred to as simple TGA or isolated TGA. Before birth, oxygenation of the fetus is nearly normal, but after birth, once the ductus begins to close, the minimal mixing of systemic and pulmonary blood via the patent foramen ovale is usually insufficient and severe hypoxemia ensues, generally within the 1st few days of life.

CLINICAL MANIFESTATIONS. Cyanosis and tachypnea are most often recognized within the 1st hrs or days of life. Untreated, the vast majority of these infants would not survive the neonatal period. Hypoxemia is usually severe, but heart failure is less common. This condition is a medical emergency, and only early diagnosis and appropriate intervention can avert the development of prolonged severe hypoxemia and acidosis, which lead to death. Physical findings associated with cyanosis may be nonspecific. The precordial impulse may be normal, or a parasternal heave may be present. The 2nd heart sound is usually single and loud, although occasionally it may be split. Murmurs may be absent, or a soft systolic ejection murmur may be noted at the midleft sternal border.

DIAGNOSIS. The electrocardiogram shows the normal neonatal right-sided dominant pattern. Roentgenograms of the chest may show mild cardiomegaly, a narrow mediastinum (hence an egg-shaped heart), and normal to increased pulmonary blood flow. In the early newborn period, the chest roentgenogram is generally normal. As pulmonary vascular resistance drops during the 1st wk or two of life, evidence of increased pulmonary blood flow is apparent. Arterial PO_2 is low and does not rise appreciably after the patient breathes 100% oxygen (hyperoxia test), although this test may not be totally reliable. Echocardiography confirms the transposed ventricular-arterial connections (Fig. 431-2). In addition, the size of the interatrial communication and the ductus arteriosus can be visualized; the degree of mixing is assessed by pulsed and color Doppler examination. The presence of any associated lesion, such as left ventricular outflow tract obstruction or a VSD, can also be assessed. The origins of the coronary arteries can usually be imaged, although echocardiography is not as accurate as catheterization for this purpose. Cardiac catheterization is occasionally performed in patients for whom noninvasive imaging is diagnostically inconclusive or in patients who require emergency balloon atrial septostomy (see later). Catheterization will show right ventricular pressure to be systemic because this ventricle is supporting the systemic circulation. The blood in the left ventricle and pulmonary artery has higher oxygen saturation than that in the aorta. Depending on the age at catheterization, left ventricular and pulmonary arterial pressure can vary from systemic level to <50% of systemic-level pressure. Right ventriculography demonstrates the anterior and rightward aorta originating from the right ventricle, as well as the intact ventricular septum. **Anomalous coronary arteries** are noted in 10–15% of patients. Left ventriculography shows that the pulmonary artery arises exclusively from the left ventricle.

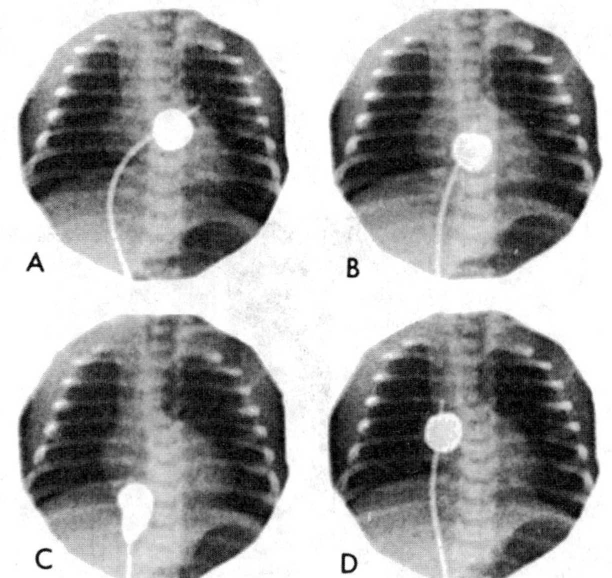

Figure 431-3. Rashkind balloon atrial septostomy. Four frames from a continuous cineangiogram show the creation of an atrial septal defect in a hypoxemic newborn infant with transposition of the great arteries and an intact ventricular septum. *A,* Balloon inflated in the left atrium. *B,* The catheter is jerked suddenly so that the balloon ruptures the foramen ovale. *C,* Balloon in the inferior vena cava. *D,* Catheter advanced to the right atrium to deflate the balloon. The time from A to C is <1 sec.

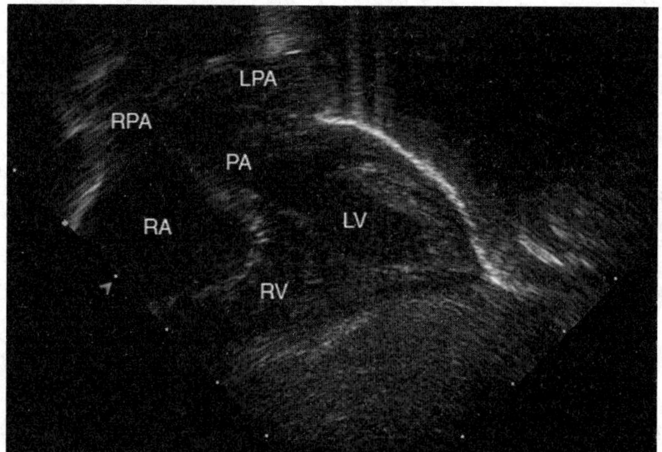

Figure 431-2. Subcostal four-chamber two-dimensional echocardiographic demonstration of d-transposition of the great arteries. The pulmonary artery (PA) can be seen arising directly from the left ventricle (LV). The immediate bifurcation of this great vessel into the branch pulmonary arteries differentiates it from the aorta, which branches more distally from the heart. LPA, left pulmonary artery; RA, right atrium; RPA, right pulmonary artery; RV, right ventricle.

TREATMENT. When transposition is suspected, an infusion of prostaglandin E_1 should be initiated immediately to maintain patency of the ductus arteriosus and improve oxygenation (dosage, 0.01–0.20 μg/kg/min). Because of the risk of apnea associated with prostaglandin infusion, an individual skilled in neonatal endotracheal intubation should be available. Hypothermia intensifies the metabolic acidosis resulting from hypoxemia, and thus the patient should be kept warm. Prompt correction of acidosis and hypoglycemia is essential.

Infants who remain severely hypoxic or acidotic despite prostaglandin infusion should undergo **Rashkind balloon atrial septostomy** (Fig. 431-3). A Rashkind atrial septostomy is usually performed in all patients in whom any significant delay in surgery is necessary. At most centers, the arterial switch (**Jantene**) operation is performed within the 1st 2 wk of life. If the arterial switch is planned during this time frame, catheterization and atrial septostomy may often be avoided.

A successful Rashkind atrial septostomy should result in a rise in PaO_2 to 35–50 mm Hg and elimination of any pressure gradient across the atrial septum. Some patients with TGA and VSD

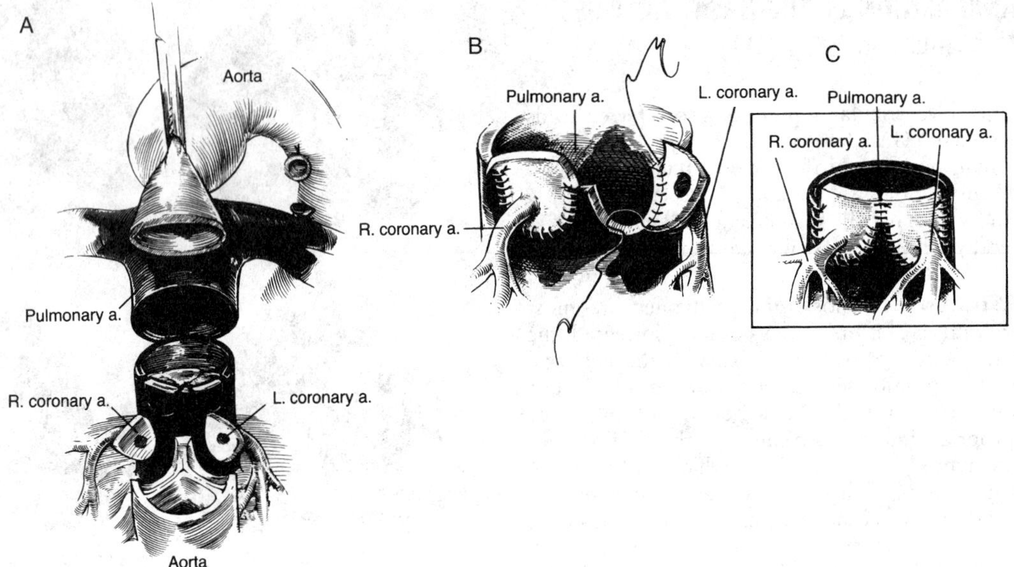

Figure 431-4. Method for translocating the coronary arteries in the arterial switch (Jantene) procedure. *A,* The aorta (anterior) and the pulmonary artery (posterior) have been transected to allow visualization of the left and right coronary arteries. The coronaries have been excised from their respective sinuses, including a large flap (button) of arterial wall. Equivalent segments of the wall of the pulmonary artery (which will become the neoaorta) are also removed. *B,* The aortocoronary buttons are sutured into the proximal portion of the neoaorta. With this technique all sutures are placed in the button of aortic wall rather than directly on the coronary arteries. *C,* Completed anastomosis of the left and right coronary arteries to the neoaorta. (Adapted from Castañeda AR, Jonas RA, Mayer JE Jr, Hanley FL: *Cardiac Surgery of the Neonate and Infant.* Philadelphia, WB Saunders, 1994.)

may require balloon atrial septostomy because of poor mixing, even though the VSD is large. Others may benefit from decompression of the left atrium to alleviate the symptoms of increased pulmonary blood flow and left-sided heart failure.

The **arterial switch (Jantene) procedure** is the surgical **treatment of choice** for neonates with d-TGA and an intact ventricular septum and is usually performed within the 1st 2 wk of life. The reason for this urgency is that as pulmonary vascular resistance declines after birth, pressure in the left ventricle (connected to the pulmonary vascular bed) also declines. This drop in pressure results in a decrease in left ventricular mass in the 1st few weeks of life. If the arterial switch operation is attempted after left ventricular pressure has declined too far, the left ventricle will be unable to generate adequate pressure to pump blood to the systemic circulation. The operation involves dividing the aorta and pulmonary artery just above the sinuses and re-anastomosing them in their correct anatomic positions. The coronary arteries are then removed from the old aortic root along with a button of aortic wall and reimplanted in the old pulmonary root (the "neoaorta"). By using a button of great vessel tissue, the surgeon avoids having to suture directly onto the coronary artery (Fig. 431-4). Rarely, a two-stage arterial switch procedure, with initial placement of a pulmonary artery band, may be used in patients older than 3–4 wk who already have a reduction in left ventricular muscle mass and pressure.

The arterial switch procedure has a survival rate of 90–95% for uncomplicated d-TGA. It restores the normal physiologic relationships of systemic and pulmonary arterial blood flow and eliminates the long-term complications of the atrial switch procedure.

Previous operations for d-TGA consisted of some form of **atrial switch procedure** (**Mustard** or **Senning** operation). In older infants, these procedures produced excellent early survival (≈85–90%), but significant long-term morbidity. Atrial switch procedures reverse blood flow patterns at the atrial level by the surgical creation of an intra-atrial baffle that allows systemic venous blood to be directed to the left atrium and the left ventricle and then, via the pulmonary artery, into the lungs. The same baffle also permits oxygenated pulmonary venous blood to cross over to the right atrium, right ventricle, and aorta. Atrial switch procedures involve significant atrial surgery and may result in the late development of atrial conduction disturbances, sick sinus syndrome with bradyarrhythmia and tachyarrhythmia, atrial flutter, sudden death, superior or inferior vena cava syndrome, edema, ascites, and protein-losing enteropathy. The atrial switch procedure leaves the right ventricle as the systemic pumping chamber and, often, these systemic right ventricles begin to fail in young adulthood. Atrial switch operations are reserved for patients whose anatomy is such that they are not candidates for the arterial switch procedure (TGA and severe pulmonic stenosis).

431.3 • Transposition of the Great Arteries with Ventricular Septal Defect

If the VSD associated with TGA is small, the clinical manifestations, laboratory findings, and treatment are similar to those described previously for transposition with an intact ventricular septum. A harsh systolic murmur is audible at the lower left sternal border and results from flow through the defect. Many of these small defects eventually close spontaneously and are often not addressed at the time of surgery.

When the VSD is large and not restrictive to ventricular ejection, significant mixing of oxygenated and deoxygenated blood usually occurs and clinical manifestations of cardiac failure are seen. The onset of cyanosis may be subtle and frequently delayed, and its intensity is variable. Cyanosis can generally be recognized within the 1st mo of life, but it may remain undiagnosed in some infants for several months. The murmur is holosystolic and generally indistinguishable from that produced by a large VSD in patients with normally related great arteries. The heart is usually significantly enlarged.

Cardiomegaly, a narrow mediastinal waist, and increased pulmonary vascularity are demonstrated on the chest roentgenogram. The electrocardiogram shows prominent P waves and isolated right ventricular hypertrophy or biventricular hypertrophy. Occasionally, dominance of the left ventricle is present. Usually, the QRS axis is to the right, but it is sometimes normal or even to the left. The diagnosis can be confirmed by echocardiography, and the extent of pulmonary blood flow can also be assessed by the degree of enlargement of the left atrium and ventricle. In equivocal cases, the diagnosis can be confirmed by cardiac catheterization. Right and left ventriculography indicate the presence of arterial transposition and demonstrate the site and size of the VSD. Peak systolic pressure is equal in the two ventricles, the aorta, and the pulmonary artery. Left atrial pressure may be much higher than right atrial pressure, a finding indicative of a restrictive communication at the atrial level. At the time of cardiac catheterization, Rashkind balloon atrial septostomy may be performed to decompress the left atrium, even when adequate mixing is occurring at the ventricular level.

Surgical treatment is advised soon after diagnosis, usually within the 1st months of life, because heart failure and failure to thrive are difficult to manage and pulmonary vascular disease can develop unusually rapidly. Management includes diuretics and, possibly, digitalis to lessen the symptoms of heart failure while awaiting surgical repair.

Patients with TGA and a VSD without pulmonic stenosis can be managed with an arterial switch procedure combined with VSD closure. In these patients, the arterial switch operation can be safely performed after the 1st 2 wk of life because the VSD results in equal pressure in both ventricles and prevents regression of left ventricular muscle mass. At major centers, however, there is no reason to delay repair, as results are excellent whether the surgery is performed in the neonatal period or later.

Without treatment, the prognosis is poor; most patients succumb in the 1st yr of life because of heart failure, hypoxemia, and pulmonary hypertension. In the past, some survived infancy with medical therapy alone, but pulmonary vascular disease often developed. The clinical picture and treatment of these patients are similar to those described with Eisenmenger syndrome secondary to an isolated large VSD (see Chapter 433.2).

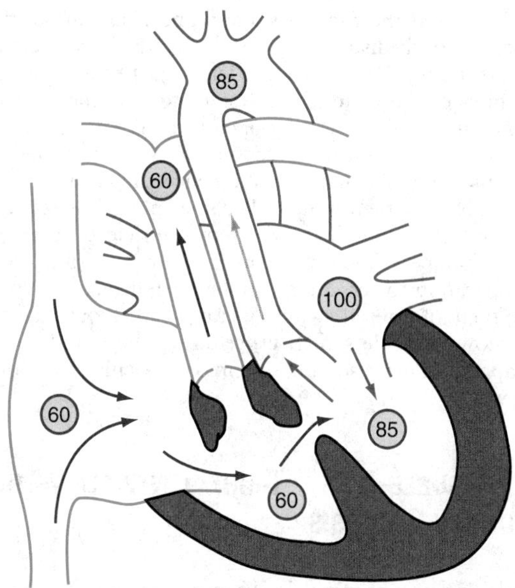

Figure 431-5. Physiology of l- or corrected transposition of the great arteries (l-TGA) with a ventricular septal defect and pulmonic stenosis (VSD + PS). *Circled numbers* represent oxygen saturation values. Right atrial (mixed venous) oxygen saturation is decreased secondary to systemic hypoxemia. Blood from the right atrium flows through the mitral valve into the "inverted" left ventricle. The left ventricle is, however, attached to the transposed pulmonary artery. Therefore, despite the anomalies, desaturated blood still winds up in the pulmonary circulation. Saturated blood returns to the left atrium, traverses the tricuspid valve into the "inverted" right ventricle, and is pumped into the transposed aorta. This circulation would be totally "corrected" were it not for the frequent association of other congenital anomalies, in this case, VSD + PS. Because of the stenotic pulmonary valve, some left ventricular blood flow crosses the VSD and into the right ventricle and the ascending aorta, and systemic desaturation results.

431.4 • L-Transposition of the Great Arteries (Corrected Transposition)

In l-transposition, the atrioventricular relationships are discordant, with the right atrium connected to the left ventricle and the left atrium to the right ventricle (ventricular inversion). The great arteries are also transposed, with the aorta arising from the right ventricle and the pulmonary artery from the left. The aorta arises to the left of the pulmonary artery (hence the designation *l* for levotransposition). The aorta may be anterior to the pulmonary artery; usually, they are nearly side by side. Desaturated systemic venous blood is returned to a normally positioned right atrium, from which it passes through a bicuspid atrioventricular (mitral) valve into a right-sided ventricle that has the architecture and smooth wall morphologic features of the normal left ventricle (Fig. 431-5). Because transposition is also present, desaturated blood ejected from this left ventricle enters the transposed pulmonary artery and flows into the lungs. Oxygenated pulmonary venous blood returns to a normally positioned left atrium, passes through a tricuspid atrioventricular valve into a left-sided ventricle, which has the trabeculated morphologic features of a normal right ventricle, and is then ejected into the transposed aorta. The double inversion of the atrioventricular and ventriculoarterial relationships results in desaturated right atrial blood reaching the lungs and oxygenated pulmonary venous blood appropriately flowing to the aorta. The circulation is physiologically "corrected." Without other defects, the hemodynamics would be nearly normal. In most patients, however, associated anomalies coexist: VSD, Ebstein-like abnormalities of the left-sided atrioventricular (tricuspid) valve, pulmonary valvular or subvalvular stenosis (or both), and atrioventricular conduction disturbances (complete heart block, accessory pathways such as Wolff-Parkinson-White syndrome).

CLINICAL MANIFESTATIONS. Symptoms and signs are widely variable and are determined by the associated lesions. If pulmonary outflow is unobstructed, the clinical signs are similar to those of an isolated VSD. If the TGA is associated with pulmonary stenosis and a VSD, the clinical signs are similar to those of tetralogy of Fallot.

DIAGNOSIS. The chest roentgenogram may suggest the abnormal position of the great arteries; the ascending aorta occupies the upper left border of the cardiac silhouette and has a straight profile. In addition to atrioventricular conduction disturbances, the electrocardiogram may show abnormal P waves; absent Q waves in V_6; abnormally present Q waves in leads III, aVR, aVF, and V_1; and upright T waves across the precordium. The echocardiogram is diagnostic. The characteristic features of the right ventricle (moderator band, coarser trabeculations, tricuspid valve that sits more inferiorly compared to the bicuspid mitral valve, and a smooth muscular conus or infundibulum separating the atrioventricular valve from the semilunar valve) allow the echocardiographer to determine the presence of atrioventricular discordance (right atrium connected to left ventricle; left atrium to right ventricle).

Surgical treatment of the associated anomalies, most often the VSD, is complicated by the position of the bundle of His, which can be injured at the time of surgery and result in heart block. Identification of the usual course of the bundle in corrected transposition (running superior to the defect) has been accomplished by mapping of the conduction system so that the surgeon can avoid the bundle of His during open heart repair.

Because simple surgical correction leaves the right ventricle as the systemic pumping chamber, and hence vulnerable to late ventricular failure, surgeons have become more aggressive about trying operations that leave the left ventricle as the systemic pumping chamber. This is accomplished by performing an atrial switch operation to reroute the systemic and pulmonary venous returns, then an arterial switch operation to reroute the ventricular outflows (**double switch procedure**). The long-term benefit of this approach in preserving systemic ventricular function is not yet known.

431.5 • Double-Outlet Right Ventricle Without Pulmonary Stenosis

In double-outlet right ventricle without pulmonary stenosis, both the aorta and the pulmonary artery arise from the right ventricle. The only outlet from the left ventricle is through a VSD. The clinical manifestations closely simulate those of an uncomplicated VSD with a large left-to-right shunt, although mild systemic desaturation may be present because of mixing of oxygenated and deoxygenated blood in the right ventricle. The electrocardiogram usually shows biventricular hypertrophy. Echocardiography is diagnostic and shows the right ventricular origin of both great vessels and their anteroposterior relationship, as well as the position of the VSD. Cardiac catheterization demonstrates the proximity of the VSD to the aorta, which results in most of the left ventricular blood being ejected directly into the systemic circulation. The angiogram also confirms the lack of mitral-aortic fibrous continuity and shows the aortic valve displaced superiorly and at the same level as the pulmonary valve. It is important to differentiate this condition from a simple VSD.

Surgical correction is accomplished by creation of an intracardiac tunnel. Blood is then ejected from the left ventricle via the VSD into the aorta. Pulmonary arterial banding may be required in infancy, followed by surgical correction when the child is bigger. When associated pulmonary stenosis is present, the cyanosis is more marked and pulmonary blood flow is decreased (see Chapter 430).

431.6 • Double-Outlet Right Ventricle with Transposition of the Great Arteries (Taussig-Bing Anomaly)

In double-outlet right ventricle with TGA, the VSD is located above the crista supraventricularis (subarterial VSD) and is either directly subpulmonary or related to both the pulmonary and aortic valves (doubly committed VSD). Patients experience cardiac failure early in infancy and are at risk for the development of pulmonary vascular disease and cyanosis. Cardiomegaly is usual, and a parasternal systolic ejection murmur is audible, sometimes preceded by an ejection click and loud closure of the pulmonary valve. Left-sided obstructive lesions are frequent, including coarctation of the aorta, interruption of the aortic arch, and a restrictive VSD, which obstructs left ventricular ejection. The electrocardiogram shows right axis deviation and right, left, or biventricular hypertrophy. The roentgenogram documents cardiomegaly, a large left atrium, and prominence of the pulmonary artery and pulmonary vasculature. The anatomic features of the anomaly and associated abnormalities are best demonstrated by a combination of echocardiography and selective right and left ventriculography. Palliation may be achieved by pulmonary arterial banding in infancy and surgical correction at a later age, which may be accomplished by a Rastelli procedure (see Chapter 430) or by an arterial switch procedure (see Chapter 431.2).

431.7 • Total Anomalous Pulmonary Venous Return

PATHOPHYSIOLOGY. Abnormal development of the pulmonary veins may result in either partial or complete anomalous drainage into the systemic venous circulation. Partial anomalous pulmonary venous return is usually an acyanotic lesion (see Chapter 426.4). Total anomalous pulmonary venous return (TAPVR) allows total mixing of systemic venous and pulmonary venous blood flow within the heart and thus produces cyanosis.

In TAPVR, the heart has no direct pulmonary venous connection into the left atrium. The pulmonary veins may drain above the diaphragm into the right atrium directly, into the coronary sinus, or into the superior vena cava via a "vertical vein," or they may drain below the diaphragm and join into a "descending vein" that enters into the inferior vena cava or one of its major tributaries, often via the ductus venosus. This latter form of anomalous venous drainage is most commonly associated with obstruction, usually as the ductus venosus closes soon after birth, although supracardiac anomalous veins may also become obstructed. Occasionally, the drainage may be mixed, with some veins draining above and others below the diaphragm.

All forms of TAPVR involve mixing of oxygenated and deoxygenated blood before or at the level of the right atrium (total mixing lesion). Right atrial blood either passes into the right ventricle and pulmonary artery or passes through an atrial septal defect (ASD) or patent foramen ovale into the left atrium. The right atrium and ventricle and the pulmonary artery are generally enlarged, whereas the left atrium and ventricle may be normal or small. The manifestations of TAPVR depend on the presence or absence of obstruction of the venous channels (Table 431-1). If pulmonary venous return is obstructed, severe pulmonary congestion and pulmonary hypertension develop; rapid deterioration occurs without surgical intervention. Obstructed TAPVR is a pediatric cardiac surgical emergency because prostaglandin therapy is usually not effective.

CLINICAL MANIFESTATIONS. Three major clinical patterns of TAPVR are seen. Some are manifested in the neonatal period as severe obstruction to pulmonary venous return, most prevalent in the infracardiac group (see Table 431-1). Cyanosis and severe tachypnea are prominent, but murmurs may not be present. Infants are severely ill and fail to respond to mechanical ventilation. Rapid diagnosis and surgical correction are necessary for survival. Another group is characterized by heart failure in early life, but these infants have only mild or moderate obstruction to pulmonary venous return and a large left-to-right shunt. Because

TABLE 431-1. Anomalous Pulmonary Venous Return

% AND SITE OF CONNECTION	% WITH SEVERE OBSTRUCTION
Supracardiac (50)	
Left superior vena cava (40)	40
Right superior vena cava (10)	75
Cardiac (25)	
Coronary sinus (20)	10
Right atrium (5)	5
Infracardiac (20)	95–100
Mixed (5)	

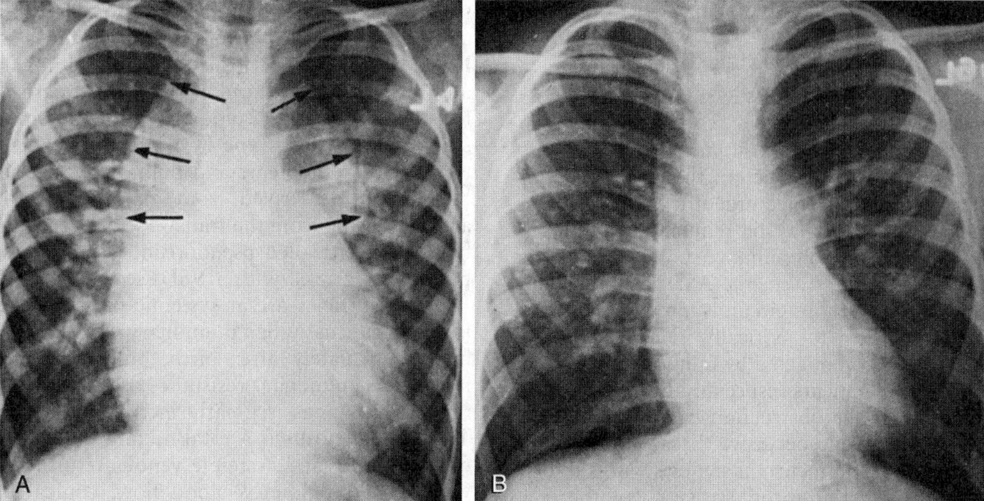

Figure 431-6. Chest x-ray of total anomalous pulmonary venous return to the left superior vena cava. *A,* Preoperative image. *Arrows* point to the supracardiac shadow, which produces the snowman or figure 8 configuration. Cardiomegaly and increased pulmonary vascularity are evident. *B,* Postoperative image showing a decrease in the size of the heart and the supracardiac shadow.

pulmonary artery hypertension is present, these infants are severely ill. Systolic murmurs are audible along the left sternal border, and a gallop rhythm may be present. A continuous murmur is occasionally heard along the upper left sternal border over the pulmonary area. Cyanosis is mild. The third group of patients with TAPVR consists of those in whom pulmonary venous obstruction is not present; these patients have total mixing of systemic venous and pulmonary venous blood and a large left-to-right shunt. Pulmonary hypertension is absent, and these patients are less likely to be severely symptomatic during infancy. Clinical cyanosis is usually mild.

DIAGNOSIS. The electrocardiogram demonstrates right ventricular hypertrophy (usually a qR pattern in V_3R and V_1, and the P waves are frequently tall and spiked). Roentgenograms are pathognomonic in older children if the anomalous pulmonary veins enter the innominate vein and persistent left superior vena cava (Fig. 431-6). A large supracardiac shadow can be seen, which together with the normal cardiac shadow forms a **"snowman"** appearance. This appearance is not helpful for diagnosis in early infancy because of the thymus. In most cases without obstruction, the heart is enlarged, the pulmonary artery and right ventricle are prominent, and pulmonary vascularity is increased. In neonates with marked pulmonary venous obstruction, the chest roentgenogram demonstrates a perihilar pattern of pulmonary edema and a small heart. This appearance can be confused with primary pulmonary disease. The differential diagnosis includes persistent pulmonary hypertension of the newborn, respiratory distress syndrome, pneumonia (bacterial, meconium aspiration), pulmonary lymphangiectasia, and other heart defects (hypoplastic left heart syndrome).

The echocardiogram demonstrates a large right ventricle and usually identifies the pattern of abnormal pulmonary venous connections (Fig. 431-7). The demonstration of a vessel in the abdomen with Doppler venous flow away from the heart is pathognomonic of TAPVR below the diaphragm. Shunting occurs almost exclusively from right to left at the atrial level.

Cardiac catheterization shows that the oxygen saturation of blood in both atria, both ventricles, and the aorta is more or less similar, indicative of a total mixing lesion. An increase in systemic venous saturation occurs at the site of entry of the abnormal pulmonary venous channel. In older patients, pulmonary arterial and right ventricular pressure may be only moderately elevated, but in infants with pulmonary venous obstruction, pulmonary hypertension is usual. Selective pulmonary arteriography shows the anatomy of the pulmonary veins and their point of entry into the

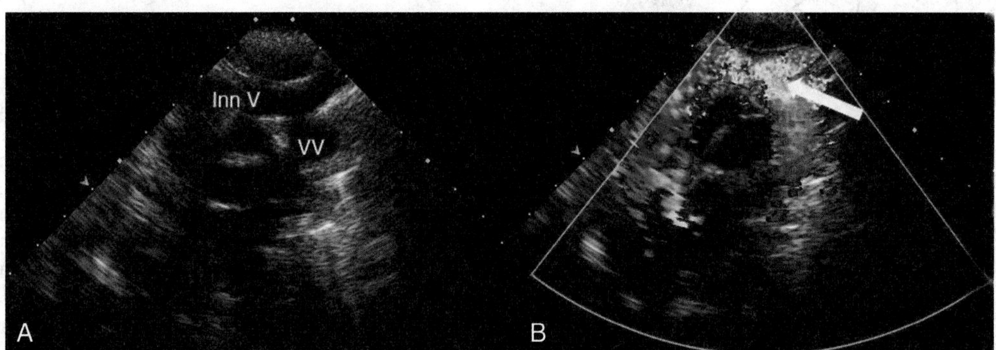

Figure 431-7. Suprasternal two-dimensional echocardiographic views demonstrating supracardiac total anomalous pulmonary venous return (type I). *A,* The large vertical ascending vein can be seen entering the innominate vein. There is a moderate narrowing where the anomalous vein enters the upper body venous system. *B,* Color Doppler examination shows a venous flow signal *(red color)* indicating that blood is moving away toward the transducer and thus from the heart (all venous flow should normally return toward the heart), diagnostic of anomalous pulmonary venous return. The turbulent acceleration of flow can be seen *(arrow)* where the vertical vein enters the innominate. Inn V, innominate vein; VV, vertical vein.

systemic venous circulation. MRI and CT may be alternative methods of confirming the diagnosis.

TREATMENT. Surgical correction of TAPVR is indicated during infancy. Before surgery, infants may be stabilized with prostaglandin E_1 to dilate the ductus venosus and the ductus arteriosus, although with significant obstruction this is usually not effective. If surgery cannot be performed urgently, extracorporeal membrane oxygenation (ECMO) may be required to maintain oxygenation. Surgically, the common pulmonary venous trunk is anastomosed directly to the left atrium, the ASD is closed, and the connection to the systemic venous circuit is interrupted. Early results are generally good, even for critically ill neonates. The postoperative period may be complicated by pulmonary vascular hypertensive crises. In some patients, especially those in whom the diagnosis was delayed or the obstruction was severe, recurrent stenosis and pulmonary veno-occlusive disease may occur. Attempts have been made to treat recurrent stenosis with surgery, balloon angioplasty, stents, and antiproliferative chemotherapy. To date, the long-term prognosis in these patients is poor and **heart-lung transplantation** may be the only option (see Chapter 443.2).

431.8 • Truncus Arteriosus

PATHOPHYSIOLOGY. In truncus arteriosus, a single arterial trunk (truncus arteriosus) arises from the heart and supplies the systemic, pulmonary, and coronary circulations. A VSD is always present, with the truncus overriding the defect and receiving blood from both the right and left ventricles (Fig. 431-8). The number of truncal valve cusps varies from two to as many as six. The pulmonary arteries may arise together from the posterior left side of the persistent truncus arteriosus and then divide into left and right pulmonary arteries (**type I truncus arteriosus**). In **types II** and **III** truncus arteriosus, no main pulmonary artery is present, and the right and left pulmonary arteries arise from separate orifices in the posterior (**type II**) or lateral (**type III**) aspects of the truncus arteriosus. **Type IV** truncus has no identifiable connection between the heart and pulmonary arteries, and pulmonary blood flow is derived from major aortopulmonary collateral arteries arising from the transverse or descending aorta; this form has also been called pseudotruncus but is essentially a form of pulmonary atresia with a VSD (see Chapter 430.2).

Both ventricles are at systemic pressure and both eject blood into the truncus. When pulmonary vascular resistance is relatively high immediately after birth, pulmonary blood flow may be normal; as pulmonary resistance drops in the 1st mo of life, blood flow to the lungs is greatly increased and heart failure ensues. Truncus arteriosus is a total mixing lesion with total admixture of pulmonary and systemic venous return. Because of the large volume of pulmonary blood flow, clinical cyanosis is usually minimal. If the lesion is left untreated, pulmonary resistance eventually increases, pulmonary blood flow decreases, and cyanosis becomes more apparent (Eisenmenger physiology; see Chapter 433.2). The truncal valve is occasionally incompetent, which significantly complicates medical and surgical management.

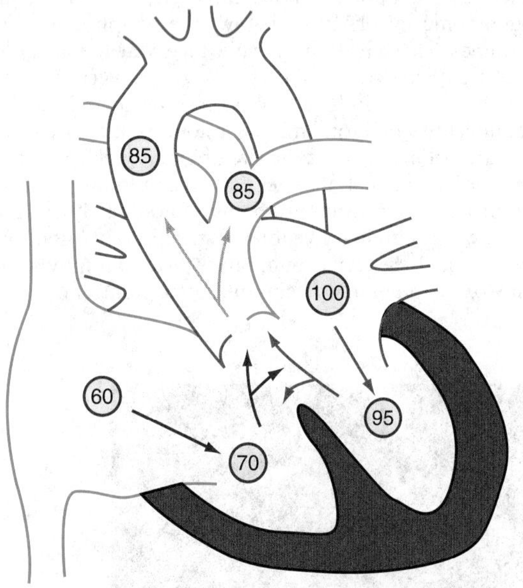

Figure 431-8. Physiology of truncus arteriosus. *Circled numbers* represent oxygen saturation values. Right atrial (mixed venous) oxygen saturation is decreased secondary to systemic hypoxemia. Desaturated blood enters the right atrium, flows through the tricuspid valve into the right ventricle, and is ejected into the truncus. Saturated blood returning from the left atrium enters the left ventricle and is also ejected into the truncus. The common aortopulmonary trunk gives rise to the ascending aorta and to the main or branch pulmonary arteries. Oxygen saturation in the aorta and pulmonary arteries is usually the same (definition of a total mixing lesion). As pulmonary vascular resistance decreases in the 1st few weeks of life, pulmonary blood flow increases dramatically and mild cyanosis and congestive heart failure result.

CLINICAL MANIFESTATIONS. The clinical signs of truncus arteriosus vary with age and depend on the level of pulmonary vascular resistance. In the immediate newborn period, signs of heart failure are usually absent; a murmur and minimal cyanosis are the initial signs. In most older infants, pulmonary blood flow is torrential and the clinical picture is dominated by heart failure. Cyanosis is minimal. Runoff of blood from the truncus to the pulmonary circulation may result in a wide pulse pressure and bounding pulses. These findings may be further exaggerated if truncal valve insufficiency is present. The heart is usually enlarged, and the precordium is hyperdynamic. The 2nd heart sound is loud and single. A systolic ejection murmur, sometimes accompanied by a thrill, is generally audible along the left sternal border. The murmur is frequently preceded by an early systolic ejection click. In the presence of truncal valve insufficiency, a high-pitched early diastolic decrescendo murmur is heard at the midleft sternal border. An apical mid-diastolic rumbling murmur caused by increased flow through the mitral valve is audible with the bell of the stethoscope. In older children with restricted pulmonary blood flow secondary to pulmonary vascular obstructive disease, progressive cyanosis, polycythemia, and clubbing develops. Truncus arteriosus is a conotruncal malformation and may be associated with **DiGeorge syndrome,** which has been linked to a deletion of chromosome 22q11.

DIAGNOSIS. The electrocardiogram shows right, left, or combined ventricular hypertrophy. The chest roentgenogram also shows considerable variation. The cardiac enlargement is due to prominence of both ventricles. The truncus may produce a prominent shadow that follows the normal course of the ascending aorta and aortic knob; the aortic arch is to the right in 50% of patients. Sometimes a high bulge left of the aortic knob is produced by the main or left pulmonary artery. Pulmonary vascularity is increased after the 1st few weeks of life. Echocardiography demonstrates the large truncal artery overriding the VSD and the pattern of origin of the branch pulmonary arteries (Fig. 431-9). Associated anomalies such as an interrupted aortic arch may be noted. Pulsed and color Doppler studies are used to evaluate truncal valve regurgitation. If required, cardiac catheterization shows a left-to-right shunt at the ventricular level, with right-to-left shunting into the truncus. Systolic pressure in both ventricles and the truncus is similar. Angiography reveals the large truncus arteriosus and more precisely defines the origin of the pulmonary arteries.

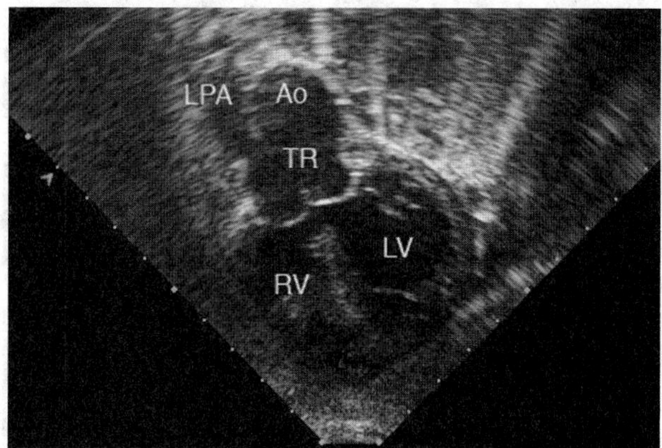

Figure 431-9. Subcostal two-dimensional echocardiographic demonstration of truncus arteriosus. The large truncal valve can be seen overriding the ventricular septal defect. In this case, only the left pulmonary artery (LPA) arises from the truncus (TR). The pulmonary arteries are discontinuous and the right pulmonary artery arises from the descending aorta via the ductus arteriosus (not shown). Ao, aorta; LV, left ventricle; RV, right ventricle.

PROGNOSIS AND COMPLICATIONS. Without surgery, many of these patients succumb during infancy or by the 1st or 2nd yr of life. If pulmonary blood flow is restricted by the development of pulmonary vascular disease, the patient may survive into early adulthood. Surgical results have been very good, and many patients with repaired truncus are entering young adulthood. When truncus arteriosus is associated with DiGeorge syndrome, the associated endocrine, immunologic, facial, and pulmonary abnormalities may complicate recovery.

TREATMENT. In the 1st few weeks of life, many of these infants can be managed with anticongestive medications; as pulmonary vascular resistance falls, heart failure symptoms worsen and surgery is indicated, usually in the next few weeks. Delay of surgery much beyond 4–8 wk may increase the likelihood of pulmonary vascular disease; some centers advocate neonatal repair at the time of diagnosis. At surgery, the VSD is closed, the pulmonary arteries are separated from the truncus, and continuity is established between the right ventricle and the pulmonary arteries with a homograft conduit (**Rastelli repair**). Immediate surgical results are excellent, but after repair the conduit must be replaced, often several times, as the child grows. In older patients who already have pulmonary vascular obstruction, routine surgical treatment is contraindicated and **heart-lung transplantation** is the only option.

431.9 • Single Ventricle (Double-Inlet Ventricle, Univentricular Heart)

PATHOPHYSIOLOGY. With a single ventricle, both atria empty through a common atrioventricular valve or via two separate valves into a single ventricular chamber, with total mixing of systemic and pulmonary venous return. This chamber may have left, right, or indeterminate ventricular anatomic characteristics. The aorta and pulmonary artery both arise from this single chamber, although one of the great vessels may originate from a rudimentary outflow chamber. The aorta may be posterior, anterior (malposition), or side by side with the pulmonary artery and either to the right or to the left. Pulmonary stenosis or atresia is common.

CLINICAL MANIFESTATIONS. The clinical picture is variable and depends on the associated intracardiac anomalies. If pulmonary outflow is obstructed, the findings may be similar to those of tetralogy of Fallot: marked cyanosis without heart failure. If pulmonary outflow is unobstructed, the findings are similar to those of transposition with VSD: minimal cyanosis with marked heart failure.

In patients with pulmonary stenosis, cyanosis is present in infancy and increases in intensity during childhood, when clubbing and polycythemia appear. Dyspnea and fatigue are frequent, cardiomegaly is mild or moderate, a left parasternal lift is palpable, and a systolic thrill is common. The systolic ejection murmur is usually loud; an ejection click may be audible, and the 2nd heart sound is single and loud.

Patients with unobstructed pulmonary outflow have torrential pulmonary blood flow and are initially seen in early infancy with tachypnea, dyspnea, failure to thrive, and recurrent pulmonary infections. Cyanosis is only mild or moderate. Cardiomegaly is generally marked, and a left parasternal lift is palpable. The systolic ejection murmur is not usually intense, and the 2nd heart sound is loud and closely split. A 3rd heart sound is common and may be followed by a short mid-diastolic rumbling murmur caused by increased flow through the atrioventricular valves. The eventual development of pulmonary vascular disease reduces pulmonary blood flow so that the cyanosis increases and signs of cardiac failure appear to improve (Eisenmenger physiology; see Chapter 433.2).

DIAGNOSIS. Findings on the electrocardiogram are nonspecific. P waves are normal, spiked, or bifid. The precordial lead pattern suggests right ventricular hypertrophy, combined ventricular hypertrophy, or sometimes left ventricular dominance. The initial QRS forces are usually to the left and anterior. Roentgenographic examination confirms the degree of cardiomegaly. If present, a rudimentary outflow chamber may produce a bulge on the upper left border of the cardiac silhouette in the posteroanterior projection. In the absence of pulmonary stenosis, pulmonary vasculature is increased, whereas in the presence of pulmonary stenosis, pulmonary vasculature is diminished. Absence or near absence of the ventricular septum is the principal echocardiographic sign. The echocardiogram can usually determine whether the single ventricle has right, left, or mixed morphologic features. The presence of a rudimentary outflow chamber under one of the great vessels can be identified, and pulsed Doppler can be used to determine whether flow through this communication (bulboventricular foramen) is obstructed.

If cardiac catheterization is performed, arterial oxygen saturation is seen to be decreased in the presence of severe pulmonary stenosis or obstructive pulmonary hypertension, but it may be near normal when pulmonary blood flow is unimpeded. The pressure in the ventricular chamber is at systemic level; a gradient may be demonstrated across the entrance to a rudimentary outflow chamber. Pressure measurements and angiography demonstrate whether pulmonary stenosis is present. Severe pulmonary hypertension may be demonstrated in older patients in the absence of pulmonary stenosis.

PROGNOSIS AND COMPLICATIONS. Unoperated, some patients succumb during infancy from heart failure. Others may survive to adolescence and early adult life but finally succumb to the effects of chronic hypoxemia or, in the absence of pulmonary stenosis, to the effects of pulmonary vascular disease. Patients with moderate pulmonary stenosis have the best prognosis because pulmonary blood flow, though restricted, is still adequate.

TREATMENT. If pulmonary stenosis is severe, a **Blalock-Taussig aortopulmonary shunt** is indicated (see Chapter 430.1). If pulmonary blood flow is unrestricted, pulmonary arterial banding is used to control heart failure and prevent progressive pulmonary vascular disease. The **bidirectional Glenn shunt** followed by a **modified Fontan operation** (cavopulmonary isolation procedure, see Chapter 430.4) is the ultimate treatment of choice. If subaortic stenosis is present because of a restrictive connection to a rudimentary outflow chamber, surgical relief can be provided by anastomosing the proximal pulmonary artery to the side of the ascending aorta (**Damus-Stansyl Kaye operation**).

431.10 • Hypoplastic Left Heart Syndrome

PATHOPHYSIOLOGY. The term hypoplastic left heart is used to describe a related group of anomalies that include underdevelopment of the left side of the heart (atresia of the aortic or mitral orifice) and hypoplasia of the ascending aorta. The left ventricle may be small and nonfunctional or totally atretic; the right ventricle maintains both the pulmonary and systemic circulation (Fig. 431-10). Pulmonary venous blood passes through an atrial defect or dilated foramen ovale from the left to the right side of the heart, where it mixes with systemic venous blood (**total mixing lesion**). When the ventricular septum is intact, which is usually the case, all the right ventricular blood is ejected into the main pulmonary artery; the descending aorta is supplied via the ductus arteriosus, with flow from the ductus also filling the ascending aorta and coronary arteries in a retrograde fashion. In the presence of a VSD and a patent but small aortic orifice, right ventricular blood is ejected into the small left ventricle and ascending aorta, as well as the pulmonary artery. The major hemodynamic abnormalities are inadequate maintenance of the systemic circulation and, depending on the size of the atrial-level communication, either pulmonary venous hypertension (restrictive foramen ovale) or pulmonary overcirculation (moderate or large ASD).

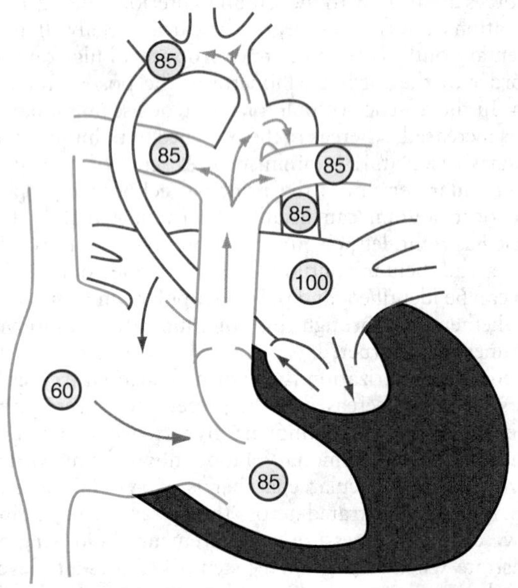

Figure 431-10. Physiology of hypoplastic left heart syndrome (HLHS). *Circled numbers* represent oxygen saturation values. HLHS is not a single lesion but a constellation of different degrees of hypoplasia of the left-sided heart structures. This drawing shows a patent mitral valve, a small left ventricular cavity, and a diminutive ascending aorta. Right atrial (mixed venous) oxygen saturation is decreased secondary to systemic hypoxemia. Desaturated blood enters the right atrium, flows through the tricuspid valve into the right ventricle, and is ejected into the pulmonary artery. Because of the markedly decreased left ventricular compliance, most of the pulmonary venous blood returning to the left atrium shunts left to right at the atrial level. A small amount of left atrial blood will cross the mitral valve and be ejected into the tiny ascending aorta. The right ventricular oxygen saturation represents a mixing of desaturated systemic venous blood and saturated pulmonary venous blood. Pulmonary artery blood flows into the pulmonary arteries as well as right to left across the patent ductus arteriosus (PDA) into the aorta. Ductal blood flows prograde to the descending aorta as well as retrograde to the ascending aorta, where it supplies the head and neck vessels in addition to the coronary arteries (which arise off the small ascending aorta). Closure of the PDA results in profound hypoxia and circulatory collapse.

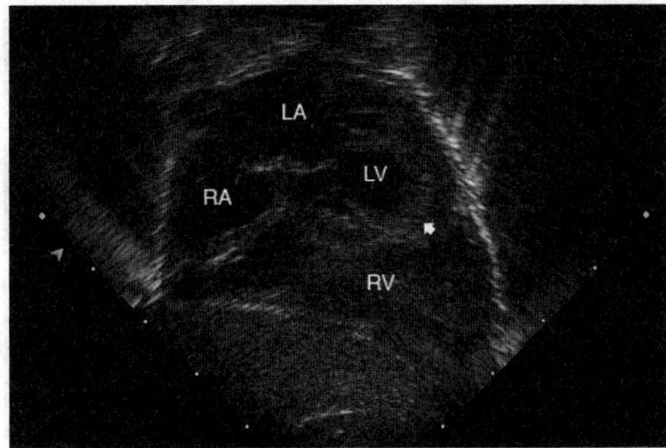

Figure 431-11. Subcostal two-dimensional echocardiographic diagnosis of hypoplastic left heart syndrome. The small left ventricular chamber can be seen, the apex of which *(arrowhead)* does not form the apex of the heart. The atrial septum can be seen bowing from the left to the right, indicating that the communication between the two atria is pressure restrictive. LA, left atrium; LV, left ventricle; RA, right atrium; RV, right ventricle.

CLINICAL MANIFESTATIONS. Although cyanosis may not always be obvious in the 1st 48 hr of life, a grayish-blue color of the skin is soon apparent and denotes a mix of cyanosis and poor perfusion. The condition is diagnosed in most infants in the 1st few hours or days of life. If the ductus arteriosus partially closes, signs of poor systemic perfusion and shock predominate. Signs of heart failure usually appear within the 1st few days or weeks of life and include dyspnea, hepatomegaly, and low cardiac output. All of the peripheral pulses may be weak or absent. Cardiac enlargement is usual, with a palpable right ventricular parasternal lift. A nondescript systolic murmur is generally audible. Extracardiac anomalies, particularly of the kidneys and central nervous system, may be present.

DIAGNOSIS. On the chest roentgenogram, the heart is variable in size in the 1st days of life, but cardiomegaly develops rapidly and is associated with increased pulmonary vascularity. The initial electrocardiogram may show only the normal right ventricular dominance with poor ventricular voltage, but later, P waves become prominent and right ventricular hypertrophy is usual. The echocardiogram is diagnostic and demonstrates absence or hypoplasia of the mitral valve and aortic root, a variably small left atrium and left ventricle, and a large right atrium and right ventricle (Fig. 431-11). The size of the atrial communication, by which pulmonary venous blood leaves the left atrium, can be assessed directly and by pulsed and color flow Doppler studies. Suprasternal notch views identify the small ascending aorta and transverse aortic arch and may also show a discrete coarctation of the aorta in the juxtaductal area. Doppler echocardiography demonstrates the absence of anterograde flow in the ascending aorta, which is supplied by retrograde flow via the ductus arteriosus. The diagnosis of hypoplastic left heart syndrome can usually be made without need for cardiac catheterization. If catheterization is necessary, the hypoplastic ascending aorta can be demonstrated by angiography.

PROGNOSIS AND COMPLICATIONS. Untreated patients most often succumb during the 1st months of life, usually during the 1st or 2nd wk. Occasionally, unoperated patients may live for months or rarely years. One third of infants with hypoplastic left heart syndrome have evidence of either a major or minor central nervous system abnormality. Other dysmorphic features may be found in up to 40% of patients. Thus, careful preoperative evaluation (genetic, neurologic, and ophthalmologic) should be performed in patients being considered for either standard surgical therapy or cardiac transplantation.

TREATMENT. Surgical therapy for hypoplastic left heart syndrome has been associated with survival rates as high as 95% for the 1st-stage palliation in many centers. Management options include the **Norwood procedure** (Fig. 431-12) or the **Sano procedure,** which is similar to the Norwood procedure, but instead of using a Blalock-Taussig shunt to provide pulmonary blood flow, the surgeon inserts a right ventricle to pulmonary artery homograft, essentially creating a double-outlet right ventricle. Primary heart transplantation, previously advocated by several centers, is less common due to the substantially improved survival rates with standard surgery.

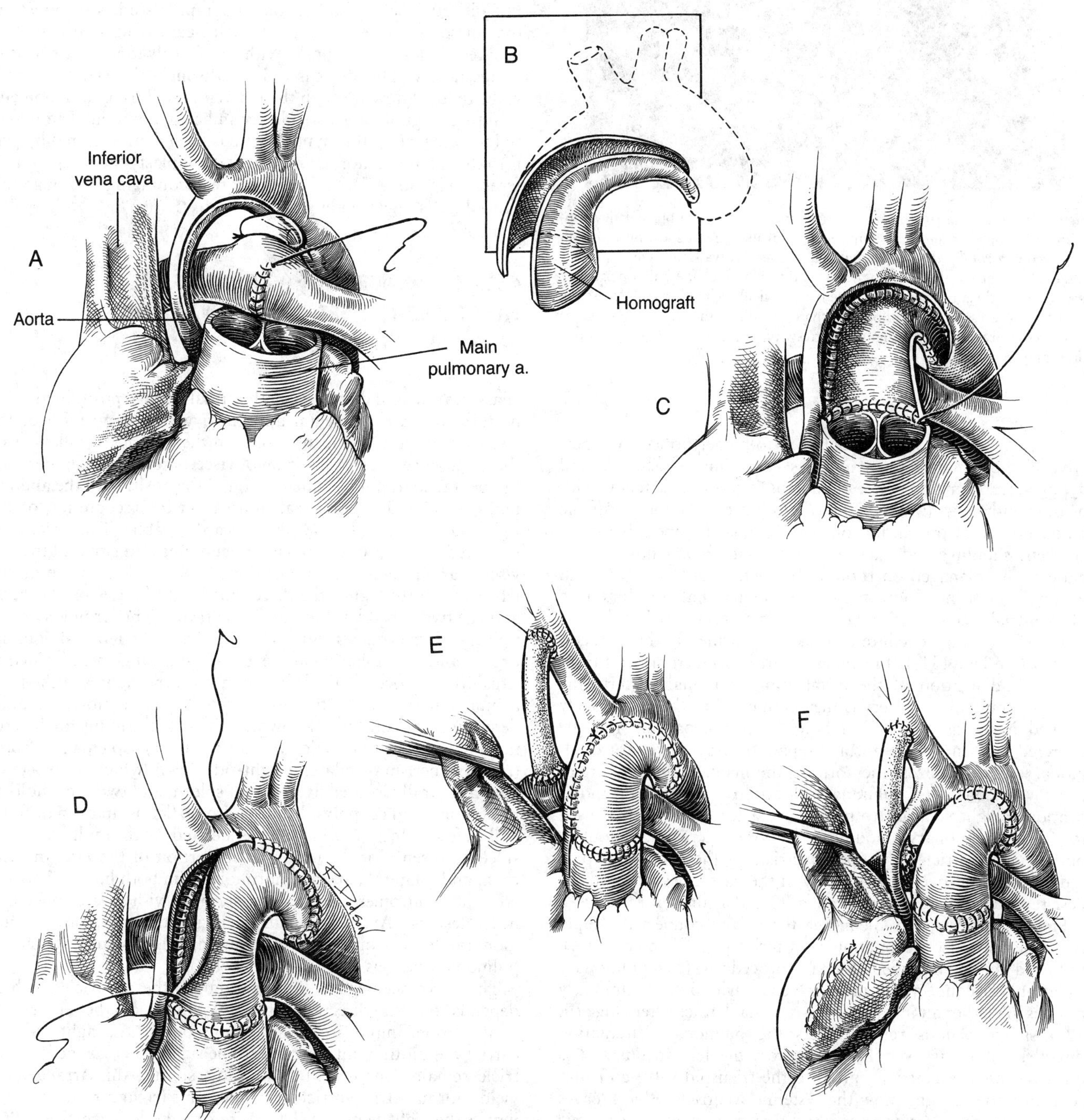

Figure 431-12. The Norwood procedure, one of the two current techniques for 1st-stage palliation of hypoplastic left heart syndrome. *A,* Incisions used for the procedure incorporate a cuff of arterial wall allograft. The distal divided main pulmonary artery may be closed by direct suture or with a patch. *B,* Dimensions of the cuff of the arterial wall allograft. *C,* The arterial wall allograft is used to supplement the anastomosis between the proximal divided main pulmonary artery and the ascending aorta, aortic arch, and proximal descending aorta. *D* and *E,* The procedure is completed by an atrial septectomy and a 3.5 mm modified right Blalock shunt. *F,* When the ascending aorta is particularly small, an alternative procedure involves placement of a complete tube of arterial allograft. The tiny ascending aorta may be left in situ, as indicated, or implanted into the side of the neoaorta. (From Castañeda AR, Jonas RA, Mayer JE Jr, Hanley FL: Single-ventricle tricuspid atresia. In *Cardiac Surgery of the Neonate and Infant.* Philadelphia, WB Saunders, 1994.)

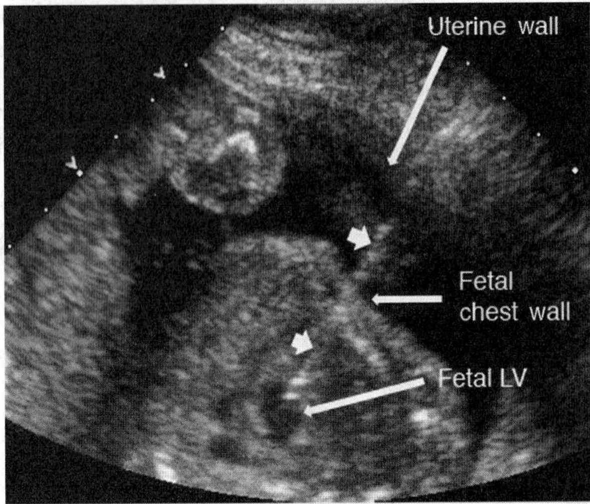

Figure 431-13. Fetal treatment of critical aortic stenosis to prevent development of hypoplastic left heart syndrome. Fetal ultrasound showing insertion of a needle *(arrowheads)* via the maternal abdominal wall, through the uterus and the fetal chest wall, and into the fetal left ventricle (LV). A balloon catheter is next inserted via the needle into the left ventricular chamber and across the stenotic aortic valve. The balloon is inflated to dilate the valve, the catheter and needle are removed. (Figure courtesy of Dr. Stanton Perry, Stanford University, Stanford, CA).

If a Norwood or Sano procedure is to be performed, preoperative medical management includes correction of acidosis and hypoglycemia, maintenance of ductus arteriosus patency with prostaglandin E_1 (0.01–0.20 mg/kg/min) to support systemic blood flow, and prevention of hypothermia. Preoperative management should avoid excessive pulmonary blood flow; often, patients are managed on room air or with a FIO_2 of 18% with nitrogen gas blended into the oxygen source. Balloon dilatation of the atrial septum may be indicated if surgery is delayed.

The Norwood procedure is usually performed in three stages. **Stage I** (see Fig. 431-12) includes an atrial septectomy and transection and ligation of the distal main pulmonary artery; the proximal pulmonary artery is then connected to the transversely opened hypoplastic aortic arch to form a neoaorta, and the coarcted segment of the aorta is repaired. A synthetic aortopulmonary shunt connects the aorta to the main pulmonary artery to provide controlled pulmonary blood flow. In the Sano modification, a right ventricle to pulmonary artery homograft is used to provide pulmonary blood flow, temporarily creating a double-outlet right ventricle. The operative risk for these 1st-stage procedures has improved dramatically in the past 2 decades and the best reported results demonstrate a 90–95% survival rate.

Stage II consists of a Glenn anastomosis to connect the superior vena cava to the pulmonary arteries (see Chapter 431.4), followed by a modified Fontan procedure (cavopulmonary isolation) to connect the inferior vena cava to the pulmonary arteries via either an intra-atrial or external baffle. After **stage III**, all systemic venous return enters the pulmonary circulation directly. Pulmonary venous flow enters the left atrium and is directed across the atrial septum to the tricuspid valve and subsequently to the right (now the systemic) ventricle. Blood leaves the right ventricle via the neoaorta, which supplies the systemic circulation. The old aortic root now attached to the neoaorta provides coronary blood flow. The risks associated with stages II and III are even less than those of stage I; the long-term results of the Norwood and Sano procedures remain to be demonstrated.

An alternative therapy is **cardiac transplantation,** either in the immediate neonatal period, thereby obviating stage I of the Norwood procedure, or after a successful stage I Norwood procedure is performed as a bridge to transplantation. After transplantation, patients usually have normal cardiac function and no symptoms of heart failure; however, these patients have the chronic risk of organ rejection and lifelong immunosuppressive therapy (see Chapter 443.1). The combination of donor shortage and improved results with standard surgical procedures has caused most centers to stop recommending transplantation except when associated lesions make the Norwood operation an exceptionally high-risk procedure.

PREVENTION. Serial fetal echocardiographic studies demonstrate that in some fetuses, hypoplastic left heart syndrome may be a progressive lesion, beginning with simple valvar aortic stenosis in midgestation. The decreased flow through the stenotic aortic valve reduces flow through the left ventricle during development, resulting in gradual ventricular chamber hypoplasia. The potential for preventing this hypoplasia has been demonstrated by performing in utero aortic balloon valvuloplasty in midgestation fetuses (Fig. 431-13). Early results are encouraging, although this procedure is regarded as experimental.

431.11 • Abnormal Positions of the Heart and the Heterotaxy Syndromes (Asplenia, Polysplenia)

Classification and diagnosis of abnormal cardiac position are best performed via a segmental approach, with the position of the viscera and atria first identified, then the ventricles, followed by the great vessels. Determination of **visceroatrial situs** can be made by roentgenographic demonstration of the position of the abdominal organs and the tracheal bifurcation for recognition of the right and left bronchi and by echocardiography. The atrial situs is related to the situs of the viscera and lungs. In situs solitus, the viscera are in their normal positions (stomach and spleen on the left, liver on the right), the three-lobed right lung is on the right, and the two-lobed left lung on the left; the right atrium is on the right, and the left atrium is on the left. When the abdominal organs and lung lobation are reversed, an arrangement known as situs inversus occurs, the left atrium is on the right and the right atrium on the left. If the visceroatrial situs cannot be readily determined, a condition known as situs indeterminus or heterotaxia exists. The two major variations are (1) **asplenia syndrome** (right isomerism or bilateral right-sidedness), which is associated with a centrally located liver, absent spleen, and two morphologic right lungs; and (2) **polysplenia syndrome** (left isomerism or bilateral left-sidedness), which is associated with multiple small spleens, absence of the intrahepatic portion of the inferior vena cava, and bilateral left lung morphology (in both lungs). The heterotaxia syndromes are usually associated with severe congenital heart lesions: ASD, VSD, atrioventricular septal defect, pulmonary stenosis or atresia, and anomalous systemic venous or pulmonary venous return (Table 431-2).

The next segment is localization of the ventricles, which depends on the direction of development of the embryonic cardiac loop. Initial protrusion of the loop to the right (d-loop) carries the future right ventricle to the right, whereas the left ventricle remains on the left. With situs solitus, this arrangement yields normal atrioventricular connections (right atrium connecting to the right ventricle, left atrium to the left ventricle). Protrusion of the loop to the left (l-loop) carries the future right ventricle to the left and the left ventricle to the right. In this case, in the presence of situs solitus, the right atrium connects with the left ventricle and the left atrium with the right ventricle (ventricular inversion).

The final segment is that of the great vessels. With each type of cardiac loop, the ventricular-arterial relationships may be

TABLE 431-2. Comparison of Cardiosplenic Heterotaxy Syndromes

FEATURE	ASPLENIA (RIGHT ISOMERISM)	POLYSPLENIA (LEFT ISOMERISM)
Spleen	Absent	Multiple
Sidedness (isomerism)	Bilateral right	Bilateral left
Lungs	Bilateral trilobar with eparterial bronchi	Bilateral bilobar with hyparterial bronchi
Sex	Male (65%)	Female ≥ male
Right-sided stomach	Yes	Less common
Symmetric liver	Yes	Yes
Partial intestinal rotation	Yes	Yes
Dextrocardia (%)	30–40	30–40
Pulmonary blood flow	Decreased (usually)	Increased (usually)
Severe cyanosis	Yes	No
Transposition of great arteries (%)	60–75	15
Total anomalous pulmonary venous return (%)	70–80	Rare
Common atrioventricular valve (%)	80–90	20–40
Single ventricle (%)	40–50	10–15
Absent inferior vena cava with azygos continuation	No	Characteristic
Bilateral superior vena cava	Yes	Yes
Other common defects	PA, PS	Partial anomalous pulmonary venous return, ventricle septal defect, double-outlet right ventricle
Risk of sepsis	Yes	No
Howell-Jolly and Heinz bodies, pitted erythrocytes	Yes	No
Absent gallbladder; biliary atresia	No	Yes

PA, pulmonary atresia; PS, pulmonary stenosis.

regarded as either normal (right ventricle to the pulmonary artery, left ventricle to the aorta) or transposed (right ventricle to the aorta, left ventricle to the pulmonary artery). A further classification can be based on the position of the aorta (normally to the right and posterior) relative to the pulmonary artery. In transposition, the aorta is usually anterior and either to the right of the pulmonary artery (d-transposition) or to the left (l-transposition). These segmental relationships can be determined by echocardiographic and angiographic studies demonstrating both atrioventricular and ventriculoarterial relationships. The clinical manifestations of these syndromes of abnormal cardiac position are determined primarily by their associated cardiovascular anomalies.

Dextrocardia occurs when the heart is in the right side of the chest; levocardia (the normal situation) is present when the heart is in the left side of the chest. Dextrocardia without associated situs inversus and levocardia in the presence of situs inversus are most often complicated by severe malformations that include various combinations of single ventricle, arterial transposition, pulmonary stenosis, ASDs and VSDs, atrioventricular septal defect, anomalous pulmonary venous return, tricuspid atresia, and pulmonary arterial hypoplasia or atresia. Surveys of older children and adults indicate that dextrocardia with situs inversus and normally related great arteries ("mirror-image" dextrocardia) is often associated with a functionally normal heart, although congenital heart disease of a less severe nature is common.

Anatomic or functional abnormalities of the lungs, diaphragm, and thoracic cage may result in displacement of the heart to the right (dextroposition). In this case, however, the cardiac apex is pointed normally to the left. This anatomic position is less often associated with congenital heart lesions, although hypoplasia of a lung may be accompanied by anomalous pulmonary venous return from that lung (**scimitar syndrome**).

The electrocardiogram is difficult to interpret in the presence of lesions with discordant atrial, ventricular, and great vessel anatomy. Diagnosis usually requires detailed echocardiographic and cardiac catheterization studies. The prognosis and treatment of patients with one of the cardiac positional anomalies are determined by the underlying defects. Asplenia increases the risk of serious infections such as bacterial sepsis and thus requires daily antibiotic prophylaxis.

Transposition of the Great Arteries

Bellinger DC, Wypij D, duDuplessis AJ, et al: Neurodevelopmental status at eight years in children with dextro-transposition of the great arteries: The Boston Circulatory Arrest Trial. *J Thorac Cardiovasc Surg* 2003;126:1385–1396.

Blume ED, Wernovsky G: Long-term results of arterial switch repair of transposition of the great vessels. *Semin Thorac Cardiovasc Surg Pediatr Card Surg Annu* 1998;1:129–138.

Dearani JA, Danielson GK, Puga FJ, et al: Late results of the Rastelli operation for transposition of the great arteries. *Semin Thorac Cardiovasc Surg Pediatr Card Surg Annu* 2001;4:3–15.

Dunbar-Masterson C, Wypij D, Bellinger DC, et al: General health status of children with D-transposition of the great arteries after the arterial switch operation. *Circulation* 2001;104(Suppl 1):I138–I142.

Hayes CJ, Gersony WM: Arrhythmias after the Mustard operation for transposition of the great arteries: A long-term study. *J Am Coll Cardiol* 1986;7:133–137.

Hovels-Gurich HH, Konrad K, Wiesner M, et al: Long term behavioural outcome after neonatal arterial switch operation for transposition of the great arteries. *Arch Dis Child* 2002;87:506–510.

Losay J, Touchot A, Serraf A, et al: Late outcome after arterial switch operation for transposition of the great arteries. *Circulation* 2001;104(Suppl 1):I121–I126.

Total Anomalous Pulmonary Venous Return

Choe YH, Lee HJ, Kim HS, et al: MRI of total anomalous pulmonary venous connections. *J Comput Assist Tomogr* 1994;18:243–249.

Duff DG, Nihill MR, McNamara DG: Infradiaphragmatic total anomalous pulmonary venous return. Review of clinical and pathological findings and results of operation in 28 cases. *Br Heart J* 1977;39:619–626.

Huhta J, Gutgesell HP, Nihill MR: Cross sectional echocardiographic diagnosis of total anomalous pulmonary venous connection. *Br Heart J* 1985;53:525–534.

Kirshbom PM, Flynn TB, Clancy RR, et al: Late neurodevelopmental outcome after repair of total anomalous pulmonary venous connection. *J Thorac Cardiovasc Surg* 2005;129:1091–1097.

Truncus Arteriosus

Reddy VM, Hanley F: Late results of repair of truncus arteriosus. *Semin Thorac Cardiovasc Surg Pediatr Card Surg Annu* 1998;1:139–146.

Reddy VM, McElhinney DB, Sagrado T, et al: Results of 102 cases of complete repair of congenital heart defects in patients weighing 700 to 2500 grams. *J Thorac Cardiovasc Surg* 1999;117:324–331.
Thompson LD, McElhinney DB, Reddy M, et al: Neonatal repair of truncus arteriosus: Continuing improvement in outcomes. *Ann Thorac Surg* 2001;72:391–395.
Wilson DI, Burn J, Scambler P, et al: DiGeorge syndrome: Part of CATCH 22. *J Med Genet* 1993;30:852–856.

Hypoplastic Left Heart Syndrome

Chiavarelli M, Gundry SR, Razzouk AJ, et al: Cardiac transplantation for infants with hypoplastic left heart syndrome. *JAMA* 1993;270:2944–2947.
Connor JA, Arons RR, Figueroa M, et al: Clinical outcomes and secondary diagnoses for infants born with hypoplastic left heart syndrome. *Pediatrics* 2004;114:e160–e165.
Daebritz SH, Nollert GD, Zurakowski D, et al: Results of Norwood stage I operation: Comparison of hypoplastic left heart syndrome with other malformations. *J Thorac Cardiovasc Surg* 2000;119:358–367.
Forbess JM, Visconti KJ, Bellinger DC, et al: Neurodevelopmental outcomes in children after the Fontan operation. *Circulation* 2001;104(Suppl 1):I127–I132.
Sano S, Ishino K, Kado H, et al: Outcome of right ventricle-to-pulmonary artery shunt in first-stage palliation of hypoplastic left heart syndrome: A multi-institutional study. *Ann Thorac Surg* 2004;78:1951–1958.
Theilen U, Shekerdemian L: The intensive care of infants with hypoplastic left heart syndrome. *Arch Dis Fetal Neonatal Ed* 2005;90:F97–F102.
Tworetzky W, Wilkins-Haug L, Jennings RW, et al: Balloon dilation of severe aortic stenosis in the fetus: Potential for prevention of hypoplastic left heart syndrome: Candidate selection, technique, and results of successful intervention. *Circulation* 2004;110:2125–2131.

Dextrocardia and Levocardia

Britz-Cunningham SH, Shah MM, Zuppan CW, et al: Mutation of the connexin 43 gap-junction gene in patients with heart malformations and defects of laterality. *N Engl J Med* 1995;332:1323–1329.
Rose V, Izukawa T, Moes CAF: Syndromes of asplenia and polysplenia: A review of cardiac and non-cardiac malformations in 60 cases with special reference to diagnosis and prognosis. *Br Heart J* 1975;37:840–852.
Wa MH, Wang JK, Lue HC: Sudden death in patients with right isomerism (asplenism) after palliation. *J Pediatr* 2002;140:93–96.

Chapter 432 ■ Other Congenital Heart and Vascular Malformations

432.1 • Anomalies of the Aortic Arch

RIGHT AORTIC ARCH

In this abnormality, the aorta curves to the right and, if it descends on the right side of the vertebral column, is usually associated with other cardiac malformations. It is found in 20% of cases of tetralogy of Fallot and is also common in truncus arteriosus. A right aortic arch without other cardiac anomalies is not associated with symptoms. It can often be visualized on the chest roentgenogram. The trachea is deviated to the left of the midline rather than to the right, as in the presence of a normal left arch. On a barium esophagogram, the esophagus is indented on its right border at the level of the aortic arch.

VASCULAR RINGS

Congenital abnormalities of the aortic arch and its major branches result in the formation of vascular rings around the trachea and esophagus with varying degrees of compression (Table 432-1). The origin of these lesions can best be appreciated by reviewing the embryology of the aortic arch (see Fig. 420-2). The most common anomalies include (1) double aortic arch (Fig. 432-1*A*), (2) right aortic arch with a left ligamentum arteriosum, (3) anomalous innominate artery arising farther to the left on the arch than usual, (4) anomalous left carotid artery arising farther to the right than usual and passing anterior to the trachea, and (5) anomalous left pulmonary artery (vascular sling). In the latter anomaly, the abnormal vessel arises from an elongated main pulmonary artery or from the right pulmonary artery. It courses between and compresses the trachea and the esophagus. Associated congenital heart disease may be present in 5–50% of patients, depending on the vascular anomaly.

CLINICAL MANIFESTATIONS. If the vascular ring produces compression of the trachea and esophagus, symptoms are frequently present during infancy. Chronic wheezing is exacerbated by crying, feeding, and flexion of the neck. Extension of the neck tends to relieve the noisy respiration. Vomiting may also be a component. Affected infants may have a brassy cough, pneumonia, or sudden death from aspiration.

DIAGNOSIS. Roentgenographic examination of the barium-filled esophagus (Fig. 432-2) and aortography identify the anomaly. An aberrant right subclavian artery is commonly seen but does not cause compression of the trachea. The diagnosis is confirmed by two-dimensional echocardiography, MRI, or CT. Cardiac catheterization is reserved for cases with associated anomalies or in rare cases where these other modalities are not diagnostic. Bronchoscopy is helpful in more severe cases to determine the extent of airway narrowing.

TREATMENT. Surgery is advised for symptomatic patients who have roentgenographic evidence of tracheal compression. The anterior vessel is usually divided in patients with a double aortic arch (see Fig. 432-1*B*). Compression produced by a right aortic arch and left ligamentum arteriosum is relieved by division of the latter. Anomalous innominate or carotid arteries cannot be divided; attaching the adventitia of these vessels to the sternum usually relieves the tracheal compression. An anomalous left pulmonary artery is corrected by division at its origin and reanastomosis to the main pulmonary artery after it has been brought in front of the trachea. Severe tracheomalacia, if present, may require reconstruction of the trachea as well.

432.2 • Anomalous Origin of the Coronary Arteries

ANOMALOUS ORIGIN OF THE LEFT CORONARY ARTERY FROM THE PULMONARY ARTERY (ALCAPA)

In anomalous origin of the left coronary artery from the pulmonary artery, the blood supply to the left ventricular myocardium is severely compromised. Soon after birth, as pulmonary arterial pressure falls, perfusion pressure to the left coronary artery becomes inadequate; myocardial ischemia, infarction, and fibrosis result. In some cases, interarterial collateral anastomoses develop between the right and left coronary arteries. Blood flow in the left coronary artery is then reversed, and it empties into the pulmonary artery, a condition known as the **"myocardial steal"** syndrome. The left ventricle becomes dilated, and performance is decreased. Mitral insufficiency is a frequent complication secondary to a dilated valve ring or infarction of a papillary muscle. Localized aneurysms may also develop in the left ventricular free wall. Occasional patients have adequate

TABLE 432-1. Vascular Rings

LESION	SYMPTOMS	PLAIN FILM	BARIUM SWALLOW	BRONCHOSCOPY	MRI/ECHOCARDIOGRAPHY	TREATMENT
Double arch	Stridor Respiratory distress Swallowing dysfunction Reflex apnea	AP—wider base of heart Lat.—narrowed trachea displaced forward at C3-C4	Bilateral indentation of esophagus	Bilateral tracheal compression—both pulsatile	Diagnostic	Ligate and divide smaller arch (usually left)
Right arch and ligamentum/ductus	Respiratory distress Swallowing dysfunction	AP—tracheal deviation to left (right arch)	Bilateral indentation of esophagus R > L	Bilateral tracheal compression—r. pulsatile	Diagnostic	Ligate ligamentum or ductus
Anomalous innominate	Cough Stridor Reflex apnea	AP—normal Lat.—anterior tracheal compression	Normal	Pulsatile anterior tracheal compression	Unnecessary	Conservative Apnea, then suspend
Aberrant right subclavian	Occasional swallowing dysfunction	Normal	AP—oblique defect upward to right Lat.—small defect on right posterior wall	Usually normal	Diagnostic	Ligate artery
Pulmonary sling	Expiratory stridor Respiratory distress	AP—low l. hilum, r. emphysema/atelectasis Lat.—anterior bowing of right bronchus and trachea	±Anterior indentation above carina between esophagus and trachea	Tracheal displacement to left Compression of right main bronchus	Diagnostic	Detach and reanastomose to main pulmonary artery in front of trachea

AP, anteroposterior; L and l., left; Lat., lateral; MRI, magnetic resonance imaging; R and r., right.
From Kliegman RM, Greenbaum LA, Lye PS: *Practical Strategies in Pediatric Diagnosis and Therapy*, 2nd ed. Elsevier, Philadelphia, 2004, p 88.

myocardial blood flow during childhood and, later in life, a continuous murmur and a small left-to-right shunt via the dilated coronary system (aorta to right coronary to left coronary to pulmonary artery).

CLINICAL MANIFESTATIONS. Evidence of heart failure becomes apparent within the 1st few months of life, and is often precipitated by respiratory infection. Recurrent attacks of discomfort, restlessness, irritability, sweating, dyspnea, and pallor with or without mild cyanosis occur and probably represent angina pectoris. Cardiac enlargement is moderate to massive. A gallop rhythm is common. Murmurs may be of the nonspecific, ejection type or may be holosystolic due to mitral insufficiency. Older patients with abundant intercoronary anastomoses may have continuous murmurs and minimal left ventricular dysfunction. During adolescence, they may experience angina during exercise. Rare patients with an anomalous right coronary artery may also have such clinical findings.

DIAGNOSIS. Roentgenographic examination confirms the cardiomegaly. The electrocardiogram resembles the pattern described in lateral wall myocardial infarction in adults. A QR

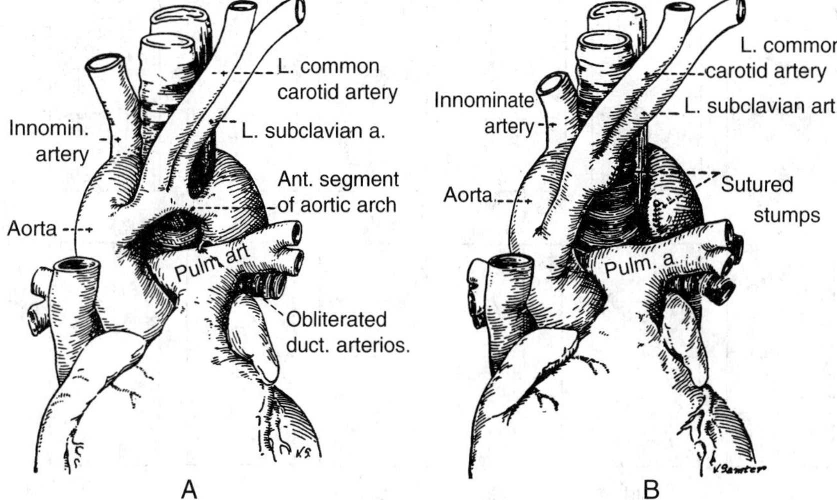

Figure 432-1. Double aortic arch. *A*, Small anterior segment of the double aortic arch (most common type). *B*, Operative procedure for release of the vascular ring.

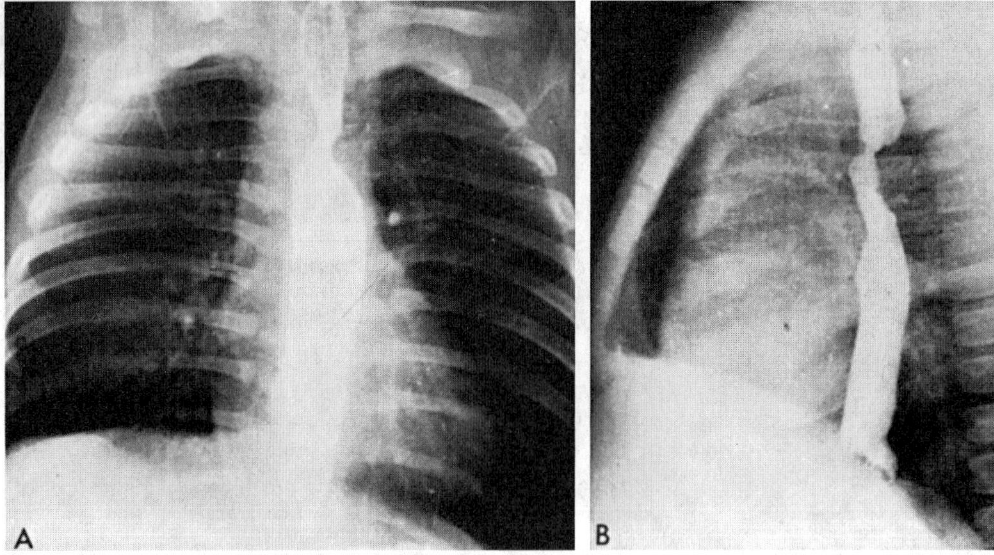

Figure 432-2. Double aortic arch in an infant aged 5 mo. *A*, Anteroposterior view. The barium-filled esophagus is constricted on both sides. *B*, Lateral view. The esophagus is displaced forward. The anterior arch was the smaller and was divided at surgery.

pattern followed by inverted T waves is seen in leads I and aVL. The left ventricular surface leads (V_5 and V_6) may also show deep Q waves and exhibit elevated ST segments and inverted T waves (Fig. 432-3). In older patients, an exercise study may be helpful as ST-T wave changes or symptoms occur. Two-dimensional echocardiography can usually suggest the diagnosis; however, echocardiography is not always reliable in diagnosing this condition. On two-dimensional imaging alone, the left coronary artery may appear as though it is arising from the aorta. Color Doppler ultrasound examination has improved the accuracy of diagnosis of this lesion and may demonstrate retrograde flow in the left coronary artery. CT or MRI may be helpful in confirming the origin of the coronary arteries. Cardiac catheterization is diagnostic; aortography shows immediate opacification of the right coronary artery only. This vessel is large and tortuous. After filling of the intercoronary anastomoses, the left coronary artery is opacified, and contrast can be seen to enter the pulmonary artery. Pulmonary arteriography may also opacify the origin of the anomalous left coronary artery. Selective left ventriculography usually demonstrates a dilated left ventricle that empties poorly.

TREATMENT AND PROGNOSIS. Untreated, death often occurs from heart failure within the 1st 6 mo. Those who survive generally have abundant intercoronary collateral anastomoses. Medical management includes standard therapy for heart failure (diuretics, digoxin, captopril) and for controlling ischemia (nitrates, β-blocking agents).

Surgical treatment consists of detaching the anomalous coronary artery from the pulmonary artery and anastomosing it to the aorta to establish normal myocardial perfusion. A seriously ill infant with a tiny left coronary artery may present a difficult technical problem. Ligation of the anomalous left coronary artery at its origin was once performed to prevent runoff from the coronary circuit and possibly to increase myocardial perfusion by the collateral circulation. As surgical experience with switching coronary arteries in neonates has expanded, this option has largely been abandoned. In patients who have already sustained a sig-

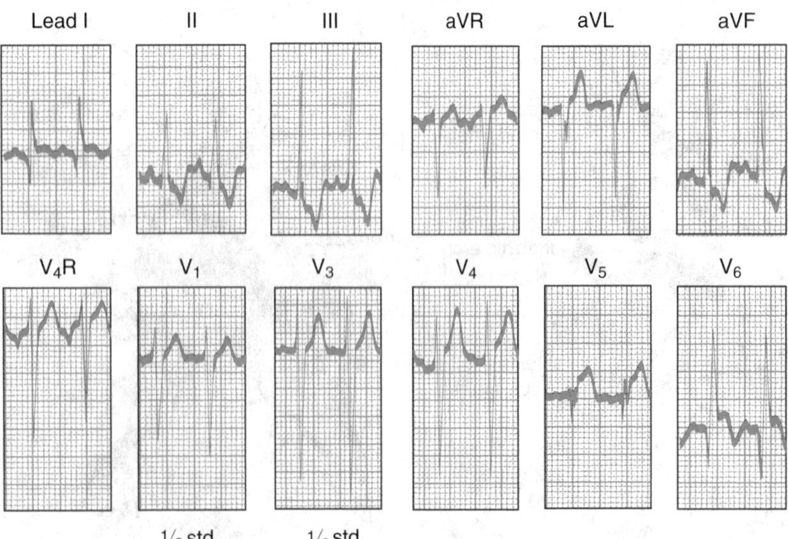

Figure 432-3. Electrocardiogram of a 3 mo old child with anomalous origin of the left coronary artery from the pulmonary artery. Lateral myocardial infarction is present as evidenced by abnormally large and wide Q waves in leads I, V_5, and V_6; an elevated ST segment in V_5 and V_6; and inversion of TV_6.

nificant myocardial infarction, cardiac transplantation may be the best option.

ANOMALOUS ORIGIN OF THE RIGHT CORONARY ARTERY FROM THE PULMONARY ARTERY

Anomalous origin of the right coronary artery from the pulmonary artery is rarely manifested in infancy or early childhood. The left coronary artery is enlarged, whereas the right is thin-walled and mildly enlarged. In early infancy, perfusion of the right coronary artery is from the pulmonary artery, whereas later, perfusion is from collaterals of the left coronary vessels. Angina and sudden death can occur in adolescence or adulthood. When recognized, this anomaly should be repaired by re-anastomosis of the right coronary artery to the aorta.

ECTOPIC ORIGIN OF THE CORONARY ARTERY FROM THE AORTA WITH ABERRANT PROXIMAL COURSE

In ectopic origin of the coronary artery from the aorta with an aberrant proximal course, the aberrant artery may be a left, right, or major branch coronary artery. The site of origin may be the wrong sinus of Valsalva or a proximal coronary artery. The ostium may be hypoplastic, slitlike, or of normal caliber. The aberrant vessel may pass anteriorly, posteriorly, or between the aorta and right ventricular outflow tract; it may tunnel in the conal or interventricular septal tissue. Obstruction resulting from hypoplasia of the ostia, tunneling between the aorta and right ventricular outflow tract or interventricular septum, and acute angulation produces focal myocardial fibrosis or myocardial infarction. Unobstructed vessels produce no symptoms. Patients with this extremely rare abnormality are often initially seen with severe myocardial infarction, ventricular arrhythmias, angina pectoris, or syncope; sudden death may occur, especially in young athletes.

Diagnosis should include an electrocardiogram, stress testing, two-dimensional echocardiography, CT or MRI, and cardiac catheterization with selective coronary angiography.

Treatment is indicated for obstructed vessels and consists of aortoplasty with re-anastomosis of the aberrant vessel or, occasionally, coronary artery bypass grafting. The management of asymptomatic infants with these forms of ectopic coronary origin remains controversial.

432.3 • Pulmonary Arteriovenous Fistula

Fistulous vascular communications in the lungs may be large and localized or multiple, scattered, and small. The most common form of this unusual condition is the **Osler-Weber-Rendu syndrome** (hereditary hemorrhagic telangiectasia type I), which is also associated with angiomas of the nasal and buccal mucous membranes, gastrointestinal tract, or liver. Mutations in the endoglin gene, a cell surface component of the transforming growth factor-β receptor complex causes this syndrome. The usual communication is between the pulmonary artery and pulmonary vein; direct communication between the pulmonary artery and left atrium is extremely rare. Desaturated blood in the pulmonary artery is shunted through the fistula into the pulmonary vein, thus bypassing the lungs, and then enters the left side of the heart; this aberrant direction of flow results in systemic arterial desaturation and, sometimes, clinical cyanosis. The shunt across the fistula is at low pressure and resistance, so pulmonary arterial pressure is normal; cardiomegaly and heart failure are not present.

The clinical manifestations depend on the magnitude of the shunt. Large fistulas are associated with dyspnea, cyanosis, clubbing, a continuous murmur, and polycythemia. Hemoptysis is rare, but when it occurs, it may be massive. Features of the Osler-Weber-Rendu syndrome are seen in ≈50% of patients (or other family members) and include recurrent epistaxis and gastrointestinal tract bleeding. Transitory dizziness, diplopia, aphasia, motor weakness, or convulsions may result from cerebral thrombosis, abscess, or paradoxical emboli. Soft systolic or continuous murmurs may be audible over the site of the fistula. The electrocardiogram is normal. Roentgenographic examination of the chest may show opacities produced by large fistulas; multiple small fistulas may be visualized by fluoroscopy (as abnormal pulsations), MRI, or CT. Selective pulmonary arteriography demonstrates the site, extent, and distribution of the fistulas.

Treatment consisting of excision of solitary or localized lesions by lobectomy or wedge resection results in complete disappearance of symptoms. In most instances, fistulas are so widespread that surgery is not possible. Direct communication between the pulmonary artery and the left atrium, if present, can be obliterated by division and suture.

Patients who have undergone a **Glenn cavopulmonary** anastomosis for cyanotic congenital heart disease are also at risk for the development of pulmonary arteriovenous malformations. In these patients, the arteriovenous malformations are usually multiple and the risk increases over time after the Glenn procedure. These malformations rarely occur after the heart disease is fully palliated by completion of the Fontan operation. This finding suggests that the pulmonary circulation requires an as yet undetermined hepatic factor to suppress the development of arteriovenous malformations. The hallmark of the development of these malformations is a decrease in the patient's oxygen saturation. The diagnosis can often be made with contrast echocardiography; cardiac catheterization is the definitive test. Completion of the Fontan circuit, so that inferior vena cava blood flow (containing hepatic venous drainage) is routed through the lungs, usually results in improvement or resolution of the malformations.

432.4 • Ectopia Cordis

In the most common thoracic form of ectopia cordis, the sternum is split and the heart protrudes outside the chest. In other forms, the heart protrudes through the diaphragm into the abdominal cavity or may be situated in the neck. Associated intracardiac anomalies are common. Death occurs in the 1st days of life in most, usually from infection, cardiac failure, or hypoxemia. Surgical therapy for neonates without overwhelmingly severe cardiac anomalies consists of covering the heart with skin without compromising venous return or ventricular ejection. Palliation of associated defects is also often necessary. Occasional patients with the abdominal type have survived to adulthood.

432.5 • Diverticulum of the Left Ventricle

In this rare anomaly, a diverticulum of the left ventricle protrudes into the epigastrium. The lesion may be isolated or associated with complex cardiovascular anomalies. A pulsating mass is visible and palpable in the epigastrium. Systolic or systolic-diastolic murmurs produced by blood flow into and out of the diverticulum may be audible over the lower part of the sternum and the mass. The electrocardiogram shows a pattern of complete or incomplete left bundle branch block. Roentgenograms of the chest may or may not show the mass. Associated abnormalities include defects of the sternum, abdominal wall, diaphragm, and pericardium. Surgical treatment of the diverticulum and associated cardiac defects can be performed in selected cases. Occasionally, a diverticulum may be small and not associated with clinical signs or symptoms. These small diverticula are diagnosed at the time of echocardiographic examination for other indications.

Vascular Rings

Azarow KS, Pearl RH, Hoffman MA, et al: Vascular ring: Does magnetic resonance imaging replace angiography? *Ann Thorac Surg* 1992;53:882–885.
Bertrand J-M, Chartrand C, Lamarre A, et al: Vascular ring: Clinical and physiological assessment of pulmonary function following surgical correction. *Pediatr Pulmonol* 1986;2:378–383.
Kussman BD, Geva T, McGowan FX: Cardiovascular causes of airway compression. *Paediatr Anaesth* 2004;14:60–74.
Murdison KA, Andrews BA, Chin AJ: Ultrasonographic display of complex vascular rings. *J Am Coll Cardiol* 1990;15:1645–1653.
van Son JA, Julsrud PR, Hagler DJ, et al: Imaging strategies for vascular rings. *Ann Thorac Surg* 1994;57:604–610.

Anomalous Coronary Artery

Chang RR, Allada V: Electrocardiographic and echocardiographic features that distinguish anomalous origin of the left coronary artery from pulmonary artery from idiopathic dilated cardiomyopathy. *Pediatr Cardiol* 2001;22:3–10.
Frommelt PC, Berger S, Pelech AN, et al: Prospective identification of anomalous origin of left coronary artery from the right sinus of Valsalva using transthoracic echocardiography: Importance of color Doppler flow mapping. *Pediatr Cardiol* 2001;22:327–332.
Johnsrude CL, Perry JC, Cecchin F, et al: Differentiating anomalous left main coronary artery originating from the pulmonary artery in infants from myocarditis and dilated cardiomyopathy by electrocardiogram. *Am J Cardiol* 1995;75:71–74.
Schmidt KG, Cooper MJ, Silverman NH, et al: Pulmonary artery origin of the left coronary artery: Diagnosis by two-dimensional echocardiography, pulsed Doppler ultrasound and color flow mapping. *J Am Coll Cardiol* 1988;11:396–402.

Pulmonary Arteriovenous Fistula

Feinstein JA, Moore P, Rosenthal DN, et al: Comparison of contrast echocardiography versus cardiac catheterization for detection of pulmonary arteriovenous malformations. *Am J Cardiol* 2002;89:281–285.
Freedom RM, Yoo SJ, Perrin D: The biological "scrabble" of pulmonary arteriovenous malformations: Considerations in the setting of cavopulmonary surgery. *Cardiol Young* 2004;14:417–437.
Marchuk DA: Genetic abnormalities in hereditary hemorrhagic telangiectasia. *Curr Opin Hematol* 1998;5:332–338.
Paterson A: Imaging evaluation of congenital lung abnormalities in infants and children. *Radiol Clin North Am* 2005;43:303–323.
Srivastava D, Preminger T, Lock JE, et al: Hepatic venous blood and the development of pulmonary arteriovenous malformations in congenital heart disease. *Circulation* 1995;92:1217–1222.

Chapter 433 ■ Pulmonary Hypertension

433.1 • Primary Pulmonary Hypertension

PATHOPHYSIOLOGY. Primary pulmonary hypertension is characterized by pulmonary vascular obstructive disease and right-sided heart failure. It occurs at any age, although in pediatric patients the diagnosis is initially made in adolescence. In older patients, females outnumber males 1.7:1; in younger patients, both genders are represented equally. Some patients have evidence of either an immunologic disorder or a hypercoagulable state. Mutations in the gene for bone morphogenetic protein receptor-2 (BMPR-2, a member of the transforming growth factor-β receptor family) on chromosome 2q33 have been identified in patients with autosomal dominant familial primary pulmonary hypertension (known as PPH1). This genetic variant demonstrates a female preponderance and is found in up to 25% of patients with sporadic disease. Other potential disease causing genes have been identified, including chromosome 2q31 (PPH2) and 12q13 (ALK1). Viral infection, specifically with the vasculotropic human herpesvirus 8 (HHV8), has been suggested as a trigger factor in many patients. Diet pills, particularly fenfluramine, have also been implicated. Pulmonary hypertension is associated with precapillary obstruction of the pulmonary vascular bed as a result of hyperplasia of the muscular and elastic tissues and a thickened intima of the small pulmonary arteries and arterioles. Atherosclerotic changes may be found in the larger pulmonary arteries. In children, veno-occlusive disease may account for some cases of primary pulmonary hypertension. Other causes of elevated pulmonary pressure must be eliminated (chronic pulmonary parenchymal disease, persistent obstruction of the upper airway, congenital cardiac malformations, recurrent pulmonary emboli, alveolar capillary dysplasia, liver disease, autoimmune disease, and moyamoya disease). A classification system is noted in Table 433-1. Pulmonary hypertension places an afterload burden on the right ventricle, which results in right ventricular hypertrophy. Dilatation of the pulmonary artery is present, and pulmonary valve insufficiency may occur. In the later stages of the disease, the right ventricle dilates, tricuspid insufficiency develops, and cardiac output is decreased. Arrhythmias, syncope, and sudden death are common.

CLINICAL MANIFESTATIONS. The predominant symptoms include exercise intolerance and fatigability; occasionally, precordial chest pain, dizziness, syncope, or headaches are noted. Peripheral cyanosis may be present, especially in patients with a patent foramen ovale through which blood can shunt from right to left; in the late stages of disease, patients may have cold extremities and

TABLE 433-1. The Revised World Health Organization Classification of Pulmonary Hypertension*

Group I. Pulmonary arterial hypertension
- Idiopathic (primary)
- Familial
  - Related conditions: collagen vascular disease, congenital systemic-to-pulmonary shunts, portal hypertension, HIV infection, drugs and toxins (e.g., anorexigens, rapeseed oil, L-tryptophan, methamphetamine, and cocaine); other conditions: thyroid disorders, glycogen storage disease, Gaucher disease, hereditary hemorrhagic telangiectasia, hemoglobinopathies, myeloproliferative disorders, splenectomy
- Associated with significant venous or capillary involvement
  - Pulmonary veno-occlusive disease
  - Pulmonary-capillary hemangiomatosis
- Persistent pulmonary hypertension of the newborn

Group II. Pulmonary venous hypertension
- Left-sided atrial or ventricular heart disease
- Left-sided valvular heart disease

Group III. Pulmonary hypertension associated with hypoxemia
- Chronic obstructive pulmonary disease
- Interstitial lung disease
- Sleep-disordered breathing
- Alveolar hypoventilation disorders
- Chronic exposure to high altitude
- Developmental abnormalities

Group IV. Pulmonary hypertension due to chronic thrombotic disease, embolic disease, or both
- Thromboembolic obstruction of proximal pulmonary arteries
- Thromboembolic obstruction of distal pulmonary arteries
- Pulmonary embolism (tumor, parasites, foreign material)

Group V. Miscellaneous
- Sarcoidosis, pulmonary Langerhans-cell histiocytosis, lymphangiomatosis, compression of pulmonary vessels (adenopathy, tumor, fibrosing mediastinitis)

From Farber HW, Loscalzo J: Pulmonary arterial hypertension. *N Engl J Med* 2004;351:1655–1666.

a gray appearance associated with low cardiac output. Arterial oxygen saturation is usually normal unless there is an associated intracardiac shunt. If right-sided heart failure has supervened, jugular venous pressure is elevated, and hepatomegaly and edema are present. Jugular venous *a* waves are present, and in those with functional tricuspid insufficiency, a conspicuous jugular *cv* wave and systolic hepatic pulsations are manifested. The heart is moderately enlarged, and a right ventricular heave can be noted. The 1st heart sound is often followed by an ejection click emanating from the dilated pulmonary artery. The 2nd heart sound is narrowly split, loud, and sometimes booming in quality; it is frequently palpable at the upper left sternal border. A presystolic gallop rhythm may be audible at the lower left sternal border. The systolic murmur is soft and short and is sometimes followed by a blowing decrescendo diastolic murmur caused by pulmonary insufficiency. In later stages, a holosystolic murmur of tricuspid insufficiency is appreciated at the lower left sternal border.

DIAGNOSIS. Chest roentgenograms reveal a prominent pulmonary artery and right ventricle (Fig. 433-1). The pulmonary vascularity in the hilar areas may be prominent, in contrast to the peripheral lung fields, in which pulmonary markings are decreased. The electrocardiogram shows right ventricular hypertrophy, often with spiked P waves.

At cardiac catheterization this condition must be differentiated from Eisenmenger syndrome (see Chapter 433.2), which is associated with a communication between the left and right sides of the heart or great arteries, as well as from left-sided obstructive lesions (pulmonary venous stenosis, mitral stenosis) that result in pulmonary venous hypertension (see Chapter 427). The presence of pulmonary arterial hypertension with a normal pulmonary capillary wedge pressure is diagnostic of primary pulmonary hypertension. If the wedge pressure is elevated and left ventricular end-diastolic pressure is normal, obstruction at the level of the pulmonary veins, left atrium, or mitral valve should be suspected. The risks associated with cardiac catheterization are increased in severely ill patients with primary pulmonary hypertension.

PROGNOSIS AND TREATMENT. Primary pulmonary hypertension is progressive, and no cure is currently available. Some success has been reported with oral calcium channel blocking agents such as nifedipine in children who demonstrate pulmonary vasoreactivity when these agents are administered during catheterization.

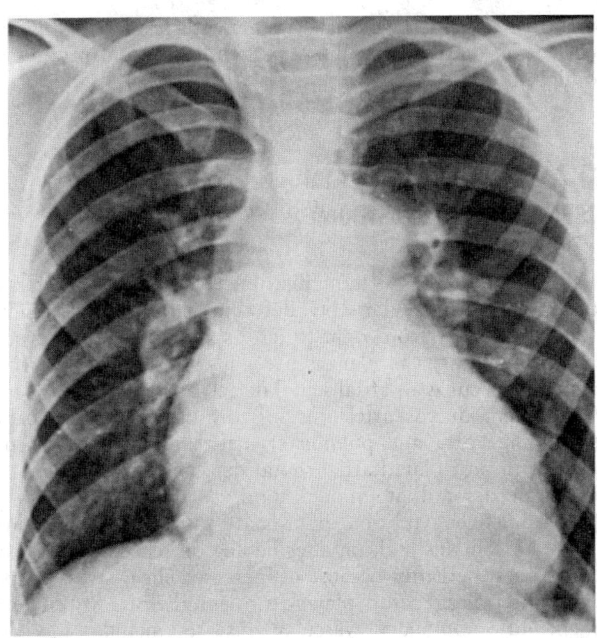

Figure 433-1. Roentgenogram in primary pulmonary hypertension. Note the moderate cardiac enlargement, dilatation of the pulmonary artery, and relative pulmonary undervascularity in the outer two thirds of the lung fields.

Continuous intravenous infusion of prostacyclin (prostaglandin I_2) provides relief as long as the infusion is continued. Despite the success of prostacyclin in reducing symptoms and improving quality of life, it slows but does not stop the progression of the disease. Continuous administration of nitric oxide via nasal cannula, nebulized forms of prostacyclin, and orally administered pulmonary vasodilators (bosentan, an antagonist of endothelin receptors; or sildenafil, a phosphodiesterase type 5 inhibitor) are all being investigated (Table 433-2). Anticoagulation may be of value in patients with previous pulmonary thromboemboli, and some of these patients will respond to balloon angioplasty of narrowed pulmonary artery segments. Despite many advances, definitive therapy is still heart-lung or lung transplantation (see Chapter 443.2). In patients with severe pulmonary hypertension and low cardiac output, the terminal event is often sudden and

TABLE 433-2. Summary of Drugs Used to Treat Pulmonary Hypertension

DRUG AND MECHANISM OF ACTION	DOSES USED IN PEDIATRIC STUDIES	COMMON SIDE EFFECTS
Epoprostenol (prostacyclin PGI_2, a potent vasodilator; also inhibits platelet aggregation)	1 nanogram/kg/min initially. Increased based on clinical course and tolerance to 20–50 nanogram/kg/min. Some patients may require even higher doses. Must be given by continuous infusion that is not interrupted.	Flushing, headache, nausea, diarrhea, hypotension, chest pain, jaw pain.
Iloprost (synthetic analogue of prostacyclin PGI_2)	2.5–5.0 μg 6–9 times daily (not more frequenctly than every 2 hours) via inhalation.	Flushing, headache, diarrhea, hypotension, jaw pain, exacerbation of pulmonary symptoms (cough, wheezing).
Treprostinil (synthetic analogue of prostacyclin)	Similar doses to epoprostenol although patients may require approximately 25% higher maximal doses. Given either i.v. or s.c. via continuous infusion. Longer half-life than epoprostenol.	Flushing, headache, diarrhea, hypotension, jaw pain. Pain at infusion site when given s.c.
Bosentan (endothelin receptor ET_A and ET_B antagonist)	10–20 kg: 31.25 mg daily for 4 wk, then increase to 32.5 mg twice daily. 20–40 kg: 31.25 mg twice a day for 4 wk, then increase to 62.5 mg twice a day. >40 kg: 62.5 mg twice a day for 4 wk, then increase to 125 mg twice a day. Other selective endothelin antagonists are currently in clinical trials.	Flushing, headache, diarrhea, hypotension, fluid retention, exacerbation of heart failure, anemia, elevated liver function tests, palpitations.
Sildenafil (inhibitor of cGMP specific phosphodiesterase PDE5)	0.5–1.0 mg/kg/dose given 3–4 times daily. Adult dose 20 mg 3 times daily. Longer acting PDE5 inhibitors are currently in clinical trials.	Flushing, headache, diarrhea, myalgia, hypotension, priapism, visual disturbance (blue coloration).
Calcium channel blockers (e.g. diltiazem, nifedipine)	Previously widely used. Now indicated only for patients who show a response to the drug during cardiac catheterization (decrease in pulmonary artery systolic pressure <40 mm Hg). Dose depends on specific agent used.	Flushing, headache, edema, arrhythmia, headache, hypotension, rash, nausea, constipation, elevated liver function tests.

s.c., subcutaneous. Note: These medications should only be administered under the direction of a specialist in pulmonary hypertension.

related to a lethal arrhythmia. Patients with primary pulmonary hypertension diagnosed in infancy often have rapid progression and high mortality.

433.2 • Pulmonary Vascular Disease (Eisenmenger Syndrome)

PATHOPHYSIOLOGY. The term **Eisenmenger syndrome** refers to patients with a ventricular septal defect in which blood is shunted partially or totally from right to left as a result of the development of pulmonary vascular disease. This physiologic abnormality can also occur with atrial septal defect, atrioventricular septal defect, patent ductus arteriosus, or any other communication between the aorta and pulmonary artery. Pulmonary vascular disease with an isolated atrial septal defect is less common and does not occur until late in adulthood.

In Eisenmenger syndrome, pulmonary vascular resistance after birth either remains high or, after having decreased during early infancy, rises thereafter because of increased shear stress on pulmonary arterioles. Factors playing a role in the rapidity of development of pulmonary vascular disease include increased pulmonary arterial pressure, increased pulmonary blood flow, and the presence of hypoxia or hypercapnia. Early in the course of disease, pulmonary hypertension (elevated pressure in the pulmonary arteries) is the result of markedly increased pulmonary blood flow (hyperkinetic pulmonary hypertension). This form of pulmonary hypertension decreases with the administration of pulmonary vasodilators or oxygen, or both. With the development of Eisenmenger syndrome, pulmonary hypertension is the result of pulmonary vascular disease (obstructive pathologic changes in the pulmonary vessels). This form of pulmonary hypertension is usually only minimally responsive to pulmonary vasodilators or oxygen or not at all.

PATHOLOGY AND PATHOPHYSIOLOGY. The pathologic changes of Eisenmenger syndrome occur in the small pulmonary arterioles and muscular arteries (<300 mm) and are graded on the basis of histologic characteristics (Heath-Edwards classification): **Grade I** changes involve medial hypertrophy alone, **grade II** consists of medial hypertrophy and intimal hyperplasia, **grade III** involves near obliteration of the vessel lumen, **grade IV** includes arterial dilatation, and **grades V and VI** include plexiform lesions, angiomatoid formation, and fibrinoid necrosis. Grades IV–VI indicate irreversible pulmonary vascular obstructive disease. Eisenmenger physiology is defined by an absolute elevation in pulmonary arterial resistance to greater than 12 Wood units (resistance units indexed to body surface area) or by a ratio of pulmonary to systemic vascular resistance of ≥1.0.

Pulmonary vascular disease occurs more rapidly in patients with trisomy 21 who have left-to-right shunts. It also complicates the natural history of patients with elevated pulmonary venous pressure secondary to mitral stenosis or left ventricular dysfunction, especially in those patients with restrictive cardiomyopathy (see Chapter 439.3). Pulmonary vascular disease can also occur in any patient with transmission of systemic pressure to the pulmonary circulation via a shunt at the interventricular or great vessel level, and in patients chronically exposed to low PO_2 (because of high altitude). Patients with cyanotic congenital heart lesions associated with unrestricted pulmonary blood flow are at particularly high risk.

CLINICAL MANIFESTATIONS. Symptoms do not usually develop until the 2nd or 3rd decade of life, although a more fulminant course may occur. Many patients survive for decades with minimal symptoms. Intracardiac or extracardiac communications that would normally shunt from left to right are converted to right-to-left shunting as pulmonary vascular resistance exceeds systemic vascular resistance. Cyanosis becomes apparent, and dyspnea, fatigue, and a tendency toward dysrhythmias begin to occur. In the late stages of the disease, heart failure, chest pain, headaches, syncope, and hemoptysis may be seen. Physical examination reveals a right ventricular heave and a narrowly split 2nd heart sound with a loud pulmonic component. Palpable pulmonary artery pulsation may be present at the left upper sternal border. A holosystolic murmur of tricuspid regurgitation may be audible along the left sternal border. An early decrescendo diastolic murmur of pulmonary insufficiency may also be heard along the left sternal border. The degree of cyanosis depends on the stage of the disease.

DIAGNOSIS. Cyanotic patients have various degrees of polycythemia that depend on the severity and duration of hypoxia. Roentgenographically, the heart varies in size from normal to greatly enlarged; the latter usually occurs late in the course of the disease. The main pulmonary artery is generally prominent, similar to primary pulmonary hypertension (see Fig. 433-1). The pulmonary vessels are enlarged in the hilar areas and taper rapidly in caliber in the peripheral branches. The right ventricle and atrium are prominent. The electrocardiogram shows marked right ventricular hypertrophy. The P wave may be tall and spiked.

The echocardiogram shows a thick-walled right ventricle and demonstrates the underlying congenital heart lesion. Two-dimensional echocardiography assists in eliminating from consideration lesions such as obstructed pulmonary veins, a supramitral membrane, and mitral stenosis. The pulmonary valve echocardiogram shows a characteristic early midsystolic closure, the "W sign." Doppler studies demonstrate the direction of the shunt and the presence of a typical hypertension waveform in the main pulmonary artery. Tricuspid and pulmonary regurgitation can be used in the Doppler examination to estimate pulmonary arterial pressure.

Cardiac catheterization usually shows a bidirectional shunt at the site of the defect. Systolic pressure is generally equal in the systemic and pulmonary circulations. Pulmonary capillary wedge pressure is normal unless a left-sided heart obstructive lesion or left ventricular failure is the cause of the pulmonary arterial hypertension. Arterial oxygen saturation is decreased because of the magnitude of the right-to-left shunt. The response to vasodilator therapy (oxygen, calcium channel blockers, prostacyclin, nitric oxide) may identify patients with hyperdynamic pulmonary hypertension. Selective angiocardiography can locate the site of the shunt, but these studies are usually avoided in such patients because of increased risk and the accuracy of echocardiography. Selective pulmonary artery injections may be necessary if pulmonary venous obstruction is suspected because of high wedge pressure and low left ventricular end-diastolic pressure.

TREATMENT. The best management for patients who are at risk for the development of late pulmonary vascular disease is prevention by early surgical elimination of large intracardiac or great vessel communications during infancy. Some patients may be missed because they have not shown early clinical manifestations. Pulmonary vascular resistance never decreases substantially at birth in some of these infants, and therefore they never acquire enough left-to-right shunting to become clinically apparent. Such delayed recognition is a particular risk in patients with congenital heart disease who live at high altitude. It is also a risk in infants with trisomy 21, who have a propensity for earlier development of pulmonary vascular disease. Because of the high incidence of congenital heart disease associated with trisomy 21, many physicians recommend routine echocardiography at the time of initial diagnosis, even in the absence of other clinical findings.

TABLE 433-3. Extracardiac Complications of Cyanotic Congenital Heart Disease and Eisenmenger Physiology

PROBLEM	ETIOLOGY	THERAPY
Polycythemia	Persistent hypoxia	Phlebotomy
Relative anemia	Nutritional deficiency	Iron replacement
CNS abscess	Right-to-left shunting	Antibiotics, drainage
CNS thromboembolic stroke	Right-to-left shunting or polycythemia	Phlebotomy
Low-grade DIC, thrombocytopenia	Polycythemia	None for DIC unless bleeding, then phlebotomy
Hemoptysis	Pulmonary infarct, thrombosis, or rupture of pulmonary artery plexiform lesion	Embolization
Gum disease	Polycythemia, gingivitis, bleeding	Dental hygiene
Gout	Polycythemia, diuretic agent	Allopurinol
Arthritis, clubbing	Hypoxic arthropathy	None
Pregnancy complications: abortion, fetal growth retardation, prematurity increase, maternal illness	Poor placental perfusion, poor ability to increase cardiac output	Bed rest, pregnancy prevention counseling
Infections	Associated asplenia, DiGeorge syndrome, endocarditis	Antibiotics
	Fatal RSV pneumonia with pulmonary hypertension	Ribavirin; RSV immunoglobulin (prevention)
Failure to thrive	Increased oxygen consumption, decreased nutrient intake	Treat heart failure; correct defect early; increase caloric intake
Psychosocial adjustment	Limited activity, cyanotic appearance, chronic disease, multiple hospitalizations	Counseling

CNS, central nervous system; DIC, disseminated intravascular coagulation; RSV, respiratory syncytial virus.

Medical treatment of Eisenmenger syndrome is primarily symptomatic (Table 433-3). Older children and adolescents with symptomatic polycythemia may be improved by cautious, repeated phlebotomies with volume replacement. Clinical trials have described benefits from chronic calcium channel blocker or intravenous prostacyclin therapy. Combined heart-lung or bilateral lung transplantation is the only surgical option for many of these patients (see Chapter 443.2).

Barst RJ: Medical therapy of pulmonary hypertension. An overview of treatment and goals. *Clin Chest Med* 2001;22:509–515.

Cool CD, Rai PR, Yeager ME, et al: Expression of human herpesvirus 8 in primary pulmonary hypertension. *N Engl J Med* 2003;349:1113–1122.

Farber HW, Loscalzo J: Pulmonary arterial hypertension. *N Eng J Med* 2004;351:1655–1666.

Feinstein JA, Goldhaber SZ, Lock JE, et al: Balloon pulmonary angioplasty for treatment of chronic thromboembolic pulmonary hypertension. *Circulation* 2001;103:10–13.

Ford K: Pulmonary artery hypertension: New drug treatment in children. *Arch Dis Child* 2005;90:ep15–ep20.

Galié N, Ghofrani HA, Torbicki A, et al: Sildenafil citrate therapy for pulmonary arteral hypertension. *N Engl J Med* 2005;353:2148–2157.

Gammie JS, Keenan RJ, Pham SM, et al: Single- versus double-lung transplantation for pulmonary hypertension. *J Thorac Cardiovasc Surg* 1998;115:397–402.

Ghofrani HA, Wiedemann R, Rose F, et al: Sildenafil for a treatment of lung fibrosis and pulmonary hypertension: A randomized controlled trial. *Lancet* 2002;360:895–900.

Mandegar M, Thistlethwaite PA, Yuan JX: Molecular biology of primary pulmonary hypertension. *Cardiol Clin* 2004;22:417–429.

McCann UD, Seiden LS, Rubin LJ, et al: Brain serotonin neurotoxicity and primary pulmonary hypertension from fenfluramine and dexfenfluramine. A systemic review of the evidence. *JAMA* 1997;278:666–672.

McLaughlin VV, Shillington A, Rich S: Survival in primary pulmonary hypertension. The impact of epoprostenol therapy. *Circulation* 2002;106:1477–1482.

McLaughlin VV, Sitbon O, Badesch DB, et al: Survival with first-line bosentan in patients with primary pulmonary hypertension. *Eur Respir J* 2005;25:244–249.

Mikhail G, Gibbs J, Richardson M, et al: An evaluation of nebulized prostacyclin in patients with primary and secondary pulmonary hypertension. *Eur Heart J* 1997;18:1499–1504.

Newman JH, Wheeler L, Lane KB, et al: Mutation in the gene for bone morphogenetic protein receptor II as a cause of primary pulmonary hypertension in a large kindred. *N Engl J Med* 2001;345:319–324.

Widlitz A, Barst RJ: Pulmonary arterial hypertension in children. *Eur Respir J* 2003;21:155–176.

Chapter 434 ■ General Principles of Treatment of Congenital Heart Disease

Most patients who have mild congenital heart disease require no treatment. The parents and child should be made aware that a normal life is expected and that no restriction of the child's activities is necessary. Overprotective parents may use the presence of a mild congenital heart lesion or even a functional heart murmur as a means to exert excessive control over their child's activities. Although fears may not be expressed overtly, the child may become anxious regarding early death or debilitation, especially when an adult member of the family acquires symptomatic heart disease. The family may have an unexpressed fear of sudden death, and the rarity of this manifestation should be emphasized in discussions directed at improving their understanding of the child's congenital heart defect. The difference between congenital heart disease and degenerative coronary disease in adults should be emphasized. General health maintenance, including a well-balanced, "heart-healthy" diet, aerobic exercise, and avoidance of smoking, should be encouraged.

Even patients with moderate to severe heart disease need not be markedly restricted in physical activity. **Physical education** should be modified appropriately to the child's capacity to participate. The extent of such modification can generally be determined best by exercise testing. Competitive sports for most of these patients should be discouraged. Patients with severe heart disease and decreased exercise tolerance usually tend to limit their own activities. Dyspnea, headache, and fatigability in cyanotic patients may be a sign of increasing hypoxemia and may require some limitation of activity in those for whom specific medical or surgical treatment is not available. **Routine immunizations** should be given, with the inclusion of influenza vaccine; patients who might be considered candidates for heart or heart-lung transplantation should not receive live-virus vaccinations just before transplantation.

Bacterial infections should be treated vigorously, but the presence of congenital heart disease is not an appropriate reason to use antibiotics indiscriminately. Prophylaxis against infective endocarditis should be carried out during dental procedures, during instrumentation of the urinary tract, and before lower gastrointestinal tract manipulation (see Table 437-2).

Cyanotic patients need to be monitored for a multitude of noncardiac manifestations of oxygen deficiency (Table 434-1). Treatment of iron deficiency anemia is important in cyanotic

TABLE 434-1. Systems Approach to Postoperative Care After Surgery for Congenital Heart Disease

SYSTEM AND PROBLEM	ETIOLOGY	TREATMENT OR PREVENTION
NERVOUS SYSTEM		
Coma	Global ischemia	Monitor and treat increased intracranial pressure
	Prolonged anesthetic effect	Reverse anesthesia
	Hypoglycemia	Glucose
Focal lesions	Emboli (air, thrombi)	
Seizures	Metabolic (hyponatremia, hypoglycemia), ischemic, embolic disturbances	Phenytoin, correct metabolic disturbances
Diaphragm paralysis	Phrenic nerve injury	Respiratory care
Vocal cord paralysis	Traction on recurrent laryngeal nerve	Respiratory care
Horner syndrome	Dissection of subclavian artery with sympathetic chain injury	None
Paraplegia	Postcoarctation repair with spinal artery ischemia	Avoid ischemia
Pain	Surgical trauma	Fentanyl, morphine
Anxiety	Stress	Midazolam (Versed), diazepam (Valium)
RESPIRATORY SYSTEM		
ARDS postpump syndrome	Unknown; possible release of vasoactive substances by cardiopulmonary bypass	PEEP, mechanical ventilation, oxygen
Pulmonary edema	Heart failure, left-sided obstructions, fluid overload	Diuresis, PEEP, mechanical ventilation, inotropic agents
Pleural effusions	Hemothorax	Thoracocentesis
	Early serous effusion	Thoracocentesis
	Delayed postpericardiotomy syndrome	Anti-inflammatory agents
Chylothorax	Injury to thoracic duct	NPO or medium-chain triglyceride diet Rarely surgical ligation of thoracic duct
Atelectasis	Hypoventilation, poor cough	Chest physiotherapy, PEEP
Pneumonia	Aspiration, nosocomial, bacteremia	Identify bacterial-viral (respiratory syncytial virus) cause; specific antimicrobial therapy
Pulmonary hypertension	Repair of TAPVR, Norwood 1st stage, trisomy 21; prior preoperative pulmonary hypertension	Hyperventilation, hyperoxia, nitric oxide, ECMO
Stridor	Vocal cord edema, paralysis	Steroids, rarely tracheotomy
CARDIOVASCULAR SYSTEM		
Bradycardia, sick sinus syndrome, atrioventricular block	Injury to interatrial or interventricular conduction system	Atropine, isoproterenol, pacemaker
Right bundle branch block	Right ventriculotomy	Atrial approach to ventricular septal defect repair or tetralogy of Fallot
Tachyarrhythmias	Supraventricular, junctional tachycardia	Antiarrhythmic agents
	Ventricular tachycardia	Defibrillation, antiarrhythmic agents
Poor cardiac output	Cardiogenic—right ventriculotomy or cardiac "stun" (prolonged pump and cross-clamp time) or infarction	Inotropic agents, support preload, reduce afterload, LVAD, ECMO
	Hypocalcemia	Calcium
	Hypovolemia	Support preload with fluids
Pericardial tamponade	Pericardial effusion, acute hemorrhage	Pericardiocentesis
	Serous postpericardiotomy syndrome	Anti-inflammatory agents
Hypertension	Stress or pain	Analgesia
	Postcoarctectomy syndrome	Nitroprusside
Mesenteric arteritis	Postcoarctectomy syndrome	NPO, nitroprusside
RENAL-METABOLIC SYSTEM		
Prerenal oliguria	Hypovolemia	Fluid administration
	Poor cardiac output	Inotropic agents
Renal failure	Hypotension, prolonged pump—cross-clamp time, acute tubular necrosis	Improve blood pressure, diuretics, dialysis
Edema	Fluid resuscitation, capillary leak, poor cardiac output, elevated systemic venous pressure	Diuresis, inotropic agents
Hyponatremia	Dilutional SIADH	Fluid restriction
	Diuretics	Fluid restriction
Hyperglycemia	Hypothermia, inhibition of insulin	None needed (usually), insulin
Hypoglycemia	Rebound following hyperglycemia, hepatic failure	Glucose infusion
HEMATOLOGIC SYSTEM		
Hemorrhage	Abnormal PT, PTT, thrombocytopenia	Correct coagulopathy
	Surgical leak	Reoperation, suture
Shunt thrombosis	Poor cardiac output, hypovolemia	Fluids, heparin, reoperation
Anemia (usually reflecting reduced blood volume)	Hemorrhage, hemolysis	Transfuse packed red blood cells
Graft vs host disease	Infusion of viable leukocytes to patients with DiGeorge syndrome	Irradiate blood products
INFECTIOUS DISEASES		
Wound infection (cutaneous, costochondral, sternotomy, mediastinitis, vascular lines, chest tubes)	Contamination in operating room	Antibiotics
Endocarditis	*Staphylococcus epidermidis, Corynebacterium*, contamination in operating room	Antibiotics
Cystitis, pyelonephritis	Contamination of indwelling urinary catheter	Antibiotics, remove, catheter
Hepatitis	Blood-borne: cytomegalovirus, Epstein-Barr virus, hepatitis B and C viruses	Screen blood products
Postperfusion syndrome (fever, hepatosplenomegaly, atypical lymphocytes, lymphadenopathy, transient rash)	Cytomegalovirus, Epstein-Barr virus	Screen blood products
PSYCHOSOCIAL CONDITIONS		
Anxiety, separation	Age related, fears, etc.	Preparedness (videotape, play acting); parent visitation, sedation

ARDS, acute respiratory distress syndrome; ECMO, extracorporeal membrane oxygenation; LVAD, left ventricular assist device; NPO, nothing per os (by mouth); PEEP, positive end-expiratory pressure; PT, prothrombin time; PTT, partial thromboplastin time; SIADH, syndrome of inappropriate antidiuretic hormone; TAPVR, total anomalous pulmonary venous return.

patients who show improved exercise tolerance and general well-being with adequate hemoglobin levels. These patients should also be carefully observed for excessive polycythemia. Cyanotic patients should avoid situations in which dehydration may occur, which leads to increased viscosity and increases the risk of stroke. Diuretics may need to be decreased or temporarily discontinued during episodes of acute gastroenteritis. High altitudes and sudden changes in the thermal environment should also be avoided. Phlebotomy with volume replacement should be carried out in symptomatic patients with severe **polycythemia** (hematocrit >65%); the use of routine phlebotomy in the absence of symptoms is controversial. Patients with severe congenital heart disease or a history of rhythm disturbance should be carefully monitored during anesthesia for even routine surgical procedures. Women with nonrepaired severe congenital heart disease should be counseled on the risks associated with childbearing and on the use of contraceptives and tubal ligation. Pregnancy may be dangerous for patients with chronic cyanosis or pulmonary arterial hypertension. Women with mild to moderate heart disease and many of those who have had corrective surgery can have normal pregnancies, although those with residual hemodynamic derangements or with systemic right ventricles should optimally be followed by a high-risk perinatologist and a cardiologist with expertise in adults with congenital heart disease.

POSTOPERATIVE MANAGEMENT. After successful open heart surgery, the severity of the congenital heart defect, the age and condition (nutritional status) of the patient before surgery, the events in the operating room, and the quality of the postoperative care influence the patient's course. Intraoperative factors that influence survival and that should be noted when a patient returns from the operating room include the duration of cardiopulmonary bypass, the duration of aortic cross-clamping (the time during which the heart is not being perfused), and the duration of profound hypothermia (generally used in infants: the period during which the entire body is not being perfused).

Immediate postoperative care should be provided in an intensive care unit staffed by a team of physicians, nurses, and technicians experienced with the unique problems encountered after open heart surgery. In most major centers, this occurs in a specialized pediatric cardiovascular intensive care unit. Preparation for postoperative monitoring begins in the operating room, where the anesthesiologist or surgeon places an arterial catheter to allow direct arterial pressure measurements and arterial sampling for blood gas determination. A central venous catheter is also placed for measuring central venous pressure and for infusions of cardioactive medications. In more complex cases, left atrial or pulmonary artery catheters may be inserted directly into these cardiac structures and used for pressure monitoring purposes. Flow-directed thermodilution monitoring (Swan-Ganz) catheters are sometimes used for monitoring pulmonary capillary wedge pressure and the cardiac index. Temporary pacing wires are placed on the atrium or ventricle, or both, in case temporary heart block occurs. Transcutaneous oximetry provides for continuous monitoring of arterial oxygen saturation.

Functional failure of one organ system may cause profound physiologic and biochemical changes in another (see Table 434-1). Respiratory insufficiency, for example, leads to hypoxia, acidosis, and hypercapnia, which, in turn, compromise cardiac, vascular, and renal function. The latter problems cannot be managed successfully until adequate ventilation is re-established. Thus, it is essential that the primary source of each postoperative problem be identified and treated.

Respiratory failure is a serious postoperative complication encountered after open heart surgery. Cardiopulmonary bypass carried out in the presence of pulmonary congestion results in decreased lung compliance, copious tracheal and bronchial secretions, atelectasis, and increased breathing effort. Because fatigue and, subsequently, hypoventilation and acidosis may rapidly ensue, mechanical positive pressure endotracheal ventilation may be continued after open heart surgery for a minimum of several hours in relatively stable patients and for up to 2–3 days or longer in severely ill patients, especially infants. Patients with certain congenital heart lesions, particularly those with DiGeorge syndrome, may also have airway abnormalities (tracheomalacia, bronchomalacia) that could make extubation more difficult.

The electrocardiogram should be monitored continuously during the postoperative period. A change in heart rate may be the first indication of a serious complication such as hemorrhage, hypothermia, hypoventilation, or heart failure. **Cardiac rhythm disorders** must be diagnosed quickly because a prolonged untreated arrhythmia may add a severe hemodynamic burden to the heart in the critical early postoperative period (see Chapter 435). Injury to the heart's conduction system during surgery can result in postoperative complete heart block. This complication is usually temporary and is treated with surgically placed pacing wires that can later be removed. Occasionally, complete heart block is permanent. If heart block persists beyond 10–14 days postoperatively, insertion of a permanent pacemaker is required. Tachyarrhythmias are a more common problem in postoperative patients. Junctional ectopic tachycardia (JET) can be a particularly troublesome rhythm to manage (see Chapter 435), although it usually responds to intravenous amiodarone.

Heart failure with poor cardiac output (see Table 434-1) after cardiac surgery may be secondary to respiratory failure, serious arrhythmias, myocardial injury, blood loss, hypervolemia or hypovolemia, or a significant residual hemodynamic abnormality. Treatment specific to the cause should be instituted. Catecholamines, phosphodiesterase inhibitors, nitroprusside and other afterload-reducing agents, and diuretics are the cardioactive agents most often used in patients with myocardial dysfunction in the early postoperative period (see Chapter 442). Postoperative pulmonary hypertension can be managed with hyperventilation and inhaled nitric oxide. In patients who are unresponsive to standard pharmacologic treatment, various ventricular assist devices are available, depending on the patient's size. If pulmonary function is adequate, a left ventricular assist device may be used. If pulmonary function is inadequate, extracorporeal membrane oxygenation (ECMO) may be used. These extraordinary measures are helpful in maintaining the circulation until cardiac function improves, usually within 2–3 days. They have also been used with some success as a bridge to transplantation in patients with severe nonremitting postoperative cardiac failure.

Acidosis secondary to low cardiac output, renal failure, or hypovolemia must be prevented or promptly corrected. Serial monitoring of arterial blood gases and lactate concentrations is performed. An arterial pH <7.3 may result in a decrease in cardiac output with an increase in lactic acid production and may be the forerunner of a series of arrhythmias or cardiac arrest.

Renal function may be compromised by congestive heart failure and further impaired by prolonged cardiopulmonary bypass (see Table 434-1). Blood and fluid replacement, cardiac inotropic agents, and sometimes vasodilators will usually re-establish normal urine flow in patients with hypovolemia or cardiac failure. Dopamine is a useful inotropic agent because it also increases renal blood flow directly. Renal failure secondary to tubular injury may require temporary peritoneal dialysis or hemofiltration.

Neurologic abnormalities can develop after cardiopulmonary bypass, especially in the neonatal period. Seizures may occur when the patient awakens from sedation and can usually be controlled with phenytoin or phenobarbital. In the absence of other neurologic signs, isolated seizures in the immediate postoperative period usually carry a good prognosis. Thromboembolism and stroke are rare but serious complications of open heart surgery. In the long term, both subtle and more substantial learning disabilities may develop. Patients who have undergone surgery entailing the use of cardiopulmonary bypass, especially in the newborn period, should be watched carefully during their early school years for signs of learning disabilities, which are often amenable to early remedial intervention. The risk is higher in patients who have undergone repair using hypothermic total circulatory arrest.

The **postpericardiotomy syndrome** may occur toward the end of the 1st postoperative week or may sometimes be delayed until weeks or months after surgery. This febrile illness is characterized by fever, decreased appetite, listlessness, nausea, and vomiting. Chest pain is not always present, so a high index of suspicion should be maintained in any recently postoperative patient. Echocardiography is diagnostic. In most instances, the postpericardiotomy syndrome is self-limited; however, when pericardial fluid accumulates rapidly, the potential danger of cardiac tamponade should be recognized (see Chapter 440). Rarely, arrhythmias may also occur. Symptomatic patients usually respond to salicylates or indomethacin and bed rest. Occasionally, steroid therapy or pericardiocentesis is required. Late recurrences can occur but are less usual.

Hemolysis of mechanical origin is seen, although rarely, after repair of certain cardiac defects, for example, atrioventricular septal defects, or after the insertion of a mechanical prosthetic valve. It is due to unusual turbulence of blood at increased pressure. Reoperation may be necessary in rare patients with severe and progressive hemolysis who require frequent blood transfusions, but in most instances the problem slowly regresses.

Infection is another potentially serious postoperative problem. Patients usually receive a broad-spectrum antibiotic for the initial postoperative period. Potential sites of infection include the lungs (generally related to postoperative atelectasis), the subcutaneous tissues at the incision site, the sternum, and the urinary tract (especially after an indwelling catheter has been in place). Sepsis with infective endocarditis is an infrequent complication, but it can be difficult to manage (see Chapter 437).

Booth KL, Roth SJ, Thiagarajan RR, et al: Extracorporeal membrane oxygenation support of the Fontan and bidirectional Glenn circulations. *Ann Thorac Surg* 2004;77:1341–1348.

Dunbar-Masterson C, Wypij D, Bellinger DC, et al: General health status of children with D-transposition of the great arteries after the arterial switch operation. *Circulation* 2001;104(Suppl 1):I138–I142.

Hoffman TM, Bush DM, Wernovsky G, et al: Postoperative junctional ectopic tachycardia in children: Incidence, risk factors, and treatment. *Ann Thorac Surg* 2002;74:1607–1611.

Hoffman TM, Wernovsky G, Atz AM, et al: Efficacy and safety of milrinone in preventing low cardiac output syndrome in infants and children after corrective surgery for congenital heart disease. *Circulation* 2003; 107:996–1002.

Limperopoulos C, Majnemer A, Shevell MI, et al: Predictors of developmental disabilities after open heart surgery in young children with congenital heart defects. *J Pediatr* 2002;141:51–58.

Limperopoulos C, Majnemer A, Shevell MI, et al: Functional limitations in young children with congenital heart defects after cardiac surgery. *Pediatrics* 2001;108:1325–1331.

Mou SS, Giroir BP, Molitor-Kirsch EA, et al: Fresh whole blood versus reconstituted blood for pump priming in heart surgery in infants. *N Engl J Med* 2004;351:1635–1644.

Nieminen H, Sairanen H, Tikanoja T, et al: Long-term results of pediatric cardiac surgery in Finland: Education, employment, marital status, and parenthood. *Pediatrics* 2003;112:1345–1350.

Ravishankar C, Tabbutt S, Wernovsky G: Critical care in cardiovascular medicine. *Curr Opin Pediatr* 2003;15:443–453.

Todd JL, Todd NW: Conotruncal cardiac anomalies and otitis media. *J Pediatr* 1997;131:215–219.

Visconti KJ, Bichell DP, Jonas RA, et al: Developmental outcome after surgical versus interventional closure of secundum atrial septal defect in children. *Circulation* 1999;100(Suppl):II145–II150.

Wernovsky G, Stiles KM, Gauvreau K, et al: Cognitive development after the Fontan operation. *Circulation* 2000;102:883–889.

434.1 • The Adult with Congenital Heart Disease • Daniel Murphy

The extraordinary success of surgical repair of congenital heart defects has dramatically improved outcomes for children born with congenital heart disease. Prior to the advent of surgical repair, >50% of such individuals died before reaching adulthood. There may now be more adults than children with congenital heart disease alive in the United States; the number of adults with congenital heart disease will continue to increase as outcomes improve. With the emergence of a substantial population of adults with congenital heart disease, a subspecialty has arisen, with caregivers drawn from pediatric cardiology, internal medicine cardiology, and cardiovascular surgical disciplines. National and international cardiovascular experts recognize the unique needs of this population and have published recommendations regarding physician training, regionalization of care, follow-up of patients, and other pertinent concerns.

All individuals born with congenital heart defects require both primary medical care and routine cardiac follow-up. The coordination of care between primary and specialty providers is particularly important during adolescence, because of new medical and social issues that arise and affect medical care.

THE ROLE OF THE PEDIATRICIAN

As individuals with chronic, lifelong health care needs, adolescents with congenital heart disease should have access to a "Medical Home" as defined by the AAP "Medical Home Policy Statement." Several aspects of the Medical Home are relevant to the population of adolescents with congenital heart disease. Most important is "provision of care coordination services . . . to implement a specific care plan as an organized team." This practice is especially important for patients with multiple medical problems. Examples of issues for patients with congenital heart disease that require care coordination are listed in Table 434-2.

Physical fitness and exercise are generally recommended for all patients. Restrictions may be placed, however, on certain patients with respect to competitive athletics and high-intensity aerobic activities. Published consensus documents address participation in competitive athletics (Chapter 685). These recommendations serve as a starting point for the discussion between the primary care provider, the cardiac specialist, and the patient. Competitive athletic participation should not be approved without recommendations from the cardiologist.

As with all adolescent patients, issues of contraception and pregnancy should be discussed at the appropriate age and in the proper setting. For some patients with congenital heart disease, specific methods of contraception may be preferred over others, such as the avoidance of intrauterine devices due to the increased

TABLE 434-2. Issues That Require Coordination of Care Between the Cardiologist and the Primary Care Physician
Antibiotic prophylaxis for endocarditis
Medications and drug interactions
Anticoagulation with prosthetic valves
Exercise and sports participation
Educational and vocational planning
Contraception and pregnancy
Drug, alcohol, and tobacco use
Noncardiac surgical planning
Anesthetic issues
New symptoms or acute illnesses
Coexistent medical conditions
Travel

risk of infective endocarditis. Although successful pregnancy is possible for most young women with congenital heart disease, there are conditions in which the risks of pregnancy are significantly increased, such as persistent cyanotic congenital heart disease or pulmonary hypertension (Table 434-3). In addition to the original cardiac lesion and surgical history, prior cardiac events, poor functional class, or ventricular dysfunction can be used to predict maternal and neonatal outcomes. For many women with congenital heart disease, pregnancy is possible but entails some increased risk and requires pre-conception planning and/or very careful evaluation and surveillance during the pregnancy. Anticipatory counseling and education are key aspects to care of the adolescent with regard to contraception and pregnancy.

The primary physician should maintain an accessible, comprehensive, central record that contains all pertinent information about the child, preserving confidentiality. In preparation for adolescent transition to adult care, the medical record must accompany the patient to the new site of care. The coordinating physician should also transmit appropriate primary care and subspecialty reports to other consultants and to the patient and his or her family. This process of sharing medical information is essential in avoiding the possibility of multiple specialists functioning independently without knowledge of each other's activities. Patient and family involvement and education act as safeguards against fractionation of medical care.

ADOLESCENT TRANSITION

In addition to consistent pediatric primary care, the Medical Home policy recommends, "transitions, including those . . . into the adult healthcare system, should be planned and organized with the child and family." Fulfillment of this aspect of the Medical Home requires planning for transition to adult care and identification of both primary care and cardiac care providers. The process should be undertaken by the pediatrician in concert with the managing pediatric cardiologist. It is well recognized that, as part of the process of obtaining independence, adolescents or young adults must develop a forward-looking, independent approach to their medical care. For children with heart disease, the transition process must begin during early adolescence and should be encouraged by both the primary care provider and the pediatric cardiologist, who must identify an appropriate adult congenital heart program to which transition and transfer will be made at an appropriate time.

TABLE 434-3. Lesion Specific Risks of Maternal and Neonatal Complications of Pregnancy

No additional risk	Small septal defects Surgically closed ASD, VSD, PDA Mild to moderate aortic regurgitation Mild to moderate pulmonary stenosis
Slightly increased risk	Postoperative repair of tetralogy of Fallot Transposition of the great arteries, s/p arterial switch procedure
Moderate risk	Transposition of the great arteries, s/p atrial switch procedure Congenitally corrected transposition of the great arteries Single ventricle physiology, s/p Fontan procedure
Severe risk	Cyanotic congenital heart disease, unoperated or palliated Marfan syndrome Prosthetic valves Obstructive lesions including coarctation
Pregnancy contraindicated	Severe pulmonary hypertension Severe obstructive lesions Marfan syndrome, aortic root >40 mm

ASD, atrial septal defect; PDA, patent ductus arteriosus; s/p, status post (after); VSD, ventricular septal defect.

TABLE 434-4. Risks in Adults Who Have Congenital Heart Disease

RHYTHM DISORDER
Supraventricular tachycardia
Right bundle branch block
Heart block
Ventricular tachycardia
Sudden death

COARCTATION OF AORTA
Essential hypertension
Recoarctation
Aneurysm formation

RESIDUAL LESIONS (SHUNTS)
VSD
ASD
PDA

ACQUIRED LESIONS
SBE
Subvalvular stenosis
Supravalvular stenosis
Valvular insufficiency
Valvular restenosis

EISENMENGER COMPLEX

PREGNANCY RISK
See Table 434-3

ASD, atrial septal defect; PDA, patent ductus arteriosus; SBE, subacute bacterial endocarditis; VSD, ventricular septal defect.

A successful transition program includes the following elements:

- **Development of a written transition plan that should begin by the age of 14 yr.**
- **Because adolescents and young adults are frequently unaware of the details of their cardiac diagnosis and history, a complete, concise, portable medical record, including all pertinent aspects of cardiac care, should be shared with adolescents and their families and prepared for transmittal to the eventual adult care destination.**
- **The primary care provider and cardiologist must address unique adolescent medical issues as they impact the cardiovascular system. In addition to medical problems, education, vocational planning, psychosocial issues, and access to medical care are all topics that should be discussed with adolescents and their families.**

Although the majority of adolescents and young adults born with complex congenital heart defects undergo surgical "repair" during infancy or childhood, such individuals are rarely "cured" of their underlying cardiac abnormality. In fact, there are large numbers of residua and sequelae that confront this population and produce a variety of potential medical problems throughout adult life (Table 434-4). Therefore, it is critical to recognize the need for ongoing primary medical care and cardiac follow-up throughout adolescence and into young adulthood. There is a tendency for young adults to avoid medical care due to lack of education, denial, or difficulty with access to the medical care system. Thus, a critical goal of the adolescent transition process is to identify an appropriate site for ongoing medical care and ensure maintenance of the medical record and continuity of care for the young adult. The site of care for a young adult with congenital heart disease may be a pediatric program or facility, or may be a specialized center or program for the adult with congenital heart disease. The critical issues are the continuity of care, the preparation of the patient, and the patients participation in the process.

American Academy of Pediatrics: Medical Home Initiatives for Children with Special Needs Project Advisory Committee. Policy statement: The Medical Home. *Pediatrics* 2004;113:1545–1547.

American Academy of Pediatrics: A consensus statement of health care transitions for young adults with special health care needs. *Pediatrics* 2002;110:1304–1306.

Deanfield J, Thaulow E, Warnes C, et al: Management of grown up congenital heart disease. *Eur Heart J* 2003;24:1035–1084.
Maron BJ, Zipes DP: 36th Bethesda Conference: Eligibility recommendations for competitive athletes with cardiovascular abnormalities. *J Am Coll Cardiol* 2005;45:1313–1375.
Perloff JK, Warnes CA: Challenges posed by adults with repaired congenital heart disease. *Circulation* 2001;103:2637–2643.
Siu SC, Sermer M, Colman JM, et al: Prospective multicenter study of pregnancy outcomes in women with heart disease. *Circulation* 2001;104:515–521.
Therrien J, Webb G: Clinical update on adults with congenital heart disease. *Lancet* 2003;362:1305–1313.
Tong EM, Kools S: Health care transitions for adolescents with congenital heart disease: Patient and family perspectives. *Nurs Clin North Am* 2004;39:727–740.
Webb GD, Williams RG: 32nd Bethesda Conference: Care of the adult with congenital heart disease. *J Am Coll Cardiol* 2001;37:1161–1198.

Section 4 — Cardiac Arrhythmias — Anne Dubin

Chapter 435 ■ Disturbances of Rate and Rhythm of the Heart

Pediatric arrhythmias may be transient or permanent, congenital (in a structurally normal or abnormal heart) or acquired (rheumatic fever, myocarditis), caused by a toxin (diphtheria) or by proarrhythmic or antiarrhythmic drugs. They may be a sequela of surgical correction of congenital heart disease, a result of congenital metabolic disorders of mitochondria, or fetal inflammation as in maternal systemic lupus erythematosus (SLE). The major risk of any arrhythmia is either severe tachycardia or bradycardia leading to decreased cardiac output or degeneration into a more critical arrhythmia such as ventricular fibrillation. These complications may lead to syncope, which itself can be dangerous under certain circumstances (swimming, driving), or to sudden death. When a patient has an arrhythmia, it is vital to determine whether the particular rhythm is prone to deteriorate into a life-threatening tachyarrhythmia or bradyarrhythmia. Some rhythm abnormalities, such as single premature atrial and ventricular beats, are common in children without heart disease and in the great majority of instances do not pose a risk to the patient.

A number of powerful pharmacologic agents are available for treating arrhythmias in adults; many have not been studied extensively in children. Problems with frequency of administration, compliance, side effects, drug interactions, and variable responses remain, and selection of an appropriate agent involves empiricism. Fortunately, the majority of rhythm disturbances in children can be reliably controlled with a single agent (Table 435-1). Transcatheter radiofrequency ablation is used not only for resistant tachyarrhythmias but also for elective definitive treatment of arrhythmias. For patients with bradyarrhythmias, implantable pacemakers are small enough for use in premature infants. Implantable cardioverter-defibrillators (ICDs) are available for use in high-risk patients with malignant ventricular arrhythmias and an increased risk of sudden death.

435.1 • Principles of Antiarrhythmic Therapy

When considering drug therapy in the pediatric population, it is important to recognize that there are marked differences in pharmacokinetics for children vs adults. Children may have immature absorption, slow gastric empyting, and differing sizes of drug tissue compartments affecting the volume of distribution. Hepatic metabolism and renal excretion may be very different among the pediatric populations (premature and term neonate, toddler, child, adolescent) as well as in comparison to adults. When specifically considering antiarrhythmic therapy, it is important to recognize that the arrhythmia substrate is extremely different for the pediatric vs adult population, and that differing mechanisms are at work.

There are multiple antiarrhythmic agents available for rhythm control. The majority have not been approved by the U.S. Food and Drug Administration (FDA) for use in children. Pediatric cardiologists have tested these drugs, however, and there are relatively well-recognized guidelines regarding dosing, safety, and efficacy.

With the availability of potentially curative ablation procedures, medical therapy has become more complicated, with physicians accepting fewer drug side effects and expecting higher drug efficacy. Intolerable side effects, as well as the potential for proarrhythmia, can seriously limit medical therapy and will lead the physician and family toward a potentially curative ablation procedure.

Antiarrhythmic drugs are commonly categorized using the Vaughan Williams classification system. This system comprises four classes: Class I is the sodium channel blockers, class II the β-blockers, class III is the repolarization blockers, and Class IV the calcium channel blockers. Class I is further divided by use-dependence and electrocardiogram (ECG) changes (see Table 435-1).

435.2 • Sinus Arrhythmias and Extrasystoles

Sinus arrhythmia represents a normal physiologic variation in impulse discharges from the sinus node related to respirations. The heart rate slows during expiration and accelerates during inspiration. Occasionally, if the sinus rate becomes slow enough, an escape beat arises from the atrioventricular (AV) junction region (Fig. 435-1). Irregularities in sinus rhythm, especially

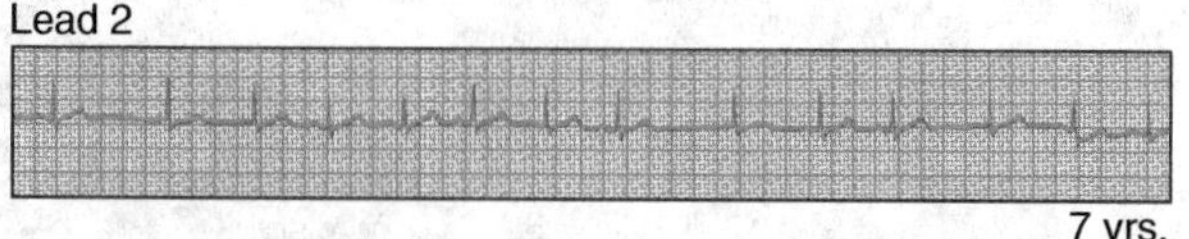

Figure 435-1. Sinus arrhythmia with a junctional escape beat. Note the variation in P-P interval with little change in P morphology or P-R interval. When the sinus rate is slow enough, the atrioventricular junction takes over and produces escape beats. This rhythm is normal.

TABLE 435-1. Antiarrhythmic Drugs Commonly Used in Pediatric Patients, by Class

DRUG	INDICATIONS	DOSING	SIDE EFFECTS	DRUG INTERACTIONS	DRUG LEVEL
CLASS IA: INHIBITS NA$^+$ FAST CHANNEL, PROLONGS REPOLARIZATION					
Quinidine	SVT, atrial fibrillation, atrial flutter, VT, AV nodal blockade (digoxin, verapamil, propranolol) must be given first to prevent 1 : 1 conduction in atrial flutter	Oral: 20–60 mg/kg/24 hr divided q 6 h (sulfate) or q 8 h (gluconate) Max dose: 2.4 g/24 hr	Nausea, vomiting, diarrhea, fever, cinchonism, QRS and QT prolongation, AV nodal block, asystole syncope, thrombocytopenia, hemolytic anemia, SLE, blurred vision, convulsions, allergic reactions, exacerbation of periodic paralysis	Enhances digoxin, may increase PTT when given with warfarin	2–7 μg/mL
Procainamide	SVT, atrial fibrillation, atrial flutter, VT	Oral: 15–50 mg/kg/24 hr divided q 4 h Max dose: 4 g/24 hr IV: 3–6 mg/kg over 5 min, repeat to 15 mg/kg load followed by 20–80 μg/kg/min Max dose: 2 g/24 hr	PR, QRS, QT interval prolongation, anorexia, nausea, vomiting, rash, fever, agranulocytosis, thrombocytopenia, Coombs-positive hemolytic anemia, SLE, hypotension, exacerbation of periodic paralysis, proarrhythmia	Toxicity increased by amiodarone and cimetidine	4–10 μg/mL
Disopyramide	SVT, atrial fibrillation, atrial flutter	Oral: <2 yrs: 20–30 mg/kg/24 hr divided q 6 h or q 12 h (long-acting form) 2–10 yrs 9–24 mg/kg/24 hr divide q 6 h or q 12 hr (long-acting form) 11 yr 5–13 mg/kg/24 hr divided q 6 h or q 12 hr (long-acting) Max dose: 1.2 g/24 hr	Anticholinergic effects, urinary retention, blurred vision, dry mouth, QT and QRS prolongation, hepatic toxicity, negative inotropic effects, agranulocytosis, psychosis, hypoglycemia, proarrhythmia		2–5 μg/mL
CLASS IB: INHIBITS NA$^+$ FAST CHANNEL, SHORTENS REPOLARIZATION					
Lidocaine	PVC, VT, VF	IV: 1 mg/kg repeat q 5 min 2 times followed by 20–50 μg/kg/min (Max dose: 3 mg/kg)	CNS effects, confusion, convulsions, high degree AV block, asystole, coma, parasthesias, respiratory failure	Propranol Cimetadine, increases toxicity	1–5 μg/mL
Mexilitene	VT, PVC	Oral: 6–15 mg/kg/24 hr divided q 8 h	GI upset, skin rash, neurologic	Cimetidine	
Phenytoin	Digitalis intoxication	Oral: 3–6 mg/kg/24 hr divided q 12 h Max dose: 600 mg IV: 10–15 mg/kg over 1 hour load	Rash, gingival hyperplasia, ataxia, lethargy, vertigo, tremor, macryocytic anemia, bradycardia with rapid push	Amiodarone, oral anticoagulants, cimetidine, nifedipine, disopyramide, increase toxicity	10–20 μg/mL
CLASS IC: INHIBITS NA$^+$ CHANNEL					
Flecainide	SVT, atrial tachycardia, VT	Oral: 3–10 mg/kg/24 hr divided q 8 h	Blurred vision, nausea, decrease in contractility, proarrhythmia	Amiodarone increases toxicity	0.2–1 μg/mL
Propafenone	SVT, atrial tachycardia, atrial fibrillation, VT	Oral: 150–300 mg/m^2/24 hr divided q 8 h	Hypotension, decreased contractility, hepatic toxicity, parasthesia, headache, proarrhythmia	Increase digoxin levels	0.2–1 μg/mL
CLASS II: β-BLOCKERS					
Propranolol	SVT, PVC, Long QT	Oral: 1–4 mg/kg/24 hr divided q 6 h Max dose: 60 mg/24 hr IV: 0.1–0.15 mg/kg over 5 minutes Max dose: 10 mg	Bradycardia, loss of concentration or memory, bronchospasm, hypoglycemia, hypotension, heart block, CHF	Use with disopyramide or verapamil exacerbates or precipitates CHF	
CLASS III: PROLONGS REPOLARIZATION					
Amiodarone	SVT, JET, VT	Oral: 10 mg/kg/24 hr in 1–2 divided doses for 4–14 days; reduce to 5 mg/kg/24 hr for several weeks; if no recurrence, reduce to 2.5 mg/kg/24 hr may be given 5 of 7 days IV: 2.5–5 mg/kg over 30–60 min, may repeat 3 times, then 2–10 mg/kg/24 q 24 hr	Hypothyroidism or hyperthyroidism, elevated triglycerides, hepatic toxicity, pulmonary fibrosis	Digoxin (increases levels) flecainide, procainamide, quinidine, warfarin, phenytoin	0.5–2.5 mg/L
CLASS IV: MISCELLANEOUS					
Digoxin	SVT (not WPW), atrial flutter, atrial fibrillation	Oral: Load: Premature: 20 μg/kg Newborn: 30 μg/kg >6 mo: 40 μg/kg Give 1/2 total dose followed by 1/4 q 8–12 h X2 doses Maintenance: 10 μg/kg/24 hr divide q 12 hr Max dose: 0.5 mg IV: 3/4 PO dose Max dose: 0.5 mg	PAC, PVC, bradycardia, AV block, nausea, vomiting, anorexia, prolongs PR interval	Quinidine Amiodarone, verapamil, increase digoxin levels	1–2 mg/mL
Verapamil	SVT (not WPW)	Oral: 2–7 mg/kg/24 hr divided q 8 hr Max dose: 480 mg IV: 0.1–0.2 mg/kg q 20 min X2 doses Max dose: 5–10 mg	Bradycardia, asystole, high degree AV block, PR prolongation, hypotension, CHF	Use with β-blocker or disopyramide exacerbates CHF, increases digoxin level and toxicity	
Adenosine	SVT	IV: 50–300 μg/kg begins with 50 μg/kg and increase by 50–100 μg/kg/dose; if no effect, need rapid IV push Max dose: 12 mg	Chest pain, flushing, dyspnea, bronchospasm, bradycardia, asystole		

AV, atrioventricular; CHF, congestive heart failure, CNS, central nervous systems; IV, intravenous; JET, junctional ectopic tachycardia; LQT, long QT syndrome, PAC, premature atrial contraction; PO, oral; PTT, partial thromboplastin time; PVC, premature ventricular contractions; SLE, systemic lupus erythematosus–like illness; antinuclear antibody positive; SVT, supraventricular tachycardia; VT, ventricular tachycardia; WPW, Wolff-Parkinson-White syndrome.

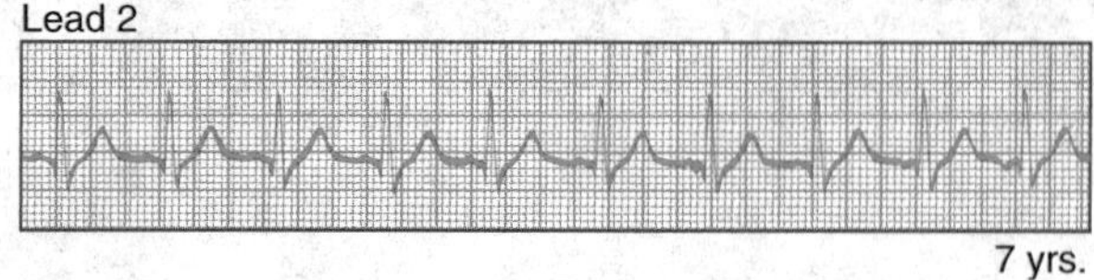

Figure 435-2. Wandering atrial pacemaker. Note the change in P-wave configuration in the 7th, 9th, and 10th beats. The 7th P wave may represent a fusion between the sinus P and the ectopic atrial pacemaker seen in the 10th beat.

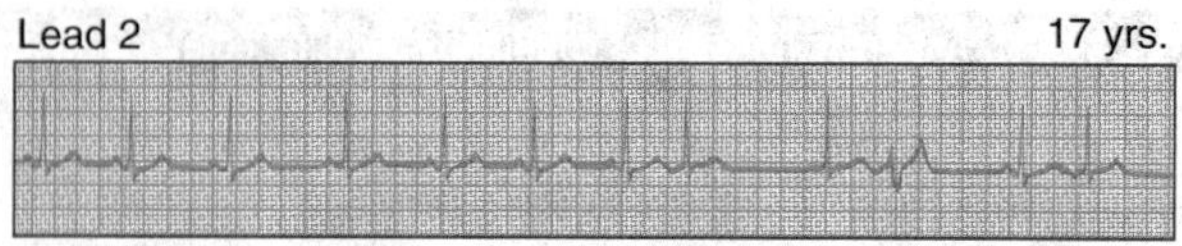

Figure 435-3. Premature atrial contraction (PAC). QRS complexes—the 8th, 10th, and final—in this strip are preceded by a P wave that is inverted, indicative of an ectopic origin of atrial depolarization. Note that the 8th and final QRS complexes resemble those of sinus origin, whereas the 10th is aberrantly conducted. This shift in origin is a function of the preceding cycle length, which influences the refractory period of the bundle branches. The fact that the pause after the PAC is longer than two P-P intervals implies that the premature atrial depolarization has invaded and discharged the sinus node and then reset it so that it fires later.

bradycardia associated with periodic apnea, are commonly seen in premature infants. Sinus arrhythmia is exaggerated during febrile illnesses and by drugs that increase vagal tone, such as digitalis; it is usually abolished by exercise.

Sinus bradycardia is due to slow discharge of impulses from the sinus node. A sinus rate <90 beats/min in neonates and <60 beats/min thereafter is considered to be sinus bradycardia. It is commonly seen in well-trained athletes; in healthy individuals, it is without significance. Sinus bradycardia may occur in systemic disease, for example, myxedema, and it resolves when the disorder is under control. Sinus bradycardia must be differentiated from sinoatrial and AV block. Children with sinus bradycardia are able to increase their heart rate with exercise to a much higher rate than 100 beats/min, whereas patients with AV block are usually unable to do so. Low birthweight infants display great variation in sinus rate. Sinus bradycardia is common in these infants in conjunction with apnea, and may be associated with junctional escape beats. Premature atrial contractions are also frequent. These rhythm changes, especially bradycardia, appear more commonly during sleep and are not associated with symptoms. Usually, no therapy is necessary.

Wandering atrial pacemaker (Fig. 435-2) is defined as an intermittent shift in the pacemaker of the heart from the sinus node to another part of the atrium. It is not uncommon in childhood and usually represents a normal variant, but it may also be seen in patients with central nervous system disturbances, for example, subarachnoid hemorrhage.

Extrasystoles are produced by the discharge of an ectopic focus that may be situated anywhere in atrial, junctional, or ventricular tissue. Usually, isolated extrasystoles are of no clinical or prognostic significance. Under certain circumstances, however, premature beats may be due to organic heart disease (inflammation, ischemia, fibrosis) or to drug toxicity, especially from digitalis.

Premature atrial complexes are common in childhood, even in the absence of cardiac disease. Depending on the degree of prematurity of the beat (coupling interval) and the preceding R-R interval (cycle length), premature atrial complexes may result in a normal, a prolonged (aberrancy), or an absent (blocked premature atrial complex) QRS complex. The last occurs when the premature impulse is conducted to the ventricle while the specialized ventricular conducting system is partially refractory (Fig. 435-3). Atrial extrasystoles must be distinguished from premature ventricular complexes (PVCs). Careful scrutiny of the electrocardiogram for a premature P wave preceding the QRS that has a different contour from that of the other sinus P waves is essential for diagnosis. Atrial premature complexes often reset the sinus node pacemaker (lack of a compensatory pause), but this feature is not regarded as a reliable means of differentiating atrial from ventricular premature complexes.

PVCs may arise in any region of the ventricles. They are characterized by premature, widened, bizarre QRS complexes that are not preceded by a P wave (Fig. 435-4). When all premature beats have identical contours, they are classified as unifocal in origin. When PVCs vary in contour, they are designated as multifocal. Ventricular extrasystoles are often, but not always followed by a compensatory pause. The presence of fusion beats, that is, complexes with morphologic features that are intermediate between those of normal sinus beats and those of PVCs, is a clue to the ventricular origin of the extrasystole. Extrasystoles produce a smaller stroke and pulse volume than normal and, if quite premature, may not be audible with a stethoscope or palpable at the radial pulse. When frequent, extrasystoles may assume a definite rhythm, for example, alternating with normal beats (**bigeminy**) or occurring after two normal beats (**trigeminy**). Most patients are unaware of single premature ventricular contractions, although some may be aware of a "skipped beat" over the precordium. This sensation is due to the increased stroke volume of the normal beat after a compensatory pause. Anxiety, a febrile illness, or ingestion of various drugs or stimulants may cause premature ventricular beats.

It is important to distinguish PVCs that are benign from those that are likely to degenerate into more severe arrhythmias. The former usually disappear during the tachycardia of exercise. If they persist or become more frequent during exercise, the arrhythmia may have greater significance. The following criteria are indications for further investigation of PVCs that could require **suppressive therapy:** (1) two or more ventricular premature beats in a row, (2) multifocal origin, (3) increased ventricular ectopic activity with exercise, (4) R on T phenomenon (premature ventricular depolarization occurs on the T wave of the preceding beat), and (5) presence of underlying heart disease. The basis of therapy for benign PVCs is reassurance that the arrhythmia is not life-threatening. Malignant PVCs are usually secondary to another medical problem (electrolyte imbalance, hypoxia, drug toxicity, cardiac injury, or an intraventricular catheter). Successful treatment includes correction of the underlying abnormality. An intravenous lidocaine bolus and drip is the 1st line of therapy, with more powerful drugs such as amiodarone reserved for refractory cases or for patients with hemodynamic compromise.

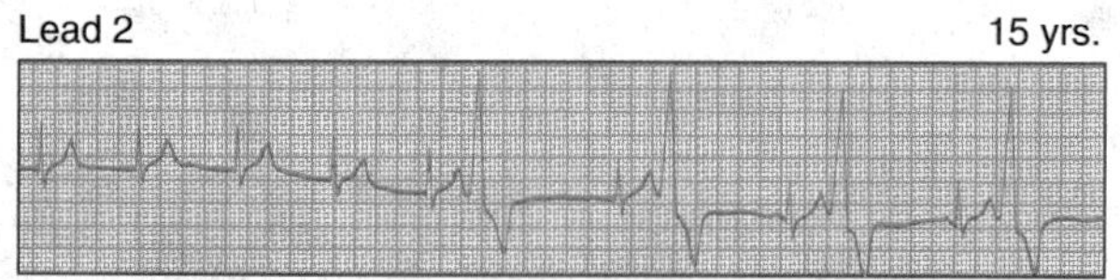

Figure 435-4. Premature ventricular contractions (PVCs) induced by hyperventilation. Note that the premature beat is wide and has a completely different morphology from that of the sinus beat. The fact that the premature beat is not preceded by a P wave and the pause following it is fully compensatory (i.e., the P-P interval containing the PVC equals two sinus cycles) indicates that the sinus mechanism has not been disturbed by the premature beats.

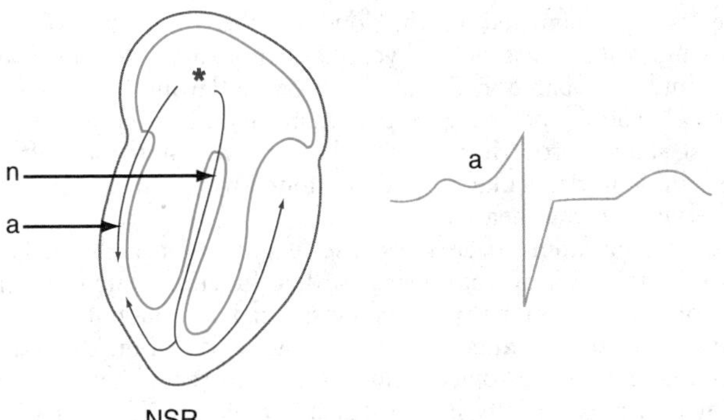

Figure 435-5. Schematic representation of the heart with a right-sided anomalous pathway. The *asterisk* indicates initiation of the sinus beat. The *arrows* indicate the direction and spread of excitation. The electrocardiographic complex shown represents a fusion beat that combines activation over the normal *(n)* and accessory *(a)* pathways. The latter inscribes the delta wave. NSR, normal sinus rhythm.

435.3 • Supraventricular Tachycardia

Supraventricular tachycardias (SVTs) involve components of the conduction system within or above the bundle of His and can be divided into three major categories: re-entrant tachycardias using an accessory pathway, re-entrant tachycardias without an accessory pathway, and ectopic or automatic tachycardias. Re-entry using an accessory pathway is the most common mechanism of SVT in infants, with an increasing incidence of AV nodal re-entry noted in childhood. The tachycardia is initiated by a premature atrial beat that is most often conducted to the ventricle through the normal AV nodal pathway (**orthodromic conduction**). The ventricular response finds the AV nodal pathway refractory, but the bypass tract, readily able to conduct in a retrograde fashion, returns to the atrium as an echo beat, which, in turn, transmits back to the ventricle, and so on (Fig. 435-5). Atrial and junctional ectopic tachycardias are more commonly associated with abnormal hearts (cardiomyopathy) or with postoperative congenital heart disease.

CLINICAL MANIFESTATIONS. Re-entrant SVT is characterized by an abrupt onset and cessation; it may be precipitated by an acute infection and usually occurs when the patient is at rest. Attacks may last only a few seconds or may persist for hours. The heart rate usually exceeds 180 beats/min and may occasionally be as rapid as 300 beats/min (Fig. 435-6). The only complaint may be awareness of the rapid heart rate. Many children tolerate these episodes extremely well, and it is unlikely that short paroxysms are a danger to life. If the rate is exceptionally rapid or if the attack is prolonged, precordial discomfort and heart failure may supervene. SVT may occur in the presence of unoperated congenital heart disease (Ebstein anomaly). In children, SVT may be precipitated by exposure to the sympathomimetic amines contained in over-the-counter decongestants.

In young infants, the diagnosis may be more obscure because of the inability to communicate their symptoms. The heart rate at this age is normally rapid and, even in the absence of tachyarrhythmia, it increases greatly with crying. Infants with SVT are often initially seen in heart failure because the tachycardia goes unrecognized for a long time. The heart rate during paroxysms is frequently in the range of 200–300 beats/min. If the attack lasts 6–24 hr or more with an extremely fast heart rate, the infant may become acutely ill, have an ashen color, and be restless and irritable. Tachypnea and hepatomegaly are the prominent signs of cardiac failure, and fever and leukocytosis may be present. When tachycardia occurs in the fetus, it can cause severe heart failure and hydrops fetalis.

In neonates, SVT is usually manifested as a narrow QRS complex (<0.08 sec). The P wave is visible on a standard electrocardiogram in only 50–60% of neonates with SVT, but it is detectable with a transesophageal lead in most patients. **Differentiation from sinus tachycardia** may be difficult; if the rate is >230 beats/min with an abnormal P-wave axis (a normal P wave is positive in leads I and aVF), SVT is more likely. The heart rate in SVT also tends to be unvarying, whereas in sinus tachycardia the heart rate varies with changes in vagal and sympathetic tone. Differentiation from ventricular tachycardia is critical because digoxin can precipitate ventricular fibrillation in patients with ventricular tachycardia. The absence of ventricular-to-atrial conduction (and thus only intermittent P waves), the presence of fusion beats, and wide QRS complexes that are dissimilar to the QRS complex during sinus rhythm are diagnostic of ventricular tachycardia.

AV re-entrant tachycardia uses a bypass tract that may either be able to conduct antegrade (**Wolff-Parkinson-White [WPW] syndrome**) or remain concealed. Patients with WPW syndrome have a small, but real risk of sudden death. If the accessory pathway rapidly conducts in antegrade fashion, the patient is at risk for atrial fibrillation begetting ventricular fibrillation. Risk stratification, including 24 hr Holter monitoring and exercise study, can help differentiate patients at higher risk for sudden death from WPW. Concurrently, any patient with syncope and WPW syndrome should have an electrophysiology study.

The typical electrocardiographic features of the Wolff-Parkinson-White syndrome are usually seen when the patient is not having the tachycardia. These features include a short P-R interval and slow upstroke of the QRS (delta wave) (Fig. 435-7). Though most often present in patients with a normal heart, this syndrome may also be associated with Ebstein anomaly and other congenital heart lesions. The anatomic substrates included in the re-entrant circuit are the AV node and an accessory pre-excitation pathway consisting of a muscular bridge connecting atrium to ventricle on either the right or the left side of the AV ring (see Fig. 435-5). During sinus rhythm, the impulse is carried over both the AV node and the accessory pathway; it produces some degree of fusion of the two depolarization fronts that results in an abnormal QRS. During tachycardia, an impulse is usually carried in anterograde fashion through the AV node (**orthodromic conduction**), which results in a normal QRS complex, and in retrograde fashion through the accessory pathway to the atrium, thereby perpetuating the tachycardia. In these cases, only after

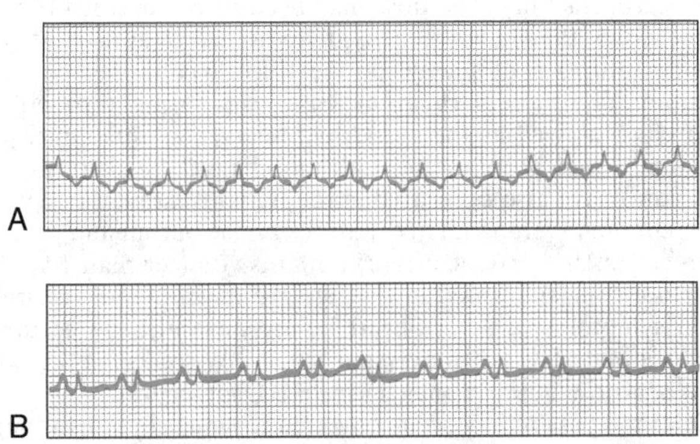

Figure 435-6. *A*, Paroxysmal supraventricular or atrial tachycardia with a ventricular rate of 230 beats/min. *B*, Sinus rhythm after DC cardioversion. Note that during the tachycardia the T wave is deformed by an inverted, presumably retrograde P wave. The QRS morphology is unchanged during the tachycardia. The low voltage is due to peripheral edema in a 1 day old infant who had intrauterine tachycardia and hydrops fetalis.

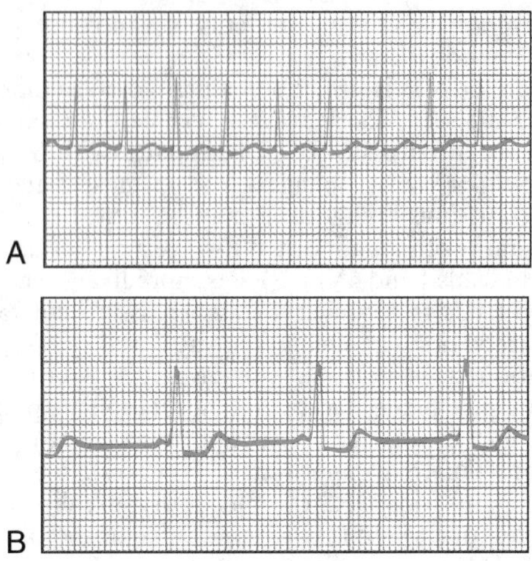

Figure 435-7. *A,* Supraventricular tachycardia in a child with Wolff-Parkinson-White (WPW) syndrome. Note the normal QRS complexes during the tachycardia. *B,* Later, the typical features of WPW syndrome are apparent (short P-R interval, delta wave, and wide QRS).

cessation of the tachycardia are the typical features of WPW syndrome recognized (see Fig. 435-7). When rapid anterograde conduction occurs through the pre-excitation pathway during tachycardia and the retrograde re-entry pathway to the atrium is via the AV node (**antidromic conduction**), the tachycardiac complexes are wide and the potential for more serious arrhythmias (ventricular fibrillation) is greater, especially if atrial fibrillation occurs.

AV nodal re-entrant tachycardia involves the use of two pathways within the AV node. This arrhythmia is more commonly seen in adolescence. It is one of the few SVTs that is frequently associated with syncope. This arrhythmia is usually amenable to antiarrhythmic therapy, such as digoxin or propranolol, or to radiofrequency ablation therapy.

TREATMENT. Vagal stimulation by submersion of the face in iced saline (in older children) or by placing an ice bag over the face (in infants) may abort the attack. To abolish the paroxysm, older children may be taught vagotonic maneuvers such as the Valsalva maneuver, straining, breath holding, drinking ice water, or adopting a particular posture. When these measures fail, several pharmacologic alternatives are available (see Table 435-1). In stable patients, adenosine by rapid intravenous push is the **treatment of choice** because of its rapid onset of action and minimal effects on cardiac contractility. The dose may need to be repeated rapidly. Other drugs that have been used for initial treatment of SVT include infusions of phenylephrine (Neo-Synephrine) or edrophonium (Tensilon), which increase vagal tone through the baroreflex, as well as the antiarrhythmic agents quinidine, procainamide, and propranolol. Calcium channel blockers such as verapamil have also been used in the initial treatment of SVT in older children. Verapamil may reduce cardiac output and produce hypotension and cardiac arrest in infants younger than 1 yr; it is therefore contraindicated in this age group. In urgent situations when symptoms of severe heart failure have already occurred, synchronized DC cardioversion (0.5–2 W-sec/kg) is recommended as the initial management (see Chapter 66).

Once the patient has been converted to sinus rhythm, a longer acting agent is selected for maintenance therapy. In patients without an antegrade accessory pathway, digoxin or propranolol is the mainstay of therapy. In children with evidence of pre-excitation (WPW syndrome), digoxin or calcium channel blockers may increase the rate of anterograde conduction of impulses through the bypass tract and should be avoided. These patients are usually managed in the long term with propranolol. In patients with resistant tachycardias, procainamide, quinidine, flecainide, propafenone, sotalol, and amiodarone have all been used. It should be recognized that most antiarrhythmic agents could have proarrhythmic and negative inotropic effects. Flecainide in particular should be limited to use in patients with otherwise normal hearts.

If cardiac failure occurs because of prolonged tachycardia in an infant with a normal heart, cardiac function usually returns to normal after sinus rhythm is reinstituted, although it may take days to weeks. Infants with SVT diagnosed within the 1st 3–4 mo of life have a lower incidence of recurrence than do those in whom it is initially diagnosed at a later age. These patients have a 40% chance of resolution; if medical therapy is required; it can be tapered within a year and the patient watched for signs of recurrence.

Twenty-four hour electrocardiographic (Holter) recordings are useful in monitoring the course of therapy and in detecting brief runs of asymptomatic tachycardia. A brief assessment of arrhythmia control can be made at the bedside with **transesophageal pacing.** More detailed electrophysiologic studies performed in the cardiac catheterization laboratory are often indicated in patients with refractory SVTs. During an **electrophysiologic study,** multiple electrode catheters are placed in different locations in the heart and can aid in pinpointing an ectopic focus or bypass tract. Pacing can induce the tachyarrhythmia, and different pharmacologic agents can be tested for their ability to inhibit the arrhythmia. These studies are necessary prerequisites to radiofrequency ablation.

Radiofrequency ablation of an accessory pathway is another treatment option commonly used in patients with re-entrant rhythms. It is often used electively in children and teenagers, as well as in patients who require multiple agents or find drug side effects intolerable or for whom arrhythmia control is poor. The overall initial success rate ranges from approximately 80% to 95%, depending on the location of the bypass tract or tracts. Surgical ablation of bypass tracts may also be successful in selected patients.

Atrial ectopic tachycardia is an uncommon tachycardia in childhood. It is characterized by a variable rate (seldom >200 beats/min), identifiable P waves with an abnormal axis, and chronicity in either a sustained or intermittent tachycardia. This form of atrial tachycardia has a single automatic focus rather than the more usual re-entry mechanism. Identification of this mechanism is aided by monitoring the electrocardiogram while initiating vagal or pharmacologic therapy. Re-entry tachycardias "break" suddenly, whereas automatic tachycardias gradually slow down and then gradually speed up again. Atrial ectopic tachycardias are usually more difficult to control pharmacologically than the more common re-entrant tachycardias are. If pharmacologic therapy with a single agent is unsuccessful, catheter ablation is suggested and has a success rate >90%.

Chaotic or multifocal atrial tachycardia are characterized by three or more ectopic P waves with three or more different ectopic P-P cycles, frequent blocked P waves, and varying P-R intervals of conducted beats. This arrhythmia occurs most often in infants younger than 1 yr, usually without cardiac disease, although some evidence suggests an association with viral myocarditis. Drug treatment may not be effective, and multiple agents are often required. Fortunately, when this arrhythmia occurs in infancy, it usually terminates spontaneously by 3 yr of age.

Accelerated junctional ectopic tachycardia (JET) is an automatic (non-re-entry) arrhythmia in which the junctional rate exceeds that of the sinus node and AV dissociation results. This arrhythmia is most often recognized in the early postoperative period after cardiac surgery and may be extremely difficult to control. Reduction of the infusion rate of catecholamines and control of fever are important adjuncts to management. JET in the absence of surgery carries a more guarded prognosis. Junctional tachycardia may also be a sign of digitalis intoxication; when intoxication occurs, the drug should be discontinued. Intravenous amiodarone is effective in the treatment of postoperative JET. Patients who require chronic therapy may respond to amiodarone or sotalol.

Atrial flutter, also known as intra-atrial re-entrant tachycardia, is a regular or regularly irregular tachycardia characterized by atrial activity at a rate of 250–400 beats/min. These contractions are thought to be due to a re-entrant or circus rhythm originating in the atria and involving a micro-re-entrant loop within the atrial tissue and some form of anatomic obstacle that creates a discontinuity in conduction (fibrosis, surgical suture site, valve annulus). Because the AV node cannot transmit such rapid impulses, some degree of **AV block** is virtually always present, and the ventricles respond to every 2nd–4th atrial beat. Occasionally, the response is variable and the rhythm appears irregular.

In older children, atrial flutter usually occurs in the setting of congenital heart disease; neonates with atrial flutter frequently have normal hearts. Atrial flutter may occur during acute infectious illnesses but is most often seen in patients with large stretched atria, such as those associated with long-standing mitral or tricuspid insufficiency, tricuspid atresia, Ebstein anomaly, or rheumatic mitral stenosis. Atrial flutter can also occur after palliative or corrective intra-atrial surgery. Uncontrolled atrial flutter may precipitate heart failure. Vagal maneuvers (such as carotid sinus pressure or iced saline submersion) or adenosine generally produce a temporary slowing of the heart rate. The **diagnosis** is confirmed by electrocardiography, which demonstrates the rapid and regular atrial saw-toothed flutter waves. Atrial flutter usually converts immediately to sinus rhythm by **synchronized DC cardioversion,** which is most often the **treatment of choice.** Patients with chronic atrial flutter in the setting of congenital heart disease may be at increased risk for **thromboembolism** and stroke and should thus undergo anticoagulation before elective cardioversion. Digitalis slows the ventricular response in atrial flutter by prolonging conduction time through the AV node. After digitalization, a type I agent such as quinidine or procainamide is usually needed to maintain adequate control. Type III agents such as amiodarone and sotalol have shown promise and may be useful in patients refractory to type I agents. Other modalities, including radiofrequency and surgical ablation, have been used in older patients with congenital heart disease with moderate success. Neonates with normal hearts who respond to digoxin may be treated for 6–12 mo, after which the medication can often be discontinued.

Atrial fibrillation is much less common in children and rare in infants. The atrial excitation is chaotic and more rapid (300–700 beats/min) and produces an irregularly irregular ventricular response and pulse (Fig. 435-8). This rhythm disorder is most often the result of a chronically stretched atrial myocardium. Atrial fibrillation occurs most frequently in older children with rheumatic mitral valve disease. It is also seen rarely as a complication of intra-atrial surgery, in patients with left atrial enlarge-

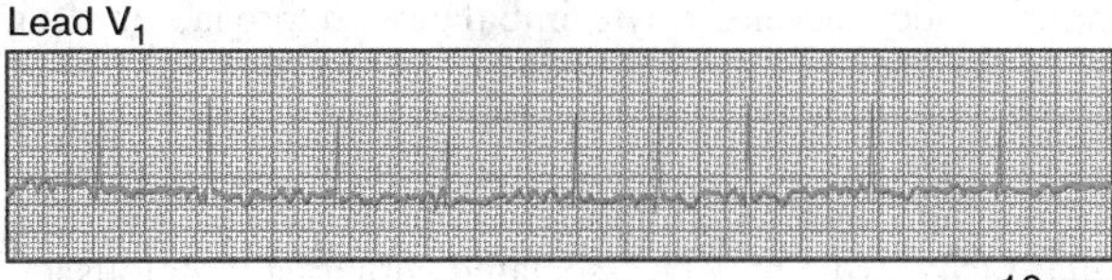

Figure 435-8. Atrial fibrillation, characterized by the absence of P waves; presence of fibrillatory waves, which are grossly irregular, rapid undulations; and an irregular ventricular response. Fibrillatory waves may not be visible in all leads and should be carefully sought in every tracing with irregular R-R intervals. (The coexisting qR in V_1 is diagnostic of right ventricular hypertrophy in this patient with Eisenmenger syndrome.)

ment secondary to left AV valve insufficiency, in conditions producing atrial flutter, and in patients with WPW syndrome. Thyrotoxicosis, pulmonary emboli, and pericarditis should be suspected in a previously normal older child or adolescent with atrial fibrillation. Atrial fibrillation may be familial. The best initial treatment is **digitalization,** which restores the ventricular rate to normal, although the atrial fibrillation usually persists. Digoxin is not given if WPW syndrome is present. Normal sinus rhythm may then be restored with a type I agent (quinidine or procainamide), with amiodarone, or by DC cardioversion. Patients with chronic atrial fibrillation are at risk for the development of thromboemboli and stroke and should undergo anticoagulation with warfarin. Patients being treated by elective cardioversion should also undergo anticoagulation.

435.4 • Ventricular Tachyarrhythmias

Ventricular tachycardia (VT) is less common than SVT in pediatric patients. VT is defined as at least three PVCs at >120 beats/min. It may be paroxysmal or incessant. VT may be associated with myocarditis, anomalous origin of a coronary artery, arrhythmogenic right ventricular dysplasia, mitral valve prolapse, primary cardiac tumors, or cardiomyopathy. It has been seen with prolonged Q-T interval of either congenital or acquired (proarrhythmic drugs) causation, WPW syndrome, and drug use (cocaine, amphetamines). It may develop years after intraventricular surgery (tetralogy of Fallot, ventricular septal defect) or occur without obvious organic heart disease. VT must be distinguished from SVT with aberrancy or rapid conduction over an accessory pathway (Table 435-2). The presence of capture and fusion beats helps confirm the diagnosis. Although some children tolerate rapid ventricular rates for many hours, this arrhythmia should be promptly treated because hypotension and degeneration into ventricular fibrillation may result. For patients who are hemodynamically stable, intravenous amiodarone, lidocaine, or procainamide are the initial drugs of choice. If treatment is to be successful, it is critical to search for and correct any underlying

TABLE 435-2. Diagnosis of Tachyarrhythmias

ELECTROCARDIOGRAPHIC FINDINGS				
	HEART RATE (BEATS/MIN)	P WAVE	QRS DURATION	REGULARITY
Sinus tachycardia	<225	Always present normal axis	Normal	Rate varies with respiration
Atrial tachycardia	180–320	Present—50% Superior axis common	Normal or prolonged (RBBB pattern)	Regular
Atrial fibrillation	120–180	Fibrillatory waves	Normal or prolonged (RBBB pattern)	Irregularly irregular
Atrial flutter	Atrial: 250–400 Ventricular response variable: 100–320	Saw-toothed flutter waves	Normal or prolonged (RBBB pattern)	Regular ventricular response (e.g., 2:1, 3:1, 3:2, and so on)
Ventricular tachycardia	120–240	Absent or atrioventricular dissociation	Usually prolonged	Slightly irregular

RBBB, right bundle branch block.

abnormalities such as electrolyte imbalance, hypoxia, or drug toxicity. Amiodarone is the **treatment of choice** during cardiac arrest (see Chapter 66.1). Overdrive ventricular pacing may also be effective, although it may occasionally cause the arrhythmia to deteriorate into ventricular fibrillation. In the neonatal period, ventricular tachycardia may be associated with an anomalous left coronary artery (see Chapter 432.2) or a myocardial tumor.

Unless a clearly reversible cause is identified, electrophysiologic study is usually indicated for patients in whom VT has developed.

Ventricular fibrillation is a chaotic dysrhythmia that results in death unless an effective ventricular beat is rapidly re-established. A thump on the chest may occasionally restore sinus rhythm. Usually, external cardiac massage with artificial ventilation and DC defibrillation is necessary. If defibrillation is ineffective or fibrillation recurs, amiodarone or lidocaine may be given intravenously and defibrillation repeated (see Chapter 66). After recovery from ventricular fibrillation, a search should be made for the underlying cause. **Electrophysiologic study** is usually indicated for patients in whom ventricular fibrillation has developed unless a clearly reversible cause is identified. If WPW syndrome is noted, ablation should be performed. For patients in whom no correctable abnormality can be found, an ICD should be strongly considered because of the high risk of sudden death.

435.5 • Long Q-T Syndromes

Long Q-T syndromes (LQTS) are genetic abnormalities of ventricular repolarization. They present as a long Q-T interval on the surface ECG and are associated with malignant ventricular arrhythmias (torsade de pointes). They are a cause of syncope and sudden death and may be associated with sudden infant death syndrome or drowning. About 50% of cases are familial: Romano-Ward syndrome (RWS) is a common form of LQTS that exhibits autosomal dominant transmission with low penetrance. Jervell and Lange-Nielsen syndrome (JLNS) is an uncommon form of LQTS, has autosomal recessive transmission, and is associated with congenital deafness. The remainder of cases are sporadic. Asymptomatic (presymptomatic) patients carrying the gene mutation may not all have a prolonged Q-T duration. This may become apparent with exercise or during catecholamine infusions.

Genetic studies have identified mutations in cardiac potassium and sodium channels. In LQT1, the gene is on chromosome 11p15.5 and encodes a potassium channel (KVLQT1). LQT2 gene is on chromosome 7q35-36, which encodes HERG (human-ether-a-go-go-related gene), a potassium channel. LQT3 is a defect on chromosome 3p21-24 and encodes a sodium channel (SCN5A). The cause of LQT4 is unknown. LQT5 is a mutation on chromosome 21q22.1 and encodes a regulator (minK) of potassium channels. LQT6 is on chromosome 21q22.1 and is a minK-related peptide. JLNS has been seen in patients who have homozygous mutations of KVLQT1 and minK, whereas the heterozygous state is manifested as RWS. Genotype may predict clinical manifestations; for example, **LQT1 events are stress induced,** whereas events in **LQT3 occur during sleep.** LQT2 events have an intermediate pattern. LQT3 has the highest probability for sudden death, followed by LQT2 and then LQT1. Drugs may prolong the QT interval directly (terfenadine, astemizole, cisapride, droperidol), but more often do so when drugs such as erythromycin or ketoconazole inhibit their metabolism.

The **clinical manifestation** of LQTS in children is most often a syncopal episode brought on by exercise, fright, or a sudden startle; some events occur during sleep (LQT3). Patients can initially be seen with seizures, presyncope, or palpitations; about 10% are initially in cardiac arrest. The diagnosis is based on electrocardiographic and clinical criteria. Not all patients with long Q-T intervals have LQTS, and patients with normal Q-T intervals on a resting electrocardiogram may have LQTS. A heart rate–corrected Q-T interval of >0.47 sec is highly indicative, whereas a Q-T interval of >0.44 sec is suggestive. Other features include notched T waves, T wave alternans, a low heart rate for age, a history of syncope (especially with stress), and a familial history of either LQTS or unexplained sudden death. Twenty-four hour Holter monitoring and exercise testing are adjuncts to the diagnosis.

Treatment of LQTS includes the use of **β-blocking agents** at doses that blunt the heart rate response to exercise. Some patients require a **pacemaker** because of drug-induced profound bradycardia. In patients with continued syncope despite treatment, an implantable cardiac defibrillator is indicated for those who do not respond to β-blocking drugs and those who have experienced cardiac arrest.

435.6 • Sinus Node Dysfunction

Sinus arrest and **sinoatrial block** may cause a sudden pause in the heartbeat. The former is presumably caused by failure of impulse formation within the sinus node and the latter by a block between the sinus impulse and the surrounding atrium. These arrhythmias are rare in childhood except as manifestations of digitalis intoxication or in patients who have had extensive atrial surgery.

Sick sinus syndrome is the result of abnormalities in the sinus node or atrial conduction pathways, or both. This syndrome may occur in the absence of congenital heart disease and has been reported in siblings, but it is most commonly seen after surgical correction of congenital heart defects, especially the atrial switch (Mustard or Senning) operation for transposition of the great arteries. Clinical manifestations depend on the heart rate. Most patients remain asymptomatic without treatment, but dizziness and syncope can occur during periods of marked sinus slowing with failure of junctional escape (Fig. 435-9). Pacemaker therapy is indicated in patients who experience symptoms.

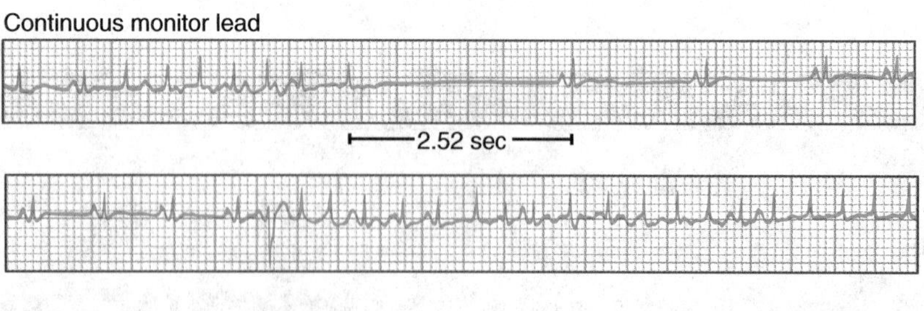

Figure 435-9. Complete atrioventricular (AV) block. The ventricular rate is regular at 53 beats/min. The atrial rate varied from 65 to 95 beats/min. The QRS morphology is normal, which is usual in congenital AV block.

Patients with sinus node dysfunction may also have episodes of SVT (**bradycardia-tachycardia syndrome**) with symptoms of palpitations, exercise intolerance, or dizziness. Treatment must be individualized. Drug therapy to control tachyarrhythmias (propranolol, quinidine, procainamide) may suppress sinus and AV node function to such a degree that further symptomatic bradycardia may be produced. Therefore, insertion of a pacemaker in conjunction with drug therapy is usually necessary for symptomatic patients.

435.7 • AV Block

AV block may be divided into three forms. In **1st-degree block,** the P-R interval is prolonged, but all the atrial impulses are conducted to the ventricle. In **2nd-degree block,** some impulses are not conducted to the ventricle. In one variant of 2nd-degree block known as the **Wenckebach type** (also called **Mobitz type I**), the P-P interval remains constant and the P-R interval increases progressively until a P wave is not conducted. In the cycle following the dropped beat, the P-R interval is again shorter (Fig. 435-10). In **Mobitz type II,** the P-R interval does not change, but an occasional atrial beat does not conduct to the ventricle. This conduction defect is uncommon but has more potential to cause syncope and may be progressive. In **3rd-degree block (complete heart block),** no impulses from the atria reach the ventricles.

Congenital complete AV block in children is most often caused by autoimmune injury of the fetal conduction system by maternally derived IgG antibodies (anti-SSA/Ro, anti-SSB/La) in a mother with overt or, more often, asymptomatic SLE or Sjögren syndrome. Autoimmune disease accounts for 60–70% of all cases of congenital complete heart block and ≈80% of cases in which the heart is structurally normal. Complete heart block is also seen in patients with complex congenital heart disease and abnormal embryonic development of the conduction system. It has been associated with myocardial tumors and myocarditis. It is a known complication of myocardial abscess secondary to endocarditis. It is also seen in genetic abnormalities including LQTS and Kearn-Sayre syndrome. It is also a complication of congenital heart disease repair.

The incidence of congenital complete heart block is 1/20,000–25,000 live births; a high fetal loss rate may cause an underestimation of its true incidence. In some infants of mothers with SLE, complete heart block is not present at birth but develops within the 1st 3–6 mo after birth. The arrhythmia is often diagnosed in the fetus (secondary to the dissociation between atrial and ventricular contractions seen on fetal echocardiography) and may produce hydrops fetalis. Infants with associated congenital heart disease and heart failure have a high mortality rate.

In older children with otherwise normal hearts, the condition is commonly asymptomatic, although syncope and sudden death may occur. Infants and toddlers may have night terrors, tiredness with frequent naps, and irritability. The peripheral pulse is prominent as a result of the compensatory large ventricular stroke volume and peripheral vasodilation; systolic blood pressure is elevated. Jugular venous pulsations occur irregularly and may be large when the atrium contracts against a closed tricuspid valve (cannon wave). Exercise and atropine may produce an acceleration of ≥10–20 beats/min. Systolic murmurs are frequently audible along the left sternal border, and apical mid-diastolic murmurs are not unusual. Heart block results in enlargement of the heart on the basis of increased diastolic ventricular filling.

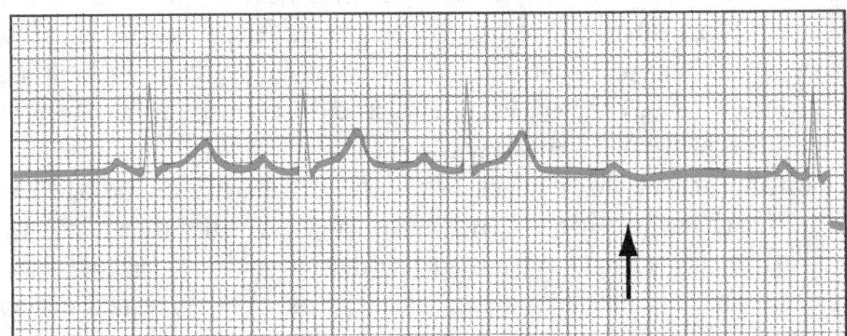

Figure 435-10. Sick sinus syndrome with bradytachycardia. Note the bursts of supraventricular tachycardia, probably multifocal in origin, followed by long periods of sinus arrest and by sinus bradycardia.

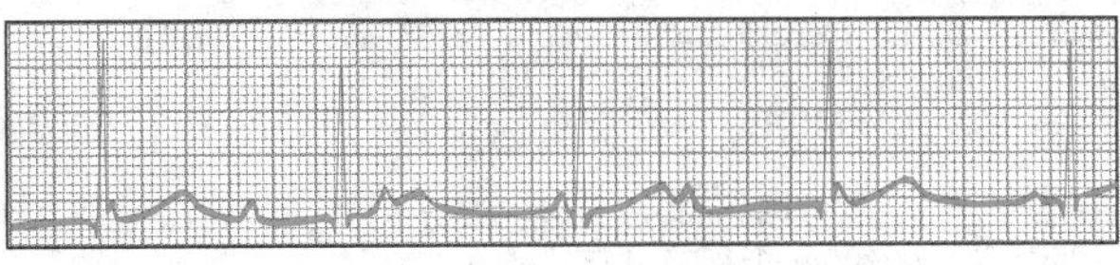

Figure 435-11. Wenckebach phenomenon (Mobitz I). The P-R interval gradually lengthens until the 4th P wave in the cycle is not conducted to the ventricle *(arrow)*. The ensuing P-R interval is once again normal.

The **diagnosis** is confirmed by electrocardiography; the P waves and QRS complexes have no constant relationship (Fig. 435-11). The QRS duration may be prolonged, or it may be normal if the heartbeat is initiated high in the AV node or bundle of His.

The **prognosis** for congenital complete heart block is usually favorable; patients who have been observed to the age of 30–40 yr have lived normal, active lives. Some patients have episodes of exercise intolerance, dizziness, and syncope (Stokes-Adams attacks); this symptom requires the implantation of a permanent cardiac pacemaker. Pacemaker implantation should be considered for patients who develop symptoms such as progressive cardiac enlargement, prolonged pauses, or awake heart rates of ≤40 beats/min.

Cardiac pacing is recommended in neonates with low ventricular rates (≤50 beats/min), evidence of heart failure, wide complex rhythms, or congenital heart disease. Isoproterenol, atropine, or epinephrine may be used to try to increase the heart rate temporarily until pacemaker placement can be arranged. Transthoracic epicardial pacemaker implants have traditionally been used in infants; transvenous placement of pacemaker leads is available for young children.

Postsurgical complete AV block can occur after any open heart procedure requiring suturing near the AV valves or crest of the ventricular septum. Postoperative heart block is initially managed with temporary pacing wires. The likelihood of a return to sinus rhythm after 10–14 days is low; a permanent pacemaker is recommended after that time.

Ackerman MJ: Molecular basis of congenital and acquired long QT syndromes. *J Electrocardiol* 2004;37(Suppl):1–6.

Bar-Cohen Y, Walsh EP, Love BA, Cecchin F: First appropriate use of automated external difibrillator in an infant. *Resuscitation* 2005;67:135–137.

Benson DW Jr, Smith WM, Dunnigan A, et al: Mechanisms of regular, wide QRS tachycardia in infants and children. *Am J Cardiol* 1982;49:1778–1788.

Buyon JP, Friedman DM: Autobody associated congenital heart block: The clinical perspective. *Curr Rheumatol Rep* 2003;5:374–378.

Chun TU, Van Hare GF: Advances in the approach to treatment of supraventricular tachycardia in the pediatric population. *Curr Cardiol Rev* 2004;6:322–326.

Delacrètaz E: Superventricular tachycardia. *N Engl J Med* 2006;354: 1039–1050.

Dunnigan A, Benson DW Jr, Banditt DG: Atrial flutter in infancy: Diagnosis, clinical features, and treatment. *Pediatrics* 1985;75:725–729.

Eronen M, Siren MK, Ekblad H, et al: Short- and long-term outcome of children with congenital complete heart block diagnosed in utero as a newborn. *Pediatrics* 2000;106:86–91.

Esberger D, Jones S, Morris F, et al: Junctional tachycardias. *Br Med J* 2002; 324:662–665.

Goldberger Z, Lampert R: Implantable cardioverter-defibrillators. *JAMA* 2006;295:809–818.
Goodacre S, McLeod K: Paediatric electrocardiography. *Br Med J* 2002;324:1382–1385.
Kaultman H, Shah M: Evaluation of the child with an arrhythmia. *Pediatr Clin North Am* 2004;51:1537–1551.
Kirk CR, Gibbs JL, Thomas R: Cardiovascular collapse after verapamil in supraventricular tachycardia. *Arch Dis Child* 1987;62:1265–1266.
Miller MD, Porter CJ, Ackerman MJ: Diagnostic accuracy of screening electrocardiograms in long QT syndrome I. *Pediatrics* 2001;108:8–12.
Perry JC, Garson A Jr: Supraventricular tachycardia due to Wolff-Parkinson-White syndrome in children: Early disappearance and late recurrence. *J Am Coll Cardiol* 1990;16:1215–1220.
Roden DM: Drug-induced prolongation of the QT interval. *N Engl J Med* 2004;350:1013–1022.
Trohman RG, Kim MH, Pinski SL: Cardiac pacing: The state of the art. *Lancet* 2004;364:1701–1718.
Van Hare GF, Dubin AM, Collins KK: Invasive electrophysiology in children: State of the art. *J Electrocardiol* 2002;35(Suppl):165–174.
Walsh EP, Cecchin F: Recent advances in pacemaker and implantable defibrillator therapy for young patients. *Curr Opin Cardiol* 2004;19:91–96.
Wellens HJJ: Catheter ablation for cardiac arrhythmias. *N Engl J Med* 2004;351:1172–1174.

Chapter 436 ■ Sudden Death

Sudden death other than sudden infant death syndrome (SIDS; see Chapter 372) is rare in children younger than 18 yr. Sudden death can be divided into either traumatic or nontraumatic origin. Traumatic causes of sudden death are the most common in children; these include motor vehicle crashes, violent deaths, recreational deaths, and occupational deaths. Nontraumatic sudden deaths are often due to specific cardiac causes. The incidence of sudden death varies from 0.8 to 6.2 per 100,000 per year in children and adolescents as opposed to the higher incidence of sudden cardiac death in adults of 1 per 1,000. Approximately 65% of sudden deaths are due to heart-related problems in patients with either normal or congenitally (corrected, palliated, or unoperated) abnormal hearts. Competitive high-school sports (basketball, football) are high-risk environmental factors. The most common cause of death in competitive athletes is hypertrophic cardiomyopathy. Other potential causes are listed in Table 436-1. These can be classified as structural abnormalities, including aortic stenosis and coronary artery abnormalities; myocardial disease, such as myocarditis; conduction system disease, including long QT syndrome (LQTS); and miscellaneous causes, including pulmonary hypertension and commotio cordis. Symptoms may be absent before the event but, if present, include syncope, chest pain, dyspnea, and palpitations. Patients may have a family history of heart disease (dilated or hypertrophic cardiomyopathy, long Q-T interval, right ventricular dysplasia, mitral valve prolapse, Marfan syndrome) or sudden death. Death often follows exertion or exercise.

MECHANISM OF SUDDEN DEATH

There are three mechanisms of sudden death: arrhythmic, nonarrhythmic cardiac (circulatory and vascular causes), and noncardiac. Ventricular fibrillation (VF), while the most common final cause of sudden death in adults, is only the final cause in 10–20% of children with sudden cardiac death. More commonly, bradycardia leads either to VF or asystole (see Chapter 435).

TABLE 436-1. Potential Causes of Sudden Death in Infants, Children, and Adolescents

SIDS AND SIDS "MIMICS"
SIDS
Long Q-T syndromes*
Inborn errors of metabolism
Child abuse
Myocarditis
Duct-dependent congenital heart disease
CORRECTED OR UNOPERATED CONGENITAL HEART DISEASE
Aortic stenosis
Tetralogy of Fallot
Transposition of great vessels (postoperative atrial switch)
Mitral valve prolapse
Hypoplastic left heart syndrome
Eisenmenger syndrome
CORONARY ARTERIAL DISEASE
Anomalous origin*
Anomalous tract (tunneled)
Kawasaki disease
Periarteritis
Arterial dissection
Marfan syndrome (rupture of aorta)
Myocardial infarction
MYOCARDIAL DISEASE
Myocarditis
Hypertrophic cardiomyopathy*
Dilated cardiomyopathy
Arrhythmogenic right ventricular dysplasia
CONDUCTION SYSTEM ABNORMALITY/ARRHYTHMIA
Long Q-T syndromes*
Brugada syndrome
Proarrhythmic drugs
Pre-excitation syndromes
Heart block
Commotio cordis
Idiopathic ventricular fibrillation
Arrhythmogenic right ventricular dysplasia
Heart tumor
MISCELLANEOUS
Pulmonary hypertension
Pulmonary embolism
Heat stroke
Cocaine
Anorexia nervosa
Electrolyte disturbances

*common.
SIDS, sudden infant death syndrome.

CONGENITAL HEART DISEASE

Valvar aortic stenosis is the congenital defect most commonly associated with sudden death in children. Approximately 5% of children with this disease die. A history of syncope, chest pain, and evidence of severe obstruction and left ventricular hypertrophy are risk factors (see Chapter 427.5).

Coronary artery anomalies are also commonly associated with sudden death in children and adolescents. The most common abnormality associated with sudden death is the origin of the left main coronary artery from the right sinus of Valsava. The coronary artery therefore courses between the aorta and pulmonary artery. Exercise results in a rise in pulmonary and aortic pressure, which compresses the left main coronary artery and results in ischemia.

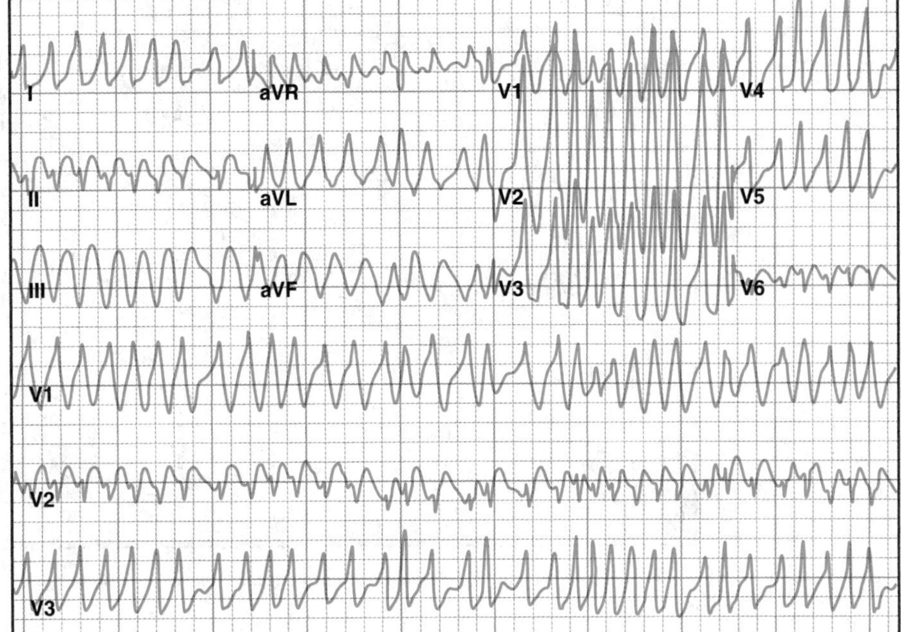

Figure 436-1. Atrial fibrillation in a patient with Wolff-Parkinson-White (WPW) syndrome and rapid conduction to the ventricle. Note the irregularly irregular rhythm.

CARDIOMYOPATHY

All three major types of cardiomyopathies (hypertrophic, dilated, and restrictive) are associated with sudden death in the pediatric population; sudden death may be the initial manifestation of the cardiomyopathy (see Chapter 439).

Hypertrophic cardiomyopathy (HCM) is the most common cause of sudden death in the athletic adolescent. The annual risk of sudden death in young patients with HCM is 2% per year. Risk factors for sudden death include a family history of sudden death, symptoms, ventricular arrhythmias, and presentation at an early age. Many patients with HCM have obstruction to the left ventricular outflow tract. The mechanism of sudden death may be secondary to development of dynamic obstruction with exercise and resultant loss of cardiac output, or may be related to cardiac ischemia.

Dilated cardiomyopathies are also associated with sudden cardiac death. Arrhythmogenic right ventricular dysplasia (ARVD) is a specific form of dilated cardiomyopathy associated with exercise-induced ventricular arrhythmias and sudden death. The diagnosis can be difficult; MRI or endomyocardial biopsy is used with limited reliability. Pathology includes fatty replacement of right ventricular myocytes, with patchy areas of fibrosis.

Myocarditis has been found on pathology in as high as 42% of patients with sudden death. Symptoms are far ranging and can include overt heart failure to subtle findings such as a high heart rate. Pediatric patients may have complete heart block or ventricular arrhythmias with this disease.

CARDIAC ARRHYTHMIA

A primary conduction system disease may result in sudden death. Causes include Wolff-Parkinson-White (WPW) syndrome and long Q-T syndrome. Besides causing supraventricular tachycardia (SVT), WPW syndrome can result in atrial fibrillation with rapid conduction across the accessory pathway leading to ventricular fibrillation and sudden death (Fig. 436-1) [see Chapter 435]. This, however, is extremely rare in pediatric patients, with an incidence of sudden death in asymptomatic patients of 1 per 1,000 patient-years. As digoxin and verapamil can augment conduction across accessory pathways, these drugs are contraindicated in WPW syndrome.

Long Q-T syndrome (see Chapter 435), a group of channelopathies that affect ventricular repolarization, is also associated with sudden death (Fig. 436-2). The mechanism of sudden death is polymorphic VT (torsades de pointes) [Fig. 436-3]. An initial presentation of sudden cardiac death is found in 9% of patients. Thus, treatment of asymptomatic patients with a long Q-T interval on electrocardiogram (ECG) and positive family history is advised.

Acquired long Q-T intervals may be seen in patients with marked electrolyte abnormalities, CNS injury, or starvation (including bulimia and anorexia nervosa). Medications can also result in prolongation of the Q-T interval. These patients are also at risk of malignant ventricular arrhythmias, and correction of the underlying problem may be necessary to reduce the risk of sudden death.

MISCELLANEOUS CAUSES

Commotio cordis is a nearly universally fatal condition that follows blunt nonpenetrating trauma to the chest (e.g., from a baseball or hockey puck). Occasionally, innocent-appearing chest blows incurred at home or at a playground may be fatal. Patients experience immediate ventricular fibrillation in the absence of identifiable cardiac trauma (contusion, hematoma, lacerated coronary artery). Death results from ventricular fibrillation that is unresponsive to all resuscitative efforts in 85–90% of children.

EVALUATION AND THERAPY FOR RESUSCITATED PATIENTS

It is important to focus therapy on potentially reversible causes of sudden death. These include correction of major hemodynamic defects, pacing therapy for a patient with bradycardia, or supportive therapy for myocarditis. Unfortunately, reversible causes are rarely found in young cardiac arrest survivors. Added to this dilemma is the fact that there is a limited ability to predict antiar-

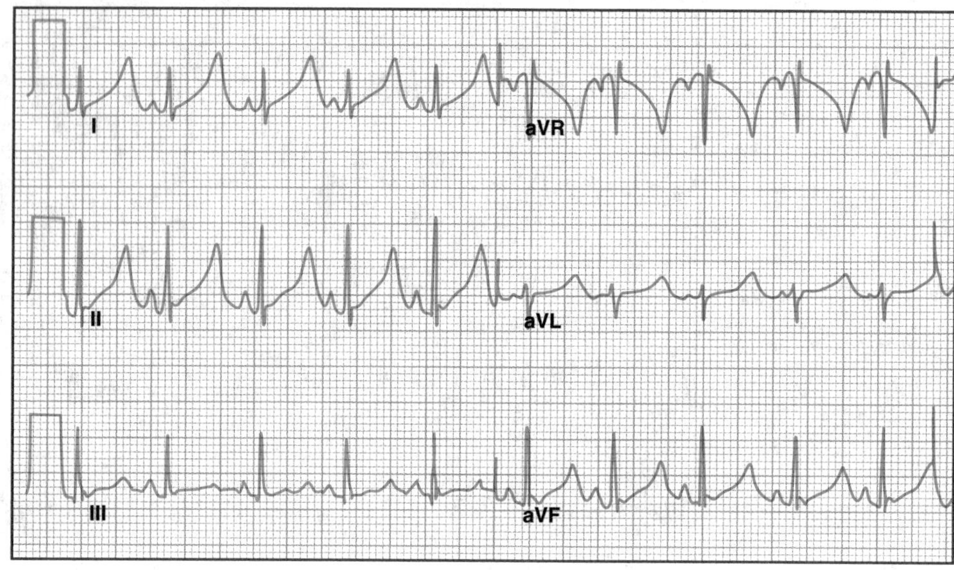

Figure 436-2. Long Q-T syndrome in a neonate. QTc is markedly prolonged. T waves are also peaked.

rhythmic drug response or risk of recurrence. Thus, the implantable cardioverter defibrillator has become the **therapy of choice** for survivors of arrhythmic sudden death.

PREVENTION OF SUDDEN DEATH

The probability of survival to hospital discharge for a young patient who experiences an out-of-hospital cardiac arrest is <20%. The presence of immediate portable external defibrillators, when combined with standard cardiopulmonary resuscitation at the site of exercise (gym, track, basketball, or football arena), may improve survival substantially. Thus, identifying patients at risk is extremely important.

Many of the more common causes of sudden death in children and adolescents can be identified from the patient's history (prodromal symptoms), the family history, and physical examination.

Patient avoidance of high-risk behavior (cocaine use, anorexia nervosa) and acquisition of knowledge of drug side effects (tricyclic antidepressants) or drug interactions (terfenadine [Seldane] and erythromycin) is critical. Chest-protecting equipment may not prevent commotio cordis. Prompt cardiopulmonary resuscitation and rapid defibrillation by an automatic external defibrillator or by an emergency medical services rescue team improves survival. Family survivors of victims of sudden death should be evaluated for genetic causes such as LQTS and hypertrophic cardiomyopathy.

Atkins DL, Kenney MA: Automated external defibrillators: Safety and efficacy in children and adolescents. *Pediatr Clin North Am* 2004;51:1443–1462.

Bar-Cohen Y, Walsh EP, Love BA, Cecchin F: First appropriate use of automated external defibrillator in an infant. *Resuscitation* 2005;67:135–137.

Behr E, Wood DA, Wright M, et al: Cardiological assessment of first-degree relatives in sudden arrhythmic death syndrome. *Lancet* 2003; 362:1457–1459.

Chun TU, Collins KK, Dubin AM: Implantable cardioverter defibrillators in children. *Expert Rev Cardiovasc Ther* 2004;2:561–571.

Doolan A, Langlois N, Semsarian C: Causes of sudden cardiac death in young Australians. *Med J Aust* 2004;180:110–112.

Geddes LA, Roeder RA: Evolution of our knowledge of sudden death due to commotio cordis. *Am J Emerg Med* 2005;23:67–75.

Gemayel C, Pelliccia A, Thompson PD: Arrhythmogenic right ventricular cardiomyopathy. *J Am Coll Cardiol* 2001;38:1773–1781.

Kumpf M, Sieverding L, Gass M, et al: Anomalous origin of left coronary artery in young athletes with syncope. *BMJ* 2006;332:1139–1141.

Kusumoto FM, Goldschlager N: Device therapy for cardiac arrhythmias. *JAMA* 2002;287:1848–1852.

Lee A, Ackerman MJ: Sudden unexplained death: Evaluation of those left behind. *Lancet* 2003;362:1429–1430.

Maron BJ: Sudden death in young athletes. *New Eng J Med* 2003;349:404–10.

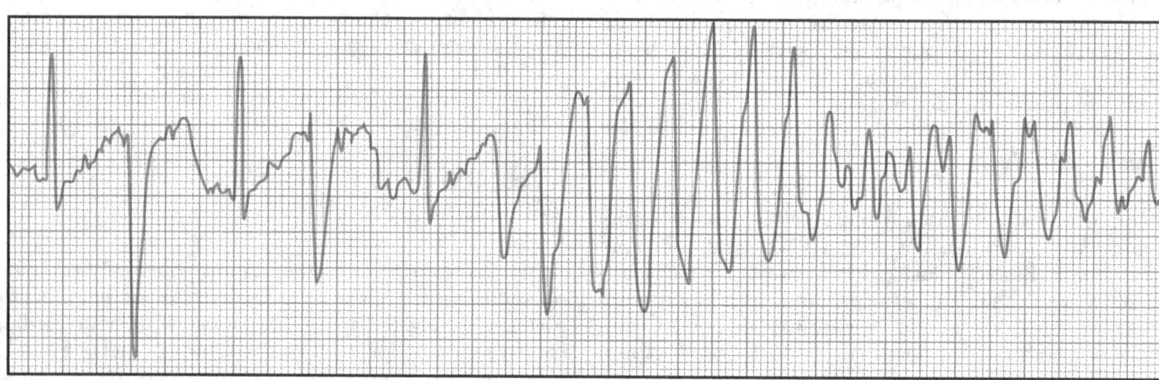

Figure 436-3. Episode of torsades de pointes in a patient with long Q-T syndrome.

Maron BJ, Gohman TE, Kyle SB, et al: Clinical profile and spectrum of commotio cordis. *JAMA* 2002;287:1142–1146.

Plunkett A, Hulse JA, Gill MJ: Variable presentation of Brugada syndrome: Lesions from three generations with syncope. *Br Med J* 2003; 326:1078–1079.

Shaddy RA: Cardiomyopathies in adolescents: Dilated, hypertrophic and restrictive. *Adolesc Med* 2001;12:35–45.

Thompson PD, Levine BD: Protecting athletes from sudden cardiac death. *JAMA* 2006;296:1648–1650.

Towbin JA: Molecular genetic basis of sudden cardiac death. *Pediatr Clin North Am* 2004;51:1229–1255.

Weinstock J, Maron BJ, Song C, et al: Failure of commercially available chest wall protectors to prevent sudden cardiac death induced by chest wall blows in an experimental model of commotio cordis. *Pediatrics* 2006; 117:e656–e662.

Williams RG, Chen AY: Identifying athletes at risk for sudden death. *J Am Coll Cardiol* 2003;42:1964–66.

Wren C: Sudden death in children and adolescents. *Heart* 2002;88:426–431.

Section 5 — Acquired Heart Disease — Daniel Bernstein

Chapter 437 ■ Infective Endocarditis

Infective endocarditis includes acute and subacute bacterial endocarditis, as well as nonbacterial endocarditis caused by viruses, fungi, and other microbiologic agents. It is a significant cause of morbidity and mortality in children and adolescents despite advances in the management and prophylaxis of the disease with antimicrobial agents. The inability to eradicate infective endocarditis by prevention or early treatment stems from several factors. The nature of the infecting organism may change; physicians, dentists, and the public are not sufficiently aware of the risk of infective endocarditis and the preventive measures available; diagnosis may be difficult when delayed; and special risk groups have emerged, including intravenous drug users, survivors of cardiac surgery, patients taking immunosuppressant medications, and patients who require chronic intravascular catheters. Many patients get endocarditis on what was thought to be a previously healthy native valve. Furthermore, endocarditis from oral flora may occur without a preceding dental procedure.

ETIOLOGY. Viridans-type streptococci (α-hemolytic streptococci) and *Staphylococcus aureus* are the leading causative agents for endocarditis in pediatric patients. Other organisms cause endocarditis less frequently and, in ≈6% of cases, blood cultures are negative for any organisms (Table 437-1). Many patients with culture-negative endocarditis have Q fever *(Coxiella burnetii)* or *Bartonella* species. No relationship exists between the infecting organism and the type of congenital defect, the duration of illness, or the age of the child. Staphylococcal endocarditis is more common in patients with no underlying heart disease; viridans group streptococcal infection is more common after dental procedures; group D enterococci are seen more often after lower bowel or genitourinary manipulation; *Pseudomonas aeruginosa* or *Serratia marcescens* is seen more frequently in intravenous drug users; and fungal organisms are encountered after open heart surgery. Coagulase-negative staphylococci are common in the presence of an indwelling central venous catheter.

TABLE 437-1. Bacterial Agents in Pediatric Infective Endocarditis

COMMON: NATIVE VALVE OR OTHER CARDIAC LESIONS
Viridans group streptococci (*S. mutans, S. sanguis, S. mitis*)
Staphylococcus aureus
Group D streptococcus (enterococcus) (*S. bovis, S. faecalis*)

UNCOMMON: NATIVE VALVE OR OTHER CARDIAC LESIONS
Streptococcus pneumoniae
Haemophilus influenzae
Coagulage-negative staphylococci
Coxiella burnetii (Q fever)*
Neisseria gonorrhoeae
*Brucella**
*Chlamydia psittaci**
*Chlamydia trachomatis**
*Chlamydia pneumoniae**
*Legionella**
*Bartonella**
HACEK group†
*Streptobacillus moniliformis**
*Pasteurella multocida**
Campylobacter fetus
Culture negative (6% of cases)

PROSTHETIC VALVE
Staphylococcus epidermidis
Staphylococcus aureus
Viridans group streptococcus
Pseudomonas aeruginosa
Serratia marcescens
Diphtheroids
Legionella species*
HACEK group†
Fungi‡

*These fastidious bacteria plus some fungi may produce culture-negative endocarditis. Detection may require special media, incubation for more than 7 days, or serologic tests.
†The HACEK group includes *Haemophilus* species (*H. paraphrophilus, H. parainfluenzae, H. aphrophilus*), *Actinobacillus actinomycetemcomitans, Cardiobacterium hominis, Eikenella corrodens,* and *Kingella species.*
‡*Candida* species, *Aspergillus* species, *Pseudallescheria boydii, Histoplasma capsulatum.*

EPIDEMIOLOGY. Infective endocarditis is often a complication of congenital or rheumatic heart disease but can also occur in children without any abnormal valves or cardiac malformations. In developed countries, congenital heart disease is the overwhelming predisposing factor. Endocarditis is rare in infancy; in this age group, it usually follows open heart surgery or is associated with a central venous line.

Patients with congenital heart lesions in which blood is ejected at high velocity through a hole or stenotic orifice are most susceptible to endocarditis. Vegetations usually form at the site of the endocardial or intimal erosion that results from the turbulent flow. Children with ventricular septal defects (VSDs), left-sided valvular disease such as aortic stenosis, tetralogy of Fallot, and systemic-pulmonary arterial communications (patent ductus arteriosus or Blalock-Taussig shunts) are at highest risk. In older patients, congenital bicuspid aortic valves and mitral valve prolapse with regurgitation pose additional risks for endocarditis. Surgical correction of congenital heart disease may reduce but does not eliminate the risk of endocarditis, with the exception of repair of a simple atrial septal defect or patent ductus arteriosus.

Children who have undergone valve replacement or valved conduit repair are also at high risk.

In ≈30% of patients with infective endocarditis, a predisposing factor is recognized. A surgical or dental procedure can be implicated in ≈65% of cases in which the potential source of bacteremia is identified. Poor dental hygiene in children with cyanotic heart disease results in a greater risk for endocarditis. Primary bacteremia with *Staphylococcus aureus* is another risk for endocarditis (10% risk). The occurrence of endocarditis directly after heart surgery is relatively low, but it is frequently an antecedent event.

CLINICAL MANIFESTATIONS (TABLE 437-2). Early manifestations are usually mild, especially when viridans group streptococci are the infecting organisms. Prolonged fever without other manifestations (except, occasionally, weight loss) that persists for as long as several months may be the only symptom. Alternatively, the onset may be acute and severe, with high, intermittent fever and prostration. Usually, the onset and course vary between these two extremes. The symptoms are often nonspecific and consist of low-grade fever with afternoon elevations, fatigue, myalgia, arthralgia, headache, and, at times, chills, nausea, and vomiting. **New or changing heart murmurs** are common, particularly with associated heart failure. Splenomegaly and petechiae are relatively common. Serious neurologic complications such as embolic strokes, cerebral abscesses, mycotic aneurysms, and hemorrhage are most often associated with staphylococcal disease and may be late manifestations. Meningismus, increased intracranial pressure, altered sensorium, and focal neurologic signs are manifestations of these complications. Myocardial abscesses may occur with staphylococcal disease and may damage the cardiac conducting system, causing heart block, or may rupture into the pericardium and produce purulent pericarditis. Pulmonary and other systemic emboli are infrequent, except with fungal disease. Many of the classic skin findings develop late in the course of the disease; they are seldom seen in appropriately treated patients. Such manifestations include **Osler nodes** (tender, pea-sized intradermal nodules in the pads of the fingers and toes), **Janeway lesions** (painless small erythematous or hemorrhagic lesions on the palms and soles), and **splinter hemorrhages** (linear lesions beneath the nails). These lesions may represent vasculitis produced by circulating antigen-antibody complexes.

Identification of infective endocarditis is most often based on a high index of suspicion during evaluation of an infection in a child with an underlying contributory factor.

TABLE 437-2. Manifestations of Infective Endocarditis

HISTORY
Prior congenital or rheumatic heart disease
Preceding dental, urinary tract, or intestinal procedure
Intravenous drug use
Central venous catheter
Prosthetic heart valve
SYMPTOMS
Fever
Chills
Chest and abdominal pain
Arthralgia, myalgia
Dyspnea
Malaise
Night sweats
Weight loss
CNS manifestations (stroke, seizures, headache)
SIGNS
Elevated temperature
Tachycardia
Embolic phenomena (Roth spots, petechiae, splinter nail bed hemorrhages, Osler nodes, CNS or ocular lesions)
Janeway lesions
New or changing murmur
Splenomegaly
Arthritis
Heart failure
Arrhythmias
Metastatic infection (arthritis, meningitis, mycotic arterial aneurysm, pericarditis, abscesses, septic pulmonary emboli)
Clubbing
LABORATORY
Positive blood culture
Elevated erythrocyte sedimentation rate; may be low with heart or renal failure
Elevated C-reactive protein
Anemia
Leukocytosis
Immune complexes
Hypergammaglobulinemia
Hypocomplementemia
Cryoglobulinemia
Rheumatoid factor
Hematuria
Renal failure: azotemia, high creatinine (glomerulonephritis)
Chest radiograph: bilateral infiltrates, nodules, pleural effusions
Echocardiographic evidence of valve vegetations, prosthetic valve dysfunction or leak, myocardial abscess, new-onset valve insufficiency

CNS, central nervous system.

TABLE 437-3. Diagnostic Approach to Uncommon Pathogens Causing Endocarditis

PATHOGEN	DIAGNOSTIC PROCEDURE
Brucella spp	Blood cultures; serology; culture, immunohistology, and PCR of surgical material
C burnetti	Serology (IgG phase I > 1 in 800); tissue culture, immunohistology, and PCR of surgical material
Bartonella spp	Blood cultures; serology; culture, immunohistology, and PCR of surgical material
Chlamydia spp	Serology; culture, immunohistology, and PCR of surgical material
Mycoplasma spp	Serology; culture, immunohistology, and PCR of surgical material
Legionella spp	Blood cultures; serology; culture, immunohistology, and PCR of surgical material
T whipplei	Histology and PCR of surgical material

PCR, polymerase chain reaction.
From Moreillon P, Que YA: Infective endocarditis. *Lancet* 2004;363:139–148.

DIAGNOSIS. The critical information for appropriate treatment of infective endocarditis is obtained from blood cultures. All other laboratory data are secondary in importance (see Table 437-2). Blood specimens for culture should be obtained as promptly as possible, even if the child feels well and has no other physical findings. Three to five separate blood collections should be obtained after careful preparation of the phlebotomy site. Contamination presents a special problem inasmuch as bacteria found on the skin may themselves cause infective endocarditis. The timing of collections is not important because bacteremia can be expected to be relatively constant. In 90% of cases of endocarditis, the causative agent is recovered from the 1st two blood cultures. The laboratory should be notified that endocarditis is suspected so that, if necessary, the blood can be cultured on enriched media for longer than usual (>7 days) to detect nutritionally deficient and fastidious bacteria or fungi. Antimicrobial pretreatment of the patient reduces the yield of blood cultures to 50–60%. The microbiology laboratory should be notified if the patient has received antibiotics so that more sophisticated methods can be used to recover the offending agent. Other specimens that may be cultured include scrapings from cutaneous lesions, urine, synovial fluid, abscesses, and, in the presence of manifestations of meningitis, cerebrospinal fluid. Serologic diagnosis is necessary in patients with unusual or fastidious microorganisms (Table 437-3).

TABLE 437-4. Therapy of Native Valve Endocarditis Caused by Highly Penicillin-Susceptible Viridans Group Streptococci and *Streptococcus bovis*

REGIMEN	DOSAGE* AND ROUTE	DURATION, WK	COMMENTS
Aqueous crystalline penicillin G sodium	12–18 million U/24 h IV either continuously or in 4 or 6 equally divided doses	4	Preferred in patients with impairment of 8th cranial nerve function or renal function
or			
Ceftriaxone sodium	2 g/24 h IV/IM in 1 dose ***Pediatric dose***[†]**:** penicillin 200,000 U/kg per 24 h IV in 4–6 equally divided doses; ceftriaxone 100 mg/kg per 24 h IV/IM in 1 dose	4	
Aqueous crystalline penicillin G sodium	12–18 million U/24 h IV either continuously or in 6 equally divided doses	2	2 wk regimen not intended for patients with known cardiac or extracardiac abscess or for those with creatinine clearance of <20 mL/min, impaired 8th cranial nerve function, or *Abiotrophia, Granulicatella,* or *Gemella* spp infection; gentamicin dosage should be adjusted to achieve peak serum concentration of 3–4 μg/mL and trough serum concentration of <1 μg/mL when 3 divided doses are used; nomogram used for single daily dosing
or			
Ceftriaxone sodium	2 g/24 h IV/IM in 1 dose	2	
plus			
Gentamicin sulfate[‡]	3 mg/kg per 24 h IV/IM in 1 dose, or 3 equally divided doses ***Pediatric dose:*** penicillin 200,000 U/kg per 24 h IV in 4–6 equally divided doses; ceftriaxone 100 mg/kg per 24 h IV/IM in 1 dose; gentamicin 3 mg/kg per 24 h IV/IM in 1 dose or 3 equally divided doses[‖]	2	
Vancomycin hydrochloride[¶]	30 mg/kg per 24 h IV in 2 equally divided doses not to exceed 2 g/24 h unless concentrations in serum are inappropriately low ***Pediatric dose:*** 40 mg/kg per 24 h IV in 2–3 equally divided doses	4	Vancomycin therapy recommended only for patients unable to tolerate penicillin or ceftriaxone; vancomycin dosage should be adjusted to obtain peak (1 h after infusion completed) serum concentration of 30–45 μg/mL and a trough concentration range of 10–15 μg/mL

Minimum inhibitory concentration ≤0.12 μg/mL.
*Dosages recommended are for patients with normal renal function.
[†]Pediatric dose should not exceed that of a normal adult.
[‡]Other potentially nephrotoxic drugs (e.g., nonsteroidal antiinflammatory drugs) should be used with caution in patients receiving gentamicin therapy.
[‖]Data for once-daily dosing of aminoglycosides for children exist, but no data for treatment of infective endocarditis exist.
[¶]Vancomycin dosages should be infused during course of at least 1 h to reduce risk of histamine-release "red man" syndrome.
From Baddour LM, Wilson WR, Bayer AS, et al: Infective endocarditis: Diagnosis, antimicrobial therapy, and management of complications. *Circulation* 2005;111:e394–e433 and correction *Circulation* 2005;112:2373.

The index of suspicion should be high when evaluating infection in a child with an underlying contributing factor. The combination of transthoracic and transesophageal echocardiography enhances the ability to diagnose endocarditis. Two-dimensional echocardiography can identify the size, shape, location, and mobility of the lesion; when combined with Doppler studies, the presence of valve dysfunction (regurgitation, obstruction) can be determined and its effect on left ventricular performance quantified. Echocardiography may also be helpful in predicting embolic complications, given that lesions >1 cm and fungating masses are at greatest risk for embolization. The absence of vegetations does not exclude endocarditis, and vegetations are often not visualized in the early phases of the disease or in patients with complex congenital heart lesions.

The **Duke criteria** help in the diagnosis of endocarditis. **Major criteria** include (1) positive blood cultures (two separate cultures for a usual pathogen, two or more for less typical pathogens) and (2) evidence of endocarditis on echocardiography (intracardiac mass on a valve or other site, regurgitant flow near a prosthesis, abscess, partial dehiscence of prosthetic valves, or new valve regurgitant flow). **Minor criteria** include predisposing conditions, fever, embolic-vascular signs, immune complex phenomena (glomerulonephritis, arthritis, rheumatoid factor, Osler nodes, Roth spots), a single positive blood culture or serologic evidence of infection, and echocardiographic signs not meeting the major criteria. Two major criteria, one major and three minor, or five minor criteria suggest definite endocarditis. A modification of the Duke criteria may increase sensitivity while maintaining specificity. The following minor criteria are added to those already listed: the presence of newly diagnosed clubbing, splenomegaly, splinter hemorrhages, and petechiae; a high erythrocyte sedimentation rate; a high C-reactive protein level; and the presence of central nonfeeding lines, peripheral lines, and microscopic hematuria.

PROGNOSIS AND COMPLICATIONS. In the pre-antibiotic era, infective endocarditis was a fatal disease. Despite the use of antibiotic agents, mortality remains at 20–25%. Serious morbidity occurs in 50–60% of children with documented infective endocarditis; the most common is heart failure caused by vegetations involving the aortic or mitral valve. Myocardial abscesses and toxic myocarditis may also lead to heart failure without characteristic changes in auscultatory findings and, occasionally, to life-threatening arrhythmias. Systemic emboli, often with central nervous system manifestations, are a major threat. Pulmonary emboli may occur in children with VSD or the tetralogy of Fallot, although massive life-threatening pulmonary embolization is rare. Other complications include mycotic aneurysms, rupture of a sinus of Valsalva, obstruction of a valve secondary to large vegetations, acquired VSD, and heart block as a result of involvement (abscess) of the conduction system. Additional complications include meningitis, osteomyelitis, arthritis, renal abscess, and immune complex–mediated glomerulonephritis.

TREATMENT. Antibiotic therapy should be instituted immediately once a definitive diagnosis is made. When virulent organisms are responsible, small delays may result in progressive endocardial damage and are associated with a greater likelihood of severe complications. The choice of antibiotics, method of administration, and length of treatment are outlined in Tables 437-4 to 437-13. High serum bactericidal levels must be maintained long enough to eradicate organisms that are growing in relatively inaccessible avascular vegetations. Between 5 and 20 times the minimal in vitro inhibiting concentration must be produced at the site of infection to destroy bacteria growing at the core of these lesions. Several weeks are required for a vegetation to organize completely; therapy must be continued through this period so that recrudescence can be avoided. A total of 4–6 wk of treatment is recommended, with serumcidal levels by tube dilution of at least 1:8 after a dose of antibiotic. Depending on the clinical and laboratory responses, antibiotic therapy may require modification and, in some instances, more prolonged treatment is required. With highly sensitive viridans group streptococcal infections, shortened regimens that include oral penicillin for some portion have been recommended. In nonstaphylococcal disease, bacteremia usually resolves in 24–48 hr, whereas fever resolves in 5–6 days with appropriate antibiotic therapy. Resolution with staphylococcal disease takes longer.

TABLE 437-5. Therapy of Native Valve Endocarditis Caused by Strains of Viridans Group Streptococci and *Streptococcus bovis* Relatively Resistant to Penicillin

REGIMEN	DOSAGE* AND ROUTE	DURATION, WK	COMMENTS
Aqueous crystalline penicillin G sodium	24 million U/24 h IV either continuously or in 4–6 equally divided doses	4	Patients with endocarditis caused by penicillin-resistant (MIC >0.5 μg/mL) strains should be treated with regimen recommended for enterococcal endocarditis (see Table 437-9)
or			
Ceftriaxone sodium	2 g/24 h IV/IM in 1 dose	4	
plus			
Gentamicin sulfate†	3 mg/kg per 24 h IV/IM in 1 dose, or 3 equally divided doses ***Pediatric dose‡:*** penicillin 300 000 U/24 h IV in 4–6 equally divided doses; ceftriaxone 100 mg/kg per 24 h IV/IM in 1 dose; gentamicin 3 mg/kg per 24 h IV/IM in 1 dose or 3 equally divided doses	2	
Vancomycin hydrochloride‡	30 mg/kg per 24 h IV in 2 equally divided doses not to exceed 2 g/24 h, unless serum concentrations are inappropriately low ***Pediatric dose:*** 40 mg/kg 24 h in 2 or 3 equally divided doses	4	Vancomycin§ therapy recommended only for patients unable to tolerate penicillin or ceftriaxone therapy

Minimum inhibitory concentration (MIC) >0.12 μg/mL–≤0.5 μg/mL.
*Dosages recommended are for patients with normal renal function.
†See Table 437-4 for appropriate dosage of gentamicin.
‡Pediatric dose should not exceed that of a normal adult.
§See Table 437-4 for appropriate dosage of vancomycin.
From Baddour LM, Wilson WR, Bayer AS, et al: Infective endocarditis: Diagnosis, antimicrobial therapy, and management of complications. *Circulation* 2005;111:e394–e433 and correction *Circulation* 2005;112:2373.

Digitalis, salt restriction, and diuretic therapy are used for the treatment of heart failure. Surgical intervention for infective endocarditis is indicated for severe aortic or mitral valve involvement with intractable heart failure. Rarely, a mycotic aneurysm, rupture of an aortic sinus, or dehiscence of an intracardiac patch requires an emergency operation. Other surgical indications include failure to sterilize the blood despite adequate antibiotic levels, myocardial abscess, recurrent emboli, new heart block, and increasing size of vegetations while receiving therapy. Although antibiotic therapy should be administered for as long as possible before surgical intervention, active infection is not a contraindication if the patient is critically ill as a result of severe hemodynamic deterioration from infective endocarditis. Removal of vegetations and, in some instances, valve replacement may be lifesaving, and sustained antibiotic administration will most often prevent reinfection. Replacement of infected prosthetic valves carries a higher risk.

Fungal endocarditis is difficult to manage and has a poorer prognosis. It has been encountered after cardiac surgery, in severely debilitated or immunosuppressed patients, and in patients on prolonged courses of antibiotics. The drugs of choice are amphotericin B (liposomal or standard preparation) and 5-fluorocytosine. Surgery to excise infected tissue is occasionally attempted, though often with limited success. Recombinant tissue

TABLE 437-6. Therapy for Endocarditis of Prosthetic Valves or Other Prosthetic Material Caused by Viridans Group Streptococci and *Streptococcus bovis*

REGIMEN	DOSAGE* AND ROUTE	DURATION, WK	COMMENTS
PENICILLIN-SUSCEPTIBLE STRAIN (MINIMUM INHIBITORY CONCENTRATION ≤0.12 μg/ml)			
Aqueous crystalline penicillin G sodium	24 million U/24 h IV either continuously or in 4–6 equally divided doses	6	Penicillin or ceftriaxone together with gentamicin has not demonstrated superior cure rates compared with monotherapy with penicillin or ceftriaxone for patients with highly susceptible strain; gentamicin therapy should not be administered to patients with creatinine clearance of <30 mL/min
or			
Ceftriaxone	2 g/24 h IV/IM in 1 dose	6	
with or without			
Gentamicin sulfate†	3 mg/kg per 24 h IV/IM in 1 dose, or 3 equally divided doses ***Pediatric dose‡:*** penicillin 300,000 U/kg per 24 h IV in 4–6 equally divided doses; ceftriaxone 100 mg/kg IV/IM once daily; gentamicin 3 mg/kg per 24 h IV/IM, in 1 dose or 3 equally divided doses	2	
Vancomycin hydrochloride§	30 mg/kg per 24 h IV in 2 equally divided doses ***Pediatric dose:*** 40 mg/kg per 24 h IV or in 2 or 3 equally divided doses	6	Vancomycin therapy recommended only for patients unable to tolerate penicillin or ceftriaxone
PENICILLIN RELATIVELY OR FULLY RESISTANT STRAIN (MINIMUM INHIBITORY CONCENTRATION >0.12 μg/ml)			
Aqueous crystalline penicillin sodium	24 million U/24 h IV either continuously or in 4–6 equally divided doses	6	
or			
Ceftriaxone	2 g/24 h IV/IM in 1 dose	6	
plus			
Gentamicin sulfate	3 mg/kg per 24 h IV/IM in 1 dose ***Pediatric dose:*** penicillin 300 000 U/kg per 24 h IV in 4–6 equally divided doses	6	
Vancomycin hydrochloride	30 mg/kg per 24 h IV in 2 equally divided doses ***Pediatric dose:*** 40 mg/kg per 24 h IV in 2 or 3 equally divided doses	6	Vancomycin therapy is recommended only for patients unable to tolerate penicillin or ceftriaxone

*Dosages recommended are for patients with normal renal function.
†See Table 437-4 for appropriate dosage of gentamicin.
‡Pediatric dose should not exceed that of a normal adult.
§See text and Table 437-4 for appropriate dosage of vancomycin.
From Baddour LM, Wilson WR, Bayer AS, et al: Infective endocarditis: Diagnosis, antimicrobial therapy, and management of complications. *Circulation* 2005;111:e394–e433 and corrections *Circulation* 2005;112:2373.

TABLE 437-7. Therapy for Endocarditis Caused by Staphylococci in the Absence of Prosthetic Materials

REGIMEN	DOSAGE* AND ROUTE	DURATION	COMMENTS
OXACILLIN-SUSCEPTIBLE STRAINS			
Nafcillin or oxacillin[†]	12 g/24 h IV in 4–6 equally divided doses	6 wk	For complicated right-sided IE and for left-sided IE; for uncomplicated right-sided IE, 2 wk
with			
Optional addition of gentamicin sulfate[‡]	3 mg/kg per 24 h IV/IM in 2 or 3 equally divided doses ***Pediatric dose***[§]: Nafcillin or oxacillin 200 mg/kg per 24 h IV in 4–6 equally divided doses; gentamicin 3 mg/kg per 24 h IV/IM in 3 equally divided doses	3–5 d	Clinical benefit of aminoglycosides has not been established
For penicillin-allergic (nonanaphylactoid type) patients:			Consider skin testing for oxacillin-susceptible staphylococci and questionable history of immediate-type hypersensitivity to penicillin
Cefazolin	6 g/24 h IV in 3 equally divided doses	6 wk	Cephalosporins should be avoided in patients with anaphylactoid-type hypersensitivity to β-lactams; vancomycin should be used in these cases§
with			
Optional addition of gentamicin sulfate	3 mg/kg per 24 h IV/IM in 2 or 3 equally divided doses ***Pediatric dose:*** cefazolin 100 mg/kg per 24 h IV in 3 equally divided doses; gentamicin 3 mg/kg per 24 h IV/IM in 3 equally divided doses	3–5 d	Clinical benefit of aminoglycosides has not been established
OXACILLIN-RESISTANT STRAINS			
Vancomycin[‖]	30 mg/kg per 24 h IV in 2 equally divided doses ***Pediatric dose:*** 40 mg/kg per 24 h IV in 2 or 3 equally divided doses	6 wk	Adjust vancomycin dosage to achieve 1 h serum concentration of 30–45 μg/mL and trough concentration of 10–15 μg/mL

IE: infective endocarditis.
*Dosages recommended are for patients with normal renal function.
[†]Penicillin G 24 million U/24 h IV in 4 to 6 equally divided doses may be used in place of nafcillin or oxacillin if strain is penicillin susceptible (minimum inhibitory concentration ≤0.1 μg/mL) and does not produce β-lactamase.
[‡]Gentamicin should be administered in close temporal proximity to vancomycin, nafcillin, or oxacillin dosing.
[§]Pediatric dose should not exceed that of a normal adult.
[‖]For specific dosing adjustment and issues concerning vancomycin, see Table 437-4 footnotes.
From Baddour LM, Wilson WR, Bayer AS, et al: Infective endocarditis: Diagnosis, antimicrobial therapy, and management of complications. *Circulation* 2005;111:e394–e433 and corrections *Circulation* 2005;112:2373.

TABLE 437-8. Therapy for Prosthetic Valve Endocarditis Caused by Staphylococci

REGIMEN	DOSAGE* AND ROUTE	DURATION, WK	COMMENTS
OXACILLIN-SUSCEPTIBLE STRAINS			
Nafcillin or oxacillin	12 g/24 h IV in 6 equally divided doses	≥6	Penicillin G 24 million U/24 h IV in 4–6 equally divided doses may be used in place of nafcillin or oxacillin if strain is penicillin susceptible (minimum inhibitory concentration ≤0.1 μg/mL) and does not produce β-lactamase; vancomycin should be used in patients with immediate-type hypersensitivity reactions to β-lactam antibiotics (see Table 437-4); cefazolin may be substituted for nafcillin or oxacillin in patients with non-immediate-type hypersensitivity reactions to penicillins
plus			
Rifampin	900 mg per 24 h IV/PO in 3 equally divided doses	≥6	
plus			
Gentamicin[†]	3 mg/kg per 24 h IV/IM in 2 or 3 equally divided doses ***Pediatric dose***[‡]: nafcillin or oxacillin 200 mg/kg per 24 h IV in 4–6 equally divided doses; rifampin 20 mg/kg per 24 h IV/PO in 3 equally divided doses; gentamicin 3 mg/kg per 24 h IV/IM in 3 equally divided doses	2	
OXACILLIN-RESISTANT STRAINS			
Vancomycin	30 mg/kg 24 h in 2 equally divided doses	≥6	Adjust vancomycin to achieve 1-h serum concentration of 30–45 μg/mL and trough concentration of 10–15 μg/mL (see text for gentamicin alternatives)
plus			
Rifampin	900 mg/24 h IV/PO in 3 equally divided doses	≥6	
plus			
Gentamicin	3 mg/kg per 24 h IV/IM in 2 or 3 equally divided doses ***Pediatric dose***: vancomycin 40 mg/kg per 24 h IV in 2 or 3 equally divided doses; rifampin 20 mg/kg per 24 h IV/PO in 3 equally divided doses (up to adult dose); gentamicin 3 mg/kg per 24 h IV or IM in 3 equally divided doses	2	

*Dosages recommended are for patients with normal renal function.
[†]Gentamicin should be administered in close proximity to vancomycin, nafcillin, or oxacillin dosing (see Table 437-4).
[‡]Pediatric dose should not exceed that of a normal adult.
From Baddour LM, Wilson WR, Bayer AS, et al: Infective endocarditis: Diagnosis, antimicrobial therapy, and management of complications. *Circulation* 2005;111:e394–e433 and corrections *Circulation* 2005;112:2373.

TABLE 437-9. Therapy for Native Valve or Prosthetic Valve Enterococcal Endocarditis Caused by Strains Susceptible to Penicillin, Gentamicin, and Vancomycin

REGIMEN	DOSAGE* AND ROUTE	DURATION, WK	COMMENTS
Ampicillin sodium *or*	12 g/24 h IV in 6 equally divided doses	4–6	Native valve: 4 wk therapy recommended for patients with symptoms of illness ≤3 mo; 6 wk therapy recommended for patients with symptoms >3 mo
Aqueous crystalline penicillin G sodium ***plus***	18–30 million U/24 h IV either continuously or in 6 equally divided doses	4–6	Prosthetic valve or other prosthetic cardiac material: minimum of 6 wk of therapy recommended
Gentamicin sulfate[†]	3 mg/kg per 24 h IV/IM in 3 equally divided doses ***Pediatric dose***[‡]: ampicillin 300 mg/kg per 24 h IV in 4–6 equally divided doses; penicillin 300 000 U/kg per 24 h IV in 4–6 equally divided doses; gentamicin 3 mg/kg per 24 h IV/IM in 3 equally divided doses	4–6	
Vancomycin hydrochloride[§] ***plus***	30 mg/kg 24 h in 2 equally divided doses	6	Vancomycin therapy recommended only for patients unable to tolerate penicillin or ampicillin
Gentamicin sulfate	3 mg per 24 h IV/IM in 3 equally divided doses ***Pediatric dose***: vancomycin 40 mg/kg per 24 h IV in 2 or 3 equally divided doses; gentamicin 3 mg/kg per 24 h IV/IM in 3 equally divided doses	6	6 wk of vancomycin therapy recommended because of decreased activity against enterococci

*Dosages recommended are for patients with normal renal function.
[†]Dosages of gentamicin should be adjusted to achieve peak serum concentration of 3–4 μg/mL and a trough concentration of <1 μg/mL (see Table 437-4 for dosing of gentamicin).
[‡]Pediatric dose should not exceed that of a normal adult.
[§]See Table 437-4 for appropriate dosing of vancomycin.
From Baddour LM, Wilson WR, Bayer AS, et al: Infective endocarditis: Diagnosis, antimicrobial therapy, and management of complications. *Circulation* 2005;111:e394–e433 and corrections *Circulation* 2005;112:2373.

TABLE 437-10. Therapy for Native or Prosthetic Valve Enterococcal Endocarditis Caused by Strains Susceptible to Penicillin, Streptomycin, and Vancomycin and Resistant to Gentamicin

REGIMEN	DOSAGE* AND ROUTE	DURATION, WK	COMMENTS
Ampicillin sodium *or*	12 g/24 h IV in 6 equally divided doses	4–6	Native valve: 4 wk therapy recommended for patients with symptoms of illness <3 mo; 6 wk therapy recommended for patients with symptoms >3 mo
Aqueous crystalline penicillin G sodium ***plus***	24 million U/24 h IV continuously or in 6 equally divided doses	4–6	
Streptomycin sulfate	15 mg/kg per 24 h IV/IM in 2 equally divided doses ***Pediatric dose***[†]: ampicillin 300 mg/kg per 24 h IV in 4–6 equally divided doses; penicillin 300 000 U/kg per 24 h IV in 4–6 equally divided doses; streptomycin 20–30 mg/kg per 24 h IV/IM in 2 equally divided doses	4–6	Prosthetic valve or other prosthetic cardiac material: minimum of 6 wk of therapy recommended
Vancomycin hydrochloride[‡] ***plus***	30 mg/kg per 24 h in 2 equally divided doses	6	Vancomycin therapy recommended only for patients unable to tolerate penicillin or ampicillin
Streptomycin sulfate	15 mg/kg per 24 h IV/IM in 2 equally divided doses ***Pediatric dose***: vancomycin 40 mg/kg per 24 h IV in 2 or 3 equally divided doses; streptomycin 20–30 mg/kg per 24 h IV/IM in 2 equally divided doses	6	

*Dosages recommended are for patients with normal renal function.
[‡]See Table 437-4 for appropriate dosing of vancomycin.
From Baddour LM, Wilson WR, Bayer AS, et al: Infective endocarditis: Diagnosis, antimicrobial therapy, and management of complications. *Circulation* 2005;111:e394–e433 and corrections *Circulation* 2005;112:2373.

TABLE 437-11. Therapy for Native or Prosthetic Valve Enterococcal Endocarditis Caused by Strains Resistant to Penicillin and Susceptible to Aminoglycoside and Vancomycin

REGIMEN	DOSAGE* AND ROUTE	DURATION, WK	COMMENTS
β-LACTAMASE-PRODUCING STRAIN			
Ampicillin-sulbactam ***plus***	12 g/24 h IV in 4 equally divided doses	6	Unlikely that the strain will be susceptible to gentamicin; if strain is gentamicin resistant, then >6 wk of ampicillin-sulbactam therapy will be needed
Gentamicin sulfate[†]	3 mg/kg per 24 h IV/IM in 3 equally divided doses ***Pediatric dose***[‡]: ampicillin-sulbactam 300 mg/kg per 24 h IV in 4 equally divided doses; gentamicin 3 mg/kg per 24 h IV/IM in 3 equally divided doses	6	
Vancomycin hydrochloride[§] ***plus***	30 mg/kg per 24 h IV in 2 equally divided doses	6	Vancomycin therapy recommended only for patients unable to tolerate ampicillin-sulbactam
Gentamicin sulfate[†]	3 mg/kg per 24 h IV/IM in 3 equally divided doses ***Pediatric dose***: vancomycin 40 mg/kg per 24 h in 2 or 3 equally divided doses; gentamicin 3 mg/kg per 24 h IV/IM in 3 equally divided doses	6	
INTRINSIC PENICILLIN RESISTANCE			
Vancomycin hydrochloride[‡] ***plus***	30 mg/kg 24 h IV in 2 equally divided doses	6	Consultation with a specialist in infectious diseases recommended
Gentamicin sulfate[†]	3 mg/kg per 24 h IV/IM in 3 equally divided doses ***Pediatric dose***: vancomycin 40 mg/kg per 24 h IV in 2 or 3 equally divided doses; gentamicin 3 mg/kg per 24 h IV/IM in 3 equally divided doses	6	

*Dosages recommended are for patients with normal renal function.
[†]See Table 437-4 for appropriate dosing of gentamicin.
[‡]Pediatric dose should not exceed that of a normal adult.
[§]See Table 437-4 for appropriate dosing of vancomycin.
From Baddour LM, Wilson WR, Bayer AS, et al: Infective endocarditis: Diagnosis, antimicrobial therapy, and management of complications. *Circulation* 2005;111:e394–e433 and corrections *Circulation* 2005;112:2373.

TABLE 437-12. Therapy for Native or Prosthetic Valve Enterococcal Endocarditis Caused by Strains Resistant to Penicillin, Aminoglycoside, and Vancomycin

REGIMEN	DOSAGE* AND ROUTE	DURATION, WK	COMMENTS
E faecium			
Linezolid	1200 mg/24 h IV/PO in 2 equally divided doses	≥8	Patients with endocarditis caused by these strains should be treated in consultation with an infectious diseases specialist; cardiac valve replacement may be necessary for bacteriologic cure; cure with antimicrobial therapy alone may be <50%; severe, usually reversible thrombocytopenia may occur with use of linezolid, especially after 2 wk of therapy; quinupristin-dalfopristin only effective against *E faecium* and can cause severe myalgias, which may require discontinuation of therapy; only small no. of patients have reportedly been treated with imipenem/cilastatin-ampicillin or ceftriaxone + ampicillin
or			
Quinupristin-dalfopristin	22.5 mg/kg per 24 h IV in 3 equally divided doses	≥8	
E faecalis			
Imipenem/cilastatin	2 g/24 h IV in 4 equally divided doses	≥8	
plus			
Ampicillin sodium	12 g/24 h IV in 6 equally divided doses	≥8	
or			
Ceftriaxone sodium	4 g/24 h IV/IM in 2 divided doses	≥8	
plus			
Ampicillin sodium	12 g/24 h IV in 6 equally divided doses	≥8	
	Pediatric dose[†]: Linezolid 30 mg/kg per 24 h IV/PO in 3 equally divided doses; quinupristin-dalfopristin 22.5 mg/kg per 24 h IV in 3 equally divided doses; imipenem/cilastatin 60–100 mg/kg per 24 h IV in 4 equally divided doses; ampicillin 300 mg/kg per 24 h IV in 4–6 equally divided doses; ceftriaxone 100 mg/kg per 24 h IV/IM in 2 equally divided doses		

Decreasing order of preference based on published data.
*Dosages recommended are for patients with normal renal function.
[†]Pediatric dose should not exceed that of a normal adult.
From Baddour LM, Wilson WR, Bayer AS, et al: Infective endocarditis: Diagnosis, antimicrobial therapy, and management of complications. *Circulation* 2005;111:e394–e433 and correction *Circulation* 2005;112:2373.

TABLE 437-13. Therapy for Both Native and Prosthetic Valve Endocarditis Caused by HACEK* Microorganisms

REGIMEN	DOSAGE AND ROUTE	DURATION, WK	COMMENTS
Ceftriaxone[†] sodium	2 g/24 h IV/IM in 1 dose	4	Cefotaxime or another 3rd- or 4th-generation cephalosporin may be substituted
or			
Ampicillin-sulbactam[‡]	12 g/24 h IV in 4 equally divided doses	4	
or			
Ciprofloxacin[‡§]	1000 mg/24 h PO or 800 mg/24 h IV in 2 equally divided doses ***Pediatric dose***[‖]: Ceftriaxone 100 mg/kg per 24 h IV/IM once daily; ampicillin-sulbactam 300 mg/kg per 24 h IV divided into 4 or 6 equally divided doses; ciprofloxacin 20–30 mg/kg per 24 h IV/PO in 2 equally divided doses	4	Fluoroquinolone therapy recommended only for patients unable to tolerate cephalosporin and ampicillin therapy; levofloxacin, gatifloxacin, or moxifloxacin may be substituted; fluoroquinolones generally not recommended for patients <18 y old Prosthetic valve: patients with endocarditis involving prosthetic cardiac valve or other prosthetic cardiac material should be treated for 6 wk

**Haemophilus parainfluenzae, H aphrophilus, Actinobacillus actinomycetemcomitans, Cardiobacterium hominis, Eikenella corrodens,* and *Kingella kingae.*
[†]Patients should be informed that IM injection of ceftriaxone is painful.
[‡]Dosage recommended for patients with normal renal function.
[§]Fluoroquinolones are highly active in vitro against HACEK microorganisms. Published data on use of fluoroquinolone therapy for endocarditis caused by HACEK are minimal.
[‖]Pediatric dose should not exceed that of a normal adult.
From Baddour LM, Wilson WR, Bayer AS, et al: Infective endocarditis: Diagnosis, antimicrobial therapy, and management of complications. *Circulation* 2005;111:e394–e433 and correction *Circulation* 2005;112:2373.

TABLE 437-14. Recommendations for Prophylaxis Against Bacterial Endocarditis

DENTAL AND ORAL PROCEDURES OR SURGERY OF THE UPPER RESPIRATORY TRACT OR ESOPHAGUS		GASTROINTESTINAL AND GENITOURINARY TRACT SURGERY AND INSTRUMENTATION	
For most patients	Oral amoxicillin Adults, 2.0 g, children, 50 mg/kg 1 hr before procedure	High-risk patients	IM or IV ampicillin Adults, 2.0 g, children, 50 mg/kg *plus*
For patients unable to take oral medication	IM or IV ampicillin Adults, 2.0 g, children, 50 mg/kg given within 30 min before procedure		IM or IV gentamicin 1.5 mg/kg (maximal dose, 120 mg) given within 30 min before procedure *plus 6 hr later*
Ampicillin- and amoxicillin-allergic patients	Oral clindamycin Adults, 600 mg, children, 20 mg/kg 1 hr before procedure *or*		IM or IV ampicillin or oral amoxicillin Adults, 1 g, children, 25 mg/kg
	Oral cephalexin* or cefadroxil* Adults, 2.0 g, children, 50 mg/kg 1 hr before procedure *or* Oral azithromycin *or* clarithromycin Adults, 500 mg, children, 15 mg/kg 1 hr before procedure	High-risk patients allergic to ampicillin and amoxicillin	IV vancomycin Adults, 1.0 g, children, 20 mg/kg given over 1–2 hr *plus* IM or IV gentamicin 1.5 mg/kg (maximal dose, 120 mg); complete injection/infusion within 30 min before starting procedure
Ampicillin- and amoxicillin-allergic patients unable to take oral medications	IV clindamycin Adults, 600 mg, children, 20 mg/kg given within 30 min before procedure *or* IV cefazolin Adults, 1.0 g, children, 25 mg/kg given within 30 min before procedure		

*Cephalosporins should not be used in patients with an immediate-type hypersensitivity reaction to penicillins.

High-risk patients: prosthetic heart valves (including homografts), previous endocarditis, complex unrepaired cyanotic congenital heart disease (e.g., transposition of great vessels, tetralogy of Fallot, single ventricle), systemic-to-pulmonary artery shunts or conduits. Repaired congenital heart defect with prosthetic material (surgery or catheter placed) 6 mo after procedure. Repaired congenital defects with residual defects. Cardiac transplantation if valvulopathy develops.

Negligible-risk patients (prophylaxis not recommended): isolated secundum ASD; surgical repair of ASD, VSD, or PDA (without residua and beyond 6 mo after repair); previous coronary artery bypass surgery; functional heart murmurs; previous Kawasaki disease or rheumatic fever without valve dysfunction; cardiac pacemakers; implantable defibrillators.

The risk of mitral valve prolapse is controversial. Mitral valve prolapse with regurgitation or thickened leaflets, or both, is categorized as a moderate risk; mitral valve prolapse without regurgitation is categorized as negligible risk.

ASD, atrial septal defect; IM, intramuscularly; IV, intravenously; PDA, patent ductus arteriosus; VSD, ventricular septal defect.

Adapted from Dajani AS, Taubert KA, Wilson W, et al: Prevention of bacterial endocarditis. Recommendations by the American Heart Association. *JAMA* 1997; 277:1794–1801 and Wilson W, Taubert KA, Gewitz M, et al: Prevention of infective endocarditis. Guidelines from the American Heart Association. *Circulation* 2007;DOI:10.1161/circulationaha.106.183095.

plasminogen activation may help lyse intracardiac vegetations and avoid surgery in some high-risk patients.

PREVENTION. Antimicrobial prophylaxis before various procedures and other forms of dental manipulation may reduce the incidence of infective endocarditis in susceptible patients (Tables 437-14 and 437-15). Continuing education regarding prophylaxis is important, especially in teenagers and young adults, who often have poor knowledge of their own congenital heart lesion. Proper general dental care and oral hygiene are most important in decreasing the risk of infective endocarditis in susceptible individuals. Vigorous treatment of sepsis and local infections and careful asepsis during heart surgery and catheterization reduce the incidence of infective endocarditis.

Ashrafian H, Bogle RG: Antimicrobial prophylaxis for endocarditis: emotion or science? *Heart* 2007;93:5–6.

Ayres NA, Miller-Hance W, Fyfe DA, et al: Indications and guidelines for performance of transesophageal echocardiography in the patient with pediatric acquired or congenital heart disease: Report from the task force of the Pediatric Council of the American Society of Echocardiography. *J Am Soc Echocardiogr* 2005;18:91–98.

Baddour LM, Wilson WR, Bayer AS, et al: Infective endocarditis: Diagnosis, antimicrobial therapy, and management of complications. *Circulation* 2005;111:e394–e433.

Bouza E, Menasalvas A, Munoz P, et al: Infective endocarditis—a prospective study at the end of the twentieth century. *Medicine (Baltimore)* 2001; 80:298–307.

Dajani AS, Taubert KA, Wilson W, et al: Prevention of bacterial endocarditis. Recommendations by the American Heart Association. *JAMA* 1997; 277:1794–1801.

Ellis ME, Al-Abdely H, Sandridge A, et al: Fungal endocarditis: Evidence in the world literature, 1965–1995. *Clin Infect Dis* 2001;32:50–62.

Ferrieri P, Gewitz MH, Berger M, et al: Unique features of infective endocarditis in childhood. *Pediatrics* 2002;109:931–943.

Hartzell JD, Torres D, Kim P, et al: Incidence of bacteremia after routine tooth brushing. *Am J Med Sci* 2005;329:178–180.

Hoen B, Alla F, Selton-Suty C, et al: Changing profile of infective endocarditis. Results of a 1-year survey in France. *JAMA* 2002;288:75–80.

Houpikian P, Raoult D: Blood culture-negative endocarditis in a reference center: Etiologic diagnosis of 348 cases. *Medicine (Baltimore)* 2005; 84:162–173.

Lamas CC, Eykyn SJ: Blood culture negative endocarditis: Analysis of 63 cases presenting over 25 years. *Heart* 2003;89:258–262.

Levitas A, Zucker N, Zalzstein E, et al: Successful treatment of infective endocarditis with recombinant tissue plasminogen activator. *J Pediatr* 2003; 143:649–652.

Martin JM, Neches WH, Wald ER: Infective endocarditis: 35 years of experience at a children's hospital. *Infect Dis* 1997;24:669–675.

Milazzo AS Jr, Li JS: Bacterial endocarditis in infants and children. *Pediatr Infect Dis J* 2001;20:799–801.

Moreillon P, Que YA: Infective endocarditis. *Lancet* 2004;363:139–148.

Morris CD, Reller MD, Menashe VD: Thirty-year incidence of infective endocarditis after surgery for congenital heart disease. *JAMA* 1998; 279:599–603.

Tissieres P, Gervaix A, Beghetti M, et al: Value and limitations of the von Reyn, Duke, and modified Duke criteria for the diagnosis of infective endocarditis in children. *Pediatrics* 2003;112:e467.

Valente AM, Jain R, Scheurer M, et al: Frequency of infective endocarditis among infants and children with *Staphylococcus aureus* bacteremia. *Pediatrics* 2005;115:e15–e19.

Wilson W, Taubert KA, Gewitz M, et al: Prevention of infective endocarditis. Guidelines from the American Heart Association. *Circulation* 2007;DOI: 10.1161/circulationaha.106.183095.

TABLE 437-15. Procedures and Endocarditis Prophylaxis

ENDOCARDITIS PROPHYLAXIS RECOMMENDED*	ENDOCARDITIS PROPHYLAXIS NOT RECOMMENDED
Dental	**Dental**
Tooth extractions	Restorative dentistry[‡] (operative and prosthodontic) with or without retraction cord[§]
Periodontal procedures, including surgery, scaling and root planing, probing, and recall maintenance	Local anesthesia injections (non-intraligamentary)
Dental implant placement and re-implantation of avulsed teeth	Intracanal endodontic treatment, after placement and buildup
Endodontic (root canal) instrumentation or surgery only beyond the apex	Placement of rubber dams
Subgingival placement of antibiotic fibers or strips	Postoperative suture removal
Initial placement of orthodontic bands but not brackets	Placement of removable prosthodontic or orthodontic appliances
Intraligamentary local anesthesia injections	Taking of oral impressions
Prophylactic cleaning of teeth or implants when bleeding is anticipated	Fluoride treatments
Respiratory Tract	Taking of oral radiographs
Tonsillectomy or adenoidectomy, or both	Orthodontic appliance adjustment
Surgical operations that involve respiratory mucosa	Shedding of primary teeth
Bronchoscopy with a rigid broncoscope or biopsy	**Respiratory Tract**
Gastrointestinal Tract[†]	Endotracheal intubation
Sclerotherapy for esophageal varices	Bronchoscopy with a flexible bronchoscope without biopsy[§]
Esophageal stricture dilatation	Tympanostomy tube insertion
Endoscopic retrograde cholangiography with biliary obstruction	**Gastrointestinal Tract**
Biliary tract surgery	Transesophageal echocardiography[§]
Surgical operations that involve intestinal mucosa	Endoscopy with or without gastrointestinal biopsy[§]
	Genitourinary Tract
	Cystoscopy
	Vaginal delivery[§]
	Cesarean section
	In uninfected tissue:
	Urethral catheterization
	Uterine dilatation and curettage
	Therapeutic abortion
	Sterilization procedures
	Insertion or removal of intrauterine devices
	Other
	Cardiac catheterization, including balloon angioplasty
	Implanted cardiac pacemakers, implanted defibrillators, and coronary stents
	Incision or biopsy of surgically scrubbed skin
	Circumcision

*Prophylaxis is recommended for patients with high- or moderate-risk heart conditions.
[†]Prophylaxis is recommended for high-risk patients; optional for medium-risk patients.
[‡]Includes restoration of decayed teeth (filling cavities) and replacement of missing teeth.
[§]Prophylaxis is optional for high-risk patients.

Chapter 438 ■ Rheumatic Heart Disease

Rheumatic involvement of the valves and endocardium is the most important manifestation of rheumatic fever (see Chapters 156 and 182.1). The valvular lesions begin as small verrucae composed of fibrin and blood cells along the borders of one or more of the heart valves. The mitral valve is affected most often, followed in frequency by the aortic valve; right-sided heart manifestations are rare. As the inflammation subsides, the verrucae tend to disappear and leave scar tissue. With repeated attacks of rheumatic fever, new verrucae form near the previous ones, and the mural endocardium and chordae tendineae become involved.

PATTERNS OF VALVULAR DISEASE

MITRAL INSUFFICIENCY

Pathophysiology. Mitral insufficiency is the result of structural changes that usually include some loss of valvular substance and shortening and thickening of the chordae tendineae. During acute rheumatic fever with severe cardiac involvement, heart failure is caused by a combination of mitral insufficiency coupled with inflammatory disease of the pericardium, myocardium, endocardium, and epicardium. Because of the high volume load and inflammatory process, the left ventricle becomes enlarged. The left atrium dilates as blood regurgitates into this chamber. Increased left atrial pressure results in pulmonary congestion and symptoms of left-sided heart failure. Spontaneous improvement usually occurs with time, even in patients in whom mitral insufficiency is severe at the onset. The resultant chronic lesion is most often mild or moderate in severity, and the patient is asymptomatic. More than half of patients with acute mitral insufficiency no longer have the mitral murmur 1 yr later. In patients with severe chronic mitral insufficiency, pulmonary arterial pressure becomes elevated, the right ventricle and atrium become enlarged, and right-sided heart failure subsequently develops.

Clinical Manifestations. The physical signs of mitral insufficiency depend on its severity. With mild disease, signs of heart failure are not present, the precordium is quiet, and auscultation reveals a high-pitched holosystolic murmur at the apex that radiates to the axilla. With severe mitral insufficiency, signs of chronic heart failure may be noted. The heart is enlarged, with a heaving apical left ventricular impulse and often an apical systolic thrill. The 2nd heart sound may be accentuated if pulmonary hypertension is present. A 3rd heart sound is generally prominent. A holosystolic murmur is heard at the apex with radiation to the axilla. A short mid-diastolic rumbling murmur is caused by increased blood flow across the mitral valve as a result of the insufficiency. Auscultation of a diastolic murmur does not necessarily mean that mitral stenosis is present. The latter lesion takes many years to develop and is characterized by a diastolic murmur of greater length with presystolic accentuation.

The electrocardiogram and roentgenograms are normal if the lesion is mild. With more severe insufficiency, the electrocardiogram shows prominent bifid P waves, signs of left ventricular hypertrophy, and associated right ventricular hypertrophy if pulmonary hypertension is present. Roentgenographically, prominence of the left atrium and ventricle can be seen. Congestion of perihilar vessels, a sign of pulmonary venous hypertension, may also be evident. Calcification of the mitral valve is rare in children. Echocardiography shows enlargement of the left atrium and ventricle, and Doppler studies demonstrate the severity of the mitral regurgitation. Heart catheterization and left ventriculography are considered only if diagnostic questions are not totally resolved by noninvasive assessment. The degree of opacification of the left atrium during left ventriculography is used as a qualitative assessment of the severity of mitral insufficiency.

Complications. Severe mitral insufficiency may result in cardiac failure that may be precipitated by progression of the rheumatic process, the onset of atrial fibrillation, or infective endocarditis. The effects of chronic mitral insufficiency may become manifest after many years and include right ventricular failure and atrial and ventricular arrhythmias.

Treatment. In patients with mild mitral insufficiency, prophylaxis against recurrences of rheumatic fever is all that is required. Treatment of complicating heart failure (see Chapter 442), arrhythmias (see Chapter 435), and infective endocarditis (see Chapter 437) is described elsewhere. Afterload-reducing agents (ACE inhibitors) may reduce the regurgitant volume and preserve left ventricular function. Surgical treatment is indicated for patients who despite adequate medical therapy have recurrent episodes of heart failure, dyspnea with moderate activity, and progressive cardiomegaly, often with pulmonary hypertension. Although annuloplasty provides good results in some children and adolescents, valve replacement may be required. Prophylaxis against bacterial endocarditis is warranted in these patients for dental or other surgical procedures. The routine antibiotics taken by these patients for rheumatic fever prophylaxis are insufficient to prevent endocarditis.

MITRAL STENOSIS

Pathophysiology. Mitral stenosis of rheumatic origin results from fibrosis of the mitral ring, commissural adhesions, and contracture of the valve leaflets, chordae, and papillary muscles over time. It takes 10 yr or more for the lesion to become fully established, although the process may occasionally be accelerated. Rheumatic mitral stenosis is seldom encountered before adolescence and is not usually recognized until adult life. Significant mitral stenosis results in increased pressure and enlargement and hypertrophy of the left atrium, pulmonary venous hypertension, increased pulmonary vascular resistance, and pulmonary hypertension. Right ventricular and atrial dilatation and hypertrophy ensue and are followed by right-sided heart failure.

Clinical Manifestations. Generally, the correlation between symptoms and the severity of obstruction is good. Patients with mild lesions are asymptomatic. More severe degrees of obstruction are associated with exercise intolerance and dyspnea. Critical lesions can result in orthopnea, paroxysmal nocturnal dyspnea, and overt pulmonary edema, as well as atrial arrhythmias. When pulmonary hypertension has developed, right ventricular dilatation may result in functional tricuspid insufficiency, hepatomegaly, ascites, and edema. Hemoptysis caused by rupture of bronchial or pleurohilar veins and, occasionally, by pulmonary infarction may occur.

Jugular venous pressure is increased in severe disease with heart failure, tricuspid valve disease, or severe pulmonary hypertension. In mild disease, heart size is normal; however, moderate cardiomegaly is usual with severe mitral stenosis. Cardiac enlargement can be massive when atrial fibrillation and heart failure supervene. A parasternal right ventricular lift is palpable when pulmonary pressure is high. The principal auscultatory findings are a loud 1st heart sound, an opening snap of the mitral valve, and a long, low-pitched, rumbling mitral diastolic murmur with presystolic accentuation at the apex. The mitral diastolic murmur may be virtually absent in patients who are in heart failure. A holosystolic murmur secondary to tricuspid insufficiency may be audible. In the presence of pulmonary hypertension, the pulmonic component of the 2nd heart sound is accentuated. An early diastolic murmur may be caused by associated aortic insufficiency or secondary pulmonary valvular insufficiency.

Electrocardiograms and roentgenograms are normal if the lesion is mild; as the severity increases, prominent and notched P waves and varying degrees of right ventricular hypertrophy become evident. Atrial fibrillation is a common late manifestation. Moderate or severe lesions are associated with roentgenographic signs of left atrial enlargement and prominence of the pulmonary artery and right-sided heart chambers; calcifications may be noted in the region of the mitral valve. Severe obstruction is associated with a redistribution of pulmonary blood flow so that the apices of the lung have greater perfusion (the reverse of normal). Echocardiography shows distinct narrowing of the mitral orifice during diastole and left atrial enlargement, and Doppler can estimate the transmitral pressure gradient. Cardiac catheterization quantitates the diastolic gradient across the mitral valve, allows for the calculation of valve area, and assesses the degree of elevation of pulmonary arterial pressure.

Treatment. Intervention is indicated in patients with clinical signs and hemodynamic evidence of severe obstruction but before the severe manifestations outlined earlier. Surgical valvotomy or balloon catheter mitral valvuloplasty generally yields good results; valve replacement is avoided unless absolutely necessary. Balloon valvuloplasty is indicated for symptomatic, stenotic, pliable, noncalcified valves of patients without atrial arrhythmias or thrombi.

AORTIC INSUFFICIENCY. In chronic rheumatic aortic insufficiency, sclerosis of the aortic valve results in distortion and retraction of the cusps. Regurgitation of blood leads to volume overload with dilatation and hypertrophy of the left ventricle. Combined mitral and aortic insufficiency is more common than aortic involvement alone.

Clinical Manifestations. Symptoms are unusual except in severe aortic insufficiency. The large stroke volume and forceful left ventricular contractions may result in palpitations. Excessive sweating and heat intolerance are related to vasodilation. Dyspnea on exertion can progress to orthopnea and pulmonary edema; angina may be precipitated by heavy exercise. Nocturnal attacks with sweating, tachycardia, chest pain, and hypertension may occur.

The pulse pressure is wide with bounding peripheral pulses. Systolic blood pressure is elevated, and diastolic pressure is lowered. In severe aortic insufficiency, the heart is enlarged, with a left ventricular apical heave. A diastolic thrill may be present. The typical murmur begins immediately with the 2nd heart sound and continues until late in diastole. The murmur is heard over the upper and midleft sternal border with radiation to the apex and the aortic area. Characteristically, it has a high-pitched blowing quality and is easily audible in full expiration with the diaphragm of the stethoscope placed firmly on the chest and the patient leaning forward. A systolic ejection murmur is frequent because of the increased stroke volume. An apical presystolic murmur (**Austin Flint murmur**) resembling that of mitral stenosis is sometimes heard and is a result of the large regurgitant aortic flow in diastole that prevents the mitral valve from opening fully.

Roentgenograms show enlargement of the left ventricle and aorta. The electrocardiogram may be normal, but in advanced cases it reveals signs of left ventricular hypertrophy and strain with prominent P waves. The echocardiogram shows a large left ventricle and diastolic mitral valve flutter or oscillation caused by regurgitant flow hitting the valve leaflets. Doppler studies demonstrate the degree of aortic runoff into the left ventricle. Magnetic resonance angiography (MRA) can be useful in quantitating regurgitant volume. Cardiac catheterization is necessary only when the echocardiographic data are equivocal.

Prognosis and Treatment. Mild and moderate lesions are well tolerated. Many adolescents with severe regurgitation are symptom free and tolerate advanced lesions into the 3rd–4th decades. Unlike mitral insufficiency, aortic insufficiency does not regress. Patients with combined lesions during the episode of acute rheumatic fever may have only aortic involvement 1–2 yr later. Treatment consists of afterload reducers (ACE inhibitors) and prophylaxis against recurrence of acute rheumatic fever and the development of infective endocarditis. Surgical intervention (valve replacement) should be carried out well in advance of the onset of heart failure, pulmonary edema, or angina, when signs of decreasing myocardial performance become evident as manifested by increasing left ventricular dimensions on the echocardiogram. Surgery is considered when early symptoms are present, ST-T wave changes are seen on the electrocardiogram, or evidence of decreasing left ventricular ejection fraction is noted.

TRICUSPID VALVE DISEASE. Primary tricuspid involvement is rare after rheumatic fever. Tricuspid insufficiency is more common secondary to right ventricular dilatation resulting from unrepaired left-sided lesions. The signs produced by tricuspid insufficiency include prominent pulsations of the jugular veins, systolic pulsations of the liver, and a blowing holosystolic murmur at the lower left sternal border that increases in intensity during inspiration. Concomitant signs of mitral or aortic valve disease, with or without atrial fibrillation, are frequent. Signs of tricuspid insufficiency decrease or disappear when heart failure produced by the left-sided lesions is successfully treated. Tricuspid valvuloplasty may be required in rare cases.

PULMONARY VALVE DISEASE. Pulmonary insufficiency usually occurs on a functional basis secondary to pulmonary hypertension and is a late finding with severe mitral stenosis. The murmur (Graham Steell murmur) is similar to that of aortic insufficiency, but peripheral arterial signs (bounding pulses) are absent. The correct diagnosis is confirmed by two-dimensional echocardiography and Doppler studies.

Camara EJ, Neubauer C, Camara GF, et al: Mechanisms of mitral valvar insufficiency in children and adolescents with severe rheumatic heart disease: An echocardiographic study with clinical and epidemiological correlations. *Cardiol Young* 2004;14:527–532.

Cilliers A: Treating acute rheumatic fever. *Br Med J* 2003;327:631–632.

Fesslova V, Bardare M: Rheumatic fever in the 21st century. *Cardiol Young* 2004;14:465; author reply 465–466.

Figueroa FE, Fernandez MS, Valdes P, et al: Prospective comparison of clinical and echocardiographic diagnosis of rheumatic carditis: Long term follow up of patients with subclinical disease. *Heart* 2001;85:407–410.

Griffiths SP, Gersony WM: Acute rheumatic fever in New York City (1969 to 1988): A comparative study of two decades. *J Pediatr* 1990;116:882–887.

Holmes DR, Nishimura RA, Reeder GS: Aortic and mitral balloon valvuloplasty: Emergence of a new percutaneous technique. *Int J Cardiol* 1987;16:227–233.

Narula J, Chandrasekhar Y, Rahimtoola S: Diagnosis of active rheumatic carditis. *Circulation* 1999;100:1576–1581.

Stollerman GH: Rheumatic fever in the 21st century. *Clin Infect Dis* 2001;33:806–814.

Section 6 — Diseases of the Myocardium and Pericardium — Daniel Bernstein

Chapter 439 ■ Diseases of the Myocardium

In most children with congenital heart disease, myocardial function is relatively unimpaired early in life. In some congenital lesions, such as left-to-right shunts, the myocardium may even be functioning at a supranormal level (**high-output state**). Children with unoperated congenital heart disease, however, and those with a previous surgical correction or palliation and residual hemodynamic abnormalities, may experience long-standing volume overload, pressure overload, or chronic hypoxia. These residua can eventually lead to the development of myocardial dysfunction. This is especially true in those patients with systemic right ventricles, particularly as they reach adolescence and young adulthood. Therefore, the preservation of myocardial function is one of the key goals in the medical and surgical management of congenital heart disease.

There are other children with primary diseases of the myocardium, known broadly as the cardiomyopathies. **Cardiomyopathies** can be divided based on etiology (Table 439-1) into **primary** (those resulting from genetic abnormalities of cardiac muscle) and **secondary** (those resulting from infections, endocrine disorders, metabolic and nutritional diseases, neuromuscular diseases, blood diseases, and tumors). Others are classified as **idiopathic;** advances in molecular diagnostics have allowed cardiologists to identify specific causes in many patients who were previously classified as "idiopathic." In some, genetic studies have identified specific gene defects; in others, the polymerase chain reaction (PCR) has been used to detect the presence of viral genome, suggesting previous viral myocarditis. A second useful scheme for classifying cardiomyopathies is based on the predominant structural and functional abnormalities (Table 439-2): **dilated cardiomyopathy** (primarily systolic dysfunction), **hypertrophic cardiomyopathy** (primarily diastolic dysfunction), and **restrictive cardiomyopathy** (primarily diastolic but often combined with systolic dysfunction). The annual incidence is just over 1 per 100,000 children, being greater in males than in

TABLE 439-1. Etiology of Myocardial Disease

FAMILIAL-HEREDITARY
Familial dilated cardiomyopathy
Familial hypertrophic cardiomyopathy
Familial restrictive cardiomyopathy
Isolated noncompaction of the left ventricle
Muscular dystrophies
 Duchenne muscular dystrophy
 Other muscular dystrophies (Becker, limb girdle)
Myotonic dystrophy
Kearns-Sayre syndrome (progressive external ophthalmoplegia)
Friedreich ataxia
Hemochromatosis
Fabry disease
Primary endocardial fibroelastosis
Arrhythmogenic right ventricular dysplasia (familial and nonfamilial)
Noonan syndrome
Barth syndrome

INFECTIOUS
Viral myocarditis: adenovirus, coxsackievirus A and B, HIV, echovirus, rubella, varicella, influenza, mumps, Epstein-Barr virus, measles, poliomyelitis, smallpox vaccine
Rickettsiae: psittacosis, Coxiella, Rocky Mountain spotted fever, typhus
Bacteria: diphtheria, mycoplasma, meningococcus, leptospirosis, Lyme disease, typhoid fever, tuberculosis, streptococcus, listeriosis
Parasites: Chagas disease, toxoplasmosis, *Loa loa*, *Toxocara canis*, schistosomiasis, cysticercosis, echinococcus, trichinosis
Fungi: histoplasmosis, coccidioidomycosis, actinomycosis

METABOLIC, NUTRITIONAL, ENDOCRINE
Mitochondrial fatty acid oxidation disorders
 Carnitine transporter (OCTN2), carnitine palmitoyl transferase-I (CPT-I), carnitine translocase (CACT), carnitine palmitoyl transferase-II (CPT-II), short-chain acyl CoA dehydrogenase (SCAD), very long-chain acyl CoA dehydrogenase (VLCAD), ETF dehydrogenase (ETF-DH), electron transport flavoprotein-α and β (α and β-ETF), short-chain L-3-hydroxyacyl CoA dehydrogenase (SCHAD), mitochondrial trifunctional protein (MTP), long-chain 3-ketoacyl-CoA thiolase (LKAT).*
Pompe disease (Glycogen storage disease)
Mucopolysaccharidosis
Beriberi (thiamine deficiency)
Keshan disease (selenium deficiency)
Kwashiorkor
Hyperthyroidism
Carcinoid
Pheochromocytoma
Hypercholesterolemia
Infant of diabetic mother
Beckwith-Wiedemann syndrome
Sphingolipidoses
Propionic acidemia
3-Methylglutaconic aciduria type II

CONNECTIVE TISSUE–GRANULOMATOUS DISEASE—INFILTRATIVE
Systemic lupus erythematosus (SLE)
Infant of mother with SLE
Scleroderma
Churg-Strauss vasculitis
Rheumatoid arthritis
Rheumatic fever
Sarcoidosis
Amyloidosis
Dermatomyositis
Periarteritis nodosa
Leukemia

DRUGS-TOXINS
Doxorubicin (Adriamycin)
Cyclophosphamide
Chloroquine
Ipecac (Emetine)
Sulfonamides
Mesalezine
Chloramphenicol
Hypersensitivity reaction
Alcohol
Envenomations
Irradiation
Herbal remedy (blue cohosh)

CORONARY ARTERY DISEASE
Kawasaki disease
Medial necrosis
Anomalous left coronary artery from the pulmonary artery (ALCAPA)
Other congenital coronary anomalies (anomalous right coronary, coronary ostial stenosis)

OTHER
Anemia
Sickle cell anemia
Hypereosinophilic syndrome (Löffler syndrome)
Endomyocardial fibrosis
Ischemia-hypoxia
Peripartum cardiomyopathy
Uhl right ventricular anomaly
Histiocytoid (oncocytic, lipidotic) cardiomyopathy
Acute eosinophilic necrotizing myocarditis
Restrictive cardiomyopathy
Chronic tachyarrhythmias

*List of fatty acid oxidation disorders adapted from Shekhawat PS, Matern D, Strauss AW: Fetal fatty acid oxidation disorders, their effect on maternal health and neonatal outcome: Impact of expanded newborn screening on their diagnosis and management. *Pediatr Res* 2005;57:78R–86R.

females and in infants younger than 1 yr. The prevalence of cardiomyopathy in the newborn period is 10/100,000 live births, whereas for all children the prevalence is 36/100,000 for dilated cardiomyopathy and 2/100,000 for hypertrophic and restrictive cardiomyopathy.

439.1 • Dilated Cardiomyopathy

PATHOPHYSIOLOGY. Dilated cardiomyopathy is characterized by varying degrees of dilatation of the ventricles, most prominently the left. A component of compensatory ventricular hypertrophy may also be present, thought to be due to growth factors induced in the myocytes by increased wall stress. The cause in the majority of pediatric cases is unknown (idiopathic dilated cardiomyopathy), but an increasing percentage have either a genetic basis or are the sequelae of viral myocarditis.

In 20–50% of cases, the disease is recognized as **familial.** Autosomal dominant inheritance is most commonly encountered and mutations in several cardiac structural or metabolic genes have been identified (see Table 439-2). In patients with dilated cardiomyopathy associated with **conduction defects,** mutations in the lamin A/C gene have been implicated. X-linked inheritance accounts for 5–10% of cases of familial dilated cardiomyopathy. Mutations in the dystrophin gene, causing the muscular dystrophies, are the most common in this group. Mutations in the gene encoding *tafazzin* are associated with **Barth syndrome** as well as some cases of isolated noncompaction of the left ventricle, a form of dilated cardiomyopathy. Autosomal recessive inheritance has been associated with a mutation in cardiac troponin I.

Mitochondrial myopathies may be due to mutations of enzymes of the electron transport chain or those of fatty acid oxidation, which follow a recessive pattern of inheritance. Some disorders of fatty acid oxidation present with systemic derangements of metabolism (hypoketotic hypoglycemia, acidosis, liver dys-

TABLE 439-2. Cardiomyopathies

	DILATED	HYPERTROPHIC	ARRHYTHMOGENIC RIGHT VENTRICULAR DYSPLASIA	RESTRICTIVE
Prevalence	50/100,000	1/500	Unknown	Unknown
Familial	25–50% AD, AR, X-L, Mt	50% AD	30% AD, rare AR (Naxos disease)	Unknown
Genes	AD: cardiac actin, desmin, δ-sarcoglycan, β-myosin heavy chain, cardiac troponin C and T, α-tropomyosin, titin, metavinculin, myosin-binding protein C, muscle LIM protein, α-actinin-2, phospholamban, cypher/LIM binding domain 3, α-myosin heavy chain, SUR2A (regulatory subunit of K_{ATP} channel), lamin A/C X-linked: dystrophin, tafazzin AR: troponin I	β-myosin heavy chain, troponin T or I, α-tropomyosin, myosin-binding protein C, myosin light chain 1 or 2, titin, PRKAG2, 2 α-galactosidase	Plakoglobin, desmoplakin, ryanodine receptor	Cardiac troponin I Desminopathies (α-B-crystallin)
Sudden death	Yes	Depends on gene 0.7–11%/yr, associated with exercise	Yes	1.5%/yr
Arrhythmias	Atrial, ventricular, and conduction disturbances	Atrial and ventricular	Ventricular and conduction disturbances	Atrial fibrillation
Ventricular function	Systolic and diastolic dysfunction	Diastolic dysfunction Dynamic systolic outflow obstruction	Normal to reduced systolic function Reduced diastolic function	Severely reduced diastolic function Normal to reduced systolic function
Diagnosis	Dilated left ventricular cavity with normal to thin wall thickness	Asymmetric, concentric or apical left ventricular hypertrophy	Right ventricular fibrofatty replacement on MRI or biopsy, right ventricular dilatation	Normal or small ventricular cavity size, marked biatrial enlargement
Medical Management	ACE inhibitors Diuretics (Lasix, Spironolactone) Digitalis β2-Blocking agents	Propranolol Pacemaker	β2-Blocking agents Class III antiarrhythmic agents	Antiarrhythmic agents Careful use of diuretics, milrinone
Surgical and Interventional Management	ICD, resynchronization biventricular pacing Transplantation	ICD Septal myomyectomy alcohol ablation (in adults) Transplantation	Catheter ablation ICD Transplantation	ICD Transplantation

ACE, angiotensin-converting enzyme; AD, autosomal dominant inheritance; AR, autosomal recessive inheritance; ICD, implantable cardioverter-defibrillator; Mt, mitochondrial inheritance; X-L, X-linked inheritance.

function), some with peripheral myopathy and neuropathy, and others with sudden death, mistakenly attributed to sudden infant death syndrome (SIDS). If the mother is heterozygous for the enzyme defect, complications can occur during the pregnancy, including intrauterine growth restriction in the fetus and preeclampsia, acute fatty liver of pregnancy (AFLP), or the combination of hemolysis, elevated liver enzymes, and low platelets (HELLP syndrome) in the mother (see Chapter 86).

Prior **viral myocarditis** is a leading cause of dilated cardiomyopathy. Because viral titers are usually nondiagnostic, in most cases (often previously classified as idiopathic), viral genome is detected in an endomyocardial biopsy sample using the polymerase chain reaction (PCR). A remote history of viral illness may be elicited. Active myocarditis is identified in only a minority (2–15%) of patients.

Patients with dilated cardiomyopathy may have infectious causes other than viral infection, endocrine disorders such as hypothyroidism, metabolic disorders such as storage disease, nutritional deficiency, exposure to cardiotoxic agents such as doxorubicin, and systemic disorders such as connective tissue disease. Specific cardiac causes of dilated cardiomyopathy include congenital and acquired (Kawasaki disease) abnormalities of the coronary arteries, tachyarrhythmias, and familial hypercholesterolemia.

CLINICAL MANIFESTATIONS. All age groups may be affected. Usually, the onset is insidious, but sometimes symptoms of heart failure occur suddenly. Irritability, anorexia, abdominal pain, cough from pulmonary congestion, and dyspnea with exertion are common. Infants and younger children tend to have respiratory symptoms and failure to thrive, whereas older children and adolescents often initially have primarily abdominal complaints such as nausea and anorexia. Although the typical sign of pulmonary edema is the presence of rales, younger infants can exhibit wheezing. When the disease is fully established, the skin is cool and pale, the arterial pulse is decreased, pulse pressure is narrow, and tachycardia is present. Jugular venous pressure is increased, and hepatomegaly and edema are common. The heart is enlarged, and holosystolic murmurs of mitral and tricuspid insufficiency may be present. A summation gallop rhythm is usually audible.

In the newborn period, systemic involvement (hypoglycemia, acidosis, liver failure) suggests the presence of an inborn error of metabolism. In older patients, peripheral muscle involvement suggests either one of the muscular dystrophies or a mitochondrial disorder. A family history of unexplained heart failure, sudden death, or SIDS suggests a genetic/metabolic disorder.

DIAGNOSIS. The electrocardiogram shows a combination of atrial enlargement, varying degrees of left or right ventricular hypertrophy, and nonspecific T-wave abnormalities. The chest roentgenogram confirms the presence of cardiomegaly and allows evaluation of the degree of pulmonary congestion and the presence of pleural effusions. Often, the initial diagnosis of dilated cardiomyopathy is suspected when a chest roentgenogram is performed on a child with respiratory distress to evaluate a suspected pneumonia. The echocardiogram is diagnostic and shows dilatation of the left atrium and ventricle and poor contractility (Fig. 439-1). The right ventricle may also be affected. Doppler studies show decreased flow velocity through the aortic valve and mitral regurgitation. In long-standing cases, evidence of pulmonary hypertension may exist.

Myocardial biopsy early in the disease process may be useful; a specific cause is rarely found when biopsy samples are obtained after long-standing disease, in which case the histologic findings consist mainly of areas of fibrosis and compensatory hypertrophy. Viral origin of many of these "idiopathic" cases may be detected with PCR. A complete family history is important, and unless a viral diagnosis is confirmed, 1st-degree family members should be screened for subclinical cardiomyopathy by echocar-

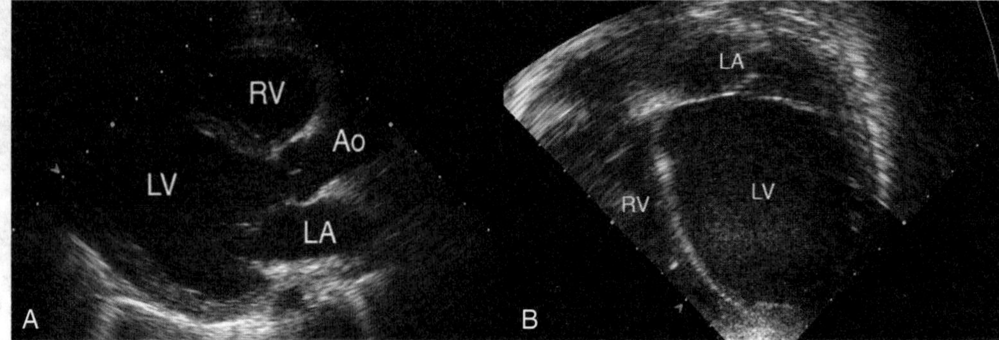

Figure 439-1. Echocardiogram of a patient with dilated cardiomyopathy. *A*, Parasternal long-axis view showing the enlarged left ventricle. *B*, Apical four-chamber view showing the large left ventricle compressing the right ventricle. Ao, ascending aorta; LA, left atrium; LV, left ventricle; RV, right ventricle.

diography. Siblings with normal echocardiograms should undergo repeat studies at regular intervals as the time of presentation of ventricular dysfunction may vary considerably even in a single family. DNA studies on both affected and nonaffected family members may help determine the specific gene defect. Newborn screening using tandem mass spectrometry is available for the detection of the mitochondrial disorders of fatty acid oxidation.

PROGNOSIS AND MANAGEMENT. The course of the disease is usually progressively downhill, although some patients may remain stable for years. Vigorous treatment of heart failure (see Chapter 442) may result in temporary remission, but relapses are common and, in time, patients tend to become resistant to therapy. Once this point is reached, the prognosis for survival beyond a year is poor. Serious complications include ventricular arrhythmias leading to syncope and sudden death, pulmonary or systemic emboli from intracardiac thrombi, and the development of pulmonary vascular disease from chronically elevated left atrial pressure. Patients with severely depressed myocardial function should be monitored closely for arrhythmias and, if present, treated aggressively with antiarrhythmic agents or an implantable cardioverter-defibrillator (ICD). They should also receive systemic anticoagulation, preferably with warfarin. The use of β-adrenergic blocking agents such as metoprolol and carvedilol in adults with cardiomyopathy has resulted in improvement in exercise capacity and a reduction in hospitalization and mortality. The initial experience with these drugs in children is encouraging. A trial of oral carnitine (100–200 mg/kg/day) may be worthwhile while awaiting the results of definitive metabolic screening tests. When medical therapy fails, heart transplantation is very effective in infants and children with dilated cardiomyopathy (see Chapter 443.1). Because of the scarcity of pediatric donor organs, patients with cardiomyopathy should be referred to a pediatric heart transplant center for an initial evaluation early in the course of their disease.

NEUROMUSCULAR DISEASES. Heart disease is common in patients with Friedreich ataxia (see Chapter 597.1), which chiefly affects the left ventricle and results in a dilated or restrictive cardiomyopathy. In some patients, exercise intolerance, chest pain, and heart failure have been the initial symptoms. Arrhythmias may also occur and consist of atrial tachycardia, fibrillation, or extrasystoles. In Duchenne muscular dystrophy (see Chapter 608.1), at least 50% of children have postmortem evidence of myocardial involvement similar to that of the striated muscle. Cardiac symptoms were previously overshadowed by peripheral muscular and pulmonary problems; with recent improvements in pulmonary support, more patients are being identified with cardiac failure. Separating disability caused by cardiac failure from that caused by peripheral muscle or pulmonary complications can be difficult. The electrocardiogram may reveal tachycardia, abnormalities in P waves, a short P-R interval, and abnormal Q and T waves. Minimal evidence of right or left ventricular hypertrophy may also be noted. In the less severe forms of muscular dystrophy (Becker dystrophy), cardiac involvement may be more prominent and the primary cause of exercise intolerance and respiratory symptoms. Other X chromosome linked dilated cardiomyopathies have been described without associated skeletal muscle involvement. Some limited experience with heart transplantation exists in patients with the milder Becker dystrophy.

KAWASAKI DISEASE (SEE CHAPTER 165). The arteritis associated with Kawasaki disease initially involves small arterioles, but in the 2nd and 3rd wk of illness, medium-sized arteries become inflamed and aneurysmal dilatation of the coronary arteries may occur. During the healing phase, areas of both coronary dilatation and stenosis may result and can lead to future myocardial infarction and death. Myocarditis is a less common sequela of Kawasaki disease but, when present, is manifested as heart failure early in the course.

AUTOIMMUNE DISEASES. Rheumatic carditis is described in Chapters 156 and 438. The cardiovascular manifestations of juvenile rheumatoid arthritis, systemic lupus erythematosus, periarteritis nodosa, dermatomyositis, and scleroderma are described in Chapters 157–159. Infants born to mothers with autoimmune disease such as systemic lupus erythematosus can develop a cardiomyopathy, usually associated with persistence of anti-Ro and anti-La antibodies.

ENDOCRINE DISORDERS. **Hyperthyroidism** (see Chapter 569) produces tachycardia, vasodilation, a wide pulse pressure, cardiac enlargement, and, occasionally, atrial fibrillation. **Hypothyroidism** can produce cardiac dysfunction in adults but seldom produces gross cardiac involvement in children. The electrocardiogram is characterized by bradycardia, low voltage of all complexes (especially the P and T waves), left axis deviation, and prolonged electrical systole. These signs usually disappear within 1 mo after initiation of adequate thyroid therapy. Diabetic cardiomyopathy is rare in children; however, infants of diabetic mothers can experience cardiac hypertrophy and dilatation. Cardiomyopathy may be caused by chronic exposure to elevated catecholamines in patients with pheochromocytoma.

METABOLIC AND NUTRITIONAL DISEASES. Among the vitamin deficiency diseases, **beriberi** (see Chapter 46) causes the most conspicuous cardiac damage. In patients with malnutrition such as

kwashiorkor, the deficiencies are often multiple, and it may be difficult to separate the cardiac lesion of one nutritional disease from that of another (see Chapter 43). Other nutritional and metabolic causes of cardiac dysfunction include **selenium** (see Chapter 51), taurine, and carnitine deficiencies (see Chapter 86.1). In children suffering from malabsorption because of their primary illness, nutritional cardiomyopathies may develop as well.

HEMATOLOGIC DISEASES. In infants and children, severe anemia may be associated with cardiac involvement. Although cardiac output increases when the hemoglobin content is less than about 7 g/dL, significant cardiac enlargement occurs with an extreme reduction in hemoglobin (≤3–4 g). The heart rate is rapid, pulse pressure is widened, and venous pressure is increased. A systolic flow murmur at the apex or along the left sternal border is usual; diastolic murmurs may occur in the same areas, and a gallop rhythm is also common. Electrocardiographic changes include depressed ST segments and flat T waves. In patients with congenital heart lesions, anemia can place extra stress on the heart's ability to maintain adequate oxygen delivery and can result in considerable worsening of heart failure symptoms. Treatment is directed toward the cause of the anemia. If blood transfusions are indicated in the presence of cardiomegaly or heart failure, only small volumes (5 mL/kg) of packed red blood cells should be administered at any one time and followed by a dose of diuretic (see Chapter 470). Sometimes, exchange transfusion may be prudent to avoid an acute increase in blood volume.

DISORDERS OF THE CORONARY ARTERIES. Anomalous origin of the left coronary artery from the pulmonary artery is one of the major causes of myocardial ischemia in infants (see Chapter 432.2). Anomalous origin of one of the coronaries from the aorta may result in its course running between the aorta and pulmonary artery ("suicide coronary") and lead to myocardial ischemia and infarction with exercise. Coronary calcinosis is a rare disorder in infants and children in which the coronary arteries are tortuous and calcareous. Other blood vessels may be similarly involved. The onset of cardiac failure is sudden; death usually occurs in infancy. Rare coronary artery malformations include coronary ostial stenosis and coronary artery stenosis in the setting of supravalvular aortic stenosis (see Chapter 427.5). Patients with homozygous familial hypercholesterolemia may have a propensity for coronary atherosclerosis at an early age. Patients who have undergone heart transplantation are at risk for the development of graft coronary artery disease (see Chapter 443.1).

DOXORUBICIN (ADRIAMYCIN) CARDIOTOXICITY. This chemotherapeutic agent can occasionally cause acute myocarditis but more often results in chronic dilated cardiomyopathy. The most common manifestation is a severe, chronic, dose-dependent cardiomyopathy, which occurs in about 30% of patients when the total cumulative dose exceeds 550 mg/m^2 but may be seen occasionally in patients after doses as low as 200 mg/m^2. One study has shown abnormalities in the echocardiographic indices of left ventricular function (wall stress) in as many as 65% of children receiving doses >220 mg/m^2. When radiation therapy is combined with doxorubicin, the risk of cardiac damage is even greater.

Cardiomyopathy may become manifest months or even years after doxorubicin treatment. Cardiomegaly is principally due to left ventricular and left atrial enlargement. T-wave flattening or inversion is nonspecific evidence of cardiac involvement. Acute electrocardiographic changes, including a long Q-T interval, may be present in 40% of patients immediately after a single dose. Early changes in cardiac function, even in the absence of symptoms, may be detected by serial echocardiograms or radionuclide (MUGA [multigated acquisition]) scans, but no method is totally able to predict which patients are at risk. The child's condition may remain clinically stable for many years, even with decreased fractional shortening. Once symptoms of heart failure develop, the case fatality rate is as high as 30–50%. Cardiac transplantation has been used with success in these patients (see Chapter 443.1).

Acute doxorubicin myocarditis is less common and typically occurs in the course of administration of the drug. It is frequently reversible, and the long-term prognosis may be somewhat better. Supportive treatment consists of anticongestive medications such as digoxin, diuretics, and afterload-reducing agents.

IPECAC CARDIAC TOXICITY. Cardiac toxicity can occur with chronic intentional ipecac abuse secondary to anorexia nervosa or bulimia nervosa. Manifestations include chest pain, tachycardia, dyspnea, hypotension, arrhythmias, flattening and inversion of T waves, ST segment abnormalities, prolongation of the Q-T and P-R intervals, cardiac failure, and, potentially, death. Differentiating the cardiac abnormalities caused by ipecac from those of chronic starvation, abnormal diets, and electrolyte abnormalities may be difficult.

439.2 • Hypertrophic Cardiomyopathy

PATHOPHYSIOLOGY. Hypertrophic cardiomyopathies in children may be either primary, due to a mutation in one of several genes that encode protein components of the sarcomere, or secondary, due to the sequelae of obstructive congenital heart disease (critical aortic stenosis, coarctation of the aorta) or to an inborn error of metabolism (glycogen storage disease or mucopolysaccharidosis). Familial or primary hypertrophic cardiomyopathy is the most common genetic cardiovascular disorder, occurring in ≈1/500 individuals.

In primary hypertrophic cardiomyopathy, abnormal ventricular hypertrophy of varying degrees characterizes the disease, and may be encountered in several anatomic variations. Most commonly the ventricular septum is disproportionately involved compared to the left ventricular free wall, also referred to as hypertrophic obstructive cardiomyopathy (HOCM), idiopathic hypertrophic subaortic stenosis (IHSS), or asymmetric septal hypertrophy (ASH). Many patients have concentric left ventricular hypertrophy; a less common variant affects predominantly the left ventricular apex. Some children, particularly infants, may have involvement of both left and right ventricles. The mitral valve is displaced anteriorly by hypertrophy of the papillary muscles, and the left ventricular cavity is distorted by the massive generalized hypertrophy. Varying degrees of myocardial fibrosis may be present. Microscopically, patchy areas of abnormally thick and short muscle fibers are arranged in circular collections and interspersed among normal as well as hypertrophied muscle fibers. Electron microscopy shows a disarray of myofibrils and myofilaments.

The hypertrophic and fibrosed muscle has **decreased distensibility (compliance)**, so resistance to left ventricular filling occurs; systolic pumping function remains intact (or may even be hyperdynamic) until late in the course of the disease. Obstruction to left ventricular outflow develops in 25% of patients. Varying degrees of mitral valve insufficiency are also common.

EPIDEMIOLOGY AND GENETICS. Hypertrophic cardiomyopathy is most often inherited in an autosomal dominant pattern with wide variability in penetrance; many cases represent de novo mutations. Manifestations can begin at any age. Siblings of the proband may not be affected as children but may show evidence of the disease as they reach adolescence and adulthood. Mutations in 10 genes have been implicated to date, all of which encode proteins of the cardiac sarcomere, either components of the thick or thin fibers or associated regulatory subunits. Mutations of the genes encoding cardiac β-myosin heavy-chain and myosin-binding protein C are the most common (see Table 439-2). Other known mutations of sarcomeric genes include the genes encoding cardiac troponin T and I, α-tropomyosin, regulatory and essential myosin light chains, titin, and α-myosin heavy chain. Non-sarcomeric protein mutations include γ-2-regulatory subunit of AMP-activated protein kinase (PRKAG2) and the lysosome-associated membrane protein 2α-galactosidase, which is responsible for Danon disease, a form of glycogen storage disease. Over 200 mutations have been identified in the 10 most common genes and some patients may carry mutations in more than one gene. Genetic testing is available and, in combination with family history, may help predict which patients are more likely to have arrhythmias and sudden death.

When diagnosed in early childhood (early-onset disease), hypertrophic cardiomyopathy is associated with more severe heart failure and increased mortality. In contrast, many patients with proven gene mutations will have normal echocardiograms in childhood, only to first manifest signs of hypertrophy in mid to late adolescence. Some patients will not show signs of hypertrophy until middle age (late-onset disease).

CLINICAL MANIFESTATIONS. Many children are asymptomatic and ≈50% of cases are first evaluated because of a heart murmur or because another family member has come to medical attention. In symptomatic children, the clinical pattern is dominated by weakness, fatigue, dyspnea on effort, palpitations, angina pectoris, dizziness, and syncope. Even asymptomatic children are at risk of sudden death. The pulse can be brisk because of the early systolic ejection of blood from the ventricle. A prominent left ventricular lift and double apical impulse may be noted. The 1st and 2nd heart sounds are usually normal. The rarity of systolic ejection clicks helps differentiate hypertrophic cardiomyopathy from valvular aortic stenosis. The systolic murmur is ejection in type and of medium intensity; it is heard maximally at the left sternal edge and apex. The murmur may increase shortly after exercise is discontinued, during the **Valsalva maneuver,** or on assumption of the erect position.

DIAGNOSIS. The electrocardiogram (ECG) shows left ventricular hypertrophy with variable degrees of ST segment depression and T-wave inversion. ECG changes may predate echocardiographic findings. Signs of the **Wolff-Parkinson-White syndrome** and other intraventricular conduction defects may be present. Roentgenograms demonstrate mild cardiomegaly with prominence of the left ventricle. The echocardiogram shows left ventricular hypertrophy that is asymmetric, concentric, or apical (Fig. 439-2). There is usually systolic anterior motion of the anterior leaflet of the mitral valve. Doppler studies demonstrate the presence of a left ventricular outflow tract gradient, which usually occurs in mid to late systole, when the muscular obstruction to outflow is maximal. Doppler flow studies may demonstrate diastolic dysfunction before the development of hypertrophy.

Echocardiography has replaced cardiac catheterization for initial diagnosis, although catheterization can be useful in assessing a patient's candidacy for surgery. Many patients who do not have a left ventricular outflow tract gradient at rest may acquire a significant gradient after the administration of isoproterenol, amyl nitrite, or nitroglycerin. Left ventriculography shows encroachment on the left ventricular cavity by the hypertrophied muscle, especially by the interventricular septum. Midsystolic cavity obliteration occurs in more severe cases. Mitral insufficiency is common. A discrete subaortic obstruction with secondary muscular hypertrophy should be ruled out because surgical management of discrete subaortic stenosis is much more effective (see Chapter 427.5).

The prognosis of hypertrophic cardiomyopathy in an individual patient is unpredictable. Asymptomatic patients may remain stable for years. Some patients progress to chronic heart failure, whereas others are at risk for sudden death from arrhythmia. The clinical course of other affected family members and the results of genetic testing may be of some use in stratifying risk in an affected child.

TREATMENT. No standardized therapy has been established that definitively protects patients from the risk of sudden death. Competitive sports and strenuous physical activity should be prohibited because most sudden deaths occur during or immediately after vigorous physical exertion, especially in adolescents and young adults. Digitalis or aggressive diuresis is **contraindicated** in most patients because of the potential to increase left ventricular outflow obstruction. Infusion of isoproterenol or other inotropic agents should also be avoided other than for diagnostic purposes in the controlled environment of the catheterization laboratory. β-Adrenergic blocking agents (propranolol) and calcium channel blocking agents (verapamil, nifedipine) are used with some success in decreasing the degree of outflow obstruction and may slow the development of ventricular hypertrophy; these drugs do not necessarily affect the long-term prognosis and have not been shown to reduce the incidence of sudden death. Calcium channel blockers should not be used during infancy because of the increased risk of cardiovascular collapse. Patients with documented arrhythmias or a history of unexplained syncope should be treated aggressively, usually with an **implantable cardioverter-defibrillator (ICD).** Pacemakers have been used to alter septal depolarization in some patients, although this modality is less effective in reducing outflow gradients and is generally reserved for older adults who are high surgical risks. **Surgery treatment,**

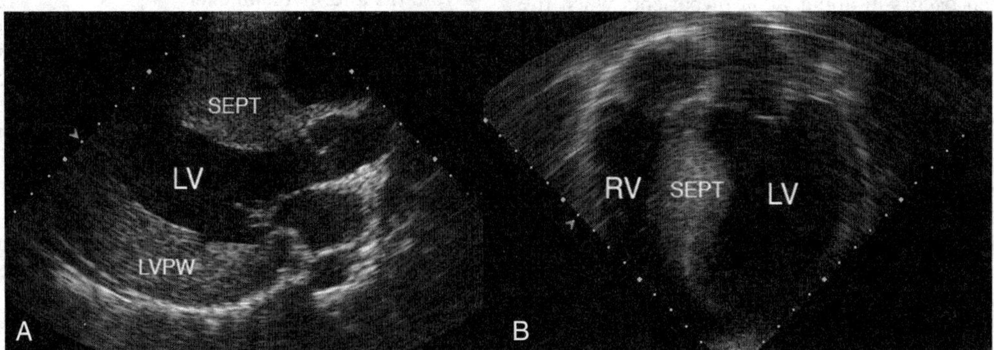

Figure 439-2. Echocardiograms demonstrating hypertrophic cardiomyopathy. *A,* Parasternal long-axis view of a patient with severe concentric left ventricular hypertrophy. *B,* Four-chamber view of a patient with asymmetric septal hypertrophy. LV, left ventricle; LVPW, left ventricular posterior wall; RV, right ventricle; SEPT, septum.

performing a ventricular **septal myotomy,** has been employed in a subgroup of patients with disabling angina or syncope associated with left ventricular outflow tract obstruction (resting or provoked gradient of ≥50 mm Hg). Although surgical reduction of the outflow tract gradient may improve symptoms, it has not been shown to reduce the risk of sudden death. Rarely, mitral valve replacement may be needed if the obstruction cannot be alleviated. In adults, some centers perform ventricular septal ablation procedures, in which the coronary artery branch supplying the hypertrophied septum is injected with alcohol. This procedure has not been utilized in children.

When a positive family history is elicited, screening consists of an ECG and echocardiogram. These are repeated every few years in children <12 yr of age, then yearly between the ages of 12 and 18–21, which is the time of greatest risk of disease. Afterwards, screening can be performed every 5 yr or at more frequent intervals if the family history suggests a particularly malignant phenotype. Genetic testing is available in a few laboratories and will be a useful adjunct to these clinical studies; however, up to 20% of cases of hypertrophic cardiomyopathy will not demonstrate mutations in the commonly tested panel of genes.

HYPERTROPHIC CARDIOMYOPATHY IN INFANTS OF DIABETIC MOTHERS. In infants of diabetic mothers, a transient form of hypertrophic cardiomyopathy may be encountered with or without left ventricular outflow tract obstruction. The increased left ventricular mass usually regresses within several months (see Chapter 107.1).

CORTICOSTEROIDS IN PREMATURE INFANTS. Premature infants who are receiving corticosteroids for chronic lung disease may also experience transient hypertrophic cardiomyopathy, which usually resolves rapidly with cessation of steroid therapy, although it may recur if steroids are reintroduced.

GLYCOGEN STORAGE DISEASE. Cardiac as well as skeletal muscles are affected in the generalized form of glycogen storage disease known as type II or Pompe disease (see Chapter 87.1). The cardiomegaly is massive, but murmurs are insignificant. Pulmonary atelectasis with secondary infection is common and related to compression by the enlarged heart. The electrocardiogram is characteristic and shows prominent P waves, a short P-R interval, massive QRS voltage, signs of isolated left or biventricular hypertrophy, and intraventricular conduction delays. Roentgenograms confirm the striking cardiomegaly with prominence of the left ventricle. The echocardiogram shows severe ventricular hypertrophy. The prognosis is poor. Recombinant enzyme replacement therapy holds some promise to improve the outcome.

439.3 • Restrictive Cardiomyopathy

Poor ventricular compliance is the major abnormality in restrictive cardiomyopathies, and inadequate filling of the ventricular cavities occurs during diastole and results in clinical manifestations that closely simulate those of constrictive pericarditis (see Chapter 440). Systolic function may be maintained until later in the course of the disease. Restrictive cardiomyopathy results in dyspnea, edema, ascites, hepatomegaly, increased venous pressure, and pulmonary congestion. Because of the high left atrial filling pressures, these patients are at risk of developing pulmonary vascular disease, often quite rapidly after diagnosis. The heart is only mildly or moderately enlarged and murmurs are nonspecific. If pulmonary hypertension exists, the pulmonic component of the second heart sound is loud. The electrocardiogram shows markedly prominent P waves, often normal QRS voltage, ST segment depression, and T-wave inversion. Roentgenographic examination shows mild to moderate cardiomegaly. The echocardiogram shows markedly enlarged atria (which may be two- to threefold larger than the ventricles) and small to normal-sized ventricles with often preserved systolic function but highly abnormal filling characteristics by Doppler echocardiography (Fig. 439-3). Differential diagnosis from constrictive pericarditis is critical, though difficult, because the latter can be treated surgically. MRI scan is useful in diagnosing a thickened pericardium in this later condition. Restrictive cardiomyopathy may be **idiopathic,** or it may be associated with a **systemic disease** such as scleroderma, amyloidosis, or sarcoidosis; an inborn error of metabolism (**mucopolysaccharidosis**); hypereosinophilic syndrome; malignancies; or radiation therapy. It may also result from a congenital abnormality such as isolated **noncompaction of the left ventricular myocardium.** The prognosis for restrictive cardiomyopathy is poor, and clinical deterioration can be rapid. **Treatment** is directed toward relief of heart failure, although these patients may show a poor response to standard heart failure management (see Chapter 442). Diuretics, used judiciously, can relieve fluid retention early in the course of the disease. Antiarrhythmic agents are used as required, and anticoagulation with aspirin or warfarin is indicated for lesions such as noncompaction with an increased risk of mural thrombosis and stroke. Cardiac transplantation has been used effectively in patients with restrictive cardiomyopathy as long as multiple organ involvement from systemic disease is not present. Referral to a transplant center should be considered immediately once a diagnosis of restrictive cardiomyopathy is made, as these patients can develop rapidly progressive pulmonary vascular disease or clinical deterioration.

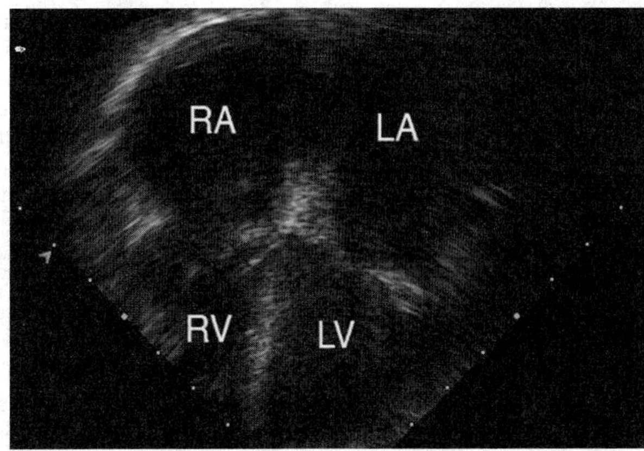

Figure 439-3. Echocardiogram of a patient with restrictive cardiomyopathy. The apical four-chamber view shows the markedly enlarged right and left atria, compared to the normal sized left and right ventricular chambers. LA, left atrium; LV, left ventricle; RA, right atrium; RV, right ventricle.

LÖFFLER HYPEREOSINOPHILIC SYNDROME. This disorder produces severe multisystem dysfunction (skin, lungs, nervous system, liver), and the predominant cause of death is restrictive cardiomyopathy with endocardial fibrosis of the mitral and tricuspid valves and the right and left ventricles. The subsequent formation of endocardial thrombi results in embolization. Löffler syndrome should be distinguished from nonrestrictive, nonfibrotic acute eosinophilic necrotizing myocarditis, an acute rapidly fatal illness, and from **hypersensitivity myocarditis** (characterized by fever, rash, tachycardia, eosinophilia, drug allergy, and arrhythmias). Steroids and cytotoxic agents may be beneficial in the hypereosinophilic syndromes. Anticoagulant therapy may reduce the incidence of thromboembolism.

MUCOPOLYSACCHARIDOSIS. In these disorders most commonly Hurler syndrome, mucopolysaccharides accumulate in many organs, including the heart and great vessels (see Chapter 88). The most pronounced lesions are found in the valves and coronary arteries, but abnormalities in the pericardium and aorta are not uncommon. The heart may be moderately enlarged, with electrocardiographic signs of left ventricular hypertrophy. Cardiac murmurs may result from insufficiency and stenosis of the mitral and aortic valves. Sometimes the pulmonary and tricuspid valves are also involved. Coronary arterial disease may result in angina, which perhaps explains the frequent occurrence of sudden death. The prognosis is poor.

ISOLATED NONCOMPACTION OF THE LEFT VENTRICLE. This cardiomyopathy of unknown cause results in elements of both left ventricular dilatation and restriction. The condition may be diagnosed at any age, from infancy to young adulthood, and the severity of heart failure varies. The echocardiogram is diagnostic and shows a specific pattern of left ventricular hypertrophy with deep muscular crypts. Patients may be at risk for ventricular arrhythmias and sudden death, as well as mural thromboses and stroke. Although some patients may remain stable for years, others may deteriorate rapidly. Cardiac transplantation has been used successfully in this group of patients.

439.4 • Myocarditis

Myocarditis refers to inflammation, necrosis, or myocytolysis and may be caused by many infectious, connective tissue, granulomatous, toxic, or idiopathic processes affecting the myocardium with or without associated systemic manifestations of the disease process or involvement of the endocardium or pericardium (see Table 439-1). Coronary pathology is uniformly absent. The most common manifestation is heart failure, although arrhythmias and sudden death may be the 1st detectable signs. Viral infections are the most common cause.

ETIOLOGY AND EPIDEMIOLOGY. The true incidence of viral myocarditis in children is unknown because many mild cases go undetected. Viral myocarditis is typically a sporadic, but occasionally an epidemic illness. Its manifestations are to some degree age dependent: in early infancy, viral myocarditis often occurs as an acute, fulminant disease; in toddlers and young children, it occurs as an acute, but less fulminant myopericarditis; and in older children and adolescents, it is often asymptomatic and comes to clinical attention primarily as a precursor to idiopathic dilated cardiomyopathy. The most common causative agents in children are adenovirus, coxsackievirus B, and other enteroviruses, although most known viral agents have been implicated.

PATHOPHYSIOLOGY. Acute viral myocarditis may produce a fulminant inflammatory process characterized by cellular infiltrates, cell degeneration and necrosis, and subsequent fibrosis. Viral myocarditis may also become a chronic process with persistence of viral RNA or DNA (but not infectious virus particles) in the myocardium. Chronic inflammation is then perpetuated by the host immune response, which includes T lymphocytes activated against viral-host antigenic alterations. Such cytotoxic lymphocytes and natural killer cells, together with persistent and possibly defective viral replication, may impair myocyte function without obvious cytolysis. Alternatively, the persistent viral infection may alter the expression of major histocompatibility complex antigens, with resultant exposure of neoantigens to the immune system. In addition, some viral proteins may share antigenic epitopes with host cells, which results in autoimmune damage to the antigenically related myocyte. Cytokines such as tumor necrosis factor-α and interleukin 1 may be released and participate in initiation of the altered immune response. The net final result of chronic viral-associated inflammation is often **dilated cardiomyopathy.**

CLINICAL MANIFESTATIONS. Signs and symptoms depend on the patient's age and the acute or chronic nature of the infection. A neonate may initially have fever, severe heart failure, respiratory distress, cyanosis, distant heart sounds, weak pulses, tachycardia out of proportion to the fever, mitral insufficiency caused by dilatation of the valve annulus, a gallop rhythm, acidosis, and shock. Evidence of viral hepatitis, aseptic meningitis, and an associated rash may be present. In the most fulminant form, death may occur within 1–7 days of the onset of symptoms. The chest roentgenogram demonstrates an enormously enlarged heart and pulmonary edema; the electrocardiogram reveals sinus tachycardia, reduced QRS complex voltage, and ST segment and T-wave abnormalities. Arrhythmias may be the first clinical manifestation and, in the presence of fever and a large heart, strongly suggest acute myocarditis.

An older patient with acute myocarditis may also initially be seen with acute congestive heart failure; however, more commonly, patients have a gradual onset of congestive heart failure or a sudden onset of ventricular arrhythmias. In these patients, the acute infectious phase has usually passed and an idiopathic dilated cardiomyopathy is present (see Chapter 439.1).

DIAGNOSIS. The sedimentation rate, heart enzymes (creatine phosphokinase, lactate dehydrogenase), and brain natriuretic peptide (BNP) may be elevated in acute or chronic myocarditis. If positive, serum viral titers are helpful; negative titers do not eliminate the diagnosis. Paired studies involving PCR of ventricular biopsy and serum samples have shown viral genome routinely present in cardiac samples yet absent in peripheral blood. Echocardiography demonstrates poor ventricular function and often a pericardial effusion, mitral valve regurgitation, and the absence of coronary artery or other congenital heart lesions. Myocarditis can be confirmed by endomyocardial biopsy. Biopsy is performed during cardiac catheterization and can also be used to detect other causes of cardiomyopathy (storage disease, mitochondrial defects). PCR can identify specific viral RNA or DNA.

DIFFERENTIAL DIAGNOSIS. The predominant diseases mimicking acute myocarditis include carnitine deficiency, hereditary mitochondrial defects, idiopathic dilated cardiomyopathy, pericarditis, fibroelastosis of the endocardium, and anomalous origin of the left coronary artery (see Table 439-1).

TREATMENT. The approach to treating acute myocarditis involves supportive measures for severe congestive heart failure or cardiogenic shock (see Chapter 442). Dopamine, epinephrine, and milrinone may be helpful in those with poor cardiac output and systemic hypoperfusion. All inotropic agents, including digoxin, should be used with caution because patients with myocarditis are susceptible to the arrhythmogenic properties of these agents. When used, digoxin is often started at half the normal dosage. Pericardiocentesis should be performed in patients with evidence of cardiac tamponade, and culture of pericardial fluid may yield the offending viral agent. Arrhythmias should be treated aggressively and may require the use of intravenous amiodarone to achieve adequate control. For infants and children in cardiogenic shock, extracorporeal membrane oxygenation (ECMO) may be indicated. Implantation of a left ventricular assist device (LVAD) can be performed, usually as a bridge to heart transplantation, which is the **treatment of choice** in those with refractory heart failure (see Chapter 443.1). The role of specific treatments of viral myocarditis is controversial. Intravenous immunoglobulin (IVIG) has been used at 2 g/kg. Corticosteroids have also been utilized and, in several small series of pediatric patients, treatment with prednisone (2 mg/kg daily, tapered to 0.3 mg/kg daily over a period of 3 mo) was effective in reducing myocardial inflammation and improving cardiac function. Relapse has been noted to occur when immunosuppression is discontinued in some patients. Clinical trials of steroids in adult patients have shown mixed results, however. Specific antiviral therapy for enterovirus (pleconaril) or Epstein-Barr virus (acyclovir) is being evaluated.

PROGNOSIS. The outcome of symptomatic neonates with acute viral myocarditis has been poor. Patients with lesser symptoms have a better prognosis, and complete resolution has been described. The outcome of older patients who have progressed to chronic dilated cardiomyopathy is also poor without therapy. These patients continue to have dilatation, fibrosis, and deteriorating cardiac function. Spontaneous resolution has occurred in various adult studies in 10–50% of patients. As many as 50% of untreated older patients die within 2 yr of diagnosis, however, and 80% within 8 yr without heart transplantation.

439.5 • Nonviral Causes of Myocarditis

BACTERIAL INFECTIONS. In diphtheria (see Chapter 186), the toxin of the bacillus may produce peripheral circulatory failure or toxic myocarditis within the 1st 2 wk of the disease. In addition to therapy for diphtheria, treatment of cardiogenic shock is essential. Diphtheritic toxic myocarditis is characterized by the development of atrioventricular block, bundle branch block, or extrasystoles. Heart failure occurs later and is associated with cardiac enlargement and a gallop rhythm. In addition to the arrhythmia, the electrocardiogram shows ST segment depression and T-wave inversion in most leads. The immediate prognosis is grave (about 50% mortality). Treatment includes strict bed rest until all signs of myocarditis have disappeared, as well as management of fluid retention and arrhythmias, including cardiac pacing.

In many systemic bacterial infections, circulatory involvement is manifested as peripheral circulatory collapse or toxic myocarditis. Toxic myocarditis, as evidenced by tachycardia, a gallop rhythm, and cardiac enlargement, may complicate pneumonia, infective endocarditis, and septicemia. A myocardial depressant factor may produce an acute toxic cardiomyopathy. The prognosis depends on the ability to control the primary infection.

RICKETTSIAL DISEASES. Rocky Mountain spotted fever (see Chapter 225.1) may be complicated by hypotension and peripheral vascular collapse. This complication has been attributed to the general vasculitis characteristic of the disease, but acute myocarditis may be a contributing factor.

PARASITIC AND FUNGAL INFECTIONS. Lesions in the myocardium have been described in association with histoplasmosis, coccidioidomycosis, toxoplasmosis, and trichinosis. In these conditions, the cardiac lesion seldom produces clinical signs of myocarditis. Actinomycosis may involve the pericardium and myocardium by direct contiguity to a pulmonary abscess. Hydatid cysts of the pericardium may be found on routine roentgenograms of the chest and usually produce symptoms only when they rupture. Schistosomiasis may result in pulmonary hypertension and cor pulmonale. Cruz trypanosomiasis (Chagas disease) may produce either acute or subacute myocarditis and is a leading cause of chronic dilated cardiomyopathy in Central and South America.

439.6 • Endocardial Fibroelastosis

Endocardial fibroelastosis (EFE) has been called fetal endocarditis, endocardial fibrosis, prenatal fibroelastosis, elastic tissue hyperplasia, and endocardial sclerosis. In primary EFE, no apparent predisposing valvular lesion or other congenital heart abnormality can be found. In secondary EFE, severe congenital heart disease of the left-sided obstructive type (aortic stenosis or atresia, forms of hypoplastic left heart syndrome, or severe coarctation of the aorta) is present. In secondary EFE, the ventricular cavity is often contracted, whereas with primary disease, a dilated left ventricular chamber is seen, usually during infancy. In young adults, however, a contracted form of primary EFE has been observed. No cause for primary EFE has been firmly established, although an association with mumps infection has been implied through analysis of affected myocardial specimens by PCR.

Pathologically, a white, opaque fibroelastic thickening of the endocardium is present, usually in the left ventricle, and it frequently obscures the trabeculation of the inner surfaces of the cardiac chamber. The lesion may spread to involve the valves. Microscopically, the lesion consists of fibroelastic thickening of the endocardium and may result in subendocardial degeneration or necrosis of muscle with vacuolation of muscle fibers. The involved valve leaflets are characterized by myxomatous proliferation with an increase in collagenous elements.

The clinical manifestations are variable. Infants, usually those younger than 6 mo who had apparently been in good health, experience severe congestive heart failure, often precipitated by a respiratory infection. Affected infants may manifest dyspnea, cough, anorexia, hepatomegaly, edema, failure to thrive, and recurrent pulmonary infections. Chronic heart failure can be controlled for some time by digitalis and diuretics; however, most patients eventually succumb. Infants in whom valvular lesions or associated congenital cardiovascular defects are predominant usually expire in the 1st mo of life. Roentgenograms confirm significant cardiac enlargement (Fig. 439-4). The electrocardiogram is abnormal, with changes indicative of left atrial and left ventricular hypertrophy with strain. The echocardiogram shows a bright-appearing endocardial surface and a dilated, poorly func-

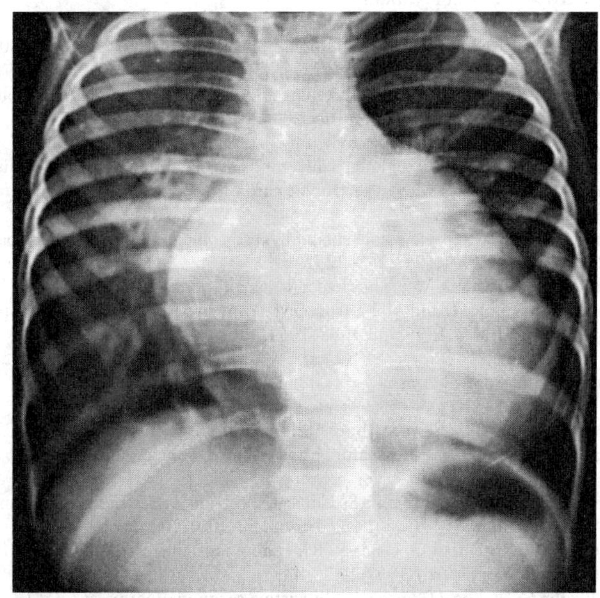

Figure 439-4. Chest x-ray of a 7 mo old girl with endocardial fibroelastosis. Note the enlargement of the heart, without a distinctive contour and clear lung fields.

tioning left ventricle. MRI may also delineate the fibrotic endomyocardial surface.

Treatment is directed toward alleviation of congestive heart failure and prevention of intercurrent infections. End-stage EFE, with signs of heart failure despite maximal medical treatment, is an indication for heart transplantation (see Chapter 443.1).

Cardiomyopathy (General)

Lipshultz SE, Sleeper LA, Towbin JA, et al: The incidence of pediatric cardiomyopathy in two regions of the United States. *N Engl J Med* 2003;348:1647–1655.

Maron BJ, Chaitman BR, Ackerman MJ, et al: Recommendations for physical activity and recreational sports participation for young patients with genetic cardiovascular diseases. *Circulation* 2004;109:2807–2816.

Nugent AW, Daubeney PEF, Chondros P, et al: The epidemiology of childhood cardiomyopathy in Australia. *N Engl J Med* 2003;348:1639–1646.

Dilated Cardiomyopathy

Barbaro G, Lipshultz SE: Pathogenesis of HIV-associated cardiomyopathy. *Ann N Y Acad Sci* 2001;946:57–81.

Brown CA, O'Connell JB: Myocarditis and idiopathic dilated cardiomyopathy. *Am J Med* 1995;99:309–314.

Burkett EL, Hershberger RE: Clinical and genetic issues in familial dilated cardiomyopathy. *J Am Coll Cardiol* 2005;45:969–981.

Forleo C, Resta N, Sorrentino S, et al: Association of beta-adrenergic receptor polymorphisms and progression to heart failure in patients with idiopathic dilated cardiomyopathy. *Am J Med* 2004;117:451–458.

Lipshultz SE, Colan SD, Gelber RD, et al: Late cardiac effects of doxorubicin therapy for acute lymphoblastic leukemia in childhood. *N Engl J Med* 1991;324:808–815.

Schonberger J, Seidman CE: Many roads lead to a broken heart: The genetics of dilated cardiomyopathy. *Am J Hum Genet* 2001;69:249–260.

Shaw T, Elliott P, McKenna WJ: Dilated cardiomyopathy: A genetically heterogeneous disease. *Lancet* 2002;360:654–655.

Shekhawat PS, Matern D, Strauss AW: Fetal fatty acid oxidation disorders, their effect on maternal health and neonatal outcome: Impact of expanded newborn screening on their diagnosis and management. *Pediatr Res* 2005;57:78R–86R.

Towbin JA, Solaro RJ: Genetics of dilated cardiomyopathy: More genes that kill. *J Am Coll Cardiol* 2004;44:2041–2043.

Weiford BC, Subbarao VD, Mulhern KM: Noncompaction of the ventricular myocardium. *Circulation* 2004;109:2965–2971.

Hypertrophic Cardiomyopathy

Elliott P, McKenna WJ: Hypertrophic cardiomyopathy. *Lancet* 2004;363:1881–1891.

MacRae CA, Ellinor PT: Genetic screening and risk assessment in hypertrophic cardiomyopathy. *J Am Coll Cardiol* 2004;44:2326–2328.

Maron BJ: Hypertrophic cardiomyopathy. *JAMA* 2002;287:1308–1320.

Maron BJ, Seidman JG, Seidman CE: Proposal for contemporary screening strategies in families with hypertrophic cardiomyopathy. *J Am Coll Cardiol* 2004;44:2125–2132.

Roberts R, Sigwart U: New concepts in hypertrophic cardiomyopathies, part II. *Circulation* 2001;104:2249–2252.

Watkins H, McKenna WJ, Thierfelder L, et al: Mutations in the genes for cardiac troponin T and alpha-tropomyosin in hypertrophic cardiomyopathy. *N Engl J Med* 1995;332:1058–1064.

Restrictive Cardiomyopathy

Cetta F, O'Leary PW, Seward JB, et al: Idiopathic restrictive cardiomyopathy in childhood: Diagnostic features and clinical course. *Mayo Clin Proc* 1995;70:634–640.

Chen SC, Balfour IC, Jureidini S: Clinical spectrum of restrictive cardiomyopathy in children. *J Heart Lung Transplant* 2001;20:90–92.

Denfield SW, Rosenthal G, Gajarski RJ, et al: Restrictive cardiomyopathies in childhood. *Tex Heart J* 1997;24:38–44.

Kushwaha SS, Fallon JT, Fuster V: Restrictive cardiomyopathy. *N Engl J Med* 1997;336:267.

Taur Y, Frishman WH: The cardiac ryanodine receptor (RyR2) and its role in heart disease. *Cardiol Rev* 2005;13:142–146.

Myocarditis

Batra AS, Lewis AB: Acute myocarditis. *Curr Opin Pediatr* 2001;13:234–239.

Chen RT, Lane JM: Myocarditis: The unexpected return of smallpox vaccine adverse events. *Lancet* 2003;362:1345–1346.

Drucker NA, Colan SD, Lewis AB, et al: Gamma-globulin treatment of acute myocarditis in the pediatric population. *Circulation* 1994;89:252–257.

Feldman AM, McNamara D: Myocarditis. *N Engl J Med* 2000;343:1388–1398.

Hrobon P, Kuntz KM, Hare JM: Should endomyocardial biopsy be performed for detection of myocarditis? A decision analytic approach. *J Heart Lung Transplant* 1998;17:479–486.

Kleinert S, Weintraub RG, Wilkinson JL, et al: Myocarditis in children with dilated cardiomyopathy: Incidence and outcome after dual therapy immunosuppression. *J Heart Lung Transplant* 1997;16:1248–1254.

Levi D, Alejos J: Diagnosis and treatment of pediatric viral myocarditis. *Curr Opin Cardiol* 2001;16:77–83.

Liu PP, Mason JW: Advances in the understanding of myocarditis. *Circulation* 2001;104:1076–1082.

Chapter 440 ■ Diseases of the Pericardium

Major diseases that involve the pericardium are noted in Table 440-1. In some diseases, pericardial involvement is one manifestation of a generalized illness; prominence of the pericardial component varies with the disease.

440.1 • Acute Pericarditis

PATHOPHYSIOLOGY. Pericardial inflammation results in an accumulation of fluid in the pericardial space. The fluid varies according to the cause of the pericarditis and may be serous, fibrinous, purulent, or hemorrhagic. **Cardiac tamponade** occurs when the amount of pericardial fluid reaches a level that compromises cardiac function. In a healthy child, 10–15 mL of fluid is normally found in the pericardial space, whereas in an adolescent with pericarditis, fluid in excess of 1,000 mL may accumulate. For every small increment of fluid, pericardial pressure rises slowly; once a critical level is reached, pressure rises rapidly and culminates in severe cardiac compression. Inhibition of ventricular filling during diastole, elevated systemic and pulmonary venous pressure, and, if untreated, eventual compromised cardiac output and shock occur.

CLINICAL MANIFESTATIONS. The first symptom of pericardial disease is often precordial pain. The major complaint is a sharp, stabbing sensation over the precordium and often the left shoulder and back; the pain may be exaggerated by lying supine and relieved by sitting, especially leaning forward. Because of the absence of sensory innervation of the pericardium, the pain is probably referred pain from diaphragmatic and pleural irritation. Cough, dyspnea, abdominal pain, vomiting, and fever may also occur. In younger children these atypical symptoms may predominate. The presence of symptoms or signs associated with other organ involvement depends on the cause of the pericarditis.

Many of the findings on physical examination are related to the degree of fluid accumulation in the pericardial sac. The presence of a **friction rub** is helpful but is a variable sign in acute pericarditis; it usually becomes apparent when the effusion is small. When the effusion is larger, muffled heart sounds may be the only

TABLE 440-1. Etiology of Pericardial Disease

CONGENITAL ANOMALIES
Absence (partial, complete)
Cysts
Mulibrey nanism (muscle, liver, brain, eye) with congenital pericardial thickening and constriction
INFECTIOUS
Viral (coxsackievirus B, Epstein-Barr virus influenza, adenovirus)
Bacterial (streptococcus, pneumococcus, staphylococcus, meningococcus, mycoplasma, tularemia, listeria, leptospirosis)
Immune complex (meningococcus, *Haemophilus influenzae*)
Tuberculosis
Fungal (histoplasmosis, actinomycosis)
Parasitic (toxoplasmosis, echinococcosis)
CONNECTIVE TISSUE DISEASES
Rheumatoid arthritis
Rheumatic fever
Systemic lupus erythematosus
Systemic sclerosis
Sarcoidosis
Wegener granulomatosis
METABOLIC-ENDOCRINE
Uremia
Hypothyroidism
Chylopericardium
HEMATOLOGY-ONCOLOGY
Bleeding diathesis
Malignancy (primary, metastatic)
Radiotherapy-induced
OTHER
Trauma (penetrating or blunt injury)
Iatrogenic (catheter related)
Postpericardiotomy (cardiac surgery)
Aortic dissection
Idiopathic
Familial Mediterranean fever
Smallpox vaccination
Pancreatitis
Löffler syndrome

auscultatory finding. Narrow pulses, tachycardia, neck vein distention, and increased pulsus paradoxus suggest significant fluid accumulation.

Pulsus paradoxus is caused by the normal slight decrease in systolic arterial pressure during inspiration. With cardiac tamponade, this normal phenomenon is exaggerated, probably because of decreased filling of the left side of the heart with the inspiratory phase of respiration. The degree of pulsus paradoxus is determined with a mercury manometer. The patient is told to breathe normally without exaggeration. By allowing the manometer to fall slowly, the 1st Korotkoff sound will initially be heard intermittently (varying with respirations). This 1st point is noted, and the manometer is then allowed to fall until the 1st Korotkoff sound is heard continuously. The difference between these two systolic pressures is the pulsus paradoxus. A pulsus paradoxus >20 mm Hg in a child with pericarditis is an indicator of the presence of cardiac tamponade; a 10–20 mm Hg change is equivocal. Increased pulsus paradoxus may also be seen in patients with severe dyspnea of any cause, in patients with pulmonary disease (emphysema or asthma), in obese individuals, or in patients being ventilated with a positive pressure respirator. In these patients, the paradoxical pulse is due to a marked increase in intrathoracic pressure. The cause of a paradoxical pulse in a child maintained on a ventilator after heart surgery may therefore be difficult to assess.

DIAGNOSIS. The specific findings depend on the underlying disease. The effects of pericarditis on the electrocardiogram are multiple. Low voltage of the QRS complexes results from a damping effect of pericardial fluid. Pressure on the myocardium by fluid or exudate produces a current of injury that results in mild elevation of ST segments. Generalized T-wave inversion occurs as a consequence of associated myocardial inflammation. The ST segment and T-wave changes with pericarditis are more generalized than those seen with myocardial infarction, and the ST segment elevations tend to precede the T-wave changes. **Electrical alternans** may be present and is demonstrated by a variable QRS complex amplitude. An interval when the electrocardiogram is in a transitional phase and appears to be normal may occur during the acute phase of the illness before diagnosis. In some instances, clear-cut abnormalities are never identified.

A relatively large pericardial effusion must be present to cause an enlarged cardiac shadow with the usual "water bottle" configuration on a chest roentgenogram (Fig. 440-1). In most instances, the lung fields are clear. With constrictive pericardial disease, the heart is relatively small and pericardial calcification may be present.

The echocardiogram is the most sensitive technique for evaluating the size and progression of pericardial effusions (Fig. 440-2). Normally, the pericardium is closely adherent to the epicardium, and the two layers can only be narrowly separated by the ultrasound beam. In patients with pericardial effusion, a clear, echo-free space is recorded between the epicardium and pericardium. A posterior effusion is recorded behind the left ventricular epicardium and ends at the junction of the left ventricle and left atrium. An anterior effusion will be recorded between the chest wall and the anterior right ventricular wall. The presence of both anterior and posterior effusion generally indicates a

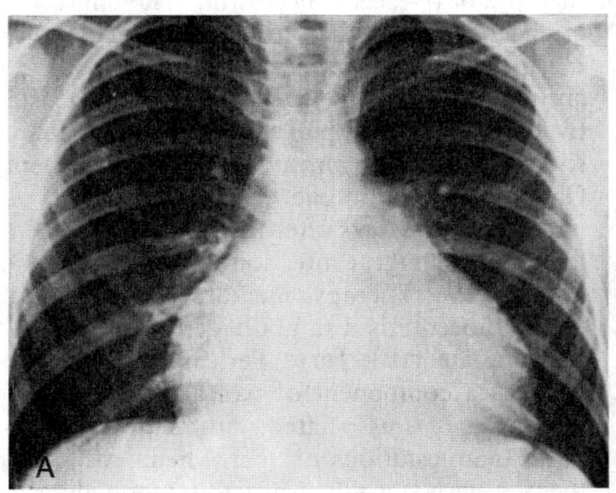

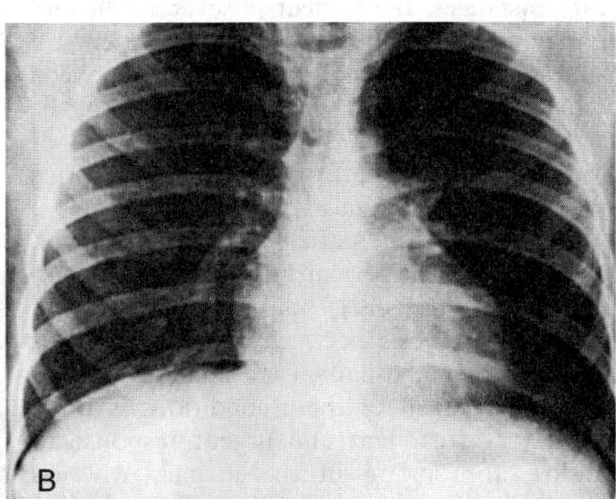

Figure 440-1. Chest x-rays in acute nonspecific pericarditis. *A*, Increase in cardiopericardial shadow caused by pericardial effusion. *B*, One month later after complete recovery.

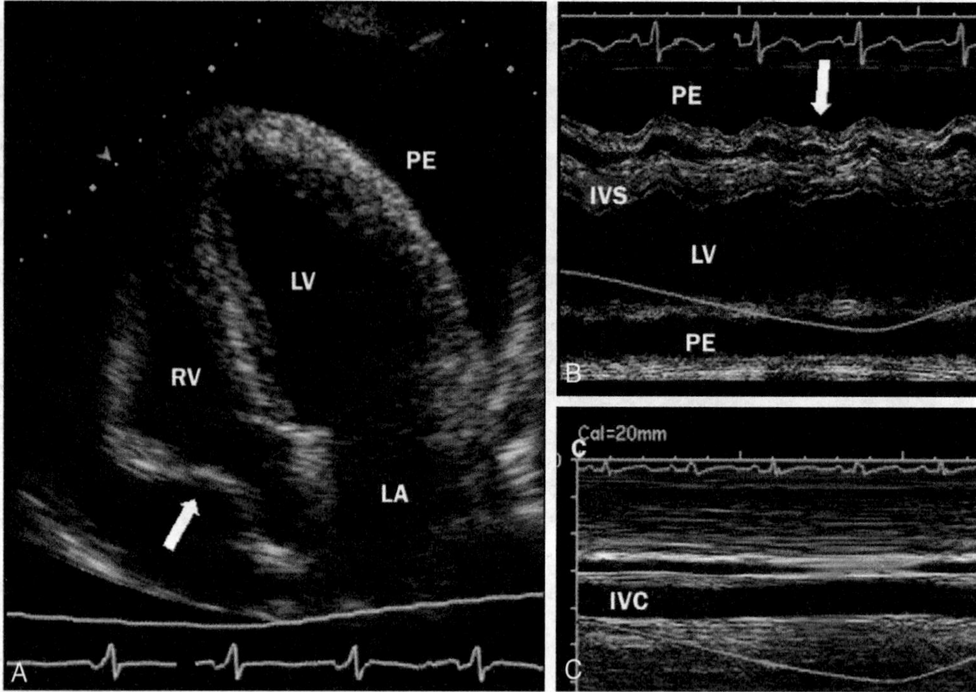

Figure 440-2. Echocardiographic images of large pericardial effusion with features of tamponade. *A*, Apical four-chamber view of LV, LA, and RV that shows large PE with diastolic right-atrial collapse *(arrow)*. *B*, M-mode image with cursor placed through RV, IVS, and LV in parasternal long axis. The view shows circumferential PE with diastolic collapse of RV free wall *(arrow)* during expiration. *C*, M-mode image from subcostal window in same patient that shows IVC plethora without inspiratory collapse. IVC, inferior vena cava; IVS, interventricular septum; LA, left atrium; LV, left ventricle; PE, pericardial effusion; RV, right ventricle. (From Troughton RW, Asher CR, Klein AL: Pericarditis. *Lancet* 2004;363:717–727.)

large collection of fluid. Flattening of septal motion and collapse of right ventricular outflow during diastole are signs of pericardial tamponade.

DIFFERENTIAL DIAGNOSIS.

Viral and Acute Benign Pericarditis. These entities are considered synonymous because most episodes of acute benign pericarditis follow or coincide with viral illness. Viruses recognized to cause pericarditis include coxsackievirus B, influenza, echovirus, and adenovirus. The pathogenesis is unclear but may be related to a hypersensitivity reaction to the viral disease. Pericardial inflammation is not necessarily the precursor of a generalized inflammatory process. Most cases are mild, and recovery occurs within several weeks. Only symptomatic treatment is indicated, usually with nonsteroidal anti-inflammatory agents such as indomethacin. In rare instances, the patient is severely ill, and cardiac tamponade may ensue. In addition, in some patients, a chronic relapsing illness occurs. Differential diagnosis between these patients and those with collagen vascular disease may be difficult. The latter patients respond dramatically to corticosteroids or nonsteroidal anti-inflammatory agents; milder forms may be controlled with aspirin. The clinical course may vary from months to 1–2 yr, during which time patients are dependent on drug therapy for suppression of the pericarditis. Ultimately, these patients improve, and the prognosis is good.

The clinical differential diagnosis between acute pericarditis and myocarditis may be difficult; usually, each includes a component of the other. Management of these conditions is quite different: anti-inflammatory treatment and urgent response to cardiac tamponade are appropriate in the former, whereas therapy for heart failure is required in the latter. The echocardiogram can demonstrate the size of the pericardial effusion and also indicate the presence of myocardial dysfunction.

Purulent Pericarditis. This condition is most often associated with bacterial infections such as pneumonia, epiglottitis, meningitis, or osteomyelitis. Generally, signs and symptoms of the primary infection are present. Once the purulent process is established, if untreated, the course is fulminant and terminated by acute cardiac tamponade and death. Open pericardial drainage is required along with appropriate intravenous antibiotics. Although closed pericardial aspiration provides a sample of the exudate for diagnostic purposes and may be lifesaving in the face of severe cardiac compression, without open drainage and removal of adhesions, tamponade almost invariably recurs. Open pericardial drainage has significantly increased survival. Rarely, with infections that are identified extremely early and with pericardial fluid that is more of a transudate than an exudate, multiple pericardial taps with placement of a drain and antibiotic therapy have been successful. The most common organisms implicated in purulent pericarditis are *Staphylococcus aureus, Haemophilus influenzae* type b, and *Neisseria meningitidis*. (For antimicrobial treatment, see Chapters 180, 192, and 190, respectively.) Tuberculous pericarditis rarely occurs in children. Extensive treatment with antituberculous chemotherapy is required (see Chapter 212). Immune complex–mediated pericarditis (sterile) may occur 5–7 days after the initiation of therapy for severe systemic or meningeal infection with meningococcus or *H. influenzae type b*. Therapy includes anti-inflammatory agents and pericardiocentesis if tamponade develops.

Acute Rheumatic Fever. Pericarditis occurs in acute rheumatic fever as a component of pancarditis (see Chapters 156, 182.1, and 430). It is associated with acute valvulitis. Pericarditis and other manifestations of acute rheumatic pancarditis respond to therapy with steroids. Cardiac tamponade is extremely rare.

Juvenile Rheumatoid Arthritis. Pericarditis is a common manifestation of juvenile rheumatoid arthritis (see Chapter 154).

Rarely, it may be the only manifestation and precede the onset of arthritis by months or even years. Differentiation of rheumatoid pericarditis from that seen with other collagen vascular disease, particularly lupus erythematosus, may be difficult. Treatment consists of steroids or salicylates, which may be needed on a long-term basis.

Uremia. Uremic pericarditis occurs only in the presence of prolonged severe renal failure and results from chemical irritation of the pericardium secondary to the metabolic abnormalities. It may culminate in cardiac tamponade or cause recurrent hypotension during hemodialysis. If adequate relief of uremic pericarditis does not occur with hemodialysis, pericardiectomy is recommended.

Neoplastic Disease. Neoplastic pericardial effusion is seen in patients with Hodgkin disease, lymphosarcoma, and leukemia, and it results from direct neoplastic invasion of the pericardium. Cardiac tamponade may occur late in the course of the illness. Rarely, pericardial infiltration is the initial manifestation of neoplastic disease. Patients with malignancy may also acquire pericarditis as a result of radiation therapy to the mediastinum.

Postpericardiotomy Syndrome (see Chapter 434). Pericardial effusions may be seen 1–2 wk or longer after open heart surgery and in some echocardiographic series are diagnosed in 15–23% of postoperative patients. The syndrome is a nonspecific hypersensitivity reaction to trauma to the pericardium and the epicardial surface of the heart. High titers of antiheart antibodies have been reported to correlate with clinical signs of the syndrome. Patients may initially have low-grade fever, lethargy, loss of appetite, or abdominal pain. Precordial or pleural chest pain may or may not be present. A high index of suspicion should accompany any acute illness in a child within the 1st 4–6 weeks after cardiac surgery. In most children, the syndrome responds well to therapy with aspirin or other nonsteroidal anti-inflammatory agents. Corticosteroids may be needed for more severe cases, and progression to tamponade can occur if untreated. Treatment is maintained for 1–3 mo, but recurrences may be seen as long as 1 yr postoperatively and require reinstitution of therapy.

440.2 • Constrictive Pericarditis

In most instances, constriction occurs months or years after the initial pericarditis, but it may occasionally be an acute, rapidly progressive process. Constrictive pericarditis most often occurs without an immediately preceding illness or generalized systemic disease.

Clinical manifestations occur as a result of impaired diastolic ventricular filling, compromised myocardial contractility, and resultant depression of cardiac function. Hepatomegaly and ascites may be out of proportion to the other signs and symptoms and thus suggest chronic liver disease. Liver function studies are only mildly abnormal; careful physical examination reveals other subtle findings of constriction, including neck vein distention, narrow pulses, quiet precordium, distant heart sounds, a faint pericardial friction rub, and increased pulsus paradoxus. Typical findings become apparent gradually and may be overlooked. The auscultatory presence of an early pericardial knock and the appearance of calcification of the pericardium on chest roentgenograms are the more obvious manifestations. Protein-losing enteropathy with hypoproteinemia and lymphopenia may be seen in association with severe constriction.

Constrictive pericarditis may be difficult to distinguish from restrictive cardiomyopathy (see Chapter 439.3). Impaired myocardial function occurs with both conditions. The myocardial disease of constrictive pericarditis is usually reversible with pericardiectomy. At times, a definite diagnosis can be made only by exploratory thoracotomy and direct examination of the pericardium.

Radical pericardiectomy with decortication of the pericardium over a wide area of the heart, including the systemic and pulmonary veins, is the only effective treatment of constrictive pericarditis. In most patients, surgical intervention elicits a rapid response characterized by increased cardiac output and prompt diuresis. The long-term prognosis is usually excellent.

Demmler GJ: Infectious pericarditis in children. *Pediatr Infect Dis J* 2006;25:165–166.

Goldstein JA: Cardiac tamponade, constrictive pericarditis, and restrictive cardiomyopathy. *Curr Probl Cardiol* 2004;29:503–567.

Lange RA, Hillis LD: Clinical practice. Acute pericarditis. *N Engl J Med* 2004;351:2195–2202.

Levy PY, Corey R, Berger P, et al: Etiologic diagnosis of 204 pericardial effusions. *Medicine* 2003;82:385–391.

Rienmuller R, Groll R, Lipton MJ: CT and MR imaging of pericardial disease. *Radiol Clin North Am* 2004;42:587–601.

Sinzobahamvya N, Ikeogu MO: Purulent pericarditis. *Arch Dis Child* 1987;62:696–699.

Troughton RW, Asher CR, Klein AL: Pericarditis. *Lancet* 2004;363:717–727.

Chapter 441 ■ Tumors of the Heart

Primary tumors of the heart are rare in infancy and childhood and are most often benign. Clinical manifestations depend primarily on the location of the tumor and, to a lesser extent, on the histologic type.

The most common benign cardiac tumors in children are rhabdomyomas, fibromas, and myxomas. **Rhabdomyomas** occur as single or, usually, multiple nodules embedded in chamber walls. They often remain clinically unimportant and regress with age, but they may cause mechanical obstruction, heart failure, or arrhythmias. They may be familial and are often found in association with Gorlin syndrome or tuberous sclerosis. Most rhabdomyomas are seen in infants younger than 1 yr. Incessant ventricular tachycardia in a child younger than 2 yr should raise suspicion of a small endocardial or epicardial rhabdomyoma or Purkinje cell tumor. Fibromas are usually solitary, nonencapsulated nodules located in the ventricles; they can be massive. Treatment of rhabdomyomas and fibromas depends on their location and size. Small asymptomatic tumors in the myocardial wall or ventricular septum may be observed for growth or regression. Rhabdomyomas associated with **tuberous sclerosis** often resolve as the child grows older. Large tumors that show signs of obstructing blood flow and those producing ventricular arrhythmias should be removed. Large and diffuse tumors may interfere with cardiac performance. Removal of large lesions is often difficult because insufficient normal myocardium may remain. Heart transplantation may be the only recourse for patients with extensive tumors.

Myxomas develop in intracavitary locations, most frequently in the left atrium (75%) and most often in females (75%). These tumors are solid, smooth, pedunculated masses (1–8 cm) that attach to the interatrial septum, protrude into the atrial chamber, and, by their position relative to the mitral or tricuspid valve, cause intermittent obstruction and a clinical picture consistent with stenosis (syncope, heart failure, atrial fibrillation). A myxoma should be considered in patients with fainting spells, a positional character (supine vs erect) of the murmur, or evidence of systemic or pulmonary embolization. Atrial myxomas can also cause fever, malaise, arthralgias, and systemic emboli mimicking **endocarditis**, rheumatic fever, or systemic lupus erythematosus.

Laboratory features include a high sedimentation rate, hematuria, and echocardiographic evidence of the tumor. Atrial myxomas may be associated with multiple pigmented skin lesions (lentiginosis), myxoid fibroadenomas of the breast, cutaneous myxomas, and adrenal pigmented nodules. Some are associated with various cutaneous and connective tissue lesions and testicular tumors or pituitary adenomas (Carney syndrome). Treatment consists of surgical excision, which must include the entire base of the tumor to prevent recurrence.

Other benign tumors include papillomas, which are attached to valve leaflets and may occur in neonates; lipomas, which are situated in ventricular walls; and mesotheliomas, which may involve the atrioventricular node and cause abnormalities in electrical conduction, including complete heart block.

Primary malignant cardiac tumors in children are almost exclusively sarcomas. These tumors are usually located in the right side of the heart, atrial septum, right atrial wall, or root of the pulmonary artery. They may extend either into the adjacent chamber and cause obstruction to blood flow or into the pericardial cavity and produce effusion or tamponade. The heart may also be involved in metastatic dissemination of a noncardiac malignancy, such as leukemia or lymphoma, or in Wilms tumor by direct extension of the tumor into the right atrium via the inferior vena cava. Physical examination may reflect the location and size of the tumor if it interferes with blood flow. Conduction system involvement can be assessed by electrocardiography. Two-dimensional echocardiography is diagnostic and allows excellent visualization of the location and extent of the tumor. Doppler studies evaluate the extent of blood flow obstruction caused by the tumor. Cardiac catheterization may provide further information about the anatomy of the tumor and its hemodynamic effects. When indicated, surgical intervention is directed toward complete removal of the tumor, relief of obstruction, and control of any arrhythmias. The long-term outcome depends on the type of tumor, the completeness of surgical removal, and postsurgical integrity of the normal heart structures and myocardium. For tumors that are unresectable because of an inability to separate them from normal heart tissue, heart transplantation is an effective treatment.

Butany J, Nair V, Naseemuddin A, et al: Cardiac tumours: Diagnosis and management. *Lancet* 2005;6:219–228.

Isaacs H Jr: Fetal and neonatal cardiac tumors. *Pediatr Cardiol* 2004;25:252–273.

Shapiro LM: Cardiac tumours: Diagnosis and management. *Heart* 2001;85:218–222.

Stratakis CA, Kirschner LS, Carney JA: Clinical and molecular features of the Carney complex: Diagnostic criteria and recommendations for patient evaluation. *J Clin Endocrinol Metab* 2001;86:4041–4046.

Section 7 — Cardiac Therapeutics — Daniel Bernstein

Chapter 442 ■ Heart Failure

Heart failure occurs when the heart cannot deliver adequate cardiac output to meet the metabolic needs of the body. In the early stages of heart failure, various compensatory mechanisms are evoked to maintain normal metabolic function. When these mechanisms become ineffective, increasingly severe clinical manifestations result (see Chapter 68).

PATHOPHYSIOLOGY. The heart can be viewed as a pump with an output proportional to its filling volume and inversely proportional to the resistance against which it pumps. As ventricular end-diastolic volume increases, a healthy heart increases cardiac output until a maximum is reached and cardiac output can no longer be augmented (the Frank-Starling principle; Fig. 442-1). The increased stroke volume obtained in this manner is due to stretching of myocardial fibers, but it also results in increased wall tension, which elevates myocardial oxygen consumption. Hearts working under various types of stress function along different Frank-Starling curves. Cardiac muscle with compromised intrinsic contractility requires a greater degree of dilatation to produce increased stroke volume and does not achieve the same maximal cardiac output as normal myocardium does. If a cardiac chamber is already dilated because of a lesion causing increased preload (e.g., a left-to-right shunt or valvular insufficiency), there is little room for further dilatation and augmentation of cardiac output. The presence of lesions that result in increased afterload to the ventricle (aortic or pulmonic stenosis, coarctation of the aorta) decreases cardiac performance, thereby resulting in a depressed Frank-Starling relationship. The ability of an immature heart to increase cardiac output in response to increased preload is less than that of a mature heart. Premature infants are more compromised by a left-to-right shunt than full-term infants are.

Systemic oxygen transport is calculated as the product of cardiac output and systemic oxygen content. **Cardiac output** can be calculated as the product of heart rate and stroke volume. The primary determinants of stroke volume are the afterload (pressure work), preload (volume work), and contractility (intrinsic myocardial function). Abnormalities in heart rate can also compromise cardiac output and produce both bradyarrhythmias and tachyarrhythmias; the latter shorten the diastolic time interval for ventricular filling. Alterations in the oxygen-carrying capacity of blood (e.g., anemia or hypoxemia) also lead to a decrease in systemic oxygen transport and, if compensatory mechanisms are inadequate, can result in decreased delivery of substrate to tissues.

In some cases of heart failure, cardiac output is normal or increased, yet because of decreased systemic oxygen content (secondary to anemia) or increased oxygen demands (secondary to hyperventilation, hyperthyroidism, or hypermetabolism), an inadequate amount of oxygen is delivered to meet the body's needs. This condition, high-output failure, results in the development of signs and symptoms of heart failure when there is no basic abnormality in myocardial function and cardiac output is greater than normal. It is also seen with large systemic arteriovenous fistulas. These conditions reduce peripheral vascular resistance and cardiac afterload and increase myocardial contractility. Heart "failure" results when the demand for cardiac output exceeds the ability of the heart to respond. Chronic severe

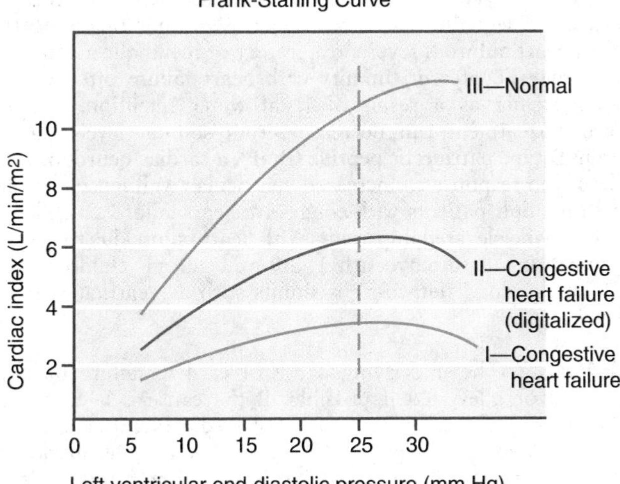

Figure 442-1. The Frank-Starling relationship. As left ventricular end-diastolic pressure (LVED) increases, the cardiac index increases, even in the presence of congestive heart failure, until a critical level of LVED is reached. Adding an inotropic agent (digoxin) shifts the curve from I and II. (From Gersony WM, Steep CN. In Dickerman JD, Lucey JF [editors]: *Smith's The Critically Ill Child: Diagnosis and Medical Management,* 3rd ed. Philadelphia, WB Saunders, 1984.)

high-output failure may eventually result in a decrease in myocardial performance as the metabolic requirements of the myocardium are not met.

There are multiple systemic compensatory mechanisms used by the body to adapt to chronic heart failure. Some are mediated at the molecular/cellular level, such as up- or downregulation of various metabolic pathway components leading to changes in efficiency of oxygen and other substrate utilization. Others are mediated by neurohormones such as the renin-angiotensin system and the sympathoadrenal axis. One of the principal mechanisms for increasing cardiac output is an increase in sympathetic tone secondary to increased adrenal secretion of circulating epinephrine and increased neural release of norepinephrine. The initial beneficial effects of sympathetic stimulation include an increase in heart rate and myocardial contractility, mediated by these hormones' action on cardiac β-adrenergic receptors; both serve to increase cardiac output. Because of localized vasoconstriction, mediated by these hormones' action on peripheral arterial α-adrenergic receptors, blood flow may be redistributed from the cutaneous, visceral, and renal beds to the heart and brain. Whereas these acute effects are beneficial, chronically increased sympathetic stimulation can have deleterious effects, including hypermetabolism, increased afterload, arrhythmogenesis, and increased myocardial oxygen requirements. Peripheral vasoconstriction can result in decreased renal, hepatic, and gastrointestinal tract function. Chronic exposure to circulating catecholamines leads to a decrease in the number of cardiac β-adrenergic receptors (downregulation or tachyphylaxis) and also causes direct myocardial cell damage. Thus, therapeutic agents for heart failure are directed at restoring balance to these neuroendocrine systems. Single nucleotide differences (known as polymorphisms [SNPs]) in the genes encoding proteins involved in sympathetic signaling can alter the patients response to medical therapy and predict risk of worsening heart failure, hospitalization, or death. These pharmacogenomic studies may soon allow us to tailor our therapies to the individual patient, based on their genetic makeup.

CLINICAL MANIFESTATIONS. The clinical manifestations of heart failure depend on the degree of the child's cardiac reserve. A critically ill infant or child who has exhausted the compensatory mechanisms to the point that cardiac output is no longer sufficient to meet the basal metabolic needs of the body will be symptomatic at rest. Other patients may be comfortable when quiet but are incapable of increasing cardiac output in response to even mild activity without experiencing significant symptoms. Conversely, it may take rather vigorous exercise to compromise cardiac function in children who have less severe heart disease. A thorough history is extremely important in making the diagnosis of heart failure and in evaluating the possible causes. Parents who observe their child on a daily basis may not recognize subtle changes that have occurred in the course of days or weeks. Gradually worsening perfusion or increasing cyanosis may not be recognized as an abnormal finding. Edema may be passed off as normal weight gain, and exercise intolerance as lack of interest in an activity. The history of a young infant should also focus on feeding (see Chapter 422). An infant with heart failure often takes less volume per feeding, becomes dyspneic while sucking, and may perspire profusely. Eliciting a history of fatigue in an older child requires detailed questions about activity level and its course over several months.

In children, the signs and symptoms of heart failure may be similar to those in adults and include fatigue, effort intolerance, anorexia, abdominal pain, dyspnea, and cough. Many children, however, especially adolescents, may have primarily abdominal symptoms and a surprising lack of respiratory complaints. Attention to the cardiovascular system may come only after an abdominal roentgenogram unexpectedly shows the lower end of an enlarged heart. The elevation in systemic venous pressure may be gauged by clinical assessment of jugular venous pressure and liver enlargement. Orthopnea and basilar rales are variably present; edema is usually discernible in dependent portions of the body, or anasarca may be present. Cardiomegaly is invariably noted. A gallop rhythm is common; when ventricular dilatation is advanced, the holosystolic murmur of mitral or tricuspid valve regurgitation may be heard.

In infants, heart failure may be difficult to identify. Prominent manifestations include tachypnea, feeding difficulties, poor weight gain, excessive perspiration, irritability, weak cry, and noisy, labored respirations with intercostal and subcostal retractions, as well as flaring of the alae nasi. The signs of cardiac-induced pulmonary congestion may be indistinguishable from those of bronchiolitis; wheezing is prominent. Pneumonitis with or without atelectasis is common, especially in the right middle and lower lobes; it is due to bronchial compression by the enlarged heart. Hepatomegaly usually occurs, and cardiomegaly is invariably present. In spite of pronounced tachycardia, a gallop rhythm can frequently be recognized. The other auscultatory signs are those produced by the underlying cardiac lesion. Clinical assessment of jugular venous pressure in infants may be difficult because of the shortness of the neck and the difficulty of observing a relaxed state. Edema may be generalized and usually involves the eyelids as well as the sacrum and less often the legs and feet. The differential diagnosis is age dependent (Table 442-1).

DIAGNOSIS. Roentgenograms of the chest show cardiac enlargement. Pulmonary vascularity is variable and depends on the cause of the heart failure. Infants and children with large left-to-right shunts have exaggeration of the pulmonary arterial vessels to the periphery of the lung fields, whereas patients with cardiomyopathy may have a relatively normal pulmonary vascular bed early in the course of disease. Fluffy perihilar pulmonary markings suggestive of venous congestion and acute pulmonary edema are seen only with more severe degrees of heart failure. Cardiac enlargement is often noted as an unexpected finding on a chest roentgenogram performed to evaluate for a possible pulmonary infection, bronchiolitis, or asthma.

Chamber hypertrophy noted by electrocardiography may be helpful in assessing the cause of heart failure but does not estab-

TABLE 442-1. Etiology of Heart Failure

FETAL
Severe anemia (hemolysis, fetal-maternal transfusion, parvovirus B19–induced anemia, hypoplastic anemia)
Supraventricular tachycardia
Ventricular tachycardia
Complete heart block
Severe Ebstein anomaly or other severe right-sided lesions
Myocarditis
PREMATURE NEONATE
Fluid overload
Patent ductus arteriosus
Ventricular septal defect
Cor pulmonale (bronchopulmonary dysplasia)
Hypertension
Myocarditis
Genetic cardiomyopathy
FULL-TERM NEONATE
Asphyxial cardiomyopathy
Arteriovenous malformation (vein of Galen, hepatic)
Left-sided obstructive lesions (coarctation of aorta, hypoplastic left heart syndrome)
Large mixing cardiac defects (single ventricle, truncus arteriosus)
Myocarditis
Genetic cardiomyopathy
INFANT-TODDLER
Left-to-right cardiac shunts (ventricular septal defect)
Hemangioma (arteriovenous malformation)
Anomalous left coronary artery
Genetic or metabolic cardiomyopathy
Acute hypertension (hemolytic-uremic syndrome)
Supraventricular tachycardia
Kawasaki disease
Myocarditis
CHILD-ADOLESCENT
Rheumatic fever
Acute hypertension (glomerulonephritis)
Myocarditis
Thyrotoxicosis
Hemochromatosis-hemosiderosis
Cancer therapy (radiation, doxorubicin)
Sickle cell anemia
Endocarditis
Cor pulmonale (cystic fibrosis)
Genetic or metabolic cardiomyopathy (hypertrophic, dilated)

lish the diagnosis. In cardiomyopathies, left or right ventricular ischemic changes may correlate well with clinical and other noninvasive parameters of ventricular function. Low-voltage QRS morphologic characteristics with ST-T wave abnormalities may also suggest myocardial inflammatory disease but can be seen with pericarditis as well. The electrocardiogram is the best tool for evaluating rhythm disorders as a potential cause of heart failure.

Echocardiographic techniques are most useful in assessing ventricular function. The most commonly used parameter in children is fractional shortening (a single dimensional variable), determined as the difference between end-systolic and end-diastolic diameter divided by end-diastolic diameter. Normal fractional shortening is between 28% and 40%. In adults, the most commonly used parameter is ejection fraction (which uses two-dimensional data to calculate a three-dimensional volume) and the normal range is 55–65%. In children with right ventricular enlargement or other cardiac pathology resulting in flattening of the interventricular septum, ejection fraction is used since fractional shortening will not be accurate. Doppler studies can be used to estimate cardiac output. Magnetic resonance angiography (MRA) can be useful in quantifying left and right ventricular function and mass. If valvar regurgitation is present, MRA can quantify the regurgitant fraction.

Arterial oxygen levels may be decreased when ventilation-perfusion inequalities occur secondary to pulmonary edema. When heart failure is severe, respiratory or metabolic acidosis, or both, may be present. Infants with heart failure often display hyponatremia as a result of renal water retention. Chronic diuretic treatment can decrease serum sodium levels further. **Serum B-type natriuretic peptide (BNP),** a cardiac neurohormone released in response to increased ventricular wall tension, is elevated in adult patients with congestive heart failure. In children, BNP may be elevated in patients with heart failure due to systolic dysfunction (cardiomyopathy) as well as in children with volume overload (left-to-right shunts such as ventricular septal defect).

TREATMENT. The underlying cause of cardiac failure must be removed or alleviated if possible. If the cause is a congenital cardiac anomaly amenable to surgery, medical treatment is indicated to prepare the patient for surgery and in the immediate postoperative period while the heart is recovering from the effects of cardiopulmonary bypass. With excellent outcomes of primary surgical repair of congenital heart defects, even in the neonatal period, few children require aggressive heart failure management to "grow big enough for surgery." In contrast, if the cause of heart failure is cardiomyopathy, medical management provides temporary relief from symptoms and may allow the patient to recover if the insult is reversible (myocarditis). If the lesion is not reversible, heart failure management usually allows the child to return to normal activities for some period and delay, sometimes for years, consideration for heart transplantation.

General Measures. Strict bed rest is rarely necessary except in extreme cases, but it is important that the child be allowed to rest during the day as needed and sleep adequately at night. Some older patients feel better sleeping in a semi-upright position, using several pillows (orthopnea). For infants with heart failure, an infant chair may be advisable. After patients begin to respond to treatment, restrictions on activities can often be modified within the context of the specific diagnosis and the patient's ability. Competitive and strenuous sports activities are usually contraindicated. Formal cardiopulmonary exercise testing can be used to assess the patient's ability to perform exercise in a controlled environment and is useful for recommending rational exercise restrictions. For patients with pulmonary edema, positive pressure ventilation may be required along with other drug therapy. For those in low-output heart failure, positive pressure ventilation can significantly reduce total body oxygen consumption by eliminating the work of breathing, and help to reverse a metabolic acidosis. β-Adrenergic agonists such as dopamine, epinephrine, and dobutamine are usually used in combination with phosphodiesterase inhibitors such as milrinone. If the blood pressure will allow, afterload-reducing agents (nitroprusside, angiotensin-converting enzyme [ACE] inhibitors) may be beneficial. These agents are usually initiated in an intensive care setting, with proper invasive monitoring of central venous and arterial blood pressure.

Diet. Infants with heart failure may fail to thrive because of increased metabolic requirements and decreased caloric intake. Increasing daily calories is an important aspect of their management. Increasing the number of calories per ounce of infant formula (or supplementing breast-feeding) may be beneficial. Many infants do not tolerate an increase beyond 24 calories/oz because of diarrhea or because these formulas provide too large a solute load for compromised kidneys.

Severely ill infants may lack sufficient strength for effective sucking because of extreme fatigue, rapid respirations, and generalized weakness. In these circumstances, nasogastric feedings may be helpful. In many children with cardiac enlargement, gastroesophageal reflux is a major problem. The use of continuous drip nasogastric feedings at night, administered by pump, may improve caloric intake while decreasing problems with reflux.

Occasionally, especially in children with heart failure due to complex congenital heart disease, medical or surgical intervention to correct reflux is necessary (Nissen fundoplication). Continued malnutrition may be an important factor in the decision to undertake earlier surgical intervention in patients who have an operable congenital heart lesion or for listing for transplantation in patients with cardiomyopathy.

The use of low sodium formulas in the routine management of infants with heart failure is not recommended because these preparations are often poorly tolerated and may exacerbate diuretic-induced hyponatremia. Human breast milk is the ideal low sodium nutritional source. The use of more potent diuretic agents allows more palatable standard formulas to be used for nutrition while controlling salt and water balance by chronic diuretic administration. Most older children can be managed with "no added salt" diets and abstinence from foods containing large amounts of sodium. A strict, extremely low sodium diet is rarely required.

Digitalis. Digoxin, once the mainstay of heart failure management in both children and adults, is currently used less, as a result of the introduction of newer therapies and the recognition of its potential toxicities. Many cardiologists will use digitalis as an adjunct to ACE inhibitors and diuretics in patients with symptomatic heart failure, whereas others have moved away from its use altogether. Despite multiple clinical studies, predominantly in adults, the controversy over digitalis remains.

Digoxin is the digitalis glycoside used most often in pediatric patients. Its half-life of 36 hr is long enough to allow daily or twice-daily administration and short enough to limit toxic effects from overdosage. It is absorbed well by the gastrointestinal tract (60–85%), even in infants. Absorption is greater with the elixir than with tablets. An initial effect can be seen as early as 30 min after administration, and the peak effect for oral digoxin occurs at ≈2–6 hr. When the drug is administered intravenously, the initial effect is seen in 15–30 min, and the peak effect occurs at 1–4 hr. The drug crosses the placenta, and therefore a fetus with heart failure (secondary to arrhythmia) can be treated by administering digoxin to the mother. The kidney eliminates digoxin, so dosing must be adjusted according to the patient's renal function. The rate of excretion is proportional to the glomerular filtration rate. After intravenous administration, 50–70% is excreted unchanged in the urine. The half-life of digoxin may be up to 6 days in patients with anuria because slower hepatic excretion pathways are used in these patients.

Rapid digitalization of infants and children in heart failure may be carried out intravenously. The dose depends on the patient's age (Table 442-2). The recommended digitalization schedule is to give half the total digitalizing dose immediately and the succeeding two one-quarter doses at 12 hr intervals later. The electrocardiogram must be closely monitored and rhythm strips obtained before each of the three digitalizing doses. Digoxin should be discontinued if a new rhythm disturbance is noted. Prolongation of the P-R interval is not necessarily an indication to withhold digitalis, but a delay in administering the next dose or a reduction in the dosage should be considered, depending on the patient's clinical status. Serum digoxin determination is helpful when digitalis toxicity is suspected, although it may be less reliable in infants. ST segment or T-wave changes are commonly noted with digitalis administration and should not affect the digitalization regimen. Baseline serum electrolyte levels should be measured before and after digitalization. Hypokalemia and hypercalcemia exacerbate digitalis toxicity. Because hypokalemia is relatively common in patients receiving diuretics, potassium levels should be monitored closely in those receiving a potassium-wasting diuretic (e.g., furosemide) in combination with digitalis. In patients with active myocarditis, some cardiologists recommend avoiding digitalization altogether and starting maintenance digitalis at half the normal dose due to the increased risk of arrhythmia in these patients.

TABLE 442-2. Dosage of Drugs Commonly Used for the Treatment of Congestive Heart Failure

DRUG	DOSAGE
	DIGOXIN
Digitalization (1/2 initially, followed by 1/4 q12h × 2)	Premature: 20 μg/kg Full-term neonate (up to 1 mo): 20–30 μg/kg Infant or child: 25–40 μg/kg Adolescent or adult: 0.5–1 mg in divided doses NOTE: These doses are PO; IV dose is 75% of po dose
Maintenance digoxin	5–10 μg/kg/day, divided q12h Trough serum level: 1.5–3.0 ng/mL <6 mo old; 1–2 ng/mL >6 mo old NOTE: These doses are PO; IV dose is 75% of po dose
	DIURETICS
Furosemide (Lasix)	IV: 1–2 mg/dose prn PO: 1–4 mg/kg/day, divided qd–qid
Bumetanide (Bumex)	IV: 0.01–0.1 mg/kg/dose PO: 0.005–0.1 mg/kg/day, divided q6–8h
Chlorothiazide (Diuril)	PO: 20–40 mg/kg/day, divided bid or tid
Spironolactone (Aldactone)	PO: 1–3 mg/kg/day, divided bid or tid
Nesiritide (B-type natriuretic peptide)	IV: 0.001–0.03 μg/kg/min
	ADRENERGIC AGONISTS (ALL IV)
Dobutamine	2–20 μg/kg/min
Dopamine	2–30 μg/kg/min
Isoproterenol	0.01–0.5 μg/kg/min
Epinephrine	0.1–1.0 μg/kg/min
Norepinephrine	0.1–2.0 μg/kg/min
	PHOSPHODIESTERASE INHIBITORS (ALL IV)
Amrinone	3–10 μg/kg/min
Milrinone	0.25–1.0 μg/kg/min
	AFTERLOAD-REDUCING AGENTS
Captopril (Capoten), all PO	Prematures: start at 0.01 mg/kg/dose Infants: 0.1–0.5 mg/kg/dose q8–12h (maximum, 4 mg/kg/day) Children: 0.1–2 mg/kg/day q8–12h (adult dose is 6.25–25 mg/dose)
Enalapril (Vasotec), all PO	0.08–0.5 mg/kg/dose q12–24h (maximum, 0.5 mg/kg/day)
Hydralazine (Apresoline)	IV: 0.1–0.5 mg/kg/dose (maximum, 20 mg) PO: 0.25–1.0 mg/kg/dose q6–8h (maximum, 200 mg/day)
Nitroglycerin	IV: 0.25–5 μg/kg/min
Nitroprusside (Nipride)	IV: 0.5–8 μg/kg/min
Prazosin	PO: 0.005–0.025 mg/kg/dose q6–8h (maximum, 0.1 mg/kg/dose)
	β-ADRENERGIC BLOCKERS
Carvedilol (Coreg)	PO: initial dose 0.1 mg/kg/day (maximum 6.5 mg) divided bid, increase gradually (usually 2 wk intervals) to maximum of 0.5–1 mg/kg/day over 8–12 wk as tolerated; adult maximal dose, 50–100 mg/day
Metoprolol (Lopressor, Toprol-XL)	PO, non-extended release form: 0.2 mg/kg/day divided bid, increase gradually (usually 2 wk intervals) to maximum dose 1–2 mg/kg/day PO, extended release form (Toprol-XL) is given once daily; adult initial dose 25 mg/day, maximum dose is 200 mg/day

Note: Pediatric doses based on weight should not exceed adult doses. Because recommendations may change, these doses should always be double-checked. Doses may also need to be modified in any patient with renal or hepatic dysfunction. bid, twice daily; IV, intravenously; PO, by mouth; prn, as necessary; qd, every day; qid, three times per day.

Maintenance digitalis therapy is started ≈12 hr after full digitalization. The daily dosage is divided in two and given at 12 hr intervals for more consistent blood levels and more flexibility in case of toxicity. The dosage is one quarter of the total digitalizing dose. For patients who are initially given digitalis intravenously, maintenance digoxin can be given orally once oral feedings are tolerated. Because absorption from the gastrointestinal tract is less certain, the oral maintenance dose is usually 20–25% higher than when digoxin is used parenterally (see Table 442-2). The normal daily dose of digoxin for older children (>5 yr of age) calculated by body weight should not exceed the usual adult dose of 0.2–0.5 mg/24 hr.

Patients who are not critically ill may be given digitalis initially by the oral route, and in most instances digitalization is completed within 24 hr. When slow digitalization is desirable, for example, in the immediate postoperative period, initiation of a maintenance digoxin schedule without a previous loading dose achieves full digitalization in 7–10 days. Often, the schedule can be completed on an outpatient basis.

Measurement of **serum digoxin levels** is useful under several circumstances: (1) when an unknown amount of digoxin has been administered or ingested accidentally, (2) when renal function is impaired or if drug interactions are possible, (3) when questions regarding compliance are raised, and (4) when a toxic response is suspected. Blood is usually drawn immediately before a dose but at a minimum of 4 hr after the last dose to ensure that tissue-plasma equilibration has occurred. An appropriate blood level is ≈2–4 ng/mL in infants and 1–2 ng/mL in older children. Exceeding these levels does not generally add significantly to the management of heart failure and only increases the risk of toxicity. In suspected toxicity, elevated serum digoxin levels are not in themselves diagnostic of toxicity but must be interpreted as an adjunct to other clinical and electrocardiographic findings (rhythm and conduction disturbances). Nausea and vomiting are less frequent in pediatric patients. Hypokalemia, hypomagnesemia, hypercalcemia, cardiac inflammation secondary to myocarditis, and prematurity may all potentiate digitalis toxicity. A cardiac arrhythmia that develops in a child who is taking digitalis may also be related to the primary cardiac disease rather than the drug. Any form of arrhythmia occurring after the institution of digitalis therapy must be considered to be drug related until proved otherwise. Succeeding doses should be withheld until the issue is resolved.

Diuretics. These agents interfere with reabsorption of water and sodium by the kidneys, which results in a reduction in circulating blood volume and thereby reduces pulmonary fluid overload and ventricular filling pressure. Diuretics are most often used in conjunction with digitalis therapy in patients with severe congestive heart failure.

Furosemide is the most commonly used diuretic in patients with heart failure. It inhibits the reabsorption of sodium and chloride in the distal tubules and the loop of Henle. Patients requiring acute diuresis should be given intravenous or intramuscular furosemide at an initial dose of 1–2 mg/kg, which usually results in rapid diuresis and prompt improvement in clinical status, particularly if symptoms of pulmonary congestion are present. Chronic furosemide therapy is then prescribed at a dose of 1–4 mg/kg/24 hr given between one and four times a day. Careful monitoring of electrolytes is necessary with long-term furosemide therapy because of the potential for significant loss of potassium. Potassium chloride supplementation is usually required unless the potassium-sparing diuretic spironolactone is given concomitantly. When furosemide is administered every other day, dietary potassium supplementation may be adequate to maintain normal serum potassium levels. Chronic administration of furosemide may cause contraction of the extracellular fluid compartment and result in "contraction alkalosis" (see Chapter 52.7). Diuretic-induced hyponatremia may become difficult to manage in patients with severe heart failure.

Spironolactone is an inhibitor of aldosterone and enhances potassium retention, often eliminating the need for oral potassium supplementation, which is frequently poorly tolerated. This drug is usually given orally in two to three divided doses of 2–3 mg/kg/24 hr. Combinations of spironolactone and chlorothiazide are commonly used for convenience. Adults with heart failure have improved survival when an aldosterone inhibitor is included in the diuretic regimen.

Chlorothiazide is used occasionally for diuresis in children with less severe chronic heart failure. It is less immediate in action and less potent than furosemide, and it affects the reabsorption of electrolytes in the renal tubules only. The usual dose is 20–40 mg/kg/24 hr in two divided doses. Potassium supplementation is often required if this agent is used alone.

Afterload-Reducing Agents and ACE Inhibitors. This group of drugs reduces ventricular afterload by decreasing peripheral vascular resistance and thereby improving myocardial performance. Some of these agents also decrease systemic venous tone, which significantly reduces preload. Afterload reducers are especially useful in children with heart failure secondary to cardiomyopathy and in patients with severe mitral or aortic insufficiency. They may also be effective in patients with heart failure caused by left-to-right shunts. They are not generally used in the presence of stenotic lesions of the left ventricular outflow tract. ACE inhibitors may have additional beneficial effects on cardiac remodeling independent of their influence on afterload. In adult patients with dilated cardiomyopathy, the addition of an ACE inhibitor to standard medical therapy reduces both morbidity and mortality. Afterload-reducing agents and ACE inhibitors are most often used in conjunction with other anticongestive drugs such as digoxin and diuretics.

Intravenously administered agents such as nitroprusside should be administered only in an intensive care setting and for as short a time as possible. Nitroprusside's short intravenous half-life makes it ideal for titrating the dose in critically ill patients. Peripheral arterial vasodilation and afterload reduction are the major effects, but venodilation causing a decrease in venous return to the heart may also be beneficial. Blood pressure must be continuously monitored because sudden hypotension can occur. Nitroprusside is contraindicated in patients with preexisting hypotension. As the drug is metabolized, small amounts of circulating cyanide are produced and detoxified in the liver to thiocyanate, which is excreted in urine. When high doses of nitroprusside are administered for several days, toxic symptoms related to thiocyanate poisoning may occur (fatigue, nausea, disorientation, acidosis, and muscular spasm). If nitroprusside use is prolonged, blood thiocyanate levels should be monitored; values greater than 10 g/dL are consistent with clinical symptoms of toxicity. Phosphodiesterase inhibitors (see later) are also excellent afterload-reducing agents.

The orally active ACE inhibitor captopril produces arterial dilatation by blocking the production of angiotensin II, thereby resulting in significant afterload reduction. Venodilation and consequent preload reduction have also been reported. In addition, this agent interferes with aldosterone production and therefore also helps control salt and water retention. ACE inhibitors have additional beneficial effects on cardiac structure and function that may be independent of their effect on afterload. The oral dose is 0.3–6 mg/kg/24 hr given in two to three divided doses. Adverse reactions to captopril include hypotension and its sequelae (syncope, weakness, dizziness, hyperkalemia). A maculopapular pruritic rash is encountered in 5–8% of patients, but the drug may be continued because the rash often disappears spontaneously with time. Neutropenia, renal toxicity, and chronic cough also occur. Enalapril is a longer acting ACE inhibitor that can be taken once or twice daily. Angiotensin II receptor blocking drugs have recently been introduced into management protocols for adults with heart failure; however, data on these agents in children with heart failure are limited.

α- and β-Adrenergic Agonists. These drugs are usually administered in an intensive care setting, where the dose can be carefully titrated to hemodynamic response. Continuous determinations of arterial blood pressure and heart rate are performed; measuring cardiac output at the bedside with a pulmonary thermodilution (Swan-Ganz) catheter may also be helpful in assessing drug efficacy. Though extremely efficacious in the acute intensive care setting, some evidence indicates that long-term administration of adrenergic agonists may in certain cases increase morbidity and mortality in patients with heart failure.

Dopamine is a predominantly β-adrenergic receptor agonist, but it has α-adrenergic effects at higher doses. Dopamine has less chronotropic and arrhythmogenic effect than the pure β-agonist isoproterenol does. In addition, it results in selective renal vasodilation because of its interaction with renal dopamine receptors, which is particularly useful in patients with the compromised kidney function that is often associated with low cardiac output. At a dose of 2–10 μg/kg/min, dopamine results in increased contractility with little peripheral vasoconstrictive effect. If the dose is increased beyond 15 μg/kg/min, however, its peripheral α-adrenergic effects may result in vasoconstriction. Fenoldopam is a dopamine DA1 receptor agonist and is used at a low dose (0.03 mcg/kg/min) to increase renal blood flow and urine output. It can cause hypotension, so blood pressure should be carefully monitored.

Dobutamine, a derivative of dopamine, is useful in treating low cardiac output. It causes direct inotropic effects with a moderate reduction in peripheral vascular resistance. Dobutamine can be used as an adjunct to dopamine therapy to avoid the vasoconstrictive effects of high-dose dopamine. Dobutamine is also less likely to cause cardiac rhythm disturbances than isoproterenol is. The usual dose is 2–20 μg/kg/min.

Isoproterenol is a pure β-adrenergic agonist that has a marked chronotropic effect; it is most effective in patients with slow heart rates and should be used with caution in those who already have significant tachycardia. Children receiving isoproterenol must be carefully monitored for arrhythmias.

Epinephrine is a mixed α- and β-adrenergic receptor agonist that is usually reserved for patients with cardiogenic shock and low arterial blood pressure. Although epinephrine can raise blood pressure effectively, it also increases systemic vascular resistance and therefore increases the afterload against which the heart has to work.

Phosphodiesterase Inhibitors. **Milrinone** is useful in treating patients with low cardiac output who are refractory to standard therapy and has been shown to be highly effective in managing low-output state in children after open heart surgery. It works by inhibition of phosphodiesterase, which prevents the degradation of intracellular cyclic adenosine monophosphate. Milrinone has both positive inotropic effects on the heart and significant peripheral vasodilatory effects and has generally been used as an adjunct to dopamine or dobutamine therapy in the intensive care unit. It is given by intravenous infusion at 0.25–1 μg/kg/min, sometimes with an initial loading dose of 50 μg/kg. A major side effect is hypotension secondary to peripheral vasodilation, especially when a loading dose is used. The hypotension can generally be managed by the administration of intravenous fluids to restore adequate intravascular volume. Amrinone, another phosphodiesterase inhibitor, can cause thrombocytopenia; the severity appears to be related to both the rate of infusion and the duration of therapy. It is reversible when use of the drug is discontinued.

Chronic Treatment with β-Blockers. Studies in adults with dilated cardiomyopathy show that β-adrenergic blocking agents, introduced gradually as part of a comprehensive heart failure treatment program, improve exercise tolerance, decrease hospitalizations, and reduce overall mortality. The agents most often used are metoprolol, a β_1-adrenergic receptor selective antagonist, and carvedilol, an agent with both α- and β-adrenergic receptor blocking as well as free radical scavenging effects. β blockers are used for the chronic treatment of patients with heart failure and should not be administered when patients are still in the acute phase of heart failure (i.e., receiving intravenous adrenergic agonist infusions). Preliminary noncontrolled studies in children show that β blockers are well tolerated and appear to be efficacious; a multicenter controlled trial of carvedilol in pediatric patients has just been completed.

ELECTROPHYSIOLOGIC APPROACHES TO HEART FAILURE MANAGEMENT. Significant improvements in symptomatology and functional capacity have been achieved in adult patients with cardiomyopathy using biventricular resynchronization pacing (BiVP). This technique improves cardiac output by restoring normal synchrony between right and left ventricular contraction, which is often lost in patients with dilated cardiomyopathy (these patients usually manifest a left bundle branch block on electrocardiogram). There is limited experience with BiVP in children; however, small series have reported early success in patients with left ventricular failure (in the setting of cardiomyopathy), right ventricular failure (in the setting of previously repaired tetralogy of Fallot), and single ventricular failure (in the setting of complex congenital heart disease).

One of the leading causes of sudden death in patients with severe cardiomyopathy (both dilated and hypertrophic) is arrhythmia. Although antiarrhythmic medications can sometimes reduce this risk, for patients at particularly high risk (those who have already experienced a "missed sudden death" episode), use of an implantable cardioverter-defibrillator (ICD) can be lifesaving (see Chapter 435).

442.1 • Cardiogenic Shock

Cardiogenic shock (see Chapter 68) may occur as a complication of (1) severe cardiac dysfunction before or after cardiac surgery, (2) septicemia, (3) severe burns, (4) anaphylaxis, (5) cardiomyopathy, (6) myocarditis, (7) myocardial infarction or stunning, and (8) acute central nervous system disorders. It is characterized by low cardiac output and hypotension and therefore results in inadequate tissue perfusion.

Treatment is aimed at reinstitution of adequate cardiac output and peripheral perfusion to prevent the untoward effects of prolonged ischemia on vital organs, as well as management of the underlying cause. Under physiologic conditions, cardiac output is increased as a result of sympathetic discharge, which increases the heart rate. In the presence of cardiogenic shock with marked tachycardia, however, the heart rate will not increase further, and cardiac output may be reduced because of decreased diastolic filling time. Cardiac output must be increased by increasing stroke volume. If the rate of fluid administration is increased, central venous pressure and ventricular filling pressure (preload) increase, and the Frank-Starling mechanism results in increased stroke volume. Optimal filling pressure is variable and depends on a number of extracardiac factors, including ventilatory support with high positive end-expiratory pressure, peak inspiratory pressure, and intra-abdominal pressure. The increased pressure necessary to fill a relatively noncompliant ventricle should also be considered, particularly after open heart surgery. If carefully administered incremental fluid administration does not result in improved cardiac output, abnormal myocardial contractility or an abnormally high afterload, or both, must be implicated as the cause of the low cardiac output.

Myocardial contractility improves when treatment of the basic cause of shock is instituted, hypoxia is eliminated, and acidosis is corrected. Dopamine, epinephrine, and dobutamine improve cardiac contractility, increase the heart rate, and ultimately increase cardiac output.

The use of cardiac glycosides to treat acute low cardiac output states should be avoided. Digoxin has a slower effect than catecholamines do, even with intravenous administration. In addition, adverse effects may result from larger doses, and toxicity is less predictable and depends on myocardial and serum potassium and calcium levels. It is common for patients in cardiovascular shock to have compromised renal perfusion, so administration of digoxin may result in high persistent blood levels because the kidneys excrete it. When digoxin is required for these patients, a lower and less frequent dosage should be used, and serum digoxin levels must be monitored frequently.

TABLE 442-3. Treatment of Cardiogenic Shock*

	DETERMINANTS OF STROKE VOLUME		
	Preload	**Contractility**	**Afterload**
Parameters measured	CVP, PCWP, LAP, cardiac chamber size on echocardiography	CO, BP, fractional shortening on echocardiography, MV O_2 saturation	BP, peripheral perfusion, SVR
Abnormal physiologic manifestations	Low CVP, PCWP, or LAP ↓CO ↓BP	High CVP, PCWP, or LAP; low MVO_2 saturation ↓CO ↓BP	High CVP, PCWP, LAP or SVR ↓CO → or ↑ BP
Treatment to improve cardiac output	Volume expansion (crystalloid, colloid, blood)	β-Adrenergic agonists, phosphodiesterase inhibitors	Afterload-reducing agents: nitroprusside, ACE inhibitors

*The goal is to improve peripheral perfusion by increasing cardiac output: cardiac output = heart rate × stroke volume.
↓, decreased; ↑, increased; →, normal; BP, blood pressure; CO, cardiac output (measured with a thermodilation catheter); CVP, central venous pressure; LAP, left atrial pressure (measured with an indwelling LA line); MV O_2 saturation, mixed venous oxygen saturation (measured with central venous catheter); PCWP, pulmonary capillary wedge pressure; SVR, systemic vascular resistance (calculated from CO and mean BP).

Patients in cardiogenic shock may have a marked increase in systemic vascular resistance resulting in high afterload and poor peripheral perfusion. If the increased systemic vascular resistance is persistent and the administration of positive inotropic agents alone does not improve tissue perfusion, the use of afterload-reducing agents may be appropriate, for example, nitroprusside or milrinone in combination with dopamine. In these patients, the use of a pulmonary thermodilution catheter to measure the cardiac index and to calculate systemic vascular resistance can be indispensable in guiding therapeutic decisions.

Sequential evaluation and management of cardiovascular shock are mandatory (see Chapter 68). Table 442-3 outlines the general treatment principles for acute cardiac circulatory failure under most circumstances. Treatment of infants and children with low cardiac output after cardiac surgery depends on the nature of the operative procedure and the patient's status after surgery (see Chapter 434).

Patients with deteriorating cardiogenic shock may benefit from a left ventricular assist device (LVAD). These devices have been used successfully in children and adolescents as a bridge to cardiac transplantation. Some devices are small enough to be capable of supporting young infants. In some cases, both right and left ventricular assist is necessary (BiVAD). Once implanted, assist devices allow patients to recover sufficiently to be extubated, become ambulatory, and often leave the intensive care setting while awaiting transplantation. Patients with reversible ventricular failure, for example, those in the immediate postoperative state or those with acute myocarditis, may also benefit from extracorporeal membrane oxygenation (ECMO). When ventricular function is not expected to recover, heart transplantation should be considered (see Chap. 443.1).

Aurigemma GP, Gaasch WH: Diastolic heart failure. *N Engl J Med* 2004;351:1097–1105.

Bristow M: Antiadrenergic therapy of chronic heart failure: Surprises and new opportunities. *Circulation* 2003;107:1100–1102.

Bristow MR, Saxon LA, Boehmer J, et al: Cardiac-resynchronization therapy with or without an implantable defibrillator in advanced chronic heart failure. *N Engl J Med* 2004;350:2140–2150.

Bruns LA, Chrisant MK, Lamour JM, et al: Carvedilol as therapy in pediatric heart failure: An initial multicenter experience. *J Pediatr* 2001;138:505–511.

Clark BJ III: Treatment of heart failure in infants and children. *Heart Dis* 2000;2:354–361.

Dubin AM, Berul CI, Bevilacqua LM, et al: The use of implantable cardioverter-defibrillators in pediatric patients awaiting heart transplantation. *J Card Fail* 2003;9:375–379.

Hoffman TM, Wernovsky G, Atz AM, et al: Efficacy and safety of milrinone in preventing low cardiac output syndrome in infants and children after corrective surgery for congenital heart disease. *Circulation* 2003; 107:996–1002.

Jessup M, Brozena S: Heart failure. *N Engl J Med* 2003;348:2007–2018.

Kay JD, Colan SD, Graham TP Jr: Congestive heart failure in pediatric patients. *Am Heart J* 2001;142:923–928.

Liggett SB: Polymorphisms of beta-adrenergic receptors in heart failure. *Am J Med* 2004;117:525–527.

Maisel AS, Krishnaswamy P, Nowak RM, et al: Rapid measurement of B-type natriuretic peptide in the emergency diagnosis of heart failure. *N Engl J Med* 2002;347:161–166.

McMurphy JJV: Heart failure. *Lancet* 2005;365:1877–1889.

Murphy MB, Murray C, Shorten GD: Fenoldopam—a selective peripheral dopamine-receptor agonist for the treatment of severe hypertension. *N Engl J Med* 2001;345:1548–1557.

Neubauer S: The failing heart: an engine out of fuel. *N Engl J Med* 2007; 356:1140–1150.

Port JD, Bristow MR: Altered beta-adrenergic receptor gene regulation and signaling in chronic heart failure. *J Mol Cell Cardiol* 2001;33:887–905.

Rosenthal D, Chrisant MR, Edens E, et al: International Society for Heart and Lung Transplantation: Practice guidelines for management of heart failure in children. *J Heart Lung Transplant* 2004;23:1313–1333.

Shaddy RE: Optimizing treatment for chronic congestive heart failure in children. *Crit Care Med* 2001;29(Suppl):237–240.

Westerlind A, Wahlander H, Lindstedt G, et al: Clinical signs of heart failure are associated with increased levels of natriuretic peptide types B and A in children with congenital heart defects or cardiomyopathy. *Acta Paediatr* 2004;93:340–345.

Chapter 443 ■ Pediatric Heart and Heart-Lung Transplantation

443.1 • Pediatric Heart Transplantation

Pediatric heart transplantation is standard therapy for children with end-stage cardiomyopathy and other lesions not amenable to surgical repair. As of 2004, >5,300 heart transplants had been performed on children in the United States, with ≈325 transplants annually. Survival rates among children compare favorably with those of adults (78% at 1 yr and 68% at 5 yr). For children transplanted between 1982 and 1988, 1 yr survival is 75%, whereas for those transplanted after 1999, 1 yr survival is 90%; during the same periods, the survival half-life (time at which 50% of patients are still alive) has improved from 8.3 yr to 11.0 yr (Fig. 443-1). A growing number of children are reaching their 15, 20, and 25 yr post-transplant anniversaries.

INDICATIONS. Heart transplantation is performed in infants and children with end-stage cardiomyopathy who have become refractory to medical therapy, in patients with previously repaired or palliated congenital heart disease who have developed ventricular dysfunction or other nonoperable late-term complications, and (less frequently) in patients with complex congenital heart disease (pulmonary atresia with intact septum and coronary arterial stenoses, some forms of hypoplastic left heart syndrome) for whom standard surgical procedures are extremely high risk. Cardiomyopathies account for >50% of heart transplants in pediatric patients older than 1 yr, although the percentage of patients with previously repaired complex congenital lesions (≈30%) is gradually increasing. In infants younger than 1 yr, congenital heart lesions used to represent >80% of transplants, this fraction

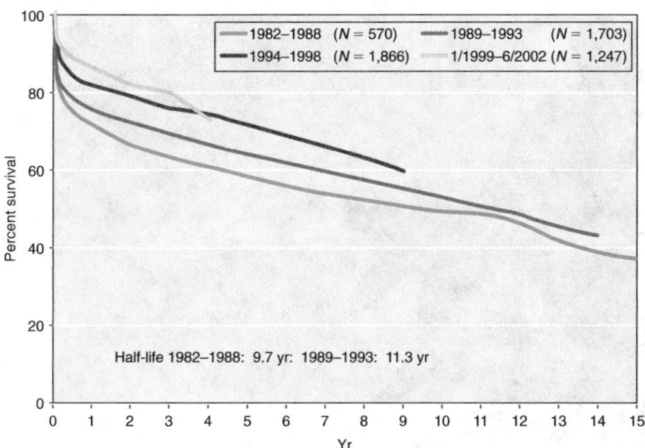

Figure 443-1. Survival after pediatric heart transplantation comparing current and past eras, based on >5,300 patients who received heart transplants from 1982 through 2002, as listed with the Registry of the International Society for Heart and Lung Transplantation. Survival was significantly improved over each successive time period: 1999–2002 vs all other eras ($p < 0.0001$); 1982–1988 vs 1994–1998 ($p < 0.0001$); 1989–1993 vs 1994–1998 ($p < 0.0001$). (Adapted from Boucek et al: Registry for the International Society for Heart and Lung Transplantation: Seventh official pediatric report—2004. *J Heart Lung Transplant* 2004;23:933–947. © 2004 International Society for Heart and Lung Transplantation.)

has dropped to 65% as surgical results for complex congenital heart disease (hypoplastic left heart syndrome) have improved.

RECIPIENT AND DONOR SELECTION. Potential heart transplant recipients must be free of serious noncardiac medical problems such as neurologic disease, systemic infection, severe hepatic or renal disease, or severe malnutrition. Many children with ventricular dysfunction may have pulmonary hypertension and even pulmonary vascular disease, which would preclude heart transplantation; pulmonary vascular resistance must be measured at cardiac catheterization, both at rest and in response to vasodilators. Patients with fixed elevated pulmonary vascular resistance (>6–8 Wood units) are at higher risk for heart transplantation and may be considered candidates for either heterotopic heart transplantation (see below) or heart-lung transplantation (see Chapter 443.2). A comprehensive social services consultation is an important component of the recipient evaluation. Because of the complex post-transplantation medical regimen, the family must have a history of compliance. Detailed informed consent must be obtained.

Donor shortage is a serious problem for both adults and children. At the national registry of transplant recipients in the United States (the United Network for Organ Sharing [UNOS]), allografts are matched by ABO blood group and body weight. HLA matching is not currently performed nor is it easily feasible for heart transplantation; with modern immunosuppression, it may offer only minimal advantage. ABO matching is not required for young infants; the exact age at which ABO tolerance develops has not yet been determined. **Contraindications** to organ donation include prolonged cardiac arrest with moderate to severe ongoing cardiac dysfunction, ongoing systemic illness or infection, and pre-existing severe cardiac disease. Physicians caring for a patient who may be a potential donor should always contact the organ donor coordinator at their institution, who can best judge the appropriateness of organ donation and has experience in interacting with donor families. A history of resuscitation alone or reparable congenital heart disease is not an automatic exclusion for donation.

The decision of when to place a patient on the transplant waiting list is based on many factors, including extremely poor ventricular function (left ventricular fractional shortening <10%; normal is 28–40%), poor exercise tolerance as determined by cardiopulmonary exercise testing (see Chapter 423.5), poor response to medical anticongestive therapy, multiple hospitalizations for heart failure, arrhythmia, progressive deterioration in renal or hepatic function, early stages of pulmonary vascular disease, and poor nutritional status. In patients awaiting transplantation, those with poor left ventricular function (fractional shortening <15%) are usually started on a regimen of anticoagulation, preferably with warfarin, to reduce the risk of mural thrombosis and thromboembolism. Patients with cardiogenic shock unresponsive to standard pharmacologic treatment may be candidates for placement of left ventricular (LVAD) or biventricular (BiVAD) assist devices, or for extracorporeal membrane oxygenation (ECMO) support, which can stabilize hemodynamics and serve as a bridge to transplantation (see Chapter 442).

PERIOPERATIVE MANAGEMENT. In the classic operation, both donor and recipient hearts are excised so that the posterior portions of the atria containing the venae cavae and pulmonary veins are left intact. The aorta and pulmonary artery are divided above the level of the semilunar valves. The anterior portion of the donor's atria is then connected to the remaining posterior portion of the recipient's atria, thereby avoiding the need for delicate suturing of the venae cavae or pulmonary veins. The donor and recipient great vessels are connected via end-to-end anastomoses. A bicaval anastomosis is usually used, with the donor right atrium left intact; the left atrial connection is still performed as in the classic procedure. **Heterotopic heart transplantation** has been used for patients with left ventricular cardiomyopathy and elevated pulmonary vascular resistance. In this operation, the donor and recipient hearts are connected in parallel, so that the recipient right ventricle (which has hypertrophied over time due to the elevated pulmonary pressures) pumps mostly to the lungs, and the donor left ventricle pumps mostly to the body (Fig. 443-2). This operation is preferable to heart-lung transplant for appropriate candidates (patients with pulmonary hypertension but without parenchymal lung disease, without evidence of right ventricular failure, and without serious congenital heart disease), as it is associated with a greater survival at all post-transplant time points.

In the immediate postoperative period, **immunosuppression** is most commonly achieved with a triple-drug regimen, although some centers use steroid-free regimens. The most common combinations are a calcineurin inhibitor (either cyclosporine or tacrolimus), a white blood cell enzyme inhibitor (mycophenolate mofetil or azathioprine), and prednisone. Some centers are using one of the cell-cycle inhibitors that act on the protein mTOR (target of rapamycin) instead of mycophenolate because of their potential benefit in reducing graft coronary artery disease. In many centers, an antilymphocyte preparation is added in the 1st wk, either antithymocyte globulin, monoclonal murine antihuman T-lymphocyte antibody (OKT3), or one of the humanized anti–interleukin 2 receptor antibodies (daclizumab, basiliximab). In children who do not experience significant graft rejection, steroids can be gradually eliminated after the 1st 6–12 mo. In centers that do not use steroids routinely, they are used as bolus treatment for acute rejection episodes.

Most pediatric heart transplant recipients can be extubated within the 1st 48 hr after transplantation and are out of bed within 3–4 days. These patients are often discharged within the 1st 2 wk after transplantation. In patients with pre-existing high-risk factors, postoperative recovery may be considerably prolonged. For those with preoperative pulmonary hypertension, the use of nitric oxide (NO) in the postoperative period can buy time to allow the donor right ventricle to hypertrophy in response to elevated pulmonary artery pressures. Occasionally, these patients will require right ventricular assist device (RVAD) support.

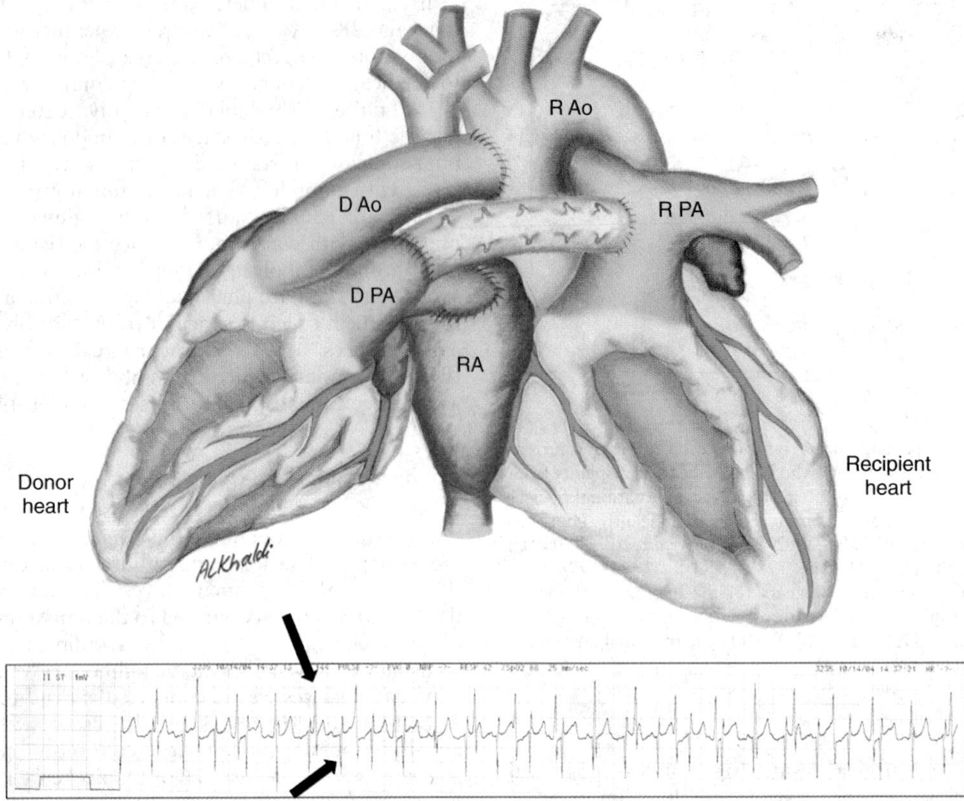

Figure 443-2. Heterotopic heart transplantation. The donor and recipient hearts are connected in parallel: the two right atria are attached; the donor pulmonary artery is anastomosed to the recipient's pulmonary artery; the two left atria are attached; the donor aorta is anastomosed to the recipient's aorta. RA, right atrium; D PA, donor pulmonary artery; R PA, recipient pulmonary artery; R Ao, donor aorta; R Ao, recipient aorta. Below the figure is an electrocardiogram from a 22 month old infant after a heterotopic heart transplant. The separate donor and recipient QRS complexes can be seen *(arrows)*. (Illustration courtesy of Dr. Aziz Alkhaldi, Stanford University, Stanford, CA).

DIAGNOSIS AND MANAGEMENT OF ACUTE GRAFT REJECTION. Post-transplantation management consists of adjusting medications to maintain a balance between the risk of rejection and the side effects of over-immunosuppression. Along with infection, acute graft rejection is a leading cause of death in adult and pediatric heart transplant recipients. The incidence of acute rejection is greatest in the 1st 3 mo after transplantation and decreases considerably thereafter. Many pediatric patients experience at least one episode of acute rejection in the 1st 2 yr after transplantation, although modern immunosuppressive regimens have decreased the frequency of serious rejection episodes. Because the symptoms of rejection can mimic many routine pediatric illnesses (pneumonia, gastroenteritis), it is mandatory that the transplant center be notified whenever a heart transplant recipient is seen in the pediatrician's office or emergency room for any acute illness.

Clinical manifestations of **acute rejection** may include fatigue, fluid retention, fever, diaphoresis, abdominal symptoms, and a gallop rhythm. The electrocardiogram may show reduced voltage, atrial or ventricular arrhythmias, or heart block, but is most usually nondiagnostic. Roentgenographic examination may show an enlarged heart, effusions, or pulmonary edema, but usually only in the more advanced stages of rejection. Most rejection episodes occur without any detectable clinical symptoms. On echocardiography, indices of systolic left ventricular function may be decreased; however, these usually do not deteriorate until rejection is at least moderately severe. Techniques to evaluate wall thickening and left ventricular diastolic function, which appeared to be promising, have not fulfilled their promise as predictors of early rejection. Most transplant centers do not rely on echocardiography alone in rejection surveillance.

Myocardial biopsy is the most reliable method of monitoring patients for rejection. Biopsy specimens are taken from the right ventricular side of the interventricular septum and can be harvested relatively safely, even in small infants. In older children, myocardial biopsies may be performed as often as every 1–4 wk during the 1st 3–6 mo after transplantation. The frequency is then reduced to 2 or 4 biopsies per year unless the patient has an episode of rejection. In infants, surveillance biopsies are usually performed less often and may be as infrequent as once or twice per year. Children may have clinically unsuspected rejection episodes even 5–10 yr after transplantation; most pediatric transplant centers continue routine surveillance biopsies, albeit at less frequent intervals (every 6–12 mo).

Criteria for **grading cardiac rejection** are based on a system developed by the International Society for Heart and Lung Transplantation (ISHLT); these criteria take into account the degree of cellular infiltration and whether myocyte necrosis is present. ISHLT rejection grades 1A, 1B, and 2 are usually mild enough to not warrant immediate treatment, and >50% of these episodes may resolve spontaneously. A repeat biopsy specimen is usually obtained within several weeks. For patients with ISHLT grade 3A rejection, treatment is instituted with either intravenous methylprednisolone or a "bump and taper" of oral prednisone. Asymptomatic patients >3 mo post-transplant and with normal echocardiograms are often treated as outpatients. Patients with grades 3B or 4, or anyone with hemodynamic instability, are admitted to the hospital for intravenous steroid and potentially more aggressive anti-rejection therapy. For rejection episodes resistant to steroid therapy, additional therapeutic regimens include a repeat course of an antilymphocyte preparation

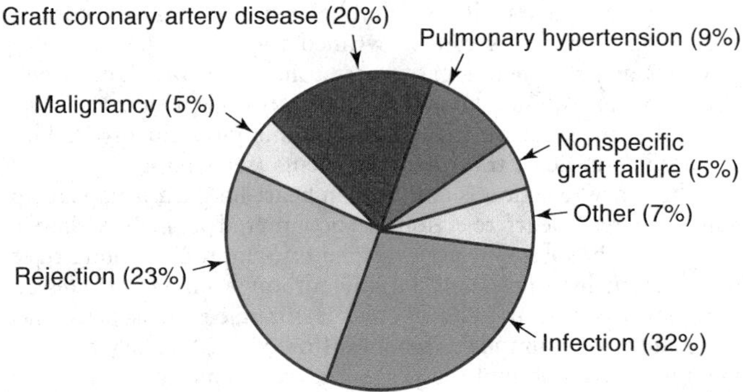

Figure 443-3. Major causes of death after pediatric heart transplantation. (Data from Stanford University, Stanford, CA.)

(daclizumab, OKT3, antithymocyte globulin), methotrexate, or total lymphoid irradiation. Patients with repeated episodes of rejection may also benefit from being switched from cyclosporine to tacrolimus (or vice versa). Rare patients with refractory rejection require retransplantation.

Some rejection episodes are not associated with a cellular infiltrate on biopsy. These cases of acellular or humoral rejection are presumably mediated by circulating antibodies and can be detected by immunostaining of the biopsy specimen for the complement component C4d and other immune markers. Humoral rejection is less responsive to standard immunnosuppresion (bolus steroids) and has been treated with plasmapheresis, photopheresis, intravenous immunoglobulin, methotrexate, and the anti-CD20 monoclonal antibody rituximab.

COMPLICATIONS OF IMMUNOSUPPRESSION.

Infection. Infection is one of the two leading causes of death in pediatric transplant patients (Fig. 443-3). The incidence of infection is greatest in the 1st 3 mo after transplantation when immunosuppressive doses are highest. Viral infections are the most common, especially cytomegalovirus, which accounts for as many as 25% of infectious episodes. Cytomegalovirus infection may occur as a primary infection in patients without previous exposure to the virus or as a reactivation. Severe cytomegalovirus infection can be disseminated or associated with pneumonitis and may provoke an episode of acute graft rejection or graft coronary disease. Many centers use intravenous ganciclovir or cytomegalovirus immune globulin (CytoGam), or both, as prophylaxis in any patient receiving a heart from a donor who is positive for cytomegalovirus or in any recipient who has serologic evidence of previous cytomegalovirus disease. Polymerase chain reaction (PCR) enhances the ability to diagnose cytomegalovirus infection and to monitor the efficacy of therapy serially. Oral preparations of ganciclovir with improved absorption profiles are available for chronic therapy.

Most normal childhood viral illnesses are well tolerated and do not usually require special treatment. Otitis media and routine upper respiratory tract infections can be treated in the outpatient setting, although fever or symptoms that last beyond the usual course require further investigation. Gastroenteritis, especially with vomiting, can result in markedly reduced absorption of immunosuppressive medications and provoke a rejection episode. In this setting, drug levels should be closely monitored and the use of intravenous medications considered. Varicella exposure is treated with varicella immune globulin, and if the patient acquires clinical varicella infection, treatment with intravenous acyclovir attenuates the illness.

Bacterial infections are the next most frequent, with the lung being the most common site of infection (35%), followed by the blood, the urinary tract, and, less commonly, the sternotomy site. Other sources of post-transplantation infection include fungi (14%) and protozoa (6%). Many centers use nystatin mouthwash to decrease fungal colonization and trimethoprim/sulfamethoxazole (Bactrim, Septra) prophylaxis to prevent *Pneumocystis carinii* infection. The incidence of serious infection is lower in children who can be managed without steroids.

Growth Retardation. Patients requiring chronic steroid administration usually have decreased linear growth, thus most pediatric transplant programs aim for steroid-free immunosuppression within 1–2 yr post-transplant. In those patients who experience rejection when steroids are withdrawn, alternate-day steroid regimens result in improved linear growth. Total lymphoid irradiation has shown promise as a steroid-sparing protocol. Long-term survivors of pediatric heart transplantation have normal growth in 75% of patients.

Hypertension. Hypertension is common in patients treated with cyclosporine. It is due to a combination of plasma volume expansion and defective renal sodium excretion. Corticosteroids usually potentiate cyclosporine-induced hypertension. Patients are typically managed with a combination of a diuretic and a vasodilator. Agents that work via calcium channel blockade have the additional advantage of possibly attenuating graft coronary disease. The incidence of hypertension may be slightly lower in patients treated with tacrolimus.

Renal Function. Chronic administration of cyclosporine or tacrolimus can lead to a tubulointerstitial nephropathy in adults, but severe renal dysfunction is rare in children. Most pediatric patients gradually have an increase in serum creatinine in the 1st yr after transplantation; if renal dysfunction occurs, it usually responds to a decrease in cyclosporine dosage. Long-term patients rarely require renal transplantation.

Neurologic Complications. Neurologic side effects of cyclosporine and tacrolimus include tremor, myalgias, paresthesias, and, rarely, seizures. These complications can be treated with reduced doses of medication and occasionally with oral magnesium supplementation. Intracranial infections pose a significant risk, especially because some of the more frequent signs (nuchal rigidity) may be absent in immunosuppressed patients. Potential organisms include *Aspergillus, Cryptococcus neoformans,* and *Listeria monocytogenes.* Aseptic meningitis can be seen days or weeks after OKT3 administration and is usually self-limited.

Tumors. One of the serious complications limiting long-term survival in pediatric heart transplant patients is the risk of neoplastic disease. The most common is post-transplant lymphoproliferative disease (PTLD), a condition associated with Epstein-Barr virus infection. PTLD usually responds to a reduction in immunosuppression and antiviral therapy with acyclovir and only occasionally requires chemotherapy. A monoclonal antibody directed against the CD20 antigen on activated lymphocytes (rituximab) shows promise against some forms of PTLD. An increased risk of skin cancer requires that children use appropriate precautions when exposed to sunlight.

Chronic Rejection. Graft **coronary artery disease** (CAD) is a manifestation of chronic graft rejection that occurs in ≈20% of children. The cause is still unclear, although it is thought to be a form of immunologically mediated vessel injury. Hypercholesterolemia and hyperglycemia increase the risk of this disease. Unlike native coronary atherosclerosis, graft CAD is a diffuse process with a high degree of distal vessel involvement. Because the transplanted heart has been denervated, patients do not experience symptoms such as angina pectoris during ischemic episodes, and the initial manifestation may be cardiovascular collapse or sudden death. Most centers perform coronary angiography annually to screen for coronary abnormalities; some also perform coronary intravascular ultrasound (IVUS). Standard coronary artery bypass procedures are not usually helpful because of the diffuse nature of the process, although transcatheter stenting is sometimes effective for isolated lesions. For severe cases, repeat heart transplantation has been the only effective treatment.

Thus, prevention has been the focus of most current research. The cell cycle inhibitors sirolimus and everolimus have been shown to decrease coronary arterial intimal thickening at 2 yr post-transplant in adult patients. Other drugs that have been shown to reduce the risk of graft coronary artery disease include the calcium channel blockers (such as diltiazem) and the cholesterol-lowering HMG-CoA (3-hydroxy-3-methyl-coenzyme A) reductase inhibitors (such as pravastatin or atorvastatin).

Other Complications. Corticosteroids usually result in cushingoid facies, steroid acne, and striae. Cyclosporine can cause a subtle change in facial features such as hypertrichosis and gingival hyperplasia. These cosmetic features can be particularly disturbing to adolescents and may be the motivation for noncompliance. Many of these complications are dose related and improve as immunosuppressive medications are weaned. Osteoporosis and aseptic necrosis are additional reasons for reducing the steroid dosage as soon as possible. Diabetes and pancreatitis are rare but serious complications.

Rehabilitation. Despite the potential risks of immunosuppression, the prospect for rehabilitation in pediatric heart transplant recipients is excellent. More than 95% of pediatric heart transplant recipients have no functional limitations in their daily lives. The majority of patients do not require rehospitalization for transplant-related problems.

Pediatric heart transplant recipients can attend daycare or school and participate in non-collision competitive sports and other age-appropriate activities. Standardized measurements of ventricular function are close to normal. Because the transplanted heart is denervated, the increase in heart rate and cardiac output during exercise is slower in transplant recipients, and maximal heart rate and cardiac output responses are mildly attenuated. These subtle abnormalities are rarely noticeable by the patient.

Growth of the transplanted heart is excellent, although a mild degree of ventricular and septal hypertrophy is commonly seen, even years after transplantation. The sites of atrial and great vessel anastomoses grow without the development of obstruction. In neonates who undergo transplantation for hypoplastic left heart syndrome, however, juxtaductal aortic coarctation may recur.

As assessed by standardized psychologic testing, the psychologic adjustment to heart transplantation in children is usually good. A serious problem with noncompliance often occurs once patients reach adolescence, and life-threatening rejection may result. Early intervention by social workers, counselors, and psychologists may be able to reduce this risk.

443.2 • Heart-Lung and Lung Transplantation

More than 700 heart-lung and lung (single or double) transplants have been performed in children in the United States, with ≈60 procedures performed annually. Primary indications for heart-lung transplantation include cystic fibrosis, primary pulmonary hypertension, complex congenital heart disease with pulmonary hypoplasia or Eisenmenger syndrome, congenital lung abnormalities, and end-stage parenchymal lung disease (bronchopulmonary dysplasia, chronic lung disease, and interstitial fibrosis). Many of these patients with normal hearts may also be candidates for single- or double-lung transplantation if right ventricular function is preserved. In some patients with Eisenmenger physiology, double-lung transplantation can be performed in combination with repair of intracardiac defects. Patients with cystic fibrosis are not candidates for single-lung grafts because of the risk of infection from the diseased contralateral lung. Patients are selected according to many of the same criteria as for heart transplant recipients (see Chapter 443.1).

Post-transplant immunosuppression is usually achieved with a triple-drug regimen, similar to that used for heart transplantation. Unlike patients with isolated heart transplants, few patients with lung transplants can be weaned totally off steroids. Prophylaxis against pneumocystis carinii infection is achieved with trimethoprim-sulfamethoxazole or aerosolized pentamidine. Ganciclovir and cytomegalovirus immune globulin prophylaxis are used as in heart transplant recipients (see Chapter 443.1).

Pulmonary rejection is common in heart-lung transplant recipients, whereas heart rejection is encountered less often than in patients with isolated heart transplants. Symptoms of lung rejection may include fever and fatigue, although many episodes are minimally symptomatic. Surveillance for rejection is performed by monitoring pulmonary function (forced vital capacity; forced expiratory volume in 1 sec [FEV_1]; forced expiratory flow, mid-expiratory phase [$FEF_{25-75\%}$]), systemic arterial oxygen tension, and chest roentgenograms and by serial transbronchial biopsy. Because of technical limitations, biopsies are not usually performed in infants, who are monitored by clinical criteria alone.

Actuarial survival rates after heart-lung or lung transplantation in children are currently 75% at 1 yr and 50% at 5 yr; improved patient selection and postoperative management are continually improving these survival statistics. Graft failure and infection are the leading cause of early death, whereas a form of chronic rejection known as **bronchiolitis obliterans (OB)** accounts for nearly 50% of late mortality. Other causes of early morbidity and mortality include tracheal complications, pulmonary venous obstruction, donor lung dysfunction, bleeding, and acute rejection. Additional late complications include the development of airway stenosis, accelerated graft CAD (though less common than in isolated heart transplantation), and other side effects of chronic immunosuppression.

Postoperative indices of cardiopulmonary function and exercise capacity show significant improvement. More than 95% of patients are without activity limitations at 2 yr follow-up. Problems of donor availability are even more severe with lung transplantation. Living related lung transplantation, in which a lobe from a parent is transplanted into a child, may partially alleviate this problem.

Heart Transplantation

Boucek MM, Edwards LB, Keck BM, et al: Registry for the International Society for Heart and Lung Transplantation: Seventh official pediatric report—2004. *J Heart Lung Transplant* 2004;23:933–947.

Burch M, Aurora P: Current status of paediatric heart, lung, and heart-lung transplantation. *Arch Dis Child* 2004;89:386–389.

Canter C, Naftel D, Caldwell R, et al: Survival and risk factors for death after cardiac transplantation in infants. A multi-institutional study. The Pediatric Heart Transplant Study. *Circulation* 1997;96:227–231.

Chin C, Gamberg P, Miller J, et al: Efficacy and safety of atorvastatin after pediatric heart transplantation. *J Heart Lung Transplant* 2002; 21:1213–1217.

Fan X, Ang A, Pollock-Barziv SM, et al: Donor-specific B-cell tolerance after ABO-incompatible infant heart transplantation. *Nat Med* 2004; 10:1227–1233.

Hornung TS, de Goede C, O'Brien C, et al: Renal function after pediatric cardiac transplantation: The effect of early cyclosporine dosage. *Pediatrics* 2001;107:1346–1350.

Hotson JR, Enzmann DR: Neurologic complications of cardiac transplantation. *Neurol Clin* 1988;6:349–365.

Mazariegos GV, Reyes J, Webber SA, et al: Cytokine gene polymorphisms in children successfully withdrawn from immunosuppression after liver transplantation. *Transplantation* 2002;73:1342–1345.

Pahl E, Zales VR, Fricker FJ, et al: Posttransplant coronary artery disease in children. A multicenter national survey. *Circulation* 1994;90:II56–II60.

Pollock-BarZiv SM, Anthony SJ, et al: Quality of life and function following cardiac transplantation in adolescents. *Transplant Proc* 2003;35: 2468–2470.

Ringewald JM, Gidding SS, Crawford SE, et al: Nonadherence is associated with late rejection in pediatric heart transplant recipients. *J Pediatr* 2001;139:75–78.

Rosenthal DN, Chin C, Nishimura K, et al: Identifying cardiac transplant rejection in children: Diagnostic utility of echocardiography, right heart catheterization and endomyocardial biopsy data. *J Heart Lung Transplant* 2004;23:323–329.
Russo LM, Webber SA: Pediatric heart transplantation: Immunosuppression and its complications. *Curr Opin Cardiol* 2004;19:104–109.
Schowengerdt KO, Naftel DC, Seib PM, et al: Infection after pediatric heart transplantation: Results of a multi-institutional study. The Pediatric Heart Transplant Study Group. *J Heart Lung Transplant* 1997;16:1207–1216.
Shirali GS, Ni J, Chinnock RE, et al: Association of viral genome with graft loss in children after cardiac transplantation. *N Engl J Med* 2001;344:1498–1503.
Sigfusson G, Fricker FJ, Bernstein D, et al: Long term survivors of pediatric heart transplantation: A multicenter report of 68 children who have survived greater than five years. *J Pediatr* 1997;130:862–871.
Webber SA: Immunology of pediatric heart transplantation: A clinical update. *Semin Thorac Cardiovasc Surg Pediatr Card Surg Annu* 2001;4:158–184.
Webber SA, Naftel DC, Fricker FJ, et al: Lymphoproliferative disorders after pediatric heart transplantation: a multi-institutional study. *Lancet* 2006;367:233–239.
West LJ, Pollock-Barziv SM, Dipchand AI, et al: ABO-incompatible heart transplantation in infants. *N Engl J Med* 2001;344:793–800.

Lung Transplantation

Conte JV, Robbins RC, Reichenspurner H, et al: Pediatric heart-lung transplantation: Intermediate-term results. *J Heart Lung Transplant* 1996;15:692–699.
Mendeloff EN, Huddleston CB, Mallory GB, et al: Pediatric and adult lung transplantation for cystic fibrosis. *J Thorac Cardiovasc Surg* 1998;115:404–413.
Moffatt SD, Demers P, Robbins RC, et al: Lung transplantation: A decade of experience. *J Heart Lung Transplant* 2005;24:145–151.
Sritippayawan S, Keens TG, Horn MV, et al: What are the best pulmonary function test parameters for early detection of post-lung transplant bronchiolitis obliterans syndrome in children? *Pediatr Transplant* 2003;7:200–203.
Starnes VA, Bowdish ME, Woo MS, et al: A decade of living lobar lung transplantation: Recipient outcomes. *J Thorac Cardiovasc Surg* 2004;127:114–122.
Sweet SC, Spray TL, Huddleston CB, et al: Pediatric lung transplantation at St. Louis Children's Hospital, 1990–1995. *Am J Respir Crit Care Med* 1997;155:1027–1035.
Webber SA, McCurry K, Zeevi A: Heart and lung transplantation in children. *Lancet* 2006;368:53–68.

Section 8 — Diseases of the Peripheral Vascular System — Daniel Bernstein

Chapter 444 ■ Disease of the Blood Vessels (Aneurysms and Fistulas)

444.1 • Kawasaki Disease (see also Chapter 165)

Aneurysms of the coronary or systemic arteries may complicate Kawasaki disease and are the leading cause of morbidity in this disease (Figs. 444-1 and 444-2). Other than in Kawasaki disease, aneurysms are not common in children and occur most frequently in the aorta in association with coarctation of the aorta, patent ductus arteriosus, and Marfan syndrome and in intracranial vessels (see Chapter 601). They may also occur secondary to an infected embolus; infection contiguous to a blood vessel; trauma; congenital abnormalities of vessel structure, especially the medial wall; and arteritis, for example, polyarteritis nodosa and Takayasu arteritis (see Chapter 166.2).

444.2 • Arteriovenous Fistulas

Arteriovenous fistulas may be limited to small cavernous hemangiomas or may be extensive (see Chapters 505 and 649). The most common sites in infants and children are within the cranium, in the liver, in the lung, in the extremities, and in vessels in or near the thoracic wall. These fistulas, though usually congenital, may follow trauma or be a manifestation of hereditary hemorrhagic telangiectasia (Osler-Weber-Rendu disease). Femoral arteriovenous fistulas are a rare complication of percutaneous femoral catheterization.

CLINICAL MANIFESTATIONS. Clinical symptoms occur only in association with large arteriovenous communications when arterial blood flows into a low-pressure venous system; local venous pressure is increased, and arterial flow distal to the fistula is decreased. Systemic arterial resistance falls because of the runoff of blood through the fistula. Compensatory mechanisms include tachycardia and increased stroke volume so that cardiac output

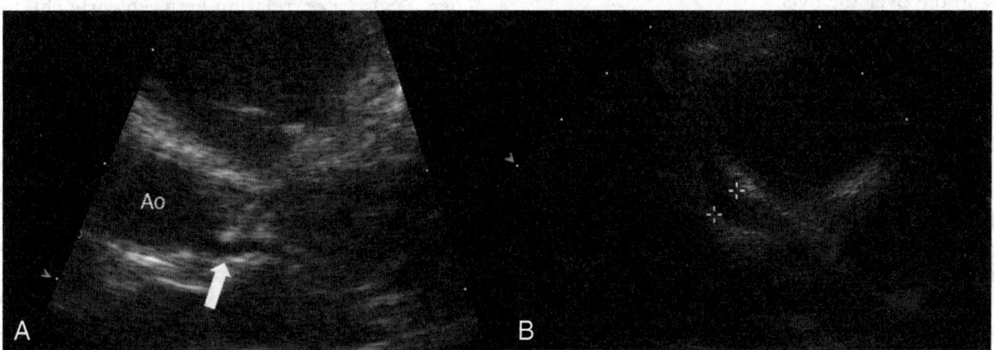

Figure 444-1. Two-dimensional echocardiogram comparing a normal left main coronary artery (*arrow* in figure on left) with a giant coronary artery aneurysm (outlined by *cross marks* in figure on right) in a patient with Kawasaki disease. Ao, aorta.

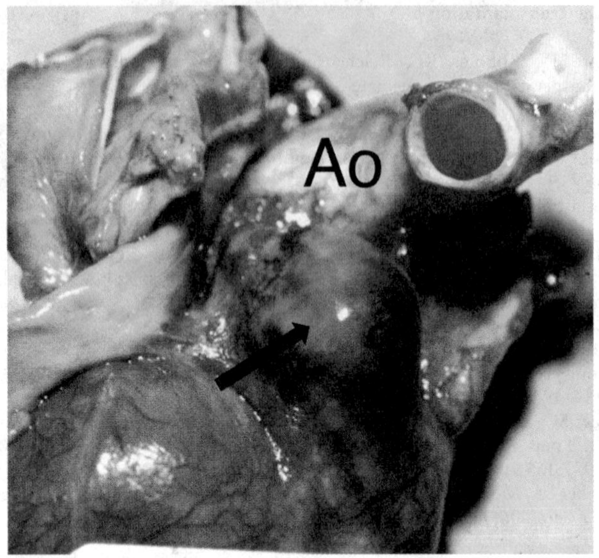

Figure 444-2. Pathologic specimen showing giant aneurysm of left main coronary artery *(arrow)*. Ao, ascending aorta.

rises. Total blood volume is also increased. In large fistulas, left ventricular dilatation, a widened pulse pressure, and heart failure occur. Injection of contrast material into an artery proximal to the fistula confirms the diagnosis.

Large intracranial arteriovenous fistulas most often occur in newborn infants in association with a **vein of Galen malformation**. The large intracranial left-to-right shunt results in heart failure secondary to the demand for high cardiac output. Patients with smaller communications may not have cardiovascular manifestations but may later be disposed to hydrocephalus (see Chapter 592.11) or seizure disorders. A newborn infant with a large symptomatic intracranial arteriovenous fistula has a grave prognosis; some survive with medical management but are subject to later complications caused by the intracranial mass. The diagnosis can often be made by auscultation of a continuous murmur over the cranium. Older children with more diffuse intracranial arteriovenous malformations may be recognized on the basis of intracranial calcification and high cardiac output without cardiac failure.

Hepatic arteriovenous fistulas may be generalized or localized in the liver and may be hemangioendotheliomas or cavernous hemangiomas. The fistula may be located between the hepatic artery and the ductus venosus or portal vein. Congenital hemorrhagic telangiectasia may also be present. Large arteriovenous fistulas are associated with increased cardiac output and heart failure. Hepatomegaly is usual, and systolic or continuous murmurs may be audible over the liver.

Peripheral arteriovenous fistulas generally involve the extremities and are associated with disfigurement, swelling of the extremity, and visible hemangiomas. Some are located in areas that result in upper airway obstruction. Because only a small minority results in large arterial runoff, cardiac failure is uncommon.

TREATMENT. Medical management of heart failure is initially helpful in neonates with these conditions; with time, the size of the shunt may diminish and symptoms spontaneously regress. Hemangiomas of the liver often eventually disappear completely. Large liver hemangiomas have been treated with steroids, ε-aminocaproic acid, interferon, local compression, embolization, or local irradiation; the beneficial effects of these management options are not firmly established because individual patients display marked variation in clinical course without treatment. Catheter embolization is becoming the treatment of choice for many patients with a symptomatic arteriovenous fistula. Embolic agents that have been used include detachable balloons, steel (Gianturco) coils, and liquid tissue adhesives (cyanoacrylate). Often, multiple procedures are necessary before flow is significantly reduced. Surgical removal of a large fistula may be attempted in patients with severe cardiac failure and lack of improvement with medical treatment. Surgical treatment may be contraindicated or unsuccessful when the lesion is extensive and diffuse or is located in a position where adjoining tissue may be injured during the surgery or related procedures.

Abernethy LJ: Classification and imaging of vascular malformations in children. *Eur Radiol* 2003;13:2483–2497.

Faughnan ME, Thabet A, Mei-Zahav M, et al: Pulmonary arteriovenous malformations in children: Outcomes of transcatheter embolotherapy. *J Pediatr* 2004;145:826–831.

Fong LV, Lee SH, Salmon AP: Diagnosis of cerebral arteriovenous malformations by colour Doppler examination. *Eur Heart J* 1992;13:415–417.

Ford EG, Stanley P, Tolo V, et al: Peripheral congenital arteriovenous fistulae: Observe, operate, or obturate? *J Pediatr Surg* 1992;27:714–719.

Friedman DM, Verma R, Madrid M, et al: Recent improvement in outcome using transcatheter embolization techniques for neonatal aneurysmal malformations of the vein of Galen. *Pediatrics* 1993;91:583–586.

Chapter 445 ■ Systemic Hypertension

Systemic hypertension occurs commonly in adults and, if untreated, is a major risk factor for myocardial infarction, stroke, and renal failure. In a pooled analysis of several adult hypertension studies, a 5 mm Hg increase in diastolic blood pressure increased the risk of coronary artery disease by 20% and the risk of stroke by 35%. Hypertension is implicated in the etiology of nearly 50% of adults with end-stage renal disease. The prevalence of hypertension increases with age, ranging from 15% in young adults to 60% in individuals older than 65 yr.

In infants and younger children, systemic hypertension is uncommon, with a prevalence of <1%, but when present, it is usually indicative of an underlying disease process (**secondary hypertension**). In contrast, adolescents may develop primary or essential hypertension (with no underlying cause). Essential hypertension during childhood may track into adulthood, as demonstrated by several large clinical studies. Children with blood pressure >90th percentile have a 2.4-fold greater risk of having hypertension as adults. Similarly, nearly half of hypertensive adults had a blood pressure >90th percentile as children. There is also a correlation between early childhood hypertension and early atherosclerosis.

Accurate blood pressure measurements should be part of the routine annual physical examination of all children 3 yr or older. A complete family history of hypertension should be elicited. Accurate measurement of blood pressure requires careful attention to the comfort of the patient and is highly dependent on proper use of the equipment, whether it be a simple sphygmomanometer or a state-of-the-art automated device. Obtaining an accurate blood pressure measurement in infants is often the most difficult and time-consuming part of the physical examination. Patients of any age have some level of anxiety associated with measurement of blood pressure that may lead to a false diagnosis of hypertension. Blood pressure can be measured with the patient either seated or supine; infants may be held in the lap of a parent. Subsequent measurements taken for comparison should be obtained with the patient in the same position. Careful attention to cuff size is necessary to avoid overdiagnosis. A wide variety of bladder sizes should be available in any medical office where children are routinely seen. The cuff should completely encircle the upper part of the arm to ensure uniform compression; the inflatable bladder should cover at least ⅔ of the upper arm length and 80–100% of its circumference. A cuff that is too short or narrow artificially increases blood pressure readings. Blood pressure should be obtained in all 4 extremities to detect coarctation of the aorta (see Chapter 427.6).

Systolic pressure is indicated by appearance of the 1st Korotkoff sound. Diastolic pressure has been defined by consensus as the 5th, rather than the 4th, Korotkoff sound. Palpation is useful for rapid assessment of systolic blood pressure, although the palpated pressure is generally about 10 mm Hg less than that obtained via auscultation. Doppler is an extremely accurate method of measuring systolic blood pressure; it is less so for diastolic pressure. Oscillometric techniques are used frequently in infants and young children, but they are susceptible to artifacts and are best for measuring mean blood pressure.

Blood pressure increases gradually with age; the 1st age-related norms were developed by a task force of the National Heart Lung and Blood Institutes in 1977, and have been revised to account for differences based on sex and height, most recently in 1996. Therefore, standard nomograms are necessary for interpretation of blood pressure values (see Figs. 422-1 and 422-2). If mild hypertension is found, it is imperative that the measurement be repeated twice more over a period of 6 wk. Anxiety usually decreases as the patient becomes more comfortable with the procedure; thus, repeated measurements are necessary to avoid inappropriately labeling a patient as hypertensive. Blood pressure that is consistently above the 95th percentile for age requires further evaluation. Ambulatory blood pressure monitoring may be especially useful in adolescents who have borderline hypertension in the office setting.

ETIOLOGY AND PATHOPHYSIOLOGY. Blood pressure is the product of cardiac output and peripheral vascular resistance. An increase in either cardiac output or peripheral resistance results in an increase in blood pressure; if one of these factors increases while the other decreases, blood pressure may not increase. When hypertension is the result of another disease process, it is referred to as **secondary hypertension.** When no identifiable cause can be found, it is referred to as **primary** or **essential hypertension.** Many factors, including heredity, diet, stress, and obesity, may play a role in the development of essential hypertension.

Secondary hypertension is most common in infants and younger children. Many childhood diseases can be responsible for both acute and chronic elevation of blood pressure (Tables 445-1 and 445-2). The most likely cause varies with age. Hypertension in the **newborn** is most often associated with umbilical artery catheterization and renal artery thrombosis. Hypertension during early **childhood** may be due to renal disease, coarctation of the aorta, endocrine disorders, or medications. In **adolescents,** essential hypertension becomes increasingly common. The severity of hypertension is also helpful in distinguishing secondary from primary hypertension; children and adolescents with essential hypertension usually have blood pressure values at or only slightly above the 95th percentile for age.

Renal and **renovascular hypertension** accounts for the majority of children with secondary hypertension. A history of urinary tract infection is present in 25–50% of these patients and is often related to an obstructive lesion of the urinary tract. Renovascular hypertension may be associated with sodium retention and increased renin secretion. Other renal parenchymal lesions associated with hypertension are detailed in Tables 445-1 and 445-2. The reduced glomerular filtration rate in patients with nephritis results in salt and water retention, whereas mass lesions (cysts, solid tumors, hematoma) may impair renal perfusion and stimulate renin production by the juxtaglomerular apparatus. Both Wilms tumor and juxtaglomerular cell tumor (hemangiopericytoma) may secrete renin or other pressors without feedback control.

Lesions such as renal artery stenosis cause hypertension through stimulation of the renin-angiotensin-aldosterone system. Renin is a proteolytic enzyme secreted by juxtaglomerular cells that converts angiotensinogen to angiotensin I. Renin secretion is affected by afferent arteriolar perfusion pressure in the kidney, sodium concentration in plasma and tubular urine, sympathetic nervous system activation, and other factors such as prostaglandins, potassium intake, and atrial natriuretic peptides. Angiotensin I possesses little physiologic activity and is rapidly converted to angiotensin II by angiotensin-converting enzyme (ACE). This enzyme is also responsible for the metabolic degradation of vasodilating kinins. Angiotensin II is a potent vasoconstrictor and also stimulates aldosterone secretion, which leads to salt and water retention.

TABLE 445-1. Conditions Associated with Transient or Intermittent Hypertension in Children

RENAL
Acute postinfectious glomerulonephritis
Anaphylactoid (Henoch-Schönlein) purpura with nephritis
Hemolytic-uremic syndrome
Acute tubular necrosis
After renal transplantation (immediately and during episodes of rejection)
After blood transfusion in patients with azotemia
Hypervolemia
After surgical procedures on the genitourinary tract
Pyelonephritis
Renal trauma
Leukemic infiltration of the kidney
Obstructive uropathy associated with Crohn disease
DRUGS AND POISONS
Cocaine
Oral contraceptives
Sympathomimetic agents
Amphetamines
Phencyclidine
Corticosteroids and adrenocorticotropic hormone
Cyclosporine or sirolimus treatment post-transplantation
Licorice (glycyrrhizic acid)
Lead, mercury, cadmium, thallium
Antihypertensive withdrawal (clonidine, methyldopa, propranolol)
Vitamin D intoxication
CENTRAL AND AUTONOMIC NERVOUS SYSTEM
Increased intracranial pressure
Guillain-Barré syndrome
Burns
Familial dysautonomia
Stevens-Johnson syndrome
Posterior fossa lesions
Porphyria
Poliomyelitis
Encephalitis
MISCELLANEOUS
Preeclampsia
Fractures of long bones
Hypercalcemia
After coarctation repair
White cell transfusion
Extracorporeal membrane oxygenation
Chronic upper airway obstruction

TABLE 445-2. Conditions Associated with Chronic Hypertension in Children

RENAL
Chronic pyelonephritis
Chronic glomerulonephritis
Hydronephrosis
Congenital dysplastic kidney
Multicystic kidney
Solitary renal cyst
Vesicoureteral reflux nephropathy
Segmental hypoplasia (Ask-Upmark kidney)
Ureteral obstruction
Renal tumors
Renal trauma
Rejection damage following transplantation
Postirradiation damage
Systemic lupus erythematosus (other connective tissue diseases)
VASCULAR
Coarctation of thoracic or abdominal aorta
Renal artery lesions (stenosis, fibromuscular dysplasia, thrombosis, aneurysm)
Umbilical artery catheterization with thrombus formation
Neurofibromatosis (intrinsic or extrinsic narrowing for vascular lumen)
Renal vein thrombosis
Vasculitis
Arteriovenous shunt
Williams-Beuren syndrome
Moyamoya disease
Takayasu arteritis
ENDOCRINE
Hyperthyroidism
Hyperparathyroidism
Congential adrenal hyperplasia (11β-hydroxylase and 17-hydroxylase defect)
Cushing syndrome
Primary aldosteronism
Dexamethasone-suppressible hyperaldosteronism
Pheochromocytoma
Other neural crest tumors (neuroblastoma, ganglioneuroblastoma, ganglioneuroma)
Diabetic nephropathy
Liddle syndrome
CENTRAL NERVOUS SYSTEM
Intracranial mass
Hemorrhage
Residual following brain injury
Quadriplegia
ESSENTIAL HYPERTENSION
Low renin
Normal renin
High renin

Several **endocrinopathies** are associated with hypertension, usually those involving the thyroid, parathyroid, and adrenal glands. Systolic hypertension and tachycardia are common in hyperthyroidism; diastolic pressure is not usually elevated. Hypercalcemia, whether secondary to hyperparathyroidism or other causes, often results in mild elevation in blood pressure because of an increase in vascular tone. Adrenocortical disorders (aldosterone-secreting tumors, congenital adrenal hyperplasia, Cushing syndrome) may produce hypertension in patients with increased mineralocorticoid secretion. Pheochromocytomas are catecholamine-secreting tumors that give rise to hypertension because of the cardiac and peripheral vascular effects of epinephrine and norepinephrine. Children with pheochromocytoma usually have sustained rather than intermittent or exercise-induced hypertension (see Chapter 581). Pheochromocytoma develops in ≈5% of patients with neurofibromatosis. Altered sympathetic tone can be responsible for acute or intermittent elevation of blood pressure in children with Guillain-Barré syndrome, poliomyelitis, burns, and Stevens-Johnson syndrome. Sympathetic outflow from the central nervous system is also affected by intracranial lesions.

In adolescents, a number of **drugs of abuse,** therapeutic agents, and toxins may cause hypertension. Cocaine may provoke a rapid increase in blood pressure and can result in seizures or intracranial hemorrhage. Phencyclidine causes transient hypertension that may become persistent in chronic abusers. Tobacco use may also increase blood pressure. Sympathomimetic agents used as nasal decongestants, appetite suppressants, and stimulants for attention deficit disorder produce peripheral vasoconstriction and varying degrees of cardiac stimulation. Individuals vary in their susceptibility to these effects. Oral contraceptives should be suspected as a cause of hypertension in adolescent girls, although the incidence is low with the use of low-estrogen preparations. Immunosuppressant agents such as cyclosporine and tacrolimus cause hypertension in organ transplant recipients, and the effect is exacerbated by the co-administration of steroids. Blood pressure may be elevated in patients with poisoning by a heavy metal.

Essential hypertension is the most common form of hypertension in adults, and it is recognized more often in adolescents than in younger children. It is often accompanied by a strong family history. The cause of essential hypertension is likely to be multifactorial; obesity, genetic alterations in calcium and sodium transport, vascular smooth muscle reactivity, the renin-angiotensin system, and insulin resistance have been implicated in this disorder. Normotensive children of hypertensive parents may show abnormal physiologic responses that are similar to those of their parents. When subjected to stress or competitive tasks, the offspring of hypertensive adults, as a group, respond with greater increases in heart rate and blood pressure than do children of normotensive parents. Similarly, some children of hypertensive parents may excrete higher levels of urinary catecholamine metabolites or may respond to sodium loading with greater weight gain and increases in blood pressure than do those without a family history of hypertension. The abnormal responses in children with affected parents tend to be greater in the black population than among white individuals. Erythrocyte sodium transport, the free calcium concentration in platelets and leukocytes, urine kallikrein excretion, and sympathetic nervous system receptors have been investigated as other possible markers for the subsequent development of hypertension.

Categorization of essential hypertension according to the level of plasma renin activity (high, normal, low) has been useful in understanding the pathophysiology and in developing treatment regimens for adults; similar large studies have not been conducted in adolescents with primary hypertension. A large number of adult patients with essential hypertension appear to be especially sensitive to salt intake. The mechanism of salt sensitivity is not clear and may involve the chloride ion rather than sodium. A subgroup of salt-sensitive individuals appears to have impaired ability for urinary excretion of a sodium load. Atrial natriuretic peptides stimulate sodium excretion by the kidneys; their role in maintenance of normal blood pressure and development of hypertension is being investigated.

Tracking of blood pressure is the process by which individuals maintain their relative ranking of blood pressure over time with respect to their peers. Children and young adolescents with blood pressure greater than the 90th percentile for age have a nearly threefold greater likelihood of becoming adults with hypertension than do children with blood pressure at the 50th percentile. Adolescents with essential hypertension may progress from high cardiac output and normal systemic vascular resistance to the adult pattern of normal cardiac output with elevated systemic vascular resistance. Racial differences have been noted: black adults with hypertension have greater elevations in peripheral

TABLE 445-3. Findings to Look For on Physical Examination

PHYSICAL FINDINGS	POTENTIAL RELEVANCE
GENERAL	
Pale mucous membranes, edema, growth retardation	Chronic renal disease
Elfin facies, poor growth, retardation	Williams syndrome
Webbing of neck, low hairline, widespread nipples, wide carrying angle	Turner syndrome
Moon face, buffalo hump, hirsutism, truncal obesity, striae	Cushing syndrome
HABITUS	
Thinness	Pheochromocytoma, renal disease, hyperthyroidism
Virilization	Congenital adrenal hyperplasia
Rickets	Chronic renal disease
SKIN	
Café au lait spots, neurofibromas	Neurofibromatosis, pheochromocytoma
Tubers, "ash-leaf" spots	Tuberous sclerosis
Rashes	SLE, vasculitis (HSP), impetigo with acute nephritis
Pallor, evanescent flushing, sweating	Pheochromocytoma
Needle tracks	Illicit drug use
Bruises, striae	Cushing syndrome
EYES	
Extraocular muscle palsy	Nonspecific, chronic, severe
Fundal changes	Nonspecific, chronic, severe
Proptosis	Hyperthyroidism
HEAD AND NECK	
Goiter	Thyroid disease
CARDIOVASCULAR SIGNS	
Absent of diminished femoral pulses, low leg pressure relative to arm pressure	Aortic coarctation
Heart size, rate, rhythm; murmurs; respiratory difficulty, hepatomegaly	Aortic coarctation, congestive heart failure
Bruits over great vessels	Arteritis or arteriopathy
Rub	Pericardial effusion secondary to chronic renal disease
PULMONARY SIGNS	
Pulmonary edema	Congestive heart failure, acute nephritis
Picture of bronchopulmonary dysplasia (BPD)	BPD-associated hypertension
ABDOMEN	
Epigastric bruit	Primary renovascular disease or in association with Williams syndrome, neurofibromatosis, fibromuscular dysplasia, or arteritis
Abdominal masses	Wilms tumor, neuroblastoma, pheochromocytoma, polycystic kidneys, hydronephrosis
NEUROLOGIC SIGNS	
Neurologic deficits	Chronic or severe acute hypertension with stroke
GENITALIA	
Ambiguous, virilized	Congenital adrenal hyperplasia

HSP, Henoch-Schönlein purpura; SLE, systemic lupus erythematosus.
From Kliegman RM, Greenbaum LA, Lye PS: *Practical Strategies in Pediatric Diagnosis and Therapy*, 2nd ed, Philadelphia, Elsevier, 2004, p 200.

resistance, whereas hypertensive white adults predominantly show an increase in cardiac output.

CLINICAL MANIFESTATIONS. Children and adolescents with essential hypertension are usually asymptomatic; the blood pressure elevation is usually mild and is detected during a routine examination or evaluation before athletic participation. These children may have mild to moderate obesity.

Children with secondary hypertension can have blood pressure elevations ranging from mild to severe. Unless the pressure has been sustained or is rising rapidly, hypertension does not usually produce symptoms. Therefore, clinical manifestations of the underlying disease, such as growth failure in children with chronic renal disease, are the most frequent reasons for detecting the hypertension. Helpful features of the physical examination are noted in Table 445-3. With substantial hypertension headache, dizziness, epistaxis, anorexia, visual changes, and seizures may occur. **Hypertensive encephalopathy** is suggested by the presence of vomiting, temperature elevation, ataxia, stupor, and seizures. Regardless of the cause, end-organ (cardiac and renal) dysfunction occurs in the face of marked hypertension.

Young children and infants with unexplained heart failure or seizures should have their blood pressure measured. Such patients often cannot communicate symptoms such as headache, and their behavior may not be considered abnormal until the complications of hypertension are present. After blood pressure has been lowered, parents of hypertensive infants often comment in retrospect that their child had been increasingly irritable before the hypertension was recognized.

DIAGNOSIS. The diagnosis of essential hypertension is suggested by the patient's age (usually adolescent), level of blood pressure elevation (usually mild), weight (mild to moderate obesity), positive family history, and the paucity of signs and symptoms of underlying disease. It is uncommon to make this diagnosis in children younger than 10 yr. Obesity is associated with essential hypertension, but except for disorders of the adrenal cortex, patients with secondary hypertension are rarely obese. Heredity is also a strong determinant of blood pressure; therefore, an adolescent with mild elevation of pressure and a strong family history of essential hypertension is less likely to have an underlying disease. Adolescents suspected of having essential hypertension require regular measurement of blood pressure to determine the course of the elevation over time. If blood pressure continues to rise over several weeks or months of observation, additional diagnostic studies to eliminate secondary hypertension are indicated.

The diagnosis of secondary hypertension is also suggested by the patient's age (younger), level of blood pressure elevation

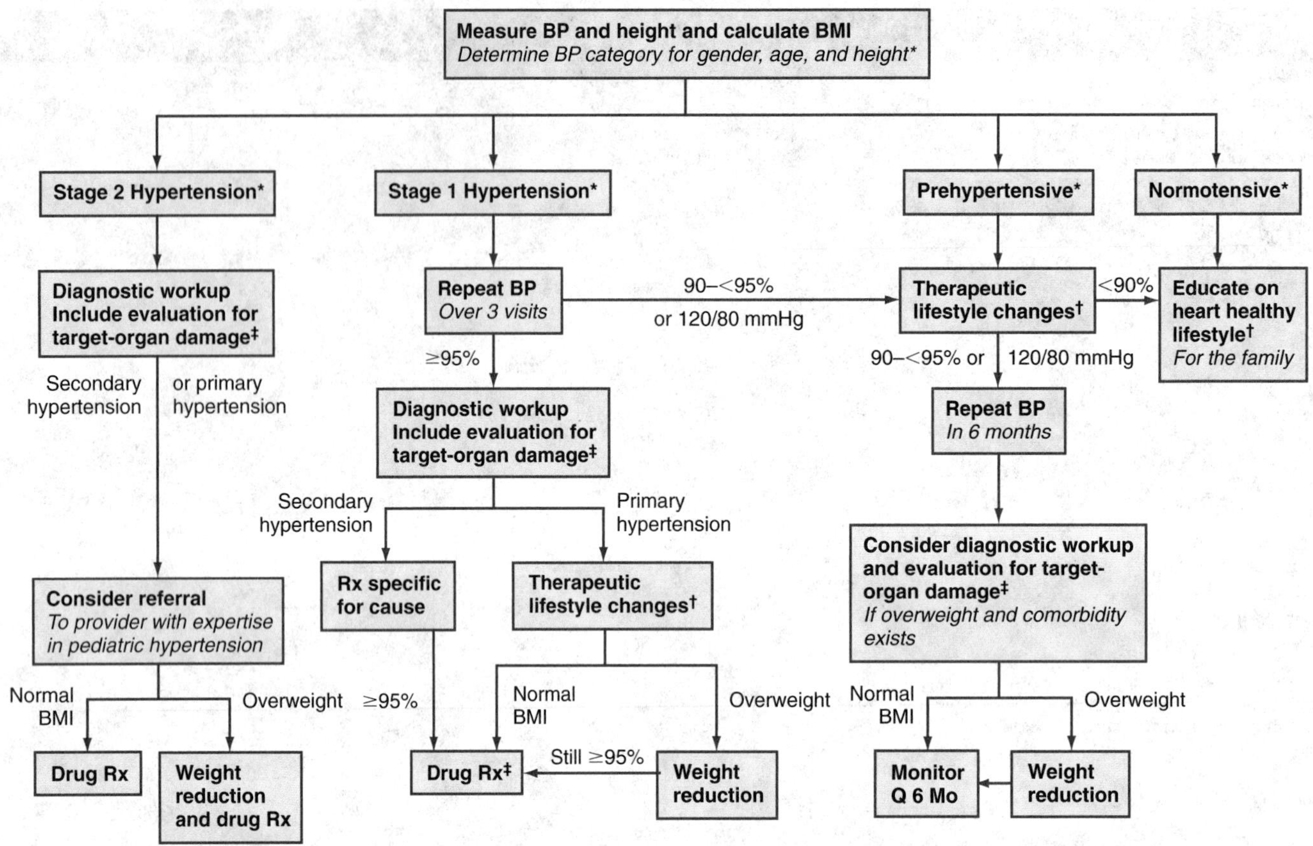

Figure 445-1. Management algorithm. BMI, body mass index; BP, blood pressure; Q, every; Rx, prescription; † diet modification and physical activity; ‡ especially if younger, very high BP, little or no family history, diabetic, or other risk factors. (From National High Blood Pressure Education Program Working Group on High Blood Pressure in Children and Adolescents: The fourth report on the diagnosis, evaluation, and treatment of high blood pressure in children and adolescents. *Pediatrics* 2004;114:555–576.)

(varying from mild to extreme), and presence of symptoms. The history may include intermittent febrile illnesses, which might suggest recurring infection of the urinary tract (reflux nephropathy). A family history of renal disease or premature cardiovascular disease should be elicited. Careful measurement of height and weight are important because they are often less than normal in children with chronic disease. Physical examination should determine the presence of flank masses or abdominal bruits. Examination should always include palpation of pulses in all extremities and blood pressure in both arms and 1 leg to evaluate for possible coarctation of the aorta. Systolic blood pressure in the lower limbs of children should be 10–20 mm Hg higher than that in the upper limbs. **Screening tests** should include a complete blood count, urinalysis, and determination of serum electrolyte, blood urea nitrogen, serum creatinine, calcium, and uric acid levels. Urine culture should be performed even if the sediment is unremarkable. A lipid panel is indicated if the family history is suggestive or if primary hypertension is suspected. Echocardiography is helpful in assessing the chronicity of the hypertension, which, if long-standing, should lead to left ventricular hypertrophy.

Renal ultrasonography provides a comparison of kidney size and a view of the anatomy of the collecting system. A radionuclide scan is helpful in distinguishing variation in perfusion or scarring of the two kidneys. Renal Doppler ultrasonography and angiography can demonstrate lesions in the main arteries or in the segmental branches; if angiography is performed, venous blood samples should be collected from both renal veins and the inferior vena cava for assay of plasma renin activity. Doppler ultrasonography may demonstrate abnormal arterial and venous blood flow.

Peripheral plasma renin activity is a useful screening test for both renovascular and renal parenchymal disease. Normal values gradually decrease with age and vary among laboratories. A suppressed value suggests excess mineralocorticoid effect, and an elevated value is associated with renal or renovascular involvement. Urinary catecholamines should be measured as well as plasma and urinary steroids. One approach to an adolescent with hypertension is summarized in Figure 445-1. A pregnancy test may be useful in a sexually active female who is noted to be hypertensive (preeclampsia). An initial diagnostic approach to hypertension is noted in Figure 445-2.

COURSE AND PROGNOSIS. The natural history of essential hypertension that is initially detected during childhood or adolescence is under investigation in several large long-term population studies. Many of these children continue to have essential hypertension as adults, although the correlation is not perfect. In adults with essential hypertension, drug therapy has been shown to be beneficial in reducing the incidence of congestive heart failure, renal failure, and stroke.

The prognosis of a child with secondary hypertension is primarily determined by the nature of the underlying disease and its responsiveness to specific therapy. Survival in patients with underlying chronic renal disease is determined by the patient's response to dialysis and the success of renal transplantation. In patients with renovascular disease, the degree of elevation in renal vein renin activity may help predict response to therapy. A discrepancy in renin secretion between the 2 kidneys of more than 1.5:1 suggests that the kidney producing the higher level is primarily responsible for the hypertension. In this case, surgical cor-

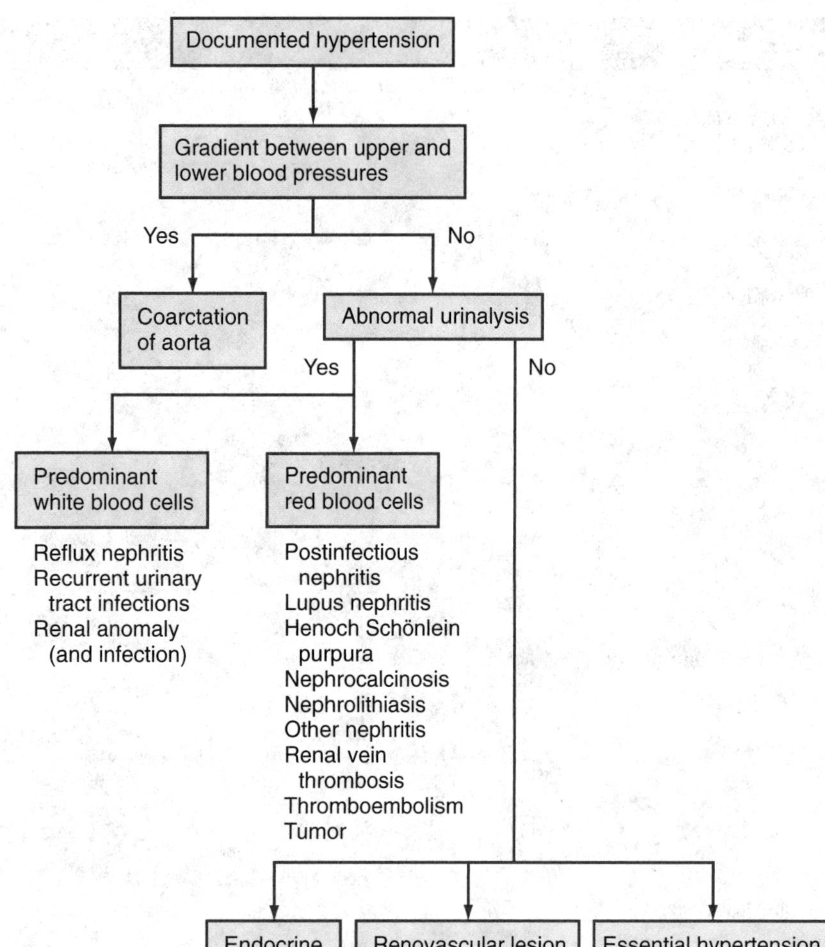

Figure 445-2. Initial diagnostic algorithm in the evaluation of hypertension. From Kliegman RM, Greenbaum LA, Lye PS: *Practical Strategies in Pediatric Diagnosis and Therapy,* 2nd ed., Philadelphia, Elsevier, 2004, p. 222

rection yields a high probability of marked improvement or resolution of the hypertension. The prognosis after surgical repair of coarctation of the aorta is variable and partly dependent on the age at which the correction is performed. Most patients operated on during infancy and childhood establish normal systemic blood pressure after surgery unless the coarctation recurs; patients in whom the diagnosis is made during adolescence, however, are at risk for persistently elevated pressure. The long-term outcome is favorable for neonates who experience hypertension as a complication of umbilical artery catheterization. Few of these infants require therapy beyond 12 mo of age, and most show marked improvement in renal perfusion.

PREVENTION. Prevention of high blood pressure may be viewed as part of the prevention of cardiovascular disease and stroke, the leading cause of death in adults in the United States. Other risk factors for cardiovascular disease include obesity, elevated serum cholesterol levels, high dietary sodium intake, a sedentary lifestyle, and alcohol and tobacco use. Beginning in childhood and continuing through adolescence, it is especially important to discourage cigarette smoking because of the pulmonary and cardiovascular consequences. The increase in arterial wall rigidity and blood viscosity that is associated with exposure to the components of tobacco may cause or exacerbate hypertension. Population approaches to prevention of essential hypertension include a reduction in sodium intake and an increase in physical activity through school-based programs.

TREATMENT. The goal of therapy for hypertension should be to reduce blood pressure below the 95th percentile for age. Both nonpharmacologic and pharmacologic approaches to treatment are useful in managing children with elevated blood pressure. Adolescents with essential hypertension are usually best managed initially with nonpharmacologic therapy. Intervention should focus on the risk factors that were cited as important in prevention. Because many patients with mild elevation of pressure are obese, weight reduction may result in a 5–10 mm Hg reduction in systolic pressure. A reduction in sodium intake often lowers pressure by a similar amount, although it is less effective in children than in adults. A consistent program of aerobic exercise also reduces blood pressure in patients with mild essential hypertension. Exercise must be continued to be effective long-term. In view of these benefits and the undesirable effects of many antihypertensive drugs, a well-supervised program of nonpharmacologic therapy should be enthusiastically prescribed for most young patients with essential hypertension. Adolescents should be counseled about the adverse effects of tobacco and alcohol on blood pressure. When the patient is unable to cooperate with the nonpharmacologic approach or the reduction in blood pressure is insufficient, antihypertensive agents should be considered. Adolescents who are poorly compliant with changes in lifestyle are also unlikely to be compliant with a long-term drug regimen.

For many children with secondary hypertension and for selected patients with essential hypertension, pharmacologic therapy is required. There is a general consensus that children

TABLE 445-4. Antihypertensive Drugs

DRUG	MECHANISM OF ACTION	DOSAGE RANGE	ROUTE	DURATION	SIDE EFFECTS
ARTERIAL VASODILATORS					
Hydralazine	Relax arteriolar smooth muscle	0.1–0.4 mg/kg/dose	IV	4–6 hr	Tachycardia, nausea
		0.25–1 mg/kg/dose and increase to max 200 mg/24 hr	PO	6–12 hr	Drug-induced lupus
Sodium Nitroprusside	Dilatation of arterioles and venules	0.3–8.0 μg/kg/min	IV	With infusion	Thiocyanate production, rarely hypothyroidism
Minoxidil	Arteriolar dilatation	Initial 0.1–0.2 mg/kg/24 hr, max 5 mg. Increase gradually to 0.25–1.0 mg/kg/24 hr, max 50 mg.	PO	12–24 hr	Hypertrichosis, fluid retention
ADRENERGIC BLOCKERS					
Esmolol	β-Adrenergic blockade	50–300 μg/kg/min	IV	With infusion	Hypotension, bronchospasm
Phentolamine	α-Receptor blockade	0.05–0.1 mg/kg/dose, max 20 mg	IV	1–2 hr	Tachycardia, dizziness, nasal congestion, chest pain
Phenoxybenzamine	α-Receptor blockade	0.2–2.0 mg/kg/24 hr, max single dose 40 mg	PO	8–12 hr	Nasal congestion, dizziness, tachycardia, arrhythmia
Prazosin	α-Receptor blockade	0.005–0.1 mg/kg/dose	PO	6–12 hr	First-dose orthostatic hypotension
Propranolol	β-Receptor blockade	0.01–0.1 mg/kg/dose	IV slow push	6–8 hr	Bronchospasm, bradycardia, vivid dreams
	Reduces renin release	0.5–8.0 mg/kg/24 hr	PO		
Atenolol	β-Blockade	1–2 mg/kg/24 hr	PO	24 hr	Bronchospasm, bradycardia
Labetalol	α- and β-Blockade	0.2–1.0 mg/kg/dose (max 20 mg dose)	IV bolus	With infusion	Orthostasis, dizziness, bronchospasm
		0.25–2.0 mg/kg/hr	IV continuous		
		1–3 mg/kg/24 hr	PO	6–12 hr	
Clonidine	CNS α_2-agonist	0.005–0.025 mg/kg/24 hr initial Max 0.9 mg/24 hr	PO	6–12 hr	Sedation, constipation, rebound withdrawal, hypertension
RENIN-ANGIOTENSIN INHIBITORS					
Captopril	Angiotensin-converting enzyme (ACE) inhibition	Neonates <2 mos: 0.05–0.1 mg/kg/dose up to 0.5 mg/kg/dose	PO	8–24 hr	Proteinuria, neutropenia, rash, dysgeusia, chronic cough
		Infants and children: 0.15–0.5 mg/kg/dose up to 6 mg/kg/24 hr	PO	8–12 hr	
		Older children and adolescents: 6.25–25 mg/dose up to 450 mg/24 hr	PO	8–12 hr	
Enalaprilat	ACE inhibition	0.005–0.010 mg/kg/dose adults 0.625–1.25 mg/dose	IV over 5 min	8–24 hr	Transient hypotension
Enalapril	ACE inhibition	Children: 0.1–0.5 mg/kg/24 hr Adolescents: 2.5–5 mg/24 hr up to 40 mg/24 hr	PO	12–24 hr	Hypotension
CALCIUM CHANNEL BLOCKERS					
Nifedipine	Calcium channel blocker	Children: 0.25–0.5 mg/kg/dose, max 5 mg/dose, max 1–2 mg/kg/24 hr	PO, SL	Repeat q 4–6 h	Facial flushing, tachycardia
		Adolescents: 10–30 mg (capsules) or 30–120 mg q.d. (sustained release)	PO PO	6–8 hr 24 hr	
Nicardipine	Calcium channel blocker	1–3 μg/kg/min	IV	With infusion	Tachycardia, hypotension, headache
Amlodipine	Calcium channel blocker	0.1–0.6 mg/kg/24 hr, max 5 mg/24 hr	PO	24 hr	Edema, dizziness, flushing, palpitations
DIURETIC AGENTS					
Hydrochlorothiazide	Diuresis	1–2 mg/kg/24 hr max 200 mg/24 hr	PO	12–24 hr	Hypokalemia, hyperuricemia, hypercalcemia
Furosemide	Diuresis	1 mg/kg/dose	IV	4–6 hr	Hypokalemia, alkalosis
		1–2 mg/kg/dose up to 6 mg/kg/24 hr	PO	6–12 hr	
Bumetanide	Diuresis	0.015–0.1 mg/kg/dose max 10 mg/24 hr	PO	6–24 hr	Hypokalemia, hyperglycemia, hyperuricemia

Note: Pediatric doses based on weight should not exceed adult doses. As recommendations may change, these doses should always be double checked. Doses may also need to be modified in any patient with renal or hepatic dysfunction.
IV, intravenous; PO, by mouth; SL, Sublingual.

with essential hypertension whose blood pressure recordings are persistently above the 99th percentile should be treated. There is less agreement on the approach to children with essential hypertension whose blood pressures are between the 95th and 99th percentiles. A number of antihypertensive drugs are available for both hypertensive emergencies and chronic therapy (Table 445-4). Determining the long-term effectiveness of antihypertensive medication in adolescents is difficult, given the decades-long follow-up required to examine effects on cardiovascular disease. Several surrogate end-points, such as left ventricular hypertrophy, endothelial dysfunction, carotid artery intimal-medial thickness, coronary artery calcification (on CT scan), and the presence of microalbuminuria, may prove useful in clinical trials. When determining whether to initiate pharmacologic treatment, it should be remembered that it is still not known whether starting antihypertensive medications earlier in life reduces the risk of later cardiovascular disease compared with starting medication during adulthood. Most antihypertensive agents have not been fully tested in children and the risks of using these drugs may be higher in children, given the longer lifetime of administration and exposure during a time of growth and development.

In response to a **hypertensive crisis,** it is important to select an agent with a rapid and predictable onset of action and to monitor blood pressure carefully as it is being reduced. Because hypertensive encephalopathy is a possible complication of hypertensive emergencies, antihypertensive agents with minimal central nervous system side effects should be chosen to avoid confusion between symptoms of disease and adverse effects of the drug. Intravenous administration is often preferred so that the fall in blood pressure can be carefully titrated. Because too rapid a reduction in blood pressure may interfere with adequate organ perfusion, a stepwise reduction in pressure should be planned. In general, the pressure should be reduced by about ⅓ of the total planned reduction during the 1st 6 hr and the remaining amount over the following 48–72 hr.

In most hypertensive emergencies, the **drugs of choice** are intravenous **labetalol** or **sodium nitroprusside** or sublingual **nifedipine.** Labetalol blocks both α- and β-adrenergic receptors;

with a single dose followed by continuous infusion, controlled reduction of blood pressure can be achieved. Similar control is possible with an infusion of nitroprusside. Nifedipine has a rapid onset of action, but its short duration of action must be anticipated. Because nifedipine is available only as a liquid within a capsule, administration to younger children has presented some difficulty. Although the drug has often been placed in the sublingual space to achieve rapid absorption, gastrointestinal absorption is also sufficiently rapid to be effective in a hypertensive crisis. Other agents useful for hypertensive emergencies include esmolol and nicardipine. Most children with hypertensive crisis have chronic or acute renal disease; in these patients, management of blood pressure also requires careful attention to fluid balance, as well as diuresis. Intravenous furosemide is usually effective, even though glomerular filtration may be impaired.

In selecting a drug regimen for long-term use, an understanding of the underlying pathophysiology is helpful. Drugs with different sites and mechanisms of action are available so that therapy can be tailored to the specific pathologic condition. For example, excessive activity of the renin-angiotensin-aldosterone system may be treated effectively with a β-blocking drug (propranolol) for suppression of renin secretion, an ACE inhibitor (captopril or enalapril), or, rarely, an aldosterone antagonist (e.g., spironolactone). ACE inhibitors are useful, not only in patients with high-renin hypertension that is secondary to renovascular or renal parenchymal disease but also in patients with high-renin essential hypertension. Excess angiotensin production is the probable cause of most hypertension in neonates after partial occlusion of a renal vessel by thrombus. Captopril or enalapril are effective agents in most of these patients, but must be used with careful attention to renal function. α-Adrenergic blocking agents (phentolamine, phenoxybenzamine) are beneficial in patients with neural crest tumors who have high circulating levels of catecholamines. In such patients, β-blocking drugs are also needed to control the heart rate, or an agent with dual blocking action (labetalol) may be used. Sympathetic blockade with labetalol is likewise efficacious in patients who experience marked stimulation of the cardiovascular system from high doses of cocaine.

Young patients with essential hypertension who require drug therapy may be treated initially with a diuretic or a β-blocking agent. Patients with volume-dependent hypertension usually have an adequate response to diuretics; those with high-renin, high cardiac output physiology respond best to β blockers. If the pressure is not lowered adequately, a calcium channel blocker may be added to the diuretic, and an ACE inhibitor may replace the β blocker. Chronic use of diuretics may result in elevation of serum lipids, which may increase the risk of ischemic heart disease in adults with hypertension. Long-term investigations of this side effect in children are not available. β-Blocking agents have also been associated with changes in serum lipids, and some studies suggest a mild reduction in exercise tolerance in patients treated with propranolol. Patients with reactive airway disease are often not able to tolerate a β-blocking agent.

Because of these side effects, ACE inhibitors and calcium channel blockers may be considered for initial therapy in an adolescent with significant hypertension. Although captopril has been used more often in young patients, enalapril has a longer duration of action and thus requires less frequent administration.

In patients with long-standing or poorly controlled hypertension, the underlying pathophysiology is often complex. Such patients frequently require trials of combinations of antihypertensive agents to gain control of markedly elevated or labile pressure. The basic principle of combination antihypertensive therapy is the co-administration of drugs with different sites or mechanisms of action. Because compliance may become a problem, the drug regimen should be as simple as possible and should take advantage of longer acting agents that can be administered once or twice daily, when available. Drug calendars, parental supervision, and close patient-physician communication also help ensure compliance.

In patients with renal artery stenosis secondary to fibromuscular dysplasia, percutaneous balloon angioplasty may cure as many as 50%. Angioplasty is not successful for renal artery stenosis because of atherosclerotic plaques. If angioplasty is unsuccessful, placement of an intravascular stent or surgery may be indicated.

Bartosh SM, Aronson AJ: Childhood hypertension. An update on etiology, diagnosis, and treatment. *Pediatr Clin North Am* 1999;46:235–252.

Blaszak RT, Savage JA, Ellis EN: The use of short-acting nifedipine in pediatric patients with hypertension. *J Pediatr* 2001;139:34–37.

Chesney RW, Jones DP: Is there a role for β-adrenergic blockers in treating hypertension in children? *J Pediatr* 2007;150:121–122.

Choi Y, Kang BC, Kim KJ, et al: Renovascular hypertension in children with moyamoya disease. *J Pediatr* 1997;131:258–263.

Egger DW, Deming DD, Hamada N, et al: Evaluation of the safety of short-acting nifedipine in children with hypertension. *Pediatr Nephrol* 2002;17:35–40.

Flynn JT: What's new in pediatric hypertension? *Curr Hypertens Rep* 2001;3:503–510.

Flynn JT, Pasko DA: Calcium channel blockers: Pharmacology and place in therapy of pediatric hypertension. *Pediatr Nephrol* 2000;15:302–316.

Kay JD, Sinaiko AR, Daniels SR: Pediatric hypertension. *Am Heart J* 2001;142:422–432.

Lurbe E, Sorof JM, Daniels SR: Clinical and research aspects of ambulatory blood pressure monitoring in children. *J Pediatr* 2004;144:7–16.

[no authors listed]: Athletic participation by children and adolescents who have systemic hypertension. American Academy of Pediatrics Committee on Sports Medicine and Fitness. *Pediatrics* 1997;99:637–638.

[no authors listed]: Initial therapy of hypertension. *Med Lett Drugs Ther* 2004;46:53–55.

[no authors listed]: Update on the 1987 Task Force Report on High Blood Pressure in Children and Adolescents: A working group report from the National High Blood Pressure Education Program. National High Blood Pressure Education Program Working Group on Hypertension Control in Children and Adolescents. *Pediatrics* 1996;98:649–658.

Sinaiko AR: Hypertension in children. *N Engl J Med* 1996;335:1968–1973.

Tyagi S, Kaul UA, Satsangi DK, et al: Percutaneous transluminal angioplasty for renovascular hypertension in children: Initial and long-term results. *Pediatrics* 1997;99:44–49.

Wolfish NM, Delbrouck NF, Shanon A, et al: Prevalence of hypertension in children with primary vesicoureteral reflux. *J Pediatr* 1993;123:559–563.

Part XX ■ Diseases of the Blood

Section 1 — The Hematopoietic System

Chapter 446 ■ Development of the Hematopoietic System

Robin K. Ohls and Robert D. Christensen

Hematopoietic regulation in the human fetus differs from that in the adult. In the adult, homeostatic maintenance is a prime function of hematopoietic regulation, whereas in the embryo and fetus, constant and marked growth characterizes all phases of hematopoiesis. During developmental erythropoiesis, the constant growth of the fetus and the resultant need to increase the red cell mass necessitates an extraordinary erythropoietic effort. In addition, the relatively low oxygen tensions but high metabolic rates of fetal tissues demand a system of oxygen delivery very different from that in adults. During developmental granulopoiesis, the sterile intra-amniotic environment results in a low demand for neutrophils and obviates the need for maintenance of a large neutrophil reserve.

Developmental hematopoiesis occurs in three anatomic stages: mesoblastic, hepatic, and myeloid. **Mesoblastic hematopoiesis** occurs in extraembryonic structures, principally in the yolk sac, and begins between the 10th and 14th days of gestation. By 6–8 wk of gestation the liver replaces the yolk sac as the primary site of blood cell production, and by 10–12 wk extraembryonic hematopoiesis has essentially ceased. **Hepatic hematopoiesis** occurs in the liver throughout the remainder of gestation, although production begins to diminish during the second trimester as bone marrow (**myeloid**) **hematopoiesis** increases. The liver remains the predominant hematopoietic organ through wk 20–24 of gestation.

Each hematopoietic organ houses distinct hematopoietic populations. At 18–20 wk of gestation, >85% of the cells in the fetal liver are erythroid and virtually no neutrophils are present. In contrast, at the same time, <40% of the cells within the bone marrow are erythroid and ≤15% are neutrophils. The subpopulations of leukocytes present in the liver and marrow also differ with gestation. Macrophages precede the presence of granulocytes in both the liver and marrow, and the ratio of macrophages to granulocytes decreases as gestation progresses. Regardless of gestational age or anatomic location, production of all hematopoietic tissues begins with **pluripotent stem cells** that are capable of both self-renewal and clonal maturation into all blood cell lineages. **Progenitor cells** differentiate under the influence of hematopoietic growth factors (Table 446-1) produced by the fetus (Fig. 446-1). Fetal hematopoietic growth factor production is independent of maternal growth factor production.

Erythroid and granulocytic blood cell indices change during gestation and continue to change through the first year of life. Circulating erythrocyte and granulocyte concentrations increase gradually during the second and third trimesters (Table 446-2). In parallel with increasing erythrocyte concentrations, hematocrits increase from 30–40% during the second trimester and continue to increase to term values over the latter part of the third trimester. Term hematocrits range from 50–63%, with variability due to delayed clamping of the umbilical cord and the sampling site. Unlike the blood concentrations of erythrocytes and neutrophils, platelet concentrations remain constant from 18 wk of gestation through term, with a range of 150,000–450,000/µL.

Mean cell volumes usually are inversely proportional to gestation and to the life span of the cell. The *mean cell volume* (MCV) of erythrocytes is >180 fL in the embryo, falls to ≈130 by midgestation, then decreases to 110 fL by 40 wk of gestation (see Table 446-2). *Mean platelet volumes* (MPV) range from 8–10 fL at birth and sometimes can be helpful in determining whether diminished platelet counts are caused primarily by decreased production (normal MPV) or increased destruction (large MPV).

GRANULOCYTOPOIESIS. Neutrophils are first observed in the human fetus about 5 wk postconception as small clusters of cells around the aorta. These cells contain myeloperoxidase, and they mature into cells with segmented nuclei, but other similarities between them and the neutrophils of adults have not been reported. The fetal bone marrow space begins to develop around the 8th week postconception. From 8–10 wk the bone marrow space enlarges, but no neutrophils are apparent in this space until 10.5 wk. These first marrow neutrophils have round nuclei, contain myeloperoxidase, and express cell surface characteristics of **myeloblasts** and **promyelocytes.** From 14 wk through term, the most common granulocytic cell type found in the fetal bone marrow space is the neutrophil.

In children and adults, neutrophils and macrophages originate from a common progenitor cell. It is not clear whether this is the case in the fetus, because neutrophils and macrophages appear at different times and in different anatomic locations. Macrophages first appear in the yolk sac, liver, lung, and brain, before the bone marrow cavity is formed.

Granulocyte colony-stimulating factor (G-CSF) and **macrophage colony-stimulating factor** (M-CSF) are likely to be involved, as they are in adults, because both are expressed in developing fetal bone as early as 6 wk post conception and both are expressed in the fetal liver as early as 8 wk (see Fig. 446-1). **Granulocyte-macrophage colony-stimulating factor** (GM-CSF) and **stem cell factor** (SCF) also are distributed widely in human fetal tissues. However, no changes in mRNA expression of any of these factors, or of their specific receptors, or in the concentrations of proteins (as judged by immunohistochemical staining) appear to be the signal for fetal production of neutrophils or macrophages. The precise signals have not yet been identified.

Few neutrophils are found in the circulation before the third trimester. The mean circulating neutrophil count is $190/mm^3$ (range, $0–490/mm^3$, mode concentration of zero) in fetuses of 20 wk gestation. Although mature neutrophils are scarce, progenitor cells with the capacity to generate neutrophil clones are relatively abundant in fetal blood. When these fetal progenitor cells are cultured in vitro in the presence of recombinant G-CSF, they mature into large colonies of neutrophils. The physiologic role of G-CSF includes upregulation of neutrophil production, and this appears to be the case for the fetus and neonate as well as for adults. Thus, the low quantities of circulating and storage neu-

TABLE 446-1. Characteristics of Hematopoietic Growth Factors

GROWTH FACTOR	MOLECULAR MASS (KD)	CHROMOSOMAL LOCATION	PRINCIPAL TARGET CELL
ERYTHROPOIETIN	30–39	7q11–12	CFU-E, fetal BFU-E
COLONY-STIMULATING FACTORS			
G-CSF	18–22	17q11.2–21	CFU-G, CFU-MIX, mature neutrophil
GM-CSF	18–30	5q23–31	CFU-MIX, CFU-GM, BFU-E, monocyte, mature neutrophil
M-CSF	45–70 dimer of 2 subunits	5q33.1	CFU-M, macrophage
SCF	36	12	CFU-MIX, BFU-E, CFU-GM, mast cell
INTERLEUKINS			
IL-1	17	Alpha 2q13 Beta 2q13–21	Hepatocyte, macrophage, lymphocyte
IL-2	15–20	4q26–27	T cell, cytotoxic lymphocyte
IL-3	14–30	5q23–31	CFU-MIX, CFU-Meg, CFU-GM, BFU-E, macrophage
IL-4	16–20	5q23–31	T cell, B cell
IL-5	46 (dimer of 2 subunits)	5q23-31	CFU-Eo, B cell
IL-6	19–26	7p21–24	CFU-MIX, CFU-GM, BFU-E, monocyte, B cell, T cell, cytotoxic lymphocyte
IL-7	35	8q12–13	B cell
IL-8	8–10	4	Neutrophil, endothelia cell, T cell
IL-9	16	5q31–32	BFU-E, CFU-MIX
IL-10	18.7	1	Macrophage, lymphocyte
IL-11	23	19q13	CFU-Meg, B cell, keratinocyte
IL-12	70–75 dimer of subunits	p35/p40	3 (p35) and 11 (p40) T cells, NK cells, macrophages
IL-13	9	5q23–31	Pre-B lymphocyte, macrophage
IL-14	53	5q31	B cells
IL-15	14–15	4q25–35	B cells, T cells
IL-16	12–14		T cell
IL-17	20–30	2q31	Marrow stromal cells
IL-18	24	9p13	$CD4^+$ T cells, NK cells
IL-21			T cells
IL-23	Dimer of subunits	p19/IL–12p40	$CD4^+$ T cells
THROMBOPOIETIN	35–38	3q27–28	Megakaryocyte progenitor, megakaryocyte

BFU-E, burst-forming units–erythroid; CFU-E, colony-forming units–erythroid; CFU-Eo, colony-forming units–eosinophil; CFU-G, colony-forming units–granulocyte; CFU-GM, colony-forming units–granulocyte macrophage; CFU-M, colony-forming units–macrophage; CFU-Meg, colony-forming units–megakaryocyte; CFU-MIX, colony-forming units–mixed; G-CSF, granulocyte colony-stimulating factor; GM-CSF, granulocyte-macrophage colony-stimulating factor; IL, interleukin; M-CSF, macrophage colony-stimulating factor; NK, natural killer; SCF, stem cell factor.

trophils in the mid-trimester human fetus may be due in part to low production of G-CSF. Monocytes isolated from the blood of adults produce G-CSF when stimulated with a variety of inflammatory mediators such as **bacterial lipopolysaccharide** (LPS) or **interleukin-1** (IL-1). In contrast, monocytes isolated from the umbilical cord blood of preterm infants, and from the liver and bone marrow of aborted fetuses up to 24 wk gestation, generate only small quantities (10–100× less per cell) of G-CSF protein and mRNA after LPS or IL-1 stimulation. Despite this low capacity for generating G-CSF, G-CSF receptors on the surface of neutrophils of newborn infants are equal in number and affinity to those on adult neutrophils.

In the fetus, the actions of G-CSF, M-CSF, GM-CSF, and SCF are not limited to hematopoiesis. Receptors for each of these factors are located in distinct areas of the fetal central nervous system and gastrointestinal tract, where their patterns of expression change with development. Important developmental roles exist for these factors beyond those known for hematopoiesis.

THROMBOPOIESIS. The marrow megakaryocyte compartment can be conceptualized as consisting of two pools of cells: megakaryocyte progenitors and megakaryocytes. **Megakaryocytes** are identified by their morphologic characteristics, as they undergo **endoreduplication,** which results in large cells with polyploid nuclei.

Megakaryocyte progenitors can be subcategorized into two populations: *burst-forming unit-megakaryocytes* (BFU-MK), which are primitive megakaryocyte progenitors, and *colony-forming unit-megakaryocytes* (CFU-MK), which are more differentiated cells. BFU-MK produce large multifocal colonies containing ≥50 megakaryocytes, whereas CFU-MK generate smaller (3–50 cells/colony), unifocal colonies. BFU-MK express CD34 but not HLA-DR, whereas CFU-MK express CD34 and HLA-DR. The colonies generated by BFU-MK of fetal origin contain significantly more megakaryocytes than do those of adult origin and on that basis are thought to represent somewhat more primitive cells.

Megakaryocytes, unlike megakaryocyte progenitors, do not have the capacity to generate clones. Rather, they undergo maturation, progressing from small mononuclear cells to large polyploid cells. The modal megakaryocyte ploidy in normal adult marrow is 16N. In the fetus and neonate, modal ploidy is lower, and megakaryocyte size is smaller. However, umbilical cord blood has a higher concentration of megakaryocytes than does adult blood. Large megakaryocytes generate more platelets than do small megakaryocytes; thus, it is assumed that megakaryocytes of neonates produce fewer platelets than do their adult counterparts.

The processes of platelet production and release from megakaryocytes are not well understood. It has been speculated that small buds, proplatelets, are formed on marrow megakaryocytes and that these are released from the marrow as platelets. An alternate possibility is that platelets are principally released from megakaryocytes in the lungs, as a consequence of shear forces. That theory is supported by the observation that megakaryocytes are abundant in the lungs.

Thrombopoietin (TPO) is the physiologic regulator of platelet production and acts as a potent stimulator of all stages of megakaryocyte growth and development. The gene that encodes TPO is located on the long arm of human chromosome 3. TPO-mRNA is expressed primarily in liver and kidney and, to a lesser extent, in bone marrow stroma. TPO is a primary, but not exclusive, regulator of platelet production. TPO stimulates the proliferation and survival not only of megakaryotic progenitors but also of erythroid, myeloid, and multipotent progenitors. Phase I

TABLE 446-2. Blood Cell Indices During Gestation and at Birth

WK OF GESTATION	TOTAL WBC COUNT* ($\times 10^9$/L)	CORRECTED WBC COUNT ($\times 10^9$/L)	PLATELETS ($\times 10^9$/L)	RBC ($\times 10^{12}$/L)	HB (G/DL)	(%) HCT	(fL) MCV
18–21	4.68 ± 2.96	2.57 ± 0.42	234 ± 57	2.85 ± 0.36	11.69 ± 1.27	37.3 ± 4.3	131.1 ± 11.0
22–25	4.72 ± 2.84	3.73 ± 2.17	247 ± 59	3.09 ± 0.34	12.2 ± 1.6	38.6 ± 3.9	125.1 ± 7.8
26–29	5.16 ± 2.53	4.08 ± 0.84	242 ± 69	3.46 ± 0.41	12.91 ± 1.38	40.9 ± 4.4	118.5 ± 8.0
>30	7.71 ± 4.99	6.40 ± 2.99	232 ± 87	3.82 ± 0.64	13.64 ± 2.21	43.6 ± 7.2	114.4 ± 9.3
Term		18.1 (9.0–30.0)	290 ± 100	4.70 ± 0.40	16.5 ± 1.5	51.0 ± 4.5	108.0 ± 5.0

*Including normoblasts.

Hb, hemoglobin; Hct, hematocrit; MCV, mean cell volume; RBC, red blood cells; WBC, white blood cell.

Adapted from Forestier F, Daffors F, Catherine N, et al: Developmental hematopoiesis in normal human fetal blood. *Blood* 1991;77:2361.

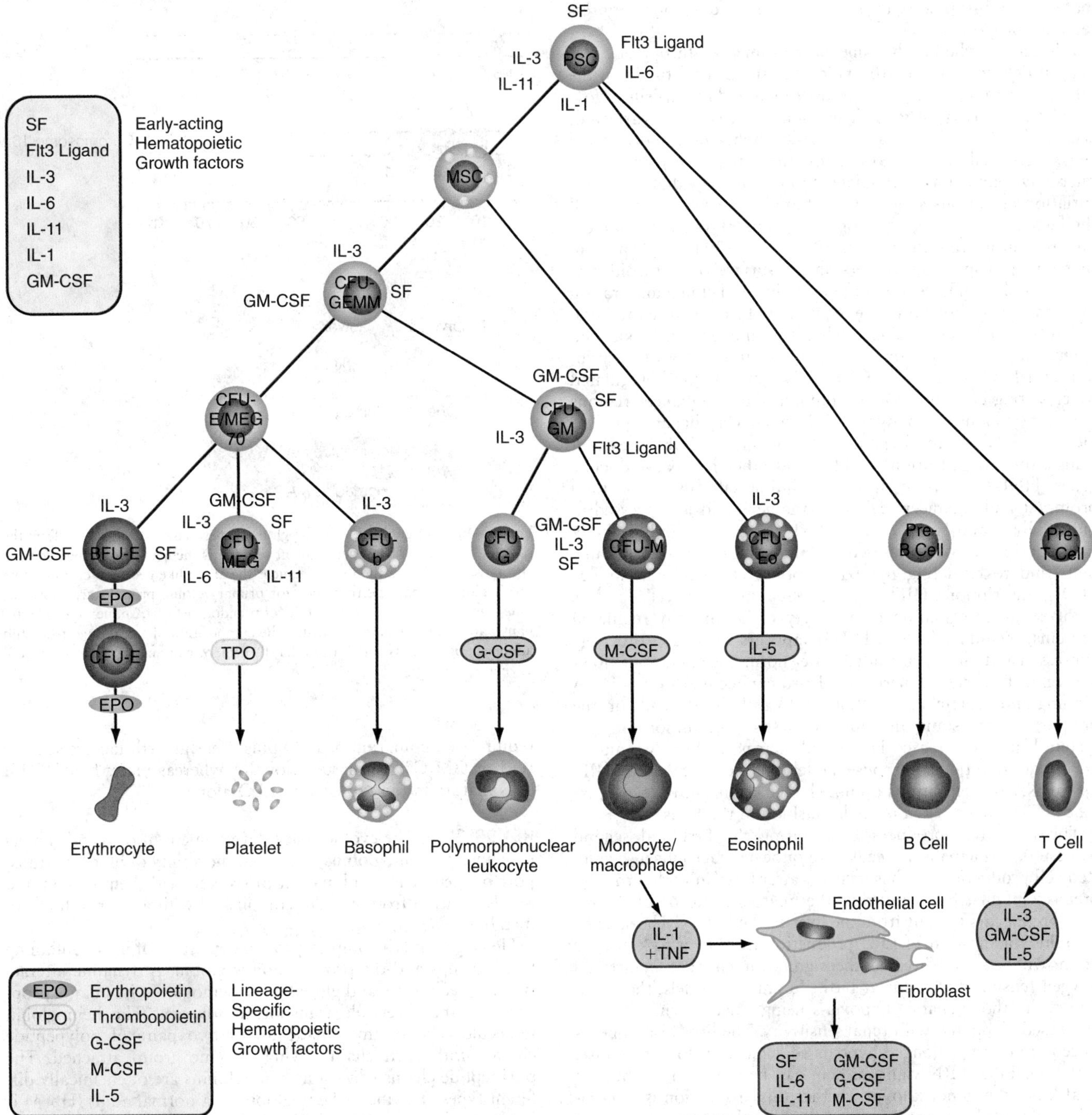

Figure 446-1. Major cytokine sources and actions to promote hematopoiesis. Cells of the bone marrow microenvironment, such as macrophages, endothelial cells, and reticular fibroblasts, produce macrophage colony-stimulating factor (M-CSF), granulocyte-macrophage colony-stimulating factor (GM-CSF), and granulocyte colony-stimulating factor (G-CSF) after stimulation. These cytokines and others listed in the text have overlapping interactions during hematopoietic differentiation, as indicated; for all lineages, optimal development requires a combination of early- and late-acting factors. BFU, burst forming unit; CFU, colony forming unit; EPO, erythropoietin; MSC, myeloid stem cells; PSC, pluripotent stem cell. (From Sieff CA, Nathan DG, Clark SC: The anatomy and physiology of hematopoiesis. In Orkin SH, Nathan DG [editors]: *Hematology of Infancy and Childhood,* 5th ed. Philadelphia, WB Saunders, 1998, p 168.)

and II human trials have demonstrated that rTPO stimulates platelet production in nonthrombocytopenic adults and in patients with chemotherapy-induced thrombocytopenia. Recombinant TPO supports the growth of megakaryocytic colonies of neonates and children. Progenitors of preterm neonates are more sensitive to rTPO than are progenitors of term neonates.

Nothing is known about the benefits and risks of rTPO administration in neonates and children. Recent clinical studies have reported evidence of anti-TPO antibody production in patients receiving rTPO, and further studies have been put on hold.

ERYTHROPOIESIS. Erythropoiesis in utero is controlled by erythroid growth factors produced solely by the fetus. Erythropoietin (EPO) does not cross the placenta in humans; therefore, stimulation of maternal EPO production does not result in stimulation of fetal red cell production. Moreover, suppression of maternal erythropoiesis by hypertransfusion does not suppress fetal erythropoiesis.

It is unclear whether the same mechanism of erythropoietic regulation defining adult erythropoiesis exists in the fetus or in the infant born prematurely. The production of red blood cells is governed by a variety of growth factors produced by a variety of accessory cells such as macrophages, lymphocytes, and stromal cells. These cells and growth factors make up the erythropoietic microenvironment and stimulate maturation, growth, and differentiation at various stages of red blood cell production. Of all the factors stimulating erythropoiesis, none plays a more important regulatory role than EPO. **EPO** is a 30–39 kd glycoprotein that binds to specific receptors on the surface of erythroid precursors and stimulates their differentiation and clonal maturation into mature erythrocytes. The regulation of EPO gene expression involves an oxygen-sensing mechanism, and both hypoxia and anemia stimulate erythropoiesis by stimulating mRNA transcription and EPO production. EPO mRNA production is regulated by cis-acting elements in the promoter and 3′ enhancer regions that are responsive to hypoxia. Two factors, hepatic nuclear factor 4 (HNF-4) and hypoxic inducible factor (HIF-1), exhibit transcriptional activation for EPO and other hypoxia-inducible genes. HNF-4 has been shown to bind specifically to the EPO promoter and enhancer regions of the gene and is expressed in kidney, liver, and Hep3B cells. HIF-1 is a basic helix-loop-helix transcription factor composed of HIF-1α and HIF-1β subunits that bind to cis-acting hypoxia-response elements and induce EPO transcription. HIF-1 is expressed in many cells and is involved in upregulation of a variety of hypoxically regulated proteins, including VEG-F. HIF-1α appears to be constitutively expressed and rapidly degraded under normoxic conditions. Regulation of the heterodimeric HIF-1 protein occurs through DNA binding and protein stabilization. RNA stability depends on the ubiquitin proteasome degradation system; inhibition of this system leads to increased HIF-1 and increased EPO, even under normoxic conditions. In mouse models exposed to hypoxia, HIF-1α mRNA concentrations do not change significantly. It appears that HIF-1α operates in a similar fashion in the fetus.

The fetal liver produces EPO during the first and second trimesters, principally by cells of monocyte/macrophage origin. Red cell production reaches its nadir after birth in both term and preterm infants; following this, the anatomic site of EPO production appears to shift from the liver to the kidney. The specific stimulus for the shift of EPO production from liver to kidney is unknown but may involve the significant changes in arterial oxygen tension that occur at birth. In animal models, the sensitivity of the hepatic hypoxia-sensing mechanism appears decreased compared with renal sensitivity. The liver also appears to require more prolonged hypoxia to achieve an EPO response. Although EPO mRNA and protein can be found in the human fetal kidney, it is not known whether this production is biologically relevant. However, it appears that renal production of EPO is not essential for normal fetal erythropoiesis, as evidenced by the normal serum EPO concentrations and normal hematocrits of anephric fetuses.

When bone marrow cells are placed in semi-solid media culture systems for 5–7 days, the EPO-sensitive precursors, termed **colony-forming units-erythroid** (CFU-E) clonally mature into clusters containing 30–100 normoblasts (see Fig. 446-1). Erythroid-specific progenitors that are less well differentiated than CFU-E, and consequently are more primitive cells, are termed *burst-forming units-erythroid* (BFU-E). Twelve to 14 days after these cells are placed in culture, BFU-E cells develop into large clusters of normoblasts, each containing 200–10,000 cells. BFU-E cells from human fetuses respond in a slightly different fashion than BFU-E cells isolated from adults. Specifically, BFU-E cells of fetal origin usually develop into erythroid clones more rapidly and generally develop substantially more normoblasts than do BFU-E cells of adult origin. BFU-E cells from adult bone marrow require a combination of EPO plus other growth factors such as IL-3 or GM-CSF to mature clonally, whereas many fetal BFU-E cells mature in the presence of EPO alone.

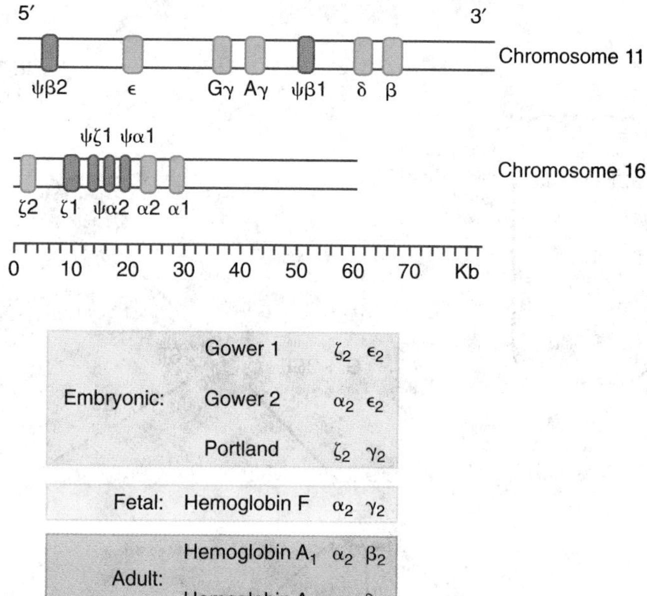

Figure 446-2. Organization of the globin genes. The bottom line reflects the scale in kilobases. The upper segment represents the beta-like globin genes on chromosome 11, and the lower segment the alpha-like genes on chromosome 16. Regions of the gene that code for primary globin proteins are shown as *blue* segments, and regions that code for pseudogenes ("ψ," nonexpressed remnants) are shown as *pink* segments. The composition of embryonic, fetal, and adult hemoglobins is listed. α, alpha; β, beta; γ, gamma; δ, delta; ε, epsilon; ζ, zeta.

HEMOGLOBIN. The evolutionary development of oxygen-carrying proteins, the **hemoglobins,** increased the ability of blood to transport oxygen. The combination of oxygen with hemoglobin and its dissociation from it are accomplished without expenditure of metabolic energy.

Hemoglobin is a complex protein consisting of iron-containing heme groups and the protein moiety globin. A dynamic interaction between heme and globin gives hemoglobin its unique properties in the reversible transport of oxygen. The hemoglobin molecule is a tetramer made up of two pairs of polypeptide chains, with each chain having a heme group attached. The polypeptide chains of various hemoglobins are of chemically different types. The major hemoglobin of a normal adult (Hb A) is made up of one pair of alpha (α) and one pair of beta (β) polypeptide chains, represented as $\alpha_2\beta_2$. The major hemoglobin in the fetus (Hb F), which is made up of two alpha and two gamma globin chains, is represented by $\alpha_2\gamma_2$.

The various globin chains differ in both the number and sequence of amino acids, and their synthesis is directed by separate genes (Fig. 446-2). Two sets of genes for the α chains are located on human chromosome 16. Two pairs of alleles provide the genetic information for the structure of the α chain. The β, γ, δ genes are closely linked on chromosome 11.

Within the red blood cell (RBC) mass of an embryo, fetus, child, and adult, six different hemoglobins may normally be detected: the **embryonic hemoglobins,** Gower-1, Gower-2, and Portland; the **fetal hemoglobin,** Hb F; and the **adult hemoglobins,** Hb A and Hb A_2. The electrophoretic mobilities of hemoglobins vary with their chemical structures. The time of appearance and quantitative relationships among the hemoglobins are determined by complex developmental processes (Fig. 446-3).

Embryonic Hemoglobins. The blood of early human embryos contains two slowly migrating hemoglobins, *Gower-1* and *Gower-2*, and *Hb Portland*, which has Hb F–like mobility. The zeta (ζ) chains of Hb Portland and Gower-1 are structurally quite similar to α chains. Both Gower hemoglobins contain a unique type of polypeptide chain, the epsilon (ε) chain. Hb Gower-1 has the structure $\zeta_2\varepsilon_2$, while Gower-2 has the structure $\alpha_2\varepsilon_2$. Hb Portland has the structure $\zeta_2\gamma_2$. In embryos of 4–8 wk gestation, the Gower hemoglobins predominate, but by the 3rd month they have disappeared.

Fetal Hemoglobin. Hb F contains γ polypeptide chains in place of the β chains of Hb A. Its resistance to denaturation by strong alkali is the basis for determining the presence of fetal RBCs in the maternal circulation (the **Kleihauer-Betke test**). After the 8th gestational wk, Hb F is the predominant hemoglobin; at 24 wk gestation it constitutes 90% of the total hemoglobin. During the 3rd trimester, a gradual decline occurs, so that at birth Hb F averages 70% of the total. Synthesis of Hb F decreases rapidly postnatally, and by 6–12 mo of age only a trace is present. Less than 2.0% can be detected by alkali denaturation in older children and adults. Hb F is heterogeneous because of two types of γ chains, whose synthesis is directed by two sets of genes. The chains differ at position 136 in the presence of either a glycine (Gγ) or an alanine (Aγ) residue. In newborns, the relative ratio of Gγ to Aγ chain is 3:1.

Adult Hemoglobins. Some Hb A ($\alpha_2\beta_2$) can be detected in even the smallest embryos. Accordingly, it is possible as early as 16–20 wk gestation to make a prenatal diagnosis of major β-chain hemoglobinopathies, such as thalassemia major (see Chapter 462.9). Prenatal diagnosis is based on techniques that examine the rates of synthesis of β chains or the structure of newly synthesized β chains. Earlier diagnosis is possible using molecular biology techniques and sampling of chorionic villus tissue or amniotic fluid if DNA structural defects are a cause of the hemoglobinopathies. Gene deletion disorders such as the α-thalassemias can be detected using the same method.

By the 24th wk of gestation, 5–10% of Hb A is present. A steady increase follows, so that at term, Hb A averages 30%. By 6–12 mo of age, the normal Hb A pattern appears. The minor Hb A component Hb A_2 contains delta (δ) chains and has the structure $\alpha_2\delta_2$. It is seen only when significant amounts of Hb A are also present. At birth, <1.0% of Hb A_2 is seen, but by 12 mo of age the normal level of 2.0–3.4% is attained. Throughout life, the normal ratio of Hb A to A_2 is about 30:1.

Normal Relationships Among the Hemoglobins. During fetal life and early childhood, the rates of synthesis of γ and β chains and the amounts of Hb A and Hb F are inversely related. This relationship has been attributed to a "switch mechanism" similar to genetic regulatory mechanisms in bacteria, but the genetic, biologic, and developmental processes that direct a switchover from predominantly γ-chain synthesis *in utero* to predominantly β-chain synthesis after birth are unclear. It is not certain whether the mechanisms involve selective genetic inhibition or facilitation. The increase in the α_1/α_2 globin ratio occurring after 36 wk gestation corresponds with a rapid decline in γ-globin synthesis, suggesting that these changes could be regulated by a coordinated molecular mechanism. Differential selection and amplified production of RBC precursors derived from BFU-E cells result in con-

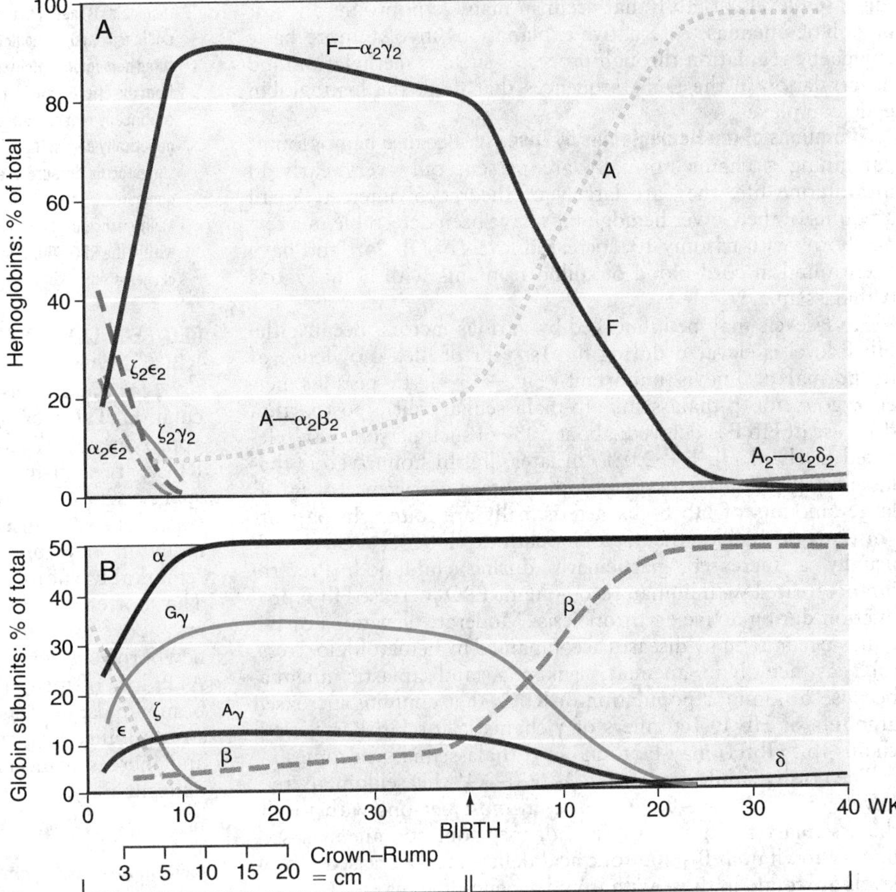

Figure 446-3. Changes in hemoglobin tetramers *(A)* and in globin subunits *(B)* during human development from embryo to early infancy. (From Polin RA, Fox WW: *Fetal and Neonatal Physiology*, 2nd ed. Philadelphia, WB Saunders, 1998, p 1769.)

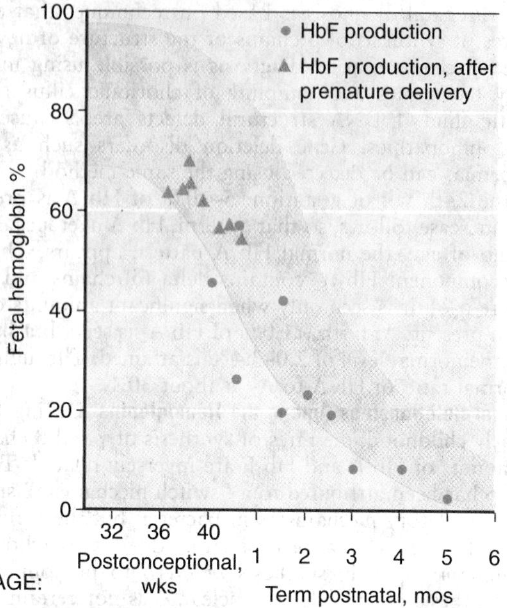

Figure 446-4. Pre- and postnatal changes in the percentage of total hemoglobin represented by fetal hemoglobin (Hb F) *(yellow)*. The *triangles* represent postnatal production by reticulocytes in premature infants, and the *circles* represent cord blood and postnatal reticulocyte production in term infants. (From Brown MS: Fetal and neonatal erythropoiesis. In Stockman JA, Pochedly C [editors]: *Developmental and Neonatal Hematology.* New York, Raven Press, 1988.)

siderable Hb F production. This may be the basis for the increased levels of Hb F that occur in many hypoproliferative or hemolytic anemias. Alternative explanations involve more basic epigenetic regulation through processes such as methylation and deacetylation in the DNA sequences that flank the hemoglobin gene complexes.

Alterations of the Hemoglobins by Disease. Because hemoglobins containing ε chains normally are present only very early in intrauterine life, they are largely of theoretical interest. Small amounts of the Gower hemoglobins have been detectable in a few newborns with trisomy 13. Increased levels of Hb Portland have been found in cord blood of stillborn infants with homozygous α-thalassemia.

Hb F levels may be influenced by various factors. Because the Hb F level is elevated during the 1st year of life, knowledge of its normal decline is important (Fig. 446-4). In persons heterozygous for β-thalassemia (β-thalassemia trait), postpartum decrease of Hb F is delayed; about 50% of such persons have elevated levels of Hb F (>2.0%) in later life. In homozygous thalassemia (Cooley anemia) and in hereditary persistence of Hb F, large amounts of Hb F characteristically are found. In patients with major β-chain hemoglobinopathies (Hb SS, SC), Hb F usually is increased, particularly during childhood. Preterm infants treated with human recombinant EPO increase Hb F production during active erythropoiesis. Moderate elevations of Hb F may occur in many diseases accompanied by hematologic stress, such as hemolytic anemias, leukemia, and aplastic anemia, because of a minor population of RBCs that contains increased amounts of Hb F. Tetramers of γ chains (γ_4 or Hb Barts) or β chains (β_4, Hb H) may be found in α-thalassemia syndromes.

The normal adult level of Hb A_2 (2.0–3.4%) is seldom altered. Levels of Hb A_2 >3.4% are found in most persons with the β-thalassemia trait and in those with megaloblastic anemias secondary to vitamin B_{12} and folic acid deficiency. Decreased Hb A_2 levels are found in those with iron-deficiency anemia (see Chapter 455) and α-thalassemia (see Chapter 462).

METABOLISM OF THE RBC. The nucleated RBCs in bone marrow participate in various metabolic functions, including active protein synthesis. After extrusion of the nucleus, most of this metabolic ability is lost, including the ability to synthesize proteins. Loss of the nucleus makes the RBC a better vessel for oxygen transport, but it imposes a finite life span on the RBC, because the cell cannot replace or repair its vital enzymatic proteins. Mature RBCs contain >40 enzymes. Many of these are essential for cellular viability, but genetically determined deficiencies of others, such as catalase, do not interfere with normal survival.

Mature RBCs have no mitochondria; adenosine triphosphate (ATP) cannot be generated by oxidative phosphorylation in Krebs cycle reactions. Rather, glucose is taken up and lactic acid produced mostly by anaerobic glycolysis *(Embden-Meyerhof pathway)*; about 10% of glucose is metabolized oxidatively through the pentose phosphate pathway. At least 5 functions for ATP generated by glucose metabolism are essential to normal cell viability:

- **Maintenance of electrolyte gradients.** The principal intracellular cation of RBCs is potassium, whereas that in plasma is sodium. Reversal of the constant tendency for sodium to enter the RBCs and concomitantly for potassium to leak out, with preservation of normal ionic gradients, is accomplished by an energy (ATP)–dependent membrane mechanism, the cation pump. When the cation pump fails, sodium and water enter the RBCs, causing them to swell and ultimately to hemolyze. Energy also is used to maintain low intracellular levels of calcium ion.
- **Initiation of energy production.** ATP is required for the initial reaction of glycolysis involving phosphorylation of glucose to glucose-6-phosphate.
- **Maintenance of RBC membrane and shape.** Energy is required to maintain the complex phospholipid structure of the RBC membrane. Maintenance of the biconcave shape probably is energy dependent as well.
- **Maintenance of heme iron in the reduced (ferrous) form.** Oxidative potentials within the RBC may cause oxidation of the iron of hemoglobin. Hemoglobin containing ferric iron (methemoglobin) is ineffective in oxygen transport. If peroxides and other oxidant substances are not inactivated, hemoglobin may be denatured and precipitated. Cells containing such denatured hemoglobin (Heinz bodies) are removed from the circulation rapidly. Protection of RBCs from the effects of oxidation ultimately depends on NADPH and NADH. These compounds are continually regenerated by activities of the glycolytic pathway and pentose shunt. In many genetically determined deficiencies of glycolytic and pentose pathway enzymes, hemolytic states occur because the energy necessary to perform these vital functions cannot be generated.
- **Maintenance of the levels of organic phosphates such as 2,3-diphosphoglycerate and ATP within the RBCs.** These compounds interact with hemoglobin and have profound effects on oxygen affinity.

RED CELL LIFE SPAN. The differences in physical properties of RBCs derived from term and preterm infants may account, in part, for the decreased life span of neonatal RBCs within the circulation. The average life span for a neonatal RBC is 60–90 days, approximately ½ to ⅔ that of an adult RBC. When neonatal RBCs are transfused into adults, they exhibit a shortened life span, owing to alterations intrinsic to the neonatal RBC. In contrast, cells transfused from adult donors appear to survive normally in newborns. With increasing degrees of prematurity, remarkably shorter red cell life spans (35–50 days) are found. The shortened red cell life span of the preterm and term neonate may be explained by some of the characteristics specific to newborn cells: a rapid decline in intracellular enzyme activity and ATP; loss of membrane surface area by internalization of membrane lipids; decreased levels of intracellular carnitine, increased susceptibility of membrane lipids and proteins to peroxidation, and increased mechanical fragility due to increased membrane deformability.

Bain BJ: Diagnosis from the blood smear. *N Engl J Med* 2005;353:498–507.
Calhoun DA, Christensen RD: Human developmental biology of granulocyte colony-stimulating factor. *Clin Perinatol* 2000;27:559–576.

Dame C, Juul S: The switch from fetal to adult erythropoiesis. *Clin Perinatol* 2000;27:507–526.
Deutsch VR, Toner A: Megakaryocyte development and platelet production. *Br J Haematol* 2006;134:453–466.
Kaushansky K: Lineage-specific hematopoietic growth factors. *N Engl J Med* 2006;354:2034–2045.
Kaushansky K: Thrombopoietin and hematopoietic stem cell development. *Ann NY Acad Sci* 1999;30:314–341.
Ohls RK, Li Y, Abdel-Mageed A, et al: Neutrophil pool sizes and granulocyte colony-stimulating factor production in human mid-trimester fetuses. *Pediatr Res* 1995;37:806–811.
Slayton WB: Development of the immune system in the human fetus. In Christensen RD (editor): *Hematologic Problems of the Neonate.* Philadelphia, WB Saunders, 2000, pp 21–42.
Sola MC, Dame C, Christensen RD: Toward a rational use of recombinant thrombopoietin in the neonatal intensive care unit. *J Pediatr Hematol Oncol* 2001;23:179–184.
Szilvassy SJ: Haematopoietic stem and progenitor cell-targeted therapies for thrombocytopenia. *Expert Opin Bio Ther* 2006;6:983–992.
Vats A, Bielby RC, Tolley NS, et al: Stem cells. *Lancet* 2005;366:592–602.

Chapter 447 ■ The Anemias Bertil Glader

Anemia is defined as a reduction of the red blood cell (RBC) volume or hemoglobin concentration below the range of values occurring in healthy persons. Table 447-1 lists the means and ranges for hemoglobin and hematocrit values by age groups of well-nourished children. There appear to be racial differences in hemoglobin levels. Black children have levels about 0.5 g/dL lower than those of white and Asian children of comparable age and socioeconomic status, perhaps in part as a result of the high incidence of α-thalassemia in blacks.

Although a reduction in the amount of circulating hemoglobin decreases the oxygen-carrying capacity of the blood, few clinical disturbances occur until the hemoglobin level falls below 7–8 g/dL. Below this level, pallor becomes evident in the mucous membranes. Physiologic adjustments to anemia include increased cardiac output, increased oxygen extraction (increased arteriovenous oxygen difference), and a shunting of blood flow toward vital organs and tissues. In addition, the concentration of 2,3-diphosphoglycerate (2,3-DPG) increases within the RBC. The resultant "shift to the right" of the oxygen dissociation curve, reducing the affinity of hemoglobin for oxygen, results in more complete transfer of oxygen to the tissues. The same shift in the oxygen dissociation curve also may occur at high altitude. When moderately severe anemia develops slowly, surprisingly few symptoms or objective findings may be evident. Weakness, tachypnea, shortness of breath on exertion, tachycardia, cardiac dilatation, and congestive heart failure ultimately result from increasingly severe anemia, regardless of its cause.

When oxygen delivery by RBCs to tissues is decreased, various mechanisms, including expanded cardiac output, increased production of 2,3-DPG in RBCs, and higher levels of erythropoietin (EPO) help the body compensate for the deficiency. RBC production by the bone marrow in response to EPO may expand several-fold, thereby compensating for mild to moderate reductions in the life span of RBCs. In some anemias, the bone marrow loses its usual capacity for sustained production and expansion of the RBC mass; and, in these instances, absolute reticulocyte numbers in the peripheral blood are decreased. The normal reticulocyte percentage of total RBCs during most of childhood is about 1.0%, with an absolute reticulocyte count of 25,000–75,000/mm^3. In the presence of anemia, EPO production and the absolute number of reticulocytes should rise. A normal or low absolute number or percentage of reticulocytes in response to anemia indicates relative bone marrow failure or ineffective erythropoiesis (e.g., megaloblastic anemia, thalassemia). Measurement of the serum transferrin receptor (TfR) level or examination of the bone marrow distinguishes between these possibilities, because TfR is elevated in ineffective erythropoiesis (or in iron deficiency) and decreased in marrow RBC hypoproliferation.

Anemia is not a specific entity but, rather, the result of many underlying pathologic processes. RBC size changes with age; and before an anemia can be specifically characterized with respect to RBC size, normal developmental changes in the mean corpuscular volume (MCV) must be understood (see Table 447-1). It is important for pediatricians to recognize the MCV variations in childhood, because many laboratories use only adult normal values, which differ considerably. For every child with significant anemia, it also is essential to review the appearance of RBCs on a peripheral blood smear (Fig. 447-1). Specific morphologic features may point to the underlying diagnosis. In addition, the presence of *polychromatophilia,* which usually correlates with the degree of reticulocytosis, indicates that the marrow is able to respond to RBC loss or destruction.

COMMON CAUSES OF ANEMIA. Figure 447-2 presents a useful approach to assessing the common causes of anemia in children.

ASSOCIATION OF ANEMIA WITH OTHER HEMATOLOGIC ABNORMALITIES. Thrombocytopenia, abnormalities in white blood cell numbers, or the presence of abnormal leukocytes often indicates bone marrow failure caused by aplastic anemia, leukemia, or other malignant marrow disease. These disorders can be differentiated by careful review of screening hematologic studies and close attention to the child's medical history and physical examination.

TABLE 447-1. Hematologic Values During Infancy and Childhood

	HEMOGLOBIN (G/DL)		HEMATOCRIT (%)		RETICULOCYTES (%)	MCV (FL)	LEUKOCYTES (WBC/MM³)		NEUTROPHILS (%)		LYMPHOCYTES (%)	EOSINOPHILS (%)	MONOCYTES (%)
AGE	Mean	Range	Mean	Range	Mean	Lowest	Mean	Range	Mean	Range	Mean*	Mean	Mean
Cord blood	16.8	13.7–20.1	55	45–65	5.0	110	18,000	(9,000–30,000)	61	(40–80)	31	2	6
2 wk	16.5	13.0–20.0	50	42–66	1.0		12,000	(5,000–21,000)	40		63	3	9
3 mo	12.0	9.5–14.5	36	31–41	1.0		12,000	(6,000–18,000)	30		48	2	5
6 mo–6 yr	12.0	10.5–14.0	37	33–42	1.0	70–74	10,000	(6,000–15,000)	45		48	2	5
7–12 yr	13.0	11.0–16.0	38	34–40	1.0	76–80	8,000	(4,500–13,500)	55		38	2	5
Adult													
Female	14	12.0–16.0	42	37–47	1.6	80	7,500	(5,000–10,000)	55	(35–70)	35	3	7
Male	16	14.0–18.0	47	42–52		80							

*Relatively wide range.
fL, femtoliters; MCV, mean corpuscular volume; WBC, white blood cells.

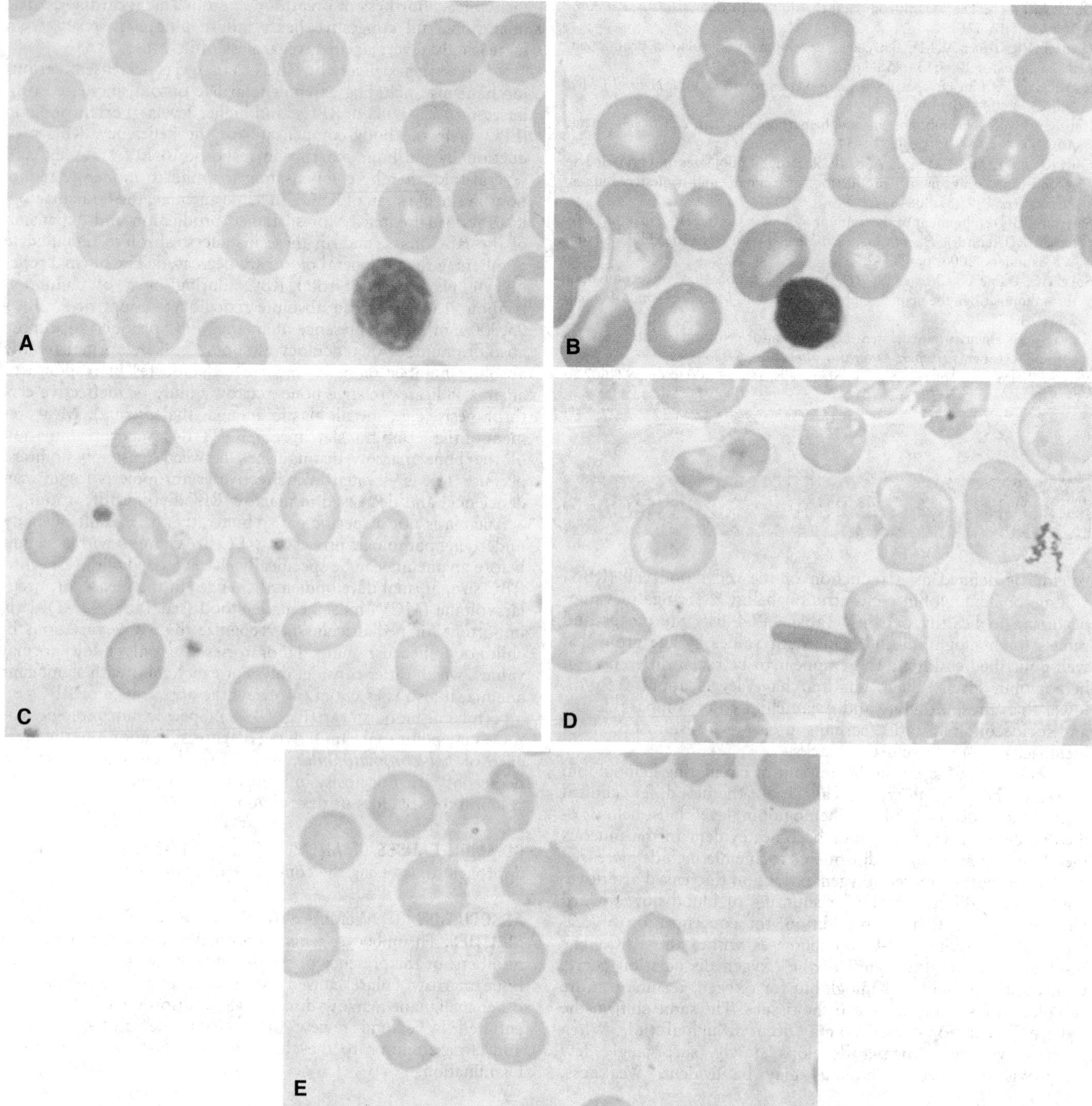

Figure 447-1. Morphologic abnormalities of the red blood cell. *A*, Normal. *B*, Macrocytes (folic acid or vitamin B_{12} deficiency). *C*, Hypochromic microcytes (iron deficiency). *D*, Target cells (Hb CC disease). *E*, Schizocytes (hemolytic-uremic syndrome). (Courtesy of Dr. E. Schwartz.)

ASSOCIATION OF ANEMIA WITH RETICULOCYTOSIS. In anemic children with an appropriate reticulocyte response, the anemia usually is a consequence of bleeding or ongoing hemolysis. The most characteristic feature of hemolysis is reticulocytosis with indirect hyperbilirubinemia and, often, increased serum lactate dehydrogenase as indicators of accelerated erythrocyte destruction. Review of the peripheral blood smear to identify abnormal RBC morphology (e.g., spherocytes, sickle forms, microangiopathy) often is helpful in ascertaining the cause of hemolysis.

ASSOCIATION OF ANEMIA WITH RETICULOCYTOPENIA. Anemia in children with a less than appropriate reticulocyte response reflects an impairment of normal erythropoiesis; in this group, analysis of red blood cell size (mean corpuscular volume [MCV]) is particularly useful.

Presence of Microcytic Red Blood Cells. Almost all children with anemia and reticulocytopenia have defects in hemoglobin synthesis from *iron deficiency* (see Chapter 455), *thalassemia trait, hemoglobin E disorders,* or *hemoglobin C* (see Chapter 462).

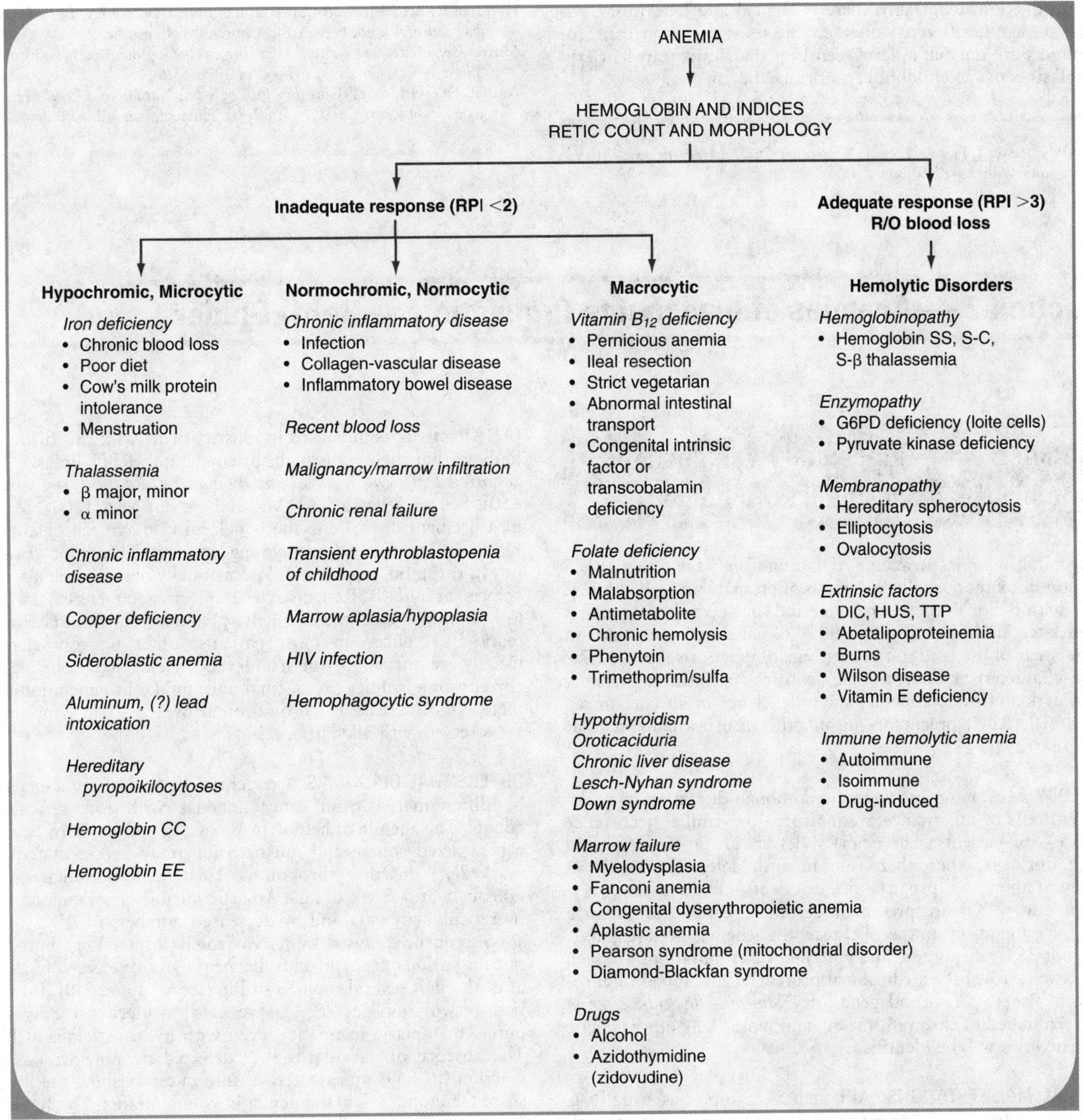

Figure 447-2. Use of the complete blood count, reticulocyte count, and blood smear in the diagnosis of anemia. DIC, disseminated intravascular coagulation; G6PD, glucose-6-phosphate dehydrogenase; HUS, hemolytic uremic syndrome; RPI, reticulocyte production index; TTP, thrombotic thrombocytopenic purpura. (From Kliegman RM, Marcdante KJ, Jenson HJ, et al: *Nelson Essentials of Pediatrics*, 5th ed. Philadelphia, Elsevier/Saunders, 2006, p 694.

Thalassemia trait disorders and other hemoglobinopathies are considered in patients of Mediterranean, Near Eastern, African, or Asian background. A distinguishing feature of thalassemia trait conditions and hemoglobin E is that the RBC count often is higher than normal despite the presence of a mild anemia and microcytosis, in contrast to iron deficiency, in which the RBC count usually decreases along with the reduced hemoglobin and MCV.

Macrocytic Red Blood Cells. The anemia seen in children with macrocytic blood cells sometimes is megaloblastic (see Chapter 454), a result of impaired DNA synthesis and nuclear development, and the formation of other blood cells also is affected. The peripheral blood smear in megaloblastic anemias contains large macrovalocytes, and often the neutrophils show nuclear hypersegmentation. The varied major causes of megaloblastic anemia include folate deficiency, vitamin B_{12} deficiency, and rare inborn errors of metabolism. However, not all macrocytic anemias are megaloblastic; one such non-megaloblastic condition in children is Diamond-Blackfan anemia.

Normocytic Red Blood Cells. Normocytic anemia, low reticulocyte count, and normal bilirubin levels characterize a large number of anemias. The *anemia of chronic disease* (see Chapter 451) usually is normocytic. Occasionally it may be slightly microcytic, and in these cases there usually is clinical evidence of associated inflammatory disease or chronic illness. The anemia of renal failure is normocytic and is caused by reduced erythropoietin production. Invariably, there is clinical and laboratory evidence of significant renal disease. The most common cause of acquired pure red cell aplasia seen in pediatrics is transient erythroblastopenia of childhood, a normocytic anemia.

Greer JP, Foerster J, Lukens J, et al: *Wintrobe's Clinical Hematology,* 11th ed. Baltimore, Williams & Wilkins, 2004.
Hoffman R, Benz EJ, Shattil SJ, et al (editors): *Hematology: Basic Principles and Practice,* 4th ed. New York, Churchill Livingstone, 2005.
Morris CR, Singer ST, Walters MC: Clinical hemoglobinopathies: iron, lungs and new blood. *Curr Opin Hematol* 2006;13(6):407–418.
Nathan DG, Orkin SH, Ginsburg O, Look AT: *Nathan and Oski's Hematology of Infancy and Childhood,* 6th ed. Philadelphia, WB Saunders, 2003.

Section 2 — Anemias of Inadequate Production — Bertil Glader

Chapter 448 ■ Congenital Hypoplastic Anemia (Diamond-Blackfan Anemia)

Congenital hypoplastic anemia (Diamond-Blackfan anemia) is a rare condition that usually becomes symptomatic in early infancy, often with pallor in the neonatal period, but occasionally is first noted later in childhood. Over 90% of cases are recognized in the 1st year of life, and the average age of diagnosis is 3 mo. The most characteristic hematologic features are anemia, usually macrocytic, reticulocytopenia, and a deficiency or absence of red blood cell (RBC) precursors in an otherwise normally cellular bone marrow.

ETIOLOGY. Most cases are sporadic, although dominant or recessive patterns of inheritance are indicated by familial occurrence in ≈15% of patients. The primary defects are in the erythroid progenitor cells, where there is an intrinsic defect that results in increased apoptosis (programmed cell death). High levels of erythropoietin (EPO) are present in serum and urine, although a search for mutations in the EPO receptor gene has been negative. In about 25% of sporadic and inherited cases mutations are seen in a gene *(DBA1)* for a ribosomal protein S19, mapped to chromosome 19q13. A second gene for *Diamond-Blackfan anemia* has been linked to chromosome 8p, and most likely other genetic abnormalities will be identified.

CLINICAL MANIFESTATIONS. Although hematopoiesis usually is adequate in fetal life, some affected infants appear pale at birth or in the first days after birth; rarely, hydrops fetalis occurs (see Chapter 103). Profound anemia usually becomes evident by 2–6 mo of age, occasionally somewhat later. More than 50% of affected children have congenital anomalies, including short stature, craniofacial dysmorphism (snub nose, wide-set eyes, thick upper lip), or defects of the upper extremities (weak radial pulse, flattening of thenar eminence), including triphalangeal thumbs. Thumb anomalies may be bilateral or unilateral and also include bifid, subluxed, absent, or supernumerary thumbs. The abnormalities are diverse, with no specific pattern emerging among most of those affected.

LABORATORY FINDINGS. The RBCs usually are macrocytic for age, but there is no hypersegmentation of neutrophils or other peripheral blood characteristics of megaloblastic anemia. Folic acid and vitamin B_{12} levels are normal. Chemical evaluation of RBCs reveals an enzyme pattern similar to a "fetal" RBC population, and there is also elevated fetal hemoglobin (Hb F) and increased expression of "i" antigen. Erythrocyte adenosine deaminase (ADA) activity is increased in most patients with this disorder, a finding that helps distinguish congenital RBC aplasia from acquired *transient erythroblastopenia of childhood* (see Chapter 450). Because elevated ADA activity is not a fetal RBC feature, measurement of this enzyme is helpful in diagnosing Diamond-Blackfan anemia in very young infants. Thrombocytosis or, rarely, thrombocytopenia and occasionally neutropenia also may be present initially. Reticulocytes rarely are characteristically very low despite severe anemia. RBC precursors in the marrow are markedly reduced in most patients; other marrow elements usually are normal. Serum iron levels are elevated. Bone marrow chromosome studies are normal and, unlike in Fanconi anemia, there is no increase in chromosomal breaks when lymphocytes are stressed with alkylating agents.

DIFFERENTIAL DIAGNOSIS. Congenital hypoplastic anemia must be differentiated from other anemias with low reticulocyte counts. The anemia of hemolytic disease of the newborn can have a protracted course and, on occasion, may be associated with markedly reduced erythropoiesis. This usually terminates spontaneously at 5–8 wk of age. Aplastic anemic crises characterized by reticulocytopenia and by decreased numbers of RBC precursors, frequently caused by parvovirus B19 infections, may complicate various types of chronic hemolytic disease, but usually after the first several months of life (see Chapter 450). Infection with parvovirus B19 (see Chapter 248) in utero also may cause pure RBC aplasia in infancy, even with hydrops fetalis at birth. The absence of parvovirus B19 detected by polymerase chain reaction (PCR) is an essential feature in establishing the diagnosis of Diamond-Blackfan anemia in young infants. The syndrome of transient erythroblastopenia of childhood may be differentiated from Diamond-Blackfan syndrome by its relatively late onset, although it may occasionally develop in infants younger than 6 mo (see Chapter 450). In very young infants whose RBCs have many fetal features, a determination of elevated erythrocyte ADA activity is particularly useful because this increased enzyme activity is not a characteristic of fetal RBCs.

TREATMENT. Corticosteroid therapy is beneficial in ¾ of patients who respond initially. The mechanism of its effect is unknown. Prednisone in three divided doses totaling 2 mg/kg/24 hr is used as an initial trial. An increase in RBC precursors is seen in the bone marrow 1–3 wk after therapy is begun, and this is followed by peripheral reticulocytosis. The hemoglobin may reach normal levels in 4–6 wk, although the rate of response is quite variable. Once it is established that the hemoglobin concentration is increasing, the dose of corticosteroid may be reduced gradually by tapering divided doses and then by eliminating all except a single, lowest effective daily dose. This dose should then be doubled, used on alternate days, and tapered still further while maintaining the hemoglobin level at 9 g/dL or above. In some patients, very small amounts of prednisone, as low as 2.5 mg twice a week, may be sufficient to sustain adequate erythropoiesis. Overall, 60% of children with Diamond-Blackfan anemia initially started on corticosteroids stop taking the drug, usually because of unacceptable corticosteroid side effects or evolution of corticosteroid refractoriness at acceptable doses. Occasionally, there is spontaneous remission of anemia.

In patients who do not respond to corticosteroid therapy, transfusions at intervals of 4–8 wk are necessary to sustain normal growth and activities. Chelation therapy for iron overload, with deferoxamine administered subcutaneously through a portable pump, is started when excess iron accumulation is reflected by serum ferritin levels >1,500 mg/dL. Deferasirox has completed clinical trials and has been approved by the FDA as an iron chelator for use in iron overload states. This agent is dissolved in water or juice and taken as a drink. It is anticipated that the use of oral deferasirox will replace the usage of parenteral deferoxamine. Other therapies, including androgens, cyclosporine, cyclophosphamide, antithymocyte globulin (ATG), high-dose intravenous immunoglobulin, high-dose methylprednisolone, EPO, and interleukin-3 have not had a consistent beneficial effect and may have a high incidence of side effects. Splenectomy may rarely be needed to decrease the need for transfusion if hypersplenism or isoimmunization develops. **Stem cell transplantation** from a related histocompatible donor has a role in children who do not respond to corticosteroids and who have demonstrated a several-year need for RBC transfusions. The survival results for matched related donors have been very encouraging, but the responses have been considerably less successful with the use of partially mismatched siblings or matched unrelated donors.

PROGNOSIS. Median survival is probably >40 yr of age, although definitive data are lacking. The Diamond-Blackfan Anemia Registry (DBAR) is accumulating data to ascertain responses to therapy and survival (http://www.dbar.org/). The outlook is best in those who respond to corticosteroid therapy. About ½ of patients are long-term responders. In the others, survival depends on transfusions. Some children in each group eventually may have spontaneous remissions (≈20%), and most of these remissions occur in the first decade. In children who receive regular transfusions, total body iron increases and hemosiderosis ensues. The complications of chronic transfusions in Diamond-Blackfan anemia are similar to those in β-thalassemia major; prevention and treatment of iron overload should be equally aggressive in both groups of transfused patients. Diamond-Blackfan anemia may be a premalignant syndrome, with acute leukemia (usually myeloid) and myelodysplasia occurring in a small proportion (<5%) of patients. Solid tumor malignancies also are reported, especially osteosarcoma. Other significant causes of death include complications associated with stem cell transplantation, corticosteroid therapy (opportunistic infections), and iron overload.

Costa LD, Willig TN, Fixler J, et al: Diamond-Blackfan anemia. *Curr Opin Pediatr* 2001;13:10.

Freedman MH: Diamond-Blackfan anemia. *Baillieres Clin Haematol* 2000;13:391.

Gazda HT, Sieff CA: Recent insights into the pathogenesis of Diamond-Blackfan anaemia. *Br J Haematol* 2006 Oct;135:149–157. Epub 2006 Aug 31.

Gustavsson P, Willig TN, van Haeringen A, et al: Diamond-Blackfan anaemia: Genetic homogeneity for a gene on chromosome 19q13 restricted to 1.8 Mb. *Nat Genet* 1997;16:368.

Lipton JM: Diamond blackfan anemia: New paradigms for a "not so pure" inherited red cell aplasia. *Semin Hematol* 2006;43:167–177.

Vlachos A, Klein GW, Lipton JM: The Diamond Blackfan anemia registry: Tool for investigating the epidemiology and biology of Diamond-Blackfan anemia. *J Pediatr Hematol Oncol* 2001;23:377–382.

Willig TN, Niemeyer CM, Leblanc T, et al: Identification of new prognosis factors from the clinical and epidemiologic analysis of a registry of 229 Diamond-Blackfan anemia patients. *Pediatr Res* 1999;46:553.

Chapter 449 ■ Pearson Marrow-Pancreas Syndrome

Pearson marrow-pancreas syndrome is a form of congenital hypoplastic anemia that initially may be confused with Diamond-Blackfan syndrome or transient erythroblastopenia of childhood. The marrow failure usually appears in the neonatal period and is characterized by a macrocytic anemia and, occasionally, neutropenia and thrombocytopenia. The level of hemoglobin F is elevated. There are vacuolated erythroblasts and myeloblasts in the marrow. This very rare disorder is considered a unique variant of congenital sideroblastic anemia because the marrow also contains ringed sideroblasts. Other clinical features are failure to thrive, pancreatic fibrosis with insulin-dependent diabetes and exocrine pancreatic deficiency, muscle and neurologic impairment, and, frequently, early death. This multiorgan disorder is caused by mitochondrial DNA deletions, with heterogeneity in different tissues and between patients. The heterogeneity accounts for the variable clinical picture, and a change in proportions of mtDNA types in tissues over time may result in spontaneous improvement of red blood cell hypoproliferation (see Chapters 80 and 346). Therapy includes transfusions of red blood cells as needed. Filgrastim (granulocyte colony-stimulating factor) may reverse episodes of severe neutropenia.

Fleming MD: The genetics of inherited sideroblastic anemias. *Semin Hematol* 2002;39:270–281.

Knerr I, Metzler M, Niemeyer CM, et al: Hematologic features and clinical course of an infant with Pearson syndrome caused by a novel deletion of mitochondrial DNA. *J Pediatr Hematol Oncol* 2003;25:948–951.

Rotig A, Bourgeron T, Chretien D, et al: Spectrum of mitochondrial DNA rearrangements in the Pearson marrow-pancreas syndrome. *Hum Mol Genet* 1995;4:1327–1330.

Chapter 450 ■ Acquired Pure Red Blood Cell Anemias

TRANSIENT ERYTHROBLASTOPENIA OF CHILDHOOD. The most common acquired red cell aplasia occurring in children, transient erythroblastopenia of childhood (TEC) is more common than congenital hypoplastic anemia. This syndrome of severe, transient hypoplastic anemia occurs mainly in previously healthy children between 6 mo and 3 yr of age, with most of the children older than 12 mo at onset. Only 10% are >3 yr of age. The cause of this decrease in red blood cell (RBC) production is a transient immunologic suppression of erythropoiesis. It often follows a viral illness, although no specific virus has been identified. Parvovirus B19 infections (see Chapter 248), which may cause hypoplasia in children with chronic hemolytic anemia (see Chapter 469), are not responsible for TEC. Reticulocytes and bone marrow erythroid precursors are markedly decreased, although examination of the bone marrow rarely is needed to make the diagnosis. Some degree of neutropenia may occur in up to 20% of cases while platelet numbers are normal or elevated. Similar to the situation observed in iron-deficiency anemia and other RBC hypoplasias, thrombocytosis presumably is caused by increased erythropoietin, which is known to have some homology with thrombopoietin. Mean corpuscular volume (MCV) is characteristically normal for age, and fetal hemoglobin (Hb F) levels are normal before the recovery phase. RBC adenosine deaminase (ADA) levels are normal in this disorder; they are elevated in a majority of children with congenital hypoplastic anemia (Table 450-1). Differentiation from the latter disease sometimes may be difficult, but differences in age at onset and in age-related MCV, Hb F, and ADA usually are helpful. The peak occurrence of TEC coincides with that of iron-deficiency anemia in infants receiving milk as their main caloric source; differences in MCV clearly distinguish these two disorders.

Virtually all children recover within 1–2 mo. RBC transfusions may be necessary for severe anemia in the absence of signs of early recovery. The anemia develops slowly, and marked symptoms usually develop only with severe anemia. Corticosteroid therapy is of no value in this disorder. Any child with presumed TEC who requires more than one transfusion should be re-evaluated for another possible diagnosis. In rare instances, a prolonged case of apparent TEC may be caused by parvovirus-induced RBC aplasia, occurring in children with congenital or acquired immunodeficiencies.

RED CELL APLASIA ASSOCIATED WITH CHRONIC HEMOLYSIS. Parvovirus B19 is the best-documented viral cause of RBC aplasia in the fetus, immunocompromised patients, or those with chronic hemolysis; it is the cause of fifth disease or erythema infectiosum (see Chapter 248). The virus is particularly infective and cytotoxic for erythroid progenitor cells in the marrow, interacting specifically with the RBC P antigen as a receptor. Characteristic nuclear inclusions in erythroblasts and giant pronormoblasts can be seen with light microscopy of bone marrow. Because infection with this virus usually is transient, with recovery occurring in <2 wk, anemia is not present or not noticed in otherwise normal children, in whom the life span of peripheral RBCs is 100–120 days. However, in patients with hemolysis, such as that caused by hereditary spherocytosis or sickle cell disease, in whom the life span of RBCs is much shorter, a brief cessation of erythropoiesis from parvovirus infection may cause severe anemia, the so-called **aplastic crisis** occurring in these diseases. Recovery from moderate to severe anemia usually is spontaneous, heralded by a wave of nucleated RBCs and subsequent reticulocytosis in the peripheral blood. An RBC transfusion occasionally is necessary for marked symptoms caused by anemia. In children with chronic hemolysis, aplastic crisis from parvovirus usually occurs only once. In families with more than one child affected with a hemolytic disorder, parents should be warned that a similar RBC aplastic episode could occur in the other children if they have not previously been exposed to parvovirus.

TABLE 450-1. Comparison of Diamond-Blackfan Anemia and Transient Erythroblastopenia of Childhood

	DBA	TEC
No. of reported patients	>700	>500
Male/female	1.1	1.3
Age at diagnosis, male (mo)		
Mean	10	26
Median	2	23
Range	0–408	1–120
Age at diagnosis, female (mo)		
Mean	14	26
Median	3	23
Range	0–768	1–192
Males >1 yr	9%	82%
Females >1 yr	12%	80%
Etiology	Genetic	Acquired
Antecedent history	None	Viral illness
Physical examination abnormal	25%	0%
Laboratory		
Hemoglobin (g/dL)	1.2–14.8	2.2–12.5
WBCs < 5000/μL	15%	20%
Platelets > 400,000/μL	20%	45%
Adenosine deaminase	Increased	Normal
MCV increased at diagnosis	80%	5%
During recovery	100%	90%
In remission	100%	0%
Hb F increased at diagnosis	100%	20%
During recovery	100%	100%
In remission	85%	0%
i Antigen increased	100%	20%
During recovery	100%	60%
In remission	90%	0%

DBA, Diamond-Blackfan anemia; Hb F, fetal hemoglobin; MCV, mean cell volume; TEC, transient erythroblastopenia of childhood; WBCs, white blood cells.

From Nathan DG, Orkin SH, Ginsburg D, et al (editors): *Nathan and Oski's Hematology of Infancy and Childhood*, 6th ed., Vol. 1. Philadelphia, WB Saunders, 2003, p 329. Adapted from Alter BP: The bone marrow failure syndromes. In Nathan DG, Oski FA (editors): *Hematology of Infancy and Childhood*, 3rd ed. Philadelphia, WB Saunders, 1987, p 159; and Link MP, Alter BP: Fetal erythropoiesis during recovery from transient erythroblastopenia of childhood (TEC). *Pediatr Res* 1981; 15:1036.

RED CELL APLASIA ASSOCIATED WITH IMMUNODEFICIENCY. Persistence of parvovirus infection rarely may occur in patients unable to mount an adequate antibody response to the virus, as in children with congenital immunodeficiency diseases, those being treated with immunosuppressive agents, and those with AIDS. The resultant pure RBC aplasia may be severe, and affected children often are thought to have TEC. This type of RBC aplasia differs from TEC in that there is no spontaneous recovery and more than one transfusion needs to be given. The diagnosis of parvovirus infection is made by detecting viral particles (by polymerase chain reaction) because the usual serologic responses are impaired in these immunodeficient children. The viral infection in chronically infected patients may be treated with high doses of intravenous immunoglobulin (IVIG), which contains neutralizing antibody to parvovirus.

RED CELL APLASIA WITH MISCARRIAGE AND HYDROPS FETALIS. Different clinical manifestations of infection with parvovirus and destruction of erythroid precursors occur with infections in utero, in which there is increased fetal wastage in the first and second trimesters, and infants may be born with hydrops fetalis (see Chapter 103) and viremia. The presence of persistent congenital parvovirus infection is detected by polymerase chain reaction of peripheral blood and/or marrow DNA, because immunologic tolerance to the virus may prevent the usual development of specific antibodies.

OTHER RED CELL APLASIAS IN CHILDREN. Adult types of red cell aplasia usually are chronic antibody-mediated and often are associated with disorders such as chronic lymphocytic leukemia, lymphoma, thymoma, lymphoproliferative disorders, and systemic lupus erythematosus. This chronic antibody-mediated type of RBC aplasia is extremely rare in childhood. Alemtuzumab (humanized anti CD52 antibody) has been used to treat adult-onset pure red cell aplasia when treatment with corticosteroids and other immunosuppressive agents was unsuccessful. Certain drugs such as chloramphenicol also can inhibit erythropoiesis in a dose-dependent manner. Reticulocytopenia, erythroid hypoplasia, and vacuolated pronormoblasts in the marrow are reversible effects of this drug, and these effects are distinct from the idiosyncratic and rare development of severe aplastic anemia in recipients of chloramphenicol.

Acquired antibody-mediated pure red cell aplasia is a rare complication seen in patients chronically treated with recombinant human erythropoietin primarily for chronic renal failure. Treatment includes immunosuppression and renal transplantation as well as discontinuing the EPO.

CONGENITAL DYSERYTHROPOIETIC ANEMIA. (SEE CHAPTER 452).

Au WY, Lam CCK, Chim CS, et al: Alemtuzumab induced complete remission of therapy-resistant pure red cell aplasia. *Leukemia Res* 2005;29:1213–1215.

Bennett CL, Luminari S, Nissenson AR, et al: Pure red-cell aplasia and epoetin therapy. *N Engl J Med* 2004;351:1403–1408.

Cherrick I, Karayalcin G, Lanzkowsky P: Transient erythroblastopenia of childhood. *Am J Pediatr Hematol Oncol* 1994;16:320.

Heimpel H: Congenital dyserythropoietic anemias: Epidemiology, clinical significance, and progress in understanding their pathogenesis. *Ann Hematol* 2004; 83:613–621.

Intalapaporn P, Poovorawan Y, Suankratay C: Immune reconstitution syndrome associated with parvovirus B19-induced pure red cell apalasia during highly active antiretroviral therapy. *J Infect* 2006;53:e79–e82.

Verhelst D, Rossert J, Casadevall N, et al: Treatment of erythropoietin-induced pure red cell aplasia: A retrospective study. *Lancet* 2004;363:1768–1771.

Wickramasinghe SN, Wood WG: Advances in the understanding of the congenital dyserythropoietic anemias. *Brit J Haematol* 2005;131:431–446.

Chapter 451 ■ Anemia of Chronic Disease and Renal Disease

451.1 • Anemia of Chronic Disease (ACD)

The anemia of chronic disease (ACD) complicates a number of chronic systemic diseases associated with infection, inflammation, or tissue breakdown, such as chronic pyogenic infections (e.g., bronchiectasis, osteomyelitis), and chronic inflammatory processes (e.g., rheumatoid arthritis, systemic lupus erythematosus, ulcerative colitis). Despite diverse underlying causes, the erythroid abnormalities are similar, although incompletely understood. The red blood cell (RBC) life span is mildly decreased, but this increased hemolysis is not the major problem. More importantly, there is a relative failure of bone marrow to respond adequately to the anemia. This impaired erythropoietic response is associated with a blunted response to erythropoietin (EPO), despite the fact that EPO levels are modestly increased. A major feature of ACD is decreased iron availability. The serum iron is low, although tissue macrophages have abundant iron, and it is thought these abnormalities are due to retention of iron in macrophages as well as decreased intestinal iron absorption. One hypothesis has been that the underlying medical conditions cause the release of inflammatory cytokines, interleukin-1 (IL-1), tumor necrosis factor (TNF), and interleukin-6 (IL-6), which lead to the production of interferon-beta (IFN-β) and interferon-gamma (IFN-γ). This hypothesis is supported by the observation that IFN-β and IFN-γ, when given to experimental animals, cause a disorder similar to the anemia of chronic disease. Some studies have found that IL-6 induces the production of hepcidin, an iron regulatory protein that seems to be responsible for many of the major features of this disorder. Hepcidin, which is made in the liver, decreases intestinal iron absorption and also blocks release of iron from macrophages.

CLINICAL MANIFESTATIONS. Although the important symptoms and signs are those of the underlying disease, the mild to moderate anemia that accompanies it may affect the patient's quality of life.

LABORATORY FINDINGS. Hemoglobin concentrations usually are 6–9 g/dL. The anemia usually is normochromic and normocytic, although some patients may have modest hypochromia and microcytosis. Absolute reticulocyte counts are normal or low, and leukocytosis is common. The serum iron level is low, without the increase in total iron-binding capacity (serum transferrin) that occurs in iron deficiency. This pattern of low serum iron and low to normal iron-binding protein (serum transferrin) is a regular and valuable diagnostic feature. The serum ferritin level may be elevated. The bone marrow has normal cellularity; the RBC precursors are low to adequate, marrow hemosiderin may be increased, and granulocytic hyperplasia may be present. A common clinical challenge is to identify concomitant iron deficiency in patients with an inflammatory disease. Measurement of the TfR/ferritin ratio may be useful, because it is elevated in patients with iron deficiency (see Chapters 447 and 455). A trial of iron therapy also may help resolve the issue, although there may be no response when inflammation caused by the primary disease persists.

TREATMENT AND PROGNOSIS. Because these anemias are secondary to other disease processes, they do not respond to iron or hematinics unless there is concomitant deficiency. Transfusions raise the hemoglobin concentration temporarily, but they rarely are indicated. If the underlying systemic disease can be controlled, the anemia will resolve. Recombinant human EPO can increase the hemoglobin level and improve activity and the sense of well-being in patients with cancer and in those with anemia of chronic inflammation. Treatment with iron usually is necessary for an optimal EPO effect.

451.2 • Anemia of Renal Disease

Although the anemia seen in chronic renal disease shares some features with the anemia of chronic disease, such as a mild degree of hemolysis, the major component of this anemia is decreased EPO production because of damage to the renal cells that produce this hormone. Hemoglobin concentration is variable (6–10 g/dL), depending on the degree of uremia. The anemia usually is normocytic, and the absolute reticulocyte count is normal or low. Iron studies are normal. There is laboratory evidence of renal failure. Recombinant human EPO is useful given in conjunction with iron.

Andrews NC: Anemia of inflammation: The cytokine-hepcidin link. *J Clin Invest* 2004;113:1251–1253.

Cazzola M, Ponchio L, de Benedetti F, et al: Defective iron supply for erythropoiesis and adequate endogenous erythropoietin production in the anemia associated with systemic-onset juvenile chronic arthritis. *Blood* 1996;87:4824–4830.

Means RT: Hepcidin and anaemia. *Blood Reviews* 2004;18:219–225.

Weiss G, Goodnough LT: Anemia of chronic disease. *N Engl J Med* 2005; 352:1011–1023.

Chapter 452 ■ Congenital Dyserythropoietic Anemias

The congenital dyserythropoietic anemias (CDA) are a class of hemolytic disorders characterized by unique morphologic abnormalities in marrow erythroblasts: multinuclearity, abnormal nuclear fragments, and intrachromatin bridges between cells. Glycosylation of membrane proteins is impaired, and patients have an accumulation of red blood cell (RBC) glycolipids. The cause of both of these abnormalities is thought to be a deficiency of *N*-acetyl-glucosaminyltransferase II, a red blood cell enzyme responsible for membrane protein glycosylation. Clinically, these disorders are characterized by variable degrees of anemia, despite the fact that there is increased marrow erythroid activity (ineffective erythropoiesis). CDA has been reported in newborn infants with hydrops fetalis. Three major types of CDA (types I, II, and III) have been defined (Table 452-1).

Type I CDA is a rare autosomal recessive disorder in which the onset of macrocytic anemia and/or jaundice may be noted at any age, although most cases are first recognized in the neonatal period. Some patients have bone abnormalities, primarily syndactyly. The reticulocyte count is less than expected for the degree of anemia. White blood cells and platelets are normal. Indirect bilirubin levels are slightly elevated, haptoglobin levels are low, and transferrin is saturated with iron (i.e., the serum iron level approximates the total iron-binding capacity concentration). The marrow exhibits erythroid hyperplasia, shown by megaloblastic erythroblasts in the absence of vitamin B_{12} or folate deficiency. A small number of erythroblasts manifest dyserythropoietic features with interchromatin bridges between cells. **Treatment** of this disorder has been unsuccessful with the usual hematinics (vitamins and corticosteroids), but some improvement has been achieved with interferon-α. Although splenomegaly is common, splenectomy is not helpful. The most important long-term complication is hemosiderosis caused by increased intestinal absorption of iron and ineffective erythropoiesis. The gene for CDA type I has been mapped to chromosome 15q15.1; the gene *CDAN1* has been cloned; and several different mutations have been identified. The cellular role of codanin-1, encoded by *CDAN1*, is unknown.

Type II CDA, an autosomal recessive disorder, is the most common variant of CDA. The gene for type II CDA has been mapped to chromosome 20q11.2. The clinical and laboratory features are similar to those of type I CDA, but the anemia usually is more severe. Many more late marrow erythroblasts (up to 50%) may be abnormal, as manifested by binuclearity, multinuclearity, and abnormal lobulation. The pathognomonic findings in type II CDA are that the patient's RBCs are lysed by acidified serum. Type II CDA is known by the acronym **HEMPAS** (*h*ereditary *e*rythroblastic *m*ultinuclearity with a *p*ositive *a*cidified *s*erum test) because it features both erythroblast multinuclearity and circulating RBCs that are sensitive to lysis by acidified normal serum. Patients with severe anemia require blood transfusions. Iron overload results from both transfusions and increased intestinal absorption (even in untransfused patients), and iron chelation therapy should be considered as clinically indicated. In contrast to type I CDA, splenectomy is useful in patients with type II CDA, and, as in hereditary spherocytosis, RBC survival is normal following surgery even though abnormal RBCs continue to circulate. Splenectomy does not prevent further iron overloading, even in those patients whose hemoglobin is normalized; this is believed to reflect ongoing ineffective erythropoiesis in the bone marrow. Most patients can lead a normal life and have a normal life expectancy if complications and consequences are managed appropriately.

Type III CDA, the least common type of CDA, is a mild to moderate macrocytic anemia. Transfusions usually are not required. In contrast to other CDA types, iron overload is not a clinically significant issue; this disorder is inherited as an autosomal dominant defect. A characteristic bone marrow feature is erythroid hyperplasia, with many multinucleated erythroblasts containing up to 12 nuclei. The gene for type III CDA has been mapped to chromosome 15q21 near the *CDAN1* gene.

TABLE 452-1. Types of Congenital Dyserythropoietic Anemias

FEATURE	TYPE I	TYPE II	TYPE III
Reported patients	130	200	60
Male : female ratio	1 : 1	0 : 9	0 : 8
Anemia	Mild to moderate	Moderate	Mild to moderate
Red cell size	Macrocytic	Normo- or macrocytic	Macrocytic
Bone marrow erythroblasts	Megaloblastoid, binucleated (2–5%), chromatin bridges	Bi- and multinucleated (10–40%), karyorrhexis	Gigantoblasts (10–40%)
Inheritance	Recessive	Recessive	Dominant
Acid serum hemolysis	Negative	Positive	Negative
Reaction			
Anti-i	Slight	Strong	Slight
Anti-I	Slight	Strong	Slight
Effect of splenectomy	50%	96%	100%
Gene locus*	15q15.1–15.3	20q11.2	15q21–25
Gene nomenclature	*CDAI*	*CDAII*	*CDAIII*

*Gene locus for some but not all patients in each category.

From Nathan DG, Orkin SH, Ginsburg D, et al: *Nathan and Oski's Hematology of Infancy and Childhood*, 6th ed., Vol. 1. Philadelphia, WB Saunders, 2003, p 332.

Chrobak L: Successful treatment of iron overload with phlebotomies in two siblings with congenital dyserythropoietic anemias-type II (CDA II). *Acta Medica (Hradee Krabue)* 2006;49:193–195.

Heimpel H, Wilts H, Hirschmann WD, et al: Aplastic crisis as a complication of Congenital Dyserythropoietic Anemia Type II. *Acta Haematol* 2006;117:115–118.

Wickramasinghe SN, Wood WB: Advances in the understanding of the congenital dyserythropoietic anaemias. *Br J Haematol* 2005;131:431–446.

Chapter 453 ■ Physiologic Anemia of Infancy

DESCRIPTION AND ETIOLOGY. Although normal full-term newborn infants have higher hemoglobin and hematocrit levels with larger red blood cells (RBCs) than older children and adults, within the first week of life, a progressive decline in hemoglobin level begins and persists for 6–8 wk. The result of this decline is referred to as **physiologic anemia of infancy.** Several factors are involved. With the onset of respiration at birth, considerably more oxygen is available for binding to hemoglobin, and the hemoglobin-oxygen saturation increases from 50 to 95% or more. The normal developmental switch from fetal to adult hemoglobin synthesis actively replaces high-oxygen-affinity fetal hemoglobin with lower-oxygen-affinity adult hemoglobin, which can deliver a greater fraction of hemoglobin-bound oxygen to the tissues. Immediately after birth the increase in blood oxygen content and tissue oxygen delivery downregulates erythropoietin (EPO) production and, as a consequence, erythropoiesis is suppressed. In the absence of erythropoiesis, hemoglobin levels decrease, because the aged RBCs are not replaced as they are normally removed from the circulation. Iron from degraded RBCs is stored for future hemoglobin synthesis. The hemoglobin concentration continues to decrease until tissue oxygen needs are greater than oxygen delivery. Normally, this point is reached between 8–12 wk of age, when the hemoglobin concentration is 9–11 g/dL. As hypoxia is detected by renal or hepatic oxygen sensors, EPO production increases and erythropoiesis resumes. The iron previously stored in reticuloendothelial tissues can then be used for hemoglobin synthesis. The supply of stored iron is sufficient for hemoglobin synthesis, even in the absence of dietary iron intake, until approximately 20 wk of age. This "anemia" should be viewed as a physiologic adaptation to extrauterine life, reflecting the excess capability for oxygen delivery relative to tissue oxygen requirements. There is no hematologic problem, and no therapy is required.

Premature infants also develop a physiologic anemia, but the decline in hemoglobin level is both more extreme and more rapid. Minimal hemoglobin levels of 7–9 g/dL commonly are reached by 3–6 wk of age, and levels may be even lower in very small premature infants (see Chapters 97 and 103.1). The cause of this anemia is multifaceted. The same factors are operative as in term infants, but they are exaggerated. An important component in the first few weeks of life is blood loss as a result of sampling for the many laboratory tests necessary to stabilize the clinical status of these infants, particularly those with cardiorespiratory problems. The erythropoietic response to anemia also is suboptimal, a significant problem because demands on erythropoiesis are heightened by the short survival of the RBCs of premature infants (40–60 days instead of the 120 days in adults) and the rapid expansion of the RBC mass that accompanies growth. The basis for suboptimal erythropoiesis in prematurity appears to be inadequate synthesis of EPO in response to hypoxia. Because the liver is the predominant source of EPO during fetal life, it has been proposed that relative insensitivity of the hepatic oxygen sensor to hypoxia explains the blunted EPO response seen in premature infants. The spontaneous resolution of the anemia that occurs by approximately 40 wk gestational age is in keeping with a developmental switch from the relatively insensitive hepatic oxygen sensor to the renal oxygen sensor, which is exquisitely sensitive to hypoxia, because by this time the predominant site of EPO synthesis has shifted to the kidneys.

The magnitude of the physiologic anemia of infancy can be modified by other ongoing processes. A late hyporegenerative anemia, with absence of reticulocytes, may occur in infants with mild hemolytic disease of the newborn, requiring only phototherapy to effectively decrease the bilirubin concentration. The persistence of maternally derived anti-RBC antibodies in the infant's circulation can lead to a low-grade hemolytic anemia for several weeks, and this may present as an exaggeration of the physiologic anemia of infancy. It also might reflect an impaired EPO response. Another observation is the lower than expected hemoglobin at the "physiologic" nadir seen in infants after intrauterine or neonatal RBC transfusions. When premature infants are transfused with adult blood containing Hb A, the shift of the oxygen dissociation curve as a result of the presence of Hb A facilitates delivery of oxygen to the tissues. Accordingly, the definition of anemia and the need for transfusion in premature infants must be based not only on hemoglobin level but also on oxygen requirements and the ability of an infant's circulating hemoglobin to release oxygen.

Dietary factors also may aggravate physiologic anemia. Deficiency of folic acid superimposed on the physiologic process may result in more severe anemia. Vitamin E deficiency and therapy do not appear to have a role in anemia of prematurity, despite early suggestions to the contrary. A controlled and blinded study of oral administration of vitamin E (25 IU/dL α-tocopherol, colloidal aqueous solution) to infants weighing <1,500 g showed no difference in hemoglobin levels, reticulocytes, RBC morphology, or platelet counts. Breast milk and modern infant formulas appear to provide adequate vitamin E (see Chapter 49). Oral vitamin C supplementation (50 mg/24 hr) does not cause hemolysis in premature infants. Supplemental iron starting at approximately 4 mg/kg/24 hr for preterm babies 4–8 wk old and by 4 mo in full-term infants should not cause significant hemolysis due to oxidation.

Unless perinatal blood loss has been significant, iron deficiency should not be considered as a cause of anemia in term infants in the first 4 mo of life. Assuming an infant is born with adequate iron stores, dietary iron deficiency cannot be a cause of anemia until these iron stores have been exhausted. In the absence of blood loss, this does not occur until the birthweight has approximately doubled.

TREATMENT. Physiologic anemia requires no therapy beyond ensuring that the diet of the infant contains essential nutrients for normal hematopoiesis, especially folic acid and iron. The optimal level of hematocrit for premature infants has not been established (see Chapter 470). Premature infants who are feeding well and growing normally rarely need transfusion unless iatrogenic blood loss has been significant. In otherwise healthy premature infants, hemoglobin levels as low as 6.5 g/dL usually are well tolerated. Assessment of the overall clinical condition, including growth rate, and monitoring of hematocrit are the best guides for determining whether transfusion of RBCs is necessary. RBC transfusions do not appear to affect the course of apneic spells and bradycardia. When transfusions are necessary, an RBC volume of 10–15 mL/kg is recommended. The number of donors for an infant should be minimized. In early preterm infants (<1,250 g), the half-life of transfused RBCs is about 30 days.

Anemia in very-low-birthweight preterm infants may be related to a relative deficiency of EPO, and clinical trials indicate that premature infants who do not have severe illnesses and are treated with recombinant human EPO (rHuEPO) and iron during the first 6 wk of life require fewer transfusions. The optimal timing for initiation of rHuEPO therapy and the optimal dose have yet to be determined. To achieve the best results, supplemental oral iron at a dose of at least 4–6 mg/kg/day needs to be administered. The cost of rHuEPO treatment currently is higher than that of RBC transfusion; however, EPO treatment may have a significant role to play in the management of infants whose parents refuse to allow blood transfusions on religious grounds.

Bednarek FJ, Weisberger S, Richardson DK, et al: Variations in blood transfusions among newborn intensive care units. *J Pediatr* 1998;133:601–607.

Fain J, Hilsenrath P, Widness JA, et al: A cost analysis comparing erythropoietin and red cell transfusions in the treatment of anemia of prematurity. *Transfusion* 1995;35:936–943.

Meyer MP, Haworth C, Meyer JH: A comparison of oral and intravenous iron supplementation in preterm infants receiving recombinant erythropoietin. *J Pediatr* 1996;129:258–263.

Ohls RK: The use of erythropoietin in neonates. *Clin Perinatol* 2000;27:681–696.

Chapter 454 ■ Megaloblastic Anemias

The megaloblastic anemias have in common certain abnormalities of red blood cell (RBC) morphology and maturation. The RBCs are larger than normal at every stage of development and have an open, finely dispersed nuclear chromatin and an asynchrony between the maturation of nucleus and cytoplasm, with the delay in nuclear progression becoming more evident with further cell divisions. Giant metamyelocytes and bands also are present in the marrow. All megaloblastic anemias are characterized by ineffective erythropoiesis, a kinetic term that describes active erythropoiesis with premature death of cells, a decreased output of RBCs from the marrow, and, consequently, anemia. In the peripheral blood, RBCs are large (increased mean corpuscular volume [MCV]) and often oval. Hypersegmented neutrophils also are characteristic, with many neutrophils having >5 lobes. Almost all cases of childhood megaloblastic anemia result from a deficiency of folic acid or vitamin B_{12}; rarely, they may be caused by inborn errors of metabolism. Both vitamin B_{12} and folate are required in the synthesis of nucleoproteins; deficiencies result in defective synthesis of DNA and, to a lesser extent, RNA and protein. Megaloblastic anemias resulting from malnutrition are relatively uncommon in the U.S. but are important worldwide (see Chapters 1 and 43).

454.1 • Folic Acid Deficiency

Folates are abundant in many foods, including green vegetables, fruits, and animal organs (e.g., liver, kidney). Folates are heat labile and water soluble, and consequently boiling or heating folate sources leads to decreased amounts of vitamin. Naturally occurring folates are in a polyglutamated form and are absorbed less efficiently than the monoglutamate species (i.e., folic acid). Folate conjugase activity in the intestinal brush border aids the conversion of polyglutamates to the monoglutamate and thereby enhances absorption. Folic acid is absorbed throughout the small intestine, and there is an active enterohepatic circulation. Much of the folate in plasma is loosely bound to albumin. Folic acid is not biologically active. It is reduced by dihydrofolate reductase to tetrahydrofolate, which is transported into tissue cells and polyglutamated. Body stores of folate are limited, and megaloblastic anemia occurs after 2–3 mo on a folate-free diet.

CLINICAL MANIFESTATIONS. Mild megaloblastic anemia has been reported in very-low-birthweight infants, and folic acid supplementation is advised. Although rare nowadays, megaloblastic anemia due to folate deficiency has its peak incidence at 4–7 mo of age, somewhat earlier than iron deficiency anemia, although both conditions may be present concomitantly in infants with poor nutrition. Besides having the usual clinical features of anemia, affected infants with folate deficiency are irritable, have inadequate weight gain, and have chronic diarrhea. Hemorrhages from thrombocytopenia occur in advanced cases. In older children with folate deficiency the signs and symptoms are related to anemia and to any underlying pathologic process responsible for the vitamin deficiency. Folic acid deficiency may accompany kwashiorkor, marasmus, or sprue.

ETIOLOGY. Folic acid deficiency can occur as a consequence of inadequate folate intake, decreased folate absorption, or acquired and congenital disorders of folate metabolism.

Inadequate Folate Intake. Anemia due to decreased folate intake usually becomes manifest under clinical conditions that have increased vitamin requirements (e.g., pregnancy, growth in infancy, chronic hemolysis). The normal infant daily requirement is 25–35 μg/day. The weight-based requirements are higher in children than adults because of children's increased needs for growth. Human breast milk, pasteurized cow's milk, and infant formulas provide adequate amounts of folic acid. Goat's milk is deficient, so folic acid supplementation must be given when it is the child's main food. Unless supplemented, powdered milk also may be a poor source of folic acid.

Folate requirements increase markedly during pregnancy, in part to meet fetal needs. Decreases in serum and RBC folate levels occur in as many as 25% of pregnant women at term and may be aggravated by infection. Folate supplementation of at least 400 μg/day is recommended from the start of pregnancy to prevent neural tube defects and to meet growth needs of the developing fetus. Mothers with folate deficiency may have infants with normal folate stores, due to selective transfer of folate to the fetus via placental folate receptors.

Decreased Folate Absorption. Malabsorption due to chronic diarrheal states or diffuse inflammatory disease can lead to folate deficiency. Megaloblastic anemia due to folic acid deficiency can occur in celiac disease or chronic infectious enteritis, and in association with enteroenteric fistulas. With both inflammatory bowel disease and diarrhea, some of the decreased folate absorption may be caused by impaired folate conjugase activity. Chronic diarrhea also interferes with the enterohepatic circulation of folate, thereby enhancing folate losses because of rapid intestinal passage. Previous intestinal surgery is another potential cause of decreased folate absorption.

Certain anticonvulsant drugs (e.g., phenytoin, primidone, phenobarbital) can impair absorption of folic acid, and many patients treated with these drugs have low serum levels of folic acid. Frank megaloblastic anemia is rare, however, and responds to folic acid therapy even when administration of the offending drug is continued.

Congenital Abnormalities in Folate Metabolism. Megaloblastic anemia resulting from congenital dihydrofolate reductase deficiency is a very rare disorder that is due to an inability to form biologically active tetrahydrofolate. Affected individuals have developed severe megaloblastic anemia in early infancy. These patients were treated successfully with large doses of folic acid or folinic acid. Deficiency of methylene tetrahydrofolate reductase has been described in some patients with homocystinuria without hematologic abnormalities.

Drug-Induced Abnormalities in Folate Metabolism. A number of drugs have anti–folic acid activity as their primary pharmacologic effect and regularly produce megaloblastic anemia. Methotrexate binds to dihydrofolate reductase and prevents formation of tetrahydrofolate, the active form. Pyrimethamine, used in the therapy of toxoplasmosis, and trimethoprim, used for treatment of various infections, may induce folic acid deficiency and, occasionally, megaloblastic anemia. Therapy with folinic acid (5-formyltetrahydrofolate) usually is beneficial.

LABORATORY FINDINGS. The anemia is macrocytic (mean corpuscular volume >100 fL). Variations in RBC shape and size are common (see Fig. 447-1*B*). The reticulocyte count is low, and nucleated RBCs demonstrating megaloblastic morphology often are seen in the blood. Neutropenia and thrombocytopenia rarely may be present, particularly in patients with long-standing and severe deficiencies. The neutrophils are large, some with hypersegmented nuclei. Normal serum folic acid levels are 5–20 ng/mL; with deficiency, levels are <3 ng/mL. Levels of RBC folate are a better indicator of chronic deficiency. The normal RBC folate level is 150–600 ng/mL of packed cells. Levels of iron and vitamin B_{12} in serum usually are normal or elevated. Serum activity of lactate dehydrogenase (LDH), a marker of ineffective erythropoiesis, is markedly elevated. The bone marrow is hypercellular because of erythroid hyperplasia, and megaloblastic changes are prominent. Large, abnormal neutrophilic forms (giant metamyelocytes) with cytoplasmic vacuolation also are seen.

TREATMENT. When the diagnosis of folate deficiency is established, folic acid may be administered orally or parenterally at 0.5–1.0 mg/day. If the specific diagnosis is in doubt, smaller doses of folate (0.1 mg/day) may be used for 1 week as a diagnostic test, because a hematologic response can be expected within 72 hr. Doses of folate >0.1 mg can correct the anemia of vitamin B_{12} deficiency but may aggravate any associated neurologic abnormalities. In most medical settings in developed countries, this therapeutic trial to distinguish the different causes of megaloblastic anemia rarely is necessary because vitamin B_{12} and folate blood levels usually are readily available. Transfusions are indicated only when the anemia is severe or the child is very ill. Folic acid therapy (0.5–1.0 mg/day) should be continued for 3–4 wk until a definite hematologic response has occurred. Maintenance therapy with a multivitamin (containing 0.2 mg of folate) is adequate.

454.2 • Vitamin B_{12} (Cobalamin) Deficiency

Vitamin B_{12} is derived from cobalamin in food (mainly animal sources) secondary to production by microorganisms. Humans cannot synthesize vitamin B_{12}. The cobalamins are released by the acidity of the stomach and combine there with R proteins and intrinsic factor (IF); traverse the duodenum, where pancreatic proteases break down the R proteins; and are absorbed in the distal ileum via specific receptors for IF-cobalamin. In addition, some vitamin B_{12} from large doses may diffuse through mucosa in the intestine and mouth. In the plasma, cobalamin binds to a transport protein, transcobalamin II (TC-II), which carries the vitamin B_{12} to the liver, bone marrow, and other tissue storage sites. TC-II enters cells by receptor-mediated endocytosis, and cobalamin is converted to active forms (methylcobalamin and adenosylcobalamin) important in the transfer of methyl groups and DNA synthesis. Plasma also contains two other vitamin B_{12}–binding proteins, transcobalamin I and III (TC-I and TC-III). These latter two forms of transcobalamin have no specific transport role but are known to reflect vitamin B_{12} tissue stores. In fact, almost all vitamin B_{12} in plasma is bound to TC-I and TC-III, and thus the measurement of serum B_{12} concentration reflects the storage of this vitamin. In contrast to folate stores, older children and adults have sufficient vitamin B_{12} stores to last 3–5 yr. However, in young infants born to mothers with low vitamin B_{12} stores, clinical signs of cobalamin deficiency can become apparent in the first 6–18 months of life.

ETIOLOGY. Vitamin B_{12} deficiency may result from inadequate dietary intake of vitamin, lack of IF secretion by the stomach, impaired intestinal absorption of IF-cobalamin, or absence of vitamin B_{12} transport protein.

Inadequate Vitamin B_{12} Intake. Because vitamin B_{12} is present in many foods, dietary deficiency is rare. It may occur in cases of extreme dietary restriction (e.g., strict vegetarians or vegans) in which no animal products are consumed. Vitamin B_{12} deficiency is not common in kwashiorkor or infantile marasmus. In children, megaloblastic anemia from inadequate intake of vitamin B_{12} occurs in breast-fed infants whose mothers are vegans or themselves have pernicious anemia. Maternal pernicious anemia may be manifest by reduced serum vitamin B_{12} with or without macrocytic anemia in the mother. This cause of childhood megaloblastic anemia can appear in the first year of life.

Lack of Intrinsic Factor. Congenital pernicious anemia is a rare autosomal recessive disorder due to an inability to secrete gastric IF or secretion of functionally abnormal IF. It differs from the typical disease in adults in that the stomach secretes acid normally and is histologically normal. There are no antibodies to parietal cells and no associated endocrine disorders. The symptoms of juvenile pernicious anemia become prominent at around 1 yr of age. This interval is consistent with exhaustion of the stores of vitamin B_{12} acquired in utero. As the anemia becomes severe, weakness, irritability, anorexia, and listlessness occur. The tongue is smooth, red, and painful. Neurologic manifestations include ataxia, paresthesias, hyporeflexia, Babinski responses, and clonus. Juvenile pernicious anemia is another rare disorder occurring in older children. It is an immunologic disorder akin to adult-type pernicious anemia. There may be atrophy of the gastric mucosa, achlorhydria, and antibodies in serum against IF and parietal cells. These children may have additional immunologic abnormalities, cutaneous candidiasis, hypoparathyroidism, and other endocrine deficiencies. An abnormal Schilling result is corrected by addition of exogenous IF. Parenteral vitamin B_{12} should be administered regularly to these patients. Gastric surgery can lead to intrinsic factor deficiency, and susceptible individuals need lifelong parenteral vitamin B_{12} supplementation.

Impaired Vitamin B_{12} Absorption. Patients with inflammatory diseases such as regional enteritis or neonatal necrotizing enterocolitis may have impaired absorption of vitamin B_{12}. When the terminal ileum has been surgically removed, lifelong parenteral administration should be used if there is evidence that vitamin B_{12} is not absorbed. An overgrowth of intestinal bacteria within diverticula or duplications of the small intestine may cause vitamin B_{12} deficiency by consumption of (or competition for) the vitamin or by splitting of its complex with IF. In these cases, hematologic response may follow appropriate antibiotic therapy. Similar mechanisms may operate when the fish tapeworm *Diphyllobothrium latum* infests the upper small intestine. When megaloblastic anemia occurs in these situations, the serum vitamin B_{12} level is low, the gastric juice contains intrinsic factor, and the abnormal Schilling test result is not corrected by addition of exogenous IF.

Rare cases of megaloblastic anemia due to vitamin B_{12} deficiency have been reported as a result of defects of the receptor for IF-B_{12} in the terminal ileum, in some instances associated with proteinuria (Imerslund-Grasbeck syndrome). This autosomal recessive disorder is caused by defects in the *CUBN* gene on chromosome 10p12.1, resulting in decreased expression of the IF-B_{12} receptor cubilin. Parenteral treatment with vitamin B_{12} monthly corrects the deficiency.

Absence of Vitamin B_{12} Transport Protein. Transcobalamin II (TC-II) deficiency is a rare cause of megaloblastic anemia due to decreased utilization of cobalamin. TC-II is the principal physiologic transport vehicle for vitamin B_{12}. The role of TC-II in B_{12} transport is similar to that of transferrin (Tf) for iron; specific receptors for TC-II and Tf exist on cells needing vitamin B_{12} or iron. A congenital deficiency is inherited as an autosomal recessive condition, with failure to absorb and transport vitamin B_{12}. Most patients lack TC-II, but some have functionally defective forms. Serum vitamin B_{12} levels are normal because the storage forms of cobalamin, TC-I and TC-III, are not affected. This disorder usually manifests in the first weeks of life. Characteristically, there is failure to thrive, diarrhea, vomiting, glossitis, neurologic abnormalities, and megaloblastic anemia. The diagnosis of this disorder is suggested by the presence of severe megaloblastic anemia with normal serum vitamin B_{12} and folate levels and no evidence of any other inborn errors of metabolism. The diagnosis is made by specific tests for TC-II. The serum vitamin B_{12} levels must be kept high to utilize cobalamin. Hence, the therapy for this disorder is large parenteral doses of vitamin B_{12} given twice a week for life. These frequent and large doses of cobalamin appear to overcome the transport deficiency. Most children with this disorder die if treatment is not provided in infancy.

CLINICAL MANIFESTATIONS. Children with cobalamin deficiency often present with nonspecific manifestations such as weakness, fatigue, failure to thrive, or irritability. Other common findings include pallor, glossitis, vomiting, diarrhea, and icterus. Neurologic symptoms also occur, and these can include paresthesias, sensory deficits, hypotonia, seizures, developmental delay, developmental regression, and neuropsychiatric changes. Neurologic problems from vitamin B_{12} deficiency can occur in the absence of any hematologic abnormalities.

LABORATORY FINDINGS. The hematologic manifestations of folate and cobalamin deficiency are identical. The anemia resulting from cobalamin deficiency is macrocytic, with prominent macro-ovalocytosis of the RBCs (see Fig. 447-1*B*). The neutrophils may be large and hypersegmented. In advanced cases, neutropenia and thrombocytopenia can occur, simulating aplastic anemia or leukemia. Serum vitamin B_{12} levels are low while the serum concentrations of methylmalonic acid and homocysteine usually are elevated. Concentrations of serum iron and serum folic acid are normal or elevated. Serum LDH activity is markedly increased, a reflection of the ineffective erythropoiesis. Moderate elevations (2–3 mg/dL) of serum bilirubin levels also may be found. Excessive excretion of methylmalonic acid in the urine (normal amount, 0–3.5 mg/24 hr) is a reliable and sensitive index of vitamin B_{12} deficiency.

DIAGNOSIS. The specific cause of vitamin B_{12} deficiency often is apparent from the clinical history. In cases where there is a reasonable explanation for decreased vitamin B_{12} absorption (previous gastric or ileal surgery) it may be reasonable to start appropriate therapy without further evaluation. In very young children in whom dietary insufficiency may be a factor, evaluation of the mother for anemia and serum vitamin B_{12} often is rewarding. If there is no obvious cause for decreased serum vitamin B_{12}, absorption of vitamin B_{12} can be assessed by the Schilling test. When a normal person ingests a small amount of vitamin B_{12} into which cobalt 57 has been incorporated, the radioactive vitamin combines with the IF in stomach secretions and passes to the terminal ileum, where absorption occurs. Because the absorbed vitamin is bound to TC-II and incorporated into tissues, little or none normally is excreted in the urine. If a large dose (1 mg) of nonradioactive vitamin B_{12} is injected parenterally after 2 hr ("flushing dose"), 10–30% of the previously absorbed radioactive vitamin appears in the urine in 24 hr. Children with pernicious anemia usually excrete ≤2% under these conditions. To confirm that absence of IF is the basis of the vitamin B_{12} malabsorption, IF is given with a second dose of radioactive vitamin B_{12}. Normal amounts of radioactive vitamin should now be absorbed and flushed out in the urine. On the other hand, when vitamin B_{12} malabsorption results from absence of ileal receptor sites or other intestinal causes, no improvement in absorption occurs with IF. The Schilling test result remains abnormal in patients with pernicious anemia, even when therapy has completely reversed the hematologic and neurologic manifestations of the disease.

TREATMENT. A prompt hematologic response follows parenteral administration of vitamin B_{12} (1 mg), usually with reticulocytosis in 2–4 days, unless there is concurrent inflammatory disease. The physiologic requirement for vitamin B_{12} is 1–5 µg/day, and hematologic responses have been observed with these small doses, indicating that administration of a minidose may be used as a therapeutic test when the diagnosis of vitamin B_{12} deficiency is in doubt. If there is evidence of neurologic involvement, 1 mg should be injected intramuscularly daily for at least 2 wk. Maintenance therapy is necessary throughout a patient's life; monthly intramuscular administration of 1 mg of vitamin B_{12} is sufficient. Oral therapy may succeed because of mucosal diffusion with high doses, but it is not generally advisable, owing to uncertainty of absorption.

454.3 • Other Rare Megaloblastic Anemias

Oroticaciduria is a rare autosomal recessive disorder that usually appears in the first year of life and is characterized by growth failure, developmental retardation, megaloblastic anemia, and increased urinary excretion of orotic acid (see Chapter 89). This defect, the most common metabolic error in the de novo synthesis of pyrimidines, therefore affects nucleic acid synthesis. The usual form of hereditary orotic aciduria is caused by a deficiency (in all body tissues) of both orotic phosphoribosyl transferase (OPT) and orotidine-5-phosphate decarboxylase (ODC), two sequential enzymatic steps in pyrimidine nucleotide synthesis. The diagnosis of this disorder is suggested by the presence of severe megaloblastic anemia with normal serum B_{12} and folate levels and no evidence of TC-II deficiency. A presumptive diagnosis is made by finding increased urinary orotic acid. Confirmation of the diagnosis, however, requires assay of the transferase and decarboxylase enzymes in the patient's erythrocytes. Physical and mental retardation often accompany this condition. The anemia is refractory to vitamin B_{12} or folic acid but responds promptly to administration of uridine (100–150 µg/kg/24 hr). Megaloblastic anemia also can occur in the Lesch-Nyhan syndrome, in which regeneration of purine nucleotides is blocked (see Chapter 89).

Thiamine-responsive megaloblastic anemia (TRMA) is characterized by megaloblastic anemia, sensorineural deafness, diabetes mellitus, and, occasionally, cardiomyopathy and optic nerve atrophy. Previously, it had been observed that the megaloblastic anemia in some patients responded to high doses of thiamine, and it now is known that the defect in this disorder is due to an abnormality in a thiamine transport gene located on chromosome 1. TRMA is an autosomal recessive disorder that presents in childhood and occurs in several ethnically distinct populations.

Deficiency of adenosylcobalamin and methylcobalamin along with megaloblastic anemia has been encountered in a few children with inability to convert cobalamin to its biologically active metabolites. These disorders are characterized by neurologic abnormalities and methylmalonic aciduria or homocystinuria, or both. Abnormalities usually are noted in the early weeks of life and include failure to thrive, lethargy, hypotonia, macrocytosis with megaloblastic bone marrow changes and anemia or pancytopenia, and hepatic dysfunction. The megaloblastic changes may reverse and other symptoms may improve with hydroxycobalamin treatment, 1 mg/24 hr IM initially, gradually changed to a dose two to three times per week, then once a month.

Carmel R, Green R, Rosenblatt DS, et al: Update on cobalamin, folate and homocysteine. *Hematology Am Soc Hematol Educ Program* 2003;62–81.

Grasbeck R: Imerslund-Grasbeck syndrome (selective vitamin B12 malabsorption with proteinuria). *Orphanet J Rare Dis* 2006 19;1:17.

Monagle PT, Tauro GP: Infantile megaloblastosis secondary to maternal vitamin B_{12} deficiency. *Clin Lab Haematol* 1997;19:23–25.

Rasmussen SA, Fernhoff PM, Scanlon KS: Vitamin B_{12} deficiency in children and adolescents. *J Pediatr* 2001;138:10–17.

Rosenblatt DS, Whitehead VM: Cobalamin and folate deficiency: Acquired and hereditary disorders in children. *Semin Hematol* 1999;36:19–34.

Xu D, Kozyraki R, Newman TC, et al: Genetic evidence of an accessory activity required specifically for cubilin brush-border expression and intrinsic factor–cobalamin absorption. *Blood* 1999;94:3604–3606.

Chapter 455 ■ Iron-Deficiency Anemia

Anemia resulting from lack of sufficient iron for synthesis of hemoglobin is the most common hematologic disease of infancy and childhood. It is estimated that 30% of the global population suffers from iron-deficiency anemia; most of those affected live in developing countries. Iron-deficiency anemia is associated with numerous deleterious health conditions (Table 455-1) [see Chapter 51].

The frequency of iron-deficiency anemia is related to certain basic aspects of iron metabolism and nutrition; to maintain positive iron balance in childhood, about 1 mg of iron must be absorbed each day. The body of a newborn infant contains about 0.5 g of iron, whereas the adult content is estimated to be 5 g. To

TABLE 455-1. Collective Judgment about the Strength of Causal Evidence Linking Iron Deficiency or Anemia to Health and Development Outcomes

A significant body of causal evidence exists for:*

1. Iron-deficiency anemia and work productivity
2. Severe anemia and child mortality
3. Severe anemia and maternal mortality
4. Iron-deficiency anemia and child development

Causal evidence is lacking or contradictory for:

- Iron-deficiency anemia and low birthweight, including preterm birth
- Iron-deficiency anemia and infectious disease, either protective or adverse effects
- Mild to moderate anemia and maternal mortality
- Mild to moderate anemia and child mortality

*Numbering reflects the relative strength of evidence, not the potential magnitude of iron's effect in public health terms.

From Stoltzfus RJ: Iron-deficiency anemia: Reexamining the nature and magnitude of the public health problem: Summary. Implications for research and programs. *J Nutr* 2001; 131(2 Suppl 2): 698S.

get from one point to the other, an average of 0.8 mg of iron must be absorbed each day during the first 15 yr of life. In addition to this growth requirement, a small amount is necessary to balance normal losses of iron by shedding of cells.

Absorption of dietary iron is assumed to be about 10%; a diet containing 8–10 mg of iron daily is necessary for optimal nutrition. Iron is absorbed in the proximal small intestine, mediated in part by a variety of duodenal proteins. Iron is absorbed 2 to 3 times more efficiently from human milk than from cow's milk. Breast-fed infants may, therefore, require less iron from other foods. During the first years of life, because relatively small quantities of iron-rich foods are eaten, it often is difficult to attain adequate iron consumption. For this reason, the diet should include such foods as infant cereals or formulas that have been fortified with iron; both of these are very effective in preventing iron deficiency. Formulas with 7–12 mg Fe/L for full-term infants and premature infant formulas with 15 mg/L for infants <1,800 g at birth are effective. Infants breast-fed exclusively should receive iron supplementation from 4 mo of age. An infant is in a precarious situation with respect to iron. Should the diet become inadequate or external blood loss occur, anemia ensues rapidly.

Adolescents also are susceptible to iron deficiency because of high requirements due to the growth spurt, dietary deficiencies, and menstrual blood loss. In the United States, about 9% of 1 to 2 yr old children are iron deficient; 3% have anemia. Of adolescent girls, 9% are iron deficient and 2% have anemia.

ETIOLOGY. Low birthweight and unusual perinatal hemorrhage are associated with decreases in neonatal hemoglobin mass and stores of iron. As the high hemoglobin concentration of the newborn infant falls during the first 2–3 mo of life, considerable iron is reclaimed and stored. These reclaimed stores usually are sufficient for blood formation in the first 6–9 mo of life in term infants. In low-birthweight infants or those with perinatal blood loss, stored iron may be depleted earlier, and dietary sources become of paramount importance. Delayed clamping of the umbilical cord (~2 min) in developing countries may reduce the incidence of iron deficiency. In term infants, anemia caused solely by inadequate dietary iron is unusual before 6 mo and usually occurs at 9–24 mo of age. Thereafter, it is relatively uncommon. The usual dietary pattern observed in infants with iron-deficiency anemia is prolonged consumption of large amounts of cow's milk (>24 oz/day) and of foods not supplemented with iron.

Blood loss must be considered as a possible cause in every case of iron-deficiency anemia, particularly in older children. Chronic iron-deficiency anemia from occult bleeding may be caused by a lesion of the gastrointestinal tract, such as milk protein–induced inflammatory colitis, peptic ulcer, Meckel diverticulum, polyp, or hemangioma, or by inflammatory bowel disease. In some geographic areas, hookworm infestation is an important cause of iron deficiency; in others it is associated with *Helicobacter pylori* infection. Pulmonary hemosiderosis may be associated with unrecognized bleeding in the lungs and recurrent iron deficiency after treatment with iron. Chronic diarrhea in early childhood may be associated with considerable unrecognized blood loss. Some infants in the U.S. with severe iron deficiency have chronic intestinal blood loss induced by exposure to a heat-labile protein in whole cow's milk. Loss of blood in the stools each day can be prevented either by reducing the quantity of whole cow's milk to ≤1 pint/24 hr, by using heated or evaporated milk, or by feeding a milk substitute. This gastrointestinal reaction is not related to enzymatic abnormalities in the mucosa, such as lactase deficiency, or to typical milk allergy. Occasionally, cow's milk–induced colitis presents with edema and anemia; the edema is due to a **protein-losing enteropathy.** Involved infants characteristically develop anemia that is more severe and occurs earlier than would be expected simply from an inadequate intake of iron.

Histologic abnormalities of the mucosa of the gastrointestinal tract, such as blunting of the villi, are present in advanced iron-deficiency anemia and may cause leakage of blood and decreased absorption of iron, further compounding the problem.

Intense exercise conditioning, as occurs in competitive athletics in high school, may result in iron depletion in girls; this occurs less commonly in boys.

CLINICAL MANIFESTATIONS. Pallor is the most important sign of iron deficiency; in fact, the World Health Organization recommends use of palmar pallor as a screening measure for anemia. There are, however, high rates of false-positive and false-negative results for palmar, nailbed, and conjunctival pallor, which vary according to the degree of anemia. In mild to moderate iron deficiency (i.e., hemoglobin levels of 6–10 g/dL), compensatory mechanisms, including increased levels of 2,3-diphosphoglycerate (2,3-DPG) and a shift of the oxygen dissociation curve, may be so effective that few symptoms of anemia are noted, although affected children may be irritable. **Pagophagia,** the desire to ingest unusual substances such as ice or dirt, may be present. In some children, ingestion of lead-containing substances may lead to concomitant **plumbism** (see Chapter 709). When the hemoglobin level falls to <5 g/dL, irritability and anorexia are prominent. Tachycardia and cardiac dilation occur, and systolic murmurs are often present.

Children with iron-deficiency anemia may be obese or may be underweight, with other evidence of poor nutrition. The irritability and anorexia characteristic of advanced cases may reflect deficiency in tissue iron, because iron therapy often produces striking improvement in behavior before significant hematologic improvement is noted.

Iron deficiency may have effects on neurologic and intellectual function. Iron-deficiency anemia, and even iron deficiency without significant anemia, affects attention span, alertness, and learning in both infants and adolescents. Adolescent girls with serum ferritin levels of ≤12 ng/L but without anemia have demonstrated improved verbal learning and memory after taking iron for 8 wk.

LABORATORY FINDINGS. In progressive iron deficiency, a sequence of biochemical and hematologic events occurs. First, the tissue iron stores represented by bone marrow hemosiderin disappear. The level of **serum ferritin,** an iron-storage protein, provides a relatively accurate estimate of body iron stores in the absence of inflammatory disease. Normal ranges are age-dependent, and decreased levels accompany iron deficiency. Next, serum iron level decreases (also age-dependent), the iron-binding capacity of the serum (serum transferrin) increases, and the percent saturation (transferrin saturation) falls below normal. When the availability of iron becomes rate-limiting for hemoglobin synthesis, free erythrocyte protoporphyrins (FEP) accumulate. As the deficiency progresses, the red blood cells (RBCs) become smaller than normal, and their hemoglobin content decreases. The morphologic characteristics of RBCs are best quantified by the determination of mean corpuscular hemoglobin (MCH) and mean corpuscular volume (MCV). Developmental changes in MCV require the use of age-related standards for diagnosis of microcytosis (see Table 447-1). With increasing deficiency, the RBCs become deformed and misshapen and present characteristic microcytosis, hypochromia, poikilocytosis, and increased RBC distribution width (RDW) [see Fig. 447-1C]. The reticulocyte percentage may be normal or moderately elevated, but absolute reticulocyte counts indicate an insufficient response to anemia. Nucleated RBCs occasionally are seen in the peripheral blood if the anemia is severe. White blood cell counts are normal. Sometimes there is a striking thrombocytosis (600,000–1 million/mm^3). Thrombocytosis is believed to be caused by increased erythropoietin, which is known to have some structural homology with thrombopoietin. Very severe iron-deficiency anemia occasionally may be associated with thrombocytopenia, and this can confuse the diagnosis with bone marrow failure disorders. The bone marrow is hypercellular, with erythroid hyperplasia. The normoblasts may have scanty, fragmented cytoplasm with poor hemoglobination. Leukocytes and megakaryocytes are normal. There is no stainable iron in marrow reticulum cells. In about ⅓ of cases, occult blood can be detected in the stool.

DIFFERENTIAL DIAGNOSIS. Iron deficiency must be differentiated from other hypochromic microcytic anemias. The most common scenario is the need to distinguish iron deficiency from α- and β-thalassemia trait and other hemoglobinopathies, particularly those related to hemoglobin E (see Chapter 462). A simple distinguishing feature of the latter conditions is that the RBC count often is elevated above normal despite the presence of a mild anemia and microcytosis; this is in marked contrast to iron deficiency, in which the RBC count usually decreases along with the reduced hemoglobin and MCV. Another difference between α- and β-thalassemia trait and iron deficiency is that the **RDW is elevated in iron deficiency.**

β-Thalassemia trait occurs in people from the Mediterranean area, Africa, and Asia. It is a mild microcytic anemia characterized by elevated levels of hemoglobin A_2 and/or increased fetal hemoglobin concentration; serum iron, total iron-binding capacity (transferrin), and ferritin are normal; and no abnormal hemoglobin is seen on electrophoresis. Homozygous β-thalassemia (or thalassemia major), with its pronounced erythroblastosis and severe hemolytic component, should present no diagnostic confusion.

α-Thalassemia trait occurs in persons of African, Chinese, and Southeast Asian descent. This mild microcytic disorder is caused by a deletion of 2 of the 4 genes that regulate α-globin production. In the usual clinical setting, the diagnosis of α-thalassemia trait can be assumed when a patient with a familial hypochromic microcytic anemia has normal results of iron studies (including ferritin), normal levels of Hb A_2 and Hb F, and a normal hemoglobin electrophoresis. In the usual clinical situation, α-thalassemia trait is a diagnosis of exclusion except during the newborn period, when infants with α-thalassemia trait have 3–10% hemoglobin Barts (γ_4) [see Chapter 462]. A specific diagnosis for α-thalassemia disorders is possible using molecular diagnostic strategies, but these studies usually are done only when the information is necessary for genetic counseling and prenatal diagnosis.

Hb H disease, another form of α-thalassemia, results from deletion of 3 of the 4 α-globin genes. It also is characterized by hypochromia and microcytosis, but in addition there is a mild hemolytic component due to the instability of β-chain tetramers (Hb H) resulting from a deficiency of α-globin chains. Beyond infancy, Hb H is readily identified by hemoglobin electrophoresis. During the newborn period, the moderately severe α-globin deficiency allows for the accumulation of more γ chains, and the concentration of hemoglobin Barts is >20%. In many states in the U.S., the newborn hemoglobin screen detects infants with Hb H disease, and this information is forwarded to the patient's physician.

The anemia of chronic disease (ACD) and infection usually is normocytic, although occasionally it may be slightly microcytic (see Chapter 451). In contrast to iron-deficiency anemia, in these inflammatory conditions both the serum iron level and iron-binding capacity (transferrin) are reduced, and serum ferritin levels are normal or elevated (ferritin is an acute phase reactant). The serum transferrin receptor (TfR) level is useful in the distinction between iron-deficiency anemia and anemia of chronic disease because it is not affected by inflammation. The concentration of TfR is elevated in iron deficiency and is within the normal range in anemia of chronic disease.

Lead poisoning (see Chapter 709) and iron-deficiency anemia both are associated with elevations of FEP. In cases of lead poisoning associated with iron deficiency, the RBCs are morphologically similar, but coarse basophilic stippling of the RBCs often is prominent. Elevated blood lead, FEP, and urinary coproporphyrin levels are seen.

TREATMENT. The regular response of iron-deficiency anemia to adequate amounts of iron is an important diagnostic and therapeutic feature. Oral administration of simple ferrous salts (e.g., sulfate, gluconate, fumarate) provides inexpensive and satisfactory therapy. No evidence shows that addition of any trace metal, vitamin, or other hematinic substance significantly increases the response to simple ferrous salts. One problem encountered with administration of oral iron to young children is that liquid $FeSO_4$ has an unpleasant taste, but sometimes the taste can be camouflaged by mixing with flavored syrup. Other, better-tasting preparations are available over the counter, but these are much more expensive than simple liquid $FeSO_4$. Aside from the unpleasant taste, intolerance to oral iron is uncommon in young children, although older children and adolescents sometimes have gastrointestinal complaints. Problems with constipation can be minimized by increasing water and fiber intake. For some children, abdominal discomfort can be minimized by administering iron with food, recognizing that this may decrease iron absorption to some extent. The therapeutic dose should be calculated in terms of elemental iron; ferrous sulfate is 20% elemental iron by weight. A daily total dose of 4–6 mg/kg of elemental iron in 3 divided doses provides an optimal amount of iron for the stimulated bone marrow to use. A parenteral iron preparation (iron dextran) is an effective form of iron when given in a properly calculated dose, but the response to parenteral iron is no more rapid or complete than that obtained with proper oral administration of iron, unless malabsorption is a factor. An occasional complication of iron dextran has been anaphylaxis. The risk of anaphylaxis is much less with ferric gluconate given IV, the parenteral form of choice.

While adequate iron medication is given, the family must be educated about the patient's diet, and the milk consumption should be limited to a reasonable quantity, preferably 500 mL (1 pint)/24 hr or less. This reduction has a dual effect: The amount of iron-rich foods is increased, and blood loss from intolerance to cow's milk proteins are reduced. When the reeducation of child and parent is not successful, parenteral iron medication rarely may be indicated. Iron deficiency can be prevented in high-risk populations by providing iron-fortified formula or cereals during infancy. Iron deficiency in adolescent females secondary to abnormal uterine blood flow loss is treated with iron and hormone therapy (see Chapter 115).

Within 72–96 hr after administration of iron to an anemic child, peripheral reticulocytosis is noted (Table 455-2). The height of this response is inversely proportional to the severity of the anemia. Reticulocytosis is followed by a rise in the hemoglo-

TABLE 455-2. Responses to Iron Therapy in Iron-Deficiency Anemia

TIME AFTER IRON ADMINISTRATION	RESPONSE
12–24 hr	Replacement of intracellular iron enzymes; subjective improvement; decreased irritability; increased appetite
36–48 hr	Initial bone marrow response; erythroid hyperplasia
48–72 hr	Reticulocytosis, peaking at 5–7 days
4–30 days	Increase in hemoglobin level
1–3 mo	Repletion of stores

bin level, which may increase as much as 0.5 g/dL/24 hr. Iron medication should be continued for 8 wk after blood values are normal. Failures of iron therapy occur when a child does not receive the prescribed medication, when iron is given in a form that is poorly absorbed, or when there is continuing unrecognized blood loss, such as intestinal or pulmonary loss, or loss with menstrual periods. Therapeutic failure of iron medication may indicate that the original diagnosis of nutritional iron deficiency was incorrect.

Because a rapid hematologic response can be confidently predicted in typical iron deficiency, blood transfusion is indicated only when the anemia is very severe or when superimposed infection may interfere with the response. Rapid correction of severe anemia by transfusion is generally not needed; the procedure may be dangerous because of associated high-output cardiac failure. Packed or sedimented RBCs should be administered slowly in an amount sufficient to raise the hemoglobin to a safe level at which the response to iron therapy can be awaited. In general, severely anemic children with hemoglobin values <4 g/dL should be given only 2–3 mL/kg of packed cells at any one time (furosemide also may be administered as a diuretic). If there is evidence of frank heart failure, a modified exchange transfusion using fresh-packed RBCs may be considered, although diuretics followed by slow infusion of packed RBCs usually suffice.

Baggett HC, Parkinson AJ, Muth PT, et al: Endemic iron deficiency associated with *Helicobacter pylori* infection among school-aged children in Alaska. *Pediatrics* 2006;117:e396–404.

Brotanek JM, Halterman JS, Auinger P, et al: Iron deficiency, prolonged bottle-feeding and racial/ethnic disparities in young children. *Arch Pediatr Adolesc* 2005;159:1038–1042.

Chaparro CM, Neufeld LM, Alvarez GT, et al: Effect of timing of umbilical cord clamping on iron status in Mexican infants: a randomized controlled trial. *Lancet* 2006;367:1997–2004.

Galloway MJ, Smellie WS: Investigating iron status in microcytic anaemia. *BMJ* 2006;333:791–793.

Lozoff B, Jimenez E, Smith JB: Double burden of iron deficiency in infancy and low socioeconomic status. *Arch Pediatr Adoless Med* 2006;160:1108–1112.

Mercer J, Erickson-Owens D: Delayed cord clamping increases infants' iron stores. *Lancet* 2006;367:1956–1957.

Moy RJ: Prevalence, consequences and prevention of childhood nutritional iron deficiency: a child public health perspective. *Clin Lab Haematol* 2006;28:291–298.

Panagiotou JP, Douros K: Clinicolaboratory findings and treatment of iron-deficiency anemia in childhood. *Pediatr Hematol Oncol* 2004;21:521–534. Review.

Sutcliffe TL, Khambalia A, Westergard S, et al: Iron depletion is associated with daytime bottle-feeding in the second and third years of life. *Arch Pediatr Adolesc Med* 2006;160:1114–1120.

Chapter 456 ■ Other Microcytic Anemias

SIDEROBLASTIC ANEMIAS. Sideroblastic anemias result from acquired and hereditary disorders of heme synthesis. The anemias are characterized by hypochromic microcytic red blood cells (RBCs) mixed with normal RBCs, thus giving an overall picture of a dimorphic population of erythrocytes, and the complete blood cell count indicates an extremely high RBC distribution width (RDW). The serum iron concentration usually is elevated, and the transferrin saturation of iron is increased. In all cases of sideroblastic anemia, regardless of the specific cause, impaired heme synthesis leads to retention of iron within the mitochondria. Morphologically, this is seen in marrow nucleated RBCs with iron granules (aggregates of iron in mitochondria) that have a perinuclear distribution. These unusual cells, known as ringed sideroblasts (Fig. 456-1), are found only in pathologic states and are distinct from the sideroblasts (RBC precursors that contain diffuse cytoplasmic ferritin granules) in the marrow of normal subjects. Sideroblastic anemias most commonly occur in adulthood, and these acquired disorders can be idiopathic or secondary to drugs, alcohol, or myelodysplastic disorders. A few sideroblastic anemias are seen in children.

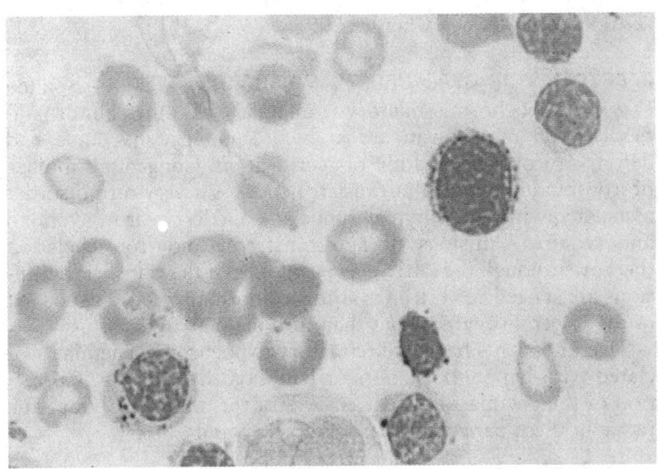

Figure 456-1. Ring sideroblast in myelodysplastic syndrome (refractory anemia with ring sideroblasts)—iron stain. (From Ryan DH, Cohen HJ: Bone marrow examination. In Hoffman R, Benz EJ Jr, Shattil SJ, et al [editors]: *Hematology*, 4th ed. Philadelphia, Churchill Livingstone, 2005.)

Congenital Sideroblastic Anemia. Congenital sideroblastic anemia is rare and conforms to an X-linked pattern of inheritance. It usually occurs in males, although skewed lyonization has resulted in affected females. Autosomal dominant and sporadic cases also occur. Hereditary sideroblastic anemias result from abnormalities of the erythrocytic isozyme for 5-aminolevulinic acid synthetase (ALAS), the rate-limiting enzyme reaction in heme synthesis. An important cofactor for ALAS is pyridoxal phosphate. The gene for the erythrocyte-specific ALAS *(ALAS2)* is located on the X chromosome, and >25 different missense mutations have been identified. Several of these mutations occur near the binding site for pyridoxal phosphate.

Severe anemias are recognized in infancy or early childhood, whereas milder cases may not become apparent until early adulthood or later. **Clinical findings** include pallor, icterus, and moderate splenomegaly and/or hepatomegaly. The severity of the anemia varies such that some patients require no therapy while others need regular RBC transfusions. A subset of patients with hereditary sideroblastic anemia manifest a hematologic response to pharmacologic doses of pyridoxine. Iron overload as manifested by elevated serum ferritin, elevated serum iron, and increased transferrin saturation is a major complication of this disorder. Clinical evidence of iron overload (e.g., diabetes mellitus, liver dysfunction) may be found in some patients who have little or no anemia. Stem cell transplantation has been used to treat affected children who were dependent on RBC transfusions.

A unique variant of congenital sideroblastic anemia is **Pearson syndrome,** characterized by the early onset of transfusion-dependent anemia, neutropenia, and thrombocytopenia. In addition to the usual marrow abnormalities of sideroblastic anemia, children with this syndrome also have vacuolization of RBC and myeloid precursors. In contrast to other sideroblastic anemias, which are microcytic, this is a macrocytic anemia and, consequently, it sometimes is confused with Diamond-Blackfan anemia (see Chapters 448 and 449).

LEAD POISONING. See Chapter 709.

RARE TYPES OF HYPOCHROMIC MICROCYTIC ANEMIA. Isolated cases of hypochromic microcytic anemia with other abnormalities of iron metabolism are known; some patients have had defects in iron mobilization or reutilization. Congenital absence of iron-binding protein (atransferrinemia) is a very rare disorder associated with severe hypochromic anemia despite iron overload and requires infusions of apo-transferrin and iron chelation therapy, although the latter may be avoided if the transferrin infusions are started early. Iron is absorbed normally and is deposited in the visceral organs rather than in bone marrow.

Several patients have had refractory hypochromic anemia associated with lymphatic tumors or lymphoid hyperplasia. Correction of the anemia followed removal of the abnormal lymphatic tissue in these patients (see Chapters 489 and 506).

Alcindor T, Bridges KR: Sideroblastic anaemias. *Br J Haematol* 2002;116:733–743.

Ayas M, Al-Jefri A, Mustafa MM, et al: Congenital sideroblastic anaemia successfully treated using allogeneic stem cell transplantation. *Br J Haematol* 2001;113:938.

Chalco JP, Huicho L, Alamo C, et al: Accuracy of clinical pallor in the diagnosis of anemia in children: A meta-analysis. *BMC Pediatrics* 2005;5:46.

Fleming MD: The genetics of inherited sideroblastic anemias. *Semin Hematol* 2002;39:270–281.

Moy RJ: Prevalence, consequences and prevention of childhood nutritional iron deficiency: a child public health perspective. *Clin Lab Haematol* 2006;28:291–298.

Panagiotou JP, Douros K: Clinicolaboratory findings and treatment of iron-deficiency anemia in childhood. *Pediatr Hematol Oncol* 2004;21:521–534, Review.

Sandoval C, Jayabose S, Eden AN: Trends in diagnosis and management of iron deficiency during infancy and early childhood. *Hematol Oncol Clin North Am* 2004;18:1423–1438, x.

Walter T: Effect of iron-deficiency anemia on cognitive skills and neuromaturation in infancy and childhood. *Food Nutr Bull* 2003;24(4 Suppl):S104–S110.

Section 3 — Hemolytic Anemias

Chapter 457 ■ Definitions and Classification of Hemolytic Anemias

George B. Segel

Hemolysis is defined as the premature destruction of red blood cells (RBCs). Anemia results when the rate of destruction exceeds the capacity of the marrow to produce RBCs. Normal RBC survival time is 110–120 days (half-life, 55–60 days), and approximately 0.85% of the most senescent RBCs are removed and replaced each day. During hemolysis, RBC survival is shortened, the RBC count falls, erythropoietin is increased, and the stimulation of marrow activity results in heightened RBC production. This is reflected in an increased percentage of reticulocytes in the blood. Thus, hemolysis should be suspected as a cause of anemia if an elevated reticulocyte count is present. The reticulocyte count also may be elevated as a response to acute blood loss or for a short period after replacement therapy for iron, vitamin B_{12}, or folate deficiency. The marrow can increase its output 2- to 3-fold acutely, with a maximum of 6- to 8-fold in long-standing hemolysis. The reticulocyte percentage can be corrected to measure the magnitude of marrow production in response to hemolysis as follows:

$$\text{Reticulocyte index} = \text{reticulocyte \%} \times \frac{\text{Observed hematocrit}}{\text{Normal hematocrit}} \times \frac{1}{\mu}$$

where μ is a maturation factor of 1–3 related to the severity of the anemia (Fig. 457-1). The normal reticulocyte index is 1.0; therefore, the index measures the fold increase in erythropoiesis (e.g., 2-fold, 3-fold).

As anemia becomes more severe, the erythropoietin concentration increases and reticulocytes are released from the marrow earlier; they are identifiable as reticulocytes in the blood for >1 day. Because the reticulocyte index is essentially a measure of RBC production per day, the maturation factor, μ, provides this correction (see Fig. 457-1). The usual marrow response in acute hemolytic anemia is reflected by a reticulocyte index of 2–3, whereas in long-standing chronic hemolysis, the increase in erythropoiesis is approximately 6-fold.

The erythroid hyperplasia resulting from chronic hemolytic anemia in children, especially thalassemia, may be so extensive that the medullary spaces expand at the expense of the cortical bone. These changes may be evident on physical examination or on radiographs of the skull and long bones (see Fig. 462-7). A propensity to fracture long bones can also occur.

Direct assessment of the severity of hemolysis requires measurement of RBC survival time using RBCs tagged with the

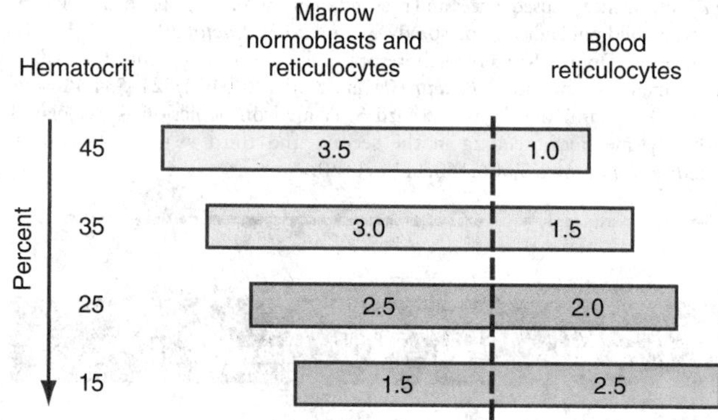

Figure 457-1. Number of days for maturation of reticulocytes to mature erythrocytes in the marrow and blood. The duration of maturation as blood reticulocytes is taken as μ, which is used in the correction equation in this chapter. (Modified from Hillman RS, Finch CA: *Red Cell Manual.* Philadelphia, FA Davis, 1983.)

TABLE 457-1. Hemolytic Anemias and Their Treatment

DIAGNOSIS	DEFECT	LABORATORY TESTS	TREATMENT
CELLULAR DEFECTS			
Membrane Defects			
Hereditary spherocytosis	Cytoskeletal protein defects Frequently involve vertical interactions of spectrin ankyrin, protein 3	Spherocytes on blood film Negative Coombs test eliminates immune hemolysis Increased incubated osmotic fragility Abnormal cytoskeletal protein analysis	If Hb > 10 g/dL and reticulocyte count < 10%—none If severe anemia, poor growth, aplastic crises, and age <2 yr—transfusion Folic acid, 1 mg qd
Hereditary elliptocytosis	Cytoskeletal protein defects Frequently involve horizontal interactions of spectrin, protein 4.1, and glycophorin c	Elliptocytes on blood film RBCs mildly heat-sensitive Abnormal cytoskeletal protein analysis	Mild types—no treatment Chronic hemolysis—transfusion and splenectomy as recommended for spherocytosis (see above) Folic acid, 1 mg qd
Hereditary pyropoikilocytosis	Cytoskeletal protein defects Homozygous or double heterozygous abnormality in horizontal interactions of α spectrin	Extreme variation in RBC size and shape on blood film Thermal sensitivity—fragmentation at 45°C for 15 min	Transfusion and splenectomy as recommended for spherocytosis (see above) Folic acid, 1 mg qd
Hereditary stomatocytosis	Cytoskeletal protein defects Decreased protein 7.2b (1 subset) Abnormal RBC cation and water content	Stomatocytes on blood film	Splenectomy should be avoided (see text) Folic acid, 1 mg qd
Paroxysmal nocturnal hemoglobinuria	Primary acquired marrow disorder RBCs unusually sensitive to complement-mediated lysis	Decreased WBC CD55 and CD59 or decreased RBC CD59 by flow cytometry Ham's test, sucrosis lysis test Marrow aspirate and biopsy to assess cellularity Decreased decay-accelerating factor	Folic acid, 1 mg qd Mild cytopenias—no treatment Chronic hemolysis and other cytopenias—prednisone, 60 mg qd initially, then taper if possible; maintenance therapy 15–40 mg qod Iron for secondary iron deficiency Androgens—fluoxymesterone Anticoagulation Marrow transplant for pancytopenia
Enzyme Deficiencies			
Pyruvate kinase deficiency	Decreased or abnormal enzyme	Pyruvate kinase assay—decreased V_{max} or rarely high *Km* variant	If severe anemia with symptoms, poor growth and age <2 yr—transfusion Splenectomy > age 6 yr, but earlier if necessary Folic acid, 1 mg qd
G6PD deficiency	A^- type: age-labile enzyme Mediterranean type: no enzyme activity in circulating RBCs	G6PD	Avoid oxidant stress to RBCs Transfusion if acute anemia is symptomatic
Hemoglobin Abnormalities ***(For discussion of hemoglobinopathies, see sections on these topics)***			
EXTRACELLULAR DEFECTS			
Autoimmune			
Autoimmune hemolytic anemia "Warm" antibody	Alteration in membrane surface antigen (Rh) or abnormal response of B lymphocytes, causing autoantibody formation	Spherocytes on blood film Positive direct Coombs test to IgG "warm" antibody antibody directed against RBCs Positive indirect Coombs test and antibody detectable in plasma Thermal amplitude 35–40°C Some complement (C3b) may be detected on RBCs Tests for underlying disease	If Hb < 10 g/dL and reticulocyte count > 10%—none Severe anemia may require transfusion Prednisone, 2 mg/kg/24 hr IVIG Danazol Splenectomy Immunosuppressives Folic acid, 1 mg/24 hr if chronic
"Cold" antibody	"Cold" or IgM autoantibody directed against I/i antigen system	Agglutination or rouleaux on blood film Positive direct Coombs test to complement (C3b) Tests for underlying disease Serology for infectious mononucleosis; anti-i present Serology for *Mycoplasma pneumoniae;* anti-I present	If Hb > 10 g/dL and reticulocyte count < 10%—none Severe anemia may require transfusion Avoid exposure to cold If severe—immunosuppressives and plasmapheresis Prednisone is less effective Splenectomy is not useful Folic acid, 1 mg/24 hr if chronic
Fragmentation Hemolysis			
DIC, TTP, HUS	Direct damage to RBC membrane	Fragments on blood film	Treat underlying condition Transfusion, but transfused cells also will have shortened life span
Extracorporeal membrane oxygenation	Direct damage to RBC membrane	Fragments on blood film	Supportive Transfusion until ECMO is discontinued
Prosthetic heart valve	Direct damage to RBC membrane	Fragments on blood film	Folic acid, 1 mg/24 hr Iron for secondary iron deficiency
Burns—thermal injury	Direct damage to RBC membrane	Spherocytes on blood film	Supportive Transfusion
Hypersplenism	Effects of sequestration, ↓ pH, lipases and other enzymes, and macrophages on RBCs	Thrombocytopenia and neutropenia	Treat underlying condition—cytopenias all usually mild Splenectomy if complicating other anemia (e.g., thalassemia major) Folic acid, 1 mg/24 hr
Plasma Factors			
Liver disease	Alteration in plasma cholesterol and phospholipids	Target cells or speculated RBCs on blood film Abnormal liver function tests	Treat underlying condition Transfusion, but transfused cells also will have shortened life span Folic acid, 1 mg/24 hr
Abetalipoproteinemia	Absence of apolipoprotein β Vitamin E deficiency and heightened sensitivity to oxidative damage	Acanthocytes on blood film Absent chylomicrons, VLDL, and LDL	Vitamin E (A, K, and D) Folic acid, 1 mg/24 hr Dietary restriction of triglycerides
Infections	Toxic effects on RBCs	Associated symptoms and signs Cultures	Antibiotics Supportive
Wilson Disease	Effect of copper on RBC membrane, usually self-limited	Spherocytes on blood film Copper, ceruloplasmin Penicillamine challenge and urine copper excretion	Penicillamine Supportive Transfusion if acute anemia is symptomatic

DIC, disseminated intravascular coagulation; ECMO, extracorporeal membrane oxygenation; G6PD, glucose-6-phosphate dehydrogenase; Hb, hemoglobin; HUS, hemolytic uremic syndrome; IVIG, intravenous immunoglobulin; LDL, low density lipoprotein; RBC, red blood cell; TTP, thrombotic thrombocytopenic purpura; VLDL, very low density lipoprotein; WBC, white blood cell.

Modified from Asselin BL, Segel GB: In Rakel R (editor): *Conn's Current Therapy*. Philadelphia, WB Saunders, 1994, pp 338–339.

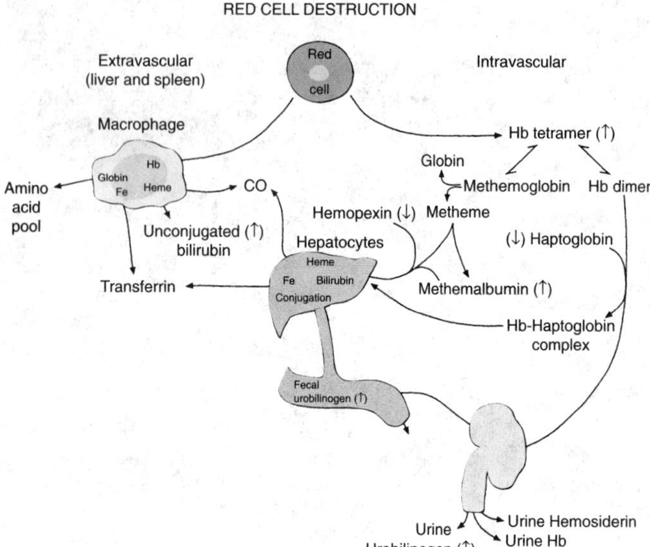

Figure 457-2. Red cell destruction and catabolism of hemoglobin (Hb) based on the description by Hillman and Finch. Fe, iron. (From Hillman RS, Finch CA: *Red Cell Manual.* Philadelphia, FA Davis, 1983.)

radioisotope $Na_2{}^{51}CrO_4$. The normal half-life of chromium 51 is 25–35 days. This value is less than the expected half-life of 55–60 days because of the elution of chromium 51 from the labeled RBCs at the rate of approximately 1% day. Techniques to measure RBC survival using RBC biotin labeling have been tested in animals and do not require the use of isotopes.

Several other plasma, urinary, or fecal chemical alterations reflect the presence of hemolysis. The exaggerated degradation rate of hemoglobin results in increased biliary excretion of heme pigment derivatives and increased urinary and fecal urobilinogen (Fig. 457-2). Gallstones composed of calcium bilirubinate may be formed in children with chronic hemolysis as young as 4 yr of age. Elevations of serum unconjugated bilirubin and lactic dehydrogenase also may accompany hemolysis.

Three heme-binding proteins in the plasma are altered during hemolysis (see Fig. 457-2). Hemoglobin binds to haptoglobin and hemopexin, both of which are cleared more rapidly as conjugates, and their plasma concentration is decreased. Oxidized heme binds to albumin to form methemalbumin, which is increased in the plasma. When the capacity of these binding molecules is exceeded, free hemoglobin appears in the plasma, and the pink color can be seen if the plasma is partitioned after centrifugation in a capillary hematocrit tube. If present, free hemoglobin in the plasma is prima facie evidence of intravascular hemolysis. Free hemoglobin dissociates into dimers and is filtered by the kidneys. When the tubular reabsorptive capacity of the kidneys for hemoglobin is exceeded, free hemoglobin appears in the urine. Even in the absence of hemoglobinuria, iron loss may result from reabsorbed hemoglobin and the shedding of renal epithelial cells in which the iron from hemoglobin is stored as hemosiderin. This may lead to iron deficiency during chronic intravascular hemolysis. When hemoglobin is degraded, an α-methene bridge is broken in the cyclic tetrapyrrole of the heme moiety, with release of carbon monoxide (CO) [see Fig. 457-2]. The amount of CO in the blood or expired air provides a dynamic measure of the hemolytic rate; end-tidal CO is not available in most clinical laboratories to measure hemolysis.

The hematocrit level is dependent on the severity of hemolysis and on the erythropoietic response. The shortened RBC life span and heightened RBC production result in a marked susceptibility to aplastic or hypoplastic crises, characterized by erythroid marrow failure and reticulocytopenia, accompanied by a rapid further reduction in hemoglobin and hematocrit to extremely low levels. The most common cause of aplastic crisis is parvovirus B19, which is erythrocytotropic (see Chapters 248, 450, 458, and 462.1). An aplastic crisis may produce a precipitous and life-threatening decline in hematocrit, that usually lasts 10–14 days. Such transient erythroid marrow failure has only a mild effect on those with a normal RBC life span, but has a proportionately greater effect if the RBC life span is shortened by hemolysis. A 2nd infection with parvovirus is uncommon, but other infections may compromise erythroid marrow output, resulting in various degrees of hypoplasia or hypoplastic crises.

Hemolytic anemias may be classified as either (1) cellular, resulting from intrinsic abnormalities of the membrane, enzymes, or hemoglobin; or (2) extracellular, resulting from antibodies, mechanical factors, or plasma factors. Most cellular defects are inherited (paroxysmal nocturnal hemoglobinuria is acquired), and most extracellular defects are acquired (abetalipoproteinemia with acanthocytosis is inherited). Table 457-1 shows the most common hemolytic anemias, their underlying defects, the diagnostic laboratory tests, and the current recommendations for treatment.

Chapter 458 ■ Hereditary Spherocytosis

George B. Segel

Hereditary spherocytosis is a common cause of hemolysis and hemolytic anemia, with a wide spectrum of severity and with a prevalence of approximately 1/5,000 in people of Northern European descent. It is the most common inherited abnormality of the red blood cell (RBC) membrane. Affected individuals may be asymptomatic, without anemia and with minimal hemolysis, or may have severe hemolytic anemia. Hereditary spherocytosis has been described in most ethnic groups, but is most common among persons of Northern European origin.

ETIOLOGY. Hereditary spherocytosis usually is transmitted as an autosomal dominant and, less frequently, as an autosomal recessive disorder. As many as 25% of patients have no previous family history. Of these patients, most represent new mutations, and a few cases result from recessive inheritance or represent nonpaternity. The most common molecular defects are abnormalities of spectrin or ankyrin, which are major components of the cytoskeleton responsible for RBC shape. A recessive defect has been described in α-spectrin; dominant defects, in β-spectrin and protein 3; and dominant and recessive defects, in ankyrin (Table 458-1). A deficiency in spectrin, protein 3, or ankyrin results in uncoupling in the "vertical" interactions of the lipid bilayer skeleton and the loss of membrane microvesicles (Fig. 458-1). The loss of membrane surface area without a proportional loss of cell volume causes sphering of the RBCs and an associated increase in cation permeability, cation transport,

TABLE 458-1. Common Gene Mutations in Hereditary Spherocytosis (HS)

PROTEIN	BAND ON GEL	GENE	PROPORTION OF PATIENTS WITH HS	INHERITANCE
Ankyrin	2.1	*ANK1*	50–67%	Dom and Rec
Band 3	3	*AE1 (SLC4A1)*	15–20%	Mostly Dom
β Spectrin	2	*SPTB*	15–20%	Dom
α Spectrin	1	*SPTA1*	<5%	Rec
Protein 4.2	4.2	*EPB42*	<5%	Rec

Dom, dominant; Rec, recessive.

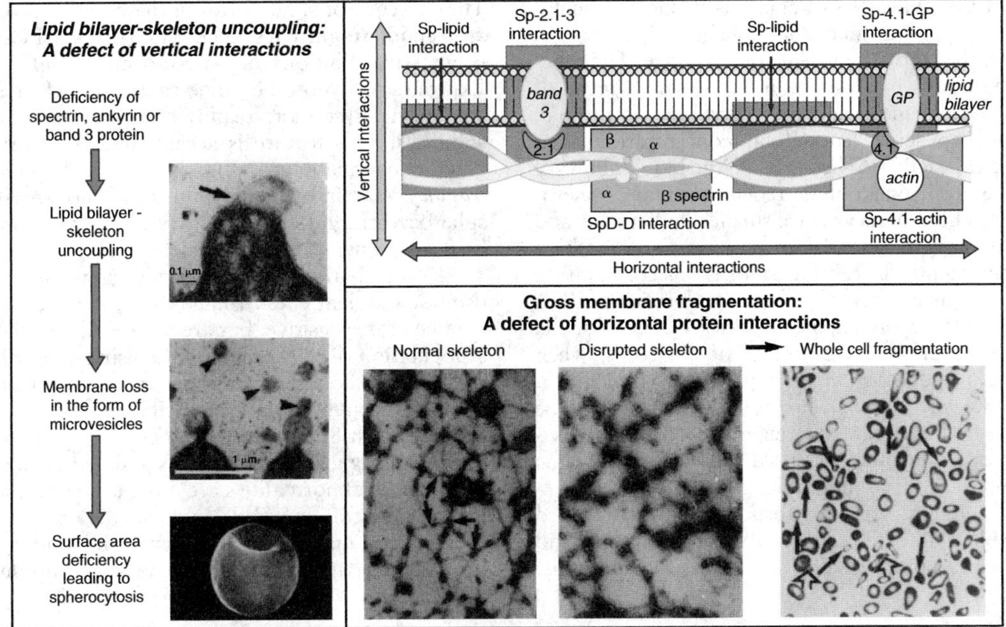

Figure 458-1. Vertical and horizontal interactions of membrane proteins and the pathobiology of the red cell lesion in hereditary spherocytosis (HS) and hereditary elliptocytosis/hereditary pyropoikilocytosis (HE/HPP). *Left,* A defect of vertical or transverse interactions as exemplified by the red cell membrane lesion in HS. Partial deficiencies of spectrin, ankyrin (band 2.1), or band 3 protein lead to uncoupling of the membrane lipid bilayer from the underlying skeleton *(arrow),* followed by formation of spectrin-free microvesicles that are 0.2–0.5 µm in diameter *(arrowheads).* These vesicles can be visualized by transmission electron microscopy, but they are not seen during examination of blood films. The subsequent loss of cell surface and a decrease in the surface/volume ratio leads to spherocytosis. *Right,* Defect of horizontal or parallel interactions of skeletal proteins, as exemplified by the membrane lesion in hemolytic forms of HE associated with a defect of spectrin heterodimer self-association. The molecular lesion involving a weakened self-association of spectrin heterodimers to tetramers represents a horizontal defect of the stress-supporting protein interactions. It leads to a disruption of the membrane skeletal lattice and, consequently, whole cell destabilization, followed by red cell fragmentation and poikilocytosis. Such fragments are readily seen on stained blood films. Sp, spectrin; Sp-D, spectrin dimer; GP, glycophorin. (Modified from Palek J, Jarolim P: Clinical expression and laboratory detection of red blood cell membrane protein mutations. *Semin Hematol* 1993;30:249.)

adenosine triphosphate use, and glycolysis. The decreased deformability of the spherocytic RBCs impairs cell passage from the splenic cords to the splenic sinuses, and the spherocytic RBCs are destroyed prematurely in the spleen. Splenectomy markedly improves RBC life span and cures the anemia.

CLINICAL MANIFESTATIONS. Hereditary spherocytosis may be a cause of hemolytic disease in the newborn and may present as anemia and hyperbilirubinemia sufficiently severe to require phototherapy or exchange transfusions. Hemolysis may be more prominent in the newborn because hemoglobin F binds 2,3-diphosphoglycerate poorly, and the increased level of free 2,3-diphosphoglycerate destabilizes spectrin-actin-protein 4.1 interactions in the RBC membrane (see Fig. 458-1). The severity of symptoms in infants and children is variable. Some children remain asymptomatic into adulthood, but others may have severe anemia, with pallor, jaundice, fatigue, and exercise intolerance. Severe cases may be marked by expansion of the diploë of the skull and the medullary region of other bones, but to a lesser extent than in thalassemia major. After infancy, the spleen is usually enlarged, and pigmentary (bilirubin) gallstones may form as early as age 4–5 yr. At least 50% of unsplenectomized patients ultimately form gallstones, although they may be asymptomatic. Because of the high RBC turnover and heightened erythroid marrow activity, children with hereditary spherocytosis are susceptible to aplastic crisis, primarily as a result of parvovirus infection, and to hypoplastic crises associated with various other infections (Fig. 458-2). The erythroid marrow failure may result rapidly in profound anemia (hematocrit <10%), high-output heart failure, hypoxia, cardiovascular collapse, and death. White blood cell and platelet counts may also fall (see Fig. 458-2).

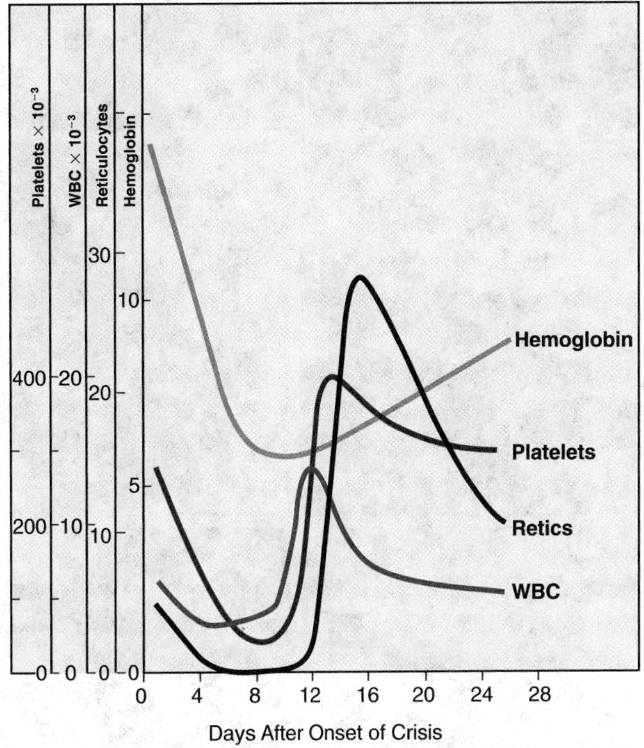

Figure 458-2. Parvovirus-induced aplastic crisis. Progression of the changes in blood count is shown for a patient with hereditary spherocytosis and infection with parvovirus. Note that the fall in baseline reticulocytosis is associated with a rapid fall in hemoglobin. White blood cells (WBC) and platelets are also affected. (Modified from Nathan DG, Orkin SH, Ginsburg D, et al [editors]: *Hematology of Infancy and Childhood,* 6th ed. Philadelphia, WB Saunders, 2003.).

LABORATORY FINDINGS. Evidence of hemolysis includes reticulocytosis and indirect hyperbilirubinemia. The hemoglobin level usually is 6–10 g/dL, but it can be in the normal range. The reticulocyte percentage often is increased to 6–20%, with a mean of approximately 10%. The mean corpuscular volume is normal, although the mean corpuscular hemoglobin concentration often is increased (36–38 g/dL RBCs). The RBCs on the blood film vary in size and include polychromatophilic reticulocytes and spherocytes (Fig. 458-3*A*). The spherocytes are smaller in diameter and appear hyperchromic on the blood film as a result of the high hemoglobin concentration. The central pallor is less conspicuous than in normal cells. Spherocytes may be the predominant cell or may be relatively sparse, depending on the severity of the disease, but they usually account for >15–20% of the cells when hemolytic anemia is present. Erythroid hyperplasia is evident in the marrow aspirate or biopsy. Marrow expansion may be evident on routine roentgenographic examination. Other evidence of hemolysis may include decreased haptoglobin and the presence of gallstones on ultrasonography.

The diagnosis of hereditary spherocytosis usually is established clinically from the blood film, which shows many spherocytes and reticulocytes, from the family history, and from splenomegaly. The presence of spherocytes in the blood can be confirmed with an osmotic fragility test (Fig. 458-4). The RBCs are incubated in progressive dilutions of an iso-osmotic buffered salt solution. Exposure to hypotonic saline causes the RBCs to swell, and the spherocytes lyse more readily than biconcave cells in hypotonic solutions. This feature is accentuated by depriving the cells of glucose overnight at 37°C, known as the *incubated osmotic fragility test*. Unfortunately, this test is not specific for hereditary spherocytosis, and results may be abnormal in immune and other hemolytic anemias. A normal test result also may be found in 10–20% of patients. Other tests, such as the cryohemolysis test, osmotic gradient ektacytometry, and the eocin-5-maleimide test, may be more sensitive, but are not readily available. Detection of a population of hyperdense RBCs using a laser-based instrument or a Coulter counter may prove more conveniently diagnostic.

As a research tool, the specific protein abnormality can be established in 80% of these patients by RBC membrane protein analysis using gel electrophoresis and densitometric quantitation. The protein abnormalities are more evident in patients who have had a splenectomy. Studies to define the underlying defects in the cytoskeleton may require assessment of protein synthesis, stability, assembly, and binding to the other membrane proteins. Mol-

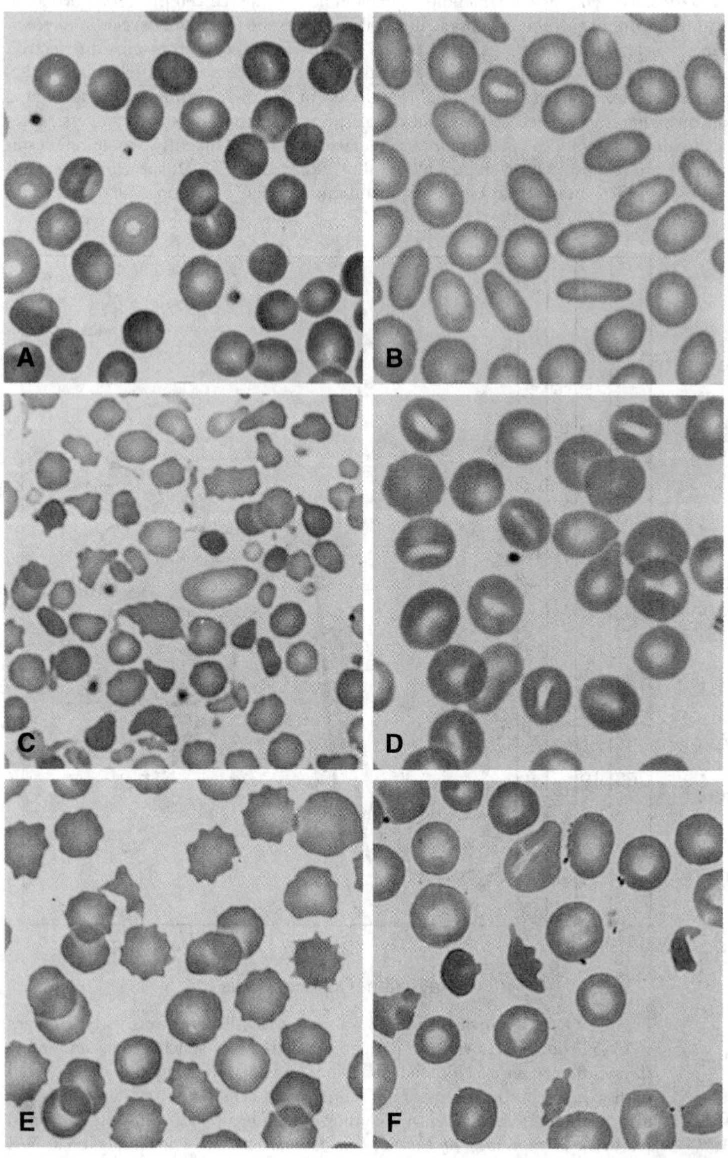

Figure 458-3. Morphology of abnormal red cells. *A*, Hereditary spherocytosis; *B*, hereditary elliptocytosis; *C*, hereditary pyropoikilocytosis; *D*, hereditary stomatocytosis; *E*, acanthocytosis; *F*, fragmentation hemolysis.

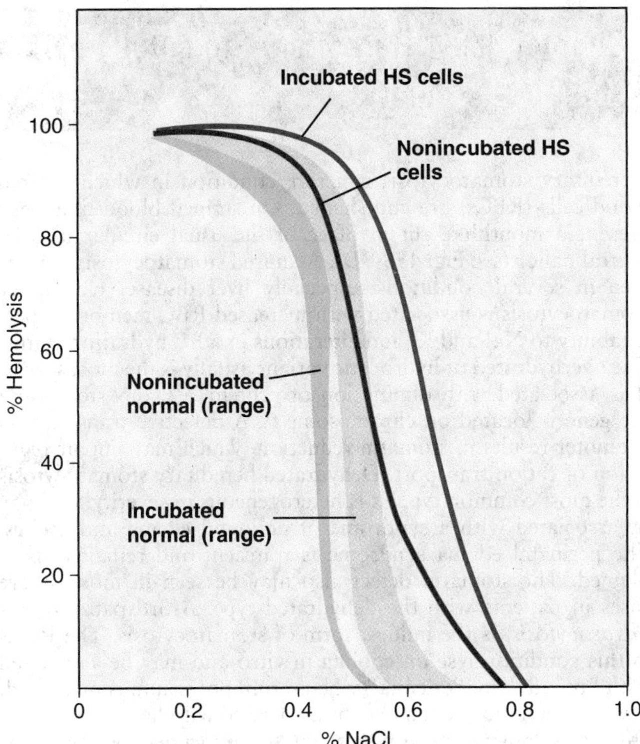

Figure 458-4. Osmotic fragility of normal red cells and red cells from a patient with hereditary spherocytosis (HS). The accentuation of the osmotic sensitivity, particularly of the HS cells, is shown after incubation overnight without glucose. (From Reich PR [editor]: *Hematology: Pathophysiologic Basis for Clinical Practice,* 2nd ed. Boston, Little, Brown, 1984, with permission.)

ecular diagnosis also is possible. Most patients have family-specific private mutations that can be detected by DNA analysis. De novo mutations in the β-spectrin and ankyrin genes have been described in 50% of patients with unaffected parents.

DIFFERENTIAL DIAGNOSIS. The major alternative considerations when large numbers of spherocytes are seen on the blood film are isoimmune and autoimmune hemolysis. Isoimmune hemolytic disease of the newborn, particularly due to ABO incompatibility, mimics hereditary spherocytosis. The detection of antibody on an infant's RBCs using a direct antiglobulin (Coombs) test should establish the diagnosis of immune hemolysis. Autoimmune hemolytic anemias also are characterized by spherocytes, and there may be evidence of previously normal values for hemoglobin, hematocrit, and reticulocyte count. Rare causes of spherocytosis include thermal injury, clostridial septicemia with exotoxemia, and Wilson disease, each of which may present as transient hemolytic anemia (see Table 457-1).

TREATMENT. Because the spherocytes in hereditary spherocytosis are destroyed almost exclusively in the spleen, splenectomy eliminates most of the hemolysis associated with this disorder. After splenectomy, osmotic fragility often improves because of diminished splenic conditioning and less RBC membrane loss; the anemia, reticulocytosis, and hyperbilirubinemia then resolve. Whether all patients with hereditary spherocytosis should undergo splenectomy is controversial. Some do not recommend splenectomy for patients whose hemoglobin values exceed 10 g/dL and whose reticulocyte percentage is <10%. Folic acid, 1 mg daily, should be administered to prevent deficiency and the resultant decrease in erythropoiesis. For patients with more severe anemia and reticulocytosis or those with hypoplastic or aplastic crises, poor growth, or cardiomegaly, splenectomy is recommended after age 5–6 yr to avoid the heightened risk of postsplenectomy sepsis in younger children. Laparoscopic splenectomy decreases the length of hospital stay and has replaced open splenectomy for many patients. Vaccines (conjugated and/or capsular) for encapsulated organisms, such as pneumococcus, meningococcus, and *Haemophilus influenzae* type b, should be administered before splenectomy, and prophylactic oral penicillin V (age <5 yr, 125 mg twice daily; age 5 yr through adulthood, 250 mg twice daily) administered thereafter. Postsplenectomy thrombocytosis is commonly observed, but needs no treatment and usually resolves spontaneously. Partial splenectomy also may be useful in children younger than age 5 yr and can provide some increase in hemoglobin and reduction in the reticulocyte count, with potential maintenance of splenic phagocytic and immune function.

Bader-Meunier B, Gauthier F, Archambaud F, et al: Long-term evaluation of the beneficial effect of subtotal splenectomy for management of hereditary spherocytosis. *Blood* 2001;97:399–403.

Bolton-Maggs PBH, Stevens RF, Dodd NJ, et al: Guidelines for the diagnosis and management of hereditary spherocytosis. *Br J Haematol* 2004;126: 455–474.

Delhommeau F, Cynober T, Schischmanoff PO, et al: Natural history of hereditary spherocytosis during the first year of life. *Blood* 2000;95:393–397.

Eber S, Lux SE: Hereditary spherocytosis: Defects in proteins that connect the membrane skeleton to the lipid bilayer. *Semin Hematol* 2004;41:118–141.

Iolascon A, Perrotta S, Stewart GW: Red cell membrane defects. *Rev Clin Exp Hematol* 2003;7:22–56.

Minkes RK, Lagzdins M, Langer JC, et al: Laparoscopic versus open splenectomy in children. *J Pediatr Surg* 2000;35:699–700.

Chapter 459 ■ Hereditary Elliptocytosis

George B. Segel

Hereditary elliptocytosis is a less common disorder than spherocytosis that also varies markedly in severity. Mild hereditary elliptocytosis produces no symptoms; more severe varieties may result in neonatal poikilocytosis (shape variation) and hemolysis, chronic or sporadic hemolytic anemia, or hereditary pyropoikilocytosis (HPP), which is a severe disorder with microspherocytosis and poikilocytosis. Hereditary elliptocytosis is rare in Western populations; it is more common among West Africans.

ETIOLOGY. Hereditary elliptocytosis is inherited as a dominant disorder. In the rare instances when 2 abnormal alleles are inherited (HPP), the patient exhibits particularly severe hemolytic anemia. Various molecular defects have been described in hereditary elliptocytosis; these produce abnormalities of α- and β-spectrin and defective spectrin heterodimer self-association (see Fig. 458-1). The abnormalities (spectrin mutations) may provide resistance to malarial infection. Such defects in horizontal protein interactions result in gross membrane fragmentation, particularly in homozygous HPP. Less commonly, mutations in protein 4.1 and glycophorin C may produce elliptocytosis.

CLINICAL MANIFESTATIONS. Elliptocytosis may be an incidental finding on a blood film examination and may not be associated with clinically significant hemolysis (see Fig. 458-3*B*). The diagnosis of hereditary elliptocytosis is established by the findings on the blood film, the autosomal dominant inheritance pattern, and the absence of other causes of elliptocytosis, such as deficiencies of iron, folic acid, or vitamin B_{12}. Hemolytic elliptocytosis may produce neonatal jaundice, even though characteristic elliptocytosis may not be evident at that time. The blood of the affected newborn may show bizarre poikilocytes and pyknocytes. Transient augmented fragmentation and hemolysis in the newborn may result from the presence of hemoglobin F that binds poorly to the glycolytic intermediate 2,3-diphosphoglycerate. The increased 2,3-diphosphoglycerate tends to destabilize the spectrin-actin-protein 4.1 complex, leading to membrane instability (see Fig. 458-1). The usual features of a chronic hemolytic process with elliptocytosis are manifested later as anemia, jaundice, splenomegaly, and osseous changes. Cholelithiasis may occur in later childhood; aplastic crises have been reported. The most severe form is HPP, which is characterized by extreme microcytosis (mean corpuscular volume, 50–60 fL/cell), extraordinary variation in cell size and shape, and primarily microspherocytic rather than elliptocytic cells (see Fig. 458-3*C*). These patients usually inherit a mutant spectrin from one parent, who has mild or no elliptocytosis, and a partial spectrin deficiency from the other parent, who is hematologically normal.

Ovalocytes, in contrast to elliptocytes, are less elongated and may reflect a condition known as *Southeast Asian ovalocytosis* (SAO). SAO is associated with an abnormal protein 3, which functions as an anion exchanger. This disorder may produce neonatal hyperbilirubinemia, but causes little hemolysis later. It may offer protection against *Plasmodium falciparum* malaria because normal protein 3 is one of the malarial receptors. Protein 3 as an anion exchanger is also expressed in renal tubular cells and may cause distal renal tubular acidosis in association with SAO.

LABORATORY FINDINGS. The blood film is the most important test to establish hereditary elliptocytosis (see Fig. 458-3*B*). The red blood cells (RBCs) show various degrees of elongation and may actually be rod-shaped. In hereditary elliptocytosis, other abnormal RBC shapes may be present, depending on the severity of hemolysis. They include microcytes, spherocytes, and other poikilocytes. The reticulocyte percentage reflects the severity of hemolysis; erythroid hyperplasia and indirect hyperbilirubinemia may be present. Increased thermal instability is characteristic of HPP; hence, its name. The abnormal spectrin denatures and the cells lyse at 45–46°C instead of the usual 49–50°C. The specific protein abnormality can be established by protein separation and analysis techniques. Molecular defects are defined only in research laboratories.

TREATMENT. If hereditary elliptocytosis represents a morphologic abnormality on the blood film without evident hemolysis, no treatment is necessary. Patients with chronic hemolysis should receive folic acid, 1 mg daily, to prevent secondary folic acid deficiency. Splenectomy decreases the hemolysis and should be considered if the hemoglobin is <10 g/dL and the reticulocyte count is >10%. The RBCs on the blood film may be more abnormal after splenectomy, even though hemoglobin increases and reticulocytes decrease. The hematologic features of SAO do not require treatment beyond the newborn period.

Benet A, Khong TY, Uru A, et al: Placental malaria in women with southeast Asian ovalocytosis. *Am J Trop Med Hyg* 2006;75:597–604.

Gallagher PG: Hereditary elliptocytosis: Spectrin and protein 4.1R. *Semin Hematol* 2004;41:142–164.

Vasuvattakul S, Yenchitsomanus PT, Vachuanichsanong P, et al: Autosomal recessive distal renal tubular acidosis associated with Southeast Asian ovalocytosis. *Kidney Int* 1999;56:1674–1682.

Chapter 460 ■ Hereditary Stomatocytosis

George B. Segel

Hereditary stomatocytosis is a rare condition in which the red blood cells (RBCs) are cup-shaped. On stained blood film, they present a mouthlike slit in place of the usual circular area of central pallor (see Fig. 458-3*D*). Acquired stomatocytosis may be seen in several conditions, especially liver disease. Hereditary stomatocytosis is associated with increased RBC membrane permeability to Na^+ and K^+ and alterations in RBC hydration status. The **overhydrated** or **hydrocytic** variant usually is the most severe. It is associated with diminution of protein 7.2, or "stomatin"; the gene is located on chromosome 9. A defective transcription promoter results in stomatin reduction, which may impair regulation of cation transport. **Dehydrated** hereditary stomatocytosis is the most common type; it is heterogeneous in severity and may be associated with a syndrome of **perinatal edema** and **ascites.** The perinatal edema syndrome is transient and remains unexplained. The stomatin defect also may be seen in more severe cases in patients with the dehydrated type. A 3rd pattern, *cryohydrocytosis,* is the mildest form of stomatocytosis. The RBCs in this condition lyse on cooling in vitro and may be associated with "pseudohyperkalemia" when serum potassium is measured. Severe hemolytic anemia may be associated with hereditary stomatocytosis, but splenectomy is not recommended because it is ineffective; persistent symptomatic thrombocytosis may follow splenectomy when hemolysis is not decreased. Some patients have a life-threatening tendency toward in situ thrombosis after splenectomy because of the abnormal adherence of stomatocytic RBCs to the vascular endothelium in conjunction with the post-splenectomy thrombocytosis.

Delaunay J: The hereditary stomatocytoses: Genetic disorders of the red cell membrane permeability to monovalent cations. *Semin Hematol* 2004;41:165–172.

Delaunay J, Stewart G, Iolascon A: Hereditary dehydrated and overhydrated stomatocytosis: Recent advances. *Curr Opin Hematol* 1999;6:110–114.

Stewart GW, Amess JA, Eber SW, et al: Thrombo-embolic disease after splenectomy for hereditary stomatocytosis. *Br J Haematol* 1997;93:301–310.

Chapter 461 ■ Other Membrane Defects

George B. Segel

PAROXYSMAL NOCTURNAL HEMOGLOBINURIA

ETIOLOGY. Paroxysmal nocturnal hemoglobinuria (PNH) reflects an abnormality of marrow stem cells that affects each blood cell lineage. The disease is not inherited; it is an acquired disorder of hematopoiesis characterized by a defect in proteins of the cell membrane that renders the red blood cells (RBCs) and other cells susceptible to damage by normal plasma complement protein. The deficient membrane-associated proteins include decay-accelerating factor, the C8 binding protein, and other proteins that normally impede complement lysis at various steps. The underlying defect involves the glycolipid anchor that maintains these protective proteins on the cell surface. Various mutations in the *PIGA* gene that are involved in glycosylphosphatidylinositol biosynthesis have been identified in patients with PNH. More than one *PIGA* gene mutation often occurs in an individual patient, suggesting multiclonality. Furthermore, glycosylphosphatidylinositol-deficient cells are found at low frequency in normal persons. This suggests that injury to the normal marrow stem cells provides a selective advantage to the PNH clones in the genesis of this disease.

CLINICAL MANIFESTATIONS. Particularly in children, PNH is a rare disorder, but 26 patients with a mean age of 13 yr (range, 0.8–21.4 yr) were diagnosed at Duke University Medical Center between 1966 and 1991. Approximately 60% of these patients had marrow failure, and the remainder had either intermittent or chronic anemia, often with prominent intravascular hemolysis. Nocturnal and morning hemoglobinuria is a classic finding in adults if hemolysis is worse during sleep. However, chronic hemolysis is more common in PNH, despite its name. In addition to chronic hemolysis, thrombocytopenia and leukopenia are often characteristic. **Thrombosis** and **thromboembolic** phenomena are serious complications that may be related to altered glycoproteins on the platelet surface and resultant platelet activation. Abdominal, back, and head pain may be prominent. Hypoplastic or aplastic **pancytopenia** may precede or follow the onset of PNH; PNH rarely progresses to acute myelogenous leukemia. Among 220 patients of all ages identified in French medical centers from 1950–95, at the time of presentation, 93% had some blood abnormality (including 33% with anemia alone, 17% with anemia and thrombocytopenia, 7% with anemia and neutropenia, and 32% with pancytopenia), 13% had abdominal pain, and 6% had thrombosis. The mortality in PNH is related primarily to the development of aplastic anemia or thrombotic complications. The predicted survival rate for children is 80% at 5 yr, 60% at 10 yr, and 28% at 20 yr.

LABORATORY FINDINGS. The diagnosis of PNH was established classically by a positive result on either the acidified serum hemolysis (Ham) test or the sucrose lysis test. These tests activate the alternative and classic pathways of complement lysis, respectively. Hemosiderinuria is common and reflects chronic intravascular hemolysis. Markedly reduced levels of RBC acetylcholinesterase activity and decay-accelerating factor also are found. **Flow cytometry** is the diagnostic test of choice for PNH. With the use of anti-CD59 for RBCs and anti-CD55 and anti-CD59 for granulocytes, flow cytometry is more sensitive than the classic RBC lysis tests in detecting the reduced glycolipid-bound membrane proteins. Fluorescent aerolysin testing may heighten the sensitivity of detection by binding selectively to glycosylphosphatidylinositol anchors.

TREATMENT. Splenectomy is not indicated. Glucocorticoids, such as prednisone (2 mg/kg/24 hr), have been used to treat acute hemolytic episodes; their dosage should be tapered as soon as the hemolysis abates. Prolonged anticoagulation therapy may be of benefit when thromboses occur; heparin and low molecular weight heparin may inhibit complement-mediated hemolysis. Because of chronic urinary loss of iron as hemosiderin, iron therapy may be necessary. Androgens, such as fluoxymesterone (Halotestin), antithymocyte globulin, cyclosporine, and growth factors, such as erythropoietin and granulocyte colony-stimulating factor, have been used to treat marrow failure. Bone marrow transplantation is successful in treating some cases; nonmyeloablative transplantation may reduce transplant-related mortality and morbidity. Eculizumab, a humanized monoclonal antibody against complement protein C5, stabilizes hemoglobin levels, reduces the number of transfusions, and decreases the rate of hemolysis in treated adults with PNH. Retroviral transfer of the *PIGA* gene restores the glycolipid anchor in cultured cells and may be the basis for future gene therapy.

ACANTHOCYTOSIS

Acanthocytosis is characterized by RBCs with irregular circumferential pointed projections (see Fig. 458-3*E*). This morphologic finding is seen with alterations in the cholesterol/phospholipid ratio in some patients with liver disease and in congenital abetalipoproteinemia associated with malabsorption, neuromuscular abnormalities, and retinitis pigmentosa (see Chapters 86.3 and 629). It also is associated with the rare X-linked McLeod syndrome, which includes absence of the Kx (Kell) antigen, late-onset myopathy, neurologic abnormalities such as chorea, splenomegaly, and hemolysis with acanthocytosis.

Brodsky RA: New insights into paroxysmal nocturnal hemoglobinuria. *Hematology Am Soc Hematol Educ Program* 2006;24–28.

Gold MM, Shifteh K, Bello JA, et al: Chorea–acanthocytosis: A mimicker of Huntington disease. Case report and review of the literature. *Neurologist* 2006;12:327–329.

Hillmen P, Young NS, Shubert J, et al: The complement inhibitor eculizumab in paroxysmal nocturnal hemoglobinuria. *N Engl J Med* 2006;355:1233–1243.

Rosse WF, Nishimura J: Clinical manifestations of paroxysmal nocturnal hemoglobinuria: Present state and future problems. *Int J Hematol* 2003;77:113–120.

Smith LJ: Paroxysmal nocturnal hemoglobinuria. [Review.] *Clin Lab Sci* 2004;17:172–177.

Socie G, Mary JY, de Gramont A, et al: Paroxysmal nocturnal haemoglobinuria: Long-term follow-up and prognostic factors. *Lancet* 1996;348:573–577.

Suenaga K, Kanda Y, Niiya H, et al: Successful application of nonmyeloablative transplantation for paroxysmal nocturnal hemoglobinuria. *Exp Hematol* 2001;29:639–642.

Van den Heuvel-Eibrink MM, Bredius RG, te Winkel ML, et al: Childhood paroxysmal nocturnal hemoglobinuria (PHH): A report of 11 cases in the Netherlands. *Br J Haematol* 2005;128:571–577.

Chapter 462 ■ Hemoglobinopathies

Michael R. DeBaun and Elliott Vichinsky

Hemoglobin is a tetramer consisting of 2 pairs of globin chains. Abnormalities in these proteins are referred to as **hemoglobinopathies.** There are approximately 800 variant hemoglobins. The most common and useful clinical classification of hemoglobinopathies is based on nomenclature associated with alteration of the involved globin chain. Two hemoglobin gene clusters are involved in the production of hemoglobin and are located at the end of the short arm of chromosomes 16 and 11, respectively. Their control is complex, including an upstream locus control region on each respective chromosome as well as an X-linked control site. On chromosome 16, there are 3 genes within the alpha (α) gene cluster: zeta (ζ) and 2 α genes (α_1, α_2). On chromosome 11, there are 5 genes within the beta (β) gene cluster: epsilon (ε), delta (δ), beta (β), and 2 gamma (γ) genes. The order of gene expression within each cluster roughly follows the order of expression during the embryonic period, the fetal period, and eventually childhood. After 8 wk of fetal life, the embryonic hemoglobins are formed: Gower-1 ($\zeta_2\varepsilon_2$), Gower-2 ($\alpha_2\varepsilon_2$), and Portland ($\zeta_2\gamma_2$). At 9 wk of fetal life, the major hemoglobin (Hb) is Hb F ($\alpha_2\gamma_2$). At approximately 1 mo of fetal life, Hb A ($\alpha_2\beta_2$) appears, but does not become the dominant hemoglobin until after birth, when Hb F levels start to decline. A minor hemoglobin, Hb A_2 ($\alpha_2\delta_2$) appears shortly before birth and remains at a low level after birth. The final hemoglobin distribution pattern that occurs in childhood is not achieved until at least 6 mo of age, and sometimes later. The normal hemoglobin pattern is ≥95% Hb A, ≤3.5 Hb A_2, and <2.5% Hb F.

462.1 • Sickle Cell Disease

Hemoglobin S (Hb S) is the result of a single base pair change, thymine for adenine, at the 6th codon of the β-globin gene. This change encodes valine instead of glutamine in the 6th position in the β-globin molecule. **Sickle cell anemia,** homozygous Hb S, occurs when both β-globin genes have the sickle cell mutation. **Sickle cell disease** refers not only to individuals with sickle cell anemia, but also to compound heterozygotes where one β-globin gene mutation includes the sickle cell mutation and the 2nd β-globin includes a gene mutation in the β-globin gene other than the sickle cell mutation, such as mutations associated with Hb C, Hb β-thalassemia, Hb D, and Hb O Arab. In sickle cell anemia, Hb S is commonly as high as 90% of the total hemoglobin. In sickle cell disease, Hb S is >50% of all hemoglobin.

In the U.S., sickle cell disease is the most common genetic disease identified through the state-mandated newborn screening program, occurring in 1/2,647 births, exceeding the incidence of primary congenital hypothyroidism (1/3,000), cystic fibrosis (1/3,900), and clinically significant hyperphenylalaninemia (1/14,000). Sickle cell disease in the U.S. occurs among African-Americans at a rate of 1/396 births; among Hispanics at a rate of 1/36,000 births; among those of Middle Eastern descent no cases were identified among 22,000 screened; and among Asian Indians at a rate of 1/16,000 screened.

Children with sickle cell disease should be followed by experts in the management of this disease, most often by pediatric hematologists. Comprehensive medical care, with evidence-based strategies delivered by experts in sickle cell disease and anticipatory guidance of the parents about the most common complications, has dramatically decreased sickle cell disease–related mortality and morbidity over the last 20 yr. Medical care provided by a pediatric hematologist is associated with decreased frequency of emergency department visits and shorter hospital stay when compared with patients who were not seen by a hematologist within the last yr. When available, children with sickle cell disease should be followed by experts in sickle cell disease or by a physician familiar with the medical care of children with the disease and co-managed with a pediatric hematologist.

SICKLE CELL ANEMIA (HOMOZYGOUS HEMOGLOBIN S) OR S β-THALASSEMIA

CLINICAL MANIFESTATIONS AND TREATMENT. Infants with sickle cell anemia have abnormal immune function. As early as 6 mo of age, some children, and by 5 yr of age, most children have functional asplenia. Bacterial sepsis is one of the greatest causes of morbidity and mortality in this patient population. Children with sickle cell anemia also have deficient levels of serum opsonins of the alternate complement pathway against pneumococci. Regardless of age, all patients with sickle cell anemia are at increased risk for infection and death as a result of bacterial infection, particularly with encapsulated organisms, such as *Streptococcus pneumoniae* (see Chapter 181) and *Haemophilus influenzae* type B (see Chapter 192). Children with sickle cell anemia should receive prophylactic oral penicillin VK at least until 5 yr of age (125 mg twice daily up to age 3 yr, then 250 mg twice daily). No established guidelines exist for penicillin prophylaxis beyond 5 yr of age. Some clinicians continue penicillin prophylaxis, whereas others recommend discontinuation. Continuation of penicillin prophylaxis should be considered for children beyond 5 yr of age when there is a previous diagnosis of pneumococcal infection due to the increased risk of a recurrent infection. An alternative for children who are allergic to penicillin is erythromycin ethyl succinate 10 mg/kg twice daily. In addition to penicillin prophylaxis, routine childhood immunizations and annual administration of influenza vaccine are highly recommended.

Human parvovirus B19 (see Chapter 248) poses a unique threat for patients with sickle cell anemia because such infections limit the production of reticulocytes. Any child with reticulocytopenia should be considered as having parvovirus B19 until proven otherwise. Acute infection with parvovirus B19 is usually associated with red cell aplasia (**aplastic episode**), fever, and pain, in addition to splenic sequestration, acute chest syndrome (ACS), glomerulonephritis, and stroke. **Treatment** requires packed red blood cell transfusions for hemodynamic instability.

The **management of fever** in a child with sickle cell anemia is a medical emergency that requires prompt medical evaluation and delivery of antibiotics because of the high risk of bacterial infection and the concomitant high fatality rate when infected. Several clinical management strategies have been developed, ranging from admitting all patients with a fever for IV antimicrobial therapy to administering a parenteral long-acting 3rd-generation cephalosporin in an outpatient setting to clinically well-appearing febrile patients without any of the previous established risk factors for bacteremia (Table 462-1). Given the observation that the average time for a positive pathogenic blood culture is <20 hr in children with sickle cell anemia, admission for 24 hr is probably the most prudent strategy for children of families with a history of poor compliance or without a telephone or transportation. For patients with a positive blood culture, pathogen-specific therapy (1st empirically, then based on sensitivities) must be initiated. If *Salmonella* or *Staphylococcus* bacteremia occurs, strong consideration should be given to evaluation of osteomyelitis with a bone scan or an MRI, given the higher risk of osteomyelitis in children with sickle cell anemia compared with the general population.

Dactylitis, often referred to as *hand-foot syndrome,* is frequently the 1st manifestation of pain in children with sickle cell anemia, occurring in 50% of children by 2 yr of age. Dactylitis often presents with symmetric swelling of the hands and/or feet (Fig. 462-1). Unilateral dactylitis can be confused with osteomyelitis and requires careful consideration, with ongoing evaluation, because treatment of the former requires palliation with pain medication, often acetaminophen with codeine, whereas osteomyelitis requires at least a 4–6 wk course of IV antibiotics (see Chapter 683).

TABLE 462-1. Clinical Factors Associated with Increased Risk of Bacteremia Requiring Admission in Febrile Children with Sickle Cell Disease
Seriously ill appearance
Hypotension (systolic blood pressure of <70 mm Hg at 1 yr of age or <70 mm Hg + 2 × the age in yr for older children)
Poor perfusion (capillary refill time > 4 sec)
Temperature > 40.0°C (104°F)
A corrected white cell count >30,000 mm^3 or <500 mm^3
Platelet count <100,000 mm^3
History of pneumococcal sepsis
Severe pain
Dehydration (poor skin turgor, dry mucous membranes, history of poor fluid intake, or decreased output of urine)
Infiltration of a segment or a larger portion of the lung
Hemoglobin level <5.0 g dL

Adapted from Wilimas JA, Flynn PM, Harris S, et al: A randomized study of outpatient treatment with ceftriaxone for selected febrile children with sickle cell disease. *N Engl J Med* 1993;329:472–476.

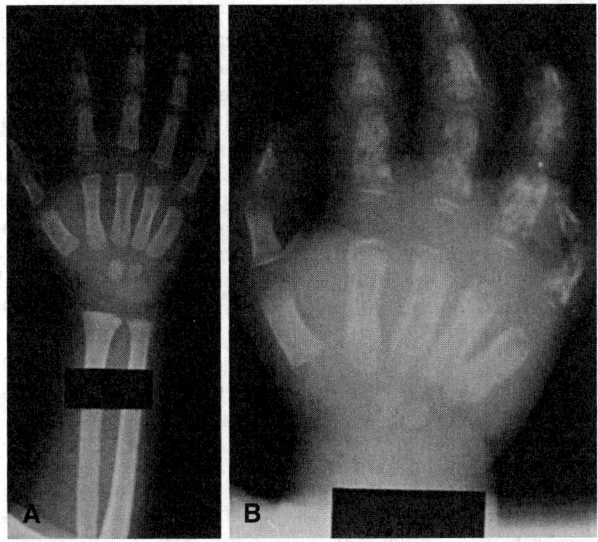

Figure 462-1. Roentgenograms of an infant with sickle cell anemia and acute dactylitis. *A,* The bones appear normal at the onset of the episode. *B,* Destructive changes and periosteal reaction are evident 2 wk later.

Acute **splenic sequestration** is a life-threatening complication occurring primarily in infants, and may occur as early as 5 wk of age. Approximately 30% of children with sickle cell anemia have significant splenic sequestration episodes; although the presentation may be variable, a significant percentage of cases can be fatal. The etiology of splenic sequestration episodes is unknown. Clinically, these events are associated with engorgement of the spleen, with a subsequent increase in spleen size, evidence of hypovolemia, and a decline in hemoglobin of at least 2.0 g/dL from baseline. Reticulocytosis and a decrease in the platelet count may be present. These events can be accompanied by upper respiratory tract infections, bacteremia, or viral infection. **Treatment** is early intervention and maintenance of hemodynamic stability that may require either isotonic fluid or blood transfusions. Repeated episodes of splenic sequestration are common, occurring in approximately 50% of patients. The majority of recurrent events occur within 6 mo of the previous event. Prophylactic splenectomy performed after the acute episode has resolved is the only effective strategy for prevention of future life-threatening episodes. Parents can be taught to palpate the spleen when the child appears ill and to seek medical care if it is enlarged. Blood transfusion therapy has been used to prevent subsequent episodes, but evidence indicates that this strategy does not reduce the risk of recurrent splenic sequestration episodes compared with no treatment.

The cardinal clinical feature of sickle cell anemia is pain from **vaso-occlusive episode.** No written definition can describe the visual picture of a child who has sickle cell anemia and is in pain. The pain is characterized as unremitting discomfort that may occur in any part of the body, but most often occurs in the chest, abdomen, or extremities. These painful episodes are often abrupt and can disrupt daily life activities and cause anguish for children and their families. The only measure of the intensity of pain is the patient. Although pain scales have proven useful for some children, others require pre-negotiated activities that determine when opioid therapy should be initiated, decreased, or discontinued. Sleeping through the night might be an indication for decreasing the pain medication by 20% the next morning. The majority of painful episodes in patients with sickle cell anemia are managed at home with comfort measures (heating blanket, relaxation techniques, massage) and pain medication. A patient with sickle cell anemia usually has approximately 1 painful episode per yr that requires medical attention.

The pathogenesis of pain is disruption of blood flow in the microvasculature by sickle cells, resulting in tissue ischemia. Precipitating causes of painful episodes can include physical stress, infection, dehydration, hypoxia, local or systemic acidosis, exposure to cold, and swimming in non-heated water for prolonged periods. Successful treatment of painful episodes requires education of both the parents and the patient regarding the symptoms and management strategy. Given the absence of any reliable objective laboratory or clinical parameter associated with pain, trust between the patient and the treating physician is paramount to a successful clinical management strategy. Specific therapies for pain vary, but generally include the use of acetaminophen or a nonsteroidal agent early in the course of pain, followed by acetaminophen with codeine and short- or long-acting oral opioids, or hospitalization with IV administration of morphine or morphine derivatives (see Chapter 77). The incremental increase and decrease in the use of medication to relieve pain roughly parallels the 8 phases associated with a chronology of pain and comfort (Table 462-2). In phase 1 (baseline), the patient is free of pain. Phase 2 involves no pain, but the child may show prodromal signs and symptoms of painful episodes, such as scleral

TABLE 462-2. Summary of the Chronology of Pain in Children with Sickle Cell Disease

PHASE	PAIN CHARACTERISTICS	SUGGESTED COMFORT MEASURES USED
1 (Baseline)	No vaso-occlusive pain. Pain or complications may be present, such as that connected with avascular necrosis of the hip.	No comfort measures are used.
2 (Pre-pain)	No vaso-occlusive pain. Pain or complications may be present, and prodromal signs of an impending vaso-occlusive episode may appear, e.g., "yellow eyes" and/or fatigue.	Comfort measures are used. Caregivers may encourage the child to increase fluids.
3 (Pain start point)	First signs of vaso-occlusive pain appear, usually in mild form.	A mild oral analgesic is often given and fluids are increased. The child usually maintains normal activities.
4 (Pain acceleration)	Intensity of pain increases from mild to moderate. Some children may skip this level or move quickly from phase 3 to phase 5.	Stronger oral analgesics are given. Rubbing, heat, or other activities are often used. Child usually stays in school until the pain becomes more severe, then stays home and limits activities. The child is usually in bed.
5 (Peak pain experience)	Pain accelerates to high moderate or severe levels and plateaus. Pain may remain elevated for an extended period. The child's appearance, behavior, and mood are significantly different from normal.	Oral analgesics are given around the clock at home. A combination of comfort measures is used. The family may avoid going to the hospital. If pain is very distressing to the child, the parent will take the child to the hospital. After the child enters the hospital, families often turn over comforting activities to health care providers and wait to see if the analgesics work. Family caregivers are often tired from the effort of caring for the child for several days with little or no rest.
6 (Pain decrease start point)	Pain finally begins to decrease in intensity from the peak pain level.	Family caregivers again become active in comforting the child, but not as intensely as during phases 4 and 5.
7 (Steady pain decline)	Pain decreases more rapidly and becomes more tolerable for the child. The child and family are more relaxed.	Health care providers begin to wean the child from the IV analgesic. Oral opioids are given, and discharge planning is started. Children may be discharged before they are pain-free
8 (Pain resolution)	Pain intensity is at a tolerable level, and discharge is imminent. The child looks and acts like his or her "normal" self. Mood improves.	The child may receive oral analgesics.

Adapted from Beyer JE, Simmons LE, Woods GM, et al: A Chronology of pain and comfort in children with sickle cell disease. *Arch Pediatr Adolesc Med* 1999;153:913–920.

icterus or fatigue. During this phase, comfort measures can be used. Phases 3–7 involve increasing and then decreasing levels of pain, including the pain start point, phase 3, when acetaminophen with codeine or nonsteroidal inflammatory agents may be used. Pain acceleration, phase 4, is often associated with administering short- or long-acting morphine derivatives. Peak pain experience, phase 5, is the point at which IV morphine may be started and the patient is often admitted to the hospital. The average hospital stay for children admitted for pain is 3–5 days. The pain starts to decrease during phases 6 and 7, and the pain medication is slowly decreased. In general, decreasing the opioid medication by 20% of the starting dose should occur during the early morning hours, when the caretaker, physician, or house staff is available to assess the effect of the change in dose. Decreasing opioid administration in the afternoon or late at night is not advisable because pain is often worse at night and the primary health care provider is often not available to assess the effect of the change in dose administration. In phase 8, pain resolution, the pain decreases to a manageable level so that the child can be discharged from the hospital. The American Pain Society recommendations are comprehensive and represent a starting point for treating pain (*http://www.ampainsoc.org/pub/sc.htm*).

Several myths exist about the treatment of pain in sickle cell anemia. The concept that painful episodes in children should be managed without opioids is without foundation and results in unwarranted suffering on the part of the patient. There is no evidence that blood transfusion therapy during an existing painful episode decreases the intensity or duration of the episode. Blood transfusion should be reserved for patients who have a decrease in hemoglobin, resulting in hemodynamic compromise, and for patients with respiratory distress or a dropping hemoglobin concentration with no expectation that a safe nadir will be reached. IV hydration does not relieve or prevent pain and is appropriate when the patient is dehydrated or is unable to drink as a result of severe pain. Concern about opioid dependency in children with sickle cell anemia must never be used as a reason not to treat a child in pain. Patients with multiple painful episodes requiring hospitalization within 1 yr or those whose pain episodes require hospital stays of longer than 7 days should be evaluated for comorbidities and psychosocial stressors that may contribute to the frequency or duration of pain.

Hydroxyurea, a myelosuppressive agent, is the only effective drug proven to reduce the frequency of painful episodes. Hydroxyurea raises the level of Hb F and the hemoglobin level. Hydroxyurea usually decreases the rate of painful episodes by 50%; it also decreases the rate of ACS episodes and blood transfusions by approximately 50% in adults. In children with sickle cell anemia, only a safety and feasibility trial of hydroxyurea has been conducted. This study demonstrated that hydroxyurea was safe and well tolerated in children older than 5 yr of age. No clinical adverse events were identified. The primary laboratory toxicities were limited to myelosuppression, which was reversed on cessation of the drug. Given the short-term safety profile of hydroxyurea in children and its established efficacy in adults, hydroxyurea is commonly used in children with multiple painful episodes. Hydroxyurea treatment begun in infancy may preserve splenic function, improve growth, and reduce the incidence of ACS. The long-term toxicity associated with hydroxyurea in children has not been established, and there are theoretical concerns about the potential risk of leukemia and unknown complications. The typical starting dose of hydroxyurea is 15–20 mg/kg daily, with an increase in dose every 8 wk of 2.5–5.0 mg/kg, if no toxicities occur, up to a maximum dose of 35 mg/kg. The therapeutic effect of hydroxyurea may require several mo of treatment. Monitoring children who are receiving hydroxyurea is labor-intensive, with initial visits every 2 wk and then monthly, after a therapeutic dose has been identified. Close monitoring of the patient requires a commitment by the parents and the patient as well as diligence by a physician to monitor toxicity.

Priapism, a common problem in sickle cell anemia, is an involuntary penile erection lasting longer than 30 min. The persistence of a painful erection beyond several hours is suggestive of a diagnosis of priapism. Although typically the ventral portion of the penis and the glans are not involved, if they are involved, urology consultation should occur, based on the poor prognosis for spontaneous resolution. Priapism occurs in 2 patterns, **stuttering** and **refractory,** with both types occurring in patients from early childhood to adulthood. No formal definitions have been established for these terms, but generally, *stuttering priapism* is defined as self-limiting intermittent bouts of priapism with several episodes over a defined period. *Refractory priapism* is defined as prolonged priapism beyond several hours. Approximately 20% of patients 5–20 yr of age report having at least 1 episode of priapism lasting at least 30 min. The majority of episodes occur between 3 A.M. and 9 A.M. The mean age at the initial episode is 12 yr, the mean number of episodes per patient is approximately 16, and the mean duration of an episode is approximately 2 hr. The actuarial probability of a patient experiencing priapism is approximately 90% by 20 yr of age. The optimal **treatment** is unknown, but treatment strategies can be divided into acute treatment and preventive therapy. For acute treatment of priapism, supported therapy, such as a sitz bath or pain medication, is commonly used. If the priapism lasts longer than 4 hr, then aspiration of blood from the corpora cavernosa, followed by irrigation with dilute epinephrine, is effective in producing immediate and sustained detumescence. Urology consultation is required to initiate this procedure with appropriate hematology consultation. Although blood transfusion therapy (either simple or exchange) has been advocated for acute treatment of priapism, limited data support this approach, and some evidence suggests that exchange transfusion therapy is not effective in achieving detumescence. For the prevention of recurrent priapism, **hydroxyurea** appears to have promise; however, no trial has been undertaken to demonstrate the benefit of hydroxyurea vs no therapy. The long-term effect of recurrent or prolonged priapism episodes in prepubertal children is not known, but in older patients, it may result in sexual dysfunction.

Neurologic complications associated with sickle cell anemia are varied and complex. Among children with sickle cell anemia, approximately 11% and 20% will have either **overt** or **silent** strokes, respectively, before their 18th birthday. An *overt stroke* is defined as a focal neurologic deficit that lasts >24 hr; this definition is outdated because many individuals with sickle cell anemia are treated with blood therapy that may hasten their recovery to baseline. A more functional definition is the presence of a focal neurologic deficit that lasts >24 hr and/or a lesion on the T2 weighted MRI of the brain indicative of a cerebral infarct and corresponding with the focal neurologic deficit (Fig. 462-2). A *silent stroke* is the absence of a focal neurologic deficit lasting >24 hr in the presence of a lesion on T2 weighted MRI indicative of a cerebral infarct. Presentation of strokes may occur as young as 1 yr of age. Stroke may run in particular families. Other neurologic complications include headaches that may or may not be related to sickle cell anemia, seizures, cerebral venous thrombosis, and reversible posterior leukoencephalopathy syndrome (RPLS).

For patients who present with an acute focal neurologic deficit, a prompt pediatric neurologic evaluation is recommended. **Treatment** of stroke includes oxygen administration to maintain oxygen saturation at >96% and simple blood transfusion therapy as quickly and safely as possible with a goal of transfusion within 1 hr of presentation, with a goal of increasing the hemoglobin to a maximum of 11.0 g/dL. Exceeding this hemoglobin threshold may limit oxygen delivery to the brain because hyperviscosity of the blood may decrease oxygen delivery. Subsequently, strong consideration should be given to prompt treatment with an exchange transfusion, either manually or with erythrocytapheresis, to reduce Hb S to at least <50%, if not 30%. CT to exclude

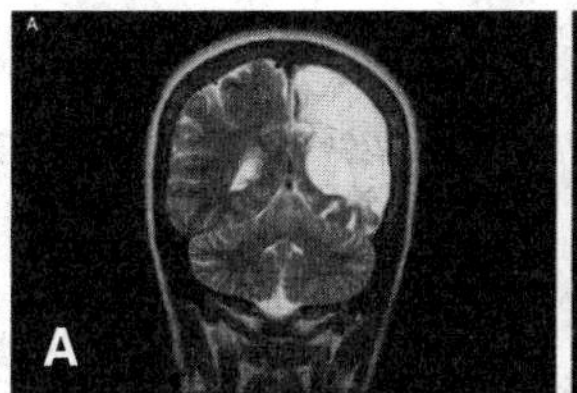

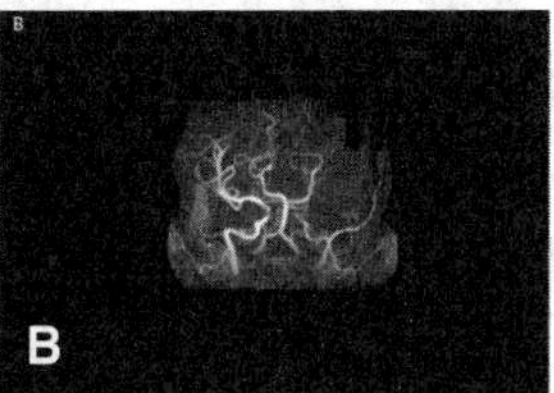

Figure 462-2. T2 weighted MRI and magnetic resonance angiography (MRA) of the brain. *A*, T2 weighted MRI shows remote infarction of the territories of the left anterior cerebral artery and middle cerebral artery. *B*, MRA shows occlusion of the left internal carotid artery siphon distal to the takeoff of the ophthalmic artery.

cerebral hemorrhage should be done as soon as possible; if available, MRI of the brain with diffusion-weighted imaging should be done to distinguish between ischemic infarcts and RPLS (Fig. 462-3). Magnetic resonance venography is also useful because of the possibility of cerebral venous thrombosis. The clinical presentation of RPLS or venous thrombosis may mimic that of a stroke. The diagnosis of either RPLS or cerebral venous thrombosis will result in a different course of treatment than a stroke. For both RPLS and cerebral venous thrombosis, the optimal management has not been defined in patients with sickle cell anemia; intervention requires consultation with a pediatric neurologist and a hematologist for case management.

Primary prevention of strokes can be accomplished by transcranial Doppler (TCD) assessment of the blood velocity in the terminal portion of the internal carotid and the proximal portion of the middle cerebral artery. In patients with a time-averaged mean maximum blood flow velocity of ≥200 cm/sec, the transfusion threshold, prophylactic blood transfusion therapy is instituted to maintain Hb S levels of <30%. This strategy results in an 85% reduction in the rate of overt strokes. Once initiated, patients may receive this therapy for an indefinite period. The optimal age to start and end TCD measurement in children with sickle cell anemia has not been established; many hematologists initiate TCD screening at 2–3 yr of age, the age at which most children do not require sedation. If a time-averaged mean maximum measurement is <200 cm/sec, but ≥180 cm/sec, a conditional threshold, then a repeat measurement is suggested within several months because of the high rate of converting to a blood velocity of >200 cm/sec.

Secondary prevention of stroke is accomplished by blood transfusion therapy aimed at maintaining the maximum Hb S concentration at <30% in the 1st 2 yr after a stroke and <50% thereafter. Despite regular blood transfusion therapy, approximately 20% of patients have a 2nd stroke and 30% have a 3rd stroke. The major toxic effect of blood transfusion therapy is excessive iron stores that can result in irreversible organ damage and premature death. A unit of blood contains approximately 200 mg of iron. In the U.S., the most commonly used iron chelating agent was deferoxamine. Optimal administration is 40 mg/kg subcutaneously for 5–7 nights for 10 hr. An oral chelating agent (deferasirox) is approved by the U.S. Food and Drug Administration for patients >2 yr of age with transfusional hemosiderosis. The initial dose of 20 mg/kg/day is adjusted after 3–6 mo of therapy, based on the serum ferritin level (if ferritin is <500, the drug may be temporarily stopped). Three methods of blood transfusion therapy are available: erythrocytapheresis, manual exchange transfusion (phlebotomy of a set amount of blood followed by rapid administration of blood), and simple transfusion. Of these methods **erythrocytapheresis** is the preferred method, followed by manual exchange transfusion. Simple transfusion therapy is less preferable because the strategy results in the highest net positive iron balance after the procedure. Despite being the preferred method, erythrocytapheresis is less frequently performed because of the requirement for the necessary technical expertise, large venous access, and access to a pheresis machine. For patients who either will not or cannot continue blood transfusion therapy to prevent subsequent strokes, hydroxyurea therapy may be a reasonable alternative. The efficacy and toxicity of hydroxyurea as an option for secondary stroke prevention must be established in a newly initiated clinical trial before blood transfusion therapy is replaced with hydroxyurea for children with strokes. Human leukocyte antigen (HLA)–matched sibling donor bone marrow transplant is a reasonable approach for patients with strokes, although only a few children have suitable donors.

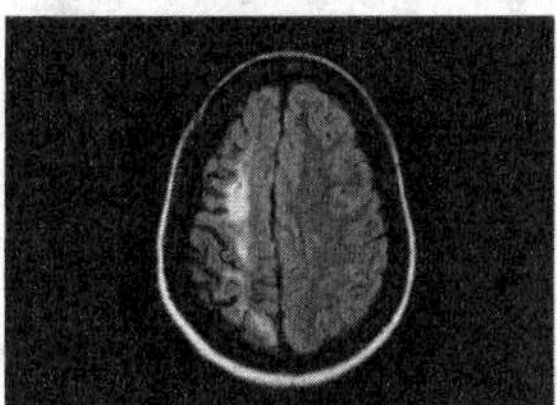

Figure 462-3. Fast fluid-attenuated inversion-recovery–sequence (FLAIR) MRI of the brain showing a right hemisphere border-zone cerebral infarction in a child with sickle cell anemia. (From Switzer JA, Hess DC, Nichols F, et al: Pathophysiology and treatment of stoke in sickle-cell disease: Present and future. *Lancet Neurol* 2006;5:501–512.)

Lung disease in children with sickle cell anemia is the 2nd most common reason for admission to the hospital and a common cause of death. **Acute chest syndrome (ACS)** is a constellation of findings including a new radiodensity on chest radiograph, fever, respiratory distress, and pain that often occurs in the chest, but may include only the back and/or the abdomen. Even when no respiratory symptoms are present, all patients with fever should receive a chest radiograph to identify ACS because clinical examination alone is insufficient to identify patients with new radiodensities on chest radiograph; in addition, early detection of ACS will alter the clinical management. The radiographic findings in ACS are variable and can progress quite rapidly. Radiographs may show single-lobe involvement, most often the left lower lobe, and when multiple lobes are involved, usually both lower lobes are affected. Pleural effusions, either unilateral or bilateral, may not be present initially (or may be minimal in size), but may progress rapidly to a total whiteout (Fig. 462-4).

Given the clinical overlap between ACS and common pulmonary complications, such as bronchiolitis, asthma (which is also common in children with sickle cell anemia), and pneumonia, a wide range of therapeutic strategies have been used. **Treatment** of ACS includes oxygen administration and simple or exchange blood transfusion therapy (manual or automated). Oxygen should be administered when the oxygen saturation is <90%. The decision as to when to give blood and whether simple or exchange transfusion should be used is less clearly defined. Blood transfusion is given when at least one of the following clinical features is present: decreasing oxygen saturation; increasing work of breathing; rapid change in respiratory effort, with or without a worsening chest radiograph; or a history of severe ACS requiring admission to the intensive care unit.

The majority of patients with ACS do not have an identifiable cause, although infection is believed to be the most common identifiable cause. The most common illness preceding ACS is a painful episode requiring opioids. The type of opioids (morphine is a greater risk than nalbuphine hydrochloride) and the route of administration of the opioid (oral is a greater risk than IV) is directly associated with an increase in the risk of ACS. Under no circumstance should opioid administration be limited because of concern about preventing ACS; rather, care must be taken to prevent ACS from occurring. In patients with chest pain, regular use of an **incentive spirometer** can significantly reduce the fre-

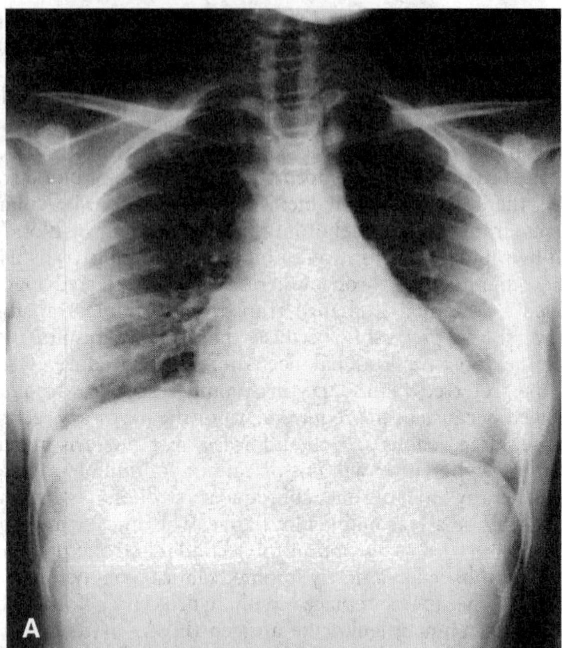

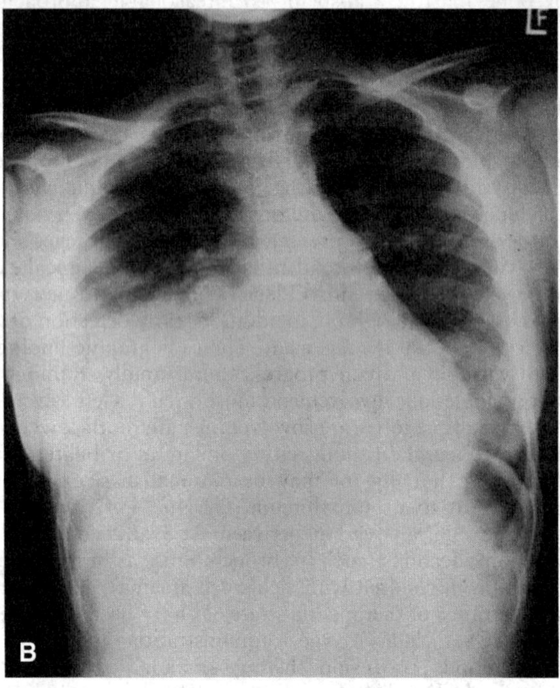

Figure 462-4. Probable pulmonary infarction in a 15 yr old patient with sickle cell anemia. *A*, Frontal radiograph shows consolidation and a small pleural effusion posteriorly in the right lower lobe. *B*, Radiograph obtained <24 hr later shows massive right middle and lower lobe consolidation and effusion. No organisms could be cultured. The diagnosis of probable pulmonary infarction was established clinically. (Courtesy of Dr. Thomas L. Slovis, Children's Hospital of Michigan, Detroit, MI. From Kuhn JP, Slovis TL, Haller JO: *Caffey's Pediatric Diagnostic Imaging,* Vol. 1, 10th ed. Philadelphia, Mosby, 2004, p 1087.)

quency of subsequent episodes of acute chest pain; the use of 10–12 breaths every 2 hr is an effective method to prevent ACS. Fat emboli have also been implicated as a cause of ACS. Fat emboli are believed to arise from infarcted bone marrow, and they can be life-threatening if large amounts are released to the lungs.

As a result of the clinical overlap between pneumonia and ACS, all episodes should be treated promptly with antimicrobial therapy that includes at least a macrolide and a 3rd-generation cephalosporin to treat the most common pathogens associated with ACS *(S. pneumoniae, Mycoplasma pneumoniae, Chlamydia pneumoniae)*. A previous diagnosis of asthma should prompt treatment with steroids and bronchodilators, even when the patient does not have evidence of wheezing (Table 462-3).

Pulmonary hypertension is a major risk factor for death in adults with sickle cell anemia. As many as 60% of adults with sickle cell anemia may have clinically unsuspected obliterative pulmonary vascular disease. Pulmonary hypertension has also been reported in other chronic hemolytic anemias (thalassemia, hereditary spherocytosis, paroxysmal nocturnal hemoglobinuria), suggesting that chronic hemolysis itself contributes to the pulmonary vascular changes, perhaps through reduced nitric oxide availability, independently of pulmonary vaso-occlusive episodes. The natural history of pulmonary hypertension in children with sickle cell anemia is unknown; therefore, the optimal diagnostic and therapeutic strategy for pulmonary hypertension has not been identified. Elevated levels of N-terminal pro-brain natriuretic peptide is associated with hemolysis-related pulmonary hypertension in adults with sickle cell anemia. Inhaled nitric oxide treatment of vaso-occlusive crisis may have a role in managing pulmonary hypertension.

Renal disease in patients with sickle cell anemia is a major comorbid condition that can lead to premature death. Seven sickle cell anemia nephropathies have been identified: (1) gross hematuria, (2) papillary necrosis, (3) nephrotic syndrome, (4) renal infarction, (5) hyposthenuria, (6) pyelonephritis, and (7) renal medullary carcinoma. The presentation of these entities may include hematuria, proteinuria, renal insufficiency, concentrating defects, or hypertension. Angiotensin-converting enzyme inhibitors are beneficial in the management of patients with proteinuria. Suspicion of renal medullary carcinoma, an aggressive malignant epithelial neoplasm, is important because most patients present with late-stage disseminated disease that responds poorly to chemotherapy and radiation therapy.

As with any child with a chronic illness, good health maintenance must include psychologic and social assessment. Ongoing evaluation of the family unit and the resources available to cope with a chronic illness are critical for optimal management. Children with sickle cell anemia are at great risk for academic failure and have a poor high school graduation rate (approximately 20%); approximately ⅓ of children with sickle cell anemia have

TABLE 462-3. Overall Strategies for the Management of Acute Chest Syndrome

PREVENTION
Incentive spirometry and periodic ambulation in patients admitted for vaso-occlusive crises, surgery, or febrile episodes
Watchful waiting in any hospitalized child or adult with sickle cell disease (pulse oximetry monitoring and frequent respiratory assessments)
Avoidance of overhydration
Intense education and optimum care of patients with sickle cell anemia with asthma

DIAGNOSTIC TESTING AND LABORATORY MONITORING
Blood cultures
Nasopharyngeal samples for viral culture (respiratory syncytial virus, influenza)
Blood counts every day and appropriate chemistries
Continuous pulse oximetry
Chest radiographs

TREATMENT
Blood transfusion (simple or exchange)
Supplemental O_2 for drop in pulse oximetry by 4% over baseline, or values <90%
Empirical antibiotics (cephalosporin and macrolide)
Continued respiratory therapy (incentive spirometry and chest physiotherapy as necessary)
Bronchodilators and steroids for patients with asthma
Optimum pain control and fluid management

had cerebral infarcts, either silent or overt strokes. Children with cerebral infarcts require ongoing cognitive and school performance assessment so that educational resources can be directed to optimize educational attainment. Relevant support groups and attendance at group activities, such as camps for children with sickle cell anemia, may be of direct benefit for improving self-esteem and establishing peer relationships.

In addition to the previously mentioned organ dysfunctions, patients with sickle cell anemia can have other significant complications. These complications include sickle cell retinopathy, delayed onset of puberty, avascular necrosis of the femoral head and humerus, and leg ulcers. Optimal treatment of each of these entities has not been determined, and individual management requires consultation with the disease-specific specialist, a hematologist, and the primary care physician.

Surgical preparation for children with sickle cell anemia requires a coordinated effort between the hematologist, surgeon, and primary care provider. ACS and pain are the 2 most common postoperative complications, with the former being a significant risk factor for postoperative death. Blood transfusion before surgery for children with sickle cell anemia designed to raise the hemoglobin level preoperatively to 10.0 g/dL is desirable; however, achieving a level of at least 10.0 g/dL is not necessary for a child to benefit from a simple transfusion. When a child is being prepared for surgery with a simple blood transfusion, caution must be used to avoid elevating the hemoglobin beyond 10.5 g/dL because of the risk of hyperviscous syndrome. Exchange transfusion before surgery is of no greater benefit than simple blood transfusion therapy and carries significantly higher risk of red blood cell alloimmunization.

DIAGNOSIS OF SICKLE CELL DISEASE. Virtually all states in the U.S. have instituted mandatory newborn screening program for sickle cell disease. Such programs identify newborns with the disease, provide prompt diagnosis and anticipatory guidance for the parents, and make possible the initiation of treatment with penicillin before 4 mo of age.

The most commonly used procedures for newborn diagnosis include thin-layer/isoelectric focusing and high-performance liquid chromatography. A 2-step system is recommended, in which all initially abnormal screens are retested during the 1st clinical visit and again after 6 mo of age to determine the final hemoglobin phenotype. A complete blood cell count as well as hemoglobin analysis is recommended on both parents to confirm the diagnosis and provide an opportunity for genetic counseling. In affected patients, the red blood cell morphology after 3–6 mo of life is helpful for sickle cell disease and other hemoglobinopathies (see Fig. 462-3). Table 462-4 describes the initial hemoglobin phenotype at birth, with the corresponding hemoglobinopathy, baseline hemoglobin range, and requirement for a hematologist.

Newborn screening programs 1st report the hemoglobin with the greatest quantity, followed by the other hemoglobins in decreasing quantity. In newborns with a hemoglobin analysis consistent with a diagnosis of sickle cell disease, the FS pattern is supportive of Hb SS, Hb hereditary persistent fetal hemoglobin (Hb S/β^0). The FSA pattern is supportive of the diagnosis of Hb S/β^+. The diagnosis of Hb S/β^+ is confirmed if at least 50% of hemoglobin is Hb S, Hb A is present, and an elevated amount of Hb A_2 is present (typically >3.5%). In newborns with a hemoglobin analysis of FSC, the pattern is supportive of a diagnosis of Hb SC. In newborns with a hemoglobin analysis of FAS, the pattern is supportive of a diagnosis of Hb AS (**sickle cell trait**). A newborn with a hemoglobin analysis of AFS may have been transfused with red blood cells before the laboratory test because the amount of Hb A is greater than the amount of Hb F, or an error was made. The patient may have either sickle cell disease (Hb SS, or Hb S/β^+) or sickle cell trait, and should be given penicillin prophylaxis until the final diagnosis can be determined.

TABLE 462-4. Various Newborn Sickle Cell Disease Screening Results with Baseline Hemoglobin and Requirement for Pediatric Hematologist or Expert in the Care of Sickle Cell Disease

NEWBORN SCREENING RESULTS: SICKLE CELL DISEASE	POSSIBLE HEMOGLOBIN PHENOTYPE*	BASELINE HEMOGLOBIN: RANGE	EXPERTISE IN HEMATOLOGY CARE REQUIRED
FS	SCD-SS	6–11 g/dL	Yes
	SCD-S/β^0 thal	6–10 g/dL	Yes
	SCD-S/β^+ thal	9–12 g/dL	Yes
	SCD-S/$\delta\beta^-$ thal	10–12 g/dL	Yes
	S HPFH	12–14 g/dL	Yes
FSC	SCD-SC	10–15 g/dL	Yes
FSA	SCD-S/β^0 thal	6–10 g/dL	Yes
FS other	SCD-SD, SO^{Arab}, SC^{Harlem}, S Lepare	6–10 g/dL, 6–9 g/dL, 7–13 g/dL	Yes
AFS	SCD-SS, SCD-S/β^+ thal, SCD-S/β^0 thal (impossible to determine the diagnosis because the infant received a blood transfusion before testing)	Variable	Yes

*Requires confirmatory hemoglobin analysis after at least 6 mo of age and, if possible, hemoglobin analysis from both parents for an accurate diagnosis of the hemoglobin phenotype.

Given the implications of a diagnosis of either sickle cell disease or sickle cell trait in a newborn, the importance of repeating the hemoglobin analysis in the patient, as well obtaining the hemoglobin analysis and complete blood counts for evaluation of the smear and red blood cell parameters in the parents for genetic counseling, cannot be overemphasized. Mistakes do occur in state newborn screening programs. Newborns who had the initial phenotype of Hb FS, but whose final true phenotype included Hb S/β^+, have been described as one of the more common errors identified in the newborn screening hemoglobinopathy programs.

OTHER SICKLE CELL SYNDROMES. The most commonly occurring sickle cell syndromes besides Hb SS are Hb SC, Hb S/β^0-thalassemia, and Hb S/β^+-thalassemia. The other syndromes, SD, SO, Arab, S hereditary persistence of fetal hemoglobin (HPFH), and other variants, are much less common. Individuals with Hb S/β^0-thalassemia have a clinical course similar to that of Hb SS. Red blood cells with Hb SC do not polymerize like Hb SS, but the crystals of Hb C interact with the membrane ion transport, dehydrating the cell and inducing sickling. Children who have Hb SC disease can experience the same symptoms and complications as those with severe Hb SS disease, but the frequency is less. Children with Hb SC also have an increased incidence of retinopathy, chronic hypersplenism, splenic sequestration, and renal medullary carcinoma. The natural history of each of these sickle cell syndromes is variable and hard to predict due to the lack of systematic evaluation. Currently, there is no valid model that can predict the clinical course of an individual with sickle cell disease. Management of end-organ dysfunction in children with sickle cell syndromes requires the same general principles as the management of patients with sickle cell anemia; each situation should be managed on a case-by-case basis and requires consultation with a pediatric hematologist.

462.2 • Sickle Cell Trait (Hb AS)

The prevalence of **sickle cell trait** varies throughout the world; in the U.S., the incidence is 7–10% of African-Americans. The amount of Hb S in individuals with sickle cell trait is <50%. The life span of people with sickle cell trait is normal, and serious complications are very rare. The complete blood count is within the normal range. Hemoglobin analysis is diagnostic, revealing a predominance of Hb A, typically >50%. Complications of sickle cell trait include sudden death during rigorous exercise, splenic infarcts at high altitude, hematuria, hyposthenuria, and bacteriuria, susceptibility to eye injury with formation of a hyphema, and renal medullary carcinoma. Renal medullary carcinoma associated with sickle cell trait occurs predominantly in young adults and children. Children with sickle cell trait should not have any restrictions on activities.

462.3 • Other Hemoglobinopathies

HEMOGLOBIN C. The mutation for Hb C is at the same site as Hb S, with lysine instead of valine substituted for glutamine. In the U.S., Hb AC occurs in 1/50 and Hb CC occurs in 1/5,000 African-Americans. Hb AC is asymptomatic. Hb CC may result in mild anemia, splenomegaly, and cholelithiasis; rare cases of spontaneous splenic rupture have been reported. Sickling does not occur. This condition is usually diagnosed through newborn screening programs. Hb C crystallizes, disrupting the red cell membrane.

HEMOGLOBIN E. Hemoglobin E/β is the 2nd most common globin mutation worldwide. In California, Hb E/β-thalassemia is found almost exclusively in Southeast Asians, with a prevalence of 1/2,600 births.

HEMOGLOBIN D. At least 16 variants of Hb D exist; only 1, D Punjab (Los Angeles), in combination with Hb S, produces symptoms of sickle cell disease. This rare hemoglobin is seen in 1–3% of Western Indians and in some Europeans with a tie to India. Heterozygous D is clinically silent. Homozygous D produces mild to moderate anemia with splenomegaly.

462.4 • Unstable Hemoglobin Disorders

At least 200 rare unstable hemoglobins have been identified; the most common is Hb Köln. Most individuals seem to have de novo mutations rather than inherited hemoglobin disorders. The most studied are those whose mutation causes unstable heme binding that eventually leads to denaturation of the hemoglobin molecule. The denatured hemoglobin can be visualized during severe hemolysis or after splenectomy as Heinz bodies. Unlike the Heinz bodies that are seen after toxic exposure, in unstable hemoglobins, Heinz bodies are present in reticulocytes and older red cells (see Fig. 462-5*D*). Heterozygotes are asymptomatic.

Children with homozygous gene mutations can present in early childhood with anemia and splenomegaly or with unexplained hemolytic anemia. Hemolysis is increased with febrile illness and with some unstable hemoglobins and the ingestion of oxidant medications (similar to glucose-6-phosphate dehydrogenase). If the spleen is functional, the blood smear may appear almost normal or may have only hypochromasia and basophilic stippling. A diagnosis may be made by demonstrating Heinz bodies, hemoglobin instability, or abnormal analysis (although some unstable hemoglobins have normal mobility).

Treatment is supportive. Transfusion may be required during hemolytic episodes in severe cases. Oxidative drugs should be avoided, and folate supplementation provided. Splenectomy has been performed, but the complications of splenectomy, including bacterial sepsis and the possibility of pulmonary hypertension, should be considered before this therapy is administered.

462.5 • Abnormal Hemoglobins with Increased Oxygen Affinity Causing Erythrocytosis

More than 110 high-affinity hemoglobins have been characterized. These mutations affect the state of configuration of hemoglobin during oxygenation and deoxygenation. Hemoglobin changes structure when in the oxygenated vs the deoxygenated state. The deoxygenated state is termed the T (tense) state and is stabilized by 2,3-diphosphoglycerate. When fully oxygenated, hemoglobin assumes the R (relaxed) state. The exact molecular interactions between these two states are not known. The high-affinity hemoglobins contain mutations that either stabilize the R form or destabilize the T form. The interactions between these two forms are complex, and the mechanisms of the mutations are not known. In most cases, the hemoglobins can be identified by hemoglobin analysis; approximately 20% must be characterized by measurements of P_{50}, which will be lower than normal (normal, 23–29 mm Hg). Because of a decrease in P_{50}, most of these hemoglobins cause erythrocytosis of 17.0–20.0 g/dL of hemoglobin. P_{50} is the oxygen tension at half oxygen saturation of blood. The lower the P_{50} the higher the oxygen affinity. Levels of erythropoietin and 2,3-diphosphoglycerate are normal. Patients are usually asymptomatic and do not need phlebotomy. If phlebotomy is performed, oxygen delivery could be problematic because of decreased hemoglobin.

462.6 • Abnormal Hemoglobins Causing Cyanosis

These hemoglobin variants are rare. The major group is the M hemoglobins, of which there are 7. Hemoglobin M variants have mutations in either the α or the β chain, all in the heme pocket of the hemoglobin molecule. Of the 7 variants, 6 have a tyrosine residue that covalently bonds with the heme iron, stabilizing it in the oxidized form. These unstable hemoglobins lead to a hemolytic anemia that is most pronounced in the β forms. These children are cyanotic from birth without other signs or symptoms of disease if the tyrosine is on the α chain (Hb M Boston, Iwate). Infants with β-chain mutations become cyanotic later in infancy because of the fetal hemoglobin switch (Hb M Saskatoon, Hyde Park, Milwaukee). The abnormal hemoglobins are autosomal dominant and are diagnosed by hemoglobin analysis using special techniques and high-performance liquid chromatography. There is no treatment; children with the β form should avoid oxidant drugs.

Low-affinity hemoglobins are associated with less cyanosis than the M hemoglobins. The amino acid substitutions destabilize the oxyhemoglobin and lead to decreased oxygen saturation. The best characterized are Hb Kansas and Hb Beth Israel.

462.7 • Hereditary Methemoglobinemia

The iron in hemoglobin is normally in the ferrous state (Fe^{2+}), which is essential for its oxygen-transporting function. Under physiologic conditions, there is a slow, constant loss of electrons to released oxygen and the ferric (Fe^{3+}) form combines with water, producing methemoglobin (MHg). The predominant intracellular mechanism for the reduction of MHg is cytochrome 5b. This mechanism is >100-fold more efficient than the production of MHg, and only 1% of hemoglobin is in the ferric state normally.

An increase in MHg in red blood cells may occur as a result of exposure to toxic substances (Table 462-5) or absence of reductive pathways (nicotinamide-adenine dinucleotide [NADH]

TABLE 462-5. Known Etiologies of Acquired Methemoglobinemia

MEDICATIONS
Benzocaine
Chloroquine
Dapsone
EMLA (Eutectic Mixture of Local Anesthetics) topical anesthetic (lidocaine 2.5% and prilocaine 2.5%)
Flutamide
Lidocaine
Metoclopramide
Nitrates
Nitric oxide
Nitroglycerin
Nitroprusside
Nitrous oxide
Phenazopyridine
Prilocaine
Primaquine
Riluzole
Silver nitrate
Sodium nitrate
Sulfonamides
MEDICAL CONDITIONS
Pediatric gastrointestinal infection, sepsis
Recreational drug overdose with amyl nitrate ("poppers")
Sickle cell disease-related painful episode
MISCELLANEOUS
Aniline dyes
Fume inhalation (automobile exhaust, burning of wood and plastics)
Herbicides
Industrial chemicals: nitrobenzene, nitroethane (found in nail polish, resins, rubber adhesives)
Pesticides
Gasoline octane booster

From Ash-Bernal R, Wise R, Wright SM: Acquired methemoglobinemia. *Medicine* 2004;83:265–273.

cytochrome b5 reductase deficiency). Toxic methemoglobinemia is much more common than hereditary methemoglobinemia. Infants are particularly vulnerable to hemoglobin oxidation because they have 50% less cytochrome b5 reductase than adults do, fetal hemoglobin is more susceptible to oxidation than Hb A, and the more alkaline infant gastrointestinal tract may promote the growth of nitrite-producing gram-negative bacteria. Methemoglobinemia has been described in infants who ingested foods and water high in nitrates, in those who were exposed to aniline teething gels or other chemicals, and in some infants with severe gastroenteritis and acidosis. An MHg level of 15% is associated with visible cyanosis; a level of 70% MHg is lethal. The level is usually reported as a percent of normal hemoglobin, and the toxic level is lower at a lower hemoglobin level. MHg may color the blood brown (Fig. 462-5). Oxygen saturation will be low, but the arterial blood gas will show a normal or high (if receiving oxygen therapy) PaO_2.

HEREDITARY METHEMOGLOBINEMIA WITH A DEFICIENCY OF NADH CYTOCHROME B5 REDUCTASE. Hereditary methemoglobinemia with a deficiency of NADH cytochrome b5 reductase is a rare disorder that is classified into 4 types. In **type I** (the most common), NADH cytochrome b5 activity is deficient only in the red cells. In **type II,** the enzyme deficiency is present in all tissues and is characterized in infancy by encephalopathy, mental retardation, spasticity, microcephaly, and growth retardation. In **type III,** the deficiency occurs in leukocytes, platelets, and red cells; and in **type IV,** there is deficiency of only red cell cytochrome b5.

Cyanosis may vary in intensity with season and diet. The blood appears brown. The time of onset of cyanosis also varies; in some patients, it appears at birth, whereas in others, it appears as late as adolescence. Although as much as 50% of the total circulating hemoglobin may be in the form of nonfunctional MHg, little or no cardiorespiratory distress occurs in these patients, except on exertion.

Daily oral treatment with ascorbic acid (200–500 mg daily in divided doses) gradually reduces the MHg to approximately 10% of the total pigment and alleviates the cyanosis as long as therapy is continued. Chronic high doses of ascorbic acid have been associated with hyperoxaluria and renal stone formation. Ascorbic acid should not be used for the treatment of toxic methemoglobinemia. **Methylene blue** given IV (1–2 mg/kg initially) is used to treat toxic methemoglobinemia. An oral dose can be administered (3–5 mg/kg/24 hr) as maintenance therapy. Methylene blue should not be used in patients with glucose-6-dehydrogenase deficiency. This treatment is ineffective and can cause severe oxidant hemolysis.

462.8 • Syndromes of Hereditary Persistence of Fetal Hemoglobin

Syndromes of HPFH are a form of thalassemia; a mutation is associated with a decrease in the production of either or both β- and δ-globins. There is an imbalance in the α:non-α synthetic ratio (see Chapter 462.9) characteristic of thalassemia. More than 20 variants of HPFH have been described. They are deletional, $\delta\beta^0$ (Black, Ghanaian, Italian), nondeletional (Tunisian, Japanese, Australian), linked to the β-globin gene cluster (British, Italian-Chinese, Black), or unlinked to the β-globin gene cluster (Atlanta, Czech, Seattle). The $\delta\beta^0$ forms have deletions of the entire δ- and β-globin gene sequences, with the most common in the U.S. being the Black (HPFH-1) variant. As a result of the δ and β gene deletions, there is production only of γ-globin and formation of Hb F. In the homozygous form, there are no manifestations of thalassemia. There is only Hb F, with very mild anemia and slight microcytosis. When inherited with other variant hemoglobins, Hb F is elevated in the 20–30% range; when inherited with Hb S, there is an amelioration of sickle hemoglobinopathy, with far fewer complications.

462.9 • Thalassemia Syndromes

Thalassemias are genetic disorders in globin chain production. In individuals with **β-thalassemia,** there is either a complete absence of β-globin gene production (β^0-thalassemia) or a partial reduction (β^+-thalassemia). In **α-thalassemia,** α-globin gene production is either absent or partially reduced. The primary pathology in thalassemia stems from the quantity of globin gene production, whereas in sickle cell disease, the primary pathology is the quality of globin production.

EPIDEMIOLOGY. Although β-thalassemia has >200 mutations, most are rare. Approximately 20 common alleles constitute 80% of the known thalassemias worldwide; 3% of the world's population carries genes for β-thalassemia, and in Southeast Asia, 5–10% of the population carries genes for α-thalassemia. In a particular area there are fewer common alleles. In the U.S., an estimated 2,000 individuals have β-thalassemia.

PATHOPHYSIOLOGY. Two major features contribute to the pathogenesis of sequelae of β-thalassemia: inadequate β-globin gene production, leading to decreased levels of normal hemoglobin (Hb A), and an imbalance in α- and β-globin chain production. Selected features of the thalassemias can be seen in Table 462-6. In bone marrow, thalassemic mutations disrupt the maturation of red blood cells, resulting in ineffective erythropoiesis; the

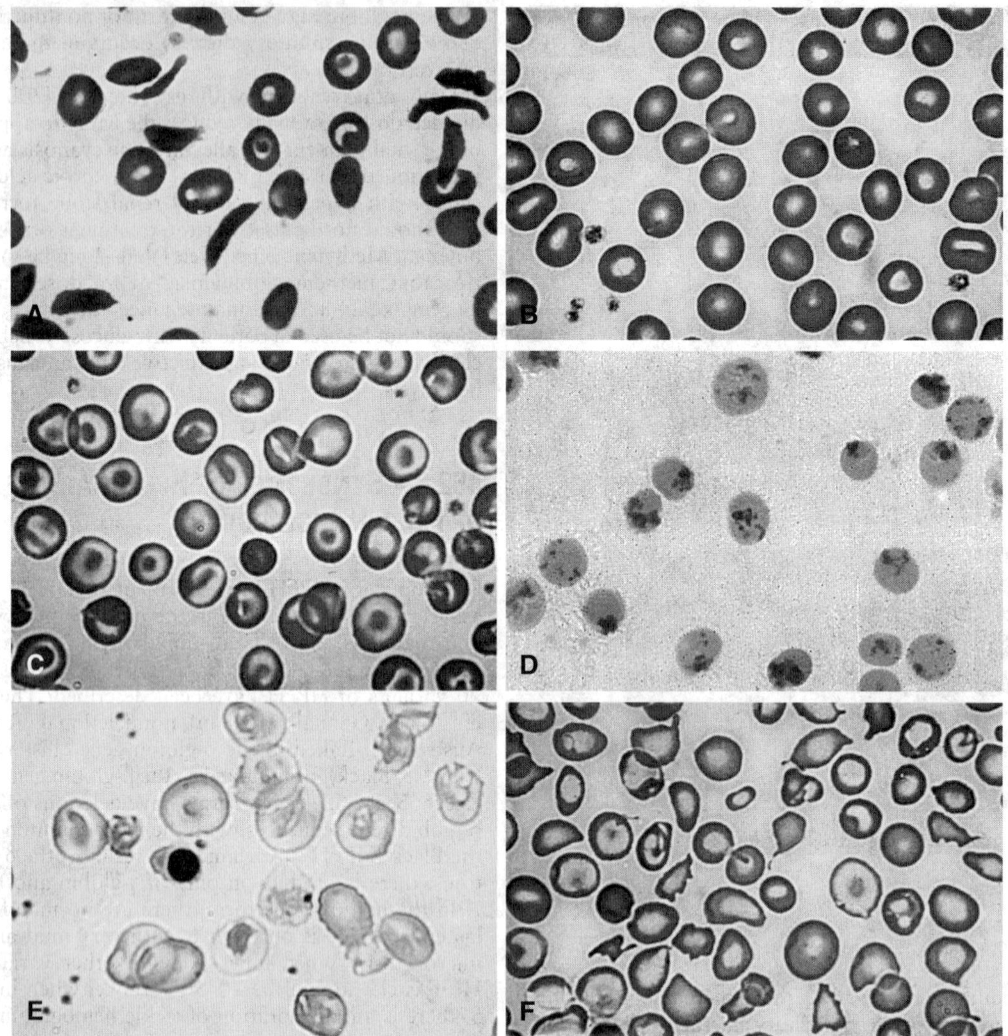

Figure 462-5. Red blood cell (RBC) morphology associated with hemoglobin disorders. *A,* Sickle cell anemia (Hb SS): target cells and fixed (irreversibly sickled) cells. *B,* Sickle cell trait (Hb AS): normal RBC morphology. *C,* Hemoglobin CC: target cells and occasional spherocytes. *D,* Congenital Heinz body anemia (unstable hemoglobin): RBCs stained with supravital stain (brilliant cresyl blue) shows intracellular inclusions. *E,* Homozygous β^0-thalassemia: severe hypochromia with deformed RBCs and normoblasts. *F,* Hemoglobin F disease (α-thalassemia): anisopoikilocytosis with target cells. (Courtesy of Dr. John Bolles, The ASH Collection, University of Washington, Seattle.)

marrow is hyperactive, but the patient has relatively few reticulocytes and severe anemia. In β-thalassemias, there is an excess of α-globin chains relative to β- and γ-globin chains; α-globin tetramers (α_4) are formed, and these inclusions interact with the red cell membrane and shorten red cell survival, leading to anemia and increased erythroid production. The γ-globin chains are produced in increased amounts, leading to an elevated Hb F ($\alpha_2\gamma_2$). The δ-globin chains are also produced in increased amounts, leading to an elevated Hb A_2 ($\alpha_2\delta_2$) in β-thalassemia.

In α-thalassemia, there are relatively fewer α-globin chains and an excess of β- and γ-globin chains. These excess chains form **Bart's hemoglobin** (γ_4) in fetal life and Hb H (β_4) after birth. These abnormal tetramers are not as lethal, but lead to extravascular hemolysis. Prenatally, a fetus with α-thalassemia may become symptomatic because Hb F requires sufficient α-globin gene production, whereas postnatally, infants with β-thalassemia become symptomatic because Hb A requires adequate production of β-globin genes.

HOMOZYGOUS β-THALASSEMIA (THALASSEMIA MAJOR, COOLEY ANEMIA)

CLINICAL MANIFESTATIONS. If not treated, children with β-thalassemia usually become symptomatic as a result of progressive hemolytic anemia, with profound weakness and cardiac decompensation during the 2nd 6 mo of life. Depending on the mutation and the degree of fetal hemoglobin production, transfusions in patients with thalassemia major are necessary in the 2nd mo of life or the 2nd yr of life, but rarely later. The decision to transfuse depends on the child's ability to compensate for the degree of anemia. Most infants and children have cardiac decompensation when the hemoglobin is 4.0 g/dL or less. Fatigue, poor appetite, and lethargy are late findings of severe anemia in an infant or child and were common before transfusions were standard therapy. The classic findings in children with severe thalassemia, including typical facies (maxillary hyperplasia, flat nasal

TABLE 462-6. The Thalassemias

THALASSEMIA	GLOBIN GENOTYPE	FEATURES	EXPRESSION	HEMOGLOBIN ELECTROPHORESIS
α-THALASSEMIA				
1 gene deletion	-,α/α,α	Normal	Normal	Newborn: Bart 1–2%
2 gene deletion trait	-,α/-,α-,-/α,α	Microcytosis, mild hypochromasia	Normal, mild anemia	Newborn: Bart 5–10%
3 gene deletion hemoglobin H	-,-/-,α	Microcytosis, hypochromic	Mild anemia, transfusions not required	Newborn: Bart 20–30%
2 gene deletion + Constant Spring	$-,-/\alpha,\alpha^{Constant\ Spring}$	Microcytosis, hypochromic	Moderate to severe anemia, transfusion, splenectomy	2–3% Constant Spring, 10–15% hemoglobin H
4 gene deletion	-,-/-,-	Anisocytosis, poikilocytosis	Hydrops fetalis	Newborn: 89–90% Bart with Gower 1 and 2 and Portland
Nondeletional	$\alpha,\alpha/\alpha,\alpha^{variant}$	Microcytosis, mild anemia	Normal	1–2% variant hemoglobin
β-THALASSEMIA				
β^0 or β^+ heterozygote: trait	$\beta^0/A, \beta^+/A$	Variable microcytosis	Normal	Elevated A_2, variable elevation of F
β^0-Thalassemia	$\beta^0/\beta^0, \beta^+/\beta^0, E/\beta^0$	Microcytosis, nucleated RBCs	Transfusion-dependent	F 98%, A_2 2% E 30–40%
β^+-Thalassemia severe	β^+/β^+	Microcytosis, nucleated RBCs	Transfusion-dependent/thalassemia intermedia	F 70–95%, A_2 2%, trace A
Silent	β^+/A	Microcytosis	Normal with only microcytosis	A_2 3.3–3.5%
	β^+/β^+	Hypochromic, microcytosis	Mild to moderate anemia	A_2 2–5%, F 10–30%
Dominant (rare)	B^0/A	Microcytosis, abnormal RBCs	Moderately severe anemia, splenomegaly	Elevated F and A_2
δ-Thalassemia	A/A	Normal	Normal	A_2 absent
$(\delta\beta)^0$-Thalassemia	$(\delta\beta)^0/A$	Hypochromic	Mild anemia	F 5–20%
$(\delta\beta)^+$-Thalassemia Lepore	β^{Lepore}/A	Microcytosis	Mild anemia	Lepore 8–20%
Lepore	$\beta^{Lepore}/\beta^{Lepore}$	Microcytic, hypochromic	Thalassemia intermedia	F 80%, Lepore 20%
γδβ-Thalassemia	$(\gamma^A\delta\beta)^0/A$	Microcytosis, microcytic, hypochromic	Moderate anemia, splenomegaly, homozygote: thalassemia intermedia	Decreased F and A_2 compared with δβ-thalassemia
γ-Thalassemia	$(\gamma^A\gamma^G)^0/A$	Microcytosis	Insignificant unless homozygote	Decreased F
HEREDITARY PERSISTENCE OF FETAL HEMOGLOBIN				
Deletional	A/A	Microcytic	Mild anemia	F 100% homozygotes
Nondeletional	A/A	Normal	Normal	F 20–40%

RBCs, red blood cells.

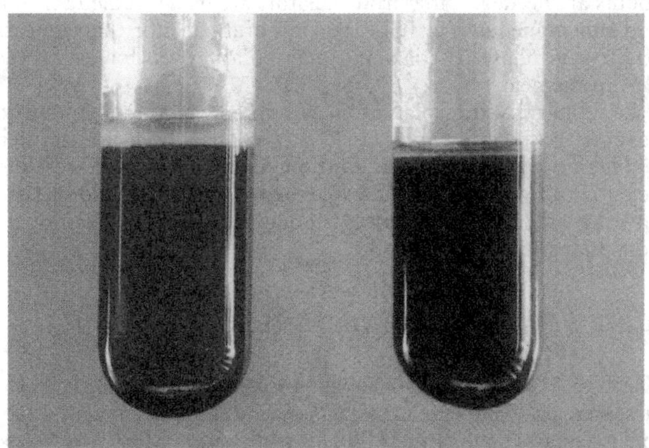

Figure 462-6. Normal arterial blood vs methemoglobulinemia. Arterial whole blood with 1% methemoglobin *(left)* vs arterial whole blood with 72% methemoglobin *(right)* [methods described later]. Note the characteristic chocolate-brown color of the sample with an elevated methemoglobin level. Both samples were briefly exposed to 100% oxygen and shaken. This quick analysis is a good bedside test for methemoglobulinemia. The sample on the *left* turned bright red, whereas the sample on the *right* remained chocolate-brown. Methods: Whole blood samples were drawn at the same time from the same person. The measured hemoglobin concentration was 11.7 g/dL. Calculated concentration of methemoglobin: 11.7 g/dL × 0.01 = 0.117 g/dL *(left)* and 11.7 g/dL × 0.72 = 8.42 g/dL *(right)*. An elevated methemoglobin level was made in vitro by adding 0.1 mL of a 0.144 molar solution of sodium nitrate *(right)*, and 0.1 mL of normal saline was added as a control *(left)*. Co-oximetry measurements were taken on both samples shortly after the blood was drawn and 20 min after the addition of sodium nitrate solution. Both blood samples were exposed to 100% oxygen before the 2nd measurement. (Protocol based on personal communication with Dr. Ali Mansouri, December 2002.)

bridge, frontal bossing), pathologic bone fractures, marked hepatosplenomegaly, and cachexia, are primarily seen in developing countries. The spleen may become so enlarged that it causes mechanical discomfort and secondary hypersplenism. Features of ineffective erythropoiesis include expanded medullary spaces (with massive expansion of the marrow of the face and skull), extramedullary hematopoiesis, and a huge caloric need (Fig. 462-7). Hepatosplenomegaly may interfere with nutritional support. Pallor, hemosiderosis, and jaundice may combine to produce a greenish brown complexion. As a result of the anemia, there is also an increase in iron absorption from the gastrointestinal tract, with toxicity leading to further complications. Many of these features became less severe and less frequent with transfusion therapy, but the creation of excessive iron stores associated with hemosiderosis is a major concern in individuals with β-thalassemia. Many of the complications of thalassemia seen in developed countries today are the result of increased iron deposition from repeated blood transfusions. Complications can be avoided by the consistent use of an iron chelator. However, chelation therapy also has associated complications. Endocrine and cardiac pathology is often associated with excessive iron stores in patients with thalassemia major who are chronically transfused. Endocrine dysfunction may include hypothyroidism, gonadal failure, hypoparathyroidism, and diabetes mellitus. Congestive heart failure and cardiac arrhythmias are potentially lethal complications of iron stores in individuals with thalassemia.

LABORATORY FINDINGS. The infant is born only with Hb F or, in some cases, Hb F and Hb E (heterozygosity for β^0-thalassemia). Eventually, patients with β-thalassemia have severe anemia, few reticulocytes, numerous nucleated red cells, and microcytosis, with almost no normal-appearing red cells on the smear (see Fig. 462-5*E*). The hemoglobin level falls progressively to <5.0 g/dL unless transfusions are given. The reticulocyte count is commonly <8% and is inappropriately low compared with the degree of anemia because of ineffective erythropoiesis. The unconjugated

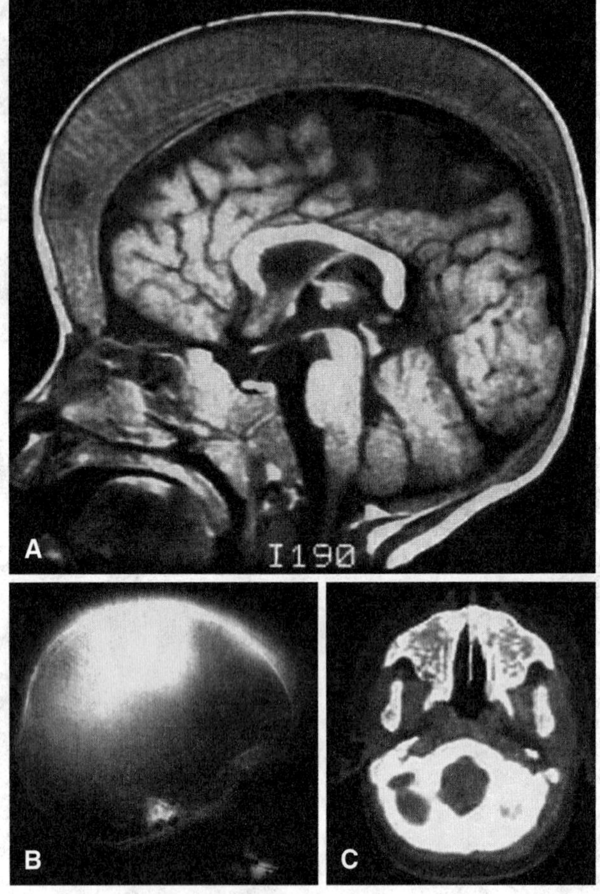

Figure 462-7. Ineffective erythropoiesis in an untransfused 3 yr old patient with thalassemia major. *A,* Massive widening of the diploic spaces of the skull as seen on MRI. *B,* Radiographic appearance of the trabeculae as seen on plain radiograph, and *C,* obliteration of the maxillary sinuses with hematopoietic tissue as seen on CT scan.

serum bilirubin level is usually elevated, but other chemistry values may be normal at an early stage. Even if the patient is untransfused, eventually there is iron accumulation, with an elevated serum ferritin level and saturation of transferrin. Bone marrow hyperplasia can be seen on radiographs (see Fig. 462-7).

TREATMENT. Before chronic transfusions are initiated, the diagnosis of β^0-thalassemia should be confirmed and the parents counseled about this lifelong therapy. Initiating transfusion and chelation therapy can be difficult for parents to face early in their child's life. Before transfusion therapy is begun, a red cell phenotype is obtained; blood products that are leukoreduced and phenotypically matched for the Rh and Kell antigens are required for transfusion. If there is the possibility of a bone marrow transplant, the blood should be negative for cytomegalovirus and irradiated. Transfusion therapy promotes general health and well-being and avoids the consequences of ineffective erythropoiesis. A transfusion program generally requires monthly transfusions, with the pretransfusion hemoglobin level >9.5 and <10.5 g/dL. In patients with cardiac disease, higher pretransfusion hemoglobin levels may be beneficial. Some blood centers have donor programs that pair donors and recipients, decreasing the exposure to multiple red cell antigens.

Transfusional hemosiderosis causes many of the complications of thalassemia major. Accurate assessment of excessive iron stores is essential to optimal therapy. The serum ferritin level is useful in assessing iron balance trends, but does not accurately predict quantitative iron stores. Undertreatment or overtreatment of presumed excessive iron stores can occur when a patient is managed based on the serum ferritin level alone. Measurement of the iron level by liver biopsy is the standard method for accurately determining the iron store. A ferritometer and specialized MRI software are emerging alternatives for liver biopsies. Although quantitative liver iron measurement accurately guides the use of iron chelators, it may not reflect cumulative changes in cardiac iron. Patients can have cardiac iron overload at the time of a safe liver iron measurement. Many thalassemia centers monitor cardiac iron with T2 weighted MRI imaging, but routine application of this technology has not been implemented across all sites.

Transfusional hemosiderosis can be prevented by the use of deferoxamine (Desferal). Deferoxamine chelates iron and some other divalent cations, allowing their excretion in urine and stool. Deferoxamine is given subcutaneously over 10–12 hr, 5–6 days a week. Side effects include ototoxicity with high-frequency hearing loss, retinal changes, and bone dysplasia with truncal shortening. The number of hours deferoxamine is used daily is more important than the daily dose. High-dose, short-term infusions increase toxicity with little efficacy. Plasma non-transferrin-bound iron (NTBI) is most likely responsible for the serious iron injury. When deferoxamine is infusing, it binds NTBI. When deferoxamine is stopped, there are rebound increases in NTBI levels, with a risk of injury. The 24 hr deferoxamine infusion has been shown to reverse cardiomyopathy in patients with excessive iron stores in the heart that result in symptomatic congestive heart failure.

Deferiprone is a new iron chelator approved by the U.S. Food and Drug Administration for children >2 yr of age (see Chapter 462.1). Deferiprone may not be as effective as deferoxamine in total body iron chelation, but may be more effective in removing cardiac iron. Side effects include neutropenia, and weekly blood counts are needed. Other iron chelators are being studied for oral and subcutaneous use. ICL670 is an oral chelator that appears effective in phase III trials and may be approved for use in the U.S. in the near future.

Bone marrow transplantation has cured >1,000 patients who have thalassemia major. Most success has been in children younger than 15 yr of age without excessive iron stores and hepatomegaly who have HLA-matched siblings. All children who have an HLA-matched sibling should be offered the option of bone marrow transplantation.

OTHER β-THALASSEMIA SYNDROMES

The β-thalassemia syndromes are broken into 6 groups: β-thalassemia, δβ-thalassemias, γ-thalassemias, δ-thalassemias, εγδβ-thalassemias, and the HPFH syndrome. Most of these thalassemias are relatively rare, with some found only in family groups. The β-thalassemias can also be classified clinically as thalassemia trait and as thalassemia minima, minor, intermedia, and major, reflecting the degree of anemia. The genetic classification does not necessarily define the phenotype, and the degree of anemia does not always predict the genetic classification.

Thalassemia intermedia can be any combination of β-thalassemia mutations (β^0/β^+, $\beta^0/\beta^{variant}$, E/β^0) that will lead to a phenotype of microcytic anemia with a hemoglobin level of approximately 7.0 g/dL. There is controversy about whether to transfuse these children. They will have a degree of medullary hyperplasia, nutritional hemosiderosis that may require chelation, splenomegaly, and other complications of thalassemia associated with excessive iron stores. Extramedullary hematopoiesis can occur in the vertebral canal, compressing the spinal cord and causing neurologic symptoms; the latter is a medical emergency requiring immediate local radiation therapy to halt erythropoiesis. Although transfusion will alleviate the thalassemic manifestations, the decision to transfuse must be balanced against the future need for chelation therapy.

Splenectomy may be indicated for patients with thalassemia intermedia who have a falling steady-state hemoglobin level and for transfused patients with a rising transfusion requirement. Splenectomy may have serious infectious consequences. All patients should be fully immunized against encapsulated bacteria before splenectomy, and subsequently they should receive long-term penicillin prophylaxis with appropriate instructions for fever management.

The **thalassemias** classified as **minima** and **minor** are usually heterozygotes (β^0/β, β^+/β^+), with a phenotype more severe than that of thalassemia trait, but not as severe as that of thalassemia intermedia. The genotype should be determined, and these children should be monitored for iron accumulation. The β-thalassemias are influenced by the presence of α-thalassemia, with α-thalassemia trait leading to less severe anemia. Duplicated α genes (ααα/α α) leading to more severe thalassemia. Frequently, these individuals require transfusions in adolescence or adulthood; some may be candidates for chemotherapy, such as hydroxyurea.

Thalassemia trait is frequently misdiagnosed as iron deficiency in children because the two are similar hematologically and iron deficiency is much more prevalent. A short course of iron and re-evaluation is all that is required to identify children who will need further evaluation. Children who have β-thalassemia trait have a persistent red cell distribution width, and on hemoglobin analysis, they have elevated Hb F and diagnostically elevated Hb A_2. There are "silent" forms of thalassemia trait, and if the family history is suggestive, further studies may be indicated.

α-THALASSEMIA

Infants are identified in the newborn period by the increased production of **Bart's hemoglobin** (γ_4) during fetal life and its presence at birth. These thalassemias occur most frequently in Southeast Asia. Deletion mutations are common in α-thalassemia. In addition to these deletional mutations, there are nondeletional α-globin gene mutations, the most common being Constant Spring ($\alpha^{CS}\alpha$). There are four α-globin genes and four deletional α-thalassemia phenotypes.

The deletion of 1 α-globin gene (silent trait) is not identifiable hematologically. No alterations are noted in the mean corpuscular volume and mean corpuscular hemoglobin. Individuals with this deletion are usually diagnosed after the birth of a child with a 2-gene deletion, or Hb H (β_4). During the newborn period, typically <3% Bart's hemoglobin is observed. The deletion of 1 α-globin gene is common in African-Americans.

The deletion of 2 α-globin genes results in α-thalassemia trait. The globin genes can be lost in *trans,* such a -α/-α, or in *cis,* such as $\alpha,\alpha/^{-SEA}$. The *trans* or *cis* mutations, combined with other mutations, can lead to Hb H, or α-thalassemia major. In individuals from Africa or of African descent, the most common α-globin gene deletion is in *trans,* whereas in individuals from Asia or the Mediterranean region, the *cis* deletion is most common. The α-thalassemia traits present as a microcytic anemia that can be mistaken for iron-deficiency anemia (see Fig. 462-5*F*). The hemoglobin analysis is normal, except during the newborn period, when Bart's hemoglobin is commonly <8%, but >3%. Children with deletion of 2 α-globin genes are commonly considered as having iron deficiency, given the presence of both low mean corpuscular volume and mean corpuscular hemoglobin. The simplest way to distinguish between iron deficiency and α-thalassemia trait is with a good dietary history. Children with iron-deficiency anemia often have a diet that is low in iron. Alternatively, a brief course of iron supplementation, along with monitoring of the red blood cell parameters, may make the diagnosis of iron deficiency, or α-globin gene deletion analysis may be necessary.

The deletion of 3 α-globin genes leads to the diagnosis of Hb H disease. In California, which has a large Asian population, approximately 1/15,000 newborns has Hb H disease. The simplest manner of diagnosing Hb H disease is during the newborn period, when the Bart's hemoglobin level is commonly >25%. In addition, supporting evidence must be obtained from the parents (at least 1 parent must have α-thalassemia trait). Later in childhood, there is an excess of β-globin chain tetramers that results in Hb H. A definitive diagnosis of Hb H disease requires DNA analysis with supporting evidence. Brilliant cresyl blue can stain Hb H, but it is rarely used for diagnosis. Individuals with Hb H disease have marked microcytosis, anemia, mild splenomegaly, and occasionally, scleral icterus or cholelithiasis. Transfusion is not commonly used for therapy because the range of hemoglobin is 7.0–11.0 g/dL, with a mean corpuscular volume of 51–73 fl.

The deletion of all 4 α-globin genes causes profound anemia during fetal life, resulting in hydrops fetalis; the ζ-globin gene must be present for fetal survival. There are no normal hemoglobins present at birth (primarily Bart's hemoglobin, with Gower-1, Gower-2, and Portland). If the fetus survives, immediate exchange transfusion is indicated. These infants with α-thalassemia major are transfusion-dependent, and bone marrow transplant is the only cure.

The presence of a nondeletional α-globin mutation with a 2-gene deletion results in more severe anemia than deletion type of α-globin thalassemia, increased hepatosplenomegaly, increased jaundice, and a much more severe clinical course than Hb H disease. Hb H Constant Spring is the most common form ($-\alpha/\alpha,\alpha^{CS}$).

Treatment of the α-thalassemia deletion syndromes consists of folate supplementation, possible splenectomy (with the attendant risks), intermittent transfusion during severe anemia for the non-deletion Hb H diseases, and chronic transfusion therapy or bone marrow transplant for survivors of hydrops fetalis. These children also should not be exposed to oxidant medications.

Sickle Cell Anemia

Alonso MH: Gallbladder abnormalities in children with sickle cell disease: Management with laparoscopic cholecystectomy. *J Pediatr* 2004;145: 580–581.

Beyer JE, Simmons LE, Woods GM, et al: A chronology of pain and comfort in children with sickle cell disease. *Arch Pediatr Adolesc Med* 1999; 153:913–920.

Boyd JH, Strunk RC, Morgan WJ: The outcomes of sickle cell disease in adulthood are clear, but the origins and progression of sickle cell anemia-induced problems in the heart and lung in childhood are not. *J Pediatr* 2006;149: 3–4.

Buchanan ID, Woodward M, Reed GW: Opioid selection during sickle cell pain crisis and its impact on the development of acute chest syndrome. *Pediatr Blood Cancer* 2005;45:716–724.

Claster S, Vichinsky EP: Managing sickle cell disease. *BMJ* 2003;327: 1151–1155.

De Montalembert M, Maunoury C, Acar P, et al: Myocardial ischaemia in children with sickle cell disease. *Arch Dis Child* 2004;89:359–362.

Dhar M, Bellevue R, Carmel R: Pernicious anemia with neuropsychiatric dysfunction in a patient with sickle cell anemia treated with folate supplementation. *N Engl J Med* 2003;348:2204–2207.

Driscoll MC, Hurlet A, Styles L, et al: Stroke risk in siblings with sickle cell anemia. *Blood* 2003;101:2401–2404.

Geva A, Clark JJ, Zhang Y, et al: Hemoglobin Jamaica plain: A sickling hemoglobin with reduced oxygen affinity. *N Engl J Med* 2004;351:1532–1538.

Gladwin MT, Sachdev V, Jison ML, et al: Pulmonary hypertension as a risk factor for death in patients with sickle cell disease. *N Engl J Med* 2004; 350:886–895.

Hankins JS, Ware RE, Rogers ZR, et al: Long-term hydroxyurea therapy for infants with sickle cell anemia: The HUSOFT extension study. *Blood* 2005;106:2269–2275.

Henderson JN, Noetzel MJ, McKinstry RC, et al: Reversible posterior leukoencephalopathy syndrome and silent cerebral infarcts are associated with severe acute chest syndrome in children with sickle cell disease. *Blood* 2003;101:415–419.

Kizito ME, Mworozi E, Ndugwa C, Serjeant GR: Bacteraemia in homozygous sickle cell disease in Africa: Is pneumococcal prophylaxis justified? *Arch Dis Child* 2007;92:21–23.

Kopecky EA, Jacobson S, Joshi P, et al: Systemic exposure to morphine and the risk of acute chest syndrome in sickle cell disease. *Clin Pharmacol Ther* 2004;75:140–146.

Machado RF, Anthi A, Steinberg MH, et al: N-terminal pro-brain natriuretic peptide levels and risk of death in sickle cell disease. *JAMA* 2006;296: 310–318.

Makis AC, Hatzimichael EC, Stebbing J: The genomics of new drugs in sickle cell disease. *Pharmacogenomics* 2006;7:909–917.

McCarthy LJ, Vattuone J, Weidner J, et al: Do automated red cell exchanges relieve priapism in patients with sickle cell anemia? *Ther Apher* 2000; 4:256–258.

Morris CR, Kato GJ, Poljakovic M, et al: Dysregulated arginine metabolism hemolysis-associated pulmonary hypertension, and mortality in sickle cell disease. *JAMA* 2005;294:81–90.

Neumayr L, Lennette E, Kelly D, et al: *Mycoplasma* disease and acute chest syndrome in sickle cell disease. *Pediatrics* 2003;112:87–95.

Norris CF, Smith-Whitley K, McGowan KL: Positive blood cultures in sickle cell disease: Time to positivity and clinical outcome. *J Pediatr Hematol Oncol* 2003;25:390–395.

Optimizing Primary Strike Prevention in Sickle Cell Anemia (STOP2) Investigators: Discontinuing prophylactic transfusions used to prevent stroke in sickle cell disease. *N Engl J Med* 2005;353:2769–2778.

Panepinto JA, Brousseau DC, Hillery CA, et al: Variation in hospitalization and hospital length of stay in children with vaso-occlusive crises in sickle cell disease. *Pediatr Blood Cancer* 2005;44:182–186.

Pirich LM, Chou P, Walterhouse DO: Prolonged survival of a patient with sickle cell trait and metastatic renal medullary carcinoma. *J Pediatr Hematol/Oncol* 1999;21:67–69.

Powars DR, Chan LS, Hiti A, et al: Outcome of sickle cell anemia: A 4-decade observational study of 1056 patients. *Medicine* 2005;84:363–376.

Quinn CT, Rogers ZR, Buchanan GR: Survival of children with sickle-cell disease. *Blood* 2004;103:4023–4027.

Qureshi N, Lubin B, Walter MC: The prevention and management of stroke in sickle cell anemia. *Expert Opin Biol Ther* 2006;6:1087–1098.

Saad ST, Lajolo C, Gilli S, et al: Follow-up of sickle cell disease patients with priapism treated by hydroxyurea. *Am J Hematol* 2004;77:45–49.

Scothorn DJ, Price C, Schwartz D, et al: Risk of recurrent stroke in children with sickle cell disease receiving blood transfusion therapy for at least five years after initial stroke. *J Pediatr* 2002;140:348–354.

Sebire G, Tabarki B, Saunders DE, et al: Cerebral venous sinus thrombosis in children: Risk factors, presentation, diagnosis and outcome. *Brain* 2005; 128:477–489; Epub 2005 Feb 7.

Smith LA, Oyeku SO, Homer C, Zuckerman B: Sickle cell disease: a question of equity and quality. *Pediatrics* 2006;117:1763–1770.

Smith-Whitley K, Zhao H, Hodinka RL, et al: Epidemiology of human parvovirus B19 in children with sickle cell disease. *Blood* 2004;103:422–427.

Strouse JJ, Hulbert ML, DeBaun MR, et al: Primary hemorrhagic stroke in children with sickle cell disease is associated with recent transfusion and use of corticosteroids. *Pediatrics* 2006;118:1916–1924.

Stuart MJ, Nagel RL: Sickle cell disease. *Lancet* 2004;364:1343–1360.

Switzer JA, Hess DC, Nichols FT, et al: Pathophysiology and treatment of stroke in sickle-cell disease: Present and future. *Lancet Neurol* 2006;5:501–512.

Sylvester KP, Patey RA, Milligan P, et al: Impact of acute chest syndrome on lung function of children with sickle cell disease. *J Pediatr* 2006;149:17–22.

Talano JAM, Hillery CA, Gottschall JL, et al: Delayed hemolytic transfusion reaction/hyperhemolysis syndrome in children with sickle cell disease. *Pediatrics* 2003;111:e661–e665.

Uong EC, Henderson Boyd J, DeBaun MR: Daytime pulse oximeter measurements do not predict incidence of pain and acute chest syndrome episodes in sickle cell anemia. *J Pediatr* 2006;149:707–709.

Vargas-Gonzalez R, Sotelo-Avila C, Coria AS: Case report: Renal medullary carcinoma in a six-year-old boy with sickle cell trait. *Pathol Oncol Res* 2003;9:193–195.

Vichinsky EP, Neumayr LD, Earles AN, et al: Causes and outcomes of the acute chest syndrome in sickle cell disease. *N Engl J Med* 2000;342:1855–1865.

Ware RE, Zimmerman SA, Sylvestre PB, et al: Prevention of secondary stroke and resolution of transfusional iron overload in children with sickle cell anemia using hydroxyurea and phlebotomy. *J Pediatr* 2004;145:346–352.

Weiner DL, Hibberd PL, Betit P, et al: Preliminary assessment of inhaled nitric oxide for acute vaso-occlusive crisis in pediatric patients with sickle cell disease. *JAMA* 2003;289:1136–1142.

Zarrouk V, Habibi A, Zahar JR, et al: Bloodstream infection in adults with sickle cell disease. *Medicine* 2006;85:43–48.

Methemoglobinemia

Ash-Bernal R, Wise R, Wright SM: Acquired methemoglobinemia: A retrospective series of 138 cases at 2 teaching hospitals. *Medicine* 2004;83: 265–273.

Moore TJ, Walsh CS, Cohen MR: Reported adverse event cases of methemoglobinemia associated with benzocaine products. *Arch Intern Med* 2004;164:1192–1196.

Rehman HU: Methemoglobinemia. *West J Med* 2001;175:193–196.

Sanchez-Echaniz J, Benito-Fernandez J, Mintegui-Raso S: Methemoglobinemia and consumption of vegetables in infants. *Pediatrics* 2001;107:1024–1028.

Thalassemia

Aessopos A, Tsironi M, Vassiliadis I, et al: Exercise-induced myocardial perfusion abnormalities in sickle beta-thalassemia: Tc-99m tetrofosmin gated SPECT imaging study. *Am J Med* 2001;111:355–360.

Berkovitch M, Bistritzer T, Milone SD, et al: Iron deposition in the anterior pituitary in homozygous beta-thalassemia: MRI evaluation and correlation with gonadal function. *J Pediatr Endocrinol Metab* 2000;13:179–184.

Chen FE, Ooi C, Ha SY, et al: Genetic and clinical features of hemoglobin H disease in Chinese patients. *N Engl J Med* 2000;343:544–550.

Chern JP, Lin KH, Lu MY, et al: Abnormal glucose tolerance in transfusion-dependent beta-thalassemic patients. *Diabetes Care* 2001;24:850–854.

Chui DHK, Fuchareon S, Chan V: Hemoglobin H disease: Not necessarily a benign disorder. *Blood* 2003;101:791–800.

Eldor A, Rachmilewitz EA: The hypercoagulable state in thalassemia. *Blood* 2002;99:36–43.

Gallanello R, Piga A, Forri GL, et al: Phase II clinical evaluation of defarasirov, a once-daily oral chelating agent in pediatric patients with beta-thalassemia major. *Hematologica* 2006;91:1343–1351.

Gulati R, Bhatia V, Agarwal SS: Early onset of endocrine abnormalities in beta-thalassemia major in a developing country. *J Pediatr Endocrinol Metab* 2000;13:651–656.

Hahalis G, Manolis AS, Gerasimidou I, et al: Right ventricular diastolic function in beta-thalassemia major: Echocardiographic and clinical correlates. *Am Heart J* 2001;141:428–434.

Kattamis AC, Antoniadis M, Manoli I, et al: Endocrine problems in ex-thalassemic patients. *Transfus Sci* 2000;23:251–252.

Lorey F, Cunningham G, Vichinsky EP, et al: Universal newborn screening for Hb H disease in California. *Genet Test* 2001;5:93–100.

Rund D, Rachmilewitz E: β-Thalassemia. *N Engl J Med* 2005;353:1135–1146.

Telfer PT, Prestcott E, Holden S, et al: Hepatic iron concentration combined with long-term monitoring of serum ferritin to predict complications of iron overload in thalassaemia major. *Br J Haematol* 2000;110:971–977.

Weatherall DJ: Introduction to the problem of hemoglobin E–beta thalassemia. *J Pediatr Hematol Oncol* 2000;22:551.

Winichagoon P, Fucharoen S, Chen P, et al: Genetic factors affecting clinical severity in beta-thalassemia syndromes. *J Pediatr Hematol Oncol* 2000;22: 573–580.

Wonke B: Clinical management of beta-thalassemia major. *Semin Hematol* 2001;38:350–359.

Iron Overload Disorders

Andrews NC: Inherited iron overload disorders. *Curr Opin Pediatr* 2000; 12:596–602.

Deferasirox (Exjade): A new iron chelator. *Med Lett Drugs Ther* 2006;48:35–36.

McCullen MA, Crawford DH, Hickman PE: Screening for hemochromatosis. *Clin Chim Acta* 2002;315:169–186.

Murray KF, Kowdley KV: Neonatal hemochromatosis. *Pediatrics* 2001;108: 960–964.

Roy CN, Andrews NC: Recent advances in disorders of iron metabolism: Mutations, mechanisms and modifiers. *Hum Mol Genet* 2001;10: 2181–2186.

Sanchez AM, Schreiber GB, Bethel J, et al: Prevalence, donation practices, and risk assessment of blood donors with hemochromatosis. *JAMA* 2001; 286:1475–1481.

Vohra P, Haller C, Emre S, et al: Neonatal hemochromatosis: The importance of early recognition of liver failure. *J Pediatr* 2000;136:537–541.

Chapter 463 ■ Enzymatic Defects

George B. Segel

DEFICIENCIES OF ENZYMES OF THE GLYCOLYTIC PATHWAY

Various red blood cell (RBC) enzymatic defects produce hemolytic anemias. These anemias generally do not have a prominent morphologic alteration. Inherited deficiencies of most of the enzymes in both the anaerobic Embden-Meyerhof pathway and the oxidative hexose monophosphate (pentose) shunt have been described (Fig. 463-1). The most common glycolytic enzyme defect as a cause of hemolytic anemia is the rare occurrence of pyruvate kinase (PK) deficiency.

463.1 • Pyruvate Kinase Deficiency

Congenital hemolytic anemia occurs in persons homozygous for an autosomal recessive gene that causes either a marked reduction in RBC PK or production of an abnormal enzyme with decreased activity. Generation of adenosine triphosphate (ATP) within RBCs is impaired, and low levels of ATP, pyruvate, and the oxidized form of nicotinamide-adenine dinucleotide (NAD^+) are found (see Fig. 463-1). The concentration of 2,3-diphosphoglycerate is increased; 2,3-diphosphoglycerate is beneficial in facilitating oxygen release from hemoglobin, but detrimental in inhibiting hexokinase and enzymes of the hexose monophosphate shunt. In addition, an unexplained decrease occurs in the sum of the adenine (ATP, adenosine diphosphate, and adenosine monophosphate) and pyridine (NAD^+ and the reduced form of NAD) nucleotides; this further impairs glycolysis. As a consequence of decreased ATP, RBCs cannot maintain the potassium and water content; the cells become rigid, and their life span is considerably reduced.

ETIOLOGY. There are 2 mammalian PK genes, but only the *PKLR* gene is expressed in red cells. The human *PKLR* gene is located on chromosome 1q21; 133 mutations are reported in this structural gene, which codes for a 574–amino acid protein that forms a functional tetramer. Most affected patients are compound heterozygotes for 2 different PK gene defects. The many possible combinations likely account for the variability in clinical severity. The mutations 1456 C to T and 1529 G to A are the most common mutations in the white population.

CLINICAL MANIFESTATIONS AND LABORATORY FINDINGS. The clinical manifestations vary from severe neonatal hemolytic anemia to mild, well-compensated hemolysis first noted in adulthood. Severe jaundice and anemia may occur in the neonatal period; kernicterus has been reported. The hemolysis in older children and adults varies in severity, with hemoglobin values ranging from 8–12 g/dL associated with some pallor, jaundice, and splenomegaly. These patients usually do not require transfusion. A severe form of the disease has a relatively high incidence among the Amish of the Midwestern United States.

Polychromatophilia and mild macrocytosis reflect the elevated reticulocyte count. Spherocytes are uncommon, but a few spiculated **pyknocytes** are found. Non-incubated osmotic fragility is normal. Diagnosis relies on demonstration of a marked reduction

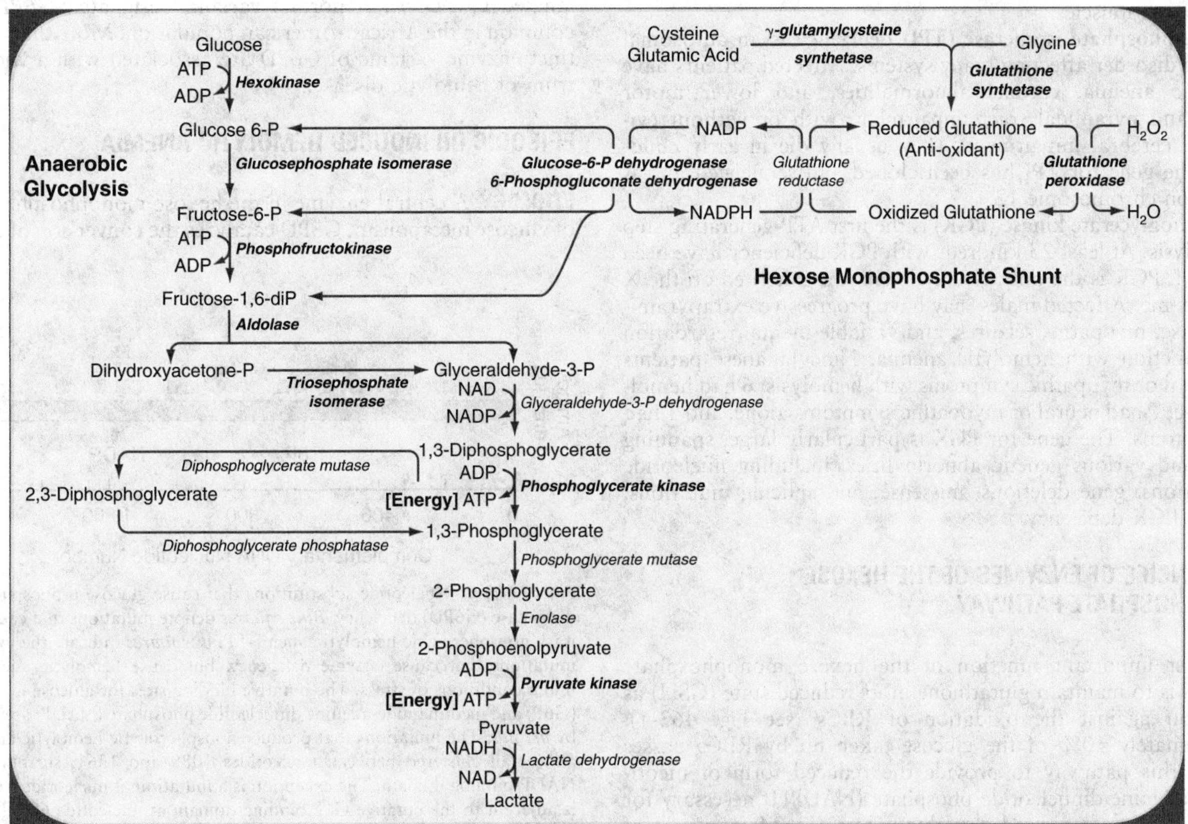

Figure 463-1. Red cell metabolism. Glycolysis and the hexose monophosphate pathway. The enzyme deficiencies clearly associated with hemolysis are shown in *bold* type. ATP, adenosine triphosphate; ADP, adenosine diphosphate; NADP, nicotinamide-adenine dinucleotide phosphate; reduced form of NADP.

of RBC PK activity or an increase in the Michaelis-Menten dissociation constant (K_m) for its substrate, phosphoenolpyruvate. Other RBC enzyme activity is normal or elevated, reflecting the reticulocytosis. No abnormalities of hemoglobin are noted. The white cells have normal PK activity and must be rigorously excluded from the hemolysates used to measure PK activity. Heterozygous carriers usually have moderately reduced levels of PK activity.

TREATMENT. Exchange transfusions may be indicated for hyperbilirubinemia in newborns. Transfusions of packed RBCs are necessary for severe anemia or for aplastic crises. If the anemia is consistently severe or if frequent transfusions are required, splenectomy should be performed after 5–6 yr of age. Although it is not curative, splenectomy may be followed by higher hemoglobin levels and by strikingly high (30–60%) reticulocyte counts. Death resulting from overwhelming pneumococcal sepsis has followed splenectomy; thus, immunization with vaccines for encapsulated organisms should be given before splenectomy, and prophylactic penicillin should be administered after splenectomy.

463.2 • Other Glycolytic Enzyme Deficiencies

Chronic nonspherocytic hemolytic anemias of varying severity have been associated with deficiencies of other enzymes in the glycolytic pathway, including hexokinase, glucose phosphate isomerase, and aldolase, which are inherited as autosomal recessive disorders. **Phosphofructokinase deficiency** occurs primarily in Ashkenazi Jews in the U.S. and results in hemolysis associated with a myopathy classified as glycogen storage disease type VII (see Chapter 87.1). Clinically, hemolytic anemia is complicated by muscle weakness, exercise intolerance, cramps, and possibly myoglobinuria. Enzyme assays for phosphofructokinase are low in RBCs and muscle.

Triose phosphate isomerase (TPI) deficiency is an autosomal recessive disorder affecting many systems. Affected patients have hemolytic anemia, cardiac abnormalities, and lower motor neuron and pyramidal tract impairment, with or without evidence of cerebral impairment. They usually die in early childhood. The gene for TPI has been cloned and sequenced and is located on chromosome 12.

Phosphoglycerate kinase (PGK) is the first ATP-generating step in glycolysis. At least 23 kindreds with PGK deficiency have been described. PGK is the only glycolytic enzyme inherited on the X chromosome. Affected males may have progressive extrapyramidal disease, myopathy, seizures, and variable mental retardation in conjunction with hemolytic anemia. Nine Japanese patients had neural or myopathic symptoms with hemolysis; 6 had hemolysis alone, 7 had neural or myopathic symptoms alone, and 1 had no symptoms. The gene for PGK is particularly large, spanning 23 kb, and various genetic abnormalities, including nucleotide substitutions, gene deletions, missense, and splicing mutations, result in PGK deficiency.

DEFICIENCIES OF ENZYMES OF THE HEXOSE MONOPHOSPHATE PATHWAY

The most important function of the hexose monophosphate pathway is to maintain glutathione in its reduced state (GSH) as protection against the oxidation of RBCs (see Fig. 463-1). Approximately 10% of the glucose taken up by RBCs passes through this pathway to provide the reduced form of nicotinamide-adenine dinucleotide phosphate (NADPH) necessary for the conversion of oxidized glutathione to GSH. Maintenance of GSH is essential for the physiologic inactivation of oxidant compounds, such as hydrogen peroxide, that are generated within RBCs. If glutathione, or any compound or enzyme necessary for maintaining it in the reduced state, is decreased, the SH groups of the RBC membrane are oxidized and the hemoglobin becomes denatured and may precipitate into **RBC inclusions called Heinz bodies.** Once Heinz bodies have formed, an acute hemolytic process results from damage to the RBC membrane by the precipitated hemoglobin, the oxidant agent, and the action of the spleen. The damaged RBCs then are rapidly removed from the circulation.

463.3 • Glucose-6-Phosphate Dehydrogenase and Related Deficiencies

Glucose-6-phosphate dehydrogenase (G6PD) deficiency is the most important disease of the hexose monophosphate pathway and is responsible for 2 clinical syndromes, episodic hemolytic anemia induced by infections, certain drugs or, rarely, fava beans, and spontaneous chronic nonspherocytic hemolytic anemia. This X-linked enzyme deficiency affects more than 200 million people worldwide; it represents an example of "balanced polymorphism" in which there is an evolutionary advantage of resistance to falciparum malaria in heterozygous females that outweighs the small negative effect of affected hemizygous males.

The deficiency is caused by inheritance of any of a large number of abnormal alleles of the gene responsible for the synthesis of the G6PD protein. The gene for G6PD has been cloned and sequenced. A web-accessible data base catalogs G6PD mutations *(www.bioinf.org.uk/g6pd)*. Some of these mutations that cause episodic vs chronic hemolysis are shown in Figure 463-2. Milder disease is associated with mutations near the amino terminus of the G6PD molecule, and chronic nonspherocytic hemolytic anemia is associated with mutations clustered near the carboxyl terminus. The normal enzyme found in most populations is designated *G6PD B*$^+$. A normal variant, designated *G6PD A*$^+$, is common in the African-American population. More than 100 distinct enzyme variants of G6PD are associated with a wide spectrum of hemolytic disease.

EPISODIC OR INDUCED HEMOLYTIC ANEMIA

ETIOLOGY. A central enzyme in the hexose monophosphate shunt of glucose metabolism, G6PD catalyzes the conversion of glucose-

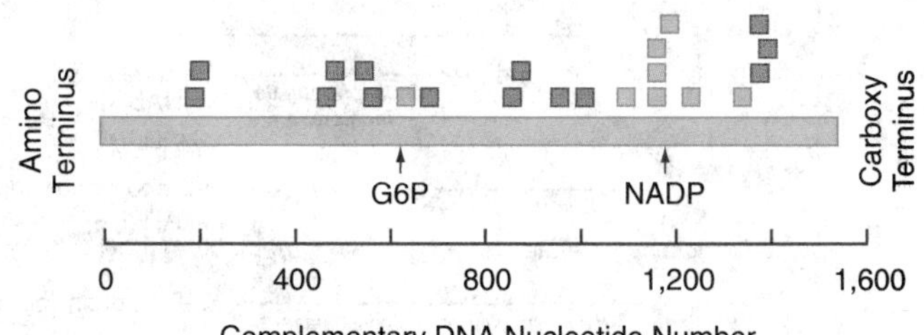

Figure 463-2. Nucleotide substitutions that cause glucose-6-phosphate dehydrogenase (G6PD) deficiency. *Blue squares* denote mutations that cause hereditary nonspherocytic hemolytic anemia. *Pink squares* indicate the location of mutations that cause enzyme deficiency, but cause hemolytic anemia only under conditions of stress. The putative binding sites for glucose-6-phosphate (G6P) and nicotinamide-adenine dinucleotide phosphate (NADP) are indicated by *arrows*. The mutations that produce nonspherocytic hemolytic anemia are almost all clustered between nucleotides 1089 and 1361, surrounding the NADP-binding domain. The exception is a mutation at nucleotide 637, which is adjacent to the putative G6P binding domain at nucleotide 605. (Modified from Beutler E: Glucose-6-phosphate deficiency. *N Engl J Med* 1991;324:169.) G6P, glucose-6-phosphate; NADP, nicotinamide-adenine dinucleotide phosphate.

6-phosphate to 6-phosphogluconic acid to produce NADPH and maintain glutathione in the reduced state (see Fig. 463-1).

Synthesis of RBC G6PD is determined by a gene on the X chromosome. Diseases involving this enzyme therefore occur more frequently in males than in females. Approximately 13% of male African-Americans have a mutant enzyme (**G6PD A⁻**) that results in a deficiency of RBC G6PD activity (≤5–15% of normal). Italians, Greeks, and other Mediterranean, Middle Eastern, African, and Asian ethnic groups also have a high incidence, ranging from 5–40%, of a variant designated **G6PD B⁻ (G6PD Mediterranean)**. In these variants, the G6PD activity of homozygous females or hemizygous males is <5% of normal. Heterozygous females have intermediate enzymatic activity and have 2 populations of RBCs: one is normal, and the other is deficient in G6PD activity. Most heterozygous females do not have clinical hemolysis after exposure to oxidant drugs. Rarely, the majority of RBCs are G6PD deficient in heterozygous females because of random inactivation (Lyon hypothesis) of the normal X chromosome.

Considerable variation in the defect is noted among various racial groups. The defect in Americans of African descent is less severe than in affected Americans of European descent. In Americans of African descent, the electrophoretically distinct enzyme variant is unstable in vivo, and its activity is decreased primarily in the older RBCs in the circulation. The enzyme activity of RBCs containing the variant enzyme (G6PD B⁻) in Americans of European descent is very low, often <1% of normal. A 3rd common mutant enzyme with markedly reduced activity (**G6PD Canton**) occurs in approximately 5% of the Chinese population. A large number of other rare enzyme variants have been associated with drug-induced hemolysis.

CLINICAL MANIFESTATIONS. In the usual pattern of G6PD deficiency, symptoms develop 24–48 hr after a patient has ingested a substance that has oxidant properties. Drugs that have these properties include aspirin, sulfonamides, and antimalarials, such as primaquine (Table 463-1). In some patients, ingestion of fava beans, a Mediterranean dietary staple, may also produce an acute, severe hemolytic syndrome called *favism*. This results from oxidative products derived from 2 glycosidic compounds, vicine and convicine, which are hydrolyzed to divicine and isouramil, ultimately producing hydrogen peroxide and other reactive oxygen products.

TABLE 463-1. Agents Precipitating Hemolysis in Glucose-6-Phosphate Dehydrogenase Deficiency

MEDICATIONS	CHEMICALS
Antibacterials	Phenylhydrazine
Sulfonamides	Benzene
Trimethoprim-sulfamethoxazole	Naphthalene
Nalidixic acid	**ILLNESS**
Chloramphenicol	Diabetic acidosis
Nitrofurantoin	Hepatitis
Antimalarials	Sepsis
Primaquine	
Pamaquine	
Chloroquine	
Quinacrine	
Others	
Phenacetin	
Vitamin K analogs	
Methylene blue	
Probenecid	
Acetylsalicylic acid	
Phenazopyridine	

Reproduced from Asselin BL, Segel GB. In Rakel R (editor): *Conn's Current Therapy*. Philadelphia, WB Saunders, 1994, p 341.

The degree of hemolysis varies with the inciting agent, the amount ingested, and the severity of the enzyme deficiency. In severe cases, hemoglobinuria and jaundice result, and the hemoglobin concentration may fall precipitously and may be life-threatening. In the **A⁻ variety** (Americans of African descent), the stability of the folded protein dimer is impaired, and this defect is accentuated as RBCs age. Thus, some spontaneous recovery of the hemolysis may be observed, even if administration of the drug is continued. This recovery is a result of the age-labile enzyme, which is abundant and more stable in younger RBCs. The associated reticulocytosis produces a compensated hemolytic process. Infection may be the most common cause of hemolysis, and significant but insidious hemolysis may occur in patients hospitalized for other illnesses, even when no exposure to drugs can be documented. In A⁻ G6PD deficiency, spontaneous hemolysis may occur in premature infants, but not in term infants. In Greek and Chinese newborns with the **G6PD B⁻ and Canton varieties**, the deficiency of G6PD is an important cause of hyperbilirubinemia and potential kernicterus. In a group of Sephardic Jewish female newborn heterozygotes, there is increased hyperbilirubinemia, particularly if the variant promoter *(UGT1A1)* of uridine 5c-diphosphate-glucuronyl transferase seen in Gilbert syndrome is present. When a pregnant woman ingests oxidant drugs, they may be transmitted to her G6PD-deficient fetus, and hemolytic anemia and jaundice may be apparent at birth.

LABORATORY FINDINGS. The onset of acute hemolysis results in a precipitous fall in hemoglobin and hematocrit. If the episode is severe, the hemoglobin-binding proteins, such as haptoglobin, are saturated, and free hemoglobin may appear in the plasma and subsequently in the urine (see Fig. 457-2). Unstained or supravital preparations of RBCs reveal **Heinz bodies** (precipitated hemoglobin), which are not visible on the Wright-stained blood film. Because cells containing these inclusions are rapidly removed from the circulation, they are not seen after the first 3–4 days of illness. The blood film reveals a few fragmented and polychromatophilic cells (bluish, large RBCs), representing reticulocytosis, which may be substantial (5–15%).

DIAGNOSIS. The diagnosis depends on direct or indirect demonstration of reduced G6PD activity in RBCs. By direct measurement, enzyme activity in affected persons is ≤10% of normal, and the reduction of enzyme activity is more extreme in Americans of European descent and in Asians than in Americans of African descent. Satisfactory screening tests are based on decoloration of methylene blue, reduction of methemoglobin, or fluorescence of NADPH. Immediately after a hemolytic episode, reticulocytes and young RBCs predominate. These young cells have significantly higher enzyme activity than do older cells in the A⁻ variety. Testing may therefore have to be deferred for a few weeks before a diagnostically low level of enzyme can be shown. The diagnosis can be suspected when G6PD activity is within the low-normal range in the presence of a high reticulocyte count. G6PD variants also can be detected by electrophoretic analysis.

PREVENTION AND TREATMENT. Prevention of hemolysis constitutes the most important therapeutic measure. When possible, males belonging to ethnic groups with a significant incidence of G6PD deficiency (e.g., Greeks, southern Italians, Sephardic Jews, Filipinos, southern Chinese, Americans of African descent, and Thais) should be tested for the defect before known oxidant drugs are given. The usual doses of aspirin and trimethoprim-sulfamethoxazole do not cause clinically relevant hemolysis in the A⁻ variety. However, aspirin administered in doses used for acute rheumatic fever (60–100 mg/kg/24 hr) may produce a severe hemolytic episode. When hemolysis has occurred, supportive therapy may require blood transfusions, although recovery is the rule when the oxidant agent is discontinued.

CHRONIC HEMOLYTIC ANEMIAS ASSOCIATED WITH DEFICIENCY OF G6PD OR RELATED FACTORS

Chronic nonspherocytic hemolytic anemia has been associated with profound deficiency of G6PD caused by enzyme variants, particularly those defective in quantity, activity, or stability. The gene defects leading to chronic hemolysis are located primarily in the region of the NADP binding site near the carboxyl terminus of the protein (see Fig. 463-2). These include the Loma Linda, Tomah, Iowa, Beverly Hills, Nashville, Riverside, Santiago de Cuba, and Andalus variants. Persons with G6PD B⁻ (Mediterranean) enzyme deficiency occasionally have chronic hemolysis, and the hemolytic process may worsen after ingestion of oxidant drugs. Splenectomy is of little value in these types of chronic hemolysis.

Other enzyme defects may impair the regeneration of GSH as an oxidant "sump" (see Fig. 463-1). Mild, chronic nonspherocytic anemia has been reported in association with decreased RBC GSH, resulting from γ-glutamylcysteine or glutathione synthetase deficiencies. Deficiency of 6-phosphogluconate dehydrogenase (6PDG) has been associated primarily with drug-induced hemolysis, and hemolysis with hyperbilirubinemia has been related to a deficiency of glutathione peroxidase in newborn infants.

Beutler E: Glucose-6-phosphate dehydrogenase deficiency. *N Engl J Med* 1994;331:169–173.

Fujii H, Miwa S: Other erythrocyte enzyme deficiencies associated with non-haematological symptoms: Phosphoglycerate kinase and phosphofructokinase deficiency. *Baillieres Best Pract Res Clin Haematol* 2000;13:141–148.

Kaplan M, Beutler E, Vreman HJ, et al: Neonatal hyperbilirubinemia in glucose-6-phosphate dehydrogenase-deficient heterozygotes. *Pediatrics* 1999;104:68–74.

Kaplan M, Muraca M, Hammerman C, et al: Bilirubin conjugation, reflected by conjugated bilirubin fractions, in glucose-6-phosphate dehydrogenase-deficient neonates: A determining factor in the pathogenesis of hyperbilirubinemia. *Pediatrics* 1998;102:E37.

Martinov MV, Plotnikov AG, Vitvitsky VM, et al: Deficiencies of glycolytic enzymes as a possible cause of hemolytic anemia. *Biochim Biophys Acta* 2000;1474:75–87.

McMullin MF: The molecular basis of disorders of red cell enzymes. *J Clin Pathol* 1999;52:241–244.

Min-Oo G, Gros P: Erythrocyte variants and the nature of their malaria protective effect. *Cell Microbiol* 2005;7:753–763.

Valentin C, Pissard S, Martin J, et al: Triose phosphate isomerase deficiency in 3 French families: Two novel null alleles, a frameshift mutation (TPI Alfortville) and an alteration in the initiation codon (TPI Paris). *Blood* 2000;96:1130–1135.

Zanella A, Bianchi P: Red cell pyruvate kinase deficiency: From genetics. *Baillieres Best Pract Res Clin Haematol* 2000;13:57–81.

Zanella A, Fermo E, Bianchi P, Valentini G: Red cell pyruvate kinase deficiency: Molecular and clinical aspects. *Br J Haematol* 2005;130:11–25.

Chapter 464 ■ Hemolytic Anemias Resulting from Extracellular Factors

George B. Segel

AUTOIMMUNE HEMOLYTIC ANEMIAS

A number of extrinsic agents and disorders may lead to premature destruction of red blood cells (RBCs) [see Table 457-1]. Among the most clearly defined are antibodies associated with immune hemolytic anemias. The hallmark of this group of diseases is a positive direct antiglobulin (Coombs) test, which detects a coating of immunoglobulin or components of complement on the RBC surface. The most important immune hemolytic disorder in pediatric practice is hemolytic disease of the newborn (erythroblastosis fetalis), caused by transplacental transfer of maternal antibody active against the RBCs of the fetus, that is, isoimmune hemolytic anemia (see Chapter 103.2). Various other immune hemolytic anemias are autoimmune (Table 464-1) and may be idiopathic or related to various infections (Epstein-Barr virus, rarely HIV, cytomegalovirus, and mycoplasma), immunologic diseases (systemic lupus erythematosus [SLE], rheumatoid arthritis), immunodeficiency diseases (agammaglobulinemia, autoimmune lymphoproliferative disorder, dysgammaglobulinemias), neoplasms (lymphoma, leukemia, and Hodgkin disease), or drugs (methyldopa, L-dopa). Other drugs (penicillins, cephalosporins) cause immune hemolysis that is not "autoimmune." The antibodies are "drug-dependent" and usually (although not always) have no "specificity" for RBC membrane antigens.

TABLE 464-1. Diseases Characterized by Immune-mediated Red Blood Cell Destruction

AUTOIMMUNE HEMOLYTIC ANEMIA DUE TO WARM REACTIVE AUTOANTIBODIES
Primary (idiopathic)
Secondary
Lymphoproliferative disorders
Connective tissue disorders (especially systemic lupus erythematosus)
Nonlymphoid neoplasms (e.g., ovarian tumors)
Chronic inflammatory diseases (e.g., ulcerative colitis)
AUTOIMMUNE HEMOLYTIC ANEMIA DUE TO COLD REACTIVE AUTOANTIBODIES (CRYOPATHIC HEMOLYTIC SYNDROMES)
Primary (idiopathic) cold agglutinin disease
Secondary cold agglutinin disease
Lymphoproliferative disorders
Infections (*Mycoplasma pneumoniae*, Epstein-Barr virus)
Paroxysmal cold hemoglobinuria
Primary (idiopathic)
Viral syndromes (most common)
Congenital or tertiary syphilis
DRUG-INDUCED IMMUNE HEMOLYTIC ANEMIA (SEE TABLE 464-2)
Hapten/drug adsorption (e.g., penicillin)
Ternary (immune) complex (e.g., quinine or quinidine)
True autoantibody induction (e.g., methyldopa)

Modified from Packman CH: Autoimmune hemolytic anemias. In Rakel R (editor): *Conn's Current Therapy*. Philadelphia, WB Saunders, 1995, p 305.

AUTOIMMUNE HEMOLYTIC ANEMIAS ASSOCIATED WITH "WARM" ANTIBODIES

ETIOLOGY. In the autoimmune hemolytic anemias, abnormal antibodies are directed against RBCs, but the pathogenetic mechanisms are uncertain. The autoantibody may be produced as an inappropriate immune response to an RBC antigen or to another antigenic epitope similar to an RBC antigen, known as *molecular mimicry.* Alternatively, an infectious agent may alter the RBC membrane so that it becomes "foreign" or antigenic to the host. The antibodies usually react to epitopes (antigens) that are "public" or common to all human RBCs, such as Rh proteins.

In most instances of warm antibody hemolysis, no underlying cause can be found; this is the primary or idiopathic type (see Table 464-1). If the autoimmune hemolysis is associated with an underlying disease, such as a lymphoproliferative disorder, SLE, or immunodeficiency, it is secondary. In as many as 20% of cases of immune hemolysis, drugs may be implicated (Table 464-2).

Drugs (penicillin or sometimes cephalosporins) that cause hemolysis via the "hapten" mechanism (immune but not autoimmune) bind tightly to the RBC membrane (see Table 464-1). Anti-

TABLE 464-2. Selected Drugs that Cause Immune-mediated Hemolysis

MECHANISM	DRUG ABSORPTION (HAPTEN)	IMMUNE COMPLEX	AUTOANTIBODY
Direct antiglobulin test	Positive anti-IgG	Positive anti-C3	Positive anti-IgG
Site of hemolysis	Extravascular	Intravascular	Extravascular
Medications	Penicillin	Quinidine	α Methyldopa
	Ampicillin	Phenacetin	Mefenamic acid (Ponstel)
	Methicillin	Hydrochlorothiazide	L-dopa
	Carbenicillin	Rifampin (Rifadin)	Procainamide
	Cephalothin (Keflin)*	Sulfonamides	Ibuprofen
	Cephaloridine (Loridine)*	Isoniazid	Diclofenac (Voltaren)
		Quinine	Interferon alfa
		Insulin	
		Tetracycline	
		Melphalan (Alkeran)	
		Acetaminophen	
		Hydralazine (Apresoline)	
		Probenecid	
		Chlorpromazine (Thorazine)	
		Streptomycin	
		Fluorouracil (Adrucil)	
		Sulindac (Clinoril)	

*Not available in the United States.

Adapted with permission in *American Family Physician* (see below) from Schwartz RS, Berkman EM, Silberstein LE: Autoimmune hemolytic anemias. In Hoffman R, Benz EJ Jr, Schattil SJ, et al (editors): *Hematology: Basic Principles and Practice*, 3rd ed. Philadelphia, Churchill Livingstone, 2000, p 624. Reproduced with permission from Dhaliwal G, Cornett PA, Tierney LM: Hemolytic anemia. *Am Family Physician* 2004;69:2603.

bodies to the drug, either newly or previously formed, bind to the drug molecules on RBCs, mediating their destruction in the spleen. In other cases, certain drugs, such as quinine and quinidine, do not bind to RBCs, but rather form part of a "ternary complex," consisting of the drug, an RBC membrane antigen, and an antibody that recognizes both (see Table 464-1). Methyldopa and sometimes cephalosporins may, by unknown mechanisms, incite true autoantibodies to RBC membrane antigens, so that the presence of the drug is not required to cause hemolysis.

CLINICAL MANIFESTATIONS. Autoimmune hemolytic anemias may occur in either of 2 general clinical patterns. The first, an acute transient type lasting 3–6 mo and occurring predominantly in children ages 2–12 yr, accounts for 70–80% of patients. It is frequently preceded by an infection, usually respiratory. Onset may be acute, with prostration, pallor, jaundice, pyrexia, and hemoglobinuria, or more gradual, with primarily fatigue and pallor. The spleen is usually enlarged and is the primary site of destruction of immunoglobulin G (IgG)–coated RBCs. Underlying systemic disorders are unusual. A consistent response to glucocorticoid therapy, a low mortality rate, and full recovery are characteristic of the acute form. The other clinical pattern involves a prolonged and chronic course, which is more frequent in infants and in children older than 12 yr. Hemolysis may continue for many months or years. Abnormalities involving other blood elements are common, and the response to glucocorticoids is variable and inconsistent. The mortality rate is approximately 10%, and death is often attributable to an underlying systemic disease.

LABORATORY FINDINGS. In many cases, anemia is profound, with hemoglobin levels <6 g/dL. Considerable spherocytosis and polychromasia are present. More than 50% of the circulating RBCs may be reticulocytes, and nucleated RBCs usually are present. In some cases, a low reticulocyte count may be present, particularly early in the episode. Leukocytosis is common. The platelet count is usually normal, but concomitant immune thrombocytopenic purpura sometimes occurs (**Evans syndrome**). The prognosis for patients with Evans syndrome is guarded, because many have chronic disease, including SLE or an autoimmune lymphoproliferative disorder.

Results of the direct antiglobulin test are strongly positive, and free antibody can sometimes be demonstrated in the serum (indirect Coombs test). These antibodies are active at 35–40°C ("warm" antibodies) and most often belong to the IgG class. They do not require complement for activity and usually do not produce agglutination in vitro; the latter feature is referred to as an *incomplete* antibody. Antibodies from the serum and those eluted from the RBCs react with the RBCs of many persons, in addition to those of the patient. They often have been regarded as nonspecific panagglutinins, but careful studies have revealed specificity for RBC antigens of the Rh system in 70% (≈50% adults) of patients. Complement, particularly C3b, may be detected on the RBCs in conjunction with IgG. The Coombs test result is occasionally negative because of the limited sensitivity of the Coombs reaction. A minimum of 260–500 molecules of IgG per cell is necessary on the RBC membrane to produce a positive reaction. Special tests are required to detect the antibody in cases of "Coombs-negative" autoimmune hemolytic anemia. Warm antibody hemolysis may be IgG-positive, both IgG- and complement (C3b)-positive, or solely complement-positive if the IgG is < the detection limit of the anti-IgG Coombs reagent.

TREATMENT. Transfusions usually are only of transient benefit, but may be required initially because of the severity of the anemia until the effect of other treatment is observed. It may be extremely difficult to find compatible blood; blood in which the RBCs give the least positive in vitro reaction by the Coombs technique should be chosen. It is sometimes necessary to give blood that is "incompatible" as judged by cross matching. Failure to transfuse a profoundly anemic infant or child may lead to serious morbidity and even death.

Patients with mild disease and compensated hemolysis may not require any treatment. If the hemolysis is severe and results in significant anemia or symptoms, treatment with glucocorticoids is initiated. Glucocorticoids decrease the rate of hemolysis by blocking macrophage function by downregulating Fcγ receptor expression, decreasing the production of the autoantibody, and perhaps by enhancing the elution of antibody from the RBCs. Prednisone or its equivalent is administered at a dose of 2 mg/kg/24 hr. In some patients with severe hemolysis, doses of prednisone of up to 6 mg/kg/24 hr may be required to reduce the rate of hemolysis. Treatment should be continued until the rate of hemolysis decreases, and then the dose is gradually reduced. If relapse occurs, resumption of the full dosage may be necessary. The disease tends to remit spontaneously within a few wk or mo. The Coombs test result may remain positive, even after hemolysis has subsided. When hemolytic anemia remains severe despite glucocorticoid therapy, or if very large doses are necessary to maintain a reasonable hemoglobin level, IV immunoglobulin may be tried. Rituximab, a monoclonal antibody that targets B lymphocytes, the source of antibody production, has been useful in chronic cases refractory to conventional therapy. Plasmapheresis has been used in refractory cases, but generally is not helpful. Splenectomy may be beneficial, but is complicated by a heightened risk of infection with encapsulated organisms, particularly in patients younger than 2 yr. Prophylaxis is indicated with appropriate vaccines (pneumococcal, meningococcal, and *Haemophilus influenzae* type b) before splenectomy and with oral penicillin after splenectomy.

COURSE AND PROGNOSIS. Acute idiopathic autoimmune hemolytic disease in childhood varies in severity, but is self-limited; mortality from untreatable anemia is rare. Approximately 30% of patients have chronic hemolysis, often associated with an underlying disease, such as SLE, lymphoma, or leukemia. In adults, the presence of antiphospholipid antibodies in patients with immune hemolysis predisposes to thrombosis. Mortality in chronic cases depends on the primary disorder.

AUTOIMMUNE HEMOLYTIC ANEMIAS ASSOCIATED WITH "COLD" ANTIBODIES

"Cold" antibodies are RBC antibodies that are more active at low temperatures and agglutinate RBCs at temperatures <37°C. They are primarily of the IgM class and require complement for activity. The range of temperature associated with RBC agglutination is called the *thermal amplitude*. A higher thermal amplitude results in hemolysis with less severe exposure to a cold environment. High antibody titers are associated with a high thermal amplitude.

COLD AGGLUTININ DISEASE. Cold antibodies usually have specificity for the oligosaccharide antigens of the I/i system. They may occur in primary or idiopathic cold agglutinin disease, secondary to infections such as those from *Mycoplasma pneumoniae* and Epstein-Barr virus, or secondary to lymphoproliferative disorders. After *M. pneumoniae* infection, the anti-I levels may increase considerably, and occasionally, enormous increases may occur to titers of ≥1:30,000. The antibody has specificity for the I antigen and thus reacts poorly with human cord RBC, which possess the i antigen, but exhibit low levels of I. Patients with infectious mononucleosis occasionally have cold agglutinin disease, and the antibodies in these patients often have anti-i specificity. This antibody causes less hemolysis in adults than in children because adults have fewer i molecules on their RBCs. Spontaneous RBC agglutination is observed in the cold, and RBC aggregates are seen on the blood film. Mean corpuscular volume may be spuriously elevated because of cell agglutination. The severity of the hemolysis is related to the thermal amplitude of the antibody, which itself is partly dependent on the IgM antibody titer.

When very high titers of cold antibodies are present and active near body temperature, severe intravascular hemolysis with hemoglobinemia and hemoglobinuria may occur and be heightened on a patient's exposure to cold (external temperature or ingested foods). Each IgM molecule has the potential to activate a C1 molecule so that large amounts of complement are found on the RBCs in cold agglutinin disease. These sensitized RBCs may undergo intravascular complement lysis or may be destroyed in the liver and spleen.

Cold agglutinin disease is less common in children than in adults, and it more frequently results in an acute, self-limited episode of hemolysis. Glucocorticoids are much less effective in cold agglutinin disease than in disease with warm antibodies. Patients should avoid exposure to cold and should be treated for underlying disease. In the infrequent patients with severe hemolytic disease, treatment includes immunosuppression and plasmapheresis. Successful treatment of cold agglutinin disease has been reported with the monoclonal antibody rituximab, which effectively depletes B lymphocytes. Splenectomy is not useful in cold agglutinin disease.

PAROXYSMAL COLD HEMOGLOBINURIA. This form of hemolytic anemia is mediated by the Donath-Landsteiner hemolysin, which is an IgG cold-reactive autoantibody with anti-P specificity. This antibody fixes large amounts of complement in the cold, and the RBCs lyse as the temperature is increased. Most reported cases are self-limited and usually are associated with nonspecific viral infections. They are now rarely found in association with congenital or acquired syphilis. This disorder may account for 30% of immune hemolytic episodes among children. Treatment includes transfusion for severe anemia and avoidance of cold ambient temperatures.

Flores G, Cunningham-Rundles C, Newland AC, et al: Efficacy of intravenous immunoglobulin in the treatment of autoimmune hemolytic anemia: Results in 73 patients. *Am J Hematol* 1993;44:237–242.

Gehrs BC, Friedberg RC: Autoimmune hemolytic anemia. *Am J Hematol* 2002;69:258–271.

King KE, Ness PM: Treatment of hemolytic anemia. *Semin Hematol* 2005;42:131–136.

Packman CH: Acquired hemolytic anemia due to warm-reacting autoantibodies. In Beutler E, Lichtman MA, Coller BS, et al (editors): *Williams Manual of Hematology*, 6th ed. New York, McGraw-Hill, 2001, pp 639–648.

Petz L: Treatment of autoimmune hemolytic anemias. *Curr Opin Hematol* 2001;8:411–416.

Ramanathan S, Koutts J, Hertzberg MS: Two cases of refractory warm autoimmune hemolytic anemia treated with rituximab. *Am J Hematol* 2005;78:123–126.

Sparling TG, Andricevic M, Wass H: Remission of cold hemagglutinin disease induced by rituximab therapy. *CMAJ* 2001;164:1405.

Chapter 465 ■ Hemolytic Anemias Secondary to Other Extracellular Factors

George B. Segel

FRAGMENTATION HEMOLYSIS. See Table 457-1. Red blood cell (RBC) destruction may occur in hemolytic anemias because of mechanical injury as the cells traverse a damaged vascular bed. Damage may be microvascular, when RBCs are sheared by fibrin in the capillaries during intravascular coagulation or when renovascular disease accompanies hemolytic-uremic syndrome (see Chapter 518) or thrombotic thrombocytopenic purpura. Larger vessels may be involved in Kasabach-Merritt syndrome (giant hemangioma and thrombocytopenia; see Chapter 505) or when a replacement heart valve is poorly epithelialized. The blood film shows many "schistocytes," or fragmented cells, as well as polychromatophilia, reflecting the reticulocytosis (see Fig. 458-3*F*). Secondary iron deficiency may complicate the intravascular hemolysis because of urinary hemoglobin and hemosiderin iron loss (see Fig. 457-2). Treatment should be directed toward the underlying condition, and the prognosis depends on the effectiveness of this treatment. The benefit from transfusion is transient because the transfused cells are destroyed as quickly as those produced by the patient.

THERMAL INJURY. Extensive burns may directly damage the RBCs and cause hemolysis that results in the formation of spherocytes. Blood loss and marrow suppression may contribute to anemia and require blood transfusion. Erythropoietin (EPO) has been used as treatment for diminished RBC production.

RENAL DISEASE. The anemia of uremia is multifactorial in origin. EPO production may be decreased and the marrow suppressed by toxic metabolites. Furthermore, the RBC life span often is shortened owing to retention of metabolites and organic acidemia. The use of EPO in chronic renal disease has markedly decreased the need for blood transfusion.

LIVER DISEASE. A change in the ratio of cholesterol to phospholipids in the plasma may result in changes in the composition of the RBC membrane and shortening of the RBC life span. Some patients with liver disease have many target RBCs on the blood film, whereas others have a preponderance of spiculated cells.

TOXINS AND VENOMS. Bacterial sepsis due to *Haemophilus influenzae,* staphylococci, and streptococci may be complicated by accompanying hemolysis. Particularly severe hemolytic anemia has been observed in clostridial infections and results from a hemolytic clostridial toxin. Large numbers of spherocytes may be seen on the blood film. Spherocytic hemolysis also may be noted after bites by various snakes, including cobras, vipers, and rattlesnakes, which have phospholipases in their venom. Large numbers of bites by insects, such as bees, wasps, and yellow jackets, also may cause spherocytic hemolysis by a similar mechanism (see Chapter 714).

WILSON DISEASE. See Chapter 354.2. An acute and self-limited episode of hemolytic anemia may precede by years the onset of hepatic or neurologic symptoms in Wilson disease. This appears to result from the toxic effects of free copper on the RBC membrane. The blood film often (but not always) shows large numbers of spherocytes, and the Coombs test result is negative. Because early diagnosis of Wilson disease permits prophylactic treatment with penicillamine and prevention of hepatic and neurologic disease, correct assessment of this rare type of hemolysis is important.

Grudeva-Popova JG, Spasova MI, Chepileva KG, Zaprianov ZH: Acute hemolytic anemia as an initial clinical manifestation of Wilson's disease. *Folia Med (Plovdiv)* 2000;42:42–46.

Sakuri J, Nagahama M, Oda M: Clostridium perfringens alpha-toxin: Characterization and mode of action. *J Biochem (Tokyo)* 2004;136:569–574.

Section 4 — Polycythemia (Erythrocytosis) — Karen Burns and Bruce M. Camitta

Chapter 466 ■ Primary Polycythemia (Polycythemia Rubra Vera)

Polycythemia exists when the red blood cell (RBC) count, hemoglobin level, and total RBC volume all exceed the upper limits of normal. In postpubertal individuals, an RBC mass >25% above the mean normal value (based on body surface area), or hematocrit >60 (in males) or >56 (in females) indicates absolute erythrocytosis. A decrease in plasma volume, such as occurs in acute dehydration and burns, may result in a high hemoglobin value. These situations are more accurately designated as *hemoconcentration* because the RBC mass is not increased and normalization of the plasma volume restores hemoglobin to normal levels.

TABLE 466-1. Diagnosis of Polycythemia Vera

MAJOR CRITERIA

1. Increased red cell mass (see text)
2. Arterial O_2 saturation of ≥92%*
3. Palpable splenomegaly

MINOR CRITERIA

1. Platelet count of >400 × 10^9/L
2. Leukocytosis of >12 × 10^9/L
3. Increased leukocyte alkaline phosphatase
4. Increased vitamin B_{12} (>900 pg/mL) or unbound B_{12} binding capacity (>2,200 pg/mL)

DIAGNOSIS

All 3 major criteria

1, 2, and 2 minor criteria

*Absent causes of secondary polycythemia

PATHOGENESIS. Polycythemia vera, a panmyeloproliferative disorder, has been reported in only a few children. A gain of function mutation of *JAK2* has been shown in 75% of affected patients. The erythropoietin receptor is normal, and in vitro cultures of erythroid precursors of affected persons do not require added erythropoietin to stimulate growth. Serum erythropoietin levels are normal or low. Diagnostic criteria are listed in Table 466-1.

CLINICAL MANIFESTATIONS. Patients with polycythemia vera usually have hepatosplenomegaly. Erythrocytosis may cause hypertension, headache, shortness of breath, or neurologic symptoms. Granulocytosis may cause diarrhea or pruritus from histamine release. Thrombocytosis (with or without platelet dysfunction) may cause thrombosis or hemorrhage.

TREATMENT. Phlebotomy is the initial treatment of choice. Iron supplementation should be given to prevent viscosity problems from microcytosis. Antiplatelet agents (aspirin) may reduce the risks of thrombosis and abnormal bleeding in patients with marked thrombocytosis. If this is unsuccessful, antiproliferative treatments (hydroxyurea, anagrelide, interferon-α) may be helpful. The risk of transformation of the disease into myelofibrosis or acute leukemia has diminished with discontinuation of the use of alkylating agents and radioactive phosphorus. Prolonged survival is not unusual.

Cario H: Childhood polycythemias/erythrocytoses: Classification, diagnosis, clinical presentation, and treatment. *Ann Hematol* 2005;84:137–145. Epub 2004 Dec 15.

Gregg XT, Prchal JT: Recent advances in the molecular biology of congenital polycythemias and polycythemia vera. *Current Hematol Rep* 2005;4: 238–242.

Klippel S, Strunck E, Temprinac S, et al: Quantification of PRV-1 mRNA distinguishes polycythemia vera from secondary erythrocytosis. *Blood* 2003;102:3569–3574.

Kralovics R, Passamonti F, Buser AS, et al: A gain of function mutation of *JAK2* in myeloproliferative disorders. *N Engl J Med* 2005;352:1779–1790.

Kwaan HC, Wang I: Hyperviscosity in polycythemia vera and other red cell abnormalities. *Semin Thromb Hemostasis* 2003;29:451–458.

Schaefer AI: Molecular basis of the diagnosis and treatment of polycythemia vera and essential thrombocythemia. *Blood* 2006;107:4214–4222.

Spivak JL: Polycythemia vera: Myths, mechanisms, and management. *Blood* 2002;100:4272–4290.

Chapter 467 ■ Secondary Polycythemia

PATHOGENESIS. Secondary polycythemia is diagnosed when true polycythemia is caused by another physiologic process (Table 467-1). Polycythemia may be present in any clinical situation associated with chronic arterial oxygen desaturation. Cardiovascular defects involving right-to-left shunts and pulmonary diseases interfering with proper oxygenation are the most common causes of hypoxic polycythemia. Clinical findings usually include cyanosis, hyperemia of the sclerae and mucous membranes, and clubbing of the fingers. As the hematocrit rises to >65%, clinical manifestations of hyperviscosity, such as headache and hypertension, may require phlebotomy (see Chapter 103.3). Living at high altitudes also causes hypoxic polycythemia; the hemoglobin level increases approximately 4% for each rise of 1,000 M in altitude. Partial obstruction of a renal artery rarely results in polycythemia.

More subtle forms of hypoxia may also cause polycythemia. Congenital methemoglobinemia resulting from a deficiency of cytochrome b5 reductase may cause cyanosis and polycythemia (see Chapter 462.7). This condition is transmitted as an autosomal recessive trait. Most affected individuals are asymptomatic. Neurologic abnormalities may be present in patients whose enzyme deficit is not limited to hematopoietic cells. Dominantly transmitted polycythemia is caused by hemoglobins that have increased oxygen affinity. Cyanosis may occur in the presence of as little as 1.5 g/dL of methemoglobin, but is uncommon in other hemoglobin variants unless hyperviscosity results in localized hypoxemia (see Chapter 103.3).

Polycythemia has also been associated with benign and malignant tumors that secrete erythropoietin. Exogenous or endogenous excess of anabolic steroids also may cause polycythemia.

TABLE 467-1. Differential Diagnosis of Polycythemia

POLYCYTHEMIA VERA
SECONDARY
Familial
Hemoglobinopathy
High–oxygen affinity variants
Methemoglobin reductase deficiency
Chronic carbon monoxide exposure
Hormonal
Adrenal disease
Virilizing hyperplasia, Cushing syndrome
Anabolic steroid therapy
Malignant tumors
Adrenal, cerebellar, hepatic, other
Renal disease
Cysts, hydronephrosis
Hypoxia
Altitude
Cardiac disease
Lung disease
Central hypoventilation
Metabolic
2,3-diphosphoglycerate deficiency
Neonatal
Normal intrauterine environment
Twin-twin or maternal-fetal hemorrhage
Infants of diabetic mothers
Intrauterine growth retardation
Trisomy 13, 18, or 21
Adrenal hyperplasia
Thyrotoxicosis
SPURIOUS (PLASMA VOLUME DECREASE)

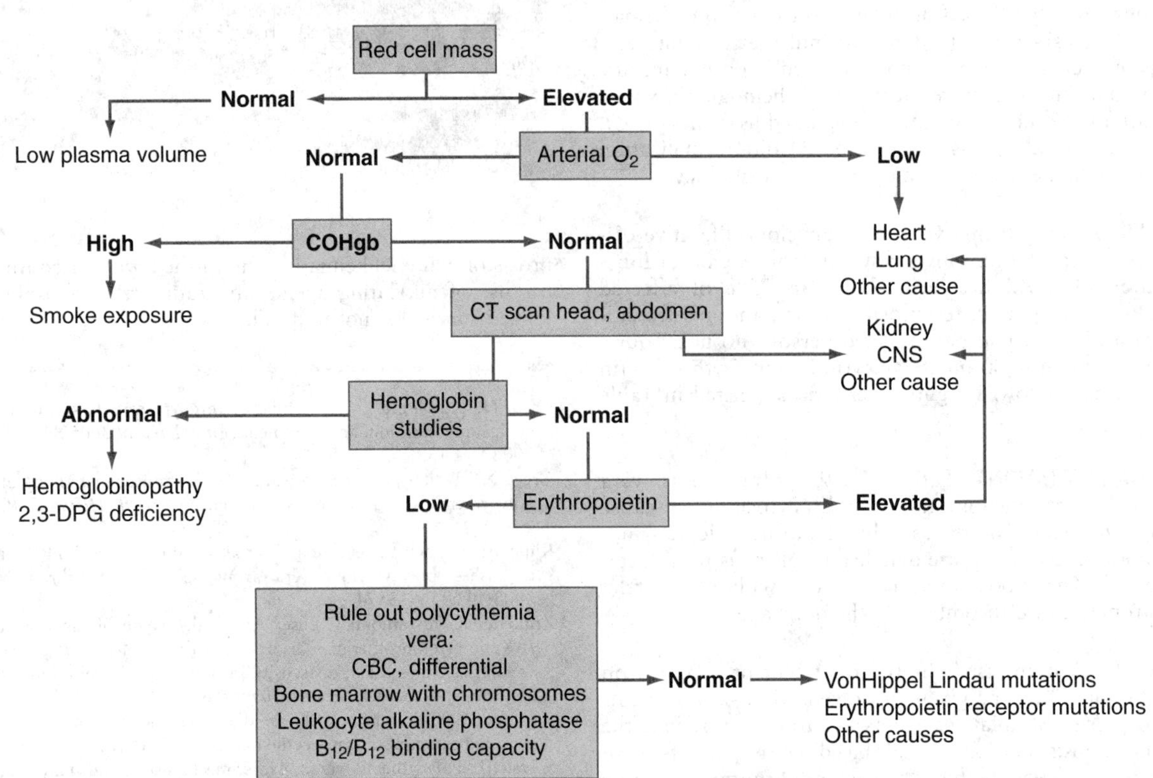

Figure 467-1. Sequential studies to evaluate polycythemia. COHgb, carboxyhemoglobin; CNS, central nervous system; 2,3-DPG, 2,3-diphosphoglycerate; CBC, complete blood count.

Polycythemias have been transmitted as dominant or recessive conditions. In some families, there is an abnormality of the erythropoietin receptor or the von-Hippel Lindau gene.

DIAGNOSIS. Sequential studies to evaluate polycythemia are outlined in Figure 467-1.

TREATMENT. For mild disease, observation is sufficient. When hematocrit is >65–70% (hemoglobin >23 g/dL), blood viscosity markedly increases. Periodic phlebotomy may prevent or decrease symptoms. Apheresed blood should be replaced with plasma or saline to prevent hypovolemia in patients accustomed to a chronically elevated total blood volume. Increased demand for red blood cell production may cause iron deficiency. Iron-deficient microcytic red cells are more rigid, further increasing the risk of intracranial and other thromboses in patients with polycythemia. Periodic assessment of iron status, with treatment of iron deficiency, should be performed.

Cario H: Childhood polycythemias/erythrocytoses: Classification, diagnosis, clinical presentation, and treatment. *Ann Hematol* 2005;84:137–145.

Pappas A, Delaney-Black V: Differential diagnosis and management of polycythemia. *Pediatr Clin North Am* 2004;51:1063–1086.

Percy MJ, McMullin MF, Jowit TT, et al: Chuvash-type congenital polycythemia in 4 families of Asian and Western European ancestry. *Blood* 2003;102:1097–1099.

Prchal JT: Pathogenetic mechanisms of polycythemia vera and congenital polycythemia disorders. *Semin Hematol* 2001;38(Suppl 2):10–20.

Van Maerken T, Hunnick K, Callewaert L, et al: Familial and congenital polycythemias: A diagnostic approach. *J Pediatr Hematol Oncol* 2004;26:407–416.

Section 5 — The Pancytopenias

Chapter 468 ■ The Constitutional Pancytopenias

Melvin H. Freedman

Pancytopenia refers to a reduction below normal values of all 3 peripheral blood lineages: leukocytes, platelets, and erythrocytes. Pancytopenia requires microscopic examination of a bone marrow biopsy specimen and a marrow aspirate to assess overall cellularity and morphology. **Hypocellular marrow** on biopsy is seen with constitutional (inherited) marrow failure syndromes, acquired aplastic anemia of varied etiologies (see Chapter 469), and the hypoplastic variant of myelodysplastic syndrome (MDS; see Chapter 134). **Cellular marrow** is seen with primary bone marrow disease: acute leukemia (see Chapter 495), MDS, myelofibrosis, osteopetrosis (see Chapter 697), and hemophagocytic lymphohistiocytosis (see Chapter 507). Cellular marrow is also seen secondary to systemic disease: autoimmune (systemic lupus erythematosus; see Chapter 157), vitamin B_{12} or folate deficiency (see Chapter 46), storage disease (Gaucher and Niemann-Pick diseases; see Chapter 86), overwhelming infection, metastatic solid tumors, sarcoidosis, and hypersplenism.

THE CONSTITUTIONAL PANCYTOPENIAS

Constitutional pancytopenia is defined as decreased marrow production of the 3 major hematopoietic lineages on an inherited basis, resulting in anemia, neutropenia, and thrombocytopenia. These conditions (Table 468-1) can be inherited in mendelian fashion by mutant genes with patterns of autosomal dominant, autosomal recessive, or X-linked types. Acquired factors may also be operative. Constitutional pancytopenias account for approximately ⅓ of cases of pediatric marrow failure. Fanconi anemia is the most common constitutional disorder.

FANCONI (APLASTIC) ANEMIA

Etiology and Epidemiology. This syndrome is inherited in an autosomal recessive manner in almost every case; it occurs in all racial and ethnic groups. At presentation, patients may have: (1) typical physical anomalies, but normal hematologic findings; (2) normal physical features, but abnormal hematologic findings; or (3) physical anomalies and abnormal hematologic findings, the classic phenotype (39% of cases). There can be sibling discordance in clinical and hematologic findings, even in affected monozygotic twins. Approximately 75% of patients are 3–14 yr of age at the time of diagnosis (mean age, 8–9 yr; range, 0–48 yr).

Pathology. All patients have abnormal chromosome fragility seen in metaphase preparations of peripheral blood lymphocytes cultured with phytohemagglutinin and enhanced by adding clastogenic agents such as **diepoxybutane (DEB)**. Cell fusion of Fanconi cells with normal cells or with cells from unrelated patients with Fanconi anemia produces a corrective effect on chromosomal fragility, a process called *complementation.* This allows subtyping of patients into discrete complementation groups. Twelve complementation groups have been identified, which led to the cloning of 11 mutant Fanconi (*FANC*) genes. The protein products of wild-type *FANC* genes are involved in the DNA damage repair biochemical pathway. Mutant gene proteins lead to genomic instability, chromosome fragility, and Fanconi anemia. An inability of the Fanconi cell to remove oxygen-free radicals, resulting in oxidative damage, is a contributing factor in the pathogenesis. Additional factors are also operative. Leukocyte telomere length is significantly shortened, but telomerase activity is increased, suggesting a high proliferative rate of marrow progenitors, ultimately leading to their pre-

TABLE 468-1. Constitutional (Inherited) Pancytopenia Syndromes
Fanconi anemia
Shwachman-Diamond syndrome
Dyskeratosis congenita
Amegakaryocytic thrombocytopenia
Other genetic syndromes
Down syndrome
Dubowitz syndrome
Seckel syndrome
Reticular dysgenesis
Schimke immuno-osseous dysplasia
Familial aplastic anemia (non-Fanconi)
Pearson syndrome
Reticular dysgenesis
Noonan syndrome

mature senescence. Increased marrow cell apoptosis occurs and is mediated by Fas, a membrane glycoprotein receptor containing an integral death domain. A consistent finding is diminished interleukin 6 production and markedly heightened tumor necrosis factor-α generation.

Clinical Manifestations. The most common anomaly is hyperpigmentation of the trunk, neck, and intertriginous areas, as well as café-au-lait spots and vitiligo, alone or in combination (Fig. 468-1 and Table 468-2). Most patients have short stature. Growth failure may be associated with abnormal growth hormone secretion, or with hypothyroidism. Absent radii and hypoplastic, supernumerary, bifid, or absent thumbs are common. Anomalies of the feet, congenital hip dislocation, and leg abnormalities are seen. Males may have an underdeveloped penis; undescended, atrophic, or absent testes; and hypospadias or phimosis. Females can have malformations of the vagina, uterus, and ovary. Many patients have a Fanconi "facies," including microcephaly, small eyes, epicanthal folds, and abnormal shape, size, or positioning of the ears (see Fig. 468-1). Approximately 10% of patients are mentally retarded. Ectopic, pelvic, or horseshoe kidneys are detected by imaging, as well as duplicated, hypoplastic, dysplastic, or absent organs.

Laboratory Findings. Marrow failure usually ensues in the 1st decade of life. Thrombocytopenia often appears initially, with subsequent onset of granulocytopenia and then **macrocytic anemia.** Severe aplasia develops in most cases, but its full expres-

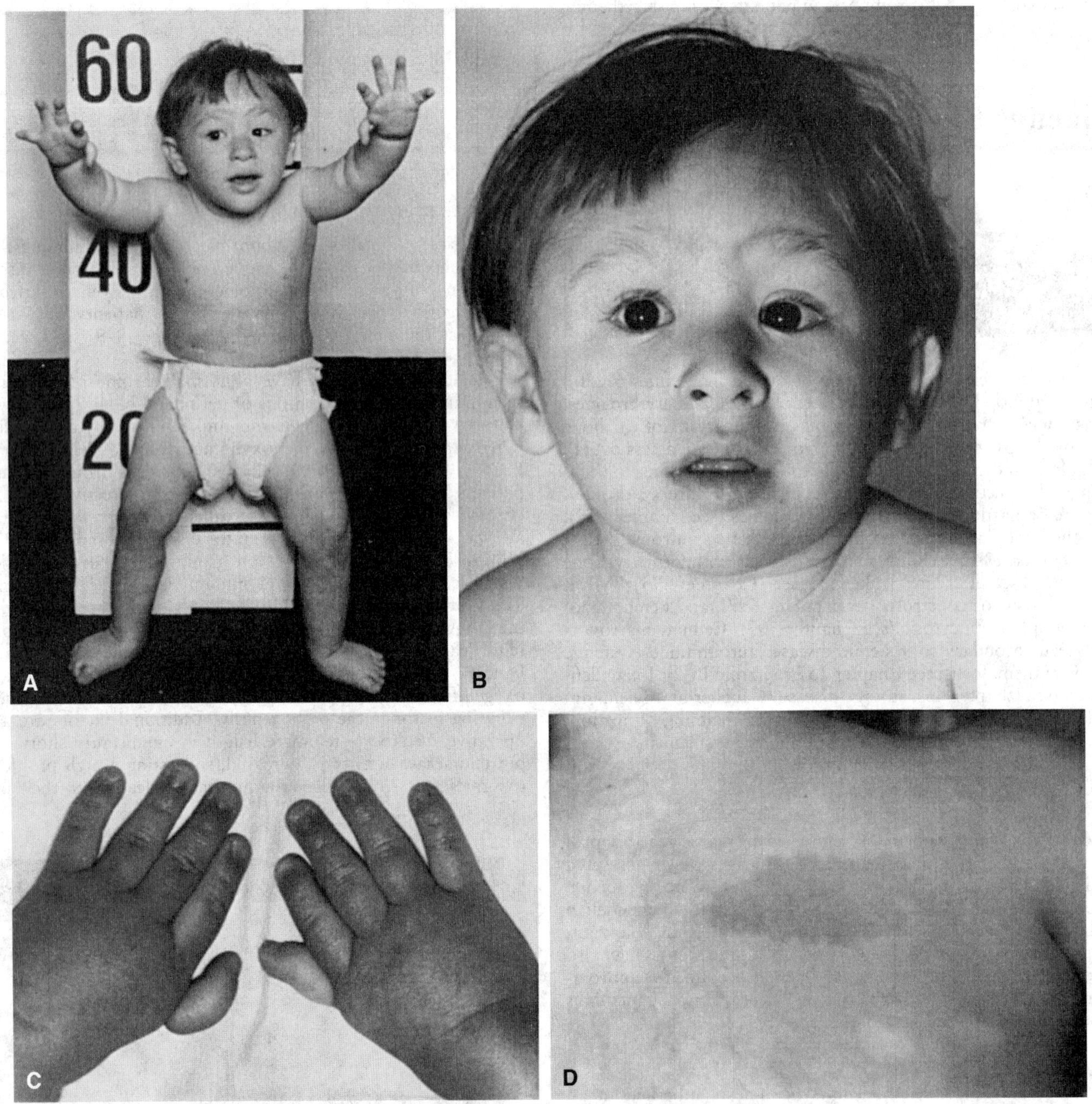

Figure 468-1. A 3 yr old male with Fanconi anemia who exhibits several classic phenotype features. *A*, Front view. *B*, Face. *C*, Hands. *D*, Back right shoulder. The features to be noted include short stature, dislocated hips, microcephaly, a broad nasal base, epicanthal folds, micrognathia, thumbs attached by a thread, and café-au-lait spots with hypopigmented areas beneath. (From Nathan DC, Orkin SH, Ginsburg D, et al [editors]: *Nathan and Oski's Hematology of Infancy and Childhood*, 6th ed., Vol. I. Philadelphia, WB Saunders, 2003, p 285.)

TABLE 468-2. Characteristic Physical Anomalies in Fanconi Anemia

ANOMALY	APPROXIMATE FREQUENCY (% OF PATIENTS)
Skin pigment changes	65
Short stature	60
Upper limb abnormalities (thumbs, hands, radii, ulnas)	50
Hypogonadal and genital changes (mostly male)	40
Other skeletal findings (head/face, neck, spine)	30
Eye/lid/epicanthal fold anomalies	25
Renal malformations	25
Ear anomalies (external and internal), deafness	10
Hip, leg, foot, toe abnormalities	10
Gastrointestinal/cardiopulmonary malformations	10

sion is variable and evolves over a period of mo to yr. The marrow becomes progressively hypocellular and fatty, similar to severe acquired aplastic anemia. Chromosome fragility is indicated by spontaneously occurring chromatid breaks, rearrangements, gaps, endoreduplications, and chromatid exchanges. Cultured skin fibroblasts also show this, underscoring the constitutional nature of the disorder. Fragility is strikingly enhanced in patients compared with controls if DEB is added to the cultures. Abnormal chromosome breakage can be tested on amniotic fluid cells or with chorionic villus biopsy to make a prenatal diagnosis. Most patients have stable, elevated levels of serum α-fetoprotein expressed constitutively, independent of liver complications and of certain therapies, such as androgens. This can be used as a rapid screening diagnostic test.

Complications. A major long-term feature of the phenotype is the propensity for cancer. The most frequent solid tumors are carcinomas of the head, neck, and upper esophagus, followed by carcinomas of the vulva and/or anus and lower esophagus. Some patients have oral cancer after bone marrow transplantation. Benign and malignant liver tumors occur (hepatomas, adenomas) and are usually associated with androgen therapy for aplastic anemia. Androgens are also implicated in the etiology of **peliosis hepatis** (blood-filled empty spaces in the liver). Peliosis hepatis is reversible when androgen therapy is discontinued, and tumors may regress. Approximately 15% of patients with Fanconi anemia have acute leukemia or MDS.

Diagnosis. Abnormal hematologic findings and characteristic physical anomalies suggest the diagnosis, which is confirmed with a chromosomal breakage study using DEB. No other constitutional pancytopenia is associated with an abnormal chromosomal breakage study.

Treatment. A hematologist using a multidisciplinary approach should supervise patients. If the hematologic findings are stable and there are no transfusion requirements, observation is indicated. Subspecialty consultations can be arranged during this interval. If growth velocity is below expectations, endocrine evaluation is needed to identify growth hormone deficiency or hypothyroidism. Glucose intolerance and hyperinsulinemia should be screened for annually or biannually, depending on the degree of hyperglycemia found on initial testing. Patients should be assessed for cancer at least annually.

Hematopoietic stem cell transplantation (HSCT; see Chapter 134) is the only curative therapy for the hematologic abnormalities. Patients with Fanconi anemia who undergo transplantation with a human leukocyte antigen–identical sibling donor have a 5 yr disease-free survival rate of approximately 75%. For patients who do not have a matched sibling donor, a search for a matched unrelated donor (including a search of umbilical cord blood banks) might be initiated. Because of the heightened graft vs host response observed in patients with Fanconi anemia, the survival and cure rates have not been as good compared with matched sibling donor HSCT (≈30% survival). Molecular technology has led to preimplantation genetic diagnosis on parent-derived blastomeres to find a human leukocyte antigen–matched sibling donor without Fanconi anemia.

The potential for recombinant growth factor (cytokine) therapy has not been defined. Granulocyte colony-stimulating factor (G-CSF) can usually induce an increase in the absolute neutrophil count and occasionally may boost platelet counts and hemoglobin levels. However, there may be a heightened risk of marrow cell cytogenetic clonal expansion with monosomy 7. Combination therapy with G-CSF daily or every 2 days subcutaneously with erythropoietin subcutaneously or IV 3 times a wk results in improved neutrophil counts in almost all patients and a sustained rise in platelet count and an increase in hemoglobin levels in approximately ⅓ of patients, but most lose the response after 1 yr due to progression of marrow failure.

Androgens produce a response in 50% of patients, heralded by reticulocytosis and a rise in hemoglobin within 1–2 mo. White cell counts may increase next, followed by platelet counts, but it may take many mo to achieve the maximum response. When the response plateaus, androgens can be slowly tapered, but not stopped entirely. Oral oxymetholone is used most frequently once a day. Low-dose prednisone orally every 2nd day may be added to counter androgen-induced growth acceleration and prevent thrombocytopenic bleeding by promoting vascular stability. In many patients who are taking androgens, the disease becomes refractory as marrow failure progresses. Potential side effects include masculinization and elevated hepatic enzymes, cholestasis, peliosis hepatis, and liver tumors. Screening for these changes should be performed serially.

The premise for gene therapy in Fanconi anemia is based on the assumption that corrected hematopoietic cells offer a growth advantage. Attempts at gene therapy have been disappointing, possibly due to the type of vector, but also because of the fragility and impaired proliferative function of the hematopoietic progenitors. Encouraging preclinical data using lentiviral vectors offer hope that gene therapy will be a safe and effective treatment for Fanconi anemia. Transposons are nonviral vectors that have been used successfully for gene delivery in murine models and may hold promise for humans.

Prognosis. From cases reported in the 1990s, the projected median survival is >30 yr of age, an improvement compared with the previous decade. Successes with HSCT have dramatically improved the outlook. Careful surveillance for known complications, especially cancer, and prompt intervention on their detection have also contributed to the improved survival.

SHWACHMAN-DIAMOND SYNDROME

Etiology and Epidemiology. Shwachman-Diamond syndrome (SDS) is inherited in an autosomal recessive manner; it occurs in all racial and ethnic groups. Essential diagnostic criteria are exocrine pancreatic insufficiency and variable hematologic cytopenias due to marrow failure (see Chapter 346). Chromosomes are normal, and there is no increased breakage after DEB clastogenic stress testing.

Pathology. The mutant gene *SBDS* maps to chromosome 7q11 and is responsible for the multisystem, pleiotropic phenotype in 90% of cases. The wild-type gene protein product is involved in RNA metabolism and/or ribosome biogenesis. Pancreatic insufficiency is due to failure of pancreatic acinar development. Fatty replacement of pancreatic tissue is prominent. Bone marrow failure is characterized by a generalized marrow cell and microenvironmental dysfunction that does not support and maintain normal hematopoiesis.

Clinical Manifestations. Although most patients have symptoms of fat malabsorption from birth caused by pancreatic insufficiency, the absence of steatorrhea does not exclude a diagnosis of SDS. Approximately 50% of patients appear to exhibit a modest improvement in pancreatic enzyme secretion with advancing age. Short stature is a consistent feature of the syndrome; most patients show normal growth velocity, yet remain consistently below the 3rd percentile for height and weight. The occasional adult achieves the 25th percentile for height. The clinical picture can be dominated by complications of hematologic cytopenia. Pancytopenia is diagnosed at a mean age of 7.5 yr (range, 0–35 yr). Bacterial and fungal infections secondary to neutropenia and neutrophil dysfunction and immune deficiency can occur. Although skeletal abnormalities are variable, classic findings are delayed bone maturation, metaphyseal dysplasia, short or flared ribs, thoracic dystrophy, and bifid thumb. Most patients have dental abnormalities and poor oral health. Many have neurocognitive problems and poor social skills.

Laboratory Findings. Neutropenia is present in virtually all patients on at least 1 occasion. It can be chronic, cyclic, or intermittent. It has been identified in some neonates during an episode of sepsis. Anemia, thrombocytopenia, and pancytopenia are seen in 66%, 60%, and up to 44% of cases, respectively. Pancytopenia can be severe as a result of full-blown aplastic anemia. Bone marrow biopsy specimens and aspirates usually show varying degrees of marrow hypoplasia and fat infiltration. The fatty pancreatic replacement can be visualized by CT scan or ultrasonography. Fat malabsorption is confirmed by a 72 hr fecal fat balance study. Pancreatic function studies show markedly impaired enzyme secretion, but ductal function is preserved. Serum trypsinogen and isoamylase levels are reduced. Neutrophils may have a defect in mobility, migration, and chemotaxis due to alterations in neutrophil cytoskeletal or microtubular function. Patients may also have B-cell defects, with 1 or more of the following: low immunoglobulin G or immunoglobulin G subclasses, low percentage of circulating B lymphocytes, decreased in vitro B-cell proliferation, and lack of specific antibody production. Patients may have a low percentage of circulating T cells, subsets, or natural killer cells, and decreased in vitro T-cell proliferation.

Diagnosis. Mutational analysis for *SBDS* is definitive in 90% of cases. **Pearson syndrome** (refractory sideroblastic anemia, cytoplasmic vacuolization of bone marrow precursors, metabolic acidosis, mitochondrial DNA mutation, and exocrine pancreatic insufficiency) is similar to SDS, but the clinical course and morphologic features of the bone marrow are different. Severe anemia requiring transfusion, rather than neutropenia, is present from birth to 1 yr of age. Patients with Pearson syndrome have abnormalities of mitochondrial DNA (mtDNA). SDS shares some manifestations with Fanconi anemia, such as marrow dysfunction and growth failure, but patients with SDS are readily distinguished because of pancreatic insufficiency with fat malabsorption, fatty changes within the pancreatic body that can be visualized by imaging, characteristic skeletal abnormalities not seen in Fanconi anemia, and normal DEB clastogenic stress test results.

Complications. Patients with SDS are predisposed to MDS and leukemic transformation. The crude rate of MDS or acute leukemia in patients with SDS is 8–33%. Clonal change is often accompanied by isochromosome 7 [i(7q)] in marrow cells. This is particularly common and suggests that it is a fairly specific clonal marker of SDS and is probably related to the presence of the mutant SDS gene on 7q11. Other clonal chromosome abnormalities include monosomy 7, i(7q) combined with monosomy 7, deletions or translocations involving part of 7q, and deletions of 20q (20q).

Treatment. Fat malabsorption responds to oral pancreatic enzyme replacement and supplemental fat-soluble vitamins, following guidelines similar to those for cystic fibrosis (see Chapter 400). A long-term plan should be initiated to monitor changes in peripheral blood counts that require corrective action and to look for early evidence of malignant myeloid transformation. The latter requires serial bone marrow aspirates for smears and cytogenetics and marrow biopsy. One recommendation is to do marrow testing annually.

Daily subcutaneous G-CSF for profound neutropenia is effective in inducing a sustained increase in neutrophils. Some patients require transfusional support to manage severe anemia or thrombocytopenia. Experience with erythropoietin is limited. Small numbers of patients have been treated with corticosteroids, with hematologic improvement in approximately 50%. Some patients have received androgens plus steroids and have had improved blood counts. The only curative option for severe marrow failure in SDS is allogeneic HSCT, although experience has been limited. About 50% of transplanted SDS patients have died of complications related to the preparative therapy. The risk of cardiotoxicity has been noted.

Prognosis. Approximately 50% of patients spontaneously convert from pancreatic insufficiency to sufficiency due to improvement in pancreatic enzyme secretion. Enzyme replacement therapy is then no longer needed. Although all patients have some degree of hematologic cytopenia, the changes in most patients are mild to moderate and do not require therapeutic intervention. Severe neutropenia responds well to G-CSF, but there is concern that the predisposition to MDS and acute leukemia can be heightened by its powerful growth stimulus on marrow cells. HSCT for severe marrow failure produces a 50% survival rate. Malignant marrow transformation is ominous.

DYSKERATOSIS CONGENITA

Etiology and Epidemiology. Dyskeratosis congenita (DC) is an inherited disorder of the mucocutaneous and hematopoietic systems in association with somatic abnormalities. The diagnostic ectodermal **triad** is reticulate skin pigmentation of the upper body, mucosal leukoplakia, and nail dystrophy (Fig. 468-2). Skin and nail findings usually become apparent in the 1st 10 yr of life, whereas oral leukoplakia is seen later. These manifestations tend to progress as patients get older. DC is a constitutional pancytopenia; aplastic anemia occurs in approximately 50% of cases, usually in the 2nd decade of life. Patients also have a predisposition to cancer and MDS. Approximately 85% of patients are male, compatible with X-linked recessive inheritance. Approximately 15% of patients appear to have either autosomal dominant or autosomal recessive modes of inheritance.

Pathology. The X-linked recessive form of DC maps to Xq28, and many mutations have been identified in the *DKC1* gene, which codes for the nuclear protein dyskerin. Dyskerin may be involved in ribosomal assembly and RNA production. The autosomal dominant form is due to mutations in the *TERC* gene that encodes the RNA component of telomerase that is responsible for telomere maintenance. Short telomeres have been demonstrated in the peripheral blood cells of patients with autosomal dominant and X-linked recessive forms of the disorder and are a marker for marrow failure. The mutant autosomal recessive gene has not been identified. The marrow failure may be due to progressive attrition and depletion of hematopoietic stem cells, which manifests as pancytopenia. Alternatively, marrow dysfunction may represent a failure of replication and/or maturation of stem cells.

Clinical Manifestations. Skin pigmentation and nail changes typically appear first, mucosal leukoplakia and excessive ocular tearing appear later, and by the mid-teens, bone marrow failure and malignancy ensue. Many female patients share the same features as male patients. In males, cutaneous findings are the most consistent feature. Lacy reticulated skin pigmentation affecting the face, neck, chest, and arms is a common finding (89%). The degree of pigmentation increases with age and can involve the entire skin surface. There may also be a telangiectatic erythematous component. Nail dystrophy of the hands and feet is the next most common finding (88%). It usually starts with longitudinal ridging, splitting, or pterygium formation and may progress to complete nail loss. Leukoplakia usually involves the oral mucosa (78%), especially the tongue, but may also be seen in the conjunctiva and the anal, urethral, or genital mucosa. Hyperhidrosis of the palms and soles is common, and hair loss is sometimes seen. Eye abnormalities are observed in approximately 50% of cases. Excessive tearing (epiphora) secondary to nasolacrimal

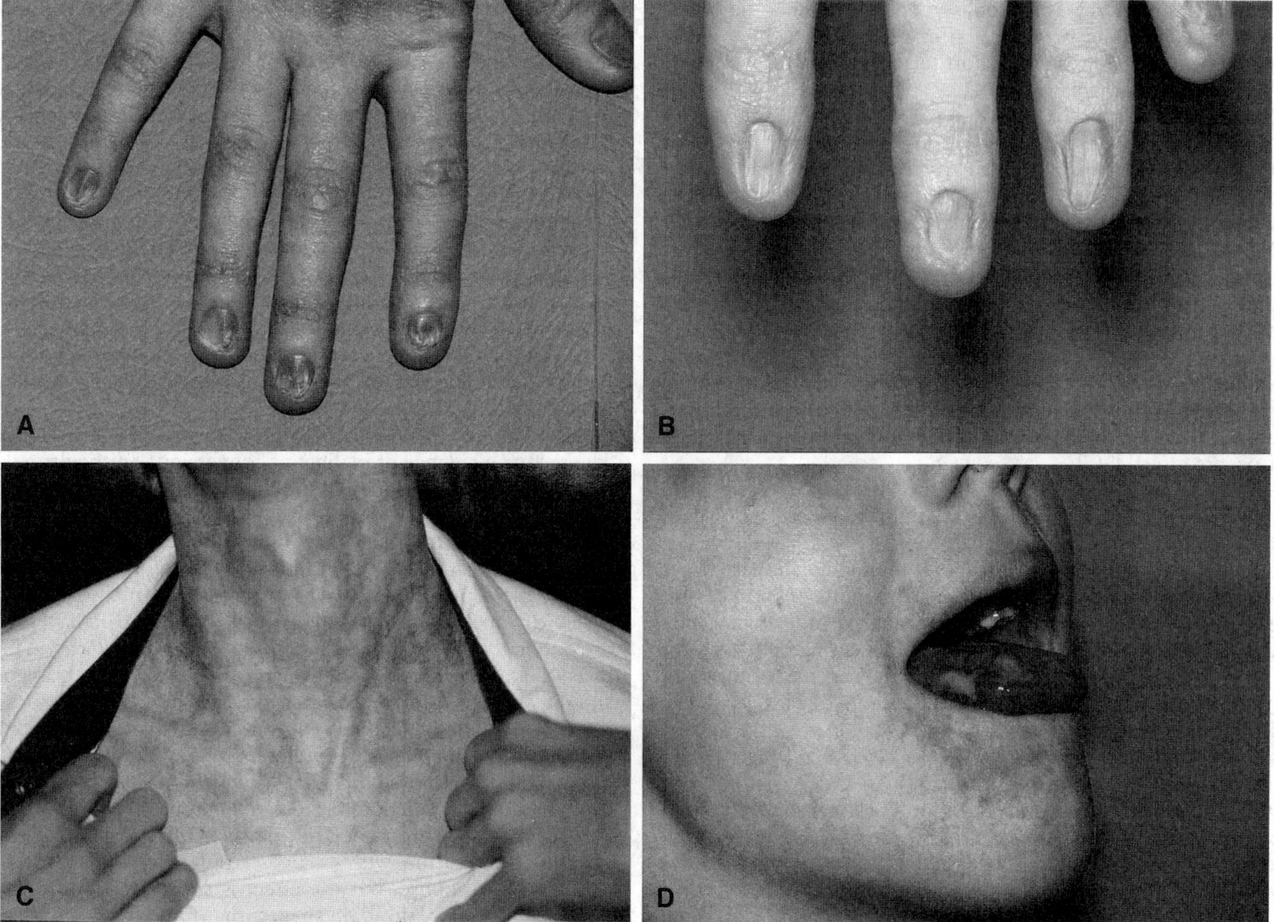

Figure 468-2. Physical findings in patients with dyskeratosis congenita. *A* and *B*, Dystrophic fingernails in 2 different patients. *C*, Lacy reticular pigmentation. *D*, Leukoplakia on the tongue. (From Nathan DG, Orkin SH, Ginsburg D, et al [editors]: *Nathan and Oski's Hematology of Infancy and Childhood,* 6th ed., Vol. I. Philadelphia, WB Saunders, 2003, p 300.)

duct obstruction is common. Other ophthalmologic manifestations include conjunctivitis, blepharitis, loss of eyelashes, strabismus, cataracts, and optic atrophy. An increased rate of dental decay and early loss of teeth are common. Skeletal abnormalities, such as osteoporosis, avascular necrosis, abnormal bone trabeculation, scoliosis, and mandibular hypoplasia, are seen in approximately 20% of cases. Genitourinary abnormalities include hypoplastic testes, hypospadias, phimosis, urethral stenosis, and horseshoe kidney. Gastrointestinal findings, such as esophageal strictures, hepatomegaly, or cirrhosis, are seen in 10% of cases. A subset of patients has pulmonary complications, with reduced diffusion capacity and/or a restrictive defect. In fatal cases, lung tissue shows pulmonary fibrosis and abnormalities of the pulmonary vasculature.

Laboratory Findings. The initial hematologic change is usually thrombocytopenia, anemia, or both, followed by full-blown pancytopenia caused by aplastic anemia. The red cells are often macrocytic, and the fetal hemoglobin can be elevated initially. Bone marrow specimens may be hypercellular, but with time, a symmetric decrease in all hematopoietic lineages ensues. Some patients have immunologic abnormalities, including reduced or elevated immunoglobulin levels, reduced B- and/or T-lymphocyte counts, and reduced or absent proliferative response to phytohemagglutinin. There is no significant difference in chromosomal breakage in mitogen-stimulated lymphocytes with or without exposure to DEB or mitomycin C between patients and controls. However, primary skin fibroblasts in culture have abnormal morphologic features and doubling rate and show numerous unbalanced chromosome rearrangements, such as dicentrics, tricentrics, and translocations in the absence of clastogenic agents. These findings provide evidence of a defect that predisposes patient cells to chromosomal rearrangements and possibly DNA damage.

Diagnosis. The following abnormalities are seen in patients with DC, but not in those with Fanconi anemia: nail dystrophy, leukoplakia, tooth abnormalities, hyperhydrosis of the palms and soles, and hair loss. There are overlap syndromes that share some of the features of DC. **Hoyerall-Hreidarsson syndrome** is a multisystem disorder that affects boys who have aplastic anemia, immunodeficiency, microcephaly, growth retardation, and cerebellar hypoplasia. The syndrome is caused by mutations in *DKC1* and hence is a variant of DC. **Revesz syndrome** consists of dystrophic nails, leukoplakia, aplastic anemia, cerebellar hypoplasia, growth retardation, microcephaly, and bilateral exudative retinopathy. The mutation has not been identified.

Complications. Cancer develops in approximately 10–15% of patients, usually in the 3rd and 4th decades of life. DC patients are predisposed to MDS as well as to solid tumors. Most cancers are squamous cell carcinoma or adenocarcinoma, and the oropharynx and gastrointestinal tract are involved most frequently.

Treatment. Androgens, usually combined with low-dose prednisone, can induce improved marrow function in approximately 50% of patients. When the response is maximal, the androgen dose can be slowly tapered, but not stopped. Patients can become refractory to androgens as the aplastic anemia progresses. There is no published information on the use of immunosuppressive therapy for this disorder. Although reports are scanty, cytokine therapy with granulocyte-macrophage colony–stimulating factor or with G-CSF alone or with erythropoietin appears to offer potential benefit, at least in the short term, especially for improving neutrophil numbers.

Allogeneic HSCT has been used to correct marrow failure, with a 50% survival rate. Vascular lesions and fibrosis involving various organs occur in both the early and the late periods after transplantation and carry a high mortality rate. Patients with DC may be more susceptible to endothelial damage that occurs after HSCT as a result of various factors, including the conditioning regimen, infectious disease, and graft vs host disease. Up to 40% of patients with DC experience early and late fatal pulmonary complications after transplantation. Additional factors with negative effects after HSCT are the subtle degree of chromosomal instability in DC with a predisposition to chromosomal rearrangements and the inherent telomere shortening that characterizes DC, combined with the accelerated telomere shortening that occurs after HSCT.

Although the mutated genes for the X-linked recessive and autosomal dominant forms of DC are known, prospects for gene therapy are not imminent.

Prognosis. Patients with autosomal dominant disease have milder clinical manifestations; those with autosomal recessive disease appear to have more physical anomalies and a higher incidence of aplastic anemia and cancer. The mean age of death for patients with DC is approximately 30 yr. The main causes of death are bone marrow failure, complications of HSCT, cancer, and fatal pulmonary problems.

AMEGAKARYOCYTIC THROMBOCYTOPENIA

Etiology and Epidemiology. Congenital amegakaryocytic thrombocytopenia (CAT or CAMT) is the rarest of the 4 major constitutional pancytopenias. It is inherited in an autosomal recessive manner. CAT presents in infancy with isolated thrombocytopenia due to reduced or absent marrow megakaryocytes, with preservation initially of granulopoietic and erythroid lineages. Pancytopenia due to **aplastic anemia** subsequently ensues in approximately 45% of patients; the mean age at onset is 3.5 yr (range, 0.4–12.5 yr). The defect in CAT is directly related to mutations in the gene for the thrombopoietin receptor c-*mpl*, which maps to chromosome 1p35. Carriers of the mutant gene have normal hematologic features; affected individuals have mutations in both alleles. Without the receptor function seen with frameshift and nonsense mutations of c-*mpl*, the growth-promoting effect of thrombopoietin is abolished and megakaryocytic growth and development ceases. Because thrombopoietin also has an anti-apoptotic effect on stem cells, impaired stem cell survival explains the evolution of CAT into aplastic anemia. Missense mutations of c-*mpl* are associated with a milder course. Plasma thrombopoietin levels in patients with CAT are consistently elevated, and the immunoreactive material detected retains full biologic activity.

Clinical Manifestations. Patients have petechial rash, bruising, or bleeding at birth or in the 1st year of life. Approximately 50% of patients have characteristic **physical anomalies;** the others have normal physical and imaging features. Some affected sibships have both normal and abnormal physical findings in the same family. The most common anomalies are neurologic and cardiac. Findings related to cerebellar and cerebral atrophy are frequent, and developmental delay is a prominent feature. Patients may also have microcephaly and an abnormal facies. Congenital heart disease occurs, including atrial septal defects, ventricular septal defects, patent ductus arteriosus, tetralogy of Fallot, and coarctation of the aorta. Some of these occur in combinations. Other anomalies include abnormal hips or feet, kidney malformations, eye anomalies, and cleft or high-arched palate.

Laboratory Findings. Thrombocytopenia is the major laboratory finding, with normal hemoglobin levels and white blood cell counts initially. Peripheral blood platelets are reduced or totally absent. As in other inherited bone marrow failure syndromes, red cells may be macrocytic. Hemoglobin F may be elevated, and there may be increased expression of i antigen. Bone marrow aspirates and biopsy specimens show normal cellularity, with markedly reduced or absent megakaryocytes. In patients who have aplastic anemia, marrow cellularity is decreased, with fatty replacement; the erythroid and granulopoietic lineages are also symmetrically reduced.

Diagnosis. If CAT presents beyond the neonatal age group, marrow aspirate and biopsy will point to the diagnosis and mutational analysis will confirm it. If CAT presents at birth or shortly after, it must be distinguished from other causes of acquired and inherited neonatal thrombocytopenia (see Chapter 484). Increased platelet destruction also occurs in newborns with giant benign hemangiomas of the skin, liver, or spleen—Kasabach-Merritt syndrome (see Chapter 505).

Complications. In some patients, CAT evolves into leukemia. The risk or incidence of malignant conversion is difficult to determine because of the rarity of the disease and the paucity of published data.

Therapy and Prognosis. The mortality rate in patients with frameshift or nonsense mutations of c-*mpl* from thrombocytopenic bleeding, complications of aplastic anemia, or malignant myeloid transformation has been very close to 100%. HSCT is the only curative option. The majority of patients with CAT who receive HSCT are cured. Pretransplantation, platelet transfusion should be used discretely. Platelet count should not be the sole indication; clinical bleeding is a more appropriate reason. Single-donor filtered platelets are preferred to minimize sensitization, and if HSCT is a possibility, all blood products should be free of cytomegalovirus. Corticosteroids do not appear to be effective for treatment of the thrombocytopenia. For aplastic anemia, androgens in combination with corticosteroids may induce a temporary partial response, but the effect is short-lived and does not prevent mortality. Pilot data suggest that interleukin 3 may be an important adjunct to the medical management of CAT. Thrombopoietin has not been tried for the treatment of CAT and would likely fail because endogenous thrombopoietin levels are markedly increased, and the autosomal recessive form of CAT has a mutated c-*mpl* receptor.

OTHER GENETIC SYNDROMES

Bone marrow failure can occur in the context of several nonhematologic syndromes and also in familial settings that do not exactly correspond to the entities already described.

DOWN SYNDROME. Down syndrome (see Chapter 81), or trisomy 21, has a unique association with aberrant hematologic findings. In addition to the propensity for acute lymphoblastic and myeloblastic leukemias, a few patients have been reported with pancytopenia due to aplastic anemia.

DUBOWITZ SYNDROME. Dubowitz syndrome is an autosomal recessive disorder characterized by a peculiar facies, infantile eczema, small stature, and mild microcephaly. The face is small, with a shallow supraorbital ridge, a nasal bridge at the same level as the forehead, short palpebral fissures, variable ptosis, and micrognathia. There is a predilection to cancer as well as to bone marrow dysfunction in these patients. Approximately 10% of patients have hematopoietic disorders, including hypoplastic anemia, moderate pancytopenia, and full-blown aplastic anemia.

SECKEL SYNDROME. Seckel syndrome, sometimes called "bird-headed dwarfism," is an autosomal recessive developmental disorder characterized by marked growth failure and mental deficiency, microcephaly, a hypoplastic face with a prominent nose, and low-set and/or malformed ears. Approximately 25%

of patients have aplastic anemia or malignancies. One locus for the syndrome maps to 3q22.1–q24. A second locus maps to 18p11.31–q11.2, demonstrating genetic heterogeneity.

RETICULAR DYSGENESIS. Reticular dysgenesis (see Chapter 125) is an immunologic deficiency syndrome coupled with congenital agranulocytosis. The mode of inheritance is probably autosomal recessive, but an X-linked mode is also possible in some cases. The disorder is a variant of severe combined immune deficiency, in which cellular and humoral immunity are absent and patients also have severe lymphopenia and neutropenia. Anemia and thrombocytopenia may also be present. Bone marrow specimens are hypocellular, with markedly reduced myeloid and lymphoid elements. The only curative therapy is HSCT.

SCHIMKE IMMUNO-OSSEOUS DYSPLASIA. Schimke immuno-osseous dysplasia is an autosomal recessive disorder caused by mutations in the chromatin remodeling protein SMARCAL1. Patients have spondyloepiphyseal dysplasia with exaggerated lumbar lordosis and a protruding abdomen. There are pigmentary skin changes and abnormally discolored and configured teeth. Renal dysfunction can be problematic, with proteinuria and nephrotic syndrome. Approximately 50% of patients have hypothyroidism, 50% have cerebral ischemia, and 10% have bone marrow failure, with neutropenia, thrombocytopenia, and anemia. Lymphopenia and altered cellular immunity are present in almost all patients. In 1 published case, a patient underwent successful bone marrow transplantation.

FAMILIAL APLASTIC ANEMIA. Bone marrow failure can cluster in families, but many of these cases cannot be readily classified into discrete diagnostic entities, such as Fanconi anemia. The phenotype of these conditions can be complex, with varying combinations of hematologic abnormalities, immunologic deficiency, physical malformations, and predisposition to leukemia. Both autosomal dominant and autosomal recessive inheritances have been observed; both patterns occur with or without associated physical anomalies. An X-linked type is described with physical anomalies; additionally, the X-linked lymphoproliferative syndrome associated with Epstein-Barr virus is associated with pancytopenia.

Alter BP: Inherited bone marrow failure syndromes. In Nathan DG, Orkin SH, Ginsburg D, et al (editors): *Hematology of Infancy and Childhood,* 6th ed. Philadelphia, WB Saunders, 2003, pp 280–365.

Dokal I: Dyskeratosis congenita in all its forms. *Br J Haematol* 2000;110:768–779.

Dror Y, Freedman, MH: Shwachman-Diamond syndrome. *Br J Haematol* 2002;118:701–713.

Freedman MH: Inherited forms of bone marrow failure. In Hoffman R, Benz EJ, Shattil SJ, et al (editors): *Hematology: Basic Principles and Practice,* 5th ed. Philadelphia, Elsevier Churchill Livingstone, 2007, in press.

Kuijpers TW, Nannenberg E, Alders M, et al: Congenital aplastic anemia caused by mutations in the SBDS gene: A rare presentation of Shwachman-Diamond syndrome. *Pediatrics* 2004;114:e387–e391.

Landmann E, Bluetters-Sawatzki R, Schindler D, et al: Fanconi anemia in a neonate with pancytopenia. *J Pediatr* 2004;145:125–127.

Levitus M, Joenje H, de Winter JP: The Fanconi anemia pathway of genomic maintenance. *Cell Oncol* 2006;28:3–29.

Lieberman L, Dror Y: Advances in understanding the genetic basis for bone-marrow failure. *Curr Opin Pediatr* 2006;18:15–21.

Mathew CG: Fanconi anaemia genes and susceptibility to cancer. *Oncogene* 2006;25:5875–5884.

Tischkowitz M, Dokal I: Fanconi anaemia and leukaemia: Clinical and molecular aspects. *Br J Haematol* 2004;126:176–191.

Vulliamy T, Dokal I: Dyskeratosis congenita. *Semin Hematol* 2006;43:157–166.

Xia B, Dorsman JC, Ameziane N, et al: Fanconi anemia is associated with a defect in the BRCA2 partner PALB2. *Nat Genet* 2007;39:159–161.

Chapter 469 ■ The Acquired Pancytopenias

Jeffrey D. Hord

ETIOLOGY AND EPIDEMIOLOGY. Drugs, chemicals, toxins, infectious agents, radiation, and immune disorders can result in pancytopenia, by direct destruction of hematopoietic progenitors, disruption of the marrow microenvironment, or immune-mediated suppression of marrow elements (Table 469-1). A careful history of exposure to known risk factors should be obtained from every child presenting with pancytopenia. Even in the absence of the classic associated physical findings, the possibility of a genetic predisposition to bone marrow failure should always be considered (see Chapter 468). The majority of cases of acquired marrow failure in childhood are "idiopathic," in that no causative agent is identified. These are probably immune-mediated through activated T lymphocytes and cytokine destruction of marrow progenitor cells. The overall incidence of acquired aplastic anemia is relatively low, with an approximate incidence in both children and adults, in the U.S. and Europe, of 2–6 cases/million/yr. The incidence is higher in Asia, with as many as 14 cases/million/yr in Japan.

Severe bone marrow suppression can develop after exposure to many different drugs and chemicals, including certain chemotherapeutic agents, insecticides, antibiotics, anticonvulsants, and nonsteroidal anti-inflammatory agents. Some of the most notable agents are benzene, chloramphenicol, and gold. The severity and duration of the pancytopenia is dependent on the extent of exposure to these agents. A genetic predisposition may exist and may increase the likelihood of pancytopenia after exposure.

A number of viruses can either directly or indirectly result in bone marrow failure. Parvovirus B19 is classically associated with isolated red cell aplasia, but in patients with sickle cell disease or immunodeficiency, it can result in transient pancytopenia (see Chapters 248 and 462). Prolonged pancytopenia can occur after infection with many of the hepatitis viruses, herpesviruses, Epstein-Barr virus (see Chapter 251), cytomegalovirus (Chapter 252), and HIV (see Chapter 273).

TABLE 469-1. Etiology of Acquired Aplastic Anemia

RADIATION DRUGS AND CHEMICALS
Predictable: chemotherapy, benzene
Idiosyncratic: chloramphenicol, antiepileptics, gold
VIRUSES
Cytomegalovirus
Epstein-Barr
Hepatitis B
Hepatitis C
Hepatitis non-A, non-B, non-C (seronegative hepatitis)
Human immunodeficiency (HIV)
IMMUNE DISEASES
Eosinophilic fasciitis
Hypoimmunoglobulinemia
Thymoma
PREGNANCY
PAROXYSMAL NOCTURNAL HEMOGLOBINURIA
MARROW REPLACEMENT
Leukemia
Myelodysplasia
Myelofibrosis
AUTOIMMUNE
OTHER
Cryptic dyskeratosis congenita (no physical stigmata)
Telomerase reverse transcriptase haploinsufficiency

Patients with evidence of bone marrow failure should also be evaluated for paroxysmal nocturnal hemoglobinuria (PNH; see Chapter 461) and collagen vascular diseases, although these are uncommon causes of pancytopenia in childhood. Pancytopenia without peripheral blasts may be caused by bone marrow replacement by leukemic blasts or neuroblastoma cells.

PATHOLOGY AND PATHOGENESIS. The hallmark of aplastic anemia is peripheral pancytopenia, coupled with hypoplastic or aplastic bone marrow. The severity of the clinical course is related to the degree of myelosuppression. **Severe aplastic anemia** is defined as a condition in which 2 or more cell components have become seriously compromised (absolute neutrophil count [ANC] of <500/mm^3, platelet count of <20,000/mm^3, reticulocyte count of <1% after correction for hematocrit) in a patient whose bone marrow biopsy material is moderately or severely hypocellular. Approximately ⅔ of patients who first present with a more **moderate form of aplastic anemia** (ANC of 500–1,500/mm^3, platelet count of 20,000–100,000/mm^3, reticulocyte count of <1%) and are only observed will eventually progress to meet the criteria for severe disease. Bone marrow failure may be a consequence of a direct cytotoxic effect on hematopoietic stem cells from a drug or chemical or may result from either cell-mediated or antibody-dependent cytotoxicity. There is strong evidence that many cases of idiopathic aplastic anemia are caused by an immune-mediated process, with increased circulating activated T lymphocytes producing cytokines (interferon-α) that suppress hematopoiesis. Shortened telomere length in granulocytic precursors and increased expression of cell surface Flt3 ligand (a member of the class III receptor tyrosine kinase family) in the lymphocytes of patients with aplastic anemia suggest that early apoptosis of hematopoietic progenitors may play a role in the pathogenesis of this disease.

CLINICAL MANIFESTATIONS, LABORATORY FINDINGS, AND DIFFERENTIAL DIAGNOSIS. Pancytopenia results in increased risks of cardiac failure, infection, bleeding, and fatigue. Acquired pancytopenia is typically characterized by anemia, leukopenia, and thrombocytopenia in the setting of elevated serum cytokine levels. Other treatable disorders, such as cancer, collagen vascular disorders, PNH, or infections that may respond to specific therapies (IV immune globulin for parvovirus) should be considered in the differential diagnosis. Careful examination of the peripheral blood smear for RBC, leukocyte, and platelet morphologic features is important. A reticulocyte count should be performed to assess erythropoietic activity. In children, the possibility of congenital pancytopenia must always be considered and chromosomal breakage analysis should be performed to evaluate for Fanconi anemia (see Chapter 468). The presence of fetal hemoglobin suggests congenital pancytopenia, but is not diagnostic. To assess for the possibility of PNH, flow cytometric analysis of erythrocytes for CD48 and CD59 is the most sensitive test. Bone marrow examination should include both aspiration and a biopsy, and the marrow should be carefully evaluated for morphologic features, cellularity, and cytogenetic findings.

TREATMENT. The treatment of children with acquired pancytopenia requires comprehensive supportive care coupled with an attempt to treat the underlying marrow failure. For patients with a human leukocyte antigen–identical sibling marrow donor, allogeneic bone marrow transplantation (BMT) offers a 90% chance of long-term survival. The risks associated with this approach include the immediate complications of transplantation, graft failure, and graft vs host disease. Late adverse effects associated with transplantation may include secondary cancers, cataracts, short stature, hypothyroidism, and gonadal dysfunction (see Chapters 136 and 138). The life-threatening problem of graft failure has diminished with the incorporation of antithymocyte globulin (ATG) and cyclophosphamide into the transplant conditioning regimen. Only 1 of 5 patients has a human leukocyte antigen–matched sibling donor, so allogeneic BMT is not an option for the majority of patients.

For patients without a sibling donor, the major form of therapy is immunosuppression with ATG combined with cyclosporine, with a response rate of 60–80%. As many as 25–30% of responders relapse after discontinuation of immunosuppression, and some patients must continue cyclosporine for several yr to maintain a hematologic response. There is an increased risk of clonal bone marrow disease, such as leukemia, myelodysplasia (MDS), or PNH, after immunosuppression. The exact risk of clonal disease after immunosuppression is probably <10%, and the abnormal karyotypes most frequently involve chromosomes 6, 7, and 8. To accelerate neutrophil recovery, a hematopoietic colony-stimulating factor (e.g., granulocyte colony-stimulating factor, granulocyte-macrophage colony–stimulating factor) is sometimes added to ATG and cyclosporine when treating patients with very severe neutropenia (<200/mm^3). For those who do not respond to immunosuppression or who relapse after immunosuppression, matched unrelated donor BMT and high-dose cyclophosphamide remain treatment options. Other therapies that have been used in the past with inconsistent results include androgens, corticosteroids, and plasmapheresis. Alternative marrow transplants continue to be studied as a therapeutic intervention in refractory aplastic anemia.

COMPLICATIONS. The major complications of severe pancytopenia are predominantly related to the risk of life-threatening bleeding from prolonged thrombocytopenia or to infection secondary to protracted neutropenia. Patients with protracted neutropenia due to bone marrow failure are at risk, not only for serious bacterial infections but also for invasive mycoses. The general principles of supportive care that have evolved from the use of chemotherapy-related myelosuppression to treat patients with cancer should be fully extended to the care of patients with acquired pancytopenia (see Chapter 177).

PROGNOSIS. Spontaneous recovery rarely occurs. Severe pancytopenia, left untreated, has an overall mortality rate of approximately 50% within 6 mo of diagnosis and of >75% overall, with infection and hemorrhage the major causes of morbidity and mortality. The majority of children with acquired severe aplastic anemia respond to allogeneic marrow transplantation or immunosuppression and cytokine, leaving them with normal or near-normal blood cell counts. For those who do not respond to first-line therapy, the prognosis remains poor.

PANCYTOPENIA CAUSED BY MARROW REPLACEMENT

Processes that either infiltrate or replace the bone marrow can present as acquired pancytopenia. This can occur either before or during malignancy (classically, neuroblastoma or leukemia) or as a consequence of myelofibrosis, MDS, or osteoporosis. Although uncommon, evidence of hypoplastic anemia can precede, generally by a few mo, the onset of acute leukemia. This is important to appreciate in evaluating and monitoring children who present with what appears to be acquired aplastic anemia. Morphologic examination of the peripheral blood and bone marrow, as well as marrow cytogenetic studies, is critically important in making the diagnoses of leukemia, myelofibrosis, and MDS.

Although very rare in children, when it occurs, MDS has a clinical course that is more aggressive than the same category of MDS in adults. Approximately ½ of children with reported cases of MDS have had clonal abnormalities involving chromosome 7 (usually monosomy 7). The transition time from pediatric MDS to acute leukemia is relatively short, at 14–26 mo, so aggressive treatment, such as BMT, must be considered shortly after diagnosis. With conventional chemotherapy with ATG, there is a 20–25% long-term survival rate, but with allogeneic BMT, the survival rate increases to approximately 50%. One exception may be MDS and acute myelocytic leukemia in children with Down syndrome because this disease in this specific population is very responsive to conventional chemotherapy, with long-term survival rates of >80%. Ongoing clinical trials are evaluating several new therapies for MDS, including angiogenesis inhibitors, molecules affecting apoptosis, hypomethylating agents, and farnesyl transferase inhibitors.

Ades L, Mary JY, Robin M, et al: Long-term outcome after bone marrow transplantation for severe aplastic anemia. *Blood* 2004;103:2490–2497.
Bacigalupo A, Bruno B, Saracco P, et al: Antilymphocyte globulin, cyclosporine, prednisolone, and granulocyte colony-stimulating factor for severe aplastic anemia: An update of the GITMO/EBMT on 100 patients. *Blood* 2000;95:1931–1934.
Brodsky RA, Chen AR, Brodsky I, et al: High-dose cyclophosphamide as salvage therapy for severe aplastic anemia. *Exp Hematol* 2004;32:435–440.
Brodsky RA, Jones RJ: Aplastic anaemia. *Lancet* 2005;365:1647–1656.
Howard SC, Naidu PE, Hu XJ, et al: Natural history of moderate aplastic anemia in children. *Pediatr Blood Cancer* 2004;43:545–551.
Maciejewski JP, Selleri C: Evolution of clonal cytogenetic abnormalities in aplastic anemia. *Leuk Lymphoma* 2004;45:433–440.
Marsh JCW, Gordon-Smith EC: Insights into the autoimmune nature of aplastic anaemia. *Lancet* 2004;364:308–309.
Risitano AM, Maciejewski JP, Green S, et al: In-vivo dominant immune responses in aplastic anaemia: Molecular tracking of putatively pathogenetic T-cell clones by TCR beta-CDR3 sequencing. *Lancet* 2004;364:355–364.
Rosenfeld R, Follman D, Nunez O, et al: Antithymocyte globulin and cyclosporine for severe aplastic anemia. *JAMA* 2003;289:1130–1135.
Torres HA, Bodey GP, Rolston KVI, et al: Infections in patients with aplastic anemia. *Cancer* 2003;98:86–93.
Yamaguchi H, Calado RT, Ly H, et al; Mutations in *TERT,* the gene for telomerase reverse transcriptase, in aplastic anemia. *N Engl J Med* 2005;352:1413–1424.
Young NS: *Bone Marrow Failure Syndromes.* Philadelphia, WB Saunders, 2000.

Section 6 — Blood Component Transfusions — Ronald G. Strauss

Chapter 470 ■ Red Blood Cell Transfusions and Erythropoietin Therapy

Red blood cells (RBCs) are transfused to increase the oxygen-carrying capacity of the blood and, in turn, to maintain satisfactory tissue oxygenation. Guidelines for RBC transfusions in children and adolescents are similar to those for adults (Table 470-1). However, transfusions may be given more stringently to children because normal hemoglobin levels are lower in healthy children than in adults and, except in defined circumstances, children do not have the underlying cardiorespiratory and vascular diseases that develop with aging in adults. Thus, children should be better able to compensate for RBC loss. In the perioperative period, for example, it is unnecessary for most children to maintain hemoglobin levels of 80 g/L or greater, a level frequently desired for adults. There should be a compelling reason for any postoperative RBC transfusion because most children (without continued bleeding) can, over time, restore their RBC mass with iron therapy. The most important measures in the treatments of acute hemorrhage are to control the hemorrhage and to restore the circulating blood volume and tissue perfusion with crystalloid and/or colloid solutions. If the estimated blood loss is >25% of the circulating blood volume (>17 mL/kg) **and** the patient's condition remains unstable, RBC transfusions may be indicated. In acutely ill children with severe pulmonary disease requiring assisted ventilation, it is common practice to maintain the hemoglobin level close to the normal range, although the efficacy of this practice has not been documented by controlled scientific studies. In fact, some physicians in critical care settings prefer to transfuse RBCs quite conservatively and to permit modest anemia because patients with levels close to the normal range have poorer outcomes. Studies in critically ill adults demonstrated better outcomes when the hemoglobin target was 7–9 g/dL vs 10–12 g/dL. However, anemic adults with chronic congestive heart failure do better with hemoglobin of 13 g/dL vs 10 g/dL.

TABLE 470-1. Guidelines for Pediatric Red Blood Cell Transfusions*

CHILDREN AND ADOLESCENTS
Acute loss of >25% at circulating blood volume
Hemoglobin of <8.0 g/dL[†] in the perioperative period
Hemoglobin of <13.0 g/dL and *severe* cardiopulmonary disease
Hemoglobin of <8.0 g/dL and *symptomatic* chronic anemia
Hemoglobin of <8.0 g/dL and *marrow failure*
INFANTS WITHIN THE FIRST 4 MO OF LIFE
Hemoglobin of <13.0 g/dL and *severe* pulmonary disease
Hemoglobin of <10.0 g/dL and *moderate* pulmonary disease
Hemoglobin of <13.0 g/dL and *severe* cardiac disease
Hemoglobin of <10.0 g/dL and *major* surgery
Hemoglobin of <8.0 g/dL and *symptomatic* anemia

*Words in *italics* must be defined for local transfusion guidelines.
[†]Hematocrit estimated by Hb g/dL × 3.

With chronic anemia, the decision to transfuse RBCs should not be based solely on blood hemoglobin levels because children compensate well and may be asymptomatic despite low hemoglobin levels. Patients with iron-deficiency anemia are often treated successfully with oral iron alone, even at hemoglobin levels of <5 g/dL. Factors other than hemoglobin concentration to be considered in the decision to transfuse RBCs include: (1) the patient's symptoms, signs, and functional capacities; (2) the presence of cardiorespiratory, vascular, and central nervous system disease; (3) the cause and anticipated course of the anemia; and (4) alternative therapies, such as recombinant human erythropoietin (EPO) therapy, which is known to reduce the need for RBC transfusions and to improve the overall condition of children with chronic renal insufficiency (see Chapter 535.2). In anemias that are likely to be permanent, it is also important to balance the detrimental effects of anemia on growth and development vs the potential toxicity associated with repeated transfusions. RBC transfusions for disorders such as sickle cell anemia and thalassemia are discussed in Chapters 462.1 and 462.9.

For neonates, there are no clearly established and accepted indications for RBC transfusions based on results of controlled scientific studies. Generally, RBCs are given to maintain a hemoglobin value believed to be the most desirable for each neonate's clinical status (see Table 470-1). This clinical approach is imprecise, but more physiologic indications, such as measurement of RBC mass, available calculations of oxygen delivery and tissue extraction, and imaging of tissue perfusion, are too cumbersome for clinical practice. Because definitive data are limited, it is important for pediatricians to critically evaluate the need for neonatal RBC transfusions in light of the pathophysiologic need.

During the first few wk of life, all neonates experience a decline in circulating RBC mass caused both by physiologic factors and, in sick premature infants, by phlebotomy blood losses. In healthy term infants, the nadir hemoglobin value rarely falls to <11 g/dL at an age of 10–12 wk. This "physiologic" drop in RBCs does not require transfusions. In contrast, the decline occurs earlier and is more pronounced in premature infants, even in those without complicating illnesses, in which the mean hemoglobin concentration falls to approximately 8 g/dL in infants of 1.0–1.5 kg birthweight and to 7 g/dL in infants weighing <1.0 kg at birth. Most infants with birthweight of <1.0 kg need RBC transfusions. A key reason why the nadir hemoglobin values of premature infants are lower than those of term infants is the former group's relatively diminished plasma EPO level in response to anemia (see Chapters 103.1 and 446). The mechanisms responsible for low plasma EPO levels are only partially defined. One factor is the reliance of preterm infants on the liver as the primary site of EPO production during the first few wk of life. The liver is less responsive than the kidneys to anemia and tissue hypoxia. Preterm infants exhibit a sluggish EPO response to falling hematocrit values. Low plasma EPO levels provide a rationale for the use of recombinant EPO in the treatment of anemia of prematurity. Proper doses of EPO and iron effectively stimulate neonatal erythropoiesis. However, the efficacy of EPO therapy to substantially diminish the need for RBC transfusions has not been convincingly demonstrated, particularly for sick, extremely premature neonates, and recombinant EPO has not been widely accepted as a treatment for anemia of prematurity (see Chapter 103.1). In rare cases, some preparations of EPO have been associated with the development of anti-EPO antibodies that result in severe anemia.

Because of the controversies over recombinant EPO therapy, many low-birthweight preterm infants need RBC transfusions (see Table 470-1). In neonatal patients with severe respiratory disease, defined as those requiring relatively large quantities of oxygen and ventilator support, it is customary to maintain blood hemoglobin at >13 g/dL (hematocrit >40%). Proponents believe that transfused RBCs containing adult hemoglobin, with their superior interaction with 2,3-diphosphoglycerate, leading to better oxygen offloading than that of fetal hemoglobin, are likely to provide optimal oxygen delivery throughout the period of diminished pulmonary function. Although this practice is widely recommended, little evidence is available to firmly establish its efficacy or to define its optimal use (the best hemoglobin level for each degree of pulmonary dysfunction). Infants with less severe cardiopulmonary disease may require less vigorous support; hence, a lower hemoglobin level is suggested for those with only moderate disease. Consistent with the rationale for oxygen delivery in neonates with severe respiratory disease, it seems appropriate to maintain the hemoglobin value of >13 g/dL (hematocrit >40%) in neonates with severe cardiac disease leading to either cyanosis or congestive heart failure.

The optimal hemoglobin level for neonates facing major surgery has not been established by definitive studies. However, it seems reasonable to maintain the hemoglobin level at >10 g/dL (hematocrit >30%) because of the limited ability of a neonate's heart, lungs, and vasculature to compensate for anemia; the inferior offloading of oxygen because of the diminished interaction between fetal hemoglobin and 2,3-diphosphoglycerate; and the developmental impairment of neonatal renal, hepatic, and neurologic function. This transfusion guideline must be applied with flexibility to individual infants facing different kinds of surgery.

Stable neonates do not require RBC transfusion, regardless of their blood hemoglobin level, unless they exhibit clinical problems attributable to anemia. Proponents of RBC transfusions for symptomatic anemia believe that the low RBC mass contributes to tachypnea, dyspnea, tachycardia, apnea and bradycardia, feeding difficulties, and lethargy, and can be alleviated by transfusing RBCs. However, anemia is only 1 of several possible causes of these problems, and RBC transfusions should only be given when clinical problems are attributable to the anemia.

The RBC product of choice for children and adolescents is the standard suspension of RBCs separated from whole blood by centrifugation and re-suspended in an anticoagulant/preservative storage solution at a hematocrit value of approximately 60%. The usual dose is 10–15 mL/kg, but transfusion volumes vary greatly, depending on clinical circumstances (continued vs arrested bleeding, hemolysis). For neonates, many centers transfuse the same RBC product as selected for older children, whereas others prefer a packed RBC concentrate (hematocrit of 70–90%). Either is infused slowly (over 2–4 hr) at a dose of approximately 15 mL/kg. Because of the small quantity of extracellular fluid given at these relatively high hematocrit values and the slow rate of transfusion, the type of RBC anticoagulant/preservative solution used does not pose risks for premature infants. Packing RBCs by centrifugation at the time the aliquot is issued for transfusion ensures that a consistent RBC dose is infused with each transfusion, but is not mandatory and is impractical for some blood banks.

The traditional use of relatively fresh RBCs (<7 days of storage) has been halted in many centers in favor of diminishing donor exposure by using a single unit of RBCs to obtain aliquots for transfusing each infant throughout its permitted duration of storage (currently 42 days). Neonatologists who insist on transfusing only fresh RBCs generally are fearful of the rise in the plasma potassium (K^+) level that occurs in RBC units during extended storage. After 42 days of storage, plasma K^+ levels are approximately 50 mEq/L (0.05 mEq/mL), a value that, at 1st glance, seems alarmingly high. However, the actual dose of K^+ transfused in the extracellular fluid is tiny. An infant weighing 1.0 kg, given a 15 mL/kg transfusion of packed RBCs (hematocrit 80%), will receive 3 mL of extracellular fluid that contains only 0.15 mEq of K^+, and it will be transfused slowly. However, the safety of stored RBCs may not apply to large-volume (>25 mL/kg) transfusions infused rapidly, in which greater doses of K^+ may be harmful.

For children weighing >30–40 kg who are to undergo surgery, autologous RBC transfusions may be another alternative to donor allogenic RBCs. **Predeposit autologous** blood collections from the patient occur a few wk before the surgery. **Acute normovolemic hemodilution** occurs in the preoperative period, in which blood is withdrawn from the patient and replaced with saline. **Salvage autologous blood** is collected from blood loss during the operation, but is less favored due to complications.

Bratton SL, Annich GM: Packed red blood cell transfusions for critically ill pediatric patients: When and for what conditions? *J Pediatr* 2003;142:95–97.

Desmet L, Lacroix J: Transfusion in pediatrics. *Crit Care Clin* 2004;20:299–311.

Guay J, de Moerloose P, Lasne D: Minimizing perioperative blood loss and transfusions in children. *Can J Anaesth* 2006;53:559–567.

Hebert PC, McDonald BJ, Tinmouth A: Clinical consequences of anemia and red cell transfusion in the critically ill. *Crit Care Clin* 2004;20:225–235.

Hume HA, Limoges P: Perioperative blood transfusion therapy in pediatric patients. *Am J Ther* 2002;9:396–405.

Ross SD, Allen IE, Henry DH, et al: Clinical benefits and risks associated with epoetin and darbepoetin in patients with chemotherapy-induced anemia: A systematic review of the literature. *Clin Ther* 2006;28:801–831.

Savakis EC, Strauss RG: Meta-analysis of controlled clinical trials studying the efficacy of recombinant human erythropoietin in reducing blood transfusions in the anemia of prematurity. *Transfusion* 2001;41:406.

Strauss RG: Controversies in the management of the anemia of prematurity using single-donor red blood cell transfusion and/or recombinant human erythropoietin. *Transfus Med Rev* 2006;20:34–44.

Chapter 471 ■ Platelet Transfusions

Guidelines for platelet (PLT) support of children and adolescents with quantitative and qualitative PLT disorders are similar to those for adults (Table 471-1), where the risk of life-threatening bleeding after injury or occurring spontaneously can be related to the severity of thrombocytopenia. PLT transfusions should be given to patients with PLT counts of $<50 \times 10^9$/L when they are bleeding or are scheduled for an invasive procedure. Studies of patients with thrombocytopenia resulting from bone marrow failure indicate that spontaneous bleeding increases markedly when PLT levels fall to $<20 \times 10^9$/L, if serious complications (infection, organ failure, clotting abnormalities, or anemia) are present. In this setting, prophylactic PLT transfusions are given to maintain a PLT count of $>20 \times 10^9$/L. This threshold has been challenged by studies of adult patients; a lower PLT transfusion trigger of $5–10 \times 10^9$/L is recommended for stable patients. However, in practice, severe thrombocytopenia commonly occurs in association with the complications of fever, antimicrobial therapy, active bleeding, the need for an invasive procedure, disseminated intravascular coagulation, and other severe clotting abnormalities, situations in which PLT transfusions are given to maintain relatively high PLT counts. Despite the desire by some physicians, often those preparing a patient for an invasive procedure, to elevate the blood PLT count to $\geq 70 \times 10^9$/L, there are no definitive data to justify a true benefit of a PLT count of $>50 \times 10^9$/L.

Qualitative PLT disorders may be inherited or acquired (in advanced hepatic or renal insufficiency or after cardiopulmonary bypass). In such patients, PLT transfusions are justified only if significant bleeding actually occurs. Because inherited PLT dysfunction is long term and repeated transfusions may lead to alloimmunization and refractoriness, prophylactic PLT transfusions are rarely justified, unless an invasive procedure is planned. In these cases, a bleeding time of > twice the upper limit of laboratory normal or an abnormal result with the use of a more modern PLT function device may be taken as diagnostic evidence of PLT dysfunction, but bleeding time or any other laboratory test result is poorly predictive of hemorrhagic risk or the need to transfuse PLTs. Alternative therapies, particularly desmopressin acetate, should be considered to avoid PLT transfusions. Antiplatelet medications (nonsteroidal anti-inflammatory drugs) should be avoided in these patients.

In neonates, hemostasis is quantitatively and qualitatively different from that in older children, and the potential exists for either serious hemorrhage or thrombosis. Approximately 25% of neonates treated in intensive care units exhibit blood PLT counts of $<150 \times 10^9$/L at some time during admission. Multiple pathogenetic mechanisms are involved in these sick neonates, predominantly accelerated PLT destruction plus diminished PLT production, as evidenced by decreased numbers of megakaryocyte progenitors and relatively low levels of thrombopoietin in thrombocytopenic neonates, compared with thrombocytopenic children and adults.

Blood PLT counts of $<100 \times 10^9$/L pose significant clinical risks for premature neonates. Bleeding time may be prolonged at PLT counts of $<100 \times 10^9$/L in infants with birthweight of <1.5 kg; PLT dysfunction is suggested by bleeding times that are disproportionately long for the degree of thrombocytopenia, and the risk of hemorrhage may be greater in thrombocytopenic infants. The incidence of intracranial hemorrhage in thrombocytopenic infants with birthweight of <1.5 kg is 78% vs 48% for nonthrombocytopenic infants of similar size. Moreover, the extent of hemorrhage and neurologic morbidity is greater in the thrombocytopenic group. However, in a randomized trial, transfusing PLTs prophylactically whenever the PLT count fell to $<150 \times 10^9$/L to maintain the average PLT count at $>200 \times 10^9$/L vs transfusing PLTs only when the PLT count fell to $<50 \times 10^9$/L to maintain the average PLT count at approximately 100×10^9/L did not diminish the incidence of intracranial hemorrhage (28% vs 26%). Thus, there is no documented benefit to transfusing PLTs for mild thrombocytopenia (PLT count <150 but $>100 \times 10^9$/L) to sustain a blood PLT count in the normal range. Although basic questions about the relative risks of different degrees of thrombocytopenia in various clinical settings are only partially answered, guidelines acceptable to many neonatologists are listed in Table 471-1.

The goal of most PLT transfusions is to raise the PLT count to $>50 \times 10^9$/L and to increase that for neonates to $>100 \times 10^9$/L. This can be achieved consistently in children weighing up to 30 kg by infusing 10 mL/kg of standard (unmodified) PLT concentrates, obtained either from processing whole blood units or by plateletpheresis. For larger children, the appropriate dose is 3–6 pooled whole blood–derived PLT units or 1 apheresis unit. PLT concentrates should be transfused as rapidly as the patient's overall condition permits, certainly within 2 hr. Patients requiring repeated PLT transfusions should receive leukocyte-reduced blood products, including PLT concentrates, to diminish alloimmunization and PLT refractoriness and reduce the risk of transfusion-transmitted cytomegalovirus infection.

Routinely reducing the volume of PLT concentrates for infants and small children by additional centrifugation steps is both unnecessary and unwise. Transfusion of 10 mL/kg of an unmodified PLT concentrate is adequate because it adds 10×10^9 PLTs to 70 mL of blood (the blood volume of a 1-kg neonate), a number calculated (taking the usual hematocrit and post-transfusion PLT recovery values into account) to increase the PLT count by 100×10^9/L. This calculated increment is consistent with the actual increment. Moreover, 10 mL/kg is not an excessive transfusion volume, providing the intake of other IV fluids, medications, and nutrients is monitored and adjusted. It is important to minimize repeated transfusion of group O PLTs to group A or B recipients because passive anti-A or anti-B in group O plasma can lead to hemolysis. Although proven methods exist to reduce the volume of PLT concentrates when truly warranted (many transfusions are anticipated, in which the quantity of passive anti-A or anti-B might lead to hemolysis, or failure of 10 mL/kg of unmodified PLT concentrate to increase the PLT count), additional processing should be performed with great care because of

TABLE 471-1. Guidelines for Pediatric Platelet Transfusions*

CHILDREN AND ADOLESCENTS
PLTs $< 50 \times 10^9$/L and bleeding
PLTs $< 50 \times 10^9$/L and an *invasive* procedure
PLTs $< 20 \times 10^9$/L and *marrow failure* with hemorrhagic risk factors
PLTs $< 10 \times 10^9$/L and *marrow failure* without hemorrhagic risk factors
PLTs at any count, but with PLT dysfunction plus bleeding or an invasive procedure
INFANTS WITHIN THE FIRST 4 MO OF LIFE
PLTs $< 100 \times 10^9$/L and bleeding
PLTs $< 50 \times 10^9$/L and an invasive procedure
PLTs $< 20 \times 10^9$/L and *clinically stable*
PLTs $< 100 \times 10^9$/L and *clinically unstable*
PLTs at any count, but with PLT dysfunction plus bleeding or an invasive procedure

*Words in *italics* must be defined for local transfusion guidelines.
PLTs, platelets.

probable PLT loss, clumping, and dysfunction caused by the additional handling, all of which could diminish the efficacy and increase the toxicity of PLT transfusions.

Chakravorty S, Murray N, Roberts I: Neonatal thrombocytopenia. *Early Hum Dev* 2005;81:35–41.

Murray NA: Evaluation and treatment of thrombocytopenia in the neonatal intensive care unit. *Acta Paediatr Suppl* 2002;91:74–81.

Strauss RG: Low-dose prophylactic platelet transfusions: Time for further study, but too early for routine clinical practice. *Transfusion* 2004;44: 1680–1682.

Chapter 472 ■ Neutrophil (Granulocyte) Transfusions

Guidelines for granulocyte transfusion (GTX) are listed in Table 472-1. Although GTX has been used sparingly in the past, the ability to collect markedly higher numbers of neutrophils from donors stimulated with recombinant granulocyte colony-stimulating factor (G-CSF) has led to renewed interest, particularly for recipients of hematopoietic progenitor cell transplantation. GTX should be reconsidered at institutions where neutropenic patients continue to die of progressive bacterial and fungal infections despite the optimal use of antimicrobial agents and recombinant myeloid growth factors.

The role of GTX added to antibiotics for patients with severe neutropenia ($<0.5 \times 10^9$/L) due to bone marrow failure is similar for adults and children. Infected neutropenic patients usually respond to antibiotics alone, provided bone marrow function recovers early during the infection. Because children with newly diagnosed leukemia respond rapidly to induction chemotherapy, they are rarely candidates for GTX. In contrast, infected children with sustained bone marrow failure (malignant neoplasms resistant to treatment, aplastic anemia, and hematopoietic progenitor cell transplant recipients) may benefit when GTX is added to antibiotics. The use of GTX for bacterial sepsis unresponsive to antibiotics in patients with severe neutropenia ($<0.5 \times 10^9$/L) is supported by many controlled studies (see Chapter 177).

Children with qualitative neutrophil defects (neutrophil dysfunction) usually have adequate numbers of blood neutrophils, but are susceptible to serious infections because their cells kill pathogenic microorganisms inefficiently. Neutrophil dysfunction syndromes are rare, and no definitive studies have established the efficacy of GTX. However, several patients with progressive life-threatening infections have improved strikingly with the addition of GTX to antimicrobial therapy. These disorders are chronic, and because of the risk of inducing alloimmunization, GTX is recommended only when infections are clearly unresponsive to antimicrobial drugs.

TABLE 472-1. Guidelines for Pediatric Granulocyte Transfusions*

CHILDREN AND ADOLESCENTS
Neutrophils of $<0.5 \times 10^9$/L and bacterial infection unresponsive to appropriate antimicrobial therapy
Qualitative neutrophil defect and infection (bacterial or fungal) *unresponsive* to appropriate antimicrobial therapy
INFANTS WITHIN THE FIRST 4 MO OF LIFE
Neutrophils of $<3.0 \times 10^9$/L (1st wk of life) or $<1.0 \times 10^9$/L (thereafter) and *fulminant* bacterial infection

*Words in *italics* must be defined for local transfusion guidelines.

Neonates are unusually susceptible to severe bacterial infections, and a number of defects of neonatal body defenses may be contributing factors (see Chapter 109). These abnormalities are accentuated in sick premature neonates, and it is logical to consider GTX. Neonates exhibiting fulminant sepsis, relative neutropenia ($<3.0 \times 10^9$/L during the 1st wk of life and $<1.0 \times 10^9$/L thereafter), and a severely diminished neutrophil marrow storage pool (with <10% of nucleated marrow cells postmitotic neutrophils) are at particularly great risk of dying if treated only with antibiotics. Although some studies have shown a significant benefit from GTX, it is rarely used. Instead, some neonatologists consider alternative therapies, including IV immunoglobulin and recombinant myeloid growth factors (G-CSF or granulocyte-macrophage colony–stimulating factor). Results of studies evaluating IV immunoglobulin have been mixed, but a meta-analysis found significant benefit for neonates with proven sepsis. Current data are insufficient to determine whether recombinant myeloid growth factors have a role in treating these neonates, although both G-CSF and granulocyte-macrophage colony–stimulating factor have been demonstrated to enhance myelopoiesis and increase neutrophil counts in infants. Importantly, G-CSF is efficacious for the treatment of several types of severe congenital neutropenia.

Once the decision to provide GTX has been made, an adequate dose of fresh leukapheresis cells must be transfused. Neonates and infants weighing <10 kg should receive $1–2 \times 10^9$/kg neutrophils per GTX. Larger infants and children should receive a total dose of at least 1×10^{10} neutrophils per GTX; the preferred dose for adolescents is $5–8 \times 10^{10}$ per GTX—a dose requiring donors to be stimulated with G-CSF. GTX should be given daily until either the infection resolves or the neutrophil count exceeds 1.0×10^9/L for a few days.

Dale DC, Liles WC: Return of granulocyte transfusions. *Curr Opin Pediatr* 2000;12:18–22.

Stravss RG: Rebirth of granulocyte transfusions: Should it involve pediatric oncology and transplant patients? *J Pediatr Hematol Oncol* 1999;21: 475–478.

Chapter 473 ■ Fresh Frozen Plasma Transfusions

Guidelines for fresh frozen plasma (FFP) transfusion in children (Table 473-1) are similar to those for adults. FFP is transfused to replace clinically significant deficiencies of plasma proteins for which more highly purified concentrates are not available. Requirements for FFP vary with the specific factor being replaced, but a starting dose of 15 mL/kg is usually satisfactory. Transfusion of FFP is efficacious for the treatment of deficiencies of clotting factors II, V, X, and XI. Deficiencies of factor XIII and fibrinogen are treated with cryoprecipitate. Transfusion of FFP is not recommended for the treatment of patients with severe hemophilia A or B or for factor VII deficiency because safer factor VII, VIII, and IX concentrates are available. Moreover, mild to moderate hemophilia A and certain types of von Willebrand disease can be treated with desmopressin (see Chapter 477). An important use of FFP is for rapid reversal of the effects of warfarin in patients who are actively bleeding or who require emergency surgery (in whom functional deficiencies of factors II, VII, IX, and X cannot be rapidly reversed by vitamin K). Results of screening coagulation tests (prothrombin, activated partial

TABLE 473-1. Guidelines for Pediatric Fresh Frozen Plasma Transfusions*

INFANTS, CHILDREN, AND ADOLESCENTS
Severe clotting factor deficiency and bleeding
Severe clotting factor deficiency and an invasive procedure
Emergency reversal of warfarin effects
Dilutional coagulopathy and bleeding
Anticoagulant protein (antithrombin III, proteins C and S) replacement
Plasma exchange replacement fluid for thrombotic thrombocytopenic purpura

*Words in *italics* must be defined for local transfusion guidelines.

thromboplastin, and thrombin times) should not be assumed by themselves to reflect the integrity of the coagulation system. To justify FFP transfusion, coagulation test results must be related to the patient's clinical condition. Transfusion of FFP in patients with chronic liver disease and prolonged clotting times is not recommended unless bleeding is present or an invasive procedure is planned because correction of the clotting factor deficiencies is brief.

FFP also contains several anticoagulant proteins (antithrombin III, protein C, and protein S), whose deficiencies have been associated with thrombosis. In selected situations, FFP may be appropriate as replacement therapy, along with anticoagulant treatment, in patients with these disorders. However, when available, purified concentrates are preferred. Other indications for FFP include replacement fluid during plasma exchange in patients with thrombotic thrombocytopenic purpura or other disorders for which FFP is likely to be beneficial (plasma exchange in a patient with bleeding and severe coagulopathy). FFP is not indicated for correction of hypovolemia or as immunoglobulin replacement therapy, because safer alternatives exist (albumin or saline solutions and IV immunoglobulin, respectively).

In neonates, FFP transfusion merits special consideration. Clotting times are "physiologically" prolonged, owing to developmental deficiency of clotting proteins, and FFP should be transfused only after reference to normal values expected for the birthweight and age of the infant. The indications for FFP in neonates include: (1) reconstitution of red blood cell (RBC) concentrates to simulate whole blood for use in massive transfusions (exchange transfusion or cardiovascular surgery); (2) hemorrhage secondary to vitamin K deficiency; (3) disseminated intravascular coagulation with bleeding; and (4) bleeding in congenital coagulation factor deficiency when more specific treatment is either unavailable or inappropriate. The use of prophylactic FFP transfusion to prevent intraventricular hemorrhage in premature infants is not recommended. FFP should not be used as a suspending agent to adjust the hematocrit values of RBC concentrates before small-volume RBC transfusions to neonates because it offers no apparent medical benefit over the use of sterile solutions. Similarly, the use of FFP in partial exchange transfusion for the treatment of neonatal hyperviscosity syndrome is unnecessary because safer crystalloid or colloid solutions are available.

In the treatment of bleeding infants, cryoprecipitate is often considered because of its small infusion volume. However, cryoprecipitate contains only fibrinogen and factors VIII and XIII. Thus, it is not effective for treating the usual clinical situation in bleeding infants of multiple clotting factor deficiencies, despite the appeal and convenience of a small infusion volume. In preliminary studies, infusions of very small volumes of recombinant activated factor VII have been life-saving in patients with hemorrhage due to several mechanisms. Because the efficacy and toxicity of factor VIIa have not been fully defined in these "off-label" (not approved by the U.S. Food and Drug Administration) uses, it must be considered experimental therapy at this time.

Felderhoff-Mueser U, Buhrer C: Clinical measures to preserve cerebral integrity in preterm infants. *Early Hum Dev* 2005;81:237–244.

Goldenberg NA, Manco-Johnson MJ: Pediatric hemostasis and use of plasma components. *Best Pract Res Clin Haematol* 2006;19:143–155.

O'Shaughnessy DF, Atterbury C, Bolton Maggs P, et al: Guidelines for the use of fresh-frozen plasma, cryoprecipitate and cryosupernatant. *Br J Haematol* 2004;126:11–28.

Stanworth SJ, Brunskill SJ, Hyde CJ, et al: Is fresh frozen plasma clinically effective? A systematic review of randomized controlled trials. *Br J Haematol* 2004;126:139–152.

Chapter 474 ■ Risks of Blood Transfusions

Although the risks of allogeneic blood transfusions are low, transfusions must be given judiciously. Taking nucleic acid amplification testing (NAT) and all other donor-screening activities (antibody and epidemiology screening) into account, a current estimate of the risk of transfusion-associated HIV is approximately 1/2,000,000 donor exposures, with estimates ranging from 1/800,000–1/4,000,000 donor exposures. Similarly, with NAT, the risk of viral hepatitis C is 1/1,600,000 donor exposures. NAT identifies circulating viral genes in the window period before antibodies develop and is available for HIV, hepatitis C, and West Nile virus. Transfusion-associated cytomegalovirus can be nearly eliminated by transfusing leukocyte-reduced cellular blood products or by selecting blood from donors who are seronegative for antibody to cytomegalovirus. Both methods have compatible efficacy, and there is no documented advantage to doing both (using leukocyte-reduced blood collected from seronegative donors). Additional infectious risks include other types of hepatitis (B, E) and retroviruses (human T-cell lymphotropic virus types I and II and HIV-2), syphilis, parvovirus B19, Epstein-Barr virus, human herpesvirus 8, West Nile virus, malaria, babesiosis, and Chagas disease. Variant Creutzfeldt-Jacob disease has also been transmitted by blood transfusions in humans.

Transfusion-associated risks of a noninfectious nature that may occur include hemolytic and nonhemolytic transfusion reactions, fluid overload, graft vs host disease, electrolyte and acid-base imbalances, iron overload if chronic repeated transfusions are needed, increased susceptibility to oxidant damage, exposure to plasticizers, hemolysis with T-antigen activation of red blood cells, post-transfusion purpura, acute lung injury, immunosuppression, and alloimmunization. Immunomodulation may be reduced by leukoreduction. Transfusion reactions and alloimmunization to red blood cell and leukocyte antigens seem to be uncommon in infants. Adverse effects are seen only in massive transfusion settings, such as exchange transfusions, trauma, or surgery, when relatively large quantities of blood are needed, and are rare with the small-volume transfusions usually given. In addition, medical errors, such as transfusing the wrong blood type, occur in approximately 1/25,000 units.

Premature infants are known to have immune dysfunction, but their relative risk of post-transfusion graft vs host disease is controversial. The postnatal age of the infant, the number of immunocompetent lymphocytes in the transfusion product, the degree of human leukocyte antigen compatibility between donor and recipient, and other poorly described phenomena determine which infants are truly at risk. In utero transfusion has a high risk of graft vs host disease. Regardless, many centers caring for preterm infants transfuse exclusively γ-irradiated cellular products. Directed donations with blood drawn from blood relatives must always be irradiated because of the risk of engraftment with transfused human leukocyte antigen–homozygous haploidentical lymphocytes. Cellular blood products given as intrauterine and exchange transfusions should be γ-irradiated, as are transfusions for patients with severe congenital immunodeficiency disorders (DiGeorge syndrome requiring heart surgery) and those for recipients of hematopoietic progenitor cell transplants. Other groups who are potentially at risk, but for whom no conclusive data are available, are patients given T-cell antibody therapy (antithymocyte globulin or OKT3), those with organ allografts, those receiving immunosuppressive drug regimens, and patients infected with HIV.

Current practice uses γ-irradiation from a cesium, cobalt, or linear acceleration source at doses ranging from 2,500–5,000 cGy; a minimum dose of 2,500 cGy is required. All cellular blood components should be irradiated, but frozen "acellular" products, such as plasma and cryoprecipitate, do not require it. Leukocyte reduction cannot be substituted for γ-irradiation to prevent graft vs host disease.

Arendt A, Carmean J, Koch E, et al: Fatal bacterial infections associated with platelet transfusions—United States, 2004. *MMWR* 2005;57:168.
Blajchman MA, Vamvakas EC: The continuing risk of transfusion-transmitted infections. *N Engl J Med* 2006;355:1303–1305.
Bolton-Maggs PHB, Murphy MF: Blood transfusions. *Arch Dis Child* 2004; 89:4–7.
Busch MP, Kleinman SH, Nemo GJ: Current and emerging infectious risks of blood transfusions. *JAMA* 2003;289:959–962.
Chakravorty S, Murray N, Roberts I: Neonatal thrombocytopenia. *Early Hum Dev* 2005;81:35–41.
College of American Pathologists Task Force: Practice parameter for the use of fresh-frozen plasma, cryoprecipitate, and platelets. *JAMA* 1994;271: 777.
Goodnough LT, Shander A, Brecher ME: Transfusion medicine: Looking to the future. *Lancet* 2003;361:161–169.
Hladik W, Dollard SC, Mermin J, et al: Transmission of human herpes virus 8 by blood transfusion. *N Engl J Med* 2006;355:1331–1338.
Mohan P, Brocklehurst P: Granulocyte transfusions for neonates with confirmed or suspected sepsis and neutropenia. *Cochrane Database Syst Rev* 2003;4:CD003956.
Murray NA: Evaluation and treatment of thrombocytopenia in the neonatal intensive care unit. *Acta Paediatr Suppl* 2002;91:74–81.
Savakis EC, Strauss RG: Meta-analysis of controlled clinical trials studying the efficacy of recombinant human erythropoietin in reducing blood transfusions in the anemia of prematurity. *Transfusion* 2001;41:406.
Stramer SL, Glynn SA, Kleinman SH, et al: Detection of HIV-1 and HCV infections among antibody-negative blood donors by nucleic acid amplification testing. *N Engl J Med* 2004;351:760–768.
Strauss RG: Low-dose prophylactic platelet transfusions: Time for further study, but too early for routine clinical practice. *Transfusion* 2004;44: 1680–1682.
Strauss RG: Data-driven blood banking practices for neonatal RBC transfusions. *Transfusion* 2000;40:1528–1540.
Wilson K, Ricketts MN: A third episode of transfusion-derived VCJD. *Lancet* 2006;368:2037–2038.

Section 7 — Hemorrhagic and Thrombotic Diseases — J. Paul Scott and Robert R. Montgomery

Chapter 475 ■ Hemostasis

Hemostasis is the active process that clots blood in areas of blood vessel injury, yet simultaneously limits the clot size only to the areas of injury. Over time, the clot is lysed by the fibrinolytic system, and normal blood flow is restored. If clotting is impaired, hemorrhage occurs. If clotting is excessive, thrombotic complications ensue. The hemostatic response needs to be rapid and regulated such that trauma does not trigger a systemic reaction, but must initiate a rapid, localized response. Key to the speed and coordination of response is the fact that when a platelet adheres to a site of vascular injury, the platelet surface provides a reaction surface where clotting factors bind. The active enzyme is brought together with its substrate, accelerating reaction rates and providing activated products for reaction with clotting factors further down the coagulation cascade. Active clotting is controlled by negative feedback loops that inhibit the clotting process when the procoagulant process comes in contact with intact endothelium. The main components of the hemostatic process are the **vessel wall, platelets, coagulation proteins, anticoagulant proteins,** and **fibrinolytic system.** Most components of hemostasis are multifunctional; fibrinogen serves as the ligand between platelets during platelet aggregation and also serves as the substrate for thrombin that forms the fibrin clot. Platelets provide the reaction surface on which clotting reactions occur, form the plug at the site of vessel injury, and contract to constrict and limit clot size.

THE PROCESS. The intact vascular endothelium is the primary barrier against hemorrhage. The endothelial cells that line the vessel wall normally inhibit coagulation and provide a smooth surface that permits rapid blood flow.

After vascular injury, vasoconstriction occurs and flowing blood comes in contact with the subendothelial matrix (Fig. 475-1). In flowing blood, when exposed to subendothelial matrix proteins, von Willebrand factor (VWF) changes conformation and provides the glue to which the platelet VWF receptor binds. After adherence, platelets become activated and release storage granules containing adenosine diphosphate (ADP), thromboxane A_2, and other stored proteins. These trigger the aggregation and recruitment of other platelets to form the platelet plug. Aggregation involves the interaction of specific receptors on the platelet surface with plasma hemostatic proteins, primarily fibrinogen.

One of the subendothelial matrix proteins that is exposed after vascular injury is tissue factor. Just as exposed subendothelial matrix proteins bind VWF, tissue factor is also exposed, binds to factor VII, and activates the clotting cascade, as shown in Figure 475-2. In the cascade, inactive clotting factors, denoted by Roman numerals, become activated. The activated clotting factor then initiates the activation of the next sequential clotting factor in a systematic manner. The proteins in the cascade fall into 2 groups: serine protease zymogens that are activated into functional enzymes and cofactors that help to catalyze the clotting reactions. During the process of platelet activation, internalized platelet phospholipids (primarily phosphatidylserine) become externalized and interact at 2 specific, rate-limiting steps in the clotting process—those involving the cofactors factor VIII (X-ase

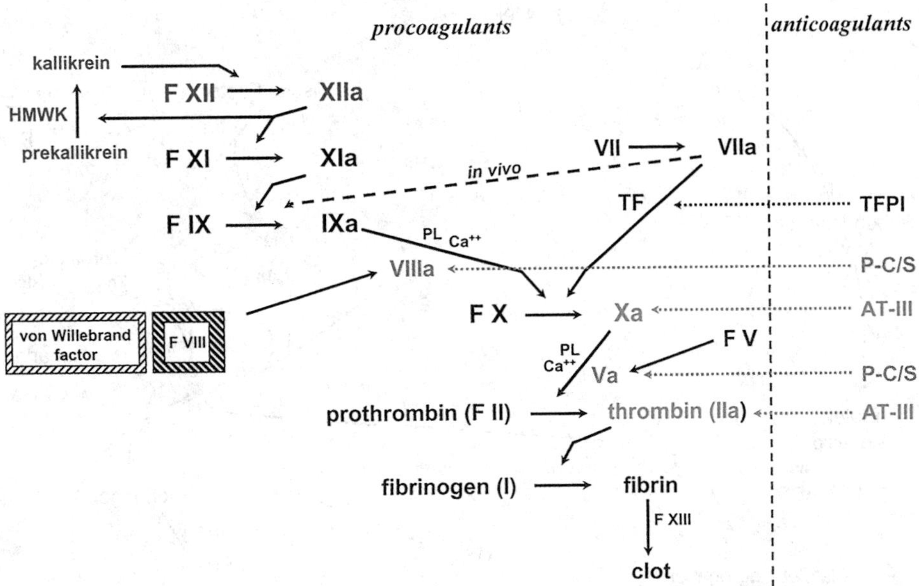

Figure 475-1. The clotting cascade, with sequential activation and amplification of clot formation. Many of the factors are activated by the clotting factor shown above them in the cascade. The activated factors (F) are designated by the addition of an *a*. On the *right side,* the major anticoagulants and the sites that they regulate are shown (tissue factor pathway inhibitor [TFPI] regulates tissue factor [TF] and factor VIIa, protein C and protein S (P-C/S) regulate factors VIII and V, and antithrombin III (AT-III) regulates factor Xa and thrombin [factor IIa]). The *dotted line* shows that, in vivo, TF and factor VIIa activate both factors IX and X, but in vitro, only the activation of factor X is measured. Unactivated factor VIII, when bound to its carrier protein, von Willebrand factor, is protected from protein C inactivation. When thrombin, or factor Xa, activates factor VIII, it becomes unbound to von Willebrand factor, where it can participate with factor IXa in the activation of factor X in the presence of phospholipid (PL) and calcium (Ca^{2+}). Factor XIIIa cross links the fibrin clot and thereby makes it more stable. Prekallikrein, high molecular weight kininogen (HMWK), and factor XII are shown in *blue* because, although they contribute to the clotting time in partial thromboplastin time (PTT), they do not have a physiologic role in coagulation.

complex) and factor V (prothrombinase complex). Both of these reactions are localized to the platelet surface and bring together the active enzyme, an activated cofactor, and the zymogen that will form the next active enzyme in the cascade. This results in amplification of the process, which supplies a burst of clotting where it is physiologically needed. In vivo, autocatalysis of factor VII generates small amounts of factor VIIa continuously, so the system is always poised to act. Near the bottom of the cascade, the multipotent enzyme thrombin is formed. Thrombin clots fibrinogen into fibrin, activates factors V, VIII, and XI, and aggregates platelets. Thrombin also activates factor XIII. The stable fibrin-platelet plug is ultimately formed through clot retraction and cross linking of the fibrin clot by factor XIIIa.

Virtually all procoagulant proteins are balanced by an anticoagulant protein that regulates or inhibits procoagulant function. There are 4 clinically important, naturally occurring anticoagulants that regulate the extension of the clotting process. These include antithrombin III (AT-III), protein C, protein S, and tissue factor pathway inhibitor (TFPI). AT-III is a serine protease inhibitor that regulates factor Xa and thrombin primarily and also, to a lesser extent, factors IXa, XIa, and XIIa. When thrombin in flowing blood encounters intact endothelium, thrombin binds to thrombomodulin, its endothelial receptor. The thrombin-thrombomodulin complex then activates protein C into activated protein C. In the presence of the cofactor protein S, activated protein C proteolyses and inactivates factor Va and factor VIIIa. Inactivated factor Va is, in fact, a functional anticoagulant that inhibits clotting. The final inhibitor is TFPI, which quickly shuts down the activation of factor X by factor VII and tissue factor and shifts the activation site of tissue factor and factor VII to that of factor IX (see Figs. 475-1 and 475-2).

Once a stable fibrin-platelet plug is formed, the fibrinolytic system limits its extension and also lyses the clot (fibrinolysis) to re-establish vascular integrity. Plasmin, generated from plasminogen by either urokinase-like or tissue-type plasminogen activator, degrades the fibrin clot. In the process of dissolving the fibrin clot, fibrin degradation products are produced. The fibrinolytic pathway is regulated by plasminogen activator inhibitors and α_2-antiplasmin. Finally, the flow of blood in and around the clot is crucial as flowing blood returns to the liver, where activated clotting factor complexes are removed and new pro- and anticoagulant proteins are synthesized to maintain homeostasis of the hemostatic system.

PATHOLOGY. Congenital deficiency of an individual procoagulant protein leads to a bleeding disorder, whereas deficiency of an anticoagulant (clotting factor inhibitor) predisposes the patient to excessive thrombosis. In acquired hemostatic disorders, there are frequently multiple problems with homeostasis that perturb and dysregulate hemostasis. A primary illness (sepsis) and its secondary effects (shock and acidosis) activate coagulation and fibrinolysis and impair the host's ability to restore normal hemostatic function. When sepsis triggers **disseminated intravascular coagulation,** procoagulant clotting factors and anticoagulant proteins are consumed, leaving the hemostatic system unbalanced and prone to bleeding or clotting. Similarly, newborn infants and patients with severe liver disease have synthetic deficiencies of both procoagulant and anticoagulant proteins. Such dysregulation causes the patient to be predisposed to both hemorrhage and thrombosis with mild or moderate triggers that result in major alterations in the hemostatic process.

In the laboratory evaluation of hemostasis, parameters are manipulated to allow assessment of isolated aspects of hemostasis and limit the multifunctionality of some of its components. The coagulation process is studied in plasma anticoagulated with

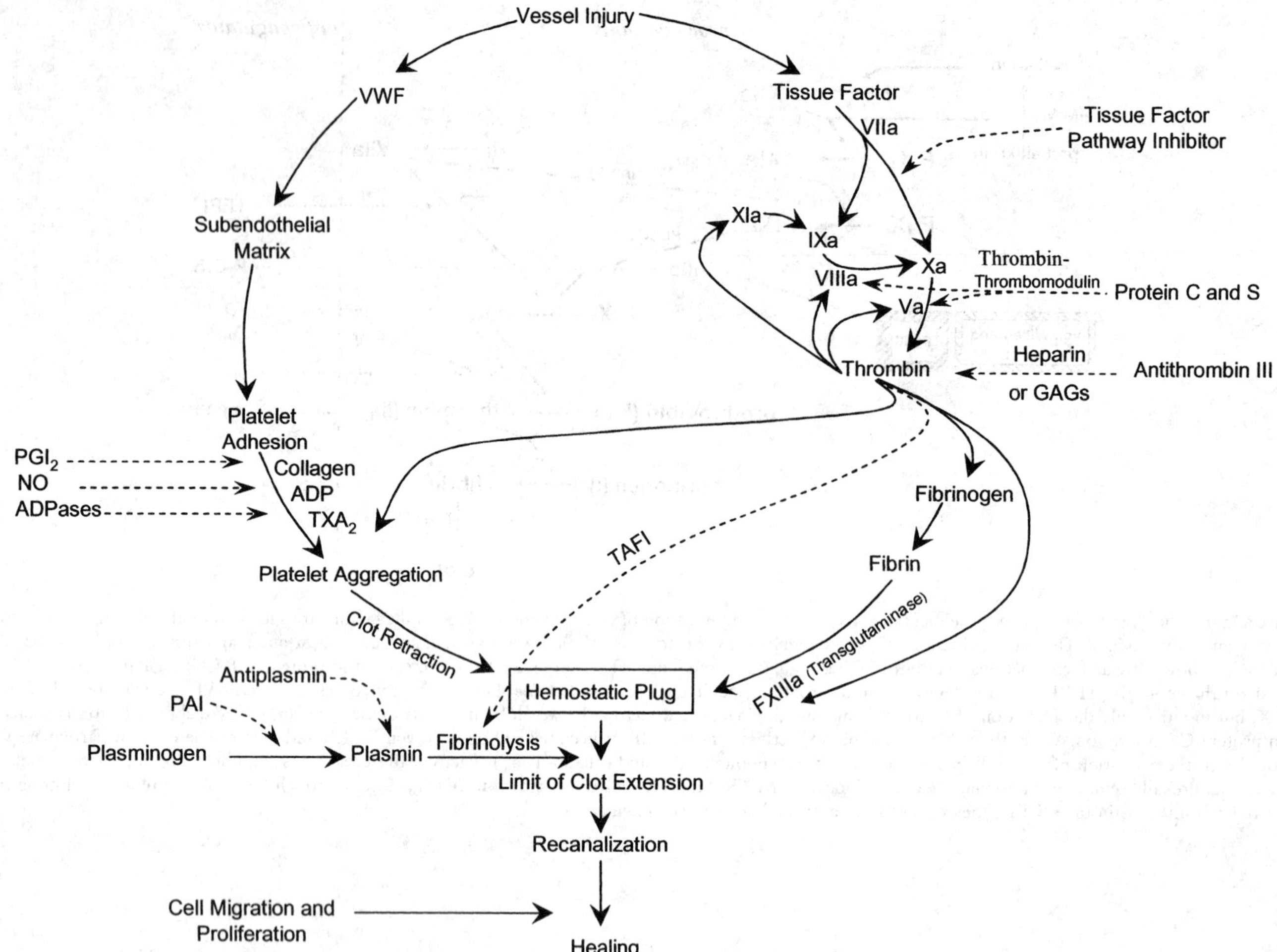

Figure 475-2. The hemostatic mechanism. ADP, adenosine diphosphate; GAGs, glycosaminoglycans; NO, nitric oxide; PGI_2, prostacyclin; PAI, plasminogen activator inhibitor; TAFI, thrombin-activated fibrinolytic inhibitor; TXA_2, thromboxane A_2; VWF, von Willebrand factor.

citrate to bind calcium, with added phospholipid to mimic the reaction surface normally provided by the platelet membrane, and with a stimulus to trigger clotting. Calcium is added to restart the clotting process. This results in anomalies such that the in vivo physiologic pathway of clotting in which factor VIIa activates factor IX is bypassed; instead, in prothrombin time (PT), factor VIIa activates factor X. If this were truly the physiologic situation, then there would be an in vivo bypass mechanism that would ameliorate severe factor VIII and factor IX deficiency, the 2 most common severe bleeding disorders.

475.1 • Clinical and Laboratory Evaluation of Hemostasis

HISTORY. For most hemostatic disorders, the clinical history provides the most useful information. For a hemorrhagic condition, the history should determine the site or sites of bleeding, the severity and duration of hemorrhage, and the age at onset. Was the bleeding spontaneous, or did it occur after trauma? Was there a previous personal or family history of similar problems? Did the symptoms correlate with the degree of injury or trauma? Does bruising occur spontaneously? Are there lumps with bruises for which there is minimal trauma? If the patient had previous surgery or significant dental procedures, was there any increased bleeding? If a child or adolescent has had surgery affecting the mucosal surfaces, such as a tonsillectomy or major dental extractions, the absence of bleeding usually rules out a hereditary bleeding disorder. Delayed or slow healing of superficial injuries may suggest a hereditary bleeding disorder. In postpubertal females, it is important to take a careful menstrual history. Because some common bleeding disorders, such as von Willebrand disease (VWD), have a fairly high prevalence, mothers and family members may have the same mild bleeding disorder and may not be cognizant that the child's menstrual history is abnormal. Women with mild VWD who have a moderate history of bruising frequently have a reduction of that bruising during pregnancy or after administration of oral contraceptives. Some medications, such as aspirin and other nonsteroidal anti-inflammatory drugs, may inhibit platelet function and increase bleeding symptoms in patients with a low platelet count or abnormal hemostasis.

Outside the neonatal period, thrombotic disorders are relatively rare until adulthood. In the neonate, physiologic deficiencies of procoagulants and anticoagulants cause the hemostatic mechanism to be dysregulated, and clinical events can lead to either hemorrhage or thrombosis. If a child or teenager presents with deep venous thrombosis or pulmonary emboli, a detailed family history must be obtained to evaluate for deep venous thrombosis, pulmonary emboli, myocardial infarction, or stroke in other family members. Even in the absence of a family history, the presence of thrombosis in the child or teenager should trigger an evaluation of the individual for a hereditary or acquired predisposition to thrombosis.

PHYSICAL EXAMINATION. The physical examination should focus on whether bleeding symptoms are primarily associated with the mucous membranes or skin (mucocutaneous bleeding) or the muscles and joints (deep bleeding). The examination should determine the presence of petechiae, ecchymoses, hematomas, hemarthroses, or mucous membrane bleeding. Patients with defects in platelet–blood vessel wall interaction (VWD or platelet function defects) usually have mucocutaneous bleeding, which may include epistaxis, menorrhagia, petechiae, ecchymoses, occasional hematomas, and less commonly, hematuria and gastrointestinal bleeding. Individuals with a clotting factor deficiency, such as hemophilia (factor VIII or factor IX deficiency), have symptoms of deep bleeding into muscles and joints, with much more extensive ecchymoses and hematoma formation. Patients with mild VWD or other mild bleeding disorders may have no abnormal findings on physical examination. Individuals with disorders of the collagen matrix and vessel wall may have loose joints and lax skin associated with easy bruising (Ehlers-Danlos syndrome).

Patients undergoing evaluation for thrombotic disorders should be asked about swollen, warm, tender extremities or internal organs (venous thrombosis), unexplained dyspnea or persistent "pneumonia," especially in the absence of fever (pulmonary emboli), and varicosities and post-phlebitic changes. Arterial thrombi usually cause an acute, dramatic impairment of organ function, such as stroke, myocardial infarction, or a painful, white, cold extremity.

LABORATORY TESTS. Patients who have a positive bleeding history or who are actively hemorrhaging should have a platelet count, PT, and partial thromboplastin time (PTT). If the results are normal, a thrombin time to evaluate fibrinogen function and VWF testing should be considered. In individuals with abnormal screening test results, further specific factor work-up should be undertaken. In a patient with an abnormal bleeding history and a positive family history, normal screening tests should not preclude further laboratory evaluation.

There are no useful routine screening tests for hereditary thrombotic disorders. If the family history is positive or clinical thrombosis is unexplained, specific anticoagulant assays should be undertaken. Thrombosis is rare in children, and when present, the possibility of a hereditary predisposition must be considered and evaluated in the laboratory.

Bleeding Time. Bleeding time assesses the function of platelets and their interaction with the vascular wall. Disposable standardized devices have been developed that control the length and depth of the skin incision. A blood pressure cuff is applied to the upper arm and inflated to 40 mm Hg for children and adults. In term newborns and younger children, a modified device has been developed and used with a lower blood pressure cuff pressure. Bleeding time is a difficult laboratory test to standardize, and there is much interlaboratory and interindividual variation. Although platelet counts of <100,000/mm^3 are associated with prolonged bleeding time, disproportionate prolongation of bleeding time may suggest a qualitative platelet defect or VWD. After an incision is made with the bleeding time device, blood is blotted from the margin of the incision at 30 sec intervals until bleeding ceases. Although each laboratory must establish its own normal range, bleeding usually stops within 4–8 min. Accurate evaluation of bleeding time requires the cooperation of the patient.

Platelet Function Analyzer. In an attempt to evaluate the early stages of hemostasis (platelet function and VWF interaction under high shear), several in vitro platelet analyzers have been developed. The greatest experience has been with the platelet function analyzer (PFA-100). The PFA-100 measures platelet adhesion-aggregation in whole blood at high shear when exposed to either collagen-epinephrine or collagen-ADP. Results are reported as the closure time measured in sec. The PFA-100 has variable sensitivity, particularly in the detection of VWD and some platelet function defects. The PFA-100 is sensitive to some variants of VWD that are characterized by a reduction in VWF antigen or activity (see Chapter 477). The sensitivity of the PFA-100 to less severe platelet function disorders is controversial, and concerns remain about its specificity. Further studies are warranted to establish whether the PFA-100 can be used as a screening tool.

Platelet Count. Platelet count is essential in the evaluation of the child with a positive bleeding history because thrombocytopenia is the most common acquired cause of a bleeding diathesis in children. Patients with a platelet count of >50,000/mm^3 rarely have significant clinical bleeding. Thrombocytosis in children is usually reactive and is not associated with bleeding or thrombotic complications. Persistent, severe thrombocytosis in the absence of an underlying illness may require evaluation for the very rare pediatric presentation of essential thrombocythemia or polycythemia vera.

PROTHROMBIN TIME AND ACTIVATED PARTIAL THROMBOPLASTIN TIME. Because clotting factors were named in the order of discovery, they do not necessarily reflect the sequential order of activation (Table 475-1). In fact, factors III, IV, and VI were not subsequently found to be independent proteins; thus, these terms are no longer used. The dual mechanisms of activating clotting have been termed the **intrinsic** (surface activation) and **extrinsic** (tissue factor-mediated) pathways. Study of the hemostatic mechanism is further complicated in that the interactions in vivo may use different pathways from those studied in clinical laboratory testing. PT measures the activation of clotting by tissue factor (thromboplastin) in the presence of calcium. Addition of tissue factor causes a burst of factor VIIa generation. The tissue factor-factor VIIa complex activates factor X. Whether factor X is activated by the intrinsic or the extrinsic pathway, factor Xa is generated. On the platelet phospholipid surface, factor Xa complexes with factor V and calcium (the "prothrombinase" complex) to activate prothrombin to thrombin (also referred to as *factor IIa*). Once thrombin is generated, fibrinogen is converted to a fibrin clot—the end-point of the reaction (see Fig. 475-2). PT is not prolonged with deficiencies of factors VIII, IX, XI,

TABLE 475-1. Coagulation Factors

CLOTTING FACTOR	SYNONYM	DISORDER
I	Fibrinogen	Congenital deficiency (afibrinogenemia) or dysfunction (dysfibrinogenemia)
II	Prothrombin	Congenital deficiency or dysfunction
V	Labile factor, proaccelerin	Congenital deficiency (parahemophilia)
VII	Stable factor or proconvertin	Congenital deficiency
VIII	Antihemophilic factor	Congenital deficiency is hemophilia A (classic hemophilia)
IX	Christmas factor	Congenital deficiency is hemophilia B
X	Stuart-Prower factor	Congenital deficiency
XI	Plasma thromboplastin antecedent	Congenital deficiency, sometimes referred to as hemophilia C
XII	Hageman factor	Congenital deficiency is not associated with clinical symptoms
XIII	Fibrin-stabilizing factor	Congenital deficiency

or XII. In most laboratories, normal PT is 10–13 sec. PT has been standardized using the **International Normalized Ratio (INR)** so that values can be compared from 1 laboratory or instrument to another. This ratio is used to determine similar degrees of anticoagulation with warfarin (Coumadin)-like medications.

Partial Thromboplastin Time. The intrinsic pathway involves the initial activation of factor XII, which is accelerated by 2 other plasma proteins, prekallikrein and high molecular weight kininogen. In the clinical laboratory, factor XII is activated using a surface (silica or glass) or a contact activator, such as ellagic acid. Factor XIIa, in turn, activates factor XI to factor XIa, which then catalyzes factor IX to factor IXa. On the platelet phospholipid surface, factor IXa complexes with factor VIII and calcium to activate factor X ("tenase" complex).

This process is accelerated by interaction with phospholipid and calcium at the steps involving factors V and VIII. An isolated deficiency of a single clotting factor may result in isolated prolongation of PT, PTT, or both, depending on the location of the factor in the clotting cascade. This is useful in determining hereditary clotting factor deficiencies; however, in acquired hemostatic disorders encountered in clinical practice, >1 clotting factor is frequently deficient, so the relative prolongation of PT and PTT must be assessed.

Measurement of PTT as performed in the clinical laboratory is actually "activated" PTT; however, most refer to it as *PTT.* This test measures the initiation of clotting at the level of factor XII through sequential steps to the final clot end-point. It does not measure factor VII, factor XIII, or anticoagulants. PTT uses a contact activator (silica, kaolin, or ellagic acid) in the presence of calcium and phospholipid. Because of differences in reagents and laboratory instruments, the normal range for PTT varies between 1 hospital laboratory and another. Normal ranges for PTT are much more variable from laboratory to laboratory than is the case for PT.

Thus, the mechanisms studied by PT and PTT allow the evaluation of clotting factor deficiencies, even though these pathways may not be the same as those occurring physiologically In vivo, factor VIIa activates factors IX and X, but as routinely studied in the clinical laboratory, the pathway through which factor VIIa activates factor IX is not evaluated. If the tissue factor–factor VIIa complex activated only factor X, it would be difficult to explain why the most severe bleeding disorders are deficiencies of factor VIII (hemophilia A) and factor IX (hemophilia B). In vivo, thrombin is generated and feeds back to activate factor XI and accelerate the clotting process. Clotting in PTT can be prolonged by deficiencies of factor XII, prekallikrein, and high molecular weight kininogen; yet, these are asymptomatic conditions.

Thrombin Time. Thrombin time measures the final step in the clotting cascade, in which fibrinogen is converted to fibrin. The normal thrombin time varies between laboratories, but is usually 11–15 sec. Prolongation of thrombin time occurs with reduced fibrinogen levels (*hypofibrinogenemia* or *afibrinogenemia*), with dysfunctional fibrinogen (*dysfibrinogenemia*), or with the use of substances that interfere with fibrin polymerization, such as heparin or fibrin split products. If heparin contamination is a potential cause of prolonged thrombin time, a reptilase time is usually ordered.

Reptilase Time. Reptilase time uses snake venom to clot fibrinogen. Unlike thrombin time, reptilase time is not sensitive to heparin and is prolonged only by reduced or dysfunctional fibrinogen and fibrin split products. Therefore, if thrombin time is prolonged but reptilase time is normal, the prolonged thrombin time is due to heparin and does not indicate the presence of fibrin split products or reduced concentration or function of fibrinogen.

Mixing Studies. If there is unexplained prolongation of PT, PTT, or thrombin time, a mixing study is usually performed. Normal plasma is added to the patient's plasma, and PT or PTT is repeated. Correction of PT or PTT by 1:1 mixing with normal plasma suggests deficiency of a clotting factor, because a 50% level of individual clotting proteins is sufficient to produce normal PT or PTT. If the clotting time is not corrected or only partially corrected, an inhibitor is usually present. An inhibitor of clotting is a chemical similar to heparin that delays coagulation or an antibody directed against a specific clotting factor or the phospholipid used in clotting tests. In the inpatient setting, the most common cause of this finding is heparin contamination of the sample. The presence of heparin in the sample can be ruled in or out using thrombin time and reptilase time, as noted earlier. If the mixing study is not corrected or if it becomes more prolonged and the patient has clinical bleeding, an inhibitor of a specific clotting factor (antibody directed against the factor), most commonly factor VIII, factor IX, or factor XI, may be present. If the patient has no bleeding symptoms and both PTT and the mixing study are prolonged, a lupus-like anticoagulant (see Chapter 482) is often present. These patients usually have a long PTT, do not bleed, and may have a clinical predisposition to excessive clotting.

Clotting Factor Assays. Each of the clotting factors can be measured in the clinical laboratory using individual factor-deficient plasmas. For most clotting factors, activity is measured against pooled normal plasma or against a standard, where 100% activity is expressed as 100 IU/dL. By definition, 1 international unit (IU) of each factor is defined as that amount in 1 mL of normal plasma referenced against a standard established by the World Health Organization (WHO). In general, severe deficiency of factor VIII or factor IX is <1 IU/dL (<1% of normal), moderate deficiency is 1–5 IU/dL, and mild deficiency is >5 IU/dL, but < the normal range (Table 475-2). For most clotting factors, the normal range is 50–150 IU/dL (50–150%).

In patients with hemophilia A or hemophilia B, inhibitors of factor VIII or factor IX may develop after exposure to replacement therapy. To quantitate the amount of inhibitor present, the standardized clinical assay of these clotting inhibitors is the Bethesda assay. One Bethesda unit is defined as the amount that will inhibit 50% of the clotting factor in normal plasma.

Platelet Aggregation. When a qualitative platelet function defect is suspected, platelet aggregation testing is usually ordered. Platelet-rich plasma from the patient is activated with 1 of a series of agonists (ADP, epinephrine, collagen, thrombin or thrombin-receptor peptide, and ristocetin). Repeat testing or testing of other symptomatic family members can help to determine the hereditary nature of the defect. Many medications, especially aspirin, other nonsteroidal anti-inflammatory drugs, and valproic acid, alter platelet function testing. Some platelet aggregometers measure specific ADP release from the platelets, as reflected in generating luminescence (lumiaggregometer), and are more sensitive in detecting abnormalities of the platelet release reaction from storage granules.

Testing for Thrombotic Predisposition. Hereditary predisposition to thrombosis is associated with a reduction of anticoagulant function (protein C, protein S, AT-III); the presence of a factor V molecule that is resistant to inactivation by protein C (factor V Leiden); elevated levels of procoagulants (a mutation of the prothrombin gene); or a deficiency of fibrinolysis (plasminogen deficiency). When patients are being screened for prothrombotic tendencies, specific tests of the natural anticoagulants are warranted. Although both immunologic and functional tests are usually available, functional assay of protein C, protein S, and AT-III is more clinically useful.

Factor V Leiden is a common mutation in factor V that is associated with a significant risk of thrombosis. A point mutation in the factor V molecule prevents the inactivation of factor Va by activated protein C and, thereby, the persistence of factor Va. This defect is also known as *activated protein C resistance* and is easily diagnosed by DNA testing.

The **prothrombin gene mutation (G20210A)** is a mutation in the noncoding portion of the prothrombin gene, with a G at position 20210 being replaced by an A. This mutation increases the

TABLE 475-2. Reference Values for Coagulation Tests in Healthy Children*

TEST	28–31 Wk GESTATION	30–36 Wk GESTATION	FULL TERM	1–5 Yr	6–10 Yr	11–18 Yr	ADULT
SCREENING TESTS							
PT (sec)	15.4 (14.6–16.9)	13.0 (10.6–16.2)	13.0 (10.1–15.9)	11 (10.6–11.4)	11.1 (10.1–12.0)	11.2 (10.2–12.0)	12 (11.0–14.0)
APTT (sec)	108 (80–168)	53.6 (27.5–79.4)[‡§]	42.9 (31.3–54.3)[‡]	30 (24–36)	31 (26–36)	32 (26–37)	33 (27–40)
BT (min)				6 (2.5–10)[‡]	7 (2.5–13)[‡]	5 (3–8)[‡]	4 (1–7)
PROCOAGULANTS							
Fibrinogen	256 (160–550)	243 (150–373)[‡§]	283 (167–399)	276 (170–405)	279 (157–400)	300 (154–448)	278 (156–40)
II	31 (19–54)	45 (20–77)[‡]	48 (26–70)[‡]	94 (71–116)[‡]	88 (67–107)[‡]	83 (61–104)[‡]	108 (70–146)
V	65 (43–80)	88 (41–144)[§]	72 (34–108)[‡]	103 (79–127)	90 (63–116)[‡]	77 (55–99)[‡]	106 (62–150)
VII	37 (24–76)	67 (21–113)[‡]	66 (28–104)[‡]	82 (55–116)[‡]	86 (52–120)[‡]	83 (58–115)[‡]	105 (67–143)
VIII procoagulant	79 (37–126)	111 (5–213)	100 (50–178)	90 (59–142)	95 (58–132)	92 (53–131)	99 (50–149)
VWF	141 (83–223)	136 (78–210)	153 (50–287)	82 (60–120)	95 (44–144)	100 (46–153)	92 (50–158)
IX	18 (17–20)	35 (19–65)[‡§]	53 (15–91)[†‡]	73 (47–104)[‡]	75 (63–89)[‡]	82 (59–122)[‡]	109 (55–163)
X	36 (25–64)	41 (11–71)[‡]	40 (12–68)[‡]	88 (58–116)[‡]	75 (55–101)[‡]	79 (50–117)	106 (70–152)
XI	23 (11–33)	30 (8–52)[‡§]	38 (40–66)[‡]	30 (8–52)[‡]	38 (10–66)	74 (50–97)[‡]	97 (56–150)
XII	25 (5–35)	38 (10–66)[‡§]	53 (13–93)[‡]	93 (64–129)	92 (60–140)	81 (34–137)[‡]	108 (52–164)
PK	26 (15–32)	33 (9–89)[‡]	37 (18–69)[‡]	95 (65–130)	99 (66–131)	99 (53–145)	112 (62–162)
HMWK	32 (19–52)	49 (9–89)[‡]	54 (6–102)[‡]	98 (64–132)	93 (60–130)	91 (63–119)	92 (50–136)
XIIIa[‖]		70 (32–108)[‡]	79 (27–131)[‡]	108 (72–143)	109 (65–151)	99 (57–140)	105 (55–155)
XIIIb[‖]		81 (35–127)[‡]	76 (30–122)[‡]	113 (69–156)[‡]	116 (77–154)[‡]	102 (60–143)	98 (57–137)
ANTICOAGULANTS							
ATIII	28 (20–38)	38 (14–62)[‡§]	63 (39–87)[‡]	111 (82–139)	111 (90–131)	106 (77–132)	100 (74–126)
Protein C		28 (12–44)[‡§]	35 (17–53)[‡]	66 (40–92)[‡]	69 (45–93)[‡]	83 (55–111)[‡]	96 (64–128)
Protein S							
Total (U/mL)		26 (14–38)[‡§]	36 (12–60)[‡]	86 (54–118)	78 (41–114)	72 (52–92)	81 (61–113)
Free (U/mL)				45 (21–69)	42 (22–62)	38 (26–55)	45 (27–61)
Plasminogen (U/mL)		170 (112–248)[‖]	195 (125–265)[‖]	98 (78–118)	92 (75–108)	86 (68–103)	99 (77–122)
TPA (ng/mL)		8.48 (3.00–16.70)	9.6 (5.0–18.9)	2.15 (1.0–4.5)[‡]	2.42 (1.0–5.0)[‡]	2.16 (1.0–4.0)[‡]	1.02 (0.68–1.36)
α_2AP (U/mL)		78 (40–116)	85 (55–115)	105 (93–117)	99 (89–110)	98 (78–118)	102 (68–136)
PAI-1		5.4 (0.0–12.2)[‡]	6.4 (2.0–15.1)	5.42 (1.0–10.0)	6.79 (2.0–12.0)[‡]	6.07 (2.0–10.0)[‡]	3.60 (0.0–11.0)

*All factors except fibrinogen are expressed as units/mL (fibrinogen in mg/mL), where pooled normal plasma contains 1 U/mL. All data are expressed as the mean followed by the upper and lower boundaries encompassing 95% of the normal population.

†Levels for 19–27 wk and 28–31 wk are from multiple sources and cannot be analyzed statistically.

‡Values are significantly different from those of adults.

§Values are significantly different from those of full-term infants.

‖Value given as CTA units/mL.

APTT, activated partial thromboplastin time; α_2AP, α_2 antiplasmin; BT, bleeding time; CTA, committee on thrombolytic agents (units); HMWK, high molecular weight kininogen; PAI-1, plasminogen activator inhibitors; PK, prekallikrein; PT, prothrombin time; TPA, tissue type plasminogen activator; VWF, von Willebrand factor.

Data from Andrew M, Paes B, Johnston M: Development of the hemostatic system in the neonate and young infant. *Am J Pediatr Hematol Oncol* 1990; 12:95; and Andrew M, Vegh P, Johnston M, et al: Maturation of the hemostatic system during childhood. *Blood* 1992; 80:1998.

amount of prothrombin messenger RNA, is associated with elevated levels of prothrombin, and causes a predisposition to thrombosis. This abnormality is easily identified using molecular diagnostic (DNA) testing.

Elevated Homocysteine. Levels of homocysteine may be increased as a result of genetic mutations, causing homocystinuria. Such patients are predisposed to arterial and venous thrombosis as well as to an increase in arteriosclerosis.

Tests of the Fibrinolytic System. Euglobulin clot lysis time is a screening test used in some laboratories to assess fibrinolysis. More specific tests are available in most laboratories to determine the levels of plasminogen, plasminogen activator, and inhibitors of fibrinolysis. An increase in fibrinolysis may be associated with hemorrhagic symptoms, and a delay in fibrinolysis is associated with thrombosis.

DEVELOPMENTAL HEMOSTASIS. The normal newborn infant has a reduced level of most procoagulants and anticoagulants (see Table 475-1). In general, there is a more marked abnormality in the preterm infant. Although major differences exist in the normal ranges for newborn and preterm infants, these ranges vary greatly between laboratories. During gestation, there is progressive maturation and increase of the clotting factors synthesized by the liver. The extremely premature infant will have prolonged PT and PTT as well as a marked reduction in anticoagulant proteins (protein C, protein S, and AT-III). Levels of fibrinogen, factors V and VIII, VWF, and platelets are near-normal throughout the later stages of gestation (see Chapter 103.4). Because protein C and protein S are physiologically reduced, the normal factors V and VIII are not balanced with their regulatory proteins. In contrast, the physiologic deficiency of vitamin K–dependent procoagulant proteins (factors II, VII, IX, and X) is partially balanced by the physiologic reduction of AT-III. The net effect is that newborns (especially premature infants) are at increased risk for complications of bleeding, clotting, or both.

Chalmers EA: Neonatal coagulation problems. *Arch Dis Child Fetal Neonatal Ed* 2004;89:F475–F478.

Coller BS, Schneiderman PI: Clinical evaluation of hemorrhagic disorders: The bleeding history and differential diagnosis of purpura. In Hoffman R, Benz EJ, Shattil SJ, et al (editors): *Hematology: Basic Principles and Practice,* 4th ed. Philadelphia, Elsevier Churchill Livingstone, 2005, pp 1975–1999.

Esmon CT: Blood coagulation. In Nathan DG, Orkin SH, Ginsburg D, et al (editors): *Hematology of Infancy and Childhood,* 6th ed. Philadelphia, WB Saunders, 2003, pp 1475–1496.

Handin RI: Blood platelets and the vessel wall. In Nathan DG, Orkin SH, Ginsburg D, et al (editors): *Hematology of Infancy and Childhood,* 6th ed. Philadelphia, WB Saunders, 2003, pp 1457–1476.

Lusher JM: Clinical and laboratory approach to the bleeding patient. In Nathan DG, Orkin SH, Ginsburg D, et al (editors): *Hematology of Infancy and Childhood,* 6th ed. Philadelphia, WB Saunders, 2003, pp 1515–1526.

Monagle P, Andrew M: Acquired disorders of hemostasis. In Nathan DG, Orkin SH, Ginsburg D, et al (editors): *Hematology of Infancy and Childhood,* 6th ed. Philadelphia, WB Saunders, 2003, pp 1631–1668.

Monagle P, Andrew M: Developmental hemostasis: Relevance to newborns and infants. In Nathan DG, Orkin SH, Ginsburg D, et al (editors): *Hematology of Infancy and Childhood,* 6th ed. Philadelphia, WB Saunders, 2003, pp 121–168.

Montgomery RR, Gill JC, Scott JP: Hemophilia and von Willebrand disease. In Nathan DG, Orkin SH, Ginsburg D, et al (editors): *Hematology of Infancy and Childhood,* 6th ed. Philadelphia, WB Saunders, 2003, pp 1547–1576.

Parmar N, Albisetti M, Berry LR, Chan AK: The fibrinolytic system in newborns and children. *Clin Lab* 2006;52:115–124. Erratum in *Clin Lab* 2006;52:324.

Peyvandi F, Jayandharan G, Chandy M, et al: Genetic diagnosis of haemophilia and other inherited bleeding disorders. *Haemophilia* 2006;12:82–89.

Scott JP: Bleeding and thrombosis. In Kliegman R, Greenbaum L, Lye P (editors): *Practical Strategies in Pediatric Diagnosis and Therapy,* 2nd ed. Philadelphia, WB Saunders, 2004, pp 240–247.

Sugar NF, Taylor JA, Feldman KW: Bruises in infants and toddlers: Those who don't cruise rarely bruise. *Arch Pediatr Adolesc Med* 1999;153:399–403.

Chapter 476 ■ Hereditary Clotting Factor Deficiencies (Bleeding Disorders)

Hemophilia A (factor VIII deficiency) and **hemophilia B** (factor IX deficiency) are the most common and serious congenital coagulation factor deficiencies. The clinical findings in hemophilia A and hemophilia B are virtually identical. **Hemophilia C** is the bleeding disorder associated with reduced levels of factor XI (see Chapter 476.2). Reduced levels of the *contact factors* (factor XII, high molecular weight kininogen, and prekallikrein) are associated with significant prolongation of activated partial thromboplastin time (APTT; also referred to as *PTT*), but are not associated with hemorrhage, as discussed in Chapter 476.3. Other coagulation factor deficiencies that are less common are briefly discussed in subsequent subchapters.

476.1 • Factor VIII or Factor IX Deficiency (Hemophilia A or B)

Deficiencies of factors VIII and IX are the most common severe inherited bleeding disorders. In 1985, the genes for both factors VIII and IX were cloned. Subsequently, recombinant factor VIII and factor IX concentrates were developed to treat patients with hemophilia and thereby avoid the infectious risk of plasma-derived transfusion-transmitted diseases.

PATHOPHYSIOLOGY. Factors VIII and IX participate in a complex required for the activation of factor X. Together with phospholipid and calcium, they form the "tenase," or factor X-activating, complex. Figure 475-2 shows the clotting process as it occurs in the test tube, with factor X being activated by either the complex of factors VIII and IX or the complex of tissue factor and factor VII. In vivo, the complex of factor VIIa and tissue factor activates factor IX to initiate clotting. In the laboratory, prothrombin time (PT) measures the activation of factor X by factor VII and is therefore normal in patients with factor VIII or factor IX deficiency.

After injury, the initial hemostatic event is formation of the platelet plug, together with the generation of the fibrin clot that prevents further hemorrhage. In hemophilia A or B, clot formation is delayed and is not robust. Inadequate thrombin generation leads to failure to form a tightly cross-linked fibrin clot to support the platelet plug. Patients with hemophilia slowly form a soft, friable clot. When untreated bleeding occurs in a closed space, such as a joint, cessation of bleeding may be the result of tamponade. With open wounds, in which tamponade cannot occur, profuse bleeding may result in significant blood loss. The clot that is formed may be friable, and rebleeding occurs during the physiologic lysis of clots or with minimal new trauma.

CLINICAL MANIFESTATIONS. Neither factor VIII nor factor IX crosses the placenta; bleeding symptoms may be present from birth or may occur in the fetus. Only approximately 2% of neonates with hemophilia sustain intracranial hemorrhages and 30% of male infants with hemophilia bleed with circumcision. Thus, in the absence of a positive family history (hemophilia has a high rate of spontaneous mutation), hemophilia may go undiagnosed in the newborn. Obvious symptoms of easy bruising, intramuscular hematomas, and hemarthroses begin when the child "begins to cruise." Bleeding from minor traumatic lacerations of the mouth (a torn frenulum) may persist for hr or days and may cause the parents to seek medical evaluation. Even in patients with severe hemophilia, only 90% have evidence of increased bleeding by 1 yr of age. Although bleeding may occur in any area of the body, the hallmark of hemophilia is **hemarthrosis.** Bleeding into the joints may be induced by minor trauma; many hemarthroses are spontaneous. The earliest joint hemorrhages appear most commonly in the ankle. In the older child and adolescent, hemarthroses of the knees and elbows are also common. Whereas the child's early joint hemorrhages are recognized only after major swelling and fluid accumulation in the joint space, older children are frequently able to recognize bleeding before the physician does. They complain of a warm, tingling sensation in the joint as the first sign of an early joint hemorrhage. After repeated bleeding episodes into the same joint, patients with severe hemophilia may develop a "target" joint. Recurrent bleeding may then become spontaneous because of the underlying pathologic changes in the joint.

Although most muscular hemorrhages are clinically evident owing to localized pain or swelling, bleeding into the iliopsoas muscle requires specific mention. Patients may lose large volumes of blood into the **iliopsoas muscle** and verge on hypovolemic shock, with only a vague area of referred pain in the groin. The hip is held in a flexed, internally rotated position due to irritation of the iliopsoas. The diagnosis is made clinically by the inability to extend the hip, but must be confirmed with ultrasonography or CT scan (Fig. 476-1). Life-threatening bleeding in the patient with hemophilia is caused by bleeding into vital structures (central nervous system, upper airway) or by exsanguination (external, gastrointestinal, or iliopsoas hemorrhage). Prompt treatment with clotting factor concentrate for these life-threatening hemorrhages is imperative. If head trauma is of sufficient concern to suggest radiologic evaluation, factor replacement should precede radiologic evaluation. Life-threatening hemorrhages require replacement therapy to achieve a level equal to that of normal plasma (100 IU/dL, or 100%).

Patients with mild hemophilia who have factor VIII or factor IX levels of >5 IU/dL usually do not have spontaneous hemorrhages. These individuals may experience prolonged bleeding after dental work, surgery, or injuries from moderate trauma.

LABORATORY FINDINGS AND DIAGNOSIS. The laboratory screening test that is affected by a reduced level of factor VIII or factor IX is PTT. In severe hemophilia, PTT is usually 2–3 times the upper limit of normal. Results of the other screening tests of the hemostatic mechanism (platelet count, bleeding time, prothrombin time, and thrombin time) are normal. Unless the patient has an inhibitor to factor VIII or IX, the mixing of normal plasma with patient plasma results in correction of PTT. The specific

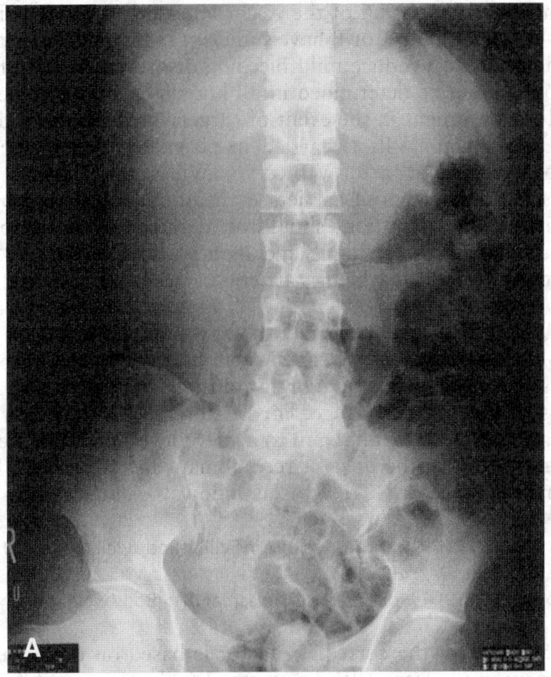

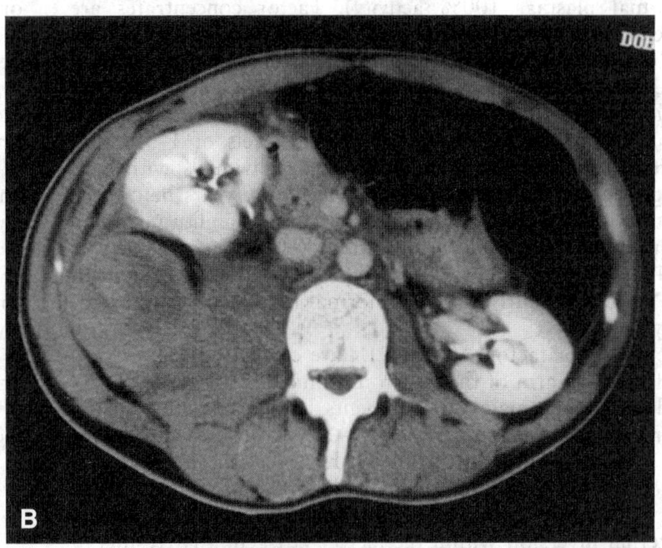

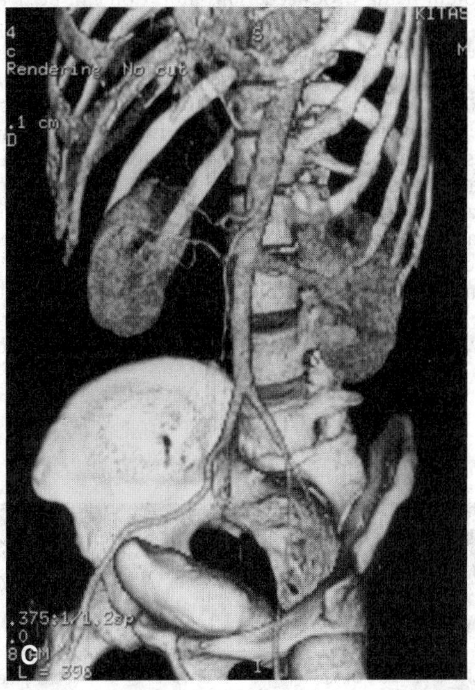

Figure 476-1. Massive hematoma into the iliopsoas muscle. CT scan shows a massive hematoma in the right iliopsoas muscle in a patient with hemophilia B. A 38-yr-old man with severe deficiency of factor IX (hemophilia B) was admitted for right lower abdominal pain of progressively increasing severity and tenderness. He had had a common cold with severe cough and loss of appetite for approximately 1 wk. *A*, Abdominal radiograph shows a positive psoas sign on the right side and left-shifted colon gas. *B*, CT scan shows massive hematoma in the right iliopsoas muscle, resulting in anterior translocation of the right kidney. C, Reconstructed 3-dimensional image shows more clearly the kidney translocation and the extended, but intact large vessels. These are useful findings for the diagnostic procedures because progressive right lower abdominal pain may closely simulate acute appendicitis. The hemorrhage was successfully managed by replacing factor IX for 1 wk without any recurrence. He did not have any inhibitors to factor IX. (From Miyazaki K, Higashihara M: Massive hemorrhage into the iliopsoas muscle. *Intern Med* 2005;44:158.)

assay for factors VIII and IX will confirm the diagnosis of hemophilia. If correction does not occur on mixing, an inhibitor may be present. In 25–35% of patients with hemophilia who receive infusions of factor VIII or factor IX, a factor-specific antibody may develop. These antibodies are directed against the active clotting site and are termed *inhibitors*. In such patients, the quantitative Bethesda assay for inhibitors should be performed to measure the antibody titer.

DIFFERENTIAL DIAGNOSIS. In young infants with severe bleeding manifestations, the differential diagnosis includes severe thrombocytopenia; severe platelet function disorders, such as Bernard-Soulier syndrome and Glanzmann thrombasthenia; type 3 (severe) von Willebrand disease; and vitamin K deficiency. Hemostatic screening tests should differentiate these entities from hemophilia.

GENETICS AND CLASSIFICATION. Hemophilia occurs in approximately 1:5,000 males, with 85% having factor VIII deficiency and 10–15% having factor IX deficiency. Hemophilia shows no apparent racial predilection, appearing in all ethnic groups. The severity of hemophilia is classified on the basis of the patient's baseline level of factor VIII or factor IX because factor levels usually correlate with the severity of bleeding symptoms. By definition, 1 international unit (IU) of each factor is defined as that amount in 1 mL of normal plasma referenced against a standard established by the World Health Organization (WHO); thus, 100 mL of normal plasma has 100 IU/dL (100% activity) of each factor. For ease of discussion, henceforth in this chapter, we will use the term *% activity* to refer to the percentage found in normal plasma (100% activity). Factor concentrates are also referenced against an international WHO standard, so treatment doses are usually referred to in international units (IU). **Severe hemophilia** is characterized by having <1% activity of the specific clotting factor, and bleeding is often spontaneous. Patients with **moderate hemophilia** have levels of 1–5% and require mild trauma to induce bleeding. Individuals with **mild hemophilia** have levels of >5%, may go many years before the condition is diagnosed, and frequently require significant trauma to cause bleeding. The hemostatic level for factor VIII is >30–40%, and for factor IX, it is >25–30%. The lower limit of levels for factors VIII and IX in normal individuals is approximately 50%.

The genes for factors VIII and IX are carried near the terminus of the long arm of the X chromosome and are therefore X-linked traits. The majority of patients have a reduction in the amount of clotting factor protein; 5–10% of those with hemophilia A and 40–50% of those with hemophilia B make a dysfunctional protein. Approximately 45–50% of patients with severe hemophilia A have the same mutation, in which there is an internal inversion within the factor VIII gene that results in no protein being produced. This mutation can be detected in the blood of patients or carriers and in the amniotic fluid by molecular techniques. Because of the multiple genetic causes of either factor VIII or factor IX deficiency, most patients are classified based on the amount of factor VIII or factor IX clotting activity. In the newborn, factor VIII levels may be artificially elevated because of the acute-phase response elicited by the birth process. This may cause a mildly affected patient to have normal or near-normal levels of factor VIII. Patients with severe hemophilia will not have detectable levels. In contrast, factor IX levels are physiologically low in the newborn. If severe hemophilia is present in the family, an undetectable level of factor IX is diagnostic of severe hemophilia B. In some patients with mild factor IX deficiency, the presence of hemophilia can be confirmed only after several wk of life.

Through lyonization of the X chromosome, some **female carriers** of hemophilia A or B have sufficient reduction of factor VIII or factor IX to produce mild bleeding disorders. Levels of these factors should be determined in all known carriers to assess the need for treatment in the event of surgery or clinical bleeding.

Because factor VIII is carried in plasma by von Willebrand factor, the ratio of factor VIII to von Willebrand factor is sometimes used to diagnose carriers of hemophilia. When possible, specific genetic mutations should be identified in the propositus and used to test other family members who are at risk for either having hemophilia or being carriers.

TREATMENT. Early, appropriate therapy is the hallmark of excellent hemophilia care. When mild to moderate bleeding occurs, levels of factor VIII or factor IX must be raised to hemostatic levels in the 35–50% range. For life-threatening or major hemorrhages, the dose should aim to achieve levels of 100% activity.

Calculation of the dose of recombinant factor VIII (FVIII) or recombinant factor IX (FIX) is as follows:

$$\text{Dose of FVIII (IU)} = \%\ \text{desired (rise in FVIII)} \times \text{Body weight (kg)} \times 0.5$$

$$\text{Dose of FIX (IU)} = \%\ \text{desired (rise in plasma FIX)} \times \text{Body weight (kg)} \times 1.4$$

For factor VIII, the correction factor is based on the volume of distribution of factor VIII. For factor IX, the correction factor is based on the volume of distribution and the observed rise in plasma level after infusion of recombinant factor IX.

Table 476-1 summarizes the treatment of some common types of hemorrhage in a patient with hemophilia.

With the availability of recombinant replacement products, **prophylaxis** has become the standard of care for most children with severe hemophilia to prevent spontaneous bleeding and early joint deformities. The results of prophylaxis have been impressive in the prevention of chronic joint disease. If target joints develop, "secondary" prophylaxis is often initiated.

With mild factor VIII hemophilia, the patient's endogenously produced factor VIII can be released by the administration of

TABLE 476-1. Treatment of Hemophilia

TYPE OF HEMORRHAGE	HEMOPHILIA A	HEMOPHILIA B
Hemarthrosis*	40 IU/kg factor VIII concentrate† on day 1; then 20 IU/kg on days 2, 3, 5 until joint function is normal or back to baseline. Consider additional treatment every other day for 7–10 days. Consider prophylaxis.	60–80 IU/kg on day 1; then 40 IU/kg on days 2, 4. Consider additional treatment every other day for 7–10 days. Consider prophylaxis.
Muscle or significant subcutaneous hematoma	20 IU/kg factor VIII concentrate; may need every-other-day treatment until resolved.	40 IU/kg factor IX concentrate‡; may need treatment every 2–3 days until resolved.
Mouth, deciduous tooth, or tooth extraction	20 IU/kg factor VIII concentrate; antifibrinolytic therapy; remove loose deciduous tooth.	40 IU/kg factor IX concentrate‡; antifibrinolytic therapy§; remove loose deciduous tooth.
Epistaxis	Apply pressure for 15–20 min; pack with petrolatum gauze; give antifibrinolytic therapy; 20 IU/kg factor VIII concentrate if this treatment fails.**	Apply pressure for 15–20 min; pack with petrolatum gauze; antifibrinolytic therapy; 30 IU/kg factor IX concentrate‡ if this treatment fails.
Major surgery, life-threatening hemorrhage	50–75 IU/kg factor VIII concentrate, then initiate continuous infusion of 2–4 IU/kg/hr to maintain factor VIII > 100 IU/dL for 24 hr, then give 2–3 IU/kg/hr continuously for 5–7 days to maintain the level at > 50 IU/dL and an additional 5–7 days at a level of > 30 IU/dL.	120 IU/kg factor IX concentrate‡, then 50–60 IU/kg every 12–24 hr to maintain factor IX at > 40 IU/dL for 5–7 days, and then > 30 IU/dL for 7 days.
Iliopsoas hemorrhage	50 IU/kg factor VIII concentrate, then 25 IU/kg every 12 hr until asymptomatic, then 20 IU/kg every other day for a total of 10–14 days.‖	120 IU/kg factor IX concentrate‡; then 50–60 IU/kg every 12–24 hr to maintain factor IX at > 40 IU/dL until asymptomatic, then 40–50 IU every other day for a total of 10–14 days.‖¶
Hematuria	Bed rest; 11/2 × maintenance fluids; if not controlled in 1–2 days, 20 IU/kg factor VIII concentrate; if not controlled, give prednisone (unless HIV-infected).	Bed rest; 11/2 × maintenance fluids; if not controlled in 1–2 days, 40 IU/kg factor IX concentrate‡; if not controlled, give prednisone (unless HIV-infected).
Prophylaxis	20–40 IU/kg factor VIII concentrate every other day to achieve a trough level of ≥ 1%.	30–50 IU/kg factor IX concentrate‡ every 2–3 days to achieve a trough level of ≥ 1%.

*For hip hemarthrosis, orthopedic evaluation for possible aspiration is advisable to prevent avascular necrosis of the femoral head.

**OTC coagulant-promoting products may be helpful.

†For mild or moderate hemophilia, a desmopressin, 0.3 μg/kg, should be used instead of factor VIII concentrate, if the patient is known to respond with a hemostatic level of factor VIII; if repeated doses are given, monitor factor VIII levels for tachyphylaxis.

‡Stated doses apply for recombinant factor IX concentrate; for plasma-derived factor IX concentrate, use 70% of the stated dose.

§Do not give antifibrinolytic therapy until 4–6 hr after a dose of prothrombin complex concentrate.

‖Repeat radiologic assessment should be performed before discontinuation of therapy.

¶If repeated doses of factor IX concentrate are required, use highly purified, specific factor IX concentrate.

Adapted from Montgomery RR, Gill JC, Scott JP: Hemophilia and von Willebrand disease. In Nathan DG, Orkin SH (editors): *Nathan and Oski's Hematology of Infancy and Childhood*, 5th ed. Philadelphia, WB Saunders, 1998.

desmopressin acetate. In patients with moderate or severe factor VIII deficiency, the stored levels of factor VIII in the body are inadequate, and desmopressin treatment is ineffective. The risk of exposing the patient with mild hemophilia to transfusion-transmitted diseases and the cost of recombinant products warrant the use of desmopressin, if it is effective. A concentrated intranasal form of **desmopressin acetate (Stimate)** can also be used to treat patients with mild hemophilia A. The dose is 150 µg (1 puff) for children weighing <50 kg and 300 µg (2 puffs) for children and young adults weighing >50 kg. Most centers administer a trial of desmopressin to determine the level of factor VIII achieved after its infusion. Desmopressin is not effective in the treatment of factor IX–deficient hemophilia.

PROPHYLAXIS. Many patients are now given lifelong prophylaxis to prevent spontaneous joint bleeding. Usually, such programs are initiated with the first joint hemorrhage. Young children often require the insertion of a central catheter to ensure venous access. Such programs, although expensive, are highly effective in preventing or greatly limiting the degree of joint pathology. Treatment is usually provided every 2–3 days to maintain a measurable plasma level of clotting factor (1–2%) when assayed just before the next infusion (trough level). Because gene therapy may be available within the lifetime of pediatric patients, keeping joints normal through prophylaxis is a logical priority. If moderate arthropathy develops, prevention of future bleeding will require higher plasma levels of clotting factors. In the older child who is not given primary prophylaxis, secondary prophylaxis is frequently initiated if a target joint develops.

SUPPORTIVE CARE. Although it is easy to advise parents that their child should avoid trauma, this advice is practically useless. Toddlers are active, are curious about everything, and injure themselves easily. Effective measures include anticipatory guidance, including the use of car seats, seatbelts, and bike helmets, and the importance of avoiding high-risk behaviors. Older boys should be counseled to avoid violent contact sports, but this is a challenge. Boys with severe hemophilia often sustain hemorrhages in the absence of known trauma. Early psychosocial intervention helps the family to achieve a balance between overprotection and permissiveness. Patients with hemophilia should avoid aspirin and other nonsteroidal anti-inflammatory drugs that affect platelet function. The child with a bleeding disorder should receive the appropriate vaccinations against hepatitis B, even though recombinant products may avoid exposure to transfusion-transmitted diseases. Patients exposed to plasma-derived products should be screened periodically for hepatitis B and C, HIV, and abnormalities in liver function.

CHRONIC COMPLICATIONS. Long-term complications of hemophilia A and B include chronic arthropathy, the development of an inhibitor to either factor VIII or factor IX, and the risk of transfusion-transmitted infectious diseases. Although an aggressive, or prophylactic, approach to treatment has reduced the problems of chronic arthropathy, these problems have not been eliminated.

Historically, chronic arthropathy has been the major long-term disability associated with hemophilia. The natural history of untreated hemophilia is one of cyclic recurrent hemorrhages into specific joints, including hemorrhages into the same (target) joint. In young children, the joint distends easily and a large volume of blood may fill the joint until tamponade ensues or therapy intervenes. After joint hemorrhage, proteolytic enzymes are released by white blood cells into the joint space and heme iron induces macrophage proliferation, leading to inflammation of the synovium. The synovium thickens and develops frondlike projections into the joint that are susceptible to being pinched and may induce further hemorrhage. The cartilaginous surface becomes eroded and ultimately may even expose raw bone, leaving the joint susceptible to articular fusion. In the older patient with advanced arthropathy, bleeding into the target joint, with its thickened synovium, causes severe pain because the joint may have little space to accommodate blood. Once a target joint is seen to be developing, the patient is usually given short-or long-term prophylaxis to prevent progression of the arthropathy and reduce inflammation.

Infusion of the deficient clotting factor may initiate an immune response in patients with either factor VIII or factor IX deficiency. **Inhibitors** are antibodies directed against factor VIII or factor IX that block the clotting activity. Failure of a bleeding episode to respond to appropriate replacement therapy is usually the first sign of an inhibitor. Less often, inhibitors are identified during routine follow-up testing. Inhibitors develop in approximately 25–35% of patients with hemophilia A; the percentage is somewhat lower in patients with hemophilia B, many of whom make an inactive dysfunctional protein that renders them less susceptible to an immune response. Highly purified factor IX or recombinant factor IX seems to increase the frequency of inhibitor development, and some anti-factor IX inhibitors induce anaphylaxis. Many patients who have an inhibitor lose this inhibitor with continued regular infusions. Others have a higher titer of antibody with subsequent infusions and may need to go through **desensitization** programs, in which high doses of factor VIII or factor IX are infused in an attempt to saturate the antibody and permit the body to develop tolerance. Factor IX immune tolerance programs have resulted in nephrotic syndrome in some patients. Rituximab has been used, off label, as an alternate therapy for patients with high titer inhibitors who have failed immune tolerance programs. If desensitization fails, bleeding episodes are treated with either recombinant factor VIIa or activated prothrombin complex concentrates. The use of these products bypasses the inhibitor in many instances, but may increase the risk of thrombosis. Patients with inhibitors require referral to a center that cares for many such patients and has a comprehensive hemophilia program.

In the past, plasma-derived treatment products transmitted hepatitis B and C as well as HIV to large numbers of patients with hemophilia. In the era of recombinant products, the risk of acquiring such infections should be minimal, but patients should receive appropriate immunizations against hepatitis B. Those who are exposed to blood products should be monitored for hepatitis B and C as well as HIV.

COMPREHENSIVE CARE. Today, patients with hemophilia are best managed through comprehensive hemophilia care centers. Such centers are dedicated to patient and family education as well as to the prevention and/or treatment of the complications of hemophilia, including chronic joint disease and inhibitor development as well as infection, such as hepatitis C and HIV. Such centers involve a team of physicians, nurses, orthopedists, physical therapists, and psychosocial workers, among others. Education remains crucial in hemophilia care because patients who are receiving prophylaxis may be less "experienced" in recognizing bleeding episodes than affected children from previous eras.

476.2 • Factor XI Deficiency (Hemophilia C)

Factor XI deficiency is an autosomal deficiency associated with mild to moderate bleeding symptoms. It is frequently encountered in Ashkenazi Jews, but has been found in many other ethnic groups. In Israel, 1–3/1,000 are homozygous for this deficiency. Sephardic Jews are rarely affected.

The bleeding tendency is not as severe as in factor VIII or factor IX deficiency. The bleeding associated with factor XI deficiency is not correlated with the amount of factor XI. Some patients with severe deficiency may have minimal or no symptoms at the time of major surgery. Unless the patient previously had surgery without bleeding, replacement therapy should be considered and given preoperatively, depending on the nature of the surgical procedure. There is no approved concentrate of factor XI available in the United States; therefore, the physician must use fresh frozen plasma (FFP).

Bleeding during minor surgery can be controlled with local pressure; patients undergoing dental extractions can be monitored closely and treated only if hemorrhage occurs. In a patient with homozygous deficiency of factor XI, PTT is often longer than it is in patients with either severe factor VIII or factor IX deficiency. The paradox of fewer clinical symptoms in combination with longer PTT is surprising, but it occurs because factor VIIa can activate factor IX in vivo. The deficiency of factor XI can be confirmed by specific factor XI assays. Plasma infusions of 1 IU/kg usually increase the plasma concentration by 2%. Thus, infusion of plasma at 10–15 mL/kg will result in a plasma level of 20–30%, a level usually sufficient to control moderate hemorrhage. Frequent infusions of plasma would be necessary to achieve higher levels of factor XI. Because the half-life of factor XI is usually ≥ 48 hr, maintaining adequate levels of factor XI usually is not difficult.

Chronic joint bleeding is rarely a problem, and for most patients, factor XI deficiency is a concern only at the time of major surgery unless there is a second underlying hemostatic defect (e.g., von Willebrand disease).

476.3 • Deficiencies of the Contact Factors (Nonbleeding Disorders)

Deficiency of the “contact factors” (factor XII, prekallikrein, and high molecular weight kininogen) causes prolonged PTT, but no bleeding symptoms. Because these contact factors function at the step of initiation of the intrinsic clotting system by the reagent used to determine PTT, the PTT is markedly prolonged when these factors are absent. Thus, there is the paradoxical situation in which PTT is extremely prolonged, but there is no evidence of clinical bleeding. It is important that these individuals be well informed about the meaning of their clotting factor deficiency because they do not need treatment, even for major surgery.

476.4 • Factor VII Deficiency

Factor VII deficiency is a rare bleeding disorder that is usually detected only in the homozygous state. Individuals with this deficiency may have spontaneous intracranial hemorrhage and frequent mucocutaneous bleeding. Such patients have markedly prolonged PT but normal PTT. Factor VII assays show a marked reduction of factor VII. Because the plasma half-life of factor VII is 2–4 hr, therapy with FFP is difficult and is often complicated by fluid overload. A commercial concentrate of recombinant factor VIIa has been shown in case reports to be effective in treating some patients with factor VII deficiency; this use has not been approved by the FDA.

DEFICIENCIES IN THE FACTORS OF THE COMMON PATHWAY (FACTORS I, II, V, AND X) CAUSING PROLONGATION OF BOTH PT AND PTT

476.5 • Factor X Deficiency

Factor X deficiency is a rare autosomal disorder that results in mucocutaneous and post-traumatic bleeding. Factor X deficiency is the result of either a quantitative deficiency or a dysfunctional molecule. A reduced factor X level is associated with prolongation of both PT and PTT. In patients with hereditary factor X deficiency, factor X levels can be increased using either FFP or prothrombin complex concentrate. The half-life of factor X is approximately 30 hr, and its volume of distribution is similar to that of factor IX. Thus, 1 U/kg will increase the plasma level of factor X by 1%.

Although it is rarely a problem in pediatric patients, systemic amyloidosis may be associated with factor X deficiency owing to the adsorption of factor X on the amyloid protein. In the setting of amyloidosis, transfusion therapy often is not successful because of the rapid clearance of factor X.

476.6 • Prothrombin (Factor II) Deficiency

Prothrombin deficiency is caused either by a markedly reduced prothrombin level (hypoprothrombinemia) or by functionally abnormal prothrombin (dysprothrombinemia). Laboratory testing in homozygous patients shows prolonged PT and PTT. Factor II, or prothrombin, assays show a markedly reduced prothrombin level. Patients are treated with either prothrombin complex concentrates or FFP. In prothrombin deficiency, FFP is useful, because the half-life of prothrombin is 3.5 days. Administration of 1 IU/kg of prothrombin will increase the plasma activity by 1%.

476.7 • Factor V Deficiency

Deficiency of factor V is an autosomal recessive, mild to moderate bleeding disorder that has also been termed **parahemophilia.** Hemarthroses occur rarely; mucocutaneous bleeding and hematomas are the most common symptoms. Severe menorrhagia is a frequent symptom in women. Laboratory evaluation shows prolonged PTT and PT. Specific assays for factor V show a reduction in factor V levels. FFP is the only currently available therapeutic product that contains factor V. Factor V is lost rapidly from stored FFP. Patients with severe factor V deficiency are treated with infusions of FFP at 10 mL/kg every 12 hr. Rarely, a patient with a negative family history of bleeding has an acquired antibody to factor V. Often, these patients do not bleed because the factor V in platelets prevents excessive bleeding.

476.8 • Combined Deficiency of Factors V and VIII

Combined deficiency of factors V and VIII occurs secondary to the absence of an intracellular transport protein, ERGIC-53, that is responsible for transporting factors V and VIII from the endoplasmic reticulum to the Golgi compartments. ERGIC-53 is encoded on chromosome 18. The deficiency of factors V and VIII is not related to defective genes for this protein, but is secondary to a deficiency of a transport protein. This explains the paradoxical deficiency of 2 factors, one encoded on chromosome 1 and the other on the X chromosome.

476.9 • Fibrinogen Deficiency (Factor I)

Congenital afibrinogenemia is a rare autosomal recessive disorder in which there is an absence of fibrinogen. These patients do not bleed as frequently as patients with hemophilia, and they rarely have hemarthroses. Affected patients may present in the neonatal period with gastrointestinal hemorrhage or hematomas after vaginal delivery. In addition to marked prolongation of PT and PTT, thrombin time is prolonged. In the absence of consumptive coagulopathy, an unmeasurable fibrinogen level is diagnostic. In addition to the quantitative deficiency of fibrinogen, a number of dysfunctional fibrinogens have been reported (**dysfibrinogenemia**). Currently, no fibrinogen concentrates are commercially available. Because the plasma half-life of fibrinogen is 2–4 days, treatment with either FFP or cryoprecipitate is effective. The hemostatic level of fibrinogen is >60 mg/dL. Each bag of cryoprecipitate contains 100–150 mg of fibrinogen. Some clinical assays for fibrinogen are inhibited by high doses of heparin. Thus, markedly prolonged thrombin time, associated with a low fibrinogen level, should be evaluated with determination of reptilase time. Prolonged reptilase time confirms that functional levels of fibrinogen are low and that heparin is not present.

476.10 • Factor XIII Deficiency (Fibrin-Stabilizing Factor or Transglutaminase Deficiency)

Because factor XIII is responsible for the cross linking of fibrin to stabilize the fibrin clot, symptoms of delayed hemorrhage are secondary to instability of the clot. Typically, patients have trauma 1 day and then have a bruise or hematoma the next day. Clinical symptoms include mild bruising, delayed separation of the umbilical stump beyond 4 wk, poor wound healing, and recurrent spontaneous abortions in women. Results of the usual screening tests for hemostasis are normal in patients with factor XIII deficiency. Screening tests for factor XIII deficiency are based on the observation that there is increased solubility of the clot because of the failure of cross linking. The normal clot remains insoluble in the presence of 5 M urea, whereas in a patient with XIII deficiency, the clot dissolves. More specific assays for factor XIII are immunologic. Because the half-life of factor XIII is 5–7 days and the hemostatic level is 2–3% activity, infusion of FFP or cryoprecipitate will correct the deficiency in these patients. Plasma contains 1 IU/dL, and cryoprecipitate contains 75 IU/bag. In patients with significant bleeding symptoms, prophylaxis can be achieved with infusion of cryoprecipitate every 3–4 wk.

476.11 • Antiplasmin or Plasminogen Activator Inhibitor Deficiency

Deficiency of either antiplasmin or plasminogen activator inhibitor, which are antifibrinolytic proteins, results in increased plasmin generation and premature lysis of fibrin clots. Patients have mucocutaneous bleeding, but rarely have joint hemorrhages. Because results of the usual hemostatic tests are normal, further work-up of a patient with a positive bleeding history should include euglobulin clot lysis time (if available), which measures fibrinolytic activity and is shortened in the presence of these deficiencies. Specific assays for α_2-antiplasmin and plasminogen activator inhibitor are available. Patients are treated with FFP.

Abshire T: An approach to target joint bleeding in hemophilia: Prophylaxis for all or individualized treatment? *J Pediatr* 2004;145:581–583.

Bauer KA: Rare hereditary coagulation factor abnormalities. In Nathan DG, Orkin SH, Ginsburg D, et al (editors): *Hematology of Infancy and Childhood,* 6th ed. Philadelphia, WB Saunders, 2003, pp 1577–1582.

Bolton-Maggs PH: Factor XI deficiency and its management. *Haemophilia* 2000;6(Suppl 1):100–109.

Bolton-Maggs PH, Perry DJ, Chalmers EA, et al: The rare coagulation disorders: Review with guidelines for management from the United Kingdom Haemophilia Centre Doctors' Organisation. *Haemophilia* 2004;10:593–628.

Bolton-Maggs PH, Stobart K, Smyth RL: Evidence-based treatment of haemophilia. *Haemophilia* 2004;10(Suppl 4):20–24.

Chalmers EA: Haemophilia and the newborn. *Blood Rev* 2004;18:85–92.

Dunn AL, Abshire TC: Recent advances in the management of the child who has hemophilia. *Hematol Oncol Clin North Am* 2004;18:1249–1276.

Funk M, Schmidt H, Escuriola-Ettingshausen C, et al: Radiological and orthopedic score in pediatric hemophilic patients with early and late prophylaxis. *Ann Hematol* 1998;77:171–174.

Hedner U: Recombinant factor VIIa (NovoSeven) as a hemostatic agent. *Semin Hematol* 2001;38(4 Suppl 12):43–47.

Kern M, Blanchette V, Stain AM, et al: Clinical and cost implications of target joints in Canadian boys with severe hemophilia A. *J Pediatr* 2004;145:628–634.

Key NS: Inhibitors in congenital coagulation disorders. *Br J Haematol* 2004;127:379–391.

Manco-Johnson M: Hemophilia management: Optimizing treatment based on patient needs. *Curr Opin Pediatr* 2005;17:3–6.

Montgomery RR, Gill JC, Scott JP: Hemophilia and von Willebrand Disease. In Nathan DG, Orkin SH, Ginsburg D, et al (editors): *Hematology of Infancy and Childhood,* 6th ed. Philadelphia, WB Saunders, 2003, pp 1547–1576.

O'Connell NM: Factor XI deficiency. *Semin Hematol* 2004;41(1 Suppl 1):76–81.

Oldenburg J, Ananyeva NM, Saenko EL: Molecular basis of haemophilia A. *Haemophilia* 2004;10(Suppl 4):133–139.

Chapter 477 ■ von Willebrand Disease

The most common hereditary bleeding disorder is von Willebrand disease (VWD), and some reports suggest that it is present in 1–2% of the general population. VWD is inherited autosomally, but most centers report more affected women than men. Because menorrhagia is a major symptom, women may be more likely to seek treatment and thus to be diagnosed. VWD is classified on the basis of whether the protein is quantitatively reduced, but not absent (type 1); qualitatively abnormal (type 2); or absent (type 3) [Fig. 477-1]. Mutations in different loci that code for different functional domains of the von Willebrand factor (VWF) protein cause the different variants of VWD.

PATHOPHYSIOLOGY. A large multimeric glycoprotein that is synthesized in megakaryocytes and endothelial cells, VWF is stored in platelet α-granules and endothelial cell Weibel-Palade bodies. The highest molecular weight multimers of VWF are responsible for the normal interaction of VWF with the subendothelial matrix and platelets. During normal hemostasis, VWF adheres to the subendothelial matrix after vascular damage. When VWF binds to the subendothelial matrix, the conformation of VWF is changed so that it causes platelets to adhere to VWF through their glycoprotein IB (GPIb) receptor. These platelets are then activated, causing the recruitment of additional platelets and exposing phosphatidylserine, which is an important regulatory step for factor V- and factor VIII–dependent steps in the clotting cascade. VWF also serves as the carrier protein for plasma factor VIII. A severe deficiency of VWF causes a secondary deficiency in factor VIII, even though the gene for factor VIII is normal. This is the cause of autosomal deficiency of factor VIII, now known to be a molecular abnormality of VWF and known as *type 2N VWD.*

	Normal	Type 1	Type 3	Type 2A	Type 2B	Type 2N	Type 2M	PT-VWD	BSS
VWF:Ag	N	↓	absent	↓	↓	N or ↓	↓ or N	↓	N
VWF:RCo	N	↓	absent	↓↓↓	↓	N or ↓	↓↓↓	↓	N
FVIII	N	↓ or N	1-3%	N or ↓	N or ↓	↓↓	N	N	N
RIPA	N	often normal	absent	↓	often normal	N	↓	N	absent
LD-RIPA	absent	absent	absent	absent	↑↑↑	absent	absent	↑↑↑	absent
PFA	N	↑	↑↑↑	↑	↑	N	↑	↑	↑↑↑
BT	N	N or ↑	↑↑↑	↑	↑	N	↑	↑	↑↑↑
Platelet count	N	N	N	N	↓	N	N	↓	↓
Usual Tx		DDAVP VWF conc	VWF conc	VWF conc (DDAVP)	VWF conc (DDAVP)	VWF conc (DDAVP)	VWF conc (DDAVP)	platelets	platelets
Response to DDAVP		good	none	variable	decreases platelets	variable	variable	decreases platelets	none or modest
Response to VWF Conc		good	good	good	good	good	good	decreases platelets	no response
Frequency in general population		? (reported 1-2%)	very rare 1:250,000	rare	rare	rare	rare	rare	rare
VWF multimers	N	N but ↓	absent	abnormal	abnormal	N but ↓	N but ↓	abnormal	normal
			absent						

Figure 477-1. Common variants of von Willebrand disease (VWD) and other related disorders. Laboratory testing is listed on the *left*, and the results most commonly identified in patients with these conditions are shown. N, normal; ↑, degree of increase; ↓, degree of decrease. A graphic representation of von Willebrand factor (VWF) multimers is shown at the *bottom* of each column. A *lighter shade* illustrates a reduction in staining intensity, and *figure length* represents the relative size of the multimers. PT-VWD, platelet-type pseudo-VWD; BSS, Bernard Soulier syndrome; FVIII, factor VIII; VWF:Ag, von Willebrand antigen; VWF:RCo, ristocetin cofactor activity; BT, bleeding time; PFA, platelet function analyzer; VWF conc, VWF concentrate; Tx, treatment. RIPA, ristocetin reduced platelet aggregation to standard dose ristocetin; DDVAP, desmopressin; LD-RIPA, ristocetin induced platelet aggregation to low dose ristocetin.

CLINICAL MANIFESTATIONS. Patients with VWD usually have symptoms of **mucocutaneous hemorrhage,** including excessive bruising, epistaxis, menorrhagia, and postoperative hemorrhage, particularly after mucosal surgery, such as tonsillectomy or wisdom tooth extraction. Because a teenager's menstrual history is usually put in the context of other family members, excessive menstrual bleeding is not always recognized as being abnormal, because others in the family may be affected with the same disorder. If a menstruating female has iron deficiency, a detailed history of bruising and other bleeding symptoms should be elicited and further hemostatic evaluation undertaken.

Because VWF is an acute-phase protein, stress will increase its level. Thus, patients may not bleed with procedures that incur major stress, such as appendectomy and childbirth, but may bleed excessively at the time of cosmetic or mucosal surgery. Bruising symptoms may diminish during pregnancy because VWF levels may double or triple during pregnancy. Rarely, patients with VWD may have gastrointestinal telangiectasia. This combination results in major bleeding and accounts for numerous hospital admissions for patients with severe disease. In patients with type 3, or homozygous, VWD, bleeding symptoms are much more profound. These patients are usually diagnosed early in life and may have severe epistaxis or menorrhagia that results in major blood loss and possibly shock. Patients with severe type 3 VWD may have joint hemorrhages or spontaneous central nervous system hemorrhages.

LABORATORY FINDINGS. Although historically patients with VWD were described as having a long bleeding time and a long partial thromboplastin time, these findings are frequently normal in patients with type 1 VWD. Normal results on screening tests do not preclude the diagnosis of VWD. Because there is no single assay that has demonstrated the ability to rule out VWD, if the history is suggestive of a mucocutaneous bleeding disorder, VWD testing should be undertaken, including a quantitative assay for VWF antigen, testing for VWF activity (ristocetin cofactor activity), testing for plasma factor VIII activity, determination of VWF structure (VWF multimers), and a platelet count. Although the platelet count is usually normal in most patients, those with type 2B disease or platelet-type disease (pseudo-VWD) may have lifelong thrombocytopenia. Figure 477-1 lists the variants of VWD and summarizes their laboratory findings. Levels of VWF vary with blood type (type O < A < B < AB), which can confound the clinical diagnosis of hereditary VWD. In addition, there is controversy regarding the clinical definition of "true" VWD. Molecular genetics may clarify the diagnosis of type 1 VWD, but other genetic modifiers may exist outside the gene for VWF and significantly influence the diagnosis. The milder the patient's phenotype, the greater the difficulty in diagnosis.

GENETICS. Chromosome 12 contains the gene for VWF. In each of the type 2 variants listed in Figure 477-1, specific areas of the molecule are affected. The phenotype can guide the genetic diagnosis of the specific mutation. Investigations are underway to clarify whether all cases of type I VWD are related to mutations in the VWF gene on chromosome 12 or if there are genetic modifiers, such as blood type, that cause phenotypic VWD. Clinical genetic testing for VWD variants is only available in a few referral laboratories.

VON WILLEBRAND DISEASE VARIANTS

Type 1 VWD is the most common form and accounts for 85% of cases. Bleeding symptoms include epistaxis, bruising, and menorrhagia. If bleeding is excessive, desmopressin (DDAVP) administration at a dose of 0.3 µg/kg IV will increase the level of VWF and factor VIII by 3- to 5-fold. Intranasal DDAVP (Stimate) is particularly helpful for the outpatient treatment of bleeding episodes. The dose is 150 µg (1 puff) for children weighing <50 kg and 300 µg (2 puffs) for those weighing >50 kg.

Type 2A VWD is caused by the abnormal proteolysis of VWF, with only the smallest VWF multimers being present. This results in a reduction in VWF antigen with a much greater reduction in VWF activity. Although DDAVP is safe in these patients, it is not always effective, because normal multimers are not maintained in plasma. Significant bleeding should be treated with VWF replacement therapy.

Type 2B VWD may be caused by one of several mutations resulting in "hyperactive" VWF. The abnormal VWF binds spontaneously to platelets, with resulting rapid clearance of VWF and platelets. The higher molecular weight multimers of VWF are preferentially cleared from the circulation, and moderate to severe thrombocytopenia is common. The laboratory diagnosis is based on the finding that the hyperactive 2B VWF binds to platelets and agglutinates them at low concentrations of ristocetin, a concentration that would not agglutinate normal platelets. If DDAVP is given to these patients, the abnormal hyperactive 2B VWF will be released and more profound thrombocytopenia might occur. Patients with 2B VWD usually respond to the infusion of VWF.

Type 2M VWD is caused by mutations that result in reduction of the platelet-binding function of VWF. Thus, levels of VWF activity are significantly lower than the levels of VWF antigen. Binding of this protein to factor VIII is normal; thus, factor VIII levels are similar to those of VWF antigen. DDAVP will increase VWF and factor VIII levels, but the released type 2M VWF may not have sufficient activity to cause cessation of bleeding. Thus, VWF replacement therapy may need to be used.

Type 2N VWD is caused by the reduction of factor VIII binding by VWF. This disorder has also been termed **autosomal hemophilia.** With this variant, platelet interaction with VWF is normal, but type 2N VWF binds weakly (or not at all) to factor VIII, resulting in rapid clearance of factor VIII that is weakly complexed to VWF. Thus, the factor VIII level is reduced much more than VWF levels. Commonly, patients who have symptomatic bleeding are compound heterozygotes who have inherited a gene for type 1 VWD from 1 parent and a gene for type 2N VWD from the other. Rarely, type 2N mutations are inherited from both parents and VWF levels are normal. In the patient who is compound heterozygous for types 1 and 2N, 1 allele makes no protein and the other allele makes a functionally abnormal protein, and as a result, all of the VWF is dysfunctional. Although DDAVP will release type 2N VWF, sustained factor VIII levels occasionally may be inadequate for normal hemostasis. A trial of DDAVP is indicated to assess the response and half-life of VWF and factor VIII after infusion. VWF replacement therapy is usually effective.

Platelet-type (pseudo-) VWD is actually an abnormality of the GPIb receptor on platelets. This can be considered the converse abnormality of type 2B, in that the GPIb receptor on platelets is hyperfunctional and binds plasma VWF spontaneously. This results in **thrombocytopenia** and a loss of high molecular weight VWF multimers, which are indistinguishable from those seen in type 2B VWD. Specific testing, however, shows that this is a platelet abnormality rather than a plasma abnormality.

Type 3 VWD is the homozygous or compound heterozygous inheritance of VWF deficiency. Patients exhibit undetectable plasma levels of VWF and low, but measurable, levels of factor VIII. These patients will have major hemorrhage, but only rarely have joint hemorrhages. This severe, very rare form occurs in approximately 1:250,000 individuals. Intracranial hemorrhage, major epistaxis, and menorrhagia in women are the major features. Bleeding episodes require treatment with VWF-containing concentrates. VWF is both a plasma and a platelet protein.

Because treatment with VWF-containing concentrate only corrects the plasma VWF level, patients with severe bleeding may need to be transfused with platelet concentrates to correct the deficiency of platelet VWF. DDAVP is not effective in type 3 VWD.

DIAGNOSIS AND DIFFERENTIAL DIAGNOSIS. The diagnosis of VWD is dependent on the finding of a low level of at least 1 of the laboratory measures of VWF noted in Figure 477-1. The differential diagnosis of mucocutaneous bleeding includes abnormalities of platelet number, platelet function, or the vessel wall (see Chapter 484). In caring for children, it is important to remember that the most common cause of such findings is trauma, especially nonaccidental trauma—child abuse.

COMPLICATIONS. Complications of bleeding due to VWD are rare. In adolescent females, blood loss due to menorrhagia can lead to severe anemia, either acutely, with signs and symptoms of hypovolemia, or chronically, caused by iron deficiency. Individuals with type 3 VWD can manifest joint or muscle bleeding similar to individuals with hemophilia.

TREATMENT. Treatment of VWD is directed toward increasing the plasma level of VWF and factor VIII. Because the gene for factor VIII is normal in patients with VWD, elevating the plasma concentration of VWF permits normal recovery and survival of endogenously produced factor VIII. The most common form of VWD is type 1. In these patients, the synthetic drug DDAVP induces the release of VWF from endothelial cells. In some patients with type 2 variants, DDAVP may be similarly effective, but in other circumstances, the released VWF is dysfunctional. Patients with VWD may not respond adequately to DDAVP because they release an abnormal VWF molecule (most type 2 variants); because they have type 3 disease, in which there is no VWF to be released; or because they have accelerated clearance of released VWF. A small subset of children and adults, especially infants, do not release VWF in response to DDAVP. In these cases, replacement therapy must be used. Current replacement therapy uses plasma-derived VWF containing concentrates that also contain factor VIII. VWF distributes only to the intravascular space, because it is so large. During plasma fractionation, VWF multimers are altered to a variable extent. Therefore, 1 U/kg will increase the plasma level by 1.5%. The plasma half-life of both factor VIII and VWF is 12 hr, but the alteration of VWF during fractionation results in half-lives of 8–10 hr when concentrates are infused. Purified or recombinant VWF concentrates (containing no factor VIII) may become available in the near future. These will be useful in prophylaxis or in presurgical management. When used for acute bleeding, however, these VWF concentrates, which contain little or no factor VIII, may need to be supplemented by an infusion of recombinant factor VIII for the 1st infusion. Both VWF and factor VIII are required for normal hemostasis. If only VWF is replaced, endogenous correction of the factor VIII level takes 12–24 hr. Dental extractions and sometimes nosebleeds can be managed with both DDAVP and an antifibrinolytic agent, such as ε-aminocaproic acid (Amicar).

Favaloro EJ, Lillicrap D, Lazzari MA, et al: von Willebrand disease: Laboratory aspects of diagnosis and treatment. *Haemophilia* 2004;10:164–168.

Federici AB: Clinical diagnosis of von Willebrand disease. *Haemophilia* 2004;10(Suppl 4):169–176.

Gill JC: Diagnosis and treatment of von Willebrand disease. *Hematol Oncol Clin North Am* 2004;18:1277–1299.

Mannucci PM: Treatment of von Willebrand's disease. *N Engl J Med* 2004;351:683–694.

Mannucci PM: Desmopressin (DDAVP) in the treatment of bleeding disorders: The first 20 years. *Blood* 1997;90:2515–2521.

Montgomery RR, Gill JC, Scott JP: Hemophilia and von Willebrand disease. In Nathan DG, Orkin SH, Ginsburg D, et al (editors): *Hematology of Infancy and Childhood,* 6th ed. Philadelphia, WB Saunders, 2003, pp 1547–1576.

Sadler JE: Von Willebrand disease type 1: A diagnosis in search of a disease. *Blood* 2003;101:2089–2093.

Shankar M, Lee CA, Sabin CA, et al: von Willebrand disease in women with menorrhagia: A systematic review. *BJOG* 2004;111:734–740.

Werner EJ: von Willebrand disease in children and adolescents. *Pediatr Clin North Am* 1996;43:683–707.

White GC, Sadler EA: Von Willebrand disease: Clinical aspects and therapy. In Hoffman R, Benz EJ, Shattil SJ, et al (editors): *Hematology: Basic Principles and Practice,* 4th ed. Philadelphia, Elsevier Churchill Livingstone, 2005, pp 2121–2135.

Chapter 478 ■ Hereditary Predisposition to Thrombosis

Thromboses in children are frequently associated with a hereditary or acquired prothrombotic state. A significant number of hereditary causes of thrombosis are identified (Tables 478-1 and 478-2). The newborn infant, because of the physiologic deficiency of various regulatory proteins, is particularly predisposed to both hemorrhage and thrombosis. For both anticoagulant proteins and most procoagulant factors, the more premature the infant, the greater the deficiency. The sick newborn infant is particularly at risk because interventions to provide support often include placement of large indwelling catheters into major veins or arteries. Those with hereditary deficiencies of anticoagulants may have major symptoms. After the neonatal period, young children seem to have some resistance to clinical thrombosis, even if they have a heterozygous hereditary deficiency of an anticoagulant protein. When a thrombus is identified in the young child, particularly when the family history is abnormal, a thrombotic evaluation should be initiated. In children and teenagers, thromboses are often triggered by major medical or surgical challenges.

PATHOPHYSIOLOGY AND CLINICAL MANIFESTATIONS. The principal physiologic anticoagulants are illustrated in Figures 475-1 and 475-2. A hereditary predisposition to thrombosis can be caused by deficiencies of the regulatory proteins protein C, protein S, antithrombin III, and plasminogen; synthesis of a procoagulant protein unable to be inhibited by its regulatory protein, factor V Leiden; elevated levels of procoagulant protein; prothrombin mutation (G20210A); and elevated levels of a toxic organic acid, homocystinemia.

The hereditary mutation of factor V, **factor V Leiden,** results in a factor V molecule that, when activated, is not subsequently inactivated by activated protein C. This leaves the patient with unregulated "active" factor V and so-called resistance to activated protein C. Furthermore, after proteolysis by activated protein C–inactivated factor Va (Vai) is a functional anticoagulant that inhibits clotting. Individuals with the prothrombin mutation (G20210A) have a mutation in the 3′-untranslated end of the messenger RNA for prothrombin that results in increased levels of prothrombin synthesis. Children with these hereditary mutations have an increased frequency of venous thrombosis. Young women are at increased risk for venous thrombosis during pregnancy or while receiving oral contraceptive agents. There is

TABLE 478-1. Common Prothrombotic States

CONGENITAL
Deficiency of Anticoagulants
AT-III, protein C or protein S, plasminogen
Resistance to Cofactor Proteolysis
Factor V Leiden
High Levels of Procoagulants
Prothrombin 20210 mutation
Elevated factor VIII levels
Damage to Endothelium
Homocystinemia
ACQUIRED
Obstruction to Flow
Indwelling lines
Pregnancy
Polycythemia/dehydration
Immobilization
Injury
Trauma, surgery
Inflammation
IBD, vasculitis, infection, Behçet syndrome
Hypercoagulability
Pregnancy
Malignancy
Antiphospholipid syndrome
Nephrotic syndrome
Oral contraceptives
L-Asparaginase
Elevated factor VIII levels
RARE OTHER ENTITIES
Congenital
Dysfibrinogenemia
Acquired
Paroxysmal nocturnal hemoglobinuria
Thrombocythemia
Vascular grafts

AT-III, antithrombin III; IBD, inflammatory bowel disease.

also an increased risk of recurrent abortions. In young adults with thrombosis, factor V Leiden and the prothrombin mutation (G20210A) are the most common associated abnormalities. Factor V Leiden is found in approximately 5% of whites and the prothrombin gene mutation is found in 1–2%; the prevalence of these mutations in other ethnic populations is lower.

Heterozygous deficiency of anticoagulant proteins, protein C, protein S, or antithrombin III, induces a tendency toward venous thromboembolic disease at an early age. The special case of neonatal purpura fulminans, characterized by necrotic purpura of the skin and thromboses of major vessels, is caused by homozygous protein C deficiency. Such infants were probably overlooked in the past because the symptoms were believed to be secondary to sepsis and disseminated intravascular coagulation. Because the newborn is physiologically deficient in protein C, its absence is difficult to determine, except in a laboratory that has established normal ranges for neonates and preterm infants. If an individual has undetectable levels of protein C, this is most likely a hereditary disorder. However, the physiologic deficiency of protein C in the newborn, coupled with true sepsis, may also lead to nearly undetectable levels of protein C.

LABORATORY FINDINGS. There are no screening tests for a hereditary predisposition to thrombosis; thus, specific testing is required for protein C, protein S, antithrombin III, factor V Leiden, and prothrombin 20210. A careful family history may reveal thromboembolic diseases in family members at a young age, but the absence of a positive history does not rule out a hereditary predisposition to thrombosis. If hereditary deficiency of anticoagulant or regulatory proteins is suspected, specific assays should be undertaken. Techniques that quantitate the amount and function of antithrombin III, protein C, and free protein S are well established. Molecular testing for the factor V Leiden and the prothrombin mutation (G20210A) genes is more sensitive and specific than clotting-based tests.

TREATMENT. Homozygous deficiency of protein C presents with purpura fulminans in the first few hr of life. Fresh frozen plasma (FFP) is the only immediately available source of protein C. Amelioration of symptoms usually requires 10–15 mL/kg of FFP every 8–12 hr. Clinical trials are in progress using a plasma protein C concentrate, which eliminates the need for large amounts of FFP. A recombinant activated protein C concentrate (drotrecogin-α) has been approved for the treatment of adult sepsis, but it has not been approved for treating hereditary deficiency. There are a few case reports wherein activated protein C concentrate has been successfully used to treat homozygous protein C deficiency. After the infant's symptoms have improved, the amount of FFP or protein C concentrate is adjusted by monitoring of protein C levels. When the infant is beyond the neonatal period, high-dose warfarin (to achieve an **International Normalized Ratio** of 3–5) may prevent most of the thrombotic problems, but acute intermittent thromboses require additional FFP or protein C concentrate (see also Chapter 479).

Patients who sustain a thrombosis associated with a hereditary predisposition to clotting should be treated with anticoagulants (see Chapter 479). Replacement therapy is usually not indicated. Individuals with homocystinuria should receive anticoagulation

TABLE 478-2. Inherited Thrombotic Disorders

CLASSIFICATION AND DISORDERS	INHERITANCE	CLINICAL FEATURES
DEFICIENCY OR QUALITATIVE ABNORMALITIES OF INHIBITORS OF ACTIVATED COAGULATION FACTORS		
AT deficiency	AD	Venous thromboembolism (usual and unusual sites), heparin resistance
TM deficiency	AD	Venous thromboembolism
Protein C deficiency	AD	Venous thromboembolism
Protein S deficiency	AD	Venous and arterial thromboembolism
APC resistance	AD	Venous and arterial thromboembolism
IMPAIRED CLOT LYSIS		
Dysfibrinogenemia	AD	More venous thrombosis than arterial thrombosis
Plasminogen deficiency	AD, AR	Venous thromboembolism
TPA deficiency	AD	Venous thromboembolism
Excess PAI-1 activity	AD	Venous thromboembolism and arterial thrombosis
METABOLIC DEFECT		
Hyperhomocysteinemia	Not known	Venous thromboembolism and premature atherosclerotic vascular disease
ABNORMALITY OF COAGULATION ZYMOGEN OR COFACTOR		
Prothrombin mutation	AD	Venous thromboembolism
Elevated factor VIII levels	Not known	Venous thromboembolism
Elevated factor IX levels	Not known	Venous thromboembolism
Elevated factor X levels	Not known	Venous thromboembolism
Elevated factor XI levels	Not known	Venous thromboembolism

AD, autosomal dominant; APC, activated protein C; AR, autosomal recessive; AT, antithrombin; PAI-1, plasminogen activator inhibitor-1; TM, thrombomodulin; TPA, tissue plasminogen activator.

From Robetorye RS, Rodgers GM: Update on selected inherited venous thrombic disorders. *Am J Hematol* 2001;68:256–268. Modified with permission from Rodgers GM, Chandler WL: Laboratory and clinical aspects of inherited thrombotic disorders. *Am J Hematol* 1992;41:113–122. Reprinted with permission of Wiley-Liss, Inc., a subsidiary of John Wiley & Sons, Inc.

in addition to management of their primary disease (see Chapter 85.3).

Bhojwani D, Hart D: Thrombophilia in childhood. *Curr Probl Pediatr Adolesc Health Care* 2004;34:190–212.
Chalmers EA: Heritable thrombophilia and childhood thrombosis. *Blood Rev* 2001;15:181–189.
David M, Andrew M: Venous thromboembolic complications in children. *J Pediatr* 1993;123:337–346.
de Moerloose P, Alhenc-Gelas M, Boehlen F, et al: Deep venous thrombosis and thrombophilia: Indications for testing and clinical implications. *Semin Vasc Med* 2001;1:89–96.
Esmon CT: Blood coagulation. In Nathan DG, Orkin SH, Ginsburg D, et al (editors): *Hematology of Infancy and Childhood,* 6th ed. Philadelphia, WB Saunders, 2003, pp 1475–1496.
Heller C, Nowak-Gottl U: Maternal thrombophilia and neonatal thrombosis. *Best Pract Res Clin Haematol* 2003;16:333–345.
Hoppe C, Matsunaga A: Pediatric thrombosis. *Pediatr Clin North Am* 2002;49:1257–1283.
Langlois NJ, Wells PS: Risk of venous thromboembolism in relatives of symptomatic probands with thrombophilia: A systematic review. *Thromb Haemost* 2003;90:17–26.
Male C, Kuhle S, Mitchell L: Diagnosis of venous thromboembolism in children. *Semin Thromb Hemost* 2003;29:377–390.
Monagle P, Chan A, Massicotte P, et al: Antithrombotic therapy in children: The Seventh ACCP Conference on Antithrombotic and Thrombolytic Therapy. *Chest* 2004;126:645S–687S.
Monagle P, Andrew M: Acquired disorders of hemostasis. In Nathan DG, Orkin SH, Ginsburg D, et al (editors): *Hematology of Infancy and Childhood,* 6th ed. Philadelphia, WB Saunders, 2003, pp 1631–1668.
Robetorye RS, Rodgers GM: Update on selected inherited venous thrombotic disorders. *Am J Hematol* 2001;68:256–268.
Scott JP: Bleeding and thrombosis. In Kliegman R, Greenbaum L, Lye P (editors): *Practical Strategies in Pediatric Diagnosis and Therapy,* 2nd ed. Philadelphia, WB Saunders, 2004, pp 240–247.
Seligsohn U, Lubetsky A: Genetic susceptibility to venous thrombosis. *N Engl J Med* 2001;344:1222–1231.

Chapter 479 ■ Acquired Thrombotic Disorders

Occlusion of a blood vessel with a platelet plug or fibrin clot may occur in vessels of any size. A large number of systemic disorders are associated with occlusion of arterial or venous vessels of diverse caliber, including vasculitic diseases, such as systemic lupus erythematosus (see Chapter 157) and Kawasaki disease (see Chapter 165); metabolic defects, such as homocystinuria (see Chapter 85); and hemoglobinopathies, such as sickle cell anemia (see Chapter 462) and polycythemia (see Chapters 466 and 467). Activation of clotting as a complication of disseminated intravascular coagulation can cause microvascular and macrovascular thrombosis (see Chapter 483). Medical interventions themselves can cause a predisposition to thrombosis, such as when sick newborns have indwelling catheters placed in major vessels or when children with acute lymphoblastic leukemia receive the chemotherapeutic agent L-asparaginase, which depletes anticoagulant proteins. In addition to vessel injury, mechanisms that lead to thrombosis include one or more of the following: *abnormal platelet adhesiveness-aggregation, an activated coagulation mechanism, a defective or deficient anticoagulant system, a dysfunctional fibrinolytic mechanism,* and *reduced blood flow.* Arterial thrombosis appears to depend on vascular injury and platelet activation under high shear, whereas venous thrombosis generally occurs in low-flow (low-shear) conditions associated with activation of the coagulation mechanism or with an impaired inhibitor-fibrinolytic system.

EPIDEMIOLOGY. Although acquired thrombotic and embolic events are uncommon in otherwise healthy children, thromboembolism is a common complication in sick newborns and in patients with specific diseases (see Table 478-1). In the United States, the prevalence of thromboembolic disease at the time of hospital discharge is approximately 10/100,000 children/yr, but it varies significantly with the age of the child. Infants and older teens have the highest rates.

CLINICAL MANIFESTATIONS. Arterial thromboses usually present with striking organ dysfunction due to ischemia (cold, pulseless extremity). Such findings can be triggered by thrombi formed at the site of vascular damage or caused by emboli. Venous events usually present as a warm, swollen, or distended tender organ or extremity. A deep venous thrombosis (DVT) may be asymptomatic and present only after the development of pulmonary emboli. In general, vascular occlusive events in children have an acute or sudden onset.

DIAGNOSIS. The diagnosis of thrombosis is made by Doppler ultrasonography or magnetic resonance angiography. In special cases (upper extremity thromboses), radiocontrast angiography may be necessary. Routine coagulation screening studies are rarely helpful in diagnosing a thromboembolic event. Studies in adults have suggested that a quantitative assay of **D-dimer** (formed when cross-linked fibrin is proteolysed by plasmin) is a sensitive screening tool for DVT and especially for pulmonary emboli (see Chapter 406). In acute disseminated intravascular coagulation, screening test results are strikingly abnormal, characterized by thrombocytopenia, hypofibrinogenemia, prolongation of prothrombin time (PT) and partial thromboplastin time (PTT), and elevated D-dimer levels (see Chapter 483).

Disorders commonly associated with thromboses are presented in Table 478-1. The **lupus anticoagulant** is a special case in which an apparent inhibitor of clotting causes a predisposition to thrombosis. In the laboratory, the lupus anticoagulant causes prolongation of PTT that does not correct on 1:1 mixing with normal plasma. The antibody is directed against the phospholipid used as a reagent in PTT. Specific assays confirm the presence of an antiphospholipid antibody. Although PTT is prolonged, the patient with an isolated lupus anticoagulant is usually not at increased risk for bleeding. Paradoxically, 5–20% of such individuals may develop arterial or venous thromboses. The lupus anticoagulant, either alone or as a component of the antiphospholipid syndrome, may be primary (idiopathic) or associated with systemic lupus erythematosus; infection, especially HIV; drug reactions; or other autoimmune diseases. Associated features include livedo reticularis, thrombocytopenia, recurrent fetal loss, and thrombosis (arterial, venous, or both). Some children may have a transient lupus anticoagulant after a viral illness. Treatment of thromboses associated with the lupus anticoagulant includes heparin and warfarin, with or without aspirin.

The **differential diagnosis** of thromboembolic disease is dependent on the affected organ and the type of vessel. For arterial disorders, the most common alternative diagnosis is some form of arteritis (Kawasaki disease or systemic lupus erythematosus). For venous thrombosis of the extremities, trauma and infection may cause similar clinical findings. A pulmonary infiltrative process of any cause may lead to respiratory symptoms and other findings similar to those of a pulmonary embolus.

COMPLICATIONS. Acute arterial occlusion causes severe organ dysfunction due to ischemia. Complications of venous thromboembolic disease are more often related to long-term venous stasis changes, with swelling, skin changes, and discomfort of the affected extremity. Such findings in the upper extremities have been recently appreciated as a common, long-term complication of indwelling central venous catheters.

TREATMENT

Venous Thrombosis and Thrombophlebitis. Superficial thrombophlebitis is treated with anti-inflammatory drugs (nonsteroidal anti-inflammatory agents), heat compresses, rest, and elevation of the affected part. Patients with DVT or thrombophlebitis are treated with anticoagulation and rarely with thrombolytic agents. Heparin anticoagulation using standard unfractionated heparin or low molecular weight (LMW) heparin should be used in a full dose for 3–5 days, with warfarin added for an additional 6 mo in patients with proximal (above the knee) venous thrombosis. The use of thrombolytic therapy should probably be limited to life- or limb-threatening situations. The optimal treatment of patients with isolated calf vein thrombosis is unclear, but short-term anticoagulation may hasten recovery and prevent progression.

Pulmonary Embolism. The patient with acute pulmonary embolism can be treated with heparin or, less often, with thrombolytic drugs (see Chapter 406). Most patients should receive heparin and, later, warfarin, as described in Table 479-1. Thrombolytic therapy should be reserved for life-threatening pulmonary emboli ("saddle thrombus") because thrombolytic therapy in adults produces more rapid clinical improvement than heparin therapy, but overall survival and long-term pulmonary function abnormalities appear to be the same in both treatment groups. Embolectomy is used rarely when there is a large embolism and no benefit is derived from thrombolytic or anticoagulant therapy.

Arterial Thrombosis. Fibrinolytic therapy with recombinant tissue-type plasminogen activator, followed by heparin anticoagulation, has been used successfully to treat acute arterial thromboses of recent onset. Rarely, surgical removal of the clot is performed if lytic therapy is not successful or if the thrombosis affects a major organ or limb. Thrombolytic therapy should not be used if there has been recent surgery or central nervous system thrombosis or hemorrhage.

Stroke. Ischemic stroke commonly presents with hemiparesis, loss of consciousness, or seizures. Arterial occlusion in the brain may occur as a component of a systemic disorder (sickle cell disease) or after embolization either from a damaged vessel (carotid aneurysm after trauma) or from venous thrombi that enter the arterial circulation via a patent foramen ovale (see Chapter 601). Often strokes are idiopathic. The most common identified cause of stroke in children is sickle cell disease. Venous thrombosis of the cerebral vessels (sinovenous thrombosis) can be seen in those with cyanotic heart disease, inflammatory or infectious lesions of the brain or surrounding tissues, hyperviscosity states, or congenital thrombophilia. The therapeutic approach to arterial or venous stroke is controversial. Antiplatelet therapy with aspirin is safe. Heparin therapy may improve the outcome of stroke in adults, although the risk of hemorrhagic infarction may be increased. Sinovenous thrombosis in the absence of hemorrhage is usually treated with heparin. The presence of a hemorrhagic infarct is a **contraindication** to anticoagulant therapy. It is not known whether thrombolytic therapy is effective or safe in children with nonhemorrhagic strokes; but, if used, it should only be instituted in patients within 3 hr of the onset of symptoms.

479.1 • Anticoagulant and Thrombolytic Therapy

Table 479-1 provides an outline of commonly used anticoagulant agents.

UNFRACTIONATED (STANDARD) HEPARIN. Heparin enhances the rate by which antithrombin III neutralizes the activity of several activated clotting proteins, especially factor Xa and thrombin. The average half-life of heparin administered IV is approximately 60 min in adults and can be as short as 30 min in the newborn. Heparin does not cross the placenta. The half-life of heparin is dose-dependent; the higher the dose, the longer the circulating half-life. In thrombotic disease, the half-life may be shorter than normal in patients with significant thromboembolism (pulmonary embolism) and longer than normal in patients with cirrhosis and uremia.

Anticoagulation with heparin is **contraindicated** in the following circumstances: a recent central nervous system hemorrhage; bleeding from inaccessible sites; malignant hypertension; bacterial endocarditis; recent surgery of the eye, brain, or spinal cord; and current administration of regional or lumbar block anesthesia. A pre-existing coagulation defect or bleeding abnormality is a relative contraindication. Despite these precautions, the frequency of bleeding in patients given heparin anticoagulation is 0.2–1.0%.

TABLE 479-1. Comparison of Antithrombotic Agents

	THROMBOLYTIC THERAPY	UNFRACTIONATED HEPARIN*	WARFARIN	LMW HEPARIN (ENOXAPARIN)
Indication	Recent onset of life- or limb-threatening thrombus	Thrombus of indeterminate age	Long-term oral anticoagulation	Thrombus of indeterminate age
Dose	rTPA 0.1–0.2 mg/kg/hr IV	75 U/kg/bolus, 20–28* U/kg/hr by continuous infusion IV	0.1–0.2 mg/kg/day PO	1.0–1.5* mg/kg q12hr SC
Adjustment	Increase dose for lack of clinical effect	↑ dose by 5–10% q6hr until adequate level or PTT is achieved	↑ dose q 2 days by 20–30% until appropriate, stable INR	↑ or ↓ by 10–20%
Course	6–12 hr	5–14 days	Weeks to months	5 days–6 mo
Monitors/goal	"Lytic state": FDP or D-dimer (TPA)	PTT 2–2½ times control; thrombin time infinity; heparin level 0.3–0.7 U/mL	INR 2.0–3.0	LMW heparin level 4 hr after 4th dose = 0.5–1.0 U/mL
Mechanism	Activation of plasminogen to plasmin	Accelerates AT-III-dependent inactivation of thrombin, FXa	Impairs vitamin K-dependent carboxylation of FII, VII, IX, X, proteins C and S	Accelerates AT-III-dependent inactivation of FXa and thrombin
Risk of bleeding	Medium to high	Low	Low	Low

*Higher dose is required in newborns.

AT-III, antithrombin III; F, factor; FDP, fibrin degradation product; INR, international normalized ratio; LMW, low molecular weight; PTT, partial thromboplastin time; rTPA, recombinant tissue-type plasminogen activator; U, unit.

Aspirin is the only commonly used antiplatelet agent, and the usual dose is 80 mg/day (1 baby aspirin daily). There is no need to monitor aspirin therapy.

Guidelines for therapy using unfractionated heparin are shown in Table 479-1. In newborns with low levels of clotting factors, in patients with a lupus inhibitor, or in patients with elevated levels of factor VIII (as a result of stress or surgery), PTT may not reflect the correct degree of anticoagulation, and specific heparin levels should be obtained so that the heparin level is 0.35–0.70 Unit/mL by anti-factor Xa assay or 0.2–0.4 unit/mL by protamine sulfate assay.

Heparin can be neutralized immediately by using protamine sulfate. Because of the rapid clearance rate of heparin, however, stopping the infusion is adequate treatment for most patients. One milligram of protamine sulfate neutralizes 90–110 Units of heparin. Because heparin has rapid in vivo metabolic decay, only ½ of the total dose of protamine should be administered. A clotting test is performed to determine whether adequate neutralization has occurred; if not, the additional protamine can be given. Protamine itself is an anticoagulant; thus, if too much is given, clotting time may be prolonged. Although excess protamine has an anticoagulant effect, it rarely (if ever) is a cause of clinical bleeding. Once heparin is neutralized, the patient is returned to the original "prothrombotic" state.

LOW MOLECULAR WEIGHT HEPARIN. Low molecular weight (LMW) heparin is an effective, convenient alternative to standard heparin therapy, and its use is described in Table 479-1. Several heparins and heparinoids are undergoing clinical trials. Most pediatric experience is with enoxaparin. Adult patients receiving LMW heparin rarely need to have their heparin levels monitored, but in pediatric patients, there is more diversity of response. Monitoring is critical to ensure that a therapeutic level is achieved. PTT cannot be used to monitor LMW heparin; a specific assay should be used. Once a therapeutic range is achieved, routine monitoring is not required or is required only infrequently. When LMW heparin is used for prophylaxis against thrombosis, the dose is 0.5 mg/kg q12hr subcutaneously, with the goal of achieving a level of 0.3 Unit/mL 4 hr after injection.

WARFARIN. Coumarin derivatives are oral anticoagulant drugs that act by decreasing the functional levels of the vitamin K–dependent coagulation factors: II, VII, IX, and X, as well as protein C and protein S (vitamin K–dependent anticoagulants). These drugs inhibit vitamin K–dependent carboxylation of the precursor coagulation proteins. Warfarin probably acts by competitively inhibiting vitamin K metabolism. After the administration of warfarin, levels of factors II, VII, IX, and X decrease gradually, according to each factor's plasma half-life. Because factor VII has the shortest half-life, its level is the 1st to decrease, followed by factors IX and X, and finally, factor II. It generally takes 4–5 days to reduce the levels of all 4 coagulation factors consistent with effective anticoagulation.

Prothrombin time (PT) is the clotting test used to assess warfarin anticoagulation. Current recommendations are based on the International Normalized Ratio (INR), which permits comparison of PT using a wide variety of reagents or instruments. The INR for standard treatment of thrombosis is 2.0–3.0. Table 479-1 provides guidelines for the administration of warfarin to children. For patients with mechanical heart valves and those with homozygous protein C deficiency, the INR should be 3.0–4.0.

The most serious side effect of warfarin is hemorrhage. This is often related to changes in the dose or metabolism of the drug. The addition or removal of certain drugs in the patient's therapeutic regimen can have significant effects on oral anticoagulation. The effect of warfarin can be enhanced by the administration of antibiotics, salicylates, anabolic steroids, chloral hydrate, laxatives, allopurinol, vitamin E, and methylphenidate hydrochloride; its effect can be diminished by barbiturates, vitamin K, oral contraceptives, phenytoin, and other agents. Warfarin-induced bleeding is treated by discontinuation of the drug and oral administration of vitamin K. Generally, the amount of vitamin K given is equal to the amount of the daily warfarin dose. Vitamin K can be administered orally, subcutaneously, or IV (not IM), but the parenteral forms have a much longer half-life and may overshoot the correction. Correction of coagulopathy begins within 6–8 hr and should be complete in 24–48 hr. If the patient is having a significant or life-threatening hemorrhage, fresh frozen plasma (15 mL/kg) should be given when the vitamin K is administered.

Contraindications to coumarin anticoagulants are essentially the same as those for heparin therapy. The oral anticoagulants are teratogenic, cross the placenta, and should not be given during pregnancy, particularly during the 1st trimester. Although breast milk contains warfarin, the quantity is insignificant and the drug can be used to treat the lactating mother without a significant effect on the infant.

THROMBOLYTIC THERAPY. Thrombolytic agents, such as recombinant tissue-type plasminogen activator (rTPA), activate plasminogen to lyse blood clots by enzymatic digestion; rTPA is most often used in pediatrics for thrombolytic therapy, as described in Table 479-1. For this therapy to be effective, the patient should have a relatively fresh clot (<3–5 days old), the clot must be accessible to the lytic agent, and there must be an adequate amount of plasminogen. Once plasmin has been formed, it lyses fibrin. Relatively more fibrin-specific than the older thrombolytic agents urokinase and streptokinase, rTPA activates plasminogen within or on a fibrin clot. Clinical trials with rTPA suggest that it rarely produces a systemic hyperfibrinolytic state. The initial dose of rTPA is 0.1 mg/kg/hr. It may be useful to monitor for a therapeutic effect by looking for an increase in the concentration of D-dimers or fibrin degradation products. Higher doses or more prolonged courses of thrombolytic therapy are likely to be associated with an increased risk of bleeding complications. Low doses of rTPA have been efficacious in restoring patency in occluded vascular access catheters.

PREVENTION

There have been no formal trials of prevention of venous thromboembolic disease in children. Children with known prothrombotic conditions who are going to be immobilized for a protracted time probably should receive prophylactic treatment with enoxaparin 0.5 mg/kg q12hr while immobile. More controversial is the use of such therapy for children who are immobilized for a prolonged period due to a severe medical illness, especially if it is associated with inflammation or trauma.

Anton N, Massicotte MP: Venous thromboembolism in pediatrics. *Semin Vasc Med* 2001;1:111–122.

Bauer KA: Role of thrombophilia in deciding on the duration of anticoagulation. *Semin Thromb Hemost* 2004;30:633–637.

Chan AK, Deveber G, Monagle P, et al: Venous thrombosis in children. *J Thromb Haemost* 2003;1:1443–1455.

Christiansen SC, Cannegieter SC, Koster T, et al: Thrombophilia, clinical factors and recurrent venous thrombotic events. *JAMA* 2005;293:2352–2361.

Di Nisio M, Middeldorp S, Buller HR: Direct thrombin inhibitors. *N Engl J Med* 2005;353:1028–1040.

Goldenberg NA, Knapp-Clevenger R, Manco-Johnson MJ: Elevated plasma factor VIII and D-dimer levels as predictors of poor outcomes of thrombosis in children. *N Engl J Med* 2004;351:1081–1088.

Jilma B, Kamath S, Lip GY: ABC of antithrombotic therapy: Antithrombotic therapy in special circumstances. II—In children, thrombophilia, and miscellaneous conditions. *BMJ* 2003;326:93–96.

Johnson MC, Parkerson N, Ward S, et al: Pediatric sinovenous thrombosis. *J Pediatr Hematol Oncol* 2003;25:312–315.
Kyrle PA, Eichinger S: Deep vein thrombosis. *Lancet* 2005;365:1163–1174.
Lim W, Crowther MA, Eikelboom JW: Management of antiphospholipid antibody syndrome. *JAMA* 2006;295:1050–1057.
Male C, Kuhle S, Mitchell L: Diagnosis of venous thromboembolism in children. *Semin Thromb Hemost* 2003;29:377–390.
Monagle P, Chan A, Massicotte P, et al: Antithrombotic therapy in children: The Seventh ACCP Conference on Antithrombotic and Thrombolytic Therapy. *Chest* 2004;126(3 Suppl):645S–687S.
Nowak-Gottl U, Straeter R, Sebire G, et al: Antithrombotic drug treatment of pediatric patients with ischemic stroke. *Paediatr Drugs* 2003;5:167–175.
Ozturk MA, Haznedaroglu IC, Turgut M, et al: Current debates in antiphospholipid syndrome: The acquired antibody-mediated thrombophilia. *Clin Appl Thromb Hemost* 2004;10:89–126.
Rieder MJ, Reiner AP, Gage BF, et al: Effect of VKORC1 haplotypes on transcriptional regulation and warfarin dose. *N Engl J Med* 2005;352: 2285–2292.
Streif W, Goebel G, Chan AKC, et al: Use of low molecular mass heparin (enoxaparin) in newborn infants: A prospective cohort study of 62 patients. *Arch Dis Child Fetal Neonatal Ed* 2003;88:F365–F370.
Sutor AH, Chan AK, Massicotte P: Low-molecular-weight heparin in pediatric patients. *Semin Thromb Hemost* 2004;30(Suppl 1):31–39.
Watson LI, Armon MP: Thrombolysis for acute deep vein thrombosis. *Cochrane Database Syst Rev* 2004; Oct 18(4):CD002783.
Wells PS, Anderson DR, Rodger M, et al: Excluding pulmonary embolism at the bedside without diagnostic imaging: Management of patients with suspected pulmonary embolism presenting to the emergency department by using a simple clinical model and D-dimer. *Ann Intern Med* 2001;135: 98–107.

Chapter 480 ■ Postneonatal Vitamin K Deficiency

Although "late" hemorrhagic disease has been reported in breastfed children, vitamin K deficiency occurring after the neonatal period is usually secondary to a lack of oral intake of vitamin K, alterations in the gut flora due to the long-term use of broad-spectrum antibiotics, or malabsorption of vitamin K. Intestinal malabsorption of fats may accompany cystic fibrosis or biliary atresia and result in a deficiency of fat-soluble dietary vitamin, with reduced synthesis of vitamin K–dependent clotting factors (factors II, VII, IX, and X, and protein C and protein S). Prophylactic administration of water-soluble vitamin K orally is indicated in these cases (2–3 mg/24 hr for children and 5–10 mg/24 hr for adolescents and adults), or vitamin K may be administered at 1–2 mg IV. In patients with advanced cirrhosis, synthesis of many of the clotting factors may be reduced because of hepatocellular damage. In these patients, vitamin K may be ineffective. The anticoagulant properties of warfarin (Coumadin) and related anticoagulants depend on interference with vitamin K, with a concomitant reduction of factors II, VII, IX, and X. Rat poison (superwarfarin) produces a similar deficiency; vitamin K is a specific antidote.

Bolton-Maggs P, Brook L: The use of vitamin K for reversal of over-warfarinization in children. *Br J Haematol* 2002;118:839–840.
Monagle P, Andrew M: Acquired disorders of hemostasis. In Nathan DG, Orkin SH, Ginsburg D, et al (editors): *Hematology of Infancy and Childhood,* 6th ed. Philadelphia, WB Saunders, 2003, pp 1631–1668.

Chapter 481 ■ Liver Disease

Because all of the clotting factors are produced exclusively in the liver except factor VIII, coagulation abnormalities are very common in patients with severe liver disease. Only 15% of such patients have significant clinical bleeding states. The severity of the coagulation abnormality appears to be directly proportional to the extent of hepatocellular damage. The most common mechanism causing the defect is decreased synthesis of coagulation factors. Patients with severe liver disease characteristically have normal to increased (not reduced) levels of factor VIII activity in plasma. In some instances, disseminated intravascular coagulation (see Chapter 483) or hyperfibrinolysis may complicate liver disease, making laboratory differentiation of severe liver disease from disseminated intravascular coagulation difficult.

Treatment of the coagulopathy of liver disease consists of replacement with fresh frozen plasma (FFP) or cryoprecipitate. FFP (10–15 mL/kg) contains all clotting factors, but replacement of fibrinogen for severe hypofibrinogenemia may require cryoprecipitate at a dose of 1 bag/5 kg body weight. Because a reduction in vitamin K–dependent coagulation factors is common in those with acute or chronic liver disease, vitamin K therapy can be given as a trial. Vitamin K can be given orally, subcutaneously, or IV (not IM) at a dose of 1 mg/24 hr for infants, 2–3 mg/24 hr for children, and 5–10 mg/24 hr for adolescents and adults. Inability to correct coagulopathy with vitamin K indicates that the coagulopathy may be caused by reduced levels of clotting factors that are not vitamin K–dependent and/or by inadequate production of precursor vitamin K proteins. In severe liver disease, it is often difficult to attain correction of abnormal clotting studies despite vigorous therapy with FFP and cryoprecipitate. Some patients with bleeding due to liver disease have responded to therapy with desmopressin, and others have responded to treatment with recombinant factor VIIa.

Frequently, severe liver disease is associated with moderate prolongation of bleeding time that is not corrected by either vitamin K or plasma replacement. Desmopressin (0.3 µg/kg IV) has been found to be effective in shortening bleeding time and has been used effectively to augment hemostasis before liver biopsy.

Atkison PR, Jardine L, Williams S, et al: Use of recombinant factor VIIa in pediatric patients with liver failure and severe coagulopathy. *Transplant Proc* 2005;37:1091–1093.
Kaul V, Munoz SJ: Coagulopathy of liver disease. *Curr Treat Options Gastroenterol* 2000;3:433–438.
Monagle P, Andrew M: Acquired disorders of hemostasis. In Nathan DG, Orkin SH, Ginsburg D, et al (editors): *Hematology of Infancy and Childhood,* 6th ed. Philadelphia, WB Saunders, 2003, pp 1631–1668.

Chapter 482 ■ Acquired Inhibitors of Coagulation

Acquired circulating anticoagulants (inhibitors) are antibodies that react or cross react with clotting factors or components used in coagulation screening tests (phospholipids), thereby prolonging screening tests, such as prothrombin time and partial thromboplastin time. Some of these anticoagulants are autoantibodies that react with phospholipid and thereby interfere with clotting in vitro, but not in vivo. The most common form of these antiphospholipid antibodies has been referred to as the *lupus anticoagulant* (see Chapter 479). This anticoagulant is found in patients with systemic lupus erythematosus (see Chapter 157), in those with other collagen-vascular diseases, and sometimes after common viral infections, including HIV. Spontaneous lupus-like inhibitors have developed transiently in children after incidental viral infection. These transient inhibitors are usually not associated with thrombosis.

Although the classic lupus anticoagulant is more often associated with a predisposition to thrombosis than with bleeding symptoms, bleeding symptoms in a patient with the lupus anticoagulant may be caused by thrombocytopenia, as a manifestation of the antiphospholipid syndrome or of lupus itself, or rarely, by a coexistent specific autoantibody against prothrombin (factor II). This antiprothrombin antibody does not inactivate prothrombin, but causes accelerated clearance of the protein, resulting in low levels of prothrombin.

Rarely, antibodies may arise spontaneously against a specific clotting factor, such as factor VIII or von Willebrand factor, similar to those seen more frequently in elderly patients. These patients are prone to excessive hemorrhage and may require specific treatment. In patients with a hereditary deficiency of a clotting factor (factor VIII or factor IX), antibodies may develop after exposure to transfused factor concentrates. These hemophilic inhibitory antibodies are discussed in Chapter 476.

LABORATORY FINDINGS. Inhibitors against specific coagulation factors usually affect factors VIII, IX, and XI, or rarely, prothrombin. Depending on the target of the antibody, prothrombin time, partial thromboplastin time, or both may be prolonged. The mechanism by which the inhibitory antibody functions determines whether mixing patient plasma with normal plasma will normalize (correct) the clotting time. Patient plasma containing antibodies directed against the active site of the clotting factor (factor VIII or factor IX) will not correct on 1:1 mixing with normal plasma, whereas antibodies that lead to increased clearance of the factor (prothrombin) will correct on 1:1 mixing. Specific factor assays are used to determine which factor is involved.

TREATMENT. Management of the patient with an inhibitor against a specific coagulation factor is the same as for the patient with hemophilia who has an alloantibody against factor VIII or factor IX. Infusions of recombinant factor VIIa or activated prothrombin complex concentrate may be needed to control significant bleeding. Spontaneous inhibitors that arise after a viral infection tend to disappear within a few wk to mo. Inhibitors seen with an underlying disease often disappear when the primary disease is treated. The lupus anticoagulant often disappears after appropriate treatment of systemic lupus erythematosus.

Bernini JC, Buchanan GR, Ashcraft J: Hypoprothrombinemia and severe hemorrhage associated with lupus anticoagulant. *J Pediatr* 1993;123:937–939.

Levine JS, Branch DW, Rauch J: The antiphospholipid syndrome. *N Engl J Med* 2002;346:752–763.

Monagle P, Andrew M: Acquired disorders of hemostasis. In Nathan DG, Orkin SH, Ginsburg D, et al (editors): *Hematology of Infancy and Childhood,* 6th ed. Philadelphia, WB Saunders, 2003, pp 1631–1668.

Moraca RJ, Ragni MV: Acquired anti-FVIII inhibitors in children. *Haemophilia* 2002;8:28–32.

Roberts HR, Monroe DM, White GC: The use of recombinant factor VIIa in the treatment of bleeding disorders. *Blood* 2004;104:3858–3864. Epub 2004;Aug 24.

Savage WJ, Kickler TS, Takemoto CM: Acquired coagulation factor inhibitors in children after topical bovine thrombin exposure. *Pediatr Blood Cancer* 2006;Mar 8.

Chapter 483 ■ Disseminated Intravascular Coagulation

Thrombotic microangiopathy refers to a heterogeneous group of conditions, including disseminated intravascular coagulation (DIC), that result in consumption of clotting factors, platelets, and anticoagulant proteins. Consequences of this process include widespread intravascular deposition of fibrin, leading to tissue ischemia and necrosis, a generalized hemorrhagic state, and hemolytic anemia.

ETIOLOGY. Any life-threatening pathologic process associated with hypoxia, acidosis, tissue necrosis, shock, and/or endothelial damage may trigger DIC; a large number of conditions have been reported to be associated with DIC, including septic shock (especially meningococcemia), incompatible blood transfusion, rickettsial infection, snakebite, purpura fulminans, giant hemangioma, and malignancy, especially acute promyelocytic leukemia (Table 483-1). Although the clinical symptoms are primarily hemorrhagic, the initiating event is usually excessive activation of clotting that consumes both the physiologic anticoagulants (protein C, protein S, and antithrombin III) and procoagulants, resulting in a deficiency of factor V, factor VIII, prothrombin, fibrinogen, and platelets. Commonly, the clinical result of this sequence of events is hemorrhage. The hemostatic dysregulation may also result in thromboses in the skin, kidneys, and other organs.

CLINICAL MANIFESTATIONS. Usually, DIC accompanies a severe systemic disease process. Bleeding frequently first occurs from sites of venipuncture or surgical incision. The skin may show petechiae and ecchymoses. Tissue necrosis may involve many organs and can be most spectacularly seen as infarction of large areas of skin, subcutaneous tissue, or kidneys. Anemia caused by hemolysis may develop rapidly owing to microangiopathic hemolytic anemia.

LABORATORY FINDINGS. There is no well-defined sequence of events. Certain coagulation factors (factors II, V, and VIII, and fibrinogen) and platelets may be consumed by the ongoing intravascular clotting process, with resultant prolongation of the prothrombin, partial thromboplastin, and thrombin times. Platelet counts may be profoundly depressed. The blood smear may contain fragmented, burr-, and helmet-shaped red blood cells (schistocytes). In addition, because the fibrinolytic mechanism is activated, fibrinogen degradation products (FDPs, D-dimers) appear in the blood. The D-dimer is formed by fibrinolysis of a cross-linked fibrin clot. The D-dimer assay is as sensitive as the FDP test and more specific for activation of coagulation and fibrinolysis.

TREATMENT. The first 2 steps in the treatment of DIC are the most critical: (1) treat the trigger that caused DIC and (2) restore normal homeostasis by correcting the shock, acidosis, and hypoxia that usually complicate DIC. If the underlying problem can be controlled, bleeding quickly ceases, and there is improvement of the abnormal laboratory findings. Blood components are used for replacement therapy in patients with hemorrhage. This may consist of platelet infusions (for thrombocytopenia), cryoprecipitate (for hypofibrinogenemia), and/or fresh frozen plasma (for replacement of other coagulation factors and natural inhibitors).

In DIC associated with sepsis, a controlled trial of drotrecogin-α (activated protein C concentrate [APC]) in adults with sepsis showed a statistically significant survival advantage in those

TABLE 483-1. Causes of Disseminated Intravascular Coagulation

INFECTIOUS
Meningococcemia (purpura fulminans)
Other gram-negative bacteria (*Haemophilus, Salmonella, Escherichia coli*)
Gram-positive bacteria (group B streptococci, staphylococci)
Rickettsia (Rocky Mountain spotted fever)
Virus (cytomegalovirus, herpes simplex, hemorrhagic fevers)
Malaria
Fungus
TISSUE INJURY
Central nervous system trauma (massive head injury)
Multiple fractures with fat emboli
Crush injury
Profound shock or asphyxia
Hypothermia or hyperthermia
Massive burns
MALIGNANCY
Acute promyelocytic leukemia
Acute monoblastic or myelocytic leukemia
Widespread malignancies (neuroblastoma)
VENOM OR TOXIN
Snake bites
Insect bites
MICROANGIOPATHIC DISORDERS
"Severe" thrombotic thrombocytopenic purpura or hemolytic-uremic syndrome
Giant hemangioma (Kasabach-Merritt syndrome)
GASTROINTESTINAL DISORDERS
Fulminant hepatitis
Severe inflammatory bowel disease
Pancreatitis
HEREDITARY THROMBOTIC DISORDERS
Antithrombin-III deficiency
Homozygous protein C deficiency
NEWBORN
Maternal toxemia
Group B streptococcal infections
Abruptio placentae
Severe respiratory distress syndrome
Necrotizing enterocolitis
Congenital viral disease (cytomegalovirus, herpes simplex)
Erythroblastosis fetalis
Fetal demise of a twin
MISCELLLANEOUS
Severe acute graft rejection
Acute hemolytic transfusion reaction
Severe collagen-vascular disease
Kawasaki disease
Heparin-induced thrombosis
Infusion of "activated" prothrombin complex concentrates
Hyperpyrexia/encephalopathy, hemorrhagic shock syndrome
Placental abruption

Modified from Montgomery RR, Scott JP: Hemostasis: Diseases of the fluid phase. In Nathan DG, Oski FA (editors): *Hematology of Infancy and Childhood*, 4th ed., Vol. 2. Philadelphia, WB Saunders, 1993.

treated with APC. Clinical trials using protein C concentrate in purpura fulminans and APC in children with sepsis syndrome have not shown a statistically significant improvement. The role of these agents in childhood remains to be defined.

The role of heparin in DIC is limited to patients who have vascular thrombosis in association with DIC. Such individuals should be treated as outlined in Chapter 479, with careful attention to replacement therapy to maintain an adequate platelet count and thus limit bleeding complications.

The prognosis of patients with DIC is primarily dependent on the outcome of the treatment of the primary disease and prevention of end-organ damage.

Bernard GR, Vincent JL, Laterre PF, et al: Efficacy and safety of recombinant human activated protein C or severe sepsis. *N Engl J Med* 2001;344:699–709.

Fourrier F: Recombinant human activated protein C in the treatment of severe sepsis: An evidence-based review. *Crit Care Med* 2004;32(11 Suppl):S534–S541.

Franchini M, Manzato F: Update on the treatment of disseminated intravascular coagulation. *Hematology* 2004;9:81–85.

Levi M, Ten Cate H: Disseminated intravascular coagulation. *N Engl J Med* 1999;341:586–592.

Liebman HA, Weitz IC: Disseminated intravascular coagulation. In Hoffman R, Benz EJ, Shattil SJ, et al (editors): *Hematology: Basic Principles and Practice*, 4th ed. Philadelphia, Elsevier Churchill Livingstone, 2005, pp 2169–2182.

Monagle P, Andrew M: Acquired disorders of hemostasis. In Nathan DG, Orkin SH, Ginsburg D, et al (editors): *Hematology of Infancy and Childhood*, 6th ed. Philadelphia, WB Saunders, 2003, pp 1631–1668.

Sparrow A, Willis F: Management of septic shock in childhood. *Emerg Med Australas* 2004;16:125–134.

Toh CH, Dennis M: Disseminated intravascular coagulation: Old disease, new hope. *BMJ* 2003;327:974–977.

Chapter 484 ■ Platelet and Blood Vessel Disorders

MEGAKARYOPOIESIS. Platelets are non-nucleated cellular fragments produced by megakaryocytes within the bone marrow and other tissues. Megakaryocytes are large polyploid cells. When the megakaryocyte approaches maturity, budding of the cytoplasm occurs and large numbers of platelets are liberated. Platelets circulate with a life span of 10–14 days. **Thrombopoietin** (TPO) is the primary growth factor that controls platelet production. Levels of TPO appear to correlate inversely with platelet number and megakaryocyte mass. Levels of TPO are highest in the thrombocytopenic states associated with decreased marrow megakaryopoiesis and may be variable in states of increased platelet production.

The platelet plays multiple hemostatic roles. The platelet surface possesses a number of important receptors for adhesive proteins, including von Willebrand factor (VWF) and fibrinogen, as well as receptors for agonists that trigger platelet aggregation, such as thrombin, collagen, and adenosine diphosphate (ADP). After injury to the blood vessel wall, subendothelial collagen binds VWF. VWF undergoes a conformational change that induces binding of the platelet glycoprotein Ib (GPIb) complex (the VWF receptor). This process is called *platelet adhesion*. Platelets then undergo activation. During the process of activation, the platelets generate thromboxane A_2 from arachidonic acid via the enzyme cyclo-oxygenase. After activation, they release agonists, such as ADP, adenosine triphosphate (ATP), Ca^{2+}, serotonin, and coagulation factors, into the surrounding milieu. Circulating fibrinogen binds to its receptor on the activated platelets, the glycoprotein IIb-IIIa (GPIIb-IIIa) complex, linking platelets together in a process called *aggregation*. This series of events forms a hemostatic plug at the site of vascular injury. The serotonin and histamine that are liberated during activation increase local vasoconstriction. In addition to acting in concert with the vessel wall to form the platelet plug, the platelet provides the catalytic surface on which coagulation factors assemble and eventually generate thrombin through a sequential series of enzymatic cleavages. Last, the platelet contractile proteins and cytoskeleton mediate clot retraction.

THROMBOCYTOPENIA. The normal platelet count is 150–450 × 10^9/L. *Thrombocytopenia* refers to a reduction in platelet count to <150 × 10^9/L. Causes of thrombocytopenia include: (1) decreased production on either a congenital or an acquired basis; (2) sequestration of the platelets within an enlarged spleen or other organ; and (3) increased destruction of normally synthesized platelets on either an immune or a nonimmune basis (see also Chapters 468, 469, and 483) [Tables 484-1 and 484-2 and Fig. 484-1].

TABLE 484-1. Differential Diagnosis of Thrombocytopenia in Children and Adolescents

DESTRUCTIVE THROMBOCYTOPENIAS
Primary Platelet Consumption Syndromes
- Immune thrombocytopenias
  - Acute and chronic ITP
  - Autoimmune diseases with chronic ITP as a manifestation
    - Cyclic thrombocytopenia
    - Autoimmune lymphoproliferative syndrome and its variants
    - Systemic lupus erythematosus
    - Evans syndrome
    - Antiphospholipid antibody syndrome
    - Neoplasia-associated immune thrombocytopenia
  - Thrombocytopenia associated with HIV
  - Neonatal immune thrombocytopenia
    - Alloimmune
    - Autoimmune (e.g., maternal ITP)
  - Drug-induced immune thrombocytopenia (including heparin-induced thrombocytopenia)
  - Post-transfusion purpura
  - Allergy and anaphylaxis
  - Post-transplant thrombocytopenia
- Nonimmune thrombocytopenias
  - Thrombocytopenia of infection
    - Bacteremia or fungemia
    - Viral infection
    - Protozoan
  - Thrombotic microangiopathic disorders
    - Hemolytic-uremic syndrome
    - Thrombotic thrombocytopenic purpura
    - Bone marrow transplantation–associated microangiopathy
    - Drug-induced
  - Platelets in contact with foreign material
  - Congenital heart disease
  - Drug-induced via direct platelet effects (ristocetin, protamine)
  - Type 2B VWD or platelet-type VWD

Combined Platelet and Fibrinogen Consumption Syndromes
- Disseminated intravascular coagulation
- Kasabach-Merritt syndrome
- Virus-associated hemophagocytic syndrome

IMPAIRED PLATELET PRODUCTION
- Hereditary disorders (see Chapter 40)
- Acquired disorders
  - Aplastic anemia
  - Myelodysplastic syndrome
  - Marrow infiltrative process
  - Osteopetrosis
  - Nutritional deficiency states (iron, folate, vitamin B_{12}, anorexia nervosa)
  - Drug- or radiation-induced thrombocytopenia
  - Neonatal hypoxia or placental insufficiency

SEQUESTRATION
- Hypersplenism
- Hypothermia
- Burns

HIV, human immunodeficiency virus; ITP, immune thrombocytopenic purpura; VWD, von Willebrand disease.
From Nathan DG, Orkin SH, Ginsburg D: *Nathan and Oskis Hematology of Infancy and Childhood*, 6th ed., Vol. 2. Philadelphia, WB Saunders, 2003, p 1598.

TABLE 484-2. Classification of Fetal and Neonatal Thrombocytopenias*

	CONDITION
Fetal	**Alloimmune condition**
	Congenital infection (e.g., CMV, toxoplasma, rubella, HIV)
	Aneuploidy (e.g., trisomy 18, 13, or 21, or triploidy)
	Autoimmune condition (e.g., ITP, SLE)
	Severe Rh hemolytic disease
	Congenital/inherited (e.g., Wiskott-Aldrich syndrome)
Early-onset neonatal (<72 hr)	**Placental insufficiency** (e.g., PET, IUGR, diabetes)
	Perinatal asphyxia
	Perinatal infection (e.g., *Escherichia coli*, GBS, *Haemophilus influenzae*),
	DIC
	Alloimmune condition
	Autoimmune condition (e.g., ITP, SLE)
	Congenital infection (e.g., CMV, toxoplasma, rubella, HIV)
	Thrombosis (e.g., aortic, renal vein)
	Bone marrow replacement (e.g., congenital leukemia)
	Kasabach-Merritt syndrome
	Metabolic disease (e.g., proprionic and methylmalonic acidemia)
	Congenital/inherited (e.g., TAR, CAMT)
Late-onset neonatal (>72 hr)	**Late-onset sepsis**
	NEC
	Congenital infection (e.g., CMV, toxoplasma, rubella, HIV)
	Autoimmune
	Kasabach-Merritt syndrome
	Metabolic disease (e.g., proprionic and methylmalonic acidemia)
	Congenital/inherited (e.g., TAR, CAMT)

CAMT, congenital amegakaryocytic thrombocytopenia; CMV, cytomegalovirus; DIC, disseminated intravascular coagulation; GBS, group B streptococcus; ITP, idiopathic thrombocytopenic purpura; IUGR, intrauterine growth restriction; NEC, necrotizing enterocolitis; PET, pre-eclampsia; SLE, systemic lupus erythematosus; TAR, thrombocytopenia with absent radii.
*The most common conditions are shown in bold.
From Roberts I, Murray NA: Neonatal thrombocytopenia: Causes and management. *Arch Dis Child Fetal Neonatal Ed* 2003;88:F359–F364.

484.1 • Idiopathic Thrombocytopenic Purpura

The most common cause of acute onset of thrombocytopenia in an otherwise well child is (autoimmune) idiopathic thrombocytopenic purpura (ITP).

ETIOLOGY. In a small number of children, 1–4 wk after exposure to a common viral infection, an autoantibody directed against the platelet surface develops. The exact antigenic target for most such antibodies in most cases of acute ITP remains undetermined. After binding of the antibody to the platelet surface, circulating antibody-coated platelets are recognized by the Fc receptor on the splenic macrophages, ingested, and destroyed. A recent history of viral illness is described in 50–65% of cases of childhood ITP. The reason why some children respond to a common infection with an autoimmune disease remains unknown. Most common infectious viruses have been described in association with ITP, including Epstein-Barr virus (see Chapter 251) and HIV (see Chapter 273). Epstein-Barr virus–related ITP is usually of short duration and follows the course of infectious mononucleosis. HIV-associated ITP is usually chronic.

CLINICAL MANIFESTATIONS. The classic presentation of ITP is that of a previously healthy 1–4 yr old child who has sudden onset of generalized petechiae and purpura. The parents often state that the child was fine yesterday and now is covered with bruises and purple dots. Often there is bleeding from the gums and mucous membranes, particularly with profound thrombocytopenia (platelet count <10 × 10^9/L). There is a history of a preceding viral infection 1–4 wk before the onset of thrombocytopenia. Findings on physical examination are normal, other than the finding of petechiae and purpura. Splenomegaly is rare, as is lym-

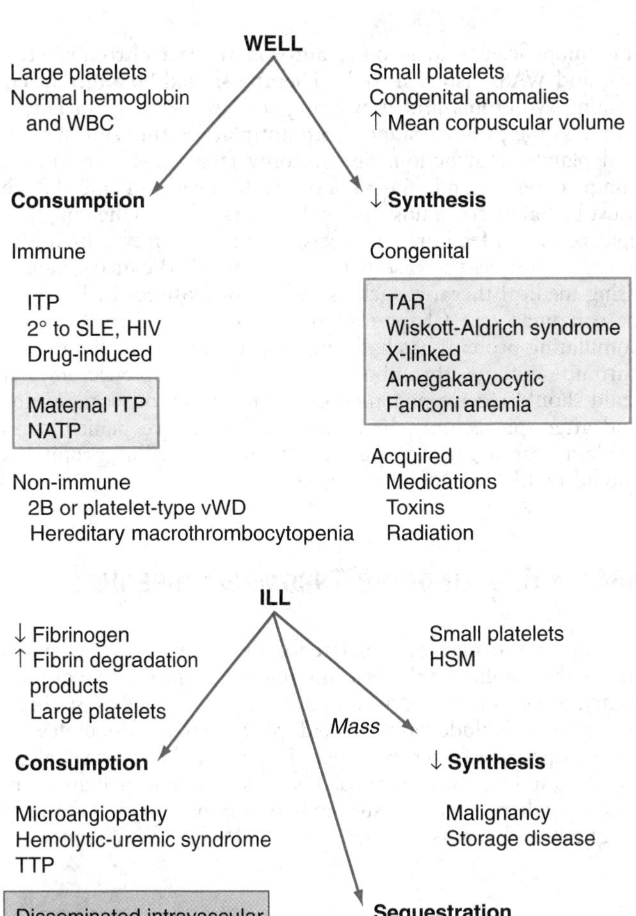

Figure 484-1. Differential diagnosis of childhood thrombocytopenic syndromes. The syndromes initially are separated by their clinical appearance. Clues leading to the diagnosis are shown in *italics*. The mechanisms and common disorders leading to these findings are shown in the *lower part* of the figure. Disorders that commonly affect neonates are listed in the *shaded boxes*. WBC, white blood cell; ITP, idiopathic immune thrombocytopenic purpura; SLE, systemic lupus erythematosus; NATP, neonatal alloimmune thrombocytopenic purpura; TAR, thrombocytopenia-absent radius; VWD, von Willebrand disease; HSM, hepatosplenomegaly; TTP, thrombotic thrombocytopenic purpura; UAC, umbilical artery catheter. (From Scott JP: Bleeding and thrombosis. In Kliegman RM [editor]: *Practical Strategies in Pediatric Diagnosis and Therapy*. Philadelphia, WB Saunders, 1996, p 849. From Kliegman RM, Marcdante KJ, Jenson HB, et al [editors]: *Nelson Essentials of Pediatrics*, 5th ed. Philadelphia, Elsevier/Saunders, 2006, p 716.)

phadenopathy or pallor. An easy to use classification system has been proposed from the U.K. to characterize the severity of bleeding in ITP on the basis of symptoms and signs, but not platelet count:

1. **No symptoms**
2. **Mild symptoms: bruising and petechiae, occasional minor epistaxis, very little interference with daily living**
3. **Moderate: more severe skin and mucosal lesions, more troublesome epistaxis and menorrhagia**
4. **Severe: bleeding episodes—menorrhagia, epistaxis, melena—requiring transfusion or hospitalization, symptoms interfering seriously with the quality of life**

The presence of abnormal findings, such as hepatosplenomegaly or remarkable lymphadenopathy, suggests other diagnoses (leukemia). When the onset is insidious, especially in an adolescent, chronic ITP or the possibility that thrombocytopenia is a manifestation of a systemic illness, such as systemic lupus erythematosus (SLE), is more likely.

In 70–80% of children who present with acute ITP, spontaneous resolution occurs within 6 mo. Therapy does not appear to affect the natural history of the illness. Fewer than 1% of patients have intracranial hemorrhage. Those who favor interventional therapy argue that the objective of early therapy is to raise the platelet count to $>20 \times 10^9$/L and prevent the rare development of intracranial hemorrhage. Approximately 20% of children who present with acute ITP go on to have chronic ITP.

LABORATORY FINDINGS. Severe thrombocytopenia (platelet count $<20 \times 10^9$/L) is common, and platelet size is normal or increased, reflective of increased platelet turnover. In acute ITP, the hemoglobin value, white blood cell (WBC) count, and differential count should be normal. Hemoglobin may be decreased if there have been profuse nosebleeds or menorrhagia. Bone marrow examination shows normal granulocytic and erythrocytic series, with characteristically normal or increased numbers of megakaryocytes. Some of the megakaryocytes may appear to be immature and are reflective of increased platelet turnover. **Indications for bone marrow** aspiration include an abnormal WBC count or differential or unexplained anemia as well as findings suggestive of bone marrow disease on history and physical examination. Other laboratory tests should be done as indicated by the history and physical examination. In adolescents with new-onset ITP, an antinuclear antibody test should be done to evaluate for SLE. HIV studies should be done in at-risk populations, especially sexually active teens. Platelet antibody testing is seldom useful in acute ITP. A Coombs test should be done if there is unexplained anemia to rule out Evans syndrome (autoimmune hemolytic anemia and thrombocytopenia) [see Chapter 464] or before instituting therapy with IV anti-D.

DIFFERENTIAL DIAGNOSIS. The well-appearing child with moderate to severe thrombocytopenia, an otherwise normal complete blood cell count (CBC), and normal findings on physical examination has a limited differential diagnosis that includes exposure to medication that induces drug-dependent antibodies, splenic sequestration due to previously unappreciated portal hypertension, and rarely, early aplastic processes, such as Fanconi anemia (see Chapter 468). Other than congenital syndromes, such as amegakaryocytic thrombocytopenia and thrombocytopenia-absent radius (TAR) syndrome, most marrow processes that interfere with platelet production also cause abnormal synthesis of red blood cells (RBCs) and WBCs and therefore manifest diverse abnormalities on the CBC. Disorders that cause increased platelet destruction on a nonimmune basis are usually serious systemic illnesses with obvious clinical findings (e.g., hemolytic-uremic syndrome [HUS], disseminated intravascular coagulation [DIC]) [see Table 484-1 and Fig. 484-1]. Isolated enlargement of the spleen suggests the potential for hypersplenism owing to either liver disease or portal vein thrombosis. Autoimmune thrombocytopenia may be an initial manifestation of SLE, HIV infection, or rarely, lymphoma. Wiskott-Aldrich syndrome (WAS; see Chapter 125.2) must be considered in young males found to have low platelet counts, particularly if there is a history of eczema and recurrent infection.

TREATMENT. There are no data showing that treatment affects either short- or long-term clinical outcome of ITP. Many patients with new-onset ITP have mild symptoms, with findings limited to petechiae and purpura on the skin, despite severe thrombocytopenia. Compared with untreated control subjects, treatment appears to be capable of inducing a more rapid rise in platelet count to the theoretically safe level of >20 × 10^9/L, although there are no data indicating that early therapy prevents intracranial hemorrhage. Antiplatelet antibodies bind to transfused platelets as well as they do to autologous platelets. Thus, platelet transfusion in ITP is usually contraindicated unless life-threatening bleeding is present. Initial approaches to the management of ITP include the following:

1. No therapy other than education and counseling of the family and patient for patients with minimal, mild, and moderate symptoms, as defined earlier. This approach emphasizes the usually benign nature of ITP and avoids the therapeutic roller coaster that ensues once interventional therapy is begun. This approach is far less costly, and side effects are minimal.
2. Intravenous immunoglobulin (IVIG). IVIG at a dose of 0.8–1.0 g/kg/day for 1–2 days induces a rapid rise in platelet count (usually >20 × 10^9/L) in 95% of patients within 48 hr. IVIG appears to induce a response by downregulating Fc-mediated phagocytosis of antibody-coated platelets. IVIG therapy is both expensive and time-consuming to administer. Additionally, after infusion, there is a high frequency of headaches and vomiting, suggestive of IVIG-induced aseptic meningitis.
3. Intravenous anti-D therapy. For Rh positive patients, IV anti-D at a dose of 50–75 µg/kg causes a rise in platelet count to >20 × 10^9/L in 80–90% of patients within 48–72 hr. When given to Rh positive individuals, IV anti-D induces mild hemolytic anemia. RBC-antibody complexes bind to macrophage Fc receptors and interfere with platelet destruction, thereby causing a rise in platelet count. IV anti-D is ineffective in Rh negative patients.
4. Prednisone. Corticosteroid therapy has been used for many years to treat acute and chronic ITP in adults and children. Doses of prednisone of 1–4 mg/kg/24 hr appear to induce a more rapid rise in platelet count than in untreated patients with ITP. Whether bone marrow examination should be performed to rule out other causes of thrombocytopenia, especially acute lymphoblastic leukemia, before institution of prednisone therapy in acute ITP is controversial. Corticosteroid therapy is usually continued for 2–3 wk or until a rise in platelet count to >20 × 10^9/L has been achieved, with a rapid taper to avoid the long-term side effects of corticosteroid therapy, especially growth failure, diabetes mellitus, and osteoporosis.

Each of these medications may be used to treat exacerbations of ITP, which commonly occur several wk after an initial course of therapy.

In the special case of intracranial hemorrhage, multiple modalities should be used, including platelet transfusion, IVIG, high-dose corticosteroids, and prompt surgical consultation, with plans for emergency splenectomy.

Currently, there is no consensus regarding the management of acute childhood ITP. The American Society of Hematology has published treatment guidelines for adults with ITP, but there is significant disagreement within the field. The only consensus is that patients who are bleeding significantly should be treated, and these may represent only 5% of children with ITP. Intracranial hemorrhage remains rare, and there are no data showing that treatment actually reduces its incidence.

The role of splenectomy in ITP should be reserved for 1 of 2 circumstances. The older child (≥ 4 yr) with severe ITP that has lasted >1 yr (chronic ITP) and whose symptoms are not easily controlled with therapy is a candidate for splenectomy. Splenectomy must also be considered when life-threatening hemorrhage (intracranial hemorrhage) complicates acute ITP, if the platelet count cannot be corrected rapidly with transfusion of platelets and administration of IVIG and corticosteroids. Splenectomy is associated with a lifelong risk of overwhelming postsplenectomy infection caused by encapsulated organisms.

CHRONIC IDIOPATHIC THROMBOCYTOPENIC PURPURA. Approximately 20% of patients who present with acute ITP have persistent thrombocytopenia for **>6 mo** and are said to have chronic ITP. At that time, a careful re-evaluation for associated disorders should be performed, especially for autoimmune disease, such as SLE; chronic infectious disorders, such as HIV; and nonimmune causes of chronic thrombocytopenia, such as type 2B and platelet-type von Willebrand disease, X-linked thrombocytopenia, autoimmune lymphoproliferative syndrome, common variable immunodeficiency syndrome, autosomal macrothrombocytopenia, and WAS (also X-linked). Therapy should be aimed at controlling symptoms and preventing serious bleeding. In ITP, the spleen is the primary site of both antiplatelet antibody synthesis and platelet destruction. Splenectomy is successful in inducing complete remission in 64–88% of children with chronic ITP. This must be balanced against the lifelong risk of overwhelming postsplenectomy infection. This decision is often affected by lifestyle issues as well as the ease with which the child can be managed using medical therapy, such as IVIG, corticosteroids, IV anti-D, or rituximab (see Chapter 464). AMG 531, a thrombopoiesis-stimulating protein, has had some success in treating adults with chronic immune thrombocytopenia. Before splenectomy, the child should receive pneumococcal and meningococcal vaccines, and after splenectomy, he or she should receive penicillin prophylaxis for a number of yr. Whether penicillin prophylaxis should be lifelong is controversial.

484.2 • Drug-Induced Thrombocytopenia

A number of drugs are associated with immune thrombocytopenia as the result of either an immune process or megakaryocyte injury. Some common drugs used in pediatrics that cause thrombocytopenia include valproic acid, phenytoin, sulfonamides, and trimethoprim-sulfamethoxazole. Heparin-induced thrombocytopenia (and rarely, thrombosis) is seldom seen in pediatrics, but it occurs when, after exposure to heparin, the patient has an antibody directed against the heparin-platelet factor 4 complex.

484.3 • Nonimmune Platelet Destruction

The syndromes of DIC (see Chapter 483), HUS (see Chapter 518), and thrombotic thrombocytopenic purpura (TTP) share the hematologic picture of a thrombotic microangiopathy in which there is RBC destruction and consumptive thrombocytopenia caused by platelet and fibrin deposition in the microvasculature. The microangiopathic hemolytic anemia is characterized by the presence of RBC fragments, including helmet cells, schistocytes, spherocytes, and burr cells.

484.4 • Hemolytic-Uremic Syndrome

See also Chapter 518. HUS, an acute disease of infancy and early childhood, usually follows an episode of acute gastroenteritis, often triggered by *Escherichia coli* 0157:H7. Shortly thereafter, signs and symptoms of hemolytic anemia, thrombocytopenia, and acute renal failure ensue. Sometimes neurologic symptoms are associated with these findings. *E. coli* 0157:H7 produces a specific toxin (verotoxin) that binds to and damages renal endothelial cells preferentially.

The hemolytic anemia is characterized by morphologically abnormal RBCs, with the presence of helmet cells, spherocytes, schistocytes, burr cells, and other distorted forms. Thrombocytopenia despite normal numbers of megakaryocytes in the marrow indicates excessive platelet destruction. Results of tests for DIC are usually normal, except for elevated levels of D-dimer. Evaluation of the urine shows protein, RBCs, and casts. Anuria and severe azotemia indicate grave renal damage. Treatment of most cases of HUS involves institution of careful fluid management and prompt appropriate dialysis. Treatment using plasmapheresis is usually reserved for patients with HUS associated with major neurologic complications.

484.5 • Thrombotic Thrombocytopenic Purpura

Thrombotic thrombocytopenic purpura (TTP) is a rare pentad of **fever, microangiopathic hemolytic anemia, thrombocytopenia, abnormal renal function,** and **central nervous system changes** that is clinically similar to HUS, although TTP usually presents in adults and occasionally in adolescents. Microvascular thrombi within the central nervous system cause subtle, shifting neurologic signs that vary from changes in affect and orientation to aphasia, blindness, and seizures. Initial manifestations are often nonspecific (weakness, pain, emesis); prompt recognition of this disorder is critical. **Laboratory findings** provide important clues to the diagnosis and show microangiopathic hemolytic anemia characterized by morphologically abnormal RBCs, with schistocytes, spherocytes, helmet cells, and an elevated reticulocyte count in association with thrombocytopenia. Coagulation studies are usually nondiagnostic. Blood urea nitrogen and creatinine are usually elevated. The treatment of TTP is plasmapheresis (plasma exchange), which is effective in 80–95% of cases. Corticosteroids and splenectomy are reserved for refractory cases.

The majority of cases of TTP are caused by an acquired deficiency of a metalloproteinase (ADAMTS-13) that is responsible for cleaving the high molecular weight multimers of VWF and appears to play a pivotal role in the evolution of the thrombotic microangiopathy. In contrast, levels of the metalloproteinase in HUS are usually normal. Congenital deficiency of the metalloproteinase causes rare familial cases of TTP, usually manifested as recurrent episodes of thrombocytopenia and hemolytic anemia, with or without neurologic changes that often present in infancy. The deficiency can be treated by repeated infusions of fresh frozen plasma.

484.6 • Kasabach-Merritt Syndrome

See also Chapter 505. The association of a giant hemangioma with localized intravascular coagulation causing thrombocytopenia and hypofibrinogenemia is called *Kasabach-Merritt syndrome.* In most patients, the site of the hemangioma is obvious, but retroperitoneal and intra-abdominal hemangiomas may require body imaging for detection. Inside the hemangioma there is platelet trapping and activation of coagulation, with fibrinogen consumption and generation of fibrin(ogen) degradation products. Arteriovenous malformation within the lesions can cause heart failure. Some authors contend that Kasabach-Merritt syndrome is really a kaposiform hemangioendothelioma rather than a simple hemangioma. The peripheral blood smear shows microangiopathic changes. Multiple modalities have been used to treat Kasabach-Merritt syndrome, including surgical excision (if possible), laser photocoagulation, high-dose corticosteroids, local radiation therapy, and antiangiogenic agents, such as interferon-α_2. Over time, most patients who present in infancy have regression of the hemangioma. Treatment of the associated coagulopathy may benefit from a trial of antifibrinolytic therapy with ε-aminocaproic acid (Amicar).

484.7 • Sequestration

Thrombocytopenia develops in individuals with massive splenomegaly because the spleen acts as a sponge for platelets and sequesters large numbers. Most such patients also have mild leukopenia and anemia on CBC. Individuals who have thrombocytopenia caused by splenic sequestration should undergo a work-up to diagnose the etiology of splenomegaly, including infectious, inflammatory, infiltrative, neoplastic, obstructive, and hemolytic causes.

484.8 • Congenital Thrombocytopenic Syndromes

See Table 484-2. **Congenital amegakaryocytic thrombocytopenia** is caused by a rare defect in hematopoiesis that usually manifests within the first few days to wk of life, when the child presents with petechiae and purpura caused by profound thrombocytopenia. Other than skin and mucous membrane findings, findings on physical examination are normal. Examination of the bone marrow shows an absence of megakaryocytes. These patients often progress to marrow failure (aplasia) over time. Amegakaryocytic thrombocytopenia is caused by a mutation in the stem cell TPO receptor that is essential for the development of all hematopoietic cell lines. Bone marrow transplantation is curative.

Thrombocytopenia-absent radius (TAR) syndrome consists of thrombocytopenia (absence or hypoplasia of megakaryocytes) that presents in early infancy with bilateral radial anomalies of variable severity, ranging from mild changes to marked limb shortening (Fig. 484-2). Many such individuals also have other skeletal abnormalities of the ulna, radius, and lower extremities. Thumbs are present. Intolerance to cow's milk formula (present in 50%) may complicate management by triggering gastrointestinal bleeding, increased thrombocytopenia, eosinophilia, and a leukemoid reaction. The thrombocytopenia of TAR syndrome frequently remits over the first few yr of life. The molecular basis of TAR syndrome remains to be defined, but is suggestive of an autosomal recessive disorder.

Wiskott-Aldrich syndrome (WAS) is characterized by thrombocytopenia, with tiny platelets, eczema, and recurrent infection due to immune deficiency (see Chapter 125.2). WAS is inherited as an X-linked disorder, and the gene for WAS has been sequenced. The WAS protein appears to play an integral role in regulating the cytoskeletal architecture of both platelets and T lymphocytes in response to receptor-mediated cell signaling. The WAS protein is common to all cells of hematopoietic lineage. Molecular analysis of families with X-linked thrombocytopenia has shown that many affected members have a point mutation within the WAS gene, whereas individuals with the full manifestation of WAS have large gene deletions. Examination of the bone marrow in WAS shows the normal number of megakaryocytes, although they may have bizarre morphologic features. Transfused platelets have a normal life span. Splenectomy often corrects the thrombocytopenia, suggesting that the platelets formed in WAS have accelerated destruction. After splenectomy, these patients are at increased risk for overwhelming infection and require lifelong antibiotic prophylaxis against encapsulated organisms. Approximately 5% of patients with WAS develop lymphoreticular malignancies. Successful bone marrow transplantation cures WAS.

A diverse number of **hereditary thrombocytopenia syndromes,** given names such as Sebastian, Epstein, May-Hegglin, and Fechtner syndromes, are characterized by autosomal dominant macrothrombocytopenia, neutrophil inclusion bodies, and a variety of physical anomalies, including deafness, renal disease, and/or eye disease. These have all been shown to be due to different mutations in the nonmuscle myosin heavy chain 9 gene. Some other individuals with recessively inherited macrothrombocytopenia have abnormalities in chromosome 22q11. The thrombocytopenia is usually mild and is not progressive.

484.9 • Neonatal Thrombocytopenia

See also Chapter 103.4. Thrombocytopenia in the newborn rarely is indicative of a primary disorder of megakaryopoiesis, but more often is the result of either systemic illness or transfer of mater-

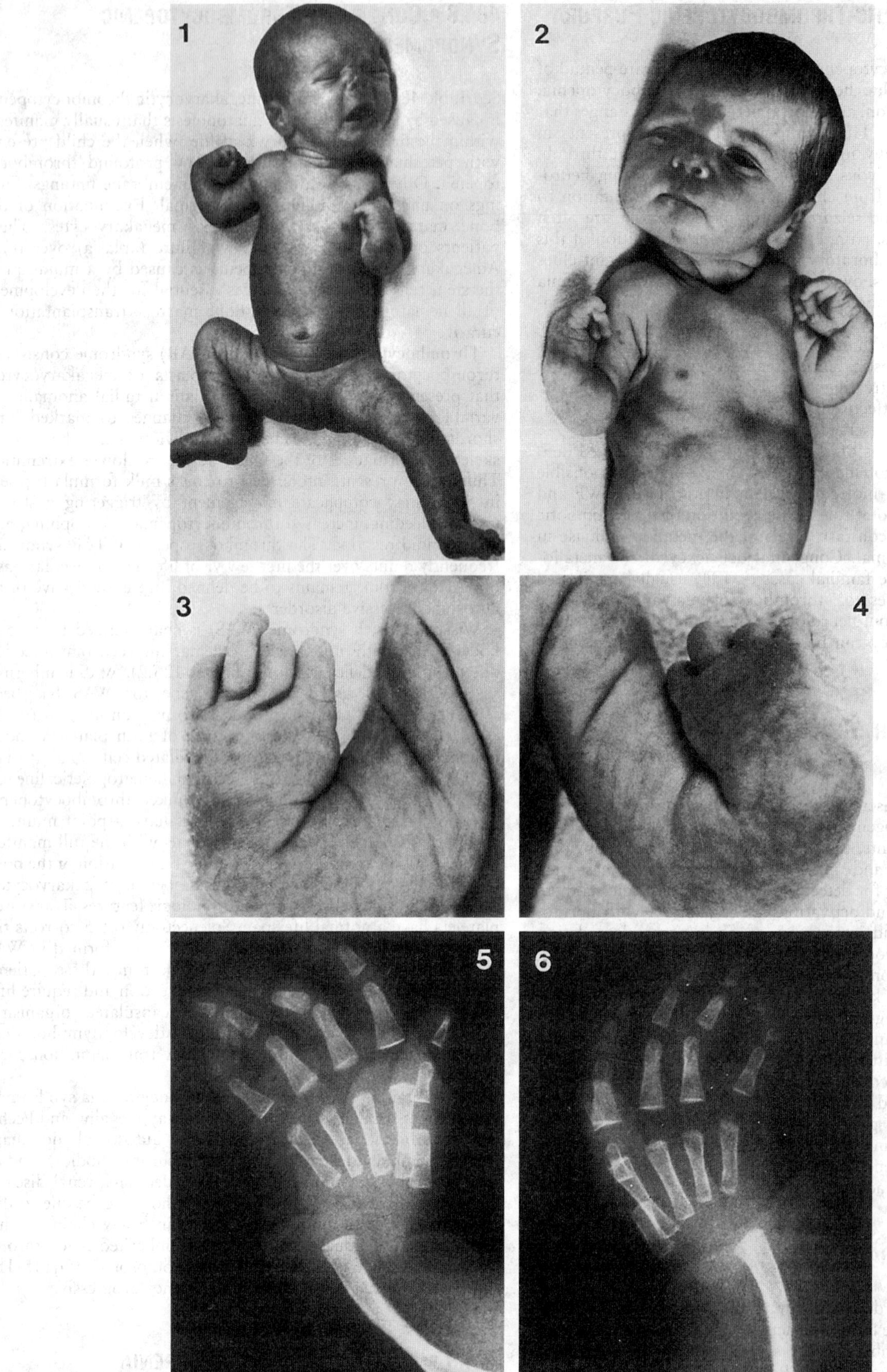

Figure 484-2. A newborn, the 1st child of young, healthy parents, with fully expressed thrombocytopenia-absent radius syndrome, including thrombocytopenia, hypereosinophilia, and anemia. Hypoplasia of the distal humeri and the shoulder girdles, bilateral hip dysplasia, mild talipes calcaneus, and clinodactyly of both little fingers are seen. This patient had a pronounced allergy to cow's milk, with exposure followed by diarrhea, vomiting, and decreased weight and platelet count, making a cow's milk–free diet mandatory. A persistent depressed nasal bridge and development of pronounced bowed legs are seen. (From Wiedemann H-R, Kunze J, Grosse F-R [editors]: *Clinical Syndromes,* 3rd ed. [English translation]. London, Mosby-Wolfe, 1997, p 430.)

nal antibodies directed against fetal platelets (see Table 484-2). Thrombocytopenia may occur in various fetal and neonatal infections and may be responsible for severe spontaneous bleeding. Neonatal thrombocytopenia often occurs in association with congenital viral infection, especially rubella and cytomegalovirus; protozoal infection, such as toxoplasmosis; syphilis; and bacterial infection, especially those caused by gram-negative bacilli. The constellation of marked thrombocytopenia and abnormal abdominal findings is common in necrotizing enterocolitis and other causes of necrotic bowel. Thrombocytopenia in an ill child requires a prompt search for viral and bacterial pathogens.

Antibody-mediated thrombocytopenia in the newborn occurs because of transplacental transfer of maternal antibodies directed against fetal platelets. Neonatal alloimmune thrombocytopenic purpura (NATP) is caused by the development of maternal antibodies against antigens present on fetal platelets that are shared with the father and recognized as foreign by the maternal immune system. This is the platelet equivalent of Rh disease of the newborn. The incidence of NATP is 1/4,000–5,000 live births. The clinical manifestations of NATP are those of an apparently well child who, within the 1st few days after delivery, has generalized petechiae and purpura. Laboratory studies show a normal maternal platelet count, yet moderate to severe thrombocytopenia in the newborn. Detailed review of the history should show no evidence of maternal thrombocytopenia. Up to 30% of infants with severe NATP may have intracranial hemorrhage, either prenatally or in the perinatal period. Unlike Rh disease, first pregnancies may be severely affected. Subsequent pregnancies may be even more severely affected than the first.

The **diagnosis** of NATP is made by checking for the presence of maternal alloantibodies directed against the father's platelets. Specific studies can be done to identify the target alloantigen. The most common cause is incompatibility for the platelet alloantigen HPA-1a. Specific DNA sequence polymorphisms have been identified that permit informative prenatal testing to identify at-risk pregnancies. The differential diagnosis of NATP includes transplacental transfer of maternal antiplatelet autoantibodies (maternal ITP), and more commonly, viral or bacterial infection.

Treatment of NATP requires the administration of IVIG prenatally to the mother. Therapy usually begins in the 2nd trimester and is continued throughout the pregnancy. Fetal platelet count can be monitored by percutaneous umbilical blood sampling. Delivery should be performed by cesarean section. After delivery, if severe thrombocytopenia persists, transfusion of 1 unit of platelets that share the maternal alloantigens (e.g., washed maternal platelets) will cause a rise in platelet counts to provide effective hemostasis. After there has been 1 affected child, genetic counseling is critical to inform the parents of the high risk of thrombocytopenia in subsequent pregnancies.

Children born to mothers with ITP (**maternal ITP**) appear to have a lower risk of serious hemorrhage than infants born with NATP, although severe thrombocytopenia occurs. The mother's pre-existing platelet count may have some predictive value in that severe maternal thrombocytopenia before delivery appears to predict a higher risk of fetal thrombocytopenia. In mothers who have had splenectomy for ITP, the maternal platelet count may be normal and is not predictive of fetal thrombocytopenia.

Treatment includes prenatal administration of corticosteroids to the mother and administration of IVIG and sometimes corticosteroids to the infant after delivery. Thrombocytopenia in an infant, whether due to NATP or maternal ITP, usually resolves within 2–4 mo after delivery. The period of highest risk is the immediate perinatal period.

Two syndromes of congenital failure of platelet production often present in the newborn period. In **amegakaryocytic thrombocytopenia,** the newborn manifests petechiae and purpura shortly after birth. Findings on physical examination are otherwise normal. Megakaryocytes are absent from the bone marrow. This syndrome is caused by a mutation in the megakaryocyte TPO receptor that is essential for development of all hematopoietic cell lines. Pancytopenia eventually develops, and hematopoietic stem cell transplantation is curative. **TAR syndrome** consists of thrombocytopenia that presents in early infancy, with bilateral radial anomalies of variable severity, ranging from mild changes to marked limb shortening. Thumbs are present. In many such individuals, there are also other skeletal abnormalities of the lower extremities. Intolerance to cow's milk formula is present in 50% of patients. TAR syndrome frequently remits over the first few yr of life (see Chapter 484.8) [see Fig. 484-2].

484.10 • Thrombocytopenia Due to Acquired Disorders Causing Decreased Production

Disorders of the bone marrow that inhibit megakaryopoiesis usually affect RBC and WBC production. Infiltrative disorders, including malignancies, such as acute lymphocytic leukemia, histiocytosis, lymphomas, and storage disease, usually cause either abnormalities on physical examination (lymphadenopathy, hepatosplenomegaly, or masses) or abnormalities of the WBC count, or anemia. Aplastic processes may present as isolated thrombocytopenia, although there are usually clues on the CBC (leukopenia, neutropenia, anemia, or macrocytosis). Children with constitutional aplastic anemia (Fanconi anemia) often have abnormalities on examination, including radial anomalies, other skeletal anomalies, short stature, microcephaly, and hyperpigmentation. Bone marrow examination should be done when thrombocytopenia is associated with abnormalities found on physical examination or on examination of the other blood cell lines.

484.11 • Platelet Function Disorders

Bleeding time and the platelet function analyzer (PFA-100) are the only commonly available tests to screen for abnormal platelet function. Bleeding time measures the interaction of platelets with the blood vessel wall and thus is affected by both platelet count and platelet function. The predictive value of bleeding time is problematic because bleeding time is dependent on a number of other factors, including the skill of the technician and the cooperation of the patient. A normal bleeding time does not rule out a mild platelet function defect in a clinically symptomatic individual. The PFA-100 measures platelet adhesion and aggregation in whole blood at high shear when the blood is exposed to either collagen-epinephrine or collagen-ADP. Results are reported as the closure time measured in sec. The PFA-100 appears to be more sensitive than bleeding time, and many clinical laboratories have replaced bleeding time with the use of the PFA-100. Although the PFA-100 value is prolonged in VWD as well as in congenital and acquired platelet function defects, the use of the PFA-100 as a screening test remains controversial. Both bleeding time and the PFA-100 detect moderate to severe von Willebrand disease and platelet function defects. Both are variably insensitive to mild platelet function abnormalities. Bleeding time is the only commonly available test to assess platelet-vessel wall interaction.

Platelet function in the clinical laboratory is currently measured using platelet aggregometry. In the aggregometer, agonists, such as collagen, ADP, ristocetin, arachidonic acid, and thrombin, are added to platelet-rich plasma, and the clumping of platelets over time is measured by an automated machine. At the same time, other instruments measure the release of granular contents, such as ATP, from the platelets after activation. The ability of platelets to aggregate and their metabolic activity can be assessed simultaneously.

484.12 • Acquired Disorders of Platelet Function

A number of systemic illnesses are associated with platelet dysfunction, most commonly, liver disease, kidney disease (uremia), and disorders that trigger increased amounts of fibrin degradation products. These disorders frequently cause prolonged bleeding time and are often associated with other abnormalities of the coagulation mechanism. The most important element of management is to treat the primary illness. If treatment of the primary process is not feasible, infusions of desmopressin have been helpful in augmenting hemostasis and correcting bleeding time. In some patients, transfusions of platelets and/or cryoprecipitate have also been helpful in improving hemostasis.

Many drugs alter platelet function. The most commonly used drug in adults that alters platelet function is acetylsalicylic acid (aspirin). Aspirin irreversibly acetylates the enzyme cyclo-oxygenase, which is critical in the formation of thromboxane A_2. Aspirin usually causes moderate platelet dysfunction that becomes more prominent if there is another abnormality of the hemostatic mechanism. Other commonly used drugs that affect platelet function include other nonsteroidal anti-inflammatory drugs, valproic acid, and high-dose penicillin. When a patient is being evaluated for possible platelet dysfunction, it is critically important to exclude the presence of other exogenous agents and to study the patient, if possible, off all medications for 2 wk.

484.13 • Congenital Abnormalities of Platelet Function

Severe platelet function defects usually present with petechiae and purpura shortly after birth, especially after vaginal delivery. Defects in the platelet GPIb complex (the VWF receptor) or the GPIIb-IIIa complex (the fibrinogen receptor) cause severe congenital platelet dysfunction.

Bernard-Soulier syndrome, a severe congenital platelet function disorder, is caused by absence or severe deficiency of the VWF receptor (GPIb complex) on the platelet membrane. This syndrome is characterized by thrombocytopenia, with giant platelets and markedly prolonged bleeding time (>20 min). Platelet aggregation tests show absent ristocetin-induced platelet aggregation, but normal aggregation to all other agonists. Ristocetin induces the binding of VWF to platelets and agglutinates platelets. Results of studies of VWF are normal. The GPIb complex interacts with the platelet cytoskeleton; a defect in this interaction is believed to be the cause of the large platelet size. Bernard-Soulier syndrome is inherited as an autosomal recessive disorder. Genetic mutations causing Bernard-Soulier syndrome are usually identified in the genes forming the GPIb complex of glycoproteins IBα, IBβ, and IX.

Glanzmann thrombasthenia is a congenital disorder associated with severe platelet dysfunction that yields prolonged bleeding time and a normal platelet count. Platelets have normal size and morphologic features on the peripheral blood smear, and bleeding time is markedly prolonged. Aggregation studies show abnormal or absent aggregation with all agonists used except ristocetin, because ristocetin agglutinates platelets and does not require a metabolically active platelet. This disorder is caused by deficiency of the platelet fibrinogen receptor GPIIb-IIIa, an integrin complex on the platelet surface that undergoes conformational changes when platelets are activated. Fibrinogen binds to this complex when the platelet is activated and causes platelets to aggregate. Caused by identifiable mutations in the genes for GPIIb or GPIIIa, this disorder is inherited in an autosomal recessive manner.

Hereditary deficiency of platelet storage granules occurs in 2 well-characterized, but rare syndromes that involve deficiency of intracytoplasmic granules. **Dense body deficiency** is characterized by absence of the granules that contain ADP, ATP, Ca^{2+}, and serotonin. This disorder is diagnosed by the finding that ATP is not released on platelet aggregation studies and ideally is characterized by electron microscopic studies. **Gray platelet syndrome** is caused by the absence of platelet α granules, resulting in platelets that appear gray on Wright stain of peripheral blood. In this rare syndrome, aggregation and release are absent with most agonists other than thrombin and ristocetin. Electron microscopic studies are diagnostic.

OTHER HEREDITARY DISORDERS OF PLATELET FUNCTION. Abnormalities in the pathways of platelet activation and release of granular contents cause a heterogeneous group of platelet function defects that are usually manifested as increased bruising, epistaxis, and/or menorrhagia. Symptoms may be subtle and are often made more obvious by high-risk surgery, such as tonsillectomy or adenoidectomy, or by administration of nonsteroidal anti-inflammatory drugs. In the laboratory, bleeding time is variable and closure time as measured by the PFA-100 is frequently, but not always, prolonged. Platelet aggregation studies show deficient aggregation with 1 or 2 agonists and/or abnormal release of granular contents.

The formation of thromboxane from arachidonic acid after the activation of phospholipase is critical to normal platelet function. Deficiency or dysfunction of enzymes, such as cyclo-oxygenase and thromboxane synthase, which metabolize arachidonic acid, causes abnormal platelet function. In the aggregometer, platelets from such patients do not aggregate in response to arachidonic acid.

The most common platelet function defects are those characterized by variable bleeding time and abnormal aggregation with 1 or 2 agonists, usually ADP and/or collagen. These patients have normal aggregation with thrombin. Some of these individuals have only decreased release of ATP from intracytoplasmic granules. This selective release defect is a common cause of mild platelet function defects.

TREATMENT OF PLATELET FUNCTION DEFECTS. Successful treatment depends on the severity of both the diagnosis and the hemorrhagic event. In all but severe platelet function defects, desmopressin 0.3 μg/kg IV may be used for mild to moderate bleeding episodes. In addition to its effect on stimulating levels of VWF and factor VIII, desmopressin corrects bleeding time and provides normal hemostasis in many individuals with mild to moderate platelet function defects. For individuals with Bernard-Soulier syndrome or Glanzmann thrombasthenia, platelet transfusions of 1 U/5–10 kg corrects the defect in hemostasis and may be lifesaving. Rarely, antibodies develop to the deficient platelet protein, rendering the patient refractory to the transfused platelets. In such patients, the off labeled use of recombinant factor VIIa has been effective, and this treatment is undergoing clinical trials. In both conditions, stem cell transplantation would be expected to be curative.

484.14 • Disorders of the Blood Vessels

HENOCH-SCHÖNLEIN PURPURA. Henoch-Schönlein purpura (HSP) is characterized by the sudden development of a purpuric rash, arthritis, abdominal pain, and renal involvement (see Chapter 166.1). The characteristic rash, consisting of petechiae and often palpable purpura, usually involves the lower extremities and buttocks. Results of coagulation studies are normal. The pathologic lesions in the skin, intestines, and synovium are leukocytoclastic angiitis, inflammatory damage to the endothelium of the capillary and postcapillary venules mediated by WBCs and macrophages. The trigger for HSP is unknown. In the kidney, the lesion is focal glomerulonephritis with deposition of immunoglobulin A. Results of coagulation studies as well as platelet count are normal in HSP.

EHLERS-DANLOS SYNDROME. Ehlers-Danlos syndrome is a common disorder of collagen structure that causes easy bruising and poor wound healing (see Chapter 658). Suggestive findings on physical examination include soft, velvety skin that is hyperelastic; lax joints that are easily subluxed; and unusual scarring. More than 10 variants of Ehlers-Danlos syndrome have been described. The most serious forms have been associated with sudden rupture of visceral organs. Results of coagulation screening tests are usually normal, although bleeding time may be mildly prolonged. Results of platelet aggregation studies are either normal or mildly abnormal, with deficient aggregation to collagen.

ACQUIRED DISORDERS. Scurvy, chronic corticosteroid therapy, and severe malnutrition are associated with "weakening" of the collagen matrix that supports the blood vessels. Therefore, these factors are associated with easy bruising, and particularly in the case of scurvy, bleeding gums and loosening of the teeth. Lesions of the skin that initially appear to be petechiae and purpura may be seen in vasculitic syndromes, such as SLE.

Andrews RK, Berndt MC: Platelet physiology and thrombosis. *Thromb Res* 2004;114:447–453.
Aronis S, Platokouki H, Avgeri M, et al: Retrospective evaluation of long-term efficacy and safety of splenectomy in chronic idiopathic thrombocytopenic purpura in children. *Acta Paediatr* 2004;93:638–642.
Beck CE, Nathan PC, Parkin PC, et al: Corticosteroids versus intravenous immune globulin for the treatment of acute immune thrombocytopenic purpura in children: A systematic review and meta-analysis of randomized controlled trials. *J Pediatr* 2005;147:521–527.
Bengston KL, Skinner MA, Ware RE: Successful use of anti-CD20 (rituximab) in severe, life-threatening childhood immune thrombocytopenic purpura. *J Pediatr* 2003;143:67–73.
Blanchette V: Childhood chronic immune thrombocytopenic purpura (ITP). *Blood Rev* 2002;16:23–26.
Bussel JB, Kuter DJ, George JN, et al: AMG 531, a thrombopoiesis-stimulating protein, for chronic ITP. *N Engl J Med* 2006;355:1672–1681.
Bussel JB, Zabusky MR, Berkowitz RL, et al: Fetal alloimmune thrombocytopenia. *N Engl J Med* 1997;337:22–26.
Coppo P, Bengoufa D, Veyradier A, et al: Severe ADAMTS13 deficiency in adult idiopathic thrombotic microangiopathies defines a subset of patients characterized by various autoimmune manifestations, lower platelet count, and mild renal involvement. *Medicine (Baltimore)* 2004;83:233–244.
de Alarcon PA: Immune or idiopathic thrombocytopenic purpura (ITP) in childhood: What are the risks and who should be treated? *J Pediatr* 2003;143:287–289.
de Paepe A, Malfait F: Bleeding and bruising in patients with Ehlers-Danlos syndrome and other collagen vascular disorders. *Br J Haematol* 2004;127:491–500.
Geddis AE, Kaushansky K: Inherited thrombocytopenias: Toward a molecular understanding of disorders of platelet production. *Curr Opin Pediatr* 2004;16:15–22.
Horton TM, Stone JD, Yee D, et al: Case series of thrombotic thrombocytopenic purpura in children and adolescent. *J Pediatr Hematol Oncol* 2003;25:336–339.
Iyori H, Bessho F, Ookawa H, et al: Intracranial hemorrhage in children with immune thrombocytopenic purpura: Japanese Study Group on Childhood ITP. *Ann Hematol* 2000;79:691–695.
Kokame K, Miyata T: Genetic defects leading to hereditary thrombotic thrombocytopenic purpura. *Semin Hematol* 2004;41:34–40.
Kuhne T, Buchanan GR, Zimmerman S, et al: A prospective comparative study of 2,540 infants and children with newly diagnosed idiopathic thrombocytopenic purpura (ITP) from the Intercontinental Childhood ITP Study Group. *J Pediatr* 2003;143:605–608.
Posan E, McBane RD, Grill DE, et al: Comparison of PFA-100 testing and bleeding time for detecting platelet hypofunction and von Willebrand disease in clinical practice. *Thromb Haemost* 2003;90:483–490.
Ramasamy I: Inherited bleeding disorders: Disorders of platelet adhesion and aggregation. *Crit Rev Oncol Hematol* 2004;49:1–35.
Roberts I, Murray NA: Neonatal thrombocytopenia: Causes and management. *Arch Dis Child Fetal Neonatal Ed* 2003;88:F359–F364.
Seri M, Pecci A, Di BF, et al: MYH9-related disease: May-Hegglin anomaly, Sebastian syndrome, Fechtner syndrome, and Epstein syndrome are not distinct entities but represent a variable expression of a single illness. *Medicine (Baltimore)* 2003;82:203–215.
Snapper SB, Rosen FS: A family of WASPs. *N Engl J Med* 2003;348:350–351.
Tarrantino MD, Young G, Bertolone SJ, et al: Single dose of anti-D immune globulin at 75 µg/kg is as effective as intravenous immune globulin at rapidly raising the platelet count in newly diagnosed immune thrombocytopenic purpura in children. *J Pediatr* 2006;148:489–494.
Wang J, Wiley JM, Luddy R, et al: Chronic immune thrombocytopenic purpura in children: Assessment of rituximab treatment. *J Pediatr* 2005; 146:217–221.

Section 8 — The Spleen — Bruce M. Camitta

Chapter 485 ■ Anatomy and Function of the Spleen

ANATOMY. The splenic precursor is recognizable by 5 wk of gestation. At birth, the spleen weighs approximately 11 g. Thereafter, it enlarges until puberty, reaching an average weight of 135 g before diminishing in size during adulthood. The major splenic components are a lymphoid compartment (*white pulp*) and a filtering system (*red pulp*). The white pulp consists of periarterial lymphatic sheaths of T cells with embedded germinal centers containing B cells. The red pulp has a skeleton of fixed reticular cells, mobile macrophages, partially collapsed endothelial passages (cords of Billroth), and splenic sinuses. A *marginal zone* rich in dendritic (antigen-presenting) cells separates the red pulp from the white pulp. The splenic capsule contains smooth muscle and contracts in response to epinephrine. Approximately 10% of the blood delivered to the spleen flows rapidly through a closed vascular network. The other 90% flows more slowly through an open system (the *splenic cords*), where it is filtered through 1–5 µm slits before entering the splenic sinuses.

FUNCTION. The unique anatomy and blood flow of the spleen enable it to perform reservoir, filtering, and immunologic functions. The spleen receives 5–6% of the cardiac output, but normally contains only 25 mL of blood. It can retain much more when it enlarges. Hematopoiesis is a major splenic function at 3–6 mo of fetal life, but then it disappears. Splenic hematopoiesis can be resumed in patients with myelofibrosis or severe hemolytic anemia. Factor VIII and platelets are stored in the spleen and can be released by stress or epinephrine injection. Thrombocytosis and leukocytosis occur with loss of the splenic reservoir function. A high platelet count after the loss of splenic function is not associated with an increased risk of thrombosis in children.

Slow blood flow past macrophages and through small openings in the sinus walls facilitates the filtering functions of the spleen. Excess membrane is removed from young red blood cells (RBCs); loss of this function is characterized by target cells, poikilocytosis, and decreased osmotic fragility. The spleen is the primary site for destruction of old RBCs; this function is assumed by other reticuloendothelial cells after splenectomy. The spleen also removes damaged and abnormal cells, such as spherocytes and antibody-coated RBCs. Intracytoplasmic inclusions may be removed from RBCs without cell lysis. Functional or anatomic hyposplenia is characterized by continued circulation of cells containing nuclear remnants (**Howell-Jolly bodies**), denatured hemoglobin (**Heinz bodies**), and other debris in RBCs. This debris may appear as "**pits**" on indirect microscopy.

Immunoglobulins, properdin, and tuftsin are produced in the spleen. The spleen has a minor role in antibody response to intramuscularly or subcutaneously injected antigens, but is required for early antibody production after exposure to intravenous antigens. Young (nonimmune) or hyposplenic individuals are at increased risk for **sepsis** caused by pneumococci and other encapsulated bacteria. The spleen can also use phagocytosis to trap and destroy intracellular parasites. The spleen may be an important site of antibody production in immune thrombocytopenia purpura.

Chadburn A: The spleen: Anatomy and anatomical function. *Semin Hematol* 2000;37(Suppl 1):13–21.

Steininger B, Barth P: Microanatomy and function of the spleen. *Adv Anat Embryol Cell Biol* 2000;151:1–101.

TABLE 486-1. Differential Diagnosis of Splenomegaly by Pathophysiology

ANATOMIC LESIONS
Cysts, pseudocysts
Hamartomas
Polysplenia syndrome
Hemangiomas and lymphangiomas
Hematoma or rupture (traumatic)
Hamartoma

HYPERPLASIA CAUSED BY HEMATOLOGIC DISORDERS
Acute and Chronic Hemolysis*
Hemoglobinopathies (sickle cell disease in infancy with or without sequestration crisis and sickle variants, thalassemia major, unstable hemoglobins)
Erythrocyte membrane disorders (hereditary spherocytosis, elliptocytosis, pyropoikilocytosis)
Erythrocyte enzyme deficiencies (severe G6PD deficiency, pyruvate kinase deficiency)
Immune hemolysis (autoimmune and isoimmune hemolysis)
Paroxysmal nocturnal hemoglobinuria

Chronic Iron Deficiency
Extramedullary hematopoiesis
Severe hemolytic anemias
Myeloproliferative diseases: chronic myelogenous leukemia (CML), juvenile CML, myelofibrosis with myeloid metaplasia, polycythemia vera
Osteopetrosis
Patients receiving granulocyte and granulocyte-macrophage colony-stimulating factors

INFECTIONS[†]
Bacterial
Acute sepsis: *Salmonella typhi, Streptococcus pneumoniae, Haemophilus influenzae* type b, *Staphylococcus aureus*
Chronic infections: infective endocarditis, chronic meningococcemia, brucellosis, tularemia, cat-scratch disease
Local infections: splenic abscess (*S. aureus*, streptococci, less often *Salmonella* species, polymicrobial species), pyogenic liver abscess (anaerobic bacteria, gram-negative enteric bacteria), cholangitis

Viral*
Acute viral infections, especially in children
Congenital cytomegalovirus (CMV), herpes simplex, rubella
Hepatitis, A, B, and C; CMV
Epstein-Barr virus (EBV)
Viral hemophagocytic syndromes: CMV, EBV, HHV-6
Human immunodeficiency virus (HIV)

Spirochetal
Syphilis, especially congenital syphilis
Leptospirosis

Rickettsial
Rocky Mountain spotted fever
Q fever
Typhus

Fungal/Mycobacterial
Miliary tuberculosis
Disseminated histoplasmosis
South American blastomycosis
Systemic candidiasis (in immunosuppressed patients)

Parasitic
Malaria
Toxoplasmosis, especially congenital
Toxocara canis, Toxocara cati (visceral larva migrans)
Leishmaniasis (kala-azar)
Schistosomiasis (hepatic-portal involvement)
Trypanosomiasis
Fascioliasis

IMMUNOLOGIC AND INFLAMMATORY PROCESSES*
Systemic lupus erythematosus
Rheumatoid arthritis
Mixed connective tissue disease
Systemic vasculitis
Serum sickness
Drug hypersensitivity, especially to phenytoin
Graft vs host disease
Sjögren syndrome
Cryoglobulinemia
Amyloidosis
Sarcoidosis
Large granular lymphocytosis and neutropenia
Histiocytosis syndromes
Hemophagocytic syndromes (nonviral, familial)

MALIGNANCIES
Primary: leukemia (acute, chronic), lymphoma, angiosarcoma, Hodgkin disease
Metastatic

STORAGE DISEASES
Lipidosis (Gaucher disease, Niemann-Pick disease, infantile GM_1 gangliosidosis)
Mucopolysaccharidoses (Hurler, Hunter-type)
Mucolipidosis (I-cell disease, sialidosis, multiple sulfatase deficiency, fucosidosis)
Defects in carbohydrate metabolism: galactosemia, fructose intolerance
Sea-blue histiocyte syndrome

CONGESTIVE*
Heart failure
Intrahepatic cirrhosis or fibrosis
Extrahepatic portal (thrombosis), splenic, and hepatic vein obstruction (thrombosis, Budd-Chiari syndrome)

*Common.
[†]Chronic or recurrent infection suggests underlying immunodeficiency.
G6PD, glucose-6-phosphate dehydrogenase; HHV-6, human herpesvirus 6.
From Kliegman RM, Greenbaum LA, Lye PS: *Practical Strategies in Pediatric Diagnosis and Therapy*, 2nd ed. Philadelphia, Elsevier, 2004, p 347.

Chapter 486 ■ Splenomegaly

CLINICAL MANIFESTATIONS. A soft, thin spleen may be palpable in 15% of neonates, 10% of normal children, and 5% of adolescents. In most individuals, the spleen must be 2–3 times its normal size before it is palpable. The spleen is best examined in a supine patient by palpating across the abdomen toward the left costal margin from below as the patient inspires deeply. An enlarged spleen might descend into the pelvis; when splenomegaly is suspected, the abdominal examination should begin at a lower starting point. Superficial abdominal venous distention may be present when splenomegaly is a result of portal hypertension. Radiologic detection or confirmation of splenic enlargement is done with ultrasonography, CT, or technetium-99 sulfur colloid scan. The latter also assesses splenic function.

DIFFERENTIAL DIAGNOSIS. Specific causes of splenomegaly are listed in Table 486-1. Unique problems are discussed next.

Pseudosplenomegaly. Abnormally enlarged mesenteric connections may produce a wandering or ptotic spleen. An enlarged left lobe of the liver, a left upper quadrant mass, or a splenic hematoma may be mistaken for splenomegaly. Splenic cysts may contribute to splenomegaly or mimic it; these may be congenital (epidermoid) or acquired (pseudocyst) after trauma or infarction. Cysts are usually asymptomatic and are found on radiologic evaluation. Splenosis after splenic rupture or an accessory spleen (present in 10% of normal individuals) may also mimic splenomegaly; most are not palpable. The syndrome of congenital polysplenism includes cardiac defects, left-sided organ anomalies, bilobed lungs, biliary atresia, and pseudosplenomegaly (see Chapter 431.11).

Hypersplenism. Increased splenic function (sequestration or destruction of circulating cells) results in peripheral blood cytopenia, increased bone marrow activity, and splenomegaly. It is usually secondary to another disease and may be cured by treatment of the underlying condition or, if absolutely necessary, moderated by splenectomy.

Congestive Splenomegaly (Banti Syndrome). Splenomegaly may result from obstruction in the hepatic, portal, or splenic veins. Wilson disease (see Chapter 354.2), galactosemia (see Chapter 87.2), biliary atresia (see Chapter 353), and α-antitrypsin deficiency (see Chapter 354.6) may result in hepatic inflammation, fibrosis, and vascular obstruction. Congenital abnormalities of the portal (absent or hypoplastic) or splenic veins may cause vascular obstruction. Septic omphalitis or thrombophlebitis may be spontaneous or may occur as a result of umbilical venous catheterization in neonates and may also result in secondary obliteration of these vessels. Splenic venous flow may be obstructed by masses of sickled erythrocytes. When the spleen is the site of vascular obstruction, splenectomy cures hypersplenism. However, the obstruction usually is in the hepatic or portal systems. In these latter cases, portocaval shunting may be more helpful, because both portal hypertension and thrombocytopenia contribute to variceal bleeding.

Aslanidou E, Fotoulaki M, Tsitouridis I, Nousia-Arvanitakis S: Partial splenic embolization: Successful treatment of hypersplenism, secondary to biliary cirrhosis and portal hypertension in cystic fibrosis. *J Cyst Fibrosis* 2006;Dec 6. E pub ahead of print.

Subhasis RC, Rajiv C, Kumar SA, et al: Surgical treatment of massive splenomegaly and severe hypersplenism secondary to extrahepatic portal venous obstruction in children. *Surg Today* 2007;37:19–23.

Chapter 487 ■ Hyposplenism, Splenic Trauma, and Splenectomy

HYPOSPLENISM. Congenital absence of the spleen is associated with complex cyanotic heart defects, dextrocardia, bilateral trilobed lungs, and heterotopic abdominal organs (**Ivemark syndrome;** see Chapter 431.11). Splenic function is usually normal in children with **congenital polysplenia. Functional hyposplenism** may occur in normal neonates, especially premature infants. Children with sickle cell hemoglobinopathies (see Chapter 462.1) may have splenic hypofunction as early as 6 mo of age. Initially, this is caused by vascular obstruction, which can be reversed with red blood cell (RBC) transfusion. The spleen eventually autoinfarcts and becomes fibrotic and permanently nonfunctioning. Functional hyposplenism may also occur in malaria (see Chapter 285), after irradiation to the left upper quadrant, and when the reticuloendothelial function of the spleen is overwhelmed (as in severe hemolytic anemia or metabolic storage disease). Splenic hypofunction has been reported occasionally in patients with vasculitis, nephritis, inflammatory bowel disease, celiac disease, Pearson syndrome, Fanconi anemia, and graft vs host disease.

Splenic hypofunction is characterized by RBC inclusions in peripheral blood smears, "**pits**" on interference microscopy, and poor uptake of technetium on spleen scan. Patients with functional hyposplenism or asplenia are at increased risk for sepsis from encapsulated organisms (pneumococcus).

TRAUMA. Injury to the spleen may occur with abdominal trauma. Small splenic capsular tears may cause abdominal or referred left shoulder pain as a result of peritoneal irritation by blood. Larger tears result in more severe blood loss, with similar pain and signs of hypovolemia. Previously enlarged spleens (as in patients with a history of infectious mononucleosis) are more likely to rupture with minor trauma. CT scan with IV contrast is the best imaging modality to assess for splenic trauma.

Treatment of a small capsular injury should include careful observation, with attention to changes in vital signs or abdominal findings, serial hemoglobin determinations, and the availability of prompt surgical intervention should a patient's condition deteriorate (see Chapter 71). RBC transfusion requirements should be minimal (<25 mL/kg/48 hr). These patients are usually hospitalized for 10–14 days and have their activities restricted for months. Laparotomy, with or without splenectomy, is indicated for more marked abdominal bleeding, in patients who have clinical instability or deterioration, or when other organ damage is suspected. Partial splenectomy and splenic repair should be substituted for total splenectomy when feasible.

SPLENECTOMY. Splenectomy should be limited to specific indications where medical therapy is (or has been) ineffective. These include traumatic splenic rupture, anatomic defects, severe hemolytic anemia, immune cytopenia, metabolic storage disease, and secondary hypersplenism. The major long-term risk of splenectomy is sudden, overwhelming bacterial infection (sepsis or meningitis). This risk is especially high in children younger than 5 yr at the time of surgery. The risk of sepsis is less when splenectomy is performed for trauma, RBC membrane defects, and immune thrombocytopenia (2–4%) than when there is pre-existing immune deficiency (Wiskott-Aldrich syndrome, Hodgkin disease) or reticuloendothelial blockade (storage disease, severe hemolytic anemia) [8–30%]. The use of laparoscopic splenectomy has decreased morbidity and hospitalization time.

Encapsulated bacteria, such as *Streptococcus pneumoniae* (>60% of cases), *Haemophilus influenzae,* and *Neisseria meningitidis,* account for >80% of cases of postsplenectomy sepsis. Because the spleen is responsible for filtering the blood and for early antibody responses, sepsis (with or without meningitis) can progress rapidly, leading to death within 12–24 hr of onset. Febrile splenectomized patients should be treated promptly with an antibiotic. This treatment should be initiated at home if access to definitive medical care will be delayed. A broad-spectrum cephalosporin (cefotaxime 50 mg/kg q8hr) or vancomycin (10 mg/kg q6hr) to cover penicillin-resistant pneumococci is recommended until specific antibiotic susceptibility is known. Splenectomized patients are also at increased for contracting protozoal infections, such as malaria and babesiosis.

Preoperative, intraoperative, and postoperative management may decrease the risk of postsplenectomy infection. It is important to be certain of the need for splenectomy and, if possible, to postpone the operation until the patient is 5 yr of age or older. Pneumococcal, meningococcal, and *H. influenzae* vaccines given before splenectomy may reduce postsplenectomy sepsis. However, the efficacy of unconjugated vaccine is lower in children younger than 2 yr of age and in immune-suppressed patients. In patients with traumatic injury, splenic repair or partial splenectomy should be considered in an attempt to preserve splenic function. Partial splenectomy or partial splenic embolization may be sufficient to ameliorate some forms of hemolytic anemia. Up to 50% of children whose spleen is removed because of trauma have spontaneous splenosis; surgical splenosis (distributing small pieces of spleen throughout the abdomen) may decrease the risk of sepsis in patients whose splenectomy is necessitated by trauma. However, in both of these settings, the splenic tissue that regrows frequently has inadequate function. Prophylaxis with oral penicillin V (125 mg twice daily for children younger than 5 yr; 250 mg twice daily for children 5 yr or older) should be given for at least 2 yr after splenectomy (to at least 6 yr of age). Prophylaxis may be continued into adulthood for higher-risk patients. Penicillin reduces the risk of pneumococcal sepsis in younger patients with hemoglobin SS, but other populations have not been well studied. Although the greatest risk is in the immediate postoperative period, reports of deaths occurring many yr after splenectomy suggest that the risk (and the need for prophylaxis) may be lifelong. Other postoperative measures include patient and family education, use of a medical information bracelet, and prompt evaluation and treatment of fevers.

Bader-Meunier B, Gauthier F, Archambaud F, et al: Long-term evaluation of the beneficial effect of subtotal splenectomy for management of hereditary spherocytosis. *Blood* 2001;97:399–403.

Castagnola E, Fioredda F: Prevention of life-threatening infections due to encapsulated bacteria in children with hyposplenia or asplenia: A brief review of current recommendations for practical purposes. *Eur J Haematol* 2003;71:319–326.

Hansen K, Singer DB: Asplenic-hyposplenic overwhelming sepsis: Postsplenectomy sepsis revisited. *Pediatr Dev Pathol* 2001;4:105–121.

Upadhyaya P: Conservative management of splenic trauma: History and current trends. *Pediatr Surg Int* 2003;19:617–627.

Section 9 — The Lymphatic System

Chapter 488 ■ Anatomy and Function of the Lymphatic System

The lymphatic system includes circulating lymphocytes, lymphatic vessels, lymph nodes, spleen, tonsils, adenoids, Peyer patches, and thymus. Lymph, an ultrafiltrate of blood, is collected by lymphatic capillaries that are present in all organs except the brain and the heart. These join to form progressively larger vessels that drain regions of the body. During their course, the lymphatic vessels carry lymph to the lymph nodes. In the nodes, lymph is filtered through sinuses, where particulate matter and infectious organisms are phagocytosed, processed, and presented as antigens to surrounding lymphocytes. These actions stimulate antibody production, T-cell responses, and cytokine secretion (see Chapter 122).

The composition of lymph can vary with the site of lymph drainage. It is usually clear, but lymph drained from the intestinal tract may be milky (chylous) because of the presence of fats. The protein content is intermediate between that of an exudate and that of a transudate. The protein level may be increased with inflammation and in lymph drained from the liver or intestines. Lymph also contains variable numbers of lymphocytes.

Chapter 489 ■ Abnormalities of Lymphatic Vessels

Abnormalities of the lymph vessels may be congenital or acquired. Signs and symptoms may result from increased lymphatic tissue mass or from leakage of lymph. **Lymphangiectasia** is dilation of the lymphatics. Pulmonary lymphangiectasia causes respiratory distress (see Chapter 392). Involvement of the intestinal lymphatics causes hypoproteinemia and lymphocytopenia secondary to loss of lymph into the intestines (see Chapter 335.1). **Lymphangioma** (cystic hygroma) is a mass of dilated lymphatics. Some of these lesions also have a hemangiomatous component (see Chapter 505). Surgical treatment is complicated by a high incidence of recurrence. Intralesional sclerosing with OK-432, a streptococcal derivative, has been used successfully in selected patients. Macrocystic lesions appear to respond better than microcystic lymphangiomas to sclerotherapy. **Lymphatic dysplasia** may cause multisystem problems. These include lymphedema, chylous ascites, chylothorax, and lymphangiomas of the bone, lung, or other sites.

Lymphedema is caused by obstruction of lymph flow. Congenital lymphedema may be found in Turner syndrome, Noonan syndrome, and the autosomal dominantly inherited Milroy disease. Several families with Milroy disease have mutations in *FLT4*, which encodes the vascular endothelial growth factor receptor-3 gene. Autosomal recessive and X-linked inheritance has also been reported. **Lymphedema praecox** (Meige disease) causes progressive lower extremity edema, usually in females during the peripubertal period or during pregnancy. Lymphedema has also been found in association with intestinal lymphangiectasia, cerebrovascular malformation, ptosis, yellow dystrophic nails, distichiasis, and cholestasis. Mutations in *FOXC2* are associated with lymphedema-distichiasis syndrome, which has a pubertal onset of lymphedema. Acquired obstruction of the lymphatics can result from tumor, postirradiation fibrosis, and postinflammatory scarring. Filariasis is an important cause of lymphedema in Africa, Asia, and Latin America; of the estimated 120 million infected persons, approximately 40 million (primarily older adolescents and adults) are believed to have lymphedema or hydrocele. Injury to the major lymphatic vessel can cause collection of lymph fluid in the abdomen (chylous ascites) or chest (chylothorax).

Lymphangitis is an inflammation of the lymphatics that drain an area of infection. Tender, erythematous streaks extend proximally from the infected area. Regional nodes may also be tender. Group A streptococci and *Staphylococcus aureus* are the most frequent pathogens.

Addiss DG, Beach MJ, Streit TG, et al: Randomised placebo-controlled comparison of ivermectin and albendazole alone and in combination for *Wuchereria bancrofti* microfilaraemia in Haitian children. *Lancet* 1997;350:480–484.

Banieghbal B, Davies MR: Guidelines for successful treatment of lymphangioma with OK-432. *Eur J Pediatr Surg* 2003;13:103–107.

Fischer P, Supali T, Maizels RM: Lymphatic filariasis and *Brugia timori*: Prospects for elimination. *Trends Parasitol* 2004;20:351–355.

Giguere CM, Bauman NM, Smith RJ: New treatment options for lymphangioma in infants and children. *Ann Otol Rhinol Laryngol* 2002;111:1066–1075.

Levinson KL, Feingold E, Ferell R, et al: Age of onset in hereditary lymphedema. *J Pediatr* 2003;142:704–708.

Mulliken JB, Fishman SJ, Burrows PE: Vascular anomalies. *Curr Pediatr Surg* 2000;37:527–584.

Orvidas LJ, Kasperbauer JL: Pediatric lymphangioma of the head and neck. *Ann Otol Rhinol Laryngol* 2000;109:411–421.

Schuster T, Grantzow R, Nicolai T: Lymphangioma colli: A new classification contributing to prognosis. *Eur J Pediatr Surg* 2003;13:97–102.

Chapter 490 ■ Lymphadenopathy

Most lymph nodes are not usually palpable in the newborn. With antigenic exposure, lymphoid tissue increases in volume so that the cervical, axillary, and inguinal nodes are often palpable during childhood. They are not considered enlarged until their diameter exceeds 1 cm for cervical and axillary nodes and 1.5 cm for inguinal nodes. Other lymph nodes usually are not palpable or visualized with plain radiographs.

DIAGNOSIS. Lymph node enlargement is caused by proliferation of normal lymphoid elements or by infiltration with malignant or phagocytic cells. In most patients, a careful history and a complete physical examination suggest the proper diagnosis. Nonlymphoid masses (cervical rib, thyroglossal cyst, branchial cleft cyst or infected sinus, cystic hygroma, goiter, sternomastoid muscle tumor, thyroiditis, thyroid abscess, neurofibroma) occur frequently in the neck and less often in other areas. Acutely infected nodes are usually tender. There may also be erythema and warmth of the overlying skin. Fluctuance suggests abscess formation. Tuberculous nodes may be matted. With chronic infection, many of the above signs are not present. Tumor-bearing nodes are usually firm and nontender, and may be matted or fixed to the skin or underlying structures.

Generalized adenopathy (enlargement of >2 noncontiguous node regions) is caused by systemic disease (Table 490-1) and is often accompanied by abnormal physical findings in other systems. In contrast, regional adenopathy is most frequently the result of infection in the involved node and/or its drainage area (Table 490-2). When due to infectious agents other than bacteria, adenopathy may be characterized by atypical anatomic areas, a prolonged course, a draining sinus, lack of prior pyogenic infection, and unusual clues in the history (cat scratches, tuberculosis exposure, venereal disease). A firm, fixed node should always raise the question of malignancy, regardless of the presence or absence of systemic symptoms or other abnormal physical findings.

TREATMENT. Evaluation and treatment of lymphadenopathy is guided by the probable etiologic factor, as determined from the history and physical examination. Many patients with cervical adenopathy have a history compatible with viral infection and need no intervention. If bacterial infection is suspected, antibiotic treatment covering at least streptococci and staphylococci is indicated. Those who do not respond to oral antibiotics, as demonstrated by persistent swelling and fever, require IV antistaphylococcal antibiotics. If there is no response in 1–2 days or if there are signs of airway obstruction or significant toxicity, CT or ultrasound of the neck should be obtained. If pus is present, it may be aspirated, with CT or ultrasound guidance, or if it is extensive, it will require incision and drainage. Gram stain and culture of the pus should be obtained. Surgical drainage is required for an abscess. The sizes of involved nodes should be documented before treatment. Failure to decrease in size within 10–14 days also suggests the need for further evaluation. This may include a complete blood cell count with differential; Epstein-Barr virus, cytomegalovirus, *Toxoplasma,* and cat scratch

TABLE 490-1. Differential Diagnosis of Systemic Generalized Lymphadenopathy

INFANT	CHILD	ADOLESCENT
COMMON CAUSES		
Syphilis	Viral infection	Viral infection
Toxoplasmosis	EBV	EBV
CMV	CMV	CMV
HIV	HIV	HIV
	Toxoplasmosis	Toxoplasmosis
		Syphilis
RARE CAUSES		
Chagas disease (congenital)	Serum sickness	Serum sickness
Congenital leukemia	SLE, JRA	SLE, JRA
Congenital tuberculosis	Leukemia/lymphoma	Leukemia/lymphoma/Hodgkin disease
Reticuloendotheliosis	Tuberculosis	Lymphoproliferative disease
Lymphoproliferative disease	Measles	Tuberculosis
Metabolic storage disease	Sarcoidosis	Histoplasmosis
Histiocytic disorders	Fungal infection	Sarcoidosis
	Plague	Fungal infection
	Langerhan cell histiocytosis	Plague
	Chronic granulomatous disease	Drug reaction
	Sinus histiocytosis	Castleman disease
	Drug reaction	

CMV, cytomegalovirus; EBV, Epstein-Barr virus; HIV, human immunodeficiency virus; JRA, juvenile rheumatoid arthritis (as Still disease); SLE, systemic lupus erythematosus.

From Kliegman RM, Greenbaum LA, Lye PS: *Practical Strategies in Pediatric Diagnosis and Therapy*, 2nd ed. Philadelphia, Elsevier, 2004, p 863.

TABLE 490-2. Sites of Local Lymphadenopathy and Associated Diseases

CERVICAL
Oropharyngeal infection (viral or group A streptococcal, staphylococcal)
Scalp infection
Mycobacterial lymphadenitis (tuberculosis and nontuberculous mycobacteria)
Viral infection (EBV, CMV, HHV-6)
Cat-scratch disease
Toxoplasmosis
Kawasaki disease
Thyroid disease
Kikuchi disease
Sinus histiocytosis
Autoimmune lymphoproliferative disease
ANTERIOR AURICULAR
Conjuctivitis
Other eye infection
Oculoglandular tularemia
Facial cellulitis
Otitis media
Viral infection (especially rubella, parvovirus)
SUPRACLAVICULAR
Malignancy or infection in the mediastinum (right)
Metastatic malignancy from the abdomen (left)
Lymphoma
Tuberculosis
EPITROCHLEAR
Hand infection, arm infection*
Lymphoma†
Sarcoid
Syphilis
INGUINAL
Urinary tract infection
Venereal disease (especially syphilis or lymphogranuloma venereum)
Other perineal infections
Lower extremity suppurative infection
Plague
HILAR (NOT PALPABLE, FOUND ON CHEST RADIOGRAPH OR CT)
Tuberculosis†
Histoplasmosis†
Blastomycosis†
Coccidioidomycosis†
Leukemia/lymphoma†
Hodgkin disease†
Metastatic malignancy*
Sarcoidosis†
Castleman disease
AXILLARY
Cat-scratch disease
Arm or chest wall infection
Malignancy of chest wall
Leukemia/lymphoma
Brucellosis
ABDOMINAL
Malignancies
Mesenteric adenitis (measles, tuberculosis, Yersinia, group A streptococcus)

*Unilateral.
†Bilateral.
CMV, cytomegalovirus; CT, computed tomography; EBV, Epstein-Barr virus; HHV-6, human herpesvirus 6.
From Kliegman RM, Greenbaum LA, Lye PS: *Practical Strategies in Pediatric Diagnosis and Therapy*, 2nd ed. Philadelphia, Elsevier 2004, p 864.

disease titers; antistreptolysin O or anti-DNAse serologic tests; tuberculin skin test; and chest radiograph. If these are not diagnostic, consultation with an infectious disease or oncology specialist may be helpful. Biopsy should be considered if there is persistent or unexplained fever, weight loss, night sweats, hard nodes, or fixation of the nodes to surrounding tissues. Biopsy may also be indicated if there is an increase in size over baseline in 2 wk, no decrease in size in 4–6 wk, or no regression to "normal" in 8–12 wk, or if new signs and symptoms develop.

Haberman TM, Steensma PA: Lymphadenopathy. *Mayo Clin Proc* 2000; 75:723–732.
Nield LS, Kamat D: Lymphadenopathy in children: When and how to evaluate. *Clin Pediatr* 2004;43:25–33.
Peters TR, Edwards KM: Cervical lymphadenopathy and adenitis. *Pediatr Rev* 2000;21:399–405.
Soldes OS, Younger JG, Hirschl RB: Predictors of malignancy in childhood peripheral lymphadenopathy. *J Pediatr Surg* 1999;34:1447–1452.
Tokuda Y, Kishaba Y, Kato J, Nakazato N: Assessing the validity of a model to identify patients for lymph node biopsy. *Medicine* 2003;82:414–418.
Twist CJ, Link MP: Assessment of lymphadenopathy in children. *Pediatr Clin North Am* 2002;49:1009–1025.

490.1 • Kikuchi-Fujimoto Disease (Histiocytic Necrotizing Lymphadenitis)

Kikuchi-Fujimoto disease is a rare, self-limiting disease that is most commonly seen in children and young adults of Asian heritage. Presentation may include fever of unknown origin, but more often, it occurs in children 8–16 yr of age as unilateral posterior cervical adenitis, fever, malaise, and leukopenia. Nodes range in size from 0.5–6.0 cm, are painful or tender in 50% of cases, may be multiple, and must be differentiated from lymphoma.

The etiology is unknown, and the diagnosis is made if the histologic features of the node show crescentic plasmacytoid monocytes and an absence of neutrophils. The disease resolves within 6 mo, although systemic lupus erythematosus may develop in some patients.

490.2 • Sinus Histiocytosis with Massive Lymphadenopathy (Rosai-Dorfman Disease)

This uncommon, benign, and usually self-limited disease of unknown etiology has a worldwide distribution, but is more common in Africa and the Caribbean. Children and adolescents present with massive symmetric, painless, cervical adenopathy, along with fever, leukocytosis, a high erythrocyte sedimentation rate, and polyclonal elevation of immunoglobulin G. It rarely occurs at birth or in siblings, and males are affected more often than females.

Occasionally, it is associated with autoantibodies to erythrocytes or the synovium, and extranodal involvement may occur. Sites include the skin, nasal cavity and sinuses, palate, orbit, bone, and central nervous system. Diagnosis requires a biopsy, which demonstrates pale histiocytes containing engulfed lymphocytes. The differential diagnosis includes Langerhan cell histiocytosis and lymphoma.

Therapy is usually not needed for this self-limited disease, although extranodal or persistent disease or exacerbations and remissions may respond to prednisone. Refractory cases have been treated with surgical excision or radiation.

490.3 • Castleman Disease

This uncommon lymphoproliferative disease, also called *angiofollicular lymph node hyperplasia,* is of unknown etiology, but has an association with human herpesvirus 8 and presents in adolescents and young adults with localized or multicentric forms. Human herpesvirus 8 may stimulate excessive production of interleukin 6 (IL-6). Enlargement of a single node, most often in the mediastinum or abdomen, is the most common localized presentation. Some of these patients may have fever, night sweats, weight loss, and fatigue. Management includes surgery and/or radiation therapy.

Multicentric Castleman disease is a systemic disorder that causes lymphadenopathy, hepatosplenomegaly, fever, anemia, and polyclonal hypergammaglobulinemia. Multicentric Castleman disease may be associated with HIV infection, autoimmune disease–associated lymphadenopathy, POEMS syndrome (polyneuropathy, organomegaly, endocrinopathy, M-proteins and skin lesions) and non-Hodgkin lymphoma. Treatment includes steroids, monoclonal antibodies to IL-6, anti-IL-6–receptor antibodies (tocilizumab), antiviral agents, and interferon-α. Chemotherapy for diffuse large B-cell lymphoma may be beneficial in some patients.

Bosch X, Guilabert A, Miquel R, et al: Enigmatic Kikuchi-Fujimoto disease. *Am J Clin Pathol* 2004;122:141–152.

Carbone A, Passannante A, Gloghini A, et al: Review of sinus histiocytosis with massive lymphadenopathy (Rosai-Dorfman disease) of head and neck. *Ann Otol Rhinol Laryngol* 1999;108:1095–1104.

Casper C: The aetiology and management of Castleman disease at 50 years: Translating pathophysiology to patient care. *Br J Haematol* 2005;129:3–17.

Chuang CH, Yan DC, Chiu CH, et al: Clinical and laboratory manifestations of Kikuchi's disease in children and differences between patients with and without prolonged fever. *Pediatr Infect Dis J* 2005;24:551–554.

Dispenzieri A, Gertz MA: Treatment of Castleman's disease. *Curr Treat Options Oncol* 2005;6:255–266.

Guihot A, Couderc LJ, Agbalika F, et al: Pulmonary manifestations of multicentric Castleman's disease in HIV infection: A clinical, biological and radiological study. *Eur Respir J* 2005;26:118–125.

Herrada J, Cabanillas F, Rice L, et al: The clinical behavior of localized and multicentric Castleman disease. *Ann Intern Med* 1998;128:657–662.

Kojima M, Nakamura S, Nishikawa M, et al: Idiopathic multicentric Castleman's disease: A clinicopathologic and immunohistochemical study of five cases. *Pathol Res Pract* 2005;201:325–332.

Lin HC, Su CY, Huang SC: Kikuchi's disease in Asian children. *Pediatrics* 2005;115:e92–e96.

Nishimoto N: Clinical studies in patients with Castleman's disease, Crohn's disease, and rheumatoid arthritis in Japan. *Clin Rev Allergy Immunol* 2005;28:221–229.

Parez N, Bader-Meunier B, Roy CC, et al: Paediatric Castleman disease: Report of seven cases and review of the literature. *Eur J Pediatr* 1999;158:631–637.

Pulsoni A, Anghel G, Falcucci P, et al: Treatment of sinus histiocytosis with massive lymphadenopathy (Rosai-Dorfman disease): Report of a case and literature review. *Am J Hematol* 2002;69:67–71.

Raveenthiran V, Dhanalakshmi M, Rao PVH, et al: Rosai-Dorfman disease: Report of a 3-year-old girl with critical review of treatment options. *Eur J Pediatr Surg* 2003;13:350–354.

Scagni P, Peisino MG, Bianchi M, et al: Kikuchi-Fujimoto disease is a rare cause of lymphadenopathy and fever of unknown origin in children. *J Pediatr Hematol Oncol* 2005;27:337–340.

Part XXI ■ Cancer and Benign Tumors

Chapter 491 ■ Epidemiology of Childhood and Adolescent Cancer*

Nina S. Kadan-Lottick

Cancer in individuals ≤19 yr of age is uncommon, with an age-adjusted annual incidence rate of 16.5/100,000, representing only about 1% (12,400 cases/yr) of all new cancer cases in the USA. Although relative 5-yr survival rates have improved from 56% in 1974 to >81% in 2000 (Fig. 491-1), malignant neoplasms remain the second most common cause of all deaths (12.8%) among persons 1–14 yr of age in the USA. Multi-institutional cooperative clinical trials investigating novel therapies and investigating ways to improve survival rates even further are currently underway. Because increasingly more patients survive their disease, clinical investigation also is focusing on the quality of life among survivors and the late outcomes of therapy experienced by pediatric and adult survivors of childhood cancer. The National Cancer Institute estimates that, in 1997, there were 269,700 individuals alive (in all age groups) who had survived childhood cancer, corresponding to 1 in 810 of individuals <20 yr of age and 1 in 1000 of individuals 20–39 yr of age in the US population.

Pediatric cancers differ markedly from adult malignancies in both prognosis and distribution by histology and tumor site. Lymphohematopoietic cancers (i.e., acute lymphoblastic leukemia, lymphomas) account for approximately 40%, nervous system cancers for approximately 30%, and embryonal and sarcomas for approximately 10% each among the broad categories of childhood cancers (Table 491-1). In contrast, epithelial tumors of organs such as lung, colon, breast, and prostate are most common among adults. Unlike incidence patterns in adults, where cancer rates tend to increase rapidly with increasing age, a relatively wide age range exists in the pediatric age group, with two peaks—the first in early childhood and the second in adolescence (Fig. 491-2). During the first year of life, **embryonal tumors** such as neuroblastoma, nephroblastoma (Wilms tumor), retinoblastoma, rhabdomyosarcoma, hepatoblastoma, and medulloblastoma are most common (Fig. 491-3). These tumors are much less common in older children and adults after cell differentiation processes have slowed considerably. Embryonal tumors, acute leukemias, non-Hodgkin lymphomas, and gliomas peak in incidence from 2–5 yr of age. As children age, bone malignancies, Hodgkin disease, gonadal germ cell malignancies (testicular and ovarian carcinomas), and other carcinomas increase in incidence. Adolescence is a transitional period between the common early childhood malignancies and characteristic carcinomas of adulthood.

Childhood neoplasms include a diverse array of malignant tumors, termed "cancers," and nonmalignant tumors arising from disorders of genetic processes involved in control of cellular growth and development. Although many genetic conditions are associated with increased risks for childhood cancer, such conditions are believed to account for <5% of all occurrences (see Chapter 492). The most notable genetic conditions that impart childhood cancer susceptibility are neurofibromatosis types 1 and 2, Down syndrome, Beckwith-Wiedemann syndrome, tuberous sclerosis, von Hippel-Lindau disease, xeroderma pigmentosum, ataxia-telangiectasia, nevus basal cell carcinoma syndrome, and Li-Fraumeni (P53) syndrome. The varying incidence patterns of individual childhood cancers around the world imply additional genetic and epidemiologic risk factors that remain uncharacterized.

Compared with adult epithelial tumors, an extremely small fraction of pediatric cancers appear to be explained by known environmental exposures (Table 491-2). Ionizing radiation exposure and several chemotherapeutic agents explain only a small number of pediatric cases (see Chapter 706). The association between fetal exposures and pediatric cancer is largely unestablished, with the exception of maternal diethylstilbestrol intake during pregnancy and subsequent vaginal adenocarcinoma in adolescent daughters. Environmental exposures that have been studied without convincing evidence for a causal role include non-ionizing power frequency electromagnetic fields, pesticides, parental occupational chemical exposures, dietary factors, and environmental cigarette smoke. Viruses have been associated with certain pediatric cancers, such as polyomaviruses (BK, JC, SV40) associated with brain cancer and Epstein-Barr virus with non-Hodgkin lymphoma, but the etiologic importance remains unclear. Because the etiology of cancer in children still is poorly understood, for the most part, epidemiology studies have recognized that the likely mechanism is multifactorial, possibly resulting from potential interactions between genetic susceptibility traits and environmental exposures. Ongoing studies are investigating the role of polymorphisms of genes encoding enzymes, which function in the activation or metabolism of xenobiotics; protection of cells against oxidative stress; DNA repair; and/or immune modulation.

Curative therapy with chemotherapy, radiation, and/or surgery may adversely affect a child's development and result in serious long-term medical and psychosocial effects in both childhood and adulthood. Potential adverse **late effects** include subsequent malignancy, early mortality, infertility, reduced stature, cardiomyopathy, pulmonary fibrosis, osteoporosis, neurocognitive impairment, affective mood disorders, and altered social functioning. Much has been learned about the incidence of late effects from large, multi-site cohort studies such as the Childhood Cancer Survivor Study, an ongoing study of medical and psychosocial outcomes in survivors (http://www.cancer.umn.edu/ltfu).

Given the relative rarity of specific types of childhood cancer and the sophisticated technology and expertise required for diagnosis, treatment, and monitoring of late effects, all children with cancer should be treated on standardized clinical protocols in pediatric clinical research settings whenever possible. Promoting such treatment, the **Children's Oncology Group** is a multi-institutional research consortium that facilitates cooperative clinical, biologic, and epidemiologic research in more than 200 affiliated institutions in the United States, Canada, and other countries (http://www.curesearch.org/). Coordinated participation in such research trials has been a major factor in the increased survival for many children with cancer. Such ongoing efforts are critical to better understand the etiology of childhood cancers, improve survival for malignancies with a poor prognosis, and maximize the quality of life for survivors.

*The author would like to acknowledge the work of James G. Gurney and Melissa L. Bondy on Chapter 483, "Epidemiology of Childhood and Adolescent Cancer," in the previous edition of this work.

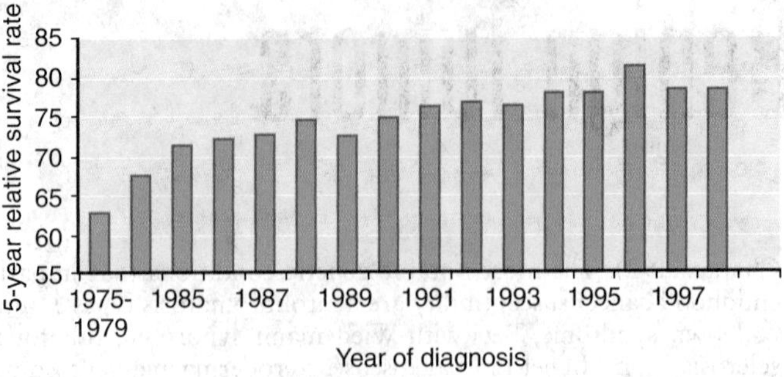

Figure 491-1. Five-year relative survival rates (%) by year of diagnosis of all cancers in children ≤19 yr of age. Rates based on follow-up of patients into 2003. (From Ries LAG, Harkins D, Krapcho M, et al (editors): *SEER Cancer Statistics Review, 1975–2003*. Bethesda, MD, National Cancer Institute. http://seer.cancer.gov/csr/1975_2003/, based on November 2005 SEER data submission, posted to the SEER web site, 2006.)

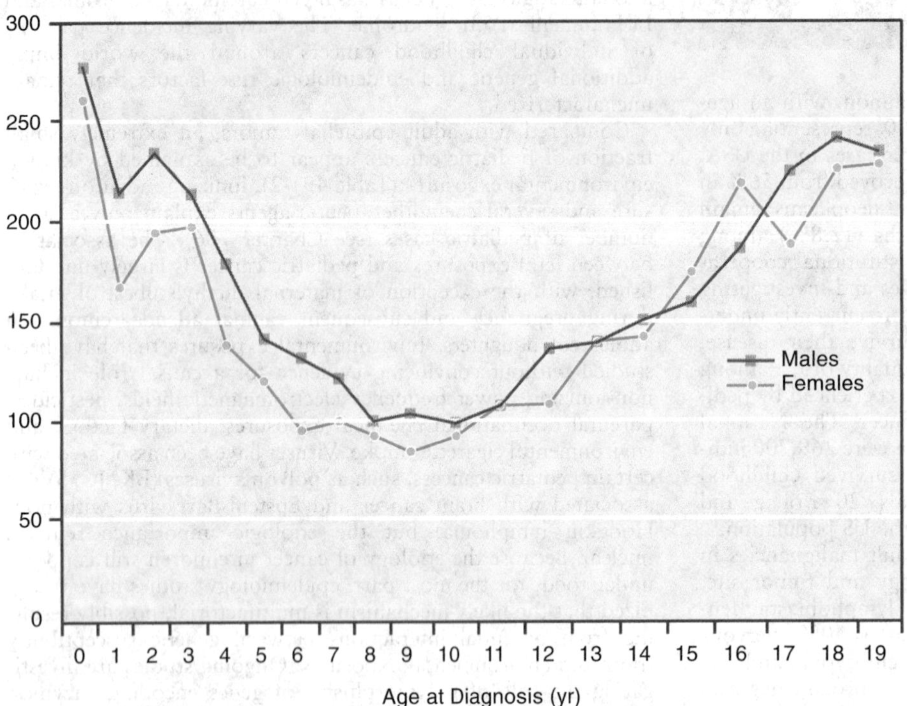

Figure 491-2. Age- and sex-specific cancer incidence rates per million children in the USA. (From Ries LAG, Smith MA, Gurney JG, et al (editors): *Cancer Incidence and Survival Among Children and Adolescents: United States SEER Program 1975–1995*. Bethesda, MD, National Cancer Institute, SEER Program, 1999.)

TABLE 491-1. Incidence and Survival Rates of Malignant Neoplasms by Age Among US Children

	ANNUAL INCIDENCE RATES PER MILLION CHILDREN, 2000–2003							5-YR SURVIVAL, ≤19 YR OF AGE AT DIAGNOSIS, 1996–2000 (%)
	≤14 YR	≤19 YR	≤1 YR	≤4 YR	5–9 YR	10–14 YR	15–19 YR	
All malignancies combined	147.8	163.2	230.8	205.1	111.9	124.2	209.1	77.9
Leukemias	47.8	43.2	45.2	86.3	38.4	28.3	29.6	75.2
Acute lymphoid	37.9	32.7	19.6	79.4	31.9	19.7	17.1	81.4
Acute myeloid	7.5	8.0	18.5	9.0	4.7	7.2	9.2	50.5
Lymphomas	15.1	23.4	8.5	8.4	13.7	22.8	48.1	86.9
Hodgkin disease	5.3	11.4	—	1.1	4.1	10.7	29.5	94.6
Non-Hodgkin lymphomas	6.2	8.4	—	3.7	6.3	8.9	15.1	79.4
Central nervous system and miscellaneous intracranial and intraspinal tumors	31.9	28.9	32.3	40.7	31.9	25.0	19.9	71.7
Astrocytoma	15.6	14.3	12.5	19.1	15.5	13.6	10.4	82.6
Embryonal tumors	7.5	6.6	11.3	10.4	7.5	4.6	3.8	67.3
Ependymomas and choroid plexus tumors	3.0	2.6	4.4	5.2	2.2	1.7	1.4	73.5
Neuroblastoma and other peripheral nervous cell tumors	9.9	7.6	50.5	19.2	3.4	1.7	—	68.9
Retinoblastoma	3.9	3.0	23.8	8.7	—	—	—	97.0
Renal tumors	7.8	6.2	17.1	18.7	4.7	1.1	1.3	87.1
Nephroblastoma	7.5	5.7	17.1	18.5	4.3	—	—	88.3
Hepatic tumors	2.5	2.1	12.5	4.4	0.9	0.7	0.9	47.1
Hepatoblastoma	2.1	1.6	11.8	4.3	—	—	—	59.2
Bone tumors	6.3	8.5	—	1.4	5.0	12.4	15.1	65.1
Osteosarcoma	3.9	5.2	—	—	3.1	8.0	9.0	65.8
Ewing tumor and related sarcomas	2.0	2.5	—	1.0	1.5	3.6	4.0	59.0
Soft tissue sarcomas	10.7	12.1	17.5	10.7	7.9	12.2	16.3	69.2
Rhabdomyosarcoma	5.3	4.9	5.1	8.3	4.4	3.8	3.8	61.0
Germ cell tumors	5.5	11.5	20.8	3.9	2.1	7.4	29.1	89.7
Carcinomas and melanoma	5.7	16.2	—	1.8	3.1	12.1	47.5	89.2

Based on the International Classification of Childhood Cancer (ICCC). Rates are per 1,000,000 children and are age-adjusted to the 2000 US standard population. — = rate could not be calculated with <6 cases for the age interval.

From Ries LAG, Harkins D, Krapcho M, et al (editors): *SEER Cancer Statistics Review, 1975–2003*. Bethesda, MD, National Cancer Institute. http://seer.cancer.gov/csr/1975_2003/, based on November 2005 SEER data submission, posted to the SEER web site, 2006.

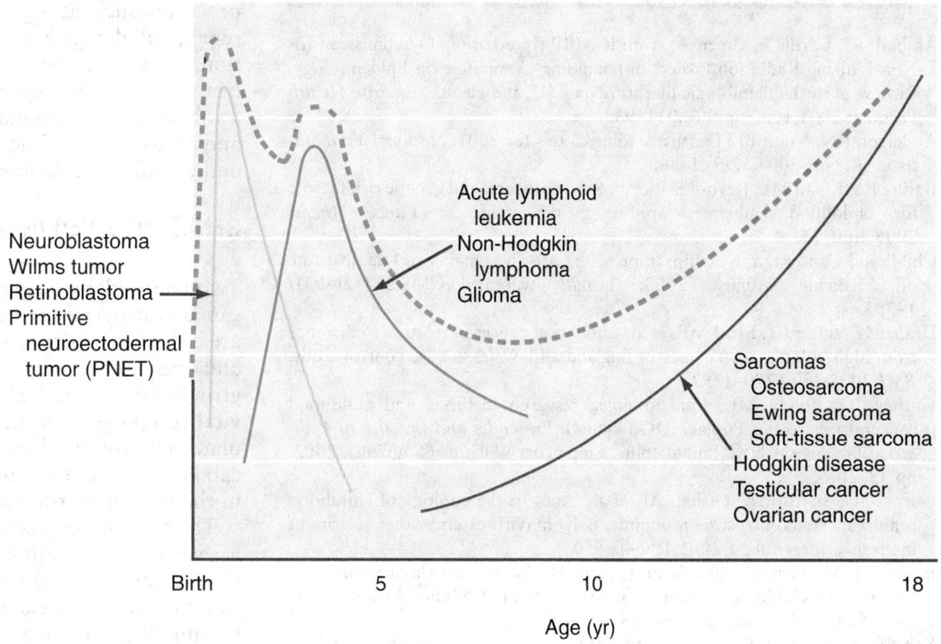

Figure 491-3. Generalized incidence of the most common types of cancer in children by age. The cumulative incidence of all cancers is shown as a dashed line. (Courtesy of Archie Bleyer, MD.)

INFLUENCING THE INCIDENCE OF CANCER

Pediatricians have a unique opportunity to educate children and adolescents, and their parents, regarding means of preventing cancer. There are only a few recognized environmental causes of childhood cancer that can be avoided. One example is immunization against hepatitis B, which does decrease the incidence of hepatoblastoma in adolescence and adulthood. An objective of pediatric medicine is to teach children how to adopt healthy lifestyles to reduce their risk of cancer during adulthood, such as avoiding tobacco, alcohol, high-fat diets, and obesity. The earlier these habits are instilled the greater the lifelong benefit and the more likely it is to be present and sustained during adulthood.

TABLE 491-2. Known Risk Factors for Selected Pediatric Cancers

CANCER TYPE	RISK FACTOR	COMMENTS
Acute lymphoid leukemia	Ionizing radiation	Although primarily of historical significance, prenatal diagnostic x-ray exposure increases risk.
		Therapeutic irradiation for cancer treatment also increases risk.
	Race	White children have a 2-fold higher rate than black children in the USA.
	Genetic factors*	Down syndrome is associated with an estimated 10- to 20-fold increased risk.
		Neurofibromatosis type 1, Bloom syndrome, ataxia-telangiectasia, and Langerhans' cell histiocytosis, among others, are associated with an elevated risk.
Acute myeloid leukemias	Chemotherapeutic agents	Alkylating agents and epipodophyllotoxins increase risk.
	Genetic factors*	Down syndrome and neurofibromatosis type 1 are strongly associated. Familial monosomy 7 and several other genetic syndromes are also associated with increased risk.
Brain cancers	Therapeutic ionizing radiation to the head	With the exception of cancer radiation therapy, higher risk from radiation treatment is essentially of historical importance.
	Genetic factors*	Neurofibromatosis type 1 is strongly associated with optic gliomas, and, to a lesser extent, with other central nervous system tumors. Tuberous sclerosis and several other genetic syndromes are associated with increased risk.
Hodgkin disease	Family history	Monozygotic twins and siblings are at increased risk.
	Infections	Epstein-Barr virus is associated with increased risk.
Non-Hodgkin lymphoma	Immunodeficiency	Acquired and congenital immunodeficiency disorders, and immunosuppressive therapy, increase risk.
	Infections	Epstein-Barr virus is associated with Burkitt lymphoma in Africa.
Osteosarcoma	Ionizing radiation	Cancer radiation therapy and high radium exposure increase risk.
	Chemotherapy	Alkylating agents increase risk.
	Genetic factors*	Increased risk is apparent with Li-Fraumeni syndrome and hereditary retinoblastoma.
Ewing sarcoma	Race	White children have about a 9-fold higher incidence rate than black children in the USA.
Neuroblastoma		No established risk factors.
Retinoblastoma	Genetic factors*	No established other risk factors.
Wilms tumor	Congenital anomalies	Aniridia, Beckwith-Wiedemann syndrome, and other congenital and genetic conditions are associated with increased risk.
	Race	Asian children reportedly have about half the rates of white and black children.
Renal medullary carcinoma	Sickle cell trait	Etiology unknown
Rhabdomyosarcoma	Congenital anomalies and genetic conditions	Li-Fraumeni syndrome and neurofibromatosis type 1 are believed to be associated with increased risk. There is some concordance with major birth defects.
Hepatoblastoma	Genetic factors*	Beckwith-Wiedemann syndrome, hemihypertrophy, Gardner syndrome, and family history of adenomatous polyposis are associated with increased risk.
Leiomyosarcoma	Immunosuppression and EBV infection	Epstein-Barr virus is associated with leiomyosarcoma for all forms of congenital and acquired immunosuppression but not leiomyosarcoma among immunocompetent persons
Malignant germ cell tumors	Cryptorchidism	Cryptorchidism is a risk factor for testicular germ cell tumors.

From Gurney JG, Bondy ML: Epidemiologic research methods and childhood cancer. In Pizzo PA, Poplack DG (editors): *Principles and Practice of Pediatric Oncology*, 4th ed. Philadelphia, Lippincott Williams & Wilkins, 2001, pp 13–20.
*See Table 492-2.

Ahlbom IC, Cardis E, Green A, et al: ICNIRP (International Commission for Non-Ionizing Radiation Protection) Standing Committee on Epidemiology: Review of the epidemiologic literature on EMF and Health. *Environ Health Perspect* 2001;109(Suppl 6):911–933.

Anderson RN, Smith BL: Deaths: leading causes for 2001. *National Vital Statistics Report* 2003;52(9):1–86.

Buffler PA, Kwan ML, Reynolds P, et al: Environmental and genetic risk factors for childhood leukemia: appraising the evidence. *Cancer Invest* 2005;1:60–75.

Childhood Cancer Survivorship: Improving Care and Quality of Life. Institute of Medicine, August 2003. http://www.iom.edu/CMS/28312/4931/14782.aspx

Draper G, Vincent T, Kroll ME, et al: Childhood cancer in relation to distance from high voltage power lines in England and Wales: a case-control study. *BMJ* 2005;330:1290–1292.

Gurney JG, Bondy ML: Epidemiologic research methods and childhood cancer. In Pizzo PA, Poplack DG (editors): *Principles and Practice of Pediatric Oncology,* 4th ed. Philadelphia, Lippincott Williams & Wilkins, 2002, pp 13–20.

Gurney JG, Smith MA, Olshan AF, et al: Clues to the etiology of childhood brain cancer: N-nitroso compounds, polyomaviruses and other factors of interest. *Cancer Invest* 2001;19:640–650.

Hudson MM, Mertens AC, Yasui Y, et al: Health status of adult long-term survivors of childhood cancer: A report from the Childhood Cancer Survivor Study. *JAMA* 2003;290:1583–1592.

Kaatsch P, Steliarova-Foucher E, Crocetti E, et al: Time trends of cancer incidence in European children (1978–1997): Report from the automated childhood cancer information system project. *Eur J Cancer* 2006;42:1961–1971.

Merks JHM, Caron HN, Hennekam RCM: High incidence of malformation syndromes in a series of 1,073 children with cancer. *Am J Med Genetics* 2005;134A:132–143.

Ness KK, Mertens AC, Hudson MM, et al: Limitations on physical performance and daily activities among long-term survivors of childhood cancer. *Ann Intern Med* 2005;143:639–647.

Ries LAG, Harkins D, Krapcho M, et al (editors): *SEER Cancer Statistics Review, 1975–2003.* Bethesda, MD, National Cancer Institute. http://seer.cancer.gov/csr/1975_2003/, based on November 2005 SEER data submission, posted to the SEER web site, 2006.

Ries LAG, Smith MA, Gurney JG, et al (editors): *Cancer Incidence and Survival Among Children and Adolescents: United States SEER Program 1975–1995.* Bethesda, MD, National Cancer Institute, SEER Program, 1999.

Steliarova-Foucher E, Stiller C, Kaatsch P, et al: Geographical patterns and time trends of cancer incidence and survival among children and adolescents in Europe since the 1970s (the ACCIS project): An epidemiological study. *Lancet* 2004 Dec 11;364(9451):2097–2105.

Chapter 492 ■ Molecular and Cellular Biology of Cancer

Laura L. Worth

Cancer is a complex of diseases arising from alterations that can occur in a wide variety of genes. Alterations in normal cellular processes such as signal transduction, cell cycle control, DNA repair, cellular growth and differentiation, translational regulation, senescence and apoptosis (programmed cell death) can result in a malignant phenotype. In addition, cancer stem cells may have a role in certain malignancies such as CML, AML, ALL, gliomas, and breast cancer. These tumor-initiating cells have self renewal and proliferative properties similar to nonmalignant stem cells.

GENES INVOLVED IN ONCOGENESIS

Two major classes of genes are implicated in the development of cancer: oncogenes and tumor suppressor genes. **Proto-oncogenes** are cellular genes that are important for normal cellular function and code for various proteins, including transcriptional factors, growth factors, and growth factor receptors. These proteins are vital components in the network of signal transduction that regulate cell growth, division, and differentiation. Proto-oncogenes can be altered to form **oncogenes** that, when translated, can result in the malignant transformation of a cell.

The three main mechanisms by which proto-oncogenes can be activated include amplification, point mutation, and translocation (Table 492-1). *MYC* codes for a protein that regulates transcription and is an example of a proto-oncogene that is activated by amplification (Fig. 492-1). Patients with neuroblastoma in which the *MYC* gene is amplified 10- to 300-fold have a poorer outcome (Fig. 492-2). Point mutations also can activate proto-oncogenes. The *NRAS* proto-oncogene codes for a guanine nucleotide-binding protein with guanosine triphosphatase activity that is important in signal transduction and is mutated in 25–30% of acute nonmyelogenous leukemias, resulting in a constitutively active protein. The *RET* gene encodes a transmembrane tyrosine kinase receptor that is important in signal transduction. A point mutation in the *RET* gene results in the constitutive activation of a tyrosine kinase, as found in multiple neoplasia syndromes and familial thyroid carcinoma. The third mechanism by which proto-oncogenes become activated is chromosomal translocations. In some leukemias and lymphomas, transcription factor controlling sequences are relocated in front of T-cell receptors or immunoglobulin genes, resulting in unregulated transcription of the genes and leukemogenesis. Chromosomal translocations also can result in **fusion genes;** transcription of the fusion gene can result in the production of a chimeric protein with new and potentially oncogenic activity. Cancers associated with fusion genes include the childhood solid tumors, such as Ewing sarcoma [t(11;22)] and alveolar rhabdomyosarcoma [t(2;13) or t(1;13)]. The translocations result in novel proteins that are useful as diagnostic markers. The best described translocation in leukemia is the **Philadelphia chromosome t(9;22),** which results in the BCR/ABL protein found in chronic myelogenous leukemia. This translocation results in a tyrosine kinase protein that is constitutively activated. In addition, the protein is localized to the cytoplasm instead of the nucleus, exposing the kinase to a new spectrum of substrates.

Alteration in the regulation of tumor suppressor genes is another mechanism involved in oncogenesis. Tumor suppressor

TABLE 492-1. Oncogene Activators of Pediatric Tumors

MECHANISM	CHROMOSOME	GENES	PROTEIN FUNCTION	TUMOR
Chromosomal translocation	t(9;22)	*BCR-ABL*	Chimeric tyrosine kinase	Acute lymphocytic leukemia, chronic myelocytic leukemia
	t(1:19)	*E2A-PBX1*	Chimeric transcription factor	Pre-B acute lymphocytic leukemia
	t(14:18)	*CMYC*	Transcription factor	Burkitt lymphoma
	t(15;17)	*APL-RARα*	Chimeric transcription factor	Acute promyelocytic leukemia
Gene amplification	Amplicon	*NMYC*	Transcription factor	Neuroblastoma
	Amplicon	*EGFR*	Growth factor kinase, tyrosine kinase	Glioblastoma
Point mutation	1p	*NRAS*	GTPase	Acute myelocytic leukemia
	10q	*RET*	Tyrosine kinase	Multiple endocrine neoplasia, type 2

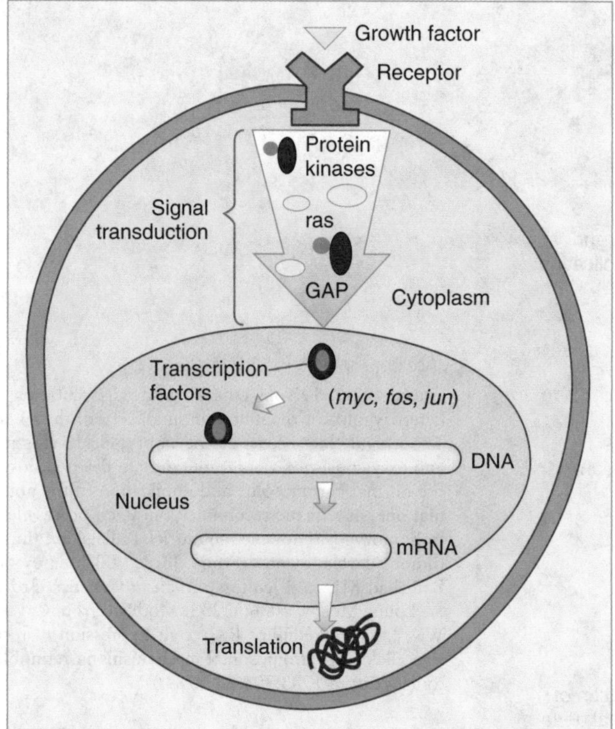

Figure 492-1. The major features of cellular regulation. External *growth factors* (proteins and steroid hormones such as epidermal growth factor) bind to membrane-spanning *growth factor receptors* on the cell surface, activating *signal-transduction* pathways in which genes such as *RAS* participate. Components of the signal-transduction pathway in turn interact with *nuclear transcription factors,* such as *MYC* and *FOS,* which can bind to regulatory regions in DNA. (From Jorde LB, Carey JC, Bamshad MJ, et al [editors]: *Medical Genetics,* 3rd ed. St. Louis, Mosby, 2006, p 231.)

genes are important regulators of cellular growth and programmed cell death or apoptosis. They have been called *recessive oncogenes* because the inactivation of both alleles of a tumor suppressor gene is required for expression of a malignant phenotype. Knudson's **"two-hit" model of cancer development** was based on observation of the behavior of the tumor suppressor gene *RB*. In sporadic cases of retinoblastoma, both alleles of the *RB* gene must be inactivated (Fig. 492-3). However, in familial cases, children inherit an inactivated allele from one parent, and consequently require the inactivation of the only remaining normal allele. This helps explain why familial cases of retinoblastoma present earlier in childhood than sporadic cases, since only one "hit" is required.

Another major tumor suppressor protein is p53, which is known as the "guardian of the genome" because it detects the presence of chromosomal damage and prevents the cell from dividing until repairs have been made. In the presence of damage beyond repair, p53 initiates apoptosis and the cell dies. More than 50% of all tumors have abnormal p53 proteins. Mutations in the *P53* gene are important in many cancers, including breast, colorectal, lung, esophageal, stomach, ovarian, and prostatic carcinomas as well as gliomas, sarcoma, and some leukemias.

SYNDROMES PREDISPOSING TO CANCER

Several syndromes are associated with an increased risk of developing malignancies, which can be characterized by different mechanisms (Table 492-2). One mechanism involves the **inactivation of tumor suppressor genes,** such as *RB* in familial retinoblastoma. Interestingly, a patient with retinoblastoma in which one of the alleles is inactivated throughout all of his or her cells is at a very high risk for developing osteosarcoma. A familial syndrome, Li-Fraumeni syndrome, in which one mutant *P53* allele is inherited, also has been described in patients who can develop sarcomas, leukemias, and cancers of the breast, bone, lung, and brain. Neurofibromatosis is characterized by the proliferation cells of neural crest origin, leading to neurofibromas. These patients are at a higher risk of developing malignant schwannomas and pheochromocytomas. Neurofibromatosis often is inherited in an autosomal dominant fashion, although 50% of the cases present without a family history and develop because of the high rate of spontaneous mutations of the *NF1* gene.

A second mechanism responsible for an inherited predisposition to develop cancer involves **defects in DNA repair.** Syndromes associated with an excessive number of broken chromosomes due to repair defects include Bloom syndrome (short stature, photosensitive telangiectatic erythema), ataxia-telangiectasia (childhood ataxia with progressive neuromotor degeneration), and Fanconi anemia (short stature, skeletal and renal anomalies, pancytopenia). Due to the decreased ability to repair chromosomal defects, cells accumulate abnormal DNA that results in significantly increased rates of cancer, especially leukemia. Xeroderma pigmentosum likewise increases the risk of skin cancer, owing to defects in repair to DNA damaged by ultraviolet light. These disorders display an autosomal recessive pattern.

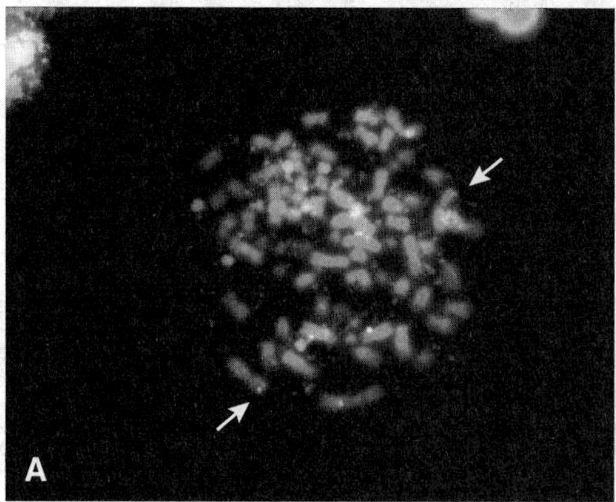

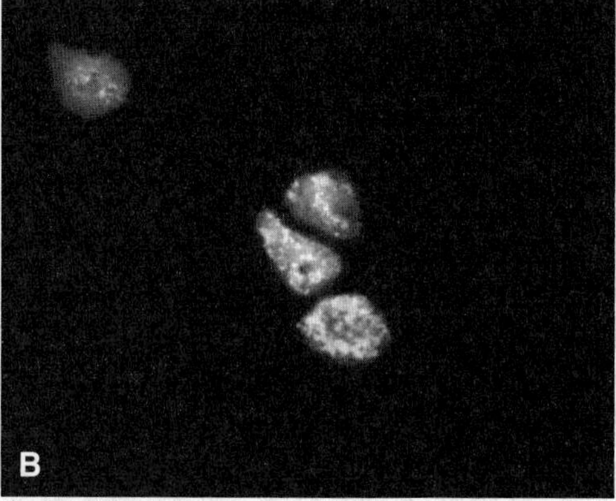

Figure 492-2. Fluorescence in situ hybridization with *MYCN* probe in advanced neuroblastoma. *A,* Metaphase spread of a tetraploid neuroblastoma cell showing double minutes. Intensity of fluorescent signal varies according to the size of the double minute and the number of *MYCN* copies it contains. White arrows point to fluorescent signal arising from the normal *MYCN* locus on distal chromosome 2p. *B,* Interphase nuclei of neuroblastoma cells showing varying degrees of fluorescent intensity arising from double minute chromosomes. (Photograph courtesy of J. Biegel, Children's Hospital of Philadelphia. Previously published in Nussbaum RL, McInnes RR, Willard HF [eds]: *Thompson and Thompson Genetics in Medicine,* 6th ed. Philadelphia, WB Saunders, 2004, p 331.)

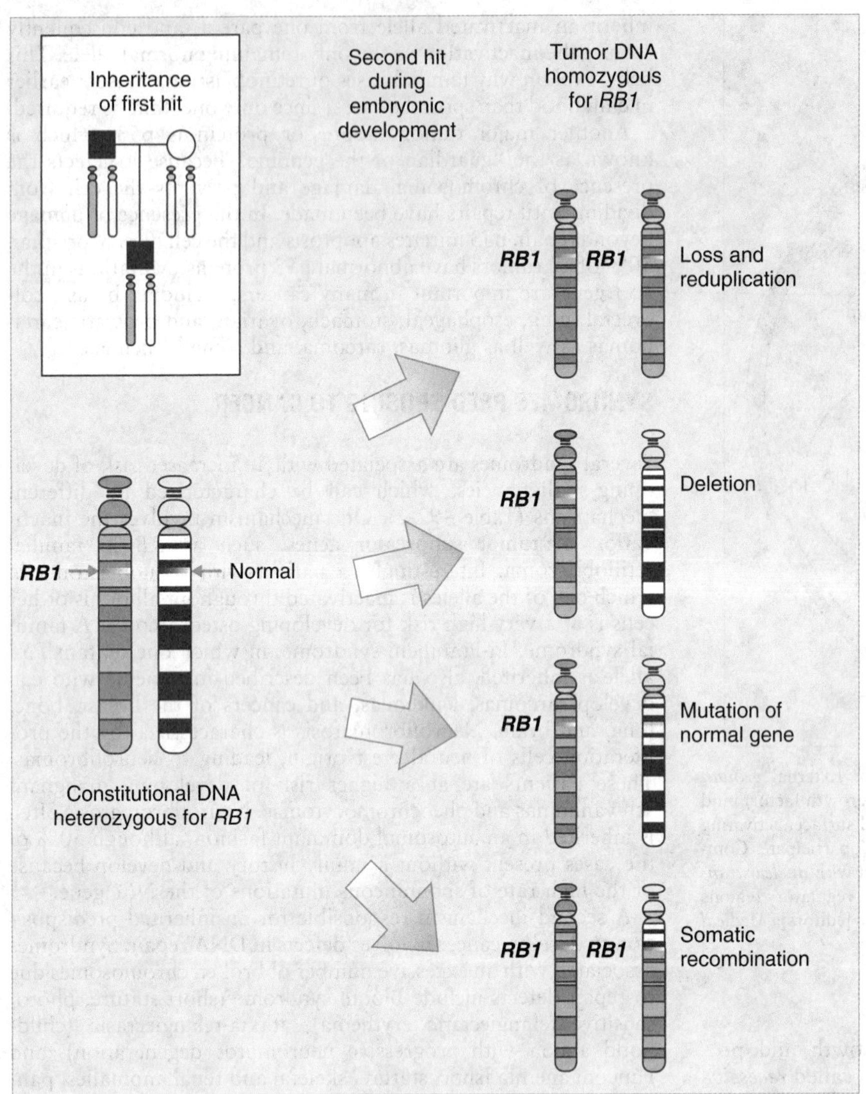

Figure 492-3. Persons inheriting an *RB1* mutation are heterozygous for the mutation in all cells of their body. The second "hit" occurs during embryonic development and may consist of a point mutation, a deletion, loss of the normal chromosome and duplication of the abnormal one, or somatic recombination. Each process leads to homozygosity for the mutant *RB1* allele and thus to tumor development. (From Jorde LB, Carey JC, Bamshad MJ, et al [editors]: *Medical Genetics*, 3rd ed. St. Louis, Mosby, 2006, p 233. Modified from Cavenee WK, Dryja TP, Phillips RA, et al: Expression of recessive alleles by chromosomal mechanisms in retinoblastoma. *Nature* 1983;305:779–784.)

TABLE 492-2. Familial or Genetic Susceptibility to Malignancy

DISORDER	TUMOR/CANCER	COMMENT
CHROMOSOMAL SYNDROMES		
Chromosome 11p- (deletion) with sporadic aniridia	Wilms tumor	Associated with genitourinary anomalies, mental retardation, *WT1* gene
Chromosomal 13q- (deletion)	Retinoblastoma Sarcoma	Associated with mental retardation, skeletal malformations; autosomal dominant (bilateral) or sporadic new mutations in the *RB1* gene
Trisomy 21	Lymphocytic or nonlymphocytic leukemia, especially megakaryocytic leukemia Transient leukemoid reaction	Risk of acute lymphocytic leukemia is increased 20%; risk of acute myelocytic leukemia is increased 400%; patients have an increased sensitivity to chemotherapy
Klinefelter syndrome (47,XXY)	Breast cancer Extragonadal germ cell tumors	—
Trisomy 8	Preleukemia	—
Noonan syndrome	Juvenile myelomonocytic leukemia	Autosomal dominant; mutations in *PTPN11* gene
Monosomy 5 or 7	Myelodysplastic syndrome	Recurrent infections may precede neoplasia.
CHROMOSOMAL INSTABILITY		
Xeroderma pigmentosum	Basal cell and squamous cell carcinomas Melanoma	Autosomal recessive; failure to repair UV-damaged DNA. Mutations in *XP* gene on chromosome 3p25
Fanconi anemia	Leukemia Myelodysplastic syndrome Liver neoplasias Rare head and neck tumors Gastrointestinal and genitourinary cancers	Autosomal recessive; chromosome fragility; positive diepoxybutane test result; mutations in *FANCX* gene family.
Bloom syndrome	Leukemia Lymphoma Solid tumors	Autosomal recessive; increased sister chromatid exchange; mutations in *BLM* gene, a member of the RecQ helicase gene family.

TABLE 492-2. Familial or Genetic Susceptibility to Malignancy—cont'd

DISORDER	TUMOR/CANCER	COMMENT
Ataxia-telangiectasia	Lymphoma Leukemia Central nervous system and non-neural solid tumors (less commonly)	Autosomal recessive; sensitive to x-irradiation, radiomimetic drugs; mutation in *ATM* tumor suppressor gene
Dysplastic nevus syndrome	Melanoma	Autosomal dominant; some cases associated with mutations in *CDKN2A* gene
Rothmund-Thompson syndrome	Osteosarcoma Skin cancers	Autosomal recessive; mutation in RecQ helicase gene family
Werner syndrome (premature aging)	Soft tissue sarcomas	Autosomal recessive; mutation in the *WRN* gene—member of the RecQ helicase gene family
IMMUNODEFICIENCY SYNDROMES		
Wiskott-Aldrich syndrome	Lymphoma, leukemia	X-linked recessive; *WAS* gene mutation (Xp11.22-23); WASp protein functions in signal transduction associated with cytoskeletal actin filament rearrangement
X-linked immunodeficiency (Duncan syndrome)	Lymphoproliferative disorder	X-linked; Epstein-Barr viral infection may be fatal; mutation in *SH2D1A* gene locus
X-linked agammaglobulinemia (Bruton disease)	Lymphoma, leukemia	X-linked; mutation in *BKT* gene resulting in absence of mature B cells
Severe combined immunodeficiency	Leukemia, lymphoma	X-linked; mutations in *ADA* gene
OTHERS		
Neurofibromatosis type 1	Neurofibroma Optic glioma Acoustic neuroma Astrocytoma Meningioma Pheochromocytoma Sarcoma	Autosomal dominant, mutation in tumor suppressor gene, *NF1*
Neurofibromatosis type 2	Bilateral acoustic neuromas Meningiomas	Autosomal dominant; mutation in tumor suppressor gene *NF2*
Tuberous sclerosis	Fibroangiomatous nevi Myocardial rhabdomyoma	Autosomal dominant
Gorlin-Goltz syndrome (nevus basal cell carcinoma syndrome)	Multiple basal cell carcinomas Medulloblastoma	Autosomal dominant; mutation in *PTCH* gene
Li-Fraumeni syndrome	Bone Soft tissue sarcoma Breast	Mutation of *P53* tumor-suppressor gene, autosomal dominant
Retinoblastoma	Sarcoma	Autosomal recessive; Increased risk of secondary malignancy 10–20 yr later, mutation in *RB* tumor suppressor gene
Hemihypertrophy ± Beckwith syndrome	Wilms tumor Hepatoblastoma Adrenal carcinoma	*WT1* gene. 25% develop tumor, most in first 5 yr of life
von Hippel-Lindau disease	Hemangioblastoma of the cerebellum and retina Pheochromocytoma Renal cancer	Autosomal dominant, mutation of tumor-suppressor gene, *VHL* gene
Multiple endocrine neoplasia syndrome, type 1 (Wermer syndrome)	Parathyroid, pancreatic islet, and pituitary tumors	Autosomal dominant; mutation in *PYGM* tumor suppressor gene
Multiple endocrine neoplasia syndrome, type 2A (Sipple syndrome)	Medullary carcinoma of the thyroid Hyperparathyroidism Pheochromocytoma	Autosomal dominant; mutations in Cys rich regions of the *RET* gene activates this proto-oncogene. *RET* codes for a tyrosine kinase; monitor calcitonin and calcium levels
Multiple endocrine neoplasia type 2B (multiple mucosal neuroma syndrome)	Mucosal neuroma Pheochromocytoma Medullary thyroid carcinoma Marfan habitus Neuropathy	Autosomal dominant; mutation in catalytic site (codon 883 or 914) activates proto-oncogene. *RET* codes for a tyrosine kinase.
Familial adenomatous polyposis	Colorectal and thyroid carcinoma Duodenal and periampullar carcinomas Pediatric hepatoblastoma	Autosomal dominant; mutation in *APC* gene
Familial juvenile polyposis	Colorectal carcinoma	Autosomal dominant; mutation in *SMAD4* gene
Hereditary nonpolyposis colon cancer (Lynch syndrome, NHPCC)	Colon cancer	Autosomal dominant; mutation in mismatch repair genes; *hMSH2, hMLH1, PMS1, PMS2, hMSH6, hMSG3*
Turcot syndrome	Pediatric brain tumors Increased risk of colon carcinoma and polyps	Mutation in the *APC* gene
Familial adenomatous polyposis coli	Adenocarcinoma of colon	Autosomal dominant, *APC* gene
Gardner syndrome	Adenocarcinoma of colon Skull and soft tissue tumors	Autosomal dominant, *APC* gene
Peutz-Jeghers syndrome	Gastrointestinal carcinoma Ovarian neoplasia	Autosomal dominant, *LKB1* gene codes for a Ser/Thr kinase that regulates cell cycle, metabolism, cell polarity
Hemochromatosis	Hepatocellular carcinoma	Autosomal dominant; malignancy associated with cirrhotic liver
Glycogen storage disease 1 (von Gierke disease)	Hepatocellular carcinoma	Autosomal recessive; malignancy associated with cirrhotic liver. Mutation in glucose-6-phosphatase or glucose 6-phosphatase translocase gene
Tyrosinemia, galactosemia	Hepatocellular carcinoma	Autosomal recessive; tumor associated with cirrhotic liver
BRCA1 and BRCA2	Breast and ovarian cancers	DNA repair defect
Sickle cell trait	Renal medullary carcinoma	Etiology unknown

The third category of inherited cancer predisposition is characterized by **defects in immune surveillance.** This group includes patients with Wiskott-Aldrich syndrome, severe combined immunodeficiency, common variable immunodeficiency, and the X-linked lymphoproliferative syndrome. The most common types of malignancy in these patients are lymphoma and leukemia. Cure rates for immunodeficient children with cancer are much poorer than for nonimmunodeficient children with similar malignancies, suggesting a role for the immune system in cancer treatment as well as in cancer prevention.

OTHER FACTORS ASSOCIATED WITH ONCOGENESIS

VIRUSES. Several viruses have been implicated in the pathogenesis of malignancy. The association between the **Epstein-Barr virus (EBV)** and Burkitt lymphoma and nasopharyngeal carcinoma was identified >30 yr ago, although EBV infection alone is not sufficient for malignant transformation. EBV also is associated with mixed cellularity and lymphocyte-depleted Hodgkin disease, as well as some T-cell lymphomas, which is particularly intriguing because EBV normally does not infect T lymphocytes. The most conclusive evidence for a role of EBV in lymphogenesis is the direct causal role of EBV for B-cell lymphoproliferative disease in immunocompromised persons, especially those with AIDS. EBV also is associated with leiomyosarcoma in immunocompromised persons.

In children with chronic **hepatitis B** infection (HBsAg-positive), the risk of developing hepatocellular carcinoma is increased >200-fold. In adults, the latency period between viral infection and the development of hepatocellular carcinoma approaches 20 yr. However, in children who acquire the viral infection through perinatal transmission, the latency period can be as short as 6–7 yr. The additional factors that are required for the malignant transformation of the virally infected hepatocytes have not been determined. **Hepatitis C virus** infection also is a risk factor for hepatocellular carcinoma and is associated with splenic lymphoma.

Nearly all cervical carcinomas contain **human papillomavirus (HPV).** Papillomaviruses type 16 and 18 are highly associated with cervical cancer. Types 31, 33, 35, 45, and 56 are less likely to cause cervical cancer. The low-risk papillomaviruses, including types 6 and 11, which commonly are found in genital warts, rarely are associated with malignancies. Like other virus-associated cancers, the presence of HPV alone is not sufficient to cause malignant transformation. The mechanism by which HPV 19 induces malignant transformation is thought to involve *P53* and *RB* tumor suppressor gene, which regulate cell cycle by acting as gatekeepers of the G1/S and G2/M checkpoints. By interfering with these proteins, HPV alters the regulation of cell growth.

Human herpesvirus 8 (HHV8) is associated with Kaposi's sarcoma, primary effusion B-cell lymphoma, and the plasma cell variant of Castleman disease, all of which occur primarily among persons with AIDS. **Human T-cell leukemia virus 1 (HTLV-1)** is associated with adult T-cell leukemia and lymphoma.

GENOMIC IMPRINTING. The development of cancer also has been linked to genomic imprinting, which is the selective inactivation of one of two alleles of a certain gene. Which gene is inactivated is determined by whether the gene is inherited from the mother or father. Normally the maternal *IGF2* (insulin-like growth factor receptor 2) gene is inactivated. The inactivation is thought to be secondary to methylation of specific CpG sequences upstream of the *IGF2* promoter, which interferes with the transcription of the *IGF2* gene. In some Wilms tumors, there is loss of methylation in the upstream area of the maternal gene, which, in turn, allows transcript expression of the maternal *IGF2* gene. At the same time the *H19* gene (whose function is not yet clear), a previously actively transcribed maternal gene, is silenced by methylation. Beckwith-Weidemann syndrome, an overgrowth syndrome characterized by macrosomia, macroglossia, hemihypertrophy, omphalocele, and renal anomalies also is associated with an increased risk of Wilms tumor, hepatoblastoma, rhabdomyosarcoma, neuroblastoma, and adrenal cortical carcinoma. The increased risk of developing cancer is associated with changes in the methylation pattern of genes on the 11p15 chromosome. In vitro fertilization has been associated with imprinting defects and the development of some cases of Beckwith-Weidemann syndrome-associated Wilm tumor and retinoblastoma.

TELOMERASE. Telomeres are a series of tens to thousands of TTAGGG repeats at the ends of chromosomes that are important for stabilizing the chromosomal ends and limiting breakage, translocation, and loss of DNA material. With DNA replication there is a progressive shortening of telomere length, which is a hallmark of cellular aging and may be a senescence signal. In some instances **telomerase,** an enzyme that adds telomeres to the ends of chromosomes, becomes active. The addition of telomeres can be found in immortalized cell lines and most tumor types, and as a consequence, these cells may have a survival advantage that allows them to undergo additional cell divisions. Therapy aimed at inhibition of telomerase activity may result in cell death.

Attiyeh EF, London WB, Mosse YP, et al: Chromosome 1p and 11q deletions and outcome in neuroblastoma. *N Engl J Med* 2005;353:2243–2253.

Blackburn E: Telomeres and telomerase; their mechanisms of action and the effects of altering their functions. *FEBS Letters* 2005;579:859–862.

Hitchens MP, Wong JJL, Suthers G, et al: Inheritance of a cancer-associated MLHI germ-line epimutation. *N Engl J Med* 2007;356:697–705.

Jordan CT, Guzman ML, Noble M: Cancer stem cells. *N Engl J Med* 2006;355:1253–1260.

Messahel B, Hing S, Nash R, et al: Clinical features of molecular pathology of solid tumours in childhood. *Lancet Oncol* 2005;6:421–430.

Mitelman F, Johansson B, Mertens F: Fusion genes and rearranged genes as a linear function of chromosome aberrations in cancer. *Nature Genetics* 2004;36:331–334.

Moll AC, Imhof SM, Cruysberg JRM, et al: Incidence of retinoblastoma in children born after in-vitro fertilization. *Lancet* 2003;361:309–310.

Prawitt D, Enklar T, Gartner-Rupprecht B, et al: Microdeletion and IGF2 loss of imprinting in a cascade causing Beckwith-Wiedemann syndrome with Wilms' tumor. *Nature Genetics* 2005;37:785–786.

Quackenbush J: Microarray analysis and tumor classification. *N Engl J Med* 2006;354:2463–2472.

Reinhart B, Chaillet JR: Genomic imprinting: cis-acting sequences and regional control. *Int Rev Cytol* 2005:243;173–213.

Schiavi F, Boedeker CC, Bausch B, et al: Predictors and prevalence of paraganglioma syndrome associated with mutations of the SDHC gene. *JAMA* 2005;294:2057–2062.

Windschwendter M, Fiegl H, Egle D, et al: Epigenetic stem cell signature in cancer. *Nat Genet* 2007;39:157–164.

Chapter 493 ■ Principles of Diagnosis Archie Bleyer

Symptoms and physical findings are important in the recognition of malignant diseases and life-threatening benign tumors in children and adolescents. In addition to the classic manifestations, any persistent, unexplained symptom or sign should be evaluated as potentially emanating from a cancerous or precancerous condition. As part of the diagnostic evaluation, the pediatrician and

TABLE 493-1. The Most Common Signs and Symptoms of Cancer in Children and Adults

ADULTS*
Change in bowel or bladder habits
Blood in stool
Lump in breast or elsewhere
Hoarseness or nagging cough
Difficulty in swallowing
Sore that will not heal
Change in wart or mole
CHILDREN†
Abdominal mass
Persistent lymphadenopathy
>1 abnormal hematopoietic lineage
Specific neurologic deficit
Increased intracranial pressure
Diffuse enlargement of pons
Proptosis
White pupillary reflex
Unilateral knee or shoulder pain/swelling
Vaginal bleeding or mass

*Developed by the American Cancer Society in the 1950s.
†Developed by the University of Texas M.D. Anderson Cancer Center.

pediatric oncologist must convey the diagnosis to the patient and family in a sensitive and informative manner.

SIGNS AND SYMPTOMS. In contrast to the classic warning signs of cancer in adults (Table 493-1), there is no established set of symptoms and signs of cancer in children, for a number of reasons. The symptoms and signs of cancer are more variable and nonspecific in pediatric than adult patients. The types of cancer that occur during the first 20 yr of life vary dramatically as a function of age—more so than at any other comparable age range (see Chapter 491). Unlike cancers in adults, childhood cancers usually originate from the deeper, visceral structures and from the parenchyma of organs rather than from the epithelial layers that line the ducts and glands of organs and compose the skin. In children, metastases are present at diagnosis in approximately 80% of cases, whereas only about 20% of adults have evidence of metastases at diagnosis. In children, therefore, the presenting symptoms or signs are more likely to be caused by metastases than the primary tumor. Infants and young children cannot express or localize their symptoms as clearly as adults, and diagnostic tests may not have the utility or precision of those that can be applied to adults. Another factor is the variability in the physiology and biology of the host related to growth and development during infancy, childhood, and adolescence.

As a result, the signs of cancer in children often are attributed to other causes before the malignancy is recognized. Delays in diagnosis are particularly problematic during late adolescence, and are due to a variety of factors prominent in this age group, including loss of health insurance coverage.

Although there is no clearly established set of warning signs of cancer in young people, the most common cancers in children suggest some guidelines that may be helpful in early recognition of signs and symptoms of cancer (Table 493-2; see also Table 493-1). Most of the symptoms and signs are not specific and may represent other possibilities in a differential diagnosis. Nonetheless, these hints encompass the common cancers of childhood and have been very useful in early detection. In addition, there are many additional but less common signs and symptoms of cancer in children (Table 493-3).

PHYSICAL EXAMINATION. The most common pediatric cancers may be classified into 5 categories on the basis of the involved tissue or organ system: the lymphohematopoietic system; the nervous system; the embryonal group; connective tissue; and gonadal system. Accordingly, paying particular attention during physical examination to "blood, brain, belly, and bone" manifestations—the *four Bs*—is helpful in eliciting evidence of malignancy.

Abnormalities of the hematopoietic system manifest as pallor, which indicates anemia; bleeding from orifices, petechiae,

TABLE 493-2. Common Manifestations of Childhood Malignancies

SIGNS AND SYMPTOMS	SIGNIFICANCE	EXAMPLE
HEMATOLOGIC		
Pallor, anemia	Bone marrow infiltration	Leukemia, neuroblastoma
Petechiae, thrombocytopenia	Bone marrow infiltration	Leukemia, neuroblastoma
Fever, pharyngitis, neutropenia	Bone marrow infiltration	Leukemia, neuroblastoma
SYSTEMIC		
Bone pain, limp, arthralgia	Primary bone tumor, metastasis to bone	Osteosarcoma, Ewing sarcoma, leukemia, neuroblastoma
Fever of unknown origin, weight loss, night sweats	Lymphoreticular malignancy	Hodgkin disease, non-Hodgkin lymphoma
Painless lymphadenopathy	Lymphoreticular malignancy, metastatic solid tumor	Leukemia, Hodgkin disease, non-Hodgkin lymphoma, Burkitt lymphoma, thyroid carcinoma
Cutaneous lesion	Primary or metastatic disease	Neuroblastoma, leukemia, Langerhans cell histiocytosis, melanoma
Abdominal mass	Adrenal-renal tumor	Neuroblastoma, Wilms tumor, lymphoma
Hypertension	Sympathetic nervous system tumor	Neuroblastoma, pheochromocytoma, Wilms tumor
Diarrhea	Vasoactive intestinal polypeptide	Neuroblastoma, ganglioneuroma
Soft tissue mass	Local or metastatic tumor	Ewing sarcoma, osteosarcoma, neuroblastoma, thyroid carcinoma, rhabdomyosarcoma, eosinophilic granuloma
Diabetes insipidus, galactorrhea, poor growth	Neuroendocrine involvement of hypothalamus or pituitary gland	Adenoma, craniopharyngioma, prolactinoma, Langerhans' cell histiocytosis
Emesis, visual disturbances, ataxia, headache, papilledema, cranial nerve palsies	Increased intrathecal pressure	Primary brain tumor; metastasis
OPHTHALMOLOGIC SIGNS		
Leukokoria	White pupil	Retinoblastoma
Periorbital ecchymosis	Metastasis	Neuroblastoma
Miosis, ptosis, heterochromia	Horner syndrome: compression of cervical sympathetic nerves	Neuroblastoma
Opsomyoclonus, ataxia	Neurotransmitters? Autoimmunity?	Neuroblastoma
Exophthalmos, proptosis	Orbital tumor	Rhabdomyosarcoma, lymphoma
THORACIC MASS		
Anterior mediastinal	Cough, stridor, pneumonia, tracheal-bronchial compression	Germ cell tumor, T cell lymphoma, Hodgkin disease
Posterior mediastinal	Vertebral or nerve root compression; dysphagia	Neuroblastoma, neuroenteric cyst

From Kliegman RM, Marcdante KJ, Jenson HB, et al (editors): *Nelson Essentials of Pediatrics,* 5th ed. Philadelphia, WB Saunders, 2006, p 729.

TABLE 493-3. Uncommon Signs and Symptoms of Cancer in Children

RELATED DIRECTLY TO TUMOR
Superior vena caval syndrome
Subcutaneous nodules
Leukemoid reaction
Myasthenia gravis
Heterochromia
NOT RELATED DIRECTLY TO TUMOR GROWTH
Chronic diarrhea
Polymyoclonus-opsoclonus
Failure to thrive
Cushing syndrome
Pseudomuscular dystrophy

Modified from Vietti TJ, Steuber CP: Clinical assessment and differential diagnosis of the child with suspected cancer. In Pizzo PA, Poplack DG (editors): *Principles and Practice of Pediatric Oncology,* 4th ed. Philadelphia, Lippincott Williams & Wilkins, 2002, pp 149–160.

purpura, and ecchymosis, which indicate thrombocytopenia or disseminated intravascular coagulation; cellulitis or other evidence of infection, which indicates leukopenia; skin nodules, which indicate leukocytosis; and other abnormalities of the formed elements of the blood. Abnormalities of the lymphatic system include lymphadenopathy (Fig. 493-1), superior vena cava syndrome, or respiratory distress when the patient is in a supine position, suggesting an upper anterior mediastinal mass or thymic enlargement (Fig. 493-2). Enlargement of the cervical lymph nodes is common in children with infection and in patients with lymphoma. Persistent or progressive enlargement of lymph nodes, often painless, is suggestive of lymphoma and indicates the need for biopsy.

Abnormalities of the central nervous system that indicate cancer include decreased level of consciousness, paresis of cranial nerve VI, seizures, ptosis, decreased visual activity, and increased intracranial pressure, which may be diagnosed by the presence of papilledema (Fig. 493-3). Any focal neurologic deficit in the motor or sensory system, especially a decrease in cranial nerve function, should prompt further investigation for malignancy.

Abnormalities of the embryonal system usually are apparent on physical examination as organomegaly or an abdominal mass. However, an unexplained mass in any area of the body should be considered malignant until proven otherwise. Diffuse enlargement of the pons is a radiographic finding, usually revealed on an MRI scan (Fig. 493-4), that nearly always indicates malignant disease and may be considered pathognomonic. Diffuse, not local, enlargement of the pons is considered astrocytoma and treated accordingly without tissue biopsy, in part because of the risk and difficulty of a surgical procedure on this part of the brain. Retinoblastoma usually manifests as a white pupillary reflex (Fig. 493-5) rather than the usual red reflection from incident light. A white pupillary reflex is essentially pathognomonic for retinoblastoma, although astrocytic hamartomas, Coats disease, and persistent hypertrophy of the primary vitreous may mimic this finding. In neonates, "blueberry muffin" spots on the skin may be neuroblastoma. A sacrococcygeal mass usually is a teratoma that may undergo malignant transformation if it is not removed.

AGE-RELATED MANIFESTATIONS. Because various types of cancer in children occur at specific ages, the physician should tailor the history and physical examination based on the age of the child. The embryonal tumors, including neuroblastoma, usually occur during the first 2 yr of life (see Fig. 491-3). From 2–5 yr of age, acute lymphoblastic leukemias, non-Hodgkin lymphoma, and gliomas peak in incidence. During adolescence, bone tumors, Hodgkin disease, and the gonadal and connective tissue tumors predominate. Hence, for infants and toddlers, special attention should be paid to the possibility of embryonal and intra-abdominal tumors (e.g., Wilms tumor, retinoblastoma, teratoma, neuroblastoma, and liver tumors). Preschool-aged and early school-aged children showing compatible signs and symptoms should be specifically evaluated for leukemia, lymphoma, and brain tumors. Adolescents require assessment for sarcomas and genital or gonadal malignancies, as well as for Hodgkin disease.

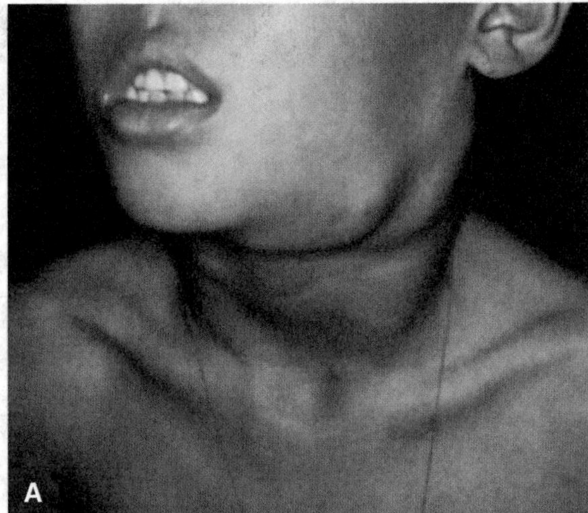

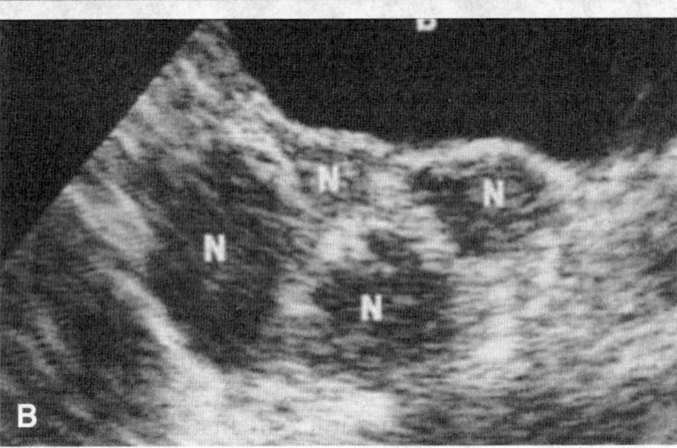

Figure 493-1. Cervical lymphadenopathy. Manifestations on physical examination (*A*) and on ultrasound examination (*B*). N, abnormally enlarged lymph nodes. (From Sinniah D, D'Angio GJ, Chatten J, et al: *Atlas of Pediatric Oncology.* London, Arnold, 1996.)

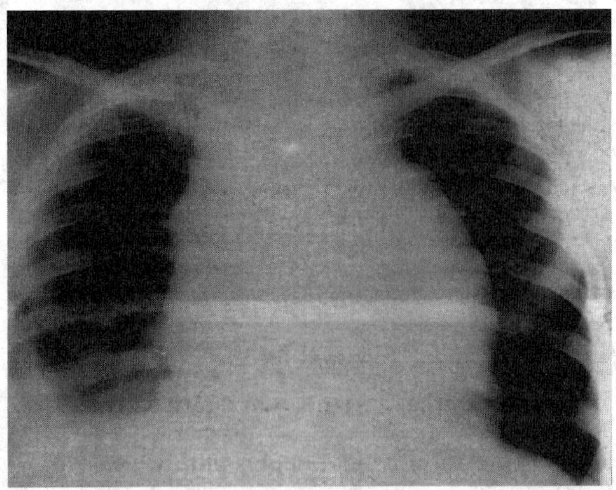

Figure 493-2. Anterior upper mediastinal mass from non-Hodgkin lymphoma. (From Sinniah D, D'Angio GJ, Chatten J, et al: *Atlas of Pediatric Oncology.* London, Arnold, 1996.)

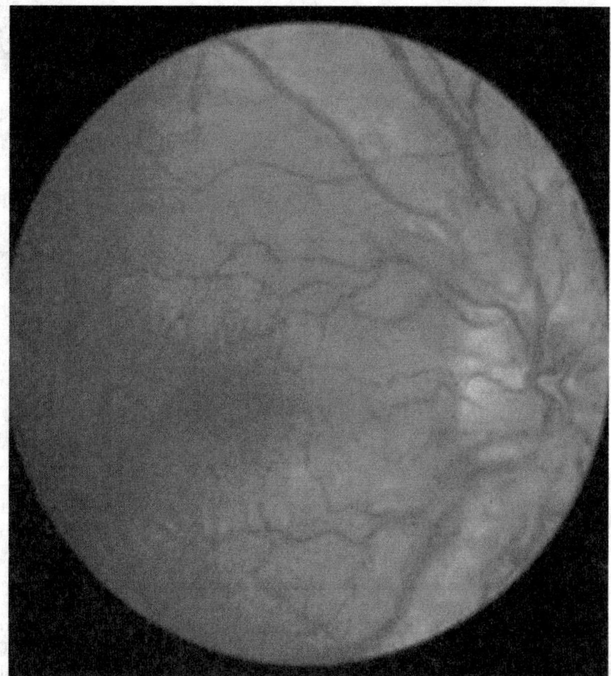

Figure 493-3. Papilledema on funduscopic examination. (From Sinniah D, D'Angio GJ, Chatten J, et al: *Atlas of Pediatric Oncology.* London, Arnold, 1996.)

EARLY DETECTION

Because most childhood cancers are curable, early detection is crucial. In addition, for several types of childhood cancer, less aggressive therapy is indicated for early-stage disease than for advanced disease. In fact, early detection often minimizes the amount and duration of treatment required for cure and, therefore, may not only lead to a higher potential for cure but also spare the patient intensive or prolonged therapy.

The prognosis of malignancy in children depends primarily on tumor type, extent of disease at diagnosis, and rapidity of response to treatment. Early diagnosis helps to ensure that appropriate therapy is given in a timely fashion and, hence, optimizes the chances of cure. Because most physicians in general practice rarely encounter children with undiagnosed cancer, they should remember to investigate the possibility of malignancy, especially when they encounter an atypical course of a common childhood condition, unusual manifestations that do not fit common conditions, and any persistent symptom that defies diagnosis.

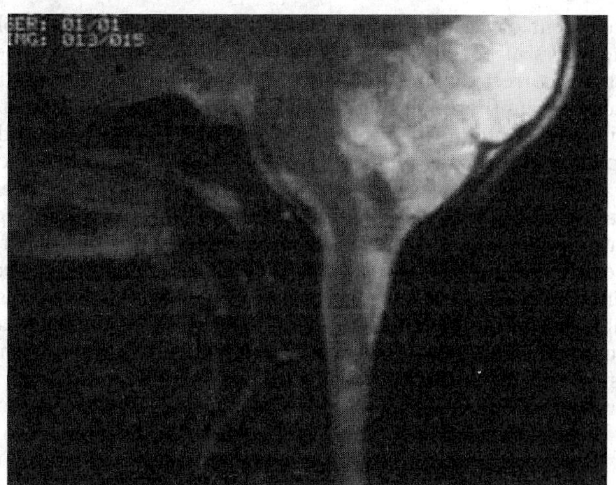

Figure 493-4. Brain stem tumor apparent on MRI. (From Sinniah D, D'Angio GJ, Chatten J, et al: *Atlas of Pediatric Oncology.* London, Arnold, 1996.)

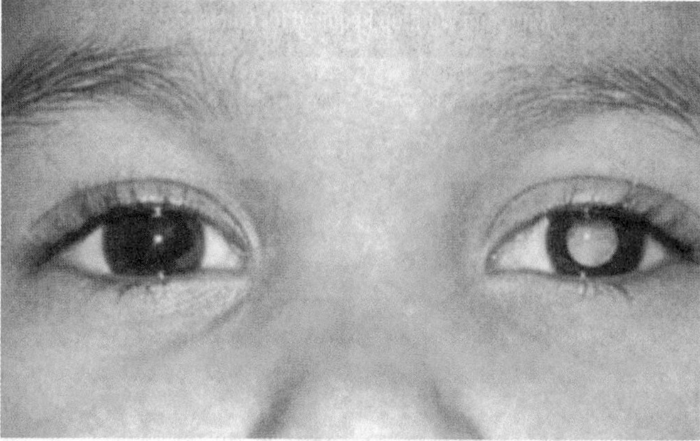

Figure 493-5. White pupillary reflex in the left eye. (From Sinniah D, D'Angio GJ, Chatten J, et al: *Atlas of Pediatric Oncology.* London, Arnold, 1996.)

Delays in diagnosis are particularly likely in certain clinical situations. The cardinal symptom of both osteosarcoma and Ewing sarcoma is localized and usually persistent pain. Because these tumors occur during the second decade of life, a time of increased physical activity, patients often assume the pain results from trauma. Prompt radiologic evaluation can help confirm the diagnosis. Tumors of the nasopharynx or middle ear may mimic infection. Prolonged, unexplained ear pain, nasal discharge, retropharyngeal swelling, and trismus should be investigated as possible signs of malignancy.

Early symptoms of leukemia may be limited to low-grade fever or bone and joint pain. Blood counts, with particular attention to normocytic anemia or mild thrombocytopenia, may indicate the need for bone marrow examination, even when leukemic blast cells are not seen in the blood smear. Malignancy can also occur in neonates and should be considered in children with masses in any area or with "blueberry muffin" spots on their skin; the latter sign is indicative of neuroblastoma.

STAGING

When a malignant neoplasm is suspected, the immediate goal is to determine its type and extent. A tentative diagnosis often can be established on the basis of the patient's age, presenting symptoms, and the location of a suspected mass. A thorough search for metastatic disease usually precedes biopsy of a suspicious lesion (Table 493-4). The surgeon can make a more informed choice between an attempt at complete resection and a more limited procedure when the presence or likelihood of disseminated disease is known. The appropriate preoperative studies depend on the tentative diagnosis. CT and MRI are noninvasive techniques that may be useful in evaluating patients for the presence of metastatic lesions; bone marrow aspiration, biopsy, or both also may be needed. These studies also are used in assessing the disease stage, information that is critical in determining the prognosis and developing a treatment plan. In addition to traditional methods, DNA microarray analysis may help identify gene expression patterns of many tumors, which adds to more accurate staging and tumor classification.

HISTOPATHOLOGY

Central to the diagnosis of any tumor is histologic examination of specimens. The initial specimen of tumor tissue should be obtained under conditions that allow for a full range of pathologic studies. In some cases, such as suspected lymphomas, fresh

TABLE 493-4. Minimum Work-up Required for Common Pediatric Malignancies to Assess Primary Tumor and Potential Metastases*

	BONE MARROW ASPIRATE/BIOPSY	CHEST X-RAY	CT SCAN	MRI	BONE SCAN	CSF ANALYSIS	SPECIFIC MARKERS	OTHER TESTS
Leukemia	Yes	Yes	—	—	—	Yes	—	—
Non-Hodgkin lymphoma	Yes	Yes	Yes	—	Yes	Yes	—	—
Hodgkin disease	Yes	Yes	Yes	—	Yes	—	—	Gallium scan
CNS tumors	—	—	—	Yes	—	Yes	—	—
Neuroblastoma	Yes	—	Yes	—	Yes	—	VMA, HVA	MIBG scan
Wilms tumor	—	Yes	Yes	—	—	—	—	—
Rhabdomyosarcoma	Yes	Yes	Yes	—	Yes	Yes (for parameningeal tumors only)	—	—
Osteosarcoma	—	Yes	Yes (of chest)	Yes (for primary tumors)	Yes	—	—	—
Ewing sarcoma	Yes	Yes	Yes (of chest)	Yes (for primary tumors)	Yes	—	—	—
Germ cell tumors	—	Yes	Yes	Consider MRI of brain	—	—	AFP, HCG	—
Liver tumors	—	Yes	Yes	—	—	—	AFP	—
Retinoblastoma	±**	—	Yes, if MRI not available	Yes (of brain)	±	Yes	—	Retinoblastoma gene analysis

*Individual cases may require additional studies.
**If marrow involvement is suspected.
From Kliegman RM, Marcdante KJ, Jenson HB, et al (editors): *Nelson Essentials of Pediatrics,* 5th ed. Philadelphia, WB Saunders, 2006, p 730.
AFP, alpha-fetoprotein; CNS, central nervous system; CSF, cerebrospinal fluid; HCG, human chorionic gonadotropin; HVA, homovanillic acid; MIBG, metaiodobenzylguanidine; VMA, vanillylmandelic acid.

tissue may be required for special studies. Some of these studies are time-consuming, which precludes discussing the specific diagnosis with the patient's family immediately after surgery.

All too often, malignancy is not suspected prior to a surgical procedure and the course of subsequent events requires reoperation to obtain the appropriate diagnostic test, assess the extent of disease (staging), and remove residual tumor, transforming the initial surgical procedure into a cancer operation.

In many cases, the diagnosis can be confirmed by means of a fine-needle biopsy, thus eliminating the need for an incision or major operation. However, making a diagnosis based on the results of a fine-needle biopsy requires an experienced radiologist and an experienced cytologist, so that this option usually is available only at major medical centers. Minimally invasive surgery using endoscopic techniques usually is performed in patients with abdominal and thoracic masses. At the time of biopsy, definitive excision, or exploration the surgeon must search carefully for evidence of regional dissemination to lymph node groups or to adjacent organs. Sentinal nodes may be identified by scintigraphy and/or dye injection adjacent to the primary tumor. Node biopsy will be limited to the principal draining nodes if histologically negative for tumor cells. If total resection is attempted, the pathologist must examine the margins carefully for microscopic residual tumor, because this information is needed for determining subsequent treatment.

DISCUSSING THE DIAGNOSTIC EVALUATION

The diagnostic and treatment plan must be carefully explained to parents and, if the child is old enough to understand, to the patient. An honest discussion of the facts is the best policy. Children should be given as much information as they can understand and would find useful or that they express a desire or wish to know. Effects of treatment, such as the possible need to amputate a limb, loss of hair during chemotherapy, and possible temporary or permanent functional impairment must be anticipated and fully discussed. The possibility and probability of death from cancer should be covered in an age-appropriate manner. It usually is necessary to repeat explanations several times before distraught family members fully understand. Throughout treatment, parents, patients, siblings, and medical staff will need help in expressing feelings of anxiety, depression, guilt, and anger. Experienced professionals, including pediatric social workers, child psychologists and psychiatrists, child life specialists, and schoolteachers with special expertise in managing students with cancer should be called on by the pediatrician, pediatric oncologist, and nurses to assist when needed.

Guillerman RP, Braverman RM, Parker BR: Imaging studies in the diagnosis and management of pediatric malignancies. In Pizzo PA, Poplack DG (editors): *Principles and Practice of Pediatric Oncology,* 5th ed. Philadelphia, Lippincott Williams & Wilkins, 2006; pp 256–289.

Malogolowkin M, Quinn JJ, Vietti TJ, Steuber CP: Clinical assessment and differential diagnosis of the child with suspected cancer. In Pizzo PA, Poplack DG (editors): *Principles and Practice of Pediatric Oncology,* 5th ed. Philadelphia, Lippincott Williams & Wilkins, 2006; pp 145–159.

Quackenbush J: Microarray analysis and tumor classification. *N Engl J Med* 2006;354:2463–2472.

Sinniah D, D'Angio GJ, Chatten J, et al: *Atlas of Pediatric Oncology.* London, Arnold, 1996.

Triche TJ, Sorenson PHB: Molecular pathology of pediatric malignancies. In Pizzo PA, Poplack DG (editors): *Principles and Practice of Pediatric Oncology,* 4th ed. Philadelphia, Lippincott Williams & Wilkins, 2002, pp 161–204.

Chapter 494 ■ Principles of Treatment

Archie Bleyer

Treatment of children with cancer is one of the most complex endeavors in pediatrics. It begins with an absolute requirement for the correct diagnosis (including subtype), proceeds through accurate and thorough staging of the extent of disease and determination of prognostic subgroup, provides appropriate multidisciplinary and usually multimodal therapy, and requires assiduous evaluation of the possibilities of recurrent disease and of adverse late effects of the disease and the therapies rendered. Throughout treatment, every child with cancer should have the benefit of the expertise of specialized teams of providers of pediatric cancer care, including pediatric oncologists, pathologists, radiologists, surgeons, radiotherapists, nurses, and various support staff, including nutritionists, social workers, psychologists, pharmacists, other medical specialists, and teachers trained to work with seriously ill children.

The best chance for cure of cancer is during the initial course of treatment; as with adults, the cure rates for patients with recurrent disease are much lower than those for patients with primary disease. All patients with cancer should be referred to an appropriate specialized center as soon as possible when the diagnosis

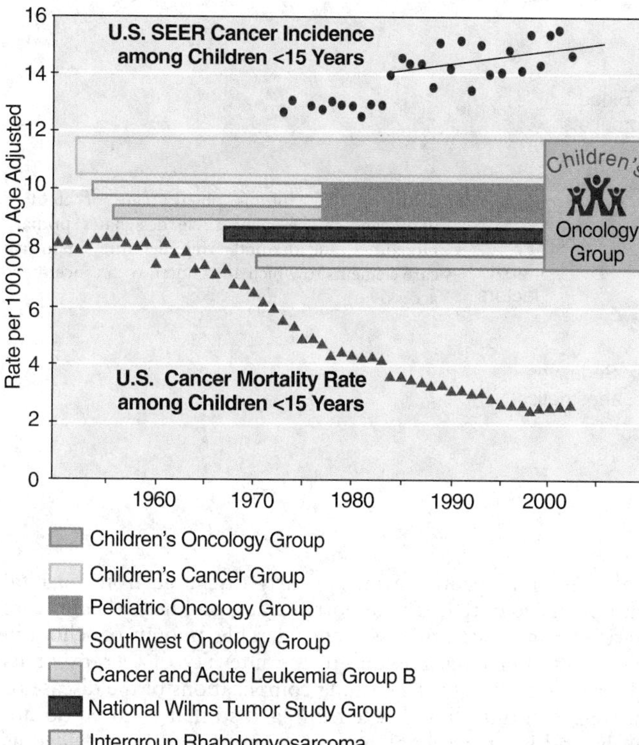

Figure 494-1. Reduction in the national cancer mortality rate among children <15 yr of age (triangles) in the USA as a direct consequence of the National Cooperative Group Program sponsored by the National Cancer Institute, and in comparison to the rising incidence of cancer before age 15 yr (circles). The horizontal bars indicate the duration of the existence of the national pediatric cancer cooperative groups, beginning with the Children's Cancer Group (CCG) in 1955. Other groups are the Pediatric Oncology Group (POG), which was derived from the Pediatrics Divisions of the Southwest Oncology Group and the Cancer and Acute Leukemia Group B, the National Wilms Tumor Study Group, and the Intergroup Rhabdomyosarcoma Study Group. In 2000, the four pediatric cooperative groups merged into the Children's Oncology Group. (Incidence and mortality rate data from Ries LAG, Eisner MP, Kosary CL, et al [editors]: *SEER Cancer Statistics Review, 1975–2002,* National Cancer Institute, Bethesda, MD; *http://seer.cancer.gov/csr/1975_2002/*, based on November 2004 SEER data submission, posted to the SEER web site 2005. The mortality rate data are national rates, and the incidence data are derived from the SEER program, representing about 15% of the USA.)

of cancer is suspected. All such centers in North America are identified on the Children's Oncology Group website (www.childrensoncologygroup.org) and on the National Cancer Institute cancer trials website (www.clinicaltrials.gov). The remarkable increases in cure rates for childhood malignancies over the past 30 yr would not have occurred without the collective participation of patients and their physicians in clinical research programs at these centers. In the USA, the National Cancer Institute's Clinical Trials Cooperative Groups Program has been associated with a >80% reduction in the incidence of mortality due to cancer among children <15 yr of age despite an overall increase in cancer incidence during this interval (Fig. 494-1). This remarkable achievement represents the effects of an effective multimodal, multi-institutional, multidisciplinary collaboration.

DIAGNOSIS AND STAGING

Accurate diagnosis and staging of the extent of disease is imperative, especially for childhood cancers that have high cure rates, because the nature of therapy depends strongly on the type of cancer. In addition, **prognostic subgroups** based on the stage of disease have been established for most cancers that occur in children. Accordingly, children with a better prognosis are treated with less intensive therapy, including lower doses of chemotherapy or radiation therapy, a shorter duration of treatment, or elimination of at least one treatment modality (radiation therapy, chemotherapy, surgery). Accurate staging thus reduces the risk of excessive acute adverse effects and long-term complications of therapy in patients whose prognosis indicates that less therapy is required for cure. Overtreatment of patients with a more favorable prognosis is a definite risk if the patient is not referred to a cancer treatment center for management of adverse effects of such treatment. Conversely, undertreatment also is a clear risk if the diagnosis and stage are not correct, resulting in a compromise of an otherwise high potential for cure.

Diagnostic imaging is a critical phase of evaluation in most children with solid tumors (i.e., cancers other than leukemia). MRI, CT, ultrasonography, scintigraphy (nuclear medicine scans), positron emission tomography, and spectroscopy, as appropriate, all serve a clear purpose in the evaluation of children with cancer, not only before treatment to determine the extent of disease and the appropriate therapy but also during follow-up to determine whether the therapy was effective. In addition, the rapidity and completeness of response to treatment of an increasing number of malignant diseases in children are being evaluated, with imaging techniques used to quantify the magnitude of the response and to guide appropriate changes in the therapy if it is not adequate. Competence in the sedation of children for diagnostic imaging also is critical.

Expertise in pathology and laboratory medicine provides critical diagnostic support and guides therapy in most children with cancer. Fine-needle aspiration cytology avoids the need for open biopsies of masses in most locations of the body and can be performed in pediatric centers with appropriate expertise in diagnostic imaging, cytology, analgesia, and local anesthesia. **Sentinel node mapping** is increasingly being applied in the staging of children's cancers. Determining the adequacy of surgery by evaluation of frozen sections of the surgical margins for tumor cells is essential in many tumor operations.

A MULTIMODAL, MULTIDISCIPLINARY APPROACH

Many pediatric subspecialties are involved in the evaluation, treatment, and management of children with cancer, including provision of primary modalities and multiple supportive care services (Fig. 494-2). More than two of the primary modalities are often used together, with chemotherapy being the most widely used, followed, in order of use, by surgery, radiation therapy, and biologic agent therapy (Fig. 494-3).

The leukemias that occur in childhood usually are managed with chemotherapy alone, with a small proportion of patients receiving cranial or craniospinal radiation therapy for prevention or treatment of overt central nervous system leukemia. Most children with non-Hodgkin lymphoma also are treated with chemotherapy alone. Exceptions include bulky nonlymphoblastic non-Hodgkin tumors, for which radiation therapy often is beneficial, and resectable primary Burkitt tumor in the abdomen, for which surgery alone can be curative. Localized therapy with surgery or irradiation, or both, is an important component of treatment of most solid tumors, including Hodgkin disease, but systemic multiagent chemotherapy usually is necessary because tumor dissemination generally is present even if undetectable. Chemotherapy alone usually is not adequate to eradicate gross residual tumors. Hence, it is not unusual for children with malignant tumors to require treatment with all three modalities (see Fig. 494-3). Unfortunately, most treatments that are effective in children with cancer have a narrow therapeutic index (a low ratio of efficacy to toxicity). The acute and chronic adverse effects of these treatments can be minimized but not entirely avoided.

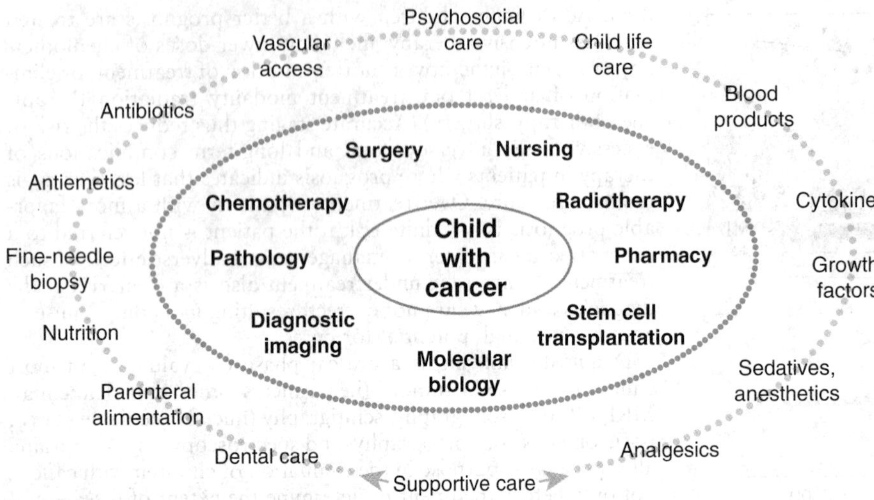

Figure 494-2. Multidisciplinary care of children with cancer. The inner circle designates primary modalities, and the outer ring identifies supportive care elements to which all children with cancer have access.

Over the past 10 yr, biologic agent therapy has become an important modality in a few childhood cancers (see Fig. 494-3). This type of treatment generally refers to immunotherapy, biologic response modifiers, or endogenously occurring molecules that have therapeutic effects in supraphysiologic doses. Examples are retinoic acid therapy in acute progranulocytic leukemia, monoclonal antibody therapy for certain non-Hodgkin lymphomas, imatinib mesylate for chronic myelogenous and Philadelphia chromosome–positive leukemias, and radioactive meta-iodobenzylguanidine therapy for neuroblastoma.

Chemotherapy is used more widely in children than in adults because children better tolerate the acute adverse effects and the malignant diseases that occur in childhood are more responsive to chemotherapy than are malignant diseases of adults. Radiation therapy is used sparingly in children because they are more vulnerable than adults to its late adverse effects.

Whenever possible, treatment is given on an outpatient basis. Children should remain living at home and in school as much as possible throughout treatment. Increasingly, pediatric cancer therapies are being administered to ambulatory patients, with the advent of such innovations as programmable infusion pumps, oral chemotherapeutic regimens, early discharge from hospital with intensive outpatient supportive care, and home health care services. Some patients miss a considerable amount of school in the 1st yr after diagnosis due to the intensity of therapy or its adverse effects and to the ensuing complications of the disease or therapy. Tutoring should be encouraged so that children do not fall behind in their schooling; counseling should be provided as appropriate. In-hospital school services should be provided for those patients who must spend much of their time as inpatients receiving therapy for disease or for managing adverse effects.

Development of selective, highly effective therapy for cancer in both children and adults had been hindered by a lack of understanding of the molecular mechanisms that underlie malignant transformation. Ongoing discoveries of molecular and cellular mechanisms that explain the cancer process have led to increasingly specific antineoplastic therapies, generally referred to as **molecularly targeted therapies.** Their most prominent feature is a relative lack of normal tissue toxicity, such that the additional therapeutic benefit occurs with minimum additional toxicity. Many of the new biologic agent therapies, such as imatinib and rituximab, fall into this category (Table 494-1). **Complementary**

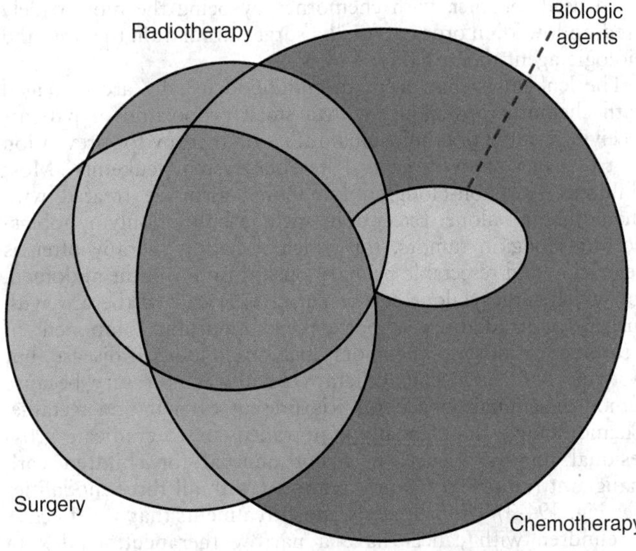

Figure 494-3. The primary modalities of therapy used in the treatment of children with cancer. The relative sizes of the circles designate the approximate proportion of overall role in the management of pediatric cancers.

TABLE 494-1. Protein Tyrosine Kinase Inhibitors and Monoclonal Antibodies

AGENT	KINASE	MALIGNANCY
Imatinib	BCR-ABL	CML T-cell ALL
	PDGFRα	Hypereosinophilic syndrome Systemic mastocytosis
	PDGFRβ	CML
	cKIT	Systemic mastocytosis Gastrointestinal stromal
Dasatinib	BCR-ABL	CML Philadelphia chromosome–positive ALL
Nilotinib	BCR-ABL	CML Philadelphia chromosome–positive ALL
Gefitinib	EGFR	Non–small cell lung cancer Glioblastoma
Erlotinib	EGFR	Non–small cell lung cancer Glioblastoma
Trastuzumab	ERBB2/HER-2	Breast cancer
Cetuximab	EGFR	Non–small cell lung cancer Squamous cell cancer of head/neck
Bevacizumab	VEGFR-1, -2	Non–small cell lung cancer Breast cancer Renal cell carcinoma

ALL, acute lymphoblastic leukemia; CML, chronic myelogenous leukemia.

TABLE 494-2. Mechanism of Drug Resistance for the Anticancer Drugs Commonly Used in the Treatment of Pediatric Cancers

DRUG	MECHANISM OF ACTION
ALKYLATING AGENTS	
Cyclophosphamide/ifosfamide	↑ DNA repair, ↑ free radical scavengers, ↑ aldehyde dehydrogenase (catabolism)
Dacarbazine	↑ DNA repair
Cisplatin	↓ uptake, ↑ DNA repair, ↑ free radical scavengers
Carboplatin	↓ uptake, ↑ DNA repair, ↑ free radical scavengers
ANTIMETABOLITES	
Methotrexate	↓ transport, ↑ DHFR (target), ↓ affinity of DHFR, ↓ polyglutamation
Mercaptopurine	↓ activation, ↑ catabolism
Cytarabine	↓ deoxycytidine kinase (activation), ↑ dCTP, ↓ transport, ↑ cytidine deaminase (catabolism)
Fluorouracil	↓ activation, ↑ thymidylate synthase (target), ↓ affinity of thymidylate synthase
ANTITUMOR ANTIBIOTICS	
Anthracyclines	MDR, ↓ topoisomerase II activity, ↑ free radical scavengers
Dactinomycin	MDR
PLANT ALKALOIDS	
Vinca alkaloids	↓ affinity of tubulin (target), MDR
Epipodophyllotoxins	↑ DNA repair, MDR, ↓ topoisomerase II activity
Paclitaxel	MDR
MISCELLANEOUS	
Corticosteroids	Loss or alteration of glucocorticoid receptor
L-Asparaginase	↓ asparagine synthetase in lymphoblasts

↑, increased; ↓, decreased; DHFR, dihydrofolate reductase; dCTP, deoxycytidine triphosphate; MDR, multidrug resistance mediated by ↑ membrane P-170 glycoprotein.

From Nathan DG, Orkin SH, Ginsburg D, Look AT (eds): *Nathan & Oski's Hematology of Infancy and Childhood,* 6th ed. Philadelphia, WB Saunders, 2003, p 1295.

and **alternative remedies** are increasingly being provided by parents to their children with cancer, with or without knowledge of the medical professionals entrusted with the child's care (see Chapter 59). Many of these have not been evaluated by rigorous testing and most are ineffective; some are toxic or interfere with the metabolism of other drugs. De novo or acquired resistance to chemotherapy and radiation therapy remains an obstacle (Table 494-2). Dramatic advances in the discipline have reduced the empiricism of therapy for cancer, but much remains to be discovered.

CHEMOTHERAPY

The most widely used modality in pediatric cancer therapy is chemotherapy (see Fig. 494–3). Therapy nearly always involves combinations of drugs, such as VAC (vincristine, doxorubicin [Adriamycin] or dactinomycin [Actinomycin D], and cyclophosphamide) and CHOP (cyclophosphamide, doxorubicin [Adriamycin], vincristine [Oncovin], and prednisone). Historically, sequential single-drug therapy rarely resulted in complete responses, and partial responses usually were infrequent and transient and grew progressively shorter in duration with each drug used. Combination chemotherapy became the standard when combinations of drugs with different mechanisms of action and nonoverlapping toxicities (e.g., POMP [mercaptopurine, vincristine (Oncovin), methotrexate, and prednisone], VAMP [vincristine, doxorubicin (Adriamycin), methotrexate, and prednisone], and MOPP [nitrogen mustard, vincristine (Oncovin), prednisone, and procarbazine] were first demonstrated to be effective in childhood leukemia. Most of the cytotoxic drugs for childhood cancer are selected from several classes of agents, including alkylating agents, antimetabolites, antibiotics, hormones, plant alkaloids, and topoisomerase inhibitors (Table 494-3). The increased metabolic and cell cycle activity of malignant cells makes them more susceptible to the cytotoxic effects of these types of agents (Fig. 494-4).

Because most antineoplastic agents are cell cycle–dependent, their adverse effects usually are related to the proliferation kinetics of individual cell populations. Most susceptible are those tissues or organs with high rates of cell turnover: bone marrow, oral and intestinal mucosa, epidermis, liver, and spermatogonia. The most common acute adverse effects are myelosuppression (with neutropenia and thrombocytopenia being the most problematic), immunosuppression, nausea and vomiting, hepatic dysfunction, upper and lower gastrointestinal mucositis, dermatitis, and alopecia. Fortunately, the tissues affected also recover relatively quickly, such that the acute adverse effects are nearly always reversible. Life-threatening effects of many chemotherapy agents include severe neutropenia with infection, fungemia or fungal pneumonia due to immunosuppression, and septicemia, not infrequently linked to indwelling intravascular devices (Table 494-4; see Chapters 177 and 178). Cardiomyopathy caused by anthracyclines (e.g., doxorubicin and daunorubicin) and renal failure from platinum-containing agents also may be life-threatening and often disabling.

Least susceptible to chemotherapy and radiation therapy are cells that do not replicate or that replicate slowly, such as neurons, muscle cells, connective tissue, and bone. However, children are not exempt from toxicities of these tissues, probably because they are still undergoing proliferation, albeit at a slower pace than other tissues, during growth and growth spurts. Certain chemotherapeutic agents are particularly toxic to these tissues, but more so in adults than children; for instance, children are spared the neurotoxic effects of vincristine and methotrexate and the cardiotoxic effect of anthracyclines that occur in adults.

Physically, children can endure the acute adverse effects of chemotherapy better than adults can, in many ways. The maximum tolerated dose in children, when expressed on the basis of body surface area or body weight, commonly is greater than that in adults. A comparison of anticancer drugs tested in phase I trials in both adult and pediatric patients showed that the maximum tolerated dose in children was greater than that in adults for 70% of the agents, equal to that in adults for 15% of the agents, and less than the adult dose for only 15% of the agents. For all the drugs that were compared, the mean pediatric maximum tolerated dose was greater than the adult mean.

Evolving treatment approaches that have not reached general clinical application in children are specific tumor-directed therapies such as tumor antigen–specific monoclonal antibodies, tumor vaccines, antisense DNA and RNA transcripts, and antiangiogenic agents.

SURGERY

Superb pediatric surgical and anesthesia services are indispensable for children with cancer. The pediatric surgeon's role varies, depending on the type of tumor. For solid tumors, complete resection with documented evidence of negative margins often is required for cure or long-term control. Considerable prolongation of life nearly always depends on whether the tumor is resectable and on the actual extent of resection.

With the exception of brainstem tumors and retinoblastoma, all solid tumors in children require a tissue diagnosis; therefore, biopsy of the suspected neoplasm is paramount. Staging with sentinel node biopsies has become the standard of care for several pediatric malignancies. Surgical expertise is essential for implantation of vascular access devices and removal and replacement of such devices when infection or thrombosis supervenes (see Chapter 178).

Increasingly, minimally invasive endoscopic surgical techniques are being used when indicated and, if the patient's condition permits, for biopsy and resection of tumor, direct ascertainment of residual disease and assessment of response, lysis of adhesions, and splenectomy.

TABLE 494-3. Common Chemotherapeutic Agents Used in Children

DRUG	MECHANISM OF ACTION OR CLASSIFICATION	INDICATION(S)	ADVERSE REACTIONS	MONITORY DRUG LEVEL	COMMENTS
Methotrexate	Folic acid antagonist; inhibits dihydrofolate reductase	ALL non-Hodgkin lymphoma, osteosarcoma, Hodgkin lymphoma, medulloblastoma	Myelosuppression, mucositis, stomatitis, dermatitis, hepatitis With long-term administration; osteopenia and bone fractures With high-dose administration; renal and central nervous system toxicity With intrathecal administration; arachnoiditis, leukoencephalopathy, leukomyelopathy	Plasma levels must be monitored with high-dose therapy and when low doses are administered to patients with renal dysfunction and leucovorin rescue applied accordingly	Systemic administration may be Po, IM, or IV; also may be administered intrathecally
6-Mercaptopurine (Purinethol)	Purine analog; inhibits purine synthesis	ALL	Myelosuppression, hepatic necrosis, mucositis; allopurinol increases toxicity	Therapeutic drug monitoring not available or indicated	Allopurinol inhibits metabolism
Cytarabine (Ara-C)	Pyrimidine analog; inhibits DNA polymerase	ALL, AML, non-Hodgkin lymphoma, Hodgkin lymphoma	Nausea, vomiting, myelosuppression, conjunctivitis, mucositis, central nervous system dysfunction With intrathecal administration; arachnoiditis, leukoencephalopathy, leukomyelopathy	Therapeutic drug monitoring not available or indicated	Systemic administration may be Po, IM, or IV; may also be administered intrathecally
Cyclophosphamide (Cytoxan)	Alkylates guanine; inhibits DNA synthesis	ALL, non-Hodgkin lymphoma, Hodgkin lymphoma, soft tissue sarcoma, Ewing sarcoma	Nausea, vomiting, myelosuppression, hemorrhagic cystitis, pulmonary fibrosis, inappropriate ADH secretion, bladder cancer, anaphylaxis	Therapeutic drug monitoring not available or indicated	Requires hepatic activation and thus less effective in presence of liver dysfunction
Ifosfamide (Ifex)	Alkylates guanine; inhibits DNA synthesis	Non-Hodgkin lymphoma, Wilms tumor, sarcoma, germ cell and testicular tumors	Nausea, vomiting myelosuppression, hemorrhagic cystitis, pulmonary fibrosis, inappropriate ADH secretion, bladder cancer, central nervous system dysfunction, cardiac toxicity, anaphylaxis	Therapeutic drug monitoring not available or indicated	
Doxorubicin (Adriamycin) and daunorubicin (Cerubidine)	Binds to DNA, intercalation	ALL, AML, osteosarcoma, Ewing sarcoma, Hodgkin lymphoma, non-Hodgkin lymphoma, neuroblastoma	Nausea, vomiting, cardiomyopathy, red urine, tissue necrosis on extravasation, myelosuppression, conjunctivitis, radiation dermatitis, arrhythmia	Therapeutic drug monitoring not available or indicated	
Dactinomycin	Binds to DNA, inhibits transcription	Wilms tumor, rhabdomyosarcoma, Ewing sarcoma	Nausea, vomiting tissue necrosis on extravasation, myelosuppression, radiosensitizer, mucosal ulceration	Therapeutic drug monitoring not available or indicated	
Bleomycin (Blenoxane)	Binds to DNA cleaves DNA strands	Hodgkin disease, non-Hodgkin lymphoma, germ cell tumors	Nausea, vomiting, pneumonitis, stomatitis, Raynaud phenomenon, pulmonary fibrosis, dermatitis	Therapeutic drug monitoring not available or indicated	
Vincristine (Oncovin)	Inhibits microtubule formation	ALL, non-Hodgkin lymphoma, Hodgkin disease, Wilms tumor, Ewing sarcoma, neuroblastoma rhabdomyosarcoma	Local cellulitis, peripheral neuropathy, constipation, ileus, jaw pain, inappropriate ADH secretion, seizures, ptosis, minimal myelosuppression	Therapeutic drug monitoring not available or indicated	IV administration only; must not be allowed to extravasate
Vinblastine (Velban)	Inhibits microtubule formation	Hodgkin disease; Langerhans' cell histiocytosis	Local cellulitis, leukopenia	Therapeutic drug monitoring not available or indicated	IV administration only; must not be allowed to extravasate
L-Asparaginase	Depletion of L-asparagine	ALL; AML, when used in combination with asparaginase	Allergic reaction pancreatitis, hyperglycemia, platelet dysfunction and coagulopathy, encephalopathy	Therapeutic drug monitoring not available or indicated	PEG-asparaginase now preferred to L-asparaginase
Pegaspargase (Pegaspar)	Polyethylene glycol conjugate of L-asparagine	ALL	Indicated for prolonged asparagine depletion and for patients with allergy to L-asparaginase	Therapeutic drug monitoring not available or indicated	
Prednisone and Dexamethasone (Decadron)	Lymphatic cell lysis	ALL; Hodgkin disease, non-Hodgkin lymphoma	Cushing syndrome, cataracts, diabetes, hypertension, myopathy, osteoporosis, infection, peptic ulceration, psychosis	Therapeutic drug monitoring not available or indicated	
Carmustine (nitrosourea)	Carbamylation of DNA; inhibits DNA synthesis	CNS tumors, non-Hodgkin lymphoma, Hodgkin disease	Nausea, vomiting, delayed myelosuppression (4–6 wk); pulmonary fibrosis, carcinogenic stomatitis	Therapeutic drug monitoring not available or indicated	Phenobarbital increases metabolism, decreases activity
Carboplatin and cisplatin (Platinol)	Inhibits DNA synthesis	Gonadal tumors; osteosarcoma, neuroblastoma, CNS, tumors, germ cell tumors	Nausea, vomiting, renal dysfunction, myelosuppression, ototoxicity, tetany, neurotoxicity, hemolytic-uremic syndrome, anaphylaxis	Therapeutic drug monitoring not available or indicated	Aminoglycosides may increase nephrotoxicity
Etoposide (VePesid)	Topoisomerase inhibitor	ALL, non-Hodgkin lymphoma, germ cell tumor	Nausea, vomiting, myelosuppression, secondary leukemia	Therapeutic drug monitoring not available or indicated	
Etretinate (Tegison) (vitamin A analog) and tretinoin	Enhances normal differentiation	Acute progranulocytic leukemia; neuroblastoma	Dry mouth, hair loss, pseudotumor cerebri, premature epiphyseal closure	Therapeutic drug monitoring not available or indicated	

ADH, antidiuretic hormone; ALL, acute lymphoblastic leukemia; AML, acute myelogenous leukemia; CNS, central nervous system; IM, intramuscular; IV, intravenous; Po, oral.

RADIATION THERAPY

Radiation therapy is used sparingly in children, who are more susceptible than are adults to the adverse delayed effects of ionizing radiation. A major advance in pediatric radiation therapy has been the application of **conformal irradiation** to children with cancer. This technique, most commonly applied as **intensity modulated radiation therapy (IMRT)**, spares normal tissue by conforming the radiation volume to the shape of the tumor, thereby enabling delivery of higher doses to the tumors with lower exposure of normal tissue adjacent to the tumor or in the path of the radiation beam. Another example is proton beam therapy, which has just begun to be more widely available for children with cancer. With more focused beams and better sedation and immobilization techniques, radiation therapy is becoming more frequently used in children. Acute adverse effects from radiation therapy are less severe than those from chemotherapy and depend on which part of the body is irradiated and the means of administration. Dermatitis is the most common general adverse effect, because skin is always in the treatment field. Nausea and diar-

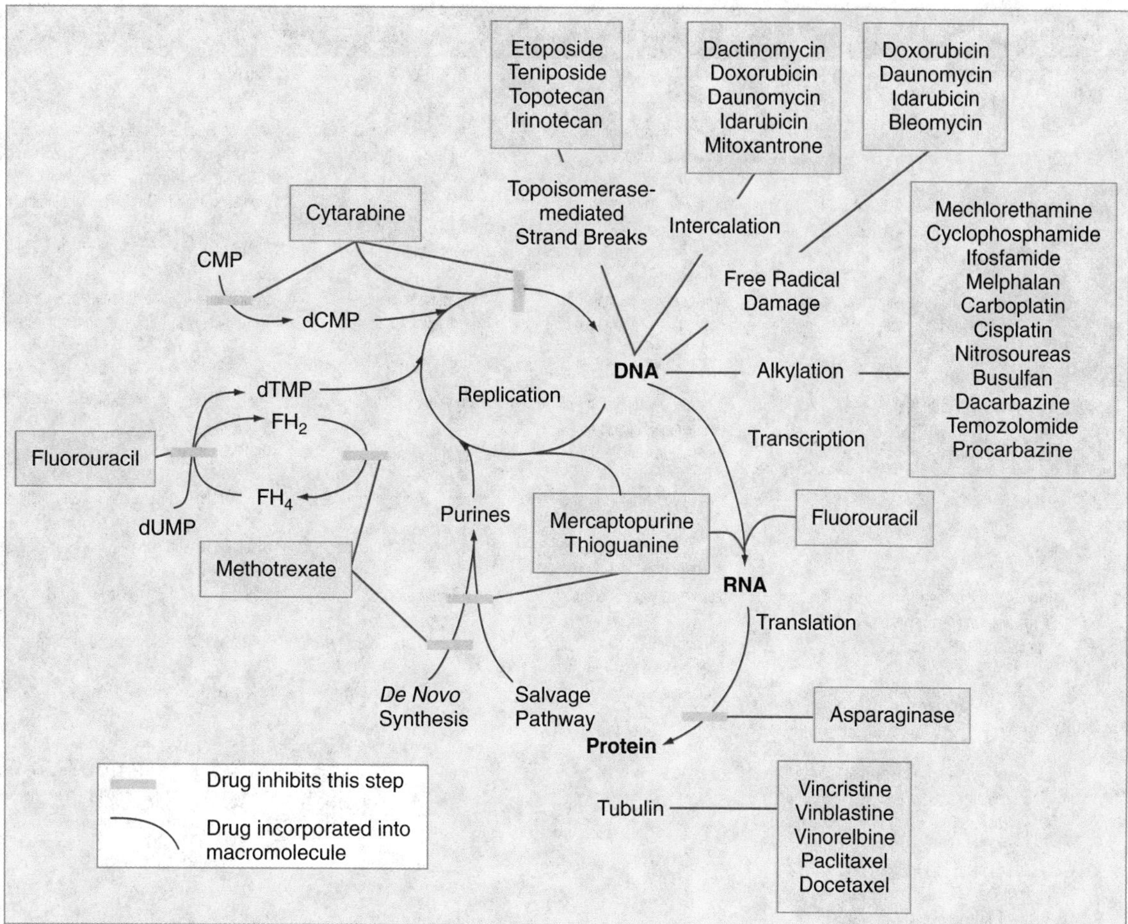

Figure 494-4. Site of action of the commonly used anticancer drugs. CMP, cytidine monophosphate; dCMP, deoxycytidine monophosphate; dTMP, deoxythymidine monophosphate; dUMP, deoxyuridine monophosphate; FH_2, dihydrofolate; FH_4, tetrahydrofolate. (Redrawn from Balis FM, Holcenberg JS, Blaney SM: General principles of chemotherapy. In Pizzo PA, Poplack DG [editors]: *Principles and Practice of Pediatric Oncology*, 4th ed. Philadelphia, Lippincott Williams & Wilkins, 2002, p 241.)

rhea are common subacute adverse effects with abdominal radiation therapy. Mucositis nearly always occurs to some extent whenever oral or intestinal mucosa is in the treatment volume. Somnolence is common with cranial irradiation. Alopecia occurs where hair is in the radiation port.

Most radiation therapy schedules require treatment 5 days/wk for 4–7 wk, depending on the dose needed to control the tumor and on the amount and nature of normal tissue in the field. Most adverse effects are not noted until the second half of the course of irradiation. Late effects may occur months to years after radiation therapy and usually are dose-limiting manifestations. The type of delayed toxicity also depends on the site of irradiation. Examples are impaired growth resulting from cranial or vertebral irradiation, endocrine dysfunction from midbrain irradiation, pulmonary or cardiac insufficiency from chest irradiation, strictures and adhesions from abdominal irradiation, and infertility from pelvic irradiation.

ACUTE TOXIC EFFECTS AND SUPPORTIVE CARE

Adverse treatment effects that occur early in therapy include metabolic disorders, bone marrow suppression, and immunosuppression (Table 494-5). Patients with a large tumor burden may have had substantial breakdown of tumor cells, which, in some cases, causes renal function impairment, owing to tubular

TABLE 494-4. Infectious Complications of Malignancy

PREDISPOSING FACTOR	ETIOLOGY	SITE OF INFECTION	INFECTIOUS AGENTS
Neutropenia	Chemotherapy, bone marrow infiltration	Sepsis, shock, pneumonia, soft tissue, proctitis, mucositis	*Staphylococcus aureus, Staphylococcus epidermidis, Escherichia coli, Pseudomonas aeruginosa, Candida, Aspergillus*, anaerobic oral and rectal bacteria
Immunosuppression, lymphopenia, lymphocyte-monocyte dysfunction	Chemotherapy, prednisone	Pneumonia, meningitis, disseminated viral infection	*Pneumocystis carinii, Cryptococcus neoformans, Mycobacterium, Nocardia, Listeria monocytogenes, Candida, Aspergillus, Strongyloides, Toxoplasma*, varicella-zoster virus, cytomegalovirus, herpes simplex
Splenectomy	Staging of Hodgkin disease	Sepsis, shock, meningitis	Pneumococcus, *Haemophilus influenzae*, meningococcus
Indwelling central venous catheter	Nutrition, administration of chemotherapy	Line sepsis, tract of tunnel, exit site	*S. epidermidis, S. aureus, Candida albicans, P. aeruginosa, Aspergillus, Corynebacterium* JK, *Streptococcus faecalis, Mycobacterium fortuitum, Propionibacterium acnes*

From Kliegman RM, Marcdante KJ, Jenson HB, et al (editors): *Nelson Essentials of Pediatrics*, 5th ed. Philadelphia, WB Saunders, 2006, p 733.

TABLE 494-5. Oncologic Emergencies

CONDITION	MANIFESTATIONS	ETIOLOGY	MALIGNANCY	TREATMENT
METABOLIC				
Hyperuricemia	Uric acid nephropathy; gout	Tumor lysis syndrome	Lymphoma, leukemia	Allopurinol, alkalinize urine; hydration and diuresis, rasburicase
Hyperkalemia	Arrhythmias, cardiac arrest	Tumor lysis syndrome	Lymphoma, leukemia	Kayexalate, sodium bicarbonate, glucose, and insulin; check for pseudohyperkalemia from leukemic cell lysis in test tube
Hyperphosphatemia	Hypocalcemic tetany; metastatic calcification, photophobia, pruritus	Tumor lysis syndrome	Lymphoma, leukemia	Hydration, forced diuresis; stop alkalinization; oral aluminum hydroxide to bind phosphate
Hyponatremia	Seizure, lethargy, asymptomatic	SIADH; fluid, sodium losses in vomiting	Leukemia, CNS tumor	Restrict free water for SIADH; replace sodium if depleted
Hypercalcemia	Anorexia, nausea, polyuria, pancreatitis, gastric ulcers; prolonged PR, shortened QT interval	Bone resorption; ectopic parathormone, vitamin D, or prostaglandins	Metastasis to bone, rhabdomyosarcoma	Hydration and furosemide diuresis; corticosteroids; mithramycin; calcitonin, diphosphonates
HEMATOLOGIC				
Anemia	Pallor, weakness, heart failure	Bone marrow suppression or infiltration; blood loss	Any with chemotherapy	Packed red blood cell transfusion
Thrombocytopenia	Petechiae, hemorrhage	Bone marrow suppression or infiltration	Any with chemotherapy	Platelet transfusion
Disseminated intravascular coagulation	Shock, hemorrhage	Sepsis, hypotension, tumor factors	Promyelocytic leukemia, others	Fresh frozen plasma; platelets, treat infection
Neutropenia	Infection	Bone marrow suppression or infiltration	Any with chemotherapy	If febrile, administer broad-spectrum antibiotics, and G-CSF if appropriate
Hyperleukocytosis (>50,000/mm^3)	Hemorrhage, thrombosis; pulmonary infiltrates, hypoxia; tumor lysis syndrome	Leukostasis; vascular occlusion	Leukemia	Leukapheresis; chemotherapy
Graft-versus-host disease	Dermatitis, diarrhea, hepatitis	Immunosuppression and nonirradiated blood products; bone marrow transplantation	Any with immunosuppression	Corticosteroids; cyclosporine; antithymocyte globulin
SPACE-OCCUPYING LESIONS				
Spinal cord compression	Back pain ± radicular *Cord above T10:* symmetric weakness, increased deep tendon reflex; sensory level present; toes up *Conus medullaris (T10-L2):* symmetric weakness, increased knee reflexes; decreased ankle reflexes; saddle sensory loss; toes up or down *Cauda equina (below L2):* asymmetric weakness; loss of deep tendon reflex and sensory deficit; toes down	Metastasis to vertebra and extramedullary space	Neuroblastoma; medulloblastoma	MRI or myelography for diagnosis; corticosteroids; radiotherapy; laminectomy; chemotherapy
Increased intracranial pressure	Confusion, coma, emesis, headache, hypertension, bradycardia, seizures, papilledema, hydrocephalus; cranial nerve III and VI palsies	Primary or metastatic brain tumor	Neuroblastoma, astrocytoma; glioma	CT or MRI for diagnosis; corticosteroids; phenytoin; ventriculostomy tube; radiotherapy; chemotherapy
Superior vena cava syndrome	Distended neck veins plethora, edema of head and neck, cyanosis, proptosis, Horner syndrome	Superior mediastinal mass	Lymphoma	Chemotherapy; radiotherapy
Tracheal compression	Respiratory distress	Mediastinal mass compressing trachea	Lymphoma	Radiation, corticosteroids

From Kliegman RM, Marcdante KJ, Jenson HB, et al (editors): *Nelson Essentials of Pediatrics*, 5th ed.
CNS, central nervous system; G-CSF, granulocyte colony-stimulating factor; SIADH, syndrome of inappropriate antidiuretic hormone secretion.

precipitates of uric acid crystals. This effect occurs most often in patients with leukemia and lymphoma (particularly Burkitt lymphoma) but also can occur in patients with large solid tumors (e.g., hepatoblastoma, germ cell tumors, neuroblastoma). Before therapy is initiated, the serum levels of uric acid and creatinine should be measured and adequate hydration ensured; allopurinol (a xanthine oxidase inhibitor) or, more often, rasburicase (an enzyme that degrades uric acid) can be given, if necessary, to lower uric acid levels to within the normal range. In the metabolic **tumor lysis syndrome,** phosphates and potassium are released into the circulation in large quantities as cells are lysed by treatment. Symptomatic hyperkalemia and hyperphosphatemia with subsequent hypocalcemia may develop in the setting of inadequate renal function.

Virtually all chemotherapy regimens can produce **myelosuppression,** as can tumors that invade and replace bone marrow. Anemia can be corrected by transfusions of packed erythrocytes, and thrombocytopenia by platelet infusions. Patients receiving immunosuppressive therapy should receive irradiated blood products to prevent graft-versus-host disease. Granulocytopenia (granulocyte counts <500/mm^3) poses a risk of life-threatening infection. Febrile granulocytopenic patients should be hospitalized and treated with empirical broad-spectrum intravenous antimicrobial therapy pending the results of appropriate cultures of blood, urine, or any obvious sites of infection (see Chapter 177). Treatment is continued until fever resolves and the granulocyte count rises. If fever persists for >1 wk while the patient is receiving broad-spectrum antibiotics, the possibility of fungal infection must be considered. Fungal infections caused by *Candida* and *Aspergillus* are common in immunosuppressed patients. Opportunistic organisms such as *Pneumocystis carinii* can produce fatal pneumonia. Prophylactic treatment with trimethoprim-sulfamethoxazole is given when severe or prolonged immunosuppression is anticipated.

Viruses of low pathogenicity can produce serious disease in the setting of immunosuppression caused by malignancy or its treatment. Patients should not be given live virus vaccines. Children who are receiving chemotherapy and who are exposed to chickenpox should receive varicella-zoster immunoglobulin and, if clinical disease develops, should be hospitalized and treated with intravenous acyclovir.

Adequate **pain management** is critical. The World Health Organization (WHO) guidelines are particularly useful in the management of pain associated with cancer and cancer therapy (see Chapter 77).

It is common for patients undergoing cancer therapy to lose >10% of body weight. Patients sometimes reduce their food intake because of temporary, treatment-associated nausea, stomatitis, and vomiting. Appetite loss is not a cause for alarm. Malnutrition is a particular risk in patients receiving radiation therapy involving the abdomen or the head and neck, intensive chemotherapy, or total body irradiation and high-dose chemotherapy before marrow transplantation. If oral supplementation proves inadequate, such patients may require enteral tube feedings or parenteral hyperalimentation.

LATE ADVERSE EFFECTS

Injury to tissues with low repair potential often results in long-lasting or permanent deficit. For example, a brain or spinal tumor can leave the child with a permanent paresis or autonomic dysfunction, anthracycline-induced cardiomyopathy usually produces refractory cardiac dysfunction, and the leukoencephalopathy caused by intrathecal methotrexate and by central nervous system radiation therapy often is only partially reversible. The potential types of late adverse effects depend on the child's age at the time of treatment, the location(s) of the cancer, and the therapy administered. A good resource for the pediatrician, patient, and family who have to anticipate the possibilities is available at *www.survivorshipguidelines.org*.

Late adverse effects of therapy can cause substantial morbidity (Tables 494-6 and 494-7). Successful surgical resection may result in loss of important functional structures. Irradiation can produce irreversible organ damage, with symptoms and functional limitations depending on the organ involved and the severity of the damage. Many radiation therapy-related problems do not become obvious until the patient is fully grown, such as asymmetry between irradiated and nonirradiated areas or extremities. Irradiation of fields that include endocrine organs can cause hypothyroidism, pituitary dysfunction, or infertility. In sufficient doses, cranial irradiation can produce neurologic dysfunction and spinal irradiation can produce growth retardation.

Chemotherapy also carries the risk of long-lasting organ damage. Of particular concern are leukoencephalopathy after high-dose methotrexate therapy; infertility in male patients treated with alkylating agents (e.g., cyclophosphamide); myocardial damage caused by anthracyclines; pulmonary fibrosis caused by bleomycin; pancreatitis caused by asparaginase; renal dysfunction due to ifosfamide, nitrosourea, or platinum agents; and hearing loss from cisplatin. Development of these sequelae may be dose-related and usually is irreversible. Appropriate baseline and intermittent testing should be performed before these drugs are administered to ensure that there is no pre-existing damage to the organs likely to be affected and to permit monitoring of the adverse effects of treatment-induced changes.

Perhaps the most serious late adverse effect is the occurrence of **second cancers** in patients successfully cured of a first malignancy. The risk appears to be cumulative, increasing by about

TABLE 494-6. General Guidelines for Late Effects Assessment and Management: Radiation Late Effects

SYSTEM	POTENTIAL EFFECTS	MONITORING GUIDELINES
Central nervous system	Precocious puberty, growth hormone deficiency and other pituitary and hypothalamic dysfunction	Neuroendocrine monitoring, including growth and gonadal status
	Cognitive dysfunction, leukencephalopathy, second CNS tumors (worsens with increased dose)	Neurocognitive and psychological testing Neurologic examination
	Stroke, ototoxicity, myelitis, blindness, peripheral neuropathy	Auditory and ophthalmic evaluation Neurologic examination
Eye	Cataracts Cornea, lacrimal duct, retina, conjunctiva, sclera, optic neuropathy	Ophthalmic examination
Cardiac	Cardiomyopathy Pericarditis Coronary artery disease Valvular disease	ECG, echocardiogram, Holter or cardiac stress dependent on dose, age at time of treatment, symptoms or anthracycline exposure
Pulmonary	Pulmonary fibrosis	Pulmonary function tests
Thyroid	Overt or compensated hypothyroidism Thyroid nodules or cancer Hyperthyroidism	Thyroid function tests
Gonadal	Ovarian failure Oligospermia/azospermia Leydig cell dysfunction	LH, FSH Estradiol or testosterone Reproductive counseling or endocrinology evaluation Gynecologic evaluation Sperm analysis Tanner staging Menstrual history
Second malignancies	Sarcomas CNS tumors Breast cancer Melanoma Non-melanoma skin cancer Thyroid cancer Other solid tumors	Complete physical examinations annually Attention paid to organs in radiation field Mammography to screen for female breast cancer
Any	Any organ within the field of radiation may develop dysfunction, or may be at risk for development of a second cancer	Routine tests of organ function for organs at risk

From Friedman DL, Meadows AT: Late effects of childhood cancer therapy. *Pediatr Clin North Am* 2002;49, p 1084.
CNS, central nervous system; ECG, electrocardiogram; FSH, follicle-stimulating hormone; LH, luteinizing hormone.

TABLE 494-7. General Guidelines for Late Effects Assessment and Management: Chemotherapy Late Effects

SYSTEM	AGENTS	POTENTIAL EFFECTS	MONITORING GUIDELINES
Central nervous system	Intrathecal chemotherapy High-dose methotrexate	Cognitive dysfunction Leukencephalopathy (risk increases with increased dose)	Neurocognitive evaluation Neurologic evaluation
Cardiac	Anthracyclines	Cardiomyopathy Arrhythmias	ECG, echocardiogram, Holter or cardiac stress dependent on dose, age at time of treatment, symptoms, or radiation exposure
Hearing	Platinums	Hearing loss	Audiology evaluation
Pulmonary	Bleomycin Nitrosureas	Restrictive lung disease	Pulmonary function tests
Urologic	Cyclophosphamide Ifosfamide	Chronic hemorrhagic cystitis Second bladder cancers	Urinalysis
Hepatic	Methotrexate Thioguanine Mercaptopurine Dactinomycin Busulfan	Hepatic dysfunction Venoocclusive disease (Dactinomycin, busulfan, thioguanine)	Liver function tests Doppler ultrasound
Renal	Platinums High-dose methotrexate Ifosfamide	Renal insufficiency or failure Renal electrolyte wasting/ insufficiency	Urinalysis Renal function tests Creatinine clearance
Gonadal	Alkylating agents Nitrosureas	Ovarian failure; early menopause Testicular failure; Leydig cell dysfunction	LH, FSH Estradiol or testosterone Reproductive counseling or endocrinology evaluation Gynecologic evaluation Sperm analysis Tanner staging Menstrual history
Second malignancies	Alkylating agents: Mechlorethamine > others Topoisomerase II inhibitors Platinums	Leukemia	Complete blood count
	Cyclophosphamide	Transitional bladder carcinoma	Urinalysis

From Friedman DL, Meadows AT: Late effects of childhood cancer therapy. *Pediatr Clin North Am* 2002;49:1085.
ECG, electrocardiogram; FSH, follicle-stimulating hormone; LH, luteinizing hormone.

0.5% per year, resulting in approximately a 12% incidence at 25 yr after treatment. Patients who have been treated for childhood cancer should be examined annually, with particular attention to possible late adverse effects of therapy, including second malignancies.

PALLIATIVE CARE

At all stages of caring for children with cancer, principles of palliative care should be applied to relieve pain and suffering and to provide comfort (see Chapter 40). Pain is a serious cause of suffering among patients with cancer. It may be the result of organ obstruction or compression or bone metastasis, or it may be neuropathic. Pain should be managed in a stepwise manner, as recommended by the WHO, in accordance with the principles of selecting the appropriate analgesic, prescribing the appropriate dosage, administering the drug by the appropriate route, and choosing an appropriate dosing schedule to prevent persistent pain and to relieve breakthrough pain (see Chapter 77). In addition, the dosage should be titrated aggressively while attempts are made to prevent, anticipate, and manage side effects. Adjuvant drugs and sequential trials of analgesic drugs should be considered.

The goals in the care of dying patients are to avoid distress for the patient, family, and caregivers; to provide care consistent with the patient's and family's wishes; and to comply with and advocate for clinical, cultural, and ethical standards.

Bradlyn AS: Health-related quality of life in pediatric oncology: current status and future challenges. *J Pediatr Oncol Nurs* 2004;21:137–140.

Cardous-Ubbink MC, Heinen RC, Langeveld NE, et al: Long-term cause-specific mortality among five-year survivors of childhood cancer. *Pediatr Blood Cancer* 2004;42:563–573.

Dickerman JD: The late effects of childhood cancer therapy. *Pediatrics* 2007;119:554–568.

Eshelman D, Landier W, Sweeney T, et al: Facilitating care for childhood cancer survivors: integrating children's oncology group long-term follow-up guidelines and health links in clinical practice. *J Pediatr Oncol Nurs* 2004;21:271–280.

Fallon M, Hanks G, Cherny N: Principles of control of cancer pain. *BMJ* 2006;332:1022–1024.

Harris MB: Palliative care in children with cancer: which child and when? *J Natl Cancer Inst Monogr* 2004;(32):144–149.

Hoffer FA: Interventional radiology in pediatric oncology. *Eur J Radiol* 2005;53:3–13.

Hudson MM, Mertens AC, Yasui Y, et al: Health status of adult long-term survivors of childhood cancer. *JAMA* 2003;290:1583–1592.

Joensuu A: Sunitinib for imatinib-resistant GIST. *Lancet* 2006;368:1303–1304.

Juweid ME, Cheson BD: Positron-emission tomography and assessment of cancer therapy. *N Engl J Med* 2006;354:496–507.

Kelly KM: Complementary and alternative medical therapies for children with cancer. *Eur J Cancer* 2004;40:2041–2046.

Krause DS, Van Etten RA: Tyrosine kinases as targets for cancer therapy. *N Engl J Med* 2005;353:172–187.

Lobo RA: Potential options for preservation of fertility in women. *N Engl J Med* 2005;353:64–73.

Mack JW, Grier HE. The Day One Talk. *J Clin Oncol* 2004;22:563–566.

Mocellin S, Mandruzzato S, Bronte V, et al: Part 1: Vaccines for solid tumours. *Lancet Oncol* 2004;5:681–689.

Mocellin S, Semenzato G, Mandruzzato S, et al: Part II: Vaccines for haematological malignancy disorders. *Lancet Oncol* 2004;5:727–737.

Nathan PC, Furlong W, Barr RD: Challenges to the measurement of health-related quality of life in children receiving cancer therapy. *Pediatr Blood Cancer* 2004;43:215–223.

Oeffinger KC, Mertens AC, Sklar AC, et al: Chronic health conditions in adult survivors of childhood cancer. *N Engl J Med* 2006;355:1572–1582.

Offit K, Sagi M, Hurley K: Preimplantation genetic diagnosis for cancer syndromes. *JAMA* 2006;296:2727–2730.

Patenaude AF, Kupst MJ: Psychosocial functioning in pediatric cancer. *J Pediatr Psychol* 2005;30:9–27.

Pollock BH, Knudson AG: Preventing cancer in adulthood: Advice for the pediatrician. In Pizzo PA, Poplack DG (editors): *Principles and Practice of Pediatric Oncology,* 5th ed. Philadelphia, Lippincott Williams & Wilkins, 2006;pp 1617–1628.

Prasad D, Schiff D: Malignant spinal-cord compression. *Lancet Oncol* 2005;6:15–24.

Pui CH, Relling MV: Can the genotoxicity of chemotherapy be predicted? *Lancet* 2004;364:917–918.

Reaman GH: Pediatric cancer research from past successes through collaboration to future transdisciplinary research. *J Pediatr Oncol Nurs* 2004;21:123–127.

Ross L, Johansen C, Dalton SO, et al: Psychiatric hospitalization among survivors of cancer in childhood or adolescence. *N Engl J Med* 2003;349:650–656.

Shamberger RC, Jaksic T, Ziegler MM: General principles of surgery. In Pizzo PA, Poplack DG (editors): *Principles and Practice of Pediatric Oncology,* 5th ed. Philadelphia, Lippincott Williams & Wilkins, 2006; pp 405–420.

Sharma R, Tobin P, Clarke SJ: Management of chemotherapy-induced nausea, vomiting, oral mucositis, and diarrhoea. *Lancet Oncol* 205;6:93–102.

Spielberger R, Stiff P, Bensinger W, et al: Palifermin for oral mucositis after intensive therapy for hematologic cancers. *N Engl J Med* 2004;351: 2590–2598.

Steward AF: Hypercalcemia associated with cancer. *N Engl J Med* 2005;352:373–378.

Tarbell NJ, Yock Kooy TH: General principles of radiation oncology. In Pizzo PA, Poplack DG (editors): *Principles and Practice of Pediatric Oncology,* 6th ed. Philadelphia, Lippincott Williams & Wilkins, 2006; pp 421–432.

Uren A, Toretsky JA: Pediatric malignancies provide unique cancer therapy targets. *Curr Opin Pediatr* 2005;17:14–19.

Chapter 495 ■ The Leukemias

David G. Tubergen and Archie Bleyer

The leukemias are the most common malignant neoplasms in childhood, accounting for about 41% of all malignancies that occur in children <15 yr of age. In 2002, approximately 2,500 children <15 yr of age were diagnosed with leukemia in the USA, an annual incidence of 4.5 cases per 100,000 children. Acute lymphoblastic leukemia (ALL) accounts for about 77% of cases of childhood leukemia, acute myelogenous leukemia (AML) for about 11%, chronic myelogenous leukemia (CML) for 2–3%, and juvenile chronic myelogenous leukemia (JCML) for 1–2%. The remaining cases consist of a variety of acute and chronic leukemias that do not fit classic definitions for ALL, AML, CML, or JCML.

The leukemias may be defined as a group of malignant diseases in which genetic abnormalities in a hematopoietic cell give rise to an unregulated clonal proliferation of cells. The progeny of these cells have a growth advantage over normal cellular elements, because of their increased rate of proliferation, and a decreased rate of spontaneous apoptosis. The result is a disruption of normal marrow function and, ultimately, marrow failure. The clinical features, laboratory findings, and responses to therapy vary depending on the type of leukemia.

Pizzo PA and Poplack DG (editors): *Principles and Practice of Pediatric Oncology,* 5th ed. Philadelphia, Lippincott Williams & Wilkins, 2005.

495.1 • Acute Lymphoblastic Leukemia

Childhood ALL was the first disseminated cancer shown to be curable and consequently has represented the model malignancy for the principles of cancer diagnosis, prognosis, and treatment. It actually is a heterogeneous group of malignancies with a number of distinctive genetic abnormalities that result in varying clinical behaviors and responses to therapy.

EPIDEMIOLOGY. Approximately 2,000 children <15 yr of age are diagnosed with ALL in the USA each year. It has a striking peak incidence between 2–6 yr of age and occurs more frequently in boys than in girls, at all ages. This peak age incidence was apparent decades ago in white populations in advanced socioeconomic countries, but has since been confirmed in the black population of the USA as well. The disease is more common in children with certain chromosomal abnormalities, such as Down syndrome, Bloom syndrome, ataxia-telangiectasia, and Fanconi syndrome. Among identical twins, the risk to the second twin if one develops leukemia is greater than that in the general population. The risk is >70% if the first twin is diagnosed during the first year of life and the twins shared the same (monochorionic) placenta. If the first twin develops ALL by 5–7 yr of age, the risk to the second twin is at least twice that in the general population, regardless of zygosity.

ETIOLOGY. In virtually all cases, the etiology of ALL is unknown, although several genetic and environmental factors are associated with childhood leukemia (Table 495-1). Exposure to medical diagnostic radiation both in utero and in childhood has been associated with an increased incidence of ALL. In addition, published descriptions and investigations of geographic clusters of cases have raised concern that environmental factors may increase the incidence of ALL. Thus far, no such factors other than radiation have been identified in the USA. In certain developing countries, there has been an association between B-cell ALL and Epstein-Barr viral infections.

PATHOGENESIS. The classification of ALL depends on characterizing the malignant cells in the bone marrow to determine the morphology, phenotypic characteristics as measured by cell membrane markers, and cytogenetic and molecular genetic features. **Morphology** alone usually is adequate to establish a diagnosis, but the other studies are essential for disease classification, which may have a major influence on both the prognosis and the choice of appropriate therapy. The most important distinguishing morphologic feature is the French-American-British (FAB) L3 subtype, which is evidence of a mature B-cell leukemia. The L3 type, also known as Burkitt leukemia, is one of the most rapidly growing cancers in humans and requires a different therapeutic approach. Phenotypically, surface markers show that about 85% of cases of ALL are derived from progenitors of B cells, about 15% are derived from T cells, and about 1% are derived from B cells. A small percentage of children diagnosed with leukemia have a disease characterized by surface markers of both lymphoid and myeloid derivation. Immunophenotypes often correlate to disease manifestations (Table 495-2).

Chromosomal abnormalities are found in most patients with ALL (Table 495-3, Fig. 495-1). The abnormalities, which may be related to chromosomal number, translocations, or deletions, provide important prognostic information. The identification of the leukemia-specific fusion-gene sequences in archived neonatal blood spots of some children who develop ALL at a later date indicates the importance of in utero events in the initiation of the malignant process, but the long lag period before the onset of the disease in some children, reported to be as long as 14 yr, supports the concept that additional genetic modifications also are required for disease expression. Specific chromosomal findings, such as the t(9;22) translocation, which expresses BCR-ABL fusion protein, suggest a need for additional, molecular genetic

TABLE 495-1. Factors Predisposing to Childhood Leukemia

GENETIC CONDITIONS
Down syndrome
Fanconi syndrome
Bloom syndrome
Diamond-Blackfan anemia
Schwachman syndrome
Klinefelter syndrome
Turner syndrome
Neurofibromatosis type 1
Ataxia-telangiectasia
Severe combined immune deficiency
Paroxysmal nocturnal hemoglobinuria
Li-Fraumeni syndrome
ENVIRONMENTAL FACTORS
Ionizing radiation
Drugs
Alkylating agents
Nitrosourea
Epipodophyllotoxin
Benzene exposure
Advanced maternal age

TABLE 495-2. Correlation of Immunophenotype with Clinical Characteristics

	PRO-B, CD10$^-$	EARLY PRE-B, CD10$^+$	PRE-B	MATURE B	T-CELL
No. patients	52	635	156	39	124
Sex (% male)	39	53	50	85	75
Age (years)					
<1 (%)	33	1	6	3	1
1–<10 (%)	50	82	80	64	62
≥10 (%)	17	17	14	33	37
Leukocyte count < 100 × 10^9/L					
Median	38	33	42	77	87
≤20 (%)	38	75	53	69	23
>50 (%)	44	11	21	5	57
Platelet count < 100 × 10^9 L (%)	77	75	81	56	56
Hemoglobin ≤8 g/dL (%)	58	40	60	21	15
Splenomegaly (%)*	50	34	46	28	57
Hepatomegaly (%)*	56	46	48	36	61
Mediastinal mass (%)	0	0	1	0	72
Lymphadenopathy	35	36	41	54	78
CNS disease	10	1	1	0	11

CNS, central nervous system.
*>4 cm below the costal margin.
From Nathan DG, Orkin SH, Ginsburg D, et al (editors): *Nathan & Oski's Hematology of Infancy and Childhood,* 6th ed. Philadelphia, WB Saunders, 2003, p. 1139. Data from Reiter A, Schrappe M, Ludwig WD, et al: Chemotherapy in 998 unselected childhood acute lymphoblastic leukemia patients. Results and conclusions of the multicenter trial ALL-BFM 86. *Blood* 1994;84:3122–3123.

TABLE 495-3. Common Chromosomal Abnormalities in the Acute Leukemias of Childhood

DISEASE	SUBTYPE	CHROMOSOMAL ABNORMALITY	INFLUENCE ON PROGNOSIS
ALL	Pre-B	Trisomy 4 and 10	Favorable
		t(12;21)	
	Pre-B	t(4;11)	Unfavorable
	Pre-B	t(9;22)	Unfavorable
	B-cell	t(8;14)	None
	General	Hyperdiploidy	Favorable
	General	Hypodiploidy	Unfavorable
AML	M1*	t(8;21)	Favorable
	M4*	inv(16)	Favorable
	M3*	t(5;17)	Favorable
	General	del(7)	Unfavorable
	Infant	t(4;11)	Unfavorable

*Per the French-American-British classification of acute myelogenous leukemia (see Table 495-4).
ALL, acute lymphoblastic leukemia; AML, acute myelogenous leukemia.

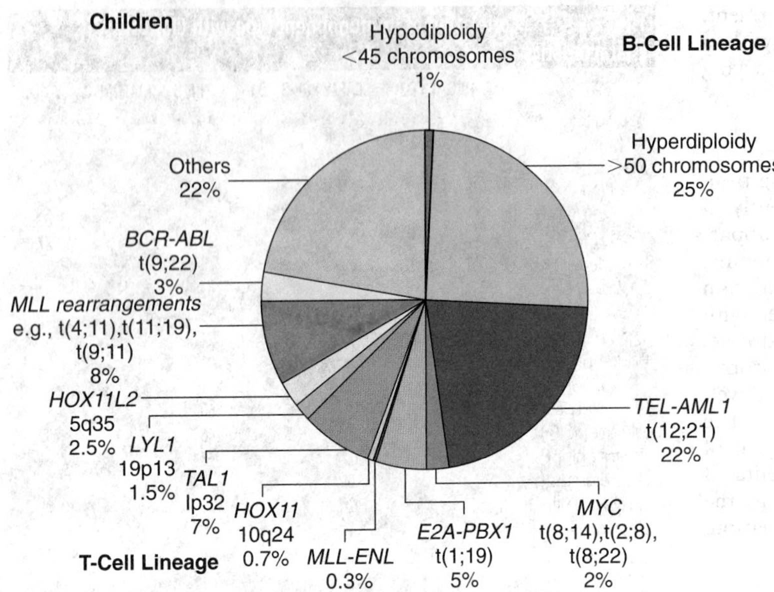

Figure 495-1. Estimated frequency of specific genotypes of acute lymphoblastic leukemia (ALL) in children. The genetic lesions that are exclusively seen in cases of T-cell-lineage leukemias are indicated in purple. All other genetic subtypes are either exclusively or primarily seen in cases of B-cell-lineage ALL. (From Pui CH, Relling MV, Downing JR: Acute lymphoblastic leukemia. *N Engl J Med* 2004;350:1535–1548.)

studies. The polymerase chain reaction and fluorescence in situ hybridization techniques, for example, offer the ability to pinpoint molecular genetic abnormalities and to detect small numbers of malignant cells during follow-up; however, the clinical utility of these findings has yet to be firmly established. The development of DNA microanalysis makes it possible to analyze the expression of thousands of genes in the leukemic cell. This technique promises to further enhance the understanding of the fundamental biology and to provide clues to the therapeutic approach of ALL.

CLINICAL MANIFESTATIONS. The initial presentation of ALL usually is nonspecific and relatively brief. Anorexia, fatigue, and irritability often are present, as is an intermittent, low-grade fever. Bone or, less often, joint pain, particularly in the lower extremities, may be present. Patients often have a history of an upper respiratory tract infection in the preceding 1–2 mo. Less commonly, symptoms may be of several months' duration, may be localized predominantly to the bones or joints, and may include joint swelling. Bone pain is severe and may wake the patient at night. As the disease progresses, signs and symptoms of bone marrow failure become more obvious with the occurrence of pallor, fatigue, bruising, or epistaxis, as well as fever, which may be caused by infection.

On **physical examination,** findings of pallor, listlessness, purpuric and petechial skin lesions, or mucous membrane hemorrhage may reflect bone marrow failure (see Chapter 493). The proliferative nature of the disease may be manifested as lymphadenopathy, splenomegaly, or, less commonly, hepatomegaly. In patients with bone or joint pain, there may be exquisite tenderness over the bone or objective evidence of joint swelling and effusion. Nonetheless, with marrow involvement, deep bone pain may be present but tenderness will not be elicited. Rarely, patients show signs of increased intracranial pressure that indicate leukemic involvement of the central nervous system (CNS). These include papilledema (see Fig. 493-3), retinal hemorrhages, and cranial nerve palsies. Respiratory distress usually is related to anemia but may occur in patients with an obstructive airway problem due to a large anterior mediastinal mass (e.g., in the thymus or nodes). This problem is most typically seen in adolescent boys with T-cell ALL. T-cell ALL also has a higher leukocyte count.

Early pre–B-cell ALL ($CD10^+$ or $CALLA^+$) is the most common immunophenotype (see Table 495-2), with onset between 1–10 yr of age. The median leukocyte count at presentation is 33,000, although 75% of patients have counts <20,000; thrombocytopenia is seen in 75% of patients, and hepatosplenomegaly is seen in 30–40% of patients. In all types of leukemia, CNS symptoms are seen at presentation in 5% of patients (10–20% have blasts in the CSF). Testicular (20%) and ovarian (30%) involvement occurs but does not require a biopsy.

DIAGNOSIS. The diagnosis of ALL is strongly suggested by peripheral blood findings indicative of bone marrow failure. Anemia and thrombocytopenia are seen in most patients. Leukemic cells often are not observed in the peripheral blood in routine laboratory examinations. Many patients with ALL present with total leukocyte counts of <10,000/μL. In such cases, the leukemic cells often are reported initially to be atypical lymphocytes, and it is only on further evaluation that the cells are found to be part of a malignant clone. When the results of an analysis of peripheral blood suggest the possibility of leukemia, a bone marrow examination should be done promptly to establish the diagnosis. Bone marrow aspiration alone usually is sufficient, but sometimes a bone marrow biopsy is needed to provide adequate tissue for study or to exclude other possible causes of bone marrow failure.

ALL is diagnosed by a bone marrow evaluation that demonstrates >25% of the bone marrow cells as a homogeneous population of lymphoblasts. Staging of ALL is based partly on a cerebrospinal fluid (CSF) examination. If lymphoblasts are found and the CSF leukocyte count is elevated, overt CNS or meningeal leukemia is present. This finding reflects a worse stage and indicates the need for additional CNS and systemic therapies. The staging lumbar puncture may be performed in conjunction with the first dose of intrathecal chemotherapy if the diagnosis of leukemia has been previously established from bone marrow evaluation.

DIFFERENTIAL DIAGNOSIS. Acute lymphoblastic leukemia must be differentiated from acute myelogenous leukemia (AML). Other malignant diseases that invade the bone marrow and cause marrow failure include neuroblastoma, rhabdomyosarcoma, Ewing sarcoma, and retinoblastoma; and causes of primary bone marrow failure, such as aplastic anemia (congenital, acquired) and myelofibrosis. Failure of a single cell line, as in transient erythroblastic anemia, immune thrombocytopenia, and congenital or acquired neutropenia, sometimes produces a clinical picture that is difficult to distinguish from ALL and that may require

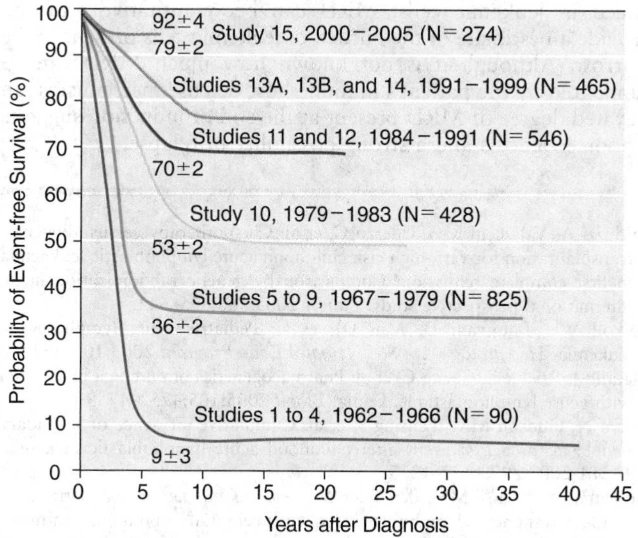

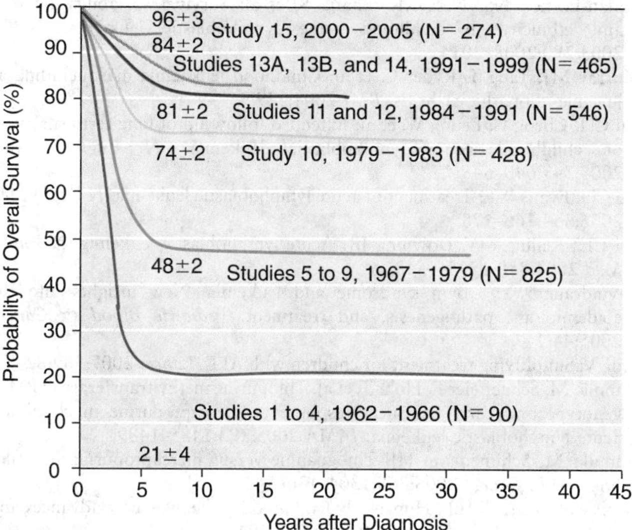

Figure 495-2. Kaplan-Meier analyses of event-free survival (*A*) and overall survival (*B*) in 2628 children with newly diagnosed ALL. The patients participated in 15 consecutive studies conducted at St. Jude Children's Research Hospital from 1962–2005. The 5-year event-free and overall survival estimates (±SE) are shown, except for Study 15, for which preliminary results at 4 years are provided. The results demonstrate steady improvement in clinical outcome over the past 4 decades. The difference in event-free and overall survival rates has narrowed in the more recent periods, suggesting that relapses or second cancers that occur after contemporary therapy are more refractory to treatment. (From Pui CH, Evans WE: Treatment of acute lymphoblastic leukemia. *N Engl J Med* 2006;354:166–178.)

bone marrow examination. A high index of suspicion is required to differentiate ALL from infectious mononucleosis in patients with acute onset of fever and lymphadenopathy and from rheumatoid arthritis in patients with fever and joint swelling. These presentations also may require bone marrow examination.

TREATMENT. The single most important prognostic factor in ALL is the treatment: without effective therapy, the disease is fatal. The survival rates of children with ALL over the past 40 yr have improved as the results of clinical trials have improved the therapies and outcomes (Fig. 495-2).

The choice of treatment of ALL is based on the estimated clinical risk of relapse in the patient, which varies widely among the subtypes of ALL. Three of the most important predictive factors are the age of the patient at the time of diagnosis, the initial leukocyte count, and the speed of response to treatment (i.e., how rapidly the leukemic cells can be cleared from the marrow or peripheral blood). Different study groups use various factors to define risk, but age between 1–10 yr and a leukocyte count of <50,000/μL are widely used to define average risk. Children who are >10 yr of age or who have an initial leukocyte count of >50,000/μL are considered to be at higher risk. The outcome for patients at higher risk can be improved by administration of more intensive therapy despite the greater toxicity of such therapy. Infants with ALL, along with patients who present with specific chromosomal abnormalities such as t(9;22) or t(4;11), have an even higher risk of relapse despite intensive therapy. Clinical trials have demonstrated that the prognosis for patients with a slower response to initial therapy may be improved by therapy that is more intensive than the therapy considered necessary for patients who respond more rapidly.

Most children with ALL are treated on clinical trials conducted by national or international cooperative groups. In general, the initial therapy is designed to eradicate the leukemic cells from the bone marrow; this is known as **remission induction.** During this phase, therapy usually is given for 4 wk and consists of vincristine weekly, a corticosteroid such as dexamethasone or prednisone, and either repeated doses of native L-asparaginase or a single dose of a long-acting, pegylated asparaginase preparation. Intrathecal cytarabine or methotrexate, or both, also may be given. Patients at higher risk also receive daunomycin at weekly intervals. With this approach, 98% of patients are in **remission,** as defined by <5% blasts in the marrow and a return of neutrophil and platelet counts to near-normal levels after 4–5 wk of treatment. Intrathecal chemotherapy is usually given at the start of treatment and once more during induction.

The second phase of treatment focuses on **CNS therapy** in an effort to prevent later CNS relapses. Intrathecal chemotherapy is given repeatedly by lumbar puncture in conjunction with intensive systemic chemotherapy. The likelihood of later CNS relapse is thereby reduced to <5%. A small proportion of patients with features that predict a high risk of CNS relapse may receive irradiation to the brain and spinal cord. This includes those patients who, at the time of diagnosis, have lymphoblasts in the CSF and either an elevated CSF leukocyte count or physical signs of CNS leukemia, such as cranial nerve palsy.

After remission has been induced, many regimens provide 14–28 wk of multiagent therapy, with the drugs and schedules used varying depending on the risk group of the patient. Finally, patients are given daily mercaptopurine and weekly methotrexate, usually with intermittent doses of vincristine and a corticosteroid. This period, known as the **maintenance phase** of therapy, lasts for 2–3 yr, depending on the protocol used. Many patients benefit from administration of a delayed intensive phase of treatment (delayed intensification), approximately 5–7 mo after the beginning of therapy, and after a relatively nontoxic phase of treatment (interim maintenance) to allow recovery from the initial intensive therapy. A small number of patients with particularly poor prognostic features, principally those with the t(9;22) translocation known as the Philadelphia chromosome, may undergo bone marrow transplantation during the first remission. In ALL, this chromosome is similar but not identical to the Philadelphia chromosome of chronic myelogenous leukemia (CML).

Treatment also may be stratified by gene expression profiles of leukemic cells. In particular, gene expression arrays induced by exposure to the chemotherapeutic agent can predict which patients have drug-resistant ALL (see Chapter 494). Furthermore, **pharmacogenetic testing** of the thiopurine S-methyltransferase gene, which converts mercaptopurine or thioguanine (both prodrugs) into active chemotherapeutic agents, can identify rapid metabolizers (associated with toxicity) or slow metabolizers (associated with treatment failure), thus optimizing drug dosing (see Chapter 56).

The major impediment to a successful outcome is relapse of the disease. Relapse occurs in the bone marrow in 15–20% of patients with ALL and carries the most serious implications, especially if it occurs during or shortly after completion of therapy. Intensive chemotherapy with agents not previously used in the patient followed by allogeneic stem cell transplantation can result in long-term survival for a few patients with bone marrow relapse (see Chapter 134).

Patients with relapse in the CNS usually present with signs and symptoms of increased intracranial pressure and may present with isolated cranial nerve palsies. The diagnosis is confirmed most readily by demonstrating the presence of leukemic cells in the CSF and, rarely, by imaging studies. The treatment includes intrathecal medication and craniospinal irradiation. Systemic chemotherapy also must be used, because these patients are at high risk for subsequent bone marrow relapse. Most patients with leukemic relapse confined to the CNS do well, especially those in whom the CNS relapse occurs after chemotherapy has been completed or during the latter phase of chemotherapy.

Testicular relapse occurs in 1–2% of boys with ALL, usually after completion of therapy. Such relapse presents as painless swelling of one or both testes. The diagnosis is confirmed by biopsy of the affected testis. Treatment includes systemic chemotherapy and local irradiation. A high proportion of boys with a testicular relapse can be successfully re-treated, and the survival rate of these patients is good.

SUPPORTIVE CARE. Close attention to the medical supportive care needs of the patients is essential in successfully administering aggressive chemotherapeutic programs. Patients with a large tumor burden are prone to tumor lysis syndrome as therapy is initiated. The renal failure associated with very high levels of serum uric acid can be prevented with the use of urate oxidase. Chemotherapy often produces severe myelosuppression, which may require erythrocyte and platelet transfusion and which always requires a high index of suspicion and aggressive empirical antimicrobial therapy for sepsis in febrile children with neutropenia. Patients must receive prophylactic treatment for *Pneumocystis carinii* pneumonia during chemotherapy and for several months after completing treatment.

The success of therapy has changed ALL from an acute disease with a high mortality rate to a chronic disease. However, such chronic treatment can incur substantial academic, developmental, and psychosocial costs for children with ALL and considerable financial costs and stress for their families. Because of the intensity of therapy, long-term and acute toxicity effects may occur. An array of cancer care professionals with training and experience in addressing the myriad of problems that may arise is essential to minimize the complications and achieve an optimal outcome.

PROGNOSIS. Most children with ALL can now be expected to have long-term survival, with the survival rate >80% at 5 yr from diagnosis (see Fig. 495-2). The most important prognostic factor is the choice of appropriate risk-directed therapy, with the type of treatment chosen according to the type of ALL, the stage of disease, the age of the patient, and the rate of response to initial therapy (favorable if the patient responds in <1 mo). Characteristics generally believed to adversely affect outcome include age <1 yr or >10 yr at diagnosis, a leukocyte count of >100,000/µL at diagnosis, or a slow response to initial therapy. Chromosomal abnormalities, including hypodiploidy, the Philadelphia chromosome, and MLL gene rearrangements and translocations [t(1:19) or t(4;11)], portend a poorer outcome. More favorable characteristics include a rapid response to therapy, hyperdiploidy, trisomy of specific chromosomes, and rearrangements of the TEL/AML1 genes.

Minimal residual disease (MRD) can be detected with specific molecular probes to translocations and other DNA markers contained in leukemic cells. MRD can be quantitative and can provide an estimate of the burden of leukemic cells present in the marrow. Although it is not known how much MRD can be eliminated by the patient's immune host defense mechanisms, an elevated degree of MRD present at the end of induction suggests a poor prognosis and a strong possibility of relapse.

Balduzzi A, Valsecchi MG, Uderzo C, et al: Chemotherapy versus allogeneic transplantation for very-high-risk childhood acute lymphoblastic leukaemia in first complete remission: Comparison by genetic randomization in an international prospective study. *Lancet* 2005;366:635–642.

Carroll WL, Bhojwani D, Min DJ, et al: Pediatric acute lymphoblastic leukemia. *Hematology Am Soc Hematol Educ Program* 2003:102–131.

Claudio J, Rocha C, Cheng C, et al: Pharmacogenetics of outcome in children with acute lymphoblastic leukemia. *Blood* 2005;105:4752–4758.

Hijiya N, Hudson MM, Lensing S, et al: Cumulative incidence of secondary neoplasms as a first event after childhood acute lymphoblastic leukemia. *JAMA* 2007;297:1207–1215.

Holleman A, Cheok MH, den Boer ML, et al: Gene-expression patterns in drug-resistant acute lymphoblastic leukemia cells and response to treatment. *N Engl J Med* 2004;351:533–542.

Kadan-Lottick NS, Ness KK, Bhatia S, et al: Survival variability by race and ethnicity in childhood acute lymphoblastic leukemia. *JAMA* 2003;290:2008–2014.

Murray MJ, Tang T, Ryder C, et al: Childhood leukaemia masquerading as juvenile idiopathic arthritis. *BMJ* 2004;329:959–961.

Pui CH, Cheng C, Leung W, et al: Extended follow-up of long-term survivors of childhood acute lymphoblastic leukemia. *N Engl J Med* 2003;349:640–648.

Pui CH, Evans WE: Treatment of acute lymphoblastic leukemia. *N Engl J Med* 2006;354:166–178.

Pui CH, Relling MV, Downing JR: Acute lymphoblastic leukemia. *N Engl J Med* 2004;350:1535–1548.

Ravindranath Y: Down syndrome and leukemia: New insights into the epidemiology, pathogenesis, and treatment. *Pediatric Blood & Cancer* 2005;44:1–7.

Saha V: Simplifying treatment for children with ALL. *Lancet* 2007;369:82–83.

Stanulla M, Schaeffeler E, Flohr T, et al: Thiopurine methyltransferase (TPMT) genotype and early treatment response to mercaptopurine in childhood acute lymphoblastic leukemia. *JAMA* 2005;293:1485–1489.

Stanulla M, Schünemann HJ: Thioguanine versus mercaptopurine in childhood ALL. *Lancet* 2006;368:1304–1306.

Winick NJ, Carroll WL, Hunger SP: Childhood leukemia—new advances and challenges. *N Engl J Med* 2004;351:601–604.

495.2 • Acute Myelogenous Leukemia

EPIDEMIOLOGY. AML accounts for 11% of the cases of childhood leukemia in the USA, with approximately 370 children diagnosed with AML annually. One subtype, acute promyelocytic leukemia (APL), is more common in certain other regions of the world, but incidence of the other types is generally uniform. Several chromosomal abnormalities associated with AML have been identified, but no predisposing genetic or environmental factors can be identified in most patients (see Table 495-3). Nonetheless, a number of risk factors have been identified, including ionizing radiation, chemotherapeutic agents (e.g., alkylating agents, epipodophyllotoxin), organic solvents, paroxysmal nocturnal hemoglobinuria, and certain syndromes: Down syndrome, Fanconi anemia, Bloom syndrome, Kostmann syndrome, Shwachman-Diamond syndrome, Diamond-Blackfan syndrome, Li-Fraumeni syndrome, and neurofibromatosis type 1.

PATHOGENESIS. The characteristic feature of AML is that >30% of bone marrow cells on bone marrow aspiration or biopsy touch preparations constitute a fairly homogeneous population of blast cells, with features similar to those that characterize early differentiation states of the myeloid-monocyte-megakaryocyte series of blood cells. The most common classification of the subtypes of AML is the FAB system (Table 495-4). Although this system is based on morphologic criteria alone, current practice also requires the use of flow cytometry for identification of cell surface antigens and of chromosomal and molecular genetic techniques for additional diagnostic precision and also to aid the choice of therapy.

CLINICAL MANIFESTATIONS. The production of symptoms and signs of AML, as in ALL, is due to replacement of bone marrow by malignant cells and to secondary bone marrow failure. Thus, patients with AML may present with any or all of the findings associated with **marrow failure** in ALL. In addition, patients with AML present with signs and symptoms that are uncommon in ALL, including **subcutaneous nodules** or "blueberry muffin" lesions, infiltration of the gingiva, signs and laboratory findings of **disseminated intravascular coagulation** (especially indicative of acute promyelocytic leukemia), and discrete masses, known as **chloromas** or **granulocytic sarcomas.** These masses may occur in the absence of apparent bone marrow involvement and typically are associated with the M2 subcategory of AML with a t(8;21) translocation. Chloromas also may be seen in the orbit and epidural space. CNS symptoms are more common in AML than ALL.

DIAGNOSIS. Analysis of bone marrow aspiration and biopsy specimens of patients with AML typically reveals the features of a hypercellular marrow consisting of a rather monotonous pattern of cells with features that permit FAB subclassification of disease. Special stains assist in identification of myeloperoxidase-containing cells, thus confirming both the myelogenous origin of the leukemia and the diagnosis. Some chromosomal abnormalities and molecular genetic markers are characteristic of specific subtypes of disease (see Table 495-2).

TREATMENT. Aggressive multiagent chemotherapy is successful in inducing remission in about 80% of patients. Targeting therapy to genetic markers may be beneficial (Table 495-5). Up to 10% of patients die of either infection or bleeding before a remission can be achieved. Matched-sibling bone marrow or stem cell transplantation after remission has been shown to achieve long-term disease-free survival in 60–70% of patients. Continued chemotherapy for patients who do not have a matched donor is less effective than marrow transplantation but, nevertheless, is curative in some patients. Matched, unrelated marrow or stem cell transplants may be effective therapy but have the risk of significant graft-versus-host disease as well as the complications associated with intensive myeloablative therapy. One factor that favors allogeneic transplantation is that **graft-versus-leukemia** effect is known to occur in AML, whereas it has been difficult to demonstrate that this immunologic antileukemic process occurs when patients with ALL undergo allogeneic hematopoietic stem cell transplantation.

TABLE 495-4. French-American-British (FAB) Classification of Acute Myelogenous Leukemia

SUBTYPE	COMMON NAME
M1	Acute myeloblastic leukemia without maturation
M2	Acute myeloblastic leukemia with maturation
M3	Acute promyeloblastic leukemia
M4	Acute myelomonocytic leukemia
M5	Acute monocytic leukemia
M6	Erythroleukemia
M7	Acute megakaryocytic leukemia

Acute promyelocytic leukemia, characterized by a gene rearrangement involving the retinoic acid receptor, is very responsive to **retinoic acid** combined with anthracyclines. The success of this therapy makes marrow transplantation in first remission unnecessary for patients with this disease.

The supportive care needs of patients with AML are basically the same as those for patients with ALL. The very intensive therapy required in AML produces prolonged bone marrow suppression with a very high incidence of serious infections.

Clark JJ, Smith FO, Arceci RJ: Update in childhood acute myeloid leukemia: Recent developments in the molecular basis of disease and novel therapies. *Curr Opin Hematol* 2003;10:31–39.

Cushing T, Clericuzio C, Wilson C, et al: Risk for leukemia in infants without Down syndrome who have transient myeloproliferative disorder. *J Pediatr* 2006;148:687–689.

Kantarjian H, Giles F, Wunderle L, et al: Nilotinib in imatinib-resistant CML and Philadelphia chromosome-positive ALL. *N Engl J Med* 2006;354:2542–2550.

Kolb EA, Pan Q, Ladanyi M, et al: Imatinib mesylate in Philadelphia chromosome-positive leukemia of childhood. *Cancer* 2003;98:2643–2650.

Linabery AM, Olshan AF, Gamis AS, et al: Exposure to medical test irradiation and acute leukemia among children with Down Syndrome: A report from the children's oncology group. *Pediatrics* 2006;118:e1499–e1508.

Pui CH, Relling MV, Downing JR: Acute lymphoblastic leukemia. *N Engl J Med* 2004;350:1535–1548.

Ross ME, Mahfouz R, Onciu M et al: Gene expression profiling of pediatric acute myelogenous leukemia. *Blood* 2004;104:3679–3687.

Talpaz M, Shah NP, Kantarjian H, et al: Dasatinib in imatinib-resistant Philadelphia chromosome-positive leukemias. *N Engl J Med* 2006;354: 2531–2540.

Woods WG, Barnard DR, Alonzo TA, et al: Prospective study of 90 children requiring treatment for juvenile myelomonocytic leukemia or myelodysplastic syndrome. *J Clin Oncol* 2002;20:434–440.

Woods WG, Neudorf S, Gold S, et al: A comparison of allogeneic bone marrow transplantation, autologous bone marrow transplantation, and aggressive chemotherapy in children with acute myeloid leukemia in remission. *Blood* 2001;97:56–62.

TABLE 495-5. Therapeutic Implications of Common Chromosomal Abnormalities in Pediatric Acute Myelogenous Leukemia and Myelodysplastic Syndromes

CHROMOSOMAL ABNORMALITY	ALTERED GENES	USUAL MORPHOLOGY	PROGNOSIS	RECOMMENDED TREATMENT
t(8;21)	*AML1-ETO*	FAB AML-M2	Favorable	Intensive chemotherapy, including high-dose cytarabine
inv(16), t(16;16)	*CBFB-MYHII*	FAB AML-M4Eo	Favorable	Intensive chemotherapy, including high-dose cytarabine
t(15;17)	*PML-RARA*	FAB AML-M3	Favorable	Intensive chemotherapy, including ATRA and anthracyclines
t(11;17)	*PLZF-RARA*	FAB AML-M3	Favorable	Intensive chemotherapy, including ATRA and anthracyclines
11q23 abnormalities	*MLL* rearrangements	FAB AML-M4 or AML-M5	Unfavorable	Intensive chemotherapy, with high-dose cytarabine and MRD HSCT
t(3;v)	*EVI1*	MDS/AML	Unfavorable	Intensive chemotherapy with or without HSCT
t(3;5)	*NPM-MLF*	MDS/AMS	Unfavorable	Intensive chemotherapy with or without HSCT
del(7q), −7	Unknown	MDS/FAB AML-M0	Unfavorable	Intensive chemotherapy with or without HSCT
del(5q), −5	Unknown	MDS/FAB AML-M0	Unfavorable	Intensive chemotherapy with or without HSCT

From Nathan DG, Orkin SH, Ginsburg D, et al (editors): *Nathan and Oski's Hematology of Infancy and Childhood,* 6th ed. Philadelphia, WB Saunders, 2003, p. 1177.

AML, acute myelogenous leukemia; ATRA, all-*trans* retinoic acid; FAB, French-American-British; HSCT, hematopoietic stem cells transplantation; MDS, myelodysplastic syndromes; MRD, matched related donor.

495.3 • Down Syndrome and Acute Leukemia and Myeloproliferation

Acute leukemia occurs about 14 times more frequently in children with Down syndrome than in the general population (see Chapter 81). The ratio of ALL to AML in patients with Down syndrome is the same as that in the general population. In children with Down syndrome who have ALL, the expected outcome of treatment is the same as that for other children. However, patients with Down syndrome demonstrate a remarkable sensitivity to methotrexate and other antimetabolites, which can result in substantial toxicity if standard doses are administered. In AML, however, patients with Down syndrome have much better outcomes, with a >80% long-term survival rate, than do children who do not have Down syndrome. After induction therapy, these patients require less intensive therapy to achieve better results.

Approximately 10% of neonates with Down syndrome may develop a transient leukemia or **myeloproliferative** syndrome characterized by high leukocyte counts, blast cells in the peripheral blood, and associated anemia, thrombocytopenia, and hepatosplenomegaly. These features usually resolve within days to a few weeks after onset. Although these neonates may require temporary transfusion support, they do not require chemotherapy. However, patients who have Down syndrome and who develop this transient leukemia or myeloproliferative syndrome require close follow-up, because 20–30% will develop typical leukemia (often acute megakaryocytic leukemia) by 3 yr of life (mean onset 16 mo). *GATA1* mutations (a transcription factor that controls megakaryopoiesis) are present in blasts from patients with Down syndrome who have transient myeloproliferative disease and also in those with leukemia. Transient myeloproliferative disease also may occur in patients who do not have phenotypic features of Down syndrome. Blasts from these patients may be trisomy 21, suggesting a mosaic state.

495.4 • Chronic Myelogenous Leukemia

CML is a clonal disorder of the hematopoietic tissue that accounts for 2–3% of all cases of childhood leukemia. About 99% of the cases are characterized by a specific translocation, t(9;22)(q34;q11), known as the **Philadelphia chromosome.** The disease has been associated with exposure to ionizing radiation, but very few children with CML have a history of such exposure. The disease is characterized clinically by an initial chronic phase in which the malignant clone produces an elevated leukocyte count with a predominance of mature forms but with increased numbers of immature granulocytes. The **spleen** often is greatly enlarged, often resulting in pain in the left upper quadrant of the abdomen. In addition to leukocytosis, blood counts may reveal mild anemia and thrombocytosis.

Typically, the chronic phase terminates 3–4 yr after onset, when the CML moves into the accelerated or "blast crisis" phase. At this point, the blood counts rise dramatically and cannot be controlled with drugs such as hydroxyurea. Additional manifestations may occur, including hyperuricemia and neurologic symptoms, which are related to increased blood viscosity with decreased CNS perfusion.

The presenting symptoms of CML are nonspecific and may include fever, fatigue, weight loss, and anorexia. Splenomegaly also may be present. The diagnosis is suggested by increased numbers of myeloid cells with differentiation to mature forms in the peripheral blood and bone marrow and is confirmed by cytogenetic studies that demonstrate the presence of the characteristic Philadelphia chromosome. Molecular techniques usually demonstrate the **BCR-ABL** gene rearrangement. This translocation, although characteristic of CML, also is found in a small percentage of patients with ALL or AML.

Imatinib mesylate, an agent designed specifically to inhibit the BCR-ABL tyrosine kinase, has been used in adults and has shown an ability to produce major cytogenetics responses in over 70% of patients (see Table 494-1). Limited experience in children suggests it can be used safely with results comparable to those seen in adults. While waiting for a response with imatinib, disabling or threatening signs and symptoms of CML can be controlled during the chronic phase with hydroxyurea, which will gradually return the leukocyte count to normal. Prolonged morphologic and cytogenetics responses are expected, but the opportunity for cure is enhanced by allogeneic stem cell or marrow transplant, with up to 80% of children achieving a cure.

495.5 • Juvenile Chronic Myelogenous Leukemia

Juvenile chronic myelogenous leukemia (JCML), also known as juvenile myelomonocytic leukemia, is a clonal proliferation of hematopoietic stem cells that typically affects children <2 yr of age. Patients with this disease do not have the Philadelphia chromosome that is characteristic of CML. Patients with JCML present with rashes, lymphadenopathy, and splenomegaly. Analysis of the peripheral blood often shows an elevated leukocyte count and also may show thrombocytopenia and the presence of erythroblasts. The bone marrow shows a myelodysplastic pattern, with blasts accounting for <30% of cells. No distinctive cytogenetic abnormalities are seen. JCML is rare, constituting <2% of all cases of childhood leukemia. Therapeutic reports are largely anecdotal. Patients with neurofibromatosis type 1 have a predilection for this type of leukemia. Stem cell transplantation offers the best opportunity for cure, but much less so than for classic CML.

495.6 • Infant Leukemia

About 2% of cases of leukemia during childhood occur before the age of 1 yr. In contrast to older children, the ratio of ALL to AML is 2 : 1. Some cases may be due to maternal exposure to naturally occurring DNA topoisomerase II inhibitors. Several unique biologic features and a particularly poor prognosis are characteristic of ALL during infancy. More than two thirds of the cases demonstrate rearrangements of the MLL gene, found at the site of the 11q23 band translocation; this subset of patients largely accounts for the very high relapse rate. These patients often present with hyperleukocytosis and extensive tissue infiltration producing organomegaly, including CNS disease. Subcutaneous nodules, known as **leukemia cutis,** and tachypnea due to diffuse pulmonary infiltration by leukemic cells are observed more often in infants than in older children. The leukemic cell morphology is usually that of large irregular lymphoblasts (FAB L2), with a phenotype negative for the CD10 (cALLa) marker.

Very intensive chemotherapy programs including stem cell transplantation are being explored in infants with rearrangement of MLL in band 11q23, but none has yet proved satisfactory. Infants with leukemia who lack the 11q23 rearrangements have a prognosis similar to that of older children with ALL. Infants with AML often present with CNS or skin involvement and have the FAB M4 subtype, which is commonly known as **acute myelomonocytic leukemia.** The treatment may be the same as that for older children with AML. Meticulous supportive care is necessary because of the young age and aggressive therapy needed in these patients.

Bajwa RPS, Skinner R, Windebank KP, et al: Demographic study of leukaemia presenting within the first 3 months of life in the Northern Health Region of England. *J Clin Pathol* 2004;57:186–188.

Chapter 496 ■ Lymphoma

Mitchell S. Cairo and M. Brigid Bradley

Lymphoma is the third most common cancer among children in the USA, with an annual incidence of 15 per million children ≤14 yr of age. The two broad categories of lymphoma, Hodgkin disease (HD) and non-Hodgkin lymphoma (NHL), have different clinical manifestations and treatments.

496.1 • Hodgkin Disease

HD is a malignant process of the lymphoreticular system that constitutes 6% of childhood cancers. In the USA, HD accounts for about 5% of cancers in persons ≤14 yr of age and for about 15% in persons 15–19 yr of age. It is rare in children <10 yr of age.

EPIDEMIOLOGY. The incidence of HD is bimodal with regard to age. In industrialized countries, the early peak occurs in the middle to late 20s, with a second peak after 50 yr of age. In developing countries, the early peak occurs before adolescence. A male : female predominance is found among young children, with a ratio of 4 : 1 for children 3–7 yr of age, 3 : 1 for children 7–9 yr of age, and 1.3 : 1 for children >10 yr of age. Clustering of cases in families or races may suggest a genetic predisposition to the disease or a common exposure to an etiologic agent. The risk is 100-fold for an unaffected monozygotic twin of an affected twin; there is no increased risk for dizygotic twins. Studies of families suggest an increased association of HD with specific HLA antigens. Several studies suggest that infectious agents may be involved, such as human herpesvirus 6, cytomegalovirus, and Epstein-Barr virus (EBV). The role of EBV is supported by prospective serologic studies. The large proportion of patients with HD who have high EBV antibody titers suggests that enhanced activation of EBV may precede the development of HD, a possibility that also is supported by in situ hybridization evidence of the EBV genomes in Reed-Sternberg cells. EBV antigens have been demonstrated in HD tissues, although EBV status is not prognostic of outcome. HD may represent a common result of multiple pathologic processes that include viral infection and exposure of a genetically susceptible host to a sensitizing agent. Pre-existing immunodeficiency, either congenital, such as ataxia-telangiectasia, or acquired, such as HIV infection, increases the risk of HD.

ETIOLOGY. The **Reed-Sternberg cell** (Fig. 496-1E) is a large cell (15–45 μm in diameter) with multiple or multilobulated nuclei. This cell type is considered the hallmark of HD, although similar cells are seen in infectious mononucleosis, NHL, and other conditions. The Reed-Sternberg cell is clonal in origin and arises from the germinal center B cells. HD is characterized by a variable number of Reed-Sternberg cells surrounded by an inflammatory infiltrate of lymphocytes, plasma cells, and eosinophils in different proportions, depending on the HD histologic subtype. Other features that distinguish the histologic subtypes include various degrees of fibrosis and the presence of collagen bands, necrosis, or malignant reticular cells.

The **Rye classification system** (Table 496-1) defines four major histologic subtypes: lymphocyte predominant (**LP**) (see Fig. 496-1A and B), nodular sclerosing (**NS**) (see Fig. 496-1C), mixed cellularity (**MC**) (see Fig. 496-1D), and lymphocyte depleted (**LD**). LP affects 10–15% of patients, is more common among male and younger patients, and usually presents as localized disease. MC is observed in 30% of patients, is more common among children ≤10 yr of age, and often presents as advanced disease with extranodal extension. LD is rare in children but is common in patients with HIV infection patients. NS is the most common subtype, affecting 40% of younger patients and 70% of adolescents with HD.

The **Revised European-American Classification of Lymphoid Neoplasms (REAL) classification system** (see Table 496-1) includes two modifications of the older Rye system. In addition to classical HD, it defines lymphocyte predominance (LPHD) but also anaplastic large cell lymphoma Hodgkin-like. The lymphocyte predominance subtype closely resembles a low-grade B-cell lymphoma in clinical behavior and Reed-Sternberg cell phenotype. Most patients with LPHD present with early disease and have an excellent prognosis. Anaplastic large cell lymphoma Hodgkin-like has a poor response to conventional HD chemotherapy and has been reported to respond better to aggressive NHL therapy regimens. HD appears to arise in lymphoid tissue and spreads to adjacent lymph node areas in a relatively orderly fashion. Hematogenous spread also occurs, leading to involvement of the liver, spleen, bone, bone marrow, or brain, and usually is associated with systemic symptoms. Levels of various **cytokines** have been shown to be elevated in patient sera or are produced by cultured cell lines or HD tissue. They may be responsible for the systemic symptoms of fever and night sweats (interleukin-1 or -2) and weight loss (tissue necrosis factor [TNF]), in addition to influencing the proliferation of Reed-Sternberg cells and inducing immunosuppression (transforming growth factor-β). Various degrees of **cellular immune impairment** can be identified in most newly diagnosed cases of HD. The severity of the immune defect varies with the extent of disease and persists even after successful curative therapy. Whether it predisposes to the disease or results from it is unknown.

CLINICAL MANIFESTATIONS. Patients commonly present with painless, non-tender, firm, rubbery, cervical or supraclavicular lymphadenopathy. Affected lymph nodes are firmer than inflammatory nodes. Most patients present with some degree of mediastinal involvement. Clinically detectable hepatosplenomegaly rarely is encountered. Depending on the extent and location of nodal and extranodal disease, patients may present with symptoms and signs of airway obstruction (dyspnea, hypoxia, cough), pleural or pericardial effusion, hepatocellular dysfunction, or

TABLE 496-1. Classification Systems for Hodgkin Disease

RYE CLASSIFICATION
Lymphocyte predominance
Mixed cellularity
Nodular sclerosis
Lymphocyte depletion
NEW WHO/REAL CLASSIFICATION
Nodular lymphocyte predominance
Classical Hodgkin lymphoma
Lymphocyte rich
Mixed cellularity
Nodular sclerosis
Lymphocyte depletion
Anaplastic large cell lymphoma Hodgkin-like

REAL, Revised European-American Classification of Lymphoid Neoplasms; WHO, World Health Organization.

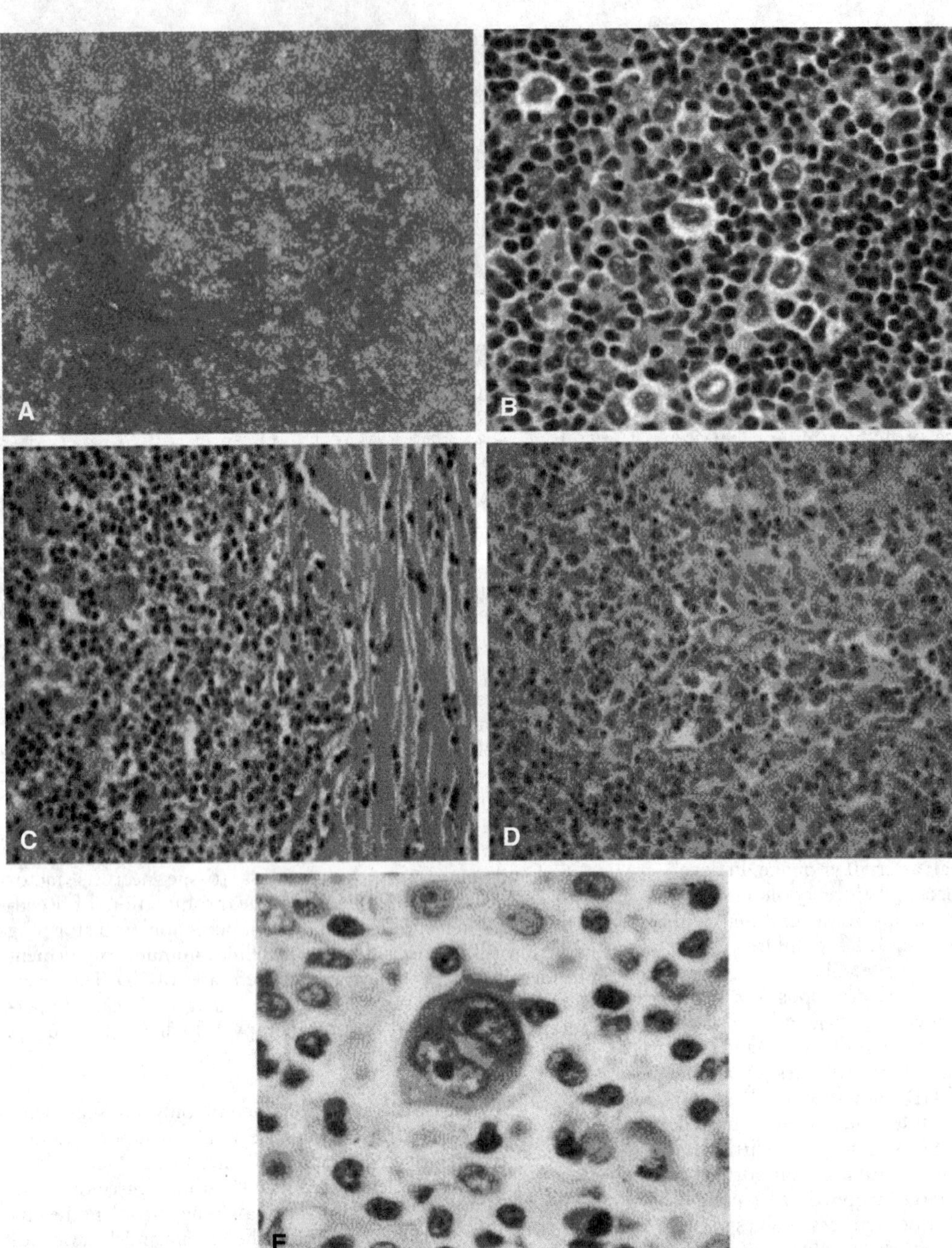

Figure 496-1. Histological subtypes of Hodgkin lymphoma. *A,* Hematoxylin and eosin stains of lymphocyte-predominant Hodgkin lymphoma (NLPHL) demonstrating a nodular proliferation with a motheaten appearance. *B,* High-power view demonstrating the neoplastic L and H cells found in NLPHL. *C,* Classic Hodgkin lymphoma, nodular sclerosis subtype. Large mononuclear and binucleate Reed-Sternberg cells are seen admixed in the inflammatory cell background. *D,* Classic Hodgkin lymphoma, mixed cellularity subtype, demonstrating increased numbers of Reed-Sternberg cells in a mixed inflammatory background without sclerotic changes. *E,* High-power view of a classic Reed-Sternberg cell showing binucleate cells with prominent eosinophilic nucleoli and relatively abundant cytoplasm.

bone marrow infiltration (anemia, neutropenia, or thrombocytopenia). Disease presenting below the diaphragm is rare and occurs in approximately 3% of all cases. **Systemic symptoms,** classified as **B symptoms** that are considered important in staging, are unexplained fever >39°C, weight loss >10% total body weight over 3 mo, or drenching night sweats. Some present as a fever of unknown origin. Less common and not considered of prognostic significance are symptoms of pruritus, lethargy, anorexia, or pain that worsens after ingestion of alcohol. Patients also exhibit immune system abnormalities that often persist during and after therapy. They include anergy to delayed-hypersensitivity skin tests, abnormal cellular immune response, slightly decreased CD4:CD8 ratio, and reduced natural killer cell cytotoxicity. Humoral immunity also can be impaired following treatment.

DIAGNOSIS. Any patient with persistent, unexplained lymphadenopathy unassociated with an obvious underlying inflammatory or infectious process should have a chest radiograph to identify the presence of a mediastinal mass before undergoing node biopsy (Fig. 496-2). Unless signs or symptoms dictate otherwise, additional laboratory studies can be delayed until the biopsy results are available. Patients with persistently enlarged lymph nodes, even after serologically proven infectious mononucleosis, also should be considered for biopsy. Formal excisional biopsy is preferred over needle biopsy to ensure that adequate tissue is obtained, both for light microscopy and for appropriate immunocytochemical and molecular studies, culture, and cytogenetic analysis if routine studies fail to provide a firm diagnosis. HD rarely is diagnosed with certainty on frozen section. Ideally, a portion of the biopsy specimen should be frozen and stored to allow for additional studies. Once the diagnosis of HD is established, extent of disease (stage) should be determined to select appropriate therapy (Table 496-2). **Evaluation includes** history, physical examination, and imaging studies, including chest radi-

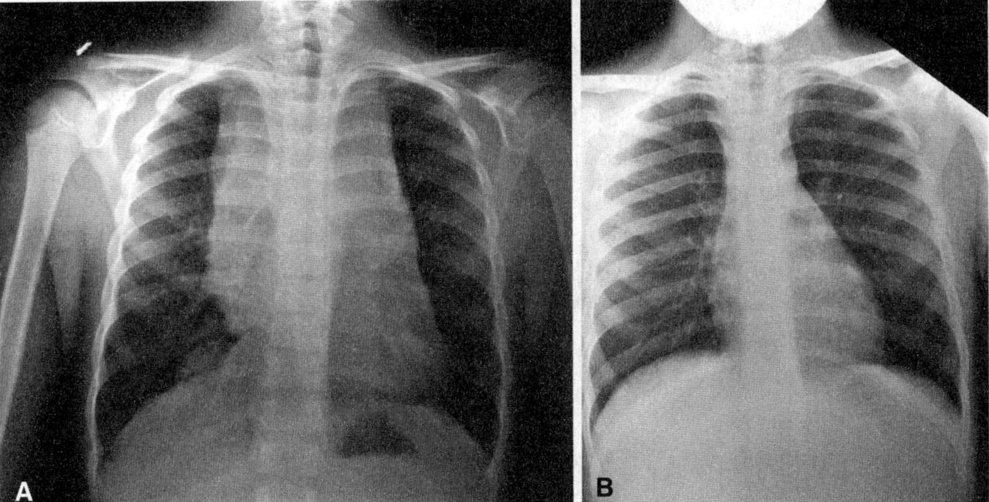

Figure 496-2. *A,* Anterior mediastinal mass in a patient with Hodgkin disease before therapy. *B,* After 2 mo of chemotherapy, the mediastinal mass has disappeared.

ograph; CT scans of the chest, abdomen and pelvis; gallium scan; and positron emission tomography (PET) scan. **Laboratory studies** include a complete blood cell count (CBC) to identify abnormalities that might suggest marrow involvement, erythrocyte sedimentation rate (ESR), and serum copper and serum ferritin levels, which are of some prognostic significance and, if abnormal at diagnosis, serve as a baseline to evaluate the effects of treatment. Liver function tests, although not particularly sensitive to the presence of liver involvement, can influence treatment and treatment complications. A chest radiograph is particularly important for measuring the size of the mediastinal mass in relation to the maximal diameter of the thorax. Chest CT more clearly defines the extent of a mediastinal mass if present and identifies hilar nodes and pulmonary parenchymal involvement, which may not be evident on chest radiographs. Abdominal CT or MRI can identify gross subdiaphragmatic involvement of nodes and enlargement and defects in the liver and spleen. Bone marrow aspiration and biopsy should be performed in patients with advanced disease (stage III or IV) or B symptoms (fever, weight loss, night sweats). Bone scans are performed in patients with bone pain and/or elevated alkaline phosphatase. Lymphangiograms, used in the past to evaluate involvement of the abdominal lymph nodes, rarely are used today. More false-positives occur in children than in adults, and the studies are technically difficult to perform. Gallium-67 scan is particularly helpful in identifying areas of increased uptake, which can then be re-evaluated at the end of treatment, especially in patients with mediastinal masses that do not resolve completely on chest radiographs or CT. Fluorodeoxyglucose (FDG)-PET has advantages over gallium-67 scanning because the scan is a 1-day procedure with higher resolution, better dosimetry, and less intestinal activity and has a quantitation potential. However, its false-positive and false-negative rates are still under investigation in childhood HD.

When standard-dose radiation therapy was an acceptable treatment strategy for patients with early-stage HD, exploratory laparotomy with splenectomy was performed to determine the presence and extent of abdominal involvement. There is no longer any role for surgical staging laparotomies in the treatment of pediatric HD patients. The staging classification currently used for HD was adopted at the Ann Arbor Conference in 1971 and was revised in 1989 (see Table 496-2). HD can be subclassified into A or B categories: *A* is used to identify asymptomatic patients and *B* is for patients who exhibit any B symptoms. Extralymphatic disease resulting from direct extension of an involved lymph node region is designated by category E. A complete response in HD is defined as the complete resolution of disease on clinical examination and imaging studies or at least 70–80% reduction of disease and a change from initial positivity to negativity on either gallium or PET scanning because residual fibrosis in common.

TABLE 496-2. Ann Arbor Staging Classification for Hodgkin Disease

STAGE	DEFINITION
I	Involvement of a single lymph node (1) or of a single extralymphatic organ or site (I_E)
II	Involvement of two or more lymph node regions on the same side of the diaphragm (II) or localized involvement of an extralymphatic organ or site and one or more lymph node regions on the same side of the diaphragm (II_E)
III	Involvement of lymph node regions on both sides of the diaphragm (III), which may be accompanied by involvement of the spleen (III_S) or by localized involvement of an extralymphatic organ or site (III_E) or both (III_{SE})
IV	Diffuse or disseminated involvement of one or more extralymphatic organs or tissues with or without associated lymph node involvement

The absence or presence of fever >38°C for 3 consecutive days, drenching night sweats, or unexplained loss of ≥10% of body weight in the 6 months preceding admission are to be denoted in all cases by the suffix letters A or B, respectively.

From Lister TA, Crowther D, Sutcliffe SB, et al: Report of a committee convened to discuss the evaluation and staging of patients with Hodgkin's disease: Cotswolds meeting. *J Clin Oncol* 1989;7:1630–1636.

TREATMENT. Chemotherapy and radiation therapy are effective in the treatment of HD. Current treatment of HD in pediatric patients involves the use of combined chemotherapy with or without low-dose involved field radiation therapy. Treatment is determined largely by disease stage, age at diagnosis, presence or absence of B symptoms, and the presence of hilar lymphadenopathy or bulky nodal disease. Radiation therapy alone, at standard doses of 3,500–4,000 cGy, initially was used and resulted in prolonged remission and cure rates of 40–95% in patients with surgically low-staged HD. This treatment approach, however, resulted in significant long-term morbidity in pediatric patients, including growth retardation, thyroid dysfunction, and cardiac and pulmonary toxicity. The **MOPP** regimen (mechlorethamine [nitrogen mustard], vincristine, procarbazine, and prednisone) introduced in 1964 was the first combination chemotherapy regimen used in the treatment of HD and was a major milestone in the treatment of advanced stage HD. It resulted in a complete response rate of 70–80% and cure rate of 40–50% at 10 yr in patients with advanced stage disease. This regimen also resulted, however, in significant acute and long-term toxicity. The desire to reduce side effects has stimulated attempts to reduce the intensity of chemotherapy and radiation dose and volume.

Chemotherapy agents commonly used to treat children and adolescents with HD include cyclophosphamide, procarbazine,

TABLE 496-3. Chemotherapy Regimens Commonly Used for Children and Young Adults With Hodgkin Disease

CHEMOTHERAPY REGIMENS	CORRESPONDING AGENTS
ABVD	Doxorubicin (Adriamycin), bleomycin, vinblastine, dacarbazine
ABVE (DBVE)	Doxorubicin (Adriamycin), bleomycin, vincristine, etoposide
VAMP	Vincristine, doxorubicin (Adriamycin), methotrexate, prednisone
OPPA ± COPP (females)	Vincristine (Oncovin), prednisone, procarbazine, doxorubicin (Adriamycin), cyclophosphamide, vincristine (Oncovin), prednisone, procarbazine
OEPA ± COPP (males)	Vincristine (Oncovin), etoposide, prednisone, doxorubicin (Adriamycin), cyclophosphamide, vincristine (Oncovin), prednisone, procarbazine
COPP/ABV	Cyclophosphamide, vincristine (Oncovin), prednisone, procarbazine, doxorubicin (Adriamycin), bleomycin, vinblastine
BEACOPP (advanced stage)	Bleomycin, etoposide, doxorubicin (Adriamycin), cyclophosphamide, vincristine (Oncovin), prednisone, procarbazine
COPP	Cyclophosphamide, vincristine (Oncovin), prednisone, procarbazine
CHOP	Cyclophosphamide, doxorubicin (Adriamycin), vincristine (Oncovin), prednisone
ABVE-PC (DBVE-PC)	Doxorubicin (Adriamycin), bleomycin, vincristine, etoposide, prednisone, cyclophosphamide

vincristine or vinblastine, prednisone or dexamethasone, doxorubicin, bleomycin, dacarbazine, etoposide, methotrexate, and cytosine arabinoside. The combination chemotherapy regimens in current use are based on **COPP** (cyclophosphamide, vincristine [Oncovin], procarbazine, and prednisone) or **ABVD** (doxorubicin [Adriamycin], bleomycin, vinblastine, and dacarbazine), with **BEACOPP** (bleomycin, etoposide, doxorubicin, cyclophosphamide, vincristine, procarbazine, prednisone) typically used for patients with advanced stage disease (Table 496-3). Different combination regimens to reduce potential toxicities have been developed. The **COPP/ABV** (cyclophosphamide, vincristine, procarbazine, prednisone/doxorubicin, bleomycin and vinblastine) regimen is an example. Originally, a minimum of six cycles of chemotherapy was given, with significant cumulative toxicity, including second malignancies, sterility, and cardiac and pulmonary dysfunction. "Risk-adapted" protocols are based on staging criteria as well as rapidity of response to initial chemotherapy. The aim is to reduce total drug doses and treatment duration and even eliminate radiation therapy.

RELAPSE. Most relapses occur within the first 3 yr from diagnosis but relapses as late as 10 yr have been reported. Relapse cannot be predicted accurately with this disease. Poor prognostic features include tumor bulk, stage at diagnosis, and presence of B symptoms. Patients who never achieve remission or relapse <12 mo after initiation of therapy are candidates for myeloablative chemotherapy and **autologous stem cell transplant** with or without the addition of radiation therapy. This treatment is most successful in patients with chemoresponsive disease. Myeloablative **allogeneic stem cell transplantation** reduces the relapse rate in patients with high-risk relapsed or refractory HD. However, there was no improvement in overall survival in the studies reported, due to a high transplant-related mortality. These results, however, do suggest a graft-versus-HD effect. The use of nonmyeloablative nontoxic regimens to reduce regimen-related morbidity and mortality associated with myeloablative allogeneic stem cell transplantation but still achieve a graft-versus-HD effect is under investigation.

PROGNOSIS. Using current therapeutic regimens, patients with favorable prognostic factors and early-stage disease have an event-free survival (EFS) of 85–90% and an overall survival (OS) at 5 yr of 95%. Patients with advanced stage disease have an EFS and OS of 80–85% and 90%, respectively. Prognosis after relapse depends on the time from completion of treatment to recurrence, site of relapse (nodal vs. extranodal), and presence of B symptoms at relapse. Patients who relapse >12 mo after chemotherapy alone or combined modality therapy have the best prognosis and usually respond to additional standard therapy, resulting in a long-term survival of 60–70%. A myeloablative autologous stem cell transplant in patients with refractory disease or relapse within 12 mo of therapy results in a long-term survival rate of 40–50%. Long-term complications are related to radiation or chemotherapy; these include secondary malignancy (e.g., acute myelogenous leukemia, breast, lung, thyroid, non-Hodgkin lymphoma), sepsis (e.g., splenectomy or splenic irradiation), sterility, short stature, hypothyroidism, dental caries, subclinical pulmonary dysfunction, and ischemic heart disease.

Claviez A, Klingebiel T, Beyer J, et al: Allogeneic peripheral blood stem cell transplantation following fludarabine-based conditioning in six children with advanced Hodgkin disease. *Ann Hematol* 2004;83:237–241.

Hjalgrim HH, Askling J, Rostgaard K, et al: Characteristics of Hodgkin's lymphoma after infectious mononucleosis. *N Engl J Med* 2003;349:1324–1332.

Hudson MM, Donaldson SS: Hodgkin disease. In Pizzo PA, Poplack DG (editors): *Principles and Practice of Pediatric Oncology,* 4th ed. Philadelphia, Lippincott Williams & Wilkins, 2002, pp 637–660.

Hueltenschmidt B, Sautter-Bihl ML, Lang O, et al: Whole body positron emission tomography in the treatment of Hodgkin disease. *Cancer* 2001;91:302–310.

Peggs KS, Hunter A, Chopra R, et al: Clinical evidence of a graft-versus-Hodgkin's-lymphoma effect after reduced-intensity allogeneic transplantation. *Lancet* 2005;365:1934–1940.

Pileri SA, Ascani S, Leoncini L, et al: Hodgkin lymphoma: the pathologist's viewpoint. *J Clin Pathol* 2002;55:162–176.

Schwartz CL: The management of Hodgkin disease in the young child. *Curr Opin Pediatr* 2003;15:10–16.

Thomson AB, Wallace WH: Treatment of paediatric Hodgkin disease. A balance of risks. *Eur J Cancer* 2002;38:468–477.

Yung L, Linch D: Hodgkin's lymphoma. *Lancet* 2003;361:943–950.

496.2 • Non-Hodgkin Lymphoma (NHL)

NHL accounts for approximately 60% of all lymphomas in children and adolescents. It represents 8–10% of all malignancies in children between 5–19 yr of age, with an annual incidence in the USA of 750–800 cases per year in children ≤19 yr of age. Although >70% of patients present with advanced disease at diagnosis, the prognosis has improved dramatically, with survival rates of 90–95% for localized disease and 60–90% with advanced disease.

EPIDEMIOLOGY. While most children and adolescents with NHL present with de novo disease, a small number of patients develop NHL secondary to specific etiologies, including inherited or acquired immune deficiencies (e.g., severe combined immunodeficiency syndrome, Wiskott-Aldrich syndrome), viral etiologies (e.g., HIV, EBV) or as part of genetic syndromes (e.g., ataxia-telangiectasia, Bloom syndrome). Most children who develop NHL, however, have no obvious genetic or environmental etiology.

PATHOGENESIS. The four major pathological subtypes of childhood and adolescent NHL are Burkitt lymphoma (BL), constituting 40% of NHL; lymphoblastic lymphoma (LL), accounting for 30%; diffuse large B-cell lymphoma (DLBCL), constituting 20%; and anaplastic large cell lymphoma (ALCL), accounting for 10% (Fig. 496-3). Most childhood and adolescent NHLs are high-grade tumors with an aggressive clinical behavior compared to those of adult NHL, which usually are low- to intermediate-grade indolent tumors. Almost all childhood and adolescent NHL is derived from germinal center aberrations. Almost all forms of

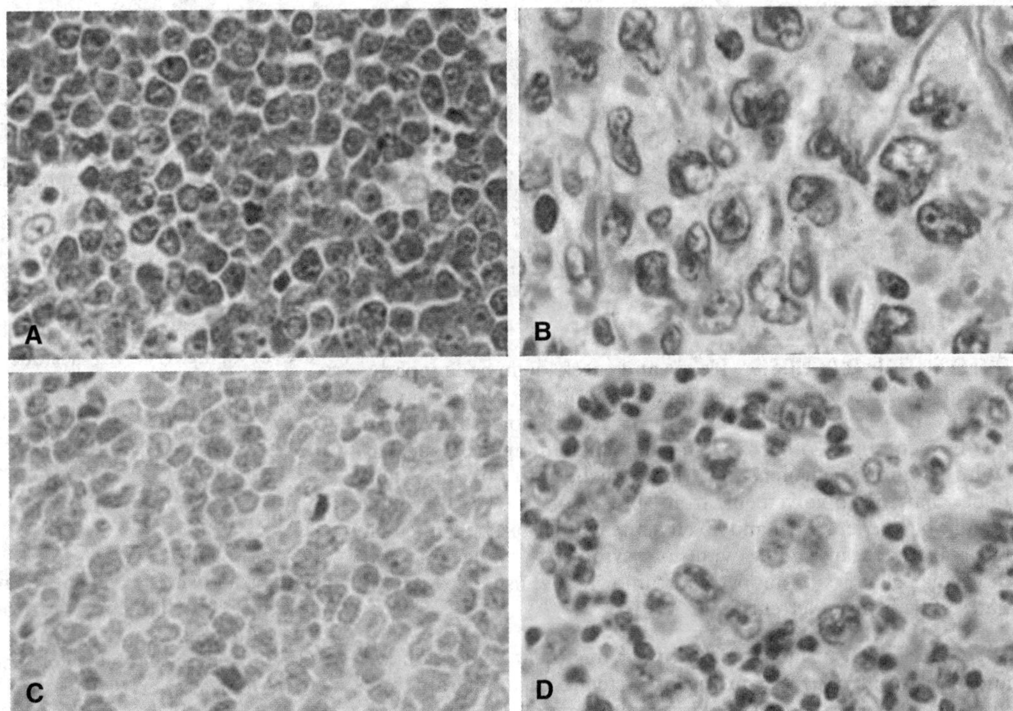

Figure 496-3. Distribution of childhood and adolescent non-Hodgkin lymphoma. Hematoxylin and eosin stains showing morphology of Burkitt lymphoma (*A*, high power), diffuse large B-cell lymphoma (*B*, high power), precursor T-lymphoblastic lymphoma (*C*, high power), and anaplastic large cell lymphoma (*D*, high power). (From Cairo MS, Raetz E, Lim MS, et al: Childhood and adolescent non-Hodgkin lymphoma: New insights in biology and critical challenges for the future. *Pediatr Blood Cancer* 2005;45:753–769.)

BL and DLBCL are of B cell origin; cases of LL are 80% T cell and 20% B cell; and cases of ALCL are 70% T cell, 20% null cell, and 10% B cell in origin. Some pathological subtypes have specific cytogenetic aberrations. Children with BL commonly have a t(8;14) translocation (90%) or, less commonly, a t(2;8) or t(8;22) translocation (10%). Patients with ALCL commonly have a t(2;5) translocation (≥5%). Patients with DLBCL and LL have a variety of different cytogenetic abnormalities.

CLINICAL MANIFESTATIONS. The clinical manifestations of childhood and adolescent NHL depend primarily on pathological subtype and primary and secondary sites of involvement. NHLs are rapidly growing tumors and can cause symptoms based on size and location. Approximately 70% present with advanced disease of stages III or IV (Table 496-4), including extranodal disease that manifests as gastrointestinal, bone marrow, and central nervous system (CNS) involvement. **BL commonly presents** with abdominal (sporadic type) or head and neck (endemic type) disease with involvement of the bone marrow or CNS. **LL commonly presents** with an intrathoracic or mediastinal supradiaphragmatic mass, and also has a predilection for spreading to the bone marrow and CNS. **DLBCL commonly presents** with either an abdominal or mediastinal primary and, rarely, dissemination to the bone marrow or CNS. **ALCL presents** either with a primary cutaneous manifestation (10%) or with systemic disease (fever, weight loss) with dissemination to liver, spleen, lung, mediastinum, or skin; spread to the bone marrow or CNS is rare.

TABLE 496-4. St. Jude Staging System for Childhood Non-Hodgkin Lymphoma

STAGE	DESCRIPTION
I	A single tumor (extranodal) or single anatomic area (nodal), with the exclusion of mediastinum or abdomen
II	A single tumor (extranodal) with regional node involvement
	Two or more nodal areas on the same side of the diaphragm
	Two single (extranodal) tumors with or without regional node involvement on the same side of the diaphragm
	A primary gastrointestinal tract tumor, usually in the ileocecal area, with or without involvement of associated mesenteric nodes only, which must be grossly (>90%) resected
III	Two single tumors (extranodal) on opposite sides of the diaphragm
	Two or more nodal areas above and below the diaphragm
	Any primary intrathoracic tumor (mediastinal, pleural, or thymic)
	Any extensive primary intra-abdominal disease
IV	Any of the above, with initial involvement of central nervous system or bone marrow at time of diagnosis

From Murphy SB: Classification, staging and end results of treatment of childhood non-Hodgkin's lymphomas: Dissimilarities from lymphomas in adults. *Semin Oncol* 1980;7:332–339.

Site-specific manifestations include painless, rapid lymph node enlargement; cough, superior vena cava (SVC) syndrome, dyspnea with thoracic involvement; abdominal (massive and rapidly enlarging) mass, intestinal obstruction, intussusception-like symptoms, ascites with abdominal involvement; nasal stuffiness, earache, hearing loss, tonsil enlargement with Waldeyer ring involvement; and localized bone pain (primary or metastatic).

Three clinical manifestations that require special alternative treatment strategies include SVC syndrome secondary to a large mediastinal mass obstructing various blood flow or respiratory airways; acute paraplegias secondary to spinal cord or central nervous system compression from neighboring localized NHL; and tumor lysis syndrome (TLS) secondary to severe metabolic abnormalities, including hyperuricemia, hyperphosphatemia, hyperkalemia, and hypocalcemia from massive tumor cell lysis.

LABORATORY FINDINGS. Recommended laboratory and radiologic testing includes: complete blood count (CBC); electrolytes, uric acid, calcium, phosphorus, bilirubin urea nitrogen, creatinine, alanine aminotransferase, and aspartate aminotransferase; bilateral bone marrow aspiration and biopsies; lumbar puncture with CSF cytology, cell count and protein; chest x-ray; and neck, chest, abdominal, and pelvic CT scans, PET scan and bone scan (optional), and head CT scan (optional) (Table 496-5). The tumor tissue (i.e., biopsy, bone marrow, CSF, or pleural/paracentesis fluid) should be tested by flow cytometry for immunophenotypic origin (T, B, or null) and cytogenetics (karyotype). Additional tests might include fluorescent in situ hybridization (FISH) or quantitative RT-PCR for specific genetic translocations, T and B cell gene rearrangement studies, and molecular profiling by oligonucleotide microarray.

TABLE 496-5. Pretreatment Studies for Staging Pediatric Non-Hodgkin Lymphoma
Complete blood cell count
Serum electrolytes, uric acid, lactate dehydrogenase, creatinine, calcium, phosphorus
Liver function tests (ALT, AST)
Chest radiograph
Neck, chest, abdominal, pelvic CT
Positive emission tomography scan
Bilateral bone marrow aspirate and biopsy
Cerebrospinal fluid cytology, cell count, protein

ALT, alanine aminotransferase; AST, aspartate aminotransferase.

DIFFERENTIAL DIAGNOSIS. Head and neck lymphadenopathy should be differentiated from infectious nodal etiologies; mediastinal masses from HD and germ cell tumors; abdominal involvement from other abdominal malignant masses such as Wilms tumor, neuroblastoma, and rhabdomyosarcoma; and bone marrow involvement from precursor B (Pre-B) acute lymphoblastic leukemia and T-cell acute lymphoblastic leukemia. CT and PET scans, along with flow cytometry, cytogenetic and molecular genetics on biopsy and tumor tissue, usually differentiate NHL from other entities.

TREATMENT. The primary modality of treatment for childhood and adolescent NHL is multiagent systemic chemotherapy and intrathecal chemotherapy. Surgery is used mainly for diagnostic and/or biologic specimens and staging but rarely is used for debulking large masses. Radiation therapy is rarely, if ever, used, except in special circumstances such as CNS involvement in LL or occasionally BL, acute SVC, and acute paraplegias. Patients at diagnosis and at risk of TLS, especially advanced/bulky BL or LL, require vigorous hydration and either a xanthine oxidase inhibitor (allopurinol, 10 mg/kg/day PO divided tid) or, more often, recombinant urate oxidase (rasburicase, 0.2 mg/kg/day PO once daily for 1–3 days).

Specific treatment for localized and advanced disease is similar for BL and DLBCL. Localized BL and DLBCL require 6 wk to 6 mo of multiagent chemotherapy. Common regimens include COPAD (cyclophosphamide, vincristine, prednisone and doxorubicin), as demonstrated by the recent international B-NHL study (FAB/LMB 96 [French-American-British Lymphoma, mature B cell]) or COMP (cyclophosphamide, vincristine, methotrexate, 6-mercaptopurine and prednisone). Advanced disease usually is treated by 4–6 mo of multiagent chemotherapy such as FAB/LMB 96 protocol therapy or BFM (Berlin Frankfurt Munich) NHL90 protocol therapy.

Localized and advanced LL usually require almost 24 mo of therapy. The best results in advanced LL have been obtained using the BFM NHL 90 protocol, which uses therapeutic approaches similar to those for childhood acute leukemia, which includes an induction cycle of chemotherapy, consolidation phase, interim maintenance phase, reinduction phase (advanced disease only), and a year of maintenance therapy with 6-mercaptopurine and methotrexate.

Localized ALCL may require only cutaneous excision or more aggressive therapy similar to that for advanced ALCL. Advanced ALCL commonly is treated with a BFM NHL 90 protocol or with a COG protocol of APO (doxorubicin, prednisone and vincristine) with additional VP-16, Ara-C, or vinblastine.

Intrathecal chemotherapy is administered to moderate to advanced disease in all subtypes of childhood and adolescent NHL and may include intrathecal methotrexate, hydrocortisone, or Ara-C.

Patients with NHL who develop progressive or relapsed disease require reinduction chemotherapy and either allogeneic or autologous stem cell transplantation. The specific reinduction regimen or transplant depends on the pathologic subtype, previous therapy, site or reoccurrence, and stem cell donor availability.

SUPPORTIVE CARE

Some patients require G-CSF prophylaxis to prevent fever and neutropenia following myelosuppressive chemotherapy and prophylactic antibiotics to prevent infections. Indwelling central venous catheters routinely are placed to facilitate frequent blood draws, chemotherapy and transfusion administration, and parenteral nutrition to prevent weight loss and nutritional debilitation.

COMPLICATIONS

Patients receiving multiagent chemotherapy for advanced disease are at acute risk for serious mucositis, infections, cytopenias requiring red cell and platelet blood product transfusions, electrolyte imbalance, and poor nutrition. Long-term complications may include growth retardation, cardiac toxicity, gonadal toxicity with infertility, and secondary malignancies.

PROGNOSIS

The prognosis is excellent for most forms of childhood and adolescent NHL. Patients with localized disease have a 90–100% chance of survival, and patients with advanced disease have a 60–95% chance of survival. The variation in survival depends on pathological subtype, tumor burden at diagnosis as reflected in serum LDH level, presence or absence of CNS disease, and specific sites of metastatic spread. Specific cytogenetic and molecular genetic subtyping also may be important in predicting outcome and influencing specific therapeutic strategies.

Cairo MS, Bishop M: Tumour lysis syndrome: new therapeutic strategies and classification. *Br J Haematol* 2004;127:3–11.

Cairo MS, Sposto R, Hoover-Regan M, et al: Childhood and adolescent large-cell lymphoma (LCL): A review of the Children's Cancer Group experience. *Am J Hematol* 2003;72:53–63.

Cairo MS, Sposto R, Perkins SL, et al: Burkitt's and Burkitt-like lymphoma in children and adolescents: A review of the Children's Cancer Group experience. *Br J Haematol* 2003;120:660–670.

Dave SS, Wright G, Tan B, et al: Prediction of survival in follicular lymphoma based on molecular features of tumor-infiltrating immune cells. *N Engl J Med* 2004;351:2159–2169.

Hummel M, Bentink S, Berger H, et al: A biologic definition of Burkitt's lymphoma from transcriptional and genomic profiling. *N Engl J Med* 2006;354:2419–2430.

Patte C, Auperin A, Michon J, et al: The Societe Francaise d'Oncologie Pediatrique LMB89 protocol: highly effective multiagent chemotherapy tailored to the tumor burden and initial response in 561 unselected children with B-cell lymphomas and L3 leukemia. *Blood* 2001;97:3370–3379.

Peniket AJ, Ruiz de Elvira MC, Taghipour G, et al: An EBMT registry matched study of allogeneic stem cell transplants for lymphoma: allogeneic transplantation is associated with a lower relapse rate but a higher procedure-related mortality rate than autologous transplantation. *Bone Marrow Transplant* 2003;31:667–678.

Reiter A, Schrappe M, Tiemann M, et al: Improved treatment results in childhood B-cell neoplasms with tailored intensification of therapy: A report of the Berlin-Frankfurt-Munster Group Trial NHL-BFM 90. *Blood* 1999;94:3294–3306.

Chapter 497 ■ Brain Tumors in Childhood

John F. Kuttesch, Jr. and Joann L. Ater

Primary central nervous system (CNS) tumors are a heterogeneous group of diseases that are, collectively, the second most

TABLE 497-1. Familial Syndromes Associated with Pediatric Brain Tumors

SYNDROME	CNS MANIFESTATIONS	CHROMOSOME	GENE
Neurofibromatosis type 1 (autosomal dominant)	Optic pathway gliomas, astrocytoma, malignant peripheral nerve sheath tumors, neurofibromas	17q11	*NF1*
Neurofibromatosis type 2 (autosomal dominant)	Vestibular schwannomas, meningiomas, spinal cord ependymoma, spinal cord astrocytoma, hamartomas	22q12	*NF2*
von Hippel-Lindau (autosomal dominant)	Hemangioblastoma	3p25-26	*VHL*
Tuberous sclerosis (autosomal dominant)	Subependymal giant cell astrocytoma, cortical tubers	9q34	*TSC1*
		16q13	*TSC2*
Li-Fraumeni (autosomal dominant)	Astrocytoma, primitive neuroectodermal tumor	17q13	*TP53*
Cowden (autosomal dominant)	Dysplastic gangliocytoma of the cerebellum (Lhermitte-Duclos disease)	10q23	*PTEN*
Turcot (autosomal dominant)	Medulloblastoma	5q21	*APC*
	Glioblastoma	3p21	*hMLH1*
		7p22	*hPSM2*
Nevoid basal cell carcinoma (autosomal dominant)	Medulloblastoma	9q31	*PTCH*

Modified from Kleihues P, Cavenee WK: *World Health Organization Classification of Tumors: Pathology and Genetics of Tumors of the Nervous System.* Lyon, IARC Press, 2000.

frequent malignancy in childhood and adolescence. The overall mortality among this group approaches 45%. These patients have the highest morbidity, primarily neurologic, of all childhood malignancies. Outcomes have improved over time with innovations in neurosurgery and radiation therapy as well as introduction of chemotherapy as a therapeutic modality. The treatment approach for these tumors is multimodal. Surgery with complete resection, if feasible, is the foundation, with radiation therapy and chemotherapy used based on the diagnosis, patient age, and other factors.

ETIOLOGY. The etiology of pediatric brain tumors is not well defined. A male predominance is noted in the incidence of medulloblastoma and ependymoma. Familial and hereditary syndromes associated with increased incidence of brain tumors account for approximately 5% of cases (Table 497-1). Cranial exposure to ionizing radiation also is associated with an increased incidence of brain tumors. There are sporadic reports of brain tumors within families without evidence of a heritable syndrome. The molecular events associated with tumorigenesis of pediatric brain tumors are not known.

EPIDEMIOLOGY. Approximately 2,200 primary brain tumors are diagnosed each year in children and adolescents, with an overall annual incidence of 28 cases per million children <19 yr of age. The incidence of CNS tumors is higher in infants and young children ≤7 yr of age (≈36 cases/million children) compared with older children and adolescents (≈21 cases/million children) [Fig. 497-1].

PATHOGENESIS. Among the >100 histologic categories and subtypes of primary brain tumors described in the World Health Organization (WHO) classification of tumors of the CNS and meninges, 5 categories constitute 80% of all pediatric brain tumors: juvenile pilocytic astrocytoma; medulloblastoma/primitive neuroectodermal tumor (PNET); diffuse astrocytomas: ependymoma; and craniopharyngioma (Table 497-2).

The Childhood Brain Tumor Consortium reported a slight predominance of infratentorial tumor location (43.2%), followed by the supratentorial location (40.9%), spinal cord (4.9%), and multiple sites (11%). There are age-related differences in primary location of tumor (Fig. 497-2). Within the first year of life, supratentorial tumors predominate and include, most commonly, choroid plexus complex tumors and teratomas. From 1–10 yr of age, infratentorial tumors predominate, owing to the high incidence of juvenile pilocytic astrocytoma and medulloblastoma. After 10 yr of age, supratentorial tumors again predominate, with diffuse astrocytomas most common. Tumors of the optic pathway and hypothalamus region, the brainstem, and pineal-midbrain region are more common in children and adolescents than in adults.

CLINICAL MANIFESTATIONS. The clinical presentation of patients with brain tumors depends on the tumor location, the tumor type, and the age of the child. Signs and symptoms are related to obstruction of cerebrospinal fluid (CSF) drainage paths by the tumor, leading to **increased intracranial pressure (ICP)** or causing focal brain dysfunction. Subtle changes in personality, mentation, and speech may precede these classic signs and symptoms; these often occur with supratentorial (cortical) lesions. In young children, the diagnosis of a brain tumor may be delayed because their symptoms are similar to those of more common illnesses such as gastrointestinal disorders. Infants with open cranial sutures may present with signs of increased ICP such as vomiting, lethargy, and irritability, as well as the later finding of macrocephaly. The **classic triad** of headache, nausea and vomiting, and papilledema is associated with midline or infratentorial tumors. Disorders of

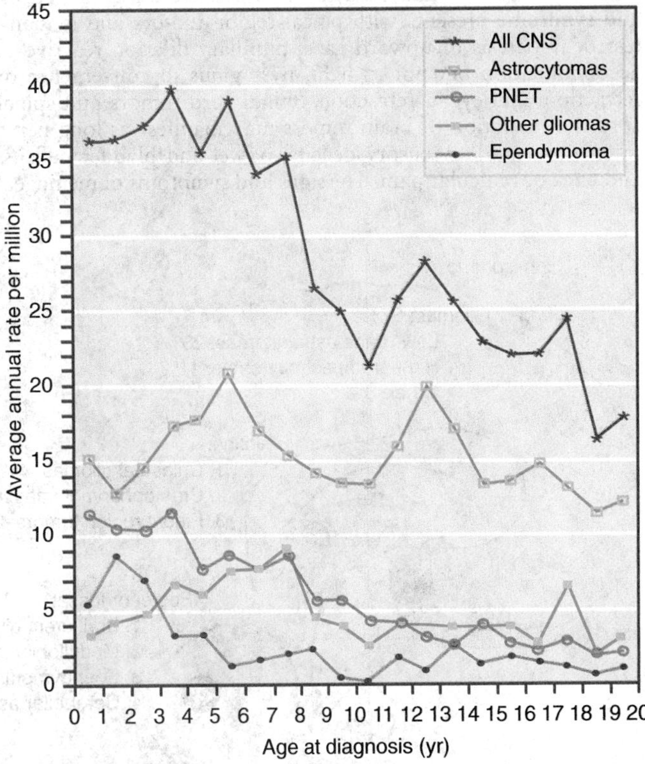

Figure 497-1. Age-specific incidence rates of malignant brain tumors of childhood from SEER 1986–1994. CNS, central nervous system; PNET, primitive neuroectodermal tumor. (Redrawn from Gurney JC, Smith MA, Bunin GR: *National Cancer Institute SEER Program.* NIH publication No. 99–4649. Bethesda, MD, National Cancer Institute, 1999, pp 51–63.)

TABLE 497-2. Distribution of Childhood Brain Tumors Based on Histology

HISTOLOGY	DISTRIBUTION (% OF TOTAL)
Medulloblastoma/primitive neuroectodermal tumor	20
Juvenile pilocytic astrocytoma	20
Low-grade astrocytoma	15
High-grade astrocytoma	7
Ependymoma	7
Craniopharyngioma	7
Unclassified primary tumors	7
Choroid plexus tumors, germ cell tumors, oligodendroglioma, meningioma, mixed tumors, pineal parenchymal tumors	1–2 (each histologic group)

Adapted from Fuller GN: Central nervous system tumors. In Parham DM (editor): *Pediatric Neoplasia: Morphology and Biology.* Philadelphia, Lippincott-Raven, 1996, pp 153–204.

equilibrium, gait, and coordination occur with infratentorial tumors. **Torticollis** may result in cerebellar tonsil herniation. Blurred vision, diplopia, and nystagmus also are associated with infratentorial tumors. Tumors of the brainstem region may be associated with gaze palsy, multiple cranial nerve palsies, and upper motor neuron deficits (e.g., hemiparesis, hyperreflexia, clonus). **Supratentorial tumors** more commonly are associated with focal disorders such as motor weaknesses, sensory changes, speech disorders, seizures, and reflex abnormalities. Infants with supratentorial tumors may present with hand preference. Optic pathway tumors present with visual disturbances such as decreased visual acuity, Marcus Gunn pupil (afferent papillary defect), nystagmus, and/or visual field defects. Suprasellar region tumors and third ventricular region tumors may present initially with **neuroendocrine deficits** such as diabetes insipidus, galactorrhea, precocious puberty, delayed puberty, and hypothyroidism. The **diencephalic syndrome** presents with failure to thrive, emaciation, increased appetite, and euphoric affect, and occurs in infants and young children with tumors in these regions. **Parinaud syndrome** presents with pineal region tumors and is manifested by paresis of upward gaze, pupillary dilation reactive to accommodation but not to light, nystagmus to convergence or retraction, and eyelid retraction. Spinal cord tumors and spinal cord dissemination of brain tumors may manifest as long nerve tract motor and/or sensory deficits, bowel and bladder deficits, and back or radicular pain. The signs and symptoms of meningeal metastatic disease from brain tumors or leukemia are similar to those of infratentorial tumors.

DIAGNOSIS. The evaluation of a patient suspected of having a brain tumor is an emergency. Initial evaluation should include a complete history, physical (including ophthalmic) examination, and neurologic assessment with neuroimaging. For primary brain tumors, **MRI** is the neuroimaging standard. Tumors in the pituitary/suprasellar region, optic path, and infratentorium are better delineated with MRI than with CT. Patients with tumors of the midline and the pituitary/suprasellar/optic chiasmal region should undergo evaluation for **neuroendocrine dysfunction.** Formal ophthalmologic examination is beneficial in patients with optic path region tumors to document the impact of the disease on oculomotor function, visual acuity, and fields of vision. The suprasellar region and pineal region are preferential sites for germ cell tumors. Both serum and CSF measurements of **β-human chorionic gonadotropin** and **α-fetoprotein** can assist in the diagnosis of germ cell tumors. In tumors with a propensity for spreading to the leptomeninges, such as medulloblastoma/PNET, ependymoma, and germ cell tumors, lumbar puncture and cytologic analysis of the CSF is indicated; lumbar puncture is contraindicated in individuals with newly diagnosed hydrocephalus secondary to CSF flow obstruction or in individuals with infratentorial tumors. Lumbar puncture in these individuals may lead to brain herniation, resulting in neurologic compromise and death. Therefore, in children with newly diagnosed intracranial tumors and signs of increased ICP, the lumbar puncture usually is delayed until surgery or shunt placement.

SPECIFIC TUMORS

ASTROCYTOMAS. Astrocytomas are a heterogeneous group of pediatric CNS tumors that account for approximately 40% of cases. These tumors occur throughout the CNS.

Low-grade astrocytomas (LGAs) are the predominant group of astrocytomas in childhood and are characterized by an indolent clinical course. **Juvenile pilocytic astrocytoma (JPA)** is the most common astrocytoma in children, accounting for 20% of all brain tumors (Fig. 497-3). Based on clinicopathologic features using the WHO Classification System, JPA is classified as a WHO grade I tumor. Although JPA can occur anywhere in the CNS, the

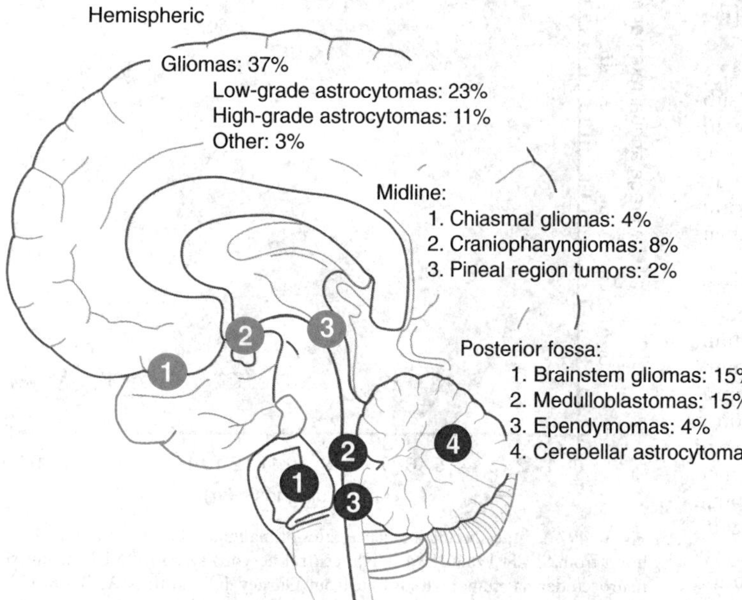

Figure 497-2. Childhood brain tumors occur at any location within the central nervous system. The relative frequency of brain tumor histologic types and the anatomic distribution are shown. (Redrawn from Albright AL: Pediatric brain tumors. *CA Cancer J Clin* 1993;43:272–288.)

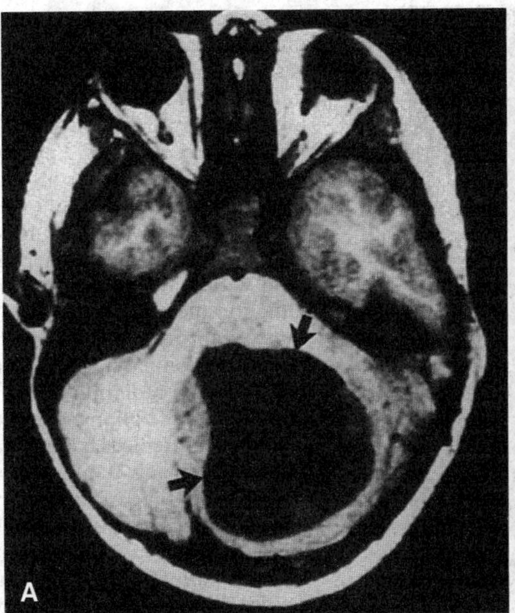

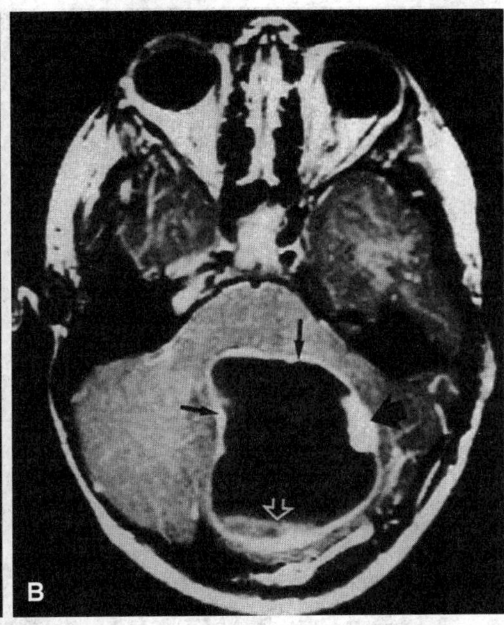

Figure 497-3. *A*, Axial T1-weighted MRI of a patient with cerebellar pilocytic astrocytoma, demonstrating predominantly cystic (hypointense) component *(arrows)* involving the left cerebellar hemisphere and vermis. *B*, Gadolinium-enhanced axial T1-weighted MRI in the same child demonstrates enhancement of the solid component *(large arrow)*, enhancement of the capsule *(small arrows)*, and layering of contrast material *(open arrow)* at the bottom of the cyst. (From Kuhn JP, Slovis TL, Haller JO: *Caffey's Pediatric Diagnostic Imaging,* 10th ed. Philadelphia, Mosby, 2004, p 576.)

classic site of presentation is the **cerebellum.** Other common sites include the hypothalamic/third ventricular region and the optic nerve and chiasmal region. The classic but not exclusive neuroradiologic findings of JPA are the presence of a contrast medium-enhancing nodule within the wall of a cystic mass (see Fig. 497-3). The microscopy findings exhibit a biphasic appearance of bundles of compact fibrillary tissue interspersed with loose microcystic, spongy areas. The presence of **Rosenthal fibers,** which are condensed masses of glial filaments occurring in the compact areas, helps establish the diagnosis. JPA has a low metastatic potential and rarely is invasive. A small proportion of these tumors can progress and develop leptomeningeal spread, particularly tumors occurring in the optic path region. JPA very rarely undergoes malignant transformation to a more aggressive tumor. JPA of the optic nerve and chiasmal region is a relatively common finding in patients with neurofibromatosis type 1 (15% incidence). Unlike diffuse fibrillary astrocytomas, there are no characteristic cytogenetic abnormalities in JPA nor are there any known molecular abnormalities. Other tumors occurring in the pediatric age group with clinicopathologic characteristics similar to those of JPA include pleomorphic xanthoastrocytoma, desmoplastic cerebral astrocytoma of infancy, and subependymal giant cell astrocytoma.

The second most common astrocytoma is **fibrillary infiltrating astrocytoma,** a group of tumors characterized by a pattern of diffuse infiltration of tumor cells among normal neural tissue and potential for anaplastic progression. Based on their clinicopathologic characteristics, they are grouped as low-grade astrocytomas (WHO grade II), malignant astrocytomas (anaplastic astrocytoma, WHO grade III), and glioblastoma multiforme (GBM, WHO grade IV). Of this group, the fibrillary LGA is the second most common astrocytoma in children, accounting for 15% of brain tumors. Histologically, these low-grade tumors demonstrate increased cellularity compared with normal brain parenchyma, with few mitotic figures, nuclear pleomorphism, and microcysts. The characteristic MRI finding is the lack of enhancement after contrast agent infusion. Molecular genetic abnormalities found among low-grade diffuse infiltrating astrocytomas include mutations of P53 and overexpression of platelet-derived growth factor α-chain and platelet-derived growth factor receptor-α. These tumors have the potential to evolve into malignant astrocytomas, a development that is associated with cumulative acquisition of multiple molecular abnormalities.

The **clinical management** of LGAs focuses on a multimodal approach incorporating surgery as the primary treatment as well as radiation therapy and chemotherapy. The outcome of JPA is better than with fibrillary LGAs. With complete surgical resection the overall survival approaches 80–100%. In patients with partial resection (<80% resection), overall survival varies from 50–95%, depending on the anatomic location of the tumor. In patients with partial resection and stable neurologic status, the current approach is to follow the patient closely by examination and imaging. With evidence of progression, surgical re-resection should be considered. In patients in whom second surgery was less than complete or is not feasible, radiation therapy is beneficial. Radiation therapy is delivered to the tumor bed at a total cumulative dose ranging from 50–55 Gy given on a daily schedule over 6 wk. Historically, patients with deep midline tumors were treated empirically without surgery or biopsy using radiation therapy, with variable survival rates from 33–75%. However, modern surgical techniques and innovative radiation therapy methodology may have a positive impact on the survival and clinical outcome of these patients. The role of chemotherapy in the management of LGAs is evolving. Because of concerns regarding morbidity from radiation therapy in young children, several chemotherapy approaches have been evaluated, especially in children <5 yr of age. Complete response to chemotherapy is low; however, these approaches have yielded prolonged disease control in 70–100% of patients. Patients with midline tumors in the hypothalamic/optic chiasmatic region have tended to do less well. Taken together, the chemotherapy approaches have permitted delay and, potentially, avoidance of radiation therapy. In a national trial currently underway, investigators are comparing the effectiveness and tolerance of a carboplatin-based chemotherapy schedule with a lomustine (CCNU)-based schedule in children <10 yr of age with a progressive LGA. Clinical trials investigating either temozolomide or vinblastine also are underway. Observation is the primary approach in clinical management of selective patients with LGAs that are biologically indolent. One group includes patients with neurofibromatosis type 1, who may develop an LGA of the optic chiasm/optic pathway or brainstem that is found incidentally. Another group includes patients with midbrain astrocytomas who have resolution of clinical symptoms after ventricular shunting and do not require further intervention.

Malignant astrocytomas are much less common in children and adolescents than in adults, accounting for 7–10% of all child-

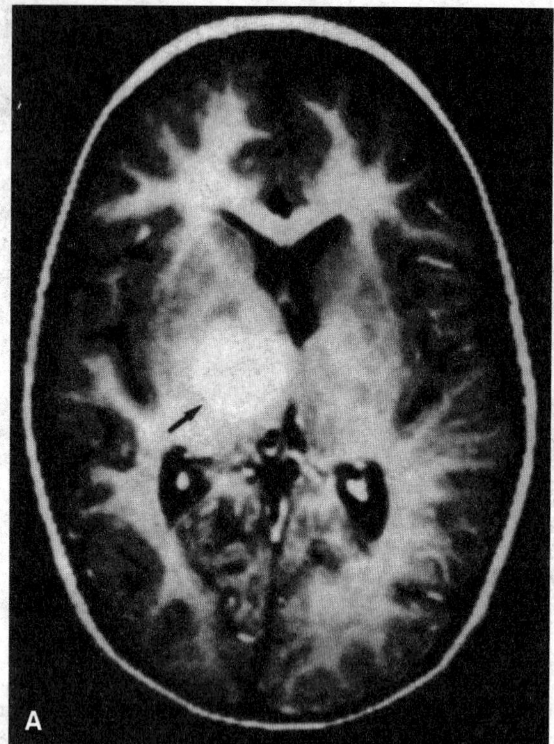

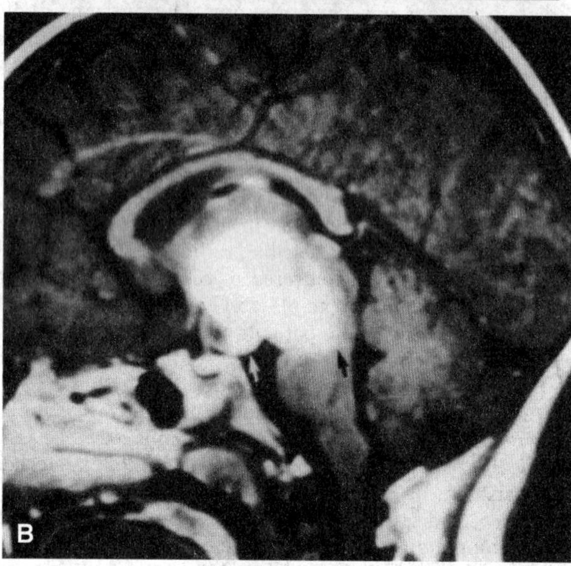

Figure 497-4. *A,* Gadolinium-enhanced axial T1-weighted MRI of grade III astrocytoma of the right thalamus demonstrating diffuse enhancement *(arrow). B,* Gadolinium-enhanced sagittal T1-weighted MRI showing enhancement of grade III astrocytoma of the thalamus with extension into the midbrain *(black arrow)* and hypothalamus *(white arrow).* (From Kuhn JP, Slovis TL, Haller JO: *Caffey's Pediatric Diagnostic Imaging,* 10th ed. Philadelphia, Mosby, 2004, p. 595.)

hood tumors. Among this group, **anaplastic astrocytoma** (WHO grade III) [Fig. 497-4] is more common than **glioblastoma multiforme** (WHO grade IV). The histopathology of anaplastic astrocytomas demonstrates increased cellularity compared with low-grade diffuse astrocytomas, cellular and nuclear atypia, presence of mitoses, and, variably, microvascular proliferation. Characteristic histopathology findings in glioblastoma multiforme include dense cellularity, high mitotic index, microvascular proliferation, and foci of tumor necrosis. Limited information is available regarding the molecular abnormalities in malignant astrocytomas of children. Overexpression of P53 in malignant astrocytomas of children is an adverse prognostic factor. The frequency of mutations in P53 in childhood malignant astrocytomas is similar to that noted in adults, although the frequency of such mutations in malignant astrocytomas of children <3 yr of age is lower. This suggests differing mechanisms of oncogenesis between younger and older children. Optimal therapeutic approaches for malignant astrocytomas have yet to be defined. Standard therapy continues to be surgical resection followed by involved-field radiation therapy, usually followed by a nitrosourea-containing chemotherapy regimen. A pediatric trial showed improved survival with lomustine and vincristine after radiation compared to radiation alone. A study of adult glioblastoma showed significantly improved survival with temozolomide during and after radiation, compared to radiation alone. This combined temozolomide and radiation currently is under investigation for pediatric high-grade gliomas.

Oligodendrogliomas are uncommon tumors of childhood. These infiltrating tumors occur predominantly in the cerebral cortex and originate in the white matter. Histologically, oligodendrogliomas consist of rounded cells with little cytoplasm and microcalcifications. Observation of a **calcified cortical mass** on CT in a patient presenting with a seizure is suggestive of oligodendroglioma. Treatment approaches are similar to those for infiltrating astrocytomas.

MIXED GLIOMAS. Mixed gliomas are composed of two or more distinct glial cell types—astrocytoma, oligodendroglioma, and ependymoma—and are rare in pediatric patients.

EPENDYMAL TUMORS. Ependymal tumors are derived from the ependymal lining of the ventricular system. Ependymoma (WHO grade II) is the most common of these neoplasms, occurring predominantly in childhood and accounting for 10% of childhood tumors. Approximately 70% of ependymomas in childhood occur in the posterior fossa. The mean age of patients is 6 yr, with approximately 30% of cases occurring in children <3 yr of age. The incidence of leptomeningeal spread approaches 10% overall. Clinical presentation depends on the anatomic location of the tumor. MRI demonstrates a well-circumscribed tumor with variable and complex patterns of gadolinium enhancement, with or without cystic structures (Fig. 497-5). These tumors usually are noninvasive, extending into the ventricular lumen and/or displacing normal structures. Histologic characteristics include perivascular pseudorosettes, ependymal rosettes, monomorphic nuclear morphology, and occasional nonpalisading foci of necrosis. Surgery is the primary treatment modality, with extent of surgical resection a major prognostic factor. Two other major prognostic factors are age, with younger children having poorer outcomes, and tumor location, with localization in the posterior fossa, which often is seen in young children, associated with poorer outcomes. Surgery alone rarely is curative. Multimodal therapy incorporating radiation with surgery has resulted in long-term survival in approximately 40% of patients after gross total resection. Recurrence is predominantly local. Radiation therapy of the involved field is recommended for most children with ependymoma and anaplastic ependymoma. Ependymoma is sensitive to a spectrum of chemotherapeutic agents; however, the role of chemotherapy in multimodal therapy of ependymoma is still unclear. Several limited trials have shown no benefit of high-dose chemotherapy with peripheral blood stem cell rescue in ependymoma. Current investigations are directed toward identification of optimal radiation dose, surgical questions addressing the use of second-look procedures after chemotherapy, and further evaluation of classic as well as novel chemotherapeutic agents. There are no characteristic cytogenetic or molecular genetic alterations in ependymoma. However, preliminary studies suggest that there are genetically distinct subtypes, exemplified by an association between alterations in the NF2 gene and spinal ependymoma.

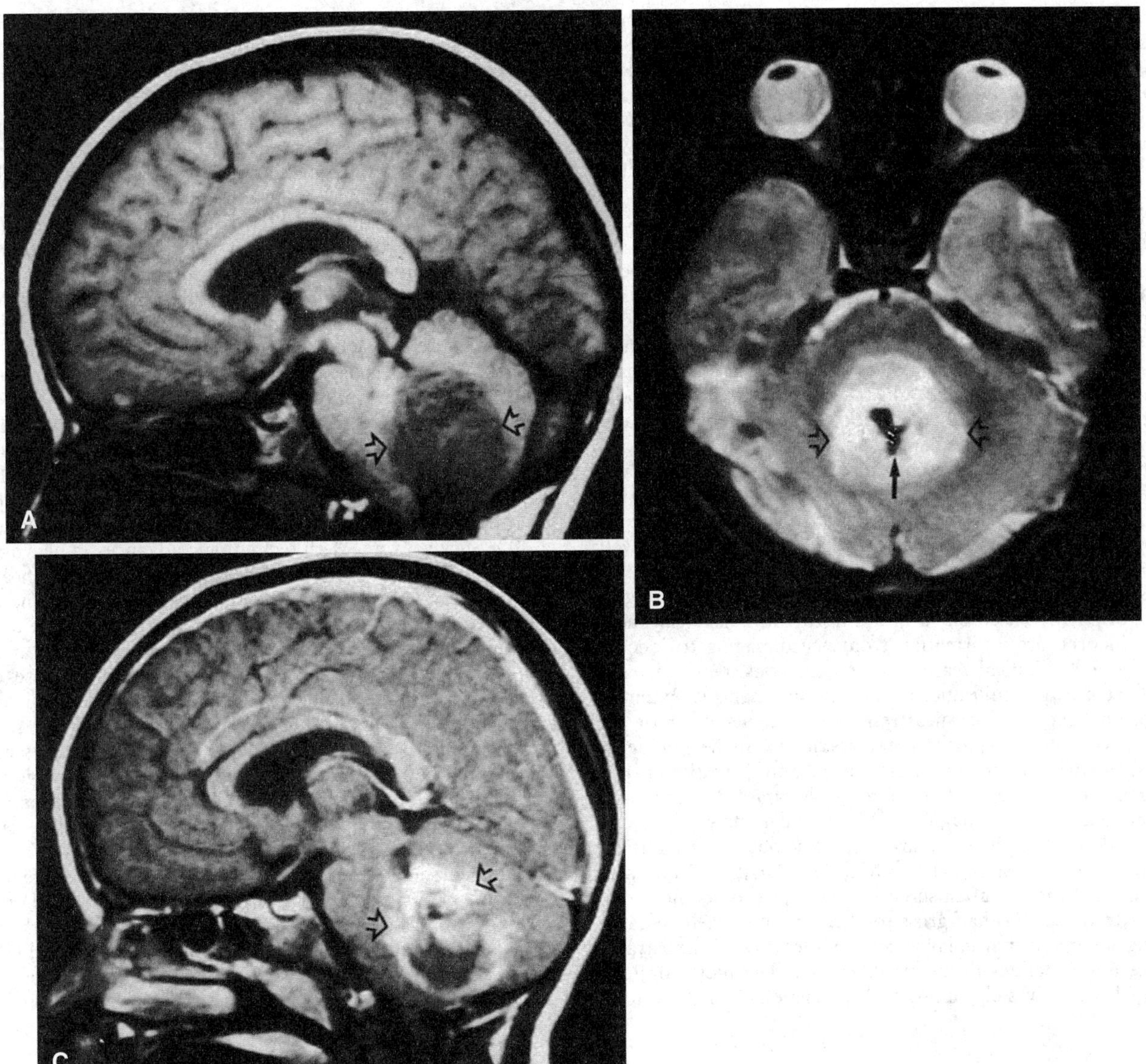

Figure 497-5. *A*, Sagittal T1-weighted MRI of a patient with ependymoma, demonstrating a hypointense mass *(arrows)* within the fourth ventricle. *B*, Axial T2-weighted image of an ependymoma showing a hyperintense mass *(open arrows)* and a hypointense central area of calcification *(closed arrow)* within the fourth ventricle. *C*, Gadolinium-enhanced sagittal T1-weighted image demonstrating an ependymoma *(arrows)*. (From Kuhn JP, Slovis TL, Haller JO: *Caffey's Pediatric Diagnostic Imaging,* 10th ed. Philadelphia, Mosby, 2004, p 579.)

Anaplastic ependymoma (WHO grade III) is much less common in childhood, and these tumors are characterized by a high mitotic index and histologic features of microvascular proliferation and pseudopalisading necrosis. Myxopapillary ependymoma (WHO grade I) is a slow-growing tumor arising from the filum terminale and conus medullaris.

CHOROID PLEXUS TUMORS. Choroid plexus tumors account for 2–4% of childhood CNS tumors. They are the most common CNS tumor in children <1 yr of age and account for 10–20% of CNS tumors occurring in infancy. These tumors are intraventricular epithelial neoplasms arising from choroid plexus. Children present with signs and symptoms of increased ICP. Infants may present with macrocephaly and focal neurologic deficits. In children, these tumors occur predominantly supratentorially in the lateral ventricles. **Choroid plexus papilloma** (WHO grade I), the most common of this group, is a well-circumscribed lesion by neuroimaging and closely resembles normal choroid plexus histologically. **Choroid plexus carcinoma** (WHO grade III) is a malignant tumor with metastatic potential to seed into the CSF pathways. This malignancy has histologic characteristics of nuclear pleomorphism, high mitotic index, and increased cell density. Immunopositivity for transthyretin (prealbumin) is useful in confirming the diagnosis of these tumors. These tumors are associated with the **Li-Fraumeni syndrome. Simian virus 40 (SV40)** may play an etiologic role in choroid plexus tumors. After complete surgical resection, outcome for choroid plexus papilloma approaches 100%, whereas outcome for choroid plexus carcinoma approaches 20–40%. Reports suggest that radiation therapy and/or chemotherapy may lead to better disease control for choroid plexus carcinoma.

EMBRYONAL TUMORS. Embryonal tumors or **primitive neuroectodermal tumors (PNET)** are the most common group of malignant CNS tumors of childhood, accounting for 20–25% of pediatric CNS tumors. These tumors have the potential to metastasize to the neuraxis. This group includes medulloblastoma, supratentorial PNET, ependymoblastoma, medulloepithelioblastoma, and atypical teratoid/rhabdoid tumor (ATRT), all of which are histologically classified as WHO grade IV tumors.

Medulloblastoma, accounting for 90% of embryonal tumors, is a cerebellar tumor occurring predominantly in males and at a median age of 5–7 yr. Most of these tumors occur in the midline cerebellar vermis; however, older patients may present with tumors in the cerebellar hemisphere. CT and MRI demonstrate a solid, homogeneous, contrast medium-enhancing mass in the posterior fossa causing 4th ventricular obstruction and hydrocephalus. Up to 30% of patients present with neuroimaging evidence of leptomeningeal spread. Among a variety of diverse histologic patterns of this tumor, the most common is a monomorphic sheet of undifferentiated cells classically noted as small, blue, round cells. Neuronal differentiation is more common among these tumors and is characterized histologically by the presence of Homer Wright rosettes and by immunopositivity for synaptophysin. An anaplastic variant may be associated with worse prognosis. Patients present with signs and symptoms of increased ICP (i.e., headache, nausea, vomiting, mental status changes, and hypertension) and cerebellar dysfunction (i.e., ataxia, poor balance, dysmetria). Standard clinical staging evaluation includes MRI of the brain and spine, both preoperatively and postoperatively, as well as lumbar puncture after the increased ICP has resolved (Fig. 497-6). The Chang staging system, originally based on surgical information, has been modified to incorporate information from neuroimaging to identify risk categories. Clinical features that have consistently demonstrated prognostic significance include age at diagnosis, extent of disease, and extent of surgical resection. Patients <4 yr of age have a poor outcome, partly as the result of a higher incidence of disseminated disease on presentation and past therapeutic approaches that have used less intense therapies. Patients with disseminated disease at diagnosis (M>0), including positive CSF cytology alone (M1), have a markedly worse outcome than those patients with no dissemination (M0). Similarly, patients with gross residual disease after surgery have worse outcomes compared with those who had gross total resection of their disease.

Cytogenetic and molecular genetic studies have demonstrated multiple abnormalities in medulloblastoma. The most common abnormality involves chromosome 17p deletions, which occur in 30–40% of all cases. These deletions are not associated with P53 mutations. Two new risk stratification systems for medulloblastoma combining molecular markers with clinical factors have been proposed. One system is based on retrospective analysis of information about histological variants (classic, nodular desmoplastic, anaplastic large cell); TRKC, MYCC, ERBB2, and MYCC expression; and clinical characteristics in children with medulloblastoma. One study found that the combination of clinical characteristics and ERBB2 expression provided a highly accurate means of discriminating disease risk. Another study found that gene expression profiling predicted medulloblastoma outcome independent of clinical variables. Both approaches still must be validated in larger prospective studies. With the evolution of gene array technology, preliminary studies have identified clusters of genes/gene expression that appear to be associated with metastatic medulloblastoma and outcome.

A multimodal treatment approach is pursued in medulloblastoma, with surgery the starting point of treatment. Medulloblastoma is sensitive to both chemotherapy and radiation therapy. Historically, surgery alone was ineffective. In the 1940s radiation therapy was found to be effective, improving overall outcome to a 30% survival rate. With technologic advances in neurosurgery, neuroradiology, and radiation therapy, as well as identification of chemotherapy as an effective modality, overall outcome among all patients approaches 60–70%. Standard radiation treatment in medulloblastoma incorporates craniospinal radiation at a total cumulative dose of 30–36 Gy, with a cumulative dose of 50–55 Gy to the tumor bed. Craniospinal radiation at this dose in children <3 yr of age results in severe late neurologic sequelae, including microcephaly, learning disabilities, mental retardation, neuroendocrine dysfunction (growth failure, hypothyroidism, hypogonadism, and absent/delayed puberty), and/or second malignancies. Similarly, in older children, late sequelae, such as learning disabilities, neuroendocrine dysfunction, and/or second malignancies, can occur. These observations have resulted in stratification of treatment approaches into three strata: (1) patients <3 yr of age; (2) standard risk patients >3 yr of age with surgical total resection and no disease dissemination (M0); and (3) high-risk patients >3 yr of age with disease dissemination (M>0) and/or bulky residual disease after surgery. With the risk-based

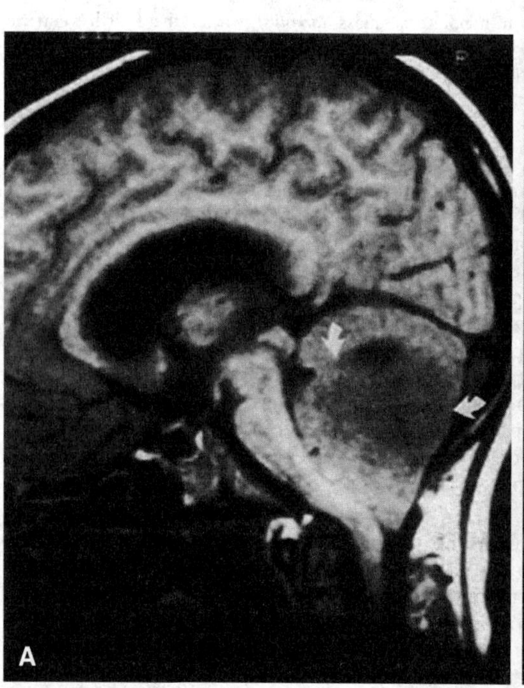

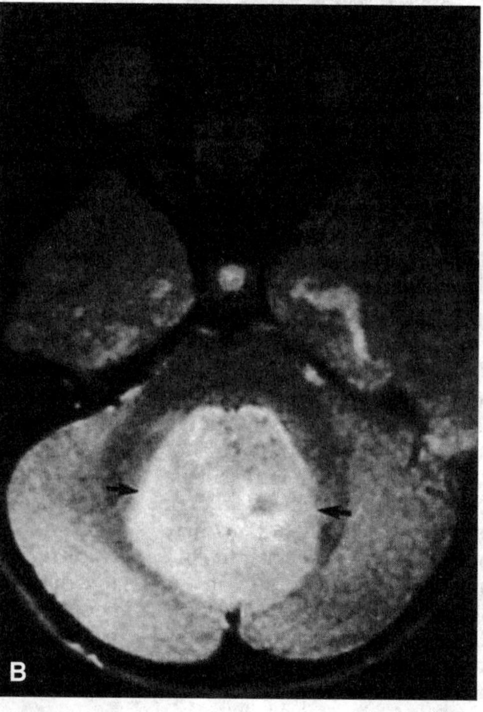

Figure 497-6. MRI scan of medulloblastoma. *A,* Sagittal T1-weighted image shows hypointense mass involving the vermis *(arrows)*. *B,* Axial T2-weighted image shows hyperintense mass *(arrows)* with areas of hypointensity representing acute hemorrhagic infarction within the medulloblastoma involving the vermis. (From Kuhn JP, Slovis TL, Haller JO: *Caffey's Pediatric Diagnostic Imaging,* 10th ed. Philadelphia, Mosby, 2004, p 574.)

approach to treatment, children with high-risk medulloblastoma receive full-dose cranial-spinal radiation with chemotherapy during and after radiation therapy.

In children with nonmetastatic medulloblastoma and gross total tumor resection, chemotherapy alone (methotrexate, cyclophosphamide, vincristine, carboplatin, etoposide) results in an overall survival of 90%. The presence of residual tumor (56% survival) or metastases (38%) confers a poor prognosis.

Supratentorial primitive neuroectodermal tumors (SPNET) account for 2–3% of childhood brain tumors, primarily in children within the first decade of life. These tumors are similar histologically to medulloblastoma and are composed of undifferentiated or poorly differentiated neuroepithelial cells. Historically, patients with SPNET have had poorer outcomes than those with medulloblastoma after combined modality therapy. In current clinical trials, children with these tumors are considered among the high-risk group and receive dose-intense chemotherapy with craniospinal radiation therapy.

Atypical teratoid/rhabdoid tumor (ATRT) is a very aggressive embryonal malignancy that occurs predominantly in children <5 yr of age and can occur at any location in the neuraxis. The histology demonstrates a heterogeneous pattern of cells, including rhabdoid cells that express epithelial membrane antigen and neurofilament antigen. The characteristic cytogenetic pattern is partial or complete deletion of chromosome 22q that has been associated with mutation in the INI1 gene. The relation between this mutation and tumorigenesis is unclear. Outcome after combined modality therapy with intensive chemotherapy is very poor, but long-term survival has been reported in some children.

Ependymoblastoma and **medullomyoblastoma** are rare, highly malignant embryonal tumors of early childhood and infancy.

PINEAL PARENCHYMAL TUMORS. The pineal parenchymal tumors are the second most common malignancies, after germ cell tumors, that occur in the pineal region. These include pineoblastoma, occurring predominantly in childhood, pineocytoma, and the mixed pineal parenchymal tumors. The therapeutic approach in this group of diseases is multimodal. In the past, there was significant concern regarding the location of these masses and the potential complications of surgical intervention. With recent developments in neurosurgical technique and surgical technology, the morbidity and mortality associated with these approaches have markedly decreased. Stereotactic biopsy of these tumors may be adequate to establish diagnosis; however, consideration should be pursued for total resection of the lesion before institution of additional therapy. Pineoblastoma is the more malignant variant and is considered a subgroup of childhood PNET. Chemotherapy regimens incorporate cisplatin, cyclophosphamide (Cytoxan), etoposide (VP-16), and vincristine and/or lomustine. Data have shown that survival outcome of pineal region PNET with combined modality therapy of chemotherapy and radiation approaches 70% at 5 yr, similar to that noted for medulloblastoma. Pineocytoma usually is approached with surgical resection.

NEURONAL/MIXED NEURONAL–GLIAL TUMORS. Neuronal and mixed neuronal–glial tumors are a heterogeneous group of tumors that are slow-growing and of low malignant progression. They are associated with favorable outcome after surgical resection. They are categorized as WHO grade I or WHO grade II tumors. Diseases in this category include ganglioglioma, dysembryoplastic neuroepithelial tumor, desmoplastic infantile astrocytoma, and desmoplastic infantile ganglioglioma.

CRANIOPHARYNGIOMA. Craniopharyngioma (WHO grade I) is a common tumor of childhood, accounting for 7–10% of all childhood tumors. The adamantinomatous variant of craniopharyngioma predominates in childhood. These tumors are solid with cystic components and occur within the suprasellar region. They are minimally invasive, adhere to adjacent brain parenchyma, and engulf normal brain structures. MRI demonstrates the solid tumor with cystic structures containing fluid of intermediate density. CT may show calcifications associated with the solid and cystic wall components. Surgery is the primary treatment modality, with gross total resection curative in small lesions. Controversy exists regarding the relative roles of surgery and radiation therapy in large, complex tumors. There is significant morbidity (panhypopituitarism, growth failure, visual loss) associated with these tumors and their therapy owing to the anatomic location. There is no role for chemotherapy in craniopharyngioma.

MENINGEAL TUMORS. Meningiomas are uncommon tumors of childhood. These tumors arise from the arachnoid layer of the meninges and usually are very slow-growing. Among children, a large proportion of these tumors can be associated with either a genetic disposition such as neurofibromatosis type 2 or basal cell nevus syndrome or prior radiation exposure (secondary malignancy).

GERM CELL TUMORS. Germ cell tumors of the CNS are a heterogeneous group of tumors that are primarily tumors of childhood arising predominantly in midline structures of the pineal and suprasellar regions. They account for 1–2% of pediatric brain tumors. The peak incidence of these tumors is 10–12 yr of age. Overall, there is a male preponderance, although there is a female preponderance for suprasellar tumors. These tumors occur multifocally in 5–10% of cases. This group of tumors is much more prevalent in Asian populations than European populations. As in peripheral germ cell tumors, the analysis of protein markers, **α-fetoprotein**, and **β-human chorionic gonadotropin** may be useful in establishing the diagnosis and monitoring treatment response. Surgical biopsy is recommended to establish the diagnosis; however, nongerminomatous germ cell tumors may be diagnosed based on protein marker elevations. Therapeutic approaches to germinomas and mixed germ cell tumors are different. The survival proportion among patients with pure germinoma exceeds 90%. The postsurgical treatment of pure germinomas is somewhat controversial in defining the relative roles of chemotherapy and radiation therapy. Excellent outcomes are reported in patients who have received local field doses of radiation of >40 Gy and craniospinal radiation therapy. Similarly, groups have reported excellent outcomes when chemotherapy has been incorporated in regimens that utilize reduced doses of radiation therapy (24 Gy to the local field alone). More recently, clinical trials have investigated the use of chemotherapy and reduced-dose radiation after surgery in pure germinomas. The therapeutic approach in nongerminomatous germ cell tumors is more aggressive, combining more intense chemotherapy regimens with craniospinal radiation therapy. Survival rates among these tumors are markedly less than noted in germinoma, ranging from 40–70% at 5 yr. Trials have shown benefit using high doses of chemotherapy with blood stem cell rescue. If confirmed in larger studies, future approaches may test the use of high doses of chemotherapy with dose-reduced radiation therapy.

TUMORS OF THE BRAINSTEM. Tumors of the brainstem are a heterogeneous group of tumors that account for 10–15% of childhood primary CNS tumors. Outcome depends on tumor location, imaging characteristics, and the patient's clinical status. Patients with these tumors may present with motor weakness, cranial nerve deficits, cerebellar deficits, and/or signs of increased ICP. Based on MR evaluation and clinical findings, tumors of the brainstem can be classified into four types: focal (5–10% of patients); dorsally exophytic (5–10%); cervicomedullary (5–10%); and diffuse intrinsic tumors (70–85%) [Figs. 497-7 and 497-8]. Surgical resection is the primary treatment approach for focal and dorsally exophytic tumors and leads to a favorable

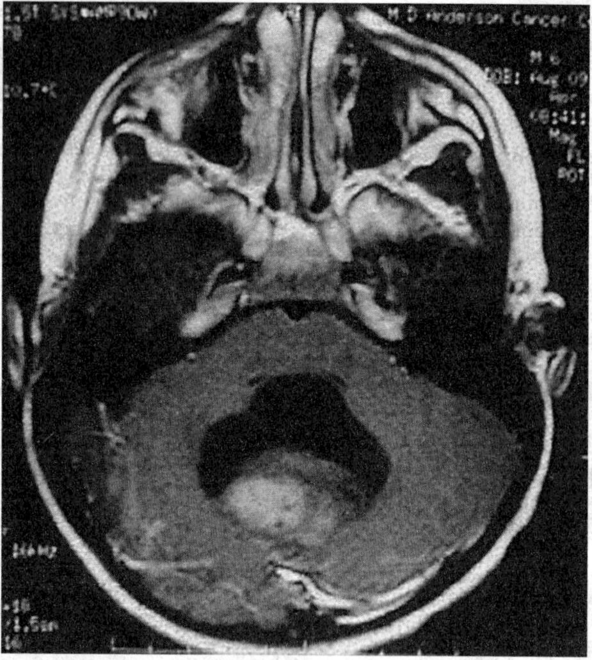

Figure 497-7. T1-weighted sequence post-gadolinium MRI (sagittal image) of a pontine diffuse infiltrating glioma in a 10-yr-old girl presenting with headache, cranial nerve palsies, and left-sided weakness.

outcome. Histologically, these two groups usually are low-grade gliomas. Cervicomedullary tumors, owing to their location, may not be amenable to surgical resection but are sensitive to radiation therapy. Diffuse intrinsic tumors, characterized by the diffuse infiltrating pontine glioma, are associated with very poor outcome independent of histologic diagnosis. These tumors are not amenable to surgical resection. Biopsy in children with MR findings of a diffuse intrinsic tumor is controversial and is not recommended unless there is suspicion of another diagnosis, such as infection, demyelination, vascular malformation, multiple sclerosis, or metastatic tumors. These diagnoses are much more common in adults. The standard approach for treatment in diffuse infiltrating pontine gliomas has been radiation therapy, and median survival with this treatment is 12 mo, at best. Use of chemotherapy, including high-dose chemotherapy with blood stem cell rescue, has not yet been of survival benefit in this group of patients. Current approaches include evaluation of investigational agents alone or in combination with radiation therapy, similar to approaches being pursued in patients with malignant gliomas.

METASTATIC TUMORS. Metastatic spread of other childhood malignancies to the brain is uncommon. Childhood acute lymphoblastic leukemia and non-Hodgkin lymphoma can spread to the leptomeninges, causing symptoms of communicating hydrocephalus. **Chloromas,** which are collections of myeloid leukemia cells, can occur throughout the neuraxis. Rarely, brain parenchymal metastases occur from lymphoma, neuroblastoma, rhabdomyosarcoma, Ewing sarcoma, osteosarcoma, and clear cell sarcoma of the kidney. Therapeutic approaches are based on the specific histologic diagnosis and may incorporate radiation therapy, intrathecal administration of chemotherapy, and/or systemic administration of chemotherapy. Medulloblastoma is the childhood brain tumor that most commonly metastasizes extraneuronally. Less commonly, extraneuronal metastases from malignant glioma, PNET, and ependymoma can occur. Ventriculoperitoneal shunts have been known to allow extraneural metastases, primarily within the peritoneal cavity but also systemically.

COMPLICATIONS AND LONG-TERM MANAGEMENT

Data from the National Cancer Institute SEER Program indicate that >70% of patients with childhood brain tumors will be long-term survivors. At least $^1/_2$ of these survivors will experience chronic problems as a direct result of their tumor and treatment. These problems include chronic neurologic deficits such as focal motor and sensory abnormalities, seizure disorders, neurocognitive deficits (e.g., developmental delays, learning disabilities), and neuroendocrine deficiencies (e.g., hypothyroidism, growth failure, delayed or absent puberty). These patients also are at significant risk of secondary malignancies. Supportive multidisciplinary interventions for children with brain tumors both during

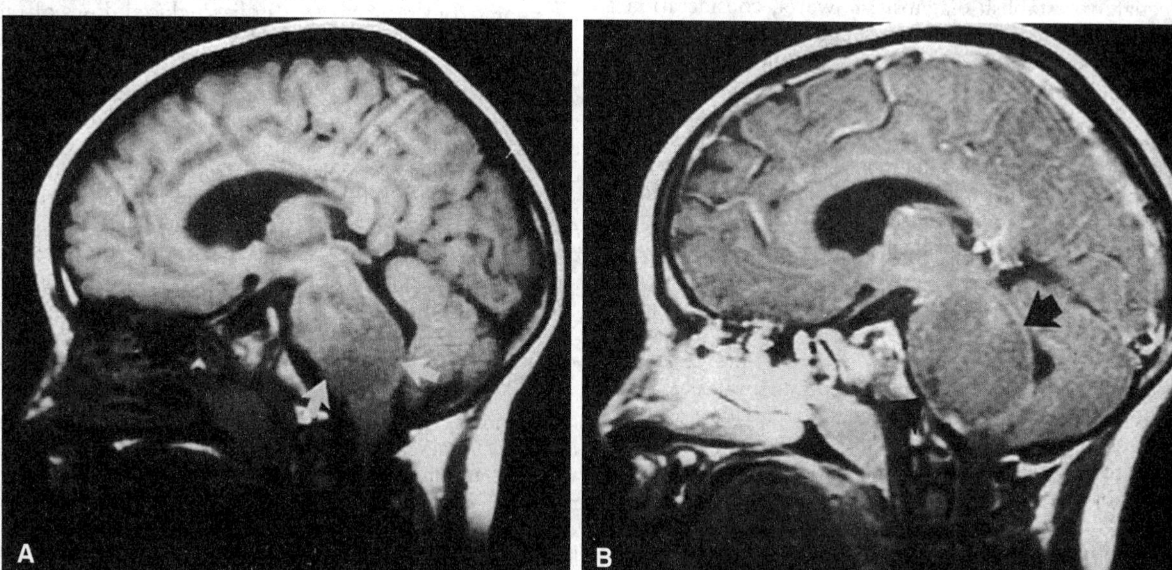

Figure 497-8. *A,* Sagittal T1-weighted MRI demonstrating brainstem astrocytoma with enlargement of the pons by a slightly hypointense mass *(arrows). B,* Gadolinium-enhanced sagittal T1-weighted image demonstrating brainstem astrocytoma, without enhancement, and slightly hypointense mass *(arrows)* enlarging the pons. (From Kuhn JP, Slovis TL, Haller JO: *Caffey's Pediatric Diagnostic Imaging,* 10th ed. Philadelphia, Mosby, 2004, p 577.)

and after therapy may help improve their ultimate outcome. Optimal seizure management, physical therapy, endocrine management with timely growth hormone and thyroid replacement therapy, tailored educational programs, and vocational interventions may enhance the childhood brain tumor survivor's quality of life.

Fernandez-Teijeiro A, Betensky RA, Sturla LM, et al: Combining gene expression profiles and clinical parameters for risk stratification in medulloblastomas. *J Clin Oncol* 2004; 22:994–998.

Freeman CR, Perilongo G: Chemotherapy for brain stem gliomas. *Childs Nerv Syst* 1999;15:545–553.

Gajjar A, Hernan R, Kocak M, et al: Clinical, histopathologic, and molecular markers of prognosis: Toward a new disease risk stratification system for medulloblastoma. *J Clin Oncol* 2004;22:984–993.

Grill J, Sainte-Rose C, Jouvet A, et al: Treatment of medulloblastoma with postoperative chemotherapy alone: An SFOP prospective trial in young children. *Lancet Oncol* 2005;6:573–580.

Gurney JC, Smith MA, Bunin GR: In Reis LAG, Smith MA, Gurney JC, et al (editors): *Cancer Survival and Incidence Among Children and Adolescents: United States SEER Program 1975–1995*. Bethesda, MD, National Cancer Institute SEER Program. NIH publication No. 99–4649, 1999, pp 51–63.

Kleihues P, Cavenee WK: *World Health Organization Classification of Tumours: Pathology and Genetics of Tumours of the Nervous System*. Lyon, IARC Press, 2000.

Mellinghoff IK, Wang MY, Vivanco I, et al: Molecular determinations of the response of glioblastomas to EGFR kinase inhibitors. *N Engl J Med* 2005;353:2012–2024.

Merchant TE, Mulhern RK, Krasin MJ, et al: Preliminary results from a phase II trial of conformal radiation therapy and evaluation of radiation-related CNS effects for pediatric patients with localized ependymoma. *J Clin Oncol* 2004;15:3156–3162.

Packer RJ, Cohen BH, Coney K: Intracranial germ cell tumors. *Oncologist* 2000;5:312–320.

Pollack IF, Finkelstein SD, Woods J, et al: Expression of p53 and prognosis in children with malignant gliomas. *N Engl J Med* 2002;346:420–426.

Rutkowski S, Bode U, Deinlein F, et al: Treatment of early childhood medulloblastoma by postoperative chemotherapy alone. *N Engl J Med* 2005;352:978–986.

Shaw EG, Wisoff JH: Prospective clinical trials of intracranial low-grade glioma in adults and children. *Neurooncol* 2003;5:153–160.

Strother DR, Pollac IF, Fisher PG, et al: Tumors of the central nervous system. In Pizzo PA, Poplack DG (editors): *Principles and Practice of Pediatric Oncology*, 5th ed. Philadelphia, Lippincott Williams & Wilkins, 2006.

Stupp R, Mason WP, van den Bent MJ, et al: Radiotherapy plus concomitant and adjuvant temozolomide for glioblastoma. *N Engl J Med* 2005;352:987–996.

Zebrack BJ, Gurney JG, Oeffinger K, et al: Psychological outcomes in long-term survivors of childhood brain cancer: A report from the Childhood Cancer Survivors Study. *J Clin Oncol* 2004;22:999–1006.

Chapter 498 ■ Neuroblastoma

Joann L. Ater

Neuroblastoma (NB) is an embryonal cancer of the peripheral sympathetic nervous system with heterogeneous clinical presentation and course. The clinical spectrum of NB varies, ranging from spontaneous regression in some types to very aggressive tumors unresponsive to multimodality therapy in others. It is now recognized that more than one type of NB exists.

EPIDEMIOLOGY. NB is the third most common pediatric cancer, accounting for about 8% of childhood malignancies. About 500 new cases are diagnosed each year in the USA. NB is the most commonly diagnosed neoplasm in infants, accounting for 28–39% of neonatal malignancies. The median age at diagnosis is 2 yr, and 90% of cases are diagnosed by 5 yr of age. The incidence is slightly higher in boys and in whites.

PATHOLOGY. NB includes a spectrum of tumors with variable degrees of neural differentiation, ranging from undifferentiated small round cells (neuroblastoma) to tumors containing mature ganglion cells (ganglioneuroblastoma or ganglioneuroma). The tumors may resemble other **small round cell tumors,** such as rhabdomyosarcoma, Ewing sarcoma, and non-Hodgkin lymphoma. The prognosis varies with the histologic definition of tissue pattern (Shimada classification). Prognostic factors include the amount of stroma, degree of tumor cell differentiation, presence of enlarged and prominent nucleoli, and the mitosis-karyorrhexis index.

PATHOGENESIS. The genetic event that initially triggers formation of NB is not known. The pathogenesis is likely to be related to a succession of mutational events, prenatally and perinatally, that may be caused by environmental and genetic factors. Increased incidence of NB is associated with some maternal and paternal occupational chemical exposures, work in farming, and work related to electronics. Familial NB is found in 1–2% of cases. Neuroblastoma and congenital cardiovascular malformations also may be associated.

Genetic characteristics of NB tumor tissue that are of prognostic importance and currently are used along with clinical factors to determine treatment include amplification of the MYCN (N-myc) proto-oncogene and hyperdiploidy of tumor cell DNA content (Table 498-1). Amplification of MYCN has prognostic importance independent of stage and age and is strongly associated with advanced tumor stage and poor outcome. Hyperdiploidy confers better prognosis if the child is <1 yr of age at diagnosis. Genetic abnormalities, including loss of heterozygosity (LOH) of 1p, 11q, and 14q, and gain of 17q, commonly are found in NB tumor tissue. In addition, other biologic factors that correlate with prognosis include the level of nerve growth factor receptor (Trk-A) expression, multidrug-resistance-associated protein, and telomerase activity. These factors are under investigation in clinical trials to determine whether they can be used to further refine risk-based therapy. Thus, therapy can be reduced for children predicted to fare well with minimal therapy and intensified in those predicted to be at high risk of relapse.

CLINICAL MANIFESTATIONS. NB can mimic many other disorders and may be difficult to diagnose. NB may develop at any site of sympathetic nervous system tissue. The signs and symptoms of NB reflect the tumor site and extent of disease. Most cases of NB arise in the abdomen, either in the adrenal gland or in retroperitoneal sympathetic ganglia. Usually a firm, nodular mass that is palpable in the flank or midline is causing abdominal discomfort.

TABLE 498-1. Neuroblastoma Risk Groups

RISK GROUP	INSS STAGE	AGE	MYCN STATUS	SHIMADA HISTOLOGY	SURVIVAL
Low	1	All	Any	Any	90–100%
	2	<1 yr	Any	Any	
	2	>1 yr	Any	Favorable	
	4S	<1 yr	<10 copies	Favorable	
Average	3	>1 yr	<10 copies	Favorable	75–98%
	3 and 4	<1 yr	<10 copies	Any	
	4S	<1 yr	<10 copies	Unfavorable	
High	2	>1 yr	Any	Unfavorable	20–60%
	3	All	>10 copies	Any	
	4	<1 yr	>10 copies	Any	
	4	>1 yr	Any	Any	

INSS, International Neuroblastoma Staging System.

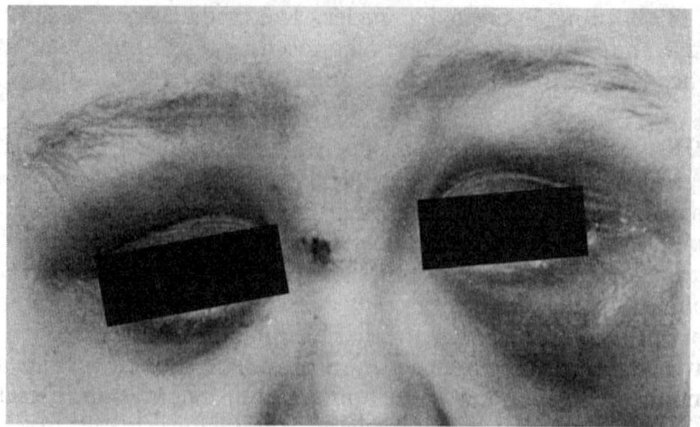

Figure 498-1. Periorbital metastases of neuroblastoma with proptosis and ecchymoses.

On plain radiography or CT the mass often contains calcification and hemorrhage. Wilms tumor, another common flank mass in a young child, usually does not calcify. NB originates from cervical, thoracic, or pelvic ganglia in 30% of cases. Metastatic disease can be associated with myriad signs and symptoms, including fever, irritability, failure to thrive, bone pain, bluish subcutaneous nodules, orbital proptosis, and periorbital ecchymoses (see Fig. 498-1). The most common sites of metastasis are the long bones and skull, bone marrow, liver, lymph nodes, and skin. Lung metastases are rare, occurring in <3% of cases. Prenatal diagnosis of NB sometimes is possible on maternal ultrasound scans.

Less commonly, children present first with neurologic signs and symptoms. Location in the superior cervical ganglion can result in **Horner syndrome.** Paraspinal NB can invade the neural foramina, producing symptoms of spinal cord and nerve root compression. NB can present as a paraneoplastic syndrome of autoimmune origin manifesting as ataxia or **opsomyoclonus** ("dancing eyes and dancing feet"). In such cases, the primary tumor is in the chest or abdomen, and the brain is negative for tumor. Some tumors produce catecholamines that can cause increased sweating and hypertension, and some release vasoactive intestinal peptide, causing a secretory diarrhea. Children <1 yr of age also can present with a unique stage, 4S, which often includes subcutaneous tumor nodules, massive liver involvement, and a small primary tumor without bone involvement.

DIAGNOSIS. NB usually is discovered as a mass or multiple masses on plain radiographs, CT, or MRI (Fig. 498-2). Tumor markers, including homovanillic acid (HVA) and vanillylmandelic acid (VMA) in urine, are elevated in 95% of cases and help to confirm the diagnosis. A pathologic diagnosis is established from tumor tissue obtained by biopsy. NB can be diagnosed in a typical presentation without a primary tumor biopsy if the patient has neuroblasts observed in bone marrow (Fig. 498-3) and elevated VMA or HVA in the urine.

Evaluations for metastatic disease should include bone scan to detect cortical bone involvement and bone marrow aspirates and biopsies to detect marrow disease. On experimental protocols, positron emission tomography and iodine 131 or **iodine 123 meta-iodobenzylguanidine (I-123 MIBG)** studies also may be used to better define the extent of disease. The clinical extent of disease and the patient's age, together with cytogenetic and molecular marker testing performed on the tumor tissue, are used to estimate the prognosis and to guide the choice of which risk-directed therapy. Although several staging systems have been used in the past, the **International Neuroblastoma Staging System (INSS)** now is universally used (Table 498-2). In the INSS, stage 1 includes tumors confined to the organ or structure of origin. Stage 2 tumors extend beyond the structure of origin but not across the midline, with (stage 2B) or without (stage 2A) ipsilateral lymph node involvement. Stage 3 tumors extend beyond the midline, with or without bilateral lymph node involvement. Stage 4 tumors are disseminated to distant sites (e.g., bone, bone marrow, liver, distant lymph nodes, other organs). Stage 4S refers to children <1 yr of age with dissemination to liver, skin, or bone marrow without bone involvement and with a primary tumor that would otherwise be stage 1 or 2.

TREATMENT. The most important clinical and biologic prognostic factors currently used to determine treatment are the age of the patient at diagnosis, stage of disease, MYCN status, and Shimada histology (see Table 498-1). The prognosis has improved with current treatment regimens. The usual treatment for low-risk NB is surgery for stages 1 and 2 and observation for stage

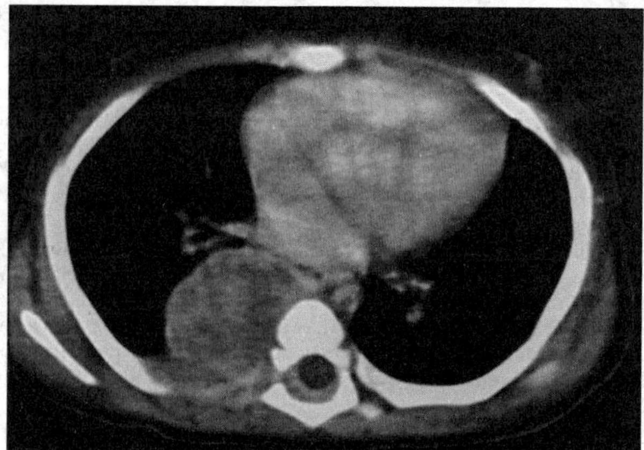

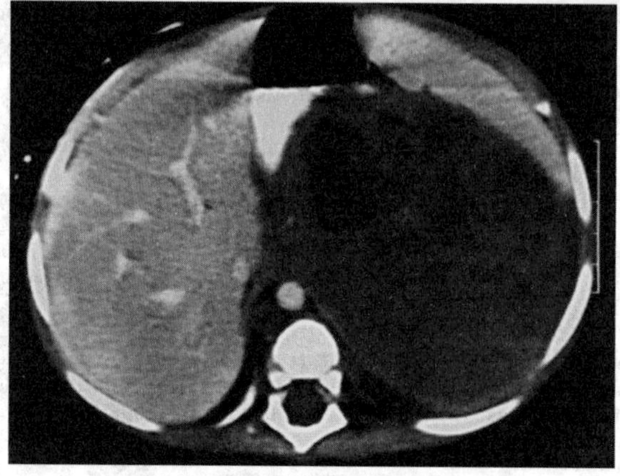

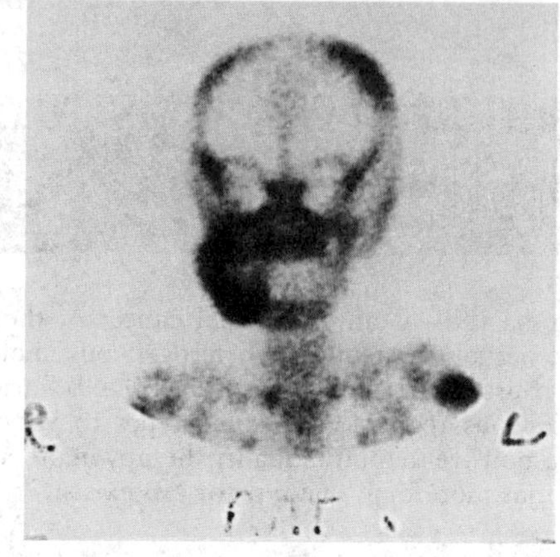

Figure 498-2. *Top,* CT scan of a thoracic neuroblastoma with intraspinal extension at diagnosis. *Middle,* CT scan of adrenal primary with extensive lymph node involvement. *Bottom,* Bone scintigraphy with technetium diphosphonate demonstrating diffuse skeletal involvement.

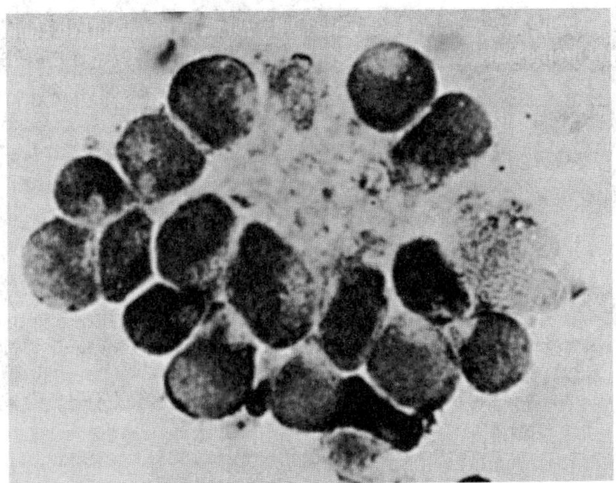

Figure 498-3. Neuroblastoma cells aspirated from the bone marrow. Clumps of cells often contain ≥3 cells with or without evidence of rosette formation. Rosettes of cells surrounding an inner mass of fibrillary material are characteristic of neuroblastoma.

4S. Even in stage 2 with small amounts of residual tumor, the cure rate is >90% without further therapy. Treatment with chemotherapy or radiation for the rare child with local recurrence still can be curative. Children with spinal cord compression at diagnosis also may require urgent treatment with chemotherapy, surgery, or radiation to avoid neurologic damage. Stage 4S has a very favorable prognosis, with nearly 100% survival with supportive care only, because the tumor regresses spontaneously. Chemotherapy or resection of the primary tumor does not improve survival. Infants <2 mo of age with stage 4S are more at risk if they have massive liver involvement and respiratory compromise. In such infants, low-dose cyclophosphamide or very-low-dose hepatic radiation may be recommended to alleviate symptoms. For children with stage 4S NB who require treatment for symptoms, the survival rate is 81%.

Treatment of intermediate-risk NB includes surgery, chemotherapy, and, in some cases, radiation therapy. The chemotherapy usually includes moderate doses of cisplatin or carboplatin, cyclophosphamide, etoposide, and doxorubicin given for several months. Radiation therapy is used for tumors with incomplete response to chemotherapy. Children with stage 3 disease and infants with stage 4 disease and favorable characteristics have an excellent prognosis of >90% survival with this moderate treatment. In this intermediate-risk group, obtaining adequate diagnostic material for determination of the Shimada pathologic classification and for MYCN amplification is critical, so that children with unfavorable characteristics can receive more aggressive treatment and those with favorable features can be spared excessive toxic therapy.

The usual treatment for high-risk NB (see Table 498-1) is induction chemotherapy to achieve complete response or very good partial response. With partial response, resection of the primary tumor followed by focal radiation to residual tumor is recommended. Induction is then followed by high-dose chemotherapy and autologous stem cell transplantation (SCT). A national randomized study showed significantly improved survival with SCT compared with chemotherapy without SCT. The addition of *cis*-retinoic acid after SCT for 1 yr further improved the 5-yr event-free survival to 50%, compared with 20% for those treated with chemotherapy without SCT or *cis*-retinoic acid.

Better therapy is needed for most patients with high-risk NB. New therapies currently under investigation include new chemotherapeutic agents, high-dose chemotherapy with multiple stem cell rescues, monoclonal antibodies combined with growth factors, and antitumor vaccines. It also is hoped that biologic studies of NB eventually will lead to new genetic targets for therapy.

PREVENTION. Currently there is no recognized way to prevent neuroblastoma. A worldwide attempt to improve survival by early detection through infant catecholamine screening has proven to be ineffective.

Attiyeh EF, London WB, Mosse YP, et al: Chromosome 1p and 11q deletions and outcome in neuroblastoma. *N Engl J Med* 2005;353:2243–2253.

Blaes F, Fuhlhuber V, Korfei M, et al: Surface-binding autoantibodies to cerebellar neurons in opsoclonus syndrome. *Ann Neurol* 2005;58:313–317.

Brodeur GM: Neuroblastoma: Biological insights into a clinical enigma. *Nature Rev Cancer* 2003;3:203–216.

De Roos AJ, Olshan AF, Teschke K, et al: Parental occupational exposures to chemicals and incidence of neuroblastoma in offspring. *Am J Epidemiol* 2001;154:106–114.

George RE, Lipshultz SE, Lipsitz SR, et al: Association between congenital cardiovascular malformations and neuroblastoma. *J Pediatr* 2004;144:444–448.

Goldsby RE, Matthay KK: Neuroblastoma: Evolving therapies for a disease of many faces. *Paediatr Drugs* 2004;6:107–122.

TABLE 498-2. International Neuroblastoma Staging System

STAGE	DEFINITION	INCIDENCE (%)	SURVIVAL AT 5 YR*
1	Localized tumor with complete gross excision, with or without microscopic residual disease; representative ipsilateral lymph nodes negative for tumor microscopically (nodes attached to and removed with the primary tumor may be positive)	5	≥90%
2A	Localized tumor with incomplete gross excision; representative ipsilateral nonadherent lymph nodes negative for tumor microscopically	10	70–80%
2B	Localized tumor with or without complete gross excision, with ipsilateral nonadherent lymph nodes positive for tumor. Enlarged contralateral lymph nodes must be negative microscopically	10	70–80%
3	Unresectable unilateral tumor infiltrating across the midline,[†] with or without regional lymph node involvement; or localized unilateral tumor with contralateral regional lymph node involvement; or midline tumor with bilateral extension by infiltration (resectable) or by lymph node involvement	25	40–70%
4	Any primary tumor with dissemination to distant lymph nodes; bone, bone marrow, liver, skin, and other organs (except as defined for stage 4S)	60	85–90% if age at diagnosis is <18 mo 30–40% if age at diagnosis is >18 mo
4S	Localized primary tumor (as defined for stage 1, 2A, or 2B), with dissemination limited to skin, liver, and bone marrow[‡] (limited to infants <1 yr of age)	5	>80%

*Survival is influenced by other characteristics such as *MYCN* amplification. Percentages are approximate.

[†]The midline is defined as the vertebral column. Tumors originating on one side and crossing the midline must infiltrate to or beyond the opposite side of the vertebral column.

[‡]Marrow involvement in stage 4S should be minimal (i.e., <10% of total nucleated cells identified as malignant on bone marrow biopsy or on marrow aspirate). More extensive marrow involvement would be considered stage 4. The MIBG scan (if performed) should be negative in the marrow.

From Kliegman RM, Marcdante KJ, Jenson HB, et al (editors): *Nelson Essentials of Pediatrics*, 5th ed. Philadelphia, WB Saunders, 2006, p 746. Modified from Brodeur GM et al: Revisions of the International Criteria for Neuroblastoma Diagnosis, Staging, and Response to Treatment. *J Clin Oncol* 1993;11:1466–1477.

MIBG, meta-iodobenzylguanidine.

Inagaki J, Yasui M, Sakata N, et al: Successful treatment of chemoresistant stage 3 neuroblastoma using irinotecan as a single agent. *J Pediatr Hematol Oncol* 2005;27:604–606.
Matthay KK, Villablanca JG, Seeger RC, et al: Treatment of high-risk neuroblastoma with intensive chemotherapy, radiotherapy, autologous bone marrow transplantation, and 13-cis-retinoic acid. *N Engl J Med* 1999;341:1165–1173.
Nickerson HJ, Matthay KK, Seeger RC, et al: Favorable biology and outcome of stage IV-S neuroblastoma with supportive care or minimal therapy: A Children's Cancer Group study. *J Clin Oncol* 2000;18:477–486.
Perez CA, Matthay KK, Atkinson JB, et al: Biological variables in the outcome of stages I and II neuroblastoma treated with surgery as primary therapy: A Children's Cancer Group Study. *J Clin Oncol* 2000;18:18–26.
Rudnick E, Khakoo Y, Antunes NL, et al: Opsoclonus-myoclonus-ataxia syndrome in neuroblastoma: Clinical outcome and antineuronal antibodies: A report from the Children's Cancer Group Study. *Med Pediatr Oncol* 2001;36:612–622.
Schmidt ML, Lukens JN, Seeger RC, et al: Biologic factors determine prognosis in infants with stage IV neuroblastoma: A prospective Children's Cancer Group Study. *J Clin Oncol* 2000;18:1260–1268.
Van Noesel MM, Versteeg R: Pediatric neuroblastomas: Genetic and epigenetic 'Danse Macabre.' *Gene* 2004; 325:1–15.
Woods WG: Screening for neuroblastoma: The final chapters. *J Pediatr Hematol Oncol* 2003;25:3–4.

Chapter 499 ■ Neoplasms of the Kidney

Norman Jaffe and Vicki Huff

499.1 • Wilms Tumor

ETIOLOGY. Wilms tumor, also known as **nephroblastoma,** is a complex mixed embryonal neoplasm of the kidney composed of three elements: blastema, epithelia, and stroma. Most cases of Wilms tumor are sporadic, although 1–2% of patients have a family history. Familial predisposition to Wilms tumor is inherited in an **autosomal dominant manner.** Familial cases are associated with a lower age at diagnosis and an increased frequency of bilateral disease, although these features are not observed in all families. Congenital anomalies are absent in most families. Nephrogenic rests often are associated with Wilms tumor.

One **Wilms tumor gene,** WT1 located at 11p13, has been isolated among the genetic alterations observed with Wilms tumor (Table 499-1). WT1 encodes a zinc finger transcription factor, which is critical for normal kidney development. Roughly 20% of all Wilms tumors carry WT1 mutations, and most of these mutations are tumor-specific. Patients with Wilms tumor who have associated congenital anomalies often carry germline WT1 mutations. Familial predisposition to Wilms tumor usually is not associated with WT1 alterations; familial predisposition genes have been localized to 19q13 and 17q.

TABLE 499-1. Genetic Alterations Observed in Wilms Tumors

GENE	WILMS TUMOR CHARACTERISTIC	FREQUENCY	TYPE OF ALTERATION
WT1	Unselected	~20%	Deletions, truncating mutations, missense mutations in zinc finger-encoding exons
β-catenin	Unselected	~15%	Missense mutations or deletions affecting protein phosphorylation sites
	Tumors with WT1 mutations (~20% of total)	~50%	—
p53	Anaplastic histology (~5% of total)	~80%	Missense and truncating mutations

TABLE 499-2. Syndromes Associated with Wilms Tumor and Their Clinical and Chromosomal Characteristics

SYNDROME	CLINICAL CHARACTERISTICS	CHROMOSOME OR OTHER ABNORMALITIES
WAGR	Aniridia, genitourinary abnormalities, mental retardation	Del 11p13 (*WT1* and *PAX6* loci)
Denys-Drash	Early-onset renal failure with renal mesangial sclerosis, male pseudohermaphrodism, increased risk of Wilms tumor	*WT1* mutations
Beckwith-Wiedemann	Organomegaly (liver, kidney, adrenal, pancreas), macroglossia omphalocele, hemihypertrophy	Uniparental paternal disomy, duplication 11p15.5, loss of imprinting, mutation of p57KIP57 have been described. Del 11p15.5 (*WT2* locus) May also involve *IGF2* and/or *H19* genes

Several syndromes and congenital abnormalities commonly are reported in patients with Wilms tumor (Table 499-2). **WAGR syndrome** is a contiguous gene deletion syndrome that consists of Wilms tumor, aniridia, genitourinary abnormalities (cryptorchidism, streak ovaries, bicornate uterus, ambiguous genitalia), and mental retardation. Patients with this syndrome have a constitutional deletion of chromosome 11p13 where the Wilms tumor gene, WT1, and the aniridia gene, PAX6, are located. **Denys-Drash syndrome** is characterized by male pseudohermaphrodism, early-onset renal failure characterized by mesangial sclerosis, and an increased risk of Wilms tumor. Patients with this syndrome typically carry a missense mutation in the WT1 gene. **Beckwith-Wiedemann syndrome** is characterized by hemihypertrophy, macroglossia, and visceromegaly, with a 3–5% risk of developing Wilms tumor. A variety of 11p15.5 abnormalities have been reported in patients with this syndrome, and it is postulated that a second Wilms tumor gene, WT2, is located in this region. Loss of imprinting of the insulin-like growth factor 2 gene, an epigenetic process, also is associated with Wilms tumor. Other syndromes or conditions with an increased risk of Wilms tumor include hemihypertrophy, sporadic aniridia, genitourinary anomalies, Pearlman syndrome, Sotos syndrome, neurofibromatosis (von Recklinghausen disease), and von Willebrand disease. The genitourinary anomalies most commonly associated with Wilms tumor are hypoplasia, fusion and ectopia of the kidney, duplications of the collecting systems, hypospadias, and cryptorchidism.

EPIDEMIOLOGY. The incidence of Wilms tumor is approximately 8 cases per million children <15 yr of age. It usually occurs in children between 2–5 yr of age, although it has also been encountered in neonates, adolescents, and adults. It accounts for approximately 6% of pediatric cancers and is the second most common malignant abdominal tumor in childhood. It may arise in one or both kidneys; the incidence of bilateral Wilms tumor is 7%. It may be associated with hemihypertrophy, aniridia, and other congenital anomalies, usually of the genitourinary tract. It also has been described in association with a variety of syndromes.

PATHOGENESIS. Two broad categories of Wilms tumor have been recognized: favorable and unfavorable. The favorable form is the more common form and usually carries a good prognosis. It is characterized by blastema, epithelia, and stroma devoid of ectopia or anaplasia. Small amounts of sarcomatous elements in the stroma in an otherwise favorable type apparently do not adversely influence the prognosis. The unfavorable form is characterized by marked enlargement of the nuclei, hyperchromatism of the enlarged nuclei, and multipolar mitotic figures. Areas of anaplasia may be focal or diffuse and predict probable high rates of tumor relapse and death. It tends to occur in older, non-white patients. Clear cell sarcoma is a subtype of the unfavorable form, and usually metastasizes to bone. Rhabdoid tumor, which may metastasize to the brain, is no longer classified as a subtype of Wilms tumor.

Nodal or other potential metastatic sites usually are the best areas for identifying anaplasia, which is extremely uncommon in children <2 yr of age. A high index of suspicion and more thorough sampling techniques are appropriate if anaplasia is detected, particularly in older children. The phenomenon usually is not found once chemotherapy has been administered. Anaplasia related to skeletal muscle cells does not appear to be associated with an increased incidence of relapse.

CLINICAL MANIFESTATIONS. Wilms tumor usually presents as an abdominal mass. It generally is discovered fortuitously, and it is not uncommon for the parent to notice it while bathing the infant. It also may be identified during a well child examination. These renal masses vary in size, usually are smooth and firm, and occasionally may cross the midline. Some patients may present with abdominal pain and vomiting, and hematuria is seen in 12–25% of patients. Hypertension also has been described and probably is due to renal ischemia. Occasionally, rapid abdominal enlargement and anemia may occur due to bleeding into the renal parenchyma or pelvis. Tumor growth into the renal veins or vena cava may embolize to the heart or lungs, with grave consequences.

DIAGNOSIS. Any abdominal mass in a child must be considered malignant until diagnostic imaging and laboratory findings define its true nature. If there is any doubt, biopsy or excision and histological verification is the final arbiter. Wilms tumor must be differentiated from a variety of malignant abdominal and pelvic tumors (Table 499-3). Once an abdominal mass is discovered, a complete physical examination should be performed, followed by a complete blood count, liver and kidney function studies, and a search for specific tumor markers secreted by the suspected tumor. Imaging studies include a flat plate of the abdomen, ultrasonography, and CT and/or MRI.

CT scanning provides confirmation of the intrarenal origin of the mass (Fig. 499-1). It also may provide information on the extent of tumor, growth into the inferior vena cava, and integrity

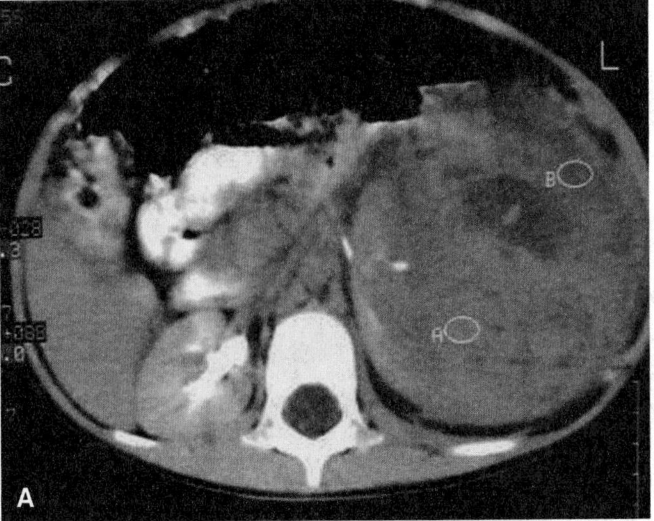

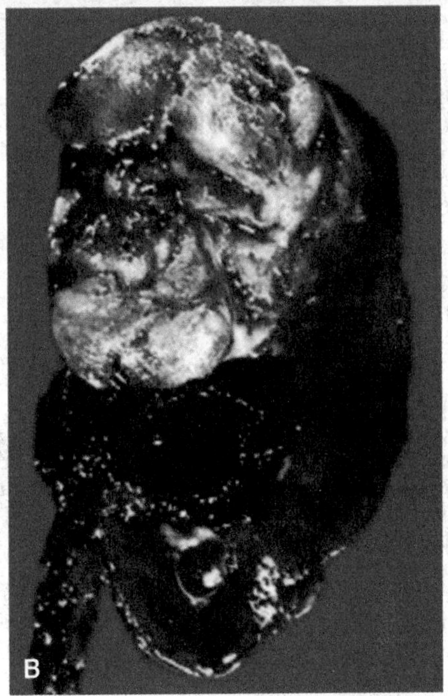

Figure 499-1. *A*, CT scan of the abdomen demonstrating a massive left Wilms tumor. *B*, Morbid anatomic view of the resected tumor seen in *A*.

of the contralateral kidney. Tumors enhance slightly after injection of contrast medium, which is useful for determining the function of the uninvolved kidney in the event that nephrectomy is required. MRI also helps to define the extent of tumor. Ultrasonography also may contribute to identification of the tumor and provide information regarding the integrity of the inferior vena cava as well as the presence of tumor in the renal vein or vena cava. Occasionally, angiography may be requested to plan the surgical procedure. Bone scans are obtained for clear cell sarcoma of the kidney and MRI or CT of the brain in a malignant rhabdoid tumor.

Radiographic examination of the chest is required to determine the presence of pulmonary metastases. CT scans of the lungs are not routinely obtained, because pulmonary metastases from Wilms tumor can be identified on conventional radiograph. Occasionally a CT scan demonstrates isolated nodules in patients with normal chest radiographs; the true nature of these nodules is uncertain.

TABLE 499-3. Differential Diagnosis of Abdominal and Pelvic Tumors in Infants and Children

TUMOR	AGE	CLINICAL SIGNS	LABORATORY FINDINGS
Wilms	Preschool	Unilateral flank mass, aniridia, hemihypertrophy	Hematuria; bone scintigraphy (clear cell sarcoma)
Neuroblastoma	Preschool	GI/GU obstruction, raccoon eyes, myoclonus-opsoclonus, diarrhea, skin nodules (infants)	Increased VMA; increased HVA; increased ferritin; stippled calcification in mass. Bone marrow positive
Non-Hodgkin lymphoma	>1 yr	Intussusception in >2-yr-old	Increased urate; bone marrow positive
Rhabdomyosarcoma	All	GI/GU obstruction, sarcoma botryoides, vaginal bleeding, paratesticular mass	
Germ cell/teratoma	Preschool, teens	Girls: abdominal pain, vaginal bleeding Boys: testicular mass, new-onset "hydrocele" Sacrococcygeal mass/dimple	Increased hCG; Increased AFP
Hepatoblastoma	Birth–3 yr	Large, firm liver	Increased AFP
Hepatoma	School age, teens	Large, firm liver; hepatitis B, cirrhosis	Increased AFP

AFP, α-fetoprotein; GI, gastrointestinal; GU, genitourinary; hCG, human chorionic gonadotropin; HVA, homovanillic acid; VMA, vanillylmandelic acid.

TABLE 499-4. Staging System Developed by the Third National Wilms Tumor Study

STAGE	DESCRIPTION
Stage I	Tumor is limited to kidney and is completely excised. Capsular surface intact; no tumor rupture; no residual tumor apparent beyond margins of excision
Stage II	Tumor extends beyond kidney but is completely excised. Regional extension of tumor; vessel infiltration; tumor biopsied or local spillage of tumor confined to the flank. No residual tumor apparent at or beyond margins of excision
Stage III	Residual non-hematogenous tumor confined to the abdomen. Lymph node involvement of hilus, periaortic chains, or beyond; diffuse peritoneal contamination by tumor spillage; peritoneal implants of tumor, tumor extends beyond surgical margins microscopically or macroscopically; tumor not completely removable because of local infiltration into vital structures
Stage IV	Deposits beyond stage III (e.g., lung, liver, bone, brain)
Stage V	Bilateral renal involvement at diagnosis

Modified from National Wilms' Tumor Study Committee: Wilms' tumor: status report, 1990. *J Clin Oncol* 1991;9:877–887.

STAGING. The staging system most often used was developed by the National Wilms Tumor Study group (Table 499-4) and the stage correlates with prognosis (Table 499-5). Stage I Wilms tumor is confined to the kidney and, by definition, is excised completely with the capsular surface intact. Stage II Wilms tumor also is confined to the kidney, although the capsule is penetrated or tumor is present in the perirenal soft tissue. Stage III Wilms tumor has postsurgical residual non-hematogenous extension. Spread is confined to the abdomen and may involve the perirenal bed, draining lymph nodes, or the surrounding tissue and organs by contiguity. Stage IV Wilms tumor is characterized by hematogenous metastases. The metastases usually involve the lungs and occasionally the liver. Stage V Wilms tumor is characterized by bilateral renal involvement.

TREATMENT. Controversial issues in the management of Wilms tumor include the use of preoperative chemotherapy and radiation therapy, and also the composition of chemotherapeutic agents. The intent is to reduce the incidence and nature of late effects while providing optimum therapy. Indications for partial nephrectomy must still be defined, as must the role of surgery alone in patients with low-risk Wilms tumor. The optimal preoperative imaging approach to assess the nature of the disease in the presenting kidney and contralateral kidney for bilateral Wilms tumor also has not yet been determined.

Surgical extirpation of the tumor should be performed. The patency of the inferior vena cava should be established prior to the resection; if it is not patent, preoperative chemotherapy should be administered. During the operation the contralateral kidney should be examined to exclude bilateral Wilms tumor. The liver should be inspected for possible metastases, although CT, MRI, or ultrasonography may have identified metastases preoperatively. The retroperitoneal lymph nodes should be examined and suspicious nodes biopsied for tumor involvement. Every attempt should be made to avoid spillage of tumor.

TABLE 499-5. Wilms Tumor: Survival by Histology and Stage

	SURVIVAL	
HISTOLOGY/STAGE	2 Yr (%)	4 Yr (%)
Favorable I	98	97
Favorable II	96	94
Favorable III	91	88
Favorable IV	88	82
Anaplastic I	89	89
Anaplastic II–IV	56	54

Modified from National Wilms' Tumor Study Committee: Wilms' tumor: status report, 1990. *J Clin Oncol* 1991;9:877–887.

Most centers follow chemotherapy guidelines provided by the National Wilms Tumor Study Group. For stage I and II tumors with favorable histology, vincristine and actinomycin D are administered. For stage III tumors with favorable histology, vincristine, actinomycin D, and doxorubicin are administered, and radiation therapy also is administered to the tumor bed. For stage IV tumors with favorable histology, vincristine, actinomycin D, and doxorubicin are administered, and radiation therapy also is administered to all the sites of known disease, particularly the lungs. If tumor in the liver is present, surgical resection rather than radiation therapy may be considered. Resistant tumors that fail to respond to chemotherapy and radiation therapy, or tumors that recur, may be considered for surgical resection and alternate, investigational chemotherapy.

For tumors with unfavorable histology, vincristine, actinomycin D, doxorubicin, and cyclophosphamide are administered, and radiation therapy also is administered to all the known sites of disease. Clear cell sarcoma of bone has responded to a combination of cisplatin, doxorubicin, and radiation therapy. Additional therapy with cyclophosphamide or ifosfamide also may be considered.

Most patients tolerate treatment extremely well, although therapy may cause both acute and chronic adverse effects. Most acute adverse effects consist of nausea, vomiting, and myelosuppression with possible superimposed infection. Antiemetics usually are administered for transient nausea and vomiting. Actinomycin D and doxorubicin may cause mouth ulcers, which usually are mild and inconsequential. Vincristine may cause constipation and abdominal pain. Chronic adverse effects may involve the gastrointestinal, hepatic, cardiac, reproductive, and skeletal systems. Intestinal obstruction may result from adhesions, fibrosis, or volvulus. Rarely, radiation therapy enteritis or malabsorption may supervene. Severe hepatic damage may occur with veno-occlusive disease, which usually is caused by the concomitant administration of actinomycin D with radiation therapy to the liver.

Congestive cardiac failure may occur after treatment with doxorubicin, particularly if administered in combination with radiation therapy to the lungs. The cumulative dose of doxorubicin usually is limited, to prevent cardiac damage, to 200–300 mg/m^2, particularly in patients with pulmonary metastases who will subsequently receive pulmonary radiation therapy.

Radiation therapy to the chest can affect breast maturation, and treatment to the uterus may result in low birthweight infants. Radiation therapy to the ovaries may result in premature menopause and reproductive dysfunction. Kyphoscoliosis also may occur after radiation therapy if it is administered to the hemiabdomen with only part of the vertebral column included in the radiation portal, but usually can be avoided with modern techniques.

Recurrent tumors and pulmonary metastases may develop within the first 2 yr after diagnosis. A variety of follow-up schedules have been implemented for early detection and treatment, such as monthly follow-up with a clinical evaluation and chest radiograph for the first 2 years. The interval between visits over the next 3 yr is extended, and at the 5th year the visits are annual. Ultrasonography of the abdomen is performed after completion of treatment to detect the presence of recurrent tumor and establish the integrity of the contralateral kidney, and is then obtained annually. It also is important for long-term survivors to have systematic follow-up with measurements of blood pressure, urine protein, serum creatinine, renal clearance, and renal size, especially if they were treated for bilateral Wilms tumor.

Inoperable Wilms Tumor. Chemotherapy is administered for all Wilms tumors that appear inoperable. In these circumstances the diagnosis usually is established by percutaneous needle biopsy, with the selection of chemotherapy dictated by histologic criteria. For tumors with favorable histology, vincristine and actinomycin D are used for stages I and II, with vincristine, actinomycin D, and doxorubicin for tumors of stages III and IV. For tumors with unfavorable histology, treatment involves a combination of vincristine, actinomycin D, doxorubicin, and cyclophosphamide. In most instances a reduction in tumor size is obtained. The prognosis for inoperable tumors treated with chemotherapy, surgery, and, if required, radiation therapy, usually is favorable, with survival rates of >50%.

Bilateral Wilms Tumor. Chemotherapy for bilateral Wilms tumor is identical to that employed for inoperable tumors, and is given to render the tumor amenable to surgical extirpation, which may include unilateral nephrectomy and contralateral partial nephrectomy or bilateral partial nephrectomies. These maneuvers permit ablation of viable neoplasm and conservation of renal tissue. Surgical procedures are dictated by the extent of tumor and response to chemotherapy. Postoperatively, chemotherapy and, often, radiation therapy are administered. Occasionally, preoperative radiation also is utilized. These therapeutic strategies have yielded survival rates of 60–85%.

Salvage Chemotherapy. Patients with relapse during or following treatment with conventional therapy often respond to alternate treatment, particularly those with tumors of favorable histology. In these circumstances, combination chemotherapy with vincristine, doxorubicin, cyclophosphamide, and actinomycin D or ifosfamide, carboplatin, and etoposide may be used. High-dose chemotherapy with bone marrow rescue also has been employed. A multidisciplinary salvage strategy with surgery, radiation therapy, and chemotherapy usually yields the best result.

PROGNOSIS. There is remarkable correlation among the DNA content in the cells of Wilms tumor, histologic subtype, and treatment outcome. Stem lines of both the primary tumor and metastases are in the diploid and low aneuploid (hyperdiploid) range. Tumors with hyperdiploid content also are characteristic of the anaplastic (unfavorable) varieties and have enormous complex translocations. They respond poorly to chemotherapy. The prognosis is worse with a larger tumor (>500 g), advanced stage (III and IV), and an unfavorable histologic subtype.

Wilms tumor is a paradigm of successful multidisciplinary treatment, and >60% of patients with all stages generally survive. Stages I through III have a cure rate of >90%.

499.2 • Other Kidney Tumors In Children

CONGENITAL MESOBLASTIC NEPHROMA. Congenital mesoblastic nephroma is a unique congenital neoplasm of the infant kidney that rarely metastasizes. It occurs more often in boys and has been noted to produce renin. The tumor is a massive, firm, infiltrative, solitary renal mass. Grossly and microscopically it resembles a leiomyoma or a low-grade leiomyosarcoma with trapped nephrons. Microscopy reveals fibroblast or myofibroblast cells. The tumor accounts for the majority of **congenital renal tumors.** Most cases are considered benign, and opinion is divided regarding the utility of chemotherapy. One report noted that vincristine and actinomycin administered as adjuvant therapy did not prevent metastases. In another report, metastatic disease apparently responded to vincristine, doxorubicin, and cyclophosphamide.

NEPHROGENIC RESTS. The term "nephrogenic rests," or **nodular renal blastema** or **nephroblastomatosis,** refers to the abnormal persistence of embryonal renal tissue. The favorable survival and response rate of bilateral Wilms tumor suggests a strong relation to the nephrogenic rests. It has been suggested that a brief course of relatively nontoxic chemotherapy, such as vincristine and actinomycin D, may be beneficial for nephrogenic rests by reducing the large volume of the kidneys. Persistent blastema and nephroblastic abnormalities appear to remain in the kidneys of many, if not all, treated patients, despite the reduction in renal volume. Nephrogenic nests detected in one kidney should prompt a careful evaluation of the contralateral kidney. Radiographic follow-up with CT scanning also may be indicated. Whether chemotherapy reduces the subsequent development of Wilms tumor is unknown.

MULTICYSTIC NEPHROBLASTOMA. Tumors of the kidney occasionally may contain cysts, some of which may be linked to Wilms tumor. Several diagnostic terms may be applied to such tumors, including **cystic partially differentiated nephroblastoma (CPDN), polycystic nephroblastoma,** and **multilocular nephroma.** Most cases of multicystic nephroblastoma occur in patients <1 yr of age. This type of tumor biology indicates a benign process. However, if there is definite evidence of Wilms tumor, treatment with chemotherapy is justified.

RENAL CELL CARCINOMA. Renal cell carcinoma is rare in the first decades of life, but occasionally has been reported in children and teenagers. It usually presents as an abdominal mass and/or hematuria. Complete resection may achieve cure. Occasionally, adjuvant treatment with interferon and 5-fluorouracil has been recommended.

RENAL MEDULLARY CARCINOMA. This is a rare, highly aggressive tumor associated with sickle cell trait, presenting with hematuria and a flank mass. Metastasis is usually present at the time of diagnosis. The prognosis is poor.

Blakely ML, Ritchey ML: Controversial issues in the maintenance of Wilms' tumor. *Semin Pediatr* 2001;10:127–131.

de Kraker J, Graf N, van Tinteren H, et al: Reduction of postoperative chemotherapy in children with stage 1 intermediate-risk and anaplastic Wilms' tumour (SIOP 93–01 trial): A randomized controlled trial. *Lancet* 2004;364:1229–1235.

Dome JS, Liu T, Krasin M, et al: Improved survival for patients with recurrent Wilms tumor: The experience at St. Jude Children's Research Hospital. *J Pediatr Hematol Oncol* 2002;24:192–198.

Firoozi F, Kogan BA: Follow-up and management of recurrent Wilms' tumor. *Urol Clin North Am* 2003;30:869–879.

Fischbach BV, Trout KL, Lewis J, et al: WAGR syndrome: A clinical review of 54 cases. *Pediatrics* 2005;116:984–988.

Fukuzawa R, Breslow NE, Morison IM, et al: Epigenetic differences between Wilms' tumours in white and east-Asian children. *Lancet* 2004;363: 446–451.

Gronskov K, Olsen JH, Sand A, et al: Population-bases risk estimates of Wilms tumor in sporadic aniridia. *Hum Genet* 2001;109:11–18.

Kalapurakal JA, Dome JS, Perlman EJ, et al: Management of Wilms' tumour: Current practice and future goals. *Lancet Oncol* 2004;5:37–46.

Malcolm AW, Jaffe N, Folkman MJ, et al: Bilateral Wilms' tumor. *Int J Radiat Oncol Biol Phys* 1980;6:167–174.

Patel K, Livni N, Macdonald D: Renal medullary carcinoma, a rare cause of haematuria in sickle cell trait. *Br J Haematol* 2006;132:1.

Pirich LM, Chou P, Walterhouse DO: Prolonged survival of a patient with sickle cell trait and metastatic renal medullary carcinoma. *J Pediatr Hematol Oncol* 1999;21:67–69.

Pritchard-Jones K, Pritchard J: Success of clinical trials in childhood Wilms' tumour around the world. *Lancet* 2004;364:1468–1470.

Ritchey ML: The role of preoperative chemotherapy for Wilms' tumor: The NWTSG perspective. Wilms' Tumor Study Group. *Semin Urol Oncol* 1999;17:21–27.

Shamberger RC: Pediatric renal tumors. *Semin Surg Oncol* 1999;16:105–120.

Chapter 500 ■ Soft Tissue Sarcomas

Carola A. S. Arndt

The annual incidence of soft tissue sarcomas is 8.4 cases per million white children <14 yr of age. Rhabdomyosarcoma accounts for more than $^1/_2$ of soft tissue sarcomas. The prognosis most strongly correlates with extent of disease at diagnosis, primary tumor site, and type of treatment.

RHABDOMYOSARCOMA

EPIDEMIOLOGY. The most common pediatric soft tissue sarcoma, rhabdomyosarcoma, accounts for ~3.5% of childhood cancers. These tumors may occur at virtually any anatomic site but usually are found in the head and neck (25%), genitourinary tract (22%), extremities (18%); retroperitoneal and other sites account for the remainder of primary sites. The incidence at each anatomic site is related to both patient age and tumor type. Extremity lesions are more likely to occur in older children and to have alveolar histology. Rhabdomyosarcoma occurs with increased frequency in patients with neurofibromatosis and has been associated with maternal breast cancer in the Li-Fraumeni syndrome, suggesting a genetic influence.

PATHOGENESIS. Rhabdomyosarcoma is thought to arise from the same embryonic mesenchyme as striated skeletal muscle. On the basis of light microscopic appearance, it belongs to the group of small round cell tumors that includes Ewing sarcoma, neuroblastoma, and non-Hodgkin lymphoma. Definitive diagnosis of a pathologic specimen may require immunohistochemical studies using antibodies to skeletal muscle (desmin, muscle-specific actin, Myo-D) and electron microscopy.

Determination of the specific histologic subtype is important in treatment planning and assessment of prognosis. There are four recognized histologic subtypes. The **embryonal type** accounts for about 60% of all cases and has an intermediate prognosis. The **botryoid type,** a variant of the embryonal form in which tumor cells and an edematous stroma project into a body cavity like a bunch of grapes, is found most often in the vagina, uterus, bladder, nasopharynx, and middle ear. The **alveolar type** accounts for about 15% of cases and often is characterized by 2;13 or 1;13 chromosomal translocations. The tumor cells tend to grow in cores that often have cleft-like spaces resembling alveoli. Alveolar tumors occur most often in the trunk and extremities and carry the poorest prognosis. The **pleomorphic type** (adult form) is rare in childhood and accounts for only 1% of cases.

CLINICAL MANIFESTATIONS. The most common presenting feature is a mass that may or may not be painful. Symptoms are caused by displacement or obstruction of normal structures (Table 500-1). Origin in the nasopharynx may be associated with nasal congestion, mouth breathing, epistaxis, and difficulty with swallowing and chewing. Regional extension into the cranium can produce cranial nerve paralysis, blindness, and signs of increased intracranial pressure with headache and vomiting. When the tumor develops in the face or cheek there may be swelling, pain, trismus, and, as extension occurs, paralysis of cranial nerves. Tumors in the neck can produce progressive swelling with neurologic symptoms after regional extension. Orbital primary tumors usually are diagnosed early in their course because of associated proptosis, periorbital edema, ptosis, change in visual acuity, and local pain. When the tumor arises in the middle ear, the most common early signs are pain, hearing loss, chronic otorrhea, or a mass in the ear canal; extensions of tumor produce cranial nerve paralysis and signs of an intracranial mass on the involved side. An unremitting croupy cough and progressive stridor can accompany rhabdomyosarcoma of the larynx. Because most of these signs and symptoms also are associated with common childhood conditions, clinicians must be alert to the possibility of tumor.

TABLE 500-1. Common Clinical Symptoms of Rhabdomyosarcoma

REGION	SYMPTOMS
Head and neck	Asymptomatic mass, may mimic enlarged lymph node
Orbit	Proptosis, chemosis, ocular paralysis, eyelid mass
Nasopharynx	Snoring, nasal voice, epistaxis, rhinorrhea, local pain, dysphagia, cranial nerve palsies
Paranasal sinuses	Swelling, pain, sinusitis, obstruction, epistaxis, cranial nerve palsies
Middle ear	Chronic otitis media, hemorrhagic discharge, cranial nerve palsies, extruding polypoid mass
Larynx	Hoarseness, irritating cough
Trunk	Asymptomatic mass (usually)
Biliary tract	Hepatomegaly, jaundice
Retroperitoneum	Painless mass, ascites, gastrointestinal or urinary tract obstruction, spinal cord symptoms
Bladder/prostate	Hematuria, urinary retention, abdominal mass, constipation
Female genital tract	Polypoid vaginal extrusion of mucosanguineous tissue, vulval nodule
Male genital tract	Painful or painless scrotal mass
Extremity	Painless mass, may be very small but with secondary lymph node involvement
Metastatic	Nonspecific symptoms, associated with the diagnosis of leukemia

From McDowell HP: Update on childhood rhabdomyosarcoma. *Arch Dis Child* 2003;88:354–357.

Rhabdomyosarcoma of the trunk or extremities often is first noticed after trauma and initially may be regarded as a hematoma. If the swelling does not resolve or increases, malignancy should be suspected. Involvement of the genitourinary tract can produce hematuria, obstruction of the lower urinary tract, recurrent urinary tract infections, incontinence, or a mass detectable on abdominal or rectal examination. Paratesticular tumors usually present as a painless, rapidly growing mass in the scrotum. Vaginal rhabdomyosarcoma may present as a grapelike mass of tumor tissue bulging through the vaginal orifice, known as **sarcoma botryoides,** and can cause urinary tract or large bowel symptoms. Vaginal bleeding or obstruction of the urethra or rectum may occur. Similar findings can be noted with uterine primaries.

Tumors in any location may disseminate early and present with symptoms of pain or respiratory distress associated with pulmonary metastases. Extensive bone involvement can produce symptomatic hypercalcemia. In such cases, it may be difficult to identify the primary lesion.

DIAGNOSIS. Early diagnosis of rhabdomyosarcoma requires a high index of suspicion. The microscopic appearance is of a small round blue cell tumor. Neuroblastoma, lymphoma, and Ewing sarcoma also are **small round blue cell tumors.** The differential diagnosis depends on the site of presentation. Definitive diagnosis is established by biopsy, microscopic appearance, and results of immunohistochemical stains. A lesion in an extremity may be thought to be a hematoma or hemangioma, an orbital lesion resulting in proptosis may be treated as an orbital cellulitis, or bladder obstructive symptoms may be missed. Adolescents may ignore paratesticular lesions for a long time. Unfortunately, several months often elapse between the initial symptoms and biopsy. Diagnostic procedures are determined mainly by the area of involvement. CT or MRI is necessary for evaluation of the primary tumor site. With signs and symptoms in the head and neck area, radiographs should be examined for evidence of a tumor mass and for indications of bony erosion. CT or MRI should be performed to identify intracranial extension and also may reveal bony involvement or erosion at the base of the skull. For abdominal and pelvic tumors, ultrasound, CT with contrast, or MRI can help delineate the tumor (Fig. 500-1). A radionuclide bone scan, chest CT, and bilateral bone marrow aspirate and

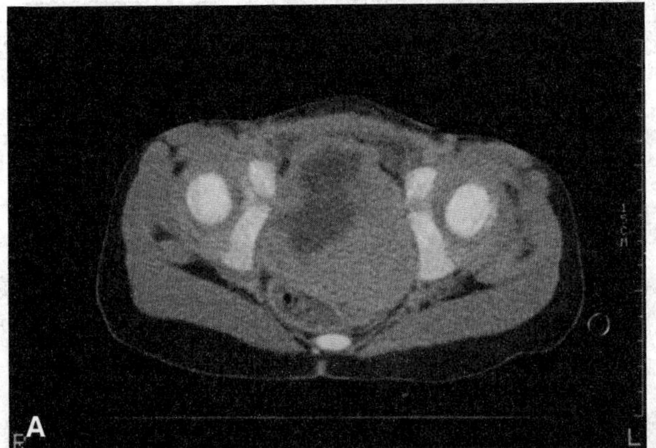

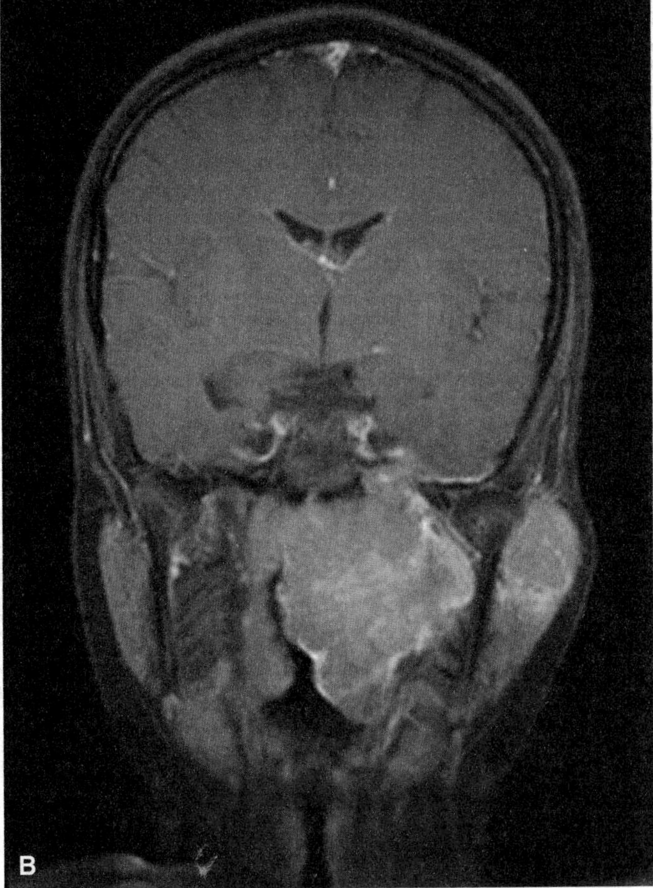

Figure 500-1. *A*, Pelvic CT of a child with a bladder rhabdomyosarcoma. *B*, MRI of a child with a parameningeal rhabdomyosarcoma.

biopsy should be performed to evaluate the patient for the presence of metastatic disease to plan treatment. The most critical element of the diagnostic work-up is examination of tumor tissue, which includes the use of special histochemical stains and immunostains. Cytogenetics and molecular genetics may be helpful in detecting specific chromosomal translocations of fusion proteins present in alveolar rhabdomyosarcoma. Lymph nodes also should be sampled for presence of disease spread, especially in tumors of the extremities.

TREATMENT. Patients with completely resected tumors have the best prognosis. Unfortunately, most rhabdomyosarcomas are not completely resectable. At the initial surgery, tumor margins should be carefully defined and an appropriate search for regional or metastatic disease to adjacent structures or regional lymph nodes should be completed, even if the procedure is limited to biopsy. Treatment is based on the primary tumor location and disease stage, which defines the clinical group. Most patients are given preoperative chemotherapy in an attempt to reduce the extent of surgery required and to preserve vital organs, particularly of the genitourinary tract. Group I tumors are treated with complete local excision followed by chemotherapy to reduce the likelihood of subsequent metastases. Group II tumors (microscopic residual tumor) are treated with surgery followed by local irradiation and systemic chemotherapy. Group III tumors (gross residual tumor) are treated with systemic chemotherapy followed by irradiation and, if possible, surgery. Group IV rhabdomyosarcoma (metastatic) is treated principally with systemic chemotherapy and irradiation. Standard chemotherapeutic agents include vincristine, dactinomycin, and cyclophosphamide. Topotecan and irinotecan are being evaluated in therapeutic trials.

PROGNOSIS. Prognostic factors include stage, histology, and primary site. Among patients with resectable tumor, 80–90% have prolonged disease-free survival. Unresectable tumor localized to certain favorable sites, such as the orbit, also has a high likelihood of cure. About 70% of patients with incompletely resected tumor also achieve long-term disease-free survival. Patients with disseminated disease have a poor prognosis; only about $^1/_2$ achieve remission, and fewer than $^1/_2$ of these are cured. Older children have a poorer prognosis than younger children. For all patients, surveillance for late effects of cancer treatment (such as impaired bone growth secondary to radiation, sterility from cyclophosphamide, and second malignancies) is important.

OTHER SOFT TISSUE SARCOMAS

The non-rhabdomyosarcoma soft tissue sarcomas (NRSTS) constitute a heterogeneous group of tumors that account for 3% of all childhood malignancies (Table 500-2). Because they are relatively rare in children, much of the information about their natural history and treatment has been derived from studies of adult patients. In children, the median age at diagnosis is 12 yr, with a male:female ratio of 2.3 : 1. These tumors commonly arise in the trunk or lower extremities. The most common histologic types are synovial sarcoma (42%), fibrosarcoma (13%), malignant fibrous histiocytoma (12%), and neurogenic tumors (10%). Molecular genetic studies often prove useful in diagnosis, as several of these tumors have characteristic chromosomal translocations.

Surgery remains the mainstay of therapy, but a careful search for lung and bone metastases should be undertaken before surgical excision. Lymph node spread is rare, and routine dissection is not recommended. Chemotherapy and radiation therapy should be considered for large, high-grade, and unresectable tumors. The role of chemotherapy for non-rhabdomyosarcomatous tumors is not as well defined as for rhabdomyosarcoma. Patients with unresectable or metastatic disease are treated with multiagent chemotherapy in addition to radiation and/or surgery. Tumor size, stage (clinical group), invasiveness, and histologic grade correlate with survival.

Arndt CAS, Crist WM: Medical progress: Common musculoskeletal tumors of childhood and adolescence. *N Engl J Med* 1999;341:342–352.

Baker KS, Anderson JR, Lind MP, et al: Benefit of intensified therapy for patients with local or regional embryonal rhabdomyosarcoma: Results from the Intergroup Rhabdomyosarcoma Study IV. *J Clin Oncol* 2000;18:2427–2434.

Crist WM, Anderson JR, Meza JL, et al: Intergroup rhabdomyosarcoma study: IV. Results for patients with nonmetastatic disease. *J Clin Oncol* 2001;19:3091–3102.

TABLE 500-2. Features of Most Common Types of Nonrhabdomyocarcoma Soft Tissue Sarcomas

TISSUE TYPE	TUMOR	NATURAL HISTORY AND BIOLOGY
Adipose	Liposarcoma	A very rare tumor. Usually arises in the extremities or retroperitoneum; associated with a nonrandom translocation, t(12;16) (q13;p11). Tends to be locally invasive and rarely metastasizes; wide local excision is the treatment of choice. The role of radiation therapy and chemotherapy in treating gross residual or metastatic disease is not established.
Fibrous	Fibrosarcoma	Most common soft tissue sarcoma in children <1 yr. Congenital fibrosarcoma is a low-grade malignancy that commonly arises in the extremities or trunk and rarely metastasizes. Surgical excision is treatment of choice; dramatic responses to preoperative chemotherapy may occur. In children >4 yr, the natural history is similar to that in adults (a 5-yr survival rate of 60%); wide surgical excision and preoperative chemotherapy are commonly used.
	Malignant fibrous histiocytoma	Most commonly arises in the trunk and extremities, deep in the subcutaneous layer. Histologically subdivided into storiform, giant cell, myxoid, and angiomatoid variants. The angiomatoid type tends to affect younger patients and is curable with surgical resection alone. Wide surgical excision is the treatment of choice. Chemotherapy has produced objective tumor regressions.
Vascular	Hemangiopericytoma	Often arises in the lower extremities or retroperitoneum; may present with hypoglycemia and hypophosphatemic rickets. Both benign and malignant histology. Nonrandom translocations t(12;19) (q13;q13) and t(13;22) (q22;q11) have been described. Complete surgical excision is the treatment of choice. Chemotherapy and radiation therapy may produce responses.
	Angiosarcoma	Rare in children; 33% arise in skin, 25% in soft tissue, and 25% in liver, breast, or bone. Associated with chronic lymphedema and exposure to vinyl chloride in adults. Survival rate is poor (12% at 5 yr) despite some responses to chemotherapy/radiation therapy.
	Hemangioendothelioma	Can occur in soft tissue, liver, and lung. Localized lesions have a favorable outcome; lesions in lung and liver often are multifocal and have a poor prognosis.
Peripheral nerves	Neurofibrosarcoma	Also known as the malignant peripheral nerve sheath tumor. Develops in up to 16% of patients with NF1; almost 50% occur in patients with NF1. Deletions of chromosome 22q11-q13 or 17q11 and p53 mutations have been reported. Commonly arises in trunk and extremities and usually is locally invasive. Complete surgical excision is necessary for survival; response to chemotherapy is suboptimal.
Synovium	Synovial sarcoma	The most common NRSTS in some series. Often presenting in the 3rd decade, but 33% of patients are <20 yr. Typically arises around the knee or thigh and is characterized by a nonrandom translocation t(X;18) (p11;q11). Wide surgical excision is necessary. Radiation therapy is effective in microscopic residual disease, and ifosfamide-based therapy is active in advanced disease.
Unknown	Alveolar soft part sarcoma	Slow-growing tumor; tends to recur or metastasize to lung and brain years after diagnosis. Often arises in the extremities and head and neck. A myogenic origin has been proposed. Resection of primary and metastatic sites, when possible, is recommended.
Smooth muscle	Leiomyosarcoma	Often arises in the gastrointestinal tract and may be associated with a t(12;14) (q14;q23) translocation. Associated with Epstein-Barr virus in immunodeficiency syndromes (including AIDS). Complete surgical excision is the treatment of choice.

NF, neurofibromatosis; NRSTS, nonrhabdomyosarcoma soft tissue sarcoma.

McDowell HP: Update on childhood rhabdomyosarcoma. *Arch Dis Child* 2003;88:354–357.

Meyer WH, Spunt SL: Soft tissue sarcomas of childhood. *Cancer Treat Rev* 2004;30:269–280.

Spunt SL, Poquette CA, Hurt YS, et al: Prognostic factors for children and adolescents with surgically resected nonrhabdomyosarcoma soft tissue sarcoma: An analysis of 121 patients treated at St. Jude Children's Research Hospital. *J Clin Oncol* 1999;17:3697—3705.

Stevens MCG: Treatment for childhood rhabdomyosarcoma: The cost of cure. *Lancet Oncol* 2005;6:77–84.

Chapter 501 ■ Neoplasms of Bone

Carola A. S. Arndt

501.1 • Malignant Tumors of Bone

The annual incidence of malignant bone tumors in the USA is approximately 7 cases per million white children <14 yr of age, with a slightly lower incidence in African-American children. Osteosarcoma is the most common primary malignant bone tumor in children and adolescents, followed by Ewing sarcoma (Table 501-1; Fig. 501-1). In children <10 yr of age, Ewing sarcoma is more common than osteosarcoma. Both tumor types are most likely to occur in the second decade of life.

OSTEOSARCOMA

EPIDEMIOLOGY. The annual incidence of osteosarcoma in the USA is 5.6 cases per million children <15 yr of age. The highest risk period for development of osteosarcoma is during the adolescent growth spurt, suggesting an association between rapid bone growth and malignant transformation. Patients with osteosarcoma are taller than their peers of similar age.

PATHOGENESIS. Although the cause of osteosarcoma is unknown, certain genetic or acquired conditions predispose patients to development of osteosarcoma. Patients with **hereditary retinoblastoma** have a significantly increased risk of developing osteosarcoma. The sites of osteosarcoma in these patients initially were thought to be located only in previously irradiated areas, but more recently they have been shown to arise in sites far from the radiation field. Predisposition to development of osteosarcoma in these patients may be related to loss of heterozygosity of the RB gene. Osteosarcoma also occurs in the **Li-Fraumeni**

TABLE 501-1. Comparison of Features of Osteosarcoma and the Ewing Family of Tumors

FEATURE	OSTEOSARCOMA	EWING FAMILY OF TUMORS
Age	Second decade	Second decade
Race	All races	Primarily whites
Sex (M : F)	1.5 : 1	1.5 : 1
Cell	Spindle cell–producing osteoid	Undifferentiated small round cell, probably of neural origin
Predisposition	Retinoblastoma, Li-Fraumeni syndrome, Paget disease, radiotherapy	None known
Site	Metaphyses of long bones	Diaphyses of long bones, flat bones
Presentation	Local pain and swelling; often, history of injury	Local pain and swelling; fever
Radiographic findings	Sclerotic destruction (less commonly lytic); sunburst pattern	Primarily lytic, multilaminar periosteal reaction ("onion skinning")
Differential diagnosis	Ewing sarcoma, osteomyelitis	Osteomyelitis, eosinophilic granuloma, lymphoma, neuroblastoma, rhabdomyosarcoma
Metastasis	Lungs, bones	Lung, bones
Treatment	Chemotherapy Ablative surgery of primary tumor	Chemotherapy Radiotherapy and/or surgery of primary tumor
Outcome	Without metastases: 70% cured; with metastases at diagnosis, ≤20% survival	Without metastases: 60% cured; with metastases at diagnosis, 20–30% survival

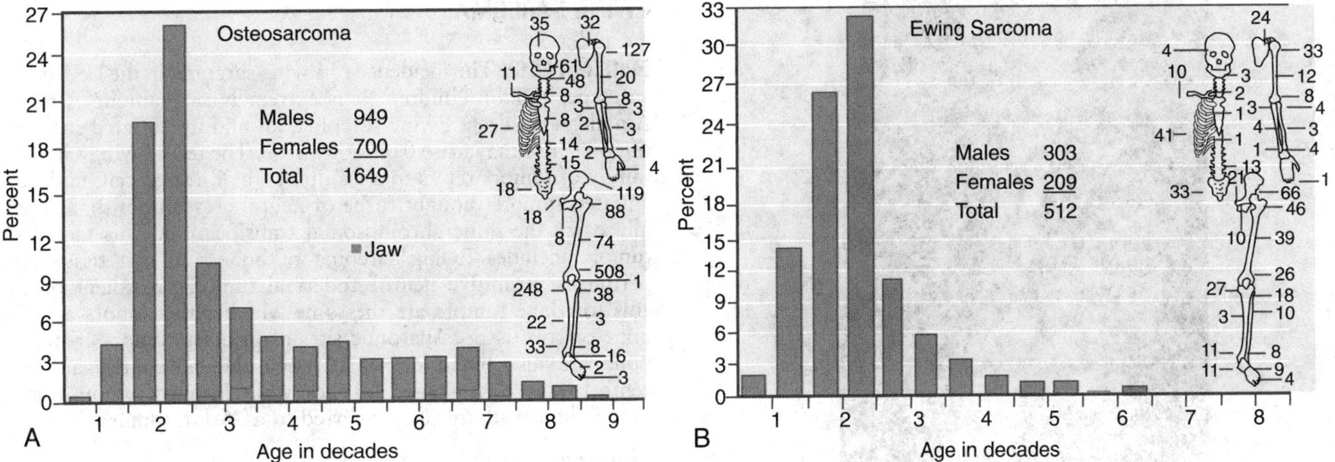

Figure 501-1. *A*, Age and skeletal distribution of 1,649 cases of osteosarcoma in the Mayo Clinic files. *B*, Age and skeletal distribution of 512 cases of Ewing sarcoma in the Mayo Clinic files. (From Unni KK [editor]: *Dahlin's Bone Tumors: General Aspects and Data on 11,087 Cases*, 5th ed. Philadelphia, Lippincott-Raven, 1996. Reprinted by permission of the Mayo Foundation.)

syndrome, which is a familial cancer syndrome associated with germline mutations of the p53 gene. Kindreds with **Li-Fraumeni syndrome** have a spectrum of malignancies in 1st-degree relatives, including carcinoma of the breast, soft tissue sarcomas, brain tumors, leukemia, adrenal cortical carcinoma, and other malignancies. **Rothmund-Thomson syndrome** is a rare syndrome associated with short stature, skin telangiectasia, small hands and feet, hypoplastic or absent thumbs, and a high risk of osteosarcoma. Osteosarcoma also can be induced by irradiation for Ewing sarcoma, craniospinal irradiation for brain tumors, or high-dose irradiation for other malignancies. Other benign conditions that can be associated with malignant transformation to osteosarcoma include Paget disease, enchondromatosis, multiple hereditary exostoses, and fibrous dysplasia.

The pathologic diagnosis of osteosarcoma is made by demonstration of a highly malignant, pleomorphic, spindle cell neoplasm associated with the formation of malignant osteoid and bone. There are four pathologic subtypes of conventional high-grade osteosarcoma: osteoblastic, fibroblastic, chondroblastic, and telangiectatic. No significant differences in outcome are associated with the various subtypes, although the chondroblastic component of that subtype may not respond as well to chemotherapy. The role in prognosis of various genes such as drug resistance-related genes, tumor suppressor genes, and genes related to apoptosis is being evaluated.

Telangiectatic osteosarcoma may be confused with aneurysmal bone cyst because of its lytic appearance radiographically. High-grade osteosarcoma typically arises in the diaphyseal region of long bones and invades the medullary cavity. It also may be associated with a soft tissue mass. Two variants of osteosarcoma, parosteal and periosteal osteosarcoma, should be distinguished from conventional osteosarcoma because of their characteristic clinical features. **Parosteal osteosarcoma** is a low-grade, well-differentiated tumor that does not invade the medullary cavity and most commonly is found in the posterior aspect of the distal femur. Surgical resection alone often is curative in this lesion, which has a low propensity for metastatic spread. **Periosteal osteosarcoma** is a rare variant that arises on the surface of the bone but has a higher rate of metastatic spread than the parosteal type and an intermediate prognosis.

CLINICAL MANIFESTATIONS. Pain, limp, and swelling are the most common presenting manifestations of osteosarcoma. Because these tumors occur most often in active adolescents, initial complaints may be attributed to a sports injury or sprain; any bone or joint pain not responding to conservative therapy within a reasonable amount of time should be investigated thoroughly. Additional clinical findings may include limitation of motion, joint effusion, tenderness, and warmth. Results of routine laboratory tests, such as a complete blood cell count and chemistry panel, usually are normal, although alkaline phosphatase or lactic dehydrogenase levels may be elevated.

DIAGNOSIS. Bone tumor should be suspected in a patient who presents with deep bone pain, often causing nighttime awakening, a palpable mass, and a radiograph demonstrating a lesion. The lesion may be mixed lytic and blastic in appearance, but new bone formation usually is visible. The classic radiographic appearance of osteosarcoma is the **sunburst pattern** (Fig. 501-2). When osteosarcoma is suspected, the patient should be referred to a center with experience in managing bone tumors. The biopsy and the surgery should be performed by the same surgeon so that the incisional biopsy site can be placed in a manner that will not compromise the ultimate limb salvage procedure. Tissue usually is obtained for molecular and biologic studies at the time of the initial biopsy. Before biopsy, MRI of the primary lesion and the entire bone should be performed to evaluate the tumor for its proximity to nerves and blood vessels, soft tissue and joint extension, and skip lesions. The metastatic work-up should be performed before biopsy and includes CT of the chest and radionuclide bone scan to evaluate for lung and bone metastases, respectively. The **differential diagnosis** of a lytic bone lesion includes histiocytosis, Ewing sarcoma, lymphoma, and bone cyst.

TREATMENT. With chemotherapy and surgery, the 5-yr disease-free survival rate of patients with nonmetastatic extremity osteosarcoma is 65–75%. Complete surgical resection of the tumor is important for cure. The current approach is to treat patients with preoperative chemotherapy in an attempt to facilitate limb salvage operations and to treat micrometastatic disease immediately. Up to 80% of patients are able to undergo limb salvage operations after initial chemotherapy. Some institutions use intra-arterial chemotherapy to infuse chemotherapy directly into an artery feeding the tumor, although this has not been shown to be better than conventional intravenous chemotherapy. It is important to resume chemotherapy as soon as possible after surgery. Lung metastases present at diagnosis should be resected by thoracotomies at some time during the course of treatment. Active agents currently in use in multidrug chemotherapy regi-

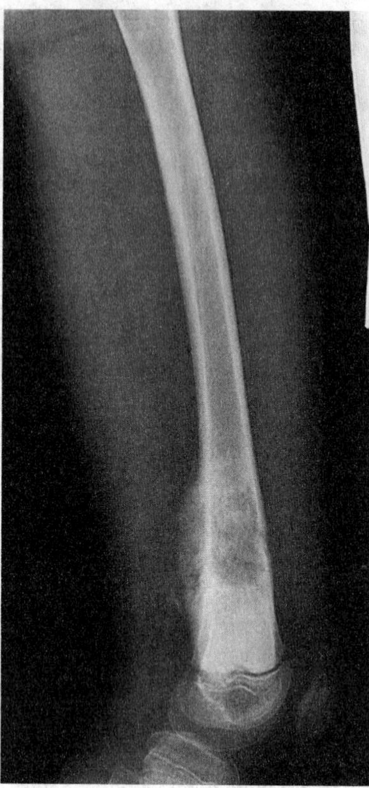

Figure 501-2. Radiograph of an osteosarcoma of the femur with typical "sunburst" appearance of bone formation.

mens for conventional osteosarcoma include doxorubicin, cisplatin, methotrexate, and ifosfamide.

One of the most important prognostic factors in osteosarcoma is the histologic response to chemotherapy. An international cooperative group is evaluating a randomized trial of the postoperative addition of high-dose ifosfamide with etoposide to standard three-drug therapy with cisplatin, doxorubicin, and methotrexate to improve the outcome of patients with a poor histologic response. Good histologic responders will be randomized to the addition of PEGylated interferon α2b. After limb salvage surgery, intensive rehabilitation and physical therapy is necessary to ensure maximal functional outcome.

For patients who require amputation, early prosthetic fitting and gait training is essential to enable them to resume activities as normally as possible. Before definitive surgery, patients with tumors on weight-bearing bones should be instructed to use crutches to avoid stressing the weakened bone and causing a pathologic fracture. The role of chemotherapy in parosteal and periosteal osteosarcoma is not well defined.

PROGNOSIS. Surgical resection alone is curative only for patients with parosteal osteosarcoma. Conventional osteosarcoma requires multiagent chemotherapy. Up to 75% of patients with nonmetastatic extremity osteosarcoma are cured with current multiagent treatment protocols. The prognosis is not as favorable for patients with pelvic tumors as for those with primary tumors in an extremity. From 20–30% of patients who have limited numbers of pulmonary metastases also can be cured with aggressive chemotherapy and resection of lung nodules. Patients with bone metastases and those with widespread lung metastases have an extremely poor prognosis. Long-term follow-up of patients with osteosarcoma is important to monitor for late effects of chemotherapy such as cardiotoxicity from anthracycline. Patients who develop late, isolated lung metastases may be cured with surgical resection alone.

EWING SARCOMA

EPIDEMIOLOGY. The incidence of Ewing sarcoma in the USA is 2.1 cases per million children. It is extremely rare among African-American children. Ewing sarcoma, an undifferentiated sarcoma of bone, also may arise from soft tissue. The term **Ewing sarcoma family of tumors** refers to a group of small, round cell, undifferentiated tumors thought to be of neural crest origin that generally carry the same chromosomal translocation. This family of tumors includes Ewing sarcoma of bone and soft tissue and peripheral **primitive neuroectodermal tumor.** Treatment protocols for these tumors are the same whether the tumors arise in bone or soft tissue. Anatomic sites of primary tumors arising in bone are distributed evenly between the extremities and the central axis (pelvis, spine, and chest wall). Primary tumors arising in the chest wall are often referred to as **Askin tumors.**

PATHOGENESIS. Immunohistochemical staining assists in the diagnosis of Ewing sarcoma to differentiate it from **small round blue cell tumors** such as lymphoma, rhabdomyosarcoma, and neuroblastoma. Histochemical stains may react positively with certain neural markers on tumor cells (neuron-specific enolase and S-100), especially in peripheral primitive neuroectodermal tumor. Reactivity with muscle markers (e.g., desmin, actin) is absent. Additionally, the cell surface glycoprotein MIC-2 usually is positive. A specific chromosomal translocation, t(11;22), or a variant thereof is found in most of the Ewing sarcoma family of tumors. Analysis for the translocation by routine cytogenetics or polymerase chain reaction analysis for the chimeric fusion gene products EWS/FLI1 or EWS/ERG can be helpful in confirming the diagnosis in extremely undifferentiated tumors.

CLINICAL MANIFESTATIONS. Symptoms of Ewing sarcoma are similar to those of osteosarcoma. Pain, swelling, limitation of motion, and tenderness over the involved bone or soft tissue are common presenting symptoms. In the case of huge chest wall primary tumors, patients may present with respiratory distress. Patients with paraspinal or vertebral primary tumors may present with symptoms of cord compression. Ewing sarcoma often is associated with **systemic manifestations** such as fever or weight loss; patients may have undergone treatment for a presumptive diagnosis of osteomyelitis. Patients also may have a delay in diagnosis when their pain or swelling is attributed to a sports injury.

DIAGNOSIS. The diagnosis of Ewing sarcoma should be suspected in a patient who presents with pain and swelling, with or without systemic symptoms, and with a radiographic appearance of a primarily lytic bone lesion with periosteal reaction, the characteristic **onion-skinning** (Fig. 501-3). A large associated soft tissue mass often is visualized on MRI or CT (Fig. 501-4). The **differential diagnosis** includes osteosarcoma, osteomyelitis, Langerhans' cell histiocytosis, primary lymphoma of bone, metastatic neuroblastoma, or rhabdomyosarcoma in the case of a pure soft tissue lesion. Patients should be referred to a center with experience in managing bone tumors for evaluation and biopsy. Thorough evaluation for metastatic disease includes CT of the chest, radionuclide bone scan, and bone marrow aspirate and biopsy specimens from at least two sites. MRI of the tumor and the entire length of involved bone should be performed to determine the exact extension of the soft tissue and bony mass and the proximity of tumor to neurovascular structures. To avoid compromising an ultimate potential for limb salvage by a poorly planned biopsy incision, the same surgeon should perform the biopsy and the surgical procedure. CT-guided biopsy of the lesion often provides diagnostic tissue. It is important to obtain adequate tissue for special stains, cytogenetics, and molecular studies.

TREATMENT. Tumors of the Ewing sarcoma family are best managed with a comprehensive multidisciplinary approach

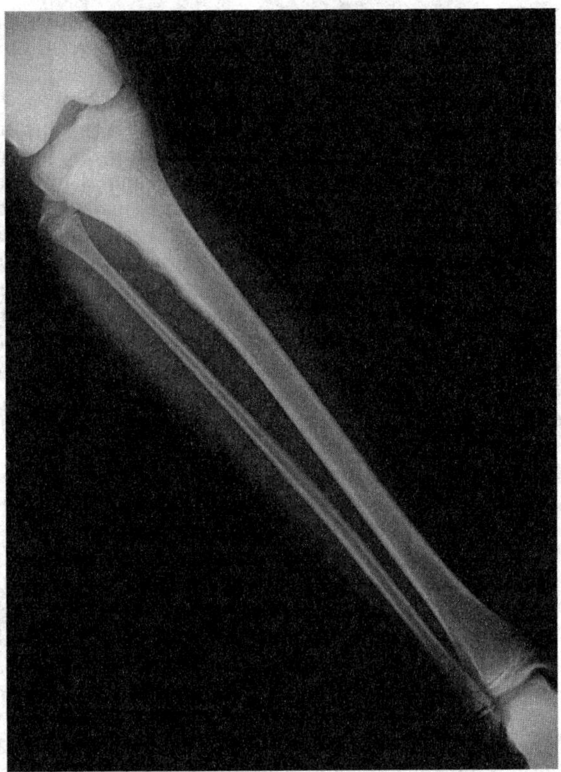

Figure 501-3. Radiograph of tibial Ewing sarcoma showing periosteal elevation or "onion-skinning."

incorporating the surgeon, chemotherapist, and radiation oncologist in planning therapy. Multiagent chemotherapy is important because it can shrink the tumor rapidly and usually is given before local control is attempted. The addition of ifosfamide and etoposide to the conventional agents of vincristine, doxorubicin, and cyclophosphamide improves the outcome of nonmetastatic Ewing sarcoma. Chemotherapy usually causes dramatic shrinkage of the soft tissue mass and rapid, significant pain relief. Current randomized studies of chemotherapy in Ewing sarcoma are evaluating the role of dose intensity for both metastatic and nonmetastatic Ewing sarcoma. An international cooperative group trial is evaluating whether myeloablative chemotherapy and stem cell rescue is superior to chemotherapy with lung irradiation for patients with pulmonary metastases. Myeloablative chemotherapy for patients with extremely high risk disease (bone and marrow metastases) also is being studied, as are approaches using angiogenesis inhibitors on a standard chemotherapy backbone. Ewing sarcoma is considered a radiosensitive tumor, and local control may be achieved with radiation or surgery. Radiation therapy is associated with a risk of radiation-induced second malignancies, especially osteosarcoma, as well as failure of bone growth in skeletally immature patients. Many centers prefer surgical resection, if possible, to achieve local control. It is important to provide patients with crutches if the tumor is in a weight-bearing bone to avoid a pathologic fracture before definitive local control. Chemotherapy should be resumed as soon as possible after surgery.

PROGNOSIS. Patients with small, nonmetastatic, distally located extremity tumors have the best prognosis, with a cure rate of up to 75%. The type of chromosomal translocation may be related to prognosis. Patients with pelvic tumors have, until recently, had a much worse outcome. Patients with metastatic disease at diagnosis, especially bone or bone marrow metastases, have a poor prognosis, with <30% surviving long term. New approaches, such as very intensive chemotherapy with peripheral blood stem cell rescue, are being investigated in these patients.

Long-term follow-up of patients with Ewing sarcoma is important because of the potential for late effects of treatment such as anthracycline cardiotoxicity; second malignancies, especially in the radiation field; and late relapses, even as long as 10 yr after initial diagnosis.

501.2 • Benign Tumors and Tumor-like Processes of Bone

Benign bone lesions in children are common in comparison with the relatively rare malignant neoplasms of bone and present diagnostic challenges. Some, although histologically benign, can be life-threatening. No single element in the history or diagnostic test is sufficient to rule out malignancies or suggest nonneoplastic conditions. A broad range of diagnostic possibilities must be considered when confronted with an unknown bone lesion. Benign lesions may be painless or painful, especially if a pathologic fracture is impending. Night pain that awakens a child is suggestive of malignancy; relief of such pain with aspirin is common with benign lesions such as osteoid osteomas. Rapidly enlarging lesions usually are associated with malignancy, but several benign lesions, such as aneurysmal bone cysts, may enlarge faster than most malignancies. Several conditions, such as osteomyelitis, may simulate the appearance of benign bone tumors.

Many benign bone tumors are diagnosed incidentally or after pathologic fracture. Management of these fractures is similar to that of nonpathologic fractures in the same location. It is unusual

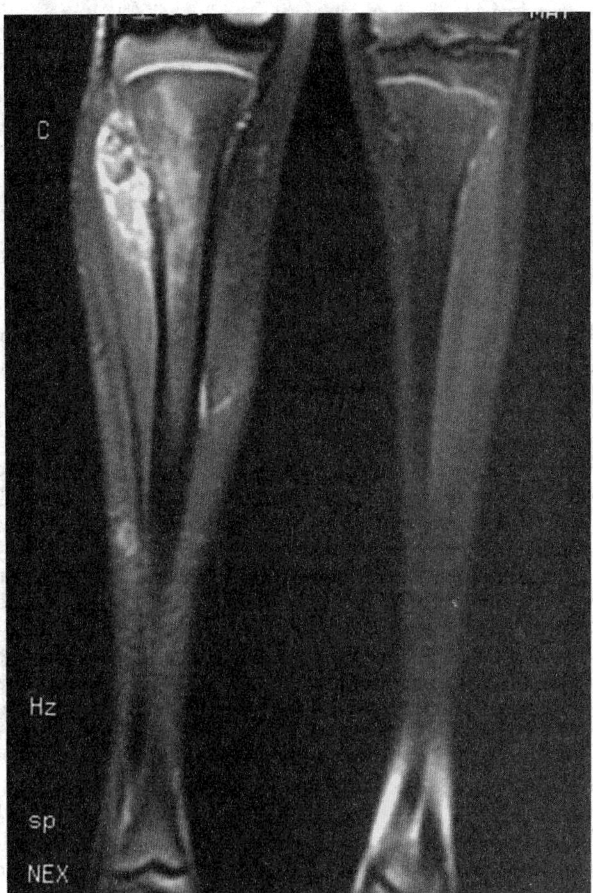

Figure 501-4. MRI of tibial Ewing sarcoma showing a large associated soft tissue mass.

for benign bone tumors to interfere with fracture healing. Likewise, the fractures rarely result in changes or healing of these tumors, which usually are treated after the fracture has healed.

Radiographs of any suspected bone lesion should always be obtained in two planes. Additional studies may be necessary to help arrive at the correct diagnosis and to guide treatment. Although these lesions are benign, many do require intervention.

Osteochondroma (exostosis) is one of the most common benign bone tumors in children. Because many are completely asymptomatic and unrecognized, the true incidence of this lesion is unknown. Most osteochondromas develop in childhood, arising from the metaphysis of a long bone, particularly the distal femur, proximal humerus, and proximal tibia. The lesion enlarges with the child until skeletal maturity. Most are discovered from 5–15 yr of age when the child or parent notices a bony, nonpainful mass. Some are discovered because they are irritated by pressure during athletic or other activities. Osteochondromas appear radiographically as stalks or broad-based projections from the surface of the bone, usually in a direction away from the adjacent joint. Invariably, the lesion is radiographically smaller than suggested by palpation because the cartilage "cap" covering the lesion is not seen. This cartilage cap may be up to 1 cm thick. Both the cortex of the bone and the marrow space of the involved bone are continuous with the lesion. Malignant degeneration to a chondrosarcoma is rare in children but may occur in as many as 1% of adults. Routine removal is not performed unless the lesion is large enough to cause symptoms or if rapid lesion growth occurs.

Multiple hereditary exostoses is a related but rare condition characterized by the presence of multiple osteochondromas. Severely involved children may have short stature, limb-length inequality, premature partial physeal arrests, and deformity of both the upper and lower extremities. These individuals must be monitored carefully during growth.

Enchondroma is a benign lesion of hyaline cartilage that occurs centrally in the bone. Most of these lesions are asymptomatic and occur in the hands. Most are discovered incidentally, although pathologic fractures often lead to the diagnosis. Radiographically, the lesions occupy the medullary canal, are radiolucent, and are sharply marginated. Punctate or stippled calcification may be present within the lesion, but this is much more common in adults than in children. Almost all enchondromas are solitary. Most can simply be observed, with curettage and bone grafting reserved for those lesions that are symptomatic or large enough to weaken the bone structurally. Multifocal involvement is referred to as **Ollier disease** and may result in bony dysplasia, short stature, limb-length inequality, and joint deformity. Surgery may be necessary to correct or prevent such deformities. When multiple enchondromas are associated with angiomas of the soft tissue, the condition is referred to as **Maffucci syndrome.** A high rate of malignant transformation has been reported in both of these multifocal conditions.

Chondroblastoma is a rare lesion usually found in the epiphysis of long bones. Most patients present in the second decade with complaints of mild to moderate pain in the adjacent joint. Common sites include the hip, shoulder, and knee. Muscle atrophy and local tenderness may be the only clinical findings. The lesion appears radiographically as a sharply marginated radiolucency within the epiphysis or apophysis, occasionally with metaphyseal extension across the physis. Proximity to the joint may cause deformity of the subchondral bone, an effusion, or erosion into the joint. Recognition is important because most lesions can be cured with curettage and bone grafting before joint destruction occurs.

Chondromyxoid fibroma is an uncommon benign bone tumor in children. This metaphyseal lesion usually causes pain and local tenderness. The lesion occasionally may be asymptomatic. Chondromyxoid fibroma appears radiographically as eccentric, lobular, metaphyseal radiolucency with sharp, sclerotic, and scalloped margins. The lower extremity is involved most often. Treatment usually consists of curettage and bone grafting or en bloc resection.

Osteoid osteoma is a small benign bone tumor. Most of these tumors are diagnosed between 5–20 yr of age. The clinical pattern is characteristic, consisting of unremitting and gradually increasing pain that often is worst at night and is relieved by aspirin. Males are affected more often than females. Any bone can be involved, but the most common sites are the proximal femur and tibia. Vertebral lesions may cause scoliosis or symptoms that mimic a neurologic disorder. Examination may reveal a limp, atrophy, and weakness when the lower extremity is involved. Palpation and range of motion do not alter the discomfort. Radiographs are distinctive, showing a round or oval metaphyseal or diaphyseal lucency (0.5–1.0 cm diameter) surrounded by sclerotic bone. The central lucency, or nidus, shows intense uptake on bone scan. About 25% of osteoid osteomas are not visualized on plain radiographs but can be identified with CT. Because of the small size of the lesion and its location adjacent to thick cortical bone, MRI is poor at detecting osteoid osteomas. Treatment is directed at removing the lesion. This may involve en bloc excision, curettage, or percutaneous CT-guided ablation of the nidus. Patients with mild pain may be treated with salicylates. Some lesions resolve spontaneously after skeletal maturity.

Osteoblastoma is a locally destructive, progressively growing lesion of bone with a predilection for the vertebrae, although almost any bone may be involved. Most patients note the insidious onset of dull aching pain, which may be present for months before they seek medical attention. Spinal lesions may cause neurologic symptoms or deficits. The radiographic appearance is variable and less distinctive than that of other benign bone tumors. About 25% show features suggesting a malignant neoplasm, making biopsy necessary in many cases. Expansile spinal lesions often involve the posterior elements. Treatment involves curettage and bone grafting or en bloc excision, taking care to preserve nerve roots when treating spinal lesions. Surgical stabilization of the spine may be necessary.

Fibromas (nonossifying fibroma, fibrous cortical defect, metaphyseal fibrous defect) are fibrous lesions of bone that occur in 40% of children >2 yr of age. They most likely represent a defect in ossification rather than a neoplasm and usually are asymptomatic. Most are discovered incidentally when radiographs are taken for other reasons, usually to rule out a fracture after trauma. Occasional pathologic fractures can occur through rare large lesions. Physical examination usually is unrevealing. Radiographs show a sharply marginated eccentric lucency in the metaphyseal cortex. Lesions may be multilocular and expansile, with extension from the cortex into the medullary bone. The long axis of the lesion runs parallel to that of the bone. Approximately 50% are bilateral or multiple. Because of the characteristic radiographic appearance, most lesions do not require biopsy or treatment. Spontaneous regression can be expected after skeletal maturity. Curettage and bone grafting may be recommended for lesions occupying more than 50% of the bone diameter because of the risk of a pathologic fracture.

Unicameral bone cysts can occur at any age in childhood but are rare in children <3 yr of age and after skeletal maturity. The cause of these fluid-filled lesions is unknown. Some resolve spontaneously after skeletal maturity is reached. Most are asymptomatic until diagnosis, which usually follows a pathologic fracture. Such fractures may occur with relatively minor trauma, such as with throwing or catching a ball. Unicameral bone cysts appear radiographically as solitary, centrally located lesions within the medullary portion of the bone. These cysts are most common in the proximal humerus or femur. They often extend to (but not through) the physis and are sharply marginated. Thinning and expansion of the cortex occurs but does not exceed the width of the adjacent physis. Treatment involves allowing the pathologic fracture to heal, followed by aspiration and injection with methylprednisolone or bone marrow. Repeat injections, curettage, and bone grafting occasionally are necessary to treat recurrent lesions.

Aneurysmal bone cyst is a reactive lesion of bone seen in persons <20 yr of age. The lesion is characterized by cavernous spaces filled with blood and solid aggregates of tissue. Although the femur, tibia, and spine are most commonly involved, this progressively growing, expansile lesion develops in any bone. Pain and swelling are common. Spinal involvement may lead to cord or nerve root compression and associated neurologic symptoms, including paralysis. Radiographs show eccentric lytic destruction and expansion of the metaphysis surrounded by a thin sclerotic rim of bone. Posterior elements of the spine are involved more commonly than the vertebral body. Unlike most other benign bone tumors, which usually are confined to a single bone, aneurysmal bone cysts may involve adjacent vertebrae. Rapid growth is characteristic and may lead to confusion with malignant neoplasms. Treatment consists of curettage and bone grafting or excision. Spinal lesions may require stabilization after excision. As with other benign tumors, attempts are made to preserve nerve roots and other vital structures. Recurrence after surgical treatment occurs in 20–30% of patients, is more common in younger than older children, and usually occurs in the first 1–2 yr after treatment.

Fibrous dysplasia is a developmental abnormality characterized by fibrous replacement of cancellous bone. Lesions may be solitary or multifocal (polyostotic), relatively stable, or progressively more severe. Most children are asymptomatic, although those with skull involvement may have swelling or exophthalmos. Pain and limp are characteristic of proximal femoral involvement. Limb-length discrepancy, bowing of the tibia or femur, and pathologic fractures may be presenting complaints. The triad of polyostotic disease, precocious puberty, and cutaneous pigmentation is known as Albright syndrome. Radiographic features of fibrous dysplasia include a lytic or ground-glass expansile lesion of the metaphysis or diaphysis. The lesion is sharply marginated and often is surrounded by a thick rim of sclerotic bone. Bowing, especially of the proximal femur, may be present. Treatment usually involves observation. Surgery is indicated for patients with progressive deformity, pain, or impending pathologic fractures. Bone grafting is not as successful in the treatment of fibrous dysplasia as with other benign tumors because the lesion often recurs within the grafted bone. Reconstructive surgical techniques often are necessary to provide stability.

Osteofibrous dysplasia affects children 1–10 yr of age. This lesion usually involves the tibia. It is clinically, radiographically, and histologically distinct from fibrous dysplasia. Most children present with anterior swelling or enlargement of the leg. Progression is unlikely after 10 yr of age. Radiographs show solitary or multiple lucent, cortical, diaphyseal lesions surrounded by sclerosis. Anterior bowing of the tibia often is present. The radiographic appearance closely resembles that of adamantinoma, a malignant neoplasm, making biopsy more common than with other benign bone tumors. Treatment involves observation. Some lesions heal spontaneously. Excision and bone grafting should be delayed until the child is >10 yr of age because of a high recurrence rate before this age. Pathologic fractures heal with immobilization.

Eosinophilic granuloma is a monostotic or polyostotic disease with no extraskeletal involvement. This latter finding distinguishes eosinophilic granuloma from the other forms of Langerhans' cell histiocytosis (Hand-Schüller-Christian or Letterer-Siwe variants), which may have a less favorable prognosis (see Chapter 507). Eosinophilic granuloma usually occurs during the first 3 decades of life and is most common in boys 5–10 yr of age. The skull is most commonly affected, but any bone may be involved. Patients usually present with local pain and swelling. Marked tenderness and warmth often are present in the area of the involved bone. Spinal lesions may cause pain, stiffness, and occasional neurologic symptoms. The radiographic appearance of the skeletal lesions is similar in all forms of Langerhans' cell histiocytosis but is variable enough to mimic many other benign and malignant lesions of bone. The radiolucent lesions have well-defined or irregular margins with expansion of the involved bone and periosteal new bone formation. Spine involvement may cause uniform compression or flattening of the vertebral body. A skeletal survey is warranted because polyostotic involvement and the typical skull lesions strongly suggest the diagnosis of eosinophilic granuloma. Biopsy often is necessary to confirm the diagnosis because of the broad radiographic differential diagnosis. Treatment includes curettage and bone grafting, low-dose radiation therapy, or corticosteroid injection. Observation for symptomatic lesions is reasonable because most osseous lesions heal spontaneously and do not recur. Children with bone lesions should be evaluated for visceral involvement because treatment of Hand-Schüller-Christian disease and Letterer-Siwe disease is more complex and often systemic.

Arndt CAS, Crist WM: Common musculoskeletal tumors of childhood and adolescence. *N Engl J Med* 1999;341:342–352.

Campanacci M, Capanna R, Picci P: Unicameral and aneurysmal bone cysts. *Clin Orthop Relat Res* 1986;204:25–36.

Campanacci M, Laus M: Osteofibrous dysplasia of the tibia and fibula. *J Bone Joint Surg Am* 1981;63:367–375.

Dahlin DC, Ivins JC: Benign chondroblastoma: A study of 125 cases. *Cancer* 1972;30:401–413.

De Alava E, Gerald WL: Molecular biology of the Ewing's sarcoma/primitive neuroectodermal tumor family. *J Clin Oncol* 2000;18:204–213.

Freiberg AA, Loder RT, Heidelberger KT: Aneurysmal bone cysts in young children. *J Pediatr Orthop* 1994;14:86–91.

Ginsberg JP, Woo SY, Johnson ME, et al: Ewing's sarcoma family of tumors. In Pizzo PA, Poplack DG (editors): *Principles and Practice of Pediatric Oncology,* 4th ed. Philadelphia, Lippincott Williams & Wilkins, 2002, pp 973–1016.

Gorlick R, Anderson P, Andrulis I, et al: Biology of childhood osteogenic sarcoma and potential targets for therapeutic development: meeting summary. *Clin Cancer Res* 2003;9:5442–5453.

Grier H, Krailo M, Tarbell N, et al: Addition of ifosfamide and etoposide to standard chemotherapy for Ewing's sarcoma and primitive neuroectodermal tumor of bone. *N Engl J Med* 2003;348:694–701.

Grier RJ: Surgical options for children with osteosarcoma. *Lancet Oncol* 2005;6:85–92.

Kneisl JS, Simon MA: Medical management compared with operative treatment for osteoid osteoma. *J Bone Joint Surg Am* 1992;74:179–185.

Marina N, Gebhardt M, Teot L, et al: Biology and therapeutic advances for pediatric osteosarcoma. *Oncologist* 2004;9:422–441.

Rodriguez-Galindo C, Sount SL, Pappo AS: Treatment of Ewing sarcoma family of tumors: Current status and outlook for the future. *Med Pediatr Oncol* 2003;40:276–287.

Schmale GA, Conrad EU III, Raskind WH: The natural history of hereditary multiple exostoses. *J Bone Joint Surg Am* 1994;76:986–992.

Chapter 502 ■ Retinoblastoma

Cynthia E. Herzog

EPIDEMIOLOGY. Retinoblastoma occurs at a rate of 3.7 cases per million in the USA, with no racial or gender predilection. Overall, about 60% of cases are unilateral and nonhereditary, 15% are unilateral and hereditary, and 25% are bilateral and hereditary. Bilateral involvement at presentation is found in 42% of cases <1 yr of age, 21% of cases in children who are 1 yr of age, and less commonly in children presenting at older ages.

The hereditary form is associated with inactivation of the **retinoblastoma gene (RB1),** which is located on chromosome 13q14 and encodes the **retinoblastoma protein (pRb),** a tumor suppressor protein that controls cell-cycle phase transition and has roles in apoptosis and cell differentiation. Many types of mutations have been found, including translocations, deletions, insertions, point mutations, and epigenetic mutations such as hypermethylation of the promoter region. The nature of the predisposing mutation affects the penetrance and expressivity of retinoblastoma development. Hereditary cases usually are multifocal and bilateral, whereas nonhereditary cases tend to have unilateral, unifocal involvement.

According to the "two-hit" model of oncogenesis, two mutational events are required for tumor development (see Chapter 492). In the inherited form of retinoblastoma, the first mutation in the RB1 gene is inherited through germinal cells and a second mutation occurs subsequently in somatic retinal cells. Second mutations that lead to retinoblastoma often result in the loss of the normal allele and concomitant loss of heterozygosity. Many children with heritable retinoblastoma have new germinal mutations, and both parents are normal. Heterozygous carriers of oncogenic RB1 mutations demonstrate variable phenotypic expression. In the nonhereditary form of retinoblastoma, the two mutations occur in somatic retinal cells.

PATHOGENESIS. Histologically, retinoblastoma appears as a small round blue cell tumor with rosette formation. It may arise in any of the nucleated layers of the retina, exhibits various degrees of differentiation, and tends to outgrow its blood supply, resulting in necrosis and calcification.

Endophytic tumors arise from the inner surface of the retina, grow into the vitreous, and may result in **vitreous seeding** to other areas of the retina. Exophytic tumors grow from the outer retinal layer and may cause retinal detachment. These tumors can spread by direct extension to the choroid or along the optic nerve beyond the lamina cribrosa, or by hematogenous or lymphatic spread to distant sites.

CLINICAL MANIFESTATIONS. Only about 10% of retinoblastomas are detected by routine ophthalmologic screening in the context of a positive family history. Retinoblastoma classically presents with **leukocoria,** a white pupillary reflex (Fig. 502-1), which often is first noticed when a red reflex is not present at routine newborn or well-child examination or in a flash photograph of the child. Strabismus often is the initial presenting complaint. Orbital inflammation, hyphema, or pupil irregularity occurs with advancing disease. Pain usually is a feature if secondary glaucoma is present.

DIAGNOSIS. The diagnosis is established by the characteristic ophthalmologic findings. Biopsy is contraindicated. Evaluation usually requires an examination under general anesthesia by an ophthalmologist to obtain complete visualization of both eyes, which also facilitates photographing and mapping of the tumors. Retinal detachment or vitreous hemorrhage can complicate the evaluation.

Orbital ultrasonography and CT or MRI are used to evaluate the extent of intraocular disease and extraocular spread. Occasionally, a pineal area tumor is detected, a phenomenon known as **trilateral retinoblastoma.** MRI allows for better evaluation of optic nerve involvement. Bone scan, cerebrospinal fluid evaluation, and bone marrow evaluation are required only if indicated by other clinical, laboratory, or imaging findings.

The **differential diagnosis** includes hyperplastic primary vitreous, Coats disease, cataract, visceral larva migrans, choroidal coloboma, and retinopathy of prematurity.

TREATMENT. Treatment is determined by the size and location of the tumor. The primary goal is cure; the secondary goal is preserving vision. As newer modalities for local control of intraocular tumor and more effective systemic chemotherapy have emerged, primary enucleation is being performed less often.

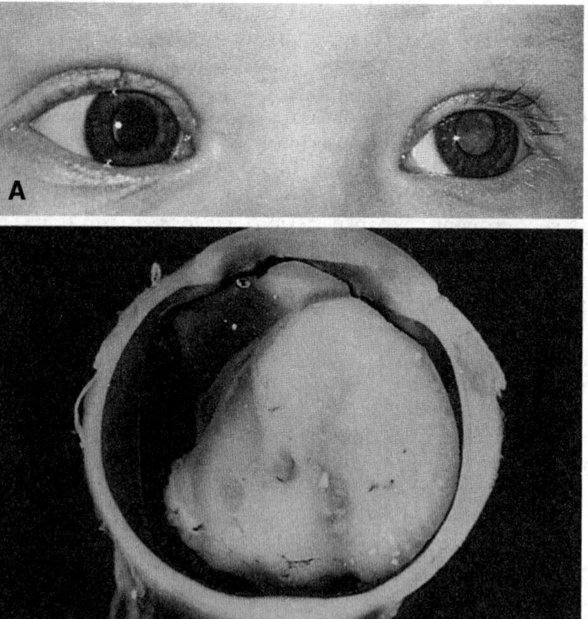

Figure 502-1. *A,* Leukocoria noted in the left eye of a child presenting with retinoblastoma. *B,* A large white tumor mass noted within the posterior chamber of the enucleated eye. (From Shields JA, Shields CL: Current management of retinoblastoma. *Mayo Clin Proc* 1994;69:50–56.)

Most unilateral disease presents as a solitary, large tumor. Enucleation is performed if there is no potential for useful vision. With bilateral disease, chemoreduction in combination with **focal therapy** (laser photocoagulation or cryotherapy) has replaced the traditional approach of enucleation of the more severely affected eye and irradiation of the remaining eye. If feasible, small tumors can be treated with focal therapy with careful follow-up for evidence of recurrence or new tumor growth. Larger tumors often respond to multiagent chemotherapy including carboplatin, vincristine, and etoposide. If this approach fails, external-beam irradiation should be considered, although this approach may result in significant orbital deformity and increased incidence of second malignancies in patients with germ line mutations. Brachytherapy, or episcleral plaque radiotherapy, if feasible, is an alternative with less morbidity. Enucleation may be required for unresponsive or recurrent tumors.

All first-degree relatives of children with retinoblastoma should have retinal examinations to identify retinomas or retinal scars, which may suggest a predisposition to retinoblastoma even though malignant retinoblastoma did not develop.

PROGNOSIS. Approximately 95% of retinoblastomas in the USA, where extraocular extension rarely is seen, are cured. Current efforts using chemotherapy in combination with focal therapy are intended to preserve useful vision and avoid irradiation or enucleation. Routine ophthalmologic examinations should continue until about 6 yr of age to detect new lesions. The prognosis for patients with metastases is poor.

Children with germ line RB1 mutations are at significant risk for development of second malignancies, especially osteosarcoma and also soft tissue sarcomas and malignant melanoma. The risk of cancers of the brain, nasal cavities, and eye and orbit is further increased by the use of radiation therapy. Other radiation-related late adverse effects include cataracts, orbital growth deformities, lacrimal dysfunction, and late retinal vascular injury.

Abramson DH, Schefler AC: Update on retinoblastoma. *Retina* 2004;24:828–848.
Classon M, Harlow E: The retinoblastoma tumour suppressor in development and cancer. *Nat Rev Cancer* 2002:2:910–917.
Kleinerman R, Tucker MA, Tarone RF, et al: Risk of new cancers after radiotherapy in long-term survivors of retinoblastoma: An extended follow-up. *J Clin Oncol* 2005;23:2272–2279.
Lohman DR, Gallie BL: Retinoblastoma: Revisiting the model prototype of inherited cancer. *Am J Med Genet C (Semin Med Genet)* 2004;129:23–28.
Richter S, Vandezande K, Chen N, et al: Sensitive and efficient detection of *RB1* gene mutations enhances care of families with retinoblastoma. *Am J Hum Genet* 2003;72:253–269.
Rodriguez-Galindo C, Wilson MW, Haik BG, et al: Treatment of metastatic retinoblastoma. *Ophthalmology* 2003;110:1237–1240.

Chapter 503 ■ Gonadal and Germ Cell Neoplasms

Cynthia E. Herzog

EPIDEMIOLOGY. Malignant germ cell tumors (GCTs) and gonadal tumors are rare, with an incidence of 12 cases per million persons <20 yr of age. Most malignant tumors of the gonads in children are GCTs. The incidence varies according to age and sex. Sacrococcygeal tumors occur predominantly in infant girls. Testicular GCTs occur predominantly before age 4 yr and after puberty. Testicular GCTs occur much more often in whites than in blacks, whereas ovarian GCTs have a slight predominance in blacks. Klinefelter syndrome is associated with an increased risk of mediastinal GCTs; Down syndrome, undescended testes, infertility, testicular atrophy and inguinal hernias are associated with an increased risk of testicular cancer. The risk of testicular GCT is increased in first-degree relatives, and is highest among monozygotic twins.

PATHOGENESIS. The GCTs and non-GCTs arise from primordial germ cells and coelomic epithelium, respectively. Testicular and sacrococcygeal GCTs arising during early childhood characteristically have deletions at chromosome arms 1p and 6q and gains at 1q, and lack the isochromosome 12p that is highly characteristic of malignant GCTs of adults. Testicular GCT also may demonstrate loss of imprinting. Because GCTs may contain benign and malignant elements in different areas of the tumor, extensive sectioning is essential to confirm the correct diagnosis. The many histologically distinct subtypes of GCTs include teratoma (mature and immature), endodermal sinus tumor, and embryonal carcinoma (Fig. 503-1). Non-GCTs of the ovary include epithelial (serous and mucinous) and sex cord/stromal tumors; non-GCTs of the testicle include sex cord/stromal tumors (e.g., Leydig cell, Sertoli cell).

CLINICAL MANIFESTATIONS AND DIAGNOSIS. The clinical presentation of germ cell neoplasms depends on location. Ovarian

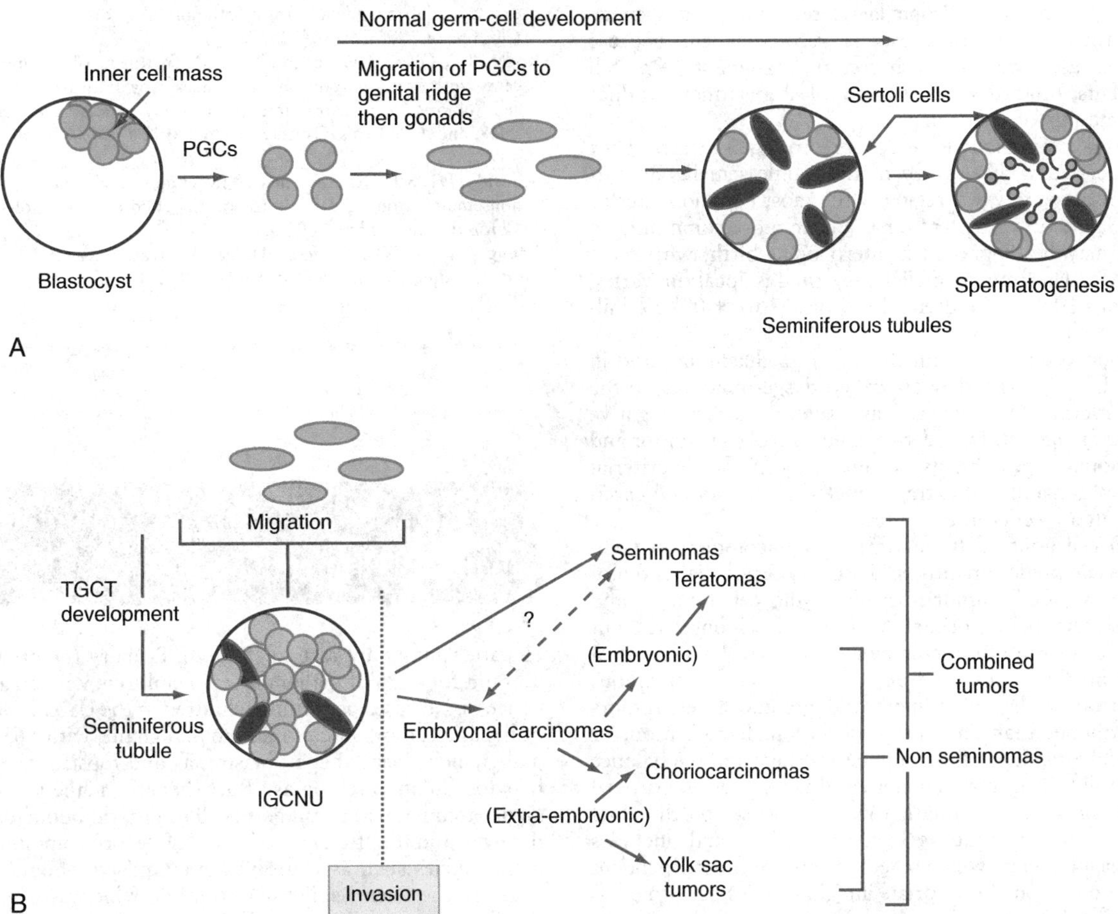

Figure 503-1. *A*, Normal germ cell development. *B*, Model for the origin and histogenesis of different subtypes of testicular germ cell tumors. IGCNU, intratubular germ cell neoplasia unclassified; PGC, primary germ cell; TGCT, testicular germ cell tumor(s).

tumors often are quite large by the time they are diagnosed. Extragonadal GCTs occur in the midline, including the suprasellar region, pineal region, neck, mediastinum, and retroperitoneal and sacrococcygeal areas. Symptoms relate to mass effect, but the intracranial GCTs often present with anterior and posterior pituitary deficits (see Chapter 497).

The **serum α-fetoprotein (AFP)** level is elevated with endodermal sinus tumors and may be minimally elevated with teratomas. Infants have higher levels of AFP, which fall to normal adult levels by about 8 mo; therefore, high AFP levels must be interpreted with caution in this age group. Elevation of the β subunit of **human chorionic gonadotropin (β-hCG)** is seen with choriocarcinoma and germinomas. Lactate dehydrogenase (LDH), although nonspecific, may be a useful marker. If elevated, these markers provide important confirmation of the diagnosis and provide a means to monitor the patient for tumor response and recurrence. Both serum and cerebrospinal fluid should be assayed for these markers in patients with intracranial lesions.

Diagnosis begins with physical examination and imaging studies, including plain radiographs of the chest and ultrasonography of the abdomen. CT or MRI can further delineate the primary tumor. If germ cell malignancy is strongly suggested, preoperative staging with CT of the chest and bone scan is appropriate. Primary surgical resection is indicated for tumors deemed resectable. The exception is intracranial lesions, where the diagnosis can be established with imaging and AFP or β-hCG determinations.

Gonadoblastomas often occur in patients with gonadal dysgenesis and all or parts of a Y chromosome. Gonadal dysgenesis is characterized by failure to fully masculinize the external genitalia. If this syndrome is diagnosed, imaging of the gonad with ultrasonography or CT is performed, and surgical resection of the tumor usually is curative. Prophylactic resection of dysgenetic gonads at the time of diagnosis is recommended, because gonadoblastomas, some of which contain malignant germ cell tumor elements, often develop. Gonadoblastomas may produce abnormal amounts of estrogen.

Teratomas occur in many locations, presenting as masses. They are not associated with elevated markers unless malignancy is present. The sacrococcygeal region is the most common site for teratomas. Sacrococcygeal teratomas occur most commonly in infants and may be diagnosed in utero or at birth, with most found in girls. The rate of malignancy in this location varies, ranging from <10% in children <2 mo of age to >50% in children >4 mo of age.

Germinomas occur intracranially, in the mediastinum, and in the gonads. In the ovary, they are called **dysgerminomas;** in the testis, **seminomas.** They usually are tumor marker negative despite being malignant. Endodermal sinus or yolk sac tumor and choriocarcinoma appear highly malignant by histologic criteria. Both occur at gonadal and extragonadal sites. Embryonal carcinoma most often occurs in the testes.

Non-germ cell gonadal tumors are very uncommon in pediatrics and occur predominantly in the ovary. Epithelial carcinomas (usually an adult tumor), Sertoli-Leydig cell tumors, and granulosa cell tumors may occur in children. Carcinomas account for about $^{1}/_{3}$ of ovarian tumors in females <20 yr of age; most of these occur in older teens and are of the serous or mucinous subtype. Sertoli-Leydig cell tumors and granulosa cell tumors produce hormones that can cause virilization, feminization, or precocious puberty, depending on pubertal stage and the balance between Sertoli (estrogen production) and Leydig cells (androgen production). Diagnostic evaluation usually focuses on the chief complaint of inappropriate sex steroid effect and includes hormone measurements, which reflect gonadotropin-independent sex steroid production. Appropriate imaging also is performed to rule out a functioning gonadal tumor. Surgery usually is curative. No effective therapy for nonresectable disease has been found.

TREATMENT. Complete surgical excision of the tumor usually is indicated, except for patients with intracranial tumors, where the primary therapy consists of radiation therapy and chemotherapy. For testicular tumors, an inguinal approach is indicated. When complete excision cannot be accomplished, preoperative chemotherapy is indicated, with second-look surgery. For teratomas, both mature and immature, and completely resected malignant tumors, surgery alone is the treatment. Cisplatin-based chemotherapy regimens usually are curative in GCTs that cannot be completely resected, even if metastases are present. Except for GCTs of the central nervous system, radiation therapy is limited to those tumors that are not amenable to complete excision and are refractory to chemotherapy.

PROGNOSIS. The overall cure rate for children with GCTs is >80%. Age is the most predictive factor of survival for extragonadal GCTs. Children >12 yr of age have a 4-fold higher risk of death, and a 6-fold higher risk if the tumor is thoracic. Histology has little effect on prognosis. Nonresected extragonadal GCTs have a slightly worse prognosis.

Cushing B, Giller R, Cullen JW, et al: Randomized comparison of combination chemotherapy with etoposide, bleomycin, and either high-dose or standard-dose cisplatin in children and adolescents with high risk malignant germ cell tumors: A pediatric intergroup study—Pediatric Oncology Group 9049 and Children's Cancer Group 8882. *J Clin Oncol* 2004;22:2691–2700.

Horwich A, Shipley J, Huddart R: Testicular germ-cell cancer. *Lancet* 2006;367:754–764.

Marina N, London WB, Frazier L, et al: Prognostic factors in children with extragonadal malignant germ cell tumors: A pediatric intergroup study. *J Clin Oncol* 2006;24:2544–2548.

Rogers PC, Olson TA, Cullen JW, et al: Treatment of children and adolescents with stage I testicular and stages I or II ovarian malignant germ cell tumors: A pediatric intergroup study—Pediatric Oncology Group 9048 and Children's Cancer Group 8891. *J Clin Oncol* 2004;22:563–569.

Schneider DT, Schuster AE, Fritsch MK, et al: Genetic analysis of mediastinal nonseminomatous germ cell tumors in children and adolescents. *Genes Chromosomes Cancer* 2002;3:115–125.

Young JL, Wu XC, Roffers SD, et al: Ovarian cancer in children and young adults in the United States, 1992–1997. *Cancer* 2003;97:2694–2700.

Chapter 504 ■ Neoplasms of the Liver

Cynthia E. Herzog

Hepatic tumors are rare in children. Primary tumors of the liver account for ≈1% of malignancies in children, with an annual incidence of 1.6 cases per million children in the USA. From 50–60% of hepatic tumors in children are malignant, with >65% of these malignancies being hepatoblastomas and most of the remainder hepatocellular carcinomas. Rare hepatic malignancies include angiosarcoma, malignant germ cell tumor, rhabdomyosarcoma of the liver, and undifferentiated sarcoma. More common childhood malignancies such as neuroblastoma and lymphoma can metastasize to the liver. Benign liver tumors, which usually present in the first 6 mo of life, include hemangiomas, hamartomas, and hemangioendotheliomas.

HEPATOBLASTOMA

EPIDEMIOLOGY. Hepatoblastoma occurs predominantly in children <3 yr of age. The etiology is unknown. Hepatoblastomas are associated with familial adenomatous polyposis. Alterations in the antigen-presenting cell (APC)/β-catenin pathway have been found in most of the tumors evaluated. Hepatoblastoma also is associated with Beckwith-Wiedemann syndrome, which can show a similar loss of genomic imprinting of the insulin-like growth factor-2 gene. Low birthweight is associated with increased incidence of hepatoblastoma, with the risk increasing as birthweight decreases.

PATHOGENESIS. Hepatoblastoma can be epithelial type, containing fetal or embryonal malignant cells (either as a mixture or as pure elements), or the mixed type, containing mesenchymal and epithelial elements. Pure fetal histology predicts a more favorable outcome.

CLINICAL MANIFESTATIONS. Hepatoblastoma usually presents as a large, asymptomatic abdominal mass. It arises from the right lobe 3 times more often than the left and usually is unifocal. As the disease progresses, weight loss, anorexia, vomiting, and abdominal pain may ensue. Metastatic spread of hepatoblastoma most commonly involves regional lymph nodes and the lungs.

A valuable serum tumor marker, **α-fetoprotein (AFP)**, is used in the diagnosis and monitoring of hepatic tumors. AFP level is elevated in almost all hepatoblastomas. Bilirubin and liver enzymes usually are normal. Anemia is common, and thrombocytosis occurs in about $^1/_3$ of patients. Hepatitis B and C serology should be obtained but usually are negative in hepatoblastoma.

Diagnostic imaging should include plain radiographs and ultrasonography of the abdomen to characterize the hepatic mass. Ultrasonography can differentiate malignant hepatic masses from benign vascular lesions. Either CT or MRI is an accurate method of defining the extent of intrahepatic tumor involvement and the potential for surgical resection. Evaluation for metastatic disease should include CT of the chest and bone scan.

TREATMENT. In general, the cure of malignant hepatic tumors in children depends on complete resection of the primary tumor (Fig. 504-1). As much as 85% of the liver can be resected, with hepatic regeneration noted within 3–4 mo after surgery. Cisplatin in combination with vincristine and 5-fluorouracil or doxorubicin is effective treatment for hepatoblastoma and increases the chances of cure after complete surgical resection. In low-stage tumors, survival rates >90% can be achieved with multimodal treatment, including surgery and adjuvant chemotherapy. With tumors unresectable at diagnosis, survival rates of approximately 60% can be obtained. Metastatic disease further reduces survival, but complete regression of disease often can be obtained with chemotherapy and surgical resection of the primary tumor and isolated pulmonary metastatic disease, resulting in survival rates of about 25%. Liver transplant is a viable option for unresectable primary hepatic malignancies and results in good long-term survival. Pretransplant medical condition is an important predictor of outcome, and thus transplant is much more effective as the primary surgery than as salvage therapy.

HEPATOCELLULAR CARCINOMA

EPIDEMIOLOGY. Hepatocellular carcinoma occurs mostly in adolescents and often is associated with hepatitis B or C infection. It is more common in East Asia and other areas where hepatitis B is endemic, and is already showing decreased incidence following the introduction of hepatitis B vaccination. In these areas it also tends to occur in a bimodal pattern, with the younger age peak overlapping the age of hepatoblastoma presentation. It also occurs in the chronic form of hereditary tyrosinemia, galactosemia, glycogen storage disease, α_1-antitrypsin deficiency, and biliary cirrhosis. Aflatoxin B contamination of food is another risk factor.

PATHOGENESIS. Hepatocellular carcinoma usually presents as a multicentric, invasive tumor consisting of large pleomorphic cells with a lack of underlying cirrhosis. The fibrolamellar variant of hepatocellular carcinoma occurs more often in adolescent and young adult patients. Although previous reports have suggested that the fibrolamellar type has a better prognosis, more recent data analysis refutes this.

CLINICAL MANIFESTATIONS. Hepatocellular carcinoma usually presents as a hepatic mass, abdominal distention, and symptoms of anorexia, weight loss, and abdominal pain. Hepatocellular carcinoma can present as an acute abdominal crisis with rupture of the tumor and hemoperitoneum. The AFP level is elevated in approximately 60% of children with hepatocellular carcinoma. Evidence of hepatitis B and C infection usually is found in endemic areas, but not in Western countries or with the fibrolamellar type. Bilirubin usually is normal, but liver enzymes may be abnormal.

Diagnostic imaging should include plain radiographs and ultrasonography of the abdomen to characterize the hepatic mass. Ultrasonography can differentiate malignant hepatic masses from benign vascular lesions. Either CT or MRI is an accurate method of defining the extent of intrahepatic tumor involvement and the potential for surgical resection. Evaluation for metastatic disease should include CT of the chest and bone scan.

TREATMENT. Because of the multicentric origin of hepatocellular carcinoma, complete resection of this tumor is accomplished in only 30–40% of cases. Even with complete surgical resection, only 30% of children are long-term survivors. Chemotherapy, including cisplatin, doxorubicin, etoposide, and 5-fluorouracil, has shown some activity against this tumor, but improved long-term outcome has been difficult to achieve. Other techniques such as chemoembolization and liver transplantation are under study as therapy for hepatocellular carcinomas.

Austin MT, Leys CM, Feurer ID, et al: Liver transplantation for childhood hepatic malignancy: A review of the United Network for Organ Sharing (UNOS) database. *J Pediatr Surg* 2006;41:182–186.

Darbari A, Sabin KM, Shapiro CN, et al: Epidemiology of primary hepatic malignancies in U.S. children. *Hepatology* 2003;38:560–566.

Katzenstein HM, Krailo MD, Malogolowkin MH, et al: Hepatocellular carcinoma in children and adolescents: Results from the Pediatric Oncology Group and Children's Cancer Group Intergroup Study. *J Clin Oncol* 2002;20:2789–2797.

Katzenstein HM, Krailo MD, Malogolowkin MH, et al: Fibrolamellar hepatocellular carcinoma in children and adolescents. *Cancer* 2003;97:2006–2012.

Llovet JM, Burroughs A, Bruix J: Hepatocellular carcinoma. *Lancet* 2003;362:1907–1916.

Otte JB, Pritchard J, Aronson DC, et al: Liver transplantation for hepatoblastoma: Results from the International Society of Pediatric Oncology (SIOP) study SIOPEL-1 and review of the world experience. *Pediatr Blood Cancer* 2004;42:74–83.

Schnater JM, Kohler SE, Lamers WH, et al: Where do we stand with hepatoblastoma? A review. *Cancer* 2003;98:668–678.

Tiao GM, Bobey N, Allen S, et al: The current management of hepatoblastoma: A combination of chemotherapy, conventional resection, and liver transplantation. *J Pediatr* 2005;146:204–211.

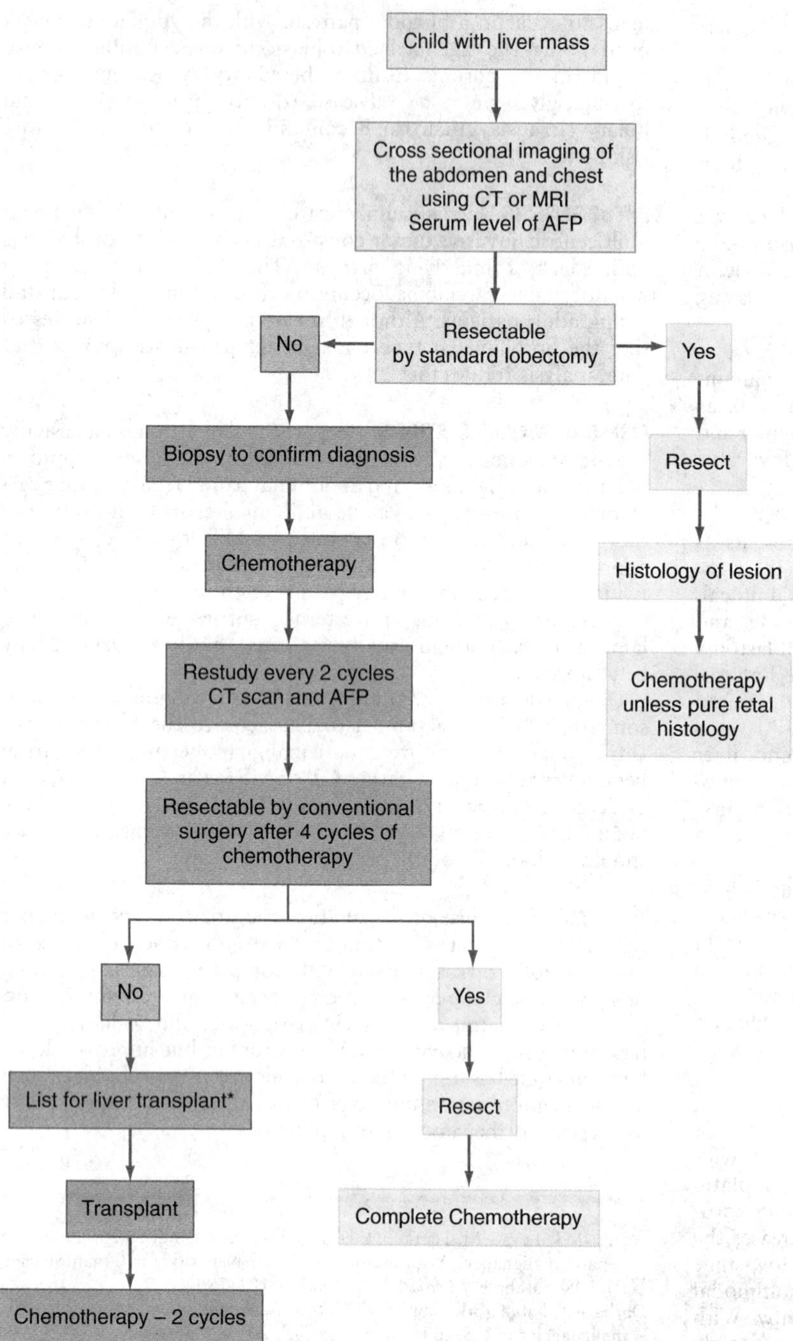

Figure 504-1. Algorithm for the management of a child who presents with a hepatoblastoma. AFP, α-fetoprotein. (From Tiao GM, Bobey N, Allen S, et al: The current management of hepatoblastoma: A combination of chemotherapy, conventional resection, and liver transplantation. *J Pediatr* 2005;146:204–211.)

Chapter 505 ■ Benign Vascular Tumors

Cynthia E. Herzog

505.1 • Hemangiomas

Hemangiomas, the most common benign tumors of infancy, occur in about 10% of term infants (see Chapter 649). The risk of hemangioma is 3–5 times higher in girls than boys. The risk is doubled in premature infants and 10 times higher in offspring of women who had chorionic villus sampling. Hemangiomas can be present at birth but usually arise shortly after birth and grow rapidly during the first year of life, with slowing of growth in the next 5 yr and involution by 10–15 yr of age.

CLINICAL MANIFESTATIONS. More than ½ of all hemangiomas are located in the head and neck region. Most are solitary lesions, but the presence of more than one cutaneous lesion increases the likelihood of visceral hemangiomas. The liver is the primary site of visceral involvement; other involved organs include the brain, intestines, and lung. Most hemangiomas require no therapy, but approximately 10% of hemangiomas cause significant impairment and 1% are life-threatening because of their location. Hemangiomas around the airway can cause airway obstruction, and those around the eyes can result in loss of vision. Ulceration is a common complication and can lead to secondary infection. Large hepatic hemangiomas or hemangioendotheliomas may result in hepatomegaly, anemia, thrombocytopenia, and high-output heart failure.

Kasabach-Merritt syndrome is characterized by a rapidly enlarging lesion, thrombocytopenia, microangiopathic hemolytic anemia, and coagulopathy as a result of platelet and red blood cell trapping and activation of the clotting system within the vasculature of the hemangioma. This syndrome has been shown to be associated with kaposiform hemangioendotheliomas or tufted hemangiomas.

Cutaneous lesions usually can be diagnosed by typical appearance and rapid proliferation. Segmental hemangiomas, or those with geographic localization and some plaquelike features, recently have been shown to have a higher risk of complications and association with developmental abnormalities. A deep lesion may require imaging studies to help differentiate it from a lymphangioma. The presence of a midline hemangioma in the lumbosacral area indicates the need for an MRI to search for underlying asymptomatic neurologic abnormalities. Location also may dictate the need for an ophthalmologic or surgical consultation. An ultrasonographic scan or MRI of the liver should be performed if multiple cutaneous lesions are present.

TREATMENT. Most hemangiomas require no specific therapy beyond reassurance of the parents. For hemangiomas that are life-threatening or that threaten vital functions such as eyesight, treatment is warranted. Prednisone (1–3 mg/kg/day PO) typically is the initial therapy; higher doses or intralesional corticosteroids sometimes are used. Approximately 30% of hemangiomas respond dramatically to corticosteroids and begin to regress within 1 wk; 40% of hemangiomas stabilize or show minimal response; and the remaining tumors do not respond. Interferon (IFN)-α (1–3 MU/m^2/day) also has been used as initial therapy and in patients who do not respond to corticosteroid therapy. Although response rates of up to 70% have been reported, the risk of neurologic adverse effects in 10–20% of patients necessitates caution in using IFN-α. Laser therapy has been used in some situations.

Treatment of patients with Kasabach-Merritt syndrome usually consists of supportive care while also beginning therapy with corticosteroids or IFN-α. Heparin therapy is contraindicated, and platelet transfusions should be avoided in the absence of life-threatening hemorrhage, because they may exacerbate the bleeding. The use of aminocaproic acid or tranexamic acid may be beneficial. Failure to respond to therapy warrants the use of less conventional treatments, such as irradiation, embolization, or surgical resection.

Bruckner AL, Frieden IJ: Hemangiomas of infancy. *J Am Acad Dermatol* 2003;48:477–496.

Chiller KG, Passaro D, Frieden IJ: Hemangiomas of infancy: Clinical characteristics, morphologic subtypes, and their relationship to race, ethnicity, and sex. *Arch Dermatol* 2002;138:1567–1576.

505.2 • Lymphangiomas and Cystic Hygromas

Lymphatic malformations, including lymphangiomas and cystic hygromas, which arise in the embryonic lymph sac, are the second most common benign vascular tumors in children. About half are located in the head and neck area. Approximately 50% are present at birth, with most presenting by 2 yr of age. There is no gender predisposition. Spontaneous regression has been reported but is not typical.

Lymphatic malformations present as soft, painless masses that transilluminate if superficial. Intrathoracic lymphatic malformation can present as symptoms related to a mediastinal mass or pericardial or pleural effusion. Rapid enlargement can occur with infection or hemorrhage. Localized lesions may be surgically resected, but this can be difficult, owing to their infiltrative nature. Recurrence is common with incompletely resected lesions. Aspiration can provide temporary relief in an emergency, such as in the presence of dyspnea, but reaccumulation will occur. Treatment by injection of sclerosing agents, laser therapy, and systemic IFN therapy also has been used. The streptococcal immunotherapeutic agent OK-432 (Picibanil) is the sclerosing agent of choice, avoiding the need for surgery in most cases. It appears to be especially effective for the treatment of macrocystic lymphangiomas of the head and neck.

Brewis C, Pracy JP, Albert DM: Treatment of lymphangiomas of the head and neck in children by intralesional injection of OK-432 (Picibanil). *Clin Otolaryngol* 2000;25:130–134.

Giguere CM, Bauman NM, Sato Y, et al: Treatment of lymphangiomas with OK-432 (Picibanil) sclerotherapy: A prospective multi-institutional trial. *Arch Otolaryngol Head Neck Surg* 2002;128:1137–1144.

Chapter 506 ■ Rare Tumors

Cynthia E. Herzog

506.1 • Thyroid Tumors

The incidence of thyroid cancer in patients <20 yr of age in the USA is 4.9 cases per million. Most thyroid cancers in this age group occur among adolescent females (see Chapter 570). Thyroid cancer is about 4 times more common in females than males and 2.5 times more common in whites than blacks. The greatest risk factor for thyroid cancer is prior radiation exposure, especially following head and neck irradiation. Thyroid cancer accounts for about 10% of second malignancies among cancer survivors, especially survivors of Hodgkin lymphoma, due to treatment not only with radiation but also with alkylating agents. Almost all are differentiated carcinomas (papillary or follicular). Medullary thyroid carcinoma (MTC) may occur in familial cases, especially with **multiple endocrine neoplasia** (MEN type 2). In MEN type 2a, MTC usually occurs in older children or adults and may be associated with pheochromocytoma and parathyroid hyperplasia. MEN type 2b is associated with onset of MTC at a very early age. Other findings of MEN 2b include mucosal neuromas and marfanoid habitus. MEN type 2 is associated with mutations in the *RET* proto-oncogene, whereas genetic translocations involving *RET* are found in about half of pediatric thyroid cancers with differentiated histology. Patients with a family history of MTC should undergo genetic testing and prophylactic total thyroidectomy. Specific *RET* mutations are associated with specific disease phenotypes and risk of developing MTC at an earlier age. Therefore, the age at which thyroidectomy is performed depends on the specific RET mutation, but it should be done before age 2 yr in patients with MEN 2b. The patient will then require lifelong thyroid hormone replacement therapy.

Patients present with a thyroid mass and/or cervical lymphadenopathy; symptoms related to abnormal hormone levels are rare. About 20% of thyroid nodules in young children are malignant, compared with about 10% in adolescents and adults. Fine-needle aspiration (FNA) commonly is used to assess thyroid nodules in adults, but the use of FNA in the pediatric population has not been firmly established, especially in preadolescent patients; surgical resection of nodules is recommended for these patients. Evaluation should include determination of thyroid hormone levels, thyroid scan, chest radiography, and CT of the chest. Total thyroidectomy for disease confined to one lobe has been controversial in pediatrics owing to good prognosis and the risk of complications such as hypoparathyroidism. However, total or near-total thyroidectomy reduces the risk of local recurrence. Routine lymph node dissection is not indicated, but should be done if cervical lymph nodes are involved. Treatment with iodine 131 is then used to eradicate residual disease and treat pulmonary metastases, which occur in 6–10% of cases. Pulmonary metastases are best detected with radioiodine after resection of bulk disease.

Hung W, Sarlis NJ: Current controversies in the management of pediatric patients with well-differentiated nonmedullary thyroid cancer: A review. *Thyroid* 2002;12:683–702.

Machens A, Holzhausen H-j, Thanh PN, et al: Malignant progression from C-cell hyperplasia to medullary thyroid carcinoma in 167 carriers of RET germline mutations. *Surgery* 203;134:425–31.

Sherman SI: Thyroid carcinoma. *Lancet* 2003;361:501–510.

Szinnai G, Meier C, Komminoth P, et al: Review of multiple endocrine neoplasia type 2A in children: Therapeutic results of early thyroidectomy and prognostic value of codon analysis. *Pediatrics* 203;111:e132–e139.

506.2 • Melanoma

The incidence of melanoma in persons <20 yr of age in the USA is 4.2 cases per million, with almost all of these cases occurring in adolescents (see Chapter 650). Melanoma is more common among adolescent females than males. Incident rates of melanoma in younger age groups have remained stable in the USA, but the incidence is rapidly increasing in adults. Although sun exposure is a well-known risk factor for melanoma in adults, its role in pediatric melanoma is less clear. Pediatricians should counsel patients regarding avoidance of sun exposure to decrease the risk of later development of melanoma. Patients with fair skin and a family history of melanoma are at particularly high risk. Known risk factors for children are giant hairy nevus (>20 cm), dysplastic nevus syndrome, and xeroderma pigmentosum.

Findings of a rapidly enlarging nevus that is dark, has changed colors, has irregular borders, or bleeds easily should raise a concern of melanoma. However, many of the melanomas diagnosed in children have none of these features. Diagnosis is based on pathology. However, extra care must be taken in the diagnosis of melanoma in children because making the distinction from other lesions, particularly Spitz nevus, can be difficult.

Treatment recommendations are based on adult data. The primary treatment is local excision with lymph node mapping and sentinel node biopsy for all but the most superficial melanomas. If the sentinel node is positive, a formal lymph node dissection is recommended. High-dose adjuvant interferon has shown some efficacy in the treatment of adult melanoma, while chemotherapy in combination with biologic agents and vaccine therapy has been used for treatment of distant metastases. Whether the outcome is better for children than adults is unclear.

Mones JM, Ackerman AB: Melanomas in prepubescent children: Review comprehensively, critique historically, criteria diagnostically, and course biologically. *Am J Dermatopathol* 2003;25:223–238.

Pappo AS: Melanoma in children and adolescents. *Eur J Cancer* 2003;39: 2651–2661.

506.3 • Nasopharyngeal Carcinoma

Nasopharyngeal carcinoma is rare in the pediatric population, but is one of the most common nasopharyngeal tumors in pediatric patients. In adults, the incidence is highest in South China, but it is also high among the Inuit people and in North Africa and Northeast India. In China, it is rare in the pediatric population, but in other populations a substantial proportion of cases occur in the pediatric age group, primarily in adolescents. It occurs in males twice as often as in females and is more common in blacks. In the pediatric population the tumors are more commonly of undifferentiated histology and associated with Epstein-Barr virus (EBV). Nasopharyngeal carcinoma has been associated with specific HLA types.

Most pediatric patients present with advanced locoregional disease manifesting as cervical lymphadenopathy. Epistaxis, trismus, and cranial nerve deficits also may be present. The diagnosis is established from biopsy of the nasopharynx or cervical lymph nodes. In most cases the lactate dehydrogenase level is elevated, but this finding is nonspecific. CT or MRI evaluation of the head and neck is performed to determine the extent of locoregional disease. Chest radiography, CT, bone scan, and liver scan are used to evaluate for metastatic disease. Monitoring EBV IgA and ZEBRA (antibodies to the Epstein-Barr virus Bam H1Z transactivator protein) protein levels also may be useful.

Treatment is a combination of chemotherapy and irradiation. Cisplatin-based chemotherapy is given before or concurrent with irradiation. The outcome depends on the extent of disease; patients with distant metastases have a very poor prognosis. The use on intensity-modulated radiation therapy (IMRT) has improved local control and reduced the late adverse effects associated with radiation therapy, including hormonal dysfunction, dental caries, fibrosis, and second malignancies.

Ayan I, Kaytan E, Ayan N: Childhood nasopharyngeal carcinoma: From biology to treatment. *Lancet Oncol* 2003;4:13–21.

Tsao SW, Lo KW, Huang DP: Nasopharyngeal carcinoma. In Tselis A, Jenson HB (editors): *Epstein-Barr Virus*. New York, Taylor and Francis, 2006, pp 273–295.

506.4 • Adenocarcinoma of the Colon and Rectum

Colorectal carcinoma is rare in the pediatric population. There is a male predominance in children, as compared with a female predominance in adults. Even in patients with predisposing conditions, such as familial adenomatous polyposis and Peutz-Jeghers syndrome, cancer usually does not present until adulthood, although genetic testing is available and screening should begin during childhood or adolescence.

Hereditary nonpolyposis colon cancer (HNPCC), an autosomal dominant disorder, may present with early-onset colon cancer as well as a predisposition to cancers in other tissues (e.g., ovarian, brain, renal, uterine). Germline mutations in DNA mismatch repair genes *(MMR)* cause DNA repair errors and microsatellite instability.

Presenting symptoms include bloody stools or melena, abdominal pain, weight loss, and changes in bowel patterns. Signs often are vague, often resulting in a delay in diagnosis and advanced disease. The histologic subtype differs from that seen in adults, with the majority of pediatric tumors being mucinous. Treatment consists of surgical resection when possible, with chemotherapy for unresectable tumors. Radiation therapy is useful in the treatment of rectal carcinomas.

Grady WM: Genetic testing for high-risk colon cancer patients. *Gastroenterology* 2003;124:1574–1594.

Marcos I, Borrego S, Urioste M, et al: Mutations in the DNA mismatch repair gene *MLH1* associated with early onset colon cancer. *J Pediatr* 2006;148: 837–839.

506.5 • Adrenocortical Carcinoma

Adrenocortical carcinoma is rare but is associated with the Li-Fraumeni and Beckwith-Wiedemann syndromes. Due to the rarity of adrenocortical carcinoma in children and the association with Li-Fraumeni syndrome, the diagnosis of adrenocortical carcinoma should prompt consultation for genetic testing. The tumor may occur at any age during childhood but is more common during the first few years of life, and more common in females. In Brazil, childhood adrenocortical carcinoma is 10 times more common than in the USA. Younger children typically present with virilization, whereas adolescents present either with no endocrine symptoms or with Cushing syndrome. Prognosis depends on tumor size, extent of tumor, and resectability. Although it does respond to mitotane- and cisplatin-based chemotherapy, the prognosis is poor for unresectable or metastatic disease.

Michalkiewicz E, Sandrini R, Figueiredo B, et al: Clinical and outcome characteristics of children with adrenocortical tumors: A report from the International Pediatric Adrenocortical Tumor Registry. *J Clin Oncol* 2004;5:838–845.

506.6 • Desmoplastic Small Round Cell Tumor

Desmoplastic small round cell tumor (DSRCT) is a recently recognized tumor that occurs predominantly in adolescent males. It is associated with a translocation between the Ewing tumor gene and the Wilms tumor gene, t(11;22)(p13;q12). Patients typically present with diffuse abdominal disease with no definitive primary, although disease outside the abdomen is possible. Aggressive treatment with surgery, chemotherapy, and radiation has resulted in almost universally poor outcome.

Gerald WL, Ladanyi M, de Alava E: Clinical, pathologic, and molecular spectrum of tumors associated with t(11;22)(p13;q12): Desmoplastic small round-cell tumor and its variants. *J Clin Oncol* 1998;16:3028–3036.

Chapter 507 ■ Histiocytosis Syndromes of Childhood

Stephan Ladisch

The childhood histiocytoses constitute a diverse group of disorders, which, although individually rare, may be severe in their clinical expression. These disorders are grouped together because they have in common a prominent proliferation or accumulation of cells of the monocyte-macrophage system of bone marrow origin. Although these disorders sometimes are difficult to distinguish clinically, accurate diagnosis is essential nevertheless for facilitating progress in treatment. A systematic classification of the childhood histiocytoses is based on histopathologic findings (Table 507-1). A thorough, comprehensive evaluation of a biopsy specimen obtained at the time of diagnosis is essential. This evaluation includes studies such as electron microscopy and immunostaining that may require special sample processing.

CLASSIFICATION AND PATHOLOGY. Three classes of childhood histiocytosis are recognized, based on histopathologic findings. The most well-known childhood histiocytosis, previously known as **histiocytosis X,** constitutes class I and includes the clinical entities of eosinophilic granuloma (see Chapter 501), **Hand-Schüller-Christian disease,** and **Letterer-Siwe disease.** The name **Langerhans' cell histiocytosis** (LCH) has been applied to the class I histiocytoses. The normal Langerhans' cell is an antigen-presenting cell (APC) of the skin. The hallmark of LCH in all forms is the presence of a clonal proliferation of cells of the monocyte lineage containing the characteristic electron microscopic findings of a Langerhans' cell. This is the **Birbeck granule,** a tennis racket–shaped bilamellar granule that, when seen in the cytoplasm of lesional cells in LCH, is diagnostic of the disease. The Birbeck granule expresses a newly characterized antigen, langerin (CD207), which is involved in antigen presentation to T lymphocytes. The definitive diagnosis of LCH also can be established by demonstrating CD1a-positivity of lesional cells, which now can be done using fixed tissue. The lesions may contain various proportions of these Langerhans' granule-containing cells, lymphocytes, granulocytes, monocytes, and eosinophils.

TABLE 507-1. Classification of the Childhood Histiocytoses

CLASS	DISEASE	CELLULAR CHARACTERISTICS OF LESIONS	TREATMENT
I	Langerhans' cell histiocytosis	Langerhans' cells (CD1a-positive) with Birbeck granules	Local therapy for isolated lesions; chemotherapy for disseminated disease
II	Familial erythrophagocytic lymphohistiocytosis* Infection-associated hemophagocytic syndrome†	Morphologically normal reactive macrophages with prominent erythrophagocytosis	Chemotherapy; allogeneic bone marrow transplantation
III	Malignant histiocytosis Acute monocytic leukemia	Neoplastic proliferation of cells with characteristics of monocytes/macrophages or their precursors	Antineoplastic chemotherapy, including anthracyclines

*Also called familial hemophagocytic lymphohistiocytosis (FHLH).
†Also called secondary hemophagocytic lymphohistiocytosis.

TABLE 507-2. Infections Associated with Hemophagocytic Syndrome

VIRAL
Adenovirus
Cytomegalovirus
Dengue virus
Epstein-Barr virus
Herpes simplex virus
Human immunodeficiency virus
Parvovirus B19
Varicella-zoster virus

BACTERIAL
Babesia microti
Brucella abortus
Enteric gram-negative rods
Haemophilus influenzae
Mycoplasma pneumoniae
Staphylococcus aureus
Streptococcus pneumoniae

FUNGAL
Candida albicans
Cryptococcus neoformans
Histoplasma capsulatum

MYCOBACTERIAL
Mycobacterium tuberculosis

RICKETTSIAL
Coxiella brunetii

PARASITIC
Leishmania donovani

From Nathan DG, Orkin SH, Ginsburg D, et al (editors): *Nathan and Oski's Hematology of Infancy and Childhood,* 6th ed. Philadelphia, WB Saunders, 2003, p 1381.

In contrast to the prominence of an APC (the Langerhans' cell) in the class I histiocytoses, the **class II histiocytoses** are nonmalignant proliferative disorders that are characterized by accumulation of antigen-processing cells (macrophages). **Hemophagocytic lymphohistiocytoses** (HCH) are the result of uncontrolled hemophagocytosis and uncontrolled activation (upregulation) of inflammatory cytokines similar to the macrophage activation syndrome (see Table 154-5). Tissue infiltration by activated CD8 T lymphocytes and activated macrophages as well as hypercytokinemia are classic features. With the characteristic morphology of normal macrophages by light microscopy, these phagocytic cells lack the two markers (Birbeck granules and CD1a-positivity) characteristic of the cells found in LCH. The two major diseases among the class II histiocytoses have indistinguishable pathologic findings. One is **familial hemophagocytic lymphohistiocytosis** (FHLH), previously called familial erythrophagocytic lymphohistiocytosis FEL, which is the only inherited form of histiocytosis and is autosomal recessive. Specific genes involved with FEL include mutations of perforin, Munc 13-4, and Syntaxin-11. The other is the **infection-associated hemophagocytic syndrome (IAHS),** also called secondary hemophagocytic lymphohistiocytosis (Table 507-2). Both diseases are characterized by disseminated lesions that involve many organ systems. The lesions are characterized by infiltration of the involved organ with activated phagocytic macrophages and lymphocytes, in which the lymphocyte defects are considered to be the primary abnormality. These diseases are grouped together under the term **hemophagocytic lymphohistiocytosis** (HLH) [Table 507-3].

The mixed cellular lesions of both the class I and class II histiocytoses suggest that these may be disorders of immune regulation, resulting from either an unusual and unidentified antigenic stimulation or an abnormal and somehow defective cellular immune response. Mutations in the perforin (PRF1) gene or the Munc 13-4 gene cause defective function of the cytotoxic lymphocytes whose activity is inhibited in FHLH.

The **class III histiocytoses,** in contrast, are unequivocal malignancies of cells of monocyte-macrophage lineage. By this definition, acute monocytic leukemia and true malignant histiocytosis are included among the class III histiocytoses (see Chapter 495). The existence of neoplasms of Langerhans' cells is controversial. Some cases of LCH demonstrate clonality.

507.1 • Class I Histiocytoses

CLINICAL MANIFESTATIONS. LCH has an extremely variable presentation. The skeleton is involved in 80% of patients and may be the only affected site, especially in children >5 yr of age. Bone lesions may be single or multiple and are seen most commonly in the skull (Fig. 507-1). Other sites include the pelvis, femur, vertebra, maxilla, and mandible. They may be asymptomatic or associated with pain and local swelling. Involvement of the spine may result in collapse of the vertebral body, which can be seen radiographically, and may cause secondary compression of the spinal cord. In flat and long bones, osteolytic lesions with sharp borders occur and no evidence exists of reactive new bone formation until the lesions begin to heal. Lesions that involve weight-bearing long bones may result in pathologic fractures. Chronically draining, infected ears are commonly associated with destruction in the mastoid area. Bone destruction in the mandible and maxilla may result in teeth that, on radiographs, appear to be free floating. With response to therapy, healing may be complete.

About 50% of patients experience skin involvement at some time during the course of disease, usually as a hard-to-treat scaly, papular, seborrheic dermatitis of the scalp, diaper, axillary, or posterior auricular regions). The lesions may spread to involve

TABLE 507-3. Distinguishing Characteristics of the Reactive Lymphohistiocytoses

	GENETIC HISTORY	VIRUS INFECTION	CELLULAR IMMUNE FUNCTION	MISCELLANEOUS
HLH, genetic	Autosomal recessive	Possibly associated	↓ CMI ↓ NK cell activity ↓ Monocyte killing ↓ CMI	Perforin deficiency Hypertriglyceridemia, Perforin (PRF1), Munc 13-4 mutations
Secondary infection–associated	Sporadic	Yes	↓ CMI NL or ↑ NK cell in instances associated with EBV ↓ Anomalous EBV-related killing	Coagulopathy early in the course of the disease
XLP	X-linked sporadic	EBV	NL or ↑ NK cell NL or ↑ anomalous EBV-related killing	*SH2DIA* mutation Severe, often fatal hepatitis
SHML	Sporadic	?EBV	Not reported	Autoimmune phenomena
LG	Sporadic	EBV	↓ CMI	Lymphoma development

From Nathan DG, Orkin SH, Ginsburg D, et al (editors): *Nathan and Oski's Hematology of Infancy and Childhood,* 6th ed. Philadelphia, WB Saunders, 2003, p 1387.
CMI, cell-mediated immunity; EBV, Epstein-Barr virus; HLH, hemophagocytic lymphohistiocytosis; LG, lymphomatoid granulomatosis; NK, natural killer; NL, normal; SHML, sinus histiocytosis with massive lymphadenopathy; XLP, X-linked lymphoproliferative syndrome.

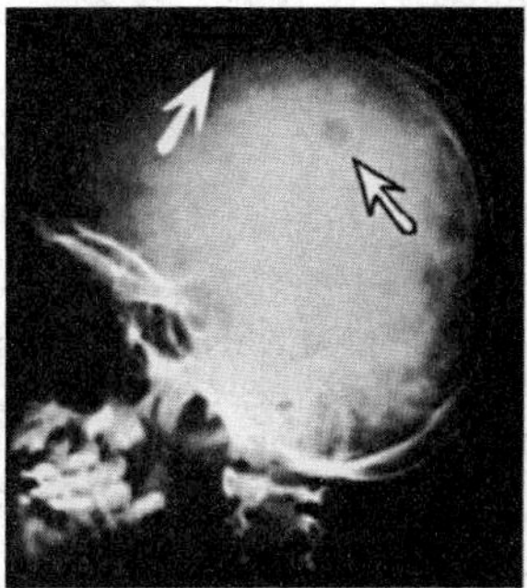
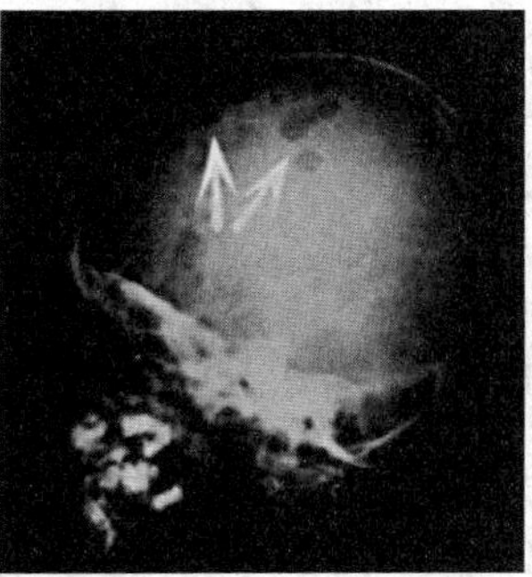

Figure 507-1. Two skull radiographs from patients with Langerhans' cell histiocytosis (LCH). *Left,* The patient was >2 yr of age and had involvement limited to isolated bone lesions *(arrows)*. She had a good recovery. *Right,* The patient was <2 yr of age and had extensive bone disease *(arrows),* a febrile course, anemia, severe skin eruption, generalized lymphadenopathy, hepatosplenomegaly, pulmonary infiltrates, and a fatal outcome despite antitumor chemotherapy. These patients represent opposite ends of the clinical spectrum of LCH.

the back, palms, and soles. The exanthem may be petechial or hemorrhagic, even in the absence of thrombocytopenia. Localized or disseminated lymphadenopathy is present in approximately 33% of patients. Hepatosplenomegaly occurs in approximately 20% of patients. Various degrees of hepatic malfunction may occur, including jaundice and ascites.

Exophthalmos, when present, often is bilateral and is caused by retro-orbital accumulation of granulomatous tissue. Gingival mucous membranes may be involved with infiltrative lesions that appear superficially like candidiasis. Otitis media is present in 30–40% of patients; deafness may follow destructive lesions of the middle ear. In 10–15% of patients, pulmonary infiltrates are found on radiography. The lesions may range from diffuse fibrosis and disseminated nodular infiltrates to diffuse cystic changes. Rarely, pneumothorax may be a complication. If the lungs are severely involved, tachypnea and progressive respiratory failure may result.

Pituitary dysfunction or hypothalamic involvement may result in growth retardation. In addition, patients may have diabetes insipidus; patients suspected of having LCH should demonstrate the ability to concentrate their urine before going to the operating room for a biopsy. Rarely, panhypopituitarism may occur. Primary hypothyroidism due to thyroid gland infiltration also may occur.

Patients who are affected more severely may have systemic manifestations, including fever, weight loss, malaise, irritability, and failure to thrive. Bone marrow involvement may cause anemia and thrombocytopenia. Two uncommon but serious and unusual manifestations of LCH are hepatic involvement (leading to cirrhosis) and a peculiar central nervous system (CNS) involvement characterized by ataxia, dysarthria, and other neurologic symptoms. Hepatic involvement is associated with multisystem disease that is often already present at the time of diagnosis. In contrast, the CNS involvement, which is progressive and histopathologically characterized by gliosis, and for which no treatment is known, may be observed only many years after the initial diagnosis of LCH, which may have consisted only of mild bone disease. Neither of these manifestations evidences Langerhans' cells or Birbeck granules.

After tissue biopsy, which is diagnostic and is easiest to perform on skin or bone lesions, a thorough clinical and laboratory evaluation should be undertaken. This should include a series of studies in all patients (complete blood cell count, liver function tests, coagulation studies, skeletal survey, chest radiograph, and measurement of urine osmolality). In addition, detailed evaluation of any organ system that has been shown to be involved by physical examination or by these studies should be performed to establish the extent of disease before initiation of treatment.

TREATMENT AND PROGNOSIS. The clinical course of single-system disease (usually, bone, lymph node, or skin) usually is benign, with a high chance of spontaneous remission. Therefore, treatment should be minimal and should be directed at arresting the progression of a bone lesion that could result in permanent damage before it resolves spontaneously. Curettage or, less often, low-dose local radiation therapy (5–6 Gy) may accomplish this goal. Multisystem disease, in contrast, should be treated with systemic multiagent chemotherapy. Several different regimens have been proposed, but a central element is the inclusion of either vinblastine or etoposide, both of which have been found to be very effective in treating LCH. Treatment of multisystem LCH includes therapy with multiple agents, designed to reduce reactivation of disease and long-term consequences. The response rate to therapy, contrary to previous belief, may be high, especially if the diagnosis is made accurately and expeditiously. Experimental therapies, suggested only for unresponsive disease (often in very young children with multisystem disease and organ dysfunction who have not responded to initial treatment), include immunosuppressive therapy with cyclosporine/antithymocyte globulin and possibly certain new agents and modalities, such as imatinib, 2-chlorodeoxyadenosine, and stem cell transplantation. Current treatment approaches and experimental protocols for both class I and class II histiocytoses can be obtained at the website for the Histiocyte Society: www.histio.org/society.

507.2 • Class II Histiocytoses: Hemophagocytic Lymphohistiocytosis

See "Classification and Pathology" above.

CLINICAL MANIFESTATIONS. The major forms of HLH, familial hemophagocytic lymphohistiocytosis (FHLF) and secondary HLH, have a remarkably similar presentation consisting of a generalized disease process, most often with fever, maculopapular and/or petechial rash, weight loss, and irritability (Table 507-4). FHLH also is characterized by severe immunodeficiency. Children with FHLH always are <4 yr of age, whereas children with secondary HLH may present at an older age. **Physical examination** often reveals hepatosplenomegaly, lymphadenopathy, respiratory distress, and symptoms of CNS involvement, unlike that of aseptic meningitis in which the cerebrospinal fluid cells are the same phagocytic macrophages as found in the peripheral blood or bone marrow. The diagnosis rests on the pathologic findings

TABLE 507-4. Diagnostic Criteria for Hemophagocytic Lymphohistiocytosis

Fever >38.5°C and lasting ≥7 days
Splenomegaly >3 cm
TWO OF THE FOLLOWING HEMATOLOGIC ABNORMALITIES:
Anemia (>9 g/dL hemoglobin)
Thrombocytopenia (>100,000 cells/µL)
Neutropenia (<1000 neutrophils/µL)
ONE OF THE FOLLOWING ABNORMALITIES:
Hypertriglyceridemia >2.0 nmol/L
Hypofibrinogenemia <150 mg/dL
and
Hemophagocytosis in bone marrow, spleen, or lymph node
No evidence of marrow hyperplasia or malignant neoplasia

From Nathan DG, Orkin SH, Ginsburg D, et al (editors): *Nathan and Oski's Hematology of Infancy and Childhood,* 6th ed. Philadelphia, WB Saunders, 2003, p 1379. Adapted from MacMahon HE, Bedizel M, Ellis CA: Familial erythrophagocytic lymphohistiocytosis. *Pediatrics* 1963;32:868–879.

in skin or bone marrow biopsy. Associated laboratory findings in both forms of HLH include hyperlipidemia, hypofibrinogenemia, elevated levels of hepatic enzymes, extremely elevated levels of circulating soluble interleukin-2 receptors released by the activated lymphocytes, very high levels of serum ferritin (often >10,000), and cytopenias (especially pancytopenia from hemophagocytosis in the marrow). No absolute clinical or laboratory distinction can be made between FHLH and secondary HLH, although genetic markers for FHLH can complement a positive family history for other affected children. HLH may be present in the absence of genetic mutations of the perforin or Munc 13-4 genes and the presence of 5 of the following: fever, splenomegaly, cytopenia of 2 cell lines, hypertriglyceridemia or hypofibrinogenemia, hyperferritinemia, elevated SCD25 (interleukin-2 receptor), reduced or absent NK cells, and bone marrow, cerebrospinal fluid or lymph node evidence of hemophagocytosis.

TREATMENT AND PROGNOSIS. The diagnostic distinction between FHLH and secondary HLH sometimes can be based on the acute onset of secondary HLH in the presence of a documented infection. In this case, treatment of the underlying infection, coupled with supportive care, is critical. If the diagnosis is made in a setting of iatrogenic immunodeficiency, immunosuppressive treatment should be withdrawn and supportive care should be instituted along with specific therapy for underlying infection. When FHLH (gene mutations in perforin or Munc 13-4 proteins) is diagnosed or suspected and when an infection cannot be documented, therapy currently includes etoposide, corticosteroids, and intrathecal methotrexate. Some recommend antithymocyte globulin and cyclosporine for maintenance therapy. Nevertheless, even with chemotherapy, FHLH remains ultimately fatal, often after a relapse of the disease. Allogeneic **stem cell transplantation** is effective in curing approximately 60% of patients with FHLH.

In contrast, in secondary HLH, when an infection can be documented and effectively treated, the prognosis is good without any other specific treatment. When a treatable infection cannot be documented, which is the case in most patients presumed to have secondary HLH, the prognosis may be as poor as that of FHLH, and an identical chemotherapeutic approach, including etoposide, is recommended. It is theorized that, by its cytotoxic effect on macrophages, etoposide interrupts cytokine production, the hemophagocytic process, and the accumulation of macrophages, all of which may contribute to the pathogenesis of IAHS. A broad spectrum of infectious agents, viruses (e.g., cytomegalovirus, Epstein-Barr virus, human herpesvirus 6), fungi, protozoa, and bacteria may trigger secondary HLH, usually in the setting of immunodeficiency (see Table 507-2). A thorough evaluation for infection should be undertaken in immunodeficient patients with hemophagocytosis. Rarely, the same syndrome may be identified in conjunction with a rheumatologic disorder (e.g., systemic lupus erythematosus, Kawasaki disease) or a neoplasm (leukemia); in this case, treatment of the underlying disease may cause resolution of the hemophagocytosis. In some patients, interferon and intravenous immunoglobulin have been effective.

507.3 • Class III Histiocytoses

Acute monocytic leukemia and true malignant histiocytosis are included among the class III histiocytoses (see Chapter 495), because they are unequivocal malignancies of the monocyte-macrophage lineage.

Arico M, Danesino C, Pende D, et al: Pathogenesis of haemophagocytic lymphohistiocytosis. *Br J Haematol* 2001;114:761–769.

Arico M, Imashuku S, Clementi R, et al: Hemophagocytic lymphohistiocytosis due to germline mutations in SH2D1A, the X-linked lymphoproliferative disease gene. *Blood* 2001;97:1131–1133.

Broadbent V, Gadner, H: Current therapy for Langerhans cell histiocytosis. *Hematol Oncol Clin North Am* 1998;12:327–328.

Domachowske JB: Infectious triggers of hemophagocytic syndrome in children. *Pediatr Infect Dis J* 2006;25:1067–1068.

Durken M, Finckenstein FG, Janka GE: Bone marrow transplantation in hemophagocytic lymphohistiocytosis. *Leuk Lymphoma* 2001;41:89–95.

Feldmann J, Callebaut I, Raposo G, et al: Munc 13–4 is essential for cytolytic granules fusion and is mutated on a form of familial hemophagocytic lymphohistiocytosis (FHL3). *Cell* 2003;115:461–473.

Gadner H, Grois N, Arico M, et al: A randomized trial of treatment for multisystem Langerhans' cell histiocytosis. *J Pediatr* 2001;138:728–734.

Hait E, Liang M, Degar B, et al: Gastrointestinal tract involvement in Langerhans cell histiocytosis: case report and literature review. *Pediatrics* 2006; 118:e1593–e1599.

Horne A, Janka G, Egeler R, et al: Hematopoietic stem cell transplantation in haemophagocytic lymphohistiocytosis. *Br J Haematol* 2005;129:622–630.

Kogawa K, Lee SM, Villanueva J, et al: Perforin expression in cytotoxic lymphocytes from patients with hemophagocytic lymphohistiocytosis and their family members. *Blood* 2002;99:61–66.

Lee SM, Sumegi J, Villanueva J, et al: Patients of African ancestry with hemophagocytic lymphohistiocytosis share a common haplotype of PRFI with a 50 delt mutation. *J Pediatr* 2006;149:134–137.

Leonidas JC, Guelfguat M, Valderrama E: Langerhans' cell histiocytosis. *Lancet* 2003;361:1293–1295.

Montella L, Insabato L, Palmieri G: Imatinib mesylate for cerebral Langerhans'-cell histiocytosis. *N Engl J Med* 2004;351:1034–1035.

Ouachee-Chardin M, Elie C, de Saint Basile G, et al: Hematopoietic stem cell transplantation in hemophagocytic lymphohistiocytosis: A single-center report of 48 patients. *Pediatrics* 2006;117:e743–e750.

Palazzi DL, McClain KL, Kaplan SL: Hemophagocytic syndrome in children: An important diagnostic consideration in fever of unknown origin. *Clin Infect Dis* 2003;36:306–312.

Valladeau J, Dezutter-Dambuyant C, Saeland S: Langerin/CD207 sheds light on formation of Birbeck granules and their possible function in Langerhans cells. *Immunol Res* 2003;28:93–107.

Writing Group of the Histiocyte Society: Histiocytosis syndromes in childhood. *Lancet* 1987;1:208–209.

Part XXII ▪ Nephrology

Section 1 — Glomerular Disease — Ira D. Davis and Ellis D. Avner

Chapter 508 ▪ Introduction to Glomerular Diseases

508.1 • Anatomy of the Glomerulus

The kidneys lie in the retroperitoneal space slightly above the level of the umbilicus. They range in length and weight, respectively, from approximately 6 cm and 24 g in a full-term newborn to 12 cm or more and 150 g in an adult. The kidney (Fig. 508-1) has an outer layer, the cortex, that contains the glomeruli, proximal and distal convoluted tubules, and collecting ducts and an inner layer, the medulla, that contains the straight portions of the tubules, the loops of Henle, the vasa recta, and the terminal collecting ducts (Fig. 508-2).

The blood supply to each kidney usually consists of a main renal artery that arises from the aorta; multiple renal arteries may occur. The main artery divides into segmental branches within the medulla and these into interlobar arteries that pass through the medulla to the junction of the cortex and medulla. At this point, the interlobar arteries branch to form the arcuate arteries, which run parallel to the surface of the kidney. Interlobular arteries originate from the arcuate arteries and give rise to the afferent arterioles of the glomeruli. Specialized muscle cells in the wall of the afferent arteriole and the macula densa within the distal tubule next to the glomerulus form the juxtaglomerular apparatus that controls the secretion of renin. The afferent arteriole divides into the glomerular capillary network, which then merges into the efferent arteriole (Fig. 508-3). The efferent arterioles of glomeruli next to the medulla (juxtamedullary glomeruli) are larger than those in the outer cortex and provide the blood supply (vasa recta) to the tubules and medulla.

Each kidney contains approximately 1 million nephrons (glomeruli and associated tubules). In humans, formation of nephrons is complete at birth, but functional maturation with tubular growth and elongation continues during the first decade of life. Because new nephrons cannot be formed after birth, progressive loss of nephrons may lead to renal insufficiency. Decreased nephron number at birth may be associated with hypertension in adulthood, presumably related to hyperfiltration and "premature" sclerosis of overworked nephron units. This provocative hypothesis, if proven, could identify a major risk factor for hypertension and its associated cardiovascular complications in the newborn period.

The glomerular network of specialized capillaries serves as the filtering mechanism of the kidney. The glomerular capillaries are lined by endothelial cells (Fig. 508-4) and have very thin cytoplasm that contains many holes (fenestrations). The glomerular basement membrane (GBM) forms a continuous layer between the endothelial and mesangial cells on one side and the epithelial cells on the other. The membrane has 3 layers: (1) a central electron-dense lamina densa; (2) the lamina rara interna, which lies between the lamina densa and the endothelial cells; and (3) the lamina rara externa, which lies between the lamina densa and the epithelial cells. The visceral epithelial cells cover the capillary and project cytoplasmic "foot processes," which attach to the lamina rara externa. Between the foot processes are spaces or filtration slits. The mesangium (mesangial cells and matrix) lies between the glomerular capillaries on the endothelial cell side of the GBM and forms the medial part of the capillary wall. The mesangium may serve as a supporting structure for the glomerular capillaries and probably has a role in the regulation of glomerular blood flow and filtration and in the removal of macromolecules (such as immune complexes) from the glomerulus, either through intracellular phagocytosis or by transport through intercellular channels to the juxtaglomerular region. Bowman's capsule, which surrounds the glomerulus, is composed of (1) a basement membrane, which is continuous with the basement membranes of the glomerular capillaries and the proximal tubules, and (2) the parietal epithelial cells, which are continuous with the visceral epithelial cells.

Fogo A: Renal pathology. In Avner ED, Harmon WE, Niaudet P (editors): *Pediatric Nephrology*, 5th ed. Baltimore, Lippincott Williams & Wilkins, 2004, pp 475–500.

Kon V, Ichikawa I: In Avner ED, Harmon WE, Niaudet P (editors): *Pediatric Nephrology*, 5th ed. Baltimore, Lippincott Williams & Wilkins, 2004, pp 25–44.

508.2 • Glomerular Filtration

As the blood passes through the glomerular capillaries, the plasma is filtered through the glomerular capillary walls. The ultrafiltrate, which is cell free, contains all the substances in the plasma (electrolytes, glucose, phosphate, urea, creatinine, peptides, low molecular weight proteins) except proteins (such as albumin and the globulins) having a molecular weight of ≥68 kd. The filtrate is collected in Bowman's space and enters the tubules, where its composition is modified by solute and fluid secretion and absorption in accordance with tightly regulated tubular homeostatic mechanisms until it leaves the kidney as urine.

Glomerular filtration is the net result of opposing forces across the capillary wall. The force for ultrafiltration (glomerular capillary hydrostatic pressure) is a result of systemic arterial pressure, modified by the tone of the afferent and efferent arterioles. The major force opposing ultrafiltration is the glomerular capillary oncotic pressure, which is created by the gradient between the high concentration of plasma proteins within the capillary and the almost protein-free ultrafiltrate in Bowman's space. Filtration may be modified by the rate of glomerular plasma flow, the hydrostatic pressure within Bowman's space, and the permeability of the glomerular capillary wall.

Although glomerular filtration begins around the 9th wk of fetal life, kidney function is not necessary for normal intrauterine homeostasis because the placenta serves as the major fetal excretory organ. After birth, the glomerular filtration rate (GFR) increases until growth ceases toward the end of the 2nd decade of life. To facilitate the comparison of the GFRs of children and adults, the GFR is standardized to the surface area (1.73 m^2) of a 70-kg adult. Even after correction for surface area, the GFR of a child does not approximate adult values until the 3rd yr of life (Fig. 508-5).

The GFR may be estimated by measurement of the serum creatinine level (Fig. 508-6). Creatinine is derived from muscle metabolism. Its production is relatively constant, and its excretion is primarily through glomerular filtration, although tubular secretion may become important in renal insufficiency. In contrast to the concentration of blood urea nitrogen, which is affected by state of hydration and nitrogen balance, the serum creatinine level is primarily influenced by the level of glomerular function. The serum creatinine is of value only in estimating the GFR in the steady state. A patient may have a normal creatinine level without effective renal function very shortly after the onset of acute renal failure with anuria. In this clinical setting, serum creatinine may be an insensitive measure of decreased renal function because its level does not rise above normal until the GFR falls by 30–40%. Cystatin C, a 13.6-kd protease inhibitor produced by nucleated cells, is an endogenous marker that may be more reliable than serum creatinine measurements in estimating the GFR since serum levels are unaffected by gender, height, muscle mass, bilirubin, or red blood cell hemolysis.

The precise measurement of the GFR is accomplished by quantitating the "clearance" of a substance that is freely filtered across the capillary wall and that is neither reabsorbed nor secreted by the tubules. The clearance (C_s) of such a substance is that volume of plasma that, when completely "cleared" of the contained substance, would yield a quantity of that substance equal to that excreted in the urine over a specified time. The clearance is represented by the following formula C_s (mL/min) = U_s (mg/mL) × V (mL/min)/P_s (mg/mL), where C_s equals the clearance of substance s, U_s reflects the urinary concentration of s, V represents the urinary flow rate, and P_s equals the plasma concentration of s. To correct the clearance for body surface area, the formula is

$$\text{Corrected clearance}\,(\text{mL/min}/1.73\,\text{m}^2) = \text{Cs}(\text{mL/min}) \times \frac{1.73}{\text{Surface area}\,(\text{M}^2)}$$

The GFR is optimally measured by the clearance of inulin, a fructose polymer having a molecular weight of approximately 5 kd. Because the inulin clearance technique is cumbersome, the GFR is commonly estimated by the clearance of endogenous creatinine. When the GFR is relatively normal, the creatinine clearance closely approximates the inulin clearance. As the GFR declines, an increasing proportion of the total creatinine in the urine is secreted by tubules, resulting in a creatinine clearance that progressively overestimates the actual GFR. Therefore, changes in renal function should be monitored by serum creatinine concentration when the serum creatinine level exceeds 2.0 mg/dL (180 µmol/L).

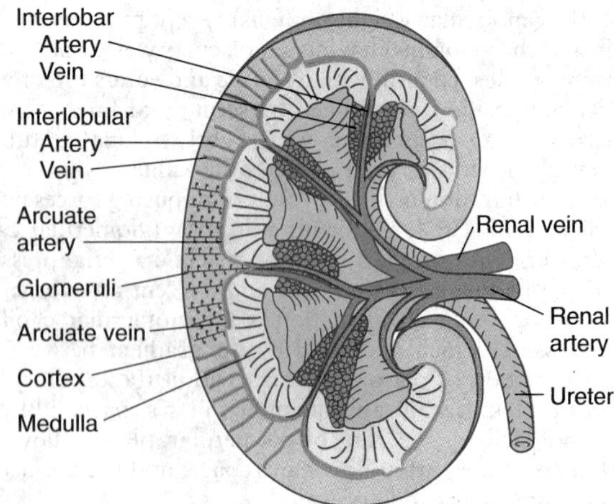

Figure 508-1. Gross morphology of the renal circulation. (From Pitts RF: *Physiology of the Kidney and Body Fluids,* 3rd ed. Chicago, Year Book Medical Publishers, 1974.)

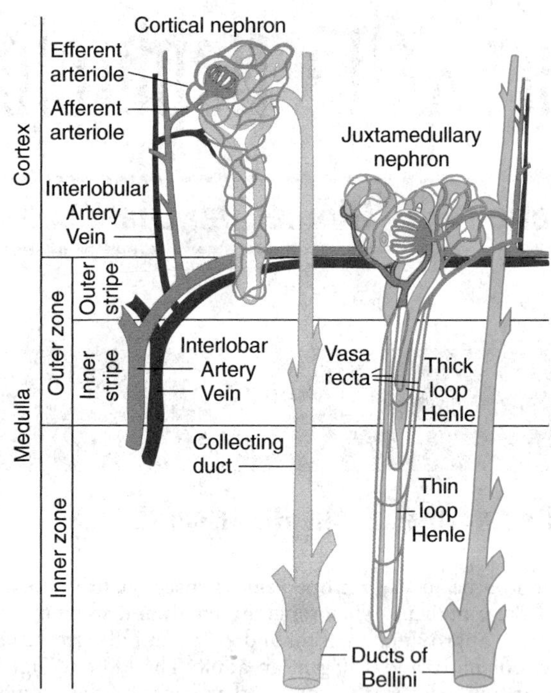

Figure 508-2. Comparison of the blood supplies of cortical and juxtamedullary nephrons. (From Pitts RF: *Physiology of the Kidney and Body Fluids,* 3rd ed. Chicago, Year Book Medical Publishers, 1974.)

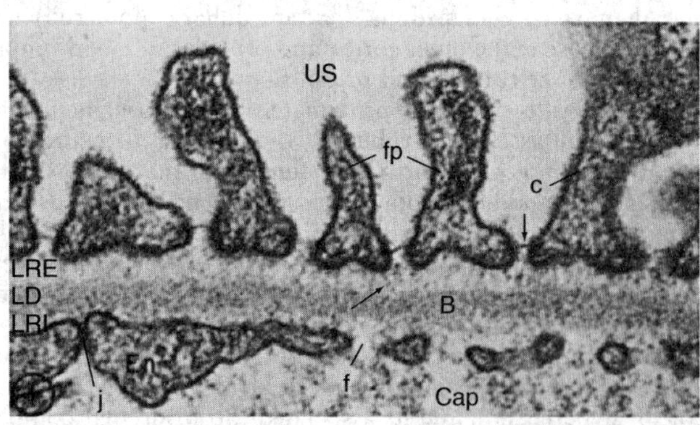

Figure 508-3. Electron micrograph of the normal glomerular capillary (Cap) wall demonstrating the endothelium (En) with its fenestrations (f), the glomerular basement membrane (B) with its central dense layer, the lamina densa (LD), and adjoining lamina rara interna (LRI) and externa (LRE) *(long arrow)* and the epithelial cell foot processes (fp) with their thick cell coat (c). The glomerular filtrate passes through the endothelial fenestrae, crosses the basement membrane, and passes through the filtration slits *(short arrow)* between the epithelial cell foot processes to reach the urinary space (US) (×60,000). J is the junction between two endothelial cells. (From Farquhar MG, Kanwar YS: Functional organization of the glomerulus: State of the science in 1979. In Cummings NB, Michael AF, Wilson CB (editors): *Immune Mechanisms in Renal Disease.* New York, Plenum, 1982.)

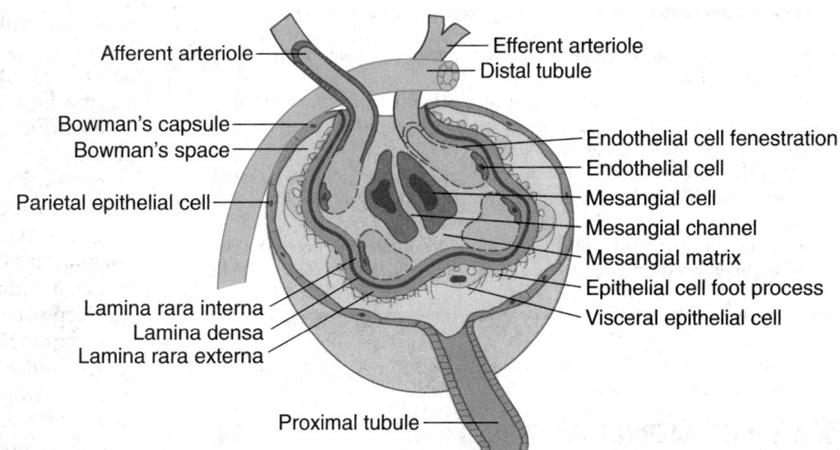

Figure 508-4. Schematic depiction of the glomerulus and surrounding structures.

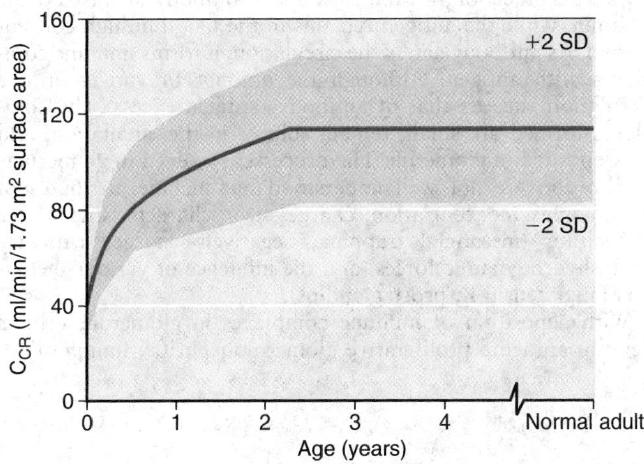

Figure 508-5. Changes in the normal value of the glomerular filtration rate, as measured by the creatinine clearance (CCR), when standardized to mL/min/1.73 m^2 of body surface area. The *solid line* depicts the mean, and the *shaded area* includes two standard deviations. (From McCrory W: *Developmental Nephrology.* Cambridge, MA, Harvard University Press, 1972.)

The absence of plasma proteins larger than the size of albumin from the glomerular filtrate confirms the effectiveness of the glomerular capillary wall as a filtration barrier. Major factors restricting the filtration of these and other macromolecules include their size and their ionic charge.

Clearance studies of macromolecules in animals have shown no restriction to the filtration of molecules up to the size of inulin. As size increases farther, filtration diminishes progressively, approaching zero for substances the size of albumin. Morphologic studies suggest that the size-selective filtration barrier resides within the GBM.

The endothelial cell, basement membrane, and epithelial cell of the glomerular capillary wall possess strong negative ionic charges. These charges are a consequence of two negatively charged moieties: proteoglycans (heparan sulfate) and glycoproteins containing sialic acid. Proteins in the blood have a relatively low isoelectric point and carry a net negative charge. Consequently, they are repelled by the negatively charged sites in the glomerular capillary wall, thus restricting filtration.

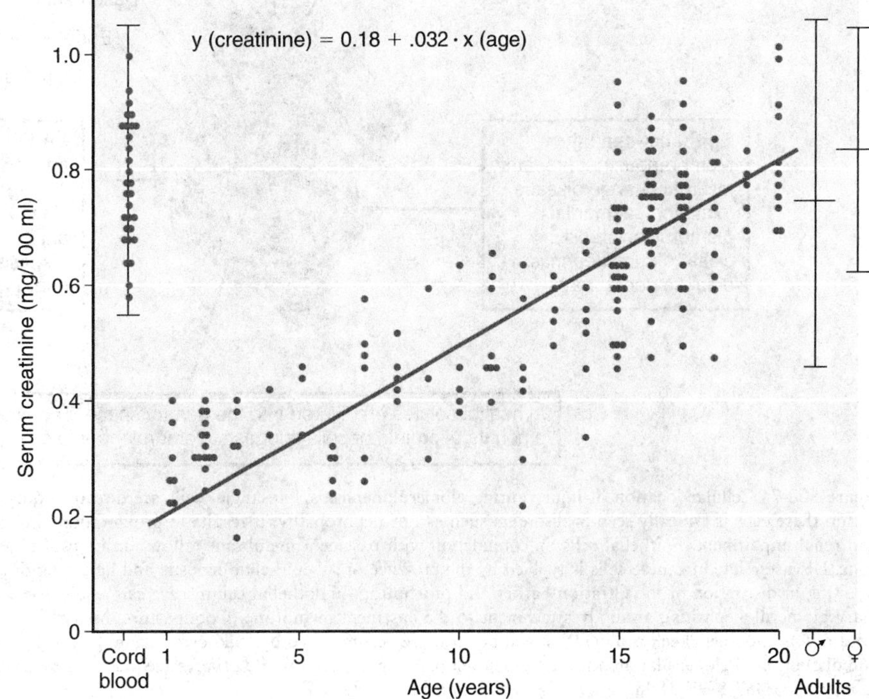

Figure 508-6. The serum creatinine in relation to age. (From McCrory W: *Developmental Nephrology.* Cambridge, MA, Harvard University Press, 1972.)

Arant BS Jr: Postnatal development of renal function during the first year of life. *Pediatr Nephrol* 1987;1:308–313.

Finney H, Newman DJ, Thakkar H, et al: Reference ranges for plasma cystatin C and creatinine measurements in premature infants, neonates, and older children. *Arch Dis Child* 2000;82:71–75.

Kon V, Ichikawa I: In Avner ED, Harmon WE, Niaudet P (editors): *Pediatric Nephrology,* 5th ed. Baltimore, Lippincott Williams & Wilkins, 2004, pp 25–44.

Schwartz GJ, Haycock GB, Spitzer A: Plasma creatinine and urea concentration in children: Normal values for age and sex. *J Pediatr* 1976;88:828–837.

508.3 • Glomerular Diseases

PATHOGENESIS. Glomerular injury may be a result of genetic, immunologic, or coagulation disorders. Genetic disorders of the glomerulus result from (1) mutations in the exons of DNA encoding transcriptional units that undergo translation in the ribosomes forming proteins located within the glomerulus, interstitium, or tubular epithelium; (2) mutations in the regulatory genes controlling DNA transcription; (3) abnormal post-transcriptional modification of RNA transcripts; or (4) abnormal post-translational modification of proteins. Immunologic injury is the most common cause and results in **glomerulonephritis,** which is a generic term for several diseases and a histopathologic term signifying inflammation of the glomerular capillaries. Evidence that glomerulonephritis is caused by immunologic injury includes (1) morphologic and immunopathologic similarities to experimental immune-mediated glomerulonephritis; (2) the demonstration of immune reactants (immunoglobulin, complement) in glomeruli; and (3) abnormalities in serum complement and the finding of autoantibodies (anti-GBM) in some of these diseases (Fig. 508-7). There appear to be 2 major mechanisms of immunologic injury: (1) glomerular deposition of circulating antigen-antibody immune complexes and (2) interaction of antibody with local antigen in situ. In the latter circumstance, the antigen may be a normal component of the glomerulus (the noncollagenous domain [NC-1] of type IV collagen, a putative antigen in human anti-GBM nephritis) or an antigen that has been deposited in the glomerulus.

In **immune complex–mediated** diseases, antibody is produced against and combines with a circulating antigen that is usually unrelated to the kidney (see Fig. 508-7). The immune complexes accumulate in GBMs and activate the complement system, leading to immune injury. Acute serum sickness in rabbits is produced by a single intravenous injection of bovine albumin. Within 1 wk after injection, a rabbit produces antibody against bovine albumin, while the antigen remains in the blood in high concentration. As antibody enters the circulation, it forms immune complexes with antigen. Although the amount of antigen in the circulation exceeds that of antibody (antigen excess), the complexes formed are small, remain soluble in the circulation, and are deposited in glomeruli. The processes involved in glomerular localization are not well understood but include attributes of the complex (concentration, charge, size), characteristics of the glomerulus (mesangial trapping, negatively charged capillary wall), hydrodynamic forces, and the influence of various mediators (angiotensin II, prostaglandins).

With deposition of immune complexes in glomeruli, rabbits develop an acute proliferative glomerulonephritis. Immunofluo-

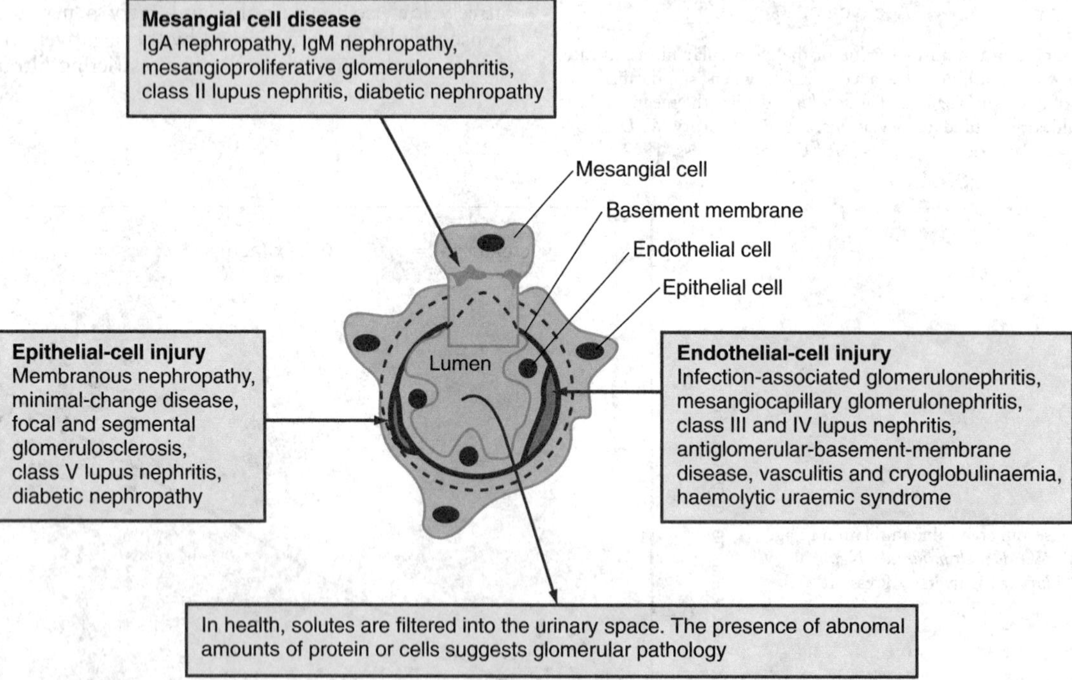

Figure 508-7. Cellular location of injury during glomerulonephritis. Mesangial cells are directly exposed to the circulation. Deposition of immune complexes within these cells is typically seen in disorders such as IgA nephropathy; it results in proliferation and expansion of the cells leading to hematuria, proteinuria, and renal impairment. Epithelial cells, in conjunction with basement membrane, allow filtration of plasma solutes but retard passage of cells and plasma proteins. Disease related to these cells is typified by the presence of subepithelial deposits and flattening of the foot processes that engage the basement membrane, resulting in disruption of the filtration barrier and proteinuria. Endothelial cell disease can result from immune complex deposition (as occurs in mesangiocapillary glomerulonephritis), antibody attachment to the basement membrane (Goodpasture disease), or trauma and activation of coagulation (hemolytic uremic syndrome). Endothelial cell proliferation and necrosis are accompanied by leukocyte accumulation, and rupture of the basement membrane, crescent formation, and disruption of glomerular architecture can develop. A nephritic or rapidly progressive presentation ensues. (From Chadban SJ, Atkins RC: Glomerulonephritis. *Lancet* 2005;365:1797–1806.)

rescence microscopy demonstrates granular (**"lumpy-bumpy"**) deposits containing immunoglobulin and complement in the glomerular capillary wall. Electron microscopic studies show these deposits to be on the epithelial side of the GBM and in the mesangium. For the next few days, as additional antibody enters the circulation, the antigen is ultimately removed from the circulation and the glomerulonephritis subsides.

An example of in situ antigen-antibody interaction is **anti-GBM antibody disease,** in which antibody reacts with antigen(s) of the GBM. Immunopathologic studies reveal linear deposition of immunoglobulin and complement on the GBM, similar to that in Goodpasture disease and certain types of rapidly progressive glomerulonephritis.

The inflammatory reaction that follows immunologic injury results from activation of one or more mediator pathways. The most important of these is the complement system, which has two initiating sequences: (1) the classic pathway, which is activated by antigen-antibody immune complexes, and (2) the alternative or properdin pathway, which is activated by polysaccharides and endotoxin. These pathways converge at C3; from that point on, the same sequence leads to lysis of cell membranes (see Chapter 132). The major noxious products of complement activation are produced after activation of C3 and include anaphylatoxin (which stimulates contractile proteins within vascular walls and increases vascular permeability) and chemotactic factors (C5a) that direct neutrophils and perhaps macrophages to the site of complement activation, where the cells release substances that damage vascular cells and basement membranes.

The coagulation system may be activated directly, after endothelial cell injury, which exposes the thrombogenic subendothelial layer (initiating the coagulation cascade), or indirectly, after complement activation. Fibrin deposits may occur within glomerular capillaries or within the Bowman space in crescents. Activation of the coagulation process may activate the kinin system, which also produces chemotactic and anaphylatoxin-like factors.

PATHOLOGY. The glomerulus may be injured by several mechanisms but has only a limited number of histopathologic responses; accordingly, different disease states may produce similar microscopic changes.

Proliferation of glomerular cells occurs in most forms of glomerulonephritis and may be generalized, involving all glomeruli, or focal, involving only some glomeruli while sparing others. Within a single glomerulus, proliferation may be diffuse, involving all parts of the glomerulus, or segmental, involving only some areas but not others. Proliferation commonly involves the endothelial and mesangial cells and is frequently associated with an increase in the mesangial matrix (see Fig. 508-7). Mesangial proliferation may result from immune complex deposition within the mesangium. The resultant increase in cell size and number and in mesangial matrix may increase glomerular size and narrow the lumens of glomerular capillaries, leading to renal insufficiency.

Crescent formation in Bowman's space (capsule) is a result of proliferation of parietal epithelial cells. Crescents develop in several forms of glomerulonephritis (termed **rapidly progressive**) and are thought to be a response to fibrin deposited in Bowman's space. New crescents contain fibrin, the proliferating epithelial cells of Bowman's space, basement membrane-like material produced by these cells, and macrophages that may have a role in the genesis of glomerular injury. In days to weeks, the crescent is invaded by connective tissue (fibroepithelial crescent); this generally results in glomerular obsolescence. Crescent formation is frequently associated with glomerular cell death. The necrotic glomerulus has a characteristic eosinophilic appearance and usually contains nuclear remnants. Crescent formation is usually associated with generalized proliferation of the mesangial cells and with either immune complex or anti-GBM antibody deposition in the glomerular capillary wall.

Certain forms of acute glomerulonephritis show glomerular exudation of blood cells, including neutrophils, eosinophils, basophils, and mononuclear cells. The thickened appearance of GBM may result from a true increase in the width of the membrane (as seen in membranous glomerulopathy), from massive deposition of immune complexes that have staining characteristics similar to the membrane (as seen in systemic lupus erythematosus), or from the interposition of mesangial cells and matrix into the subendothelial space between the endothelial cells and the GBM. The latter may give the basement membrane a split appearance, as seen in type I membranoproliferative glomerulonephritis and other diseases.

Sclerosis refers to the presence of scar tissue within the glomerulus. Occasionally, pathologists use this term to refer to an increase in mesangial matrix.

Tubulointerstitial fibrosis is present in all patients with glomerular disease who develop progressive renal injury. This fibrosis is initiated by injury to the renal tubules, resulting in mononuclear cell infiltrates that release soluble factors that have fibrosis-promoting effects. Additionally, matrix proteins of the renal interstitium begin to accumulate, leading to eventual destruction of renal tubules and peritubular capillaries. The actual transformation of tubular epithelium to mesenchymal tissue may contribute to progressive tubulointerstitial fibrosis.

Chadban SJ, Atkins RC: Glomerulonephritis. *Lancet* 2005;365:1797–1806.

Fogo A: Renal pathology. In Avner ED, Harmon WE, Niaudet P (editors): *Pediatric Nephrology,* 5th ed. Baltimore, Lippincott Williams & Wilkins, 2004, pp 475–500.

Stevens LA, Coresh J, Greene T, Levey AS: Assessing kidney function-measured and estimated glomerular filtration rate. *N Engl J Med* 2006;354:2473–2483.

Section 2 — Conditions Particularly Associated with Hematuria — Ira D. Davis and Ellis D. Avner

Chapter 509 ■ Clinical Evaluation of the Child with Hematuria

Hematuria is defined as the presence of at least 5 red blood cells (RBCs) per microliter of urine and occurs with a prevalence of 0.5–2.0% among school-aged children. Quantitative studies demonstrate that normal children may excrete more than 500,000 RBCs per 12-hr period; this increases with fever and/or exercise. In the clinical setting, qualitative estimates are provided by a urinary "dipstick" that uses a very sensitive peroxidase-like chemical reaction between hemoglobin (or myoglobin) and a chemical indicator compound impregnated on the dipstick. Chemstrip (Boehringer Mannheim), a common commercially available dipstick, is capable of detecting 3–10 RBCs/μL of unspun urine with significant hematuria suggested by the presence of >50 RBCs/μL. False-negative results may occur in the presence of formalin (used as a urine preservative) or high urinary concentrations of ascorbic acid. False-positive results may be seen in a child with fever or after exercise or in the presence of menstrual blood or alkaline urine with a pH >9 or contamination with oxidizing agents such as hydrogen peroxide used to clean the perineum before obtaining a specimen. Microscopic analysis of 10–15 mL of freshly centrifuged urine is essential in confirming the diagnosis of hematuria suggested by a positive dipstick. Screening urinalyses should be obtained during well child care visits at 5 yr and once during the 2nd decade of life (see Chapter 5).

Red urine **without** RBCs is seen in a number of conditions (Table 509-1). Heme-positive urine without RBCs is caused by the presence of either hemoglobin or myoglobin. Hemoglobinuria without hematuria may occur in the presence of hemolysis. Myoglobinuria without hematuria occurs in the presence of rhabdomyolysis syndrome resulting from skeletal muscle injury and is generally associated with a fivefold increase in the plasma concentration of creatine kinase. Rhabdomyolysis may occur secondary to viral myositis, crush injury, severe electrolyte abnormalities (hypernatremia, hypophosphatemia), hypotension, disseminated intravascular coagulation, toxins (drugs, venom), and prolonged seizures. Heme-negative urine may appear red, cola colored, or burgundy, owing to ingestion of various drugs, foods (blackberries, beets), or food dyes, whereas dark brown (or black) urine may result from various urinary metabolites (see Table 509-1).

Evaluation of the child with hematuria begins with a careful history, physical examination, and urinalysis. This information is used to determine the level of hematuria (upper vs lower urinary tract) and to determine the urgency of the evaluation based on symptomatology. Special consideration needs to be given to family history, identification of anatomic abnormalities/malformation syndromes, and the presence of gross hematuria.

Causes of hematuria are listed in Table 509-2. Upper urinary tract sources of hematuria originate within the nephron (glomerulus, convoluted/collecting tubules, and interstitium). Lower urinary tract sources of hematuria originate from the pelvocalyceal system, ureter, bladder, or urethra. Hematuria from within the glomerulus is frequently associated with brown, cola-colored, or burgundy urine, proteinuria >100 mg/dL via dipstick, urinary microscopic findings of RBC casts, and deformed urinary RBCs (particularly acanthocytes). Hematuria originating within the convoluted or collecting tubules may be associated with the presence of leukocyte or renal tubular epithelial cell casts. Lower urinary tract sources of hematuria may be associated with gross hematuria, terminal hematuria (onset of gross hematuria occurring at the end of the urine stream), blood clots, normal urinary RBC morphology, by microscopy, and minimal proteinuria on dipstick (<100 mg/dL).

Patients with hematuria may present with a number of symptoms suggestive of specific disorders. Tea or cola-colored urine, facial/body edema, hypertension, and oliguria suggest the acute nephritic syndrome. Diseases commonly presenting as acute nephritic syndrome include postinfectious glomerulonephritis, IgA nephropathy, membranoproliferative glomerulonephritis, Henoch-Schönlein purpura (HSP) nephritis, systemic lupus erythematosus (SLE) nephritis, Wegener granulomatosis, microscopic polyarteritis nodosa, Goodpasture syndrome, and hemolytic-uremic syndrome. A history of recent upper respiratory, skin, or gastrointestinal infection suggests acute glomerulonephritis, hemolytic-uremic syndrome, or HSP nephritis. Rash and joint complaints suggest HSP nephritis or SLE nephritis. Frequency, dysuria, and unexplained fevers suggest a urinary tract infection, whereas renal colic suggests nephrolithiasis. A flank mass may signal hydronephrosis, cystic disease, renal vein thrombosis, or tumor. Hematuria associated with headache, visual changes, epistaxis, or heart failure suggests significant hypertension. Patients with a history of trauma require immediate evaluation. Child abuse must always be suspected in the child presenting with unexplained bruising and hematuria.

A careful family history is critical in the initial assessment of the child with hematuria in view of numerous genetic causes of renal disorders. Hereditary glomerular diseases include hereditary nephritis (Alport syndrome), thin glomerular basement membrane disease, SLE nephritis, and IgA nephropathy (Berger disease). Other hematuric renal disorders with a hereditary component include polycystic kidney disease, urolithiasis, and sickle cell disease/trait.

Physical examination is critical in assessing the cause of hematuria. Hypertension, body edema, hepatosplenomegaly, or signs of heart failure suggest acute glomerulonephritis. Several malformation syndromes are associated with renal disease including VATER (*v*ertebral body anomalies, *a*nal atresia, *t*racheo-*e*sophageal fistula, and *r*enal dysplasia) syndrome. Abdominal masses may be caused by posterior urethral valves, ureteropelvic junction obstruction, polycystic kidney disease, or Wilms tumor. Hematuria seen in patients with neurologic or cutaneous abnormalities may be the result of renal cystic disease or tumors associated with several syndromes, including tuberous sclerosis, von Hippel-Lindau syndrome, and Zellweger (cerebrohepatorenal) syndrome. Anatomic abnormalities of the external genitalia may be associated with renal disease.

Patients with gross hematuria present additional challenges because of the associated parental anxiety. This entity must be distinguished from urethrorrhagia, which refers to urethral bleeding (in the absence of urine) associated with dysuria and blood spots on underwear after voiding. This condition, which often occurs in prepubertal boys at intervals several months apart over a period of many years, has a benign self-limited course. Common causes of gross hematuria are listed in Table 509-3. The most common cause of gross hematuria is either documented or sus-

TABLE 509-1. False Positive Tests for Hematuria

HEME POSITIVE
Hemoglobin
Myoglobin
HEME NEGATIVE
Drugs
Chloroquine
Deferoxamine
Ibuprofen
Iron sorbitol
Metronidazole
Nitrofurantoin
Phenazopyridine (Pyridium)
Phenolphthalein
Phenothiazines
Rifampin
Salicylates
Sulfasalazine
Dyes (Vegetable/Fruit): Beets, Blackberries, Food Coloring
Metabolites
Homogentisic acid
Melanin
Methemoglobin
Porphyrin
Tyrosinosis
Urates

pected urinary tract infections. Less than 10% of patients have evidence of glomerulonephritis. Recurrent episodes of gross hematuria suggest IgA nephropathy, Alport syndrome, thin glomerular basement membrane disease, hypercalciuria, or urolithiasis.

A general approach to the laboratory and radiologic evaluation of the patient with glomerular or extraglomerular hematuria is outlined in Figure 509-1. Asymptomatic patients with isolated microscopic hematuria should not undergo diagnostic evaluation until at least 2 additional urine specimens collected over a 1- to 2-wk period demonstrate an abnormal number of RBCs. This will reduce the number of unnecessary evaluations by 10- to a 100-fold.

The child with persistent asymptomatic isolated microscopic hematuria of longer than a 2-wk duration poses a dilemma in regard to the degree of further diagnostic testing that should be performed (Table 509-4). Significant disease of the urinary tract is infrequent with this clinical presentation. The initial evaluation of these children should include a urine culture followed by a spot urine for calcium and creatinine concentration in culture-negative patients. In African-American patients, a sickle cell screen should be included. If these studies are normal, urinalysis of all first-degree relatives is indicated. Renal and bladder ultrasonography should be considered to rule out structural lesions such as tumor, cystic disease, hydronephrosis, or urolithiasis. Ultrasonography of the urinary tract is most informative in patients presenting with gross hematuria, abdominal pain, flank pain, or trauma. If these initial studies are normal, assessment of serum creatinine and electrolytes is recommended.

The finding of certain hematologic abnormalities may narrow the differential diagnosis. Anemia in this setting may be caused by (1) intravascular dilution secondary to hypervolemia associated with acute renal failure; (2) decreased RBC production in chronic renal failure; (3) hemolysis from hemolytic-uremic syndrome or SLE; and (4) blood loss from pulmonary hemorrhage as seen in Goodpasture syndrome or melena in patients with Henoch-Schönlein purpura or hemolytic-uremic syndrome. Inspection of the peripheral blood smear may reveal a microangiopathic process consistent with the hemolytic-uremic syndrome, renal vein thrombosis, vasculitis, or SLE. In the latter, the presence of autoantibodies may result in a positive Coombs test, the presence of antinuclear antibody, leukopenia, and multisystem disease. Thrombocytopenia may result from decreased platelet production (malignancies) or increased platelet consumption (SLE, idiopathic thrombocytopenic purpura, hemolytic-uremic syndrome, renal vein thrombosis). Although urinary RBC morphology may be normal with lower tract bleeding and dysmorphic from glomerular bleeding, cell morphology does not reliably correlate with the site of hematuria. The best screening test for a bleeding diathesis is a thorough history. Coagulation studies are not routinely obtained unless personal or family history suggests a bleeding tendency.

TABLE 509-2. Causes of Hematuria in Children

GLOMERULAR HEMATURIA
Isolated Renal Disease
IgA nephropathy (Berger disease)
Alport syndrome (hereditary nephritis)
Thin glomerular basement membrane nephropathy
Postinfectious GN (poststreptococcal GN)
Membranous nephropathy
Membranoproliferative GN
Focal segmental glomerulosclerosis
Antiglomerular basement membrane disease
Multisystem Disease
Systemic lupus erythematosus nephritis*
Henoch-Schönlein purpura nephritis
Wegener granulomatosis
Polyarteritis nodosa
Goodpasture syndrome
Hemolytic-uremic syndrome
Sickle cell glomerulopathy
HIV nephropathy
EXTRAGLOMERULAR HEMATURIA
Upper Urinary Tract
Tubulointerstitial
Pyelonephritis
Interstitial nephritis
Acute tubular necrosis
Papillary necrosis
Nephrocalcinosis
Vascular
Arterial/venous thrombosis
Malformations (aneurysms, hemangiomas)
Nutcracker syndrome
Crystalluria
Calcium
Oxalate
Uric acid
Hemoglobinopathy (sickle cell trait/disease, SC hemoglobin)
Anatomic
Hydronephrosis
Cystic kidney disease
Polycystic kidney disease
Multicystic dysplasia
Tumor (Wilms, rhabdomyosarcoma, angiomyolipoma)
Trauma
Lower Urinary Tract
Inflammation (infectious and noninfectious)
Cystitis
Urethritis
Urolithiasis
Trauma
Coagulopathy
Heavy exercise
Munchausen syndrome/Munchausen syndrome by proxy

*Denotes glomerulonephritides presenting with hypocomplementemia.
GN, glomerulonephritis.

TABLE 509-3. Common Causes of Gross Hematuria

Urinary tract infection
Meatal stenosis
Perineal irritation
Trauma
Urolithiasis/hypercalciuria
Coagulopathy
Tumor
Glomerular
IgA nephropathy
Alport syndrome (hereditary nephritis)
Thin glomerular basement membrane disease
Postinfectious glomerulonephritis
Henoch-Schönlein purpura nephritis
Systemic lupus erythematosus nephritis

A voiding cystourethrogram is only required in patients with a urinary tract infection, renal scarring, hydroureter, or pyelocaliectasis. Cystoscopy is an unnecessary and costly procedure in patients with hematuria that carries the associated risks of anesthesia. This procedure should be reserved for the evaluation of the rare child with a bladder mass noted on ultrasound, urethral abnormalities caused by trauma, posterior urethral valves, or tumor. Unilateral gross hematuria localized by cystoscopy is rarely encountered in the pediatric patient.

Referral to a pediatric nephrologist is recommended for patients with nephritis (glomerulonephritis, tubulointerstitial nephritis), hypertension, renal insufficiency, urolithiasis/nephrocalcinosis, or a family history of renal disease such as polycystic kidney disease or hereditary nephritis. Renal biopsy is indicated for children with persistent microscopic hematuria or recurrent gross hematuria associated with decreased renal function, proteinuria, or hypertension.

Children with persistent asymptomatic isolated hematuria and a normal evaluation should have their serum creatinine values checked annually and their blood pressure and urine checked every 3 mo until the hematuria resolves. Diagnoses to be considered in this situation include resolving postinfectious glomerulonephritis, thin basement membrane disease, IgA nephropathy, or heavy exercise/trauma. Referral to a pediatric nephrologist should be considered for patients with persistent asymptomatic hematuria greater than 1-yr duration.

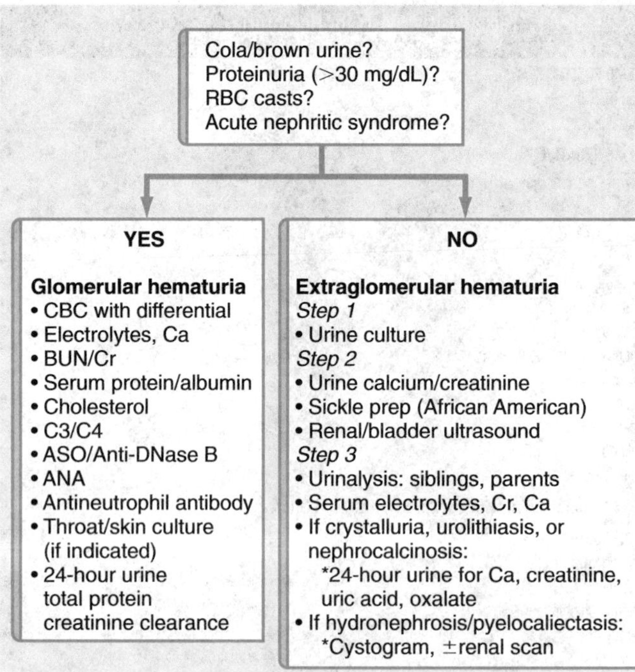

Figure 509-1. Algorithm of the general approach to the laboratory and radiologic evaluation of the patient with glomerular or extraglomerular hematuria. ANA, antinuclear antibody; ASO, antistreptolysin O; BUN, blood urea nitrogen; C3/C4, complement; CBC, complete blood cell count; Cr, creatinine; RBC, red blood cell.

TABLE 509-4. Differential Diagnosis of Symptomatic and Asymptomatic Hematuria

CONFIRM THE PRESENCE OF RED BLOOD CELLS
Symptomatic
Renal symptoms
Urinary tract infections
Nephrolithiasis
Urethrorrhagia
Systemic symptoms
Henoch-Schönlein purpura
Tuberous sclerosis
Asymptomatic
Hypercalciuria
Cystic disease
Obstruction
Vascular
Arteriovenous malformation
Thrombosis
Trauma
Tumor
Hemoglobinopathies
Coagulopathies
Exercise-induced hematuria
Benign familial hematuria (thin basement membrane)
Glomerulonephritis (resolving)
Acute postinfectious nephritis
Immunoglobulin A nephropathy
Henoch-Schönlein purpura

From Kliegman RM, Greenbaum LA, Lyle PS: *Practical Strategies in Pediatric Diagnosis and Therapy,* 2nd ed. Philadelphia, Elsevier, 2004.

Bergstein J, Leiser J, Andreoli S: The clinical significance of asymptomatic gross and microscopic hematuria in children. *Arch Pediatr Adolesc Med* 2005;159:353–355.

Cohen RA, Brown RS: Microscopic hematuria. *N Engl J Med* 2003;348:2330–2338.

Feld LG, Waz WR, Perez LM, et al: Hematuria. An integrated medical and surgical approach. *Pediatr Clin North Am* 1997;44:1191–1210.

Meyers KE: Evaluation of hematuria in children. *Urol Clin North Am* 2004;3:559–573.

Chapter 510 ■ Isolated Glomerular Diseases with Recurrent Gross Hematuria

Approximately 10% of children with gross hematuria have either an acute or chronic form of glomerulonephritis that may be associated with a systemic illness. The gross hematuria, which is usually characterized by brown or cola-colored urine, may be painless or associated with vague flank or abdominal pain. Presentation with gross hematuria is common within 1–2 days after the onset of an apparent viral upper respiratory tract infection in many forms of glomerulonephritis, such as IgA nephropathy, and typically resolves within 5 days. This relatively short period contrasts to a latency period of 7–21 days occurring between the onset of a streptococcal pharyngitis or impetiginous skin infection and the development of poststreptococcal acute glomerulonephritis. Gross hematuria in these circumstances may last as long as 4–6 wk. Gross hematuria may also be seen in children with glomerular basement membrane (GBM) disorders such as hereditary nephritis (Alport syndrome [AS]) and thin GBM disease. These glomerular diseases may also present as microscopic hematuria and/or proteinuria without gross hematuria.

510.1 • IgA Nephropathy (Berger Nephropathy)

IgA nephropathy is the most common chronic glomerular disease worldwide. It is characterized by a predominance of IgA within mesangial deposits of the glomerulus in the absence of systemic diseases such as systemic lupus erythematosus or Henoch-Schönlein purpura. Other diseases with prominent IgA mesangial deposition include rheumatoid arthritis, ankylosing spondylitis, reactive arthritis, inflammatory bowel disease, celiac disease, dermatitis herpetiformis, HIV, and hepatic cirrhosis.

PATHOLOGY AND PATHOLOGIC DIAGNOSIS. Focal and segmental mesangial proliferation and increased mesangial matrix are seen in the glomerulus (Fig. 510-1). Some children display generalized mesangial proliferation that may be associated with crescent formation and scarring. IgA is the predominant immunoglobulin deposited in the mesangium (Fig. 510-2), but lesser amounts of IgG, IgM, C3, and properdin are common. Electron-dense mesangial deposits are seen in most patients; they may also be seen in the subendothelial and subepithelial regions of the GBM.

IgA nephropathy is an immune complex disease that appears to be caused by abnormalities in the IgA immune system. Familial clustering of IgA nephropathy cases suggests the importance of genetic factors. Genome-wide linkage analysis suggest the linkage of IgA nephropathy to 6q22-23 in multiplex IgA nephropathy kindreds.

CLINICAL AND LABORATORY MANIFESTATIONS. A majority of children with IgA nephropathy in the United States and Europe present with gross hematuria, whereas microscopic hematuria and/or proteinuria is a more common presentation in Japan. Other types of presentation include acute nephritic syndrome, nephrotic syndrome, or a combined nephritic-nephrotic syndrome. IgA nephropathy is seen more often in males than in females. Gross hematuria often occurs in association with an upper respiratory or gastrointestinal infection and may be associated with loin pain. Proteinuria is frequently less than 1000 mg/24 hr in patients with asymptomatic microscopic hematuria. Mild to moderate hypertension is most often seen in patients with nephritic or nephrotic syndrome but is rarely severe enough to result in hypertensive emergencies. Normal serum levels of C3 in IgA nephropathy help to distinguish this disorder from poststreptococcal glomerulonephritis. Serum IgA levels have no diagnostic value because they are elevated in only 15% of patients.

PROGNOSIS AND TREATMENT. Although IgA nephropathy does not lead to significant kidney damage in most children, progressive disease develops in 20–30% of children at 15–20 yr after disease onset. Therefore, most children with IgA nephropathy will not display progressive renal dysfunction until adulthood, prompting the need for careful long-term follow-up. Poor prognostic indicators include persistent hypertension, diminished renal function, and heavy or prolonged proteinuria. A worse prognosis is suggested by histologic evidence of diffuse mesangial proliferation, extensive glomerular crescents, glomerulosclerosis, and tubulointerstitial changes, including inflammation and fibrosis.

The primary treatment of IgA nephropathy is proper blood pressure control. Fish oil, which contains anti-inflammatory omega-3 polyunsaturated fatty acids, decreases the rate of renal progression in adults. Immunosuppressive therapy with alternate-day corticosteroids or more intensive multidrug regimens may be beneficial in some patients. Angiotensin-converting enzyme inhibitors and angiotensin II receptor antagonists are effective in reducing proteinuria and retarding the rate of renal progression when used as single agents or in combination. Tonsillectomy may reduce the frequency of gross hematuria and the rate of renal disease progression. Patients with IgA nephropathy may undergo successful renal transplantation. Although recurrent disease is frequent, allograft loss caused by IgA nephropathy occurs in only 15–30% of patients.

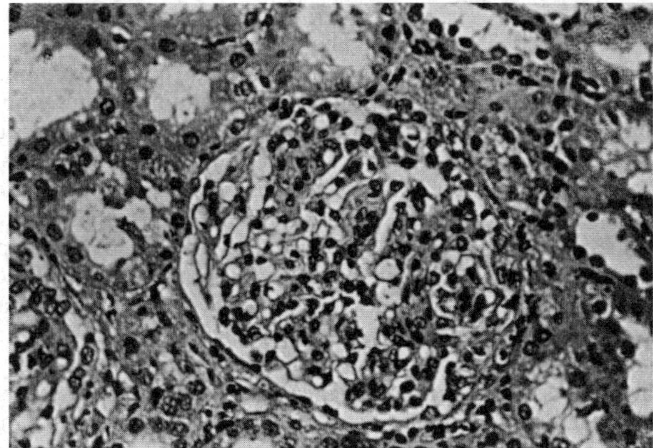

Figure 510-1. Light microscopy of IgA nephropathy demonstrating segmental mesangial proliferation and increased matrix (×180).

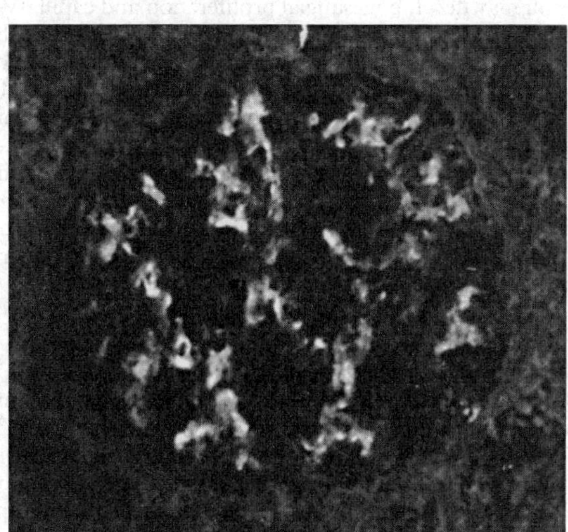

Figure 510-2. Immunofluorescence microscopy of the biopsy specimen from a child with episodes of gross hematuria demonstrating mesangial deposition of immunoglobulin A (×150).

Bartosik LP, Lajoie, Sugar L, et al: Predicting progression in IgA nephropathy. *Am J Kidney Dis* 2001;38:728–735.
Delos Santos NM, Wyatt RJ: Pediatric IgA nephropathies: Clinical aspects and therapeutic approaches. *Semin Nephrol* 2004;24:269–286.
Dillon JJ: Angiotensin-converting enzyme inhibitors and angiotensin receptor blockers for IgA nephropathy. *Semin Nephrol* 2004;24:218–224.
Donadio JV, Grande JP: The role of fish oil/omega-3 fatty acids in the treatment of IgA nephropathy. *Semin Nephrol* 2004;3:225–243.
Gharavi AG, Yan Y, Scolari F, et al: IgA nephropathy, the most common cause of glomerulonephritis is linked to 6q22-23. *Nat Genet* 2000;26:354–357.
Samuels JA, Strippoli GF, Craig JC, et al: Immunosuppressive treatments for immunoglobulin A nephropathy: A meta-analysis of randomized controlled trials. *Nephrology (Carlton)* 2004;4:177–185.
Wang AY, Lai FM, Yu AW, et al: Recurrent IgA nephropathy in renal transplant allografts. *Am J Kidney Dis* 2001;38:588–596.
Wyatt RJ, Hogg RJ: Evidence-based assessment of treatment options for children with IgA nephropathies. *Pediatr Nephrol* 2001;16:156–167.
Xie Y, Chen X, Nishi S, et al: Relationship between tonsils and IgA nephropathy as well as indications of tonsillectomy. *Kidney Int* 2004;65:1135–1144.

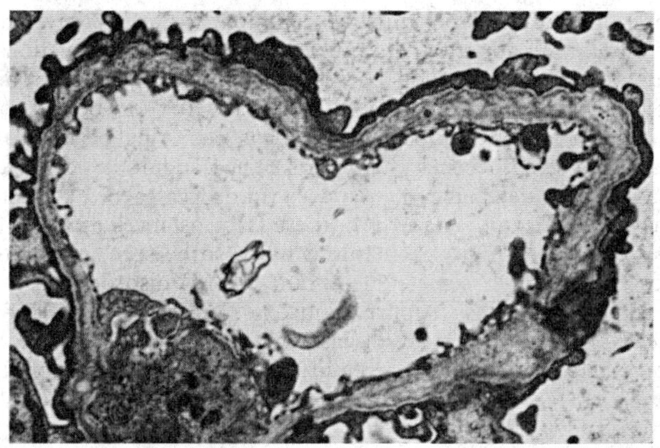

Figure 510-3. Electron micrograph of a biopsy specimen from a child with Alport syndrome depicting thickening, thinning, splitting, and layering of the glomerular basement membrane (×1,650). (From Yum M, Bergstein JM: Basement membrane nephropathy. *Hum Pathol* 1983;14:996–1003.)

510.2 • Alport Syndrome (AS)

AS, hereditary nephritis, is a genetically heterogeneous disease caused by mutations in the genes coding for type IV collagen, a major component of basement membranes. These genetic alterations are associated with marked variability in clinical presentation, natural history, and histologic abnormalities.

GENETICS. Approximately 85% of patients have X-linked disease caused by a mutation in the *COL4A5* gene encoding the α5 chain of type IV collagen. Patients with a subtype of X-linked AS and diffuse leiomyomatosis demonstrate a contiguous mutation within the *COL4A5* and *COL4A6* genes that encodes the α5 and α6 chains, respectively, of type IV collagen. Autosomal recessive forms of AS are caused by mutations in the *COL4A3* and *COL4A4* genes on chromosome 2 encoding the α3 and α4 chains, respectively, of type IV collagen. An autosomal dominant form of AS linked to the *COL4A3-COL4A4* gene locus occurs in 5% of cases.

PATHOLOGY. Kidney biopsy specimens during the 1st decade of life may show few changes on light microscopy. Later, the glomeruli may develop mesangial proliferation and capillary wall thickening, leading to progressive glomerular sclerosis. Tubular atrophy, interstitial inflammation and fibrosis, and presence of lipid containing tubular or interstitial cells, referred to as foam cells, develop as the disease progresses. Immunopathologic studies are usually nondiagnostic.

In most patients, electron microscopic studies reveal diffuse thickening, thinning, splitting, and layering of the basement membranes of the glomeruli (Fig. 510-3) and tubules. However, ultrastructural analysis of the GBM may be completely normal, display nonspecific alterations, or demonstrate only uniform thinning in families that have the typical clinical manifestations of AS.

CLINICAL MANIFESTATIONS. All patients with AS have asymptomatic microscopic hematuria, which may be intermittent in girls and younger boys. Single or recurrent episodes of gross hematuria commonly occurring 1–2 days after an upper respiratory infection are seen in approximately 50% of patients. Proteinuria is frequently seen in males but may be absent, mild, or intermittent in females. Progressive proteinuria, often exceeding 1 g/24 hr, is common by the 2nd decade of life and can be severe enough to cause nephrotic syndrome.

Extrarenal manifestations of AS include hearing deficits and ocular abnormalities. Bilateral sensorineural hearing loss, which is never congenital in onset, occurs in 90% of hemizygous males with X-linked AS, 10% of heterozygous females with X-linked AS, and 67% of individuals with autosomal recessive AS. This deficit begins in the high-frequency range but progresses to involve conversational speech, prompting the need for hearing aids. Ocular abnormalities, which occur in 30–40% of patients with X-linked AS, include anterior lenticonus (extrusion of the central portion of the lens into the anterior chamber), macular flecks, and corneal erosions. Leiomyomatosis of the esophagus, tracheobronchial tree, and female genitals and platelet abnormalities are rarely seen.

DIAGNOSIS. A careful family history, a screening urinalysis of first-degree relatives, an audiogram, and an ophthalmologic examination are critical in making the diagnosis of AS. The presence of anterior lenticonus is pathognomonic. AS is highly likely in the patient with hematuria and at least two of the following characteristic clinical features: macular flecks, recurrent corneal erosions, GBM thickening and thinning, and sensorineural deafness. Absence of epidermal basement membrane staining for the α5 chain of type IV collagen in male hemizygotes and discontinuous epidermal basement membrane staining in female heterozygotes is pathognomonic for X-linked AS. Mutation screening or linkage analysis is not readily available for routine clinical use. Prenatal diagnosis is available for families with X-linked AS individuals who carry an identified mutation.

PROGNOSIS AND TREATMENT. The risk of progressive renal dysfunction leading to end-stage renal disease (ESRD) is highest among hemizygotes and autosomal recessive homozygotes. ESRD occurs before age 30 yr in approximately 75% of hemizygotes with X-linked AS. The risk of ESRD in X-linked heterozygotes is 12% by age 40 and 30% by age 60. Risk factors for progression are gross hematuria during childhood, nephrotic syndrome, and prominent GBM thickening. Intrafamilial variation in phenotypic expression results in significant differences in the age of ESRD among family members. No specific therapy is available to treat AS, although some studies suggest that cyclosporine and angiotensin-converting enzyme inhibitors may slow the rate of renal progression. Careful management of renal failure complications such as hypertension, anemia, and electrolyte imbalance is critical. Patients with ESRD are treated with dialysis and successful kidney transplantation (Chapter 535.3). Approximately 5% of renal transplant recipients develop anti-GBM nephritis, which occurs primarily in males with X-linked AS who develop ESRD before age 30 yr.

Jais JP, Knebelmann B, Giatras I, et al: X-linked Alport syndrome: Natural history and genotype-phenotype correlations in girls and women belonging to 195 families: A "European Community Alport Syndrome Concerted Action" study. *J Am Soc Nephrol* 2003;14:2603–2610.

Kashtan CE: Familial hematuria due to type IV collagen mutations: Alport syndrome and thin basement membrane nephropathy. *Curr Opin Pediatr* 2004;16:177–181.

Proesmans W, Van Dyck M: Enalapril in children with Alport syndrome. *Pediatr Nephrol* 2004;19:271–275.

Wang YY, Rana K, Tonna S, et al: COL4A3 mutations and their clinical consequences in thin basement membrane nephropathy (TBMN). *Kidney Int* 2004;65:786–790.

510.3 • Thin Glomerular Basement Membrane Disease

Thin GBM disease (TGBMD) is defined by the presence of persistent microscopic hematuria and isolated thinning of the GBM on electron microscopy. Isolated hematuria in multiple family members without renal dysfunction is referred to as benign familial hematuria.

TGBMD may be sporadic or transmitted as an autosomal dominant trait. Mutations in the *COL4A3* and *COL4A4* genes among heterozygotes with benign familial hematuria have been reported. Family kindreds with isolated GBM thinning and no identified mutations within the type IV collagen genes have also been reported.

Microscopic hematuria is usually persistent and often initially observed during childhood. Hematuria may initially present in adulthood and may be intermittent. Episodic gross hematuria may also be present, particularly after a respiratory illness. There is no treatment. Progressive renal insufficiency, hypertension, proteinuria, and extrarenal manifestations of TGBMD are rare and suggest the presence of AS. GBM thinning may also be seen in IgA nephropathy.

Savige J, Rana K, Tonna S, et al: Thin basement membrane nephropathy. *Kidney Int* 2003;64:1169–1178.

Chapter 511 ■ Glomerulonephritis Associated with Infections

511.1 • Acute Poststreptococcal Glomerulonephritis

This is a classic example of the **acute nephritic syndrome** characterized by the sudden onset of gross hematuria, edema, hypertension, and renal insufficiency. Acute poststreptococcal glomerulonephritis is one of the most common glomerular causes of gross hematuria in children, surpassed only by IgA nephropathy.

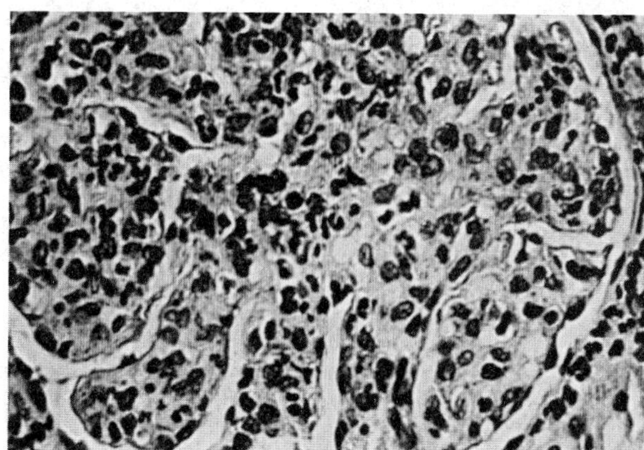

Figure 511-1. Glomerulus from a patient having poststreptococcal glomerulonephritis appearing enlarged and relatively bloodless and showing mesangial proliferation and exudation of neutrophils (×400).

ETIOLOGY AND EPIDEMIOLOGY. Acute poststreptococcal glomerulonephritis follows infection of the throat or skin by certain "nephritogenic" strains of group A β-hemolytic streptococci. The factors that allow only certain strains of streptococci to be nephritogenic remain unclear. Poststreptococcal glomerulonephritis commonly follows streptococcal pharyngitis during cold weather months and streptococcal skin infections or pyoderma during warm weather months. Although epidemics of nephritis have been described in association with both throat (serotype 12) and skin (serotype 49) infections, this disease is most commonly sporadic.

PATHOLOGY. The kidneys appear symmetrically enlarged. All glomeruli appear enlarged and relatively bloodless and show diffuse mesangial cell proliferation with an increase in mesangial matrix (Fig. 511-1). Polymorphonuclear leukocytes are common in glomeruli during the early stage of the disease. Crescents and interstitial inflammation may be seen in severe cases. These changes are not specific for poststreptococcal glomerulonephritis. Immunofluorescence microscopy reveals lumpy-bumpy deposits of immunoglobulin and complement on the glomerular basement membrane (GBM) and in the mesangium. On electron microscopy, electron-dense deposits, or "humps," are observed on the epithelial side of the GBM (Fig. 511-2).

PATHOGENESIS. Although morphologic studies and a depression in the serum complement (C3) level strongly suggest that poststreptococcal glomerulonephritis is mediated by immune complexes, the precise mechanisms by which nephritogenic streptococci induce complex formation remain to be determined. Despite clinical and histologic similarities to acute serum sickness in rabbits, the finding of circulating immune complexes in poststreptococcal glomerulonephritis is not uniform and complement activation is primarily through the alternative rather than the classic (immune complex–activated) pathway.

CLINICAL MANIFESTATIONS. Poststreptococcal glomerulonephritis is most common in children aged 5–12 yr and uncommon before the age of 3 yr. The typical patient develops an acute nephritic syndrome 1–2 wk after an antecedent streptococcal pharyngitis or 3–6 wk after a streptococcal pyoderma. The severity of renal involvement varies from asymptomatic microscopic hematuria with normal renal function to acute renal failure. Depending on the severity of renal involvement, patients may develop various degrees of edema, hypertension, and oliguria. Patients may develop encephalopathy and/or heart failure owing to hypertension or hypervolemia. Encephalopathy may also possibly result from the direct toxic effects of the streptococcal bacteria on the central nervous system. Edema typically results from salt and water retention; nephrotic syndrome may develop in 10–20% of cases. Nonspecific symptoms such as malaise, lethargy, abdominal or flank pain, and fever are common. Acute subglottic edema and airway compromise have been reported. The acute phase generally resolves within 6–8 wk. Although urinary protein excretion and hypertension usually normalize by 4–6 wk after onset, persistent microscopic hematuria may persist for 1–2 yr after the initial presentation.

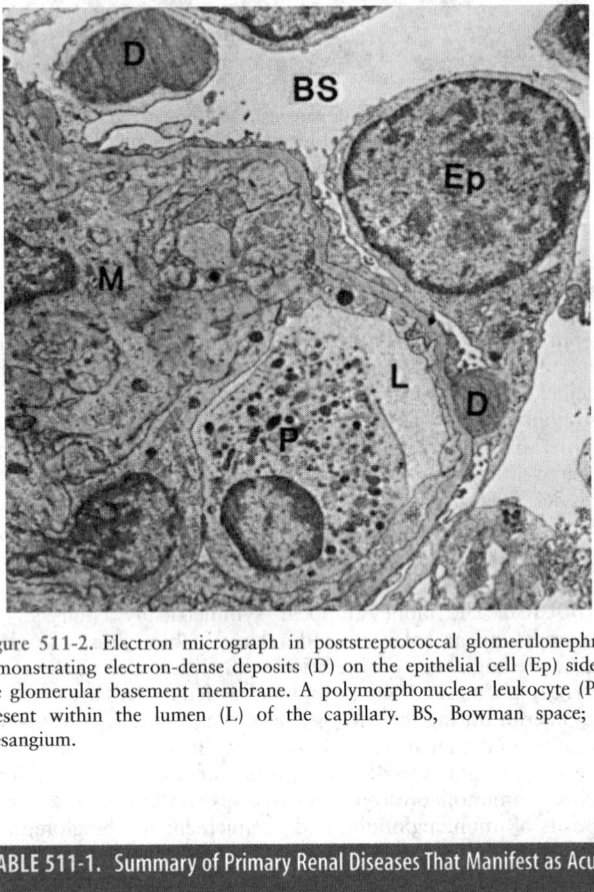

Figure 511-2. Electron micrograph in poststreptococcal glomerulonephritis demonstrating electron-dense deposits (D) on the epithelial cell (Ep) side of the glomerular basement membrane. A polymorphonuclear leukocyte (P) is present within the lumen (L) of the capillary. BS, Bowman space; M, mesangium.

DIAGNOSIS. Urinalysis demonstrates red blood cells (RBCs), frequently in association with RBC casts, proteinuria, and polymorphonuclear leukocytes. A mild normochromic anemia may be present from hemodilution and low-grade hemolysis. The serum C3 level is usually reduced in the acute phase and returns to normal 6–8 wk after onset.

Confirmation of the diagnosis requires clear evidence of invasive streptococcal infection. A positive throat culture report may support the diagnosis or may simply represent the carrier state. On the other hand, a rising antibody titer to streptococcal antigen(s) confirms a recent streptococcal infection. Importantly, the antistreptolysin O titer is commonly elevated after a pharyngeal infection but rarely increases after streptococcal skin infections. The best single antibody titer to document cutaneous streptococcal infection is the anti-deoxyribonuclease (DNase) B level. The Streptozyme test (Wampole Laboratories, Stamford, CT) is a useful and simple diagnostic test that detects antibodies to streptolysin O, DNase B, hyaluronidase, streptokinase, and nicotinamide-adenine dinucleotidase using a slide agglutination test.

The clinical diagnosis of poststreptococcal glomerulonephritis is quite likely in a child presenting with acute nephritic syndrome, evidence of recent streptococcal infection, and a low C3 level. However, it is important to consider other diagnoses such as systemic lupus erythematosus and an acute exacerbation of chronic glomerulonephritis. Renal biopsy should be considered only in the presence of acute renal failure, nephrotic syndrome, absence of evidence of streptococcal infection, or normal complement levels. In addition, renal biopsy is considered when hematuria and proteinuria, diminished renal function, and/or a low C3 level persist more than 2 mo after onset.

The differential diagnosis of poststreptococcal glomerulonephritis includes many of the causes of hematuria listed in Table 509-2 and Table 511-1. Acute glomerulonephritis may also follow infection with coagulase-positive and coagulase-negative staphylococci, *Streptococcus pneumoniae*, and gram-negative bacteria. Bacterial endocarditis may produce a hypocomple-

TABLE 511-1. Summary of Primary Renal Diseases That Manifest as Acute Glomerulonephritis

DISEASES	POSTSTREPTOCOCCAL GLOMERULONEPHRITIS	IGA NEPHROPATHY	GOODPASTURE SYNDROME	IDIOPATHIC RAPIDLY PROGRESSIVE GLOMERULONEPHRITIS (RPGN)
Clinical manifestations				
Age and sex	All ages, mean 7 yr, 2 : 1 male	10–35 yr, 2 : 1 male	15–30 yr, 6 : 1 male	Adults, 2 : 1 male
Acute nephritic syndrome	90%	50%	90%	90%
Asymptomatic hematuria	Occasionally	50%	Rare	Rare
Nephrotic syndrome	10–20%	Rare	Rare	10–20%
Hypertension	70%	30–50%	Rare	25%
Acute renal failure	50% (transient)	Very rare	50%	60%
Other	Latent period of 1–3 wk	Follows viral syndromes	Pulmonary hemorrhage; iron deficiency anemia	None
Laboratory findings	↑ ASO titers (70%) Positive streptozyme (95%) ↓C3–C9; normal C1, C4	↑ Serum IgA (50%) IgA in dermal capillaries	Positive anti-GBM antibody	Positive ANCA in some
Immunogenetics	HLA-B12, D"EN" (9)*	HLA-Bw 35, DR4 (4)*	HLA-DR2 (16)*	None established
Renal pathology				
Light microscopy	Diffuse proliferation	Focal proliferation	Focal → diffuse proliferation with crescents	Crescentic GN
Immunofluorescence	Granular IgG, C3	Diffuse mesangial IgA	Linear IgG, C3	No immune deposits
Electron microscopy	Subepithelial humps	Mesangial deposits	No deposits	No deposits
Prognosis	95% resolve spontaneously 5% RPGN or slowly progressive	Slow progression in 25–50%	75% stabilize or improve if treated early	75% stabilize or improve if treated early
Treatment	Supportive	Uncertain (options include steroids, fish oil, and ACE inhibitors)	Plasma exchange, steroids, cyclophosphamide	Steroid pulse therapy

*Relative risk.
ACE, angiotensin-converting enzyme; ANCA, antineutrophil cytoplasmic antibody; ASO, anti-streptolysin O; GBM, glomerular basement membrane; GN, glomerulonephritis; HLA, human leukocyte antigen; Ig, immunoglobulin.
From Kliegman RM, Greenbaum LA, Lye PS: *Practical Strategies in Pediatric Diagnosis and Therapy*, 2nd ed. Philadelphia, Elsevier, 2004, p 427.

mentemic glomerulonephritis with renal failure. Acute glomerulonephritis may occur after certain fungal, rickettsial, and viral diseases, particularly influenza.

COMPLICATIONS. Acute complications of this disease result from hypertension and acute renal dysfunction. Hypertension is seen in 60% of patients and may be associated with hypertensive encephalopathy in 10% of cases. Other potential complications include heart failure, hyperkalemia, hyperphosphatemia, hypocalcemia, acidosis, seizures, and uremia.

PREVENTION. Early systemic antibiotic therapy for streptococcal throat and skin infections does not eliminate the risk of glomerulonephritis. Family members of patients with acute glomerulonephritis should be cultured for group A β-hemolytic streptococci and treated if culture positive.

TREATMENT. Management is directed at treating the acute effects of renal insufficiency and hypertension (Chapter 535.1). Although a 10-day course of systemic antibiotic therapy with penicillin is recommended to limit the spread of the nephritogenic organisms, antibiotic therapy does not affect the natural history of glomerulonephritis. Sodium restriction, diuresis usually with intravenous Lasix, and pharmacotherapy with calcium channel antagonists, vasodilators, or angiotensin-converting enzyme inhibitors are standard therapies used to treat hypertension.

PROGNOSIS. Complete recovery occurs in more than 95% of children with acute poststreptococcal glomerulonephritis. Mortality in the acute stage can be avoided by appropriate management of acute renal failure, cardiac failure, and hypertension. Infrequently, the acute phase may be severe and lead to glomerular hyalinization and chronic kidney disease. However, the diagnosis of acute poststreptococcal glomerulonephritis must be questioned in patients with chronic kidney disease because other diagnoses such as membranoproliferative glomerulonephritis may be present. Recurrences are extremely rare.

Clark G, White RHR, Glasgow EF, et al: Poststreptococcal glomerulonephritis in children: Clinicopathological correlations and long-term prognosis. *Pediatr Nephrol* 1988; 2:381–388.

Dodge WF, Spargo BH, Travis LB, et al: Poststreptococcal glomerulonephritis in children: A prospective study. *N Engl J Med* 1972;286:273–278.

Potter EV, Lipschultz SA, Abidh S, et al: Twelve to fifteen-year follow-up of patients with poststreptococcal acute glomerulonephritis in Trinidad. *N Engl J Med* 1982;307:725–729.

White AV, Hoy WE, McCredie DA: Childhood post-streptococcal glomerulonephritis as a risk factor for chronic renal disease in later life. *Med J Aust* 2001;10:492–496.

511.2 • Other Chronic Infections

Occurrence of glomerulonephritis has been recognized during the course of various chronic infections, including bacterial endocarditis caused by viridans streptococcus and other organisms, ventriculoatrial shunts for hydrocephalus infected with *Staphylococcus epidermidis,* syphilis, hepatitis B virus, hepatitis C virus, and candidiasis. Parasitic infections associated with glomerular disease include malaria, schistosomiasis, leishmaniasis, filariasis, hydatid disease, trypanosomiasis, and toxoplasmosis. In each condition, the infecting organism has low virulence and the host is chronically infected with foreign antigen. In the presence of high levels of circulating antigen, the host's antibody response leads to formation of immune complexes that deposit in the kidneys and initiate glomerular inflammation.

The histopathologic findings may resemble poststreptococcal, membranous, or membranoproliferative glomerulonephritis. The clinical manifestations are generally those of an acute nephritic or nephrotic syndrome. The complement C3 level is frequently depressed.

Eradication of the infection before severe glomerular injury occurs usually results in resolution of the glomerulonephritis. Progression to end-stage renal failure has been described, but is uncommon.

Chesney RW, O'Regan S, Guyda HJ, et al: *Candida* endocrinopathy syndrome with membranoproliferative glomerulonephritis: Demonstration of glomerular *Candida* antigen. *Clin Nephrol* 1976;5:232–238.

Connor FL, Rosenberg AR, Kennedy SE, et al: HBV associated nephrotic syndrome: Resolution with oral lamivudine. *Arch Dis Child* 2003;88:446–449.

Hendrickse RG, Adeniyi A: Quartan malarial nephrotic syndrome in children. *Kidney Int* 1979;16:64–74.

Hunte W, Al-Ghraoui F, Cohen RJ: Secondary syphilis and the nephrotic syndrome. *J Am Soc Nephrol* 1993;3:1351–1355.

Meyers CM, Seeff LB, Stehman-Breen CO, et al: Hepatitis C and renal disease: An update. *Am J Kidney Dis* 2003;42:631–657.

Neugarten J, Baldwin DS: Glomerulonephritis in bacterial endocarditis. *Am J Med* 1984;77:297–304.

Ozdamar SO, Gucer S, Tinaztepe K: Hepatitis-B virus associated nephropathies: A clinicopathological study in 14 children. *Pediatr Nephrol* 2003;181:23–28.

Ray PE, Xu L, Rakusan T, Liu XH: A 20-year history of childhood HIV-associated nephropathy. *Pediatr Nephrol* 2004;10:1075–1092.

Vella J, Carmody M, Campbell E, et al: Glomerulonephritis after ventriculoatrial shunt. *Q J Med* 1995;88:911–918.

Walters S, Levin M: Infectious diseases and the kidney. In Barratt TM, Avner ED, Harmon WE (editors): *Pediatric Nephrology,* 4th ed. Baltimore, Lippincott Williams & Wilkins, 1999, pp 1079–1102.

Chapter 512 ■ Membranous Glomerulopathy (Glomerulonephritis)

Although membranous glomerulopathy is the most common cause of nephrotic syndrome in adults, it is an uncommon cause of hematuria in children. Membranous glomerulopathy typically presents as an isolated renal disease. However, it may be associated with systemic illnesses, including autoimmune diseases such as systemic lupus erythematosus or chronic immune thrombocytopenic purpura, sarcoidosis, neuroblastoma, gonadoblastoma, gold or penicillamine therapy, syphilis, and hepatitis B and C virus infections. These secondary causes of membranous glomerulopathy are more common in children compared to adults. Furthermore, identification of these secondary causes of membranous glomerulopathy is important because treatment of these diseases may lead to resolution of the glomerular lesions.

PATHOLOGY. The glomeruli show diffuse thickening of the glomerular basement membrane (GBM), without significant proliferative changes (Fig. 512-1). The thickening presumably results from the production of membrane-like material by the visceral epithelial cells in response to immune complexes deposited on the epithelial side of the membrane. This new material may in certain areas resemble spikes on the epithelial side of the GBM. Immunofluorescent microscopy demonstrates granular deposits

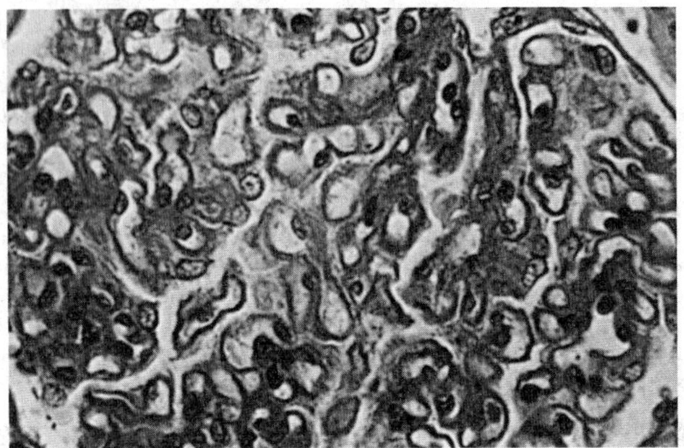

Figure 512-1. Glomerulus from a patient having membranous glomerulopathy demonstrating diffuse thickening of the glomerular basement membrane in the absence of cellular proliferation (×400).

of IgG and C3 located on the epithelial side of the GBM when viewed under electron microscopy. Linear staining of IgG, IgA, and C3 along the tubular basement membrane may be seen on immunofluorescence.

PATHOGENESIS. Morphologic studies suggest that membranous glomerulopathy is an immune complex–mediated disease. The molecular pathogenesis of membranous nephropathy in humans remains unknown. Genetic factors may influence disease susceptibility and/or disease progression. Neonatal-onset membranous glomerulopathy is characterized by maternal anti–neutral endopeptidase (NEP) antibodies, which cross the placenta from mothers genetically deficient in the NEP antigen. NEP is a membrane metalloendopeptidase that is absent in antibody-producing mothers. Alloimmunization by fetal NEP produces maternal antibodies that cross the placenta, initiating membranous glomerulopathy.

CLINICAL MANIFESTATIONS. In children, membranous glomerulopathy is most common in the 2nd decade of life. The disease usually presents as nephrotic syndrome and accounts for 2–6% of childhood nephrotic syndrome cases (see Chapter 527). Most patients have microscopic hematuria and occasionally demonstrate gross hematuria. Approximately 20% of children present with hypertension. C3 levels are normal except in cases of systemic lupus erythematosus, in which levels may be depressed.

DIAGNOSIS. The diagnosis of membranous nephropathy is confirmed only by kidney biopsy, as there is no specific diagnostic laboratory test. The usual indications for biopsy include the presentation of nephrotic syndrome in a child, usually older than 10 yr, or the presence of unexplained hematuria and proteinuria. Patients with membranous glomerulopathy are at an increased risk of **renal vein thrombosis.**

PROGNOSIS AND TREATMENT. The clinical course of membranous glomerulopathy is variable. Children presenting with asymptomatic low-grade proteinuria may achieve a spontaneous remission. Follow-up studies of 1–14 yr suggest that 20% of children progress to chronic renal failure, whereas 40% continue with active disease. The nephrotic state is best controlled with salt restriction and diuretic agents (see Chapter 527). Proteinuria may be decreased by angiotensin-converting enzyme inhibitors or angiotensin II receptor antagonists (alone or in combination). Immunosuppressive therapy with prednisone in conjunction with chlorambucil or cyclophosphamide may be beneficial in adults in slowing the rate of progressive renal disease, particularly in patients with severe or prolonged proteinuria, renal insufficiency, or hypertension. There are no controlled data on the use of these agents in children with membranous nephropathy. Rituximab, a monoclonal antibody to the B-cell CD20 antigen, has been effective therapy in a small number of adult patients.

Cattran DC: Idiopathic membranous glomerulonephritis. *Kidney Int* 2000;59:1983–1994.

Debiec H, Nauta J, Coulet F, et al: Role of truncating mutations in *MME* gene in fetomaternal alloimmunization and antenatal glomerulopathies. *Lancet* 2004;364:1252–1259.

Eddy AA, Symons JM: Nephrotic syndrome in childhood. *Lancet* 2003;362:629–639.

Louis CU, Morgenstern BZ, Butani L: Thrombotic complications in childhood-onset idiopathic membranous nephropathy. *Pediatr Nephrol* 2003;18:1298–1300.

Makker SP: Treatment of membranous nephropathy in children. *Semin Nephrol* 2003;23:379–385.

Pape L, Mengel M, Offner G, et al: Cyclosporin A-induced remission of primary membranous glomerulonephritis in a child. *Nephrol Dial Transplant* 2004;19:3207.

Remuzzi G, Chiurchiu C, Abbate M, et al: Rituximab for idiopathic membranous nephropathy. *Lancet* 2002;360:923–924.

Chapter 513 ■ Membranoproliferative (Mesangiocapillary) Glomerulonephritis

The term **chronic glomerulonephritis** implies continuing glomerular injury that frequently leads to glomerular destruction and end-stage renal failure. Membranoproliferative glomerulonephritis (MPGN) is the most common cause of chronic glomerulonephritis in older children and young adults.

PATHOLOGY AND PATHOGENESIS. MPGN was initially distinguished from other forms of chronic glomerulonephritis by the finding of hypocomplementemia in most patients. In some patients, hypocomplementemia results from an antibody, referred to as C3 nephritic factor, that activates the alternative complement pathway. Three histologic types of MPGN are described.

Type I MPGN is the most common form. The glomeruli reveal an accentuation of the lobular pattern owing to a generalized increase in mesangial cells and matrix (Fig. 513-1). The glomerular capillary walls appear thickened, often containing regions of duplication or splitting from interposition of mesangial cytoplasm and matrix between the endothelial cells and glomerular basement membrane (GBM). Crescents may be present and indicate a poor prognosis when detected in a high percentage of glomeruli. Immunofluorescent microscopy reveals C3 and lesser amounts of immunoglobulin in the mesangium and along the peripheral capillary walls in a lobular pattern (Fig. 513-2). Electron microscopy confirms the presence of immune complex–like deposits in the mesangial and subendothelial regions.

In **type II disease,** the mesangial changes are less prominent than in type I. The capillary walls demonstrate irregular ribbon-like thickening owing to the deposition of electron-dense deposits. Splitting of the membrane is rare, but crescents are common. On electron microscopy, the dense deposits are seen as thickenings of the GBM in a region distinct from the lamina densa. The deposits are also found in the Bowman capsule, mesangium, and tubular basement membranes. Immunofluores-

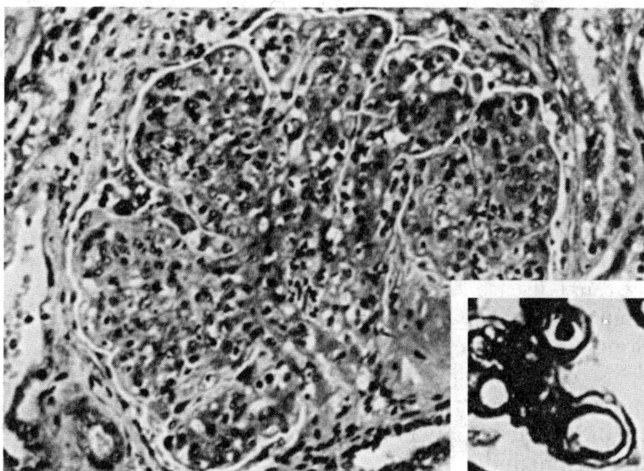

Figure 513-1. Glomerulus from a patient with type I membranoproliferative glomerulonephritis demonstrating an accentuated lobular pattern, a generalized increase in mesangial wall and matrix, and "splitting" of the glomerular capillary wall (inset) (×250). (From Kim Y, Michael F: Idiopathic membranoproliferative glomerulonephritis. *Annu Rev Med* 1980;31:273–288.)

cent studies show C3 and minimal immunoglobulin along the margin of the dense deposit material.

In **type III disease,** the light and immunofluorescent microscopic findings resemble those found in type I disease. Electron microscopy reveals contiguous subepithelial and subendothelial deposits associated with disruption and layering of the lamina densa portion of the GBM.

CLINICAL MANIFESTATIONS. MPGN is most common in the 2nd decade of life. The majority of patients present with nephrotic syndrome (see Chapter 527). Others may present with an acute nephritic syndrome characterized by gross hematuria or asymptomatic microscopic hematuria and proteinuria. Renal function may be normal or decreased. Hypertension is common. The serum C3 complement level may be decreased.

DIAGNOSIS AND DIFFERENTIAL DIAGNOSIS. The diagnosis of MPGN is made by renal biopsy. Indications for biopsy include nephrotic syndrome in a child older than 10 yr, significant proteinuria with microscopic hematuria, and hypocomplementemia lasting longer than 8 wk in a child with acute nephritis.

Both MPGN and poststreptococcal glomerulonephritis may be associated with gross hematuria, hypertension, low C3 levels, and elevated antistreptococcal antibody titers. Patients with poststreptococcal glomerulonephritis improve within 2 mo of onset, whereas nephritic syndrome, proteinuria, and hypocomplementemia persist in children with MPGN, generally mandating a kidney biopsy.

PROGNOSIS AND TREATMENT. Although some patients recover completely, approximately 50% of patients with MPGN progress to end-stage renal disease 10 yr after their initial presentation. Factors associated with a poor prognosis include nephrotic syndrome at time of presentation, histologic presence of type II MPGN, and decreased glomerular filtration rate 1 yr following the initial presentation. Recurrence of MPGN in the allograft following kidney transplantation occurs in approximately 30% of patients with type I and 90% of patients with type II MPGN, suggesting the presence of a systemic disorder. No definitive therapy exists, although stabilization of the clinical course has been reported in many patients receiving 3–7 yr of alternate-day prednisone therapy.

Bergstein JM, Andreoli SP: Response of type I membranoproliferative glomerulonephritis to pulse methylprednisolone and alternate-day prednisone therapy. *Pediatr Nephrol* 1995;9:268–271.

Cansick JC, Lennon R, Cummins CL, et al: Prognosis, treatment and outcome of childhood mesangiocapillary (membranoproliferative) glomerulonephritis. *Nephrol Dial Transplant* 2004;19:2769–2777.

McEnery PT: Membranoproliferative glomerulonephritis: The Cincinnati experience—cumulative renal survival from 1957 to 1989. *J Pediatr* 1990;116:S109–S114.

Tarshish P, Bernstein J, Tobin JN, et al: Treatment of mesangiocapillary glomerulonephritis with alternate-day prednisone—a report of The International Study of Kidney Disease in Children. *Pediatr Nephrol* 1992;6:123–130.

Yanagihara T, Hayakawa M, Yoshida J, et al: Long-term follow-up of diffuse membranoproliferative glomerulonephritis type I. *Pediatr Nephrol* 2005;20:585–590.

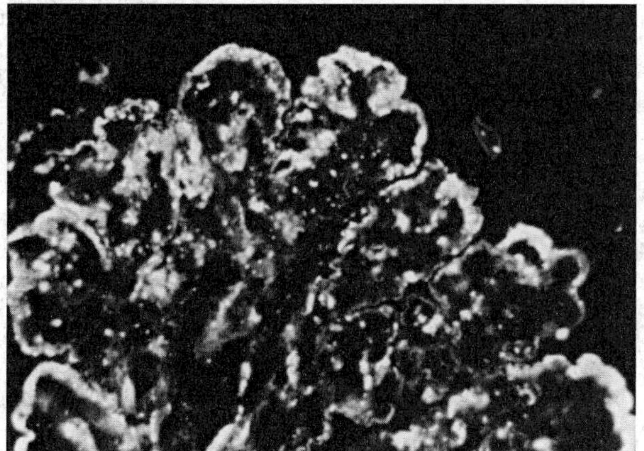

Figure 513-2. Immunofluorescence microscopy in type I membranoproliferative glomerulonephritis demonstrating granular deposition of C3 along the glomerular basement membrane and in the mesangium. (From Kim Y, Michael F: Idiopathic membranoproliferative glomerulonephritis. *Annu Rev Med* 1980;31:273–288.)

Chapter 514 ■ Glomerulonephritis Associated with Systemic Lupus Erythematosus

Systemic lupus erythematosus (SLE) is characterized by fever, weight loss, rash, hematologic abnormalities, arthritis, and involvement of the heart, lungs, central nervous system, and kidneys (see Chapter 157). Kidney disease, one of the most common features of SLE in childhood, may occasionally be the only manifestation.

PATHOGENESIS AND PATHOLOGY. The clinical manifestations of SLE are mediated by immune complexes. Aberrations in both B- and T-cell function are noted.

The classification of lupus nephritis of the World Health Organization (WHO) is based on a combination of light microscopy, immunofluorescence, and electron microscopy features. In patients with **WHO class I nephritis,** no histologic abnormalities are detected. In **WHO class II nephritis** (mesangial lupus nephritis), glomeruli demonstrate mesangial deposits containing immunoglobulin and complement; light microscopy may show mild (**class II-A**) or moderate mesangial hypercellularity and increased matrix (**class II-B**).

In **WHO class III nephritis** (focal segmental lupus glomerulonephritis), mesangial deposits occur in almost all glomeruli and subendothelial deposits are noted between the endothelial cells and glomerular basement membrane. In addition to focal and segmental mesangial proliferation, occasional glomeruli show capillary wall necrosis, crescent formation, and sclerosis.

WHO class IV nephritis (diffuse proliferative lupus nephritis) is the most common and most severe form of lupus nephritis. All glomeruli contain significant mesangial and subendothelial deposits of immunoglobulin and complement. All glomeruli show mesangial proliferation. The capillary walls are frequently thickened secondary to subendothelial deposits (creating the "wire-loop" lesion) and often demonstrate necrosis, crescent formation, and scarring.

WHO class V nephritis (membranous lupus nephritis) is the least common. It histologically resembles idiopathic membranous glomerulopathy, except for the presence of mild to moderate mesangial proliferation.

Transformation of the histologic lesion from one class to another is common. This is more likely to occur among inadequately treated patients and usually results in progression to a more severe histologic lesion.

CLINICAL MANIFESTATIONS. The majority of children with SLE are adolescent females. Clinical evidence of renal disease occurs in 30–70% of children. The clinical findings in patients having the milder forms (all class II, some class III) of lupus nephritis include hematuria, normal renal function, and proteinuria of <1 g/24 hr. Some patients with class III and all patients with class IV nephritis have hematuria and proteinuria, reduced renal function, nephrotic syndrome, or acute renal failure. In rare patients with proliferative glomerulonephritis, the urinalysis may be completely normal. Patients with class V nephritis commonly present with nephrotic syndrome.

DIAGNOSIS. The diagnosis of SLE is suggested by the detection of circulating antinuclear antibodies and is confirmed by demonstrating antibodies that react with native double-stranded DNA. In most patients with active disease, C3 and C4 levels are depressed. In view of the lack of a clear correlation between the clinical manifestations and the severity of the renal involvement, renal biopsy should be performed in all patients with SLE. These results are used to guide the selection of immunosuppressive therapies.

TREATMENT. Children with SLE should be treated by pediatric specialists in medical centers where both medical and psychological support can be given to both patients and their families. Immunosuppressive therapy in lupus nephritis is aimed at establishing a clinical and serologic remission, defined as normalization of anti-DNA, C3, and C4 levels. Therapy is initiated in all patients with prednisone at a dose of 1–2 mg/kg/day divided into 2 or 3 doses followed by a slow steroid taper over 4–6 mo beginning 4–6 wk after achieving a serologic remission. For patients having more severe forms of nephritis (WHO classes III and IV), 6 consecutive monthly intravenous infusions of cyclophosphamide at a dose of 500–1,000 mg/m^2 followed by dosing every 3 mo for 18 mo appears to reduce the risk of progressive renal dysfunction. Azathioprine at a single daily dose of 1.5–2.0 mg/kg may be used as a steroid-sparing agent in patients with WHO class I or II lupus nephritis. Single-center case reports also suggest the potential benefit of mycophenolate mofetil in patients with mild lupus nephritis. Rituximab, a chimeric monoclonal antibody specific for human CD20, may be effective in patients with WHO type IV lupus nephritis resistant to conventional immunosuppressive therapies.

PROGNOSIS. Aggressive immunosuppressive therapy improves the prognosis of SLE in childhood. Renal survival without the need for dialysis is seen in 80% of patients 10 yr after the diagnosis of SLE nephritis. Patients with diffuse proliferative WHO class IV lupus nephritis exhibit the highest risk for progression to end-stage renal disease. Concerns regarding the side effects of chronic immunosuppressive therapy and the risk of recurrent disease are lifelong. Special care must be taken to minimize the risks of osteoporosis, obesity, hypertension, and diabetes mellitus associated with chronic steroid therapy. The risk of malignancy or infertility is increased in patients receiving a cumulative dose of >20 g cyclophosphamide.

Baqi N, Moazami S, Singh A, et al: Lupus nephritis in children: A longitudinal study of prognostic factors and therapy. *J Am Soc Nephrol* 1996;7:924–929.

Bogdanovic R, Nikolic V, Pasic S, et al: Lupus nephritis in childhood: A review of 53 patients followed at a single center. *Pediatr Nephrol* 2004;19:36–44.

Edelbauer M, Jungraithmayr T, Zimmerhackl LB: Rituximab in childhood systemic lupus erythematosus refractory to conventional immunosuppression. *Pediatr Nephrol* 2005;20:811–813.

Hagelberg S, Lee Y, Bargman J, et al: Longterm followup of childhood lupus nephritis. *J Rheumatol* 2002;29:2635–2642.

Illei GG, Austin HA, Crane M, et al: Combination therapy with pulse cyclophosphamide plus pulse methylprednisolone improves long-term renal outcome without adding toxicity in patients with lupus nephritis. *Ann Intern Med* 2001;135:296–298.

Perfumo F, Martini A: Lupus nephritis in children. *Lupus* 2005;14:83–88.

Chapter 515 ■ Henoch-Schönlein Purpura Nephritis

Henoch-Schönlein purpura (HSP) nephritis (anaphylactoid purpura) is a small vessel vasculitis characterized by a purpuric rash, arthritis, abdominal pain, and glomerulonephritis (see Chapter 166.1). HSP nephritis and IgA nephropathy demonstrate identical renal pathologic findings, but systemic findings are only seen in HSP nephritis.

PATHOLOGY AND PATHOGENESIS. Glomerular and tubulointerstitial abnormalities on light, immunofluorescence, and electron microscopy in HSP nephritis are virtually indistinguishable from the pathologic findings in IgA nephropathy. Crescent formation is more common and more extensive in patients with HSP nephritis. Although the pathogenesis of HSP nephritis remains unknown, this disease appears to be mediated by the formation of immune complexes containing polymeric IgA1 within capillaries of the skin, intestines, and glomerulus.

CLINICAL AND LABORATORY MANIFESTATIONS. The symptoms and signs of HSP nephritis typically appear 1–3 wk after an upper respiratory tract infection (see Chapter 166.1). The diagnosis of HSP is based on the constellation of clinical findings. Whereas gross hematuria is seen in 20–30% of cases, patients may also present with isolated microscopic hematuria, hematuria and proteinuria; acute nephritic syndrome, nephrotic syndrome, and acute renal insufficiency are less common. Renal manifestations of HSP nephritis occur up to 12 wk after the initial presentation of HSP. An uncommon urologic manifestation of this disease is **ureteritis**, which is associated with loin pain and renal colic. Ureteritis is usually seen in children younger than 5 yr of age and frequently leads to ureteral stenosis with subsequent hydronephrosis, which requires surgical correction.

PROGNOSIS AND TREATMENT. The prognosis in HSP nephritis is generally favorable, although the risk of chronic kidney disease is 2–5%. Presentation with isolated microscopic hematuria alone carries the best prognosis, whereas presentation with acute nephritic and/or nephrotic syndrome carries the highest risk of developing hypertension, pregnancy-induced hypertension, hematuria, or chronic renal failure.

There are no controlled data demonstrating that steroids, cytotoxic agents, or anticoagulants alter the course of HSP nephritis. Uncontrolled studies suggest the potential value of high-dose corticosteroid and cytotoxic therapy with cyclophosphamide or azathioprine in patients with crescentic glomerulonephritis or significant proteinuria. Addition of dipyridamole and/or heparin/warfarin may provide additional benefit in patients with severe forms of nephritis. Some studies suggest that short courses of low-dose prednisone initiated at diagnosis reduce the subsequent risk of developing any clinical signs of nephritis. There are no controlled data suggesting that any therapy reduces the risk of progression to severe renal disease. Tonsillectomy does not appear to alter the course of HSP nephritis. Children with more severe forms of HSP nephritis remain at risk of chronic kidney disease into adulthood.

Algoet C, Proesmans W: Renal biopsy 2–9 years after Henoch Schonlein purpura. *Pediatr Nephrol* 2003;18:471–473.

Foster BJ, Bernard C, Drummond K, et al: Effective therapy for severe Henoch-Schönlein purpura nephritis with prednisone and azathioprine: A clinical and pathologic study. *J Pediatr* 2000;136:370–375.

Halling S, Soderberg M, Berg U: Henoch Schonlein nephritis: Clinical findings related to renal function and morphology. *Pediatr Nephrol* 2005;20:46–51.

Niaudet P, Habib R: Methylprednisolone pulse therapy in the treatment of severe forms of Henoch-Schönlein purpura nephritis. *Pediatr Nephrol* 1998;12:238–243.

Ronkainen J, Nuutinen M, Koskimies O: The adult kidney 24 years after childhood Henoch-Schonlein purpura: A retrospective cohort study. *Lancet* 2002;360:666–670.

Tarshish P, Bernstein J, Edelmann CM Jr: Henoch-Schonlein purpura nephritis: Course of disease and efficacy of cyclophosphamide. *Pediatr Nephrol* 2004;19:51–56.

Chapter 516 ■ Rapidly Progressive (Crescentic) Glomerulonephritis

Rapidly progressive describes the clinical course of several forms of glomerulonephritis (GN) whose unifying abnormality is the histopathologic finding of crescents in the majority of glomeruli. The natural history in most forms is rapid progression to end-stage renal failure.

TABLE 516-1. Classification of Rapidly Progressive (Crescentic) Glomerulonephritis (RPGN)

TYPE OF RPGN	FREQUENCY
ANTI-GBM ANTIBODY–MEDIATED RPGN	20%
Goodpasture syndrome	
Idiopathic anti-GBM nephritis	
Membranous nephropathy with crescents	
RPGN ASSOCIATED WITH GRANULAR IMMUNE DEPOSITS	40%
Postinfectious	
Poststreptococcal glomerulonephritis	
Bacterial endocarditis	
"Shunt" nephritis	
Visceral abscesses, other nonstreptococcal infections	
Noninfectious	
Systemic lupus erythematosus	
Henoch-Schönlein purpura	
Mixed cryoglobulinemia	
Solid tumors	
Primary Renal Disease	
Membranoproliferative glomerulonephritis	
IgA nephropathy	
Idiopathic immune-complex nephritis	
RPGN WITHOUT GLOMERULAR IMMUNE DEPOSITS	40%
Vasculitis	
Polyarteritis	
Hypersensitivity vasculitis	
Wegener granulomatosis	
Idiopathic RPGN	

GBM-glomerular basement membrane.
From Kliegman RM, Greenbaum LA, Lye PS: *Practical Strategies in Pediatric Diagnosis and Therapy*, 2nd ed. Philadelphia, Elsevier, 2004, p 426.

CLASSIFICATION. Crescents may be found in several well-defined types of GN including (1) the immune complex–mediated forms of GN: poststreptococcal GN, lupus nephritis, membranoproliferative GN, and Henoch-Schönlein purpura/IgA nephritis; (2) anti–glomerular basement membrane–mediated GN such as Goodpasture disease; and (3) antineutrophil cytoplasmic antibody (ANCA)–mediated GN: microscopic polyarteritis nodosa and Wegener granulomatosis (Table 516-1). The typical findings on light, immunofluorescence, and electron microscopy examinations are maintained despite crescent formation. These histologic findings, in conjunction with clinical features and appropriate laboratory studies, reveal the underlying disease. A small group of patients do not have a clearly identified underlying GN and/or considered to have "idiopathic" rapidly progressive (crescentic) GN.

PATHOLOGY AND PATHOGENESIS. Crescents are found on the inside of the Bowman capsule and are composed of proliferating epithelial cells of the capsule, fibrin, basement membrane–like material, and macrophages (Fig. 516-1). The stimulus for crescent formation is presumed to be the deposition of fibrin in the Bowman space, probably because of necrosis or disruption of the glomerular capillary wall. Many patients display capillary wall immune-complex deposits or linear IgG antibody staining against glomerular basement membrane. Immunofluorescence and electron microscopy studies in patients with ANCA-mediated forms of GN typically show no evidence of immunologic injury. The complement C3 level is normal.

CLINICAL MANIFESTATIONS. Most patients develop acute renal failure associated with acute nephritic and/or nephrotic syn-

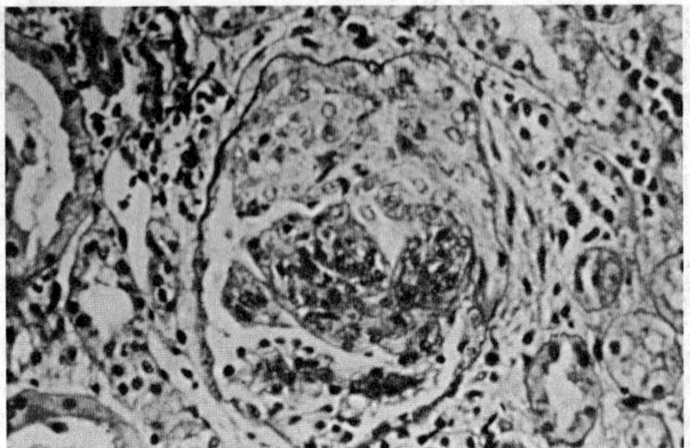

Figure 516-1. Light micrograph of a biopsy specimen from a child with Henoch-Schönlein purpura glomerulonephritis demonstrating a crescent overlying the glomerulus (×180).

drome. Progression to end-stage renal failure usually occurs within weeks to months after onset.

DIAGNOSIS AND DIFFERENTIAL DIAGNOSIS. Appropriate serologic studies such as antinuclear antibody, C3, and anti-deoxyribonucleotidase B titers should be obtained to delineate specific types of GN. Rare forms of vasculitis, such as Wegener granulomatosis and microscopic polyarteritis nodosa, may be suggested by the detection of ANCA antibodies to either myeloperoxidase or serine proteinase-3 within the neutrophil cytoplasm. The diagnosis is confirmed by kidney biopsy.

PROGNOSIS AND TREATMENT. Children with a rapidly progressive course associated with poststreptococcal GN usually recover spontaneously. Excellent therapeutic response using a combination of corticosteroids and cytotoxic therapy with cyclophosphamide often occurs in patients with systemic lupus erythematosus, IgA nephropathy, and Henoch-Schönlein purpura nephritis. Renal outcomes in other diseases causing rapidly progressive GN are less favorable, with end-stage renal disease occurring within 2–3 yr. Therapy combining pulse methylprednisolone and oral cyclophosphamide may be effective, particularly in patients with Wegener granulomatosis. Plasmapheresis or lymphocytapheresis has been effective in case reports.

Bacon PA: The spectrum of Wegener's granulomatosis and disease relapse. *N Engl J Med* 2005;352:330–332.

Frosch M, Foell D: Wegener granulomatosis in childhood and adolescence. *Eur J Pediatr* 2004;163:425–434.

Furuta T, Hotta O, Yusa N, et al: Lymphocytapheresis to treat rapidly progressive glomerulonephritis: A randomized comparison with steroid-pulse treatment. *Lancet* 1998;352:203–204.

Hattori M, Kurayama H, Koitabashi Y: Antineutrophil cytoplasmic autoantibody-associated glomerulonephritis in children. *J Am Soc Nephrol* 2001;12:1493–1500.

Savage J, Davies D, Falk RJ, et al: Antineutrophil cytoplasmic antibodies and associated diseases: A review of the clinical and laboratory features. *Kidney Int* 2000;57:846–862.

Valentini RP, Smoyer WE, Sedman AB, et al: Outcome of antineutrophil cytoplasmic autoantibodies-positive glomerulonephritis and vasculitis in children: A single-center experience. *J Pediatr* 1998;132:325–328.

von Vigier RO, Trummler SA, Laux-End R, et al: Pulmonary renal syndrome in childhood: A report of twenty-one cases and a review of the literature. *Pediatr Pulmonol* 2000;29:382–388.

Chapter 517 ■ Goodpasture Disease

Goodpasture disease is characterized by pulmonary hemorrhage and glomerulonephritis associated with antibodies commonly directed against specific epitopes of type IV collagen within the alveolar basement membrane of the lung and glomerular basement membrane (GBM) of the glomerulus. The etiology of these antibodies is unknown. This entity should be distinguished from **Goodpasture syndrome,** which is a clinical picture of pulmonary hemorrhage and glomerulonephritis that may be seen with several disorders, including systemic lupus erythematosus, Henoch-Schönlein purpura, polyarteritis nodosa, and Wegener's granulomatosis. In some patients, anti-GBM nephritis occurs without pulmonary hemorrhage and presents as rapidly progressive glomerulonephritis. Antineutrophil cytoplasmic antibodies are also present in 25% of patients with Goodpasture syndrome and may be a vasculitis variant.

PATHOLOGY. In most patients, the changes on light microscopy resemble those of rapidly progressive glomerulonephritis. Immunofluorescent microscopy demonstrates a continuous linear pattern of IgG along the GBM (Fig. 517-1).

CLINICAL MANIFESTATIONS. Goodpasture disease is rare in childhood. Patients usually present with hemoptysis associated with pulmonary hemorrhage that can be life-threatening. Renal manifestations include acute nephritic syndrome with hematuria, proteinuria, and hypertension. Progressive renal dysfunction occurs within days to weeks. The serum complement C3 level is normal.

DIAGNOSIS. The diagnosis is suggested by kidney biopsy. Serum antibodies to the GBM confirm the diagnosis and rule out other disorders associated with Goodpasture syndrome.

PROGNOSIS AND TREATMENT. Patients who survive pulmonary hemorrhage commonly progress to end-stage renal failure. Rates of survival and recovery of renal function have improved with pulse methylprednisolone, oral cyclophosphamide, and plasmapheresis therapy, though controlled data are not available.

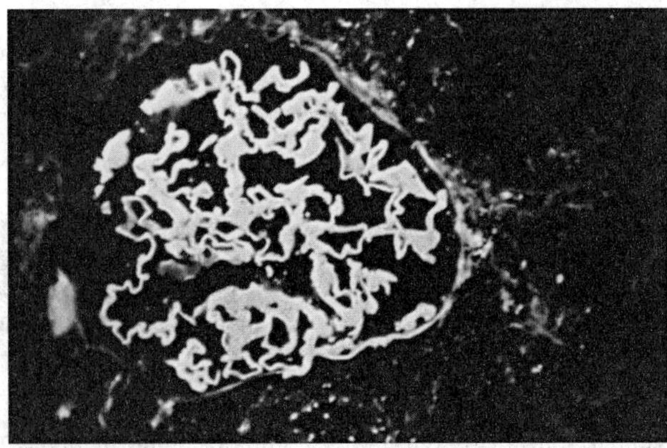

Figure 517-1. Immunofluorescence micrograph demonstrating the continuous linear staining of IgG along the glomerular basement membrane, as found in diseases mediated by antiglomerular basement membrane antibody (×250).

Gittins N, Basu A, Eyre J, et al: Cerebral vasculitis in a teenager with Goodpasture's syndrome. *Nephrol Dial Transplant* 2004;19:3168–3171.
Hudson BG: The molecular basis of Goodpasture and Alport syndromes: Beacons for the discovery of the collagen IV family. *J Am Soc Nephrol* 2004;15:2514–2527.
Levy JB, Turner N, Rees AJ, et al: Long-term outcome of anti-glomerular basement membrane antibody disease treated with plasma exchange and immunosuppression. *Ann Intern Med* 2001;134:1033–1042.
McCarthy LJ, Cotton J, Danielson C, et al: Goodpasture's syndrome in childhood: Treatment with plasmapheresis and immunosuppression. *J Clin Apher* 1994;9:116.

Chapter 518 ■ Hemolytic-Uremic Syndrome

The hemolytic-uremic syndrome (HUS) is the most common cause of acute renal failure in young children. It is classically characterized by the triad of microangiopathic hemolytic anemia, thrombocytopenia, and uremia. HUS has features common to thrombotic thrombocytopenic purpura, except that the latter tends to occur in young adult women as a relapsing illness with fever, serious central nervous system involvement, and thrombocytopenia.

ETIOLOGY. An acute enteritis with diarrhea caused by Shiga-like toxin–producing *Escherichia coli* 0157:H7 precedes 80% or more of HUS cases in developed countries. The reservoir of this organism is the intestinal tract of domestic animals. It is usually transmitted by undercooked meat or unpasteurized milk. Outbreaks have usually followed ingestion of undercooked hamburger at fast food restaurants. Outbreaks also occur with diarrheal epidemics after swimming in contaminated ponds, lakes, or pools as well as eating contaminated milk, cheese, lettuce, or apple cider; from contaminated buildings, day care centers, child care centers, dairy or petting farms; and by person-to-person contact. The organism produces a Shiga-like verotoxin that is absorbed from the intestines and initiates endothelial cell injury. HUS is also associated with *Shigella* and less commonly with other bacterial (*Salmonella, Campylobacter, Streptococcus pneumoniae, Bartonella*) and viral (coxsackievirus, echovirus, influenza, varicella, HIV, Epstein-Barr) infections. HUS may also develop with the use of oral contraceptives, mitomycin, or cyclosporine or exposure to pyran copolymer, which induces interferon production. In addition, a clinical picture similar to that of HUS has been reported in diseases with significant endothelial cell injury such as systemic lupus erythematosus, malignant hypertension, preeclampsia, postpartum renal failure, and radiation nephritis. Several reports describe its occurrence in more than one member of a family. Familial occurrences are usually not associated with diarrhea and may be autosomal recessive or dominant disorders. Mutations in complement component H (inhibits activation of the alternate complement pathway) are noted in 10–20% of familial cases. Complete deficiency of the von Willebrand factor metalloprotease (cleaves multimers of von Willebrand factor) and of membrane cofactor protein is responsible for other familial cases.

PATHOLOGY. Initial glomerular changes include thickening of the capillary walls, narrowing of the capillary lumens, and widening of the mesangium. These changes are the result of subendothelial and mesangial deposition of a granular, amorphous material of unknown origin. Fibrin thrombi can be found in glomerular capillaries and arterioles and may lead to cortical necrosis.

Severely involved glomeruli progress to partial or total sclerosis. Severe vascular involvement may render other glomeruli obsolescent because of ischemia. In severely involved small arteries and arterioles, concentric intimal proliferation leads to vascular occlusion.

PATHOGENESIS. The primary event in the pathogenesis of the syndrome is endothelial cell injury. Capillary and arteriolar endothelial injury in the kidney leads to localized clotting. Evidence of disseminated intravascular coagulation is unusual. Microangiopathic anemia results from mechanical damage to red blood cells (RBCs) as they pass through the altered vasculature. Thrombocytopenia is caused by intrarenal and diffuse microvascular platelet adhesion or damage. Damaged RBCs and platelets are removed from circulation by the liver and spleen. Nondiarrheal and sporadic recurrent familial cases of HUS are associated with low complement (C3) levels due to complement dysregulation and activation following an inciting injury to the endothelial cell.

CLINICAL MANIFESTATIONS. HUS is most common in children younger than 4 yr of age. The onset is usually preceded by a gastroenteritis characterized by fever, vomiting, abdominal pain, and diarrhea that is initially watery but then becomes bloody. Less commonly, patients may present after an upper respiratory tract infection. Sudden onset of pallor, irritability, weakness, lethargy, and oliguria usually occurs 5–10 days after the initial gastrointestinal or respiratory illness. Physical examination may reveal dehydration, edema, petechiae, hepatosplenomegaly, and marked irritability.

DIAGNOSIS AND DIFFERENTIAL DIAGNOSIS. The diagnosis is supported by the findings of a microangiopathic hemolytic anemia, thrombocytopenia, and acute renal failure (Tables 518-1 and 518-2). The hemoglobin value is commonly in the 5–9 g/dL range. The blood peripheral smear reveals helmet cells, burr cells, and fragmented RBCs (see Chapter 447). Plasma hemoglobin levels are elevated, whereas plasma haptoglobin levels are diminished. The reticulocyte count is moderately elevated, and the Coombs test result is negative. Leukocytosis is significant, and commonly the leukocyte count may exceed 30,000/mm^3. Thrombocytopenia (20,000–100,000/mm^3) occurs in more than 90% of patients. Findings on urinalysis are surprisingly mild and usually consist of low-grade microscopic hematuria and proteinuria. Partial thromboplastin time and prothrombin time are usually normal. Prolongation of coagulation studies is more commonly caused by vitamin K deficiency than by disseminated intravascular coagulation. Renal manifestations vary from mild renal insufficiency to acute oliguric or anuric renal failure requiring dialysis. Barium contrast studies reveal colonic spasm and transient early filling defects, and colitis may appear as "thumb-printing" on radiographs. Intestinal strictures are rare sequelae.

HUS should always be considered in the child with a sudden onset of acute renal failure. The typical history, clinical picture, and laboratory findings confirm the diagnosis in most patients. Other causes of acute renal failure, especially those that can be associated with a microangiopathic hemolytic anemia such as systemic lupus erythematosus and malignant hypertension, should be excluded. A renal biopsy is rarely indicated.

Patients with bilateral renal vein thrombosis (see Chapter 519.7) may be difficult to distinguish from those with HUS. Both disorders may be preceded by a gastrointestinal disorder associated with dehydration, pallor, and evidence of microangiopathic hemolytic anemia, thrombocytopenia, and acute renal failure. Marked renal enlargement and absence of renal vein flow by renal Doppler ultrasonography is consistent with renal vein thrombosis.

TABLE 518-1. Definition of Postdiarrheal Hemolytic Uremic Syndrome: Centers for Disease Control and Prevention, 1996

CLINICAL DESCRIPTION

Hemolytic uremic syndrome (HUS) is characterized by the acute onset of microangiopathic hemolytic anemia, renal injury, and a low platelet count. Thrombotic thrombocytopenic purpura (TTP) also is characterized by these features but can include central nervous system (CNS) involvement and fever and may have a more gradual onset. Most cases of HUS (but few cases of TTP) occur after an acute gastrointestinal illness (usually diarrheal).

LABORATORY CRITERIA FOR DIAGNOSIS

The following are both present at some time during the illness:

- Anemia (acute onset) with microangiopathic changes (i.e., schistocytes, burr cells, or helmet cells) on peripheral blood smear; and
- Renal injury (acute onset) evidenced by either hematuria, proteinuria, or elevated creatinine level (i.e., ≥1.0 mg/dL in a child younger than 13 yr or ≥1.5 mg/dL in a person 13 yr or older or ≥50% increase over baseline).

Note: A low platelet count can usually, but not always, be detected early in the illness, but it may then become normal or even high. If a platelet count obtained within 7 days after onset of the acute gastrointestinal illness is not <150,000/mm^3, other diagnoses should be considered.

CASE CLASSIFICATION

Probable

- An acute illness diagnosed as HUS or TTP that meets the laboratory criteria in a patient who does not have a clear history of acute or bloody diarrhea in the preceding 3 wk, or
- An acute illness diagnosed as HUS or TTP that (a) has onset within 3 wk after onset of an acute or bloody diarrhea and (b) meets the laboratory criteria except that microangiopathic changes are not confirmed.

Confirmed

An acute illness diagnosed as HUS or TTP that both meets the laboratory criteria and began within 3 wk after onset of an episode of acute or bloody diarrhea.

COMMENT

Some investigators consider HUS and TTP to be part of a continuum of disease. Therefore, criteria for diagnosing TTP on the basis of CNS involvement and fever are not provided because cases diagnosed clinically as postdiarrheal TTP also should meet the criteria for HUS. These cases are reported as postdiarrheal HUS.

From Elliott EJ, Robins-Browne RM: Hemolytic uremic syndrome. *Curr Probl Pediatr Adolesc Health Care* 2005;35:305–344.

COMPLICATIONS. Complications include anemia, acidosis, hyperkalemia, fluid overload, heart failure, hypertension, and uremia. Extrarenal manifestations of the central nervous system, gastrointestinal tract, heart, and skeletal muscles may be life-threatening. Central nervous system dysfunction includes irritability, seizures, infarcts of the basal ganglion and cerebral cortex, cortical blindness, and coma. Gastrointestinal manifestations include ischemic or inflammatory colitis, intestinal perforation, intussusception, and hepatitis. Focal pancreatic necrosis may result in acute pancreatitis, glucose intolerance, insulin-dependent diabetes mellitus, and elevated lipase levels. Pericarditis, myocardial dysfunction, and arrhythmias may be seen in cases with cardiac involvement. Other complications such as skin necrosis, parotitis, adrenal dysfunction, and rhabdomyolysis have been reported.

TABLE 518-2. Classification of Hemolytic Uremic Syndrome (HUS)

TYPE OF HUS	ETIOLOGY
TYPICAL (POSTDIARRHEAL) HUS	
Postgastrointestinal infection	Shiga toxin–producing organisms, usually enterohemorrhagic *Escherichia coli* and *Shigella dysenteriae*
ATYPICAL HUS	
Urinary tract infection	Shiga toxin–producing *E. coli*
Postinfectious	Infection outside the gastrointestinal tract (e.g., lungs, central nervous system) with neuraminidase-producing organisms, usually *Streptococcus pneumoniae*
Familial (autosomal dominant or recessive)	Abnormal regulation of complement pathway (e.g., genetic defect in control of factor H, factor I, or membrane cofactor protein production)
	Abnormal regulation of coagulation (e.g., gene defect or autoantibodies resulting in decreased activity of ADAMTS-13)
Associated with drug use	Immunosuppressants (e.g., cyclosporine, FK-506, OKT3, mitomycin C); other (e.g., ganciclovir, oral contraceptive pill, crack cocaine, quinine)
Rare reported associations	Systemic lupus erythematosus, systemic sclerosis, post–bone marrow transplantation, leukemia, nail-patella syndrome, post-streptococcal glomerulonephritis

From Elliott EJ, Robins-Browne RM: Hemolytic uremic syndrome. *Curr Probl Pediatr Adolesc Health Care* 2005;35:305–344.

PROGNOSIS AND TREATMENT. Supportive care with meticulous attention to fluid and electrolytes, control of hypertension, aggressive nutrition, and early institution of dialysis has been responsible for a decrease in the mortality from this disease from 80% to less than 10% over the past 30 yr. Antibiotics should be avoided in patients with acute enteritis presumed secondary to *E. coli* 0157:H7 as they may increase the risk of developing HUS. Nephroprotection in the early phase of HUS may be possible by prevention of dehydration with intravenous fluids. Antithrombotic therapy has no proven therapeutic benefit in HUS. Prospective controlled studies assessing the value of plasmapheresis in HUS with a diarrheal prodrome are not available. However, plasmapheresis or administration of fresh frozen plasma may be beneficial in thrombotic thrombocytopenic purpura or HUS that is **not** associated with a diarrheal prodrome or in children with familial recurrent HUS or with severe central nervous system involvement. Plasmapheresis or administration of fresh frozen plasma may exacerbate HUS caused by *S. pneumoniae* and should be avoided when this infection is present. Peritoneal dialysis controls fluid and electrolyte abnormalities, maintains a normal intravascular volume, and provides the opportunity for aggressive nutritional support. Peritoneal dialysis may contribute to the dissolution of vascular thrombi by removing fibrinolysis inhibitors and circulating plasminogen activating inhibitor-1, thereby activating normal endogenous fibrinolytic pathways. Shiga toxin–binding resin was ineffective in diminishing the prevalence of death or serious extrarenal events. In vitro studies using more potent multivalent synthetic inhibitors of Shiga toxin or genetically engineered bacteria that neutralize large amounts of the Shiga toxin show promise in reducing the incidence of diarrhea-associated HUS.

With aggressive management of acute renal failure, more than 90% of patients survive the acute phase of HUS with a diarrheal prodrome. Death or end-stage renal disease affects 12% (0–30% of patients in various studies). Hypertension, proteinuria, or low glomerular filtration rates (<80 mL/min/1.73 m^2) affects 25%. The overall prognosis of HUS is associated with negative long-term renal outcomes when central nervous symptoms (coma, stroke, seizures) are present during the acute illness and dialysis is required. Other predictive factors for acute or chronic severity include a white blood cell count >20,000, ischemic colitis, and hypertension. Patients recovering from the acute phase of HUS require long-term follow-up because complications such as hypertension, chronic renal insufficiency, and proteinuria may not be apparent for up to 20 yr. Kidney transplantations in patients with HUS can be successful, although there may be disease recurrence, particularly in familial or non–diarrhea-associated cases. Combined liver and renal transplantation may be an option for those familial cases associated with compliment factor H mutations.

Ake JA, Jelacic S, Ciol MA, et al: Relative nephroprotection during *Escherichia coli* O157:H7 infections: Association with intravenous volume expansion. *Pediatrics* 2005;115:e673–e680.

Banatvala N, Griffin PM, Greene KD, et al: The United States national prospective hemolytic-uremic syndrome study: Microbiologic, serologic, clinical, and epidemiologic findings. *J Infect Dis* 2001;183:1063–1070.

Bonnardeaux A, Pichette V: Complement dysregulation in haemolytic uraemic syndrome. *Lancet* 2003;362:1514–1516.

Cabrera GR, Fortenberry JD, Warshaw BL, et al: Hemolytic-uremic syndrome associated with invasive *Streptococcus pneumoniae* infection. *Pediatrics* 1998;101:699–703.

Centers for Disease Control and Prevention: Laboratory-confirmed non-0157 shiga toxin—producing *escherichia coli*—Connecticut, 2000–2005. *MMWR* 2007;56:29–31.
Centers for Disease Control and Prevention: *Escherichia coli* 0157:H7 infection associated with drinking raw milk—Washington and Oregon, November–December 2005. *MMWR* 2007;56:165–167.
Coppo P, Bussel A, Charrier S, et al: High-dose plasma infusion versus plasma exchange as early treatment of thrombotic thrombocytopenic purpura/hemolytic-uremic syndrome. *Medicine* 2003;82:27–38.
Crump JA, Sulka AC, Langer AJ, et al: An outbreak of *Escherichia coli* O157:H7 infections among visitors to a dairy farm. *N Engl J Med* 2002;347:555–560.
DeCaluwe H, Harrison LM, Mariscalco MM, et al: Procalcitonin in children with *Escherichia coli* O157:H7 associated hemolytic uremic syndrome. *Pediatr Res* 2006;59:579–583.
Eliott EJ, Robins-Browne RM: Hemolytic uremic syndrome. *Curr Probl Pediatr Adolesc Health Care* 2005;35:305–344.
Garg AX, Suri RS, Barrowman N, et al: Long-term renal prognosis of diarrhea-associated hemolytic uremic syndrome. *JAMA* 2003;290:1360–1370.
Noris M, Brioschi S, Caprioli J, et al: Familial haemolytic uraemic syndrome and an *MCP* mutation. *Lancet* 2003;362:1542–1546.
Oakes RS, Siegler RL, Me Reynolds MA, et al: Predicters of fatality in post-diarrheal hemolytic uremic syndrome. *Pediatrics* 2006;117:1656–1662.
Olie KH, Florquin S, Groothoff JW, et al: Atypical relapse of hemolytic uremic syndrome after transplantation. *Pediatr Nephrol* 2004;19:1173–1176.
Remuzzi G, Ruggenenti P, Codazzi D, et al: Combined kidney and liver transplantation for familial haemolytic uraemic syndrome. *Lancet* 2002;359:1671–1672.
Spizzirri FD, Rahman RC, Bibiloni N, et al: Childhood hemolytic-uremic syndrome in Argentina: Long-term follow-up and prognostic features. *Pediatr Nephrol* 1997;11:156–160.
Tarr PI, Gordon CA, Chandler WL: Shiga-toxin-producing *Escherichia coli* and haemolytic uraemic syndrome. *Lancet* 2005;365:1073–1086.
Trachtman H, Cnaan A, Christen E, et al: Effect of an oral Shiga toxin-binding agent on diarrhea-associated hemolytic uremic syndrome in children. *JAMA* 2003;290:1337–1344.
Wong CS, Jelacic S, Habeeb RL, et al: The risk of the hemolytic-uremic syndrome after antibiotic treatment of *Escherichia coli* O157:H7 infections. *N Engl J Med* 2000; 342:1930–1936.

Chapter 519 ■ Upper Urinary Tract Causes of Hematuria

519.1 • Interstitial Nephritis (See Chapter 532)

519.2 • Toxic Nephropathy (See Chapter 533)

519.3 • Cortical Necrosis (See Chapter 534)

519.4 • Pyelonephritis (See Chapter 538)

519.5 • Nephrocalcinosis (See Chapter 547)

519.6 • Vascular Abnormalities

Hemangiomas, angiomyomas, and arteriovenous malformations of the kidneys and lower urinary tract are rare causes of hematuria. They usually present as gross hematuria and the passage of blood clots. Renal colic may develop if the upper tract is involved. The diagnosis is confirmed by angiography.

Unilateral bleeding of varicose veins of the left ureter, resulting from compression of the left renal vein between the aorta and superior mesenteric artery, is referred to as the **nutcracker syndrome.** Patients with this syndrome typically present with persistent microscopic hematuria (occasionally recurrent gross hematuria) that may be accompanied by proteinuria, lower abdominal pain, flank pain, or orthostatic hypotension. Diagnosis is confirmed by Doppler ultrasonography, CT, or magnetic resonance angiography.

Shin JI, Park JM, Lee SM, et al: Factors affecting spontaneous resolution of hematuria in childhood nutcracker syndrome. *Pediatr Nephrol* 2005;20: 609–613.
Chang CT, Hung CC, Ng KK, et al: Nutcracker syndrome and left unilateral haematuria. *Nephrol Dial Transplant* 2005;20:460–461.

519.7 • Renal Vein Thrombosis

EPIDEMIOLOGY. Renal vein thrombosis (RVT) occurs in two distinct clinical situations. In newborns and infants, RVT is commonly associated with asphyxia, dehydration, shock, sepsis, congenital hypercoagulable states, and infants born to mothers with diabetes mellitus. In older children, RVT is seen in patients with nephrotic syndrome, cyanotic heart disease, inherited hypercoagulable states, and following exposure to angiographic contrast agents.

PATHOGENESIS. RVT begins in the intrarenal venous circulation and may spread to the main renal vein and inferior vena cava. Thrombus formation is mediated by endothelial cell injury resulting from hypoxia, endotoxin, or contrast media. Other contributing factors include (1) hypercoagulability from either nephrotic syndrome or mutations in genes that encode clotting factors (like the gene that produces factor V Leiden); (2) hypovolemia and diminished vascular blood flow associated with septic shock, dehydration, or nephrotic syndrome; and (3) intravascular sludging due to polycythemia.

CLINICAL MANIFESTATIONS. The development of RVT is usually heralded by the sudden onset of gross hematuria and unilateral or bilateral flank masses. Patients may also present with microscopic hematuria, flank pain, hypertension, or oliguria. RVT is usually unilateral. Bilateral RVT results in acute renal failure.

DIAGNOSIS. The diagnosis of RVT is suggested by the development of hematuria and flank masses in a patient with predisposing clinical factors. Patients may also have a microangiopathic hemolytic anemia and thrombocytopenia. Ultrasonography shows marked enlargement, whereas radionuclide studies reveal little or no renal function in the affected kidney(s). Doppler flow studies of the inferior vena cava and renal vein confirm the diagnosis. Contrast studies should be avoided to minimize the risk of further vascular damage.

DIFFERENTIAL DIAGNOSIS. The differential diagnosis of RVT includes other causes of hematuria that are associated with microangiopathic hemolytic anemia or renal enlargement. These include hemolytic-uremic syndrome, hydronephrosis, polycystic kidney disease, Wilms tumor, abscess, or hematoma. All patients should be evaluated for congenital, and in older children acquired, hypercoagulable states.

TREATMENT. The primary treatment of RVT consists of supportive care including correction of fluid and electrolyte imbalance and treatment of renal insufficiency. Treatment with anticoagulation or thrombolytic agents including streptokinase, urokinase, or recombinant tissue plasminogen activator is common but remains controversial. Patients with thrombosis of the inferior vena cava may require surgical thrombectomy. Children with severe hypertension refractory to antihypertensive medications may require nephrectomy.

PROGNOSIS. Perinatal mortality from RVT has decreased significantly over the past 20 yr. However, partial or complete renal atrophy is a common sequela of RVT in the neonate leading to renal insufficiency, renal tubular dysfunction, and systemic hypertension. These complications are also seen in older children, although recovery of renal function is common in children with RVT due to nephrotic syndrome or cyanotic heart disease.

Bokenkamp A, von Kries R, Nowak-Gottl U, et al: Neonatal renal venous thrombosis in Germany between 1992 and 1994: Epidemiology, treatment and outcome. *Eur J Pediatr* 2000;159:44–48.

Kosch A, Kuwertz-Broking E, Heller C, et al: Renal venous thrombosis in neonates: Prothrombotic risk factors and long-term follow-up. *Blood* 2004;104:1356–1360.

Kuhle S, Massicotte P, Chan A, et al: Data from the 1-800-NO-CLOTS Registry. A case series of 72 neonates with renal vein thrombosis. *Thromb Haemost* 2004;92:729–733.

519.8 • Idiopathic Hypercalciuria

This entity, which may be inherited as an autosomal dominant disorder, may present as recurrent gross hematuria, persistent microscopic hematuria, dysuria, or abdominal pain in the absence of stone formation. Hypercalciuria may be caused by conditions resulting in hypercalcemia, such as hyperparathyroidism, vitamin D intoxication, immobilization, and sarcoidosis. Hypercalciuria may be associated with Cushing syndrome, corticosteroid therapy, tubular dysfunction secondary to Fanconi syndrome (Wilson disease, oculocerebrorenal syndrome), Williams syndrome, distal renal tubular acidosis, or Bartter syndrome. Hypercalciuria may also be seen in patients with **Dent disease,** which is an X-linked form of nephrolithiasis associated with hypophosphatemic rickets. Although microcrystal formation and consequent tissue irritation are believed to mediate symptoms, the precise mechanism by which hypercalciuria causes hematuria or dysuria is unknown.

DIAGNOSIS. Hypercalciuria is diagnosed by a 24-hr urinary calcium excretion exceeding 4 mg/kg. A screening test for hypercalciuria in patients who cannot collect a timed urine specimen may be performed on a random urine specimen by measuring the calcium and creatinine concentrations. A spot urine calcium to creatinine ratio (mg/mg) exceeding 0.2 suggests hypercalciuria, although normal ratios may be as high as 0.8 in infants younger than 7 mo of age.

TREATMENT. If untreated, hypercalciuria leads to nephrolithiasis in approximately 15% of cases. Oral thiazide diuretics may normalize urinary calcium excretion by stimulating calcium reabsorption in the proximal and distal tubule. Such therapy may halt the gross hematuria or dysuria and prevent nephrolithiasis. However, the precise indications for thiazide treatment remain controversial. In patients with persistent gross hematuria or dysuria, therapy is initiated with hydrochlorothiazide at a dose of 1–2 mg/kg/24 hr as a single morning dose. The dose is titrated upward until the 24-hr urinary calcium excretion is <4 mg/kg and the clinical manifestations resolve. After 1 yr of treatment, hydrochlorothiazide is usually discontinued but may be resumed if gross hematuria, nephrolithiasis, or dysuria recurs. During hydrochlorothiazide therapy, the serum potassium level should be monitored periodically to avoid hypokalemia. **Potassium citrate** at a dose of 1 mEq/kg/24 hr may also be beneficial, particularly in patients with low urinary citrate excretion and symptomatic dysuria. Sodium restriction is important because calcium excretion parallels sodium excretion. Importantly, dietary calcium restriction is not recommended (except in children with massive calcium intake by dietary history) because of the obligate requirement for growth and lack of evidence demonstrating a relationship between decreased calcium intake and decreased urinary calcium levels.

Bhimma R, Robbs J: Nutcracker. *Lancet* 2005;365:1280–1281.

Kari JA, Farouq M, Alshaya HO: Familial hypomagnesemia with hypercalciuria and nephrocalcinosis. *Pediatr Nephrol* 2003;18:506–510.

Knohl SJ, Scheinman SJ: Inherited hypercalciuric syndromes: Dent's disease (CLC-5) and familial hypomagnesemia with hypercalciuria (paracellin-1). *Semin Nephrol* 2004;24:55–60.

Magen D, Adler L, Mandel H, et al: Autosomal recessive renal proximal tubulopathy and hypercalciuria: A new syndrome. *Am J Kidney Dis* 2004;43:600–606.

Polito C, Iolascon G, Nappi B, et al: Growth and bone mineral density in long-lasting idiopathic hypercalciuria. *Pediatr Nephrol* 2003;18:545–547.

Polito C, LaManna A, Cioce F, et al: Clinical presentation and natural course of idiopathic hypercalciuria in children. *Pediatr Nephrol* 2000;15:211–214.

So NP, Osorio AV, Simon SD, et al: Normal urinary calcium/creatinine ratios in African-American and Caucasian children. *Pediatr Nephrol* 2001;16:133–139.

Stapleton FB: Childhood stones. *Endocrinol Metab Clin North Am* 2002;31:1001–1015.

Vachvanichsanong P, Malagon M, Moore ES: Recurrent abdominal and flank pain in children with idiopathic hypercalciuria. *Acta Paediatr* 2001;90:643–648.

Chapter 520 ■ Hematologic Diseases Causing Hematuria

520.1 • Sickle Cell Nephropathy

Gross or microscopic hematuria may be seen in children with sickle cell disease or sickle trait. Signs and symptoms resolve spontaneously in the majority of patients (see Chapter 462.1). The hematuria presumably results from microthrombosis secondary to sickling in the relatively hypoxic, acidic, hypertonic renal medulla where vascular stasis is present. Ischemia, papillary necrosis, and interstitial fibrosis may also be present in these patients. Additional clinical manifestations of sickle cell nephropathy include polyuria caused by a urinary concentrating defect, renal tubular acidosis, and proteinuria associated with a glomerular lesion resembling focal segmental glomerulosclerosis or membranoproliferative glomerulonephritis. Angiotensin-converting enzyme inhibitors, such as enalapril, are often used to achieve a reduction in urine protein excretion in patients with daily urine protein excretions exceeding 500 mg. Hydroxyurea may also be beneficial in reducing urinary protein excretion. Sickle cell nephropathy may eventually lead to hypertension and renal insufficiency that may progress to end-stage renal disease.

Fitzhugh CD, Wigfall DR, Ware RE: Enalapril and hydroxyurea therapy for children with sickle nephropathy. *Pediatr Blood Cancer* 2005;45:982–985.
Pham PT, Pham PC, Wilkinson AH, et al: Renal abnormalities in sickle cell disease. *Kidney Int* 2000;57:1–8.
Scheinman JI: Sickle cell disease and the kidney. *Semin Nephrol* 2003;23:66–76.

520.2 • Coagulopathies and Thrombocytopenia

Gross or microscopic hematuria may be associated with inherited or acquired disorders of coagulation (hemophilia, disseminated intravascular coagulation, thrombocytopenia). In these cases, however, hematuria is not usually the presenting complaint but develops after other manifestations (see Part XX, Section 7).

Chapter 521 ■ Anatomic Abnormalities Associated with Hematuria

521.1 • Congenital Anomalies

Gross or microscopic hematuria may be associated with many types of different malformations of the urinary tract. The sudden onset of gross hematuria after minor trauma to the flank is frequently associated with ureteropelvic junction obstruction or cystic kidneys (see Chapter 537).

521.2 • Autosomal Recessive Polycystic Kidney Disease

Also known as **infantile polycystic disease,** autosomal recessive polycystic kidney disease (ARPKD) is an autosomal recessive disorder occurring with an incidence of 1:10,000 to 1:40,000. The gene for ARPKD encodes fibrocystin, a large protein (>4,000 amino acids) with multiple motifs. The function of fibrocystin in normal kidney development and the pathophysiology of its abnormal expression in ARPKD are unknown.

PATHOLOGY. Both kidneys are markedly enlarged and grossly show innumerable cysts throughout the cortex and medulla. Microscopic studies demonstrate microcysts radiating from the medulla to the cortex located primarily within the collecting tubules and ducts, although transient proximal tubule cysts have been reported in the fetus. Development of progressive interstitial fibrosis and tubular atrophy during advanced stages of disease eventually leads to renal failure. Liver involvement is characterized by a basic ductal plate abnormality that leads to bile duct proliferation and ectasia, as well as hepatic fibrosis, and is indistinguishable from congenital hepatic fibrosis or Caroli disease.

CLINICAL MANIFESTATIONS. The typical child presents with bilateral flank masses during the neonatal period or early infancy. ARPKD may be associated with oligohydramnios, pulmonary hypoplasia, respiratory distress, and spontaneous pneumothorax in the neonatal period. Potter facies and other components of the oligohydramnios complex including low-set ears, micrognathia, flattened nose, limb-positioning defects, and growth deficiency may be present. Hypertension is usually noted within the first few weeks of life and is often severe. Urine output is usually not diminished, although oliguria and acute renal failure may be seen. Transient hyponatremia, often in the presence of acute renal failure, is common in the neonatal period and frequently responds to diuresis. Renal function is usually impaired but may be initially normal in 20–30% of patients. Infrequently, ARPKD presents beyond infancy with renal insufficiency, hypertension, or hepatosplenomegaly related to hepatic fibrosis.

In the newborn, clinical evidence of liver disease by radiologic or clinical laboratory assessment is present in about 45% of children. It is believed to be universal by microscopic evaluation. Patients with ARPKD are at risk of developing (1) ascending cholangitis, varices, and hypersplenism related to portal hypertension and (2) progressive liver dysfunction, which rarely leads to overt liver failure and cirrhosis. A subset of older children with ARPKD may present with hepatosplenomegaly and display mild renal disease that is discovered incidentally during imaging studies of the abdomen.

DIAGNOSIS. The diagnosis of ARPKD is strongly suggested by bilateral palpable flank masses in an infant with pulmonary hypoplasia, oligohydramnios, and hypertension and the absence of renal cysts by sonography of the parents. Markedly enlarged and uniformly hyperechogenic kidneys with poor corticomedullary distinction are commonly seen on ultrasonography (Fig. 521-1). The diagnosis is supported by clinical/laboratory signs of hepatic fibrosis, pathologic findings of ductal plate abnormalities seen on liver biopsy, anatomic and pathologic proof of ARPKD in a sibling, or parental consanguinity. The differential diagnosis includes other causes of bilateral renal enlargement, such as multicystic dysplasia, hydronephrosis, Wilms tumor, and bilateral renal vein thrombosis. Prenatal diagnostic

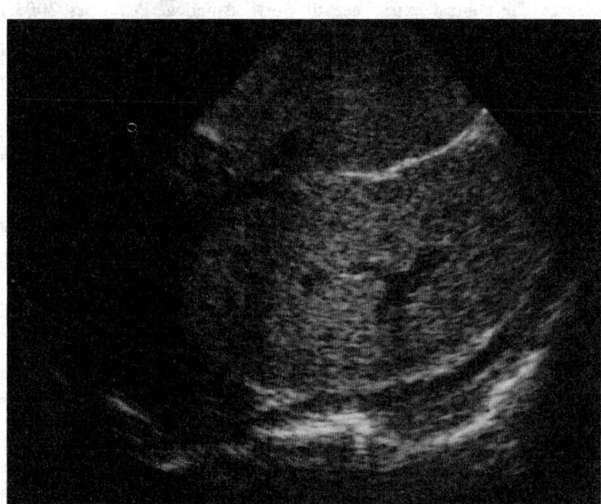

Figure 521-1. Ultrasound examination of a neonate with autosomal recessive polycystic kidney disease demonstrating renal enlargement (9 cm) and increased diffuse echogenicity with complete loss of corticomedullary differentiation resulting from multiple small cystic interfaces.

testing using genetic linkage analysis or direct mutation analysis is available in families with at least 1 affected child.

TREATMENT. The treatment of ARPKD is supportive. Aggressive ventilatory support is often necessary in the neonatal period secondary to pulmonary hypoplasia, hypoventilation, and the many respiratory illnesses of prematurity (which are common). Careful management of hypertension, fluid and electrolyte abnormalities, and clinical manifestations of renal insufficiency is essential. Children with severe respiratory failure or feeding intolerance from enlarged kidneys may require unilateral or bilateral nephrectomies, prompting the need for renal replacement therapy.

PROGNOSIS. Mortality has improved dramatically, although approximately 30% of patients die in the neonatal period of complications from pulmonary hypoplasia. Neonatal respiratory support and renal replacement therapies have increased the 10-yr survival of children surviving beyond the 1st year of life to >80%. Fifteen-year survival is estimated at 70–80%. End-stage renal disease is seen in >50% of children and usually occurs during the 1st decade of life. As a result, dialysis and renal transplantation have become standard therapies for these children. Morbidity and mortality in the older child are related to complications from chronic renal failure and liver disease.

Adeva M, El-Youssef M, Rossetti S, et al: Clinical and molecular characterization defines a broadened spectrum of autosomal recessive polycystic kidney disease (ARPKD). *Medicine* 2006;85:1–21.

Bergmann C, Senderek J, Kupper F, et al: PKHD1 mutations in autosomal recessive polycystic kidney disease (ARPKD). *Hum Mutat* 2004;23:453–463.

Davis ID, Ho M, Hupertz V, et al: Survival of childhood polycystic kidney disease following renal transplantation: The impact of advanced hepatobiliary disease. *Pediatr Transplant* 2003;7:364–369.

Dell KM: Cystic and dysplastic disorders: Polycystic kidney diseases. In Kaplan BS, Meyers KM (editors): *Requisites in Pediatrics: Nephrology/Urology.* St. Louis, Harcourt, 2004.

Dell KM, Avner ED: Autosomal recessive polycystic kidney disease. In GeneClinics: Clinical Genetic Information Resource [database online]. University of Washington, Seattle. Available at http://www.geneclinics.org/.

Guay-Woodford LM: Autosomal recessive polycystic kidney disease (ARPKD): New insights from the identification of the ARPKD gene, PKHD1. *Pediatr Res* 2002;52:830–831.

Guay-Woodford LM, Desmond RA: Autosomal recessive polycystic kidney disease: The clinical experience in North America. *Pediatrics* 2003;111:1072–1080.

Roy S, Dillon MJ, Trompeter RS, et al: Autosomal recessive polycystic kidney disease: Long-term outcome of neonatal survivors. *Pediatr Nephrol* 1997;11:302–306.

Zerres K, Rudnik-Schoneborn S, Deget F, et al: Autosomal recessive polycystic kidney disease in 115 children: Clinical presentation, course and influence of gender. *Acta Paediatr* 1996;85:437–445.

521.3 • Autosomal Dominant Polycystic Kidney Disease

Autosomal dominant polycystic kidney disease (ADPKD) is the most common hereditary human kidney disease. The autosomal dominant pattern of inheritance occurs with an incidence of 1/500 to 1/1,000. Approximately 85% of patients with ADPKD map to the *PKD1* gene on the short arm of chromosome 16, which encodes polycystin, a transmembrane glycoprotein. Another 10–15% of ADPKD map to the *PKD2* gene on the long arm of chromosome 4, which encodes polycystin 2, a proposed nonselective cation channel. Remaining patients may map to other loci yet to be determined.

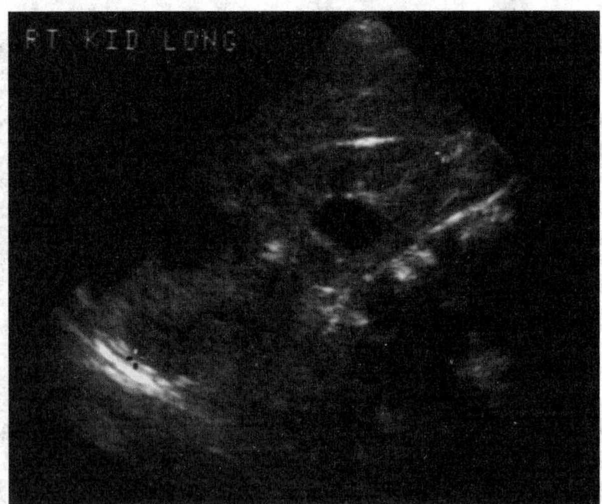

Figure 521-2. Ultrasound examination of an 18 mo old boy with autosomal dominant polycystic kidney disease demonstrating renal enlargement (10 cm) and two large cysts.

PATHOLOGY. Both kidneys are enlarged and show cortical and medullary cysts originating from all regions of the nephron.

CLINICAL PRESENTATION. Although symptomatic ADPKD commonly presents in the 4th or 5th decade of life, symptoms, including gross or microscopic hematuria, bilateral flank pain, abdominal masses, hypertension, and urinary tract infection, may be seen in children and neonates. Renal ultrasonography usually demonstrates multiple bilateral macrocysts (Fig. 521-2), although unilateral disease may be seen in the early phase of the disease.

ADPKD is a systemic disorder affecting many organ systems. Cysts may be present within the liver, pancreas, spleen, and ovaries. **Intracranial aneurysms,** which appear to cluster within certain families, are an important cause of mortality in adults but are rarely reported in children. Mitral valve prolapse is seen in approximately 12% of children. Hernias and intestinal diverticula may also occur in these children.

DIAGNOSIS. ADPKD is confirmed by the presence of enlarged kidneys with bilateral macrocysts in a patient with an affected first-degree relative. Absence of a family history of ADPKD does not preclude this diagnosis because affected family members may have silent disease or the affected child may have a new mutation that occurs in 5–10% of cases. Among patients with genetically defined ADPKD, screening renal ultrasonography results may be normal in up to 20% by 20 yr of age and <5% by 30 yr of age.

Prenatal diagnosis is suggested from the presence of enlarged kidneys with or without cysts on ultrasonography in families with known ADPKD. Prenatal DNA testing is available in families with affected members whose disease is caused by identified mutations in the *PKD1* or *PKD2* genes.

The differential diagnosis includes renal cysts associated with glomerulocystic kidney disease, tuberous sclerosis, and von Hippel-Lindau disease, which may be inherited in an autosomal dominant pattern. The neonatal manifestations of ADPKD and ARPKD may be indistinguishable.

TREATMENT AND PROGNOSIS. Treatment of ADPKD is primarily supportive. Control of blood pressure is critical because the rate of disease progression in ADPKD correlates with the presence of hypertension. Angiotensin-converting enzyme inhibitors and/or angiotensin II receptor antagonists are agents of choice.

Although neonatal ADPKD may be lethal, long-term patient and renal survival is possible for children surviving the neonatal period. Presentation of ADPKD in older children has a favorable prognosis, with normal renal function during childhood seen in >80% of children.

Davis ID, MacRae DK, Sweeney WS, et al: Can progression of autosomal dominant or autosomal recessive polycystic kidney disease be prevented? *Semin Nephrol* 2001;21:430–440.

Dell KM, McDonald R, Watkins S, et al: Polycystic kidney disease. In Avner ED, Harmon W, Niaudet P (editors): *Pediatric Nephrology,* 5th ed. Philadelphia, Lippincott Williams & Wilkins, 2004, pp 675–699.

Fick GM, Duley IT, Johnson AM, et al: The spectrum of autosomal dominant polycystic disease in children. *J Am Soc Nephrol* 1994;4:1654–1660.

Fick-Brosnahan GM, Tran ZV, Johnson AM, et al: Progression of autosomal-dominant polycystic kidney disease in children. *Kidney Int* 2001;59:1979–1980.

Kelleher CL, McFann KK, Johnson AM, et al: Characteristics of hypertension in young adults with autosomal dominant polycystic kidney disease compared with the general U.S. population. *Am J Hypertens* 2004;17:1029–1034.

Kubo S, Nakajima M, Fukuda K, et al: A 4-year-old girl with autosomal dominant polycystic kidney disease complicated by a ruptured intracranial aneurysm. *Eur J Pediatr* 2004;163:675–677.

Martinez-Vea A, Bardaj A, Gutierrez C, et al: Exercise blood pressure, cardiac structure, and diastolic function in young normotensive patients with polycystic kidney disease: A prehypertensive state. *Am J Kidney Dis* 2004;44:216–223.

Ong AC, Harris PC: Molecular pathogenesis of ADPKD: The polycystin complex gets complex. *Kidney Int* 2005;67:1234–1247.

Perrone RD: Extrarenal manifestations of ADPKD. *Kidney Int* 1997;51:2022–2036.

Rossetti S, Chauveau D, Kubly V, et al: Association of mutation position in polycystic kidney disease 1 (PKD1) gene and development of a vascular phenotype. *Lancet* 2003;361:2196–2101.

521.4 • Trauma

Infants and children are more susceptible to renal injury following blunt or penetrating injury to the back or abdomen due to the decreased muscle mass "protecting" the kidney. Gross or microscopic hematuria, flank pain, and abdominal rigidity may occur; associated injuries may be present. Urethral trauma may result from crush injury, frequently associated with a fractured pelvis or from direct injury. Such injury is suspected when gross blood appears at the external urethral meatus.

Buckley JC, McAninch JW: Pediatric renal injuries: Management guidelines from a 25-year experience. *J Urol* 2004;172:687–690.

Dreitlein DA, Suner S, Basler J: Genitourinary trauma. *Emerg Med Clin North Am* 2001;19:569–590.

Grantham JJ, Torres VE, Chapman AB, et al: Volume progression in polycystic kidney disease. *N Engl J Med* 2006;354:2122–2130.

521.5 • Renal Tumors (see Chapter 498 and 499)

Chapter 522 ■ Lower Urinary Tract Causes of Hematuria

522.1 • Infectious Causes of Cystitis and Urethritis

Gross or microscopic hematuria may be associated with bacterial, mycobacterial, or viral infections of the bladder (see Chapter 538). The occurrence of hematuria may be related to the depth and severity of the inflammatory reaction within the bladder wall.

Urethritis may present as gross or microscopic hematuria, usually in conjunction with urgency and pyuria. Urine cultures occasionally reveal bacteria, *Ureaplasma,* or *Chlamydia* but are usually negative. A history of trauma should be sought. The disorder frequently resolves spontaneously. In children older than 8 yr of age, a 10-day course of doxycycline is the treatment of choice in conjunction with a urinary analgesic such as phenazopyridine for relief of pain. If conservative management fails, cystoscopy may be required to determine the nature of any underlying abnormality such as ulceration or inflammation.

522.2 • Hemorrhagic Cystitis

Hemorrhagic cystitis (see also Chapter 259) is defined as acute or chronic bleeding of the bladder. Patients with hemorrhagic cystitis often present with gross hematuria and dysuria. In severe forms, bleeding may lead to a decrease in blood hemoglobin levels. Hemorrhagic cystitis may occur in response to chemical toxins (cyclophosphamide, penicillins, busulfan, thiotepa, dyes, insecticides), viruses (adenovirus types 11 and 21, polyoma BK virus, influenza A), radiation, and amyloidosis. Hydration and the use of MESNA disulfide (350 mg/m^2 every 6 hr), which inactivates cyclophosphamide metabolites, helps to protect the bladder from the chemical irritation related to the use of IV cyclophosphamide for many disorders. Administration of oral cyclophosphamide in the morning followed by aggressive oral hydration throughout the remainder of the day is very effective in minimizing the risk of hemorrhagic cystitis. Bladder irrigation with saline, alum, silver nitrate, or aminocaproic acid may be necessary in more severe forms of this disorder. Gross hematuria associated with viral hemorrhagic cystitis usually resolves within 1 wk.

DeVries CR, Freiha FS: Hemorrhagic cystitis: A review. *J Urol* 1990;143:1–9.

Hale GA, Rochester RJ, Heslop HE, et al: Hemorrhagic cystitis after allogeneic bone marrow transplantation in children: Clinical characteristics and outcome. *Biol Blood Marrow Transplant* 2003;9:698–705.

Pahari A, Rees L: BK virus-associated renal problems—clinical implications. *Pediatr Nephrol* 2003;18:743–748.

522.3 • Heavy Exercise

Gross or microscopic hematuria may follow vigorous exercise. Exercise hematuria is rare in females and can be associated with dysuria. The color of the urine may vary from red to black. Blood clots may be present in the urine. Findings on urine culture, intravenous pyelography, voiding cystourethrography, and cystoscopy are normal in most patients. This seems to be a benign condition, and the hematuria generally resolves within 48 hr after cessation of exercise. The absence of red blood cell casts or evidence of renal disease and the presence of dysuria and blood clots in some patients suggest that the source of bleeding lies in the lower urinary tract. Rhabdomyolysis with myoglobinuria or hemoglobinuria must be considered in the differential diagnosis when associated with symptoms in the appropriate clinical context.

Abarbanel J, Benet AE, Lask D, et al: Sports hematuria. *J Urol* 1990;143:887–890.

Gambrell RC, Blount BW: Exercise-induced hematuria. *Am Fam Physician* 1996;53:905–911.

Siegel AJ, Hennekens CH, Solomon HS, et al: Exercise-related hematuria. *JAMA* 1979;241:391–392.

522.4 • Munchausen Syndrome by Proxy (See Chapter 36.2)

Section 3 — Conditions Particularly Associated with Proteinuria — Beth A. Vogt and Ellis D. Avner

Chapter 523 ■ Introduction to the Child with Proteinuria

The demonstration of proteinuria on a routine screening urinalysis is common; 10% of children aged 8–15 yr will test positive for proteinuria by urinary dipstick at some time. The challenge is to differentiate the child with proteinuria related to renal disease from the otherwise healthy child with transient or other benign forms of proteinuria.

The urine dipstick test offers a qualitative assessment of urinary protein excretion. Dipsticks primarily detect albuminuria and are less sensitive for other forms of proteinuria (low molecular weight proteins, Bence Jones protein, gamma globulins). Visual changes in the color of the dipstick are a semiquantitative measure of increasing urinary protein concentration. The dipstick is reported as negative, trace (10–20 mg/dL), 1+ (30 mg/dL), 2+ (100 mg/dL), 3+ (300 mg/dL), and 4+ (1000–2000 mg/dL).

False-negative test results may occur in patients with dilute urine (specific gravity <1.005) or in disease states in which the predominant urinary protein is not albumin. False-positive test results may be seen in patients with gross hematuria, contamination with antiseptic agents (chlorhexidine, benzalkonium chloride), urinary pH >7.0, or phenazopyridine therapy. The dipstick may be falsely positive in patients with highly concentrated urine. A dipstick should be considered positive for protein if it registers ≥1+ (30 mg/dL) in a urine sample in which the specific gravity is ≤1.015. If the specific gravity is >1.015, the dipstick must read ≥2+ to be considered clinically significant.

Because the dipstick reaction offers only a qualitative measurement of urinary protein excretion, children with persistent proteinuria should have proteinuria quantitated with the more precise spot urine protein/creatinine ratio (UPr/UCr). This ratio is calculated by dividing the UPr (mg/dL) concentration by the UCr (mg/dL) concentration and is best performed on a first morning voided urine specimen to eliminate the possibility of orthostatic (postural) proteinuria (see Chapter 525). Ratios <0.5 in children younger than 2 yr of age and <0.2 in children 2 yr of age or older suggest normal protein excretion. A ratio >3 suggests nephrotic-range proteinuria. UPr/UCr ratios have been shown to have a high correlation with protein excretion determinations by timed urine collection.

Timed (24-hr) urine collections offer more precise information regarding UPr excretion but are more cumbersome to obtain and highly inaccurate and have largely been replaced by the spot protein-to-creatinine ratio. A reasonable upper limit of normal protein excretion in healthy children is 150 mg/24 hr (0.15 g/24 hr). More specifically, normal protein excretion in children is defined as ≤4 mg/m^2/hr; abnormal is defined as 4–40 mg/m^2/hr; and nephrotic range is defined as >40 mg/m^2/hr.

Abitbol C, Zilleruelo G, Freundlich M, et al: Quantitation of proteinuria with urinary protein/creatinine ratios and random testing with dipsticks in nephrotic syndrome. *J Pediatr* 1990;116:243–247.

D'Amico G, Bazzi C: Pathophysiology of proteinuria. *Kidney Int* 2003;63:809–825.

Hogg R, Portman RJ, Milliner D, et al: Evaluation and management of proteinuria and nephrotic syndrome in children: Recommendations from a pediatric nephrology panel established at the National Kidney Foundation Conference of Proteinuria, Albuminuria, Risk, Assessment, Detection, and Elimination. *Pediatrics* 2000;105:1242–1249.

Tryggvason K, Patrakka J, Wartiovaara J: Hereditary proteinuria syndromes and mechanisms of proteinuria. *N Engl J Med* 2006;354:1387–1401.

Vehaskari VM, Rapola J: Isolated proteinuria: Analysis of a school-age population. *J Pediatr* 1982;101:661–668.

Chapter 524 ■ Transient Proteinuria

The majority of children found to have a positive urinary dipstick for protein will have normal dipstick values on repeated measurements. Of the 10% of children found to have proteinuria by a single dipstick measurement, only 1% had persistent proteinuria when measured on 4 separate occasions. This phenomenon, called **transient proteinuria,** may be caused by a temperature >38.3°C (101°F) (see Chapter 174), exercise (see Chapter 685), dehydration, cold exposure, heart failure, seizures, or stress. The proteinuria usually does not exceed 2+ on the dipstick. The mechanism of transient proteinuria is unknown. No evaluation or therapy is needed for children with this benign condition.

Jensen H, Henriksen K: Proteinuria in non-renal infectious disease. *Acta Med Scand* 1974;196:75–82.
Marks MI, McLaine PN, Drummond KN: Proteinuria in children with febrile illnesses. *Arch Dis Child* 1970;45:250–253.
Poortmans JR: Post-exercise proteinuria in humans. *JAMA* 1985;253:236–240.
Vehaskari VM, Rapola J: Isolated proteinuria: Analysis of a school-age population. *J Pediatr* 1982;101:661–668.

Chapter 525 ■ Orthostatic (Postural) Proteinuria

Orthostatic proteinuria is the most common cause of persistent proteinuria in school-aged children and adolescents, occurring in up to 60% of children with persistent proteinuria. Children with this condition are usually asymptomatic, and the condition is discovered on routine urinalysis. Individuals with orthostatic proteinuria excrete normal or minimally increased amounts of protein in the supine position. In the upright position, urinary protein excretion is increased up to 10-fold, up to 1,000 mg/24 hr (1 g/24 hr). Hematuria, hypertension, hypoalbuminemia, edema, and renal dysfunction are absent.

In a child with persistent asymptomatic proteinuria, the first step in evaluation is to rule out orthostatic proteinuria by obtaining a complete urinalysis and spot protein/creatinine ratio on a first morning urine sample. It is important that the child fully empties his or her bladder prior to going to bed and collects the first voided urine sample immediately upon arising in the morning. The absence of proteinuria (dipstick negative or trace for protein and UPr/Cr ratio <0.2) in the first morning urine sample for 3 consecutive days confirms the diagnosis of orthostatic proteinuria. No further evaluation is necessary, and the patient and family should be reassured of the benign nature of this condition. On the other hand, if there are other abnormalities in the urinalysis (hematuria) or the UPr/Cr ratio >0.2, the patient should be referred to a pediatric nephrologist for evaluation.

The cause of orthostatic proteinuria is unknown, although altered renal hemodynamics and partial renal vein obstruction in the upright position are possible causes. Long-term follow-up studies in adults suggest that orthostatic proteinuria is a benign process, but similar data are not available for children. Therefore, long-term follow-up of children is prudent to monitor patients for evidence of renal disease, including hematuria, hypertension, edema, diminished renal function, or proteinuria exceeding 1,000 mg/24 hr.

Cho BS, Choi YM, Kang MI, et al: Diagnosis of nutcracker phenomenon using renal Doppler ultrasound in orthostatic proteinuria. *Nephrol Dial Transplant* 2001;16:1620–1625.
Devarajan P: Mechanisms of orthostatic proteinuria: Lessons from a transplant donor. *J Am Soc Nephrol* 1993;4:36–39.
Springberg PD, Garrett LE Jr, Thompson AL, et al: Fixed and reproducible orthostatic proteinuria: Results of a 20-year follow-up study. *Ann Intern Med* 1982;97:516.

Chapter 526 ■ Fixed Proteinuria

Individuals found to have significant proteinuria on a first morning urine sample on 3 consecutive days (>1+ on dipstick, or protein/creatinine ratio >0.2) have fixed proteinuria. Fixed proteinuria indicates renal disease and may be caused by either glomerular or tubular disorders.

526.1 • Glomerular Proteinuria

A variety of renal diseases are characterized by increased permeability of the glomerular capillary wall, leading to glomerular proteinuria (Table 526-1). Glomerular proteinuria may range from <1 g to >30 g/24 hr. Glomerular proteinuria may be termed *selective* (loss of plasma proteins of molecular weight up to and

TABLE 526-1. Causes of Proteinuria

TRANSIENT PROTEINURIA
Fever
Exercise
Dehydration
Cold exposure
Congestive heart failure
Seizure
Stress
ORTHOSTATIC (POSTURAL) PROTEINURIA
GLOMERULAR DISEASES CHARACTERIZED BY ISOLATED PROTEINURIA
Focal segmental golmerulosclerosis
Mesangial proliferative glomerulonephritis
Membranous nephropathy
Membranoproliferative glomerulonephritis
Amyloidosis
Diabetic nephropathy
Sickle cell nephropathy
GLOMERULAR DISEASES WITH PROTEINURIA AS A FEATURE
Acute postinfectious glomerulonephritis
IgA nephropathy
Henoch-Schönlein purpura nephritis
Lupus nephritis
Alport syndrome
TUBULAR DISEASES
Cystinosis
Wilson disease
Lowe syndrome
Galactosemia
Tubulointerstitial nephritis
Heavy metal poisoning
Acute tubular necrosis
Renal dysplasia
Polycystic kidney disease
Reflux nephropathy

including albumin) or *nonselective* (loss of albumin and of larger molecular weight proteins such as IgG). The determination of urinary protein selectivity is of little clinical value because of the considerable overlap among various forms of renal disease. It can, however, when "selective," identify nephrotic patients most likely to respond to corticosteroids (see Chapter 527).

Glomerular proteinuria should be suspected in any patient with a first morning urine protein/creatinine ratio >1.0, or proteinuria of any degree, accompanied by hypertension, hematuria, edema, or renal dysfunction. Disorders characterized primarily by proteinuria include focal segmental glomerulosclerosis, mesangial proliferative glomerulonephritis, membranous nephropathy, membranoproliferative glomerulonephritis, amyloidosis, diabetic nephropathy, and obesity-related glomerulopathy. Other renal disorders that may include proteinuria as a prominent feature include acute postinfectious glomerulonephritis, IgA nephropathy, lupus nephritis, Henoch-Schönlein purpura nephritis, and Alport syndrome.

Initial evaluation of a child with fixed proteinuria should include measurement of serum creatinine and electrolyte panel, first morning urine protein/creatinine ratio, serum albumin level, and C3 level. The child should be referred to a pediatric nephrologist for further evaluation and management. Renal biopsy is often necessary to establish a diagnosis and guide therapy.

In asymptomatic patients with low-grade proteinuria (protein/creatinine ratio 0.2–1.0) in whom all other findings are normal, renal biopsy may not be indicated because the underlying process may be either transient/resolving or because specific pathologic features of a chronic kidney disease may not yet be apparent. Such patients should have periodic re-evaluation (q 4–6 mo unless symptomatic) consisting of a physical examination and blood pressure determination, urinalysis, and measurement of serum creatinine and first morning voided urine protein/creatinine ratio. Indications for renal biopsy include increasing proteinuria (protein/creatinine >1.0) and/or the development of hematuria, hypertension, or diminished renal function.

Bergstein JM: A practical approach to proteinuria. *Pediatr Nephrol* 1999;13:697–700.

Mahan, JD, Turman MA, Mentser MI: Evaluation of hematuria, proteinuria, and hypertension in adolescents. *Pediatr Clin North Am* 1997; 44:1573–1589.

Roy S: Proteinuria. *Pediatr Ann* 1996;25:277–282.

Wilmer WA, Rovin BH, Hebert CJ, et al: Management of glomerular proteinuria: A commentary. *J Am Soc Nephrol* 2003;14:3217–3232.

526.2 • Tubular Proteinuria

A variety of renal disorders that primarily involve the tubulointerstitial compartment of the kidney may cause low-grade fixed proteinuria (protein/creatinine ratio <1.0). In the healthy state, large amounts of proteins of lower molecular weight than albumin are filtered by the glomerulus and reabsorbed in the proximal tubule. Injury to the proximal tubules may result in diminished reabsorptive capacity and the loss of these low molecular weight proteins in the urine.

Tubular proteinuria (see Table 526-1) may be seen in acquired and inherited disorders and may be associated with other defects of proximal tubular function, such as glycosuria, phosphaturia, bicarbonate wasting, and aminoaciduria. Tubular proteinuria rarely presents a diagnostic dilemma because the underlying disease is usually detected before the proteinuria is detected.

Asymptomatic patients having persistent proteinuria generally have glomerular rather than tubular proteinuria. In occult cases, glomerular and tubular proteinuria can be distinguished by electrophoresis of the urine. In tubular proteinuria, little or no albumin is detected, whereas in glomerular proteinuria the major protein is albumin.

Alt JM, Von der Heyde D, Assel E, et al: Characteristics of protein excretion in glomerular and tubular disease. *Contrib Nephrol* 1981;24:115–121.

Chapter 527 ■ Nephrotic Syndrome

Nephrotic syndrome is primarily a pediatric disorder and is 15 times more common in children than adults. The incidence is 2–3/100,000 children per year; and the majority of affected children will have steroid-sensitive minimal change disease. The characteristic features of nephrotic syndrome are heavy proteinuria (>3.5 g/24 hr in adults or 40 mg/m^2/hr in children), hypoalbuminemia (<2.5 g/dL), edema, and hyperlipidemia.

ETIOLOGY. Most children (90%) with nephrotic syndrome have a form of the idiopathic nephrotic syndrome. Causes of idiopathic nephrotic syndrome include minimal change disease (85%), mesangial proliferation (5%), and focal segmental glomerulosclerosis (10%). The remaining 10% of children with nephrotic syndrome have secondary nephrotic syndrome related to systemic (Table 527-1) or glomerular diseases such as membranous nephropathy or membranoproliferative glomerulonephritis (Table 527-2).

PATHOPHYSIOLOGY. The underlying abnormality in nephrotic syndrome is an increase in permeability of the glomerular capillary wall, which leads to massive proteinuria and hypoalbuminemia. The cause of the increased permeability is not well understood. In minimal change disease, it is possible that T-cell dysfunction leads to alteration of cytokines, which causes a loss of negatively charged glycoproteins within the glomerular capillary wall. In focal segmental glomerulosclerosis, a plasma factor, perhaps produced by lymphocytes, may be responsible for the increase in capillary wall permeability. Alternately, mutations in podocyte proteins (podocin, α-actinin 4) are associated with focal segmental glomerulosclerosis (Table 527-3). Steroid-resistant nephrotic syndrome is associated with mutations in *NPHS2* (podocin) and *WT1* genes.

Although the mechanism of edema formation in nephrotic syndrome is incompletely understood, it seems likely that, in most instances, massive urinary protein loss leads to hypoalbuminemia, which causes a decrease in the plasma oncotic pressure and transudation of fluid from the intravascular compartment to the interstitial space. The reduction in intravascular volume decreases renal perfusion pressure, activating the renin-angiotensin-aldosterone system, which stimulates tubular reabsorption of sodium. The reduced intravascular volume also stimulates the release of antidiuretic hormone, which enhances the reabsorption of water in the collecting duct.

This theory does not apply to all patients with nephrotic syndrome because some patients actually have increased intravascular volume with diminished plasma levels of renin and aldosterone. Therefore, other factors, including a primary renal avidity for sodium and water, may be involved in the formation of edema in some patients with nephrotic syndrome.

TABLE 527-1. Causes of Childhood Nephrotic Syndrome*

GENETIC DISORDERS

Nephrotic Syndrome Typical
Finnish-type congenital nephrotic syndrome
Focal segmental glomerulosclerosis
Diffuse mesangial sclerosis
Denys-Drash syndrome
Schimke immuno-osseous dysplasia

Proteinuria with or without Nephrotic Syndrome
Nail-patella syndrome
Alport syndrome

Multisystem Syndromes with or without Nephrotic Syndrome
Galloway-Mowat syndrome
Charcot-Marie-Tooth disease
Jeune syndrome
Cockayne syndrome
Laurence-Moon-Biedl-Bardet syndrome

Metabolic Disorders with or without Nephrotic Syndrome
Alagille syndrome
α_1 Antitrypsin deficiency
Fabry disease
Glutaric acidemia
Glycogen storage disease
Hurler syndrome
Lipoprotein disorders
Mitochondrial cytopathies
Sickle cell disease

IDIOPATHIC NEPHROTIC SYNDROME
Minimal change disease
Focal segmental glomerulosclerosis
Membranous nephropathy

SECONDARY CAUSES

Infections
Hepatitis B, C
HIV-1
Malaria
Syphilis
Toxoplasmosis

Drugs
Penicillamine
Gold
Nonsteroidal anti-inflammatory drugs
Pamidronate
Interferon
Mercury
Heroin
Lithium

Immunologic or Allergic Disorders
Castleman disease
Kimura disease
Bee sting
Food allergens

Associated with Malignant Disease
Lymphoma
Leukemia

Glomerular Hyperfiltration
Oligomeganephronia
Morbid obesity
Adaptation to nephron reduction

*May also be consequence of inflammatory glomerular disorders, normally associated with features of nephritis, e.g., vasculitis, lupus nephritis, membranoproliferative glomerulonephritis, IgA nephropathy.
From Eddy AA, Symons JM: Nephrotic syndrome in childhood. *Lancet* 2003; 362:629–638.

TABLE 527-2. Summary of Primary Renal Diseases That Present as Idiopathic Nephrotic Syndrome

	MINIMAL CHANGE NEPHROTIC SYNDROME	FOCAL SEGMENTAL GLOMERULOSCLEROSIS	MEMBRANOUS NEPHROPATHY	MEMBRANOPROLIFERATIVE GLOMERULONEPHRITIS Type I	MEMBRANOPROLIFERATIVE GLOMERULONEPHRITIS Type II
FREQUENCY*					
Children	75%	10%	<5%	10%	10%
Adults	15%	15%	50%	10%	10%
Clinical Manifestations					
Age (yr)	2–6, some adults	2–10, some adults	40–50	5–15	5–15
Sex	2 : 1 male	1.3 : 1 male	2 : 1 male	Male-female	Male-female
Nephrotic syndrome	100%	90%	80%	60%	60%
Asymptomatic proteinuria	0	10%	20%	40%	40%
Hematuria	10–20%	60–80%	60%	80%	80%
Hypertension	10%	20% early	Infrequent	35%	35%
Rate of progression to renal failure	Does not progress	10 yr	50% in 10–20 yr	10–20 yr	5–15 yr
Associated conditions	Allergy? Hodgkin disease, usually none	None	Renal vein thrombosis, cancer, SLE, hepatitis B	None	Partial lipodystrophy
Laboratory Findings	Manifestations of nephrotic syndrome ↑ BUN in 15–30%	Manifestations of nephrotic syndrome ↑ BUN in 20–40%	Manifestations of nephrotic syndrome	Low C1, C4, C3–C9	Normal C1, C4, low C3–C9
Immunogenetics	HLA-B8, B12 (3.5)†	Mutations in podocin, α-actinin-4, other genes	HLA-DRw3 (12–32)†	Not established	C3 nephritic factor Not established
Renal Pathology					
Light microscopy	Normal	Focal sclerotic lesions	Thickened GBM, spikes	Thickened GBM, proliferation	Lobulation
Immunofluorescence	Negative	IgM, C3 in lesions	Fine granular IgG, C3	Granular IgG, C3	C3 only
Electron microscopy	Foot process fusion	Foot process fusion	Subepithelial deposits	Mesangial and subendothelial deposits	Dense deposits
Response to Steroids	90%	15–20%	May be slow progression	Not established	Not established

*Approximate frequency as a cause of idiopathic nephrotic syndrome. About 10% of adult nephrotic syndrome is due to various diseases that usually present as acute glomerulonephritis.
†Relative risk.
BUN, blood urea nitrogen; C, complement; GBM, glomerular basement membrane; HLA, human leukocyte antigen; Ig, immunoglobulin; SLE, systemic lupus erythematosus; hepatitis B, hepatitis B virus; ↑, elevated.
Modified from Couser WG: Glomerular disorders. In Wyngaarden JB, Smith LH, Bennett JC (editors): *Cecil Textbook of Medicine,* 19th ed. Philadelphia, WB Saunders, 1992, p 560.

In the nephrotic state, serum lipid levels (cholesterol, triglycerides) are elevated for two reasons. Hypoalbuminemia stimulates generalized hepatic protein synthesis, including synthesis of lipoproteins. In addition, lipid catabolism is diminished, as a result of reduced plasma levels of lipoprotein lipase, related to increased urinary losses of this enzyme.

Nephrotic syndrome in children: Prediction of histopathology from clinical and laboratory characteristics at time of diagnosis. A report of the International Study of Kidney Disease in Children. *Kidney Int* 1978;13:159.

Van de Walle JGJ, Donckerwolcke RA: Pathogenesis of edema formation in the nephrotic syndrome. *Pediatr Nephrol* 2001;16:283.

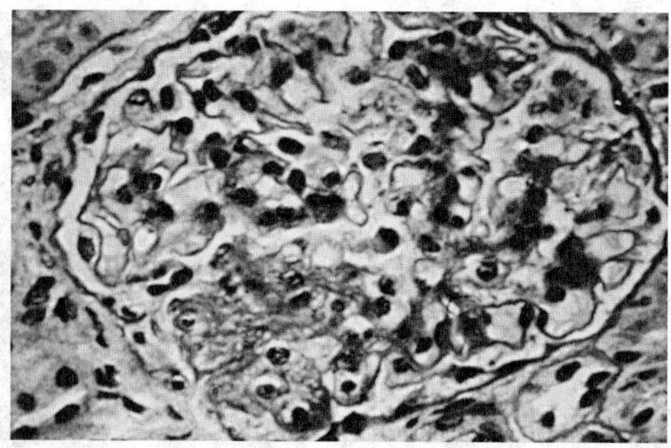

Figure 527-1. Glomerulus from a patient with steroid-resistant nephritic syndrome showing mesangial hypercellularity and an area of sclerosis in the lower portion (×250).

527.1 • Idiopathic Nephrotic Syndrome

Approximately 90% of children with nephrotic syndrome have idiopathic nephrotic syndrome. Idiopathic nephrotic syndrome includes 3 histologic types: minimal change disease, mesangial proliferation, and focal segmental glomerulosclerosis. These 3 disorders may represent 3 separate diseases with a similar clinical presentation; alternately, these disorders may represent a spectrum of a single disease.

PATHOLOGY. In **minimal change nephrotic syndrome** (MCNS) (85% of total cases of nephrotic syndrome in children), the glomeruli appear normal or show a minimal increase in mesangial cells and matrix. Findings on immunofluorescence microscopy are typically negative, and electron microscopy simply reveals effacement of the epithelial cell foot processes. More than 95% of children with minimal change disease respond to corticosteroid therapy.

Mesangial proliferation (5% of total cases) is characterized by a diffuse increase in mesangial cells and matrix on light microscopy. Immunofluorescence microscopy may reveal trace to 1+ mesangial IgM and/or IgA staining. Electron microscopy reveals increased numbers of mesangial cells and matrix as well as effacement of the epithelial cell foot processes. Approximately 50% of patients with this histologic lesion respond to corticosteroid therapy.

In **focal segmental glomerulosclerosis (FSGS)** (10% of total cases), glomeruli show mesangial proliferation and segmental scarring on light microscopy (Fig. 527-1, Table 527-2). Immunofluorescence microscopy shows IgM and C3 staining in the areas of segmental sclerosis. Electron microscopy shows segmental scarring of the glomerular tuft with obliteration of the glomerular capillary lumen. A similar lesion may be seen with HIV infection, vesicoureteral reflux, and intravenous heroin abuse. Only 20% of patients with FSGS respond to prednisone. The disease is frequently progressive, ultimately involving all glomeruli, and leads to end-stage renal disease in most patients.

CLINICAL MANIFESTATIONS. The idiopathic nephrotic syndrome is more common in males than in females (2:1) and most commonly appears between the ages of 2 and 6 yr. It has been reported as early as 6 mo of age and throughout adulthood. MCNS is present in 85–90% of patients <6 yr of age; FSGS develops in older children. Twenty to 30% of adolescents have MCNS. The incidence of FSGS may be increasing; it may be more common in African-American or Hispanic patients. The initial episode and subsequent relapses may follow minor infections and, occasionally, reactions to insect bites, bee stings, or poison ivy. Children usually present with mild edema, which is initially noted around the eyes and in the lower extremities. Nephrotic syndrome may initially be misdiagnosed as an allergic disorder because of the periorbital swelling that decreases throughout the day. With time, the edema becomes generalized, with the development of ascites, pleural effusions, and genital edema. Anorexia, irritability, abdominal pain, and diarrhea are common; hypertension and gross hematuria are uncommon. The differential diagnosis of the child with marked edema includes protein-losing enteropathy, hepatic failure, congestive heart failure, acute or chronic glomeru-

TABLE 527-3. Nephrotic Syndrome in Children Due to Genetic Disorders of the Podocyte

GENE	NAME	LOCATION	INHERITANCE	RENAL DISEASE
STEROID-RESISTANT NEPHROTIC SYNDROME				
NPHS1	Nephrin	19q13.1	Recessive	Finnish-type congenital nephrotic syndrome
NPHS2	Podocin	1q25	Recessive	FSGS
FSGS1	α-actinin-4 (α*ACTN4*)	19q13	Dominant	FSGS
FSGS2	Unknown	11q21–22	Dominant	FSGS
WT1	Wilms tumor-suppressor gene	11p13	Dominant	Denys-Drash syndrome with diffuse mesangial sclerosis Frasier's syndrome with FSGS
LMX1B	LIM-homeodomain protein	9q34	Dominant	Nail-patella syndrome
SMARCAL1	SW1/SNF2-related, matrix-associated, actin-dependent regulator of chromatin, subfamily a-like 1	2q35	Recessive	Schimke immuno-osseous dysplasia with FSGS*
STEROID-RESPONSIVE NEPHROTIC SYNDROME				
Unknown	Unknown	Unknown	Recessive	MCNS

*Podocyte expression of *SMARCAL1* presumptive but not yet established. Mutations in another protein, CD2-AP or NEPH1 (novel protein structurally related to nephrin), cause congenital nephrotic syndrome in mice. A mutational variant in the *CD2AP* gene has been identified in a few patients with steroid-resistant nephrotic syndrome.

From Eddy AA, Symons JM: Nephrotic syndrome in childhood. *Lancet* 2003; 362:629–638.

lonephritis, and protein malnutrition. A diagnosis other than MCNS should be considered in the presence of age <1 yr, a family history, extrarenal findings (arthritis, rash, anemia), hypertension or pulmonary edema, acute or chronic renal insufficiency, and hematuria.

DIAGNOSIS. The urinalysis reveals 3+ or 4+ proteinuria; microscopic hematuria may be present in 20% of children. Spot urine protein/creatinine ratio exceeds 2.0 and urinary protein excretion exceeds 3.5 g/24 hr in adults and 40 mg/m^2/hr in children. The serum creatinine value is usually normal, but it may be increased because of diminished renal perfusion resulting from contraction of the intravascular volume. The serum albumin level is generally <2.5 g/dL, and the serum cholesterol and triglyceride levels are elevated. C3 and C4 levels are normal. Renal biopsy is not required for diagnosis in most children.

TREATMENT. Children having the first episode of nephrotic syndrome and mild to moderate edema may be managed as outpatients. Affected children may attend school and participate in physical activities as tolerated. The pathophysiology and treatment of nephrotic syndrome should be carefully reviewed with the family to enhance their understanding of their child's disease. Sodium intake should be reduced by the initiation of a low-sodium diet and may be normalized when the child enters remission. Although there are no data to support their safety or efficacy, oral diuretics are used by many clinicians for children with nephrotic syndrome. Because of the possibility of increasing the risk of thromboembolic complications, diuretic use should be reserved for patients with severe symptoms and must be closely monitored.

Children with severe symptomatic edema, including large pleural effusions, ascites, or severe genital edema, should be hospitalized. In addition to sodium restriction, fluid restriction may be necessary if the child is hyponatremic. A swollen scrotum may be elevated with pillows to enhance the removal of fluid by gravity. Diuresis may be augmented by administration of chlorothiazide (10 mg/kg/dose IV every 12 hr) or metolazone (0.1 mg/kg/dose PO bid) followed by furosemide 30 min later (1–2 mg/kg/dose IV q 12 hr).

IV administration of 25% human albumin (0.5 g/kg/dose q 6–12 hr administered over 1–2 hr) followed by furosemide (1–2 mg/kg/dose IV) is often necessary when fluid restriction and parenteral diuretics are not effective. Such therapy mandates close monitoring of volume status, serum electrolyte balance, and renal function. Symptomatic volume overload, with hypertension and heart failure, is a potential complication of parenteral albumin therapy, particularly with rapid infusions.

Children with onset of nephrotic syndrome between 1 and 8 yr of age are likely to have steroid-responsive MCNS; steroid therapy may be initiated without diagnostic renal biopsy. Children with features that make MCNS less likely (hematuria, hypertension, renal insufficiency, hypocomplementemia, age <1 yr or >8 yr) should be considered for renal biopsy before treatment.

In children with presumed MCNS, prednisone should be administered (after confirming a negative PPD test) at a dose of 60 mg/m^2/day (maximum daily dose, 80 mg divided into 2–3 doses) for at least 4 consecutive weeks. There is good evidence that an initial 6-wk course of **daily** steroid treatment may lead to a lower relapse rate, although the frequency of steroid-induced side effects is higher. Eighty to 90% of children will respond to steroid therapy (urine trace or negative for protein for 3 consecutive days), by 2 wk. The vast majority of children who will respond to prednisone therapy will do so within the first 4 wk of treatment.

After the initial 6-wk course, the prednisone dose should be tapered to 40 mg/m^2/day given every other day as a single morning dose. The **alternate-day** dose is then slowly tapered and discontinued over the next 2–3 mo. Children who continue to have proteinuria (2+ or greater) after 8 wk of steroid therapy are considered steroid resistant, and a diagnostic renal biopsy should be performed.

Many children with nephrotic syndrome will experience at least 1 relapse (3–4+ proteinuria plus edema). Although relapse rates of 60–80% have been noted in the past, the relapse rate in children treated with longer initial steroid courses may be as low as 30–40%.

Relapses should be treated with daily divided-dose prednisone at the doses noted earlier until the child enters remission (urine trace or negative for protein for 3 consecutive days). The prednisone dose is then changed to alternate-day dosing and tapered over 1–2 mo.

A subset of patients will relapse while on alternate-day steroid therapy or within 28 days of stopping prednisone therapy. Such patients are termed **steroid dependent.** Patients who respond well to prednisone therapy but relapse ≥4 times in a 12-mo period are termed **frequent relapsers.** Children who fail to respond to prednisone therapy within 8 wk are termed **steroid resistant.** Steroid-resistant nephrotic syndrome is usually FSGS (80%), MCNS (20%), and rarely mesangial proliferative.

Steroid-dependent patients, frequent relapsers, and steroid-resistant patients may be candidates for alternative agents, particularly if the child suffers severe corticosteroid toxicity (cushingoid appearance, hypertension, cataracts, and/or growth failure). **Cyclophosphamide** prolongs the duration of remission and reduces the number of relapses in children with **frequently relapsing** and **steroid-dependent** nephrotic syndrome. The potential side effects of the drug (neutropenia, disseminated varicella, hemorrhagic cystitis, alopecia, sterility, increased risk of future malignancy) should be carefully reviewed with the family before initiating treatment. The dose of cyclophosphamide is 2–3 mg/kg/24 hr given as a single oral dose, for a total duration of 8–12 wk. Alternate-day prednisone therapy is often continued during the course of cyclophosphamide administration. During cyclophosphamide therapy, the white blood cell count must be monitored weekly and the drug should be withheld if the count falls below 5,000/mm^3.

An additional option for the child with complicated nephrotic syndrome is **high-dose pulse methylprednisolone.** Methylprednisolone is usually given as a 30-mg/kg bolus (maximum 1,000 mg), with the first 6 doses given every other day, followed by a tapering regimen for periods up to 18 mo. Cyclophosphamide may be added to this regimen in selected patients.

Cyclosporine (3–6 mg/kg/24 hr divided q 12 hr) or **tacrolimus** (0.15 mg/kg/24 hr divided q 12 hr) are also effective in maintaining prolonged remissions in children with nephrotic syndrome and are useful as steroid-sparing agents. Children must be monitored for side effects, including hypertension, nephrotoxicity, hirsutism, and gingival hyperplasia. **Mycophenolate** may maintain remission in children with steroid-dependent or frequently relapsing nephrotic syndrome. Most children who respond to cyclosporine, tacrolimus, or mycophenolate therapy tend to relapse when the medication is discontinued. Angiotensin-converting enzyme (ACE) inhibitors and angiotensin II blockers may be helpful as adjunct therapy to reduce proteinuria in steroid-resistant patients.

COMPLICATIONS. Infection is the major complication of nephrotic syndrome. Children in relapse have increased susceptibility to bacterial infections because of urinary losses of immunoglobulins and properdin factor B, defective cell-mediated immunity, immunosuppressive therapy, malnutrition, and edema/ascites acting as a potential "culture medium." **Spontaneous bacterial peritonitis** is the most frequent type of infection, although sepsis, pneumonia, cellulitis, and urinary tract infections may also be seen. Although *Streptococcus pneumoniae* is the most common organism causing peritonitis, gram-negative bacteria such as *Escherichia coli* may also be encountered. Because fever and physical findings may be minimal in the presence of corticosteroid therapy, a high index of suspicion, prompt evaluation (including cultures of blood and peritoneal fluid), and early initiation of antibiotic therapy are critical. The role of prophylactic antibiotic therapy during nephrotic syndrome relapse is controversial.

All children with nephrotic syndrome should receive polyvalent pneumococcal vaccine (if not previously immunized), ideally administered when the child is in remission and off daily prednisone therapy. Children with a negative varicella titer should be given varicella vaccine when in remission or on a low dose of alternate-day steroids. Nonimmune nephrotic children in relapse exposed to varicella should receive varicella-zoster immunoglobulin within 72 hr of exposure. Influenza vaccine should be given on a yearly basis.

Children with nephrotic syndrome are also at increased risk of thromboembolic events. The incidence of this complication in children is 2–5%, which represents a much lower risk than that of adults with nephrotic syndrome. Both arterial and venous thromboses may be seen, including renal vein thrombosis, pulmonary embolus, sagittal sinus thrombosis, and thrombosis of indwelling arterial and venous catheters. The risk of thrombosis is related to increased prothrombotic factors (fibrinogen, thrombocytosis, hemoconcentration, relative immobilization) and decreased fibrinolytic factors (urinary losses of antithrombin III, proteins C and S). Prophylactic anticoagulation is not recommended in children unless they have had a previous thromboembolic event. Overaggressive diuresis should be avoided and use of indwelling catheters limited because these factors may increase the likelihood of clotting complications.

Hyperlipidemia, particularly in complicated patients with nephrotic syndrome, may be a risk factor for cardiovascular disease; myocardial infarction is a rare complication in children. It has been suggested that consideration be given to the use of 3-hydroxy-3-methylglutaryl coenzyme A (HMG-CoA) reductase–inhibiting drugs to treat the hyperlipidemia seen in nephrotic syndrome.

PROGNOSIS. The majority of children with steroid-responsive nephrotic syndrome have repeated relapses, which generally decrease in frequency as the child grows older. Although there is no proven way to predict an individual child's course, those children who respond to steroids rapidly and those who have no relapses during the first 6 mo after diagnosis are likely to follow an infrequently relapsing course. It is important to indicate to the family that the child with steroid-responsive nephrotic syndrome is unlikely to develop chronic kidney disease, that the disease is generally not hereditary, and that the child (in the absence of prolonged cyclophosphamide therapy) will remain fertile. To minimize the psychological effects of the condition, the physician should emphasize that the child should be considered normal when in remission and may have unrestricted diet and activity, without the need for urine testing for protein.

Children with steroid-resistant nephrotic syndrome, most often caused by FSGS, generally have a much poorer prognosis. These children develop progressive renal insufficiency, ultimately leading to end-stage renal disease requiring dialysis or renal transplantation. Recurrent nephrotic syndrome develops in 30–50% of transplant recipients with FSGS. Plasmapheresis, plasma protein absorption onto protein A–based columns, high-dose cyclosporine or tacrolimus, and ACE inhibitors may reduce proteinuria in these patients.

Barletta GM, Smoyer WE, Bunchman TE, et al: Use of mycophenolate mofetil in steroid-dependent and -resistant nephrotic syndrome. *Pediatr Nephrol* 2003;18:833–837.

Cattran DC, Appel GB, Hebert LA, et al., for the North America Nephrotic Syndrome Study Group: A randomized trial of cyclosporine in patients with steroid-resistant focal segmental glomerulosclerosis. *Kidney Int* 1999; 56:2220–2226.

Constantinescu AR, Shah HB, Foote EF, et al: Predicting first-year relapses in children with nephrotic syndrome. *Pediatrics* 2000;105:492–495.

Eddy AA, Symons JM: Nephrotic syndrome in childhood. *Lancet* 2003;362:629–639.

Hinkes B, Wiggins RC, Gbadegesin R, et al: Positional cloning uncovers mutations in PLCEI responsible for a nephrotic syndrome variant that may be reversible. *Nat Genet* 2006;38:1397–1405.

Hogg R, Portman RJ, Milliner D, et al: Evaluation and management of proteinuria and nephrotic syndrome in children: Recommendations from a pediatric nephrology panel established at the National Kidney Foundation Conference of Proteinuria, Albuminuria, Risk, Assessment, Detection, and Elimination. *Pediatrics* 2000;105:1242–1249.

Leonard MB, Feldman HI, Shults J, et al: Long-term, high-dose glucocorticoids and bone mineral content in childhood glucocorticoid-sensitive nephrotic syndrome. *N Engl J Med* 2004;351:868–875.

Loeffler K, Gowrishankar M, Yiu V: Tacrolimus therapy in pediatric patients with treatment-resistant nephrotic syndrome. *Pediatr Nephrol* 2004; 19:281–287.

Mao J, Zhang Y, Du L, et al: NPHS1 and NPHS2 gene mutations in Chinese children with sporadic nephrotic syndrome. *Pediatr Res* 2007;61:117–122.

Mucha B, Ozaltin F, Hinkes BG, et al: Mutations in the Wilms' tumor 1 gene cause isolated steroid resistant nephrotic syndrome and occur in exons 8 and 9. *Pediatr Res* 2006;59:325–331.

527.2 • SECONDARY NEPHROTIC SYNDROME

Nephrotic syndrome also occurs as a secondary feature of many forms of glomerular disease. Membranous nephropathy, membranoproliferative glomerulonephritis, postinfectious glomerulonephritis, lupus nephritis, and Henoch-Schönlein purpura nephritis may all have a nephrotic component (see Tables 527-1 and 527-2). Secondary nephrotic syndrome should be suspected in patients with age >8 yr, hypertension, hematuria, renal dysfunction, extrarenal symptomatology (rash, arthralgias, fever), or depressed serum complement levels.

In certain areas of the world, malaria and schistosomiasis are the leading causes of nephrotic syndrome. Other infectious agents associated with nephrotic syndrome include hepatitis B virus, hepatitis C virus, filaria, leprosy, and HIV.

Nephrotic syndrome has been associated with malignancy, particularly in the adult population. In patients with solid tumors, such as carcinomas of the lung and gastrointestinal tract, the renal pathology often resembles membranous glomerulopathy. Immune complexes composed of tumor antigens and tumor-specific antibodies presumably mediate the renal involvement. In patients with lymphomas, particularly Hodgkin lymphoma, the renal pathology most often resembles MCNS. The proposed mechanism of the nephrotic syndrome is that the lymphoma produces a lymphokine that increases glomerular capillary wall permeability. Nephrotic syndrome may develop before or after the malignancy is detected, may resolve as the tumor regresses, and may return if the tumor recurs.

Nephrotic syndrome has also developed during therapy with numerous drugs and chemicals. The histologic picture may resemble membranous glomerulopathy (penicillamine, captopril, gold, nonsteroidal anti-inflammatory drugs, mercury compounds), MCNS (probenecid, ethosuximide, methimazole, lithium), or proliferative glomerulonephritis (procainamide, chlorpropamide, phenytoin, trimethadione, paramethadione).

Barsoum RS: Schistosomal glomerulopathies. *Kidney Int* 1993;44:1–12.

Herman ES, Klotman PE: HIV-associated nephropathy: Epidemiology, pathogenesis, and treatment. *Semin Nephrol* 2003;23:200–208.

Ronco PM: Paraneoplastic glomerulopathies: New insights into an old entity. *Kidney Int* 1999;56:355–377.

Sitprija V: Nephropathy in falciparum malaria. *Kidney Int* 1998;34:867.

527.3 • Congenital Nephrotic Syndrome

Infants who develop nephrotic syndrome within the first 3 mo of life are considered to have congenital nephrotic syndrome. The most common cause of this syndrome is Finnish-type congenital nephrotic syndrome, an autosomal recessive disorder that is most common in populations of Scandinavian descent (1:8,000 incidence). Congenital nephrotic syndrome may be caused by mutations in 1 of 2 genes, *NPHS1* and *NPHS2,* which encode the proteins nephrin and podocin, respectively. Nephrin and podocin are key components of the slit diaphragm of the glomerular epithelial cell and are thought to play an essential role in the normal function of the glomerular filtration barrier. The major pathologic features of the Finnish type of this syndrome are dilatation of the proximal tubules, mesangial hypercellularity, and glomerular sclerosis.

Infants with the Finnish type of congenital nephrotic syndrome present with massive proteinuria (detectable in utero by increased α-fetoprotein), a large placenta, and marked edema. Additional clinical features include prematurity, respiratory distress, and separation of the cranial sutures. The natural history of the disease is one of persistent edema, recurrent infections, and progressive renal failure with death by the age of 5 yr. Corticosteroids and immunosuppressive agents are of no value.

ACE inhibitors, indomethacin, and unilateral nephrectomy may diminish proteinuria and ameliorate the nephrotic state. Patients uniformly require aggressive nutritional support, and ultimately chronic dialysis and kidney transplantation. In families at risk of the Finnish type of congenital nephrotic syndrome, antenatal diagnosis is suggested by an elevated amniotic fluid α-fetoprotein level and the diagnosis may be confirmed by DNA analysis.

Other causes of congenital nephrotic syndrome include congenital infections such as syphilis, toxoplasmosis, rubella, and cytomegalovirus. HIV and hepatitis B have also been reported to cause nephrotic syndrome in the neonatal period (Table 527-4). The nephrotic state, which is generally less severe than the Finnish type of congenital nephrotic syndrome, may improve or resolve with treatment of the underlying infection.

Diffuse mesangial sclerosis is a rare glomerular disease seen in a minority of children with congenital nephrotic syndrome. The characteristic pathologic finding is progressive sclerosis of the glomerular mesangium, and the clinical picture is one of rapid loss of renal function, with end-stage renal disease developing within months to years. Diffuse mesangial sclerosis may occur as an isolated disease or as part of **Denys-Drash syndrome,** a condition also characterized by Wilms tumor and male pseudohermaphroditism, caused by a mutation in the Wilms tumor gene *(WT1)* on chromosome 11.

TABLE 527-4. Causes of Nephrotic Syndrome in Infants Younger than 1 Year
SECONDARY CAUSES
Infections
Syphilis
Cytomegalovirus
Toxoplasmosis
Rubella
Hepatitis B
HIV
Malaria
Drug reactions
Toxins
Mercury
Systemic lupus erythematosus
Syndromes with associated renal disease
Nail-patella syndrome
Lowe syndrome
Nephropathy associated with congenital brain malformation
Drash syndrome–Wilms tumor
Hemolytic uremic syndrome
PRIMARY CAUSES
Congenital nephrotic syndrome
Diffuse mesangial sclerosis
Minimal change disease
Focal segmental sclerosis
Membranous nephropathy

From Kliegman RM, Greenbaum LA, Lye PS: *Practical Strategies in Pediatric Diagnosis and Therapy,* 2nd ed. Philadelphia, Elsevier, 2004, p 418.

Holmberg C, Tryqqvason K, Kestila MK, Jalanko HJ: Congenital nephrotic syndrome. In Avner E, Harmon W, Niaudet P (editors): *Pediatric Nephrology,* 5th ed. Philadelphia, Lippincott Williams & Wilkins, 2004, pp 503–516.

Lenkkeri U, Mannikko M, McCready P, et al: Structure of the gene for congenital nephrotic syndrome of the Finnish type *(NPHS 1)* and characterization of mutations. *Am J Hum Genet* 1999;64:51–61.

Mannikko M, Kestila M, Lenkkeri U, et al: Improved prenatal diagnosis of the congenital nephrotic syndrome of the Finnish type based on DNA analysis. *Kidney Int* 1997;51:868.

McTaggart SJ, Algar E, Chow CW, et al: Clinical spectrum of Denys-Drash and Frasier syndrome. *Pediatr Nephrol* 2001;16:335–339.

Papez KE, Smoyer WE: Recent advances in congenital nephrotic syndrome. *Curr Opin Pediatr* 2004;16:165–170.

Patrakka J, Martin P, Salonen R, et al: Proteinuria and prenatal diagnosis of congenital nephrosis in fetal carriers of nephrin gene mutations. *Lancet* 2002;359:1575–1576.

Section 4 — Tubular Disorders

Chapter 528 ■ Tubular Function

Katherine MacRae Dell and
Ellis D. Avner

Water and electrolytes are freely filtered at the level of the glomerulus. Thus, the electrolyte content of "ultrafiltrate" at the beginning of the proximal tubule is similar to that of plasma. Carefully regulated processes of tubular reabsorption and/or tubular secretion determine final water content and electrolyte composition of urine. "Bulk" movement of solute tends to occur in the proximal portions of the nephron, whereas fine adjustments tend to occur distally (see also Chapter 52.).

SODIUM. Sodium is essential in maintaining extracellular fluid balance and, thus, volume status. The kidney is capable of effecting large changes in sodium excretion in a variety of normal and pathologic states. There are 4 main sites of sodium transport. Approximately 60% of sodium is absorbed in the proximal tubule by coupled transport with glucose or amino acids, 25% in the ascending loop of Henle (mediated by NKCC2, the bumetanide-sensitive sodium-potassium 2 chloride transporter), and 15% in the distal tubule (mediated by NCCT, the thiazide-sensitive sodium chloride cotransporter) and collecting tubule (mediating by EnaC, the epithelial sodium channel). The urinary excretion of sodium normally approximates the sodium intake of 2–6 mEq/kg/24 hr for a child consuming a typical American diet, minus 1–2 mEq/kg/24 hr required for normal metabolic processes. However, in states of volume depletion (dehydration, blood loss) or decreased effective circulating blood volume (septic shock, hypoalbuminemic states, heart failure), there may be a dramatic decrease in urinary sodium excretion to as low as 1 mEq/L. Changes in volume status are detected by baroreceptors in the atria, afferent arteriole, and the carotid sinus and by the macula densa, which detects changes in chloride delivery. The major hormonal mechanisms mediating sodium balance include the renin-angiotensin-aldosterone axis, atrial natriuretic factor, and norepinephrine. Angiotensin II and aldosterone increase sodium reabsorption in the proximal tubule and distal tubules, respectively. Norepinephrine, released in response to volume depletion, does not directly act on tubular transport mechanisms but affects sodium balance by decreasing renal blood flow and thus decreasing the filtered load of sodium as well as stimulating renin release. With more severe volume depletion, antidiuretic hormone is also released (see Chapter 530). Sodium excretion is promoted by atrial natriuretic factor and suppression of renin.

POTASSIUM. Extracellular potassium homeostasis is regulated because small changes in plasma potassium concentrations have dramatic effects on cardiac, neural, and neuromuscular function (see Chapter 52.4). Essentially all filtered potassium is fully reabsorbed in the proximal tubule. Therefore, urinary excretion of potassium is completely dependent on tubular secretion by potassium channels present in the principal cells of the collecting tubule. Factors that promote potassium secretion include aldosterone, increased sodium delivery to the distal nephron, and increased urine flow rate.

CALCIUM. A significant portion of filtered calcium (70%) is reabsorbed in the proximal tubule. Additional calcium is reabsorbed in the ascending loop of Henle (20%) and the distal tubule and collecting duct (5–10%). Calcium is reabsorbed by passive movement between cells (paracellular absorption) in a process driven by sodium chloride reabsorption and potassium recycling into the lumen. In addition, calcium uptake is actively regulated by calcium receptors, specific transporters, and calcium channels. Factors that promote calcium reabsorption include parathyroid hormone (released in response to hypocalcemia), calcitonin, vitamin D, thiazide diuretics, and volume depletion (see Chapter 571). Factors that promote calcium excretion include volume expansion, increased sodium intake, and diuretics such as mannitol and furosemide.

PHOSPHATE. The majority of filtered phosphate is reabsorbed in the proximal tubule by active transport. Reabsorption is increased by dietary phosphorus restriction, volume contractions, and growth hormone. Parathyroid hormone and volume expansion increase phosphate excretion.

MAGNESIUM. About 25% of filtered magnesium is reabsorbed in the proximal tubule. Modulation of renal magnesium excretion occurs primarily in the ascending loop of Henle, with some contribution of the distal convoluted tubule. Although specific magnesium transporters have been identified, the precise mechanisms by which they are regulated remain unclear.

ACIDIFICATION AND CONCENTRATING MECHANISMS. These are addressed in the sections on renal tubular acidosis and nephrogenic diabetes insipidus (see Chapters 529 and 530).

DEVELOPMENTAL CONSIDERATIONS. Tubular transport capabilities of neonates (especially premature infants) and young infants are less than those of adults. Although nephrogenesis (the formation of new glomerular/tubular units) is complete by about 36 wk of gestation, significant tubular maturation occurs during infancy. Renal tubular immaturity, reduced glomerular filtration rate, decreased concentrating gradient, and diminished responsiveness to antidiuretic hormone are characteristic of young infants. These factors can contribute to impaired regulation of water, solute and electrolyte and acid-base homeostasis, particularly during times of acute illness.

Baum M, Quigley R, Satlin L: Maturational changes in renal tubular transport. *Curr Opin Nephrol Hypertens* 2003;12:521–526.

Jones DP, Chesney RW: Tubular function: In Avner ED, Harmon WE, Niaudet P (editors): *Pediatric Nephrology,* 5th ed. Philadelphia, Lippincott Williams & Wilkins, 2004, pp 45–72.

Schrier RW (editor): *Renal and Electrolyte Disorders,* 6th ed. Philadelphia, Lippincott Williams & Wilkins, 2003.

Van't Hoff WG: Molecular developments in renal tubulopathies. *Arch Dis Child* 2000;83:189–191.

Chapter 529 ■ Renal Tubular Acidosis

Katherine MacRae Dell and
Ellis D. Avner

Renal tubular acidosis (RTA) is a disease state characterized by a normal anion gap metabolic acidosis resulting from either impaired bicarbonate reabsorption or impaired urinary acid (hydrogen ion) excretion. Both inherited and acquired primary and secondary forms exist. There are 3 main forms of RTA: proximal (type II) RTA, distal (type I) RTA, and hyperkalemic (type IV) RTA. Mixed lesions (those with elements of type I and II RTA), which occur primarily in patients with inherited carbonic anhydrase deficiency, are designated as type III RTA by some authors.

NORMAL URINARY ACIDIFICATION. Urinary acidification involves 2 processes: bicarbonate reabsorption and hydrogen ion excretion. Bicarbonate reabsorption results in reclamation of the filtered bicarbonate but does not result in net acid secretion. Approximately 85% of the filtered bicarbonate is reabsorbed in the proximal tubule. In infants, bicarbonate reabsorption is less efficient, and renal bicarbonate excretion may occur at serum concentrations <22 mmol/L. Bicarbonate itself is not directly absorbed through a specific transporter but instead is absorbed by an indirect process. Proximal tubule reabsorption of bicarbonate begins with secretion of a hydrogen ion in exchange for a sodium ion. The hydrogen ion in the tubular lumen binds with bicarbonate and, under the influence of carbonic anhydrase, is converted to carbon dioxide and water. Carbon dioxide then diffuses into the proximal tubular cell, where a series of chemical reactions result in the creation of a bicarbonate molecule (which enters the peritubular capillary) and a hydrogen ion, which can participate in further buffering of bicarbonate in the tubular lumen. The remaining 15% of bicarbonate is reabsorbed distally. Secretion of the daily acid load (approximately 1 mEq/kg/24 hr produced during normal cellular processes) is accomplished by hydrogen ion secretion (mediated by a H^+ ATPase present in the intercalated cells of the collecting tubule), ammoniagenesis, and formation of titratable acids (formed when H^+ ions are buffered by organic acids such as phosphate).

529.1 • Proximal (Type II) Renal Tubular Acidosis

PATHOGENESIS. Proximal RTA results from impaired proximal tubule bicarbonate reabsorption. Isolated forms of inherited or acquired proximal RTA occur, although they are rare. Isolated autosomal dominant forms, as well as an autosomal recessive form associated with ocular abnormalities, have been reported. Proximal RTA usually occurs as a component of global proximal tubular dysfunction or **Fanconi syndrome,** which is characterized by low molecular weight proteinuria, glycosuria, phosphaturia, aminoaciduria, and proximal RTA. Both autosomal dominant and autosomal recessive forms of primary Fanconi syndrome occur. Secondary Fanconi syndrome may occur as a component of one of several inherited renal tubular disorders or in acquired disease states. The causes of proximal RTA and Fanconi syndrome are outlined in Table 529-1. Many of these causes are inherited disorders. Two diseases, **cystinosis** and **Lowe syndrome,** are addressed further in this section. Other inherited forms of Fanconi syndrome include **galactosemia** (see Chapter 87.2), **hereditary fructose intolerance** (see Chapter 87.3), **tyrosinemia** (see Chapter 85.2), and **Wilson disease** (see Chapter 354.2). **Dent disease,** or X-linked nephrolithiasis, is discussed in Chapter 531.3. In children, an important form of secondary Fanconi syndrome is exposure to ifosfamide, a component of many treatment regimens for Wilms tumor and other solid tumors.

Cystinosis is a systemic disease caused by a defect in the metabolism of cystine, which results in accumulation of cystine crystals

TABLE 529-1. Classification of Renal Tubular Acidosis

PROXIMAL (TYPE II)
- Isolated
  - Sporadic
  - Hereditary
- Fanconi syndrome
- Primary
  - Sporadic
  - Hereditary
    - Cystinosis
    - Lowe syndrome
    - Galactosemia
    - Tyrosinemia
    - Hereditary fructose intolerance
    - Fanconi-Bickel syndrome
    - Wilson disease
    - Mitochondrial diseases
    - Dent disease (X-linked nephrolithiasis)
- Secondary
  - Heavy metals (lead, cadmium, mercury)
  - Outdated tetracycline
  - Gentamicin
  - Ifosfamide
  - Cyclosporine/tacrolimus

DISTAL (TYPE I)
- Primary
  - Sporadic
  - Hereditary
- Secondary
  - Interstitial nephritis
  - Obstructive uropathy
  - Vesicoureteral reflux
  - Pyelonephritis
  - Transplant rejection
  - Sickle cell nephropathy
  - Ehlers-Danlos syndrome
  - Lupus nephritis
  - Nephrocalcinosis
  - Medullary sponge kidney
  - Hepatic cirrhosis
- Toxins/medications
  - Amphotericin B
  - Lithium
  - Toluene
  - Cisplatin

HYPERKALEMIC (TYPE IV)
- Primary
  - Sporadic
  - Hereditary
- Secondary
  - Hypoaldosteronism
  - Addison disease
  - Congenital adrenal hyperplasia
  - Prolonged heparinization
  - Pseudo hypoaldosteronism (type I or II)
  - Obstructive uropathy
  - Pyelonephritis
  - Interstitial nephritis
  - Diabetes mellitus
  - Sickle cell nephropathy
  - Trimethoprim/sulfamethoxazole
  - Angiotensin-converting enzyme inhibitors
  - Cyclosporine

in most of the major organs of the body, notably the kidney, liver, eye, and brain. It occurs at an incidence of 1 : 100,000–1 : 200,000. In certain populations, such as French Canadians, the incidence is much higher. At least 3 clinical patterns have been described. Young children with the most severe form of the disease (*infantile* or *nephropathic cystinosis*) present in the first 2 yr of life with severe tubular dysfunction and growth failure. If the disease is not treated, the children develop end-stage renal disease by the end of their 1st decade. A milder form of the disease presents in adolescents and is characterized by less severe tubular abnormalities and a slower progression to renal failure. A benign adult form with no renal involvement also exists. Cystinosis is caused by mutations in the *CTNS* gene, which encodes a novel protein, cystinosin. Cystinosin is thought to be an H^+-driven lysosomal cystine transporter. Genotype-phenotype studies demonstrate that patients with severe nephropathic cystinosis carry mutations that lead to complete loss of cystinosin function. Patients with milder clinical disease have mutations that lead to expression of partially functional protein. Patients with nephropathic cystinosis present with **clinical manifestations** reflecting their pronounced tubular dysfunction and Fanconi syndrome, including polyuria and polydipsia, growth failure, and rickets. Fever, caused by dehydration or diminished sweat production, is common. Patients are typically fair skinned and blond because of diminished pigmentation. Photophobia occurs. With progressive tubulointerstitial fibrosis, renal insufficiency is invariant. Retinopathy and impaired visual acuity occur, as well as hypothyroidism, hepatosplenomegaly, and delayed sexual maturation.

The **diagnosis** of cystinosis is suggested by the detection of cystine crystals in the cornea and confirmed by measurement of increased leukocyte cystine content. Prenatal testing is available for at-risk families.

Treatment is directed at correcting the metabolic abnormalities associated with Fanconi syndrome or chronic renal failure. In addition, specific therapy is available with **cysteamine**, which binds to cystine and converts it to cysteine. This facilitates lysosomal transport and decreases tissue cystine. Oral cysteamine does not achieve adequate levels in ocular tissues, so additional therapy with cysteamine eyedrops is required. Early initiation of the drug may prevent or delay deterioration of renal function. Patients with growth failure that does not improve with cysteamine may benefit from treatment with growth hormone. Renal transplantation is a viable option in patients with renal failure; with prolonged survival, additional complications may become evident, including central nervous system abnormalities, muscle weakness, swallowing dysfunction, and pancreatic insufficiency. It is unclear whether long-term cysteamine therapy will decrease these complications.

Lowe syndrome *(oculocerebrorenal syndrome of Lowe)* is a rare X-linked disorder characterized by congenital cataracts, mental retardation, and Fanconi syndrome. The disease is caused by mutations in the *OCRL1* gene, which encodes the phosphatidylinositol polyphosphate 5-phosphatase protein. The abnormalities seen in Lowe syndrome are thought to be due to abnormal transport of vesicles within the Golgi apparatus. Kidneys show nonspecific tubulointerstitial changes. Thickening of glomerular basement membrane and changes in proximal tubule mitochondria are also seen.

Patients with Lowe syndrome typically present in infancy with cataracts, progressive growth failure, hypotonia, and Fanconi syndrome. Significant proteinuria is common. Blindness and renal insufficiency often develop. Characteristic behavioral abnormalities are also seen, including tantrums, stubbornness, stereotypy (repetitive behaviors), and obsessions. There is no specific therapy for the renal disease or neurologic deficits. Cataract removal is generally required.

CLINICAL MANIFESTATIONS OF PROXIMAL RTA AND FANCONI SYNDROME. Patients with isolated, sporadic, or inherited proximal RTA present with growth failure in the 1st year of life. Additional symptoms may include polyuria, dehydration (due to sodium losses), anorexia, vomiting, constipation, and hypotonia. Patients with primary Fanconi syndrome will have additional symptoms secondary to phosphate wasting such as rickets. Those with systemic diseases will present with additional signs and symptoms specific to their underlying disease. A non-anion gap metabolic acidosis will be present. Urinalysis in patients with isolated proximal RTA is generally unremarkable. The urine pH is acidic (<5.5) because distal acidification mechanisms are intact in these patients. Urinary indices in patients with Fanconi syndrome demonstrate varying degrees of phosphaturia, aminoaciduria, glycosuria, uricosuria, and elevated urinary sodium or potassium. Depending on the nature of the underlying disorder, laboratory evidence of chronic renal insufficiency, including elevated serum creatinine, may be present.

529.2 • Distal (Type I) Renal Tubular Acidosis

PATHOGENESIS. Distal RTA occurs as the result of impaired distal urinary acidification (hydrogen ion secretion). Primary or secondary causes can result in damaged or impaired functioning of one or more transporters or proteins involved in the acidification process, including the H^+/ATPase, the HCO_3^-/Cl^- anion exchangers, or the components of the aldosterone pathway. Because of impaired hydrogen ion excretion, urine pH cannot be reduced below 5.5, despite the presence of severe metabolic acidosis. Loss of sodium bicarbonate results in hyperchloremia and hypokalemia. **Hypercalciuria** is usually present and may lead to nephrocalcinosis or nephrolithiasis. Chronic metabolic acidosis also impairs urinary citrate excretion. **Hypocitraturia** further increases the risk of calcium deposition in the tubules. Bone disease is common, resulting from mobilization of organic components from bone to serve as buffers to chronic acidosis. Both primary sporadic or inherited forms occur. As with proximal RTA, distal RTA can also occur as a complication of either inherited or acquired diseases of the distal tubules.

CLINICAL MANIFESTATIONS. Patients with distal RTA share common features with those of proximal RTA, including non-anion gap metabolic acidosis and growth failure. However, distinguishing features of distal RTA include nephrocalcinosis and hypercalciuria. The phosphate and massive bicarbonate wasting characteristic of proximal RTA is generally absent.

Causes of primary and secondary distal RTA are listed in Table 529-1. Although rare, 3 specific inherited forms of distal RTA have been identified, including an autosomal recessive form associated with sensorineural deafness.

Medullary sponge kidney is a relatively rare sporadic disorder in children, although not uncommon in adults. It is characterized by cystic dilatation of the terminal portions of the collecting ducts as they enter the renal pyramids. Ultrasonographically, patients often have medullary nephrocalcinosis (Fig. 529-1). Although patients with this condition typically maintain normal renal function through adulthood, complications include nephrolithiasis, pyelonephritis, hyposthenuria (inability to concentrate urine), and distal RTA. Associations of medullary sponge kidney with Beckwith-Wiedemann syndrome or hemihypertrophy have been reported.

529.3 • Hyperkalemic (Type IV) Renal Tubular Necrosis

PATHOGENESIS. Type IV RTA occurs as the result of impaired aldosterone production (hypoaldosteronism) or impaired renal

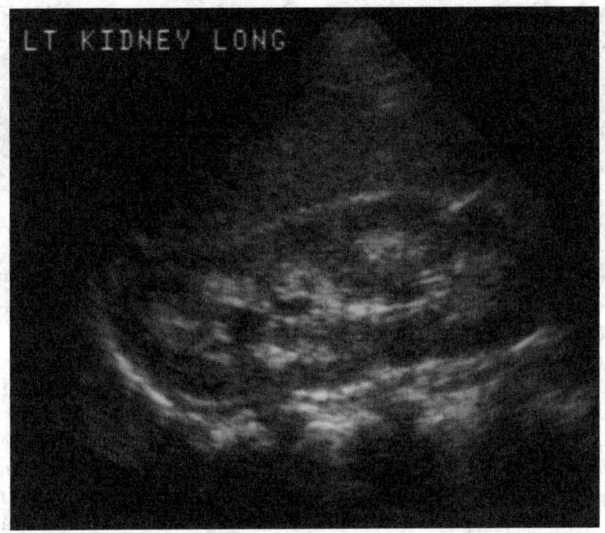

Figure 529-1. Ultrasound examination of a child with distal renal tubular acidosis demonstrating medullary nephrocalcinosis.

responsiveness to aldosterone ("pseudo" hypoaldosteronism). Because aldosterone has a direct effect on the H^+/ATPase responsible for hydrogen secretion, acidosis results. In addition, aldosterone is a potent stimulant for potassium secretion in the collecting tubule. Loss of aldosterone effect results in hyperkalemia. This further affects acid-base status by inhibiting ammoniagenesis and, thus, hydrogen ion excretion. Aldosterone deficiency typically occurs as a result of adrenal gland disorders such as Addison disease or some forms of congenital adrenal hyperplasia. In children, aldosterone unresponsiveness is a more common cause of type IV RTA. This may occur transiently, during an episode of acute pyelonephritis or acute urinary obstruction, or chronically, particularly in infants and children with a history of obstructive uropathy. The latter patients may have significant hyperkalemia, even in instances when renal function is normal or only mildly impaired. Rare examples of inherited forms of type IV RTA have been identified.

CLINICAL MANIFESTATIONS. Patients with type IV RTA, like those with type I and II RTA, may present with growth failure in the first few years of life. Polyuria and dehydration (from salt wasting) are common. Rarely, patients (especially those with pseudo hypoaldosteronism type 1) will present with life-threatening hyperkalemia. Patients with obstructive uropathies may present acutely with signs and symptoms of pyelonephritis, such as fever, vomiting, and foul-smelling urine. Laboratory tests reveal a hyperkalemic non-anion gap metabolic acidosis. Urine may be alkaline or acidic. Elevated urine sodium levels with inappropriately low urine potassium levels reflect the absence of aldosterone effect.

DIAGNOSTIC APPROACH TO RTA

The first step in the evaluation of a patient with suspected RTA is to confirm the presence of a normal anion gap metabolic acidosis, identify electrolyte abnormalities, assess renal function, and rule out other causes of bicarbonate loss such as diarrhea (see Chapter 52). Metabolic acidosis associated with diarrheal dehydration is extremely common, and acidosis will generally improve with correction of volume depletion. Patients with protracted diarrhea may deplete their total-body bicarbonate stores and may have persistent acidosis despite apparent restoration of volume status. In those instances in which a patient has a recent history of severe diarrhea, full evaluation for RTA should be delayed for several days to permit adequate time for reconstitution of total-body bicarbonate stores. If acidosis persists beyond a few days in this setting, additional studies are indicated.

Serum electrolytes, blood urea nitrogen, calcium, phosphorus, and creatinine and pH should be obtained by venous puncture. Traumatic blood draws (such as heel stick specimens) small volumes of blood in "adult-size" specimen collection tubes, or prolonged specimen transport time at room temperature can lead to falsely low bicarbonate levels, often in association with an elevated serum potassium value. True hyperkalemic acidosis is consistent with type IV RTA, whereas the finding of normal or low potassium suggests type I or II. The **blood anion gap** should be calculated using the formula $[Na^+] - [Cl^- + HCO_3^-]$. Values of <12 demonstrate the absence of an anion gap. Values of >20 are highly suggestive of the presence of an anion gap. If such an anion gap is found, then other diagnoses (lactic acidosis, inborn errors of metabolism, ingestions) should be investigated. If tachypnea is noted, an arterial blood gas analysis may be obtained to rule out the possibility of a mixed acid-base disorder primarily involving both respiratory and metabolic components. A detailed history, with particular attention to growth and development, recent or recurrent diarrheal illnesses, and any family history of mental retardation, failure to thrive, end-stage renal disease, infant deaths, or miscarriages is essential. Physical examination should determine growth parameters and volume status as well as the presence of dysmorphic features suggesting an underlying syndrome.

Once the presence of a non-anion gap metabolic acidosis is confirmed, urine pH may help distinguish distal from proximal causes. A urine pH <5.5 in the presence of acidosis suggests proximal RTA, whereas patients with distal RTA typically have a urine pH >6.0. The **urine anion gap** ([urine Na^+ + urine K^+] − urine Cl^-) is sometimes calculated to confirm the diagnosis of distal RTA. A positive gap suggests a deficiency of ammoniagenesis and, thus, the possibility of a distal RTA. A negative gap is consistent with proximal tubule bicarbonate wasting (gastrointestinal bicarbonate wasting). A urinalysis should also be obtained to determine the presence of glycosuria, proteinuria, or hematuria, suggesting the possibility of more global tubular damage or dysfunction. Random or 24-hr urine calcium and creatinine measurements will identify hypercalciuria. Renal ultrasonography should be performed to identify underlying structural abnormalities such as obstructive uropathies as well as to determine the presence of nephrocalcinosis.

TREATMENT AND PROGNOSIS OF RTA

The mainstay of therapy in all forms of RTA is bicarbonate replacement. Patients with proximal RTA often require large quantities of bicarbonate, up to 20 mEq/kg/24 hr in the form of sodium bicarbonate or sodium citrate solution (Bicitra or Stohl solution). The base requirement for distal RTAs is generally in the range of 2–4 mEq/kg/24 hr, although patient requirements may vary. Patients with Fanconi syndrome usually require phosphate supplementation. Patients with distal RTA should be monitored for the development of hypercalciuria. Those with symptomatic hypercalciuria (recurrent episodes of gross hematuria), nephrocalcinosis, or nephrolithiasis may require thiazide diuretics to decrease urine calcium excretion. Patients with type IV RTA may require chronic treatment for hyperkalemia with sodium-potassium exchange resin (Kayexalate).

Prognosis is dependent to a large part on the nature of any underlying disease, if present. Patients with treated isolated proximal or distal RTA will generally demonstrate improvement in growth, provided serum bicarbonate levels can be maintained in the normal range. Patients with systemic illness and Fanconi syndrome may have ongoing morbidity with growth failure, rickets, and signs and symptoms related to their underlying disease.

529.4 • Rickets Associated with Renal Tubular Acidosis • Russell W. Chesney

Rickets may be present in primary RTA, particularly in type II or proximal RTA. Hypophosphatemia and phosphaturia are common in these syndromes, which are also characterized by hyperchloremic metabolic acidosis, various degrees of bicarbonaturia, and, frequently, hypercalciuria and hyperkaluria. Bone demineralization without overt rickets usually is detected in type I and distal RTA. This metabolic bone disease may be characterized by bone pain, growth retardation, osteopenia, and, occasionally, pathologic fractures. Although acute metabolic acidosis in vitamin D–deficient animals may impair the conversion of 25-hydroxyvitamin D (25[OH]D) to 1,25-dihydroxyvitamin D (1,25[OH]$_2$D), resulting in reduced levels of this active metabolite, the circulating levels of 1,25(OH)$_2$D in patients with either type of RTA are normal. If patients with RTA have chronic renal insufficiency, serum 1,25(OH)$_2$D levels are often reduced.

Bone demineralization in distal RTA probably relates to dissolution of bone because the calcium carbonate in bone serves as a buffer against the metabolic acidosis due to the hydrogen ions retained by patients with RTA.

Administration of sufficient bicarbonate to reverse acidosis stops bone dissolution and the hypercalciuria that is common in distal RTA. Proximal RTA is treated with both bicarbonate and oral phosphate supplements to heal rickets. Doses of phosphate similar to those used in familial hypophosphatemia or Fanconi syndrome may be necessary. Vitamin D is indicated to offset the secondary hyperparathyroidism that complicates oral phosphate therapy. Following therapy, growth in patients with type II (proximal) RTA is greater than in patients with primary Fanconi syndrome.

Hsu SY, Tsai IJ, Tsau YK: Comparison of growth in primary Fanconi syndrome and proximal renal tubular acidosis. *Pediatr Nephrol* 2005;20:460.

Alper SL: Genetic diseases of acid-base transporters. *Annu Rev Physiol* 2002;64:899–923.

Gahl WA: Early oral cysteamine therapy for nephropathic cystinosis *Eur J Pediatr* 2003;162 (Suppl 1):S38–S41.

Chan JCM, Scheinman JI, Roth KS: Renal tubular acidosis. *Pediatr Rev* 2001;22:277–286.

Izzedine H, Launay-Vacher V, Isnard-Bagnis C, et al: Drug-induced Fanconi's syndrome. *Am J Kidney Dis* 2003;41:292–309.

Kalatzis V, Antignac C: New aspects of the pathogenesis of cystinosis. *Pediatr Nephrol* 2003:18:207–215.

Nicoletta JA, Schwartz GJ: Distal renal tubular acidosis. *Curr Opin Pediatr* 2004;16:194–198.

Rodriguez-Soriano J: New insights into the pathogenesis of renal tubular acidosis—from functional to molecular studies. *Pediatr Nephrol* 2000; 14:1121–1136.

Wappner RS: Lowe syndrome. In GeneClinics: Clinical Genetic Information Resource [database online]. Seattle, University of Washington, July 2001 (updated September 2003). Available at *http://www.geneclinics.org/*.

Wuhl E, Haffner D, Offner G, et al: Long-term treatment with growth hormone in short children with nephropathic cystinosis. *J Pediatr* 2001;138:880–887.

Chapter 530 ■ Nephrogenic Diabetes Insipidus Katherine MacRae Dell and Ellis D. Avner

Congenital nephrogenic diabetes insipidus (NDI) is a rare disorder of water metabolism characterized by an inability to concentrate urine, even in the presence of antidiuretic hormone (ADH). The most common pattern of inheritance is as an X-linked recessive disorder. Rarely, affected females are seen, presumably secondary to unfavorable X-chromosome inactivation. Rare autosomal recessive forms have also been described, with males and females affected equally. The clinical phenotype of autosomal recessive forms is similar to that of the X-linked form. Secondary (acquired), either partial or complete, forms of NDI may be seen in disorders affecting renal tubular function including obstructive uropathies, acute or chronic renal failure, renal cystic diseases, interstitial nephritis, nephrocalcinosis, or toxic nephropathy due to hypokalemia, hypercalcemia, lithium, or amphotericin B.

PATHOGENESIS. The ability to concentrate urine (and thus absorb water) requires the presence of an intact concentrating gradient in the renal medulla and the ability to modulate water permeability in the collecting tubule. The latter is mediated by ADH (also called arginine vasopressin [AVP]), which is synthesized in the hypothalamus and stored in the posterior pituitary. Under basal situations, the collecting tubule is impermeable to water. However, in response to increased serum osmolarity (as detected by osmoreceptors in the hypothalamus) and/or severe volume depletion, ADH is released into the systemic circulation. It then binds to its receptor, vasopressin V2 (AVPR2), on the basolateral membrane of the collecting tubule cell. Binding of the hormone to its receptor activates a cyclic adenosine monophosphate–dependent cascade that results in movement of preformed water channels (aquaporin 2 [AQP2]) to the luminal membrane of the collecting duct, rendering it permeable to water. Defects in the *AVPR2* gene cause the more common X-linked form of NDI. Mutations in the *AQP2* gene have been identified in patients with the rarer autosomal recessive form. Prenatal testing is available for families at risk for X-linked NDI. Patients with secondary forms of NDI may have ADH resistance owing to defective aquaporin expression (lithium intoxication). Secondary ADH resistance usually occurs as the result of loss of the hypertonic medullary gradient due to solute diuresis or tubular damage, resulting in the inability to absorb sodium or urea.

CLINICAL MANIFESTATIONS. Patients with congenital NDI typically present in the newborn period with massive polyuria, volume depletion, hypernatremia, and hyperthermia. Irritability and crying are common features. Constipation and poor weight gain are also seen. After multiple episodes of hypernatremic dehydration, patients may have developmental delay and mental retardation. Enuresis, caused by large urine volumes, is common. Because of the need to consume large volumes of water during the day, patients often have diminished appetite and poor food intake. However, even with adequate caloric supplementation, patients still exhibit growth abnormalities. Patients with congenital NDI also exhibit behavioral problems, including hyperactivity and short-term memory problems. Patients with the secondary form generally present later in life, primarily with hypernatremia and polyuria. Associated symptoms such as developmental delay and behavioral abnormalities are less common in this latter group.

DIAGNOSIS. The diagnosis is suggested in a male infant with polyuria, hypernatremia, and dilute urine. Simultaneous serum and urine osmolality measurements should be obtained. If the serum osmolality value is 290 mOsm/kg or higher with a urine osmolality value of less than 290 mOsm/kg, a formal water deprivation test is not necessary. Because the differential diagnosis includes causes of **central diabetes insipidus,** the inability to respond to ADH (and thus the presence of NDI) should then be confirmed by the administration of vasopressin (10–20 µg intranasally) followed by serial urine and serum osmolality measurements hourly for 4 hr. In patients with possible "partial" or secondary diabetes insipidus, in whom the initial serum osmolality value may be <290 mOsm/kg, a water deprivation test should be considered. Fluids should be withheld and urine and serum osmolalities measured periodically until the serum osmolality value is >290 mOsm/kg; vasopressin is then given as before. Criteria for premature termination of a water deprivation test include a decrease in body weight of more than 3%. If NDI is confirmed or suspected, additional evaluation should include a detailed history to assess possible toxic exposures, determination of renal function by serum creatinine and blood urea nitrogen levels, and renal ultrasonography to identify obstructive uropathies or cystic disease. Because of massive urine output, patients with congenital NDI may have nonobstructive hydronephrosis of varying severity.

TREATMENT AND PROGNOSIS. Treatment of NDI includes (1) maintenance of adequate fluid intake and access to free water; (2) minimizing urine output by limiting solute load with a low-osmolar, low-sodium diet; and (3) administering medications directed at decreasing urine output. For infants, human milk or a low solute formula, such as Similac PM 60/40, is preferred. Most infants with congenital NDI require gastrostomy or nasogastric feedings to ensure adequate fluid administration throughout the day and night. Sodium intake in older patients should be <0.7 mEq/kg/24 hr. **Thiazide diuretics** (2–3 mg/kg/24 hr of hydrochlorothiazide) effectively induce sodium loss and stimulate proximal tubule reabsorption of water. Potassium-sparing diuretics, in particular, amiloride (0.3 mg/kg/24 hr in 3 divided doses), are often indicated. Patients who have an inadequate response to diuretics alone may benefit from the addition of **indomethacin** (2 mg/kg/24 hr), which has an additive effect in reducing water excretion in some patients. Renal function must be monitored closely in such patients because indomethacin may cause deterioration in renal function over time. Patients with secondary NDI may not require medications but should have access to free water. Such patients should have serum electrolytes and volume status monitored closely, particularly during times of superimposed acute illnesses.

Prevention of recurrent dehydration and hypernatremia in patients with congenital NDI has significantly improved the neurodevelopmental outcome of these patients. However, behavioral issues remain a significant problem. In addition, chronic use of nonsteroidal anti-inflammatory drugs may predispose patients to renal insufficiency. Prognosis of patients with secondary NDI generally depends on the nature of the underlying disease.

Bonilla-Felix M: Development of water transport in the collecting duct. *Am J Physiol Renal Physiol* 2004;287:F1093–F1101.

Knoers NV: Nephrogenic diabetes insipidus. In GeneClinics: Clinical Genetic Information Resource [database online]. Seattle, University of Washington, February 2000 (updated January 2005). Available at *http://www.geneclinics.org/*.

Saborio P, Tipton GA, Chan JCM: Diabetes insipidus. *Pediatr Rev* 2000;21:122–129.

Chapter 531 ■ Bartter/Gitelman Syndromes and Other Inherited Tubular Transport Abnormalities

Katherine MacRae Dell and Ellis D. Avner

531.1 • Bartter Syndrome

Bartter syndrome is a rare form of hypokalemic metabolic alkalosis with hypercalciuria, with an autosomal recessive pattern of inheritance (see Chapter 52). Two distinct clinical subtypes of Bartter syndrome are seen. **Antenatal** Bartter syndrome (also called hyperprostaglandin E syndrome) typically presents in infancy and has a more severe phenotype than "classic" Bartter syndrome, including polyhydramnios, salt wasting, and severe dehydration. The milder phenotype, **classic** Bartter syndrome, presents in childhood with failure to thrive and a history of recurrent episodes of dehydration. A phenotypically related disease, Gitelman syndrome has a distinct genetic defect and is discussed in Chapter 531.2. A genetically distinct variant of antenatal Bartter syndrome associated with sensorineural deafness and chronic renal insufficiency has also been reported.

PATHOGENESIS. The biochemical features of Bartter syndrome, including hypokalemic metabolic alkalosis with hypercalciuria, resemble those seen with chronic loop diuretic use and reflect a defect in sodium, chloride, and potassium transport in the ascending loop of Henle. The loss of sodium and chloride, with resultant volume contraction, stimulates the renin/angiotensin II/aldosterone axis. Aldosterone promotes sodium uptake and potassium secretion, exacerbating the hypokalemia. It also stimulates hydrogen ion secretion distally, worsening the metabolic alkalosis. Hypokalemia stimulates prostaglandins, which further activate the renin/angiotensin II/aldosterone axis. Bartter syndrome has been associated with 3 distinct genetic defects in loop of Henle transporters. Each contributes, in some manner, to sodium and chloride transport. Mutations in the genes that encode the sodium potassium 2 chloride transporter NKCC2 (the site of action of furosemide) or the luminal potassium channel ROMK cause neonatal Bartter syndrome. Defects in the genes that produce the basolateral chloride channel ClC-Kb cause classic Bartter syndrome.

CLINICAL MANIFESTATIONS. A history of polyhydramnios may be elicited. Dysmorphic features, including triangular facies, protruding ears, large eyes with strabismus, and drooping mouth may be present on physical examination. Consanguinity suggests the presence of an autosomal recessive disorder. Older children may have a history of recurrent episodes of dehydration, failure to thrive, and the classic biochemical abnormalities of a hypokalemic metabolic alkalosis. Urinary calcium levels are typically elevated, as are urinary potassium and sodium levels. Serum renin, aldosterone, and prostaglandin E levels are often markedly elevated, particularly in the more severe antenatal form. Blood pressure is usually normal, although patients with the antenatal form may have severe salt wasting, resulting in dehydration and hypotension. Renal function is typically normal. Nephrocalcinosis, resulting from hypercalciuria, may be seen on ultrasound examination.

DIAGNOSIS. The diagnosis is usually made based on clinical presentation and laboratory findings. The diagnosis in the neonatal infant is suggested by severe hypokalemia, usually <2.5 mmol/L, with metabolic alkalosis. Hypercalciuria is typical; hypomagnesemia is seen in a minority of patients but is more common in Gitelman syndrome. Because features of Bartter syndrome resemble chronic loop diuretic use, diuretic abuse should be considered in the differential diagnosis, even in young children. Chronic vomiting may also give a similar clinical picture but can be distinguished by **measurement of urinary chloride,** which is elevated in Bartter syndrome and low in patients with chronic vomiting. Histologically, kidneys demonstrate hyperplasia of the juxtaglomerular apparatus. Renal biopsy samples are rarely performed to diagnose this condition.

TREATMENT AND PROGNOSIS. Treatment of Bartter syndrome is directed at preventing dehydration, maintaining nutritional status, and correcting hypokalemia. Potassium supplementation, often at very high doses, is required. Even with appropriate therapy, serum potassium values may not normalize, particularly in patients with the neonatal form. Infants and young children may require sodium supplementation as well. Indomethacin, a prostaglandin inhibitor, may also be effective. With close attention to electrolyte balance, volume status, and growth, the long-term prognosis is generally good. In a small minority of patients, chronic hypokalemia, nephrocalcinosis, and chronic indomethacin therapy can lead to chronic interstitial nephritis and chronic renal failure.

531.2 • Gitelman Syndrome

Gitelman syndrome (often called a Bartter syndrome variant) is also a rare autosomal recessive cause of hypokalemic metabolic alkalosis, with distinct features of **hypocalciuria** and **hypomagnesemia.** Patients with Gitelman syndrome typically present later in childhood or early adulthood.

PATHOGENESIS. The biochemical features of Gitelman syndrome resemble those of chronic thiazide diuretic use. Thiazides act on the sodium chloride co-transporter NCCT, present in the distal convoluted tubule. Through linkage analysis and mutational studies, defects in the gene encoding NCCT have been demonstrated in patients with Gitelman syndrome.

CLINICAL MANIFESTATIONS. Patients with Gitelman syndrome typically present at a later age than those with Bartter syndrome. Patients often have a history of recurrent muscle cramps and spasms, presumably caused by low serum magnesium levels. They typically do not have a history of recurrent episodes of dehydration. Biochemical abnormalities include hypokalemia, metabolic alkalosis, and hypomagnesemia. The urinary calcium level is usually very low (in contrast to the elevated urinary calcium level often seen in Bartter syndrome), and the urinary magnesium level is elevated. Renin and aldosterone levels are usually normal, and prostaglandin E secretion is not elevated. Growth failure is less prominent in Gitelman syndrome than in Bartter syndrome, but it may be present.

DIAGNOSIS. The diagnosis of Gitelman syndrome is suggested in an adolescent or adult presenting with hypokalemic metabolic alkalosis, hypomagnesemia, and hypocalciuria.

TREATMENT. Therapy is directed at correcting hypokalemia and hypomagnesemia with supplemental potassium and magnesium. Sodium supplementation or treatment with prostaglandin inhibitors is generally not necessary because patients typically do not have episodes of volume depletion or elevated prostaglandin E excretion.

531.3 • Other Inherited Tubular Transport Abnormalities

Inherited abnormalities in distinct transporters in each segment of the nephron have now been identified and the molecular defects characterized. Renal tubular acidosis and nephrogenic diabetes insipidus are discussed in detail in Chapters 529 and 530, respectively. **Cystinuria** is an autosomal recessive disorder seen primarily in patients of Middle Eastern descent and is characterized by recurrent stone formation. The disease is caused by a defective high-affinity transporter for L-cystine and dibasic amino acids present in the proximal tubule.

X-linked nephrolithiasis (Dent disease) is a disease characterized by recurrent stone formation and progression to Fanconi syndrome. Consistent with the X-linked recessive inheritance, it is seen almost exclusively in males. Dent disease is caused by mutations in the gene that encodes the voltage-gated chloride channel CLN5, present throughout the nephron. In the loop of Henle, activating and inactivating mutations in the calcium receptor gene, which mediates parathyroid hormone–induced calcium uptake, cause severe hypoparathyroidism or hyperparathyroidism, respectively.

In the collecting duct, gain of function mutations of the gene that encodes the epithelial sodium channel, causes an inherited form of hypertension, **Liddle syndrome.** Patients with this disorder have constitutive sodium uptake in the collecting duct, with hypokalemia and suppressed aldosterone. Conversely, loss of function mutations causes pseudo hypoaldosteronism, characterized by severe sodium wasting and hyperkalemia. A variant of the latter disorder is associated with systemic abnormalities, including defects in sweat chloride and may resemble cystic fibrosis.

Hebert SC: Bartter syndrome. *Curr Opin Nephrol Hypertens* 2003;12:527–532.

Jeck N, Reinalter SC, Henne T, et al: Hypokalemic salt-losing tubulopathy with chronic renal failure and sensorineural deafness. *Pediatrics* 2001;108:E5.

Kleta R, Bockenhauer D: Bartter syndrome and other salt-losing tubulopathies. *Nephron Physiol* 2006;104:73–80.

Thakker RV: Pathogenesis of Dent's disease and related syndromes of X-linked nephrolithiasis. *Kidney Int* 2000;57:787–793.

Vehaskari VM: Inherited Na transport disorders: The taming of the syndromes. *Curr Opin Pediatr* 2004;16:182–187.

Chapter 532 ■ Tubulointerstitial Nephritis

Katherine MacRae Dell and Ellis D. Avner

Tubulointerstitial nephritis (TIN, also called interstitial nephritis) is the term applied to conditions characterized by tubulointerstitial inflammation and damage with relative sparing of glomeruli and vessels. Both acute and chronic primary forms exist. Interstitial nephritis can also be present with primary glomerular diseases as well as systemic diseases affecting the kidney.

ACUTE TUBULOINTERSTITIAL NEPHRITIS

PATHOGENESIS AND PATHOLOGY. The hallmarks of acute TIN are lymphocytic infiltration of the tubulointerstitium, tubular edema, and varying degrees of tubular damage. Eosinophils may be present, especially in drug-induced TIN; occasionally, granulomas occur. The pathogenesis is not fully understood, but a T cell–mediated immune mechanism has been postulated. A large number of medications, especially antimicrobials, anticonvulsants, and analgesics, have been implicated as etiologic agents (Table 532-1). Other causes include infections, primary glomerular diseases, and systemic diseases such as systemic lupus erythematosus (SLE).

CLINICAL MANIFESTATIONS. The classic presentation of acute TIN is fever, rash, and arthralgia in the setting of a rising serum creatinine value. Although the full "triad" may be noted in drug-induced TIN, many patients with acute TIN do not have all the typical features. The rash, if present, may vary from maculopapular to urticarial and is often transient. Patients often have nonspecific constitutional symptoms of nausea, vomiting, fatigue, and weight loss. Flank pain may be present from stretching of the renal capsule from acute inflammatory kidney enlargement. If acute TIN is caused by a systemic disease such as SLE, clinical presentation will be consistent with specific signs and symptoms of the underlying disease. Unlike the typical presentation of oliguric acute renal failure seen with glomerular diseases, 30–40% of patients with acute TIN are nonoliguric. Peripheral eosinophilia may occur, especially with drug-induced TIN. Some degree of microscopic hematuria is invariably present, but significant hematuria or proteinuria is uncommon. One exception is patients with TIN caused by nonsteroidal anti-inflammatory drugs (NSAIDs) that may present with the nephrotic syndrome. Urinalysis may reveal white blood cells and granular or hyaline casts, but red blood cell casts, characteristic of glomerular disease, are rarely seen. The presence of urine eosinophils is neither sensitive nor specific.

DIAGNOSIS. The diagnosis is usually made based on clinical presentation and laboratory findings. A careful history of the timing of disease onset in relation to drug exposure is essential in suspected drug-induced TIN. Because of the immune-mediated nature of TIN, signs or symptoms generally appear 1–2 wk after exposure. In children, antimicrobials are a common inciting agent. NSAIDs are an important cause of acute TIN in children. Urinalysis and serial measurements of serum creatinine and electrolytes should be monitored. Renal ultrasonography is not diagnostic, but may demonstrate enlarged, echogenic kidneys. Removal of a suspected offending agent followed by spontaneous improvement in renal function is highly suggestive of the diagnosis, and additional testing is generally not performed. In more severe cases, in which the cause is unclear or the patient's renal function deteriorates rapidly, a renal biopsy may be indicated.

TREATMENT AND PROGNOSIS. Treatment is generally supportive and directed at addressing complications of acute renal failure such as hyperkalemia or volume overload. Several uncontrolled studies suggest that patients with significant renal impairment may benefit from a trial of corticosteroids, although other uncontrolled studies have failed to demonstrate similar outcomes. In those patients who show rapid improvement in renal function without treatment, prognosis is excellent. However, in cases with prolonged renal insufficiency, the prognosis is guarded. Severe acute TIN from any cause that does not resolve may progress to chronic TIN.

CHRONIC TUBULOINTERSTITIAL NEPHRITIS

In children, chronic TIN most commonly occurs as the result of an underlying congenital renal disease, such as obstructive uropathy or vesicoureteral reflux (see Table 532-1). Chronic TIN can occur as an idiopathic disease, although this is more common in

TABLE 532-1. Etiology of Interstitial Nephritis

ACUTE
Drugs
Antimicrobials
Penicillin derivatives
Cephalosporins
Sulfonamides
Trimethoprim-sulfamethoxazole
Ciprofloxacin
Tetracyclines
Erythromycin derivatives
Amphotericin B
Anticonvulsants
Carbamazapine
Phenobarbital
Phenytoin
Sodium valproate
Other drugs
Diuretics
Allopurinol
Cimetidine
Cyclosporine
Nonsteroidal anti-inflammatory drugs
Protease inhibitors
Proton pump inhibitors
Infections
Bacteria associated with acute pyelonephritis
Streptococcal species
Cytomegalovirus
Epstein-Barr virus
Hepatitis B virus
Histoplasmosis
Human immunodeficiency virus
Hantavirus
Adenovirus
Toxoplasma gondii
Disease-associated
Glomerulonephritis (e.g., systemic lupus erythematosus)
Acute allograft rejection
Tubulointerstitial nephritis and uveitis syndrome
Sarcoidosis
Idiopathic
CHRONIC
Drugs and Toxins
Analgesics
Cyclosporine
Lithium
Heavy metals
Infections (see Acute)
Disease-associated
Metabolic/hereditary
Cystinosis
Oxalosis
Fabry disease
Wilson disease
Sickle cell nephropathy
Alport syndrome
Juvenile nephronophthisis/medullary cystic disease
Polycystic kidney disease
Immunologic
Systemic lupus erythematosus
Chronic allograft rejection
Tubulointerstitial nephritis and uveitis syndrome
Urologic
Posterior urethral valves
Eagle-Barrett syndrome
Ureteropelvic junction obstruction
Vesicoureteral reflux
Miscellaneous
Balkan nephropathy
Chinese herb nephropathy
Radiation
Sarcoidosis
Neoplasm
Idiopathic

adults. **The juvenile nephronophthisis (JN)/medullary cystic kidney disease complex** (MCKD) is a group of inherited cystic renal diseases that share a common histologic phenotype of chronic TIN. JN is generally inherited as an autosomal recessive trait. Although rare in the United States, JN causes 10–20% of end-stage renal disease in Europe. Patients with JN typically present with polyuria, growth failure, "unexplained" anemia, and chronic renal failure in late childhood or adolescence. Variants of JN with extrarenal involvement include **Senior-Løken syndrome** (retinitis pigmentosa), **Joubert syndrome,** and **oculomotor apraxia type Cogan.** MCKD is an autosomal dominant disease that typically presents in adulthood. **Tubulointerstitial nephritis with uveitis** is a rare autoimmune syndrome of chronic TIN with anterior uveitis and bone marrow granulomas that occurs primarily in adolescent females. Chronic TIN is seen in all forms of progressive renal disease, regardless of the underlying cause, and the severity of interstitial disease is the single most important factor predicting progression to end-stage renal disease.

PATHOGENESIS AND PATHOLOGY. The pathophysiology of chronic TIN is undefined, but data suggest that it is immune mediated. Grossly, kidneys may appear pale and small for age. Microscopically, tubular atrophy and "dropout" with interstitial fibrosis and a patchy lymphocytic interstitial inflammation are seen. Patients with JN often have characteristic small cysts in the corticomedullary region. In primary chronic TIN, glomeruli are relatively spared until late in the disease course. Patients with chronic TIN secondary to a primary glomerular disease will have histologic evidence of the primary disease.

CLINICAL MANIFESTATIONS. The clinical features of chronic TIN are often nonspecific and may reflect signs and symptoms of chronic renal insufficiency (see Chapter 535). Fatigue, growth failure, polyuria, polydipsia, and enuresis are often present. Anemia is common and is a particularly prominent feature of juvenile nephronophthisis. Because tubular damage often leads to renal salt wasting, significant hypertension is unusual.

DIAGNOSIS. The diagnosis is suggested by signs or symptoms of renal tubular damage such as polyuria and an elevated serum creatinine value, coupled with a history suggestive of a chronic disease, such as long-standing enuresis or the presence of anemia resistant to iron therapy. Radiographic studies, in particular ultrasonography, may give additional evidence of chronicity, such as small, echogenic kidneys, corticomedullary cysts suggestive of JN, or findings of obstructive uropathy. A vesicocystourethrogram may demonstrate the presence of vesicoureteral reflux or bladder abnormalities. If JN is suspected, molecular diagnosis is available. In those instances in which the cause is unclear, a renal biopsy may be performed. In cases of advanced disease, a renal biopsy may not be diagnostic. Many end-stage kidney diseases display a common histologic appearance of tubular fibrosis and inflammation.

TREATMENT AND PROGNOSIS. Therapy is directed at maintaining fluid and electrolyte balance and avoiding further exposure to nephrotoxic agents. Patients with obstructive uropathies may require salt supplementation and treatment with potassium binding resin (Kayexalate). Prevention of infection by antibiotic prophylaxis is also important in slowing progression of renal damage in those patients. Prognosis in patients with chronic TIN is dependent, in large part, on the nature of the underlying disease. Patients with obstructive uropathy or vesicoureteral reflux may have a variable degree of renal damage and thus a variable course. End-stage renal disease, if it occurs, may develop over months to years. Patients with JN uniformly progress to end-stage renal disease by adolescence.

Alon U: Tubulointerstitial nephritis. In Avner ED, Harmon WE, Niaudet P (editors): *Pediatric Nephrology,* 5th ed. Philadelphia, Lippincott Williams & Wilkins, 2004, pp 817–831.

Clarkson MR, Giblin L, O'Connell FP, et al: Acute interstitial nephritis: Clinical features and response to corticosteroid therapy. *Nephrol Dial Transplant* 2004;19:2778–2883.

Harris DC: Tubulointerstitial nephritis. *Curr Opin Nephrol Hypertens* 2001;10:303–313.

Hildebrandt F, Omram H: New insights: Nephronophthisis—medullary cystic kidney disease. *Pediatr Nephrol* 2001;16:168–176.

Rossert J: Drug-induced acute interstitial nephritis. *Kidney Int* 2001; 60:804–817.

Section 5 — Toxic Nephropathies-Renal Failure

Chapter 533 ■ Toxic Nephropathy

Beth A. Vogt and Ellis D. Avner

Medications, diagnostic agents (iodinated radiographic contrast media), and chemicals may alter the kidneys directly (through reduction of renal blood flow, acute tubular necrosis, intratubular obstruction) or indirectly (through induction of an allergic or hypersensitivity reaction in the vessels or interstitium). In addition, marine animals, reptiles, and insects produce a number of biologic nephrotoxins that result in acute renal failure, often through induction of rhabdomyolysis (snake venom). Common nephrotoxic agents and their clinical manifestations are listed in Table 533-1. Nephrotoxicity is frequently reversible if the noxious agent is promptly removed.

Useful agents should not be withheld because of potential nephrotoxicity, but the following preventive measures may reduce the risks of nephrotoxicity: (1) substitution of ultrasonography, MRI, or radionuclide scans for studies using contrast media in patients with pre-existing renal disease; (2) substitution of non-nephrotoxic agents for nephrotoxic agents; (3) use of the lowest effective dose of the agent in conjunction with monitoring of the blood level; (4) appropriate reduction of all drug dosing in patients with renal insufficiency, guided by well-developed nomograms; and (5) avoidance of simultaneous use of several nephrotoxic agents. When possible, at-risk patients should be well hydrated before a procedure or drug therapy; acetylcysteine before and during a radiocontrast procedure pre-

TABLE 533-1. Renal Syndromes Produced by Nephrotoxins

NEPHROTIC SYNDROME
Angiotensin-converting enzyme inhibitors
Gold salts
Interferon
Mercury compounds
Nonsteroidal anti-inflammatory drugs
Penicillamine

NEPHROGENIC DIABETES INSIPIDUS
Amphotericin B
Colchicine
Demeclocycline
Lithium
Methoxyflurane
Propoxyphene
Vinblastine

RENAL VASCULITIS
Hydralazine
Isoniazid
Propylthiouracil
Sulfonamides
Numerous other drugs that may cause a hypersensitivity reaction

NEPHROCALCINOSIS OR NEPHROLITHIASIS
Allopurinol
Bumetanide
Ethylene glycol
Furosemide
Methoxyflurane
Topiramate
Vitamin D

ACUTE RENAL FAILURE
Acetaminophen
Acyclovir
Aminoglycosides
Amphotericin B
Angiotensin-converting enzyme inhibitors
Biologic toxins (snake, spider, bee, wasp)
Cisplatin
Cyclosporine
Ethylene glycol
Halothane
Heavy metals
Ifosfamide
Lithium
Methoxyflurane
Nonsteroidal anti-inflammatory drugs
Radiocontrast agents
Tacrolimus
Vancomycin

FANCONI SYNDROME
Aminoglycosides
Chinese herbs (aristolochic)
Cisplatin
Heavy metals (cadmium, lead, mercury, and uranium)
Ifosfamide
Lysol
Outdated tetracycline

RENAL TUBULAR ACIDOSIS
Amphotericin B
Lithium
Toluene

INTERSTITIAL NEPHRITIS
Amidopyrine
p-Aminosalicylate
Carbon tetrachloride
Cephalosporins
Cimetidine
Cisplatin
Colistin
Copper
Cyclosporine
Ethylene glycol
Foscarnet
Gentamicin
Gold salts
Indomethacin
Interferon-α
Iron
Kanamycin
Lithium
Mannitol
Mercury salts
Mitomycin C
Neomycin
Nonsteroidal anti-inflammatory drugs
Penicillins (especially methicillin)
Pentamidine
Phenacetin
Phenylbutazone
Poisonous mushrooms
Polymyxin B
Radiocontrast agents
Rifampin
Salicylate
Streptomycin
Sulfonamides
Tacrolimus
Tetrachloroethylene
Trimethoprim-sulfamethoxazole

vents deterioration of renal function if the patients are also well hydrated.

Aronoff GR, Berns JS, Brier ME, et al (editors): *Drug Prescribing in Renal Failure,* 4th ed. Philadelphia, American College of Physicians, 1999.

Chesney RW, Jones DW: Nephrotoxins. In Avner E, Harmon W, Niaudet P (editors): *Pediatric Nephrology,* 5th ed. Philadelphia, Lippincott Williams & Wilkins, 2004, pp 987–1004.

Kay J, Chow WH, Chan TM, et al: Acetylcysteine for prevention of acute deterioration of renal function following elective coronary angiography and intervention. *JAMA* 2003;289:553–558.

O'Brien KL, Selanikio JD, Hecdivert C, et al: Epidemic of pediatric deaths from acute renal failure caused by diethylene glycol poisoning. *JAMA* 1998;279:1175–1180.

Perazella MA: Crystal-induced acute renal failure. *Am J Med* 1999;106: 459–465.

Schwartz A, Perez-Canto A: Nephrotoxicity of antiinfective drugs. *Int J Clin Pharmacol Ther* 1998;35:164–167.

Sturmer T, Elseviers MM, De Broe ME: Nonsteroidal anti-inflammatory drugs and the kidney. *Curr Opin Nephrol Hypertens* 2001;10:161–163.

Timmer RH, Sands JM: Lithium intoxication. *J Am Soc Nephrol* 1999;10: 666–674.

Chapter 534 ■ Cortical Necrosis

Beth A. Vogt and Ellis D. Avner

Renal cortical necrosis represents a final common result of several types of renal injury. It usually affects both kidneys and may be patchy or involve the entire cortex.

ETIOLOGY. In newborns, cortical necrosis is most commonly associated with hypoxic/ischemic insults caused by perinatal asphyxia, placental abruption, and twin-twin or fetal-maternal transfusion. Other causes include renal vascular thrombosis and severe congenital heart disease. After the neonatal period, cortical necrosis is most commonly seen in children with septic shock or severe hemolytic-uremic syndrome as well as in adolescents with pregnancy-related acute renal failure. Less common causes of cortical necrosis include snakebites, infectious endocarditis, and therapy with antifibrinolytic drugs (tranexamic acid).

PATHOLOGY. Involved portions of the renal cortex show infarction, with congestion of the glomeruli, thrombosis of the arterioles, and necrosis of the tubules.

PATHOGENESIS. Cortical necrosis develops when endothelial cell injury occurs in conjunction with diminished renal cortical blood flow. Toxins or other mediators that presumably develop during shock, hemolytic-uremic syndrome, or sepsis may injure the endothelial cells and initiate intrarenal coagulation, leading to thrombosis and cortical necrosis.

CLINICAL MANIFESTATIONS. Cortical necrosis presents as acute renal failure developing in individuals having the previously mentioned predisposing causes. Urine output is diminished and gross and/or microscopic hematuria may be present. Hypertension is common, and thrombocytopenia may be present, as a result of renal microvascular injury.

DIAGNOSIS. Early in the course, the diagnosis is supported by ultrasonographic detection of normal-sized or enlarged, nonobstructed kidneys. Sequential ultrasound evaluations show a progressive decrease in renal size, suggestive of renal atrophy. Radionuclide renal scans show decreased or absent renal perfusion with delayed or absent function. The differential diagnosis includes other causes of acute renal failure (see Table 535-1).

TREATMENT AND PROGNOSIS. Therapy is supportive and involves volume repletion, correction of asphyxia, and treatment of sepsis. Medical management of the complications of acute renal failure and supportive dialysis may be necessary. Children with cortical necrosis may have partial or no renal recovery, and the prognosis depends on the amount of surviving renal cortex. Those children with partial recovery are at increased risk of the subsequent development of chronic kidney disease.

Agraharkar M, Fahlen M, Siddiqui M, et al: Waterhouse-Friderichsen syndrome and bilateral renal cortical necrosis in meningococcal sepsis. *Am J Kidney Dis* 2000;36:396–400.

Lerner GR, Kurnetz R, Bernstein J, et al: Renal cortical and renal medullary necrosis in the first 3 months of life. *Pediatr Nephrol* 1992;6:516–518.

Manley HJ, Bailie GR, Eisele G: Bilateral renal cortical necrosis associated with cefuroxime axetil. *Clin Nephrol* 1998;49:268–270.

Palapattu GS, Barbaris Z, Raijfer J: Acute bilateral renal cortical necrosis as a cause of postoperative renal failure. *Urology* 2001;58:281.

Chapter 535 ■ Renal Failure

Beth A. Vogt and Ellis D. Avner

535.1 • Acute Renal Failure

Acute renal failure (ARF) is a clinical syndrome in which a sudden deterioration in renal function results in the inability of the kidneys to maintain fluid and electrolyte homeostasis. ARF occurs in 2–3% of children admitted to pediatric tertiary care centers and in as many as 8% of infants in the neonatal intensive care unit.

PATHOGENESIS. ARF has been conventionally classified into 3 categories: prerenal, intrinsic renal, and postrenal (Table 535-1).

Prerenal ARF, also called prerenal azotemia, is characterized by diminished effective circulating arterial volume, which leads to inadequate renal perfusion and a decreased glomerular filtration rate (GFR). Evidence of kidney damage is absent. Common causes of prerenal ARF include dehydration, sepsis, hemorrhage, severe hypoalbuminemia, and cardiac failure. If the underlying cause of the renal hypoperfusion is reversed promptly, renal function returns to normal. If hypoperfusion is sustained, intrinsic renal parenchymal damage may develop.

Intrinsic renal ARF includes a variety of disorders characterized by renal parenchymal damage, including sustained hypoperfusion/ischemia. Many forms of **glomerulonephritis,** including postinfectious glomerulonephritis, lupus nephritis, Henoch-Schönlein purpura nephritis, membranoproliferative glomerulonephritis, and anti–glomerular basement membrane nephritis, may cause ARF.

Hemolytic-uremic syndrome (HUS) has been described as the most common cause of intrinsic ARF in the United States

TABLE 535-1. Common Causes of Acute Renal Failure
PRERENAL
Dehydration
Hemorrhage
Sepsis
Hypoalbuminemia
Cardiac failure
INTRINSIC RENAL
Glomerulonephritis
Postinfectious/poststreptococcal
Lupus erythematosus
Henoch-Schönlein purpura
Membranoproliferative
Anti–glomerular basement membrane
Hemolytic-uremic syndrome
Acute tubular necrosis
Cortical necrosis
Renal vein thrombosis
Rhabdomyolysis
Acute interstitial nephritis
Tumor infiltration
Tumor lysis syndrome
POSTRENAL
Posterior urethral valves
Ureteropelvic junction obstruction
Ureterovesicular junction obstruction
Ureterocele
Tumor
Urolithiasis
Hemorrhagic cystitis
Neurogenic bladder

(see Chapter 518). The cardinal features of HUS include ARF, microangiopathic hemolytic anemia, and thrombocytopenia. Although HUS has been linked to numerous factors, the most common cause in underdeveloped countries is *Shigella* toxin–induced endothelial cell damage. In developed countries, HUS is most commonly associated with *Escherichia coli* (OI57:H7).

Acute tubular necrosis (ATN) occurs most often in critically ill infants and children who have been exposed to nephrotoxic and/or ischemic insults. The typical pathologic process of ATN is tubular cell necrosis, although significant histologic changes are not consistently seen in patients with clinical ATN. The mechanisms of injury in ATN may include alterations in intrarenal hemodynamics, tubular obstruction, and passive backleak of the glomerular filtrate across injured tubular cells into the peritubular capillaries.

Tumor lysis syndrome is a specific form of ARF related to spontaneous or chemotherapy-induced cell lysis in patients with lymphoproliferative malignancies. This disorder is primarily caused by obstruction of the tubules by uric acid crystals (see Chapters 495 and 499).

Acute interstitial nephritis is an increasingly common cause of ARF and is usually a result of a hypersensitivity reaction to a therapeutic agent or various infectious agents (see Chapter 532).

Postrenal ARF includes a variety of disorders characterized by obstruction of the urinary tract. In neonates and infants, congenital conditions such as posterior urethral valves and bilateral ureteropelvic junction obstruction account for the majority of cases of ARF. Other conditions such as urolithiasis, tumor (intra-abdominal or within the urinary tract), hemorrhagic cystitis, and neurogenic bladder may cause ARF in older children and adolescents. In a patient with 2 functioning kidneys, obstruction must be bilateral to result in ARF. Relief of the obstruction usually results in recovery of renal function except in patients with associated renal dysplasia or prolonged urinary tract obstruction.

CLINICAL MANIFESTATIONS AND DIAGNOSIS. A carefully taken history is critical in defining the cause of ARF. An infant with a 3-day history of vomiting and diarrhea most likely has prerenal ARF caused by volume depletion. A 6 yr old child with a recent pharyngitis who presents with periorbital edema, hypertension, and gross hematuria most likely has intrinsic ARF related to acute postinfectious glomerulonephritis. A critically ill child with a history of protracted hypotension and exposure to nephrotoxic medications most likely has ATN. A neonate with a history of hydronephrosis on prenatal ultrasound and a palpable bladder and prostate most likely has congenital urinary tract obstruction, probably related to posterior urethral valves.

The physical examination must be thorough, with careful attention to volume status. Tachycardia, dry mucous membranes, and poor peripheral perfusion suggest inadequate circulating volume and the possibility of prerenal ARF (see Chapters 54 and 55). Peripheral edema, rales, and a cardiac gallop suggest volume overload and the possibility of intrinsic ARF from glomerulonephritis or ATN. The presence of a rash and arthritis may suggest systemic lupus erythematosus (SLE) or Henoch-Schönlein purpura nephritis. Palpable flank masses may suggest renal vein thrombosis, tumors, cystic disease, or urinary tract obstruction.

LABORATORY FINDINGS. Laboratory abnormalities may include anemia (the anemia is usually dilutional or hemolytic, as in SLE, renal vein thrombosis, HUS); leukopenia (SLE); thrombocytopenia (SLE, renal vein thrombosis, HUS); hyponatremia (dilutional); metabolic acidosis; elevated serum concentrations of blood urea nitrogen, creatinine, uric acid, potassium, and phosphate (diminished renal function); and hypocalcemia (hyperphosphatemia).

The serum C3 level may be depressed (postinfectious glomerulonephritis, SLE, or membranoproliferative glomerulonephritis), and antibodies may be detected in the serum to streptococcal (poststreptococcal glomerulonephritis), nuclear (SLE), neutrophil cytoplasmic (Wegener granulomatosis, microscopic polyarteritis), or glomerular basement membrane (Goodpasture disease) antigens.

The presence of hematuria, proteinuria, and red blood cell or granular urinary casts suggests intrinsic ARF, in particular glomerular disease. The presence of white blood cells and white blood cell casts, with low-grade hematuria and proteinuria, suggests tubulointerstitial disease. Urinary eosinophils may be present in children with drug-induced tubulointerstitial nephritis.

Urinary indices may be useful in differentiating prerenal ARF from intrinsic ARF (Table 535-2). Patients whose urine shows an elevated specific gravity (>1.020), elevated urine osmolality (UOsm > 500 mOsm/kg), low urine sodium (UNa < 20 mEq/L), and fractional excretion of sodium (FENa) <1% (<2.5% in neonates) most likely have prerenal ARF. Those with a specific gravity of <1.010, low urine osmolality (UOsm < 350 mOsm/kg), high urine sodium (UNa > 40 mEq/L), and FENa greater than 2% (>10% in neonates) most likely have intrinsic ARF.

$$\mathrm{FENa}\,(\%) = \frac{\mathrm{UNa} \times \mathrm{PCr}}{\mathrm{PNa} \times \mathrm{UCr}} \times 100$$

Chest radiography may reveal cardiomegaly and pulmonary congestion (fluid overload). Renal ultrasonography may reveal hydronephrosis and/or hydroureter, which are suggestive of urinary tract obstruction. Renal biopsy may ultimately be required to determine the precise cause of ARF in patients who do not have clearly defined prerenal or postrenal ARF.

In high-risk patients (trauma, surgery), early detection of acute renal failure (before an increase in blood urea nitrogen or crea-

TABLE 535-2. Urinalysis, Urine Chemistries, and Osmolality in Acute Renal Failure

	HYPOVOLEMIA	ACUTE TUBULAR NECROSIS	ACUTE INTERSTITIAL NEPHRITIS	GLOMERULONEPHRITIS	OBSTRUCTION
Sediment	Bland	Broad, brownish granular casts	White blood cells, eosinophils, cellular casts	Red blood cells, red blood cell casts	Bland or bloody
Protein	None or low	None or low	Minimal but may be increased with NSAIDs	Increased, >100 mg/dL	Low
Urine sodium, mEq/L*	<20	>30	>30	<20	<20 (acute) >40 (few days)
Urine osmolality, mOsm/kg	>400	<350	<350	>400	<350
Fractional excretion of sodium%†	<1	>1	Varies	<1	<1 (acute) >1 (few days)

*The sensitivity and specificity of urine sodium of <20 in differentiating prerenal azotemia from acute tubular necrosis are 90% and 82%, respectively.

†Fractional excretion of sodium is the urine to plasma (U/P) of sodium divided by U/P of creatinine × 100. The sensitivity and specificity of fractional excretion of sodium of <1% in differentiating prerenal azotemia from acute tubular necrosis are 96% and 95%, respectively.

NSAIDs, nonsteroidal anti-inflammatory drugs.

From Singri N, Ahya SN, Levin ML: Acute renal failure. *JAMA* 2003;289:747–751.

tinine levels) may be determined by measuring serum or urine neutrophil gelatinase–associated lipocalin, which accumulates in the kidneys after acute ischemic renal injury.

TREATMENT

MEDICAL MANAGEMENT. In infants and children with urinary tract obstruction, such as in a newborn with suspected posterior ureteral valves, a bladder catheter should be placed immediately to ensure adequate drainage of the urinary tract. The placement of a bladder catheter may also be considered in nonambulatory older children and adolescents to accurately monitor urine output during ARF.

Determination of the volume status is of critical importance when initially evaluating a patient with ARF. If there is no evidence of volume overload or cardiac failure, intravascular volume should be expanded by intravenous administration of isotonic saline, 20 mL/kg over 30 min. In the absence of blood loss or hypoproteinemia, colloid-containing solutions are not required for volume expansion. Severe hypovolemia may require additional fluid boluses (see Chapters 53 and 68). Determination of the central venous pressure may be helpful if adequacy of the blood volume is in question. After volume resuscitation, hypovolemic patients generally void within 2 hr; failure to do so points toward the presence of intrinsic or postrenal ARF.

Diuretic therapy should be considered only after the adequacy of the circulating blood volume has been established. Mannitol (0.5 g/kg) and furosemide (2–4 mg/kg) may be administered as a single IV dose. Bumetanide (0.1 mg/kg) may be given as an alternative to furosemide. If urine output is not improved, then a continuous diuretic infusion may be considered. To increase renal cortical blood flow, many clinicians administer dopamine (2–3 µg/kg/min) in conjunction with diuretic therapy, although no controlled data support this practice. There is little evidence that diuretics or dopamine can prevent ARF or hasten recovery. Mannitol may be effective in pigment (myoglobin, hemoglobin)-induced renal failure.

If there is no response to a diuretic challenge, diuretics should be discontinued and fluid restriction becomes essential. Patients with a relatively normal intravascular volume should initially be limited to 400 mL/m^2/24 hr (insensible losses) plus an amount of fluid equal to the urine output for that day. Extrarenal (blood, gastrointestinal tract) fluid losses should be replaced, milliliter for milliliter, with appropriate fluids. Markedly hypervolemic patients may require further fluid restriction, omitting the replacement of insensible fluid losses, urine output, and extrarenal losses to diminish the expanded intravascular volume. Fluid intake, urine and stool output, body weight, and serum chemistries should be monitored on a daily basis.

In ARF, rapid development of **hyperkalemia** (serum potassium level >6 mEq/L) may lead to cardiac arrhythmia, cardiac arrest, and death. The earliest electrocardiographic change seen in patients with developing hyperkalemia is the appearance of peaked T waves. This may be followed by widening of the QRS intervals, ST segment depression, ventricular arrhythmias, and cardiac arrest (see Chapter 52.4). Procedures to deplete body potassium stores should be initiated when the serum potassium value rises above 6.0 mEq/L. Exogenous sources of potassium (dietary, intravenous fluids, total parenteral nutrition) should be eliminated. Sodium polystyrene sulfonate resin (Kayexalate), 1 g/kg, should be given orally or by retention enema. This resin exchanges sodium for potassium and may take several hours to take effect. A single dose of 1 g/kg can be expected to lower the serum potassium level by about 1 mEq/L. Resin therapy may be repeated every 2 hr, the frequency being limited primarily by the risk of sodium overload.

More severe elevations in serum potassium (>7 mEq/L), especially if accompanied by electrocardiographic changes, require emergency measures in addition to Kayexalate. The following agents should be administered:

- **Calcium gluconate 10% solution, 1.0 mL/kg IV, over 3–5 min**
- **Sodium bicarbonate, 1–2 mEq/kg IV, over 5–10 min**
- **Regular insulin, 0.1 U/kg, with glucose 50% solution, 1 mL/kg, over 1 hr**

Calcium gluconate counteracts the potassium-induced increase in myocardial irritability but does not lower the serum potassium level. Administration of sodium bicarbonate and insulin and glucose lowers the serum potassium level by shifting potassium from the extracellular to the intracellular compartment. A similar effect has been reported with the acute administration of β-adrenergic agonists in adults, but there are no controlled data in pediatric patients. Because the duration of action of these emergency measures is just a few hours, persistent hyperkalemia should be managed by dialysis.

Mild **metabolic acidosis** is common in ARF because of retention of hydrogen ions, phosphate, and sulfate, but it rarely requires treatment. If acidosis is severe (arterial pH <7.15; serum bicarbonate <8 mEq/L) or contributes to hyperkalemia, treatment is required. The acidosis should be corrected partially by the intravenous route, generally giving enough bicarbonate to raise the arterial pH to 7.20 (which approximates a serum bicarbonate level of 12 mEq/L). The remainder of the correction may be accomplished by oral administration of sodium bicarbonate after normalization of the serum calcium and phosphorus levels. Correction of metabolic acidosis with intravenous bicarbonate may precipitate tetany in patients with renal failure as rapid correction of acidosis reduces the ionized calcium concentration (see also Chapter 52).

Hypocalcemia is primarily treated by lowering the serum phosphorus level. Calcium should not be given intravenously, except in cases of tetany, to avoid deposition of calcium salts into tissues. Patients should be instructed to follow a low phosphorus diet, and phosphate binders should be orally administered to bind any ingested phosphate and increase gastrointestinal phosphate excretion. Common agents include sevelamer (Renagel), calcium carbonate (Tums tablets or Titralac suspension), and calcium acetate (PhosLo). Aluminum-based binders, commonly employed in the past, should be avoided because of the clear risk of aluminum toxicity.

Hyponatremia is most commonly a dilutional disturbance that must be corrected by fluid restriction rather than sodium chloride administration. Administration of hypertonic (3%) saline should be limited to those patients with symptomatic hyponatremia (seizures, lethargy) or those with a serum sodium level <120 mEq/L. Acute correction of the serum sodium to 125 mEq/L (mmol/L) should be accomplished using the following formula:

$$\text{mEq NaCl required} = 0.6 \times \text{weight (kg)} \times [125 - \text{serum sodium (mEq/L)}]$$

ARF patients are predisposed to **gastrointestinal bleeding** because of uremic platelet dysfunction, increased stress, and heparin exposure if on hemodialysis or continuous renal replacement therapy. Oral or intravenous H_2 blockers such as ranitidine are commonly administered to prevent this complication.

Hypertension may result from hyperreninemia associated with the primary disease process and/or expansion of the extracellular fluid volume and is most common in ARF patients with acute glomerulonephritis or HUS. Salt and water restriction is critical, and diuretic administration may be useful (see Chapter 445). Isradipine (0.05–0.15 mg/kg per dose, maximum dose 5 mg qid) may be administered for relatively rapid reduction in blood pressure. Longer acting agents such as calcium channel blockers (amlodipine, 0.1–0.6 mg/kg/24 hr qd or divided bid) or β blockers (propranolol, 0.5–8 mg/kg/24 hr divided bid or tid; labetalol, 4–40 mg/kg/24 hr divided bid or tid) may be helpful in maintaining control of blood pressure. Children with severe symptomatic hypertension (hypertensive urgency/emergency) should be treated with continuous infusions of sodium nitroprusside (0.5–10 μg/kg/min), labetalol (0.25–3.0 mg/kg/hr), or esmolol (150–300 μg/kg/min) and converted to intermittently dosed antihypertensives when more stable.

Neurologic symptoms in ARF may include headache, seizures, lethargy, and confusion. Potential etiologic factors include hyponatremia, hypocalcemia, hypertension, cerebral hemorrhage, cerebral vasculitis, and the uremic state. Diazepam is the most effective agent in controlling seizures, and therapy should be directed toward the precipitating cause.

The **anemia** of ARF is generally mild (hemoglobin 9–10 g/dL) and primarily results from volume expansion (hemodilution). Children with HUS, SLE, active bleeding, or prolonged ARF may require transfusion of packed red blood cells if their hemoglobin level falls below 7 g/dL. In hypervolemic patients, blood transfusion carries the risk of further volume expansion, which may precipitate hypertension, heart failure, and pulmonary edema. Slow (4–6 hr) transfusion with packed red blood cells (10 mL/kg) diminishes the risk of hypervolemia. The use of fresh, washed red blood cells minimizes the risk of hyperkalemia. In the presence of severe hypervolemia or hyperkalemia, blood transfusions are most safely administered during dialysis/ultrafiltration.

Nutrition is of critical importance in children who develop ARF. In most cases, sodium, potassium, and phosphorus should be restricted. Protein intake should be restricted moderately while maximizing caloric intake to minimize the accumulation of nitrogenous wastes. In critically ill patients with ARF, parenteral hyperalimentation with essential amino acids should be considered.

DIALYSIS. Indications for dialysis in ARF include the following:

- **Volume overload with evidence of hypertension and/or pulmonary edema refractory to diuretic therapy**
- **Persistent hyperkalemia**
- **Severe metabolic acidosis unresponsive to medical management**
- **Neurologic symptoms (altered mental status, seizures)**
- **Blood urea nitrogen greater than 100–150 mg/dL (or lower if rapidly rising)**
- **Calcium/phosphorus imbalance, with hypocalcemic tetany**

An additional indication for dialysis is the inability to provide adequate nutritional intake because of the need for severe fluid restriction. In patients with ARF, dialysis support may be necessary for days or for up to 12 wk. Many patients with ARF require dialysis support for 1–3 wk. The advantages and disadvantages of the 3 types of dialysis are shown in Table 535-3.

Intermittent hemodialysis is useful in patients with relatively stable hemodynamic status. This highly efficient process accomplishes both fluid and electrolyte removal in 3- to 4-hr sessions using a pump-driven extracorporeal circuit and large central venous catheter. Intermittent hemodialysis may be performed 3 to 7 times per week based on the patient's fluid and electrolyte balance.

Peritoneal dialysis is most commonly employed in neonates and infants with ARF, although this modality may be used in children and adolescents of all ages. Hyperosmolar dialysate is infused into the peritoneal cavity via a surgically or percutaneously placed peritoneal dialysis catheter. The fluid is allowed to dwell for 45–60 min and is then drained from the patient by gravity (manually or with the use of a cycler machine), accomplishing both fluid and electrolyte removal. Cycles are repeated for 8–24 hr/day based on the patient's fluid and electrolyte balance. Anticoagulation is not necessary; peritoneal dialysis is contraindicated in patients with significant abdominal pathology.

Continuous renal replacement therapy (CRRT) is useful in patients with unstable hemodynamic status, concomitant sepsis, or multiorgan failure in the intensive care setting. CRRT is an extracorporeal therapy in which fluid, electrolytes, and small- and medium-sized solutes are continuously removed from the blood (24 hr/day) using a specialized pump-driven machine. Usually, a double-lumen catheter is placed into the subclavian, internal jugular, or femoral vein. The patient is then connected to the pump-driven CRRT circuit, which continuously passes the patient's blood across a highly permeable filter.

TABLE 535-3. Peritoneal Dialysis (PD) vs Intermittent Hemodialysis (IHD) vs Continual Renal Replacement Therapy (CRRT)

	PD	IHC	CRRT
BENEFITS			
Fluid removal	+	++	++
Urea and creatinine clearance	+	++	+
Potassium clearance	++	++	+
Toxin clearance	+	++	+
COMPLICATIONS			
Abdominal pain	+	–	–
Bleeding	–	+	+
Dysequilibrium	–	+	–
Electrolyte imbalance	+	+	+
Need for heparinization	–	+	+
Hyperglycemia	+	–	–
Hypotension	+	++	+
Hypothermia	–	–	+
Central line infection	–	+	+
Inguinal/abdominal hernia	+	–	–
Peritonitis	+	–	–
Protein loss	+	–	–
Respiratory compromise	+	–	–
Vessel thrombosis	–	+	+

Adapted from Rogers MC: *Textbook of Pediatric Intensive Care.* Baltimore, Williams & Wilkins, 1992.

CRRT may be performed in 3 basic fashions. In continuous venovenous hemofiltration (CVVH), a large amount of fluid moves by pressure across the filter, bringing with it by convection other molecules such as urea, creatinine, phosphorus, and uric acid. The blood volume is reconstituted by IV infusion of a replacement fluid having a desirable electrolyte composition similar to that of blood. Continuous venovenous hemofiltration dialysis (CVVH-D) uses the principle of diffusion by circulating dialysate in a countercurrent direction on the ultrafiltrate side of the membrane. No replacement fluid is used. Continuous hemodiafiltration (CVVH-DF) employs both replacement fluid and dialysate, offering the most effective solute removal of all forms of CRRT.

PROGNOSIS. The mortality rate in children with ARF is variable and depends entirely on the nature of the underlying disease process rather than on the renal failure itself. Children with ARF caused by a renal-limited condition such as postinfectious glomerulonephritis have a very low mortality rate (<1%); those with ARF related to multiorgan failure have a very high mortality rate (>90%).

The prognosis for recovery of renal function depends on the disorder that precipitated ARF. Recovery of renal function is likely after ARF resulting from prerenal causes, HUS, ATN, acute interstitial nephritis, or tumor lysis syndrome. Recovery of renal function is unusual when ARF results from most types of rapidly progressive glomerulonephritis, bilateral renal vein thrombosis, or bilateral cortical necrosis. Medical management may be necessary for a prolonged period to treat the sequelae of ARF, including chronic renal insufficiency, hypertension, renal tubular acidosis, and urinary concentrating defect.

Andreoli SP: Acute renal failure in the newborn. *Semin Perinatol* 2004;28:112–123.

Bellomo R, Chapman M, Finfer S, et al: Low-dose dopamine in patients with early renal dysfunction: A placebo-controlled randomized trial. Australian and New Zealand Intensive Care Society (ANZICS) Clinical Trials Group. *Lancet* 2000;356:2139–2143.
Bunchman TE, McBryde KD, Mottes TE, et al: Pediatric acute renal failure: Outcome by modality and disease. *Pediatr Nephrol* 2001;16:1067–1071.
Chan JCM, Williams DM, Roth KS: Kidney failure in infants and children. *Pediatr Rev* 2002;23:47–59.
Herget-Rosenthal S: One step forward in the early detection of acute renal failure. *Lancet* 2005;365:1205–1206.
Lamiere N, Van Biesen W, Vanholder R: Acute renal failure. *Lancet* 2005;365:417–430.
Lamiere N, Vanholder R, Vab Biesen W: Loop diuretics for patients with acute renal failure. *JAMA* 2002;288:2599–2600.
Manns M, Sigler MH, Teehan BP: Continuous renal replacement therapies: An update. *Am J Kidney Dis* 1998;32:185–207.
Singri N, Ahya SN, Levin ML: Acute renal failure. *JAMA* 2003;289:747–751.
Williams DM, Sreedhar SS, Mickell JJ, Chan JCM: Acute kidney failure. *Arch Pediatr Adolesc Med* 2002;156:893–900.

535.2 • Chronic Kidney Disease

Chronic kidney disease (CKD) is defined as either renal injury (proteinuria) and/or a glomerular filtration rate <60 mL/min/1.73 m^2 for >3 mo. The prevalence of CKD in the pediatric population is approximately 18 per 1 million. The prognosis for the infant, child, or adolescent with CKD has improved dramatically over the past 4 decades because of improvements in medical management (aggressive nutritional support, recombinant erythropoietin, recombinant growth hormone), dialysis techniques, and renal transplantation.

ETIOLOGY. In children, CKD may be the result of congenital, acquired, inherited, or metabolic renal disease, and the underlying cause correlates closely with the age of the patient at the time when the CKD is first detected. CKD in children younger than 5 yr is most commonly a result of congenital abnormalities such as renal hypoplasia, dysplasia, and/or obstructive uropathy. Additional causes include congenital nephrotic syndrome, prune belly syndrome, cortical necrosis, focal segmental glomerulosclerosis, polycystic kidney disease, renal vein thrombosis, and hemolytic uremic syndrome.

After 5 yr of age, acquired diseases (various forms of glomerulonephritis including lupus nephritis) and inherited disorders (familial juvenile nephronophthisis, Alport syndrome) predominate. CKD related to metabolic disorders (cystinosis, hyperoxaluria) and certain inherited disorders (polycystic kidney disease) may present throughout the childhood years.

PATHOGENESIS. In addition to progressive injury with ongoing structural/metabolic genetic diseases, renal injury may progress despite removal of the original insult.

Hyperfiltration injury may be an important final common pathway of glomerular destruction, independent of the underlying cause of renal injury. As nephrons are lost, the remaining nephrons undergo structural and functional hypertrophy characterized by an increase in glomerular blood flow. The driving force for glomerular filtration is thereby increased in the surviving nephrons. Although this compensatory hyperfiltration temporarily preserves total renal function, it may cause progressive damage to the surviving glomeruli, possibly by a direct effect of the elevated hydrostatic pressure on the integrity of the capillary wall and/or the toxic effect of increased protein traffic across the capillary wall. Over time, as the population of sclerosed nephrons increases, the surviving nephrons suffer an increased excretory burden, resulting in a vicious cycle of increasing glomerular blood flow and hyperfiltration injury.

Proteinuria itself may contribute to renal functional decline, as evidenced by studies that have shown a beneficial effect of reduction in proteinuria. Proteins that traverse the glomerular capillary wall may exert a direct toxic effect and recruit monocytes/macrophages, enhancing the process of glomerular sclerosis and tubulointerstitial fibrosis. Uncontrolled **hypertension** may exacerbate disease progression by causing arteriolar nephrosclerosis as well as by increasing the hyperfiltration injury described earlier.

Hyperphosphatemia may increase progression of disease by leading to calcium-phosphate deposition in the renal interstitium and blood vessels. Hyperlipidemia, a common condition in CKD patients, may adversely affect glomerular function through oxidant-mediated injury.

CKD may be viewed as a continuum of disease with increasing biochemical and clinical manifestations as renal function deteriorates. The pathophysiologic manifestations of CKD are outlined in Table 535-4. The terminology to describe the stages of chronic kidney disease is standardized (Table 535-5).

End-stage renal disease (ESRD) is an administrative term in the USA, defining all patients treated with dialysis or kidney trans-

TABLE 535-4. Pathophysiology of Chronic Kidney Disease

MANIFESTATION	MECHANISMS
Accumulation of nitrogenous waste products	Decrease in glomerular filtration rate
Acidosis	Decreased ammonia synthesis Impaired bicarbonate reabsorption Decreased net acid excretion
Sodium retention	Excessive renin production Oliguria
Sodium wasting	Solute diuresis Tubular damage
Urinary concentrating defect	Solute diuresis Tubular damage
Hyperkalemia	Decrease in glomerular filtration rate Metabolic acidosis Excessive potassium intake Hyporeninemic hypoaldosteronism
Renal osteodystrophy	Impaired renal production of 1,25-dihydroxycholecalciferol Hyperphosphatemia Hypocalcemia Secondary hyperparathyroidism
Growth retardation	Inadequate caloric intake Renal osteodystrophy Metabolic acidosis Anemia Growth hormone resistance
Anemia	Decreased erythropoietin production Iron deficiency Folate deficiency Vitamin B_{12} deficiency Decreased erythrocyte survival
Bleeding tendency	Defective platelet function
Infection	Defective granulocyte function Impaired cellular immune functions Indwelling dialysis catheters
Neurologic symptoms (fatigue, poor concentration, headache, drowsiness, memory loss, seizures, peripheral neuropathy)	Uremic factor(s) Aluminum toxicity Hypertension
Gastrointestinal symptoms (feeding intolerance, abdominal pain)	Gastroesophageal reflux Decreased gastrointestinal motility
Hypertension	Volume overload Excessive renin production
Hyperlipidemia	Decreased plasma lipoprotein lipase activity
Pericarditis/cardiomyopathy	Uremic factor(s) Hypertension Fluid overload
Glucose intolerance	Tissue insulin resistance

TABLE 535-5. Standardized Terminology for Stages of Chronic Kidney Disease

STAGE	DESCRIPTION	GFR (mL/min/1.73 m²)
Stage 1	Kidney damage with normal or increased GFR	>90
Stage 2	Kidney damage with mild decrease in GFR	60–89
Stage 3	Moderate decrease in GFR	30–59
Stage 4	Severe decrease in GFR	5–29
Stage 5	Kidney failure	<15 or on dialysis

GFR, glomerular filtration rate.

plantation. Patients with ESRD are a subset of the patients with Stage 5 CKD.

CLINICAL MANIFESTATIONS. The clinical presentation of CKD is quite varied and dependent on the underlying renal disease. Children and adolescents with CKD from chronic glomerulonephritis (membranoproliferative glomerulonephritis) may present with edema, hypertension, hematuria, and proteinuria. Infants and children with congenital disorders such as renal dysplasia and obstructive uropathy may present in the neonatal period with failure to thrive, polyuria dehydration, urinary tract infection, or overt renal insufficiency. Many infants with congenital kidney disease are identified with prenatal ultrasonography, allowing early diagnostic and therapeutic intervention. Children with familial juvenile nephronophthisis may have a very subtle presentation with nonspecific complaints such as headache, fatigue, lethargy, anorexia, vomiting, polydipsia, polyuria, and growth failure over a number of years.

The physical examination in patients with CKD may reveal pallor and a sallow appearance. Patients with long-standing untreated CKD may have short stature and the bony abnormalities of renal osteodystrophy (see also Chapters 529.3 and 529.4). Children with CKD due to chronic glomerulonephritis (or children with advanced renal failure from any cause) may have edema, hypertension, and other signs of extracellular fluid volume overload.

Laboratory findings include elevations in blood urea nitrogen and serum creatinine. In children, the degree of renal dysfunction may be determined by applying the following formula, which provides an estimation of the patient's GFR:

$$\text{GFR (mL/min/1.73 m}^2) = \frac{k \times \text{height (cm)}}{\text{serum creatimine (mg/dL)}}$$

where k is 0.33 for low-birthweight infants younger than 1 yr, 0.45 for term AGA infants younger than 1 yr, 0.55 for children and adolescent females, and 0.70 for adolescent males.

Laboratory findings may also reveal hyperkalemia, hyponatremia (if volume overloaded), acidosis, hypocalcemia, hyperphosphatemia, and an elevation in uric acid. Patients with heavy proteinuria may have hypoalbuminemia. A complete blood cell count usually shows a normochromic, normocytic anemia. Serum cholesterol and triglyceride levels are usually elevated. In children with CKD caused by glomerulonephritis, the urinalysis shows hematuria and proteinuria. In children with CKD from congenital lesions such as renal dysplasia, the urinalysis usually has a low specific gravity and minimal abnormalities.

TREATMENT

The treatment of CKD is aimed at (1) replacing absent/diminished renal functions, which progressively deteriorate in parallel with the progressive loss of GFR, and (2) slowing the progression of renal dysfunction. Children with CKD should be treated at a medical center capable of supplying multidisciplinary services, including medical, nursing, social service, nutritional, and psychological support.

The management of CKD requires close monitoring of a patient's clinical and laboratory status. Blood studies to be followed routinely include serum electrolytes, blood urea nitrogen, creatinine, calcium, phosphorus, albumin, alkaline phosphatase, and hemoglobin levels. Periodic measurement of intact parathyroid hormone (PTH) levels and roentgenographic studies of bone may be of value in detecting early evidence of renal osteodystrophy. Echocardiography should be performed periodically to identify left ventricular hypertrophy and cardiac dysfunction that may occur as a consequence of the complications of CKD.

FLUID AND ELECTROLYTE MANAGEMENT. Most children with CKD maintain normal sodium and water balance with the sodium intake derived from an appropriate diet. Infants and children whose CKD is a consequence of renal dysplasia may be polyuric with significant urinary sodium losses. These children may benefit from high volume, low caloric density feedings with sodium supplementation. Children with high blood pressure, edema, or heart failure may require sodium restriction and diuretic therapy. Fluid restriction is rarely necessary in children with CKD until the development of end-stage renal disease (ESRD) requires the initiation of dialysis.

In most children with CKD, potassium balance is maintained until renal function deteriorates to the level at which dialysis is initiated. Hyperkalemia may develop, however, in patients with moderate renal insufficiency who have excessive dietary potassium intake, severe acidosis, or hyporeninemic hypoaldosteronism (related to destruction of the renin-secreting juxtaglomerular apparatus). Hyperkalemia may be treated by restriction of dietary potassium intake, administration of oral alkalinizing agents, and/or treatment with Kayexalate.

ACIDOSIS. Metabolic acidosis develops in almost all children with CKD as a result of decreased net acid excretion by the failing kidneys. Either Bicitra (1 mEq sodium citrate/mL) or sodium bicarbonate tablets (650 mg equals 8 mEq of base) may be used to maintain the serum bicarbonate level >22 mEq/L.

NUTRITION. Patients with CKD usually require progressive restriction of various dietary components as their renal function declines. Dietary phosphorus, potassium, and sodium should be restricted according to the individual patient's laboratory studies and fluid balance. In infants with CKD, formulas containing a reduced amount of phosphate (Similac PM 60/40) are commonly employed.

The optimal caloric intake in patients with CKD is unknown, but it is recommended to provide at least the recommended dietary allowance of caloric intake for age. Protein intake should be 2.5 g/kg/24 hr and should consist of proteins of high biologic value that are metabolized primarily to usable amino acids rather than to nitrogenous wastes. The proteins of highest biologic value are those of eggs and milk, followed by meat, fish, and fowl.

Dietary intake should be adjusted according to response, optimally through consultation with a dietitian with expertise in childhood CKD. Caloric intake may be enhanced in infants by supplementing the formula with modular components of carbohydrates (Polycose), fat [medium chain triglycerides (MCT) oil], and protein (pro-Mod) as tolerated by the patient. In older children and adolescents, commercial enteral products (Boost) may be helpful. If oral caloric intake remains inadequate and/or weight gain and growth velocity suboptimal, enteral tube feedings should be considered. Supplemental feedings may be provided via a nasogastric, gastrostomy, or gastrojejunal tube. Continuous overnight infusions with or without daytime bolus administrations are commonly employed.

Children with CKD may become deficient in water-soluble vitamins either because of inadequate dietary intake or dialysis losses. These should be routinely supplied, using preparations such as Nephrocaps (Fleming, Fenton, MO). Zinc and iron supplements should be added only if deficiencies are confirmed. Supplementation with fat-soluble vitamins A, E, and K is usually not required.

GROWTH. Short stature is a significant long-term sequela of childhood CKD. Children with CKD have an apparent growth hormone (GH)-resistant state with elevated GH levels but decreased insulin-like growth factor 1 levels and major abnormalities of insulin-like growth factor–binding proteins.

Children with CKD who remain less than −2 SD for height despite optimal medical support (adequate caloric intake and effective treatment of renal osteodystrophy, anemia, and metabolic acidosis) may benefit from treatment with pharmacologic doses of recombinant human GH (rHuGH). Treatment may be initiated with rHuGH (0.05 mg/kg/24 hr) subcutaneously, with periodic adjustment in the dose to achieve a goal of normal height velocity for age.

Treatment with rHuGH continues until the patient (1) reaches the 50th percentile for midparental height, (2) achieves a final adult height, or (3) undergoes renal transplantation. Long-term rHuGH treatment significantly improves final adult height and induces persistent catch-up growth; some patients achieve normal adult height.

RENAL OSTEODYSTROPHY. The term renal osteodystrophy is used to indicate a spectrum of bone disorders seen in patients with CKD. The most common condition seen in children is high-turnover bone disease caused by secondary hyperparathyroidism. The skeletal pathologic finding in this condition is osteitis fibrosa cystica.

The **pathophysiology** of renal osteodystrophy is complex. Early in the course of CKD, when the GFR declines to approximately 50% of normal, the decrease in functional renal mass leads to a decline in renal 1α-hydroxylase activity, with decreased production of activated vitamin D (1,25-dihydroxycholecalciferol). This deficiency in activated vitamin D results in decreased intestinal calcium absorption, hypocalcemia, and increased parathyroid gland activity. Excessive parathyroid hormone (PTH) secretion attempts to correct the hypocalcemia by effecting an increase in bone resorption. Later in the course of CKD, when the GFR declines to 20–25% of normal, compensatory mechanisms to enhance phosphate excretion become inadequate, resulting in hyperphosphatemia, which further promotes hypocalcemia and increased PTH secretion.

Clinical manifestations of renal osteodystrophy include muscle weakness, bone pain, and fractures with minor trauma. In growing children, rachitic changes, varus and valgus deformities of the long bones, and slipped capital femoral epiphyses may be seen. Laboratory studies may demonstrate a decreased serum calcium level, increased serum phosphorus level, increased alkaline phosphatase, and a normal PTH level. Radiographs of the hands, wrists, and knees show subperiosteal resorption of bone with widening of the metaphyses.

The goals of **treatment** are to prevent bony deformity and normalize growth velocity using both dietary and pharmacologic interventions. Children and adolescents should follow a low phosphorus diet, and infants should be provided with a low-phosphorus formula such as Similac PM 60/40. Because it is impossible to fully restrict phosphorus intake, phosphate binders are used to enhance fecal phosphate excretion. Although calcium carbonate (Tums) and calcium acetate (PhosLo) have historically been the most commonly used phosphate binders, newer, non–calcium-based binders such as sevelamer (Renagel) are increasing in use, particularly in patients prone to hypercalcemia. Because aluminum may be absorbed from the gastrointestinal tract and can lead to aluminum toxicity, aluminum-based binders should be avoided.

The cornerstone of therapy for renal osteodystrophy is vitamin D administration. **Vitamin D therapy** is indicated in patients with (1) 25-hydroxy-vitamin D levels below the established goal range for his or her particular stage of CKD or (2) PTH levels above the established goal range for CKD stage. Patients with low 25-hydroxy-vitamin D levels should be treated with ergocalciferol. Patients with a normal 25-hydroxy-vitamin D level but elevated PTH level should be treated with 0.01–0.05 µg/kg/24 hr of calcitriol (Rocaltrol, 0.25-µg capsules or 1 µg/mL suspension). Newer activated vitamin D analogues such as paracalcitol and doxecalciferol are increasingly used, especially in patients predisposed to hypercalcemia. Phosphate binders and vitamin D should be adjusted to maintain the PTH level within the designated goal range and the serum calcium and phosphorus levels within the normal range for age. Many nephrologists also attempt to maintain the calcium/phosphorus product ($Ca \times PO_4$) at <55 to minimize the possibility of tissue deposition of calcium phosphorus salts.

ADYNAMIC BONE DISEASE. Adynamic bone disease (low-turnover bone disease) has been recognized in both children and adults with CKD. The pathologic finding is osteomalacia and is associated with oversuppression of PTH, perhaps related to the widespread use of calcium-containing phosphate binders and vitamin D analogues.

ANEMIA. Anemia in patients with CKD is primarily the result of inadequate erythropoietin production by the failing kidneys and usually becomes manifest in patients with stages 3–4 CKD.

Other possible contributory factors include iron deficiency, folic acid or vitamin B_{12} deficiency, and decreased erythrocyte survival. Recombinant human erythropoietin (rHuEPO) therapy has decreased the need for transfusion in patients with CKD. Erythropoietin is usually initiated when the patient's hemoglobin concentration falls below 10 g/dL, at a dose of 50–150 mg/kg/dose subcutaneously 1–3 times weekly. The dose is adjusted to maintain the hemoglobin concentration between 12 and 13 g/dL. All patients receiving rHuEPO therapy should be provided with either oral or intravenous iron supplementation. Patients who appear to be resistant to rHuEPO should be evaluated for iron deficiency, occult blood loss, chronic infection/inflammatory state, vitamin B_{12} or folate deficiency, and bone marrow fibrosis related to secondary hyperparathyroidism. The merits of erythropoietin therapy are summarized in Table 535-6. An alternative option is darbopoeitin alfa (Aranesp), a

TABLE 535-6. Merits of Recombinant Human Erythropoietin or Darbopoietin Therapy

BENEFITS
Avoidance/minimization of blood transfusions
Reduced sensitization to histocompatibility antigens
Reduced exposure to infectious diseases
Less chance of chronic iron overload
Improved appetite
Enhanced exercise tolerance
Improved sleep
Improved well-being
POTENTIAL COMPLICATIONS
Iron deficiency
Hypertension
Seizures
Clotting of vascular access
Pure red cell aplasia (reported in adults due to recombinant human erythropoietin antibodies)

longer-acting agent administered at a dose of 0.45 μg/kg/wk. The chief advantage to this agent is that it may be dosed once weekly to once monthly because of its extended duration of action.

HYPERTENSION. Children with CKD may have sustained hypertension related to volume overload and/or excessive renin production related to glomerular disease. Hypertensive children with suspected volume overload should follow a salt-restricted diet (2–3 g/24 hr) and may benefit from diuretic therapy. Thiazide diuretics (hydrochlorothiazide 2 mg/kg/24 hr divided bid) are the initial diuretic class of choice for children with mild renal dysfunction (CKD stages 1–3). However, when a patient's estimated GFR falls into stage 4 CKD, thiazides are less effective and loop diuretics (furosemide 1–2 mg/kg/dose bid or tid) become the diuretic class of choice. **Angiotensin-converting enzyme (ACE) inhibitors** (enalapril, lisinopril) and angiotensin II blockers (losartan) are the antihypertensive medications of choice in all children with proteinuric renal disease because of their potential ability to slow the progression to ESRD. Extreme care must be taken when using these agents, however, to monitor renal function and electrolyte balance, particularly in those children with advanced CKD. Calcium channel blockers (amlodipine), β blockers (propranolol, atenolol), and centrally acting agents (clonidine) may be useful as adjunctive agents in children with CKD whose blood pressure cannot be controlled using dietary sodium restriction, diuretics, and ACE inhibitors.

IMMUNIZATIONS. Children with CKD should receive all standard immunizations according to the schedule used for healthy children. An exception must be made in withholding live vaccines from children with CKD related to glomerulonephritis during treatment with immunosuppressive medications. It is critical, however, to make every attempt to administer live virus vaccines [MMR (mumps, measles, rubella), varicella] before renal transplantation because these vaccines are not advised for use in immunosuppressed patients. All children with CKD should receive a yearly influenza vaccine. Data suggest that children with CKD may respond suboptimally to immunizations.

ADJUSTMENT IN DRUG DOSE. Because many drugs are excreted by the kidneys, their dosing may need to be adjusted in patients with CKD to maximize effectiveness and minimize the risk of toxicity (see Chapter 716). Strategies in dose adjustment include lengthening of the interval between doses, decreasing the absolute dose, or both.

PROGRESSION OF DISEASE. Although there are no definitive treatments to improve renal function in children or adults with CKD, there are several strategies that may be effective in slowing the rate of progression of renal dysfunction. Optimal control of hypertension (maintaining the blood pressure at lower than the 75th percentile and perhaps even lower) is critical in all patients with CKD. ACE inhibitors or angiotensin II receptor blockers should be the antihypertensive drugs of choice in hypertensive children with chronic proteinuric renal disease. Such agents should also be strongly considered in children with CKD who have significant proteinuria, even in the absence of hypertension. Serum phosphorus should be maintained within the normal range for age and the calcium-phosphorus product <55 to minimize renal calcium-phosphorus deposition. Prompt treatment of infectious complications and episodes of dehydration may minimize additional loss of renal parenchyma.

Other potentially beneficial recommendations include correction of anemia with erythropoietin or darbopoietin alfa therapy, control of hyperlipidemia, avoidance of cigarette smoking, prevention of obesity, and minimization of use of nonsteroidal anti-inflammatory medications. Although dietary protein restriction has been shown to be useful in adults, this recommendation is generally not suggested for children with CKD because of the concern of adverse effects on growth and development.

535.3 • End-Stage Renal Disease

ESRD represents the state in which a patient's renal dysfunction has progressed to the point at which homeostasis and survival can no longer be sustained with native kidney function and maximal medical management. At this point, renal replacement therapy (dialysis or renal transplantation) becomes necessary. The ultimate goal for children with ESRD is successful kidney transplantation (see Chapter 536) because it provides the most normal lifestyle and possibility for rehabilitation for the child and family.

Seventy-five percent of U.S. children with ESRD require a period of dialysis before transplantation can be performed. It is recommended that plans for renal replacement therapy be initiated when a child reaches stage 4 CKD. The optimal time to actually initiate dialysis, however, is based on a combination of the biochemical and clinical characteristics of the patient including refractory fluid overload, electrolyte imbalance, acidosis, growth failure, or uremic symptoms, including fatigue, nausea, and impaired school performance. In general, most nephrologists attempt to initiate dialysis early enough to prevent the development of severe fluid and electrolyte abnormalities, malnutrition, and uremic symptoms. Pre-emptive transplantation before initiation of dialysis is increasingly being used.

The selection of dialysis modality must be individualized to fit the needs of each child. In the United States, two thirds of children with ESRD are treated with peritoneal dialysis, whereas one third are treated with hemodialysis. Age is a defining factor in dialysis modality selection: 88% of infants and children from birth to 5 yr of age are treated with peritoneal dialysis, whereas 54% of children older than 12 yr of age are treated with hemodialysis.

Peritoneal dialysis is a technique that employs the patient's peritoneal membrane as a dialyzer. Excess body water is removed by an osmotic gradient created by the high dextrose concentration in the dialysate; wastes are removed by diffusion from the peritoneal capillaries into the dialysate. Access to the peritoneal cavity is achieved by a surgically inserted, tunneled Tenckhoff catheter.

Peritoneal dialysis may be provided either as continuous ambulatory peritoneal dialysis or as any of several forms of automated therapies using a cycler (continuous cyclic peritoneal dialysis, intermittent peritoneal dialysis, or nocturnal intermittent peritoneal dialysis). The majority of U.S. children treated with peritoneal dialysis use cycler-driven therapy, which allows the child and family to be free of dialysis demands during the waking hours. The exchanges are performed automatically during sleep by machine. This permits an uninterrupted day of activities, a reduction in the number of dialysis catheter connections and disconnections (which should decrease the risk of peritonitis), and a reduction in the time required by patients and parents to perform dialysis, reducing the risk of fatigue and burnout. Because peritoneal dialysis is not as efficient as hemodialysis, it must be performed daily rather than 3 times weekly as in hemodialysis. The merits of peritoneal dialysis are outlined in Table 535-7.

Hemodialysis, unlike peritoneal dialysis, is usually performed in a hospital setting. Children and adolescents typically have three 3- to 4-hr sessions per week during which fluid and solute wastes are removed. Access to the child's circulation is achieved by a surgically created arteriovenous fistula, graft, or indwelling subclavian or internal jugular catheter.

TABLE 535-7. Merits of Peritoneal Dialysis in Pediatric Patients with End-Stage Renal Disease

ADVANTAGES
Ability to perform dialysis treatment at home
Technically easier than hemodialysis, especially in infants
Ability to live a greater distance from medical center
Freedom to attend school and after-school activities
Less restrictive diet
Less expensive than hemodialysis
Independence (adolescents)
DISADVANTAGES
Catheter malfunction
Catheter-related infections (peritonitis, exit site)
Impaired appetite (due to full peritoneal cavity)
Negative body image
Caregiver burnout

Brouhard BH, Donaldson LA, Lawry KW, et al: Cognitive functioning in children on dialysis and post-transplantation. *Pediatr Transplant* 2000;4:261–267.

Coulthard MG, Crosier J: Outcome of reaching end stage renal failure in children under 2 years of age. *Arch Dis Child* 2002;87:511–517.

El Nahas AM, Bello AK: Chronic kidney disease: The global challenge. *Lancet* 2005;365:331–340.

Neu AM, Fivush BA: Immunizations for pediatric dialysis patients. *Adv Ren Replace Ther* 2000;7:239–246.

Goodman WG, Goldin J, Kuizon BD, et al: Coronary artery calcification in young adults with end-stage renal disease who are undergoing dialysis. *N Engl J Med* 2000;342:1478–1483.

Haffner D, Schaefer F, Nissel R, et al: Effect of growth hormone treatment on the adult height of children with chronic renal failure. *N Engl J Med* 2000;343:923–930.

Hebert LA, Wilmer WA, Falkenhain ME, et al: Renoprotection: One or many therapies? *Kidney Int* 2001;59:1211–1226.

Hogg RJ, Furth S, Lemley KV, et al: National Kidney Foundation's Kidney Disease Outcomes Quality Initiative clinical practice guidelines for chronic kidney disease in children and adolescents: Evaluation, classification, and stratification. *Pediatrics* 2003;111:1416–1421.

Hingorani S, Watkins SL: Dialysis for end-stage renal disease. *Curr Opin Pediatr* 2000;12:140–145.

Lewis EJ, Hunsicker LG, Clarke WR, et al: Renoprotective effect of the angiotensin-receptor antagonist irbesartan in patients with nephropathy due to type 2 diabetes. *N Engl J Med* 2001;345:851–860.

Martin KJ, Olgaard K, Coburn JW, et al: Diagnosis, assessment, and treatment of bone turnover abnormalities in renal osteodystrophy. *Am J Kidney Dis* 2004;43:558–565.

McDonald SP, Craig JC: Long-term survival of children with end-stage renal disease. *N Engl J Med* 2004;350:2654–2662.

Parekh RS, Carroll CE, Wolfe RA, et al: Cardiovascular mortality in children and young adults with end-stage kidney disease. *J Pediatr* 2002; 141:197–207.

Parekh RS, Flynn JT, Smoyer WE, et al: Improved growth in young children with severe chronic renal insufficiency who use specified nutritional therapy. *J Am Soc Nephrol* 2001;12:2418–2426.

Sanchez CP: Prevention and treatment of renal osteodystrophy in children with chronic renal insufficiency and end-stage renal disease. *Semin Nephrol* 2001;21:441–450.

Seikaly MG, Ho PL, Emmett L, et al: Chronic renal insufficiency in children: The 2001 Annual Report of the NAPRTCS. *Pediatr Nephrol* 2003; 18:796–804.

Warady BA, Alexander SR, Watkins S, et al: Optimal care of the pediatric end-stage renal disease patient on dialysis. *Am J Kidney Dis* 1999; 33:567–583.

Warady BA, Belden B, Kohaut E: Neurodevelopmental outcome of children initiating peritoneal dialysis in early infancy. *Pediatr Nephrol* 1999; 13:759–765.

Chapter 536 ■ Renal Transplantation

Rodrigo E. Urizar

Optimal treatment for children with end-stage renal disease (ESRD) is early renal transplantation (RT) from a living related donor (LRD-RT). Technical advantages, supportive strategies, and particularly the use of efficacious immunosuppressive substances also allows highly successful living nonrelated and cadaveric (CAD)-RT in children.

EPIDEMIOLOGY. The U.S. Renal Data System documents 20 new ESRD cases per million children yearly, peaking at about age 11–15 yr. Before 1 yr of age, the incidence is 0.2 patient/million per year. The North American Pediatric Renal Transplant Cooperative Study (NAPRTCS) reported the registration and sequential follow-up, through January 2003, of over 80% of American and Canadian children with chronic renal insufficiency, dialysis, transplantation, and post-transplant events. Of 13,341 registered children, 7,651 (57.3%) received their first (index) transplant; 1,713 of 8,399 primary transplantations were done preemptively (without previous dialysis; 24%). Of the remaining, 3,646 had chronic renal insufficiency (27.3%), whereas 1,519 (11.5%) of the 13,341 are on dialysis awaiting transplantation. Fifty-one percent of allografts came from a living donor, fewer recipients are younger than 6 yr old, and fewer donors are younger than 10 yr old.

A well-functioning graft (LRD or CAD) may fully rehabilitate a patient. The expectant graft recipient and relatives must realize that RT is not a permanent cure for ESRD. Furthermore, a poorly functioning transplanted kidney (uncontrollable progressive rejection) is associated with serious morbidity, mortality, and prospective return to long-term dialysis. The transiency of renal grafts has committed transplantation programs to many engraftments per patient, a goal seriously hampered by the limited availability of CAD kidneys. The latter may reflect reticence of the general public, nurses, and physicians toward organ donation. Because of the large disproportion among the yearly increments in the need for RT (22%), and the number of transplantations performed in the same period (8%), it is estimated that 100,000 kidneys will be required to be distributed among 180,000 dialysis patients in the United States alone. With the present state of organ procurement, the gap between kidney availability and transplantation will widen progressively, unless living related and cadaveric donation is increased; more kidneys are obtained from donors younger than 15 yr old who are brain dead; and other measures such as xenotransplantation (between different species, now sporadically used in fields other than RT, as a temporary measure) become more acceptable. Criteria for RT are noted in Table 536-1.

TABLE 536-1. Criteria for Performing Living Related Donor or Cadaveric Renal Transplantation in Pediatric Patients

Renal failure, chronic or end-stage renal disease of any etiology
Age, weight dependent to accommodate adult kidney
Good nutritional condition
Absence of
Active infection
Severe mental retardation
Obstructed urinary tract (ileal loops, colonic diversions and bladder augmentation procedures are helpful in many instances)
Gastrointestinal, liver, pancreas, or cardiovascular disease
Serious psychosocial or behavioral problems, and noncompliance with medication and dietary regimen
Sensitization in recipient
Massive obesity

From Mauer SM, Nevins TE, Ascher N: Renal transplantation in children. In Edelman CM Jr (editor): *Pediatric Kidney Disease.* Boston, Little, Brown, 1992, pp 941–981.

TABLE 536-2. Distribution of the Most Frequent Conditions Leading to End-Stage Renal Disease in Children

	N	%
GROUP 1		
Congenital, metabolic, genetic		
Obstructive uropathy (PUV)		
Aplasia/dysplasia/hypoplasia	4,113 (all combined)	53.9 (all combined)
Reflux nephropathy		
Genetic and metabolic diseases (cystinosis, oxalosis, PCKD, nail-patella, Alport syndrome, medullary cystic, nephronophthisis complex)		
GROUP 2		
Glomerulonephritides (all acute and chronic immunologically mediated processes)	1,015	13.3
GROUP 3		
FSGS	873	11.4
GROUP 4		
Infrequent conditions		
Wilms tumor	43	0.6
Other immunologic processes	30	0.4
HUS	206	2.7
IDDM nephropathy	8	0.1
Pyelo/interstitial nephropathy	146	1.9
Renal infarct	119	1.6
Membranous nephropathy	36	0.5
GROUP 5		
Other	596	7.8
Unknown	466	6.1
Total	7,651	100

FSGS, focal segmental glomerular sclerosis; HUS, hemolytic-uremic syndrome; IDDM = insulin-dependent diabetes mellitus; PCKD, polycystic kidney disease (infantile and adult types); PUV, posterior urethral valves.
Post-infections, IgA nephritides (Henoch-Schönlein purpura and Berger nephritis), systemic lupus nephritis; all types of membranoproliferative nephritis (types I–II and III), Goodpasture syndrome and variants (no lung involvement), vasculitides (polyarteritis nodosa, Wegener).
Modified from North American Pediatric Renal Transplant Cooperative Study, 2003 Annual Report; section 1:1–5.

Causes of ESRD vary with the patient's age and include very young to older children in decreasing frequency: congenital renal diseases (53%), glomerulonephritides (20%), focal segmental glomerulosclerosis (12%), metabolic diseases (10%), and miscellaneous (5%) (Table 536-2). Although the glomerulopathies constitute a significant proportion of this population (particularly in 13–17 yr olds), congenital and obstructive processes predominate in the very young (<5 yr) (see Chapter 535.2).

TREATMENT. Children weighing <15–20 kg should have a transperitoneal graft via a midline incision; in those weighing >20 kg, the kidney is placed retroperitoneally in the right iliac fossa. Renal vessels are anastomosed to the recipient iliac vessels, and the ureter is reimplanted in the bladder (ureteroneocystostomy). The extraperitoneal kidney facilitates access for future percutaneous biopsies. The donor and recipient's clinical laboratory evaluations before RT are summarized in Table 536-3. Very young age of the recipient may be an obstacle to RT. For both LRD and CAD recipients, younger than 24 mo of age is associated with decreased graft survival; similar results have been documented in children transplanted with small kidneys, from very young donors.

Although in general, LRD-RT fares better than CAD-RT, marked improvement in the latter has been observed overtime (Table 536-4). However, approximately 80% of LRD-RTs are functioning by 5 yr, while CAD-RTs do so in 65.9%.

Approximately 50% of graft failure is due to rejection, which is acute in 14% of cases; 33% is chronic. Recurrence of the original disease has remained stable at about 6.3% (Table 536-5). Thrombosis-related renal graft failure occurs in approximately 11% of cases, more frequently in CAD-RT, independent of the recipient's age. In very young recipients, thrombotic episodes are

TABLE 536-3. Clinical and Laboratory Evaluation of Prospective Living Related Kidney Donor and Recipient

RECIPIENT

Complete history and physical examination—updated immunizations, including pneumococcal and hepatitis B
Transplantation orientation session: patient (if old enough), parents, prospective donors, transplantation surgeon or representative, nephrologist or representative, social worker
Laboratory data
- Blood group (ABO)
- Tissue typing (HLA-A, -B, -C, -D/DR), MLC
- Hepatitis, cytomegalovirus, varicella, Epstein-Barr virus panel
- CBC, complement (C3, C4), ANA, quantitative Ig
- Serum creatinine, electrolytes, cholesterol, liver function tests, coagulation profile, blood sugar
- Urinalysis, urine and throat cultures
- Chest radiograph (two-position), bone age films (if not previously available)
- Neurologic consult and EEG and CT scan of brain (for infants)
- Dental evaluation
- Cultures: exit site of all catheters and peritoneal fluid in patients undergoing CAPD
- Complete urologic evaluation for those with obstructive or congenital urinary tract problems
- 24-hr protein excretion

DONOR

Complete history and physical examination
Chest radiographs
Electrocardiogram
Renal ultrasonography (IVP if necessary)
Laboratory
- CBC, ESR, ABO blood groups, HLA and MLC testing
- Coagulation profile
- Serum creatinine and electrolytes, liver function tests, blood sugar
- Urinalysis, urine culture, 24-hr urine protein and creatinine excretion
- Hepatitis, cytomegalovirus, herpes, Epstein-Barr virus antibody titers
- Renal angiogram

CAPD, continuous ambulatory peritoneal dialysis; CBC, complete blood cell count; EEG, electroencephalogram; ESR, erythrocyte sedimentation rate; HLA, human leukocyte antigen; IVP, intravenous pyelogram.
From Mauer SM, Nevins TE, Ascher N: Renal transplantation in children. In Edelman CM Jr (editor): *Pediatric Kidney Disease.* Boston, Little, Brown, 1992, pp 941–981.

TABLE 536-4. One-Year Renal Graft Survival by Donor Source and Annual Cohort Groups

YEARS	LIVING DONOR (%)	CADAVERIC (%)
1987–1990	89.3	75.2
1991–1994	91.8	85.0
1995–1998	93.9	90.3
1999–2002	95.6	91.8

Modified from North American Pediatric Renal Transplant Cooperative Study, 2003 Annual Report; Graft Function, 5-3.

TABLE 536-5. Rate of Recurrence of Glomerulopathies in Allografts and Graft Loss

GLOMERULOPATHY	% RECURRENCE	% GRAFT DAMAGE/LOSS
FSGS (with NS)	20–40	25
IgA	50	5–10
HSP	30–80	10
MN	20	5–10
MPGN I	25	5–10
MPGN II	90	20
HUS	10–50	10–50
WG	5–20	5–20
AGBM	<10 (rare in children)	<1 (uncertain)
SLEGN	5–10	<5
HYPEROX	High	High losses
Cystinosis	Graft handles cystine load	Loss to rejection
IGN (de novo MPGN)	Uncertain	Uncertain

AGBM, anti-glomerular basement membrane nephritis; FSGS, focal segmental glomerulosclerosis; HSP, Henoch-Schönlein purpura; HUS, hemolytic-uremic syndrome; HYPEROX, hyperoxalosis/oxaluria; IgA, immunoglobulin A nephritis; IGN, idiopathic glomerulonephritis; MN, membranous nephropathy; MPGN I and II, membranoproliferative glomerulonephritis type I and type II; SLEGN, systemic lupus erythematosus glomerulonephritis; WG, Wegener granulomatosis.
Modified from Denton MC, Singh AK: Recurrent and de novo glomerulonephritis in the renal allograft. *Semin Nephrol* 2000; 20: 164–75; and Mauer SM, Nevins TE, Ascher N: Renal transplantation in children. In Edelman CM Jr (editor): *Pediatric Kidney Disease.* Boston, Little Brown, 1992, pp 941–981.

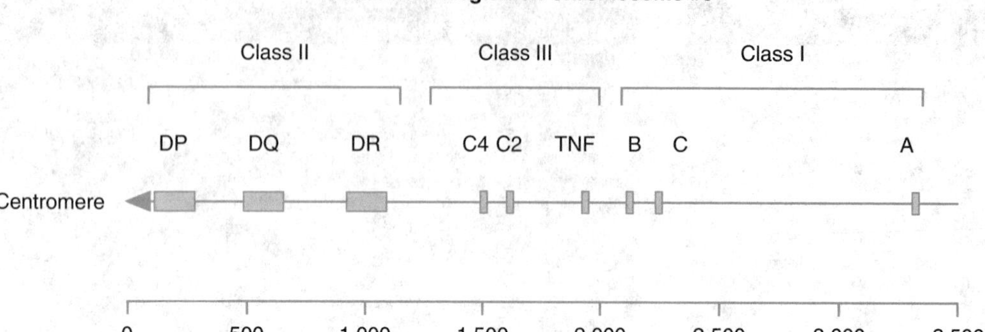

Figure 536-1. Organization of human leukocyte antigen (HLA) region of chromosome 6. The loci for HLA-A, -B, and -C are found in the class I region. The loci encoding HLA-DR, -DQ, and -DP are found in the class II region, centrometric to class I. In between classes I and II are the so-called class III genes, which encode some of the complement proteins as well as some cytokines. (From Grimm PC, Laufer J, Ettenger RB: The immunobiology of renal transplantation. In Edelman CM Jr (editor): *Pediatric Kidney Disease.* Boston, Little, Brown, 1992.)

related to volume and fluid imbalances created by the demands of usually large grafts. In older children, acute graft failure is frequently caused by acute tubular necrosis (ATN). The risks for graft loss include recipient age younger than 2 yr, cadaveric donor younger than 6 yr old, previous RT, delayed graft function (ATN), and lack of antilymphocyte gamma globulin (ATGAM) or OKT3 therapy.

HISTOCOMPATIBILITY. The major histocompatibility complex (MHC) genes, present on the short arm of chromosome 6, encode the human leukocyte antigens (HLA) (Fig. 536-1). These are composed of class I proteins (tissue transplantation antigens) and cell-mediated immunotoxicity; class II proteins that control induction of immune response; and class III proteins, which include tumor necrosis factor (TNF) and complement components (C2 and C4). Each chromosome 6 contains all 3 classes of proteins: HLA-A, -B, and -C for class I; HLA-DP, -DQ, and -DR for class II; and C2, C4, and TNF for class III. Multiple and codominant alleles (polymorphism) exist for each protein, while the A, B, DR, are considered the most important in clinical transplantation. Haplotypes, the chromosome 6 area where HLA genes are located, are inherited as a group, so that an individual will receive a haplotype from each parent concurrently, thus determining the offspring's HLA profile. The parent donor and child recipient share 50% of the haplotypes; thus, he or she will have one representative antigen from class I, II, and III loci of each parent, whereas among siblings, all, some, or no haplotypes may be shared (2 haplotypes, 1 haplotype, or 0 haplotype match). A child is a 1 haplotype match to each parent and inheritance of haplotypes follows codominant mendelian pattern (Fig. 536-2). In the genetically related donor/recipient pair, the probability of a good HLA match increases and graft loss due to rejection reaction (RR), decreases.

REJECTION REACTION. In the acute and chronic RR, both cellular and humoral mechanisms damage the graft. Preformed or T cell–induced antibodies mediate accelerated (hyperacute) RR, a condition seldom seen nowadays (Fig. 536-3).

RR is manifested by graft tenderness and swelling, fever, oliguria, hypertension, and progressive elevation of serum creatinine level. Renal ultrasonography may reveal an enlarged graft with cortical hyperechogenicity, and a renal scan demonstrates decreased blood flow. Graft biopsy material shows signs of rejection with relatively intact glomeruli, mild ultrastructural pathology, and negative glomerular immunofluorescence. Differentiation among RR, ATN, cyclosporine, or other drug toxicity and recurrence of the original renal disease in the graft require a kidney biopsy. Because pre-transplantation, crossmatching detects the presence of pre-existing anti-HLA antibodies, hyperacute RR very rarely occurs. In this condition,

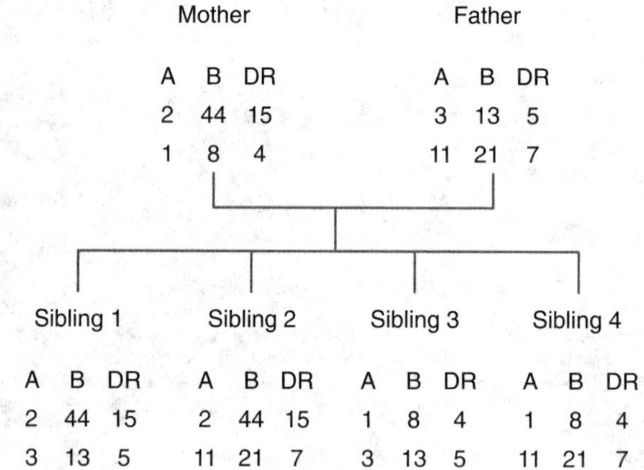

Figure 536-2. Inheritance of haplotypes and HLA profile in four theoretical siblings. Sibling 1 is a 1 haplotype match to siblings 2 and 3 and a 0 haplotype match to sibling 4. (From Terasaki PI, Park MA, Danovitch GM: Histocompatibility testing, crossmatching and allocation of cadaveric kidney transplants. In Danovitch GM (editor): *Handbook of Kidney Transplantation.* Boston, Little, Brown, 1992.)

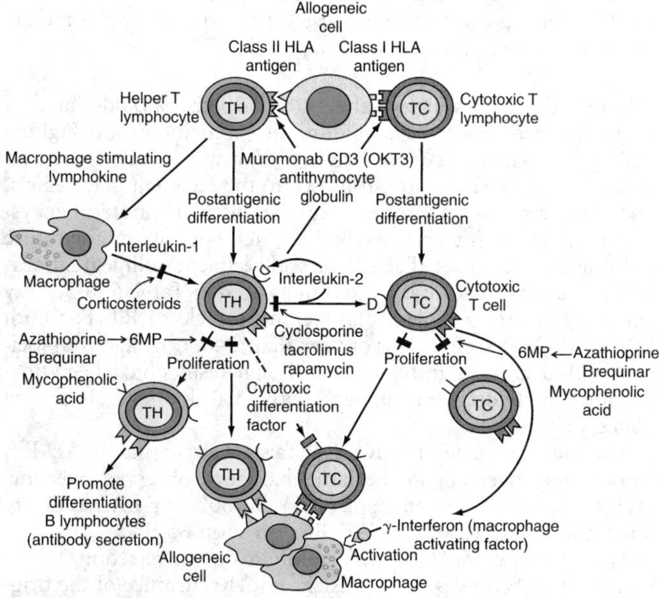

Figure 536-3. A representation of allograft rejection and the proposed sites of action for immunosuppressive medications. (From Shaefer MA, Collier DS: Immunosuppression for solid organ transplantation. *Dial Transplant* 1993; 22:542.)

anti-HLA antibodies bind to endothelium, leading to intravascular clotting causing glomerular and peritubular capillary necrosis. Conversely, chronic RR thickens and obstructs graft arterioles, which display parietal immunoglobulin deposits while glomeruli undergo hyalinization. Concurrently, the interstitium fills with activated mononuclear cells, some of which can be detected in the urine.

Histocompatibility testing is of paramount importance in prolonging the survival of LRD and CAD-RT. Having HLA-A, -B, -C, and -D/DR identical with a nonstimulatory MHC sibling donor produces the best graft survival results. The second best is the sibling or parent donor who has 1 haplotype match.

PRINCIPLES OF IMMUNOSUPPRESSION AND THERAPY OF REJECTION REACTION. Immune system stimulation by foreign protein (renal graft) results in activation of cell-mediated and humoral-mediated immune inflammation with cell destruction or RR (see Fig. 536-3) (see also Chapter 135). To subdue or control this process, immunosuppressive medications are required to avoid graft loss. The current clinically used immunosuppressives and those undergoing clinical trials are listed in Table 536-6 and Figure 536-3. Sequential immunosuppression with azathioprine, cyclosporine, and low-dose corticosteroids was the most frequently used antirejection protocol. However, new corticosteroid and calcineurin inhibitor–sparing protocols have been designed to avoid growth failure and other prednisone effects, and nephrotoxicity from cyclosporin A (hypertension, renal damage, serum creatinine elevation). Acute RR occurred in 52.5% of all 8,398 NAPRTCS-registered patients; no acute RR was documented in 4,004 (47.8%) RT cases. Acute RR is reversible in over 60% of cases, whereas only 30% can be reversed when 4 or more crises have occurred. Conversely, chronic RR is unrelenting and unresponsive to therapy; because immunosuppressive therapy renders patients more susceptible to infection, these children are at high risk of graft loss, death, or both.

TABLE 536-7. Post-transplantation Complications in Pediatric Patients

Acute tubular necrosis
Rejection reaction
Technical: vascular, urologic
Recurrence of original renal disease
Drug toxicity (immunosuppressives, antibiotics)
Infection (particularly viral, systemic); wound or urinary tract infection
Bleeding
Pancreatitis
Lymphocele
Urinoma
Bowel obstruction

From Mauer SM, Nevins TE, Ascher N: Renal transplantation in children. In Edelman CM Jr (editor): *Pediatric Kidney Disease*. Boston, Little, Brown, 1992, pp 941–981.

COMPLICATIONS (TABLE 536-7). Infection is the most common cause of death during the first year after RT. Epstein-Barr virus (EBV) and cytomegalovirus (CMV) infections are particularly frequent; antibody titers to both are routinely screened in the donor and recipient. CMV may be primary, transmitted by the graft

TABLE 536-6. Most Frequently Used Immunosuppressive Substances Used in Pediatric Renal Transplantation

MEDICATION	MECHANISM(S) OF ACTION	DOSAGE	TOXICITY
GLUCOCORTICOIDS			
(prednisone and derivatives)	Anti-inflammatory; block immune reaction: TNF-α and IL-2/IL-6 depletion; also depletes T cells (arrests cell reproductive cycle): decreases cellular immunity	1–2 mg/kg/24 hr (or 60 mg/m²/24 hr) PO or IV may be as high as 30 mg/kg when given as IV emergency bolus	Electrolyte imbalance, growth stunting, IDDM arterial hypertension, cataracts, pancreatitis
SMALL MOLECULE DRUGS			
Cyclosporin A* and derivatives ISA (TX) 247	Immunophilin/cyclophilin binding; inhibit calcineurin phosphatase	4–6 mg/kg/24 hr	Hirsutism, hypertension, arteriolitis, RTID, CNS damage, acute renal failure
TK506 (tacrolimus or Prograf)	Immunophilin/cyclophilin binding; inhibit calcineurin phosphatase (macrolide antibiotic)	0.15–0.2 mg/kg/24 hr	Renal failure
Mycofenolate mofetil* (Cellcept)	Blocks purine synthesis; stops activation of T and B cells; alters cell membrane glycosylation	1–3 g/24 hr (or 600 mg/m²; max 2 g/24 hr)	Acute renal failure post-transplantation IDDM; HTN; gastritis, diarrhea, PTLD
Azathioprine (Imuran)	Antimetabolite, blocks protein synthesis (6-thioguanine incorporated into DNA as fraudulent base)	2–3 mg/kg/24 hr orally, alone; combined: 1–2 mg/kg/24 hr	Bone marrow suppression, liver damage, PTLD
Target of rapamycin inhibitors: sirolimus* (Rapamune) and everolimus	Block cytokine—driven cell proliferation and maturation	7.5 mg/m²/5 days; 5 mg/m² when combined (Rapamune)	Thrombocytopenia, hyperlipidemia
PROTEIN DRUGS			
Deplete antibodies against B and T cells or both: equine and rabbit Ig (Atgam)	Bind opsonizing cell-surface receptors, inhibiting complement-mediated lysis and phagocytosis	Atgam: 1.5 mg/kg/24 hr, central IV only with filter, over 4–6 hr; thymoglobulin: peripheral or central IV over 6 hr, 1.5 mg/kg; both 14–21 days	Profound peripheral T-lymphocyte count (<150–<50/mm³), chills, fever, arthralgias, thrombocytopenia, general leukopenia, CMVI, PTLD, and other tumors
Mouse monoclonal anti-CD3 antibody (muromonab CD3, or orthoclone OKT3)	Bind opsonizing cell-surface receptors, inhibiting complement-mediated lysis and phagocytosis	IV only; <30 kg 2.5 mg/24 hr; >30 kg, 5 mg; bolused daily 10–14 days (to decrease CD3 cell count to <25/mm³)	Profound peripheral T-lymphocyte count (<150–<50/mm³), chills, fever, arthralgias, thrombocytopenia, general leukopenia, CMVI, PTLD, and other tumors
Do not deplete antibodies and fusion proteins: humanized/chimeric monoclonal anti-CD25 Antibodies: daclizumab (Zenapax), basiliximab (Simulect)	Monoclonal antibody to IL-2 receptor prevents cell activation; no cytokine release syndrome; no neutralizing antibodies	Dose 1: 1 mg/kg IV peripherally/centrally, over 15 min 24 hr before transplantation; same 4 remaining doses at 14-day intervals (Zenapax); <35 kg, 2 doses of 10 mg each, 1st dose 2 hr before transplantation; 2nd dose 4 days after; >35 kg, 2 doses of 20 mg each, as above (Simulect)	Abdominal pain, diarrhea, lower extremities, edema, tremor, dizziness, IDDM, poor wound healing, rash, puruitis, hirsutism, blurred vision, hyperkalemia, dyspnea, hypertension, arrythmias, arthralgias, neuropathies, paresthesias, proteinuria

*Require through blood level measurements to adjust dose. Many other immunosuppressive medications are available; however, these are not commonly used in pediatrics yet or presently are undergoing experimental trials: FK778, mizoribine, leflunomide, FTY720, alemtuzumab, and rituximab (monoclonal antibodies to CD52 and CD20 cells, respectively) and fusion proteins with natural binding properties: CTLA-4-Ig (LEA29).

CMV, cytomegalovirus; CNS, central nervous system; HTN, hypertensive nephropathy; IDDM, insulin–dependent diabetes mellitus; IL, interleukin; PTLD, post-transplantation lymphoproliferative disorder; RTID, renal tubular-interstitial disease; TNF, tumor necrosis factor.

TABLE 536-8. Types of Cytomegalovirus in the Pediatric Renal Transplant Recipient

TYPE OF INFECTION	TYPE OF PATIENT	SYMPTOMATIC	PREVENTION
Primary	Seronegative with seropositive kidney, transfusion of leukocytes, blood products transfusion	60%	Avoidance of CMV infection or use active immunization (live attenuated vaccine: Towne strain; not very effective)
Reactivation	Seropositive before transplantation	<20%	High titer human hyperimmune anti-CMV globulin (CytoGam)
Superinfection	Seropositive patient transplanted with CMV + kidney	40%	Human IgG concentrates (CMV nonspecific Gammagard or Polygam)

CMV, cytomegalovirus.
From Snydman DR: Prevention of cytomegalovirus-associated diseases with immunoglobulin. *Transplant Proc* 1991; 23:131.

TABLE 536-9. Consequences of EBV Growth and High-Risk Factors for the Development of PTLD in Immunosuppressed Patients

CLINICAL SYNDROMES
Mononucleosis
Meningoencephalitis
Hairy, oral leukoplakia
Smooth muscle cell tumors
T-cell lymphomas
Post-transplantation lymphoproliferative disorder (PTLD, uncontrolled proliferation of EBV-infected and transformed B cells, in a polyclonal, oligoclonal, and monoclonal fashion)
Non-Hodgkin lymphoma

HIGH RISK FOR PTLD
High EBV load
Primary EBV infection
High-dose immunosuppression (cyclosporin A, tacrolimus, antilymphocyte antibodies and steroid pulses alone or combinations)
Cardiac treatment is most commonly affected.

EBV, Epstein-Barr virus.

or by blood transfusions, or reactivated within 1–3 mo by the immunosuppressives in a seropositive patient (Table 536-8). Eighty-five to 90% of cases may be asymptomatic and self-limited but 5–10% lead to death; CMV results in direct tissue damage and may trigger RR and graft loss. Lower doses of immunosuppressives, IV treatment with ganciclovir, and infusions of anti-CMV immunoglobulin may control the infection. In addition, continued use of ganciclovir for 3–5 mo is done routinely post-engraftment in most transplantation centers. Protocol percutaneous graft biopsies are used in many centers, along with clinical data to diagnose infections and early RR. Immunosuppressives must be discontinued in CMV with systemic, multiorgan involvement (lung, liver, brain in addition to kidney), and the kidney lost if the RR is unresponsive. Other viral infections, the polyoma BK virus (BKV), varicella-zoster, herpes simplex, and hepatitis are associated with transplant nephropathy. In children, acquisition of BKV is most likely a primary infection as opposed to reactivation of virus latent in renal tubules. This primary BKV infection of children may manifest minor fever, myalgias, and gastroenteritis prior to allograft dysfunction. BKV may also present with florid acute RR or with interstitial nephritis–like and obstructive uropathy–like syndromes with graft losses fluctuating from 45 to 80%. Treatment of BKV infection follows the same principles as those of EBV and CMV, reduction or discontinuation of immunosuppressives, steroids may be continued, and antiviral therapy (ganciclovir, cidofovir, leflunomide, IV immunoglobulin).

Pneumocystis carinii infection is less common with the use of trimethoprim-sulfamethoxazole preventively. In 2003, the NAPRTCS reported documented deaths of 463 patients out of a total of 7,651 LRD-RTs and CAD-RTs (6.1%). Of these deaths, 141 (30.5%) were due to infection; viral disease was responsible for about 30%. The 5-yr post-transplantation patient survival for LRD-RT it is 95.9, while for CAD-RT it is 95.5.

MALIGNANCIES. Although immunosuppression remains an unavoidable requisite for transplantation, it may result in increased EBV replication leading to aggressive and potentially lethal post-transplantation lymphoproliferative disorder (PTLD) in 1–2% of RTs. In 2003, the NAPRTCS reported 203 malignancies out of 7,898 RTs (2.6%, with grafts functioning 30 days or more). Of the 203 malignancies, 150 were PTLD (73%), with a median time from transplantation to malignancy (with confirmed diagnosis) of 14 mo (range 1–20 mo). PTLD, a rare pre- and fully malignant condition, still is a major cause of serious morbidity and mortality in children after the 1st year post-transplantation. This disorder should be diagnosed as early as

TABLE 536-10. FSGS: Clinical Characteristics and Effects on the Allograft

EFFECTS ON NATIVE KIDNEY	EFFECTS ON ALLOGRAFT	FORMS OF THERAPY
Severe progressive FSGS and hypercellularity; clinically, nephrotic syndrome, chronic renal failure with progression to ESRD in 60% of cases	Histologic recurrence of FSGS in graft 20–40%; recurrent nephrotic syndrome, renal failure, ESRD in 25%.	Avoid living related donor and high cyclosporin A dose; to treat, use plasmapheresis exchange and immunoadsorption, cyclophosphamide, and OKT3; pretransplantation bilateral nephrectomy should not be done; forms of treatment seem purely palliative
Dialysis and transplantation needed	Favor recurrence: <6 yr, rapidly progressive renal failure, glomerular hypercellularity, previous recurrence, closely matched living related donor, familial distribution of FSGS, presence of assayable high levels of permeability factor in recipient's blood	

ESRD, end-stage renal disease; FSGS, focal segmental glomerulosclerosis.

possible in the febrile transplant recipient with lymphadenopathy, gastrointestinal manifestations (abdominal mass, bleeding, pain, obstruction, perforation, ascites), seizures or other central nervous system abnormalities, and asymptomatic chest and/or mediastinal masses. Definitive diagnosis of PTLD, an EBV-CMV driven condition, should be sought by tissue sampling and other laboratory means. The clinical consequences of EBV growth and the high risks for the development of PTLD in the immunosuppressed patient are listed in Table 536-9. PTLD patients at less than 1 yr post-transplantation exhibit a more benign prognosis and may regress by simple reduction of the immunosuppressive medication. The use of full antitumor treatment (cyclophosphamide, doxorubicin, vincristine, and prednisone), in more severe cases, has shown no nephrotoxicity and no evidence of RR in a significant number of patients, while they were maintained on low or no specific immunosuppressive therapy.

RENAL TRANSPLANTATION IN THE HIV-INFECTED PATIENT. With the development of effective antiretroviral therapy, prognosis of the HIV-infected child has improved enough to consider RT in these cases on an individual basis. The conditions for performing an RT or retransplantation in HIV-infected patients require that the candidate is free of opportunistic infections for 2 yr and is on a stable and well-tolerated anti-HIV/*Pneumocystis* regimen. Good compliance, undetectable viral load (by polymerase chain reaction), acceptable CD4 lymphocyte count, and no complicating illnesses are mandatory.

RECURRENCE OF GLOMERULAR DISEASE IN THE GRAFT. Potentially all glomerulopathies can redevelop in the transplant, with 5–10% of all grafts lost through this mechanism. Of these, membranoproliferative glomerulopathy type II and focal segmental glomerulosclerosis are some of the most frequent and most difficult to treat (Tables 536-5 and 536-10).

The postinfectious hemolytic-uremic syndrome (HUS) does not recur; however, the genetically nondiarrhea transmitted varieties may develop de novo in 1–3% of cases. Additionally, HUS may happen in association with calcineurin inhibitor treatment (cyclosporine and others), although more frequently in bone marrow engraftment than in RTs. Important predictors for the development of noninfection-related HUS occurrence in the renal graft include familial disease (autosomal dominant or recessive), transplantation done before 6 mo to 1 yr after primary disease remitted completely, and use of high doses of cyclosporine. In familial cases of LRD-RT, treatment with oral contraceptives and the use of ATGAM and OKT3 are questionable and perhaps should not be recommended in the genetic forms of HUS. Combined hepatic transplantation and RT may be a more appropriate approach to patients with familial HUS (see Chapter 518).

GROWTH AND RENAL TRANSPLANTATION. Stunted linear growth and overt malnutrition occur frequently in ESRD patients despite dialysis (see Chapter 535). Supportive care (dialysis and the appropriate medications) improves stamina and induces a sense of well-being. A successful RT corrects these abnormalities and rehabilitates patients.

In most children younger than 5 yr of age awaiting their index RT or on those with more than 1 RT, growth retardation reaches −2.8 and −3.2 SD, respectively. RT growth acceleration lasting 6–12 mo is observed in younger children; in adolescents, treatment with growth hormone (*rh*GH) induces prepubertal growth roughly equal to that of normal untreated children. Final height of *rh*GH-treated children is significantly increased.

Daily use of corticosteroids is usually the norm in RT treatment protocols. Daily prednisone therapy retards growth even at relatively small doses; it is therefore necessary to minimize this highly frequent untoward effect of prednisone in children. Alternate-day prednisone treatment may maximize growth potential. Complete steroid avoidance attempts to significantly decrease or withdraw steroids but may increase the risk of RR. Judicious use of *rh*GH before and after RT along with alternate-day or no steroid therapy, with the use of immunosuppressives (daclizumab, tacrolimus, mycophenolate), may offer a distinct advantage to children requiring RT.

Abouna GM: The use of marginal-suboptimal donor organs: A practical solution for organ shortage. *Adv Transpl* 2004;9:62–66.

Acott PD, Pernica JM: Growth hormone therapy before and after pediatric renal transplant. *Pediatr Transplant* 2003;7:426–440.

Ahsan N: Induction immunotherapy with I L-2Ra monoclonal antibody in kidney transplantation. *Min Urol Nefrol* 2003;55:67–79.

Benfield MR: Current status of kidney transplant: Update 2003. *Pediatr Clin North Am* 2003;50:1301–1334.

Bennett WM, Vella JP: Transplantation. In Glassock RJ (editor): Nephrology Self Assessment Program (Neph sap) 2005;4:1–63.

Charpenter B: Tacrolimus in renal transplantation: A review of recent data. *Min Urol Nefrol* 2003;55:25–32.

Dharnidharka V, Sullivan EK, Stablein DM, et al: Risk factors for post-transplant lymphoproliferative disorder (PTLD) in pediatric kidney transplantation: A report of the North American Pediatric Transplant Cooperative Study (NAPRTCS). *Transplantation* 2001;71:1065–1068.

Doyle AM, Lechler RI, Turka LA: Organ transplantation: Halfway through the first century. *J Am Soc Nephrol* 2004;15:2965–2971.

El Sayegh S, Keller MJ, Shrish H, et al: Solid organ transplantation in HIV-infected recipients. *Pediatr Transplant* 2004;8:214–221.

Fine RN, Alonso EM, Fischel JE, et al: Pediatric transplantation of the kidney, liver, and heart: Summary report. *Pediatr Transplant* 2004;8:75–86.

Halloran PF: Immunosuppressive drugs for kidney transplantation. *N Engl J Med* 2004;351:2715–2729.

Kaplan B, Herwic-Ulf MK: Renal transplantation: A half century of success and the long road ahead. *J Am Soc Nephrol* 2004;15:3270–3271.

Quist E, Jalanko H, Holmberg C: Psychosocial adaptation after solid organ transplantation in children. *Pediatr Clin North Am* 2003;50:1505–1519.

Ramos EL, Drachenberg CB: BK virus: Life cycle and interactions with host cells. *Transplant Immunol Lett* 2004;20:4–13.

Samsonov D, Briscoe DM: Long-term care of pediatric renal transplant patients: From bench to beside. *Curr Opin Pediatr* 2002;14:205–210.

Sarwal MM, Yorgin PD, Alexander S, et al: Promising early outcomes with a novel complete steroid avoidance immunosuppression protocol in pediatric renal transplantation. *Transplantation* 2001;72:13–21.

Seikali MG: Recurrence of primary disease on children after renal transplantation: An evidence based update. *Pediatr Transplant* 2004;8:113–119.

Swiatecka-Urban A: Anti-interleukin-2 receptor antibodies for prevention of rejection in pediatric renal transplant patients. Current status. *Pediatr Drugs* 2003;5:699–716.

Tsuzuki K: Role of mizoribine in renal transplantation. *Pediatr Int* 2002; 44:224–231.

United States Renal Data System: *Atlas of End Stage Renal Disease in the United States. 16th Annual Report 2004. Pediatric ESRD.* Bethesda, MD, National Institutes of Health-National Institute of Diabetes & Digestive & Kidney Diseases—Division of Kidney, Urologic & Hematologic Diseases, 2004, pp 154–166.

Vats A, Randhawa PS, Shapiro R: BK virus-associated transplant nephropathy: Diagnosis and treatment. *Transplant Immunol Lett* 2004;20:5–12.

Vitko S, Margreiter R, Weimar W, et al: Everolimus (certican) 12 month safety and efficacy versus mycophenolate mofetil in de novo renal transplant recipients. *Transplantation* 2004;78:1532–1540.

Weber LT, Hocker B, Mehl O, et al: Mycophenolate mofetil in pediatric renal transplantation. *Min Urol Nefrol* 2003;55:91–99.

Part XXIII ▪ Urologic Disorders in Infants and Children

Chapter 537 ▪ Congenital Anomalies and Dysgenesis of the Kidneys Jack S. Elder

EMBRYONIC DEVELOPMENT

The kidney is derived from the ureteral bud and the metanephric blastema. During the 5th wk of gestation, the ureteral bud arises from the mesonephric (wolffian) duct and penetrates the metanephric blastema, which is an area of undifferentiated mesenchyme on the nephrogenic ridge. The ureteral bud undergoes a series of approximately 15 generations of divisions and by the 20th wk of gestation forms the entire collecting system: the ureter, renal pelvis, calyces, papillary ducts, and collecting tubules. Signals from the mesenchymal cells induce ureteric bud formation from the wolffian duct as well as ureteric bud branching. Reciprocal signals from the ureteric bud and, later, from its branching tips induce mesenchymal cells to condense, proliferate, and convert into epithelial cells. Under the inductive influence of the ureteral bud, nephron differentiation begins during the 7th wk of gestation. By the 20th wk of gestation, when the collecting system is developed, approximately 30% of the nephrons are present. Nephrogenesis continues at a nearly exponential rate and is complete by the 36th wk of gestation. To date, at least 16 signaling agents have been identified that regulate renal development. Defects in any of the signaling activities could cause a kidney not to form (**renal agenesis**), to differentiate abnormally (**renal dysgenesis**), or to develop **cysts.**

The fetal kidneys play a minor role in the maintenance of fetal salt and water homeostasis. The rate of urine production increases throughout gestation and, at term, volumes have been reported to be 51 mL/hr. The glomerular filtration rate is 25 mL/min/1.73 m^2 at term and triples by 3 mo of age. The increase in glomerular filtration rate is caused by a reduction in intrarenal vascular resistance and redistribution of intrarenal blood flow to the cortex, where more nephrons are located.

Dysgenesis of the kidney includes aplasia, dysplasia, hypoplasia, and cystic disease.

RENAL AGENESIS. *Renal agenesis,* or absent kidney development, can occur secondary to a defect of the wolffian duct, ureteric bud, or metanephric blastema. Unilateral renal agenesis has an incidence of 1 in 450 to 1,000 births. Unilateral renal agenesis often is discovered during the course of an evaluation for other congenital anomalies (see VATER syndrome in Chapter 108). Its incidence is increased in newborns with a single umbilical artery. In true agenesis, the ureter and the ipsilateral bladder hemitrigone are absent. The contralateral kidney undergoes compensatory hypertrophy, to some degree prenatally but primarily after birth. Approximately 15% of these children have contralateral vesicoureteral reflux, and most males have an ipsilateral absent vas deferens because the wolffian duct is absent. Because the wolffian and müllerian ducts are contiguous, müllerian abnormalities in girls also are common. The **Mayer-Rokitansky-Kuster-Hauser** syndrome refers to a group of associated findings that includes unilateral renal agenesis or ectopia, ipsilateral müllerian defects, and vaginal agenesis.

Renal agenesis is distinguished from aplasia, in which a nubbin of nonfunctioning tissue is seen capping a normal or abnormal ureter. Clinically, this distinction may be difficult. Some individuals are diagnosed as having unilateral renal agenesis based on the finding of an absent kidney on ultrasonography or excretory urography. Some of these patients, however, actually were born with a hypoplastic kidney or a multicystic dysplastic kidney that underwent complete cyst regression. Although the specific diagnosis is not critical, if the finding of an absent kidney is based on an ultrasonogram, a functional imaging study such as an excretory urogram or renal scan should be performed because some of these patients may have an ectopic kidney. If there is a normal contralateral kidney, renal function should remain normal over time.

Bilateral renal agenesis is incompatible with extrauterine life and is termed **Potter syndrome.** Death occurs shortly after birth from pulmonary hypoplasia. The newborn has a characteristic facial appearance, termed *Potter facies* (Fig. 537-1). The eyes are widely separated with epicanthic folds, the ears are low set, the nose is broad and compressed flat, the chin is receding, and there are limb anomalies. Bilateral renal agenesis should be suspected when maternal ultrasonography demonstrates **oligohydramnios,** nonvisualization of the bladder, and absent kidneys. The incidence of this disorder is 1 in 3,000 births, with a male predominance, and represents 20% of newborns with the Potter phenotype. Other common causes of neonatal renal failure associated with the Potter phenotype include cystic renal dysplasia and obstructive uropathy. Less common causes are autosomal recessive polycystic kidney disease (infantile), renal hypoplasia, and medullary dysplasia. Neonates with bilateral renal agenesis die of pulmonary insufficiency from pulmonary hypoplasia rather than renal failure (see Chapter 101).

The term **familial renal adysplasia** describes families in which renal agenesis, renal dysplasia, multicystic kidney (dysplasia), or a combination, occurs in a single family. This disorder has an autosomal dominant inheritance pattern with a penetrance of 50–90% and variable expression. Because of this association, some clinicians advise screening first-degree relatives of individuals identified with renal agenesis or dysplasia, but it is not standard practice to do so.

Whether individuals with a solitary kidney should avoid contact sports such as football and karate is unresolved. The arguments favoring participation are that there are other solitary organs, e.g., the spleen, liver, and brain, that do not preclude contact sport participation, and there have been few reports of individuals losing a kidney from sports injuries. The arguments against such participation are that the contralateral normal kidney is hypertrophic and not as well protected by the ribs, and a serious renal injury could have devastating life-long consequences. The American Academy of Pediatrics recommends an "individual assessment for contact, collision, and limited-contact sports."

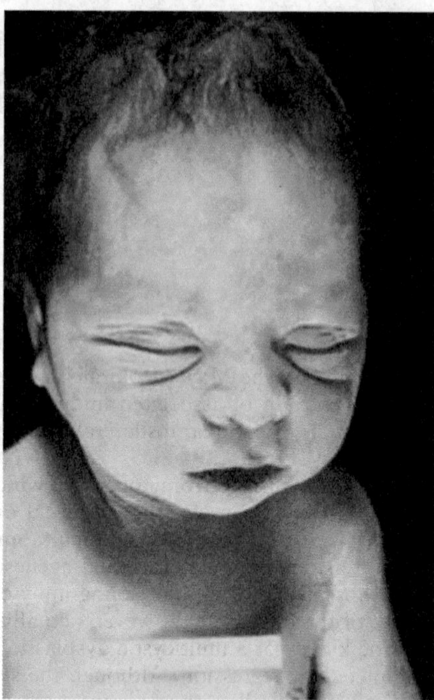

Figure 537-1. Stillborn infant with renal agenesis exhibiting characteristic Potter facies.

RENAL DYSGENESIS: DYSPLASIA, HYPOPLASIA, AND CYSTIC ANOMALIES. *Renal dysgenesis* refers to maldevelopment of the kidney that affects its size, shape, or structure. The 3 principal types of dysgenesis are dysplastic, hypoplastic, and cystic. Although dysplasia always is accompanied by a decreased number of nephrons (hypoplasia), the converse is not true; hypoplasia may occur in isolation. When both conditions are present, the term **hypodysplasia** is preferred. The term **dysplasia** is technically a histologic diagnosis and refers to focal, diffuse, or segmentally arranged primitive structures, specifically primitive ductal structures, resulting from abnormal metanephric differentiation. Nonrenal elements, such as cartilage, also may be present. The condition may affect all or only part of the kidney. If cysts are present, the condition is termed **cystic dysplasia.** If the entire kidney is dysplastic with a preponderance of cysts, the kidney is referred to as a **multicystic dysplastic kidney** (Fig. 537-2). The pathogenesis of dysplasia is multifactorial. The "bud" theory proposes that if the ureteral bud arises in an abnormal location, such as an ectopic ureter, there is abnormal penetration and induction of the metanephric blastema, which causes abnormal kidney differentiation, resulting in dysplasia. Renal dysplasia also may occur with severe obstructive uropathy early in gestation, as with the most severe cases of posterior urethral valves or in a multicystic dysplastic kidney, in which a portion of the ureter is absent or atretic.

A multicystic kidney is a congenital condition in which the kidney is replaced by cysts and does not function, and may result from ureteral atresia. Renal size is highly variable. The incidence is approximately 1 in 2,000. Some clinicians assume incorrectly that the terms *multicystic kidney* and *polycystic kidney* are synonymous. However, polycystic kidney disease is an inherited disorder that may be autosomal recessive or autosomal dominant and affects both kidneys (see Chapter 521). Multicystic kidney usually is unilateral and is not inherited. Bilateral multicystic kidneys are incompatible with life.

Multicystic dysplastic kidney is the most common cause of an abdominal mass in the newborn. In most cases it is discovered incidentally during prenatal sonography. In some individuals, the cysts are identified prenatally or postnatally, but no renal tissue is identified because of cyst regression in utero. Contralateral hydronephrosis is present in 5–10% of patients. Sonography shows the characteristic appearance of a kidney replaced by multiple cysts of varying sizes that do not communicate, and no identifiable parenchyma is present; the diagnosis should be confirmed with a renal scan, which should demonstrate nonfunction. Obtaining a voiding cystourethrogram also is advisable, because 15% of patients have contralateral reflux. Management is controversial. There have been a few reports of renin-mediated hypertension and Wilms tumor arising in these kidneys. Because neoplasms arise from the stromal rather than the cystic component, even if the cysts regress completely, the likelihood that the kidney could develop a neoplasm is not altered. The risk of hypertension is 0.2–1.2%, and the risk of Wilms tumor is 1 in 333. Because of the occult nature of these potential problems, many clinicians advise annual follow-up with sonography and blood pressure measurement. If there is an abdominal mass, the cysts enlarge, the stromal core increases in size, or hypertension develops, nephrectomy is recommended. In lieu of follow-up screening, laparoscopic nephrectomy may be performed.

Renal hypoplasia refers to a small nondysplastic kidney that has fewer than the normal number of calyces and nephrons. The term encompasses a group of conditions with an abnormally small kidney and should be distinguished from aplasia, in which the kidney is rudimentary. If the condition is unilateral, the diagnosis usually is made incidentally during evaluation for another urinary tract problem or hypertension. Bilateral hypoplasia usually presents with the manifestations of chronic renal failure and is a leading cause of end-stage renal disease during the first decade of life. A history of polyuria and polydipsia is common. Urinalysis results may be normal. In a rare form of

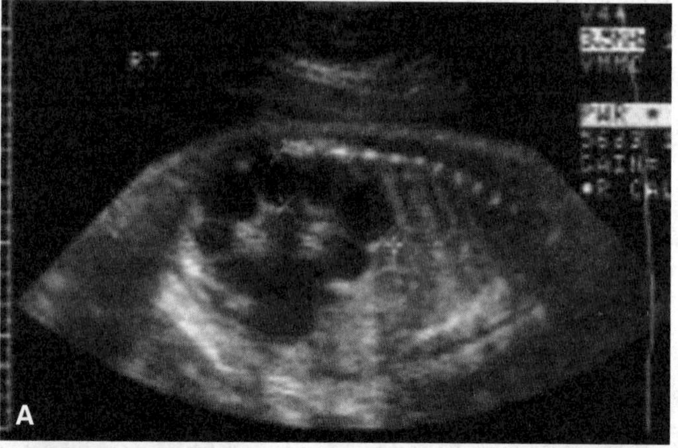

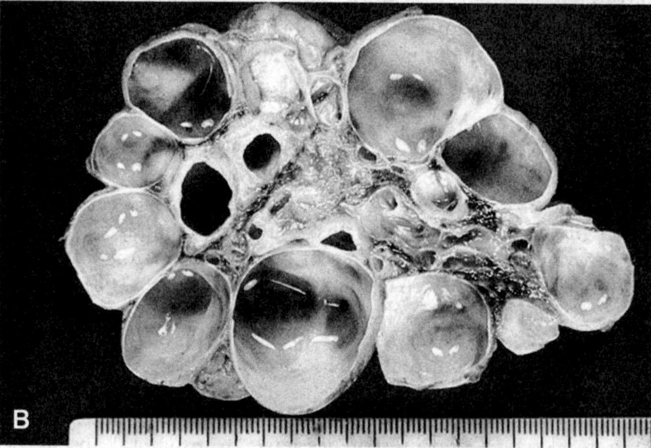

Figure 537-2. *A*, Prenatal sonogram demonstrating multicystic dysplastic kidney. *B*, Surgical specimen.

bilateral hypoplasia called **oligomeganephronia,** the number of nephrons is markedly reduced and those present are markedly hypertrophied.

The **Ask-Upmark kidney,** also termed **segmental hypoplasia,** refers to small kidneys, usually weighing not more than 35 g, with one or more deep grooves on the lateral convexity, underneath which the parenchyma consists of tubules resembling those in the thyroid gland. It is unclear whether the lesion is congenital or acquired. Most patients are 10 yr or older at diagnosis and have severe hypertension. Nephrectomy usually controls the hypertension.

ANOMALIES IN SHAPE AND POSITION. During renal development the kidneys normally ascend from the pelvis into their normal position behind the ribs. The normal process of ascent and rotation of the kidney may be incomplete, resulting in renal ectopia or nonrotation. The ectopic kidney may be in a pelvic, iliac, thoracic, or contralateral position. If the ectopia is contralateral, in 90% of individuals there is fusion of the two kidneys. The incidence of renal ectopia is approximately 1 in 900.

Renal fusion anomalies are common. The lower poles of the kidneys may fuse in the midline, resulting in a horseshoe kidney (Fig. 537-3); the fused portion is termed the *isthmus* and may be thick parenchyma or a thin fibrous strand. Horseshoe kidneys occur in 1 in 400 to 500 births but are seen in 7% of patients with Turner syndrome. Horseshoe kidney is one of the many renal anomalies that occur in 30% of patients with Turner syndrome (see Chapter 587). Wilms tumors are four times more common in children with horseshoe kidneys than in the general population. Stone disease and hydronephrosis secondary to ureteropelvic junction obstruction are other potential late complications. The increased incidence of multicystic dysplastic kidney affecting one of the two sides of a horseshoe kidney also appears to be increased. With crossed fused ectopia, one kidney crosses over to the other side and the parenchyma of the two kidneys fuse. Renal function usually is normal. In the most common finding, the left kidney may cross over and fuse with the lower pole of the right kidney. The insertion of the ureter to the bladder does not change, and the adrenal glands remain in their normal positions. The clinical significance of this anomaly is that if renal surgery is necessary, the blood supply is variable and may make partial nephrectomy more difficult.

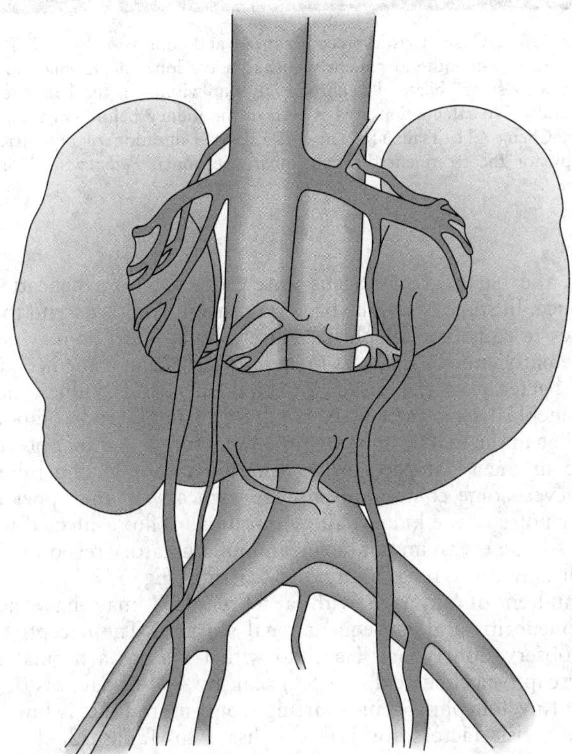

Figure 537-3. Horseshoe kidney.

ASSOCIATED PHYSICAL FINDINGS. Upper urinary tract anomalies are more common in children with certain physical findings. The incidence of renal anomalies is increased if there is a single umbilical artery and an abnormality of another organ system (congenital heart disease). External ear anomalies (particularly if the child has multiple congenital anomalies), imperforate anus, and scoliosis are associated with renal anomalies. Infants with these physical findings should undergo a renal sonogram.

Aslam M, Watson AR: Unilateral multicystic dysplastic kidney: long term outcomes. *Arch Dis Child* 2006;91:820–823.

Cheng AM, Phan V, Geary DF, et al: Outcome of isolated antenatal hydronephrosis. *Arch Pediatr Adolesc Med* 2004;158:38–40.

Coplen DE, Austin PF: Outcome analysis of prenatally detected ureteroceles associated with multicystic dysplasia. *J Urol* 2004;172:1637–1639.

Damen-Elias HA, Stoutenbeek PH, Visser GH, et al: Concomitant anomalies in 100 children with unilateral multicystic kidney. *Ultrasound Obstet Gynecol* 2005;25:384–388.

Elder JS: Sports recommendations for children with solitary kidneys and other genitourinary abnormalities. In Baskin LS, Kogan BA (editors), *Handbook of Pediatric Urology*, 2nd ed. Philadelphia, Lippincott Williams & Wilkins, 2005, pp 271–277.

Grinsell MM, Showalter S, Gordon KA, Norwood VF: Single kidney and sports participation: perception versus reality. *Pediatrics* 2006;118(3):1019–1027.

Guarino N, Cassamassima MG, Tadini B, et al: Natural history of vesicoureteral reflux associated with kidney anomalies. *Urology* 2005;65:1208–1211.

Guarino N, Tadini B, Camardi P, et al: The incidence of associated urological abnormalities in children with renal ectopia. *J Urol* 2004;172:1757–1759.

Ismaili K, Avni FE, Alexander M, et al: Routine voiding cystourethrography is of no value in neonates with unilateral multicystic dysplastic kidney. *J Pediatr* 2005;146:759–763.

Merrot T, Lumenta CB, Tercier S, et al: Multicystic dysplastic kidney with ipsilateral abnormalities of genitourinary tract: Experience in children. *Urology* 2006;67:603–607.

Miller DC, Rumohr JA, Dunn RL, et al: What is the fate of the refluxing contralateral kidney in children with multicystic dysplastic kidney? *J Urol* 2004;172:1630–1634.

Narchi H: Risk of hypertension with multicystic kidney disease: A systematic review. *Arch Dis Child* 2005;90:921–924.

Narchi H: Risk of Wilms' tumour with multicystic kidney disease: A systematic review. *Arch Dis Child* 2005;90:147–149.

Rabelo EA, Oliveira EA, Gilva GS, et al: Predictive factors of ultrasonographic involution of prenatally detected multicystic dysplastic kidney. *BJU Int* 2005;95:868–871.

Welch TR, Wacksman J: The changing approach to multicystic dysplastic kidney in children. *J Pediatr* 2005;146:723–725.

Yamatake A, Satake S, Kaneko K, et al: Outcome and cost analysis of laparoscopic or open surgery versus conservative management for multicystic dysplastic kidney. *J Laparoendosc Adv Surg Tech A* 2005;15:190–193.

Chapter 538 ■ Urinary Tract Infections

Jack S. Elder

See also Chapter 519.4.

PREVALENCE AND ETIOLOGY. Urinary tract infections (UTIs) occur in 3–5% of girls and 1% of boys. In girls, the first UTI usually occurs by the age of 5 yr, with peaks during infancy and toilet training. After the first UTI, 60–80% of girls will develop a second UTI within 18 mo. In boys, most UTIs occur during the 1st yr of life; UTIs are much more common in uncircumcised boys. The prevalence of UTIs varies with age. During the 1st yr of life, the male : female ratio is 2.8–5.4 : 1. Beyond 1–2 yr, there is a striking female preponderance, with a male : female ratio of 1 : 10.

UTIs are caused mainly by colonic bacteria. In females, 75–90% of all infections are caused by *Escherichia coli,* followed by *Klebsiella* spp. and *Proteus* spp. Some series report that in males older than 1 yr of age, *Proteus* is as common a cause as *E. coli;* others report a preponderance of gram-positive organisms in males. *Staphylococcus saprophyticus* and enterococcus are pathogens in both sexes. Viral infections, particularly adenovirus, also may occur, especially as a cause of cystitis.

UTIs have been considered an important risk factor for the development of renal insufficiency or end-stage renal disease in children. Some researchers have questioned the importance of UTI as a risk factor, because only 2% of children with renal insufficiency report a history of UTI. This paradox may be secondary to better recognition of the risks of UTI and prompt diagnosis and therapy.

CLINICAL MANIFESTATIONS AND CLASSIFICATION. The 3 basic forms of UTI are pyelonephritis, cystitis, and asymptomatic bacteriuria.

Clinical **pyelonephritis** is characterized by any or all of the following: abdominal or flank pain, fever, malaise, nausea, vomiting, and, occasionally, diarrhea. Newborns may show nonspecific symptoms such as poor feeding, irritability, and weight loss. Pyelonephritis is the most common serious bacterial infection in infants <24 mo of age who have fever without a focus (see Chapter 175). These symptoms are an indication that there is bacterial involvement of the upper urinary tract. Involvement of the renal parenchyma is termed *acute pyelonephritis,* whereas if there is no parenchymal involvement, the condition may be termed *pyelitis.* Acute pyelonephritis may result in renal injury, termed *pyelonephritic scarring.*

Acute lobar nephronia (acute lobar nephritis) is a localized renal bacterial infection involving >1 lobe that represents either a complication of pyelonephritis or an early stage in the development of a renal abscess. Manifestations are identical to pyelonephritis; renal imaging demonstrates the abnormality (Fig. 538-1). **Renal abscess** may occur following a pyelonephritis or may be secondary to a primary bacteremia *(S. aureus).* **Perinephric abscesses** may be secondary to contiguous infection in the perirenal area (e.g., vertebral osteomyelitis, psoas abscess) or pyelonephritis that dissects to the renal capsule.

Cystitis indicates that there is bladder involvement; symptoms include dysuria, urgency, frequency, suprapubic pain, incontinence, and malodorous urine. Cystitis does not cause fever and does not result in renal injury. Malodorous urine, however, is not specific for a UTI.

Asymptomatic bacteriuria refers to a condition that results in a positive urine culture without any manifestations of infection. It is most common in girls. The incidence is 1–2% in preschool and school-age girls and 0.03% in boys. The incidence declines with increasing age. This condition is benign and does not cause renal injury, except in pregnant women, in whom asymptomatic bacteriuria, if left untreated, can result in a symptomatic UTI. Some girls are mistakenly identified as having asymptomatic bacteriuria, whereas they actually are symptomatic, experiencing day or night incontinence or perineal discomfort.

PATHOGENESIS AND PATHOLOGY. Virtually all UTIs are ascending infections. The bacteria arise from the fecal flora, colonize the perineum, and enter the bladder via the urethra. In uncircumcised boys, the bacterial pathogens arise from the flora beneath the prepuce. In some cases, the bacteria causing cystitis ascend to the kidney to cause pyelonephritis. Rarely, renal infection may occur by hematogenous spread, as in endocarditis or in some neonates.

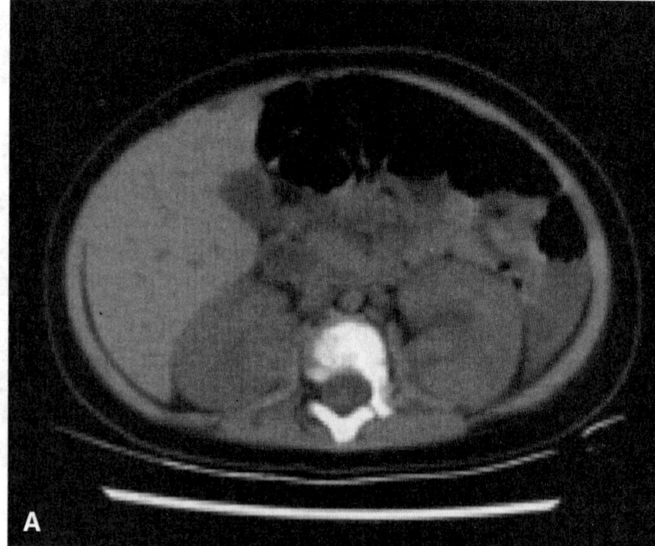

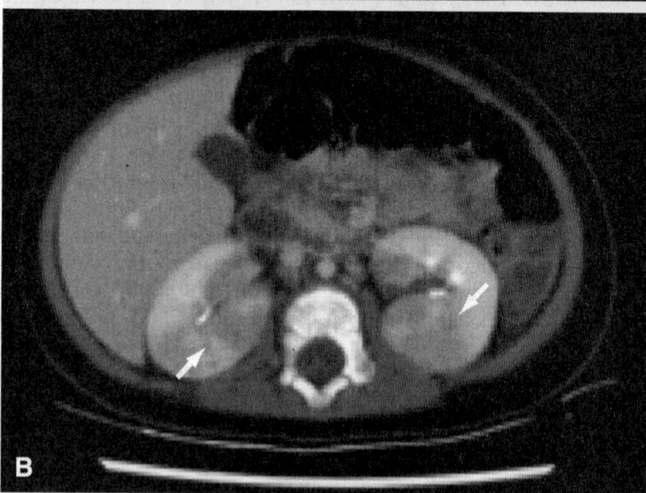

Figure 538-1. Characteristic precontrast *(A)* and contrast-enhanced *(B)* CT scans for an 8-month-old patient who had acute lobar nephronia and presented with severe bilateral nephromegaly but without a focal mass sonographically. No attenuation area is seen in the kidney before enhancement. (From Cheng CH, Tsau YK, Lin TY: Effective duration of antimicrobial therapy for the treatment of acute lobar nephronia. *Pediatrics* 2006;117:e84–e89.)

If bacteria ascend from the bladder to the kidney, acute pyelonephritis may occur. Normally the simple and compound papillae in the kidney have an antireflux mechanism that prevents urine in the renal pelvis from entering the collecting tubules. However, some compound papillae, typically in the upper and lower poles of the kidney, allow intrarenal reflux. Infected urine then stimulates an immunologic and inflammatory response. The result may cause renal injury and scarring (Fig. 538-2).

Children of any age with a febrile UTI may have acute pyelonephritis and subsequent renal scarring. The exception to this observation is that if a child with UTIs has a normal 2,3-dimercaptosuccinic acid (DMSA) scan by 4 yr of age, his or her risk of pyelonephritogenic scarring from future UTIs is low.

Host risk factors for UTI are listed in Table 538-1. Vesicoureteral reflux is discussed in Chapter 539. In girls, UTIs often occur at the onset of toilet training because of voiding dysfunc-

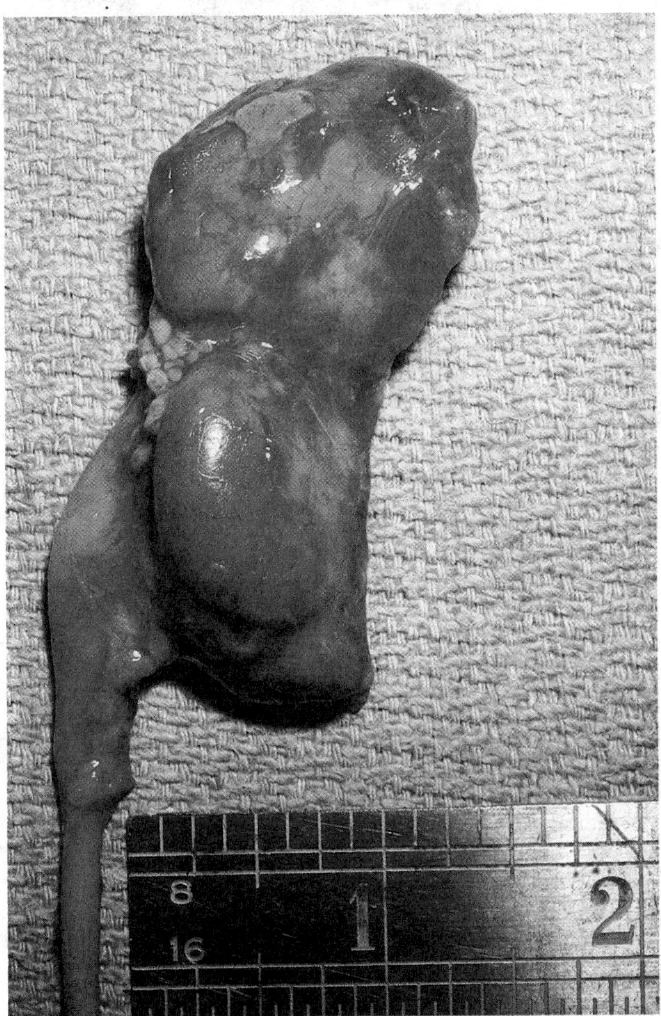

Figure 538-2. Scarred kidney from recurrent pyelonephritis.

tion that occurs at that age. The child is trying to retain urine to stay dry, yet the bladder may have uninhibited contractions forcing urine out. The result may be high-pressure, turbulent urine flow or incomplete bladder emptying, both of which increase the likelihood of bacteriuria. Voiding dysfunction may occur in the toilet-trained child who voids infrequently. Similar problems may arise in school-age children who refuse to use the school bathroom. Obstructive uropathy resulting in hydronephrosis increases the risk of UTI because of urinary stasis. Urethral instrumentation during a voiding cystourethrogram or nonsterile catheterization may infect the bladder with a pathogen. Constipation can increase the risk of UTI because it may cause voiding dysfunction.

TABLE 538-1. Risk Factors for Urinary Tract Infection

Female gender
Uncircumcised male
Vesicoureteral reflux*
Toilet training
Voiding dysfunction
Obstructive uropathy
Urethral instrumentation
Wiping from back to front in females
Bubble bath?
Tight clothing (underwear)
Pinworm infestation
Constipation
Bacteria with P fimbriae
Anatomic abnormality (labial adhesion)
Neuropathic bladder
Sexual activity
Pregnancy

*Risk increased for clinical pyelonephritis, not cystitis.

The pathogenesis of UTI is based in part on the presence of bacterial pili or fimbriae on the bacterial surface. There are two types of fimbriae, type I and type II. Type I fimbriae are found on most strains of *E. coli.* Because attachment to target cells can be blocked by D-mannose, these fimbriae are referred to as "mannose-sensitive." They have no role in pyelonephritis. The attachment of type II fimbriae is not inhibited by mannose, and these are known as "mannose-resistant." These fimbriae are expressed by only certain strains of *E. coli.* The receptor for type II fimbriae is a glycosphingolipid that is present on both the uroepithelial cell membrane and red blood cells. The Gal 1–4 Gal oligosaccharide fraction is the specific receptor. Because these fimbriae can agglutinate by P blood group erythrocytes, they are known as P fimbriae. Bacteria with P fimbriae are more likely to cause pyelonephritis. Between 76–94% of pyelonephritogenic strains of *E. coli* have P fimbriae, compared with 19–23% of cystitis strains.

Other host factors for UTI include anatomic abnormalities precluding normal micturition, such as a labial adhesion. This lesion acts as a barrier and causes vaginal voiding. A neuropathic bladder may cause UTIs if there is incomplete bladder emptying or detrusor-sphincter dyssynergia, or both. Sexual activity is associated with UTIs in girls, in part because of incomplete bladder emptying. From 4–7% of pregnant women have asymptomatic bacteriuria, which can develop into a symptomatic UTI. The incidence of UTI in infants who are breastfed is lower than in those fed with formula.

Xanthogranulomatous pyelonephritis is a rare type of renal infection characterized by granulomatous inflammation with giant cells and foamy histiocytes. It may present clinically as a renal mass or an acute or chronic infection. Renal calculi, obstruction, and infection with *Proteus* spp. or *E. coli* contribute to the development of this lesion, which usually requires total or partial nephrectomy.

DIAGNOSIS. A UTI may be suspected based on symptoms or findings on urinalysis, or both, but a urine culture is necessary for confirmation and appropriate therapy. The correct diagnosis of UTI depends on having the proper sample of urine. There are several ways to obtain a urine sample; some are more accurate than others.

In toilet-trained children, a midstream urine sample usually is satisfactory. Most studies have failed to show any benefit to formally cleansing the introitus before obtaining the specimen. If the culture shows >100,000 colonies of a single pathogen, or if there are 10,000 colonies and the child is symptomatic, the child is considered to have a UTI. In uncircumcised males, the prepuce must be retracted; if the prepuce is not retractable, this method of urine collection may be unreliable.

In infants, the application of an adhesive, sealed, sterile collection bag after disinfection of the skin of the genitals can be useful, particularly if the culture is negative. A positive culture may reflect a contaminant, particularly in girls and uncircumcised boys. In such cases, if the urinalysis result is positive, the patient is symptomatic, and there is a single organism cultured with a colony count greater than 100,000, there is a presumed UTI. If any of these criteria are not met, confirmation of infection with a catheterized sample is recommended.

When greater accuracy regarding the possibility of infection is needed, a catheterized specimen must be obtained. Proper skin preparation and good catheterization technique are important. Use of a No. 5 French polyethylene feeding tube in infants or a No. 8 French tube with proper lubrication in older children minimizes the chance of urethral trauma and contamination. Only a few milliliters need to be aspirated with a syringe to obtain the urine sample. Catheterization shortly after spontaneous voiding produces a measure of the residual urine in the bladder and helps assess problems related to bladder emptying.

Prompt plating of the urine sample is important, because if the urine sits at room temperature for more than 60 min, overgrowth of a minor contaminant may suggest a UTI when the urine may not, in fact, be infected. Refrigeration is a reliable method of storing the urine until it can be cultured.

A urinalysis should be obtained from the same specimen that was cultured. **Pyuria** (leukocytes in the urine) suggests infection, but infection can occur in the absence of pyuria; consequently, this finding is more confirmatory than diagnostic. Conversely, pyuria can be present without UTI. Nitrites and leukocyte esterase usually are positive in infected urine. Microscopic hematuria is common in acute cystitis. White blood cell casts in the urinary sediment suggest renal involvement, but in practice these are rarely seen. If the child is asymptomatic and the urinalysis result is normal, it is unlikely that there is a UTI. However, if the child is symptomatic, a UTI is possible, even if the urinalysis result is negative.

With acute renal infection, leukocytosis, neutrophilia, and elevated erythrocyte sedimentation rate and C-reactive protein are common. The latter two are nonspecific markers of bacterial infection, and their elevation does not mean that the child has acute pyelonephritis. With a renal abscess, the white blood cell count is markedly elevated to >20,000–25,000/mm^3. Because sepsis is common in pyelonephritis, particularly in infants and in any child with obstructive uropathy, blood cultures should be considered.

Acute hemorrhagic cystitis often is caused by *E. coli;* it also has been attributed to adenovirus types 11 and 21. Adenovirus cystitis is more common in males; it is self-limiting, with hematuria lasting approximately 4 days.

Eosinophilic cystitis is a rare form of cystitis of obscure origin that occasionally is found in children. The usual symptoms are those of cystitis with hematuria, ureteral dilation with occasional hydronephrosis, and filling defects in the bladder caused by masses that consist histologically of inflammatory infiltrates with eosinophils. Children with eosinophilic cystitis may have been exposed to an allergen. Bladder biopsy often is necessary to exclude a neoplastic process. Treatment usually includes antihistamines and nonsteroidal anti-inflammatory agents, but in some cases intravesical dimethyl sulfoxide instillation is necessary.

Interstitial cystitis is characterized by irritative voiding symptoms such as urgency, frequency, and dysuria, and bladder and pelvic pain relieved by voiding with a negative urine culture. The disorder is most likely to affect adolescent girls and is idiopathic (see Chapter 519.1). Diagnosis is made by cystoscopic observation of mucosal ulcers with bladder distention. Treatments have included bladder hydrodistention and laser ablation of ulcerated areas, but no treatment provides sustained relief.

TREATMENT. Acute cystitis should be treated promptly to prevent possible progression to pyelonephritis. If the symptoms are severe, a specimen of bladder urine is obtained for culture, and treatment is started immediately. If the symptoms are mild or the diagnosis is doubtful, treatment can be delayed until the results of culture are known, and the culture can be repeated if the results are uncertain. For example, if a midstream culture grows between 10^4 and 10^5 colonies of a gram-negative organism, a second culture may be obtained by catheterization before treatment is initiated. If treatment is initiated before the results of a culture and sensitivities are available, a 3- to 5-day course of therapy with trimethoprim-sulfamethoxazole is effective against most strains of *E. coli.* Nitrofurantoin (5–7 mg/kg/24 hr in 3 to 4 divided doses) also is effective and has the advantage of being active against *Klebsiella-Enterobacter* organisms. Amoxicillin (50 mg/kg/24 hr) also is effective as initial treatment but has no clear advantages over sulfonamides or nitrofurantoin.

In acute febrile infections suggestive of **pyelonephritis,** a 10- to 14-day course of broad-spectrum antibiotics capable of reaching significant tissue levels is preferable. Children who are dehydrated, are vomiting, or are unable to drink fluids, are ≤1 mo of age, or in whom urosepsis is a possibility should be admitted to the hospital for intravenous rehydration and intravenous antibiotic therapy. Parenteral treatment with ceftriaxone (50–75 mg/kg/24 hr, not to exceed 2 g) or ampicillin (100 mg/kg/24 hr) with an aminoglycoside such as gentamicin (3–5 mg/kg/24 hr in 1 to 3 divided doses) is preferable. The potential ototoxicity and nephrotoxicity of aminoglycosides should be considered, and serum creatinine and trough gentamicin levels must be obtained before initiating treatment, as well as daily thereafter as long as treatment continues. Treatment with aminoglycosides is particularly effective against *Pseudomonas* spp., and alkalinization of urine with sodium bicarbonate increases their effectiveness in the urinary tract. Oral 3rd-generation cephalosporins such as cefixime are as effective as parenteral ceftriaxone against a variety of gram-negative organisms other than *Pseudomonas,* and these medications are considered by some authorities to be the treatment of choice for oral therapy. Nitrofurantoin should not be used routinely in children with a febrile UTI because it does not achieve significant renal tissue levels. The oral fluoroquinolone ciprofloxacin is an alternative agent for resistant microorganisms, particularly *Pseudomonas,* in patients older than 17 yr. It also has been used in younger children with cystic fibrosis and pulmonary infection secondary to *Pseudomonas* and is used on occasion for short-course therapy in children with *Pseudomonas* UTI. However, the clinical use of fluoroquinolones in children should be restricted because of potential cartilage damage that has been seen in research with immature animals. The safety and efficacy of oral ciprofloxacin in children is under study. In some children with a febrile UTI, intramuscular injection of a loading dose of ceftriaxone followed by oral therapy with a 3rd-generation cephalosporin is effective. A urine culture 1 wk after the termination of treatment of a UTI ensures that the urine is sterile; in most children, this is unnecessary, because the cultures often are negative.

Children with a renal or perirenal abscess or with infection in obstructed urinary tracts often require surgical or percutaneous drainage in addition to antibiotic therapy and other supportive measures.

In a child with recurrent UTIs, identification of predisposing factors is beneficial. Many school-aged girls have **voiding dysfunction;** treatment of this condition often reduces the likelihood of recurrent UTI. Some children with urinary tract infections void infrequently, and many also have severe constipation. Counseling of parents and patients to try to establish more normal patterns of voiding and defecation may be helpful in controlling recurrences. Prophylaxis against reinfection, using sulfamethoxazole-trimethoprim, trimethoprim, or nitrofurantoin at ⅓ of the normal therapeutic dose once a day, often is effective. Prophylaxis with amoxicillin or cephalexin also may be effective, but the risk of breakthrough UTI may be higher because bacterial resistance may be induced. Other indications for long-term prophylaxis (e.g., neurogenic bladder, urinary tract stasis and obstruction, reflux, calculi) are discussed in other chapters. There is interest in probiotic therapy, which replaces normal vaginal flora, and cranberry juice, which prevents bacterial adhesion and biofilm formation, but these agents have not proved beneficial in preventing UTI.

The main consequences of chronic renal damage caused by pyelonephritis are arterial hypertension and renal insufficiency; when they are found they should be treated appropriately (see Chapters 445 and 535).

IMAGING STUDIES. The goal of imaging studies in children with a UTI is to identify anatomic abnormalities that predispose to

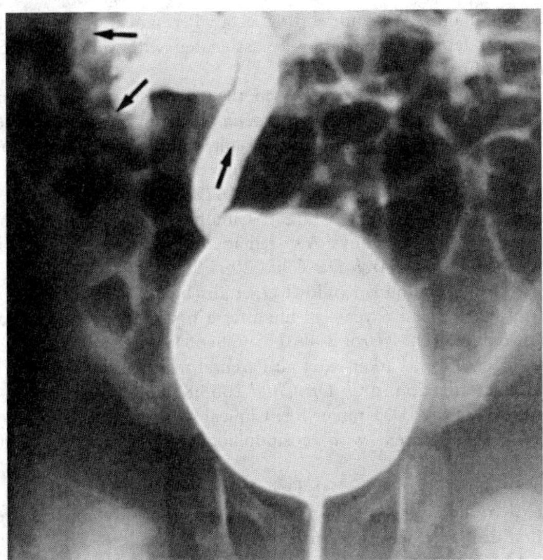

Figure 538-3. Intrarenal reflux. Voiding cystourethrogram in an infant boy with a past history of a urinary tract infection. Note the right vesicoureteral reflux with ureteral dilatation, with opacification of the renal parenchyma representing intrarenal reflux.

infection. In children with clinical pyelonephritis (febrile UTI), a renal sonogram should be obtained to rule out hydronephrosis and structural urinary abnormalities; sonography also may suggest acute pyelonephritis by demonstrating an enlarged kidney. Power Doppler sonography has been slightly more sensitive but is unreliable in identifying all cases. Sonography demonstrates many but not all renal scars. Normally, the difference in renal lengths between the two kidneys is less than 1 cm, and a larger disparity may be an indication of impaired renal growth. One should remember that in a child with acute pyelonephritis, a small kidney may be enlarged because of the infection, giving the erroneous impression that the kidneys are equal in size. Renal sonography also is sensitive for detecting nephronia and pyonephrosis, a condition that may require prompt drainage of the collecting system by percutaneous nephrostomy.

Indications for a voiding cystourethrogram (VCUG) are controversial and are changing. Most clinicians recommend it for all children with a febrile UTI. A VCUG also is recommended in girls who have had 2 or 3 UTIs in a period of 6 mo, and for boys with more than one UTI. A VCUG also should be obtained if the renal sonogram shows any significant abnormality, such as hydronephrosis, disparity in renal length, or bladder wall thickening. The most common finding is vesicoureteral reflux, which is identified in approximately 40% of patients (Fig. 538-3). Timing of the VCUG is controversial. Although in some centers the study is delayed for 2–6 wk to allow inflammation in the bladder to resolve, the incidence of reflux is identical, regardless of whether the VCUG is obtained during treatment of the UTI or after 6 wk. Consequently, obtaining the VCUG before the child is discharged from the hospital is appropriate and ensures that the evaluation is complete. If available, a radionuclide VCUG rather than a contrast VCUG can be used in girls; this technique causes less radiation exposure to the gonads than does the contrast study. However, the radioisotopic VCUG does not provide anatomic definition of the bladder, allow precise grading of reflux, demonstrate a paraureteral diverticulum, or show whether reflux is occurring into a duplicated collecting system or an ectopic ureter. In boys, radiographic definition of the urethra is important; consequently, contrast VCUG is recommended for the initial work-up.

Because of concern that the VCUG may be traumatic to the child, some parents question the need for a VCUG if the ultrasonogram is normal. Ultrasonography is insensitive in detecting reflux; only 40% of children with reflux have any abnormality on the ultrasonogram. The VCUG should not be performed routinely using general anesthesia, because the study is incomplete without a voiding phase and it subjects the child unnecessarily to the risk and cost of anesthesia. In selected cases, oral or nasal midazolam (up to 0.5 mg/kg oral route, 0.2 mg/kg nasal route), which causes anterograde amnesia and anxiolysis, may be used. Vital signs are monitored and pulse oximetry is used; no anesthesiologist is present.

When the diagnosis of acute pyelonephritis is uncertain, **renal scanning** with technetium-labeled DMSA or glucoheptonate is useful. The presence of photopenia supports the diagnosis of pyelonephritis, and experienced radiologists can differentiate between an acute and a chronic process. In approximately 50% of children with a febrile UTI, irrespective of age, the DMSA scan demonstrates parenchymal involvement. Among children with grade III, IV, or V reflux and a febrile UTI, 80–90% show acute pyelonephritis. If the DMSA scan shows acute pyelonephritis, approximately 50% of children will acquire a scar in that site over the following 5 mo. However, if the DMSA scan is normal during a febrile UTI, no scarring will result from that particular infection. Computed tomography is another diagnostic tool that can diagnose acute pyelonephritis, but clinical experience with DMSA is much greater. An alternative and rational imaging algorithm has been proposed for children with a febrile UTI: renal sonogram and DMSA renal scan, with a VCUG performed if the DMSA shows acute pyelonephritis. Whether this approach is optimal awaits the results of prospective trials.

A DMSA scan (Fig. 538-4) often is performed in the presence of vesicoureteral reflux to assess whether renal scarring is present. The DMSA is the most sensitive and accurate study for demonstrating scarring. Excretory urography is not as sensitive as the DMSA scan in demonstrating renal scarring; in addition, visualization of the collecting system in infants and young children often is suboptimal, there is a slight risk of a contrast allergy, and it can take 1–2 yr for a renal scar to appear on the urogram. CT scanning also has been used to evaluate the upper urinary tract, because it is effective in demonstrating renal scarring (Fig. 538-5).

In the past, cystoscopy and measurements of urethral caliber often were performed in girls with UTIs, but these studies contribute nothing to the therapeutic decisions to be made in children with UTIs and are contraindicated. Narrowing of the female urethra was once postulated to be a contributing factor in the development of UTIs, but the urethras of girls with recurrent UTIs have been found not to be narrower than those of girls without infections.

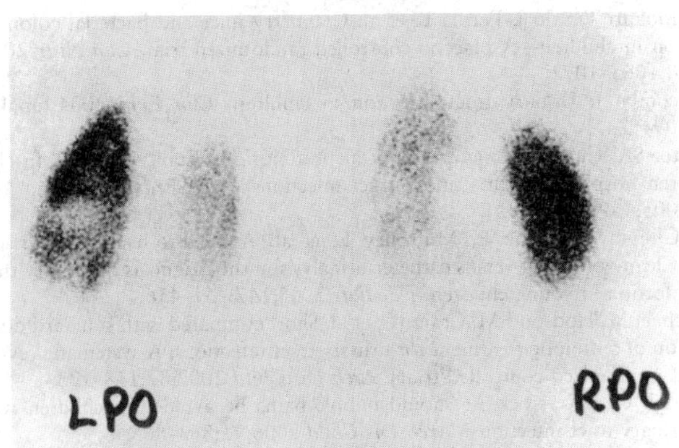

Figure 538-4. DMSA renal scan showing bilateral photopenic areas indicative of acute pyelonephritis and renal scarring.

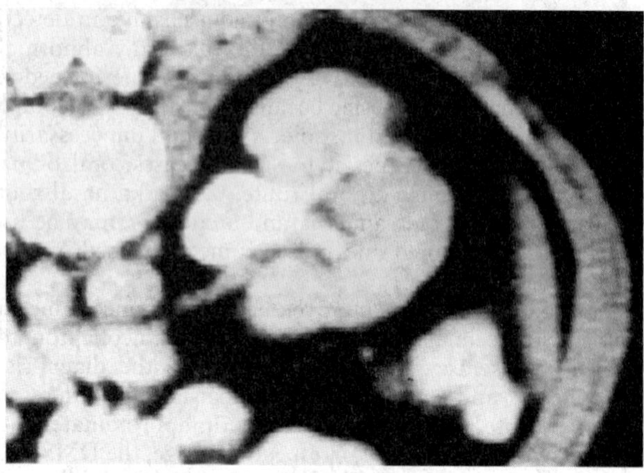

Figure 538-5. CT scan showing an area of parenchymal thinning corresponding to an underlying calyx, characteristic of pyelonephritic scarring or reflux nephropathy.

Beattie TJ: Imaging guidelines for urinary tract infection in childhood; time for change? *Arch Dis Child* 2004; 89:398–399.

Beetz R: May we go on with antibacterial prophylaxis for urinary tract infections? *Pediatr Nephrol* 2006;21:5–13.

Bloomfield P, Hodson EM, Craig J: Antibiotics for acute pyelonephritis in children. *Cochrane Database Syst Rev* 2005;25:CD003772.

Bratalavsky G, Feustel PJ, Aslan AR, et al: Recurrence risk in infants with urinary tract infections and a negative radiographic evaluation. *J Urol* 2004;172:1610–1613.

Chen L, Hasio AL, Moore CL, et al: Utility of bedside bladder ultrasound before urethral catheterization in young children. *Pediatrics* 2005;115: 108–111.

Cheng CH, Tsau YK, Lin TY: Effective duration of antimicrobial therapy for the treatment of acute lobar nephronia. *Pediatrics* 2006;117:e84–e89.

Craig JC, Hodson EM: Treatment of acute pyelonephritis in children. *BMJ* 2004;328:179–180.

Currie ML, Mitz L, Raasch CS, et al: Follow-up urine cultures and fever in children with urinary tract infection. *Arch Pediatr Adolesc Med* 2003;157:1237–1240.

Freedman AL: Urologic diseases in North America Project: Trends in resource utilization for urinary tract infections in children. *J Urol* 2005; 173:949–954.

Giorgi LJ Jr, Bratalavsky G, Kogan BA: Febrile urinary tract infections in infants: Renal ultrasound remains necessary. *J Urol* 2005;173:568–570.

Grady RW: Systemic quinolone antibiotics in children: A review of the use and safety. *Expert Opin Drug Saf* 2005;4:623–630.

Hoberman A, Charron M, Hickey RW, et al: Imaging studies after a first febrile urinary tract infection in young children. *N Engl J Med* 2003;348:195–202.

Jahnukainen T, Chen M, Celsi G: Mechanisms of renal damage owing to infection. *Pediatr Nephrol* 2005;20:1043–1053.

Jahnukainen T, Honkinen O, Ruuskanen O, et al: Ultrasonography after the first febrile urinary tract infection in children. *Eur J Pediatr* 2006;165:556–559. Epub 2006 Mar 25.

Kontiokari T, Salo J, Eerola E, et al: Cranberry juice and bacterial colonization in children—A placebo-controlled randomized trial. *Clin Nutr* 2005; 24:1065–1072.

Larcombe J: Urinary tract infection in children. *Clin Evid* 2004;Jun(11): 509–523.

Lutter SA, Currie ML, Mitz LB, et al: Antibiotic resistance patterns in children hospitalized for urinary tract infections. *Arch Pediatr Adolesc Med* 2005;159:924–928.

McGillivray D, Mok E, Mulroney E, et al: A head-to-head comparison: "Clean-void" bag versus catheter urinalysis in the diagnosis of urinary tract infection in young children. *J Pediatr* 2005;147:451–456.

Michael M, Hodson EM, Craig JC, et al: Short compared with standard duration of antibiotic treatment for urinary tract infections: A systematic review of randomized controlled trials. *Arch Dis Child* 2002;87:118–123.

Modgil G, Baverstock A: Should bubble baths be avoided in children with urinary tract infections? *Arch Dis Child* 2006;91:863–865.

Peratoner L, Pennesi M, Bordugo A, et al: Kidney length and scarring in children with urinary tract infection: Importance of ultrasound scans. *Abdom Imaging* 2005;30:780–785.

Polito C, Rambaldi PF, Signoriello G, et al: Permanent renal parenchymal defects after febrile UTI are closely associated with vesicoureteric reflux. *Pediatr Nephrol* 2006;21:521–526.

Shah G, Upadhyay J: Controversies in the diagnosis and management of urinary tract infections in children. *Paediatr Drugs* 2005;7:339–346.

Shaikh N, Abedin S, Docimo SG: Can ultrasonography or uroflowmetry predict which children with voiding dysfunction will have recurrent urinary tract infections? *J Urol* 2005;174:1620–1622.

Singh-Grewal D, Macdessi J, Craig J: Circumcision for the prevention of urinary tract infection in boys: A systematic review of randomised trials and observational studies. *Arch Dis Child* 2005;90:853–858.

Siomou E, Papadopoulou F, Kollios KD, et al: Duplex collecting system diagnosed during the first 6 years of life after a first urinary tract infection: A study of 63 children. *J Urol* 2006;175:678–681.

Struthers S, Scanlon J, Parker K, et al: Parental reporting of smelly urine and urinary tract infection. *Arch Dis Child* 2003;88:250–252.

Thompson RH, Dicks D, Kramer SA: Clinical manifestations and functional outcomes in children with eosinophilic cystitis. *J Urol* 2005;174: 2347–2349.

Tseng MH, Lin WJ, Lo WT, et al: Does a normal DMSA obviate the performance of voiding cystourethrography in evaluation of young children after their first urinary tract infection? *J Pediatr* 2007;150:96–99.

Westwood ME, Whiting PF, Cooper J, et al: Further investigation of confirmed urinary tract infection (UTI) in children under five years: A systematic review. *BMC Pediatr* 2005;5:2.

Zamir G, Sakran W, Horowitz Y, et al: Urinary tract infection: Is there a need for routine renal ultrasonography? *Arch Dis Child* 2004;89:466–468.

Zhanel GG, Hisanaga TL, Laing NM, et al: Antibiotic resistance in outpatient urinary isolates: Final results from the North American Urinary Tract Infection Collaborative Alliance (NAUTICA). *Int J Antimicrob Agents* 2005; 26:380–388.

Zorc JJ, Levine DA, Platt SL, et al: Clinical and demographic factors associated with urinary tract infection in young febrile infants. *Pediatrics* 2005;116:644–648.

Chapter 539 ■ Vesicoureteral Reflux

Jack S. Elder

Retrograde flow of urine from the bladder to the ureter and renal pelvis is referred to as **vesicoureteral reflux.** The ureter normally is attached to the bladder in an oblique direction, perforating the bladder muscle (detrusor) laterally and proceeding between the bladder mucosa and detrusor muscle, creating a flap-valve mechanism that prevents reflux (Fig. 539-1). Reflux occurs when the submucosal tunnel between the mucosa and detrusor muscle is short or absent. Reflux usually is congenital, occurs in families, and affects approximately 1% of children.

Reflux predisposes to renal infection (pyelonephritis) by facilitating the transport of bacteria from the bladder to the upper

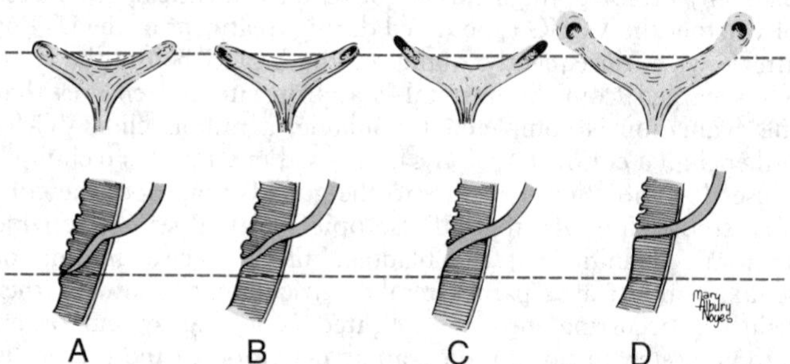

Figure 539-1. Normal and abnormal configuration of the ureteral orifices. Shown from left to right, progressive lateral displacement of the ureteral orifices and shortening of the intramural tunnels. *Top,* Endoscopic appearance. *Bottom,* Sagittal view through the intramural ureter.

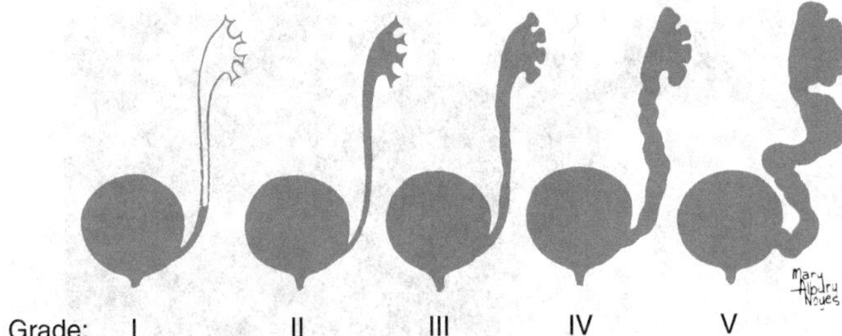

Figure 539-2. Grading of vesicoureteral reflux. Grade I: reflux into a nondilated ureter. Grade II: reflux into the upper collecting system without dilatation. Grade III: reflux into dilated ureter and/or blunting of calyceal fornices. Grade IV: reflux into a grossly dilated ureter. Grade V: massive reflux, with significant ureteral dilatation and tortuosity and loss of the papillary impression.

urinary tract (see Chapter 538). The inflammatory reaction caused by a pyelonephritic infection may result in renal injury or scarring, also termed **reflux nephropathy.** Extensive renal scarring impairs renal function and may result in renin-mediated hypertension (see Chapter 445), renal insufficiency or end-stage renal disease (see Chapter 535), impaired somatic growth, and morbidity during pregnancy. Reflux nephropathy once accounted for as much as 15–20% of end-stage renal disease in children and young adults. With greater attention to the management of urinary tract infections (UTIs) and a better understanding of reflux, end-stage renal disease secondary to reflux nephropathy is uncommon. Reflux nephropathy remains one of the most common causes of hypertension in children. Reflux in the absence of infection or elevated bladder pressure does not cause renal injury.

CLASSIFICATION. Reflux severity is graded using the International Study Classification of I to V and is based on the appearance of the urinary tract on a contrast voiding cystourethrogram (VCUG) (Figs. 539-2 and 539-3). The higher the reflux grade, the greater the likelihood of renal injury. Reflux severity is an indirect indication of the degree of abnormality of the ureterovesical junction.

Reflux may be primary or secondary (Table 539-1). Primary vesicoureteral reflux results from an anatomic deformity of the ureterovesical junction (see Fig. 539-1). Bladder instability can precipitate reflux or worsen pre-existing reflux if there is a marginally competent ureterovesical junction. In the most severe cases, there is such massive reflux into the upper tracts that the bladder becomes overdistended. This condition, the **megacystis-megaureter syndrome,** occurs primarily in males and may be unilateral or bilateral (Fig. 539-4). Reimplantation of the ureters into the bladder to correct reflux resolves the condition.

Approximately 1 in 125 children have a **duplication** of the upper urinary tract in which two ureters rather than one drain the kidney. Duplication may be partial or complete. In partial duplication, the ureters join above the bladder and there is one ureteral orifice. In complete duplication, the attachment of the lower pole ureter to the bladder is superolateral to the upper pole ureter. The valve-like mechanism for the lower pole ureter often is marginal, and reflux into the lower ureter occurs in as many as 50% of cases. Reflux occurs into both the lower and upper systems in some individuals (Fig. 539-5). With a duplication anomaly, some patients have an ectopic ureter, in which the upper pole ureter drains outside the bladder (see Chapter 540). If the ectopic ureter drains into the bladder neck, typically it is obstructed and refluxes. Duplication anomalies also are common in children with a ureterocele, which is a cystic swelling of the intramural portion of the distal ureter. In these patients there often is reflux into the associated lower pole ureter or the contralateral ureter. Reflux also typically is present when the ureter enters a bladder diverticulum (Fig. 539-6).

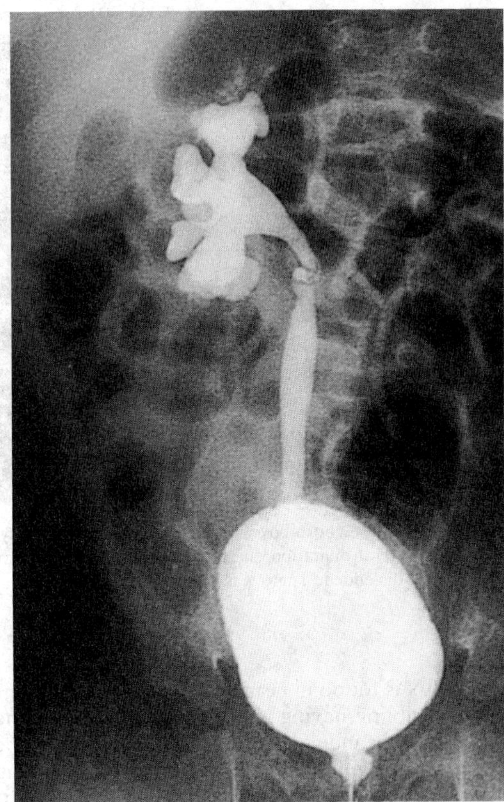

Figure 539-3. Voiding cystourethrogram (VCUG) showing grade IV right vesicoureteral reflux with intrarenal reflux.

Reflux is present at birth in 25% of children with **neuropathic bladder,** as occurs in myelomeningocele, sacral agenesis, and many children with a high imperforate anus. Reflux also is seen in 50% of boys with posterior urethral valves. Clinically, reflux with increased intravesical pressure (as in detrusor-sphincter dyssynergia or bladder outlet obstruction) can result in renal injury, even in the absence of infection.

Primary reflux occurs in association with several congenital urinary tract abnormalities. For example, 15% of children with a multicystic dysplastic kidney or renal agenesis have reflux into the contralateral kidney, and 10–15% of children with a ureteropelvic junction obstruction have reflux into either the hydronephrotic kidney or the contralateral kidney.

Reflux appears to be an autosomal dominant inherited trait. Approximately 35% of siblings of children with reflux also have

TABLE 539-1. Classification of Vesicoureteral Reflux

TYPE	CAUSE
Primary	Congenital incompetence of the valvular mechanism of the vesicoureteral junction
Primary associated with other malformations of the ureterovesical junction	Ureteral duplication Ureterocele with duplication Ureteral ectopia Paraureteral diverticula
Secondary to increased intravesical pressure	Neuropathic bladder Non-neuropathic bladder dysfunction Bladder outlet obstruction
Secondary to inflammatory processes	Severe bacterial cystitis Foreign bodies Vesical calculi Clinical cystitis
Secondary to surgical procedures involving the ureterovesical junction	Surgery

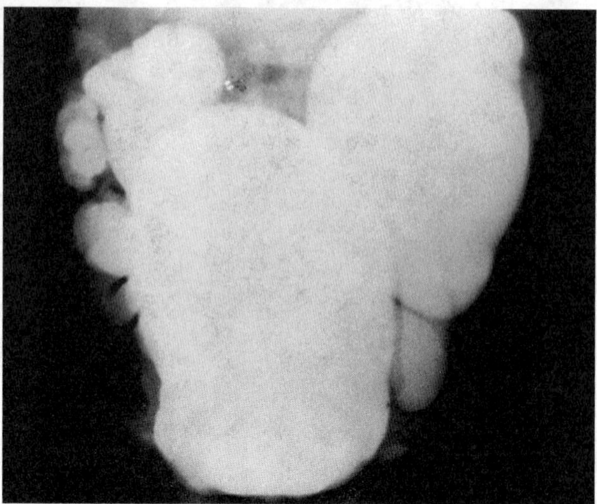

Figure 539-4. VCUG in newborn boy with megacystis-megaureter syndrome. Note the massive ureteral dilatation due to high-grade vesicoureteral reflux. The bladder is very distended. There was no urethral obstruction or neuropathic dysfunction.

reflux, and reflux is found in nearly half of newborn siblings. The likelihood of a sibling having reflux is independent of the grade of reflux or sex of the index child. Approximately 12% of asymptomatic siblings with reflux have evidence of renal scarring. Consequently, many believe that siblings of children with reflux should be screened even if they have not had a UTI. In addition, 50% of children born to women with a history of reflux also have reflux. Screening with a radionuclide cystogram of all siblings 3 yr or younger and any sibling with a UTI is appropriate. However, there are no general guidelines on sibling or offspring screening. Older siblings may undergo a renal sonogram, and if an abnormality such as hydronephrosis or disparity in renal length is found, a VCUG is recommended. Primary reflux is less common in African-Americans.

CLINICAL MANIFESTATIONS. Reflux usually is discovered during an evaluation for a UTI (see Chapter 538). Among children with reflux, 80% are female, and the average age at diagnosis is 2–3 yr. In other children, VCUG is performed during evaluation

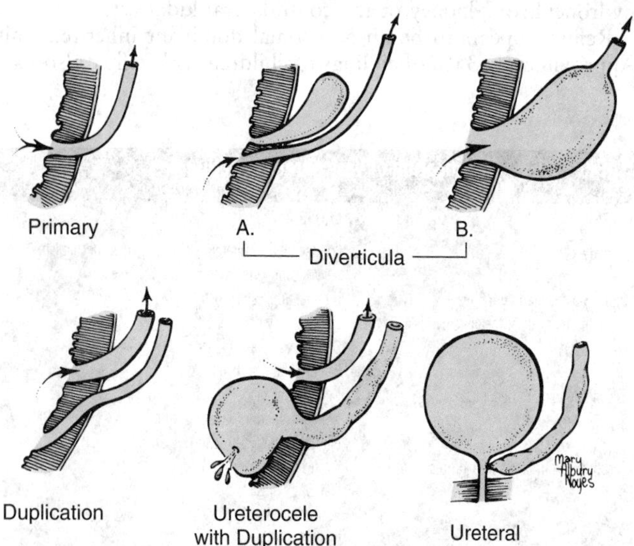

Figure 539-5. Various anatomic defects of the ureterovesical junction associated with vesicoureteral reflux.

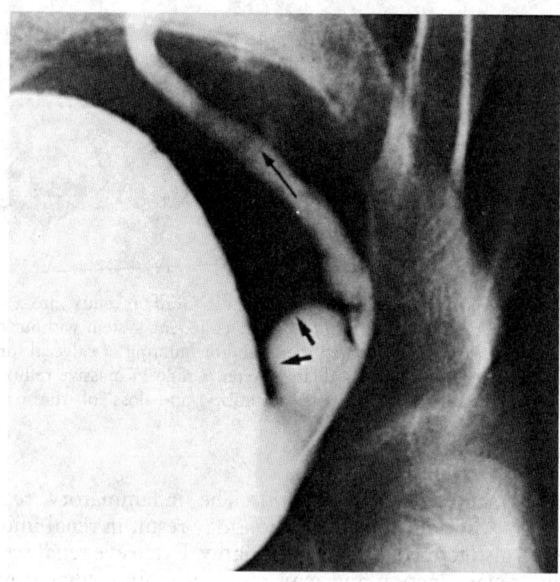

Figure 539-6. Reflux and bladder diverticulum. The voiding cystourethrogram demonstrates left vesicoureteral reflux and a paraureteral diverticulum.

of voiding dysfunction, renal insufficiency, hypertension, or other suspected pathologic process of the urinary tract. Primary reflux also may be discovered during evaluation for prenatal hydronephrosis. In this select population, 80% of affected children are male, and the reflux grade usually is higher than in females diagnosed following a UTI. Reflux resolves in most prenatally diagnosed patients after birth. Nonetheless, repeated renal ultrasonographic examinations are indicated after birth to demonstrate resolution of the hydronephrosis.

DIAGNOSIS. Diagnosis of reflux usually requires catheterization of the bladder, instillation of a solution containing iodinated contrast or a radiopharmaceutical, and radiologic imaging of the lower and upper urinary tract—a contrast VCUG or radionuclide VCUG, respectively. The bladder and upper urinary tracts are imaged during bladder filling and voiding. Reflux occurring during bladder filling is termed *low-pressure* or *passive* reflux; reflux during voiding is termed *high-pressure* or *active* reflux. Children with passive reflux are less likely to show spontaneous reflux resolution than are children who exhibit only active reflux. Radiation exposure during radionuclide VCUG is significantly less than that from a contrast VCUG. However, the contrast study provides more anatomic information, such as demonstration of a duplex collecting system, ectopic ureter, paraureteral (bladder) diverticulum, bladder outlet obstruction in boys, upper urinary tract stasis, and signs of voiding dysfunction, such as a "spinning top" urethra in girls. The reflux grading system is based on the appearance on VCUG. Consequently, the VCUG is used as the initial study in most centers. For follow-up evaluation, the radionuclide cystogram often is preferred because of the lower radiation exposure (Fig. 539-7), although it may be difficult to determine whether the reflux severity has changed.

Children undergoing cystography may be psychologically traumatized by the catheterization. Careful preparation by caregivers or administration of oral or nasal midazolam (for sedation and amnesia) or propofol before the study can result in a less distressing experience.

Indirect cystography is a technique of detecting reflux without catheterization that involves injecting an intravenous radiopharmaceutical that is excreted by the kidneys, waiting for it to be excreted into the bladder, and imaging the lower urinary tract while the patient voids. This technique detects only 75% of reflux cases, however. Another technique, which avoids radiation exposure, involves the instillation of sonographic contrast medium

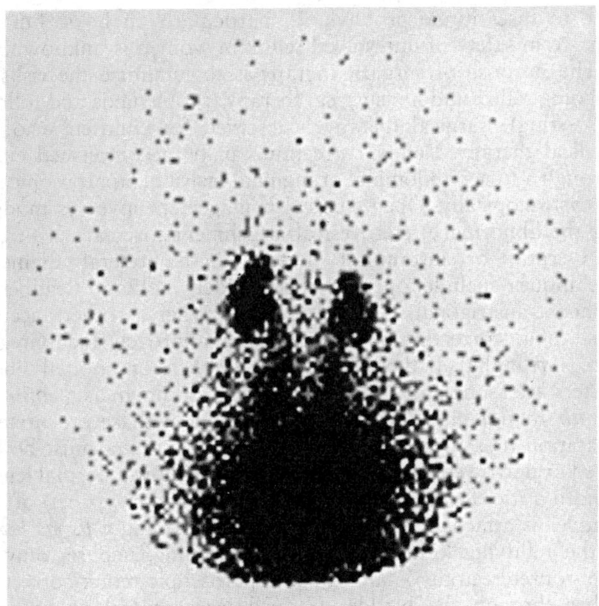

Figure 539-7. Radionuclide cystogram shows bilateral reflux.

through a urethral catheter. The kidneys are imaged sonographically. The advantage of this technique is the absence of radiation, but it is less accurate than contrast VCUG and reflux cannot be graded.

After reflux is diagnosed, graded, and determined to be primary or secondary, it is important to assess the upper urinary tract. The goal of upper tract imaging is to assess whether renal scarring and associated urinary tract anomalies are present. Renal imaging can be performed by a renal sonogram, renal scintigraphy, excretory urogram (intravenous pyelogram [IVP]), or CT scan. Renal sonography can demonstrate whether significant renal scarring is present or whether there is an anatomic condition that predisposes to UTI, such as a ureteropelvic junction or ureterovesical junction obstruction, or renal duplication anomaly with an obstructed ureter. Sonography also allows the clinician to monitor renal growth over time. Renal scintigraphy usually is performed with dimercaptosuccinic acid (DMSA), which displays renal cortical detail well and is reliable in demonstrating virtually all renal scarring as well as acute renal parenchymal infection. However, it is unreliable in demonstrating hydronephrosis. The IVP involves injection of an iodinated contrast agent and provides good anatomic detail of the kidneys, but this study is performed infrequently in children because it rarely adds additional information. On occasion a CT scan is performed during evaluation for a UTI. This study provides similar information to the studies discussed, but involves significant radiation exposure.

The child should be evaluated for voiding dysfunction, including urgency, frequency, diurnal incontinence, infrequent voiding, or a combination of these. Bowel habits should be assessed. Children with bladder instability often undergo a regimen of bladder training (timed voiding) and, on occasion, anticholinergic therapy in addition to antimicrobial prophylaxis.

After diagnosis, the child's height, weight, and blood pressure should be measured and monitored. If upper tract imaging shows renal scarring, a serum creatinine measurement should be obtained. The urine should be assessed for infection and proteinuria. Cystoscopy is of no value in determining the prognosis or selecting treatment. Urethral dilatation is not beneficial.

NATURAL HISTORY. The incidence of renal scarring or reflux nephropathy increases with the grade of reflux. With bladder growth and maturation, there is a tendency for reflux to resolve or improve over time. Lower grades of reflux are much more likely to resolve than are higher grades. For grades 1 and 2 reflux, the likelihood of resolution is similar regardless of age at diagnosis and whether it is unilateral or bilateral. For grade 3, a younger age at diagnosis and unilateral reflux usually are associated with a higher rate of spontaneous resolution (Fig. 539-8). Bilateral grade 4 reflux is much less likely to resolve than is unilateral grade 4 reflux. Grade 5 reflux rarely resolves. The mean age at reflux resolution is 6 yr. Although reflux is unlikely to cause renal injury in the absence of infection, in situations with high-pressure reflux, as in children with posterior urethral valves, neuropathic bladder, and non-neurogenic neurogenic bladder (i.e., Hinman syndrome), sterile reflux can cause significant renal damage. Children with high-grade reflux who acquire a UTI are at significant risk for pyelonephritis and renal scarring.

TREATMENT. The goals of treatment are to prevent pyelonephritis, renal injury, and other complications of reflux. Medical therapy is based on the principle that reflux often resolves over time and that the morbidity or complications of reflux may be prevented without surgery. The basis for surgical therapy is that, in selected children, ongoing reflux has caused or has significant potential for causing renal injury or other reflux-related complications and that elimination of reflux minimizes the likelihood of these problems.

Based on a few early studies demonstrating the effectiveness of antimicrobial prophylaxis in reducing the risk of complications of reflux, daily prophylaxis has been the cornerstone in the initial

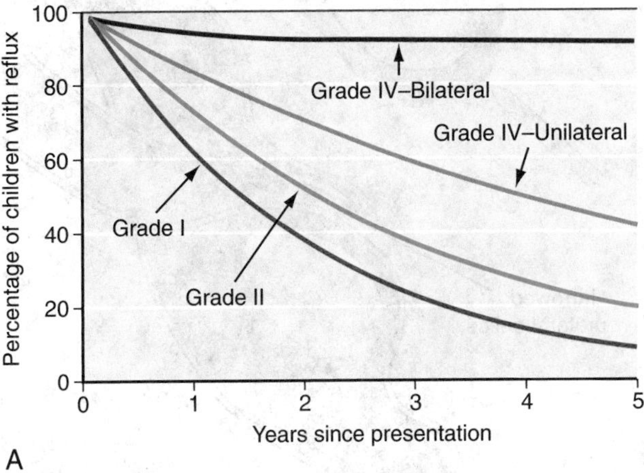

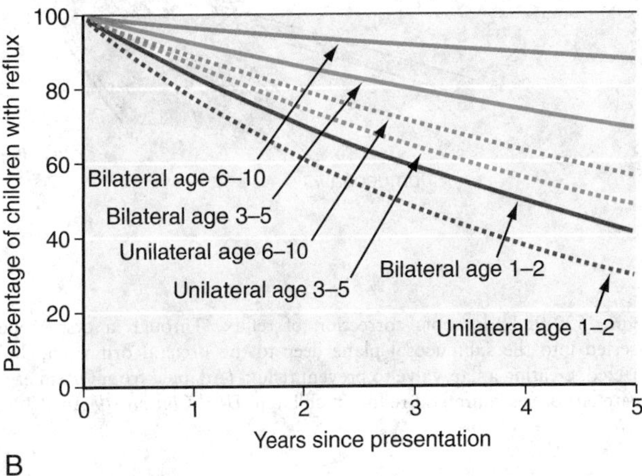

Figure 539-8. *A,* Percent chance of reflux persistence, grades I, II, and IV, for 1–5 yr after presentation. *B,* Percent chance of reflux persistence by age at presentation, grade III, for 1–5 yr after presentation. (From Elder JS, Peters CA, Arant BS Jr, et al: Pediatric Vesicoureteral Reflux Guidelines Panel Summary Report on the management of primary vesicoureteral reflux in children. *J Urol* 1997;157:1846–1851.)

management of children with reflux. Drugs commonly used for prophylaxis include sulfamethoxazole-trimethoprim, trimethoprim alone, and nitrofurantoin, generally administered once daily at a dose of ¼ to ⅓ of the dose necessary to treat an acute infection. Prophylaxis usually is continued until reflux resolves or until the risk of reflux to the individual is considered to be low. The child's voiding and defecation habits are assessed, and any voiding dysfunction and constipation should be treated (see Chapter 543). A urine culture should be performed if there are symptoms or signs of a UTI. VCUG (contrast or radionuclide) is performed every 12–18 mo. Periodic upper tract imaging should be done to monitor the status of the upper urinary tracts. Follow-up clinical evaluation should be performed at least annually, at which time the child's height, weight, and blood pressure should be recorded.

Concerns have been raised regarding the risks as well as the effectiveness of antimicrobial prophylaxis compared with intermittent therapy (close monitoring and prompt antimicrobial therapy for UTI). Whether intermittent therapy is safe is unproven; prospective clinical trials are being conducted through the NIH, as well as in Sweden. Nonrandomized retrospective studies have demonstrated that discontinuing antibiotics in children with persistent low-grade reflux and normal bladder function usually is safe in the short term, but longitudinal studies into adulthood, particularly in women, have not been performed.

Medical management is considered successful if the child remains free of infection and has no new renal scarring and if the reflux resolves spontaneously. Breakthrough UTI, development of new renal scars, and failure of reflux to resolve indicate failed medical management. Noncompliance, allergic reaction, or side effects to the prescribed medication may preclude medical management or lead to its failure. In older children with persistent low-grade reflux and a normal voiding pattern, it is considered safe to discontinue prophylaxis, particularly in boys, but the long-term safety of unresolved reflux in women is unknown.

The purpose of surgical therapy is to minimize the risks of ongoing reflux and nonsurgical therapy (prophylaxis and follow-up testing). Surgical therapy is reserved for children who fail medical therapy. Reflux correction can be accomplished either through a lower abdominal or inguinal incision, laparoscopically, or cystoscopically. Open surgical management involves modifying the abnormal ureterovesical attachment to create a 4 : 1 to 5 : 1 ratio of intramural ureter length : ureteral diameter. Techniques include opening the bladder (Politano-Leadbetter, Cohen transtrigonal, Glenn-Anderson), whereas others accomplish reflux correction by an extravesical approach (Lich-Gregoir detrusorrhaphy). If there is a simple duplication anomaly, both ureters are reimplanted together, in what is known as a *common sheath reimplant*. When reflux associated with severe ureteral dilatation (i.e., megaureter) is corrected, the ureter must be tailored or narrowed to a more normal size to allow a normal length : width ratio for the intramural tunnel, and a corner of the bladder is attached to the psoas tendon, forming a *psoas hitch*. If the refluxing kidney is poorly functioning, nephrectomy or nephroureterectomy is indicated. Laparoscopic reflux correction either through the bladder (termed *vesicoscopic*) or with an extravesical approach is being evaluated.

Open surgical repair is performed in children who fail medical management, including those with breakthrough UTI, persistent reflux, and grade 4 or 5 reflux. Blood loss is minimal, and the hospital stay averages 1–2 days. The success rate in children with primary reflux is greater than 95–98% for grades 1–4, with 2% experiencing persistent reflux and 1% having ureteral obstruction that requires correction. The success rate is so high that many pediatric urologists do not perform a postoperative VCUG unless the child develops clinical pyelonephritis. For grade 5 reflux, the

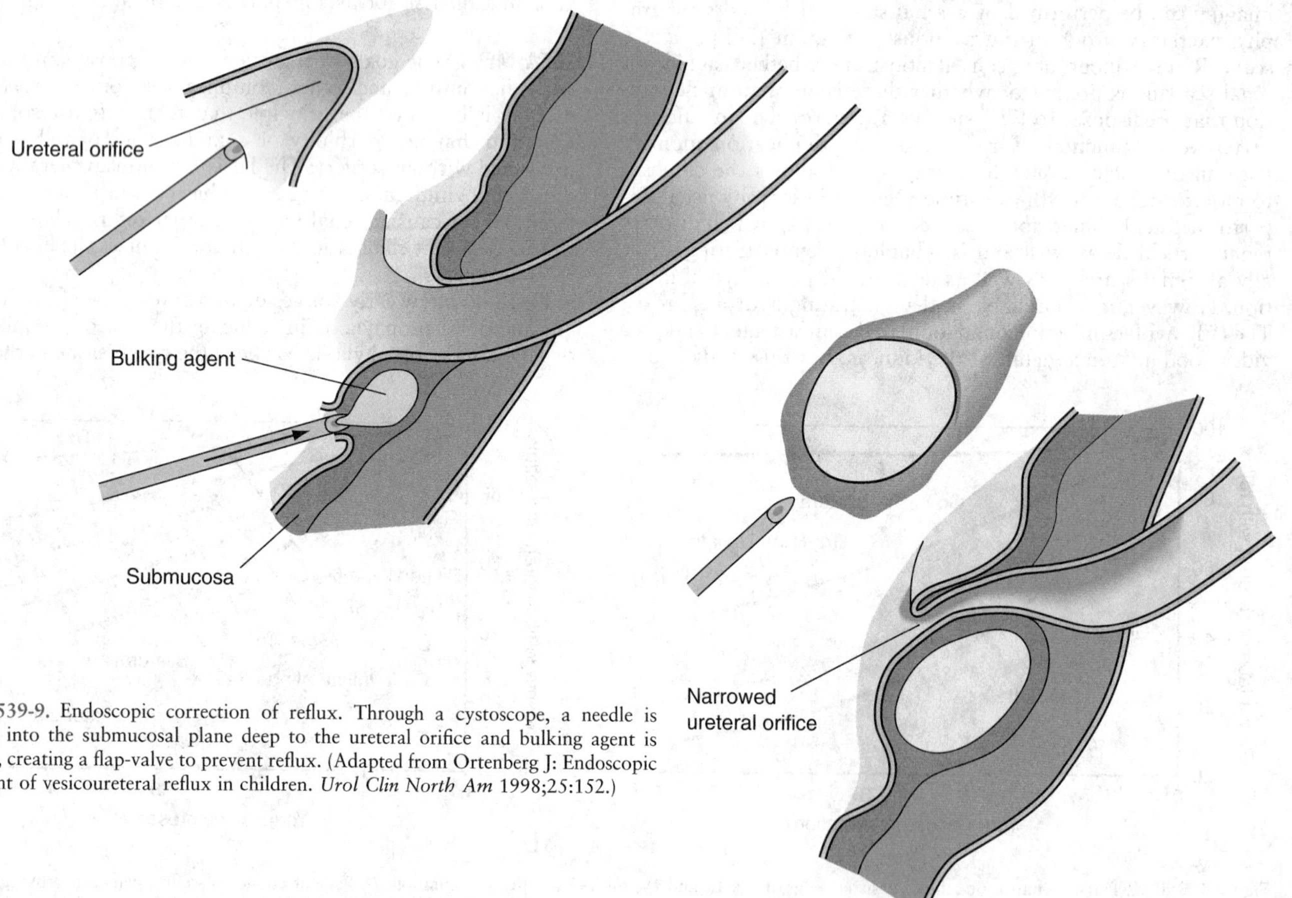

Figure 539-9. Endoscopic correction of reflux. Through a cystoscope, a needle is inserted into the submucosal plane deep to the ureteral orifice and bulking agent is injected, creating a flap-valve to prevent reflux. (Adapted from Ortenberg J: Endoscopic treatment of vesicoureteral reflux in children. *Urol Clin North Am* 1998;25:152.)

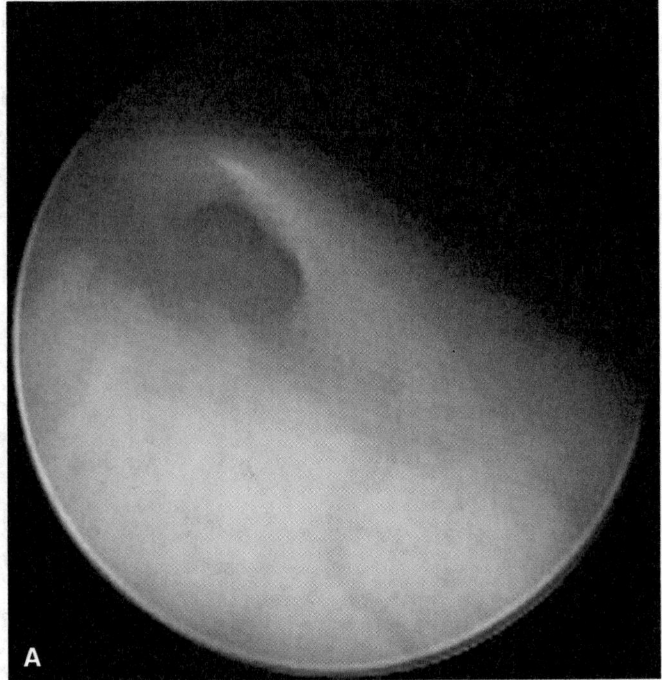

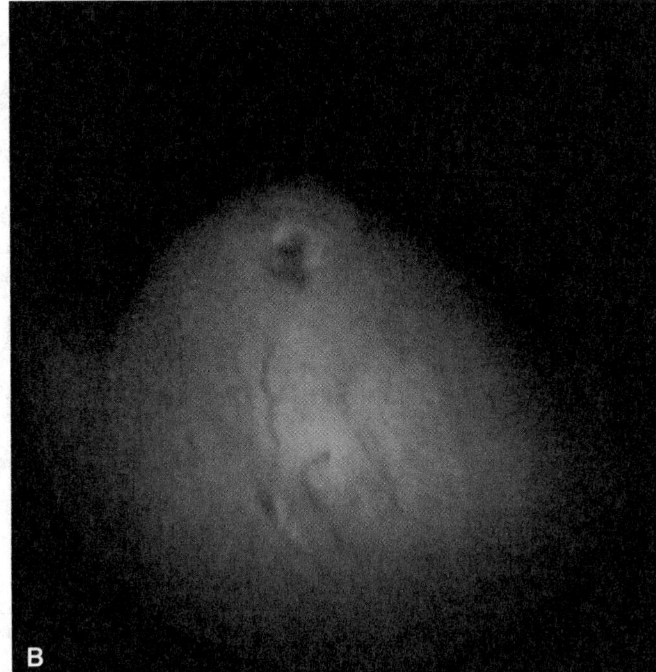

Figure 539-10. *(A)* Endoscopic view of right refluxing ureter. *(B)* The same ureter after subureteral injection of dextranomer microspheres.

success rate is approximately 80%. In lower grades of reflux, a failed reimplantation is most likely to occur in children with undiagnosed voiding dysfunction. In children with secondary reflux (posterior urethral valves, neuropathic bladder), the success rate is slightly lower than with primary reflux.

Endoscopic repair of reflux involves injection of a bulking agent via a cystoscope just beneath the ureteral orifice, creating an artificial flap-valve (Fig. 539-9). The advantage of subureteral injection is that it is a noninvasive, outpatient procedure (performed under general anesthesia) with no recovery time. The success rate is 70–80% and is highest for lower grades of reflux. If the first injection is unsuccessful, one or two repeat injections can be performed. In October 2001, the U.S. Food and Drug Administration (FDA) approved the use of a biodegradable material, dextran microspheres suspended in hyaluronic acid (Deflux), for subureteral injection. The reflux recurrence rate is approximately 10%. In the U.S., more than 40% of antireflux surgery is performed with this procedure (Fig. 539-10).

The International Reflux Study showed that in children with grades 3–4 reflux, after 5 yr of medical or surgical therapy, similar results occurred with regard to new renal scarring and renal function. However, the incidence of clinical pyelonephritis was 2.5 times higher in the children managed medically; at the end of the study, more than half of the medically managed children still had reflux and were receiving antimicrobial prophylaxis.

Evidence-based guidelines pertaining to the treatment of reflux diagnosed after a UTI were published in 1997 by the American Urological Association (Table 539-2). These guidelines were written before an endoscopic FDA-approved implant became available. A guide for parents based on the report is available to assist the physician in discussing treatment options with the parents. The decision whether to recommend observation, medical, or surgical therapy is based on the risk of reflux to the patient, the likelihood of spontaneous resolution, and parental-patient preferences.

TABLE 539-2. Treatment Recommendations for Vesicoureteral Reflux Diagnosed Following a Urinary Tract Infection*

GRADE	AGE (YR)	SCARRING	INITIAL TREATMENT	FOLLOW-UP
I–II	Any	Yes/No	Antibiotic prophylaxis	No consensus
III–IV	0–5	Yes/No	Antibiotic prophylaxis	Surgery
III–IV	6–10	Yes/No	Unilateral: antibiotic prophylaxis Bilateral: surgery	Surgery
V	<1	Yes/No	Antibiotic prophylaxis	Surgery
V	1–5	No	Unilateral: antibiotic prophylaxis	Surgery
V	1–5	No	Bilateral: surgery	
V	1–5	Yes	Surgery	
V	6–10	Yes/No	Surgery	

*Summary of guidelines developed by American Urological Association; age refers to age at diagnosis.

Afshar K, Papanikolaou F, Malek R, et al: Vesicoureteral reflux and complete ureteral duplication. Conservative or surgical management? *J Urol* 2005;173:1725–1727.

Al-Sayyad AJ, Pike JG, Leonard MP: Can prophylactic antibiotics safely be discontinued in children with vesicoureteral reflux? *J Urol* 2005; 174:1587–1589.

Charbonneau SG, Tackett LD, Gray EH, et al: Is long-term sonographic follow-up necessary after uncomplicated ureteral reimplantation in children? *J Urol* 2005;174:1429–1431.

Chen HW, Yuan SSF, Lin CJ: Ureteral reimplantation for vesicoureteral reflux: Comparison of minimally invasive extravesical with transvesical and conventional extravesical techniques. *Urology* 2004;63:364–368.

Edmondson JD, Maizels M, Alpert SA, et al: Multi-institutional experience with PIC cystography—Incidence of occult vesicoureteral reflux in Children with febrile urinary tract infections. *Urology* 2006;67:608–611.

Elder JS: Imaging for vesicoureteral reflux—Is there a better way? *J Urol* 2005; 74:7–8.

Elder JS, Diaz M, Caldamone AA, et al: Endoscopic therapy for vesicoureteral reflux: A meta-analysis. I. Reflux resolution and urinary tract infection. *J Urol* 2006;175:716–722.

Elder JS, Peters CA, Arant BS Jr, et al: Pediatric Vesicoureteral Reflux Guidelines Panel Summary Report on the management of primary vesicoureteral reflux in children. *J Urol* 1997;157:1846–1851.

Fanos V, Cataldi L: Antibiotics or surgery for vesicoureteric reflux in children. *Lancet* 2004;364:1720–1722.

Garin EH, Olavarria F, Garcia Nieto V, et al: Clinical significance of primary vesicoureteral reflux and urinary antibiotic prophylaxis after acute pyelonephritis: A multicenter, randomized, controlled study. *Pediatrics* 2006;117:626–632.

Georgaki-Angelaki H, Kostaridou S, Daikos GL, et al: Long-term follow-up of children with vesicoureteral reflux with and without antibiotic prophylaxis. *Scand J Infect Dis* 2005;37:842–845.

Giel DW, Noe HN, Williams MA: Ultrasound screening of asymptomatic siblings of children with vesicoureteral reflux: A long-term follow-up study. *J Urol* 2005;174:1602–1604.

Hollowell JG: Screening siblings for vesicoureteral reflux. *J Urol* 2002; 168:2138–2141.

Ismaili K, Hall M, Piepsz A, et al: Primary vesicoureteral reflux detached in neonates with a history of fetal renal pelvis dilation: A prospective clinical and imaging study. *J Pediatr* 2006;148:222–227.

Jodal U, Smellie JM, Lax H, et al: Ten-year results of randomized treatment of children with severe vesicoureteral reflux. Final report of the International Reflux Study in Children. *Pediatr Nephrol* 2006;2006:785–792.

Kajbafzadeh AM, Habibi Z, Tajik P, et al: Endoscopic subureteral Urocol injection for the treatment of vesicoureteral reflux. *J Urol* 2006;175: 1480–1483.

Leroy S, Marc E, Adamsbaum C, et al: Prediction of vesicoureteral reflux after a first febrile urinary tract infection in children: Validation of a clinical decision rule. *Arch Dis Child* 2006;91:241–244.

Moorthy I, Easty M, McHigh K, et al: The presence of vesicoureteric reflux does not identify a population at risk for renal scarring following a first urinary tract infection. *Arch Dis Child* 2005;90:733–736.

Putman S, Wicher C, Wayment R, et al: Unilateral extravesical ureteral reimplantation in children performed on an outpatient basis. *J Urol* 2005;174:1987–1989.

Routh JC, Vandersteen DR, Pfefferle H, et al: Single center experience with endoscopic management of vesicoureteral reflux in children. *J Urol* 2006;175:1889–1892.

Thompson M, Simon SD, Sharma V, et al: Timing of follow-up voiding cystourethrogram in children with primary vesicoureteral reflux: Development and application of a clinical algorithm. *Pediatrics* 2005;115:426–434.

Tombesi M, Ferrari CM, Bertolotti JJ: Renal damage in refluxing and non-refluxing siblings of index children with vesicoureteral reflux. *Pediatr Nephrol* 2005;20:1201–1202.

Van Capelle JW, De Haan T, El Sayed W, et al: The long-term outcome of the endoscopic subureteric implantation of polydimethylsiloxane for treating vesico-ureteric reflux in children: A retrospective analysis of the first 195 consecutive patients in two European centres. *BUJ Int* 2004;94:1348–1351.

Venhola M, Huttunen MP, Uhari M: Meta-analysis of vesicoureteral reflux and urinary tract infection in children. *Scand J Urol Nephrol* 2006; 40:98–102.

Wheeler D, Vimalachandra D, Hodson EM, et al: Antibiotics and surgery for vesicoureteric reflux: A meta-analysis of randomized controlled trials. *Arch Dis Child* 2003;88:688–694.

Yeung CK, Sihoe JD, Borzi PA: Endoscopic cross-trigonal ureteral reimplantation under carbon dioxide bladder insufflation: A novel technique. *J Endourol* 2005;19:295–299.

Chapter 540 ■ Obstruction of the Urinary Tract Jack S. Elder

Obstruction of the urinary tract can be either congenital (anatomic) or caused by trauma, neoplasia, calculi, inflammatory processes, or surgical procedures, although most childhood obstructive lesions are congenital. Obstructive lesions occur at any level from the urethral meatus to the calyceal infundibula (Table 540-1). The pathophysiologic effects of obstruction depend on its level, the extent of involvement, the child's age at onset, and whether it is acute or chronic.

ETIOLOGY. Ureteral obstruction occurring early in fetal life results in renal dysplasia, ranging from multicystic kidney, which is associated with ureteral or pelvic atresia (see Fig. 537-2), to various degrees of histologic renal cortical dysplasia that are seen with less severe obstruction. Chronic ureteral obstruction in late fetal life or after birth results in dilation of the ureter, renal pelvis, and calyces, with alterations of renal parenchyma ranging from minimal tubular changes to dilation of Bowman's space, glomerular fibrosis, and interstitial fibrosis. After birth, infections often complicate obstruction and may increase renal damage.

TABLE 540-1. Types and Causes of Urinary Tract Obstruction

LOCATION	CAUSE
Infundibula	Congenital
	Calculi
	Inflammatory (tuberculosis)
	Traumatic
	Postsurgical
	Neoplastic
Renal pelvis	Congenital (infundibulopelvic stenosis)
	Inflammatory (tuberculosis)
	Calculi
	Neoplasia (Wilms tumor, neuroblastoma)
Ureteropelvic junction	Congenital stenosis
	Calculi
	Neoplasia
	Inflammatory
	Postsurgical
	Traumatic
Ureter	Congenital obstructive megaureter
	Midureteral structure
	Ureteral ectopia
	Ureterocele
	Retrocaval ureter
	Ureteral fibroepithelial polyps
	Ureteral valves
	Calculi
	Postsurgical
	Extrinsic compression
	Neoplasia (neuroblastoma, lymphoma, and other retroperitoneal or pelvic tumors)
	Inflammatory (Crohn disease, chronic granulomatous disease)
	Hematoma, urinoma
	Lymphocele
	Retroperitoneal fibrosis
Bladder outlet and urethra	Neurogenic bladder dysfunction (functional obstruction)
	Posterior urethral valves
	Anterior urethral valves
	Diverticula
	Urethral strictures (congenital, traumatic, or iatrogenic)
	Urethral atresia
	Ectopic ureterocele
	Meatal stenosis (males)
	Calculi
	Foreign bodies
	Phimosis
	Extrinsic compression by tumors
	Urogenital sinus anomalies

CLINICAL MANIFESTATIONS. Obstruction of the urinary tract generally causes **hydronephrosis,** which typically is asymptomatic in its early phases. An obstructed kidney secondary to a ureteropelvic junction (UPJ) or ureterovesical junction obstruction may present as a mass or cause upper abdominal or flank pain on the affected side. Pyelonephritis may occur because of urinary stasis. An upper urinary tract stone may occur, causing abdominal and flank pain and hematuria. With bladder outlet obstruction, the urinary stream may be weak; urinary tract infection (UTI) is common. Many of these lesions are identified by antenatal ultrasonography; an abnormality involving the genitourinary tract is suspected in as many as 1 in 100 fetuses.

Obstructive renal insufficiency can manifest itself by failure to thrive, vomiting, diarrhea, or other nonspecific signs and symptoms. In older children, infravesical obstruction can be associated with overflow urinary incontinence or a poor urinary stream. Acute ureteral obstruction causes flank or abdominal pain; there may be nausea and vomiting. Chronic ureteral obstruction can be silent or can cause vague abdominal or typical flank pain with increased fluid intake.

DIAGNOSIS. Often, urinary tract obstruction is diagnosed prenatally by ultrasonography, typically showing hydronephrosis. More complete evaluation, including imaging studies, should be undertaken in these children in the neonatal period. Urinary tract obstruction is often silent. In the newborn infant, a palpable abdominal mass most commonly is a hydronephrotic or multicystic dysplastic kidney. With posterior urethral valve, which is an infravesical obstructive lesions in boys, a walnut-sized mass representing the bladder, is palpable just above the pubic symphysis. A patent draining urachus also may suggest urethral obstruction. Urinary ascites in the newborn usually is caused by renal or bladder urinary extravasation secondary to posterior urethral valves. Infection and sepsis may be the first indications of an obstructive lesion of the urinary tract. The combination of infection and obstruction poses a serious threat to infants and children and generally requires parenteral administration of antibiotics and drainage of the obstructed kidney. Renal ultrasonography should be performed in all children during the acute stage of febrile urinary tract infections.

IMAGING STUDIES

RENAL ULTRASONOGRAPHY. The presence of a dilated urinary tract is the most common characteristic of obstruction. Hydronephrosis is a common ultrasonographic finding (Fig. 540-1). Dilation is not always indicative of obstruction and may persist after surgical correction of an obstructive lesion. Dilation may result from vesicoureteral reflux, or it may be a manifestation of abnormal development of the urinary tract, even when there is no obstruction. Renal length, degree of caliectasis and parenchymal thickness, and presence or absence of ureteral dilation should be assessed. Ideally, the severity of hydronephrosis should be graded from 1 to 4 using the Society for Fetal Urology grading scale (Table 540-2). The clinician should ascertain that the contralateral kidney is normal, and the bladder should be imaged to see whether the bladder wall is thickened, the lower ureter is dilated, and bladder emptying is complete. In acute or intermittent obstruction, the dilation of the collecting system may be minimal and ultrasonography may be misleading.

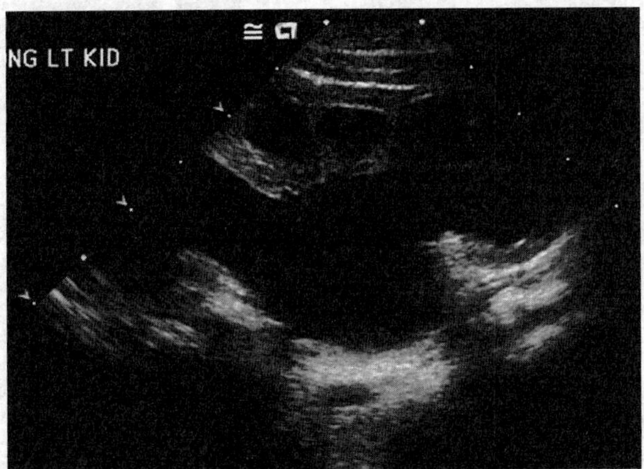

Figure 540-1. Ultrasonographic image of the left kidney with marked pelvic and calyceal dilatation (grade 4 hydronephrosis) in a boy with ureteropelvic junction obstruction.

TABLE 540-2. Society for Fetal Urology Grading System for Hydronephrosis

GRADE OF HYDRONEPHROSIS	RENAL IMAGE: CENTRAL RENAL COMPLEX	RENAL IMAGE: RENAL PARENCHYMAL THICKNESS
0	Intact	Normal
1	Slight splitting	Normal
2	Evident splitting, complex confined within renal border	Normal
3	Wide splitting pelvis dilated outside renal border, calyces uniformly dilated	Normal
4	Further dilatation of pelvis and calyces (calyces may appear convex)	Thin

After Maizels M, Mitchell B, Kass E, et al: Outcome of nonspecific hydronephrosis in the infant: A report from the registry of the Society for Fetal Urology. *J Urol* 1994;152:2324.

VOIDING CYSTOURETHROGRAM. In all cases of congenital hydronephrosis and in any child with ureteral dilatation, a voiding cystourethrogram (VCUG) should be obtained, because the dilation is secondary to vesicoureteral reflux in 15% of cases. In boys, the VCUG also is necessary to rule out urethral obstruction, particularly in cases of suspected posterior urethral valves. In infravesical obstruction in infants, the bladder may be palpable because of chronic distention and incomplete emptying. In older children, the urinary flow rate can be measured noninvasively with a urinary flowmeter; decreased flow with a normal bladder contraction is suggestive of infravesical obstruction. When the urethra cannot be catheterized to obtain a VCUG, the clinician should suspect a urethral stricture or an obstructive urethral lesion. Retrograde urethrography with contrast medium injected into the urethral meatus helps delineate the anatomy of the urethral obstruction.

RADIOISOTOPE STUDIES. Renal scintigraphy is used to assess renal anatomy and function. The two most commonly used radiopharmaceuticals are mercaptoacetyl triglycine (MAG-3) and technetium-99m-labeled dimercaptosuccinic acid (DMSA). MAG-3, which is excreted by renal tubular secretion, is used to assess differential renal function, and, when furosemide is administered, drainage also can be measured. An alternative to MAG-3 is diethylene tetrapentaacetic acid (DTPA), which is cleared by glomerular filtration. The background activity of DTPA is much higher than that of MAG-3. DMSA is a renal cortical imaging agent and is used to assess differential renal function and to demonstrate whether renal scarring is present. It is used infrequently in children with obstructive uropathy.

In a MAG-3 diuretic renogram, a small dose of technetium-labeled MAG-3 is injected intravenously (Figs. 540-2 and 540-3). During the first 2–3 min, renal parenchymal uptake is analyzed and compared, allowing computation of differential renal function. Subsequently, excretion is evaluated. After 20–30 min, furosemide is injected intravenously, and the rapidity and pattern of drainage from the kidneys to the bladder are analyzed. If no obstruction is present, half of the radionuclide should be cleared from the renal pelvis within 10–15 min, termed the *half-life* ($t^1\!/_2$). If there is significant upper tract obstruction, the $t^1\!/_2$ usually is >20 min. A $t^1\!/_2$ between 15–20 min is indeterminate. The images generated usually provide an accurate assessment of the site of obstruction. Numerous variables affect the outcome of the diuretic renogram. Newborn kidneys are functionally immature, and, in some cases, normal kidneys may not demonstrate normal drainage after diuretic administration. Dehydration prolongs parenchymal transit and can blunt the diuretic response. Giving an insufficient dose of furosemide may result in inadequate drainage. If vesicoureteral reflux is present, continuous catheter drainage is mandatory to prevent the radionuclide from refluxing from the bladder into the dilated upper tract, which would prolong the washout phase. In response to the numerous

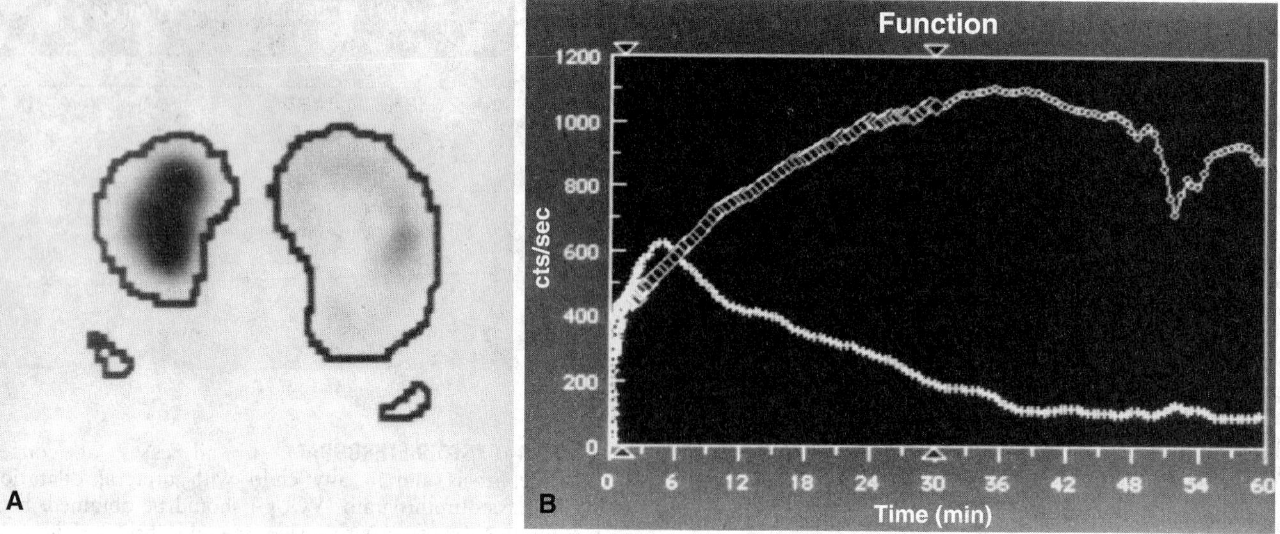

Figure 540-2. MAG-3 diuretic renogram in a 6 wk old infant with right hydronephrosis detected by prenatal ultrasonography. The right kidney is on the right side of the image. *A*, Differential renal function: left kidney 70%, right kidney 30%. *B*, After administration of furosemide, drainage from the left kidney was normal and drainage from the right kidney was slow, consistent with right ureteropelvic junction obstruction. Pyeloplasty was performed on the right kidney.

variables, the Society for Fetal Urology and the Pediatric Nuclear Medicine Club jointly developed a standardized method for performing diuretic renography in infants and children, termed the *well-tempered renogram.*

The MAG-3 diuretic renogram is considered superior to the excretory urogram in infants and children with hydronephrosis, because bowel gas and immaturity of renal function often cause the intravenous pyelogram (IVP) images to be suboptimal. In addition, the diuretic renogram provides an objective assessment of the relative function of each kidney.

EXCRETORY UROGRAM. Although used infrequently for imaging the urinary tract in children, the IVP is useful in selected cases (Fig. 540-4). The plain film of the abdomen should be inspected for calculi, spinal abnormalities, and an abnormal intestinal gas pattern or severe constipation. In infravesical obstruction, the bladder wall is irregular or trabeculated because of detrusor hypertrophy. A postvoid film may show residual bladder urine. In ureteral obstruction, the collecting system is dilated above the obstruction and the calyces are blunted. Concentration of the radiopaque medium on the obstructed side is impaired, and the appearance of contrast medium in the collecting system may be delayed, with progressive increase in concentration at the point of obstruction when delayed radiographs are obtained. In high-grade obstruction, the contrast agent may remain in the collecting system after 24 hr.

Urinary extravasation can be detected in the early or delayed films of a urographic study as well as on an MAG-3 renogram. When intermittent obstruction is suspected, intravenous urography during an acute episode of pain is often the most valuable diagnostic study.

MR UROGRAPHY. The newest study used to evaluate suspected upper urinary tract pathology is MR urography. The child is hydrated and given intravenous furosemide. Next, gadolinium-DTPA is injected and routine T1-weighted and fat-suppressed fast spin-echo T2-weighted imaging is performed through the kidneys, ureters, and bladder. This study provides superb images of the pathology, and methodology is being developed to allow assessment of differential renal function.

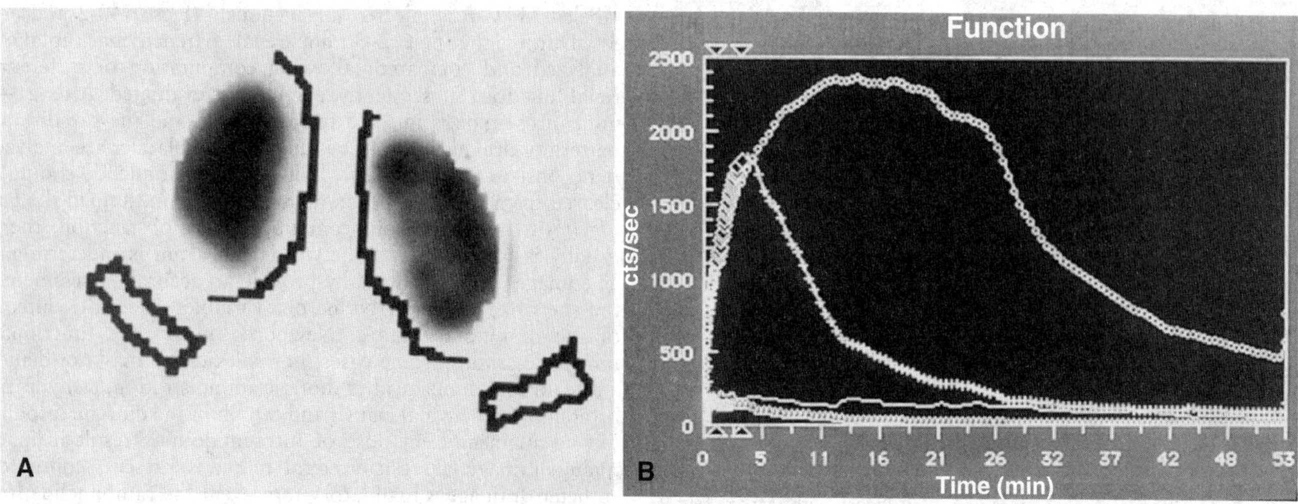

Figure 540-3. Same patient as in Figure 540-2. *A*, MAG-3 diuretic renogram at 14 mo of age shows equal function in the two kidneys and *B*, prompt drainage after the administration of furosemide.

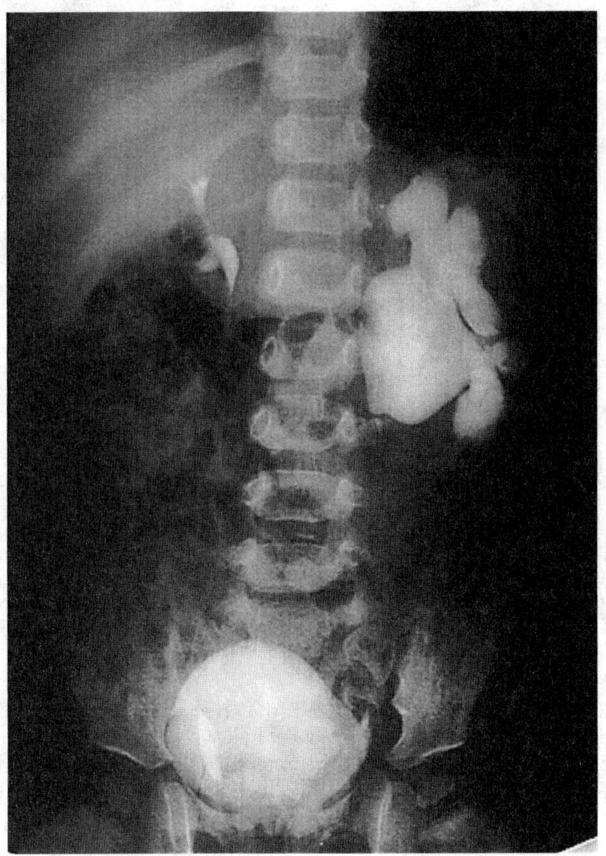

Figure 540-4. Excretory urogram in a boy, showing dilatation of the left renal pelvis and blunting of the calyces characteristic of a ureteropelvic junction obstruction.

COMPUTED TOMOGRAPHY. In children with a suspected ureteral calculus, noncontrast spiral CT of the abdomen and pelvis is a standard method of demonstrating whether a calculus (or calculi) is present, its location, and whether there is significant proximal hydronephrosis. This study is the initial study of choice in these patients.

ANCILLARY STUDIES. In unusual cases, an **antegrade pyelogram** (insertion of a percutaneous nephrostomy tube and injection of contrast agent), can be performed to assess the anatomy of the upper urinary tract. This procedure usually requires general anesthesia. In addition, an **antegrade pressure-perfusion flow study** ("Whitaker test") may be performed, in which fluid is infused at a measured rate, usually 10 mL/min. The pressures in the renal pelvis and the bladder are monitored during this infusion, and pressure differences exceeding 20 cm H_2O are suggestive of obstruction. In other cases, cystoscopy with retrograde pyelography provides excellent images of the upper urinary tract (Fig. 540-5).

SPECIFIC TYPES OF URINARY TRACT OBSTRUCTION AND THEIR TREATMENT

HYDROCALYCOSIS. The term *hydrocalycosis* refers to a localized dilatation of the calyx caused by obstruction of its infundibulum, termed *infundibular stenosis*. Such obstruction can be developmental in origin or secondary to inflammatory processes, such as UTI. When the abnormality is not discovered by antenatal ultrasonography or incidentally, it usually is discovered during evaluation for pain or UTI. The diagnosis of infundibular stenosis is usually established by IVP or CT scan with contrast.

URETEROPELVIC JUNCTION OBSTRUCTION. Ureteropelvic junction (UPJ) obstruction is the most common obstructive lesion in childhood and usually is caused by intrinsic stenosis (see Figs. 540-1 through 540-4). An accessory artery to the lower pole of the kidney also may cause extrinsic obstruction. The typical appearance on ultrasonography is grade 3 or 4 hydronephrosis without a dilated ureter. UPJ obstruction most commonly presents (1) on maternal ultrasonography revealing fetal hydronephrosis; (2) as a palpable renal mass in a newborn or infant; (3) as abdominal, flank, or back pain; (4) as a febrile UTI; or (5) as hematuria after minimal trauma. Approximately 60% of cases occur on the left side, and the male : female ratio is 2 : 1. In 10% of cases UPJ obstruction is bilateral. In kidneys with UPJ obstruction, renal function may be significantly impaired from pressure atrophy, but approximately half of affected kidneys have relatively normal function. The anomaly is corrected by performing a pyeloplasty, in which the stenotic segment is excised and the normal ureter and renal pelvis are reattached. Success rates are 91–98%. In many institutions pyeloplasty is performed using laparoscopic techniques, often robotic-assisted.

Lesser degrees of UPJ obstruction may cause mild hydronephrosis, which usually is nonobstructive, and typically these kidneys function normally. The spectrum of UPJ abnormalities has been referred to as *anomalous UPJ*. Another cause of mild hydronephrosis is fetal folds of the upper ureter, which also are nonobstructive.

The diagnosis can be difficult to establish in an asymptomatic infant in whom dilatation of the renal pelvis is found incidentally in a prenatal ultrasonogram. After birth, the sonographic study is repeated to confirm the prenatal finding. A VCUG is necessary because 10–15% of patients have ipsilateral vesicoureteral reflux. Because neonatal oliguria may cause temporary decompression of a dilated renal pelvis, it is ideal to perform the first postnatal

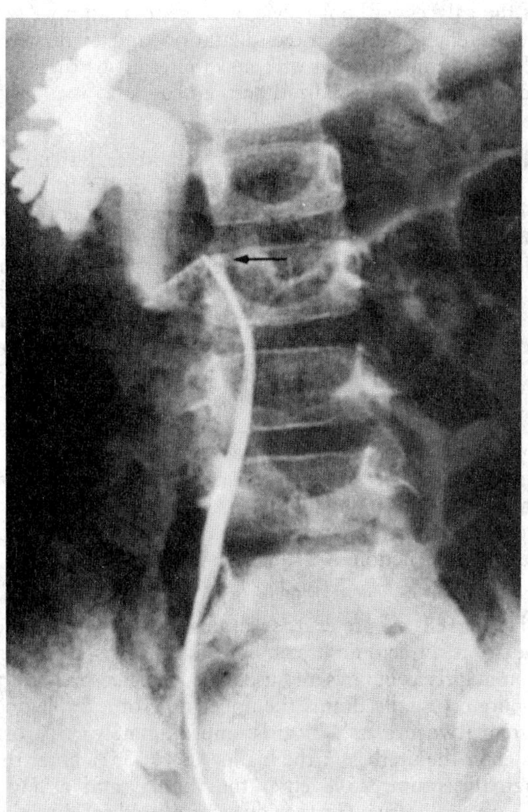

Figure 540-5. Retrograde pyelogram showing medial deviation of a dilated upper ureter to the level of the 3rd lumbar vertebra, characteristic of a retrocaval ureter.

sonogram after the 3rd day of life. However, delaying the sonogram may be impractical. If no dilation is found on the initial sonogram, a repeat study should be performed at 1 mo of age. If the kidney shows grade 1 or 2 hydronephrosis and the renal parenchyma appears normal, a period of observation usually is appropriate, with sequential renal ultrasonograms to monitor the severity of hydronephrosis, and the hydronephrosis usually disappears. The child should receive **antibiotic prophylaxis,** usually trimethoprim-sulfamethoxazole or trimethoprim, although amoxicillin is preferable before 2 mo of age. If the hydronephrosis is grade 3 or 4, spontaneous resolution is less likely and obstruction is more likely to be present, particularly if the renal pelvic diameter is 2 cm. A diuretic renogram with MAG-3 is performed at 4–6 wk of age. If there is poor upper tract drainage or the differential renal function is poor, pyeloplasty is recommended. After pyeloplasty the differential renal function often improves, and improved drainage with furosemide stimulation is expected.

If the differential function on renography is normal, and drainage is satisfactory, the infant can be followed with serial ultrasonograms, even with grade 4 hydronephrosis. If the hydronephrosis remains severe with no improvement, a repeat diuretic renogram after 6–12 mo may help in the decision between continued observation and surgical repair. Prompt surgical repair is indicated in infants with an abdominal mass, bilateral severe hydronephrosis, a solitary kidney, or diminished function in the involved kidney. In unusual cases in which the differential renal function is less than 10% but the kidney definitely has some function, insertion of a percutaneous nephrostomy tube allows drainage of the hydronephrotic kidney for a few weeks to allow reassessment of renal function. In older children who present with symptoms, the diagnosis of UPJ obstruction usually is established by ultrasonography and diuretic renography.

The following entities should be considered in the **differential diagnosis:** (1) megacalycosis, a congenital nonobstructive dilatation of the calyces without pelvic or ureteric dilatation; (2) vesicoureteral reflux with marked dilatation and kinking of the ureter; and (3) midureteral or distal ureteral obstruction when the ureter is not well visualized on the urogram.

MIDURETERAL OBSTRUCTION. Congenital ureteral stenosis or a ureteral valve in the midureter is rare. It is corrected by excision of the strictured segment and reanastomosis of the normal upper and lower ureteral segments. A retrocaval ureter is an anomaly in which the upper right ureter travels posterior to the inferior vena cava. In this anomaly, the vena cava may cause extrinsic compression and obstruction. An IVP shows the right ureter to be medially deviated at the level of the 3rd lumbar vertebra. The diagnosis may be confirmed by retrograde pyelography (see Fig. 540-5). Surgical treatment consists of transection of the upper ureter, moving it anterior to the vena cava, and reanastomosing the upper and lower segments. Repair is necessary only when obstruction is present. Retroperitoneal tumors, fibrosis caused by surgical procedures, inflammatory processes (as in chronic granulomatous disease), and radiation therapy can cause acquired midureteral obstruction.

ECTOPIC URETER. A ureter that drains outside the bladder is referred to as an **ectopic ureter.** This anomaly is three times as common in girls as in boys and usually is detected prenatally. The ectopic ureter usually drains the upper pole of a duplex collecting system (two ureters). In girls, approximately 35% of these ureters enter the urethra at the bladder neck, 35% enter the urethrovaginal septum, 25% enter the vagina, and a few drain into the cervix, uterus, Gartner duct, or a urethral diverticulum. Often the terminal aspect of the ureter is narrowed, causing hydroureteronephrosis. With the exception of the ectopic ureter entering the bladder neck, in girls an ectopic ureter causes continuous urinary incontinence from the affected renal moiety. UTI is common because of urinary stasis. In boys, ectopic ureters enter the posterior urethra (above the external sphincter) in 47%, the prostatic utricle in 10%, the seminal vesicle in 33%, the ejaculatory duct in 5%, and the vas deferens in 5%. Consequently, in boys, an ectopic ureter does not cause incontinence, and most patients present with a UTI or epididymitis. Evaluation includes a renal sonogram, VCUG, and renal scan, which demonstrates whether the affected segment has significant function. The sonogram shows the affected hydronephrotic kidney or dilated upper pole and ureter down to the bladder (Fig. 540-6). If the ectopic ureter drains into the bladder neck (female), a VCUG usually shows reflux into the ureter. Otherwise, there is no reflux into the ectopic ureter, but there may be reflux into the ipsilateral lower pole ureter or contralateral collecting system.

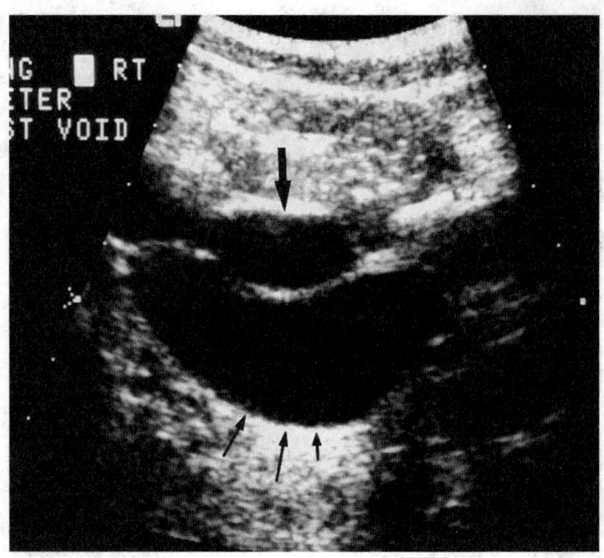

Figure 540-6. Ultrasonographic image of the right dilated ureter *(thin arrows)* extending behind and caudal to a nearly empty bladder *(arrow)* in a girl with urinary incontinence and ectopic ureter draining into the vagina.

Treatment depends on the status of the renal unit drained by the ectopic ureter. If there is satisfactory function, ureteral reimplantation into the bladder or ureteroureterostomy (anastomosing the ectopic upper pole ureter into the normally inserting lower pole ureter) is indicated. If function is poor, partial or total nephrectomy is indicated. In many centers this procedure is done laparoscopically.

URETEROCELE. A ureterocele is a cystic dilatation of the terminal ureter and is obstructive because of a pinpoint ureteral orifice. Ureteroceles are much more common in girls than in boys. Affected children usually are discovered by prenatal ultrasonography, but some may present with a UTI. Ureteroceles may be ectopic, in which case the cystic swelling extends through the bladder neck into the urethra, or orthotopic, in which case the ureterocele is entirely within the bladder. Both orthotopic and ectopic ureteroceles can be bilateral.

In girls, ureteroceles nearly always are associated with ureteral duplication (Fig. 540-7), whereas in 50% of affected boys there is only one ureter. When associated with a duplication, the ureterocele drains the upper renal moiety, which commonly functions poorly or is dysplastic because of congenital obstruction. The lower pole ureter drains into the bladder superior and lateral to the upper pole ureter and frequently refluxes.

An **ectopic ureterocele** extends submucosally into the urethra. Rarely, large ectopic ureteroceles may cause bladder outlet obstruction and retention of urine with bilateral hydronephrosis; in girls, the ureterocele may prolapse from the urethral meatus.

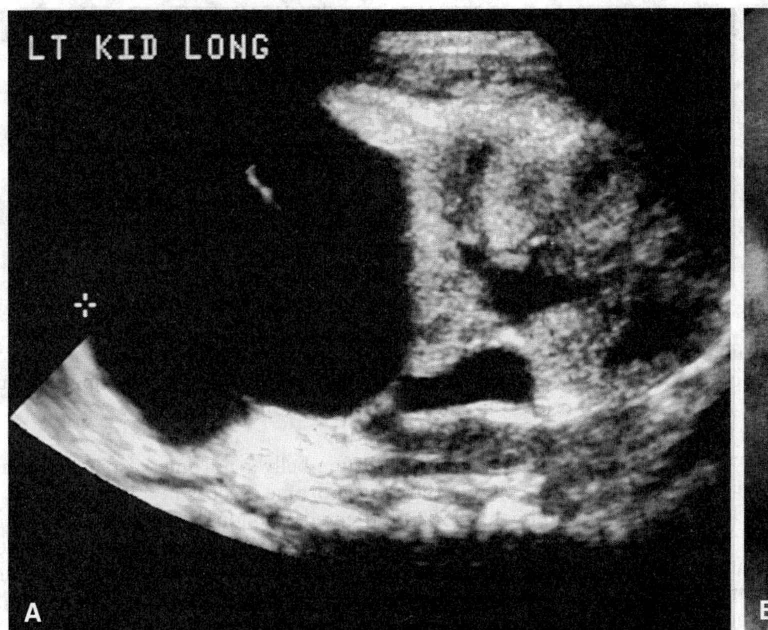

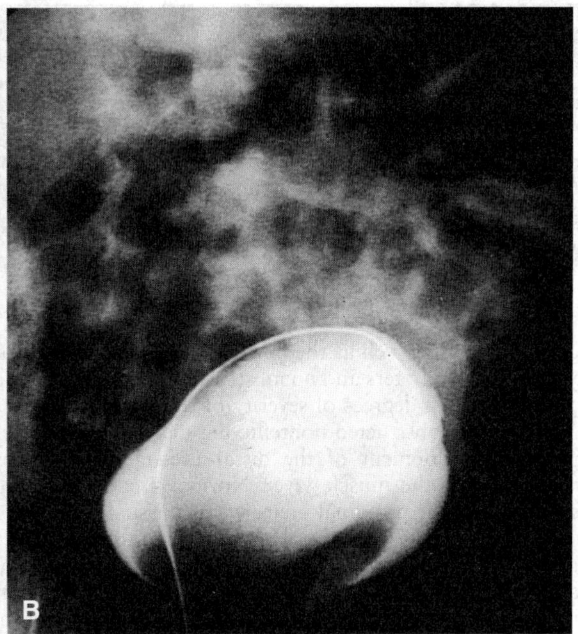

Figure 540-7. *A*, Infant with ectopic ureterocele. Sonogram of the left kidney shows massive dilation of the upper pole and a normal lower pole. *B*, VCUG shows large ureterocele, draining the left upper pole, in the bladder. No reflux is present.

Ultrasonography is effective in demonstrating the ureterocele and whether the associated obstructed system is duplicated or single. VCUG usually shows a filling defect in the bladder, sometimes large, corresponding to the ureterocele, and often shows reflux into the adjacent lower pole collecting system with typical findings of a "drooping lily" appearance to the kidney. Nuclear renal scintigraphy is most accurate in demonstrating whether the affected renal moiety has significant function.

Treatment of ectopic ureteroceles varies among different medical centers and depends on whether the upper pole functions on renal scan and whether there is reflux into the lower pole ureter. If there is non-function of the upper pole and there is no reflux, treatment usually involves laparoscopic or open excision of the obstructed upper pole and most of the associated ureter. If there is function in the upper pole or significant reflux into the lower pole ureter, or if the patient is septic from infection of the hydronephrotic kidney, then transurethral incision with cautery or the holmium : YAG laser is appropriate initial therapy to decompress the ureterocele. However, reflux into the incised ureterocele is common, and subsequent excision of the ureterocele and ureteral reimplantation usually is necessary.

Orthotopic ureteroceles are associated with duplicated or single collecting systems, and the orifice is in the expected location in the bladder (Fig. 540-8). These anomalies usually are discovered during an investigation for prenatal hydronephrosis or a UTI. Ultrasonography is sensitive for detecting the ureterocele in the bladder and hydroureteronephrosis. IVP reveals varying degrees of ureteral and calyceal dilatation, and there is a round filling defect in the bladder. In delayed films, cystic dilatation of the ureter may be clearly visible and full of contrast material. Transurethral incision of the ureterocele effectively relieves the obstruction, but it may result in vesicoureteral reflux, necessitating ureteral reimplantation later. Some prefer open excision of the ureterocele and reimplantation as the initial form of treatment. Small, simple ureteroceles discovered incidentally without upper tract dilatation may not require treatment.

MEGAURETER. Table 540-3 presents a classification of megaureters (dilated ureter). Numerous disorders can cause ureteral dilation, and many are nonobstructive.

Megaureters usually are discovered through screening ultrasonography of the kidneys and bladder because of either a prenatal diagnosis of hydronephrosis or postnatal UTI, hematuria, or abdominal pain. A careful history, physical examination, and VCUG identify causes of secondary megaureters and reflux-

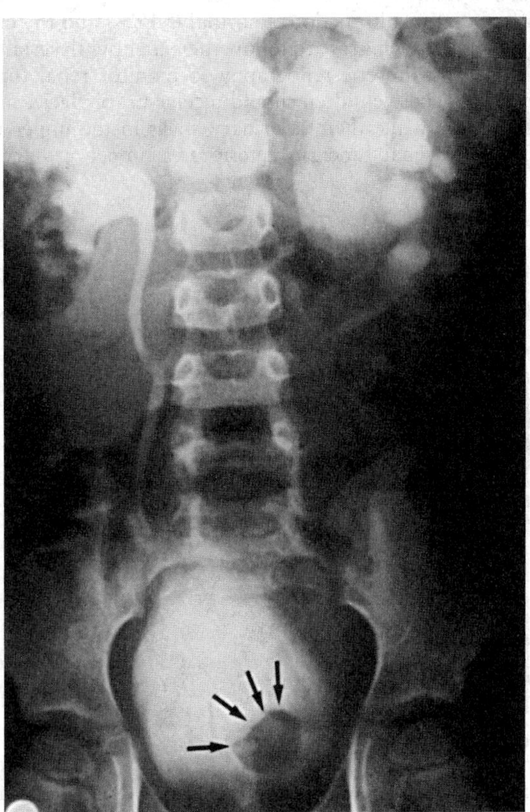

Figure 540-8. Simple intravesical ureterocele. The excretory urogram shows left hydronephrosis and a round filling defect on the left side of the bladder corresponding to a simple ureterocele causing left ureteral obstruction. This lesion was treated by transurethral incision and drainage of the ureterocele.

TABLE 540-3. Classification of Megaureter

REFLUXING		OBSTRUCTED		NONREFLUXING AND NONOBSTRUCTED	
PRIMARY	SECONDARY	PRIMARY	SECONDARY	PRIMARY	SECONDARY
Primary reflux	Neuropathic bladder	Intrinsic (primary obstructed megaureter)	Neuropathic bladder	Nonrefluxing, nonobstructive	Diabetes insipidus
Megacystic-megaureter syndrome	Hinman syndrome	Ureteral valve	Hinman syndrome		Infection
Ectopic ureter	Posterior urethral valves	Ectopic ureter	Posterior urethral valves		Persistent after relief of obstruction
Prune-belly syndrome	Bladder diverticulum	Ectopic uretocele	Ureteral calculus		
	Postoperative		Extrinsic		
			Postoperative		

ing megaureters as well as the "prune-belly" syndrome. Primary obstructed megaureters and nonobstructed megaureters probably represent varying degrees of severity of the same anomaly.

The primary obstructed nonrefluxing megaureter results from abnormal development of the distal ureter, with collagenous tissue replacing the muscle layer. Normal ureteral peristalsis is disrupted, and the proximal ureter widens. Usually there is not a true stricture. On IVP, the distal ureter is more dilated in its distal segment and tapers abruptly at or above the junction of the bladder (Fig. 540-9). The lesion may be unilateral or bilateral. Dilation of the upper collecting system and calyceal blunting are suggestive of obstruction. Megaureter predisposes to UTI, urinary stones, hematuria, or flank pain because of urinary stasis. In most cases, diuretic renography and sequential sonographic studies can differentiate obstructed from nonobstructed megaureters reliably. In most nonobstructed megaureters, the hydroureteronephrosis diminishes gradually (Fig. 540-10). Truly obstructed megaureters require surgical treatment, with excision of the narrowed segment, ureteral tapering, and reimplantation of the ureter. The results of surgical reconstruction usually are good, but the prognosis depends on pre-existing renal function and whether complications develop.

If differential renal function is normal (>45%) and the child is asymptomatic, it seems safe to follow the patient with serial ultrasonography and diuretic renography to monitor renal function and drainage. These children should receive prophylactic antimicrobial therapy while there is urinary stasis in the upper ureter and kidney. If renal function deteriorates, upper urinary tract drainage slows, or UTI occurs, ureteral reimplantation is recommended. From 20–30% of children with a nonrefluxing megaureter undergo ureteral reimplantation.

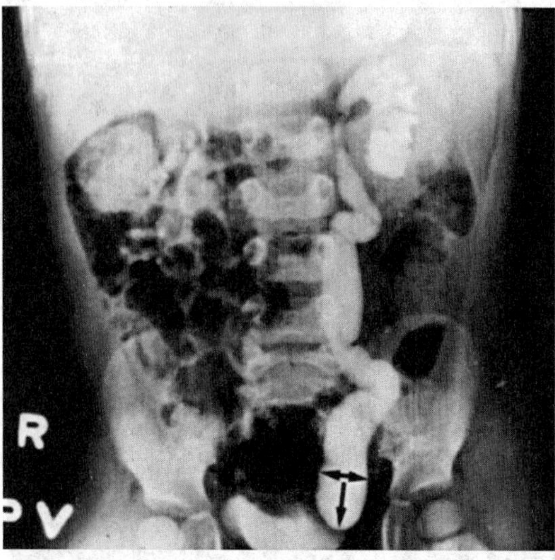

Figure 540-9. Obstructed nonrefluxing megaureter. Excretory urogram in a girl with a history of a febrile urinary tract infection. The right side is normal. The left side reveals hydroureteronephrosis with predominant dilatation of the distal ureter. Note the characteristic appearance of the distal ureter. There was no vesicoureteral reflux. The diagnosis of obstruction was confirmed by diuretic renography.

PRUNE-BELLY SYNDROME. Prune-belly syndrome, also called **triad syndrome** or **Eagle-Barrett syndrome,** occurs in approximately 1 in 40,000 births; 95% of affected individuals are male. The characteristic association of deficient abdominal muscles, undescended testes, and urinary tract abnormalities probably results from severe urethral obstruction in fetal life (Fig. 540-11). Oligohydramnios and pulmonary hypoplasia are common complications in the perinatal period. Many affected infants are stillborn. Urinary tract abnormalities include massive dilatation of the ureters and upper tracts and a very large bladder, with a patent urachus or a urachal diverticulum. Most patients have vesicoureteral reflux. The prostatic urethra usually is dilated, and the prostate is hypoplastic. The anterior urethra may be dilated, resulting in a megalourethra. Rarely, there is urethral stenosis or atresia. The kidneys usually show various degrees of dysplasia, and the testes usually are intra-abdominal. Malrotation of the bowel often is present. Cardiac abnormalities occur in 10% of cases; more than 50% have abnormalities of the musculoskeletal system, including limb abnormalities and scoliosis. In girls, anomalies of the urethra, uterus, and vagina usually are present.

Many neonates with prune-belly syndrome have difficulty with effective bladder emptying because the bladder musculature is poorly developed, and the urethra may be narrowed. When no obstruction is present, the goal of treatment is the prevention of urinary tract infection with antibiotic prophylaxis. When obstruction of the ureters or urethra is demonstrated, temporary drainage procedures, such as a vesicostomy, may help to preserve renal function until the child is old enough for surgery. Some children with prune-belly syndrome have been found to have classic or atypical posterior urethral valves. Urinary tract infections occur often and should be treated promptly. Correction of the undescended testes by orchidopexy can be difficult in these children because the testes are located high in the abdomen and is best accomplished in the first 6 mo of life. Reconstruction of the abdominal wall offers cosmetic and functional benefits.

The prognosis ultimately depends on the degree of pulmonary hypoplasia and renal dysplasia. One-third of children with prune-belly syndrome are stillborn or die in the first few months of life because of pulmonary complications. As many as 30% of the long-term survivors develop end-stage renal disease from dysplasia or complications of infection or reflux and eventually require renal transplantation. Renal transplantation in these children offers good results.

BLADDER NECK OBSTRUCTION. Bladder neck obstruction usually is secondary to ectopic ureterocele, bladder calculi, or a tumor of the prostate (rhabdomyosarcoma). The manifestations include difficulty voiding, urinary retention, urinary tract infection, and bladder distention with overflow incontinence. Apparent bladder neck obstruction is common in cases of posterior urethral valves, but it seldom has any functional significance. Primary bladder neck obstruction is extremely rare.

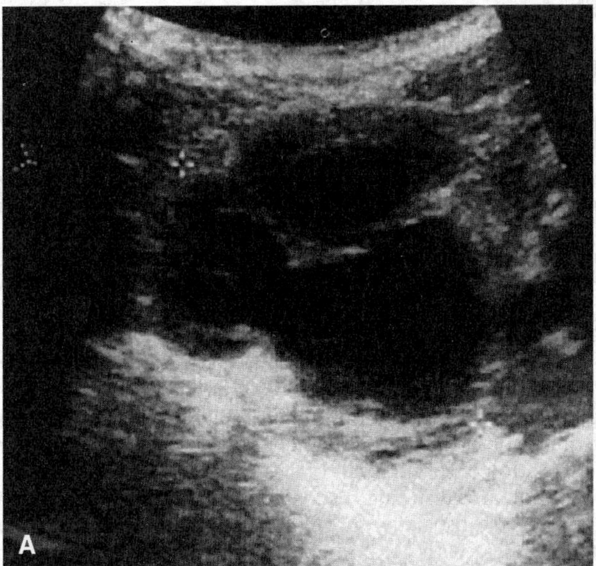

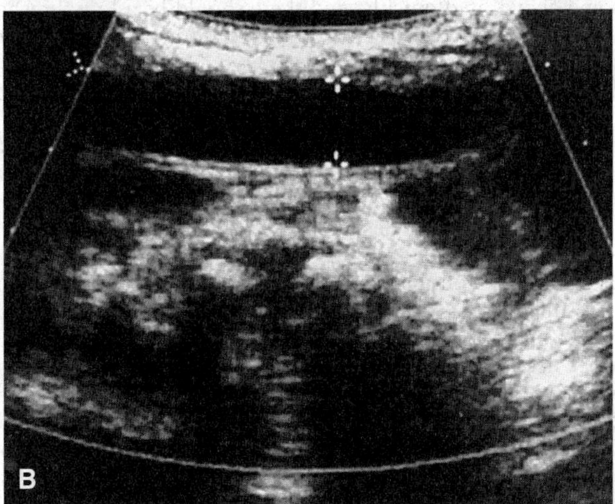

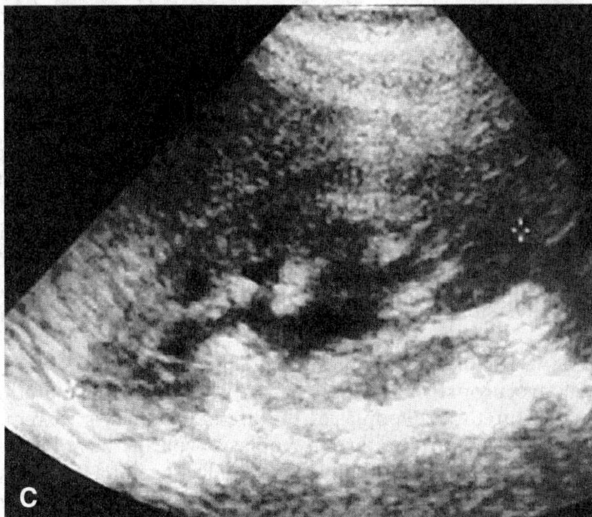

Figure 540-10. Neonate with primary nonrefluxing megaureter. *A,* Renal sonogram shows grade 4 hydronephrosis. *B,* Dilated ureter. Renal scan showed equal function with the contralateral kidney and satisfactory drainage with diuresis stimulation. *C,* Follow-up sonogram at 10 months shows complete resolution of hydronephrosis.

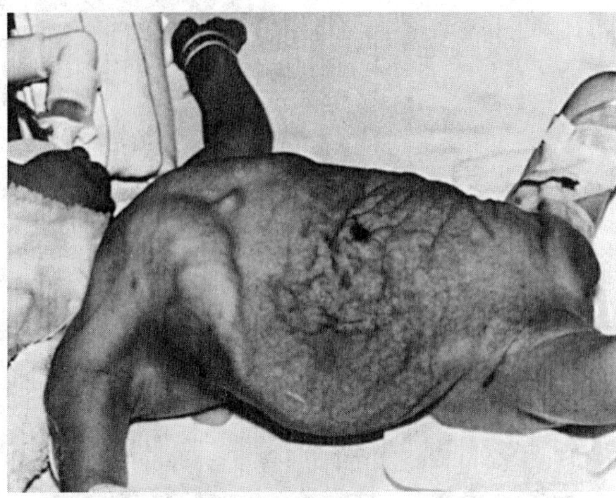

Figure 540-11. Photograph of a 1,600-g newborn with the prune-belly syndrome. Note the lack of tonicity of the abdominal wall and the wrinkled appearance of the skin.

POSTERIOR URETHRAL VALVES. The most common cause of severe obstructive uropathy in children is posterior urethral valves, affecting 1 in 8,000 boys. The urethral valves are tissue leaflets fanning distally from the prostatic urethra to the external urinary sphincter. A slit-like opening usually separates the leaflets. Valves are of unclear embryologic origin and cause varying degrees of obstruction. Approximately 30% of patients experience end-stage renal disease or chronic renal insufficiency. The prostatic urethra dilates, and the bladder muscle undergoes hypertrophy. Vesicoureteral reflux occurs in 50% of patients, and distal ureteral obstruction may result from a chronically distended bladder or bladder muscle hypertrophy. The renal changes range from mild hydronephrosis to severe renal dysplasia; their severity probably depends on the severity of the obstruction and its time of onset during fetal development. As in other cases of obstruction or renal dysplasia, there may be oligohydramnios and pulmonary hypoplasia.

Affected boys with posterior urethral valves are discovered prenatally when maternal ultrasonography reveals bilateral hydronephrosis, a distended bladder, and, if the obstruction is severe, oligohydramnios. Prenatal bladder decompression by percutaneous vesicoamniotic shunt or open fetal surgery has been reported. Experimental and clinical evidence of the possible benefits of fetal intervention is lacking, and few affected fetuses are candidates. Prenatally diagnosed posterior urethral valves, particularly when discovered in the second trimester, carry a poorer prognosis than those detected after birth. In the male neonate, posterior urethral valves are suspected when there is a palpably **distended bladder** and the **urinary stream is weak.** If the obstruction is severe and goes unrecognized during the neonatal period, infants may present later in life with failure to thrive due to uremia or sepsis caused by infection in the obstructed urinary tract. With lesser degrees of obstruction, children present later in life with difficulty in achieving diurnal urinary continence or with UTI. The diagnosis is established with a VCUG (Fig. 540-12) or by perineal ultrasonography.

After the diagnosis is established, renal function and the anatomy of the upper urinary tract should be carefully evaluated. In the healthy neonate, a small polyethylene feeding tube (No. 5 or No. 8 French) is inserted in the bladder and left for several days. Passing the feeding tube may be difficult, because the tip of the tube may coil in the prostatic urethra. A sign of this problem is that urine drains around the catheter rather than through it. A Foley (balloon) catheter should not be used, because the balloon may cause severe bladder spasm, which may produce severe ureteral obstruction.

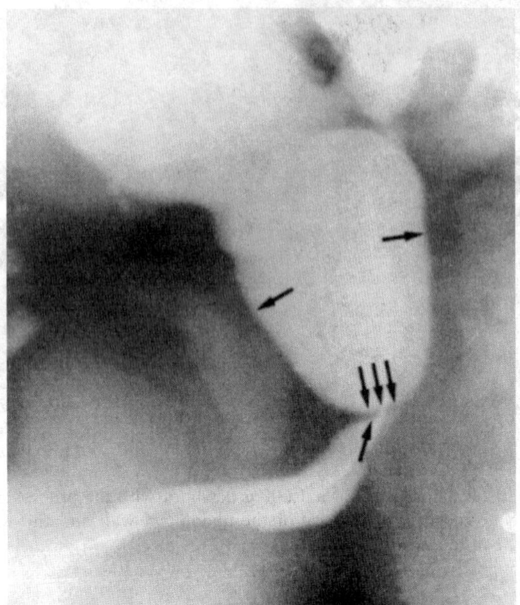

Figure 540-12. Voiding cystourethrogram in an infant with posterior urethral valves. Note the dilation of the prostatic urethra and the transverse linear filling defect corresponding to the valves.

If the serum creatinine level remains normal or returns to normal, treatment consists of transurethral ablation of the valve leaflets, which is performed endoscopically under general anesthesia. If the urethra is too small for transurethral ablation, temporary vesicostomy is preferred, in which the dome of the bladder is exteriorized on the lower abdominal wall. When the child is older, the valves may be ablated and the vesicostomy closed.

If the serum creatinine level remains high or increases despite bladder drainage by a small catheter, secondary ureteral obstruction, irreversible renal damage, or renal dysplasia should be suspected. In such cases, a vesicostomy should be performed. Cutaneous pyelostomy rarely affords better drainage when compared with cutaneous vesicostomy, and the latter also allows continued bladder growth and gradual improvement in bladder wall compliance.

In the septic and uremic infant, lifesaving measures must include prompt correction of the electrolyte imbalance and control of the infection by appropriate antibiotics. Drainage of the upper tracts by percutaneous nephrostomy and hemodialysis may be necessary. After the patient's condition becomes stable, evaluation and treatment can be undertaken. Some older boys are diagnosed with valves because of a poor stream, diurnal incontinence, or a UTI; these boys generally are treated by primary valve ablation.

Favorable prognostic factors include a normal prenatal ultrasonogram between 18 and 24 wk of gestation, a serum creatinine level <0.8–1.0 mg/dL after bladder decompression, and visualization of the corticomedullary junction on renal sonography. In several situations, a "popoff valve" may occur during urinary tract development, which preserves the integrity of one or both kidneys. For example, 15% of boys with posterior urethral valves have unilateral reflux into a nonfunctioning dysplastic kidney, termed the **VURD syndrome** (*v*alves, *u*nilateral *r*eflux, *d*ysplasia). In these boys, the high bladder pressure is dissipated into the nonfunctioning kidney, allowing normal development of the contralateral kidney. In newborn boys with urinary ascites, the urine generally leaks out from the obstructed collecting system through the renal fornices, allowing normal renal development. Unfavorable prognostic factors include the presence of oligohydramnios in utero, identification of hydronephrosis before 24 wk of gestation, a serum creatinine level >1.0 mg/dL after bladder decompression, identification of cortical cysts in both kidneys, and persistence of diurnal incontinence beyond 5 yr of age.

The prognosis in the newborn is related to the child's degree of pulmonary hypoplasia and potential for recovery of renal function. Severely affected infants often are stillborn. Of those who survive the neonatal period, approximately 30% retain some degree of renal insufficiency, and many eventually require renal transplantation. In some series, renal transplantation in children with posterior urethral valves has a lower success rate than does transplantation in children with normal bladders, presumably because of the adverse influence of altered bladder function on graft function and survival.

After valve ablation, antimicrobial prophylaxis is beneficial in preventing UTI, because hydronephrosis to some degree often persists for many years. These boys should be evaluated annually with a renal ultrasonogram, physical examination including assessment of somatic growth and blood pressure, urinalysis, and determination of serum levels of electrolytes. Many boys have significant polyuria resulting from a concentrating defect secondary to prolonged obstructive uropathy. If these children acquire a systemic illness with vomiting or diarrhea, or both, urine output cannot be used to assess the child's hydration status. They can become dehydrated quickly, and there should be a low threshold for hospital admission for intravenous rehydration. Some of these patients have renal tubular acidosis, requiring oral bicarbonate therapy. If there is any significant degree of renal dysfunction, growth impairment, or hypertension, they should be followed closely by a pediatric nephrologist. When vesicoureteral reflux is present, expectant treatment and prophylactic doses of antibacterial drugs are advisable. If breakthrough UTI occurs, surgical correction should be undertaken.

After treatment, boys with urethral valves often do not achieve diurnal urinary continence as early as other boys. Incontinence may result from a combination of factors, including uninhibited bladder contractions, poor bladder compliance, bladder atonia, bladder neck dyssynergia, or polyuria. Often these boys require urodynamic evaluation with urodynamics or videourodynamics to plan therapy. Boys with noncompliance are at significant risk for ongoing renal damage, even in the absence of infection. Overnight catheter drainage has been shown to be beneficial in boys with polyuria and may help preserve renal function. Urinary incontinence usually improves with age, particularly after puberty. Meticulous attention to bladder compliance, emptying, and infection may improve results in the future.

URETHRAL ATRESIA. The most severe form of obstructive uropathy in boys is urethral atresia. In utero there is a distended bladder, bilateral hydroureteronephrosis, and oligohydramnios. In most cases, these infants are stillborn or succumb to pulmonary hypoplasia. Some boys with prune-belly syndrome also have urethral atresia. If the urachus is patent, oligohydramnios is unlikely and the infant usually survives. Urethral reconstruction is difficult, and most patients are managed with continent urinary diversion.

URETHRAL HYPOPLASIA. Urethral hypoplasia is a rare form of obstructive uropathy in boys that is less severe than urethral atresia. In urethral hypoplasia, the urethral lumen is extremely small. Neonates with urethral hypoplasia typically have bilateral hydronephrosis and a distended bladder. Passage of a small pediatric feeding tube through the urethra is difficult or impossible. Usually a cutaneous vesicostomy must be performed to relieve upper urinary tract obstruction, and the severity of renal insufficiency is variable. The most severely affected boys have end-stage renal disease. Treatment includes urethral reconstruction, gradual urethral dilatation, or continent urinary diversion.

URETHRAL STRICTURES. Urethral strictures in males usually result from urethral trauma, either iatrogenic (catheterization, endoscopic procedures, previous urethral reconstruction) or accidental (straddle injuries, pelvic fractures). Because these lesions may develop gradually, the decrease in force of the urinary stream is seldom noticed by the child or the parents. More commonly, the obstruction causes symptoms of bladder instability, hematuria, or dysuria. Catheterization of the bladder usually is impossible. The diagnosis is made by a voiding film obtained during intravenous urography or retrograde urethrography. Ultrasonography also has been used to diagnose urethral strictures. Endoscopy is confirmatory. Endoscopic treatment of short strictures by direct vision urethrotomy is often successful and results in a profoundly improved urinary stream. Longer strictures surrounded by periurethral fibrosis often require urethroplasty. Repeated endoscopic procedures should generally be avoided, because they may cause additional urethral damage. Noninvasive measurement of the urinary flow rate and pattern is useful for diagnosis and follow-up.

In females, true urethral strictures are exceptional. because the female urethra is protected from trauma, particularly in childhood. In the past it was thought that a distal urethral ring commonly caused obstruction of the female urethra and urinary tract infection and that affected girls benefited from urethral dilatation. The diagnosis was suspected when a "spinning top" deformity of the urethra was found in the VCUG (see Fig. 543-4) and was confirmed by urethral calibration. There is no correlation between the radiologic appearance of the urethra in the VCUG and the urethral caliber and no significant difference in urethral caliber between females with recurrent cystitis and normal age-matched controls. The finding usually is secondary to detrusor-sphincter dyssynergia. Consequently, urethral dilatation in girls rarely is indicated.

ANTERIOR URETHRAL VALVES AND URETHRAL DIVERTICULA IN THE MALE. Anterior urethral valves are rare. The obstruction is not obstructing valve leaflets, as occurs in the posterior urethra. Rather, it is a urethral diverticulum in the penile urethra that expands during voiding. Distal extension of the diverticulum causes extrinsic compression of the distal penile urethra, causing urethral obstruction. Typically there is a soft mass on the ventral surface of the penis at the penoscrotal junction. In addition, the urinary stream often is weak, and the physical findings associated with posterior urethral valves often are present. The diverticulum may be small and minimally obstructive, or, in other cases, may be severely obstructive and cause renal insufficiency. The diagnosis is suspected on physical examination and is confirmed by the VCUG. Treatment involves open excision of the diverticulum or transurethral excision of the distal urethral cusp. Urethral diverticula occasionally occur after extensive hypospadias repair.

Fusiform dilatation of the urethra or **megalourethra** may result from underdevelopment of the corpus spongiosum and support structures of the urethra. This condition is commonly associated with the prune-belly syndrome.

MALE URETHRAL MEATAL STENOSIS. See Chapter 544 for information on urethral meatal stenosis in males.

Ashmead GG, Mercer B, Herbst M, et al: Fetal bladder outlet obstruction due to ureterocele: In utero "colander" therapy. *J Ultrasound Med* 2004;23:565–568.

Biard JM, Johnson MP, Carr MC, et al: Long-term outcomes in children treated by prenatal vesicoamniotic shunting for lower urinary tract obstruction. *Obstet Gynecol* 2005;106:503–508.

Capello SA, Kogan BA, Giorgi LJ Jr, et al: Prenatal ultrasound has led to earlier detection and repair of ureteropelvic junction obstruction. *J Urol* 2005; 74:1425–1428.

Chertin B, Pollack A, Koulikov D, et al: Conservative treatment of ureteropelvic junction obstruction in children with antenatal diagnosis of hydronephrosis: Lessons learned after 16 years of follow-up. *Eur Urol* 2006; 49:734–739.

DeFoor W, Minevich E, Reddy P, et al: Results of tapered ureteral reimplantation for primary megaureter: Extravesical versus intravesical approach. *J Urol* 2004;172:1640–1643.

Direnna T, Leonard MP: Watchful waiting for prenatally detected ureteroceles. *J Urol* 2006;175:1493–1495.

Fefer S, Ellsworth P: Prenatal hydronephrosis. *Pediatr Clin North Am* 2006;53:429–447.

Gundeti MS, Ransley PG, Duffy PG, et al: Renal outcome following heminephrectomy for duplex kidney. *J Urol* 2005;173:1743–1744.

Holmdahl G, Sillen U: Boys with posterior urethral valves: Outcome concerning renal function, bladder function and paternity at ages 31 to 44 years. *J Urol* 2005;174:1031–1034.

Hwang AH, McAleer IM, Shapiro E, et al: Congenital mid ureteral strictures. *J Urol* 2005;174:1999–2002.

Hwang WY, Peters CA, Zurakowski D, et al: Renal biopsy in congenital ureteropelvic junction obstruction: Evidence for parenchymal maldevelopment. *Kidney Int* 2006;69:137–143.

Krishnan A, deSouza A, Konijeti R, et al: The anatomy and embryology of posterior urethral valves. *J Urol* 2006;175:1214–1220.

Lee RS, Retik AB, Borer JG, et al: Pediatric robot assisted laparoscopic dismembered pyeloplasty: Comparison with a cohort of open surgery. *J Urol* 2006;175:683–687.

McDaniel BB, Jones RA, Scherz H, et al: Dynamic contrast-enhanced MR urography in the evaluation of pediatric hydronephrosis: Part 2, anatomic and functional assessment of ureteropelvic junction obstruction. *AJR Am J Roentgenol* 2005;185:1608–1614.

Narasimhan KL, Mahajan JK, Kaur B, et al: The vesicoureteral reflux dysplasia syndrome in patients with posterior urethral valves. *J Urol* 2005;174:1433–1435.

Nguyen MT, Pavlock CL, Zderic SA, et al: Overnight catheter drainage in children with poorly compliant bladders improves post-obstructive diuresis and urinary incontinence. *J Urol* 2005;174:1633–1636.

Perez-Brayfield MR, Baseman A, Kirsch AJ: Adolescent urology. *Adolesc Med Clin* 2005;16:215–227.

Piaggio L, Franc-Guimond J, Figueroa TE, et al: Comparison of laparoscopic and open partial nephrectomy for duplication anomalies in children. *J Urol* 2006;175:2269–2273.

Shukla AR, Cooper J, Patel RP, et al: Prenatally detected primary megaureter: A role for extended follow-up. *J Urol* 2005;173:1353–1356.

Sty JR, Pan CG: Genitourinary imaging techniques. *Pediatr Clin North Am* 2006;53 339–361.

Tsai JD, Huang FY, Lin CC, et al: Intermittent hydronephrosis secondary to ureteropelvic junction obstruction: Clinical and imaging features. *Pediatrics* 2006;117:139–146.

Yee DS, Shanberg AM, Duel BP, et al: Initial comparison of robotic-assisted laparoscopic versus open pyeloplasty in children. *Urology* 2006;67:599–602.

Chapter 541 ■ Anomalies of the Bladder

Jack S. Elder

BLADDER EXSTROPHY

Exstrophy of the urinary bladder occurs about once in every 35,000–40,000 births. The male : female ratio is 2 : 1. The severity ranges from simple epispadias to complete exstrophy of the cloaca involving exposure of the entire hindgut and the bladder.

CLINICAL MANIFESTATIONS. Anomalies of the bladder are hypothesized to result when the mesoderm fails to invade the cephalad extension of the cloacal membrane; the extent of this failure determines the degree of the anomaly. In classic bladder exstrophy (Fig. 541-1), the bladder protrudes from the abdominal wall and its mucosa is exposed. The umbilicus is displaced downward, the pubic rami are widely separated in the midline, and the rectus muscles are separated. In **males,** there is complete epispadias with dorsal chordee, and the overall penile length is approximately

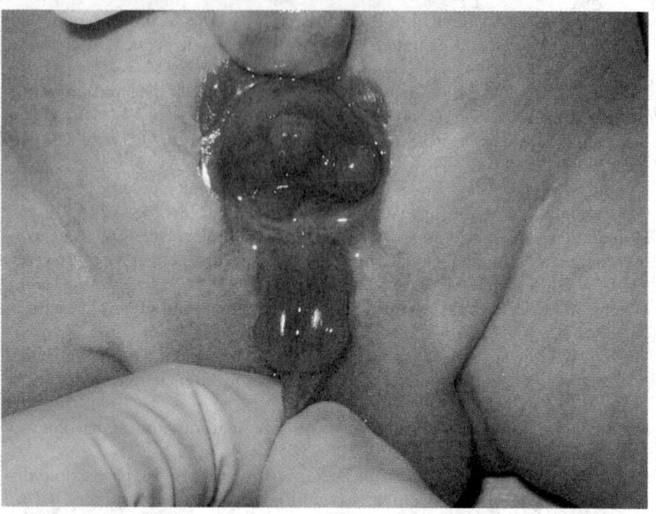

Figure 541-1. Classic bladder exstrophy in a newborn boy. The bladder is exposed in the midline; the umbilical cord is displaced caudad; the penis is epispadiac; and the scrotum is broad.

half of unaffected boys. The scrotum typically is separated slightly from the penis and is wide and shallow. Undescended testes and inguinal hernias are common. **Females** also have epispadias, with separation of the two halves of the clitoris and wide separation of the labia. The anus is displaced anteriorly in both sexes, and there may be rectal prolapse. The pubic rami are widely separated. Individuals with exstrophy tend to be shorter than normal. The consequences of untreated bladder exstrophy are total urinary incontinence and an increased incidence of bladder cancer, usually adenocarcinoma. The genital deformities can produce sexual disability in both sexes, particularly in males. The wide separation of the pubic rami causes a characteristic broad-based gait but no significant disability. In classic bladder exstrophy, the upper urinary tracts usually are normal.

TREATMENT. Management of bladder exstrophy should start at birth. The bladder should be covered with plastic wrap to keep the bladder mucosa moist. *Application of gauze or petroleum-gauze to the bladder mucosa should be avoided, as significant inflammation will result.* The infant should be transferred promptly to a center equipped for the treatment of such anomalies. Conventional therapy has included a series of staged reconstructive procedures, but a single-stage complete reconstruction in the neonatal infant has gained popularity. These individuals are prone to **latex allergy,** so latex precautions should be practiced in their care.

Prompt closure of the exstrophic bladder is the preferred treatment. During this procedure the abdominal wall is mobilized and the pubic rami are brought together in the midline. If the bladder closure is performed during the first 48 hr of life, often there is sufficient mobility of the pubic rami to allow approximation of the pubic symphysis. If the procedure is delayed, the pelvic bones must be broken (pelvic osteotomy) to allow the pubic rami to be brought together and create a pubic symphysis to support the bladder closure. Early bladder closure can be applied to almost all neonates with classic bladder exstrophy. Treatment should be deferred in selected situations when surgical therapy would be excessively risky or complex, such as in a premature baby or when it would have to be performed by inexperienced surgeons.

Total reconstruction includes closure of the bladder, closure of the abdominal wall, and, in boys, correction of epispadias using a technique of penile disassembly, in which the two corpora cavernosa and the midline urethra are mobilized separately into three parts. Postoperatively, the infant's upper urinary tract is monitored closely for the possible development of hydronephrosis and infection. Most infants with bladder exstrophy have vesicoureteral reflux and should receive antibiotic prophylaxis. In boys, if the epispadias is not corrected at birth, epispadias repair usually is performed between 1–2 yr of age. At this point the child has total urinary incontinence because there is no external urinary sphincter.

The final stage of reconstruction involves creation of a sphincter muscle for bladder control and correction of the vesicoureteral reflux. At this point the child is 3–6 yr old, the bladder capacity should be at least 80–90 mL, and the child must have gained rectal control. Typically. bladder capacity is monitored every 12–24 mo using cystoscopy under anesthesia.

At puberty, often the pubic hair is distributed to the sides of the external genitals. A monsplasty is performed to provide a more normal escutcheon.

PROGNOSIS. This plan of treatment has yielded a continence rate of 60–70% in a few centers, with less than 15% deterioration of the upper urinary tract. This continence rate reflects not only the successful reconstruction but also the quality and size of the bladder. The reconstructed bladder neck does not relax during voiding as in a normal child; instead the patient must void by Valsalva. Children who undergo reconstructive surgery as newborns have a greater chance of obtaining a normally functioning bladder. Children who remain incontinent for more than 1 yr after bladder neck reconstruction or those who are not eligible for bladder neck reconstruction because of a small bladder capacity are candidates for an alternative reconstructive procedure to achieve dryness. In selected cases, cystoscopic injection of dextranomer or polydimethylsiloxane microspheres into the bladder neck may provide sufficient bladder neck coaptation to establish continence. Alternatively, if the child is not a candidate for endoscopic therapy, options include (1) augmentation cystoplasty, in which the bladder is enlarged with a patch of small or large bowel to increase its capacity; (2) creation of a neobladder out of small and large bowel with placement of a continent abdominal stoma through which clean intermittent catheterization can be performed; (3) placement of an artificial urinary sphincter, with possible augmentation cystoplasty; (4) ureterosigmoidostomy, in which the ureters are detached from the bladder and sutured to the sigmoid colon; individuals void urine and stool from the rectum and rely on their anal sphincter for continence; and (5) Mainz II procedure, in which the sigmoid colon is reconfigured into a "bladder" into which the ureters are connected, and the patient voids 3 to 6 times daily through the rectum, and the stool tends to be more solid. Ureterosigmoidostomy carries a significant risk of chronic pyelonephritis, upper urinary tract damage, metabolic acidosis resulting from absorption of hydrogen ion and chloride in the intestine, and at least a 15% long-term risk of colon carcinoma. Patients from undeveloped countries often undergo the Mainz II procedure because the continence rate is high and pyelonephritis and upper tract changes are uncommon.

Late follow-up has shown that although men with exstrophy have a penis that is half normal length, they usually experience satisfactory sexual function. Fertility has been low, possibly because of iatrogenic injury to the secondary sexual organs during reconstruction. With artificial reproductive technology, nearly all men can be fertile. In women, fertility is not affected, but uterine prolapse during pregnancy is a problem. In addition, in women who have undergone a continent urinary diversion, delivery by cesarean section may be necessary.

OTHER EXSTROPHY ANOMALIES

Children with more complex cases of **cloacal exstrophy,** which has an incidence of 1 in 400,000, have an omphalocele and severe abnormalities of the colon and the rectum and often have short bowel syndrome, the most devastating anomaly managed by pediatric urologists. Approximately 50% of patients have an upper urinary tract anomaly, and 50% have spina bifida. No child with cloacal exstrophy has achieved normal urinary or stool continence. Current reconstructive techniques result in a satisfactory outcome in most patients with permanent urinary diversion (either ileal conduit or continent urinary diversion) and a colostomy. Because the penis in boys with cloacal exstrophy usually is diminutive, genital reconstruction in males with cloacal exstrophy has been unsatisfactory. In the past, most specialists recommended assigning a female gender to such infants, but currently there is debate whether these children, who have a 46,XY karyotype and androgen imprinting in utero, can have a satisfactory female gender identity. Decisions regarding gender assignment should be made jointly by the physicians caring for the infant (surgical team, pediatric endocrinologist, child psychiatrist, and ethicist) and family.

Epispadias is in the spectrum of exstrophy anomalies, affecting approximately 1 in 117,000 boys and 1 in 480,000 girls. In boys, the diagnosis is obvious because the prepuce is distributed primarily on the ventral aspect of the penile shaft and the urethral meatus is on the dorsum of the penis. Distal epispadias in boys usually is associated with normal urinary control and normal upper urinary tracts and should be repaired by 6–12 mo of age. In girls, the clitoris is bifid and the urethra is split dorsally. In more severely affected boys and in all girls with epispadias, there is total urinary incontinence because the sphincter is incompletely formed, and there is wide separation of the pubic rami. These children require surgical reconstruction procedures analogous to those of the 2nd and 3rd stages of management of patients with classic bladder exstrophy.

BLADDER DIVERTICULA

Bladder diverticula usually occur at the ureterovesical junction and are associated with vesicoureteral reflux (Fig. 541-2), because the diverticulum interferes with the normal flap-valve attachment between the ureter and bladder. Congenital diverticula also occur in other locations. Bladder diverticula also commonly are associated with distal urethral obstruction such as posterior urethral valves or neurogenic bladder dysfunction. Small diverticula require no treatment other than that of the primary disease, whereas large diverticula may contribute to inefficient voiding, residual urine, urinary stasis, and urinary tract infections and should be excised.

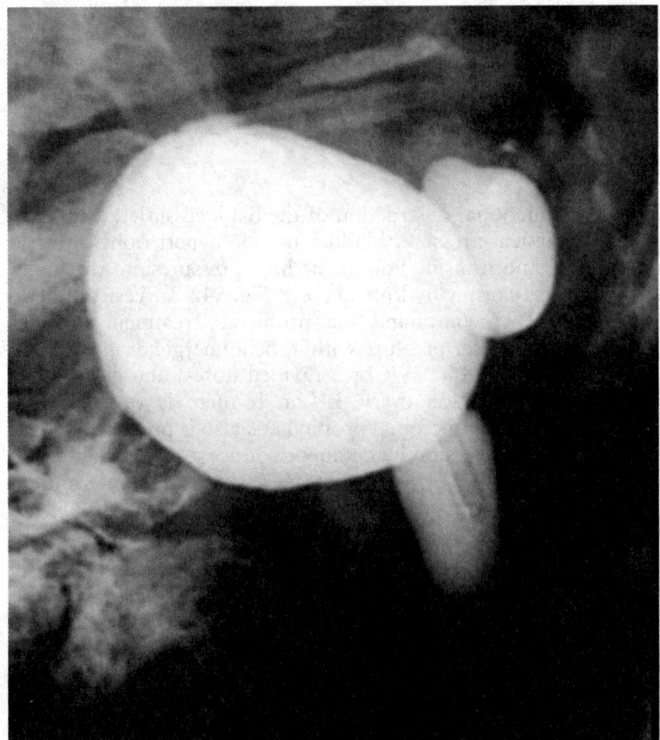

Figure 541-2. Bladder diverticulum demonstrated on voiding cystourethrogram in a newborn boy with posterior urethral valves.

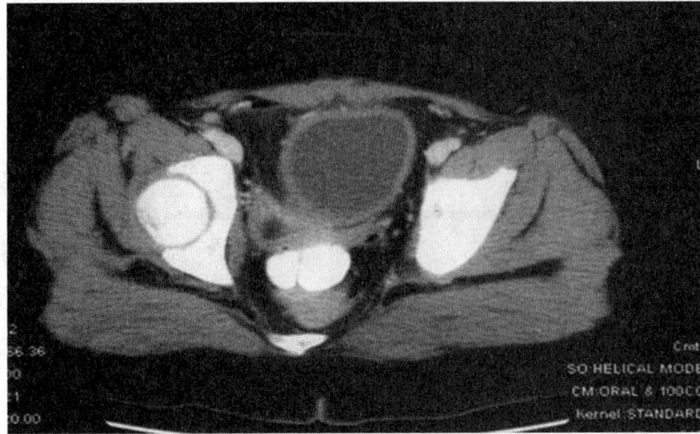

Figure 541-3. CT scan demonstrating infected urachal abscess in an 8 yr old girl. The condition was managed by drainage and excision.

URACHAL ANOMALIES

Urachal abnormalities are more common in males than in females. A patent urachus can occur as an isolated anomaly; it may be associated with prune-belly syndrome or posterior urethral valves. In this condition there is continuous urinary drainage from the umbilicus. The tract should be excised surgically. Another urachal anomaly is the urachal cyst, which can become infected. Typical symptoms and physical findings include suprapubic pain, fever, irritative voiding symptoms, and an infraumbilical mass, which can be erythematous. Diagnosis is made by ultrasonography or CT (Fig. 541-3). Treatment is intravenous antibiotic therapy and drainage and excision. Other urachal anomalies include the urachal diverticulum, which is a diverticulum of the bladder dome, and external urachal sinus, which is a blind external sinus that opens at the umbilicus. These lesions should be excised.

Allen JW, Song J, Velcek FT: Acute presentation of infected urachal cysts: Case report and review of diagnosis and therapeutic interventions. *Pediatr Emerg Care* 2004;20:108–111.

Borer JG, Gargollo PC, Hendren WH, et al: Early outcome following complete primary repair of bladder exstrophy in the newborn. *J Urol* 2005;174:1674–1678.

Borer JG, Gargollo PC, Kinnamon DD, et al: Bladder growth and development after complete primary repair of bladder exstrophy in the newborn with comparison to staged approach. *J Urol* 2005;174:1553–1557.

Gearhart JP, Baird AD: The failed complete repair of bladder exstrophy: Insights and outcomes. *J Urol* 2005;174:1669–1672.

Husmann DA, Gearhart JP: Loss of the penile glans and/or corpora following primary repair of bladder exstrophy using the complete penile disassembly technique. *J Urol* 2004;172:1696–1700.

Lottmann HB, Margarayan M, Bernuy M, et al: Long-term effects of dextranomer endoscopic injections for treatment of urinary incontinence: An update of a prospective study of 31 patients. *J Urol* 2006;175:1485–1489.

Meyer-Bahlburg HF: Gender identity outcome in female-raised 46,XY persons with penile agenesis, cloacal exstrophy of the bladder, or penile ablation. *Arch Sex Behav* 2005;34:423–438.

Mitchell ME: Bladder exstrophy repair: Complete primary repair of exstrophy. *Urology* 2005;65:5–8.

Nelson CP, Dunn RL, Wei JT, et al: Surgical repair of bladder exstrophy in the modern era: Contemporary practice patterns and the role of hospital case volume. *J Urol* 2005;174:1099–1102.
Pahernik S, Beetz R, Schede J, et al: Rectosigmoid pouch (Mainz pouch II) in children. *J Urol* 2006;175:284–287.
Reiner WG, Kropp BP: A 7-year experience of genetic males with severe phallic inadequacy assigned female. *J Urol* 2004;172:2395–2398.

Chapter 542 ■ Neuropathic Bladder

Jack S. Elder

Neuropathic bladder dysfunction in children usually is congenital and may result from neural tube defects or other spinal abnormalities (see Chapter 592). Acquired diseases and traumatic lesions of the spinal cord are less common. Central nervous system tumors, sacrococcygeal teratoma, and spinal abnormalities associated with imperforate anus (see Chapter 341) also can result in abnormal innervation of the bladder or sphincter, or both.

NEURAL TUBE DEFECTS. Neural tube defects are various abnormal conditions of the vertebral column that affect spinal cord function, including myelomeningocele and meningocele (see Chapter 592). As a result of folic acid supplementation and antenatal screening, the incidence of neural tube defects is decreasing in the U.S. and in many countries. In Newfoundland the incidence has decreased from 4.67 per 1,000 total births in 1992–1996 to 1.01 per 1,000 total births in 1998–2002. Still, it remains high in many parts of the world; in Shanxi Province, China, for example, the rate is 13.87/1,000 births. A few medical centers in the U.S. have been performing antenatal myelomeningocele closure, but follow-up studies of the urinary tract have not shown a definite improvement in lower urinary tract function. Trials randomizing mothers to antenatal verses postnatal myelomeningocele closure to assess urologic, neurologic, and quality-of-life outcomes are ongoing to address this issue further.

CLINICAL MANIFESTATIONS AND DIAGNOSIS. The most important urologic consequences of neuropathic bladder dysfunction associated with neural tube defects are urinary incontinence (see Chapter 543), urinary tract infections (UTIs; see Chapter 538), and hydronephrosis from vesicoureteral reflux or detrusor-sphincter dyssynergia. Pyelonephritis (Chapter 519.4) and renal functional deterioration (see Chapter 535) are common causes of premature death of affected individuals.

In the neonate, renal ultrasonography, assessment of postvoid residual urine volumes, and a voiding cystourethrogram are performed after closure of the myelomeningocele. From 10–15% of patients have hydronephrosis, and 25% have vesicoureteral reflux. A urodynamic study also should be performed. This study involves filling the bladder with saline, measuring the bladder volume and pressure, and assessing sphincter tone. During bladder filling, the bladder may show uninhibited (premature) contractions at low volumes; normal bladder volume with contraction at an appropriate volume; or atonia (lack of bladder contraction). Bladder compliance or elasticity also may be reduced. The sphincter may show normal tone with relaxation during bladder contraction, reduced or absent tone, or normal or increased tone that increases during bladder contraction (termed detrusor-sphincter dyssynergia) (Fig. 542-1).

RENAL DAMAGE. Renal damage usually results from failure of the sphincter to relax during a bladder contraction. This dyssynergia

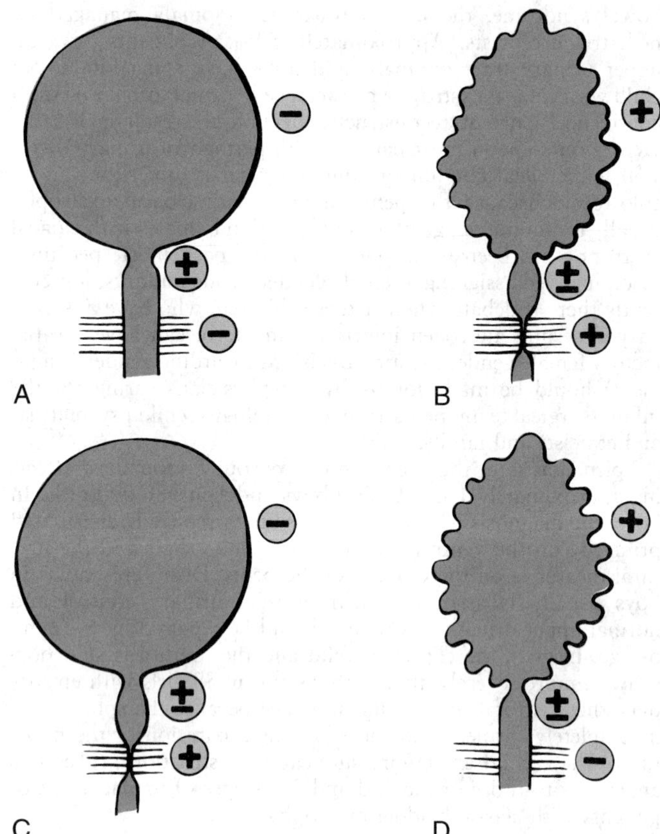

Figure 542-1. Grouping of neurogenic bladder dysfunction according to the innervation, tonicity, and coordination of the detrusor and sphincters described by Guzman. This grouping is based on data from imaging studies, cystometrography, and electromyography of the sphincters. Patients in group B are at risk of developing reflux and hydronephrosis. For guidance in the treatment of incontinence, group A benefits from procedures that increase outlet resistance, group B from anticholinergics or bladder augmentation surgery, and group C from intermittent catheterization and group D requires both increased outlet resistance and pharmacologic or surgical bladder enlargement. Most patients require intermittent catheterization to empty. (Modified from Gonzalez R: Urinary incontinence. In Kelalis PK, King LR, Belman AB (editors): *Clinical Pediatric Urology.* Philadelphia, WB Saunders, 1992, p 387.)

results in functional obstruction of the bladder outlet, leading to high intravesical pressure, bladder muscle hypertrophy and trabeculation, and transmission of the high pressure into the upper urinary tracts causing hydronephrosis (Fig. 542-2). Vesicoureteral reflux and UTI compound the problem. Treatment includes reduction of bladder pressure with anticholinergic drugs (oxybutynin, 0.2 mg/kg/24 hr in 2 or 3 divided doses) and clean intermittent catheterization every 3–4 hr. If there is vesicoureteral reflux or UTIs, antimicrobial prophylaxis also is prescribed. Temporary urinary diversion by cutaneous vesicostomy is an alternative in the newborn or infant with severe reflux, if intermittent catheterization is difficult, or anticholinergic medications are not well tolerated. Other options in the child with severe detrusor-sphincter dyssynergia are urethral overdilation or transurethral injection of botulinum toxin (Botox) into the sphincter. The latter procedure requires general anesthesia and results in sphincteric incompetence for 4–6 mo. Clean intermittent catheterization and anticholinergic therapy cure the reflux in up to 80% of children with grade 1 or 2 reflux. In children with upper tract changes, continuous overnight bladder catheterization allows significant bladder relaxation and can reduce bladder wall thickening. Children with more severe reflux often require endoscopic reflux correction or open antireflux surgery followed by intermittent

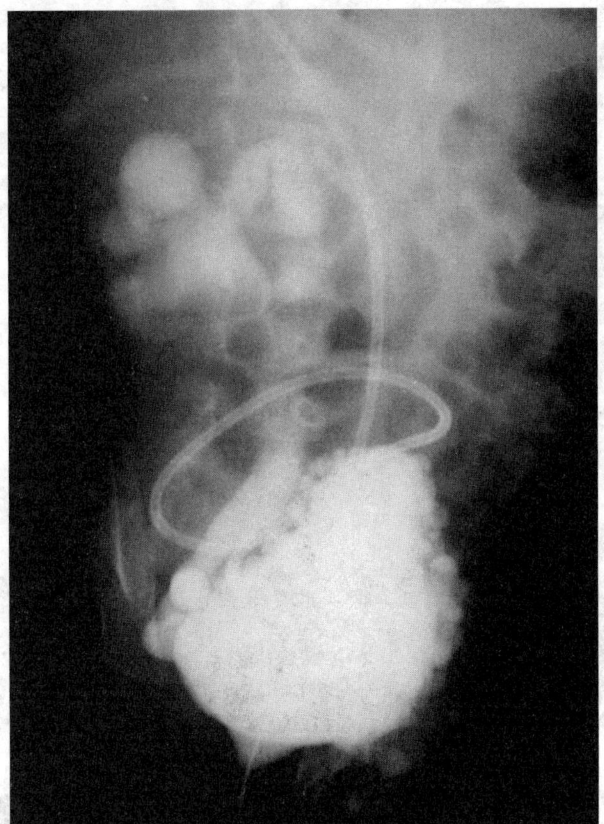

Figure 542-2. Voiding cystourethrogram in an infant with myelodysplasia shows a severely trabeculated bladder with multiple diverticula and grade V (out of V) right vesicoureteral reflux. Evaluation showed severe detrusor-sphincter dyssynergia.

catheterization and anticholinergic drugs. In older children with myelomeningocele with high-grade reflux, UTI, and hydronephrosis, augmentation enterocystoplasty with intermittent catheterization may be necessary.

URINARY INCONTINENCE. Incontinence in the child with neuropathic bladder can result from total or partial denervation of the sphincter, bladder hyperreflexia, poor bladder compliance, chronic urinary retention, or a combination of these factors.

Incontinence often is addressed around 4 yr of age and is tailored to the individual child. Nearly all children require clean intermittent catheterization to stay dry. This technique allows efficient bladder emptying with minimal risk of symptomatic UTI. The urinary tract should be re-evaluated with renal ultrasonography, a voiding cystourethrogram, and a urodynamic study, including bladder capacity. If the sphincter tone is sufficient and the bladder has adequate compliance, intermittent catheterization every 3–4 hr usually is successful in keeping the child dry. If there are unstable bladder contractions, an anticholinergic medication such as oxybutynin chloride, hyoscyamine, or tolterodine is prescribed to increase bladder capacity. If there is sphincter incompetence, α-adrenergic medications are prescribed to enhance outlet resistance. Bacteriuria is seen in up to 50% of children using intermittent self-catheterization, but it seldom causes symptoms. In the absence of reflux, there seems to be little cause for concern. Antibacterial prophylaxis often can be effective in keeping the urine sterile while intermittent catheterization is used. Performing intermittent catheterization with a new catheter (hydrophilic or standard silicone) each time also is quite effective in preventing bacteriuria and avoids the need for antibiotic prophylaxis. With this treatment plan, 40–85% of patients are dry, depending on their definition of continence. Some children wear a pad in their underwear or a diaper but state that they are dry.

If there is persistent incontinence despite these measures, reconstructive urinary tract surgery nearly always can provide complete or satisfactory continence. If urethral resistance is low, implantation of an artificial sphincter usually is successful. This sphincter consists of an inflatable cuff that is placed around the bladder neck, a pressure-regulating balloon implanted in the extraperitoneal space, and a pumping mechanism that is implanted in the scrotum of males and in the labia majora of females. Alternatively, bladder neck reconstructive procedures such as a periurethral sling often are successful. If the bladder capacity or bladder compliance is low, or if there are persistent uninhibited contractions despite anticholinergic therapy, enlargement of the bladder with a patch of small or large intestine or stomach, termed **augmentation cystoplasty** or **enterocystoplasty,** is effective. These patients still need to perform clean intermittent catheterization. If urethral catheterization is difficult, a continent stoma may be incorporated into the urinary tract reconstruction. A common method is the **Mitrofanoff procedure,** in which the appendix is isolated from the cecum on its vascular pedicle and is interposed between the bladder and abdominal wall to allow intermittent catheterization through a dry stoma.

Complications. Several potential complications may arise with enterocystoplasty.

URINARY TRACT INFECTIONS. The urine usually is colonized with gram-negative bacteria, and attempts to sterilize the urine for prolonged periods usually fail. There is no evidence that chronic bacteriuria in patients who have had enterocystoplasty is associated with renal damage, however; therefore, only symptomatic UTIs should be treated.

ACIDOSIS. The enteric mucosal surface in contact with the urine absorbs ammonium, chloride, and hydrogen ions and loses potassium. Hyperchloremic metabolic acidosis can result, possibly requiring medical treatment (see Chapter 52). Chronic acidosis may compromise skeletal growth. This complication is most common in patients with compromised renal function and in those in whom colon has been used to enlarge the bladder. To overcome this limitation of enterocystoplasty in patients with chronic renal insufficiency, a gastric segment can be used instead of a segment of the small or large intestine. The stomach secretes chloride and hydrogen ions; thus, pre-existing metabolic acidosis remains stable or improves. However, the possibility of intractable metabolic alkalosis and peptic ulceration of the augmentation has diminished enthusiasm for this procedure. A composite augmentation using stomach and small or large bowel results in few metabolic complications.

PERFORATION. Perforation of the augmented bladder is a life-threatening complication that results most often from acute or chronic overdistention of the augmented bladder. Patients with this complication typically present with severe abdominal pain and signs of peritonitis. Prompt diagnosis and treatment with exploratory laparotomy and bladder closure are necessary. Meticulous adherence to the prescribed program of intermittent catheterization to avoid bladder overdistention is important.

BLADDER CALCULI. Bladder calculi have developed in as many as 70% of children followed for 10 yr after enterocystoplasty. The calculi develop in response to mucus that accumulates in the bladder and acts as a nidus for stone formation. This complication can be prevented by daily irrigation of the bladder with sterile saline.

INVASIVE TRANSITIONAL CELL CARCINOMA. Invasive transitional cell carcinoma has been reported in nearly 2% of patients undergoing enterocystoplasty. The pathogenesis is uncertain but is speculated that it is related to bacteriuria and the bowel–bladder contact. It is prudent to advise yearly endoscopic examinations or urine cytologic studies beginning in the 10th postoperative year.

CONSTIPATION. Many patients with spina bifida also have bowel problems with constipation, and some benefit from a procedure known as the *Malone antegrade continence enema procedure,* in which the appendix is brought out to the skin to allow a catheter to be inserted into the cecum for antegrade enema. The stoma is continent, and an antegrade enema can be performed with tap water each day. This form of management allows the patient to be continent of stool and more self-sufficient.

LATEX ALLERGY. Latex allergy (see Chapter 148) is a very serious problems encountered by as many as half of individuals with spina bifida and other urologic conditions who require clean intermittent catheterization and urinary tract reconstructive procedures. This IgE-mediated allergy is acquired and is secondary to repeated exposure to the latex allergen. Latex allergy may manifest as watery eyes, sneezing, itching, hives, or anaphylaxis when blowing up a balloon or if an examiner is using latex gloves. Intraoperatively, a sensitized individual can experience anaphylactic shock. A latex-free environment should be provided for all children with spina bifida in the office, during hospitalization, and during operative procedures. Affected children also should wear a medical alert bracelet.

OCCULT SPINAL DYSRAPHISM. Approximately 1/4,000 patients have occult spinal dysraphism, a category that includes lipomeningocele, intradural lipoma, diastematomyelia, tight filum terminale, dermoid cyst-sinus, aberrant nerve roots, anterior sacral meningocele, and cauda equina tumor (see Chapter 592). More than 90% of patients have a cutaneous abnormality overlying the lower spine, including a small dimple, tuft of hair, dermal vascular malformation, or a subcutaneous lipoma (Fig. 542-3). Often these children have high-arched feet, discrepancy in muscle size and strength between the legs, and a gait abnormality. Newborns and young infants often have a normal neurologic examination. Older children often have absent perineal sensation and back pain. Lower urinary tract function is abnormal in 40% of patients, including incontinence, recurrent UTI, and fecal soiling. The likelihood of a normal examination is inversely related to the child's age at surgical correction of the spinal lesion. In infants with abnormal urodynamics, 60% revert to normal; in older children, only 27% become normal. Management of the urinary tract in other children is similar to that described earlier for neural tube defects.

SACRAL AGENESIS. Sacral agenesis is defined as the absence of part or all of two or more lower vertebral bodies. This condition is more common in the offspring of women with diabetes. These children have a flattened buttock and a low, short gluteal cleft but usually have no orthopedic deformity, although some have high-arched feet. Palpation of the coccygeal area detects the absent vertebrae. Approximately 20% of cases are undetected until the age of 3–4 yr; many are diagnosed after unsuccessful toilet training. Urodynamic studies in these children show a variety of patterns, and most need clean intermittent catheterization and pharmacotherapy to stay dry.

IMPERFORATE ANUS. Between 30–45% of children with a high imperforate anus have a neuropathic bladder, often because of sacral agenesis. Newborns with imperforate anus should undergo a spinal ultrasound during their initial evaluation; and if these children have difficulty with toilet training, complete urologic evaluation with upper and lower urinary tract imaging and urodynamics should be performed. See Chapter 341 for further details.

CEREBRAL PALSY. Children with cerebral palsy (see Chapter 598.1) have reasonable bladder control. However, they achieve continence at a later age than unaffected children. Overall,

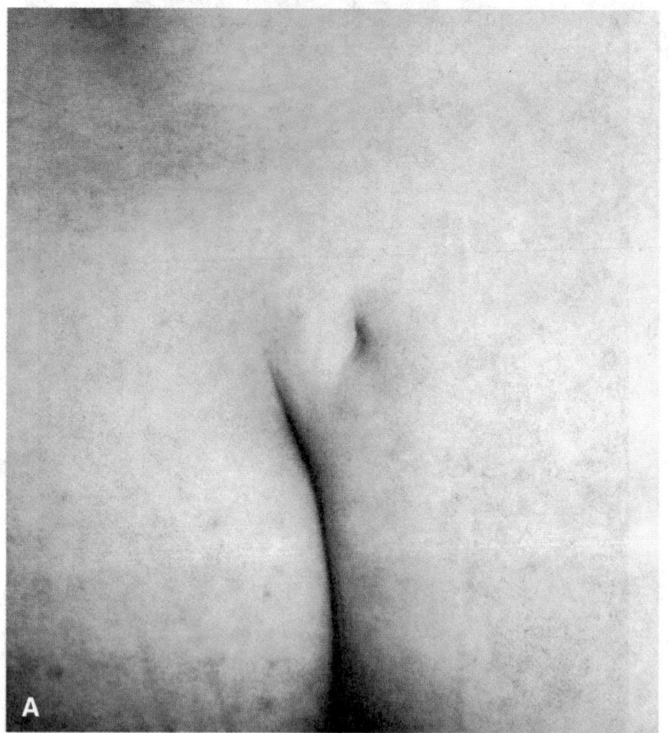

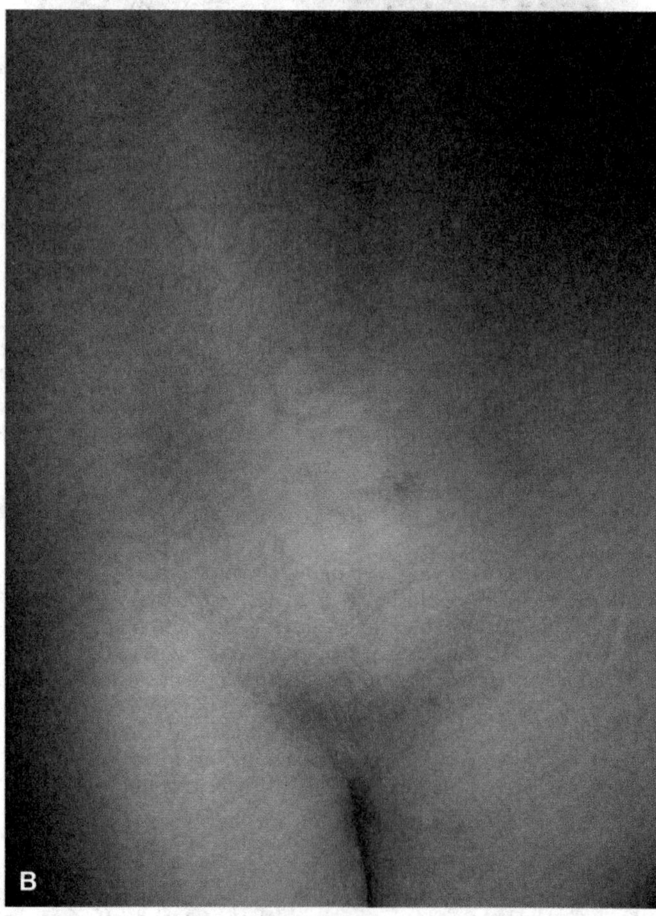

Figure 542-3. *A,* Buttocks of teenage boy with tethered cord secondary to lipomeningocele. Note sacral dimple and deviation of gluteal fold to the left. *B,* Fat deposit over sacrum in girl with tethered cord secondary to lipomeningocele.

25–50% are incontinent, and the risk is directly related to the severity of physical impairment. Their upper urinary tracts usually are normal. Urodynamic studies have shown that most have uninhibited bladder contractions. Timed voiding and anticholinergic therapy are usually effective. Clean intermittent catheterization rarely is necessary.

Alpert SA, Cheng EY, Zebold KF, et al: Clean intermittent catheterization in genitally sensate children: Patient experience and health related quality of life. *J Urol* 2005;174:1616–1619.

Altaweel W, Jednack R, Bilodeau C, et al: Repeated intradetrusor botulinum toxin type A in children with neurogenic bladder due to myelomeningocele. *J Urol* 2006;175:1102–1105.

Elder JS: Latex allergy: Time for a change. *J Urol* 2006;175:1193–1194.

Gilbert SM, Hensle TW: Metabolic consequences and long-term complications of enterocystoplasty. *J Urol* 2005;173:1080–1086.

Joseph DB: Bladder rehabilitation in children with spina bifida: State of the art. *J Urol* 2005;173:1850–1851.

Kaufman BA: Neural tube defects. *Pediatr Clin North Am* 2004;51:389–419.

Lottmann HB, Margaryan M, Bernuy M, et al: Long-term effects of dextranomer endoscopic injections for treatment of urinary incontinence: An update of a prospective study of 31 patients. *J Urol* 2006;175:1485–1489.

Metcalfe PD, Casale AJ, Kiefer MA, et al: Spontaneous bladder perforations: A report of 500 augmentations in children and analysis of risk. *J Urol* 2006;175:1466–1471.

Nguyen MT, Pavlock CL, Zderic, SA, et al: Overnight catheter drainage in children with poorly compliant bladders improves post-obstructive diuresis and urinary incontinence. *J Urol* 2005;174:1633–1636.

Nogueira M, Greenfield SP, Wan J, et al: Tethered cord in children: A clinical classification with urodynamic correlation. *J Urol* 2004;172:1677–1680.

Ozkan KU, Bauer SB, Khoshbin S, et al: Neurogenic bladder dysfunction after sacrococcygeal teratoma resection. *J Urol* 2006;175:292–296.

Snodgrass WT, Adams R: Initial urologic management of myelomeningocele. *Urol Clin North Am* 2004;31:427–434.

Soergel TM, Cain MP, Misseri R, et al: Transitional cell carcinoma of the bladder following augmentation cystoplasty for the neuropathic bladder. *J Urol* 2004;172:1649–1651.

Tanaka ST, Stone AR, Kurzrock EA: Transverse myelitis in children: Long-term urological outcomes. *J Urol* 2006;175:1865–1868.

Thomas J, Elder JS: Neuropathic bladder in children. *AUA Update Series*, 2007.

Chapter 543 ■ Voiding Dysfunction

Jack S. Elder

NORMAL VOIDING AND TOILET TRAINING

The fetus voids by reflex bladder contraction in concert with simultaneous contraction of the bladder and relaxation of the sphincter. Urine storage consists of sympathetic and pudendal nerve-mediated inhibition of detrusor contractile activity accompanied by closure of the bladder neck and proximal urethra with increased activity of the external sphincter.

The infant has coordinated reflex voiding as often as 15–20 times per day. Over time, bladder capacity increases. In children up to the age of 14 yr, the mean bladder capacity in ounces is equal to the age (in years) plus 2.

At 2–4 yr, the child is developmentally ready to begin toilet training. To achieve conscious bladder control, several conditions must be present: awareness of bladder filling; cortical inhibition (suprapontine modulation) of reflex (unstable) bladder contractions; ability to consciously tighten the external sphincter to prevent incontinence; normal bladder growth; and motivation by the child to stay dry. The transitional phase of voiding refers to the period when children are acquiring bladder control. Girls typically acquire bladder control before boys, and bowel control typically is achieved before urinary control.

NOCTURNAL ENURESIS

By 5 yr of age, 90–95% of children are nearly completely continent during the day and 80–85% are continent at night. Nocturnal enuresis (see Chapter 22.3) refers to the occurrence of involuntary voiding at night after 5 yr, the age when volitional control of micturition is expected. Enuresis may be primary (estimated 75–90% of children with enuresis; nocturnal urinary control never achieved) or secondary (10–25%; the child was dry at night for at least a few months and then enuresis developed). In addition, 75% of children with enuresis are wet only at night, whereas 25% are wet day and night. This distinction is important, because children with both forms are more likely to have abnormalities of the urinary tract.

EPIDEMIOLOGY. Approximately 60% of children with nocturnal enuresis are boys. Family history is positive in 50% of cases. Although primary nocturnal enuresis may be polygenetic, candidate genes have been localized to chromosomes 12 and 13. If one parent was enuretic, each child has a 44% risk of enuresis; if both parents were enuretic, each child has a 77% likelihood of enuresis. Nocturnal enuresis without overt daytime voiding symptoms affects up to 20% of children at the age of 5 yr; it ceases spontaneously in approximately 15% of involved children every year thereafter. Its frequency among adults is less than 1%.

PATHOGENESIS. The pathogenesis of nocturnal enuresis (normal daytime voiding habits) is multifactorial (Table 543-1).

CLINICAL MANIFESTATIONS AND DIAGNOSIS. A careful history should be obtained, especially with respect to fluid intake at night and pattern of nocturnal enuresis. Children with diabetes insipidus (see Chapter 559), diabetes mellitus (see Chapter 590), and chronic renal disease (see Chapter 535) may have a high obligatory urinary output and a compensatory polydipsia. The family should be asked whether the child snores loudly at night. A complete physical examination should include palpation of the abdomen and rectal examination after voiding to assess the possibility of a chronically distended bladder. The child with nocturnal enuresis should be examined carefully for neurologic and spinal abnormalities. There is an increased incidence of bacteriuria in enuretic girls, and, if found, it should be investigated and treated (see Chapter 538), although this does not always lead to resolution of bed-wetting. A urine sample should be obtained after an overnight fast and evaluated for specific gravity or osmolality, or both, to exclude polyuria as a cause of frequency and incontinence and to ascertain that the concentrating ability is

TABLE 543-1. Causes of Nocturnal Enuresis

Delayed maturation of the cortical mechanisms that allow voluntary control of the micturition reflex
Sleep disorders
- "Deep sleeping" (no specific sleep pattern identified)
- Enuresis can occur in any stage of sleep.
- All children are most difficult to arouse in the 1st third of the night, easiest to awaken in the last third, but enuretic children are more difficult to arouse than those with normal bladder control.

Reduced antidiuretic hormone production at night, resulting in an increased urine output
- Enuretic children often are described as "soaking the bed."

Genetic factors, with chromosomes 12 and 13q the likely sites of the gene for enuresis
- Family history in enuretic children often positive for enuresis

Organic factors, such as urinary tract infection (UTI) or obstructive uropathy
Psychologic factors
- More often implicated in secondary enuresis

Sleep apnea (snoring) secondary to enlarged adenoids.

normal. The absence of glycosuria should be confirmed. If there are no daytime symptoms, the physical examination and urinalysis are normal, and the urine culture is negative, further evaluation for urinary tract pathology generally is not warranted. A renal ultrasonogram is reasonable in an older child with enuresis or in children who do not respond appropriately to therapy.

TREATMENT. The best approach to treatment is to reassure parents that the condition is self-limited and to avoid punitive measures that may affect the child's psychological development adversely. Fluid intake should be restricted to 2 oz after 6 or 7 o'clock in the evening if the child weighs less than 75 lb, 3 oz if the child weighs 75–100 lb, and 4 oz if the child weighs more than 100 lb. The parents should be certain that the child voids at bedtime. Avoiding extraneous sugar and caffeine after 4 P.M. also is beneficial. If the child snores and the adenoids are enlarged, referral to an otolaryngologist should be considered, because adenoidectomy may cure the enuresis.

Active treatment should be avoided in children younger than age 6 yr, because enuresis is extremely common in younger children. Treatment is more likely to be successful in children approaching puberty compared with younger children.

The simplest initial measure is **motivational therapy** and includes a star chart for dry nights. Waking children a few hours after they go to sleep to have them void often allows them to awaken dry, although this measure is not curative. Some have recommended that children try holding their urine for longer periods during the day, but there is no evidence that this approach is beneficial. **Conditioning therapy** involves use of a loud auditory or vibratory alarm attached to a wetness sensor in the underwear. The alarm sounds when voiding occurs and is intended to awaken children and alert them to void. This form of therapy is considered curative and has a reported success of 30–60%. Often the auditory alarm wakes up other family members and not the enuretic child; persistence for several months often is necessary. Conditioning therapy tends to be most effective in older children. Another form of therapy to which some children respond is self-hypnosis. The primary role of psychological therapy is to help the child deal with enuresis psychologically and help motivate the child to void at night if he or she awakens with a full bladder.

Pharmacologic therapy is intended to treat the symptom of enuresis and thus is regarded as second-line and is not curative. As noted in Chapter 22.3, direct comparisons of the bell and bed compared to pharmacologic therapy favor the former because of lower relapse rates, although initial response rates are equivalent. One form of treatment is desmopressin acetate, a synthetic analog of antidiuretic hormone that reduces urine production overnight. It is available as a tablet, with a dosage of 0.2–0.6 mg at bedtime. In the past it was used as a nasal spray, with a dosage of 10 μg (1 spray) to 40 μg (4 sprays total) at bedtime. The lowest effective dose should be used. In children with rhinorrhea, the nasal spray is not absorbed and, consequently, is ineffective. Fluid restriction at night is important, and the drug should not be used if the child has a systemic illness with vomiting or diarrhea. Hyponatremia has been reported in a few children using the nasal spray, primarily those who were not using the medication properly. It has not been reported in children using the tablets. Desmopressin acetate is effective in as many as 40% of children. If effective, it should be used for 3–6 mo, and then an attempt should be made to taper the dosage. If tapering results in recurrent enuresis, the child should return to the higher dosage. No adverse events have been reported with the long-term use of desmopressin acetate. Another pharmacologic agent is imipramine, which is a tricyclic antidepressant. This medication has mild anticholinergic and α-adrenergic effects, reduces urine output slightly, and also may alter the sleep pattern. The dosage of imipramine is 25 mg in children age 6–8 yr, 50 mg in children age 9–12 yr, and 75 mg in teenagers. Reported success rates are 30–60%. Side effects include anxiety, insomnia, and dry mouth, and heart rhythm may be affected. In addition, the drug is one of the most common causes of poisoning by prescription medication in younger siblings. Oxybutynin chloride, a pure anticholinergic agent, has been used in some children with primary nocturnal enuresis, but the response rate is low, in part because the duration of action is only 6 hr.

In unsuccessful cases, combining therapies often is effective. For example, alarm therapy plus desmopressin is more successful than either one alone. In addition, the combination of oxybutynin chloride and desmopressin is more successful than either one alone. Desmopressin and imipramine should not be combined.

DIURNAL INCONTINENCE

Daytime incontinence not secondary to neurologic abnormalities is common in children. At age 5 yr, 95% have been dry during the day at some time and 92% are dry. At 7 yr, 96% are dry, although 15% have significant urgency at times. At 12 yr, 99% are dry during the day. The most common cause of daytime incontinence is a **pediatric unstable bladder** (also termed uninhibited or overactive bladder, bladder spasms). Table 543-2 lists the causes of diurnal incontinence in children.

Important points in the history include the pattern of incontinence, including the frequency, the volume of urine lost during incontinent episodes, whether the incontinence is associated with urgency or giggling, whether it occurs after voiding, and whether the incontinence is continuous. The frequency of voiding and whether there is nocturnal enuresis, a strong, continuous urinary stream, or sensation of incomplete bladder emptying should be assessed. A diary of when the child voids and whether they were wet or dry is helpful. Other urologic problems such as urinary tract infections (UTIs), reflux, neurologic disorders, or a family history of duplication anomalies should be assessed. Bowel habits also should be evaluated, because incontinence is common in children with constipation or encopresis, or both. Diurnal incontinence may occur in girls with a history of sexual abuse. Physical examination is directed at identifying signs of organic causes of incontinence: short stature, hypertension, enlarged kidneys or bladder or both, constipation, labial adhesion, ureteral ectopy (Figs. 543-1 to 543-3), back or sacral anomalies (see Fig. 542-3), and neurologic abnormalities. A urinalysis or culture, or both, should be performed to check for infection. In some cases, assessing the postvoid residual urine volume or urinary flow rate is appropriate. Imaging is reserved for children who have significant physical findings, a family history of urinary tract anomalies, UTIs, or those who do not respond to therapy appropriately. A renal ultrasonogram with or without a voiding cystourethrogram is indicated. Urodynamics should be performed if there is evi-

TABLE 543-2. Causes of Urinary Incontinence in Childhood
Pediatric unstable bladder (uninhibited bladder)
Infrequent voiding
Detrusor-sphincter dyssynergia
Non-neurogenic neurogenic bladder (Hinman syndrome)
Vaginal voiding
Giggle incontinence
Cystitis
Bladder outlet obstruction (posterior urethral valves)
Ectopic ureter and fistula
Sphincter abnormality (epispadias, exstrophy, urogenital sinus abnormality)
Neurogenic
Overflow incontinence
Traumatic
Iatrogenic
Behavioral
Combination

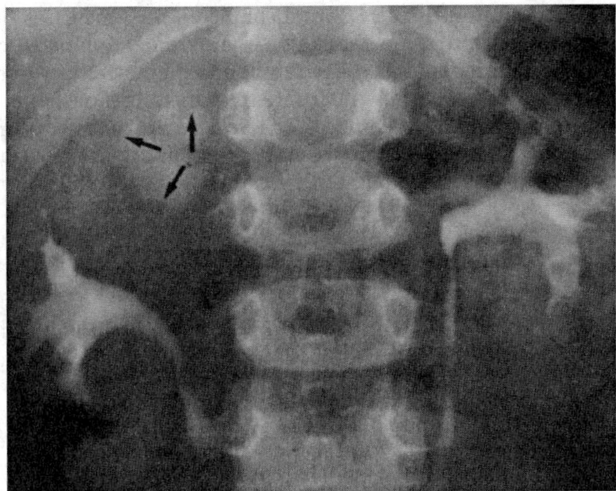

Figure 543-1. Duplication of the right collecting system with ectopic ureter. Excretory urogram in a female presenting with a normal voiding pattern and constant urinary dribbling. The left kidney is normal, and the right side, well visualized, is the lower collecting system of a duplicated kidney. On the upper pole opposite the first and second vertebral bodies, note the accumulation of contrast material corresponding with a poorly functioning upper pole drained by a ureter opening in the vestibule.

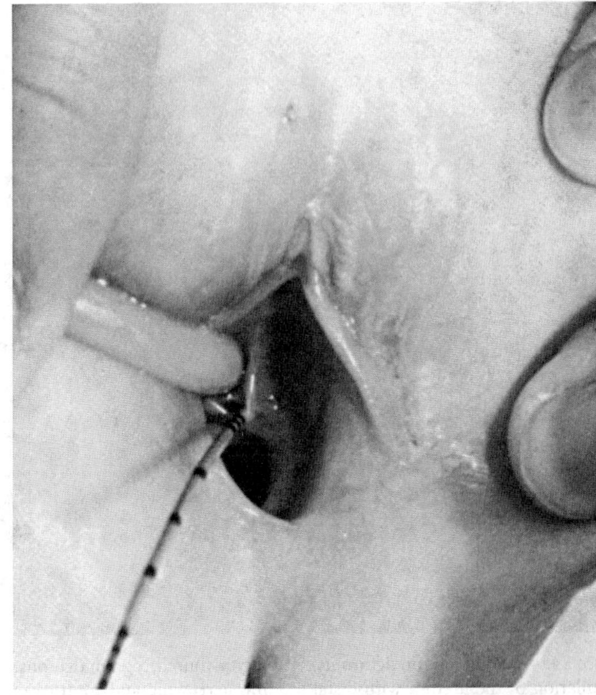

Figure 543-2. The photograph shows an ectopic ureter entering the vestibule next to the urethral meatus. The thin ureteral catheter with transverse marks has been introduced into this ectopic ureter. This girl had a normal voiding pattern and constant urinary dribbling.

dence of neurologic disease and may be helpful if empirical therapy is ineffective.

PEDIATRIC UNSTABLE (OVERACTIVE) BLADDER

Children with an overactive bladder typically exhibit urinary frequency, urgency, and urge incontinence. Often girls will squat down on their foot to try to prevent incontinence (termed **"Vincent's curtsy"**). The bladder in these children is smaller than normal and exhibits strong uninhibited contractions. Approximately 25% of children with nocturnal enuresis also have symptoms of an overactive bladder. Many children indicate they do not feel the need to urinate, even just before they are incontinent. In females, a history of recurrent UTI is common, but incontinence may persist long after infections are brought under control. It is not clear in these cases if the voiding dysfunction is a sequel of the UTIs or if the voiding dysfunction predisposes to recurrent UTIs. In girls, voiding cystourethrography often shows a dilated urethra ("spinning top deformity"; Fig. 543-4) and narrowed bladder neck with bladder wall hypertrophy. The urethral finding results from inadequate relaxation of the external urinary sphincter. Constipation is common.

The overactive bladder nearly always will resolve, but the time to resolution is highly variable, sometimes not until the teenage years. Initial therapy is timed voiding, every 1.5–2.0 hr. In addition, treatment of constipation and UTIs is important. Another treatment is biofeedback, in which children are taught pelvic floor

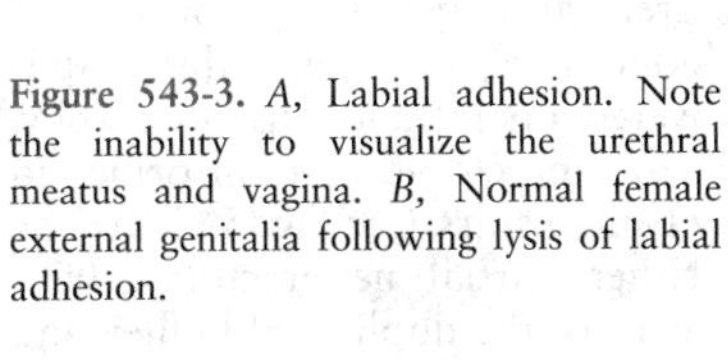

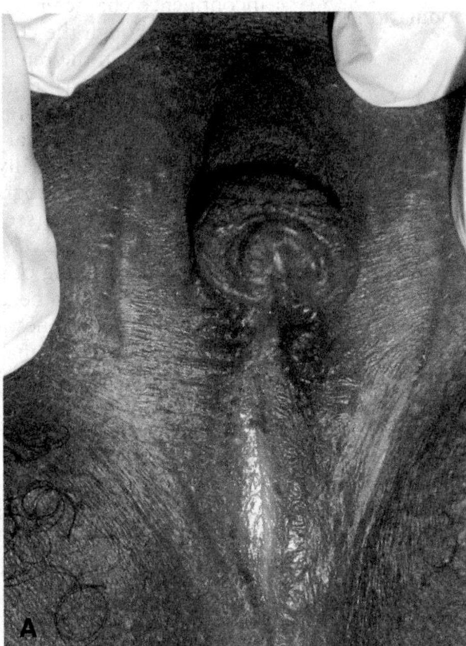

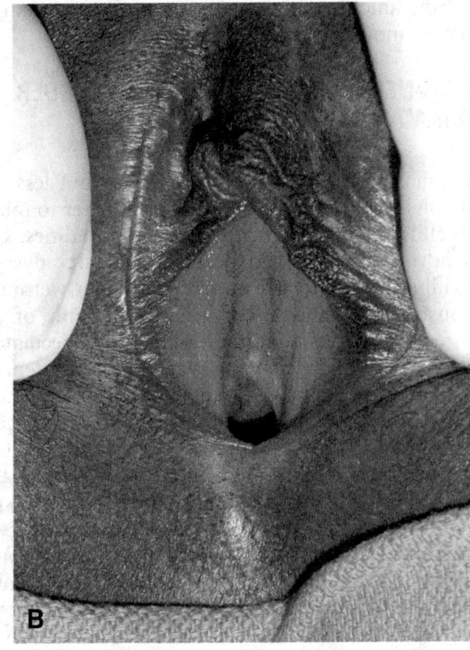

Figure 543-3. *A,* Labial adhesion. Note the inability to visualize the urethral meatus and vagina. *B,* Normal female external genitalia following lysis of labial adhesion.

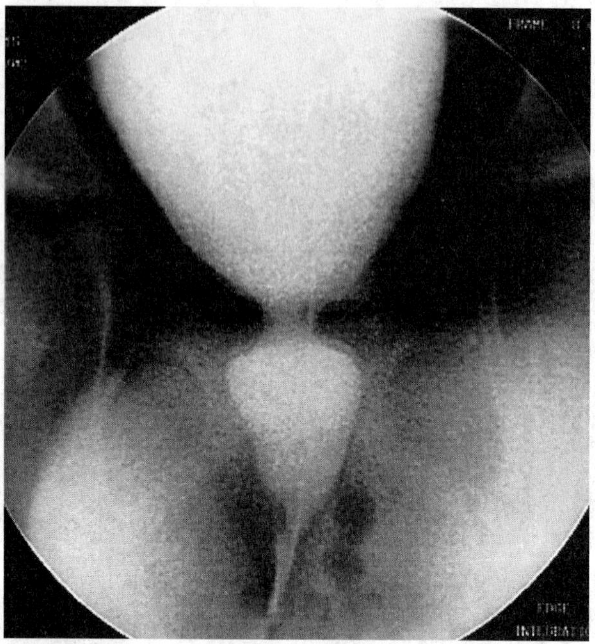

Figure 543-4. Spinning top deformity. Voiding cystourethrogram demonstrating dilation of the urethra with distal urethral narrowing and contraction of the bladder neck.

exercises (**Kegel exercises**), because there is evidence that daily performance of these exercises may reduce or eliminate unstable bladder contractions. Biofeedback also may include periodic uroflow studies with sphincter electromyography to be certain that the pelvic floor relaxes during voiding, and assessment of postvoid residual urine volume by sonography. Anticholinergic therapy with oxybutynin chloride, hyoscyamine, or tolterodine reduces bladder overactivity and may help the child achieve dryness. Treatment with an alpha blocker such as terazosin or doxazosin may aid in bladder emptying by promoting bladder neck relaxation; alpha blockers also have mild anticholinergic properties. If pharmacologic therapy is successful, the dosage should be tapered periodically to determine its continued need. Children who do not respond to therapy should be evaluated urodynamically to rule out other possible forms of bladder or sphincter dysfunction. In refractory cases sacral neuromodulation is a newer modality that has shown promise.

NON-NEUROGENIC NEUROGENIC BLADDER (HINMAN SYNDROME)

Hinman syndrome is a more serious but less common disorder involving failure of the external sphincter to relax during voiding in children without neurologic abnormalities. Children with this syndrome, also called **detrusor-sphincter dyssynergia**, typically exhibit a staccato stream, day and night wetting, recurrent UTIs, constipation, and encopresis. Evaluation of affected children often reveals vesicoureteral reflux, a trabeculated bladder, and a decreased urinary flow rate with an intermittent pattern. In severe cases, hydronephrosis, renal insufficiency, and even end-stage renal disease can occur. The pathogenesis of this syndrome is thought to involve learning abnormal voiding habits during toilet training; the syndrome is rarely seen in infants. Urodynamic studies and magnetic resonance imaging of the spine are indicated to rule out a neurologic cause for the bladder dysfunction. The treatment usually is complex and may include anticholinergic and alpha blocker therapy, timed voiding, treatment of constipation, behavioral modification, and encouragement of relaxation during voiding. Biofeedback has been used successfully in older children to teach relaxation of the external sphincter. In some cases botulinum toxin (Botox) injection into the external sphincter can provide temporary sphincteric paralysis and thereby reduce outlet resistance. In severe cases, intermittent catheterization is necessary to ensure bladder emptying. In selected patients, external urinary diversion is necessary to protect the upper urinary tract. These children require long-term treatment and careful follow-up.

INFREQUENT VOIDING

Infrequent voiding is a common disorder of micturition, usually associated with urinary tract infections. Affected children, usually girls, void only twice a day rather than the normal four to seven times. With bladder overdistention and prolonged retention of urine, bacterial growth can lead to recurrent UTIs. Some of these children are constipated. Some also have occasional episodes of incontinence due to overflow or urgency. The disorder is behavioral. If the child has UTIs, treatment includes antibacterial prophylaxis and encouragement of frequent voiding and complete emptying of the bladder by double voiding until a normal pattern of micturition is re-established.

VAGINAL VOIDING

In girls with vaginal voiding, incontinence typically occurs after urination after the girl stands up. Usually the volume of urine is 5–10 mL. One of the most common causes is labial adhesion (see Fig. 543-3). This lesion is seen in young girls and can be managed either by topical application of estrogen cream to the adhesion or lysis in the office. Some girls experience vaginal voiding because they do not separate their legs widely during urination. These girls usually are overweight or do not pull their underwear down to their ankles when they urinate. Management involves encouraging the girl to separate the legs as widely as possible during urination. The most effective way to do this is to have the child sit backward on the toilet seat during micturition.

OTHER CAUSES OF INCONTINENCE IN GIRLS

Ureteral ectopia, usually associated with a duplicated collecting system in girls, refers to a urine that drains outside the bladder, often into the vagina or distal urethra. It can produce urinary incontinence characterized by constant urinary dripping all day long, even though the child voids regularly. Sometimes the urine production from the renal segment drained by the ectopic ureter is small, and urinary drainage is confused with watery vaginal discharge. Children with a history of vaginal discharge or incontinence and an abnormal voiding pattern require careful study. The ectopic orifice usually is difficult to find. On ultrasonography or intravenous urography, one may suspect duplication of the collecting system (see Fig. 543-1), but the upper collecting system drained by the ectopic ureter usually has poor or delayed function. CT scanning of the kidneys helps rule out subtle duplication that may not be discovered on intravenous urography. Examination under anesthesia for an ectopic ureteral orifice in the vestibule or the vagina may be necessary (see Fig. 543-2). The treatment in these cases is either partial nephrectomy, with removal of the upper pole segment of the duplicated kidney and its ureter down to the pelvic brim, or ipsilateral ureteroureterostomy, in which the upper pole ectopic ureter is anastomosed to the normally positioned lower pole ureter.

Giggle incontinence typically affects girls between 7–15 yr of age. The incontinence occurs suddenly during giggling, and the entire bladder volume is lost. The pathogenesis is thought to be sudden relaxation of the urinary sphincter. Anticholinergic medication and timed voiding rarely are effective. The most effective treatment is low-dose methylphenidate.

Total incontinence in girls may be secondary to **epispadias.** This condition, which affects only 1 of 480,000 females, is characterized by separation of the pubic symphysis, separation of the right and left sides of the clitoris, and a patulous urethra. Treatment is bladder neck reconstruction or placement of an artificial urinary sphincter to repair the incompetent urethra.

A short, incompetent urethra may be associated with certain urogenital sinus malformations. The diagnosis of these malformations requires a high index of suspicion and a careful physical examination of all incontinent girls. In these cases, urethral and vaginal reconstruction can often restore continence.

VOIDING DISORDERS WITHOUT INCONTINENCE

Some children have abrupt onset of severe urinary frequency, voiding as often as every 10–15 min during the day, without dysuria, UTI, daytime incontinence, or nocturia. The most common age for these symptoms to occur is 4–6 yr, after the child is toilet-trained, and the vast majority are boys. This condition is termed the **daytime frequency syndrome of childhood** or **pollakiuria.** The condition is functional; no anatomic problem is detected. Often the symptoms occur just before a child starts kindergarten or if the child is having emotional family stress-related problems. These children should be checked for UTIs, and the clinician should ascertain that the child is emptying the bladder satisfactorily. Occasionally, pinworms can cause these symptoms. The condition is self-limited, and symptoms generally resolve within 2–3 mo. Anticholinergic therapy rarely is effective.

Some children have the **dysuria–hematuria syndrome,** in which the child has dysuria without UTI and microscopic or gross hematuria. This condition affects children who are toilet-trained and often is secondary to hypercalciuria. A 24-hr urine sample should be obtained and calcium and creatinine excretion assessed. A 24-hr calcium excretion of more than 4 mg/kg is abnormal and deserves treatment with thiazides, because some of these children may be at risk for urolithiasis.

Akbal C, Genc Y, Burbu B, et al: Dysfunctional voiding and incontinence scoring system: Quantitative evaluation of incontinence symptoms in pediatric population. *J Urol* 2005;173:969–973.

Ayan S, Kaya K, Topsakal K, et al: Efficacy of tolterodine as a first-line treatment for non-neurogenic voiding dysfunction in children. *BJU Int* 2005; 96:411–414.

Bower WF, Yip SK, Yeung CK: Dysfunctional elimination symptoms in childhood and adulthood. *J Urol* 2005;174:1623–1627.

Feldman AS, Bauer SB: Diagnosis and management of dysfunctional voiding. *Curr Opin Pediatr* 2006;18:139–147.

Firoozi F, Batniji R, Aslan AR, et al: Resolution of diurnal incontinence and nocturnal enuresis after adenotonsillectomy in children. *J Urol* 2006; 175:1885–1888.

Fitzgerald MP, Thom DH, Wassel-Fyr C, et al: Childhood urinary symptoms predict adult overactive bladder symptoms. *J Urol* 2006;175:989–993.

Glazener CM, Evans JH, Cheuk DK: Complementary and miscellaneous interventions for nocturnal enuresis in children. *Cochrane Database Syst Rev* 2005 Apr 18:CD005230.

Glazener CM, Evans JH, Peto RE: Alarm interventions for nocturnal enuresis in children. *Cochrane Database Syst Rev* 2005 Apr 18:CD002911.

Hjalmas K, Arnold T, Bower W, et al: Nocturnal enuresis: An international evidence based management strategy. *J Urol* 2004;171:2545–2561.

Humphreys MR, Reinberg YE: Contemporary and emerging drug treatments for urinary incontinence in children. *Paediatr Drugs* 2005;7:151–162.

Joinson C, Heron J, Butler U, et al: Psychological differences between children with and without soiling problems. *Pediatrics* 2006;117:1575–1583.

Kilic N, Balkan E, Akgoz S, et al: Comparison of the effectiveness and side-effects of tolterodine and oxybutynin in children with detrusor instability. *Int J Urol* 2006;13:105–108.

Klijn AJ, Asselman M, Vijverberg MA, et al: The diameter of the rectum on ultrasonography as a diagnostic tool for constipation in children with dysfunctional voiding. *J Urol* 2004;172:1986–1988.

Kramer SA, Rathbun SR, Elkins D, et al: Double-blind placebo controlled study of alpha-adrenergic receptor antagonists (doxazosin) for treatment of voiding dysfunction in the pediatric population. *J Urol* 2005;173: 2121–2124.

Neveus T, von Gontard A, Hoebeke P, et al: The standardisation of terminology of lower urinary tract function in children and adolescents: Report from the Standardisation Committee of the International Children's Continence Society (ICCS). *J Urol* 2006;176:314–324.

Nguyen MT, Pavlock CL, Zderic SA, et al: Overnight catheter drainage in children with poorly compliant bladders improves post-obstructive diuresis and urinary incontinence. *J Urol* 2005;174:1633–1636.

Robson WL, Leung AK, Van Howe R: Primary and secondary nocturnal enuresis: Similarities in presentation. *Pediatrics* 2005;115:956–959.

Sommer BR, O'Hara R, Askari N, et al: The effect of oxybutynin treatment on cognition in children with diurnal incontinence. *J Urol* 2005;173: 2125–2127.

Thumfart J, Roehr CC, Kapelari K, et al: Desmopressin associated symptomatic hyponatremic hypervolemia in children. Are there predictive factors? *J Urol* 2005;174:294–298.

Van de Walle JG, Bogaert GA, Mattsson S, et al: A new fast-melting oral formulation of desmopressin: A pharmacodynamic study in children with primary nocturnal enuresis. *BJU Int* 2006;97:603–609.

Yagci F, Kibar Y, Akay O, et al: The effect of biofeedback treatment on voiding and urodynamic parameters in children with voiding dysfunction. *J Urol* 2005;174:1994–1997.

Chapter 544 ■ Anomalies of the Penis and Urethra

Jack S. Elder

HYPOSPADIAS

The term **hypospadias** refers to a urethral opening that is on the ventral surface of the penile shaft, a condition that affects 1 in 250 male newborns. There is incomplete development of the prepuce, called a **dorsal hood,** in which the foreskin is on the sides and dorsal aspect of the penile shaft and absent ventrally. Some boys with hypospadias, particularly those with proximal hypospadias, have **chordee,** in which there is ventral penile curvature during erection. It has been speculated that the incidence of hypospadias is increasing, possibly because of in utero exposure to estrogenic or antiandrogenic endocrine-disrupting chemicals (e.g., polychlorobiphenyls, phytoestrogens).

CLINICAL MANIFESTATIONS. Hypospadias is classified according to the position of the urethral meatus after taking into account whether chordee is present (Fig. 544-1). The deformity is described as glanular (on the glans penis), coronal, subcoronal, midpenile, penoscrotal, scrotal, or perineal. Approximately 60% of cases are distal, 25% are subcoronal or midpenile, and 15% are proximal. In the most severe cases, the scrotum is bifid and sometimes extends to the dorsal base of the penis (scrotal engulfment). There also is a megameatal variant, in which the foreskin is developed normally, but there is either distal or subcoronal hypospadias with a "fish mouth" meatus. These cases may not be diagnosed until after a circumcision is performed.

Hypospadias usually is an isolated anomaly, but it also is common in boys with multiple congenital anomalies. Approximately 10% of boys with hypospadias have an undescended testis; inguinal hernias also are common. In the newborn, the differential diagnosis of proximal hypospadias associated with an undescended testis should include forms of ambiguous genitalia, particularly female virilization (congenital adrenal hyperplasia) and mixed gonadal dysgenesis. A karyotype should be obtained in patients with midpenile or proximal hypospadias and cryp-

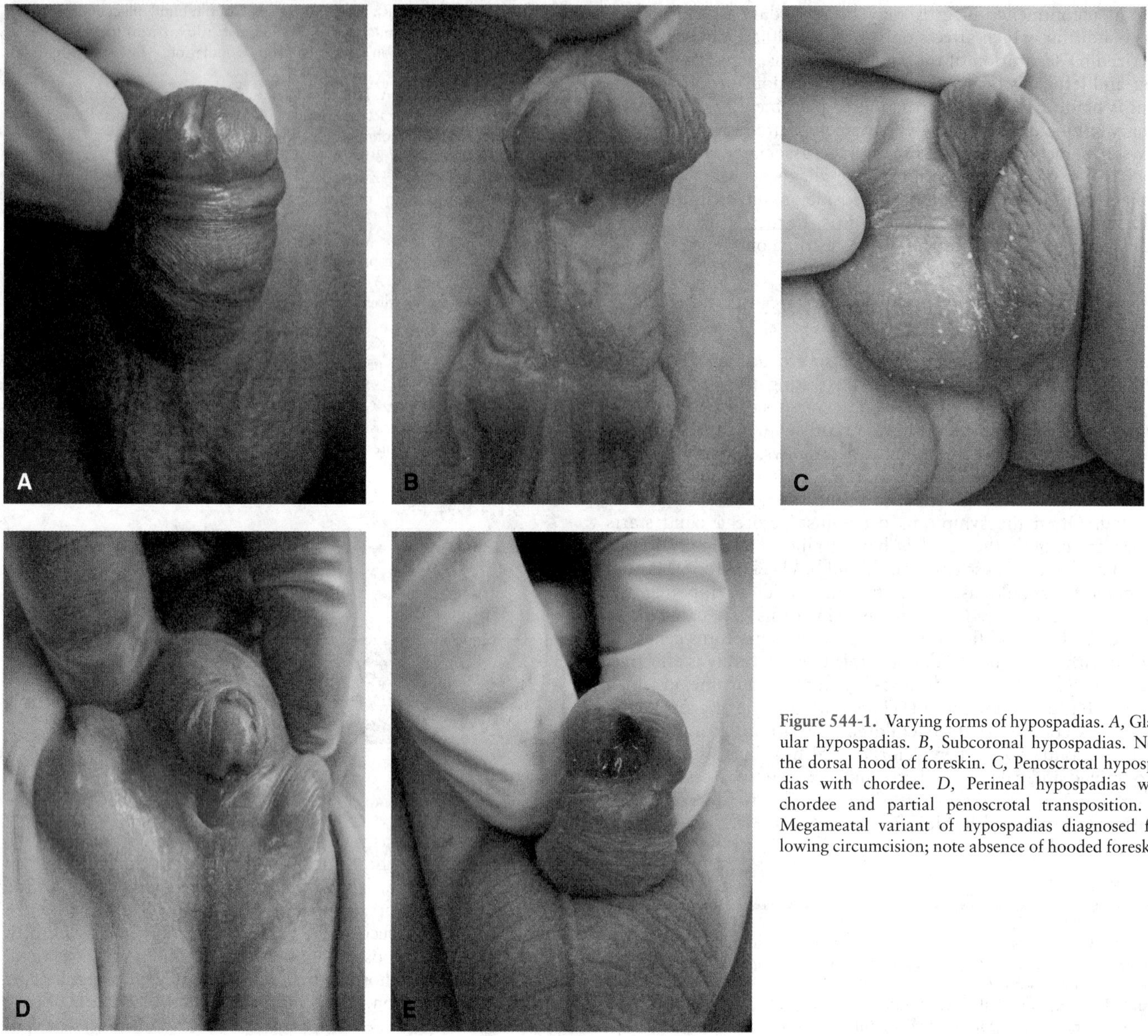

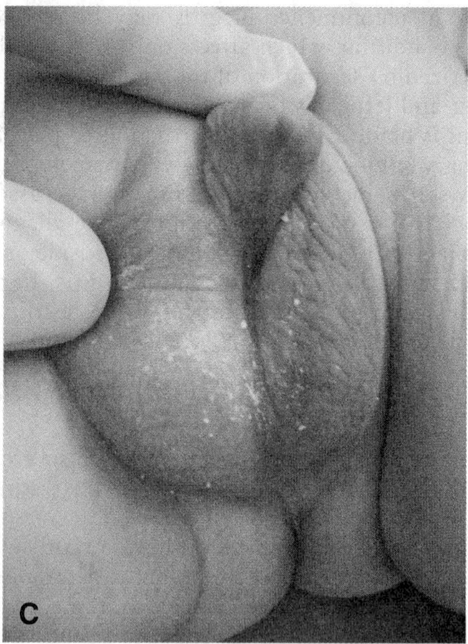

Figure 544-1. Varying forms of hypospadias. *A,* Glanular hypospadias. *B,* Subcoronal hypospadias. Note the dorsal hood of foreskin. *C,* Penoscrotal hypospadias with chordee. *D,* Perineal hypospadias with chordee and partial penoscrotal transposition. *E,* Megameatal variant of hypospadias diagnosed following circumcision; note absence of hooded foreskin.

torchidism (see Chapter 584). In boys with penoscrotal hypospadias, a voiding cystourethrogram should be considered because 5–10% of these children have a dilated prostatic utricle, which is a remnant of the müllerian system (see Chapter 554). The incidence of other anomalies of the genitourinary tract in boys with hypospadias is low.

Complications of untreated hypospadias include (1) deformity of the urinary stream, either ventral deflection or severe splaying; (2) sexual dysfunction secondary to penile curvature; (3) infertility if the urethral meatus is proximal; and (4) meatal stenosis (congenital), which is rare. The goal of hypospadias surgery is to correct the functional and cosmetic deformities. Whereas hypospadias repair is recommended for boys with midpenile and proximal hypospadias, some boys with distal hypospadias will have no functional abnormality and do not need any surgical correction.

TREATMENT. Management begins in the newborn period. Circumcision should be avoided, because the foreskin often is used in the repair. The ideal age for repair in a healthy infant is 6–12 mo, because there is no greater risk of general anesthesia at this age compared to 2–3 yr; penile growth over the next several years is slow; the child does not remember the surgical procedure; and postoperative analgesic needs are less than in older children. With the exception of proximal hypospadias, virtually all cases are repaired in a single operation on an ambulatory basis. The most common repair involves tubularization of the urethral plate distal to the urethral meatus, in which it is covered by a vascularized flap from the pedicle to the foreskin, termed a *tubularized incised plate* (TIP) repair. More proximal cases often require a 2-stage repair. The complication rate is low: 5% for distal hypospadias, 10% for midpenile hypospadias, and 15–20% for proximal hypospadias. The most common complications include urethrocutaneous fistula and meatal stenosis. Other complications include a deformed urinary stream and urethra. Treatment of these complications generally is straightforward. Repair of hypospadias is a technically demanding operation and should be performed by a surgeon with special training in pediatric urology and extensive experience.

CHORDEE WITHOUT HYPOSPADIAS

In some boys there is ventral penile curvature (**chordee**) and incomplete development of the foreskin (**dorsal hood**), but the

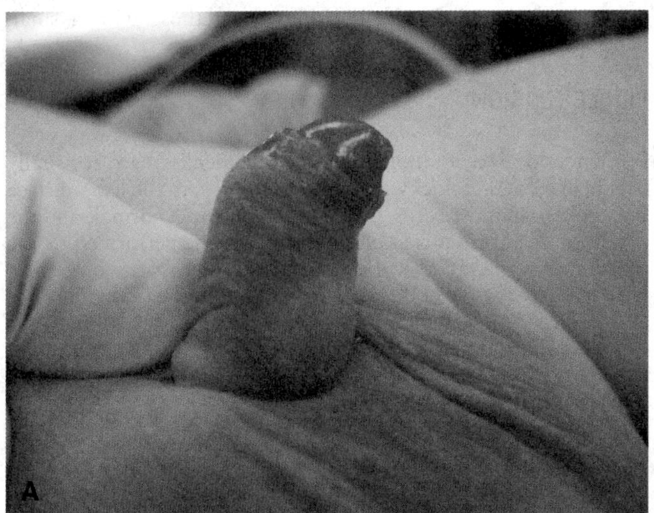

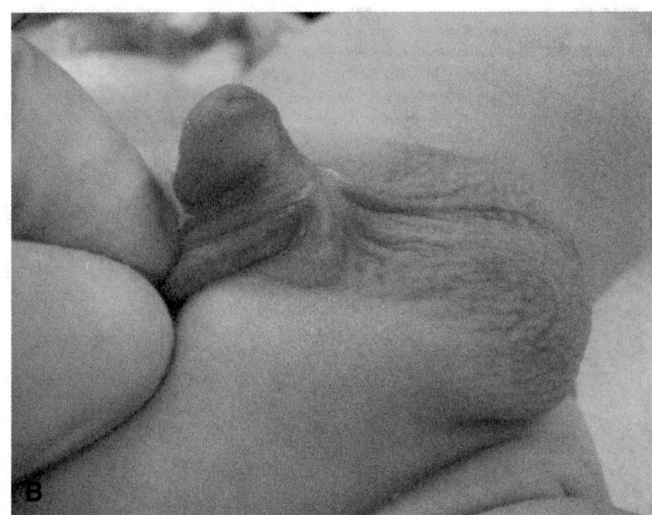

Figure 544-2. *A* and *B,* Two examples of chordee without hypospadias. Note hooded foreskin and normal location of urethral meatus.

urethral meatus is at the tip of the glans (Fig. 544-2). In most of these boys, the urethra is normal but there is insufficient ventral penile skin or prominent, inelastic ventral bands of dartos fascia that prevent a straight erection. In some cases, however, the urethra is short and hypoplastic, and a formal urethroplasty is necessary for repair. The only sign of this anomaly in the neonate may be the hooded foreskin, and delayed repair under general anesthesia at 6 mo of age is recommended.

PHIMOSIS AND PARAPHIMOSIS

Phimosis refers to the inability to retract the prepuce. At birth, phimosis is physiologic. Over time, the adhesions between the prepuce and glans lyse and the distal phimotic ring loosens. In 90% of uncircumcised males the prepuce becomes retractable by the age of 3 yr. Accumulation of epithelial debris under the infant prepuce is physiologic and does not mandate circumcision. In older boys, phimosis may be physiologic, may be pathologic from inflammation and scarring at the tip of the foreskin (Fig. 544-3), or may occur after circumcision. The prepuce may have been retracted forcefully on one or two occasions in the past, which can result in a cicatricial scar that prevents subsequent foreskin retraction. In boys with persistent physiologic or pathologic phimosis, application of corticosteroid cream to the foreskin three times daily for 1 mo loosens the phimotic ring in two-thirds of cases. If there is ballooning of the foreskin during voiding or phimosis beyond 10 yr of age and topical corticosteroid therapy is ineffective, circumcision is recommended.

Paraphimosis occurs when the foreskin is retracted past the coronal sulcus and the prepuce cannot be pulled back over the glans (Fig. 544-4). Painful venous stasis in the retracted foreskin results. with edema leading to severe pain and inability to reduce the foreskin (pull it back over the glans). Treatment includes lubricating the foreskin and glans and then simultaneously compressing the glans and placing distal traction on the foreskin to try to push the phimotic ring past the coronal sulcus. In rare cases, emergency circumcision under general anesthesia is necessary.

CIRCUMCISION

Whether newborn boys should undergo circumcision is controversial. In the U.S., circumcision usually is performed for cultural reasons. Reasons given in support of circumcision include reducing the risk of urinary tract infection (UTI) and sexually transmitted infections and prevention of penile cancer, phimosis, HIV infection, and balanitis. When performing a neonatal circumcision, local analgesia, such as a dorsal nerve block or application of EMLA cream (lidocaine 2.5% and prilocaine 2.5%), is recommended.

UTIs are 10 to 15 times more common in uncircumcised infant boys than in circumcised infants, with the urinary pathogens arising from bacteria that colonize the space between the prepuce and glans. The risk of febrile UTI (see Chapter 538) is highest between birth and 6 mo, but there is an increased risk of UTI through at least 5 yr of age. Many recommend circumcision in infants who are predisposed to UTI, such as those with congenital hydronephrosis and vesicoureteral reflux. Circumcision

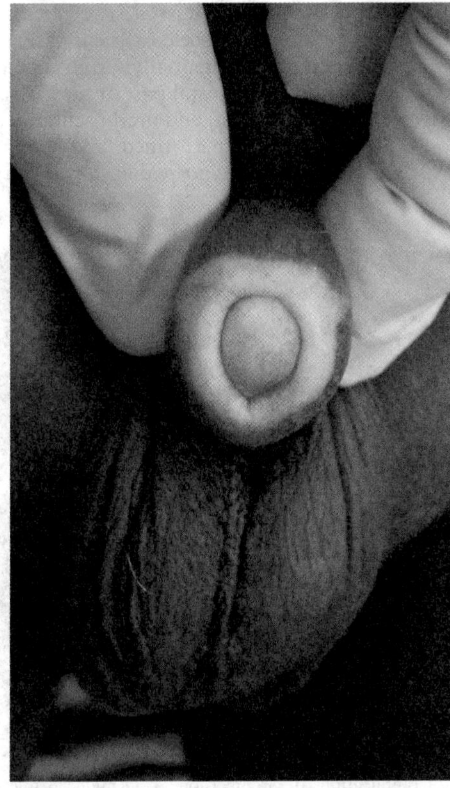

Figure 544-3. Balanitis xerotica obliterans. Note whitish cicatricial plaque.

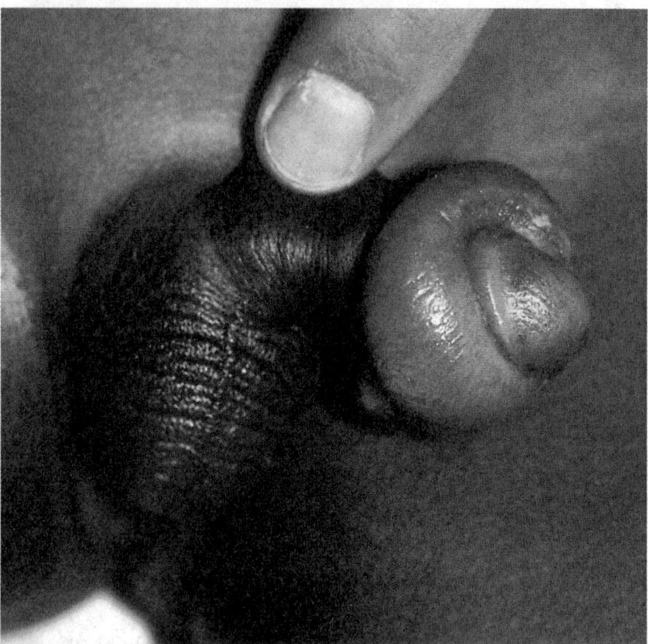

Figure 544-4. Paraphimosis. The foreskin has been retracted proximal to the glans penis and has become markedly swollen secondary to venous congestion.

reduces the risk of sexually transmitted infections in adults (see Chapter 119), in particular AIDS (see Chapter 273). There have been only a handful of reports of adult men who were circumcised at birth and subsequently acquired penile carcinoma, but in Scandinavian countries, where few men are circumcised and hygiene is good, the incidence of penile cancer is low.

Complications after neonatal circumcision include bleeding, wound infection, meatal stenosis, secondary phimosis, removal of insufficient foreskin, and dense penile adhesions (skin bridge; Fig. 544-5); 0.2–3.0% of patients have a subsequent operative procedure. Boys with a large hydrocele or hernia are at particular risk for secondary phimosis. Potentially serious complications include sepsis, amputation of the distal part of the glans, removal of an excessive amount of foreskin, and urethrocutaneous fistula. Circumcision should not be performed in neonates with hypospadias, chordee without hypospadias, or a dorsal hood deformity (relative contraindication) or in those with a small penis (Fig. 544-6).

PENILE TORSION

Penile torsion is a rotational defect of the penile shaft. It usually occurs in a counterclockwise direction, that is, to the left side (see Fig. 544-6). In most cases, penile development is normal, and the condition is unrecognized until circumcision is performed or the foreskin is retractable. Penile torsion also occurs in some boys with hypospadias. The defect has primarily cosmetic significance and correction is unnecessary if the rotation is less than 60 degrees from the midline.

INCONSPICUOUS PENIS

The term *inconspicuous penis* refers to a penis that appears to be small. A **webbed penis** is a condition in which the scrotal skin extends onto the ventrum of the penis. This deformity represents an abnormality of the attachment between the penis and scrotum. Although the deformity may appear mild, if a routine circumcision is performed, the penis may retract into the scrotum and can result in secondary phimosis (**trapped penis**). The concealed (**hidden or buried**) penis is a normally developed penis that is camouflaged by the suprapubic fat pad (Fig. 544-7). This anomaly may be congenital, iatrogenic after circumcision, or a result of obesity. Surgical correction is indicated for cosmetic reasons or if there is a functional abnormality with a splayed stream. A **trapped penis** is an acquired form of inconspicuous penis and refers to a phallus that becomes embedded in the suprapubic fat pad after circumcision (Fig. 544-8). This deformity may occur after neonatal circumcision in an infant who has significant scrotal swelling from a large hydrocele or inguinal hernia or after routine circumcision in an infant with a webbed penis. This complication can predispose to UTIs and may cause urinary retention. Initial treatment of a trapped penis should include topical corticosteroid cream, which often loosens the phimotic ring. In some cases secondary repair is necessary at 6 to 9 mo.

MICROPENIS

Micropenis is defined as a normally formed penis that is at least 2.5 standard deviations below the mean in size (Fig. 544-9). Typ-

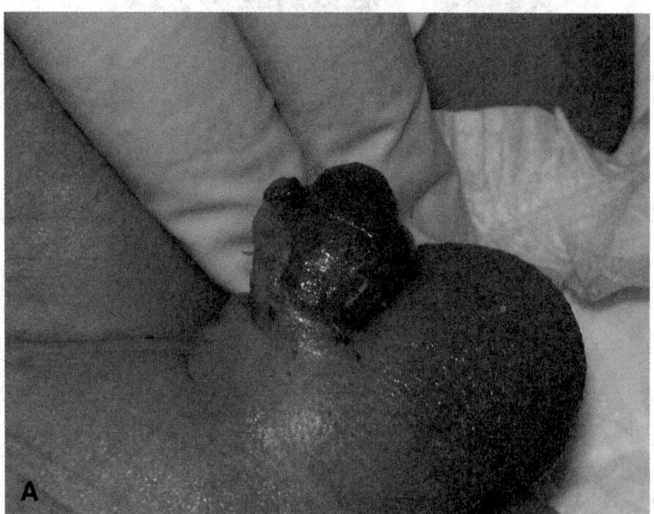

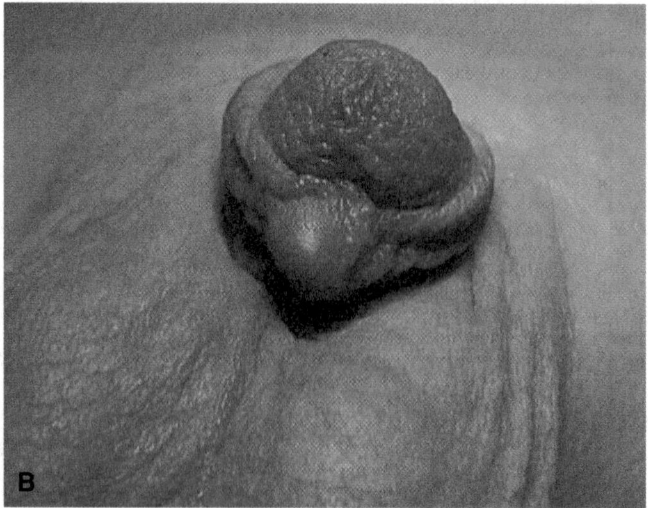

Figure 544-5. Complications of circumcision. *A,* Denuded penile shaft. With local care, the penis healed and appeared normal. *B,* Midline epithelial inclusion cyst.

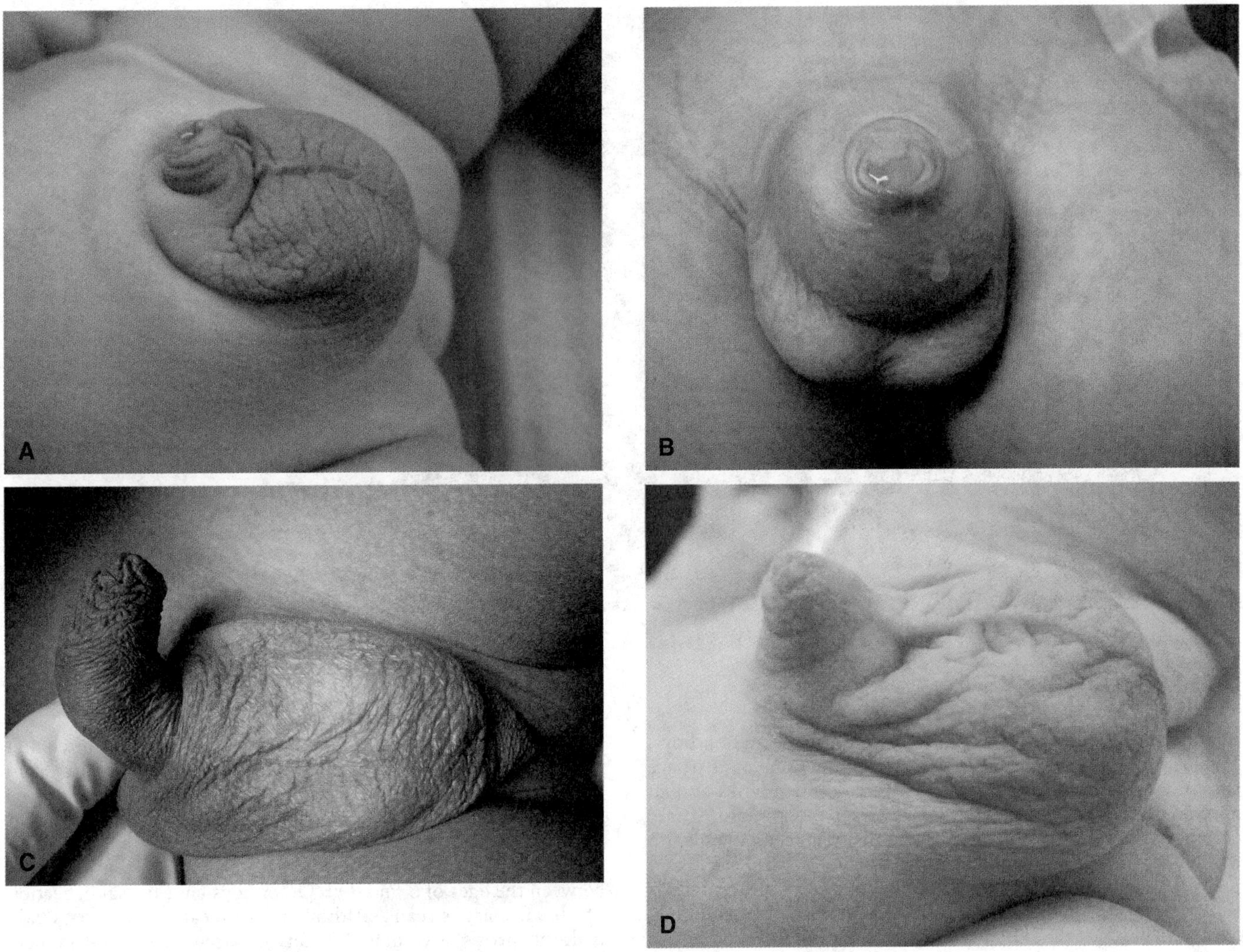

Figure 544-6. Examples of congenital deformities in which neonatal circumcision is contraindicated. *A*, Hidden penis. *B*, Megaprepuce. *C*, Penile torsion to left side. *D*, Webbed penis; note scrotal attachment to penile shaft.

ically, the ratio of the length of the penile shaft to its circumference is normal. The pertinent measurement is the **stretched penile length,** which is measured by stretching the penis and measuring the distance from the penile base under the pubic symphysis to the tip of the glans. The mean length of the term newborn penis is 3.5 ± 0.7 cm and the diameter is 1.1 ± 0.2 cm. The diagnosis of micropenis is made if the stretched length is less than 1.9 cm. Micropenis results from a hormonal abnormality that occurs after 14 wk of gestation. Common causes include hypogonadotropic hypogonadism, hypergonadotropic hypogonadism (primary testicular failure), and idiopathic micropenis. If growth hormone deficiency also is present, neonatal hypoglycemia may occur. The most common cause of micropenis is failure of the hypothalamus to produce an adequate amount of gonadotropin-releasing hormone, as typically occurs in Kallmann syndrome (see Chapter 584), Prader-Willi syndrome (see Chapter 108), and Lawrence-Moon-Biedl syndrome. In some cases, there is growth hormone deficiency. Primary testicular failure may result from gonadal dysgenesis or rudimentary testes syndrome and also occurs in **Robinow syndrome** (characterized by hypoplastic genitalia, shortening of the forearms, frontal bossing, hypertelorism, wide palpebral fissures, short broad nose, long philtrum, small chin, brachydactyly, and a normal karyotype). A pediatric endocrinologist and pediatric urologist should examine all children with these syndromes. **Evaluation** includes a karyotype, assessment of anterior pituitary function and testicular function, and MRI to determine the anatomic integrity of the hypothalamus and the anterior pituitary gland as well as the midline structure of the brain. One of the difficult questions is whether androgen therapy is essential during childhood, because androgenic stimulation of penile growth in a prepubertal boy may limit the growth potential of the penis in puberty. Studies of small groups of men with micropenis suggest that many, although not all, have satisfactory sexual function. Consequently, a decision for gender reassignment is made infrequently.

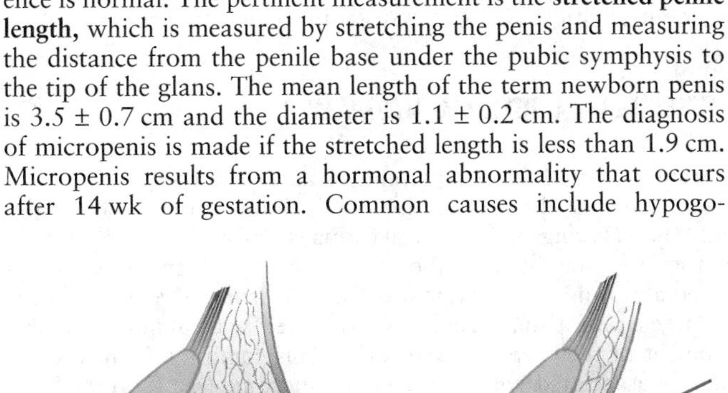

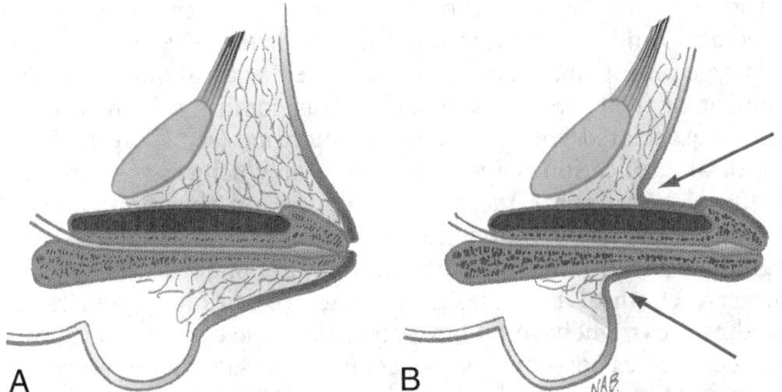

Figure 544-7. Concealed penis *(A)*, which may be visualized by retracting skin lateral to penile shaft *(B)*. (From Wein AJ, Kavoussi LR, Novick AC, et al [editors]: *Campbell-Walsh Urology*, Chapter 126, Fig. 126-4, p. 2339.)

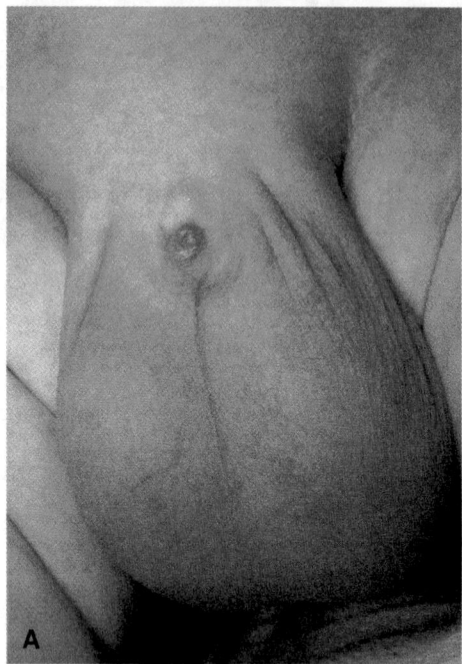

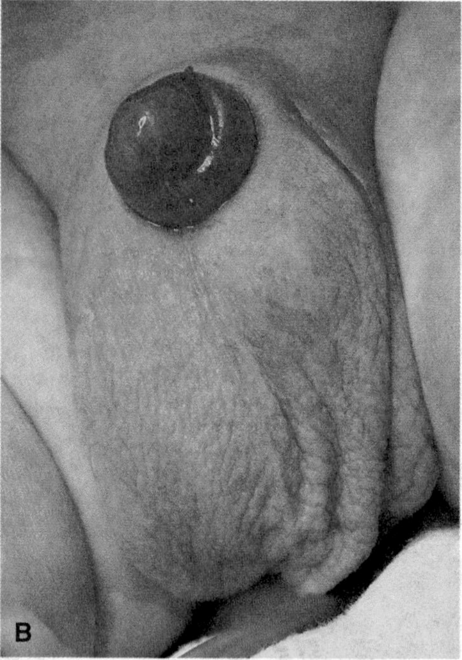

Figure 544-8. *A,* Trapped (concealed) penis resulting from circumcision. *B,* Same patient after revision of circumcision. (From Wein AJ, Kavoussi LR, Novick AC, et al [editors]: *Campbell-Walsh Urology,* Fig. 126-2a and b, p. 2340.)

OTHER PENILE ANOMALIES

Agenesis of the penis affects approximately 1 in 10 million boys. The karyotype is almost always 46,XY, and the usual appearance is that of a well-developed scrotum with descended testes and an absent penile shaft. Upper urinary tract abnormalities are common. In most cases, gender reassignment is recommended in the newborn period. **Diphallia** ranges from a small accessory penis to complete duplication. **Lateral penile curvature** usually is caused by overgrowth or hypoplasia of a corporal (erectile) body and usually is congenital. Surgical repair is recommended at age 6–12 mo.

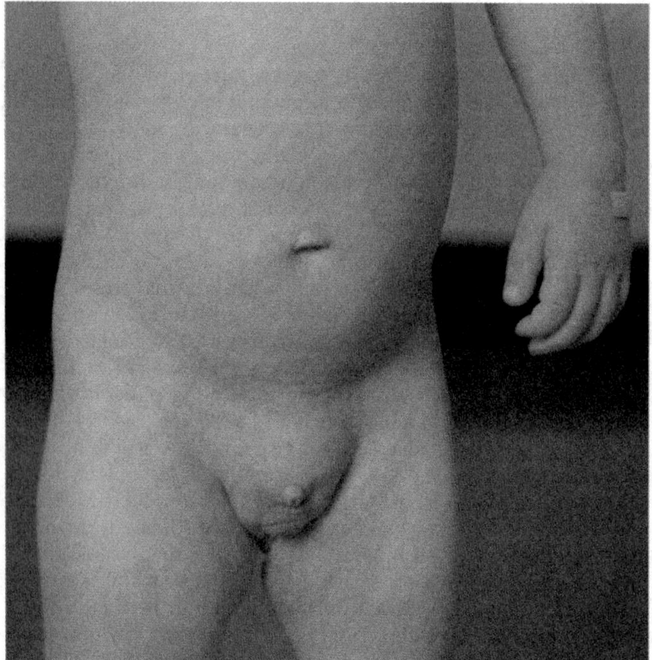

Figure 544-9. Micropenis secondary to hypopituitarism in an 8-year-old boy. (From Wein AJ, Kavoussi LR, Novick AC, et al [editors]: *Campbell-Walsh Urology* color photo Fig. 126-5A, p. 2341.)

MEATAL STENOSIS

Meatal stenosis is a condition that almost always is acquired and occurs after neonatal circumcision. It probably results from severe inflammation of the denuded glans. If the meatus is pinpoint, boys void with a forceful, fine stream that goes a great distance. These boys may experience dysuria, frequency, or hematuria, or a combination of these conditions, without UTI, between the ages of 3 and 8 yr. Other boys have dorsal deflection of the urinary stream. Although the meatus may be small, hydronephrosis or voiding difficulty is extremely rare unless there is associated **balanitis xerotica obliterans** (chronic dermatitis of unknown etiology, generally involving the glans and prepuce, occasionally extending into the urethra). **Treatment** is meatoplasty, in which the urethral meatus is opened surgically; this procedure can be performed either under anesthesia as an outpatient or in the office using local anesthesia (EMLA cream) with or without sedation. Routine cystoscopy is unnecessary.

OTHER MALE URETHRAL ANOMALIES

Parameatal urethral cyst presents as an asymptomatic small cyst on one side of the urethral meatus. Treatment is excision under anesthesia. **Congenital urethral fistula** is a rare deformity in which a fistula is present from the penile urethra. It usually is an isolated abnormality. Treatment is fistula closure. **Megalourethra** is a large urethra that usually is associated with abnormal development of the corpus spongiosum. This condition is most commonly associated with prune-belly syndrome (see Chapter 540). **Urethral duplication** is a rare condition in which the two urethral channels lie in the same sagittal plane, and the more normal urethra is the one positioned more ventrally. Some children have significant obstructive uropathy and require major reconstructive surgery. **Urethral hypoplasia** is a rare condition in which the urethra is extremely small but patent. In some cases, a temporary cutaneous vesicostomy is necessary for satisfactory urinary drainage. Either gradual enlargement of the urethra or major urethroplasty is necessary. **Urethral atresia** refers to nondevelopment of the urethra and nearly always is fatal unless the urachus remains patent throughout gestation.

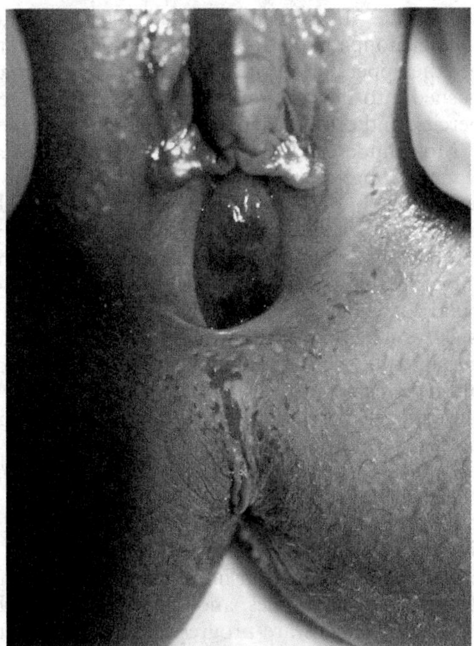

Figure 544-10. Urethral prolapse in a 4-yr-old black girl who had bloody spotting on her underwear.

URETHRAL PROLAPSE (FEMALE)

Urethral prolapse is encountered predominantly in black girls between 1 and 9 yr of age. The most common signs are bloody spotting on the underwear or diaper, although dysuria or perineal discomfort also may occur (Fig. 544-10). An inexperienced examiner may mistake the finding for sexual abuse. The usual therapy consists of application of estrogen cream two to three times daily for 3–4 wk and sitz baths. Surgical excision and reapproximation of the mucosal edges is curative.

OTHER FEMALE URETHRAL LESIONS

Paraurethral cyst results from retained secretions in the Skene glands secondary to ductal obstruction (Fig. 544-11). These lesions are present at birth, and most regress in size during the first 4–8 wk, although occasionally incision and drainage is necessary. A **prolapsed ectopic ureterocele** appears as a cystic mass protruding from the urethra and is a presenting symptom in 10% of girls with a ureterocele, which is a cystic swelling of the terminal ureter (Fig. 544-12). Ultrasonography should be performed to visualize the upper urinary tracts to confirm the diagnosis. Usually, either the ureterocele is incised or an upper urinary tract reconstructive procedure is necessary.

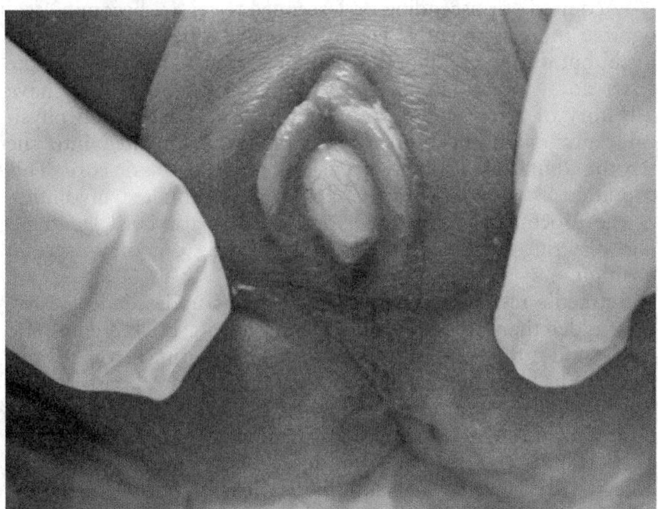

Figure 544-11. Paraurethral cyst in a newborn girl.

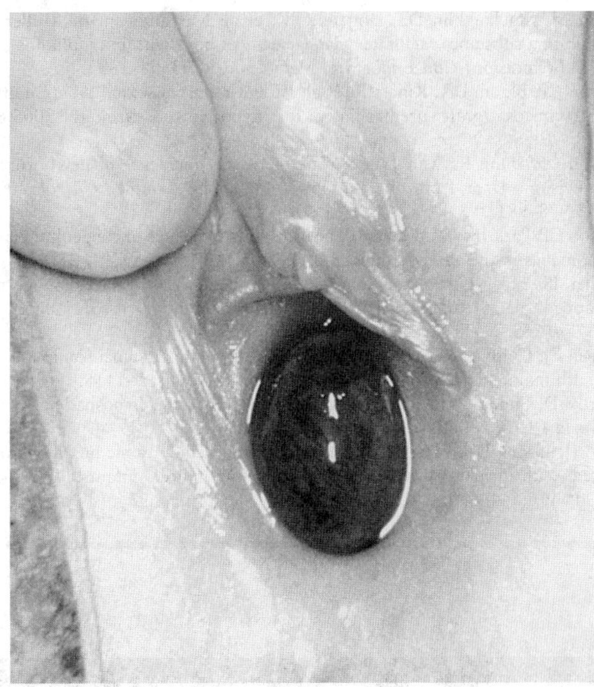

Figure 544-12. Prolapsed ectopic ureterocele in a female infant. She had a nonfunctioning upper pole collecting system connected to the ureterocele.

American Academy of Pediatrics, Task Force on Circumcision: Circumcision policy statement. *Pediatrics* 1999;103:686–693.

Auvert B, Taljaard D, Lagarde E, et al: Randomized, controlled intervention trial of male circumcision for reduction of HIV infection risk: The ANRS 1265 Trial. *PLoS Med* 2005;2:e298. Epub 2005 Oct 25.

Baskin LS, Ebbers MB: Hypospadias: Anatomy, etiology, and technique. *J Pediatr Surg* 2006;41:463–472.

Carmichael SL, Shaw GM, Laurent C, et al: Maternal progestin intake and risk of hypospadias. *Arch Pediatr Adolesc Med* 2005;159:957–962.

Castellsague X, Bosch X, Munoz N, et al: Male circumcision, penile human papillomavirus infection, and cervical cancer in female partners. *N Engl J Med* 2002;346:1105–1112.

Elder JS: Abnormalities of the genitalia in boys and their surgical management. In Wein AJ, Kavoussi LR, Novick AC, et al (editors): *Campbell-Walsh Urology,* 9th ed. Philadelphia, Elsevier, in press.

Gargollo PC, Kozakewich HP, Bauer SB, et al: Balanitis xerotica obliterans in boys. *J Urol* 2005;174:1409–1412.

Horowitz M, Sulzhauer E: The "learning curve" in hypospadias surgery. *BJU Int* 2006;97:593–596.

Husmann DA: The androgen insensitive micropenis: Long-term follow-up into adulthood. *J Pediatr Endocrinol Metab* 2004;17:1037–1041.

Kurzrock EA, Karpman E: Hypospadias: Pathophysiology and etiologic theories. *Pediatr Endocrinol Rev* 2004;1:288–295.

Lee PA, Houk CP: Outcome studies among men with micropenis. *J Pediatr Endocrinol Metab* 2004;17:1043–1053.

Lund L, Wai KH, Mui LM, et al: An 18-month follow-up study after randomized treatment of phimosis in boys with topical steroid versus placebo. *Scand J Urol Nephrol* 2005;39:78–81.

Meau-Petit V, Marcou V, Trivin C, et al: Idiopathic male pseudohermaphroditism: Variations in presentation and management. *J Pediatr Endocrinol Metab* 2005;18:569–575.

Misra M, Maclaughlin DT, Donahoe PK, et al: Measurement of Müllerian inhibiting substance facilitates management of boys with microphallus and cryptorchidism. *J Clin Endocrinol Metab* 2002;87:3598–3602.
Nelson CP, Bloom DA, Kinast R, et al: Patient-reported sexual function after oral mucosa graft urethroplasty for hypospadias. *Urology* 2005;66:1086–1089.
Nelson CP, Dunn R, Wan J, et al: The increasing incidence of newborn circumcision: Data from the nationwide inpatient sample. *J Urol* 2005;173:978–981.
Nelson CP, Park JM, Wan J, et al: The increasing incidence of congenital penile anomalies in the United States. *J Urol* 2005;174:1573–1576.
Palmer JS, Elder JS, Palmer LS: The use of betamethasone to manage the trapped penis following neonatal circumcision. *J Urol* 2005;174:1577–1578.
Schoen EJ, Colby CJ, To TT: Cost analysis of neonatal circumcision in a large health maintenance organization. *J Urol* 2006;175:1111–1115.
Wilcox D, Snodgrass W: Long-term outcome following hypospadias repair. *World J Urol* 2006;24:248–253.
Zorc JJ, Levine DA, Platt SL, et al: Clinical and demographic factors associated with urinary tract infection in young febrile infants. *Pediatrics* 2005;116:644–648.

Chapter 545 ■ Disorders and Anomalies of the Scrotal Contents Jack S. Elder

UNDESCENDED TESTES

Failure to find the testis in the scrotum indicates that the testis is undescended, absent, or retractile.

EPIDEMIOLOGY. An undescended (**cryptorchid**) testis is the most common disorder of sexual differentiation in boys. At birth, approximately 4.5% of boys have an undescended testis. Because testicular descent occurs late in gestation, 30% of premature male infants have an undescended testis; the incidence is 3.4% at term. The majority of undescended testes descend spontaneously during the first 3 mo of life, and by 6 mo the incidence decreases to 0.8%. If the testis has not descended by 4 mo, it will remain undescended. Cryptorchidism is bilateral in 10% of cases. There is some evidence that the incidence of cryptorchidism is increasing. Although cryptorchidism usually is considered to be a congenital condition, an increasing number of older boys are being diagnosed with an undescended testis. Typically these boys have a scrotal testis that "ascends" to a low inguinal position, and therefore require an orchiopexy. Some boys have secondary cryptorchidism after repair of an inguinal hernia. This complication is most common in neonates and young infants and affects as many as 1–2% of patients undergoing hernia repair.

PATHOGENESIS. The process of testicular descent is regulated by an interaction between hormonal and mechanical factors, including testosterone, dihydrotestosterone, müllerian-inhibiting factor, the gubernaculum, intra-abdominal pressure, and the genitofemoral nerve. The testis develops at 7–8 wk of gestation. At 10–11 wk, the Leydig cells produce testosterone, which stimulates differentiation of the wolffian (mesonephric) duct into the epididymis, vas deferens, seminal vesicle, and ejaculatory duct. At 32–36 wk, the testis, which is anchored at the internal inguinal ring by the gubernaculum, begins its process of descent. The gubernaculum distends the inguinal canal and guides the testis into the scrotum. Following testicular descent, the patent processus vaginalis (hernia sac) normally involutes.

CLINICAL MANIFESTATIONS. Undescended testes can be classified as **abdominal** (nonpalpable), **peeping** (abdominal but can be pushed into the upper part of the inguinal canal), **inguinal, gliding** (can be pushed into the scrotum but retracts immediately to the pubic tubercle), and **ectopic** (superficial inguinal pouch or, rarely, perineal). Most undescended testes are in or just distal to the inguinal canal. Approximately 10% of cryptorchid boys have a nonpalpable testis; in these boys the testis is present and abdominal or inguinal in 50%, and it is absent secondary to perinatal testicular torsion in 50%. In a newborn phenotypic male with bilateral nonpalpable testes, one should consider the possibility that the child could be a virilized female with congenital adrenal hyperplasia (see Chapter 577). In a boy with an undescended testis and midpenile or proximal hypospadias, an intersex condition should be considered.

The **consequences of cryptorchidism** include infertility, testicular malignancy, associated hernia, torsion of the cryptorchid testis, and the possible psychologic effects of an empty scrotum.

The undescended testis is normal at birth histologically, but pathologic changes can be demonstrated by 6–12 mo. Delayed germ cell maturation, reduction in germ cell number, hyalinization of the seminiferous tubules, and reduced Leydig cell number are typical; these changes are progressive over time if the testis remains undescended. Similar, although less severe, changes are found in the contralateral descended testis after 4–7 yr. After treatment for a unilateral undescended testis, 85% of patients are fertile, which is slightly less than the 90% rate of fertility in an unselected population of male adults. In contrast, following bilateral orchiopexy, only 50–65% of patients are fertile.

The risk of a **germ cell malignancy** (see Chapter 503) developing in an undescended testis is 4 to 10 times higher than that in the general population and is approximately 1 in 80 with a unilateral undescended testis and 1 in 40 to 1 in 50 for bilateral undescended testes. The peak age for developing a testis tumor is 15–45 yr. The most common tumor developing in an undescended testis is a **seminoma** (65%); in contrast, after orchiopexy, seminomas represent only 30% of testis tumors. Whether orchiopexy reduces the risk of developing cancer of the testis is controversial, but it is uncommon for testis tumors to occur after orchiopexy performed before the age of 2 years.

Indirect inguinal hernias usually accompany congenital undescended testes but rarely are symptomatic. Torsion and infarction of the undescended testis also is uncommon, but can occur because of excessive mobility of such testes. Consequently, inguinal pain and/or swelling in a boy with an undescended testis should raise the suspicion of an incarcerated hernia or testicular torsion of the undescended testis.

"Acquired" or **ascending undescended testes** are becoming recognized more frequently. These boys have a descended testis at birth, but during childhood, usually between 4–10 yr of age, the testis does not remain in the scrotum. Such boys often have a history of a retractile testis. With testicular ascent, on physical examination the testis often can be manipulated into the scrotum, but there is obvious tension on the spermatic cord. This condition is speculated to result from incomplete involution of the processus vaginalis, restricting spermatic cord lengthening, resulting in the testis gradually moving out of its scrotal position.

Retractile testes may be misdiagnosed as undescended testes. Boys older than 1 yr of age frequently have a brisk cremasteric reflex; and if the child is anxious or ticklish during scrotal examination, the testis may be difficult to manipulate into the scrotum. Boys should be examined with their legs in a relaxed frog-leg position, and if the testis can be manipulated into the scrotum comfortably, it is probably retractile. It should be monitored every 6–12 mo with follow-up physical examinations, because it could be an acquired undescended testis. Overall, at least one third of boys with a retractile testis will develop an acquired undescended testis, and boys <7 yr of age at diagnosis of a retractile testis are at greatest risk. Most think that boys with a retractile testis are not at increased risk for infertility or malignancy.

On **physical examination** of the scrotum, it is important to have the child entirely undressed, to help him relax. If the testis is difficult to palpate, the "soap test" often is useful; soap is applied to the inguinal canal and the examiner's hand, significantly reducing friction and facilitating identification of an inguinal testis. One "soft" sign that a testis is absent is contralateral testicular hypertrophy, but this finding is not 100% diagnostic.

TREATMENT. The congenital undescended testis should be treated surgically no later than 9–15 mo. With anesthesia by a pediatric anesthesiologist, surgical correction at 6 mo is appropriate, because spontaneous descent of the testis will not occur after 4 mo of age. Most testes can be brought down to the scrotum with an orchiopexy, which involves an inguinal incision, mobilization of the testis and spermatic cord, and correction of the indirect inguinal hernia. The procedure is typically performed on an outpatient basis and has a success rate of 98%. In some boys with a testis that is close to the scrotum, a Bianchi or prescrotal orchiopexy can be performed. In this procedure, the entire operation is performed through an incision along the edge of the scrotum. Often the associated inguinal hernia also can be corrected with this incision. Advantages of this approach over the inguinal approach include shorter operative time and less postoperative discomfort.

Hormonal treatment is used infrequently. The theory is that because testicular descent is under androgen regulation, human chorionic gonadotropin (which stimulates Leydig cell production of testosterone) or luteinizing hormone–releasing hormone (LHRH) may stimulate testicular descent. Although hormonal treatment has been used in Europe, randomized controlled trials have not shown either of these hormonal preparations to be effective in stimulating testicular descent. There has been some preliminary evidence that an LHRH analog, buserelin, may be helpful in increasing germ cell number and normalizing testicular histologic features.

In approximately 50% of boys in whom the testis is nonpalpable, there is an intra-abdominal testis or a testis that is located high in the inguinal canal; in the remaining 50%, the testis is absent (atrophic) secondary to perinatal testicular torsion, termed a **vanishing testis.** Imaging has been suggested as a method of determining whether the testis is present. Ultrasound has been demonstrated to be ineffective in "localizing" the nonpalpable testis. In contrast, CT scanning is relatively accurate in demonstrating the presence of the testis. MRI is even more accurate, but the disadvantage is that heavy sedation is necessary in most children. Because imaging has not been proven to be 100% reliable in demonstrating whether the testis is present, diagnostic laparoscopy is performed in most centers. This procedure allows safe and rapid assessment of whether the testis is intra-abdominal. In most cases, orchiopexy of the intra-abdominal testis located immediately inside the internal inguinal ring is successful, but orchiectomy should be considered in more difficult cases or when the testis appears to be atrophic. A two-stage orchiopexy sometimes is needed in boys with a high abdominal testis. Boys with abdominal testes are managed with laparoscopic techniques at many institutions. Testicular prostheses are available for older children and adolescents when the absence of the gonad in the scrotum may have an undesirable psychological effect. The U.S. Food and Drug Administration (FDA) has approved a saline testicular implant. A solid silicone "carving block" implant currently is undergoing FDA trials. Placement of testicular prostheses early in childhood is recommended for boys with anorchia (absence of both testes).

TABLE 545-1. Differential Diagnosis of Scrotal Masses in Boys and Adolescents

PAINFUL	PAINLESS
Testicular torsion	Hydrocele
Torsion of appendix testis	Inguinal hernia*
Epididymitis	Varicocele*
Trauma: ruptured testis, hematocele	Spermatocele*
Inguinal hernia (incarcerated)	Testicular tumor*
Mumps orchitis	Henoch-Schönlein purpura*
	Idiopathic scrotal edema

*May be associated with discomfort.

SCROTAL SWELLING

Scrotal swelling may be acute or chronic, and painful or painless. Abrupt onset of painful scrotal swelling necessitates prompt evaluation, because some conditions, such as testicular torsion and incarcerated inguinal hernia, require emergency surgical management. The differential diagnosis is shown in Tables 545-1 and 545-2.

CLINICAL MANIFESTATIONS. A detailed history is helpful in determining the cause of the swelling and includes (1) onset of pain—with testicular torsion the pain often is sudden in onset and may be associated with exercise or minor genital trauma; (2) duration of pain; (3) radiation of pain—inguinal discomfort is common with testicular torsion, inguinal hernia, or epididymitis, and associated flank pain may occur with passage of a ureteral calculus; (4) previous episodes of similar pain, which are common in boys with intermittent testicular torsion or inguinal hernia; (5) nausea and vomiting, which are associated with testicular torsion and inguinal hernia; and (6) irritative urinary symptoms, such as dysuria, urgency, and frequency, which are indicative of a urinary tract infection that can cause epididymitis. Boys with lower urinary tract pathology such as urethral stricture or neuropathic bladder may be prone to epididymitis.

Physical examination may be difficult in boys with a painful scrotum. Some have advocated performing a spermatic cord block or administering intravenous analgesia to facilitate the examination, but such measures usually are unnecessary. Scrotal wall erythema is common in testicular torsion, epididymitis, torsion of the appendix testis, and an incarcerated hernia. In boys with a normal cremasteric reflex, testicular torsion is unlikely. Absence of a cremasteric reflex, however, is nondiagnostic.

LABORATORY FINDINGS AND DIAGNOSIS. Pertinent laboratory studies include a urinalysis and culture. A positive urinalysis is suggestive of epididymitis. Serum studies are not helpful in establishing a diagnosis, unless a tumor of the testis is suspected. After initial evaluation, imaging studies may be helpful in establishing the diagnosis, because they assess whether testicular blood flow is normal, reduced, or increased. Imaging studies include color Doppler ultrasonography and a radionuclide testicular flow scan. In addition, if a hydrocele is present and the testis is nonpalpa-

TABLE 545-2. Differential Diagnosis of Scrotal Swelling in Newborns

Hydrocele
Inguinal hernia (reducible)
Inguinal hernia (incarcerated)*
Testicular torsion*
Scrotal hematoma
Testicular tumor
Meconium peritonitis
Epididymitis*

*May be associated with discomfort.

ble, or if an abnormality of the testis is found, ultrasonography may be helpful. Imaging studies are not 100% accurate; they should not be used to decide whether a boy with testicular pain should be referred for urologic care.

Color Doppler ultrasonography is performed most commonly and allows assessment of testicular blood flow and testicular morphologic features. Accuracy is 95% if the ultrasonographer is experienced. A false-negative study (demonstrates normal testicular blood flow) may occur in a boy with testicular torsion if the degree of torsion is less than 360 degrees and the duration of torsion is short, because there may be continued testicular perfusion. In addition, in prepubertal boys blood flow may be difficult to demonstrate in as many as 30% of normal testes.

The ^{99m}Tc-pertechnetate testicular flow scan can demonstrate whether there is blood flow to the testis. After intravenous injection of the radionuclide, flow and static images are obtained. Testicular torsion usually appears as a "cold spot" of absent flow to the affected testis. Inflammatory conditions usually cause hyperemia. Accuracy in demonstrating blood flow is approximately 95%. A false-negative scan may occur in a boy with testicular torsion if the degree of torsion is less than 360 degrees. The test often can be obtained on an emergent basis during the day, but at night it may take 2–3 hr to perform and interpret the study.

TESTICULAR (SPERMATIC CORD) TORSION

ETIOLOGY. Testicular torsion requires prompt diagnosis and treatment to save the testis. Torsion is the most common cause of testicular pain in boys 12 yr and older and is uncommon in boys younger than 10 yr. It is caused by inadequate fixation of the testis within the scrotum, resulting from a redundant tunica vaginalis, allowing excessive mobility of the testis. The abnormal attachment has been termed a *bell clapper deformity* and often is bilateral. Shortly after torsion occurs, venous congestion begins; subsequently, arterial flow is interrupted. The likelihood of testis survival depends on the duration and severity of torsion. Within 4–6 hr of absent blood flow to the testis, irreversible loss of spermatogenesis may occur.

DIAGNOSIS. Testicular torsion produces acute pain and swelling of the scrotum. On examination, the scrotum is swollen, and the testis is exquisitely tender and often difficult to examine. The cremasteric reflex nearly always is absent. The condition can be differentiated from an incarcerated hernia because swelling in the inguinal area often is absent. If the pain has lasted less than 4–6 hr, manual detorsion may be attempted. In ⅔ of cases the torsed testis rotates inward, so detorsion should be attempted in the opposite direction (e.g., the left testis is rotated clockwise). Successful manual detorsion results in dramatic pain relief.

TREATMENT. Treatment is prompt surgical exploration and detorsion. If the testis is explored within 6 hr of torsion, as many as 90% of the gonads will survive. Survival decreases rapidly with a delay of more than 6 hr. If the degree of torsion is 360 degrees or less, the testis may have sufficient arterial flow to allow the gonad to survive, even after 24–48 hr. The testis is then fixed in the scrotum with nonabsorbable sutures, termed *scrotal orchiopexy,* to prevent torsion in the future. The contralateral testis also should be fixed in the scrotum because the anatomic predisposing anatomical condition often is bilateral. If the testis appears nonviable, orchiectomy is performed (Fig. 545-1).

Testicular torsion also can occur in the fetus or neonate. It results from incomplete attachment of the tunica vaginalis to the scrotal wall and is "extravaginal." When torsion occurs in utero, the baby usually is born with a large, firm, nontender testis. Usually the ipsilateral hemiscrotum is ecchymotic (Fig. 545-2). In these cases, the testis rarely is viable because torsion was a remote event. However, the contralateral testis is at increased risk for torsion until 1 mo beyond term. Many pediatric urologists recommend exploration to establish the diagnosis, remove the necrotic testis, and anchor the contralateral testis. In other cases, the initial examination is normal, and acute scrotal swelling is recognized subsequently. In such cases, the testis occasionally may be saved.

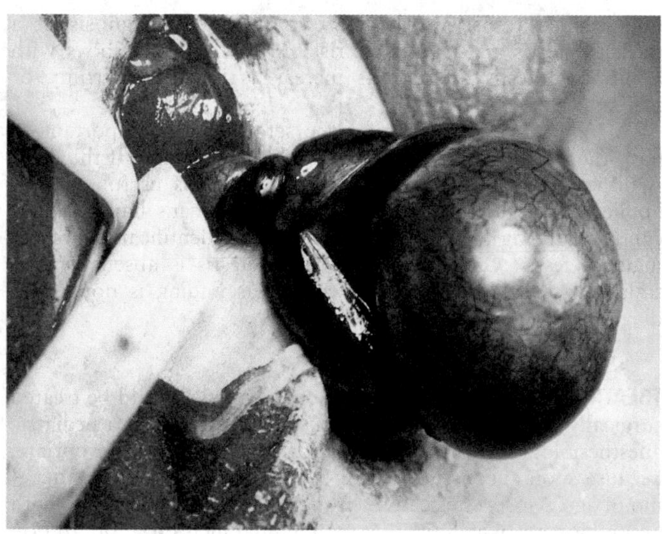

Figure 545-1. Left testicular torsion in an adolescent; the testis is necrotic.

TORSION OF THE APPENDIX TESTIS

Torsion of the appendix testis is the most common cause of testicular pain in boys between 2–10 yr but is rare in adolescents. The appendix testis is a stalk-like structure that is a vestigial embryonic remnant of the müllerian (paramesonephric) ductal system that is attached to the upper pole of the testis. When it undergoes torsion, progressive inflammation and swelling of the testis and epididymis occurs, resulting in testicular pain and scrotal erythema. The onset of pain usually is gradual. Palpation of the testis usually reveals a 3- to 5-mm tender indurated mass on the upper pole (Fig. 545-3). In some cases, the appendage that has undergone torsion may be visible through the scrotal skin, in the "blue dot" sign. In some boys, distinguishing torsion of the appendix from testicular torsion is difficult. In such cases, a testicular flow scan or color Doppler ultrasonography may be helpful because testicular blood flow will be normal or increased. In such cases, the radiologist often will recognize epididymal enlargement and make the diagnosis of epididymitis.

The natural history of torsion of the appendix testis is for the inflammation to resolve in 3–10 days. Nonoperative treatment is recommended, including bed rest and analgesia with nonsteroidal anti-inflammatory medication for 5 days. If the diagnosis is uncertain, scrotal exploration is recommended.

EPIDIDYMITIS

Acute inflammation of the epididymis is an ascending retrograde infection from the urethra, through the vas into the epididymis. This condition causes acute scrotal pain, erythema, and swelling. It is rare before puberty and should raise the question of a congenital abnormality of the wolffian duct, such as an ectopic ureter entering the vas. In younger males, the responsible organism often is *Escherichia coli.* After puberty, epididymitis becomes progressively more common and is the principal cause of acute painful scrotal swelling in young, sexually active men. Urinalysis usually reveals pyuria. Epididymitis can be infectious (usually gonococcus or **chlamydia**), but often the organism remains undetermined.

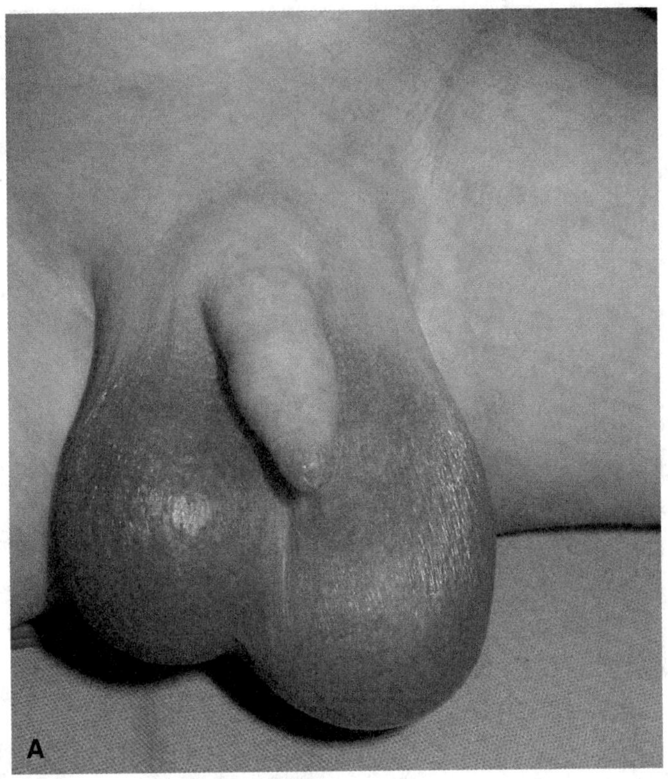

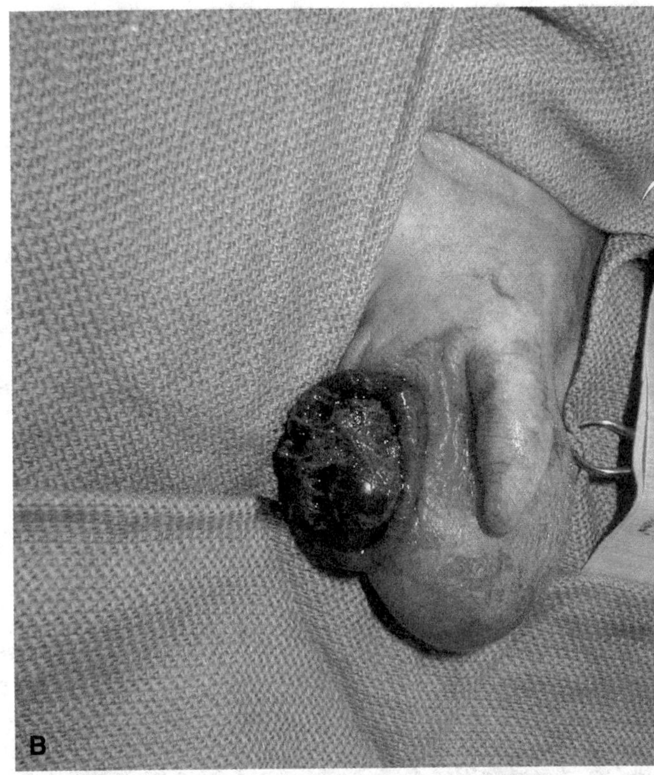

Figure 545-2. Right testicular torsion in a newborn. The right hemiscrotum is darker, and the testis was indurated and enlarged.

Additional etiologies include Henoch-Schönlein purpura, familial Mediterranean fever, enterovirus, and adenoviruses. Treatment consists of bed rest and antibiotics (see Chapter 119). Differentiation from torsion can be difficult, and surgical exploration usually is required in children.

VARICOCELE

A varicocele is a congenital condition in which there is abnormal dilation of the pampiniform plexus in the scrotum (Fig. 545-4). Dilation of the pampiniform venous plexus results from valvular incompetence of the spermatic vein. Approximately 15% of adult men have a varicocele; of these men, approximately 15% are subfertile. Varicocele is the most common (and virtually the only) surgically correctable cause of subfertility in men. A varicocele is found in 5–15% of adolescent boys, but it rarely is diagnosed in boys younger than 10 yr old, because the varicocele becomes distended only after the increased blood flow associated with puberty occurs. Varicoceles occur predominantly on the left side, are bilateral in 10% of cases, and rarely involve the right side only. A varicocele in a boy <10 yr or one on the right side may be indicative of an abdominal or retroperitoneal mass; an abdominal sonogram or CT scan should be performed in such cases.

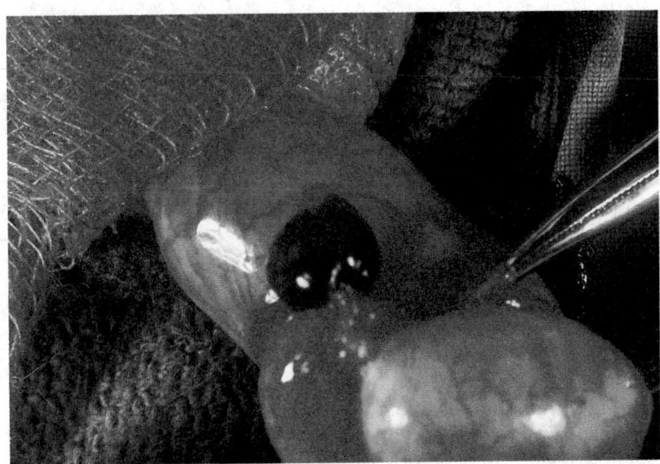

Figure 545-3. Torsion of the appendix testis; the testis is necrotic *(arrow)*.

A varicocele typically is a painless paratesticular mass, often described as a "bag of worms." Occasionally patients describe a dull ache in the affected testis. Usually the varicocele is not apparent when the patient is supine because it is decompressed; in contrast, the varicocele becomes prominent when the patient is standing and enlarges with a Valsalva maneuver. Studies have shown that most pediatricians do not routinely screen male adolescents for a varicocele. Varicoceles typically are graded from 1 to 3: **grade 1** is palpable only with Valsalva; **grade 2** is palpable without Valsalva but is not visible on inspection; and **grade 3** is visible with inspection. Boys with a grade 3 varicocele are at greatest risk for testicular growth arrest. Testicular size should be documented with calipers, an orchiometer, or scrotal sonography, because if the affected left testis is significantly smaller than the right testis, spermatogenesis probably has been adversely affected.

The goal of varicocelectomy is to maximize chances for fertility. Surgical treatment of varicoceles in children and adolescents is indicated in boys with a significant disparity in testicular size or pain in the affected testis, or if the contralateral testis is diseased or absent. Typically the involved testis enlarges and catches up with the normal testis over the following 1–2 yr. Varicocelectomy should also be considered in boys with a large grade 3 varicocele, even without a disparity in testicular size. Surgical repair is accomplished with a variety of techniques by ligation of the veins of the pampiniform plexus through an inguinal or subinguinal incision (with or without an operating microscope) or by ligating the internal spermatic vein in the retroperitoneum. Laparoscopic repair is becoming more popular. The operation is performed on an ambulatory basis.

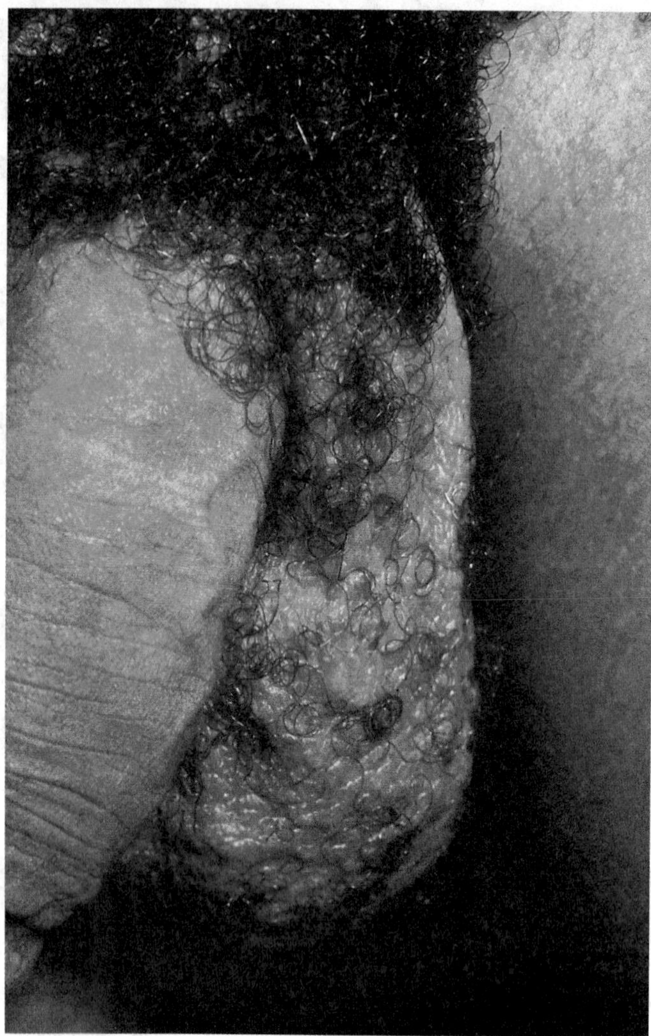

Figure 545-4. Left varicocele in an adolescent boy.

SPERMATOCELE

A spermatocele is a cystic lesion containing sperm that is attached to the upper pole of the sexually mature testis. Spermatoceles usually are painless and are incidental findings on physical examination. Enlargement of the spermatocele or pain is an indication for removal.

HYDROCELE

ETIOLOGY. A hydrocele is an accumulation of fluid in the tunica vaginalis (Fig. 545-5). From 1–2% of male neonates have a hydrocele. In most cases, the hydrocele is noncommunicating (the processus vaginalis was obliterated during development). In such cases, the hydrocele fluid disappears by 1 yr of age. If there is a persistently patent processus, the hydrocele persists and becomes progressively larger during the day and is small in the morning. A rare variant of a hydrocele is the abdominoscrotal hydrocele, in which there is a large, tense hydrocele that extends into the lower abdominal cavity. In some older boys, a noncommunicating hydrocele may result from an inflammatory condition within the scrotum, such as testicular torsion, torsion of the appendix testis, epididymitis, or testicular tumor. The long-term risk of a communicating hydrocele is the development of an inguinal hernia. Some older boys and male adolescents also develop a hydrocele. In some cases they develop acutely after an episode of scrotal

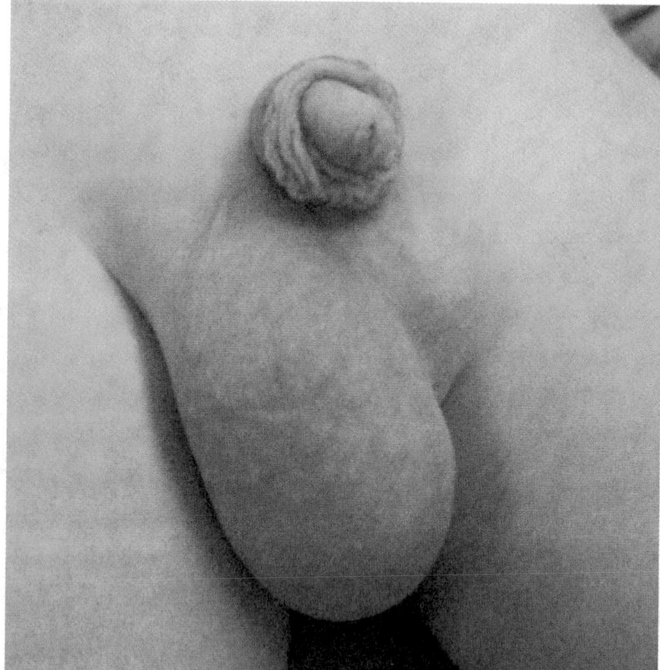

Figure 545-5. Newborn with large right hydrocele.

trauma or epididymo-orchitis, whereas others develop more insidiously.

DIAGNOSIS. On examination, hydroceles are smooth and nontender. Transillumination of the scrotum confirms the fluid-filled nature of the mass. It is important to palpate the testis, as some young men develop a hydrocele in association with a testis tumor. If compression of the fluid-filled mass completely reduces the hydrocele, an inguinal hernia/hydrocele is the likely diagnosis.

TREATMENT. Most congenital hydroceles resolve by 12 mo of age following reabsorption of the hydrocele fluid. If the hydrocele is large and tense, however, early surgical correction should be considered, because it is difficult to verify that the child does not have a hernia, and large hydroceles rarely disappear spontaneously. Hydroceles persisting beyond 12–18 mo usually are communicating and should be repaired. Surgical correction is similar to a herniorrhaphy (see Chapter 343). Through an inguinal incision, the spermatic cord is identified, the hydrocele fluid is drained, and a high ligation of the processus vaginalis is performed. If an older boy has a large hydrocele, often diagnostic laparoscopy can be performed to determine whether there is a patent processus vaginalis, and if the internal ring is closed, then the hydrocele may be corrected with a scrotal incision.

INGUINAL HERNIA

Inguinal hernia is discussed in Chapter 343.

TESTICULAR TUMOR

Testicular and paratesticular tumors can occur at any age, even in the newborn. Approximately 35% of prepubertal testis tumors are malignant; most commonly they are yolk sac tumors, although rhabdomyosarcoma and leukemia also may occur in this age group. In male adolescents, 98% of painless solid testicular masses are malignant (see Chapter 503). Most present as a painless, hard testicular mass that does not transilluminate.

Scrotal ultrasonography should be performed to confirm the finding of a testicular mass and may help to delineate the type of testis tumor. Serum tumor markers, including **α-fetoprotein** and **β-human chorionic gonadotropin,** should be drawn. Definitive therapy includes surgical exploration through an inguinal incision. In most cases a radical orchiectomy, consisting of removal of the entire testis and spermatic cord, is performed. In a prepubertal boy, if the ultrasonographic study or surgical exploration suggests that the tumor is localized and benign, such as a teratoma or epidermoid cyst, testis-sparing surgery with removal only of the mass may be appropriate.

Agarwal PK, Diaz M, Elder JS: Retractile testis—Is it really a normal variant? *J Urol* 2006;175:1496–1499.

Alukal JP, Zurakowski D, Atala A, et al: Testicular hypotrophy does not correlate with grade of adolescent varicocele. *J Urol* 2005;174:2367–2370.

Barthold JS: Is adjuvant hormonal therapy indicated in cryptorchidism? *Nat Clin Pract Urol* 2005;2:366–367.

Barthold JS, Gonzalez R. The epidemiology of congenital cryptorchidism, testicular ascent and orchiopexy. *J Urol* 2003;170:2396.

Caroppo E, Niederberger C, Elhanby C, et al: Effect of cryptorchidism and retractile testes on male factor infertility: A multicenter, retrospective, chart review. *Fertil Steril* 2005;83:1581–1584.

Cayan S, Acar D, Ulger S, et al: Adolescent varicocele repair: Long-term results and comparison of surgical techniques according to optical magnification use in 100 cases at a single university hospital. *J Urol* 2005;174:2003–2006.

De Kretser DM: Differences in the prevalence of cryptorchidism. *Lancet* 2004;363:1250–1252.

Eaton SH, Cendron MA, Estrada CA, et al: Intermittent testicular torsion: Diagnostic features and management outcomes. *J Urol* 2005;174: 1532–1535.

Eggener SE, Lotan Y, Cheng EY: Magnetic resonance angiography for the nonpalpable testis: A cost and cancer risk analysis. *J Urol* 2005;173:1745–1749.

Hack WW, Meijer RW, van der Voort-Doedens LM, et al: Natural course of acquired undescended testis in boys. *Br J Surg* 2003;90:728–731.

Husmann DA: Cryptorchidism and its relationship to testicular neoplasia and microlithiasis. *Urology* 2005;66:424–426.

Hutson JM, Hasthorpe S: Testicular descent and cryptorchidism: The state of the art in 2004. *J Pediatr Surg* 2005;40:297–302.

Kollin C, Hesser U, Ritzen EM, et al: Testicular growth from birth to two years of age, and the effect of orchiopexy at age nine months: A randomized, controlled study. *Acta Paediatr* 2006;95:318–324.

Lam WW, Yap TL, Jacobsen AS, et al: Colour Doppler ultrasonography replacing surgical exploration for acute scrotum: Myth or reality? *Pediatr Radiol* 2005;35:597–600.

Lee PA: Fertility after cryptorchidism: Epidemiology and other outcome studies. *Urology* 2005;66:427–431.

Livne PM, Sivan B, Karmazyn B, et al: Testicular torsion in the pediatric age group: Diagnosis and treatment. *Pediatr Endocrinol Rev* 2003;1:128–133.

Mansbach JM, Forbes P, Peters C: Testicular torsion and risk factors for orchiectomy. *Arch Pediatr Adolesc Med* 2005;159:1167–1171.

Mouriquand P: The normal testis. *Arch Dis Child* 2007;92:3.

Pierik FH, Burdorf A, de Muinck Keizer-Schrama SM, et al: The cryptorchidism prevalence among infants in the general population of Rotterdam, the Netherlands. *Int J Androl* 2005;28:248–252.

Rajimwale A, Brant WO, Koyle MA: High scrotal (Bianchi) single-incision orchiopexy: A "tailored" approach to the palpable undescended testis. *Pediatr Surg Int* 2004;20:618–622.

Salzhauer EW, Sokol A, Glassberg KI: Paternity after adolescent varicocele repair. *Pediatrics* 2004;114:1631–1633.

Sandlow J: Pathogenesis and treatment of varicoceles. *BMJ* 2004;328: 967–968.

Schwentner C, Oswald L, Kreczy A, et al: Neoadjuvant gonadotropin-releasing hormone therapy before surgery may improve the fertility index in undescended testes: A prospective randomized trial. *J Urol* 2005;173: 974–977.

Skakkebaek NE, Jorgensen N, Main KM, et al: Is human fecundity declining? *Int J Androl* 2006;29:2–11.

Somekh E, Gorenstein A, Serour F: Acute epididymitis in boys: Evidence of a post-infectious etiology. *J Urol* 2004;171:391–394.

Yang DM, Lim JW, Kim JE, et al: Torsed appendix testis: Gray scale and color Doppler sonographic findings compared with normal appendix testis. *J Ultrasound Med* 2005;24:87–91.

Yerkes EB, Robertson FM, Gitlin J, et al: Management of perinatal torsion: Today, tomorrow or never? *J Urol* 2005;174:1579–1582.

Chapter 546 ■ Trauma to the Genitourinary Tract

Jack S. Elder

ETIOLOGY. Injuries to the genitourinary tract in children usually result from blunt trauma during falls, athletic activities, or motor vehicle accidents (see Chapter 71). In more than half of cases there also are major injuries to the brain, spinal cord, skeleton, lungs, or abdominal organs. Children are at greater risk of blunt renal injury than are adults, because they have less body fat and because the kidneys are not located directly behind the ribs. Children with a pre-existing renal anomaly such as hydronephrosis secondary to a ureteropelvic junction obstruction, horseshoe kidney, or renal ectopia also are at increased risk for renal injury. Blunt abdominal or flank trauma often causes a renal injury. Falling may cause a deceleration injury that results in an injury to the renal pedicle, interrupting blood flow to the kidney. If the bladder is full, blunt lower abdominal trauma may cause a bladder rupture. Rupture of the membranous urethra occurs in 5% of pelvic fractures. Straddle injuries usually are associated with trauma to the bulbous urethra. Symptoms and signs of urinary tract injury include gross or microscopic hematuria, bleeding from the urethral meatus, abdominal or flank pain, a flank mass, fractured lower ribs or lumbar transverse processes, and a perineal or scrotal hematoma.

DIAGNOSIS. Evaluation of the patient begins after an adequate airway has been established and the patient is hemodynamically stable (see Chapter 66). With significant abdominal injury, gross hematuria or >50 red blood cells per high-power field, or suspicion of renal injury (deceleration injury, flank pain or bruise), renal imaging is indicated. In addition, the bladder should be catheterized, unless blood is dripping from the urethral meatus, which is an indication of potential urethral injury. Passing the catheter in the presence of a urethral injury may increase the extent of the damage and convert a partial membranous urethral tear into a total disruption. In these patients, a retrograde urethrogram should be performed by injecting radiopaque contrast medium into the urethral meatus under fluoroscopy. Oblique radiographs demonstrate the extent of the injury and whether urethral continuity is preserved or has been disrupted.

A **3-phase spiral CT scan** should be performed to evaluate the kidneys, ureters, and bladder. The delayed images are important to detect renal extravasation of blood or urine. Prompt function of both kidneys without extravasation usually excludes significant renal injury. Renal injuries are classified according to the grading scale presented in Table 546-1. Minor renal injuries are most common; these include contusion of the renal parenchyma and shallow cortical lacerations not involving the collecting system. Major renal injuries include deep lacerations involving the collecting system, the shattered kidney, and renal pedicle injuries (Fig. 546-1). Complete absence of function of one kidney without contralateral compensatory hypertrophy (indicative of congenital absence) should be regarded as an indication of major injury to the renal pedicle. Renal angiography, once used for further evaluation of renal injuries, particularly if a renal pedicle injury is suspected, now is rarely used because such patients are often hemodynamically unstable, and management is not significantly affected by the findings. In some cases, a pre-existing renal anomaly may be demonstrated on the study. A ruptured uretero-

TABLE 546-1. American Association for the Surgery of Trauma Organ Injury Severity Scale for the Kidney

GRADE*	TYPE	DESCRIPTION
I	Contusion	Microscopic or gross hematuria, urologic studies normal
	Hematoma	Subcapsular, nonexpanding without parenchymal laceration
II	Hematoma	Nonexpanding perirenal hematoma confined to renal retroperitoneum
	Laceration	Parenchymal depth of renal cortex without urinary extravasation <1 cm
III	Laceration	Parenchymal depth of renal cortex without collecting system rupture or urinary extravasation >1 cm
IV	Laceration	Parenchymal laceration extending through renal cortex, medulla, and collecting system
	Vascular	Main renal artery or vein injury with contained hemorrhage
V	Laceration	Completely shattered kidney
	Vascular	Avulsion of renal hilum, devascularizing the kidney

*Advance one grade for bilateral injuries up to grade III.

Adapted from Moore EE, Shackford SR, Pachter HL, et al: Organ injury scaling: Spleen, liver, and kidney. *J Trauma* 1989;29:1664–1666.

pelvic junction obstruction may be apparent if the kidney is intact but the distal ureter is not visualized.

TREATMENT. Minor renal injuries such as contusions are managed by bed rest and monitoring of vital signs until abdominal or flank discomfort and gross hematuria has resolved. Children with a major renal injury usually are admitted to an intensive care unit for continuous monitoring of vital signs and urine output. Intravenous antibiotics are also administered. These injuries also are managed nonoperatively, because Gerota's fascia often causes tamponade of bleeding from the kidney, and dramatic healing of the injured parenchyma can occur even with significant urinary extravasation. Approximately 10% of children with a major renal injury undergo surgical exploration because of hemodynamic instability, persistent extravasation, or persistent hematuria, or to correct a congenital renal deformity. It can be difficult to identify normal and devitalized parenchyma, and the likelihood of having to perform a nephrectomy is significant. If the child is undergoing exploration for other abdominal injuries, the injured kidney is examined. If there is persistent extravasation because of intermittent ureteral obstruction from a blood clot, passage of a temporary double-J stent endoscopically between the bladder and kidney may allow resolution. If there is a renal pedicle injury, nephrectomy is necessary. The kidney can be salvaged by emergency renal revascularization only if the kidney is explored within 2–3 hr of the injury. All penetrating injuries of the kidneys should be explored. In addition to loss of renal function, the main long-term complication of renal injury is renin-mediated hypertension. Children who sustain renal injuries must have periodic measurement of blood pressure.

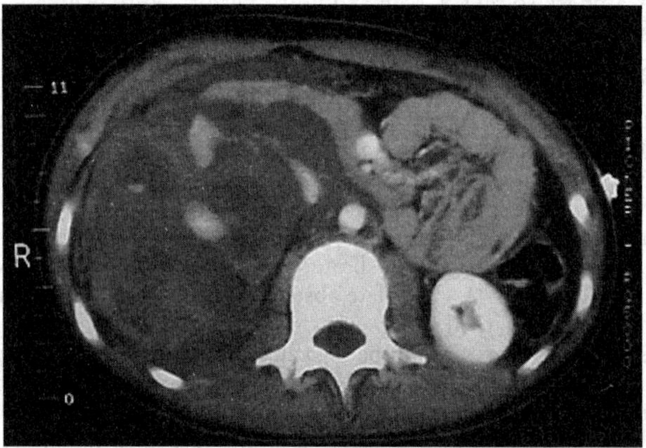

Figure 546-1. CT scan of a girl who sustained major renal injury when she fell off a bicycle. The scan demonstrates a ruptured right kidney with urinary extravasation.

Ureteral injuries usually are iatrogenic. Injuries of the ureter by blunt or penetrating trauma require immediate surgical attention.

When the bladder can be catheterized, a static cystogram is obtained, infusing a contrast solution through the catheter by gravity, ideally using fluoroscopy. Flat and oblique views are often obtained; a postvoid film also should be obtained because, in some cases, extravasation may be hidden by the full bladder.

Bladder ruptures can be intraperitoneal or extraperitoneal. All intraperitoneal ruptures require surgical repair. Minor extraperitoneal near-ruptures might be treated by catheter drainage but generally require surgical treatment.

Treatment of a membranous urethral injury is controversial. Erectile dysfunction, urethral stricture, and urinary incontinence are the major late complications of rupture of the membranous urethra, and therapy is directed at minimizing the risk of these problems. A large pelvic hematoma with tamponade often is present, and an immediate attempt to repair the injury can be technically difficult and result in significant hemorrhage. Many such injuries are managed initially by temporary suprapubic cystostomy, with continuous bladder drainage for 3–6 mo. Subsequently, open or endoscopic urethroplasty can be performed. Alternatively, some try to achieve urethral continuity under anesthesia and leave a urethral catheter for several months. These patients typically require subsequent open or endoscopic urethroplasty.

Penile injury is uncommon. Some boys who are in the process of toilet training sustain an injury to the glans penis if the lid of the toilet falls while they are urinating. These boys often have a hematoma covering the distal half of the glans. Typically, they have no difficulty urinating and do not need extensive evaluation. Some male infants will develop an inadvertent hair coil tourniquet or strangulation injury. Typically a very narrow constriction is noted with severe distal penile swelling and pain. Identification and incision of the hair allows prompt resolution of the edema. The urethra and penile vascularity should be assessed after release of the hair coil. Adolescent boys who indulge in extremely vigorous sexual intercourse may sustain rupture of one of the corporal bodies. These boys have severe swelling of the penile shaft and require emergency exploration and repair. Boys with penetrating injuries of the penis also require emergency debridement and repair.

Testicular injuries are relatively uncommon in children because of the small size of the testes and their mobility within the scrotum. Such injuries usually result from blunt trauma during athletic activity. Typically, these boys have significant scrotal swelling, testicular pain, and tenderness. Ultrasonography demonstrates rupture of the tunica albuginea, which is the capsule of the testis, and surrounding hemorrhage. Prompt surgical treatment of testicular injuries increases the salvage rate.

An uncommon injury is the zipper injury, which can affect either the scrotum or foreskin. This problem generally occurs in boys who do not wear underwear. The zipper can be cut with either bone or metal cutters. Sedation generally is unnecessary.

American Academy of Pediatrics, Committee on Sports Medicine and Fitness: Medical conditions affecting sports participation. *Pediatrics* 2001;107:1205–1209.

Buckley JC, McAninch JW: The diagnosis, management, and outcomes of pediatric renal injuries. *Urol Clin North Am* 2006;33:33–40.

Buckner BJ, Parousis V, Tarry W, et al: Strangulation injuries of the glans penis: A case series. *W V Med J* 2004;100:187–188.

Holmes JH 4th, Wiebe DJ, Tataria M, et al: The failure of nonoperative management in pediatric solid organ injury: A multi-institutional experience. *J Trauma* 2005;59:1309–1313.

Inoue N, Crook SC, Yamamoto LG: Comparing 2 methods of emergent zipper release. *Am J Emerg Med* 2005;23:480–482.

Johnson B, Christensen C, Dirusso S, et al: A need for reevaluation of sports participation recommendations for children with a solitary kidney. *J Urol* 2005;17:686–689.
Mohr AM, Pham AM, Lavery RF, et al: Management of trauma to the male external genitalia: The usefulness of American Association for the Surgery of Trauma organ injury scales. *J Urol* 2003;170:2311–2315.
Muram D, Levitt CJ, Frasier LD, et al: Genital injuries. *J Pediatr Adolesc Gynecol* 2003;16:149–155.
Nance ML, Lutz N, Carr MC, et al: Blunt renal injuries in children can be managed nonoperatively: Outcome in a consecutive series of patients. *J Trauma* 2004;57:474–478.
Onen A, Ozturk H, Yayla M, et al: Genital trauma in children: Classification and management. *Urology* 2005;65:986–990.
Onen A, Subasi M, Arslan H, et al: Long-term urologic, orthopedic, and psychological outcome of posterior urethral rupture in children. *Urology* 2005;66:174–179.
Otgun I, Karnak I, Senocak ME, et al: Late urodynamic findings after treating traumatic rupture of the posterior urethra in boys. *BJU Int* 2006;97:367–370.
Rogers CG, Knight V, MacUra KJ, et al: High-grade renal injuries in children—Is conservative management possible? *Urology* 2004;64: 574–579.
Wan J, Corvino TF, Greenfield SP, et al: Kidney and testicle injuries in team and individual sports: Data from the national pediatric trauma registry. *J Urol* 2003;170:1528–1523.

Chapter 547 ■ Urinary Lithiasis

Jack S. Elder

Urinary lithiasis in children is less common in the U.S. than in other parts of the world. The wide geographic variation in the incidence of lithiasis in childhood is related to climatic, dietary, and socioeconomic factors. Approximately 7% of urinary calculi occur in children younger than 16 yr of age. In the U.S., many children with stone disease have a metabolic abnormality. The exceptions are patients with a neuropathic bladder (see Chapter 542), who are prone to infection-initiated renal stones, and those who have urinary tract reconstruction with intestine, which predisposes to bladder calculi. Metabolic stones are twice as common in boys as in girls and are rare in African-Americans. In Southeast Asia, urinary calculi are endemic and are related to dietary factors.

STONE FORMATION. The composition and site of urinary calculi vary, depending on the pathogenesis. Most "spontaneous" stones are composed of calcium, oxalate, or phosphate crystals; others are due to uric acid, cystine, or ammonium crystals, or phosphate crystals, or a combination of these substances (Table 547-1). The risk of stone formation increases in the presence of increasing concentrations of these crystals and is reduced with increasing concentrations of inhibitors. Renal calculi develop from crystals that form on the calyx and aggregate to form a calculus. Bladder calculi may be stones that formed in the kidney and traveled down the ureter, or they may form primarily in the bladder.

Stone formation depends on four factors: matrix; precipitation-crystallization; epitaxy; and the absence of inhibitors of stone formation in the urine. **Matrix** is a mixture of protein, non-amino sugars, glucosamine, water, and organic ash that makes up 2–9% of the dry weight of urinary stones and is arranged within the stones in organized concentric laminations. **Precipitation-crystallization** refers to supersaturation of the urine with specific ions comprising the crystal. Crystals aggregate by chemical and electrical forces. Increasing the saturation of urine with respect to the ions increases the rate of nucleation, crystal growth, and aggregation and increases the likelihood of stone formation and growth. **Epitaxy** refers to the aggregation of crystals of different composition but similar lattice structure, thus forming stones of a heterogeneous nature. The lattice structures of calcium oxalate and monosodium urate have similar structures, and calcium oxalate crystals can aggregate on a nucleus of monosodium urate crystals. Urine also contains **inhibitors of stone formation,** including citrate, diphosphonate, and magnesium ion.

TABLE 547-1. Classification of Urolithiasis

CALCIUM STONES (CALCIUM OXALATE AND CALCIUM PHOSPHATE)*
Hypercalciuria
Absorptive
Renal leak
Resorptive
Distal renal tubular acidosis, type 1 (calcium phosphate)
Hyperparathyroidism
Sarcoidosis
Furosemide administration
Vitamin D excess
Immobilization
Corticosteroid administration
Cushing disease
Hyperuricosuria
Heterozygous cystinuria
Hyperoxaluria (calcium oxalate)
Primary hyperoxaluria, types 1 and 2
Secondary hyperoxaluria
Enteric hyperoxaluria
Hypocitruria
Renal tubular acidosis
CYSTINE STONES
Cystinuria
STRUVITE STONES (MAGNESIUM AMMONIUM PHOSPHATE)
Urinary tract infection (urea-splitting organism)
Foreign body
Urinary stasis
URIC ACID STONES
Hyperuricosuria
Lesch-Nyhan syndrome
Myeloproliferative disorders
After chemotherapy
Inflammatory bowel disease
INDINAVIR STONES
NEPHROCALCINOSIS

*Most common.

CLINICAL MANIFESTATIONS. Children with urolithiasis usually have gross or microscopic hematuria. If the calculus is in the renal pelvis, calyx, or ureter and causes obstruction, then severe abdominal or flank pain (renal colic) occurs. Typically the pain radiates anteriorly to the scrotum or labia. Often the pain is intermittent, corresponding to periods of obstruction of urine flow, which increases the pressure in the collecting system. If the calculus is in the distal ureter, the child may have irritative symptoms of dysuria, urgency, and frequency. If the stone passes into the bladder, the child usually is asymptomatic. If the stone is in the urethra, dysuria and difficulty voiding may result. Some children pass small amounts of gravel-like material.

DIAGNOSIS. Approximately 90% of urinary calculi are calcified to some degree and, consequently, are radiopaque on a plain abdominal film. Some calculi are only a few millimeters in diameter and may not be obvious, particularly if they are in the ureter. Struvite (magnesium ammonium phosphate) stones are radiopaque. Cystine, xanthine, and uric acid calculi may be radiolucent but often are slightly opacified. Some children have **nephrocalcinosis,** which is calcification of the renal tissue itself.

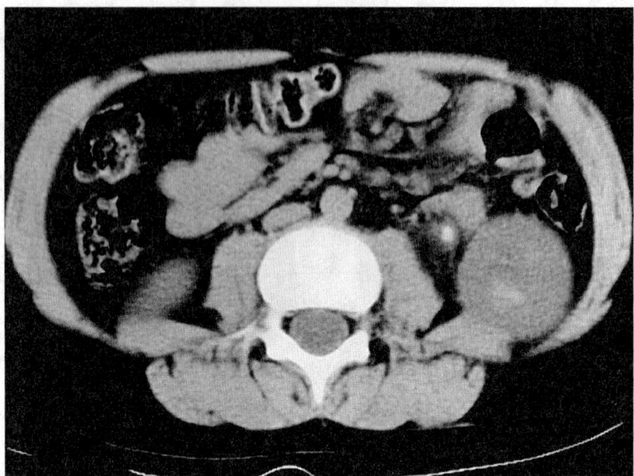

Figure 547-1. Noncontrast CT scan of the mid-abdomen shows an enlarged left kidney with soft calcification in the renal pelvis and a thickened ureter with an impacted small calcium oxalate stone. (From Kuhn JP, Slovis T, Haller J [editors]: *Caffey's Pediatric Diagnostic Imaging,* 10th ed. Philadelphia, Mosby, 2003, p 1799.)

TABLE 547-2. Laboratory Tests Suggested for Evaluation of Urolithiasis

SERUM
- Calcium
- Phosphorus
- Uric acid
- Electrolytes and anion gap
- Creatinine
- Alkaline phosphatase

URINE
- Urinalysis
- Urine culture
- Calcium:creatinine ratio
- Spot test for cystinuria
- 24-hr collection for:
  - Creatinine clearance
  - Calcium
  - Phosphate
  - Oxalate
  - Uric acid
  - Dibasic amino acids (if cystine spot test result is positive)

Nephrocalcinosis is seen most commonly in premature neonates receiving furosemide, which causes hypercalciuria, and in children with medullary sponge kidney.

In a child with suspected renal colic, a **nonenhanced spiral CT scan** of the abdomen and pelvis is performed (Fig. 547-1). This study takes only a few minutes to perform, is accurate in delineating the number and location of calculi, and demonstrates whether the involved kidney is hydronephrotic. Less often, an excretory urogram is performed. This test demonstrates a delay in visualization of the collecting system compared with the normal side; and if there is a ureteral calculus, there is columnization of contrast medium down to the stone. If the calculus is radiolucent or small, the urogram may not demonstrate the stone. Consequently, the noncontrast spiral CT scan is preferred. Another alternative is to obtain a plain radiograph of the abdomen and pelvis plus a renal ultrasonogram. However, if a small calculus is in the ureter, it may not be demonstrated by these two studies; and if the calculus is not causing impaired urinary flow at the time of the study, the renal ultrasonogram may not show hydronephrosis. In a child who has already been diagnosed with a calculus, serial plain x-rays or renal ultrasonography can be used to follow the status of the calculus, such as whether it has grown or diminished in size or moved. If a child has a renal pelvic calculus, a ureteropelvic junction obstruction should be suspected. In some cases, it can be difficult to determine whether hydronephrosis in such a child is secondary to an obstructing stone or the ureteropelvic junction obstruction, or both.

Any material that resembles a calculus should be sent for analysis by a laboratory that specializes in the identification of the components of urinary calculi.

Metabolic Evaluation. A metabolic evaluation for the most common predisposing factors should be undertaken in all children with urolithiasis, bearing in mind that structural, infectious, and metabolic factors often coexist. This evaluation should not be undertaken in a child who is in the process of passing a stone, because the altered diet and hydration status, as well as the effect of obstruction on the kidney, may alter the results of the study. The basic laboratory studies required are listed in Table 547-2, and the normal values for 24-hr urine collections are shown in Table 547-3. In children with hypercalciuria, further studies of calcium excretion with dietary calcium restriction and calcium loading are necessary.

PATHOGENESIS OF SPECIFIC RENAL CALCULI

CALCIUM OXALATE AND CALCIUM PHOSPHATE CALCULI. Most urinary calculi in children in the U.S. are composed of calcium oxalate or calcium phosphate, or both. The most common meta-

TABLE 547-3. Urine Chemistry: Normal Values

URINE CONSTITUENT	AGE	RANDOM	TIMED	COMMENTS
Calcium	0–6 mo	<0.8 mg/mg creat	<4 mg/kg/24 hr	Prandial variation
	7–12 mo	<0.6 mg/mg creat		Sodium-dependent
	≥2 yr	<0.21 mg/mg creat		
Oxalate*	<1 yr	0.15–0.26 mmol/mmol creat	≥2 yr; <0.5 mmol/1.73 m^2/24 hr	Random urine mmol/mmol highly age-dependent
	1–<5 yr	0.11–0.12 mmol/mmol creat		Excretion rate/1.73 m^2 constant through childhood and adulthood
	5–12 yr	0.006–0.15 mmol/mmol creat		
	>12 yr	0.002–0.083 mmol/mmol creat		
Uric acid	Term infant	3.3 mg/dL GFR[†]	<815 mg/1.73 m^2/24 hr	Excretion rate/1.73 m^2 from >1 yr age constant through childhood
	>3 yr	<0.53 mg/dL GFR		
Magnesium	>2 yr	<0.12 mg/mg creat	<88 mg/1.73 m^2/24 hr	Excretion rate/1.73 m^2 constant through childhood
Citrate		>400 mg/g creat		Limited data available for children
Cystine		<75 mg/g creat	<60 mg/1.73 m^2/24 hr	Cystine >250 mg/g creat suggests homozygous cystinuria

*Oxalate oxidase assay.

[†](mg/dL uric acid) (serum creatinine concentration/urine creatinine concentration).

creat, creatinine; GFR, glomerular filtration rate.

From Milliner DS: Urolithiasis. In Avner ED, Harmon WE, Naiudet P (editors): *Pediatric Nephrology,* 5th ed. Philadelphia, Lippincott Williams & Wilkins, 2004, p. 1103, with permission.

bolic abnormality in these individuals is normocalcemic **hypercalciuria.** Between 30–60% of children with calcium stones have hypercalciuria without hypercalcemia. Other metabolic aberrations that predispose to stone disease include hyperoxaluria, hyperuricosuria, hypocitruria, heterozygous cystinuria, hypomagnesuria, hyperparathyroidism, and renal tubular acidosis (see Chapter 529).

Hypercalciuria may be absorptive, renal, or resorptive. The primary disturbance in absorptive hypercalciuria is intestinal hyperabsorption of calcium. In some children, an increase in 1,25-dihydroxyvitamin D is associated with the increased calcium absorption, and in others the process is independent of vitamin D. **Renal hypercalciuria** refers to impaired renal tubular reabsorption of calcium (see Chapter 519.8). Renal leak of calcium causes mild hypocalcemia, which triggers an increased production of parathyroid hormone, with increased intestinal absorption of calcium and increased mobilization of calcium stores. Resorptive hypercalciuria is uncommon and is found in patients with primary hyperparathyroidism. Excess parathyroid hormone secretion stimulates intestinal absorption of calcium and mobilization of calcium stores. A brief summary of the metabolic evaluation of children with hypercalciuria is shown in Table 547-4.

Hyperoxaluria is another potentially important cause of calcium stones. Oxalate increases the solubility product of calcium oxalate crystallization 7–10 times more than calcium. Consequently, hyperoxaluria significantly increases the likelihood of calcium oxalate precipitation. Oxalate is found in high concentration in tea, coffee, spinach, and rhubarb. Primary hyperoxaluria is a rare autosomal recessive disorder that can be subclassified into glycolic aciduria and L-glyceric aciduria. Most patients with primary hyperoxaluria have glycolic aciduria; oxalic and glycolic acids are increased in the urine of affected individuals. Both defects cause increased endogenous production of oxalate, with hyperoxaluria, urolithiasis, nephrocalcinosis, and renal injury. Death from renal failure occurs by age 20 yr in untreated patients. **Oxalosis,** defined as extrarenal deposition of calcium oxalate, occurs when renal insufficiency is present with elevated plasma oxalate. Calcium oxalate deposits appear first in blood vessels and bone marrow, and with time they appear throughout the body. Secondary hyperoxaluria is more common and can occur in patients with increased intake of oxalate and oxalate precursors such as vitamin C, in those with pyridoxine deficiency, and in children with intestinal malabsorption.

Enteric hyperoxaluria refers to disorders such as inflammatory bowel disease (see Chapter 333), pancreatic insufficiency (see Chapter 347), and biliary disease, in which there is gastrointestinal malabsorption of fatty acids, which bind intraluminal calcium and form salts that are excreted in the feces. Normally, calcium forms a complex with oxalate to reduce oxalate absorption, but if calcium is unavailable, there is increased absorption of unbound oxalate.

Hypocitruria refers to a low excretion of citrate, which is an inhibitor of calcium stone formation. Citrate acts as an inhibitor of calcium urolithiasis by forming complexes with calcium, increasing the solubility of calcium in the urine, and inhibiting the aggregation of calcium phosphate and calcium oxalate crystals. Disorders such as chronic diarrhea, intestinal malabsorption, and renal tubular acidosis may cause hypocitruria. It may also be idiopathic.

Renal tubular acidosis (RTA) is a syndrome involving a disturbance of acid-base balance within the kidney that can be classified into three types, one of which predisposes to renal calculi that typically are calcium phosphate (see Chapter 529). In type 1, the distal nephron does not secrete hydrogen ion into the distal tubule. The urine pH is never less than 5.8, and hyperchloremic hypokalemic acidosis results. Patients acquire nephrolithiasis, nephrocalcinosis, muscle weakness, and osteomalacia. Type 1 RTA can be an autosomal dominant disorder, but more often it is acquired and associated with systemic diseases such as Sjögren syndrome, Wilson disease, primary biliary cirrhosis, and lymphocytic thyroiditis, or it results from amphotericin B, lithium, or toluene (an organic solvent associated with glue sniffing).

From 5–8% of individuals with **cystic fibrosis** (see Chapter 400) have urolithiasis. Typically the stones are calcium, and they often become manifest in adolescence or young adulthood. Microscopic nephrocalcinosis also occurs in younger children with the disease. These patients do not have hypercalciuria, and the propensity for urolithiasis has been speculated to result from an inability to excrete a sodium chloride load or from intestinal malabsorption.

Other disorders may play a role in causing calcium stones. **Hyperuricosuria** may be related to the epitactic growth of calcium oxalate crystals around a nucleus of uric acid crystals or to the action of uric acid as a counter inhibitor of urinary mucopolysaccharides, which inhibit calcium oxalate crystallization. **Heterozygous cystinuria** is found in some patients with calcium stones. The mechanism is unknown but may be similar to that of uric acid. Sarcoidosis causes an increased sensitivity to vitamin D_3 and thus an increased absorption of calcium from the gastrointestinal tract. In Lesch-Nyhan syndrome there is excessive uric acid synthesis. These patients are more likely to form uric acid stones, but some of these stones may be calcified. **Immobility** may cause hypercalciuria by mobilization of calcium stores. High-dose corticosteroids may cause hypercalciuria and calcium oxalate precipitation. Furosemide, which is administered in the neonatal intensive care unit, also can cause severe hypercalciuria, urolithiasis, and nephrocalcinosis.

In some children, calcium calculi are idiopathic. A complete metabolic evaluation must be performed before this diagnosis is made.

CYSTINE CALCULI. Cystinuria accounts for 1% of renal calculi in children. The condition is a rare autosomal recessive disorder of the epithelial cells of the renal tubule that prevents absorption of the four dibasic amino acids (cystine, ornithine, arginine, lysine) and results in excessive urinary excretion of these products. The only known complication of this familial disease is the formation of calculi, because of the low solubility of cystine. The patients usually have acidic urine, which leads to a higher rate of precipitation. In the homozygous patient, the daily excretion of cystine usually exceeds 500 mg, and stone formation occurs at an early age. Heterozygotes excrete 100–300 mg/day and typically do not have clinical urolithiasis. The sulfur content of cystine gives these stones their faint radiopaque appearance.

STRUVITE CALCULI. Urinary tract infections (see Chapter 538) caused by urea-splitting organisms (most often *Proteus* spp., and

TABLE 547-4. Metabolic Evaluation of Children with Hypercalciuria

	SERUM CALCIUM	RESTRICTED CALCIUM (URINE)	FASTING CALCIUM (URINE)	CALCIUM LOAD (URINE)	PARATHYROID HORMONE (SERUM)
Absorptive	N	N or I	N	I	I
Renal	N	I	I	I	N
Resorptive	I	I	I	I	I

I, increased; N, normal.

occasionally *Klebsiella* spp., *Escherichia coli, Pseudomonas* spp., and others) result in urinary alkalinization and excessive production of ammonia, which can lead to the precipitation of magnesium ammonium phosphate (struvite) and calcium phosphate. In the kidney, the calculi often have a staghorn configuration, filling the calyces. The calculi act as foreign bodies, causing obstruction, perpetuating infection, and causing gradual renal damage. Patients with struvite stones also may have metabolic abnormalities that predispose to stone formation. These stones often are seen in children with neuropathic bladder dysfunction, particularly those who have undergone an ileal conduit procedure (see Chapter 542). Struvite stones may form in the reconstructed bladder of children who have undergone urinary tract reconstruction with augmentation cystoplasty or continent diversion, or both.

URIC ACID CALCULI. Calculi containing uric acid represent less than 5% of all cases of lithiasis in children in the U.S. but are more common in less developed areas of the world. Hyperuricosuria with or without hyperuricemia is the common underlying factor in most cases. The stones are radiolucent. The diagnosis should be suspected when there is a persistently acid urine and urate crystalluria.

Hyperuricosuria may result from various inborn errors of purine metabolism that lead to overproduction of uric acid, the end product of purine metabolism in humans. Children with the Lesch-Nyhan syndrome and patients with glucose-6-phosphatase deficiency form urate calculi as well. In children with short-bowel syndrome, and particularly those with ileostomies, chronic dehydration and acidosis sometimes are complicated by uric acid lithiasis.

One of the most common causes of uric acid lithiasis is the rapid turnover of purine with some tumors and myeloproliferative diseases. The risk of uric acid lithiasis is especially great when treatment of these diseases causes rapid breakdown of nucleoproteins. Uric acid calculi or "sludge" can fill the entire upper collecting system and cause renal failure and even anuria. Urates also are present within calcium-containing stones. In these cases, more than one predisposing factor for stone formation may exist. A related disorder is 2,8-dihydroxyadeninelithiasis, which results from a deficiency in adenine phosphoribosyltransferase. The stones are radiolucent and can be differentiated from uric acid calculi by mass spectrometry but not by routine chemical analysis. In contrast to uric acid, which is soluble in alkaline urine, the solubility of 2,8-dihydroxyadenine changes little within physiologic pH ranges.

INDINAVIR CALCULI. Indinavir sulfate is a protease inhibitor approved for the treatment of HIV infection. As many as 4% of patients acquire symptomatic nephrolithiasis. Most of the calculi are radiolucent and are composed of indinavir-based monohydrate, although calcium oxalate or phosphate, or both, have been present in some. After each dose, 12% of the drug is excreted unchanged in the urine. The urine in these patients often contains crystals of characteristic rectangles and fan-shaped or starburst crystals. Indinavir is soluble at a pH of less than 5.5. Consequently, dissolution therapy by urinary acidification with ammonium chloride or ascorbic acid should be considered.

NEPHROCALCINOSIS. Nephrocalcinosis refers to calcium deposition within the renal tissue. Often nephrocalcinosis is associated with urolithiasis. The most common causes are furosemide (administered to premature neonates), distal RTA, hyperparathyroidism, medullary sponge kidney, hypophosphatemic rickets, sarcoidosis, cortical necrosis, hyperoxaluria, prolonged immobilization, Cushing syndrome, hyperuricosuria, and renal candidiasis.

TABLE 547-5. Primary Surgical Treatment Options Versus Stone Size and Location

STONES	SHOCK WAVE LITHOTRIPSY	URETEROSCOPY	PERCUTANEOUS NEPHROLITHOTOMY
RENAL			
<1 cm	Most common	Optional	Optional
1–2 cm	Most common	Optional	Optional
>2 cm	Optional	Rare	Most common
LOWER POLE			
<1 cm	Most common	Optional	Optional
>1 cm	Optional	Optional	Most common
URETERAL			
Proximal	Most common	Optional	Occasional
Distal	Optional	Most common	Rare

After Durkee CT, Balcom A: Surgical management of urolithiasis. *Pediatr Clin North Am* 2006; 53: 465–477, with permission.

TREATMENT

In a child with a renal or ureteral calculus, the decision whether to remove the stone depends on its location, size, and composition (if known), and whether obstruction or infection, or both, is present. Small ureteral calculi often pass spontaneously, although the child may experience severe renal colic. The narrow parts of the ureter include the ureteropelvic junction and the midureter, where it crosses the common iliac artery; the narrowest segment is the ureterovesical junction. **Alpha-adrenergic blockers,** such as tamsulosin, terazosin, and doxazosin, have been shown to facilitate stone passage in adults by decreasing ureteral pressure below the stone and decreasing the frequency of the peristaltic contractions of the obstructed ureter. Similar positive effects have been noted with calcium channel blocking agents with or without steroids. Although these agents have been used in children with ureteral calculi, their safety and efficacy have not been demonstrated. In some cases, passage of a **ureteral stent** past the stone endoscopically allows relief of pain and dilates the ureter sufficiently to allow the calculus to pass. In cases such as children with a uric acid calculus or an infant with a furosemide-associated calculus, dissolution therapy may be effective.

If the calculus does not pass or seems unlikely to pass or if there is associated urinary tract infection, removal is necessary (Table 547-5). **Lithotripsy** of bladder, ureteral, and small renal pelvic calculi using the holmium laser through a flexible or rigid ureteroscope is quite effective. Extracorporeal shock wave lithotripsy has been successfully applied to children with renal and ureteral stones, with a success rate of more than 75%.

In children with urolithiasis, the underlying metabolic disorder should be addressed (Table 547-6). Because lithiasis results from

TABLE 547-6. Suggested Therapy for Urolithiasis Caused by Metabolic Abnormalities

METABOLIC ABNORMALITY	INITIAL TREATMENT	SECOND-LINE TREATMENT
Hypercalciuria	Reduction of dietary Na^+ Dietary calcium at RDA Thiazides	Potassium citrate Neutral phosphate
Hyperoxaluria	Adjustment of dietary oxalate Potassium citrate	Neutral phosphate* Magnesium Pyridoxine*
Hypocitric aciduria	Potassium citrate Bicarbonate	
Hyperuricosuria	Alkalinization	Allopurinol
Cystinuria	Alkalinization Reduction of dietary Na^+	Tiopronin (Thiola) D-penicillamine Captopril

*Initial therapy in primary hyperoxaluria.
RDA, recommended dietary allowance.
From Milliner DS: Urolithiasis. In Avner ED, Harmon WE, Niaudet P (editors): *Pediatric Nephrology,* 5th ed. Philadelphia, Lippincott Williams & Wilkins, 2004, p 1104, with permission.

too high a concentration of specific substances in the urine, maintaining a continuous high urine output by maintaining a high fluid intake often is an effective method of preventing further stones. The high fluid intake should be continued at night, and usually it is necessary for the child to get up at least once at night to urinate and drink more water.

In children with hypercalciuria, some reduction in calcium and sodium intake is necessary, but caution is urged in the growing child. Thiazide diuretics also reduce renal calcium excretion. Addition of potassium citrate, an inhibitor of calcium stones, with a dosage of 1–2 mEq/kg/24 hr is beneficial. An excellent source of citrate is lemonade, because 4 oz of lemon juice contains 84 mEq of citric acid. A daily mixture of 4 oz of reconstituted lemon juice in 2 L of water and sweetened to taste should significantly increase the urinary citrate level. In difficult cases, neutral orthophosphate should be given also, although it is poorly tolerated.

In patients with uric acid stones, allopurinol is effective. Allopurinol is an inhibitor of xanthine oxidase and is effective in reducing the production of both uric acid and 2,8-dihydroxyadenine and can help control recurrence of both types of stones. In addition, urinary alkalinization with sodium bicarbonate or sodium citrate is beneficial. The urine pH should be at least 6.5 and can be monitored at home by the family.

Maintaining a high urine pH can also prevent recurrence of cystine calculi. Cystine is much more soluble when the urinary pH is greater than 7.5, and alkalinization of urine with sodium bicarbonate or sodium citrate is effective. Another important medication is D-penicillamine, which is a chelating agent that binds to cysteine or homocystine, increasing the solubility of the product. Although poorly tolerated by many patients, it has been reported to be effective in dissolving cystine stones and in preventing recurrences when hydration and urinary alkalinization fail. N-Acetylcysteine appears to have low toxicity and may be effective in controlling cystinuria, but long-term experience with it is lacking.

Treatment of type 1 RTA involves correction of the metabolic acidosis and replacement of potassium and sodium loss. Sodium or potassium citrate therapy, or both, is necessary. When the metabolic acidosis is corrected, the urinary citrate excretion returns to normal.

Treatment of primary hyperoxaluria involves hepatic transplantation because the defective enzymes are hepatic. Ideally, this procedure should be performed before renal failure occurs. In the most severe cases, renal transplantation is also necessary.

Afshar K, McLorie G, Papanikolaou F, et al: Outcome of small residual stone fragments following shock wave lithotripsy in children. *J Urol* 2004;172:1600–1603.

Borghi L, Schianchi T, Meschi T, et al: Comparison of two diets for the prevention of recurrent stones in idiopathic hypercalciuria. *N Engl J Med* 2002;346:77–84.

Cameron MA, Sakhaee K, Moe OW: Nephrolithiasis in children. *Pediatr Nephrol* 2005;20:1587–1592.

DeFoor W, Dharamsi N, Smith P, et al: Use of mobile extracorporeal shock wave lithotripter: Experience in a pediatric institution. *Urology* 2005;65:778–781.

Durkee CT, Balcom A: Surgical management of urolithiasis. *Pediatr Clin North Am* 2006;53:465–477.

Holdgate A, Pollock T: Systematic review of the relative efficacy of non-steroidal anti-inflammatory drugs and opioids in the treatment of acute renal colic. *BMJ* 2004;328:1401–1404.

Hollingsworth JM, Rogers MAM, Kaufman SR, et al: Medical therapy to facilitate urinary stone passage: a meta-analysis. *Lancet* 2006;368:1171–1179.

Lande MB, Varade W, Erkan E, et al.: Role of urinary supersaturation in the evaluation of children with urolithiasis. *Pediatr Nephrol* 2005;20:491–494.

Minevich E, DeFoor W, Reddy P, et al: Ureteroscopy is safe and effective in prepubertal children. *J Urol* 2005;174:276–279.

Moe OW: Kidney stones: Pathophysiology and medical management. *Lancet* 2006;367:333–334.

Nicoletta JA, Lande MB: Medical evaluation and treatment of urolithiasis. *Pediatr Clin North Am* 2006;53:479–491.

Palmer JS, Donaher ER, O'Riordan MA, et al: Diagnosis of pediatric urolithiasis: Role of ultrasound and computerized tomography. *J Urol* 2005;174:1413–1416.

Parmar MS: Kidney stones. *BMJ* 2004;328:1420–1424.

Preminger GM, Assimos DG, Lingeman JE, et al: Chapter 1: AUA guideline on management of staghorn calculi: Diagnosis and treatment recommendations. *J Urol* 2005;173:1991–2000.

Prie D, Huart V, Bakouh N, et al: Nephrolothiasis and osteoporosis associated with hypophosphatemia caused by mutations in the type 2a sodium-phosphate cotransporter. *N Engl J Med* 2002;347:983–991.

Yilmaz E, Batislam E, Basar MM, et al: The comparison and efficacy of 3 different (alpha) 1-adrenergic blockers for distal ureteral stones. *J Urol* 2005;173:2010–2012.

PART XXIV ▪ Gynecologic Problems of Childhood

Chapter 548 ▪ History and Physical Examination Joseph S. Sanfilippo

NEONATAL INFANT. Following a general physical examination, the initial gynecologic assessment of newborn infants begins with the breast examination. Commonly, as a result of maternal endogenous estrogen production, breast tissue enlarges transiently in neonates; a milklike nipple discharge may be noted. Persistent unilateral enlargement with tenderness and fever should suggest mastitis or, rarely, a breast abscess. The abdomen is gently palpated for evidence of organomegaly, and the external genitalia are assessed for any ambiguity. The labia should be gently separated, allowing inspection of the introital-hymenal area. Abducting the hips with the labia gently retracted frequently facilitates inspection of the introital area. A normal protuberant hymen with associated thin white mucoid discharge from the vagina is often perceptible. In the first few weeks of life, a small amount of vaginal bleeding may occur, reflecting the decline of circulating levels of maternal estrogens. On completion of the inspection segment of the examination, a rectal examination is performed. A midline structure, indicative of the uterus, is usually palpable, but the adnexa should not be palpable at this time.

PREPUBERTAL CHILD. A pediatric or adolescent patient undergoing her first gynecologic examination should be treated with particular care because the initial encounter may well set the stage for all future gynecologic examinations. If the examination is painful or uncomfortable or if there is significant lack of rapport between the patient and the examiner, the child may suffer lasting psychologic consequences. A gentle, caring attitude by the health care provider will go far in enabling the patient to relax.

The history is obtained primarily from the parent(s), who should be integrally involved in the physical examination of a child in this age group. Patients should have a sense of control over the examination, be involved, and should experience no discomfort. Providing an adequate explanation before the examination facilitates these goals.

Much information can be obtained by inspection of the vulvovaginal area. Ideally, the patient is placed in a frog-leg position. This is followed by the knee-chest position with a Valsalva maneuver allowing adequate assessment of the introital lower-third vaginal area. Magnification often can be accomplished with use of a colposcope or hand-held magnifying glass; appropriate documentation is also important. Visualizing the vestibule permits assessment of any discharge. Aspiration of any fluid in the vagina and lavage should be carried out with aseptic technique. An intravenous tube (butterfly) is passed into a soft number 12 bladder catheter, all of which is then attached to a 1-mL tuberculin syringe. Wet mounts can be obtained and evaluated as indicated. Cultures should be taken for evaluation of vulvovaginitis. Other instrumentation used for the genital examination includes an otoscope or Cameron-Myers vaginoscope. Gentle traction on the labia upward and outward further exposes the vaginal introitus for assessment. Calcium alginate (Calgi) swabs are also useful, especially for obtaining cultures from the vagina. A number of variations of the normal-appearing hymen occur, and care must be taken to determine whether a patient has an imperforate, microperforate, or septate hymen. If an inadequate examination is accomplished in an office-clinic setting, then sedation or examination under anesthesia should be considered.

ADOLESCENT. Obtaining a history in this age group may initially take place in the presence of the patient's parents. However, an adolescent should be made aware of the concept of confidentiality and be given the opportunity to provide her own history, one on one, without the parents' being present. This can be accomplished in the examination room before the physical examination. Concern for the presence of vaginal discharge, the potential for sexually transmitted infections, pregnancy, or menstrual aberration should be explored. Physicians should gain the confidence of the adolescent, provide a relaxed atmosphere for the examination, and communicate one's availability for consultation. Indications for the first pelvic examination in adolescents are presented in Table 548-1.

If an adolescent does not have one of the criteria listed in Table 548-1, the American College of Obstetricians and Gynecologists recommends that the first "gynecologic encounter" be between the age of 13 and 15 yr (Table 548-2). This encounter does not necessitate a pelvic examination but is an opportunity for the physician to provide education for the adolescent.

One suggestion for the adolescent interview is the use of HEADSS is VG (see Chapter 111). This mnemonic is outlined below:

Home—Household, family dynamics and relationships, living arrangements.

Education—School attendance, failed a grade, grades as compared to last year's grades, attitude toward school, most difficult and best subjects, goals: college, career.

Activities—Physical activity, sports, exercise, hobbies, friends, after school, weekends.

Drugs—Cigarettes/smokeless tobacco, alcohol, and/or other drugs: use at school or parties; use by friends, self; frequency and quantity used.

Sexuality—Sexual feelings: opposite or same sex, sexual intercourse: age at first intercourse, number of lifetime and current partners, recent change in partners, contraception, sexually transmitted infection, prior pregnancies, abortions.

Suicide/depression—Feelings about self, history of depression or other mental health problems, prior suicidal thoughts, prior suicide attempts, sleep problems.

Violence—How are conflicts handled in the home (i.e., late for curfew), school, work, guns in the home, weapon carrying, nonconsensual sex, physical contact.

Gangs—Member, friends in gangs, number present in high school, gang markings on skin should be noted.

The most important factor with respect to the interview is to establish rapport. During this time, the rules of confidentiality should be emphasized with the patient. Sufficient time is to be

TABLE 548-1. Suggested Indications for Pelvic Examination in Adolescents

Age 21, not sexually active
Sexually active within 3 yr of initiating coitus
Menstrual irregularities, acute phase
Severe dysmenorrhea
Unexplained abdominal pain
Unexplained dysuria
Abnormal vaginal discharge

Modified from The adolescent obstetric-gynecologic patient. *ACOG Technical Bull* 1990;145:3.

allowed for the office visit. This segment of the interview process (history) should be one-on-one between patient and physician.

PELVIC EXAMINATION. The teenage patient, with a specific problem necessitating a pelvic examination (abnormal uterine bleeding, vulvovaginitis, first Pap smear related to 3 yr after initiation of coitus), should be involved in the pelvic examination process. The examination is best performed in the absence of the parents, but a female chaperone should be present and may serve to neutralize any adverse psychosocial aspects of the situation. Communication should occur between the physician and the patient throughout the examination. The examination should be performed in the dorsal lithotomy position with an effort made to maintain eye contact. Appropriate-sized specula should be available, including the small Pedersen (8 cm in depth). The 4–5 cm speculum is best avoided because it usually results in inadequate visualization; however, the pediatric-sized Huffman speculum is appropriate.

Inspection of the vulva is followed by palpation of the Bartholin's-urethral Skene's glands. The clitoris, which is normally 2–4 mm wide, is then assessed. A clitoris wider than 10 mm, especially in the presence of other signs of virilization, is abnormal. The hymenal configuration should also be evaluated. A patient should be told immediately prior to the insertion of the speculum that she will experience a pressure sensation. Before touching the introitus, it is useful to touch the inner thigh with the speculum. Trauma to the urethra should be avoided, and displacement of the fourchette posteriorly further facilitates proper speculum placement. Discussion with the adolescent about techniques to relax the perineal musculature is often helpful.

Once the speculum portion of the examination is complete, a bimanual examination is undertaken. In a virginal female, a single-digit examination with an appropriately lubricated, gloved finger allows proper palpation of the vaginal walls and cervix and bimanual assessment of the uterus and the adnexa. The cul-de-sac is also assessed.

A number of resources for education of adolescents regarding their first pelvic examination are available. These include

North American Society for Pediatric and Adolescent Gynecology (http://www.naspag.org)
The Society for Adolescent Medicine (http://www.adolescent.health.org)
Association of Reproductive Health Professionals (http://www.arhp.org)
GYN101 (http://www.gyn101.com)

TABLE 548-2. Recommendations for First Gynecological Evaluation

Between 13 and 15 yr of age
"First gynecological encounter" not necessarily a pelvic examination
First pelvic examination with Pap smear within 3 yr of initiating coitus (coitarche) or 21 yr of age

American College of Obstetricians and Gynecologists Teen Tool Kit, 2003.

A "tool kit" is available through the American College of Obstetricians and Gynecologists; it includes information on how to establish an office-friendly environment for the adolescent gynecologic evaluation, tools for adolescent assessment, suggestions about how to talk with teens, handouts for adolescents, and a number of resources for health care professionals (address: 409 12th Street, SW, PO Box 96920, Washington, DC 20090-6920).

Cavanaugh R: Obtaining a personal and confidential history from adolescents. An opportunity for prevention. *J Adolesc Health Care* 1986;72:118–122.
Elford K, Spence J: The forgotten female: Pediatric and adolescent gynecological concerns and their reproductive consequences. *J Pediatr Adolesc Gynecol* 2002;15:65–77.
Farrington PF: Pediatric vulvo-vaginitis. *Clin Obstet Gynecol* 1997;40:135–140.
Kass-Wolff JH, Wilson EE: Pediatric gynecology: Assessment strategies and common problems. *Semin Reprod Med* 2003;21:329–338.
Phillips S, Bohannon W, Heald F: Teenagers' choices regarding the presence of family members during the examination of genitalia. *J Adolesc Health Care* 1986;7:245–249.
Pokorny SF, Stormer J: Atraumatic removal of secretions from the prepubertal vagina. *Am J Obstet Gynecol* 1987;156:581–582.
Ricciardi R: First pelvic examination in the adolescent. *Nurse Pract Forum* 2000;11:161–169.
Saipik R: Adolescent contraception. In Sanfilippo JS, Muram D, Dewhurst J, et al. (editors): *Pediatric Adolescent Gynecology,* 2nd ed. Philadelphia, WB Saunders, 2001, pp 305–317.
Sanders JM Jr, DuRant RH, Chastain DO: Pediatricians' use of chaperones when performing gynecologic examinations on adolescent females. *J Adolesc Health Care* 1989;10:110–114.
Talbot CW: The gynecologic examination of the pediatric patient. *Pediatr Ann* 1986;15:501–505, 508.

Chapter 549 ■ Vulvovaginitis

Joseph S. Sanfilippo

Vulvovaginitis is the most common childhood and adolescent gynecologic problem. The main clinical manifestations, in order of frequency, include vaginal discharge, erythema, tenderness, and pruritus. Dysuria and bleeding may occur but are less common. Vulvovaginal irritation results from the lack of labial fat pads and pubic hair for protection of the external genitalia. The labia minora tend to open when a child squats; this, in turn, causes exposure of the sensitive tissues within the hymenal ring. The close proximity of the anal orifice to the vagina allows transfer of fecal bacteria to the vulvovaginal area. Masturbation may also be a contributing factor.

In the relatively low estrogenic prepubertal environment, the thin atrophic vaginal epithelium is susceptible to bacterial invasion. Recurrent vulvovaginitis, especially nonspecific, usually ceases once a girl reaches puberty, estrogen increases, and the pH of the vagina becomes more acidic. In part, this change results from increased production of acetic and lactic acids, a phenomenon accompanied by an increase in superficial cell proliferation and glycogen as well as by enhancement of normal bacterial flora (Table 549-1).

Vaginal culture, cytology, and vaginoscopy may be indicated for evaluation of pediatric patients with vulvovaginitis. Leukocyte esterase dipsticks are a rapid screening test for vaginitis and cervicitis. The technique has been used to identify trichomonads, *Candida*, and bacterial vaginosis and to evaluate cervical secretions for identification of gonococcal and chlamydial infections.

TABLE 549-1. Specific Vulvovaginitis

ORGANISM	PRESENTATION	DIAGNOSIS	TREATMENT
Enterobiasis (pinworms)	Perineal pruritus (nocturnal); gastrointestinal symptoms; variable vulvovaginal contamination from feces	Adult worms in stool or eggs on perianal skin	Mebendazole; repeat in 3 wk if necessary
Giardiasis	Asymptomatic fecal contaminant, vaginal discharge, diarrhea, malabsorption syndrome	Protozoal flagellate (cyst or trophozoites) in feces	Metronidazole or quinacrine
Molluscum contagiosum	Vulvar lesions, nodules with umbilicated area; white core of curdlike material	Isolation of poxvirus	Dermal curettage of papule
Phthirus pubis (pediculosis pubis)	Pruritus, excoriation, sky-blue macules; inner thigh or lower abdomen	Nits on hair shafts, lice—skin or clothing	Lindane lotion (Kwell); also see Chapter 667
Sarcoptes scabiei (scabies)	Nocturnal pruritus, pruritic vesicles, pustules in runs	Mites; black ova, dots of feces (microscopic)	1% lindane
Shigella species (shigellosis)	Fever, malaise, fecal contamination, diarrhea; blood and mucus, cramps, pus in stool	Stools; white blood cells and red blood cells, positive for *Shigella*	Trimethoprim and sulfamethoxazole; ampicillin or tetracycline
Staphylococcus and *Streptococcus*	Vaginal discharge to vulvovaginal area; spread from primary lesion	Positive culture results of appropriate organism	Penicillin, a cephalosporin, or clindamycin

From Sanfilippo JS: Adolescent girls with vaginal discharge. *Pediatr Ann* 1986;15:509–512, 516–519.

PHYSIOLOGIC LEUKORRHEA. This discharge reflects circulating estrogen levels. Treatment consists of reassurance that this normal process is self-limited.

PATHOLOGIC VAGINAL DISCHARGE. Vaginal discharge is a common presenting complaint in pediatric patients. It is often the primary symptom of vulvitis, vaginitis, or vulvovaginitis. Pruritus, frequent urination, dysuria, or enuresis may be associated signs and symptoms. Vulvitis is manifested primarily by dysuria and pruritus and is associated with erythema of the vulva. It commonly has a more protracted course than vaginitis; the latter is characterized by discharge without associated dysuria, pruritus, or erythema. Vulvovaginitis involves a combination of these manifestations. The color, odor, and duration of the discharge should be noted. Although there are a number of causes of vulvovaginitis in pediatric patients, the more common ones include poor perineal hygiene, *Candida* infection, and a foreign body.

NONSPECIFIC VULVOVAGINITIS. Patients with poor perineal hygiene often develop a condition known as nonspecific vulvovaginitis. This condition accounts for 70% of all pediatric vulvovaginitis cases. The discharge is characteristically brown or green, has a fetid odor, and is associated with a vaginal pH of 4.7–6.0. In 68% of reported cases, this vaginitis is associated with coliform bacteria secondary to fecal contamination. The next most common bacterial organisms associated with nonspecific vulvovaginitis are hemolytic streptococcus and coagulase-positive staphylococcus. These organisms are often transmitted manually from the nasopharynx. Clothing, chemicals, cosmetics, and soap products or detergents used for bathing or laundry may also cause irritation that leads to nonspecific vulvovaginitis. Tight-fitting clothing, such as jeans, leotards, and tights, and rubber pants or plastic-coated paper diapers have also been implicated. Nonspecific vulvovaginitis occasionally can result in chronic infection, which may cause significant psychological consequences for a child and her parents alike. The physical examination should emphasize the importance of avoiding "vaginal fixation," while encouraging proper perineal hygiene.

Successful treatment of nonspecific vulvovaginitis should include instruction in perineal hygiene, switching from tight-fitting underwear, the use of sitz baths with mild soap, and air-drying the vulva. Patients should be instructed in appropriate bowel and bladder habits, emphasizing the need to wipe fecal material away from the vulvovaginal area. Recurrent vulvovaginitis should be treated with systemic antibiotics such as amoxicillin or a cephalosporin. Topical estrogen cream or polymyxin (Polysporin) ointment is often helpful.

SPECIFIC VULVOVAGINITIS. *Gardnerella vaginalis* is the most common organism cultured in pediatric or adolescent patients with vulvovaginitis, followed by *Candida*. Other identified organisms include enterococci and anaerobic bacteria such as *Peptococcus, Peptostreptococcus, Veillonella parvula, Eubacterium, Propionibacterium*, and *Bacteroides* species. Protozoa, helminths, and viruses should also be considered as etiologic agents. Treatment depends on the offending organism (see Table 549-1).

VAGINAL CYSTS. These cysts are uncommon and frequently incidental findings. They represent rests of the wolffian or müllerian ducts or an epithelial inclusion cyst. Management depends on their location and appearance; they are usually observed, but resection is recommended if they become symptomatic.

GARTNER DUCT CYST. These represent a rudimentary portion of wolffian duct. In girls, the duct usually regresses completely. However, it may have remnants along the anterolateral walls of the vagina. The cysts have been associated with dyspareunia in sexually active adolescents. This symptomatology warrants surgical resection.

CLITORAL SYNECHIAE. These are often associated with pruritus involving the clitoral area and may result from rubbing of the anterior genital area during ambulation. Erythema is variable. If the clitoral hood appears to be agglutinated to the glans clitoris, it may be painful when evaluated. Treatment consists of applying estrogen cream to the periclitoral area daily over a 1–2 wk period. This usually suffices; rarely is surgical intervention warranted.

LABIAL ADHESIONS. In this disorder, the labia minora have a central line of adherence from an area immediately inferior to the clitoris to the fourchette (Fig. 549-1). Labial adhesions are commonly seen in patients younger than 6 yr of age, and the condition is often asymptomatic. The lesions usually are associated with local inflammation and the hypoestrogenic state of preadolescents. Pooling of urine in the vagina and recurrent vulvovaginitis provide a continuous nidus for recurrent urinary tract infections. These urinary symptoms occur in 20–40% of patients and should be treated.

Topical estrogen cream applied each evening for 1 wk is the treatment of choice and is effective in >90% of cases. Cleansing followed by periodic application of a bland ointment such as petrolatum or zinc oxide should continue for 1–2 mo after the adhesions separate to prevent recurrence. Mechanical separation of the adhesions is advisable only if the adhesions appear to separate easily and if it does not cause significant trauma. Once the

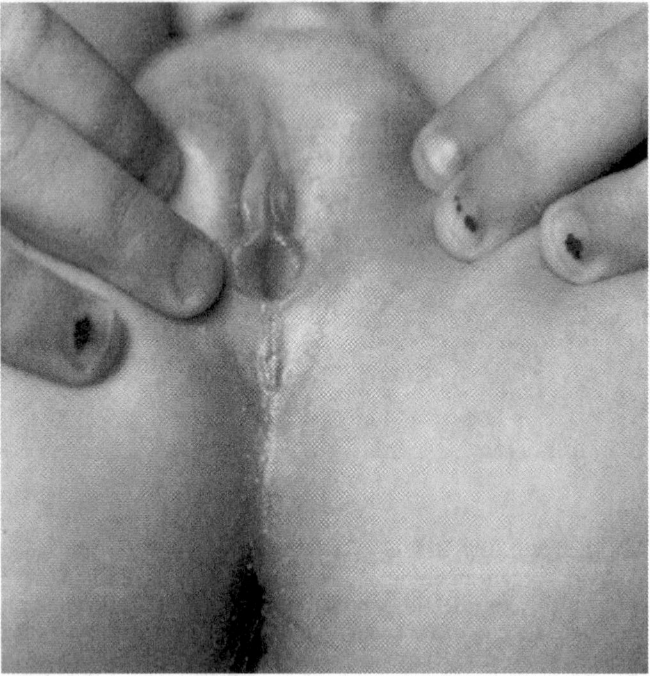

Figure 549-1. Labial adhesions.

adhesions are separated, the patient should be re-examined for any predisposing cause, such as the presence of a vaginal septum.

CANDIDIASIS. *Candida* infection is often associated with a diaper rash. *Candida* vulvovaginitis, although rare in children, must be considered, especially for girls with chronic mucocutaneous candidiasis. The presence of *Candida*-infected tissue may be indicative of significant immunosuppression. Underlying factors such as diabetes mellitus should be considered. Treatment with an imidazole cream (clotrimazole) is frequently effective, except in cases of chronic mucocutaneous candidiasis.

MOLLUSCUM CONTAGIOSUM. This common infection of the skin is caused by molluscum contagiosum virus, or poxvirus. Molluscum contagiosum presents as an umbilicated, dome-shaped papule. The central umbilication is usually associated with a pulpy core. Vulvar lesions appear to result from autoinoculation or from close contact (sexual or nonsexual) with an infected individual. The incubation period is 2–7 wk. Diagnosis is confirmed by light microscopic visualization of viral inclusions (molluscum bodies) in the central core. Treatment is expectant; if lesions persist, they may be eliminated by gentle curettage. Other methods of therapy include cryosurgery or electrocautery (see Chapter 666).

INTERTRIGO. Intertrigo can occur in the genitocrural areas in association with friction, obesity, and moisture in the area. Miliaria and secondary infection can also occur in association with intertrigo. The affected areas are red and macerated. Careful hygiene, combined with bland emollients and sometimes a mild corticosteroid, is an effective treatment.

IMPETIGO. This entity is commonly identified during the first several weeks of life. It is usually caused by *Staphylococcus aureus,* often phage group II, type 71, which may be acquired from the mother, other relatives, or staff. Impetigo tends to affect the vulva and periumbilical areas, causing lesions or blisters that later become crusted. Extensive spread and complications may ensue if treatment with antibiotics is not promptly instituted.

MALASSEZIA FURFUR. This condition is caused by *Pityrosporum orbiculare* and is manifested by scaly macules on the trunk in postpubertal patients, but lesions have been reported on the face and genital area. The diagnosis is established by visualization of hyphae and spores on wet preparation with 10% potassium hydroxide. Treatment requires application of topical imidazoles (clotrimazole).

HERPES SIMPLEX VIRUS. Herpes simplex virus (HSV) types 1 and 2 involve the vulvar area. The types are not exclusively site specific, but type 2 is commonly responsible for genital lesions and type 1, in general, for facial-oral lesions. The infection is characterized by papules that become vesicles, with the virus affecting the dorsal root ganglia. Differential diagnoses include any eroded or blistering lesions as well as herpes zoster. Culturing the virus or visualizing it via electron microscopy establishes a definitive diagnosis. Treatment with topical acyclovir reduces viral shedding and accelerates healing (see Chapter 249).

HUMAN PAPILLOMAVIRUS (HPV). HPV is associated with a number of serotypes, including 6, 11, 16, and 18, which usually are noted in the anogenital region. Types 16 and 18 are particularly associated with malignant and premalignant lesions of the vulva and cervix. Differential diagnoses include molluscum contagiosum, condyloma acuminatum, and vulvar intraepithelial neoplasia. The possibility of child sexual abuse must be strongly considered when these lesions are identified. Treatment is based on presenting signs and symptoms.

LICHEN SCLEROSUS. This is a chronic atrophic skin disease characterized by small, pink to ivory, flat-topped papules that are several millimeters in diameter. The papules appear to coalesce into plaques that become wrinkled and atrophic. The anogenital lesions frequently resemble an hourglass or a figure 8 (Fig. 549-2). Vesicles and bullae may spread over the vulva with associated hemorrhage. Lichen sclerosus commonly presents in the prepubertal patient; 10–15% of all cases of lichen sclerosus occur in children.

The onset of lichen sclerosus in most children usually occurs before 7 yr of age. The youngest reported patient was an infant several wk old. The onset of menarche often results in spontaneous improvement of the lesions, but the process usually continues. Patients are often intermittently symptomatic, and there is no relationship between menarche and symptomatic improvement or resolution of the disease. Atrophy of the labia minora

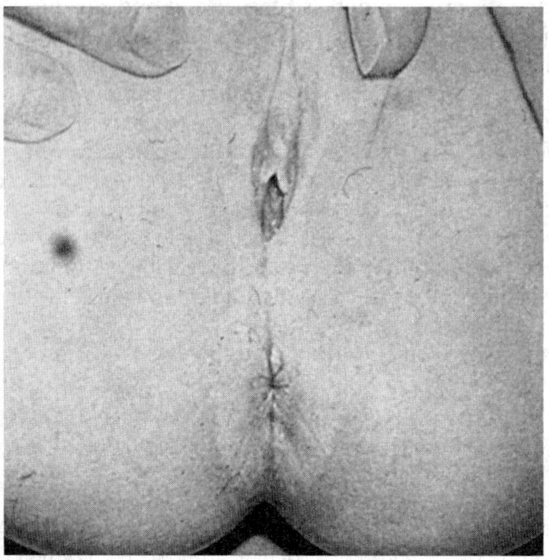

Figure 549-2. Lichen sclerosus.

and clitoral phimosis, as well as contracture of the introitus, may occur.

The cause of lichen sclerosus is unknown, but it is believed to be related to an autoimmune disorder. There is an association with certain HLA types. Family clusters have now been documented. There may be a relationship between lichen sclerosus and morphea (localized scleroderma). Decreased 5α- reductase activity has also been proposed as a possible cause for lichen sclerosus. Positive immunofluorescence for fibrin, serum complement (C3), or immunoglobulin M (IgM) in the involved area has been demonstrated in 75% of patients.

Treatment is symptomatic; emollients and topical corticosteroids usually provide relief. Corticosteroids are the treatment of choice for lichen sclerosus in adults and have been efficacious in children as well. Initially, 1–2% hydrocortisone cream is used. If there is failure to respond, a short course of betamethasone dipropionate 0.05% or clotrimazole is recommended. Minimal side effects are associated with this treatment. After the initial response, a milder topical corticosteroid may be used to prevent recurrence. Topical estrogens and androgens also have been advocated, but these agents may produce a vaginal discharge as well as other secondary problems, such as breast development and clitoral enlargement. Secondary infections should be treated with antibiotics. Some affected individuals demonstrate the Koebner phenomenon; these individuals should avoid tight-fitting clothing and genital trauma. Laser therapy has also been advocated.

LICHEN PLANUS. Vulvar lichen planus is often associated with oral mucosal and subcutaneous lesions. The vulvar lesions are characterized by angular violaceous, flat-topped papules and may simulate leukoplakia. In addition, the oral lesions consist of minute white papules that form a lacy pattern and usually are located on the buccal mucosa. The lesions are intensely pruritic and may become excoriated and macerated; erosions and ulcerations may occur in severe cases. Diagnosis requires biopsy. Exacerbation or recurrence of the lesions is common.

Treatment consists of topical intralesional corticosteroids and antihistamines to control the pruritus. Squamous cell carcinoma may occur with long-standing, hypertrophic, vulvar lichen planus; therefore, long-term follow-up and histologic examination of any changes or otherwise suspicious areas are advisable.

LICHEN SIMPLEX CHRONICUS (NEURODERMATITIS). This is a chronic, lichenified plaque that causes pruritus. It results from persistent rubbing and scratching of the vulvar skin; excoriations and fissuring occur. The labia have the appearance of white, hypertrophic, edematous lesions. The changes can occur on the mons pubis and the labia majora. Scratching and inflammation may result, causing a vicious cycle. The condition is rare in children. Treatment with antihistamines and topical or intralesional corticosteroids is recommended. Triamcinolone (5–10 mg/mL) has been used for intralesional injection.

SEBORRHEIC DERMATITIS. This presents as erythematous, oily, circumscribed patches that can be found on the face, scalp, and chest as well as on the intertriginous areas of the body. There may also be fissures and associated secondary infection around the vulva; secondary bacterial or candidal infection is quite common, causing pain, pruritus, dysuria, and vaginal bleeding. Acute episodes are best treated with sitz bath or topical aluminum acetate solution (Burow solution). Exacerbating factors, such as tight clothing or rubber pants, should be eliminated. Systemic antibiotics with appropriate topical antifungal medication should be administered for secondary infection.

ATOPIC DERMATITIS (ECZEMA). This affects 3% of all children. Patients present with hay fever or asthma or both, and generally a family history is noted. The vulvar lesion is characterized as a chronic condition accompanied by intense pruritus, erythema, papules, and vesicles, with oozing and crusting of the involved areas. Associated circumscribed, lichenified scaly patches may be seen on the vulvar area. Pruritus often causes scratching, which results in excoriation of the lesions. Secondary bacterial or candidal infection is common.

Antihistamines are necessary for control of pruritus. Sitz baths with mild soap and lubricants are helpful. Topical corticosteroids such as 1% hydrocortisone are also effective. Secondary bacterial, viral, or candidal infections require specific treatment (see Chapter 144).

DERMATITIS. In either allergic or irritant contact dermatitis, the vulva may be affected by edematous, erythematous, oozing lesions that are sometimes accompanied by vesicles or pustules. Chronic contact dermatitis is often associated with thickened and lichenified lesions. The clue to correct diagnosis of this condition is the limitation of the dermatitis to the area of contact with the etiologic agent. There may also be a secondary candidal or bacterial infection. Some common etiologic agents are soaps, powders, bubble baths, feminine hygiene sprays, topical medications, toilet paper, rubber, and certain types of clothing.

Treatment should include avoidance of the offending agents and sitz baths and compresses with topical aluminum acetate solution (Burow solution) during acute episodes. Mild topical corticosteroids such as 0.5–1% hydrocortisone cream applied several times daily may further aid healing and alleviate vulvar irritation. Recurrence can be prevented by removal of the offending etiologic agent.

FOLLICULITIS. This can occur either spontaneously or secondary to shaving or other depilatory methods such as waxing. It results in a papulopustular eruption secondary to inflammation of the hair follicle. It may occur in any hair-bearing skin. On physical examination, pustules are identified ranging in size from 2 to 10 mm. The pustules may be pierced in the center by a visible hair. The pustules become replaced by red papules. *S. aureus* is the most common agent; however, *Pseudomonas aeruginosa* can also occur and is associated with "hot tub folliculitis." Treatment includes sitz baths and cleansing with povidone-iodine solution once or twice daily. When staphylococcal infections do not respond, treatment is with clindamycin, a cephalosporin, or erythromycin.

VULVAR PSORIASIS. This is frequently associated with lesions of other parts of the body and is characterized by violaceous papules or plaques with a thick, adherent, silvery scale (Fig. 549-3). The intertriginous areas may show "inverse" psoriasis, a variation that does not occur on the extremities. Vulvar lesions are poorly demarcated and may present as scaly patches, most commonly on the mons pubis. The vulvar lesions are often resistant to therapy. A corticosteroid cream (1% hydrocortisone) should be used in conjunction with control of secondary infection and pruritus.

ENTEROBIASIS. Pinworms *(Enterobius vermicularis)* are helminths that may carry colonic bacteria to the perineum, causing recurrent vulvovaginitis. Female pinworms emerge from the anus to deposit eggs. Vulvovaginitis develops in about 20% of girls infected with *E. vermicularis*. The plastic tape test should be used to search for the organism if it is suspected or in cases of undiagnosed recurrent vulvovaginitis. Victims typically have pruritus and nocturnal episodes of scratching. Treatment consists of pyrantel pamoate (see Table 549-1).

SHIGELLOSIS. *Shigella flexneri* and *Shigella sonnei* cause various gastrointestinal symptoms in association with vaginitis. Forty-seven per cent of patients present with a bloody vaginal discharge

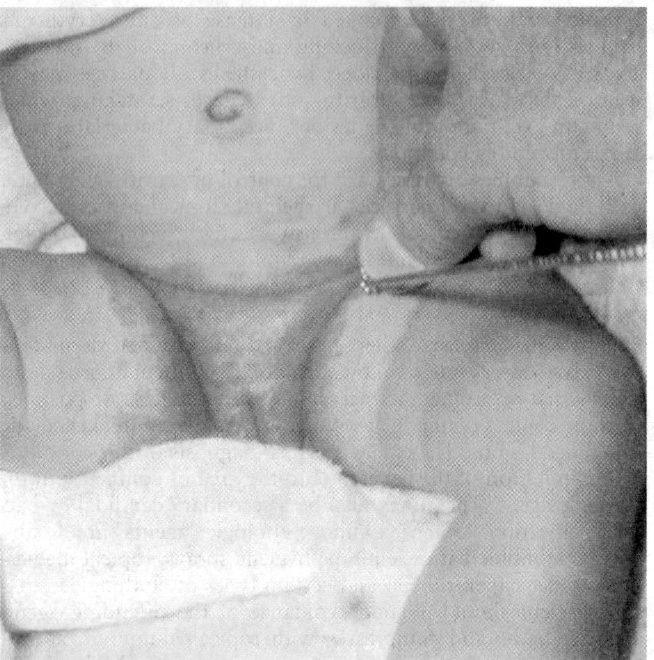

Figure 549-3. Vulvar psoriasis.

and 2% with diarrhea. Systemic antibiotics are the treatment of choice. Bowel colonization with shigella can result in subclinical gastrointestinal symptoms in 10% of household members.

VITILIGO. This presents as sharply demarcated pink to ivory patches that tend to spread and coalesce (Fig. 549-4). The skin on the patch is smooth and shows no palpable changes. It may be differentiated from lichen sclerosus because the hyperpigmented patches are asymptomatic. No treatment is necessary unless cosmetic problems result.

APHTHOUS ULCERS. Aphthous ulcers of the genital region as well as oral mucosa range in size from 1 to 10 mm and have a grayish-yellow base. These ulcers may recur and last at least 7–10 days.

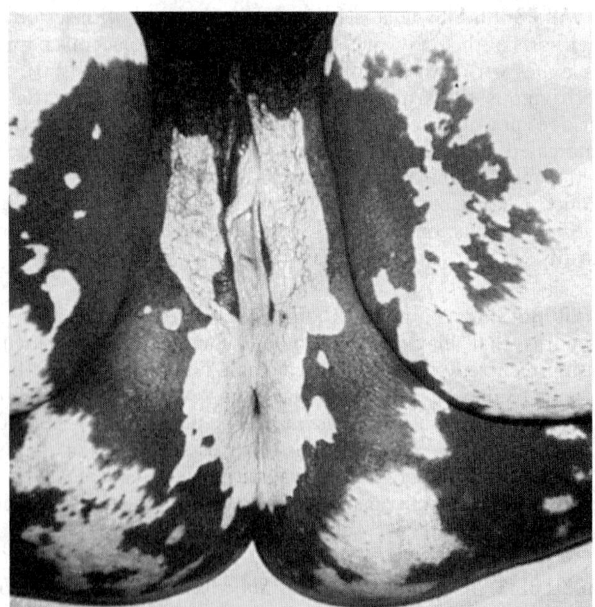

Figure 549-4. Vitiligo.

The etiology remains unclear. Vulva lesions can be treated with topical corticosteroids and if necessary topical anesthetics.

DRUG REACTIONS ASSOCIATED WITH VULVAR LESIONS. Erythema multiforme can present with genital ulcers complementing lesions on the palms, soles, and other parts of the body. The lesions usually persist for approximately 1 wk. They may represent an allergic reaction to a medication or a preceding flare-up of herpes simplex.

STEVENS-JOHNSON SYNDROME. This is a variant of erythema multiforme with more severe mucosal membrane involvement. Medications that cause Stevens-Johnson syndrome include nonsteroidal anti-inflammatory agents, sulfonamides, and some anticonvulsive drugs. *Mycoplasma pneumoniae* can also cause this syndrome. In general, the prodromal period is 1–14 days and is characterized by fever, headaches, sore throat, and malaise. There may also be vomiting and diarrhea. The oral mucosa and the eyes can be affected simultaneously (see Chapter 653).

TOXIC EPIDERMAL NECROLYSIS. These lesions are secondary to a number of medications; 20–30% of patients die. The skin appears to be scalded; vulvar erosion and ulceration can be extensive. Resulting vulvar synechiae and atrophy can produce dyspareunia.

LABIAL HYPERTROPHY. Hypertrophy of the labia minora is uncommon. It may occur either unilaterally or bilaterally. Occasionally, it is symptomatic; the patient complains of irritation or discomfort with walking, riding, biking, or intercourse. In the asymptomatic patient, treatment includes reassurance. However, in the symptomatic patient, the excessive tissue can be excised and the skin re-approximated with interrupted sutures or a subcuticular closure. The patient may require a Foley catheter immediately postoperatively.

CROHN DISEASE. This is a chronic noncaseating granulomatous disease involving the gastrointestinal tract. Gynecologic problems occur in up to 24% of women. These manifestations include erythema, edema, and subsequent ulcer formation. Cutaneous ulcers of the vulva are slitlike, deep, and multiple. Secondary infection may occur. The diagnosis must be distinguished from other defects such as sarcoidosis, condyloma acuminata, condyloma lata, and hidradenitis suppurativa. Biopsy confirms the diagnosis. Treatment of the gastrointestinal problem with steroids and antibiotics is the primary objective of management. Vulvar lesions are treated with local application of steroids and systemic antibiotics for secondary infections.

BEHÇET DISEASE. This is a rare chronic multisystem disease associated with occlusive vasculitis. It is a multiorgan system problem characterized by recurrent oral and genital aphthous ulcers and uveitis, cutaneous vasculitis, synovitis, and meningoencephalitis. Genital ulcers occur in 58–78% of patients. They are painful, red macular lesions. Symptomatic treatment includes topical anesthetics such as lidocaine jelly. Intralesional steroids may be necessary for symptomatic ulcers. In severe forms of the disease, treatment has included colchicine or methotrexate.

Brown MR, Cartwright PC, Snow BW: Common office problems in pediatric urology and gynecology. *Pediatr Clin North Am* 1997;44:1091–1115.

Fisher G, Rogers M: Treatment of childhood vulvar lichen sclerosus with potent topical corticosteroid. *Pediatr Dermatol* 1997;14:235–238.

Fivozinsky KB, Laufer MR: Vulvar disorders in adolescence. A literature review. *J Reprod Med* 1998;43:763–773.

Joishy M, Ashtekar CS, Jain A, et al: Do we need to treat vulvovaginitis in prepubertal girls? *Br Med J* 2005;330:186–188.

Kokotos F: Vulvovaginitis. *Pediatr Rev* 2006;27:116–117.
Koumantakis EE, Hassan EA, Deligeoroglou EK, et al: Vulvovaginitis during childhood and adolescence. *J Pediatr Adolesc Gynecol* 1997;10:39–43.
Leung AK, Robson WL, Tay-Uyboco J: The incidence of labial fusion in children. *J Paediatr Child Health* 1993;29:235–236.
Powell J, Wojnarowska F. Childhood vulvar lichen sclerosus: an increasingly common problem. *J Am Acad Dermatol* 2001;44:803–806.
Quint EH, Smith YR: Vulvar disorders in adolescent patients. *Pediatr Clin North Am* 1999;46:593–606, ix.
Rau F, Muram D: Vulvovaginitis in children. In Sanfilippo JS, Muram D, Dewhurst J, et al. (editors): *Pediatric Adolescent Gynecology,* 2nd ed. Philadelphia, WB Saunders, 2001, p 199.
Ridley C: Dermatologic conditions of the vulva. In Sanfilippo JS, Muram D, Dewhurst J, et al. (editors): *Pediatric Adolescent Gynecology,* 2nd ed. Philadelphia, WB Saunders 2001, p 216.
Schroeder B: Vulvar disorders in adolescents. *Obstet Gynecol Clin North Am* 2000;27:35–48.
Styed TS, Braverman P: Vaginitis in adolescents. *Adolesc Med Clin* 2004; 15:235–251.
Stricker T, Navratil F, Sennhauser FH: Vulvovaginitis in prepubertal girls. *Arch Dis Child* 2003;88:324–326.

Chapter 550 ■ Bleeding

Joseph S. Sanfilippo

The entities responsible for isolated vaginal bleeding in the pediatric patient include exposure to exogenous sex steroids, a foreign body, hemorrhagic cystitis, hypothyroidism, precocious puberty, an ovarian cyst, trauma that may or may not be associated with sexual abuse, urethral prolapse, vulvovaginitis, neoplasms, as well as other less common causes. See Chapter 115 for discussion of menstrual problems.

FOREIGN BODY. A foreign body is commonly responsible for vaginal bleeding in pediatric patients. A foul-smelling discharge associated with vaginal bleeding suggests this possibility. Wadded toilet paper is the most common foreign body identified in the vagina. Plain radiography or ultrasonography of the pelvis is often helpful. A vaginal foreign body was found in 18% of preadolescent girls with vaginal bleeding with or without discharge and in 50% of those with bleeding and no discharge.

URETHRAL PROLAPSE. Vulvar bleeding can be associated with urethral prolapse. This uncommon disorder is characterized by the urethral mucosa protruding through the meatus and forming a sensitive vulvar mass that bleeds easily. The "mass" is separate from the vagina. Patients may have difficulty with urination depending on the size of the mass and whether it occludes the urethral meatus. The entity responds to topical application of estrogens because the distal urethra is estrogen sensitive. Urethral prolapse is often misdiagnosed when there is urogenital bleeding.

GENITAL TRAUMA. Although most injuries to this area are accidental, the possibility of physical or sexual abuse must be considered. Blunt injury may cause blood vessels beneath the perineal skin to rupture. Blood accumulating under the skin forms a hematoma, which may present as a round, tense, tender mass. Contusion of the vulva usually does not require treatment. A small vulvar hematoma often can be controlled by pressure with an ice pack. Analgesics may be required.

Penetrating injuries to the vaginal area warrant further careful evaluation, including serious consideration of the possibility of sexual abuse (Chapter 36). A detailed examination is necessary, especially in the presence of active bleeding. The potential for bowel or bladder trauma must also be considered.

GENITAL TUMORS. Benign and malignant tumors of the vulva should be considered when vaginal bleeding occurs in pediatric patients. A broad spectrum of entities, ranging from capillary hemangiomas through malignancies such as rhabdomyosarcoma, requires appropriate tissue diagnosis and treatment. The most common malignant tumors include endodermal carcinoma, which occurs most often in young children; mesonephric carcinoma, which arises in a remnant of a mesonephric duct and occurs more often in girls 3 yr of age or older; and clear cell adenocarcinoma, which is often associated with a history of antenatal exposure to diethylstilbestrol.

CAPILLARY VENOUS MALFORMATION OF THE LABIA MAJORA. Capillary venous malformation has been reported as a cause of vaginal bleeding in pediatric patients with expansion in vaginal volume on response to hormonal changes at puberty. The differential diagnosis includes hemangioma and other vascular malformation(s). Diagnosis is based on an evaluation that includes ultrasonography, MRI, and abdominal arteriography. The malformation can be locally excised.

Anveden-Hertzberg L, Gauderer MW, Elder JS: Urethral prolapse: An often misdiagnosed cause of urogenital bleeding in girls. *Pediatr Emerg Care* 1995;11:212–214.
Hickey M, Balen A: Menstrual disorders in adolescence: investigation and management. *Hum Reprod Update* 2003;9:493–504.
Imai A, Horibe S, Tamaya T: Genital bleeding in premenarcheal children. *Int J Gynaecol Obstet* 1995;49:41–45.
Kanbur N, Derman O, Kutluk T, et al: Coagulation disorders as the cause of menorrhagia in adolescents. *J Adolesc Med Health* 2004;16:183–185.
Kempinaire A, De Raeve L, Roseeuw D, et al: Capillary-venous malformation in the labia majora of a 12-year-old girl. *Dermatology* 1997;194:405–407.
Lavin C: Dysfunctional uterine bleeding in adolescents. *Curr Opin Pediatr* 1996;8:328–332.
Minjarez D: Abnormal bleeding in adolescents. *Semin Reprod Med* 2003;21:363–373.
Strickland JL, Wall J: Abnormal uterine bleeding in adolescents. *Obstet Gynecol Clin North Am* 2003;30:321–335.
Strickland JL: Management of abnormal bleeding in adolescents. *Mo Med* 2004;101:38–41.
Templeman C, Hertweck SP, Muram D, et al: Vaginal bleeding in childhood and menstrual disorders in adolescence. In Sanfilippo JS, Muram D, Dewhurst J, et al. (editors): *Pediatric and Adolescent Gynecology,* 2nd ed. Philadelphia, WB Saunders, 2001, pp 237–247.

Chapter 551 ■ Breast Disorders

Joseph S. Sanfilippo

Beginning at approximately 6 wk of gestation, epidermal cells migrate to the mesenchyme and form the mammary ridges. Breast buds, lactiferous ducts, and fully developed mammary glands eventually form. Breast development normally occurs in girls between the ages of 8½ and 13 yr of age. The rate of breast growth varies, and development is often asymmetric. Complete development may not occur until a woman is in her early 20s.

BREAST SELF-EXAMINATION (BSE). Early diagnosis is central to improving health care for breast abnormalities, including carcinoma. While controversy exists, instruction in BSE merits con-

TABLE 551-1. How to Do Breast Self-Examination

1. Lie down. Flatten your right breast by placing a pillow under your right shoulder. If your breasts are large, use your right hand to hold your right breast while you do the examination with your left hand.
2. Use the sensitive pads of the middle three fingers on your left hand. Feel for lumps using a rubbing motion.
3. Press firmly enough to feel different breast tissues.
4. Completely feel all the breast and chest area to cover breast tissue that extends toward the shoulder. Allow enough time for a complete examination. Women with small breasts need at least 2 min to examine each breast. Larger breasts take longer.
5. Use the same pattern to feel every part of the breast tissue. Choose the method easiest for you. The three patterns preferred by women and their doctors are the circular, clock, or oval pattern; the vertical strip; and the wedge.
6. After you have completely examined your right breast, then examine your left breast using the same method. Compare what you have felt in one breast with the other.
7. You may also want to examine your breasts while bathing, when your skin is wet and lumps may be easier to feel.
8. You can check your breasts in a mirror; look for any change in size or contour, dimpling of the skin, or spontaneous nipple discharge.

Reproduced with permission of the American Cancer Society.

sideration in adolescents (Table 551-1). BSE is especially indicated in girls, beginning at age 20 years when they are positive for *BRCA1* and/or *BRCA2* genes.

CONGENITAL ANOMALIES. Complete absence of breast, amastia, is rare; it is usually unilateral and often associated with other abnormalities, such as Poland syndrome (aplasia of the pectoralis muscles, rib deformities, webbed fingers, and radial nerve aplasia). Amastia can be iatrogenic, as a result of inadvertent excision of a breast bud. Athelia is defined as absence of 1 or both nipples. This condition is also rare and may not be associated with absent breast tissue. Both abnormalities require surgical correction.

Supernumerary breasts (polymastia) and supernumerary nipples (polythelia) are relatively common (Fig. 551-1); they occur along the milk lines and are usually asymptomatic. There is an association between polythelia and anomalies of the urinary and cardiovascular systems. In general, surgical excision of the accessory breasts or nipples is not necessary. However, if the aberrant breasts or nipples become symptomatic, excision may be indicated.

Hypoplasia of the breasts varies in degree from a nearly total absence of breast tissue to well-formed breasts that are considered by the patient to be too small. There are 3 general causes for poor or absent breast development: (1) The onset of breast development may be delayed, and the breasts develop slowly but are normal in all other respects; (2) a patient's family history may include late breast development; (3) ovarian function may have failed or been suppressed. Treatment depends on the underlying cause.

Breast atrophy is seen occasionally in adolescents and is almost uniformly secondary to dietary changes such as occurring with anorexia nervosa. Correction of the underlying problem results in re-establishment of breast tissue.

NEONATAL BREAST ABNORMALITIES. Bilateral breast hypertrophy may occur as a result of elevated circulating maternal endogenous steroid hormones in late gestation. It may be associated with discharge from the nipples known as "witch's milk." Repeated manipulation of the breast can exacerbate the condition. On occasion, the hypertrophy is associated with mastitis caused by a staphylococcal or streptococcal infection; antibiotics should be administered.

MASTODYNIA. Painful breast engorgement (mastodynia) usually is associated with ovulatory cycles; this is uncommon in adolescents until approximately 18 mo after menarche, the time that may be necessary to establish ovulatory cycles. There is frequently a cyclic pattern of the breast discomfort. Analgesics such as nonsteroidal anti-inflammatory drugs, including ibuprofen, and the use of a good support bra are often helpful in alleviating discomfort.

BREAST MASSES. A retrospective review of breast disease in adolescent females revealed that about 54% have fibroadenomas and 13% have virginal hypertrophy. Fibrocystic or proliferative breast disease occurs in about 24%. Primary rhabdomyosarcoma, metastatic rhabdomyosarcoma, metastatic neuroblastoma, and non-Hodgkin lymphoma occur in 2–3% of all breast masses in this age group. Other diagnoses include polythelia, accessory breast tissue, mastitis, hemangioma, fat necrosis, and intramammary lymph nodes. Breast masses during adolescence may stem from several causes:

- Fibroadenoma
- Fibrocystic disease
- Breast cyst
- Abscess/mastitis
- Intraductal papilloma
- Fat necrosis/lipoma
- Cystosarcoma phyllodes
- Adenomatous hyperplasia
- Rare lesions (hemangiomas, lymphangiomas, lymphoma)
- Normal breast tissue
- Cancer

A thorough history and physical examination are recommended for any pediatric or adolescent patient who has a breast mass. The clinical problem should be reviewed with a radiologist

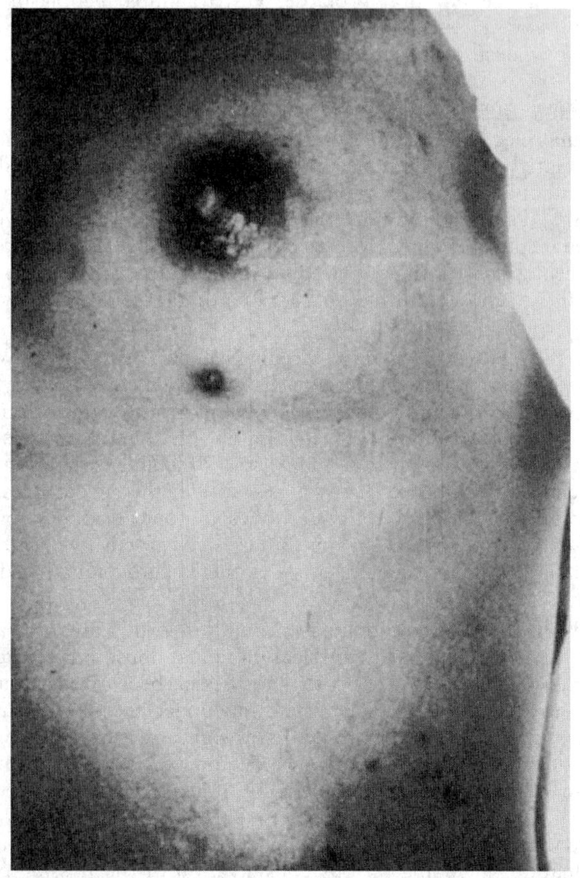

Figure 551-1. Polythelia.

before initiating any radiologic assessment. Needle aspiration and biopsy are often essential for evaluation of palpable breast abnormalities. Large breast tumors also occur in adolescents. Although malignancy is often suspected because of rapid growth of the mass and skin ulceration, the incidence is very low. Breast tumors can have varied presentations. Giant fibroadenomas in adolescence may be treated by simple enucleation.

MALIGNANT TUMORS. Although rare, <1% occur in females younger than 30 yr of age, and breast cancer does occur in adolescents. Early menarche in association with anovulatory cycles is a risk factor. The estrogen-to-androgen ratio appears to be critical, with androgens having a protective effect.

Cystosarcoma phyllodes, an uncommon breast tumor in adults, may occur in adolescents. It is characterized by asymmetric breast enlargement in association with a firm, mobile, circumscribed mass. It can mimic a giant fibroadenoma. The tumor often increases rapidly in size and can become quite large. Fixation of the tumor to the skin or chest wall is rare. The majority of these tumors are benign, but malignant cystosarcoma phylloides with metastases has been reported. Excision is the preferred initial therapy in adolescent patients, regardless of the histologic classification of the lesion. *Malignant cystosarcoma* is more likely to recur than is a benign lesion. Fatal metastatic cystosarcoma phylloides in an adolescent has occurred.

Breast tumors also may be the first manifestation of relapse (extramedullary) in acute lymphoblastic leukemia. Reports in the literature include a case of radiation-induced sarcoma of the breast in a female adolescent and a case of liposarcoma in a 17-yr-old black female who previously had a total mastectomy.

MACROMASTIA (VIRGINAL HYPERTROPHY). The cause of massive breast enlargement during puberty and early adolescence is unknown, but the condition probably represents an end-organ increased sensitivity to circulating estrogens. It is bilateral, often occurs over a brief period, and most commonly affects girls 13–17 yr old. Physical and psychological problems may occur in adolescents with macromastia. Posture problems and discomfort often result. Reduction mammoplasty is the treatment of choice but should be delayed until late adolescence to allow for complete breast development. Surgical intervention often necessitates relocation of the nipple, which may result in decreased sensation and altered lactation. In addition, strong emotional support should be provided.

TUBEROUS BREASTS. This deformity results in breasts that are reminiscent of a tuberous root plant. It may be the result of exogenous steroid use, especially with induction of pubertal development. Surgical intervention is required for correction.

MASTITIS AND ABSCESS. Mastitis and breast abscess may require antibiotic therapy as well as incision and drainage. Mastitis is estimated to occur frequently after breast piercing, with estimated rates of infection as high as 10–20%. It is common in the postpartum period.

TRAUMA AND INFLAMMATION. Breast trauma in adolescent females has become more common because of the increased number of young women participating in contact sports. The trauma usually takes the form of contusion or hematoma and often resolves with either late cystic changes in the breast or fibrosis with retraction of skin or the nipple over the injured area. These late changes may mimic those associated with malignancy; biopsy may be the only means of differentiating the two.

MAMMARY DYSPLASIA. This common lesion is characterized by changes associated with the menstrual cycle. Hormonal imbalance may cause exaggerated responses in the breast tissue, especially in the upper and outer quadrants during the premenstrual phase of the cycle. The extent of treatment depends on the degree of symptoms; ibuprofen is often helpful. In addition, methylxanthines and caffeine (coffee, tea, carbonated drinks) should be eliminated from the diet.

TABLE 551-2. Differential Diagnosis of Nipple Discharge

TYPE	DIFFERENTIAL DIAGNOSIS (IN ORDER OF FREQUENCY)
Milky	Galactorrhea
Multicolored/sticky	Duct ectasia
Purulent	Mastitis
Watery	Papilloma Cancer
Serous/serosanguineous	Intraductal papilloma Fibrocystic changes Cancer Duct ectasia

From Neinstein LS: Breast masses in adolescents. *Adolesc Pediatr Gynecol* 1994;7:119.

NIPPLE DISCHARGE. This must be carefully evaluated and a distinction made between the presence of galactorrhea (spontaneous flow of milk), blood, or other discharge (Table 551-2). Evaluation of galactorrhea in children is the same as for adults. Serum prolactin levels are obtained to rule out the presence of a pituitary prolactinoma. If a pituitary tumor or adenoma is suspected based on markedly elevated serum prolactin, appropriate radiologic (CT, MRI) assessment is necessary. Another cause of galactorrhea is hypothyroidism in association with elevated levels of thyroid-releasing hormone, which also stimulates prolactin release. Medications may also cause galactorrhea (Table 551-3). Treatment of galactorrhea (nonthyroid related) consists primarily of dopamine agonists such as bromocriptine or cabergoline. Surgical intervention, usually transsphenoidal hypophysectomy, is rarely required. Galactorrhea secondary to chest wall surgery in an adolescent has also been reported; the galactorrhea occurred for 2 mo and was associated with transient amenorrhea.

Bloody nipple discharge can be indicative of duct ectasia. Cytologic assessment and surgical consultation are indicated. Nipple discharge in association with Montgomery tubercles also has been reported. These secretions can be episodic and vary in color from clear to brown, but they are usually not milky. This discharge evolves over a period of 3–5 wk, may be associated with breast lumps, and is a benign, self-limited problem. Intraductal breast papillomas have occurred in adolescents.

BREAST ASYMMETRY. Beginning in the neonate there may be unilateral breast development. In adolescents, it is not uncommon for approximately 25% of patients to have an element of breast asymmetry that persists after the age of 18. Asymmetry is common especially between Tanner stages 2 and 4.

TABLE 551-3. Medications that Cause Galactorrhea

Amitriptyline	Estrogens	Narcotics
Amphetamines	Fluphenazine	Prostaglandins
Androgens	Haloperidol	Reserpine
Anesthetics	Meprobamate	Sulpiride
Chlorpromazine	Methyldopa	Trifluoperazine
Cimetidine	Metoclopramide	
Domperidone	Monoamine oxidase inhibitors	

Adapted from Yazigi RA, Quintero CH, Salameh WA: Prolactin disorders. *Fertil Steril* 1997;67:215–225, reprinted with permission of the American Society for Reproductive Medicine.

Dufos C, Plo-Bureau G, Thibaud E, et al: Breast diseases in adolescents. *Endocr Dev* 2004;7:183–196.
Faden H: Mastitis in children from birth to 17 years. *Pediatr Infect Dis J* 2005;24:1113.
Jacobs VR, Golombeck K, Jonat W, et al: Mastitis nonpuerperalis after nipple piercing: Time to act. *J Fertil Womens Med* 2003;48:226–231.
Michels KB, Willett WC: Breast cancer—early life matters. *N Engl J Med* 2004;351:1679–1681.
Neinstein L: Breast disease in adolescents and young women. *Pediatr Clin North Am* 1999;46:607–629.
Ogletree RJ, Hammig B, Drolet JC, et al: Knowledge and intentions of ninth-grade girls after a breast self examination program. *J Sch Health* 2004;74:365–369.
Quint E, Simmons P: Breast masses in a teenage patient: *J Pediatr Adolesc Gynecol* 2001;14:47–48.
Shannon C, Smith IE: Breast cancer in adolescents and young women. *Eur J Cancer* 2003;39:2632–2642.
Templeman C, Hertweck SP: Breast disorders in the pediatric and adolescent patient. *Obstet Gynecol Clin North Am* 2000;27:19–34.

Chapter 552 ■ Hirsutism and Polycystic Ovarian Syndrome

Joseph S. Sanfilippo

Hirsutism (excessive hair growth) must be distinguished from virilization. The latter involves increased body hair, acne, deepening of the voice, change in body habitus due to increased muscle mass, and clitoromegaly. Premature pubarche is defined as the appearance of genital hair or axillary hair or both before age 8 yr. Adrenarche, the output of increased androgen from the adrenal glands, usually occurs between ages 12 and 18 yr and is discussed in Chapter 575.3.

Polycystic ovarian syndrome (PCOS) is believed to have its origin at puberty. Teenagers usually present with menstrual disturbances with or without hirsutism (Table 552-1). Additional features include severe acne, scalp hair loss, and obesity. Adults may be infertile and are at increased risk for Type 2 diabetes and cardiovascular complications. Ultrasonographic assessment often identifies multicystic ovaries, with a characteristic "pearl necklace" appearance. The prevalence of polycystic ovaries increases throughout puberty and may reach as high as 26% by 15 yr of age.

PCOS (polycystic ovaries, chronic anovulation, and Stein-Leventhal syndrome) is the most commonly diagnosed ovarian cause of hirsutism; controversy exists about whether the basic defect is central (hypothalamic or pituitary regulation of gonadotropins), ovarian (defect in a peptide hormone, perhaps inhibin, with resultant abnormal feedback to the pituitary gland), or insulin resistance. The usual hormonal pattern of PCOS begins with altered luteinizing hormone (LH) release (a ratio of LH to follicle-stimulating hormone of 2:1 or 3:1, shortened pulse frequency, and slightly increased pulse amplitude of LH); in addition, higher circulating levels of testosterone and androstenedione occur. Adolescents with hyperandrogenism display an exaggerated LH pulsatility similar to that found in adults with PCOS. The incidence of PCOS in women between 18 and 25 yr of age is 8–26%, depending on the diagnostic criteria. The criteria for the diagnosis of PCOS include oligomenorrhea, clinical and/or serum levels indicative of hyperandrogenemia, and sonographic evidence of multiple small follicles (9–10 mm in diameter).

Family history of PCOS is important in that it is more common in first-degree relatives of women with PCOS. Evaluation should include the following: serum androgens (testosterone, androstenedione, and dehydroepiandrosterone), thyroid-stimulating hormone, thyroxine, prolactin, fasting blood glucose and insulin, and 17-hydroxyprogesterone (17OHP).

TABLE 552-1. Causes of Hirsutism

PERIPHERAL
Idiopathic
Partial androgen insensitivity (5α-reductase deficiency)
HAIR-AN syndrome (hirsutism, androgenization, insulin resistance, and acanthosis nigricans)
Hyperprolactinemia
GONADAL
Polycystic ovary syndrome (polycystic ovaries, chronic anovulation)
Ovarian neoplasm (Sertoli-Leydig cell, granulosa cell, thecoma, gynandroblastoma, lipoid cell, luteoma, hypernephroma, Brenner tumor)
Gonadal dysgenesis (Turner mosaic with XY or H-Y antigen positive)
ADRENAL
Cushing syndrome
Adrenal hyper-responsiveness
Congenital adrenal hyperplasia (classic, cryptic, adult onset)
21-Hydroxylase deficiency
11-Hydroxylase deficiency
3β-Hydroxysteroid deficiency
17α-Hydroxylase deficiency
Adrenal neoplasm (adenoma, cortical carcinoma)
EXOGENOUS
Minoxidil
Dilantin
Cyclosporine
Anabolic steroids
Acetazolamide (Diamox)
Penicillamine
Oral contraceptives with androgenic progestins
Danazol
Androgenic steroids
Psoralens
Hydrochlorothiazide
Phenothiazines
CONGENITAL ANOMALIES
Trisomy 18 (Edwards syndrome)
Cornelia de Lange syndrome
Hurler syndrome
Juvenile hypothyroidism

Adapted from Bailey-Pridham DD, Sanfilippo JS: Hirsutism in the adolescent female. *Pediatr Clin North Am* 1989;36:581–599.

Patients with PCOS should be distinguished from those with *adult-onset congenital adrenal hyperplasia* (AOCAH). This population has a markedly elevated fasting 17OHP level (see below).

PCOS is associated with peripheral insulin resistance in addition to excessive levels of LH, resulting in increased ovarian androgen production. Hyperinsulinemia is associated with increased bioavailable insulin-like growth factor-1 (IGF-1) and depressed production of IGF-1 carrier protein (IGFBP-1). Activation of IGF-1 receptor may also be involved in increased ovarian androgen production. Peripheral conversion of ovarian androstenedione to testosterone contributes to the commonly identified increase in total serum testosterone levels that are an integral part of the PCOS hormonal pattern. In addition to their hyperinsulinemic state, these patients have long-term cardiovascular risks of hypertension and coronary artery disease. This patient population often also has increases in total triglyceride levels.

The insulin resistance is an integral part of the **HAIR-AN syndrome,** which consists of **h**irsutism, **androgenization,** insulin resistance, and acanthosis **n**igricans. Insulin receptor mutation as well as circulating antibodies to the insulin receptor and postreceptor defects occurs in this syndrome. Defects in glucose transport as well as high levels of insulin stimulate the activity of cytochrome P450c 17β, an enzyme actively involved in the pro-

TABLE 552-2. Drug Treatments*

AGENT	MECHANISM OF ACTION	ADVANTAGES OR DISADVANTAGES	EXAMPLES	USES			
				HIRSUTISM, ACNE	OLIGOMENORRHEA OR AMENORRHEA	OVULATION INDUCTION	INSULIN LOWERING
Combinations of estrogen and progestin	Increase SHBG, suppress LH and FSH, suppress ovarian androgen production; progestin can act as an antiandrogen	Cyclic exposure of endometrium to estrogen and progestin; effective for hirsutism and acne; may increase risk of thrombosis and metabolic abnormalities; beneficial antiandrogenic effects of drospirenone	Ethinyl estradiol and norgestimate (Ortho-Cyclen); ethinyl estradiol and desogestrel (Orthocept); ethinyl estradiol and drospirenone (Yasmin)	X	X		
Antiandrogens	Inhibit androgens from binding to the androgen receptor	Effective for hirsutism and acne; risk of hyperkalemia (spironolactone) or hepatitis (flutamide)	Cyproterone acetate, spironolactone, flutamide	X			
Glucocorticoids	Suppress corticotropin and thus adrenal androgen production	Attenuate adrenal component of androgen excess; long-term risks of glucose intolerance, insulin resistance, osteopenia, weight gain	Prednisone, dexamethasone	X	X	X	
5α-Reductase inhibitors	Inhibit 5α-reductase	Do not specifically target the isoenzyme of 5α-reductase in the pilosebaceous unit	Finasteride (Propecia)	X			
Ornithine decarboxylase inhibitors	Inhibit ornithine decarboxylase	Minimal documented efficacy; used topically	Eflornithine hydrochloride (Vaniqa)	X			
Antiestrogen	Induces rise in FSH, LH	Moderately effective as monotherapy, less effective in obese patients; may be useful in conjunction with insulin-lowering therapies	Clomiphene citrate			X	
Biguanide	Reduces hepatic glucose production, secondarily lowering insulin levels; may have direct effects on ovarian steroidogenesis	Substantial efficacy in restoration of menstrual cycling, less effective for hirsutism; usually associated with initial weight loss; may have untoward gastrointestinal effects	Metformin (Glucophage, Glucophage XR)	X	X	X	X
Thiazolidinediones	Enhance insulin action at target-tissue level (adipocyte, muscle); may have direct effects on ovarian steroidogenesis	Extremely effective at lowering levels of insulin and androgens, modest effects on hirsutism; associated with weight gain	Pioglitazone (Actos), rosiglitazone (Avandia)	X	X	X	X

* FSH, follicle-stimulating hormone; LH, luteinizing hormone; SHBG, sex hormone–binding globulin.
From Ehrmann DA: Polycystic ovary syndrome. *N Engl J Med* 2005;352:1223–1236.

duction of androgens by the ovary. With PCOS, there is also dysregulation of the cytochrome P450c 17β enzyme system.

Hirsutism in adolescents can also be due to a heterozygous form of 21-hydroxylase deficiency. This has been called AOCAH. Various other forms of congenital adrenal hyperplasia and congenital anomalies are also associated with hirsutism. Clinically, it may be difficult to distinguish between PCOS and AOCAH.

Ovarian hyperthecosis, which can be familial, is a variant of PCOS. Hyperthecosis is defined as isolated islands of luteinized cells within the ovary contributing to increased androgen production. Ovarian androgen production and its peripheral effects are similar to those associated with PCOS.

Medications, radiation, and chronic irritation (the placement of a cast) can also initiate localized, nonendocrinologic hair growth.

TREATMENT OF HIRSUTE PATIENTS. Hirsutism secondary to hyperprolactinemia is best treated with bromocriptine. In patients with multicystic (polycystic) ovaries and primary hypothyroidism, the polycystic ovaries resolve rapidly with adequate doses of thyroid replacement therapy. If an exogenous cause such as a medication is producing hirsutism, the exogenous agent should be eliminated. Even when the increased tissue androgen effect is reversed by appropriate treatment, hair follicles converted to terminal hair may still produce that type of hair. Electrolysis may provide an improved cosmetic appearance, with the assurance that if the underlying abnormality is controlled, no new hair growth should ensue. Cushing syndrome or disease, androgen-producing tumors, and congenital adrenal hyperplasia are discussed in Chapters 577 and 578. Metformin, an insulin-sensitizing agent, is recommended for hyperinsulinemic patients with PCOS. The objective is to have more effective circulating insulin levels, which is associated with decreases in serum LH and testosterone with PCOS, within 4–8 wk. It is imperative that treated patients have pretherapy as well as periodic evaluation of liver function.

Metformin works best in the presence of weight loss in obese patients. Additional therapies include estrogen-dominant (nonandrogenic) oral contraceptive pills or, if these are not well tolerated, GNRH agonists. Hirsutism is managed with an antiandrogen (spironolactone, cyproterone) plus an oral contraceptive (Table 552-2).

Long-term adverse effects of PCOS include an increased incidence of Type 2 diabetes mellitus, hyperlipidemia, and cardiovascular disease.

Cedars M: Polycystic ovarian syndrome: What is it and how should we treat it? *J Pediatr* 2004;144:4–6.

Driscoll D: Polycystic ovarian syndrome in adolescence *Ann N Y Acad Sci* 2003;997:49–55.

Ehrmann DA: Polycystic ovary syndrome. *N Engl J Med* 2005; 352:1223–1236.

Elmer KB, George RM: HAIR-AN syndrome: A multisystem challenge. *Am Fam Physician* 2001;15:2385–2390.

Fraser IS, Kovacs G: Current recommendations for the diagnostic evaluation and follow-up of patients presenting with symptomatic polycystic ovary syndrome. *Best Pract Res Clin Obstet Gynaecol* 2004;18:813–823.

Homburg R, Lambalk CB: Polycystic ovary syndrome in adolescence—a therapeutic conundrum. *Hum Reprod* 2004;19:1039–1042.

Legro R: Detection of insulin resistance and its prognosis in adolescent polycystic ovarian syndrome. *J Pediatr Endocrinol Metab* 2002;15 Suppl 5:1367–1378.

Mulchahey K: In support of metformin use in adolescent polycystic ovarian syndrome. *J Pediatr Adolesc Gynecol* 2002;15:109–111.
Ploufee L Jr: Disorders of excessive hair growth in the adolescent. *Obstet Gynecol Clin North Am* 2000;27:79–99.
Salmi DJ, Zisser HC, Jovanovic L: Screening for and treatment of polycystic ovary syndrome in teenagers. *Exp Biol Med* 2004;229:369–377.

Chapter 553 ■ Neoplasms and Abnormal Pap Smear Management

Joseph S. Sanfilippo

The most common gynecologic neoplasm found in children is of ovarian origin and usually presents as an abdominal mass. Ovarian neoplasms constitute 1% of all childhood malignancies, and 8% of all malignant and abdominal tumors in children are of ovarian origin (Chapter 503). Furthermore, 10–30% of the ovarian neoplasms operated on during childhood or adolescence are malignant. Paraovarian tumors are next in frequency, followed by uterine neoplasms. The vagina or vulva may also be the site of a benign or malignant lesion in children. Cervical dysplasia may occur in adolescents. Breast masses are discussed in Chapter 551.

Chemotherapy for any tumor, especially with alkylating agents (cyclophosphamide, busulphan, chlorambucil, and nitrogen mustard), is associated with germ cell damage in the postpubertal ovary. The prepubertal ovary, on the other hand, is markedly resistant to chemotherapeutic damage of germ cells. The effect of combined oral contraceptive therapy to protect the ovary during chemotherapy in adolescents remains controversial.

Survivors of childhood cancer who previously underwent abdominal or gonadal irradiation have an increased rate of spontaneous abortions. However, the incidence of congenital malformations is not increased in comparison with the general population. Patients who have evidence of premature ovarian failure may be candidates for assisted reproductive technology with the use of donor ova.

OVARIES

NEONATAL AND PEDIATRIC OVARIAN CYSTS. Most often the clinical manifestations of ovarian tumors are abdominal pain, mass, or both. Functional ovarian cysts rarely persist beyond the neonatal period. In adolescents, the most common neoplasm is the teratoma, which is usually benign; malignant teratomas may occur. Calcification on an abdominal radiograph is often a hallmark of a benign teratoma. During surgery, the opposite ovary should be evaluated, and if there is any question about the possibility of a neoplasm, a biopsy specimen should be obtained. Ovarian adenomas are the second most common benign tumor.

Ovarian cancers are extremely uncommon in children, responsible for 1 : 500 ovarian malignancies (Table 553-1). Ovarian cancers affect 4% of women. Germ cell tumors are the most common. Primordial germ cells can develop into dysgerminoma, malignant teratomas, endodermal sinus tumors, embryonal carcinomas, mixed cell neoplasms, and gonadoblastomas. Immature teratomas and endodermal sinus tumors are more aggressive malignancies than dysgerminomas and occur in a significantly higher proportion of younger girls (<10 yr of age). In this age group, 10-yr survival rates were reported as 73% for epithelial carcinomas, 44% for sex cord stromal tumors, 73% for dysgerminomas, 33% for malignant teratomas, 39% for endodermal sinus tumors, 25% for embryonal carcinomas, 30% for other germ cell neoplasms, and 100% for gonadoblastomas. Dysgerminomas usually are associated with XY gonadal dysgenesis; Y-DNA probes are important in their diagnosis. Tumor markers such as α-fetoprotein (AFP), carcinoembryonic antigen, and the antigen CA 125 are also used to assess ovarian malignancy (Tables 553-1 and 553-2). The germ cell tumors are associated with positive AFP, human chorionic gonadotropin (HCG), and chorioembryonic antigen.

Treatment consists of surgical excision followed by postoperative chemotherapy; radiotherapy is often necessary. Staging at the beginning of therapy is of the utmost importance. In many cases, a second-look procedure is indicated in order to decide about subsequent treatment of these neoplasms.

EMBRYONAL CARCINOMA. This cancer accounts for 6% of pediatric ovarian neoplasms and 8% of all germ cell tumors. The patient presents with progressive increase in abdominal pain and distention. The embryonal cell carcinoma is highly malignant with an average age of detection between 13 and 15 yr. Overall, 60% of patients have endocrinologic signs and symptoms, which may include precocious pseudopuberty, abnormal vaginal bleeding, and hirsutism. Both HCG and AFP are produced by embryonal cell carcinoma. Treatment involves unilateral salpingo-oophorectomy for stage I disease.

TABLE 553-1. Malignant Ovarian Tumors in Adolescents

GERM CELL (MOST COMMON)
Dysgerminoma
Immature teratoma
Endodermal sinus tumor
Choriocarcinoma
Embryonal carcinoma
SEX CORD STROMAL TUMORS
Granulosa stroma cell tumor
Sertoli-Leydig cell tumor
Lipoid cell tumor
Gynandroblastoma
EPITHELIAL TUMORS

TABLE 553-2. Serum Tumor Markers

MARKER	ASSOCIATED TUMOR
CA 125	Epithelial tumors (especially serous)
	Immature teratoma (rare)
α-Fetoprotein	Endodermal sinus tumors
	Embryonal carcinomas
	Mixed germ cell tumors
	Immature teratoma (rare)
	Polyembryoma (rare)
Human chorionic gonadotropins	Choriocarcinoma
	Embryonal carcinomas
	Mixed germ cell tumors
	Polyembryoma
	Dysgerminoma (rare)
Lactate dehydrogenase	Dysgerminoma
	Mixed germ cell tumors
Estradiol	Thecomas
	Adult granulosa cell tumors
Testosterone	Sertoli cell tumors
	Leydig (hilus) cell tumors
F9 embryoglycan	Embryonal carcinoma
	Yolk sac tumor
	Choriocarcinoma
	Immature teratoma
Inhibin	Granulosa—theca cell tumor
Müllerian-inhibiting substance	Granulosa—theca cell tumor

ENDODERMAL SINUS TUMOR. These tumors are the most lethal of all ovarian cancers. The median age at presentation is 19 yr. The endodermal sinus tumor produces AFP as a useful tumor marker. These tumors are radiosensitive. They may be treated surgically if they are stage I, for which a unilateral salpingo-oophorectomy is performed. Chemotherapy may be necessary independent of the stage of the disease.

CHORIOCARCINOMA. Primary choriocarcinoma of the ovary is extremely rare and often fatal; 0.6% of germ cell tumors are choriocarcinomas.

MIXED GERM CELL TUMOR. The frequency of mixed germ cell tumors is 4% of all ovarian neoplasms in children.

SEX CORD STROMAL TUMOR. Sex cord stromal tumors comprise 5% of ovarian neoplasms, of which the granulosa cell tumor is the most common. Isosexual precocity and occasionally virilization may be observed in the juvenile variety. The characteristic histologic features include nodular architecture, follicle formation, microcysts, cell necrosis, and increased mitotic activity.

SERTOLI-LEYDIG CELL TUMOR. This tumor is also termed a sex cord stromal tumor and accounts for 2% of pediatric ovarian tumors. Sertoli-Leydig cell tumors are rare in prepubertal girls. The patient presents with evidence of virilization. Treatment includes unilateral salpingo-oophorectomy for stage I disease.

OVARIAN FOLLICULAR CYSTS. These cysts occur from birth to puberty and usually disappear spontaneously. On ultrasound examination, the cyst presents as a nonechogenic area, frequently >20 mm at its greatest diameter; diffuse swelling of the ovarian parenchyma and follicular enlargement of the cortical zone are also noted.

POLYCYSTIC OVARIAN SYNDROME (PCOS). This syndrome presents with menstrual dysfunction and signs and symptoms of androgen excess often at the time of puberty. The menstrual irregularity can range from amenorrhea to oligomenorrhea (Chapter 552).

FUNCTIONAL AND HEMORRHAGIC OVARIAN CYSTS. These cysts are an integral part of follicular development during the menstrual cycle. On occasion, a cyst may persist and increase in diameter. Following ovulation, it is termed a corpus hemorrhagicum. These are often symptomatic and best evaluated by ultrasonography. Expectant management for a presumed functional cyst is appropriate, with follow-up ultrasound imaging. Monophasic oral contraceptives can facilitate suppression of functional cysts.

OVARIAN TORSION. Torsion of an adnexum is a complication that should always be considered in the differential diagnosis of ovarian tumors or abdominal pain in a female patient; prompt surgical intervention is necessary. Torsion often presents with intermittent sharp abdominal pain that, in many cases, radiates down the ipsilateral extremity. Bilateral ovarian torsion also may occur in infancy. When unilateral torsion is diagnosed, oophoropexy (plication) of the contralateral adnexa may be indicated.

The incidence of ovarian torsion in 1 series was 25% (16 of 63 benign ovarian masses). Color Doppler flow studies can facilitate the diagnosis. Adnexal torsion can often be evaluated and managed with the use of Doppler flow studies and laparoscopy. The underlying cause is usually an associated ovarian cyst or neoplasm. Recovery of ovarian function after laparoscopic detorsion has been reported with identification of normal follicle development on ultrasonography. Therefore, it is recommended that adnexal torsion be managed conservatively.

TABLE 553-3. Bethesda 2001 Classification of Pap Smears

SPECIMEN TYPE

Indicate conventional smear (Pap smear) vs liquid based vs other

SPECIMEN ADEQUACY

Satisfactory for evaluation (describe presence or absence of endocervical/transformation zone component and any other quality indicators, e.g., partially obscuring blood, inflammation)

Unsatisfactory for evaluation . . . (specify reason)

- Specimen rejected/not processed (specify reason)
- Specimen processed and examined, but unsatisfactory for evaluation of epithelial abnormality because of (specify reason)

GENERAL CATEGORIZATION (OPTIONAL)

Negative for intraepithelial lesion or malignancy

Epithelial cell abnormality: see Interpretation/Result (specify squamous or glandular as appropriate)

Other: see Interpretation/Result (e.g., endometrial cells in a woman 40 years of age and older)

AUTOMATED REVIEW

If case examined by automated device, specify device and result.

ANCILLARY TESTING

Provide a brief description of the test methods and report the result so that it is easily understood by the clinician.

INTERPRETATION/RESULT

Negative for intraepithelial lesion or malignancy (when there is no cellular evidence of neoplasia, state this in the General Categorization above and/or in the Interpretation/Result section of the report, whether or not there are organisms or other non-neoplastic findings)

Organisms

Trichomonas vaginalis

Fungal organisms morphologically consistent with *Candida* species

Shift in flora suggestive of bacterial vaginosis

Bacteria morphologically consistent with *Actinomyces* species

Cellular changes consistent with herpes simplex virus

Other Non-neoplastic Findings (Optional to report; list not inclusive)

Reactive cellular changes associated with

- Inflammation (includes typical repair)
- Radiation
- Intrauterine contraceptive device

Glandular cells status post-hysterectomy

Atrophy

OTHER

Endometrial cells (in a woman 40 years of age and older)

(Specify whether negative for squamous intraepithelial lesion)

EPITHELIAL CELL ABNORMALITIES

Squamous Cell

Atypical squamous cells

- Of undetermined significance (ASC-US)
- Cannot exclude high-grade squamous intraepithelial lesion (ASC-H)
- Low-grade squamous intraepithelial lesion encompassing human papillomavirus/mild dysplasia/cervical intraepithelial neoplasia 1
- High-grade squamous intraepithelial lesion encompassing moderate and severe dysplasia, CIS/cervical intraepithelial neoplasia 2 and cervical intraepithelial neoplasia 3
  - with features suspicious for invasion (if invasion is suspected)
- Squamous cell carcinoma

Glandular Cell

Atypical

- Endocervical cells (not otherwise specified or specify in comments)
- Endometrial cells (not otherwise specified or specify in comments)
- Glandular cells (not otherwise specified or specify in comments)

Atypical

- Endocervical cells, favor neoplastic
- Glandular cells, favor neoplastic

Endocervical adenocarcinoma in situ

Adenocarcinoma

- Endocervical
- Endometrial
- Extrauterine
- Not otherwise specified

OTHER MALIGNANT NEOPLASMS: (SPECIFY)

EDUCATIONAL NOTES AND SUGGESTIONS (OPTIONAL)

Suggestions should be concise and consistent with clinical follow-up guidelines published by professional organizations (references to relevant publications may be included)

From http://www.bethesda2001.cancer.gov/terminology.html.

CIS, carcinoma in situ.

AUTOAMPUTATION OF THE OVARY. This entity presents as a small, calcified, free-floating mass associated with absent adnexa. The child may be asymptomatic, and ultrasonography is often helpful in establishing the diagnosis. It has been hypothesized that antenatal or subclinical ovarian torsion leads to necrosis, calcification, and separation of the adnexa from its blood supply.

JUVENILE GRANULOSA CELL TUMORS OF THE OVARY (JGCT). JGCT account for 1–2% of all ovarian tumors. The median age at presentation is 7.6 yr, with a range of 6 mo to 17.5 yr. The majority of patients have abdominal distention and sexual precocity. Patients appear to have increasingly better prognosis with the advent of multidrug chemotherapy, including cisplatin-based regimens. However, neurotoxicity, especially ototoxicity, and bone marrow depression are serious complications.

PREMATURE OVARIAN FAILURE IN ASSOCIATION WITH CHEMOTHERAPY AND/OR RADIATION THERAPY. The incidence of premature ovarian failure has increased with the increased survival of children and adolescent patients having neoplasms. Hormone replacement therapy in an approach similar to that for menopause, i.e., physiologic estrogen replacement therapy with the addition of progestins, provides the patient with secondary sex characteristics as well as regular menses.

CERVIX

The prevalence of dysplasia and carcinoma in situ is 18.8/1,000 for those 15–19 yr of age, and biopsy-proven cases of all grades of cervical intraepithelial neoplasia (CIN) in the teenage population have a prevalence of 13.3/1,000. The Bethesda Classification System with the Pap smear is widely used for diagnosis (Table 553-3). The overall frequency of abnormal Pap smear results in the adolescent population is 3.8%, and 1% of all abnormal Pap smears are associated with CIN. Papillomavirus infection (Chapter 263) and altered vaginal flora are consistent findings in patients with CIN. Abnormal Pap smear results in adolescents also correlate with significant CIN and should be followed with low-grade lesion (Fig. 553-1). When there is a more advanced lesion (high-grade squamous intraepithelial lesion [ASC-H]), this patient should be referred for further evaluation. Human papillomavirus vaccine appears to lower the incidence of CIN. Other pathologic abnormalities of the cervix include cervical polyps and mixed mesodermal tumors. The latter may represent a mixed, heterologous, or homologous sarcoma of the uterine cervix.

UTERUS (BENIGN AND MALIGNANT TUMORS OF THE UTERINE CORPUS)

Adenocarcinoma of the corpus is rare in children and adolescents. Vaginal bleeding not associated with sexual precocity is a frequent presenting sign. Treatment consists of hysterectomy, with removal of the ovaries, followed by adjunctive radiotherapy or chemotherapy or both, depending on the operative findings. Mixed mesodermal tumors and leiomyomas of the uterus should be included in the differential diagnosis of a pelvic mass in an adolescent. Leiomyosarcoma, although extremely rare, has also been noted in an adolescent; the presentation is variable, but abnormal vaginal bleeding usually is present.

VAGINA

A Gartner duct (mesonephric) cyst is a common vaginal wall abnormality. It usually is an incidental finding and requires no specific therapy. In sexually active patients, excision may be necessary if there is associated dyspareunia. Paramesonephric (müllerian) duct cysts often become symptomatic at menarche when the cavity fills with menstrual blood.

Sarcoma botryoides, a vaginal carcinoma that occurs primarily in pediatric patients, is best treated by surgical excision. Chemotherapy is usually administered postoperatively. Any questionable vulvar lesion should be submitted for histologic examination. Liposarcoma of the vulva has been reported in a 15 yr old girl. Malignant melanoma of the vulva has also been described in a 14 yr old patient.

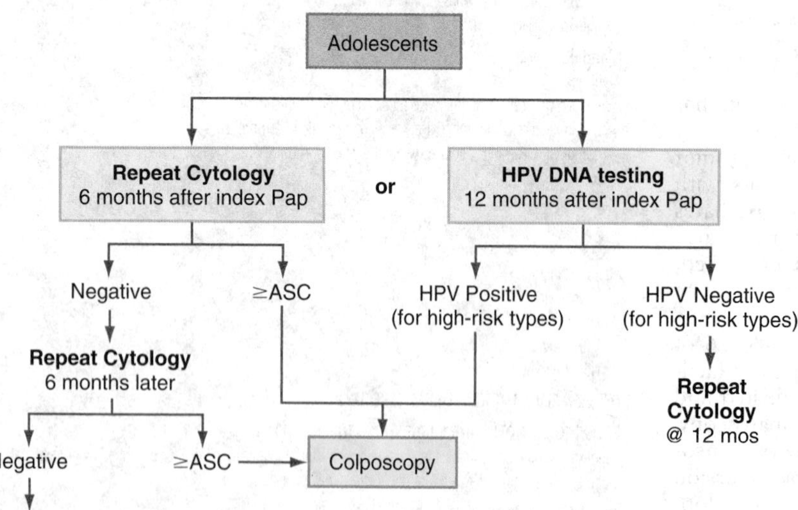

Figure 553-1. Management of a low-grade squamous intraepithelial lesion in the adolescent patient. Due to the high rate of human papillomavirus (HPV) in the adolescent population and the lack of cervical cancer screening, colposcopy may be delayed. A repeat Pap test conducted 6 mo after the initial Pap test or an HPV test alone 12 mo after the incident Pap test are acceptable alternatives to colposcopy. If the result is normal for 2 subsequent Pap tests, the adolescent may return to annual screening. It should be noted that the HPV test performed at 12 mo is conducted without a Pap test. The addition of a Pap test does not increase the sensitivity of detecting a high-grade lesion, but increases the number of patients who require colposcopy. The delay in obtaining the HPV test for 12 mo is designed to allow enough time for the resolution of infection. (From Guido R. Guidelines for screening and treatment of cervical disease in the adolescent. *J Pediatr Adolesc Gynecol* 2004;17:303–311. © 2004 The North American Society for Pediatric & Adolescent Gynecology.)

Calaminus G, Wessalowski R, Harms D, et al: Juvenile granulosa cell-tumors of the ovary in children and adolescents: Results from 33 patients registered in a prospective cooperative study. *Gynecol Oncol* 1997;64:447–452.
Falcone T, Bedaiwy MA: Fertility preservation and pregnancy outcome after malignancy. *Curr Opin Obstet Gynecol* 2005;17:21–26.
Fields KR, Neinstein LS: Uterine myomas in adolescents: Case reports and a review of the literature. *J Pediatr Adolesc Gynecol* 1996;9:195–198.
Guido R: Guidelines for screening and treatment of cervical disease in the adolescent. *J Pediatr Adolesc Gynecol* 2004;17:301–311.
Guido R, Schiffman M, Solomon D, et al, ASCUS LSIL Triage Study (ALTS) Group: Postcolposcopy management strategies for women referred with low-grade squamous intraepithelial lesions or human papillomavirus DNA-positive atypical squamous cells of undetermined significance: A two-year prospective study. *Am J Obstet Gynecol* 2003;188:1401–1405.
Kozlowski K: Ovarian masses. *Adolesc Med* 1999;10:337–350, vii.
Owens K, Honebrink A: Gynecologic care of medically complicated adolescents. *Pediatr Clin North Am* 1999;46:631–642, ix.
Ozcan C, Celik A, Ozok G, et al: Adnexal torsion in children may have a catastrophic sequel: Asynchronous bilateral torsion. *J Pediatr Surg* 2002;37:1617–1620.
Parker-Jones K: Gynecologic issues in pediatric oncology. Clin Obstet Gynecol 1997;40:200–209.
Pienkowski C, Baunin C, Gayrard M, et al: Ovarian masses in adolescent girls. *Endocr Dev* 2004;7:163–182.
Piippo S, Mustaniemi L, Lenko H, et al: Surgery for ovarian masses during childhood and adolescence: A report of 79 cases. *J Pediatr Adolesc Gynecol* 1999;12:223–227.
Pomeranz A, Sabnis S: Misdiagnosis of ovarian masses in children and adolescents. *Pediatr Emerg Care* 2004;20:172–174.

Chapter 554 ■ Vulvovaginal and Müllerian Anomalies

Joseph S. Sanfilippo

EMBRYOLOGY. The uterus is formed by fusion of the caudal elements of the müllerian ducts, a process that occurs at 8 wk of gestation. The fusion begins from the caudal end (Müller tubercle) and is completed at the upper level of the fundus. A median septum is present until the end of the 1st trimester of gestation.

The vagina is formed from the terminal portion of the uterovaginal canal (Müller tubercle). The tissue is of combined urogenital and müllerian duct origin and is known as the vaginal epithelial plate. Bilateral evaginations of the vaginal epithelial plate encircle the caudal aspect and form the uterine canal. Canalization of the vaginal plate occurs and proceeds in a caudal direction to form the vagina. The process elongates the vaginal structure, leaving the cranial ⅔ of müllerian origin and the caudal ⅓ of urogenital origin.

The paramesonephric system is responsible for müllerian tract development. Failure of lateral fusion or lack of resorption of the vertical midline septum results in a müllerian anomaly. Because of the intimate anatomic and embryologic development of the urinary and genital systems, the urinary tract is often also affected; skeletal defects, including spina bifida occulta, occur as well. Common müllerian duct anomalies and associated heritable disorders are presented in Tables 554-1 and 554-2.

TABLE 554-1. Common Müllerian Anomalies

Hydrocolpos	Accumulation of mucus or nonsanguineous fluid in the vagina
Hemihematometra	Atretic segment of vagina with menstrual fluid accumulation
Hydrosalpinx	Accumulation of serous fluid in the fallopian tube, often an end result of pyosalpinx
Didelphic uterus	Two cervices, each associated with one uterine horn
Bicornuate uterus	One cervix associated with two uterine horns
Unicornuate uterus	Result of failure of one müllerian duct to descend

IMPERFORATE HYMEN. The patient presents with primary amenorrhea; secondary sex characteristics are normal. The imperforate hymen requires surgical intervention. The outflow tract obstruction when relieved should include evaluation of the vaginal canal for any other defects.

CONGENITAL ABSENCE OF THE VAGINA (MAYER-ROKITANSKY-KÜSTER-HAUSER SYNDROME). The incidence is reported as 1/4,000 to 1/5,000 births. The cause is unknown. Vaginal agenesis is characterized by primary amenorrhea, normal vulva, anomalies of the uterus, attenuated fallopian tubes, normal ovaries, normal female karyotype and phenotype, and associated anomalies (most frequently renal and skeletal). The anomaly is often discovered in adolescence. Absence of the vagina has significant anatomic, physiologic, and psychologic implications for the patient and family.

Treatment is usually delayed until the patient is ready to be sexually active. The nonsurgical approach includes use of dilators to create a functional vagina. The series of dilators come in progressively increasing sizes and require a commitment on the part of the patient to comply with daily use. When the ultimate size that accommodates coitus is reached, then the patient must use the dilator daily or have coitus with a frequency so as to maintain adequate length. There is also a combined laparoscopic vulvar procedure (laparoscopic vaginoplasty) in which an olive-tip with suture attached is placed at the introital area and sutures are brought up through the space of Retzius. Progressive increase in tension of the sutures brought through a device placed on the abdomen to “tighten” the sutures results in development of a functional vagina. In a series of 52 patients with vaginal agenesis, this laparoscopic vaginoplasty resulted in a 98% “functional success.” Alternatively, surgical intervention with a McIndoe procedure involving a split-thickness skin graft placed in the vagina area has proved to be a successful approach.

Lesions involving other organ systems occur in association with the Mayer-Rokitansky-Küster-Hauser syndrome. The most common are urinary tract anomalies primarily involving unilateral absence of a kidney or a ureter (27%) and skeletal anomalies (12%), which primarily involve vertebral development.

INCOMPLETE VERTICAL FUSION OF THE VAGINA. Transverse and longitudinal vaginal septa represent failure of complete canalization of the vagina. Not uncommonly, the patient presents with amenorrhea and cyclical pain, which is a result of cryptomenorrhea. Müllerian agenesis must be differentiated from androgen insensitivity (testicular feminization); serum testosterone levels are usually in the male range with the latter. Müllerian agenesis, with a reported incidence of 1/50,000 to 1/20,000, is more

TABLE 554-2. Heritable Disorders Associated with Müllerian Anomalies

MODE OF INHERITANCE	DISORDER	ASSOCIATED MÜLLERIAN DEFECT
Autosomal dominant	Camptobrachydactyly	Longitudinal vaginal septa
	Hand-foot-genital	Incomplete müllerian fusion
Autosomal recessive	Kaufan-McCusick	Transverse vaginal septa
	Johanson-Blizzard	Longitudinal vaginal septa
	Renal-genital-middle ear anomalies	Vaginal atresia
	Fraser syndrome	Incomplete müllerian fusion
	Uterine hernia syndrome	Persistent müllerian duct derivatives
Polygenic/multifactorial	Mayer-Rokitansky-Küster-Hauser syndrome	Müllerian aplasia
X linked	Uterine hernia syndrome	Persistent müllerian duct derivatives

From Shulman L, Elias S: Developmental abnormalities of the female reproductive tract: Pathogenesis and nosology. *Adolesc Pediatr Gynecol* 1988;1:232.

common than androgen insensitivity and is second in frequency to gonadal dysgenesis as a cause of primary amenorrhea.

Renal anomalies are noted in 34% and skeletal anomalies in 12% of patients with müllerian anomalies. Unilateral renal agenesis occurs in 15% of patients. The most frequent skeletal anomalies are vertebral. Klippel-Feil syndrome has been associated with müllerian agenesis. Patients usually have a normal female karyotype (46 XX), but autosomal translocation of chromosomes 12q and 14q also occurs. Affected siblings have been reported, as well as families with variable expression of defects in müllerian, renal, and skeletal systems.

A pelvic ultrasound examination is helpful in defining the anomaly; CT and MRI provide increased detail. Laparoscopy is usually reserved for evaluating a pelvic mass and associated abnormalities. Radiologic or sonographic evaluation is indicated to identify associated anomalies. A karyotype should be obtained.

Vaginoplasty is best deferred until a patient has matured and should be supported by counseling for both patient and family. The McIndoe procedure involves the use of a skin graft, usually from the buttocks, to create a vagina after appropriate dissection of the vulvovaginal area. The artificial vaginal epithelium changes cytologically to an almost normal-appearing vaginal mucosa. Other reconstructive procedures have included fasciocutaneous flaps. Various dilatation procedures may also result in an increased vaginal size, which ultimately permits intercourse. Squamous cell carcinoma of the reconstructed vagina has been reported and appears to be related to the type of tissue transplanted. Radiotherapy is usually the primary method of treatment for this squamous cell carcinoma.

TRANSVERSE VAGINAL SEPTA. The incidence of this lesion is approximately 1/80,000 females. The patient usually presents with amenorrhea, which may be associated with cyclic pelvic pain, a pelvic mass, and cryptomenorrhea. Although usually asymptomatic until puberty, hydrometrocolpos may occur in children. Transverse vaginal septa may be associated with other congenital anomalies, although this occurs less often than with müllerian agenesis. The most common site of the septum is between the middle and upper thirds of the vagina. These patients have a functional uterus, although their fertility is often compromised; 47% of affected females in 1 retrospective series had spontaneous abortions. The prognosis is worse for higher obstructions. There is also an increased incidence of endometriosis secondary to retrograde menstruation.

Evaluation of transverse vaginal septa includes careful pelvic examination and often pelvic imaging to delineate the anatomic abnormalities. **Treatment** is surgical resection of the obstruction from below. Anastomosis of the upper and lower segments should be attempted, if at all possible, to prevent stenosis. A skin graft may be necessary. A Lucite stent is often placed in the vagina to maintain patency.

DISORDERS OF LATERAL FUSION. These include a number of anatomic variations of nonobstructive longitudinal septum as well as the obstructed hemivagina. The latter may be associated with a didelphic uterus and often with a pelvic mass, which represents retrograde menstruation associated with the occluded hemivagina. Menses, often cyclic, indicates an unobstructed outflow tract from one of the uterine horns.

UTERINE ABNORMALITIES. The incidence of uterine anomalies ranges from 1/100 to 1/1,000. Anomalous development of the uterine cavity may have varied clinical manifestations. Patients may present with primary amenorrhea or with irregular or even regular menses. There may be an asymptomatic pelvic mass or dysmenorrhea. In adolescents and adults, pregnancy wastage and infertility may cause the first suspicion of a uterine anomaly.

Diagnosis should include a pelvic ultrasound examination, renal tract assessment, and skeletal inspection for anomalies. Karyotyping and diagnostic laparoscopy may be necessary, depending on the presentation and laboratory assessment.

Treatment depends on the specific anomaly, and surgical repair to date has included hysteroscopic resection. Historically, a Strassman metroplasty, Jones "wedge" metroplasty, or Tompkins metroplasty have been advocated. The obstruction to the outflow tract must also be relieved; this may necessitate creation of a vaginal window or excision of a hemivagina. Retrograde menstruation in a uterine horn must also be evaluated, and, if present, appropriate surgical correction provided.

CONGENITAL ATRESIA OF THE UTERINE CERVIX. This extremely rare anomaly often presents at puberty with cryptomenorrhea, amenorrhea, and pelvic pain. It is associated with significant renal anomalies in 5–10% of patients. On examination, complete absence of a cervix but a palpable uterus is found. Pelvic imaging is helpful in defining the abnormality. A hysterectomy may be necessary. Other associated anomalies include mesonephric cysts, which are remnants of the wolffian duct, incomplete reduplication of internal genitalia (e.g., didelphic uterus), and unilateral renal aplasia. In addition, gastrointestinal (42.9%), respiratory (47.6%), central nervous system (28.6%), cardiovascular (38.1%), and musculoskeletal abnormalities (33.3%) have been reported with this abnormality.

COMPLETE VULVAR DUPLICATION. This rare congenital anomaly presents in infancy and consists of 2 vulvas, 2 vaginas, and 2 bladders, a didelphic uterus, a single rectum and anus, and 2 renal systems.

LABIAL HYPERTROPHY. Elongation of the labia minora may be present at birth. This usually is of no consequence, but surgical revision may be indicated if there are symptoms of discomfort or bulging is noted when wearing tight-fitting garments.

CLITORAL ABNORMALITIES. Agenesis of the clitoris is rare. Clitoral duplication has been reported, often associated with pelvic organ abnormalities, including agenesis of other genital tract structures and bladder exstrophy.

HYMENAL ABNORMALITIES. An imperforate hymen may be present in pediatric patients and is often associated with mucocolpos; hydrometrocolpos may also be noted. Other hymenal abnormalities include cribriform or stenotic hymen.

CLOACAL ANOMALIES. These lesions represent a common urogenital sinus into which both urethral and anal orifices exit. The single opening (cloaca) requires surgical correction.

MANAGEMENT OF EMERGENCIES ASSOCIATED WITH CONGENITAL MALFORMATIONS OF THE FEMALE GENITAL TRACT

The clinical manifestations of müllerian anomalies are varied. There may be a pelvic mass, which may or may not be associated with symptoms. A vaginal bulging mass or hemivagina is indicative of complete or partial outflow tract obstruction. An adolescent may present with pelvic pain, either in association with primary amenorrhea or several months after the onset of menarche. Patients also may be asymptomatic until there is evidence of repeat pregnancy wastage. When presentation is acutely symptomatic, emergency management may be required.

OUTFLOW TRACT OBSTRUCTION. Obstruction may result from a number of distinct anomalies including the imperforate hymen, transverse vaginal septum, and noncommunicating rudimentary horn. As menstrual fluid accumulates proximal to the obstruction, the resulting hematocolpos, hematometra, or hematocolpometra causes cyclic pain or a pelvic mass. These obstructions are best considered according to the location of the obstruction.

DISTAL VAGINA/IMPERFORATE HYMEN. This is the most common obstructive anomaly, and familial occurrences are reported. In the newborn period and early infancy, it may be diagnosed by a bulging membrane due to a mucocolpos from maternal estrogen stimulation. If not noted at this time, it is often not diagnosed until puberty, when menstrual fluid accumulates. The clinical manifestations often are a bulging blue-black membrane, pain, primary amenorrhea, and normal secondary sex characteristics. Depending on the circumstance, patients may have cyclic abdominal pain or a pelvic mass.

Treatment requires incision/resection of the membrane, thus relieving the outflow tract obstruction. Repair should be done at time of diagnosis, if the patient is symptomatic. Although the lesion may be repaired anytime during infancy, childhood, or adolescence, surgery is facilitated by estrogen stimulation and thus ideally performed in adolescence.

PROXIMAL OR MIDVAGINAL TRANSVERSE SEPTUM. Vertical fusion defects can result in a transverse septum, which may be imperforate and associated with hematocolpos or hematometra in adolescents, or mucocolpos in children. If there is a small, pinpoint aperture, fluid accumulates in the vagina. As with an imperforate hymen, a mass may be present. The vagina appears short or blind ended. The approach to resection of the septum depends on the presence or absence of an opening. In the presence of an opening, cannulation should be attempted with resection of the septum. Postoperatively, a vaginal stent may be necessary.

RUDIMENTARY HORNS. This emergency results from the presence of a horn with a functional endometrium and outflow tract obstruction. As with other types of outflow tract obstruction, severe lower abdominal pain with a pelvic mass is the primary clinical manifestation. In contrast to other forms of outflow tract obstruction, however, primary amenorrhea is usually not present because the opposite horn is unlikely to be obstructed. Asymptomatic rupture of a rudimentary horn in an adult has been reported.

Ultrasonography is indicated for visualizing the rudimentary horn. An intravenous pyelogram or renal ultrasonogram also should be obtained because of associated anomalies. If there is evidence of a functional endometrium, surgical extirpation is recommended.

RUDIMENTARY HORN PREGNANCY. This occurs in 1/40,000 pregnancies and 1/5,000 to 15,000 ectopic pregnancies. It may be a result of a fibromuscular or fibrous band connecting the unicornuate uterus and the rudimentary horn, but 80–85% of cases are noncommunicating. The latter is probably the result of transperitoneal migration of either sperm or the fertilized ovum. In contrast to tubal pregnancies, rudimentary horn pregnancies are often not detected until the second trimester. Because of the greater muscle wall thickness of most horns, rupture typically occurs later than in tubal gestation.

Most cases are diagnosed only after rupture occurs, when patients have acute abdominal pain and peritoneal signs and are often in shock. When rupture occurs, intraperitoneal hemorrhage may be massive and life threatening and requires immediate surgical intervention. Maternal mortality is about 5%, with 90% of this occurring within 10–15 min after rupture. Fetal demise occurs in 98%.

Before rupture, diagnosis of a rudimentary horn pregnancy may be difficult. It should be suspected in any gravida with a known rudimentary horn, and these patients should be closely monitored until an intrauterine pregnancy has been documented. In those who have not been previously identified as having a rudimentary horn, findings on early pelvic examination are similar to findings of tubal ectopic pregnancy and include deviation of the cervix to one side with an adnexal mass on the opposite side. Ultrasound findings before rupture include an extrauterine gestational sac and a placenta within the horn next to a slightly enlarged uterus.

Treatment consists of surgical resection of the rudimentary horn.

ACUTE URINARY RETENTION. Outflow tract obstruction resulting in accumulation of fluid in the vagina or uterus may cause urinary retention as a result of mucocolpos in the first years of life or hematocolpos, hematometra, or hematocolpometra during the pubertal years. The retained fluid in the vagina compresses the urethra, and this is aggravated when the fluid-filled uterus applies pressure on the posterior wall of the bladder and changes the angle of the urethra. Pressure on the sacral plexus from the distended vagina may also be contributory.

The usual clinical manifestations in adolescents are lower abdominal pain and the inability to void. There also may be hesitancy and incomplete voiding for several days before presentation. Adolescents generally have primary amenorrhea, a history of cyclic lower abdominal pain, and a pelvic mass. However, if the obstruction is unilateral, as with a noncommunicating rudimentary horn or an obstructed hemivagina, the patient may have normal menses.

Temporary but immediate relief can be provided by urethral catheterization. If resistance occurs within an appropriately sized rubber catheter, a pediatric feeding tube may be used, or, if necessary, a spinal needle may be passed suprapubically to empty the bladder. Urine should be sent for urinalysis and culture because urinary stasis promotes infection. Once the acute condition has been treated, the underlying problems and the obstructing mass should be appropriately evaluated. Urinary tract infections also have been associated with müllerian anomalies. This may result from renal anomalies with vesicourethral reflux or may precede retention as a result of vaginal outflow obstruction. Antibiotic treatment is indicated.

ACUTE GENITAL TRAUMA IN THE PREMENARCHAL GIRL. Acute genital trauma in children can present as superficial genital lacerations and abrasions that do not have active bleeding and may be merely observed. Active bleeding following trauma in the genital area merits appropriate evaluation, which usually includes examination under anesthesia with surgical repair. Forensic studies may be indicated if there is any suspicion of sexual abuse. Application of topical estrogen cream appears to facilitate the healing process in the vulvovaginal area, and clinicians should consider this following surgical intervention.

American College of Obstetrics and Gynecology. Nonsurgical diagnosis and management of vaginal agenesis. *Int J Gynaecol Obstet* 2002;79:167–170.

Folch M, Pigem I, Konge J: Müllerian agenesis: Etiology, diagnosis and management. *Obstet Gynecol Surv* 2000;55:644–649.

Gell J: Mullerian anomalies. *Semin Reprod Med* 2003;21:375–388.

Lin P, Bhatnagar K, Nettleton G, et al: Female genital anomalies affecting reproduction. *Fertil Steril* 2002;78:899–915.

Merit D: Evaluating and managing acute genital trauma pre-menarche girls. *J Pediatr Adolesc Gynecol* 1999;12:237–238.

Nagele F, Langle R, Stolzlechner J, et al: Noncommunicating rudimentary horn-obstetric and gynecologic implications. *Acta Obstet Gynecol Scand* 1995;74:566–568.

Porcu E: Imaging in pediatric and adolescent gynecology. *Endocr Dev* 2004;7:9–22.

Scarsbrook AF, Moore NR: MRI appearances of mullerian duct abnormalities. *Clin Radiol* 2003;58:747–754.

Siegel MJ: Magnetic resonance imaging of the adolescent female pelvis. *Magn Reson Imaging Clin N Am* 2002;10:303–324.

Stallion A: Vaginal obstruction. *Semin Pediatr Surg* 2000;9:128–134.

Troiano RN, McCarthy SM: Mullerian duct anomalies: Imaging and clinical issues. *Radiology* 2004;233:19–34.

Yamada G, Satoh Y, Baskin LS, et al: Cellular and molecular mechanisms of development of the external genitalia. *Differentiation* 2003;71:445–460.

Yu TJ, Lin MC: Acute urinary retention in two patients with imperforate hymen. *Scand J Urol Nephrol* 1993;27:543–544.

Chapter 555 ■ Special Gynecologic Needs Joseph S. Sanfilippo

MENTALLY HANDICAPPED CHILDREN. Mentally delayed children face several gynecologic issues including varying levels of understanding of reproduction, sexuality, and contraception. Counseling programs specifically addressing this issue have been demonstrated to be of help, especially for those living in the community. Perineal hygiene is also of concern. Young women with severe mental retardation are often not able to be trained by their mothers to handle personal hygiene during menstruation; the majority of higher functioning women are eventually able to be trained, particularly those who had been toilet trained. Cyclical behavioral changes (crying, self-abusive behavior, and tantrums) prior to menstruation are common. The changes are presumed to result from pain or cramps as 65% of the patients responded to nonsteroidal anti-inflammatory drugs (NSAIDs). If treatment with NSAIDs is unsuccessful, birth control pills and depo-medroxyprogesterone acetate improved behavior in 40–66% of patients. Selective serotonin reuptake inhibitors have also been effective.

Sexual abuse is a major concern; as many as 25% of mentally impaired women have been sexually assaulted.

A number of medical approaches can be considered to suppress menses. Depo-medroxyprogesterone acetate, usually prescribed at a dose of 150 mg, may be administered every 3 mo. Alternatively, oral contraceptives or the contraceptive patch do not produce amenorrhea but result in a decrease in the menstrual flow. Thorough discussion with parents or custodians and, ideally, consultation with an ethics advisory committee should be undertaken prior to any decision-making about sterilizing mentally handicapped patients. The parents of children with profound developmental disability may elect sterilization plus high-dose estrogen therapy (before the onset of puberty) to attenuate the child's growth.

Chamberlain A, Rauth J, Passer A, et al: Issues in fertility control for mentally retarded female adolescents: 1. Sexual activity, sexual abuse, and contraception. *Pediatrics* 1984;73:445–450.

Elkins TE, Gafford LS, Wilks CS, et al: A model clinic approach to the reproductive health concerns of the mentally handicapped. *Obstet Gynecol* 1986;68:185–188.

Elkins TE, Kope S, Ghaziuddin M, et al: Integration of a sexuality counseling service into a reproductive health program for persons with mental retardation. *J Pediatr Adolesc Gynecol* 1997;10:24–27.

Gunther DF, Dickema DS: Attenuating growth in children with profound developmental disability. *Arch Pediatr Adolesc Med* 2006;160:1013–1017.

Owens K, Honebrink A: Gynecologic care of mentally complicated adolescents. *Pediatr Clin North Am* 1999;46:631–642, ix.

Paransky OI, Zurawin RK: Management of menstrual problems and contraception in adolescents with mental retardation: A medical, legal, and ethical review with new suggested guidelines. *J Pediatr Adolesc Gynecol* 2003;16:223–235.

Quint EH, Elkins TE, Sorg CA, et al: The treatment of cyclical behavioral changes in women with mental disabilities. *J Pediatr Adolesc Gynecol* 1999;12:139–142.

Tharinger D, Horton CB, Millea S: Sexual abuse and exploitation of children and adults with mental retardation and other handicaps. *Child Abuse Negl* 1999;14:301–312.

Chapter 556 ■ Gynecologic Imaging Joseph S. Sanfilippo

A transabdominal ultrasonic approach is most feasible in the pediatric and adolescent patient. A distended bladder serves as an imaging window and facilitates identification of the uterus and the ovaries; bladder distention with urine displaces gas-filled bowel loops out of the pelvis and enhances imaging. A 7.5 or 5.0 MHz transducer is usually used, especially with larger children and teenagers. Ultrasonography is a key screening tool, enabling appropriate diagnosis in patients presenting with ambiguous genitalia, ovarian or uterine masses, primary amenorrhea, and abdominal or pelvic pain (Table 556-1).

TABLE 556-1. Normal Ovarian and Uterine Dimensions

OVARY
Birth
15 mm long, 3 mm wide, 2.5 mm thick
Ovarian volume 0.7 cm^3*
Postpuberty
22.5–50.0 mm in length
1.5–3.0 cm in width; 0.6–1.5 cm in thickness
Ovarian volume 1.8–5.7 cm^3*
UTERUS
Neonate
Length 2.3–4.6 cm
Anteroposterior diameter 0.8–2.2 cm
Infant to 7 yr of age
Length 2.5–3.3 cm
Anteroposterior diameter 0.4–1.0 cm
Postpuberty
Length 6 cm

* Ovarian volume can be determined by using the formula: length × height × width = 0.523.

From Sanfilippo JS, Lavery JP: The spectrum of ultrasound: Antenatal to adolescent years. *Semin Reprod Endocrinol* 1988;6:45–53.

Pelvic masses can be identified at any age. Ovarian cysts and hydrocolpos or hydrometrocolpos are the most common abnormalities noted in neonates. Hydrocolpos is defined as dilatation of the vagina, which usually is associated with accumulation of serous fluid or urine (if there is a urogenital sinus). Hydrometrocolpos causes dilatation of both the uterus and the vagina. It may also be associated with vaginal or cervical atresia, stenosis, or an imperforate hymen. Most large ovarian cysts (simple cystic) in children may be safely observed with serial pelvic ultrasonography and tend to decrease in size or completely resolve. A solid mass requires a tissue diagnosis.

MRI is useful in evaluating müllerian duct anomalies. It should be used in conjunction with ultrasound assessment and, if necessary, such techniques as genitography. Three-dimensional ultrasonographic and Doppler assessment have been used with ovarian abnormalities. The three-dimensional Doppler studies more clearly differentiate benign from malignant ovarian lesions and reduce the false-positive findings with ultrasonography.

Kurjak A, Jupesic S, Sparac V, et al: Three-dimensional ultrasonographic and power Doppler characterization of ovarian lesions. *Ultrasound Obstet Gynecol* 2000;16:365–371.

Lang IM, Babyn P, Oliver GD: MR imaging of pediatric uterovaginal anomalies. *Pediatr Radiol* 1999;29:163–170.

Porcu E: Imaging in pediatric and adolescent gynecology. *Endocr Dev* 2004;7:9–22.

Siegel MJ: Magnetic resonance imaging of the adolescent female pelvis. *Magn Reson Imaging Clin N Am* 2002;10:303–324, vi.

Warner BW, Kuhn JC, Barr LL: Conservative management of large ovarian cysts in children: The value of serial pelvic ultrasonography. *Surgery* 1992;112:749–755.

Part XXV ▪ The Endocrine System

Section 1 — Disorders of the Hypothalamus and Pituitary Gland

Chapter 557 ▪ Hormones of the Hypothalamus and Pituitary

John S. Parks and Eric I. Felner

PITUITARY: THE MASTER GLAND

The pituitary gland is the major regulator of an elaborate hormonal system. The pituitary gland receives signals from the hypothalamus and responds by sending pituitary hormones to target glands. The target glands produce hormones that provide negative feedback at the level of the hypothalamus and pituitary. This feedback mechanism enables the pituitary to regulate the amount of hormone released into the bloodstream by the target glands. The pituitary's central role in this hormonal system and its ability to interpret and respond to a variety of signals have led to its designation as the "master gland."

ANATOMY OF THE PITUITARY. The pituitary gland is located at the base of the skull in a saddle-shaped cavity of the sphenoid bone: the sella turcica. The bony structure protects and surrounds the pituitary bilaterally and inferiorly. The dura, a dense layer of connective tissue, forms the roof of the sella. An external layer of the dura continues into the sella to form its lining. The pituitary is extradural and is not normally in contact with cerebrospinal fluid. The pituitary gland is connected to the hypothalamus by the pituitary stalk. The pituitary gland is composed of an anterior (**adenohypophysis**) and a posterior (**neurohypophysis**) lobe. The anterior lobe constitutes about 80% of the gland.

EMBRYOLOGY OF THE PITUITARY. The anterior pituitary gland originates from the Rathke pouch as an invagination of the oral ectoderm (Fig. 557–1). It then detaches from the oral epithelium and becomes an individual structure of rapidly proliferating cells. By 6 wk gestation, the connection between the Rathke pouch and the oropharynx is completely obliterated and the pouch establishes a direct connection with the downward extension of the hypothalamus, which gives rise to the pituitary stalk. Persistent remnants of the original connection between the Rathke pouch and the oral cavity can develop into **craniopharyngiomas**, the most common type of tumor in this area.

VASCULAR SUPPLY OF THE PITUITARY. The arterial blood supply of the pituitary gland originates from the internal carotid via the inferior, middle, and superior hypophyseal arteries. This network of vessels forms a unique portal circulation connecting the hypothalamus and pituitary. The branches of the superior hypophyseal arteries penetrate the stalk and form a network of vessels that traverse the pituitary stalk and terminate in a network of capillaries within the anterior lobe. It is through this portal venous system that hypothalamic hormones are delivered to the anterior pituitary gland. Anterior pituitary hormones, in turn, are secreted into a secondary plexus of portal veins that drain into the dural venous sinuses.

ANTERIOR PITUITARY CELL TYPES. A series of sequentially expressed transcriptional activation factors directs the differentiation and proliferation of anterior pituitary cell types (Fig. 557-1). These proteins are members of a large family of DNA-binding proteins resembling **homeobox genes.** The consequences of mutations in several of these genes are evident in human forms of multiple pituitary hormone deficiency. Five cell types in the anterior pituitary produce 6 peptide hormones. Somatotropes produce growth hormone (GH); lactotropes produce prolactin (PRL); thyrotropes make thyroid-stimulating hormone (TSH); corticotropes express pro-opiomelanocortin (POMC), the precursor of adrenocorticotropic hormone (ACTH); and gonadotropes express both luteinizing hormone (LH) and follicle-stimulating hormone (FSH).

Growth Hormone. Human GH is a 191-amino-acid single-chain polypeptide that is synthesized, stored, and secreted by somatotropes in the pituitary. Its gene *(GH1)* is the first in a cluster of 5 closely related genes on the long arm of chromosome 17 (q22-24). The 4 other genes *(CS1, CS2, GH2, CSP)* have greater than 90% sequence identity with *GH1.*

GH is secreted in a pulsatile fashion under the regulation of hypothalamic hormones. The alternating secretion of growth hormone–releasing hormone (GHRH), which stimulates GH release, and somatostatin, which inhibits GH release, accounts for the rhythmic secretion of GH. Peaks of GH occur when peaks of GHRH coincide with troughs of somatostatin. Ghrelin, a peptide produced in the arcuate nucleus of the hypothalamus and in much greater quantities by the stomach, also stimulates GH secretion. Physiologic factors also have a role in the stimulation and inhibition of GH. Sleep, exercise, physical stress, trauma, acute illness, puberty, fasting, and hypoglycemia stimulate the release of GH, whereas hyperglycemia, hypothyroidism, and glucocorticoids inhibit GH release.

GH binds to receptor molecules on the surface of target cells. The GH receptor is a 620-amino-acid single-chain molecule with an extracellular domain, a single membrane-spanning domain, and a cytoplasmic domain. Proteolytically cleaved fragments of the extracellular domain circulate in plasma and act as a GH-binding protein. The cytoplasmic domain of the GH receptor lacks intrinsic kinase activity; instead, GH binding induces receptor dimerization and activation of a receptor-associated Janus kinase (Jak2). Phosphorylation of the kinase and other protein substrates initiates a series of events that leads to alterations in nuclear gene transcription. The signal transducer and activator of transcription 5b(STAT5b) plays a critical role in linking receptor activation to changes in gene transcription.

The biologic effects of GH include increases in linear growth, bone thickness, soft tissue growth, protein synthesis, fatty acid release from adipose tissue, insulin resistance, and blood glucose levels. The mitogenic actions of GH are mediated through increases in the synthesis of insulin-like growth factor-I (IGF-I), formerly named somatomedin C, a 70-amino-acid single-chain peptide coded for by a gene on the long arm of chromosome 12.

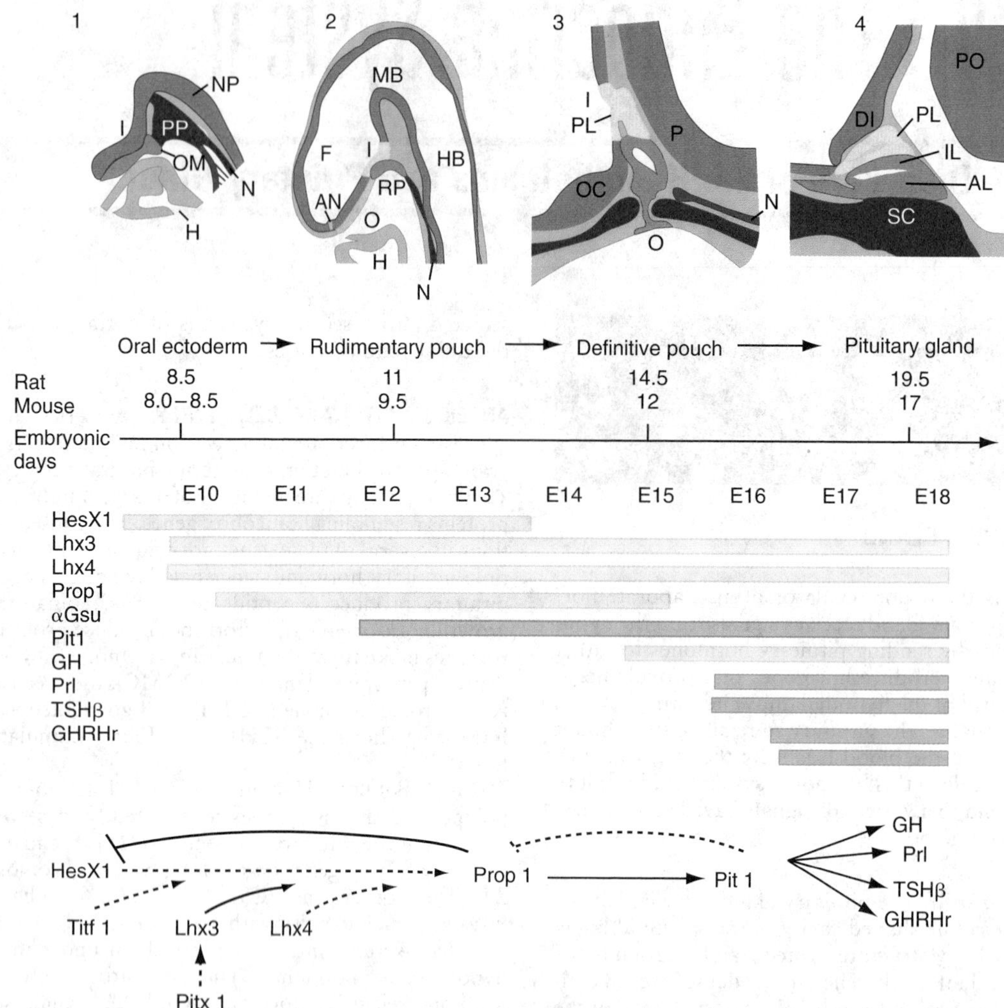

Figure 557-1. Pituitary development. *A*, Mid-sagittal or parasagittal section drawings of rat embryos showing pituitary development: (1) growth of pre-infundibular portion of neural plate and establishment of presumptive Rathke pouch area; (2) formation of a rudimentary pouch, with absence of mesoderm between pouch and floor of diencephalon; (3) formation of definitive pouch and posterior lobe with invasion of neural crest and mesenchymal tissue and separation of brain and oral cavities; (4) nascent pituitary gland. Corresponding stages in mouse development indicated. AL, anterior lobe; AN, anterior neural pore; F, forebrain; H, heart; HB, hindbrain; I, infundibulum; IL, intermediate lobe; MB, midbrain; N, notochord; NP, neural plate; O, oral cavity; OC, optic chiasm; OM, oral membrane; P, pontine flexure; PL, posterior lobe; PO, pons; PP prechordal plate; RP, Rathke pouch; SC, sphenoid cartilage. *B*, Cascade of transcription factors that regulate anterior pituitary development. The approximate timing of mRNA expression in the mouse is shown for transcription factors (green bar) and other marker genes (blue bars). Arrows represent activation; and truncated lines represent repression. Black solid arrows indicate effects supported by analysis of pituitary mutants. Broken arrows represent hypothetical interactions that might be revealed by analysis of expression in other pituitary mutants. E, embryonic day. (From Dattani M, Preece M: Growth hormone deficiency and related disorders: Insights into causation, diagnosis, and treatment. *Lancet* 2004;363: 1997–1986.)

IGF-I has considerable homology to insulin. Circulating IGF-I is synthesized primarily in the liver and formed locally in mesodermal and ectodermal cells, particularly in the growth plate of children, where its effect is exerted by paracrine or autocrine mechanisms. Circulating levels of IGF-I are related to blood levels of GH and to nutritional status. IGF-I circulates bound to several different binding proteins. The major one is a 150-kd complex (IGF-BP3), which is decreased in GH-deficient children. Human recombinant IGF-I may have therapeutic potential in conditions characterized by end organ resistance to GH such as Laron syndrome and the development of antibodies to administered GH. IGF-II is a 67-amino-acid single-chain protein that is coded for by a gene on the short arm of chromosome 11. It has homology to IGF-I. Less is known about its physiologic role, but it appears to be an important mitogen in bone cells, where it occurs in a concentration many times higher than that of IGF-I.

Prolactin. PRL is a 199-amino-acid peptide made in pituitary lactotropes. The regulation of PRL is unique because PRL is consistently secreted unless it is actively inhibited by dopamine, which is produced by neurons in the hypothalamus. Disruption of the hypothalamus or pituitary stalk can result in elevated PRL levels. Dopamine antagonists, states of primary hypothyroidism, administration of thyrotropin-releasing hormone (TRH), physiologic stress (shock) and pituitary tumors result in increased serum levels of PRL. Dopamine agonists and processes causing destruction of the pituitary cause reduced levels of PRL.

The primary physiologic role of PRL is the initiation and maintenance of lactation. PRL prepares the breasts for lactation and stimulates milk production postpartum. During pregnancy, PRL stimulates the development of the milk secretory apparatus, but lactation does not occur because of the high levels of estrogen and progesterone. After delivery, the estrogen and progesterone levels drop and physiologic stimuli such as suckling and nipple stimulation signal PRL release and initiate lactation.

Thyroid-Stimulating Hormone. TSH consists of 2 glycoprotein chains (α and β) linked by hydrogen bonding; the α-subunit is composed of 89 amino acids and is identical to other glycoproteins (FSH, LH, chorionic gonadotropin [hCG], and the β-subunit of 112 amino acids is specific for TSH).

TSH is stored in secretory granules and released into circulation primarily in response to thyrotropin-releasing hormone (TRH), which is produced by the hypothalamus. TRH is released from the hypothalamus into the hypothalamic-pituitary portal system, ultimately stimulating TSH release from pituitary thyrotropes. TSH stimulates release of thyroxine (T_4) and triiodothyronine (T_3) from the thyroid gland through the formation of cyclic adenosine monophosphate (cAMP) and the G-protein second messenger system. In addition to the negative feedback inhibition by T_3, the release of TRH and TSH are also inhibited by dopamine, somatostatin, and glucocorticoids.

Deficiency of TSH results in inactivity and atrophy of the thyroid gland, whereas excess TSH results in hypertrophy and hyperplasia of the thyroid gland.

Adrenocorticotropic Hormone. ACTH is a 39-amino-acid single-chain peptide that is derived by proteolytic cleavage from **POMC,** a 240-amino acid precursor glycoprotein product of the pituitary gland. POMC also contains the sequences for the lipotropins (LPHs), melanocyte-stimulating hormones (MSHs), and β-endorphin (β-END).

Secretion of ACTH is regulated by corticotropin-releasing hormone (CRH), a 41-amino-acid peptide found predominantly in the median eminence but also in other areas in and outside the brain. ACTH is secreted in a diurnal pattern. It acts on the adrenal cortex to stimulate cortisol synthesis and secretion. ACTH and cortisol levels are highest in the morning at the time of waking, are low in the late afternoon and evening, and reach their nadir 1–2 hr after the beginning of sleep. ACTH also appears to be the principal pigmentary hormone in humans. Similar to TRH and TSH, CRH and ACTH function through the formation of cAMP and the G-protein second messenger system. Although CRH is the primary regulator of ACTH secretion, other hormones have a role. Arginine vasopressin (AVP), oxytocin, angiotensin II, and cholecystokinin stimulate release of CRH and ACTH, whereas atrial natriuretic peptide (ANP) and opioids inhibit release of CRH and ACTH. Cortisol inhibits CRH and ACTH. Physiologic conditions such as stress, fasting, and hypoglycemia also stimulate release of CRH and ACTH.

Luteinizing Hormone and Follicle-Stimulating Hormone. Gonadotropic hormones include 2 glycoproteins: LH and FSH. They contain the same α-subunit as TSH and hCG but distinct β-subunits. Receptors for FSH on the ovarian granulosa cells and on testicular Sertoli cells mediate FSH stimulation of follicular development in the ovary and of gametogenesis in the testis. On binding to specific receptors on ovarian theca cells and testicular Leydig cells, LH promotes luteinization of the ovary and Leydig cell function of the testis. The receptors for LH and FSH belong to a class of receptors with 7 membrane-spanning protein domains. Receptor occupancy activates adenylyl cyclase through the mediation of G-proteins.

Luteinizing hormone–releasing hormone, a decapeptide, has been isolated, synthesized, and used therapeutically. Because it leads to the release of LH and FSH from the same gonadotropic cells, it appears that there is only one gonadotropin-releasing hormone.

Secretion of LH is inhibited by androgens and estrogens, and secretion of FSH is suppressed by gonadal production of inhibin, a 31-kd glycoprotein produced by the Sertoli cells. **Inhibin** consists of α- and β-subunits joined by disulfide bonds. The β-β dimer (**activin**) also occurs; its biologic effect is to stimulate FSH secretion. The biologic features of inhibin and activin are being delineated. In addition to its endocrine effect, activin has paracrine effects in the testis. It facilitates LH-induced testosterone production, indicating a direct effect of Sertoli cells on Leydig cells.

POSTERIOR PITUITARY CELL TYPES. The posterior lobe of the pituitary is part of a functional unit, the neurohypophysis, that consists of the neurons of the supraoptic and paraventricular nuclei of the hypothalamus; neuronal axons, which form the pituitary stalk; and neuronal terminals in the median eminence or in the posterior lobe. Arginine vasopressin (AVP; antidiuretic hormone [ADH]) and oxytocin are the 2 hormones produced by neurosecretion in the hypothalamic nuclei and released from the posterior pituitary. They are octapeptides and differ by only 2 amino acids.

Antidiuretic Hormone. ADH regulates water conservation at the level of the kidney by increasing the permeability of the renal collecting duct to water. ADH stimulates translocation of water channels through its interaction with vasopressin 2 (V2) receptors in the collecting duct, which act through G-proteins to increase adenylyl cyclase activity and increase permeability to water. V2 receptors also mediate the von Willebrand factor and tissue plasminogen activator. At higher concentrations, ADH activates V1 receptors in smooth muscle cells and hepatocytes and exerts pressor and glycogenolytic effects through mobilization of intracellular calcium stores. Separate V3 receptors medicate stimulation of ACTH secretion. These effects involve phosphatidylinositol hydrolysis rather than cyclic AMP production.

ADH and its accompanying protein, neurophysin II, are encoded by the same gene. A single preprohormone is cleaved, and the two are transported to neurosecretory vesicles in the posterior pituitary. The two are released in equimolar amounts.

ADH has a short half-life and responds quickly to changes in hydration. The stimuli for its release are increased plasma osmolality, perceived by osmoreceptors in the hypothalamus, and decreased blood volume, perceived by baroreceptors in the carotid sinus of the aortic arch.

Oxytocin. Oxytocin stimulates uterine contractions at the time of labor and delivery in response to distention of the reproductive tract, and it stimulates smooth muscle contraction in the breast during suckling, which results in milk let-down.

Chapter 558 ■ Hypopituitarism

John S. Parks and Eric I. Felner

Hypopituitarism denotes underproduction of growth hormone (GH) alone or in combination with deficiencies of other pituitary hormones. Affected children have postnatal growth impairment that is specifically corrected by replacement of GH. The incidence of hypopituitarism is between 1 in 4,000 and 1 in 10,000 live births. With knowledge of the genes that direct pituitary development (see Fig. 557-1) or hormone production, an increasing proportion of cases can be attributed to specific genetic disorders (Table 558-1). Mutations in these genes account for 13% of isolated growth hormone deficiency (IGHD) and 20% of multiple pituitary hormone deficiency (MPHD) cases. The likelihood of finding mutations is increased by positive family histories and decreased in cases with ACTH deficiency.

MULTIPLE PITUITARY HORMONE DEFICIENCY

GENETIC FORMS. Sequentially expressed transcriptional activation factors direct the differentiation and proliferation of anterior pituitary cell types (see Fig. 557-1). These proteins are members of a large family of DNA-binding proteins resembling homeobox genes. Mutations produce different forms of multiple pituitary hormone deficiency. The *HESX1, LHX3, LHX4,* and *PTX2* genes are expressed at early stages of pituitary development. They

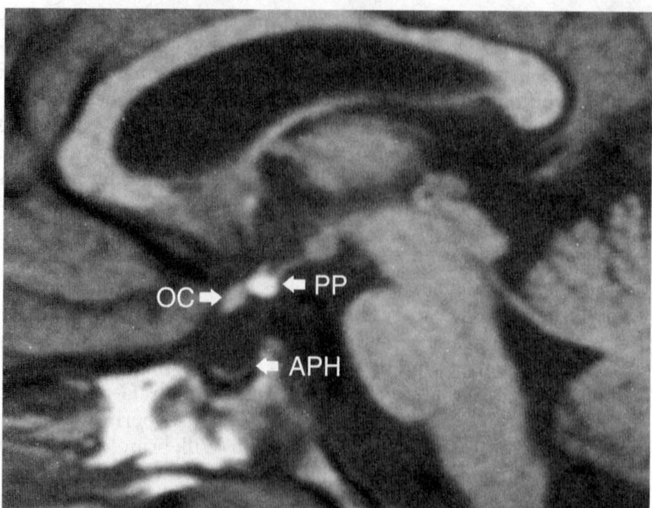

Figure 558-1. Sagittal MRI scan showing anterior pituitary hypoplasia. APH, anterior pituitary hypoplasia; OC, optic chiasm (normal here); PP, posterior pituitary (ectopic here). The infundibulum connecting the pituitary to the hypothalamus is not shown. (From Dattani MT, Preece M: Growth hormone deficiency and related disorders: Insights into causation, diagnosis, and treatment. *Lancet* 2004;363:1977–1986.)

are also expressed in other organs. Mutations in these genes tend to produce phenotypes that extend beyond hypopituitarism to include abnormalities in other organs.

HESX1. The *HESX1* gene is expressed in precursors of all 5 cell types of the anterior pituitary early in embryologic development.

TABLE 558-1. Etiologic Classification of Multiple Pituitary Hormone Deficiency

GENE OF LOCATION	PHENOTYPE	INHERITANCE
GENETIC FORMS		
POU1F1 (PIT1)	GH, TSH, PRL	R, D
PROP1	GH, TSH, PRL, LH, FSH, ±ACTH, variable AP	R
LHX3	GH, TSH, PRL, LH, FSH, variable AP, ±short neck	R
LHX4	GH, TSH, ACTH, small AP, EPP, ±Arnold-Chiari syndrome	D
TPIT	ACTH, severe neonatal form	R
HESX1	GH, variable for others, small AP, EPP	R, D
SOX3	Variable deficiencies, ±MR, EPP, small AP and stalk	XL
PTX2	Rieger syndrome	D
GLI2	Holoprosencephaly, midline defects	D
GLI3	Hall-Pallister syndrome	D
Sonic hedgehog	GH deficiency with single central incisor	D
ACQUIRED FORMS		
Idiopathic		
Irradiation	GH deficiency precedes other deficiencies	
Inflammation/Infiltrative	Histiocytosis, sarcoidosis, meningitis, encephalitis, tuberculosis	
Autoimmune	Hypophysitis	
Postsurgical	Stalk section, vascular compromise	
Tumor	Craniopharyngioma, glioma, pinealoma, adenoma, germinoma, optic glioma	
Trauma	Battering, shaken baby syndrome, motor vehicle crash, perinatal	
Hypothyroidism	Primary or acquired	
UNCERTAIN ETIOLOGY		
Idiopathic		
Congenital absence of pituitary		
Septo-optic dysplasia		
Birth trauma		
Encephalocele		
Hydrocephalus		

ACTH, adrenocorticotropic hormone; AP, anterior pituitary; D, dominant; EPP, ectopic posterior pituitary; FSH, follicle-stimulating hormone; GH, growth hormone; LH, leuteinizing hormone; PRL, prolactin; R, recessive; TSH, thyroid-stimulating hormone; XL, X-linked.

Mutations result in a complex phenotype with defects in development of the optic nerve. Heterozygotes for loss-of-function mutations show the combinations of isolated GH deficiency and optic nerve hypoplasia. Homozygotes may have full expression of **septo-optic dysplasia** (SOD), which manifests incomplete development of the septum pellucidum with optic nerve hypoplasia and other midline abnormalities. Clinical observation of nystagmus and visual impairment in infancy leads to the discovery of optic nerve and brain abnormalities. SOD is associated with anterior and/or posterior pituitary hormone deficiencies in 25% of patients. Patients often have the triad of a small anterior pituitary gland, an attenuated pituitary stalk, and an ectopic posterior pituitary bright spot. The great majority of SOD cases do not have *HESX1* mutations.

LHX3. *LHX3* activates the α-GSU promoter and acts synergistically with POU1F1 to increase transcription from the PRL, β-TSH, and POU1F1 promoters. The hormonal phenotype produced by recessive loss-of-function mutations in this gene resembles that produced by *PROP1* mutations. There are deficiencies of GH, PRL, TSH, LH, and FSH but not ACTH. It is unclear whether the deficiencies are present from birth or whether they appear later in childhood. Some affected individuals show enlargement of the anterior pituitary. The first patients to be described had the unusual findings of a short neck and a rigid cervical spine. They were able to rotate their necks only about 90 degrees compared with the normal rotation of 150–180 degrees.

LHX4. Dominantly inherited mutations in the *LHX4* gene consistently produce GH deficiency, with the variable presence of TSH and ACTH deficiencies. Additional findings may include a small, V-shaped pituitary fossa, Chiari I malformation, and an ectopic posterior pituitary.

PTX2. Rieger syndrome is a complex phenotype caused by mutations in the *PTX2* transcription factor gene. This gene is also referred to as *RIEG1*. It is expressed in multiple tissues, including the anterior pituitary gland. In addition to variable degrees of anterior pituitary hormone deficiency, children with Rieger syndrome have colobomas of the iris and abnormal development of the kidneys, gastrointestinal tract, and umbilicus.

PROP1. *PROP1* is found in the nuclei of somatotropes, lactotropes, and thyrotropes. Its roles include turning on POU1F1 expression, hence its name "prophet of PIT1." Mutations of PROP1 are the most common explanation for recessive MPHD. These mutations are 10 times as common as the combined total of mutations in other pituitary transcription factor genes. One- and two-base-pair deletions in exon 2 are most common, followed by missense, nonsense, and splice site mutations. Anterior pituitary hormone deficiencies are seldom evident in the neonatal period. Growth in the 1st yr of life is considerably better than with POU1F1 defects. The median age at diagnosis of GH deficiency is around 6 yr. Recognition of TSH deficiency is delayed relative to recognition of GH deficiency. Basal and TRH-stimulated PRL levels tend to be higher than in POU1F1 mutations. Most children with *PROP1* mutations develop LH and FSH deficiency. Some enter puberty spontaneously and then retreat from puberty. Girls experience secondary amenorrhea, and boys show regression of testicular size and secondary sexual characteristics. Partial deficiency of ACTH develops over time in about 30% of patients with *PROP1* defects. Anterior pituitary size is small in most patients, but in some there is progressive enlargement of the pituitary. A central mass originates within the sella turcica but may extend above it. The cellular content of the mass during the active phase of enlargement is not known. With time, the contents of the mass appear to degenerate, with multiple cystic areas. The mass may persist as a nonenhancing structure or may disappear completely, leaving an empty sella turcica. At different stages, MRI findings can suggest a microadenoma, macroadenoma, craniopharyngioma, or Rathke pouch cyst.

POU1F1 (PIT1). POU1F1 (formerly PIT1) was identified as a nuclear protein that binds to the GH and PRL promoters. It is necessary for emergence and mature function of somatotropes, lactotropes, and thyrotropes. Dominant and recessive mutations in POU1F1 are responsible for complete deficiencies of GH and PRL and variable TSH deficiency. Affected individuals exhibit nearly normal fetal growth but experience severe growth failure in the 1st yr of life. With normal production of LH, and FSH, puberty develops spontaneously, though at a later than normal age. These patients are not at risk for development of ACTH deficiency. Anterior pituitary size is normal to small.

Other Congenital Forms of MPHD. Severe early-onset MPHD including deficiency of ACTH is often associated with the triad of anterior pituitary hypoplasia, absence or attenuation of the pituitary stalk, and an ectopic posterior pituitary bright spot on MRI. Most cases are sporadic; there is a male predominance. Some are due to abnormalities of the *SOX3* gene, located on the X chromosome. The majority of cases have not been explained at the genetic level.

Pituitary hypoplasia can occur as an isolated phenomenon or in association with more extensive developmental abnormalities such as anencephaly or holoprosencephaly. Midfacial anomalies (cleft lip, palate) or the finding of a solitary maxillary central incisor indicate a high likelihood of GH or other anterior/posterior hormone deficiency. In the **Hall-Pallister syndrome,** absence of the pituitary gland is associated with hypothalamic hamartoblastoma, postaxial polydactyly, nail dysplasia, bifid epiglottis, imperforate anus, and anomalies of the heart, lungs, and kidneys.

Acquired Forms. Any lesion that damages the hypothalamus, pituitary stalk, or anterior pituitary may cause pituitary hormone deficiency. Because such lesions are not selective, multiple hormonal deficiencies are usually observed. The most common lesion is the craniopharyngioma (see Chapter 497). Central nervous system germinoma, eosinophilic granuloma (histiocytosis), tuberculosis, sarcoidosis, toxoplasmosis, meningitis, and aneurysms may also cause hypothalamic-hypophyseal destruction. Trauma, including shaken child syndrome, motor vehicle crash, traction at delivery, anoxia, and hemorrhagic infarction, may also damage the pituitary, its stalk, or the hypothalamus.

ISOLATED GROWTH HORMONE DEFICIENCY AND INSENSITIVITY

GENETIC FORMS OF GROWTH HORMONE DEFICIENCY. Isolated GH deficiency (IGHD) is caused by abnormalities of the GHRH receptor, growth hormone genes, and by genes located on the X chromosome (Table 558-2).

GHRH Receptor. Recessive loss-of-function mutations in the receptor for GHRH interferes with proliferation of somatotropes during pituitary development and disrupts the most important signals for release of GH. The anterior pituitary is small, in keeping with the observation that somatotropes normally account for greater than 50% of pituitary volume. There is reduction of fetal growth, followed by severe postnatal growth failure.

GH1. The *GH1* gene is one of a cluster of 5 genes on chromosome 17q22-24. This cluster arose through successive duplications of an ancestral GH gene. Unequal crossing-over at meiosis produces a variety of gene deletions. Small deletions (<10 kb) remove only the GH1 gene, whereas large deletions (45 kb) remove 1 or more of the adjacent genes *(CSL, CS1, GH2, CS2).* The growth phenotype is identical with deletion of *GH1* alone or *GH1* together with 1 or more of the adjacent genes. Loss of *CS1, GH2,* and *CS2* without loss of *GH1* causes deficiency of chorionic somatomammotropin and placental GH in the maternal circulation but does not result in fetal or postnatal growth retardation. Children who are homozygous for *GH1* gene deletions respond well to GH therapy.

Recessively transmitted mutations in the *GH1* gene produce a similar phenotype. Missense, nonsense, and frameshift mutations are described. The most common involve the 4th and final intron of the gene. These mutations eliminate the normal splice donor site and foster use of an alternative site. The abnormal mRNA encodes a protein that is longer than normal and has no biologic activity.

Autosomal dominant IGHD is also caused by mutations in *GH1*. The mutations usually involve splice site errors in intron 3. There is overproduction of a 20-kd protein that lacks the amino acids normally encoded by exon 3. Accumulation of this protein interferes with the processing, storage, and secretion of the normal 22-kd GH protein. Additional deficiencies of TSH and/or ACTH have been recognized as late complications in patients with dominant mutations in GH1.

Short stature due to biologically inactive GH is characterized by normal to high levels of circulating GH by immunoassay but by lower levels of GH when assessed by cell proliferation, receptor binding, or receptor activation assays. A well-documented example involves a child with homozygosity for a missense mutation of the *GH1* gene. Substitution of a glycine for the normal serine at position 53 prevents formation of a disulfide bridge between residues 53 and 165. The mutant molecule has subnormal activities in immunofunction, receptor binding and activation of the Jak2/Stat5 signaling pathway. Growth hormone treatment produced increases in IGF-I levels and growth rate; the patient attained a normal adult height.

X-Linked IGHD. Two loci on the X chromosome have been associated with hypopituitarism. The first lies at Xq21.3-q22 in the region of the Bruton thymidine kinase gene *(BTK).* Mutations in this region produce **hypogammaglobulinemia** as well as IGHD. The second locus maps farther out on the long arm, at Xq24-q27.1, a region containing the *SOX2* transcription factor gene. Abnormalities in this locus have been linked to IGHD with **mental retardation** as well as to MPHD with the triad of pituitary hypoplasia, missing pituitary stalk, and ectopic posterior pituitary gland.

Acquired Forms. The GH axis is more susceptible to disruption by acquired conditions than are other hypothalamic-pituitary axes. Recognized causes of acquired GH deficiency include the use of radiotherapy for malignancy, meningitis, histiocytosis, and trauma.

Children who receive radiotherapy for CNS tumors or prevention of CNS malignancies (leukemia) are at risk for developing GH deficiency. Spinal irradiation contributes to disproportionately poor growth of the trunk independent of GH status. Growth typically slows during radiation therapy or chemotherapy, improves for 1–2 yr, and then declines with the development of GH deficiency. The dose and frequency of radiotherapy are important determinants of hypopituitarism. GH deficiency is almost universal 5 yr after therapy with a total dose ≥35

TABLE 558-2. Etiologic Classification of Isolated GH Deficiency or Insensitivity

GENE OR LOCATION	PHENOTYPE		INHERITANCE
GH DEFICIENCY			
GHRH receptor	IGHD, small AP	Low GH, Low IGF-I	R
GH1	IGHD, small or normal AP	Low GH, Low IGF-I	R, D
GH1	Bioinactive GH	High GH, Low IGF-I	D
BTK (Xq21.3-q22)	IGHD, hypogammaglobulinemia	Low GH, Low IGF-I	XL
SOX3 (Xq27.1)	IGHD, MR	Low GH, Low IGF-I	XL
GH INSENSITIVITY			
GH receptor	Variable GHBP	High GH, Low IGF-I	R, D
STAT5b	Immunodeficiency	High GH, Low IGF-I	R
IGF-I	IUGR, MR, deafness	High GH, Low IGF-I	R
Acid-labile subunit	Mild short stature	Normal GH, Low IGF-1	R
IGF-I receptor	IUGR	High GH, High IGF-I	R

AP, anterior pituitary; D, dominant; EPP, ectopic posterior pituitary; IGHD, isolated growth hormone deficiency; IUGR, intrauterine growth retardation; MR, mental retardation; R, recessive; XL, X-linked.

Gy. More subtle defects are seen with doses around 20 Gy. Deficiency of GH is the most common defect, but deficiencies of TSH and ACTH may also occur. Unlike in other forms of hypopituitarism, puberty tends to be early rather than delayed. The clinician is likely to encounter children in the 8- to 10-yr age range who are growing at rates that are normal for chronological age but subnormal for stage of pubertal development.

GROWTH HORMONE INSENSITIVITY

ABNORMALITIES OF THE GROWTH HORMONE RECEPTOR. Growth hormone insensitivity is caused by disruption of pathways distal to production of GH. Laron syndrome involves mutations of the GH receptor. Children with this condition clinically resemble those with severe IGHD. Birth length tends to be about 1 SD below the mean, and severe short stature with lengths more than 4 SD below the mean is present by 1 yr of age. Resting and stimulated GH levels tend to be high, and IGF-I levels are low. The GH receptor has an extracellular GH-binding domain, a transmembrane domain, and an intracellular signaling domain. Mutations in the extracellular domain interfere with binding of GH. Serum growth hormone binding protein (GHBP) activity, representing the circulating form of the membrane receptor for GH, is generally low. Mutations in the transmembrane domain can interfere with anchoring of the receptor to the plasma membrane. In these cases, circulating GHBP activity is normal or high. Mutations in the intracellular domain interfere with JAK/STAT signaling.

POST-RECEPTOR FORMS OF GH INSENSITIVITY. Some children with severe growth failure, high GH and low IGF-I levels, and normal GHBP levels, have abnormalities distal to the GH binding and activation of the GH receptor. Several have been found to have mutations in the gene-encoding signal transducer and activator of transcription 5b (STAT5b). Disruption of this key intermediate connecting receptor activation to gene transcription produces growth failure similar to that seen in Laron syndrome. These patients also suffer from chronic pulmonary infections, consistent with important roles for STAT5b in interleukin and cytokine signaling.

IGF-I GENE ABNORMALITIES. Abnormalities of the IGF-I gene produce severe prenatal as well as postnatal growth impairment. Microcephaly, mental retardation, and deafness are present in patients with exon deletion and a missense mutation. These patients can be expected to respond to recombinant IGF-I treatment.

IGF-BINDING PROTEIN ABNORMALITIES. Mutation of the gene encoding the acid-labile subunit of the circulating 165-kd IGF-I, IGF-BP3 acid-labile subunit complex is associated with short stature. Total IGF-I levels are very low. The index case, with homozygosity for an ALS mutation, did not show an increase in IGF-I levels or an increase in growth rate during GH treatment.

IGF-I RECEPTOR GENE ABNORMALITIES. Mutations of the IGF-I receptor also compromise prenatal and postnatal growth. The phenotype does not appear to be as severe as that seen with absence of IGF-I. Adult heights are closer to the normal range, and affected individuals do not have mental retardation or deafness.

CLINICAL MANIFESTATIONS

CONGENITAL HYPOPITUITARISM. The child with hypopituitarism is usually of normal size and weight at birth although those with MPHD and genetic defects of the *GH1* or *GHR* gene have birth lengths that average 1 SD below the mean. Children with severe defects in GH production or action are more than 4 SD below the mean by 1 yr of age. Those with less severe deficiencies grow at rates below the 25% for age and gradually diverge from normal height percentiles. Delayed closure of the epiphyses permits growth beyond the normal age when growth should be complete.

Infants with congenital defects of the pituitary or hypothalamus usually present with neonatal emergencies such as apnea, cyanosis, or **severe hypoglycemia** with or without seizures. **Microphallus** in boys provides an additional diagnostic clue. Deficiency of GH may be accompanied by hypoadrenalism and hypothyroidism. Prolonged **neonatal jaundice** is common. It involves elevation of conjugated and unconjugated bilirubin and may be mistaken for neonatal hepatitis.

The head in the toddler is round, and the face is short and broad. The frontal bone is prominent, and the bridge of the nose is depressed and saddle-shaped. The nose is small, and the nasolabial folds are well developed. The eyes are somewhat bulging. The mandible and the chin are underdeveloped, and the teeth, which erupt late, are frequently crowded. The neck is short, and the larynx is small. The voice is high-pitched and remains high after puberty. The extremities are well proportioned, with small hands and feet. Weight for height is usually normal, but an excess of body fat and a deficiency of muscle mass contributes to a pudgy appearance. The genitals are usually small for age, and sexual maturation may be delayed or absent. Facial, axillary, and pubic hair usually is lacking, and the scalp hair is fine. Mainly length is affected, giving toddlers a pudgy appearance. Symptomatic hypoglycemia, usually after fasting, occurs in 10–15% of children with panhypopituitarism and those with IGHD. Intelligence is usually normal.

ACQUIRED HYPOPITUITARISM. The child initially is normal; manifestations similar to those seen in idiopathic pituitary growth failure gradually appear and progress. When complete or almost complete destruction of the pituitary gland occurs, signs of pituitary insufficiency are present. Atrophy of the adrenal cortex, thyroid, and gonads results in loss of weight, asthenia, sensitivity to cold, mental torpor, and absence of sweating. Sexual maturation fails to take place or regresses if already present. There may be atrophy of the gonads and genital tract with amenorrhea and loss of pubic and axillary hair. There is a tendency to hypoglycemia. Growth slows dramatically. Diabetes insipidus may be present early but tends to improve spontaneously as the anterior pituitary is progressively destroyed.

If the lesion is an **expanding tumor,** symptoms such as headache, vomiting, visual disturbances, pathologic sleep patterns, decreased school performance, seizures, polyuria, and growth failure may occur. Slowing of growth may antedate neurologic signs and symptoms, especially with craniopharyngiomas, but symptoms of hormonal deficit account for only 10% of presenting complaints. Evidence of pituitary insufficiency may first appear after surgical intervention. In children with craniopharyngiomas, visual field defects, optic atrophy, papilledema, and cranial nerve palsy are common.

LABORATORY FINDINGS. The diagnosis of GH deficiency is suspected in children with moderate to severe postnatal growth failure. Criteria for growth failure include height below the 1% for age and sex, or height more than 2 SD below sex-adjusted mid-parent height. Acquired GH deficiency can occur at any age; when it is of acute onset, height may be within the normal range. A strong clinical suspicion is important in establishing the diagnosis because laboratory measures of GH sufficiency lack specificity. Observation of low serum levels of IGF-I and the GH-dependent IGF-BP3 can be helpful; IGF-1 and IGF-BP3 levels should be matched to skeletal rather than chronological age normal values. Values in the upper part of the normal range for age effectively exclude GH deficiency. IGF-I values in normally growing children and those with hypopituitarism overlap during infancy and early childhood.

Definitive diagnosis of GH deficiency traditionally requires demonstration of absent or low levels of GH in response to stimulation. A variety of provocative tests have been devised that rapidly increase the level of GH in normal children. These include administration of insulin, arginine, clonidine, or glucagon. In chronic GH deficiency, the demonstration of poor linear growth, delayed skeletal age, and peak levels of GH (<10 ng/mL) in each of 2 provocative tests, are compatible with GH deficiency. In acute GH deficiency, a high clinical suspicion of GH deficiency and low peak levels of GH (<10 ng/mL) in each of 2 provocative tests are compatible with GH deficiency. This rather arbitrary cutoff is higher than the 3 or 5 ng/mL criterion used for diagnosis of adult GH deficiency. The frequency of negative GH responses to a single standard test in normally growing children is usually considered to approach 20%. Monoclonal antibody assays generally underestimate GH concentration compared with the earlier polyclonal antibody assays. There is no consensus regarding adoption of criteria that take into account age, gender, and GH assay characteristics. Stimulation with GHRH generally produces greater responses in children with GH deficiency caused by hypothalamic disorders and fails to elicit a response in those with GHRH receptor, *GH1, POU1F1, PROP1,* and *LHX3* mutations. A majority of normal prepubertal children fail to achieve GH values >10 ng/mL with 2 pharmacologic tests. Three days of estrogen priming may be needed prior to GH testing to achieve greater diagnostic specificity.

During the 3 decades in which hGH was obtained by extraction from human pituitary glands culled at autopsy, its supply was sharply limited and only patients with classic GH deficiency were treated. With the advent of an unlimited supply of recombinant GH, there has been a marked interest in redefining the criteria for GH deficiency to include children with lesser degrees of deficiency. It has become popular to evaluate the spontaneous secretion of GH by measuring its level every 20 min during a 24- or 12-hr (8 P.M. to 8 A.M.) period. Some short children with normal levels of GH when studied by provocative tests show little spontaneous GH secretion. Such children are considered to have **GH neurosecretory dysfunction.** Nonetheless, frequent GH sampling also lacks diagnostic specificity. There is a wide range of spontaneous GH secretion in normally growing prepubertal children and considerable overlap with the values observed in children with classic GH deficiency. Although the clinical and laboratory criteria for GH deficiency in patients with severe (classic) hypopituitarism are well established, the diagnostic criteria are unsettled for short children with lesser degrees of GH deficiency.

In addition to establishing the diagnosis of GH deficiency, it is necessary to examine other pituitary functions. Levels of TSH, thyroxine (T_4), ACTH, cortisol, gonadotropins, and gonadal steroids may provide evidence of other pituitary hormonal deficiencies. The defect can be localized to the hypothalamus if there is a normal response to the administration of hypothalamic-releasing hormones for TSH, ACTH, or gonadotropins. When there is a deficiency of TSH, serum levels of T_4 and TSH are low. A normal increase in TSH and PRL after stimulation with TRH places the defect in the hypothalamus, and absence of such a response localizes the defect to the pituitary. An elevated level of plasma PRL taken at random in the patient with hypopituitarism is also strong evidence that the defect is in the hypothalamus rather than in the pituitary. Some children with craniopharyngiomas have elevated PRL levels before surgery, but after surgery, PRL deficiency occurs because of pituitary damage. Antidiuretic hormone deficiency may be established by appropriate studies.

RADIOLOGIC FINDINGS. Conventional x-ray films of the skull have been replaced by computed tomography and, increasingly, by magnetic resonance imaging. CT is appropriate for recognizing suprasellar calcification associated with craniopharyngiomas and bony erosions accompanying histiocytosis. MRI provides a much more detailed view of hypothalamic and pituitary anatomy. Many cases of severe early-onset MPHD show the triad of a small anterior pituitary gland, a missing or attenuated pituitary stalk, and an ectopic posterior pituitary bright spot at the base of the hypothalamus (Fig. 558-1). Subnormal anterior pituitary height, implying a small anterior pituitary, is common in genetic and idiopathic causes of IGHD. Craniopharyngiomas are common and pituitary adenomas are rare in children with hypopituitarism. Both hypoplastic and markedly enlarged anterior pituitary glands are seen in patients with *PROP1* or *LHX3* mutations.

Skeletal maturation is delayed in patients with IGHD and may be even more delayed when there is combined GH and TSH deficiency. Dual photon x-ray absorptiometry shows deficient bone mineralization, deficiencies in lean body mass, and a corresponding increase in adiposity.

DIFFERENTIAL DIAGNOSIS. There are many causes of growth disorders (see Chapter 37). Systemic conditions such as inflammatory bowel disease, celiac disease, occult renal disease, and anemia must be considered. Patients with systemic conditions often have greater loss of weight than length. A few otherwise normal children are short (>3 SD below the mean for age) and grow 5 cm/yr or less but have normal levels of GH in response to provocative tests and normal spontaneous episodic secretion. Most of these children show increased rates of growth when treated with GH in doses comparable to those used to treat children with hypopituitarism. Plasma levels of IGF-I in these patients may be normal or low. Several groups of treated children have achieved final or near final adult heights. Different studies have found changes in adult height that range from −2.5 to +7.5 cm compared with pretreatment predictions. No methods can reliably predict which of these children will become taller as adults as a result of GH treatment and which will have compromised adult height.

Diagnostic strategies for distinguishing between permanent GH deficiency and other causes of impaired growth are imperfect. Children with a combination of genetic short stature and constitutional delay of growth have short stature, below average growth rates, and delayed bone ages. Many of these children exhibit minimal GH secretory responses to provocative stimuli. When children who have been diagnosed with idiopathic or acquired GH deficiency are treated with hGH and are retested as adults, the majority have peak GH levels within the normal range.

CONSTITUTIONAL GROWTH DELAY. Constitutional growth delay is a common variant of normal growth. Length and weight measurements of affected children are normal at birth, and growth is normal for the first 4–12 mo of life. Height is sustained at a lower percentile during childhood. The pubertal growth spurt is delayed, so their growth rates continue to decline after their classmates have begun to accelerate. Detailed questioning often reveals other family members (frequently 1 or both parents) with histories of short stature in childhood, delayed puberty, and eventual normal stature. IGF-I levels tend to be low for chronological age but within the normal range for bone age. Growth hormone responses to provocative testing tend to be lower than in children with a more typical timing of puberty. The prognosis for normal adult height in these children is guarded. Predictions based on height and bone age tend to overestimate eventual height to a greater extent in boys than in girls. Boys with more than 2 yr of pubertal delay may benefit from a short course of testosterone therapy to hasten puberty after 14 yr of age. The cause of this variant of normal growth is thought to be persistence of the relatively hypogonadotropic state of childhood (see Chapter 12).

PRIMARY HYPOTHYROIDISM. Primary hypothyroidism is more common than GH deficiency. Low total or free T_4 and elevated TSH levels establish the diagnosis. Responses to GH provocative tests may be subnormal, and enlargement of the sella may be present. Pituitary hyperplasia recedes during treatment with thyroid hormone. Because thyroid hormone is a necessary prerequisite for normal GH synthesis, it must always be assessed before GH evaluation.

PSYCHOSOCIAL DWARFISM. Emotional deprivation is an important cause of retardation of growth and mimics hypopituitarism. The condition is known as psychosocial dwarfism, maternal deprivation dwarfism, or hyperphagic short stature. The mechanisms by which sensory and emotional deprivation interfere with growth are not fully understood. Functional hypopituitarism is indicated by low levels of IGF-I and by inadequate responses of GH to provocative stimuli. Puberty may be normal or even premature in its appearance. Appropriate history and careful observations reveal disturbed mother-child or family relations and provide clues to the diagnosis (see Chapter 37). Proof may be difficult to establish because the parents or caregivers often hide the true family situation from professionals, and the children rarely divulge their plight. Emotionally deprived children frequently have perverted or voracious appetites, enuresis, encopresis, insomnia, crying spasms, and sudden tantrums. The subgroup of children with hyperphagia and a normal body mass index tends to show catch-up growth when placed in a less stressful environment.

TREATMENT. The Lawson Wilkins Pediatric Endocrine Society, Academy of Pediatrics, and GH Research Society all have published guidelines for hGH treatment. In children with classic GH deficiency, treatment should be started as soon as possible to narrow the gap in height between patients and their classmates during childhood and to have the greatest effect on mature height. The recommended dose of hGH is 0.18–0.3 mg/kg/wk during childhood. Higher doses have been used during puberty. Recombinant GH is administered subcutaneously in 6 or 7 divided doses. Maximal response to GH occurs in the 1st year of treatment. Growth velocity during this 1st yr is typically above the 95th percentile. With each successive year of treatment, the growth rate tends to decrease. If growth rate drops below the 25th percentile, compliance should be evaluated before the dose is increased. Concurrent treatment with GH and an LHRH agonist has been used in the hope that interruption of puberty will delay epiphyseal fusion and prolong growth. This strategy can increase adult height. It can also increase the discrepancy in physical maturity between GH-deficient children and their age peers and may impair bone mineralization. There have also been attempts to forestall epiphyseal fusion in boys by giving drugs that inhibit aromatase, the enzyme responsible for converting androgens to estrogens. Growth hormone therapy should be continued until near final height is achieved. Criteria for stopping treatment include a decision by the patient that he or she is tall enough, a growth rate less than 1 inch/yr and a bone age >14 yr in girls and >16 yr in boys.

Some patients develop either primary or central hypothyroidism while under treatment with GH. Similarly, there is a risk of developing adrenal insufficiency. If unrecognized, this can be fatal. Periodic evaluation of thyroid and adrenal function is indicated for all patients treated with GH.

Recombinant IGF-I is approved for use in the United States. It is given subcutaneously twice a day. The risk of hypoglycemia is reduced by giving the injections concurrently with a meal or snack. In certain situations, its use will be more efficacious than use of GH. These conditions include individuals with abnormalities of the GH receptor and *STAT5b* genes, as well as severely GH-deficient patients who have developed antibodies to administered GH. Its utility in improving growth rate and adult stature in broader categories of short children is being explored.

The doses of GH used to treat children with classic GH deficiency usually enhance the growth of many non–GH-deficient children as well. Intensive investigation is in progress to determine the full spectrum of short children who may benefit from treatment with GH. GH is currently approved in the United States for treatment of children with growth failure as a result of Turner syndrome, end-stage renal failure before kidney transplantation, Prader-Willi syndrome, intrauterine growth restriction, and idiopathic short stature. The latter indication specifies a height below the 1.2% (−2.25 SD) for age and sex, a predicted height below the 5th percentile, and open epiphyses. Studies of the effect of GH treatment on adult height suggest a median gain of 2–3 inches, depending on dose and duration of treatment.

In children with MPHD, replacement should also be directed at other hormonal deficiencies. In TSH-deficient subjects, thyroid hormone is given in full replacement doses. In ACTH-deficient patients, the optimal dose of hydrocortisone should not exceed 10 mg/m^2/24 hr. Increases are made during illness or in anticipation of surgical procedures. In patients with a deficiency of gonadotropins, gonadal steroids are given when bone age reaches the age at which puberty usually takes place. For infants with microphallus, one or two 3-month courses of monthly intramuscular injections of 25 mg of testosterone cypionate or testosterone enanthate may bring the penis to normal size without an inordinate effect on osseous maturation.

COMPLICATIONS AND ADVERSE EFFECTS OF HGH TREATMENT. Some patients treated with GH have developed leukemia. The increased risk is attributable to children with additional risk factors such as cranial irradiation. Growth hormone treatment does not increase the risk for recurrence of brain tumors or leukemia. Other reported side effects include pseudotumor cerebri, slipped capital femoral epiphysis, gynecomastia, and worsening of scoliosis. There is an increase in total body water during the first 2 wk of treatment. Fasting and postprandial insulin levels are characteristically low before treatment, and they normalize during GH replacement. Treatment does not increase risk of type 1 diabetes, but it may increase the risk of type 2 diabetes.

In the extracted pituitary GH treatment era, patients were at risk for **Creutzfeldt-Jakob** (CK) disease for at least 10–20 yr after therapy and the development of antibodies to GH. Those developing antibodies to administered GH became resistant to treatment. Use of recombinant GH over the past 2 decades has eliminated the risk for CK disease and reduced the risk of antibody formation during treatment.

Abuzzahabab MJ, Schneider A, Goddard A, et al: IGF-I receptor mutations resulting in intrauterine and postnatal growth retardation. *N Engl J Med* 2003;349:2211–2222.

Allen DB, Fost N: hGH for short stature: ethical issues raised by expanded access. *J Pediatr* 2004;144:648–652.

Amar AP, Weiss MH: Pituitary anatomy and physiology. *Neurosurg Clin North Am* 2003;14(1):11–23.

Badaru A, Wilson DM: Alternatives to growth hormone stimulation testing in children. *Trends Endocrinol Metab* 2004;15(6):252–258.

Besson A, Salemi S, Deladoey J, et al: Short stature caused by a biologically inactive mutant growth hormone. *J Clin Endocrinol Metab* 2005;90:2493–2499.

Carel JC, Ecosse E, Nicolino M, et al: Adult height after long term treatment with recombinant growth hormone for idiopathic isolated growth hormone deficiency: Observational follow up of the French population based registry. *Br Med J* 2002;25:70–73.

Committee on Drugs and Committee on Bioethics: Considerations related to the use of recombinant human growth hormone in children. *Pediatrics* 1997;99:122–129.

Dattani MT: Growth hormone deficiency and combined pituitary hormone deficiency: Does the genotype matter? *Clin Endocrinol* 2005;63:121–130.

Dattani MT, Preece M: Growth hormone deficiency and related disorders: Insights into causation, diagnosis, and treatment. *Lancet* 2004;363: 1977–1986.

Domene HM, Bengolea SV, Martinez AS, et al: Deficiency of the circulating insulin-like growth factor system associated with inactivation of the acid-labile subunit gene. *N Engl J Med* 2004;350:570–577.

Finkelstein BS, Imperiale TF, Speroff T, et al: Effect of growth hormone therapy on height in children with idiopathic short stature. *Arch Pediatr Adolesc Med* 2002;156:230–240.

Growth Hormone Research Society: Consensus guidelines for the diagnosis and treatment of growth hormone (GH) deficiency in childhood and adolescence: Summary statement of the GH Research Society. *J Clin Endocrinol Metab* 2000;85:3990–3993.

Hwa V, Little B, Adiyaman P, et al: Severe growth hormone insensitivity resulting from total absence of signal transducer and activator of transcription 5b. *J Clin Endocrinol Metab* 2005;90:4260–4266.

Kofoed EM, Hwa V, Little B, et al: Growth hormone insensitivity associated with a *STAT5b* mutation. *N Engl J Med* 2003;349:1139–1147.

Kojima M, Hosoda H, Date Y, et al: Grhelin is a growth-hormone releasing acylated peptide from stomach. *Nature* 1999;402:656–660.

Leschek EW, Rose SR, Yanovski JA, et al: Effect of growth hormone treatment on adult height in peripubertal children with idiopathic short stature: A randomized, double-blind, placebo-controlled trial. *J Clin Endocrinol Metab* 2004;89:3140–3148.

Rosenfeld RG, Rosenbloom AL, Guevara-Aguirre J: Growth hormone (GH) insensitivity due to primary GH receptor deficiency. *Endocrinol Rev* 1994;15:369–390.

Schmiegelow M, Lassen S, Weber L, et al: Dosimetry and growth hormone deficiency following cranial irradiation of childhood brain tumors. *Med Pediatr Oncol* 1999;33:564–571.

Traggiai C, Stanhope R: Endocrinopathies associated with midline cerebral and cranial malformations. *J Pediatr* 2002;140:252–255.

Woods KA, Camacho-Hubner C, Savage MO, et al: Intrauterine growth retardation and postnatal growth failure associated with deletion of the insulin-like growth factor gene. *N Engl J Med* 1996;35:1363–1367.

Yanovski JA, Rose SR, Municchi G, et al: Treatment with luteinizing hormone-releasing hormone agonist in adolescents with short stature. *N Engl J Med* 2003;348:908–917.

Chapter 559 ■ Diabetes Insipidus

David T. Breault and Joseph A. Majzoub

Diabetes insipidus (DI) presents clinically with polyuria and polydipsia and may result from either vasopressin deficiency (central DI) or vasopressin insensitivity at the level of the kidney (nephrogenic DI). Both central DI and nephrogenic DI can arise from inherited defects of congenital or neonatal onset or can be secondary to a variety of causes (Table 559-1).

TABLE 559-1. Differential Diagnosis of Polyuria and Polydipsia

DIABETES INSIPIDUS (DI)
Central DI
Genetic (autosomal dominant)
Acquired
Trauma (surgical or accidental)
Congenital malformations
Neoplasms
Infiltrative, autoimmune, and infectious diseases
Drugs
Nephrogenic DI
Genetic (X-linked, autosomal recessive, autosomal dominant)
Acquired
Hypercalcemia, hypokalemia
Drugs
Kidney disease
PRIMARY POLYDIPSIA
DIABETES MELLITUS

PHYSIOLOGY OF WATER BALANCE

The control of extracellular tonicity (osmolality) and volume within a narrow range is critical for normal cellular structure and function (see Chapter 52). Extracellular fluid tonicity is regulated almost exclusively by water intake and excretion, whereas extracellular volume is regulated by sodium intake and excretion. The control of plasma tonicity and intravascular volume involves a complex integration of endocrine, neural, behavioral, and paracrine systems (Fig. 559-1). Vasopressin, secreted from the posterior pituitary, is the principal regulator of tonicity, with its release largely stimulated by increases in plasma tonicity. Volume homeostasis is largely regulated by the renin-angiotensin-aldosterone system, with contributions from both vasopressin and the natriuretic peptide family.

Vasopressin, a 9-amino-acid peptide, has both antidiuretic and vascular pressor activity and is synthesized in the paraventricular and supraoptic nuclei of the hypothalamus. It is transported to the posterior pituitary via axonal projections, where it is stored awaiting release into the systemic circulation. The half-life of vasopressin in the circulation is 5 min. In addition to responding to osmotic stimuli, vasopressin is secreted in response to significant decreases in intravascular volume and pressure (minimum of 8% decrement) via afferent baroreceptor pathways arising from the aortic arch (carotid sinus) and volume receptor pathways in the cardiac atria and pulmonary veins. Osmotic and hemodynamic stimuli interact synergistically.

The sensation of thirst is regulated by cortical as well as hypothalamic neurons. The thirst threshold is approximately 10 mOsm/kg higher (~293 mOsm/kg) than the osmotic threshold for vasopressin release. Therefore, under conditions of hyperosmolality, vasopressin is released prior to the initiation of thirst, allowing for retention of ingested water. Chemoreceptors present in the oropharynx rapidly down-regulate vasopressin release following water ingestion.

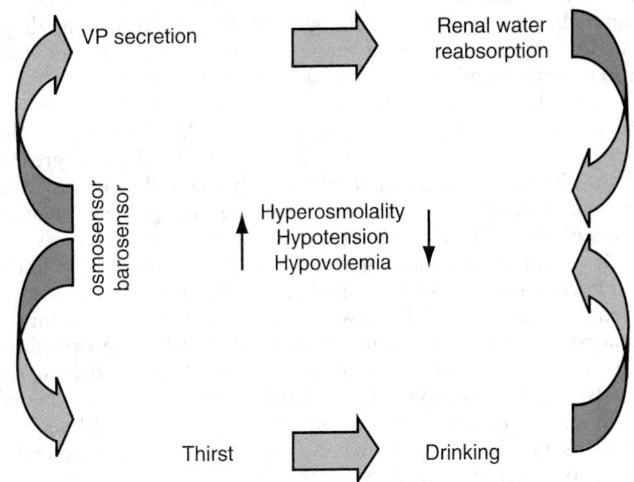

Figure 559-1. Regulation of vasopressin secretion and serum osmolality. Hyperosmolality, hypovolemia, and hypotension are sensed by osmosensors, volume sensors, and barosensors, respectively. These stimulate both vasopressin (VP) secretion and thirst. Vasopressin, acting on the kidney, causes increased reabsorption of water (antidiuresis). Thirst causes increased water ingestion. The results of these dual negative feedback loops cause a reduction in hyperosmolality or hypotension/hypovolemia. Additional stimuli for vasopressin secretion include nausea, hypoglycemia, and pain. (From Muglia LJ, Majzoub JA: Disorders of the posterior pituitary. In Sperling MA (editor): *Pediatric Endocrinology*, 2nd ed. Philadelphia, WB Saunders, 2002.)

Vasopressin exerts its principal effect on the kidney via V2 receptors located primarily in the collecting tubule, the thick ascending limb of the loop of Henle, and the peri-glomerular tubules. The human V2 receptor gene is located on the long arm of the X chromosome (Xq28) at the locus associated with **congenital, X-linked, vasopressin-resistant diabetes insipidus.** Activation of the V2 receptor results in increases in intracellular cyclic adenosine monophosphate, which leads to the insertion of the aquaporin-2 water channel into the apical (luminal) membrane. This allows water movement along its osmotic gradient into the hypertonic inner medullary interstitium from the tubule lumen and excretion of concentrated urine. In contrast to aquaporin-2, aquaporins-3 and -4 are expressed on the basolateral membrane of the collecting duct cells and aquaporin-1 is expressed in the proximal tubule. These channels may also contribute to urinary concentrating ability.

Atrial natriuretic peptide (ANP), initially isolated from cardiac atrial muscle, has a number of important effects on salt and water balance, including stimulation of natriuresis, inhibition of sodium resorption, and inhibition of vasopressin secretion. ANP is expressed in endothelial cells and vascular smooth muscle, where it appears to regulate relaxation of arterial smooth muscle. ANP is also expressed in the brain, along with other natriuretic family members; the physiologic role of these factors has yet to be defined.

APPROACH TO THE PATIENT WITH POLYURIA, POLYDIPSIA, AND HYPERNATREMIA

The cause of pathologic polyuria or polydipsia (exceeding 2 L/m^2/24 hr) may be difficult to establish in children. Infants may present with irritability, failure to thrive, and intermittent fever. Patients with suspected DI should have a careful history taken, which should quantify the child's daily fluid intake and output and establish the voiding pattern, nocturia, and primary or secondary enuresis. A complete physical examination should establish the patient's hydration status, and the physician should search for evidence of visual and central nervous system dysfunction as well as other pituitary hormone deficiencies.

If pathologic polyuria or polydipsia is present, the following should be obtained: serum for osmolality, sodium, potassium, blood urea nitrogen, creatinine, glucose, and calcium; urine for osmolality, specific gravity, and glucose determination. The diagnosis of DI is established if the serum osmolality is greater than 300 mOsm/kg and the urine osmolality is less than 300 mOsm/kg. DI is unlikely if the serum osmolality is less than 270 mOsm/kg or the urine osmolality is greater than 600 mOsm/kg. If the patient's serum osmolality is less than 300 mOsm/kg (but greater than 270 mOsm/kg) and pathologic polyuria and polydipsia are present, a water deprivation test is indicated to establish the diagnosis of DI and to differentiate central from nephrogenic causes.

In the inpatient post-neurosurgical setting, central DI is likely if hyperosmolality (serum osmolality >300 mOsm/kg) is associated with urine osmolality less than serum osmolality. It is important to distinguish between polyuria resulting from postsurgical central DI and polyuria resulting from the normal diuresis of fluids received intraoperatively. Both cases may be associated with a large volume (>200 mL/m^2/h) of dilute urine, although in patients with DI, the serum osmolality is high in comparison with patients undergoing postoperative diuresis.

559.1 • Causes of Hypernatremia (See Chapter 52.3)

CENTRAL DIABETES INSIPIDUS

Central diabetes insipidus can result from multiple etiologies, including genetic mutations in the vasopressin gene; trauma (accidental or surgical) to vasopressin neurons; congenital malformations of the hypothalamus or pituitary; neoplasms; infiltrative, autoimmune, and infectious diseases affecting vasopressin neurons or fiber tracts; and increased metabolism of vasopressin. In approximately 10% of children with central DI, the etiology is idiopathic. Other pituitary hormone deficiencies may be present (see Chapter 558).

Autosomal dominant central DI usually presents within the first 5 yr of life and results from mutations in the vasopressin gene. A number of mutations can cause gene-processing defects in a subset of vasopressin-expressing neurons. **Wolfram syndrome,** which includes DI, diabetes mellitus, optic atrophy, and deafness, also results in vasopressin deficiency. The gene for this disorder has been identified, but its function is unknown. Congenital brain abnormalities such as **septo-optic dysplasia** with agenesis of the corpus callosum, the Kabuki syndrome, holoprosencephaly, and familial pituitary hypoplasia with absent stalk may be associated with central DI and defects in thirst perception. Empty sella syndrome, possibly due to unrecognized pituitary infarction, can be associated with DI in children.

Trauma (to the base of the brain) and neurosurgical intervention (in the region of the hypothalamus or pituitary) are common causes of central DI. The **triphasic response** following surgery refers to an initial phase of transient DI, lasting 12–48 hr, followed by a 2nd phase of syndrome of inappropriate antidiuretic hormone secretion, lasting up to 10 days, which may be followed by permanent DI. The initial phase may be the result of local edema interfering with normal vasopressin secretion; the 2nd phase results from unregulated vasopressin release from dying neurons, whereas in the 3rd phase, permanent DI results if more than 90% of the neurons have been destroyed.

Given the anatomic distribution of vasopressin neurons over a large area within the hypothalamus, tumors that cause DI must either be very large and infiltrative or be strategically located near the base of the hypothalamus, where vasopressin axons converge before their entry into the posterior pituitary. Germinomas and pinealomas typically arise in this region and are among the most common primary brain tumors associated with DI. Germinomas can be very small and undetectable by MRI for several yr following the onset of polyuria. Quantitative measurement of the β–subunit of human chorionic gonadotropin, often secreted by germinomas and pinealomas, should be performed in children with idiopathic or unexplained DI in addition to serial MRI scans. Craniopharyngiomas and optic gliomas can also cause central DI when very large, although this is more often a postoperative complication of the treatment for these tumors. Hematologic malignancies, as with acute myelocytic leukemia, can cause DI via infiltration of the pituitary stalk and sella.

Langerhans cell histiocytosis and lymphocytic hypophysitis are common types of infiltrative disorders causing central DI, with **hypophysitis** as the cause in 50% of cases of "idiopathic" central DI. Infections involving the base of the brain, including meningitis (meningococcal, cryptococcal, listerial, toxoplasmal), congenital cytomegalovirus infection, and nonspecific inflammatory diseases of the brain may give rise to central DI that is often transient. Drugs associated with the inhibition of vasopressin release include ethanol, phenytoin, opiate antagonists, halothane, and α-adrenergic agents.

NEPHROGENIC DIABETES INSIPIDUS

Nephrogenic (vasopressin-insensitive) DI (NDI) can result from genetic or acquired causes. Genetic causes are less common but more severe than acquired forms of NDI. The polyuria and polydipsia associated with genetic NDI usually presents within the first several wk of life but may only become apparent after weaning or with longer periods of nighttime sleep. Many infants initially present with fever, vomiting, and dehydration. Failure to thrive may be secondary to the ingestion of large amounts of water, resulting in caloric malnutrition. Long-standing ingestion and excretion of large volumes of water may lead to nonobstructive hydronephrosis, hydroureter, and megabladder.

Congenital X-linked NDI results from inactivating mutations of the vasopressin V2 receptor. **Congenital autosomal recessive NDI** results from defects in the aquaporin-2 gene. An **autosomal dominant form of NDI** is associated with processing mutations of the aquaporin-2 gene.

Acquired nephrogenic DI may result from hypercalcemia or hypokalemia and is associated with the following drugs: lithium, demeclocycline, foscarnet, clozapine, amphotericin, methicillin, and rifampin. Impaired renal concentrating ability can also be seen with ureteral obstruction, chronic renal failure, polycystic kidney disease, medullary cystic disease, Sjögren syndrome, and sickle cell disease. Decreased protein or sodium intake or excessive water intake, as in primary polydipsia, can lead to diminished tonicity of the renal medullary interstitium and nephrogenic DI.

TREATMENT OF CENTRAL DIABETES INSIPIDUS

FLUID THERAPY. With an intact thirst mechanism and free access to oral fluids, a person with complete DI can maintain plasma osmolality and sodium in the high normal range, although at great inconvenience. Neonates and young infants are often best treated solely with fluid therapy, given their requirement for large volumes (3 L/m^2/24 hr) of nutritive fluid. The use of vasopressin analogs in patients with obligate high fluid intake is contraindicated given the risk of life-threatening hyponatremia.

Vasopressin Analogs. Treatment of central DI in older children is best accomplished with the use of the long-acting vasopressin analog dDAVP (desmopressin). dDAVP is available in an intranasal preparation (onset 5–10 min) and as tablets (onset 15–30 min). The intranasal preparation of dDAVP (10 µg/0.1 mL) can be administered by rhinal tube (allowing dose titration) or by nasal spray. The appropriate dose is determined empirically based on the desired length of antidiuresis. The nasal spray delivers 10 µg (0.1 mL) per spray and is the standard preparation used for treatment of primary enuresis in older children. Use of dDAVP in the treatment of enuresis is a temporizing measure because it does not affect the underlying condition, and it should be used with caution. To prevent water intoxication, patients should have at least 1 hr of urinary breakthrough between doses each day. dDAVP tablets are available but require at least a 10-fold increase in the dose compared with the intranasal preparation. Oral doses of 25–300 µg every 8–12 hr are safe and effective in children.

Aqueous Vasopressin. Central DI of acute onset following neurosurgery is best managed with continuous administration of synthetic aqueous vasopressin (pitressin). Under most circumstances, total fluid intake must be limited to 1 L/m^2/24 hr during antidiuresis. A typical dose for intravenous vasopressin therapy is 1.5 mU/kg/h, which results in a blood vasopressin concentration of approximately 10 pg/mL. On occasion, following hypothalamic (but not transsphenoidal) surgery, higher initial concentrations of vasopressin may be required to treat acute DI, which has been attributed to the release of a vasopressin inhibitory substance. Vasopressin concentrations greater than 1,000 pg/mL should be avoided because they may cause cutaneous necrosis, rhabdomyolysis, and cardiac rhythm disturbances. Post-neurosurgical patients treated with vasopressin infusion should be switched from intravenous to oral fluids as soon as possible to allow thirst sensation, if intact, to help regulate osmolality.

TREATMENT OF NEPHROGENIC DIABETES INSIPIDUS

The treatment of acquired NDI focuses on elimination, if possible, of the underlying disorder, such as offending drugs, hypercalcemia, hypokalemia, or ureteral obstruction. Congenital nephrogenic diabetes insipidus is often difficult to treat. The main goals are to ensure the intake of adequate calories for growth and to avoid severe dehydration. Foods with the highest ratio of caloric content to osmotic load (Na <1 mmol/kg/24 hr) should be ingested to maximize growth and to minimize the urine volume required to excrete the solute load. Even with the early institution of therapy, however, growth failure and mental retardation are common.

Pharmacologic approaches to the treatment of NDI include the use of thiazide diuretics and are intended to decrease the overall urine output. Thiazides appear to induce a state of mild volume depletion by enhancing sodium excretion at the expense of water and by causing a decrease in the glomerular filtration rate, which results in proximal tubular sodium and water reabsorption. Indomethacin and amiloride may be used in combination with thiazides to further reduce polyuria. High-dose dDAVP therapy, in combination with indomethacin, has been used in some subjects with NDI. This treatment may prove useful in patients with genetic defects in the V2 receptor associated with a reduced binding affinity for vasopressin.

Knoers N, Monnens LH: Nephrogenic diabetes insipidus: Clinical symptoms, pathogenesis, genetics and treatment. *Pediatr Nephrol* 1992; 6:476–482.

Maghnie M, Cosi G, Genovese E, et al: Central diabetes insipidus in children and young adults. *N Engl J Med* 2000; 343:988–1007.

Muglia LJ, Majzoub JA: Disorders of the posterior pituitary. In Sperling MA (editor): *Pediatric Endocrinology*, 2nd ed. Philadelphia, WB Saunders, 2002.

Chapter 560 ■ Other Abnormalities of Arginine Vasopressin Metabolism and Action

David T. Breault and Joseph A. Majzoub

Hyponatremia (serum sodium <130 mEq/L) in children is usually associated with severe systemic disorders and is most often due to (1) intravascular volume depletion, (2) excessive salt loss, or (3) hypotonic fluid overload, especially in infants (see Chapter 52). The syndrome of inappropriate antidiuretic hormone (SIADH) is an uncommon cause of hyponatremia in children.

The initial approach to the patient with hyponatremia begins with determination of the volume status. A careful review of the patient's history, physical examination, including changes in weight, and vital signs helps determine whether the patient is hypovolemic or hypervolemic. Supportive evidence includes laboratory data such as serum electrolytes, blood urea nitrogen, creatinine, uric acid, urine sodium, specific gravity, and osmolality (see Chapter 52.3) (Tables 560-1 and 560-2).

CAUSES OF HYPONATREMIA

SYNDROME OF INAPPROPRIATE ANTIDIURETIC HORMONE SECRETION. SIADH is characterized by hyponatremia, an inappropriately concentrated urine (>100 mOsm/kg), normal or slightly elevated plasma volume, normal-to-high urine sodium, and low serum uric acid. SIADH is uncommon in children, with most cases resulting from excessive administration of vasopressin in the treatment of central diabetes insipidus. It can also occur with encephalitis, with brain tumors, with head trauma, with psychiatric disease, in the postictal period after generalized seizures, after prolonged nausea, with pneumonia, with tuberculous

TABLE 560-1. Differential Diagnosis of Hyponatremia

DISORDER	INTRAVASCULAR VOLUME STATUS	URINE SODIUM
Systemic dehydration	Low	Low
Decreased effective plasma volume	Low	Low
Primary salt loss	Low	Low
Cerebral salt wasting	Low	Very high
SIADH	High	High
Decreased free water clearance	Normal or high	Normal or high
Primary polydipsia	Normal or high	Normal
Runners' hyponatremia	Low	Low
NSIAD	High	High
Pseudohyponatremia	Normal	Normal
Factitious hyponatremia	Normal	Normal

NSIAD, nephrogenic syndrome of inappropriate antidiuresis; SIADH, syndrome of inappropriate antidiuretic hormone secretion.

meningitis, and with AIDS. SIADH is the cause of the hyponatremic second phase of the triphasic response seen after hypothalamic-pituitary surgery (see Chapter 559). It is found in up to 35% of patients 1 wk after surgery and may result from retrograde neuronal degeneration with cell death and vasopressin release. Common drugs that have been shown to increase vasopressin secretion or mimic vasopressin action, resulting in hyponatremia, include oxcarbazepine, carbamazepine, chlorpropamide, vinblastine, vincristine, and tricyclic antidepressants.

NEPHROGENIC SYNDROME OF INAPPROPRIATE ANTIDIURESIS (NSIAD). Gain-of-function mutations in the V2 vasopressin receptor gene have been described in 2 male infants presenting with an SIADH-like clinical picture with undetectable vasopressin levels. Activating mutations in the aquaporin-2 gene might also give rise to the same syndrome but have not yet been described.

SYSTEMIC DEHYDRATION. The initial manifestation of systemic dehydration is often hypernatremia and hyperosmolality, which subsequently lead to the activation of vasopressin secretion and a decrease in water excretion. As dehydration progresses, hypovolemia and/or hypotension becomes a major stimulus for vasopressin release, further decreasing free water clearance. Excessive free water intake with ongoing salt losses may also produce hyponatremia. Urinary sodium excretion is low (usually <10 mEq/L) owing to a low glomerular filtration rate and concomitant activation of the renin-angiotensin-aldosterone system, unless primary renal disease or diuretic therapy is present.

PRIMARY SALT LOSS. Hyponatremia can result from the primary loss of sodium chloride as seen in specific disorders of the kidney (congenital polycystic kidney disease, acute interstitial nephritis, chronic renal failure), gastrointestinal tract, (gastroenteritis), and sweat glands (cystic fibrosis). The hyponatremia is not solely due to the salt loss, because the latter also causes hypovolemia, leading to an increase in vasopressin. Mineralocorticoid deficiency, pseudohypoaldosteronism (sometimes seen in children with urinary tract obstruction or infection), and diuretics can also result in loss of sodium chloride.

TABLE 560-2. Clinical Parameters to Distinguish Between SIADH, Cerebral Salt Wasting, and Central Diabetes Insipidus

CLINICAL PARAMETER	SIADH	CEREBRAL SALT WASTING	CENTRAL DI
Serum sodium	Low	Low	High
Urine output	Normal or low	High	High
Urine sodium	High	Very high	Low
Intravascular volume status	Normal or high	Low	Low
Serum uric acid	Low	Normal or high	High
Vasopressin level	High	Low	Low

DECREASED EFFECTIVE PLASMA VOLUME. Hyponatremia can result from decreased effective plasma volume, as found in congestive heart failure, cirrhosis, nephrotic syndrome, positive pressure mechanical ventilation, severe burns, bronchopulmonary dysplasia in neonates, cystic fibrosis with obstruction, and severe asthma. The resulting decrease in cardiac output leads to reduced water and salt excretion, as with systemic dehydration, and an increase in vasopressin secretion. In patients with impaired cardiac output and elevated atrial volume (congestive heart failure, lung disease), atrial natriuretic peptide concentrations are elevated further, leading to hyponatremia by promoting natriuresis. These patients usually have a very low urinary excretion of sodium. Unlike dehydrated patients, these patients may have excess total body sodium from activation of the renin-angiotensin-aldosterone system and may demonstrate peripheral edema as well.

PRIMARY POLYDIPSIA (INCREASED WATER INGESTION). In patients with normal renal function, the kidney can excrete dilute urine with an osmolality as low as 50 mOsm/kg. To excrete a daily solute load of 500 mOsm/m^2, the kidney must produce 10 L/m^2 of urine per day. Therefore, to avoid hyponatremia, the maximum amount of water an individual with normal renal function can consume is 10 L/m^2. Neonates, however, cannot dilute their urine to this degree, putting them at risk for water intoxication if water intake exceeds 4 L/m^2/day (approximately 60 mL/h in a newborn). Many infants develop transient but symptomatic hyponatremic seizures after being fed pure water without electrolytes rather than breast milk or formula.

DECREASED FREE WATER CLEARANCE. Hyponatremia due to decreased renal free water clearance, even in the absence of an increase in vasopressin secretion, can result from adrenal insufficiency or thyroid deficiency or can be related to a direct effect of drugs on the kidney. Both mineralocorticoids and glucocorticoids are required for normal free water clearance in a vasopressin-independent manner. In patients with unexplained hyponatremia, adrenal and thyroid insufficiency should be considered. In addition, patients with coexisting adrenal failure and diabetes insipidus may have no symptoms of the latter until glucocorticoid therapy unmasks the need for vasopressin replacement. Certain drugs may inhibit renal water excretion through direct effects on the nephron, thus causing hyponatremia; these drugs include high-dose cyclophosphamide, vinblastine, cis-platinum, and carbamazepine.

CEREBRAL SALT WASTING. Cerebral salt wasting appears to be the result of hypersecretion of atrial natriuretic peptide and is seen primarily with central nervous system disorders including brain tumors, head trauma, hydrocephalus, neurosurgery, cerebral vascular accidents, and brain death. Hyponatremia is accompanied by elevated urinary sodium excretion (often >150 mEq/L), excessive urine output, hypovolemia, normal or high uric acid, suppressed vasopressin, and elevated atrial natriuretic peptide concentrations (>20 pmol/L). Thus, it is distinguished from SIADH, in which normal or decreased urine output, euvolemia, low uric acid, only modestly elevated urine sodium concentration, and an elevated vasopressin level occur. The distinction between cerebral salt wasting and SIADH is important because the treatment of the two disorders differs markedly.

RUNNERS' HYPONATREMIA. Excess fluid ingestion during long distance running (marathon running) can result in severe hyponatremia due to hypovolemia-induced activation of AVP secretion coupled with excessive water ingestion and is correlated with weight gain, long racing time, and extremes of body mass index.

PSEUDOHYPONATREMIA AND OTHER CAUSES OF HYPONATREMIA. Pseudohyponatremia may result from hypertriglyceridemia (see

Chapter 52). Elevated lipid levels result in a relative decrease in serum water content. As electrolytes are dissolved in the aqueous phase of the serum, they appear low when expressed as a fraction of the total serum volume. As a fraction of serum water, however, electrolyte content is normal. Factitious hyponatremia can result from obtaining a blood sample proximal to the site of intravenous hypotonic fluid infusion.

Hyponatremia is also associated with hyperglycemia, which causes the influx of water into the intravascular space. Serum sodium decreases by 1.6 mEq/L for every 100 mg/dL increment in blood glucose greater than 100 mg/dL. Glucose is not ordinarily an osmotically active agent and does not stimulate vasopressin release, probably because it is able to equilibrate freely across plasma membranes. In the presence of insulin deficiency and hyperglycemia, however, glucose acts as an osmotic agent, presumably because its normal intracellular access to osmosensor sites is prevented. Under these circumstances, an osmotic gradient exists, stimulating vasopressin release.

TREATMENT OF HYPONATREMIA

Patients with systemic dehydration and hypovolemia should be rehydrated with salt-containing fluids such as normal saline or lactated Ringer solution. Because of activation of the renin-angiotensin-aldosterone system, the administered sodium is avidly conserved, and water diuresis quickly ensues as volume is restored and vasopressin concentrations decrease. Under these conditions, caution must be taken to prevent too rapid a correction of hyponatremia, which may result in central pontine myelinolysis characterized by discrete regions of axonal demyelination and the potential for irreversible brain damage.

Hyponatremia due to a decrease in effective plasma volume caused by cardiac, hepatic, renal, or pulmonary dysfunction is more difficult to reverse. The most effective therapy is the least easily achieved: treatment of the underlying systemic disorder. For example, patients weaned from positive pressure ventilation undergo a prompt water diuresis and resolution of hyponatremia as cardiac output is restored and vasopressin concentrations decrease.

Patients with hyponatremia due to primary salt loss require supplementation with sodium chloride and fluids. Initially, intravenous replacement of urine volume with fluid containing sodium chloride, 150–450 mEq/L depending on the degree of salt loss, may be necessary; oral salt supplementation may be required subsequently. This treatment contrasts with that of SIADH, in which water restriction without sodium supplementation is the mainstay.

EMERGENCY TREATMENT OF HYPONATREMIA. The development of acute hyponatremia (onset <12 hr) or a serum sodium concentration less than 120 mEq/L may be associated with lethargy, psychosis, coma, or generalized seizures, especially in younger children. Acute hyponatremia can cause cell swelling and lead to neuronal dysfunction or to cerebral herniation. The emergency treatment of cerebral dysfunction resulting from acute hyponatremia includes water restriction and may require rapid correction with hypertonic 3% sodium chloride. If hypertonic saline treatment is undertaken, the serum sodium should be raised only high enough to cause an improvement in mental status, and in no case faster than 0.5 mEq/L/hr or 12 mEq/L/24 hr.

TREATMENT OF SIADH. Chronic SIADH is best treated by oral fluid restriction. With full antidiuresis (urine osmolality of 1,000 mOsm/kg), a normal daily obligate renal solute load of 500 mOsm/m^2 would be excreted in 500 mL/m^2 water. This, plus a daily nonrenal water loss of 500 mL/m^2, would require that oral fluid intake be limited to 1,000 mL/m^2/24 hr to avoid hyponatremia. In young children, this degree of fluid restriction may not provide adequate calories for growth. In this situation, the creation of nephrogenic diabetes insipidus using demeclocycline therapy may be indicated to allow sufficient fluid intake for normal growth. Conivaptan, a V_2-receptor antagonist, decreases permeability of the collecting duct to water producing an aquaresis. It has been effective in treating SIADH in adults.

TREATMENT OF CEREBRAL SALT WASTING. Treatment of patients with cerebral salt wasting consists of restoring intravascular volume with sodium chloride and water, as for the treatment of other causes of systemic dehydration. The underlying cause of the disorder, which is usually due to acute brain injury, should also be treated if possible. Treatment involves the ongoing replacement of urine sodium losses (volume for volume).

Albanese A, Hindmarsh P, Stanhope R: Management of hyponatremia in patients with acute cerebral insults. *Arch Dis Child* 2001;85:246–251.

Almond CS, Shin AY, Fortescue EB, et al: Hyponatremia among runners in the Boston Marathon. *N Engl J Med* 2005;352:1550–1556.

Feldman BJ, Rosenthal SM, Vargas GA, et al: Nephrogenic syndrome of inappropriate antidiuresis. *N Engl J Med* 2005; 352:1884–1890.

The Medical Letter: Conivaptan (Vaprisol) for hyponatremia. *Med Lett* 2006;48:51–52.

Muglia LJ, Majzoub JA: Disorders of the posterior pituitary. In Sperling MA (editor): *Pediatric Endocrinology*, 2nd ed. Philadelphia, WB Saunders, 2002.

Chapter 561 ■ Hyperpituitarism, Tall Stature, and Overgrowth Syndromes

Pinchas Cohen and Melanie Shim

HYPERPITUITARISM

Primary hypersecretion of pituitary hormones occurs rarely in children. When it does, it usually occurs as a result of a pituitary adenoma. Primary hyperpituitarism should not be confused with **secondary hyperpituitarism,** which occurs in the setting of target hormone deficiencies resulting in decreased hormonal feedback, such as in hypogonadism, hypoadrenalism, or hypothyroidism. In some cases, long-standing hormonal hypersecretion is accompanied by sufficient hyperplasia of the pituitary to produce sellar enlargement, erosion, and rarely, increased intracranial pressure. The elevated pituitary hormone levels readily suppress to normal following replacement of end-organ hormones. Pituitary hyperplasia can also occur in response to stimulation by ectopic production of releasing hormones such as that seen occasionally in patients with Cushing syndrome secondary to corticotropin-releasing hormone excess or in children with acromegaly secondary to growth hormone–releasing hormone (GHRH) produced by a variety of systemic tumors.

The most frequently seen adenoma during childhood is the prolactinoma, followed by corticotropinoma and then somatotropinoma, which secrete prolactin, corticotropin, and growth hormone, respectively. There have been several case reports of thyrotropinoma in children. There are no pediatric reports of gonadotropinoma. The monoclonal nature of most pituitary adenomas has implied that most originate from a clonal event in a single cell. It is suspected that some pituitary tumors may result from stimulation with hypothalamic-releasing hormones and in other instances, as in McCune-Albright syndrome, the tumor is caused by constitutive activating mutation of the G-protein $G_s\alpha$

gene. The clinical presentation typically depends on the pituitary hormone that is hypersecreted. Disruption of growth regulation and/or sexual maturation is common, as a result of either hormone hypersecretion or local compression by the tumor.

TALL STATURE

The normal distribution of height predicts that 2.5% of the population will be taller than 2 SD (97.5%) above the mean. However, the social acceptability and even desirability of tallness (heightism), makes tall stature an uncommon complaint. In North America, it is extremely unusual for males to seek help regarding excessive height, although in Europe it is somewhat more common. Even in females, tall stature has become more socially acceptable although tall girls may still approach their physician with a desire to curb their growth rate.

DIFFERENTIAL DIAGNOSIS OF TALL STATURE. Table 561-1 lists the causes of tall stature in childhood and adolescence. Of these, the normal variant, familial or constitutional tall stature, is by far the most common cause. Almost invariably, a family history of tallness can be elicited, and no organic pathology is present. The child is often tall throughout childhood and enjoys excellent health. The parent of the constitutionally tall adolescent may reflect unhappily upon his or her own adolescence as a tall teenager. There are no abnormalities in the physical examination, and the laboratory studies, if obtained, are always negative.

Klinefelter syndrome (XXY syndrome) is a common (1 : 500–1000 live male births) abnormality associated with tall stature, mild mental retardation, gynecomastia, and decreased upper to lower body segment ratio. The testes are invariably small although androgen production by Leydig cells is often in the low-normal range. Spermatogenesis and Sertoli cell function are defective, and infertility results. **XYY syndrome** is associated with tall stature and possible behavioral and mental problems. **Marfan syndrome** is an autosomal dominant connective tissue disorder consisting of tall stature, increased arm span, and decreased upper to lower body segment ratio (see Chapter 700). Additional abnormalities include arachnodactyly, ocular abnormalities, and cardiac anomalies. **Homocystinuria** is an autosomal recessive inborn error of amino acid metabolism causing mental retardation when untreated, and many of its features resemble Marfan syndrome, particularly ocular manifestations (see Chapter 85). Hyperthyroidism in adolescents is associated with rapid growth but normal adult height. It is almost always caused by Graves disease and is much more common in females (see Chapter 569). Exogenous obesity is a common condition in adolescence and may be associated with rapid linear growth and early maturation; adult height is typically normal.

The purpose of the diagnostic evaluation of tall stature is to distinguish the commonly occurring normal variant constitutional variety from the rare pathologic conditions. Often, when the history is suggestive of familial tall stature and the physical examination is entirely normal, no laboratory tests are indicated. It is valuable to obtain a bone age radiograph to be able to predict adult height, which serves as a basis for discussions with the family and for management decisions. If, however, the history is suggestive for any of the above-mentioned disorders or the physical examination reveals abnormalities, additional laboratory tests should be obtained. Insulin-like growth factor-I (IGF-I) and IGF binding protein-3 (IGFBP-3) are excellent screening tests for GH excess and can be verified with a glucose suppression test. Laboratory evidence of GH excess mandates MRI evaluation of the pituitary. Chromosome analysis is useful in males, especially when the upper to lower body segment ratio is decreased or when mental retardation is present. If Marfan syndrome or homocystinuria is suspected from the physical examination, referral to a cardiologist and an ophthalmologist should be made. Thyroid function tests are useful to diagnose or rule out hyperthyroidism when this disorder is suspected.

Precocious puberty, whether mediated centrally (increased gonadotropin secretion) or peripherally (increased secretion of androgens, estrogens, or both), results initially in accelerated linear growth in childhood, mimicking the pubertal growth spurt. Because skeletal maturation is also accelerated, adult height is frequently compromised. The diagnostic evaluation and management of precocious puberty are discussed elsewhere in this book.

Although delayed puberty may be associated with short stature in childhood, as with constitutional delay, failure to eventually enter puberty and complete sexual maturation may result in sustained growth during adult life, with ultimate tall stature. The report of tall stature with open epiphyses resulting from a mutation of the estrogen receptor in a man with normal male sexual maturation underscores the fundamental role of estrogen in promoting epiphyseal fusion and termination of normal skeletal growth. Aromatase deficiency leads to tall stature through similar pathways. Furthermore, androgen insensitivity is associated with tall stature in girls, demonstrating a role for androgen in this process.

MANAGEMENT OF TALL STATURE. Reassurance of the family and the patients is the key to the management of normal-variant tall stature. The use of the bone age to predict adult height may provide some comfort, as will general supportive discussions on the social acceptability of this condition. While treatment is available for girls and boys with excessive growth, its use should be restricted to patients with (1) predicted adult height >3 SD above the mean (78 inches in males, 71 inches in females) and (2) evidence of significant psychosocial impairment. For the family that feels strongly about treatment, a trial of sex steroids may be considered. Such therapy is designed to accelerate puberty and epiphyseal fusion and is therefore of little benefit when given in late

TABLE 561-1. Differential Diagnosis of Tall Stature and Overgrowth Syndromes

FETAL OVERGROWTH
Maternal diabetes mellitus
Cerebral gigantism (Sotos syndrome)
Weaver syndrome
Beckwith-Wiedemann syndrome
Other IGF-II excess syndromes
POSTNATAL OVERGROWTH LEADING TO CHILDHOOD TALL STATURE
Familial (constitutional) tall stature
Cerebral gigantism
Beckwith-Wiedemann syndrome
Exogenous obesity
Excess GH secretion (pituitary gigantism)
McCune-Albright syndrome or MEN associated with excess GH secretion
Precocious puberty
Marfan syndrome
Klinefelter syndrome (XXY)
SHOX excess syndromes
Weaver syndrome
Fragile X syndrome
Homocystinuria
XYY
Hyperthyroidism
POSTNATAL OVERGROWTH LEADING TO ADULT TALL STATURE
Familial (constitutional) tall stature
Androgen or estrogen deficiency/estrogen resistance (in males)
Testicular feminization
ACTH/cortisol deficiency/resistance
Excess GH secretion (pituitary gigantism)
Marfan syndrome
Klinefelter syndrome (XXY)
XYY

ACTH, adrenocorticotropic hormone; GH, growth hormone; IGF, insulin-like growth factor.

puberty; therapy is initiated ideally prepubertally or in early puberty. In boys, treatment should begin before the bone age reaches 14 yr; testosterone enanthate is used at a dose of 500 mg IM every 2 wk for 6 mo. In females, oral estrogens in various doses have successfully reduced the predicted height by 5–10 cm on average. This is a direct result of the known effects of sex steroids on promoting epiphyseal fusion; therapy must begin, therefore, before the bone age has reached 12 yr. Oral ethinyl estradiol at a dose of 0.15–0.5 mg/day until cessation of growth occurs has been used successfully in girls. If necessary, a progestational agent can be added after 1 yr of unopposed estrogen. Short-term side effects of estrogen treatment for tall stature include menstrual irregularities, weight gain, nausea, limb pain, galactorrhea, benign breast disease, cholelithiasis, hypertension, and thrombosis. Reduced fertility later in life may be a potential long-term complication. The lack of extensive experience with this form of therapy and the risks involved should be carefully weighed and discussed with the family before embarking on therapy.

The mechanism of estrogen action involves effects on both GH and IGF production as well as its action on the epiphysis. Estrogen mediates epiphyseal fusion in both females and males. In prepubertal girls, adult height is reportedly decreased by as much as 5–6 cm relative to pretreatment predictions. When therapy is initiated after the onset of puberty, the decrement in adult height will not be so large.

Therapy in boys with tall stature is even more problematic. Estrogen is likely to be most efficacious in accelerating epiphyseal fusion but is obviously undesirable in boys. Androgens also accelerate skeletal maturation, presumably via aromatization, to estrogen but are associated with virilization.

PROLACTINOMA

Prolactin-secreting pituitary adenomas are the most common tumors of the pituitary in adolescents (see Chapter 497). With the advent of MRI, more of these tumors, particularly microadenomas (<1 cm), are being detected. The most common presenting manifestations are headache, amenorrhea, and galactorrhea. The disorder affects more than twice as many girls as boys; most patients have undergone normal puberty before becoming symptomatic. Only a few have delayed puberty. In some kindreds with type I multiple endocrine neoplasia (MEN), prolactinomas are the presenting feature during adolescence.

Prolactin levels may be moderately (40–50 ng/mL) or markedly (10,000–15,000 ng/mL) elevated. Most prolactinomas in children are large (macroadenomas), cause the sella to enlarge, and in some cases cause visual field defects. Approximately ⅓ of patients with macroadenomas develop hypopituitarism, particularly GH deficiency. Alternatively, prolactin-secreting adenomas may also stain for and secrete excess GH and/or TSH.

Prolactinomas should not be confused with the hyperprolactinemia and pituitary hyperplasia that may occur in patients with primary hypothyroidism, which is readily treated with thyroid hormone (see Chapter 556). Moderate elevations (<200 ng/mL) of prolactin are also associated with a variety of medications, with pituitary stalk dysfunction such as may occur with craniopharyngioma, and with other benign conditions. Treatment for most children has been surgical resection by transfrontal or transsphenoidal approach. Prolactinoma can also be effectively managed medically in most patients by treatment with bromocriptine or long-acting cabergoline. About 80% of adult patients respond with shrinkage of the tumor and marked decreases in serum prolactin levels.

CORTICOTROPINOMA

In pediatrics, corticotropinomas are the most common adenomas seen prepubertally although they occur at all ages. **Cushing's disease** refers specifically to an ACTH-producing pituitary adenoma that stimulates excess cortisol secretion. Adenomas causing Cushing's disease are significantly smaller than all other types of adenomas at presentation. The most sensitive indicator of excess glucocorticoid secretion in children is growth failure, which generally precedes other manifestations. Patients develop weight gain that tends to be centripetal rather than generalized. Pubertal arrest, fatigue, and depression are also common.

Transsphenoidal surgery is the treatment of choice for Cushing's disease in children. Initial remission rates of 70–98% of patients and long-term success rates of 50–98% have been reported. Residual transient hypoadrenalism is often observed after surgery, lasting as long as 30 months.

EXCESS GROWTH HORMONE SECRETION AND PITUITARY GIGANTISM

In young persons with open epiphyses, overproduction of GH results in **gigantism;** in persons with closed epiphyses, the result is **acromegaly.** Often, some acromegalic features are seen with gigantism, even in children and adolescents. After closure of the epiphyses, the acromegalic features become more prominent.

Pituitary gigantism is rare, and its cause is most often a pituitary adenoma, but gigantism has been observed in a 2.5 yr old boy with a hypothalamic tumor that presumably secreted GHRH. Other tumors, for example those that are part of the MEN syndromes, particularly in the pancreas, have produced acromegaly by secretion of large amounts of GHRH with resultant hyperplasia of the somatotrophs. The cardinal clinical feature of gigantism is longitudinal growth acceleration secondary to GH excess. The usual manifestations consist of coarse facial features and enlarging hands and feet. In young children, rapid growth of the head may precede linear growth. Some patients have behavioral and visual problems. In most of the recorded cases, the abnormal growth became evident at puberty, but the condition has been established as early as the newborn period in one child and at 21 mo of age in another. Giants have rarely been reported to grow to a height of over 8 ft. **Acromegalic features** consist chiefly of enlargement of the distal parts of the body, but manifestations of abnormal growth involve all portions. The circumference of the skull increases, the nose becomes broad, and the tongue is often enlarged, with coarsening of the facial features. The mandible grows excessively, and the teeth become separated. Visual field defects and neurologic abnormalities are common; signs of increased intracranial pressure appear later. The fingers and toes grow chiefly in thickness. There may be dorsal kyphosis. Fatigue and lassitude are early symptoms. GH levels are elevated and may occasionally exceed 100 ng/mL. There is usually no suppression of GH levels by the hyperglycemia of a glucose tolerance test. IGF-I and IGFBP-3 levels are consistently elevated in acromegaly, whereas other growth factors are not.

Gigantism is rare, with only several hundred reported cases to date. The presentation of gigantism is usually dramatic, unlike the insidious onset of acromegaly in adults. The tumor mass itself may cause headaches, visual changes due to optic nerve compression, and hypopituitarism. About ½ of the patients also have marked hyperprolactinemia as a result of plurihormonal adenomas that secrete GH and prolactin. This is due to the fact that mammosomatotrophs are the most common type of GH-secreting cells involved in childhood gigantism. GH-secreting tumors of the pituitary are typically eosinophilic or chromophobe adenomas. Adenomas may compromise other anterior pituitary function through growth or cystic degeneration. Secretion of gonadotropins, thyrotropin, or corticotropin may be impaired. Delayed sexual maturation or hypogonadism may occur. When GH hypersecretion is accompanied by gonadotropin deficiency, accelerated linear growth may persist for decades. In some cases, the tumor spreads outside the sella, invading the sphenoid bone, optic nerves, and brain. GH-secreting tumors in pediatric patients are more likely to be locally invasive or aggressive than are those in adults.

The etiology is uncertain although studies in acromegalics suggest that many cases result from mutations that generate constitutively activated G-proteins with reduced GTPase activity. The resultant increase in intracellular cyclic adenosine monophosphate in the pituitary leads to increased GH secretion. **McCune-Albright syndrome** (MAS), which can also be caused by mutations resulting in constitutively activated G-proteins, may also include the presence of somatotrophic tumors and excess GH secretion. Approximately 20% of patients with gigantism are those with MAS (commonly consisting of a triad of precocious puberty, café-au-lait spots, and fibrous dysplasia). GH-secreting tumors have also been reported in multiple endocrine adenomatosis and in association with neurofibromatosis, tuberous sclerosis, and Carney complex.

Activating mutations of the stimulatory $G_s\alpha$ proteins have been found in the pituitary lesions in MAS and are believed to be responsible for the other glandular adenomas observed in this condition as well. Somatic point mutations of the $G_s\alpha$ protein have also been identified in somatotrophs of up to 40% of sporadic GH-secreting pituitary adenomas.

DIAGNOSIS OF GROWTH HORMONE EXCESS. The gold standard for making the diagnosis of GH excess is the failure to suppress serum GH levels to less than 5 ng/dL after a 1.75 g/kg oral glucose challenge (maximum, 75 g). This test measures the ability of IGF-I to suppress GH secretion because the glucose load results in insulin secretion, leading to suppression of IGFBP-I, which results in an acute increase in free IGF-I levels. The increased free IGF-I suppresses GH secretion within 30–90 min. This test can be abnormal in diabetic patients. A single measurement of GH is inadequate because GH is secreted in a pulsatile manner. Therefore, the use of a random GH measurement can lead to both false-positive and false-negative results. Measurement of serum IGF-I concentration is a sensitive screening test for GH excess. An excellent linear dose-response correlation between serum IGF-I levels and 24-hr mean GH secretion has been demonstrated. An elevated IGF-I level in a patient with appropriate clinical suspicion is usually indicative of GH excess. Potential confusion may arise in the evaluation of normal adolescents, since significantly higher IGF-I levels occur during puberty than in adulthood; the IGF-I level must be age- and gender-matched. Serum IGFBP-3 levels are sensitive markers of GH elevations and may be elevated despite normal IGF-I levels. If laboratory findings suggest GH excess, the presence of a pituitary adenoma should be confirmed by MRI. In rare cases, a pituitary mass may not be identified. There may be an occult pituitary microadenoma or an ectopic tumor. CT is acceptable when MRI is unavailable.

TREATMENT OF GROWTH HORMONE OVERSECRETION. The goals of therapy are to remove or shrink the pituitary mass, to restore GH and secretory patterns to normal, to restore IGF-I and IGFBP-3 levels to normal, to retain the normal pituitary secretion of other hormones, and to prevent recurrence of disease.

For well-circumscribed pituitary adenomas, transsphenoidal surgery is the treatment of choice and may be curative. The tumor should be removed completely. The likelihood of surgical cure depends greatly on the surgeon's expertise as well as on the size and extension of the mass. Intraoperative GH measurements can improve the results of tumor resection. Transsphenoidal surgery to resect the tumors is as safe in children as in adults. At times, a transcranial approach may be necessary. The primary goal of treatment is to normalize GH levels. GH levels (<1 ng/mL within 2 hr after a glucose load) and serum IGF-I levels (age-adjusted normal range) are the best tests to define a biochemical cure.

If GH secretion is not normalized by surgery, the options include pituitary irradiation and medical therapy. Radiotherapy is recommended if GH hypersecretion is not normalized by surgery. Further growth of the tumor is prevented by irradiation in more than 99% of patients. The main disadvantage is the delayed efficacy in decreasing GH levels. GH is reduced by approximately 50% from the initial concentration by 2 yr, by 75% by 5 yr, and approaches 90% by 15 yr. Hypopituitarism is a predictable outcome, occurring in 40–50% of patients 10 yr after irradiation.

Surgery fails to cure a significant number of patients, and therefore medical therapy has an important role in the management of patients with GH excess. Treatment is effective and well tolerated with long-acting somatostatin analogs and dopamine agonists as well as by novel GH antagonists.

The **somatostatin analogs** are highly effective in the treatment of patients with GH excess. Octreotide suppresses GH to less than 2.5 ng/mL in 65% of patients with acromegaly and normalizes IGF-I levels in 70%. The effects of octreotide are well sustained over time. Tumor shrinkage also occurs with octreotide but is generally modest. Consistent GH suppression can be obtained with a continuous SC pump infusion of octreotide in a pubertal boy with pituitary gigantism. Long-acting formulations, including long-acting octreotide and lanreotide, produce consistent GH and IGF-I suppression in acromegalic patients with once monthly or biweekly IM depot injections. The sustained-release preparations have not been formally tested in children. Octreotide injection in the pediatric population has been used as doses of 1–40 µg/kg/24 hr.

For patients having both GH and prolactin oversecretion, dopamine agonists, such as **bromocriptine,** which bind to pituitary dopamine type 2 (D_2) receptors and suppress GH secretion, should be considered although their precise mechanism of action is unclear. Prolactin levels are often adequately suppressed; GH levels and IGF-I levels are rarely normalized with this treatment modality. Fewer than 20% of patients achieve GH levels below 5 ng/mL, and fewer than 10% achieve normalization of IGF-I levels. Tumor shrinkage occurs in a minority of patients. Bromocriptine is used as adjuvant medical treatment for GH excess. Its effectiveness may be additive to that of octreotide. Improved efficacy, defined by normal IGF-I concentration and reduced tumor size, also occurs with other dopamine agonists (pergolide, cabergoline). The dose of bromocriptine ranges from 10–60 mg/24 hr PO divided qid. However, only a minority of patients benefit from doses greater than 20 mg/24 hr. It has been found safe when used in children for an extended period of time, but side effects may include nausea, vomiting, abdominal pain, arrhythmias, nasal stuffiness, orthostatic hypotension, sleep disturbances, and fatigue. The dose of cabergoline is 0.25–1 mg PO 1–2 times/wk; a pediatric dose has not been established.

GH-receptor antagonists specifically block the activity of GH at its effector sites. **Pegvisomant** is an analog of GH that competes with endogenous GH for binding to the GH receptor. It effectively suppresses GH and IGF-I levels in patients with acromegaly due to pituitary tumors as well as ectopic GHRH hypersecretion. Normalization of IGF-I levels occurs in up to 90% of patients treated daily with this drug for 3 mo or longer. It has not been tested in children. The adult dose is 10–30 mg via subcutaneous injection once daily. Combined therapy with somatostatin analogs and weekly pegvisomant also is effective.

SOTOS SYNDROME (CEREBRAL GIGANTISM)

Children with cerebral gigantism (Sotos syndrome) are above the 90th percentile for both length and weight at birth; macrocrania may also be noted at that time. Sotos syndrome is caused by haploinsufficiency of the NSD1 gene (nuclear receptor SET

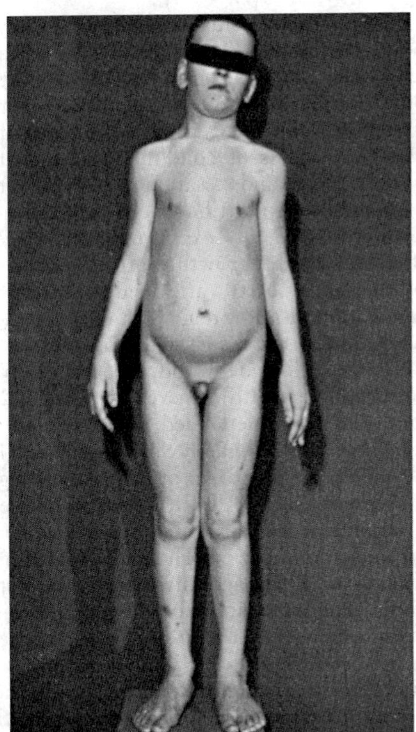

Figure 561-1. Cerebral gigantism in an 8-yr-old boy. The height age was 12 yr, and the bone age was 12 yr. IQ was 60. The electroencephalogram had abnormal findings. Note the prominence of the forehead and jaw and the large hands and feet. Sexual development was consistent with chronological age. Hormone study results were normal. The adult height was 208 cm (6 ft 10 in.); his sexual development was normal. He wears size 18 shoes.

domain–containing gene–1). Although it is characterized by rapid growth, there is no evidence that Sotos syndrome is an endocrine disorder. A hypothalamic defect has been suggested as a cause, but none has been demonstrated functionally or at necropsy. Growth is rapid, and by 1 yr of age, affected infants are greater than the 97th percentile in height. Accelerated growth continues for the first 4–5 yr and then returns to a normal rate (Fig. 561-1). Puberty usually occurs at the normal time but may occur slightly early. Adult height is usually in the upper normal range. The hands and feet are large, with thickened subcutaneous tissue. The head is large and dolichocephalic, the jaw is prominent, there is hypertelorism, and the eyes have an antimongoloid slant. Clumsiness and awkward gait are characteristic, and affected children have great difficulty in sports, in learning to ride a bicycle, and in other tasks requiring coordination. Some degree of mental retardation affects most patients; in some children, perceptual deficiencies may predominate. Osseous maturation is compatible with the patient's height. GH and IGF-I levels and results of other endocrine studies are usually normal; there are no distinctive laboratory or radiologic markers for the syndrome. Abnormal electroencephalograms are common; other studies frequently reveal a dilated ventricular system. Affected patients may be at increased risk for neoplasia; hepatic carcinoma and Wilms, ovarian, and parotid tumors have been reported.

OVERGROWTH IN THE FETUS

Maternal diabetes constitutes the most common cause of infants who are large for gestational age (LGA). Even in the absence of clinical symptoms or a family history, the birth of an excessively large infant should lead to evaluation for maternal (or gestational) diabetes.

A group of disorders associated with excessive somatic growth and growth of specific organs has been described and is collectively referred to as overgrowth syndromes. These disorders appear to be caused by excess availability of insulin-like growth factor-II (IGF-II) encoded by the gene *Igf2*. The best described of these syndromes is the **Beckwith-Wiedemann syndrome** (BWS), which is an overgrowth malformation syndrome that occurs with an incidence of 1 : 13,700 births. It manifests as a fetal overgrowth syndrome in which hypertrophy dominates the clinical picture. Typically, macroglossia, hepatosplenomegaly, nephromegaly, and hypoglycemia secondary to hyperinsulinemia due to pancreatic β-cell hyperplasia in an LGA baby make up the clinical picture at birth. These children are predisposed to a specific subset of childhood neoplasms, including Wilms tumor and adrenocortical carcinoma. Overexpression of IGF-II in BWS may be caused by a number of genetic disruptions including gene duplication, loss of heterozygosity, and relaxation or loss of imprinting of the *Igf2* gene. Various lines of investigation have localized "imprinted" genes involved in BWS and associated childhood tumors to chromosome 11p. These include, in addition to *Igf2*, the gene *H19*, which is involved in *Igf2* suppression, as well as *WT-1* (the Wilms tumor gene). Mutations in GPC3, a glypican gene (which codes for an IGF-II neutralizing membrane receptor), cause the related **Simpson-Golabi-Behmel overgrowth syndrome.**

Cannavo S, Venturino M, Curto L, et al: Clinical presentation and outcome of pituitary adenomas in teenagers. *Clin Endocrinol (Oxf)* 2003;58:519–527.

Cecconi M, Forzano F, Milani D, et al: Mutation analysis of the NSD1 gene in a group of 59 patients with congenital overgrowth. *Am J Med Genet* 2005;134:247–253.

Clemmons DR: Role of insulin-like growth factor-I in diagnosis and management of acromegaly. *Endocr Pract* 2004;10:362–371.

Colao A, Di Sarno A, Landi ML, et al: Long-term and low-dose treatment with cabergoline induces macroprolactinoma shrinkage. *J Clin Endocrinol Metab* 1997;82:3574–3579.

Colao A, Loche S, Cappabianca P, et al: Pituitary adenomas in children and adolescents: Clinical presentation, diagnosis, and therapeutic strategies. *Endocrinologist* 2000;10:314–327.

Daughaday WH: Pituitary gigantism. *Endocrinol Metab Clin North Am* 1992;21:633–647.

Feensta J, de Herder WW, Van der Beld AW, et al: Combined therapy with somatostatin analogues and weekly pegvisomant in active acromegaly. *Lancet* 2005;365:1644–1646.

Freda PU, Katznelson LO, Van der Lely AJ, et al: Long-acting somatostatin analog therapy of acromegaly: a meta-analysis. *J Clin Endocrinol Metab* 2005;90:4465–4473.

Kane LA, Leinung MC, Scheithaver BW, et al: Pituitary adenomas in childhood and adolescence. *J Clin Endocrinol Metab* 1994;79:1135–1140.

Lee JM, Howell JD: Tall girls: the social shaping of a medical therapy. *Arch Pediatr Adolesc Med* 2006;160:1035–1039.

Melmed S: Acromegaly. *N Engl J Med* 2006;355:2558–2572.

Morison IM, Becroft DM, Taniguchi T, et al: Somatic overgrowth associated with overexpression of insulin-like growth factor II. *Nature Med* 1996;2:311–316.

Rajasoorya C, Holdaway IM, Wrightson P, et al: Determinants of clinical outcome and survival in acromegaly. *Clin Endocrinol (Oxf)* 1994;41:95–102.

Serri O: Progress in management of hyperprolactinoma. *N Engl J Med* 1994;331:942–944.

Sorgo W, Scholler K, Heinze E, et al: Critical analysis of height reduction in estrogen treated tall girls. *Eur J Pediatr* 1984;142:260–265.

Sotos JF: Overgrowth: Genetic syndromes and other disorders associated with overgrowth. *Clin Pediatr* 1997;36:157–170.

Vance ML, Laws ER: Role of medical therapy in the management of acromegaly. *Neurosurgery* 2005;56:877–885.

Venn A, Bruinsma F, Werther G, et al: Oestrogen treatment to reduce the adult height of tall girls: Long-term effects on fertility. *Lancet* 2004;364:1513–1518.

Chapter 562 ■ Physiology of Puberty

Luigi Garibaldi

Between early childhood and approximately 8–9 yr of age (prepubertal stage), the hypothalamic-pituitary-gonadal axis is dormant, as reflected by undetectable serum concentrations of luteinizing hormone (LH) and sex hormones (estradiol in girls, testosterone in boys). In this phase, the activity of the hypothalamus and pituitary may be suppressed by poorly characterized neuronal restraint pathways.

One to 3 yr before the onset of clinically evident puberty, low serum levels of LH during sleep become demonstrable (peripubertal period). This sleep-entrained LH secretion occurs in a pulsatile fashion and probably reflects endogenous episodic discharge of hypothalamic gonadotropin-releasing hormone (GnRH). Nocturnal pulses of LH continue to increase in amplitude and, to a lesser extent, in frequency as clinical puberty approaches. This pulsatile secretion of gonadotropins is responsible for enlargement and maturation of the gonads and the secretion of sex hormones. The appearance of the secondary sex characteristics in early puberty is the visible culmination of the sustained, active interaction occurring among hypothalamus, pituitary, and gonads in the peripubertal period. By mid-puberty, LH pulses become evident even during the daytime and occur at about 90- to 120-min intervals.

A second critical event occurs in middle or late adolescence in girls in whom cyclicity and ovulation occur. A positive feedback mechanism develops whereby increasing levels of estrogen in mid-cycle cause a distinct increase of LH.

The factors that normally activate or restrain the hypothalamic neurons responsible for GnRH secretion (a neurosecretory unit known as the GnRH pulse generator) are unknown. In nonhuman primates, a decline in the γ-aminobutyric acid (GABA)–ergic tone in hypothalamic neurons and the resultant increase in the glutaminergic tone activate the GnRH pulse generator. Several other neurotransmitters are probably involved in humans and other primates.

It is clear that GnRH is the primary, if not the only, hormone responsible for the onset and progression of puberty because pubertal development can be reproduced in sexually immature or gonadotropin-deficient animals and humans by pulsed administration of GnRH. Mutations of the *GPR54* gene (a G protein–coupled receptor gene) cause an autosomal recessive form of hypogonadotropic hypogonadism. Defects of this receptor-ligand system do not affect GnRH neuronal migration, in contrast to the X-linked hypogonadotropic hypogonadism of Kallmann syndrome; rather they repair the activity of GnRH-secreting neurons in the hypothalamus.

Interpretation of the hormonal changes of puberty is complex because of several factors. First, pituitary gonadotropins are heterogeneous and circulate in multiple isoforms: more bioactive isoforms of LH may be preponderant during puberty. Second, LH immunoreactivity is variable in different immunoassays, and the results of LH measurements vary widely among laboratories. Third, the pulsatile secretion of gonadotropins and the synergism of follicle-stimulating hormone (FSH) and LH in promoting gonadal maturation make interpretation of single serum gonadotropin concentrations difficult. Measurement of gonadotropins in serially obtained (every 10–20 min for 12–24 hr) serum samples or timed urine collections is more meaningful. Fourth, important sex differences exist in the maturation of the hypothalamus and pituitary gland, and serum LH concentrations increase earlier in the course of the pubertal process in boys than in girls.

The effects of gonadal steroids (testosterone in boys, estradiol in girls) on bone growth and osseous maturation are critical. Both aromatase deficiency and estrogen receptor defects result in delayed epiphyseal fusion and tall stature in affected males. These observations suggest that estrogens, rather than androgens, are responsible for the process of bone maturation that ultimately leads to epiphyseal fusion and cessation of growth. Estrogens also mediate the increased production of growth hormone, which along with a direct effect of sex steroids on bone growth, is responsible for the pubertal growth spurt.

The age of onset of puberty varies and is more closely correlated with osseous maturation than with chronological age (see Chapter 12). In females, the **breast bud** is usually the first sign of puberty (10–11 yr), followed by the appearance of **pubic hair** 6–12 mo later. The interval to menarche is usually 2–2½ yr but may be as long as 6 yr. In the United States, at least one sign of puberty is present in approximately 95% of girls by 12 yr of age and in 99% of females by 13 yr of age. Peak height velocity occurs early (at breast stage II–III, typically between 11 and 12 yr of age) in girls and always precedes menarche. The mean age of menarche is about 12¾ yr. There are, however, wide variations in the sequence of changes involving growth spurt, breast bud, pubic hair, and maturation of the internal and external genitals.

In males, **growth of the testes** (>3 mL in volume or 2.5 cm in longest diameter) and thinning of the scrotum are the first signs of puberty. These are followed by pigmentation of the scrotum and growth of the penis (see Chapter 12). **Pubic hair** then appears. Appearance of **axillary hair** usually occurs in mid-puberty. In males, unlike in females, acceleration of growth begins after puberty is well under way and is maximal at genital stage IV–V (typically between 13 and 14 yr of age). In males, the growth spurt occurs approximately 2 yr later than in females, and growth may continue beyond 18 yr of age.

Genetic and environmental factors affect the onset of puberty. Following a decrease in menarcheal age in the past century, probably reflecting better nutrition and improved general health, the age of menarche has been stable for the last 30–40 yr. American black females may be more advanced in development of secondary sex characteristics for age than white females. A positive correlation between the degree of adiposity and early pubertal development in females has been reported. Conversely, ballet dancers, gymnasts, runners, and other female athletes in whom leanness and strenuous physical activity have coexisted from early childhood frequently exhibit a marked delay in puberty or menarche, and they frequently have oligomenorrhea or amenorrhea as adults (see Chapter 689). Pubertal delay is also prevalent in males who are physically very active. These observations support the thesis that the energy balance is closely related to the activity of the GnRH pulse generator and the mechanisms initiating and sustaining puberty, perhaps via hormonal signals, which may include adipokines.

Adrenocortical androgens also have a role in sexual maturation. Serum levels of dehydroepiandrosterone (DHEA) and its sulfate (DHEAS) begin to increase at approximately 6–8 yr of age, before any increase in LH or sex hormones and before the earliest physical changes of puberty are apparent; this process has been called adrenarche. DHEAS is the most abundant adrenal C-19 steroid in the blood, and its serum concentration remains fairly stable over 24 hr. A single measurement of this hormone is commonly used as a marker of adrenal androgen secretion. Although adrenarche typically antedates the onset of gonadal activity (gonadarche) by a few years, the two processes do not seem to be causally related, because adrenarche and gonadarche are dissociated in conditions such as central precocious puberty and adrenocortical failure.

Chapter 563 ■ Disorders of Pubertal Development Luigi Garibaldi

Precocious puberty is defined as the onset of secondary sexual characteristics before 8 yr of age in girls and 9 yr in boys. This definition is somewhat arbitrary because of the marked variation in the age at which puberty begins in normal children, particularly in different ethnic groups.

Precocious pubertal development may be classified as **gonadotropin dependent,** also called true or **central** precocious puberty, or **gonadotropin independent,** also called **peripheral** precocious puberty or precocious pseudopuberty (Table 563-1). True precocious puberty is always isosexual and stems from hypothalamic-pituitary-gonadal activation. The gonadotropin-mediated increase in the size and activity of the gonads leads to increasing sex hormone secretion and progressive sexual maturation. In **precocious pseudopuberty,** some of the secondary sex characteristics appear, but there is no activation of the normal hypothalamic-pituitary-gonadal interplay. In this latter group, the sex characteristics may be isosexual or heterosexual ("contrasexual") (see Chapters 584–589).

Precocious pseudopuberty may induce maturation of the hypothalamic-pituitary-gonadal axis and eventually trigger the onset of true sexual precocity. This mixed type of precocious puberty occurs commonly in conditions such as congenital adrenal hyperplasia, McCune-Albright syndrome, and familial male-limited precocious puberty, when the bone age reaches the pubertal range (10.5–12.5 yr).

TABLE 563-1. Conditions Causing Precocious Puberty

GONADOTROPIN-DEPENDENT PUBERTY (TRUE PRECOCIOUS PUBERTY)
Idiopathic
Organic brain lesions
Hypothalamic hamartoma
Brain tumors, hydrocephalus, severe head trauma, myelomeningocele
Hypothyroidism, prolonged and untreated
COMBINED GONADOTROPIN-DEPENDENT AND GONADOTROPIN-INDEPENDENT PUBERTY
Treated congenital adrenal hyperplasia
McCune-Albright syndrome, late
Familial male precocious puberty, late
GONADOTROPIN-INDEPENDENT PUBERTY (PRECOCIOUS PSEUDOPUBERTY)
Females
Isosexual (feminizing) conditions
McCune-Albright syndrome
Autonomous ovarian cysts
Ovarian tumors
Granulosa–theca cell tumor associated with Ollier disease
Teratoma, chorionepithelioma
Sex-cord tumor with annular tubules (SCTAT) associated with Peutz-Jeghers syndrome
Feminizing adrenocortical tumor
Exogenous estrogens
Heterosexual (masculinizing) conditions
Congenital adrenal hyperplasia
Adrenal tumors
Ovarian tumors
Glucocorticoid receptor defect
Exogenous androgens
Males
Isosexual (masculinizing) conditions
Congenital adrenal hyperplasia
Adrenocortical tumor
Leydig cell tumor
Familial male precocious puberty
Isolated
Associated with pseudohypoparathyroidism
hCG-secreting tumors
Central nervous system
Hepatoblastoma
Mediastinal tumor associated with Klinefelter syndrome
Teratoma
Glucocorticoid receptor defect
Exogenous androgen
Heterosexual (feminizing) conditions
Feminizing adrenocortical tumor
SCTAT associated with Peutz-Jeghers syndrome
Exogenous estrogens
INCOMPLETE (PARTIAL) PRECOCIOUS PUBERTY
Premature thelarche
Premature adrenarche
Premature menarche

563.1 • Gonadotropin-Dependent Precocious Puberty

The condition occurs at least 5- to 10-fold more frequently in girls than in boys and is usually sporadic although some cases are familial. Approximately 90% of sexual precocity in girls is idiopathic. A structural central nervous system (CNS) abnormality can, however, be demonstrated in 25–75% of boys and in 8–10% of girls with central precocious puberty. A high prevalence of idiopathic sexual precocity has been reported in girls adopted from developing countries, with the limitation that the exact date of birth may be uncertain.

CLINICAL MANIFESTATIONS. Sexual development may begin at any age and generally follows the sequence observed in normal puberty. In girls, the first sign is development of the breast; pubic hair may appear simultaneously but more often appears later. Maturation of the external genitalia, the appearance of axillary hair, and the onset of menstruation follow. The early menstrual cycles may be more irregular than they are with normal puberty. The initial cycles are usually anovulatory, but pregnancy has been reported as early as 5.5 yr of age (Fig. 563-1).

In boys, enlargement of the testes is followed by enlargement of the penis, appearance of pubic hair, and acne. Erections are common, and nocturnal emissions may occur. The voice deepens, and linear growth is accelerated. Testicular biopsies have shown stimulation of all elements of the testes, and spermatogenesis has been observed as early as 5–6 yr of age. In affected girls and boys, height, weight, and osseous maturation are advanced. The increased rate of bone maturation results in early closure of the epiphyses, and the ultimate stature is less than it would have been otherwise. Without treatment, approximately ⅓ of girls and an even larger percentage of boys achieve a height less than the 5th percentile as adults. Mental development is usually compatible with chronological age. Emotional behavior and mood swings are common, but serious psychologic problems are rare.

Although the clinical course is variable, 3 main patterns of pubertal progression can be identified. Most girls (particularly those younger than 6 yr of age at the onset) and most boys have rapidly progressive sexual precocity, characterized by rapid physical and osseous maturation, leading to a loss of height potential. Several girls (generally older than 6 yr of age at the onset) have a slowly progressive variant, characterized by parallel advancement of osseous maturation and linear growth, with preserved height potential. A slowly progressive variant of central sexual precocity also occurs in boys but is less common than in girls. A small percentage of girls have spontaneously regressive or unsustained central precocious puberty. This variability in the natural course of sexual precocity underscores the need for longitudinal observation at the onset of sexual development, before treatment is considered.

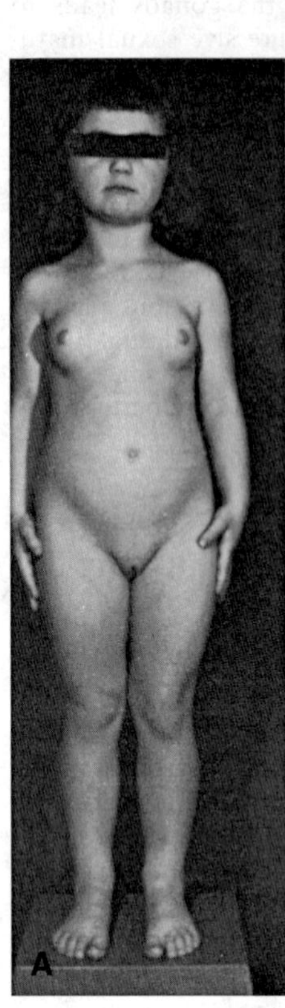

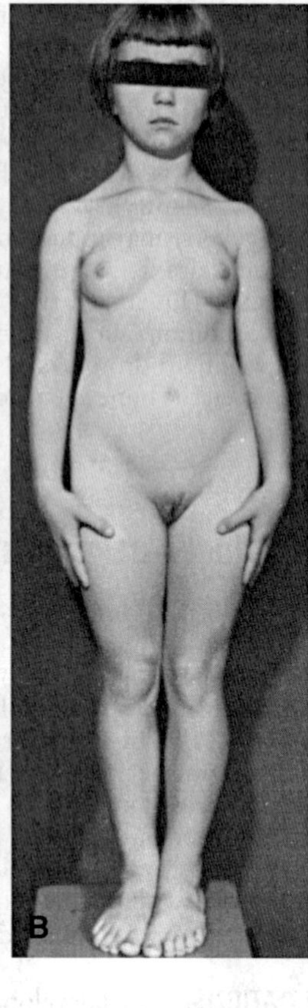

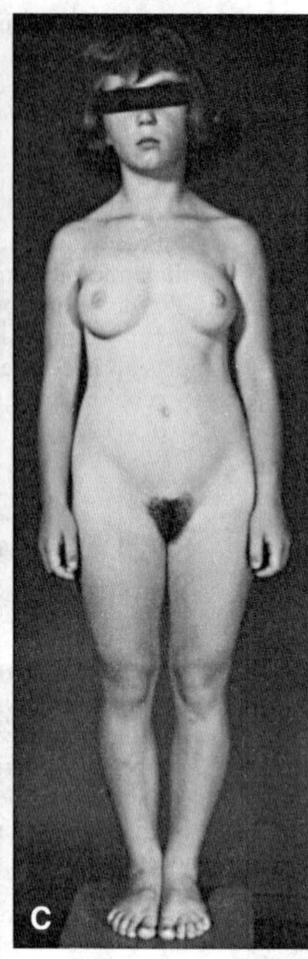

Figure 563-1. Natural course of idiopathic central precocious puberty. Patient *(A)* at $3^{11}/_{12}$, *(B)* at $5^{8}/_{12}$, and *(C)* at $8\frac{1}{2}$ yr of age. Breast development and vaginal bleeding began at $2\frac{1}{2}$ yr of age. Bone age was $7\frac{1}{2}$ yr at $3^{11}/_{12}$ and 14 yr at 8 yr of age. Intelligence and dental age were normal for chronological age. Growth was completed at 10 yr; ultimate height was 142 cm (56 in). No effective therapy was available at the time this patient sought medical attention.

LABORATORY FINDINGS. Sex hormone concentrations are usually appropriate for the stage of puberty in both sexes. Serum estradiol concentrations in girls are low or undetectable in the early phase of sexual precocity, as they are in normal puberty. In boys, serum testosterone levels are detectable or clearly elevated by the time the parents seek medical attention, particularly if an early morning blood sample is obtained. Sensitive immunometric (including immunoradiometric, immunofluorometric, and chemiluminescent) assays for luteinizing hormone (LH) have replaced the traditional LH radioimmunoassays and offer greater diagnostic sensitivity using random blood samples. With sensitive assays, serum LH concentrations are undetectable in prepubertal children but become detectable in 60–75% of girls and a higher percentage of boys with central sexual precocity. Measurement of LH in serial blood samples obtained during sleep has greater diagnostic power than measurement in a single random sample, and it typically reveals a well-defined pulsatile secretion of LH. Intravenous administration of gonadotropin-releasing hormone (GnRH stimulation test) or a GnRH agonist (leuprolide stimulation test) is a helpful diagnostic tool, particularly for boys, in whom a brisk LH response (LH peak >5–10 IU/L) with predominance of LH over follicle-stimulating hormone (FSH) occurs in the early phase of precocious puberty. In girls with sexual precocity, however, the nocturnal LH secretion and the LH response to GnRH may be quite low at breast stage II to early stage III (immunometric-LH peak, often <5 IU/L), and the LH to FSH ratio may remain low until mid-puberty. In such girls with "low" LH response, the central nature of sexual precocity can be proven by detecting pubertal levels of estradiol (>50 pg/mL), 20–24 hr after stimulation with leuprolide.

Osseous maturation is variably advanced, often more than 2–3 SD. Pelvic ultrasonography in girls reveals progressive enlargement of the ovaries, followed by enlargement of the uterus to pubertal size. An MRI scan usually demonstrates physiologic enlargement of the pituitary gland, as seen in normal puberty; it may also reveal CNS pathology (see section 563.2).

DIFFERENTIAL DIAGNOSIS. Organic CNS causes of central sexual precocity should be ruled out by MRI scans, particularly in girls with rapid breast development, in girls with estradiol greater than 30 pg/mL, in girls younger than 6 yr of age, and in all boys. However, in children presenting without neurologic signs or symptoms, the CNS lesions causing precocious puberty are rarely malignant and seldom require neurosurgical intervention or radiation therapy. Some authorities recommend MRI scans for all children with central precocious puberty.

Gonadotropin-independent causes of isosexual precocious puberty must be considered in the differential diagnosis (see Table 563-1). For girls, these include tumors of the ovaries, autonomously functioning ovarian cysts, feminizing adrenal tumors, McCune-Albright syndrome, and exogenous sources of estrogens. For boys, congenital adrenal hyperplasia, adrenal tumors, Leydig cell tumors, chorionic gonadotropin–producing tumors, and familial male precocious puberty should be considered.

TREATMENT. The observation that the pituitary gonadotropic cells require pulsatile, rather than continuous, stimulation by GnRH to maintain the ongoing release of gonadotropins provides the rationale for using GnRH agonists for treatment of central precocious puberty. By virtue of being more potent and having a longer duration of action than native GnRH, these GnRH agonists (after a brief period of stimulation) "desensitize" the gonadotropic cells of the pituitary to the stimulatory effect of endogenous GnRH and effectively halt the progression of central sexual precocity.

Virtually all boys and the large subgroup of girls with rapidly progressive precocious puberty are candidates for treatment. Girls with slowly progressive puberty do not seem to benefit in terms of height prognosis from GnRH-agonist therapy. Former low-birthweight infants may be at greater risk of short stature as adults and may require more aggressive treatment of precocious puberty. Rare patients require treatment solely for psychologic or social reasons, including great parental anxiety. Depot formulations of long-acting GnRH agonists, which maintain fairly constant serum concentration of the drug for weeks, constitute the preparations of choice for treatment of central precocious puberty. Leuprolide acetate (Lupron Depot Ped), the only depot preparation approved for this use in the United States, is given in a dose of 0.25–0.3 mg/kg (minimum 7.5 mg) intramuscularly once every 4 wk. Other long-acting preparations (D-Trp6-GnRH [Decapeptyl], goserelin acetate [Zoladex]) are approved for treatment of precocious puberty in other countries. Recurrent sterile fluid collections at the sites of injections are the most troublesome local side effect and occur in less than 3–5% of treated patients. In children with such local reactions, treatment should be changed to subcutaneous injections of aqueous leuprolide, given once or twice daily (total dose 60 mg/kg/24 hr), or intranasal administration of the GnRH agonist nafarelin (Synarel), 800 mg bid. The potential for irregular compliance with daily administration, as well as the variable absorption of the intranasal route for nafarelin, may limit the long-term benefit of the latter preparations on adult height. Preparations of depot-leuprolide with longer duration of action (90 days) are currently not FDA-approved for treatment of sexual precocity, but they appear promising. Subcutaneous implants (effect lasting up to 12–18 mo) of GnRH agonists (histrelin) have been effective in preliminary trials. GnRH antagonists are relatively new and have not been investigated sufficiently for treatment of precocious puberty. Oral GnRH antagonists are also being investigated.

Treatment results in decrease of the growth rate, generally to age-appropriate values, and an even greater decrease of the rate of osseous maturation. Some children, particularly those with greatly advanced (pubertal) bone age, may show marked deceleration of their growth rate and a complete arrest in the rate of osseous maturation. Treatment results in enhancement of the predicted height, although the actual adult height of patients followed to epiphyseal closure is approximately 1 SD less than their mid-parental height. In girls, breast development may regress in those with Tanner stage II–III development. Most commonly, the size of the breasts remains unchanged in girls with stage III–V development or may even increase slightly because of progressive adipose tissue deposition. The amount of glandular tissue decreases. Pubic hair usually remains stable in girls, or may even progress slowly during treatment, reflecting the gradual increase in adrenal androgens. Menses, if present, cease. Pelvic sonography demonstrates a decrease of the ovarian and uterine size. In boys, there is decrease of testicular size, variable regression of pubic hair, and decrease in the frequency of erections. Except for a reversible decrease in bone density (of uncertain clinical significance), no serious adverse effects of GnRH analogs have been reported in children treated for sexual precocity. If treatment is effective, the serum sex hormone concentrations decrease to prepubertal levels (testosterone, <10–20 ng/dL in boys; estradiol, <5–10 pg/mL in girls). The serum LH and FSH concentrations, as measured by sensitive immunometric assays, decrease to less than 1 IU/L in most patients, although almost never does the LH return to truly prepubertal levels (<0.1 IU/L). Moreover, the incremental FSH and LH responses to GnRH stimulation decrease to less than 1–2 IU/L. Serum LH and sex hormone levels remain suppressed for as long as therapy is continued, but puberty resumes promptly when therapy is discontinued, typically at a "pubertal" chronological age. In girls, menarche and ovulatory cycles generally appear at an average of 18 mo (range 6–24 mo) of cessation of therapy. The addition of human growth hormone (hGH) to GnRH agonists has been used in children with precocious puberty, markedly advanced bone age, and prediction of short stature. The available, albeit limited, data indicate that combined therapy may increase the adult height.

563.2 • Precocious Puberty Resulting from Organic Brain Lesions

ETIOLOGY. Hypothalamic hamartomas are the most common brain lesion causing true precocious puberty (Fig. 563-2). This congenital malformation consists of ectopically located neural tissue containing GnRH-secretory neurons and may function as an accessory GnRH pulse generator. On MRI, it appears as a small pedunculated mass attached to the tuber cinereum or the floor of the third ventricle or, less often, as a sessile mass (Fig. 563-3) that remains static in size over years. This lesion may also be associated with gelastic or psychomotor seizures. A wide variety of CNS lesions, usually involving the hypothalamus by scarring, invasion, or pressure, have been associated with gonadotropin-dependent sexual precocity. These lesions probably induce sexual maturation by interrupting poorly characterized pubertal restraint pathways. They include postencephalitic scars, tuberculous meningitis, tuberous sclerosis, severe head trauma, and hydrocephalus, either isolated or associated with myelomeningocele. Neoplasms causing precocious puberty include astrocytomas, ependymomas, and optic tract tumors. Tumors of the latter type (typically slowly progressive or indolent optic gliomas) are highly prevalent (15–20%) in children with neurofibromatosis type 1 (NF-1) and constitute the main eti-

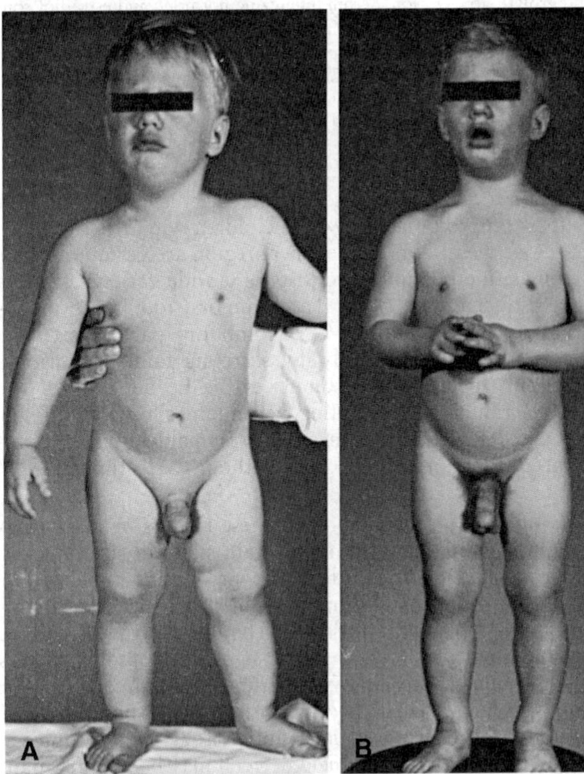

Figure 563-2. Natural course of precocious puberty with central nervous system lesion. Photographs at 1.5 *(A)* and 2.5 *(B)* yr of age. Accelerated growth, muscular development, osseous maturation, and testicular development were consistent with the degree of secondary sexual maturation. In early infancy, the patient began having frequent spells of rapid, purposeless motion; later in life, he had episodes of uncontrollable laughing with ocular movements. At 7 yr, he exhibited emotional lability, aggressive behavior, and destructive tendencies. Although a hypothalamic hamartoma had been suspected, it was not established until CT scanning became available when the patient was 23 yr of age. Epiphyses fused at 9 yr of age; final height was 142 cm (56 in). At 24 yr of age, he developed an embryonal cell carcinoma of the retroperitoneum.

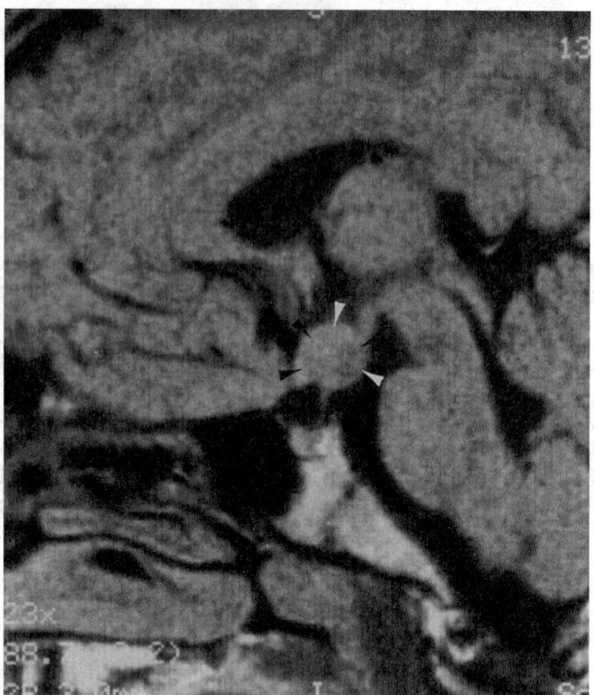

Figure 563-3. MRI of a central nervous system lesion in a child with central precocious puberty. A 6-yr-old girl was referred for stage IV breast development and growth acceleration. Serum luteinizing hormone and estradiol concentrations were in the adult range. The midsagittal T1-weighted image shows an isointense hypothalamic mass *(arrowheads)*, typical of a hamartoma. (From Sharafuddin M, Luisiri A, Garibaldi LR, et al: MR imaging diagnosis of central precocious puberty: Importance of changes in the shape and size of the pituitary gland. *Am J Roentgenol* 1994;162:1167.)

ologic factor for the central sexual precocity encountered in a small subset (approximately 3%) of children with NF-1.

About ½ of the tumors in the pineal region are germinomas or astrocytomas; the remainder consists of a wide variety of histologically distinct tumor types. These tumors, too, cause precocious puberty by interrupting CNS inhibitory pathways to the hypothalamus or, in boys only, by secreting human chorionic gonadotropin (hCG), which stimulates the Leydig cells of the testes. Intracranial hCG-secreting germinomas usually do not produce precocious puberty in girls, presumably because complete ovarian function cannot occur without FSH priming.

CLINICAL MANIFESTATIONS. Some of these tumors or malformations (hypothalamic hamartomas) remain static in size or grow slowly, producing no signs other than precocious puberty. For lesions causing neurologic symptoms, the neuroendocrine manifestations may be present for 1–2 yr before the tumor can be detected radiologically. Hypothalamic signs or symptoms such as diabetes insipidus, adipsia, hyperthermia, unnatural crying or laughing (gelastic seizures), obesity, and cachexia should suggest the possibility of an intracranial lesion. Visual signs (proptosis, decreased visual acuity, visual field defects) may be the first manifestation of an optic glioma.

The sexual precocity is always isosexual, and the endocrine patterns are generally those found in children without demonstrable organic lesions. Rapidly progressive sexual precocity in very young children suggests the likelihood of a hypothalamic hamartoma. In conditions other than hypothalamic hamartoma, growth hormone deficiency may occur and may be masked by the growth-promoting effect of the increased sex hormone levels.

TREATMENT. Regardless of the cause, therapy with GnRH agonists is as effective in children with organic brain lesions causing central precocious puberty as it is in children with idiopathic sexual precocity, and these analogs are the therapy of choice to halt premature sexual development. This includes patients with a hypothalamic hamartoma, if precocious puberty is its only manifestation. In those patients with hypothalamic hamartoma and associated intractable gelastic or psychomotor seizures, however, stereotactic radiation therapy (gamma knife surgery) is effective and less risky than neurosurgical intervention. For other neurologic lesions, therapy depends on the nature and location of the pathologic process. Combined growth hormone therapy should be considered for patients with associated growth hormone deficiency.

563.3 • Precocious Puberty Following Irradiation of the Brain

Radiation therapy, generally for leukemia or intracranial tumors, increases the risk of precocious puberty considerably, whether the irradiation is directed to the hypothalamic area or to areas of the brain anatomically distant from the hypothalamus. Low-dose radiation (18–24 Gy) hastens the onset of puberty almost exclusively in girls. High-dose radiation (25–47 Gy), conversely, appears to trigger precocious sexual development in both sexes, and the risk of sexual precocity is inversely proportional to the age of the child at the time radiation was given.

This type of sexual precocity often occurs with growth hormone deficiency and may be associated with other conditions (spinal irradiation, hypothyroidism) adversely affecting the prognosis for a reasonable adult height. Unless careful attention is paid to early signs of pubertal development in these children, the combination of growth hormone deficiency and the growth-promoting effect of sex steroids often results in a "normal" growth rate at the expense of a rapidly advancing bone age and impaired adult height potential.

TREATMENT. GnRH analogs are effective in arresting pubertal progression in this patient population. However, concomitant growth hormone deficiency (and/or thyroid hormone deficiency) should be diagnosed and treated promptly in order for the adult height prognosis to improve.

Paradoxically, hypopituitarism with gonadotropin deficiency may subsequently develop as a late effect of high-dose CNS irradiation in patients with or without a history of precocious puberty, and it may require substitution therapy with sex steroids.

563.4 • Syndrome of Precocious Puberty and Hypothyroidism

In children with untreated hypothyroidism, the onset of puberty is usually delayed until epiphyseal maturation reaches 12–13 yr of age. Precocious puberty in a child with untreated hypothyroidism and a prepubertal bone age presents a strikingly unphysiologic association, yet is common and may occur in as many as 50% of children with severe hypothyroidism of long duration. These children have the usual manifestations of hypothyroidism, including retardation of growth and of osseous maturation (see Chapter 566). The cause of the hypothyroidism is often undiagnosed lymphocytic thyroiditis and rarely thyroidectomy or overtreatment with antithyroid drugs. Sexual development in girls consists primarily of breast enlargement and menstrual bleeding; the latter may occur even in girls with minimal breast enlargement. Pelvic sonography may reveal large, multicystic ovaries. Boys have testicular enlargement associated with modest or no penile enlargement and no pubic hair development.

Enlargement of the sella, which is typical of long-standing primary hypothyroidism, may be demonstrated by skull film or MRI. Plasma levels of thyroid-stimulating hormone (TSH) are markedly elevated, often greater than 500 μU/mL, and those of prolactin are mildly elevated. Although serum FSH is low and LH is undetectable, when measured by specific assays, the massively elevated concentrations of TSH appear to interact with the FSH receptor ("specificity spillover"), thus inducing FSH-like effects in the absence of LH effects on the gonads. As a consequence, unlike in true precocious puberty, testicular enlargement occurs without substantial Leydig cell stimulation and testosterone secretion in affected boys. In affected girls, ovarian estrogen production occurs without a concomitant increase in androgens. Thus, the precocious puberty associated with hypothyroidism behaves as an incomplete form of gonadotropin-dependent puberty. Treatment of the hypothyroidism results in rapid return to normal of the biochemical and clinical manifestations. Rapid bone age advancement and progression to central puberty often occur in the months following the initiation of thyroid hormone replacement. Therapy with GnRH analogs should be initiated promptly in such patients to prevent severe impairment of the adult height. Macroorchidism (testicular volume >30 mL) may persist in adult males despite adequate thyroxine therapy.

563.5 • Gonadotropin-Secreting Tumors

HEPATIC TUMORS. Isosexual precocious puberty may be uncommonly associated with hepatoblastoma. All reported cases have been male, with the age of onset varying from 4 mo to 8 yr (average 2 yr). An enlarged liver or mass in the upper quadrant should suggest the diagnosis. The tumor cells produce hCG, which stimulates the LH receptors in the Leydig cells of the testes. The testicles are only minimally enlarged, and the testicular histology reveals interstitial cell hyperplasia and absence of spermatogenesis. Plasma levels of hCG and α-fetoprotein are usually markedly elevated; they serve as useful markers for following the effects of therapy. Plasma levels of testosterone are elevated, and the FSH and LH levels, as measured by specific, immunometric assays, are low; in the past, LH levels were falsely elevated because of cross-reaction with hCG on radioimmunoassay.

Treatment for these tumors is the same as that for other carcinomas of the liver; prognosis for survival beyond 1–2 yr from the time of diagnosis is poor.

OTHER TUMORS. Chorionic gonadotropin–secreting choriocarcinomas, teratocarcinomas, or teratomas (also called ectopic pinealomas or atypical teratomas), located in the CNS, mediastinum, gonads, or even adrenal glands, may cause precocious puberty, more commonly (10- to 20-fold) in boys than in girls. Affected patients often have marked elevations of hCG and α-fetoprotein. Mediastinal tumors, but not gonadal tumors, have been reported to cause precocious puberty in boys with Klinefelter syndrome.

PRECOCIOUS PSEUDOPUBERTY. The adrenal causes of pseudopuberty are discussed in Chapter 577, and the gonadal causes are discussed in Chapters 585 and 588.

563.6 • McCune-Albright Syndrome (Precocious Puberty with Polyostotic Fibrous Dysplasia and Abnormal Pigmentation)

This syndrome of endocrine dysfunction is associated with patchy cutaneous pigmentation and fibrous dysplasia of the skeletal system. Although sexual precocity in girls was the major recognized endocrinopathy in the past, associated pituitary, thyroid, and adrenal aberrations are also recognized. The disorder is characterized by autonomous hyperfunction of many glands and is caused by a missense mutation in the gene encoding the α-subunit of G_S, the G protein that stimulates cyclic adenosine monophosphate (cAMP) formation, resulting in the formation of the putative gsp oncoprotein. Activation of receptors (corticotropin [ACTH], TSH, FSH, and LH receptors) that operate via a cAMP-dependent mechanism, as well as cell proliferation, ensue. Because the mutation is somatic rather than genomic, it is expressed differently in different glands or tissues, hence the variability of clinical expression in different patients. Precocious puberty has been described predominantly in girls (Fig. 563-4). The average age at onset in affected girls is about 3 yr, but vaginal bleeding has occurred as early as 4 mo of age and secondary sex characteristics have occurred as early as 6 mo. Young girls have suppressed levels of LH and FSH, and there is no response to GnRH stimulation. Estradiol levels vary from normal to markedly elevated (>900 pg/mL), are often cyclic, and may correlate with the size of the cysts. In boys, precocious puberty is less common but has been reported in several instances. Unlike ovarian enlargement in girls, testicular enlargement in boys is fairly symmetric. It is followed by the appearance of phallic enlargement and pubic hair, as in normal puberty. Testicular histology has demonstrated large seminiferous tubules and no or minimal Leydig cell hyperplasia; these findings may simply reflect the fact that biopsy specimens were obtained at an early stage of pubertal development. In girls and boys, when the bone age reaches the usual pubertal age range, gonadotropin secretion begins, and the response to GnRH becomes pubertal. True (gonadotropin-dependent) precocious puberty overrides the antecedent (gonadotropin-independent) precocious pseudopuberty. In girls, menses become more regular, but often not completely, and fertility has been documented.

Pubertal progression is variable in these patients. Functioning ovarian cysts often disappear spontaneously; aspiration or surgical excision of cysts is rarely indicated. For girls with persistent estradiol secretion, agents that interfere with the final step of estrogen biosynthesis, i.e., aromatase inhibitors such as testolactone or letrozole (1.25–2.5 mg/day p.o.) or anastrozole (1 mg/day p.o.), or antiestrogens (such as tamoxifen) may limit, to a variable extent, the estrogen effects on pubertal and osseous maturation. The same compounds have also been used in boys, in combination with antiandrogens (such as spironolactone 50–100 mg bid, or flutamide 125–250 mg b.i.d.). These compounds are not approved by the U.S. FDA for this indication; tamoxifen and flutamide may be hepatotoxic, and high-dose spironolactone may rarely cause hyperkalemia. Associated therapy with long-acting analogs of GnRH is indicated only for patients whose puberty has shifted from a gonadotropin-independent to a predominantly gonadotropin-dependent mechanism.

EXTRAGONADAL MANIFESTATIONS. The hyperthyroidism that occurs in this condition differs from that characteristic of Graves disease. There is an equal distribution between male and female patients; the goiters are multinodular. Clinical hyperthyroidism is uncommon in children, but goiters, mildly elevated triiodothyronine levels, suppressed TSH levels, and abnormalities on ultrasound have been reported. Only rarely is thyroidectomy necessary.

In patients with associated Cushing syndrome, bilateral nodular adrenocortical hyperplasia has occurred in early infancy, antedating the sexual precocity. ACTH levels are low, and adrenal function is not suppressed by large doses of dexamethasone. Treatment is bilateral adrenalectomy.

Increased secretion of growth hormone occurs uncommonly and is manifested clinically by gigantism or acromegaly or by increased rates of growth even in the absence of precocious

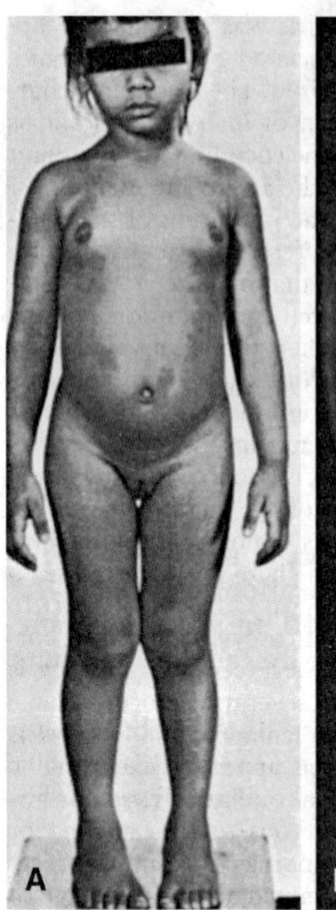

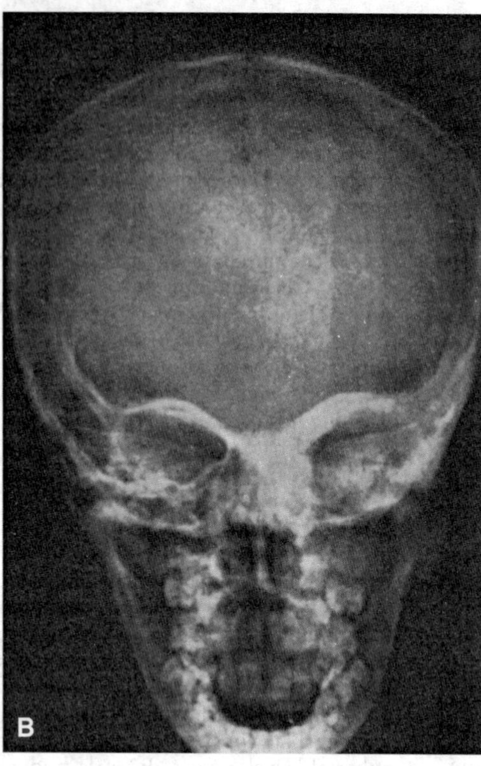

Figure 563-4. Precocious puberty associated with polyostotic fibrous dysplasia (McCune-Albright syndrome) in a girl 4.5 yr of age; at this time, her height age and bone age were normal. Menarche occurred at 4 yr of age. *A,* Note the bilateral breast development, hyperpigmented spots on the abdomen, and prominence of the left side of the face. *B,* Roentgenograms revealed fibrous dysplasia in the distal end of the left ulna and thickening of the bones about the left orbit and the maxillary portion of the frontal bones shown here.

puberty. Girls and boys are equally affected. Serum levels of growth hormone are elevated and increase during sleep; they are augmented by thyrotropin (TRH) and poorly inhibited by oral glucose. Serum levels of prolactin are increased in most patients, but fewer than ½ of the patients have a demonstrable pituitary tumor. Octreotide, a long-acting somatostatin analog, has been used to treat the hypersomatotropism. The prognosis is favorable for longevity, but deformities, repeated fractures, pain, and occasional cranial nerve compression may result from the bony lesions.

Of the extraglandular manifestations, phosphaturia, leading to rickets or osteomalacia, is the most common. Cardiovascular and hepatic involvement is rare but may be life-threatening (severe neonatal cholestasis).

563.7 • Familial Male Gonadotropin-Independent Precocious Puberty

This rare, autosomal dominant form of sexual precocity is transmitted from affected males and unaffected female carriers of the gene to their male offspring. Signs of puberty appear by 2–3 yr of age. The testes are only slightly enlarged. Testicular biopsies show Leydig cell maturation and, in some instances, marked hyperplasia. Maturation of seminiferous tubules may be present. Testosterone levels are markedly elevated to the same range seen in boys with true precocious puberty; however, baseline levels of LH are prepubertal, pulsatile secretion of LH is absent, and LH does not respond to stimulation with GnRH. The cause for activation of Leydig cells independently of gonadotropin stimulation is a missense mutation of the LH receptor leading to constitutive activation of cAMP production. Osseous maturation may be markedly advanced; when it reaches the pubertal age range, hypothalamic maturation shifts the mechanism of pubertal development to a gonadotropin-dependent one. This sequence of events is similar to that occurring in children with McCune-Albright syndrome (see earlier discussion) or in those with congenital adrenal hyperplasia (see Chapter 577.1).

Gonadotropin-independent precocious puberty has been diagnosed in a few unrelated boys with type IA pseudohypoparathyroidism who had a single mutation of the $G_s\alpha$ protein. This mutation is inactivating at normal body temperature and causes pseudohypoparathyroidism, but in the cooler temperature of the testes, it is constitutionally activating, resulting in adenyl cyclase stimulation and production of testosterone. Although this mutation differs from the constitutive LH receptor mutation, which usually causes familial male gonadotropin-independent precocious puberty, the end result is the same.

TREATMENT. Young boys have been successfully treated with ketoconazole (600 mg/24 hr in 8-hr divided doses), an antifungal drug that inhibits C-17,20-lyase and testosterone synthesis. Other investigators use a combination of antiandrogens (such as spironolactone 50–100 mg b.i.d., or flutamide 125–250 mg b.i.d.) and aromatase inhibitors (letrozole 2.5 mg/day, or anastrozole 1 mg/day), because estrogens derived from androgens stimulate bone maturation. These medications are unable to revert the serum testosterone to the normal (prepubertal) concentrations or completely offset the unfavorable effects of the elevated sex hormones. They slow down, but do not halt, the progression of puberty and may not improve the height prognosis. Boys whose GnRH pulse generator has matured require combined therapy with GnRH agonists.

563.8 • Incomplete (Partial) Precocious Development

Isolated manifestations of precocity without development of other signs of puberty are not unusual; development of the breasts in girls and growth of sexual hair in both sexes are the two most common forms.

PREMATURE THELARCHE. This term applies to a transient condition of isolated breast development that most often appears in the first 2 yr of life; in some girls, breast development is present at birth and persists. Breast development may be unilateral or asymmetric and often fluctuates in degree. Growth and osseous maturation are normal or slightly advanced. The genitals show no evidence of estrogenic stimulation. The condition is usually sporadic and rarely familial. Breast development may regress after 2 yr, often persists for 3–5 yr, and is rarely progressive. Menarche occurs at the expected age, and reproduction is normal. Basal serum levels of FSH and the FSH response to GnRH stimulation may be greater than that seen in normal controls. Plasma levels of LH and estradiol are consistently less than the limits of detection. Ultrasound examination of the ovaries reveals normal size, but a few small (<9 mm) cysts are not uncommon.

In some girls of the same age group, breast development may be associated with definite evidence of systemic estrogen effects, such as growth acceleration or bone age advancement. Pelvic sonography may reveal enlarged ovaries or uterus. This condition, referred to as **exaggerated or atypical thelarche,** differs from central sexual precocity because it has spontaneous regression. GnRH or leuprolide stimulation elicits a robust FSH response, a low LH response, and (after leuprolide only) a moderate estradiol increment at 24 hr (average 60–90 pg/mL). The pathogenesis of typical and exaggerated forms of thelarche is unclear although a delay in the transition from the activated (neonatal-infantile) to the inactive (prepubertal) pituitary-ovarian axis may underlie both conditions. Premature thelarche is a benign condition but may be the first sign of true or pseudoprecocious puberty, or it may be caused by exogenous exposure to estrogens. In addition to a detailed history, a bone age should be obtained. The serum concentrations of FSH, LH, and estradiol are generally low and not diagnostic. Pelvic ultrasound examination is rarely indicated. Continued observation is important because the condition cannot be readily distinguished from true precocious puberty. Regression and recurrence suggest functioning follicular cysts. Occurrence of thelarche in children older than 3 yr of age most often is caused by a condition other than benign precocious thelarche.

PREMATURE PUBARCHE (ADRENARCHE). This term applies to the appearance of sexual hair before the age of 8 yr in girls or 9 yr in boys without other evidence of maturation. It is much more frequent in girls than in boys and may occur more frequently in American black girls than in others. Hair appears on the mons and labia majora in girls, perineal and scrotal area in boys; axillary hair generally appears later. Adult-type axillary odor is common. Affected children are slightly advanced in height and osseous maturation. Premature adrenarche is an early maturational event of adrenal androgen production. This event coincides with precocious maturation of the zona reticularis, an associated decrease in 3β-hydroxysteroid dehydrogenase activity, and an increase in C-17,20-lyase activity. These enzymatic changes result in increased basal and ACTH-stimulated serum concentrations of the Δ^5-steroids (17-hydroxypregnenolone and DHEA) and, to a lesser extent, of the Δ^4-steroids (particularly androstenedione) compared with age-matched control subjects. The levels of these steroids and of DHEAS are usually comparable to those of older children in the early stages of normal puberty. Premature adrenarche is a slowly progressive condition that requires no therapy. However, a subset of patients with precocious pubarche has one or more features of systemic androgen effect, such as marked growth acceleration, clitoral (girls) or phallic (boys) enlargement, cystic acne, or advanced bone age (>2 SD above the mean for age). In these patients with **atypical premature adrenarche,** an ACTH stimulation test with measurement of steroid intermediates (mainly, serum 17-hydroxyprogesterone concentrations) is indicated to rule out nonclassical congenital adrenal hyperplasia due to 21-hydroxylase deficiency. Epidemiologic and molecular genetic studies have shown that the prevalence of nonclassical 21-hydroxylase deficiency is approximately 3–6% of unselected children with precocious pubarche; the prevalence of other enzyme defects (i.e., 3β-hydroxysteroid dehydrogenase or 11β-hydroxylase deficiencies) is extremely low. Although idiopathic premature adrenarche has been considered a benign condition, longitudinal observations suggest that approximately 50% of girls with premature adrenarche are at high risk for **hyperandrogenism** and **polycystic ovary syndrome,** alone or more often in combination with other components of the so-called metabolic syndrome (insulin resistance possibly progressing to type 2 diabetes mellitus, dyslipidemia, hypertension, increased abdominal fat) as adults. Whether the unfavorable progression to pubertal hyperandrogenism can be prevented by insulin-sensitizing agents (metformin 850–1000 mg/day) or lifestyle interventions (diet, exercise) remains to be proven in large studies. An increased risk of premature adrenarche and the metabolic syndrome has been documented in children born small for their gestational age. This appears to be associated with insulin resistance and decreased β-cell reserve, perhaps as a consequence of fetal undernutrition.

PREMATURE MENARCHE. This is a rare entity, much less frequent than premature thelarche or premature adrenarche, and is a diagnosis of exclusion. In girls with isolated vaginal bleeding in the absence of other secondary sexual characteristics, more common causes such as vulvovaginitis, a foreign body, or sexual abuse, and uncommon causes such as urethral prolapse and sarcoma botryoides must be carefully excluded. The majority of girls with idiopathic premature menarche have only 1–3 episodes of bleeding; puberty occurs at the usual time, and menstrual cycles are normal. Plasma levels of gonadotropins are normal, but estradiol levels may be elevated, probably owing to episodic ovarian estrogen secretion. Occasional patients are found to have ovarian follicular cysts on ultrasound.

563.9 • Medicational Precocity

A variety of medicaments can induce the appearance of secondary sexual characteristics that may be confused with precocious puberty. A careful history focused on exploring the possibility of accidental exposure to or ingestion of sex hormones is important. Precocious pseudopuberty has occurred in both boys and girls from the accidental ingestion of estrogens (including contraceptive pills) and from the administration of anabolic steroids. Estrogens in cosmetics, hair creams, and breast augmentation creams have caused breast development in girls and gynecomastia in boys; estrogens are readily absorbed through the skin. The high prevalence of premature thelarche and precocious pseudopuberty in Puerto Rico has been attributed to contamination of meats, particularly chicken, with estrogens used in animal husbandry, but has not been proved. Exogenous estrogens may produce an intense, dark brown color in the areola of the breasts that is not usually seen in endogenous types of precocity. The precocious changes disappear after cessation of exposure to the hormones. The use of testosterone gels or creams, which are applied to the skin for treatment of male hypogonadism, has resulted in virilization of children and women following skin contact at, and systemic absorption from, the area where the gel/cream was applied by their family member.

Antoniazzi F, Zamboni G, Bertoldo F: Bone development during GH and GnRH analog treatment. *Eur J Endocrinol* 2004;151:S47–54.

Carel JC, Lahlou N, Jaramillo O, et al: Treatment of central precocious puberty by subcutaneous injections of leuprorelin 3-month depot (11.25 mg). *J Clin Endocrinol Metab* 2002;87:4111–4116.

Carel JC, Lahlou N, Roger M, et al: Precocious puberty and statural growth. *Hum Reprod Update* 2004;10:135–147.

Chalumeau M, Chemaitilly W, Trivin C, et al: Central precocious puberty in girls: An evidence-based diagnosis tree to predict central nervous system abnormalities. *Pediatrics* 2002;109:61–67.

Chalumeau M, Hadjiathanasiou CG, Ng SM, et al: Selecting girls with precocious puberty for brain imaging: Validation of European evidence-based diagnosis rule. *J Pediatr* 2003;143:445–450.

Hirsch HJ, Gillis D, Strich D, et al: The histrelin implant: A novel treatment for central precocious puberty. *Pediatrics* 2005;116:e798–e802.

Ibanez L, Dimartino-Nardi J, Potau N, et al: Premature adrenarche—normal variant or forerunner of adult disease? *Endocr Rev* 2000;21:671–696.

Ibanez L, Ferrer A, Marcos MV, et al: Early puberty: Rapid progression and reduced final height in girls with low birth weight. *Pediatrics* 2000;106:E72.

Ibanez L, Ferrer A, Ong K, et al: Insulin sensitization early after menarche prevents progression from precocious pubarche to polycystic ovary syndrome. *J Pediatr* 2004;144:4–6.

Ibanez L, Potau N, Marcos MV, et al: Adrenal hyperandrogenism in adolescent girls with a history of low birthweight and precocious pubarche. *Clin Endocrinol (Oxf)* 2000;53:523–527.

Ibanez L, Potau N, Zampolli M, et al: Use of leuprolide acetate response patterns in the early diagnosis of pubertal disorders: Comparison with the gonadotropin-releasing hormone test. *J Clin Endocrinol Metab* 1994;78:30–35.

Kaplowitz PB, Slora EJ, Wasserman RC, et al: Earlier onset of puberty in girls: Relation to increased body mass and race. *Pediatrics* 2001;108:347–353.

Klein K, Barnes KM, Jones JV, et al: Increase in final height in precocious puberty after long-term treatment with LHRH agonists: The National Institutes of Health experience. *J Clin Endocrinol Metab* 2001;86: 4711–4716.

Latronico AC, Lins TS, Brito VN, et al: The effect of distinct activating mutations of the luteinizing hormone receptor gene on the pituitary-gonadal axis in both sexes. *Clin Endocrinol (Oxf)* 2000;53:609–613.

Leger J, Reynaud R, Czernichow P: Do all girls with apparent idiopathic precocious puberty require gonadotropin-releasing hormone agonist treatment? *J Pediatr* 2000;137:819–825.

Lumbroso S, Paris F, Sultan C: McCune-Albright syndrome: Molecular genetics. *J Pediatr Endocrinol Metab* 2002;15(Suppl 3):875–882.

Mul D, Oostdijk W, Drop SL: Early puberty in adopted children. *Horm Res* 2002;57:1–9.

Neville KA, Walker JL: Precocious pubarche is associated with SGA, prematurity, weight gain, and obesity. *Arch Dis Child* 2005:90:258–261.

Ng SM, Kumar Y, Cody D, et al: Cranial MRI scans are indicated in all girls with central precocious puberty. *Arch Dis Child* 2003;88:414–418.

Palmert MR, Boepple PA: Variation in the timing of puberty: Clinical spectrum and genetic investigation. *J Clin Endocrinol Metab* 2001; 86:2364–2368.

Pucarelli I, Segni M, Ortore M, et al: Combined therapy with GnRH analog plus growth hormone in central precocious puberty. *J Pediatr Endocrinol Metab* 2000;13:811–820.

Ritzen EM: Early puberty: What is normal and when is treatment indicated? *Horm Res* 2003;60:31–34.

Saenger P, Rincon M: Precocious puberty: McCune-Albright syndrome and beyond. *J Pediatr* 2003;143:9–10.

Seminara SB, Messager S, Chatzidaki EE, et al: The GPR54 gene as a regulator of puberty. *N Engl J Med* 2003;349:1614–1626.

Stanhope R: Gonadotropin-dependent precocious puberty and occult intracranial tumors: Which girls should have neuro-imaging? *J Pediatr* 2003;143:426–427.

Tanaka T, Niimi H, Matsuo N, et al: Results of long-term follow-up after treatment of central precocious puberty with leuprorelin acetate: Evaluation of effectiveness of treatment and recovery of gonadal function. *J Clin Endocrinol Metab* 2005;90:1371–1376.

Teilmann G, Pedersen CB, Kold Jensen T, et al: Prevalence and incidence of precocious pubertal development in Denmark: An epidemiologic study based on national registries. *Pediatrics* 2005;116:1323–1328.

Terasawa E, Fernandez DL: Neurobiological mechanisms of the onset of puberty in primates. *Endocr Rev* 2001;22:111–151.

Tuvemo T, Gustafsson J, Proos LA, et al: Suppression of puberty in girls with short acting intranasal versus subcutaneous depot GnRH agonist. *Horm Res* 2002;57:27–31.

Tuvemo T, Jonsson B, Gustafsson J, et al: Final height after combined growth hormone and GnRH analogue treatment in adopted girls with early puberty. *Acta Paediatr* 2004;93:1456–1462.

Van Beek JT, Sharafuddin MJ, Kao SC, et al: Prospective evaluation of pituitary size and shape on MR imaging after suppressive hormonal therapy in central precocious puberty. *Pediatr Radiol* 2000;30:444–446.

Virdis R, Street ME, Bandello MA, et al: Growth and pubertal disorders in neurofibromatosis type 1. *J Pediatr Endocrinol Metab* 2003;16:289–292.

Walvoord EC, Pescovitz OH: Combined use of growth hormone and gonadotropin-releasing hormone analogues in precocious puberty: Theoretic and practical considerations. *Pediatrics* 1999;104:1010–1014.

Section 2 — Disorders of the Thyroid Gland — Stephen LaFranchi

Chapter 564 ■ Thyroid Development and Physiology

FETAL DEVELOPMENT

The fetal thyroid bilobed shape is recognized by 7 wk of gestation, and characteristic thyroid follicle cell and colloid formation is seen by 10 wk. Thyroglobulin synthesis occurs from 4 wk, iodine trapping occurs by 8–10 wk, and thyroxine (T_4) and, to a lesser extent, triiodothyronine (T_3) synthesis and secretion occur from 12 wk of gestation. There is evidence that 4 transcription factors—TTF-1, PAX8, Foxel, and Hhex—are important in thyroid gland morphogenesis and differentiation and possibly also in its caudal migration to its final location. These factors also bind to the promoters of thyroglobulin and thyroid peroxidase genes and so influence thyroid hormone production. Hypothalamic neurons synthesize thyrotropin-releasing hormone (TRH) by 6–8 wk, the pituitary portal vessel system begins development by 8–10 wk, and thyroid-stimulating hormone (TSH) secretion is evident by 12 wk of gestation. Maturation of the hypothalamic-pituitary-thyroid axis occurs over the 2nd half of gestation, but normal feedback relationships are not mature until approximately 3 mo of postnatal life. Another transcription factor, Pit-1, is important for differentiation and growth of thyrotrophs, along with somatotrophs and lactotrophs.

THYROID PHYSIOLOGY

The main function of the thyroid gland is to synthesize T_4 and T_3. The only known physiologic role of iodine is in the synthesis of these hormones; the recommended dietary allowance of iodine is 30 µg/kg/24 hr for infants, 90–120 µg/24 hr for children, and 150 µg/24 hr for adolescents and adults.

The median iodine intake in the United States has decreased by approximately 50% between the 1970s (320 µg/L) and the 1990s (145 µg/L) although at present intake appears to have stabilized. Whatever the chemical form ingested, iodine eventually reaches the thyroid gland as iodide. Thyroid tissue has an avidity for iodine and is able to trap (with a gradient of 100 : 1), transport, and concentrate it in the follicular lumen for synthesis of thyroid hormone. Iodine transport is carried out by the sodium-iodide symporter.

Before trapped iodide can react with tyrosine, it must be oxidized; this reaction is catalyzed by **thyroidal peroxidase.** The thyroid cells also elaborate a specific thyroprotein, a globulin with approximately 120 tyrosine units **(thyroglobulin).** Iodination of tyrosine forms monoiodotyrosine and diiodotyrosine; 2 molecules of diiodotyrosine then couple to form 1 molecule of T_4, or 1 molecule of diiodotyrosine and 1 of monoiodotyrosine to form T_3. Once formed, hormones are stored as thyroglobulin in the lumen of the follicle (colloid) until ready to be delivered to the body cells. Thyroglobulin is a large globular glycoprotein with a molecular weight of about 660,000. T_4 and T_3 are liberated from thyroglobulin by activation of proteases and peptidases.

The metabolic potency of T_3 is 3 to 4 times that of T_4. In adults, the thyroid produces approximately 100 µg of T_4 and 20 µg of T_3 daily. Only 20% of circulating T_3 is secreted by the thyroid; the remainder is produced by deiodination of T_4 in the liver, kidney, and other peripheral tissues by type I 5′-deiodinase. Selenocysteine is the active center of the iodothyronine deiodinases. Thus, selenium indirectly plays a role in normal growth and development. In the pituitary and brain, approximately 80% of required T_3 is produced locally from T_4 by a different enzyme, type II 5′-deiodinase. The level of T_3 in blood is 1/50th that of T_4, but T_3 is the physiologically active thyroid hormone.

Thyroid hormones increase oxygen consumption, stimulate protein synthesis, influence growth and differentiation, and affect carbohydrate, lipid, and vitamin metabolism. The free hormones enter cells, where T_4 may be converted to T_3 by deiodination. Monocarboxylate transporter 8 is an active, specific thyroid hormone transporter that facilitates T_4 entry into cells. Mutations of the *MCT8* are associated with high T_3 levels, thyroid hormone resistance, and severe X-linked psychomotor retardation. Intracellular T_3 then enters the nucleus, where it binds to thyroid hormone receptors. Thyroid hormone receptors are members of the steroid hormone receptor superfamily that includes glucocorticoids, estrogen, progesterone, vitamin D, and retinoids. Four different isoforms of the thyroid hormone receptor (α_1, α_2 β_1, and β_2) are expressed in different tissues; the protein product of the formerly designated *c-erb* A proto-oncogene (now called *THRA2*) has been identified as the α_2 thyroid hormone receptor in the brain and hypothalamus. Thyroid hormone receptors consist of a ligand-binding domain (binds T_3), hinge region, and DNA-binding domain (zinc finger). Binding of T_3 activates the thyroid hormone receptor response element, resulting in production of an encoded mRNA and protein synthesis and of secretion specific for the target cell. In this manner, a single hormone, T_4, acting through tissue-specific thyroid hormone receptor isoforms and gene-specific thyroid response elements, can produce multiple effects in various tissues.

About 70% of the circulating T_4 is firmly bound to thyroxine-binding globulin (TBG). Less important carriers are thyroxine-binding prealbumin, called transthyretin, and albumin. Only 0.03% of T_4 in serum is not bound and comprises free T_4. Approximately 50% of circulating T_3 is bound to TBG, and 50% is bound to albumin; 0.30% of T_3 is unbound, or free, T_3. Because the concentration of TBG is altered in many clinical circumstances, its status must be considered when interpreting T_4 or T_3 levels.

THYROID REGULATION

The thyroid is regulated by TSH, a glycoprotein produced and secreted by the anterior pituitary. This hormone activates adenylate cyclase in the thyroid gland and is important in all steps of thyroid hormone biosynthesis, from trapping of iodine to release of thyroid hormones. TSH is composed of 2 noncovalently bound subunits (chains): α and β. The α subunit is common to luteinizing hormone, follicle-stimulating hormone, and chorionic gonadotropin; the specificity of each hormone is conferred by the β subunit. TSH synthesis and release are stimulated by TSH-releasing hormone (TRH), which is synthesized in the hypothalamus and secreted into the pituitary. TRH is found in other parts of the brain besides the hypothalamus and in many other organs; aside from its endocrine function, it may be a neurotransmitter. TRH is a simple tripeptide. In states of decreased production of thyroid hormone, TSH and TRH are increased. Exogenous thyroid hormone or increased thyroid hormone synthesis inhibits TSH and TRH production. Except in the neonate, levels of TRH in serum are very low.

Further control of the level of circulating thyroid hormones occurs in the periphery. In many nonthyroidal illnesses, extrathyroidal production of T_3 decreases; factors that inhibit thyroxine-type I 5′-deiodinase include fasting, chronic malnutrition, acute illness, and certain drugs. Levels of T_3 may be significantly decreased, whereas levels of free T_4 and TSH remain normal. Presumably, the decreased levels of T_3 result in decreased rates of oxygen production, of substrate use, and of other catabolic processes.

Cavalieri RD: Iodine metabolism and thyroid physiology: Current concepts. [Review.] *Thyroid* 1997;7:177–181.

De Felice M, Di Lauro F: The development of the thyroid gland: What we know and what we would like to know. *Curr Opin Endocrinol Metab* 2005;12:4.

Fisher DA, Brown RS: Thyroid physiology in the perinatal period and during childhood. In Braverman LE, Utiger RD (editors): *Werner & Ingbar's The Thyroid: A Fundamental and Clinical Text,* 8th ed. Philadelphia, Lippincott Williams & Wilkins, 2000, p 959.

Friesema ECH, Grueters A, Biebermann H, et al: Association between mutations in a thyroid hormone transporter and severe X-linked psychomotor retardation. *Lancet* 2004;364:1435–1437.

Hollowell JG, Staehling NW, Hannon WH, et al: Iodine nutrition in the United States—Trends and public health implications: Iodine excretion data from National Health and Nutrition Examination Surveys I and III (1971–1974 and 1988–1994). *J Clin Endocrinol Metab* 1998;83:3401–3408.

564.1 • Thyroid Hormone Studies

SERUM THYROID HORMONES. Methods are available to measure all the thyroid hormones in sera: T_4, free T_4, T_3, and free T_3. A metabolically inert T_3 (3,5′,3′-triiodothyronine), called reverse T_3, is also present in sera. Age must be considered in interpreting results, particularly in the neonate.

Thyroglobulin is a glycoprotein dimer that is secreted through the apical surface of the thyrocyte into the colloid. Small amounts escape into the circulation and are measurable in serum. Levels increase with TSH (also called thyrotropin) stimulation and decrease with TSH suppression. Levels are increased in the neonate, in patients with Graves disease and other forms of autoimmune thyroid disease, and in those with endemic goiter. The most marked elevations of thyroglobulin occur in patients with differentiated carcinoma of the thyroid. Athyreotic infants may have markedly reduced levels of thyroglobulin in serum.

TSH levels in serum are an extremely sensitive indicator of primary hypothyroidism. A 3rd generation of assays (chemiluminescent assays) that can measure complete suppression of TSH below the normal range is standard. After the neonatal period, normal levels of TSH are less than 6 µU/mL. These sensitive TSH assays obviate the need for TRH stimulation in the diagnosis of most patients with thyroid disorders.

FETAL AND NEWBORN THYROID. Fetal serum T_4 increases progressively from mid-gestation to approximately 11.5 μg/dL at term. Fetal levels of T_3 are low before 20 wk and then gradually increase to about 45 ng/dL at term. Reverse T_3 levels (inactive form of T_3), however, are high in the fetus (250 ng/dL at 30 wk) and decrease to 150 ng/dL at term. Serum levels of TSH gradually increase to 10 mU/L at term. Approximately ⅓ of maternal T_4 crosses the placenta to the fetus. Maternal T_4 may play a role in fetal development, especially that of the brain, before the synthesis of fetal thyroid hormones begins. The fetus of a hypothyroid mother may be at risk for neurologic damage, and a hypothyroid fetus may be partially protected by maternal T_4 until delivery. The amount of T_4 that crosses the placenta is not sufficient to interfere with a diagnosis of congenital hypothyroidism in the neonate.

At birth, there is an acute release of TSH; peak serum concentrations reach 60 mU/L in 30 min in full-term infants. A rapid decline occurs in the ensuing 24 hr and a more gradual decline within the next 5 days to less than 10 μU/mL. The acute increase in TSH produces a dramatic increase in levels of T_4 to approximately 16 μg/dL and of T_3 to approximately 300 ng/dL in about 4 hr. This T_3 seems largely derived from increased peripheral conversion of T_4 to T_3. T_4 levels gradually decrease during the 1st 2 wk of life to 12 μg/dL. T_3 levels then decline during the 1st wk of life to levels below 200 ng/mL. Serum free T_4 levels are 0.9–2.3 ng/dL in infancy and decline to 0.7–1.8 ng/dL in childhood. Serum free T_3 concentrations are approximately 540 pg/dL in infancy and decline to 210–440 pg/dL in childhood. Reverse T_3 levels are maintained for 2 wk (200 ng/dL) and decrease by 4 wk to around 50 ng/dL. In preterm infants, changes in thyroid function after birth are qualitatively similar to but quantitatively smaller than full-term infants. Serum T_4 and T_3 levels are proportional to gestational age and birth weight.

SERUM THYROXINE-BINDING GLOBULIN. The thyroid hormones are transported in plasma bound to TBG, a glycoprotein synthesized in the liver. Estimation of TBG levels is occasionally necessary because TBG is increased or decreased in a variety of clinical situations, with effects on the level of total thyroxine. TBG binds about 70% of T_4 and 50% of T_3. TBG levels increase in pregnancy, in the newborn period, and with administration of estrogens (oral contraceptives), perphenazine, or heroin, and they decrease with androgens, anabolic steroids, glucocorticoids, and L-asparaginase. These effects are the results of modulation of hepatic synthesis of TBG. Phenytoin (diphenylhydantoin) is another cause of drug-induced abnormality of thyroid function tests. Phenytoin, an inducer of hepatic enzymes, stimulates hepatic degradation of T_4 and accelerates transport of T_4 into tissues. Phenobarbital and carbamazepine have a similar effect. Some drugs, particularly phenytoin, also inhibit binding of T_4 and T_3 to TBG. Decreased or increased levels of TBG also occur as genetic traits (see Chapter 565). TBG levels may be markedly decreased owing to decreased production with liver disease or loss in the gut with protein-losing enteropathies or urine, as in the congenital nephrotic syndrome.

IN VIVO RADIONUCLIDE STUDIES. Markedly improved direct tests of thyroid function have made radioiodine uptake studies less useful. The iodine trapping or concentrating mechanism of the thyroid can be evaluated by measuring the uptake of radioactive isotope ^{123}I (half-life of 13 hr). The technology allows doses of radioiodine (0.1–0.5 mCi) that are only a fraction of those formerly used with ^{131}I. Technetium (^{99m}Tc) is a particularly useful radioisotope for children, because in contrast to iodine, it is trapped but not organified by the thyroid and has a half-life of only 6 hr. Thyroid scanning may be indicated to assess the presence of thyroid tissue in questions of thyroid agenesis and to detect ectopic thyroid tissue, and thyroid uptake may be indicated to evaluate possible "hot" thyroid nodules. These studies should be performed with ^{99m}Tc pertechnetate or ^{123}I because they have the advantages of lower radiation exposure and high-quality scintigrams. Use of ^{131}I in children should be limited to those known to have thyroid cancer.

THYROID ULTRASONOGRAPHIC STUDIES. Thyroid ultrasound examinations can determine the location, size, and shape of the thyroid gland, and they can assess the solid or cystic nature of nodules. Ultrasound is not so reliable as radionuclide studies in evaluating infants with suspected thyroid dysgenesis, particularly ectopic glands. Ultrasound examinations are useful in identifying normal thyroid gland position in children with suspected thyroglossal duct cysts. In children with autoimmune thyroiditis, ultrasound reveals scattered hypoechogenicity. Ultrasound examinations are more accurate than physical examination in estimating goiter size and assessing thyroid nodules.

Fisher DA: Physiological variations in thyroid hormones: Physiological and pathophysiological considerations. *Clin Chem* 1996;42:135–139.

Haddow JE, Palomaki GE, Allan WC, et al: Maternal thyroid deficiency during pregnancy and subsequent neuropsychological development of the child. *N Engl J Med* 1999;341:549–555.

Murphy N, Hume R, van Toor H, et al: The hypothalamic-pituitary-thyroid axis in preterm infants: Changes in the first 24 hours of postnatal life. *J Clin Endocrinol Metab* 2004;89:2824–2831.

O'Reilly DS: Thyroid function tests—Time for a reassessment. *Br Med J* 2000;320: 1332–1334.

Pop VJ, Brouwers EP, Vader HL, et al: Maternal hypothyroxinaemia during early pregnancy and subsequent child development: A 3-year follow-up study. *Clin Endocrinol (Oxf)* 2003;59:282–288.

Xu F, Sullivan K, Houston R, et al: Thyroid volumes in US and Bangladeshi schoolchildren: Comparison with European schoolchildren. *Eur J Endocrinol* 1999;140:498–504.

Chapter 565 ■ Defects of Thyroxine-Binding Globulin

Abnormalities in levels of thyroxine-binding globulin (TBG) are not associated with clinical disease and do not require treatment. They are usually uncovered by a chance finding of abnormally low or high levels of thyroxine (T_4) and may be a source of confusion in the diagnosis of hypothyroidism or hyperthyroidism.

TBG deficiency occurs as an X-linked dominant disorder. Congenital TBG deficiency is most often discovered through screening programs for neonatal hypothyroidism that use levels of T_4 as the primary screen. Affected patients have low levels of T_4 and elevated resin triiodothyronine uptake (RT_3U), but levels of free T_4 and thyroid-stimulating hormone (TSH) are normal. The diagnosis is confirmed by the finding of absent or low levels of TBG. TBG deficiency occurs in 1 in 2,400 male newborns, 36% of whom have TBG levels less than 1 mg/dL. Milder forms of TBG deficiency occur in approximately 1/42,000 heterozygous female newborns. Complete TBG deficiency (<5 μg/dL) occurs much less frequently. Three of eight families with complete TBG deficiency have been found to have a codon mutation (leucine to proline); other patients with reduced affinity of TBG for T_4 have had other point mutations that affect the tertiary structure of the protein. Acquired TBG deficiency occurs with androgen and glucocorticoid treatment, hepatic insufficiency (not hepatitis), renal disease and proteinuria, and protein-losing enteropathies.

TBG excess also is a harmless X-linked dominant anomaly, occurring in about 1 in 25,000 persons. It has been recognized primarily in adults, but neonatal screening programs uncover the condition in the neonate. The level of T_4 is elevated, T_3 is variably elevated, TSH and free T_4 are normal, and RT_3U is decreased. The elevated levels of TBG confirm the diagnosis. In neonates, levels of T_4 as high as 95 µg/dL have been found, which decrease to 20–30 µg/dL after 2–3 wk. Such high levels of T_4 may be related in part to the normally elevated levels of TBG in neonates during the 1st mo of life, presumably as an effect of maternal estrogens. Affected patients are euthyroid. Family studies may be indicated to alert other affected individuals. Acquired elevations of TBG occur with pregnancy, estrogen treatment, hepatitis, and with certain drugs (clofibrate, methadone, perphenazine).

Familial dysalbuminemic hyperthyroxinemia is an autosomal dominant disorder that may be confused with hyperthyroidism. Markedly increased binding of T_4 to an abnormal albumin variant leads to increased serum concentrations of T_4. However, the levels of free T_4, free T_3, and TSH are normal. Levels of T_3 are normal or only slightly elevated. Affected patients are euthyroid.

LaFranchi SH, Snyder DB, Sesser DE, et al: Follow-up of newborns with elevated screening T_4 concentrations. *J Pediatr* 2003;143:296–301.
Mandel SH, Hanna CE, Boston BA, et al: Thyroxine binding globulin deficiency detected by newborn screening. *J Pediatr* 1993; 122:227–230.
Refetoff S, Murata Y, Mori Y, et al: Thyroxine-binding globulin: Organization of the gene and variants. *Horm Res* 1996;45:128–138.

Chapter 566 ■ Hypothyroidism

Hypothyroidism results from deficient production of thyroid hormone or a defect in thyroid hormone receptor activity (Table 566-1). The disorder may be manifested from birth or acquired. When symptoms appear after a period of apparently normal thyroid function, the disorder may be truly "acquired" or may only appear so as a result of one of a variety of congenital defects in which the manifestation of the deficiency is delayed. The term cretinism, although often used synonymously with endemic iodine deficiency and congenital hypothyroidism, is to be avoided.

TABLE 566-1. Etiologic Classification of Congenital Hypothyroidism

CENTRAL (HYPOPITUITARY) HYPOTHYROIDISM
PIT-1 mutations
Deficiency of thyrotropin (TSH), growth hormone, and prolactin
PROP-1 mutations
Deficiency of TSH, growth hormone, prolactin, LH, FSH, ±ACTH
Thyrotropin-releasing hormone (TRH) deficiency
Isolated?
Multiple hypothalamic deficiencies (e.g., septo-optic dysplasia)
TRH unresponsiveness
Mutations in TRH receptor
TSH deficiency
Mutations in β-chain
Multiple pituitary deficiencies (e.g., craniopharyngioma)
TSH unresponsiveness
$G_s\alpha$ mutation (e.g., type IA pseudohypoparathyroidism)
Mutation in TSH receptor
PRIMARY HYPOTHYROIDISM
Defect of fetal thyroid development
Aplasia, hypoplasia, ectopia (dysgenesis)
Defect in thyroid hormone synthesis (e.g., goitrous hypothyroidism)
Iodide transport defect
Thyroid peroxidase defect
Thyroid oxidase mutations: homozygotic—permanent; heterozygotic—transient
Thyroglobulin synthesis defect
Deiodination defect
Defect in thyroid hormone transport
Iodine deficiency (endemic goiter)
Neurologic type
Myxedematous type
Maternal antibodies
Thyrotropin receptor–blocking antibody (TRBAb, also termed thyrotropin-binding inhibitor immunoglobulin)
Maternal medications
Radioiodine, iodides
Propylthiouracil, methimazole
Amiodarone

ACTH, adrenocorticotropic hormone; FSH, follicle-stimulating hormone; LH, luteinizing hormone.

CONGENITAL HYPOTHYROIDISM

Most cases of congenital hypothyroidism are not hereditary and result from thyroid dysgenesis. Some cases may be familial, usually caused by one of the inborn errors of thyroid hormone synthesis, and may be associated with a goiter. In many cases, the deficiency of thyroid hormone is severe, and symptoms develop in the early weeks of life. In others, lesser degrees of deficiency occur, and manifestations may be delayed for months.

EPIDEMIOLOGY. The prevalence of congenital hypothyroidism based on nationwide programs for neonatal screening is 1/4,000 infants worldwide; prevalence is lower in black Americans (1/32,000) and higher in Hispanics and Native Americans (1/2,000). Twice as many girls as boys are affected.

ETIOLOGY

Thyroid Dysgenesis. Some form of thyroid dysgenesis (aplasia, hypoplasia, or an ectopic gland) is the most common cause of congenital hypothyroidism, accounting for 85% of cases; 10% are caused by an inborn error of thyroxine synthesis, and 5% are the result of transplacental maternal thyrotropin-receptor blocking antibody (TRBAb). In about ⅓ of cases of dysgenesis, even sensitive radionuclide scans can find no remnants of thyroid tissue (aplasia). In the other ⅔ of infants, rudiments of thyroid tissue are found in an ectopic location, anywhere from the base of the tongue (lingual thyroid) to the normal position in the neck (hypoplasia).

The exact cause of thyroid dysgenesis is unknown in most cases. Thyroid dysgenesis occurs sporadically, but familial cases occasionally have been reported. The finding that thyroid developmental anomalies, such as thyroglossal duct cysts and hemiagenesis, are present in 8–10% of 1st-degree relatives of infants with thyroid dysgenesis supports an underlying genetic component.

Three transcription factors, TTF-1, FOXE1, and PAX-8, are important for thyroid morphogenesis and differentiation; mutations in these genes are associated with thyroid dysgenesis. In addition, genetic defects leading to absent or ineffective thyrotropin action have been described.

Another transcription factor, NKX2.1, is expressed in both the thyroid and central nervous system. Mutations in NKX2.1 have been reported to result in congenital hypothyroidism with persistent neurologic problems, including ataxia, despite early thyroid hormone treatment.

The frequent finding of thyroid dysgenesis confined to only one of a pair of monozygotic twins suggests the operation of a deleterious factor during intrauterine life. Maternal antithyroid antibodies might be that factor. Although thyroid peroxidase (TPO) antibodies have been detected in some mother-infant pairs, there is little evidence of their pathogenicity. The demonstration of thyroid growth-blocking and cytotoxic antibodies in some infants with thyroid dysgenesis, as well as in their mothers, suggests a more likely pathogenetic mechanism.

The most common form of thyroid dysgenesis is an **ectopic gland**, which may be demonstrated by a thyroid scan or ultrasonographic examination. Most cases are detected by newborn screening, but in some children ectopic thyroid tissue (lingual, sublingual, subhyoid) may provide adequate amounts of thyroid hormone for many years, or it may eventually fail in early childhood. Affected children come to clinical attention because of a growing mass at the base of the tongue or in the midline of the neck, usually at the level of the hyoid. Occasionally, ectopia is associated with thyroglossal duct cysts. It may occur in siblings. Surgical removal of ectopic thyroid tissue from a euthyroid individual usually results in hypothyroidism, because most such patients have no other thyroid tissue.

Defective Synthesis of Thyroxine (Dyshormonogenesis). A variety of defects in the biosynthesis of thyroid hormone may result in congenital hypothyroidism; these are detected in 1/30,000–50,000 live births in neonatal screening programs. These defects are transmitted in an autosomal recessive manner. A **goiter** is almost always present. When the defect is incomplete, compensation occurs, and onset of hypothyroidism may be delayed for years.

Defect of Iodide Transport. This rare defect involves mutations in the sodium-iodide symporter. Among the several cases now reported, it has been found in 9 related infants of the Hutterite sect, and about ½ the cases are from Japan. Consanguinity has occurred in about ⅓ of the families.

In the past, clinical hypothyroidism, with or without a goiter, often developed in the first few months of life; the condition has been detected in neonatal screening programs. In Japan, however, untreated patients acquire goiter and hypothyroidism after 10 yr of age, perhaps because of the very high iodine content (often 19 mg/24 hr) of the Japanese diet.

The energy-dependent mechanisms for concentrating iodide are defective in the thyroid and salivary glands. In contrast to other defects of thyroid hormone synthesis, uptake of radioiodine and pertechnetate is low; a saliva to serum ratio of ^{123}I may be required to establish the diagnosis. This condition responds to treatment with large doses of potassium iodide, but treatment with thyroxine (T_4) is preferable.

Thyroid Peroxidase Defects of Organification and Coupling. This is the most common of the T_4 synthetic defects. After iodide is trapped by the thyroid, it is rapidly oxidized to reactive iodine, which is then incorporated into tyrosine units on thyroglobulin. This process requires generation of H_2O_2, thyroid peroxidase, and hematin (an enzyme cofactor); defects can involve each of these components, and there is considerable clinical and biochemical heterogeneity. In the Dutch neonatal screening program, 23 infants were found with a complete organification defect (1/60,000), but its prevalence in other areas is unknown. A characteristic finding in all patients with this defect is a marked decrease in thyroid radioactivity when perchlorate or thiocyanate is administered 2 hr after administration of a test dose of radioiodine. In these patients, perchlorate discharges 40–90% of radioiodine compared with less than 10% in normal individuals. Several mutations in the TPO gene have been reported in children with congenital hypothyroidism. Patients with **Pendred syndrome,** a disorder comprising sensorineural deafness and goiter, also have a positive perchlorate discharge. Pendred syndrome is due to a defect in a sulfate transport protein common to the thyroid gland and the cochlea.

Thyroid oxidase 2 helps generate H_2O_2. Bi-allelic inactivating mutations produce permanent congenital hypothyroidism, whereas single-gene lesions produce transient hypothyroidism.

Defects of Thyroglobulin Synthesis. This heterogeneous group of disorders, characterized by goiter, elevated thyroid-stimulating hormone (TSH), low T_4 levels, and absent or low levels of thyroglobulin (TG), has been reported in approximately 100 patients. Molecular defects, primarily point mutations, have been described in several patients.

Defects in Deiodination. Monoiodotyrosine and diiodotyrosine released from thyroglobulin are normally deiodinated within the thyroid or in peripheral tissues by a deiodinase. The liberated iodine is recycled in the synthesis of thyroid hormones. Patients with a deficiency of this enzyme experience severe iodine loss from the constant urinary excretion of nondeiodinated tyrosines, leading to hormonal deficiency and goiter. The deiodination defect may be limited to thyroid tissue only or to peripheral tissue only, or it may be universal.

Defects in Thyroid Hormone Transport. Passage of thyroid hormone into the cell is facilitated by plasma membrane transporters. A mutation in 1 such transporter gene, monocarboxylate transporter 8 (MCT8), located on the X chromosome, has been reported in 5 boys with x-linked mental retardation. The defective transporter appears to impair passage of T3 into neurons; this syndrome is characterized by elevated serum T3 levels and psychomotor retardation.

Thyrotropin Receptor–Blocking Antibody. Maternal thyrotropin receptor–blocking antibody (TRBAb) (often measured as thyrotropin-binding inhibitor immunoglobulin), is an unusual cause of transitory congenital hypothyroidism. Transplacental passage of maternal TRBAb inhibits binding of TSH to its receptor in the neonate. The frequency is approximately 1/50,000–100,000 infants. It should be suspected whenever there is a history of maternal autoimmune thyroid disease, including Hashimoto thyroiditis, Graves disease, hypothyroidism while the patient is receiving replacement therapy, or recurrent congenital hypothyroidism of a transient nature in subsequent siblings. In these situations, maternal levels of TRBAb should be measured during pregnancy. Affected infants and their mothers may also have thyrotropin receptor–stimulating antibodies (TRSAbs) and TPO antibodies. Technetium pertechnetate and ^{125}I scans may fail to detect any thyroid tissue, mimicking thyroid agenesis, but ultrasonography will show a thyroid gland. After the condition remits, a normal thyroid gland is demonstrable by scanning following discontinuation of replacement treatment. The half-life of the antibody is 21 days, and remission of the hypothyroidism occurs in about 3–6 mo. Correct diagnosis of this cause of congenital hypothyroidism prevents unnecessary protracted treatment, alerts the clinician to possible recurrences in future pregnancies, and allows a favorable prognosis.

Radioiodine Administration. Hypothyroidism may occur as a result of inadvertent administration of radioiodine during pregnancy for treatment of Graves disease or cancer of the thyroid. The fetal thyroid is capable of trapping iodide by 70–75 days. Whenever radioiodine is administered to a woman of childbearing age, a pregnancy test must be performed before a therapeutic dose of ^{131}I is given, regardless of the menstrual history or putative history of contraception. Administration of radioactive iodine to lactating women also is contraindicated because it is readily excreted in milk.

Thyrotropin Deficiency. Deficiency of TSH and hypothyroidism may occur in any of the conditions associated with developmental defects of the pituitary or hypothalamus (see Chapter 558). More often in these conditions, the deficiency of TSH is secondary to a deficiency of thyrotropin-releasing hormone (TRH). TSH-deficient hypothyroidism is found in 1/30,000–50,000 infants; most screening programs are designed to detect primary hypothyroidism, so most of these cases are not detected by neonatal thyroid screening. The majority of affected infants have multiple pituitary deficiencies and present with hypoglycemia, persistent jaundice, and micropenis in association with septo-optic dysplasia, midline cleft lip, midface hypoplasia, and other midline facial anomalies.

Pit-1 mutations are a recessive cause of central hypothyroidism secondary to TSH deficiency. Affected children also have deficiency of growth hormone and prolactin. Pit-1, a gene transcription factor, is essential to differentiation, maintenance, and proliferation of somatotrophs, lactotrophs, and thyrotrophs. Examination of prolactin and TSH responses to TRH stimulation can detect these patients. Failure of the prolactin response to TRH should prompt examination of the Pit-1 gene.

PROP-1 is another transcription factor important in pituitary development and hormone production. Infants with a mutation in the PROP-1 gene ("prophet" of Pit-1) are reported to have not only TSH, GH, and prolactin deficiency but also LH and FSH deficiency and variable ACTH deficiency.

Isolated deficiency of TSH is a rare autosomal recessive disorder that has been reported in several sibships. DNA studies in 2 Japanese children and in 3 children in 2 related Greek families have revealed different point mutations in the TSH β subunit gene; studies in 2 German siblings revealed a mutation causing a stop codon due to a frame shift, and studies in 2 Turkish families revealed splice site mutations.

Thyrotropin Hormone Unresponsiveness. A mutation in the TSH-receptor gene has been reported in 3 siblings with elevated levels of TSH and normal levels of T_4; 2 of them had been detected during neonatal screening. Despite persistent resistance to TSH through childhood, they remained euthyroid without treatment. Patients in 3 other reports of presumed TSH-receptor gene mutations had severe hypothyroidism that required treatment. The disorder is inherited in an autosomal recessive fashion. Both homozygous and compound heterozygous mutations in the TSH receptor gene have been reported.

Mild congenital hypothyroidism has been detected in newborn infants who subsequently proved to have **type Ia pseudohypoparathyroidism.** The molecular cause of resistance to TSH in these patients is the generalized impairment of cyclic adenosine monophosphate activation caused by genetic deficiency of the α subunit of the guanine nucleotide regulatory protein G_s (see Chapter 573).

Thyrotropin-Releasing Hormone Receptor Abnormality. A patient with a TRH receptor abnormality resulting in isolated TSH deficiency and hypothyroidism has been reported. This condition was suspected because of failure of both TSH and prolactin to respond to TRH stimulation. Investigations disclosed a compound heterozygote mutation in the gene coding for the TRH receptor, resulting in inability of the receptor to bind TRH.

THYROID HORMONE UNRESPONSIVENESS. This autosomal dominant disorder is caused by mutations in the thyroid hormone receptor. Most patients have a goiter, and levels of T_4, T_3, free T_4, and free T_3 are elevated. These findings often have led to the erroneous diagnosis of Graves disease although most affected patients are clinically euthyroid. The unresponsiveness may vary among tissues. There may be subtle clinical features of hypothyroidism, including mild mental retardation, growth retardation, and delayed skeletal maturation. On the other hand, there may be clinical features compatible with hyperthyroidism, such as tachycardia and hyperreflexia. It is presumed that these patients have varying tissue resistance to thyroid hormone. One neurologic manifestation is an increased association of attention-deficit hyperactivity disorder; the converse is not true, however, because individuals with attention-deficit hyperactivity disorder do not have an increased risk of thyroid hormone resistance.

TSH levels are diagnostic in that they are not suppressed as in Graves disease but instead are moderately elevated or normal but inappropriate for the levels of T_4 and T_3 when measured by a sensitive TSH assay. A TSH response to TRH occurs in these patients, unlike the situation in Graves disease. The failure of TSH suppression indicates that the resistance is generalized and affects the pituitary gland as well as peripheral tissues. More than 40 distinct point mutations in the hormone-binding domain of the β–thyroid receptor have been identified. Different phenotypes do not correlate with genotypes. The same mutation has been observed in individuals with generalized or isolated pituitary resistance, even in different individuals of the same family. A child homozygous for the receptor mutation showed unusually severe resistance. These cases support the dominant negative effect of mutant receptors, in which the mutant receptor protein inhibits normal receptor action in heterozygotes. Elevated levels of T_4 on neonatal thyroid screening should suggest the possibility of this diagnosis. No treatment is usually required unless growth and skeletal retardation are present.

Two infants of consanguineous matings are known to have an autosomal recessive form of thyroid resistance. These infants had manifestations of hypothyroidism early in life, and genetic studies revealed a major deletion of the β–thyroid receptor in 1 individual. The resistance appears to be more severe in this form of the entity.

On rare occasions, resistance to thyroid hormone may selectively affect the pituitary gland. Because the peripheral tissues are not resistant to thyroid hormones, the patient has a goiter and manifestations of hyperthyroidism. The laboratory findings are the same as those seen with generalized thyroid hormone resistance. This condition must be differentiated from a pituitary TSH-secreting tumor. Different treatments, including D-thyroxine, TRIAC (triiodothyroacetic acid), and TETRAC (tetraiodothyroacetic acid) have been reported to be successful in some patients. Bromocriptine administration, which interferes with TSH secretion, was reported to be successful in another patient.

Iodine Exposure. Congenital hypothyroidism may result from fetal exposure to excessive iodides. Perinatal exposure may occur with the use of iodine antiseptic to prepare the skin for cesarian section or painting of the cervix prior to delivery. It has also been reported in infants born to mothers in Japan who consumed large quantities of iodine-rich seaweed. These conditions are transitory and must not be mistaken for the other forms of hypothyroidism. In the neonate, topical iodine-containing antiseptics used in nurseries and by surgeons can also cause transient congenital hypothyroidism, especially in low-birthweight infants, and can lead to abnormal results on neonatal screening tests. In older children, the usual sources of iodides are proprietary preparations used to treat asthma. In a few instances, the cause of hypothyroidism was amiodarone, an antiarrhythmic drug with high iodine content. In most of these instances, goiter is present (see Chapter 568.3).

Iodine-Deficiency Endemic Goiter. Essentially unseen in the United States, iodine deficiency or endemic goiter is the most common cause of congenital hypothyroidism worldwide. Borderline iodine deficiency is more likely to cause problems in preterm infants who depend on a maternal source of iodine for normal thyroid hormone production.

THYROID FUNCTION IN PRETERM BABIES. Postnatal thyroid function in preterm babies is qualitatively similar but quantitatively reduced compared with that of term infants. The cord serum T_4 is decreased in proportion to gestational age and birthweight. The postnatal TSH surge is reduced, and infants with complications of prematurity, such as respiratory distress syndrome, actually experience a decrease in serum T_4 in the 1st wk of life. As these complications resolve, the serum T_4 gradually increases so that generally by 6 wk of life it enters the T_4 range seen in term infants. Serum free T_4 concentrations seem less affected, and when measured by equilibrium dialysis, these levels are often normal. Preterm babies also have a higher frequency of transient TSH elevations and apparent transient primary hypothyroidism. Premature infants less than 28 wk of gestation may have problems resulting from a combination of immaturity of the hypothalamic-pituitary-thyroid axis and loss of the maternal contribution of thyroid hormone and so may be candidates for temporary thyroid hormone replacement; further studies are needed.

CLINICAL MANIFESTATIONS. Most infants with congenital hypothyroidism are asymptomatic at birth, even if there is complete agenesis of the thyroid gland. This situation is attributed to the transplacental passage of moderate amounts of maternal T_4, which provides fetal levels that are approximately 33% of normal at birth. These low serum levels of T_4 and concomitantly elevated levels of TSH make it possible to screen and detect hypothyroid neonates.

The clinician is dependent on neonatal screening tests for the diagnosis of congenital hypothyroidism. Laboratory errors occur, however, and awareness of early symptoms and signs must be maintained. Congenital hypothyroidism is twice as common in girls as in boys. Before neonatal screening programs, congenital hypothyroidism was rarely recognized in the newborn because the signs and symptoms are usually not sufficiently developed. It can be suspected and the diagnosis established during the early weeks of life if the initial but less characteristic manifestations are recognized. Birthweight and length are normal, but head size may be slightly increased because of myxedema of the brain. Prolongation of physiologic jaundice, caused by delayed maturation of glucuronide conjugation, may be the earliest sign. Feeding difficulties, especially sluggishness, lack of interest, somnolence, and choking spells during nursing, are often present during the 1st mo of life. Respiratory difficulties, due in part to the large tongue, include apneic episodes, noisy respirations, and nasal obstruction. Typical respiratory distress syndrome may also occur. Affected infants cry little, sleep much, have poor appetites, and are generally sluggish. There may be constipation that does not usually respond to treatment. The abdomen is large, and an umbilical hernia is usually present. The temperature is subnormal, often less than 35°C (95°F), and the skin, particularly that of the extremities, may be cold and mottled. Edema of the genitals and extremities may be present. The pulse is slow, and heart murmurs, cardiomegaly, and asymptomatic pericardial effusion are common. Macrocytic anemia is often present and is refractory to treatment with hematinics. Because symptoms appear gradually, the clinical diagnosis is often delayed.

Approximately 10% of infants with congenital hypothyroidism have associated congenital anomalies. Cardiac anomalies are most common, but anomalies of the nervous system and eye have also been reported.

If congenital hypothyroidism goes undetected and untreated, these manifestations progress. Retardation of physical and mental development becomes greater during the following months, and by 3–6 mo of age the clinical picture is fully developed (Fig. 566-1). When there is only partial deficiency of thyroid hormone, the symptoms may be milder, the syndrome incomplete, and the onset delayed. Although breast milk contains significant amounts of thyroid hormones, particularly T_3, it is inadequate to protect the breast-fed infant with congenital hypothyroidism, and it has no effect on neonatal thyroid screening tests.

The child's growth will be stunted, the extremities are short, and the head size is normal or even increased. The anterior and posterior fontanels are open widely; observation of this sign at birth may serve as an initial clue to the early recognition of congenital hypothyroidism. Only 3% of normal newborn infants have a posterior fontanel larger than 0.5 cm. The eyes appear far apart, and the bridge of the broad nose is depressed. The palpebral fissures are narrow and the eyelids swollen. The mouth is kept open, and the thick, broad tongue protrudes. Dentition will be delayed. The neck is short and thick, and there may be deposits of fat above the clavicles and between the neck and shoulders. The hands are broad and the fingers short. The skin is dry and scaly, and there is little perspiration. Myxedema is manifested, particularly in the skin of the eyelids, the back of the hands, and the external genitals. The skin shows general pallor with a sallow complexion. Carotenemia may cause a yellow discoloration of the skin, but the scleras remain white. The scalp is thickened, and the hair is coarse, brittle, and scanty. The hairline reaches far down on the forehead, which usually appears wrinkled, especially when the infant cries.

Development is usually retarded. Hypothyroid infants appear lethargic and are late in learning to sit and stand. The voice is hoarse, and they do not learn to talk. The degree of physical and mental retardation increases with age. Sexual maturation may be delayed or may not take place at all.

The muscles are usually hypotonic, but in rare instances generalized muscular pseudohypertrophy occurs (**Kocher-Debré-Sémélaigne syndrome**). Affected older children may have an athletic appearance because of pseudohypertrophy, particularly in the calf muscles. Its pathogenesis is unknown; nonspecific histochemical and ultrastructural changes seen on muscle biopsy return to normal with treatment. Boys are more prone to development of the syndrome, which has been observed in siblings born to a consanguineous mating. Affected patients have hypothyroidism of longer duration and severity.

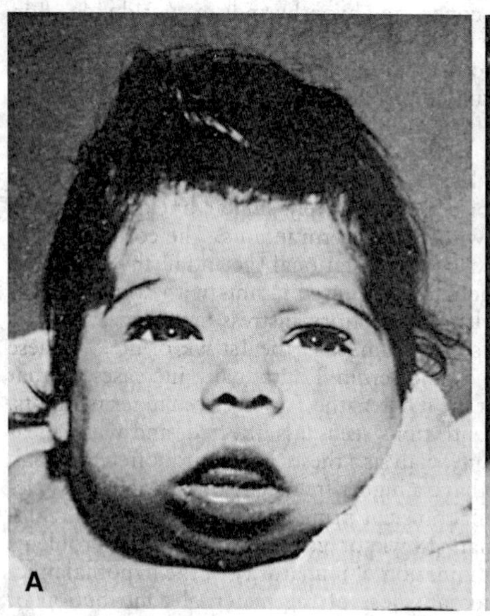

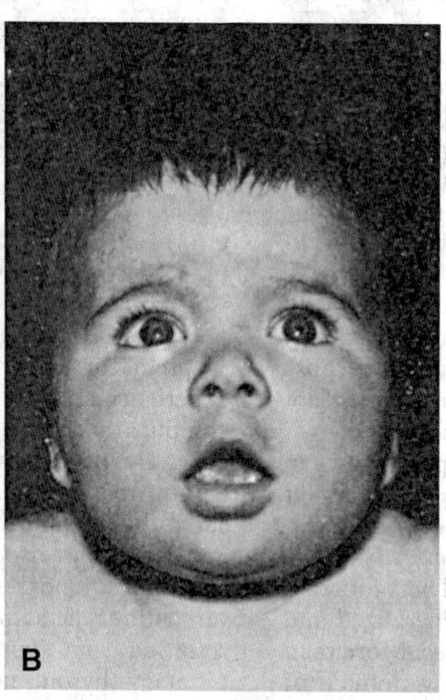

Figure 566-1. Congenital hypothyroidism in an infant 6 mo of age. The infant ate poorly in the neonatal period and was constipated. She had a persistent nasal discharge and a large tongue; she was very lethargic and had no social smile and no head control. *A,* Notice the puffy face, dull expression, and hirsute forehead. Tests revealed a negligible uptake of radioiodine. Osseous development was that of a newborn. *B,* Four months after treatment, note the decreased puffiness of the face, the decreased hirsutism of the forehead, and the alert appearance.

TABLE 566-2. Thyroid Function Tests

ANALYTE OR PROCEDURE	SPECIMEN	REFERENCE VALUES (USA)		CONVERSION FACTOR	REFERENCE VALUES (SI)	
Thyroid thyroglobulin	S	Cord blood	14.7–101.1 ng/mL	×1	14.7–101.1 μg/L	
		Birth–35 mo	10.6–92.0		10.6–92.0	
		3–11 yr	5.6–41.9		5.6–41.9	
		12–17 yr	2.7–21.9		2.7–21.9	
Thyroid stimulating hormone	S	Premature (28–36 wk)				
		1st wk of life	0.7–27.0 mIU/L	×1	0.7–27.0 mIU/L	
		Term infants				
		Birth–4 d	1.0–38.9		1.0–28.9	
		2–20 wk	1.7–9.1		1.7–9.1	
		5 mo–20 yr	0.7–6.4		0.7–6.4	
Thyroxine binding globulin (TBG)	S		mg/dL		mg/L	
		Cord blood	1.4–94	×10	14–94	
		1–4 wk	1.0–9.0		10–90	
		1–12 mo	2.0–7.6		20–76	
		1–5 yr	2.9–5.4		29–54	
		5–10 yr	2.5–5.0		25–50	
		10–15 yr	2.1–4.6		21–46	
		Adult	1.5–3.4		15–34	
Thyroxine, total	S	Full-term infants		×12.9	Full-term infants	
		1–3 day	8.2–19.9 μg/dL		1–3 d	106–256 nmol/L
		1 wk	6.0–15.9		1 wk	77–205
		1–12 mo	6.1–14.9		1–12 mo	79–192
		Prepubertal children			Prepubertal children	
		1–3 yr	6.8–13.5 μg/dL		1–3 yr	88–174 nmol/L
		3–10 yr	5.5–12.8		3–10 yr	71–165
		Pubertal children and adults			Pubertal children and adults	
			4.2–13.0 μg/dL			54–167 nmol/L
Thyroxine, free	S	Newborn infants		×12.9	Full-term infants	
		3 day	2.0–4.9 ng/dL		3 d	26–631 pmol/L
		Infants			Infants	
			0.9–2.6 ng/dL			12–33 pmol/L
		Prepubertal children			Prepubertal children	
			0.8–2.2 ng/dL			10–28 pmol/L
		Pubertal children and adults			Pubertal children and adults	
			0.8–2.3 ng/dL			10–30 pmol/L
Thyroxine, total	W	Newborn screen (filter paper)	6.2–22 μg/dL	×12.9	80–283 nmol/L	
Triidothyronine, free	S		pg/dL		pmol/L	
		Cord blood	20–240	×0.01536	0.3–0.7	
		1–3 day	200–610		3.1–9.4	
		6 wk	240–560		3.7–8.6	
		Adult (20–50 yr)	230–660		3.5–10.0	
Triiodothyronine resin uptake test (T3RU)	S				Fractional uptake	
		Newborn 26–36%		×0.01	0.26–0.36	
		Thereafter 26–35%			0.26–0.35	
Triiodothyronine, total	S		ng/dL		nmol/L	
		Cord blood	30–70	×0.0154	0.46–1.08	
		Newborn	75–260		1.16–4.00	
		1–5 yr	100–260		1.54–4.00	
		5–10 y	90–240		1.39–3.70	
		10–15 yr	80–210		1.23–3.23	
		Thereafter	115–190		1.77–2.93	

S, serum; W, whole blood.
Adapted from Nicholson JF, Pesce MA: Reference Ranges for Laboratory Tests and Procedures. In Behrman RE, Kliegman RM, Jenson HB (eds.) Nelson Textbook of Pediatrics, 17th ed. Philadelphia, Elsevier Science, 2004, pp 2412–2413.

LABORATORY FINDINGS. Most newborn screening programs in North America measure levels of T_4, followed by measurement of TSH when T_4 is low. This approach identifies infants with primary hypothyroidism, some with hypothalamic or pituitary hypothyroidism, and infants with a delayed increase in TSH levels. European and Japanese neonatal screening programs are based on a primary measurement of TSH; some North American programs are switching to primary TSH screening. This approach detects infants with primary hypothyroidism and may detect infants with subclinical hypothyroidism (normal T_4, elevated TSH), but it misses infants with delayed TSH elevation and with hypothalamic or pituitary hypothyroidism. With any of these tests, special care should be given to the normal range of values for age of the patient, particularly in the 1st weeks of life (Table 566-2). Regardless of the approach used for screening, some infants escape detection because of technical or human errors; clinicians must maintain their vigilance for clinical manifestations of hypothyroidism.

Serum levels of T_4 or free T_4 are low; serum levels of T_3 may be normal and are not helpful in the diagnosis. If the defect is primarily in the thyroid, levels of TSH are elevated, often to greater than 100 mU/L. Serum levels of prolactin are elevated, correlating with those of TSH. Serum levels of thyroglobulin are usually low in infants with thyroid agenesis or defects of thyroglobulin synthesis or secretion, whereas they may be elevated with ectopic glands and other inborn errors of thyroxine synthesis.

Special attention should be paid to identical twins; in several reported cases, neonatal screening failed to detect the discordant

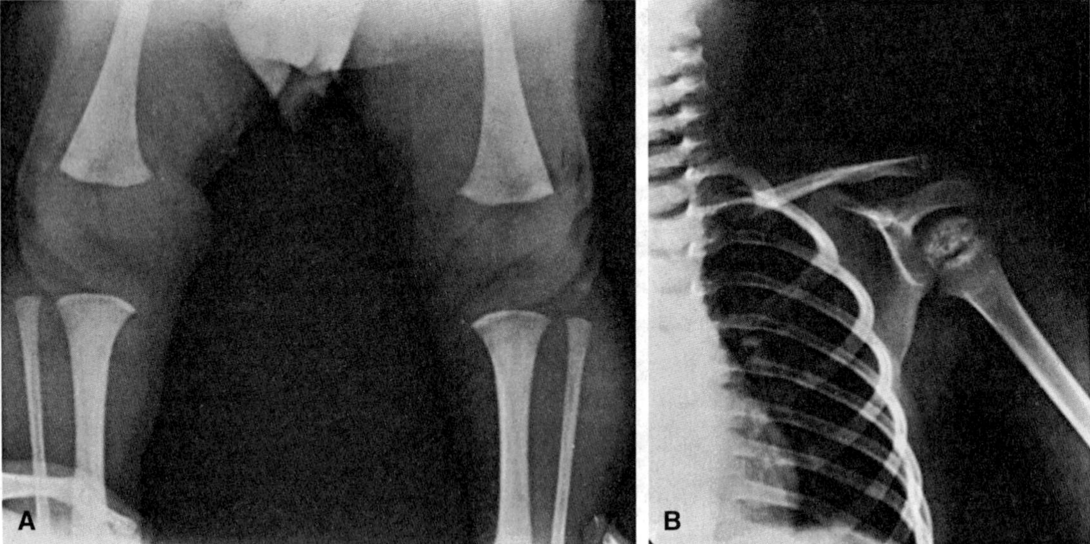

Figure 566-2. Congenital hypothyroidism. *A*, Absence of distal femoral epiphysis in a 3-mo-old infant who was born at term. This is evidence for the onset of the hypothyroid state during fetal life. *B*, Epiphyseal dysgenesis in the head of the humerus in a 9-yr-old girl who had been inadequately treated with thyroid hormone.

twin with hypothyroidism, and the diagnosis was not made until the infants were 4–5 mo of age. Apparently, transfusion of euthyroid blood from the unaffected twin normalized the serum level of T_4 and TSH in the affected twin at the initial screening.

Retardation of osseous development can be shown radiographically at birth in about 60% of congenitally hypothyroid infants and indicates some deprivation of thyroid hormone during intrauterine life. The distal femoral epiphysis, normally present at birth, is often absent (Fig. 566-2A). In undetected and untreated patients, the discrepancy between chronological age and osseous development increases. The epiphyses often have multiple foci of ossification (epiphyseal dysgenesis) [Fig. 566-2B]; deformity ("beaking") of the 12th thoracic or 1st or 2nd lumbar vertebra is common. Roentgenograms of the skull show large fontanels and wide sutures; intersutural (wormian) bones are common. The sella turcica is often enlarged and round; in rare instances, there may be erosion and thinning. Delays in formation and eruption of teeth may occur. Cardiac enlargement or pericardial effusion may be present.

Scintigraphy can help to pinpoint the underlying cause in infants with congenital hypothyroidism, but treatment should not be unduly delayed for this study. ^{123}I-sodium iodide is superior to ^{99m}Tc-sodium pertechnetate for this purpose. Ultrasonographic examination of the thyroid is helpful, but studies show it may miss some ectopic glands shown by scintigraphy. Serum levels of thyroglobulin are low with agenesis and elevated with ectopic glands and goiter, but there is a wide overlap of ranges. Demonstration of ectopic thyroid tissue is diagnostic of thyroid dysgenesis and establishes the need for lifelong treatment with T_4. Failure to demonstrate any thyroid tissue suggests thyroid aplasia, but this also occurs in neonates with TRBAb and in infants with the iodide-trapping defect. A normally situated thyroid gland with a normal or avid uptake of radionuclide indicates a defect in thyroid hormone biosynthesis. In the past, patients with goitrous hypothyroidism have required extensive evaluation, including radioiodine studies, perchlorate discharge tests, kinetic studies, chromatography, and studies of thyroid tissue, to determine the biochemical nature of the defect. Most can now be evaluated by genetic studies looking for defects in the steps along the thyroxine biosynthetic pathway.

The electrocardiogram may show low-voltage P and T waves with diminished amplitude of QRS complexes and suggest poor left ventricular function and pericardial effusion. The electroencephalogram frequently shows low voltage. In children older than 2 yr of age, the serum cholesterol level is usually elevated. Brain MRI before treatment is reportedly normal, although proton magnetic resonance spectroscopy shows high levels of choline-containing compounds, which may reflect blocks in myelin maturation.

TREATMENT. Levothyroxine given orally is the treatment of choice. Because 80% of circulating T_3 is formed by monodeiodination of T_4, serum levels of T_4 and T_3 in treated infants return to normal. This is also true in the brain, where 80% of required T_3 is produced locally from T_4. In neonates, the recommended initial starting dose is 10–15 µg/kg (37.5 to 50 µg/24 hr). Newborns with more severe hypothyroidism, as judged by a serum T4 <3 µg/dL, should be started at the higher end of the dosage range. Thyroxine tablets should not be mixed with soy protein formulas or iron, because these can bind T_4 and inhibit its absorption. Levels of T_4 or free T_4 and TSH should be monitored at recommended intervals (approximately monthly in the first 6 mo of life, and then every 2–3 mo between 6 mo and 2 yr) and maintained in the normal range for age. Children with hypothyroidism require about 4 µg/kg/24 hr, and adults require only 2 µg/kg/24 hr.

Later, confirmation of the diagnosis may be necessary for some infants to rule out the possibility of transient hypothyroidism. This is unnecessary in infants with proven thyroid ectopia or in those who manifest elevated levels of TSH after 6–12 mo of therapy because of poor compliance or an inadequate dose of T_4. Discontinuation of therapy at about 3 yr of age for 3–4 wk results in a marked increase in TSH levels in children with permanent hypothyroidism.

The only untoward effects of sodium–L-thyroxine are related to its dose. Overtreatment may risk craniosynostosis and temperament problems. An occasional older child (8–13 yr) with acquired hypothyroidism may experience pseudotumor cerebri within the first 4 mo of treatment. In older children, after catch-up growth is complete, the growth rate provides a good index of the adequacy of therapy. Parents should be forewarned about changes in behavior and activity expected with therapy, and special attention must be given to any developmental or neurologic deficits.

PROGNOSIS. With the advent of neonatal screening programs for detection of congenital hypothyroidism, the prognosis for affected infants has improved dramatically. Early diagnosis and adequate treatment from the first weeks of life result in normal linear growth and intelligence comparable with that of unaffected siblings. Some screening programs report that the most severely affected infants, as judged by the lowest T_4 levels and retarded skeletal maturation, have reduced (5–10 points) IQs and other neuropsychological sequelae, such as incoordination, hypotonia or hypertonia, short attention span, and speech problems. Approximately 20% of children have a neurosensory hearing deficit. Without treatment, affected infants are profoundly mentally deficient and growth retarded. Thyroid hormone is critical for normal cerebral development in the early postnatal months; biochemical diagnosis must be made soon after birth, and effective treatment must be initiated promptly to prevent irreversible brain damage. Delay in diagnosis, failure to correct initial hypothyroxinemia rapidly, inadequate treatment, and poor compliance in the first 2–3 yr of life result in variable degrees of brain damage. When onset of hypothyroidism occurs after 2 yr of age, the outlook for normal development is much better even if diagnosis and treatment have been delayed, indicating how much more important thyroid hormone is to the rapidly growing brain of the infant.

ACQUIRED HYPOTHYROIDISM

EPIDEMIOLOGY. Studies of school-aged children report that hypothyroidism occurs in approximately 0.3% (1/333). Acquired hypothyroidism is most commonly a result of chronic lymphocytic thyroiditis; 6% of children aged 12–19 yr have evidence of autoimmune thyroid disease, which occurs with a 2 : 1 female to male preponderance.

ETIOLOGY. The most common cause of acquired hypothyroidism (Table 566-3) is chronic lymphocytic thyroiditis (see Chapter 567). **Autoimmune thyroid disease** may be part of polyglandular syndromes; children with Down, Turner, and Klinefelter syndromes and celiac disease or diabetes are at higher risk for associated autoimmune thyroid disease (see Chapter 567). Additional autoimmune diseases with an increased risk of hypothyroidism include Sjögren syndrome, multiple sclerosis, pernicious anemia, Addison disease, and ovarian failure. Although typically seen in adolescence, it occurs as early as in the 1st yr of life. Some patients with congenital thyroid dysgenesis or with incomplete genetic defects in thyroid hormone synthesis may not display clinical manifestations until childhood and appear to have acquired hypothyroidism; these conditions are usually now detected by newborn screening programs. Subtotal thyroidectomy for thyrotoxicosis or cancer may result in hypothyroidism, as may removal of ectopic thyroid tissue. Thyroid tissue in a thyroglossal duct cyst usually constitutes the only source of thyroid hormone, and excision results in hypothyroidism. Because subhyoid glands usually mimic thyroglossal duct cysts, ultrasonographic examination or a radionuclide scan before surgery is indicated in these patients.

Children with **nephropathic cystinosis,** a disorder characterized by intralysosomal storage of cystine in body tissues, acquire impaired thyroid function. Hypothyroidism may be overt, but subclinical forms are more common, and periodic assessment of TSH levels is indicated. By 13 yr of age, ⅔ of these patients require T_4 replacement.

Histiocytic infiltration of the thyroid in children with Langerhans cell histiocytosis may result in hypothyroidism.

Irradiation of the area of thyroid that is incidental to the treatment of Hodgkin disease or other head and neck malignancies or that is administered before bone marrow transplantation often results in thyroid damage. About ⅓ of such children acquire elevated TSH levels within a yr after therapy, and 15–20% progress to hypothyroidism within 5–7 yr. Some clinicians recommend periodic TSH measurements, but others recommend treatment of all exposed patients with doses of T_4 to suppress TSH.

Protracted ingestion of **medications** containing iodides can cause hypothyroidism, usually accompanied by goiter (see Chapter 568). Amiodarone, a drug used for cardiac arrhythmias and consisting of 37% iodine by weight, causes hypothyroidism in about 20% of treated children. It affects thyroid function directly by its high iodine content as well as by inhibition of 5′-deiodinase, which converts T_4 to T_3. Children treated with this drug should have serial measurements of T_4, T_3, and TSH. Additional drugs that may produce hypothyroidism include lithium carbonate, interferon alpha, thalidomide, stavudine, and aminoglutethimide.

Hypothyroidism can occur in children with large **hemangiomas** of the liver, because of increased type 3 deiodinase activity, which catalyzes conversion of T_4 to rT_3 and T_3 to T_2. Thyroid secretion is increased, but is not sufficient to compensate for the large increase in T_4 to rT_3 degradation.

CLINICAL MANIFESTATIONS. Deceleration of growth is usually the first clinical manifestation, but this sign often goes unrecognized (Figs. 566-3 and 566-4). Goiter, which may be a presenting feature, typically is non-tender and firm, with a rubbery consistency and a pebbly surface. Myxedematous changes of the skin, constipation, cold intolerance, decreased energy, and an increased need for sleep develop insidiously. Surprisingly, schoolwork and grades usually do not suffer, even in severely hypothyroid children. Osseous maturation is delayed, often strikingly, which is an indication of the duration of the hypothyroidism. Adolescents typically have delayed puberty, whereas younger children may present with galactorrhea or pseudoprecocious puberty. Galactorrhea is a result of increased TRH stimulating prolactin secretion. The precocious puberty, characterized by breast development in girls and macro-orchidism in boys, is thought to be the result of abnormally high TSH concentrations binding to the follicle-stimulating hormone receptor with subsequent stimulation.

Some children have headaches and visual problems; they usually have hyperplastic enlargement of the pituitary gland, sometimes with suprasellar extension, after long-standing hypothyroidism; this condition, believed to be the result of thyrotroph hyperplasia, may be mistaken for a pituitary tumor (see Chapter 558). Additional features include nerve entrapment, ataxia, muscle weakness or cramps, menstrual disturbances, bradycardia, weight gain, and abnormal laboratory studies (hyponatremia, macrocytic anemia, hypercholesterolemia, elevated CPK, hyperprolactinemia). Complications seen in severe hypothyroidism are noted in Table 566-4.

TABLE 566-3. Etiologic Classification of Acquired Hypothyroidism

AUTOIMMUNE (ACQUIRED HYPOTHYROIDISM)
Hashimoto thyroiditis
Polyglandular autoimmune syndrome, types I and II
IATROGENIC
Propylthiouracil, methimazole, iodides, lithium, amiodarone
Irradiation
Radioiodine
Thyroidectomy
SYSTEMIC DISEASE
Cystinosis
Langerhans cell histiocytosis
HEMANGIOMAS (LARGE) OF THE LIVER (TYPE 3 IODOTHYRONINE DEIODINASE)
RESISTANCE TO THYROID HORMONE (ONLY OCCASIONAL CLINICAL MANIFESTATIONS OF HYPOTHYROIDISM)

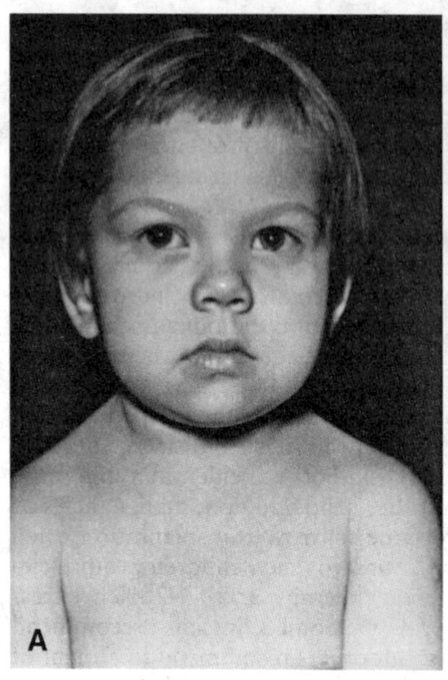

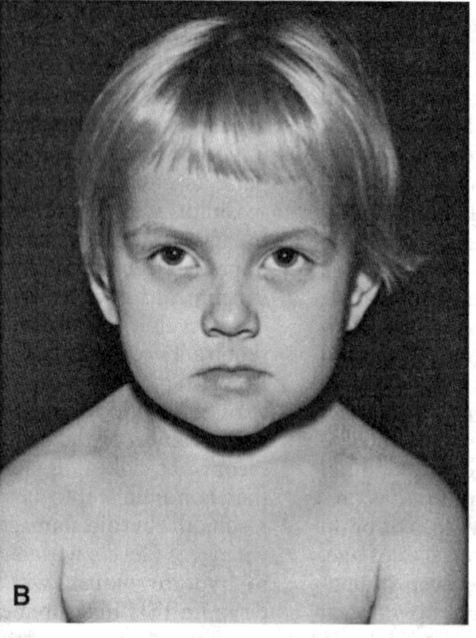

Figure 566-3. *A,* Acquired hypothyroidism in a girl 6 yr of age. She was treated with a wide variety of hematinics for refractory anemia for 3 yr. She had almost complete cessation of growth, constipation, and sluggishness for 3 yr. The height age was 3 yr; the bone age was 4 yr. She had a sallow complexion and immature facies with a poorly developed nasal bridge. Serum cholesterol, 501 mg/dL; radioiodine uptake, 7% at 24 hr; PBI, 2.8 mg/dL. *B,* After therapy for 18 mo, note the nasal development, increased luster and decreased pigmentation of hair, and maturation of the face. The height age was 5.5 yr; the bone age was 7 yr. There was a decided improvement in her general condition. Menarche occurred at 14 yr. The ultimate height was 155 cm (61 in). She graduated from high school. The disorder was well controlled with sodium–L-thyroxine daily.

All these changes return to normal with adequate replacement of T_4, but in children with long-standing hypothyroidism, catch-up growth may be incomplete (see Fig. 566-4). During the first 18 mo of treatment, skeletal maturation often exceeds expected linear growth, resulting in a loss of about 7 cm of predicted adult height; the cause is unknown.

DIAGNOSTIC STUDIES AND TREATMENT. Treatment and diagnostic studies are the same as those described for congenital hypothyroidism. Measurement of antithyroglobulin and antiperoxidase (formerly, antimicrosomal) antibodies may pinpoint autoimmune thyroiditis as the cause. Generally, there is no indication for thyroid imaging. In cases with a goiter resulting from autoimmune thyroid disease, if an ultrasound examination is carried out, it typically shows diffuse enlargement with scattered hypoechogenicity. During the 1st yr of treatment, deterioration of schoolwork, poor sleeping habits, restlessness, short attention span, and behavioral problems may ensue, but these are transient; forewarning families about these manifestations enhances appropriate management. These may be partially ameliorated by starting at sub-replacement T_4 doses and advancing slowly.

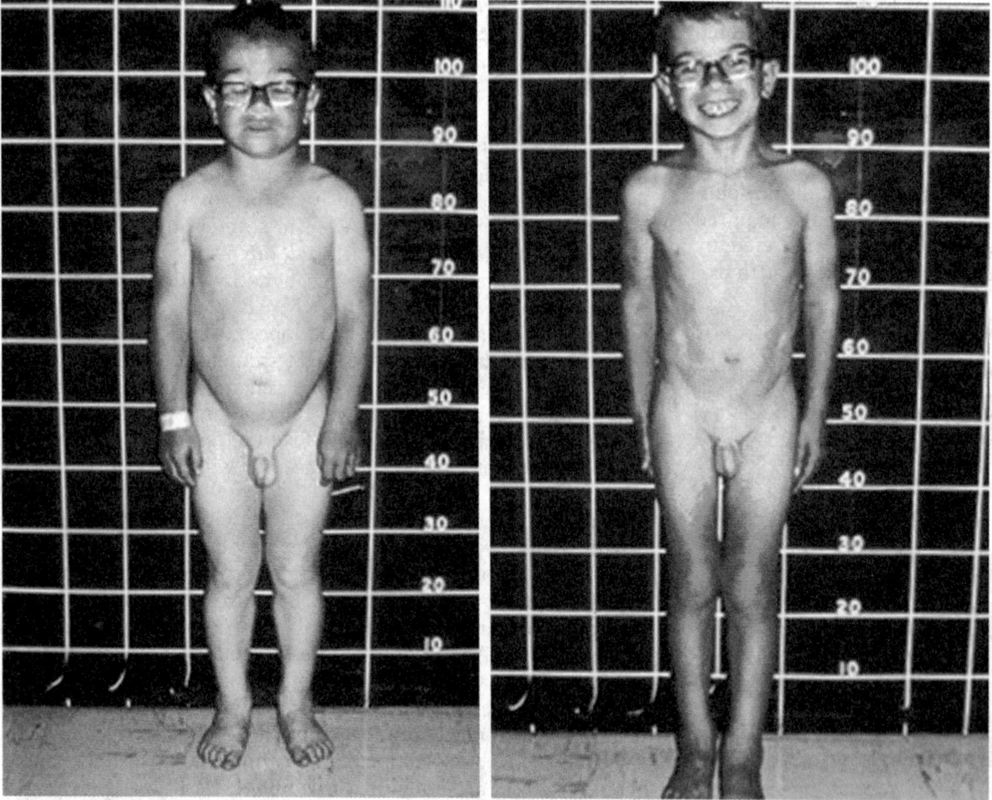

Figure 566-4. *A,* Short stature (108 cm, <3rd percentile), generalized myxedema, sleepy expression, protuberant abdomen, and coarse hair are signs of hypothyroidism in this 12-yr-old boy. Body proportions are immature for his age (1.25 : 1). *B,* Same boy 4 mo after treatment. His height increased by 4 cm; note the marked change in body habitus owing to loss of generalized myxedema, improved muscle tone, and bright facial expression. (From LaFranchi SH: Hypothyroidism. *Pediatr Clin North Am* 1979;26:44.)

TABLE 566-4. Pathogenesis of General Complications in Management of Complicated Hypothyroidism

COMPLICATION	PATHOGENESIS
Heart failure	Impaired ventricular systolic and diastolic functions and increased peripheral vascular resistance
Ventilatory failure	Blunted hypercapnoeic and hypoxic ventilatory drives
Hyponatremia	Impaired renal free water excretion and syndrome of inappropriate antidiuretic hormone secretion (SIADH)
Ileus	Bowel hypomotility
Medication sensitivity	Reduced clearance rate and increased sensitivity to sedative, analgesic, and anaesthetic agents
Hypothermia and lack of febrile response to sepsis	Decreased calorigenesis
Delirium, dementia, seizure, stupor, and coma	Decreased CNS thyroid hormone actions, and encephalopathy due to hyponatremia and hypercapnea
Adrenal insufficiency	Associated intrinsic adrenal or pituitary disease, or reversible impairment of hypothalamic-pituitary-adrenal stress response
Coagulopathy	Acquired von Willebrand syndrome (type 1), and decreased factors VIII, VII, V, IX, and X

From Roberts CG, Landenson PW: Hypothyroidism. *Lancet* 2004;363:793–803.

Adams A, Matthews C, Collingwood TH, et al: Genetic analysis of 29 kindreds with generalized and pituitary resistance to thyroid hormone. *J Clin Invest* 1994;94:506–515.

American Academy of Pediatrics; Rose SR; Section on Endocrinology and Committee on Genetics, American Thyroid Association; Brown RS; Public Health Committee, Lawson Wilkins Pediatric Endocrine Society; Foley T, Kaplowitz PB, Kaye CI, Sundararajan S, Varma SK: Update of newborn screening and therapy for congenital hypothyroidism. *Pediatrics* 2006; 117:2290–2303.

Asajura Y, Tachibana K, Adachi M, et al: Hypothalamic-pituitary hypothyroidism detected by neonatal screening for congenital hypothyroidism using measurement of thyroid-stimulating hormone and thyroxine. *Acta Paediatr* 2002;91:172–177.

Bilimoria KY, Pescovitz OH, DiMeglio LA: Autoimmune thyroid dysfunction in children with type 1 diabetes mellitus: Screening guidelines based on a retrospective analysis. *J Pediatr Endocrinol Metab* 2003;16:1111–1117.

Borck G, Topaloglu AK, Korsch E, et al: Four new cases of congenital secondary hypothyroidism due to a splice site mutation in the thyrotropin-beta gene: Phenotypic variability and founder effect. *J Clin Endocrinol Metab* 2004;89:4136–4141.

Castanet M, Park SM, Smith A, et al: A novel loss-of-function mutation in TTF-2 is associated with congenital hypothyroidism, thyroid agenesis and cleft palate. *Hum Mol Genet* 2002;11:2051–2059.

Conrad SC, Chiu H, Silverman BI: Soy formula complicates management of congenital hypothyroidism. *Arch Dis Child* 2004;89:37–40.

De Vijlder JJ: Primary congenital hypothyroidism: defects in iodine pathways. *Eur J Endocrinol* 2003;149:247–256.

Doyle DA, Gonzalez I, Thomas B, et al: Autosomal dominant transmission of congenital hypothyroidism, neonatal respiratory distress, and ataxia caused by a mutation of NKX2-1. *J Pediatr* 2004;145:190–193.

Eugene D, Djemli A, VanVliet G: Sexual dimorphism of thyroid function in newborns with congenital hypothyroidism. *J Clin Endocrinol Metab* 2005;90:2696–2700.

Eugster EA, LeMay D, Xerin JM, et al: Definitive diagnosis in children with congenital hypothyroidism. *J Pediatr* 2004;144:643–647.

Friesema EC, Grueters A, Biebermann H, et al: Association between mutations in a thyroid hormone transporter and severe X-linked psychomotor retardation. *Lancet* 2004;364:1435–1437.

Grasberger H, Ringkananont U, Lefrancois P, et al. Thyroid transcription factor 1 rescues PAX8/p300 synergism impaired by a natural PAX8 paired mutation with dominant negative activity. *Mol Endocrinol* 2005; 19:1779–1791.

Gruters A, Krude H, Biebermann H. Molecular genetic defects in congenital hypothyroidism. *Eur J Endocrinol* 2004;151(Suppl 3):U39.

Heyerdahl S, Oerbeck B: Congenital hypothyroidism: Developmental outcome in relation to levothyroxine treatment variables. *Thyroid* 2003;13: 1029–1038.

Huang SA, Tu HM, Harney JW, et al: Severe hypothyroidism caused by type 3 iodothyronine deiodinase in infantile hemangiomas. *N Engl J Med* 2000;343: 185–189.

Ishiguro H, Yasuda Y, Tomita Y, et al: Long-term follow-up of thyroid function in patients who receive bone marrow transplantation during childhood and adolescence. *J Clin Endocrinol Metab* 2004;89:5981–5986.

Karlson B, Gustafsson J, Hedov G, et al: Thyroid dysfunction in Down's syndrome: Relation to age and thyroid autoimmunity. *Arch Dis Child* 1998;79:242–245.

Kaspers S, Kordonouri O, Schober F, et al: Anthropometry, metabolic control, and thyroid autoimmunity in type 1 diabetes with celiac disease: A multicenter survey. *J Pediatr* 2004;145:790–795.

Leger J, Marinovic D, Garel C, et al: Thyroid developmental anomalies in first degree relatives of children with congenital hypothyroidism. *J Clin Endocrinol Metab* 2002;87:575–580.

Madison LD, LaFranchi S: Screening for congenital hypothyroidism: current controversies. *Curr Opin Endocrinol Metab* 2005;12:36.

Mandel SJ, Hermos RJ, Larson CA, et al: Atypical hypothyroidism and the very low birthweight infant. *Thyroid* 2000;10:693–695.

Moreno JC, Bikker H, Kempers MJE, et al: Inactivating mutations in the gene for thyroid oxidase 2 (THOX2) and congenital hypothyroidism. *N Engl J Med* 2002;347:95–102.

Murphy N, Jume R, van Toor H, et al: The hypothalamic-pituitary-thyroid axis in preterm infants: Changes in the first 24 hours of postnatal life. *J Clin Endocrinol Metab* 2004;89:2824–2831.

Nishiyama S, Mikeda T, Okada T, et al: Transient hypothyroidism or persistent hyperthyrotropinemia in neonates born to mothers with excessive iodine intake. *Thyroid* 2004;14:1077–1083.

Oerbeck B, Sundet K, Kase BF, et al: Congenital hypothyroidism: Influence of disease severity and L-thyroxine treatment on intellectual, motor, and school-associated outcomes in young adults. *Pediatrics* 2003;112:923–930.

Oerbeck B, Sundet K, Kase BF, et al: Congenital hypothyroidism: No adverse effects of high dose thyroxine treatment on adult memory, attention, and behavior. *Arch Dis Child* 2005;90:132–137.

Olivieri A, Stazi A, Mastroiacovo P, et al. A population-based study on the frequency of additional congenital malformations in infants with congenital hypothyroidism: Data from the Italian registry for congenital hypothyroidism (1991–1998). *J Clin Endocrinol Metab* 2002;87:557–562.

Roberts CG, Landenson PW: Hypothyroidism. *Lancet* 2004;363:793–803.

Rovet J: Congenital hypothyroidism: Treatment and outcome. *Curr Opin Endocrinol Diabetes* 2005;12:42.

Rovet J: Children with congenital hypothyroidism and their siblings: Do they really differ? *Pediatrics* 2005;115:e52–57.

Schoen EJ, Clapp W, To TT, et al: The key role of newborn thyroid scintigraphy with isotopic iodine (123I) in defining and managing congenital hypothyroidism. *J Pediatr* 2004;114:e683–688.

Scott DA, Wang R, Kreman VC, et al: The Pendred syndrome is caused by mutations in a putative sulphate transporter gene (PDS). *Nat Genet* 1999;17:411.

Selva KA, Harper A, Downs A, et al: Neurodevelopmental outcomes in congenital hypothyroidism: Comparison of initial T_4 dose and time to reach target T_4 and TSH. *J Pediatr* 2005;147:775–780.

Teng W, Shan Z, Teng X, et al: Effect of iodine in take on thyroid diseases in China. *N Engl J Med* 2006;354:2783–2792.

Trueba SS, Auge J, Mattei G, et al. PAX8, TITF1, and FOXE1 gene expression patterns during human development: new insight into human thyroid development and thyroid dysgenesis-associated malformations. *J Clin Endocrinol Metab* 2005;90:455–462.

Chapter 567 ■ Thyroiditis

LYMPHOCYTIC THYROIDITIS (HASHIMOTO THYROIDITIS, AUTOIMMUNE THYROIDITIS)

Lymphocytic thyroiditis is the most common cause of thyroid disease in children and adolescents and accounts for many of the enlarged thyroids formerly designated "adolescent" or "simple" goiter. It is also the most common cause of acquired hypothyroidism, with or without goiter.

One to 2% of younger school-aged children and 4–6% of adolescents have positive antithyroid antibodies as evidence of autoimmune thyroid disease.

ETIOLOGY. This typical organ-specific autoimmune disease is characterized histologically by lymphocytic infiltration of the thyroid. Early in the course of the disease, there may be hyperplasia only; this is followed by infiltration of lymphocytes and plasma cells between the follicles and by atrophy of the follicles. Lymphoid follicle formation with germinal centers is almost always present; the degree of atrophy and fibrosis of the follicles varies from mild to moderate.

Intrathyroidal lymphocyte subsets differ from those in blood. About 60% of infiltrating lymphoid cells are T cells, and about 30% express B-cell markers; the T-cell population is represented by helper ($CD4^+$) and cytotoxic ($CD8^+$) cells. The participation of cellular events in the pathogenesis is clear. Certain HLA haplotypes (HLA-DR4, HLA-DR5) are associated with an increased risk of goiter and thyroiditis, and others (HLA-DR3) are associated with the atrophic variant of thyroiditis.

A variety of different thyroid antigen autoantibodies are also involved. Thyroid antiperoxidase antibodies (TPOAbs) (formerly called "antimicrosomal antibodies") and antithyroglobulin antibodies are demonstrable in the sera of 90% of children with lymphocytic thyroiditis and in many patients with Graves disease. TPOAbs inhibit enzyme activity and stimulate natural killer cell cytotoxicity. Antithyroglobulin antibodies do not appear to play a role in the autoimmune destruction of the gland. Thyrotropin receptor-blocking antibodies are frequently present, especially in patients with hypothyroidism, and it is now believed that they are related to the development of hypothyroidism and thyroid atrophy in patients with autoimmune thyroiditis.

CLINICAL MANIFESTATIONS. The disorder is 2–4 times more frequent in girls than in boys. It may occur during the first 3 yr of life but becomes sharply more common after 6 yr of age and reaches a peak incidence during adolescence. The most common clinical manifestations are goiter and growth retardation. The goiter may appear insidiously and may be small or large. In most patients, the thyroid is diffusely enlarged, firm, and nontender. In about 30% of patients, the gland is lobular and may seem to be nodular. Most of the affected children are clinically euthyroid and asymptomatic; some may have symptoms of pressure in the neck. Some children have clinical signs of hypothyroidism, but others who appear clinically euthyroid have laboratory evidence of hypothyroidism. A few children have manifestations suggestive of hyperthyroidism, such as nervousness, irritability, increased sweating, and hyperactivity, but results of laboratory studies are not necessarily those of hyperthyroidism. Occasionally, the disorder may coexist with Graves disease. Ophthalmopathy may occur in lymphocytic thyroiditis in the absence of Graves disease.

The clinical course is variable. The goiter may become smaller or may disappear spontaneously, or it may persist unchanged for years while the patient remains euthyroid. Most children who are euthyroid at presentation remain euthyroid, although a percentage of patients acquire hypothyroidism gradually within months or years. Over several years, about ½ of children with subclinical hypothyroidism revert to euthyroidism, while the other ½ develop overt hypothyroidism. Thyroiditis is the cause of most cases of nongoitrous (atrophic) hypothyroidism.

Familial clusters of lymphocytic thyroiditis are common; the incidence in siblings or parents of affected children may be as high as 25%. Autoantibodies to thyroglobulin and thyroid peroxidase in these families appear to be inherited in an autosomal dominant fashion, with reduced penetrance in males. The concurrence within families of patients with lymphocytic thyroiditis, "idiopathic" hypothyroidism, and Graves disease provides cogent evidence for a basic relationship among these 3 conditions. The disorder has been associated with many other autoimmune disorders. Autoimmune thyroiditis occurs in 10% of patients with type I autoimmune polyglandular syndrome (APS-1), characterized by the acronym APECED, standing for autoimmune polyendocrinopathy–candidiasis–ectodermal dysplasia. APS-1 consists of 2 of the triad of hypoparathyroidism, Addison disease, and mucocutaneous candidiasis ("HAM" syndrome). This relatively rare autosomal recessive disorder presents in childhood and is caused by mutations in the autoimmune regulatory *(AIRE)* gene on chromosome 21q22.3. Autoimmune thyroiditis occurs in 70% of patients with APS-2 (Schmidt syndrome). APS-2 consists of the association of Addison disease with insulin-dependent diabetes mellitus or autoimmune thyroid disease. The etiology is unknown, and it typically presents in early adulthood. Autoimmune thyroid disease also tends to be associated with pernicious anemia, vitiligo, or alopecia. TPOAbs are found in approximately 20% of white and 4% of black children with diabetes mellitus. Autoimmune thyroid disease has an increased incidence in children with congenital rubella. Lymphocytic thyroiditis is also associated with certain chromosomal disorders, particularly Turner syndrome and Down syndrome. In children with Down syndrome, one study reported that 28% had antithyroid antibodies (predominantly anti-TPOs), 7% had subclinical hypothyroidism, 7% had overt hypothyroidism, and 5% had hyperthyroidism. In a study of girls with Turner syndrome, 41% had antithyroid antibodies (again, predominantly anti-TPOs), 18% had goiter, and 8% had subclinical or overt hypothyroidism. Another study of 75 girls with Turner syndrome found that autoimmune thyroid disease increased from the first (15%) to the third (30%) decade of life. Boys with Klinefelter syndrome are also at risk for autoimmune thyroid disease. The differential diagnosis is noted in Table 567-1.

LABORATORY FINDINGS. Thyroid function tests are often normal, although the level of thyroid-stimulating hormone (TSH) may be slightly or even moderately elevated in some individuals, termed subclinical hypothyroidism. The fact that many children with lymphocytic thyroiditis do not have elevated levels of TSH indicates that the goiter may be caused by the lymphocytic infiltrations or by thyroid growth-stimulating immunoglobulins. Young

TABLE 567-1. Characteristics of Thyroiditis Syndromes

CHARACTERISTIC	HASHIMOTO'S THYROIDITIS	PAINLESS POSTPARTUM THYROIDITIS	PAINLESS SPORADIC THYROIDITIS	PAINFUL SUBACUTE THYROIDITIS	SUPPURATIVE THYROIDITIS	RIEDEL'S THYROIDITIS
Sex ratio (F : M)	8–9 : 1	—	2 : 1	5 : 1	1 : 1	3–4 : 1
Cause	Autoimmune	Autoimmune	Autoimmune	Unknown	Infectious	Unknown
Pathologic findings	Lymphocytic infiltration, germinal centers, fibrosis	Lymphocytic infiltration	Lymphocytic infiltration	Giant cells, granulomas	Abscess formation	Dense fibrosis
Thyroid function	Hypothyroidism	Thyrotoxicosis, hypothyroidism, or both	Thyrotoxicosis, hypothyroidism, or both	Thyrotoxicosis, hypothyroidism, or both	Usually euthyroidism	Usually euthyroidism
TPO antibodies	High titer, persistent	High titer, persistent	High titer, persistent	Low titer, or absent, or transient	Absent	Usually present
ESR	Normal	Normal	Normal	High	High	Normal
24-hour ^{123}I uptake	Variable	<5%	<5%	<5%	Normal	Low or normal

ESR, erythrocyte sedimentation rate; ^{123}I, iodine 123; TPO, thyroid peroxidase.
From Pearce EN, Farwell AP, Braverman LE: Thyroiditis. *N Engl J Med* 2003;348:2646–2654.

children with lymphocytic thyroiditis have serum antibody titers to TPO, but the antithyroglobulin test for thyroid antibodies is positive in fewer than 50%. Antibodies to TPO and thyroglobulin are found equally in adolescents with lymphocytic thyroiditis. When both tests are used, approximately 95% of patients with thyroid autoimmunity are detected. Levels in children and adolescents are lower than those in adults with lymphocytic thyroiditis, and repeated measurements are indicated in questionable instances because titers may increase later in the course of the disease. Thyroid scans and ultrasonography usually are not needed. If they are done, in 50% of children, thyroid scans reveal irregular and patchy distribution of the radioisotope, and in about 60% or more, the administration of perchlorate results in a greater than 10% discharge of iodide from the thyroid gland. Thyroid ultrasonography shows scattered hypoechogenicity in most patients. The definitive diagnosis can be established by biopsy of the thyroid; this procedure is rarely clinically indicated.

Antithyroid antibodies may also be found in almost ½ the siblings of affected patients and in a significant percentage of the mothers of children with Down syndrome or Turner syndrome without demonstrable thyroid disease. They are also found in 20% of children with diabetes mellitus and in 23% of children with the congenital rubella syndrome.

TREATMENT. If there is evidence of hypothyroidism, replacement treatment with levothyroxine (50–150 µg daily) is indicated. The goiter usually shows some decrease in size but may persist for years. A large goiter in a euthyroid patient will also regress with suppressive doses of levothyroxine. Antibody levels fluctuate in both treated and untreated patients and persist for years. Because the disease may be self-limited in some instances, the need for continued therapy requires periodic reevaluation. Untreated patients should also be checked periodically. While there is some controversy about treating patients with subclinical hypothyroidism (normal T_4 or free T_4, elevated TSH), this clinician prefers to treat such children until growth and puberty are complete, and then reevaluate their thyroid function. Prominent nodules that persist despite suppressive therapy should be examined histologically, since thyroid lymphoma or carcinoma has occurred in patients with lymphocytic thyroiditis.

OTHER CAUSES OF THYROIDITIS

Specific conditions such as tuberculosis, sarcoidosis, mumps, and cat-scratch disease are rare causes of thyroiditis (see Table 567-1).

Acute suppurative thyroiditis is uncommon; it is usually preceded by a respiratory infection. The left lower lobe is affected predominantly. Abscess formation may occur. Anaerobic organisms, with or without aerobes, are the typical infectious agent. The most common organism is *Streptococcus viridans,* followed by *Staphylococcus aureus* and pneumococcus. Recurrent episodes or detection of a mixed bacterial flora suggests that the infection arises from a **thyroglossal duct** remnant or, more often, from a **piriform sinus fistula.** Exquisite tenderness of the gland, swelling, erythema, dysphagia, and limitation of head motion are characteristic findings. Fever, chills, and sore throat are not uncommon, and leukocytosis is present. Scintigrams of the thyroid often reveal decreased uptake in the affected areas, and ultrasonography may show a complex echogenic mass. Thyroid function is usually normal, but thyrotoxicosis due to escape of thyroid hormone has been encountered in a child with suppurative thyroiditis resulting from *Aspergillus.* When abscess formation occurs, incision and drainage and administration of parenteral antibiotics are indicated. After the infection subsides, a barium esophagram or CT scan with contrast is indicated to search for a fistulous tract; if one is found, surgical excision is indicated.

Subacute granulomatous thyroiditis (de Quervain disease) is rare in children. It is thought to have a viral cause and remits spontaneously. The disorder becomes manifested by an upper respiratory infection with vague tenderness over the thyroid and low-grade fever, followed by severe pain in the region of the thyroid gland. Inflammation results in leakage of preformed thyroid hormone from the gland into the circulation. Serum levels of T_4 and T_3 are elevated, and mild symptoms of hyperthyroidism may be present, but radioiodine uptake is depressed. The erythrocyte sedimentation rate is increased. The course is variable, usually passing through a euthyroid to a hypothyroid phase; remission usually occurs in several months. Occasionally, this condition is superimposed on lymphocytic thyroiditis.

Dittmar M, Kahaly GJ: Immunoregulatory and susceptibility genes in thyroid and polyglandular autoimmunity. *Thyroid* 2005;15:239–250.

Gruneiro de Papendieck L, Iorcansky S, Coco R: High incidence of thyroid disturbances in 49 children with Turner syndrome. *J Pediatr* 1987;111:258–261.

Hollowell JG, Staehling NW, Flanders D, et al: Serum TSH, T4, and thyroid antibodies in the United States Population (1988 to 1994): National Health and Nutrition Examination Survey (NHANES III). *J Clin Endocrinol Metab* 2002;87:489–499.

Jaruratanasirikul S, Leethanaporn K, Khuntigij P, et al: The clinical course of Hashimoto's thyroiditis in children and adolescents: 6 years longitudinal follow-up. *J Pediatr Endocrinol Metab* 2001;14:177–184.

Marwaha RK, Sen S, Tandon H, et al: Familial aggregation of autoimmune thyroiditis in first-degree relatives of patients with juvenile autoimmune thyroid disease. *Thyroid* 2003;13:297–300.

Nabhan ZM, Kreher NC, Eugster EA: Hashitoxicosis in children: Clinical features and natural history. *J Pediatr* 2005;146:533–536.

Pearce EN, Farwell AP, Braverman LE: Thyroiditis. *N Engl J Med* 2003;348:2646–2654.

Rallison ML, Dobyns BM, Meikle AW, et al: Natural history of thyroid abnormalities: Prevalence, incidence, and regression of thyroid diseases in adolescents and young adults. *Am J Med* 1991;91:363–370.

Rich EJ, Mendelman PM: Acute suppurative thyroiditis in pediatric patients. *Pediatr Infect Dis J* 1987;6:936–940.

Tuzsuz B, Beker DB: Thyroid dysfunction in children with Down's syndrome. *Acta Paediatr* 2001;90:1389–1393.

Chapter 568 ■ Goiter

A goiter is an enlargement of the thyroid gland. Persons with enlarged thyroids may have normal function of the gland (**euthyroidism**), thyroid deficiency (**hypothyroidism**), or overproduction of the hormones (**hyperthyroidism**). Goiter may be congenital or acquired, endemic, or sporadic.

The goiter often results from increased pituitary secretion of thyroid-stimulating hormone (TSH) in response to decreased circulating levels of thyroid hormones. Thyroid enlargement may also result from infiltrative processes that may be inflammatory or neoplastic. Goiter in patients with Graves disease and thyrotoxicosis is caused by thyrotropin receptor–stimulating antibodies (TRSAbs).

568.1 • Congenital Goiter

Congenital goiter is usually sporadic and may result from a fetal thyroxine (T_4) synthetic defect or from administration of antithyroid drugs or iodides during pregnancy for the treatment of maternal thyrotoxicosis. Goitrogenic drugs and iodides cross the placenta and at high doses may interfere with synthesis of thyroid hormone, resulting in goiter and hypothyroidism in the fetus. The concomitant administration of thyroid hormone with the goitrogen does not prevent this effect, because insufficient amounts of T_4 cross the placenta. Iodides are included in many proprietary cough preparations used to treat asthma; these preparations should be avoided during pregnancy as they have often been reported to cause congenital goiter. Amiodarone, an antiarrhythmic drug with 37% iodine content, has also caused congenital goiter with hypothyroidism. Even when the infant is clinically euthyroid, there may be retardation of osseous maturation, low levels of T_4, and elevated levels of TSH. In women with Graves disease receiving antithyroid drugs, these effects can occur when the mother takes propylthiouracil at only 100–200 mg/24 hr; all such infants should undergo thyroid studies at birth. Administration of thyroid hormone to affected infants may be indicated to treat clinical hypothyroidism, to hasten the disappearance of the goiter, and to prevent brain damage. Because the condition is rarely permanent, thyroid hormone may be safely discontinued after the antithyroid drug has been excreted by the neonate, usually after 1–2 wk.

Enlargement of the thyroid at birth may occasionally be sufficient to cause respiratory distress that interferes with nursing and may even cause death. The head may be maintained in extreme hyperextension. When respiratory obstruction is severe, partial thyroidectomy rather than tracheostomy is indicated (Fig. 568-1).

Goiter is almost always present in the congenitally hyperthyroid infant. These goiters usually are not large; the infant manifests clinical symptoms of hyperthyroidism. The mother often has a history of Graves disease; thyroid enlargement results from transplacental passage of maternal thyroid-stimulating immunoglobulin (see Chapter 569.1). TSH receptor–activating mutations are also a recognized cause of congenital goiter.

When no causative factor is identifiable, a **defect in synthesis** of thyroid hormone should be suspected. Neonatal screening programs find congenital hypothyroidism caused by such a defect in 1/30,000–50,000 live births. If the infant is hypothyroid, it is advisable to treat immediately with thyroid hormone and to postpone more detailed studies for later in life. If a specific defect is suspected, genetic tests to identify a mutation may be undertaken (see Chapter 566). Because these defects are transmitted by recessive genes, a precise diagnosis is helpful for genetic counseling. Monitoring subsequent pregnancies with ultrasonography can be useful in detecting fetal goiters (see Chapter 96).

Iodine deficiency as a cause of congenital goiter is rare in developed countries but persists in isolated endemic areas (see below). More important is the recognition that severe iodine deficiency early in pregnancy may cause neurologic damage during fetal development, even in the absence of goiter. The iodine deficiency may result in maternal and fetal hypothyroidism, preventing the partially protective transfer of maternal thyroid hormones.

When the "goiter" is lobulated, asymmetric, firm, or large to an unusual degree, a teratoma within or in the vicinity of the thyroid must be considered in the differential diagnosis (see Chapter 570).

568.2 • Endemic Goiter and Cretinism

ETIOLOGY

IODINE DEFICIENCY. The association between dietary deficiency of iodine and the prevalence of goiter or cretinism is well established. A moderate deficiency of iodine can be overcome by increased efficiency in the synthesis of thyroid hormone. Iodine liberated in the tissues is returned rapidly to the gland, which resynthesizes triiodothyronine (T_3) preferentially at a higher rate than normal. This increased activity is achieved by compensatory hypertrophy and hyperplasia (goiter), which satisfy the demands of the tissues for thyroid hormone. In geographic areas where deficiency of iodine is severe, decompensation and hypothyroidism may result. It is estimated that 1 billion individuals in developing countries live in areas of iodine deficiency.

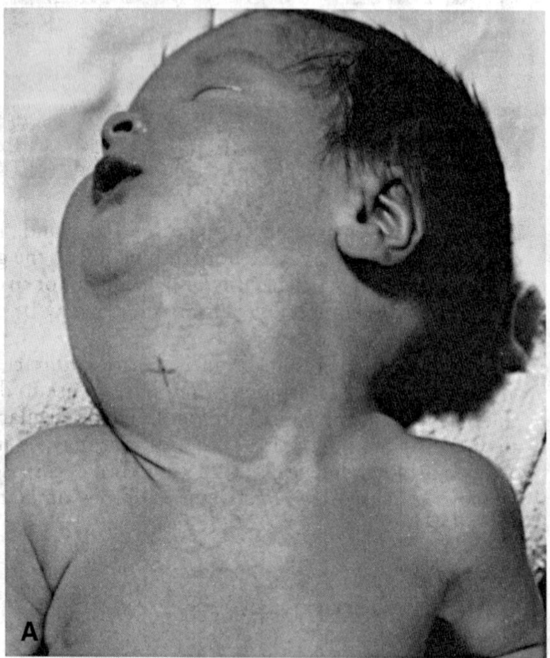

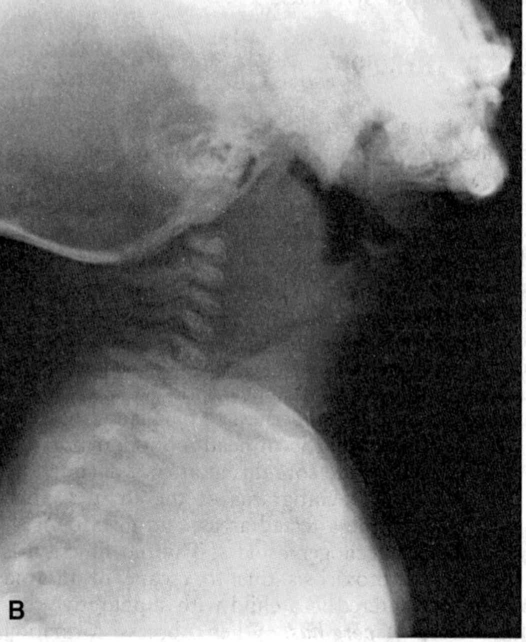

Figure 568-1. Congenital goiter in infancy. *A,* Large congenital goiter in an infant born to a mother with thyrotoxicosis who had been treated with iodides and methimazole during pregnancy. *B,* A 6-wk-old infant (not the same as in *A*) with increasing respiratory distress and cervical mass since birth. The operation revealed a large goiter that almost completely encircled the trachea. Notice the anterior deviation and posterior compression of the trachea. Partial thyroidectomy completely relieved the symptoms. It is apparent why a tracheostomy is not adequate treatment for these infants. The cause for the goiter was not found.

Seawater is rich in iodine; the iodine content of fish and shellfish is also high. Endemic goiter is therefore rare in populations living along the sea. Iodine is deficient in the water and native foods in the Pacific West and the Great Lakes areas of the United States. Deficiency of dietary iodine is even greater in certain Alpine valleys, the Himalayas, the Andes, the Congo, and the highlands of Papua New Guinea. In areas such as the United States, where iodine is provided in foods from other areas and in iodized salt, endemic goiter has disappeared. Iodized salt in the United States contains potassium iodide (100 μg/g), which provides excellent prophylaxis. Further iodine intake in the United States is contributed by iodates used in baking, iodine-containing coloring agents, and iodine-containing disinfectants used in the dairy industry. The recommended daily allowance of iodine for infants is greater than 90 μg/24 hr; this amount is exceeded in breast-fed infants and 4-fold in infants fed cow's milk in the United States.

Clinical Manifestations. If the deficiency of iodine is mild, thyroid enlargement does not become noticeable except when there is increased demand for the hormone during periods of rapid growth, as in adolescence and during pregnancy. In regions of moderate iodine deficiency, goiter observed in school children may disappear with maturity and reappear during pregnancy or lactation. Iodine-deficient goiters are more common in girls than in boys. In areas where iodine deficiency is severe, as in the hyperendemic highlands of Papua New Guinea, nearly half the population has large goiters, and endemic cretinism is common.

Serum T_4 levels are often low in individuals with endemic goiter, although clinical hypothyroidism is rare. This is true in New Guinea, the Congo, the Himalayas, and South America. Despite low serum levels of thyroid hormone, serum TSH concentrations are often normal or only moderately increased. In such patients, circulating levels of T_3 are elevated. Moreover, T_3 levels are also elevated in patients with normal T_4 levels, indicating a preferential secretion of T_3 by the thyroid in this disease.

Endemic cretinism is the most serious consequence of iodine deficiency; it occurs only in geographic association with endemic goiter. The term endemic cretinism includes 2 different but overlapping syndromes—a **neurologic type** and a **myxedematous type.** The frequency of the 2 types varies among different populations. In Papua New Guinea, the neurologic type occurs almost exclusively, whereas in Zaire, the myxedematous type predominates. Both types are found in all endemic areas, and some individuals have intermediate or mixed features.

The **neurologic syndrome** is characterized by mental retardation, deaf-mutism, disturbances in standing and gait, and pyramidal signs such as clonus of the foot, the Babinski sign, and patellar hyperreflexia. Affected individuals are goitrous but euthyroid, have normal pubertal development and adult stature, and have little or no impaired thyroid function. Individuals with the **myxedematous syndrome** also are mentally retarded and deaf and have neurologic symptoms, but in contrast to the neurologic type they have delayed growth and sexual development, myxedema, and absence of goiter. Serum T_4 levels are low, and TSH levels are markedly elevated. Delayed skeletal maturation may extend into the 3rd decade or later. Ultrasonographic examination shows thyroid atrophy.

Pathogenesis. The pathogenesis of the **neurologic syndrome** has been attributed to iodine deficiency and hypothyroxinemia during pregnancy, leading to fetal and postnatal hypothyroidism. Although some investigators have attributed brain damage to a direct effect of elemental iodine deficiency in the fetus, most believe the neurologic symptoms are caused by fetal and maternal hypothyroxinemia. There is evidence that the human fetal brain has receptors for thyroid hormone before development of the fetal thyroid, and there is also evidence of transplacental passage of maternal thyroid hormone into the fetus, which normally might ameliorate the effects of fetal hypothyroidism on the developing nervous system. Intake of iodine after birth is often sufficient for normal or only minimally impaired thyroid function. The pathogenesis of the **myxedematous syndrome** leading to thyroid atrophy is more bewildering. Searches for additional environmental factors that may provoke continuing postnatal hypothyroidism have led to incrimination of selenium deficiency, goitrogenic foods, thiocyanates, and *Yersinia.* Studies from western China suggest that thyroid autoimmunity may play a role. Myxedematous cretins with thyroid atrophy, but not euthyroid cretins, were found to have thyroid growth-blocking immunoglobulins of the kind found in infants with sporadic congenital hypothyroidism. Others are skeptical about any role of thyroid growth-blocking immunoglobulins to explain these findings.

Treatment. In many developing countries, administration of a single intramuscular injection of iodinated poppy seed oil to women prevents iodine deficiency during future pregnancies for about 5 yr. This form of therapy given to children younger than 4 yr of age with myxedematous cretinism results in a euthyroid state in 5 mo. However, older children respond poorly and adults not at all to iodized oil injections, indicating an inability of the thyroid gland to synthesize hormone; these patients require treatment with T_4. Through the efforts of the World Health Organization and its program of universal salt iodization, endemic iodine deficiency worldwide has been reduced by approximately 50%. In the Xinjiang province of China, where the usual methods of iodine supplementation had failed, iodination of irrigation water has increased iodine levels in soil, animals, and human beings.

568.3 • Acquired Goiter

Most acquired goiters are sporadic and develop from a variety of causes; patients are usually euthyroid but may be hypothyroid. The most common cause of acquired goiter is lymphocytic thyroiditis (see Chapter 567). Other causes include excess iodide ingestion and certain drugs, including amiodarone and lithium. Intrinsic biochemical defects in the synthesis of thyroid hormone are almost always associated with goiter; these may be mild and present later in childhood. The occurrence of the disorder in siblings, onset in early life, and possible association with hypothyroidism (goitrous hypothyroidism) are important clues to the diagnosis.

IODIDE GOITER. A small percentage of patients treated with iodide preparations for prolonged periods acquire goiters. Iodides are commonly included for their expectorant effect in cough medicines and in proprietary mixtures for asthma. Goiters resulting from iodide administration are firm and diffusely enlarged, and in some instances hypothyroidism may develop. In normal individuals, acute administration of large doses of iodide inhibit the organification of iodine and the synthesis of thyroid hormone (Wolff-Chaikoff effect). This effect is short-lived and does not lead to permanent hypothyroidism. When iodide administration continues, an autoregulatory mechanism in normal persons limits iodide trapping and permits the level of iodide in the thyroid to decrease and organification to proceed normally. In patients with iodide-induced goiter, this escape does not occur because of an underlying abnormality of biosynthesis of thyroid hormone. The persons most susceptible to the development of iodide goiter are those with lymphocytic thyroiditis or with a subclinical inborn error in thyroid hormone synthesis and those who have had a partial thyroidectomy.

Lithium carbonate, which is used to treat manic depression, also causes goiters. Lithium competes with iodide, resulting in decreased T_4 and T_3 synthesis and release; the mechanism producing the goiter or hypothyroidism is similar to that described earlier for iodide goiter. Lithium and iodide also act synergistically to produce goiter; their combined use should be avoided.

Amiodarone, a drug used to treat cardiac arrhythmias, can cause thyroid dysfunction with goiter because it is rich in iodine. It is also a potent inhibitor of 5′-deiodinase, preventing conversion of T_4 to T_3. It can cause hypothyroidism, particularly in patients with underlying autoimmune disease; in other patients, it may cause hyperthyroidism.

SIMPLE GOITER (COLLOID GOITER). A few children with euthyroid goiters have simple goiters, a condition of unknown cause not associated with hypothyroidism or hyperthyroidism and not caused by inflammation or neoplasia. The condition predominates in girls and has a peak incidence before and during the pubertal years. Histologic examination of the thyroid either is normal or reveals variable follicular size, dense colloid, and flattened epithelium. The goiter may be small or large. It is firm in half the patients and occasionally is asymmetric or nodular. Levels of TSH are normal or low, scintiscans are normal, and thyroid antibodies are absent. Differentiation from lymphocytic thyroiditis may not be possible without a biopsy; biopsy is usually not indicated. Therapy with thyroid hormone may help avoid progression to a large multinodular goiter, although it is difficult to separate any treatment effects from the natural history, which is for the goiter to decrease in size. Patients should be reevaluated periodically, as some may have antibody-negative lymphocytic thyroiditis and therefore at risk for changes in thyroid function (see Chapter 567).

MULTINODULAR GOITER. Rarely, a firm goiter with a lobulated surface and single or multiple palpable nodules is encountered. Areas of cystic change, hemorrhage, and fibrosis may be present. The incidence of this condition has decreased markedly with the use of iodine-enriched salt. A mild goitrogenic stimulus, acting over a long time, is thought to be the cause. Ultrasonographic examination may reveal multiple echo-free and echogenic lesions that are nonfunctioning on scintiscans. Thyroid studies are usually normal. Some children with chronic lymphocytic thyroiditis develop multinodular goiter; TSH may be elevated, and thyroid antibodies may be present. Rarely, children may develop "toxic multinodular goiter," characterized by a suppressed TSH and hyperthyroidism. The condition occurs in children with **McCune-Albright syndrome** (usually resulting in hyperthyroidism) and has been described in 3 children (including 2 siblings) with digital anomalies and cystic renal disease. Dominant nodules within a multinodular goiter, particularly those not suppressed by replacement therapy with T_4, may be an indication for evaluation by fine-needle aspiration because malignancy cannot readily be ruled out.

TOXIC GOITER (HYPERTHYROIDISM). See Chapter 569.

568.4 • Intratracheal Goiter

One of the many ectopic locations of thyroid tissue is within the trachea. The intraluminal thyroid lies beneath the tracheal mucosa and is frequently continuous with the normally situated extratracheal thyroid. The thyroid tissue is susceptible to goitrous enlargement, which involves the normally situated and the ectopic thyroid. When there is obstruction of the airway associated with a goiter, it must be ascertained whether the obstruction is extratracheal or endotracheal. If obstructive manifestations are mild, administration of sodium L-thyroxine usually causes the goiter to decrease in size. When symptoms are severe, surgical removal of the endotracheal goiter is indicated (see 568.1).

Congenital Goiter

Bikker H, den Hartog MT, Baas F, et al: A 20-base pair duplication in the human thyroid peroxidase gene results in a total iodide organification defect and congenital hypothyroidism. *J Clin Endocrinol Metab* 1994;79:248–252.

Caron P, Moya CM, Malet D, et al: Compound heterozygous mutations in the thyroglobulin gene (1143delC and 6725G → A [R2223H]) resulting in fetal goitrous hypothyroidism. *J Clin Endocrinol Metab* 2003;88: 3546–3453.

Vade A, Gottschalk ME, Yetter EM, et al: Sonographic measurements of the neonatal thyroid gland. *J Ultrasound Med* 1997;16:395–399.

Vicens-Calvet E, Potau N, Carreras E, et al: Diagnosis and treatment in utero of goiter with hypothyroidism caused by iodine overload. *J Pediatr* 1998;133:147–148.

Endemic Goiter and Cretinism

Aghini-Lombardi F, Antonangeli L, Pinchera A, et al: Effect of iodized salt on thyroid volume of children living in an area previously characterized by moderate iodine deficiency. *J Clin Endocrinol Metab* 1997;82:1136–1139.

Benmiloud M, Chaouki ML, Gutekunst R, et al: Oral iodized oil for correcting iodine deficiency: Optimal dosing and outcome indicator selection. *J Clin Endocrinol Metab* 1994;79:20–24.

Boyages SC, Halpern JP, Maberly GF, et al: A comparative study of neurological and myxedematous endemic cretinism in western China. *J Clin Endocrinol Metab* 1988;67:1262–1271.

Boyages SC, Halpern JP, Maberly GF, et al: Endemic cretinism: Possible role for thyroid autoimmunity. *Lancet* 1989;2:529–532.

Boyages SC, Halpern JP, Maberly GF, et al: Supplementary iodine fails to reverse hypothyroidism in adolescents and adults with endemic cretinism. *J Clin Endocrinol Metab* 1990;70:336–341.

DeLange F: Iodine deficiency as a cause of brain damage. *Postgrad Med J* 2001;77:217–220.

Delange F, de Benoist B, Pretell E, et al: Iodine deficiency in the world: Where do we stand at the turn of the century? *Thyroid* 2001;11:437–447.

WHO, UNICEF, and ICCIDD: Assessment of the iodine deficiency disorders and monitoring their elimination. Geneva,WHO publ.WHO/NHD/01.1, 2001;1–107.

Acquired Goiter

Brix TH, Kyvik KO, Hegedus L: Major role of genes in the etiology of simple goiter in females: A population-based twin study. *J Clin Endocrinol Metab* 1999;84:3071–3075.

Daneman D, Davy T, Mancer K, et al: Association of multinodular goiter, cystic renal disease, and digital anomalies. *J Pediatr* 1985;107:270–272.

Feuillan PP, Shawker T, Rose SR, et al: Thyroid abnormalities in the McCune-Albright syndrome: Ultrasonography and hormonal studies. *J Clin Endocrinol Metab* 1990;71:1596–1601.

Jaruratanasirkul S, Leethanaporn K, Suchat K: The natural clinical course of children with an initial diagnosis of simple goiter: A 5-year longitudinal follow-up. *J Pediatr Endocrinol Metab* 2000;13:1109–1113.

Lisboa HR, Gross JL, Orsolin A, et al: Clinical examination is not an accurate method of defining the presence of goiter in schoolchildren. *Clin Endocrinol* 1996;45:471–475.

Chapter 569 ■ Hyperthyroidism

Hyperthyroidism results from excessive secretion of thyroid hormone and, during childhood, with few exceptions, is due to Graves disease (Table 569-1). **Graves disease** is an autoimmune disorder; production of thyroid-stimulating immunoglobulin (TSI) results in diffuse toxic goiter. Germline mutations of the **thyroid-stimulating hormone (TSH) receptor** resulting in constitutively activating (gain-of-function) mutations are found in both familial (autosomal dominant) and sporadic cases of non-autoimmune hyperthyroidism. These patients, whose disease may

TABLE 569-1. Causes of Hyperthyroidism

CAUSES OF HYPERTHYROIDISM	PATHOPHYSIOLOGIC FEATURES	FREQUENCY
CIRCULATING THYROID STIMULATORS		
Graves' disease	Thyroid-stimulating immunoglobulins	Common
Neonatal Graves' disease	Thyroid-stimulating immunoglobulins	Very rare
Thyrotropin-secreting tumor	Pituitary adenoma	Rare
Hyperemesis gravidarum	Human chorionic gonadatropin secretion	Uncommon
Choriocarcinoma	Human chorionic gonadatropin secretion	Rare
Abnormal thyrotropin receptor	Human chorionic gonadatropin secretion	Very rare
THYROIDAL AUTONOMY		
Toxic multinodular goiter	Activating mutations in thyrotropin receptor or G-protein	Common
Toxic solitary adenoma	Activating mutations in thyrotropin receptor or G-protein	Common
Congenital hyperthyroidism	Activating mutations in thyrotropin receptor	Very rare
Iodine-induced hyperthyroidism (Jod-Basedow)	Unknown; excess iodine results in unregulated thyroid hormone production	Uncommon in USA and other iodine-sufficient areas
DESTRUCTION OF THYROID FOLLICLES (THYROIDITIS)		
Subacute thyroiditis	Probable viral infection	Uncommon
Painless or postpartum thyroiditis	Autoimmune	Common
Amiodarone-induced thyroiditis	Direct toxic drug effects	Uncommon
Acute (infectious) thyroiditis	Thyroid infection (bacterial, fungal, etc)	Uncommon
EXOGENOUS THYROID HORMONE		
Iatrogenic	Excess ingestion of thyroid hormone	Common
Factitious	Excess ingestion of thyroid hormone	Rare
Hamburger thyrotoxicosis	Thyroid gland included in ground beef	Probably rare
ECTOPIC THYROID TISSUE		
Struma ovarii	Ovarian teratoma containing thyroid tissue	Rare
Metastatic follicular thyroid cancer	Large tumor mass capable of secreting thyroid hormone autonomously	Rare
Pituitary resistance to thyroid hormone	Mutated thyroid hormone receptor with greater expression in the pituitary compared with peripheral tissues	Rare

From Cooper DS: Hyperthyroidism. *Lancet* 2003;362:459–468.

present in the neonatal period or in later childhood, have thyroid hyperplasia with goiter and suppressed levels of TSH. Different activating mutations have been identified in some cases of thyroid adenomas. Hyperthyroidism occurs in some patients with **McCune-Albright syndrome** as a result of an activating mutation of the α subunit of the G-protein; these patients tend to have a multinodular goiter. Other rare causes of hyperthyroidism that have been observed in children include toxic uninodular goiter (Plummer disease), hyperfunctioning thyroid carcinoma, thyrotoxicosis factitia, subacute thyroiditis, and acute suppurative thyroiditis. Suppression of plasma TSH indicates that the hyperthyroidism is not pituitary in origin. Hyperthyroidism due to excess thyrotropin secretion is rare and, in most cases, is caused by pituitary resistance to thyroid hormone. TSH-secreting pituitary tumors have been reported only in adults. In infants born to mothers with Graves disease, hyperthyroidism is almost always a transitory phenomenon; classic Graves disease during the neonatal period is rare. Choriocarcinoma, hydatidiform mole, and struma ovarii have caused hyperthyroidism in adults but have not been recognized as causes in children.

569.1 • Graves Disease

EPIDEMIOLOGY. Graves disease occurs in approximately 0.02% of children (1 : 5,000). It has a peak incidence in the 11- to 15-yr old; there is a 5 : 1 female to male ratio. Most children with Graves disease have a positive family history of some form of autoimmune thyroid disease. In Japan, familial Graves disease, defined as Graves disease in a 1st-degree relative, occurs in 2–3% of cases.

ETIOLOGY. Enlargement of the thymus, splenomegaly, lymphadenopathy, infiltration of the thyroid gland and retro-orbital tissues with lymphocytes and plasma cells, and peripheral lymphocytosis are well-established findings in Graves disease. In the thyroid gland, T helper cells ($CD4^+$) predominate in dense lymphoid aggregates; in areas of lower cell density, cytotoxic T cells ($CD8^+$) predominate. The percentage of activated B lymphocytes infiltrating the thyroid is higher than in peripheral blood. A postulated failure of T suppressor cells allows expression of T helper cells, sensitized to the TSH antigen, which interact with B cells. These cells differentiate into plasma cells, which produce thyrotropin receptor-stimulating antibody (TRSAb). TRSAb binds to the receptor for TSH and stimulates cyclic adenosine monophosphate, analogous to TSH itself. In addition to TRSAb, thyrotropin receptor-blocking antibody (TRBAb) may also be produced, and the clinical course of the disease usually correlates with the ratio between the two antibodies.

The ophthalmopathy occurring in Graves disease appears to be caused by antibodies against antigens shared by the thyroid and eye muscle. TSH receptors have been identified in retro-orbital adipocytes and may represent a target for antibodies. The antibodies that bind to the extraocular muscles and orbital fibroblasts stimulate the synthesis of glycosaminoglycans by orbital fibroblasts and produce cytotoxic effects on muscle cells.

In whites, Graves disease is associated with HLA-B8 and HLA-DR3; the latter carries a 7-fold relative risk for Graves disease. Graves disease is also associated with other HLA-D3-related disorders such as Addison disease, insulin-dependent diabetes mellitus, myasthenia gravis, and celiac disease. Systemic lupus erythematosus, rheumatoid arthritis, vitiligo, idiopathic thrombocytopenic purpura, and pernicious anemia have been described in children with Graves disease. In family clusters, the conditions associated most frequently with Graves disease are autoimmune lymphocytic thyroiditis and hypothyroidism. In Japanese children, Graves disease is associated with different HLA haplotypes: HLA-DRB1*0405 and HLA-DQB1*0401.

CLINICAL MANIFESTATIONS. About 5% of all patients with hyperthyroidism are younger than 15 yr of age; the peak incidence in these children occurs during adolescence. Graves disease has begun between 6 wk and 2 yr of age in children born to mothers without a history of hyperthyroidism. The incidence is about 5 times higher in girls than in boys.

TABLE 569-2. Major Symptoms and Signs of Hyperthyroidism and of Graves Disease and Conditions Associated with Graves Disease

MANIFESTATIONS OF HYPERTHYROIDISM
Symptoms
Hyperactivity, irritability, altered mood, insomnia, anxiety
Heat intolerance, increased sweating
Palpitations
Fatigue, weakness
Dyspnea
Weight loss with increased appetite (weight gain in 10% of patients)
Pruritus
Increased stool frequency
Thirst and polyuria
Oligomenorrhea or amenorrhea, loss of libido
Signs
Sinus tachycardia, atrial fibrillation (rare in children), supraventricular tachycardia
Fine tremor, hyperkinesis, hyperreflexia
Warm, moist skin
Palmar erythema, onycholysis
Hair loss
Osteoporosis
Hypercalcemia
Muscle weakness and wasting
High-output heart failure
Chorea
Periodic (hypokalemic) paralysis (primarily in Asian men)
Psychosis (rare)
MANIFESTATIONS OF GRAVES DISEASE
Diffuse goiter
Ophthalmopathy
A feeling of grittiness and discomfort in the eye
Retrobulbar pressure or pain
Eyelid lag or retraction
Periorbital edema, chemosis, scleral injection
Exophthalmos (proptosis)
Extraocular muscle dysfunction
Exposure keratitis
Optic neuropathy
Localized dermopathy (rare in children)
Lymphoid hyperplasia
Thyroid acropachy (rare in children)
CONDITIONS ASSOCIATED WITH GRAVES DISEASE
Type 1 diabetes mellitus
Addison disease
Vitiligo
Pernicious anemia
Alopecia areata
Myasthenia gravis
Celiac disease

Adapted from Weetman AP: Graves disease. *N Engl J Med* 2000;343:1236–1248.

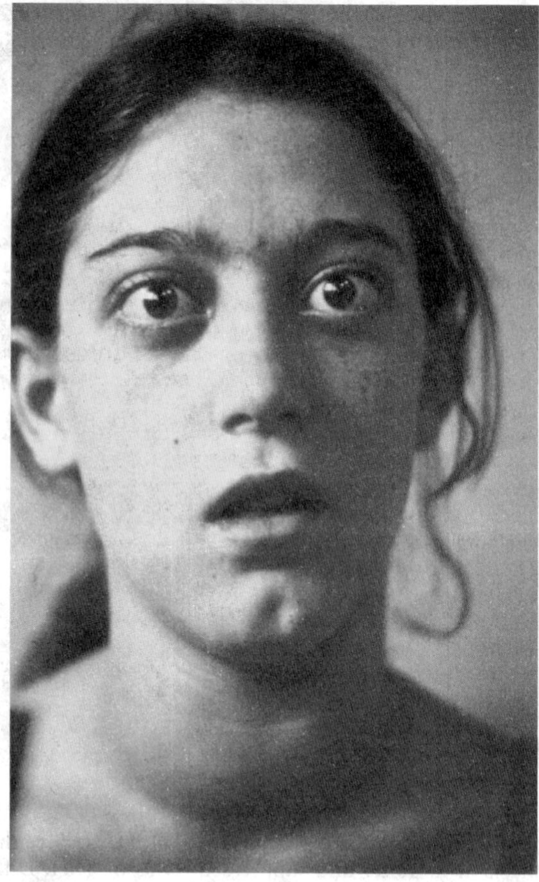

Figure 569-1. A 15-yr-old girl with classic Graves disease. Clinical features include a goiter and exophthalmos. She was treated with antithyroid drugs, to which she had a good response.

The clinical course in children is highly variable but usually is not so fulminant as in many adults (Table 569-2). Symptoms develop gradually; the usual interval between onset and diagnosis is 6–12 mo and may be longer in prepubertal children compared with adolescents. The earliest signs in children may be emotional disturbances accompanied by motor hyperactivity. The children become irritable, excitable, and cry easily because of emotional lability. They are restless sleepers and tend to kick their covers off. Their schoolwork suffers as a result of a short attention span and poor sleep. Tremor of the fingers can be noticed if the arm is extended. There may be a voracious appetite combined with loss of or no increase in weight. The size of the thyroid is variable. It may be so minimally enlarged that it initially escapes detection, but with careful examination, a diffuse goiter, soft with a smooth surface, is found in almost all patients. Exophthalmos is noticeable in most patients but is usually mild. Lagging of the upper eyelid as the eye looks downward, impairment of convergence, and retraction of the upper eyelid and infrequent blinking may be present (Figs. 569-1 and 569-2). Ocular manifestations may produce pain, lid erythema, chemosis, decreased extraocular muscle function, and decreased visual acuity (corneal or optic nerve involvement). The skin is smooth and flushed, with excessive sweating. Muscular weakness is uncommon but may be severe enough to result in clumsiness. Tachycardia, palpitations, dyspnea, and cardiac enlargement and insufficiency cause discomfort but rarely endanger the patient's life. Atrial fibrillation is a rare complication. Mitral regurgitation, probably resulting from papillary muscle dysfunction, is the cause of the apical sys-

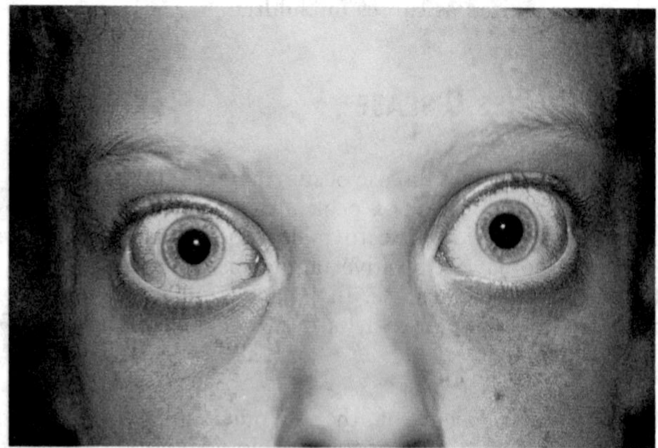

Figure 569-2. Retraction of upper eyelids in the primary gaze (Dalrymple sign). (From Kanski JJ: Systemic Diseases and the Eye: Signs and Differential Diagnosis. London, Mosby, 2001, Fig. 2.230.)

tolic murmur present in some patients. The systolic blood pressure and the pulse pressure are increased. Many of the findings in Graves disease result from hyperactivity of the sympathetic nervous system.

Thyroid "crisis," or "storm," is a form of hyperthyroidism manifested by an acute onset, hyperthermia, severe tachycardia, heart failure, and restlessness. There may be rapid progression to delirium, coma, and death. Precipitating events include trauma, parturition, infection, or surgery. **"Apathetic," or "masked," hyperthyroidism** is another variety of hyperthyroidism characterized by extreme listlessness, apathy, and cachexia. A combination of both forms may occur. These symptom complexes are rare in children.

LABORATORY FINDINGS. Serum levels of thyroxine (T_4), triiodothyronine (T_3), free T_4, and free T_3 are elevated. In some patients, levels of T_3 may be more elevated than those of T_4. Levels of TSH are suppressed to less than normal levels. Antithyroid antibodies, including thyroid peroxidase antibodies, are often present. Most patients with newly diagnosed Graves disease have measurable TRSAb; its disappearance predicts remission of the disease. Measurement of TRSAb is useful in confirming the diagnosis of Graves disease. Radioiodine is rapidly and diffusely concentrated in the thyroid, but this study is rarely necessary. Very young children or those congenitally affected with Graves disease often have advanced skeletal maturation and craniostenosis. Bone density may be reduced at diagnosis but returns to normal with treatment.

DIFFERENTIAL DIAGNOSIS. Diagnosis is rarely difficult once hyperthyroidism is considered. Elevated levels of T_4 or free T_4 and T_3 in association with suppressed levels of TSH are usually diagnostic (see Table 569-1). The presence of TRSAb establishes the cause as Graves disease.

Other causes of hyperthyroidism are uncommon. If a thyroid nodule is palpable, or if T_3 is preferentially elevated, a functional thyroid nodule must be considered. Radionuclide study is diagnostic, with uptake in the nodule and absent uptake in the rest of the gland ("hot nodule"). If precocious puberty, polyostotic fibrous dysplasia, or café-au-lait pigmentation is present, the autonomous thyroid disorder of McCune-Albright syndrome is likely. Patients with generalized thyroid hormone resistance have elevated levels of free T_4, but levels of TSH are inappropriately elevated or normal. Patients with isolated pituitary resistance to thyroid hormone also have clinical hyperthyroidism, but their levels of TSH are elevated or normal, and they must be differentiated from patients with TSH-secreting pituitary tumors who have elevated serum levels of the TSH α chain. Most other causes of hyperthyroxinemia are uncommon but may result in erroneous diagnosis. Patients with elevated thyroxine-binding globulin (TBG) levels or familial dysalbuminemic hyperthyroxinemia have normal levels of free T_4 and TSH.

When hyperthyroxinemia is caused by **exogenous thyroid hormone,** levels of free T_4 and TSH are the same as those seen in Graves disease, but the level of thyroglobulin is very low, whereas in patients with Graves disease, it is elevated.

TREATMENT. Most pediatric endocrinologists recommend initial medical therapy using antithyroid drugs rather than radioiodine or subtotal thyroidectomy, although radioiodine is gaining acceptance as initial treatment in children >10 yr of age. All therapeutic options have advantages and disadvantages (Table 569-3). The 2 antithyroid drugs in widest use are propylthiouracil (PTU) and methimazole (Tapazole). Both compounds inhibit incorporation of trapped inorganic iodide into organic compounds, and they may also suppress TRSAb levels by directly affecting intrathyroidal autoimmunity. However, there are important differences between the drugs. Methimazole is at least 10 times more potent than PTU on a weight basis and has a much longer serum half-life (6–8 hr vs 0.5 hr); PTU generally is administered 3 times daily, but methimazole can be given once daily. Unlike methimazole, PTU is heavily protein-bound and has a lesser ability to cross the placenta and to pass into breast milk; theoretically, PTU is the preferred drug during pregnancy and for nursing mothers. PTU, more than methimazole, inhibits extrathyroidal conversion of T_4 to T_3; this may be advantageous in the treatment of neonatal thyrotoxicosis.

Adverse reactions occur with both drugs; most are mild, but some are life-threatening. Minor adverse effects occur in approximately 10–20% while more severe adverse effects occur in 2–5% of children. Reactions are unpredictable and can occur after therapy of any duration. There is increasing evidence that these reactions may be fewer in patients treated with methimazole. Transient granulocytopenia (<2,000/mm^3) is common; it is asymptomatic and is not a harbinger of agranulocytosis, and it usually is not a reason to discontinue treatment. Transient urticarial rashes are common. They can be managed by a short period off therapy, restarting with the alternate antithyroid drug. The most severe reactions are hypersensitive and include agranulocytosis (0.1–0.5%), hepatitis (0.2–1%), hepatic failure, a lupus-like polyarthritis syndrome, glomerulonephritis, and an ANCA-positive vasculitis involving the skin and other organs. These reactions have been reported with both drugs, although hepatitis occurs almost exclusively with PTU. Patients with severe adverse effects should be treated with radioiodine or thyroidectomy. Cases of congenital skin defects (aplasia cutis) have been seen in infants exposed in fetal life to methimazole, but this association does not appear to be a strong one.

The initial dosage of PTU is 5–10 mg/kg/24 hr given 3 times daily, and that of methimazole is 0.25–1.0 mg/kg/24 hr given

TABLE 569-3. Treatments for Hyperthyroidism Caused by Graves Disease

TREATMENT	ADVANTAGE	DISADVANTAGE	COMMENT
Antithyroid drugs	Noninvasive Less initial cost Low risk of permanent hypothyroidism Possible remissions owing to immune effects	Cure rate (30–80%; average 40–50%) Adverse drug reactions Drug compliance required	First-line treatment in children and adolescents and in pregnancy Initial treatment in severe cases or preoperative preparation
Radioactive iodine (^{131}I)	Cure of hyperthyroidism Most cost effective	Permanent hypothyroidism almost inevitable Might worsen ophthalmopathy Pregnancy must be deferred for 6–12 months, mother cannot breast-feed; small potential risk of exacerbation of hyperthyroidism	No evidence for infertility, birth defects, cancer Best treatment for toxic nodules and toxic multinodular goiter
Surgery	Rapid, effective treatment especially in patients with large goiter	Most invasive therapy Potential complications (recurrent laryngeal nerve damage, hypoparathyroidism) Most costly therapy Permanent hypothyroidism; pain; scarring	Potential use in pregnancy if major side effect from antithyroid drugs Useful when coexisting suspicious nodule present Option for patients who refuse radioiodine

From Cooper DS: Hyperthyroidism. *Lancet* 2003;362:459–468.

TABLE 569-4. Management of Thyroid Storm in Adolescents

GOAL	TREATMENT
Inhibition of thyroid hormone formation and secretion	Propylthiouracil (PTU), 400 mg every 8 hr PO or by nasogastric tube Sodium iodide, 1 g IV in 24 hr, or saturated solution of KI, 5 drops every 8 hr
Sympathetic blockade	Propranolol, 20–40 mg every 4–6 hr, or 1 mg IV slowly (repeat doses until heart rate slows); not indicated in patients with asthma or heart failure that is not rate related
Glucocorticoid therapy	Hydrocortisone, 50–100 mg IV every 6 hr
Supportive therapy	Intravenous fluids (depending on indication: glucose, electrolytes, multivitamins) Temperature control (cooling blankets, acetaminophen; avoid salicylates) O_2 if required Digitalis for heart failure and to slow ventricular response; pentobarbital for sedation Treatment of precipitating event (e.g., infection)

From Goldman L, Ausiello D: *Cecil Textbook of Medicine,* 22nd ed, Philadelphia, WB Saunders, 2004, p 1401.

once or twice daily. Smaller initial dosages should be used in early childhood. Careful surveillance is required after treatment is initiated. Rising serum levels of TSH to greater than normal indicates overtreatment and leads to increased size of the goiter. Clinical response becomes apparent in 3–6 wk, and adequate control is evident in 3–4 mo. The dose is decreased to the minimal level required to maintain a euthyroid state.

Drug therapy may be necessary for 5 yr or longer because there appears to be a remission rate of about 25% every 2 yr. If a relapse occurs, it usually appears within 3 mo and almost always within 6 mo after therapy has been discontinued. Therapy may be resumed in case of relapse. Patients older than 13 yr of age, boys, those with a higher body mass index, and those with small goiters and modestly elevated T_3 levels appear to have earlier remissions.

A β-adrenergic blocking agent such as propranolol (0.5–2.0 mg/kg/24 hr po, given 3 times daily) is a useful supplement to antithyroid drugs in the management of severely toxic patients. Additional therapies for **thyroid storm** are listed in Table 569-4. Thyroid hormones potentiate the actions of catecholamines, including tachycardia, tremor, excessive sweating, lid lag, and stare. These symptoms abate with the use of propranolol, which does not, however, alter thyroid function or exophthalmos.

Surgery or radioiodine treatment is indicated when adequate cooperation for medical management is not possible, when adequate trial of medical management has failed to result in permanent remission, or when severe side effects preclude further use of antithyroid drugs. Subtotal thyroidectomy, a rather safe procedure when performed by an experienced team, is done only after the patient has been brought to a euthyroid state. This may be accomplished with PTU or methimazole over 2–3 mo. After a euthyroid state has been attained, a saturated solution of potassium iodide, 5 drops/24 hr, are added to the regimen for 2 wk before surgery to decrease the vascularity of the gland. Complications of surgical treatment are rare and include hypoparathyroidism (transient or permanent) and paralysis of the vocal cords. The incidence of residual or recurrent hyperthyroidism or hypothyroidism depends on the extent of the surgery. Most recommend near-total thyroidectomy. The incidence of recurrence is low but that of hypothyroidism may exceed 50%.

Radioiodine is an effective, relatively safe first or alternative therapy for Graves disease in children over 10 yr of age. Pretreatment with antithyroid drugs is unnecessary; if a patient is taking them, they should be stopped a week before radioiodine administration. Many pediatric endocrinologists prefer to select a dose of radioiodine to ensure complete ablation of thyroid tissue. A dose of 300 μCi/g of thyroid tissue, or a total dose of approximately 15 mCi, will achieve this goal. Essentially all patients treated at this dose will become hypothyroid; the time course to hypothyroidism averages 11 wk, with a range of 9 wk to 28 wk. Because the full effects of treatment may not be complete for 1–6 mo, adjunctive therapy with a β-adrenergic antagonist and lower doses of antithyroid drugs are recommended. Although there have been concerns about radiation oncogenesis and genetic damage, follow-up of treated children for as long as 50 yr has not shown this. The risk of benign adenoma may be increased (0.6–1.9% in one study). With lower treatment doses of radioiodine, hypothyroidism occurs in 10–20% of patients after the 1st year and in about 3% per year thereafter.

The **ophthalmopathy** remits gradually and usually independently of the hyperthyroidism. Severe ophthalmopathy may require treatment with high-dose prednisone, orbital radiotherapy (of questionable value), or orbital decompression surgery. Cigarette smoking is a risk factor of thyroid eye disease and should be avoided or discontinued to avoid progression of eye involvement.

569.2 • Congenital Hyperthyroidism

ETIOLOGY AND PATHOGENESIS. Neonatal Graves disease is caused by transplacental passage of TRSAb, but the clinical onset, severity, and course may be modified by the concurrent presence of TRBAb and by the transplacental passage of antithyroid drugs taken by the mother. Very high levels of TRSAb usually result in classic neonatal hyperthyroidism, but if the infant has been exposed to the antithyroid drugs, onset of symptoms is delayed by 3–4 days to allow degradation of the maternally derived antithyroid drug. If TRBAb is also present, onset of hyperthyroid symptoms may be delayed for several weeks. The mothers of these infants have active Graves disease, Graves disease in remission, or rarely hypothyroidism and a history of lymphocytic thyroiditis.

Neonatal hyperthyroidism occurs in only about 2% of infants born to mothers with a history of Graves disease. The finding of very high levels of TRSAb in these mothers usually predicts the occurrence of an affected infant. Fetal tachycardia and goiter may allow prenatal diagnosis. Unlike Graves disease at all other ages, neonatal hyperthyroidism affects boys as often as girls. The disorder usually remits spontaneously within 6–12 wk but may persist longer, depending on the levels of TRSAb. Mild asymptomatic hyperthyroxinemia also occurs. Rarely, classic neonatal Graves disease does not remit but persists for several years or longer. These children have impressive family histories of Graves disease. In these infants, TRSAb transfer from the mother apparently blends with the infantile onset of autonomous Graves disease.

CLINICAL MANIFESTATIONS. Many of the infants are premature and appear to have intrauterine growth restriction. Most have goiters. The infant is extremely restless, irritable, and hyperactive, and appears anxious and unusually alert. Microcephaly and ventricular enlargement may be present. The eyes are opened widely and appear exophthalmic (Fig. 569-3). There may be extreme tachycardia and tachypnea, and the temperature is elevated. In severely affected infants, there is a progression of symptoms; weight loss occurs despite a ravenous appetite, hepatosplenomegaly increases, and jaundice may become manifested. Severe hypertension and cardiac decompensation may occur. The infant may die if therapy is not instituted promptly. The serum level of T_4 is markedly elevated, and TSH is suppressed. Advanced bone age, frontal bossing with triangular facies, and cranial synostosis are common, especially in infants with persistent clinical manifestations of hyperthyroidism.

TREATMENT. Treatment of the neonate consists of oral administration of propranolol (1–2 mg/kg/24 hr, orally in 3 divided doses) and PTU (5–10 mg/kg/24 hr given every 8 hr) or methi-

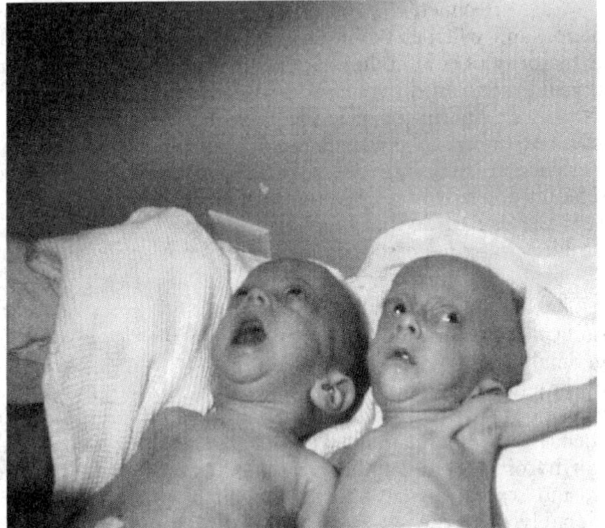

Figure 569-3. Twin boys with neonatal hyperthyroidism confirmed by abnormal thyroid function tests. Clinical features include lack of subcutaneous tissue due to a hypermetabolic state and a wide-eyed, anxious stare. They were given the diagnosis of neonatal Graves disease, but in fact, their mother did not have Graves disease; they had persistent, not transient, hyperthyroidism. At age 8 yr, they were treated with radioiodine. They are now believed to have had some other form of neonatal hyperthyroidism, such as a constitutive activation of the TSH receptor.

mazole (0.25–1.0 mg/kg/24hr given every 12 hr); Lugol solution (1 drop every 8 hr) may be added. When propranolol is used during pregnancy to treat thyrotoxicosis, it crosses the placenta and may cause respiratory depression in the newborn infant. If the thyrotoxic state is severe, parenteral fluid therapy and corticosteroids may be indicated. If heart failure occurs, digitalization is indicated. After a euthyroid state is reached, only antithyroid drug treatment is necessary. The dose should be gradually tapered to keep the infant euthyroid. Most cases remit by 3–4 mo of age.

Occasionally, neonatal hyperthyroidism does not remit but persists into childhood. These patients may have an impressive family history of hyperthyroidism. Neonatal hyperthyroidism, without evidence for autoimmune disease in mother or infant, is due to a mutation in the TSHR gene that produced constitutive activation of the receptor. Hyperthyroidism recurs when antithyroid drugs are discontinued; these children must be treated with radioiodine or surgery.

PROGNOSIS. Advanced osseous maturation, microcephaly, and mental retardation occur when treatment is delayed. Intellectual development is normal in most treated infants with neonatal Graves disease, though some may show injury from in utero hyperthyroidism. In some infants, in utero hyperthyroidism appears to suppress the hypothalamic-pituitary-thyroid feedback mechanism, and they develop permanent central hypothyroidism, requiring lifelong thyroid hormone treatment.

Akamizu T, Nakamura Y, Tamaoki A, et al: Prevalence and clinico-epidemiology of familial Graves' disease in Japan based on nationwide epidemiologic survey in 2001. *Endocrinol J* 2003;50:429–436.
Azizi F, Khamseh ME, Bahreynian M, et al: Thyroid function and intellectual development of children of mothers taking methimazole during pregnancy. *J Endocrinol Invest* 2002;25:586–589.
Birrell G, Cheetham T: Juvenile thyrotoxicosis; Can we do better? *Arch Dis Child* 204;89:745–750.
Cawood T, Moriarty P, O'Shea D: Recent developments in thyroid eye disease. *Br Med J* 2004;329:385–390.
Chan W, Wong GW, Fan DS, et al: Ophthalmopathy in childhood Graves' disease. *Br J Ophthalmol* 2002;86:740–742.
Cooper DS: Antithyroid drugs. *N Engl J Med* 2005;352:905–917.
Cooper DS: Hyperthyroidism. *Lancet* 2003;362:459–468.
Iwama S, Ikezaki A, Kikuoka N, et al: Association of HLA-DR, DQ genotypes and CTLA-4 gene polymorphism with Graves' disease in Japanese children. *Horm Res* 2005;63:55–60.
Kempers MJ, van Tijn DA, van Trotsenburg AS, et al: Central congenital hypothyroidism due to gestational hyperthyroidism: Detection where prevention failed. *J Clin Endocrinol Metab* 2003;88:5851–5857.
Kopp P, van Sande J, Parma J, et al: Brief report: Congenital hyperthyroidism caused by a mutation in the thyrotropin-receptor gene. *N Engl J Med* 1995;332:150–154.
Mastorakos G, Mitsiades NS, Doufas AG, et al: Hyperthyroidism in McCune-Albright syndrome with a review of thyroid abnormalities sixty years after the first report. *Thyroid* 1997;7:433–439.
Milham S Jr: Scalp defects in infants of mothers treated for hyperthyroidism with methimazole or carbimazole during pregnancy. *Teratology* 1985;32:321.
Nabhan Z, Kreher NC, Eugster EA: Hashitoxicosis in children: Clinical features and natural history. *J Pediatr* 2005;146:533–536.
Nesbesio TD, Siddiqui AR, Pescovitz OH, et al: Time course to hypothyroidism after fixed-dose radioablation therapy of Graves' disease in children. *J Pediatr* 2002;141:99–103.
Pearce EN: Diagnosis and management of thyrotoxicosis. *BMJ* 2006;332: 1369–1373.
Polak M: Hyperthyroidism in early infancy: Pathogenesis, clinical features and diagnosis with a focus on neonatal hyperthyroidism. *Thyroid* 1998;8:1171–1177.
Read CH, Tansey MJ, Menda Y: A 36-year retrospective analysis of the efficacy and safety of radioactive iodine in treating young Graves' patients. *J Clin Endocrinol Metab* 2004;89:4229–4233.
Rivkees SA, Cornelius EA: Influence of iodine-131 dose on the outcome of hyperthyroidism in children. *J Pediatr* 2003;111:745–749.
Skuza KA, Sills IN, Stene M, et al: Prediction of neonatal hyperthyroidism in infants born to mothers with Graves' disease. *J Pediatr* 1996;128:264–268.
Sugino K, Ito K, Mimura T, et al: Surgical treatment of Graves' disease in children. *Thyroid* 2004;14:447–452.
Weber G, Ielo V, Vigone MC, et al: Neonatal hyperthyroidism: report of eight cases. *Ital J Pediatr* 2001;27:757.
Zimmerman D, Lteif AN: Thyrotoxicosis in children. *Endocrinol Metab Clin North Am* 1998;27:109–126.

Chapter 570 ■ Carcinoma of the Thyroid

EPIDEMIOLOGY. Carcinoma of the thyroid is rare in childhood; the annual incidence in children younger than 15 yr of age is approximately 2/100,000 cases, compared with an annual incidence at all ages around the world ranging from 4–10/100,000 cases. Unlike other malignancies in childhood, thyroid cancer usually has an indolent course, even after pulmonary metastases have developed.

PATHOGENESIS. Genetic factors and radiation exposure are important factors in the pathogenesis of thyroid cancer. Rearrangements of the *RET* proto-oncogene are found in 3–33% of papillary carcinomas and 60–80% of those occurring after irradiation, as in children in Belarus exposed to radiation after the nuclear accident at Chernobyl or in those who were exposed to external therapeutic irradiation in childhood. Inactivating point mutations of the *p53* tumor-suppressor gene are rare in patients with differentiated thyroid carcinoma but are common in those with anaplastic thyroid cancer. Overall, 5–10% of cases of papillary thyroid carcinoma are familial and are usually inherited in an autosomal dominant manner.

The thyroid gland of children is unusually sensitive to exposure to external radiation. There probably is no threshold dose; 1 Gy results in a 7.7 relative risk of thyroid cancer. In the past, about 80% of children with cancer of the thyroid had received inappropriate therapeutic irradiation of the neck and adjacent areas during infancy for benign conditions such as "enlarged" thymus, hypertrophied tonsils and adenoids, hemangiomas, nevi, eczema, tinea capitis, and "cervical adenitis." With the discontinuation of irradiation for benign conditions, this cause of thyroid cancer has vanished. However, the long-term survival of children who have received appropriate therapeutic irradiation of areas of the neck for neoplastic disease has made this cause of thyroid cancer and nodules increasingly prevalent; increased dose, younger age at time of treatment, and female sex are factors that increase the risk of thyroid cancer. Long-term risk data for cancer are sparse, but 15–50% of children who have received irradiation and chemotherapy for Hodgkin disease, leukemia, bone marrow transplant, brain tumors, and other malignancies of the head and neck have elevated levels of thyroid-stimulating hormone (TSH) within the 1st yr of therapy, and 5–20% progress to hypothyroidism during the next 5–7 yr. Most large groups of treated children have a 10–30% incidence of benign thyroid nodules and an increased incidence of thyroid cancer. The latter begins to appear within 3–5 yr after radiation treatment and reaches a peak in 15–25 yr. It is unknown whether there is a period after which no more tumors develop. Administration of iodine-131 for diagnostic or therapeutic purposes does not increase the risk of thyroid cancer.

Differentiated thyroid carcinoma has been reported in patients with chronic lymphocytic thyroiditis; it is not clear whether there is an increased risk of thyroid cancer in children with autoimmune thyroid disease. Conversely, lymphocytic infiltration within the thyroid cancer carries a more favorable prognosis, perhaps as a sign of an immune response to the cancer.

Histologically, the carcinomas are papillary (80%), follicular (17%), medullary (2%), or mixed differentiated tumors. These are usually slow-growing tumors and may remain dormant for years. The type of tumor and the natural course of disease in irradiated and nonirradiated patients are the same except that multicentricity is more frequent in irradiation-induced cancer. Undifferentiated (anaplastic) thyroid neoplasms are rare in children and usually have a rapidly fatal course. Thyroid cancer, most commonly papillary cancer, has been reported in thyroglossal duct remnants in children. Lymphomas and teratomas of the thyroid are also reported in children.

CLINICAL MANIFESTATIONS. Girls are affected twice as often as boys. The average age at diagnosis is 9 yr, but the onset may be as early as the 1st yr of life. A painless nodule in the thyroid or in the neck is the usual initial evidence of disease. Large nodule size, firmness, fixation to adjacent tissues, and vocal cord paralysis are risk factors for thyroid cancer. Cervical lymph node involvement is often present at the time of initial diagnosis. Any unexplained cervical lymph node enlargement requires examination of the thyroid, which occasionally has a primary tumor too small to be felt; the diagnosis is based on biopsy results of the lymph node. The lungs are the most common site of metastases beyond the neck. There may be no clinical manifestations referable to them; radiologically, they appear as diffuse miliary or nodular infiltrations, principally in the basal portions. They may be mistaken for tuberculosis, histoplasmosis, or sarcoidosis. Other sites of metastases include the mediastinum, long bones, skull, and axilla. Almost all children are euthyroid, but rarely, the carcinoma may be functional and produce symptoms of hyperthyroidism.

DIAGNOSIS. The most helpful diagnostic test in the case of a solitary nodule is fine-needle aspiration (FNA). An ultrasonographic examination of the thyroid can provide information on the consistency of the nodule (solid vs cystic) and whether other nonpalpable nodules are present. A thyroid scan, preferably using ^{123}I or ^{99m}Tc-pertechnetate, can provide information on trapping function and whether the nodule is "cold," "warm," or "hot." The majority of cold nodules are benign. Neither ultrasound nor a thyroid scan can differentiate between a benign or malignant lesion. FNA specimens may be interpreted as benign tumor, malignant tumor, indeterminate, or inadequate specimen. FNA experience in children shows a 5–10% false-negative rate and a 1–2% false-positive rate, with an overall diagnostic accuracy of 90–95%. Tests of thyroid function are normal, but Hashimoto's thyroiditis has been associated with thyroid cancer.

TREATMENT. Because differentiated thyroid carcinoma is a chronic disease with a long survival, optimal therapy is still evolving. Small (<1 cm) papillary carcinoma, the least aggressive type, may be effectively treated by subtotal thyroidectomy and suppressive doses of thyroid hormone. However, there is increasing evidence that most patients are best managed by total or near-total thyroidectomy. Papillary carcinomas tend to be multicentric, and several studies show that half of these children have regional lymph node involvement at presentation. For larger papillary carcinomas, follicular carcinoma, or with regional lymph node involvement, total thyroidectomy with excision of regional lymph nodes is the treatment of choice. There is no role for radical neck dissection. Thyroidectomy is usually followed by an ablative dose (30–100 mCi) of ^{131}I. Only patients who have undergone total thyroidectomy can be monitored by whole body radioiodine scanning and serum thyroglobulin.

After surgery, all patients should be treated with sodium L-thyroxine in doses sufficient to suppress TSH to the lower range of normal. Serum thyroglobulin (Tg) is an excellent marker for tumor recurrence, and periodic determinations of Tg levels should be performed. Serum Tg level should be less than 3 ng/mL when thyroxine (T_4) suppressive therapy is being received. Patients with an elevated serum Tg should undergo whole-body radioactive iodine uptake and scan and ultrasound examination of the neck to locate the source of Tg and plan appropriate management.

PROGNOSIS. For any form of therapy, survival or recurrence does not appear to be different for patients with or without involvement of the cervical nodes. Even patients with cervical or pulmonary metastases have survived many years. More than 95% of patients are alive 25 yr after initial treatment if the tumor was intrathyroid, less than 2 cm in diameter, and classified as grade 1. Greater tumor size, distant spread, and greater atypia are associated with increased cumulative mortality. Thyroid carcinomas that express telomerase and the IGF-1 receptor are more likely to show aggressive clinical features, while those that express the sodium-iodide symporter are associated with a lower risk of recurrence.

570.1 • Solitary Thyroid Nodule

Solitary nodules of the thyroid are common in children. They are found by palpation in approximately 2% of children aged 11–18 yr; ultrasound examination would likely show a higher prevalence, as it does in adults. Genetic factors play an etiologic role. Most thyroid nodules in children are benign. There is an approximately 15% incidence of malignancy, perhaps because of decreasing exposure of children to irradiation (Table 570-1). Children exposed to irradiation have a high incidence of benign adenoma and carcinoma of the thyroid.

Benign disorders that may present as solitary thyroid nodules include benign adenomas (follicular, embryonal, Hürthle cell), colloid (adenomatous) nodule, a simple cyst, lymphocytic thyroiditis, a thyroid abscess, and developmental anomalies such as thyroglossal duct cyst or hemiagenesis. A suddenly appearing or

TABLE 570-1. Etiologic Classification of Solitary Thyroid Nodules

Lymphoid follicle, as part of chronic lymphocytic thyroiditis
Thyroid developmental anomalies
Hemiagenesis
Intrathyroidal thyroglossal duct cyst
Thyroid abscess (acute suppurative thyroiditis)
Simple cyst
Neoplasms
Benign
Colloid (adenomatous) nodule
Follicular adenoma
Toxic adenoma
Nonthyroidal (e.g., lymphohemangioma)
Malignant
Papillary carcinoma
Follicular carcinoma
Mixed papillary-follicular carcinoma
Undifferentiated (anaplastic)
Medullary carcinoma
Nonthyroidal
Lymphoma
Teratoma

rapidly enlarging thyroid mass may indicate hemorrhage into a cyst or benign adenoma. In most cases, the child is euthyroid, and thyroid function studies are normal. When lymphocytic thyroiditis is the cause of the nodule, T_4 may be low, TSH may be elevated, and thyroid antibodies are usually present. Radionuclide imaging, if performed, may reveal a moth-eaten appearance. Rarely, lymphocytic thyroiditis may be associated with carcinoma of the thyroid. Ultrasonography is particularly useful in detecting cystic lesions.

The diagnostic studies to delineate the underlying cause include serum thyroid function tests, antithyroid antibody determinations, ultrasonographic examination of the thyroid, and FNA. Radioiodine uptake and scan are useful when a suppressed serum TSH suggests an autonomous "hot" nodule. Response to a trial of suppressive T_4 treatment to look for shrinkage of nodule size is not reliable. Although thyroid carcinomas generally present as a solid, "cold" nodule, most "cold" nodules are benign lesions. FNA is useful in avoiding surgery for benign nodules. However, surgery without delay is indicated when the nodule is hard or has grown rapidly, when there is evidence of tracheal or vocal cord involvement, and when there is enlargement of adjacent lymph nodes. All persons with a history of head or neck irradiation should have careful examinations of the thyroid at least every 2 yr and indefinitely.

Rarely, thyroid nodules may be functional, producing hyperthyroidism (**Plummer disease**). The uptake of radionuclide is concentrated in the nodule ("hot" or "warm" nodule), and thyroid function studies indicate that the nodule is functioning autonomously. Such nodules are usually benign, but a few instances of carcinoma in such cases have been reported. T_4 levels are usually normal, but triiodothyronine (T_3) levels are elevated (T_3 toxicosis) and TSH levels are suppressed. Treatment consists of surgical removal of the nodule.

570.2 • Medullary Carcinoma

Medullary carcinoma of the thyroid arises from the parafollicular cells (C cells) of the thyroid and accounts for about 2% of thyroid malignancies. The most common symptom is goiter or a palpable thyroid nodule. X-rays may reveal dense, conglomerate, homogeneous calcification in the thyroid. Metastases to the regional lymph nodes and to the liver are common; these also may calcify. Death may result, but long survival is common.

The tumors occur sporadically, as a familial autosomal dominant disorder and as components of two distinct autosomal dominant syndromes. The susceptibility for all these disorders has been associated with germ line mutations of the *RET* proto-oncogene on chromosome 10q11.2. When the tumor occurs sporadically, it is usually unicentric, but in the familial form, it is usually multicentric, and it begins as hyperplasia of parafollicular cells. The tumors are often too small to be found by palpation, scintigraphy, or ultrasonographic examination in at-risk patients in these families. Diagnosis of medullary carcinoma should lead to a careful search for associated tumors, particularly pheochromocytoma. No clinically recognizable manifestations result from the elevated serum levels of calcitonin or from the calcitonin gene-related peptide. Nonetheless, these tests are helpful in screening and monitoring therapy.

MULTIPLE ENDOCRINE NEOPLASIA, TYPE IIA. When hyperplasia or carcinoma of C cells is associated with adrenal medullary hyperplasia or pheochromocytoma and parathyroid hyperplasia, it is known as multiple endocrine neoplasia (MEN) IIA. The inheritance pattern for MEN IIA is autosomal dominant, with a high degree of penetrance and variable expressivity. At least 19 different specific missense mutations of exon 10 or 11 of the extracellular domain of the *RET* gene have been described for MEN IIA and for cases of familial medullary thyroid carcinoma. DNA analysis permits unambiguous identification of carriers of the *RET* proto-oncogene. C-cell hyperplasia or tumors usually appear earlier than pheochromocytoma. Pheochromocytomas are frequently bilateral and may be multiple. Adrenal medullary hyperplasia is known to precede pheochromocytoma, but the detectable latent period is short. Hypercalcemia is a late manifestation and indicates hyperparathyroidism. The parathyroid glands may reveal chief-cell hyperplasia or only hypercellularity.

MULTIPLE ENDOCRINE NEOPLASIA, TYPE IIB. The distinguishing feature of MEN IIB, also called the **mucosal neuroma syndrome,** is the occurrence of multiple neuromas and a characteristic phenotype associated with medullary carcinoma and pheochromocytoma. This condition is also autosomal dominant, and 93% of families have a missense mutation of the *RET* proto-oncogene. However, the mutation is in exon 16, the tyrosine catalytic domain of *RET;* all patients have had the same point mutation.

The neuromas most often occur on the tongue, buccal mucosa, lips, and conjunctivae. Peripheral neurofibromas and café-au-lait patches may be present, and intestinal ganglioneuromatosis is common. Diffuse proliferation of nerves and ganglion cells is found in mucosal, submucosal, myenteric, and subserosal plexus involving the small and large bowel as well as the esophagus. The patients may be tall, with arachnodactyly and a Marfan-like appearance. Scoliosis, pectus excavatum, pes cavus, and muscular hypotonia are common. The eyelids may be thickened and everted, the lips patulous and blubbery, the jaw prognathic. Feeding difficulties, poor sucking, diarrhea, constipation, and failure to thrive may begin in infancy or early childhood, many years before the appearance of neuromas or endocrine symptoms.

TREATMENT. Total thyroidectomy is indicated for all children who are shown by DNA studies to carry the gene mutation. Recognition of familial forms of this tumor is critical to the early diagnosis in children at risk. Evidence suggests that thyroidectomy must be performed early because medullary carcinoma has been seen in a 6-mo-old child with MEN IIB and in a 3-yr-old child with MEN IIA. In MEN IIA, there is correlation between the specific mutation and the onset of C-cell hyperplasia or medullary carcinoma. Codon 634 mutations occur at an early age, whereas mutations at codons 618, 620, and 804 tend to occur at a later age. In young children, mutation analysis may help individualize the age of total thyroidectomy. All these children should be screened for pheochromocytoma prior to surgery. Monitoring the levels of calcitonin is useful in following the course of the disease after operation and in detecting metastatic lesions. Periodic screening for the development of pheochromocytoma and hyperparathyroidism is indicated.

Acharya S, Sarafoglou K, LaQuaglia M, et al: Thyroid neoplasms after therapeutic radiation for malignancies during childhood or adolescence. *Cancer* 2003;97:2397–2403.

Amrikachi M, Ponder TB, Wheeler TM, et al: Thyroid fine-needle aspiration biopsy in children and adolescents: Experience with 218 aspirates. *Diagn Cytopath* 2005;32:189–192.

Antonelli A, Miccoli P, Fallahi P, et al: Role of neck ultrasonography in the follow-up of children operated on for thyroid papillary cancer. *Thyroid* 2003;13:479–484.

Borson-Chazot F, Causeret S, Lifante JC, et al: Predictive factors for recurrence from a series of 74 children and adolescents with differentiated thyroid cancer. *World J Surg* 2004;28:1088–1092.

Collins BJ, Chiappetta G, Schneider AB, et al: RET expression in papillary thyroid cancer from patients irradiated in childhood for benign conditions. *J Clin Endocrinol Metab* 2002;87:3941–3946.

Degnan BM, McClellan DR, Francis GL: An analysis of fine-needle aspiration biopsy of the thyroid in children and adolescents. *J Pediatr Surg* 1996;31:903–907.

Grigsby PW, Gal-or A, Michalski JM, Doherty GM: Childhood and adolescent thyroid cancer. Cancer 2002;95:724–732.

Hansen PS, Brix TH, Bennedbaek FN, et al: The relative importance of genetic and environmental factors in the aetiology of thyroid nodularity: A study of healthy Danish twins. *Clin Endocrinol* 2005;62:380–386.

Hegedüs L: The thyroid nodule. *N Engl J Med* 2004;351:1764–1771.

Hung W, Sarlis NJ. Current controversies in the management of pediatric thyroid patients with well-differentiated nonmedullary thyroid cancer: A review. *Thyroid* 2002;8:683–702.

Lafferty AR, Batch JA: Thyroid nodules in childhood and adolescence—Thirty years of experience. *J Pediatr Endocrinol Metab* 1997;10:479–486.

Lando A, Holm K, Nysom K, et al: Serum thyroglobulin as a marker of thyroid neoplasms after childhood cancer. *Acta Paediatr* 2003;92:1284–1290.

Peretz A, Leibermann E, Kapelushnik J, et al: Thyroglossal duct carcinoma in children: Case presentation and review of the literature. *Thyroid* 2004;14:777–785.

Ries LAG, Eisner MP, Kosary CL, et al: SEER Cancer Statistics Review, 1975–2000. Bethesda, MD, National Cancer Institute, 2003. Available at *seer.cancer.gov/csr/1975_2000.*

Svensson J, Nilsson PE, Olsson C, et al: Interpretation of normative thyroid volumes in children and adolescents: Is there a need for a multivariate model? *Thyroid* 2004;14:536–543.

Szinnai G, Meier C, Komminoth P, Zumsteg UW: Review of multiple endocrine neoplasia type 2A in children: Therapeutic results of early thyroidectomy and prognostic value of codon analysis. *Pediatrics* 2003;111: E132–139.

Utiger RD: The multiplicity of thyroid nodules and carcinomas. *N Engl J Med* 2005;352:2376–2378.

Zimmerman D: Thyroid neoplasia in children. *Curr Opin Pediatr* 1997;9: 413–418.

Section 3 — Disorders of the Parathyroid — Daniel A. Doyle and Angelo M. DiGeorge

Chapter 571 ■ Hormones and Peptides of Calcium Homeostasis and Bone Metabolism

Parathyroid hormone (PTH) and vitamin D are the principal regulators of calcium homeostasis (see Chapters 48 and 701). Calcitonin and PTH-related peptide (PTHrP) are important primarily in the fetus.

PARATHYROID HORMONE. PTH is an 84-amino-acid chain (9,500 Da), but its biologic activity resides in the first 34 residues. In the parathyroid gland, a pre-pro-PTH (115-amino-acid chain) and a proparathyroid hormone (90 amino acids) are synthesized. Pre-pro-PTH is converted to pro-PTH and pro-PTH to PTH. PTH (1–84) is the major secretory product of the gland, but it is rapidly cleaved in the liver and kidney into smaller COOH-terminal, mid-region, and NH_2-terminal fragments.

The occurrence of these fragments in serum has led to the development of a variety of assays. The 1–34 amino-terminal (N-terminus) fragments possess biologic activity but are present in low amounts in the circulation; assay of these fragments is most useful for detecting acute secretory changes. The carboxy-terminal (C-terminus) and mid-region fragments, although biologically inert, are cleared more slowly from the circulation and represent 80% of plasma immunoreactive PTH; values of the C-terminal fragment are 50–500 times the level of the active hormone. The C-terminal assays are effective in detecting patients with hyperparathyroidism, but because C-terminal fragments are removed from the circulation by glomerular filtration, these assays are less useful for evaluating the secondary hyperparathyroidism characteristic of renal disease. Only certain sensitive radioimmunoassays for PTH can differentiate the subnormal concentrations that occur in hypoparathyroidism from normal levels. A sensitive 15-min immunochemiluminometric assay, developed for intraoperative use, can provide the surgeon with useful information.

When serum levels of calcium fall, the signal is transduced through the calcium-sensing receptor and secretion of PTH increases (Fig. 571-1). PTH stimulates activity of 1α-hydroxylase in the kidney, enhancing production of 1,25-dihydroxycholecalciferol ($1,25[OH]_2D_3$). The increased level of $1,25[OH]_2D_3$ induces synthesis of a calcium-binding protein (calbindin-D) in the intestinal mucosa with resultant absorption of calcium. PTH also mobilizes calcium by directly enhancing bone resorption, an effect that requires $1,25[OH]_2D_3$. The effects of PTH on bone and kidney are mediated through binding to specific receptors on the membranes of target cells and through activation of a transduction pathway involving a G-protein coupled to the adenylate cyclase system (also see Chapter 573).

The calcium-sensing receptor regulates the secretion of PTH and the reabsorption of calcium by the renal tubules in response to alterations in serum calcium concentrations. The gene for the receptor is located on chromosome 3q13.3-q21 and encodes a

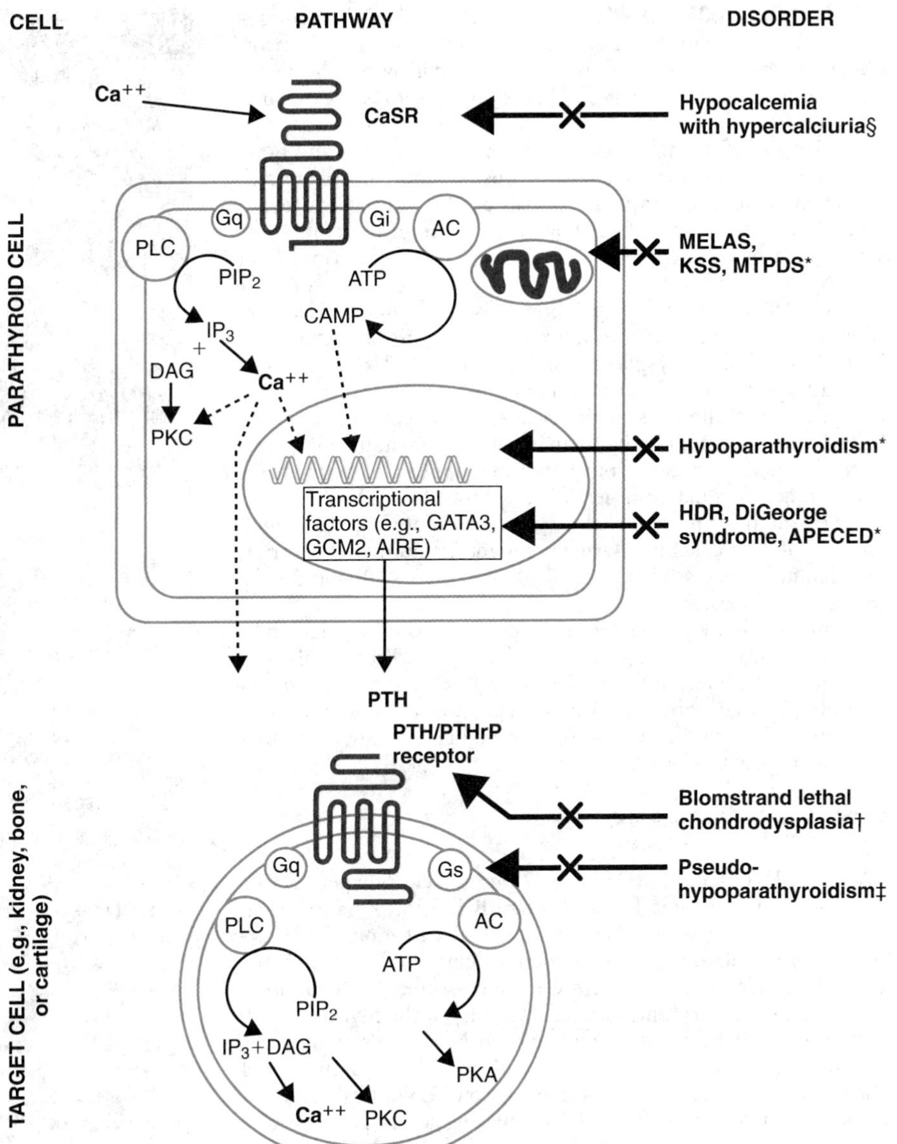

CELL | PATHWAY | DISORDER

Ca++ → CaSR ← Hypocalcemia with hypercalciuria§

PARATHYROID CELL: Gq, Gi, AC, PLC, PIP$_2$, ATP, CAMP, IP$_3$ + DAG, Ca++, PKC

MELAS, KSS, MTPDS*

Hypoparathyroidism*

Transcriptional factors (e.g., GATA3, GCM2, AIRE) ← HDR, DiGeorge syndrome, APECED*

PTH

PTH/PTHrP receptor ← Blomstrand lethal chondrodysplasia†

TARGET CELL (e.g., kidney, bone, or cartilage): Gq, Gs, PLC, AC, ATP, PIP$_2$, IP$_3$+DAG, PKA, Ca++, PKC

Gs ← Pseudo-hypoparathyroidism‡

CaSR and PTH/PTHrP-receptor mediate their effects through G protein-coupled signaling pathways, which in turn activate the adenyl cyclase (AC) and phospholipase C (PLC) systems.
Gq = G-pertussis-toxin-insensitive protein; Gi = G inhibitory protein; PIP$_2$ = phosphatidyl inositol 4,5-bisphosphate; IP$_3$ = inositol 1,4,5-triphosphate; DAG = diacylglycerol; PKC = protein kinase C.
*Disorders due to PTH deficiency.
†Defect due to defect in the PTH/PTHrP receptor.
‡Defect due to insensitivity to PTH caused by defects downstream of the PTH/PTHrP receptor.
§Defect due to altered set-point in the Ca^{++}/PTH axis, associated with a gain-of-function mutation of the CaSR.
MELAS = mitochondrial encephalopathy, stroke-like episodes, and lactic acidosis.
KSS = Kearns Sayre syndrome (progressive external opthalmoplegia, pigmentary retinopathy, heart block, and cardiomyopathy).
MTPDS = mitochondrial trifunctional protein-deficiency syndrome.
HDR = hypoparathyroidism, deafness, and renal anomalies.
APECED = autoimmune polyendocrinopathy-candidosis-ectodermal dystrophy.

Figure 571-1. Some components involved in calcium homeostasis. CaSR and PTH/PTHrP receptor mediate their effects through G-protein–coupled signaling pathways, which in turn activate the adenyl cyclase (AC) and phospholipase C (PLC) systems. APECED, autoimmune polyendocrinopathy-candidosis-ectodermal dystrophy; DAB, diacylglycerol; Gi, G inhibitory protein; Gq, G-pertussis-toxin–insensitive protein; HDR, hypoparathyroidism, deafness, and renal anomalies; IP$_3$, inositol 1,45-triphosphate; KSS, Kearns-Sayre syndrome (progressive external ophthalmoplegia, pigmentary retinopathy, heart block, and cardiomyopathy); MELAS, mitochondrial encephalopathy, stroke-like episodes, and lactic acidosis; MTPDS, mitochondrial trifunctional protein deficiency syndrome; PIP$_2$, phosphatidyl inositol 4,5-bisphosphate; PKC, protein kinase C.
*Disorders due to PTH deficiency.
†Defect due to defect in the PTH/PTHrP receptor.
‡Defect due to insensitivity to PTH caused by defects downstream of the PTH/PTHrP receptor.
§Defect due to altered set point in the Ca^{2+}/PTH axis, associated with a gain-of-function mutation of the CaSR.
(From Thakker RV: Genetic development in hypoparathyroidism. *Lancet* 2001;357:974–976, with permission.)

cell surface protein of 1,078 amino acids that is expressed in parathyroid glands and kidneys and belongs to the family of G-protein–coupled receptors. In the normally functioning calcium-sensing receptor, hypocalcemia induces increased secretion of PTH and hypercalcemia depresses PTH secretion. Loss-of-function mutations cause an increased set point with respect to serum calcium, resulting in hypercalcemia and in the conditions of **familial hypocalciuric hypercalcemia** and neonatal severe hyperparathyroidism. Acquired hypocalciuric hypercalcemia may be due to autoantibodies to the calcium-sensing receptor and manifests with hypercalcemia and hyperparathyroidism. Gain-of-function mutations result in depressed secretion of PTH in response to hypocalcemia, leading to the syndrome of familial hypocalcemia with hypercalciuria (see Fig. 571-1).

PARATHYROID HORMONE–RELATED PEPTIDE. PTHrP is homologous to PTH only in the first 13 amino acids of its amino terminus, 8 of which are identical to PTH. Its gene is on the short arm of chromosome 12 and that of PTH is on the short arm of chromosome 11.

PTHrP, like PTH, activates PTH receptors in kidney and bone cells and increases urinary cyclic adenosine monophosphate and renal production of 1,25$[OH]_2D_3$. It is produced in almost every type of cell of the body, including every tissue of the embryo at some stage of development. PTHrP is critical for normal fetal development. Inactivating mutations of the receptor for PTH/PTHrP result in a lethal bone disorder characterized by short limbs and markedly advanced bone maturation known as Blomstrand chondrodysplasia (see Fig. 571-1). PTHrP appears to have a paracrine or autocrine role because serum levels are low except in a few clinical situations. Cord blood contains levels of PTHrP that are 3-fold higher than in serum from adults; it is produced by the fetal parathyroid glands and appears to be the main agent stimulating maternal-fetal calcium transfer. PTHrP appears to be essential for normal skeletal maturation of the fetus, which requires 30 g of calcium. During pregnancy, maternal absorption of calcium increases from about 150 mg daily to 400 mg during the second trimester.

As in cord blood, PTHrP levels are increased during lactation and in patients with benign breast hypertrophy. Breast milk and pasteurized bovine milk have levels of PTHrP that are 10,000 times higher than those of normal plasma. Most instances of the hormonal hypercalcemia syndrome of malignancy are caused by elevated concentrations of PTHrP.

VITAMIN D. See Chapter 48.

CALCITONIN. Calcitonin (CT) is a 32-amino-acid polypeptide. Its gene is on chromosome 11p and is tightly linked to that of PTH. The gene for CT encodes three peptides: CT, a 21-amino-acid carboxyterminal flanking peptide (katacalcin), and a CT gene-related peptide. Katacalcin and CT are co-secreted in equimolar amounts by the parafollicular cells (C cells) of the thyroid gland. CT appears to be of little consequence in children and adults because very high levels in patients with medullary carcinoma of the thyroid (a tumor arising from the C cells) do not cause hypercalcemia. In the fetus, however, circulating levels are high and appear to augment bone metabolism and skeletal growth; these high levels are probably stimulated by the normally high fetal calcium levels. Unlike the high levels in cord blood and circulating concentrations in young children, levels in older children and adults are low. Infants and children with congenital hypothyroidism (and presumed deficiency of C cells) have lower levels of CT than do normal children.

Its action appears to be independent of PTH and vitamin D. Its main biologic effect appears to be the inhibition of bone resorption by decreasing the number and activity of bone-resorbing osteoclasts. This action of CT is the rationale for its use in treatment of Paget disease. CT is synthesized in other organs, such as the gastrointestinal tract, pancreas, brain, and pituitary. In these organs, CT is thought to behave as a neurotransmitter to impose a local inhibitory effect on cell function.

Chapter 572 ■ Hypoparathyroidism

ETIOLOGY (TABLE 572-1). Hypocalcemia is common between 12 and 72 hr of life, especially in premature infants, in infants with asphyxia, and in infants of diabetic mothers (early neonatal hypocalcemia) (see Chapter 106). After the 2nd to 3rd day and during the 1st wk of life, the type of feeding also is a determinant of the level of serum calcium (late neonatal hypocalcemia). The role played by the parathyroid glands in these hypocalcemic infants remains to be clarified, although functional immaturity of the parathyroid glands is invoked as one pathogenetic factor. In a group of infants with transient idiopathic hypocalcemia (1–8 wk of age), serum levels of parathyroid hormone (PTH) are significantly lower than those in normal infants. It is possible that the functional immaturity is a manifestation of a delay in development of the enzymes that convert glandular PTH to secreted PTH; other mechanisms are possible.

TABLE 572-1. Etiologic Classification of Hypocalcemia

PARATHYROID HORMONE (PTH) DEFICIENCY
Aplasia or hypoplasia of parathyroids
With 22q11 deletion
DiGeorge syndrome
Velocardiofacial syndrome
Conotruncal-face syndrome
With 10p13 deletion
With maternal diabetes mellitus or retinoic acid embryopathy
With X-linked isolated hypoparathyroidism
With mutation of *GCMB* (glial cell missing B), autosomal recessive
With retardation and dysmorphism (Sanjad-Sakati syndrome), autosomal recessive
With deafness and renal dysplasia (*GATA3* mutation)
With osteosclerosis (Kenny-Caffey syndrome), *TBCE* mutation
Suppression of neonatal PTH secretion due to maternal hyperparathyroidism
Preproparathyroid hormone gene mutation
Autosomal dominant
Ca^{2+}-sensing receptor activating mutation
Sporadic
Autosomal dominant
Autoimmune parathyroiditis
Isolated
With type 1 autoimmune polyendocrinopathy, APECED
Mutation of *AIRE* gene
Infiltrative lesions
Hemosiderosis (treatment of thalassemia)
Copper deposition (Wilson disease)
PTH RECEPTOR DEFECTS (PSEUDOHYPOPARATHYROIDISM)
Type 1a (inactivating mutation of Gs_α)
With gonadotropin-independent precocious puberty
Type 1b (paternal imprinting of *GNAS1*)
Type 2 (normal cAMP response)
MITOCHONDRIAL DNA MUTATIONS
Kearns-Sayre syndrome
Pearson marrow pancreas syndrome
Mutation of long-chain 3-hydroxyacylcoenzyme A dehydrogenase
MAGNESIUM DEFICIENCY
Renal magnesium loss (autosomal dominant)
Magnesium malabsorption (autosomal recessive)
Aminoglycoside therapy
EXOGENOUS INORGANIC PHOSPHATE EXCESS
Laxatives
Soft drinks with phosphoric acid
VITAMIN D DEFICIENCY
Nutritional
Vitamin D dependency (rickets)
Mutation of 1α-(OH)ase (P450)

APLASIA OR HYPOPLASIA OF THE PARATHYROID GLANDS. This is often associated with the **DiGeorge/velocardiofacial syndrome** (see Fig. 571-1). This syndrome occurs in 1/4,000 newborns. In 90% of patients, the condition is caused by a deletion of chromosome 22q11.2. Approximately 25% of these patients inherit the chromosomal abnormality from a parent. Neonatal hypocalcemia occurs in 60% of affected patients, but it is transitory in the majority; hypocalcemia may recur or may have its onset later in life. Associated abnormalities of the 3rd and 4th pharyngeal pouches are common; these include conotruncal defects of the heart in 25%, velopharyngeal insufficiency in 32%, cleft palate in 9%, renal anomalies in 35%, and aplasia of the thymus with severe immunodeficiency in 1%. This syndrome has also been reported in a small number of patients with a deletion of chromosome 10p13, in infants of diabetic mothers, and in infants born to mothers treated with retinoic acid for acne early in pregnancy.

X-LINKED RECESSIVE HYPOPARATHYROIDISM. Familial clusters of hypoparathyroidism with various patterns of transmission have been described. In two large North American pedigrees, this disorder appears to be transmitted by an X-linked recessive gene located on Xq26-q27. In these families, the onset of afebrile seizures characteristically occurs in infants from 2 wk to 6 mo of age. The absence of parathyroid tissue after detailed examination of a boy with this condition suggests a defect in embryogenesis.

AUTOSOMAL RECESSIVE HYPOPARATHYROIDISM WITH DYSMORPHIC FEATURES. This syndrome has been described in Middle Eastern children. Parental consanguinity occurred for almost all of several dozen affected patients. Profound hypocalcemia occurs early in life, and dysmorphic features include microcephaly, deep-set eyes, beaked nose, micrognathia, and large floppy ears. Intrauterine and postnatal growth retardation are severe, and mental retardation is common. The putative gene is on chromosome 1q42-43. The autosomal recessive form of hypoparathyroidism that occurs with type I polyglandular autoimmune disease is described subsequently. In a few patients with autosomal recessive inheritance of isolated hypoparathyroidism, mutations of the PTH gene have been found.

HDR SYNDROME. Hypoparathyroidism, sensorineural deafness, and renal anomaly occur owing to mutations of the *GATA3* gene. The protein encoded by this gene is essential in the development of the parathyroids, auditory system, and kidneys. The *GATA3* gene is located at chromosome 10p14 and is nonoverlapping with the DiGeorge critical region at 10p13 (see Fig. 571-1).

SUPPRESSION OF NEONATAL PTH SECRETION DUE TO MATERNAL HYPERPARATHYROIDISM. This may result in transient hypocalcemia of the newborn infant. It appears that neonatal hypocalcemia results from suppression of the fetal parathyroid glands by exposure to elevated levels of calcium in maternal and hence fetal serum. Tetany usually develops within 3 wk but may be delayed by 1 mo or more if the infant is breast-fed. Hypocalcemia may persist for weeks or months. When the cause of hypocalcemia in an infant is unknown, measurements of calcium, phosphorus, and PTH should be obtained from the mother. Most affected mothers are asymptomatic, and the cause of their hyperparathyroidism is usually a parathyroid adenoma.

AUTOSOMAL DOMINANT HYPOPARATHYROIDISM. These patients have an activating (gain-of-function) mutation of the Ca^{2+}-sensing receptor, forcing the receptor to an "on" state with subsequent depression of PTH secretion even during hypocalcemia. The patients have hypercalciuria. The hypocalcemia is usually mild and may not require treatment beyond childhood (see Fig. 571-1).

HYPOPARATHYROIDISM ASSOCIATED WITH MITOCHONDRIAL DISORDERS. Mitochondrial DNA mutations in Kearns-Sayre syndrome and in mitochondrial trifunctional protein have been associated with hypoparathyroidism. A diagnosis of mitochondrial cytopathy should be considered in patients with unexplained symptoms such as ophthalmoplegia, sensorineural hearing loss, cardiac conduction disturbances, and tetany (see Fig. 571-1).

SURGICAL HYPOPARATHYROIDISM. Removal or damage of the parathyroid glands may complicate thyroidectomy. Hypoparathyroidism has developed even when the parathyroid glands have been identified and left undisturbed at the time of operation. This may be the result of interference with the blood supply or of postoperative edema and fibrosis. Symptoms of tetany may occur abruptly postoperatively and may be temporary or permanent. In some instances, symptoms may develop insidiously and go undetected until months after thyroidectomy. Occasionally, the first evidence of surgical hypoparathyroidism may be the development of cataract. The status of parathyroid function should be carefully monitored in all patients undergoing thyroidectomy.

Deposition of iron pigment or of copper in the parathyroid glands (thalassemia, Wilson disease) may produce hypoparathyroidism.

AUTOIMMUNE HYPOPARATHYROIDISM. An autoimmune mechanism for hypoparathyroidism is strongly suggested by the finding of parathyroid antibodies and by its frequent association with other autoimmune disorders or organ-specific antibodies. Autoimmune hypoparathyroidism is often associated with Addison disease and chronic mucocutaneous candidiasis. The association of at least 2 of these 3 conditions has been tentatively classified as **autoimmune polyglandular disease type I.** It is also known as autoimmune polyendocrinopathy/candidiasis/ectodermal dystrophy. This syndrome is inherited in an autosomal recessive fashion and is not related to any single HLA-associated haplotype. One third of patients with this syndrome have all 3 components; ⅔ have only 2 of 3 conditions. The candidiasis almost always precedes the other disorders (70% of cases occur in children younger than 5 yr of age); the hypoparathyroidism (90% after 3 yr of age) usually occurs before Addison disease (90% after 6 yr of age). A variety of other disorders occur at various times and include alopecia areata or totalis, malabsorption disorder, pernicious anemia, gonadal failure, chronic active hepatitis, vitiligo, and insulin-dependent diabetes. Some of these associations may not appear until adult life. Autoimmune thyroid disease is a rare concomitant finding.

Affected siblings may have the same or different constellations of disorders (hypoparathyroidism, Addison disease). The disorder is exceptionally prevalent among Finns and Iranian Jews. The gene for this disorder is designated *AIRE* (autoimmune regulator); it is located on chromosome 21q22. It appears to be a transcription factor that plays an essential role in the development of immunologic tolerance. Patients with Addison disease as part of polyendocrinopathy syndrome type I have demonstrated adrenal-specific autoantibody reactivity directed against the side-chain cleavage enzyme.

IDIOPATHIC HYPOPARATHYROIDISM. This term should be reserved for the small residuum of children with hypoparathyroidism for whom no causative mechanism can be defined. Most children in whom onset of hypoparathyroidism occurs after the first few years of life have an **autoimmune condition.** Autoantibodies to the extracellular domain of the calcium-sensing receptor have been identified in some patients with acquired hypoparathyroidism. One should always consider incomplete forms of DiGeorge syndrome or an activating calcium-sensing receptor mutation in the differential diagnosis.

Clinical Manifestations. There is a spectrum of parathyroid deficiencies with clinical manifestations varying from no symptoms to those of complete and long-standing deficiency. Mild deficiency may be revealed only by appropriate laboratory studies. Muscular pain and cramps are early manifestations; they progress to numbness, stiffness, and tingling of the hands and feet. There may be only a positive Chvostek or Trousseau sign or laryngeal and carpopedal spasms. Convulsions with or without loss of consciousness may occur at intervals of days, weeks, or months.

These episodes may begin with abdominal pain, followed by tonic rigidity, retraction of the head, and cyanosis. Hypoparathyroidism is frequently mistaken for epilepsy. Headache, vomiting, increased intracranial pressure, and papilledema may be associated with convulsions and may suggest a brain tumor.

In patients with long-standing hypocalcemia, the teeth erupt late and irregularly. Enamel formation is irregular, and the teeth may be unusually soft. The skin may be dry and scaly, and the nails of the fingers and toes may have horizontal lines. Mucocutaneous candidiasis, when present, antedates the development of hypoparathyroidism; the candidal infection most often involves the nails, the oral mucosa, the angles of the mouth, and less often, the skin; it is difficult to treat.

Cataracts in patients with long-standing untreated disease are a direct consequence of hypoparathyroidism; other autoimmune ocular disorders such as keratoconjunctivitis may also occur. Manifestations of Addison disease, lymphocytic thyroiditis, pernicious anemia, alopecia areata or totalis, hepatitis, and primary gonadal insufficiency may also be associated with those of hypoparathyroidism.

Permanent physical and mental deterioration occur if initiation of treatment is long delayed.

Laboratory Findings. The serum calcium level is low (5–7 mg/dL), and the phosphorus level is elevated (7–12 mg/dL). Blood levels of ionized calcium (usually approximately 45% of the total) more nearly reflect physiologic adequacy but also are low. The serum level of alkaline phosphatase is normal or low, and the level of 1,25[OH]$_2$D$_3$ is usually low, but high levels have been found in some children with severe hypocalcemia. The level of magnesium is normal but should always be checked in hypocalcemic patients. Levels of PTH are low when measured by immunometric assay. Administration of the synthetic 1–34 fragment of human PTH (teriparatide acetate) results in increased urinary levels of cyclic adenosine monophosphate and phosphate. This response differentiates hypoparathyroidism from pseudohypoparathyroidism. With the advent of very sensitive PTH assays, this test is usually not necessary. Radiographs of the bones occasionally reveal an increased density limited to the metaphyses, suggestive of heavy metal poisoning, or an increased density of the lamina dura. Radiographs or CT scans of the skull may reveal calcifications in the basal ganglia. There is a prolongation of the QT interval on the electrocardiogram, which disappears when the hypocalcemia is corrected. The electroencephalogram usually reveals widespread slow activity; the tracing returns to normal after the serum calcium concentration has been within the normal range for a few weeks, unless irreversible brain damage has occurred or unless the parathyroid insufficiency is associated with epilepsy. When hypoparathyroidism occurs concurrently with Addison disease, the serum level of calcium may be normal, but hypocalcemia appears after effective treatment of the adrenal insufficiency.

Treatment. Emergency treatment of neonatal tetany consists of intravenous injections of 5–10 mL of a 10% solution of calcium gluconate at the rate of 0.5–1 mL/min while the heart rate is monitored. Additionally, 1,25-dihydroxycholecalciferol (calcitriol) should be given. The initial dosage is 0.25 µg/24 hr; the maintenance dosage ranges from 0.01–0.10 µg/kg/24 hr to a maximum of 1–2 µg/24 hr. Calcitriol has a short half-life and should be given in 2 equal divided doses; it has the advantages of rapid onset of effect (1–4 days) and rapid reversal of hypercalcemia after discontinuation in the event of overdosage (calcium levels begin to fall in 3–4 days). Calcitriol is supplied as an oral solution.

An adequate intake of calcium should be ensured. Supplemental calcium can be given in the form of calcium gluconate or calcium glubionate (Neo-Calglucon) to provide 800 mg of elemental calcium daily, but it is rarely essential. Foods with high phosphorus content such as milk, eggs, and cheese should be reduced in the diet.

Clinical evaluation of the patient and frequent determinations of the serum calcium levels are indicated in the early stages of treatment to determine the requirement for calcitriol or vitamin D$_2$. If hypercalcemia occurs, therapy should be discontinued and resumed at a lower dose after the serum calcium level has returned to normal. In long-standing cases, repair of cerebral and dental changes is not likely. Pigmentation, lowering of the blood pressure, or weight loss may indicate adrenal insufficiency, which requires specific treatment. Patients with autosomal dominant hypocalcemic hypercalciuria may develop nephrocalcinosis and renal impairment if treated with vitamin D.

Differential Diagnosis. Magnesium deficiency must be considered in patients with unexplained hypocalcemia. Concentrations of serum magnesium less than 1.5 mg/dL (1.2 mEq/L) are usually abnormal. Familial hypomagnesemia with secondary hypocalcemia has been reported in about 50 patients, most of whom developed tetany and seizures at 2–6 wk of age. Administration of calcium is ineffective, but administration of magnesium promptly corrects both calcium and magnesium levels. Oral supplements of magnesium are necessary to maintain levels of magnesium in the normal range. Two genetic forms have been described. One is caused by an autosomal recessive gene on chromosome 9, resulting in a specific defect in absorption of magnesium. The other is caused by an autosomal dominant gene on chromosome 11q23, resulting in renal loss of magnesium.

Hypomagnesemia also occurs in malabsorption syndromes such as Crohn disease and cystic fibrosis. Patients with autoimmune polyglandular disease type I and hypoparathyroidism may also have concurrent steatorrhea and low magnesium levels. Therapy with aminoglycosides causes hypomagnesemia by increasing urinary losses.

It is not clear how low levels of magnesium lead to hypocalcemia. Evidence suggests that hypomagnesemia impairs release of PTH and induces resistance to the effects of the hormone, but other mechanisms also may be operative.

Poisoning with inorganic phosphate leads to hypocalcemia and tetany. Infants administered large doses of inorganic phosphates, either as laxatives or as sodium phosphate enemas, have had sudden onset of tetany, with serum calcium levels less than 5 mg/dL and markedly elevated levels of phosphate. Symptoms are quickly relieved by intravenous administration of calcium. The mechanism of the hypocalcemia is not clear (see Chapter 52.6).

Hypocalcemia may occur early in the course of treatment of acute lymphoblastic leukemia. Hypocalcemia is usually associated with hyperphosphatemia resulting from destruction of lymphoblasts.

Episodic symptomatic hypocalcemia occurs in the **Kenny-Caffey syndrome,** which is characterized by medullary stenosis of the long bones, short stature, delayed closure of the fontanel, delayed bone age, and eye abnormalities. Idiopathic hypoparathyroidism and abnormal PTH levels have been found. Autosomal dominant and autosomal recessive modes of inheritance have been reported. Mutations of the *TBCE* gene (1q 43–44) perturb microtubule organization in diseased cells.

Chapter 573 ■ Pseudohypoparathyroidism (Albright Hereditary Osteodystrophy)

In contrast to the situation in hypoparathyroidism, in pseudohypoparathyroidism (PHP) the parathyroid glands are normal or hyperplastic and they can synthesize and secrete parathyroid hormone (PTH). Serum levels of immunoreactive PTH are elevated even when the patient is hypocalcemic and may be elevated when the patient is normocalcemic. Neither endogenous nor administered PTH raises the serum levels of calcium or lowers the levels of phosphorus. The genetic defects in the **hormone receptor adenylate cyclase system** are classified into various types depending on the phenotypic and biochemical findings.

TYPE IA. Type Ia accounts for the majority of patients with PHP. Affected patients have a genetic defect of the α subunit of the stimulatory guanine nucleotide–binding protein ($G_s\alpha$). This coupling factor is required for PTH bound to cell surface receptors to activate cyclic adenosine monophosphate (AMP). Heterogeneous mutations of the $G_s\alpha$ gene have been documented; the gene is located on chromosome 20q13.2. Deficiency of the $G_s\alpha$ subunit is a generalized cellular defect and accounts for the association of other endocrine disorders with type Ia PHP. The defect is inherited as an autosomal dominant trait, and the paucity of father-to-son transmissions is thought to be due to decreased fertility in males.

Tetany is often the presenting sign. Affected children have a short, stocky build and a round face. Brachydactyly with dimpling of the dorsum of the hand is usually present. The 2nd metacarpal is involved least often. As a result, the index finger may occasionally be longer than the middle finger. Likewise, the 2nd metatarsal is only rarely affected. There may be other skeletal abnormalities such as short and wide phalanges, bowing, exostoses, and thickening of the calvaria. These patients frequently have calcium deposits and metaplastic bone formation subcutaneously. Moderate degrees of mental retardation, calcification of the basal ganglia, and lenticular cataracts are common in patients who are diagnosed late.

Some members of affected kindreds may have the usual anatomic stigmata of PHP, but serum levels of calcium and phosphorus are normal despite reduced $G_s\alpha$ activity; however, PTH levels may be slightly elevated. Such patients have been labeled as having **pseudopseudohypoparathyroidism.** Transition from normocalcemia to hypocalcemia often occurs with increasing age of the patient. These phenotypically similar but metabolically dissimilar patients may be in the same family and have the same mutations of $G_s\alpha$ protein. It is not known what other factors cause clinically overt hypocalcemia in some affected patients and not in others. There is some evidence to suggest that the $G_s\alpha$ mutation is paternally transmitted in pseudopseudohypoparathyroidism and maternally transmitted in patients with type Ia disease. The gene may be imprinted in a tissue-specific manner.

In addition to resistance to PTH, resistance to other G protein–coupled receptors for thyroid-stimulating hormone (TSH), gonadotropins, and glucagon may result in various metabolic effects. Clinical hypothyroidism is uncommon, but basal levels of TSH are elevated and thyrotropin-releasing hormone-stimulated TSH responses are exaggerated. Moderately decreased levels of thyroxine and increased levels of TSH have been demonstrated by newborn thyroid screening programs, leading to the detection of type Ia PHP in infancy. In adults, gonadal dysfunction is common, as manifested by sexual immaturity, amenorrhea, oligomenorrhea, and infertility. Each of these abnormalities can be related to deficient synthesis of cyclic AMP secondary to a deficiency of $G_s\alpha$, but it is not clear why resistance to other G protein–dependent hormones (corticotropin, vasopressin) is much less affected.

Serum levels of calcium are low, and those of phosphorus and alkaline phosphatase are elevated. Clinical diagnosis can be confirmed by demonstration of a markedly attenuated response in urinary phosphate and cyclic AMP after intravenous infusion of the synthetic 1–34 fragment of human PTH (teriparatide acetate). Definitive diagnosis is established by demonstration of the mutated G-protein.

Type Ia with Precocious Puberty. Two boys have been reported with both type Ia PHP and gonadotropin-independent precocious puberty (see Chapter 563.6). They were found to have a temperature-sensitive mutation of the G_s protein. Thus, at normal body temperature (37°C), the G_s is degraded, resulting in PHP, but in the cooler temperature of the testes (33°C) the G_s mutation results in constitutive activation of the luteinizing hormone receptor and precocious puberty.

TYPE IB. Affected patients have normal levels of G protein activity and a normal phenotypic appearance. These patients have tissue-specific resistance to PTH but not to other hormones. Serum levels of calcium, phosphorus, and immunoreactive PTH are the same as those in patients with type Ia PHP. These patients also show no rise in cyclic AMP in response to exogenous administration of PTH. Bioactive PTH is not increased. The pathophysiology of the disorder in this group of patients is caused by paternal uniparental isodisomy of chromosome 20q and resulting *GNAS1* methylation. This, along with the loss of the maternal *GNAS1* gene, leads to PTH resistance in the proximal renal tubules, which leads to impaired mineral ion homeostasis.

TYPE II. Type II has been detected in only a few patients and differs from type I in that the urinary excretion of cyclic AMP is elevated both in the basal state and after stimulation with PTH but phosphaturia does not increase. Phenotypically, patients are normal and hypocalcemia is present. The defect appears to be distal to cyclic AMP because it is normally activated, but the cell is unable to respond to the signal.

Chapter 574 ■ Hyperparathyroidism

Excessive production of parathyroid hormone (PTH) may result from a primary defect of the parathyroid glands such as an adenoma or hyperplasia (primary hyperparathyroidism).

More often, the increased production of PTH is compensatory, usually aimed at correcting hypocalcemic states of diverse origins (secondary hyperparathyroidism). In vitamin D–deficient rickets and the malabsorption syndromes, intestinal absorption of calcium is deficient but hypocalcemia and tetany may be averted by increased activity of the parathyroid glands. In **pseudohypoparathyroidism,** PTH levels are elevated because a mutation in the $G_s\alpha$ protein interferes with response to PTH. Early in chronic renal disease, hyperphosphatemia results in a reciprocal fall in the calcium concentration with a consequent increase in PTH, but in advanced stages of renal failure, production of $1,25[OH]_2D_3$ is also decreased, leading to worsening hypocalcemia and further stimulation of PTH. In some instances, if stimulation of the parathyroid glands has been sufficiently intense and protracted, the glands may continue to secrete increased levels of PTH for months or years after renal transplantation, with resulting hypercalcemia.

ETIOLOGY. Childhood hyperparathyroidism is rare. Onset during childhood is usually the result of a single benign adenoma. It usually becomes manifested after 10 yr of age. There have been a number of kindreds in which multiple members have hyperparathyroidism transmitted in an autosomal dominant fashion. Most of the affected family members are adults, but children have been involved in about ⅓ of the pedigrees. Some affected patients in these families are asymptomatic and are detected only by careful study. In other kindreds, hyperparathyroidism occurs as part of the constellation known as the **multiple endocrine neoplasia** (MEN) syndromes or of the hyperparathyroidism/jaw tumor syndrome.

Neonatal severe hyperparathyroidism is a rare disorder. Symptoms develop shortly after birth and consist of anorexia, irritability, lethargy, constipation, and failure to thrive. Radiographs reveal subperiosteal bone resorption, osteoporosis, and pathologic fractures. Symptoms may be mild, resolving without treatment, or may have a rapidly fatal course if diagnosis and treatment are delayed. Histologically, the parathyroid glands show diffuse hyperplasia. Affected siblings have been observed in some kindreds, and parental consanguinity has been reported in several kindreds. Most cases have occurred in kindreds with the clinical and biochemical features of **familial hypocalciuric hypercalcemia.** Infants with neonatal severe hyperparathyroidism may be homozygous or heterozygous for the mutation in the Ca^{2+}-sensing receptor gene, whereas most individuals with 1 copy of this mutation exhibit autosomally dominant familial hypocalciuric hypercalcemia.

MEN type I is an autosomal dominant disorder characterized by hyperplasia or neoplasia of the endocrine pancreas (which secretes gastrin, insulin, pancreatic polypeptide, and occasionally glucagon), the anterior pituitary (which usually secretes prolactin), and the parathyroid glands. In most kindreds, hyperparathyroidism is usually the presenting manifestation, with a prevalence approaching 100% by 50 yr of age and occurring only rarely in children younger than 18 yr of age. With appropriate DNA probes, it is possible to detect carriers of the gene with 99% accuracy at birth, avoiding unnecessary biochemical screening programs.

The gene for MEN type I is on chromosome 11q13; it appears to function as a tumor suppressor gene and follows the two-hit hypothesis of tumor development. The first mutation (germinal) is inherited and is recessive to the dominant allele; this does not result in tumor formation. A second mutation (somatic) is required to eliminate the normal allele, which then leads to tumor formation.

Hyperparathyroidism/jaw tumor syndrome is an autosomal dominant disorder characterized by parathyroid adenomas and fibro-osseous jaw tumors. Affected patients may also have polycystic kidney disease, renal hamartomas, and Wilms tumor. Although the condition affects adults primarily, it has been diagnosed as early as age 10 yr.

MEN type II may also be associated with hyperparathyroidism (see Chapter 570.2).

Transient neonatal hyperparathyroidism has occurred in a few infants born to mothers with hypoparathyroidism (idiopathic or surgical) or with pseudohypoparathyroidism. In each case, the maternal disorder had been undiagnosed or inadequately treated during pregnancy. The cause of the condition is chronic intrauterine exposure to hypocalcemia with resultant hyperplasia of the fetal parathyroid glands. In the newborn, manifestations involve the bones primarily and healing occurs between 4 and 7 mo of age.

CLINICAL MANIFESTATIONS. At all ages, the clinical manifestations of hypercalcemia of any cause include muscular weakness, fatigue, headache, anorexia, abdominal pain, nausea, vomiting, constipation, polydipsia, polyuria, loss of weight, and fever. When hypercalcemia is of long duration, calcium may be deposited in the renal parenchyma (nephrocalcinosis), with progressively diminished renal function. Renal calculi may occur and may produce renal colic and hematuria. Osseous changes may produce pain in the back or extremities, disturbances of gait, genu valgum, fractures, and tumors. Height may decrease from compression of vertebrae; the patient may become bedridden. Detection of completely asymptomatic patients is increasing with the advent of automated panel assays that include serum calcium determinations.

Abdominal pain is occasionally prominent and may be associated with **acute pancreatitis.** Parathyroid crisis may occur, manifested by serum calcium levels greater than 15 mg/dL and progressive oliguria, azotemia, stupor, and coma. In infants, failure to thrive, poor feeding, and hypotonia are common. Mental retardation, convulsions, and blindness may occur as sequelae of long-standing hypercalcemia.

LABORATORY FINDINGS. The serum calcium level is elevated; 39 of 45 children with adenomas had levels greater than 12 mg/dL. The hypercalcemia is more severe in infants with parathyroid hyperplasia; concentrations ranging from 15 to 20 mg/dL are common, and values as high as 30 mg/dL have been reported. Even when the total serum calcium level is borderline or only slightly elevated, ionized calcium levels are often increased. The serum phosphorus level is reduced to about 3 mg/dL or less, and the level of serum magnesium is low. The urine may have a low and fixed specific gravity, and serum levels of nonprotein nitrogen and uric acid may be elevated. In patients with adenomas who have skeletal involvement, serum phosphatase levels are elevated, but in infants with hyperplasia the levels of alkaline phosphatase may be normal even when there is extensive involvement of bone.

Serum levels of PTH measured by carboxyterminal antisera are elevated, especially in relation to the level of calcium. Results may vary markedly from one laboratory to another, depending on the antibody used. Calcitonin levels are normal. Acute hypercalcemia can stimulate calcitonin release; but with prolonged hypercalcemia, hypercalcitoninemia does not occur.

The most consistent and characteristic radiographic finding is resorption of subperiosteal bone, best seen along the margins of the phalanges of the hands. In the skull, there may be gross trabeculation or a granular appearance resulting from focal rarefaction; the lamina dura may be absent. In more advanced disease, there may be generalized rarefaction, cysts, tumors, fractures, and deformities. About 10% of patients have radiographic signs of rickets. Radiographs of the abdomen may reveal renal calculi or nephrocalcinosis.

DIFFERENTIAL DIAGNOSIS. Other causes of hypercalcemia may result in a similar clinical pattern and must be differentiated from hyperparathyroidism (Table 574-1). A low serum phosphorus level with hypercalcemia is characteristic of primary hyperparathyroidism; elevated levels of PTH are also diagnostic. With hypercalcemia of any cause except hyperparathyroidism and familial hypocalciuric hypercalcemia, PTH levels are suppressed. Pharmacologic doses of corticosteroids lower the serum calcium level to normal in patients with hypercalcemia from other causes but generally do not affect the calcium level in patients with hyperparathyroidism.

TREATMENT. Surgical exploration is indicated in all instances. All glands should be carefully inspected; if an adenoma is discovered, it should be removed; very few instances of carcinoma are known in children. Most neonates with severe hypercalcemia require total parathyroidectomy; less severe hypercalcemia may remit spontaneously in others. A portion of a parathyroid gland may be autografted into the forearm. The patient should be carefully observed postoperatively for the development of hypocalcemia and tetany; intravenous administration of calcium gluconate may be required for a few days. The serum calcium level then gradually returns to normal, and, under ordinary circumstances, a diet high in calcium and phosphorus must be maintained for only several months after operation.

CT, real-time ultrasonography, and subtraction scintigraphy using sestamibi/Tc-pertechnetate alone and in combination have proven effective in localization of a single adenoma versus diffuse hyperplasia in 50–90% of adults. These procedures are rarely required by expert parathyroid surgeons, who now often rely on intraoperative selective venous sampling with intraoperative assay of PTH for localization and removal of the source of increased PTH secretion.

TABLE 574-1. Etiologic Classification of Hypercalcemia

PARATHYROID HORMONE (PTH) EXCESS
Primary hyperparathyroidism
Adenoma
Sporadic
Autosomal dominant
Hyperparathyroidism–jaw tumor syndrome
Hyperplasia or adenoma
Multiple endocrine neoplasia type1
Mutation in MEN1 gene (11q13)
Parathyroid hyperplasia of infancy
Inactivating mutation of Ca^{2+}-sensing receptor
Secondary to maternal hypoparathyroidism
Ectopic PTH production
Nonendocrine malignancies
PARATHYROID HORMONE–RELATED PEPTIDE (PTHrP) EXCESS
Nonendocrine malignancies
Benign hypertrophy of breasts
CA^{2+}-SENSING RECEPTOR INACTIVATING MUTATION
Heterozygous–familial hypocalciuric hypercalcemia
Neonatal severe hyperparathyroidism
ACTIVATING MUTATION OF PTH/PTHrP RECEPTOR
Autosomal dominant
Jansen-type metaphyseal chondrodysplasia
INACTIVATING MUTATION OF PTH/PTHrP RECEPTOR
Autosomal recessive
Blomstrand chondrodysplasia
VITAMIN D EXCESS
Iatrogenic
Ectopic production
Sarcoidosis, tuberculosis, granulomatous lesions, subcutaneous fat necrosis
Excessively fortified milk
UNKNOWN CAUSE
Williams syndrome (7q11.23 deletion)
OTHER
Hypophosphatasia
Mutation of tissue-nonspecific alkaline phosphatase gene
Prolonged immobilization
Thyrotoxicosis
Hypervitaminosis A
Leukemia
Acquired hypocalciuric hypercalcemia (autoantibodies to calcium-sensing receptor)

PROGNOSIS. The prognosis is good if the disease is recognized early and there is appropriate surgical treatment. When extensive osseous lesions are present, deformities may be permanent. A search for other affected family members is indicated.

574.1 • Other Causes of Hypercalcemia

FAMILIAL HYPOCALCIURIC HYPERCALCEMIA (FAMILIAL BENIGN HYPERCALCEMIA). Patients with this disorder are usually asymptomatic, and the hypercalcemia is identified by chance during routine investigation for other conditions. The parathyroid glands are normal, PTH levels are inappropriately normal, and subtotal parathyroidectomy does not correct the hypercalcemia. Serum levels of magnesium are high normal or mildly elevated. The rate of calcium to creatinine clearance is usually decreased despite hypercalcemia. The disorder is inherited in an autosomal dominant manner and is caused by a mutant gene on chromosome 3q2. Penetrance is near 100%, and affected individuals can be diagnosed early in childhood by serum and urinary calcium concentrations. Detection of other affected family members is important to avoid inappropriate parathyroid surgery. The basic defect in this condition results from inactivating mutations in the Ca^{2+}-sensing receptor gene. This G-protein–coupled receptor senses the level of free Ca^{2+} in the blood and triggers the pathway to increase extracellular Ca^{2+} in the face of hypocalcemia. This receptor functions in the parathyroid and kidney to regulate calcium homeostasis; inactivating mutations lead to an increased set point with respect to serum Ca^{2+}, resulting in mild to moderate hypercalcemia in heterozygotes.

GRANULOMATOUS DISEASES. Hypercalcemia occurs in 30–50% of children with sarcoidosis and less often in patients with other granulomatous diseases such as tuberculosis. Levels of PTH are suppressed, and levels of $1,25[OH]_2D_3$ are elevated. The source of **ectopic $1,25[OH]_2D_3$** is the activated macrophage, through stimulation by interferon-α from T lymphocytes, which are present in abundance in granulomatous lesions. Unlike renal tubular cells, the 1α-hydroxylase in macrophages is unresponsive to homeostatic regulation. Oral administration of prednisone (2 mg/kg/24 hr) lowers serum levels of $1,25[OH]_2D_3$ to normal and corrects the hypercalcemia.

HYPERCALCEMIA OF MALIGNANCY. Hypercalcemia frequently occurs in adults with a wide variety of solid tumors but is identified much less often in children. It has been reported in infants with malignant rhabdoid tumors of the kidney or congenital mesoblastic nephroma and in children with neuroblastoma, medulloblastoma, leukemia, Burkitt lymphoma, dysgerminoma, and rhabdomyosarcoma. Serum levels of PTH are rarely elevated. In most patients, the hypercalcemia associated with malignancy is caused by elevated levels of parathyroid hormone–related peptide (PTHrP) and not PTH. Rarely, tumors produce $1,25[OH]_2D_3$ or PTH ectopically.

MISCELLANEOUS CAUSES OF HYPERCALCEMIA. Hypercalcemia may occur in infants with **subcutaneous fat necrosis.** Levels of PTH are normal. In one infant, the level of $1,25[OH]_2D_3$ was elevated and biopsy of the skin lesion revealed granulomatous infiltration, suggesting that the mechanism of the hypercalcemia was akin to that seen in patients with other granulomatous disease. In another infant, although the level of $1,25[OH]_2D_3$ was normal, PTH was suppressed, suggesting the hypercalcemia was not PTH related. Treatment with prednisone is effective.

Hypophosphatasia, especially the severe infantile form, is usually associated with mild to moderate hypercalcemia (see Chapter 703). Serum levels of phosphorus are normal, and those of alkaline phosphatase are subnormal. The bones exhibit rachitic-like lesions on radiographs. Urinary levels of phosphoethanolamine, inorganic pyrophosphate, and pyridoxal 5′-phosphate are elevated; each is a natural substrate to a tissue-nonspecific (liver, bone, kidney) alkaline phosphatase enzyme. Missense mutations of the tissue-nonspecific alkaline phosphatase enzyme gene result in an inactive enzyme in this autosomal recessive disorder.

Idiopathic hypercalcemia of infancy is manifested by failure to thrive and hypercalcemia during the 1st yr of life, followed by spontaneous remission. Serum levels of phosphorus and PTH are normal. The hypercalcemia results from increased absorption of calcium. Vitamin D may be involved in the pathogenesis. Both normal and elevated levels of $1,25[OH]_2D_3$ have been reported. An excessive rise in the level of $1,25[OH]_2D_3$ in response to PTH administration years after the hypercalcemic phase suggests that vitamin D has a role in the pathogenesis. A blunted calcitonin response to intravenous calcium has also been reported.

Ten per cent of patients with **Williams syndrome** also inconsistently exhibit associated infantile hypercalcemia. The phenotype consists of feeding difficulties, slow growth, elfin facies (small mandible, prominent maxilla, upturned nose), renovascular disorders, and a gregarious "cocktail party" personality. Cardiac lesions include supravalvular aortic stenosis, peripheral pulmonic stenosis, aortic hypoplasia, coronary artery stenosis, and atrial or ventricular septal defects. Nephrocalcinosis may develop if hypercalcemia persists. The IQ score of 50–70 is curiously accompanied by enhanced quantity and quality of vocabulary, auditory memory, and social use of language. A submicroscopic deletion at chromosome 7q11.23, which includes deletion of one elastin allele, occurs in 90% of patients and seems to account for the vascular problems. Definitive diagnosis can be established by specific fluorescence in situ hybridization. The hypercalcemia and central nervous system symptoms may be caused by deletion of adjacent genes. Hypercalcemia has been successfully controlled with either prednisone or calcitonin.

Hypervitaminosis D resulting in hypercalcemia from drinking milk that has been incorrectly fortified with vitamin D has been reported. Not all patients with hypervitaminosis D develop hypercalcemia. Affected infants may manifest failure to thrive, nephrolithiasis, poor renal function, and osteosclerosis. Serum levels of 25[OH]D are a better indicator of hypervitaminosis D than levels of $1,25[OH]_2D_3$ because 25[OH]D has a longer half-life.

Prolonged immobilization may lead to hypercalcemia and occasionally to decreased renal function, hypertension, and encephalopathy. Children having hypophosphatemic rickets and undergoing surgery with subsequent long-term immobilization are at risk for hypercalcemia and should therefore have their vitamin D supplementation decreased or discontinued.

Jansen-type metaphyseal chondrodysplasia is a rare genetic disorder characterized by short-limbed dwarfism and severe but asymptomatic hypercalcemia (see Chapter 702). Circulating levels of PTH and PTHrP are undetectable. These patients have an activating PTH-PTHrP receptor mutation that results in aberrant calcium homeostasis and abnormalities of the growth plate.

Ahonen P, Myllarniemi S, Sipla I, et al: Clinical variation of autoimmune polyendocrinopathy-candidiasis-ectodermal dystrophy (APECED) in a series of 68 patients. *N Engl J Med* 1990;322:1829–1836.

Brown EM: The calcium-sensing receptor (CaR) and its disorders. *Hormones* 2002;1:10–21.

Cook JS, Stone MS, Hansen JR: Hypercalcemia in association with subcutaneous fat necrosis of the newborn: Studies of calcium-regulating hormones. *Pediatrics* 1992;90:93–96.

Cooper L, Wertheimer J, Levey R, et al: Severe primary hyperparathyroidism in a neonate with two hypercalcemic parents: Management with parathyroidectomy and heterotopic autotransplantation. *Pediatrics* 1986;78: 263–268.

Ding C, Buckingham B, Levine M: Familial isolated hypoparathyroidism caused by a mutation in the gene for the transcription factor GCMB. *J Clin Invest* 2001;108:1215–1220.

Ewart AK, Morris CA, Atkinson D, et al: Hemizygosity at the elastin locus in a developmental disorder, Williams syndrome. *Nat Genet* 1993;5:11–16.

Fedde KN, Michell MP, Whyte MP, et al: Aberrant properties of alkaline phosphatase in patients with clinical expressivity in severe forms of hypophosphatasia. *J Clin Endocrinol Metab* 1996;81:2587–2594.

Gillis D, Hirsch HJ, Peylan-Ramu N, et al: Parathyroid adenoma after radiation in an 8-year old boy. *J Pediatr* 1998;132:892–893.

Hobbs MR, Pole AR, Pidisirng GN, et al: Hyperparathyroidism-jaw tumor syndrome: The HRPT2 locus is within a 0.7-cM region on chromosome 1q. *Am J Hum Genet* 1999;64:518–525.

Irvin GL, Carneiro DM: Management changes in primary hyperparathyroidism. *JAMA* 2000;284:934–936.

Jacabus CH, Holick MF, Shao G, et al: Hypervitaminosis D associated with drinking milk. *N Engl J Med* 1992;326:1173–1177.

Kahn KT, Uma R, Farag TI, et al: Kenny-Caffey syndrome in six Bedouin sibships: Autosomal recessive inheritance is confirmed. *Am J Med Genet* 1997;69:126–132.

Key LL, Thorne M, Pitzer B, et al: Management of neonatal hyperparathyroidism with parathyroidectomy and autotransplantation. *J Pediatr* 1990;116:923–926.

Kollars J, Zarroug AE, van Heerden J, et al: Primary hyperparathyroidism in pediatric patients. *Pediatrics* 2005;115:974–980.

Kovacs CS, Kronenberg HM: Maternal-fetal calcium and bone metabolism during pregnancy, puerperium and lactation. *Endocr Rev* 1997;18:832–872.

Learoyd DL, Twigg SM, Robinson BG, et al: The practical management of multiple endocrine neoplasia. *Trends Endocrinol Metab* 1995;6:273.

Levitt M, Gessert C, Finberg L: Inorganic phosphate (laxative) poisoning resulting in tetany in an infant. *J Pediatr* 1973;82:479–481.

Li Y, Song Y-H, Muir A, et al: Autoantibodies to the extracellular domain of the calcium-sensing receptor in patients with acquired hypoparathyroidism. *J Clin Invest* 1996;97:910–914.

Liu J, Litman D, Weinstein LS, et al: A GNAS1 imprinting defect in pseudohypoparathyroidism type 1B. *J Clin Invest* 2000;107:793.

Marx SJ: Hyperparathyroid and hypoparathyroid disorders. *N Engl J Med* 2000;343:1863–1875.

McKay C, Furman WL: Hypercalcemia complicating childhood malignancies. *Cancer* 1993;72:256–260.

Miric A, Vechio JD, Levine MA: Heterogeneous mutations in the gene encoding the α-subunit of the stimulatory G protein of adenylyl cyclase in Albright hereditary osteodystrophy. *J Clin Endocrinol Metab* 1993;76: 1560–1568.

Nakamoto JM, Sandstrom AT, Van Dop C, et al: Pseudohypoparathyroidism type Ia from maternal but not paternal transmission of a $G_s\alpha$ gene mutation. *Am J Med Genet* 1998;77:261–267.

Pallais JC, Kifor O, Chen YB, et al: Acquired hypocalciuric hypercalcemia due to autoantibodies against the calcium-sensing receptor. *N Engl J Med* 2004;351:362–368.

Parvari R, Hershkovitz F, Grossman N, et al: Mutation of TBCE causes hypoparathyroidism-retardation-dysmorphism and autosomal recessive Kenny-Caffey syndrome. *Nat Genet* 2002;32:448–452.

Pearce SH: Multiple endocrine neoplasia type I (MEN 1): Recent advances (commentary). *Clin Endocrinol* 1997;47:513–514.

Pearce SH, Williamson C, Thaker RV, et al: A familial syndrome of hypocalcemia with hypercalciuria due to mutations in the calcium-sensing receptor. *N Engl J Med* 1996;335:1115–1122.

Pollak MR, WuChou YH, Marx SJ, et al: Familial hypocalciuric hypercalcemia and neonatal severe hyperparathyroidism: Effects of mutant gene dosage on phenotype. *J Clin Invest* 1994;93:1108–1112.

Ryan AK, Goodship JA, Wilson DI, et al: Spectrum of clinical features associated with interstitial chromosome 22q11 deletions: A European collaborative study. *J Med Genet* 1997;34:708–804.

Schipani E, Langman CB, Juppner H, et al: Constitutively activated receptors for parathyroid hormone and parathyroid hormone-related peptide in Jansen's metaphyseal chondrodysplasia. *N Engl J Med* 1996;335:708–714.

Shalev H, Phillip M, Landau D, et al: Clinical presentation and outcome in primary familial hypomagnesaemia. *Arch Dis Child* 1998;78:127–130.

Stewart AF: Translational implications of the parathyroid calcium receptor. *N Engl J Med* 2004;351:324–326.

Tean BT, Farnebo F, Larson C, et al: Familial isolated hyperparathyroidism maps to the hyperparathyroidism-jaw tumor locus in 1q21-q32 in a subset of families. *J Clin Endocrinol Metab* 1998;83:2114–2120.

Tengan CH, Kiyomoto BH, Moraes CT, et al: Mitochondrial encephalomyopathy and hypoparathyroidism associated with a duplication and a deletion of mitochondrial deoxyribonucleic acid. *J Clin Endocrinol Metab* 1998;83:125–129.

Thakker RV: Genetic developments in hypoparathyroidism. *Lancet* 2001;357:974–976.

Thomas BR, Bennett JD: Symptomatic hypocalcemia and hypoparathyroidism in two infants of mothers with hyperparathyroidism and familial benign hypercalcemia. *J Perinatol* 1995;15:23–26.

Toft AD: Surgery for primary hyperparathyroidism—sooner rather than later. *Lancet* 2000;355:1478–1479.

Trump D, Dixon PH, Mumm S, et al: Localization of X-linked idiopathic hypoparathyroidism to a 1.5 Mb region on Xq26-q27. *J Med Genet* 1998;35:905–909.

Van Esch H, Groenen P, Devriendt K, et al: GATA3 haplo-insufficiency causes human HDR syndrome. *Nature* 2000;406:419–422.

Walder RY, Shalev H, Sheffield VC, et al: Familial hypomagnesemia maps to chromosome 9q not to the X chromosome: Genetic linkage mapping and analysis of a balanced translocation breakpoint. *Hum Mol Genet* 1997;6:1491–1497.

Watanabe T, Bai M, Yasuda T, et al: Familial hypoparathyroidism: Identification of a novel gain of function mutation in transmembrane domain 5 of the calcium-sensing receptor. *J Clin Endocrinol Metab* 1998;83:2497–2502.

Weinstein LS, Yu S: The role of genomic imprinting of $G_s\alpha$ in the pathogenesis of Albright hereditary osteodystrophy. *Trends Endocrinol Metab* 1999;10:81–85.

Section 4 — Disorders of the Adrenal Glands — Perrin C. White

Chapter 575 ■ Physiology of the Adrenal Gland

575.1 • Histology and Embryology

The adrenal gland is composed of 2 endocrine tissues: the medulla and the cortex. The chromaffin cells of the adrenal medulla are derived from neuroectoderm, whereas the cells of the adrenal cortex are derived from mesoderm. Mesodermal cells also contribute to the development of the gonads. The adrenal glands and gonads have certain common enzymes involved in steroid synthesis; an inborn error in steroidogenesis in one tissue may also be present in the other.

The adrenal cortex consists of 3 zones: the zona glomerulosa, the outermost zone located immediately beneath the capsule; the zona fasciculata, the middle zone; and the zona reticularis, the innermost zone, lying next to the adrenal medulla. The zona fasciculata is the largest zone, constituting about ¾ of the cortex; the zona glomerulosa constitutes about 15% and the zona reticularis about 10%. Glomerulosa cells are small, with a lower cytoplasmic : nuclear ratio, an intermediate number of lipid inclusions, and smaller nuclei containing more condensed chromatin than the cells of the other two zones. The cells of the zona fasciculata are large, with a high cytoplasmic : nuclear ratio and many lipid inclusions that give the cytoplasm a foamy, vacuolated appearance. The cells are arranged in radial cords. The cells of the zona reticularis are arranged in irregular anastomosing cords. The cytoplasmic : nuclear ratio is intermediate, and the compact cytoplasm has relatively little lipid content.

The zona glomerulosa synthesizes aldosterone, the most potent natural mineralocorticoid in humans. The zona fasciculata produces cortisol, the most potent natural glucocorticoid in humans, and the zona fasciculata and zona reticularis synthesize the adrenal androgens.

The adrenal medulla consists mainly of neuroendocrine (chromaffin) cells and glial (sustentacular) cells with some connective tissue and vascular cells. Neuroendocrine cells are polyhedral with abundant cytoplasm and small, pale-staining nuclei. Under the electron microscope, the cytoplasm contains many large secretory granules that contain catecholamines. Glial cells have less cytoplasm and more basophilic nuclei.

The primordium of the fetal adrenal gland can be recognized at 3–4 wk of gestation just cephalad to the developing mesonephros. At 5–6 wk, the gonadal ridge develops into the steroidogenic cells of the gonads and adrenal cortex; the adrenal and gonadal cells separate, the adrenal cells migrate retroperitoneally, and the gonadal cells migrate caudad. At 6–8 wk of gestation, the gland rapidly enlarges, the cells of the inner cortex differentiate to form the fetal zone, and the outer subcapsular rim remains as the definitive zone. The primordium of the adrenal cortex is invaded at this time by sympathetic neural elements that differentiate into the chromaffin cells capable of synthesizing and storing catecholamines. Catechol *O*-methyltransferase, which converts norepinephrine to epinephrine, is expressed later in gestation. By the end of the 8th wk of gestation, the encapsulated adrenal gland is associated with the upper pole of the kidney. By 9–12 wk of gestation, the cells of the fetal zone are capable of active steroidogenesis. In the fetus of 2 mo, the adrenals are larger than the kidneys, but from the 4th mo, the kidneys grow rapidly, becoming twice as large as the adrenals by the end of the 6th mo. In the full-term infant, the adrenal gland is ⅓ of the size of the kidney and the combined weight of both glands is 7–9 g. At birth, the inner fetal cortex makes up about 80% of the gland and the outer "true" cortex, 20%. Within a few days the fetal cortex begins to involute, undergoing a 50% reduction by 1 mo of age. Conversely, the adrenal medulla is relatively small at birth and undergoes a proportionate increase in size over the first 6 postnatal months. By 1 yr, the adrenal glands each weigh less than 1 g. Adrenal growth thereafter results in adult adrenal glands reaching a combined weight of 8 g. The zonae fasciculata and glomerulosa are fully differentiated by about 3 yr of age. The zona reticularis is not fully developed until puberty.

Early fetal adrenal growth appears to be independent of adrenocorticotropic hormone (ACTH), but—at least from midterm until term—ACTH is essential for adrenal growth and maturation. At which stage of fetal development feedback regulation of ACTH by cortisol is established has not been fully defined, but clinical experience suggests that normal pituitary-adrenal feedback relationships are operative in the 1st trimester. Additional factors important in fetal growth and steroidogenesis include placental chorionic gonadotropins and a number of peptide growth factors produced by the placenta and fetus.

Two transcription factors are critical for the development of the adrenal glands: steroidogenic factor-1 (SF-1; NR5A1) and DAX-1 (dosage-sensitive sex reversal, adrenal hypoplasia congenita, X chromosome; NR0B1). SF-1 is also important in the transcriptional regulation of several genes coding for enzymes of steroidogenesis. Disruption of SF-1, encoded on chromosome 9q33, results in adrenal and gonadal agenesis, absence of pituitary gonadotropes, and an underdeveloped ventral medial hypothalamus. Mutations in the DAX1 gene, encoded on Xp21, result in congenital adrenal hypoplasia and hypogonadotropic hypogonadism. DAX-1 also plays an important role in regulating steroidogenesis.

575.2 • Adrenal Steroid Biosynthesis

Cholesterol is the starting substrate for all steroid biosynthesis (Fig. 575-1). Although adrenal cortex cells can synthesize cholesterol de novo from acetate, circulating plasma lipoproteins provide 80% of the cholesterol for adrenal cortex hormone formation. Specific cell surface receptors for low-density lipoprotein (LDL) bind circulating LDL and internalize it by receptor-mediated endocytosis. Cholesterol is stored as cholesteryl esters in vesicles and subsequently hydrolyzed by cholesteryl ester hydrolase to liberate free cholesterol to be used for steroid hormone synthesis.

The rate-limiting step of adrenal steroidogenesis is importation of cholesterol across the mitochondrial outer and inner membrane. This requires several proteins, including the peripheral benzodiazepine receptor and the steroidogenic acute regulatory (StAR) protein. StAR protein has a very short half-life, and its synthesis is rapidly induced by trophic factors (corticotropin); thus, it is the main short-term (min to hr) regulator of steroid hormone biosynthesis.

At the mitochondrial inner membrane, the side chain of cholesterol is cleaved to yield pregnenolone. This is catalyzed by cholesterol side-chain cleavage enzyme (cholesterol desmolase, P450scc, CYP11A1), a cytochrome P450 (CYP) enzyme. Like

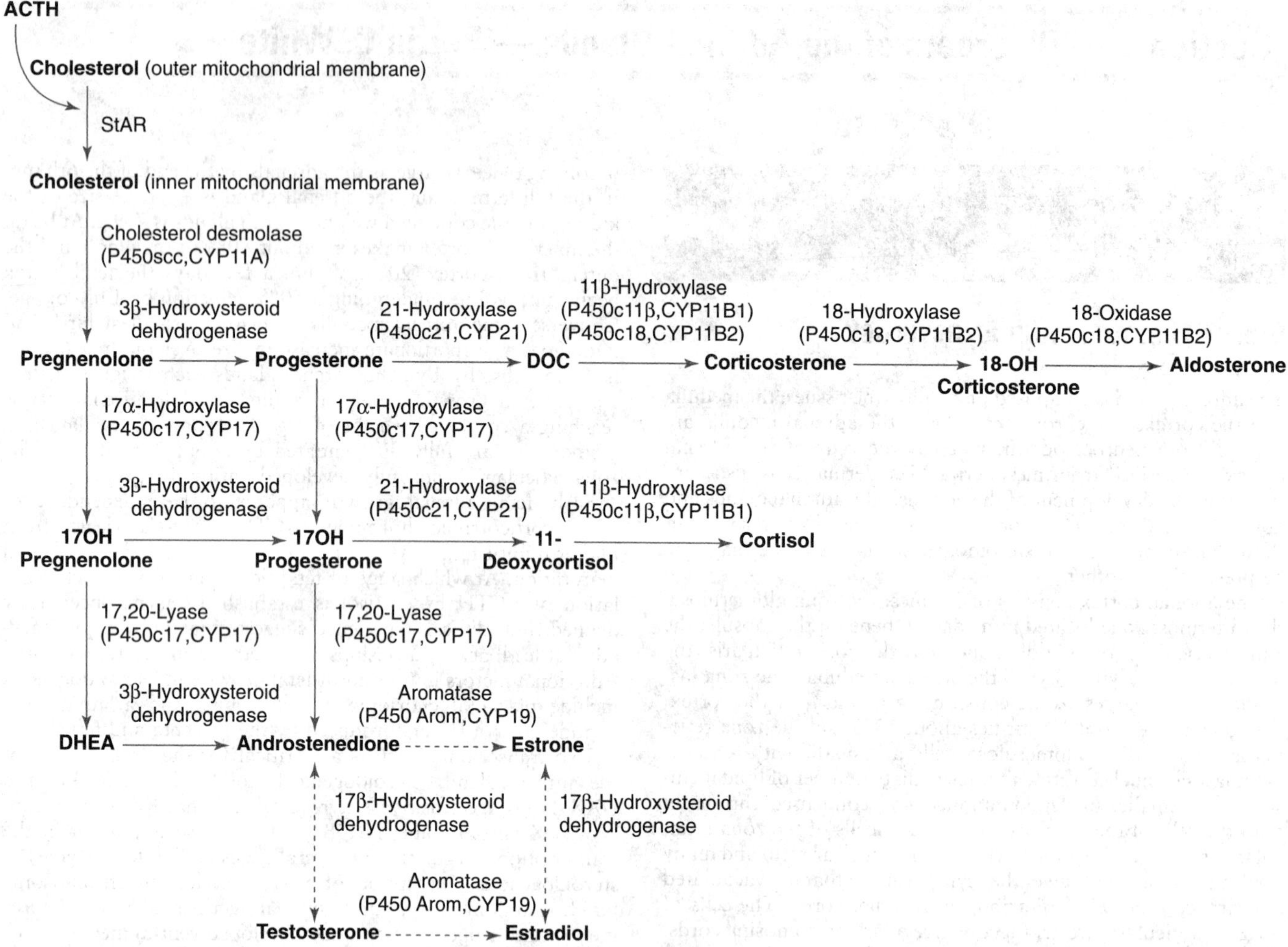

Figure 575-1. Pathways of steroid biosynthesis. The pathways for adrenal synthesis of mineralocorticoids (aldosterone), glucocorticoids (cortisol), and androgens (DHEA, androstenedione) are arranged vertically. The enzymatic activity for each bioconversion is indicated. The systematic name for the activities mediated by specific cytochromes P450 is indicated in parentheses. The reactions shown with dashed arrows occur primarily in gonads, not in adrenals. P450c11β mediates 11β-hydroxylase activity in the zona fasciculata to convert 11-deoxycorticosterone (DOC) to corticosterone and 11-deoxycortisol to cortisol. P450c18 mediates 11β-hydroxylase, 18-hydroxylase, and 18-oxidase activities in the zona glomerulosa for the conversion of DOC to aldosterone.

other P450s, this is a membrane-bound hemoprotein with a molecular mass of about 50 kDa. It accepts electrons from an NADPH-dependent mitochondrial electron transport system consisting of 2 accessory proteins, adrenodoxin reductase (a flavoprotein) and adrenodoxin (a small protein containing nonheme iron). P450 enzymes utilize electrons and O_2 to hydroxylate the substrate and form H_2O. In the case of cholesterol side-chain cleavage, 3 successive oxidative reactions are performed to cleave the C20,22 carbon bond. Pregnenolone then diffuses out of mitochondria and enters the endoplasmic reticulum. The subsequent reactions that occur depend on the zone of the adrenal cortex.

ZONA GLOMERULOSA. In the zona glomerulosa, pregnenolone is converted to progesterone by 3β-hydroxysteroid dehydrogenase (HSD3B2), an NAD^+-dependent enzyme of the "short chain dehydrogenase" type. Progesterone is converted to 11-deoxycorticosterone by steroid 21-hydroxylase (P450c21, CYP21), which is another cytochrome P450. Like other P450s in the endoplasmic reticulum, it utilizes an electron transport system with only one accessory protein, cytochrome P450 oxidoreductase.

Deoxycorticosterone then reenters mitochondria and is converted to aldosterone by aldosterone synthase (P450aldo, CYP11B2), a P450 enzyme structurally related to cholesterol desmolase. Aldosterone synthase also carries out 3 successive oxidations: 11β-hydroxylation, 18-hydroxylation, and further oxidation of the 18-methyl carbon to an aldehyde.

ZONA FASCICULATA. In the endoplasmic reticulum of the zona fasciculata, pregnenolone and progesterone are converted by 17α-hydroxylase (P450c17, CYP17) to 17-hydroxypregnenolone and 17-hydroxyprogesterone, respectively. This enzyme is not expressed in the zona glomerulosa, which consequently cannot synthesize 17-hydroxylated steroids. 17-Hydroxypregnenolone is converted to 17-hydroxyprogesterone and 11-deoxycortisol by the same 3β-hydroxysteroid and 21-hydroxylase enzymes, respectively, as are active in the zona glomerulosa. Thus, inherited disorders in these enzymes affect both aldosterone and cortisol synthesis (see Chapter 577). Finally, 11-deoxycortisol reenters mitochondria and is converted to cortisol by steroid 11β-hydroxylase (P450c11, CYP11B1). This enzyme is closely related to aldosterone synthase but has low 18-hydroxylase and nonexistent 18-oxidase activity. Thus, under normal circumstances the zona fasciculata cannot synthesize aldosterone.

ZONA RETICULARIS. In the zona reticularis and to some extent in the zona fasciculata, the 17-hydroxylase (CYP17) enzyme has an additional activity, cleavage of the 17,20 carbon-carbon bond. This converts 17-hydroxypregnenolone to dehydroepiandrosterone (DHEA). Dehydroepiandrosterone is converted to androstenedione by 3β-hydroxysteroid dehydrogenase. This may be further converted in other tissues to testosterone and estrogens.

FETOPLACENTAL UNIT. Steroid synthesis in the fetal adrenal differs from that in the postnatal gland. LDL cholesterol synthesized by the fetal liver is the major cholesterol source for steroid synthesis in the fetal adrenal gland. The fetal adrenal gland has low 3β-hydroxysteroid dehydrogenase activity and high steroid sulfokinase activity. Thus, the major steroid products of the fetal adrenal gland are DHEA and DHEA sulfate (DHEAS) and, by 16α-hydroxylation in the liver, 16α-hydroxy DHEAS. The placenta, which has high steroid sulfatase activity, uses DHEA and DHEAS as substrates for estrone and estradiol and 16α-OH DHEAS as a substrate for estriol. Placental estrone and estradiol are derived equally from fetal and maternal precursors; estriol is almost exclusively produced from substrates of fetal origin. In addition to providing substrate for the placental synthesis of estrogens, the fetal adrenal gland produces significant amounts of cortisol, much of which is converted to cortisone by the enzyme 11β-hydroxysteroid dehydrogenase. As term approaches, fetal cortisol concentration increases as a result of increased cortisol secretion and decreased conversion of cortisol to cortisone. Low levels of aldosterone are produced in mid gestation, but aldosterone secretory capacity increases near term.

575.3 • Regulation of the Adrenal Cortex

REGULATION OF CORTISOL SECRETION. Glucocorticoid secretion is regulated mainly by adrenocorticotropic hormone (corticotropin, ACTH), a 39-amino-acid peptide that is produced in the anterior pituitary. It is synthesized as part of a larger molecular weight precursor peptide known as pro-opiomelanocortin (POMC). This precursor peptide is also the source of β-lipotropin (β-LPH). ACTH and β-LPH are cleaved further to yield α- and β-melanocyte–stimulating hormone, corticotropin-like intermediate lobe peptide (CLIP), γ-LPH, β- and γ-endorphin, and enkephalin (see Chapter 557).

ACTH is released in secretory bursts of varying amplitude throughout the day and night. The normal diurnal rhythm of cortisol secretion is caused by the varying amplitudes of ACTH pulses. Pulses of ACTH and cortisol occur every 30–120 min, are highest at about the time of waking, are low in late afternoon and evening, and reach their lowest point 1 or 2 hr after sleep begins.

Corticotropin-releasing hormone (CRH), synthesized by neurons of the parvicellular division of the hypothalamic paraventricular nucleus, is the most important stimulator of ACTH secretion. Arginine vasopressin (AVP) augments CRH action. Neural stimuli from the brain cause the release of CRH and AVP (see Chapter 557). AVP and CRH are secreted in the hypophyseal-portal circulation in a pulsatile manner. This pulsatile secretion appears to be responsible for the pulsatile (ultradian) release of ACTH. The circadian rhythm of corticotropin release is probably induced by a corresponding circadian rhythm of hypothalamic CRH secretion, regulated by the suprachiasmatic nucleus with input from other areas of the brain. Cortisol exerts a negative feedback effect on the synthesis and secretion of ACTH, CRH, and AVP. ACTH inhibits its own secretion, a feedback effect mediated at the level of the hypothalamus. Thus the secretion of cortisol is a result of the interaction of the hypothalamus, pituitary, and adrenal glands and other neural stimuli.

ACTH acts through a specific G protein–coupled receptor to activate adenylate cyclase and increase levels of cyclic adenosine monophosphate (AMP). Cyclic AMP has short-term (minutes to hours) effects on cholesterol transport into mitochondria by increasing expression of steroidogenesis acute regulatory (StAR) protein. The long-term effects (hours to days) of ACTH stimulation are to increase the uptake of LDL cholesterol and the expression of genes encoding the enzymes required to synthesize cortisol. These transcriptional effects occur at least in part through increased activity of protein kinase A, which phosphorylates several transcriptional regulatory factors.

REGULATION OF ALDOSTERONE SECRETION. The rate of aldosterone synthesis, which is normally 100– to 1000–fold less than that of cortisol synthesis, is regulated mainly by the renin-angiotensin system and by potassium levels, with ACTH having only a short-term effect. In response to decreased intravascular volume, renin is secreted by the juxtaglomerular apparatus of the kidney. Renin is a proteolytic enzyme that cleaves angiotensinogen (renin substrate), an α_2-globulin produced by the liver, to yield the inactive decapeptide angiotensin I. Angiotensin-converting enzyme in the lungs and other tissues rapidly cleaves angiotensin I to the biologically active octapeptide angiotensin II. Cleavage of angiotensin II produces the heptapeptide angiotensin III. Angiotensin II and III are potent stimulators of aldosterone secretion; angiotensin II is a more potent vasopressor agent. Angiotensin II and III occupy a G protein–coupled receptor activating phospholipase C. The latter protein hydrolyzes phosphatidylinositol bisphosphate to produce inositol triphosphate and diacylglycerol, which raise intracellular calcium levels and activate protein kinase C and calmodulin-activated (CaM) kinases. Similarly, increased levels of extracellular potassium depolarize the cell membrane and increase calcium influx through voltage-gated L-type calcium channels. Phosphorylation of transcriptional regulatory factors by CaM kinases, increases transcription of the aldosterone synthase (CYP11B2) enzyme required for aldosterone synthesis.

REGULATION OF ADRENAL ANDROGEN SECRETION. The mechanisms by which the adrenal androgens, dehydroepiandrosterone and androstenedione, are regulated are not completely understood. Adrenarche is a maturational process in the adrenal gland that results in increased adrenal androgen secretion between the ages of 5 and 20 yr. The process begins before the earliest signs of puberty and continues throughout the years when puberty is occurring. Histologically, it is associated with the appearance of the zona reticularis. Whereas ACTH stimulates adrenal androgen production acutely and clearly is the primary stimulus for cortisol release (see later), additional factors have been implicated in the stimulation of the adrenal androgens. These include a relative decrease in expression of 3β-hydroxysteroid dehydrogenase in the zona reticularis and possibly increases in 17,20-lyase activity owing to phosphorylation of CYP17 or increased cytochrome b5 expression.

575.4 • Adrenal Steroid Hormone Actions

Steroid hormones act through several distinct receptors corresponding to the known biologic activities of the steroid hormones: glucocorticoid, mineralocorticoid, progestin, estrogen, and androgen. These receptors belong to a larger superfamily of nuclear transcriptional factors that include, among others, thyroid hormone and retinoic acid receptors. They have a common structure that includes a carboxyterminal ligand-binding domain and a mid-region DNA-binding domain. The latter domain contains 2 "zinc fingers," each of which consists of a loop of amino acids stabilized by 4 cysteine residues chelating a zinc ion.

Unliganded glucocorticoid and mineralocorticoid receptors are found mainly in the cytosol. Hormone molecules diffuse through the cell membrane and bind receptors, changing their conformation and causing them to be translocated to the nucleus where they bind DNA at specific hormone response elements. Bound receptors may recruit other transcriptional co-regulatory factors to DNA.

Whereas different steroids may share bioactivities because of their ability to bind to the same receptor, a given steroid may exert diverse biologic effects in different tissues. The diversity of hormonal responses is determined by the different genes that are regulated by the hormone in different tissues. Additionally, different combinations of co-regulators are expressed in different tissues, allowing each steroid hormone to have many different effects. Moreover, enzymes may increase or decrease the affinity of steroids for their receptors and thus modulate their activity. For example, 11β-hydroxysteroid dehydrogenase type 1 (HSD11B1) converts cortisone, which is not a ligand for the glucocorticoid receptor, to cortisol, which is an active glucocorticoid. This increases local glucocorticoid concentrations in several tissues, especially the liver, where glucocorticoids maintain hepatic glucose output (see below). Conversely, 11β-hydroxysteroid dehydrogenase type 2 (HSD11B2) oxidizes cortisol to cortisone, particularly in the kidney, preventing mineralocorticoid receptors from being occupied by high levels of cortisol (see below).

ACTIONS OF GLUCOCORTICOIDS. Glucocorticoids are essential for survival. The term glucocorticoid refers to the glucose-regulating properties of these hormones. However, glucocorticoids have multiple effects on carbohydrate, lipid, and protein metabolism. They also regulate immune, circulatory, and renal function. They influence growth, development, bone metabolism, and central nervous system activity.

In stress situations, glucocorticoid secretion can increase up to 10-fold. This increase is believed to enhance survival through increased cardiac contractility, cardiac output, sensitivity to the pressor effects of catecholamines and other pressor hormones, work capacity of the skeletal muscles, and capacity to mobilize energy stores.

Metabolic Effects. The primary action of the glucocorticoids on carbohydrate metabolism is to increase glucose production by increasing hepatic gluconeogenesis. Glucocorticoids also increase cellular resistance to insulin, thereby decreasing entry of glucose into the cell. This inhibition of glucose uptake occurs in adipocytes, muscle cells, and fibroblasts. In addition to opposing insulin action, glucocorticoids may work in parallel with insulin to protect against long-term starvation by stimulating glycogen deposition and production in liver. Both hormones stimulate glycogen synthetase activity and decrease glycogen breakdown. Glucocorticoid excess may cause hyperglycemia, whereas glucocorticoid deficiency may cause hypoglycemia.

Glucocorticoids increase free fatty acid levels by enhancing lipolysis, decreasing cellular glucose uptake, and decreasing glycerol production, which is necessary for re-esterification of fatty acids. This increase in lipolysis is also stimulated through the permissive enhancement of lipolytic action of other factors such as epinephrine. This action affects adipocytes differently according to their anatomic locations. In the patient with glucocorticoid excess, fat is lost in the extremities, but it is increased in the trunk (centripetal obesity), neck, and face (moon facies). This may involve effects on adipocyte differentiation.

Glucocorticoids generally exert a catabolic/antianabolic effect on protein metabolism. Proteolysis in fat, skeletal muscle, bone, lymphoid, and connective tissue increases amino acid substrates that can be used in gluconeogenesis. Cardiac muscle and the diaphragm are almost entirely spared from this catabolic effect.

Circulatory and Renal Effects. Glucocorticoids have a positive inotropic influence on the heart, increasing the left ventricular work index. Moreover, they have a permissive effect on the actions of epinephrine and norepinephrine on both the heart and the blood vessels. In the absence of glucocorticoids, decreased cardiac output and shock may develop; in states of glucocorticoid excess, hypertension is frequently observed. This may be due to activation of the mineralocorticoid receptor (see later), which occurs when renal 11β-hydroxysteroid dehydrogenase is saturated by excessive levels of glucocorticoids.

Growth. In excess, glucocorticoids inhibit linear growth and skeletal maturation in children. This results primarily from the direct inhibitory effect of glucocorticoids on the epiphyses. This may in part be mediated by decreasing levels of growth hormone and insulin-like growth factor-1 (IGF-1) and by increasing IGF binding protein-1 (IGFBP-1), which inhibits somatic growth by decreasing circulating levels of free IGF-1.

Although excess glucocorticoids clearly impair growth, they are also necessary for normal growth and development. In the fetus and neonate, they accelerate the differentiation and development of various tissues. These actions include the development of the hepatic and gastrointestinal systems, as well as the production of surfactant in the fetal lung. Glucocorticoids are often given to pregnant women at risk for delivery of premature infants in an effort to accelerate these maturational processes (see Chapter 96.8).

Immunologic Effects. Glucocorticoids play a major role in immune regulation. They inhibit synthesis of glycolipids and prostaglandin precursors and the actions of bradykinin. They also block histamine and proinflammatory cytokine (tumor necrosis factor-α, interleukin-1, and interleukin-6) secretion and effects. These actions diminish the inflammatory process. High doses of glucocorticoids deplete monocytes, eosinophils, and lymphocytes, especially T cells. They do so at least in part by inducing cell cycle arrest in the G_1 phase and by activating apoptosis through glucocorticoid receptor-mediated effects. The effects on lymphocytes are primarily exerted on T helper 1 cells and hence on cellular immunity, whereas the T helper 2 cells are spared, leading to a predominantly humoral immune response. Pharmacologic doses of glucocorticoids may also decrease the size of immunologic tissues (spleen, thymus, and lymph nodes).

Glucocorticoids increase circulating polymorphonuclear cell counts, mostly by preventing their egress from the circulation. Glucocorticoids decrease diapedesis, chemotaxis, and phagocytosis of polymorphonuclear cells. Thus, the mobility of these cells is altered such that they do not arrive at the site of inflammation to mount an appropriate immune response. High levels of glucocorticoids decrease inflammatory and cellular immune responses and increase susceptibility to certain bacterial, viral, fungal, and parasitic infections.

Effects on Skin, Bone, and Calcium. Glucocorticoids inhibit fibroblasts, leading to increased bruising and poor wound healing through cutaneous atrophy. This effect explains the thinning of the skin and striae that are seen in patients with Cushing syndrome.

Glucocorticoids have the overall effect of decreasing serum calcium and have been used in emergency therapy for certain types of hypercalcemia. This hypocalcemic effect probably results from a decrease in the intestinal absorption of calcium and a decrease in the renal reabsorption of calcium and phosphorus. Serum calcium levels, however, generally do not fall below normal because of the secondary increase in parathyroid hormone secretion.

The most significant effect of long-term glucocorticoid excess on calcium and bone metabolism is **osteoporosis.** Glucocorticoids inhibit osteoblastic activity by decreasing the number and activity of osteoblasts. Glucocorticoids also decrease osteoclastic activity but to a lesser extent, leading to low bone turnover with an overall negative balance. The tendency of glucocorticoids to lower serum calcium and phosphate levels causes secondary hyperparathyroidism. These actions decrease bone accretion and cause a net loss of bone mineral.

Central Nervous System Effects. Glucocorticoids readily penetrate the blood-brain barrier and have direct effects on brain metabolism. They decrease certain types of CNS edema and are frequently used to treat increased intracranial pressure. They stimulate appetite and cause insomnia with a reduction in rapid eye movement sleep. There is an increase in irritability and emotional lability, with an impairment of memory and ability to concentrate. Mild to moderate glucocorticoid excess for a limited period of time often causes a feeling of euphoria or well-being, but glucocorticoid excess and deficiency may both be associated with clinical depression. Glucocorticoid excess may produce **psychosis** in some patients.

Glucocorticoid effects in brain are mediated largely through interactions with both the mineralocorticoid and glucocorticoid receptors (sometimes referred to in this context as type I and type II corticosteroid receptors, respectively). Activation of type II receptors increases sensitivity of hippocampal neurons to the neurotransmitter serotonin, which may help explain the euphoria associated with high doses of glucocorticoids. Glucocorticoids suppress release of corticotropin-releasing hormone (CRH) in the anterior hypothalamus, but stimulate it in the central nucleus of the amygdala and lateral bed nucleus of the stria terminalis, where it may mediate fear and anxiety states. In addition, glucocorticoids and other steroids may have nongenomic effects by modulating activities of both γ-aminobutyric acid (GABA) and N-methyl-D-aspartate (NMDA) receptors.

ACTIONS OF MINERALOCORTICOIDS. The most important mineralocorticoids are aldosterone and, to a lesser degree, 11-deoxycorticosterone; corticosterone and cortisol are normally not important as mineralocorticoids unless secreted in excess. Mineralocorticoids have more limited actions than glucocorticoids. Their major function is to maintain intravascular volume by conserving sodium and eliminating potassium and hydrogen ions. They exert these actions in kidney, gut, and salivary and sweat glands. Aldosterone may have distinct effects in other tissues. Mineralocorticoid receptors are found in the heart and vascular endothelium, and aldosterone increases myocardial fibrosis in heart failure.

Mineralocorticoids have their most important actions in the distal convoluted tubules and cortical collecting ducts of the kidney, where they induce reabsorption of sodium and secretion of potassium. In the medullary collecting duct, they act in a permissive fashion to allow vasopressin to increase osmotic water flux. Thus, patients with mineralocorticoid deficiency may develop weight loss, hypotension, hyponatremia, and hyperkalemia, whereas patients with mineralocorticoid excess may develop hypertension, hypokalemia, and metabolic alkalosis (see Chapters 576–579).

The mechanisms of how aldosterone affects sodium excretion are unclear. Most effects of aldosterone are presumably due to changes in gene expression mediated by the mineralocorticoid receptor, and indeed levels of subunits of both the Na^+, K^+-ATPase and the epithelial sodium channel (ENaC) increase in response to aldosterone. Additionally, aldosterone increases expression of the sgk kinase, which reduces turnover of ENaC subunits and thus increases the number of open sodium channels.

The mineralocorticoid receptor has similar affinities in vitro for cortisol and aldosterone, yet cortisol is a weak mineralocorticoid in vivo. This discrepancy results from the action of 11β-hydroxysteroid dehydrogenase type 2, which converts cortisol to cortisone. Cortisone is not a ligand for the receptor, whereas aldosterone is not a substrate for the enzyme. Pharmacologic or genetic inhibition of this enzyme allows cortisol to occupy renal mineralocorticoid receptors and produce sodium retention and hypertension.

ACTIONS OF THE ADRENAL ANDROGENS. Many actions of adrenal androgens are exerted through their conversion to active androgens or estrogens such as testosterone, dihydrotestosterone, estrone, and estradiol. In adult men, less than 2% of the biologically important androgens are derived from adrenal production, whereas in women approximately 50% of androgens are of adrenal origin. The adrenal contribution to circulating estrogen levels is mainly important in pathologic conditions, such as feminizing adrenal tumors. Adrenal androgens contribute to the physiologic development of pubic and axillary hair during normal puberty. They also play an important role in the pathophysiology of congenital adrenal hyperplasia, premature adrenarche, adrenal tumors, and Cushing syndrome (see Chapters 577 and 578).

In humans, circulating levels of DHEA and DHEAS, the chief adrenal androgens, reach a peak in early adulthood and then decline. This has led to speculation that age-related physiologic changes might be reversed by DHEA administration, and beneficial effects have been suggested (but not proven) on insulin sensitivity, bone mineral density, muscle mass, cardiovascular risk, obesity, cancer risk, autoimmunity, and the central nervous system.

Synthetic Corticosteroids. Many synthetic analogs of cortisone and hydrocortisone are available. Prednisone and prednisolone are derivatives with an additional double bond in ring A. Like cortisone, prednisone is not an active steroid but it is converted to prednisolone by 11β-hydroxysteroid dehydrogenase type 1 in the liver. Prednisone and prednisolone are 4–5 times as potent in anti-inflammatory and carbohydrate activity but have slightly less effect on retention of water and sodium than cortisol. Halogenated derivatives have different effects. Betamethasone and dexamethasone have 25–40 times the glucocorticoid potency of cortisol but have little mineralocorticoid effect. These analogs are usually used in pharmacologic doses for their anti-inflammatory or immunosuppressive properties. Fludrocortisone has about 15 times greater anti-inflammatory activity than does hydrocortisone but is more than 125 times as active a mineralocorticoid; it is used to treat aldosterone deficiency.

575.5 • Adrenal Medulla

The principal hormones of the adrenal medulla are the physiologically active catecholamines: dopamine, norepinephrine, and epinephrine (Fig. 575-2). Catecholamine synthesis also occurs in the brain, in sympathetic nerve endings, and in chromaffin tissue outside the adrenal medulla. Metabolites of catecholamines are excreted in the urine, principally 3-methoxy-4-hydroxymandelic acid (VMA), metanephrine, and normetanephrine. Urinary metanephrines and catecholamines are measured to detect pheochromocytomas of the adrenal medulla and sympathetic nervous system (see Chapter 581).

The proportions of epinephrine and norepinephrine in the adrenal gland vary with age. In early fetal stages, there is practically no epinephrine; at birth, norepinephrine is predominant. In adults, norepinephrine makes up only 10–30% of the pressor amines in the medulla.

The effects of catecholamines are mediated through a series of G protein–coupled adrenergic receptors. Both epinephrine and norepinephrine raise the mean arterial blood pressure, but only epinephrine increases cardiac output. By increasing peripheral vascular resistance, norepinephrine increases systolic and diastolic blood pressures with only a slight reduction in the pulse rate. Epinephrine increases the pulse rate and, by decreasing the peripheral vascular resistance, decreases the diastolic pressure. The hyperglycemic and calorigenic effects of norepinephrine are much less pronounced than are those of epinephrine.

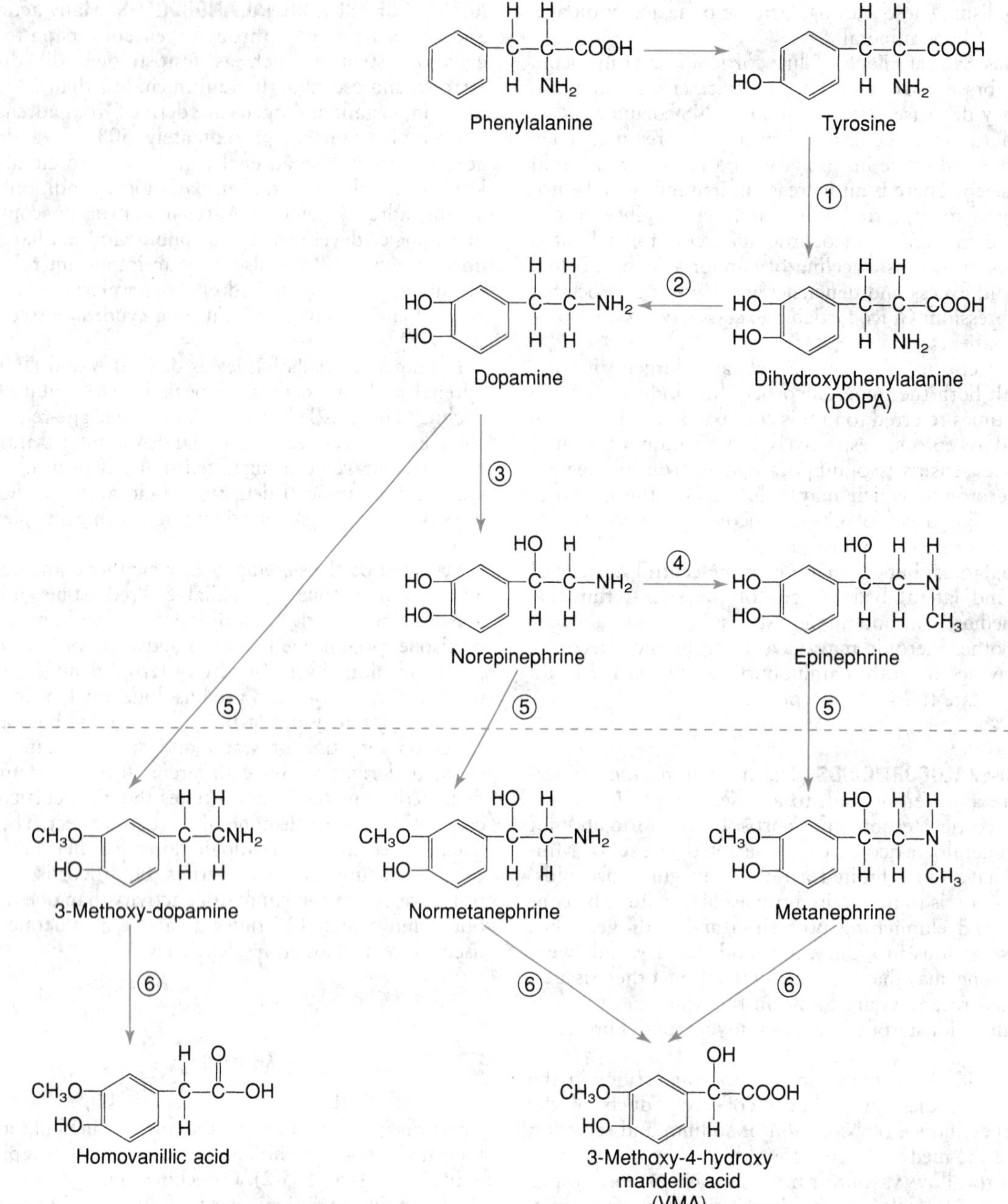

Figure 575-2. Biosynthesis (above dashed line) and metabolism (below dashed line) of the catecholamines norepinephrine and epinephrine. Enzymes: 1, tyrosine hydroxylase; 2, dopa decarboxylase; 3, dopamine β-oxidase; 4, phenylethanolamine-N-methyltransferase; 5, catechol O-methyltransferase; 6, monoamine oxidase.

Aguilera G, Rabadan-Diehl C: Vasopressinergic regulation of the hypothalamic-pituitary-adrenal axis: Implications for stress adaptation. *Regul Pept* 2000;96: 23–29.

Allen DB: Growth suppression by glucocorticoid therapy. *Endocrinol Metab Clin North Am* 1996;25:699–717.

Ashwell JD, Lu FW, Vacchio MS: Glucocorticoids in T cell development and function. *Annu Rev Immunol* 2000;18:309–345.

Bamberger CM, Schulte HM, Chrousos GP: Molecular determinants of glucocorticoid receptor function and tissue sensitivity to glucocorticoids. *Endocr Rev* 1996;17:245–261.

de Kloet ER, Vreugdenhil E, Oitzl MS, et al: Brain corticosteroid receptor balance in health and disease. *Endocr Rev* 1998;19:269–301.

Itoi K, Seasholtz AF, Watson SJ: Cellular and extracellular regulatory mechanisms of hypothalamic corticotropin-releasing hormone neurons. *Endocr J* 1998;45:13–33.

Jenkins BD, Pullen CB, Darimont BD: Novel glucocorticoid receptor coactivator effector mechanisms. *Trends Endocrinol Metab* 2001;12:122–126.

Lamberts SW, Bruining HA, de Jong FH: Corticosteroid therapy in severe illness. *N Engl J Med* 1997;337:1285–1292.

Lane NE, Lukert B: The science and therapy of glucocorticoid-induced bone loss. *Endocrinol Metab Clin North Am* 1998;27:465–483.

Lupien SJ, McEwen BS: The acute effects of corticosteroids on cognition: Integration of animal and human model studies. *Brain Res Brain Res Rev* 1997;24:1–27.

Manelli F, Giustina A: Glucocorticoid-induced osteoporosis. *Trends Endocrinol Metab* 2000;11:79–85.

Matsusaka T, Ichikawa I: Biological functions of angiotensin and its receptors. *Annu Rev Physiol* 1997;59:395–412.

Miller WL: Early steps in androgen biosynthesis: From cholesterol to DHEA. *Baillieres Clin Endocrinol Metab* 1998;12:67–81.

Peter M, Dubuis JM: Transcription factors as regulators of steroidogenic P-450 enzymes. *Eur J Clin Invest* 2000;30(Suppl 3):14–20.

Rainey WE, White PC: Functional adrenal zonation and regulation of aldosterone biosynthesis. *Curr Opin Endocrinol Diabet* 1998;5:175–182.

Stocco DM: StAR protein and the regulation of steroid hormone biosynthesis. *Annu Rev Physiol* 2001;63:193–213.
Tomlinson JW, Walker EA, Bujalska IJ, et al: 11β-Hydroxysteroid dehydrogenase type 1: A tissue-specific regulator of glucocorticoid response. *Endocr Rev* 2004;25:831–866.
Wallberg AE, Wright A, Gustafsson JA: Chromatin-remodeling complexes involved in gene activation by the glucocorticoid receptor. *Vitam Horm* 2000;60:75–122.
White PC: Genetic diseases of steroid metabolism. *Vitam Horm* 1994;49:131–195.
White PC: Abnormalities of aldosterone synthesis and action in children. *Curr Opin Pediatr* 1997;9:424–430.
White PC, Mune T, Agarwal AK: 11β-Hydroxysteroid dehydrogenase and the syndrome of apparent mineralocorticoid excess. *Endocr Rev* 1997;18:135–156.
Yanovski JA, Cutler GBJ: Glucocorticoid action and the clinical features of Cushing's syndrome. *Endocrinol Metab Clin North Am* 1994;23:487–509.

Chapter 576 ■ Adrenocortical Insufficiency

In primary adrenal insufficiency, congenital or acquired lesions of the adrenal cortex prevent production of cortisol and often aldosterone (Table 576–1). Acquired primary adrenal insufficiency is termed Addison disease. Dysfunction of the hypothalamus or anterior pituitary gland may cause a deficiency of corticotropin (ACTH) and lead to hypofunction of the adrenal cortex; this is termed secondary adrenal insufficiency (Table 576–2).

576.1 • Primary Adrenal Insufficiency

Primary adrenal insufficiency may be caused by genetic conditions that are not always manifested in infancy and by acquired problems such as autoimmune conditions. However, susceptibil-

TABLE 576-1. Causes of Primary Adrenal Insufficiency

DIAGNOSIS	CLINICAL FEATURES IN ADDITION TO ADRENAL INSUFFICIENCY	PATHOGENESIS OR GENETICS
AUTOIMMUNE ADRENALITIS		
Isolated autoimmune adrenalitis	No other features	Associations with *HLA-DR, CTLA-4*
Autoimmune adrenalitis as part of APS		
APS type 1 (APECED)	Hypoparathyroidism, chronic mucocutaneous candidiasis, other autoimmune disorders	*AIRE* gene mutations (21q22.3)
APS type 2	Thyroid disease, type 1 diabetes mellitus, other autoimmune diseases (rare in children)	Associations with *HLA-DR, CTLA-4*
APS type 4	Other autoimmune diseases, excluding thyroid disease or diabetes (rare in children)	Associations with *HLA-DR, CTLA-4*
INFECTIOUS ADRENALITIS		
Tuberculous adrenalitis	Other organ manifestations of tuberculosis	Tuberculosis
AIDS	Other AIDS-associated diseases	HIV-1, cytomegalovirus
Fungal adrenalitis	Mostly in immunosuppressed patients	Cryptococcosis, histoplasmosis, coccidioidomycosis
GENETIC DISORDERS LEADING TO ADRENAL INSUFFICIENCY		
Adrenoleukodystrophy, adrenomyeloneuropathy	Demyelination of CNS (cerebral adrenoleukodystrophy), spinal cord, or peripheral nerves (adrenomyeloneuropathy)	Mutation of the *ABCD1* gene encoding for the peroxisomal adrenoleukodystrophy protein
Congenital adrenal hyperplasia		
21-Hydroxylase deficiency	Ambiguous genitalia in girls	*CYP21* mutation
11β-Hydroxylase deficiency	Ambiguous genitalia in girls and hypertension	*CYP11B1* mutation
3β-HSD type 2 deficiency	Ambiguous genitalia in boys, postnatal virilization in girls	*HSD3B2* mutation
17α-Hydroxylase deficiency	Ambiguous genitalia in boys, lack of puberty in both sexes, hypertension	*CYP17* mutation
Congenital lipoid adrenal hypoplasia	XY sex reversal	Mutations in the steroidogenic acute regulatory protein (*STAR*) gene; mutations in *CYP11A* (encoding P450scc) POR mutation
Pyrooxidoreductase deficiency	Antley-Bixler syndrome	
Smith-Lemli-Opitz syndrome	Mental retardation, craniofacial malformations, growth failure	7-Dehydrocholesterol reductase mutations in gene *DHCR7*
Adrenal hypoplasia congenita		
X-linked	Hypogonadotropic hypogonadism	Mutation in *NROB1 (DAX1)*
Xp21 contiguous gene syndrome	Duchenne muscular dystrophy and glycerol kinase deficiency (psychomotor retardation)	Deletion of the Duchenne muscular dystrophy, glycerol kinase, and *NROB1 (DAX1)* genes
SF-1 linked	XY sex reversal	Mutation in *NR5A1 (SF1)*
IMAGe syndrome	Intrauterine growth retardation, metaphyseal dysplasia, adrenal insufficiency, and genital anomalies (IMAGe)	Unknown
Kearns-Sayre syndrome	External ophthalmoplegia, retinal degeneration, and cardiac conduction defects; other endocrinopathies	Mitochondrial DNA deletions
ACTH insensitivity syndromes (familial glucocorticoid deficiency)	Glucocorticoid deficiency, but no impairment of mineralocorticoid synthesis	
Type 1	Tall stature	ACTH receptor *(MC2R)* mutations
Type 2	No other features	Unknown
Triple A syndrome (Allgrove's syndrome)	Alacrimia, achalasia; additional symptoms, including neurologic impairment, deafness, mental retardation, hyperkeratosis	Mutations in triple A gene (*AAAS*) encoding for a WD-repeat protein
BILATERAL ADRENAL HAEMORRHAGE	Symptoms of underlying disease	Septic shock, specifically meningococcal sepsis (Waterhouse-Friderichsen syndrome); primary antiphospholipid syndrome
ADRENAL INFILTRATION	Symptoms of underlying disease	Adrenal metastases, primary adrenal lymphoma, sarcoidosis, amyloidosis, hemochromatosis
BILATERAL ADRENALECTOMY	Symptoms of underlying disease	Unresolved Cushing's syndrome
DRUG-INDUCED ADRENAL INSUFFICIENCY	No other symptoms	Treatment with mitotane, aminoglutethimide, etomidate, ketoconazole, suramin, mifepristone

HSD, 3β-hydroxysteroid dehydrogenase.
From Arlt W, Allolio B: Adrenal insufficiency. *Lancet* 2003;361:1881–1892.

TABLE 576-2. Causes of Secondary Adrenal Insufficiency

DIAGNOSIS	COMMENT
Pituitary tumors	Secondary adrenal insufficiency mostly as part of panhypopituitarism; additional symptoms (visual-field impairment): generally adenomas, carcinoma is a rarity; consequence of tumor growth, surgical treatment, or both
Other tumors of the hypothalamic-pituitary region	Craniopharyngioma, meningioma, ependymoma, and intrasellar or suprasellar metastases
Pituitary irradiation	Craniospinal irradiation in leukemia, irradiation for tumors outside the hypothalamic-pituitary axis, irradiation of pituitary tumors
Lymphocytic hypophysitis	
Isolated	Autoimmune hypophysitis; most frequently in relation to pregnancy (80%); mostly hypopituitarism, but also isolated adrenocorticotropic hormone deficiency
As part of APS	Associated with autoimmune thyroid disease and, less frequently, with vitiligo, primary gonadal failure, type 1 diabetes, and pernicious anaemia
Isolated congenital ACTH deficiency	Pro-opiomelanocortin cleavage enzyme defect?
Pro-opiomelanocortin-deficiency syndrome	Pro-opiomelanocortin gene mutations; clinical triad of adrenal insufficiency, early-onset obesity, and red hair pigmentation
Combined pituitary-hormone deficiency	Mutations in the gene encoding the pituitary transcription factor Prophet of Pit1 (*PROP1*), progressive development of panhypopituitarism in the order GH, PRL, TSH, LH/FSH, (ACTH) Mutations in the homeo box gene *HESX1*, combined pituitary hormone deficiency, optic-nerve hypoplasia, and midline brain defects (septo-optic dysplasia)
Pituitary apoplexy	Onset mainly with abrupt severe headache, visual disturbance, and nausea or vomiting
(Sheehan's syndrome)	Histiocytosis syndromes, pituitary apoplexy or necrosis with peripartal onset, e.g., due to high blood loss or hypotension
Pituitary infiltration or granuloma	Tuberculosis, actinomycosis, sarcoidosis, Wegener's granulomatosis
Head trauma	For example, pituitary stalk lesions
Previous chronic glucocorticoid excess	Exogenous glucocorticoid administration for more than 4 weeks, endogenous glucocorticoid hypersecretion due to Cushing's syndrome

FSH, follicle stimulating hormone; GH, growth hormone; LH, luteinizing hormone; PRL, prolactin; TSH, thyrotropin.
From Arlt W, Allolio B: Adrenal insufficiency. *Lancet* 2003;361:1881–1892.

ity to autoimmune conditions often has a genetic basis, and so these distinctions are not absolute.

INHERITED ETIOLOGIES

INBORN DEFECTS OF STEROIDOGENESIS. The most common causes of adrenocortical insufficiency in infancy are the salt-losing forms of congenital adrenal hyperplasia (see Chapter 577). Approximately 75% of infants with 21-hydroxylase deficiency, almost all infants with lipoid adrenal hyperplasia, and most infants with a deficiency of 3β-hydroxysteroid dehydrogenase manifest salt-losing symptoms in the newborn period because they are unable to synthesize either cortisol or aldosterone.

ADRENAL HYPOPLASIA CONGENITA. Hypoadrenalism usually presents acutely in the neonatal period but may be delayed until later childhood or even adulthood with a more insidious onset. Histologic examination of the hypoplastic adrenal cortex reveals disorganization and cytomegaly. The disorder affects primarily boys and is caused by mutation of the *DAX1 (NR0B1)* gene, a member of the nuclear hormone receptor family, located on Xp21. Boys with adrenal hypoplasia congenita (AHC) do not undergo puberty owing to hypogonadotropic hypogonadism; both AHC and hypogonadotropic hypogonadism are caused by the same mutated *DAX1* gene. **Cryptorchidism,** often noted in these boys, is probably an early manifestation of hypogonadotropic hypogonadism.

AHC also occurs as part of a **contiguous gene deletion** syndrome together with Duchenne muscular dystrophy, glycerol kinase deficiency, mental retardation, or a combination of these conditions.

SF-1 DEFICIENCY. The transcription factor SF-1 is required for adrenal and gonadal development (see Chapter 575). Very rare patients with a heterozygous mutation in SF-1 *(NR5A1)* have adrenal insufficiency despite the presence of a normal copy of the gene on the other chromosome. Males have impaired development of the testes and may appear as females, similarly to patients with lipoid adrenal hyperplasia (see Chapter 577).

ADRENOLEUKODYSTROPHY. In this disorder, adrenocortical deficiency is associated with demyelination in the central nervous system (see Chapters 86 and 599.3). High levels of very long chain fatty acids are found in tissues and body fluids, resulting from their impaired β-oxidation in the peroxisomes.

The most frequent form of ALD is an X-linked disorder with various presentations. The most common clinical picture is of a degenerative neurologic disorder appearing in childhood or adolescence and progressing to severe dementia and deterioration of vision, hearing, speech, and gait, with death occurring within a few years. A milder form of X-linked ALD is adrenomyeloneuropathy (ALM), which begins in later adolescence or early adulthood. Many patients have evidence of adrenal insufficiency at the time of neurologic presentation, but Addison disease may be present without neurologic symptoms or may precede them by many years. X-linked adrenal leukodystrophy (X-ALD) is caused by mutations in the *ABCD1* gene located on Xq28. The gene encodes a transmembrane transporter involved in the importation of very long chain fatty acids into peroxisomes. More than 400 mutations have been described in patients with X-ALD; the majority of X-ALD families have a unique mutation. Clinical phenotypes can vary even within families, perhaps owing to modifier genes or other unknown factors. There is no correlation between the degree of neurologic impairment and severity of adrenal insufficiency. Prenatal diagnosis by DNA analysis and family screening by very long chain fatty acid assays and mutation analysis are available. Women who are heterozygous carriers of the X-ALD gene may develop symptoms in midlife or later. Adrenal insufficiency is rare.

Neonatal ALD is a rare autosomal recessive disorder. Infants have neurologic deterioration and have or acquire evidence of adrenocortical dysfunction. Most patients have severe mental retardation and die before 5 yr of age. This disorder is a subset of Zellweger (cerebro-hepato-renal) syndrome, in which peroxisomes do not develop at all owing to mutations in any of several genes controlling the development of this organelle.

FAMILIAL GLUCOCORTICOID DEFICIENCY. This form of chronic adrenal insufficiency is characterized by isolated deficiency of glucocorticoids, elevated levels of ACTH, and normal aldosterone production. The salt-losing manifestations present in most other forms of adrenal insufficiency do not occur; instead, patients mainly have hypoglycemia, seizures, and increased pigmentation during the 1st decade of life. The disorder affects both sexes equally and is inherited in an autosomal recessive manner. There is marked adrenocortical atrophy with relative sparing of the zona glomerulosa. A number of mutations in the gene for the

ACTH receptor have been described in approximately 40% of these patients.

Another syndrome of ACTH resistance occurs in association with **achalasia** of the gastric cardia and **alacrima** (**triple A** or **Allgrove syndrome**). These patients often have a progressive neurologic disorder that includes autonomic dysfunction, mental retardation, deafness, and motor neuropathy. This syndrome is also inherited in an autosomal recessive fashion, and the AAAS gene has been mapped to chromosome 12q13. The encoded protein, aladin, may help regulate nucleocytoplasmic transport of other proteins.

TYPE I AUTOIMMUNE POLYENDOCRINOPATHY (APS-1)

Although autoimmune Addison disease most often occurs sporadically (see below), it may occur as a component of 2 syndromes, each consisting of a constellation of autoimmune disorders. **Type I autoimmune polyendocrinopathy (APS-1)**, also known as the autoimmune polyendocrinopathy/candidiasis/ectodermal dystrophy (APECED) syndrome, is inherited in mendelian autosomal recessive manner, whereas APS-2 (described below) has complex inheritance. **Chronic mucocutaneous candidiasis** is most often the first manifestation of APS-1, followed by hypoparathyroidism and then by Addison disease, which typically develops in early adolescence. Other closely associated autoimmune disorders include gonadal failure, alopecia, vitiligo, keratopathy, enamel hypoplasia, nail dystrophy, intestinal malabsorption, and chronic active hepatitis. Hypothyroidism and type I diabetes mellitus occur in fewer than 10% of affected patients. Some components of the syndrome continue to develop as late as the 5th decade. The presence of antiadrenal antibodies and steroidal cell antibodies in these patients usually indicates a high likelihood of the development of Addison disease or, in females, ovarian failure. Adrenal failure may evolve rapidly in APS-1; death in patients previously diagnosed and unexplained deaths in siblings of patients with APS-1 have been reported, indicating the need to closely monitor patients with APS-1 and to thoroughly evaluate apparently unaffected siblings of patients with this disorder.

Autoantibodies to the CYP21, CYP17, and CYP11A1 enzymes have been reported in patients with APS-1. The gene affected in APS-1 is designated autoimmune regulator-1 *(AIRE1)*; it has been mapped to chromosome 21q22.3. The *AIRE1* gene encodes a protein that appears to be a transcription factor having an important role in immune response. Approximately 40 different mutations in the *AIRE1* gene have been described in patients with APS-1, with 2 mutations (R257X and a 3-bp deletion) being most frequent. There has been autosomal dominant transmission in 1 kindred owing to a specific missense mutation (G228W).

DISORDERS OF CHOLESTEROL SYNTHESIS/METABOLISM. Patients with disorders of cholesterol synthesis or metabolism, including abetalipoproteinemia with deficient lipoprotein B–containing lipoproteins, and familial hypercholesterolemia, with decreased or impaired LDL receptors, have been demonstrated to have limited adrenocortical function. Adrenal insufficiency has been reported in patients with **Smith-Lemli-Opitz syndrome** (SLOS), an autosomal recessive disorder presenting with facial anomalies, microcephaly, limb anomalies, and developmental delay. Mutations in the gene coding for sterol Δ7-reductase, mapped to 11q12-q13, resulting in impairment of the final step in cholesterol synthesis with marked elevation of 7-dehydrocholesterol, abnormally low cholesterol, and adrenal insufficiency, have been identified in SLOS. **Wolman disease** is a rare autosomal recessive disorder caused by mutations in the gene encoding human lysosomal acid lipase. Cholesteryl esters accumulate in lysosomes in most organ systems, leading to organ failure. Infants during the 1st or 2nd mo of life have hepatosplenomegaly, steatorrhea, abdominal distention, and failure to thrive. Adrenal insufficiency and bilateral adrenal calcification are present, and death usually occurs in the first year of life. The gene for lysosomal acid lipase has been mapped to chromosome 10q23.2-23.3; the genetic defects in patients with Wolman disease have been elucidated.

CORTICOSTEROID-BINDING GLOBULIN (CBG) DEFICIENCY AND DECREASED CORTISOL-BINDING AFFINITY. These disorders result in low levels of plasma cortisol but normal urinary free cortisol and normal plasma ACTH levels. A high prevalence of hypotension and fatigue has been reported in some adults with abnormalities of CBG.

ACQUIRED ETIOLOGIES

AUTOIMMUNE ADDISON DISEASE. The most common cause of Addison disease is autoimmune destruction of the glands. The glands may be so small that they are not visible at autopsy, and only remnants of tissue are found in microscopic sections. Usually, the medulla is not destroyed, and there is marked lymphocytic infiltration in the area of the former cortex. In advanced disease, all adrenocortical function is lost, but early in the clinical course, isolated cortisol deficiency may occur. Most patients have antiadrenal cytoplasmic antibodies in their plasma; 21-hydroxylase (CYP21) is the most frequently occurring autoantigen.

Addison disease may occur as a component of 2 autoimmune polyendocrinopathy syndromes. Type I (APS-1) was discussed previously. **Type II autoimmune polyendocrinopathy (APS-2)** consists of Addison disease associated with autoimmune thyroid disease (Schmidt syndrome) or type 1 diabetes (Carpenter syndrome). Gonadal failure, vitiligo, alopecia, and chronic atrophic gastritis, with or without pernicious anemia, may occur. HLA-D3 and HLA-D4 are increased in these patients and appear to confer an increased risk for development of this disease; alleles at the major histocompatibility complex class I chain-related genes A and B (MICA and MICB) also have been associated with this disorder. The disorder is most common in middle-aged females and may occur in many generations of the same family. Antiadrenal antibodies, specifically antibodies to the CYP21, CYP17, and CYP11A1 enzymes, are also found in these patients.

INFECTION. Tuberculosis was a common cause of adrenal destruction in the past but is much less prevalent now. The most frequent infectious etiology for adrenal insufficiency is meningococcemia (see Chapter 190); adrenal crisis from this cause is referred to as the Waterhouse-Friderichsen syndrome. Patients with AIDS may have a variety of subclinical abnormalities in the hypothalamic-pituitary-adrenal axis, but frank adrenal insufficiency is rare. However, drugs used in the treatment of AIDS may affect adrenal hormone homeostasis.

DRUGS. Ketoconazole, an antifungal drug, can cause adrenal insufficiency by inhibiting adrenal enzymes. Rifampicin and anticonvulsive drugs such as phenytoin and phenobarbital reduce the effectiveness and bioavailability of corticosteroid replacement therapy by inducing steroid-metabolizing enzymes in the liver. Mitotane (o,p′-DDD), used in the treatment of adrenal carcinoma and refractory Cushing syndrome (see Chapters 578 and 581), is cytotoxic to the adrenal cortex and may also alter extra-adrenal cortisol metabolism. Signs of adrenal insufficiency occur in a substantial percentage of patients treated with mitotane.

HEMORRHAGE INTO ADRENAL GLANDS. This may occur in the neonatal period as a consequence of a difficult labor (especially breech presentation), or its etiology may not be apparent. An incidence rate of 3 per 100,000 live births has been suggested. The hemorrhage may be sufficiently extensive to result in death from exsanguination or hypoadrenalism. An abdominal mass, anemia, unexplained jaundice, or scrotal hematoma may be the presenting sign. Often, the hemorrhage is asymptomatic initially and is identified later by calcification of the adrenal gland. Fetal adrenal hemorrhage has also been reported. Postnatally, adrenal hemorrhage most often occurs in patients being treated with anticoagulants. It may also occur as a result of child abuse.

CLINICAL MANIFESTATIONS. Primary adrenal insufficiency leads to cortisol and often aldosterone deficiency. The signs and symptoms of adrenal insufficiency are most easily understood in the context of the normal actions of these hormones, which were discussed in Chapter 575.

Hypoglycemia is a prominent feature of adrenal insufficiency. It is often accompanied by ketosis as the body attempts to utilize fatty acids as an alternative energy source. Ketosis is aggravated by anorexia, nausea, and vomiting, all of which occur frequently.

Cortisol deficiency decreases cardiac output and vascular tone; moreover, catecholamines such as epinephrine have decreased inotropic and pressor effects in the absence of cortisol. These problems are initially manifested as orthostatic hypotension in older children and may progress to frank shock in patients of any age. They are exacerbated by aldosterone deficiency, which results in hypovolemia due to decreased resorption of sodium in the distal nephron.

Hypotension and decreased cardiac output decrease glomerular filtration and thus decrease the ability of the kidney to excrete free water. Vasopressin (AVP) is secreted by the posterior pituitary in response to hypotension and also as a direct consequence of lack of inhibition by cortisol. These factors decrease plasma osmolality and lead in particular to hyponatremia. Hyponatremia is also caused by aldosterone deficiency and may be much worse when both cortisol and aldosterone are deficient.

In addition to hypovolemia and hyponatremia, aldosterone deficiency causes hyperkalemia by decreasing potassium excretion in the distal nephron. Cortisol deficiency alone does not cause hyperkalemia.

Cortisol deficiency decreases negative feedback on the hypothalamus and pituitary, leading to increased secretion of ACTH. Hyperpigmentation is caused by ACTH and other peptide hormones (γ-melanocyte-stimulating hormone) arising from the ACTH precursor pro-opiomelanocortin. In patients with a fair complexion, the skin may have a bronze cast. Pigmentation may be more prominent in skin creases, mucosa, and scars. In dark-skinned patients, it may be most readily appreciated in the gingival and buccal mucosa.

The clinical presentation of adrenal insufficiency depends on the age of the patient, whether both cortisol and aldosterone secretion are affected, and to some extent on the underlying etiology. The most common causes in early infancy are inborn errors of steroid biosynthesis, sepsis, adrenal hypoplasia congenita, and adrenal hemorrhage. Infants have a relatively greater requirement for aldosterone than do older children, possibly owing to immaturity of the kidney and also to the low sodium content of human breast milk and infant formula. Hyperkalemia, hyponatremia, and hypoglycemia are prominent presenting signs of adrenal insufficiency in infants. Ketosis is not consistently present because infants generate ketones less well than do older children. Hyperpigmentation is not usually seen because this takes weeks or months to develop, and orthostatic hypotension is obviously difficult to demonstrate in infants.

Infants can become ill very quickly. There may be only a few days of decreased activity, anorexia, and vomiting before critical electrolyte abnormalities develop.

In older children with Addison disease, the onset is usually more gradual and is characterized by muscle weakness, malaise, anorexia, vomiting, weight loss, and orthostatic hypotension. Hyperpigmentation is often but not necessarily present. Hypoglycemia and ketosis are common, as is hyponatremia. Hyperkalemia tends to occur later in the course of the disease in older children than in infants. Thus, the clinical presentation can be easily confused with gastroenteritis or other acute infections. Chronicity of symptoms may alert the clinician to the possibility of Addison disease, but this diagnosis should be considered in any child with orthostatic hypotension, hyponatremia, hypoglycemia, and ketosis.

Salt craving is seen in primary adrenal insufficiency with mineralocorticoid deficiency. Fatigue, myalgias, fever, eosinophilia, lymphocytosis, hypercalcemia, and anemia may be noted with glucocorticoid deficiency.

LABORATORY FINDINGS. Hypoglycemia, ketosis, hyponatremia, and hyperkalemia have been discussed. An electrocardiogram is useful for quickly detecting hyperkalemia in a critically ill child. Acidosis is frequently present, and the blood urea nitrogen level is elevated if the patient is dehydrated.

Cortisol levels may sometimes be at the low end of the normal range but are invariably low when the patient's degree of illness is considered. ACTH levels are high in primary adrenal insufficiency but may take time to be reported by the laboratory. Similarly, aldosterone levels may be within the normal range but inappropriately low considering the patient's hyponatremia, hyperkalemia, and hypovolemia. Plasma renin activity is elevated. Blood eosinophils may be increased in number, but this is rarely useful diagnostically.

Urinary excretion of sodium and chloride are increased and urinary potassium is decreased, but these are difficult to assess on random urine samples. Accurate interpretation of urinary electrolytes requires more prolonged (24 hr) urine collections and knowledge of the patient's sodium and potassium intake.

The **most definitive** test for adrenal insufficiency is measurement of serum levels of cortisol before and after administration of ACTH; resting levels are low and do not increase normally after administration of ACTH. Occasionally, normal resting levels that do not increase after administration of ACTH may indicate an absence of adrenocortical reserve. A low initial level followed by a significant response to ACTH may indicate secondary adrenal insufficiency. Traditionally, this test has been performed by measuring cortisol levels before and 30 or 60 min after giving 0.250 mg of cosyntropin (ACTH 1–24) by rapid intravenous infusion. Aldosterone will transiently increase in response to this dose of ACTH and may also be measured. A low-dose test (0.5–1 μg ACTH 1–24/1.73 m^2) is a more sensitive test of pituitary-adrenal reserve but has somewhat lower specificity (more false-positive tests).

DIFFERENTIAL DIAGNOSIS. Upon presentation, Addison disease often needs to be distinguished from more acute illnesses such as gastroenteritis with dehydration or sepsis. Additional testing is directed at identifying the specific cause for adrenal insufficiency. When congenital adrenal hyperplasia is suspected, serum levels of cortisol precursors (17-hydroxyprogesterone) should be measured along with cortisol in an ACTH stimulation test (see Chapter 577). Elevated levels of very long chain fatty acids are diagnostic of adrenoleukodystrophy. The presence of antiadrenal antibodies suggests an autoimmune pathogenesis. Patients with autoimmune Addison disease must be closely observed for the development of other autoimmune disorders. In children, hypoparathyroidism is the most frequently associated disorder, and it is suspected if hypocalcemia and elevated phosphate levels are present.

Ultrasonography, CT, or MRI may help define the size of the adrenal glands.

TREATMENT. Treatment of acute adrenal insufficiency must be immediate and vigorous. If the diagnosis of adrenal insufficiency has not been established, a blood sample should be obtained before therapy for determination of electrolytes, glucose, ACTH, cortisol, aldosterone, and plasma renin activity. If the patient's condition permits, an ACTH stimulation test can be performed while initial fluid resuscitation is underway. Intravenous administration of 5% glucose in 0.9% saline solution should be given to correct hypoglycemia, hypovolemia, and hyponatremia. If hyperkalemia is severe, it may require treatment with intravenous calcium and/or bicarbonate, intrarectal potassium-binding resin (Kayexalate), or intravenous infusion of glucose and insulin. A water-soluble form of hydrocortisone, such as hydrocortisone sodium succinate, should be given intravenously. As much as 10 mg for infants, 25 mg for toddlers, 50 mg for older children, and 100 mg for adolescents should be administered at 6-hr intervals for the first 24 hr. These doses may be reduced during the next 24 hr if progress is satisfactory. Adequate fluid and sodium repletion is achieved by intravenous saline administration, aided by the mineralocorticoid effect of high doses of hydrocortisone.

Particular caution should be exercised in the rare patient with concomitant adrenal insufficiency and hypothyroidism, because thyroxine may increase cortisol clearance. Thus, an **adrenal crisis** may be precipitated if hypothyroidism is treated without first assuring adequate glucocorticoid replacement.

After the acute manifestations are under control, most patients require chronic replacement therapy for their cortisol and aldosterone deficiencies. Hydrocortisone (cortisol) may be given orally in daily doses of 10 mg/M²/24 hr in 3 divided doses; some patients require 15 mg/M²/24 hr to minimize fatigue, especially in the morning. Equivalent doses (20–25% of the hydrocortisone dose) of prednisone or prednisolone may be used and divided and given twice daily. ACTH levels may be used to monitor adequacy of glucocorticoid replacement in primary adrenal insufficiency; in congenital adrenal hyperplasia, levels of precursor hormones are used instead (see Chapter 577). During situations of stress, such as periods of infection or minor operative procedures, the dose of hydrocortisone should be increased 2- to 3-fold. Major surgery under general anesthesia requires high intravenous doses of hydrocortisone similar to those used for acute adrenal insufficiency. If aldosterone deficiency is present, fludrocortisone (Florinef), a mineralocorticoid, is given orally in doses of 0.05–0.3 mg daily. Measurements of plasma renin activity are useful in monitoring the adequacy of mineralocorticoid replacement. Chronic overdosage with glucocorticoids leads to obesity, short stature, and osteoporosis, whereas overdosage with fludrocortisone results in tachycardia, hypertension, and occasionally hypokalemia.

Replacement of dehydroepiandrosterone (DHEA) in adults remains controversial; prepubertal children do not normally secrete large amounts of DHEA. Many adults with Addison disease complain of having decreased energy, and replacing DHEA may improve this problem, particularly in women in whom adrenal androgens represent approximately ½ of total androgen secretion. However, large, well-controlled studies are lacking.

Additional therapy may be need to be directed at the underlying cause of the adrenal insufficiency in regard to infections and certain metabolic defects. Therapeutic approaches to adrenoleukodystrophy include administration of glycerol trioleate and glycerol trierucate (Lorenzo's oil), bone marrow transplantation, and lovastatin (see Chapter 599.3).

576.2 • Secondary Adrenal Insufficiency

ETIOLOGY

ABRUPT CESSATION OF ADMINISTRATION OF CORTICOSTEROIDS. Secondary adrenal insufficiency most commonly occurs when the hypothalamic-pituitary-adrenal axis is suppressed by prolonged administration of high doses of a potent glucocorticoid and that agent is suddenly withdrawn or the dose is tapered too quickly. Patients at risk for this problem include those with leukemia, asthma (particularly when patients are transitioned from oral to inhaled corticosteroids), and collagen vascular disease or other autoimmune conditions and those who have undergone tissue transplants or neurosurgical procedures. The maximal duration and dose of glucocorticoid that can be administered before encountering this problem is not known, but it is assumed that high-dose glucocorticoids (the equivalent of >10 times physiologic cortisol secretion) can be administered for at least a wk without requiring a subsequent taper of dose. On the other hand, when high doses of dexamethasone are given to children with leukemia, it can take up to 2 mo or longer after therapy is stopped before tests of adrenal function return to normal. Signs and symptoms of adrenal insufficiency are most likely in patients who are subsequently subjected to stresses such as severe infections or additional surgical procedures.

CORTICOTROPIN (ACTH) DEFICIENCY. Pituitary or hypothalamic dysfunction can cause corticotropin deficiency (see Chapter 558), usually associated with deficiencies of other pituitary hormones such as growth hormone and thyrotropin. Destructive lesions in the area of the pituitary, such as craniopharyngioma and germinoma, are the most common causes of corticotropin deficiency. In many cases the pituitary or hypothalamus is further damaged during surgical removal or radiotherapy of tumors in the midline of the brain. In rare instances, autoimmune hypophysitis is the cause of corticotropin deficiency.

Congenital lesions of the pituitary also occur. The pituitary alone may be affected, or additional midline structures may be involved, such as the optic nerves or septum pellucidum. The latter type of abnormality is termed **septo-optic dysplasia,** or de Morsier syndrome. More severe developmental anomalies of the brain, such as anencephaly and holoprosencephaly, can also affect the pituitary. These disorders are usually sporadic, although a few cases of autosomal recessive inheritance have occurred. Isolated deficiency of corticotropin has been reported, including in several sets of siblings. Patients with multiple pituitary hormone deficiencies due to mutations in the *PROP1* gene have been described with progressive ACTH/cortisol deficiency. Isolated deficiency of corticotropin-releasing hormone has been documented in an Arabic kindred as an autosomal recessive trait.

CLINICAL PRESENTATION. Aldosterone secretion is unaffected in secondary adrenal insufficiency because the adrenal gland is, by definition, intact and the renin-angiotensin system is not involved. Thus, signs and symptoms are those of cortisol deficiency. Newborns often have hypoglycemia. Older children may have orthostatic hypotension or weakness. Electrolytes are usually normal.

When secondary adrenal insufficiency is due to an inborn or acquired anatomic defect involving the pituitary, there may be signs of associated deficiencies of other pituitary hormones. The penis may be small in male infants if gonadotropins are also deficient. Infants with secondary hypothyroidism are often jaundiced. Children with associated growth hormone deficiency grow poorly after the 1st yr of life.

Some children with pituitary abnormalities have hypoplasia of the midface. Children with optic nerve hypoplasia may have obvious visual impairment. They usually have a characteristic wandering nystagmus, but this is often not apparent until several months of age.

TREATMENT. Iatrogenic secondary adrenal insufficiency (caused by chronic glucocorticoid administration) is best avoided by use of the smallest effective doses of systemic glucocorticoids for the shortest period of time. When a patient is thought to be at risk, tapering the dose rapidly to a level equivalent to or slightly less than physiologic replacement (~10 mg/M²/24 hr of hydrocortisone) and further tapering over several wk may allow the adrenal cortex to recover without development of signs of adrenal insufficiency. Patients with anatomic lesions of the pituitary should be treated indefinitely with glucocorticoids. Mineralocorticoid replacement is not required. In patients with panhypopituitarism treating cortisol deficiency may cause freewater excretion thus unmasking central diabetes insipidus. Electrolytes must be monitored carefully when initiating cortisol therapy in panhypopituitary patients.

Abdu TAM, Clayton RN: The low-dose synanthem test for the assessment of secondary adrenal insufficiency. *Curr Opin Endocrinol* 2000;7:116–121.

Arlt W, Allolio B: Adrenal insufficiency. *Lancet* 2003;361:1881–1893.

Anderson RA, Bryson GM, Parks JS: Lysosomal acid lipase mutations that determine phenotype in Wolman and cholesterol ester storage disease. *Mol Genet Metab* 1999;68:333–345.

Berberogly M, Aycan Z, Oeal G, et al: Syndrome of congenital adrenocortical unresponsiveness to ACTH: Report of six patients. *J Pediatr Endocrinol Metab* 2001;14:1113–1118.

Boles RG, Roe T, Senadheera D, et al: Mitochondrial DNA deletion with Kearns-Sayre syndrome in a child with Addison disease. *Eur J Pediatr* 1998;157:643–647.

Clark AJL, Metherell L, Swords FM, et al: The molecular pathogenesis of ACTH insensitivity syndromes. *Ann Endocrinol* 2001;62:207–211.

Cooper MS, Stewart PM: Corticosteroid insufficiency in acutely ill patients. *N Engl J Med* 2003;348:727–734.

Coursin DB, Wood KE: Corticosteroid supplementation for adrenal insufficiency. *JAMA* 2002;287:236–240.

Dickstein G: Hypothalamo-pituitary-adrenal axis testing: Nothing is sacred and caution in interpretation is needed. *Clin Endocrinol* 2001;54:15–16.

Drake AJ, Howells RJ, Shield PH, et al: Symptomatic adrenal insufficiency presenting with hypoglycaemia in asthmatic children with asthma receiving high dose inhaled fluticasone propionate. *Br Med J* 2002;324:1081–1082.

Eledrisi MS, Verghese AC: Adrenal insufficiency in HIV infection: A review and recommendations. *Am J Med Sci* 2001;321:137–144.

Fujieda K, Tajima T: Molecular basis of adrenal insufficiency. *Pediatr Res* 2005;57(5 pt 2):62R–69R.

Heino M, Peterson P, Kudoh J, et al: APECED mutations in the autoimmune regulator (AIRE) gene. *Hum Mutat* 2001;18:205–211.

Huysman MWA, Hokken-Koelega ACS, De Ridder MAJ, et al: Adrenal function in sick very preterm infants. *Pediatr Res* 2000;48:629–633.

Kemp S, Pujol A, Waterham HR, et al: ABCD1 mutations and the X-linked adrenoleukodystrophy mutation database: Role in diagnosis and clinical correlations. *Hum Mutat* 2001;18:499–515.

Krivit W, Peters C, Dusenbery K, et al: Case report: Wolman disease successfully treated by bone marrow transplantation. *Bone Marrow Transplant* 2000;26:567–570.

Moser H, Dubey P, Fatemi A: Progress in X-linked adrenoleukodystrophy. *Curr Opin Neurol* 2004;17:263–269.

Myhre AG, Undlien DE, Lovas K, et al: Autoimmune adrenocortical failure in Norway autoantibodies and human leukocyte antigen class II associations related to clinical features. *J Clin Endocrinol Metab* 2002;87:618–623.

Pearce SHS, Cheetham TD: Autoimmune polyendocrinopathy syndrome type 1: Treat with kid gloves. *Clin Endocrinol* 2001;54:433–435.

Peters C, Charnas LR, Tan Y, et al: Cerebral X-linked adrenoleukodystrophy: The international hematopoietic cell transplantation experience from 1982 to 1999. *Blood* 2004;104:881–888.

Ronghe MD, Barton J, Jardine PE, et al: The importance of testing for adrenoleukodystrophy in males with idiopathic Addison's disease. *Arch Dis Child* 2002;86:185–189.

Salvatori R: Adrenal insufficiency. *JAMA* 2005;294:2481–2488.

Sandrini F, Farmakidis C, Kirschner LS, et al: Spectrum of mutations of the AAAS gene in Allgrove syndrome: Lack of mutations in six kindreds with isolated resistance to corticotropin. *J Clin Endocrinol Metab* 2001;86:5433–5437.

Vaidya B, Pearce S, Kendall-Taylor P: Recent advances in the molecular genetics of congenital and acquired primary adrenocortical failure. *Clin Endocrinol* 2000;53:403–418.

Velaphi SC, Perlman JM: Neonatal adrenal hemorrhage: Clinical and abdominal sonographic findings. *Clin Pediatr* 2001;40:545–548.

Chapter 577 ■ Congenital Adrenal Hyperplasia and Related Disorders

Congenital adrenal hyperplasia (CAH) is a family of autosomal recessive disorders of cortisol biosynthesis (normal adrenal steroidogenesis is discussed in Chapter 575). Cortisol deficiency increases secretion of corticotropin (ACTH), which in turn leads to adrenocortical hyperplasia and overproduction of intermediate metabolites. Depending on the enzymatic step that is deficient, there may be signs, symptoms, and laboratory findings of mineralocorticoid deficiency or excess; incomplete virilization or premature puberty in affected males; and virilization or sexual infantilism in affected females (Figs. 577-1 and 577-2 and Table 577-1).

577.1 • Congenital Adrenal Hyperplasia Due to 21-Hydroxylase Deficiency

ETIOLOGY. More than 90% of CAH cases are caused by 21-hydroxylase deficiency. This P450 enzyme (CYP21, P450c21) hydroxylates progesterone and 17-hydroxyprogesterone (17-OHP) to yield 11-deoxycorticosterone (DOC) and 11-deoxycortisol, respectively (see Fig. 575-1). These conversions are required for synthesis of aldosterone and cortisol, respectively. Both hormones are deficient in the most severe, "salt wasting" form of the disease. Slightly less severely affected patients are able to synthesize adequate amounts of aldosterone but have elevated levels of androgens of adrenal origin; this is termed simple virilizing disease. These 2 forms are collectively termed classical 21-hydroxylase deficiency. Patients with nonclassical disease have relatively mildly elevated levels of androgens and may have signs of androgen excess after birth.

EPIDEMIOLOGY. Classical 21-hydroxylase deficiency occurs in about 1 in 15,000–20,000 births in most populations. Approximately 70% of affected infants have the salt-losing form, whereas 30% have the simple virilizing form of the disorder. Alaskan Yupik Eskimos have an incidence of 1 : 280; high rates are also seen in the French island of Réunion (1 : 2,100), Brazil (1 : 7,500), and the Philippines (1 : 7,000). In the United States, CAH is less common in African Americans compared with white children (1 : 42,000 vs 1 : 15,500). Nonclassical disease has a prevalence of about 1 in 1,000 in the general population but occurs more frequently in specific ethnic groups such as Ashkenazi Jews, Hispanics, and Yugoslavians.

GENETICS. There are 2 steroid 21-hydroxylase genes—*CYP21P (CYP21A1P, CYP21A)* and *CYP21 (CYP21A2, CYP21B)*—which alternate in tandem with 2 genes for the 4th component of complement (C4A and C4B) in the human leukocyte antigen (HLA) major histocompatibility complex on chromosome 6p21.3 between the HLA-B and HLA-DR loci. Many other genes are located in this cluster. *CYP21* is the active gene; *CYP21P* is 98% identical in DNA sequence to *CYP21* but is a pseudogene due to 9 different mutations. More than 90% of mutations causing 21-hydroxylase deficiency are recombinations between *CYP21* and *CYP21P*. Approximately 20% are deletions generated by unequal meiotic crossing-over between *CYP21* and *CYP21P*, whereas the remainder are nonreciprocal transfers of deleterious mutations from *CYP21P* to *CYP21*, a phenomenon termed gene conversion.

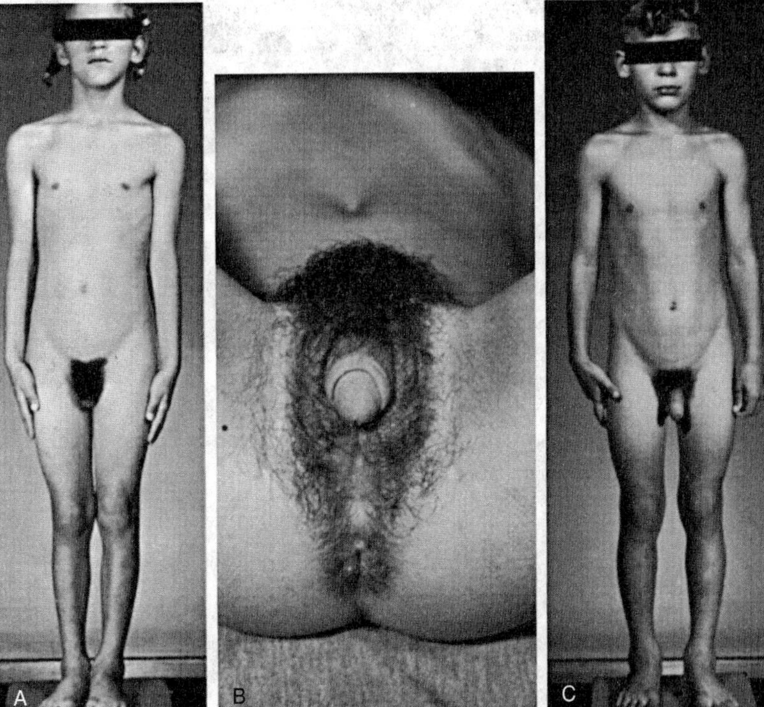

Figure 577-1. *A*, A 6-yr-old girl with congenital virilizing adrenal hyperplasia. The height age was 8.5 yr, and the bone age was 13 yr. *B*, Notice the clitoral enlargement and labial fusion. *C*, Her 5-yr-old brother was not considered to be abnormal by the parents. The height age was 8 yr, and the bone age was 12.5 yr.

The deleterious mutations in *CYP21P* have varying effects on enzymatic activity when transferred to *CYP21*. Several mutations completely prevent synthesis of a functional protein, whereas others are missense mutations (they result in amino acid substitutions) that yield enzymes with 1–50% of normal activity. Disease severity correlates well with the mutations carried by an affected individual; for example, patients with salt-wasting disease usually carry mutations on both alleles that completely destroy enzymatic activity. When patients are compound heterozygotes (which many are) for different types of mutations, the severity of disease expression is largely determined by the activity of the less severely affected of the 2 alleles.

PATHOGENESIS AND CLINICAL MANIFESTATIONS

Aldosterone and Cortisol Deficiency. Because both cortisol and aldosterone require 21-hydroxylation for their synthesis, both hormones are deficient in the most severe, "salt wasting" form of the disease. This form constitutes about 70% of cases of classical 21-hydroxylase deficiency. The signs and symptoms of cortisol and aldosterone deficiency, and the pathophysiology underlying them, are essentially those described in Chapter 576. These include progressive weight loss, anorexia, vomiting, dehydration, weakness, hypotension, hypoglycemia, hyponatremia, and hyperkalemia. These problems typically first develop in affected infants at approximately 2 wk of age. Without treatment, shock, cardiac arrhythmias, and death may occur within days or weeks.

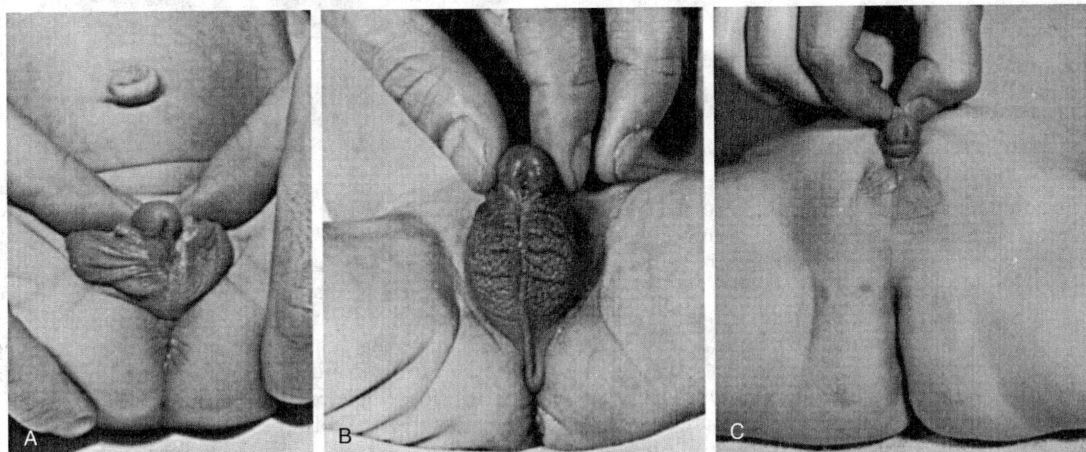

Figure 577-2. Three female pseudohermaphrodites with untreated congenital adrenal hyperplasia. All were erroneously assigned male sex at birth, and each had a normal female sex-chromosome complement. Infants *A* and *B* were salt losers and received the diagnosis early in infancy. Infant *C* was referred at 1 yr of age because of bilateral cryptorchidism. Notice the completely penile urethra; such complete degrees of masculinization in females with adrenal hyperplasia are rare; most of these infants are salt losers.

TABLE 577-1. Diagnosis and Treatment of Congenital Adrenal Hyperplasia

DISORDER	AFFECTED GENE AND CHROMOSOME	SIGNS AND SYMPTOMS	LABORATORY FINDINGS	THERAPEUTIC MEASURES
21-Hydroxylase deficiency, classical form	*CYP21* 6p21.3	Glucocorticoid deficiency	↓ Cortisol, ↑ACTH ↑↑ Baseline and ACTH-stimulated 17-hydroxy-progesterone	Glucocorticoid (hydrocortisone) replacement
		Mineralocorticoid deficiency (salt-wasting crisis)	Hyponatremia, hyperkalemia ↑ Plasma renin	Mineralocorticoid (fludrocortisone) replacement; sodium chloride supplementation
		Female pseudohermaphroditism	↑ Serum androgens	Vaginoplasty and clitoral recession
		Postnatal virilization in males and females	↑ Serum androgens	Suppression with glucocorticoids
21-Hydroxylase deficiency, nonclassical form	*CYP21* 6p21.3	Precocious adrenarche, menstrual irregularity, hirsutism, acne, infertility	↑ Baseline and ACTH-stimulated 17-hydroxyprogesterone ↑ Serum androgens	Suppression with glucocorticoids
11β-Hydroxylase deficiency	*CYP11B1* 8q24.3	Glucocorticoid deficiency	↓ Cortisol, ↑ ACTH ↑↑ Baseline and ACTH-stimulated 11-deoxycortisol and deoxycorticosterone	Glucocorticoid (hydrocortisone) administration
		Female pseudohermaphroditism	↑ Serum androgens	Vaginoplasty and clitoral recession
		Postnatal virilization in males and females	↑ Serum androgens	Suppression with glucocorticoids
		Hypertension	↓ Plasma renin, hypokalemia	Suppression with glucocorticoids
3β-Hydroxysteroid dehydrogenase deficiency, classical form	*HSD3B2* 1p13.1	Glucocorticoid deficiency	↓ Cortisol, ↑ ACTH ↑↑ Baseline and ACTH-stimulated Δ5 steroids (pregnenolone, 17-OH pregnenolone, DHEA)	Glucocorticoid (hydrocortisone) replacement
		Mineralocorticoid deficiency (salt-wasting crisis)	Hyponatremia, hyperkalemia ↑ Plasma renin	Mineralocorticoid (fludrocortisone) replacement; sodium chloride supplementation
		Male and female pseudohermaphroditism	↑ DHEA, ↓ androstenedione, testosterone, and estradiol	Surgical correction of genitals and sex hormone replacement as necessary consonant with sex of rearing
		Precocious adrenarche, disordered puberty	↑ DHEA, ↓ androstenedione, testosterone, and estradiol	Suppression with glucocorticoids
17α-Hydroxylase/17,20-lyase deficiency	*CYP17* 10q24.3	Cortisol deficiency (corticosterone is an adequate glucocorticoid)	↓ Cortisol, ↑ ACTH ↑ DOC, corticosterone Low 17α-hydroxylated steroids; poor response to ACTH	Glucocorticoid (hydrocortisone) administration
		Male pseudohermaphroditism	↓ Serum androgens; poor response to hCG	Orchidopexy or removal of intra-abdominal testes; sex hormone replacement consonant with sex of rearing
		Sexual infantilism	↓ Serum androgens or estrogens	Sex hormone replacement consonant with sex of rearing
		Hypertension	↓ Plasma renin; hypokalemia	Suppression with glucocorticoids
Congenital lipoid adrenal hyperplasia	*StAR* 8p11.2	Glucocorticoid deficiency	↑ ACTH Low levels of all steroid hormones, with decreased or absent response to ACTH	Glucocorticoid (hydrocortisone) replacement
		Mineralocorticoid deficiency (salt-wasting crisis)	Hyponatremia, hyperkalemia ↓ Aldosterone, ↑ plasma renin	Mineralocorticoid (fludrocortisone) replacement; sodium chloride supplementation
		Male pseudohermaphoditism	Decreased or absent response to hCG in male pseudohermaphroditism	Orchidopexy or removal of intra-abdominal testes; sex hormone replacement consonant with sex of rearing
		Poor pubertal development or premature ovarian failure in females	↑ FSH, ↑ LH, ↓ estradiol (after puberty)	Estrogen replacement
P450 oxidoreductase deficiency	*POR* 7q11.3	Glucocorticoid deficiency	↓ Cortisol, ↑ ACTH ↑ Pregnenolone, ↑ progesterone	Glucocorticoid (hydrocortisone) replacement
		Male and female pseudohermaphroditism	↑ Serum androgens prenatally, ↓ androgens and estrogens at puberty	Surgical correction of genitals and sex hormone replacement as necessary consonant with sex of rearing
		Maternal virilization Antley-Bixler syndrome	Decreased ratio of estrogens to androgens	

CAH differs from other causes of primary adrenal insufficiency in that precursor steroids accumulate proximal to the blocked enzymatic conversion. Because cortisol is not synthesized efficiently, ACTH levels are high, leading to hyperplasia of the adrenal cortex and levels of precursor steroids that may be hundreds of times normal. In the case of 21-hydroxylase deficiency, these precursors include 17-hydroxyprogesterone and progesterone. Progesterone and perhaps other metabolites act as antagonists of the mineralocorticoid receptor and thus may exacerbate the effects of aldosterone deficiency in untreated patients.

Prenatal Androgen Excess. The most important problem caused by accumulation of steroid precursors is that 17-hydroxyprogesterone is shunted into the pathway for androgen biosynthesis, leading to high levels of androstenedione that are converted outside the adrenal gland to testosterone. This problem begins in affected fetuses by 8–10 wk of gestation and leads to abnormal genital development in females (see Figs. 577-1 and 577-2).

The external genitals of males and females normally appear identical early in gestation (see Chapter 583). Affected females, who are exposed in utero to high levels of androgens of adrenal origin, have masculinized external genitals (see Figs. 577-1 to 577-2). This is manifested by enlargement of the clitoris and by partial or complete labial fusion. The vagina usually has a common opening with the urethra (urogenital sinus). The clitoris may be so enlarged that it resembles a penis; because the urethra opens below this organ, some affected females may be mistakenly presumed to be males with hypospadias and cryptorchidism. The severity of virilization is usually greatest in females with the salt-losing form of 21-hydroxylase deficiency. The internal genital organs are normal, because affected females have normal ovaries and not testes and thus do not secrete anti-müllerian hormone.

Prenatal exposure of the brain to high levels of androgens may influence subsequent sexually dimorphic behaviors in affected females. Girls tend to be interested in masculine toys such as cars and trucks and often show decreased interest in playing with dolls and demonstrate aggressive play behavior. Women may have decreased interest in maternal roles. There is an increased frequency of homosexuality in affected females. Nonetheless, most function heterosexually and do not have gender identity confusion or dysphoria. It is unusual for affected females to assign themselves a male role.

Male infants appear normal at birth. Thus, the diagnosis may not be made in boys until signs of adrenal insufficiency develop. Because patients with this condition can deteriorate quickly, infant boys are more likely to die than infant girls. For this reason, many states and countries have instituted newborn screening for this condition (see Newborn Screening, below).

Postnatal Androgen Excess. Untreated or inadequately treated children of both sexes develop additional signs of androgen excess after birth. Boys with the simple virilizing form of 21-hydroxylase deficiency often have delayed diagnosis because they appear normal and rarely develop adrenal insufficiency.

Signs of androgen excess include rapid somatic growth and accelerated skeletal maturation. Thus, affected patients are tall in childhood but premature closure of the epiphyses causes growth to stop relatively early, and adult stature is stunted (see Fig. 577-1). Muscular development may be excessive. Pubic and axillary hair may appear; and acne and a deep voice may develop. The penis, scrotum, and prostate may become enlarged in affected boys; however, the **testes are usually prepubertal** in size so that they appear relatively small in contrast to the enlarged penis. Occasionally, ectopic adrenocortical cells in the testes of patients become hyperplastic similarly to the adrenal glands, producing testicular adrenal rest tumors (see Chapter 585). The clitoris may become further enlarged in affected females (see Fig. 577-1). Although the internal genital structures are female, breast development and menstruation may not occur unless the excessive production of androgens is suppressed by adequate treatment.

Similar but usually milder signs of androgen excess may occur in **nonclassical 21-hydroxylase deficiency.** In this attenuated form, cortisol and aldosterone levels are normal and affected females have normal genitals at birth. Males and females may present with precocious pubarche and early development of pubic and axillary hair. Hirsutism, acne, menstrual disorders, and infertility may develop later in life. However, many females and males are completely asymptomatic.

LABORATORY FINDINGS (SEE TABLE 577-1). Patients with salt-losing disease have typical laboratory findings associated with cortisol and aldosterone deficiency, including hyponatremia, hyperkalemia, metabolic acidosis, and often hypoglycemia, but these abnormalities can take 1–2 wk or longer to develop after birth. Blood levels of **17-hydroxyprogesterone** are markedly elevated. However, levels of this hormone are high during the first 2–3 days of life, even in unaffected infants and especially if they are sick or premature. After infancy, once the circadian rhythm of cortisol is established, 17-hydroxyprogesterone levels vary in the same circadian pattern, being highest in the morning and lowest at night. Blood levels of cortisol are usually low in patients with the salt-losing type of disease. They are often normal in patients with simple virilizing disease but inappropriately low in relation to the ACTH and 17-hydroxyprogesterone levels. In addition to 17-hydroxyprogesterone, levels of androstenedione and testosterone are elevated in affected females; testosterone is not elevated in affected males because normal infant males have high testosterone levels compared with those seen later in childhood. Levels of urinary 17-ketosteroids and pregnanetriol are elevated but are now rarely used clinically because blood samples are easier to obtain than 24-hr urine collections. Corticotropin (ACTH) levels are elevated but have no diagnostic utility over 17-hydroxyprogesterone levels. Plasma levels of renin are elevated, and serum aldosterone is inappropriately low for the renin level. However, renin levels are normally high in the first few days of life.

Diagnosis of 21-hydroxylase deficiency is most reliably established by measuring 17-hydroxyprogesterone before and 30 or 60 min after an intravenous bolus of 0.125–0.25 mg of cosyntropin (ACTH 1–24). Nomograms exist that readily distinguish normals and patients with nonclassical and classical 21-hydroxylase deficiency. Heterozygous carriers of this autosomal recessive disorder tend to have higher ACTH-stimulated 17-hydroxyprogesterone levels than genetically unaffected individuals, but there is significant overlap between subjects in these 2 categories.

DIFFERENTIAL DIAGNOSIS. Intersex conditions are discussed more generally in Chapter 589. The initial step in evaluating an infant with ambiguous genitals is a thorough physical examination to define the anatomy of the genitals, locate the urethral meatus, palpate the scrotum or labia and the inguinal regions for testes (palpable gonads almost always indicate the presence of testicular tissue and thus that the infant is a genetic male), and look for any other anatomic abnormalities. Ultrasonography is helpful in demonstrating the presence or absence of a uterus and can often locate the gonads. A rapid karyotype (such as fluorescence in situ hybridization of interphase nuclei for X and Y chromosomes) can quickly determine the genetic sex of the infant. These results are all likely to be available before the results of hormonal testing and together allow the clinical team to advise the parents as to the genetic sex of the infant and the anatomy of internal reproductive structures. Injection of contrast medium into the urogenital sinus of female pseudohermaphrodites demonstrates a vagina and uterus, and most surgeons utilize this information to formulate a plan for surgical management.

PRENATAL DIAGNOSIS. Prenatal diagnosis of 21-hydroxylase is possible late in the first trimester by analysis of DNA obtained by chorionic villus sampling or during the second trimester by amniocentesis. This is usually done because the parents already have an affected child. Most often, the *CYP21* gene is analyzed for frequently occurring mutations, but closely linked, highly polymorphic microsatellite markers may be used instead if an affected child (i.e., the proband) is available for genetic comparison.

NEWBORN SCREENING. Because 21-hydroxylase deficiency is often undiagnosed in affected males until they have severe adrenal insufficiency, many American states and other countries have instituted newborn screening programs. These programs analyze **17-hydroxyprogesterone** levels in dried blood obtained by heelstick and absorbed on filter paper cards; the same cards are screened in parallel for other congenital conditions such as hypothyroidism and phenylketonuria. Potentially affected infants are typically quickly recalled for additional testing (electrolytes and repeat 17-hydroxyprogesterone determination) at approximately 2 wk of age. Infants with salt-wasting disease often have abnormal electrolytes by this age but are usually not severely ill. Thus, screening programs are effective in preventing many cases of adrenal crisis in affected males. The nonclassical form of the disease is not reliably detected by newborn screening, but this is of little clinical significance because adrenal insufficiency does not occur in this type of 21-hydroxylase deficiency.

The main difficulty with current newborn screening programs is that to reliably detect all affected infants, the cut-off 17-

hydroxyprogesterone levels for recalls are set so low that there is a very high frequency of false-positive results (i.e., the test has low positive predictive value). This problem is worst in premature infants. Genotyping for *CYP21* might improve specificity but is not routinely available.

TREATMENT

Glucocorticoid Replacement. Cortisol deficiency is treated with glucocorticoids. Treatment also suppresses excessive production of androgens by the adrenal cortex and thus minimizes problems such as excessive growth and skeletal maturation and virilization. This often requires larger glucocorticoid doses than are needed in other forms of adrenal insufficiency, typically 15–20 mg/m^2/24 hr of hydrocortisone daily administered orally in 3 divided doses. Affected infants usually require dosing at the high end of this range. Double or triple doses are indicated during **periods of stress,** such as infection or surgery. Glucocorticoid treatment must be continued indefinitely in all patients with classical 21-hydroxylase deficiency but may not be necessary in patients with nonclassical disease unless signs of androgen excess are present. Therapy must be individualized. It is desirable to maintain linear growth along percentile lines; crossing to higher height percentiles may suggest undertreatment, whereas loss of height percentiles often indicates overtreatment with glucocorticoids. Overtreatment is also suggested by excessive weight gain. Pubertal development should be monitored by periodic examination, and skeletal maturation is evaluated by serial radiographs of the hand and wrist for bone age. Hormone levels, particularly 17-hydroxyprogesterone and androstenedione, should be measured early in the morning, before taking the morning medications, or at a consistent time in relation to medication dosing. In general, desirable 17-hydroxyprogesterone levels are in the high-normal range or several times normal; low-normal levels can usually be achieved only with excessive glucocorticoid doses.

Menarche occurs at the appropriate age in most girls in whom good control has been achieved. However, it may be delayed in girls with suboptimal control.

Children with simple virilizing disease, particularly males, are frequently not diagnosed until 3–7 yr of age, at which time skeletal maturation may be 5 yr or more in advance of chronologic age. In some children, especially if the bone age is 12 yr or more, **spontaneous gonadotropin-dependent puberty** may occur when treatment is instituted, because therapy with hydrocortisone has suppressed production of adrenal androgens and stimulated release of pituitary gonadotropins if the appropriate level of hypothalamic maturation is present. This form of superimposed true precocious puberty may be treated with a gonadotropin hormone–releasing hormone analog such as leuprolide.

Males with 21-hydroxylase deficiency who have had inadequate corticosteroid therapy may develop adrenal rest testicular tumors, which usually regress with increased steroid dosage. Testicular MRI, ultrasonography, and color flow Doppler examination help define the character and extent of disease. Testis-sparing surgery for steroid-unresponsive tumors has been reported.

Mineralocorticoid Replacement. Patients with salt-wasting disease (i.e., aldosterone deficiency) require mineralocorticoid replacement with **fludrocortisone.** Infants may have very high mineralocorticoid requirements in the first few months of life, usually 0.1–0.3 mg daily in 2 divided doses but occasionally up to 0.4 mg daily, and often require sodium supplementation (sodium chloride, 1–3 g) in addition to the mineralocorticoid. Older infants and children are usually maintained with 0.05–0.1 mg daily of fludrocortisone. In some patients, simple virilizing disease may be easier to control with a low dose of fludrocortisone in addition to hydrocortisone even when these patients have normal aldosterone levels in the absence of mineralocorticoid replacement. Therapy is evaluated by monitoring of vital signs; tachycardia and hypertension are signs of overtreatment with mineralocorticoids. Serum electrolytes should be measured frequently in early infancy as therapy is adjusted. Plasma renin activity is a useful way to determine adequacy of therapy; it should be maintained in or near the normal range but not suppressed.

Additional approaches to improve outcome include an antiandrogen with an aromatase inhibitor (blocks conversion of androgens to estrogen), growth hormone with or without LHRH agonists, and adrenalectomy for poorly controlled patients.

Surgical Management of Ambiguous Genitals. Significantly virilized females usually undergo surgery between 2–6 mo of age. If there is severe clitoromegaly, the clitoris is reduced in size, with partial excision of the corporal bodies and preservation of the neurovascular bundle; however, moderate clitoromegaly may become much less noticeable even without surgery as the patient grows. Vaginoplasty and correction of the urogenital sinus usually are performed at the time of clitoral surgery; revision in adolescence is often necessary.

Risks and benefits of surgery should be fully discussed with parents of affected females. There is limited long-term follow-up of functional outcomes in patients who have undergone **modern** surgical procedures. Sex assignment of infants with **intersex conditions** (including CAH) is usually based on expected sexual functioning and fertility in adulthood with early surgical correction of the external genitals to conform with the sex assignment. Confused psychosexual identity is not common with CAH. However, lay and medical opponents of this practice for other intersex conditions state that it ignores any prenatally biased gender role predisposition and precludes the patient from having any decision as to his or her own preferred sexual identity and what surgical correction of the genitals should be performed. These individuals and groups say treatment should be aimed primarily at educating patient, family, and others about the medical condition, its treatment, and how to deal with the intersex condition. They propose that surgery should be delayed until the patient decides on what, if any, correction should be performed. Whether this would be a successful practice in our society requires long-term follow-up studies.

In adolescent and adult females with poorly controlled 21-hydroxylase deficiency (hirsutism, obesity, amenorrhea) bilateral laparoscopic adrenalectomy (with hormone replacement) may be superior to standard medical hormone replacement therapy.

Prenatal Treatment. Besides genetic counseling, the main goal of prenatal diagnosis is to facilitate appropriate prenatal treatment of affected females. Recommendations for pregnancies at risk consist of administration of dexamethasone, a steroid that readily crosses the placenta, in an amount of 20 µg/kg prepregnancy maternal weight daily in 2 or 3 divided doses. This suppresses secretion of steroids by the fetal adrenal, including secretion of adrenal androgens. If started by 6 wk of gestation, it ameliorates virilization of the external genitals in affected females. Chorionic villus biopsy is then performed to determine the sex and genotype of the fetus; therapy is continued only if the fetus is an affected female. DNA analysis of fetal cells isolated from maternal plasma for sex determination and *CYP21* gene analysis may permit earlier identification of the affected female fetus. No specific deleterious effects have been observed in children exposed to this therapy, but at present there is insufficient information to determine whether there are any long-term risks, particularly in the males and unaffected females who derive no benefit from the treatment. Maternal side effects of prenatal treatment have included edema, excessive weight gain, hypertension, glucose intolerance, cushingoid facial features, and severe striae. Prenatal treatment is therefore carried out only under institutional protocols in some locales, but it is frequently offered as a routine option by high-risk obstetricians in other communities.

577.2 • Congenital Adrenal Hyperplasia Due to 11β-Hydroxylase Deficiency

ETIOLOGY. Deficiency of 11β-hydroxylase is due to a mutation in the *CYP11B1* gene located on chromosome 8q24. *CYP11B1* mediates 11-hydroxylation of 11-deoxycortisol to cortisol. Because 11-deoxycortisol is not converted to cortisol, levels of corticotropin are high. In consequence, precursors—particularly 11-deoxycortisol and deoxycorticosterone—accumulate and are shunted into androgen biosynthesis in the same manner as occurs in 21-hydroxylase deficiency. However, the adjacent *CYP11B2* gene encoding aldosterone synthase is unaffected in this disorder, so patients are able to synthesize aldosterone normally.

EPIDEMIOLOGY. 11β-Hydroxylase deficiency accounts for ~5% of cases of adrenal hyperplasia; its incidence has been estimated as 1/250,000 to 1/100,000. More than 30 different mutations in *CYP11B1* have been identified. The disorder occurs relatively frequently in Israeli Jews of North African origin (1 in 15,000–17,000 live births); in this ethnic group almost all alleles carry an Arg448 to His (R448H) mutation. This disorder presents in a classical, severe form and very rarely in a nonclassical, milder form.

CLINICAL MANIFESTATIONS. Although cortisol is not synthesized efficiently, aldosterone synthetic capacity is normal, and some corticosterone is synthesized from progesterone by the intact aldosterone synthase enzyme. Thus, it is unusual for patients to manifest signs of adrenal insufficiency such as hypotension, hypoglycemia, hyponatremia, and hyperkalemia. Approximately two thirds of patients become **hypertensive,** although this can take several years to develop. Hypertension is probably a consequence of elevated levels of deoxycorticosterone, which has mineralocorticoid activity. Infants may transiently develop signs of mineralocorticoid deficiency after treatment with hydrocortisone is instituted. This is presumably due to sudden suppression of deoxycorticosterone secretion in a patient with atrophy of the zona glomerulosa caused by chronic suppression of renin activity.

All signs and symptoms of androgen excess that are found in 21-hydroxylase deficiency may also occur in 11-hydroxylase deficiency.

LABORATORY FINDINGS. Plasma levels of 11-deoxycortisol and deoxycorticosterone are elevated. Because deoxycorticosterone and metabolites have mineralocorticoid activity, plasma renin activity is suppressed. Consequently, aldosterone levels are low even though the ability to synthesize aldosterone is intact. Hypokalemic alkalosis occasionally occurs.

TREATMENT. Patients are treated with hydrocortisone in doses similar to those used for 21-hydroxylase deficiency. Mineralocorticoid replacement is sometimes transiently required in infancy but is rarely necessary otherwise. Hypertension often resolves with glucocorticoid treatment but may require additional therapy if it is of long standing. Calcium channel blockers may be beneficial under these circumstances.

577.3 • Congenital Adrenal Hyperplasia Due to 3β-Hydroxysteroid Dehydrogenase Deficiency

ETIOLOGY. Deficiency of 3β-hydroxysteroid dehydrogenase (3β-HSD) occurs in fewer than 2% of patients with adrenal hyperplasia. This enzyme is required for conversion of Δ5 steroids (pregnenolone, 17-hydroxypregnenolone, dehydroepiandrosterone [DHEA]) to Δ4 steroids (progesterone, 17-hydroxyprogesterone, and androstenedione). Thus, deficiency of the enzyme results in decreased synthesis of cortisol, aldosterone, and androstenedione but increased secretion of DHEA (see Fig. 575-1). The 3β-HSD enzyme expressed in the adrenal cortex and gonad is encoded by the *HSD3B2* gene located on chromosome 1p13.1. Over 30 mutations in the *HSD3B2* gene have been described in patients with 3β-HSD deficiency.

CLINICAL MANIFESTATIONS. Because cortisol and aldosterone are not synthesized in patients with the classical form of the disease, infants are prone to **salt-wasting crises.** Because androstenedione and testosterone are not synthesized, boys are incompletely virilized. Varying degrees of hypospadias may occur, with or without bifid scrotum or cryptorchidism. Because DHEA levels are elevated and this hormone is a weak androgen, girls are mildly virilized, with slight to moderate clitoral enlargement. Postnatally, continued excessive DHEA secretion can cause precocious adrenarche. During adolescence and adulthood, hirsutism, irregular menses, and polycystic ovarian disease occur in females. Males manifest variable degrees of hypogonadism, although appropriate male secondary sexual development may occur. A persistent defect of testicular 3β-HSD is demonstrated, however, by the high Δ5 to Δ4 steroid ratio in testicular effluent.

LABORATORY FINDINGS. The hallmark of this disorder is the marked elevation of the Δ5 steroids (such as 17-hydroxypregnenolone and DHEA) preceding the enzymatic block. Patients may also have elevated levels of 17-hydroxyprogesterone because of the extra-adrenal 3β-HSD activity that occurs in peripheral tissues; these patients may be mistaken for patients with 21-hydroxylase deficiency. However, the ratio of 17-hydroxypregnenolone to 17-hydroxyprogesterone is markedly elevated in 3β-HSD deficiency, in contrast to the decreased ratio in 21-hydroxylase deficiency. Plasma renin activity is elevated in the salt-wasting form.

DIFFERENTIAL DIAGNOSIS. It is not unusual for children with premature adrenarche, or women with signs of androgen excess, to have mild to moderate elevations in DHEA levels. It has been suggested that such individuals have "nonclassical 3β-HSD deficiency." However, mutations in the *HSD3B2* gene are usually not found in such individuals, and a nonclassical form of this deficiency must actually be quite rare. The activity of 3β-HSD in the adrenal zonae fasciculata and reticularis, relative to CYP17 (17-hydroxylase/17,20-lyase) activity, normally decreases during adrenarche to facilitate DHEA synthesis, and so modest elevations in DHEA in pre-teenage children or women usually represent a normal variant.

TREATMENT. Patients require glucocorticoid and mineralocorticoid replacement with hydrocortisone and fludrocortisone, respectively, as in 21-hydroxylase deficiency. Incompletely virilized genetic males in whom a male sex of rearing is contemplated may benefit from several injections of a depot form of testosterone early in infancy to increase the size of the phallus. They may also require testosterone replacement at puberty.

577.4 • Congenital Adrenal Hyperplasia Due to 17-Hydroxylase Deficiency

ETIOLOGY. Less than 1% of CAH cases are caused by 17-hydroxylase deficiency. A single polypeptide, CYP17, catalyzes 2 distinct reactions: 17-hydroxylation of pregnenolone and progesterone to 17-hydroxypregnenolone and 17-hydroxyprogesterone, respectively, and the 17,20-lyase reaction mediating conversion of 17-hydroxypregnenolone to DHEA and, to a lesser extent, 17-hydroxyprogesterone to Δ4-androstenedione. DHEA and androstenedione are steroid precursors of testosterone and estrogen (see Fig. 575-1). The enzyme is expressed in both the adrenal cortex and the gonads and is encoded by a gene on chromosome 10q24.3. Most mutations affect both the hydroxylase and lyase activities, but rare mutations can affect either activity alone.

CLINICAL MANIFESTATIONS AND LABORATORY FINDINGS. Patients with 17-hydroxylase deficiency cannot synthesize cortisol, but their ability to synthesize corticosterone is intact. Because corticosterone is an active glucocorticoid, patients do not develop adrenal insufficiency. Deoxycorticosterone, the immediate precursor of corticosterone, is synthesized in excess. This can cause **hypertension, hypokalemia,** and suppression of renin and aldosterone secretion, as occurs in 11-hydroxylase deficiency. However, in contrast to 11-hydroxylase deficiency, patients with 17-hydroxylase deficiency are unable to synthesize sex hormones. Affected **males are incompletely virilized** and present as phenotypic females (but gonads are usually palpable in the inguinal region or the labia) or with sexual ambiguity (male pseudohermaphroditism). Affected females usually present with **failure of sexual development** at the expected time of **puberty.** 17-Hydroxylase deficiency in females must be considered in the differential diagnosis of primary hypogonadism (see Chapter 587). In addition to the increased DOC, suppressed renin and aldosterone, and decreased 17-hydroxylated steroids, cortisol and sex steroids are unresponsive to stimulation with ACTH and human chorionic gonadotropin, respectively.

TREATMENT. Patients with 17-hydroxylase deficiency require cortisol replacement to suppress secretion of deoxycorticosterone and thus control hypertension. Additional antihypertensive medication may be required. Females require estrogen replacement at puberty. Genetic males may require either estrogen or androgen supplementation depending on the sex of rearing. As with androgen insensitivity syndrome (see Chapter 584), genetic males with severe 17-hydroxylase deficiency being reared as females require gonadectomy at or before adolescence because of the possibility of malignant transformation of abdominal testes.

577.5 • Lipoid Adrenal Hyperplasia

ETIOLOGY AND PATHOGENESIS. Lipoid adrenal hyperplasia is a rare disorder, reported in fewer than 100, mostly Japanese patients. There is marked accumulation of cholesterol and lipids in the adrenal cortex and gonads, associated with severe impairment of all steroidogenesis. Lipoid adrenal hyperplasia is usually caused by mutations in the gene for steroidogenic acute regulatory protein (StAR), a mitochondrial protein that promotes the movement of cholesterol from the outer to the inner mitochondrial membrane. Mutations in the *CYP114 (P450scc)* gene have been reported in 2 patients with lipoid adrenal hyperplasia.

Some cholesterol is able to enter mitochondria even in the absence of StAR, so it might be supposed that this disorder would not completely impair steroid biosynthesis. However, the accumulation of cholesterol in the cytoplasm is cytotoxic, eventually leading to death of all steroidogenic cells in which StAR is normally expressed. This occurs prenatally in the adrenals and testes. However, the ovaries do not normally synthesize steroids until puberty, so cholesterol does not accumulate and the ovaries can retain the capacity to synthesize estrogens until adolescence.

CLINICAL MANIFESTATIONS. Patients with lipoid adrenal hyperplasia are usually unable to synthesize any adrenal steroids. **Salt-losing** manifestations are usual, and many infants die in early infancy. Genetic males are unable to synthesize androgens and thus are **phenotypically female** but with gonads. Genetic females appear normal at birth and may undergo feminization at puberty with menstrual bleeding. They too, however, progress to **hypergonadotropic hypogonadism** when accumulated cholesterol kills granulosa (i.e., steroid-synthesizing) cells in the ovary.

LABORATORY FINDINGS. Adrenal and gonadal steroid hormone levels are low in lipoid adrenal hyperplasia, with a decreased or absent response to stimulation (ACTH, human chorionic gonadotropin). Plasma renin levels are increased.

Imaging studies of the adrenal gland demonstrating massive adrenal enlargement in the newborn help establish the diagnosis of lipoid adrenal hyperplasia.

TREATMENT. Patients require glucocorticoid and mineralocorticoid replacement. Genetic males are usually assigned a female sex of rearing; thus, both genetic males and females require estrogen replacement at the expected age of puberty.

577.6 • Deficiency of P450 Oxidoreductase (Antley-Bixler Syndrome)

ETIOLOGY, PATHOGENESIS, AND CLINICAL MANIFESTATIONS. P450 oxidoreductase (POR, gene located on chromosome 7q11.3) is required for the activity of all microsomal cytochrome P450 enzymes (see Chapter 575) including the adrenal enzymes CYP17 and CYP21. Thus, complete POR deficiency abolishes all microsomal P450 activity. This is embryonically lethal in mice and presumably in humans as well. Patients with mutations that decrease but do not abolish POR activity have partial deficiencies of 17-hydroxylase and 21-hydroxylase activities in the adrenals. Deficiency of 17-hydroxylase leads to incomplete masculinization in males, whereas 21-hydroxylase deficiency may lead to virilization in females. Additionally, aromatase *(CYP19)* activity in the placenta is decreased, leading to unopposed action of androgens produced by the fetal adrenal. This exacerbates virilization of female fetuses and may virilize the mother of an affected fetus as well. Although it is puzzling that affected females could be virilized despite a partial deficiency in *CYP17* (which is required for androgen biosynthesis), an alternative biosynthetic pathway may be utilized in which 17-hydroxyprogesterone is converted to 5αpregnane-3α,17α-diol-20-one, a metabolite that is a much better substrate for the 17,20-lyase activity of *CYP17* than the usual substrate, 17-hydroxypregnenolone (see Chapter 575). The metabolite is then converted in several enzymatic steps to dihydrotestosterone, a potent androgen.

Because many other P450 enzymes are affected, patients often (but not invariably) have other congenital anomalies collectively referred to as **Antley-Bixler syndrome.** These include craniosynostosis; brachycephaly; frontal bossing; severe midface hypoplasia with proptosis and choanal stenosis or atresia; humeroradial synostosis; medial bowing of ulnas; long, slender fingers with camptodactyly; narrow iliac wings; anterior bowing of femurs; and malformations of the heart and kidneys. The precise metabolic defects responsible for these anomalies are as yet uncertain but may involve defective metabolism of retinoic acid or a related teratogen, or a deficiency of lanosterol 14-demethylase *(CYP51).* The finding that similar abnormalities result from maternal exposure to ketoconazole, an antifungal drug that inhibits *CYP51,* supports the latter possibility.

EPIDEMIOLOGY. The prevalence is not known with certainty. It must be rare compared with 21-hydroxylase deficiency but might occur at similar frequencies to the other forms of CAH.

LABORATORY FINDINGS. Serum steroids that are not 17- or 21-hydroxylated are most increased, including pregnenolone and progesterone. 17-Hydroxy, 21-deoxy-steroids are also increased, including 17-hydroxypregnenolone, 17-hydroxyprogesterone, and 21-deoxycortisol. Urinary steroid metabolites may be determined by quantitative mass spectrometry. Metabolites excreted at increased levels include pregnanediol, pregnanetriol, pregnanetriolone, and corticosterone metabolites. Urinary cortisol metabolites are decreased. Genetic analysis demonstrates mutations in the *POR* gene.

DIFFERENTIAL DIAGNOSIS. This disorder must be distinguished from other forms of congenital adrenal hyperplasia, particularly 21-hydroxylase deficiency in females, which is far more common and has similar laboratory findings. Suspicion for *POR* deficiency may be raised if the mother is virilized or if the associated abnormalities of Antley-Bixler syndrome are present. Conversely, virilization of both the mother and her daughter can result from a luteoma of pregnancy, but in this case postnatal abnormalities of corticosteroid biosynthesis should not be observed. Antley-Bixler syndrome may also occur without abnormalities of steroid hormone biosynthesis, resulting from mutations in the fibroblast growth factor receptor, FGFR2.

577.7 • Aldosterone Synthase Deficiency

ETIOLOGY. This is a rare autosomal recessive disorder in which conversion of corticosterone to aldosterone is impaired; a group of Iranian Jewish patients has been the most thoroughly studied. The majority of cases result from mutations in the *CYP11B2* gene coding for aldosterone synthase; however, linkage to *CYP11B2* has been excluded in other kindreds. When not due to *CYP11B2* mutations, the disorder has been termed familial hyperreninemic hypoaldosteronism type 2; the causative gene or genes have not yet been identified.

Aldosterone synthase mediates the 3 final steps in the synthesis of aldosterone from deoxycorticosterone (11-hydroxylation, 18-hydroxylation, and 18-oxidation). Although 11-hydroxylation is required to convert deoxycorticosterone to corticosterone, this conversion can also be catalyzed by the related enzyme, CYP11B1, located in the fasciculata, which is unaffected in this disorder. For the same reason, these patients have normal cortisol biosynthesis.

The disease has previously been classified into 2 types, termed corticosterone methyloxidase deficiency types I and II. They differ only in levels of the immediate precursor of aldosterone, 18-hydroxycorticosterone; levels are low in type I deficiency and elevated in type II deficiency. These differences do not correspond in a simple way to particular mutations and are of limited clinical importance.

CLINICAL MANIFESTATIONS. Infants with aldosterone synthase deficiency may have severe electrolyte abnormalities with **hyponatremia, hyperkalemia,** and **metabolic acidosis.** However, because cortisol synthesis is unaffected, infants rarely become as ill as untreated infants with salt-losing forms of congenital adrenal hyperplasia such as 21-hydroxylase deficiency. Thus, some infants escape diagnosis. Later in infancy or in early childhood they may exhibit failure to thrive and poor growth. Adults often are asymptomatic, although they may develop electrolyte abnormalities when depleted of sodium through procedures such as bowel preparation for a barium enema.

LABORATORY FINDINGS. Infants have elevated plasma renin activity. Aldosterone levels are decreased; they may be at the lower end of the normal range but are always inappropriately low for the degree of hyperkalemia or hyperreninemia. Corticosterone levels are often elevated. As mentioned, some but not all patients have marked elevation of 18-hydroxycorticosterone, but low levels of this steroid do not exclude the diagnosis. In kindreds in which 18-hydroxycorticosterone levels are elevated in affected individuals, this biochemical abnormality persists in adults even when they have no electrolyte abnormalities.

DIFFERENTIAL DIAGNOSIS. It is important to distinguish aldosterone synthase deficiency from primary adrenal insufficiency in which both cortisol and aldosterone are affected (including salt-wasting forms of congenital adrenal hyperplasia) because the latter condition is usually associated with a much greater risk of shock and hyponatremia. This becomes apparent after the appropriate laboratory studies. Pseudohypoaldosteronism (see Chapter 52) may have similar electrolyte abnormalities and hyperreninemia, but aldosterone levels are high, and this condition usually does not respond to fludrocortisone treatment.

TREATMENT. Treatment consists of giving enough fludrocortisone (0.05–0.3 mg daily), sodium chloride, or both to return plasma renin levels to normal. With increasing age, salt-losing signs usually improve and drug therapy can often be discontinued.

577.8 • Glucocorticoid-Suppressible Hyperaldosteronism

ETIOLOGY. Glucocorticoid-suppressible aldosteronism (glucocorticoid-remediable aldosteronism, familial hyperaldosteronism type I) is an autosomal dominant form of **low-renin hypertension** in which hyperaldosteronism is rapidly suppressed by glucocorticoid administration. This unusual effect of glucocorticoids suggests that this disorder is regulated by ACTH aldosterone secretion instead of by the renin-angiotensin system. In addition to abnormally regulated secretion of aldosterone, there is marked overproduction of 18-hydroxycortisol and 18-oxocortisol. The synthesis of these steroids requires both 17-hydroxylase (CYP17) activity, which is expressed only in the zona fasciculata, and aldosterone synthase (CYP11B2) activity, which is normally expressed only in the zona glomerulosa. Together, these features imply that aldosterone synthase is being expressed in a manner similar to the closely related enzyme steroid 11-hydroxylase *(CYP11B1)*. The disorder is caused by unequal meiotic crossing over events between the *CYP11B1* and *CYP11B2* genes, which are closely linked on chromosome 8q24. An additional "hybrid" gene is produced, having regulatory sequences of *CYP11B1* juxtaposed with coding sequences of *CYP11B2*. This results in the inappropriate expression of a *CYP11B2*-like enzyme with aldosterone synthase activity in the adrenal fasciculata.

CLINICAL MANIFESTATIONS. Some affected children have no symptoms, the diagnosis being established after incidental discovery of moderate hypertension, typically about 30 mm Hg higher than unaffected family members of the same age. Others have more symptomatic hypertension with headache, dizziness, and visual disturbances. A strong family history of early-onset hypertension or early strokes may alert the clinician to the diagnosis. Some patients have chronic hypokalemia, but this is not a consistent finding and is usually mild.

LABORATORY FINDINGS. Patients have elevated plasma and urine levels of aldosterone and suppressed plasma renin activity. As mentioned, hypokalemia is not consistently present. Urinary and plasma levels of 18-oxocortisol and 18-hydroxycortisol are markedly increased. The hybrid *CYP11B1/CYP11B2* gene can be readily detected by molecular genetic methods. However, these assays are not routinely available.

DIFFERENTIAL DIAGNOSIS. This condition should be distinguished from primary aldosteronism due to bilateral hyperplasia or an aldosterone-producing adenoma (see Chapter 579). Most cases of primary aldosteronism are sporadic although rare affected kindreds have been reported. Patients with primary aldosteronism may also have elevated levels of 18-hydroxycortisol and 18-oxocortisol, and these biochemical tests should be used cautiously to distinguish primary and glucocorticoid-suppressible aldosteronism. A therapeutic trial of dexamethasone may be helpful if aldosterone secretion is suppressed, and genetic testing should identify the hybrid gene of glucocorticoid-suppressible hyperaldosteronism if it is present.

TREATMENT. Glucocorticoid-suppressible hyperaldosteronism is managed by daily administration of a glucocorticoid, usually dexamethasone, 25 μg/kg/day in divided doses. If necessary, effects of aldosterone can be blocked with a potassium-sparing diuretic such as spironolactone, eplerenone, or amiloride. Hypertension resolves in patients in whom the hypertension is not severe or of long standing. If hypertension is of long standing, additional antihypertensive medication may be required, such as a calcium channel blocker.

GENETIC COUNSELING. Because of the autosomal dominant mode of inheritance, at-risk family members should be investigated for this easily treated cause of hypertension.

Arlt W, Walker EA, Draper N, et al: Congenital adrenal hyperplasia caused by mutant P450 oxidoreductase and human androgen synthesis: Analytical study. *Lancet* 2004;363:2128–2135.

Auchus RJ: The genetics, pathophysiology, and management of human deficiencies of P450c17. *Endocrinol Metab Clin North Am* 2001;30:101–119.

Bose HS, Sato S, Aisenberg J, et al: Mutations in the steroidogenic acute regulatory protein (StAR) in six patients with congenital lipoid adrenal hyperplasia. *J Clin Endocrinol Metab* 2000;85:3636–3639.

Consensus statement on 21-hydroxylase deficiency from the Lawson Wilkins Pediatric Endocrine Society and the European Society for Paediatric Endocrinology. *J Clin Endocrinol Metab* 2002;87:4048–4053.

Dluhy RG: Glucocorticoid-remediable aldosteronism. *Endocrinologist* 2001; 11:263–268.

Fluck CE, Tajima T, Pandey AV, et al: Mutant P450 oxidoreductase causes disordered steroidogenesis with and without Antley-Bixler syndrome. *Nat Genet* 2004;36:228–230.

Giacaglia LR, Mendonca BB, Madureira G, et al: Adrenal nodules in patients with congenital adrenal hyperplasia due to 21-hydroxylase deficiency: Regression after adequate hormonal control. *J Pediatr Endocrinol Metab* 2001;14:415–419.

Gmyrek GA, New MI, Sosa RE, et al: Bilateral laparoscopic adrenalectomy as a treatment for classic congenital adrenal hyperplasia attributable to 21-hydroxylase deficiency. *Pediatrics* 2002;109:E28.

Hughes IA, Houk C, Ahmed SF, Lee PA: Consensus statement on management of intersex disorders. *Arch Dis Child* 2006;91:554–562.

Katsumata N, Ohtake M, Hojo T, et al: Compound heterozygous mutations in the cholesterol side chain cleaving enzyme (CYP11A) causing congenital adrenal insufficiency in humans. *J Clin Endocrinol Metab* 2002;87: 3808–3813.

Krege S, Walz KH, Hauffa BP, et al: Long-term follow-up of female patients with congenital adrenal hyperplasia from 21-hydroxylase deficiency, with special emphasis on the results of vaginoplasty. *BJU Int* 2000;86:253–259.

Lajic S, Nordenstrom A, Ritzen EM, et al: Prenatal treatment of congenital adrenal hyperplasia. *Eur J Endocrinol* 2004;151(Suppl 3): U63–69.

Merke DP, Bornstein SR: Congenital adrenal hyperplasia. *Lancet* 2005; 365:2125–2136.

Meyer-Bahlburg HF: Gender and sexuality in classic congenital adrenal hyperplasia. *Endocrinol Metab Clin North Am* 2001;30:155–171.

Morgan JF, Murphy H, Lacey JH, Conway G: Long term psychosocial outcome for women with congenital adrenal hyperplasia: Cross sectional survey. *Br Med J* 2005;330:340–341.

New MI: Prenatal treatment of congenital adrenal hyperplasia: The United States experience. *Endocrinol Metab Clin North Am* 2001;30:1–13.

Nordenstrom A, Wedell A, Hagenfeldt L, et al: Neonatal screening for congenital adrenal hyperplasia: 17-Hydroxyprogesterone levels and CYP21 genotypes in preterm infants. *Pediatrics* 2001;108:E68.

Pang S: Congenital adrenal hyperplasia owing to 3 beta-hydroxysteroid dehydrogenase deficiency. *Endocrinol Metab Clin North Am* 2001;30:81–99.

Rangecroft L: Surgical management of ambiguous genitalia. *Arch Dis Child* 2003;88:799–801.

Schnitzer JJ, Donahoe PK: Surgical treatment of congenital adrenal hyperplasia. *Endocrinol Metab Clin North Am* 2001;30:137–154.

Speiser PW, White PC: Congenital adrenal hyperplasia. *N Engl J Med* 2003;349:776–788.

Tajima T, Fujieda K, Kouda N, et al: Heterozygous mutation in the cholesterol side chain cleavage enzyme (P450scc) gene in a patient with 46,XY sex reversal and adrenal insufficiency. *J Clin Endocrinol Metab* 2001;86: 3820–3825.

Therrell BL: Newborn screening for congenital adrenal hyperplasia. *Endocrinol Metab Clin North Am* 2001;30:15–30.

White PC: Steroid 11-beta-hydroxylase deficiency and related disorders. *Endocrinol Metab Clin North Am* 2001;30:61–79.

Chapter 578 ■ Cushing Syndrome

Cushing syndrome is the result of abnormally high blood levels of cortisol or other glucocorticoids. This can be iatrogenic or the result of endogenous cortisol secretion, due either to an adrenal tumor or to hypersecretion of corticotropin (adrenocorticotropic hormone [ACTH]) by the pituitary (Cushing disease) or by a tumor (Table 578-1).

TABLE 578-1. Etiologic Classification of Adrenocortical Hyperfunction

EXCESS ANDROGEN
Congenital adrenal hyperplasia
21-Hydroxylase (P450c21) deficiency
11β-Hydroxylase (P450c11) deficiency
3β-Hydroxysteroid dehydrogenase defect
Tumor
Carcinoma
Adenoma
EXCESS CORTISOL (CUSHING SYNDROME)
Bilateral adrenal hyperplasia
Hypersecretion of corticotropin (Cushing disease)
Ectopic secretion of corticotropin
Exogenous corticotropin
Adrenocortical nodular dysplasia
Pigmented nodular adrenocortical disease (Carney complex)
Tumor
Carcinoma
Adenoma
EXCESS MINERALOCORTICOID (HYPERTENSIVE HYPOKALEMIC SYNDROME)
Primary hyperaldosteronism
Aldosterone-secreting adenoma
Bilateral micronodular adrenocortical hyperplasia
Glucocorticoid-suppressible aldosteronism
Tumor
Adenoma
Carcinoma
Deoxycorticosterone excess
Congenital adrenal hyperplasia
11β-Hydroxylase (P450c11)
17α-Hydroxylase (P450c17)
Tumor (carcinoma)
Apparent mineralocorticoid excess
11β-Hydroxysteroid dehydrogenase deficiency
EXCESS ESTROGEN (ADRENAL FEMINIZATION SYNDROME)
Carcinoma
Adenoma
Mixed hypercorticism and tumor

ETIOLOGY. The most common cause of Cushing syndrome is prolonged exogenous administration of glucocorticoid hormones, especially at the high doses used to treat lymphoproliferative disorders. This rarely represents a diagnostic challenge, but management of hyperglycemia, hypertension, weight gain, linear growth retardation, and osteoporosis often complicates therapy with corticosteroids.

Endogenous Cushing syndrome is most often caused in infants by a functioning adrenocortical tumor, usually a malignant carcinoma but occasionally a benign adenoma (see Chapter 580). Patients with these tumors often exhibit signs of hypercortisolism along with signs of hypersecretion of other steroids such as androgens, estrogens, and aldosterone.

Although extremely rare in infants, the most common etiology of endogenous Cushing syndrome in children older than 7 yr of age is **Cushing disease,** in which excessive ACTH secreted by a pituitary adenoma causes bilateral adrenal hyperplasia. Such adenomas are often too small to detect by imaging techniques and are termed microadenomas. They consist principally of chromophobe cells and frequently show positive immunostaining for ACTH and its precursor, pro-opiomelanocortin (POMC).

ACTH-dependent Cushing syndrome may also result from ectopic production of ACTH, although this is uncommon in children. Ectopic ACTH secretion in children has been associated with islet cell carcinoma of the pancreas, neuroblastoma or ganglioneuroblastoma, hemangiopericytoma, Wilms tumor, and thymic carcinoid. Hypertension is more common in the ectopic ACTH syndrome than in other forms of Cushing syndrome, because very high cortisol levels may overwhelm 11β-hydroxysteroid dehydrogenase in the kidney (see Chapter 575) and thus have an enhanced mineralocorticoid (salt-retaining) effect.

Primary pigmented nodular adrenocortical disease (PPNAD) is a distinctive form of ACTH-independent Cushing syndrome, usually presenting before 20 yr of age. It may occur as an isolated event or, more commonly, as a familial disorder with other manifestations. The adrenal glands are small and have characteristic multiple, small (<4 mm in diameter), pigmented (black) nodules containing large cells with cytoplasm and lipofuscin; there is cortical atrophy between the nodules. This adrenal disorder occurs as a component of **Carney complex,** an autosomal dominant disorder also consisting of centrofacial lentigines and blue nevi; cardiac and cutaneous myxomas; pituitary, thyroid, and testicular tumors; and pigmented melanotic schwannomas. Carney complex is inherited in an autosomal dominant manner, although sporadic cases occur. Genetic loci for Carney complex have been mapped to chromosome 2p16 and to the gene for the type 1α regulatory subunit of protein kinase A (PRKAR1A) on chromosome 17q22–24.

ACTH-independent Cushing syndrome with nodular hyperplasia and adenoma formation occurs rarely in cases of **McCune-Albright syndrome,** with symptoms beginning in infancy or childhood. McCune-Albright syndrome is caused by a somatic mutation of a G protein, $G_s\alpha$, resulting in inhibition of guanosine triphosphatase activity and constitutive activation of adenylate cyclase. When the mutation is present in adrenal tissue, cortisol and cell division are stimulated independently of ACTH. Other tissues in which activating mutations may occur are bone (producing fibrous dysplasia), gonads, thyroid, and pituitary. Clinical manifestations depend on which tissues are affected.

Adrenocortical lesions including diffuse hyperplasia, nodular hyperplasia, adenoma, and rarely carcinoma may occur as part of the multiple endocrine neoplasia type 1 syndrome, an autosomal dominant disorder, in which there is homozygous inactivation of the menin (**MEN1**) tumor suppressor gene on chromosome 11q13 (see Chapter 574).

CLINICAL MANIFESTATIONS. Signs of Cushing syndrome have been recognized in infants younger than 1 yr of age. The disorder appears to be more severe and the clinical findings more flagrant in infants than in older children. The face is rounded, with prominent cheeks and a flushed appearance (moon facies). Generalized obesity is common in younger children. In children with adrenal tumors, signs of abnormal masculinization occur frequently; accordingly, there may be hirsutism on the face and trunk, pubic hair, acne, deepening of the voice, and enlargement of the clitoris in girls. Growth is impaired, with length falling below the 3rd percentile, except when significant virilization produces normal or even accelerated growth. Hypertension is common and may occasionally lead to heart failure. An increased susceptibility to infection may also lead to fatal sepsis.

In older children, in addition to obesity, short stature is a common presenting feature. Gradual onset of obesity and deceleration or cessation of growth may be the only early manifestations. Older children most often have more severe obesity of the face and trunk compared with the extremities. Purplish striae on the hips, abdomen, and thighs are common. Pubertal development may be delayed, or amenorrhea may occur in girls past menarche. Weakness, headache, and emotional lability may be prominent. Hypertension and hyperglycemia usually occur; hyperglycemia may progress to frank diabetes. Osteoporosis is common and may cause pathologic fractures.

LABORATORY FINDINGS. Cortisol levels in blood are normally elevated at 8 A.M. and decrease to less than 50% by midnight except in infants and young children in whom a diurnal rhythm is not always established. In patients with Cushing syndrome this circadian rhythm is lost, and cortisol levels at midnight and 8 A.M. are usually comparable. Obtaining diurnal blood samples presents logistic difficulties as part of an outpatient evaluation, but cortisol can be measured in saliva samples, which can be obtained at home at the appropriate times of day. Elevated nighttime salivary cortisol levels raise suspicion for Cushing syndrome.

Urinary excretion of free cortisol is increased. This is best measured in a 24-hr urine sample and is expressed as a ratio of micrograms of cortisol excreted per gram of creatinine. This ratio is independent of body size and completeness of the urine collection.

A single-dose dexamethasone suppression test is often helpful; a dose of 25–30 µg/kg (maximum of 2 mg) given at 11 P.M. results in a plasma cortisol level of less than 5 µg/dL at 8 A.M. the next morning in normal individuals but not in patients with Cushing syndrome.

A glucose tolerance test is often abnormal despite elevated levels of insulin. Levels of serum electrolytes are usually normal, but potassium may be decreased, especially in patients with tumors that secrete ACTH ectopically.

After the diagnosis of Cushing syndrome has been established, it is necessary to determine whether it is caused by a pituitary adenoma, an ectopic ACTH-secreting tumor, or a cortisol-secreting adrenal tumor. ACTH concentrations are usually suppressed in patients with cortisol-secreting tumors, are very high in patients with ectopic ACTH-secreting tumors, but may be normal in patients with ACTH-secreting pituitary adenomas. After an intravenous bolus of corticotropin-releasing hormone (CRH), patients with ACTH-dependent Cushing syndrome have an exaggerated ACTH and cortisol response, whereas those with adrenal tumors show no increase in ACTH and cortisol. The 2-step dexamethasone suppression test consists of administration of dexamethasone, 30 and 120 µg/kg/24 hr in 4 divided doses, on consecutive days. In children with pituitary Cushing syndrome, the larger dose, but not the smaller dose, suppresses serum levels of cortisol. Typically, patients with ACTH-independent Cushing syndrome do not show suppressed cortisol levels with dexamethasone.

CT detects virtually all adrenal tumors larger than 1.5 cm in diameter. MRI may detect ACTH-secreting pituitary adenomas, but many are too small to be seen; the addition of gadolinium contrast increases the sensitivity of detection. Bilateral inferior petrosal blood sampling to measure concentrations of ACTH before and after CRH administration may be required to localize the tumor when a pituitary adenoma is not visualized.

DIFFERENTIAL DIAGNOSIS. Cushing syndrome is frequently suspected in children with obesity, particularly when striae and hypertension are present. Children with simple obesity are usually tall, whereas those with Cushing syndrome are short or have a decelerating growth rate. Although urinary excretion of cortisol is often elevated in simple obesity, salivary nighttime levels of cortisol are normal and cortisol secretion is suppressed by oral administration of low doses of dexamethasone.

Elevated levels of cortisol and ACTH without clinical evidence of Cushing syndrome occur in patients with generalized glucocorticoid resistance. Affected patients may be asymptomatic or exhibit hypertension, hypokalemia, and precocious pseudopuberty; these manifestations are caused by increased mineralocorticoid and adrenal androgen secretion in response to elevated ACTH levels. Mutations in the glucocorticoid receptor have been identified. Absence of cushingoid phenotype in a patient with a pituitary adenoma and biochemically proved Cushing disease has been reported. In this patient, defective cortisone to cortisol conversion resulted in increased cortisol clearance, protecting the patient from cortisol excess.

TREATMENT. Transsphenoidal pituitary microsurgery is the treatment of choice in pituitary Cushing disease in children. The overall success rate with follow-up of less than 10 yr is 60–80%. Low postoperative serum or urinary cortisol concentrations predict long-term remission in the majority of cases. Relapses are treated with re-operation or pituitary irradiation.

Cyproheptadine, a centrally acting serotonin antagonist that blocks ACTH release, has been used to treat Cushing disease in adults; remissions are usually not sustained after discontinuation of therapy. This agent is rarely used in children. Inhibitors of adrenal steroidogenesis (metyrapone, ketoconazole, aminoglutethimide) have been used preoperatively to normalize circulating cortisol levels and reduce perioperative morbidity and mortality.

If a pituitary adenoma does not respond to treatment or if ACTH is secreted by an ectopic metastatic tumor, the adrenal glands may need to be removed. This can often be accomplished laparoscopically. Adrenalectomy may lead to increased ACTH secretion by an unresected pituitary adenoma, evidenced mainly by marked hyperpigmentation; this condition is termed **Nelson syndrome.**

Benign cortical adenomas are treated with unilateral adrenalectomy. Such adenomas are occasionally bilateral; then the treatment of choice is subtotal adrenalectomy. In either instance, an excellent therapeutic result is achieved by removing the tumor. Adrenocortical carcinomas frequently metastasize, especially to the liver and lungs, and may have an unfavorable prognosis despite removal of the primary lesion. Rarely, the tumors are bilateral and require total adrenalectomy. It is often impossible to differentiate benign from malignant tumors by histologic appearance alone.

Management of patients undergoing adrenalectomy requires adequate preoperative and postoperative replacement therapy with a corticosteroid. Tumors that produce corticosteroids usually lead to atrophy of the normal adrenal tissue, and replacement with cortisol (10 mg/M^2/24 hr in 3 divided doses after the immediate postoperative period) is required until there is recovery of the hypothalamic-pituitary-adrenal axis. Postoperative complications may include sepsis, pancreatitis, thrombosis, poor wound healing, and sudden collapse, particularly in infants with Cushing syndrome. Substantial catch-up growth, pubertal progress, and increased bone density occur, but bone density remains abnormal and adult height is often compromised.

Bourdeau I, D'amour P, Hamet P, et al: Aberrant membrane hormone receptors in incidentally discovered bilateral macronodular adrenal hyperplasia with subclinical Cushing's syndrome. *J Clin Endocrinol Metab* 2001;86:5534–5540.

Devoe DJ, Miller WL, Conte FA, et al: Long-term outcome in children and adolescents after transsphenoidal surgery for Cushing's disease. *J Clin Endocrinol Metab* 1997;82:3196–3202.

Gafni RI, Papanicolaou DA, Nieman LK: Nighttime salivary cortisol measurement as a simple, noninvasive, outpatient screening test for Cushing's syndrome in children and adolescents. *J Pediatr* 2000;137:30–35.

Hiroi N, Chrousos GP, Kohn B, et al: Clinical Case Seminar: Adrenocortical-pituitary hybrid tumor causing Cushing's syndrome. *J Clin Endocrinol Metab* 2001;86:2631–2637.

Kirk JMW, Brain CE, Carson DJ, et al: Cushing's syndrome caused by nodular adrenal hyperplasia in children with McCune-Albright syndrome. *J Pediatr* 1999;134:789–792.

Lacroix A, N'Diaye N, Tremblay J, et al: Ectopic and abnormal hormone receptors in adrenal Cushing's syndrome. *Endocr Rev* 2001;22:75–110.

Lienhardt A, Grossman AB, Dacie JE, et al: Relative contributions of inferior petrosal sinus sampling and pituitary imaging in the investigation of children and adolescents with ACTH-dependent Cushing's syndrome. *J Clin Endocrinol Metab* 2001;86:5711–5714.

Newell-Price J, Bertagna X, Grossman AB, et al: Cushing's syndrome. *Lancet* 2006;367:1605–1617.

Raff H, Findling JW: A physiologic approach to diagnosis of the Cushing syndrome. *Ann Intern Med* 2003;138:980–991.

Raffin-Sanson ML, de Keyzer Y, Bertagna X: Syndromes of ectopic ACTH secretion: Recent pathophysiological progresses and their clinical implications. *Endocrinologist* 2000;10:97–106.

Stratakis CA, Kirschner LS, Carney JA: Clinical and molecular features of the Carney complex: Diagnostic criteria and recommendations for patient evaluation. *J Clin Endocrinol Metab* 2001;86:4041–4046.

Stratakis CA: Genetics of adrenocortical tumors: Gatekeepers, landscapers and conductors in symphony. *Trends Endocrinol Metab* 2003;14:404–410.

Chapter 579 ■ Primary Aldosteronism

Primary aldosteronism encompasses disorders caused by excessive aldosterone secretion independent of the renin-angiotensin system. These disorders are characterized by **hypertension, hypokalemia,** and suppression of the renin-angiotensin system.

ETIOLOGY. Aldosterone-secreting adenomas are unilateral and have been reported in children as young as 3½ yr of age; they mainly affect girls. Bilateral micronodular adrenocortical hyperplasia tends to occur in older children and is more frequent in males. Primary aldosteronism due to unilateral adrenal hyperplasia may also occur. Glucocorticoid-suppressible hyperaldosteronism is discussed in Chapter 577.

EPIDEMIOLOGY. These conditions are thought to be rare in children, but they may account for 5–10% of cases of hypertension in adults. Although usually sporadic, kindreds with several affected members have been reported.

CLINICAL MANIFESTATIONS. Some affected children have no symptoms, the diagnosis being established after incidental discovery of moderate hypertension. Others have severe hypertension (up to 240/150 mm Hg), with headache, dizziness, and visual disturbances. Chronic hypokalemia, if present, may lead to polyuria, nocturia, enuresis, and polydipsia. Muscle weakness and discomfort, tetany, intermittent paralysis, fatigue, and growth failure affect children with severe hypokalemia.

LABORATORY FINDINGS. Hypokalemia occurs frequently. Serum pH and the carbon dioxide and sodium concentrations may be elevated and the serum chloride and magnesium levels decreased. Serum levels of calcium are normal, even in children who manifest tetany. The urine is neutral or alkaline, and urinary potassium excretion is high. Plasma levels of aldosterone may be normal or elevated. Aldosterone concentrations in 24-hr urine collections are always increased. Plasma levels of renin are persistently low.

The diagnostic test of choice for primary aldosteronism is controversial. Both renin and aldosterone levels may vary by time of day, posture, and sodium intake, making it difficult to establish consistent reference ranges. It is desirable to establish a consistent sampling protocol, for example, mid-morning after the patient has been sitting for 15 min. If possible, antihypertensive drugs or other medications that can affect aldosterone or renin secretion should be avoided for several weeks prior to testing, including diuretics, β-blockers, angiotensin-converting enzyme inhibitors, angiotensin receptor blockers, clonidine and nonsteroidal anti-inflammatory agents. Patients taking these agents may need to be changed to α-adrenergic blockers or calcium channel blockers that have smaller effects on the biochemical measurements. The ratio of plasma aldosterone concentration to renin activity is always high, and this represents a cost-effective screening test for primary aldosteronism. Aldosterone does not decrease with administration of saline solution or fludrocortisone, and renin does not respond to salt and fluid restriction. Urinary and plasma levels of 18-oxocortisol and 18-hydroxycortisol may be increased but not to the extent seen in glucocorticoid-suppressible hyperaldosteronism.

DIFFERENTIAL DIAGNOSIS. Primary aldosteronism should be distinguished from glucocorticoid-suppressible hyperaldosteronism (see Chapter 577.7), which is specifically treated with glucocorticoids. An autosomal dominant pattern of inheritance should raise suspicion for the latter disorder. Glucocorticoid-suppressible hyperaldosteronism is diagnosed by dexamethasone suppression tests or by specific genetic testing. More generally, primary aldosteronism should be distinguished from other forms of hypertension by means of the testing previously discussed.

TREATMENT. The treatment of an aldosterone-producing adenoma is surgical removal. This has been performed primarily by laparotomy and adrenalectomy; successful enucleation of aldosterone-producing adenomas as well as laparoscopic adrenalectomy is reported. Hyperaldosteronism due to bilateral adrenal hyperplasia is treated with the mineralocorticoid antagonists spironolactone or eplerenone, often normalizing blood pressure and serum potassium levels. There is greater experience with spironolactone, but this agent has anti-androgenic properties that may be unacceptable in pubertal males. Eplerenone is a more specific anti-mineralocorticoid, but there is little experience with this agent in the pediatric age group. As an alternative, an epithelial sodium channel blocker such as amiloride may be used and other antihypertensive agents added as necessary. In patients whose condition cannot be controlled medically, unilateral adrenalectomy may be considered.

Gordon RD: The challenge of more robust and reproducible methodology in screening for primary aldosteronism. *J Hypertens* 2004;22:251–255.

Grim CE: Evolution of diagnostic criteria for primary aldosteronism: Why is it more common in "drug-resistant" hypertension today? *Curr Hypertens Rep* 2004;6:485–492.

Kaplan NM: The current epidemic of primary aldosteronism: Causes and consequences. *J Hypertens* 2004;22:863–869.

Chapter 580 ■ Adrenal Tumors

EPIDEMIOLOGY. Adrenocortical tumors are rare in childhood. They occur in all age groups but most commonly in children younger than 10 yr of age. In 2–10% of cases, the tumors are bilateral. Symptoms of endocrine hyperfunction are present in more than 90% of children with adrenal tumors (see Table 578-1). Tumors may be associated with hemihypertrophy, usually occurring during the first few years of life. They are also associated with the **Beckwith-Wiedemann syndrome** and other congenital defects, particularly genitourinary tract and central nervous system abnormalities and hamartomatous defects.

ETIOLOGY. Germline mutations in p53 (on chromosome 17p13.1) have been found in patients with isolated adrenal carcinoma as well as in patients with familial clustering of unusual malignancies. Loss of heterozygosity involving chromosomes 2, 4, 11, and 18 and *IGF2* gene overexpression (chromosome 11p15.5) have also been reported in sporadic adrenocortical carcinomas.

580.1 • Virilizing Adrenocortical Tumors

CLINICAL MANIFESTATIONS. Virilization is the most common presenting symptom in children with adrenocortical tumors. In males, the clinical picture is similar to that of simple virilizing congenital adrenal hyperplasia: accelerated growth velocity and muscle development, acne, penile enlargement, and the precocious development of pubic and axillary hair. In females, virilizing tumors of the adrenal gland cause masculinization of a previously normal female with clitoral enlargement, growth acceleration, acne, deepening of the voice, and premature pubic and axillary hair development.

In addition to virilization, 20–40% of children with adrenocortical tumors also have Cushing syndrome (see Chapter 578). Although virilization may occur alone (50–80%), children with adrenal tumors usually do not have Cushing syndrome alone.

LABORATORY FINDINGS. Serum levels of dehydroepiandrosterone (DHEA), DHEA sulfate, and androstenedione are usually elevated, often markedly. Serum levels of testosterone are often increased, usually as a result of peripheral conversion of androstenedione, but infants with predominantly testosterone-secreting adenomas have been reported. Urinary 17-ketosteroids (sex steroid metabolites) are also increased. Many adrenocortical tumors have a relative deficiency of 11β-hydroxylase activity and secrete increased amounts of deoxycorticosterone; these patients are hypertensive, and their tumors are often malignant.

Tumors can usually be detected by ultrasonography, CT, or MRI. Preoperatively, the presence of metastatic disease should be determined by MRI or CT of the chest, abdomen, and pelvis. Differentiation between benign and malignant tumors by histologic criteria often is not possible.

TREATMENT. The treatment is surgical. A transperitoneal approach usually has been recommended, but laparoscopic removal is possible. Some of these neoplasms are highly malignant and metastasize widely, but cure with regression of the masculinizing features may follow removal of less malignant, encapsulated tumors. Incomplete resection, tumors weighing more than 100 g, tumors larger than 200 cm^3, age greater than 3.5 yr at diagnosis, symptoms for more than 6 mo, and a marked increase in urinary 17-ketosteroids and 17-hydroxysteroids have been associated with poor prognosis. Postoperatively, patients should be closely monitored biochemically, with frequent determinations of adrenal androgen levels and imaging studies. Recurrent symptoms or biochemical abnormalities should prompt a careful search for metastatic disease. Metastases primarily involve liver, lung, and regional lymph nodes. The majority of metastatic recurrences appear within 1 yr of tumor resection. Repeat surgical resection of metastatic lesions should be performed if possible and adjuvant therapy instituted. Radiation therapy has not been generally helpful. Antineoplastic agents, such as cisplatin and etoposide, ifosfamide and carboplatin, and 5-fluorouracil and leucovorin have had limited use in children, and their success is not established. Therapy with o,p′-DDD (mitotane), an adrenolytic agent, may relieve the symptoms of hypercortisolism or virilization in recurrent disease but does not appear to improve survival. Other agents that interfere with adrenal steroid synthesis, such as ketoconazole, aminoglutethimide, and metyrapone, may also relieve symptoms of steroid excess but do not improve survival.

A neoplasm of one adrenal gland may produce atrophy of the other because excessive production of cortisol by the tumor suppresses adrenocorticotropic hormone stimulation of the normal gland. Consequently, adrenal insufficiency may follow surgical removal of the tumor. This situation can be avoided by giving 10–25 mg of hydrocortisone every 6 hr, starting on the day of operation and continuing for 3–4 days postoperatively. Adequate quantities of water, sodium chloride, and glucose also must be provided.

580.2 • Feminizing Adrenal Tumors

Feminizing adrenocortical tumors may be either carcinomas or benign adenomas. They may produce only estrogens or, in addition, androgens, cortisol, or mineralocorticoids (see Fig. 575-1). High levels of aromatase activity and expression of the *CYP19 (P450arom)* gene, absent in normal adrenal tissue, are found in these tumors.

CLINICAL MANIFESTATIONS. Such tumors may become symptomatic at any age after 6 mo. Gynecomastia in males or premature thelarche in girls is often the initial manifestation. Growth and development may be otherwise normal, or concomitant virilization may occur, evidenced by acne, deep voice, penile or clitoral enlargement, and advanced skeletal maturation. Hypertension is common in affected adults but has not been observed in children.

LABORATORY FINDINGS. In addition to elevated plasma and urinary levels of estrogens, there are often elevated levels of adrenal androgens (i.e., dehydroepiandrosterone and its sulfate) in plasma and 17-ketosteroids in urine. Plasma gonadotropin levels are suppressed, and gonadotropin-releasing hormone stimulation does not elicit a response. Tumors may appear calcified on radiographs but are usually localized by CT.

TREATMENT. If the tumor can be resected, gynecomastia regresses and hormone values return to normal.

Koch CA, Pacak K, Chrousos GP: The molecular pathogenesis of hereditary and sporadic adrenocortical and adrenomedullary tumors. *J Clin Endocrinol Metab* 2002;87:5367–5384.

Ribeiro RC, Figueiredo B: Childhood adrenocortical tumours. *Eur J Cancer* 2004;40:1117–1126.

Stratakis CA: Genetics of adrenocortical tumors: Gatekeepers, landscapers and conductors in symphony. *Trends Endocrinol Metab* 2003;14:404–410.

Chapter 581 ■ Pheochromocytoma

Pheochromocytomas, catecholamine-secreting tumors, arise from chromaffin cells. The most common site of origin (approximately 90%) is the adrenal medulla; however, tumors may develop anywhere along the abdominal sympathetic chain and are likely to be located near the aorta at the level of the inferior mesenteric artery or at its bifurcation. They also appear in the peri-adrenal area, urinary bladder or ureteral walls, thoracic cavity, and cervical region. Ten per cent occur in children, in whom they present most frequently between 6 and 14 yr of age. Tumors vary from 1 to 10 cm in diameter; they are found more often on the right side than on the left. In more than 20% of affected children, the adrenal tumors are bilateral; in 30–40% of children, tumors are found in both the adrenal and extra-adrenal areas or only in an extra-adrenal area.

Pheochromocytoma may be inherited as an autosomal dominant trait. In affected families, the ages of patients at the time of diagnosis have varied from the 1st to 5th decades of life; more than half the patients have had multiple tumors.

Pheochromocytomas may also be associated with other syndromes such as **neurofibromatosis** and **von Hippel–Lindau disease** and as a component of **multiple endocrine neoplasia** (MEN) syndromes MEN-2A and MEN-2B. The *NF1* neurofibromatosis gene is a tumor suppressor gene mapping to chromosome 17q11.2. Germline mutations of the *RET* proto-oncogene on chromosome 10 (10q11.2) have been found in families with MEN-2A and MEN-2B, and germline mutations in a tumor suppressor gene on chromosome 3p25–26 have been identified in von Hippel–Lindau syndrome. Pheochromocytoma is also associated with tuberous sclerosis, Sturge-Weber syndrome, and ataxia-telangiectasia. Somatic mutations of genes associated with familial cancer syndromes have been found in nonfamilial forms of pheochromocytoma.

CLINICAL MANIFESTATIONS. The clinical features of pheochromocytoma result from excessive secretion of epinephrine and norepinephrine. All patients have hypertension at some time. Paroxysmal hypertension should particularly suggest pheochromocytoma as a diagnostic possibility. The hypertension in children is more often sustained rather than paroxysmal, in contrast to adults. When there are paroxysms of hypertension, the attacks are usually infrequent at first but become more frequent and eventually give way to a continuous hypertensive state. Between attacks of hypertension, the patient may be free of symptoms. During attacks, the patient complains of headache, palpitations, abdominal pain, and dizziness; pallor, vomiting, and sweating also occur. Convulsions and other manifestations of hypertensive encephalopathy may occur. In severe cases, precordial pains radiate into the arms; pulmonary edema and cardiac and hepatic enlargement may develop. Symptoms may be exacerbated by exercise. The child has a good appetite but because of hypermetabolism does not gain weight, and severe cachexia may develop. Polyuria and polydipsia can be sufficiently severe to suggest diabetes insipidus. Growth failure may be striking. The blood pressure may range from 180 to 260 mm Hg systolic and from 120 to 210 mm Hg diastolic, and the heart may be enlarged. Ophthalmoscopic examination may reveal papilledema, hemorrhages, exudate, and arterial constriction.

LABORATORY FINDINGS. The urine may contain protein, a few casts, and occasionally glucose. Gross hematuria suggests that the tumor is in the bladder wall. Polycythemia is occasionally observed. The diagnosis is established by demonstration of elevated blood or urinary levels of catecholamines and their metabolites.

Pheochromocytomas produce norepinephrine and epinephrine. Normally, norepinephrine in plasma is derived from both the adrenal gland and adrenergic nerve endings, whereas epinephrine is derived primarily from the adrenal gland. In contrast to adults with pheochromocytoma in whom both norepinephrine and epinephrine are elevated, children with pheochromocytoma predominantly excrete norepinephrine. Total urinary catecholamine excretion usually exceeds 300 µg/24 hr. Urinary excretion of vanillylmandelic acid (VMA, 3-methoxy-4-hydroxymandelic acid), the major metabolite of epinephrine and norepinephrine, is increased, as is excretion of metanephrine (see Fig. 575-2). Catecholamine levels can be measured by radioimmunoassay and high-performance liquid chromatography methods. Excretion of catecholamine metabolites may be similar in children with neuroblastoma and pheochromocytoma, but neuroblastoma does not usually produce hypertension. Urinary levels of most catecholamines are higher in those with pheochromocytoma, although levels of dopamine and homovanillic acid are usually higher in neuroblastoma. Daily urinary excretion of these compounds by unaffected children increases with age, and vanilla-containing foods and fruits can produce falsely elevated levels of VMA. Certain drugs interfere with fluorometric determinations of catecholamines.

Most tumors in the area of the adrenal gland are readily localized by ultrasonography or by CT or MRI; their frequent bilateral occurrence must not be forgotten. Extra-adrenal tumors may be difficult to detect. ^{131}I-metaiodobenzylguanidine (MBIG) is taken up by chromaffin tissue anywhere in the body and is useful for localizing small tumors. Venous catheterization with sampling of blood at different levels for catecholamine determinations is now only rarely necessary for localizing the tumor.

DIFFERENTIAL DIAGNOSIS. Various causes of hypertension in children must be considered, such as renal or renovascular disease; coarctation of the aorta; hyperthyroidism; Cushing syndrome; deficiencies of 11β-hydroxylase, 17α-hydroxylase, or 11β-hydroxysteroid dehydrogenase (type 2 isozyme); primary aldosteronism; adrenocortical tumors; and essential hypertension (see Chapter 445). A nonfunctioning kidney may result from compression of a ureter or of a renal artery by a pheochromocytoma. Paroxysmal hypertension may be associated with porphyria or familial dysautonomia. Urinary excretion of VMA is low in familial dysautonomia because of a defect in release rather than in synthesis of catecholamines. Cerebral disorders, diabetes insipidus, diabetes mellitus, and hyperthyroidism must also be considered in the differential diagnosis. Hypertension in patients with neurofibromatosis may be caused by renal vascular involvement or by concurrent pheochromocytoma.

Neuroblastoma, ganglioneuroblastoma, and ganglioneuroma frequently produce catecholamines. Secreting neurogenic tumors commonly produce hypertension, excessive sweating, flushing, pallor, rash, polyuria, and polydipsia. Chronic diarrhea may be associated with these tumors, particularly with ganglioneuroma, and at times may be sufficiently persistent to suggest celiac disease.

TREATMENT. Removal of these tumors results in cure, but the operation is very high risk. Careful preoperative, intraoperative, and postoperative management is essential. Preoperative α- and β-adrenergic blockade and fluid loading are required. Because these tumors are often multiple in children, a thorough transabdominal exploration of all the usual sites offers the best opportunity to find them all. Appropriate choice of anesthesia and expansion of blood volume with appropriate fluids during surgery are critical to avoid a precipitous drop in blood pressure during operation or within 48 hr postoperatively. Manipulation and excision of these tumors result in marked increases in catecholamine secretion that increase blood pressure and heart rate. Surveillance must continue postoperatively.

Although these tumors often appear malignant histologically, the only accurate indicators of malignancy are the presence of metastatic disease, local invasiveness that precludes complete resection, or both. Approximately 10% of all adrenal pheochromocytomas are malignant. Such tumors are rare in childhood; pediatric malignant pheochromocytomas occur more frequently in extra-adrenal sites. Prolonged follow-up is indicated because functioning tumors at other sites may be manifested many years after the initial operation. Examination of relatives of affected patients may reveal other individuals harboring unsuspected tumors that may be asymptomatic.

Chapter 582 ■ Adrenal Masses

582.1 • Adrenal Incidentaloma

Adrenal masses are discovered with increasing frequency in patients undergoing abdominal imaging for reasons unrelated to the adrenal gland. The rate of detection of single adrenal masses has ranged from less than 1% to more than 4% of abdominal CT examinations in adults. The unexpected discovery of such a mass presents the clinician with a dilemma in terms of diagnostic steps to undertake and treatment interventions to recommend. The differential diagnosis of adrenal incidentaloma includes benign lesions such as cysts, hemorrhagic cysts, hematomas, and myelolipomas. These lesions can usually be identified on CT or MRI. If the nature of the lesion is not readily apparent, additional evaluation is required. Included in the differential diagnosis of lesions requiring additional evaluation are benign adenomas, pheochromocytomas, adrenocortical carcinoma, and metastasis from an extra-adrenal primary carcinoma. Benign, hormonally inactive adrenocortical adenomas make up the majority of incidentalomas. Careful history, physical examination, and endocrine evaluation must be performed to seek evidence of autonomous cortisol, androgen, mineralocorticoid, or catecholamine secretion. Functional tumors require removal. If the adrenal mass is nonfunctional and larger than 4–6 cm, recommendations are to proceed with surgical resection of the mass. Lesions of 3 cm or less should be followed clinically with periodic re-imaging. Treatment must be individualized; nonsecreting adrenal incidentalomas may enlarge and become hyperfunctioning. Nuclear scan, and occasionally fine-needle aspiration, may be helpful in defining the mass.

582.2 • Adrenal Calcification

Calcification within the adrenal glands may occur in a wide variety of situations, some serious and others of no obvious consequence. Adrenal calcifications are often detected as incidental findings in radiographic studies of the abdomen in infants and children. The physician may elicit a history of anoxia or trauma at birth. Hemorrhage into the adrenal gland at or immediately after birth is probably the most common factor that leads to subsequent calcification. Although it is advisable to assess the adrenocortical reserve of such patients, there is rarely any functional disorder.

Neuroblastomas, ganglioneuromas, cortical carcinomas, pheochromocytomas, and cysts of the adrenal gland may be responsible for calcifications, particularly if hemorrhage has occurred within the tumor. Calcification in such lesions is almost always unilateral.

In the past, tuberculosis was a common cause both of calcification within the adrenals and of Addison disease. Calcifications may also develop in the adrenal glands of children who recover from the Waterhouse-Friderichsen syndrome; such patients are usually asymptomatic. Infants with Wolman disease, a rare lipid disorder due to deficiency of lysosomal acid lipase, have extensive bilateral calcifications of the adrenal glands (see Chapter 86.2).

Agrons GA, Lonergan GJ, Dickey GE, et al: Adrenocortical neoplasms in children: Radiologic-pathologic correlation. *Radiographics* 1999;19:989–1008.

Barzon L, Boscaro M: Diagnosis and management of adrenal incidentalomas. *J Urol* 2000;163:398–407.

Bravo EL: Evolving concepts in the pathophysiology, diagnosis and treatment of pheochromocytoma. *Endocr Rev* 1994;15:356–368.

Brunt LM, Moley JF: Adrenal incidentaloma. *World J Surg* 2001;25:905–913.

Ciftci AO, Senocak ME, Tanyel FC, et al: Adrenocortical tumors in children. *J Pediatr Surg* 2001;36:549–554.

Ein SH, Weitzman S, Thorner P, et al: Pediatric malignant pheochromocytoma. *J Pediatr Surg* 1994;29:1197–1201.

Eisenhoffer G, Lenders JWM, Linehan WM, et al: Plasma normetanephrine and metanephrine for detecting pheochromocytoma in von Hippel-Lindau disease and multiple endocrine neoplasia type 2. *N Engl J Med* 1999; 340:1872–1879.

Ghazi AAM, Mofid D, Rahimi F, et al: Oestrogen and cortisol producing adrenal tumour. *Arch Dis Child* 1994;71:358–359.

Kjellman M, Roshani L, Teh BT, et al: Genotyping of adrenocortical tumors: Very frequent deletions of the MEN1 locus in 11q13 and of a 1-centimorgan region in 2p16. *J Clin Endocrinol Metab* 1999;84:730–735.

Koch CA, Vortmeyer AO, Huang SC, et al: Genetic aspects of pheochromocytoma. *Endocr Regul* 2001;35:43–52.

LaFranchi SH, Hanna CE, Mandel SH: Feminizing adrenal adenoma secreting estrone presenting as prepubertal gynecomastia. *J Pediatr Endocrinol* 1989;3:261–265.

Latronico AC, Pinto EM, Domenice S, et al: An inherited mutation outside the highly conserved DNA-binding domain of the p53 tumor suppressor protein in children and adults with sporadic adrenocortical tumors. *J Clin Endocrinol Metab* 2001;86:4970–4973.

Magill SB, Raff H, Shaker JL, et al: Comparison of adrenal vein sampling and computed tomography in the differentiation of primary aldosteronism. *J Clin Endocrinol Metab* 2001;86:1066–1071.

Mayer SK, Oligny LL, Deal C, et al: Childhood adrenocortical tumors: Case series and reevaluation of prognosis—a 24-year experience. *J Pediatr Surg* 1997;32:911–915.

Mendonca BB, Lucon AM, Menezes CAV, et al: Clinical, hormonal and pathological findings in a comparative study of adrenocortical neoplasms in childhood and adulthood. *J Urol* 1995;154:2004–2009.

Moneva MH, Gomez-Sanchez CE: Establishing a diagnosis of primary hyperaldosteronism. *Curr Opin Endocrinol Diabet* 2001;8:124–129.

Phornphutkul C, Okubo T, Wu K, et al: Aromatase P450 expression in a feminizing adrenal adenoma presenting as isosexual precocious puberty. *J Clin Endocrinol Metab* 2001;86:649–652.

Prys-Roberts C: Phaeochromocytoma—recent progress in its management. *Br J Anaesth* 2000;85:44–57.

Reincke M, Beuschlein F, Slawik M, et al: Molecular adrenocortical tumourigenesis. *Eur J Clin Invest* 2000;30:63–68.

Ross JH: Pheochromocytoma: Special considerations in children. *Urol Clin North Am* 2000;27:393–402.

Siren J, Tervahartiala P, Sivula A, et al: Natural course of adrenal incidentalomas: Seven-year follow-up study. *World J Surg* 2000;24:579–582.

Wajchenberg BL, Albergaria Pereira MA, Medonca BB, et al: Adrenocortical carcinoma: Clinical and laboratory observations. *Cancer* 2000;88:711–736.

Wilkin F, Gagne N, Paquette J, et al: Pediatric adrenocortical tumors: Molecular events leading to insulin-like growth factor II gene overexpression. *J Clin Endocrinol Metab* 2000;85:2048–2056.

Young J, Bulun SE, Agarwal V, et al: Aromatase expression in a feminizing adrenocortical tumor. *J Clin Endocrinol Metab* 1996;81:3173–3176.

Section 5 — Disorders of the Gonads — Robert Rapaport

Chapter 583 ■ Development and Function of the Gonads

EMBRYONIC GONADAL DIFFERENTIATION. The undifferentiated, bipotential fetal gonad arises from a thickening of the urogenital ridge, close to the region that forms the kidney and adrenal cortex. At 6 wk of gestation, the gonad contains germ cells—stromal cells that will become Leydig cells in testes, or theca, interstitial or hilar cells in the ovary, and supporting cells that will develop into Sertoli cells in testes or granulosa cells in ovaries. In the absence of a testis-determining factor, thought to be the SRY (sex-determining region on the Y chromosome), the gonad develops into an ovary. SRY is thought to normally suppress a putative factor 2 (not yet identified) that functions as repressor of male development.

A 46,XX complement of chromosomes is necessary for the development of **normal ovaries.** Both the long and the short arms of X chromosomes bear genes for normal ovarian development. The DSS (dosage sensitive/sex reversal) locus associated with the *DAX1* gene responsible for X-linked congenital adrenal hypoplasia and hypogonadotropic hypogonadism, a member of the nuclear receptor superfamily, acts as a repressor of male gene expression. *DAX1* acts by binding to a related nuclear receptor SF-1 (steroidogenic factor-1). The signaling gene *WNT4* in vitro up-regulates *DAX1,* resulting in the suppression of androgen synthesis in XX females. WNTs are secreted ligands that activate receptor-mediated signal transduction pathways and are involved in modulating gene expression as well as cell behavior, adhesion, and polarity. A loss-of-function mutation of the *WNT4* gene was found in an 18-yr-old 46,XX woman with absence of müllerian-derived structures (uterine and fallopian tubes), unilateral renal agenesis, and clinical signs of androgen excess. Alternative splicing of the Wilms tumor 1 *(WT1)* gene may also be involved in sex differentiation. *WT1* mutations are associated with the Denys-Drash syndrome (early-onset renal failure with abnormal external genitals and Wilms tumor). Haploinsufficiency of a 3-amino-acid (KTS) form of *WT1* has been implicated in the gonadal dysgenesis of patients with Fraser syndrome (late-onset progressive glomerulopathy and 46,XY gonadal dysgenesis). Mutations in the *FOXL2* gene are associated with ovarian failure. Autosomal genes also play a role in normal ovarian organogenesis and testicular development. Several conditions of gonadal dysgenesis are associated with chromosomal abnormalities. A deletion affecting the short arm of the X chromosome produces the typical somatic anomalies of Turner syndrome (see Chapter 81).

Development of the testis requires the short arm of the Y chromosome; a testis-determining factor at this site has been identified, and the gene for it has been cloned and designated *SRY.* During male meiosis, the Y chromosome must segregate from the X chromosome so that both X and Y chromosomes do not occur in the same spermatozoa. The major portion of the Y chromosome is composed of Y-specific sequences that do not pair with the X chromosome. However, a minor portion of the Y chromosome shares sequences with the X chromosome and pairing does occur in this region. The genes and sequences in this area recombine between the sex chromosomes, behaving like autosomal genes. Therefore, the term pseudoautosomal is used to describe the genetic behavior of these genes. The *SRY* gene is localized to the 35-kb portion proximal to this pairing and exchange (pseudoautosomal) region of the Y chromosome. It contains a high-mobility group nonhistone protein (HMG box), suggesting that *SRY* may be a transcriptional regulator of other genes involved in sex differentiation. The gonadal ridge forms at around 33 days of gestation. *SRY* is detected at 41 days, peaks at 44 days when testis cords are first visible, and persists into adulthood. These genes include *SOX9,* an *SRY*-related gene, containing a shared motif homologous with the high-mobility group box 9 (HMG box 9) of *SRY,* located on chromosome 17, that results in sex reversal and camptomelic dysplasia, steroidogenic factor 1 (SF-1) on chromosome 9q33, and the Wilms tumor genes *(WTI),* especially the -KSTiso form on chromosome 11p13 needed for early gonadal, adrenal, and renal development, fibroblast growth factor-9 (FGF-9), GATA-4, and XH-2. SOY9 also interacts with heat shock protein 70 (HSP) in testis. When recombination events extend beyond the pseudoautosomal region, X- and Y-specific DNA may be transferred between the chromosomes. Such aberrant recombinations result in X chromosomes carrying SRY, resulting in XX males, or Y chromosomes that have lost SRY, resulting in **XY females.** SRY acts as a transcriptional regulator to increase cellular proliferation, attract interstitial cells from adjacent mesonephros into the genital ridge and stimulates Sertoli cell differentiation. Sertoli cells act as organizer of steroidogenic and germ cell lines and produce **antimüllerian hormone** (AMH) that causes the female duct system to regress. They express low levels of SRY. (For additional genes involved in sex development, see Table 583-1.)

FUNCTION OF THE TESTES. In the 1st trimester of pregnancy, levels of placental chorionic gonadotropin peak (8–12 wk) and stimulate the fetal Leydig cells to secrete testosterone, the main hormonal product of the testis. This period is critical for normal virilization of the XY fetus. Defects in this process lead to different forms of atypical male development (see Chapter 589.2). After virilization occurs, fetal levels of testosterone decrease but are maintained at low levels in the latter half of pregnancy by luteinizing hormone (LH) secreted by the fetal pituitary; this is required for continued penile growth.

As part of the normal transition from intrauterine to extrauterine life, likely as a result of the abrupt withdrawal of maternal and placental hormones, the newborn experiences a transient postnatal surge of gonadotropins and sex steroids. In males, LH and testosterone peak at 1–2 mo of age and reach prepubertal levels by 4–6 mo of age. Follicle-stimulating hormone (FSH), along with inhibin B, peaks at 3 mo and declines to prepubertal levels by 9 and 15 mo, respectively. The LH rise is, however, dominant. In females, the FSH surge predominates. FSH peaks around 3–6 mo of age, declines by 12 mo, but remains detectable for 24 mo. Under LH influence, estradiol peaks at 2–6 mo of age. The inhibin B response is variable, peaking between 2–12 mo and remaining at above prepubertal levels until 24 mo. The neonatal surge may be important for postnatal maturation of the gonads, stabilization of male external genitals, and perhaps also for gender identity and sexual behaviors. The postnatal surge in LH and testosterone is absent or blunted in infants with hypopitu-

TABLE 583-1. Genes Known to Be Involved in Disorders of Sex Development (DSD)

GENE	PROTEIN	OMIM DATA BASE NO.	LOCUS	INHERITANCE	GONAD	MÜLLERIAN STRUCTURES	EXTERNAL GENITALS	ASSOCIATED FEATURES/VARIANT PHENOTYPES
46,XY DSD								
DISORDERS OF GONADAL (TESTICULAR) DEVELOPMENT: SINGLE GENE DISORDERS								
WT1	TF	607102	11p13	AD	Dysgenetic testis	±	Female or ambiguous	Wilms tumor, renal abnormalities, gonadal tumors (WAGR, Denys-Drash and Frasier syndromes)
SF1 (NR5A1)	Nuclear receptor TF	184757	9q33	AD/AR	Dysgenetic testis	±	Female or ambiguous	More severe phenotypes include primary adrenal failure; milder phenotypes have isolated partial gonadal dysgenesis
SRY	TF	480000	Yp11.3	Y	Dysgenetic testis or ovotestis	±	Female or ambiguous	
SOX9	TF	608160	17q24-25	AD	Dysgenetic testis or ovotestis	±	Female or ambiguous	Camptomelic dysplasia (17q24 rearrangements milder phenotype than point mutations)

TABLE 583-1. Genes Known to Be Involved in Disorders of Sex Development (DSD)—cont'd

GENE	PROTEIN	OMIM DATA BASE NO.	LOCUS	INHERITANCE	GONAD	MÜLLERIAN STRUCTURES	EXTERNAL GENITALS	ASSOCIATED FEATURES/VARIANT PHENOTYPES
DHH	Signaling molecule	605423	12q13.1	AR	Dysgenetic testis	+	Female	The severe phenotype of one patient included minifascicular neuropathy; other patients have isolated gonadal dysgenesis
ATRX	Helicase (?chromatin remodeling)	300032	Xq13.3	X	Dysgenetic testis	–	Female, ambiguous or male	α-Thalassemia, mental retardation
ARX	TF	3003382	Xp22.13	X	Dysgenetic testis	–	Ambiguous	X-linked lissencephaly, epilepsy, temperature instability
DISORDERS OF GONADAL (TESTICULAR) DEVELOPMENT: CHROMOSOMAL CHANGES INVOLVING KEY CANDIDATE GENES								
DMRT1	TF	602424	9p24.3	Monosomic deletion	Dysgenetic testis	±	Female or ambiguous	Mental retardation
DAX1 (NR0B1)	Nuclear receptor TF	300018	Xp21.3	dupXp21	Dysgenetic testis or ovary	±	Female or ambiguous	
WNT4	Signaling molecule	603490	1p35	dup1p35	Dysgenetic testis	+	Ambiguous	Mental retardation
DISORDERS IN HORMONE SYNTHESIS OR ACTION								
LHGCR	G-protein receptor	152790	2p21	AR	Testis	–	Female, ambiguous or micropenis	Leydig cell hypoplasia
DHCR7	Enzyme	602858	11q12-13	AR	Testis	–	Variable	Smith-Lemli-Opitz syndrome: coarse facies, second-third toe syndactyly, failure to thrive, developmental delay, cardiac and visceral abnormalities
StAR	Mitochondrial membrane protein	600617	8p11.2	AR	Testis	–	Female	Congenital lipoid adrenal hyperplasia (primary adrenal failure), pubertal failure
CYP11A1	Enzyme	118485	15q23-24	AR	Testis	–	Female or ambiguous	Congenital adrenal hyperplasia (primary adrenal failure), pubertal failure
HSD3B2	Enzyme	201810	1p13.1	AR	Testis	–	Ambiguous	CAH, primary adrenal failure, partial androgenization due to ↑ DHEA
CYP17	Enzyme	202110	10q24.3	AR	Testis	–	Female ambiguous or micropenis	CAH, hypertension due to ↑ corticosterone and 11-deoxycorticosterone (except in isolated 17,20-lyase deficiency)
POR (P450 oxidoreductase)	CYP enzyme electron donor	124015	7q11.2	AR	Testis	–	Male or ambiguous	Mixed features of 21-hydroxylase deficiency, 17α-hydroxylase/17,20-lyase deficiency and aromatase deficiency; sometimes associated with Antley-Bixler craniosynostosis
HSD17B3	Enzyme	605573	9q22	AR	Testis	–	Female or ambiguous	Partial androgenization at puberty, ↑ androstenedione : testosterone ratio
SRD5A2	Enzyme	607306	2p23	AR	Testis	–	Ambiguous or micropenis	Partial androgenization at puberty, ↑ testosterone : DHT ratio
AMH	Signaling molecule	600957	19p13.3-13.2	AR	Testis	+	Normal male	Persistent müllerian duct syndrome (PMDS); male external genitalia, bilateral cryptorchidism
AHM-receptor	Serine-threonine kinase transmembrane receptor	600956	12q13	AR	Testis	–	Normal male	
Androgen receptor	Nuclear receptor TF	3130700	Xq11-12	X	Testis	–	Female, ambiguous, micropenis, or normal male	Phenotypic spectrum from complete androgen insensitivity syndrome (female external genitalia) and partial androgen insensitivity (ambiguous) to normal male genitalia/infertility
46,XX DSD								
DISORDERS OF GONADAL (OVARIAN) DEVELOPMENT								
SRY	TF	480000	Yp11.3	translocation	Testis or ovotestis	–	Male or ambiguous	
SOX9	TF	608160	17q24	dup17q24	ND	–	Male or ambiguous	
ANDROGEN EXCESS								
HSD3B2	Enzyme	201810	1p13	AR	Ovary	+	Clitorimegaly	CAH, primary adrenal failure, partial androgenization due to ↑ DHEA
CYP21A2	Enzyme	201910	6p21-23	AR	Ovary	+	Ambiguous	CAH, phenotypic spectrum from severe salt-losing forms associated with adrenal failure to simple virilizing forms with compensated adrenal function, ↑ 17-hydroxyprogesterone
CYP11B1	Enzyme	20210	8q21-22	AR	Ovary	+	Ambiguous	CAH, hypertension due to ↑ 11-deoxycortisol and 11-deoxycorticosterone
POR (P450 oxidoreductase)	CYP enzyme electron donor	124015	7q11.2	AR	Ovary	+	Ambiguous	Mixed feature of 21-hydroxylase deficiency, 17α-hydroxylase/17,20-lyase deficiency and aromatase deficiency; associated with Antley-Bixler craniosynostosis
CYP19	Enzyme	107910	15q21	AR	Ovary	+	Ambiguous	Maternal androgenization during pregnancy, absent breast development at puberty, except in partial cases
Glucocorticoid receptor	Nuclear receptor TF	138040	5q31	AR	Ovary	+	Ambiguous	↑ ACTH, 17-hydroxyprogesterone and cortisol; failure of dexamethasone suppression (patient heterozygous for a mutation in CYP21)

ACTH, adrenocorticotropin; AD, autosomal dominant (often de novo mutation); AR, autosomal recessive; CAH, congenital adrenal hyperplasia; ND, not determined; TF, transcription factor; WAGR, Wilms, aniridia, genital anomalies, and retardation; X, X-chromosomal; Y, Y-chromosomal. Chromosomal rearrangements likely to include key genes are included.

Lee PA, Houk CP, Ahmed SF, Hughes IA: International Consensus Conference on Intersex organized by the Lawson Wilkins Pediatric Endocrine Society and the European Society for Paediatric Endocrinology. Consensus statement on management of intersex disorders. International Consensus Conference on Intersex. *Pediatrics* 2006 Aug; 118(2):e488–500.

itarism, cryptorchidism, and complete androgen insensitivity syndrome (CAIS). The development of nocturnal pulsatile secretion of LH marks the advent of puberty (see Chapter 562).

Within specific target cells, 6–8% of testosterone is converted by 5α-reductase to dihydrotestosterone, another potent androgen (Fig. 583-1) and about 0.3% is acted on by aromatase to produce estradiol (see Fig. 575-1). Approximately half of circulating testosterone is bound to sex hormone–binding globulin (SHBG) and half to albumin; only 2% circulates in the free form. Plasma levels of SHBG are low at birth, rise rapidly during the 1st 10 days of life, and then remain stable until the onset of puberty. Thyroid hormone may play a role in this physiologic increase because neonates with athyreosis have very low levels of SHBG.

Antimüllerian hormone (AMH; previously referred to as müllerian inhibitory substance [MIS]), inhibin, and activin are members of the transforming growth factor-β (TGF-β) superfamily of growth factors, which has over 45 members, including bone morphogenic proteins (BMPs). Members of the TGF-β superfamily are involved in the regulation of developmental processes and multiple human disease states, including chondrodysplasias and cancer.

AMH, a 140-kd homodimeric glycoprotein hormone, is the earliest secreted product of the Sertoli cells of the fetal testis. Produced as a prohormone, its carboxyterminal fragment needs to be removed before it is active by way of a plasma membrane receptor. The gene for AMH is on chromosome 19. Its transcription is initiated by *SOX9* acting through the HMG box while its expression is up-regulated by SF-1 binding to its promoter and further interacting with *SOX9, WTI,* and *GATA4.* Two distinct serine/threonine receptors with a single transmembrane domain have been identified. The activated type 1 receptor signals to the SMAD family of intracellular mediators.

The gene for the AMH receptor (on chromosome 12) is expressed in Sertoli cells and also in fetal müllerian duct and fetal and postnatal granulosa cells. During sexual differentiation, AMH causes involution of the embryologic precursors of the cervix, uterus, and—together with SFI—fallopian tubes (müllerian ducts).

AMH is secreted in males by Sertoli cells during both fetal and postnatal life. In females, it is secreted by granulosa cells from 36 wk of gestation to menopause but at lower levels. The serum concentration of AMH in males is highest at birth, whereas in females it is highest at puberty. After puberty, both sexes have similar serum concentrations of AMH.

Inhibin is another glycoprotein hormone secreted by the Sertoli cells of the testes and granulosa and theca cells of the ovary. Inhibin A consists of an α-subunit disulfide linked to the β-A subunit, whereas inhibin B consists of the same α subunit linked to the β-B subunit.

Activins are dimers of the B subunits, either homodimers (BA/BA, BB/BB) or heterodimers (BA/BB). Inhibins selectively inhibit whereas activins stimulate pituitary FSH secretion. By means of immunoassays specific for inhibin A or B, it has been shown that inhibin A is absent in males and is present mostly in the luteal phase in women. Inhibin B is the principal form of inhibin in males and females during the follicular phase. Inhibin B may be used as a marker of Sertoli cell function in males. FSH stimulates inhibin B secretion in females and males, but only in males is there also evidence for a gonadotropin-independent way of its regulation. Levels of inhibin B are currently being studied in children with various forms of gonadal and pubertal disorders.

Like inhibin and activin, follistatin (a single-chain glycosylated protein) is produced by gonads and other tissues such as the hypothalamus, kidney, adrenal gland, and placenta. Follistatin inhibits FSH secretion principally by binding activins, thereby blocking the effects of activins at the level of both ovary and pituitary.

An additional plethora of peptides are known to be involved as mediators of the development and function of the testis. They

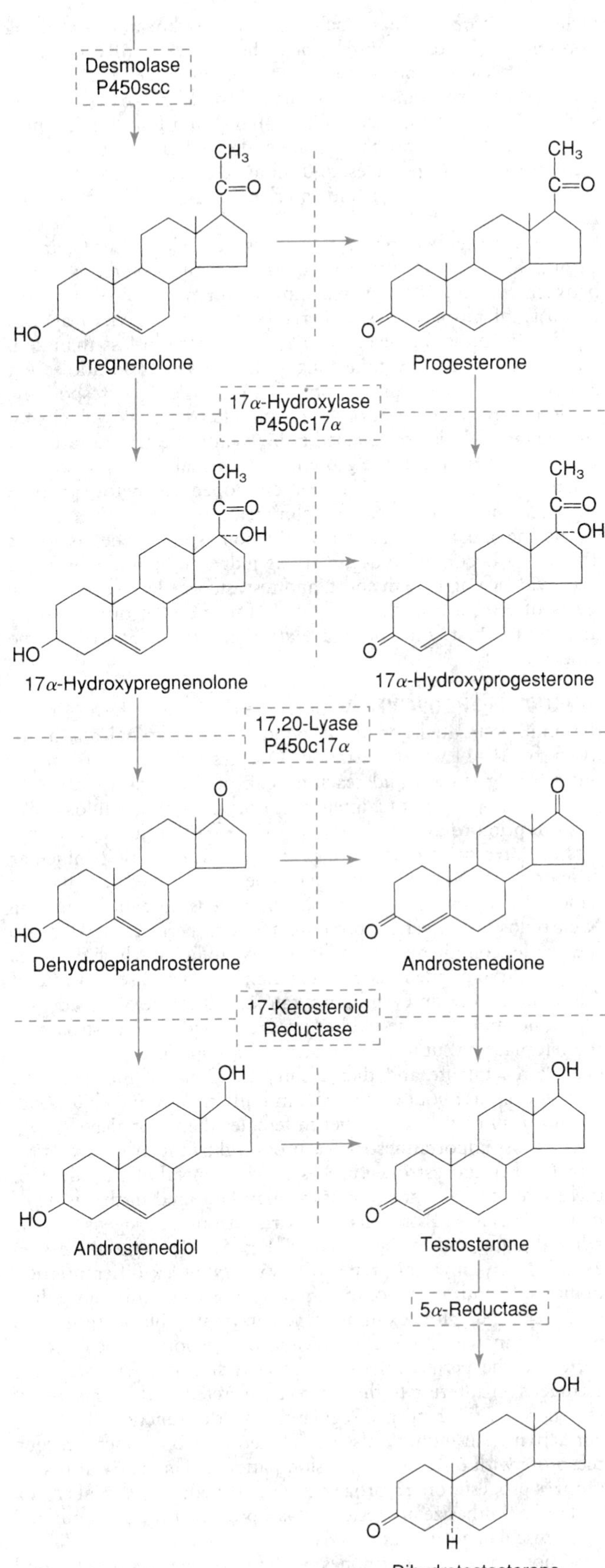

Figure 583-1. Biosynthesis of androgens. Dashed lines indicate enzymatic defects associated with 46XY disorder of sex differentiation. The vertical dashed line indicates a defect in 3β-hydroxysteroid dehydrogenase. A single polypeptide, P450c17, catalyzes both 17α-hydroxylase and 17,20-lyase activities.

include neurohormones such as growth hormone–releasing hormone, gonadotropin-releasing hormone (GnRH), corticotropin-releasing hormone, oxytocin, arginine vasopressin, somatostatin, substance P, and neuropeptide Y; growth factors such as insulin-like growth factors (IGFs) and IGF-binding proteins, TGF-β, and fibroblast, platelet-derived, and nerve growth factors; vasoactive peptides; and immune-derived cytokines such as tumor necrosis factor and interleukins IL-1, IL-2, IL-4, and IL-6.

Clinical patterns of pubertal changes vary widely (see Chapters 12 and 562). In 95% of boys, enlargement of the genitals begins between 9.5 and 13.5 yr, reaching maturity at 13–17 yr. In a minority of normal boys, puberty begins after 15 yr of age. In some boys, pubertal development is completed in less than 2 yr, but in others, it may take longer than 4.5 yr. The adolescent growth spurt occurs later in boys than in girls at corresponding levels of sexual maturation; for example, the peak velocity of change in height is not attained in boys until the genitals are well developed, but in girls the growth rate is usually at its maximum when the nipple and areola have developed but before there is any other significant breast development.

The median age of sperm production (spermarche) is 14 yr. This event occurs in mid-puberty as judged by pubic hair, testis size, evidence of growth spurt, and testosterone levels. Nighttime levels of FSH are in the adult male range at the time of spermarche; the first conscious ejaculation occurs at about the same time.

FUNCTION OF THE OVARIES. Without the presence of the *SRY* gene, the undifferentiated gonad can be identified histologically as an ovary by 10–11 wk of gestation. Oocytes are present from the 4th mo of gestation and reach a peak of 7 million by 5 mo of gestation. For normal maintenance, oocytes need granulosa cells to form primordial follicles. Functional FSH (but not LH) receptors are present in oocytes of primary follicles during follicular development. Normal X chromosomes are needed for maintenance of oocytes. In contrast to somatic cells, in which only one X chromosome is active, both are active in germ cells. At birth, the ovaries contain about 1 million active follicles, which decrease to 0.5 million by menarche. Thereafter, they decrease at a rate of 1000/mo, and at an even higher rate after the age of 35 yr.

The hormones of the fetal ovary are provided in most part by the fetoplacental unit. As in males, peak gonadotropin secretion occurs in fetal life and then again at 2–3 mo of life, with the lowest levels at about 6 yr of age. In both infancy and childhood, gonadotropin levels are higher in females than in males.

The most important estrogens produced by the ovary are estradiol-17 (E_2) and estrone (E_1); estriol is a metabolic product of these two, and all three estrogens may be found in the urine of mature females. Estrogens also arise from androgens in the adrenal gland and in the testis (see Fig. 575-1). This conversion explains why in certain types of disorders of sex differentiation in males, feminization occurs at puberty; in 17-ketosteroid reductase deficiency, for example, the enzymatic block results in markedly increased secretion of androstenedione, which is converted in the peripheral tissues to estradiol and estrone; these estrogens, in addition to those directly secreted by the testis, result in gynecomastia. Estrogen regulates a host of functionally different activities in multiple tissues. There are two distinct estrogen receptors with different expression patterns. The ovary also synthesizes progesterone, a progestational steroid; the adrenal cortex and testis synthesize progesterone as a precursor for other adrenal and testicular hormones.

A host of other hormones with autocrine, paracrine, and intracrine effects have been identified in the ovary. They include inhibins, activins, relaxin, and growth factors IGF-1, TGF-α and TGF-β, and cytokines.

Plasma levels of estradiol increase slowly but steadily with advancing sexual maturation and correlate well with clinical evaluation of pubertal development, skeletal age, and rising levels of FSH. Levels of LH do not rise until secondary sexual characteristics are well developed. Estrogens, like androgens, inhibit secretion of both LH and FSH (negative feedback). In females, estrogens also provoke the surge of LH secretion that occurs in the mid-menstrual cycle. The capacity for this positive feedback is another maturational milestone of puberty.

The average age at menarche in American girls is 12.5–13 yr, but the range of "normal" is wide, and 1–2% of "normal" girls have not menstruated by 16 yr of age. The age at onset of pubertal signs varies, with recent studies suggesting earlier ages than previously thought, especially in the United States African American population (see Chapter 12). Menarche generally correlates closely with skeletal age (see Chapters 12 and 562). Maturation and closure of the epiphyses is at least partially estrogen dependent, as demonstrated by a 28-yr-old, normally masculinized male with incomplete closure of the epiphyses who proved to have complete estrogen insensitivity owing to an estrogen-receptor defect.

DIAGNOSTIC AIDS. Improved, sensitive, and specific assays for pituitary and gonadal hormones that can be measured in small amounts of blood have contributed to rapid advances in the understanding of normal and aberrant hypothalamic-pituitary-gonadal interactions. For example, in male infants, measurements of LH, FSH, and testosterone can detect pituitary-testicular defects. Leydig cell integrity in childhood can be determined by the testosterone response following human chorionic gonadotropic administration (5,000 IU daily for 3 days). The integrity as well as the maturity of the hypothalamic-pituitary-gonadal axis in males and females can be assessed by the administration of gonadotropin-releasing hormone (GnRH) or a GnRH analog. An ultrasensitive LH assay has been shown to differentiate between boys with delayed puberty and those with complete but not partial hypogonadotropic hypogonadism.

Normal inhibin B levels have been documented in infant boys; inhibin B may be a marker of spermatogenesis and also of tumors such as granulosa cell tumors. Inhibin may be involved in tumor suppression. Estrogen-receptor assays may be clinically useful in the management of various ovarian cancers. AMH measurements are useful in the evaluation of children with nonpalpable gonads and disorders of sex development.

THERAPEUTIC AIDS. The estrogenic effects of polyhalogenated aromatic hydrocarbons (PHAHs) may in part be due to inhibition of estradiol sulfation by estrogen sulfotransferase (SULT1E1), an important pathway of estradiol inactivation. Naturally occurring estrogens administered orally are rapidly destroyed by gastrointestinal and liver enzymes; accordingly, they are usually given as conjugates or esters. The most widely used oral preparations are equine conjugated estrogens (Premarin) and ethinyl estradiol. Estrogen-containing skin patches for transdermal absorption are also used. With improvements in the understanding of estrogen and estrogen receptor interactions, a new class of compounds called selective estrogen-receptor modulators has been synthesized. For example, raloxifene, a nonsteroidal benzothiophene derivative, acts as an estrogen agonist in bone and liver and as an estrogen antagonist in breast and uterus. Androgens such as testosterone are generally injected intramuscularly as long-acting esters (enanthate or cypionate, most commonly) because of their potency and steady response. Transdermal testosterone patches applied to the scrotal or nonscrotal areas and a cutaneously applied gel have to date been used mostly in adults with hypogonadism because of the difficulty in titrating the doses needed during childhood and adolescence. Oral preparations, such as methyltestosterone or fluoxymesterone, do not produce so potent an androgenic response and may be hepatotoxic. Testosterone undecenoate, another oral preparation, is used in Europe but not in the United States. Sublingual (microspheres or pellets) and buccal (absorption via the buccal mucosa) preparations of testosterone are in development.

Bergada I, Bergada C, Campo S: Role of inhibins in childhood and puberty. *J Pediatr Endocrinol Metab* 2001;14:343–353.

Biason-Lauber A, Konrad D, Navratil F, et al: A WNT4 mutation associated with Müllerian-duct regression and virilization in a 46,XX woman. *N Engl J Med* 2005;351:792–798.

Bouvattier C, Carel JC, Lecointre C, et al: Postnatal changes of T, LH, and FSH in 46,XY infants with mutations in the AR gene. *J Pediatr Endocrinol Metab* 2002;87:29–32.

Habert R, Lejeune H, Saez J: Origin, differentiation and regulation of fetal and adult Leydig cells. *Mol Cell Endocrinol* 2001;179:47–74.

Hughes IA: Female development—all by default? *N Engl J Med* 2004;351: 748–750.

Josso N, diClemente N, Gouedard L: Anti-müllerian hormone and its receptors. *Mol Cell Endocrinol* 2001;179:25–32.

Koopman P: The genetics and biology of vertebrate sex determination. *Cell* 2001;105:843–847.

Ostrer H: Sex determination: Lessons from families and embryos. *Clin Genet* 2001;59:207–215.

Pierik FH, Vreeburg JTM, Stijnen T, et al: Serum inhibin B as a marker of spermatogenesis. *J Clin Endocrinol Metab* 1998;83:3110–3114.

Quigley CA: The postnatal gonadotropin and sex steroid surge: Insights from the androgen insensitivity syndrome. (Editorial.) *J Clin Endocrinol Metab* 2002;87:24–28.

Rajpert-De Meyts E: Expression of anti-müllerian hormone during normal and pathological gonadal development: Association with differentiation of Sertoli and granulosa cells. *J Clin Endocrinol Metab* 1999;84:3836–3844.

Rey RA, Belville C, Nihoul-Fékété C, et al: Evaluation of gonadal function in 107 intersex patients by means of serum anti-müllerian hormone measurements. *J Clin Endocrinol Metab* 1999;84:627–631.

Sequera AM, Fideleff HL, Boquete HR, et al: Basal ultra sensitive LH assay: A useful tool in the early diagnosis of male pubertal delay? *J Pediatr Endocrinol Metab* 2002;15:589–596.

Swerdloff RS, Wang C, Cunningham G, et al: Long-term pharmacokinetics of transdermal testosterone gel in hypogonadal men. *J Clin Endocrinol Metab* 2000;85:4500–4510.

Teixeira J, Maheswaran S, Donahue PK: Müllerian inhibiting substance: An instructive development hormone with diagnostic and possible therapeutic applications. *Endocr Rev* 2001;22:657–674.

Chapter 584 ■ Hypofunction of the Testes

Testicular hypofunction may be primary in the testis (primary hypogonadism) or secondary to deficiency of pituitary gonadotropic hormones (secondary hypogonadism). Patients with primary hypogonadism have elevated levels of gonadotropin (hypergonadotropic); those with secondary hypogonadism have low or absent levels (hypogonadotropic).

584.1 • Hypergonadotropic Hypogonadism in the Male (Primary Hypogonadism)

Defects of androgen production involving the fetal testis and resulting in male undervirilization are discussed in Chapter 589.2.

ETIOLOGY. Congenital anorchia occurs in 0.6% of boys with nonpalpable testes (1/20,000 males). These boys have normal external genitals, indicating that a noxious factor damaged the fetal testes of the genetic male fetus at some time after sexual differentiation had taken place (14th wk of fetal life). Hence, some refer to this condition as **vanishing testes syndrome.** The condition has been reported in monozygotic twins. Familial occurrence of this condition suggests a genetic etiology. Perhaps a more appropriate term for the condition may be **embryonic testicular regression syndrome.** Low levels of testosterone (<10 ng/dL) and markedly elevated levels of luteinizing hormone (LH) and follicle-stimulating hormone (FSH) are found in the early postnatal months; thereafter, levels of gonadotropins tend to decrease even in agonadal children, rising to very high levels as the pubertal years approach. Stimulation with human chorionic gonadotropin (hCG) fails to evoke an increase in the levels of testosterone. Serum levels of anti-müllerian hormone (AMH) are undetectable or low.

A syndrome of **rudimentary testes** has been described in which the testes are exceedingly small; this appears to be inherited as an autosomal or X-linked recessive trait. The cause is unknown. Atrophy of the testes may follow damage to the vascular supply as a result of unskillful manipulation of the testes during surgical procedures for correction of cryptorchidism or as a result of bilateral torsion of the testes. Acute orchitis in pubertal or adult males with mumps may occasionally damage the testes; usually, only the reproductive function of the testes is impaired. The routine immunization of all prepubertal males with mumps vaccine should prevent this complication.

Testicular damage is a frequent consequence of **chemotherapy** and **radiotherapy** for cancer. The frequency and extent of damage depend on the agent used, total dose, duration of therapy, and post-therapy interval of observation. Another important variable is age at therapy; germ cells are less vulnerable in prepubertal than in pubertal and postpubertal boys. Chemotherapy is most damaging if more than one agent is used. The use of alkylating agents such as cyclophosphamide in prepubertal children does not impair pubertal development, even though there may be biopsy evidence of germ cell damage. High doses of cyclophosphamide and ifosfamide are associated with infertility. Most chemotherapeutic agents produce azoospermia and infertility more commonly than Leydig cell damage. Cisplatin also causes transient azoospermia or oligospermia. Interleukin-2 can depress Leydig cell function, whereas interferon-α does not seem to affect gonadal function.

Radiation damage is dose dependent (see Chapter 706). Temporary azoospermia can be seen with doses greater than 0.1 Gy, with permanent azoospermia seen with doses greater than 2 Gy. Leydig cells are more resistant to irradiation. Mild damage as determined by elevated LH levels can be seen with up to 6 Gy; doses greater than 30 Gy cause hypogonadism in most. Whenever possible, testes should be shielded from irradiation. Testicular function should be carefully evaluated in adolescents after multimodal treatment for cancer in childhood. Replacement therapy with testosterone and counseling concerning fertility may be indicated.

The term hypogonadism has been widely used to describe aspects in children with a variety of multiple malformation syndromes. The term often refers simply to cryptorchidism, a small phallus, or a scrotal anomaly. In many of these syndromes, little is known about the function of the testes; hypergonadotropic or hypogonadotropic hypogonadism has been proved in some instances.

In patients with **Prader-Willi syndrome,** both hypogonadotropic hypogonadism and hypergonadotropic hypogonadism, perhaps secondary to cryptorchidism and its treatment, have been reported (see Chapters 80 and 81). Growth hormone treatment has resulted in improved body composition, physical and psychomotor function, as well as growth in these patients. Reports of death in few growth hormone–treated patients with Prader Willi syndrome make it imperative that extreme caution be used before such treatment is recommended. Small testes and azoospermia are seen in patients with the Sertoli cell–only syndrome (germ cell aplasia, or **Del Castillo syndrome**).

Various degrees of hypogonadism also occur in a significant percentage of patients with chromosomal aberrations such as in **Klinefelter syndrome** or in **XX males.**

CLINICAL MANIFESTATIONS. Primary hypogonadism may be suspected at birth if the testes and penis are abnormally small. Normative data are available for different populations. The condition often is not noticed until puberty, when secondary sex characteristics fail to develop. Facial, pubic, and axillary hair is scant or absent; there is neither acne nor regression of scalp hair; and the voice remains high pitched. The penis and scrotum remain infantile and may be almost obscured by pubic fat; the testes are small or absent. Fat accumulates in the region of the hips and buttocks and sometimes in the breasts and on the abdomen. The epiphyses close late in life; therefore, extremities are long. The span is several inches longer than the height, and the distance from the symphysis pubis to the soles of the feet is much greater than that from the symphysis to the vertex. The proportions of the body are described as **eunuchoid.** The upper to lower segment ratio is considerably less than 0.9. Many individuals with milder degrees of hypogonadism may be detected only by appropriate studies of the pituitary-gonadal axis. Examination of the testes should be performed routinely by pediatricians; testicular volumes as determined by comparison with standard orchidometers should be recorded.

DIAGNOSIS. Levels of serum FSH and, to a lesser extent, of LH are elevated to greater than age-specific normal values. These elevated levels indicate that even in the prepubertal child there is an active hypothalamic-gonadal feedback relationship. After the age of 11 yr, FSH and LH levels rise significantly, reaching the castrate range. Measurements of random plasma testosterone levels in prepubertal boys are not helpful because they are ordinarily low in normal prepubertal children, rising during puberty to attain adult levels. During puberty, these levels correlate better with testicular size, stage of sexual maturity, and bone age than with chronologic age. In patients with primary hypogonadism, testosterone levels remain low at all ages. There is an attenuated rise or no rise after administration of hCG, in contrast to normal males in whom hCG produces a significant rise in plasma testosterone at any stage of development. Measurements of serum AMH and inhibin levels may give an indication of gonadal presence and function.

NOONAN SYNDROME

ETIOLOGY. The term Noonan syndrome has been applied to males and females with normal karyotypes who have certain phenotypic features that occur also in females with Turner syndrome (see Chapter 81). Noonan syndrome occurs in 1 : 1000–2500 live births. The disorder is autosomal dominant with variable expression. Sporadic and autosomal recessive occurrence has been reported. Missense mutations in *PTPN11*—a gene on chromosome 12q24.1 encoding the nonreceptor protein tyrosine phosphatase SHP-2—are seen in the majority of studied cases. Mutations in the *KRAS* gene may also cause Noonan syndrome.

CLINICAL MANIFESTATIONS. The most common abnormalities are short stature, webbing of the neck, pectus carinatum or pectus excavatum, cubitus valgus, right-sided congenital heart disease, and characteristic facies. Hypertelorism, epicanthus, downward slanted palpebral fissures, ptosis, micrognathia, and ear abnormalities are common. Other abnormalities such as clinodactyly, hernias, and vertebral anomalies occur less frequently. The mean IQ of school-aged children with the condition is 86, with a range of 53 to 127. Verbal IQ tends to be better than performance IQ. High-frequency sensorineural hearing loss is common. The cardiac defect is most often pulmonary valvular stenosis, hypertrophic cardiomyopathy, or atrial septal defect. Hepatosplenomegaly and several hematologic diseases, including low clotting factors XI and XII, acute lymphoblastic leukemia, and chronic myelomonocytic leukemia, are noted. Features of both Noonan syndrome and type 1 neurofibromatosis have been reported, but linkage has been excluded. Noonan-like features can be part of the phenotypic variation of the NF1 gene mutation, suggesting the possible existence of a Noonan syndrome locus also on chromosome 17q. A few patients with NF1 and features of Noonan syndrome were subsequently reported as having Turner syndrome. Males frequently have cryptorchidism and small testes; they may be hypogonadal or normal. Puberty is delayed 2 yr; adult height is achieved by the end of the 2nd decade and usually reaches the lowest limit of the normal population. Prenatal diagnosis should be suspected in fetuses with normal karyotype, edema, or hydrops and short femur length.

TREATMENT. Human growth hormone has resulted in improvement in growth velocity comparable to that seen in patients with Turner syndrome without adverse effects on cardiac ventricular wall thickness. Improved adult height after growth hormone treatment has been reported in a few patients. Patients with Noonan syndrome and demonstrable *PTNP11* mutations grow less well and are less responsive to growth hormone treatment than those without mutations. They have lower IGF1 and higher GH levels, suggesting the possibility of partial GH resistance due to postreceptor signaling defects.

KLINEFELTER SYNDROME

Also see Chapters 81 and 561.

ETIOLOGY. Approximately 1/500 newborn males has a 47,XXY chromosome complement, representing the most common sex chromosomal aneuploidy in males. The incidence approximates 1% among the mentally retarded, clustering among patients with IQs greater than 50 and among children admitted to psychiatric hospitals or referred to psychiatric clinics. In infertile males, the incidence is 3% and in those with oligospermia or azoospermia 5–10%. The chromosomal aberration most often results from meiotic nondisjunction of an X chromosome during parental gametogenesis; the extra X chromosome is maternal in origin in 54% and paternal in origin in 46% of patients. Increased maternal age predisposes to meiotic nondisjunction and to this syndrome, but in most instances maternal age is not advanced. A national study in Denmark revealed a prenatal prevalence of 213 per 100,000 male fetuses and, standardized according to maternal age, of 153/100,000. In adult men, the prevalence was only 40/100,000, suggesting that only 1 in 4 of adult males with Klinefelter syndrome was diagnosed.

The 47,XXY complement is the most common chromosomal pattern in persons with Klinefelter syndrome (80%); some have mosaic patterns: 46,XY/47,XXY, 46,XY/48,XXYY, 45,X/46,XY/47,XXY, or 46,XX/47,XXY. Rarely, occurrence of more than two X chromosomes may result in Klinefelter variants: 48,XXXY, 49,XXXYY, 49,XXXXY, 50,XXXXYY, 47,XXY/48,XXXY, 47,XXY/ 49,XXXXY, or 48,XXYY karyotype. Even with as many as four X chromosomes, the Y chromosome determines a male phenotype. In most patients with four or five X chromosomes, all the additional chromosomes come from the same parent and are not associated with increased parental age.

CLINICAL MANIFESTATIONS. The diagnosis is rarely made before puberty because of the paucity or subtleness of clinical manifestations in childhood. Because behavioral or psychiatric disorders may often be apparent long before defects in sexual development, the condition should be considered in all boys with mental retardation and in children with psychosocial, learning, or school adjustment problems. Affected children may be anxious, immature, excessively shy, or aggressive, and they may engage in antisocial acts. Fire-setting behavior has been observed in some of these children. In a prospective study, a group of children with 47,XXY karyotypes identified at birth exhibited relatively mild deviations from normal during the first 5 yr of life. None had major physical, intellectual, or emotional disabilities; some were inactive, with poorly organized motor function and mild delay in language acquisition. Problems often first become apparent after the child begins school. Full-scale IQ scores may be normal, with verbal IQ being somewhat decreased. Verbal cognitive defects and underachievement in reading, spelling, and mathematics are common. By late adolescence, most boys with Klinefelter syndrome have generalized learning disabilities, most of which are language based, and are 4 to 5 grade levels behind. Despite these difficulties, most complete high school. High-resolution MRI has shown reduction in left temporal lobe gray matter volumes (less so in testosterone-treated subjects).

The patients tend to be tall, slim, and underweight and to have relatively long legs, but body habitus can vary markedly. The testes tend to be small for age, but this sign may become apparent only after puberty, when normal testicular growth fails to occur. The phallus tends to be smaller than average, and cryptorchidism or hypospadias may occur in a few patients.

Pubertal development may be delayed, although some children may undergo almost normal virilization. A study of 14 nonmosaic 47,XXY Finnish boys had normal onset and progression of puberty with normal increases in serum testosterone and PSA, and decrease in leptin and SHBG concentrations. Despite normal testosterone levels, serum LH and FSH concentrations and their responses to gonadotropin-releasing hormone (GnRH) stimulation were elevated starting at 13 yr of age. About 80% of adults have **gynecomastia;** they have sparser facial hair, most shaving less often than daily. The most common testicular lesions are spermatogenic arrest and Sertoli cell predominance. The sperm have a high incidence of sex chromosomal aneuploidy. Azoospermia and infertility are usual, although rare instances of fertility are known. Testicular sperm extraction followed by intracytoplasmic sperm injection can result in the birth of healthy infants. Antisperm antibodies have been detected in one quarter of tested specimens. In nonmosaic Klinefelter patients, most testicular sperm (94%) have a normal pattern of sex chromosome segregation.

The height of patients with Klinefelter syndrome tends to be increased. There is an increased incidence of pulmonary disease, varicose veins, and cancer of the breast. Among 93 unselected **male breast cancer** patients, 7.5% were found to have Klinefelter syndrome. Mediastinal germ cell tumors have been reported; some of these tumors produce hCG and cause precocious puberty in young boys. They may also be associated with leukemia, lymphoma, and other hematologic neoplasia. The highest cancer risk (relative risk 2.7) occurs in the 15–30 yr age group. A large cohort study in Britain demonstrated an overall significantly increased standardized mortality ratio (1.5) with particular increases in deaths due to diabetes, epilepsy, peripheral and intestinal vascular sufficiency, pulmonary embolism and renal disease. Mortality from ischemic heart disease was decreased. In adults, structural brain abnormalities correlate with cognitive deficits.

In adults with XY/XXY mosaicism, the features of Klinefelter syndrome are decreased in severity and frequency. Children with mosaicism have a better prognosis for virilization, fertility, and psychosocial adjustment.

Klinefelter Variants. When the number of X chromosomes exceeds 2, the clinical manifestations, including mental retardation and impairment of virilization, are more severe. The XXYY variant is the most common variant (1/50,000 male births). In most, mental retardation occurs with IQ scores between 60 and 80, but 10% have IQs greater than 110. The XXYY male phenotype is not distinctively different from that of the XXY patient, except that XXYY adults tend to be taller than the average XXY patient. The 49,XXXXY variant is sufficiently distinctive to be detected in childhood. Its incidence is estimated to be 1/80,000 to 1/100,000 male births. The disorder arises from sequential nondisjunction in meiosis. Affected patients are severely retarded and have short necks and typical coarse facies with wide-set eyes with a mild upward slant of the fissures, epicanthus, strabismus, a wide and flat upturned nose, a large open mouth, and large malformed ears. The testes are small and may be undescended, the scrotum is hypoplastic, and the penis is very small. Defects suggestive of Down syndrome (short, incurved terminal 5th phalanges, single palmar creases, and hypotonia) and other skeletal abnormalities (including defects in the carrying angle of the elbows and restricted supination) are common. The most frequent radiographic abnormalities are radioulnar synostosis or dislocation, elongated radius, pseudoepiphyses, scoliosis or kyphosis, coxa valga, and retarded osseous age. Most patients with such extensive changes have a 49,XXXXY chromosome karyotype; several mosaic patterns have also been observed: 48,XXXY/49,XXXXY (Fig. 584-1); 48,XXXY/49,XXXXY/50,XXXXXY; and 48,XXXY/49,XXXXY/50,XXXXYY. Prenatal diagnosis of a 49,XXXXY infant has been reported. The fetus had intrauterine growth retardation, edema, and cystic hygroma colli.

The 48,XXXY variant is relatively rare. The characteristic features are generally less severe than those of patients with 49,XXXXY and more severe than those of 47,XXY patients. Mild mental retardation, delayed speech and motor development, and immature but passive and pleasant behavior are associated with this condition.

Very few patients have been described with 49,XYYY and 49,XXYYY karyotypes. Dysmorphic features and mental retardation are common to both.

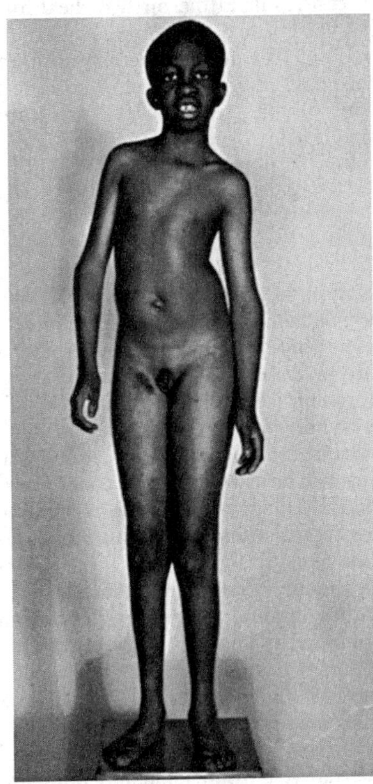

Figure 584-1. A 12-yr-old boy with 48,XXXY/49,XXXXY mosaicism who has prognathism, epicanthal folds, scoliosis, small testes, severe mental retardation, clinodactyly, and radioulnar synostoses.

LABORATORY FINDINGS. Most males with this condition go through life undiagnosed. The chromosomes should be examined in all patients suspected of having Klinefelter syndrome, particularly those attending child guidance, psychiatric, and mental retardation clinics. In infancy, inhibin B and AMH levels are normal but testosterone levels lower than in controls. Before 10 yr of age, boys with 47,XXY Klinefelter syndrome have normal basal plasma levels of FSH and LH. Responses to gonadotropin-stimulating hormone and to hCG are normal. The testes show normal growth early in puberty, but by mid-puberty the testicular growth stops, gonadotropins become elevated, and testosterone levels are slightly low. Inhibin B levels are normal in early puberty, decrease in late puberty, and are low in adults with the syndrome. Elevated levels of estradiol, resulting in a high estradiol to testosterone ratio, account for the development of gynecomastia during puberty. Despite hypogonadism, most have normal bone mass. Long androgen receptor polyglutamine (CAG) repeat length is associated with the more severe phenotype including gynecomastia, small testes, and short penile length.

Testicular biopsy before puberty may reveal only deficiency or absence of germinal cells. After puberty, the seminiferous tubular membranes are hyalinized, and there is adenomatous clumping of Leydig cells. Sertoli cells predominate. Azoospermia is characteristic, and infertility is the rule.

TREATMENT. Replacement therapy with a long-acting testosterone preparation depends on the age of the patient. It should begin at 11–12 yr of age. The enanthate ester may be used in a starting dose of 25–50 mg injected intramuscularly every 3–4 wk, with 50-mg increments every 6–9 mo until a maintenance dose for adults (200–250 mg every 3–4 wk) is achieved. At that time, testosterone patches or testosterone gel may be substituted for the injections. For older boys, larger initial doses and increments can achieve more rapid virilization. Testosterone treatment leads to an increase in prostate volume and prostate-specific antigen levels. Testicular sperm extraction followed by intracytoplasmic sperm injection can result in the birth of healthy infants. Antisperm antibodies have been detected in one quarter of tested specimens. In nonmosaic Klinefelter patients, most testicular sperm (94%) have a normal pattern of sex chromosome segregation to treatment. At one center, sperm retrieval rates are greater than 70%, with nearly 70% of men having adequate sperms found, nearly half resulting in normal live births.

XX MALES

This disorder is thought to occur in 1 in 20,000 newborn males. Affected individuals have a male phenotype, small testes, a small phallus, and no evidence of ovarian or müllerian duct tissue; they appear, therefore, to be distinct from the ovotesticular disorder of sexual development (see Chapter 589.3). This disorder resembles Klinefelter syndrome, but stature is greater in the latter. Undescended testes and hypospadias occur in a minority of patients. The histologic features of the testes are essentially the same as in Klinefelter syndrome. Patients with the condition usually come to medical attention in adult life because of hypogonadism, gynecomastia, or infertility. Hypergonadotropic hypogonadism occurs secondary to testicular failure. A few cases have been diagnosed perinatally as a result of discrepancies between prenatal ultrasonography and karyotype findings.

In 80% of XX males with normal male external genitals, one of the X chromosomes carries the *SRY* gene. The exchange from the Y to the X chromosome occurs during paternal meiosis, when the short arms of the Y and X chromosomes pair. XX males inherit one maternal X chromosome and one paternal X chromosome containing the translocated male-determining gene. Such exchanges occur because of the proximity of the SRY gene to the pseudoautosomal region where recombination between X and Y chromosomes normally occurs in meiosis. A few cases of 46,XX males with 9P translocations were identified. Most XX males who are identified before puberty have hypospadias or micropenis; this group of patients usually lacks Y-specific sequences, suggesting other mechanisms for virilization (see Chapter 576). Fluorescent in situ hybridization and primed in situ labeling (PRINS) have been used to identify small *SRY* DNA segments. Yp fragment abnormalities may result in sexually ambiguous phenotypes.

45,X MALES

Also see Chapter 583.

Of the few male patients recognized with a 45,X karyotype, Yp sequences have been translocated to an autosomal chromosome. In one instance, the terminal short arm of the Y chromosome was translocated onto an X chromosome. In another, *SRY/autosomal* translocation was postulated. A male with 45,X karyotype and Leri-Weill dyschondrosteosis, *SHOX* gene loss, and SRY to Xp translocation was also described.

47,XXX MALES

A Japanese male with poor pubic hair development, hypoplastic scrotal testes (4 mL), normal penis and normal height, gynecomastia, and severe mental retardation had 47,XXX karyotype due to abnormal X-Y interchange during paternal meiosis and X-X nondisjunction during maternal meiosis.

584.2 • Hypogonadotropic Hypogonadism in the Male (Secondary Hypogonadism)

In hypogonadotropic hypogonadism, there is deficiency of FSH or LH, or both. The primary defect may lie in the anterior pituitary or in the hypothalamus as a deficiency of GnRH. The testes are normal but remain in the prepubertal state because stimulation by gonadotropins is lacking. The disorder may be recognized in infancy, around the time of puberty, or rarely in adulthood. Several different gene defects have been described in patients with hypogonadotropic hypogonadism.

ETIOLOGY

Hypopituitarism. Most causes of hypopituitarism may be associated with deficiency of gonadotropins and hypogonadotropic hypogonadism (see Chapter 558). In patients with organic lesions in or near the pituitary, whether congenital or acquired, the gonadotropin deficiency is pituitary in origin. In most patients with "idiopathic" hypopituitarism, the defect is in the hypothalamus, caused by a deficiency of GnRH. In patients with multiple pituitary hormone deficiencies, defects in pituitary transcription factors such as PROP-1, HESX-1, and LHX-3 have been described. Microphallus (<2.5 cm) in the newborn male with growth hormone deficiency suggests the likelihood of gonadotropin deficiency.

Isolated Deficiency of Gonadotropin. Usually, this disorder involves the hypothalamus rather than the pituitary. It affects about 1/10,000 males and 1/50,000 females and encompasses a heterogeneous group of entities. GnRH deficiency may be complete or partial; it may occur sporadically or in families. A locus for an autosomal recessive form of idiopathic hypogonadotropic hypogonadism has been identified on chromosome 19p13.3.

Kallmann syndrome, one of the most frequent genetic forms of hypogonadotropic hypogonadism, is characterized by its association with **anosmia** or **hyposmia.** The X-linked disorder (KAL1) is caused by mutations of the *KAL* gene at Xp22.3. The association reflects the failure of olfactory axons and GnRH-expressing neurons to migrate from their common origin in the olfactory placode to the brain. The *KAL* gene product anosmin-1, an extracellular 95 kDa matrix glycoprotein, facilitates neuronal growth and migration. The *KAL* gene is also expressed in various parts of the brain, facial mesenchyme, and mesonephros and metanephros, thus explaining some of the associated findings in patients with Kallman syndrome, such as synkinesia, midfacial defects, and renal agenesis.

Some kindreds contain anosmic individuals with or without hypogonadism; others contain hypogonadal individuals who are anosmic. Cleft lip and palate, hypotelorism, median facial clefts, sensorineural hearing loss, unilateral renal aplasia, neurologic deficits, and other findings occur in some affected patients. When Kallmann syndrome is caused by terminal or interstitial deletions of the Xp22.3 region, it may be associated with other contiguous gene syndromes, such as steroid sulfatase deficiency, chondrodysplasia punctata, X-linked ichthyosis, or ocular albinism. Mental disorders are not seen in patients whose mutations are restricted to the KAL1 locus.

Autosomal dominant and autosomal recessive forms of Kallmann syndrome have been reported.

The autosomal dominant form of Kallman syndrome (KAL 2) occurring in 10% of patients, is due to a loss of function mutation in the fibroblast growth factor receptor 1 (FGFR1) gene. Cleft lip and palate is associated with KAL2 but not with KAL1. Oligodontia and hearing loss may occur with both KAL1 and KAL2. There is a less well described autosomal recessive form of the disease (KAL3).

Children with **X-linked congenital adrenal hypoplasia** have associated hypogonadotropic hypogonadism (HHG) owing to impaired GnRH secretion. In these patients, there is a mutation of the *DAX1* gene at Xp21.2–21.3. Conditions occasionally associated with these patients because of the **contiguous gene syndrome** include glycerol kinase deficiency, Duchenne muscular dystrophy, and ornithine transcarbamoyl transferase deficiency. Most boys with *DAX1* mutations develop HHG in adolescence, although a patient with adult-onset adrenal insufficiency and partial HHG and two females with HHG and delayed puberty have also been described, the latter as part of extended families with males with classic HHG. The *DAX1* gene defect is, however, rare in patients with delayed puberty or HHG without at least a family history of adrenal failure.

Several genetic defects involving the hypothalamic-pituitary-gonadal axis have been identified. They involve the function of either hormones or their receptors. Depending on both the level and nature of the mutation, hypogonadism, precocious puberty, or sexual ambiguity may develop. To date, eight different GnRH-receptor gene mutations, most compound heterozygotes, have been identified as the cause of HHG. The phenotype, however, varies from partial to complete hypogonadism. A mutation in the gene for the β subunit of LH at the level of the pituitary causes HHG. At the level of the gonads, LH-receptor defects have led to Leydig cell hypoplasia and undervirilization in genetic males. A boy was reported with micropenis and normal testes that did not produce testosterone even after repeated courses of hCG. Vanishing Leydig cell syndrome was thought to be a possibility (by analogy with the vanishing testes syndrome). Normally functioning Leydig cells must have been present in the first trimester of pregnancy, but because of LH receptor defect, inadequate testosterone production in the 2nd and 3rd trimesters led to an underdeveloped penis at birth. A novel mutation of the β subunit of FSH also has been described as the cause of hypogonadism in an 18-yr-old man evaluated for delayed puberty and in three women with delayed puberty and primary amenorrhea (Table 584-1). Mutations in leptin, in the leptin receptor, and in the endopeptidase prohormone convertase-1 (PC-1), have been associated with HHG.

Other Disorders. HHG has been observed in a few patients with polyglandular autoimmune syndrome, in some with elevated melatonin levels, and in those with a variety of other syndromes such as Bardet-Biedl, Prader-Willi, multiple lentigines, and several ataxia syndromes.

TABLE 584-1. Known Gene Defects Causing Hypogonadism

DEFECT	CLINICAL CONDITION	AFFECTED GENDER
GONADOTROPIN-RELEASING HORMONE		
KAL-1	Kallmann syndrome	Both
DAX-1	X-linked adrenal hypoplasia and hypogonadotropic hypogonadism	Male
Receptor	Familial hypogonadotropic hypogonadism	Both
LUTEINIZING HORMONE		
β Subunit	Pubertal delay, Leydig cell hypoplasia, infertility	Male
Receptor	Male pseudohermaphroditism, Leydig cell hypoplasia, micropenis Amenorrhea	Both
FOLLICLE-STIMULATING HORMONE		
β Subunit	Pubertal delay Amenorrhea	Both
Receptor	Ovarian failure Ovarian germ cell tumors	Female

DIAGNOSIS. Levels of gonadotropins and gonadal steroids remain in the prepubertal range, and nocturnal pulsatile secretion of LH does not occur. The gonadotropin response to stimulation with GnRH or a more potent analog of GnRH is markedly blunted. These findings are also consistent with those observed in normal adolescents with the variant known as constitutional delayed puberty; it is difficult to distinguish between the two conditions. Many different tests, including stimulation tests with GnRH, thyrotropin-releasing hormone, metoclopramide, and domperidone, have yielded inconclusive results. The measurement of a single, 8 A.M. testosterone level may be a good indicator of impending puberty. A value of more than 0.7 nmol/L (20 mg/dL) was noted in boys all of whom had an increase in testicular volume to greater than 4 mL by 15 mo and 77% by 12 mo. In contrast, of boys with testosterone levels lower than 0.7 nmol/L, only 25% entered puberty by 15 yr of age. The use of a GnRH analog or the GnRH test after 36 hr of "priming" of the hypothalamic-pituitary-gonadal axis with pulsatile GnRH administration may distinguish adolescents with hypogonadism from those with delayed puberty.

Gonadotropin deficiency is likely if the patient has evidence of another pituitary deficiency, such as a deficiency of growth hormone, particularly if it is associated with corticotropin (adrenocorticotropic hormone [ACTH]) deficiency. The presence of **anosmia** usually indicates permanent gonadotropin deficiency, but occasional instances of markedly delayed puberty (18–20 yr of age) have been observed in anosmic individuals. Although anosmia may be present in the family or in the patient from early childhood, its existence is rarely volunteered, and direct questioning is necessary in all patients with delayed puberty. MRI may detect anomalous olfactory lobes and sulci in some patients. **Prolactinomas** are increasingly recognized as a cause of delayed puberty and should be excluded by determination of serum levels of prolactin.

Probes are available to establish the diagnosis in heterozygotes and newborn infants with the X-linked form of Kallmann syndrome. During the first 3–4 mo of life, unaffected infants demonstrate the usual physiologic rise in gonadotropins and gonadal steroids, and the response to GnRH exceeds that seen in prepubertal children. Adult men with documented *KAL1* mutations have complete lack of LH pulsations.

TREATMENT. Constitutional delayed puberty should be ruled out before a diagnosis of isolated deficiency of GnRH is established and treatment is initiated. Testicular volume of less than 4 mL by 14 yr of age occurs in about 3% of boys, but true hypogonadotropic hypogonadism is a rare condition. Even relatively moderate delays in sexual development and growth may result in significant psychologic distress and require attention. Initially, an explanation of the variations characteristic of puberty and reassurance suffice for the majority of boys. If by 15 yr of age no clinical evidence of puberty is beginning and the testosterone level is less than 50 ng/dL, a brief course of testosterone is indicated. Testosterone enanthate, 100 mg intramuscularly once monthly for 4–6 mo, usually results in an increase in the signs of secondary sexual characteristics and an increase in growth velocity; it may initiate puberty and may differentiate constitutional delay in puberty from isolated gonadotropin deficiency. The age of initiation of this treatment must be individualized.

Patients with established deficiency of gonadotropins should be treated with the same program of repository testosterone as that used for those with primary testicular deficiency (see Chapter 584.1). With this therapy, the testes will remain small. Treatment with hCG, given subcutaneously or intramuscularly in doses of 500–1,000 IU, three times weekly, stimulates growth of the testes and spermatogenesis. If, after 6–12 mo of therapy, sufficient growth of the testes has not occurred, human menopausal gonadotropin may be added in a dose of 37.5–150 IU, three times weekly. It may require up to 2 yr of treatment to achieve adequate spermatogenesis in adults. Recombinantly produced gonadotropins are able to stimulate gonadal growth and function.

A more physiologic but cumbersome form of treatment consists of episodic administration (subcutaneously or intravenously) of GnRH. Long-term therapy has been provided with a programmable peristaltic infusion pump. Most patients require about 2 yr of treatment to maximize testicular growth and achieve spermatogenesis.

Acierno SA, Shagoury JK, Bo-Abbas Y, et al: A locus for autosomal recessive idiopathic hypogonadotropic hypogonadism on chromosome 19p13.3. *J Clin Endocrinol Metab* 2003;88:2730–2737.

Bahuau M, Houdayer C, Assouline B, et al: Novel recurrent nonsense mutation causing neurofibromatosis type 1 (NF1) in a family segregating both NF1 and Noonan syndrome. *Am J Med Genet* 1998;75:265–272.

Carrel AL, Myers SE, Whitman BY, et al: Growth hormone improves body composition, fat utilization, physical strength and agility, and growth in Prader-Willi syndrome: A controlled study. *J Pediatr* 2000;134:215–221.

Cotterill AM, McKenna WJ, Brady AF, et al: The short-term effects of growth hormone therapy on height velocity and cardiac ventricular wall thickness in children with Noonan syndrome. *J Clin Endocrinol Metab* 1996;81:2291–2297.

DeRoux N, Young J, Misrahi M, et al: A family with hypogonadotropic hypogonadism and mutations in the gonadotropin-releasing hormone receptor. *N Engl J Med* 1997;337:1597–1602.

Dobs AS, Hoover DR, Chen MC, et al: Pharmacokinetic characteristics, efficacy, and safety of buccal testosterone in hypogonadal males: A pilot study. *J Clin Endocrinol Metab* 1998;83:33–39.

Geschwind DH, Boone KB, Miller BL, et al: Neurobehavioral phenotype of Klinefelter syndrome. *Ment Retard Dev Disabil Res Rev* 2000;6:107–116.

Goodfellow PN, Camerino G: DAX-1, an "antitestis" gene. *EXS* 2001;91:57–69.

Hardelin J: Kallmann syndrome: Towards molecular pathogenesis. *Mol Cell Endocrinol* 2001;179:75–81.

Hultborn R, Hanson C, Kopf I, et al: Prevalence of Klinefelter's syndrome in male breast cancer patients. *Anticancer Res* 1997;17:4293–1497.

Itti E, Gaw Gonzalo IT, Pawlikowska-Haddal A, et al: The structural brain correlates of cognitive deficits in adults with Klinefelter's syndrome. *J Clin Endocrinol Metab* 2006;91:1423–1427.

Kadandale JS, Wachtel SS, Tunca Y, et al: Localization of SRY by primed in situ labeling in XX and XY sex reversal. *Am J Med Genet* 2000;95:71–74.

Khorram O, Patrizio P, Wang C, et al: Reproductive technologies for male infertility. *J Clin Endocrinol Metab* 2001;86:2373–2379.

Latronico AC, Anasti J, Arnhold IJ, et al: Brief report: Testicular and ovarian resistance to luteinizing hormone caused by inactivating mutations of the luteinizing hormone-receptor gene. *N Engl J Med* 1996;334:507–512.

Layman LC, Lee EJ, Peak DB, et al: Delayed puberty and hypogonadism caused by mutations in the follicle stimulating hormone β-subunit gene. *N Engl J Med* 1997;337:607–611.

Lee MM, Donahoe PK, Silverman BL, et al: Measurements of serum müllerian inhibiting substance in the evaluation of children with nonpalpable gonads. *N Engl J Med* 1997;336:1480–1486.

Limal J, Parfait B, Cabrol S, et al: Noonan Syndrome: Relationships between genotype, growth, and growth factors. *J Clin Endocrinol Metab* 2006;91:300–306.

Matthews CH, Borgato S, Beck-Peccoz, et al: Primary amenorrhea and infertility due to a mutation in the β-subunit of follicle-stimulating hormone. *Nat Genet* 1993;5:83–86.

McCabe ERB: Vulnerability within a robust complex system-DAX1 mutations and steroidogenic axis development. *J Clin Endocrinol Metab* 2002;87:41–43.

Merke DP, Tajima T, Baron J, et al: Hypogonadotropic hypogonadism in a female caused by an X-linked recessive mutation in the DAX1 gene. *N Engl J Med* 1999;340:1248–1252.

Meyer J, Sudbeck P, Held M, et al: Mutational analysis of the SOX9 gene in campomelic dysplasia and autosomal sex reversal: Lack of genotype/phenotype correlations. *Hum Mol Genet* 1997;6:91–98.

Muller J: Hypogonadism and endocrine metabolic disorders in Prader-Willi syndrome. *Acta Paediatr Suppl* 1997;423:58–59.

Nisbet DL, Griffin DR, Chitty LS: Prenatal features of Noonan syndrome. *Prenat Diagn* 1999;19:642–647.

Noonan JA: Noonan syndrome revisited. *J Pediatr* 1999;135:667–668.

Ogata T, Matsuo M, Muroya K, et al: 47,XXX male: A clinical and molecular study. *Am J Med Genet* 2001;98:353–356.

Patwardhan AJ, Eliez S, Bender B, et al: Brain morphology in Klinefelter syndrome: Extra X chromosome and testosterone supplementation. *Neurology* 2000;54:2218–2223.

Phillip M, Arbelle JE, Segev Y, et al: Male hypogonadism due to a mutation in the gene for the β-subunit of follicle-stimulating hormone. *N Engl J Med* 1998;338:1729–1732.

Romano AA, Blethen SL, Dana K, et al: Growth hormone treatment in Noonan syndrome: The National Cooperative Growth Study experience. *J Pediatr* 1996;128:S18–21.

Rovet J, Netley C, Keenan M, et al: The psychoeducational profile of boys with Klinefelter syndrome. *J Learn Disabil* 1996;29:180–196.

Sato N, Katsumata N, Kagami M, et al: Clinical assessment of mutation analysis of Kallman Syndrome 1 (KAL1) and fibroblast growth factor receptor 1 (FGFR1, or KAL2) in five families and 18 sporadic patients. *J Clin Endocrinol Metab* 2004;89:1079–1088.

Schiff JD, Palermo GD, Veeck LL, et al: Success of testicular sperm injection and intracytoplasmic sperm injection in men with Klinefelter Syndrome. *J Clin Endocrinol Metab* 2005;90:6263–6267.

Schubbert S, Zenker M, Rowe SL, et al: Germline KRAS mutations cause Noonan syndrome. *Nat Genet* 2006;38:331–336.

Smals AGH, Hermus ARM, Boers GHJ, et al: Predictive value of luteinizing hormone releasing hormone (LHRH) bolus testing before and after 36-hour pulsatile LHRH administration in the differential diagnosis of constitutional delay of puberty and male hypogonadotropic hypogonadism. *J Clin Endocrinol Metab* 1994;78:602–608.

Stuppia L, Calabrese G, Borrelli P, et al: Loss of the SHOX gene associated with Leri-Weill dyschondrosteosis in a 45,X male. *J Med Genet* 1999;36:711–713.

Swerdlow AJ, Higgins CD, Schoemaker MJ, et al: Mortality in patients with Klinefelter Syndrome in Britain: A cohort study. *J Clin Endocrinol Metab* 2005;90:6516–6522.

Toledo SPA, Brunner HG, Kraaij R, et al: An inactivating mutation of the luteinizing hormone receptor causes amenorrhea in a 46,XX female. *J Clin Endocrinol Metab* 1996;81:3850–3854.

VanDop C, Burstein S, Conte FA, et al: Isolated gonadotropin deficiency in boys: Clinical characteristics and growth. *J Pediatr* 1987;111:684–692.

Wu FC, Brown DC, Butler GE, et al: Early morning plasma testosterone is an accurate predictor of imminent pubertal development in prepubertal boys. *J Clin Endocrinol Metab* 1993;76:26–31.

Chapter 585 ■ Pseudoprecocity Resulting from Tumors of the Testes

Leydig cell tumors of the testes are rare causes of precocious pseudopuberty and cause asymmetric enlargement of the testes.

They account for 3% of all testicular tumors. Leydig cells are sparse before puberty; tumors derived from them are more common in the adult. The reported cases in children include one member in each of two pairs of identical twins. These tumors are usually unilateral and benign; 10% may become malignant. Reinke crystalloids are a characteristic microscopic feature but occur in fewer than 50% of Leydig cell tumors. A *gsp* mutation was described in one testicular Leydig cell tumor. In adult testes, testicular germ cell tumors, but not Sertoli cell tumors or Leydig cell tumors, exhibit bi-allelic expression of the human *H19* gene.

The **clinical manifestations** are those of puberty in the male; onset occurs usually from 5 to 9 yr of age. Gynecomastia has been described. The tumor of the testis can usually be readily felt; the contralateral unaffected testis is normal in size for the age of the patient.

Plasma levels of testosterone are markedly elevated. Follicle-stimulating hormone and luteinizing hormone levels are suppressed, and there is no response to gonadotropin-releasing hormone. Ultrasonography may aid in the detection of small nonpalpable tumors. Fine-needle aspiration biopsy may help define the diagnosis.

Treatment consists of surgical removal of the affected testis. Progression of virilization ceases, and partial reversal of the signs of precocity may occur.

Testicular adrenal rests may develop into tumors that mimic Leydig cell tumors; in the absence of Reinke crystals, these two tumors cannot be differentiated histologically. Adrenal rest tumors are usually bilateral and occur in children with congenital adrenal hyperplasia, usually salt-losing patients, during adolescence or young adult life. The stimulus for the growth of the adrenal rests is inadequate corticosteroid suppressive therapy, and treatment with adequate doses almost always results in their regression. Definite evidence of the origin of these tumors has been achieved by demonstrating their 21-hydroxylase activity. The misdiagnosis of these tumors in patients with congenital adrenal hyperplasia has led to unnecessary orchidectomy.

Fragile X syndrome is a common cause of hereditary mental retardation, with an incidence of 1/2,000 births. It is caused by the amplification of a polymorphic CGG repeat in the 5′ untranslated region of the *FMR1* gene at Xp17.3 (see Chapter 81). A cardinal characteristic of the condition is testicular enlargement (**macro-orchidism**), reaching 40–50 mL after puberty. Although the condition has been recognized in a child as young as 5 mo of age, affected boys younger than 6 yr of age rarely have testicular enlargement; by 8–10 yr of age, most have testicular volumes greater than 3 mL. The testes are enlarged bilaterally, are not nodular, and are histologically normal. Results of hormonal studies are normal. Direct DNA analysis searching for CGG repeat sequences permits definitive diagnosis (see Chapter 81).

Sex cord tumors with annular tubules of the testes can cause breast development in young boys. These tumors usually are associated with Peutz-Jeghers syndrome; they occur bilaterally, are multifocal, and are detectible by ultrasonography. Excessive production of aromatase ($P450_{arom}$) causes feminization of these boys.

In boys with unilateral cryptorchidism, the contralateral testis is about 25% larger than normal for age. Testicular enlargement has also been noted in boys with Henoch-Schönlein purpura and lymphangiectasia. Epidermoid and dermoid cysts of the testes have been reported rarely.

Assi A, Sironi M, Bacchioni AM, et al: Leydig cell tumor of the testis: A cytohistological, immunohistochemical, and ultrastructural case study. *Diagn Cytopathol* 1997;16:262–266.

Clark RV, Albertson BD, Monabi A, et al: Steroidogenic enzyme activities, morphology and receptor studies of a testicular rest in a patient with congenital adrenal hyperplasia. *J Clin Endocrinol Metab* 1990;70:1408–1413.

Coen P, Kulin H, Ballantine T, et al: An aromatase-producing sex-cord tumor resulting in prepubertal gynecomastia. *N Engl J Med* 1991;324:317–322.

Combes-Moukousky ME, Kottler ML, Valensi P, et al: Gonadal and adrenal catheterization during adrenal suppression and gonadal stimulation in a patient with bilateral testicular tumors and congenital adrenal hyperplasia. *J Clin Endocrinol Metab* 1994;79:1390–1394.

Fragoso MCBV, Latronico AC, Carvalho FM, et al: Activating mutation of the stimulatory G protein (gsp) as a putative cause of ovarian and testicular human stromal Leydig cell tumors. *J Clin Endocrinol Metab* 1998;83:2074–2078.

Nisula BC, Loriaux DL, Sherins RJ, et al: Benign bilateral testicular enlargement. *J Clin Endocrinol Metab* 1974;38:440–445.

Rosenberg T, Gilboa Y, Golik A, et al: Pseudoprecocious puberty in a young boy due to interstitial cell adenomas of the testis. *Helv Paediatr Acta* 1984;39:79–87.

Chapter 586 ■ Gynecomastia

Gynecomastia, the occurrence of mammary tissue in the male, is a common condition. True gynecomastia (the presence of granular breast tissue) needs to be distinguished from pseudogynecomastia (consisting of only adipose tissue) seen in overweight boys. Gynecomastia is usually a sign of estrogen-androgen imbalance; its cause is often obscure. It occurs in many newborn males as a result of a normal stimulation by maternal hormones; the effect disappears in a few weeks.

During early to mid-puberty, approximately two thirds of boys develop various degrees of subareolar hyperplasia of the breasts. Physiologic pubertal gynecomastia may involve only one breast, and it is not unusual for both breasts to enlarge at disproportionate rates or at different times. Tenderness of the breast is common but transitory. Spontaneous regression may occur within a few months; it rarely persists longer than 2 yr. Mean concentrations of follicle-stimulating hormone, luteinizing hormone, prolactin, testosterone, estrone, and estradiol are the same as in boys without gynecomastia. When levels are correlated with stage of puberty, a decreased ratio of testosterone to estradiol is found in boys with gynecomastia. Cultured pubic skin fibroblasts from boys with gynecomastia show excessive aromatase activity. Treatment usually consists of reassuring the boy and his family of the physiologic and transient nature of the phenomenon. When the enlargement is striking and persistent and causes serious emotional disturbance to the patient, treatment may be justified. **Medical treatment** is generally aimed at decreasing the estrogen/androgen ratio. Danazol has antiestrogenic effects but also numerous untoward side effects. Anastrozole, an aromatase inhibitor, at 1.0 mg given orally for 6 mo was no different from placebo in decreasing total breast volume by 50% or more in boys with pubertal gynecomastia.

Occasionally, breast development may mimic female breast development (to Tanner stages 3–5) and fail to regress. In such cases, **surgical** removal of the enlarged breast tissue may be indicated. One technique involves endoscopically assisted transaxillary removal of glandular tissue.

Benign, self-limited, and usually transient gynecomastia has been reported in prepubertal children during the initiation of therapy with human growth hormone.

Familial gynecomastia has occurred in several kindreds as an X-linked or autosomal dominant sex-limited trait. Levels of gonadotropins, testosterone, prolactin, and steroid-binding globulins are normal. Increased peripheral conversion of C-19 steroids to estrogens (increased aromatization) has been found in familial and sporadic cases of gynecomastia and may explain some instances of this condition.

A report of the syndrome of aromatase excess in a father and his son and daughter suggests autosomal dominant inheritance.

There was gynecomastia in the 9-yr-old boy and macromastia and isosexual precocity in his 7½-yr-old sister. Excess aromatase activity was shown in skin fibroblasts and transformed lymphocytes in vitro. This was associated with a $P450_{arom}$ polymorphism that suggested a sequence change in the $P450_{arom}$ promoter region. Dominant transmission of prepubertal gynecomastia in a large kindred with a likely mutation of the P450 aromatase gene was detected by elevated serum estrone and not by 17β-estradiol levels. In mice, disruption of the *DAX1* gene causes increased aromatase expression.

In prepubertal children with gynecomastia, an **exogenous source of estrogens** must be sought. Accidental or therapeutic exposure to small amounts of exogenous estrogens by inhalation, percutaneous absorption, or ingestion may cause gynecomastia. Three boys developed gynecomastia after indirect exposure to their mothers' custom-compounded topical estrogen-containing creams. Increased pigmentation of the nipple and areola should suggest this cause. Exposure to medications that decrease levels of androgens, especially free androgens, increase estradiol, or displace androgens from breast androgen receptors may result in gynecomastia. Lavender and certain tea oils have also been a cause of prepubertal gynecomastia.

Several other pathologic conditions may cause gynecomastia. It has been observed in children with congenital virilizing adrenal hyperplasia (**11β-hydroxylase deficiency**). It may be associated with Leydig cell tumors of the testis or with feminizing tumors of the adrenal gland. Several boys with the Peutz-Jeghers syndrome and gynecomastia had sex-cord tumors with annular tubules of the testes. The testes may not be enlarged; the tumor is usually multifocal and bilateral. Excessive aromatase production accounts for the gynecomastia. This condition occurs in patients with **Klinefelter syndrome** and with other types of testicular failure (hypergonadotropic states). It is a common finding in boys with certain types of conditions characterized by male undervirilization (particularly **Reifenstein syndrome**), with the androgen insensitivity syndromes, and with the 17-ketosteroid reductase defect. When gynecomastia is associated with galactorrhea, a **prolactinoma** should be considered. In a pubertal boy with **fibrolamellar carcinoma** of the liver, the associated gynecomastia and elevated estrogen level were attributed to increased aromatization of circulating androgens by the tumor. In an 8-yr-old boy with a calcifying Sertoli cell tumor, the gynecomastia was postulated to be the result of peripheral aromatization of androgens derived from Leydig cells newly differentiated from interstitial cells stimulated by the tumor. **Hyperthyroidism** alters the androgen to estrogen ratio by increasing bound androgen and decreasing the free testosterone and may result in gynecomastia.

In adults, gynecomastia occurs with liver cirrhosis, digitalis therapy for congestive heart failure, bronchogenic carcinoma, administration of various nonsteroidal therapeutic agents, and heavy marijuana smoking. Ketoconazole, an antifungal drug, causes gynecomastia by directly inhibiting testosterone synthesis. Spironolactone, methyldopa, phenothiazines, antidepressants, warfarin (Coumadin), digitalis, and heroin have all been associated with gynecomastia.

Binder G, Iliev DI, Dufke A, et al: Dominant transmission of prepubertal gynecomastia due to serum estrone excess: Hormonal, biochemical, and genetic analysis in a large kindred. *J Clin Endocrinol Metab* 2005;90:484–492.

Braunstein GD: Gynecomastia. *N Engl J Med* 1993;328:490–495.

Felner EI, White PC: Prepubertal gynecomastia: Indirect exposure to estrogen cream. *Pediatrics* 2000;105:1–3.

Henley DV, Lipson N, Korach KS, Bloch CA: Prepubertal gynecomastia linked to lavender and tea tree oils. *N Engl J Med* 2007;356:479–485.

Lazala C, Saenger P: Pubertal gynecomastia. *J Pediatr Endocrinol Metab* 2002;15:553–560.

Maclaren NK, Migeon CJ, Raiti S: Gynecomastia with congenital virilizing adrenal hyperplasia (11β-hydroxylase deficiency). *J Pediatr* 1975;86:579–581.

Malozowski S, Stadel BV: Prepubertal gynecomastia during growth hormone therapy. *J Pediatr* 1995;126:659–661.

Ohyama T, Takada A, Fujikawa M, et al: Endoscope-assisted transaxillary removal of glandular tissue in gynecomastia. *Ann Plast Surg* 1998;40:62–64.

Plourde PV, Reiter EO, Jou H, et al: Safety and efficacy of anastrozole for the treatment of pubertal gynecomastia: A randomized, double-blind, placebo-controlled trial. *J Clin Endocrinol Metab* 2004;89:4428–4433.

Stratakis CA, Vottero A, Brodies A, et al: The aromatase excess syndrome is associated with feminization of both sexes and autosomal dominant transmission of aberrant P450 aromatase gene transcription. *J Clin Endocrinol Metab* 1998;83:1348–1357.

Chapter 587 ■ Hypofunction of the Ovaries

Hypofunction of the ovaries may be caused by congenital failure of development, postnatal destruction (primary or hypergonadotropic hypogonadism), or lack of stimulation by the pituitary and or hypothalamus (secondary or tertiary hypogonadotropic hypogonadism). Many chronic diseases may result in hypogonadotropic hypogonadism.

587.1 • Hypergonadotropic Hypogonadism in the Female (Primary Hypogonadism)

Diagnosis of hypergonadotropic hypogonadism before puberty is difficult. Except in the case of Turner syndrome, most affected patients have no prepubertal clinical manifestations.

TURNER SYNDROME

Turner described a syndrome consisting of sexual infantilism, webbed neck, and cubitus valgus in adult females (also see Chapter 81). Ullrich described an 8-yr-old girl with short stature and many of the same phenotypic features. The term Ullrich-Turner syndrome is frequently used in Europe but rarely used in the United States. The condition is defined as the combination of the characteristic phenotypic features accompanied by complete or partial absence of the second X chromosome with or without mosaicism.

PATHOGENESIS. Half the patients with Turner syndrome have a 45,X chromosomal complement. About 15% of patients are mosaics for 45,X and a normal cell line (45,X/46,XX). Other mosaics with isochromosomes, 45,X/46,X,i(Xq); with rings, 45,X/46,X,r(X); or with fragments, 45,X/46fra, occur less often. Mosaicism is detected most commonly when more than one tissue is examined. The single X is of maternal origin in nearly 80% of 45,X patients. The mechanism of chromosome loss is unknown, and the risk for the syndrome does not increase with maternal age. The genes involved in the Turner phenotype are X-linked genes that escape inactivation. A major locus involved in the control of linear growth has been mapped within the pseudoautosomal region of the X chromosome (PAR1). *SHOX*, a homeobox-containing gene of 170 kb of DNA within the PAR1, is thought to be important for controlling growth in children with Turner syndrome, in patients having idiopathic short stature, and in the Leri-Weill syndrome. Genes for the control of normal ovarian function are postulated to be on Xp and perhaps two "supergenes" on Xq.

Turner syndrome occurs in about 1/1,500–2,500 liveborn females. The frequency of the 45,X karyotype at conception is about 3.0%, but 99% of these are spontaneously aborted, accounting for 5–10% of all abortuses. Mosaicism (45,X/46,XX) occurs in a proportion higher than that seen with any other aneuploid state, but the mosaic Turner constitution is rare among the abortuses; these findings indicate preferential survival for mosaic forms.

The normal fetal ovary contains about 7 million oocytes, but these begin to disappear rapidly after the 5th mo of gestation. At birth, there are only 2 million (1 million active follicles); by menarche, there are 400,000–500,000; and at menopause, 10,000 remain. In the absence of one X chromosome, this process is accelerated, and nearly all oocytes are gone by 2 yr of age. In aborted 45,X fetuses, the number of primordial germ cells in the gonadal ridge appears to be normal, suggesting that the normal process is accelerated in patients with Turner syndrome. Eventually, the ovaries are described as "streaks" and consist only of connective tissue, but a few germ cells may persist.

CLINICAL MANIFESTATIONS. Many patients with Turner syndrome are recognizable at birth because of a characteristic edema of the dorsa of the hands and feet and loose skinfolds at the nape of the neck. Low birthweight and decreased length are common (see Chapter 81). Clinical manifestations in childhood include webbing of the neck, a low posterior hairline, small mandible, prominent ears, epicanthal folds, high arched palate, a broad chest presenting the illusion of widely spaced nipples, cubitus valgus, and hyperconvex fingernails. The diagnosis is often first suspected at puberty when sexual maturation fails to occur.

Short stature, the cardinal finding in all girls with Turner syndrome, may be present with minimal other clinical manifestations. The growth deceleration begins in infancy and young childhood, gets progressively more pronounced in later childhood and adolescence, and results in significant adult short stature. Sexual maturation fails to occur at the expected age. The mean adult height is 143–144 cm in the United States and most of northern Europe, but 140 cm in Argentina and 147 cm in Scandinavia (Fig. 587-1). The height is well correlated with the mid-parental height (average of the parents' heights). Specific growth curves have been developed for girls with Turner syndrome.

Associated defects are common. Complete cardiologic evaluation, including echocardiography, reveals isolated nonstenotic bicuspid aortic valves in one third to one half of patients. In later life, bicuspid aortic valve disease can progress to dilatation of the aortic root. Less frequent defects include aortic coarctation (20%), aortic stenosis, mitral valve prolapse, and anomalous pulmonary venous drainage. In a study of 170/393 females with Turner syndrome in Denmark, 38% of patients with 45,X chromosomes had cardiovascular malformations compared with 11% of those with mosaic monosomy X; the most common were aortic valve abnormalities and aortic coarctation. Webbed neck in patients with or without recognized syndromes is associated with both flow- and non-flow-related heart defects. Among patients with Turner syndrome, those with webbed neck have a much greater chance of having coarctation of the aorta than do those without webbed necks. Repeat cardiac evaluation should be considered even in those without prior findings of cardiac abnormalities during adolescence, and certainly before pregnancy is contemplated. Blood pressure should be routinely monitored even in the absence of cardiac or renal lesions and especially in those with suggestions of aortic root dilatation. MRI may be a valuable tool to detect and monitor aortic root dilation.

One fourth to one third of patients have renal malformations on ultrasonographic examination (50% of those with 45,X karyotypes). The more serious defects include pelvic kidney, horseshoe kidney, double collecting system, complete absence of one kidney, and ureteropelvic junction obstruction. Idiopathic hypertension is also common. When the ovaries were examined by ultrasonography, older studies found a significant decrease in percentage of detectable ovaries from infancy to later childhood. A subsequent report found no such age-related differences in a cross-sectional and longitudinal study conducted in Italy; 27–46% of patients had detectable ovaries at various ages; 76% of those with X mosaicism and 26% of those with 45,X karyotypes had detectable ovaries.

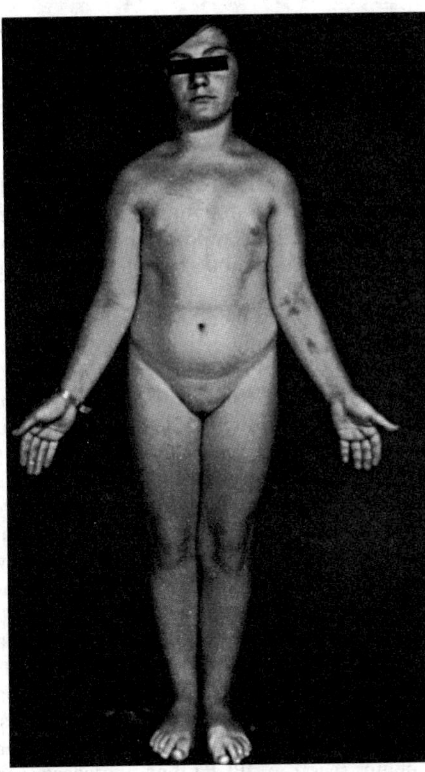

Figure 587-1. Turner syndrome in a 15-yr-old girl exhibiting failure of sexual maturation, short stature, cubitus valgus, and a goiter. There is no webbing of the neck. Karyotyping revealed 45,X/46,XX chromosome complement.

Sexual maturation usually fails to occur, but 10–20% of girls have spontaneous breast development, and a small percentage may have menstrual periods. Primary gonadal failure is associated with early onset of adrenarche (elevation in DHEA sulfate) but delayed pubarche (pubic hair development). Pregnancies have been reported for spontaneously menstruating patients with Turner syndrome. Premature menopause, increased risk of miscarriage, and offspring with increased risk of trisomy 21 have been reported in some of these women. A woman with a 45,X/46,X,r(X) karyotype treated with hormone replacement therapy had 3 pregnancies, resulting in a normal 46,XY male infant, a spontaneous abortion, and a healthy term female with Turner syndrome 45,X/46,Xr(X).

Antithyroid antibodies, thyroid peroxidase, or thyroglobulin antibodies occur in 30–50% of patients. The prevalence increases with advancing age. Ten to 30% have **autoimmune thyroid disease,** with or without the presence of a goiter. Age-dependent abnormalities in carbohydrate metabolism characterized by abnormal glucose tolerance and insulin resistance and, only rarely, frank type 2 diabetes occur in patients with Turner syndrome. Impaired insulin secretion has been described in 45,X women. Cholesterol levels are elevated in adolescence, regardless of body mass index or karyotype.

Inflammatory bowel disease, both Crohn disease and ulcerative colitis; gastrointestinal bleeding due to abnormal mesenteric vasculature; and delayed gastric emptying time have all been reported.

Sternal malformations can be detected by lateral chest radiography. An increased carrying angle at the elbow is usually not clinically significant. Scoliosis occurs in about 10% of adolescent girls. Congenital hip dysplasia occurs more commonly than in the general population. Reported eye findings include anterior segment dysgenesis and keratoconus. Pigmented nevi become more prominent with age; melanocytic nevi are common. Essential hyperhidrosis, torus mandibularis, and alopecia areata occur rarely.

Recurrent bilateral otitis media develops in about 75% of patients. Sensorineural hearing deficits are common, and the frequency increases with age. Problems with gross and fine motor-sensory integration, failure to walk before 15 mo of age, and early language dysfunction often raise questions about developmental delay, but intelligence is normal in most patients. However, mental retardation does occur in patients with 45,X/46,X,r(X); the ring chromosome is unable to undergo inactivation and leads to 2 functional X chromosomes. In adults, deficits in perceptual spatial skills are more common than they are in the general population. Some unconfirmed data suggest the existence of an imprinted X-linked locus that affects cognitive function such as verbal and higher-order executive function skills (better when X is paternal in origin).

The prevalence of mosaicism depends in large part on the techniques used for studying chromosomal patterns. The use of fluorescent in situ hybridization and reverse transcription-polymerase chain reaction (PCR) has increased the reported prevalence of mosaic patterns to as high as 60–74%.

Mosaicism involving the Y chromosome occurs in 5%. A population study of Danish women using PCR with 5 different primer sets found Y chromosome material in 12.2%. Gonadoblastoma among Y-positive patients occurred in 7–10%. Therefore, the current recommendation that prophylactic gonadectomy should be performed even in the absence of MRI or CT evidence of tumors may need to be re-evaluated in the future. The gonadoblastoma locus on the Y chromosome (GBY) maps close to the Y centromere. The presence of only the SRY (sex determining region on Y) locus is not sufficient to confer increased susceptibility for the development of gonadoblastoma. A careful study of 53 patients with Turner syndrome by nested PCR excluded low-level Y mosaicism in almost all cases. A second round of PCR detected SRY on the distal short arm of the Y chromosome in only 2 subjects. Therefore, routine PCR for Y chromosome detection for the purpose of assigning gonadoblastoma risk does not seem indicated. However, high-throughput quantitative genotyping may provide an effective and inexpensive method for the identification of X chromosome abnormalities and Y chromosome material identification.

In patients with 45,X/46,XX mosaicism, the abnormalities are attenuated and fewer; short stature is as frequent as it is in the 45,X patient and may be the only manifestation of the condition other than ovarian failure (see Fig. 587-1).

LABORATORY FINDINGS. Chromosomal analysis must be considered in all short girls. In a systematic search, using Southern blot analysis of leukocyte DNA, Turner syndrome was detected in 4.8% of girls referred to an endocrinology service because of short stature. Patients with a marker chromosome in some or all cells should be tested for DNA sequences at or near the centromere of the Y chromosome.

Ultrasonography of the heart, kidneys, and ovaries is indicated after the diagnosis is established. The most common skeletal abnormalities are shortening of the 4th metatarsal and metacarpal bones, epiphyseal dysgenesis in the joints of the knees and elbows, Madelung deformity, scoliosis, and in older patients, inadequate osseous mineralization.

Plasma levels of gonadotropins, particularly follicle-stimulating hormone (FSH), are markedly elevated to greater than those of age-matched controls during infancy; at 2–3 yr of age, a progressive decrease in levels occurs until they reach a nadir at 6–8 yr of age, and by 10–11 yr, they rise to adult castrate levels.

Thyroid antiperoxidase antibodies should be checked periodically, and if positive, levels of thyroxine and thyroid-stimulating hormone should be obtained. Extensive studies have failed to establish that growth hormone deficiency plays a primary role in the pathogenesis of the growth disorder. Defects in normal secretory patterns of growth hormone are seen in adolescents but not in younger girls with Turner syndrome. In vitro, monocytes and lymphocytes show decreased sensitivity to insulin-like growth factor-1 (IGF-1).

The American Academy of Pediatrics has published a comprehensive guide to the health supervision of children with Turner syndrome. A guide to the care of girls and women with Turner syndrome has been published in 2007.

TREATMENT. Treatment with recombinant human **growth hormone** increases height velocity and ultimate stature in most but not all children. Many girls achieve heights of greater than 150 cm with early initiation of treatment. In a large, multicenter, placebo-controlled U.S. clinical trial, 99 patients with Turner syndrome who started receiving growth hormone at a mean age of 10.9 yr at doses between 0.27 and 0.36 mg/kg/wk achieved a mean height of 149 cm, with nearly one third reaching heights greater than 152.4 cm (60 in). In the Netherlands, higher doses of growth hormone (up to 0.63 mg/kg/wk in the 3rd yr of treatment) resulted in 85% of the subjects reaching adult heights in the normal range for the Dutch reference population. Growth hormone treatment should be initiated in early childhood and/or when there is evidence of growth velocity attenuation on specific Turner syndrome growth curves. The starting dose of growth hormone is 0.375 mg/kg/wk. Growth hormone therapy does not significantly aggravate carbohydrate tolerance and does not result in marked adverse events in patients with Turner syndrome. Serum levels of IGF-1 should be routinely monitored during growth hormone treatment.

Replacement therapy with **estrogens** is indicated, but there is little consensus about the optimal age at which to initiate treatment. The psychologic preparedness of the patient to accept therapy must be taken into account. The improved growth achieved by girls treated with growth hormone in childhood permits initiation of estrogen replacement at 12–13 yr. For greater gains in height, especially for those in whom growth hormone treatment is not initiated until later in childhood or adolescence, estrogen treatment may need to be delayed until 14–15 yr of age. Careful consideration should be given to conflicting psychologic consequences of delaying estrogen therapy for the purpose of achieving better ultimate height. The effects on bone accretion should also be considered. The availability of very low dose estrogen replacement therapy in the near future may obviate the need to choose between appropriate pubertal replacement and optimization of height potential. Preliminary data suggest that very low dose parenteral monthly depot estrogen started with GH at 12 yr of age may result in improved adult height. Estrogen therapy improves verbal and nonverbal memory in girls with Turner syndrome. In young women with age-appropriate pubertal development who achieve normal height, health-related quality-of-life questionnaires have yielded normal results.

A conjugated estrogen (Premarin), 0.3–0.625 mg, or micronized estradiol (Estrace), 0.5 mg, given daily for 3–6 mo is usually effective in inducing puberty. The estrogen then is cycled (taken on days 1–23), and a progestin (Provera) is added (taken on days 10–23) in a dose of 5–10 mg daily. In the remainder of the calendar month, during which no treatment is given, withdrawal bleeding usually occurs. There are insufficient data regarding the use of transdermal and depot estrogen preparations in Turner syndrome.

Prenatal chromosome analysis for advanced maternal age has revealed a frequency of 45,X/46,XX that is 10 times higher than when diagnosed postnatally. Most of these patients have no clinical manifestations of Turner syndrome, and levels of gonadotropins are normal. Awareness of this mild phenotype is important in counseling patients.

Psychosocial support for these girls is an integral component of treatment. The Turner Syndrome Society, which has local chapters in the United States, and similar groups in Canada and other countries provide a valuable support system for these patients and their families in addition to that given by the health care team.

Successful pregnancies have been carried to term using ovum donation and in vitro fertilization. In adult women with Turner syndrome, there seems to be a high prevalence of undiagnosed bone mineral density, lipid, and thyroid abnormalities. Glucose intolerance, diminished first-phase insulin response, elevated blood pressure, and lowered fat free mass are common. Glucose tolerance worsens, but fat free mass and blood pressure and general physical fitness improve with sex hormone replacement. The neurocognitive profile of adult women is unaffected by estrogen status.

XX GONADAL DYSGENESIS

Some phenotypically and genetically normal females have gonadal lesions identical to those in 45,X patients but without somatic features of Turner syndrome; their condition is termed pure gonadal dysgenesis or pure ovarian dysgenesis.

The disorder is rarely recognized in children because the external genitals are normal, no other abnormalities are visible, and growth is normal. At pubertal age, sexual maturation fails to take place. Plasma gonadotropin levels are elevated. Delay of epiphyseal fusion results in a **eunuchoid** habitus. Pelvic ultrasonography reveals streak ovaries.

Affected siblings, parental consanguinity, and failure to uncover mosaicism all point to female-limited autosomal recessive inheritance. The disorder appears to be especially frequent in Finland (1/8,300 liveborn girls). In this population, several mutations in the FSH receptor gene (on chromosome 2p) were demonstrated as the cause of the condition. FSH receptor gene mutations were not detected in Mexican women with 46,XX gonadal dysgenesis. In some patients, XX gonadal dysgenesis has been associated with sensorineural deafness (Perrault syndrome). A patient with this condition and concomitant growth hormone deficiency and virilization has also been reported. There may be distinct genetic forms of this disorder. **Müllerian agenesis,** or the **Mayer-Rokitansky-Küster-Hauser** syndrome, which is second to gonadal dysgenesis as the most common cause of primary amenorrhea, occurring in 1 : 4,000–1 : 5,000 females, has been reported in association with 46,XX gonadal dysgenesis in a 17-yr-old adolescent with primary amenorrhea and lack of breast development. One case of dysgerminoma with syncytiotrophoblastic giant cells was reported. An 18-yr-old woman with primary amenorrhea and an absence of müllerian-derived structures, unilateral renal agenesis, and clinical signs of androgen excess—a phenotype resembling the Mayer-Rokitansky-Küster-Hauser syndrome—was found to have a loss-of-function mutation in the *WNT4* gene. Treatment consists of estrogen replacement therapy.

45,X/46,XY GONADAL DYSGENESIS

45,X/46,XY gonadal dysgenesis, also called **mixed gonadal dysgenesis,** has extreme phenotypic variability postnatally that may extend from a Turner-like syndrome to a male phenotype with a penile urethra; it is possible to delineate 3 major clinical phenotypes. Short stature is a major finding in all affected children. Ninety per cent of prenatally diagnosed cases have a normal male phenotype.

Some patients have no evidence of virilization; they have a female phenotype and often have the somatic signs of Turner syndrome. The condition is discovered prepubertally when chromosomal studies are made in short girls, or later when chromosomal studies are made because of failure of sexual maturation. Fallopian tubes and uterus are present. The gonads consist of intra-abdominal undifferentiated streaks; chromosomal study of the streak often reveals an XY cell line. The streak gonad differs somewhat from that in girls with Turner syndrome; in addition to wavy connective tissue, there are often tubular or cordlike structures, occasional clumps of granulosa cells, and frequently, mesonephric or hilar cells.

Some children have mild virilization manifested only by prepubertal clitorimegaly. Normal müllerian structures are present, but at puberty virilization occurs. These patients usually have an intra-abdominal testis, a contralateral streak gonad, and bilateral fallopian tubes.

Most children present with **frank ambiguity** of the genitals in infancy. A testis and vas deferens are found on one side in the labioscrotal fold, and a streak gonad is identified on the contralateral side. Despite the presence of a testis, fallopian tubes are often present bilaterally. An infantile or rudimentary uterus is almost always present.

Other genotypes and phenotypes have been described. About 25% of 200 analyzed patients have a dicentric Y chromosome (45,X/46,X,dic Y). In some patients, the Y chromosome may be represented by only a fragment (45,X/45,X +fra); application of Y-specific probes can establish the origin of the fragment. It is not clear why the same genotype (45,X/46,XY) can result in such diverse phenotypes. Mutations in the SRY gene have been described in some patients.

Children with a female phenotype present no problem in gender of rearing. Patients who are only slightly virilized are usually assigned a female gender of rearing before a diagnosis is established. Patients with ambiguity of the genitals are readily confused with various types of male disorders of sex development. In most but not all instances, these children are best reared as females; the short stature, the ease of genital reconstruction, and the predisposition of the gonad to the development of malignancy favor this choice. In some patients followed to adulthood, the putative normal testis proves to be dysgenetic with eventual loss of Leydig and Sertoli cell function (see also Chapter 584). In an analysis of 22 Australian patients with mixed gonadal dysgenesis, no significant associations or correlations were found between internal and external phenotypes or endocrine function and gonadal morphologic features. The sex of rearing was determined by the appearance of the external genitals. In 11 patients, basal and human chorionic gonadotropin–stimulated testosterone levels were lower than in control subjects.

Gonadal tumors, usually **gonadoblastomas,** occur in about 25% of these children. A gonadoblastoma locus has been localized to a region near the centromere of the Y chromosome (GBY). These germ cell tumors are preceded by the changes of carcinoma in situ. Accordingly, both gonads should be removed in all patients reared as girls, and the undifferentiated gonad should be removed in the patients reared as boys.

There is no correlation among the proportion of 45,X/46,XY cell lines in either blood or fibroblasts and phenotype. In the past, all patients came to clinical attention because of their abnormal phenotypes. However, 45,X/46,XY mosaicism is found in about 7% of fetuses with true chromosome mosaicism encountered prenatally. Of 76 infants with 45,X/46,XY mosaicism diagnosed prenatally, 72 had a normal male phenotype, 1 had a female phenotype, and only 3 males had hypospadias. Of 12 males whose gonads were examined, only 3 were abnormal. These data must be taken into account when counseling a family in which a 45,X/46,XY infant is discovered prenatally.

XXX, XXXX, AND XXXXX FEMALES

XXX FEMALES. The 47,XXX (trisomy) chromosomal constitution is the most frequent X chromosome abnormality in females, occurring in almost 1/1,000 liveborn females. In 68%, this condition is caused by maternal meiotic nondisjunction, but most 45,X and half of 47,XXY constitutions are caused by paternal sex chromosome errors. The phenotype is that of a normal female; affected infants and children are not recognized.

Sexual development and menarche are normal. Most pregnancies have resulted in normal infants. By 2 yr of age, delays in speech and language become evident and lack of coordination, poor academic performance, and immature behavior are seen in some. These girls tend to be tall and gangly, manifest behavior disorders, and are placed in special education classes. Using high-resolution MRI, ten 47,XXX subjects had lower amygdala volumes than 20 euploid controls; ten 47,XXY subjects had even lower amygdala volumes. In a review of 155 girls, 62% were physically normal. There is marked variability within the syndrome, and a small proportion of affected girls are well coordinated, socially outgoing, and academically superior.

XXXX AND XXXXX FEMALES. The great majority of females with these rare karyotypes have been mentally retarded. Commonly associated defects are epicanthal folds, hypertelorism, clinodactyly, transverse palmar creases, radioulnar synostosis, and congenital heart disease. Sexual maturation is often incomplete and may not occur at all. Nevertheless, three women with the tetra-X syndrome gave birth, but no pregnancies were reported in 49,XXXXX women. Most 48,XXXX women tend to be tall, with an average height of 169 cm, whereas short stature is a common feature of the 49,XXXXX phenotype.

NOONAN SYNDROME

Girls with Noonan syndrome show certain anomalies that also occur in girls with 45,X Turner syndrome, but they have normal 46,XX chromosomes. The most common abnormalities are the same as those described for males with Noonan syndrome (see Chapter 584.1). The phenotype differs from Turner syndrome in several respects. Mental retardation is often present, the cardiac defect is most often pulmonary valvular stenosis or an atrial septal defect rather than an aortic defect, normal sexual maturation usually occurs but is delayed by 2 yr on average, and premature ovarian failure has been reported.

OTHER OVARIAN DEFECTS

Some young women with no chromosomal abnormality are found to have streak gonads that may contain only occasional or no germ cells. Gonadotropins are increased. Cytotoxic drugs, especially alkylating agents such as cyclophosphamide and busulfan, procarbazine, etoposide, and exposure of the ovaries to irradiation for the treatment of malignancy are frequent causes of ovarian failure. Young women with Hodgkin disease demonstrate that combination chemotherapy and pelvic irradiation may be more deleterious than either therapy alone. Teenagers are more likely than older women to retain or recover ovarian function after irradiation or combined chemotherapy; normal pregnancies have occurred after such treatment. Current treatment regimens may result in some ovarian damage in most girls treated for cancer. The LD_{50} for the human oocyte has been estimated to be about 4 Gy; doses as low as 6 Gy have produced primary amenorrhea. Ovarian transposition before abdominal and pelvic irradiation in childhood can preserve ovarian function by decreasing the ovarian exposure to less than 4–7 Gy.

Autoimmune ovarian failure occurs in 60% of children older than 13 yr of age with type I autoimmune polyendocrinopathy (Addison disease, hypoparathyroidism, candidiasis). This condition, also known as polyglandular autoimmune disease (PGAD) type 1 is rare worldwide but not in Finland, where, as a result of a founder gene effect, it occurs in 1 : 25,000 people. The gene for this disorder is located on chromosome 21 and is associated with HLA-DR5. In patients with PGAD-1 and ovarian failure, an association with HLA-A3 has been described. Affected girls may not develop sexually, or secondary amenorrhea may occur in young women. The ovaries may have lymphocytic infiltration or appear simply as streaks. Most affected patients have circulating steroid cell antibodies and autoantibodies to 21-hydroxylase. Among patients with polyglandular autoimmune syndromes, 5% were found to have hypogonadism.

The condition also occurs in young women as an isolated event or in association with other autoimmune disorders, leading to secondary amenorrhea (premature ovarian failure, POF). It occurs in 0.2–0.9% of women younger than 40 yr of age. Premature ovarian failure is a heterogeneous disorder with many causes: chromosomal, genetic, enzymatic, infectious, and iatrogenic. When associated with autoimmune adrenal disease, steroid cell autoantibodies are always present. These antibodies react with P450scc, 17α-OH, or 21-OH enzymes. When associated with an entire host of endocrine and nonendocrine autoimmune diseases and not adrenal autoimmunity, steroid cell autoantibodies are rarely found. A second autoimmune disorder, often subclinical, is found in 10–39% of adult patients with POF. One 17-yr-old with idiopathic thrombocytopenic purpura and 47,XXX chromosomes had autoimmune POF. Patients with POF do not have the neurocognitive defects found in Turner syndrome patients.

Galactosemia, particularly the classical form of the disease, usually results in ovarian damage, beginning during intrauterine life. Levels of FSH and luteinizing hormone (LH) are elevated early in life. Ovarian damage may be due to deficient uridine diphosphate-galactose (see Chapter 87). The **Denys-Drash syndrome,** caused by a *WT1* mutation, can result in ovarian dysgenesis.

Ataxia-telangiectasia may be associated with ovarian hypoplasia and elevated gonadotropins; the cause is unknown. Gonadoblastomas and dysgerminomas have occurred in a few girls.

Hypergonadotropic hypogonadism has been postulated to also occur because of the resistance of the ovary to both endogenous and exogenous gonadotropins (Savage syndrome). This condition occurs also in women with POF. Antiovarian antibodies or FSH receptor abnormalities may cause this condition. Mutation of the FSH receptor gene has been reported as an autosomal recessive condition (see XX Gonadal Dysgenesis section). A few females with 46,XX chromosomes presenting in primary amenorrhea with elevated gonadotropin levels were found to have inactivating mutations of the LH receptor gene. This suggests that LH action is needed for normal follicular development and ovulation. Other genetic defects associated with ovarian failure include mutations in *FOXL2, GNAS, CYP17,* and *CYP19.*

587.2 • Hypogonadotropic Hypogonadism in the Female (Secondary Hypogonadism)

Hypofunction of the ovaries can result from failure to secrete normal levels of gonadotropins. The defect may lie in the anterior pituitary or, more commonly, in the hypothalamus.

ETIOLOGY

Hypopituitarism (Also See Chapter 558). Congenital or acquired lesions in or near the pituitary almost always result in impaired secretion of gonadotropins and other pituitary hormones. In children with multiple pituitary hormone defects including gonadotropin deficiency, pituitary transcription factor defects such as in PROP-1 have been described. In children with idiopathic hypopituitarism, the defect is usually found in the hypothalamus. In these patients, administration of gonadotropin-releasing hormone (GnRH) results in increased plasma levels of FSH and LH, establishing the integrity of the pituitary gland.

Isolated Deficiency of Gonadotropins. This heterogeneous group of disorders is sorted out with the help of the GnRH test. In most children, the pituitary is normal, with the defect residing in the hypothalamus.

Several sporadic instances of anosmia with hypogonadotropic hypogonadism have been reported. **Anosmic** hypogonadal females have also been reported in kindreds with Kallmann syndrome, but hypogonadism more frequently affects the males in these families. Mutations in the gene for the β-subunit of FSH and LH have been reported.

Some autosomal recessive disorders such as the Laurence-Moon-Biedl, multiple lentigines, and Carpenter syndromes appear in some instances to include gonadotropic hormone deficiency. Girls with Prader-Willi syndrome may have hypogonadotropic hypogonadism. Girls with severe thalassemia may have gonadotropin deficiency from pituitary damage caused by chronic iron overload secondary to multiple transfusions. Anorexia nervosa frequently results in hypogonadotropic hypogonadism (see Chapter 27).

DIAGNOSIS. The diagnosis may be apparent in patients with other deficiencies of pituitary tropic hormones, but, as in males, it is difficult to differentiate isolated hypogonadotropic hypogonadism from physiologic delay of puberty. Repeated measurements of FSH and LH, particularly during sleep, may reveal the rising levels that herald the onset of puberty. Stimulation testing with GnRH or one of its analogs may help establish the diagnosis.

POLYCYSTIC OVARY SYNDROME (STEIN-LEVENTHAL SYNDROME)

The classical polycystic ovary syndrome (PCOS) is characterized by obesity, hirsutism, and secondary amenorrhea, with bilaterally enlarged polycystic ovaries, but these manifestations may not all be present (also see Chapter 552). Onset usually occurs at puberty or shortly thereafter; menstrual irregularities and hirsutism are the most frequent complaints. In the reproductive years, the condition is the most common cause of anovulatory infertility. Several terms have gained acceptance in describing these patients: functional ovarian hyperandrogenism and, especially in adults, chronic hyperandrogenic anovulation. There seems to be a strong relationship between premature adrenarche and the subsequent development of PCOS. The enlarged ovaries can often be felt on combined rectal and abdominal palpation and are always demonstrable by ultrasonography (see Chapter 552).

The cause of the disorder in most patients is unsettled despite intensive investigation. PCOS is a heterogeneous condition that may be associated with several distinct entities, such as 21-hydroxylase deficiency, deficiency of 3β-hydroxysteroid dehydrogenase, and deficiency of ovarian 17-ketoreductase, the enzyme that converts androstenedione to testosterone and estrone to estradiol. Conversion of cholesterol to pregnenolone by the cholesterol side-chain cleavage enzyme P450scc, encoded by the gene *CYP11A*, occurs after cholesterol enters the mitochondria aided by the steroidogenic acute regulatory protein (StAR). *DAX1* can repress StAR gene expression, and SF-1 regulates SF-1. *CYP11A* or *DAX1* abnormalities were found in hyperandrogenic hirsute women with and without menstrual disturbances. In most patients with PCOS, the elevated plasma level of free testosterone or androstenedione is not suppressed by dexamethasone, ruling out an adrenal cause of the disorder. In some patients, serum levels of total testosterone may not be elevated but serum levels of free testosterone are, and sex hormone–binding globulins are markedly diminished. About 75% of patients have an increased ratio of LH to FSH levels, an increased amplitude and frequency of plasma LH levels, and an exaggerated response to GnRH. Inhibin B levels are high at baseline and lack normal pulsatile changes. Premenarcheal girls may have an early morning rise in LH rather than the characteristic nocturnal one. The perturbances of LH secretion are believed to bring about hyperplasia of theca cells, arrested follicular development, and impaired estradiol production. Aberrant follicular development, one of the hallmarks of PCOS, may be related to dysregulation of oocyte growth differentiation factor-9 (GDF-9) but not bone morphogenic factor-15 (BMP-15), both known oocyte growth factors. These effects lead to hyperandrogenemia and irregular cycles or amenorrhea. In children having congenital virilizing syndromes, the hypothalamic-pituitary axis appears to be programmed for hypersecretion of LH at puberty, leading to hyperandrogenism even when adrenal androgens are thought to be adequately suppressed. Several common polymorphisms in the interleukin-6 gene promoter are associated with hyperandrogenism.

There is an association between **hyperandrogenism** and **insulin resistance.** Especially in obese patients, PCOS may be associated with hyperinsulinism, insulin resistance, and acanthosis nigricans. Because of the high prevalence of PCOS, it needs to be counted among the most common conditions associated with glucose intolerance and type II diabetes. Adolescents with PCOS tend to have a higher incidence of impaired glucose tolerance. The insulin resistance seems to be related to excessive serine phosphorylation of the insulin receptor. The same process, serine phosphorylation, is important in regulating the activity of P450c17, a major enzyme involved in androgen biosynthesis. Therefore, some have postulated this defect as the single abnormality that may be responsible for both the insulin resistance and hyperandrogenism seen in PCOS. Variations in the gene encoding the cysteine protease calpain-10 may be associated with increased susceptibility to type 2 diabetes. The 112/121 haplotype is associated with both insulin levels and a 2-fold risk of PCOS in white and African American women.

For **diagnosis** of PCOS, measurements of serum LH, FSH, prolactin, free testosterone, and sex hormone–binding globulin as well as dehydroepiandrosterone sulfate (DHEAS) are helpful. Brothers of women with PCOS have elevated DHEAS levels, whereas in sisters of women with PCOS, markers of insulin resistance (elevated fasting insulin levels and decreased fasting glucose to insulin ratios) are associated with hyperandrogenemia but not menstrual irregularities. Measures of insulin resistance, however, may have significant intraindividual variations in women with PCOS. Complex stimulation and inhibitory pharmacologic manipulation have been used to distinguish between adrenal and ovarian causes of hyperandrogenism. Basal and adrenocorticotropic hormone–stimulated adrenal steroid levels may reveal subtle adrenal steroidogenic defects.

A deficiency of 17-ketoreductase is suggested when there are affected brothers or when the estrone : estradiol and androstenedione : testosterone ratios are increased. Women treated with valproate for epilepsy before 20 yr of age often have PCOS and elevated serum testosterone levels, but normal levels of LH.

Candidate genes involved in androgen regulation, biosynthesis, transport, and action that have been studied in patients with PCOS include *SF1, DAX1*, StAR protein, *CYP17, CYP11B2, CYP21, CYP19, HSD3B2, HSD17B, LHβ, FSHβ*, FSH receptor, GnRH receptor, dopamine, glucocorticoid and androgen receptors, and SHBG.

The **mainstay of therapy** is ovarian suppression with oral contraceptives containing nonandrogenic progestins such as desogestrel (Desogen). Spironolactone, in addition to oral contraceptives, has been the main pharmacologic agent available in the United States to diminish hirsutism. Further suppression can be achieved with testolactone, a compound with antiandrogen and weak progestin properties. Electrolysis and laser therapy are the main nonpharmacologic treatment modalities for hirsutism. Attention to obesity is important because its correction often leads to correction of the insulin resistance. Oral agents to treat type II diabetes are beginning to be used to improve insulin resistance in patients with PCOS. Insulin-sensitizing agents such as metformin and troglitazone decrease hyperinsulinemia and ovarian hyperandrogenism in women. Three months of metformin treatment improves insulin resistance and the exaggerated adrenal androgen responses to ACTH. D-Chiro-inositol treatment of women with PCOS improves insulin action, thereby enhancing ovarian function while decreasing serum androgen levels. This approach stimulates postreceptor insulin action. Naltrexone, an opioid antagonist, decreases insulin secretion in hyperinsulinemic patients with PCOS.

Aittomaki K, Lucena JLD, Pakarinen P, et al: Mutation in the follicle-stimulating hormone receptor gene causes hereditary hypergonadotropic ovarian failure. *Cell* 1995;82:959–968.

Arslanian SA, Lewy V, Danadian K, et al: Metformin therapy in obese adolescents with polycystic ovary syndrome and impaired glucose tolerance: Amelioration of exaggerated adrenal response to adrenocorticotropin with reduction of insulinemia/insulin resistance. *J Clin Endocrinol Metab* 2002; 87:1555–1559.

Berdahl LD, Wenstrom KD, Hanson JW: Web neck anomaly and its association with congenital heart disease. *Am J Med Genet* 1995;56:304–307.

Betterle C, Volpato M: Adrenal and ovarian autoimmunity. *Eur J Endocrinol* 1998;138:16–25.

Binder G, Kock A, Wajs E, et al: Nested polymerase chain reaction study of 53 cases with Turner syndrome: Is cytogenetically undetected Y mosaicism common? *J Clin Endocrinol Metab* 1995;80:3532–3536.

Bondy CA: Care of girls and women with Turner Syndrome: A guideline of the Turner syndrome study group. *J Clin Endo Metab* 2007;92:10–25.

Calvo RM, Asuncion M, Telleria D, et al: Screening for mutations in the steroidogenic acute regulatory protein and steroidogenic factor-1 genes, and in CYP11A and dosage-sensitive sex reversal-adrenal hypoplasia gene on the X chromosome, gene-1 (DAX-1), in hyperandrogenic hirsute women. *J Clin Endocrinol Metab* 2001;86:1746–1749.

Carel JC, Mathivon L, Gendrel C, et al: Near normalization of final height with adapted doses of growth hormone in Turner syndrome. *J Clin Endocrinol Metab* 1998;83:1462–1466.

Chang HJ, Clark RD, Bachman H: The phenotype of 45,X/46,XY mosaicism: An analysis of 92 prenatally diagnosed cases. *Am J Hum Genet* 1990; 46:156–167.

De la Chesnayae E, Canto P, Ulloa-Aguirre A, et al: No evidence of mutations in the follicle-stimulating hormone receptor gene in Mexican women with 46,XX pure gonadal dysgenesis. *Am J Med Genet* 2001;98:125–128.

Doherty E, Pakarinen P, Tiitinen A, et al: A novel mutation in the FSH receptor inhibiting signal transduction and causing primary ovarian failure. *J Clin Endocrinol Metab* 2002;87:1151–1155.

Dunaif A: Insulin resistance and the polycystic ovary syndrome: Mechanism and implications for pathogenesis. *Endocr Rev* 1997;18:774–800.

Ehrmann DA, Schwarz PEH, Hara M, et al: Relationship of calpain-10 genotype to phenotype features of polycystic ovary syndrome. *J Clin Endocrinol Metab* 2002;87:1669–1673.

Escobar-Morreale HF, Luque-Ramírez M, San Millán JL: The molecular-genetic basis of functional hyperandrogenism and the polycystic ovary syndrome. *Endocr Rev* 2005;26:251–282.

Gicquel C, Gaston V, Cabrol S, et al: Assessment of Turner syndrome by molecular analysis of the X chromosome in growth-retarded girls. *J Clin Endocrinol Metab* 1998;83:1472–1476.

Gravholt CH, Fedder J, Naeraa RW, et al: Occurrence of gonadoblastoma in females with Turner syndrome and Y chromosome material: A population study. *J Clin Endocrinol Metab* 2000;85:3199–3202.

Hoek A, Schoemaker J, Drexhage HA: Premature ovarian failure and ovarian autoimmunity. *Endocr Rev* 1997;18:107–134.

Holland CM: 47,XXX in an adolescent with premature ovarian failure and autoimmune disease. *J Pediatr Adolesc Gynecol* 2001;14:77–80.

Iezzoni JC, Kap-Herr CV, Golden W, et al: Gonadoblastomas in 45,X/46,XY mosaicism. *Am J Clin Pathol* 1997;108:197–203.

Jayagopal V, Kilpatrick ES, Holding S, et al: The biological variation of insulin resistance in polycystic ovarian syndrome. *J Clin Endocrinol Metab* 2002;87:1560–1562.

Lin AE, Lippe B, Rosenfeld RD: Further delineation of aortic dilation, dissection, and rupture in patients with Turner syndrome. *Pediatrics* 1998;102: e12.

Linssen WH, van den Bent MJ, Brunner HG, et al: Deafness, sensory neuropathy, and ovarian dysgenesis: A new syndrome or a broader spectrum of Perrault syndrome? *Am J Med Genet* 1994;51:81–82.

Mazzanti L, Cacciari E, Bergamaschi R, et al: Pelvic ultrasonography in patients with Turner syndrome: Age-related findings in different karyotypes. *J Pediatr* 1997;131:135–140.

Melner MH, Feltus FA: Autoimmune premature ovarian failure—endocrine aspects of a T-cell disease: Review. *Endocrinology* 1999;140:3401–3403.

Merke DP, Tajima T, Baron J, et al: Hypogonadotropic hypogonadism in a female caused by an X-linked recessive mutation in the Dax1 gene. *N Engl J Med* 1999;340:1248–1252.

Migeon BR, Luo S, Jani M, et al: The severe phenotype of females with tiny ring X chromosomes are associated with inability of these chromosomes to undergo X inactivation. *Am J Med Genet* 1994;55:497–504.

Nester J, Jakubowicz D, Reamer P, et al: Ovulatory and metabolic effects of D-chiro-inositol in polycystic ovary syndrome. *N Engl J Med* 1999;340: 1314–1320.

Palmert MR, Gordon CM, Kartashov AI, et al: Screening for abnormal glucose tolerance in adolescent with polycystic ovary syndrome. *J Clin Endocrinol Metab* 2002;87:1017–1023.

Pasquino AM, Passeri F, Pucarelli I, et al: Spontaneous pubertal development in Turner syndrome. *J Clin Endocrinol Metab* 1997;82:1810–1813.

Patwardham AJ, Brown WE, Bender BG, et al: Reduced size of the amygdala in individuals with 47,XXY and 47,XXX karyotypes. *Am J Med Genet* 2002;114:93–98.

Quigley CA, Crowe BJ, Anglin DG, et al: Growth hormone and low dose estrogen in Turner syndrome: Results of a United States multi-center trial to near-final height. *J Clin Endocrinol Metab* 2002;87:2033–2041.

Rongen-Westerlaken C, Corel K, van den Broeck J, et al: Reference values for height, height velocity and weight in Turner syndrome. *Acta Paediatr* 1997; 86:937–942.

Rosenfeld R, Devine N, Julius Hunold J, et al: Treatment of girls with Turner syndrome (TS) with very low doses of estrogen beginning at 12 years enhances the growth–promoting effect of GH. *J Clin Endocrinol Metab* 2005;90:6424–6430.

Ross JL, Roeltgen D, Feuillan P, et al: Use of estrogen in young girls with Turner syndrome. *Neurology* 2000;54:164–170.

Schorry EK, Lovell AM, Milatovich A, et al: Ullrich-Turner syndrome and neurofibromatosis-1. *Am J Med Genet* 1996;66:423–425.

Seashore MR, Cho S, Desposito F, et al, American Academy of Pediatrics Committee on Genetics: Health supervision for children with Turner syndrome. *Pediatrics* 1995;96:1166–1173.

Sempe M, Hansson Bodallaz C, Limoni C: Growth curves in untreated Ullrich-Turner syndrome: French reference standards 1–22 years. *Eur J Pediatr* 1996;155:862–869.

Sybert VP: Cardiovascular malformations and complications in Turner syndrome. *Pediatrics* 1998;101:E11.

Telvi L, Lebar A, DelPino O, et al: 45,X/46,XY mosaicism: Report of 27 cases. *Pediatrics* 1999;104:304–308.

Thibaud E, Ramirez M, Brauner R, et al: Preservation of ovarian function by ovarian transposition performed before pelvic irradiation during childhood. *J Pediatr* 1992;121:880–884.

Chapter 588 ■ Pseudoprecocity Due to Lesions of the Ovary

Ovarian tumors are rare in pediatrics, thought to occur at a rate of 2.6/100,000. Most ovarian masses are benign, but 10–30% may be malignant. Ovarian malignancies, the most common genital neoplasms in adolescence, account for 1% of childhood cancers. More than 60% are germ cell tumors, most of which are dysgerminomas that can secrete tumor markers and hormones (see Chapter 503). Five to 10% of them occur in phenotypic females with abnormal gonads associated with the presence of a

Y sex chromosome. Next most common are epithelial cell tumors (~20%), and nearly 10% are sex cord/stromal tumors (granulosa, Sertoli cell, and mesenchymal tumors). Multiple tumor markers can be seen in ovarian tumors, including α-fetoprotein, human chorionic gonadotropin (hCG), carcinoembryonic antigen, oncoproteins, p105, p53, *KRAS* mutations, cyclin D1, epidermal growth factor–related proteins and receptors, cathepsin B, and others. Various levels of inhibin-activin subunit gene expression were detected in ovarian tumors.

Functioning lesions of the ovary consist of benign cysts or malignant tumors. The majority synthesize estrogens; a few synthesize androgens.

ESTROGENIC LESIONS OF THE OVARY. These lesions cause isosexual precocious sexual development but account for only a small percentage of all cases of precocity. Benign ovarian follicular cysts are the most common tumors associated with isosexual precocious puberty in girls; they may rarely be gonadotropin dependent.

Juvenile Granulosa Cell Tumor. In childhood, the most common neoplasm of the ovary with estrogenic manifestations is the granulosa cell tumor, although it makes up 1–10% of all ovarian tumors. These tumors have distinctive histologic features that differ from those encountered in older women (adult granulosa cell tumor). The cells have high mitotic activity, follicles are often irregular, Call-Exner bodies are rare, and luteinization is frequent. The tumor may be solid or cystic, or both. It usually is benign. In a few instances, this tumor has been associated with multiple enchondromas (**Ollier disease**) and, in fewer still, with multiple subcutaneous hemangiomas (**Maffucci syndrome**).

Clinical Manifestations and Diagnosis. The tumor has been observed in newborns and may manifest with sexual precocity at 2 yr of age or younger; about half these tumors have occurred before 10 yr of age. The mean age at diagnosis is 7.5 yr. The tumors are almost always unilateral. The breasts become enlarged, rounded, and firm and the nipples prominent. The external genitals resemble those of a normal girl at puberty, and the uterus is enlarged. A white vaginal discharge is followed by irregular or cyclic menstruation. Ovulation, however, does not occur. The presenting manifestation may be abdominal pain or swelling. Pubic hair is usually absent unless there is mild virilization.

A mass is readily palpable in the lower portion of the abdomen in most children by the time sexual precocity is evident. The tumor may be small, however, and escape detection even on careful rectal and abdominal examination; the tumors may be detected by ultrasonography, but multidetector CT scans are most sensitive. Most such tumors (90%) are diagnosed at very early stages of malignancy (FIGO [International Federation of Gynecology and Obstetrics] stage I).

Plasma estradiol levels are markedly elevated. Plasma levels of gonadotropins are suppressed and do not respond to gonadotropin-releasing hormone (GnRH) stimulation. Levels of anti-müllerian hormone (AMH), inhibin, and α-fetoprotein may be elevated. Activating mutations of Gsα are seen in 30%, and GATA-4 expression is retained in the more aggressive tumors while AMH levels are inversely proportional to tumor size. Osseous development is moderately advanced.

Treatment and Prognosis. The tumor should be removed as soon as the diagnosis is established. Prognosis is excellent because fewer than 5% of these tumors in children are malignant. Advanced-stage tumors, however, behave aggressively and require difficult decisions regarding surgical approaches as well as the use of irradiation and chemotherapy. In adults with granulosa cell tumors, p53 expression is associated with unfavorable prognosis. Vaginal bleeding immediately after removal of the tumor is common. Signs of precocious puberty abate and may disappear within a few months after the operation. The secretion of estrogens returns to normal.

Sex cord tumor with annular tubules is a distinctive tumor, thought to arise from granulosa cells, that occurs primarily in patients with Peutz-Jeghers syndrome. These tumors are multifocal, bilateral, and usually benign. The presence of calcifications aids ultrasonographic detection. Increased aromatase production by these tumors results in gonadotropin-independent precocious puberty. Inhibin A and B levels are elevated and decrease after tumor removal. In one study, 9 of 13 sex cord/stromal tumors exhibited follicle-stimulating hormone (FSH) receptor mutations, suggesting a role for such mutation in the development of these tumors.

Chorioepithelioma has been reported only rarely. This highly malignant tumor is thought to arise from a pre-existing teratoma. The usually unilateral tumor produces large amounts of hCG, which stimulates the contralateral ovary to secrete estrogens and progesterone. Elevated levels of hCG are diagnostic.

Follicular Cyst. Small ovarian cysts (<0.7 cm in diameter) are common in prepubertal children. At puberty and in girls with true isosexual precocious puberty, larger cysts (1–6 cm) are often seen; these are secondary to stimulation by gonadotropins. However, similar larger cysts occur occasionally in young girls with precocious puberty in the absence of luteinizing hormone and FSH. Because surgical removal or spontaneous involution of these cysts results in regression of pubertal changes, there is little doubt that they are its cause. The mechanism of production of these autonomously functioning cysts is unknown. Such cysts may form only once, or they may disappear and recur, resulting in waxing and waning of the signs of precocious puberty. They may be unilateral or bilateral. The sexual precocity that occurs in young girls with **McCune-Albright syndrome** is usually associated with autonomous follicular cysts caused by a somatic-activating mutation of the G-protein occurring early in development (see Chapter 563.6). Gonadotropins are suppressed, and estradiol levels are often markedly elevated, but they may fluctuate widely and even return to normal. GnRH stimulation fails to evoke an increase in gonadotropins. Because gonadotropins are suppressed in these children, the mechanism of ovarian stimulation is unknown. Ultrasonography is the method of choice for the detection and monitoring of such cysts. A short period of observation to ascertain the lack of spontaneous resolution is advisable before cyst aspiration or cystectomy is considered. Cystic neoplasms must be considered in the differential diagnosis.

ANDROGENIC LESIONS OF THE OVARY. Virilizing ovarian tumors are rare at all ages but particularly so in prepubertal girls. The **arrhenoblastoma** has been reported as early as 14 days of age, but few cases have been reported in girls younger than 16 yr of age.

The **gonadoblastoma** occurs exclusively in dysgenetic gonads, particularly in phenotypic females who have a Y chromosome in their genotype (46,XY; 45,X/46,XY; 45,X/46,X-fra). The tumor may be bilateral. Virilization occurs with some but not all tumors. The clinical features are the same as those seen in patients with virilizing adrenal tumors and include accelerated growth, acne, clitoral enlargement, and growth of sexual hair. A palpable, abdominal mass is found in only about 50% of patients. Plasma levels of testosterone and androstenedione are elevated, and those of gonadotropins are suppressed. Ultrasonography, CT, and MRI usually localize the lesion. The dysgenetic gonad of phenotypic females with a Y chromosome should be removed prophylactically. When a unilateral tumor is removed, the contralateral dysgenetic gonad should also be removed. In an immunohistochemical study of two gonadoblastomas, expressions of WT1, p53, and MIS as well as inhibin were all demonstrated.

Virilizing manifestations occur occasionally in girls with **juvenile granulosa cell tumors.** Adrenal rests and hilum cell tumors rarely lead to virilization. Activating mutations of G-protein genes have been described in ovarian (and testicular) tumors. *GSP* mutations, usually seen in gonadal tumors associated with **McCune-Albright syndrome,** were also noted in 4 of 6 Leydig cell tumors (3 ovarian, 1 testicular). Two granulosa cell tumors and one thecoma of 10 ovarian tumors studied were found to have *GIP-2* mutations.

Sertoli-Leydig cell tumors, rare sex cord/stromal neoplasms, constitute less than 1% of ovarian tumors. The average age at diagnosis is 25 yr; less than 5% of these tumors occur before puberty. AFP levels may be mildly elevated. In one 12-mo-old with Sertoli-Leydig cell tumor presenting with isosexual precocity the only detectable tumor marker was the serum inhibin level, with elevations in both A and B subunits. Five-year survival rates are 70–90%.

Of 102 consecutive patients who underwent surgery because of ovarian masses over a 15-yr period, the presenting symptoms were acute abdominal pain in 56% and abdominal or pelvic mass in 22%. Of 9 children whose cause for surgery was presumed malignancy, 3 had dysgerminomas, 2 had teratomas, 2 had juvenile granulosa cell tumors, 1 had a Sertoli-Leydig cell tumor, and 1 had a yolk sac tumor.

Anttonen M, Unkila-Kallio L, Leminen A, et al: High GATA-4 expression associates with aggressive behavior, whereas low anti-Müllerian hormone expression associates with growth potential of ovarian granulosa cell tumors. *J Clin Endocrinol Metab* 2005;90:6529–6535.

Calaminus G, Wessalowski R, Harms D, et al: Juvenile granulosa cell tumors of the ovary in children and adolescents: Results from 33 patients registered in a prospective cooperative study. *Gynecol Oncol* 1997;65:447–452.

Cass DL, Hawkins E, Brandt ML, et al: Surgery for ovarian masses in infants, children, and adolescents: 102 Consecutive patients treated in a 15-year period. *J Pediatr Surg* 2001;36:693–699.

Choong CS, Fuller PJ, Chu S, et al: Sertoli-Leydig cell tumor of the ovary, a rare cause of precocious puberty in a 12 month-old infant. *J Clin Endocrinol Metab* 2002;87:49–56.

Fink D, Kubik-Huch RA, Wildermuth S: Juvenile granulosa cell tumor. *Abdom Imaging* 2001;26:550–552.

Fotiou SK: Ovarian malignancies in adolescence. *Ann NY Acad Sci* 1997;816:338–346.

Kalfa, N, Ecochard A, Patte C, et al: Activating mutations of the stimulatory G protein in juvenile ovarian granulosa cell tumors: A new prognostic factor? *J Clin Endocrinol Metab* 2006;91:1842–1847.

Lazar EL, Stolar CJ: Evaluation and management of pediatric solid ovarian tumors. *Semin Pediatr Surg* 1998;7:29–34.

Powell JL, Connor GP, Henderson GS: Management of recurrent juvenile granulosa cell tumor of the ovary. *Gynecol Oncol* 2001;81:113–116.

Silverman LA, Gitelman SE: Immunoreactive inhibin, müllerian inhibitory substance, and activin as biochemical markers for juvenile granulosa cell tumors. *J Pediatr* 1996;129:918–921.

Stepanian M, Cohn D: Gynecologic malignancies in adolescents. *Adolesc Med* 2004;15:549–568.

Chapter 589 ■ Disorders of Sex Development (Intersex)

SEXUAL DIFFERENTIATION (SEE ALSO CHAPTER 583). In normal differentiation, the final form of all sexual structures is consistent with normal sex chromosomes (either XX or XY). A 46,XX complement of chromosomes as well as genetic factors such as DAX1 and the signaling molecule WNT-4 are necessary for the development of normal ovaries. Development of the male phenotype is even more complex. It requires a Y chromosome and, specifically, an intact *SRY* gene, which, in association with other genes such as *SOX9, SF1,* and *WT1* and others (see Chapter 583), directs the undifferentiated gonad to become a testis. Aberrant recombinations may result in X chromosomes carrying *SRY,* resulting in XX males, or Y chromosomes that have lost *SRY,* resulting in XY females.

Anti-müllerian hormone (AMH), also known as müllerian-inhibiting substance, the first testicular hormone produced at 6–7 wk of gestation, causes the müllerian ducts to regress; in its absence, they persist. AMH activation in the testes may require the *SF1* gene for activation. By about 8 wk of gestation, the Leydig cells of the testis begin to produce testosterone. During this critical period of male differentiation, testosterone secretion is stimulated by placental human chorionic gonadotropin (hCG), which peaks at 8–12 wk. In the latter half of pregnancy, lower levels of testosterone are maintained by luteinizing hormone secreted by the fetal pituitary. Testosterone initiates virilization of the wolffian duct into the epididymis, vas deferens, and seminal vesicle. Development of the external genitals also requires dihydrotestosterone (DHT), an active metabolite of testosterone. DHT is necessary to fuse the genital folds to form the penis and scrotum. A functional androgen receptor, controlled by an X-linked gene, is required for testosterone and DHT to produce these virilizing changes.

In the XX fetus with normal long and short arms of the X chromosome, the bipotential gonad develops into an ovary by about the 10th–11th wk. This occurs only in the absence of *SRY,* testosterone, and AMH and requires a normal gene in the DSS locus DAX1, and the WNT-4 molecule. The female phenotype develops independently of the fetal gonads, but maleness is imposed on a basically female potential by the hormones of the fetal testis. Estrogen is unnecessary for normal prenatal sexual differentiation, as demonstrated by 46,XX patients with aromatase deficiency and by mice without estradiol receptors.

Intersex implies a discrepancy between the morphology of the gonads and that of the external genitals. Chromosomal aberrations may result in ambiguity of the external genitals (see Chapters 584 and 587). Conditions of aberrant sexual differentiation may also be imposed on the XX or XY genotype. The new, proposed appropriate term for what was previously called intersex is **disorders of sex development (DSD).** This term defines a condition "in which development of chromosomal, gonadal or anatomical sex is atypical." It is preferable to use the term "atypical genitalia" rather than "ambiguous genitalia." Comparison with the previous terms and a new etiologic classification are seen in Tables 589-1 and 589-2. Some of the genes involved in disorders of sex development are listed in Table 583-1.

Development of the external genitals begins with the potential to be either male or female (Fig. 589-1). Virilization of a female, the most common form of DSD, results in varying phenotypes (Fig. 589-2), which start from the basic genital appearances of the embryo (see Fig. 589-1).

TABLE 589-1. Proposed Revised Nomenclature

PREVIOUS	PROPOSED
Intersex*	Disorders of sex development (DSD)
Male pseudohermaphrodite Undervirilization of an XY male Undermasculinization of an XY male *46,XY intersex	46,XY DSD
Female pseudohermaphrodite Overvirilization of an XX female Masculinization of an XX female *46,XX intersex	46,XX DSD
True hermaphrodite *Gonadal intersex	Ovotesticular DSD
XX male or XX sex reversal	46,XX testicular DSD
XY sex reversal	46,XY complete gonadal dysgenesis

*Terms used in previous edition of this chapter.

From Lee PA, Houk CP, Ahmed SF, et al: Consensus statement on management of intersex disorders. *Pediatrics* 2006;118:e488–500.

TABLE 589-2. Etiologic Classification of Disorders of Sex Development (DSD)

46,XX-DSD
Androgen Exposure
Fetal/Fetoplacental Source
21-Hydroxylase (P450 c21) deficiency
11β-Hydroxylase (P450 c11) deficiency
3β-Hydroxysteroid dehydrogenase II (3β-HSD II) deficiency
Cytochrome p450 oxidoreductase (POR)
Aromatase ($P450_{arom}$) deficiency
Glucocorticoid receptor gene mutation
Maternal Source
Virilizing ovarian tumor
Virilizing adrenal tumor
Androgenic drugs
Disorder of Ovarian Development
XX gonadal dysgenesis
Testicular DSD (SRY+, SOX9Dup)
Undetermined Origin
Associated with genitourinary and gastrointestinal tract defects
46,XY-DSD
Defects in Testicular Development
Denys-Drash syndrome (mutation in *WT1* gene)
WAGR syndrome (Wilms tumor, aniridia, genitourinary malformation, retardation)
Deletion of 11p13
Camptomelic syndrome (autosomal gene at 17q24.3–q25.1) and SOX9 mutation
XY pure gonadal dysgenesis (Swyer syndrome)
Mutation in SRY gene
XY gonadal agenesis
Unknown cause
Deficiency of Testicular Hormones
Leydig cell aplasia
Mutation in LH receptor
Lipoid adrenal hyperplasia (P450 scc) deficiency; mutation in StAR (steroidogenic acute regulatory protein)
3β-HSD II deficiency
17-Hydroxylase/17,20-lyase (P450 c17) deficiency
Persistent müllerian duct syndrome
Gene mutations, anti-müllerian hormone
Receptor defects for anti-müllerian hormone
Defect in Androgen Action
5α-Reductase II mutations
Androgen receptor defects
Complete androgen insensitivity syndrome
Partial androgen insensitivity syndrome (Reifenstein and other syndromes)
Smith-Lemli-Opitz syndrome (Defect in conversion of 7-dehydrocholesterol to cholesterol, DHCR7)
Ovotesticular DSD
XX
XY
XX/XY chimeras

From Lee PA, Houk CP, Ahmed SF, et al: Consensus statement on management of intersex disorders. *Pediatrics* 2006;118;e488–500.

589.1 • 46,XX DSD

In this condition, the genotype is XX and the gonads are ovaries, but the external genitals are virilized. Because there is no AMH (the gonads are ovaries, not testes), the uterus, tubes, and ovaries develop. The varieties and causes of this condition are relatively few. Most instances result from exposure of the female fetus to excessive exogenous or endogenous androgens during intrauterine life. The changes consist principally of virilization of the external genitals (clitoral hypertrophy and labioscrotal fusion).

CONGENITAL ADRENAL HYPERPLASIA (SEE CHAPTER 577.1). This is the most common cause of genital ambiguity and 46,XX DSD. Females with the 21-hydroxylase and 11-hydroxylase defects are the most highly virilized, although minimal virilization also occurs with the type II 3β-hydroxysteroid dehydrogenase defect (see Fig. 589-1). Salt losers tend to have greater degrees of virilization than do non-salt-losing patients. Masculinization may be so intense that a complete penile urethra results, and the condition may mimic a male with cryptorchidism (see Chapter 577.1).

AROMATASE DEFICIENCY. In genotypic females, aromatase deficiency during fetal life leads to 46,XX DSD and results in hypergonadotropic hypogonadism at puberty because of ovarian failure to synthesize estrogen (see Fig. 575-1).

Two 46,XX infants had enlargement of the clitoris and posterior labial fusion at birth. In one instance, maternal serum and urinary levels of estrogen were very low and serum levels of androgens were high. Cord serum levels of estrogen were also extremely low, but those of androgen were elevated. The second patient also had virilization of unknown cause since birth, but the aromatase deficiency was not diagnosed until 14 yr of age, when she had further virilization and failed to go into puberty. At that time, she had elevated levels of gonadotropins and androgens but low estrogen levels, and ultrasonography revealed large ovarian cysts bilaterally. These two patients demonstrate the important role of aromatase in the conversion of androgens to estrogens. Additional female and male patients with aromatase deficiency due to mutations in the $P450_{arom}$ *(CYP19)* gene are known. Two siblings were described. The 28-yr-old XY proband was 177.6 cm tall (+2.5 SD) after having received hormonal replacement therapy; her 24-yr-old brother was 204 cm tall (+3.7 SD), and had a bone age of 14 yr. Low-dose estradiol replacement, carefully adjusted to maintain normal age-appropriate levels, may be indicated for affected females even prepubertally.

GLUCOCORTICOID RECEPTOR GENE MUTATION. A 9-yr-old girl with 46,XX disorder of sexual development, thought to be due to 21-OHase deficiency (congenital adrenal hyperplasia) since the age of 5 yr, had elevated cortisol levels at baseline and after dexamethasone, hypertension, and hypokalemia, suggestive of the diagnosis of generalized glucocorticoid resistance. A novel homozygous mutation in exon 5 of the glucocorticoid receptor was demonstrated. In this Brazilian family, the condition was autosomal recessive.

POR, cytochrome P450 oxidoreductase, encoded by a gene on 7q11.2, is a cofactor implicated in combined P450C17 and P450C21 steroidogenic defects. Girls are born with ambiguous genitals, but the virilization does not progress postnatally and androgen levels are normal or low. Boys may be born undervirilized. Both may exhibit bony abnormalities seen in **Antley-Bixler syndrome** (ABS). Conversely, in a series of ABS patients, those with ambiguous genitals and disordered steroidogenesis had POR deficiency while those without ambiguity and normal steroidogenesis had *FGFR2* mutations. The cardinal features of ABS include craniosynostosis, severe midface hypoplasia, proptosis, choanal atresia/stenosis, frontal bossing, dysplastic ears, depressed nasal bridge, radiohumeral synostosis, long bone fractures and femoral bowing, and urogenital abnormalities.

VIRILIZING MATERNAL TUMORS. Rarely, the female fetus has been virilized during fetal life by a maternal androgen-producing tumor. In a few cases, the lesion was a benign adrenal adenoma, but all others were ovarian tumors, particularly androblastomas, luteomas, and Krukenberg tumors. **Maternal virilization** may be manifested by enlargement of the clitoris, acne, deepening of the voice, decreased lactation, hirsutism, and elevated levels of androgens. In the infant, there is enlargement of the clitoris of varying degrees, often with labial fusion. Mothers of children with unexplained 46,XX DSD should undergo measurements of their own levels of plasma testosterone, dehydroepiandrosterone sulfate, and androstenedione.

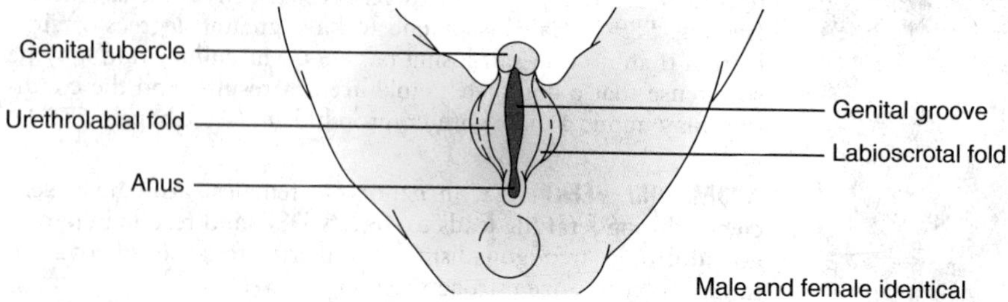

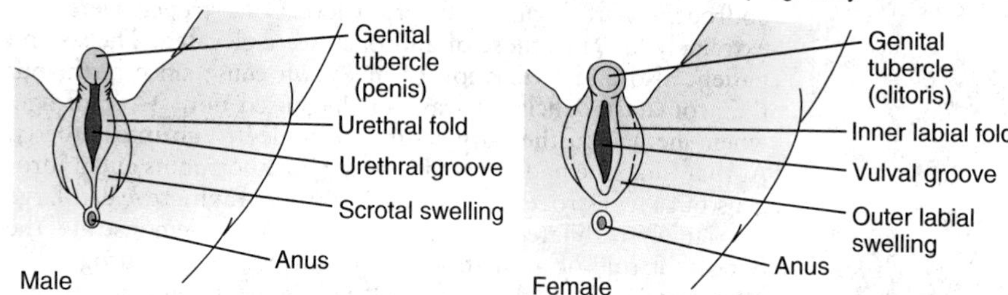

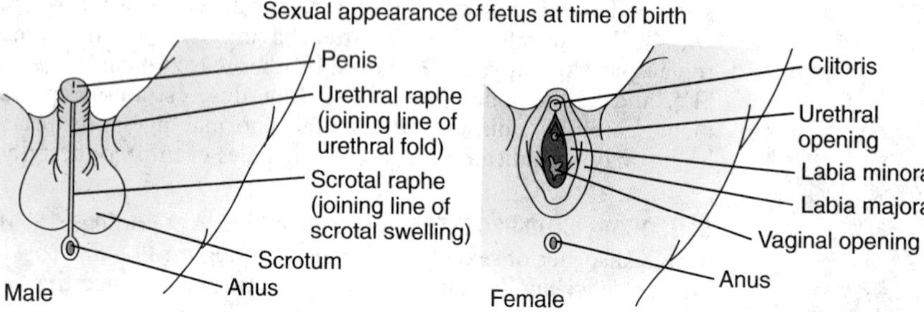

Figure 589-1. Schematic demonstration of differentiation of normal male and female genitals during embryogenesis. (From Zitelli BJ, Davis HW: *Atlas of Pediatric Physical Diagnosis,* 4th edition. St. Louis, Mosby, 2002, p 328.)

ADMINISTRATION OF ANDROGENIC DRUGS TO WOMEN DURING PREGNANCY. Testosterone and 17-methyltestosterone have been reported to cause 46,XX intersex in some instances. The greatest number of cases has resulted from the use of certain progestational compounds for the treatment of threatened abortion. These progestins have been replaced by nonvirilizing ones.

Infants with virilization and 46,XX chromosomes and caudal anomalies have been reported for whom no virilizing agent could be identified. In such instances, the disorder is usually associated with other congenital defects, particularly of the urinary and gastrointestinal tracts. Y-specific DNA sequences, including SRY, are absent. In one case, a scrotal raphe and elevated testosterone levels were found, but the cause remains unknown.

589.2 • 46,XY DSD

In this condition, the genotype is XY, but the external genitals are incompletely virilized, ambiguous, or completely female. When gonads can be found, they are invariably testes; their development ranges from rudimentary to normal. Because the process of normal virilization in the fetus is so complex, it is not surprising that there are many varieties of undervirilized 46,XY individuals.

DEFECTS IN TESTICULAR DIFFERENTIATION

The first step in male differentiation is conversion of the indifferent gonad to a testis. In the XY fetus, if there is a deletion of the short arm of the Y chromosome or of the *SRY* gene, male differentiation does not occur. The phenotype is female; müllerian ducts are well developed because of the absence of AMH, but gonads consist of undifferentiated streaks. By contrast, even extreme deletions of the long arm of the Y chromosome (Yq-) have been found in normally developed males, most of whom are azoospermic and have short stature, indicating that the long arm of the Y chromosome normally has genes that prevent these manifestations. In other syndromes in which the testes fail to differentiate, Y chromosomes are morphologically normal.

DENYS-DRASH SYNDROME. The constellation of nephropathy with ambiguous genitals and **bilateral Wilms tumor** are the major characteristics of this syndrome (see Chapter 499). Most reported cases have been 46,XY. Müllerian ducts are often present, indicating a global deficiency of fetal testicular function. Patients with 46,XX karyotype have normal external genitals. The onset of proteinuria in infancy progresses to **nephrotic syndrome** and end-stage renal failure by 3 yr of age, with focal or diffuse mesangial sclerosis being the most consistent histopathologic finding. Wilms tumor usually develops in children younger than 2 yr of age and is frequently bilateral. Gonadoblastomas have been reported.

Several mutations of the Wilms tumor gene *(WT1),* located on chromosome 11p13, have been found. *WT1* functions as a tumor-suppressor gene and transcriptional factor and is expressed in the genital ridge and fetal gonads. Nearly all reported mutations have been near or within the zinc finger–coding region. One report found a zinc finger domain mutation in the *WT1* alleles of a patient with no genitourinary abnormalities, suggesting that some cases of sporadic Wilms tumor may carry the *WT1* mutation. Dif-

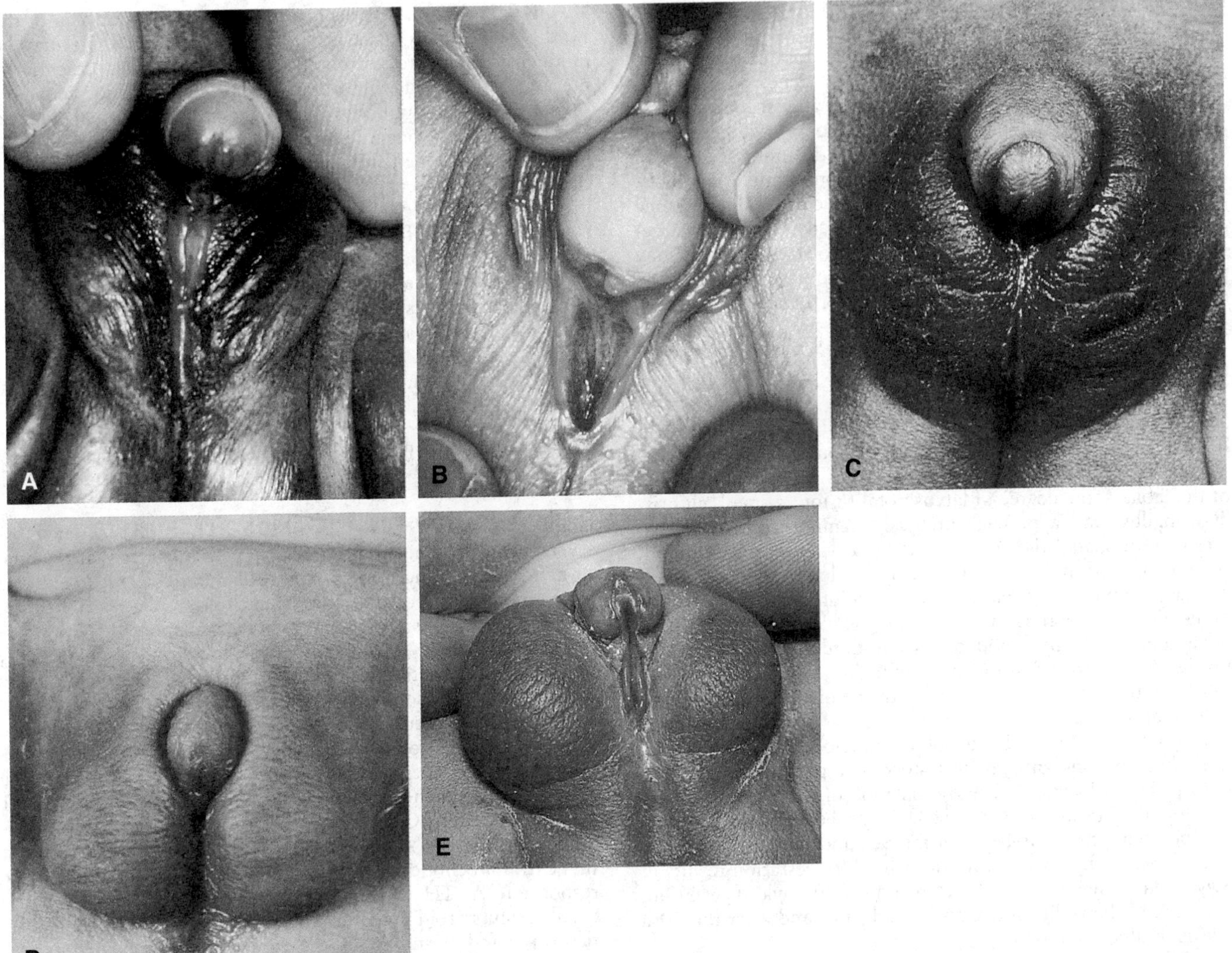

Figure 589-2. Examples of atypical genitals. These cases include ovotesticular disorder of sexual development *(A)* and congenital virilizing adrenal hyperplasia *(B–E)*. *(B–D,* courtesy of D. Becker, MD, Pittsburgh.) (From Zitelli BJ, Davis HW: *Atlas of Pediatric Physical Diagnosis,* 4th edition. St. Louis, Mosby, 2002, p 329.)

ferent mutations of the *WT1* gene, constitutional heterozygote mutations at intron 9, have been described in **Fraser syndrome,** a condition of nonspecific focal and segmental glomerulosclerosis, 46,XY gonadal dysgenesis, and frequent gonadoblastoma, all without Wilms tumor.

WAGR SYNDROME. This acronymic contiguous gene syndrome consists of Wilms tumor, aniridia, genitourinary malformations, and retardation (see Chapter 499). These children have a deletion of one copy of chromosome 11p13, which may be visible on karyotype analysis. The deleted region encompasses the aniridia gene *(PAX6)* and the Wilms tumor suppressor gene *(WT1)*. Only 46,XY males have genital abnormalities, ranging from cryptorchidism to severe deficiency of virilization. Gonadoblastomas have developed in the dysgenetic gonads. Wilms tumor usually occurs by 2 yr of age. Some cases also had unexplained obesity, raising the question of an obesity-associated gene in this region of chromosome 11 and naming the syndrome **WAGRO.**

CAMPTOMELIC SYNDROME (SEE CHAPTER 702). This form of **short-limbed dysplasia** is characterized by anterior bowing of the femur and tibia, small, bladeless scapulae, small thoracic cavities and 11 pairs of ribs, along with malformations of other organs. It is usually lethal in early infancy. About 75% of reported 46,XY patients exhibit a completely **female phenotype;** the external and internal genitals are female. Some 46,XY patients have ambiguous genitals. The gonads appear to be ovaries but histologically may contain elements of ovaries and testes.

The gene responsible for the condition is *SOX9* (SRY-related HMG-box gene) and is on 17q24–q25. This gene is structurally related to *SRY* and also directly regulates the type II collagen gene *(COL2A1)* development. The same mutations may result in different gonadal phenotypes. Gonadoblastoma was reported in a patient with this condition. The inheritance is autosomal dominant. Adrenal insufficiency and 46,XY gonadal dysgenesis was described in a patient with mutation of the *SF1* gene.

46,XY sex reversal has been described in patients with deletions of parts of autosomal loci on chromosomes 2q, 9p, and 10q.

XY PURE GONADAL DYSGENESIS (SWYER SYNDROME). The designation "pure" distinguishes this condition from forms of gonadal dysgenesis that are of chromosomal origin and associated with somatic anomalies. Affected patients have normal stature and a **female phenotype,** including vagina, uterus, and fallopian tubes, but at pubertal age, breast development and menarche fail to occur. None of the defects associated with 45,X children is present. Patients present at puberty with hypergonadotropic primary amenorrhea. Familial cases suggest an X-linked or a sex-limited dominant autosomal transmission. Most of the patients examined have had mutations of the *SRY* gene. None had a *SOX9* gene mutation. The gonads consist of almost totally undifferentiated streaks despite the presence of a cytogenetically normal Y chromosome. The primitive gonad cannot accomplish any testicular function, including suppression of müllerian ducts. There may be hilar cells in the gonad capable of producing some androgens; accordingly, some virilization, such as clitoral enlargement, may occur at the age of puberty. The streak gonads may undergo neoplastic changes, such as gonadoblastomas and dysgerminomas and should be removed shortly after diagnosis, regardless of age.

Pure gonadal dysgenesis also occurs in XX individuals (see Chapter 587).

XY GONADAL AGENESIS SYNDROME (EMBRYONIC TESTICULAR REGRESSION SYNDROME). In this rare syndrome, the external genitals are slightly ambiguous but more nearly **female.** Hypoplasia of the labia; some degree of labioscrotal fusion; a small, clitoris-like phallus; and a perineal urethral opening are present. No uterus, no gonadal tissue, and usually no vagina can be found. At the age of puberty, no sexual development occurs and gonadotropin levels are elevated. Most children have been reared as females. In several patients with XY gonadal agenesis in whom no gonads could be found on exploration, significant rises in testosterone followed stimulation with hCG, indicating Leydig cell function somewhere. Siblings with the disorder are known.

It is presumed that testicular tissue was active long enough during fetal life for AMH to inhibit development of müllerian ducts but not long enough for testosterone production to result in virilization. In one patient, no deletion of the Y chromosome was found by means of Y-specific DNA probes. Testicular degeneration seems to occur between the 8th and the 12th fetal wk. Regression of the testis before the 8th wk of gestation results in Swyer syndrome; between the 14th and the 20th wk of gestation, it results in the rudimentary testis syndrome; and after the 20th wk, it results in anorchia.

In **bilateral anorchia,** testes are absent, but the **male phenotype** is complete; it is presumed that tissue with fetal testicular function was active during the critical period of genital differentiation but that sometime later it was damaged. Bilateral anorchia in identical twins and unilateral anorchia in identical twins and in siblings suggest a genetic predisposition. Coexistence of anorchia and the gonadal agenesis syndrome in a sibship is evidence for a relationship between the disorders. *SRY* defects have not yet been reported for patients with anorchia.

A retrospective review of urologic explorations revealed absent testes in 21% of 691 testes. Of those, 73% had blind-ending cord structures with the suggested site of the vanishing testes being the inguinal canal (59%), the abdomen (21%), superficial inguinal ring (18%), and scrotum (2%). It was suggested that the presence of cord structures on laparoscopy should prompt inguinal exploration because viable testicular tissue was found in four of these children. No hormonal data (hCG stimulation tests, AMH levels) were reported.

DEFECTS IN TESTICULAR HORMONES

Five genetic defects have been delineated in the enzymatic synthesis of testosterone by fetal testis, and a defect in Leydig cell differentiation has been described. These defects produce 46,XY males with inadequate masculinization (see Fig. 583-1). Because levels of testosterone are normally low before puberty, an hCG stimulation test must be used in children to assess the ability of the testes to synthesize testosterone.

LEYDIG CELL APLASIA. Patients with aplasia or hypoplasia of the Leydig cells usually have **female phenotypes,** but there may be mild virilization. Testes, epididymis, and vas are present; the uterus and fallopian tubes are absent. There are no secondary sexual changes at puberty; pubic hair may be normal. Plasma levels of testosterone are low and do not respond to hCG; luteinizing hormone (LH) levels are elevated. The Leydig cells of the testes are absent or markedly deficient. The defect may involve a lack of receptors for LH. In children, hCG stimulation is necessary to differentiate the condition from the androgen insensitivity syndromes (AISs). There is male-limited autosomal recessive inheritance. The human LH receptor is a member of the G-protein–coupled superfamily of receptors that contains 7 transmembrane domains. Several inactivating mutations of the LH receptor have been described in males with hypogonadism suspected of having Leydig cell hypoplasia or aplasia.

High serum LH and low follicle-stimulating hormone (FSH) were noted in one male with hypogonadism owing to a mutation in the gene for the β subunit of FSH (see Table 584-1).

LIPOID ADRENAL HYPERPLASIA (ALSO SEE CHAPTER 577). The most severe form of congenital adrenal hyperplasia derives its name from the appearance of the enlarged adrenal glands resulting from accumulation of cholesterol and cholesterol esters. The rate-limiting process in steroidogenesis is the transport of free cholesterol through the cytosol to the inner mitochondrial membrane, where p450SCC acts. Cholesterol transport into mitochondria is mediated by a steroidogenetic acute regulatory protein (StAR) whose synthesis occurs via cAMP through a cyclic AMP response element–binding protein (CREB). StAR is a 30 kDa protein essential for steroidogenesis and is encoded by a gene on chromosome 8p11.2. The mitochondrial content of StAR increases between 1 and 5 hours after ACTH stimulation, long after the acute ACTH-induced increase in steroidogenesis. This has led some to suggest that extramitochondrial StAR might also be involved in the acute response to ACTH.

All serum steroid levels are low or undetectable, whereas corticotropin and plasma renin levels are elevated. The phenotype is female in genetic females and males; genetic males have no müllerian structures because the testes can produce normal AMH but no steroid. These children present with acute adrenal crisis and salt wasting in infancy. Most patients are 46,XY. In a few patients, ovarian steroidogenesis is present at puberty.

The regulatory role of StAR-independent steroidogenesis is illustrated by 46,XX 4-mo-old twins with lipoid adrenal hyperplasia. One died at 15 mo because of cardiac complications related to coarctation of the aorta. The adrenal glands had characteristic lipid deposits. The surviving twin had spontaneous puberty with feminization at 11.5 yr with menarche at 13.8 yr. When restudied at the age of 15 yr, a homozygous frameshift-inactivating mutation in her StAR gene was discovered. This and the fact that she survived as an infant until 4 mo of age without replacement therapy with detectable serum aldosterone levels supports the hypothesis that StAR-independent steroidogenesis was able to proceed until enough intracellular lipid accumulated to destroy steroidogenic activity. Partial defects in only partially virilized males and delayed onset of salt wasting have been described. Complete P450scc defects may be incompatible with life because only this enzyme can convert cholesterol to pregnenolone, which then becomes progesterone, a hormone essential for the maintenance of normal mammalian pregnancy. Heterozygous mutation in P450scc was described in a 4-yr-old with 46,XY sex reversal and late-onset form of lipoid adrenal hyperplasia. At 6–7 wk of gestation, when maternal corpus luteum progesterone synthesis stops, the placenta, which does not express StAR, produces progesterone by StAR-independent steroidogenesis using the P450scc enzyme system.

3β-HYDROXYSTEROID DEHYDROGENASE DEFICIENCY. Males with this form of congenital adrenal hyperplasia (see Chapter 577) have various degrees of **hypospadias,** with or without bifid scrotum and cryptorchidism and, rarely, a complete female phenotype. Affected infants usually acquire salt-losing manifestations shortly after birth. Incomplete defects, occasionally seen in boys with premature pubarche, as well as late-onset nonclassic forms have been reported. These children have point mutations of the gene for type II 3β-hydroxysteroid enzyme, resulting in impairment of steroidogenesis in the adrenals and gonads; the impairment may be unequal between adrenals and gonads. Normal pubertal changes in some boys could be explained by the normally present type I 3β-hydroxysteroid dehydrogenase present in many peripheral tissues. Infertility is not infrequent. More than 31 different mutations are reported. There is no correlation between degree of salt wasting and degree of phenotypic abnormality.

DEFICIENCY OF 17-HYDROXYLASE/17,20 LYASE. A single enzyme (P450c17) encoded by a single gene on chromosome 10q24.3 has both 17-hydroxylase and 17,20 lyase activities in adrenal and gonadal tissues (see Chapter 577). Many different genetic lesions have been reported. Genetic males usually have a complete female phenotype or, less often, various degrees of undervirilization from labioscrotal fusion to perineal hypospadias and cryptorchidism. Pubertal development fails to occur in both genetic sexes.

In the classical disorder, there is decreased synthesis of cortisol by the adrenals and of sex steroids by the adrenals and gonads (see Figs. 583-1 and 575-1). Levels of deoxycorticosterone (DOC) and corticosterone are markedly increased and lead to the hypertension and hypokalemia characteristic of this form of male DSD. Although levels of cortisol are low, the elevated corticotropin and corticosterone levels maintain a eucorticoid state. The renin-aldosterone axis is suppressed because of the strong mineralocorticoid effect of elevated DOC. Virilization does not occur at puberty; levels of testosterone are low, and those of gonadotropins are increased. Because fetal production of AMH is normal, no müllerian duct remnants are present. In phenotypic XY females, gonadectomy and replacement therapy with hydrocortisone and sex steroids are indicated.

The defect follows autosomal recessive inheritance. Affected XX females are usually not detected until young adult life, when they fail to experience normal pubertal changes and are found to have hypertension and hypokalemia. This condition should be suspected in patients presenting with primary amenorrhea and hypertension whose chromosomal complement is either 46,XX or 46,XY.

DEFICIENCY OF 17-KETOSTEROID REDUCTASE. This enzyme, also called 17β-hydroxysteroid dehydrogenase (17β-HSD), is the last in the testosterone biosynthetic pathway; it is necessary to convert androstenedione to testosterone and also dehydroepiandrosterone to androstenediol and estrone to estradiol. Enzymatic defects in fetal testicular tissue give rise to males with complete or near-complete female phenotype in 46,XY males. Müllerian ducts are absent, and a shallow vagina is present. The diagnosis is based on the ratio of testosterone to androstenedione; in prepubertal children, prior stimulation with hCG is necessary.

The defect is inherited in an autosomal recessive fashion. At least four different types of 17β-HSD are recognized, each coded by a different gene or different chromosomes. Type III is the enzyme defect that is especially common in a highly inbred Arab population in Gaza. The gene for the disorder is at 9q22 and is expressed only in the testes, where it converts androstenedione to testosterone. Most patients are diagnosed at puberty because of the failure to menstruate and of virilization. Testosterone levels at puberty may approach normal, presumably as a result of peripheral conversion of androstenedione to testosterone; at this time, some patients spontaneously adopt a male gender role.

Type I 17β-HSD, encoded by a gene on chromosome 17q21, converts estrone to estradiol and is found in placenta, ovary, testis, liver, prostate, adipose tissue, and endometrium. Type II, whose gene is on chromosome 16q24, has activities that are opposite to those of types I and III (convert testosterone to androstenedione and estrone to estradiol). Type IV is similar in action to type II. A late-onset form of 17-ketosteroid reductase deficiency presents as gynecomastia in young adult males.

PERSISTENT MÜLLERIAN DUCT SYNDROME. In this disorder, there is persistence of müllerian duct derivatives in otherwise completely virilized males. Cases have been reported in siblings and identical twins. **Cryptorchidism** is present in 80% of affected males; and during surgery for this or inguinal hernia, the condition is uncovered when a fallopian tube and uterus are found. The degree of müllerian development is variable and may be asymmetric. Testicular function is normal in most, but testicular degeneration has been reported. Some affected males acquire testicular tumors after puberty. In a study of 38 families, 16 families had defects in the AMH gene, located on the short arm of chromosome 19. They had low AMH levels. In 16 families with high AMH levels, the defect was in the AMH type II receptor gene, with 10/16 having identical 27-bp deletions on exon 10 in at least one allele.

Treatment consists of removal of as many of the müllerian structures as possible without causing damage to the testis, epididymis, or vas deferens.

DEFECTS IN ANDROGEN ACTION

In the following group of disorders, fetal synthesis of testosterone is normal and defective virilization results from inherited abnormalities in androgen action.

5α-REDUCTASE DEFICIENCY. Decreased production of dihydrotestosterone (DHT) in utero results in severe ambiguity of the external genitals of the affected male fetus. Biosynthesis and peripheral action of testosterone are normal.

The phenotype most commonly associated with this condition results in boys who have a small phallus, bifid scrotum, urogenital sinus with perineal hypospadias, and a blind vaginal pouch (Fig. 589-3). Testes are in the inguinal canals or labioscrotal folds and are normal histologically. There are no müllerian structures. Wolffian structures—the vas deferens, epididymis, and seminal vesicles—are present. Most affected patients have been identified as females. At puberty, virilization occurs; the phallus enlarges, the testes descend and grow normally, and spermatogenesis occurs. There is no gynecomastia. Beard growth is scanty, acne is absent, the prostate is small, and recession of the temporal hairline fails to occur. Virilization of the wolffian duct is caused by the action of testosterone itself, although masculinization of the urogenital sinus and external genitals depends on the action of DHT during the critical period of fetal masculinization. Growth of facial hair and of the prostate also appears to be DHT dependent.

The adult height reached is close to that of the father and other male siblings. There is, however, significant phenotypic heterogeneity. This has led to a classification of such patients into 5 types of steroid 5α-reductase deficiency (SRD) ranging from complete female (type 5), to partial female (type 4), ambiguous (type 3), predominantly male with micropenis (type 2), and completely male phenotype without apparent undervirilization (type 1).

Several different gene defects leading to SRD have been identified in the 5α-reductase type 2 gene, located on the short arm of chromosome 2, in patients from throughout the world. Famil-

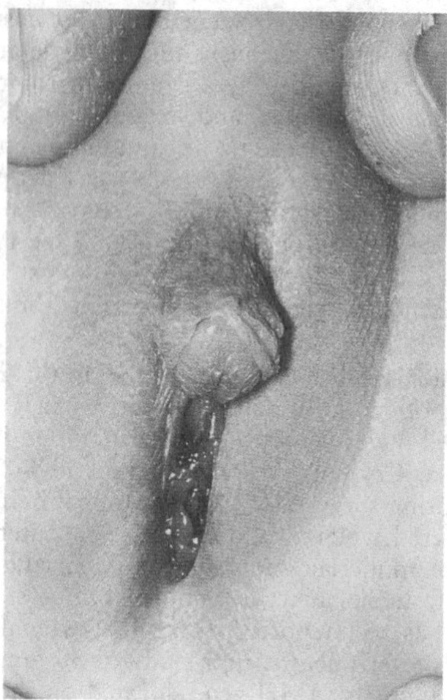

Figure 589-3. 5α-Reductase deficiency. (From Wales JKH, Wit JM, Rogol AD: *Pediatric Endocrinology and Growth,* 2nd edition. Philadelphia, Elsevier/Saunders, 2003, p 165.)

ial clusters have been reported from the Dominican Republic, Turkey, Papua New Guinea, Brazil, Mexico, and the Middle East. There is no correlation between severity of the genetic defect and phenotype.

The disorder is inherited as an autosomal recessive trait but is limited to males; normal homozygous females with normal fertility indicate that in females DHT has no role in sexual differentiation or in ovarian function later in life. The clinical diagnosis should be made as early as possible in infancy; it should be distinguished from androgen insensitivity syndrome. The biochemical diagnosis is based on finding normal serum testosterone levels, normal or low DHT levels with markedly increased basal and especially hCG-stimulated testosterone : DHT ratios (>17), and high ratios of urinary etiocholanolone to androsterone and 5α to 5α metabolites. Children with androgen insensitivity have normal hepatic 5α reduction and, thus, a normal ratio of tetrahydrocortisol to 5α-tetrahydrocortisol, as opposed to those with SRD.

Most but, importantly, not all children reared as females in childhood have changed to male around the time of puberty. It appears that exposures to testosterone in utero, neonatally, and at puberty contribute to the formation of male gender identity. Much more needs to be learned about the influences of hormones such as androgens as well as the influences of cultural, social, psychologic, genetic, and other biologic factors in gender identity and behavior. Infants with this condition should be reared as boys whenever practical. **Treatment** of male infants with DHT results in phallic enlargement.

ANDROGEN INSENSITIVITY SYNDROMES. The AISs are the most common forms of male DSD, occurring with a presumed frequency of 1/20,000 genetic males. This group of heterogeneous X-linked disorders is due to more than 150 different mutations in the androgen receptor gene, located on Xq11–12: single point mutations resulting in amino acid substitutions or premature stop codons, frameshift and premature terminations, gene deletions, and splice site mutations.

Clinical Manifestations. The clinical spectrum of patients with AISs, all of whom have a 46,XY chromosomal complement, range from phenotypic females (in complete AIS) to males with various forms of ambiguous genitals and undervirilization (partial AIS, or clinical syndromes such as **Reifenstein syndrome**) to phenotypically normal-appearing males with infertility. In addition to normal 46,XY chromosomes, the presence of testes and normal or elevated testosterone levels are common to all such children (Figs. 589-4 and 589-5).

In **complete AIS,** an extreme form of failure of virilization, genetic males appear female at birth and are invariably reared accordingly. The external genitals are female. The vagina ends blindly in a pouch, and the uterus is absent. In about one third of patients, unilateral or bilateral fallopian tube remnants are found. The testes are usually intra-abdominal but may descend into the inguinal canal; they consist largely of seminiferous tubules. Twin girls with inguinal hernias containing testes were described. At puberty, there is normal development of breasts, and the habitus is female, but menstruation does not occur and sexual hair is absent. Adult heights of these women are commensurate with those of normal males despite profound congenital deficiency of androgenic effects.

The testes of affected adult patients produce normal male levels of testosterone and DHT. Failure of normal male differentiation during fetal life reflects defective response to androgens at that time, but the absence of müllerian ducts indicates normal fetal

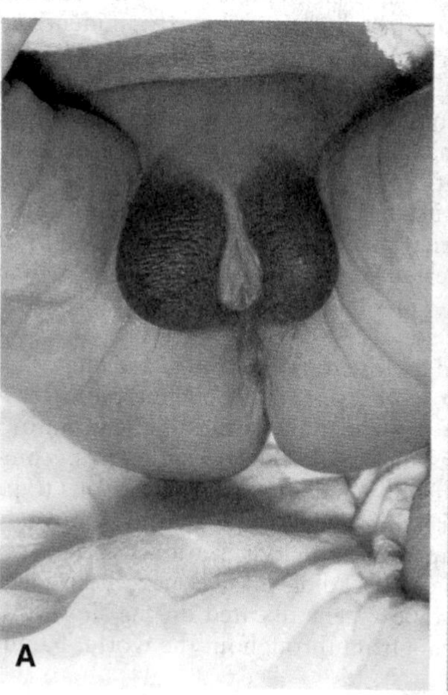

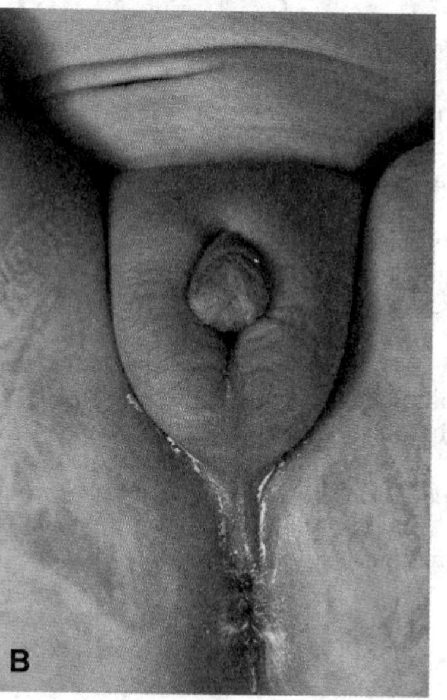

Figure 589-4. *A,* Partial androgen insensitivity with descended testes in bifid labioscrotal folds. *B,* Less severe partial androgen insensitivity with severe hypospadias and maldescent of testes. (From Wales JKH, Wit JM, Rogol AD: *Pediatric Endocrinology and Growth,* 2nd edition. Philadelphia, Elsevier/Saunders, 2003, p 165.)

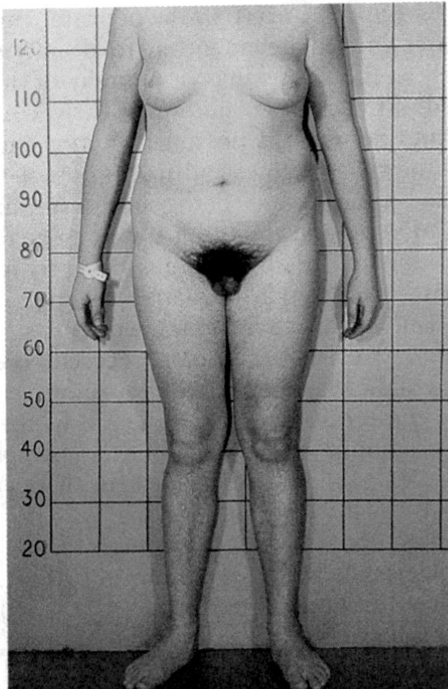

Figure 589-5. Partial androgen insensitivity syndrome at adolescence, male sex of rearing. Note gynecomastia from peripheral aromatase conversion of testosterone to estrogen. Abundant pubic hair implies only partial resistance. (From Wales JKH, Wit JM, Rogol AD: *Pediatric Endocrinology and Growth*, 2nd edition. Philadelphia, Elsevier/Saunders, 2003, p 165.)

testicular production of AMH. The absence of androgenic effects is caused by a striking resistance to the action of endogenous or exogenous testosterone at the cellular level.

Prepubertal children with this disorder are often detected when inguinal masses prove to be testes or when a testis is unexpectedly found during herniorrhaphy in a phenotypic female. About 1–2% of girls with an inguinal hernia prove to have this disorder. In infants, elevated gonadotropin levels should suggest the diagnosis. In adults, **amenorrhea** is the usual presenting symptom. In prepubertal children, the condition must be differentiated from other types of XY undervirilized males in which there is complete feminization. These include XY gonadal dysgenesis (Swyer syndrome), true agonadism, Leydig cell aplasia including LH receptor defects, and 17-ketosteroid reductase deficiency; all these conditions, unlike complete AIS, are characterized by **low levels of testosterone** as neonates and during adult life and by failure to respond to hCG during the prepubertal years. Although patients with complete AIS have unambiguously female external genitals at birth, those with **partial AIS** have a wide variety of phenotypic presentations ranging from **perineoscrotal hypospadias,** bifid scrotum, and cryptorchidism to extreme undervirilization appearing as clitoromegaly and labial fusion. Some forms of partial AIS have been known as specific syndromes. Patients with **Reifenstein syndrome** have incomplete virilization characterized by hypogonadism, severe hypospadias, and gynecomastia (see Fig. 589-5). **Gilbert-Dreyfus** and **Lubs** are additional syndromes classified as partial AIS. In all cases, abnormalities in the androgen receptor gene have been identified.

Diagnosis. The diagnosis of patients with partial AIS may be particularly difficult in infancy. The postnatal surge in testosterone and LH is diminished in those with complete AIS (CAIS) but not in those with partial AIS (PAIS). In some, especially those sufficiently virilized in infancy, the diagnosis is not suspected until puberty when there is inadequate virilization with lack of facial hair or voice change and the appearance of gynecomastia. Azoospermia and infertility are common. Increasingly, androgen receptor defects are being recognized in adults who have a small phallus and testes and infertility. A single-amino-acid substitution in the androgen receptor was reported in a large Chinese family in whom some affected members were fertile while others had gynecomastia and/or hypospadias. IGF2 and IGFBP2 but not IGFBP3 production by genital skin fibroblasts is decreased in CAIS compared with normal genital skin fibroblasts, suggesting a possible role for the IGF system in modulating androgen action.

Treatment and Prognosis. In patients with CAIS whose sexual orientation is unambiguously female, the testes should be removed as soon as they are discovered. Laparoscopic removal of Y-chromosome-bearing gonads has been performed in patients with AIS and in those with gonadal dysgenesis. In one third of patients, malignant tumors, usually seminomas, develop by 50 yr of age. Several teenaged girls have acquired seminomas. Replacement therapy with estrogens is indicated at the age of puberty.

Normal breasts develop in affected girls who have not had their testes removed by the age of puberty. In these individuals, production of estradiol results from aromatase activity. The absence of androgenic activity also contributes to the feminization of these women.

The psychosexual and surgical management of patients with partial AIS is extremely complex and depends in large part on the presenting phenotype. Osteopenia is recognized as a feature of AIS.

Molecular analyses have suggested that phenotype may depend in part on somatic mosaicism of the androgen receptor gene. This was based on the case of a 46,XY patient who had a premature stop codon in exon 1 of the AR gene but who also had evidence of virilization (pubic hair and clitoral enlargement) explained by the discovery of the wild-type alleles on careful examination of the sequencing gel. The presence of mosaicism shifts the phenotype to a higher degree of virilization than expected from the genotype of the mutant allele alone.

Genetic counseling is difficult in families with androgen receptor gene mutation. In addition to lack of genotype-phenotype correlations, there is a high rate (27%) of de novo mutations in families.

Sex hormone–binding globulin reduction after exogenous androgen administration (stanozolol) has been shown to correlate with the severity of the receptor defect and may become a useful clinical tool. Successful therapy with supplemental androgens has been reported in patients with partial AIS and various mutations of the androgen receptor in the DNA-binding domain and the ligand-binding domain.

Mutated androgen receptors are also reported in patients with spinal and bulbar muscular atrophy in whom clinical manifestations including testicular atrophy, infertility, gynecomastia, and elevated LH, FSH, and estradiol levels usually manifest between the 3rd and 5th decades of life. Androgen receptor mutations have also been described in patients with prostate cancer.

UNDETERMINED CAUSES

Other XY undervirilized males display great variability of the external and internal genitals and various degrees of phallic and müllerian development. Testes may be histologically normal or rudimentary, or there may only be one. Even the newer techniques may find no recognized cause of DSD in a substantial number of children. Some ambiguity of genitals is associated with a wide variety of chromosomal aberrations, which must always be considered in the differential diagnosis, the most common being the 45,X/46,XY syndrome (see Chapter 587.1). It may be necessary to examine several tissues to establish mosaicism. Other complex genetic syndromes, many resulting from single gene mutations, are associated with varying degrees of ambiguity of the genitals, particularly in the male. These entities must be identified on the basis of the associated extragenital malformations.

Smith-Lemli-Opitz syndrome is an autosomal recessive disorder caused by mutations in the sterol Δ7-reductase gene located on chromosome 11q12–q13. It is characterized by prenatal and postnatal growth retardation, microcephaly, ptosis, anteverted nares, broad alveolar ridges, syndactyly of the 2nd–3rd toes, and severe mental retardation (see Chapter 86.3). Its incidence is 1/20,000 to 1/60,000; 70% are male. Genotypic males usually have genital ambiguity and, occasionally, complete sex reversal with female genital ambiguity or complete sex reversal with female external genitals. Müllerian duct derivatives are usually absent. Affected 46,XX patients have normal genitals. Two types of Smith-Lemli-Opitz syndrome have been recognized: the **classical form** (type I) described earlier and the acrodysgenital syndrome, which is usually lethal within 1 yr and is associated with severe malformations, postaxial polydactyly, and extremely abnormal external genitals (type II). Pyloric stenosis is associated with Smith-Lemli-Opitz syndrome type I and Hirschsprung disease with type II. Cleft palate, skeletal abnormalities, and one case of a lipoma of the pituitary gland have been seen in **type II** cases. Some authors believe in a spectrum of disease severity rather than in the above classification. Low plasma cholesterol with elevated 7-dehydrocholesterol, its precursor, are found in types 1 and 2, and the levels do not correlate with severity. Maternal apolipoprotein E values do seem to correlate with severity. The most common prenatal expression of Smith-Lemli-Opitz syndrome is intrauterine growth retardation (see Chapter 86.3 for treatment).

46,XY DSD subjects also have been described in siblings with the α-thalassemia/mental retardation syndrome.

589.3 • Ovotesticular DSD

In ovotesticular DSD, both ovarian and testicular tissues are present, either in the same or in opposite gonads. Affected patients have ambiguous genitals, varying from normal female with only slight enlargement of the clitoris to almost normal male external genitals (see Fig. 589-2A).

About 70% of all patients have a 46,XX karyotype; 97% of affected African blacks are 46,XX. Fewer than 10% of persons with ovotesticular DSD are 46,XY. About 20% have 46,XX/46,XY mosaicism. Half of these are derived from more than one zygote and are chimeras (chi 46,XX/46,XY). The presence of paternal and both maternal alleles for some blood groups is demonstrated. An ovotesticular DSD chimera, 46,XX/46,XY, was reported as resulting from embryo amalgamation after in vitro fertilization. Each embryo was derived from an independent, separately fertilized ovum.

Examination of 46,XX ovotesticular DSD patients with Y-specific probes has detected fewer than 10% with a portion of the Y chromosome including the *SRY* gene. Ovotesticular DSD is usually sporadic, but a number of siblings have been reported. The cause of most cases of ovotesticular DSD is unknown.

The most frequently encountered gonad in ovotesticular DSD is an ovotestis, which may be bilateral; if unilateral, the contralateral gonad is usually an ovary but may be a testis. The ovarian tissue is normal, but the testicular tissue is dysgenetic. The presence and function of testicular tissue can be determined by measuring basal and hCG-stimulated testosterone levels as well as AMH levels. Patients who are highly virilized, have good testicular function, and have no uterus are usually reared as males. If a uterus exists, virilization is mild, and testicular function minimal; assignment of female sex may be indicated. Selective removal of gonadal tissue inconsistent with sex of rearing may be indicated. In a few families, 46,XY ovotesticular DSD subjects and 44,XX males have been in the same sibship.

Pregnancies with living offspring have been reported in 46,XX ovotesticular DSD individuals reared as females, but very few males with ovotesticular DSD have fathered children. About 5% of patients acquire gonadoblastomas, dysgerminomas, or seminomas.

DIAGNOSIS AND MANAGEMENT. In the neonate, ambiguity of the genitals requires immediate attention to decide on the sex of rearing as early in life as possible. The family of the infant needs to be informed of the child's condition as early, completely, compassionately, and honestly as possible. Caution must be used to avoid feelings of guilt, shame, and discomfort. Guidance needs to be provided to alleviate both short-term and long-term concerns and to allow the child to grow up in a completely supportive environment. The initial care is best provided by a team of professionals that include neonatologists and pediatric specialists, endocrinologists, radiologists, urologists, psychologists, and geneticists, all of whom remain focused foremost on the needs of the child. Management of the potential psychologic upheaval that these disorders can generate in the child or the family is of paramount importance and requires physicians and other health care professionals with sensitivity, training, and experience in this field.

While awaiting the results of chromosomal analysis, pelvic ultrasonography is indicated to determine the presence of a uterus and ovaries. Presence of a uterus and absence of palpable gonads usually suggests a virilized XX female. A search for the source of virilization should be undertaken; this includes studies of adrenal hormones to rule out varieties of congenital adrenal hyperplasia, and studies of androgens and estrogens occasionally may be necessary to rule out aromatase deficiency. Virilized XX females are generally (but not always) reared as females even when highly virilized.

The absence of a uterus, with or without palpable gonads, almost always indicates an undervirilized male and an XY karyotype. Measurements of levels of gonadotropins, testosterone, AMH, and DHT are necessary to determine whether testicular production of androgen is normal. Undervirilized males who are totally feminized may be reared as females. However, certain significantly feminized infants, such as those with 5α-reductase deficiency, may be reared as males because these children virilize normally at puberty. Sixty per cent of individuals assigned as female in infancy live as males. An infant with a comparable degree of feminization resulting from an androgen receptor defect, such as CAIS, is best reared as a female. Infants with 45,XX/46,XY karyotype whose phenotype varies from almost completely male to completely female are usually reared as females because they are generally short in stature and have a uterus; they require gonadectomy.

When receptor disorders are suspected in the XY male with a small phallus (micropenis), a course of 3 monthly intramuscular injections of testosterone enanthate (25–50 mg) may assist in the differential diagnosis as well as in treatment.

In some mammals, the female exposed to androgens prenatally or in early postnatal life exhibits nontraditional sexual behavior in adult life. Most, but not all, girls who have undergone fetal masculinization from congenital adrenal hyperplasia or from maternal progestin therapy have no such problems in sexual identity, although during childhood they may appear to prefer male playmates and activities over female playmates and feminine play with dolls in mothering roles.

It has been thought that it is more feasible to reconstruct the external genitals to create a functional female, particularly when a vagina is present, than to create a functional male phallus. Hence, in the absence of reasonable prospects for a well-functioning male phallus, such DSD infants have in the past always been assigned a female gender. Considerable controversy currently exists regarding these decisions. A poorly functioning female external genital system may be no better than a poorly functioning male phallus. In addition, sexual functioning is to a large extent more dependent on other neurohormonal and behavioral factors than the physical appearance and functional ability of the genitals. This concept is given added support by a case report of a 46,XY subject whose penis was accidentally ablated and was subsequently reared as a female. At puberty, this individual switched to male and continues to successfully live as such.

Similarly, controversy exists regarding the timing of the performance of invasive and definitive procedures, such as surgery. Whenever possible without endangering the physical or psychological health of the child, an expert multidisciplinary team should consider deferring elective surgical repairs and gonadectomies until the child can participate in the informed consent for the procedure. Long-term prospective as well as retrospective science- and evidence-based studies in sufficient numbers of individuals born with DSD are necessary to evaluate their anatomic, psychosexual, social, as well as functional status. The results of these studies can then be utilized to make informed recommendations about all aspects of the management of infants and children with DSD.

The pediatrician and pediatric endocrinologist, along with the appropriate additional specialists, should provide ongoing compassionate, supportive care to the patient and the patient's family throughout childhood, adolescence, and even young adulthood. Support groups are available for families and patients with many of the conditions discussed.

Bose HS, Pescovitz OH, Miller WL: Spontaneous feminization in a 46,XX female patient with congenital lipoid adrenal hyperplasia due to a homozygous frameshift mutation in the steroidogenic acute regulatory protein. *J Clin Endocrinol Metab* 1997;82:1511–1515.

Brinkmann AO: Molecular basis of androgen insensitivity. *Mol Cell Endocrinol* 2001;179:105–1099.

Cameron FJ, Montalto J, Byrt E, et al: Gonadal dysgenesis: Associations between clinical features and sex of rearing. *Endocr J* 1997;44:95–104.

Canto P, Vilchis F, Chavez B, et al: Mutations of the 5α-reductase type 2 gene in eight Mexican patients from six different pedigrees with 5α-reductase-2 deficiency. *Clin Endocrinol* 1997;46:155–160.

Chu J, Zhang R, Zhao Z, et al: Male fertility is compatible with an Arg840 Cys substitution in the AR in a large Chinese family affected with divergent phenotypes of AR insensitivity syndrome. *J Clin Endocrinol Metab* 2002;87:347–351.

Creighton S, Minto C: Managing intersex. *Br Med J* 2001;323:1264–1265.

Daaboul J, Frader J: Ethics and the management of the patient with intersex: A middle way. *J Pediatr Endocrinol Metab* 2001;14:1575–1583.

Damiani D, Fellous M, McElreavey K, et al: True hermaphroditism: Clinical aspects and molecular studies in 16 cases. *Eur J Endocrinol* 1997;136:201–204.

Diamond DA, Mitchell C, Lamb K, et al: Sex assignment for newborns with ambiguous genitalia and exposure to fetal testosterone: Attitudes and practices of pediatric urologists. *J Pediatr* 2006;148:445–449.

Diamond M, Sigmundson K: Sex reassignment at birth. *Arch Pediatr Adolesc Med* 1997;151:298–304.

Frade Costa EM, Bilharinho Mendonca B, Inacio M, et al: Management of ambiguous genitalia in pseudohermaphrodites: New perspectives on vaginal dilation. *Fertil Steril* 1997;67:229–232.

Geissler WM, Davis DL, Wu L, et al: Male pseudohermaphroditism caused by mutation of testicular 17β-hydroxysteroid dehydrogenase 3. *Nat Genet* 1994;7:34–39.

Gul D: Third case of WAGR syndrome with severe obesity and constitutional deletion of chromosome (11)(p12p14). *Am J Med Genet* 2002;107:70–71.

Hiort O, Sinnecker GHG, Holterbus PM, et al: Inherited and de novo androgen receptor gene mutations: Investigation of single-case families. *J Pediatr* 1998;132:939–943.

Hochberg Z, Chayen R, Reiss N, et al: Clinical, biochemical and genetic findings in a large pedigree of male and female patients with 5α-reductase 2 deficiency. *J Clin Endocrinol Metab* 1996;81:2821–2827.

Kremer H, Karaaij R, Toledo SPA, et al: Male pseudohermaphroditism due to a homozygous missense mutation of the luteinizing hormone receptor gene. *Nat Genet* 1995;9:160–164.

Krob G, Braun A, Kuhnle U: True hermaphroditism: Geographical distribution, clinical findings, chromosomes and gonadal histology. *Eur J Pediatr* 1994;153:2–10.

Lee PA, Houk CP, Ahmed SF, et al: Consensus statement on management of intersex disorders. *Pediatrics* 2006;118:e488–500.

MacLaughlin DT, Donahoe PK: Sex determination and differentiation. *N Engl J Med* 2004;350:367–378.

McPherson EW, Clemens MM, Gibbons RJ, et al: X-linked α-thalassemia/mental retardation (ATR-X) syndrome: A new kindred with severe genital anomalies and mild hematologic expression. *Am J Med Genet* 1995;55:302–306.

Mebarki F, Sanchez R, Rheaumes E, et al: Non-salt-losing male pseudohermaphroditism due to the novel homozygous N100S mutation in the type II 3 β-hydroxysteroid dehydrogenase gene. *J Clin Endocrinol Metab* 1995;80:2127–2134.

Mendonca BB, Inacio M, Costa EMF, et al: Male pseudohermaphroditism due to steroid 5α-reductase 2 deficiency. *Medicine* 1996;75:64–76.

Mendonca BB, Leite MV, DeCastro M, et al: Female pseudohermaphroditism caused by a novel homozygous mutation of the GR gene. *J Clin Endocrinol Metab* 2002;87:1805–1809.

Moisan AM, Ricketts ML, Tardy V, et al: New insight into the molecular basis of 3β-hydroxysteroid dehydrogenase deficiency: Identification of eight mutations in the HSD3 gene in eleven patients from seven new families and comparison of the functional properties of twenty-five mutant enzymes. *J Clin Endocrinol Metab* 1999;84:4410–4425.

Mongan NP, Jaaskelainen J, Green K, et al: Two de novo mutations in the AR gene cause the complete androgen insensitivity syndrome in a pair of monozygotic twins. *J Clin Endocrinol Metab* 2002;87:1057–1061.

Morishima A, Grumbach MM, Simpson ER, et al: Aromatase deficiency in male and female siblings caused by a novel mutation and the physiological role of estrogens. *J Clin Endocrinol Metab* 1995;80:3689–3698.

Mueller RF: The Denys-Drash syndrome. *J Med Genet* 1994;31:471–477.

Mullis PE, Yoshimura N, Kuhlmann B, et al: Aromatase deficiency in a female who is compound heterozygote for two new point mutations in the $P450_{arom}$ gene: Impact of estrogens on hypergonadotropic hypogonadism, multicystic ovaries, and bone densitometry in childhood. *J Clin Endocrinol Metab* 1997;82:1739–1745.

Quigley CA, French FS: Androgen insensitivity syndromes. *Curr Ther Endocrinol Metab* 1994;5:342–351.

Reardon W, Gibbons RJ, Winter RM, et al: Male pseudohermaphroditism in sibs with the α-thalassemia/mental retardation (ATR-X) syndrome. *Am J Med Genet* 1995;55:285–287.

Saenger P: New developments in congenital lipoid adrenal hyperplasia and steroidogenic acute regulatory protein. *Pediatr Clin North Am* 1997;44:397–421.

Sarafoglou K, Ostrer H: Clinical Review 111—Familial sex reversal: A review. *J Clin Endocrinol Metab* 2000;85:483–493.

Smith EP, Boyd J, Frank GR, et al: Estrogen resistance caused by a mutation in the estrogen-receptor gene in a man. *N Engl J Med* 1994;331:1056–1061.

Tajima T, Fujieda K, Kouda N, et al: Heterozygous mutation in the cholesterol side chain cleavage enzyme (P450scc) gene in a patient with 46,XY sex reversal and adrenal insufficiency. *J Clin Endocrinol Metab* 2001;86:3820–3825.

Weidemann W, Peters B, Romalo G, et al: Response to androgen treatment in a patient with partial androgen insensitivity and a mutation in the deoxyribonucleic acid-binding domain of the androgen receptor. *J Clin Endocrinol Metab* 1998;83:1173–1176.

Section 6 — Diabetes Mellitus in Children — Ramin Alemzadeh and David T. Wyatt

Chapter 590 ■ Diabetes Mellitus

590.1 • Introduction and Classification

Diabetes mellitus (DM) is a common, chronic, metabolic syndrome characterized by hyperglycemia as a cardinal biochemical feature. The major forms of diabetes are classified according to those caused by deficiency of insulin secretion due to pancreatic β-cell damage (type 1 DM, or T1DM) and those that are a consequence of insulin resistance occurring at the level of skeletal muscle, liver, and adipose tissue, with various degrees of β-cell impairment (type 2 DM, or T2DM). T1DM is the most common endocrine-metabolic disorder of childhood and adolescence, with important consequences for physical and emotional development. Individuals with T1DM confront serious lifestyle alterations that include an absolute daily requirement for exogenous insulin, the need to monitor their own glucose level, and the need to pay attention to dietary intake. Morbidity and mortality stem from acute metabolic derangements and from long-term **complications** (usually in adulthood) that affect small and large vessels resulting in retinopathy, nephropathy, neuropathy, ischemic heart disease, and arterial obstruction with gangrene of the extremities. The acute clinical manifestations are due to hypoinsulinemic hyperglycemic ketoacidosis. Autoimmune mechanisms are factors in the genesis of T1DM; the long-term complications are related to metabolic disturbances (hyperglycemia).

DM is not a single entity but rather a heterogeneous group of disorders in which there are distinct genetic patterns as well as other etiologic and pathophysiologic mechanisms that lead to impairment of glucose tolerance. A classification of diabetes and other categories of glucose intolerance is presented in Table 590-1. Three major forms of diabetes and several forms of carbohydrate intolerance are identified.

TYPE 1 DIABETES MELLITUS. Formerly called insulin-dependent diabetes mellitus (IDDM) or juvenile diabetes, T1DM is characterized by low or absent levels of endogenously produced insulin and dependence on exogenous insulin to prevent development of ketoacidosis, an acute life-threatening complication of T1DM. The natural history includes 4 distinct stages: (1) preclinical β-cell autoimmunity with progressive defect of insulin secretion, (2) onset of clinical diabetes, (3) transient remission "honeymoon period," and (4) established diabetes associated with acute and chronic complications and decreased life expectancy. The onset occurs predominantly in childhood, with median age of 7 to 15 yr, but it may present at any age. T1DM is characterized by autoimmune destruction of pancreatic islet β cells. Both genetic susceptibility and environmental factors contribute to the pathogenesis. Susceptibility to T1DM is genetically controlled by alleles of the major histocompatibility complex (MHC) class II genes expressing human leukocyte antigens (HLAs). It is also associated with autoantibodies to islet cell cytoplasm (ICA), insulin (IAA), antibodies to glutamic acid decarboxylase (GADA or GAD65), and ICA512 (IA2). T1DM is associated with other **autoimmune** diseases such as thyroiditis, celiac disease, multiple sclerosis, and Addison disease. In some children and adolescents with apparent T1DM, the β-cell destruction is not immune mediated. This subtype of diabetes occurs in patients of African or Asian origin and is distinct from known causes of β-cell destruction such as drugs or chemicals, viruses, mitochondrial gene defects, pancreatectomy, and ionizing radiation. These individuals may have ketoacidosis, but they have extensive periods of remission with variable insulin deficiency, similarly to patients with T2DM.

TYPE 2 DIABETES MELLITUS. The children and adolescents with this type of diabetes are usually obese but are not insulin dependent and infrequently develop ketosis. Some may develop ketosis during severe infections or other stresses and may then need insulin for correction of symptomatic hyperglycemia. This category includes the most prevalent form of diabetes in adults, which is characterized by insulin resistance and often a progressive defect in insulin secretion. This type of diabetes was formerly known as adult-onset diabetes mellitus, non-insulin-dependent diabetes mellitus (NIDDM), or maturity-onset diabetes of the young (MODY).

The presentation of T2DM is typically more insidious than that with T1DM. In contrast to patients with T1DM who are usually ill at the time of diagnosis, children with T2DM often seek medical care because of excessive weight gain and fatigue as a result of insulin resistance and/or an incidental finding of glycosuria during routine physical examination. A history of polyuria and polydipsia is relatively uncommon in these patients. The incidence of T2DM in children has increased by more than 10-fold in many diabetes centers, in part as a result of the epidemic of childhood obesity (see Chapter 44). Pediatric T2DM may account for as many as 30% of the new cases of diabetes, especially in obese African and Mexican American adolescents. **Acanthosis nigricans** (dark pigmentation of skin creases/flexural areas), a sign of insulin resistance, is present in the majority of patients with T2DM and is accompanied by a relative hyperinsulinemia at the time of the diagnosis (see Chapter 651). However, the serum insulin elevation is usually disproportionately lower than that of age-, weight-, and sex-matched nondiabetic children and adolescents, suggesting a state of insulin insufficiency. In some individuals, it may represent slowly evolving T1DM.

In some children with strong family history of T2DM, impaired glucose tolerance may occur in a pattern implying dominant inheritance. This pattern of diabetes has been termed **maturity-onset diabetes of the young** (MODY) and may require insulin treatment. In MODY, there is no apparent autoimmune destruction of β cells and no HLA association. This subclass of T2DM consists of specific genetic disorders involving mutations in the gene encoding either pancreatic β-cell and liver glucokinase (GK) or in the nuclear transcription factors hepatocyte nuclear factor (HNF) (1α, 4α, or 1β). A defect in the gene regulating glucose transport into the pancreatic β cell, the GLUT2 transporter, may be responsible for other forms of T2DM. The genetic basis of T2DM also includes defects in glycogen synthase, insulin receptors, Rad (Ras associated with diabetes), and possibly apolipoprotein C-III.

OTHER SPECIFIC TYPES OF SECONDARY DIABETES. Examples include diabetes secondary to exocrine pancreatic diseases (cystic fibrosis), other endocrine diseases (Cushing syndrome), and ingestion of certain drugs or poisons (the rodenticide Vacor). Certain genetic syndromes, including those with abnormalities of the

TABLE 590-1. Etiologic Classifications of Diabetes Mellitus

Type I diabetes* (β-cell destruction, usually leading to absolute insulin deficiency)
Immune mediated
Idiopathic
Type 2 diabetes* (may range from predominantly insulin resistance with relative insulin deficiency to a predominantly secretory defect with insulin resistance)
Dominant type 2 due to sulfonylurea receptor 1 mutation.
Other specific types
Genetic defects of β-cell function
Chromosome 12, HNF-1α (MODY3)
Chromosome 7, glucokinase (MODY2)
Chromosome 20, HNF-4α (MODY1)
Insulin promotor factor–1 (MODY4)
HNF-1β (MODY5)
NEUROD1 (MODY6)
Mitochondrial DNA
Others
Genetic defects in insulin action
Type A insulin resistance
Leprechaunism
Rabson-Mendenhall syndrome
Lipoatrophic diabetes
Others
Diseases of the exocrine pancreas
Pancreatitis
Trauma, pancreatectomy
Neoplasia
Cystic fibrosis
Hemochromatosis
Fibrocalculous pancreatopathy
Pancreatic resection
Others
Endocrinopathies
Acromegaly
Cushing disease
Glucagonoma
Pheochromocytoma
Hyperthyroidism
Somatostatinoma
Aldosteronoma
Others
Drug-or chemical-induced
Vacor
Pentamidine
Nicotinic acid
Glucocorticoids
Thyroid hormone
Diazoxide
β-Adrenergic agonists
Thiazides
Dilantin
β-Interferon
Others—cyclosporine, tacrolimus
Infections
Congenital rubella
Cytomegalovirus
Others—hemolytic uremic syndrome
Uncommon forms of immune-mediated diabetes
"Stiff-man" syndrome
Cytomegalovirus
Others
Other genetic syndromes sometimes associated with diabetes
Down syndrome
Klinefelter syndrome
Turner syndrome
Wolfram syndrome
Friedreich ataxia
Huntington chorea
Laurence-Moon-Biedl syndrome
Myotonic dystrophy
Porphyria
Prader-Willi syndrome
Others
Gestational diabetes mellitus
Neonatal diabetes mellitus
Transient—without recurrence
Transient—recurrence 7–20 yr later
Permanent from onset

*Patients with any form of diabetes may require insulin treatment at some stage of the disease. Such use of insulin does not, of itself, classify the patient.

TABLE 590-2. Diagnostic Criteria for Impaired Glucose Tolerance and Diabetes Mellitus

IMPAIRED GLUCOSE TOLERANCE (IGT)	DIABETES MELLITUS (DM)
Fasting glucose 110–125 mg/dL (6.1–7.0 mmol/L)	Symptoms* of DM plus random plasma glucose ≥200 mg/dL (11.1 mmol/L)
	or
2-hr plasma glucose during the OGTT <200 mg/dL (11.1 mmol/L)	Fasting plasma glucose ≥126 mg/dL (7.0 mmol/L)
	or
but ≤140 mg/dL	2-hr plasma glucose during the OGTT ≥200 mg/dL

*Symptoms include polyuria, polydipsia, and unexplained weight loss with glucosuria and ketonuria.
OGTT, oral glucose tolerance test.
From Report of the Expert Committee on the Diagnosis and Classification of Diabetes Mellitus. *Diabetes Care* 1999;20(Suppl 1):S5.

insulin receptor, also are included in this category. There are no associations with HLAs, autoimmunity, or islet cell antibodies among the entities in this subdivision.

Table 590-2 details the current criteria for the diagnosis of DM. It should be noted that a fasting blood glucose that exceeds 125 mg/dL (6.9 mmol/L) is the accepted criterion for the diagnosis of diabetes.

IMPAIRED GLUCOSE TOLERANCE. The term impaired glucose tolerance (IGT) refers to a metabolic stage that is intermediate between normal glucose homeostasis and diabetes. A fasting glucose concentration of 99 mg/dL (5.5 mmol/L) is the upper limit of "normal." This choice is near the level above which acute-phase insulin secretion is lost in response to intravenous administration of glucose and is associated with a progressively greater risk of the development of microvascular and macrovascular complications.

Many individuals with IGT (fasting glucose 100–125 mg/dL) are euglycemic in their daily lives and may have normal or nearly normal glycated hemoglobin levels. Individuals with IGT often manifest hyperglycemia only when challenged with the oral glucose load used in the standardized oral glucose tolerance test.

In the absence of pregnancy, IGT is not a clinical entity but rather a risk factor for future diabetes and cardiovascular disease. This may be observed as an intermediate stage in any of the disease processes listed in Table 590-1. IGT is often associated with the **insulin resistance syndrome** (also known as syndrome X or the metabolic syndrome), which consists of insulin resistance, compensatory hyperinsulinemia to maintain glucose homeostasis, obesity (especially abdominal or visceral obesity), dyslipidemia of the high-triglyceride or low- or high-density lipoprotein type, or both, and hypertension (see Chapter 44). Insulin resistance is directly involved in the pathogenesis of T2DM. IGT appears as a risk marker for this type of diabetes at least in part because of its correlation with insulin resistance. The diagnostic criteria for IGT are presented in Table 590-2.

590.2 • Type 1 Diabetes Mellitus (Immune Mediated)

EPIDEMIOLOGY: GENETICS AND ENVIRONMENT. The incidence of T1DM is rapidly increasing in specific regions and shows a trend toward earlier age of onset. T1DM accounts for about 10% of all diabetes, affecting 1.4 million in the United States and about 15 million in the world. It is one of the most common severe chronic childhood diseases; 40% of individuals with type 1 DM are younger than 20 yr of age. The incidence of T1DM is highly variable among different ethnic groups. The overall age-adjusted incidence of type 1 DM varies from 0.7/100,000 per year in Karachi (Pakistan) to about 40/100,000 per year in Finland (Fig.

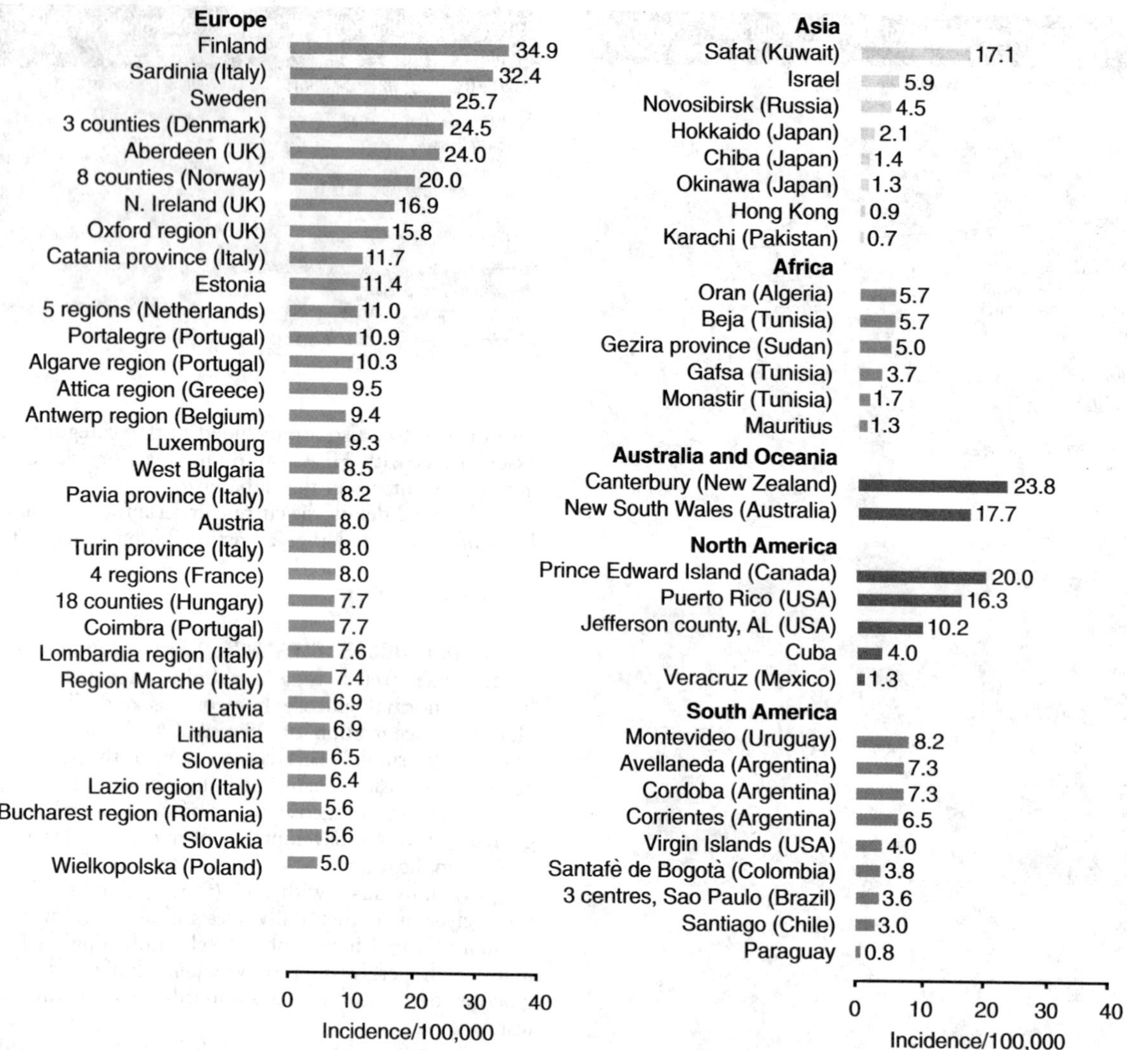

Figure 590-1. Incidence rates of type 1 diabetes mellitus by region and country. (From Karvonen M, Viik-Kajander M, Moltchanova E, et al: Incidence of type I diabetes worldwide. Diabetes Mondiale (DiaMond) Project Group. *Diabetes Care* 2000;23(10):1516–1526.)

590-1). This represents a more than 400-fold variation in the incidence among 100 populations. Often, the increased incidence is seen in nations with a previous low incidence of autoimmune diabetes; the incidence of T1DM in Thailand increased markedly from 0.2/100,000 in 1984–1985 to 1.65/100,000 10 yr later. It is predicted that the overall incidence of T1DM will be about 40% higher in 2010 than in 1997.

Data from Western European diabetes centers suggest that the annual rate increase in T1DM incidence is 3–4%, whereas some central and eastern European countries demonstrate an even more rapid increase. The increasing rate is greatest among the youngest children; rates of increase in T1DM incidence as a function of age at onset are 6.3%, 3.1%, and 2.4% in age groups of children 0–4 yr, 5–9 yr, and 10–14 yr, respectively. In the United States, the overall prevalence of diabetes among school-aged children is about 1.9/1,000. The frequency, however, is highly correlated with increasing age; the range is 1/1,430 children at 5 yr of age to 1/360 children at 16 yr. Among African Americans, the occurrence of T1DM is 30–60% of that seen in American whites. The annual incidence of new cases in the United States is about 14.9/100,000 of the child population. It is estimated that 30,000 new cases occur each year in the United States, affecting 1 in 300 children and as many as 1 in 100 adults during the lifespan. Girls and boys are almost equally affected; there is no apparent correlation with socioeconomic status. Peaks of presentation occur in 2 age groups: at 5–7 yr of age and at the time of puberty. A growing number of cases are presenting between 1 and 2 yr of age. The 1st peak may correspond to the time of increased exposure to infectious agents coincident with the beginning of school; the 2nd peak may correspond to the pubertal growth spurt induced by gonadal steroids and the increased pubertal growth hormone secretion (which antagonizes insulin). These possible cause-and-effect relationships remain to be proved.

Genes. Genes for T1DM may provide susceptibility to, or protection from, the disease. Although many chromosomal loci associated with such activities have been located, few true genes have been identified. The genetics of T1DM cannot be classified according to a specific model of inheritance. The most important genes are located within the MHC HLA class II region on chromosome 6p21, formally termed (IDDM1), accounting for about 60% genetic susceptibility for the disease. Their specific contribution to the pathogenesis of T1DM remains unclear. The importance of the class II haplotypes not only depends on the well-known risk for disease associated with HLA-DR3 and HLA-DR4 but also on additional susceptibility associated with DQ α-chains and DQ β-chains. Inheritance of HLA-DR3 or -DR4 antigens appears to confer a 2- to 3-fold increased risk for the development of T1DM. When both DR3 and DR4 are inherited, the relative risk for the development of diabetes is increased by 7- to 10-fold. Analysis of DNA polymorphisms after digestion by specific restriction endonucleases has revealed further heterogeneity in the HLA-DR region among individuals with and without diabetes despite the possession of both DR3 or DR4 markers, suggesting a yet to be defined "susceptibility" locus within these markers.

In Caucasians, at least one major susceptibility locus may reside in the DQ β_1 gene. The homozygous absence of aspartic acid at position 57 of the HLA DQ β-chain (non-Asp/non-Asp) confers an approximately 100-fold relative risk for the development of type 1 diabetes. Those who are heterozygous with a single aspartic acid at position 57 (non-Asp/Asp) are far less likely to acquire diabetes and only marginally more susceptible than individuals who have aspartic acid on both DQ β-chains, that is, homozygous Asp/Asp. Thus, the presence of aspartic acid at one or both alleles of DQ β protects against the development of autoimmune diabetes. Indeed, the incidence of type 1 DM in any given population appears to be proportional to the gene frequency of non-Asp alleles in that population. In addition, arginine at position 52 of the DQ β-chain confers marked susceptibility to T1DM. Position 57 of the DQ β and position 52 of DQ β are at critical locations of the HLA molecule that permit or prevent antigen presentation to T-cell receptors and activate the autoimmune cascade. However, type 1 DM seems unique among autoimmune diseases in that, in addition to forming susceptibility, certain MHC haplotypes provide significant protection. The HLA-DRB1*0301, HLA-DRB1*0401, HLA-DQB1*0302, and HLA-DQA1*0301 alleles of MHC (IDDM1) confer high-risk susceptibility in humans, whereas other alleles such as HLA-DRB1*0403, HLA-DQB1*0602, and HLA-DQA1*0102 are negatively associated with type 1 DM and may confer resistance. The observation that 20% of individuals from Europe or the United States carry protective HLA-DR2 haplotype, yet fewer than 1% of children with type 1 DM are DR2 (DQB1*0602) positive, highlights this important genetic component.

T1DM represents a heterogeneous and polygenic disorder. About 20 non-HLA loci contributing to disease susceptibility have been identified. The function of only 2 non-HLA loci is known. IDDM2 on chromosome 11p5.5 is a polymorphic region that maps to a variable number of tandem minisatellite repeats (VNTR), with short class I VNTR alleles predisposing to type 1 DM and the longer class III alleles providing dominant protective effect. This locus contributes about 10% toward disease susceptibility. Another locus associated with type 1 DM in some populations is IDDM12 on chromosome 2q33, which maps close to 2 T-cell markers involved in the T-cell activation: cytotoxic T lymphocyte-associated protein4 (CTLA-4) and CD28. Studies in Italian and Spanish families have shown that a polymorphism at CTL4 gene (A–G transition at position 49 of exon 1), called G allele, is preferentially transmitted to the affected siblings.

Factors other than pure inheritance of HLA markers or other genes must also be involved in producing diabetes. For example, HLA-DR3 or -DR4 is found in approximately 50% of the general population, and (non-Asp/non-Asp) is found in approximately 20% of nondiabetic whites in the United States, yet the risk for type 1 DM in these subjects is only one tenth of that in an HLA-identical sibling of an index case possessing these markers. Even siblings sharing only one haplotype have a 6- to 10-fold greater risk of development of type 1 DM compared with the normal population. In addition, about 10% of patients with T1DM do not possess either HLA-DR3 or -DR4 although most white diabetic patients lack at least one aspartic acid at position 57 of the DQ β chain. The concordance rate among identical twins is only 30–50%, suggesting either the participation of environmental triggering factors or other genetic factors such as the postnatal selection of certain autoreactive T-cell clones that bear receptors recognizing "self." This postnatal process occurs within the thymus and implies that identical twins are not identical with respect to the T-cell receptor repertoire they possess.

T1DM among African Americans is associated with the same HLA genes as it is in whites. If a sibling shares both HLA-D haplotypes with an index case, the risk for type 1 DM in that individual is 12–20%; for a sibling sharing one haplotype, the risk is 5–7%; with no haplotypes in common, the risk is only 1–2%. It can be assumed that in whites, the overall risk to siblings is approximately 6% if the proband is younger than 10 yr of age and 3% if the proband is older at the time of diagnosis. The risk to offspring of a diabetic parent is 2–5%, with the higher risk occurring in the offspring of a diabetic father. In African Americans, these risks are only one half to two thirds of those in whites.

Environment. Childhood T1DM was uncommon in the 1st half of the 20th century, but its incidence has risen rapidly over the past 50 yr. The overall proportion of newly diagnosed individuals carrying either or both of the 2 established susceptibility haplotypes DR4-DQ8 and DR3-DQ2 has not changed; there are now fewer with the highest risk DR4-DQ8/DR3-DQ2 genotype, balanced by an increase in the number of those with lower risk DR4-DQ8/X and DR3-DQ2/X genotypes. The overall proportion of DR3-DQ2/DR4-DQ8 genotype declined in children aged 0–15 yr from 47% to 35%, with a decrease in children aged under 5 yr from 63% to 42%. The rising incidence of T1DM in young children has, therefore, been confined to a genetically susceptible subgroup of the population. However, it should be pointed out that the risk of developing T1DM with DR3-DQ2/DR4-DQ8 genotype is only 4%, which makes screening for this genotype a poor screening tool for those who may be at risk. Therefore, the incidence of T1DM is increasing much faster than can be explained by genetic changes in the population.

The heightened proportion of lower risk haplotypes and decreased median age at onset of the disorder within this subgroup are consistent with a **major environmental effect** on diabetes development. Competing explanations include increasing prevalence of an old as yet undetermined adversary or decreasing prevalence of a protective factor such as breastfeeding, mild early childhood infections (hygiene theory), or herd immunity to viruses that can be transmitted transplacentally to the fetus. Possible environmental agents that trigger islet autoimmunity include cereals and dietary elements, such as toxins from tuberous vegetables, and enteroviruses.

Factors such as infections and chemicals as well as clues to environmental factors such as seasonality and geographic locations have been suspected of contributing to differences in the incidence and prevalence of T1DM in various ethnic populations. No dominant environmental agent or agents responsible for triggering T1DM have been uncovered. Environmental risk determinants that have been vigorously investigated can be classified as viral infections, early infant diet, and chemicals.

VIRAL INFECTIONS AND VACCINATIONS. Although the etiologic role of viral infections in human T1DM is controversial, coxsackie B3, coxsackie B4, cytomegalovirus, rubella, and mumps can infect human β cells. Only congenital rubella infection is associated with diabetes in later life. It is estimated that 10–12% of patients infected with congenital rubella develop T1DM and up to 40% develop impaired glucose tolerance. The diabetes induced by rubella resembles T1DM because it is associated with HLA-DR3 and HLA-DR4 and is mediated by immune responses against β-cell antigens. There has been no convincing correlation between childhood vaccinations and risk of T1DM.

SEASONAL ASSOCIATIONS. Seasonal and long-term cyclic variations occur in the incidence of IDDM. Newly recognized cases appear with greater frequency in the respective autumn and winter months in the northern and southern hemispheres. Seasonal variations are most apparent in the adolescent years. Attempts to link a pattern of long-term cyclicity with the incidence of mumps or other viral infections have not been successful. Seasonality in type 1 DM in Belgian patients above age 10 yr appears to be restricted to HLA-DQ2/DQ8–negative males.

PUBERTY. The pubertal peak in onset of type 1 DM occurs earlier in girls than boys. This sex difference might be mediated, in part, by estrogen or by genes regulated by estrogen, such as the interleukin-6 (IL6) gene, and suggests that pubertal changes may contribute to accelerated onset of type 1 DM in genetically susceptible females.

DIETARY FACTORS. Dietary factors have been implicated in the pathogenesis of T1DM, but the role of dietary factors in induction of islet autoimmunity remains controversial. Feeding cow's milk to animal models of T1DM has been associated with the development of diabetes in these animals. The likely mechanism is the molecular mimicry between a 17-amino-acid peptide of the bovine serum albumin and the islet antigen 69. Even though there appears to be a strong relationship between cow's milk consumption and national incidence of diabetes in children, the role of cow's milk in human T1DM is controversial. *N*-nitroso compounds, derived from the conversion of nitrates from dietary vegetables and meat in the gut, have also been involved in the development of diabetes. The role of these compounds as a significant risk factor in the pathogenesis of diabetes remains controversial. An initial exposure of infants to cereals before 4 mo of age or after 6 mo of age has been suggested to increase the risk of islet autoimmunity independent of HLA genotype, family history of T1DM, ethnicity, and maternal age. The risk of islet autoimmunity in both age groups is further increased in children who are positive for the HLA-DRB1*03/04,DQB8 genotype.

BODY MASS INDEX. There may be a greater risk of T1DM among individuals who were heavier as young children. The **accelerator hypothesis** predicts earlier onset in heavier people, without necessarily a change in risk, and views type 1 and T2DM as the same disorder of insulin resistance, set against different genetic backgrounds. Insulin resistance is a function of fat mass, and because increasing body weight in the industrialized world has been accompanied by earlier presentation (acceleration) of T2DM, proponents of the accelerator hypothesis suggest that the age at presentation of T1DM is also associated with adiposity. Therefore, limiting excessive weight gain may be as important for children susceptible to T1DM as for those at genetic risk for T2DM.

CHEMICALS. Drugs such as alloxan, streptozotocin (STZ), pentamidine, and Vacor are directly cytotoxic to β cells and cause diabetes in experimental animals and humans. In susceptible animals, multiple subdiabetogenic doses of STZ induce primary β-cell damage and subsequently immune responses against β cells, providing mechanistic evidence that a β-cell insult can elicit specific autoimmunity. Autoimmunity against β cells has also been reported in humans after intoxication with the human rodenticide Vacor.

Figure 590-2 summarizes current hypothetical concepts of the etiology of T1DM as an autoimmune disease, with a genetic component inherited through the HLA system, in which autoimmune destruction of β cells is triggered by an as yet unidentified agent. The slope of decline in insulin varies, and the point at which clinical features appear corresponds to an approximately 80% destruction of the insulin secretory reserve. This process may take months to years, usually in adolescent and older patients, and weeks in the very young patient. Higher titers of spontaneous autoinsulin antibodies and islet cell antibodies are characteristic of the more active islet cell destruction typically seen in the younger patient and may prove useful in predicting evolving diabetes.

Environmental agents may serve as modifiers of disease pathogenesis rather than triggers. Multiple infections during the 1st yr of life are associated with a decreased risk of T1DM. Increased risk has been associated with perinatal infections coupled with a protective effect of preschool daycare with a possible link to the age-dependent modifying effect of infections on the developing immune system. Environmental exposures could act to promote and attenuate disease during different stages of development, with effect dependent on both timing and quantity of encounters.

PATHOGENESIS

Autoimmune Injury. T1DM is a chronic, T cell–mediated autoimmune disease that results in the destruction of the pancreatic islets. Genetic predisposition and environmental factors lead to initiation of an autoimmune process against the pancreatic islets. It is also assumed that the autoimmune response needs to be sustained and diversified against multiple target proteins (epitope spreading) for prolonged periods of time to overcome protective mechanisms. The autoimmune attack on the pancreatic islets leads to a gradual and progressive destruction of β cells, with loss of insulin secretion. It is estimated that, at the onset of clinical diabetes, 80–90% of the pancreatic islets are destroyed. Regeneration of new islets has been detected at onset of T1DM, and it is thought to be responsible for the honeymoon phase (a transient decrease in insulin requirement associated with improved β-cell function). In young diabetic children, especially those of DR3/DR4 haplotypes, the destruction of β cells is almost com-

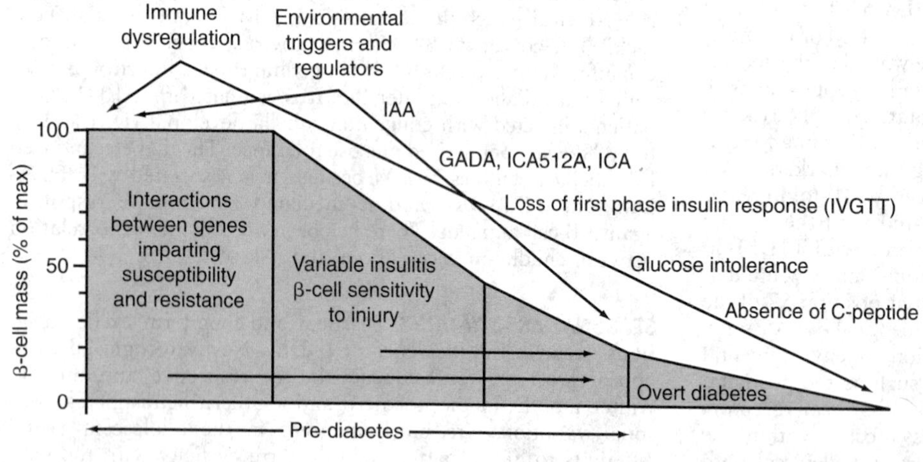

Figure 590-2. Proposed model of the pathogenesis and natural history of type 1 DM. IAA, insulin autoantibodies; GADA, glutamic acid decarboxylase antibody; ICA, islet cell antibody; IVGTT, intravenous glucose tolerance test. (Adapted from Atkinson MA, Eisenbarth GS: Type 1 diabetes: New perspectives on disease pathogenesis and treatment. *Lancet* 2001;358:221–229.)

plete during the 1st 3 yr after the onset of hyperglycemia, whereas in older patients complete β-cell destruction may take up to 10 yr. These observations indicate that the impairment of β-cell function at the onset of hyperglycemia is the consequence of both β-cell destruction and cytokine-mediated inhibition of insulin secretion. The distinction between β-cell destruction and inhibition of insulin secretion is important, since a fraction of β cells may be recovered, providing that effective therapeutic interventions can be implemented at the onset of the disease. Once islet cell autoimmunity has begun, progression to islet cell destruction is quite variable, with some patients rapidly progressing to clinical diabetes while others remain in a nonprogressive state. Antigenic/epitope spreading of the autoantibody responses is an important marker of impending progression; those with but a single autoantibody progress slowly, whereas those with autoantibodies to multiple antigens most often progress rapidly. Most individuals progressing to overt diabetes express multiple anti–islet cell antibodies (GAD65, ICA512/IA-2, and IAA) before the onset of diabetes. The autoimmune response against the pancreatic β cells is believed to consist of 4 phases: (1) environmental insult, (2) priming of T cells, (3) T-cell differentiation, and (4) β-cell destruction (Fig. 590-3).

Environment. Pathogens can initiate or precipitate the self-reactive process by 3 mechanisms. First, molecular mimicry between viral proteins and self-proteins expressed by β cells (PC2 protein of coxsackievirus and GAD65, rubella virus capsid protein and 52-kd islet protein, cytomegalovirus and 38-kd islet protein). Second, after acute β-cell infection or β-cell damage induced by cytokines during inflammatory responses against pathogens, the released proteins can be taken up by antigen-presenting cells (APCs), which present the self-peptides to T cells. Third, cytokines secreted during a viral infection can up-regulate the expression of co-stimulatory and MHC molecules on the surface of the facultative or nonfacultative APCs, enabling them to present self-peptides in immunogenic form to T cells. Induction of the cytokine interferon (IFN)-α following enteroviral infection has been implicated in the pathogenesis of T1DM. Activation of toll receptors by double-stranded RNA or poly-IC (viral mimic) through induction of IFN-α may activate or accelerate immune-mediated β-cell destruction. Several clinical case reports have implicated that IFN-α therapy may be associated with autoimmune diseases and that elevated serum IFN-α levels are associated with T1DM. Exposure to microbial and viral pathogens early in life may also be protective against the development of T1DM.

Psychosocial stress stemming from serious life events may also constitute a trigger mechanism for T1DM or the autoimmune process behind the disease. Psychosocial stress, measured as psychosocial strain in the family, has been shown to be involved in the induction, or progression, of diabetes-related autoimmunity in children during the 1st yr of life independently of family history of diabetes. It is likely that psychosocial stress in families may affect children negatively owing to a link to hormonal levels and neuronal signals that in turn influence both insulin sensitivity/insulin requirement and the immune system.

PRIMING OF T CELLS. The presentation of β-cell-specific autoantigens by APC macrophages or dendritic cells (DCs) to CD4 T helper (Th) cells in association with MHC class II molecules is considered the 1st step in the initiation of the disease process (see Fig. 590-3). Macrophages secrete interleukin (IL)-12, stimulating CD4 T cells to secret interferon (IFN)-γ and IL-2. IFN-γ stimulates other resting macrophages to release, in turn, other cytokines such as IL-1β, tumor necrosis factor (TNF)-α, and free radicals (NO_2^-, O_2^+), which are toxic to pancreatic β cells. During this process, cytokines induce the migration of β-cell autoantigen-specific CD8 cytotoxic cells. On recognizing specific autoantigens on β cells in association with class 1 molecules, these CD8 cytotoxic T cells cause β-cell damage by releasing perforin and granzyme and by Fas-mediated apoptosis of the β cells.

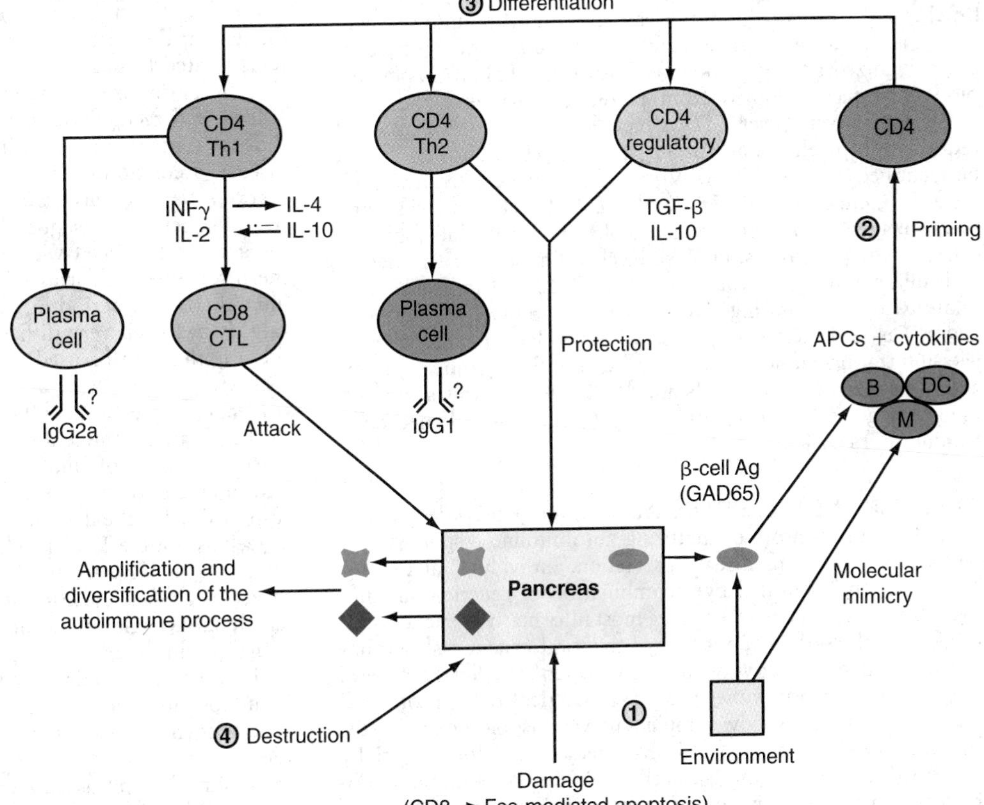

Figure 590-3. Schematic representation of the autoimmune response against pancreatic β cells. An insult to the pancreas leads to the release of β-cell antigens (GAD65), which are taken up by antigen-presenting cells (APCs) and the epitopes presented to the CD4 T cells. Type and stages of activation of APCs as well as the cytokine environment, in which the CD4 T cell priming takes place, dictate the differentiation of autoreactive T cells toward diabetogenic T helper-1 (Th1) cells, Th2 cells, or antigen-specific regulatory T cells. A predominant Th1 autoimmune response results in the recruitment and differentiation of cytotoxic CD8 cells, which attack the pancreatic β cells, leading to a massive release of β-cell antigens (Ag), epitope spreading, and destruction of the pancreatic islets. B, B lymphocyte; DC, dendritic cell; M, macrophage; CTL, cytotoxic cell; TGF-β, tumor growth factor–β; INFγ, interferon-γ; IL, interleukin. (Adapted from Casares S, Brumeanu TD: Insights into the pathogenesis of T1DM: A hint for novel immunospecific therapies. *Curr Molec Med* 2001;1:357–378).

DIFFERENTIATION OF T CELLS. Immune-mediated diabetes is associated with polyclonal populations of T cells reactive against multiple β-cell antigens. Thus, T cells reactive against specific glutamic acid decarboxylase 65 (GAD65), proinsulin, tyrosine phosphatase (ICA512/IA-2), heat-shock protein 60 (hsp60), and islet antigen 69 (ICA69) has been detected in T1DM patients. Among these antigens, GAD65 appears to be the early target of T cells. Because GAD65 is an intracellular protein, β-cell injury, which exposes the antigen, may be required to initiate the autoimmune process. The association between MHC class II and T1DM strongly suggests a pathogenic role of CD4 T cells because MHC class II molecules are required for thymic education of precursors and for restriction of CD4 T-cell responses. There is a correlation between the binding affinity of the peptide to MHC class II and antigenicity. Whereas the T1DM protective class II molecules bind self-peptides with high affinity and delete thymic precursors, T1DM-susceptible class II molecules bind self-peptides with low affinity, leading to a failure of central tolerance and escape of self-reactive T cells to periphery. T cells are differentiated into Th1 and Th2 effector cells. Th1 cells protect against intracellular microbes and parasites and mediate delayed-type hypersensitivity and acute allograft rejection, whereas Th2 cells regulate humoral immune responses (IgE and IgG1), mediate allergic reactions, and protect against organ-specific autoimmune diseases such as T1DM, multiple sclerosis, thyroiditis, and Crohn disease. CD4 Th1 cells secrete IL-2 and IFN-α and are associated with cell-mediated immunity. Th2 cells secrete IL-4 and IL-10 and are associated with humoral and anti-inflammatory responses. A subset of regulatory T cells known as natural killer T (NKT) cells prevents diabetes by secretion of IL-4 and/or IL-10. The regulatory Th3 (CD4) cells also tend to exert antidiabetogenic effect by the secretion of the suppressive cytokine tumor growth factor-β. Functional abnormalities in these regulatory cells may also play a role in the pathogenesis of T1DM. A relative functional defect in a population of regulatory T cells, known as $CD4^+CD25^+$ cells, could contribute to lack of immune self-tolerance in T1DM and may influence its pathogenesis.

β-CELL DESTRUCTION. Mononuclear cell infiltration into the pancreatic islets (insulitis) and a reduction in insulin-producing β cells are recognized as key pathologic features of T1DM. Pancreatic biopsy samples obtained from prediabetic patients and from those with recent-onset T1DM have shown various degrees of reduction in β-cell volume in all patients, yet insulitis could not be identified in about 50%. When insulitis is detected, the infiltrate is composed of CD8 and CD4 T cells, B cells, and macrophages, with a predominance of CD8 T cells. Inflamed islet cells show hyperexpression of MHC class I molecules. The degree of insulitis and hyperexpression of MHC class I molecules correlates with deteriorating glycemic control and GAD65 antibody levels. Fas is detected on β cells within inflamed cells, whereas islet-infiltrating mononuclear cells express Fas ligand. An interaction between Fas on β cells and Fas ligand on infiltrating cells might trigger selective apoptotic β-cell death in inflamed cells, leading to T1DM.

PREDICTION AND PREVENTION. Autoimmunity precedes clinical T1DM, and indicators of maturing autoimmune responses may be useful markers for disease prediction. Individuals at risk for T1DM can be identified by a combination of genetic, immunologic, and metabolic markers. The most informative genetic locus, HLA class II, confers about half of the total genetic risk but has a low positive predictive value (PPV) when used in the general population. Autoantibodies provide a practical readout of β-cell autoimmunity, are easily sampled in venous blood, and have become the mainstay of T1DM prediction efforts. Initially described in terms of the islet cell antibody (ICA) immunofluorescence assay on pancreatic sections, autoantibodies are described in terms of defined ICA target antigens, such as insulin (IAA), glutamic acid dehydrogenase (GAD65), and the tyrosine phosphatase homolog ICA512/IA-2.

Autoantibodies are useful for detecting developing T1DM in close relatives of diabetic patients whose risk for diabetes is about 3.5–5.0%. However, most cases are sporadic rather than familial, necessitating general population screening. This has been difficult, in part, because the observed autoantibody prevalence greatly exceeds the low disease prevalence in nonrelatives, leading to high false-positive rates. Single defined autoantibody (d-aab) positivity may result from persistent memory B cells in lymph nodes or bone marrow after brief transient insulitis not resulting in clinical diabetes. It has been suggested that because different d-aab appear sequentially over time during prediabetes, the presence of multiple d-aab may mark more persistent insulitis and greater diabetes risk. In the 1st-degree relatives of patients with T1DM, the number of positive d-aab can help estimate the risk of developing T1DM: low risk (single d-aab: PPV of 2–6%), moderate risk (2 d-aab: PPV of 21–40%), and high risk (>2 d-aab: PPV of 59%–80%) over a 5-yr period. In children carrying the T1DM highest-risk genotype (HLA-DQB1*0201-DQA1*05/DQB1*0302-DQA1*03), insulitis is almost 10 times more frequent (PPV 21%) than in children with other genotypes (PPV 2.2%). On the other hand, in general populations of children, some studies have suggested a very low overall PPV for single d-aab (0–0.5%), whereas overall PPV for multiple (≥2) d-aab has been reported to be as high as 19–50% (high risk) over a 2- to 8-yr period. Children at risk for T1DM develop early IAA, which may progress to multiple islet autoantibodies based on the degree of IAA affinity to insulin. High IAA affinity is associated with HLA DRB1*04, young age of IAA appearance, subsequent progression to multiple islet autoantibodies, or T1DM.

There is currently no known agent capable of preventing T1DM. There are several obstacles to finding a plausible prevention strategy. These include (1) ethical issues surrounding prediction, (2) treatment dilemma, (3) selection of populations at risk and treatment strategies, and (4) finding new preventive agents. The ability to predict future cases of T1DM, although a major benefit to knowledge about the natural history of this disease, in the absence of a preventing agent raises ethical conflicts related to induction of stress, lifestyle changes, and potential effects on insurability in healthy children and their families.

It is well recognized that the most effective interventions are those that are started early in the autoimmune process. However, disease prediction, using immunologic, genetic, and metabolic markers, is most accurate in the period close to the onset of overt diabetes. Consequently, many health care providers and researchers are faced with ethical and clinical conflicts wherein the most effective forms of therapy might involve treatment of individuals in a period in which disease prediction is least accurate. It has been very difficult to find safe and benign forms of therapy that can be used in individuals who may never develop T1DM.

Immunotherapy in New-Onset Type 1 DM. Type 1 DM is a T-cell-mediated autoimmune disease that begins, in many cases, 3–5 yr before the onset of clinical symptoms, continues after diagnosis, and can recur after islet transplantation. The effector mechanisms responsible for the destruction of β cells involve cytotoxic T cells as well as soluble T-cell products, such as IFN-γ and TNF-α. Such observations have led to clinical trials with immunomodulatory drugs such as cyclosporine, azathioprine, prednisone, and antithymocyte globulin. These agents do cause transient improvement in clinical measures of β-cell function. Unfortunately, the toxic effects of such drugs, concern about the risk associated with immunosuppression, and the need for continuous treatment in an otherwise healthy, young population severely limit the use of these agents.

Immunotherapy using modified **monoclonal antibody against CD3 hOKT3γ1** has efficacy in patients with renal-allograft rejection and has been used in limited trials with T1DM. Treatment with hOKT3γ1 infusions mitigates the deterioration in insulin production and improves metabolic control during the 1st yr of T1DM in a majority of patients. The side effects include transient fever, gastrointestinal symptoms, and pruritic rash, without any long-term toxic effects up to 2 yr. The mechanisms of action of the anti-CD3 monoclonal antibody may involve direct effects on pathogenic T cells and/or the induction of populations of regulatory cells. Short-term (6-day) CD3 monoclonal human IgG1 antibody (ChAglyCD3) therapy in patients aged 12 to 39 yr with new-onset T1DM preserved residual β-cell function for at least 18 mo in patients with recent-onset T1DM. This was associated with a moderate "flu-like" syndrome and transient symptoms of Epstein-Barr viral mononucleosis.

PATHOPHYSIOLOGY. Insulin performs a critical role in the storage and retrieval of cellular fuel. Its secretion in response to feeding is exquisitely modulated by the interplay of neural, hormonal, and substrate-related mechanisms to permit controlled disposition of ingested foodstuff as energy for immediate or future use. Insulin levels must be lowered to then mobilize stored energy during the fasted state. Thus, in normal metabolism, there are regular swings between the postprandial, high-insulin anabolic state and the fasted, low-insulin catabolic state that affect liver, muscle, and adipose tissue (Table 590-3). T1DM is a progressive low-insulin catabolic state in which feeding does not reverse but rather exaggerates these catabolic processes. With moderate insulinopenia, glucose utilization by muscle and fat decreases and postprandial hyperglycemia appears. At even lower insulin levels, the liver produces excessive glucose via glycogenolysis and gluconeogenesis, and fasting hyperglycemia begins. Hyperglycemia produces an osmotic diuresis (glycosuria) when the renal threshold is exceeded (180 mg/dL; 10 mmol/L). The resulting loss of calories and electrolytes, as well as the persistent dehydration, produce a physiologic stress with hypersecretion of stress hormones (epinephrine, cortisol, growth hormone, and glucagon). These hormones, in turn, contribute to the metabolic decompensation by further impairing insulin secretion (epinephrine), by antagonizing its action (epinephrine, cortisol, growth hormone), and by promoting glycogenolysis, gluconeogenesis, lipolysis, and ketogenesis (glucagon, epinephrine, growth hormone, and cortisol) while decreasing glucose utilization and glucose clearance (epinephrine, growth hormone, cortisol).

The combination of insulin deficiency and elevated plasma values of the counter-regulatory hormones is also responsible for accelerated lipolysis and impaired lipid synthesis, with resulting increased plasma concentrations of total lipids, cholesterol, triglycerides, and free fatty acids. The hormonal interplay of insulin deficiency and glucagon excess shunts the free fatty acids into ketone body formation; the rate of formation of these ketone bodies, principally β-hydroxybutyrate and acetoacetate, exceeds the capacity for peripheral utilization and renal excretion. Accumulation of these keto acids results in metabolic acidosis (diabetic ketoacidosis, DKA) and compensatory rapid deep breathing in an attempt to excrete excess CO_2 (Kussmaul respiration). Acetone, formed by nonenzymatic conversion of acetoacetate, is responsible for the characteristic fruity odor of the breath. Ketones are excreted in the urine in association with cations and thus further increase losses of water and electrolyte. With progressive dehydration, acidosis, hyperosmolality, and diminished cerebral oxygen utilization, consciousness becomes impaired, and the patient ultimately becomes comatose.

TABLE 590-3. Influence of Feeding (High Insulin) or of Fasting (Low Insulin) on Some Metabolic Processes in Liver, Muscle, and Adipose Tissue*

	HIGH PLASMA INSULIN (POSTPRANDIAL STATE)	LOW PLASMA INSULIN (FASTED STATE)
Liver	Glucose uptake	Glucose production
	Glycogen synthesis	Glycogenolysis
	Absence of gluconeogenesis	Gluconeogenesis
	Lipogenesis	Absence of lipogenesis
	Absence of ketogenesis	Ketogenesis
Muscle	Glucose uptake	Absence of glucose uptake
	Glucose oxidation	Fatty acid and ketone oxidation
	Glycogen synthesis	Glycogenolysis
	Protein synthesis	Proteolysis and amino acid release
Adipose tissue	Glucose uptake	Absence of glucose uptake
	Lipid synthesis	Lipolysis and fatty acid release
	Triglyceride uptake	Absence of triglyceride uptake

*Insulin is considered to be the major factor governing these metabolic processes. Diabetes mellitus may be viewed as a permanent low-insulin state that, untreated, results in exaggerated fasting.

CLINICAL MANIFESTATIONS. As diabetes develops, symptoms steadily increase, reflecting the decreasing β-cell mass, worsening insulinopenia, progressive hyperglycemia, and eventual ketoacidosis. Initially, when only insulin reserve is limited, occasional hyperglycemia occurs. When the serum glucose increases above the renal threshold, intermittent **polyuria** or **nocturia** begins. With further β-cell loss, chronic hyperglycemia causes a more persistent diuresis, often with nocturnal **enuresis,** and **polydipsia** becomes more apparent. Female patients may develop monilial vaginitis due to the chronic glycosuria. Calories are lost in the urine (glycosuria), triggering a compensatory **hyperphagia.** If this hyperphagia does not keep pace with the glycosuria, loss of body fat ensues, with clinical **weight loss** and diminished subcutaneous fat stores. An average, healthy 10-yr-old child consumes about 50% of 2,000 daily calories as carbohydrate. As that child becomes diabetic, daily losses of water and glucose may be 5 L and 250 g, respectively, representing 1,000 calories, or 50%, of the average daily caloric intake. Despite the child's compensatory increased intake of food, the body starves because unused calories are lost in the urine.

When extremely low insulin levels are reached, **keto acids accumulate.** At this point, the child quickly deteriorates. Keto acids produce abdominal discomfort, nausea, and emesis, preventing oral replacement of urinary water losses. Dehydration accelerates, causing weakness or orthostasis—but polyuria persists. As in any hyperosmotic state, the degree of dehydration may be clinically underestimated because intravascular volume is conserved at the expense of intracellular volume. Ketoacidosis exacerbates prior symptoms and leads to Kussmaul respirations (deep, heavy, rapid breathing), fruity breath odor (acetone), diminished neurocognitive function, and possible coma. About 20–40% of children with new-onset diabetes progress to DKA before diagnosis.

This entire progression happens much more quickly (over a few weeks) in younger children, probably owing to more aggressive autoimmune destruction of β cells. In infants, most of the weight loss is acute water loss because they will not have had prolonged caloriuria at diagnosis, and there will be an increased incidence of DKA at diagnosis. In adolescents, the course is usually more prolonged (over months), and most of the weight loss represents fat loss due to prolonged starvation. Additional weight loss due to acute dehydration may occur just before diagnosis. In any child, the progression of symptoms may be accelerated by the stress of an intercurrent illness or trauma, when counter-regulatory (stress) hormones overwhelm the limited insulin secretory capacity.

DIAGNOSIS. The diagnosis of T1DM is usually straightforward. Although most symptoms are nonspecific, the most important clue is an inappropriate polyuria in any child with dehydration, poor weight gain, or "the flu." Hyperglycemia, glycosuria, and ketonuria can be determined quickly. Nonfasting blood glucose greater than 200 mg/dL (11.1 mmol/L) with typical symptoms is diagnostic with or without ketonuria. In the obese child, T2DM must be considered (see Type 2 Diabetes Mellitus, below). Once hyperglycemia is confirmed, it is prudent to determine whether DKA is present (especially if ketonuria is found) and to evaluate electrolyte abnormalities—even if signs of dehydration are minimal. A baseline hemoglobin A_{1C} (HbA_{1C}) allows an estimate of the duration of hyperglycemia and provides an initial value by which to compare the effectiveness of subsequent therapy.

In the nonobese child, testing for autoimmunity to β cells is not necessary. Other autoimmunities associated with type 1 diabetes should be sought, including **celiac disease** (by tissue transglutaminase IgA and total IgA) and **thyroiditis** (by antithyroid peroxidase and antithyroglobulin antibodies). Because significant physiologic distress can disrupt the pituitary-thyroid axis, free thyroxine (T_4) and TSH levels should be checked after the child is stable for a few weeks.

Rarely, a child has transient hyperglycemia with glycosuria while under substantial physical stress. This usually resolves permanently during recovery from the stressors. However, such stress-produced hyperglycemia can reflect a limited insulin reserve temporarily revealed by counter-regulatory hormones. A child with temporary hyperglycemia should therefore be monitored for the development of symptoms of persistent hyperglycemia and tested if such symptoms occur. Formal testing in a child who remains clinically asymptomatic is not necessary.

Routine screening procedures, such as postprandial determinations of blood glucose or screening oral glucose tolerance tests, have yielded low detection rates in healthy, asymptomatic children, even among those considered at risk, such as siblings of diabetic children. Accordingly, such screening procedures are not recommended in children.

Diabetic Ketoacidosis. DKA is the end result of the metabolic abnormalities resulting from a severe deficiency of insulin or insulin effectiveness. The latter occurs during stress as counter-regulatory hormones block insulin action. DKA occurs in 20–40% of children with new-onset diabetes and in children with known diabetes who omit insulin doses or who do not successfully manage an intercurrent illness. DKA may be arbitrarily classified as mild, moderate, or severe (Table 590-4), and the range of symptoms depends on the depth of ketoacidosis. There is a large amount of ketonuria, an increased ion gap, a decreased serum bicarbonate (or total CO_2) and pH, and an elevated effective serum osmolality, indicating hypertonic dehydration.

TREATMENT. Therapy is tailored to the degree of insulinopenia at presentation. Most children with new diabetes (60–80%) have mild to moderate symptoms, have minimal dehydration with no history of emesis, and have not progressed to ketoacidosis. Once DKA has resolved in the newly diagnosed child, therapy is transitioned to that described for children with nonketotic onset. Children with previously diagnosed diabetes who develop DKA are usually transitioned to their previous insulin regimen.

New-Onset Diabetes Without Ketoacidosis. Excellent diabetes control involves many goals: to maintain a balance between tight glucose control and avoiding hypoglycemia, to eliminate polyuria and nocturia, to prevent ketoacidosis, and to permit normal growth and development with minimal effect on lifestyle. Therapy encompasses initiation and adjustment of insulin, extensive teaching of the child and caretakers, and reestablishment of the life routines. Each aspect should be addressed early in the overall care. Ideally, therapy can begin in the outpatient setting, with complete team staffing by a pediatric endocrinologist, experienced nursing staff, dietitians with training as diabetes educators, and a social worker. Close contact between the diabetes team and family must be assured. Otherwise, initial therapy should be done in the hospital setting.

Insulin Therapy. Several factors influence the initial daily insulin dose per kilogram of body weight. The dose is usually higher in pubertal children. It is higher in those who have to restore greater deficits of body glycogen, protein, and fat stores and who, therefore, have higher initial caloric capacity. On the other hand, most children with new-onset diabetes have some residual β-cell function (the "honeymoon" period), which reduces exogenous insulin needs. Children with long-standing diabetes and no insulin reserve require about 0.7 U/kg/d if prepubertal, 1.0 U/kg/d at midpuberty, and 1.2 U/kg/d by the end of puberty. A reasonable dose in the **newly diagnosed** child, then, is about 60–70% of the full replacement dose based on pubertal status. The optimal insulin dose can only be determined empirically, with frequent self-monitored blood glucose levels and insulin adjustment by the diabetes team. Residual β-cell function usually fades within a few months and is reflected as a steady increase in insulin requirements and wider glucose excursions.

The initial insulin schedule should be directed toward the optimal degree of glucose control in an attempt to duplicate the activity of the β cell. There are inherent limits to our ability to mimic the β cell. Exogenous insulin does not have a 1st pass to the liver, whereas 50% of pancreatic portal insulin is taken up by the liver, a key organ for the disposal of glucose; absorption of an exogenous dose continues despite hypoglycemia, whereas endogenous insulin release ceases and serum levels quickly lower with a normally rapid clearance; and absorption rate from an injection varies by injection site and patient activity level, whereas endogenous insulin is secreted directly into the portal circulation. Despite these fundamental physiologic differences, acceptable glucose control can be obtained with new insulin analogs used in a basal-bolus regimen, that is, with slow-onset, long-duration background insulin for between-meal glucose control and rapid-onset insulin at each meal.

All preanalog insulins form hexamers, which must dissociate into monomers subcutaneously before being absorbed into the circulation. Thus, a detectable effect for regular (R) insulin is delayed by 30–60 min after injection. This, in turn, requires delaying the meal 30–60 min after the injection for optimal effect—a delay rarely attained in a busy child's life. R has a wide peak and a long tail for bolus insulin (Figs. 590-4 and 590-5). This profile limits postprandial glucose control, produces prolonged peaks with excessive hypoglycemic effects between meals, and increases the risk of nighttime hypoglycemia. These unwanted between-meal effects often necessitate "feeding the insulin" with snacks and limiting the overall degree of blood glucose control. NPH and Lente insulins also have inherent limits because they do not create a peakless background insulin level (see Fig. 590-5C–E). This produces significant hypoglycemic effect during the midrange of their duration. Thus, it is often difficult to predict their interaction with fast-acting insulins. When R is combined with NPH or Lente (see Fig. 590-5E), the composite insulin profile poorly mimics normal endogenous insulin secretion. There are broad areas of excessive insulin effect alternating with insufficient effect throughout the day and night. Lente and Ultralente insulins have been discontinued and are no longer available.

Lispro (L) and aspart (A), insulin analogs, are absorbed much quicker because they do not form hexamers. They provide discrete pulses with little if any overlap and short tail effect. This allows better control of post-meal glucose increase and reduces

TABLE 590-4. Classification of Diabetic Ketoacidosis

	NORMAL	MILD	MODERATE	SEVERE[†]
CO_2 (mEq/L, venous)*	20–28	16–20	10–15	<10
pH (venous)*	7.35–7.45	7.25–7.35	7.15–7.25	<7.15
Clinical	No change	Oriented, alert but fatigued	Kussmaul respirations; oriented but sleepy; arousable	Kussmaul or depressed respirations; sleepy to depressed sensorium to coma

*CO_2 and pH measurement are method dependent; normal ranges may vary.
[†]Severe hypernatremia (corrected Na >150 mEq/L) would also be classified as severe DKA.

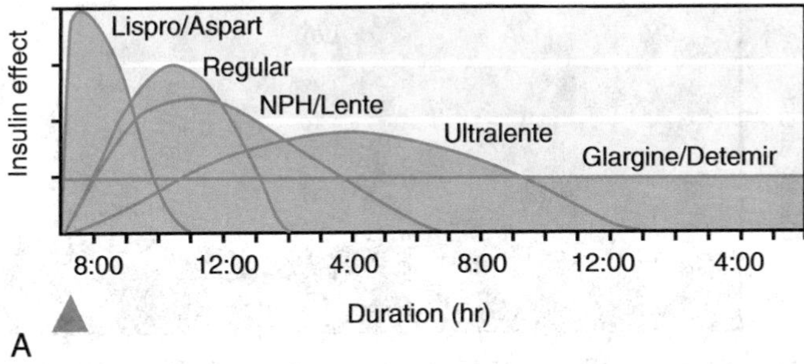

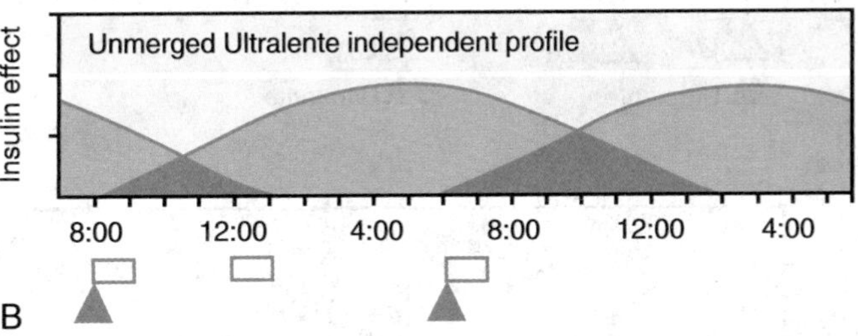

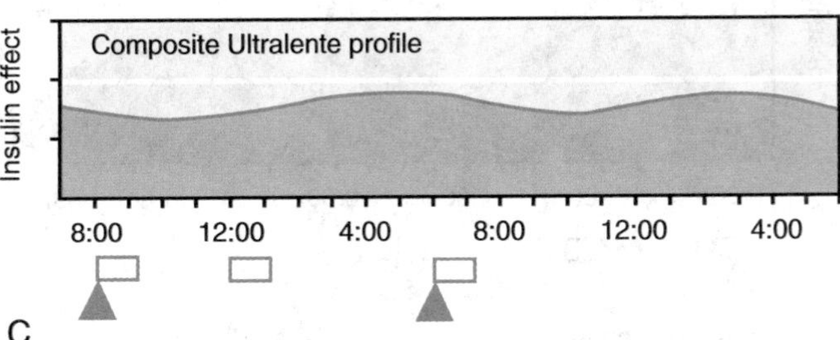

Figure 590-4. Approximate insulin effect profiles. Meals are shown as rectangles below time axis. *A,* The following relative peak effect and duration units are used: lispro/aspart, peak 20 for 4 hours; regular, peak 15 for 7 hours; NPH/Lente, peak 12 for 12 hours; Ultralente, peak 9 for 18 hours; glargine, peak 5 for 24 hours. Though Lente and Ultralente are no longer manufactured, they are shown to give historical comparison to newer insulin analogs. ▲, Injection time. *B,* Two Ultralente injections given at breakfast and supper. Note overlap of profiles. *C,* Composite curve showing approximate cumulative insulin effect for the 2 Ultralente injections. This composite view is much more useful to the patient, parents, and medical personnel because it shows important combined effects of multiple insulin injections with variable absorption characteristics and overlapping durations.

between-meal or nighttime hypoglycemia (see Fig. 590-5A). The long-acting analog glargine (G) creates a much flatter 24-hr profile, making it easier to predict the combined effect of a rapid bolus (L or A) on top of the basal insulin, producing a more physiologic pattern of insulin effect (see Fig. 590-5A). Postprandial glucose elevations are better controlled, and between-meal and nighttime hypoglycemia are reduced.

Ultralente (UL) given twice a day provided a reasonable basal profile (see Fig. 590-4C) and was quite effective when used with lispro or aspart (see Fig. 590-5B). Since UL is no longer available, G may be given every 12 hours in young children if a single daily dose of G does not produce complete 24-hr basal coverage. The basal insulin glargine should be 25–30% of the total dose in toddlers and 40–50% in older children. The remaining portion of the total daily dose is divided evenly as bolus injections for the 3 meals. A simple 3- or 4-step dosing schedule is begun based on the blood glucose level (Table 590-5). As soon as the family is taught to calculate the carbohydrate content of meals, bolus insulin can be more accurately dosed by both the carbohydrate content of the meal as well as the ambient glucose (see Table 590-5).

Frequent blood glucose monitoring and insulin adjustment are necessary in the 1st weeks as the child returns to routine activities and adapts to a new nutritional schedule, and as the total daily insulin requirements are determined. The major physiologic limit to tight control is hypoglycemia. Intensive control dramatically reduces the risk of long-term vascular complications; it is associated with a 3-fold increase in severe hypoglycemia. Use of insulin analogs moderates but does not eliminate this problem.

Some families may be unable to administer 4 daily injections. In these cases, a compromise may be needed. A 3-injection regimen combining NPH with a rapid analog bolus at breakfast, a rapid-acting analog bolus at supper, and NPH at bedtime may provide fair glucose control. Further compromise to a 2-injection regimen (NPH and rapid analog at breakfast and supper) may occasionally be needed. However, such a schedule would provide poor coverage for lunch and early morning, and would increase the risk of hypoglycemia at midmorning and early night.

Insulin Pump Therapy. Continuous subcutaneous insulin infusion (CSII) via battery-powered pumps provides a closer approximation of normal plasma insulin profiles and increased flexibility regarding timing of meals and snacks compared with conventional insulin injection regimens. Insulin pump models can be programmed with a patient's personal insulin dose algorithms, including the insulin to carbohydrate ratio and the correction scale for pre-meal glucose levels. The patient can enter his or her blood glucose level and the carbohydrate content of the meal, and the pump computer will calculate the proper insulin bolus dose. Insulin pump therapy in adolescents with T1DM is associated with improved metabolic control and reduced risk of severe hypoglycemia without affecting psychosocial outcomes. The use of overnight CSII improves the metabolic control in children aged 7–10 yr. CSII has also been useful in toddlers. CSII may not always improve metabolic control. Some studies show improvement in less than one half and worsening control (higher HbA_{1C}) in one fifth of patients. It is likely that the degree of glycemic control is mainly dependent on how closely patients adhere to the principles of diabetes self-care, regardless of the type of intensive insulin regimen. One benefit of pump therapy may be a reduction in severe hypoglycemia and associated seizures. Nonetheless, randomized trials comparing multiple daily insulin (MDI) regimen using glargine insulin and CSII in children with T1DM demonstrate similar metabolic control and frequency of hypoglycemic events.

Inhaled and Oral Insulin Therapies. Preprandial inhaled insulin is being evaluated in adults with T1DM and T2DM. The preliminary metabolic data are promising. Patients taking pre-meal inhaled insulin in combination with once daily bedtime long-acting insulin (Ultralente) injection achieved similar metabolic control compared with patients taking 2 to 3 daily injections of insulin. There was no significant difference in the frequency of

TABLE 590-5. Subcutaneous Insulin Dosing

				BOLUS[†] INSULIN	
AGE (YR)	TARGET GLUCOSE (MG/DL)	TOTAL DAILY INSULIN (U/KG/D)*	BASAL INSULIN, % OF TOTAL DAILY DOSE	Units Added per 100 mg/dL above Target	Units Added per 15 g at Meal
0–5	100–200	0.6–0.7	25–30	0.50	0.50
5–12	80–150	0.7–1.0	40–50	0.75	0.75
12–18	80–150	1.0–1.2	40–50	1.0–2.0[‡]	1.0–2.0

*Newly diagnosed children in the "honeymoon" may only need 60–70% of a full replacement dose. Total daily dose per kg increases with puberty.

[†]Newly diagnosed children who do not use carbohydrate dosing should divide the nonbasal portion of the daily insulin dose into equal doses for each meal. A dosing scale is then added for each dose. **For example**: a 6-yr-old child who weighs 20 kg needs about (0.7 units/kg/24 hr × 20 kg) = 14 units/24 hr with 7 units (50%) as basal and 7 units as total daily bolus. Give basal as glargine at hs. Give 2 units lispro or aspart before each meal if the blood glucose is within target; subtract 1 unit if below target; add 0.75 unit for each 100 mg/dL above target (round the dose to the nearest 0.5 unit).

[‡]For finer control, extra insulin may be added in 50-mg/dL increments.

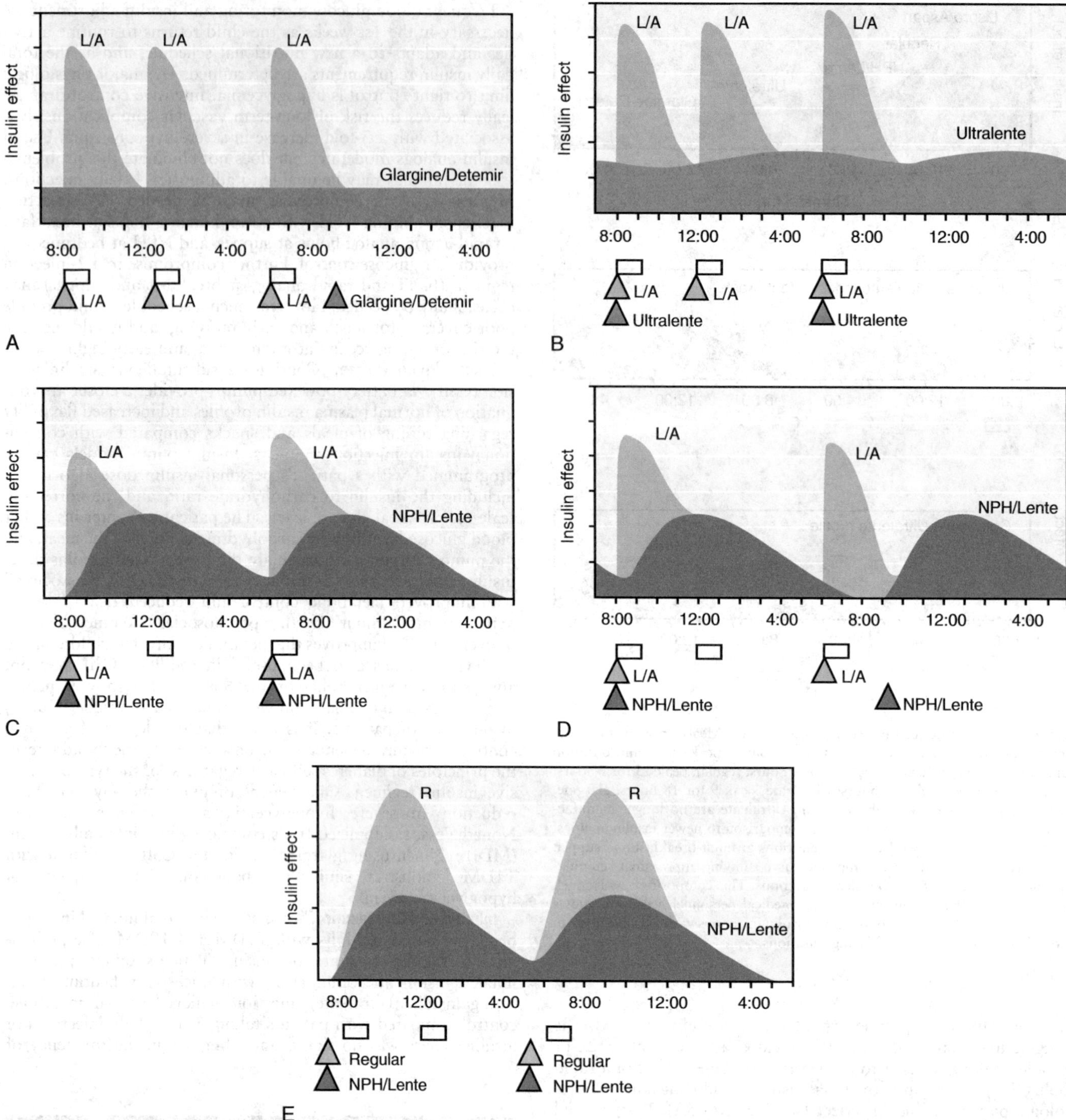

Figure 590-5. Approximate composite insulin effect profiles. Meals are shown as rectangles below time axis. Injections are shown as labeled triangles. L/A, lispro or aspart. Even though the fast- and long-acting insulins are shaded differently to show the addition of one insulin effect to another, the profile is changed to show the combined effect. For example, in the breakfast injection in C, the quick decline of L/A effect is blunted by the rising NPH/Lente effect, producing a broad tail, which slowly declines to baseline at supper. All profiles are idealized using average absorption and clearance rates. In typical clinical situations, these profiles vary among patients. A given patient has varying rates of absorption depending on the injection site, physical activity, and other variables. *A,* L or A pre-meal; glargine at bedtime. The rapid onset and short duration of L or A reduce overlap between pre-meal injections, and there is no extended nighttime action. This reduces the risk of hypoglycemia. Glargine provides a steady basal profile that simplifies prediction of bolus insulin effect. *B,* L or A pre-meal; Ultralente at breakfast and supper. Ultralente produces a basal profile similar to that seen with glargine. Some excessive insulin effect, however, is seen before supper and at nighttime. *C,* L or A pre-meal; NPH or Lente at breakfast and supper. The broad peak of NPH or Lente produces substantial risk of hypoglycemia before lunch and during the early hours of the night. The waning insulin effect before supper and breakfast may also allow breakthrough hyperglycemia. *D,* L or A pre-meal; NPH or Lente at breakfast and bedtime. Moving the evening long-acting insulin helps to cover the pre-breakfast hours, but the risk of nighttime lows persists. *E,* Regular and NPH or Lente at breakfast and supper. This produces the least physiologic profile, with large excesses before lunch and during the early night, combined with poor coverage before supper and breakfast. Though Lente and Ultralente are no longer manufactured, they are shown to give historical comparison to newer insulin analogs.

hypoglycemic episodes between the 2 groups. There have been reports of pulmonary fibrosis in a small number of patients, necessitating further monitoring and evaluation of patients taking inhaled insulin before this route of insulin administration is deemed safe. Bioavailability of inhaled insulin is increased with smoking and reduced with asthma.

Pre-meal oral insulin (Oralin) has been evaluated in comparison with oral hypoglycemic agents, mostly in patients with T2DM. The clinical data appear promising, but further evaluation of efficacy in T1DM is needed.

Basic Education. Therapy consists not only of initiation and adjustment of insulin dose but also of education of the patient and family. Teaching is most efficiently provided by experienced diabetes educators and nutritionists. In the acute phase, the family must learn the "basics," which includes monitoring the child's blood glucose and urine ketones, preparing and injecting the correct insulin dose subcutaneously at the proper time, recognizing and treating low blood glucose reactions, and having a basic meal plan. Most families are trying to adjust psychologically to the new diagnosis of diabetes in their child and thus have a limited ability to retain new information. Written materials covering these basic topics help the family during the 1st few days.

Ketoacidosis. Severe insulinopenia (or lack of effective insulin action) results in a physiologic cascade of events in 3 general pathways.

1. Excessive glucose production coupled with reduced glucose utilization raises serum glucose. This produces an osmotic diuresis, with loss of fluid and electrolytes, dehydration, and activation of the renin-angiotensin-aldosterone axis with accelerated potassium loss. If glucose elevation and dehydration are severe and persist for several hours, the risk of cerebral edema increases.
2. Increased catabolic processes result in cellular losses of sodium, potassium, and phosphate.
3. Increased release of free fatty acids from peripheral fat stores supplies substrate for hepatic keto acid production. When keto acids accumulate, buffer systems are depleted and a metabolic acidosis ensues. Therapy must address both the initiating event in this cascade (insulinopenia) and the subsequent physiologic disruptions.

Reversal of DKA is associated with inherent risks that include hypoglycemia, hypokalemia, and cerebral edema. Any protocol must be used with caution and close monitoring of the patient. Adjustments based on sound medical judgment may be necessary for any given level of DKA (Table 590-6).

Hyperglycemia and Dehydration. Insulin must be given at the beginning of therapy to accelerate movement of glucose into cells, to subdue hepatic glucose production, and to halt the movement of fatty acids from the periphery to the liver. However, an initial insulin bolus does not speed recovery and may increase the risk of hypokalemia and hypoglycemia. Therefore, insulin infusion is begun **without** a bolus at a rate of 0.1 U/kg/h. This approximates maximal insulin output in normal subjects during an oral glucose tolerance test. Rehydration also lowers glucose levels by improving renal perfusion and enhancing renal excretion. The combination of these therapies usually causes a rapid initial decline in serum glucose levels. Once glucose goes below 180 mg/dL (10 mmol/L), the osmotic diuresis stops and rehydration accelerates without further increase in the infusion rate.

Repair of hyperglycemia occurs well before correction of acidosis. Therefore, insulin is still needed to control fatty acid release after normal glucose levels are reached. To continue the insulin infusion without causing hypoglycemia, glucose must be added to the infusion, usually as a 5% solution. Glucose should be added when the serum glucose has decreased to about 250 mg/dL (14 mmol/L) so that there is sufficient time to adjust the infusion before the serum glucose falls further. The insulin infusion can also be lowered from the initial maximal rate once hyperglycemia has resolved.

Repair of fluid deficits must be tempered by the potential risk of **cerebral edema.** It is prudent to approach any child in any hyperosmotic state with cautious rehydration. The effective serum osmolality ($E_{osm} = 2 \times [Na_{uncorrected}] + [glucose]$) is an accurate index of tonicity of the body fluids, reflecting intracellular and extracellular hydration better than measured plasma osmolality. It is calculated with sodium and glucose in mmol/L. This value is usually elevated at the beginning of therapy and should steadily normalize. A rapid decline, or a slow decline to a subnormal range, may indicate an excess of free water entering the vascular space and an increasing risk of cerebral edema. Therefore, patients should not be allowed oral fluids until rehydration is well progressed and significant electrolyte shifts are no longer likely. Limited ice chips may be given as a minimal oral intake. All fluid intake and output should be closely monitored.

Calculation of fluid deficits using clinical signs is difficult in children with DKA because intravascular volume is better maintained in the hypertonic state. For any degree of tachycardia, delayed capillary refill, decreased skin temperature, or orthostatic blood pressure change, the child with DKA will be more dehydrated than the child with a normotonic fluid deficit. The protocol in Table 583-6 corrects a deficit of 85 mL/kg (8.5% dehydration) for all patients in the 1st 24 hr. Children with mild DKA rehydrate earlier and can be switched to oral intake, whereas those with severe DKA and a greater volume deficit require 30–36 hr with this protocol. This more gradual rehydration of the child with severe DKA is an inherent safety feature. The initial intravenous bolus (20 mL/kg of glucose-free isotonic sodium salt solution such as Ringer lactate or 0.9% sodium chloride) for all patients ensures a quick volume expansion and may be repeated if clinical improvement is not quickly seen. This bolus is given as isotonic saline because the patient is inevitably hypertonic, keeping most of the initial infusion in the intravascular space. Subsequent fluid is hypotonic to repair the free water

TABLE 590-6. Diabetic Ketoacidosis (DKA) Treatment Protocol

TIME	THERAPY	COMMENTS
1st hour	10–20 mL/kg IV bolus 0.9% NaCl or LR Insulin drip at 0.05 to 0.10 μ/kg/hr	Quick volume expansion; may be repeated. NPO. Monitor I/O, neurologic status. Use flow sheet. Have mannitol at bedside; 1 g/kg IV push for cerebral edema.
2nd hour until DKA resolution	0.45% NaCl: plus continue insulin drip 20 mEq/L KPhos and 20 mEq/L KAc 5% glucose if blood sugar <250 mg/dL (14 mmol/L)	$\text{IV rate} = \frac{85\,\text{mL/kg} + \text{maintenance} - \text{bolus}}{23\,\text{hr}}$ If $K < 3$ mEq/L, give 0.5 to 1.0 mEq/kg as oral K solution *OR* increase IV K to 80 mEq/L
Variable	Oral intake with subcutaneous insulin	No emesis; $CO_2 \geq 16$ mEq/L; normal electrolytes

Note that the initial IV bolus is considered part of the total fluid allowed in the first 24 hr and is subtracted before calculating the IV rate.

Maintenance (24 hr) = 100 mL/kg (for the 1st 10 kg) + 50 mL/kg (for the 2nd 10 kg) + 25 mL/kg (for all remaining kg)

Sample calculation for a 30-kg child:

1st hour = 300 mL IV bolus 0.9% NaCl or LR

$$\text{2nd and subsequent hours} = \frac{(85\,\text{mL} \times 30) + 1750\,\text{mL} - 300\,\text{mL}}{23\,\text{hr}} = \frac{175\,\text{mL}}{\text{hr}} (0.45\%\ \text{NaCl with } 20\,\text{mEq/L KPhos and } 20\,\text{mEq/L KAC})$$

I/O, input and output (urine, emesis); KAc, potassium acetate; KPhos, potassium phosphate; LR, lactated Ringer solution; NaCl, sodium chloride.

deficit, to allow intracellular rehydration, and to allow a more appropriate replacement of ongoing hypotonic urine losses.

The initial serum sodium is usually normal or low because of the osmolar dilution of hyperglycemia and the effect of an elevated sodium-free lipid fraction. An estimate of the reconstituted, or "true," serum sodium for any given glucose level above 100 mg/dL (5.6 mmol/L) is calculated as follows:

$$\frac{[Na^+] + glucose - 100 \times 1.6}{100}$$

where glucose is in mg/dL, or

$$\frac{[Na^+] + glucose - 5.6 \times 1.6}{5.6}$$

where glucose is in mmol/L.

The sodium should increase by about 1.6 mmol/L for each 100 mg/dL decline in the glucose. The corrected sodium is usually normal or slightly elevated and indicates moderate hypernatremic dehydration. If the corrected value is greater than 150 mmol/L, severe hypernatremic dehydration may be present and may require slower fluid replacement. The sodium should steadily increase with therapy. Declining sodium may indicate excessive free water accumulation and the risk of cerebral edema.

Catabolic Losses. Both the metabolic shift to a catabolic predominance and the acidosis move potassium and phosphate from the cell to the serum. The osmotic diuresis, the kaliuretic effect of the hyperaldosteronism, and the ketonuria then accelerate renal losses of potassium and phosphate. Sodium is also lost with the diuresis, but free water losses are greater than isotonic losses. With prolonged illness and severe DKA, total body losses can approach 10–13 mEq/kg of sodium, 5–6 mEq/kg of potassium, and 4–5 mEq/kg of phosphate. These losses continue for several hours during therapy until the catabolic state is reversed and the diuresis is controlled. For example, 50% of infused sodium may be lost in the urine during IV therapy. Even though the sodium deficit may be repaired within 24 hr, intracellular potassium and phosphate may not be completely restored for several days.

Although patients with DKA have a total body potassium deficit, the initial serum level is often normal or elevated. This is due to the movement of potassium from the intracellular space to the serum, both as part of the keto acid buffering process and as part of the catabolic shift. These effects are reversed with therapy, and potassium returns to the cell. Improved hydration increases renal blood flow, allowing for increased excretion of potassium in the elevated aldosterone state. The net effect is often a dramatic decline in serum potassium levels, especially in severe DKA, and can precipitate changes in cardiac conductivity, flattening of T waves, and prolongation of the QRS complex and can cause skeletal muscle weakness or ileus. The risk of myocardial dysfunction is increased with shock and acidosis. Potassium levels must be closely followed and electrocardiographic monitoring continued until DKA is substantially resolved. If needed, the parenteral potassium can be increased to 80 mEq/L or an oral supplement can be given if there is no emesis. Rarely, the IV insulin must be temporarily stopped.

It is unclear whether phosphate deficits contribute to symptoms of DKA such as generalized muscle weakness. In pediatric patients, a deficit has not been shown to compromise oxygen delivery via a deficiency of 2,3-diphosphoglycerate (2,3-DPG). Because the patient will receive an excess of chloride, which may aggravate acidosis, it is prudent to use potassium phosphate rather than potassium chloride as a potassium source. Potassium acetate is also used, because it provides an additional buffer.

Pancreatitis is occasionally seen with DKA, especially if prolonged abdominal distress is present; serum amylase may be elevated. If the serum lipase is not elevated, the amylase is likely nonspecific or salivary in origin. Serum creatinine adjusted for age may be falsely elevated owing to interference by ketones in the autoanalyzer methodology. An initial elevated value rarely indicates renal failure and should be rechecked when the child is less ketonemic. Blood urea nitrogen (BUN) may be elevated with prerenal azotemia and should be rechecked as the child is rehydrated. Mildly elevated creatine or BUN is not a reason to withhold potassium therapy if good urinary output is present.

Keto Acid Accumulation. Low insulin infusion rates (0.02–0.05 units/kg/h) are usually sufficient to stop peripheral release of fatty acids, thereby eliminating the flow of substrate for ketogenesis. Therefore, the initial infusion rate may be decreased if blood glucose levels go below 150 mg/dL (8 mmol/L) despite the addition of glucose to the infusion. Ketogenesis continues until fatty acid substrates already in the liver are depleted, but this production declines much more quickly without new substrate inflow. Bicarbonate buffers, regenerated by the distal renal tubule and by metabolism of ketone bodies, steadily repair the acidosis once keto acid production is controlled. Bicarbonate therapy is rarely necessary and may even increase the risk of hypokalemia and cerebral edema.

There should be a steady increase in pH and serum bicarbonate as therapy progresses. Kussmaul respirations should abate and abdominal pain resolve. Persistent acidosis may indicate inadequate insulin or fluid therapy, infection, or rarely lactic acidosis. Urine ketones may be positive long after ketoacidosis has resolved because the nitroprusside reaction routinely used to measure urine ketones by dipstick measures only acetoacetate. During DKA, most excess ketones are β-hydroxybutyrate, which increases the normal ratio to acetoacetate from 3 : 1 to as high as 8 : 1. With resolution of the acidosis, β-hydroxybutyrate converts to acetoacetate, which is excreted into the urine and detected by the dipstick test. Therefore, persistent ketonuria may not accurately reflect the degree of clinical improvement and should not be relied upon as an indicator of therapeutic failure.

All patients with DKA should be checked for **initiating events** that may have triggered the metabolic decompensation.

DKA Protocol (See Table 590-6). Even though DKA can be of variable severity, a common approach to all cases simplifies the therapeutic regimen and can be safely used for most children. Fluids are best calculated based on weight, not body surface area (M^2), because heights are rarely available for the calculation. The Milwaukee protocol has been used for more than 20 yr in a large clinic setting with no deaths and no neurologic sequelae in any child treated initially with this protocol. It can be used for children of all ages and with all degrees of DKA. It is designed to restore most electrolyte deficits, to reverse the acidosis, and to rehydrate the moderately ill child in about 24 hr. A standard water deficit (85 mL/kg) is assumed. This amount, when added to maintenance, yields about 4 L/M^2 for children of all sizes. Children with milder DKA recover in 10–20 hr (and need less total IV fluid before switching to oral intake), whereas those with more severe DKA require 30–36 hr with this protocol. Any child can be easily transitioned to oral intake and subcutaneous insulin when DKA has essentially resolved (total CO_2 >15 mEq/L; pH >7.30; sodium stable between 135 and 145 mEq/L; no emesis). The IV is capped, and the 1st dose of subcutaneous insulin is given with a meal. Children with mild DKA often can be discharged after a few hours of therapy in the emergency department if adequate follow-up is provided.

A flow sheet is mandatory for accurate monitoring of changes in acidosis, electrolytes, fluid balance, and clinical status, especially if the patient is transferred from the emergency department to an inpatient setting with new caretakers. This flow sheet is best implemented by a central computer system, which allows for rapid update and wide availability of results, as well as rule-driven highlighting of critical values. A paper flow sheet suffices if it stays with the patient, is kept current, and is reviewed frequently by the physician. Any flow sheet should include columns for serial electrolytes, pH, glucose, and fluid balance. Blood testing should occur every 1–2 hr for children with severe DKA and every 3–4 hr for those with mild to moderate DKA.

Even though this protocol has a long safety record, each patient must be closely monitored. For all but the mildest cases, this includes frequent neurologic checks for any signs of **increasing intracranial pressure,** such as a change of consciousness, depressed respiration, worsening headache, bradycardia, apnea, pupillary changes, papilledema, posturing, and seizures. Mannitol must be readily available for use at the earliest sign of cerebral edema. The physician must also keep informed of the laboratory changes; hypokalemia or hypoglycemia can occur rapidly. Children with moderate to severe DKA have a higher overall risk and should be treated in an intensive care environment. Finally, this protocol may not be appropriate for some patients such as the severely hypernatremic child (corrected sodium >150 mEq/L), who may need slower rehydration with a longer duration of isotonic fluids.

Some residual β-cell function is seen even in children with DKA. This function may improve as the child recovers from the effects of hyperglycemia and elevated counter-regulatory hormones. This residual secretion may necessitate a reduction in the initial total subcutaneous insulin dose used in the 1st few days of therapy.

Nonketotic Hyperosmolar Coma. This syndrome is characterized by severe hyperglycemia (blood glucose >800 mg/dL), absence of or only slight ketosis, nonketotic acidosis, severe dehydration, depressed sensorium or frank coma, and various neurologic signs that may include grand mal seizures, hyperthermia, hemiparesis, and positive Babinski signs. Respirations are usually shallow, but coexistent metabolic (lactic) acidosis may be manifested by Kussmaul breathing. Serum osmolarity is commonly 350 mOsm/kg or greater. This condition is uncommon in children; among adults, mortality rates have been high, possibly in part because of delays in recognition and institution of appropriate therapy. In children, there has been a high incidence of pre-existing neurologic damage. Profound hyperglycemia may develop over a period of days and, initially, the obligatory osmotic polyuria and dehydration may be partially compensated for by increasing fluid intake. With progression of disease, thirst becomes impaired, possibly because of alteration of the hypothalamic thirst center by hyperosmolarity and, in some instances, because of a pre-existing defect in the hypothalamic osmoregulating mechanism.

The low production of ketones is attributed mainly to the hyperosmolarity, which in vitro blunts the lipolytic effect of epinephrine and the antilipolytic effect of residual insulin; blunting of lipolysis by the therapeutic use of β-adrenergic blockers may contribute to the syndrome. Depression of consciousness is closely correlated with the degree of hyperosmolarity in this condition as well as in DKA. Hemoconcentration may also predispose to cerebral arterial and venous thromboses.

Treatment of nonketotic hyperosmolar coma is directed at rapid repletion of the vascular volume deficit and very slow correction of the hyperosmolar state. One-half isotonic saline (0.45% NaCl; some use normal saline) is administered at a rate estimated to replace 50% of the volume deficit in the 1st 12 hr, and the remainder is administered during the ensuing 24 hr. The rate of infusion and the saline concentration are titrated to result in a slow decline of serum osmolality. When the blood glucose concentration approaches 300 mg/dL, the hydrating fluid should be changed to 5% dextrose in 0.2 normal (N) saline. Approximately 20 mEq/L of potassium chloride should be added to each of these fluids to prevent hypokalemia. Serum potassium and plasma glucose concentrations should be monitored at 2-hr intervals for the 1st 12 hr and at 4-hr intervals for the next 24 hr to permit appropriate adjustments of administered potassium and insulin.

Insulin can be given by continuous IV infusion beginning with the 2nd hr of fluid therapy. Blood glucose may decrease dramatically with fluid therapy alone. The IV insulin dosage should be 0.05 U/kg/h of regular (fast-acting) rather than 0.1 U/kg/h as advocated for patients with DKA.

TABLE 590-7. Calorie Needs for Children and Young Adults

AGE	KCAL REQUIRED/KG BODY WEIGHT*
Children	
0–12 mo	120
1–10 yr	100–75
Young women	
11–15 yr	35
≥16 yr	30
Young men	
11–15 yr	80–55 (65)
16–20 yr	
Average activity	40
Very physically active	50
Sedentary	30

Numbers in parentheses are means.
*Gradual decline in calories per unit weight as age increases.
From *Nutrition Guide for Professionals: Diabetes Education and Meal Planning*. Alexandria, VA, and Chicago, IL, The American Diabetes Association and The American Dietetic Association, 1988.

Nutritional Management. Nutrition plays an essential role in the management of patients with T1DM. This is of critical importance during childhood and adolescence, when appropriate energy intake is required to meet the needs for energy expenditure, growth, and pubertal development. Nutritional treatment alone or in combination with appropriate insulin therapy averts or relieves symptoms of hyperglycemia in diabetic patients. Moreover, nutritional practices may influence the development of long-term complications of diabetes (diabetic nephropathy). There are no special nutritional requirements for the diabetic child other than those for optimal growth and development. In outlining nutritional requirements for the child on the basis of age, sex, weight, and activity, food preferences, including cultural and ethnic ones, must be considered.

Total recommended caloric intake is based on size or surface area and can be obtained from standard tables (Tables 590-7 and 590-8). The caloric mixture should comprise approximately 55% carbohydrate, 30% fat, and 15% protein. Approximately 70% of the carbohydrate content should be derived from complex carbohydrates such as starch; intake of sucrose and highly refined sugars should be limited. Complex carbohydrates require prolonged digestion and absorption so that plasma glucose levels increase slowly, whereas glucose from refined sugars, including carbonated beverages, is rapidly absorbed and may cause wide swings in the metabolic pattern; carbonated beverages should be sugar free. Priority should be given to total calories and total carbohydrate consumed rather than its source. Carbohydrate counting has become a mainstay in the nutrition education and management of patients with DM. Each carbohydrate exchange unit is 15 g. Patients and their families are provided with information regarding the carbohydrate contents of different foods and food label reading. This allows patients to adjust their insulin dosage to their mealtime carbohydrate intake. The use of carbohydrate counting and insulin to carbohydrate ratios and the use of fast-acting insulin analogs and long-acting basal insulin (detemir and glargine) provide many children with less rigid meal planning. Flexibility in the use of insulin in relation to carbohydrate content of food improves the quality of life.

Although in children there is concern about the potential cumulative effect of saccharin, available data do not support an association of moderate amounts with bladder cancer. Other non-nutritive sweeteners such as aspartame are used in a variety of products. Sorbitol and xylitol should not be used as artificial sweeteners; they are products of the polyol pathway and are implicated in some of the complications of diabetes.

TABLE 590-8. Summary of Nutrition Guidelines for Children and/or Adolescents with Type 1 Diabetes Mellitus

Nutrition Care Plan

Promotes optimal compliance.

Incorporates goals of management: normal growth and development, control of blood glucose, maintenance of optimal nutritional status, and prevention of complications. Uses staged approach.

Nutrient Recommendations and Distribution

NUTRIENT	(%) of CALORIES	RECOMMENDED DAILY INTAKE
Carbohydrate	Will vary	High fiber, especially soluble fiber; optimal amount unknown
Fiber	>20 g per day	
Protein	12–20	
Fat	<30	
Saturated	<10	
Polyunsaturated	6–8	
Monounsaturated	Remainder of fat allowance	
Cholesterol		300 mg
Sodium		Avoid excessive; limit to 3,000–4,000 mg if hypertensive

Additional Recommendations

Energy: If using measured diet, reevaluate prescribed energy level at least every 3 mo.

Protein: High-protein intakes may contribute to diabetic nephropathy. Low intakes may reverse preclinical nephropathy. Therefore, 12–20% of energy is recommended; lower end of range is preferred. In guiding toward the end of the range, a staged approach is useful.

Alcohol: Safe use of moderate alcohol consumption should be taught as routine anticipatory guidance as early as junior high school.

Snacks: Snacks vary according to individual needs (generally 3 snacks per day for children; midafternoon and bedtime snacks for junior high children or teens).

Alternative sweeteners: Use of a variety of sweeteners is suggested.

Educational techniques: No single technique is superior. Choice of educational method used should be based on patient needs. Knowledge of variety of techniques is important. Follow-up education and support are required.

Eating disorders: Best treatment is prevention. Unexplained poor control or severe hypoglycemia may indicate a potential eating disorder.

Exercise: Education is vital to prevent delayed or immediate hypoglycemia and to prevent worsened hyperglycemia and ketosis.

From Connell JE, Thomas-Doberson D: Nutritional management of children and adolescents with insulin-dependent diabetes mellitus: A review by the Diabetes Care and Education Dietetic Practice Group. *J Am Diet Assoc* 1991;91:1556.

Diets with high fiber content are useful in improving control of blood glucose. Moderate amounts of sucrose consumed with fiber-rich foods such as whole-meal bread may have no more glycemic effect than their low-fiber, sugar-free equivalents. The concept of biologic equivalence or of a "glycemic index" of foods is under investigation.

The intake of fat is adjusted so that the polyunsaturated : saturated ratio is increased to about 1.2 : 1.0, in contrast to the estimated American average of 0.3 : 1.0. Dietary fats derived from animal sources are, therefore, reduced and replaced by polyunsaturated fats from vegetable sources. Substituting margarine for butter, vegetable oil for animal oils in cooking, and lean cuts of meat, poultry, and fish for fatty meats, such as bacon, is advisable. The intake of cholesterol is also reduced by these measures and by limiting the number of egg yolks consumed. These simple measures reduce serum low-density lipoprotein cholesterol, a predisposing factor to atherosclerotic disease. Less than 10% of calories should be derived from saturated fats, up to 10% from polyunsaturated fats, and the remaining fat-derived calories from monounsaturated fats. Table 590-8 summarizes current nutritional guidelines.

The total daily caloric intake is divided to provide 20% at breakfast, 20% at lunch, and 30% at dinner, leaving 10% for each of the midmorning, midafternoon, and evening snacks, if they are desired. In older children, the midmorning snack may be omitted and its caloric equivalent added to lunch. Special brochures and pamphlets describing sample meal plans for children are usually available from regional diabetes associations; their use should be encouraged as part of the educational process. Meal plans are often based on groups of food exchanges; within each of the exchange lists of the foods that are principal sources of carbohydrates, proteins, and fats, there is a wide variety of foods that can be substituted or exchanged. There are few restrictions so that each child can select a diet based on personal taste or preferences with the help of the physician or dietitian (or both). Emphasis should be placed on regularity of food intake and on constancy of carbohydrate intake. Occasional excesses for birthdays and other parties are permissible and tolerated to not foster rebellion and stealth in obtaining desired food. Cakes and even candies are permissible on special occasions as long as the food exchange value and carbohydrate content are adjusted in the meal plan. Adjustments in meal planning must constantly be made to meet the needs as well as the desires of each child although a consistent eating pattern with appropriate supplements for exercise, the pubertal growth spurt, and pregnancy in a diabetic adolescent are important for metabolic control.

The prevalence of overweight children and adolescents with T1DM has tripled over the past 20 yr, which appears to correspond to the increasing prevalence of obesity in the general population. The authors have observed that among our patients with T1DM, normal-weight preschool children have better glycemic control than age-matched overweight children. This may mean that excess body weight status may impede achievement of therapeutic goals in this group of patients. There is also an increased frequency of eating disorders among young women with diabetes. Thus, expectations and educational advice regarding nutrition must be dealt with in a sensitive, careful manner, especially in adolescents.

Monitoring. Success in the daily management of the diabetic child can be measured by the competence acquired by the family, and subsequently by the child, in assuming responsibility for daily "diabetic care." Their initial and ongoing instruction in conjunction with their supervised experience can lead to a sense of confidence in making intermittent adjustments in insulin dosage for dietary deviations, for unusual physical activity, and even for some minor intercurrent illnesses, as well as for otherwise unexplained repeated hypoglycemic reactions and excessive glycosuria. Such acceptance of responsibility should make them relatively independent of the physician for their ordinary care. The physician must maintain ongoing interested supervision and shared responsibility with the family and the child.

Self-monitoring of blood glucose (SMBG) is an essential component of managing diabetes. Monitoring often also needs to include insulin dose, unusual physical activity, dietary changes, hypoglycemia, intercurrent illness, and other items that may influence the blood glucose. These items may be valuable in interpreting the SMBG record, prescribing appropriate adjustments in insulin doses, and teaching the family. If there are discrepancies in the SMBG and other measures of glycemic control (such as the HbA_{1C}), the clinician should attempt to clarify the situation in a manner that does not undermine their mutual confidence.

Daily blood glucose monitoring has been markedly enhanced by the availability of strips impregnated with glucose oxidase that permit blood glucose measurement from a drop of blood. A portable calibrated reflectance meter can approximate the blood glucose concentration accurately. Many meters contain a memory "chip" enabling recall of each measurement, its average over a given interval, and the ability to display the pattern on a computer screen. Such information is a useful educational tool for verifying degree of control and modifying recommended regimens. A small, spring-loaded device that automates capillary blood letting (lancing device) in a relatively painless fashion is commercially available. Parents and patients should be taught to use these devices and measure blood glucose at least 4 times daily—before breakfast, lunch, and supper and at bedtime. When insulin therapy is initiated and when adjustments are made that may affect the overnight glucose levels, SMBG should also be performed at 12 A.M. and 3 A.M. to detect nocturnal hypoglycemia. Ideally, the blood glucose concentration should range from

TABLE 590-9. Target Pre-meal and 30-Day Average Blood Glucose Ranges and the Corresponding Hemoglobin A_{1c} for each Age Group

AGE GROUP (YR)	TARGET PRE-MEAL BG RANGE (MG/DL)	30-DAY AVERAGE BG RANGE (MG/DL)	TARGET HBA_{1C} (%)
<5	100–200	180–250	7.5–9.0
5–11	80–150	150–200	6.5–8.0
12–15	80–130	120–180	6.0–7.5
16–18	70–120	100–150	5.5–7.0

In our laboratory, the nondiabetic reference range for HbA_{1c} is 4.5–5.7% (95% confidence interval).
BG, blood glucose; HBA_{1c}, hemoglobin A_{1c}.

approximately 80 mg/dL in the fasting state to 140 mg/dL after meals. In practice, however, a range of 60–220 mg/dL is acceptable, based on age of the patient (Table 590-9). Blood glucose measurements that are consistently at or outside these limits, in the absence of an identifiable cause such as exercise or dietary indiscretion, are an indication for a change in the insulin dose. If the fasting blood glucose is high, the evening dose of long-acting insulin is increased by 10–15% and/or additional fast-acting insulin (lispro or aspart) coverage for bedtime snack may be considered. If the noon glucose level exceeds set limits, the morning fast-acting insulin (lispro or aspart) is increased by 10–15%. If the pre-supper glucose is high, the noon dose of fast-acting insulin is increased by 10–15%. If the pre-bedtime glucose is high, the pre-supper dose of fast-acting insulin is increased by 10–15%. Similarly, reductions in the insulin type and dose should be made if the corresponding blood glucose measurements are consistently below desirable limits.

A minimum of 4 daily blood glucose measurements should be performed. However, some children and adolescents may need to have more frequent blood glucose monitoring based on their level of physical activity and history of frequent hypoglycemic reactions. Families should be encouraged to become sufficiently knowledgeable about managing diabetes. They can maintain near-normal glycemia for prolonged periods by self-monitoring of blood glucose levels before and 2 hr after meals, and in conjunction with multiple daily injections of insulin, adjusted as necessary, they can maintain near-normal glycemia.

A continuous glucose monitoring system (CGMS) records data obtained from a subcutaneous sensor every 5 min for up to 72 hr and provides the clinician with a continuous profile of tissue glucose levels. The interstitial glucose levels lag 13 min behind the blood glucose values at any given level. The CGMS values tend to have a high correlation coefficient for blood glucose values ranging between 40 and 400 mg/dL. CGMS is minimally invasive and entails the placement of a small, subcutaneous catheter that can be easily worn by adults and children. The system provides information that allows the patient and health care team to adjust the insulin regimen and the nutrition plan to improve glycemic control. CGMS can be helpful in detecting asymptomatic nocturnal hypoglycemia as well as in lowering HbA_{1C} values without increasing the risk for severe hypoglycemia. While there are potential pitfalls in CGMS use, including suboptimal compliance, human error, incorrect technique and sensor failure, the implementation of CGMS in ambulatory diabetes practice allows the clinician to diagnose abnormal glycemic patterns in a more precise manner.

Glucowatch Biographer uses reverse iontophoresis to analyze the glucose content of interstitial fluid, which is extracted through a membrane patch on the patient's wrist beneath the Glucowatch device. Glucowatch provides real-time interstitial fluid glucose values, in the range of 40–400 mg/dL, that are the average of blood glucose values for the preceding 20 min. Glucose values in the range of 70–280 mg/dL have the highest correlation coefficient with blood glucose values. Additionally, the Glucowatch alarm can be set for monitoring nocturnal hypoglycemia as needed. Newer generations of continuous glucose monitors not only display real-time glucose data but also the alarm can be set at below or above predetermined blood glucose thresholds. The latter safety feature can assist parents of young children to guard against nocturnal hypoglycemia.

A reliable index of long-term glycemic control is provided by measurement of glycosylated hemoglobin. HbA_{1C} represents the fraction of hemoglobin to which glucose has been nonenzymatically attached in the bloodstream. The formation of HbA_{1C} is a slow reaction that is dependent on the prevailing concentration of blood glucose; it continues irreversibly throughout the red blood cell's life span of approximately 120 days. The higher the blood glucose concentration and the longer the red blood cell's exposure to it, the higher is the fraction of HbA_{1C}, which is expressed as a percentage of total hemoglobin. Because a blood sample at any given time contains a mixture of red blood cells of varying ages, exposed for varying times to varying blood glucose concentrations, an HbA_{1C} measurement reflects the average blood glucose concentration from the preceding 2–3 mo. When measured by standardized methods to remove labile forms, the fraction of HbA_{1C} is not influenced by an isolated episode of hyperglycemia. Consequently, as an index of long-term glycemic control, a measurement of HbA_{1C} is superior to measurements of glycosuria or even multiple blood glucose determinations. (The latter can reveal important fluctuations but may not accurately reflect the average overall glycemic control.) It is recommended that HbA_{1C} measurements be obtained 3 to 4 times per yr to obtain a profile of long-term glycemic control. The more consistently lower the HbA_{1C} level, and hence the better the metabolic control, the more likely it is that microvascular complications such as retinopathy and nephropathy will be less severe, delayed in appearance, or even avoided altogether. Depending on the method used for determination, HbA_{1C} values may be spuriously elevated in thalassemia (or other conditions with elevated hemoglobin F) and spuriously lower in sickle cell disease (or other conditions with high red blood cell turnover). Although values of HbA_{1C} may vary according to the method used for measurement, in nondiabetic individuals, the HbA_{1C} fraction is usually less than 6%; in diabetics, values of 6–7.9% represent good metabolic control, values of 8.0–9.9%, fair control, and values of 10.0% or higher, poor control. Adjustments in target HbA_{1C} should be made for younger children (see Table 590-9).

Exercise. No form of exercise, including competitive sports, should be forbidden to the diabetic child. A major complication of exercise in diabetic patients is the presence of a hypoglycemic reaction during or within hours after exercise. If hypoglycemia does not occur with exercise, adjustments in diet or insulin are not necessary, and glucoregulation is likely to be improved through the increased utilization of glucose by muscles. The major contributing factor to hypoglycemia with exercise is an increased rate of absorption of insulin from its injection site. Higher insulin levels dampen hepatic glucose production so that it is inadequate to meet the increased glucose utilization of exercising muscle. Regular exercise also improves glucoregulation by increasing insulin receptor number. In patients who are in poor metabolic control, vigorous exercise may precipitate ketoacidosis because of the exercise-induced increase in the counter-regulatory hormones.

In anticipation of vigorous exercise, one additional carbohydrate exchange may be taken before exercise, and glucose from orange juice, a carbonated nondietetic beverage, or candy should be available during and after exercise. With experience and trial and error, each patient, guided by the physician, should develop an appropriate regimen for regularly planned exercise that is frequently associated with hypoglycemia; in such instances, the total dose of insulin may be reduced by about 10–15% on the day of the scheduled exercise. Prolonged exercise, such as long-distance running, may require reduction of as much as 50% or more of the usual insulin dose. It is also important to watch for delayed hypoglycemia several hours after exercise.

Benefits of Improved Glycemic Control. The Diabetes Control and Complications Trial (DCCT) established conclusively the association between higher glucose levels and long-term microvascular complications. Intensive management produced dramatic reductions of retinopathy, nephropathy, and neuropathy by 47–76%. The data from the adolescent cohort demonstrated the same degree of improvement and the same relationship between the outcome measures of microvascular complications. Adolescents gained more weight and experienced significantly more frequent episodes of severe hypoglycemia and ketoacidosis than did adults. Other studies of children and adolescents have not documented increased frequency or severity of hypoglycemia.

The beneficial effect of intensified treatment was determined by the degree of blood glucose normalization, independently of the type of intensified treatment used. Frequent blood glucose monitoring was considered an important factor in achieving better glycemic control for the intensively treated adolescents and adults. Patients who were intensively treated had individualized glucose targets, frequent adjustments based on ongoing capillary blood glucose monitoring, and a team approach that focused on the person with diabetes as the prime initiator of ambulatory care. Care was constantly adjusted toward reaching normal or near-normal glycemic goals while avoiding or minimizing severe episodes of hypoglycemia. Teaching emphasized a preventive approach to blood glucose fluctuations with constant readjustment to counterbalance any high or low blood glucose readings. Target blood glucose goals were adjusted upward if hypoglycemia could not be prevented.

Total duration of diabetes contributes to development and severity of complications. Nonetheless, many professionals have concerns about applying the results of the DCCT to preschool-aged children, who often have hypoglycemia unawareness with unique safety issues, and to prepubertal school-aged children, who were not included in the DCCT.

Current Intensive Insulin Replacement Regimens. The goal of physiologic insulin replacement for T1DM is accomplished with short-acting insulins that more closely mimic the sharp increase and short duration of pancreatic insulin secreted with nutrient intake. The rapid-acting insulin analog lispro has superior pharmacokinetic properties for the control of postprandial glucose. Improved postprandial glucose responses occur with twice-daily injections (conventional insulin, CI), multiple daily injections (MDI), or CSII. The use of lispro or aspart insulin reduces the frequency of between-meal hypoglycemic events, especially when it is carefully balanced with the carbohydrate content of meal. This has improved how insulin is given to toddlers as well as how to manage a flexible meal plan.

The carbohydrate content of food does not influence glycemic control if pre-meal rapid-acting insulin (bolus) is adjusted to the carbohydrate content of meal. Wide variations in carbohydrate intake do not modify long-acting (detemir or glargine) or basal insulin requirements. Insulin replacement strategies stress the importance of administering smaller doses of insulin throughout the day. This approach allows insulin doses to be changed as needed to correct hyperglycemia, supplement for additional anticipated carbohydrate intake, or subtract for exercise. Indeed, bolus-basal treatment with multiple injections is better adapted to the physiologic profiles of insulin and glucose and can therefore provide better glycemic control than the conventional 2- to 3-dose regimen. Age-adjusted and individualized insulin to carbohydrate ratios and insulin dosage adjustment algorithms have been developed to normalize elevated blood glucose levels and to compensate for alterations in carbohydrate intake. The use of flexible multiple daily injections (FMDIs) and CSII in children with T1DM improves glycemic control without an increase in the incidence of severe hypoglycemia.

Hypoglycemic Reactions. Hypoglycemia is the major limitation to tight control of glucose levels. Once injected, insulin absorption and action are independent of the glucose level, thus creating a unique risk of hypoglycemia from an unbalanced insulin effect. Insulin analogs may help reduce but cannot eliminate this risk. Most children with T1DM can expect mild hypoglycemia each week, moderate hypoglycemia a few times each year, and severe hypoglycemia every few years. These episodes are usually not predictable, although exercise, delayed meals or snacks, and wide swings in glucose levels increase the risk. Infants and toddlers are at higher risk because they have more variable meals and activity levels, are unable to recognize early signs of hypoglycemia, and are limited in their ability to seek a source of oral glucose to reverse the hypoglycemia. The very young have an increased risk of permanently reduced cognitive function as a long-term sequela of severe hypoglycemia. For this reason, a more relaxed degree of glucose control is necessary until the child matures (see Table 590-9).

Hypoglycemia can occur at any time of day or night. Early symptoms and signs (mild hypoglycemia) may occur with a sudden decrease in blood glucose to levels that do not meet standard criteria for hypoglycemia in nondiabetic children (see Chapter 92). The child may show pallor, sweating, apprehension or fussiness, hunger, tremor, and tachycardia, all due to the surge in catecholamines as the body attempts to counter the excessive insulin effect. Behavioral changes such as tearfulness, irritability, aggression, and naughtiness are more prevalent in children. As glucose levels decline further, cerebral glucopenia occurs with drowsiness, personality changes, mental confusion, and impaired judgment (moderate hypoglycemia), progressing to inability to seek help and seizures or coma (severe hypoglycemia). Prolonged severe hypoglycemia can result in a depressed sensorium or stroke-like focal motor deficits that persist after the hypoglycemia has resolved. Although permanent sequelae are rare, severe hypoglycemia is frightening for the child and family and can result in significant reluctance to attempt even moderate glycemic control afterward.

Important counter-regulatory hormones in children include growth hormone, cortisol, epinephrine, and glucagon. The latter two seem more critical in the older child. Many older patients with long-standing T1DM lose their ability to secrete glucagon in response to hypoglycemia. In the young adult, epinephrine deficiency may also develop as part of a general autonomic neuropathy. This substantially increases the risk of hypoglycemia because the early warning signals of a declining glucose level are due to catecholamine release. Recurrent hypoglycemic episodes associated with tight metabolic control may aggravate partial counter-regulatory deficiencies, producing a syndrome of hypoglycemia unawareness and reduced ability to restore euglycemia (hypoglycemia-associated autonomic failure). Avoidance of hypoglycemia allows some recovery from this unawareness syndrome.

The most important factors in the management of hypoglycemia are an understanding by the patient and family of the symptoms and signs of the reaction and an anticipation of known precipitating factors such as gym or sports activities. Tighter glucose control increases the risk. Families should be taught to look for typical hypoglycemic scenarios or patterns in the home blood glucose log, so that they may adjust the insulin dose and avert predictable episodes. A source of emergency glucose should be available at all times and places, including at school and during visits to friends. If possible, it is initially important to document the hypoglycemia before treating, because some symptoms may not always be due to hypoglycemia. Most families and children develop a good sense for true hypoglycemic episodes and can institute treatment before testing. Any child suspected of having a moderate to severe hypoglycemic episode should also be treated before testing. It is important not to give too much glucose; 5–10 g should be given as juice or a sugar-containing carbonated beverage or candy and the blood glucose checked 15–20 minutes later. Patients, parents, and teachers should also be instructed in the administration of glucagon when the child cannot take glucose orally. An injection kit should be kept at home and school. The intramuscular dose is 0.5 mg if the child weighs less than 20 kg and 1.0 mg if more than 20 kg. This produces a brief release of glucose from the liver. Glucagon often causes emesis, which precludes giving oral supplementation if the blood glucose declines after the glucagon effect has waned. Caretakers must then be prepared to take the child to the hospital for IV glucose administration, if necessary. Mini-dose glucagon (10 μg/yr of age up to a maximum of 150 μg subcutaneously) is effective in treating hypoglycemia in children with blood glucose less than 60 mg/dL who failed to respond to oral glucose and remained symptomatic.

Somogyi Phenomenon, Dawn Phenomenon, and Brittle Diabetes. There are several reasons that blood glucose levels increase in the early morning hours before breakfast. The most common is a simple decline in insulin levels and is seen in many children using NPH or Lente as the basal insulin at supper or bedtime. This usually results in routinely elevated morning glucose. The **dawn phenomenon** is thought to be due mainly to overnight growth hormone secretion and increased insulin clearance. It is a normal physiologic process seen in most nondiabetic adolescents, who compensate with more insulin output. A child with T1DM cannot compensate and may actually have declining insulin levels if using evening NPH or Lente. The dawn phenomenon is usually recurrent and modestly elevates most morning glucose levels.

Rarely, high morning glucose is due to the **Somogyi phenomenon,** a theoretical rebound from late night or early morning hypoglycemia, thought to be due to an exaggerated counter-regulatory response. It is unlikely to be a common cause, in that most children remain hypoglycemic (do not rebound) once nighttime glucose levels decline. Continuous glucose monitoring systems may help clarify ambiguously elevated morning glucose levels.

The term **brittle diabetes** has been used to describe the child, usually an adolescent female, with unexplained wide fluctuations in blood glucose, often with recurrent DKA, who is taking large doses of insulin. An inherent physiologic abnormality is rarely present because these children usually show normal insulin responsiveness when in the hospital environment. Psychosocial or psychiatric problems, including eating disorders, and dysfunctional family dynamics are usually present, which preclude effective diabetes therapy. Hospitalization is usually needed to confirm the environmental effect, and aggressive psychosocial or psychiatric evaluation is essential. Therefore, clinicians should refrain from using "brittle diabetes" as a diagnostic term.

Behavioral/Psychological Aspects and Eating Disorders. Diabetes in a child affects the lifestyle and interpersonal relationships of the entire family. Feelings of anxiety and guilt are common in parents. Similar feelings, coupled with denial and rejection, are equally common in children, particularly during the rebellious teenage years. Family conflict has been associated with poor treatment adherence and poor metabolic control among youths with T1DM. No specific personality disorder or psychopathology is characteristic of diabetes; similar feelings are observed in families with other chronic disorders.

COPING STYLES. Children and adolescents with T1DM are faced with a complex set of developmental changes as well as shifting burdens of the disease. Adjustment problems might affect psychological well-being and the course of the disease by contributing to poor self-management and poor metabolic control. Coping styles refer to typical habitual preferences for ways of approaching problems and might be regarded as strategies that people generally use to cope across a wide range of stressors. Problem-focused coping refers to efforts directed toward rational management of a problem, and it is aimed at changing the situation causing distress. On the other hand, emotion-focused coping implies efforts to reduce emotional distress caused by the stressful event and to manage or regulate emotions that might accompany or result from the stressor. In adolescents with diabetes, avoidance coping and venting emotions have been found to predict poor illness-specific self-care behavior and poor metabolic control. Patients who use more mature defenses and exhibit greater adaptive capacity are more likely to adhere to their regimen. Coping strategies seem to be age dependent, with adolescents using more avoidance coping than younger children with diabetes.

NONADHERENCE. Family conflict, denial, and feelings of anxiety find expression in nonadherence to instructions regarding nutritional and insulin therapy and in noncompliance with self-monitoring. Deliberate overdosage with insulin, resulting in hypoglycemia, or omission of insulin, often in association with excesses in nutritional intake and resulting in ketoacidosis, may be pleas for psychological help or manipulative attempts to escape an environment perceived as undesirable or intolerable; occasionally, they may be manifestations of suicidal intent. Frequent admissions to the hospital for ketoacidosis or hypoglycemia should arouse suspicion of an underlying emotional conflict. Overprotection on the part of parents is common and often is not in the best interest of the patient. Feelings of being different or of being alone, or both, are common and may be justified in view of the restrictive schedules imposed by testing of urine and blood, administration of insulin, and nutritional limitations. Furthermore, concern about the likelihood of complications developing and the decreased life span of patients with diabetes fosters anxiety. Unfortunately, misinformation abounds about the risks of the development of diabetes in siblings or offspring and of pregnancy in young diabetic women. Even appropriate information may cause further anxiety.

Many of these problems can be averted through continued empathic counseling based on correct information and attempts to build attitudes of normality in the patient and a feeling of being a productive member of society. Recognizing the potential impact of these problems, peer discussion groups have been organized in many locales; feelings of isolation and frustration tend to be lessened by the sharing of common problems. Summer camps for diabetic children afford an excellent opportunity for learning and sharing under expert supervision. Education about the pathophysiology of diabetes, insulin dose, technique of administration, nutrition, exercise, and hypoglycemic reactions can be reinforced by medical and paramedical personnel. The presence of numerous peers with similar problems offers new insights to the diabetic child. Residential treatment for children and adolescents with difficult to manage T1DM is an option available only in some centers.

ANXIETY AND DEPRESSION. It has been shown that there are significant correlations between poor metabolic control and depressive symptoms, a high level of anxiety, or a previous psychiatric diagnosis. In a similar way, poor metabolic control is related to higher levels of personal, social, school maladjustment, or family environment dissatisfaction. It is estimated that 20–26% of adolescent patients may develop major depressive disorder (MDD), which is similar to the occurrence rate of MDD in nondiabetic adolescents. The course characteristics of MDD in young diabetic subjects and psychiatric control subjects appear to be similar; however, eventual propensity of diabetic youths for more protracted depressions is greater and there is higher risk of recurrence among young diabetic females. Therefore, the health care providers managing a child or adolescent with diabetes should be aware of their pivotal role as counselor and advisor and should closely monitor the mental health of patients with diabetes.

FEAR OF SELF-INJECTING AND SELF-TESTING. Extreme fear of self-injecting (FSI) insulin (injection phobia) is likely to compromise glycemic control as well as emotional well-being. Likewise, fear of finger pricks can be a source of distress and may seriously hamper self-management. Children and adolescents may either omit insulin dosing or refuse to rotate their injection sites because repeated injection in the same site is associated with less pain sensation. Failure to rotate injection sites results in subcutaneous scar formation (lipohypertrophy). Insulin injection into the lipohypertrophic skin is usually associated with poor insulin absorption and/or insulin leakage with resultant suboptimal glycemic control.

EATING DISORDERS. Treatment of T1DM involves constant monitoring of food intake. In addition, improved glycemic control is commonly associated with increased weight gain. In adolescent females, these two factors, along with individual, familial, and socioeconomic factors, can lead to an increased incidence of both nonspecific and specific eating disorders, which can disrupt glycemic control and increase the risk of long-term complications. Eating disorders and subthreshold eating disorders are almost twice as common in adolescent females with T1DM as in their nondiabetic peers. The reports of the frequencies of specific (anorexia or bulimia nervosa) eating disorders vary from 1% to 6.9% among female patients with T1DM. The prevalence of nonspecific and subthreshold eating disorders is 9% and 14%, respectively. About 11% of T1DM adolescent females take less insulin than prescribed in order to lose weight. Among adolescent females with an eating disorder, about 42% of patients misuse insulin, whereas the estimates of insulin misuse prevalence in subthreshold and nondisordered eating groups are 18% and 6%, respectively. While there is little information regarding the prevalence of eating disorders among male adolescents with T1DM, available data suggest normal eating attitudes in most. Among healthy adolescent males who participate in wrestling, however, the drive to lose weight has led to the seasonal, transient development of abnormal eating attitudes and behaviors, which may lead to insulin dose omission in order to lose weight.

When behavioral/psychological problems and/or eating disorders are assumed to be responsible for poor compliance with the medical regimen, referral for psychological evaluation and management is indicated. Children and adolescents with injection phobia and fear of self-testing can be counseled by a trained behavioral therapist and benefit from such techniques as desensitization and biofeedback to attenuate pain sensation and psychological distress associated these procedures. Behavioral therapists and psychologists usually form part of the pediatric diabetes team in most centers and can help assess and manage emotional and behavioral disorders in diabetic children.

Management During Infections. Although infections are no more common in diabetic children than in nondiabetic ones, they can often disrupt glucose control and may precipitate DKA. In addition, the diabetic child is at increased risk of dehydration if hyperglycemia causes an osmotic diuresis or if ketosis causes emesis. Counter-regulatory hormones associated with stress blunt insulin action and elevate glucose levels. If anorexia occurs, however, lack of caloric intake increases the risk of hypoglycemia. Although children younger than 3 yr tend to become hypoglycemic and older children tend toward hyperglycemia, the overall effect is unpredictable. Therefore, frequent blood glucose monitoring and adjustment of insulin doses are essential elements of sick day guidelines (Table 590-10).

The overall goals are to maintain hydration, control glucose levels, and avoid ketoacidosis. This can usually be done at home if proper sick day guidelines are followed and with telephone contact with health care providers. The family should seek advice if home treatment does not control ketonuria, hyperglycemia, or hypoglycemia, or if the child shows signs of dehydration. A child with large ketonuria and emesis should be seen in the emergency department for a general examination, to evaluate hydration, and to determine whether ketoacidosis is present by checking serum electrolytes, glucose, pH, and total CO_2. A child whose blood glucose declines to less than 50–60 mg/dL (2.8–3.3 mmol/L) and who cannot maintain oral intake may need IV glucose, especially if further insulin is needed to control ketonemia.

TABLE 590-10. Guidelines for Sick Day Management

URINE KETONE STATUS	GLUCOSE TESTING AND EXTRA INSULIN	RAPID-ACTING INSULIN CORRECTION DOSES*	COMMENT
Negative or small†	q2 hr	q2 hr for glucose >250 mg/dL	Check ketones every other void.
Moderate to large‡	q1 hr	q1 hr for glucose >250 mg/dL	Check ketones each void. Go to hospital if emesis occurs.

Basal insulin: glargine or detemir basal insulin should be given at the usual dose and time. NPH and Lente should be reduced by one half if blood glucose <150 mg/dL and the oral intake is limited.
Oral fluids: sugar-free if blood glucose >250 mg/dL (14 mmol/L); sugar-containing if blood glucose <250 mg/dL.
Call physician or nurse if blood glucose remains elevated after 3 extra doses; if blood glucose remains less than 70 mg/dL and child cannot take oral supplement; if dehydration occurs.
**Give insulin based on individualized dosing schedule. Also give usual dose for carbohydrate intake if glucose >150 mg/dL.*
†For home serum ketones <1.5 mmol/L per commercial kit.
‡For home serum ketones >1.5 mmol/L.

Management During Surgery. Surgery can disrupt glucose control in the same way as can intercurrent infections. Stress hormones associated with the underlying condition as well as with surgery itself decrease insulin sensitivity. This increases glucose levels, exacerbates fluid losses, and may initiate DKA. On the other hand, caloric intake is usually restricted, which decreases glucose levels. The net effect is as difficult to predict as during an infection. Vigilant monitoring and frequent insulin adjustments are required to maintain euglycemia and avoid ketosis.

Maintaining glucose control and avoiding DKA are best accomplished with IV insulin and fluids. A simple insulin adjustment scale based on the patient's weight and blood glucose level can be used in most situations (Table 590-11). The IV insulin is continued after surgery as the child begins to take oral fluids; the IV fluids can be steadily decreased as oral intake increases. When full oral intake is achieved, the IV may be capped and subcutaneous insulin begun. When surgery is elective, it is best performed early in the day, allowing the patient maximal recovery time to restart oral intake and subcutaneous insulin therapy. When elective surgery is brief (less than 1 hr) and full oral intake is expected shortly afterward, one may simply monitor the blood glucose hourly and give a dose of insulin analog according to the child's home glucose correction scale. If glargine or detemir is used as the basal insulin, a full dose is given the evening before planned surgery. If NPH or Lente is used, one half of the morning dose is given before surgery. The child should not be discharged until blood glucose levels are stable and oral intake is tolerated.

LONG-TERM COMPLICATIONS: RELATION TO GLYCEMIC CONTROL. The increasingly prolonged survival of the diabetic child is associated with an increasing prevalence of complications. Complications of DM can be divided into 3 major categories—(1) microvascular complications, specifically, retinopathy and nephropathy; (2) macrovascular complications, particularly accelerated coronary artery disease, cerebrovascular disease, and peripheral vascular disease; and (3) neuropathies, both peripheral

TABLE 590-11. Guidelines for Intravenous Insulin Coverage During Surgery

BLOOD GLUCOSE LEVEL (MG/DL)	INSULIN INFUSION (U/KG/HR)	BLOOD GLUCOSE MONITORING
<120	0.00	1 hr
121–200	0.03	2 hr
200–300	0.06	2 hr
300–400	0.08	1 hr†
400	0.10	1 hr†

**An infusion of 5% glucose and 0.45% saline solution with 20 mEq/L of potassium acetate is given at 1.5 times maintenance rate.*
†Check urine ketones.

TABLE 590-12. Screening Guidelines

	WHEN TO COMMENCE SCREENING	FREQUENCY	PREFERRED METHOD OF SCREENING	OTHER SCREENING METHODS	POTENTIAL INTERVENTION
Retinopathy	After 5 years' duration in prepubertal children, after 2 years' in pubertal children	1–2 yearly	Fundal photography	Fluorescein angiography, mydriatic ophthalmoscopy	Improved glycemic control, laser therapy
Nephropathy	After 5 years' duration in prepubertal children, after 2 years' in pubertal children	Annually	Overnight timed urine excretion of albumin	24-h excretion of albumin, Urinary albumin/creatinine ratio	Improved glycemic control, blood pressure control, ACE inhibitors
Neuropathy	Unclear	Unclear	Physical examination	Nerve conduction, thermal and vibration threshold, pupillometry, cardiovascular reflexes	Improved glycemic control
Macrovascular disease	After age 2	Every 5 years	Lipids	Blood pressure	Statins for hyperlipidemia Blood pressure control
Thyroid disease	At diagnosis	Every 2–3 years	TSH	Thyroid peroxidase antibody	Thyroxine
Celiac disease	At diagnosis	Every 2–3 years	Tissue transglutaminase, endomysial antibody	Antigliadin antibodies	Gluten-free diet

From Glastras SJ, Mohsin F, Donaghue KC: Complications of diabetes mellitus in childhood. *Pediatr Clin North Am* 2005;52:1735–1753.

and autonomic, affecting a variety of organs and systems (Table 590-12). In addition, cataract may occur more frequently.

Diabetic retinopathy is the leading cause of blindness in the United States in adults aged 20–65 yr. The risk of diabetic retinopathy after 15 yr duration of diabetes is 98% for individuals with type 1 DM and 78% for those with T2DM. Lens opacities (due to glycation of tissue proteins and activation of the polyol pathway) are present in at least 5% of those younger than 19 yr. Although the metabolic control has an impact on the development of this complication, genetic factors also have a role, because only 50% of patients develop proliferative retinopathy. The earliest clinically apparent manifestations of diabetic retinopathy are classified as nonproliferative or background diabetic retinopathy—microaneurysms, dot and blot hemorrhages, hard and soft exudates, venous dilation and beading, and intraretinal microvascular abnormalities. These changes do not impair vision. The more severe form is proliferative diabetic retinopathy—manifested by neovascularization, fibrous proliferation, and preretinal and vitreous hemorrhages. Proliferative retinopathy, if not treated, is relentlessly progressive and impairs vision, leading to blindness. The mainstay of treatment is panretinal laser photocoagulation. In advanced diabetic eye disease—manifested by severe vitreous hemorrhage or fibrosis, often with retinal detachment—vitrectomy is an important therapeutic modality. Eventually, the eye disease becomes quiescent, a stage termed involutional retinopathy. A separate subtype of retinopathy is diabetic maculopathy, which is manifested by severe macular edema impairing central vision, for which focal laser photocoagulation may be effective.

Guidelines suggest that diabetic patients have an initial dilated and comprehensive examination by an ophthalmologist shortly after the diagnosis of diabetes is made in patients with T2DM, and within 3–5 yr after the onset of T1DM (but not before age 10 yr). Any patients with visual symptoms or abnormalities should be referred for ophthalmologic evaluation. Subsequent evaluations for both type 1 and T2DM patients should be repeated annually by an ophthalmologist who is experienced in diagnosing the presence of diabetic retinopathy and is knowledgeable about its management (see Table 590-12).

Diabetic nephropathy is the leading known cause of end-stage renal disease (ESRD) in the United States. Most ESRD from diabetic nephropathy is preventable. Diabetic nephropathy affects 20–30% of patients with T1DM and 15–20% of T2DM patients 20 yr after onset. The mean 5-yr life expectancy for patients with diabetes-related ESRD is less than 20%. The increased mortality risk in long-term T1DM may be due to nephropathy, which may account for about 50% of deaths. The risk of nephropathy increases with duration of diabetes (up until 25–30 yr duration, after which this complication rarely begins), degree of metabolic control, and genetic predisposition to essential hypertension. Only 30–40% of patients affected by type 1 DM eventually experience ESRD. The glycation of tissue proteins results in glomerular basement membrane thickening. The course of diabetic nephropathy is slow. An increased urinary albumin excretion rate (AER) of 30–300 mg/24 hr (20–200 μg/min)—so-called microalbuminuria—can be detected and constitutes an early stage of nephropathy from intermittent to persistent (incipient), which is commonly associated with glomerular hyperfiltration and blood pressure elevation. As nephropathy evolves to early overt stage with proteinuria (AER >300 mg/24 hr, or >200 μg/min), it is accompanied by hypertension. Advanced stage nephropathy is defined by a progressive decline in renal function (declining glomerular filtration rate and elevation of serum blood urea and creatinine), progressive proteinuria, and hypertension. Progression to ESRD is recognized by the appearance of uremia, the nephritic syndrome, and the need for renal replacement (transplantation or dialysis).

Screening for diabetic nephropathy is a routine aspect of diabetes care (see Table 590-12). The American Diabetes Association (ADA) recommends yearly screening for individuals with type 2 DM and yearly screening for those with type 1 DM after 5 yr duration of disease (but not before puberty). Twenty-four hour AER (urinary albumin and creatinine) or timed (overnight) urinary AER are acceptable techniques. Positive results should be confirmed by a 2nd measurement of AER because of the high variability of albumin excretion in patients with diabetes. Short-term hyperglycemia, exercise, urinary tract infections, marked hypertension, heart failure, and acute febrile illness can cause transient elevation urinary albumin excretion. There is marked day-to-day variability in albumin excretion, so at least 2 of 3 collections done in a 3- to 6-mo period should show elevated levels before microalbuminuria is diagnosed and treatment is started. Once albuminuria is diagnosed, a number of factors attenuate the effect of hyperfiltration on kidneys: (1) meticulous control of hyperglycemia, (2) aggressive control of systemic blood pressure, (3) selective control of arteriolar dilation by use of angiotensin-converting enzyme (ACE) inhibitors (thus decreasing transglomerular capillary pressure), and (4) dietary protein restriction (because high protein intake increases renal perfusion rate). Tight glycemic control will delay the progression of microalbuminuria and slow the progression of diabetic nephropathy. Previous extensive therapy of diabetes has a persistent benefit for 7–8 yr and may delay or prevent the development of diabetic nephropathy.

DIABETIC NEUROPATHY. Both the peripheral and autonomic nervous systems can be involved, and adolescents with diabetes can show early evidence of neuropathy. This complication can be traced to the metabolic effects of hyperglycemia and/or other effects of insulin deficiency on the various constituents of the peripheral nerve. The polyol pathway, nonenzymatic glycation, and/or disturbances of myoinositol metabolism affecting one or more cell types in the multicellular constituents of the peripheral nerve appear likely to have an inciting role. The role of other factors, such as possible direct neurotrophic effects of insulin, insulin-related growth factors, nitric oxide, and stress proteins, seems to be relevant. Peripheral neuropathy may first present in some adolescents with long-standing history of diabetes. Using quantitative sensory testing (QST), abnormal cutaneous thermal perception is a common finding in both upper and lower limbs in neurologically asymptomatic young diabetic patients. Heat-induced pain threshold in the hand is correlated with the duration of the diabetes. There is no correlation between QST scores and metabolic control. Subclinical motor nerve impairment as manifested by reduced sensory nerve conduction velocity and sensory nerve action potential amplitude can be detected during late puberty and after puberty in about 10% of adolescents. Poor metabolic control during puberty appears to induce deteriorating peripheral neural function in young patients. An early sign of autonomic neuropathy such as decreased heart rate variability may present in adolescents with a history of long-standing disease and poor metabolic control. A number of therapeutic strategies have been attempted with variable results. These treatment modalities include (1) improvement in metabolic control, (2) use of aldose reductase inhibitors to reduce byproducts of the polyol pathway, (3) use of α-lipoic acid (an antioxidant) that enhances tissue nitric oxide and its metabolites, and use of anticonvulsants (e.g., lorazepam, valproate, carbamazepine, tiagabine, and topiramate) for treatment of neuropathic pain.

Other complications in diabetic children include dwarfism associated with a glycogen-laden enlarged liver (**Mauriac syndrome**), osteopenia, and a syndrome of limited joint mobility associated with tight, waxy skin; growth impairment; and maturational delay. The Mauriac syndrome is related to underinsulinization; it is much less common since longer-acting insulins have become available. Clinical features of Mauriac syndrome include moon face, protuberant abdomen, proximal muscle wasting, and enlarged liver due to fat and glycogen infiltration. The syndrome of limited joint mobility is frequently associated with the early development of diabetic microvascular complications, such as retinopathy and nephropathy, which may appear before 18 yr of age.

PROGNOSIS. T1DM is a serious, chronic disease. It has been estimated that the average life span of individuals with diabetes is about 10 yr shorter than that of the nondiabetic population. Although diabetic children eventually attain a height within the normal adult range, puberty may be delayed, and the final height may be less than the genetic potential. From studies in identical twins, it is apparent that despite seemingly satisfactory control, the diabetic twin manifests delayed puberty and a substantial reduction in height when onset of disease occurs before puberty. These observations indicate that, in the past, conventional criteria for judging control were inadequate and that adequate control of T1DM was almost never achieved by routine means.

The introduction of portable devices (insulin pumps) that can be programmed to provide CSII with meal-related pulses is one approach to the resolution of these long-term problems. In selected individuals, nearly normal patterns of blood glucose and other indices of metabolic control, including HbA_{1C}, have been maintained for several years. This approach, however, should be reserved for highly motivated persons committed to rigorous self-monitoring of blood glucose who are alert to the potential complications, such as mechanical failure of the infusion device causing hyperglycemia or hypoglycemia and to infection at the site of catheter insertion.

The changing pattern of metabolic control is having a profound influence on reducing the incidence and the severity of certain complications. For example, after 20 yr of diabetes, there is a decline in the incidence of nephropathy in T1DM in Sweden among children whose disease was diagnosed in 1971–1975 compared with in the preceding decade. In addition, in most patients with microalbuminuria in whom it was possible to obtain good glycemic control, microalbuminuria disappeared. This improved prognosis is directly related to metabolic control.

PANCREAS AND ISLET TRANSPLANTATION AND REGENERATION. In an attempt to cure T1DM, transplantation of a segment of the pancreas or of isolated islets has been performed. These procedures are both technically demanding and associated with the risks of disease recurrence and complications of rejection or its treatment by immunosuppression. Complications of immunosuppression include the development of malignancy. Some antirejection drugs, notably cyclosporine and tacrolimus, are toxic to the islets of Langerhans, impairing insulin secretion and even causing diabetes. Hence, segmental pancreas transplantation is generally only performed in association with transplantation of a kidney for a patient with ESRD due to diabetic nephropathy in which the immunosuppressive regimen is indicated for the renal transplantation. Several thousand such transplants have been performed in adults. With experience and newer immunosuppressive agents, functional survival of the pancreatic graft may be achieved for up to several years, during which time patients may be in metabolic control with no or minimal exogenous insulin and reversal of some of the microvascular complications. However, because children and adolescents with DM are not likely to have ESRD from their diabetes, pancreas transplantation as a primary treatment in children cannot be recommended.

Attempts to transplant isolated islets have been equally challenging because of rejection. Research continues to improve techniques for the yield, viability, and reduction of immunogenicity of the islets of Langerhans for transplantation. An **islet transplantation** strategy (**Edmonton protocol**) infuses isolated pancreatic islets into the portal vein of a group of adults with T1DM. This therapeutic strategy also involves the use of a new generation of immunosuppressive medications that apparently have lower side-effect profiles than do other drugs. Of 36 consecutive patients with at least 2 yr of follow-up after the initial transplant, 5 (14%) were insulin independent at 2 yr. Although patients experienced minimal side effects from immunosuppressive medications, some complications associated with islet transplantation procedures were observed that included portal vein thrombosis, bleeding related to the percutaneous portal vein access, an expanding intrahepatic and subscapular hemorrhage on anticoagulation (requiring transfusion and surgery). Elevated liver function test results were found in 46% of subjects but resolved in all. However, only half of the patients remained insulin free at 2 yr. It has been suggested that positive long-term clinical outcome is dependent on islet graft composition, especially the presence of high numbers of islet progenitor (ductal-epithelial) cells. There is improved islet engraftment by the peritransplant administration of immunosuppressants, antithymocyte globulin, and etanercept. Long-term monitoring will be needed before the success of these techniques can be assessed.

Regeneration of islets is an approach that could potentially cure T1DM. It is classified into 3 categories:

1. In vitro therapy using transplanted cultured cells, including embryonic stem cells, pancreatic stem cells, and β cell lines, in conjunction with immunosuppressive therapy or immunoisolation.
2. Ex vivo regeneration therapy, in which patients' own cells, such as bone marrow stem cells, which are transiently removed and induced to differentiate into β cells in vitro. Although some investigators have reported successful transdifferentiation of embryonic stem cells into pancreatic β cells after transplantation of bone marrow cells into rodents, others have failed to observe such effects. Therefore, insulin-producing cells cannot be generated from bone marrow stem cells consistently at this time.
3. In vivo regeneration therapy, in which impaired tissues regenerate from patients' own cells in vivo. β-cell neogenesis from non-β cells and β-cell proliferation in vivo has been considered, particularly as regeneration therapies for T2DM.

Regeneration therapy of pancreatic β cells can be combined with various other therapeutic strategies, including islet transplantation, cell-based therapy, gene therapy, and drug therapy to promote β-cell proliferation and neogenesis, and it is hoped that these strategies will, in the future, provide a cure for diabetes.

590.3 • Type 2 Diabetes Mellitus

T2DM is considered a polygenic disease aggravated by environmental factors, such as low physical activity or a hypercaloric, lipid-rich diet. Obese type 2 diabetic patients show insulin resistance of skeletal muscle, enhanced hepatic glucose production, and decreased glucose-induced insulin secretion. Over time, hyperglycemia worsens, a phenomenon that has been attributed to the deleterious effect of chronic hyperglycemia (glucotoxicity) or chronic hyperlipidemia (lipotoxicity) on β-cell function and is often accompanied by increased triglyceride content and decreased insulin gene expression. Numerous studies have described T2DM in Native American youth, as well as their African American, Hispanic, and white peers. Pediatric T2DM in adolescents represents one of the most rapidly growing forms of diabetes. The incidence of T2DM among children with diabetes at one medical center increased from 4% before 1992 to 16% in 1994. In that report, among those aged 10–19 yr, T2DM accounted for one third of all newly diagnosed diabetes in children in 1994. Overall, the incidence of adolescent T2DM increased 10-fold from 0.7 to 7.2/100,000 per year in the reported Midwest metropolitan area. The mean age at presentation was 13.8 yr; most children were markedly obese. We, at Children's Hospital of Wisconsin (Milwaukee), have observed a more than 10-fold increase in incidence of T2DM (from less than 2% to about 22% of new cases of DM) in children aged 10–18 yr in the past decade. African American (almost 70% of cases), Hispanic, and white adolescents are usually affected.

The epidemic of T2DM in children and adolescents parallels the emergence of the obesity epidemic (see Chapter 44). Although obesity itself is associated with insulin resistance, diabetes does not develop until there is some degree of failure of insulin secretion. Thus, when measured, insulin secretion in response to glucose or other stimuli is always lower in persons with T2DM than in control subjects matched for age, sex, weight, and equivalent glucose concentration. Although it is generally believed that autoimmune destruction of pancreatic β cells does not occur in type 2 DM diabetes, autoimmune markers of T1DM—namely, GAD65, ICA512, and IAA—may be positive in up to one third of the cases of adolescent T2DM. These findings reflect a broad spectrum of pancreatic and peripheral abnormalities that could lead to T2DM, and the presence of these autoimmune markers does not rule out type 2 DM in children and adolescents.

In type 2 DM, insulin deficiency is rarely absolute, so patients usually do not need insulin to survive. Nevertheless, glycemic control can be improved by exogenous insulin. DKA, when it occurs, is associated with the stress of another illness such as severe infection and may resolve when the stressful illness resolves. DKA tends to be more common in African American patients than in other ethnic groups. Most patients with T2DM remain asymptomatic for months to years because hyperglycemia is so moderate that symptoms are not so dramatic as the polyuria and weight loss accompanying T1DM. Even weight gain may continue. The prolonged hyperglycemia may be accompanied, in time, by the development of microvascular and macrovascular complications.

T2DM occurs more frequently in certain ethnic or racial groups, such as Pacific Islanders, Pima Indians, and African Americans. It also occurs in individuals with hypertension and dyslipidemia. T2DM has a stronger genetic component than does T1DM. Concordance rates among identical twins are virtually 100% for type 2 and only 30–50% for type 1 DM. The genetic basis for type 2 DM is complex and incompletely defined; no single identified defect predominates as does the HLA association with T1DM. Acanthosis nigricans may be a marker for insulin resistance, hyperinsulinemia, and eventually type 2 DM. Hirsutism, associated with the polycystic ovary syndrome, premature adrenarche, or mild mutations in steroidogenic enzymes, is frequently associated with insulin resistance in children and adolescents and may be a forerunner of the future development of type 2 DM (see Chapter 587).

Type A insulin resistance with **acanthosis nigricans** is characterized by severe insulin resistance and acanthosis nigricans in the absence of obesity or lipoatrophy; affected females also have hyperandrogenism, possibly as a secondary manifestation of the hyperinsulinemia with stimulation of androgen synthesis by ovarian theca cells (see Chapter 587). Glucose intolerance is variable and includes symptomatic diabetes. The hyperandrogenism presents with clinical and biochemical findings suggestive of polycystic ovary syndrome. Some cases, predominantly in African American females with obesity, acanthosis nigricans, and accelerated growth suggestive of gigantism, may represent insulin resistance due to obesity with down-regulation of the insulin receptor. The gigantism may represent a "spillover" effect of insulin acting via the insulin growth factor 1 receptor rather than the insulin receptor.

TREATMENT. Nutritional education and an **improved exercise level** are cornerstones of therapy for children and adolescents with T2DM. These children often come from a household environment with a poor understanding of healthy eating habits. Commonly observed behaviors include skipping meals, heavy snacking, and excessive daily television viewing, video game playing, and computer use. Adolescents engage in non-appetite-based eating (i.e., emotional eating, television-cued eating, boredom) and cyclic dieting ("yo-yo" dieting). Treatment for T2DM should target weight loss and increased physical activity as an initial approach. These approaches, however, are frequently unsuccessful.

At the time of diagnosis, insulin therapy may be necessary, especially if glucose levels are high or ketones are present. With close medical follow-up, insulin doses can often be reduced, substituted, or even discontinued, usually within a few weeks after glucose control is achieved. Effective initial therapy should also include metformin (a biguanide), which decreases hepatic glucose production. The starting dose of metformin is usually 500 mg twice daily with meals. Metformin is contraindicated if there is significant renal or liver impairment; proper assessment of liver and renal function is essential before initiating therapy (Table 590-13). A class of pharmaceutical agents, the thiazolidinediones, enhances insulin action by decreasing hepatic glucose production and facilitating glucose disposal in muscle and fat. Because they act as insulin enhancers, they may be used in conjunction with exogenous insulin and metformin. However, the thiazolidinediones are not approved for use in children in the United States, and there may be undue liver toxicity. Glucagon-like peptide-1 (GLP-1) analog and amylin have become available for the management of T2DM. GLP-1 is secreted by the L cells of small bowel in the postprandial state and stimulates insulin secretion while suppressing glucagon response. However, amylin primarily inhibits glucagon secretion. Both agents decrease gastric emptying and appetite. Incretin enhancers, a class of GLP-1, known also as dipeptidylpeptidase-4 (DPP-4 or sitagliptin), have been effective in managing T_2DM in adults. Studies in T2DM adult patients have shown that GLP-1 analog, GLP-1 receptor agonists (sitagliptin), and amylin improve glycemic control when used as an adjunct with insulin and metformin. No clinical data are available in children and adolescents.

PREVENTION. The difficulties in achieving good glucose control and preventing diabetes complications make prevention a com-

TABLE 590-13. Oral Hypoglycemic Agents

DRUG	MECHANISM OF ACTION	DURATION OF BIOLOGIC EFFECT (H)	USUAL DAILY DOSE (MG)	DOSES/DAY	SIDE EFFECTS	CAUTION
Biguanide	Insulin sensitizer				Gastrointestinal disturbance, lactic acidosis	Avoid in hepatic or renal impairment
Metformin			1500–2500	2–3		
Sulfonylureas						
First generation						
Acetohexamide		12–18	500–750	1 or divided		
Chlorpropamide		27–72	250–500	1		
Tolbutamide		14–16	1000–2000	1 or divided		
Second generation						
Glipizide		14–16	2.5–10 XL: 5–10	1 or divided 1		
Gliburide		20–24+	2.5–10	1 or divided		
Glimepride		24+	2–4	1		
Glitinides	Promote insulin secretion					Titrate carefully in renal or hepatic dysfunction
Repaglinide		≤24	2–16	3		
Nateglinide		4	360	3		
α-Glucosidase inhibitors	Slow hydrolysis and absorption of complex carbohydrates		150–300	3 (with meals)	Transient gastrointestinal disturbances	
Acarbose			150–300	3 (with meals)		
Miglitol						
Thiazolidinedione	Peripheral insulin sensitizer				Upper respiratory tract infection, headache, edema, weight gain	
Rosiglitazone			4–8	1 or divided		
Pioglitazone			15–45	1		
Sitagliptin	GLP-1 receptor agonist	24	50–100	1	Upper respiratory tract infection, sore throat, diarrhea	No data in children or adolescents

From Jacobson-Dickman E, Levistky L: Oral agents in managing diabetes mellitus in children and adolescents. *Pediatr Clin North Am* 2005;52:1689–1703.

pelling strategy. This is particularly true for T2DM, which is clearly linked to modifiable risk factors (obesity, a sedentary lifestyle). The Diabetes Prevention Program (DPP) was designed to prevent or delay the development of T2DM in adult individuals at high risk by virtue of impaired glucose tolerance (IGT). DPP results demonstrated that intensified lifestyle or drug intervention in individuals with IGT prevented or delayed the onset of T2DM. The results were striking. Lifestyle intervention reduced diabetes incidence by 58%; metformin reduced the incidence by 31% compared with placebo. The effects were similar for men and women and for all racial and ethnic groups. Lifestyle interventions are believed to have similar beneficial effects in obese adolescents with IGT. Screening is indicated for at-risk patients (Table 590-14). Complications associated with T2DM are noted in Table 590-15.

IMPAIRED GLUCOSE TOLERANCE. The term impaired glucose tolerance (IGT) is suggested as a replacement for terms such as asymptomatic diabetes, chemical diabetes, subclinical diabetes, borderline diabetes, and latent diabetes in order to avoid the stigma associated with the term diabetes mellitus. Such diagnostic labels may influence the choice of vocation, eligibility for health or life insurance, and self-image. Although IGT represents a biochemical intermediate between normal glucose metabolism and that of diabetes, experience has shown that few children with IGT go on to acquire diabetes; estimates range from zero to 10%. There is disagreement about whether the degree of glucose intolerance is useful as a prognostic index of the likelihood of progression, but there is evidence that among the few instances of progression, the insulin response during glucose tolerance testing is severely impaired. Islet cell or insulin autoantibodies as well as the HLA-DR3 or -DR4 haplotype are commonly found in those who go on to develop clinical diabetes. In most obese children with IGT, insulin responses during oral glucose tolerance tests are higher than the mean for age-adjusted but not weight-adjusted control subjects; these individuals have some resistance to the effects of insulin rather than a total inability to secrete it.

In healthy nondiabetic children, the glucose response during an oral glucose tolerance test is similar at all ages. In contrast, plasma insulin responses during the test increase progressively within the age span of about 3–15 yr and are significantly higher during puberty so that interpretation of these responses requires comparison with age- and puberty-adjusted responses.

The performance of the glucose tolerance test should be standardized according to currently accepted criteria. These include at least 3 days of a well-balanced diet containing approximately 50% of calories from carbohydrates, fasting from midnight until

TABLE 590-14. Testing for Type 2 Diabetes in Children

Criteria*

Overweight (BMI > 85th percentile for age and sex, weight for height > 85th percentile, or weight > 120% of ideal for height)

Plus

Any two of the following risk factors:

Family history of type 2 diabetes in 1st- or 2nd-degree relative

Race/ethnicity (American Indian, African American, Hispanic, Asian/Pacific Islander)

Signs of insulin resistance or conditions associated with insulin resistance (acanthosis nigricans, hypertension, dyslipidemia, PCOS)

Age of initiation: age 10 years or at onset of puberty if puberty occurs at a younger age

Frequency: Every 2 years

Test: FPG preferred

*Clinical judgment should be used to test for diabetes in high-risk patients who do not meet these criteria.

From American Diabetes Association. Type 2 diabetes in children and adolescents. *Diabetes Care* 2000; 23:386. Reproduced by permission.

TABLE 590-15. Monitoring for Complications and Co-morbidities

CONDITION	SCREENING TEST	COMMENT
Hypertension	Blood pressure	
Fatty liver	AST, ALT, possibly liver ultrasound	
Polycystic ovary syndrome	Menstrual history, assessment for androgen excess with free/total testosterone, DHEA	
Microalbuminuria	Urine albumin concentration and albumin/creatinine ratios	
Dyslipidemia	Fasting lipid profile (total, LDL, HDL cholesterol, triglycerides)	Obtain at diagnosis and every 2 years
Sleep apnea	Sleep study to assess overnight oxygen saturation	

From Liu L, Hironaka K, Pihoker C: Type 2 diabetes in youth. *Curr Probl Pediatr Adolesc Health Care* 2004; 34:249–280.

the time of the test in the morning, and a dose of glucose for the test of 1.75 g/kg but not more than 75 g. Plasma samples are obtained before ingestion of the glucose and at 1, 2, and 3 hr thereafter. The arbitrarily designated response to the test that identifies IGT is a fasting plasma glucose value of less than 126 mg/dL and a value at 2 hr of more than 140 mg/dL but less than 200 mg/dL (see Table 590-2). Determination of serum insulin responses during the glucose tolerance test is not a prerequisite for reaching a diagnosis; the magnitude of the response, however, may have prognostic value.

In children with IGT but without fasting hyperglycemia, repeated oral glucose tolerance tests are not recommended. Investigations in such children indicate that the degree of impaired glucose tolerance tends to remain stable or may actually improve over a period of years, except in patients with markedly subnormal insulin responses. Consequently, apart from reduction in weight for the obese child, no therapy is indicated. In particular, the use of oral hypoglycemic agents should be restricted to investigational studies. If fasting hyperglycemia or characteristic symptoms of diabetes develop, the affected children have the characteristics of T2DM, previously known as NIDDM (see Table 590-1).

590.4 • Other Specific Types of Diabetes

GENETIC DEFECTS OF β-CELL FUNCTION

Maturity-Onset Diabetes of Youth. This subtype of DM contains a group of heterogeneous genetic and clinical entities that are characterized by early onset between the ages of 9 and 25 yr of age, autosomal dominant inheritance (AD), and a primary defect in insulin secretion (Table 590-16). Strict criteria for the diagnosis of MODY include diabetes in at least 3 generations with AD transmission and diagnosis before age 25 yr in at least one affected subject.

Mutations in the glucokinase gene responsible for MODY2 result in mild, chronic hyperglycemia due to mild reductions in pancreatic β-cell response to glucose. As a result, this is usually a relatively mild form of diabetes with mild fasting hyperglycemia and IGT in the majority of patients, which can be treated with small doses of exogenously administered insulin. Patients affected with mutations in HNF-4α or -1α show more severe abnormalities of carbohydrate metabolism varying from impaired glucose tolerance to severe diabetes and often progressing from a mild to a severe form over time. About one third of these patients will require insulin and are prone to the development of vascular complications. Patients with MODY2 and defects in the glucokinase gene may demonstrate normal insulin responses to intravenous glucose when blood glucose concentrations are maintained at greater than 7 mmol/L. Defective glucokinase activity has been likened to a defective glucose sensor in the pancreatic β cell. By contrast, patients with MODY1 and MODY3 have more severe impairment of insulin secretion, and this defect cannot be overcome by priming with glucose infusion.

TABLE 590-16. Summary of MODY Types and Special Clinical Characteristics

	GENE MUTATED	FUNCTION	SPECIAL FEATURE
MODY1	HNF4α	Transcription factor	Decreased levels of triglycerides, apolipoproteins apoAII and apoCIII
MODY2	Glucokinase (GCK)	Enzyme, glucose sensor	Hyperglycemia of early onset but mild and nonprogressive
MODY3	HNF-1α	Transcription factor	Decreased renal absorption of glucose and consequent glycosuria
MODY4	IPF-1	Necessary for pancreatic development	
MODY5	HNF-1β	Transcription factor	Nonhyperglycemic renal disease; associated with uterine abnormalities, hypospadias, joint laxity, and learning difficulties
MODY6	NEUROD1	Differentiation factor in the development of pancreatic islets	

MODY, maturity-onset diabetes of the young.
From Nakhla M, Polychronakos C: Monogenic and other unusual causes of diabetes mellitus. *Pediatr Clin North Am* 2005;52:1637–1650.

By definition, the absence of a family history suggestive of AD inheritance precludes a diagnosis of MODY. In such circumstances, the appearance of diabetes in a relatively young person would most likely represent evolving T1DM, and therefore evaluation for markers of autoimmunity are warranted. Milder, slowly evolving type 1 DM could be confused with T2DM.

Distinction among the present forms of MODY has clinical relevance in counseling because of the lesser likelihood of vascular complications in MODY2 and, therefore, the need to treat appropriately with insulin, if necessary, in patients with MODY1 and MODY3. Molecular analysis for the currently known gene mutations on chromosomes 20, 7, and 12 are currently available for routine clinical use, which can facilitate diagnosis and management. An additional form of MODY due to heterozygous mutation in a homeodomain transcription factor called insulin promoter factor-1 (IPF-1) or MODY4 has also been described, but a routine molecular screen is not available at this time. Other less common forms of MODY result from mutations in other transcription factors, including HNF-1β (MODY5) and Neuro D1 (MODY6).

Primary or secondary defects in the GLUT2 type of glucose transporter, an insulin-independent form, may also be associated with diabetes. GLUT2 rapidly transports glucose into β cells for subsequent phosphorylation by glucokinase, which eventually leads to insulin secretion. The phenomenon of glucose toxicity, in which there is a loss or reduction in the 1st-phase insulin response to a pulse of glucose, may be the result of secondary down-regulation of GLUT2 transporters.

MODY also may be a manifestation of a polymorphism in the glycogen synthase gene. This enzyme is crucially important for storage of glucose as glycogen in muscle. Patients with this defect are notable for marked resistance to insulin and hypertension as well as a strong family history of diabetes.

Mitochondrial Gene Defects. Point mutations in mitochondrial DNA are sometimes associated with DM and deafness. One mutation is identical to the mutation in MELAS (myopathy, encephalopathy, lactic acidosis, and stroke-like syndrome), but this syndrome is not associated with diabetes so that the phenotypic expression of the same defect varies. Another form of IDDM, sometimes associated with mitochondrial mutations, is the Wolfram syndrome.

Wolfram syndrome is characterized by diabetes insipidus, DM, optic atrophy, and deafness—thus, the acronym DIDMOAD. Wolfram syndrome is caused by mitochondrial dysfunction, possibly by a nuclear gene mapped to the short arm of chromosome 4. Some patients with diabetes appear to have severe insulinopenia, whereas others have significant insulin secretion as judged by C-peptide. In 2 patients who were tested, islet cell antibodies were not detected, whereas HLA typing revealed DR2, which is generally considered "protective" for diabetes. In some patients with diabetes and deafness, a mutation in mitochondrial tRNA has been detected; in others, this mutation is absent. The overall prevalence is 1/770,000. The sequence of appearance of the stigmata was as follows: nonautoimmune IDDM in the 1st decade, central diabetes insipidus and sensorineural deafness in two-thirds to three-fourths of the patients in the 2nd decade, renal tract anomalies in about one half of the patients in the 3rd decade, and neurologic complications such as cerebellar ataxia and myoclonus in one half to two thirds of the patients in the 4th decade. Other features included primary gonadal atrophy in the majority of males and a progressive neurodegenerative course with neurorespiratory death at a median age of 30 yr. Absence of maternal diabetes or deafness and absence of the previously reported mitochondrial gene defect suggests autosomal recessive inheritance.

DIABETES MELLITUS OF THE NEWBORN

Transient. Neonatal diabetes mellitus is rare, with an estimated incidence of 1 per 100,000 newborns. Onset of persistent T1DM before the age of 6 mo is most unusual. The syndrome of transient DM in the newborn infant has its onset in the 1st wk of life and persists only several weeks to months before spontaneous resolution. It occurs most often in infants who are small for gestational age and is characterized by hyperglycemia and pronounced glycosuria, resulting in severe dehydration and, at times, metabolic acidosis but with only minimal or no ketonemia or ketonuria. Insulin responses to glucose or tolbutamide are low to absent; basal plasma insulin concentrations are normal. After spontaneous recovery, the insulin responses to these same stimuli are brisk and normal, implying a functional delay in β-cell maturation with spontaneous resolution. Occurrence of the syndrome in consecutive siblings has been reported. **Abnormalities of chromosome 6 are common** in transient neonatal DM. There are also reports of patients with classic T1DM who formerly had transient diabetes of the newborn. It remains to be determined whether this association of transient diabetes in the newborn followed much later in life by classic T1DM is a chance occurrence or causally related. This syndrome should be distinguished from the severe hyperglycemia that may occur in hypertonic dehydration; this condition usually occurs in infants beyond the newborn period, who respond promptly to rehydration with a minimal requirement for insulin.

Administration of insulin is mandatory during the active phase of DM in the newborn. One to 2 U/kg/24 hr of an intermediate-acting insulin in 2 divided doses usually results in dramatic improvement and accelerated growth and gain in weight. Attempts at gradually reducing the dose of insulin may be made as soon as recurrent hypoglycemia becomes manifested or after 2 mo of age.

Permanent. DM in the newborn period may be permanent if associated with the rare syndrome of pancreatic agenesis. Long-term follow-up of a cohort of patients with neonatal diabetes revealed that almost one half had permanent diabetes, one third had transient diabetes, and about one fourth had transient diabetes that recurred when they were 7–20 yr old. The majority of all these infants were small at birth. Instances of affected twins and families with more than one affected infant have been reported. Some infants with permanent neonatal DM are initially euglycemic and the disease presents within the 1st mo of life.

Activating mutations in the *ABCC8* gene encoding the ATP-sensitive potassium-channel subunit Kir6.2 producing permanent neonatal diabetes have been described in infants. Gene sequencing of 29 patients with permanent neonatal diabetes showed that 10 of the patients had one of 6 heterozygous mutations in the gene KCNJ11, which encodes the Kir6.2 subunit of ATP-sensitive potassium channels found within the β cells of the pancreas. Dominant mutations in *ABCC8* account for about 12% of cases of neonatal diabetes. Diabetes results from a mechanism through which basal magnesium-nucleotide-dependent stimulatory action of the sulfonylurea receptor (SUR)-1 on kir pores is increased but blockade by sulfonylureas is preserved. The identified patients had severe diabetes requiring insulin therapy and did not produce insulin when stimulated with glucose or glucagon, although they did when stimulated with tolbutamide, a sulfonylurea. Therefore sulfonylurea therapy is more effective than insulin in diabetes due to ABCC8 or KCNJII mutations. Comorbidities included paresis and delayed development in 4 patients, 3 of whom also suffered from seizure disorder and mild dysmorphism.

Abnormalities of the Insulin Gene. Diabetes of variable degrees may also result from defects in the insulin gene from faulty processing of proinsulin to insulin, an autosomal dominant defect, to various amino acid substitutions that impair the effectiveness of insulin at the receptor level. However, these defects are notable for the high concentration of insulin as measured by radioimmunoassay, whereas defects in glucokinase, MODY1, MODY3, and GLUT2 are characterized by relative or absolute deficiency of insulin secretion for the prevailing glucose concentrations.

GENETIC DEFECTS OF INSULIN ACTION. Two mutations in the insulin receptor gene with relevance for children are leprechaunism and Rabson-Mendenhall syndrome.

Leprechaunism. This is a syndrome characterized by intrauterine growth retardation, fasting hypoglycemia, and postprandial hyperglycemia in association with profound resistance to insulin, whose serum concentrations may be 100-fold that of comparable age-matched infants during an oral glucose tolerance test. Various defects of the insulin receptor have been described, thereby attesting to the important role of insulin and its receptor in fetal growth and possibly in morphogenesis. However, even probable complete absence of functional insulin receptors due to homozygous inheritance of a missense mutation in the insulin-receptor gene resulted in normal organogenesis and a liveborn infant who had a severe form of leprechaunism. Most of these patients die in the 1st yr of life.

Rabson-Mendenhall Syndrome. This entity is defined by clinical manifestations that appear to be intermediate between those of acanthosis nigricans with insulin resistance type A and leprechaunism. The features include extreme insulin resistance, acanthosis nigricans, abnormalities of the teeth and nails, and pineal hyperplasia. It is not clear whether this syndrome is entirely distinct from leprechaunism; however, patients with Rabson-Mendenhall tend to live beyond the 1st yr of life. Defects in the insulin-receptor gene have been described in this syndrome.

CYSTIC FIBROSIS–RELATED DIABETES. Because of improvements in the medical care of children with cystic fibrosis (CF), many survive to the late teenage and early adult years. On the other hand, as the annual screening of patients for diabetes among CF centers has become routine, the number of CF-related diabetes (CFRD) cases has almost doubled. It is estimated that up to 25% of adolescents with CF have diabetes. The care of these patients is very different from that of patients with type 1 or type 2 DM, because CFRD patients have distinct pathophysiologic and complicated nutritional and medical problems.

Patients with CFRD are slender and have insulin deficiency. The clinical presentation is similar to that of type 2 DM in that the onset of the disease is insidious and the occurrence of ketoacidosis is rare. Islet antibody titers are negative. The prevalence of microvascular complications in CFRD in relationship to duration of diabetes, glycemic control, and pulmonary diseases is not well characterized. Macrovascular complications do not appear to be of concern in CFRD, perhaps because of the shortened life span of these patients. Several factors unique to CF influence both the onset and the course of diabetes: (1) frequent acute or chronic infections are associated with waxing and waning of insulin resistance; (2) energy needs are increased because of infection and pulmonary disease; (3) malnutrition is associated with poor survival; (4) malabsorption is caused by pancreatic exocrine insufficiency, despite enzyme supplementation; (5) altered nutrient absorption is caused by abnormal intestinal transit time; (6) liver disease is present; (7) anorexia and nausea are common as a result of illness, gastroesophageal reflux, delayed gastric emptying, intestinal obstruction, increased work of breathing, and psychosocial factors; (8) there is a wide variation in daily food intake based on the patient's acute health status; and (9) insulin and glucagon secretion are impaired.

In the pancreas, exocrine tissue is replaced by fibrosis and fat; many of the pancreatic islets are destroyed. The remaining islets demonstrate diminished numbers of β-, α-, and pancreatic polypeptide-secreting cells. Secretion of the islet hormones insulin, glucagon, and pancreatic polypeptide is impaired in patients with CF in response to a variety of secretagogues. It is possible that insulin resistance may also play a role in the development of CFRD, especially in the setting of acute infection.

In Denmark, oral glucose tolerance screening of the entire CF population demonstrated no diabetes in patients younger than 10 yr, 12% diabetes in patients aged 10–19 yr, and 48% diabetes in adults aged 20 yr and older. At a Midwestern center where routine annual oral glucose tolerance screening is performed, only about one half of children and one fourth of adults have normal glucose tolerance. Diabetes is seen in 9% of CF children, 26% of adolescents, and 35% of adults aged 20–29 yr. About one third of patients with CFRD have fasting hyperglycemia, and two thirds have CFRD without fasting hyperglycemia. The fasting hyperglycemia is exacerbated chronically, or intermittently with infection or glucocorticoid therapy in 3% of children, 11% of adolescents, and 15% of adults.

When hyperglycemia develops, the accompanying metabolic derangements are usually mild, and if insulin therapy becomes necessary, relatively low doses usually suffice for adequate management. Ketoacidosis is uncommon but may occur with progressive deterioration of islet cell function. Treatment with insulin is as outlined for T1DM, but dietary management may be limited by the constraints of the primary disturbance.

AUTOIMMUNE DISEASES. **Chronic lymphocytic thyroiditis (Hashimoto thyroiditis)** is frequently associated with T1DM in children (see Chapter 567). As many as one in 5 insulin-dependent diabetic patients may have thyroid antibodies in their serum; the prevalence is 2–20 times greater than in control populations. Only a small proportion of these patients, however, acquire clinical hypothyroidism; the interval between diagnosis of diabetes and thyroid disease averages about 5 yr. Periodic palpation of the thyroid gland is indicated in all diabetic children; if the gland feels firm or enlarged, serum measurements of thyroid antibodies and thyroid-stimulating hormone (TSH) should be obtained. A confirmed TSH level of greater than 10 μU/mL indicates existing or incipient thyroid dysfunction that warrants replacement with thyroid hormone. Deceleration in the rate of growth may also be due to thyroid failure and is, in itself, a reason for securing serum measurements of thyroxine and TSH concentrations.

When diabetes and thyroid disease coexist, the possibility of autoimmune adrenal insufficiency should be considered. It may be heralded by decreasing insulin requirements, increasing pigmentation of the skin and buccal mucosa, salt craving, weakness, asthenia and postural hypotension, or even frank addisonian crisis. This syndrome is most unusual in the 1st decade of life, but it may become apparent in the 2nd decade or later.

Celiac disease, formerly known as nontropical sprue, is another autoimmune disorder, which is due to hypersensitivity to dietary gluten, that occurs with significant frequency in children with type 1 DM (see Chapter 335.2). It is estimated that about 7.0% of children with type 1 DM develop celiac disease within the 1st 6 yr from the diagnosis. Additionally, the incidence of celiac disease is significantly higher in children under 4 yr of age and girls. Young children with type 1 DM and celiac disease usually present with gastrointestinal symptoms (abdominal cramping, diarrhea, and gastroesophageal reflux), growth failure due to suboptimal weight gain, and unexplained hypoglycemic reactions due to nutrient malabsorption; adolescents may remain asymptomatic. The diagnosis of celiac disease is considered if serum antiendomysial and/or tissue transglutaminase antibody titers are positive in the presence of normal serum total IgA level. The diagnosis is confirmed on endoscopic evaluation and biopsy of small bowel revealing characteristic atrophy of intestinal villi. Therapy consists of a gluten-free diet, which will alleviate gastrointestinal symptoms and may reduce glycemic excursions.

Circulating antibodies to gastric parietal cells and to intrinsic factor are 2–3 times more common in patients with T1DM than in control subjects. There are good correlations of antibodies to gastric parietal cells with atrophic gastritis and of antibodies to intrinsic factor with malabsorption of vitamin B_{12}. However, megaloblastic anemia is rare in children with T1DM.

A variant of the multiple endocrine deficiency syndrome is characterized by type 1 diabetes—idiopathic intestinal mucosal atrophy with associated inflammation and severe malabsorption, IgA deficiency, and circulating antibodies to multiple endocrine organs including the thyroid, adrenal, pancreas, parathyroid, and gonads. In addition, nondiabetic family members have an increased frequency of vitiligo, Graves disease, and multiple sclerosis as well as low complement levels and antibodies to endocrine tissues.

ENDOCRINOPATHIES. The endocrinopathies listed in Table 590-1 are only rarely encountered as a cause of diabetes in childhood. They may accelerate the manifestations of diabetes in those with inherited or acquired defects in insulin secretion or action.

DRUGS. High-dose oral or parenteral steroid therapy usually results in significant insulin resistance leading to glucose intolerance and overt diabetes. The immunosuppressive agents cyclosporin and tacrolimus are toxic to β cells, causing IDDM in a significant proportion of patients treated with these agents. Their toxicity to pancreatic β cells was a contributing factor in limiting their usefulness to arrest ongoing autoimmune destruction of β cells. Streptozotocin and the rodenticide Vacor also are toxic to β cells, causing diabetes.

GENETIC SYNDROMES ASSOCIATED WITH DIABETES MELLITUS. A number of rare genetic syndromes associated with IDDM or carbohydrate intolerance have been described (see Table 590-1). These syndromes represent a broad spectrum of diseases ranging from premature cellular aging, as in the Werner and Cockayne syndromes (see Chapter 90) to excessive obesity associated with hyperinsulinism, resistance to insulin action, and carbohydrate intolerance, as in the Prader-Willi syndrome (see Chapter 80). Some of these syndromes are characterized by primary disturbances in the insulin receptor or in antibodies to the insulin receptor without any impairment in insulin secretion. Although rare, these syndromes provide unique models to understand the multiple causes of disturbed carbohydrate metabolism from defective insulin secretion or from defective insulin action at the cell receptor or postreceptor level.

Epidemiology, Etiology, Pathology, Classification, and Prevention

Atkinson MA, Eisenbarth GS: Type 1 diabetes: New perspectives on disease pathogenesis and treatment. *Lancet* 2001;358:221–229.

Atkinson MA, Ellis TM: Infants' diets and insulin-dependent diabetes: Evaluating the "cows' milk hypothesis" and a role for anti-bovine serum albumin immunity. *J Am Coll Nutr* 1997;16:334–340.

Casares S, Brumeanu TD: Insights into the pathogenesis of type 1 diabetes: A hint for novel immunospecific therapies. *Curr Molec Med* 2001;1:357–378.

Daneman D: Type 1 diabetes. *Lancet* 2006;367:847–858.

Ferner RE: Drug-induced diabetes. *Baillieres Clin Endocrinol Metab* 1992;6: 849–866.

Hoppu S, Ronkainen MS, Kimpimäki T, et al: Insulin autoantibody isotypes during the prediabetic process in young children with increased genetic risk of type I diabetes. *Pediatr Res* 2004;55:236–242.

Hummel M, Bonifacio E, Schmid S, et al: Brief communication: Early appearance of islet autoantibodies predicts childhood type 1 diabetes in offspring of diabetic parents. *Ann Intern Med* 2004;140:882–886.

Lindley S, Dayan CM, Bishop A, et al: Defective suppressor function in CD4+CD25+ T-cells from patients with type diabetes. *Diabetes* 2005; 54:92–99.

Quinn M, Fleishman A, Rosner B, et al: Characteristics at diagnosis of type 1 diabetes in children younger than 6 years. *J Pediatr* 2006;148:366–371.

Rewers M, Norris J and Dabelea D: Epidemiology of type 1 diabetes mellitus. In Eisenbarth GS (editor): *Immunology of Type 1 Diabetes Mellitus*, 2nd edition. Boston, MA, Kluwer Acadamic Publishing Group, 2004.

Schatz DA, Maclaren NK: Cow's milk and insulin-dependent diabetes mellitus. *JAMA* 1996;276:647–648.

Solimena M, De Camilli P: Coxsackieviruses and diabetes. *Nat Med* 1995; 1:25–26.

Weill J, Vanderbecken S, Froguel P: Understanding the rising incidence of type 2 diabetes in adolescence. *Arch Dis Child* 2004;89:502–505.

Weir GC: A defective β-cell glucose sensor as a cause of diabetes. *N Engl J Med* 1993;328:729–731.

Yoon JW: The role of viruses and environmental factors in the induction of diabetes. *Curr Top Microbiol Immunol* 1990;164:95–123.

Genetics

Faas S, Trucco M: The genes influencing the susceptibility to IDDM in humans. *J Endocrinol Invest* 1994;17:477–495.

Ghosh S, Schork NJ: Genetic analysis of NIDDM: The study of quantitative traits. *Diabetes* 1996;45:1–14.

Johns DR: Mitochondrial DNA and disease. *N Engl J Med* 1995;333: 638–644.

Gillespie K, Bain SC, Barnett AH et al: The rising incidence of childhood type 1 diabetes and reduced contribution of high-risk HLA haplotypes. *Lancet* 2004;364:1699–1700.

Guo D, Li M, Zhang Y, et al: A functional variant of SUMO4, a new IκBα modifier, is associated with type 1 diabetes. *Nat Genet* 2004;36:837–841.

Huopio H, Otonkoski T, Vauhkonen I, et al: A new subtype of autosomal dominant diabetes attributable to a mutation in the gene for sulfonylurea receptor 1. *Lancet* 2003;361:301–307.

Velho G, Froguel P: Genetic, metabolic and clinical characteristics of maturity onset diabetes of the young. *Eur J Endocrinol* 1998;138:233–239.

Zamani M, Cassiman JJ: Reevaluation of the importance of polymorphic HLA class II alleles and amino acids in the susceptibility of individuals of different populations to type 1 diabetes. *Am J Med Genet* 1998;76:183–194.

Diabetic Ketoacidosis

Amiel SA, Alberti KGMM: Inhaled insulin. *Br Med J* 2004;228:1215–1216.

DeWitt DE, Dugdale DC: Using new insulin strategies in the outpatient treatment of diabetes. *JAMA* 2003;289:2265–2269.

Duck SC, Wyatt DT: Factors associated with brain herniation in the treatment of diabetic ketoacidosis. *J Pediatr* 1988;113:10–14.

Dunger DB, Sperling MA, Acerini CL, et al: European Society for Pediatric Endocrinology/Lawson Wilkins Pediatric Endocrine Society consensus statement on diabetic ketoacidosis in children and adolescents. *Pediatrics* 2004;113:e133–e140.

Felner EI, White PC: Improving management of diabetic ketoacidosis in children. *Pediatrics* 2001;108:735–740.

Glaser NS, Wootton-Gorges SL, Marcin JP, et al: Mechanism of cerebral edema in children with diabetic ketoacidosis. *J Pediatr* 2004;145:164–171.

Green SM, Rothrock SG, Ho JD, et al: Failure of adjunctive bicarbonate to improve outcome in severe pediatric diabetic ketoacidosis. *Ann Emerg Med* 1998;31:41–48.

Hirsch IB: Insulin analogues. *N Engl J Med* 2005;352:174–183.

Lawrence SE, Cummings EA, Gaboury I, et al: Population-based study of incidence and risk factors for cerebral edema in pediatric diabetic ketoacidosis. *J Pediatr* 2005;146;688–692.

Medical Letter: Insulin glulisine (Apidra): a new rapid-acting insulin. *Med Lett* 2006;48:33–34.

Okuda Y, Adrogue J, Field JB, et al: Counterproductive effects of sodium bicarbonate in diabetic ketoacidosis. *J Clin Endocrinol Metab* 1996;81: 314–320.

Rosenbloom AL, Hanas R: Diabetic ketoacidosis treatment guidelines. *Clin Pediatr* 1996;261–266.

Tattersall RB: Brittle diabetes revisited: The Third Arnold Bloom Memorial Lecture. *Diabet Med* 1997;14:99–110.

Management of Type 1 Diabetes in Children

Alemzadeh R, Ellis JN, Holzum MK, et al: Beneficial effects of continuous subcutaneous insulin infusion and flexible multiple daily insulin regimen using insulin glargine in type 1 diabetes mellitus. *Pediatrics* 2004;114: e91–e95.

Arslanian S, Ohki Y, Becker DJ, et al: The dawn phenomenon: comparison between normal and insulin-dependent diabetic adolescents. *Pediatr Res* 1992;31:203–206.

Berhe T, Postellon D, Wilson B, Stone R: Feasibility and safety of insulin pump therapy in children aged 2 to 7 years with type I diabetes: a retrospective study. *Pediatrics* 2006;117:2132–2137.

Bolli GB, Gerich JE: The "dawn phenomenon"—A common occurrence in both non-insulin and insulin-dependent diabetes mellitus. *N Engl J Med* 1984;310:746–750.

Bolli GB, Gottesman IS, Campbell PJ, et al: Glucose counter regulation and waning of insulin in the Somogyi phenomenon (posthypoglycemic hyperglycemia). *N Engl J Med* 1984;311:1214–1219.

Litton J, Rice A, Friedman N, et al: Insulin pump therapy in toddlers and preschool children with type 1 diabetes mellitus. *J Pediatr* 2002;141: 490–495.

Maniatis AK, Klingensmith GJ, Slover RH, et al: Continuous subcutaneous insulin infusion therapy in children and adolescents: An option for routine diabetes care. *Pediatrics* 2001;107: 351–356.

Rami B, Schober E: Postprandial glycaemia after regular and lispro insulin in children and adolescents with diabetes. *Eur J Pediatr* 1997;156:838–840.

Regan FM, Dunger DB: Use of new insulins in children. *Arch Dis Child* 2006;91:ep47–ep53.

Rutledge KS, Chase HP, Klingensmith GJ, et al: Effectiveness of postprandial Humalog in toddlers with diabetes. *Pediatrics* 1997;100:968–972.

Weinzimer S, Ahern JH, Doyle EA, et al: Persistence of benefits of continuous subcutaneous insulin infusion in very young children with type 1 diabetes: A follow-up report. *Pediatrics* 2004;114:1601–1605.

Wilson D, Buckingham B, Kunselman EL, et al: A two-center randomized controlled feasibility trial of insulin pump therapy in young children with diabetes. *Diabetes Care* 2005;28;15–19.

Zinman B: The physiologic replacement of insulin. *N Engl J Med* 1989; 321:363–370.

Long-Term Outcome of Childhood Diabetes: Relation of Control to Development of Complications

The absence of a glycemic threshold for the development of long-term complications: The perspective of the Diabetes Control and Complications Trial. *Diabetes* 1996;45:1289–1298.

Bojestig M, Arnqvist HJ, Karlberg BE: Glycemic control and prognosis in type 1 diabetic patients with microalbuminuria. *Diabetes Care* 1996;19: 313–317.

Leslie ND, Sperling MA: Relation of metabolic control to complications in diabetes mellitus. *J Pediatr* 1986;108:491–497.

Nathan DM: Long-term complications of diabetes mellitus. *N Engl J Med* 1993;328:1676–1685.

Reichard P, Nilsson BY, Rosenqvist U: The effect of long-term intensified insulin treatment on the development of microvascular complications of diabetes mellitus. *N Engl J Med* 1993;329:304–309.

Rosenbloom AL: Skeletal and joint manifestations of childhood diabetes. *Pediatr Clin North Am* 1984;31:569–589.

Sandman DD, Shore AC, Tooke JE: Relation of skin capillary pressure in patients with insulin-dependent diabetes mellitus to complications and metabolic control. *N Engl J Med* 1992;327:760–764.

Wang PH: Tight glucose control and diabetic complications. *Lancet* 1993; 342:129.

Diseases and Syndromes Associated with Diabetes

Barrett TG, Bundey SE: Wolfram (DIAMOAD) syndrome. *J Med Genet* 1997;34:838–841.

Jones KL: Non-insulin dependent diabetes in children and adolescents: The therapeutic challenge. *Clin Pediatr* 1998;37:103–110.

Krook A, Brueton L, O'Rahilly S: Homozygous nonsense mutation in the insulin receptor gene in an infant with leprechaunism. *Lancet* 1993;342: 277–278.

Low L, Chernausek SD, Sperling MA: Acromegaloid patients with type-A insulin resistance: Parallel defects in insulin and insulin-like growth factor-I receptors and biological responses in cultured fibroblasts. *J Clin Endocrinol Metab* 1989;69:329–337.

Morrison EY, McKenzie K: The Mauriac syndrome. *West Indian Med J* 1989;38:180–182.

Pinhas-Hamiel O, Dolan LM, Daniels SR: Increased incidence of non-insulin-dependent diabetes mellitus among adolescents. *J Pediatr* 1996;128: 608–615.

Rotig A, Cormier V, Chatelain P, et al: Deletion of mitochondrial DNA in a case of early-onset diabetes mellitus, optic atrophy, and deafness. *J Clin Invest* 1993;91:1095–1098.
Sullivan MM, Denning CR: Diabetic microangiopathy in patients with cystic fibrosis. *Pediatrics* 1989;84:642–647.
Taylor SI, Cama A, Accili D, et al: Mutations in the insulin receptor gene. *Endocr Rev* 1992;13:566–595.
Watkins PB, Whitcomb RW: Hepatic dysfunction associated with troglitazone. *N Engl J Med* 1998;338:916–917.
Winter WE, Maclaren NK, Riley WJ, et al: Congenital pancreatic hypoplasia: A syndrome of exocrine and endocrine pancreatic insufficiency. *J Pediatr* 1986;109:465–468.
Winter WE, Maclaren NK, Riley WJ, et al: Maturity-onset diabetes of youth in black Americans. *N Engl J Med* 1987;316:285–291.

Diabetes of the Newborn

Alcolado JC, Thomas AW: Maternally inherited diabetes mellitus: The role of mitochondrial DNA defects. *Diabet Med* 1995;12:102–108.
Babenko AP, Polak M, Cavé H, et al: Activating mutations in the ABCC8 gene in neonatal diabetes mellitus. *N Engl J Med* 2006;355:456–466.
Geffner ME, Clare-Salzler M, Kaufman DL, et al: Permanent diabetes developing after transient neonatal diabetes. *Lancet* 1993;341:1095.
Gloyn AL, Pearson ER, Antcliff AF, et al: Activating mutations in the gene encoding the ATP-sensitive potassium channel subunit Kir6.2 and permanent neonatal disease. *N Engl J Med* 2004;350:1838–1849.
Metz C, Cavé H, Bertrand AM, et al: Neonatal diabetes mellitus: Chromosomal analysis in transient and permanent cases. *J Pediatr* 2002;141:483–489.
Pagliara AS, Karl IE, Kipnis DB: Transient neonatal diabetes: Delayed maturation of the pancreatic beta cell. *J Pediatr* 1973;82:97–101.
Pearson ER, Flechtner I, Njølstad PR, et al: Switching from insulin to oral sulfonylureas in patients with diabetes due to Kir6.2 mutations. *N Engl J Med* 2006;355:467–477.
von Muhlendahl KR, Herkenhoff H: Long-term course of neonatal diabetes. *N Engl J Med* 1995;333:704–708.

Hypoglycemia and Diabetes

Amiel SA, Tamborlane WV, Simonson DC, et al: Defective glucose counter regulation after strict glycemic control of insulin-dependent diabetes mellitus. *N Engl J Med* 1987;316:1376–1383.
Bolli GB, Fanelli CG: Unawareness of hypoglycemia. *N Engl J Med* 1995; 333:1771–1772.
Cryer PE, Fisher JN, Shamoon H: Hypoglycemia. *Diabetes Care* 1994;17: 734–755.
Diabetes Control and Complications Trial Research Group: Hypoglycemia in the diabetes control and complications trial. *Diabetes* 1997;46:271–286.
Gschwend S, Ryan C, Atchinson J, et al: Effects of acute hyperglycemia on mental efficiency and counterregulatory hormones in adolescents with insulin-dependent diabetes mellitus. *J Pediatr* 1995;126:178–184.
McCrimmon RJ, Gold AE, Deary IJ, et al: Symptoms of hypoglycemia in children with IDDM. *Diabetes Care* 1995;18:858–861.
Porter PA, Keating B, Byrne G, et al: Incidence and predictive criteria of nocturnal hypoglycemia in young children with insulin-dependent diabetes mellitus. *J Pediatr* 1997;130:366–372.
Silverstein JH, Gordon G, Pollock BH, et al: Long-term glycemic control influences the onset of limited joint mobility in type I diabetes. *J Pediatr* 1998;132:944–947.
Wayne EA, Dean HJ, Booth F, et al: Focal neurologic deficits associated with hypoglycemia in children with diabetes. *J Pediatr* 1990;117:575–577.

Pancreas and Islet Transplantation

Alejandro R, Lehmann R, Ricordi C, et al: Long-term function (6 years) of islet allografts in type 1 diabetes. *Diabetes* 1997;46:1983–1989.
Hering BJ, Kandaswamy R, Ansite JD, et al: Single-donor, marginal-dose islet transplantation in patients with type 1 diabetes. *JAMA* 2005;293: 830–835.
Larsen JL, Stratta RJ: Consequences of pancreas transplantation. *J Investig Med* 1994;42:622–631.
Mitanchez D, Doiron B, Chen R, et al: Glucose-stimulated genes and prospects of gene therapy for type 1 diabetes. *Endocr Rev* 1997;18:520–540.
Robertson RP: Islet transplantation as a treatment for diabetes—a work in progress. *N Engl J Med* 2004;350:694–705.
Ryan EA, Lakey JR, Paty BW, et al: Successful islet transplantation: Continued insulin reserve provides long-term glycemic control. *Diabetes* 2002;51:2148–2157.
Shapiro AMJ, Ricordi C, Hering BJ, et al: International trial of the edmonton protocol for islet transplantation. *N Engl J Med* 2006;355:1318–1330.

Part XXVI ▪ The Nervous System

Chapter 591 ▪ Neurologic Evaluation*

Robert H. A. Haslam

The neurologic evaluation seeks to assess the integrity of the central nervous system (CNS) by means of a thorough history, physical examination, and ancillary studies to determine the location (and causes) of abnormal function.

HISTORY

The history is the most important component of the evaluation of a child with a suspected neurologic problem. The history should carefully document in chronological order the onset of symptoms and a thorough description of their frequency, duration, and associated characteristics. Most children beyond the age of 3–4 yr are capable of contributing to their history, particularly about facts relating to the present illness. It is essential to obtain a comprehensive review of the function and interaction of all organ systems, because abnormalities of the CNS may **initially** present with clinical manifestations (vomiting, pain, constipation, urinary tract disorders) implicating other systems. A detailed history might suggest that the child's vomiting is due to increased intracranial pressure (ICP), that the pain behind the eye may be caused by migraine headaches or multiple sclerosis, and that the constipation and urinary dribbling may be due to a spinal cord tumor.

It is important to start with a concise description of the chief complaint within its developmental context. Parents may be concerned that their child cannot talk. The seriousness of this problem depends on many factors, including the age of the patient, the normal range of language development for age, the parent-child interaction, functioning of the auditory system, and the intellectual level of the child. A comprehensive understanding of developmental milestones is essential in order to ascertain the relative importance of the parents' observations (see Chapters 7–15).

After the chief complaint and history of present illness are elicited, a review of the pregnancy, labor, and delivery is indicated, particularly if a congenital disorder is suspected (see Chapters 93–109). Was the mother exposed to a viral illness during the pregnancy, and what is the mother's rubella, HIV, and syphilis immune status? Were there additional concerns such as pregnancy-induced hypertension or gestational diabetes? The history should determine the number and results of ultrasound or amniocentesis studies. The review should also include information about the quantity of cigarette and alcohol consumption, toxin exposure, and the use of drugs (legal, illicit, and herbal) known to have adverse effects on fetal development. Decreased or absent fetal activity may be associated with a congenital myopathy and other neuromuscular disorders. **Seizures** in utero occasionally occur and suggest placental insufficiency or rare inborn errors of metabolism, such as pyridoxine dependence. Seizure activity in utero is difficult to evaluate, particularly in a primigravida. The fact that fetal seizures occurred during pregnancy is often realized retrospectively after the mother has had an opportunity to observe her infant's seizures. The mother's postpartum health may provide a clue to the cause of her infant's neurologic problem: maternal fever, drug dependence, cervical or vaginal vesicles (herpes simplex), hemorrhage, petechiae, or the presence of an abnormal placenta.

The **history** of the birthweight, length, and head circumference is particularly important. It may be necessary to obtain the infant's hospital records to determine the head circumference, particularly if congenital microcephaly is a consideration, and the Apgar score for suspected asphyxia. Several indicators of neurologic dysfunction during the newborn period can reliably be obtained from the history. The fact that a full-term infant was **unable to breathe spontaneously** and required ventilatory assistance may suggest a CNS abnormality. Poor, uncoordinated sucking or a full-term infant who requires an inordinate amount of time to feed suggests a neurologic disorder. If such an infant requires gavage feeding, there is almost certainly a significant problem. All of the aforementioned abnormalities may be common to a premature infant, particularly a very low birthweight infant, and do not necessarily signify a poor neurologic outcome. Additional important information in the newborn period includes the presence of **jaundice**, its degree, and management. The physician should also attempt to assess from the history the activity, sleep patterns, the nature of the cry, and the general well-being of the newborn infant.

The most important component of a neurologic history is a child's **developmental assessment** (see Chapters 6 and 15). Careful evaluation of a child's language, social skills, and motor skills (fine and gross motor) is required to distinguish global developmental delay versus delay in a particular subset of development (isolated motor delay). An abnormality in development from birth suggests an intrauterine or perinatal cause. Slowing of the rate of acquisition of skills later in infancy or childhood may imply an acquired abnormality of the nervous system. A loss of skills **(regression)** over time strongly suggests an underlying **degenerative disease** of the CNS such as an inborn error of metabolism. The ability of parents to recall the precise timing of their children's developmental milestones is extremely variable. Some are very reliably able to do so, whereas others are uncertain, particularly if the patient in question has a significant neurodevelopmental problem. Table 591-1 provides some guidelines regarding the upper range of normal skills that are usually recalled by the parents and that, if not present, should alert the physician. A comprehensive review of developmental screening tests and their interpretation are listed in Chapter 15. It is often helpful to request photographs taken at an earlier age or to review the family's baby book, because milestones for a child may have been dutifully recorded. Parents (particularly mothers) are usually aware when their children have a developmental problem, and the physician should show appropriate concern. The history should also inquire about the use of alternative therapies as many parents are reluctant to bring their use to the physician's attention.

Family history is extremely important in the neurologic evaluation of a child. Parents may be unwilling to discuss family members with debilitating neurologic disorders or may be unaware of them, particularly if they are institutionalized. Most parents are extremely cooperative in securing medical information about family members, particularly if it may have relevance for their child. The history should document the ages and

*I am grateful to child neurology fellows Drs. Michael Esser, Hannah Glass, and Adam Kirton for their review and helpful comments of Chapter 591.

TABLE 591-1. Screening Scheme for Developmental Delay: Upper Range

AGE (MO)	GROSS MOTOR	FINE MOTOR	SOCIAL SKILLS	LANGUAGE
3	Supports weight on forearms	Opens hands spontaneously	Smiles appropriately	Coos, laughs
6	Sits momentarily	Transfers objects	Shows likes and dislikes	Babbles
9	Pulls to stand	Pincer grasp	Plays pat-a-cake, peek-a-boo	Imitates sounds
12	Walks with one hand held	Releases an object on command	Comes when called	1–2 meaningful words
18	Walks upstairs with assistance	Feeds from a spoon	Mimics actions of others	At least 6 words
24	Runs	Builds a tower of 6 blocks	Plays with others	2–3 word sentences

well-being of all close relatives and the presence of neurologic disease, including epilepsy, migraine, cerebrovascular accidents, developmental delay, and inherited disorders. The sex and age at death of miscarriages or liveborn siblings, including the results of postmortem examinations, should be obtained because this information may have a direct bearing on the patient's condition. It should also be determined whether the parents are related, because the incidence of metabolic and degenerative disorders affecting the CNS is increased significantly in children of **consanguineous** marriages.

An attempt should be made to learn about the patient as a person. The child's performance in school, both academically and socially, may shed light on the diagnosis, particularly if there has been an abrupt change. A good way to get at this from the school-aged child's perspective is to have the child name his or her "best friends." Any child that is unable to name at least two or three playmates may have abnormal social development. This is especially problematic when there has been a significant change in academic performance. A description of the child's personality before and after the onset of symptoms may provide a clue to the cause of the disorder. Discussions with the daycare worker or kindergarten/schoolteacher may provide useful information that is not available from the parent.

NEUROLOGIC EXAMINATION

Neurologic examination of a child begins at the outset of the interview. **Observation** during interaction with the parents, while playing, or during the time when little attention is directed to the child can provide useful information (see Chapters 6 and 15). It may be obvious that the child has characteristic facies, an unusual posture, or an abnormality of motor function manifested by a gait disturbance or hemiparesis. Much can be learned from observing the child's **behavior** during the interview. A normally inquisitive child or toddler may play independently but soon wishes to become involved with the interview process. A child with an attention disorder may display inappropriate behaviors in the examining room, whereas a neurologically abnormal child may appear lethargic or disinterested or may show complete lack of awareness of the environment. The degree of interaction between the parent and the child should be noted. Because the neurologic examination of a newborn or premature infant requires a somewhat modified approach from that of an older child, the differences in the examination are highlighted for both age groups (see also Chapters 7 and 94).

The **examination** should be conducted in a setting that is nonthreatening and enjoyable for a child. The more it seems like a game, the greater will be the degree of cooperation. Children may be most comfortable on a parent's lap or interacting on the floor of the examination room. It is unwise to force a child to sit on the examining table or to demand that all clothes be removed at the beginning of the examination. Cooperation is essential for a comprehensive neurologic examination; as a child's confidence increases, so too does the level of participation. Several methods may be used to assess **mental status, cognitive function,** and the level of **alertness,** depending on the age of the child. Simple puzzles may be useful. A child's ability to tell a story or to draw a picture is often a powerful method for assessing cognitive function or for determining developmental level. The manner in which a child plays with toys or explores the function of a new object or game is an excellent indicator of intellectual curiosity. The level of alertness of a newborn infant depends on many factors, including the time of the last feeding, the room temperature, and the gestational age. Sequential assessment of the infant is valuable in determining changes in neurologic function. Premature infants of <28 wk of gestation do not consistently demonstrate periods of alertness, whereas gentle physical stimulation applied to a slightly older infant arouses the child from sleep and results in a brief period of alertness. Sleep and waking patterns are well developed at term. Note should also be made of particular **odors/smells** noted by parents or the examiner, as they may point to certain metabolic disorders (the "musty" smell of phenylketonuria or the "sweaty feet" smell of isovaleric academia). It is important to also determine if these smells are persistent or transient, occurring only with illnesses.

The examiner must take advantage of the opportunities provided by the patient; if the circumstances permit, evaluation of muscle power and tone or cerebellar function might precede the cranial nerve examination. If a hearing assessment is considered to be important from the historical information, attention should be directed initially to that portion of the examination so that full cooperation can be achieved before the interest and curiosity of the child are lost.

THE HEAD. The size and shape of the head should be documented carefully. A tower-head, or oxycephalic skull, suggests premature closure of sutures and is associated with various forms of inherited craniosynostosis (see Chapter 592.12). A broad forehead may indicate hydrocephalus, and a small head microcephaly. The observation of a square or a box-shaped skull should suggest chronic subdural hematomas because the long-standing presence of fluid in the subdural space causes enlargement of the middle fossa. Inspection of the scalp should include observation of the venous pattern, because increased ICP and thrombosis of the superior sagittal sinus can produce marked venous distention. Note should also be made of any cutaneous abnormalities such as cutis aplasia or abnormal hair whorls as they may suggest an underlying genetic disorder. Furthermore, a gross evaluation of anthropomorphic aspects of the face (eyes, ears, nose, lips, dentition, palate) should also be made as abnormalities may indicate a neurodevelopmental aberration.

An infant has two **fontanels** at birth: a diamond-shaped open anterior fontanel that is situated in the midline at the junction of the coronal and sagittal sutures, and a posterior fontanel between the intersection of the occipital and parietal bones that may be closed at birth or, at the most, admit the tip of a finger. The posterior fontanel is usually closed and nonpalpable after the 1st 6–8 wk of life; its persistence suggests underlying hydrocephalus or the possibility of congenital hypothyroidism. The anterior fontanel varies greatly in size, but the usual measurement approximates 2 by 2 cm. The average time of closure is 18 mo, but the fontanel may normally close as early as 9 mo. A very small or absent anterior fontanel at birth may indicate **premature fusion** of the sutures or **microcephaly,** whereas a very large fontanel could signify a variety of problems. The fontanel is normally slightly depressed and pulsatile and is best evaluated when an infant is held upright while asleep or feeding. A bulging fontanel is a reliable indicator of increased ICP, but vigorous crying can cause a protuberant fontanel in a normal infant.

Palpation of a newborn's skull characteristically shows overriding of the cranial sutures for the first several days of life as a result of the pressures exerted on the skull during its descent through the pelvis. Marked overriding of the sutures beyond a few days is cause for alarm and suggests the possibility of an underlying abnormality of the brain. Palpation may uncover cranial defects or **craniotabes,** a peculiar softening of the parietal bone so that gentle pressure produces a sensation similar to indenting a Ping-Pong ball. Craniotabes is often associated with prematurity.

Auscultation of the skull is an important adjunct to a neurologic examination. **Cranial bruits** are most prominent over the anterior fontanel, temporal region, or the orbits and are best heard through the diaphragm of the stethoscope. Soft symmetric bruits may be discovered in normal children younger than 4 yr or in association with a febrile illness. Arteriovenous malformations of the middle cerebral artery or vein of Galen may produce a loud bruit. Murmurs arising from the heart or great vessels may be transmitted to the cranium. A child with severe anemia is often found to have a skull bruit that disappears when the anemia is corrected. Increased ICP resulting from hydrocephalus, tumor, subdural effusions, or purulent meningitis may produce significant intracranial bruits. Demonstration of a loud or localized bruit is usually significant and warrants further investigation.

Correct **measurement of the head circumference** is important. It should be performed on every patient, at every visit, and should be recorded on a suitable head growth chart. A nondistensible plastic measuring tape should be used. The tape is placed over the midforehead and is extended circumferentially to include the most prominent portion of the occiput so that the greatest volume of the cranium is measured. The head circumferences of the parents and siblings should also be recorded if the patient is found to have an abnormal skull. Errors in the accurate measurement of a newborn skull are frequent and result from scalp edema, overriding of the sutures, intravenous fluid infiltration, and the presence of a cephalohematoma. The average rate of head growth in a healthy premature infant is 0.5 cm in the 1st 2 wk, 0.75 cm during the 3rd wk, and 1.0 cm in the 4th wk and thereafter until the 40th wk of development. The head circumference of a term infant at birth measures 34–35 cm, 44 cm by 6 mo, and 47 cm by 1 yr of age (see Chapters 7 and 8).

CRANIAL NERVES

Olfactory Nerve (1). **Anosmia,** loss of smell, is most commonly found in association with an upper respiratory tract infection in children and is therefore a transient abnormality. A fracture of the base of the skull and cribriform plate as well as a frontal lobe tumor may also produce anosmia. Occasionally, a child who recovers from purulent meningitis or in whom hydrocephalus develops has a diminished sense of smell. Rarely, anosmia is congenital. Although not a routine component of the examination, smell can be tested reliably as early as the 32nd wk of gestation. Care should be taken to use appropriate stimuli, such as coffee, peppermint, and other substances that are familiar to the child; strongly aromatic substances should be avoided.

Optic Nerve (2). Examination of the optic disc and retina is an important component of the neurologic examination. To visualize a good portion of the retina, dilation of the pupil is necessary. One drop of a combination of 1% cyclopentolate hydrochloride, 2.5% phenylephrine hydrochloride, and 1% tropicamide repeated three times at 15 min intervals effectively produces mydriasis. Mydriatics should not be used if a patient's pupil reaction is necessary to follow the level of consciousness or if a cataract is present. Examination of an infant's retina is enhanced by providing a nipple or soother and by placing the head on one side. The physician gently strokes the patient to maintain arousal, while examining the closest eye. An older child should be placed in the parent's lap and should be distracted by bright objects or toys that are presented during the ophthalmologic examination. The color of the optic nerve is salmon-pink in a child but is gray-white in the newborn, particularly in a blond infant. This normal finding may cause confusion and may lead to the improper diagnosis of optic atrophy.

Papilledema refers to swelling of the optic disc due to ICP. It rarely occurs in infancy because the skull sutures are capable of separating to accommodate the expanding brain. Papilledema in an older child may be recognized by the following progressive changes in the optic nerve and surrounding retina (Fig. 591-1):

1. The optic nerve becomes hyperemic.
2. The small capillaries that normally cross the optic nerve are no longer visualized as they become constricted.
3. The larger veins become dilated, and the accompanying arterioles become constricted.
4. The border of the optic nerve becomes indistinct from the surrounding retina, particularly along the temporal edge.
5. Subhyaloid, flame-shaped hemorrhages appear in the retina surrounding the optic nerve.
6. In some cases, a macular star develops owing to retinal edema in the region of the macula. Papilledema must be differentiated from **papillitis** due to inflammation of the optic nerve (optic neuritis). Visual acuity and color vision remain intact in acute papilledema, whereas there is a loss of vision in optic neuritis, but the blind spot is increased in both.

Retinal hemorrhages occur in 30–40% of all full-term newborn infants. The hemorrhages are more common after vaginal delivery than after cesarean section and are not associated with birth injury or with neurologic complications. They disappear spontaneously by 1–2 wk of age.

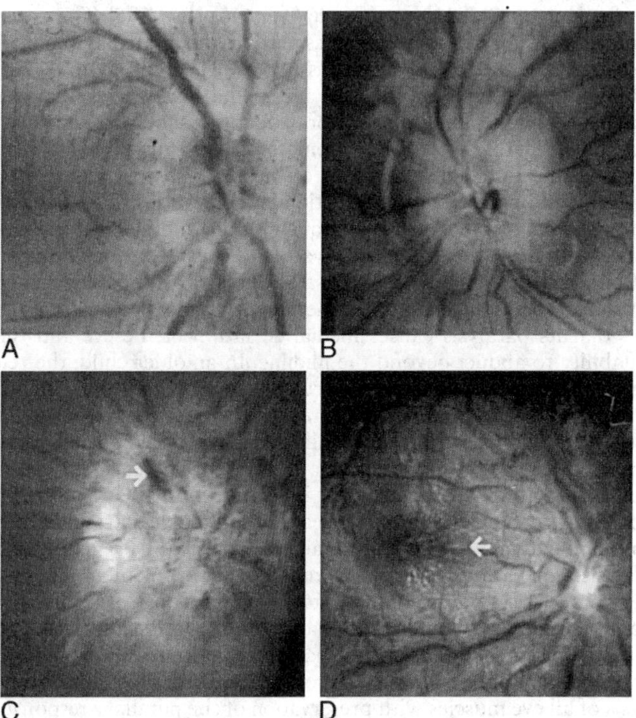

Figure 591-1. *A,* Mild papilledema. Blurred disc margins and venous congestion. *B,* Moderate papilledema. Disc edematous and raised. Vessels buried within substance of nerve tissue. *C,* Severe papilledema. Hemorrhages are evident within disc *(arrow),* and there are microinfarcts (soft exudates) in the nerve fiber layer. *D,* Macular star *(arrow)* with edema residues distributed within the Henle layer of the macula.

VISION (SEE ALSO PART XXVIII). Normal 28 wk old premature infants blink when a bright light is directed to the eyes and, by 32 wk, infants maintain eye closure until the light source is removed. At 37 wk, normal premature infants turn the head and the eyes to a soft light and, by term, visual fixation and the ability to follow a brilliant target are present. During a period of alertness, **optokinetic nystagmus** can be demonstrated in a newborn. **Visual acuity** in term infants approximates 20/150 and reaches the adult level of 20/20 by about 6 mo of age. Children who are too young to read the standard letters on the Snellen Eye Chart may learn the "E game" by pointing a finger in the direction that the E is oriented. Children as young as 2½ or 3 yr of age with normal vision identify the objects on the Allen Chart at a distance of 15–20 ft. **Visual fields** are tested in an infant by advancing a brightly colored (red) object from behind the child's head through the peripheral field of vision and noting when the child first looks at the object. Suspension of the object by a string prevents the infant from focusing on the examiner's hand and arm. The examiner should be certain that the object rather than a sound produces the visual response.

The **pupil** is difficult to examine in premature infants owing to the poorly pigmented iris and the resistance to lid opening. The pupil reacts to light by the 29th–32nd wk of gestation. The equality of the pupils, their size, and their reaction to light may be affected by drugs, a space-occupying brain lesion, metabolic disorders, and abnormalities of the midbrain and optic nerves. In evaluating the pupil, it is also important to note the existence of heterochromia or brushfield spots in the iris.

Horner syndrome is characterized by miosis, ptosis, enophthalmos, and ipsilateral anhidrosis of the face. It may be congenital or may result from a lesion involving the sympathetic nervous system in the brainstem, cervical spinal cord, or the sympathetic plexus in juxtaposition to the carotid artery. Localization of the lesion within the sympathetic nervous system is aided by the pupillary response to a series of topical drugs, including cocaine, epinephrine, hydroxyamphetamine, and phenylephrine.

Oculomotor (3), Trochlear (4), and Abducens Nerves (6). The eye is moved by the extraocular muscles that are innervated by the oculomotor, trochlear, and abducens nerves. The oculomotor nerve innervates the superior, inferior, and medial rectus as well as the inferior oblique and the levator palpebrae superioris muscles. Complete **paralysis of the oculomotor** nerve causes ptosis, dilation of the pupil, displacement of the eye outward and downward, and impairment of adduction and elevation. The **trochlear nerve** supplies the superior oblique muscle, and isolated paralysis causes the eye to deviate upward and outward, often with an associated head tilt to compensate for vertical displacement of images. The **abducens nerve** innervates the lateral rectus muscle so that its paralysis causes medial deviation of the eye and the inability to abduct beyond the midline. In an older child, the **red glass test** is used to assess extraocular palsies. A red glass is placed over one eye, and the patient is requested to follow a white light in all fields of direction. The child sees only one red/white light in the direction of normal muscle function but notes a separation of the red and white images that is greatest in the plane of action of the affected muscle. **Internuclear ophthalmoplegia** results from a lesion in the medial longitudinal fasciculus of the brainstem and consists of paralysis of medial rectus function of the adducting eye and nystagmus confined to the abducting eye. **Internal ophthalmoplegia** refers to a dilated pupil that is unreactive to light and accommodation but has normal extraocular function, and **external ophthalmoplegia** is associated with ptosis and paralysis of all eye muscles with preservation of the pupillary response. **Nystagmus** is an involuntary rapid movement of the eye that may be horizontal, vertical, rotatory, pendular, or mixed. Jerk nystagmus is used to describe a fast and slow phase and is usually normal when only present at the end-point of lateral gaze. As a general rule, horizontal nystagmus occurs with an abnormality of the peripheral labyrinth or with a lesion of the vestibular system in the brainstem or cerebellum and as a consequence of drugs, particularly phenytoin. Vertical nystagmus is indicative of brainstem dysfunction or a structural abnormality.

Complete ocular movement may be demonstrated as early as 25 wk of gestation using the **doll's eye maneuver.** This technique is used to examine horizontal and vertical eye movements in an infant or an uncooperative or comatose patient. If the head is suddenly turned to the right, the eyes look to the left in a symmetric fashion. Horizontal eye movements in the opposite direction may then be evaluated if the head is turned to the left. Vertical movements may be assessed in a similar fashion by rapid flexion and extension of the head. Normal infants and children follow a toy or interesting object in all directions. The rapid on-off occlusion ("blinking light") of a light source is a reliable test for visual following in uncooperative children. The examiner observes the completeness and flow of the eye movements and determines the presence or absence and the direction of nystagmus, diplopia, opsoclonus (chaotic, jerky oscillations of the eyes, often associated with neuroblastoma or viral infections), ocular bobbing (associated with pontine lesions), or other abnormal eye positions. Premature infants tend to have slightly disconjugate eyes at rest, with one eye horizontally displaced from the other by 1 or 2 mm. Skew deviation of the eyes (vertical displacement) is always abnormal and requires investigation. Strabismus is discussed in Chapter 622.

Trigeminal Nerve (5). The sensory distribution of the face is divided into three areas: the ophthalmic area, the maxillary area, and the mandibular area. Each region may be tested by light touch and by pinprick, and may be compared with the opposite side. The corneal response is elicited by touching the cornea with a small pledget of cotton and by observing the eye closure response. Trigeminal nerve function in premature infants is best documented by facial grimacing from a pinprick (away from the eye) or by stimulating the nostril with a cotton tip. An absent reflex may be due to a sensory defect (trigeminal nerve) or a motor deficit (facial nerve). Motor function may be tested by examination of the masseters, pterygoid, and temporalis muscles during mastication as well as by evaluation of the jaw jerk.

Facial Nerve (7). Decreased voluntary movement of the lower face with flattening of the nasolabial angle on the ipsilateral side indicates an upper motor neuron or supranuclear corticospinal lesion. A lower motor neuron lesion tends to involve upper and lower facial muscles equally. Facial nerve paralysis may be congenital or secondary to trauma, infection (Lyme disease), intracranial tumor, leukemia, histiocytosis, granulomatous diseases, hypertension, toxins, or myasthenia gravis. Taste for the anterior two thirds of the tongue may be tested in a cooperative child by placing a solution of saline or glucose on one side of the extended tongue. Normal children can identify the substance with little difficulty.

Auditory Nerve (8). Screening for hearing loss is an important component of the neurologic examination because a hearing deficit is not readily recognized by parents (see Chapter 636). Normal newborns pause briefly during sucking when a bell is presented, but after several stimuli the pauses cease as habituation occurs. Neurologically abnormal infants do not habituate. Normal hearing infants turn their head toward a bell, rattle, or crumpled paper and by 3 mo of age look in the direction of the sound source. Normally intelligent, hearing-impaired toddlers are visually alert and respond appropriately to physical stimuli. Temper tantrums and abnormal speech are common symptoms in a hearing-impaired child. Audiometry or brainstem-evoked potential testing is mandatory for any child suspected of having a hearing loss (see Chapter 636). The risk factors that indicate a need for testing during the 1st few months of life include a family history of deafness, prematurity, severe asphyxia, use of ototoxic drugs in the newborn period, hyperbilirubinemia, congenital anomalies of the head or neck, bacterial meningitis, and congenital infections due to rubella, toxoplasmosis, herpes, and cytomegalovirus. Parental concern is often a reliable indicator of hearing impairment and warrants a formal hearing assessment.

Vestibular function may be evaluated by the **caloric test.** Approximately 5 mL of ice water is delivered by syringe into the external auditory canal with the patient's head elevated 30 degrees from the horizontal position. In obtunded or comatose patients with an intact brainstem, there is prompt deviation of the eyes to the side of the stimulus. A much smaller quantity of ice water (0.5 mL) is used in alert, awake subjects. In normal subjects, introduction of ice water produces nystagmus with the quick component in the opposite direction to the stimulated labyrinth. No response implies severe dysfunction of the brainstem and medial longitudinal fasciculus. If the otoscopic examination reveals a ruptured tympanic membrane, the test should not be performed in that ear.

Glossopharyngeal Nerve (9). This nerve supplies innervation to the stylopharyngeus muscle. An isolated lesion of the 9th cranial nerve is rare. The nerve is tested by observing the gag response to tactile stimulation of the posterior pharyngeal wall. Taste for the posterior one third of the tongue is provided by the sensory portion of the glossopharyngeal nerve.

Vagus Never (10). A unilateral injury of the vagus nerve produces weakness and asymmetry of the ipsilateral soft palate and a hoarse voice due to paralysis of a vocal cord. Bilateral lesions may produce respiratory distress as a result of vocal cord paralysis as well as nasal regurgitation of fluids, pooling of secretions, and an immobile, low-lying soft palate. Isolated lesions of the vagus nerve may occur postoperatively after a thoracotomy due to separation of the recurrent laryngeal nerve, and these lesions are common during the neonatal period in children with the type II Chiari malformation. If a lesion involving the vagus nerve is suspected, visualization of the vocal cords is necessary. To test for a cough in a neonate/infant, the examiner applies gentle pressure to the trachea at the suprasternal notch.

Accessory Nerve (11). Paralysis and atrophy of the sternomastoid and trapezius muscles result from lesions of the accessory nerve. The sternomastoid muscle has two origins, sternal and clavicular, and is tested by forceful rotation of the head and neck against the examiner's hand. Motor neuron disease, myotonic dystrophy, and myasthenia gravis are the most common conditions producing weakness and atrophy of these muscles.

Hypoglossal Nerve (12). The hypoglossal nerve innervates the tongue. Examination of the tongue includes an assessment of its motility, size, and shape and the presence of atrophy or fasciculations. Malfunction of the hypoglossal nucleus or nerve produces wasting, weakness, and fasciculations of the tongue. If the injury is bilateral, tongue protrusion is not possible and dysphagia may be present. Werdnig-Hoffmann disease (infantile spinal muscular atrophy, or SMA type 1) and congenital anomalies in the region of the foramen magnum are the principal causes of hypoglossal nerve involvement.

MOTOR EXAMINATION. The motor examination includes an assessment of the integrity of the musculoskeletal system and a search for abnormal movements that may indicate a disorder of the peripheral nervous system or the CNS. The components of the motor examination include testing of strength (power), muscle bulk, tone, posture, locomotion and motility, deep tendon reflexes, and the presence of primitive reflexes, when applicable.

Strength. Testing of muscle strength is relatively straightforward in cooperative children. It may begin by requesting that the child squeeze the examiner's fingers, flex and extend the wrist and elbow, and adduct and abduct the shoulder against resistance. Shoulder girdle muscle strength may be evaluated in a newborn or infant by supporting the child by the axillae. Patients with weakness are unable to support body weight and slip through the examiner's hands. Distal power can be tested in an infant by evaluating the palmar grasp; a child with weakness does not adequately grasp or shows abnormalities in the manipulation of objects. A normal 3 to 4 yr old child cooperates in testing extension or flexion of the muscles of the foot, knee, and hip. Examination of the pelvic girdle and proximal lower extremity muscles is also performed by observing the child climb steps or stand up from a prone position. Weakness in these muscles causes the child to use the hands to "climb up" the legs in order to assume an upright position, a maneuver called *Gowers sign* (Fig. 591-2). Infants with diminished power in the lower extremities tend to have decreased spontaneous activity in the legs and refuse to support body weight when suspended by the axillae. It is important not only to assess individual muscle groups, but also to carefully compare muscle power between the upper and lower extremities as well as the opposite extremities. **Muscle power** in a cooperative child is graded on a scale of 0–5 as follows: 0 = no contraction; 1 = flicker or trace of contraction; 2 = active movement, with gravity eliminated; 3 = active movement against gravity; 4 = active movement against gravity and resistance; 5 = normal power. Examination of muscle power should include the muscles of respiration. Observation of the action of the intercostal muscles, diaphragmatic movement, and the use of accessory muscles of respiration should be documented. Evaluation of power should include an assessment of muscle bulk and nutrition. Weakness may be associated with muscle atrophy and fasciculations. Because most infants have excess body fat, muscle fasciculations and atrophy are most commonly demonstrated in the denervated tongue in this age group.

Tone. Muscle tone is tested by assessing the degree of resistance when an individual joint is moved passively. Tone undergoes considerable change and assumes different forms depending on age. A premature or newborn infant is relatively hypotonic compared with a child. Tone in this age group is tested by various maneuvers (see Chapters 94 and 97). When the upper extremity of a normal term infant is pulled gently across the chest, the elbow normally does not quite reach the midsternum (**scarf sign**). The elbow of a hypotonic infant extends beyond the midline with ease. Measurement of the popliteal angle is a useful method to document tone in the legs of a newborn. The examiner flexes the child's lower extremity on the abdomen and extends the knee. Normal term infants allow extension of the knee to ≈80 degrees. Similarly, tone can be evaluated by flexing the hip and knee to 90 degrees and then internally rotating the leg. In normal infants, the heel should not pass the umbilicus. Abnormalities of tone consist of spasticity, rigidity, and hypotonia.

Spasticity is characterized by an initial resistance to passive movement, followed by a sudden release called the **clasp-knife** phenomenon. Spasticity is most apparent in the upper extremity flexors and lower extremity extensor muscles. It is associated with brisk tendon reflexes and an extensor plantar reflex, clonus, diminished active movements, and disuse atrophy. **Clonus** may be demonstrated in the lower extremity by sudden dorsiflexion of the foot with the knee partially flexed. Whereas sustained clonus is always abnormal, 5–10 beats in a newborn is a normal finding unless the clonus is asymmetric. Spasticity results from a lesion that involves upper motor neuron tracts and may be unilateral or bilateral. **Rigidity,** the result of a basal ganglia lesion, is characterized by constant resistance to passive movement of both extensor and flexor muscles. As the extremity is undergoing passive movement, a typical **cogwheel** (caused by superimposition of an extrapyramidal tremor on rigidity) sensation may be evident. The rigidity persists with repetitive passive extension and flexion of a joint and does not give way or release, such as with spasticity. Children with spastic lower extremities drag the legs while crawling (commando style) or walk on tiptoes. Patients with marked spasticity or rigidity develop a posture of **opisthotonos,** in which the head and the heels are bent backward and the body bowed forward (Fig. 591-3). **Decerebrate** rigidity is characterized by marked extension of the extremities resulting from dysfunction or injury to the brainstem at the level of the superior colliculi. **Hypotonia** refers to abnormally diminished

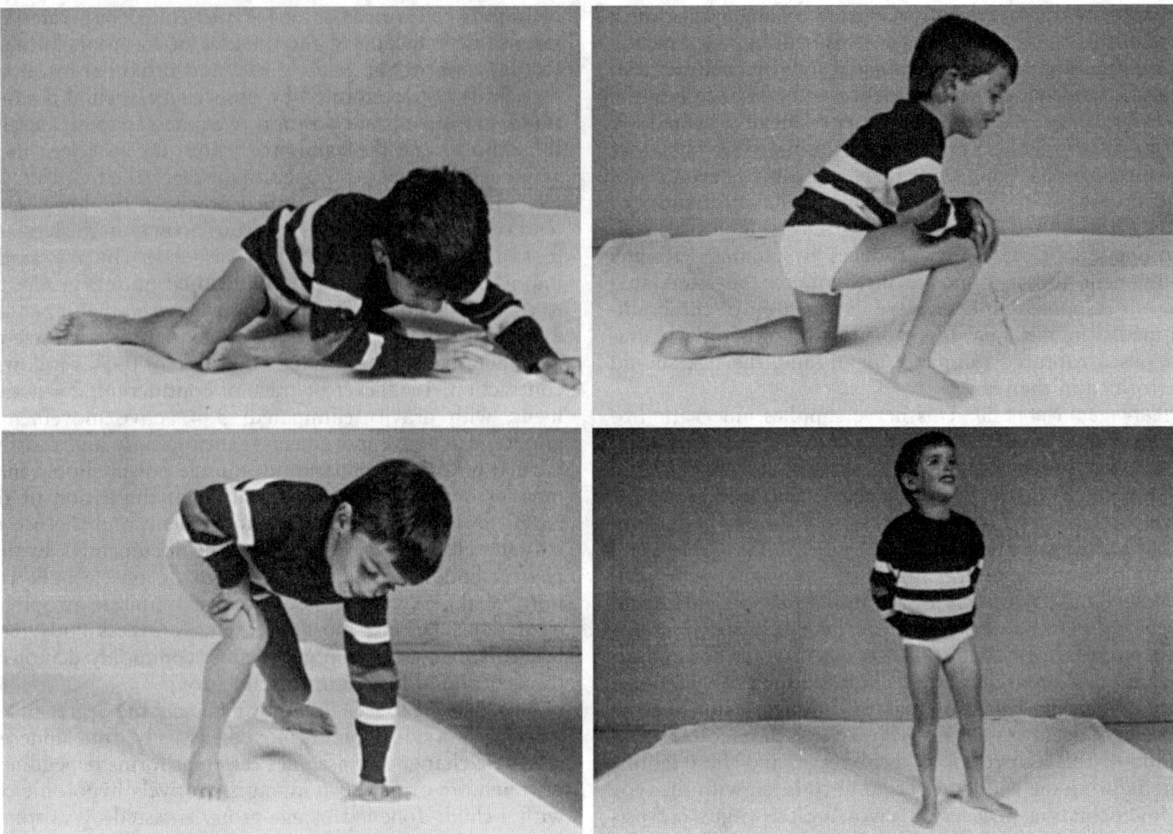

Figure 591-2. Gowers sign. A boy with hip girdle weakness due to Duchenne muscular dystrophy.

tone and is the most common abnormality of tone in neurologically compromised premature or full-term neonates. Demonstration of hypotonia may reflect pathology of the cerebral hemispheres, cerebellum, spinal cord, anterior horn cell, peripheral nerve, myoneural junction, or muscle. An unusual position or posture in an infant is a reflection of abnormal tone. A hypotonic infant is **floppy** and may have difficulty in maintaining head support or a straight back while sitting. Such infants may assume a frog-leg posture in the supine position and have significant head lag during the traction response. Premature infants of 28 wk of gestation tend to extend all extremities at rest, but by 32 wk there is evidence of flexion, particularly in the lower extremities. A

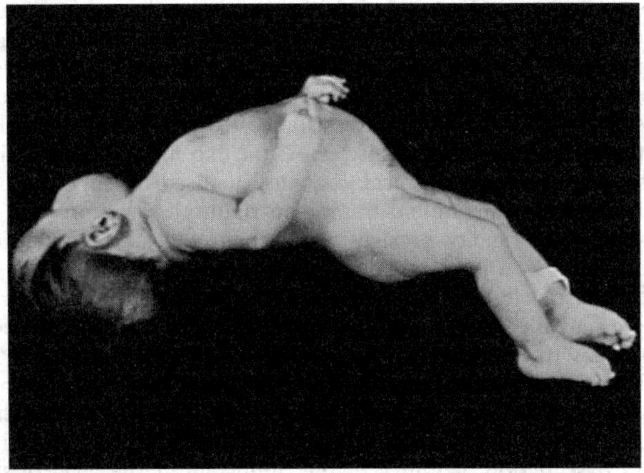

Figure 591-3. Opisthotonus in a brain-injured infant.

normal full-term infant's posture is characterized by flexion of all extremities.

Motility and Locomotion. Premature infants of <32 wk of gestation display random, slow, writhing movements interspersed with rapid, myoclonic-like activity of the extremities. Beyond 32 wk, the motor activity is primarily flexor. Observation of crawling, walking, or running in older infants and children may uncover movement disorders, most of which are likely to be apparent during motion and to disappear with rest or sleep. **Ataxia** refers to incoordination of movement or a disturbance of balance. It may be primarily truncal or may be limited to the extremities. Truncal ataxia is characterized by unsteadiness during sitting or standing and results primarily from involvement of the cerebellar vermis. Abnormalities of the cerebellar hemispheres characteristically cause intention tremor unaffected by visual attention. Ataxia may be demonstrated by the finger-to-nose and heel-to-shin tests, by heel-to-toe or tandem walking, and, in infants, by observation of reaching for or playing with toys. Additional abnormalities associated with cerebellar lesions include dysmetria (errors in measuring distances), rebound (inability to inhibit a muscular action, such as when the examiner suddenly releases the flexed arm and the patient inadvertently strikes the face), and disdiadochokinesia (diminished performance of rapid alternating movements). Hypotonia, dysarthria, nystagmus, and decreased deep tendon reflexes are common features of cerebellar abnormalities. Sensory ataxia is found with diseases of the spinal cord and peripheral nerves. In these disorders, the **Romberg sign** is positive (patient is unsteady with eyes closed, but not when they are open), and there are often related sensory findings including abnormalities in joint position and vibration sense.

Chorea is characterized by irregular involuntary movements of the major joints, trunk, and the face that are rapid and jerky. Affected children are incapable of extending their arms without producing abnormal movements. They have a tendency to pronate the arms when held above the head. The hand grip contracts and relaxes (**milkmaid sign**), the speech is explosive and inarticulate, the deep tendon reflexes of the knee are "hung up," and patients may have difficulty in maintaining protrusion of the tongue. **Athetosis** is a slow, writhing movement that is often associated with abnormalities of muscle tone. It is most prominent in the distal extremities and is enhanced by voluntary activity or emotional upset. Speech and swallowing may be affected. Chorea and athetosis are the result of basal ganglia lesions and are difficult to separate clinically. Both may be prominent in the same patient. **Dystonia** is an involuntary, slow twisting movement that primarily involves the proximal muscles of the extremities, trunk, and neck. **Motor tics** are characterized by sudden brief unsustained movements that are suppressible and usually preceded by a warning sensation. Common motor tics include eye blinking, grimacing, and brief rapid movements of the head and shoulders.

Deep Tendon Reflexes and the Plantar Response. The deep tendon reflexes are readily elicited in most infants and children. In premature and term infants, the biceps, knee, and ankle jerks are the most reliable deep tendon reflexes. They are graded from 0 (absent) to 4 (markedly hyperactive), with 2 being normal. The ankle reflex is less easy to obtain and is demonstrated by percussing the Achilles tendon. Gentle dorsiflexion of the foot and tapping the plantar surface with the reflex hammer usually elicits a response. The knee jerk in an infant may produce a **crossed adductor response** (tapping the patellar tendon in one leg causes contraction in the opposite extremity), which, if present, does not become abnormal until 6–7 mo of age. The deep tendon reflexes are absent or decreased in primary disorders of the muscle (myopathy), nerve (neuropathy), and myoneural junction and in abnormalities of the cerebellum. They are characteristically increased in upper motor neuron lesions. Asymmetry of deep tendon reflexes suggests a lateralizing lesion. The plantar response is obtained by stimulation of the external portion of the sole of the foot, beginning at the heel and extending to the base of the toes. Firm pressure from the examiner's thumb is a useful method for eliciting the response. The **Babinski reflex,** indicating an upper motor neuron lesion, is characterized by extension of the great toe and by fanning of the remaining toes. Too vigorous stimulation may produce withdrawal, which may be misinterpreted as a Babinski response. Most newborn infants show an initial flexion of the great toe on plantar stimulation. As with adults, asymmetry of the plantar response between extremities is a useful lateralizing sign in infants and children.

Primitive Reflexes. Primitive reflexes appear and disappear in sequence during specific periods of development (Table 591-2). Their absence or persistence beyond a given time frame signifies dysfunction of the CNS. Some primitive reflexes, such as the snout or **rooting reflex,** reappear during old age or with specific degenerative diseases involving the cerebral cortex. Although many primitive reflexes have been described, the Moro, grasp, tonic neck, and parachute reflexes are the most important. The **Moro reflex** is obtained by placing the infant in a semi-upright position. The head is momentarily allowed to fall backward, with immediate resupport by the examiner's hand. The child symmetrically abducts and extends the arms and flexes the thumbs, followed by flexion and adduction of the upper extremities. An asymmetric response may signify a fractured clavicle, brachial plexus injury, or a hemiparesis. Absence of the Moro reflex in a term newborn is ominous, suggesting significant dysfunction of the CNS. The **grasp response** is elicited by placing a finger or object in the open palm of each hand. Normal infants grasp the object, and with attempted removal, the grip is reinforced. The **tonic neck reflex** is produced by manually turning the head to one side while supine. Extension of the arm occurs on that side of the body corresponding to the direction of the face, while flexion develops in the contralateral extremities. An obligatory tonic neck response, by which the infant remains "locked" in the fencer's position, is always abnormal and implies a CNS disorder. The **parachute reflex** is demonstrated by suspending the child by the trunk and by suddenly producing forward flexion as if the child were to fall. The child spontaneously extends the upper extremities as a protective mechanism. The parachute reflex appears before the onset of walking.

TABLE 591-2. Timing of Selected Primitive Reflexes

REFLEX	ONSET	FULLY DEVELOPED	DURATION
Palmar grasp	28 wk	32 wk	2–3 mo
Rooting	32 wk	36 wk	Less prominent after 1 mo
Moro	28–32 wk	37 wk	5–6 mo
Tonic neck	35 wk	1 mo	6–7 mo
Parachute	7–8 mo	10–11 mo	Remains throughout life

SENSORY EXAMINATION. The sensory examination is difficult to perform on an infant or uncooperative child. Furthermore, the understanding child soon tires of the examination because it requires considerable attention to repetitious and uninteresting tasks. The more this part of the neurologic examination can be made to simulate a game, the greater is the likelihood that a child will cooperate. Disorders involving the sensory system are less common in the pediatric population than among adults. While a parent or an interesting toy distracts the infant, the examiner touches the patient with a piece of cotton or a fragment of a tongue depressor. Normal children indicate an awareness of the stimulus by pausing during play, withdrawing the extremity, crying, or looking at and touching the stimulated area. Unfortunately, a child quickly loses patience and soon begins to disregard the examiner. It is critical, therefore, that the area in question is tested efficiently and, if necessary, re-examined at an appropriate time.

Identification of a sensory level in association with a **spinal cord lesion** can be very difficult in an infant. Observation may suggest a difference in color, temperature, or perspiration, with the skin cooler and dry below the spinal cord level. Touching the skin lightly above the level evokes a response that is usually in the form of a squirming movement or physical withdrawal. The **superficial abdominal reflexes** may be absent. A child with a spinal cord lesion may have evidence of rectal sphincter incontinence that is manifested by a patulous anus, by the absence of contraction of the sphincter when the skin in the anal region is stimulated with a sharp object (anal wink), and by a lack of contraction of the anal sphincter during the rectal examination. In boys, the presence of the cremasteric reflex is also a valuable finding. Children 4–5 yr of age are capable of detailed sensory testing, including joint position, vibration, temperature, stereognosis, two-point discrimination, double simultaneous extinction, light touch, and pain. The success of the sensory examination depends on the ingenuity and the patience of the examiner.

GAIT AND STATION. Observation of a child's gait is an important aspect of a neurologic examination. The **spastic** gait is characterized by stiffness and by stepping like a tin soldier. Spastic children may walk on tiptoes because of tightness or contractures of the Achilles tendons. **Hemiparesis** is associated with a decreased arm swing on the affected side and a lateral circular motion of the leg (circumduction gait). Extrapyramidal movements, such as dystonia or chorea, may become apparent while the child is walking or running. **Cerebellar ataxia** produces a broad-based unsteady gait and, if severe, the child requires support to prevent falling. Heel-to-toe or tandem walking is performed poorly in patients with abnormalities of the cerebellum. A waddling gait results from weakness of the proximal hip girdle. Affected children often develop a compensatory lordosis and have difficulty in climbing stairs. Weakness or hypotonia of the lower extremities may result in genu recurvatum and flat feet, which causes a clumsy, tentative gait. Scoliosis may cause an abnormal gait and can result from disorders of muscle and spinal cord.

GENERAL EXAMINATION

Physical examination of other organ systems is an essential component of a neurologic examination. Cutaneous lesions suggest a neurocutaneous syndrome (see Chapter 596); hepatosplenomegaly suggests inborn errors of metabolism, storage diseases, HIV, or malignancy; and dysmorphic features suggest various syndromes (see Chapter 108). Heart murmurs raise the possibility of rheumatic fever (chorea), tuberous sclerosis (cardiac rhabdomyoma), cerebral abscess or thrombosis (cyanotic heart disease), or cerebral vascular occlusion (endocarditis). The examiner should also palpate for lymphadenopathy as well as abnormalities of the thyroid gland.

SOFT NEUROLOGIC SIGNS. These signs should be interpreted cautiously because they are present in normal children during various stages of neurodevelopment. A soft neurologic sign may be defined as a particular form of deviant performance on a motor or sensory test in the neurologic examination that is abnormal for a particular age. Testing for the presence of soft neurologic signs involves the observation of a series of timed motor tasks and a comparison of the quality and the precision of the patient's movement with normal controls of similar age and sex. The tests include repetitive and successive finger movements, hand pats, arm pronation-supination movements, foot taps, hopping, and tandem walking. There is considerable variation in the expression of these signs, depending on age, sex, and maturation of the nervous system. Minimal choreoathetoid movements in the fingers of the extended arms are normal at 4 yr of age but disappear by 7 or 8 yr of age. The neurodevelopment of girls is more accelerated than that of boys for many motor tasks, including hopping, skipping, and fine balance maneuvers. Although intellectually normal children may demonstrate a soft neurologic sign, the finding of two or more persistent soft signs correlates significantly with neurologic dysfunction, including attention deficit disorder, learning disorders, and cerebral palsy. Because specific soft signs lack association with a particular disability and can occur in a normal child, it is unwise to label a child who shows several soft neurologic signs. It is more appropriate to monitor such a patient closely and to ensure that a developmental disability has been precluded.

SPECIAL DIAGNOSTIC PROCEDURES

LUMBAR PUNCTURE AND CEREBROSPINAL FLUID EXAMINATION. Examination of the cerebrospinal fluid (CSF) is essential in confirming the diagnosis of meningitis, encephalitis, and subarachnoid hemorrhage and is often helpful in evaluating demyelinating, degenerative, and collagen vascular diseases and the presence of tumor cells within the subarachnoid space. It is the test of choice to diagnosis pseudotumor cerebri. Preparation of a patient is important in order to complete the procedure successfully. An experienced assistant has a vital role in positioning, restraining, and comforting the patient. The skin is thoroughly prepared with a cleansing agent, and the patient is placed in the lateral recumbent position. The physician should wear a mask and be gowned and gloved; the patient should be draped. The neck and legs of the patient are flexed by an assistant to enlarge the intervertebral spaces. The ideal interspace for lumbar puncture (LP) is L3-L4 or L4-L5, which is determined by drawing an imaginary horizontal line from one anterior superior spine of the ilium to the other. The skin and underlying tissue are anesthetized with a local anesthetic or by placing on the skin 30 min before the procedure a patch that contains a eutectic mixture of local anesthetics including lidocaine and prilocaine (EMLA). A 22-gauge, 1–2 in, sharp, beveled spinal needle with a properly fitting stylet is introduced into the midsagittal plane, directed slightly in the cephalic direction. The stylet is removed frequently as the needle is slowly advanced to determine whether CSF is present. A pop is felt as the needle penetrates the dura and enters the subarachnoid space. A manometer and a three-way stopcock may be attached to obtain an opening pressure. The opening pressure in the recumbent and relaxed position averages 100 mm of fluid; the range in the flexed lateral decubitus position is 60–180 mm of fluid. The most common cause of an elevated opening pressure is a crying, uncooperative, and struggling patient. The pressure is recorded most reliably with a child positioned comfortably with the head and the legs extended. Sick neonates should be placed in the upright position for a spinal tap, because decreased ventilation and perfusion abnormalities leading to respiratory arrest are more common in the recumbent position in this age group.

Contraindications for performing an LP include: (1) elevated ICP owing to a suspected mass lesion of the brain or spinal cord, (2) symptoms and signs of pending cerebral herniation in a child with probable meningitis, (3) critical illness (on rare occasions), (4) skin infection at the site of the LP, and (5) thrombocytopenia.

1. In the first instance, transtentorial herniation or herniation of the cerebellar tonsils may develop after the procedure. Inspection of the eyegrounds for the presence of papilledema and obtaining a head CT are mandatory before proceeding with an LP.
2. In the second instance, symptoms and signs include decerebrate or decorticate posture, a generalized tonic seizure, and abnormalities of pupil size and reaction, with absence of the oculocephalic response and fixed oculomotor deviation of the eyes. Pending herniation is also associated with respiratory abnormalities, including hyperventilation, Cheyne-Stokes respiration, ataxic breathing, apnea, and respiratory arrest. These children must be treated immediately with appropriate intravenous antibiotics and measures to reduce increased ICP, and transported to a critical care unit for further stabilization and cranial imaging studies before an LP is contemplated. LP is the primary diagnostic procedure in children with suspected bacterial meningitis in the absence of overwhelming sepsis or shock, or symptoms and signs of brain herniation.
3. In the third case, on rare occasions, an LP is temporarily withheld from a critically ill, moribund patient because the procedure may produce cardiorespiratory arrest. In this situation, blood cultures are drawn, antibiotics and supportive care are administered, and when the patient is stabilized, an LP may be accomplished safely under more controlled circumstances.
4. In the fourth instance, if examination of the CSF is urgent in a patient with skin infection at the site of the LP, a ventricular or cisterna magna tap performed by a skilled physician is indicated.
5. In the fifth instance, thrombocytopenia, with a platelet count $<20 \times 10^9$/L, may cause uncontrolled bleeding in the subarachnoid or subdural space. Therefore, an LP is contraindicated until the platelet count improves after platelet infusion.

Normal CSF is the color of water. Cloudy CSF results from an elevated white blood cell (WBC) or red blood cell (RBC) count. Normal CSF contains up to 5/mm^3 WBCs, and a newborn may have as many as 15/mm^3. Polymorphonuclear (PMN) cells are always abnormal in a child, but 1–2/mm^3 may be present in a normal neonate. The presence of PMN cells raises suspicion of a pathologic process. An elevated PMN count suggests bacterial meningitis or the early phase of aseptic meningitis (see Chapter 602). CSF lymphocytosis indicates aseptic, tuberculous, or fungal meningitis; demyelinating diseases; brain or spinal cord tumor; immunologic disorders including collagen vascular diseases; and chemical irritation (postmyelogram, intrathecal methotrexate).

A Gram stain of the CSF is essential in the investigation of suspected bacterial meningitis; an acid-fast stain or India ink preparation is used if tuberculous or fungal meningitis is a possibility. The fluid is placed on appropriate culture media based on the clinical findings and on the CSF analysis. Further, as indicated by the history and clinical examination, a portion of the CSF should be sent for viral (PCR or antibody) studies (HSV1 and 2, West Nile, and enteroviruses).

Normal CSF contains no RBCs. The presence of RBCs indicates a traumatic tap or a subarachnoid hemorrhage. Bloody CSF should be centrifuged immediately. The supernatant of a bloody tap is clear, but it is xanthochromic in the presence of a subarachnoid hemorrhage. Progressive clearing of bloody CSF is noted during collection of the fluid in the case of a traumatic tap. The presence of crenated RBCs does not differentiate a traumatic tap from a subarachnoid hemorrhage. Xanthochromia may also result from hyperbilirubinemia, carotenemia, and a markedly elevated CSF protein.

The normal CSF protein ranges from 10 to 40 mg/dL in a child to as high as 120 mg/dL in a neonate. The CSF protein falls to the normal childhood range by 3 mo of age. The CSF protein may be elevated in many processes, including infectious, immunologic, vascular, and degenerative diseases as well as tumors of the brain and spinal cord. The CSF protein is increased after a bloody tap by ≈1 mg/dL for every 1,000 RBCs/mm^3. Elevation of CSF immunoglobulin G (IgG), which normally represents ≈10% of the total protein, is observed in subacute sclerosing panencephalitis, postinfectious encephalomyelitis, and in some cases of multiple sclerosis. If the diagnosis of multiple sclerosis is suspected, the CSF should be tested for the presence of oligoclonal bands.

The CSF glucose content is about 60% of the blood glucose in a healthy child. To prevent a spuriously elevated blood/CSF glucose ratio in a case of suspected meningitis, it is advisable to collect the blood glucose before the LP when the child is relatively calm. Hypoglycorrhachia is found in association with diffuse meningeal disease, particularly bacterial and tuberculous meningitis. In addition, widespread neoplastic involvement of the meninges, subarachnoid hemorrhage, fungal meningitis, and, on occasion, aseptic meningitis can produce a low CSF glucose level.

The CSF may also be examined for specific antigens (latex agglutination for suspected meningitis) and metabolites in investigation of a series of metabolic diseases (lactate, amino acids, enolase determination).

SUBDURAL TAP. This procedure may be indicated to establish the diagnosis of a subdural effusion or hematoma. A blunt, short-beveled 20-gauge needle and stylet are used for the procedure. The subdural space is approached at the lateral border of the anterior fontanel or along the upper margin of the coronal suture at least 2–3 cm from the midline to prevent injury to the underlying sagittal sinus. After adequate cleansing and preparation of the skull, including shaving of the hair from the operative site, the patient is placed in the supine position and is firmly held by an attendant. After a local anesthetic, the needle and stylet are slowly advanced through the skin and underlying tissue with a z-like movement until the dura is entered with a sudden popping sensation. Considerable care is taken to prevent advancement of the needle into the cerebral cortex, which in an infant is ≈1.5 cm from the skin surface. A hemostat attached ≈5–7 mm from the beveled end of the needle should provide an adequate safeguard. The subdural fluid, which may squirt out under pressure, is collected and sent for protein analysis, cell count, and culture. The color of the fluid may be xanthochromic, bright red, or oily brown (depending on the age of the subdural collections). Bilateral subdural taps may be indicated, because subdural collections are bilateral in most cases. The amount of fluid removed with each tap should be limited to a total of 15–20 mL from each side in order to prevent rebleeding from a sudden shift of the intracranial contents. At the termination of the procedure, a sterile dressing is applied, and the child is placed in a sitting position that tends to prevent leakage of fluid from the puncture site. (See Chapter 602 for a discussion of subdural fluid associated with meningitis.)

VENTRICULAR TAP. A ventricular tap is used for the removal of CSF in the management of life-threatening increased ICP associated with hydrocephalus, when conservative measures have failed. A pediatrician should not undertake this procedure except when the patient's life is in jeopardy and a neurosurgeon is not available. For an infant, the procedure is similar to a subdural tap. A 20-gauge ventricular needle with a stylet is placed in the lateral border of the anterior fontanel and is directed toward the inner canthus of the ipsilateral eye. The needle is advanced slowly and, the stylet is removed frequently to determine the presence of CSF. The ventricle is usually encountered about 4 cm from the skin surface.

NEURORADIOLOGIC PROCEDURES. A skull roentgenogram is occasionally a useful diagnostic procedure. It may demonstrate fractures, intracranial calcification, craniosynostosis, congenital anomalies, or bony defects and evidence of increased ICP. Acute increased ICP is characterized by separation of the sutures, whereas erosion of the posterior clinoid processes, enlargement of the sella turcica, and an increase in convolutional markings indicate long-standing intracranial hypertension.

Computed tomography (CT) scanning is an important diagnostic procedure for emergencies and for less emergent disorders. It is a noninvasive and rapid procedure that uses conventional x-ray techniques. Sedation is usually required for infants and young children because a lack of head movement is essential during the study. Pentobarbital, 4 mg/kg intramuscularly 30 min before the CT scan, with a supplementary dose of 2 mg/kg intramuscularly 1–1½ hr later if necessary, is usually effective. Chloral hydrate, 50–75 mg/kg orally 45 min before the procedure, is an alternative method of sedation. CT scanning is useful in demonstrating congenital malformations of the brain, including hydrocephalus and porencephalic cysts, subdural collections, cerebral atrophy, intracranial calcification, intracerebral hematoma, brain tumors and areas of cerebral edema, infarction, and demyelination (Table 591-3). Intravenous injection of radiographic contrast medium enhances areas of increased vascular permeability due to abnormalities of the blood-brain barrier (abscess, tumor) and highlights abnormal collections of blood vessels in an arteriovenous malformation.

Magnetic resonance imaging (MRI) is a noninvasive procedure and is especially well suited for the study of neoplasms, cerebral edema, acute stroke (diffusion-weighted MRI), demyelination, degenerative diseases, and congenital anomalies, particularly of the posterior fossa and spinal cord (see Table 591-3). MRI is capable of detecting small plaques in patients with multiple sclerosis and areas of localized gliosis in children with uncontrolled seizures. MRI is routinely used in the evaluation of children who are potential candidates for epilepsy surgery. Intracerebral calcifications are not detected by MRI. The contrast agent, gadolinium-DTPA, is useful during MRI, especially to highlight lesions associated with a disrupted blood-brain barrier. **MR angiography** (MRA) and **venography** (MRV) provide detailed images of major intracranial vasculature structures and assist in the diagnosis of diseases such as stroke, vascular malformations, and cerebral venous sinus thrombosis. **Functional MRI (fMRI)** is a noninvasive technique for detecting and mapping with high

TABLE 591-3. Preferred Imaging Procedures in Neurologic Diseases

NEUROLOGIC DISEASE	IMAGING PROCEDURE
Cerebral or cerebellar ischemic infarction	CT in the 1st 12–24 hr; MRI after 12–24 hr (diffusion-weighted and perfusion-weighted MRI augments the findings, especially in the 1st 24 hr, and even before 8 hr)
Cerebral or cerebellar hemorrhage	CT in the 1st 24 hr; MRI after 24 hr; MRI and endovascular angiography for suspected arteriovenous malformation
Transient ischemic attack	MRI to identify lacunar or other small lesions; ultrasound studies of the carotid arteries; magnetic resonance angiography
Arteriovenous malformation	CT for acute hemorrhage; MRI and endovascular angiography as early as possible
Cerebral aneurysm	CT for acute subarachnoid hemorrhage; CT angiography or endovascular angiography to identify the aneurysm; TCD to detect vasospasm
Brain tumor	MRI without and with injection of contrast material
Craniocerebral trauma	CT initially; MRI after initial assessment and treatment
Multiple sclerosis	MRI without and with injection of contrast material
Meningitis or encephalitis	CT without and with injection of contrast material initially; MRI after initial assessment and treatment
Cerebral or cerebellar abscess	CT without and with injection of contrast material for initial diagnosis or, if stable, MRI instead of CT; MRI without and with injection of contrast material subsequently
Granuloma	MRI without and with injection of contrast material
Dementia	MRI; PET; SPECT
Movement disorders	MRI; PET
Neonatal and development disorders	Ultrasonography in unstable premature neonates; otherwise MRI
Epilepsy	MRI; PET; SPECT
Headache	CT in patients suspected of having structural disorders

PET, positron emission tomography; SPECT, single-photon emission computed tomography; TCD, transcranial Doppler ultrasonography.
From Gilman S: Imaging the brain. *N Engl J Med* 1998;338:812–820.

resolution the hemodynamic changes produced by localized brain activity during specific cognitive and/or sensorimotor functions. It is useful for presurgical localization of critical brain functions (and is very promising as a tool for investigating the development and plasticity of these functions).

The **radionuclide brain scan** uses a radioactive material such as ^{99}Tc, which concentrates in regions where the blood-brain barrier has been disrupted. It is useful in the investigation of herpes encephalitis and cerebral abscess. **Positron emission tomography** (PET) provides unique information on brain metabolism and perfusion by measuring blood flow, oxygen uptake, and glucose consumption. PET is an expensive technique that has been used primarily in adults, but it is increasingly used in many pediatric centers, particularly those with active epilepsy surgery programs. **Single-photon emission computed tomography** (SPECT), using ^{99m}Tc hexamethyl propylenamine oxime (Tc 99m-HMPAO), is a sensitive and inexpensive technique to study regional cerebral blood flow. SPECT is particularly useful in investigating cerebral vascular disease in children (systemic lupus erythematosus) as well as herpes encephalitis, and for localization of focal epileptiform discharges and recurrent brain tumors. **Cerebral angiography** is reserved for the study of vascular disorders. The procedure requires a general anesthetic in most children. Cerebral angiography, using subtraction techniques, is particularly useful for the delineation of arteriovenous malformations, aneurysms, arterial occlusions, and venous thrombosis. In most cases, a four-vessel study (internal carotids and vertebral arteries) is accomplished. MRA may reduce the need for contrast invasive angiography. **Cranial ultrasonography** for the detection of periventricular leukomalacia, intracranial hemorrhage, hydrocephalus, and intracranial tumors is limited to infants with a patent fontanel. The procedure is used intraoperatively in older children for placing shunts, locating small tumors, and directing needle biopsies. **Myelography** was used in the past for demonstrating congenital anomalies, tumors, and vascular malformations of the spinal cord. MRI is superior in most cases to contrast myelography and is not associated with arachnoiditis, which occasionally complicates injection of contrast material into the subarachnoid space.

ELECTROENCEPHALOGRAPHY. An electroencephalogram (EEG) provides a continuous recording of electrical activity between reference electrodes placed on the scalp. Although the genesis of the electrical activity is not certain, it likely originates from postsynaptic potentials in the dendrites of cortical neurons. Even with amplification of the electrical activity, not all potentials are recorded because there is a buffering effect of the scalp, muscles, bone, vessels, and subarachnoid fluid. The EEG waves are classified according to their frequency as delta (1–3/sec), theta (4–7/sec), alpha (8–12/sec), and beta (13–20/sec). These waves are altered by many factors, including age, state of alertness, eye closure, drugs, and disease states. High-voltage slow and sharp waves (K complexes) and sleep spindles (regular 12–14/sec waves) confined to the central regions occur during sleep in a normal EEG. Abnormalities of waveform include spikes and slow waves. Spikes are characteristically paroxysmal, sharp, and of high voltage followed by a slow wave. Spikes and slow waves are associated with epilepsy, but some normal patients may have this EEG finding. Focal spikes are often associated with irritative lesions, including cysts, slow-growing tumors, and glial scar tissue. Epileptiform activity may be enhanced by activation procedures, including hyperventilation, photic stimulation, and sleep deprivation. Slow waves may be focal, in which case, a circumscribed lesion such as a hematoma, tumor, infarction, or a localized infectious process may be considered; generalized slow waves suggest a metabolic, inflammatory, or more widespread process.

EEG/polygraphic/video monitoring provides precise characterization of seizure types, which allows for specific medical or surgical management. It facilitates more accurately differentiation of epileptic seizures from paroxysmal events that mimic epilepsy, including pseudoseizures. EEG/polygraphic/video monitoring also provides for measurement of seizure discharges and for study of the efficacy of various therapeutic regimens. Finally, EEG/polygraphic/video monitoring simultaneously records physiologic and EEG changes; this is particularly useful in neonates in whom the characterization of seizures is difficult.

Magnetoencephalography (**MEG**) detects magnetic fields associated with the intracellular current flow within neurons. **Magnetic source imaging** (**MSI**) is an advanced neurophysiologic technique that combines MEG and MRI to measure the magnetic field generated by a series of neurons. MSI is particularly useful for the investigation of patients who may be candidates for epilepsy surgery.

EVOKED POTENTIALS. An evoked potential is an electrical response that follows stimulation of the CNS by a specific stimulus of the visual, auditory, or sensory system. Clinical application of evoked potentials in infants and children has increased dramatically in the past decade. Stimulation of the visual system by a flash or patterned stimulus, such as a black-and-white checkerboard, produces **visual-evoked potentials** (VEPs), which are recorded over the occiput and averaged in a computer. Abnormal VEPs result from lesions involving the visual system from the retina to the visual cortex. Neurodegenerative diseases, such as Tay-Sachs, Krabbe, Pelizaeus-Merzbacher disease, and neuronal ceroid lipofuscinoses, show characteristic VEP abnormalities. Lesions of the optic nerve and chiasm also produce abnormalities in the VEP response. The VEP, using patterned stimuli, is particularly useful in assessing visual function in at-risk neonates. Flash VEPs are also very useful in predicting outcome in term infants after asphyxia. **Brainstem auditory-evoked potentials** (BAEPs) may be used for objective measurement of hearing acuity, particularly in a neonate or uncooperative child when routine hearing assessment techniques have failed. BAEPs are abnormal in many neurodegenerative diseases in children and are an important tool in evaluating patients with suspected tumors of the cerebellopontine angle. BAEPs are helpful in the assessment of brainstem function in comatose patients, because the waveforms are unaffected by drugs or by the level of consciousness. They are not accurate in predicting neurologic recovery and outcome. **Somatosensory-evoked potentials** (SSEPs) are obtained by stimulating a peripheral nerve (peroneal, median) and by recording the electrical response over the cervical region and contralateral parietal somatosensory cortex. The SSEP determines the functional integrity of the dorsal column–medial-lemniscal system and is useful in monitoring spinal cord function during operative procedures as in scoliosis, the repair of coarctation of the aorta, and myelomeningocele. SSEPs are abnormal in many neurodegenerative disorders in children and are the most accurate evoked potential in the assessment of neurologic outcome following a severe CNS insult.

Ellis R: Lumbar cerebrospinal fluid opening pressure measured in a flexed lateral decubitus position in children. *Pediatrics* 1994;93:622–623.

Gilman S: Imaging the brain. Parts I and II. *N Engl J Med* 1998;338:812–820, 889–896.

Haslam RH: Role of computed tomography in the early management of bacterial meningitis. *J Pediatr* 1991;119:157–159.

Mizrahi EM: Electroencephalographic/polygraphic/video monitoring in childhood epilepsy. *J Pediatr* 1984;105:1–9.

Otsubo H, Snead C: Magnetoencephalography and magnetic source imaging in children. *J Child Neurol* 2001;16:227–235.

Packer RJ, Zimmerman RA, Sutton LN, et al: Magnetic resonance imaging of spinal cord disease of childhood. *Pediatrics* 1986;78:251–256.

Piatt JH: Recognizing neurosurgical conditions in the pediatrician's office. *Pediatr Clin North Am* 2004;51:237–270.

Portnoy JM, Olson LC: Normal cerebrospinal fluid values in children: Another look. *Pediatrics* 1985;75:484–487.

Taylor MJ: Evoked potentials in paediatrics. In Halliday AM (editor): *Evoked Potentials in Clinical Testing,* 2nd ed. Edinburgh, Churchill Livingstone, 1993, p 489.

Chapter 592 ■ Congenital Anomalies of the Central Nervous System

Stephen L. Kinsman and Michael V. Johnston

592.1 • Neural Tube Defects (Dysraphism)

Neural tube defects (NTDs) account for most congenital anomalies of the central nervous system (CNS) and result from failure of the neural tube to close spontaneously between the 3rd and 4th wk of in utero development. Although the precise cause of neural tube defects remains unknown, evidence suggests that many factors, including hyperthermia, drugs, malnutrition, chemicals, maternal obesity or diabetes, and genetic determinants (mutations in folate-responsive or folate-dependent pathways) may adversely affect normal development of the CNS from the time of conception. In some cases, an abnormal maternal nutritional state or exposure to radiation before conception may increase the likelihood of a CNS congenital malformation. The major neural tube defects include spina bifida occulta, meningocele, myelomeningocele, encephalocele, anencephaly, dermal sinus, tethered cord, syringomyelia, diastematomyelia, and lipoma involving the conus medullaris and/or filum terminale.

The human nervous system originates from the primitive ectoderm that also develops into the epidermis. The ectoderm, endoderm, and mesoderm form the three primary germ layers that are developed by the 3rd wk. The endoderm, particularly the notochordal plate and the intraembryonic mesoderm, induces the overlying ectoderm to develop the neural plate in the 3rd wk of development (Fig. 592-1*A*). Failure of normal induction is responsible for most of the neural tube defects. Rapid growth of cells within the neural plate causes further invagination of the neural groove and differentiation of a conglomerate of cells, the neural crest, which migrate laterally on the surface of the neural tube (Fig. 592-1*B*). The notochordal plate becomes the centrally placed notochord, which acts as a foundation around which the vertebral column ultimately develops. With formation of the vertebral column, the notochord undergoes involution and becomes the nucleus pulposus of the intervertebral disks. The neural crest cells differentiate to form the peripheral nervous system, including the spinal and autonomic ganglia as well as the ganglia of cranial nerves V, VII, VIII, IX, and X. In addition, the neural crest forms the leptomeninges, as well as Schwann cells, which are responsible for myelinization of the peripheral nervous system. The dura is believed to arise from the paraxial mesoderm. In the region of the embryo destined to become the head, similar patterns exist. In this region, the notocord is replaced by the precordal mesoderm.

In the 3rd wk of embryonic development, invagination of the neural groove is completed and the neural tube is formed by separation from the overlying surface ectoderm (Fig. 592-1*C*). Initial closure of the neural tube is accomplished in the area corresponding to the future junction of the spinal cord and medulla and moves rapidly both caudally and rostrally. For a brief period, the neural tube is open at both ends, and the neural canal communicates freely with the amniotic cavity (Fig. 592-1*D*). Failure of closure of the neural tube allows excretion of fetal substances (α-fetoprotein [AFP], acetylcholinesterase) into the amniotic fluid, serving as biochemical markers for a neural tube defect. Prenatal screening of maternal serum for AFP in the 16th–18th wk of gestation is an effective method for identifying pregnancies at risk for fetuses with neural tube defects in utero. Normally, the rostral end of the neural tube closes on the 23rd day and the caudal neuropore closes by a process of secondary neurulation by the 27th day of development, before the time that many women realize they are pregnant.

592.2 • Spina Bifida Occulta

This common anomaly consists of a midline defect of the vertebral bodies without protrusion of the spinal cord or meninges. Most individuals are asymptomatic and lack neurologic signs, and the condition is usually of no consequence. In some cases, patches of hair, a lipoma, discoloration of the skin, or a dermal sinus in the midline of the lower back suggests a more significant malformation of the spinal cord (Fig. 592-2). A spine roentgenogram in simple spina bifida occulta shows a defect in closure of the posterior vertebral arches and laminae, typically involving L5 and S1; there is no abnormality of the meninges, spinal cord, or nerve roots. Spina bifida occulta is occasionally associated with more significant developmental abnormalities of the spinal cord, including syringomyelia, diastematomyelia, and a tethered cord. These are best identified with MRI (Fig. 592-3).

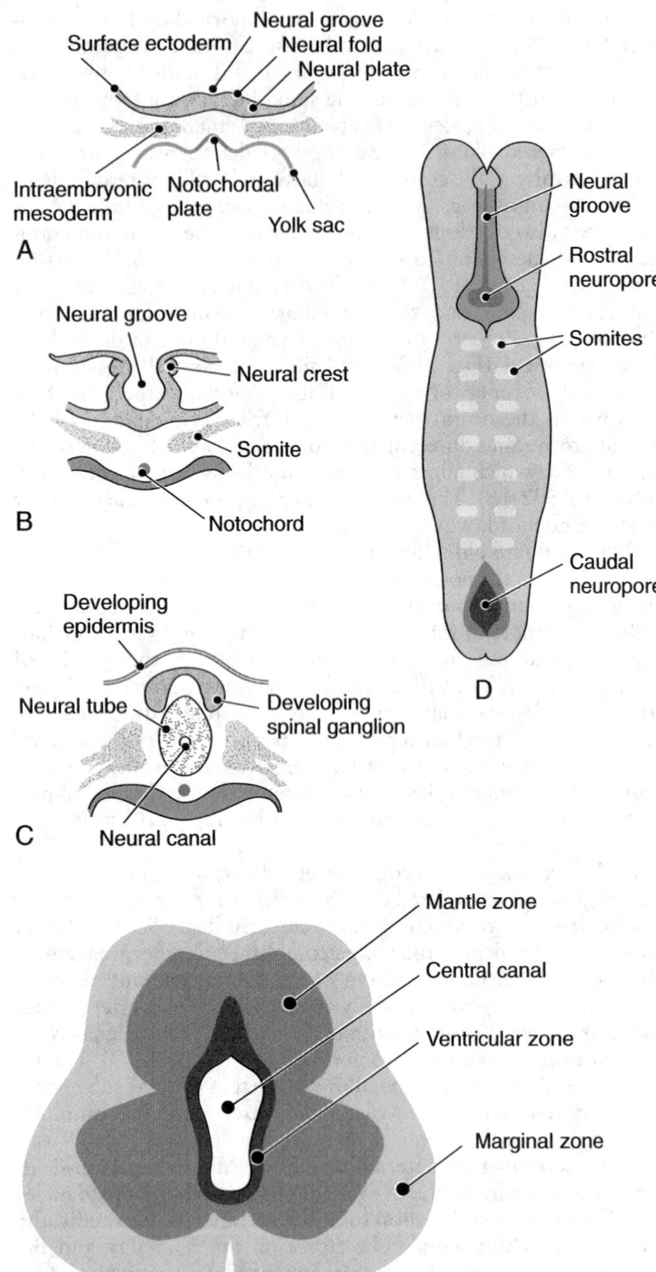

Figure 592-1. Diagrammatic illustration of the developing nervous system. *A*, Transverse sections of the neural plate during the 3rd wk. *B*, Formation of the neural groove and the neural crest. *C*, The neural tube is developed. *D*, Longitudinal drawing showing the initial closure of the neural tube in the central region. *E*, Cross-sectional drawing of the embryonic neural tube (primitive spinal cord).

Some consider the term *spina bifida occulta* to denote merely a posterior vertebral body fusion defect. This simple defect does not have an associated spinal cord malformation. Other clinically more significant forms are more correctly termed **occult spinal dysraphism.** In most of these cases, there are cutaneous manifestations such as a hemangioma, pit, lump, or hairy patch (see Fig. 592-2). A **dermoid sinus** usually forms a small skin opening, which leads into a narrow duct, sometimes indicated by protruding hairs, a hairy patch, or a vascular nevus. Dermoid sinuses occur in the midline at the site of where meningoceles or encephaloceles may occur: the lumbosacral region or occiput. Dermoid sinus tracts may pass through the dura, acting as a conduit for the spread of infection. Recurrent meningitis of occult origin should prompt careful examination for a small sinus tract in the posterior midline region, including the back of the head. Lower back sinuses are usually above the gluteal fold and are directed cephalad. Tethered spinal cord syndrome may also be an associated problem.

592.3 • Meningocele

A meningocele is formed when the meninges herniate through a defect in the posterior vertebral arches. The spinal cord is usually normal and assumes a normal position in the spinal canal, although there may be tethering, syringomyelia, or diastematomyelia. A fluctuant midline mass that may transilluminate occurs along the vertebral column, usually in the lower back. Most meningoceles are well covered with skin and pose no threat to the patient. Careful neurologic examination is mandatory. Asymptomatic children with normal neurologic findings and full-thickness skin covering the meningocele may have surgery delayed. Before surgical correction of the defect, the patient must be thoroughly examined with the use of plain roentgenograms, ultrasonography, and MRI to determine the extent of neural tissue involvement, if any, and associated anomalies, including diastematomyelia, tethered spinal cord, and lipoma. Urologic evaluation, usually including cystometrogram (CMG), will identify those children with neurogenic bladder who are at risk for renal deterioration. Those patients with leaking cerebrospinal fluid (CSF) or a thin skin covering should undergo immediate surgical treatment to prevent meningitis. A CT scan of the head is recommended for children with a meningocele because of the association with hydrocephalus in some cases. An **anterior meningocele** projects into the pelvis through a defect in the sacrum. Symptoms of constipation and bladder dysfunction develop due to the increasing size of the lesion. Female patients may have associated anomalies of the genital tract, including a rectovaginal fistula and vaginal septa. Plain roentgenograms demonstrate a defect in the sacrum, and CT scanning or MRI outlines the extent of the meningocele.

592.4 • Myelomeningocele

Myelomeningocele represents the most severe form of dysraphism involving the vertebral column and occurs with an incidence of ≈1/4,000 live births.

ETIOLOGY. The cause of myelomeningocele is unknown, but as with all neural tube closure defects, a genetic predisposition exists; the risk of recurrence after one affected child increases to 3–4% and increases to ≈10% with two previous abnormal pregnancies. Both epidemiologic evidence and the presence of substantial familial aggregation of anencephaly, myelomeningocele, and craniorachischisis indicate heredity, on a polygenic basis, as a significant contributor to the etiology of NTDs. Nutritional and environmental factors undoubtedly have a role in the etiology of myelomeningocele as well.

Folate is intricately involved in the prevention and etiology of NTDs. Folate functions in single-carbon transfer reactions and exists in many chemical forms. Folic acid (pteroylmonoglutamic acid), which is the most oxidized and stable form of folate, occurs rarely in food but is the form used in vitamin supplements and in fortified food products. Most naturally occurring folates (food folate) are pteroylpolyglutamates, which contain one to six additional glutamate molecules joined in a peptide linkage to the γ-carboxyl of glutamate. Folate coenzymes are involved in: (1)

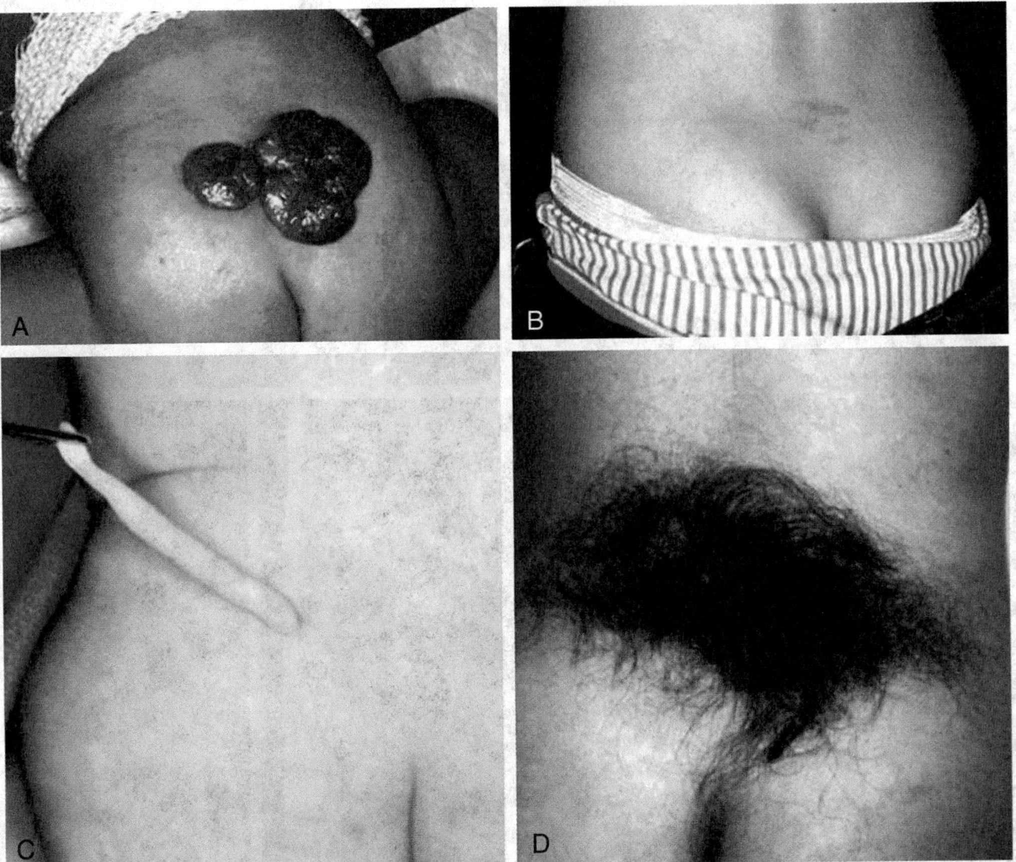

Figure 592-2. Clinical aspects of isolated or combined congenital median lumbosacral cutaneous lesions. *A*, Ulcerated hemangioma centered on a dermal sinus and deviation of the gluteal furrow. *B*, Isolated port-wine stain. *C*, Human tail. *D*, Faun tail. (From Guggisberg D, Hadj-Rabia S, Viney C, et al: Skin markers of occult spinal dysraphism. *Arch Dermatol* 2004;140:1109–1115.)

deoxyribonucleic acid (DNA) synthesis, (2) purine synthesis, (3) generation of formate into the formate pool, and (4) amino acid interconversion with the conversion of homocysteine to methionine providing methionine for the synthesis of S-adenosylmethionine (an agent important for in vivo methylation). Mutations in the genes encoding the enzymes involved in homocysteine metabolism include 5,10 methylenetetrahydrofolate reductase (MTHFR), cystathionine ß-synthase, and methionine synthase. An association between a thermolabile variant of MTHFR and mothers of children with NTDs may account for up to 15% of preventable NTDs. Maternal periconceptional use of folic acid supplementation reduces the incidence of neural tube defects in pregnancies at risk by at least 50%. To be effective, folic acid supplementation should be initiated before conception and continued until at least the 12th wk of gestation when neurulation is complete.

PREVENTION. The U.S. Public Health Service has recommended that all women of childbearing age and who are capable of becoming pregnant take 0.4 mg of folic acid daily. If, however, a pregnancy is planned in high-risk women (previously affected child), supplementation should be started with 4 mg of folic acid daily, beginning 1 mo before the time of the planned conception. The modern diet provides about half the daily requirement of folic acid. To increase folic acid intake, fortification of flour, pasta, rice, and cornmeal with 0.15 mg folic acid per 100 g was mandated in the United States and Canada in 1998. The added folic acid will be insufficient to maximize the prevention of preventable neural tube defects. Therefore, informative educational programs and folic acid vitamin supplementation remain essential for women planning a pregnancy and possibly for all women of childbearing age. In addition, women should also strive to consume food folate from a varied diet. Certain drugs, including drugs that antagonize folic acid such as trimethoprim and the anticonvulsants carbamazepine, phenytoin, phenobarbital, and primidone, increase the risk of myelomeningocele. The anticonvulsant valproic acid causes neural tube defects in ≈1–2% of pregnancies, if the drug is administered during pregnancy. Some epilepsy clinicians recommend that all female patients of childbearing potential who take anticonvulsant medications should also receive folic acid supplements.

CLINICAL MANIFESTATIONS. This condition produces dysfunction of many organs and structures, including the skeleton, skin, and gastrointestinal and genitourinary tracts, in addition to the peripheral nervous system and the CNS. A myelomeningocele may be located anywhere along the neuraxis, but the lumbosacral region accounts for at least 75% of the cases. The extent and degree of the neurologic deficit depend on the location of the myelomeningocele, as well as the associated lesions. A lesion in the low sacral region causes bowel and bladder incontinence associated with anesthesia in the perineal area but with no impairment of motor function. Newborns with a defect in the midlumbar region typically have a saclike cystic structure covered by a thin layer of partially epithelialized tissue (Fig. 592-4). Remnants of neural tissue are visible beneath the membrane, which may occasionally rupture and leak CSF. Examination of the infant shows a flaccid paralysis of the lower extremities, an absence of

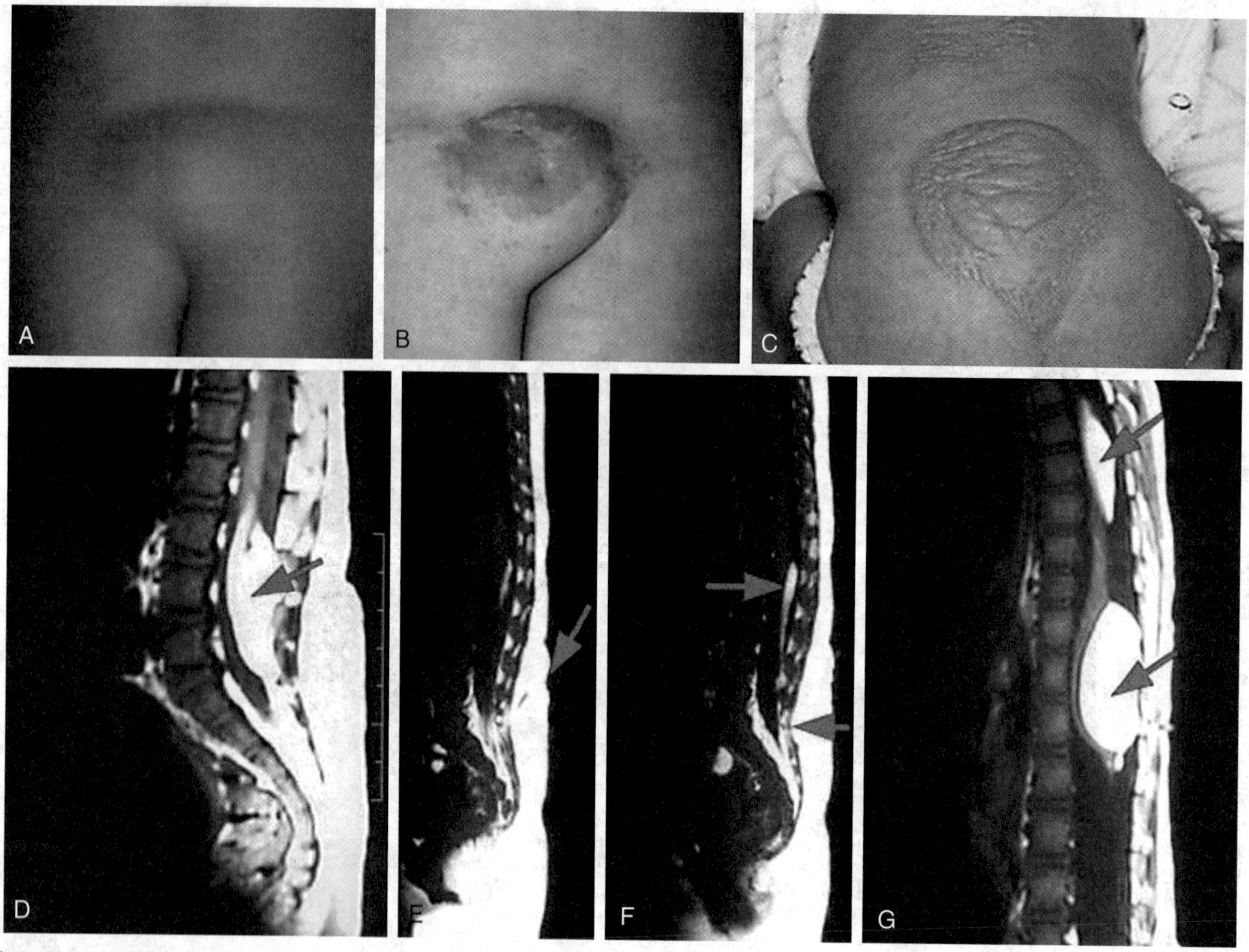

Figure 592-3. Clinical features (A–C) and corresponding occult spinal dysraphism detected by sagittal, T1 weighted magnetic resonance imaging (MRI) studies of the spinal cord (D–G). *A,* Sacral lipoma and deviated gluteal furrow (DGF). *B,* Lumbar port-wine stain, lipoma, dermal sinus, and DGF. *C,* Dorsal and lumbar unclassified hamartomas. *D,* Lipoma of the conus *(arrow)*. *E,* Dermal sinus *(arrow)*. *F,* Top of the lipoma of the filum terminale *(upper arrow)* and fistula *(lower arrow)*. *G,* Multiple lipomas of the thoracic cord *(upper arrow)* and posterior conus *(lower arrow)*. (From Guggisberg D, Hadj-Rabia S, Viney C, et al: Skin markers of occult spinal dysraphism. *Arch Dermatol* 2004;140:1109–1115.)

deep tendon reflexes, a lack of response to touch and pain, and a high incidence of lower extremity deformities (clubfeet, subluxation of the hips). Constant urinary dribbling and a relaxed anal sphincter may be evident. Other children do not leak urine and in fact have a high-pressure bladder and sphincter dyssynergy. Thus, a myelomeningocele in the midlumbar region tends to produce lower motor neuron signs due to abnormalities and disruption of the conus medullaris. Infants with myelomeningocele typically have an increasing neurologic deficit as the myelomeningocele extends higher into the thoracic region. Patients with a myelomeningocele in the upper thoracic or the cervical region usually have a very minimal neurologic deficit and, in most cases, do not have hydrocephalus.

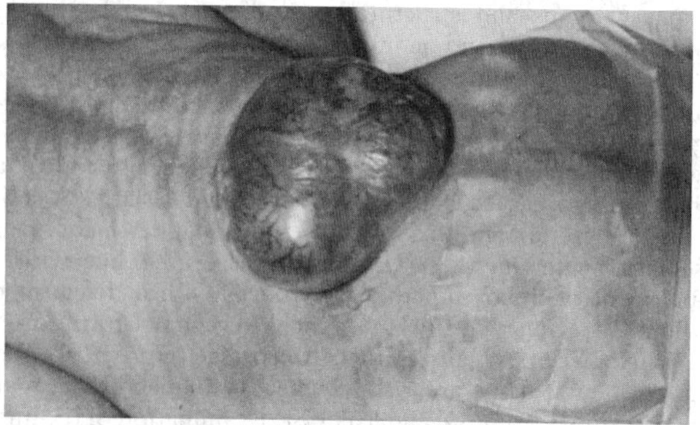

Figure 592-4. A lumbar myelomeningocele is covered by a thin layer of skin.

Hydrocephalus in association with a **type II Chiari defect** develops in at least 80% of patients with myelomeningocele. Generally, the lower the deformity in the neuraxis (sacrum), the less likely is the risk of hydrocephalus. The possibility of hydrocephalus developing should always be considered, no matter what the spinal level. Ventricular enlargement may be indolent and slow growing or may be rapid, causing a bulging anterior fontanel, dilated scalp veins, setting-sun appearance of the eyes, irritability, and vomiting associated with an increased head circumference. About 15% of infants with hydrocephalus and Chiari II malformation develop symptoms of hindbrain dysfunction, including difficulty feeding, choking, stridor, apnea, vocal cord paralysis, pooling of secretions, and spasticity of the upper extremities, which, if untreated, can lead to death. This **Chiari crisis** is due to downward herniation of the medulla and cerebellar tonsils through the foramen magnum.

TREATMENT. Management and supervision of a child and family with a myelomeningocele require a multidisciplinary team approach, including surgeons, physicians, and therapists, with one individual (often a pediatrician) acting as the advocate and coordinator of the treatment program. The news that a newborn child has a devastating condition such as myelomeningocele causes parents to feel considerable grief and anger. They need time to learn about the handicap and the associated complications and to reflect on the various procedures and treatment plans. A knowledgeable individual in an unhurried and nonthreatening setting must give the parents the facts. If possible, discussions with other parents of children with neural tube defects are helpful in resolving important questions and issues.

Surgery is often done within a day or so of birth but can be delayed for several days (except when there is a CSF leak) to allow the parents time to begin to adjust to the shock and to prepare for the multiple procedures and inevitable problems that lie ahead. Evaluation of other congenital anomalies and renal function can also be initiated before surgery. Most pediatric centers aggressively treat the majority of infants with myelomeningocele. After repair of a myelomeningocele, most infants require a shunting procedure for hydrocephalus. If symptoms or signs of hindbrain dysfunction appear, early surgical decompression of the medulla and cervical cord is indicated. Clubfeet may require casting, and dislocated hips may require operative procedures.

Careful evaluation and reassessment of the **genitourinary system** are some of the most important components of the management. Teaching the parents, and ultimately the patient, to regularly catheterize a neurogenic bladder is a crucial step in maintaining a low residual volume and bladder pressure that prevents urinary tract infections and reflux leading to pyelonephritis, hydronephrosis, and bladder damage. Latex-free catheters and gloves must be used to avoid the development of latex allergy. Periodic urine cultures and assessment of renal function, including serum electrolytes and creatinine as well as renal scans, vesiculourethrograms (VCUGs), ultrasonography, and cystometrograms (CMGs), are obtained according to the progress of the patient and the results of the physical examination. This approach to urinary tract management has greatly reduced the need for urologic diversionary procedures and significantly decreased the morbidity and mortality associated with progressive renal disease in these patients. Some children can become continent with surgical implantation of an artificial urinary sphincter (these are used less often) or bladder augmentation at a later age. Although **incontinence of fecal matter** is common and is socially unacceptable during the school years, it does not pose the same organ-damaging risks as urinary dysfunction, but occasionally fecal impaction and/or megacolon develop. Many children can be bowel-trained with a regimen of timed enemas or suppositories that allows evacuation at a predetermined time once or twice a day. Appendicostomy for antegrade enemas may also be helpful. (See also Chapter 22.4.)

Functional **ambulation** is the wish of each child and parent and may be possible, depending on the level of the lesion and on intact function of the iliopsoas muscles. Almost every child with a sacral or lumbosacral lesion obtains functional ambulation; approximately half the children with higher defects ambulate with the use of braces and canes. It should be noted that ambulation is often more difficult as adolescence approaches and body mass increases.

In utero surgical closure of a spinal lesion has been successful in a few centers. Preliminary reports suggest that there may be preservation of motor function with better motor outcomes as well as a lower incidence of hindbrain abnormalities and hydrocephalus. This suggests that the defects may be progressive in utero and that prenatal closure may prevent the development of further loss of function. In utero diagnosis is facilitated by maternal serum α-fetoprotein screening and by fetal ultrasonography (see Chapter 96).

PROGNOSIS. For a child who is born with a myelomeningocele and who is treated aggressively, the mortality rate is ≈10–15%, and most deaths occur before age 4 yr, although life-threatening complications occur at all ages. At least 70% of survivors have normal intelligence, but learning problems and seizure disorders are more common than in the general population. Previous episodes of meningitis or ventriculitis adversely affect the ultimate intelligence quotient. Because myelomeningocele is a chronic handicapping condition, periodic multidisciplinary follow-up is required for life. Renal dysfunction is one of the most important determinants of mortality.

592.5 • ENCEPHALOCELE

Two major forms of dysraphism affect the skull, resulting in protrusion of tissue through a bony midline defect, called **cranium bifidum.** A **cranial meningocele** consists of a CSF-filled meningeal sac only, and a **cranial encephalocele** contains the sac plus cerebral cortex, cerebellum, or portions of the brainstem. Microscopic examination of the neural tissue within an encephalocele often reveals abnormalities. The cranial defect occurs most commonly in the occipital region at or below the inion, but in certain parts of the world, frontal or nasofrontal encephaloceles are more prominent. These abnormalities are one tenth as common as neural tube closure defects involving the spine. The etiology is presumed to be similar to that for anencephaly and myelomeningocele; examples of each are reported in the same family.

Infants with a cranial encephalocele are at increased risk for developing hydrocephalus due to aqueduct stenosis, Chiari malformation, or the Dandy-Walker syndrome. Examination may show a small sac with a pedunculated stalk or a large cystlike structure that may exceed the size of the cranium. The lesion may be completely covered with skin, but areas of denuded skin can occur and require urgent surgical management. Transillumination of the sac may indicate the presence of neural tissue. A plain roentgenogram of the skull and cervical spine is indicated to define the anatomy of the vertebrae. Ultrasonography is most helpful in determining the contents of the sac. MRI or CT further helps define the spectrum of the lesion. Children with a cranial meningocele generally have a good prognosis, whereas patients with an encephalocele are at risk for visual problems, microcephaly, mental retardation, and seizures. Generally, children with neural tissue within the sac and associated hydrocephalus have the poorest prognosis. **Meckel-Gruber syndrome** is a rare autosomal recessive condition that is characterized by an occipital encephalocele, cleft lip or palate, microcephaly, microphthalmia, abnormal genitalia, polycystic kidneys, and polydactyly. Determination of maternal serum α-fetoprotein levels and ultrasound measurement of the biparietal diameter as well as identification of the encephalocele itself may diagnose encephaloceles in utero.

592.6 • ANENCEPHALY

An anencephalic infant presents a distinctive appearance with a large defect of the calvarium, meninges, and scalp associated with a rudimentary brain, which results from failure of closure of the rostral neuropore, the opening of the anterior neural tube. The primitive brain consists of portions of connective tissue, vessels, and neuroglia. The cerebral hemispheres and cerebellum are usually absent, and only a residue of the brainstem can be identified. The pituitary gland is hypoplastic, and the spinal cord pyramidal tracts are missing owing to the absence of the cerebral cortex. Additional anomalies include folding of the ears, cleft palate, and congenital heart defects in 10–20% of cases. Most anencephalic infants die within several days of birth. The incidence of anencephaly approximates 1/1,000 live births; the greatest frequency is in Ireland, Wales, and Northern China. The recurrence risk is ≈4% and increases to 10% if a couple has had two previously affected pregnancies. Many factors have been implicated as the cause of anencephaly (in addition to a genetic basis), including low socioeconomic status, nutritional and vitamin deficiencies, and a large number of environmental and toxic factors. It is very likely that several noxious stimuli interact on a genetically susceptible host to produce anencephaly. The frequency of anencephaly has been decreasing in the past 2 decades. Approximately 50% of cases of anencephaly have associated polyhydramnios. Couples who have had an anencephalic infant should have successive pregnancies monitored, including amniocentesis, determination of AFP levels, and ultrasound examination between the 14th and 16th wk of gestation.

Beeker T, Scheers M, Faber J, et al: Prediction of independence and intelligence at birth on meningomyelocele. *Childs New Syst* 2006;22:33–37.

Berry RJ, Li Z, Erickson JD, et al for the China-U.S. Collaborative Project for Neural Tube Defect Prevention: Prevention of neural-tube defects with folic acid in China. *N Engl J Med* 1999;341:1485–1490.

Fernandes ET, Reinberg Y, Vernier R, et al: Neurogenic bladder dysfunction in children: Review of pathophysiology and current management. *J Pediatr* 1994;124:1–7.

Guggisberg D, Hadj-Rabia S, Viney C, et al: Skin markers of occult spinal dysraphism in children. *Arch Dermatol* 2004;140:1109–1115.

Hernandez-Diaz S, Werler MM, Walker AM, et al: Folic acid antagonists during pregnancy and the risk of birth defects. *N Engl J Med* 2000;343:1608–1614.

Ickowicz V, Ewin D, Maugay-Laulom B, et al: Meckel-Gruber syndrome, sonography and pathology. *Ultrasound Obstet Gynecol* 2006;27:296–300.

Kibar Z, Torban E, McDearmid JR, et al: Mutations in VANGLI associated with neural-tube defects. *N Engl J Med* 2007;356:1432–1437.

Mazzola CA, Albright AL, Sutton LN, et al: Dermoid inclusion cysts and early spinal cord tethering after fetal surgery for myelomeningocele. *N Engl J Med* 2002;347:256–259.

Mitchell LE, Adzick NS, Melchionne J, et al: Spina bifida. *Lancet* 2004;364:1885–1895.

592.7 • Disorders of Neuronal Migration

Disorders of neuronal migration may result in minor abnormalities with little or no clinical consequence (small heterotopia of neurons) or devastating abnormalities of the CNS (mental retardation, seizures, lissencephaly, schizencephaly, particularly the open-lip form) [Fig. 592-5]. One of the most important mechanisms in the control of neuronal migration is the radial glial fiber system that guides neurons to their proper site. Migrating neurons attach to the radial glial fiber and then disembark at predetermined sites to form, ultimately, the precisely designed six-layered cerebral cortex. The product of a mouse gene called *reelin* directs the new neuron to reach its final destination in the brain. Another mouse gene *(mdab1)* may act as a signaling pathway triggered by *reelin.* Mutations of these genes in mice produce major neuronal migration abnormalities. The severity and the extent of the disorder are related to numerous factors, including the timing of a particular insult and a host of environmental and genetic factors.

The embryonic neural tube consists of three zones: ventricular, mantle, and marginal (see Fig. 592-1*E*). The ependymal layer consists of pluripotential, pseudostratified, columnar neuroepithelial cells. Specific neuroepithelial cells differentiate into primitive neurons or neuroblasts that form the mantle layer. The

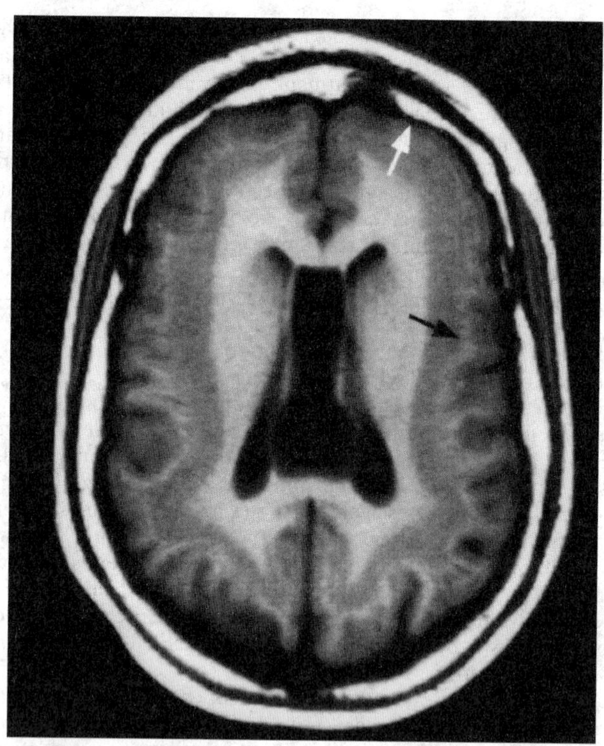

Figure 592-5. T1 weighted MRI scan demonstrating band heterotopia. A thin layer of white matter *(black arrow)* lies between the band of heterotopic gray matter and the cortical surface. Failure of cortical organization with lissencephaly is present in both frontal lobes *(white arrow).*

marginal zone is formed from cells in the outer layer of the neuroepithelium, which ultimately becomes the white matter. Glioblasts, which act as the primitive supportive cells of the CNS, also arise from the neuroepithelial cells in the ependymal zone. They migrate to the mantle and marginal zones and become future astrocytes and oligodendrocytes. It is likely that microglia originate from mesenchymal cells at a later stage of fetal development when blood vessels begin to penetrate the developing nervous system. Continued advancement of an understanding of the molecular bases of cortical development is leading to new classifications of malformations of cortical development.

LISSENCEPHALY. Lissencephaly, or **agyria,** is a rare disorder that is characterized by the absence of cerebral convolutions and a poorly formed sylvian fissure, giving the appearance of a 3–4 mo fetal brain. The condition is probably a result of faulty neuroblast migration during early embryonic life and is usually associated with enlarged lateral ventricles and heterotopias in the white matter. In some forms, there is a four-layered cortex, rather than the usual six-layered one, with a thin rim of periventricular white matter and numerous gray heterotopia visible by microscopic examination. These infants present with failure to thrive, microcephaly, marked developmental delay, and a severe seizure disorder. Ocular abnormalities are common, including hypoplasia of the optic nerve and microphthalmia. Lissencephaly can occur as an isolated finding, but it is associated with **Miller-Dieker syndrome** (MDS) in about 15% of cases. These children have characteristic facies, including a prominent forehead, bitemporal hollowing, anteverted nostrils, a prominent upper lip, and micrognathia. About 90% of children with MDS have visible or submicroscopic chromosomal deletions of 17p13.3. The gene LIS-1 (lissencephaly 1) that maps to chromosome region 17p13.3 is deleted in patients with MDS. CT and MRI scans typically show a smooth brain with an absence of sulci (Fig. 592-6).

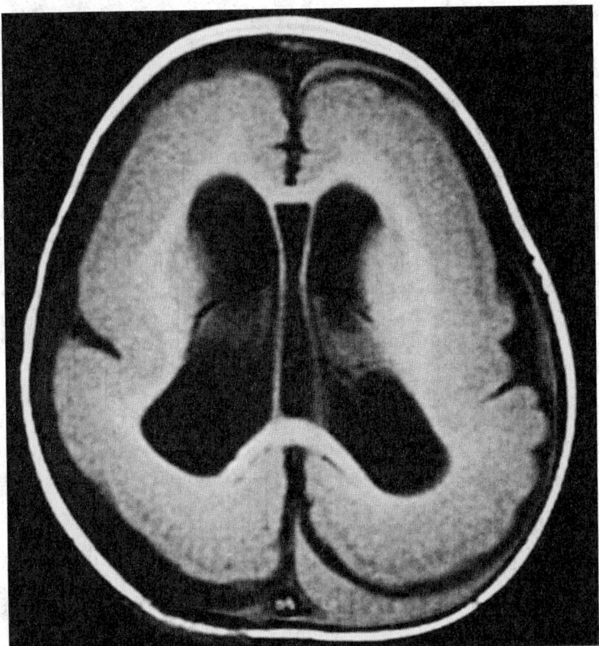

Figure 592-6. MRI of an infant with lissencephaly. Note the absence of cerebral sulci and the maldeveloped sylvian fissures associated with enlarged ventricles.

SCHIZENCEPHALY. This is the presence of unilateral or bilateral **clefts** within the cerebral hemispheres due to an abnormality of morphogenesis (Fig. 592-7). The cleft may be fused or unfused and, if unilateral and large, may be confused with a porencephalic cyst. Not infrequently, the borders of the cleft are surrounded by abnormal brain, particularly microgyria. CT scan is diagnostic and clearly demonstrates the size and extent of the cleft. Milder forms may require MRI for recognition. Many patients are severely mentally retarded, with seizures that are difficult to control, and microcephalic, with spastic quadriparesis when the clefts are bilateral. Unilateral schizencephaly is a frequent cause of **congenital hemiparesis.**

PORENCEPHALY. This is the presence of cysts or cavities within the brain that result from developmental defects or acquired lesions, including infarction of tissue. True porencephalic cysts are most frequently located in the region of the sylvian fissure and typically communicate with the subarachnoid space, the ventricular system, or both. They represent developmental abnormalities of cell migration and are often associated with other malformations of the brain, including microcephaly, abnormal patterns of adjacent gyri, and encephalocele. Affected infants tend to have many problems, including mental retardation, spastic hemi- or quadriparesis, optic atrophy, and seizures. Pseudoporencephalic cysts characteristically develop during the perinatal or postnatal period and result from abnormalities (infarction, hemorrhage) of arterial or venous circulation. These cysts extend to be unilateral, they do not communicate with a fluid-filled cavity, and they are not associated with abnormalities of cell migration or CNS malformations. Infants with pseudoporencephalic cysts present with hemiparesis and focal seizures in the 1st year of life.

HOLOPROSENCEPHALY. This developmental disorder of the brain results from defective cleavage of the prosencephalon and inadequate induction of the forebrain structures. The abnormality, which represents a spectrum of severity, is classified into three groups: alobar, semilobar, and lobar, depending on the degree of the cleavage abnormality (Fig. 592-8). A fourth type, the middle interhemispheric fusion (MIHF variant) or syntelencephaly, involves a segmental area of noncleavage of the posterior frontal and parietal lobes. **Facial abnormalities** including cyclopia, cebocephaly, single central incisor tooth, and premaxillary agenesis are common in severe cases, because the prechordal mesoderm that induces the ventral prosencephalon is also responsible for induction of the median facial structures. A lobar holoprosencephaly is characterized by a single ventricle, an absent falx, and fused basal ganglia. Care must be taken not to overdiagnose based on ventricular abnormalities alone. Evidence of noncleaved midline brain structures is the critical element.

Affected infants have high mortality rates; some live for years. Mortality and morbidity with milder types are more variable and less severe. Care must be taken not to prognosticate in these cases. The incidence of holoprosencephaly ranges from 1/5,000 to 1/16,000. A prenatal diagnosis can be confirmed by ultrasonography after the 10th wk of gestation for more severe types. The

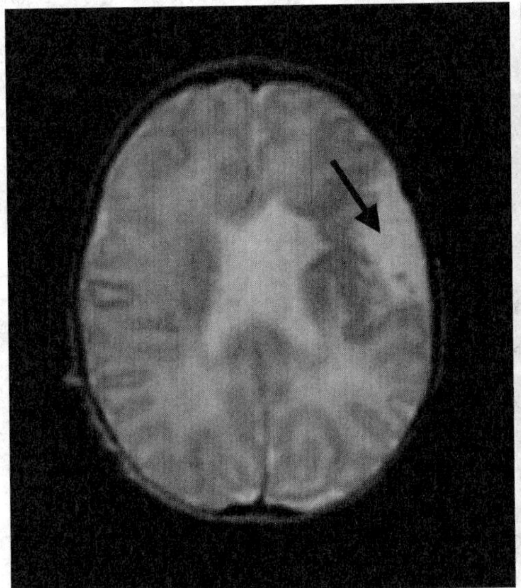

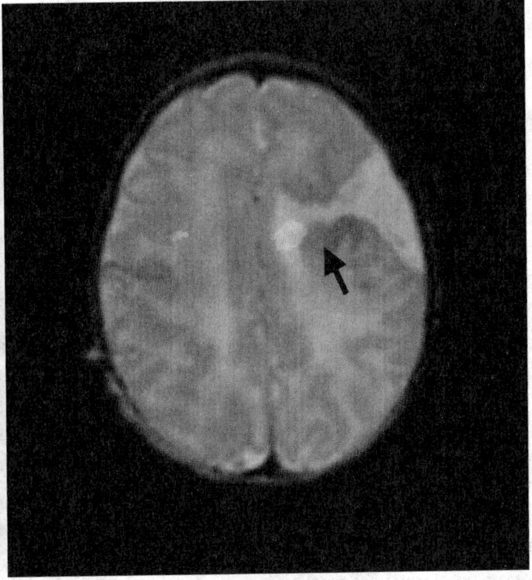

Figure 592-7. Unilateral schizencephaly shown on axial MR images of the brain. Example of an open-lip schizencephaly with a cleft communicating between the ventricle and the extra-axial cranial space (*arrow* on left panel). Many of these clefts are lined with abnormal gray matter (*arrow* on right panel).

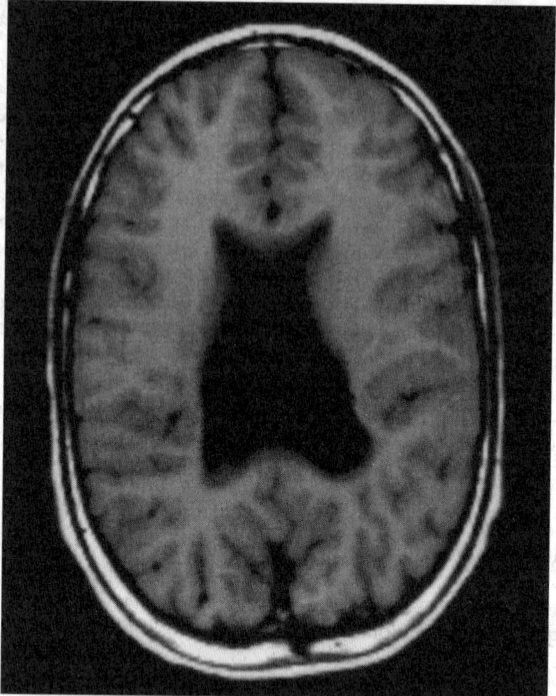

Figure 592-8. Lobar holoprosencephaly. T1 weighted MRI scan demonstrates failure of separation of the hemispheres and a persistent fused ventricle.

cause for holoprosencephaly is usually not identified, although there appears to be an association with maternal diabetes. Chromosomal abnormalities, including deletions of chromosomes 7q and 3p, 21q, 2p, 18p, and 13q, as well as trisomy 13 and 18, account for upward of 50% of all cases. Mutations in the "sonic hedgehog" gene at 7q have been shown to cause holoprosencephaly.

592.8 • Agenesis of the Corpus Callosum

Agenesis of the corpus callosum consists of a heterogeneous group of disorders that vary in expression from severe intellectual and neurologic abnormalities to the asymptomatic and normally intelligent individual (Fig. 592-9). The corpus callosum develops from the commissural plate that lies in proximity to the anterior neuropore. An insult to the commissural plate during early embryogenesis causes agenesis of the corpus callosum. When agenesis of the corpus callosum is an isolated phenomenon, the patient may be normal, whereas individuals with neurologic symptoms, including mental retardation, microcephaly, hemiparesis, diplegia, and seizures, have associated brain anomalies due to cell migration defects, such as heterotopias, microgyria, and pachygyria (broad, wide gyri) in addition to the absence of the corpus callosum. The anatomic features are best depicted on MRI or CT scan and show widely separated frontal horns with an abnormally high position of the third ventricle between the lateral ventricles. MRI precisely outlines the extent of the corpus callosum defect. Absence of the corpus callosum may be inherited as an X-linked recessive trait or as an autosomal dominant trait. The condition may be associated with specific chromosomal disorders, particularly 8-trisomy and 18-trisomy.

Aicardi syndrome represents a complex disorder that affects many systems and is typically associated with agenesis of the corpus callosum. Patients are almost all female, suggesting a genetic abnormality of the X chromosome (it may be lethal in males during fetal life). Seizures become evident during the 1st few months and are typically resistant to anticonvulsants. An electroencephalogram (EEG) shows independent activity recorded from both hemispheres as a result of the absent corpus callosum. All patients have severe mental retardation and may have abnormal vertebrae that may be fused or only partially developed (hemivertebra). Abnormalities of the retina, including circumscribed pits or lacunae and coloboma of the optic disc, are the most characteristic findings of Aicardi syndrome.

592.9 • Agenesis of the Cranial Nerves

Absence of the cranial nerves or the corresponding central nuclei has been described in several conditions and includes the optic nerve, congenital ptosis, Marcus Gunn phenomenon (sucking jaw movements causing simultaneous eyelid blinking; this congenital synkinesis results from abnormal innervation of the trigeminal and oculomotor nerves), the trigeminal and auditory nerves, and cranial nerves IX, X, XI, and XII. **Möbius syndrome** is characterized by bilateral facial weakness, which is often associated with abducens nerve paralysis. Hypoplasia or agenesis of brainstem

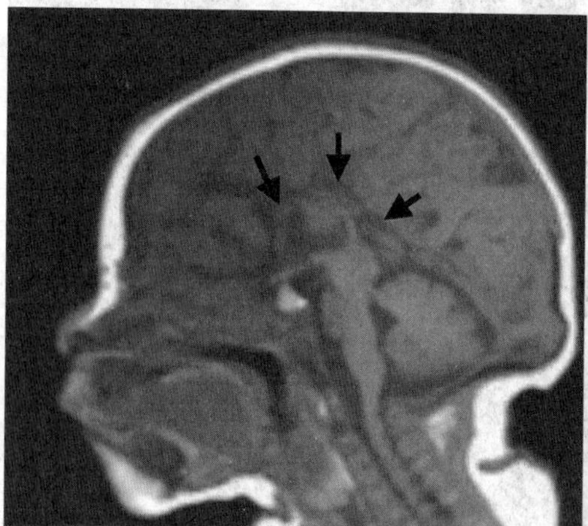

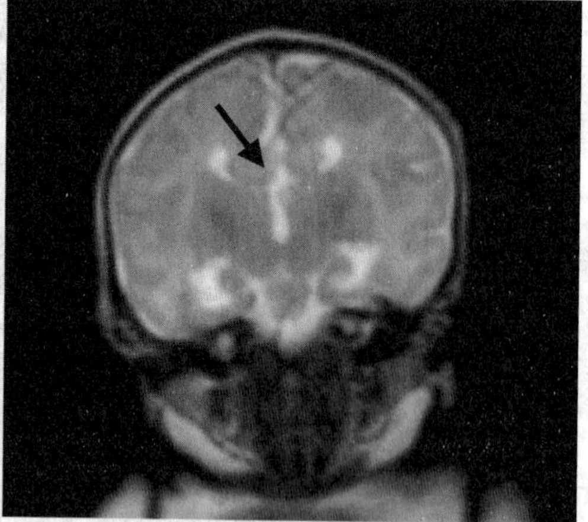

Figure 592-9. Agenesis of the corpus callosum shown on MR images of the brain. Sagittal (left panel) and coronal (right panel) views of an infant show the total absence of a midsagittal white matter structure (left panel *arrows*). The coronal view (right panel) demonstrates (despite some motion artifact) the absence of a structure bridging the two hemispheres (area under *arrow*).

nuclei as well as absent or decreased numbers of muscle fibers has been reported. Affected infants present in the newborn period with facial weakness, causing feeding difficulties due to a poor suck. The immobile, dull facies may give the incorrect impression of mental retardation; the prognosis for normal development is excellent in most cases. The facial appearance of Möbius syndrome has been improved by surgery.

592.10 • Microcephaly

Microcephaly is defined as a head circumference that measures more than three standard deviations below the mean for age and sex. This condition is relatively common, particularly among developmentally delayed children. Although there are many causes of microcephaly, abnormalities in neuronal migration during fetal development, including heterotopias of neuronal cells and cytoarchitectural derangements, are often found. Microcephaly may be subdivided into two main groups: primary (genetic) microcephaly and secondary (nongenetic) microcephaly. A precise diagnosis is important for genetic counseling and for prediction for future pregnancies.

ETIOLOGY. Primary microcephaly refers to a group of conditions that usually have no other malformations and follow a mendelian pattern of inheritance or are associated with a specific genetic syndrome. Affected infants are usually identified at birth because of a small head circumference. The more common types include familial and autosomal dominant microcephaly and a series of chromosomal syndromes that are summarized in Table 592-1. **Secondary** microcephaly results from a large number of noxious agents that may affect a fetus in utero or an infant during periods of rapid brain growth, particularly the 1st 2 yr of life.

CLINICAL MANIFESTATIONS AND DIAGNOSIS. A thorough family history should be taken, seeking additional cases of microcephaly or disorders affecting the nervous system. It is important to measure a patient's head circumference at birth. A very small head circumference implies a process that began early in embryonic or fetal development. An insult to the brain that occurs later in life, particularly beyond the age of 2 yr, is less likely to produce severe microcephaly. Serial head circumference measurements are more meaningful than a single determination, particularly when the abnormality is minimal. The head circumference of each parent and sibling should be recorded.

Laboratory investigation of a microcephalic child is determined by the history and physical examination. If the cause of the microcephaly is unknown, the mother's serum phenylalanine level should be determined. High phenylalanine serum levels in an asymptomatic mother can produce marked brain damage in an otherwise normal nonphenylketonuric infant. A karyotype is obtained if a chromosomal syndrome is suspected or if the child

TABLE 592-1. Causes of Microcephaly

CAUSES	CHARACTERISTIC FINDINGS
PRIMARY (GENETIC)	
1. Familial (autosomal recessive)	• Incidence 1/40,000 births • Typical appearance with slanted forehead, prominent nose and ears; severely mentally retarded and prominent seizures; surface convolutional markings of the brain poorly differentiated and disorganized cytoarchitecture
2. Autosomal dominant	• Nondistinctive facies, upslanting palpebral fissures, mild forehead slanting, and prominent ears • Normal linear growth, seizures readily controlled, and mild or borderline mental retardation
3. Syndromes	
Down (21-trisomy)	• Incidence 1/800 • Abnormal rounding of occipital and frontal lobes and a small cerebellum; narrow superior temporal gyrus, propensity for Alzheimer's neurofibrillary alterations, and ultrastructure abnormalities of cerebral cortex
Edward (18-trisomy)	• Incidence 1/6,500 • Low birthweight, microstomia, micrognathia, low-set malformed ears, prominent occiput, rocker-bottom feet, flexion deformities of fingers, congenital heart disease, increased gyri, heterotopias of neurons
Cri-du-chat (5 p-)	• Incidence 1/50,000 • Round facies, prominent epicanthic folds, low-set ears, hypertelorism, and characteristic cry • No specific neuropathology
Cornelia de Lange	• Prenatal and postnatal growth delay, synophrys, thin downturning upper lip • Proximally placed thumb
Rubinstein-Taybi	• Beaked nose, downward slanting of palpebral fissures, epicanthic folds, short stature with broad thumbs and toes
Smith-Lemli-Opitz	• Ptosis, scaphocephaly, inner epicanthic folds, anteverted nostrils • Low birthweight, marked feeding problems
SECONDARY (NONGENETIC)	
1. Radiation	• Microcephaly and mental retardation most severe if exposure before 15th wk of gestation
2. Congenital infections	
Cytomegalovirus	• Small for dates, petechial rash, hepatosplenomegaly, chorioretinitis, deafness, mental retardation, and seizures • Central nervous system calcification and microgyria
Rubella	• Growth retardation, purpura, thrombocytopenia, hepatosplenomegaly, congenital heart disease, chorioretinitis, cataracts, and deafness • Perivascular necrotic areas, polymicrogyria, heterotopias, subependymal cavitations
Toxoplasmosis	• Purpura, hepatosplenomegaly, jaundice, convulsions, hydrocephalus, chorioretinitis, and cerebral calcification
3. Drugs	
Fetal alcohol	• Growth retardation, ptosis, absent philtrum and hypoplastic upper lip, congenital heart disease, feeding problems, neuroglial heterotopia, and disorganization of neurons
Fetal hydantoin	• Growth delay, hypoplasia of distal phalanges, inner epicanthic folds, broad nasal ridge, and anteverted nostrils
4. Meningitis/encephalitis	• Cerebral infarcts, cystic cavitation, diffuse loss of neurons
5. Malnutrition	• Controversial cause of microcephaly
6. Metabolic	• Maternal diabetes mellitus and maternal hyperphenylalaninemia
7. Hyperthermia	• Significant fever during 1st 4–6 wk has been reported to cause microcephaly, seizures, and facial anomalies • Pathologic studies show neuronal heterotopias • Further studies showed no abnormalities with maternal fever
8. Hypoxic-ischemic encephalopathy	• Initially diffuse cerebral edema; late stages characterized by cerebral atrophy

has abnormal facies, short stature, and additional congenital anomalies. MRI is useful in identifying structural abnormalities of the brain and CT scanning is useful to detect intracerebral calcification. Additional studies include a fasting plasma and urine amino acid analysis; serum ammonia determination; *t*oxoplasmosis, *r*ubella, *c*ytomegalovirus, and *h*erpes simplex (TORCH) titers as well as HIV testing of the mother and child; and a urine sample for the culture of cytomegalovirus.

TREATMENT. Once the cause of microcephaly has been established, the physician must provide accurate and supportive genetic and family counseling. Because many children with microcephaly are also mentally retarded, the physician must assist with placement in an appropriate program that will provide for maximum development of the child (see Chapter 38.2).

Barkovich AJ, Kuzniecky RI, Jackson MD, et al: Classification system for malformations of cortical development. *Neurology* 2001;57:2168–2178.
Barr M, Cohen MM: Holoprosencephaly survival and performance. *Am J Med Genet* 1999;89:116–120.
Clark GD: The classification of cortical dysplasias through molecular genetics. *Brain Dev* 2004;26:351–362.
Denis D, Chateil JF, Brun M, et al: Schizencephaly: Clinical and imaging features in 30 infantile cases. *Brain Dev* 2000;22:475–483.
Donkelaar HJ, Lammens M, Wesseling P, et al: Development and developmental disorders of the human cerebellum. *J Neurol* 2003;250: 1025–1036.
d'Orsi G, Tinuper P, Bisulli F, et al: Clinical features and long term outcome of epilepsy in periventricular nodular heterotopia. Simple compared with plus forms. *J Neurol Neurosurg Psychiatry* 2004;75:873–878.
Hayashi N, Tsutsumi Y, Barkovich AJ: Morphological features and associated anomalies of schizencephaly in the clinical population: Detailed analysis of MR images. *Neuroradiology* 2002;44:418–427.
Hayashi N, Tsutsumi Y, Barkovich AJ: Polymicrogyria without porencephaly/schizencephaly. MRI analysis of the spectrum and the prevalence of macroscopic findings in the clinical population. *Neuroradiology* 2002;44: 647–655.
Kinsman SL, Plawner LL, Hahn JS: Holoprosencephaly: Recent advances and insights. *Curr Opin Neurol* 2000;13:127–132.
Miller SP, Shevell MI, Patenaude Y, et al: Septo-optic dysplasia plus: A spectrum of malformations of cortical development. *Neurology* 2000;54: 1701–1703.
Nerdich JA, Nussbaum RL, Packer TC, et al: Heterogeneity of clinical severity and molecular lesions in Aicardi syndrome. *J Paediatr* 1990;116: 911–917.
Parrish ML, Roessmann U, Levinsohn MW: Agenesis of the corpus callosum: A study of the frequency of associated malformations. *Ann Neurol* 1979;6:349–354.
Richards LJ, Plachez C, Ren T: Mechanisms regulating the development of the corpus callosum and its agenesis in mouse and human. *Clin Genet* 2004;66:276–289.
Sudarshan A, Goldie WD: The spectrum of congenital facial diplegia (Moebius syndrome). *Pediatr Neurol* 1985;1:180–184.
Sztriha L: Spectrum of corpus callosum agenesis. *Pediatr Neurol* 2005;32:94–101.

592.11 • Hydrocephalus

Hydrocephalus is not a specific disease; rather, it represents a diverse group of conditions that result from impaired circulation and absorption of CSF or, in the rare circumstance, from increased production by a choroid plexus papilloma (Table 592-2).

PHYSIOLOGY. The CSF is formed primarily in the ventricular system by the choroid plexus, which is situated in the lateral, 3rd, and 4th ventricles. Although most CSF is produced in the lateral ventricles, ≈25% originates from extrachoroidal sources, including the capillary endothelium within the brain parenchyma. There is active neurogenic control of CSF formation as adrenergic and cholinergic nerves innervate the choroid plexus. Stimulation of the adrenergic system diminishes CSF production, whereas excitation of the cholinergic nerves may double the normal CSF production rate. In a normal child, ≈20 mL/hr of CSF is produced. The total volume of CSF approximates 50 mL in an infant and 150 mL in an adult. Most of the CSF is extraventricular. The choroid plexus forms CSF in several stages; through a series of intricate steps, a plasma ultrafiltrate is ultimately processed into a secretion, the CSF.

CSF flow results from the pressure gradient that exists between the ventricular system and venous channels. Intraventricular pressure may be as high as 180 mm H_2O in the normal state, whereas the pressure in the superior sagittal sinus is in the range of 90 mm H_2O. Normally, CSF flows from the lateral ventricles through the foramina of Monro into the 3rd ventricle. It then traverses the narrow aqueduct of Sylvius, which is ≈3 mm long and 2 mm in diameter in a child, to enter the 4th ventricle. The CSF exits the 4th ventricle through the paired lateral foramina of Luschka and the midline foramen of Magendie into the cisterns at the base of the brain. Hydrocephalus resulting from obstruction within the ventricular system is called **obstructive** or **noncommunicating hydrocephalus.** The CSF circulates from the basal cisterns posteriorly through the cistern system and over the convexities of the cerebral hemispheres. CSF is absorbed primarily by the arachnoid villi through tight junctions of their endothelium by the pressure forces that were noted earlier. CSF is absorbed to a much lesser extent by the lymphatic channels directed to the paranasal sinuses, along nerve root sleeves, and by the choroid plexus itself. Hydrocephalus resulting from obliteration of the subarachnoid cisterns or malfunction of the arachnoid villi is called **nonobstructive** or **communicating hydrocephalus.**

PATHOPHYSIOLOGY AND ETIOLOGY. Obstructive or noncommunicating hydrocephalus develops most commonly in children

TABLE 592-2. Causes of Hydrocephalus

COMMUNICATING
Achondroplasia
Basilar impression
Benign enlargement of subarachnoid space
Choroid plexus papilloma
Meningeal malignancy
Meningitis
Posthemorrhagic
NONCOMMUNICATING
Aqueductal stenosis
Infectious*
X-linked
Chiari malformation
Dandy-Walker malformation
Klippel-Feil syndrome
Mass lesions
Abscess
Hematoma
Tumors and neurocutaneous disorders
Vein of Galen malformation
Walker-Warburg syndrome
HYDRANENCEPHALY
Holoprosencephaly
Massive hydrocephalus
Porencephaly

*Toxoplasmosis, neurocystercicosis mumps.
From Fenichel GM: *Clinical Pediatric Neurology*, 5th ed. Philadelphia, Elsevier, 2005, p 354.

because of an abnormality of the aqueduct or a lesion in the 4th ventricle. **Aqueductal stenosis** results from an abnormally narrow aqueduct of Sylvius that is often associated with branching or forking. In a small percentage of cases, aqueductal stenosis is inherited as a sex-linked recessive trait. These patients occasionally have minor neural tube closure defects, including spina bifida occulta. Rarely, aqueductal stenosis is associated with neurofibromatosis. **Aqueductal gliosis** may also give rise to hydrocephalus. As a result of neonatal meningitis or a subarachnoid hemorrhage in a premature infant, the ependymal lining of the aqueduct is interrupted and a brisk glial response results in complete obstruction. Intrauterine viral infections may also produce aqueductal stenosis followed by hydrocephalus, and mumps meningoencephalitis has been reported as a cause in a child. A vein of Galen malformation can expand to become large and, because of its midline position, obstruct the flow of CSF. Lesions or malformations of the posterior fossa are prominent causes of hydrocephalus, including posterior fossa brain tumors, Chiari malformation, and the Dandy-Walker syndrome.

Nonobstructive or communicating hydrocephalus most commonly follows a subarachnoid hemorrhage, which is usually a result of intraventricular hemorrhage in a premature infant. Blood in the subarachnoid spaces may cause obliteration of the cisterns or arachnoid villi and obstruction of CSF flow. Pneumococcal and tuberculous meningitis have a propensity to produce a thick, tenacious exudate that obstructs the basal cisterns, and intrauterine infections may also destroy the CSF pathways. Finally, leukemic infiltrates may seed the subarachnoid space and produce communicating hydrocephalus.

CLINICAL MANIFESTATIONS. The clinical presentation of hydrocephalus is variable and depends on many factors, including the age at onset, the nature of the lesion causing obstruction, and the duration and rate of increase of the intracranial pressure (ICP). In an infant, an accelerated rate of enlargement of the head is the most prominent sign. In addition, the anterior fontanel is wide open and bulging, and the scalp veins are dilated. The forehead is broad, and the eyes may deviate downward because of impingement of the dilated suprapineal recess on the tectum, producing the setting-sun eye sign. Long-tract signs including brisk tendon reflexes, spasticity, clonus (particularly in the lower extremities), and Babinski sign are common owing to stretching and disruption of the corticospinal fibers originating from the leg region of the motor cortex. In an older child, the cranial sutures are partially closed so that the signs of hydrocephalus may be subtler. Irritability, lethargy, poor appetite, and vomiting are common to both age groups, and headache is a prominent symptom in older patients. A gradual change in personality and a deterioration in academic productivity suggest a slowly progressive form of hydrocephalus. Serial measurements of the head circumference indicate an increased velocity of growth. Percussion of the skull may produce a cracked pot sound or Macewen sign, indicating separation of the sutures. A foreshortened occiput suggests Chiari malformation, and a prominent occiput suggests the Dandy-Walker malformation. Papilledema, abducens nerve palsy, and pyramidal tract signs, which are most evident in the lower extremities, are apparent in most cases.

Chiari malformation consists of two major subgroups. **Type I** typically produces symptoms during adolescence or adult life and is usually not associated with hydrocephalus. Patients complain of recurrent headache, neck pain, urinary frequency, and progressive lower extremity spasticity. The deformity consists of displacement of the cerebellar tonsils into the cervical canal (Fig. 592-10). Although the pathogenesis is unknown, a prevailing theory suggests that obstruction of the caudal portion of the 4th ventricle during fetal development is responsible. Other theories include tethering of the cord or additional anomalies (syrinx). The **type II Chiari** malformation is characterized by progressive hydrocephalus with a myelomeningocele. This lesion represents an anomaly of the hindbrain, probably due to a failure of pontine flexure during embryogenesis, and results in elongation of the 4th ventricle and kinking of the brainstem, with displacement of the inferior vermis, pons, and medulla into the cervical canal (Fig. 592-11). Approximately 10% of type II malformations produce symptoms during infancy, consisting of stridor, weak cry, and apnea, which may be relieved by shunting or by posterior fossa decompression. A more indolent form consists of abnormalities of gait, spasticity, and increasing incoordination during childhood. Plain skull radiographs show a small posterior fossa and a widened cervical canal. CT scanning with contrast and MRI display the cerebellar tonsils protruding downward into the cervical canal and the hindbrain abnormalities. The anomaly is treated by surgical decompression.

The **Dandy-Walker malformation** consists of a cystic expansion of the 4th ventricle in the posterior fossa and midline cerebellar hypoplasia, which results from a developmental failure of the roof of the 4th ventricle during embryogenesis (Fig. 592-12). Approximately 90% of patients have hydrocephalus, and a significant number of children have associated anomalies, including agenesis of the posterior cerebellar vermis and corpus callosum. Infants present with a rapid increase in head size and a prominent occiput. Transillumination of the skull may be positive. Most children have evidence of long-tract signs, cerebellar ataxia, and delayed motor and cognitive milestones, probably due to the associated structural anomalies. The Dandy-Walker malformation is managed by shunting the cystic cavity (and on occasion the ventricles as well) in the presence of hydrocephalus.

DIAGNOSIS AND DIFFERENTIAL DIAGNOSIS. Investigation of a child with hydrocephalus begins with the history. Familial cases suggest X-linked hydrocephalus secondary to aqueductal stenosis. A past history of prematurity with intracranial hemorrhage, meningitis, or mumps encephalitis is important to ascertain. Multiple café-

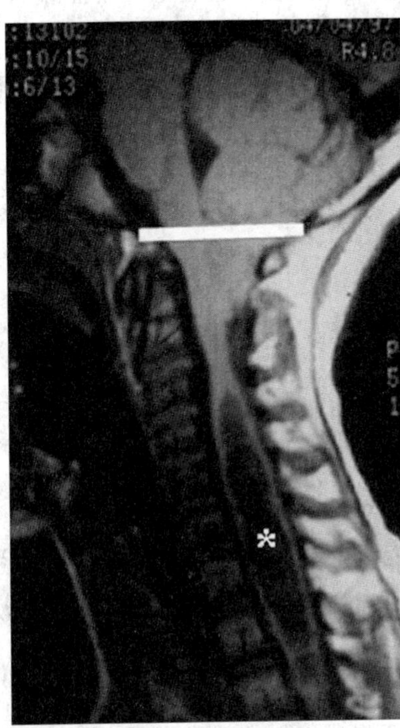

Figure 592-10. Sagittal MR scan of a patient with Chiari malformation type I. Cerebellar tonsils are displaced through the foramen magnum *(white bar)* to the lower aspect of C2 with clear crowding at the foramen. A syrinx *(white asterisk)* is visible extending from C3 to T2. (From Yassari R, Frim D: Evaluation and management of the Chiari malformation type 1 for the primary care pediatrician. *Pediatr Clin North Am* 2004;51:477–490.)

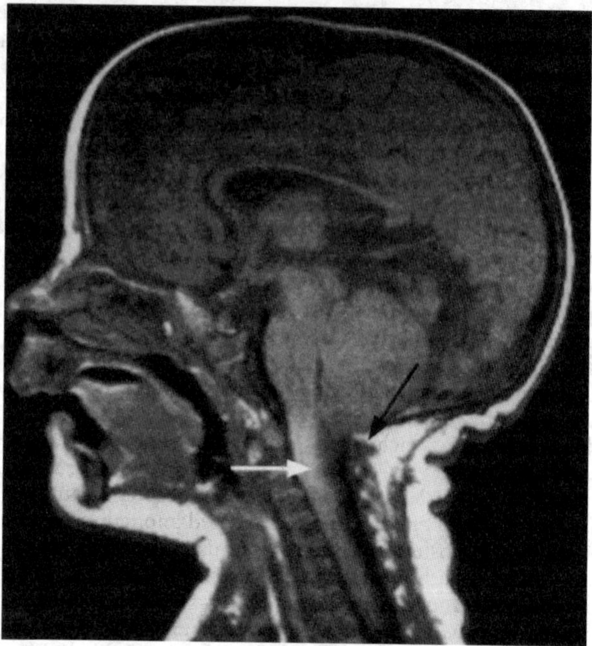

Figure 592-11. A midsagittal T1 weighted MRI of a patient with type II Chiari malformation. The cerebellar tonsils *(white arrow)* have descended below the foramen magnum *(black arrow)*. Note the small slitlike 4th ventricle, which has been pulled into a vertical position.

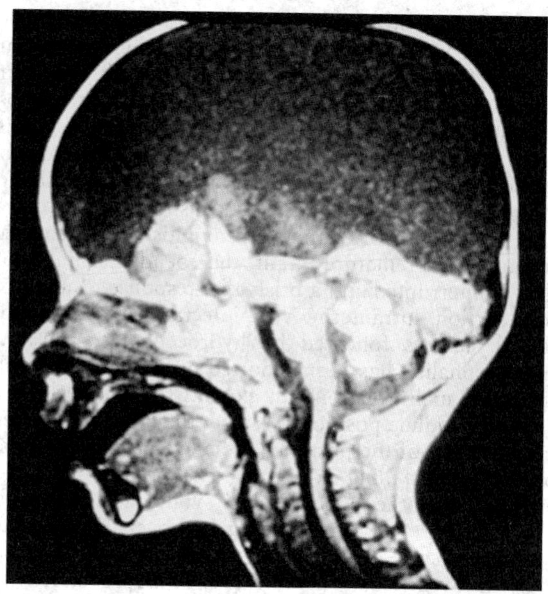

Figure 592-13. Hydranencephaly. MRI scan showing the brainstem and spinal cord with remnants of the cerebellum and the cerebral cortex. The remainder of the cranium is filled with CSF.

au-lait spots and other clinical features of neurofibromatosis point to aqueductal stenosis as the cause of hydrocephalus. Examination includes careful inspection, palpation, and auscultation of the skull and spine. The occipitofrontal head circumference is recorded and compared with previous measurements. The size and configuration of the anterior fontanel are noted, and the back is inspected for abnormal midline skin lesions, including tufts of hair, lipoma, or angioma that might suggest spinal dysraphism. The presence of a prominent forehead or abnormalities in the shape of the occiput may suggest the pathogenesis of the hydrocephalus. A cranial bruit is audible in association with many cases of vein of Galen arteriovenous malformation. Transillumination of the skull is positive with massive dilatation of the ventricular system or in the Dandy-Walker syndrome. Inspection of the eyegrounds is mandatory because the finding of chorioretinitis suggests an intrauterine infection, such as toxoplasmosis, as a cause of the hydrocephalus. Papilledema is observed in older children but is rarely present in infants because the cranial sutures separate as a result of the increased pressure. Plain skull films typically show separation of the sutures, erosion of the posterior clinoids in an older child, and an increase in convolutional markings (beaten-silver appearance) with long-standing increased ICP. The CT scan and/or MRI along with ultrasonography in an infant are the most important studies to identify the specific cause and severity of hydrocephalus.

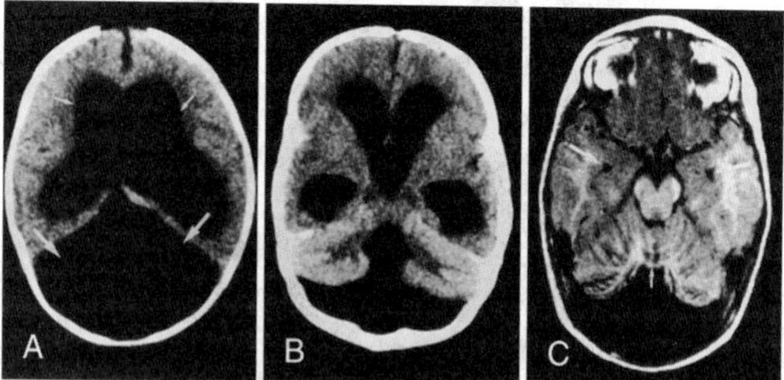

Figure 592-12. Dandy-Walker cyst. *A*, Axial CT scan (preoperative) showing large posterior fossa cyst (Dandy-Walker cyst; *large arrows*) and dilated lateral ventricles *(small arrows)*, a complication secondary to CSF pathway obstruction at the 4th ventricular outlet. *B*, Same patient, with a lower axial CT scan showing splaying of the cerebellar hemispheres by the dilated 4th ventricle (Dandy-Walker cyst). The dilated ventricles proximal to the 4th ventricle again show CSF obstruction due to the Dandy-Walker cyst. *C*, MRI of the same patient showing decreased size of the Dandy-Walker cyst and temporal horns *(arrows)* after shunting. The incomplete vermis *(small arrow)* now becomes recognizable.

The head may appear enlarged and be confused with hydrocephalus secondary to a thickened cranium resulting from chronic anemia, rickets, osteogenesis imperfecta, and epiphyseal dysplasia. Chronic subdural collections can produce bilateral parietal bone prominence. Various metabolic and degenerative disorders of the CNS produce megalencephaly due to abnormal storage of substances within the brain parenchyma. These disorders include lysosomal diseases (Tay-Sachs, gangliosidosis, and the mucopolysaccharidoses), the aminoacidurias (maple syrup urine disease), and the leukodystrophies (metachromatic, Alexander disease, Canavan disease). In addition, cerebral gigantism and neurofibromatosis are characterized by increased brain mass. Familial megalencephaly is inherited as an autosomal dominant trait and is characterized by delayed motor milestones and hypotonia but normal or near-normal intelligence. Measurement of parents' head circumference is necessary to establish the diagnosis.

Hydranencephaly may be confused with hydrocephalus. The cerebral hemispheres are absent or represented by membranous sacs with remnants of frontal, temporal, or occipital cortex dispersed over the membrane. The midbrain and brainstem are relatively intact (Fig. 592-13). The cause of hydranencephaly is unknown, but bilateral occlusion of the internal carotid arteries during early fetal development would explain most of the pathologic abnormalities. Affected infants may have a normal or enlarged head circumference at birth that grows at an excessive rate postnatally. Transillumination shows an absence of the cerebral hemispheres. The child is irritable, feeds poorly, develops seizures and spastic quadriparesis, and has little or no cognitive development. A ventriculoperitoneal shunt prevents massive enlargement of the cranium.

TREATMENT. Therapy for hydrocephalus depends on the cause. Medical management, including the use of acetazolamide and furosemide, may provide temporary relief by reducing the rate of CSF production, but long-term results have been disappointing. Most cases of hydrocephalus require extracranial shunts, particularly a ventriculoperitoneal shunt (occasionally a ventriculostomy suffices). The major complications of shunting are occlusion (characterized by headache, papilledema, emesis, mental status changes) and bacterial infection (fever, headache, meningismus), usually due to *Staphylococcus epidermidis* (see Chapter 180). With meticulous preparation, the shunt infection rate can be reduced to <5%. The results of intrauterine surgical management of fetal hydrocephalus have been poor, possibly because of the high rate of associated cerebral malformations in addition to the hydrocephalus.

PROGNOSIS. This depends on the cause of the dilated ventricles and not on the size of the cortical mantle at the time of operative intervention, except in cases in which the cortical mantle has been severely compressed and stretched. Hydrocephalic children are at increased risk for various developmental disabilities. The mean intelligence quotient is reduced compared with the general population, particularly for performance tasks as compared with verbal abilities. Many children have abnormalities in memory function. Visual problems are common, including strabismus, visuospatial abnormalities, visual field defects, and optic atrophy with decreased acuity secondary to increased ICP. The visual-evoked potential latencies are delayed and take some time to recover after correction of the hydrocephalus. Although most hydrocephalic children are pleasant and mild mannered, some children show aggressive and delinquent behavior. Accelerated pubertal development in patients with shunted hydrocephalus or myelomeningocele is relatively common, possibly because of increased gonadotropin secretion in response to increased ICP. It is imperative that hydrocephalic children receive long-term follow-up in a multidisciplinary setting.

Chumas P, Tyagi A, Livingston J: Hydrocephalus—What's new? *Arch Dis Child Fetal Neonatal Ed* 2001;85:F149–F154.

Cochrane DD, Myles ST, Nimrod C, et al: Intrauterine hydrocephalus and ventriculomegaly: Associated abnormalities and fetal outcome. *Can J Neurol Sci* 1985;12:51–59.

Fitzsimmons JS: Laryngeal stridor and respiratory obstruction in association with myelomeningocele. *Dev Med Child Neurol* 1973;15:553–556.

Greene M, Benacerraf B, Crawford J: Hydranencephaly: US appearance during in utero evolution. *Radiology* 1985;156:779–780.

Hirsch JF, Pierre-Kahn A, Renier D, et al: The Dandy-Walker malformation. *J Neurosurg* 1984;61:515–522.

Hoffman HJ, Hendrick EB, Humphreys RP: Manifestations and management of Arnold-Chiari malformations in patients with myelomeningocele. *Childs Brain* 1975;1:255–259.

Löppönen T, Saukkonen A-L, Serlo W, et al: Accelerated pubertal development in patients with shunted hydrocephalus. *Arch Dis Child* 1996;74:490–496.

Parisi MA, Dobyns WB: Human malformations of the midbrain and hindbrain: Review and proposed classification scheme. *Mol Genet Metab* 2003;80:36–53.

592.12 • Craniosynostosis

Craniosynostosis is defined as premature closure of the cranial sutures and is classified as primary or secondary. **Primary craniosynostosis** refers to closure of one or more sutures due to abnormalities of skull development, whereas **secondary craniosynostosis** results from failure of brain growth and expansion and is not discussed here. The incidence of primary craniosynostosis approximates 1/2,000 births. The cause is unknown in the majority of children; however, genetic syndromes account for 10–20% of cases.

TABLE 592-3. Commonly Used Clinical Genetic Classifications of Craniosynostoses

DIAGNOSTIC CATEGORY	NAME OF DISORDER	CAUSE
Isolated craniosynostosis	Morphologically described	Unknown, uterine constraint, or *FGFR*$_3$ mutation
Syndromic craniosynostosis	Antler-Bixler syndrome	Unknown
	Apert syndrome	Usually one of two mutations in *FGFR*$_2$
	Baere-Stevenson syndrome	Mutation in *GFGR*$_2$ or *FGFR*$_3$
	Bailler-Gerold syndrome	Mutation in *TWIST* heterogenous
	Carpenter syndrome	Unknown
	Craniofrontonasal dysplasia	Unknown gene at Xp22
	Crouzon syndrome	Numerous different mutations at *FGFR*$_2$
	Crouzonomesodermoskeletal syndrome	Mutation in *FGFR*$_3$
	Jackson-Weiss syndrome	Mutation in *FGFR*$_2$
	Muenke syndrome	Mutation in *FGFR*$_3$
	Pfeiffer syndrome	Mutation in *FGFR*$_1$ or numerous mutation in *FGFR*$_2$
	Saethre-Chotzen syndrome	Mutation in *TWIST*
	Shprintzen-Goldberg syndrome	Mutation in *FBEN*$_1$

From Ridgway EB, Weiner HL: Skull deformaties. *Pediatr Clin North Am* 2004;51:359–387.

DEVELOPMENT AND ETIOLOGY. During early development, a film of mesenchyme envelops the brain. By the 2nd mo, osseous tissue is evident in that portion of the mesenchyme corresponding to the cranium, and cartilaginous tissue is formed at the base of the skull. The bones of the cranium are well developed by the 5th mo of gestation (frontal, parietal, temporal, and occipital) and are separated by sutures and fontanels. The brain grows rapidly in the 1st several years of life and is normally not impeded because of equivalent growth along the suture lines. The cause of craniosynostosis is unknown, but the prevailing hypothesis suggests that abnormal development of the base of the skull creates exaggerated forces on the dura that act to disrupt normal cranial suture development. Genetic factors have been identified for some isolated and many syndromic causes of craniosynostosis (Table 592-3).

CLINICAL MANIFESTATIONS AND TREATMENT. Most cases of craniosynostosis are evident at birth and are characterized by a skull deformity that is a direct result of premature suture fusion. Palpation of the suture reveals a prominent bony ridge, and fusion of the suture may be confirmed by plain skull roentgenograms or bone scan in ambiguous cases (Table 592-4).

Premature closure of the sagittal suture produces a long and narrow skull, or **scaphocephaly**, the most common form of craniosynostosis. Scaphocephaly is associated with a prominent occiput, a broad forehead, and a small or absent anterior fontanel. The condition is sporadic, more common in males, and often causes difficulties during labor because of cephalopelvic disproportion. Scaphocephaly does not produce increased ICP or hydrocephalus, and results of neurologic examination of affected patients are normal.

Frontal plagiocephaly is the next most common form of craniosynostosis and is characterized by unilateral flattening of the forehead, elevation of the ipsilateral orbit and eyebrow, and a prominent ear on the corresponding side. The condition is more common in females and is the result of premature fusion of a

TABLE 592-4. Epidemiology and Clinical Characteristics of the Common Craniosynostoses

TYPE	EPIDEMIOLOGY	SKULL DEFORMITY	CLINICAL PRESENTATION
Sagittal	Most common CSO affecting a single suture, 80% male	Dolicocephaly or scaphocephaly (boat-shaped)	Frontal bossing, prominent occiput, palpable keel ridge. OFC normal and reduced biparietal diameter
Coronal	18% of CSO, more common in females Associated with Apert syndrome (with syndactly) and Crouzon disease which includes abnormal sphenoid, orbital, and facial bones (hypoplasia of the midface)	Unilateral: plagiocephaly Bilateral: brachycephaly, acrocephaly	Unilateral: flattened forehead on affected side, flat checks, nose deviation on normal side, higher supraorbital margin lead to harlequin sign on radiograph and outward rotation of orbit may result in amblyopia Bilateral: broad, flattened forehead. In Apert syndrome accompanied by syndactyly and in Crouzon disease by hypoplasia of the midface and progressive proptosis
Lambdoid	10–20% of CSO, M : F ratio 4 : 1	Lambdoid/occipital plagiocephaly; right side affected in 70% of cases	Unilateral: flattening of occiput, indentation along synostotic suture, bulging of ipsilateral forehead leading to rhomboid skull, ipsilateral ear is anterior and inferior Bilateral: brachycephaly with bilateral anteriorly and inferiorly displaced ears
Metopic	Association with 19p chromosome abnormality	Trigoncephaly	Pointed forehead and midline ridge, hypotelorism
Multiple		Oxycephaly	Tower skull with undeveloped sinuses and shallow orbits, and elevated intercranial pressure

CSO, craniosynostosis; OFC, occipital-frontal circumference.
From Ridgway EB, Weiner HL: Skull deformities. *Pediatr Clin North Am* 2004;51:359–387.

coronal and sphenofrontal suture. Surgical intervention produces a cosmetically pleasing result.

Occipital plagiocephaly is most often a result of positioning during infancy and is more common in an immobile or handicapped child, but fusion or sclerosis of the lambdoid suture can cause unilateral occipital flattening and bulging of the ipsilateral frontal bone. **Trigonocephaly** is a rare form of craniosynostosis due to premature fusion of the metopic suture. These children have a keel-shaped forehead and hypotelorism and are at risk for associated developmental abnormalities of the forebrain. **Turricephaly** refers to a cone-shaped head due to premature fusion of the coronal and often sphenofrontal and frontoethmoidal sutures. The **kleeblattschädel deformity** is a peculiarly shaped skull that resembles a cloverleaf. Affected children have very prominent temporal bones, and the remainder of the cranium is constricted. Hydrocephalus is a common complication.

Premature fusion of only one suture rarely causes a neurologic deficit. In this situation, the sole indication for surgery is to enhance the child's cosmetic appearance, and the prognosis depends on the suture involved and on the degree of disfigurement. Neurologic complications, including hydrocephalus and increased ICP, are more likely to occur when two or more sutures are prematurely fused, in which case operative intervention is essential.

The most prevalent genetic disorders associated with craniosynostosis include Crouzon, Apert, Carpenter, Chotzen, and Pfeiffer syndromes. **Crouzon syndrome** is characterized by premature craniosynostosis and is inherited as an autosomal dominant trait. The shape of the head depends on the timing and order of suture fusion but most often is a compressed back-to-front diameter or brachycephaly due to bilateral closure of the coronal sutures. The orbits are underdeveloped, and ocular proptosis is prominent. Hypoplasia of the maxilla and orbital hypertelorism are typical facial features.

Apert syndrome has many features in common with Crouzon syndrome. Apert syndrome is usually a sporadic condition, although autosomal dominant inheritance may occur. It is associated with premature fusion of multiple sutures, including the coronal, sagittal, squamosal, and lambdoid sutures. The facies tend to be asymmetric, and the eyes are less proptotic than in Crouzon syndrome. Apert syndrome is characterized by syndactyly of the 2nd, 3rd, and 4th fingers, which may be joined to the thumb and the 5th finger. Similar abnormalities often occur in the feet. All patients have progressive calcification and fusion of the bones of the hands, feet, and cervical spine.

Carpenter syndrome is inherited as an autosomal recessive condition, and the many fusions of sutures tend to produce the kleeblattschädel skull deformity. Soft tissue syndactyly of the hands and feet is always present, and mental retardation is common. Additional but less common abnormalities include congenital heart disease, corneal opacities, coxa valga, and genu valgum.

Chotzen syndrome is characterized by asymmetric craniosynostosis and plagiocephaly. The condition is the most prevalent of the genetic syndromes and is inherited as an autosomal dominant trait. It is associated with facial asymmetry, ptosis of the eyelids, shortened fingers, and soft tissue syndactyly of the 2nd and 3rd fingers.

Pfeiffer syndrome is most often associated with turricephaly. The eyes are prominent and widely spaced, and the thumbs and great toes are short and broad. Partial soft tissue syndactyly may be evident. Most cases appear to be sporadic, but autosomal dominant inheritance has been reported.

Mutations of the fibroblast growth factor receptor (FGFR) gene family have been shown to be associated with phenotypically specific types of craniosynostosis. Mutations of the $FGFR_1$ gene located on chromosome 8 result in Pfeiffer syndrome; a similar mutation of the $FGFR_2$ gene causes Apert syndrome. Identical mutations of the $FGFR_2$ gene may result in both Pfeiffer and Crouzon phenotypes.

Each of the genetic syndromes poses a risk of additional anomalies, including hydrocephalus, increased ICP, papilledema, optic atrophy due to abnormalities of the optic foramina, respiratory problems secondary to a deviated nasal septum or choanal atresia, and disorders of speech and deafness. Craniectomy is mandatory for management of increased ICP, and a multidisciplinary craniofacial team is essential for the long-term follow-up of affected children. Craniosynostosis may be surgically corrected with good outcomes and relatively low morbidity and mortality, especially for nonsyndromic infants.

Losee JE, Mason AC: Deformational plagiocephaly: Diagnosis, prevention, and treatment. *Clin Plast Surg* 2005;32:53–64.

Ridgway EB, Weiner HL: Skull deformities. *Pediatr Clin North Am* 2004;51:359–387.

Rutland P, Pulleyn LJ, Reardon W, et al: Identical mutations in the $FGFR_2$ gene cause both Pfeiffer and Crouzon syndrome phenotypes. *Nat Genet* 1995;9:173–176.

Sloan GM, Wells KC, Raffel C, et al: Surgical treatment of craniosynostosis: Outcome analysis of 250 consecutive patients. *Pediatrics* 1997;100:E2.

Speltz ML, Kapp-Simon KA, Cunningham M, et al: Single-suture craniosynostosis: A review of neurobehavioral research and theory. *J Pediatr Psychol* 2004;29(8):651–668.

Yassari R, Frim D: Evaluation and management of the Chiari malformation type 1 for the primary care pediatrician. *Pediatr Clin North Am* 2004;51:477–490.

Chapter 593 ■ Seizures in Childhood

Michael V. Johnston

A seizure or convulsion is a paroxysmal, time-limited change in motor activity and/or behavior that results from abnormal electrical activity in the brain. Seizures are common in the pediatric age group and occur in ≈10% of children. Most seizures in children are provoked by somatic disorders originating outside the brain, such as high fever, infection, syncope, head trauma, hypoxia, toxins, or cardiac arrhythmias. Other events, such as breath-holding spells and gastroesophageal reflux, can cause events that simulate seizures (see Chapter 594). A few children also exhibit pseudoseizures of psychiatric origin. Less than one third of seizures in children are caused by **epilepsy,** a condition in which seizures are triggered recurrently from within the brain. For epidemiologic classification purposes, epilepsy is considered to be present when two or more unprovoked seizures occur at an interval greater than 24 hr apart. The cumulative lifetime incidence of epilepsy is 3%; more than half of cases begin in childhood. The annual prevalence of epilepsy is lower (0.5–0.8%) because many children outgrow epilepsy. Although the outlook for most children with symptomatic seizures or those associated with epilepsy is generally good, seizures may signal a potentially serious underlying systemic or central nervous system (CNS) disorder that requires thorough investigation and management. For children with epilepsy, the prognosis is generally good, but 10–20% have persistent seizures refractory to drugs, and those cases pose a diagnostic and management challenge.

EVALUATION OF THE FIRST SEIZURE. Initial evaluation of an infant or child during or shortly after a suspected seizure should include an assessment of the adequacy of the airway, ventilation, and cardiac function as well as measurement of temperature, blood pressure, and glucose concentration. For acute evaluation of the 1st seizure, the physician should search for potentially life-threatening causes of seizures such as meningitis, systemic sepsis, unintentional and intentional head trauma, and ingestion of drugs of abuse and other toxins. The history should attempt to define factors that may have promoted the convulsion and to provide a detailed description of the seizure and the child's postictal state. Most parents vividly recall their child's initial convulsion and can describe it in detail.

The 1st step in an evaluation is to determine whether the seizure has a focal onset or is generalized. **Focal seizures** may be characterized by motor or sensory symptoms and include forceful turning of the head and eyes to one side, unilateral clonic movements beginning in the face or extremities, or a sensory disturbance such as paresthesias or pain localized to a specific area. Focal seizures in an adolescent or adult usually indicate a localized lesion, but investigation of focal seizures during childhood may be nondiagnostic. Focal seizures in a neonate may be seen in perinatal stroke. Motor seizures may be focal or generalized and tonic-clonic, tonic, clonic, myoclonic, or atonic. **Tonic seizures** are characterized by increased tone or rigidity, and **atonic seizures** are characterized by flaccidity or lack of movement during a convulsion. **Clonic seizures** consist of rhythmic muscle contraction and relaxation; **myoclonus** is most accurately described as shocklike contraction of a muscle. The duration of the seizure and state of consciousness (retained or impaired) should be documented. The history should determine whether an **aura** preceded the convulsion and the behavior of the child immediately preceding the seizure. The most common aura experienced by children consists of epigastric discomfort or pain and a feeling of fear. The posture of the patient, presence and distribution of cyanosis, vocalizations, loss of sphincter control (particularly of the urinary bladder), and postictal state (including sleep, headache, and hemiparesis) should be noted.

In addition to the assessment of cardiorespiratory and metabolic status described, examination of a child with a seizure disorder should be geared toward the search for an organic cause. The child's head circumference, length, and weight are plotted on a growth chart and compared with previous measurements. A careful general and neurologic examination should be performed. The **eyegrounds** must be examined for the presence of papilledema, retinal hemorrhages, chorioretinitis, coloboma, and macular changes, as well as retinal phakoma. The finding of unusual facial features or associated physical findings such as hepatosplenomegaly point to an underlying metabolic or storage disease as the cause of the neurologic disorder. Positive results of a search for vitiliginous lesions of tuberous sclerosis using an ultraviolet light source and examination for adenoma sebaceum, shagreen patch, multiple café-au-lait spots, a nevus flammeus, and the presence of retinal phakoma indicate a **neurocutaneous** disorder as the cause of the seizure.

Localizing neurologic signs such as a subtle **hemiparesis** with hyperreflexia, an equivocal Babinski sign, and a downward-drifting extended arm with eyes closed might suggest a contralateral hemispheric structural lesion, such as a slow-growing temporal lobe glioma, as the cause of the seizure disorder. Unilateral growth arrest of the thumbnail, hand, or extremity in a child with a focal seizure disorder suggests a chronic condition such as a porencephalic cyst, arteriovenous malformation, or cortical atrophy in the opposite hemisphere.

593.1 • FEBRILE SEIZURES

Febrile convulsions, the most common seizure disorder during childhood, generally have an excellent prognosis but may also signify a serious underlying acute infectious disease such as sepsis or bacterial meningitis. Therefore, each child with a seizure associated with fever must be carefully examined and appropriately investigated for the cause of the fever (see Chapter 175), especially when it is the 1st seizure. Febrile seizures are age dependent and are rare before 9 mo and after 5 yr of age. The peak age of onset is ≈14–18 mo of age, and the incidence approaches 3–4% of young children. A strong family history of febrile convulsions in siblings and parents suggests a genetic predisposition. Linkage studies in several large families have mapped the febrile seizure gene to chromosomes 19p and 8q13–21. An autosomal dominant inheritance pattern is demonstrated in some families.

CLINICAL MANIFESTATIONS. A simple febrile convulsion is usually associated with a core temperature that increases rapidly to ≥39°C. It is initially generalized and tonic-clonic in nature, lasts a few seconds and rarely up to 15 min, is followed by a brief postictal period of drowsiness, and occurs only once in 24 hr. A febrile seizure is described as complex or complicated when the duration is >15 min, when repeated convulsions occur within 24 hr, or when focal seizure activity or focal findings are present during the postictal period. Some children have a chronic seizure disorder with more seizures during fever. These are not febrile seizures, but are referred to as seizures with fever. Convulsive status epilepticus (one seizure lasting 30 min or multiple seizures during 30 min without regaining consciousness) is often due to central nervous system infection (viral or bacterial meningitis).

Approximately 30–50% of children have **recurrent seizures** with later episodes of fever and a small minority has numerous recurrent febrile seizures. Factors associated with increased recurrence risk include age <12 mo, lower temperature before seizure onset, a positive family history of febrile seizures, and complex features. Febrile seizures are not associated with reduction in later intellectual performance, and most children with febrile seizures have only a slightly greater risk of later epilepsy than the general population. Factors that are associated with a substantially greater risk of later epilepsy include the presence of complex features during the seizure or postictal period, a positive family history of epilepsy, an initial febrile seizure before 12 mo of age, delayed developmental milestones, or a pre-existing neurologic disorder. The risk of epilepsy is much higher than in the general population in children with one or more complex febrile seizures, especially if the seizures are focal in children with an underlying neurologic disorder. The incidence of epilepsy is >9% when several risk factors are present, compared with an incidence of 1% in children who have febrile convulsions and no risk factors.

During the acute evaluation, a physician's most important responsibility is to determine the cause of the fever and to rule out meningitis or encephalitis. *If any doubt exists about the possibility of meningitis, a lumbar puncture with examination of the cerebrospinal fluid (CSF) is indicated.* A lumbar puncture should be strongly considered in children <12 mo of age and considered in those 12–18 mo of age, especially if seizures are complex or sensorium remains clouded after a short postictal period.

Seizure-induced CSF abnormalities are rare in children and all patients with abnormal CSF after a seizure should be thoroughly evaluated for causes other than seizure. The possibility of viral meningoencephalitis should also be kept in mind, especially that caused by herpes simplex. Viral infections of the upper respiratory tract, roseola (and nonroseola human herpes virus 6 and 7 infections), and acute otitis media are most frequently the causes of febrile convulsions.

Aside from glucose determination, laboratory testing such as serum electrolytes and toxicology screening should be ordered based on individual clinical circumstances such as evidence of dehydration. An electroencephalogram (EEG) is not warranted after a simple febrile seizure but may be useful for evaluating patients with complex or atypical features or with other risk factors for later epilepsy. Similarly, neuroimaging is also not useful for children with simple febrile convulsions, but may be considered for children with atypical features, including focal neurologic signs or pre-existing neurologic deficits.

TREATMENT. Routine management of a normal infant with simple brief febrile convulsions includes a careful search for the cause of the fever and reassurance and education of the parents. Although antipyretics have not been shown to prevent seizure recurrences, active measures to control the fever, including the use of antipyretics, may reduce discomfort and are reassuring. In a setting where support for ventilation can be provided, consideration should be given to treating seizures lasting >5 min with a benzodiazepine as a first-line therapy as described in Chapter 593.8. Prolonged anticonvulsant prophylaxis for preventing recurrent febrile convulsions is controversial and no longer recommended for most children. Antiepileptics such as phenytoin and carbamazepine do not prevent febrile seizures. Phenobarbital prevents recurrent febrile seizures but may also decrease cognitive function in treated children compared with untreated children. Sodium valproate is also effective for prevention of febrile seizures, but the potential risks of the drug do not justify its use in a disorder with an excellent prognosis regardless of treatment. The incidence of fatal valproate-induced hepatotoxicity is highest in children <2 yr of age. If parental anxiety is very high, oral diazepam may be used as an effective and safe method of reducing the risk of recurrence of febrile seizures. At the onset of each febrile illness, oral diazepam, 0.3 mg/kg q8h (1 mg/kg/24 hr), is administered for the duration of the illness (usually 2–3 days). The side effects are usually minor, but symptoms of lethargy, irritability, and ataxia may be reduced by adjusting the dose. Another approach for selected patients with recurrent complex febrile seizures is to prescribe diazepam in the form of a gel that can be given rectally at the time of a seizure in a dose of approximately 0.5 mg/kg for children aged 2–5 yr. This will usually terminate the seizure and prevent recurrence over 12 hr. Preventive anticonvulsant treatment or treatment after the seizure has not been shown to reduce the risk of later epilepsy in higher risk patients.

593.2 • Unprovoked Seizures

FIRST SEIZURE. Although the occurrence of a seizure in a child without a provocative stimulus such as high fever is often considered a harbinger of a chronic seizure disorder or epilepsy, less than half of these children go on to develop a 2nd seizure. A careful history is warranted to ascertain a potential family history of epilepsy, a prior neurologic disorder, or history of seizure with fever, which may increase the likelihood of recurrence. Laboratory testing of serum electrolytes, toxicology screening, or urine and serum metabolic testing should be chosen based on individual clinical circumstances rather than on a routine basis. Serum glucose should be evaluated with the 1st afebrile seizure. In the child with a 1st nonfebrile seizure, a lumbar puncture is of limited value and should be used primarily when there is concern about possible meningitis, encephalitis, sepsis, subarachnoid hemorrhage, or a demyelinating disorder. An **EEG** is recommended as part of the neurodiagnostic evaluation of the child with an apparent 1st unprovoked seizure because it is useful for diagnosis of the event, prediction of recurrence risk, and identification of specific focal abnormalities and/or epileptic syndromes. **Neuroimaging** is generally not recommended after a 1st unprovoked seizure unless there is an indication for it on neurologic examination (focal neurologic deficits). If it is obtained, however, MRI of the brain is recommended over CT scanning. Anticonvulsant medication is generally not recommended after a single seizure. MRI may also be indicated in infants and adolescents with their 1st seizure.

RECURRENT SEIZURES. Two unprovoked seizures >24 hr apart suggest the presence of an epileptic disorder within the brain that will lead to future recurrences. It is important to perform a careful evaluation to look for the cause of the seizures as well as to assess the need for treatment with antiepileptic drugs and estimate the potential for response to treatment and remission of seizures in the future.

The **history** can provide important information about the type of seizures. Some parents can precisely act out or recreate a seizure. Children who have a propensity to develop epilepsy may experience the 1st convulsion in association with a viral illness or a low-grade fever. Seizures that occur during the early morning hours or with drowsiness, particularly during the initial phase of sleep, are common in childhood epilepsy. In retrospect, irritability, mood swings, headache, and subtle personality changes may precede a seizure by several days. Some parents can accurately predict the timing of the next seizure on the basis of changes in the child's disposition. The physical portrayal of the convulsion by the parent or caregiver is often surprisingly similar to the actual convulsion and is much more accurate than the verbal description. Aside from the description of the seizure pattern, the frequency, time of day, precipitating factors, and alternation in the type of convulsive disorder are important. Although generalized tonic-clonic seizures are readily documented, the frequency of absence seizures is often underestimated by parents. A prolonged personality change or intellectual deterioration may suggest a **degenerative disease** of the CNS, whereas constitutional symptoms, including vomiting and failure to thrive, might indicate a primary metabolic disorder or a structural lesion. It is essential to obtain details of prior anticonvulsant medication and the child's response to the regimen and to determine whether drugs that may potentiate seizures, including chlorpromazine or methylphenidate, were prescribed. The description of the seizure

TABLE 593-1. Identified Genes for Epilepsy

	FUNCTION	LOCUS	EPILEPSY SYNDROME	SEIZURE TYPES
GABRA1 GABA$_A$, α1 receptor subunit	Partial inhibition of GABA-activated currents	5q34	AD JME	TCS, mycolonic, absence
GABRG2 GABA$_A$, receptor γ2 subunit	Rapid inhibition of GABAergic neurons	5q31	FS, CAE, GEFS$^+$	Febrile, absence, TCS, myoclonic, clonic, partial
GABRD GABAA receptor δ2 subunit	Decreased GABAA receptor current amplitudes	1p36	GEFS$^-$	Febrile and afebrile seizures
SCN2A Sodium channel α2 subunit	Fast sodium influx initiation and propagation of action potential	2q24	GEFS$^-$ BFNIC	Febrile, afebrile generalized tonic and TCS
SCN1A Sodium channel α1 subunit	Somatodendritic sodium influx	2q24	GEFS$^-$ SMEI	Febrile, absence, myoclonic, TCS, partial
SCN1B Sodium channel β1 subunit	Coadjuvate and modulate α subunit	19q13	GEFS$^-$	Febrile, absence, tonic clonic, myoclonic.
KCNQ2 Potassium channel	M current interacts with *KCNQ3*	20q13	BFNC	Neonatal convulsions
KCNQ3 Potassium channel	M current interacts with *KCNQ2*	8q24	BFNC	Neonatal convulsions
ATP1A2 Na^1, K^1-ATPase pump	Dysfunction of ion transportation	1q23	BFNIC and familial hemiplegic migraine	Infantile convulsions
CHRNA4 Acetylcholine receptor α4 subunit	Nicotinic current modulation; interacts with β2 subunit	20q13	ADNFLE	Sleep-related focal seizures
CHRNB2 Acetylcholine receptor β2 subunit	Nicotinic current modulation; interacts with α4 subunit	1p21	ADNFLE	Sleep-related focal seizures
LGI1 Leucine-rich, glioma activated	Disregulates homeostasis, interactions between neurons and glia?	10q24	ADPEAF	Partial seizures with auditory or visual hallucinations
CLCN2 Voltage-gated chloride channel	Neuronal chloride efflux	3q26	IGE	TCS, myoclonic, absence
EFHC1 Protein with an EF-hand motif	Reduced mouse hippocampal induced apoptosis	6p12-p11	JME	TCS, myoclonic
BRD2 (*RING3*) Nuclear transcriptional regulator	?	6p21	JME	TCS, myoclonic

AD, autosomal dominant; ADNFLE, autosomal dominant nocturnal frontal lobe epilepsy; ADPEAF, autosomal dominant partial epilepsy with auditory features; BFNC, benign familial neonatal convulsions; BFNIC, benign familial neonatal-infantile convulsion; GEFS$^+$, generalized epilepsy with febrile seizures plus; JME, juvenile myoclonic epilepsy; MAE, myoclonic astatic epilepsy; SMEI, severe myolconic epilepsy of infancy; TCS, tonic-clonic seizures; XL, X-linked.

From Guerrini R: Epilepsy in children. *Lancet* 2006;367:499–524.

along with the family history can provide clues to the presence of possible genetic epileptic syndromes (Table 593-1). These include autosomal dominant nocturnal frontal lobe epilepsy, familial benign neonatal convulsions, familial benign infantile convulsions, autosomal dominant febrile seizures, partial epilepsy with auditory symptoms, autosomal dominant frontal lobe progressive epilepsy with mental retardation, absence epilepsy, and febrile seizures with later partial complex seizures.

The physical, ophthalmologic, and neurologic examination can provide information about the presence of increased intracranial pressure, neurocutaneous syndromes, and structural brain abnormalities including malformations, injuries, infections, or tumors.

The **EEG** is indicated in all cases of epilepsy and is useful for determining the type of epilepsy and the future prognosis. Measurement of serum electrolytes including calcium and magnesium is not recommended as a routine practice. Metabolic testing, including administration of pyridoxine or pyridoxal phosphate for suspected pyridoxine-responsive seizures, serum lactate and pyruvate, and urine organic acids, is also not recommended routinely but should be dictated by clinical circumstances. Lumbar puncture should be considered for children with repeated seizures and other evidence of neurodevelopmental disability. It may be useful for detecting low CSF glucose in the glucose transporter disorder; alterations in amino acids, neurotransmitters, or cofactors in metabolic disorders; or evidence of chronic infection. Neuroimaging with MRI is indicated during the evaluation of children with newly diagnosed epilepsy, especially for those with neurologic deficits, partial seizures, or focal EEG abnormalities that are not part of an idiopathic localization-related epilepsy syndrome. In some cases, an electrocardiogram may be warranted to rule out prolonged QT syndrome, which can, though rarely, cause seizures and syncope (see Chapter 594).

CLASSIFICATION OF SEIZURES. It is important to classify the type of seizure (Table 593-2). The seizure type may provide a clue to the cause of the seizure disorder. Precise delineation of the seizure may allow a firm basis for making a prognosis and choosing the most appropriate treatment. Anticonvulsants may readily control generalized tonic-clonic epilepsy in a child, but a patient with multiple seizure types or partial seizures may fare less well with

TABLE 593-2. International Classification of Epileptic Seizures

PARTIAL SEIZURES
- Simple partial (consciousness retained)
  - Motor
  - Sensory
  - Autonomic
  - Psychic
- Complex partial (consciousness impaired)
  - Simple partial, followed by impaired consciousness
  - Consciousness impaired at onset
- Partial seizures with secondary generalization

GENERALIZED SEIZURES
- Absences
  - Typical
  - Atypical
- Generalized tonic-clonic
- Tonic
- Clonic
- Myoclonic
- Atonic
- Infantile spasms

UNCLASSIFIED SEIZURES

the same type of therapy. Infants with benign myoclonic epilepsy have a more favorable outlook than patients with infantile spasms. Similarly, a school-aged child who has benign partial epilepsy with centrotemporal spikes (rolandic epilepsy) has an excellent prognosis and is unlikely to require a prolonged course of anticonvulsants. Clinical classification of seizures may be difficult because the manifestations of different seizure types may be similar. The clinical features of a child with absence seizures may be almost identical to those of another patient with complex partial epilepsy. An EEG is a useful adjunct to the classification of epilepsy because of the variability of seizure expressivity in this age group.

Epilepsy in children has also been classified by syndrome (Table 593-3). Using the age at onset of seizures, cognitive development and neurologic examination, description of seizure type, and EEG findings, including the background rhythm, it has been possible to classify ≈50% of childhood seizures into specific syndromes. The syndromic classification of seizures provides a distinct advantage over previous classifications by improving management with appropriate anticonvulsant medication, identifying potential candidates for epilepsy surgery, and providing patients and families with a reliable and accurate prognosis. Examples of epilepsy syndromes include infantile spasms (West syndrome), benign myoclonic epilepsy of infancy, the Lennox-Gastaut syndrome, febrile convulsions, Landau-Kleffner syndrome, benign childhood epilepsy with centrotemporal spikes (rolandic epilepsy), Rasmussen encephalitis, juvenile myoclonic epilepsy (Janz syndrome), and Lafora disease (progressive myoclonic epilepsy). Certain syndromes have a more favorable outcome (Table 593-4).

TABLE 593-3. Classification of Epilepsies and Epileptic Syndromes

LOCALIZATION-RELATED (FOCAL, PARTIAL) EPILEPSIES

Idiopathic
- Benign childhood epilepsy with centrotemporal spikes
- Childhood epilepsy with occipital paroxysms

Symptomatic
- The subclassification is determined by the anatomic location suggested by the clinical history, predominant seizure type, interictal and ictal EEG, and imaging studies; thus, SPS, CPS, or secondarily generalized seizures arising from frontal lobes, parietal, temporal, occipital, multiple lobes or an unknown focus

Localization related but uncertain symptomatic or idiopathic

GENERALIZED EPILEPSIES

Idiopathic
- Benign neonatal familial convulsions
- Benign neonatal convulsions
- Benign myoclonic epilepsy in infancy
- Childhood absence epilepsy (pyknoepilepsy)
- Juvenile absence epilepsy
- Juvenile myoclonic epilepsy (impulsive petit mal)
- Epilepsy with grand mal seizures upon awakening
- Other generalized idiopathic epilepsies that do not conform exactly to the syndromes just described

Cryptogenic or symptomatic generalized
- West syndrome (infantile spasms)
- Lennox-Gastaut syndrome
- Epilepsy with myoclonic astatic seizures
- Epilepsy with myoclonic absences
- Symptomatic
- Nonspecific cause
  - Early myoclonic encephalopathy
- Specific disease states manifesting with seizures

EPILEPSIES AND SYNDROMES UNDETERMINED AS FOCAL OR GENERALIZED

With both generalized and focal seizures
- Neonatal seizures
- Severe myoclonic epilepsy in infancy
- Epilepsy with continuous spike-and-wave patterns during slow-wave sleep
- Acquired epileptic aphasia (Landau-Kleffner syndrome)
- Without unequivocal generalized or focal features
- All cases with GTCS in which the EEG findings do not allow classification as definitely generalized or localization-related: e.g., sleep GTCS

SPECIAL SYNDROMES

Situation-related seizures
- Febrile convulsions
- Isolated seizures or isolated status epilepticus

Acute symptomatic seizures: e.g., alcohol withdrawal seizures, eclampsia, uremia

CPS, complex partial seizures; EEG, electroencephalogram; GTCS, generalized tonic-clonic seizures; SPS, simple partial seizures.
From Kliegman RM, Greenbaum LA, Lye PS: *Practical Strategies in Pediatric Diagnosis and Therapy*, 2nd ed. Philadelphia, Elsevier, 2004, p 680.

593.3 • Partial Seizures

Partial seizures account for a large proportion of childhood seizures, up to 40% in some series. Partial seizures may be classified as simple or complex; consciousness is maintained with simple seizures and is impaired in patients with complex seizures.

SIMPLE PARTIAL SEIZURES (SPS). Motor activity is the most common symptom of SPS. The movements are characterized by asynchronous clonic or tonic movements, and they tend to involve the face, neck, and extremities. Versive seizures consisting of head turning and conjugate eye movements are particularly common in SPS. Automatisms do not occur with SPS, but some patients complain of aura (chest discomfort, headache), which may be the only manifestation of a seizure. Children have difficulty in describing aura and often refer to it as "feeling funny" or "something crawling inside me." The average seizure persists for 10–20 sec. The distinguishing characteristic of SPS is that the patients remain conscious and may verbalize during the seizure. No postictal phenomenon follows the event. SPS may be confused with tics; tics are characterized by shoulder shrugging, eye blinking, and facial grimacing and primarily involve the face and shoulders (see Chapter 23). Tics can be briefly suppressed, but partial seizures cannot be controlled. The EEG may show spikes or sharp waves unilaterally or bilaterally or a multifocal spike pattern in patients with SPS.

TABLE 593-4. Childhood Epileptic Syndromes with Generally Good Prognosis

SYNDROME	COMMENT
Benign neonatal familial convulsions	Dominant, may be severe and resistant during a few days. Febrile or afebrile seizures (benign) may occur later in a minority
Infantile familial convulsions	Dominant, seizures often in clusters (overlap with benign partial complex epilepsy of infancy)
Febrile convulsions	In some families, febrile and afebrile convulsions occur in different members, the so-called GEFS. (generalized epilepsy with febrile seizures +); the old dichotomy between febrile convulsions or epilepsy does not always hold
Benign myoclonic epilepsy of infancy	Often seizures during sleep, one rare variety with reflex myoclonic seizures (touch, noise)
Partial idiopathic epilepsy with rolandic spikes	Seizures with falling asleep or on awakening; focal sharp waves with centrotemporal location on EEG; genetic
Idiopathic occipital partial epilepsy	Early childhood form with seizures during sleep and ictal vomiting, may present as status epilepticus. Later forms with migrainous symptoms; not always benign
Petit mal absence epilepsy	Cases with absences only, some have generalized seizures. 60–80% full remission; in most cases, absences disappear on therapy but there are resistant cases (unpredictable)
Juvenile myoclonic epilepsy	Adolescence onset, with early morning myoclonic seizures and generalized seizures during sleep; often history of absences in childhood

From Deonna T: Management of epilepsy. *Arch Dis Child* 2005;90:5–9.

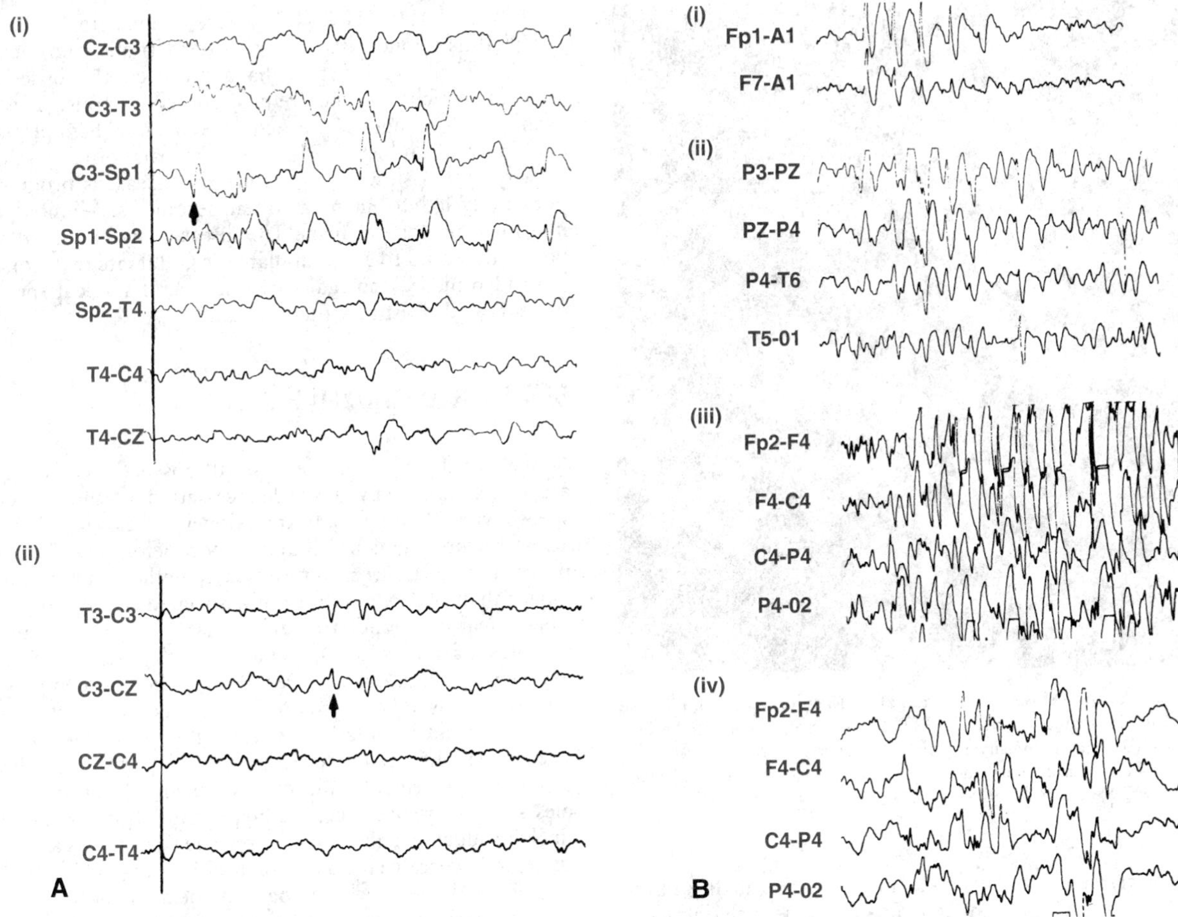

Figure 593-1. *A,* An EEG of partial seizures: (i) spike discharges from the left temporal lobe *(arrow)* in a patient with CPS, (ii) left parietal central spikes *(arrow)* characteristic of BPEC. *B,* Representative EEGs of generalized seizures: (i) 3/sec spike and wave discharge of absence seizures with normal background activity, (ii) complex myoclonic epilepsy (Lennox-Gastaut syndrome) with interictal slow spike waves, (iii) juvenile myoclonic epilepsy showing 6/sec spike and waves enhanced by photic stimulation, and (iv) hypsarrhythmia with an irregular high-voltage spike and wave activity. BPEC, benign partial epilepsy with centrotemporal spikes; CPS, complex partial seizures; EEG, electroencephalogram.

COMPLEX PARTIAL SEIZURES (CPS). A CPS may begin with a simple partial seizure with or without an aura, followed by impaired consciousness; conversely, the onset of the CPS may coincide with an altered state of consciousness. An aura consisting of vague, unpleasant feelings, epigastric discomfort, or fear is present in approximately one third of children with SPS and CPS. The presence of an aura always indicates a focal onset of the seizure. Because partial seizures are difficult to document in infants and children, the frequency of their association with CPS may be underestimated. Impaired consciousness in infants and children may be difficult to appreciate. There may be a brief blank stare or a sudden cessation or pause in activity that is frequently overlooked by the parent. Furthermore, the child is unable to communicate or to describe the periods of impaired consciousness in most cases. The periods of altered consciousness may be brief and infrequent, and only an experienced observer or an EEG may be able to identify the abnormal event.

Automatisms are a common feature of CPS in infants and children, occurring in ≈50–75% of cases; the older the child, the greater is the frequency of automatisms. Automatisms develop after the loss of consciousness and may persist into the postictal phase; they are not recalled by the child. The automatic behavior observed in infants is characterized by alimentary automatisms, including lip smacking, chewing, swallowing, and excessive salivation. These movements can represent normal infant behavior and are difficult to distinguish from the automatisms of CPS. Prolonged and repetitive alimentary automatisms associated with a blank stare or with a lack of responsiveness almost always indicate CPS in an infant. Automatic behavior in older children consists of semi-purposeful, incoordinated, and unplanned gestural automatisms, including picking and pulling at clothing or bedsheets, rubbing or caressing objects, and walking or running in a nondirective, repetitive, and often fearful fashion.

Spreading of the epileptiform discharge during CPS can result in **secondary generalization** with a tonic-clonic convulsion. During the spread of the ictal discharge throughout the hemisphere, contralateral versive turning of the head, dystonic posturing, and tonic or clonic movements of the extremities and face, including eye blinking, may be noted. The average duration of a CPS is 1–2 min, which is considerably longer than an SPS or an absence seizure.

CPSs are associated with interictal **EEG** anterior temporal lobe sharp waves or focal spikes, and multifocal spikes are a frequent finding. Approximately 20% of infants and children with CPS have a normal routine interictal EEG. In these patients, a sleep-deprived EEG study, zygomatic leads during EEG, prolonged EEG recording, or video EEG study of the hospitalized patient weaned from anticonvulsants are techniques that can be used to increase the identification of spikes and sharp waves (Fig. 593-1*A*). In addition, some children with CPS have interictal sharp waves or spikes originating from the frontal, parietal, or occipital lobes. Radiographic studies including CT scanning and

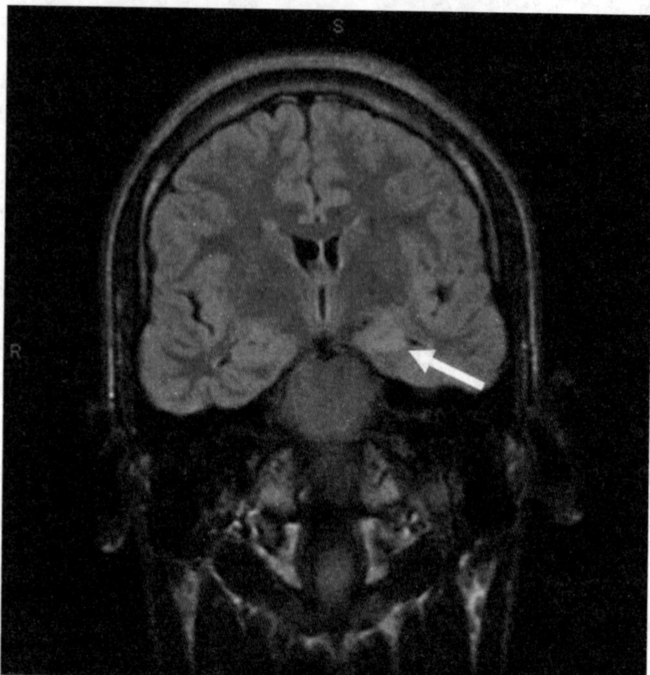

Figure 593-2. Coronal FLAIR MRI scan of a 13 yr old with intractable seizures and mesial temporal sclerosis (MTS). The *arrow* points at the hippocampus with the high-intensity signal characteristic of MTS. (From Lee JYK, Adelson PD: Neurosurgical management of pediatric epilepsy. *Pediatr Clin North Am* 2004;51:441–456.)

especially MRI are most likely to identify an abnormality in the temporal lobe of a child with CPS. These lesions include mesial temporal sclerosis, hamartoma, postencephalitic gliosis, subarachnoid cysts, infarction, arteriovenous malformations, and slow-growing glioma (Fig. 593-2).

BENIGN PARTIAL EPILEPSY WITH CENTROTEMPORAL SPIKES (BPEC). BPEC is a common type of partial epilepsy in childhood and has an excellent prognosis. The clinical features, EEG findings (rolandic foci), and lack of a neuropathologic lesion are characteristic and readily separate BPEC from CPS. BPEC occurs between the ages of 2 and 14 yr and has a peak age of onset of 9–10 yr. The disorder occurs in normal children with an unremarkable history and normal neurologic examination. There is often a positive family history of epilepsy. The seizures are usually partial, and motor signs and somatosensory symptoms are often confined to the face. **Oropharyngeal symptoms** include tonic contractions and paresthesias of the tongue, unilateral numbness of the cheek (particularly along the gum), guttural noises, dysphagia, and excessive salivation. Unilateral tonic-clonic contractures of the lower face frequently accompany the oropharyngeal symptoms, as do clonic movements or paresthesias of the ipsilateral extremities. Consciousness may be intact or impaired, and the partial seizure may proceed to secondary generalization.

Approximately 20% of children experience only one seizure, the majority has infrequent seizures, and about one fourth have repeated clusters of seizures. BPEC occurs during sleep in 75% of patients, whereas CPS tends to be observed during waking hours. The EEG pattern is diagnostic for BPEC and is characterized by a repetitive spike focus localized in the centrotemporal or rolandic area with normal background activity (see Fig. 593-1*A*). Anticonvulsants are necessary for patients who have frequent seizures but should not be prescribed automatically after the initial convulsion. **Carbamazepine** is the **preferred drug,** which is continued for at least 2 yr or until 14–16 yr of age, when spontaneous remission of BPEC usually occurs.

RASMUSSEN ENCEPHALITIS. This subacute inflammatory encephalitis is one cause of **epilepsia partialis continua.** A nonspecific febrile illness may have preceded the onset of focal seizures, which may be frequent or continuous. The onset is usually before age 10 yr. Sequelae include hemiplegia, hemianopia, and aphasia. The EEG reveals diffuse paroxysmal activity with a slow background. The disease is progressive and potentially lethal but more often becomes self-limited with significant neurologic deficits. The disease may be due to autoantibodies that bind to and stimulate the glutamate receptors. Studies have identified cytomegalovirus in several surgical specimens of patients with Rasmussen encephalitis.

593.4 • Generalized Seizures

ABSENCE SEIZURES. Simple (typical) absence (petit mal) seizures are characterized by a sudden cessation of motor activity or speech with a blank facial expression and flickering of the eyelids. These seizures, which are uncommon before age 5 yr, are more prevalent in girls, are never associated with an aura, rarely persist longer than 30 sec, and are not associated with a postictal state. These features tend to differentiate absence seizures from complex partial seizures. Children with absence seizures may experience countless seizures daily, whereas complex partial seizures are usually less frequent. Patients do not lose body tone, but their head may fall forward slightly. Immediately after the seizure, patients resume preseizure activity with no indication of postictal impairment. Automatic behavior frequently accompanies simple absence seizures. Hyperventilation for 3–4 min routinely produces an absence seizure. The EEG shows a typical 3/sec spike and generalized wave discharge (see Fig. 593-1*B*). Complex (atypical) absence seizures have associated motor components consisting of myoclonic movement of the face, fingers, or extremities and, on occasion, loss of body tone. These seizures produce atypical EEG spike and wave discharges at 2–2.5/sec.

GENERALIZED TONIC-CLONIC SEIZURES. These seizures are common and may follow a partial seizure with a focal onset (second generalization) or occur de novo. They may be associated with an **aura,** suggesting a focal origin of the epileptiform discharge. It is important to inquire about the presence of an aura, because its presence and site of origin may indicate the area of pathology. Patients suddenly lose consciousness and, in some cases, emit a shrill, piercing cry. Their eyes roll back, their entire body musculature undergoes tonic contractions, and they rapidly become cyanotic in association with apnea. The clonic phase of the seizure is heralded by rhythmic clonic contractions alternating with relaxation of all muscle groups. The clonic phase slows toward the end of the seizure, which usually persists for a few minutes, and patients often sigh as the seizure comes to an abrupt stop. During the seizure, children may bite their tongue but rarely vomit. Loss of sphincter control, particularly the bladder, is common during a generalized tonic-clonic seizure.

Tight clothing and jewelry around the neck should be loosened, the patient should be placed on one side, and the neck and jaw should be gently hyperextended to enhance breathing. The mouth should not be opened forcibly by an object or by a finger because the patient's teeth may be dislodged and aspirated, or significant injury to the oropharyngeal cavity may result. Postictally, children are initially semicomatose and typically remain in a deep sleep from 30 min to 2 hr. If patients are examined during the seizure or immediately postictally, they may demonstrate truncal ataxia, hyperactive deep tendon reflexes, clonus, and a Babinski reflex. The postictal phase is often associated with vomiting and an intense bifrontal headache.

Idiopathic seizure is a term applied when the cause of a generalized seizure cannot be ascertained. Many factors are known to precipitate generalized tonic-clonic seizures in children, including low-grade fever associated with non–central nervous system infections, excessive fatigue or emotional stress, and various drugs including psychotropic medications, theophylline, and methylphenidate, particularly if the seizures are poorly controlled by anticonvulsant drugs.

MYOCLONIC EPILEPSIES OF CHILDHOOD. This disorder is characterized by repetitive seizures consisting of brief, often symmetric muscular contractions with loss of body tone and falling or slumping forward, which has a tendency to cause injuries to the face and mouth. Myoclonic epilepsies include a heterogeneous group of conditions with multiple causes and variable outcomes. At least five distinct subgroupings can be identified; these represent the broad spectrum of myoclonic epilepsies in the pediatric population.

Benign Myoclonus of Infancy. Benign myoclonus begins during infancy and consists of clusters of myoclonic movements confined to the neck, trunk, and extremities. The myoclonic activity may be confused with infantile spasms; however, the EEG is normal in patients with benign myoclonus. The prognosis is good, with normal development and the cessation of myoclonus by 2 yr of age. An anticonvulsant is not indicated.

Typical Myoclonic Epilepsy of Early Childhood. Children who develop typical myoclonic epilepsy are near normal before the onset of seizures, with an unremarkable pregnancy, labor, and delivery and intact developmental milestones. The mean age of onset is ≈2 yr, but the range spreads from 6 mo to 4 yr. The frequency of myoclonic seizures varies; they may occur several times daily, or children may be seizure-free for weeks. A few patients have febrile convulsions or generalized tonic-clonic afebrile seizures that precede the onset of myoclonic epilepsy. Approximately half of patients occasionally have tonic-clonic seizures in addition to the myoclonic epilepsy. The EEG shows fast spike wave complexes of ≥2.5 Hz and a normal background rhythm in most cases. At least one third of the children have a positive family history of epilepsy, which suggests a genetic etiology in some cases. The long-term outcome is relatively favorable. Mental retardation develops in the minority, and >50% are seizure-free several years later. Learning and language problems and emotional and behavioral disorders occur in a significant number of these children and require prolonged follow-up by a multidisciplinary team.

Complex Myoclonic Epilepsies. These consist of a heterogeneous group of disorders with a uniformly poor prognosis. Focal or generalized tonic-clonic seizures beginning in the 1st yr of life typically antedate the onset of myoclonic epilepsy. The generalized seizure is often associated with an upper respiratory tract infection and a low-grade fever and frequently develops into status epilepticus. Approximately one third of these patients have evidence of delayed developmental milestones. A history of hypoxic-ischemic encephalopathy in the perinatal period and the finding of generalized upper motor neuron and extrapyramidal signs with microcephaly constitute a common pattern among these children. A family history of epilepsy is much less prominent in this group compared with typical myoclonic epilepsy.

Some children display a combination of frequent myoclonic and tonic seizures, and when interictal slow spike waves are evident in the EEG, the seizure disorder is classified as the **Lennox-Gastaut syndrome.** This syndrome is characterized by the triad of intractable seizures of various types, a slow spike wave EEG during the awake state, and mental retardation. Patients with complex myoclonic epilepsy routinely have interictal slow spike waves and are refractory to anticonvulsants (see Fig. 593-1*B*). The seizures are persistent, and the frequency of mental retardation and behavioral problems is ≈75% of all patients. Treatment with valproic acid or benzodiazepines may decrease the frequency or intensity of the seizures. The ketogenic diet should be considered for patients whose seizures are refractory to anticonvulsants.

Juvenile Myoclonic Epilepsy (Janz Syndrome). Juvenile myoclonic epilepsy usually begins between the ages of 12 and 16 yr and accounts for ≈5% of the epilepsies. A gene locus has been identified on chromosome 6p21. Patients note frequent myoclonic jerks on awakening, making hair combing and toothbrushing difficult. As the myoclonus tends to abate later in the morning, most patients do not seek medical advice at this stage and some deny the episodes. A few years later, early morning generalized tonic-clonic seizures develop in association with the myoclonus. The EEG shows a 4–6/sec irregular spike and wave pattern, which is enhanced by photic stimulation (see Fig. 593-1*B*). The neurologic examination is normal, and the majority responds dramatically to valproate, which is required lifelong. Discontinuance of the drug causes a high rate of recurrence of seizures.

Progressive Myoclonic Epilepsies. This heterogeneous group of rare genetic disorders uniformly has a grave prognosis. These conditions include Lafora disease, myoclonic epilepsy with ragged-red fibers (MERRF) (see Chapter 598.2), sialidosis type 1 (see Chapter 599.4), ceroid lipofuscinosis (see Chapter 599.2), juvenile neuropathic Gaucher disease, and juvenile neuroaxonal dystrophy.

Lafora disease presents in children between 10 and 18 yr with generalized tonic-clonic seizures. Ultimately, myoclonic jerks appear; these become more apparent and constant with progression of the disease. Mental deterioration is a characteristic feature and becomes evident within 1 yr of the onset of seizures. Neurologic abnormalities, particularly cerebellar and extrapyramidal signs, are prominent findings. The EEG shows polyspike-wave discharges, particularly in the occipital region, with progressive slowing and a disorganized background. The myoclonic jerks are difficult to control, but a combination of valproic acid and a benzodiazepine (clonazepam) is effective in controlling the generalized seizures. Lafora disease is an autosomal recessive disorder, and the diagnosis may be established by examination of a skin biopsy specimen for characteristic periodic acid-Schiff positive inclusions, which are most prominent in the eccrine sweat gland duct cells. The gene for Lafora disease is located on 6p24 and it encodes a protein, tyrosine phosphatase.

INFANTILE SPASMS. Infantile spasms usually begin between the ages of 4 and 8 mo and are characterized by brief symmetric contractions of the neck, trunk, and extremities. There are at least three types of infantile spasms: flexor, extensor, and mixed. Flexor spasms occur in clusters or volleys and consist of sudden flexion of the neck, arms, and legs onto the trunk, whereas extensor spasms produce extension of the trunk and extremities and are the least common form of infantile spasm. Mixed infantile spasms consisting of flexion in some volleys and extension in others, is the most common type of infantile spasm. Clusters or volleys of seizures may persist for minutes, with brief intervals between each spasm. A cry may precede or follow an infantile spasm, accounting for the confusion with colic in a few cases. The spasms occur during sleep or arousal but have a tendency to develop while patients are drowsy or immediately on awakening. The EEG that is most commonly associated with infantile spasms is referred to as hypsarrhythmia, which consists of a chaotic pattern of high-voltage, bilaterally asynchronous, slow-wave activity (see Fig. 593-1*B*) or a modified hypsarrhythmia pattern.

Infantile spasms are typically classified into two groups: **cryptogenic** and **symptomatic.** A child with cryptogenic infantile spasms has an uneventful pregnancy and birth history as well as normal developmental milestones before the onset of seizures. The neurologic examination and the CT and MRI scans of the head are normal, and there are no associated risk factors. Approximately 10–20% of infantile spasms are classified as cryptogenic, and the remainder are classified as symptomatic. Symptomatic infantile spasms are related directly to several prenatal, perinatal, and postnatal factors. Prenatal and perinatal factors include hypoxic-ischemic encephalopathy with periventricular leukomalacia, congenital infections, inborn errors of metabolism, neurocutaneous syndromes such as tuberous sclerosis, cytoarchitectural abnormalities including lissencephaly and schizencephaly, and prematurity. Postnatal conditions include CNS infections, head trauma (especially subdural hematoma and intraventricular hemorrhage), and hypoxic-ischemic encephalopathy. The fact that infantile spasms and immunizations often occur simultaneously around 6 mo of age is a coincidence of timing rather than a cause and effect of any immunization antigen.

Infants with cryptogenic infantile spasms have a good prognosis, whereas those with the symptomatic type have an 80–90% risk of mental retardation. The underlying CNS disorder has a major role in the neurologic outcome. Several theories have been advanced with regard to the pathogenesis of infantile spasms, including dysfunction of the monoaminergic neurotransmitter system in the brainstem, derangement of neuronal structures in the brainstem, and an abnormality of the immune system. One hypothesis implicates corticotropin-releasing hormone (CRH), a putative neurotransmitter, metabolized in the inferior olive. CRH acts on the pituitary to enhance the release of adrenocorticotropic hormone (ACTH); ACTH and glucocorticoids suppress the metabolism and secretion of CRH by a feedback mechanism. It is proposed that specified stresses or injury to an infant during a critical period of neurodevelopment causes CRH overproduction, resulting in neuronal hyperexcitability and seizures. The number of CRH receptors reaches a maximum in an infant's brain followed by spontaneous reduction with age, perhaps accounting for the eventual resolution of infantile spasms, even without therapy. Exogenous ACTH and glucocorticoids suppress CRH synthesis, which may account for their effectiveness in treating infantile spasms. Therapy for infantile spasms is discussed in the section on treatment.

LANDAU-KLEFFNER SYNDROME (LKS). This is a rare condition of unknown cause. It is more common in boys and has a mean onset of 5½ yr. LKS is often confused with autism, in that both conditions are associated with a loss of language function. LKS is characterized by loss of language skills in a previously normal child. At least 70% have an associated seizure disorder. Language regression may be sudden or the speech loss protracted. The **aphasia** may be primarily receptive or expressive, and auditory agnosia may be so severe that the child is oblivious to everyday sounds. Hearing is normal, but behavioral problems, including irritability and poor attention span, are particularly common. Formal testing often shows normal performance and visual-spatial skills despite poor language. The seizures are of several types, including focal or generalized tonic-clonic, atypical absence, partial complex, and, occasionally, myoclonic. High-amplitude spike and wave discharges predominate and tend to be bitemporal, but they can be multifocal or generalized. In the evolutionary stages of the condition, the EEG findings may be normal. The spike discharges are always more apparent during non–rapid eye movement (REM) sleep; thus, a child suspected of LKS should have an EEG during sleep, particularly if the awake record is normal. If the sleep EEG is normal but a high index of suspicion for the diagnosis of LKS continues, the child should be referred to a tertiary pediatric epilepsy center for prolonged EEG recording and specific neuroimaging studies. CT and MRI studies typically yield normal results, and positron emission tomography (PET) scans have demonstrated either unilateral or bilateral hypometabolism or hypermetabolism. Examination of surgical specimens has shown minimal gliosis but no evidence of encephalitis.

Valproic acid is the anticonvulsant of choice; some children require a combination of valproic acid and clobazam to control their seizures. If the seizures and aphasia persist, a trial of steroids should be considered; oral prednisone is started at 2 mg/kg/24 hr for 1 mo, tapered to 1 mg/kg/24 hr for an additional month. With clinical improvement, the prednisone is reduced further to 0.5 mg/kg/24 hr for up to 6–12 mo. It is imperative to initiate speech therapy and maintain treatment for several years, because improvement in language function occurs over a prolonged period. Some centers advocate an operative procedure subpial transection when medical management fails. Methylphenidate should be considered for patients with severe hyperactivity and inattention. Seizures, if poorly controlled, may be potentiated by methylphenidate; anticonvulsants are usually protective. Intravenous immunoglobulin may be helpful in LKS. Some children experience a recurrence of aphasia and seizures after apparent recovery. Most children with LKS have a significant abnormality of speech function in adulthood. The onset of LKS at an early age (<2 yr) uniformly tends to be associated with a poor prognosis for recovery of speech.

593.5 • MECHANISMS OF SEIZURES

Although the precise mechanisms of seizures are unknown, several physiologic factors are responsible for the development of a seizure. To initiate a seizure, there must be a group of neurons that are capable of generating a significant burst discharge and impairment of the γ-aminobutyric acid (GABA)–ergic inhibitory system. Seizure discharge transmission ultimately depends on excitatory glutamatergic synapses. Evidence suggests that excitatory amino acid neurotransmitters (glutamate, aspartate) may have a role in producing neuronal excitation by acting on specific cell receptors. Seizures may arise from areas of neuronal death, and these regions of the brain may promote development of novel hyperexcitable synapses that can cause seizures. Lesions in the temporal lobe (including slow-growing gliomas, hamartomas, gliosis, hippocampal sclerosis, and arteriovenous malformations) cause seizures, and when the abnormal tissue is removed surgically, the seizures are likely to cease. Two hypotheses have been suggested to explain the origin of seizures after brain injury. One suggests that inhibitory neurons are selectively damaged and remaining principal excitatory neurons become hyperexcitable. The other hypothesis suggests that aberrant excitatory circuits are formed as part of reorganization after injury. Convulsions may be produced in experimental animals by the phenomenon of **kindling.** In this model, repeated subconvulsive stimulation of the brain (amygdala) ultimately leads to a generalized convulsion by changes in synapses. This synaptic mechanism may also occur in humans.

Seizures are more common in infants and in immature experimental animals. Certain seizures in the pediatric population are age specific (infantile spasms); this observation suggests that the underdeveloped brain is more susceptible to specific seizures than is the brain of an older child or adult. This is consistent with basic science data indicating that the immature brain is more excitable than the mature brain, reflecting the greater influence of excitatory glutamate-containing circuits. The actions of GABA, the major inhibitory neurotransmitter, are often paradoxically excitatory in the immature brain. Enhanced excitatory activity may contribute to the developing brain's greater capacity for activity-dependent plasticity.

Genetic factors account for at least 20% of all cases of epilepsy (see Table 593-1). Using linkage analyses, the chromosomal location of several familial epilepsies has been identified, including benign neonatal convulsions (20q and 8q), juvenile myoclonic epilepsy (6p), and progressive myoclonic epilepsy (21q22.3). The genetic defect of benign familial neonatal convulsions has been characterized by the identification of submicroscopic deletion of chromosome 20q13.3. Study of the cDNAs spanning the deleted region identified one encoding a novel voltage-gated potassium channel, $KCNQ_2$. Furthermore, the substantia nigra has an integral role in the development of generalized seizures. Electrographic seizure activity spreads within the substantia nigra, causing an increase in uptake of 2-deoxyglucose in adult animals, but there is little or no metabolic activity within the substantia nigra when immature animals have a convulsion. It has been proposed that the functional immaturity of the substantia nigra may have a role in the increased seizure susceptibility of the immature brain. Additionally, the GABA-sensitive substantia nigra pars reticulata neurons play a part in preventing seizures. It is likely that substantia nigra outflow tracts modulate and regulate seizure dissemination but are not responsible for the onset of seizures.

USE OF THE EEG TO DIAGNOSE EPILEPSY. The investigation of a seizure depends on many factors, including the age of the patient, the type and frequency of the seizure, and the presence or absence of neurologic findings and constitutional symptoms. Demonstration of paroxysmal discharges on the EEG during a clinical seizure is diagnostic of epilepsy, but seizures rarely occur acutely in the EEG laboratory. A normal EEG does not preclude the diagnosis of epilepsy, because the interictal recording is normal in ≈40% of patients. Activation procedures, including hyperventilation, eye closure, photic stimulation, and, when indicated, sleep deprivation and special electrode placement (zygomatic leads), substantially increase the positive yield. Seizure discharges are more likely to be recorded in infants and children than in adolescents or adults. Patients who are taking an anticonvulsant and who are scheduled for a routine EEG should not have the medication decreased or discontinued before the study, because status epilepticus may result.

Prolonged EEG monitoring with simultaneous closed-circuit video recording is reserved for complicated cases of protracted and unresponsive seizures. It provides an invaluable method for recording ictal seizure events that are rarely obtained during routine EEG studies. This technique is extremely helpful in the classification of seizures because it can accurately determine the location and frequency of seizure discharges while recording alterations in the level of consciousness and the presence of clinical signs. Patients with pseudoseizures can be readily distinguished from those with true epilepsy, and seizure type (complex partial vs generalized) can be more precisely identified. Determination of seizure type is critical in the investigation of a child who may be a candidate for epilepsy surgery.

593.6 • Treatment of Epilepsy

The 1st step in the management of epilepsy is to ensure that the patient has a seizure disorder and not a condition that mimics epilepsy (see Chapter 594). It is sometimes difficult to be certain about the cause of a paroxysmal event in a normal child. A negative result on a neurologic examination and EEG usually supports the approach of watchful waiting rather than administration of an anticonvulsant. The true cause of the paroxysmal disorder eventually becomes apparent. Although there is not uniform agreement, most would concur that antiepileptics should be withheld from a previously healthy child with the 1st afebrile convulsion if there is a negative family history, normal results of a physical examination and EEG, and a cooperative and compliant family. Approximately 70% of these children will not experience another convulsion. Approximately 75% of those patients with two or three unprovoked seizures have additional seizures. A recurrent seizure, particularly if it occurs in close proximity to the 1st seizure, is an indication to begin an anticonvulsant. Figure 593-3 suggests an approach to a child with a suspected seizure disorder.

The 2nd step involves choosing an **anticonvulsant.** The drug of choice depends on the classification of the seizure, determined by the history and EEG findings. The goal for every patient should be the use of only one drug with the fewest possible side effects for the control of seizures. The drug is increased slowly until seizure control is accomplished or until undesirable side effects develop. The child's serum anticonvulsant level should be monitored during this stage, and the dose should be altered accordingly. Table 593-5 summarizes the common antiepileptic drugs used in childhood epilepsy and highlights the recommended daily dose, therapeutic serum levels, and common side effects. A suggested loading dose is indicated for drugs that are useful for the treatment of status epilepticus. Physicians should be familiar with the pharmacokinetics of the anticonvulsant and its toxic actions and should monitor the child on a regular basis to gauge the seizure control while watching for unwanted side effects.

Routine serum monitoring of anticonvulsant levels is not recommended because the practice is not cost-effective. There are several important indications for anticonvulsant drug monitoring: (1) at the onset of anticonvulsant therapy to confirm that the drug level is within the therapeutic range; (2) for noncompliant patients and families; (3) at the time of status epilepticus; (4) during accelerated growth spurts; (5) for patients on polytherapy, especially valproic acid, phenobarbital, and lamotrigine because of drug interactions; (6) for uncontrolled seizures or seizures that have changed in type; (7) for symptoms and signs of drug toxicity (toxicity due to a metabolite of carbamazepine, carbamazepine-10,11-epoxide); (8) for patients with hepatic or renal disease; and (9) for children with cognitive or physical disabilities, especially those taking phenytoin, in whom toxicity may be difficult to evaluate. Good clinical judgment is more reliable in achieving seizure control than over-reliance on therapeutic drug monitoring. Drug-resistant epilepsy requires trials of different drugs and may be associated with genetic polymorphisms of drug transporter mechanisms.

There is controversy about whether routine blood tests (complete blood count [CBC], liver function studies) are indicated during anticonvulsant therapy. Because most serious adverse anticonvulsant drug reactions develop during the initial 2–3 mo of therapy, monthly blood screening for the 1st 3 mo is recommended. Subsequently, routine blood tests are ordered only when clinically indicated.

Anticonvulsants that are introduced during childhood may be required during adolescence and the childbearing years. Some anticonvulsants, including phenytoin, valproic acid, carbamazepine, and primidone, are associated with the occurrence of specific **birth defects,** including facial and limb anomalies and spinal dysraphism. The pediatrician should counsel the family about the possible relationship and should avoid prescribing an anticonvulsant to a pregnant patient unless it is absolutely necessary.

If complete seizure control is accomplished by an anticonvulsant, a minimum of two seizure-free years is an adequate and safe period of treatment for a patient with no risk factors. Prominent risk factors include age >12 yr at onset, neurologic dysfunction (motor handicap, mental retardation), a history of prior neonatal seizures, and numerous seizures before control is achieved. In a child with complete seizure control for a minimum of 2 yr and low risk factors, the chance of recurrence is ≈20–25%, particularly in the 1st 6 mo after discontinuation of the anticonvulsant. Those children with the best prognosis after anticonvulsant withdrawal are those with benign epilepsy with rolandic spikes and those with idiopathic generalized seizures. CPS and juvenile myoclonic seizures are more likely to recur. When the decision is made to discontinue the drug, the weaning process should occur over 3–6 mo, because abrupt withdrawal may cause status epilepticus.

Possible sites of action, dose, and side effects of anticonvulsants are noted in Figure 593-4 and Table 593-5.

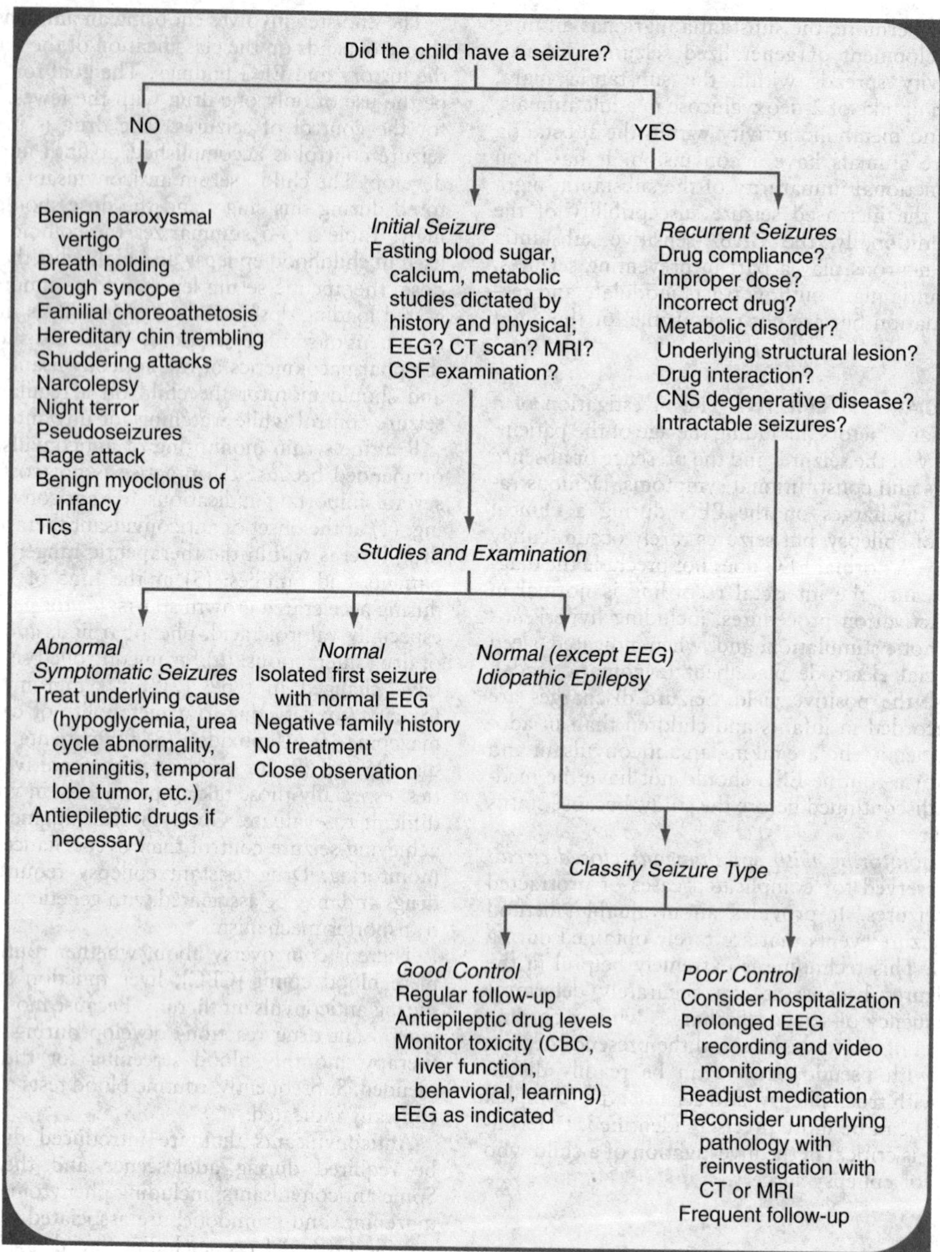

Figure 593-3. An approach to the child with a suspected convulsive disorder.

BENZODIAZEPINES. The benzodiazepines exert anticonvulsant activity by binding to a specific GABA site that enhances the opening frequency of the chloride channel without affecting open or burst duration (see Fig. 593-4). The drugs diazepam and lorazepam IV are used for initial management of status epilepticus. Rectal diazepam gel has been demonstrated to be an effective and safe treatment to abort episodes of acute repetitive seizures in children and is available as Diastat gel in 2.5, 5, and 10 mg doses for children. Buccal or nasal midazolam is also effective acutely. Clonazepam is useful for the management of the Lennox-Gastaut syndrome, myoclonic, akinetic, and absence seizures. The elimination half-life is 18–50 hr. Clonazepam may increase serum phenytoin concentrations when they are used together, and additional CNS depression may occur when clonazepam is combined with other CNS depressant drugs. Clonazepam is supplied in 0.5 and 2 mg tablets. Nitrazepam is useful for the management of myoclonic seizures. The elimination half-life is 18–57 hr. The drug may increase CNS depression when used with additional depressants. Nitrazepam is supplied in 5 and 10 mg tablets. Clobazam is indicated as adjunctive therapy for complex partial seizures. The half-life is 10–30 hr. Clobazam may increase the serum drug levels of carbamazepine, phenytoin, phenobarbital, and valproic acid when used concomitantly. Clobazam is supplied in 10 mg tablets.

CARBAMAZEPINE. This drug is effective for the management of generalized tonic-clonic and partial seizures. Carbamazepine acts similarly to phenytoin by decreasing the sustained repetitive firing of neurons by blocking sodium-dependent channels and by decreasing depolarization-dependent calcium uptake. Significant leukopenia ($<1,000$ neutrophils/mL^3) and hepatotoxicity may rarely develop, particularly during the initial 3–4 mo of therapy. Therefore, a CBC with differential and AST and ALT levels should be obtained on a monthly basis during this period,

TABLE 593-5. Common Anticonvulsant Drugs

DRUG	SEIZURE TYPE	ORAL DOSE	LOADING DOSE (IV)	THERAPEUTIC SERUM LEVEL (μG/ML)	SIDE EFFECTS AND TOXICITY
Carbamazepine (Tegretol)	Generalized tonic-clonic Partial	Begin 10 mg/kg/24 hr Increase to 20–30 mg/kg/24 hr tid	—	8–12	Dizziness, drowsiness, diplopia, liver dysfunction, anemia, neutropenia, SIADH, blood dyscrasias rare, hepatotoxic effects
Clobazam (Frisium)	Adjunctive therapy when seizures poorly controlled	0.25–1 mg/kg/24 hr bid or tid	—	—	Dizziness, fatigue, weight gain, ataxia and behavior problems
Clonazepam (Rivotril)	Absence Myoclonic Infantile spasms Partial Lennox-Gastaut Akinetic	Children <30 kg: Begin 0.05 mg/kg/24 hr Increase by 0.05 mg/kg/wk Maximum 0.2 mg/kg/24 hr bid or tid Children >30 kg: 1.5 mg/kg/24 hr tid, not to exceed 20 mg/24 hr	—	>0.013	Drowiness, irritability, agitation, behavioral abnormalities, depression, excessive salivation
Ethosuximide (Zarontin)	Absence May increase tonic-clonic seizures	Begin 20 mg/kg/24 hr Increase to maximum of 40 mg/kg/24 hr or 1.5 g/24 hr, whichever is less	—	40–100	Abdominal discomfort, skin rash, liver dysfunction, leukopenia
Gabapentin (Neurontin)	Adjuntive therapy when seizures poorly controlled	Children: 20–50 mg/kg/24 hr tid Adolescence: 900–3,600 mg/24 hr tid	—	Not necessary to monitor	Somnolence, dizziness, ataxia, headache, tremor, vomiting, nystagmus, fatigue and weight gain
Lamotrigine (Lamictal)	Adjunctive therapy when seizures poorly controlled Broad-spectrum anticonvulsant activity in various seizure types including: complex partial, absence, myoclonic, clonic, tonic-clonic, and Lennox-Gastaut	Individualized based on age and additional anticonvulsants (see Chapter 593.6)	—	—	Rash, dizziness, ataxia, somolence, diplopia, headache, nausea, vomiting
Nitrazepam (Mogadon)	Absence Myoclonic Infantile spasms	Begin 0.2 mg/kg/24 hr Increase slowly to 1 mg/kg/24 hr tid	—	—	Similar to clonazepam, hallucinations
Paraldehyde	Generalized status epilepticus	Make a 5% solution by adding 1.75 mL of paraldehyde to D5W with total volume of 35 mL	150–200 mg/kg Maintenance, 20 mg/kg/hr	10–40	
Phenobarbital	Generalized tonic-clonic Partial Status epilepticus	3–5 mg/kg/24 hr bid	20 mg/kg 20–30 mg/kg in the neonate	15–40	Hyperactivity, irritability, short attention span, temper tantrums, altered sleep pattern, Stevens-Johnson syndrome, depression of cognitive function
Phenytoin (Dilantin)	Generalized tonic-clonic Partial Status epilepticus	3–9 mg/kg/24 hr bid	20 mg/kg	10–20	Hirsutism, gum hypertrophy, ataxia, skin rash, Stevens-Johnson sydrome, nystagmus, nausea, vomiting, drowsiness, coarsening facial features, blood dyscrasias
Primidone (Mysoline)	Generalized tonic-clonic Partial	Children <8 yr: 10–25 mg/kg/24 hr tid or qid Children >8 yr: usual maintenance dose, 750–1,500 mg/24 hr tid or qid	—	5–12	Aggressive behavior, personality changes, similar to phenobarbital
Topiramate (Topimax)	Adjunctive therapy for poorly controlled seizures Refractory complex partial seizures	1–9 mg/kg/24 hr bid	—	—	Fatigue, cognitive depression
Tiagabine (Gabitril)	Adjunctive therapy for complex partial seizures	Average dose, 6 mg tid	—	—	Asthenia, dizziness, poor attention span, nervousness, tremor
Valproic acid (Depakene, Epival)	Generalized tonic-clonic Absence Myoclonic Partial Akinetic	Begin 10 mg/kg/24 hr Increase by 5–10 mg/kg/wk Usual dose, 30–60 mg/kg/24 hr tid or qid	Intravenous preparation now available Studies in children under way	50–100	Nausea, vomiting, anorexia, amenorrhea, sedation, tremor, weight gain, alopecia, hepatotoxicity
Vigabatrin (Sabril)	Infantile spasms Adjunctive therapy for poorly controlled seizures	Begin 30 mg/kg/24 hr once daily or bid Maintenance dose, 30–100 mg/kg/24 hr once daily or bid	—	—	Hyperactivity, agitation, excitement, somnolence, weight gain Note: Reports of visual field constriction, optic pallor or atrophy, and optic neuritis

SIADH, syndrome of inappropriate secretion of antidiuretic hormone.

although serious idiosyncratic drug reactions may develop despite normal liver function tests results and routine blood work. Subsequent laboratory testing is determined by the presence of adverse symptoms or signs. The parents should be informed of untoward drug effects and instructed to report them immediately to the physician. Erythromycin should be used cautiously with carbamazepine because the two drugs compete for metabolism by the liver. The plasma concentration of carbamazepine is lowered by phenytoin, phenobarbital, and valproic acid. Carbamazepine-10,11-epoxide, which is an active metabolite of carbamazepine, may produce toxicity despite therapeutic carbamazepine levels, particularly when valproic acid is added to the drug regimen. Hyponatremia has also been reported as a side effect of this drug. Carbamazepine is supplied in suspension, 20 mg/mL; chew tabs, 100 and 200 mg tablets; and controlled release (CR) form, 200 and 400 mg tablets. The half-life is 8–20 hr, and the drug should be given two or three times daily.

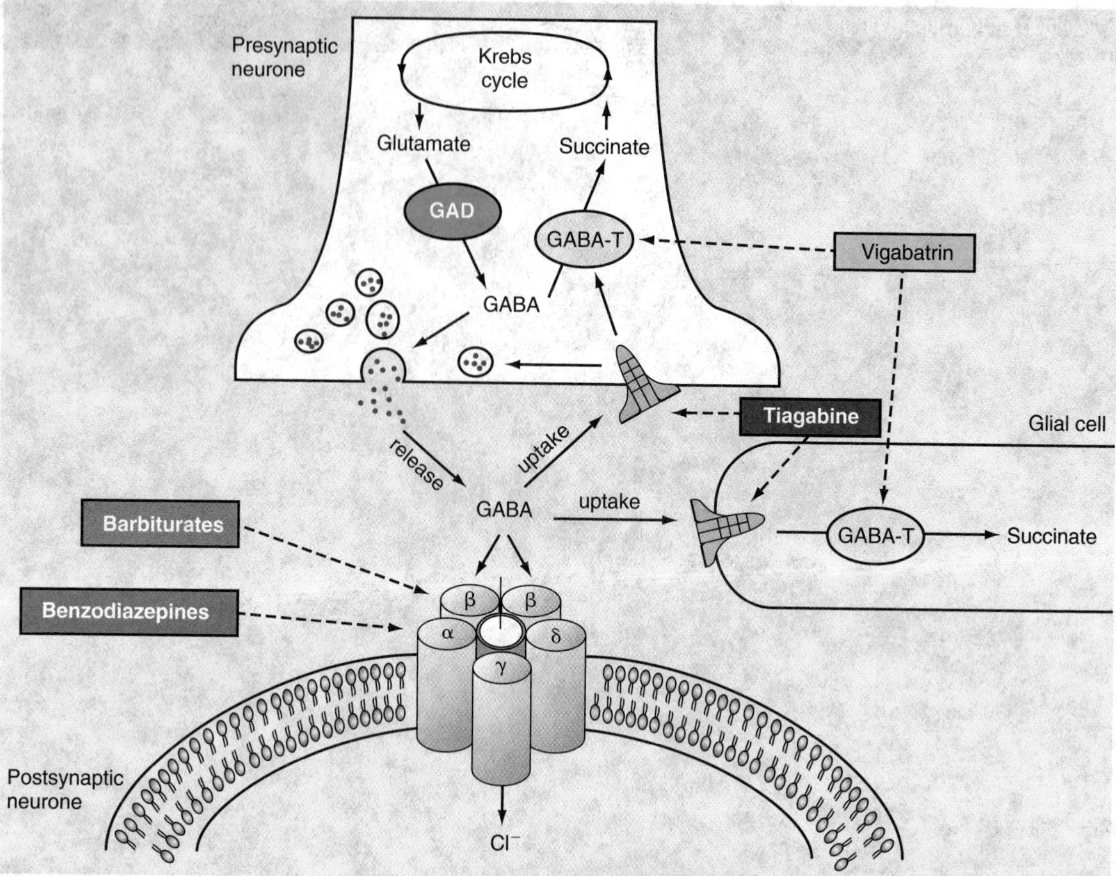

Figure 593-4. Pharmacologic effects of antiepileptic drugs at $GABA_A$ receptor. Barbiturates bind to β-subunit of $GABA_A$ receptor to potentiate action of endogenous agonist GABA and prolong opening time of chloride ion channel. Benzodiazepines bind to an α subunit of $GABA_A$ to potentiate action of GABA and increase frequency of opening of chloride ion channel. Vigabatrin irreversibly binds to GABA-T to inhibit degradation of inhibitory neurotransmitter GABA. Tiagabine blocks uptake of synaptically released GABA into both presynaptic neurons and glial cells, allowing GABA to remain at site of action for longer periods. GABA, γ-aminobutyric acid; $GABA_A$, GABA type A; GABA-T, GABA transaminase; GAD, glutamic acid decarboxylase. (From Leach JP, Brodie MJ: Tiagabine. *Lancet* 1998;351:203–207.)

ETHOSUXIMIDE. Ethosuximide provides its anticonvulsant action by blocking calcium channels associated with thalamocortical circuitry. Ethosuximide is an effective drug for the management of typical absence epilepsy and has a half-life of 60 hr. When used with phenobarbital or primidone, ethosuximide may reduce the serum levels of those anticonvulsants. Ethosuximide is supplied in syrup, 50 mg/mL, and in 250 mg capsules.

GABAPENTIN. This anticonvulsant is used as an add-on drug for patients with refractory complex partial and secondarily generalized tonic-clonic seizures. The mechanism of action results from binding of the drug to neuronal membranes (glutamate synapses) and increased brain GABA turnover. The plasma half-life of gabapentin is 5–7 hr. The drug is rapidly absorbed from the gastrointestinal tract, does not bind to plasma proteins, and is not metabolized. Gabapentin has no significant drug interactions and is relatively free of dose-related CNS adverse effects. Gabapentin is recommended for children 12 yr and older. Gabapentin is supplied in 100, 300, and 400 mg capsules.

LAMOTRIGINE. Lamotrigine is a phenyltriazine compound used as an add-on drug for the management of complex partial and generalized tonic-clonic seizures. Lamotrigine is effective as monotherapy for some children with the Lennox-Gastaut syndrome and generalized absence seizures. Pharmacologic studies suggest the drug acts at voltage-sensitive sodium channels to stabilize neuronal membranes and inhibit neuronal release, particularly glutamate. The plasma elimination half-life is 22–37 hr. In children, the recommended starting dose is 2 mg/kg/24 hr for 2 wk divided into two doses, followed by 5 mg/kg/24 hr for an additional 2 wk. The maintenance dose is 5–15 mg/kg/24 hr. If lamotrigine is added to valproate therapy, the starting dose of lamotrigine should be reduced to 0.5 mg/kg/24 hr because valproate inhibits the metabolism of lamotrigine. In this case, the maintenance dose of lamotrigine is 1–5 mg/kg/24 hr. The therapeutic serum level is 1–4 mg/L or 3.9–15.6 μmol/L. Common side effects include nausea, headache, dizziness, blurred vision, diplopia, and ataxia. A maculopapular skin rash develops in about 3% of patients. The Stevens-Johnson syndrome, angioedema, or toxic epidermal necrolysis occasionally results, usually in the 1st month of therapy, especially in association with valproate. Because these skin disorders may be fatal, the anticonvulsants must be immediately discontinued. Lamotrigine is supplied in 25, 50, 100, and 200 mg tablets.

PHENOBARBITAL AND PRIMIDONE. These are relatively safe anticonvulsants that are particularly useful for generalized tonic-clonic seizures. Approximately 25% of children undergo severe behavioral changes on these drugs. Neurologically abnormal children are at greater risk. Furthermore, there is evidence that phenobarbital may adversely affect the cognitive performance of children treated on a long-term basis. Valproic acid interferes with the metabolism of phenobarbital, causing elevated phenobarbital plasma levels and toxicity despite the usual daily doses. Phenobarbital acts on the GABA receptor to increase the chloride channel open duration (see Fig. 593-4). The plasma half-life is 48–150 hr. Phenobarbital is supplied in an elixir, 4 mg/mL; tablets, 15, 30, 60, and 100 mg; and injectable, 30 and 120 mg/mL. Primidone is prepared in a suspension, 50 mg/mL, and in 125 and 250 mg tablets. The plasma half-life of primidone is 10–21 hr. Phenobarbital is prescribed twice daily, and primidone is prescribed three times a day. Routine blood tests are not indicated for these anticonvulsants.

PHENYTOIN. Phenytoin acts by decreasing the sustained repetitive firing of single neurons by blocking sodium-dependent channels and decreasing depolarization-dependent calcium uptake. Phenytoin is used for primary and secondary generalized tonic-clonic seizures, partial seizures, and status epilepticus. The plasma half-life is 7–42 hr. Phenytoin has many drug interactions that may increase or decrease other concomitantly used anticonvulsants (see Table 593-5). Phenytoin is supplied in a suspension, 6 and 25 mg/mL; chewable tablets, 50 mg; capsules, 100 mg; and injectable, 100 mg/2 mL and 250 mg/5 mL. Fosphenytoin, a water-soluble prodrug of phenytoin for intramuscular or intravenous use, is available in a concentration of 75 mg/mL, equivalent to 50 mg/mL of phenytoin.

TIAGABINE. Tiagabine inhibits seizure activity by blocking reuptake of the neuroinhibitory transmitter GABA into neuronal and glial cells (see Fig. 593-4). The drug is effective in the management of complex partial seizures as an add-on drug. Tiagabine is supplied in 4, 12, 16, and 20 mg tablets.

TOPIRAMATE. Topiramate produces anticonvulsant action by blocking voltage-dependent sodium channels. The drug is used as adjunctive therapy for refractory complex seizures with or without secondary generalization. The elimination half-life is 21 hr. Phenytoin, carbamazepine, and valproic acid may decrease the concentration of topiramate. Topiramate is dispensed in 25, 100, and 200 mg tablets.

VALPROIC ACID. Valproic acid is a broad-spectrum anticonvulsant. It acts by blocking voltage-dependent sodium channels and increases calcium-dependent potassium conductance. The elimination half-life is 6–16 hr. This drug is useful for the management of many seizure types, including generalized tonic-clonic, absence, atypical absence, and myoclonic seizures. It rarely induces behavioral changes but is associated with mild gastrointestinal disturbances, alopecia, tremor, and hyperphagia. Two rare but serious side effects of valproate are a Reye-like syndrome and irreversible hepatotoxicity. A small number of children develop progressive lethargy and coma with elevated serum ammonia and decreased levels of serum carnitine. Valproic acid may block the metabolism of carnitine, producing the altered state of consciousness in these patients. Discontinuation of valproic acid leads to recovery over several days.

Another small group of patients, particularly children younger than 2 yr and having specific neurologic syndromes, who are treated with several anticonvulsants simultaneously are at significant risk (1 : 800) for developing an idiosyncratic potentially fatal hepatotoxic syndrome, characterized by abdominal pain, anorexia, weight loss, and retching within a few weeks to months of beginning valproate therapy. These patients have normal results of liver function studies during the initial stages; thus, significant and persistent gastrointestinal symptoms are cause for alarm during the initial few months of valproate therapy. If reduction in the valproate dose does not provide immediate relief, the physician should discontinue the drug. To decrease the risk of fatal hepatotoxicity, a series of screening tests for an underlying metabolic disorder is indicated before initiation of valproic acid therapy for a child younger than 2 yr and having a seizure disorder of unknown cause. The tests include determinations of serum ammonium, amino acids, blood gases, a lactate-pyruvate ratio, urinary organic acids, and free and total serum carnitine. The incidence of fatal valproic acid–induced hepatotoxicity has decreased dramatically in recent years due to less use of the drug in epileptic children younger than 2 yr and the knowledge that monotherapy is much less likely to result in fatal liver disease.

Valproic acid also may cause a decrease in serum-free carnitine levels by inhibition of plasmalemmal carnitine uptake. Some studies suggest that carnitine deficiency is a major cause of valproate hepatotoxicity and that supplementation with L-carnitine, 50–100 mg/kg/24 hr, may prevent this fatal complication. Until further data are available, it is recommended that L-carnitine supplementation be provided to those children at greatest risk for hepatotoxicity (see earlier). In older children on valproic acid therapy, L-carnitine supplementation should be administered if there are clinical symptoms suggestive of carnitine deficiency (weakness, lethargy, hypotonia) or if a significant decrease in the serum-free carnitine levels is measured on a periodic basis. Valproic acid is available in a syrup, 50 mg/mL; capsules, 250 and 500 mg; and tablets, 125, 250, and 500 mg. Depakote sprinkle capsules (divalproex sodium, a stable coordination compound composed of sodium valproate and valproic acid) are useful for children who are unable to tolerate valproate suspension, tablets, or capsules. The contents of the Depakote capsule are sprinkled onto soft food that does not require chewing. Depakote sprinkle is supplied in 125 mg capsules.

VIGABATRIN. This drug acts by binding to the degradative enzyme GABA transaminase receptor, causing an increase in GABA levels and inhibition of neurotransmission (see Fig. 593-4). The drug is effective in the management of infantile spasms, particularly in children with tuberous sclerosis. Vigabatrin is also useful as adjunctive therapy for poorly controlled seizures. The plasma half-life is 5–8 hr. Vigabatrin may cause a reduction in plasma phenobarbital and phenytoin levels. Visual field constrictions have also been reported. The drug is supplied in 500 mg tablets and 500 mg sachets.

LEVIRACTAM. This drug acts by an unknown mechanism and is indicated for use as an adjunctive treatment for partial seizures. Plasma half-life is ≈8 hr. It is supplied in 250, 500, and 750 mg tablets as Keppra.

OXCARBAZEPINE. This drug has some similarity to carbamazepine in its action and is useful as an adjunctive treatment for partial seizures in adults and children. The half-life of the drug is 2 hr, whereas that of its major metabolite, 10-mono-hydroxy oxcarbazepine (MHD), is 9 hr. A total of 30% of patients with allergic reactions to carbamazepine also react to oxcarbazepine; hyponatremia occurs in 2.5% of patients. Oxcarbazepine is supplied as Trileptal in tablets, 150, 300, and 600 mg, and in suspension, 300 mg/5 mL.

ZONISAMIDE. This drug is useful as an adjunctive treatment for partial seizures and may also be useful for myoclonic syndromes, but its mechanism of action is unclear. As a single drug, its half-life is 60 hr; half-life is shortened to 30 hr when used with drugs metabolized by the liver. Zonisamide has been associated with development of renal calculi. It is supplied as Zonegran in 100 mg tablets.

ACTH. This is the **preferred drug** for the management of **infantile spasms,** although the dose and duration of therapy are not uniform. Prednisone is equally effective. A common schedule includes ACTH, 20 U/day intramuscularly (IM) for 2 wk, and if no response occurs, the dosage is increased to 30 and then 40 U/day IM for an additional 4 wk. Unless seizure control is complete, ACTH is replaced with oral prednisone, 2 mg/kg/24 hr for 2 wk. If the seizures persist, prednisone is given for an additional 4 wk. The side effects of ACTH include hyperglycemia, hypertension, electrolyte abnormalities, gastrointestinal disturbances, infection (including *Pneumocystic carinii* pneumonia), and transient brain shrinkage observed by CT scanning. ACTH and prednisone are equally effective for the treatment of cryptogenic and symptomatic seizures, and control can be expected in ≈70% of patients. There is no relationship between the ease or degree of seizure control and ultimate neurologic and cognitive outcome. The response to medication is usually apparent within a few weeks of therapy, but one third of patients who respond suffer relapse when the ACTH or prednisone is discontinued.

KETOGENIC DIET. This treatment should be considered for the management of recalcitrant seizures, particularly for children with complex myoclonic epilepsy with associated tonic-clonic convulsions. The diet is also the primary therapy for infants with pyruvate dehydrogenase deficiency and glucose transporter protein deficiency and appears safe and effective for infants with epilepsy who are younger than 2 yr of age. The diet restricts the quantity of carbohydrate and protein, and most calories are provided as fat. Some children older than 2–3 yr will not tolerate this fatty, unpalatable diet. Because the diet demands precise weighing of foodstuffs and is time-consuming to prepare, it is not accepted by all families. Some children respond to a liberalized ketogenic diet that substitutes medium-chain triglycerides for the high-fat content of the former diet. Although the mechanism of action of the ketogenic diet is unknown, some evidence shows that it exerts an anticonvulsant effect secondary to elevated levels of β-hydroxybutyrate and acetoacetate resulting from the ketosis. The use of valproic acid is contraindicated in association with the ketogenic diet, because the risk of hepatotoxicity is enhanced.

SURGERY FOR EPILEPSY. Surgery should be considered for children with intractable seizures unresponsive to anticonvulsants. Certain children, particularly those with focal seizures, are candidates for surgery. Although the history and neurologic examination may suggest a focal onset of seizure activity, an EEG is critical in documenting the localization and extent of the epileptogenic discharges. Prolonged EEG recording with video monitoring, which may be frequently necessary, is essential for precise localization of the epileptogenic area. It is often helpful to decrease or discontinue the anticonvulsant in hospitalized patients to increase the probability of recording ictal and interictal epileptogenic activity. When the EEG used with sphenoidal electrodes does not adequately localize the focus, placement of subdural electrodes may provide invaluable information. Subdural electrodes are particularly useful in the investigation of epileptogenic foci in sites other than the temporal lobe. EEG studies are complemented by neuropsychologic testing, the Wada (intracarotid injection of amobarbital to establish the dominant hemisphere) test, single-photon emission CT (SPECT) or PET scanning, and neuroimaging procedures, including CT scanning, MRI, and functional MRI (fMRI). Some centers use magnetic source imaging/magnetoelectroencephalograms (MSI/MEG), which localize seizure discharges more precisely than other techniques. The results of surgery in children with a well-defined focus of epileptogenic activity supported by an identical structural lesion on CT scanning or MRI scan are extremely favorable.

VAGAL NERVE STIMULATION. Animal experiments have suggested that electrical stimulation of the left vagal nerve will interrupt or prevent seizures. In a double-blind trial of 60 children, 16 of whom were younger than 12 yr of age, left vagal nerve stimulation produced by an implanted device reduced seizures by 31–42% over 18 mo, suggesting that it may be a safe adjunctive therapy for patients refractory to other therapies.

COUNSELING THE PARENTS. Most parents are initially frightened by the diagnosis of epilepsy and require support and accurate information. Physicians should anticipate questions, including inquiries about the duration of the seizure disorder, side effects of medication and convulsions, etiology, social and academic repercussions, and parental guilt. Parents usually wish to know if restrictions should be placed on the child and whether the teacher should be informed. Others inquire about the genetic implications, including the risks for future children. Parents should be encouraged to treat their child as normally as possible. For most children with epilepsy, restriction of physical activity is unnecessary except that they must be attended by a responsible adult while bathing and swimming. The mechanism of the seizure and what epilepsy means should be explained, and the purpose and side effects of the specific anticonvulsant should be reviewed. Parents who understand the fundamental action and purpose of anticonvulsants and the need for a specific drug regimen are generally compliant. Counseling should include first-aid measures to be used if the seizure recurs. Fortunately, most parents and children readily adapt to the seizure disorder and to the requirement for long-term anticonvulsants. Most cases of epilepsy in children are well controlled with medication; the children have normal intelligence and can be expected to lead normal lives. These children require careful monitoring of their academic performance because learning disabilities are more common in children with epilepsy than in the general population. Cooperation and understanding among the parents, physician, teacher, and child enhance the outlook for patients with epilepsy.

Allen JE, Ferrie CD, Livingston JH, Feltbower RG: Recovery of consciousness after epileptic seizures in children. *Arch Dis Child* 2007;91:39–41.

Baumann RJ, Duffner PK: Treatment of children with simple febrile seizures: The AAP practice parameter. *Pediatr Neurol* 2000;23:11–17.

Berg AT, Testa FM, Levy SR, et al: Neuroimaging in children with newly diagnosed epilepsy: A community-based study. *Pediatrics* 2000;196:527–532.

Chang BS, Lowenstein DH: Epilepsy. *N Engl J Med* 2003;349:1257–1266.

Clusmann H, Kral T, Gleissner U, et al: Analysis of different types of resection for pediatric patients with temporal lobe epilepsy. *Neurosurgery* 2004;54:847–860.

Deonna T: Management of epilepsy. *Arch Dis Child* 2005;90:5–9.

French JA: First-choice drug for newly diagnosed epilepsy. *Lancet* 2007;369:970–971.

Guerrini R: Epilepsy in children. *Lancet* 2006;367:499–524.

Hamano SI, Yamashita S, Tanaka M, et al: Therapcutic efficacy and adverse effects of adrenocorticotropic hormone therapy in West syndrome: differences in dosage of adrenocorticotropic hormone, onset of age, and cause. *J Pediatr* 2006;148:485–488.

Hamano SI, Yoshinari S, Higurashi N, et al: Developmental outcomes of cryptogenic West syndrome. *J Pediatr* 2007;150:295–299.

Hirtz D, Ashwal MD, Berg A, et al: Practice parameter: Evaluating a first nonfebrile seizure in children. *Neurology* 2000;55:616–623.

Hirtz D, Berg A, Bettis D, et al: Practice parameter: Treatment of the child with a first unprovoked seizure. *Neurology* 2003;60:166–175.

Kneen R, Appleton R: Status epilepticus with fever: How common is meningitis? *Arch Dis Child* 2005;90:3–4.

LaRoche SM, Helmers SL: The new antiepileptic drugs: Scientific review. *JAMA* 2004;291:605–614.

LaRoche SM, Helmers SL: The new antiepileptic drugs: Clinical applications. *JAMA* 2004;291:615–620.

Lee JYK, Adelson PD: Neurosurgical management of pediatric epilepsy. *Pediatr Clin North Am* 2004;51:441–456.

Lux AL, Edwards SW, Hancock E, et al: The United Kingdom infantile spasms study comparing vigabatrin with prednisolone or tetracosactide at 14 days: A multicentre, randomized controlled trial. *Lancet* 2004;364:1773–1778.

Marson A, Jacoby A, Johnson A, et al: Immediate versus deferred antiepileptic drug treatment for early epilepsy and single seizures: A randomized controlled trial. *Lancet* 2005;365:2007–2012.
Murphy JV, et al: Left vagal nerve stimulation in children with medically refractory epilepsy. *J Pediatr* 1994;134:563–566.
Nordli DR, Kuroda MM, Carroll J, et al: Experience with the ketogenic diet in infants. *Pediatrics* 2001;198:129–133.
Pohlmann-Eden B, Beghi E, Camfield C, Camfield P: The first seizure and its management in adults and children. *BMJ* 2006;332:339–342.
Romanelli P, Verdecchia M, Rodas R, et al: Epilepsy surgery for tuberous sclerosis. *Pediatr Neurol* 2004;31:239–247.
Sadleir LG, Scheffer IE: Febrile seizures. *BMJ* 2007;334:307–311.
Sankar R: Initial treatment of epilepsy with antileptic drugs: Pediatric issues. *Neurology* 2004;63:S30–S39.
Shinnar S, Pellock JM: Update on the epidemiology and prognosis of pediatric epilepsy. *J Child Neurol* 2002;17:S4–S17.
Siddiqui A, Kerb R, Weale ME, et al: Association of multidrug resistance in epilepsy with a polymorphism in the drug-transporter gene *ABCB1*. *N Engl J Med* 2003;348:1442–1448.
Wang HS, Kuo MF, Chou ML, et al: Pyridoxal phosphate is better than pyridoxine for controlling idiopathic intractable epilepsy. *Arch Dis Child* 2005;90:512–515.
Warden CR, Zibulewsky J, Mace S, et al: Evaluation and management of febrile seizures in the out-of hospital and emergency department settings. *Ann Emerg Med* 2003;41:215–222.
Wiebe S, Blume WT, Girvin JP, et al: A randomized, controlled trial of surgery for temporal-lobe epilepsy. *N Engl J Med* 2001;345:311–318.
Wong M, Schlaggar BL, Landt M: Postictal cerebrospinal fluid abnormalities in children. *J Pediatr* 2001;138:373–377.

TABLE 593-6. Paroxysmal Disorders of the Neonatal Period

PAROXYSMAL NONEPILEPTIFORM DISORDERS
Jitteriness
Benign neonatal sleep myoclonus
ACUTE SYMPTOMATIC SEIZURES AND OCCASIONAL SEIZURES*
Hypoxic-ischemic encephalopathy
Intraventricular hemorrhage
Acute metabolic disorders[†]
Sepsis-meningitis
EPILEPTIC SYNDROMES
Benign idiopathic neonatal convulsions
Familial
Nonfamilial
Symptomatic focal epilepsy
Brain tumor
Malformations of cortical development
Inherited metabolic disease; mitochondrial disorders
Early-onset generalized epileptic syndromes with encephalopathy
Early myoclonic encephalopathy
Early infantile encephalopathic epilepsy

*See Table 593-7.
[†]Hypoglycemia, hypocalcemia, hypomagnesemia, hyponatremia, hypernatremia.
From Kliegman RM, Greenbaum LA, Lye PS: *Practical Strategies in Pediatric Diagnosis and Therapy*, 2nd ed. Philadelphia, Elsevier, 2004, p 680.

593.7 • Neonatal Seizures (see Chapters 97–100)

Neonates are at particular risk for the development of seizures because metabolic, toxic, structural, and infectious diseases are more likely to be manifested during this time than at any other period of life. Neonatal seizures are dissimilar from those in a child or adult because generalized tonic-clonic convulsions tend not to occur in the 1st mo of life. The arborization of axons and dendritic processes as well as myelination is incomplete in the neonatal brain. A seizure discharge, therefore, cannot readily be propagated throughout the neonatal brain to produce a generalized seizure.

CLINICAL MANIFESTATIONS AND CLASSIFICATION. **Focal seizures** consist of rhythmic twitching of muscle groups, particularly those of the extremities and face. These seizures are often associated with localized structural lesions as well as with infections and subarachnoid hemorrhage. **Multifocal clonic** convulsions are similar to focal clonic seizures but differ in that many muscle groups are involved, frequently several simultaneously. **Tonic seizures** are characterized by rigid posturing of the extremities and trunk and are sometimes associated with fixed deviation of the eyes. **Myoclonic seizures** are brief focal or generalized jerks of the extremities or body that tend to involve distal muscle groups. **Subtle seizures** consist of chewing motions, excessive salivation, and alterations in the respiratory rate including apnea, blinking, nystagmus, bicycling or pedaling movements, and changes in color.

Neonatal seizures may be difficult to recognize clinically, and some neonatal behaviors that were previously considered to be convulsions are not substantiated by the EEG recording (Table 593-6). Nonetheless, several clinical features distinguish seizures from nonepileptic activity in neonates. Autonomic changes such as tachycardia and elevation of the blood pressure are common with seizures but do not occur with nonepileptic events. Nonepileptic movements are suppressed by gentle restraint, but true seizures are not. Nonepileptic phenomena are enhanced by sensory stimuli that have no influence on seizures. Correct classification of neonatal seizures is important for appropriate selection of anticonvulsant therapy. Studies using polygraphic EEG recording with video monitoring have greatly enhanced the characterization of neonatal seizures and their medical management.

EEG CLASSIFICATION OF NEONATAL SEIZURES

CLINICAL SEIZURE WITH A CONSISTENT EEG EVENT. In this category, a clinical seizure occurs in relationship to seizure activity recorded on the EEG and includes focal clonic, focal tonic, and some myoclonic seizures. These seizures are clearly epileptic and are likely to respond to an anticonvulsant.

CLINICAL SEIZURES WITH INCONSISTENT EEG EVENTS. Neonates may have a clinical seizure without a corresponding seizure discharge. This is observed with all generalized tonic seizures and subtle seizures and with some myoclonic seizures. These infants tend to be neurologically depressed or comatose as a result of hypoxic-ischemic encephalopathy. Seizures in this category are likely to be of nonepileptic origin and may not require or respond to antiepileptics.

ELECTRICAL SEIZURES WITH ABSENT CLINICAL SEIZURES. Electrical seizures associated with a markedly abnormal background EEG may develop in comatose infants who are not on anticonvulsants. Conversely, electrical seizures may persist in patients with focal tonic or clonic seizures without clinical signs after the introduction of an anticonvulsant.

ETIOLOGIC DIAGNOSIS. The most common cause of neonatal seizures, hypoxic-ischemic encephalopathy, is discussed in Chapter 99.5. Many additional disorders are likely to cause seizures, including metabolic, infectious, traumatic, structural, hemorrhagic, embolic, and maternal disturbances (Table 593-7). Because seizures in neonates may indicate a serious, life-threatening, and potentially reversible disease, it is imperative that a timely and organized approach to the investigation of neonatal seizures be carried out.

TABLE 593-7. Causes of Neonatal Seizures

AGES 1–4 DAYS
Hypoxic-ischemic encephalopathy
Drug withdrawal, maternal drug use of narcotic or barbiturates
Drug toxicity: lidocaine, penicillin
Intraventricular hemorrhage
Acute metabolic disorders
- Hypocalcemia
  - Perinatal asphyxia, small for gestational age
  - Sepsis
  - Maternal diabetes, hyperthyroidism, or hypoparathyroidism
- Hypoglycemia
  - Perinatal insults, prematurity, small for gestational age
  - Maternal diabetes
  - Hyperinsulinemic hypoglycemia
  - Sepsis
- Hypomagnesemia
- Hyponatremia or hypernatremia
  - Iatrogenic or inappropriate antidiuretic hormone secretion

Inborn errors of metabolism
- Galactosemia
- Hyperglycinemia
- Urea cycle disorders

Pyridoxine deficiency (must be considered at any age)

AGES 4–14 DAYS
Infection
- Meningitis (bacterial), encephalitis (enteroviral, herpes simplex)

Metabolic disorders
- Hypocalcemia
  - Diet, milk formula
- Hypoglycemia, persistent
  - Inherited disorders of metabolism: galactosemia, fructosemia, leucine sensitivity
  - Hyperinsulinemic hypoglycemia
  - Anterior pituitary hypoplasia, pancreatic islet cell tumor
  - Beckwith syndrome

Drug withdrawal, maternal drug use of narcotic or barbiturates
Benign neonatal convulsions, familial and nonfamilial
Kernicterus, hyperbilirubinemia

AGES 2–8 WEEKS
Infection
- Herpes simplex or enteroviral encephalitis, bacterial meningitis

Head injury
- Subdural hematoma, child abuse

Inherited disorders of metabolism
- Aminoacidurias, urea cycle defects, organic acidurias
- Neonatal adrenoleukodystrophy

Malformations of cortical development
- Lissencephaly
- Focal cortical dysplasia

Tuberous sclerosis
Sturge-Weber syndrome

From Kliegman RM, Greenbaum LA, Lye PS: *Practical Strategies in Pediatric Diagnosis and Therapy*, 2nd ed. Philadelphia, Elsevier, 2004, p 681.

Careful neurologic examination of the infant may uncover the cause of the seizure disorder. Examination of the **retina** may show the presence of chorioretinitis, suggesting a congenital infection in which case *t*oxoplasmosis, *r*ubella, *c*ytomegalovirus, and *h*erpes simplex (TORCH) titers of mother and infant are indicated. The **Aicardi syndrome,** which occurs exclusively in infant girls, is associated with coloboma of the iris and retinal lacunae, refractory seizures, and absence of the corpus callosum. Inspection of the **skin** may show hypopigmented lesions characteristic of tuberous sclerosis or the typical crusted vesicular lesions of incontinentia pigmenti; both neurocutaneous syndromes are associated with generalized myoclonic seizures beginning early in life. An unusual body odor suggests an inborn error of metabolism.

Blood should be obtained for determinations of glucose, calcium, magnesium, electrolytes, and blood urea nitrogen. If hypoglycemia is a possibility, a serum Dextrostix testing is indicated so that treatment can be initiated immediately. See Chapter 107 for a discussion of the diagnosis and treatment of hypoglycemia. Hypocalcemia may occur in isolation or in association with hypomagnesemia. A lowered serum calcium level is often associated with birth trauma or a CNS insult in the perinatal period. Additional causes include maternal diabetes, prematurity, DiGeorge syndrome, and high-phosphate feedings. Hypomagnesemia (<1.5 mg/dL) is often associated with hypocalcemia and occurs particularly in infants of malnourished mothers. In this situation, the seizures are resistant to calcium therapy but respond to intramuscular magnesium, 0.2 mL/kg of a 50% solution of $MgSO_4$. See Chapter 106 for diagnosis and treatment of hypomagnesemia. Serum electrolyte measurement may indicate significant hyponatremia (serum sodium <135 mEq/L) or hypernatremia (serum sodium >150 mEq/L) as a cause of the seizure disorder.

A **lumbar puncture** is indicated in virtually all neonates with seizures, unless the cause is obviously related to a metabolic disorder such as hypoglycemia or hypocalcemia secondary to feeding of high concentrations of phosphate. These latter infants are normally alert interictally and usually respond promptly to appropriate therapy. The CSF findings may indicate a bacterial meningitis or aseptic encephalitis (see Chapters 109 and 602). Prompt diagnosis and appropriate therapy improve the outcome for these infants. Bloody CSF indicates a traumatic tap or a subarachnoid/intraventricular bleed. Immediate centrifugation of the specimen may assist in differentiation of the two disorders. A clear supernatant suggests a traumatic tap, and a xanthochromic color suggests a subarachnoid bleed. Mildly jaundiced normal infants may have a yellowish discoloration of the CSF that makes inspection of the supernatant less reliable in the newborn period.

Many **inborn errors of metabolism** cause generalized convulsions in the newborn period. Because these conditions are often inherited in an autosomal recessive or X-linked recessive fashion, it is imperative that a careful family history be obtained to determine whether siblings or close relatives developed seizures or died at an early age. Serum ammonia determination is useful for screening for suspected urea cycle abnormalities, such as ornithine transcarbamylase, arginosuccinic lysate, and carbamoylphosphate synthetase deficiencies. In addition to having generalized clonic seizures, these infants present during the 1st few days of life with increasing lethargy progressing to coma, anorexia and vomiting, and a bulging fontanel. If the blood gases show an anion gap and a metabolic acidosis with hyperammonemia, urine organic acids should be immediately determined to investigate the possibility of methylmalonic or propionic acidemia. Maple syrup urine disease (MSUD) should be suspected when a metabolic acidosis occurs in association with generalized clonic seizures, vomiting, and muscle rigidity during the 1st wk of life. The result of a rapid screening test using 2,4-dinitrophenylhydrazine that identifies ketoderivatives in the urine is positive in MSUD. Additional metabolic causes of neonatal seizures include nonketotic hyperglycemia, a lethal condition characterized by markedly elevated plasma and CSF glycine levels, persistent generalized seizures, and lethargy rapidly leading to coma; ketotic hyperglycinemia in which seizures are associated with vomiting, fluid and electrolyte disturbances, and a metabolic acidosis; and Leigh disease suggested by elevated levels of serum and CSF lactate or an increased lactate/pyruvate ratio. Biotinidase deficiency should also be considered. A comprehensive description of the diagnosis and management of these metabolic diseases is discussed in Part X.

Unintentional **injection of a local anesthetic** into a fetus during labor can produce intense tonic seizures. These infants are often thought to have had a traumatic delivery because they are flaccid at birth, have abnormal brainstem reflexes, and show signs of respiratory depression that sometimes requires ventilation. Examination may show a needle puncture of the skin or a perforation or laceration of the scalp. An elevated serum anesthetic level confirms the diagnosis. The treatment consists of supportive measures and promotion of urine output by administering intravenous fluids with appropriate monitoring to prevent fluid overload.

Benign familial neonatal seizures, an autosomal dominant condition, begins on the 2nd–3rd day of life, with a seizure frequency of 10–20/day. Patients are normal between seizures, which stop in 1–6 mo. **Fifth-day fits** occur on day 5 of life (4–6 days) in normal-appearing neonates. The seizures are multifocal and are present for less than 24 hr. The diagnosis requires exclusion of other causes of seizures. The prognosis is good.

Pyridoxine dependency, a rare disorder, must be considered when generalized clonic seizures begin shortly after birth with signs of fetal distress in utero. These seizures are particularly resistant to conventional anticonvulsants, such as phenobarbital or phenytoin. The history may suggest that similar seizures occurred in utero. Some cases of pyridoxine dependency are reported to begin later in infancy or in early childhood. This condition is inherited as an autosomal recessive. Although the precise biochemical defect is unknown, pyridoxine is essential for the synthesis of glutamic acid decarboxylase, which, in turn, is required for the synthesis of GABA. In affected infants, large amounts of pyridoxine are required to maintain adequate production of GABA. When pyridoxine-dependent seizures are suspected, pyridoxine, 100–200 mg or pyridoxal phosphate, should be administered intravenously during the EEG, which should be promptly completed once the diagnosis is considered. The seizures abruptly cease, and the EEG normalizes in the next few hours. Not all cases of pyridoxine dependency respond dramatically to the initial bolus of IV pyridoxine. Therefore, a 6 wk trial of oral pyridoxine (10–20 mg/day) or pyridoxal phosphate is recommended for infants in whom a high index of suspicion continues after a negative response to IV pyridoxine. In the future, measurement of CSF and plasma pyridoxal-5-phosphate may prove to be the more precise method of confirming the diagnosis of pyridoxine dependency. These children require lifelong supplementation of oral pyridoxine, 10 mg/day. Generally, the earlier the diagnosis and therapy with pyridoxine, the more favorable is the outcome. Untreated children have persistent seizures and are uniformly severely mentally retarded.

Drug withdrawal seizures can present in the newborn nursery but may take several weeks to develop because of prolonged excretion of the drug by the neonate. The incriminated drugs include barbiturates, benzodiazepines, heroin, and methadone. The infant may be jittery, irritable, and lethargic and may show myoclonus or frank clonic seizures. The mother may deny the use of drugs; a serum or urine analysis may identify the responsible agent (see Chapter 106).

Infants with focal seizures, suspected stroke or intracranial hemorrhage, and severe **cytoarchitectural abnormalities** of the brain (including lissencephaly and schizencephaly) who clinically may appear normal or microcephalic should undergo MRI or CT scan. Indeed, many recommend imaging of all neonates with seizures unexplained by serum glucose, calcium, or electrolyte disorders. Infants with chromosome abnormalities and adrenoleukodystrophy are also at risk for seizures and should be evaluated with investigation of a karyotype and serum long-chain fatty acids, respectively.

TREATMENT. Anticonvulsants should be used in the treatment of infants with seizures secondary to hypoxic-ischemic encephalopathy or an acute intracranial bleed (see Chapters 99.2 and 99.5). The dose and administration of phenobarbital, diazepam, and other medications for the treatment of neonatal seizures are discussed in Chapter 99.5. Phenytoin and phenobarbital are equally but incompletely effective as anticonvulsants in neonates, controlling seizures in less than half of cases. The greater use of EEG recording in infants with subtle seizures has identified a number of patients with abnormal movements unrelated to seizure discharges.

PROGNOSIS. This depends mainly on the primary cause of the disorder or the severity of the insult. In the case of hypoglycemic infants of a diabetic mother or hypocalcemia associated with excessive phosphate feedings, the prognosis is excellent. Conversely, a child with intractable seizures due to severe hypoxic-ischemic encephalopathy or a cytoarchitectural abnormality of the brain usually does not respond to anticonvulsants and is susceptible to status epilepticus and early death. The challenge for the physician is to identify patients who will recover with prompt treatment and to avoid delays in diagnosis that could lead to severe, irreversible neurologic damage.

Baxter P: Pyridoxine or pyridoxal phosphate for intractable seizures? *Arch Dis Child* 2005;90:441–442.

Gilman JT, Gal P, Duchowny MS, et al: Rapid sequential phenobarbital treatment of neonatal seizures. *Pediatrics* 1989;83:674–678.

Hillman L, Hillman R, Dodson WE: Diagnosis, treatment and follow-up of neonatal mepivacaine intoxication secondary to paracervical and pudendal blocks during labor. *J Pediatr* 1979;95:472–477.

Legido A, Clancy RR, Berman P: Neurologic outcome after electroencephalographically proven neonatal seizures. *Pediatrics* 1991;88:583–596.

Painter MJ, Scher MS, Stein AD, et al: Phenobarbital compared with phenytoin for treatment of neonatal seizures. *N Engl J Med* 1999;341:485–489.

Sankar R, Painter MJ: Neonatal seizures, after all these years we still love what doesn't work. *Neurology* 2005;64:776–777.

Sillanpää M, Jalava M, Kaleva O, et al: Long-term prognosis of seizures with onset in childhood. *N Engl J Med* 1998;338:1715–1722.

Volpe JJ: Neonatal seizures: Current concepts and revised classification. *Pediatrics* 1989;84:422–428.

593.8 • Status Epilepticus

Status epilepticus is defined as a **continuous** convulsion lasting longer than 20–30 min or the occurrence of **serial convulsions** between which there is no return of consciousness. Status epilepticus may be classified as generalized (tonic-clonic, absence) or partial (simple, complex, or with secondary generalization). Generalized tonic-clonic seizures predominate in cases of status epilepticus. Status epilepticus is a medical emergency that requires an organized and skillful approach to minimize the associated mortality and morbidity.

ETIOLOGY. There are three major subtypes of status epilepticus in children: prolonged febrile seizures; idiopathic status epilepticus, in which a seizure develops in the absence of an underlying CNS lesion or insult; and symptomatic status epilepticus, when the seizure occurs as a result of an underlying neurologic disorder or a metabolic abnormality. A febrile seizure lasting for >30 min, particularly in a child younger than 3 yr of age, is the most common cause of status epilepticus. The idiopathic group includes epileptic patients in whom status epilepticus followed sudden withdrawal of anticonvulsants (especially benzodiazepines and barbiturates). Epileptic children who are given anticonvulsants on an irregular basis or who are noncompliant are more likely to develop status epilepticus. Status epilepticus may also be the initial presentation of epilepsy. Sleep deprivation and an intercurrent infection tend to render epileptic patients more susceptible to status epilepticus. The mortality and morbidity among patients with prolonged febrile seizures and idiopathic status epilepticus are low.

Status epilepticus due to other causes has a much higher mortality rate, and the cause of death usually is directly attributable to the underlying abnormality. Unlike those with idiopathic status epilepticus, many of these children have not previously had a convulsion. Prolonged status epilepticus has been associated with severe damage to the hippocampus in children, so-called **hippocampal sclerosis.** A prolonged convulsion may be the initial manifestation of **encephalitis,** and epilepsy may be a long-term complication of **meningitis.** Infants with congenital malformations of the brain (lissencephaly or schizencephaly) may have recurrent episodes of status epilepticus that are frequently refractory to anticonvulsants. Inborn errors of metabolism may present with status epilepticus in newborns. Affected infants often have a progressive loss of consciousness associated with failure to thrive and excessive vomiting. Electrolyte abnormalities, hypocalcemia, hypoglycemia, drug intoxication, Reye syndrome, lead intoxication, extreme hyperpyrexia, and brain tumors, particularly in the frontal lobe, are additional causes of status epilepticus.

PATHOPHYSIOLOGY. The relationship between the neurologic outcome and the duration of status epilepticus is unknown in children and adults. Children appear to be more resistant to neuronal injury from status epilepticus than adults. In primates, pathologic changes can occur in the brain of ventilated animals after 60 min of constant seizure activity when metabolic homeostasis is maintained. Cell death may result from excessive release of the excitatory neurotransmitter glutamate and excessive stimulation of glutamate receptors, a process known as "excitotoxicity." The most vulnerable areas of the brain include the hippocampus, amygdala, cerebellum, middle cortical area, and thalamus. Characteristic acute pathologic changes consist of venous congestion, small petechial hemorrhages, and edema. Ischemic cellular changes are the earliest histologic finding, followed by neuronophagia, microglial proliferation, cell loss, and increased numbers of reactive astrocytes. Neuronal concentrations of calcium, arachidonic acid, and prostaglandins increase and may promote cell death. Prolonged generalized seizure activity may lead to dysfunction of the autonomic nervous system with hypotension and shock as well as to lactic acidosis, myoglobinuria, and acute tubular necrosis.

Several investigations have shown that seizures become more difficult to stop and the chances of neuronal injury increase when seizures persist beyond a *transitional period* that varies from 20 to 60 min in animals during constant seizure activity. Treatment of children should be directed to supporting vital functions and to controlling the convulsions as expeditiously as possible, because the precise transitional period in humans is unknown.

TREATMENT. Initial treatment of patients begins with an assessment of the respiratory and cardiovascular systems. Children should be transferred to an intensive care unit. The oral airway is secured and inspected for patency, and the pulse, temperature, respirations, and blood pressure are recorded. Excessive oral secretions are removed by gentle suction, and a properly fitting face mask attached to oxygen is applied. If patients do not respond to oxygen by mask or are difficult to ventilate by an Ambu bag, they require intubation and assisted ventilation. A nasogastric tube is placed in position, and an IV catheter is immediately inserted. If hypoglycemia is confirmed by Dextrostix, a rapid infusion of 5 mL/kg of 10% dextrose is provided. Blood is obtained for a CBC and for determination of electrolytes (including calcium, phosphorus, and magnesium), glucose, creatinine, lactate, and anticonvulsant levels, if indicated. Blood and urine may be obtained for metabolic studies and toxicology, keeping in mind that some drugs potentiate or precipitate status epilepticus (amphetamines, cocaine, phenothiazines, theophylline in toxic levels, tricyclic antidepressants). Arterial blood gases should be determined, and oxygen saturation (SaO_2) should be monitored with an oximeter. Examination of the CSF is imperative if meningitis or encephalitis is considered, unless there is a contraindication to the procedure. In this case, appropriate antibiotics should be administered, followed by imaging studies, **before** a lumbar puncture is attempted. If the seizures are refractory to the front-line anticonvulsants or if the patient is paralyzed and is on a respirator, continuous EEG monitoring is important to assess the frequency of seizure discharges, their location, and the response to anticonvulsant therapy.

A **physical and neurologic examination** should be carried out concurrently to assess the following: evidence of trauma; papilledema, a bulging anterior fontanel, or lateralizing neurologic signs suggesting increased intracranial pressure (ICP); manifestations of sepsis or meningitis; retinal hemorrhages that may indicate a subdural hematoma; Kussmaul breathing and dehydration suggestive of metabolic acidosis or irregular respirations signifying brainstem dysfunction; evidence of failure to thrive, a peculiar body odor, or abnormal hair pigmentation that suggests an inborn error of metabolism; and constriction or dilatation of pupils suggesting a toxin or drugs as the cause of the status epilepticus. A comprehensive examination should be undertaken once the seizures are under control. Further investigation of the patient including neuroradiologic studies depends on the physical and neurologic findings and on a precise history of the seizure type and frequency.

Drugs should always be administered IV in the management of status epilepticus; the IM route is unreliable because some drugs are sequestered by muscle. One of the major problems in the management of status epilepticus is the inappropriate use of anticonvulsants. An unsuitably low drug dose is too often given, and with lack of response, another antiepileptic is introduced immediately. Care should be given with regard to how the anticonvulsant is administered. Phenytoin forms a precipitate in glucose solutions and is rendered ineffective. It is essential to have resuscitation equipment at the bedside and the ability to intubate and ventilate the patient immediately if respiratory depression occurs.

A **benzodiazepine** (diazepam, lorazepam, or midazolam) should be used initially, because these are effective for immediate control of prolonged tonic-clonic seizures in most children. Diazepam should be given IV directly into the vein (not the tubing) in a dose of 0.1–0.3 mg/kg at a rate no greater than 2 mg/min for a maximum of three doses. Diazepam in the form of a rectal gel can also be given outside a hospital setting or in a hospital when IV access is not immediately available. The dose is 0.2–0.5 mg/kg.

Buccal or nasal midazolam (0.5 mg/kg) is another option when IV access is not available and can be administered safely by the emergency medical service (EMS) crew prior to arrival to the hospital. Respiratory depression and hypotension can occur, especially if administered with a barbiturate. Benzodiazepines may be as effective as pentobarbital with fewer side effects. Diazepam is effective in the management of tonic-clonic status, but the drug has a short half-life and seizures thus recur unless a longer acting anticonvulsant is administered simultaneously. Lorazepam is an equally effective short-term anticonvulsant, with a greater duration of action and decreased likelihood of producing hypotension and respiratory arrest. The recommended dose is 0.05–0.1 mg/kg IV administered slowly. The dose of midazolam is 0.15–0.3 mg/kg IV. If an IV line cannot be established or the child is some distance from a medical center, rectal diazepam or lorazepam can be used safely. Diazepam diluted in 3 mL 0.9% NaCl is placed into the rectum by a syringe and a flexible tube at a dose of 0.3–0.5 mg/kg. The effective dose of rectal lorazepam is 0.05–0.1 mg/kg. Therapeutic serum levels occur within 5–10 min. Sublingual lorazepam may be used to treat children with serial seizures that tend to develop into status epilepticus while the children are at home. The dose of sublingual lorazepam is 0.05–0.1 mg/kg. The tablet is placed under the patient's tongue and dissolves in a few seconds. Rectal diazepam gel (Diastat, pediatric doses of 2.5, 5, or 10 mg) may also be useful.

After administration of diazepam or lorazepam, several options are available for further management. If the convulsive activity ceases after diazepam or lorazepam therapy or if the seizures persist, **phenytoin** is given immediately. The loading dose of phenytoin is 15 up to 30 mg/kg IV (given in 10 mg/kg increments) at the rate of 1 mg/kg/min. The phenytoin prodrug **fosphenytoin** has advantages over the older formulation because it is water soluble, less irritating after IV injection, and well absorbed after intramuscular injection. Parenteral fosphenytoin (Cerebyx) is formulated in phenytoin equivalent (PE) units to allow the administration of the same amount of phenytoin despite its higher molecular weight (150 mg of fosphenytoin equals 100 mg of phenytoin). The dosage in PE units is the same as for the older phenytoin preparation. The older preparation of phenytoin may be safely added to half-normal or normal saline but not to glucose solutions; the undiluted drug can cause pain, irritation, and phlebitis of the vein. Electrocardiography is recommended during the loading phase to identify arrhythmias and bradycardia, a rare complication in children. Systemic hypotension may also complicate IV phenytoin. If the seizures do not recur, a maintenance dose of 3–9 mg/kg divided into two equal doses daily is begun 12–24 hr later. Serum phenytoin levels should be monitored because the maintenance dose varies considerably with age. Phenytoin is not always effective in controlling tonic-clonic status epilepticus, in which case an alternative drug is necessary. In some centers, **phenobarbital** is initiated before phenytoin. It is given in a loading dose of 15–20 mg/kg or in neonates 20–30 mg/kg IV during 10–30 min. With control of the seizures, the maintenance dose is 3–5 mg/kg/24 hr divided into two equal doses.

If the status epilepticus is not controlled by the preceding strategy, the physician must make some important therapeutic decisions, because it is likely the *transitional period* has passed. The choices for further drug management include a diazepam infusion, barbiturate coma, paraldehyde, or general anesthesia. By this stage, the patient is usually sedated and may show signs of respiratory depression, necessitating elective intubation and assisted ventilation.

Constant IV infusion of either **midazolam** (0.20 mg/kg bolus, 20–400 µg/kg/hr infusion) or **propofol** (1–2 mg/kg, 2–10 mg/kg/hr infusion) is effective in managing seizures during status epilepticus unresponsive to other anticonvulsants. If seizures continue, serious consideration is given to induction of barbiturate coma. In an intensive care unit, the patient is placed on a ventilator and a continuous EEG monitor. The initial IV loading dose of thiopental is 2–4 mg/kg and is then titrated to achieve a burst suppression EEG pattern. Barbiturate coma is continued for at least 48 hr, followed by cessation of thiopental until the serum phenobarbital level falls to the therapeutic range. Barbiturate coma requires careful monitoring because hypotension due to myocardial depression often requires pressor therapy.

Valproic acid has been an effective anticonvulsant in the management of several types of seizures. Valproic acid is available as an injectable and may be given IV. Preliminary studies recommend a loading dose of IV valproic acid, 10–15 mg/kg. IV valproic acid may become a useful drug for status epilepticus.

Paraldehyde is relatively safe for administration to children. A 5% solution of paraldehyde is prepared by adding 1.75 mL of paraldehyde (1 g/mL) to D5W to a total volume of 35 mL. The loading dose is 150–200 mg/kg IV slowly for 15–20 min, and then seizure control is maintained with an infusion of 20 mg/kg/hr in a 5% concentration in a glass bottle, because the drug is incompatible with plastic. The IV drip rate may be lowered as the seizures and EEG improve. The drug should be freshly opened, because outdated paraldehyde can deteriorate to acetylaldehyde and acetic acid.

General anesthesia is an alternative adjunct to the management of status epilepticus if conventional drug therapy is not effective or if barbiturate coma is not an option. Several agents have been used successfully, including halothane and isoflurane. General anesthesia probably acts by reversing cerebral anoxia and the concomitant metabolic abnormalities, allowing the previously administered anticonvulsants to exert their effect. The major disadvantage of general anesthesia is that it must be administered by well-trained personnel with anesthetic gas scavenging equipment for prolonged periods.

The use of anticonvulsant therapy after status epilepticus is controversial. There is little question that a long-term antiepileptic should be maintained in children with a progressive neurologic disorder or with a history of recurrent seizures before the onset of status epilepticus. It is unlikely that a lengthy period of anticonvulsant treatment is necessary after an initial attack of idiopathic status epilepticus, particularly when a prolonged febrile seizure was the cause. Anticonvulsant therapy is maintained arbitrarily for 3 mo in this case and is discontinued if the child remains asymptomatic.

PROGNOSIS. Status epilepticus produces potentially life-threatening disturbances in physiologic function, and the mortality rate of status epilepticus is ≈5%. The greatest number of deaths occur in the symptomatic group, most of whom have a serious and life-threatening CNS disorder known before the onset of status epilepticus. In the absence of a progressive neurologic insult (e.g., herpes encephalitis) or metabolic disorder, the morbidity from status epilepticus is low. The fact that long-term sequelae such as hemiplegia, extrapyramidal syndromes, mental retardation, and epilepsy are more common in children younger than 1 yr following status epilepticus is related to the fact that this group is more likely to have a premorbid underlying CNS disorder than are older children. Nevertheless, there remains considerable debate over whether prolonged status epilepticus can damage the brain as has been shown in animal experiments. It is noteworthy that febrile status epilepticus in a neurologically impaired child is a risk factor for subsequent febrile as well as nonfebrile seizures, but febrile status in an otherwise normal child does not increase the risk of seizures. MRI brain scan performed in several infants demonstrated that complex febrile convulsions can occasionally be associated with acute hippocampal injury progressing to atrophy. In some of these infants, pathology and brain imaging also demonstrated evidence of pre-existing cerebral dysgenesis. These cases suggest that hippocampal sclerosis associated with status epilepticus may reflect interaction between pre-existing and acquired processes.

Claassen J, Hirsch LJ, Emerson RG, et al: Treatment of refractory status epilepticus with pentobarbitol, propofol, or midazolam: A systemic review. *Epilepsia* 2002;43:146–153.

Hanhan UA, Fiallos MR, Orlowski JP: Status epilepticus. *Pediatr Clin North Am* 2001;48:683.

Lowenstein DH, Alldredge BK: Status epilepticus. *N Engl J Med* 1998; 338:970–976.

Maytal J, Shinnar S, Moshe SL, et al: Low morbidity and mortality of status epilepticus in children. *Pediatrics* 1989;83:323–331.

Perez ER, Maeder P, Villemure KM, et al: Acquired hippocampal damage after temporal lobe seizures in 2 infants. *Ann Neurol* 2000;48:384–387.

Riikonen R: Childhood convulsive status epilepticus. *Lancet* 2006;368:184–185.

Riviello JJ Jr., Ashwal S, Hirtz D, et al: Practice parameter: diagnostic assessment of the child with status epilepticus (an evidence-based review). *Neurology* 2006;67:1542–1550.

Sahin M, Menache CC, Holmes GL, et al: Outcome of severe refractory status epilepticus in children. *Epilepsia* 2001;42:1461–1467.

Shinnar S, Pellock JM, Berg AT, et al: Short-term outcomes of children with febrile status epilepticus. *Epilepsia* 2001;42:47S–53S.

VanLandingham KE, Heinz ER, Cavazos JE, et al: Magnetic resonance imaging evidence of hippocampal injury after prolonged focal febrile convulsions. *Ann Neurol* 1998;43:413–426.

Wiznitzer M: Buccal midazolam for seizures. *Lancet* 2005;366:182–184.

Chapter 594 ■ Conditions that Mimic Seizures Michael V. Johnston

Several conditions share common features with epilepsy. Because these disorders may be associated with altered levels of consciousness, tonic or clonic movements, or cyanosis, they are often confused with epilepsy. Affected children may be inappropriately placed on many anticonvulsants with no response and some risk; conditions that mimic epilepsy are refractory to antiepileptic drugs. The treatment of these children differs significantly from those with epilepsy. The differential diagnosis often varies with the age of the patient (Table 594-1).

BENIGN PAROXYSMAL VERTIGO. Benign paroxysmal vertigo (BPV) typically develops in toddlers and is relatively rare beyond 3 yr of age. The attacks develop suddenly and are associated with ataxia, causing the child to fall or refuse to walk or sit. **Horizontal nystagmus** may be evident during the duration of the attack. The child appears frightened and pale. Nausea and vomiting may be prominent. Consciousness and the ability to verbalize are not disturbed; lethargy or drowsiness do not follow completion of the episode. The attacks vary in duration (seconds to minutes), frequency (daily to monthly), and intensity. A rotational sensation (vertigo) is verbalized by older children with BPV. These children are susceptible to motion sickness and may develop migraine headaches several years later, suggesting a relationship between BPV and migraine. Neurologic evaluation characteristically yields negative results, except for the finding of abnormal vestibular function detected by ice water caloric testing. Patients with clusters of attacks usually respond to diphenhydramine, 5 mg/kg/24 hr with a maximum of 300 mg/24 hr orally, intramuscularly, IV, or per rectum.

NIGHT TERRORS. Night terrors are common, particularly in boys between 5 and 7 yr of age (see Chapter 18). They occur in 1–3% of children and are usually short-lived. A night terror has a sudden onset, usually between midnight and 2 A.M. during stage 3 or 4 of slow-wave sleep. The child screams and appears frightened, with dilated pupils, tachycardia, and hyperventilation. There is little or no verbalization; the child may thrash violently, cannot be consoled, and is unaware of parents or surroundings. Sleep follows in a few minutes, and there is total amnesia the following morning. Approximately one third of children with night terrors experience somnambulism. An underlying emotional disorder should be explored in children with persistent and prolonged night terrors. A short course of diazepam may be considered for treatment of protracted night terrors while the family dynamics are under investigation.

BREATH-HOLDING SPELLS. A breath-holding spell can be a frightening experience for parents because the infant becomes lifeless and unresponsive owing to cerebral anoxia at the height of the attack. There are two major types of breath-holding spells: the more common cyanotic form and the pallid form. (See also Chapter 28.)

Cyanotic Spells. A cyanotic breath-holding spell is usually predictable and is always provoked by upsetting or scolding an infant. The episode is heralded by a brief, shrill cry followed by forced expiration and apnea. There is rapid onset of generalized cyanosis and a loss of consciousness that may be associated with repeated generalized clonic jerks, opisthotonos, and bradycardia. Results of an interictal electroencephalogram (EEG) are normal. A breath-holding spell can occur repeatedly within a few hours or it can recur sporadically, but it is always stereotyped. Breath-holding spells are rare before 6 mo of age, peak at about 2 yr of

TABLE 594-1. Nonepileptic Paroxysmal Disorders

NEONATE
Jitteriness*
Benign neonatal sleep myoclonus*
INFANT
Infantile syncope*
Cyanotic breath-holding spells
Pallid syncope
Shivering attacks
Paroxysmal torticollis
Extrapyramidal drug reactions, dystonia
Gastroesophageal reflux with dystonia
Rumination
Stereotypic movements, autism; Rett syndrome, coexisting deafness and blindness
Withholding, constipation
Masturbation
Spasmus nutans
Opsoclonus
Benign paroxysmal vertigo
Myoclonus
Nonepileptic; anxiety, excitement, acute metabolic encephalopathy
Benign myoclonus of early infancy
Hyperexplexia
Alternating hemiplegia of childhood
Sleep disorders*
Jactatio capitis, head banging
CHILDREN
Breath-holding spells*
Syncope
Migraine and migraine equivalents, recurrent abdominal pain, cyclic vomiting*
Tic*
Spasmodic torticollis
Drug reactions, dystonia
Paroxysmal choreoathetosis
Gastroesophageal reflux
Benign paroxysmal vertigo
Myoclonus, nonepileptic; anxiety, excitement, acute metabolic encephalopathy
Hyperexplexia
Masturbation
Withholding, constipation*
Daydreaming, staring spells*
Stereotypic movements; autism, coexistent deafness and blindness
Munchausen syndrome by proxy
Hyperventilation
Psychogenic seizures
Transient global amnesia
Sleep disorders*
Head banging, jactatio capitis
Pavor nocturnus
Somnambulism, somniloquy
ADOLESCENTS
Syncope*
Migraine*
Psychogenic seizures
Dissociative states, conversion disorders, panic attacks, hyperventilation
Daydreaming*
Sleep disorders*
Nocturnal myoclonus, hypnic jerks
Narcolepsy
Somnambulism
Somniloquy
Episodic rage
Malingering
Paroxysmal choreoathetosis
Tremor
Tic
Drug reactions, dystonia
Transient global amnesia

*Common.

age, and abate by 5 yr of age. The management of breath-holding spells concentrates on the support and reassurance of the parents. Some parents feel that whatever the physician recommends, they must splash cold water on the face, turn the child upside down, or initiate mouth-to-mouth resuscitation and even cardiopulmonary resuscitation. A thorough examination followed by an explanation of the mechanism of breath-holding spells is reassuring for most parents. The counseling session should emphasize the need for both parents to be consistent and not reinforce the child's behavior after the child recovers from the spell. This may be accomplished by placing the child safely in bed and by refusing to cuddle, play, or hold the child for a given period of time until recovery is complete.

Pallid Spells. These spells are much less common than cyanotic breath-holding spells, but they share several characteristics. Pallid spells are typically initiated by a painful experience, such as falling and striking the head or a sudden startle. The child stops breathing, rapidly loses consciousness, becomes pale and hypotonic, and may have a tonic seizure. Bradycardia with periods of asystole of >2 sec may be recorded. The interictal EEG is normal. Pallid spells can in some cases be induced spontaneously in the laboratory by ocular compression that produces the oculocardiac reflex, afferent stimulation of the trigeminal nerve, and efferent inhibition of the heart by way of the vagus nerve. This procedure should not be attempted by an inexperienced physician, and appropriate resuscitation equipment should be readily available. Most children respond to conservative measures as outlined for cyanotic spells, but a trial of an anticholinergic, oral atropine sulfate 0.01 mg/kg/24 hr in divided doses with a maximum daily dose of 0.4 mg, which increases the heart rate by blocking the vagus nerve, may be considered in refractory cases. Atropine should not be prescribed during very hot weather because an episode of hyperpyrexia may be initiated.

SYNCOPE

SIMPLE SYNCOPE. Syncope follows an alteration in brain metabolism, the consequence of decreased cerebral blood flow, usually secondary to systemic hypotension. Decreased blood flow causes loss of consciousness, and the concomitant ischemia influences the higher cortical centers to release their inhibiting influence on the reticular formation within the brainstem. Neuronal discharges from the reticular formation then produce brief tonic contractions of the muscles of the face, trunk, and extremities in ≈50% of patients with syncope. During a syncopal episode, a child may have fixed upward deviation of the eyes that can be confused with epilepsy. Simple syncope results from vasovagal stimulation and is precipitated by pain, fear, excitement, and extended periods of standing still, particularly in a warm environment. The EEG shows transient slowing during the attack but no seizure discharges. Simple syncope is uncommon before age 10–12 yr but is quite prevalent in adolescent girls. Tilt-table testing is an effective method of producing symptoms, including hypotension, in the majority of children with unexplained syncope. Most patients with positive tilt-table test results have vasovagal syncope, which, if recurrent, responds favorably to oral β-adrenergic blocking agents. Syncope can usually be differentiated from a seizure because of its short duration, associated symptoms of nausea and perspiration, and complete orientation after the event.

COUGH SYNCOPE. This is most common in asthmatic children. It often occurs shortly after the onset of sleep, and the coughing paroxysm abruptly awakens the child. The patient's face becomes plethoric, and the child perspires, becomes agitated, and is frightened. Loss of consciousness is associated with generalized muscle flaccidity, vertical upward gaze, and clonic muscle contractions lasting for several seconds. Urinary incontinence is frequent. Recovery begins within seconds, and consciousness is usually restored a few minutes later. The child has no recollection of the attack except for the events surrounding the paroxysm of coughing. Coughing produces a marked increase in intrapleural pressure followed by a lowered venous return to the right side of the heart and an associated decrease in right ventricular output. Reduction of left ventricular filling follows, and a rapidly diminished cardiac output results in altered cerebral blood flow, cerebral hypoxia, and a loss of consciousness. The cornerstone of management for asthmatic children with cough syncope is an aggressive approach to the prevention of bronchoconstriction.

PROLONGED QT SYNDROME. The incidence of the prolonged QT syndrome is 1/10,000–1/15,000. The prolonged QT syndrome is characterized by sudden loss of consciousness during exercise or an emotional and stressful experience (see Chapter 435.5). Loss of consciousness in association with exercise or stress is rarely due to epilepsy, and in every case, a cardiac cause must be considered. The onset of the condition is typically in late childhood or adolescence, although onset in infancy may mimic sudden infant death syndrome. During the period of syncope, various cardiac arrhythmias are evident, particularly ventricular fibrillation. The child may recover within minutes or die during the event. Electrocardiography may show abnormal lengthening of the QT interval, especially during carefully monitored exercise. QT intervals corrected for heart rate of ≥0.46 msec support the diagnosis. There are at least two varieties of the syndrome: those due to acquired heart disease (myocarditis, mitral valve prolapse, electrolyte abnormalities, drug induced) and two congenital forms. The QT syndrome may be inherited as an autosomal recessive trait (Jervell and Lange-Nielsen syndrome) that is associated with deafness or as autosomal dominant (Romano-Ward syndrome). Mutations in a cardiac potassium channel gene (*KvLQT1*), linked to chromosome 11p15.5, account for about 50% of the long QT syndrome inherited as an autosomal dominant (type 1 or LQT1). LQT2 results from a mutation in a 2nd potassium channel gene (*HERG*), which is linked to chromosome 7q35-36. Type 3 long QT syndrome is the result of a mutation to a cardiac sodium channel gene (*SCN5A*) linked to chromosome 3p21-24, and a 4th type of long QT syndrome has been linked to chromosome 4q25-27. The gene for type 4 LQT has not been determined. All family members of an affected patient should have a 12-lead electrocardiogram. Further testing may include carefully supervised exercise tests or Holter monitoring. β-Adrenergic-antagonist drugs are usually effective and may be lifesaving. Permanent implantable cardiac defibrillators or left cervicothoracic sympathectomy may also be considered if drug therapy is not effective. Parents should be taught cardiopulmonary resuscitation, because exercise restriction and drug therapy may be ineffective for some children.

PAROXYSMAL KINESIGENIC CHOREOATHETOSIS. This disorder is characterized by a sudden onset of unilateral or occasionally bilateral choreoathetosis or dystonic posturing of a leg or an arm and associated facial grimacing and dysarthria. The condition is precipitated by sudden movement, particularly on rising from a sitting position, or by excitement and stress. The attacks rarely persist for longer than a minute and are never associated with loss of consciousness. The age of onset is typically between 8 and 14 yr, but the condition may begin as early as 2 yr. The child may have several attacks daily, or they may be intermittent, occurring once or twice a month. Results of neurologic examination, EEG, and neuroimaging studies are normal, and neuropathologic studies in a few cases showed no abnormalities. Most reported cases are familial, suggestive of autosomal recessive inheritance. The attacks can be prevented by the use of anticonvulsants, particularly phenytoin. The attacks of paroxysmal kinesigenic choreoathetosis tend to diminish in frequency during adulthood, and the anticonvulsant can be successfully weaned at that time.

SHUDDERING ATTACKS. Shuddering attacks have their onset at 4–6 mo of age and may persist to 6–7 yr of age. They produce an interesting posture, with sudden flexion of the head and trunk and shuddering or shivering movements similar to what must occur if ice-cold water is poured down the back of an unsuspecting individual. These children may have 100 attacks/day followed by several symptom-free weeks. Shuddering attacks may be the childhood precursor of benign essential tremor, because examination of parents and relatives reveals a high incidence of that common condition.

BENIGN PAROXYSMAL TORTICOLLIS OF INFANCY. Infants with benign paroxysmal torticollis have recurrent attacks of head tilt associated with pallor, agitation, and vomiting with an onset between 2 and 8 mo of age. During the attack, the child resists passive head movement. There is no loss of consciousness, and spontaneous remission occurs by 2–3 yr of age. As with benign paroxysmal vertigo, abnormalities in vestibular function have been documented in these patients. Children with persistent torticollis should be investigated for abnormalities of the cervical vertebrae including dislocation or fracture, or a tumor located in the posterior fossa. Some infants with benign paroxysmal torticollis develop migraine headaches later in childhood, and patients have been reported from a kindred with familial migraine linked to a calcium channel mutation.

HEREDITARY CHIN TREMBLING. Hereditary chin trembling may be confused with epilepsy due to repeated episodes of rapid 3/sec chin trembling movements. These brief attacks are precipitated by stress, anger, and frustration and are inherited as an autosomal dominant trait. Findings on the neurologic examination and EEG are normal.

NARCOLEPSY AND CATAPLEXY. (See also Chapter 18.) Narcolepsy is a disorder that rarely begins before adolescence and is characterized by paroxysmal attacks of irrepressible daytime sleep, which is sometimes associated with transient loss of muscle tone (**cataplexy**). The incidence of narcolepsy is 1/2,000. An EEG shows that the recurrent sleep attacks consist of rapid eye movement (REM) sleep. Patients with narcolepsy are easily aroused and become spontaneously alert, whereas a convulsion is followed by a deep sleep, postictal drowsiness, lethargy, and often a headache. Modafinil acetamide, 200 mg/day orally, is superior to the stimulant drugs in the management of narcolepsy and has fewer adverse side effects. Cataplexy is also occasionally confused with epilepsy. Patients with cataplexy experience sudden loss of muscle tone and fall to the floor because of laughter, stress, or frightening experiences. Cataplectic patients do not lose consciousness but lie without moving for a few minutes until normal body tone returns. Treatment may consist of scheduled naps, amphetamines, methylphenidate, tricyclic antidepressants, and counseling with respect to occupational safety and driving. The stimulant and antidepressant drugs commonly produce side effects including anxiety, euphoria, hypersomnolence, and the development of tolerance.

RAGE ATTACKS OR EPISODIC DYSCONTROL SYNDROME. The episodic dyscontrol syndrome, a nonepileptic condition, can be confused with complex partial seizures. Patients develop sudden and recurrent attacks of violent physical behavior with minimal provocation. The attacks consist of kicking, scratching, biting, and shouting (including abusive and profane language). An affected child or adolescent cannot seem to control the behavior and may seem momentarily psychotic throughout the attack. The episode is followed by fatigue, amnesia, and sincere remorse. A routine EEG may show nonspecific abnormalities in patients with the rage syndrome. The EEG in such patients during the attack remains normal; this condition is thus distinguished from complex partial seizures, which always show an abnormal EEG during an attack.

MASTURBATION. Masturbation or self-stimulation behavior may occur in girls between the ages of 2 mo and 3 yr. These children have repetitive stereotyped episodes of tonic posturing associated with copulatory movements, but without manual stimulation of the genitalia. The child suddenly becomes flushed and perspires, may grunt and breathe irregularly, but has no loss of consciousness. The masturbatory activity has a sudden onset, usually persists for a few minutes (rarely hours), and tends to occur during periods of stress or boredom. The examination should include a search for evidence of sexual abuse or abnormalities of the perineum, but in most cases, a cause is not found. Treatment consists of reassurance that the self-stimulatory activity will subside by 3 yr of age and that no specific therapy is required.

PSEUDOSEIZURES. The diagnosis of a pseudoseizure should be made only after a thorough history and physical examination and exclusion of "true" seizures by prolonged EEG recording when indicated. Pseudoseizures occur typically between 10 and 18 yr of age and are more frequent among girls. Pseudoseizures occur in many patients with a past history of epilepsy and in some with ongoing true seizures. A pseudoseizure may be quite realistic but frequently is bizarre, with unusual postures, verbalizations, and uncharacteristic tonic or clonic movements. There are several distinguishing features of a pseudoseizure, including lack of cyanosis, normal reaction of the pupil to light, no loss of sphincter control, normal plantar responses, and the absence of tongue biting or injury during the attack. Many patients moan or cry during a pseudoseizure, and some patients can be persuaded to have an attack on request by the physician. Patients with pseudoseizures are likely to have a neurotic personality documented by formal psychologic testing. It is not unusual to find a patient taking three or four anticonvulsants, which, of course, have no effect. The most reliable method of differentiating epilepsy from suspected pseudoseizures is to record an attack. The EEG shows an excess of muscle artifact during the pseudoseizure but a normal background rhythm devoid of seizure discharges. After a true epileptic seizure, there is a significant increase in serum prolactin, whereas there is no change from the baseline at the termination of a pseudoseizure.

Ackerman MJ, Clapham DE: Ion channels-basic science and clinical disease. *N Engl J Med* 1997;336:1575–1586.

Britton JW: Syncope and seizures—Differential diagnosis and evaluation. *Clin Auton Res* 2004;14:148–159.

Broughton RJ, Fleming JA, George CF, et al: Randomized double-blind placebo-controlled crossover trial of modafinil in the treatment of excessive daytime sleepiness in narcolepsy. *Neurology* 1997;49:444–451.

Fleisher DR, Morrison A: Masturbation mimicking abdominal pain or seizures in young girls. *J Pediatr* 1990;116:810–814.

Giffin NJ, Benton S, Goadsby PJ: Benign paroxysmal torticollis of infancy: Four new cases and linkage to CACNA1A mutation. *Dev Med Child Neurol* 44:490–493.

Haslam RH, Freigang B: Cough syncope mimicking epilepsy in asthmatic children. *Can J Neurol Sci* 1985;12:45–47.

Lotz T, Jankovic J: Paroxysmal kinesigenic dyskinesias. *Semin Pediatr Neurol* 2003;10:68–79.

Macleod S, Ferrie C, Zuberi SM: Symptoms of narcolepsy in children misinterpreted as epilepsy. *Epileptic Disord* 2005;7:13–17.

Chapter 595 ■ Headaches

Robert H. A. Haslam

Headache is a common problem in children. The effect of headaches on a child's academic performance, memory, personality, and interpersonal relationships, as well as school attendance, depends on their etiology, frequency, and intensity. A headache may occasionally indicate a severe underlying disorder (brain tumor), and thus careful evaluation of children with recurrent, severe, progressive, or unconventional headaches is mandatory. Infants and children respond to a headache in an unpredictable fashion. Most toddlers cannot communicate the characteristics of a headache; rather they may become irritable and cranky, vomit, prefer a darkened room because of photophobia, or repeatedly rub their eyes and head. Children are poor historians when describing a headache and its associated symptoms. The most important causes of headache in children include migraine, psychogenic factors or stress, and increased intracranial pressure (ICP). Refractive errors, strabismus, sinusitis, and malocclusion of the teeth are much less common causes of significant headaches in children. Headaches are often an associated manifestation of common head and neck infections in children.

595.1 • Migraine

Migraine is the most important and frequent type of headache in the pediatric population. Most migraine headaches are not severe and are readily managed by conservative measures without requiring medical attention. The prevalence of migraine among school-aged children between 7 and 15 yr of age was 4% in a comprehensive Swedish study and ranges from 8 to 23% in adolescents. Girls are more likely to develop migraine as adolescents, whereas boys are in the slight majority among children younger than 10 yr. More than half undergo spontaneous prolonged remission after the 10th birthday. As adults, 5–10% of men and 15–20% of women have migraine headaches.

Cortical spreading depression (CSD), a phenomenon thought to be responsible for the aura of migraine, is associated with elevation of CNS hydrogen and potassium ions, with the release of glutamate and nitrous oxide. These changes result in regional cortical oligemia and activation of the caudal portion of the trigeminal ganglion. Excitation of the trigeminal-vascular system initiates the release of vasoactive intestinal polypeptides causing vasodilation followed by extravasation of plasma proteins from the dural vessels resulting in localized inflammation of the dural vessels. Neurogenic vascular inflammation causes excitation of pain sensitive receptors and the onset of pain. CSD is considered to be an inherited physiologic response to a variety of stimuli that are responsible for triggering the migraine process.

CLASSIFICATION AND CLINICAL MANIFESTATIONS. Table 595-1 lists the various types of migraine headaches.

Migraine Without Aura. This migraine is not associated with an aura and is the most prevalent type of migraine in children. The headache is throbbing or pounding and tends to be **unilateral** at onset or throughout its duration but may also be located in the bifrontal or temporal regions. It may not be hemicranial in children and is less intense compared with the migraine in adults. The headache usually persists for 1–3 hr, although the pain may last for as long as 72 hr. The pain may inhibit daily activity, because physical activity aggravates the pain. A characteristic feature of childhood migraine is intense nausea and vomiting, which may be more bothersome than the headache. The vomiting may be associated with abdominal pain and fever; conditions such as appendicitis and a systemic infection may be erroneously confused with the primary diagnosis. Additional symptoms include extreme paleness, photophobia, light-headedness, phonophobia, osmophobia (aversion to odors), and paresthesias of the hands and feet. A positive **family history**, particularly on the maternal side, is present in ≈90% of children with migraine without aura. Considerable caution should be exercised when making the diagnosis of migraine in the absence of a positive family history.

Additional features of all migraines may include near synchrony with perimenstrual or periovulation timing, gradual appearance after sustained exercise, relief with sleep, stereotypical prodromes (hypersomnia, food craving, irritability, moodiness), precipitation by food or odors, and onset after a letdown or high period of stress. Manifestations suggestive of a more serious condition include rapid onset of the first or worst headache of the patient's life, a change in the characteristics of the headaches, a progressive headache lasting for days, headache associated with Valsalva maneuver, chronic systemic signs (weight loss, fever), persistent focal neurologic manifestations, seizures, loss of consciousness, nuchal rigidity, cranial bruits, abnormal visual fields, or papilledema (Table 595-2).

Migraine with an Aura. In this disorder, an aura precedes the onset of the headache. Visual auras are uncommonly described by young children with migraine, but when they occur they may

TABLE 595-1. 2004 International Classification of Headache Disorders*

MIGRAINE
Migraine without aura
Migraine with aura
Typical aura with migraine headache
Typical migraine with nonmigraine headache
Typical aura without headache
Familial hemiplegic migraine
Sporadic hemiplegic migraine
Basilar-type migraine
Childhood periodic syndromes that are commonly precursors of migraine
Cyclic vomiting
Abdominal migraine
Benign paroxysmal vertigo of childhood
Retinal migraine
Complications of migraine
Chronic migraine
Status migraine
Persistent aura without infarction
Migrainous infarction
Probable migraine

*Headache Classification Subcommittee of the International Headache Society: The International Classification of Headache Disorders, 2nd Edition. *Cephalalgia* 2004;24(Suppl 1):9–160.

TABLE 595-2. Indications for Neuroimaging in a Child with Headaches

Abnormal neurologic signs
Recent school failure, behavioral change, fall-off in linear growth rate
Headache awakens child during sleep; early morning headache, with increase in frequency and severity
Periodic headaches and seizures coincide, especially if seizure has a focal onset
Migraine and seizure occur in the same episode, and vascular symptoms precede the seizure (20–50% risk of tumor or arteriovenous malformation)
Cluster headaches in child; any child <5–6 yr whose principal complaint is a headache
Focal neurologic symptoms or signs developing during a headache (i.e., complicated migraine)
Focal neurologic symptoms or signs (except classic visual symptoms of migraine) develop during the aura, with fixed laterality; focal signs of the aura persisting or recurring in the headache phase
Visual graying-out occurring at the peak of a headache instead of the aura
Brief cough headache in a child or adolescent

Modified from Barlow CF: *Headaches and Migraine in Childhood.* Philadelphia, JB Lippincott, 1984, p 205.

take the form of blurred vision, scotoma (an area of depressed vision within the visual field), photopsia (flashes of light), fortification spectra (brilliant white zigzag lines), or irregular distortion of objects. Some patients also have vertigo and light-headedness during this stage of the headache. Sensory symptoms include perioral paresthesias and numbness of the hands and feet. Distortions of body image (Alice in Wonderland syndrome) may predominate as a prelude to a classic migraine headache. After the onset of the aura, the patient develops typical symptoms of a migraine as described earlier.

Hemiplegic migraine is considered a migraine aura and is characterized by the onset of unilateral sensory or motor signs during an episode of migraine. Hemisyndromes are more common in children than in adults and may be characterized by numbness of the face, arm, and leg; unilateral weakness; and aphasia. More than one attack is uncommon in the pediatric age group. The neurologic signs may be transient or may persist for days. It is unusual for a child to develop a completed stroke after a single episode. Hemiplegic migraine in an older child or adolescent has a relatively good prognosis, and a positive family history of similar hemiplegic events is often elicited. Familial hemiplegic migraine (FHM) is an autosomal dominant disorder. FHM is characterized by hemiplegia during the headache and, in some kindreds, progressive cerebellar atrophy. Mutations of the *CACNA1A* gene located on chromosome 19p3 are found in approximately ⅔ of patients with FHM1. The *CACNA1A* gene codes for the α1 subunit of a voltage-dependent calcium channel. FHM2 is due to mutations in the *ATP1A2* gene, whereas FHM3 is due to a mutation in the *SCN1A* gene, a voltage-gated sodium channel.

Basilar-type migraine is considered to represent a precursor of childhood migraine. Brainstem signs predominate in these patients because of vasoconstriction of the basilar and posterior cerebral arteries. The major symptoms include vertigo, tinnitus, diplopia, blurred vision, scotoma, ataxia, and an occipital headache. The pupils may be dilated, and ptosis may be evident. Alterations in consciousness followed by a generalized seizure may result. After the attack, there is a complete resolution of the neurologic symptoms and signs. Most affected children have a strongly positive family history of migraine. Many develop migraine with aura as adolescents or adults. Relatively minor head trauma may precipitate an episode of basilar migraine. The condition has been described in children of both sexes, with girls younger than 4 yr being at particular risk.

Childhood Periodic Syndromes That Are Common Precursors of Migraine. These variants include cyclic vomiting (see Chapter 303), abdominal migraine, and benign paroxysmal vertigo (see Chapter 594). **Cyclic vomiting** is characterized by recurrent, sometimes monthly bouts of severe vomiting that may be so intense that dehydration and electrolyte abnormalities occur, particularly in infants. Systemic manifestations such as fever, abdominal pain, and diarrhea are initially absent, but they may become prominent in association with excessive fluid losses secondary to vomiting. The vomiting may be protracted and persist for 1–5 days. Vomiting during attacks occurs at least 5 times/hr for at least 1 hr and there is complete resolution of symptoms between attacks. The child may appear pale and frightened but does not lose consciousness. After a period of deep sleep, the child awakens and resumes normal play and eating habits as if the vomiting had not occurred. Many children with cyclic vomiting have a positive family history of migraine, and as they grow older and become verbal, they describe a typical migraine headache that leaves little doubt about the diagnosis and the association of the cyclic vomiting with the condition. Cyclic vomiting is treated with rectally administered or injected antiemetics such as dimenhydrinate or ondansetron and careful attention to fluid replacement if the vomiting is excessive. Cyclic vomiting of migraine must be differentiated from gastrointestinal disorders including intestinal obstruction (malrotation, intermittent volvulus, duodenal web, duplication cysts, superior mesenteric artery compression, internal hernias), peptic ulcer, gastritis, giardiasis, chronic pancreatitis, and Crohn disease. Abnormal gastrointestinal motility and pelviureteric junction obstruction can also cause cyclic vomiting. Metabolic causes include disorders of amino acid metabolism (heterozygote ornithine transcarbamylase deficiency), organic acidurias (propionic acidemia, methylmalonic acidemia), fatty acid oxidation defects (medium-chain acyl-CoA dehydrogenase deficiency), disorders of carbohydrate metabolism (hereditary fructose intolerance), acute intermittent porphyria, and structural central nervous system (CNS) lesions (posterior fossa brain tumors, subdural hematoma or effusions).

Abdominal migraine is a recurrent disorder characterized by mid-abdominal pain with pain-free periods between each attack. The pain is usually described as "dull" and may be moderate to severe. The pain may persist from 1 to 72 hr and, although usually midline, may be periumbilical or poorly localized by the child. To meet the criteria of abdominal migraine, the child must complain at the time of the abdominal pain of at least two of the following: anorexia, nausea, vomiting, or pallor. As with cyclic vomiting, a thorough history and physical examination with appropriate laboratory studies must be completed to rule out an underlying gastrointestinal disorder as a cause of the abdominal pain.

Two conditions formerly listed as complications of migraine have been reclassified. **Alternating hemiplegia** of childhood may be caused by a metabolic or mitochondrial disorder or the result of a channelopathy. **Ophthalmoplegic migraine** is reclassified as a cranial neuralgia.

DIAGNOSIS AND DIFFERENTIAL DIAGNOSIS. A thorough history and physical examination suffice to establish the diagnosis in most cases (Table 595-3). Basilar migraine may be confused with several conditions, including congenital malformations of the skull and cervical vertebrae, posterior fossa tumors, toxins and drugs, and metabolic abnormalities including Leigh disease and

TABLE 595-3. Diagnostic Criteria for Migraine

WITHOUT AURA
A At least five attacks
B Headache attack lasts 4–72 hr (untreated or unsuccessfully treated).
C Headache has at least two of the following characteristics:
  Unilateral location
  Pulsating quality
  Moderate or severe intensity
  Aggravation by or avoidance of routine physical activity (i.e., walking or climbing stairs)
D During headache at least one of the following:
  Nausea, vomiting, or both
  Photophobia and phonophobia
E Not attributed to another disorder

WITH AURA (CLASSIC MIGRAINE)
A At least two attacks
B Migraine aura fulfills criteria for typical aura, hemiplegic aura, or basilar-type aura.
C Not attributed to another disorder

TYPICAL AURA
1 Fully reversible visual, sensory, or speech symptoms (or any combination) but no motor weakness
2 Homonymous or bilateral visual symptoms including positive features (e.g., flickering lights, spots, lines) or negative features (e.g., loss of vision), or unilateral sensory symptoms including positive features (e.g., visual loss, pins and needles) or negative features (i.e., numbness), or any combination
3 At least one of:
  a) At least one symptom develops gradually over a minimum of 5 min, or different symptoms occur in succession, or both
  b) Each symptom lasts for at least 5 min and for no longer than 60 min
4 Headache that meets criteria for migraine without aura begins during the aura or follows aura within 60 min

From Silberstein SD: Migraine. *Lancet* 2004;363:381–391.

pyruvate decarboxylase deficiency. In children with hemiplegic migraine, an arteriovenous malformation, MELAS (mitochondrial myopathy, encephalopathy, lactic acidosis, and stroke), cerebral tumor, Todd paralysis, clotting disorders, hemoglobinopathies such as sickle cell disease, and metabolic conditions including homocystinuria should be considered. A lipid profile should be obtained in children with migraine and a positive family history of premature myocardial infarction or cerebrovascular accident. Migraines may occur in patients with systemic lupus erythematosus and patients abusing cocaine. The organization of laboratory tests and radiologic studies depends on the constellation of symptoms and findings during the neurologic examination. An electroencephalogram (EEG) or neuroimaging studies (CT scan, MRI) are rarely indicated in a child unless the headache is associated with an unusual constellation of symptoms or signs or when increased ICP is suspected (see Table 595-2).

TREATMENT. The American Academy of Neurology established useful practice guidelines for the management of migraine as follows:

1. Reduction of headache frequency, severity, duration, and disability
2. Reduction of reliance on poorly tolerated, ineffective, or unwanted acute pharmacotherapies
3. Improvement in quality of life
4. Avoidance of acute headache medication escalation
5. Education and enabling of patients to manage their disease to enhance personal control of their migraine
6. Reduction of headache-related distress and psychological symptoms.

Migraine may be prevented or ameliorated by avoiding certain initiating stimuli. A few children can identify specific factors that uniformly result in a headache. The most common precipitators of migraine headaches are stress, fatigue, and anxiety. An affected child may be under undue stress because of difficulties at home or school, particularly when unrealistic pressures or demands are placed on the patient. Children who experience recurrent migraine headaches during the school year may have a learning disability or may have been placed in a too highly competitive classroom. Reassessment of the child's school placement and academic abilities may be the most important step in the management of the headache disorder. Some studies implicate certain foods as a cause of migraine, particularly nuts, chocolate, cola drinks, citrus fruits, fried foods, cheese, yogurt, hot dogs, spicy meats and processed meats, kippers, and Chinese food (monosodium glutamate). The parents may be asked to create a diary or calendar relating the onset of headache to a particular food to determine if dietary factors are responsible for the child's migraine. Elimination of the incriminating foodstuff is indicated if the history suggests a relationship between the ingestion of a particular food and the onset of headache. Avoidance of bright flashing lights, sun exposure, excessive physical exertion, mild head trauma, loud noises, hunger, fatigue, motion sickness, and drugs (including alcohol and oral contraceptives) is indicated when the history suggests a direct relationship. As sleep disorders are commonly associated with migraine, the physician should rule out that possibility during the history taking. The frequency and severity of migraine headaches are reduced significantly in at least 50% of pediatric patients who undergo a careful history and neurologic examination followed by reassurance from the physician.

Management of an acute attack of migraine should include the use of analgesics and antiemetics (Table 595-4). Most migraine headaches in children can be treated by the judicious use of *acetaminophen (15 mg/kg)* or *ibuprofen (7.5–10 mg/kg) dispensed in the gel capsule formulation,* particularly if the headaches are mild, infrequent, and of short duration. Most children either are unaware of an aura or fail to communicate the onset of the headache to their parents. An antiemetic such as *dimenhydrinate by rectal suppository,* 5 mg/kg/24 hr in four divided doses, is the mainstay of treatment when vomiting is the major symptom. Parenteral metoclopramide is also very effective. The child usually prefers to rest in a quiet, darkened room and typically awakens, refreshed and headache free, several hours later after a deep sleep. *Triptans* (e.g., *Sumatriptan*) are specific and selective 5-hydroxytryptamine receptor agonists that are effective abortive drugs in treating the acute phase of migraine with and without aura if the use of conventional analgesics is ineffective. Sumatriptan may be administered subcutaneously, nasally, or orally. The nasal spray formulation is the preferred route of administration for children. The suggested dose is 5 mg in children <25 kg, 10 mg (two sprays) in those weighing 25–50 kg, and 20 mg sumatriptan in children ≥50 kg. The dose may be repeated 2 or more hours after the initial dose, limited to two doses per 24 hr. The most common adverse effects are usually minor and transient, and include hot flushes, nausea and vomiting, fatigue, and drowsiness. Triptans should not be used for the treatment of basilar or hemiplegic migraine. The U.S. Food and Drug Administration have not approved triptan drugs for patients younger than 18 yr. Several well-designed double-blind studies in children have demonstrated that the drug is effective and safe.

Children may develop severe intractable migraine attacks or status migrainosus (persistent headache lasting longer than 3 days) that are unresponsive to conventional drug regimens. Intravenous *prochlorperazine,* 0.15 mg/kg (max 10 mg), is highly effective in aborting intractable migraine in children who have not responded to acute management of the headache.

The decision to use *continuous daily medication* (**prophylactic therapy**) is based on the severity and frequency of the headaches and on the impact of the migraine on the child's daily activities, including school attendance and performance as well as participation in recreation. The use of prophylactic drugs should be considered if a child experiences more than two to four severe episodes monthly or is unable to attend school regularly. Only two drugs have been subjected to rigorous controlled studies to test the efficacy and tolerability of these agents in reducing the severity and frequency of childhood migraine; propranolol, a β blocker, and flunarizine, a calcium channel blocking agent. The dose of propranolol is 10–20 mg tid (beginning with 10 mg/24 hr and gradually increasing the drug to the maximum dose or until the desired therapeutic effect is achieved) in children 7–8 yr and older. A common mistake is to discontinue the drug prematurely, because it often takes several weeks to a month until the drug is effective. Flunarizine (not available in the United States) also has been shown to be an effective drug for the prophylaxis of pediatric migraine. The initial dose is 5 mg at bedtime and increased if necessary to 10 mg. The most frequent side effect is drowsiness. Additional drugs that show promise for the prophylaxis of pediatric migraine include sodium valproate, toprimate, levetiracetam, gabapentin, cyproheptadine, and amitriptyline.

Behavior management is an effective method for the treatment of migraine in some children and adolescents. Biofeedback and self-hypnosis are replacing pharmacologic treatment in some centers because of the undesirable side effects of drugs and the concern that some may produce chemical dependency. Biofeedback can be mastered by most children older than 8 yr and has been effective in many clinical trials. Several studies of migrainous children show a significant decrease in frequency of headaches in those treated by self-hypnosis compared with those taking a placebo or propranolol. Many pediatric headache clinics employ social workers and psychologists skilled in pain management. Children respond favorably to being taught imagery and

TABLE 595-4. Drugs Used in the Management of Migraine Headaches in Children

DRUG	DOSE	MECHANISM	SIDE EFFECTS	COMMENTS
ACUTE MIGRAINE				
Analgesics				
Acetaminophen	15 mg/kg/dose	Inhibits prostaglandin synthesis	Overdose, fatal hepatic necrosis	
Ibuprofen	7.5–10 mg/kg/dose	Inhibits prostaglandin synthesis	abd. pain, nausea, GI bleeding	Suggest gel caplets
Triptans (not approved by FDA for children & adolescents)				
Sumatriptan Nasal spray recommended (also available oral & SC)	<25 kg: 5 mg 25–50 kg: 10 mg >50 kg: 20 mg	Selective 5-hydroxytryptamine agonist	Serious cardiac events have not been reported in children	Contraindicated in basilar and hemiplegic migraine
PROPHYLAXIS				
Calcium channel blockers				
Flunarizine*	5 mg at hs.	Calcium channel blocking agent	Headache, lethargy, dizziness	May ↑ to 10 mg at hs.
Antihypertensive				
Propranolol (contraindicated in asthma)	10–20 mg tid	Nonselective β-adrenergic blocking agent	Dizziness, lethargy	Begin 10 mg/24 hr ↑ 10 mg/wk
Anticonvulsants				
Sodium valproate	5–20 mg/kg/24 hr (begin 5 mg/kg/24 hr)	↑ brain GABA	Nausea, pancreatitis, fatal hepatotoxicity	↑ 5 mg/kg/wk
Topiramate	3–9 mg/kg/24 hr	↑ activity of GABA	Fatigue, nervousness	Begin 1–3 mg/kg/24 hr
Gabapentin	900–1200 mg/24 hr	Unknown	Somnolence, fatigue aggression, weight gain	Begin 300 mg ↑ 300 mg/wk
Antihistamines				
Cyproheptadine	0.2–0.4 mg/kg/hs	H_1 receptor & serotonin agonist	Drowsiness, thick bronchial secretions	Max 0.5 mg/kg/24 hr
Antidepressants				
Amitriptyline	Children: 0.1 mg/kg/hs Max 2 mg/kg/hs Adolescents: 25 mg hs Max 200 mg/24 hr	↑ CNS serotonin & norepinephrine	Cardiac conduction, abnormalities and dry mouth, constipation drowsiness, confusion	Do not discontinue abruptly
SEVERE INTRACTABLE				
Prochlorperazine	0.15 mg/kg/IV (max 10 mg)		Agitation, muscle stiffness	

*Not available in U.S.
GABA, γ-aminobutyric acid; GI, gastrointestinal; hs, at night; SC, subcutaneous.

can often learn to control the pain associated with migraine without the use of medication.

595.2 • Organic Headaches

A headache may be the earliest symptom of increased ICP. The headache results from tension or traction of the cerebral blood vessels and dura and occurs initially in a sporadic fashion, primarily in the early hours in the morning or shortly after the patient arises. The headache is diffuse and generalized and is more prominent over the frontal and occipital regions. Its onset may be insidious, and the pain is enhanced by any activity that elevates the ICP (coughing, sneezing, straining during a bowel movement). As the ICP increases, the child becomes lethargic and irritable, and the headache becomes constant. Early morning vomiting is often associated with increased ICP. Causes of organic headaches in children include brain tumors, particularly those located in the posterior fossa, hydrocephalus, meningitis and encephalitis, cerebral abscess, subdural hematoma, chronic lead poisoning, and pseudotumor cerebri. Additional causes of organic headaches in children that may not be associated with increased ICP include arteriovenous malformations, berry aneurysm, collagen vascular diseases affecting the CNS, hypertensive encephalopathy, acute subarachnoid hemorrhage, and stroke. The management of organic headaches depends on the cause. The initial step includes a thorough history and physical examination, including recording of the blood pressure and a funduscopic exam to identify papilledema. Ordering of laboratory tests and neuroradiologic procedures depends on the clues provided by the history and physical examination.

595.3 • Tension or Stress Headaches

Stress or tension headaches are common in the pediatric age group, particularly after the onset of puberty, and are often difficult to differentiate from migraine headaches. The two are often associated in the same patient. Tension headaches infrequently appear in the morning hours but are most apparent during the school day, particularly coinciding with a test or similarly anxiety-provoking circumstance. Although these headaches can be continuous and persist for weeks, they tend to wax and wane and build in intensity during the day. The headache is described as hurting or aching but is rarely perceived as throbbing. Most tension headaches in children are distributed in the frontal region, but they may localize over the vertex or the occipital area. Unlike migraine or headaches associated with increased ICP, tension headaches are not, as a rule, associated with nausea and vomiting.

The **diagnosis** of tension headache is made by exclusion at the completion of the history and physical examination. Studies such as an EEG or a CT scan are rarely necessary. Management consists of a search for possible underlying emotional or stressful factors. Most children have considerable insight into the origin of tension headaches and, when given the opportunity, will share concerns and conflicts. A poor self-image, fear of school failure, and lack of self-confidence are common factors. A depressed child occasionally presents with severe headaches. These patients may also complain of sudden mood changes, weight loss, anorexia, disturbed sleep, fatigue, and withdrawal from social activities. Excessive caffeine intake or acute caffeine withdrawal may be associated with headaches. Daily ingestion of cola or coffee may produce headaches. Gradual withdrawal eliminates the caffeine-induced chronic headaches.

Treatment of tension headaches begins with reassurance and an explanation about how stress may cause a headache. Anxiety and stress may unconsciously produce constant isometric contraction of the temporalis, masseter, or trapezius muscles, which leads to the characteristic dull, aching headache. Steps should be introduced to remove obvious anxiety-provoking situations. Acetaminophen and other mild analgesics are often all that are required to treat a tension headache. Sedatives and antidepressants are rarely necessary. Children with severe tension headaches may benefit from a brief hospitalization, particularly if an underlying depressive illness is under consideration. In the hospital setting, the child's interaction with other patients, nursing and medical staff, and family is observed while a plan is formulated for counseling or psychiatric intervention. In most cases, the child's headaches are considerably relieved during the period of observation. As with migraine headaches, biofeedback and self-hypnosis exercises are effective in the treatment of some patients with tension headaches.

Brandes JL, Kudrow D, Stark SR, et al: Sumatriptan-naproxen for acute treatment of migraine. *JAMA* 2007;297:1443–1454.

Brousseau DC, Duffy SJ, Anderson AC, et al: Treatment of pediatric migraine headaches: A randomized, double-blind trial of prochlorperazine versus ketorolac. *Ann Emerg Med* 2004;43:256–262.

Colman I, Brown MD, Innes GD, et al: Parenteral metoclopramide for acute migraine: Meta-analysis of randomized controlled trials. *Br Med J* 2004;329:1369–1372.

Fuller G, Kaye C: Headaches. *BMJ* 2007;334:254–256.

Goadsby PJ, Kullmann DM: Another migraine gene. *Lancet* 2005;366: S345–S346.

Goadsby PJ, Lipton RB, Ferrari MD: Migraine—Current understanding and treatment. *N Engl J Med* 2002;346:257–270.

Hämäläinen ML, Hoppu K, Santavuouri P: Sumatriptan for migraine attacks in children: A randomized placebo-controlled study. *Neurology* 1997;48:1100–1103.

Hämäläinen ML, Hoppu K, Valkeila E, et al: Ibuprofen and acetaminophen for the acute treatment of migraine in children: A double-blind, randomized, placebo controlled, crossover study. *Neurology* 1997;48:103–107.

Hering-Hanit R, Gadoth N: Caffeine-induced headache in children and adolescents. *Cephalalgia* 2003;23:332–335.

Lewis D: Practice parameter: Pharmacological treatment of migraine headache in children and adolescents. *Neurology* 2004;63:2215–2224.

Lewis DW: Toward the definition of childhood migraine. *Curr Opin Pediatr* 2004;16:628–636.

Mack KJ: What incites new daily persistent headache in children? *Pediatr Neurol* 2004;31:122–125.

Medical Letter: Topiramate (Topamax) for prevention of migraine. *Med Lett Drugs Ther* 2005;47:9–10.

Olness H, MacDonald JT, Uden DL: Comparison of self-hypnosis and propranolol in the treatment of juvenile classic migraine. *Pediatrics* 1987;79:593–597.

Silberstein SD: Migraine. *Lancet* 2004;363:381–391.

Victor S, Ryan SW: Drugs for preventing migraine headaches in children. *Cochrane Database Syst Rev* 2003;4:CD002761.

Winner P, Rothner AD, Saper J, et al: A randomized double-blind placebo-controlled study of sumatriptan nasal spray in the treatment of acute migraine in adolescents. *Pediatrics* 2000;106:989–997.

Chapter 596 ■ Neurocutaneous Syndromes

Robert H. A. Haslam

The neurocutaneous syndromes include a heterogeneous group of disorders characterized by abnormalities of both the integument and central nervous system (CNS). Most disorders are familial and believed to arise from a defect in differentiation of the primitive ectoderm. Disorders classified as neurocutaneous syndromes include neurofibromatosis, tuberous sclerosis, Sturge-Weber disease, von Hippel-Lindau disease, PHACE syndrome, ataxia telangiectasia, linear nevus syndrome, hypomelanosis of Ito (see Chapter 652), and incontinentia pigmenti (see Chapter 651).

596.1 • Neurofibromatosis

Neurofibromatosis (NF), von Recklinghausen disease, is a common autosomal dominant disorder. The condition is protean, because virtually every system and organ may be affected, and progressive because distinctive features may be present at birth, but the development of complications is delayed for decades. NF is the consequence of an abnormality of neural crest differentiation and migration during the early stages of embryogenesis (see also Chapter 651).

CLINICAL MANIFESTATIONS AND DIAGNOSIS. There are two distinct forms of NF. **NF-1** is the most prevalent type, with an incidence of 1/4,000, and is diagnosed when any two of the following seven signs are present: (1) six or more café-au-lait macules over 5 mm in greatest diameter in prepubertal individuals and over 15 mm in greatest diameter in postpubertal individuals. Café-au-lait spots are the hallmark of neurofibromatosis and are present in almost 100% of patients. They are present at birth but increase in size, number, and pigmentation, especially during the 1st few years of life. The spots are scattered over the body surface, with predilection for the trunk and extremities, and with sparing of the face. (2) Axillary or inguinal freckling consisting of multiple hyperpigmented areas 2–3 mm in diameter. (3) Two or more iris Lisch nodules. Lisch nodules are hamartomas located within the iris and are best identified by a slit-lamp examination (Fig. 596-1). They are present in >74% of patients with NF-1 but are not a component of NF-2. The prevalence of Lisch nodules increases with age, from only 5% of children <3 yr of age, to 42% among children 3–4 yr of age, and virtually 100% of adults ≥21 yr of age. (4) Two or more neurofibromas or one plexiform neurofibroma. Neurofibromas typically involve the skin, but they may be situated along peripheral nerves and blood vessels and within viscera including the gastrointestinal tract. These lesions appear characteristically during adolescence or pregnancy, suggesting a hormonal influence. They are usually small, rubbery lesions with a slight purplish discoloration of the overlying skin. Plexiform neurofibromas are usually evident at birth and result from diffuse thickening of nerve trunks that are frequently located in the orbital or temporal region of the face. The skin overlying a plexiform neurofibroma may be hyperpigmented to a greater degree than a café-au-lait spot. Plexiform neurofibromas may produce overgrowth of an extremity and a deformity of the corresponding bone. (5) A distinctive osseous lesion such as sphenoid dysplasia (which may cause pulsating exophthalmos) or cortical thinning of long bones with or without pseudoarthrosis. Scoliosis is the most common orthopedic manifestation of NF-1, although it is not specific enough to be included as a diagnostic criterion. (6) Optic gliomas are present in ≈15% of patients with

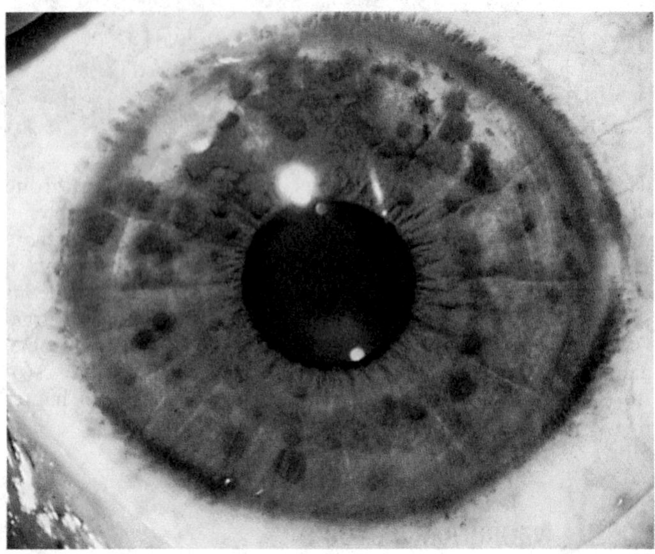

Figure 596-1. Neurofibromatosis 1 (NF-1). Pigmented hamartomas of the iris (Lisch nodules). (From Zitelli BJ, Davis HW: *Atlas of Pediatric Physical Diagnosis,* 4th ed. St. Louis, Mosby, 2002, p 507.)

NF-1. These relatively benign tumors consist of glial cells and a mucinous material. Most patients with optic gliomas are asymptomatic and have normal or near-normal vision, but ≈20% have visual disturbances or evidence of precocious sexual development secondary to tumor invasion of the hypothalamus. Symptomatic optic nerve tumors typically produce symptoms before 6 yr of age. Children are rarely aware of unilateral visual loss; thus, diagnosis may be delayed. Patients with a unilateral optic glioma typically display an afferent pupillary defect. To test for this, each eye is alternately stimulated by a bright light source (swinging flashlight test). The affected pupil dilates rather than constricts, whereas light in the unaffected eye causes both pupils to constrict equally. NF-1 and a plexiform neuroma of the eyelid have a high association with an ipsilateral optic glioma. The MRI findings of an optic glioma include diffuse thickening, localized enlargement, or a distinct focal mass originating from the optic nerve or chiasm. (7) A first-degree relative with NF-1 whose diagnosis was based on the aforementioned criteria. The majority of mutations in NF-1 occur in the paternal germ line. The NF-1 gene on chromosome region 17q11.2 encodes all mRNA of 11–13 kb containing at least 59 exons that produce a protein neurofibromin. More than 300 independent mutations have been reported in the NF-1 gene.

Children with NF-1 are susceptible to **neurologic complications.** MRI studies of selected children have shown abnormal hyperintense T2 weighted signals in the optic tracts, brainstem, globus pallidus, thalamus, internal capsule, and cerebellum. These signals, **"unidentified bright objects (UBOs),"** tend to disappear with age; most have disappeared by 30 yr of age. UBOs are thought to represent areas of dysmyelination or focal areas of increased water content and are not detected by CT scanning (Fig. 596-2). There is disagreement as to the presence and number of UBOs and their relationship to learning disabilities, attention deficit disorders, behavioral and psychosocial problems, and abnormalities of speech among affected children. These cognitive abnormalities are common and occur in 40–60% of NF-1 children. Complex partial and generalized tonic-clonic seizures are a frequent complication. Hydrocephalus is a rare manifestation secondary to aqueductal stenosis, whereas macrocephaly with normal-sized ventricles is a common finding. The cerebral vessels may develop aneurysms, or stenosis resulting in moyamoya disease (see Fig. 601-2). Neurologic sequelae of these vascular abnormalities include transient cerebrovascular ischemic attacks, hemiparesis, and cognitive defects. Psychologic disturbances are prevalent due to the seriousness and uncertainty of the disease. Precocious puberty may become evident in the presence or absence of lesions of the optic chiasm and hypothalamus. Malignant neoplasms are also a significant problem in patients with NF-1. A neurofibroma occasionally differentiates into a neurofibrosarcoma or malignant schwannoma. Patients with NF-1 are at risk for hypertension, which may result from renal vascular stenosis or a pheochromocytoma. The incidence of pheochromocytoma, rhabdomyosarcoma, leukemia, and Wilms tumor is higher than in the general population. There is an unusual association involving myeloid leukemia, juvenile xanthogranuloma, and NF-1. Tumors of the CNS (including optic gliomas, meningiomas of the brain and spinal cord, neurofibromas, astrocytomas, and neurilemmomas) account for significant morbidity and mortality, however, because of their increased frequency in patients with NF-1.

NF-2 accounts for 10% of all cases of NF, with an incidence of 1/50,000, and may be diagnosed when one of the following two features is present: (1) *bilateral eighth nerve masses* consistent with acoustic neuromas as demonstrated by CT scanning or MRI. (2) *A parent, sibling, or child with NF-2* and either unilateral eighth nerve masses or any two of the following: neurofibroma, meningioma, glioma, schwannoma, or juvenile posterior subcapsular lenticular opacities. **Bilateral acoustic neuromas** are the most distinctive feature of NF-2. Symptoms of hearing loss, facial weakness, headache, or unsteadiness may appear during childhood, although signs of a cerebellopontine angle mass are more commonly present in the 2nd and 3rd decades of life. Although café-au-lait spots and skin neurofibromas are classic findings in NF-1, they are much less common in NF-2. Posterior subcapsular lens opacities are identified in ≈50% of patients with NF-2. As with NF-1, CNS tumors, including Schwann cell and glial tumors, and meningiomas are common in patients with NF-2. Linkage analysis has shown that the gene for NF-2 is located near the center of the long arm of chromosome 22q1.11.

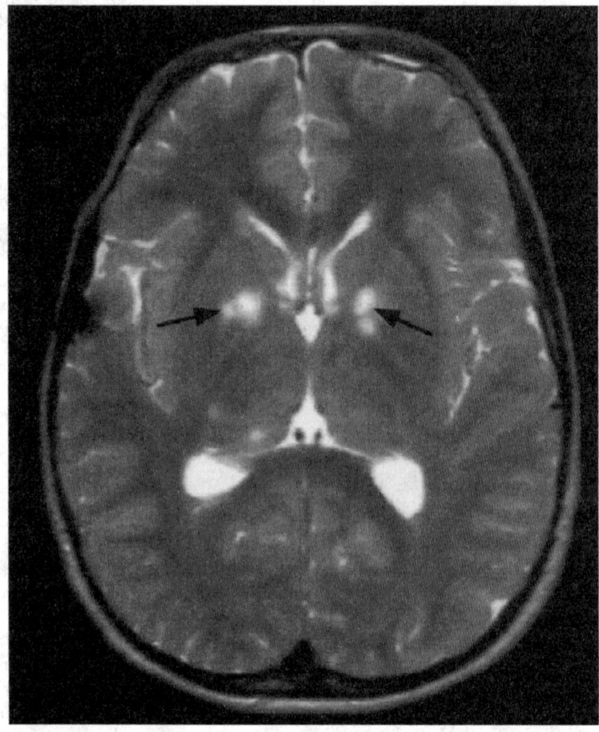

Figure 596-2. T2 weighted MRI scan of a patient with neurofibromatosis. Note the high-signal areas (UBOs) in the basal ganglia *(black arrows)*. UBOs, unidentified bright objects.

TREATMENT. Because there is no specific treatment for NF, management includes genetic counseling and early detection of treatable conditions or complications. The National Institutes of Health (NIH) consensus statement suggests that tests should be dictated by findings on clinical evaluation. In asymptomatic patients, laboratory tests, particularly evoked potentials, electroencephalogram (EEG), CT, or MRI, are unlikely to be of value. There is a lack of consensus concerning the indications for neuroimaging studies in NF-1, although there is unanimous agreement that all symptomatic cases (i.e., visual loss or disturbance, proptosis, symptoms and signs of increased intracranial pressure) must be studied without delay. The NIH Consensus Development Conference advised against routine imaging studies of the brain and optic tracts because treatment in these asymptomatic NF-1 children is rarely required. It is recommended that the child have a detailed history and physical examinations by a pediatrician and a thorough annual ophthalmologic examination by a pediatric ophthalmologist until the age of 10 yr. Thereafter, routine visual assessment is recommended. A parent with NF has a 50% chance of transmitting the disease with each pregnancy. The type of NF (NF-1 and NF-2) "breeds true" for successive generations. Because approximately half of all cases of NF result from fresh mutations, each parent should be carefully examined (including a search for Lisch nodules) before counseling for the risk of affected future pregnancies. Standard DNA diagnostic analysis is not practical for the prenatal diagnosis of the NF-1 gene because of the large size of the gene and the significant number of mutations. Prenatal diagnosis is feasible if the mutation causing the condition is known in the affected parent. The majority of NF-2 cases are the result of a mutation. Examination of fetal DNA for the characteristic single-strand conformational polymorphism of an altered DNA sequence provides accurate prenatal testing. In familial cases, when affected and unaffected family members are available, linkage can be established, making prenatal diagnosis available with a certain degree of accuracy.

596.2 • Tuberous Sclerosis

Tuberous sclerosis (TS) is inherited as an autosomal dominant trait with variable penetrance and a prevalence of 1/6,000 people. Spontaneous genetic mutations occur in up to 75% cases. Molecular genetic studies have identified two foci for the TS complex. The *TSC1* gene is located on chromosome 9q34, and the *TSC2* gene is on chromosome 16p13. The 8.6-kb *TSC1* transcript encodes a protein of 130 kd called *hamartin*. The *TSC2* gene encodes the protein *tuberin*. Hamartin and tuberin act together as a single molecular complex at the Golgi apparatus. TS is an extremely heterogeneous disease with a wide clinical spectrum varying from severe mental retardation and incapacitating seizures to normal intelligence and a lack of seizures, often within the same family. As a rule, the younger the patient presents with symptoms and signs of TS, the greater is the likelihood of mental retardation. The disease affects many organ systems other than the skin and brain, including the heart, kidney, eyes, lungs, and bone.

DIAGNOSIS

Definite TS complex is diagnosed when at least two major or one major plus two minor features are present. Major features include skin lesions, brain and eye lesions, and tumors in the heart, kidneys, or lungs. Minor features include bone cysts, rectal polyps, dental enamel pits, CNS white matter migrational abnormalities, gingival fibromas, nonrenal hamartomas, retinal achromic patches, confetti skin lesions, and multiple renal cysts.

CLINICAL MANIFESTATIONS

SKIN LESIONS. More than 90% of cases show the typical hypomelanotic macules that have been likened to an ash leaf on the trunk and extremities. Visualization of the hypomelanotic macule is enhanced by the use of a Wood ultraviolet lamp, particularly in the infant (see Chapter 553). At least three hypomelanotic macules must be present. Sebaceous adenomas develop between 4 and 6 yr of age; they appear as tiny red nodules over the nose and cheeks and are sometimes confused with acne (Fig. 596-3). Later, they enlarge, coalesce, and assume a fleshy appearance. A *shagreen patch* is also characteristic of TS and consists of a roughened, raised lesion with an orange-peel consistency located primarily in the lumbosacral region. Subungual or periungual fibromas arise from the stratum lucidum of the finger and toe in many patients with TS during adolescence.

RETINAL AND BRAIN LESIONS. Retinal lesions consist of two types: mulberry tumors that arise from the nerve head or round, flat gray lesions in the region of the disc (Fig. 596-4) and hamartoma or depigmented areas. The most common neurologic manifesta-

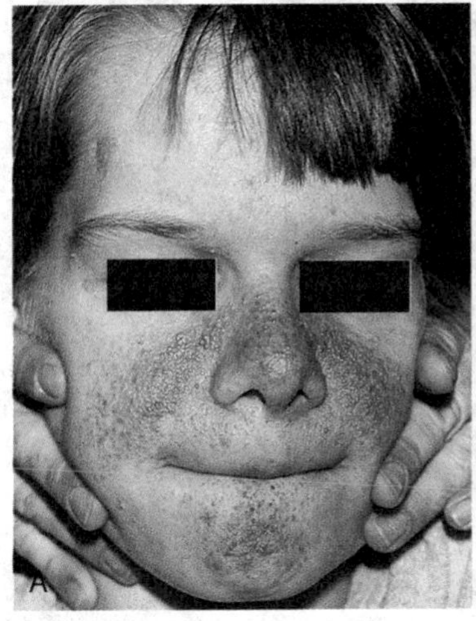

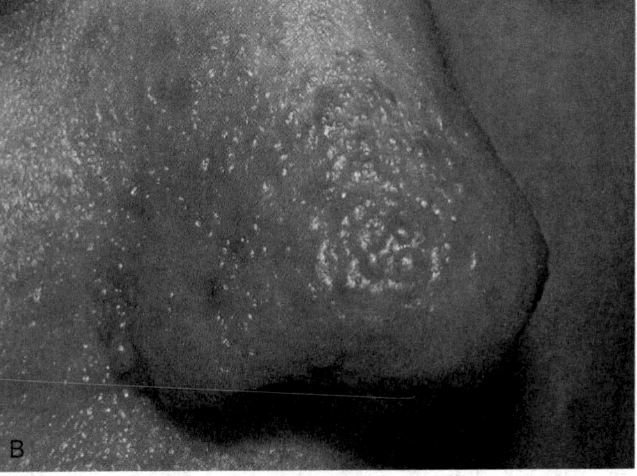

Figure 596-3. Tuberous sclerosis. *A*, This adolescent boy had adenoma sebaceum in characteristic malar distribution and chin lesions as well. *B*, Closeup view of nasal lesions is shown. (From Zitelli BJ, Davis HW: *Atlas of Pediatric Physical Diagnosis*, 4th ed. St. Louis, Mosby, 2002, p 509.)

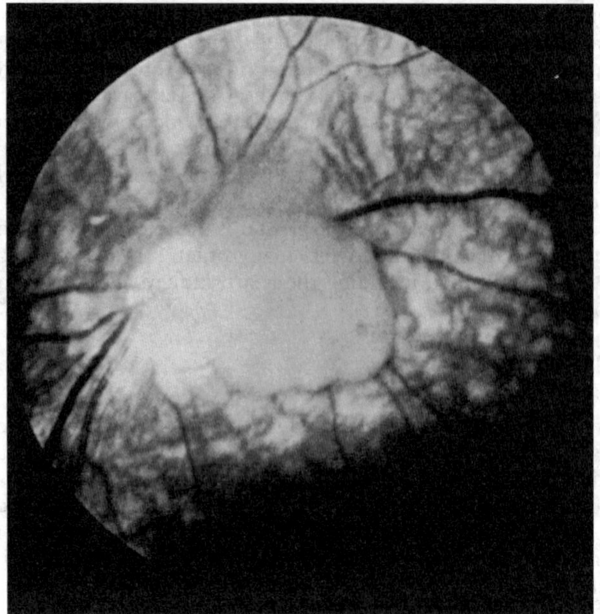

Figure 596-4. A mulberry lesion of the retina in a patient with tuberous sclerosis.

tions of TS consist of seizures, cognitive impairment, and behavioral abnormalities including autism. The characteristic brain lesion is a cortical tuber. Tubers are located in the convolutions of the cerebral hemispheres and are also present in the subependymal region, where they undergo calcification and project into the ventricular cavity, producing a candle-dripping appearance. Tubers in the region of the foramen of Monro may cause obstruction of cerebrospinal fluid (CSF) flow and hydrocephalus. The microscopic appearance of the tuber consists of decreased numbers of neurons, a proliferation of astrocytes, and the presence of oddly shaped multinucleated giant neurons. T2 weighted MRI is useful for identification of the lesions. Generally, the greater the number of tubers, the more neurologically impaired is the patient. Brain tumors are much less common in TS compared with NF, but a tuber occasionally differentiates into a malignant subependymal giant cell astrocytoma. The CT scan typically shows calcified tubers in the periventricular area, but these may not be apparent until 3–4 yr of age (Fig. 596-5). TS may present during infancy with infantile spasms and a hypsarrhythmic EEG pattern. The seizures may be difficult to control and, at a later age, they may develop into myoclonic epilepsy (see Chapter 593). In Europe and Canada, infantile spasms associated with TS are treated with vigabatrin (rather than adrenocorticotropic hormone) with good results. Vigabatrin is not available in the United States. There is a high incidence of cognitive impairment, aggressive behavior, and autism in young patients with TS and infantile spasms. Many patients with TS have normal intelligence and few, if any, neurologic abnormalities.

LESIONS IN OTHER ORGANS. Approximately 50% of children with TS have rhabdomyomas of the heart, which may be detected in a fetus at risk by an echocardiogram. The rhabdomyomas may be numerous or located at the apex of the left ventricle, and although they can cause congestive heart failure and arrhythmias, they tend to slowly resolve spontaneously. The kidneys in 75–80% of patients >10 yr of age have angiomyolipomas that are usually benign tumors. Single or multiple renal cysts are also commonly present in TS. Lymphangiomyomatosis is the classical pulmonary lesion in TS and is more common in the female patient.

DIAGNOSIS

Diagnosis of TS relies on a high index of suspicion when assessing a child with infantile spasms. A careful search for the typical skin and retinal lesions should be completed in all patients with a seizure disorder. Head CT scan or MRI confirms the diagnosis in most cases. Genetic testing for *TSC1* and *TSC2* mutations is available and may be considered when the individual patient does not meet all the clinical criteria. Prenatal testing may be offered when a known TS complex mutation exists in that family.

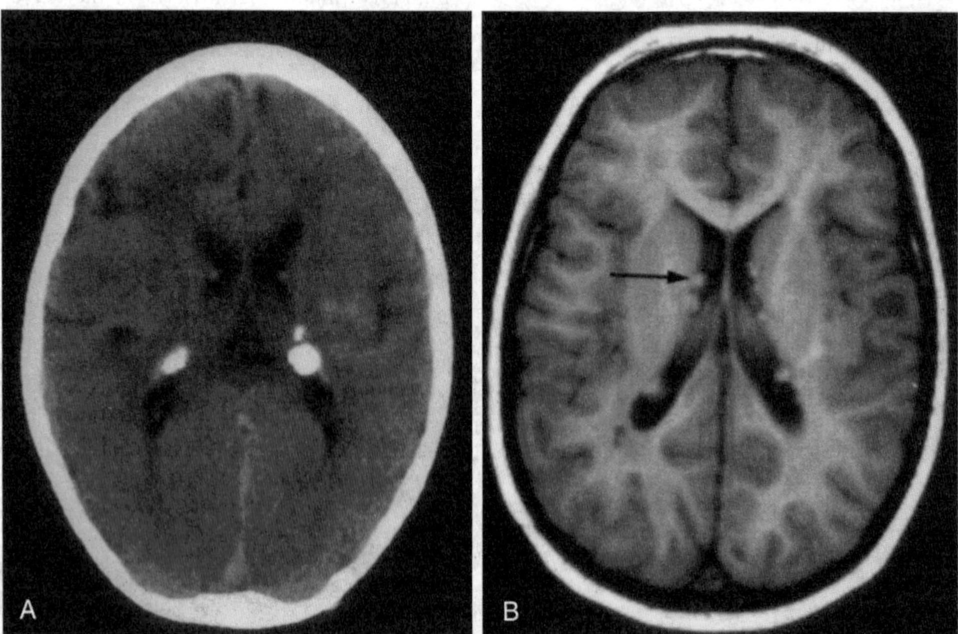

Figure 596-5. Tuberous sclerosis. *A,* CT scan with subependymal calcifications characteristic of tuberous sclerosis. *B,* The MRI demonstrates multiple subependymal nodules in the same patient *(black arrow).* Parenchymal tubers are also visible on both the CT and the MRI scan as low-density areas in the brain parenchyma.

TREATMENT

Management consists of seizure control and baseline studies, including renal ultrasonography, an echocardiogram, and a chest roentgenogram, with follow-up as indicated. Symptoms and signs of increased intracranial pressure suggest obstruction of the foramen of Monro by a tuber or malignant transformation of a tuber, and warrant immediate investigation and surgical intervention.

596.3 • Sturge-Weber Syndrome

This syndrome is a sporadic disorder and consists of a constellation of symptoms and signs including a facial nevus (port-wine stain), seizures, hemiparesis, strokelike episodes, intracranial calcifications, and, in many cases, mental retardation. It occurs sporadically with a frequency of approximately 1/50,000 live births.

ETIOLOGY. The condition is thought to result from anomalous development of the primordial vascular bed in the early stages of cerebral vascularization. At this stage, the blood supply to the brain, meninges, and face is undergoing reorganization, while the primitive ectoderm in the region differentiates into the skin of the upper face and the occipital lobe of the cerebrum. In patients with Sturge-Weber syndrome, the overlying leptomeninges are richly vascularized and the brain beneath becomes atrophic and calcified, particularly in the molecular layer of the cortex.

CLINICAL MANIFESTATIONS. The facial nevus is present at birth, tends to be unilateral, and always involves the upper face and eyelid. The nevus may also be evident over the lower face, trunk, and in the mucosa of the mouth and pharynx. Not all children with facial nevi have Sturge-Weber syndrome (see Chapter 649). Buphthalmos and glaucoma of the ipsilateral eye are common complications. Seizures develop in most patients in the 1st year of life. They are typically focal tonic-clonic and contralateral to the side of the facial nevus. The seizures may become refractory to anticonvulsants and are associated with a slowly progressive hemiparesis in many cases. Transient strokelike episodes or visual defects persisting for several days and unrelated to seizure activity are common and probably result from thrombosis of cortical veins in the affected region. Although neurodevelopment appears to be normal in the 1st year of life, mental retardation or severe learning disabilities are present in at least 50% in later childhood, probably the result of prolonged generalized seizures and increasing cerebral atrophy secondary to local hypoxia and use of numerous anticonvulsants.

DIAGNOSIS. The skull radiograph shows intracranial calcification in the occipitoparietal region in most patients. This characteristically assumes a serpentine or railroad-track appearance. The CT scan highlights the extent of the calcification that is usually associated with unilateral cortical atrophy and ipsilateral dilatation of the lateral ventricle (Fig. 596-6). MRI is a useful adjunct to CT for delineation of the size and location of the vascular malformation and the presence of white matter lesions.

TREATMENT. Management of Sturge-Weber syndrome is multifaceted and is aimed at seizure control and identification and management of behavioral or learning problems. Seizures beginning in infancy are not always associated with a poor neurodevelopmental outcome. For patients with well-controlled seizures and normal or near-normal development, management consists of anticonvulsants and surveillance for complications including glaucoma, buphthalmos, and behavioral abnormalities. If the seizures are refractory to anticonvulsant therapy, especially in infancy and the 1st 1–2 yr, and arise from primarily one hemisphere, most centers advise a hemispherectomy. Because of the risk of glaucoma, regular measurements of intraocular pressure with a tenonometer is indicated. The facial nevus is often a target for ridicule by classmates, leading to psychologic trauma. Flashlamp-pulsed laser therapy often provides excellent clearing of the port-wine stain, particularly if it is located on the forehead. Because of the high frequency of developmental disabilities, special educational facilities are frequently required.

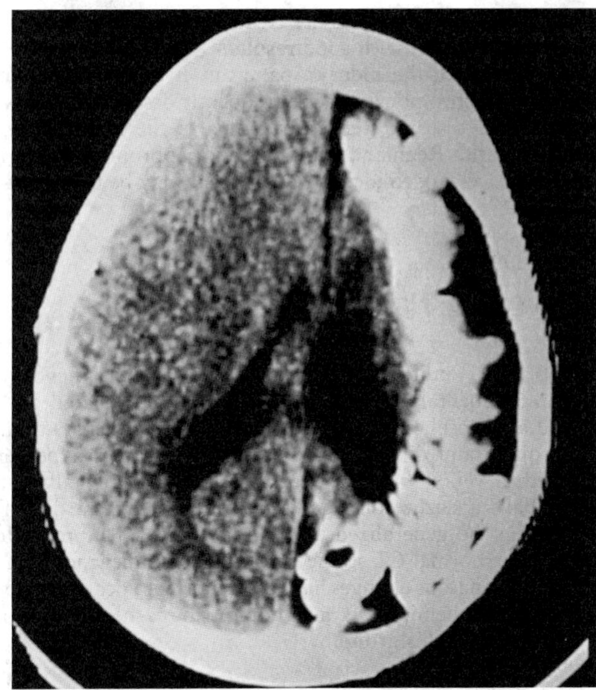

Figure 596-6. CT scan of a patient with Sturge-Weber syndrome showing unilateral calcification and underlying atrophy of a cerebral hemisphere.

596.4 • Von Hippel-Lindau Disease

As with most of the neurocutaneous syndromes, von Hippel-Lindau disease affects many organs, including the cerebellum, spinal cord, medulla, retina, kidney, pancreas, and epididymis. Von Hippel-Lindau disease is inherited as an autosomal dominant trait with variable penetrance and delayed expression with an incidence of 1/36,000 people. The disease is caused by germ line mutations in the VHL tumor suppressor gene located on 3p25–26.

The major neurologic features of the condition include cerebellar hemangioblastomas and retinal angiomata. Patients with cerebellar hemangioblastoma present in early adult life or beyond with symptoms and signs of increased intracranial pressure. A smaller number of patients have hemangioblastoma of the spinal cord, producing abnormalities of proprioception and disturbances of gait and bladder dysfunction. The CT scan and MRI typically show a cystic cerebellar lesion with a vascular mural nodule. Total surgical removal of the tumor is curative.

Approximately 25% of patients with cerebellar hemangioblastoma have retinal angiomas. Retinal angiomas are characterized by small masses of thin-walled capillaries that are fed by large and tortuous arterioles and venules. They are usually located in the peripheral retina so that vision is unaffected. Exudation in the region of the angiomas may lead to retinal detachment and visual loss. Retinal angiomas are treated with photocoagulation and cryocoagulation, with good results.

Cystic lesions of the kidneys, pancreas, liver, and epididymis as well as pheochromocytoma are frequently associated with von Hippel-Lindau disease. Renal carcinoma is the most common cause of death. Regular follow-up and appropriate imaging studies are necessary to identify lesions that may be treated at an early stage.

596.5 • Linear Nevus Syndrome

This sporadic condition is characterized by a facial nevus and neurodevelopmental abnormalities. The nevus is located on the forehead and nose and tends to be midline in its distribution. It may be quite faint during infancy but later becomes hyperkeratotic, with a yellow-brown appearance. More than half of the patients have a seizure disorder and are mentally retarded. The seizures may be generalized, myoclonic, or focal motor. Most patients have normal CT studies, although hemimeganencephaly with hamartomatous changes has been reported. Focal neurologic signs including hemiparesis and homonymous hemianopia are more common in this group.

596.6 • PHACE Syndrome

The syndrome denotes *p*osterior fossa malformations, *h*emangiomas, *a*rterial anomalies, *c*oarctation of the aorta and other cardiac defects, and *e*ye abnormalities. Large facial hemangiomas may be associated with a Dandy-Walker malformation, vascular anomalies (coarctation of aorta, aplasia or hypoplastic carotid arteries, aneurysmal carotid dilation, aberrant left subclavian artery), glaucoma, cataracts, microphthalmia, optic nerve hypoplasia, and ventral defects (sternal clefts). The facial hemangioma is typically ipsilateral to the aortic arch. There is a female predominance. Airway hemangiomas may produce obstruction. Interferon-α is of value in the management of the hemangiomas.

American Academy of Pediatrics Committee on Genetics: Health supervision for children with neurofibromatosis. *Pediatrics* 1995;96:368–372.

Cnossen MH, de Goede-Bolder A, van den Broek KM, et al: A prospective 10 year follow up study of patients with neurofibromatosis type 1. *Arch Dis Child* 1998;78:408–412.

Crino PB, Nathanson KL, Henske EP: The tuberous sclerosis complex. *N Engl J Med* 2006;355:1345–1356.

Gutmann DH, Aylsworth A, Carey JC, et al: The diagnostic evaluation and multidisciplinary management of neurofibromatosis 1 and neurofibromatosis 2. *JAMA* 1997;278:51–57.

Hofman KJ, Harris EL, Bryan RN, et al: Neurofibromatosis type 1: The cognitive phenotype. *J Pediatr* 1994;124:S1–S8.

Hurst RW, Newman SA, Cail WS: Multifocal intracranial MR abnormalities in neurofibromatosis. *AJNR Am J Neuroradiol* 1988;9:293–296.

Hymann MH, Whittemore VH: National Institutes of Health Consensus Conference: Tuberous sclerosis complex. *Arch Neurol* 2000;57:662–665.

Jozwiak S, Kawalec W, Dluzewska J, et al: Cardiac tumors in tuberous sclerosis: Their incidence and course. *Eur J Pediatr* 1994;153:155–157.

Kossoff EH, Buck C, Freeman JM: Outcomes of 32 hemispherectomies for Sturge-Weber syndrome worldwide. *Neurology* 2002;59:1735–1738.

Latif F, Tory K, Gmarra J, et al: Identification of the von Hippel-Lindau disease tumor suppressor gene. *Science* 1993;260:1317–1320.

Lazaro C, Gaona A, Ravella A, et al: Prenatal diagnosis of neurofibromatosis 1: From flanking RFLPS to intragene microsatellite markers. *Prenat Diagn* 1995;15:129–134.

Lovejoy FH, Boyle LE: Linear nevus sebaceous syndrome: Report of two cases and a review of the literature. *Pediatrics* 1973;52:382–387.

Maher ER, Kaelin WG Jr: von Hippel-Lindau disease. *Medicine* 1997;76:381–391.

Rizzo JF, Lessell S: Cerebrovascular abnormalities in neurofibromatosis type 1. *Neurology* 1994;44:1000–1002.

Roach ES, Williams MD, Laster MD: Magnetic resonance imaging in tuberous sclerosis. *Arch Neurol* 1987;44:301–303.

Seizinger BR, Martuza RL, Gusella JF: Loss of genes on chromosome 22 in tumorigenesis of human acoustic neuroma. *Nature* 1986;322:644–647.

Stumpf DA, Alksne JF, Annegers JF, et al: NIH Development Conference. Neurofibromatosis: Conference statement. *Arch Neurol* 1988;45:575–578.

Tan OT, Sherwood K, Gilchrest BA: Treatment of children with port-wine stains using the flashlamp-pulsed tunable dye laser. *N Engl J Med* 1989;320:416–421.

Chapter 597 ■ Movement Disorders

Michael V. Johnston

Movement disorders cause involuntary movements and/or abnormalities in posture, tone, balance, or fine motor control. The type of movement disorder assists in localizing the pathologic process, whereas the onset, age, and degree of abnormal motor activity and associated neurologic findings help classify the disorder and organize the investigation.

597.1 • Ataxias

Ataxia is the inability to make smooth, accurate, and coordinated movements, usually due to a disorder of the cerebellum and/or sensory pathways in the posterior columns of the spinal cord. Ataxias may be generalized or primarily affect gait or the hands and arms; they may be acute (Table 597-1) or chronic (Table 597-2). *Congenital anomalies* of the posterior fossa, including the Dandy-Walker syndrome, Chiari malformation, and encephalocele, are prominently associated with ataxia because of their destruction or replacement of the cerebellum (see Chapter 592). **Agenesis of the cerebellar vermis** presents in infancy with generalized hypotonia and decreased deep tendon reflexes. Delayed motor milestones and truncal ataxia are typical. **Joubert syndrome** is an autosomal recessive disorder marked by agenesis of the cerebellar vermis, ataxia, hypotonia, oculomotor apraxia, neonatal breathing problems, and mental retardation. Mutations have been identified in the *AHI1* gene on chromosome 6, encoding the Jouberin protein. This gene is strongly expressed in embryonic hindbrain, especially in neurons that give rise to the axons of the corticospinal tract and superior cerebellar peduncles, which fail to cross properly in Joubert syndrome. MRI is the method of choice for investigating congenital abnormalities of the cerebellum, vermis, and related structures. In Joubert syndrome, MRI reveals enlargement of the 4th ventricle at the junction between the midbrain and medulla, creating the "molar tooth sign."

The major *infectious causes of ataxia* include cerebellar abscess, acute labyrinthitis, and acute cerebellar ataxia. **Acute cerebellar ataxia** occurs primarily in children 1–3 yr of age and is a diagnosis by exclusion. The condition often follows a viral illness, such as varicella, coxsackievirus, or echovirus infection, by 2–3 wk and is thought to represent an autoimmune response to the viral agent affecting the cerebellum (see Chapters 247, 250, and 602). The onset is sudden, and the truncal ataxia can be so severe that the child is unable to stand or sit. Vomiting may occur initially, but fever and nuchal rigidity are absent. Horizontal nystagmus is evident in ≈50% of cases and, if the child is able to speak, dysarthria may be impressive. Examination of the cere-

TABLE 597-1. Acute or Recurrent Ataxia

Brain tumor
Conversion reaction
Drug ingestion
Encephalitis (brainstem)
Genetic disorders
Dominant recurrent ataxia
Episodic ataxia type 1
Episodic ataxia type 2
Hartnup disease
Maple syrup urine disease
Pyruvate dehydrogenase deficiency
Migraine
Basilar
Benign paroxysmal vertigo
Postinfectious/immune
Acute postinfectious cerebellitis (varicella)
Miller Fisher syndrome
Multiple sclerosis
Myoclonic encephalopathy/neuroblastoma
Pseudoataxia (epileptic)
Trauma
Hematoma
Postconcussion
Vertebrobasilar occlusion
Vascular disorders
Cerebellar hemorrhage
Kawasaki disease

brospinal fluid (CSF) is typically normal at the onset of ataxia; a pleocytosis of lymphocytes (10–30/mm^3) is not unusual. Later in the course, the CSF protein undergoes a moderate elevation. The ataxia begins to improve in a few weeks but may persist for as long as 2 mo. The prognosis for complete recovery is excellent; a small number have long-term sequelae, including behavioral and speech disorders as well as ataxia and incoordination. **Acute labyrinthitis** may be difficult to differentiate from acute cerebellar ataxia in a toddler. The condition is associated with middle-ear infections and intense vertigo, vomiting, and abnormalities in labyrinthine function, particularly ice water caloric testing.

Toxic causes of ataxia include alcohol, thallium (which is used occasionally in homes as a pesticide), and the anticonvulsants, particularly phenytoin when serum levels reach or exceed 30 µg/mL (120 µmol/L).

Brain tumors, including tumors of the cerebellum and frontal lobe, as well as neuroblastoma, may present with ataxia. Frontal lobe tumors may cause ataxia owing to destruction of the association fibers connecting the frontal lobe with the cerebellum. Neuroblastoma may be associated with a paraneoplastic encephalopathy characterized by progressive ataxia, myoclonic jerks, and opsoclonus (nonrhythmic horizontal and vertical oscillations of the eyes).

Several *metabolic disorders* are characterized by ataxia, including abetalipoproteinemia, arginosuccinic aciduria, and Hartnup disease. **Abetalipoproteinemia** (Bassen-Kornzweig disease) begins in childhood with steatorrhea and failure to thrive (see Chapter 86.3). A blood smear shows acanthocytosis and decreased serum levels of cholesterol and triglycerides, and the serum β-lipoproteins are absent. Neurologic signs become evident by late childhood and consist of ataxia, retinitis pigmentosa, peripheral neuritis, abnormalities in position and vibration sense, muscle weakness, and mental retardation. Vitamin E is undetectable in the serum of patients with neurologic symptoms.

Degenerative diseases of the central nervous system (CNS) represent an important group of ataxic disorders of childhood because of the genetic consequences and poor prognosis. **Ataxia-telangiectasia,** an autosomal recessive condition, is the most common of the degenerative ataxias and is heralded by ataxia beginning at about age 2 yr and progressing to loss of ambulation by adolescence (see Chapter 125.2). Ataxia-telangiectasia is caused by mutations in the *ATM* gene located at 11q22–q23. ATM is a phosphytidylinositol-3 kinase that phosphorylates proteins involved in DNA repair and cell cycle control. Oculomotor apraxia of horizontal gaze, defined as having difficulty fixating smoothly on an object and therefore overshooting the target with lateral movement of the head, followed by refixating the eyes, is a frequent finding, as is strabismus, hypometric saccade pursuit abnormalities, and nystagmus. The telangiectasia becomes evident by mid-childhood and is found on the bulbar conjunctiva, over the bridge of the nose, and on the ears and exposed surfaces of the extremities. Examination of the skin shows a loss of elasticity. Abnormalities of immunologic function that lead to frequent sinopulmonary infections include decreased serum and secretory IgA as well as diminished IgG_2, IgG_4, and IgE levels in more than 50% of patients. Children with ataxia-telangiectasia have a 50- to 100-fold greater chance over the normal population of developing lymphoreticular tumors (lymphoma, leukemia, and Hodgkin disease) as well as brain tumors. Additional laboratory abnormalities include an increased incidence of chromosome breaks, particularly of chromosome 14, and elevated levels of α-fetoprotein. Death results from infection or tumor dissemination.

Friedreich ataxia is inherited as an autosomal recessive disorder involving the spinocerebellar tracts, dorsal columns in the spinal cord, the pyramidal tracts, and the cerebellum and medulla. The majority of patients are homozygous for a GAA repeat expansion in the noncoding region of the gene coding for the mitochondrial protein frataxin. Mutations cause oxidative injury associated with excessive iron deposits in mitochondria.

TABLE 597-2. Chronic or Progressive Ataxia

Brain tumors
Cerebellar astrocytoma
Cerebellar hemangioblastoma (von Hippel-Lindau disease)
Ependymoma
Medulloblastoma
Supratentorial tumors
Congenital malformations
Basilar impression
Cerebellar aplasias
Cerebellar hemisphere aplasia
Dandy-Walker malformation
Vermal aplasia
Chiari malformation
Hereditary ataxias
Autosomal dominant inheritance
Autosomal recessive inheritance
Abetalipoproteinemia
Ataxia-telangiectasia
Ataxia without oculomotor apraxia
Ataxia with episodic dystonia
Friedreich ataxia
Hartnup disease
Juvenile GM_2 gangliosidosis
Juvenile sulfatide lipidoses
Maple syrup urine disease
Marinesco-Sjögren syndrome
Pyruvate dehydrogenase deficiency
Ramsay Hunt syndrome
Refsum disease (HSMN IV)
Respiratory chain disorders
X-linked inheritance
Adrenoleukodystrophy
Leber optic neuropathy
With adult-onset dementia
With deafness
With deafness and loss of vision

From Fenichel GM: *Clinical Pediatric Neurology,* 5th ed. Philadelphia, Elsevier, 2005, p 220.

The onset of ataxia is somewhat later than in ataxia-telangiectasia but usually occurs before age 10 yr. The ataxia is slowly progressive and involves the lower extremities to a greater degree than the upper extremities. The Romberg test result is positive; the deep tendon reflexes are absent (particularly the Achilles), and the plantar response is extensor. Patients develop a characteristic explosive, dysarthric speech, and nystagmus is present in most children. Although patients may appear apathetic, their intelligence is preserved. They may have significant weakness of the distal musculature of the hands and feet. Typically noted is a marked loss of vibration and position sense caused by degeneration of the posterior columns and indistinct sensory changes in the distal extremities. Friedreich ataxia is also characterized by skeletal abnormalities, including high-arched feet (pes cavus) and hammertoes, as well as progressive kyphoscoliosis. Results of electrophysiologic studies including visual, auditory brainstem, and somatosensory-evoked potentials are often abnormal. Hypertrophic cardiomyopathy with progression to intractable congestive heart failure is the cause of death for most patients. Antioxidant therapy with coenzyme Q10 and vitamin E has been reported to slow progression in some patients.

Several forms of *spinocerebellar ataxia* are similar to Friedreich ataxia. **Roussy-Levy disease** has, in addition, atrophy of the muscles of the lower extremity with a similar pattern of wasting observed in Charcot-Marie-Tooth disease; **Ramsay Hunt syndrome** has an associated myoclonic epilepsy. There are also more than 20 dominantly inherited spinocerebellar ataxias, some of which present in childhood. These include those associated with CAG (polyglutamine) repeats and noncoding microsatellite expansions. Dominantly inherited episodic ataxias caused by potassium or calcium channel dysfunction present as episodes of ataxia and muscle weakness. Some of these disorders may respond to acetazolamide. The dominantly inherited **olivopontocerebellar atrophies** (OPCA) include ataxia, cranial nerve palsies, and abnormal sensory findings in the 2nd or 3rd decade, but can present in children with rapidly progressive ataxia, nystagmus, dysarthria, and seizures.

Additional degenerative ataxias include **Pelizaeus-Merzbacher disease, neuronal ceroid lipofuscinoses,** and late-onset **GM_2 gangliosidosis** (see Chapter 599). Rare forms of progressive cerebellar ataxia have been described in association with **vitamin E deficiency.** A number of new inherited forms of progressive ataxia have been defined at the molecular level, including those caused by unstable trinucleotide repeat expansions.

TABLE 597-3. Etiological Classification of Choreic Syndromes

GENETIC CHOREAS
Huntington's disease
Huntington's disease-like 2 and other HD-like syndromes
Dentatorubropallidoluysian atrophy
Neuroacanthocytosis
Ataxia teleangiectasia
Benign hereditary chorea
Spinocerebellar ataxia (types 2, 3, or 17)
Paroxysmal kinesigenic choreoathetosis
STRUCTURAL BASAL-GANGLIA LESIONS
Vascular chorea in stroke
Mass lesions (eg, CNS lymphoma, metastatic brain tumours)
Multiple sclerosis plaques
Extrapontine myelinolysis
PARAINFECTIOUS AND AUTOIMMUNE DISORDERS
Sydenham's chorea
Systemic lupus erythematosus
Chorea gravidarum
Antiphospholipid antibody syndrome
Postinfectious or postvaccinal encephalitis
Paraneoplastic choreas
INFECTIOUS CHOREA
HIV encephalopathy
Toxoplasmosis
Cysticercosis
Diphtheria
Bacterial endocarditis
Neurosyphilis
Scarlet fever
Viral encephalitis (mumps, measles, varicella)
METABOLIC OR TOXIC ENCEPHALOPATHIES
Acute intermittent porphyria
Hypo/hypernatremia
Hypocalcaemia
Hyperthyroidism
Hypoparathyroidism
Hepatic/renal failure
Carbon monoxide poisoning
Manganese poisoning
Mercury poisoning
Organophosphate poisoning
DRUG-INDUCED CHOREA (SEE TABLE 597-4)

From Cardoso F, Seppi K, Mair KJ, et al: Seminar on choreas. *Lancet* 2006; 5: 589–602.

597.2 • Chorea, Athetosis, Tremor

Chorea, which means "dance" in Greek, refers to irregular, rapid, uncontrolled, involuntary movements. Choreic movements are often incorporated into semi-purposeful acts in an attempt to mask the abnormality or may result in bizarre movements of the hands and arms as well as abnormal gait. The categories of chorea are noted in Tables 597-3 and 597-4. **Sydenham chorea** is the most common acquired chorea of childhood and is the sole neurologic manifestation of rheumatic fever (see Chapter 182.1). The pathogenesis may be an autoimmune response of the CNS to group A streptococcal organisms. The majority of children with Sydenham chorea have antineuronal antibodies, which develop in response to group A β-hemolytic streptococcal infections. Antineuronal antibodies cross react with the cytoplasm of subthalamic and caudate nuclei neurons. Some pediatric patients with tics and obsessive-compulsive disorder (features also associated with Sydenham chorea) have antineuronal antibodies suggesting that some childhood neuropsychiatric disorders may be secondary to an autoimmune process. The disorder in these patients has been given the acronym **PANDAS** (pediatric autoimmune neuropsychiatric disorders associated with streptococcal infections). The primary pathologic findings, possibly the result of the cellular response to antineuronal antibodies, consist of vasculitis of the cortical arterioles with round cell infiltration of the gray and white matter in the surrounding area. The cerebral cortex, caudate nucleus, and subthalamic nuclei are most prominently involved. Chorea is likely a result of functional overactivity of the dopaminergic system.

The three major clinical manifestations of **Sydenham chorea** include chorea, hypotonia, and emotional lability. The chorea is usually symmetric, although children may have the choreic movements limited to one side of the body. The movements, which are rapid and jerky, are prominent in the face, trunk, and distal extremities and dart from one muscle group to another; they are increased by stress and disappear during sleep. The onset may be abrupt, but the chorea typically has a slowly progressive course. Hypotonia may be a prominent sign, and when combined with severe chorea, the child may be incapable of feeding, dressing, or walking. The speech is often involved and is sometimes unintelligible. Periods of uncontrollable crying and extreme mood swings are characteristic, perhaps in part as a result of the motor handicap and feelings of helplessness. Several typical signs are associated with Sydenham chorea, including the "milkmaid's grip" (relaxing and tightening hand shake), the "choreic hand" (spooning of the extended hand by flexion at the wrist and extension of the fingers), the "darting tongue" (the tongue cannot be protruded for longer than a few seconds), and the "pronator sign" (the arms and palms turn outward when held above the head). Sydenham chorea may persist for several months and as long as 1–2 yr. About 20% of children experience a recurrence of chorea within 2 yr of the initial episode. Cases with minimal signs are treated conservatively with avoidance of stress as much as possible. Incapacitating chorea is managed with a trial of diazepam followed by valproic acid, phenothiazines, or haloperidol, if the diazepam therapy is unsuccessful.

Although the phenothiazines and haloperidol are effective drugs in the treatment of Sydenham chorea, long-term use may be complicated by the development of another movement disorder, **tardive dyskinesia.** Tardive dyskinesia is characterized by stereotypical facial movements, particularly by lip smacking and protrusion and retraction of the tongue. The movement disorder may gradually disappear but in some patients persists after discontinuing the drug. Because patients with Sydenham chorea are at risk for the development of rheumatic carditis, particularly mitral stenosis, a regimen of daily penicillin prophylaxis should be instituted and maintained until adulthood. A much rarer cause of chorea during childhood, *paroxysmal kinesigenic choreoathetosis,* is discussed in Chapter 594.

Systemic lupus erythematosus (SLE) may present or be associated with neurologic symptoms and signs including seizures, organic brain syndromes (psychoses), aseptic meningitis, and various isolated neurologic signs including chorea. Chorea may be the presenting sign of SLE, particularly in children. Antiphospholipid antibodies are present in the serum in the majority of these patients. The presence of circulating antiphospholipid antibodies is associated with a high incidence of venous and arterial occlusions. Any child with chorea of unknown cause should be investigated for the possibility of antiphospholipid antibodies.

Huntington disease is a dominantly inherited degenerative disorder of the CNS caused by an expanded sequence of CAG repeats in a gene on chromosome 4p16.3, resulting in mutations in the huntingtin protein. Huntingtin forms abnormal inclusions within the nuclei of neurons and this interaction may sequester and reduce levels of proteins such as CREB binding protein (CBP) needed to activate the transcription of other genes. The onset of symptoms of progressive chorea and presenile dementia occurs most typically between 35 and 55 yr of age. Less than 1% of cases begin in children younger than 10 yr of age with rigidity, dystonia, and seizures. Mental deterioration and behavioral problems are prominent in children. Generalized tonic-clonic seizures are common and are typically resistant to anticonvulsants. Cerebellar signs are present in 50% and oculomotor apraxia occurs in ≈20% of cases. The course of the disease is more rapid in children, with an average duration of 8 yr until death compared with 14 yr in adults. CT scanning, although nondiagnostic, shows the mean bifrontal : bicaudate ratio to be decreased, indicating atrophy of the caudate nucleus and putamen. MRI shows hyperdensity of the putamen in adults with the akinetic-rigid form. There is no specific therapy for Huntington disease, but once the diagnosis is confirmed, the pediatrician should provide genetic counseling to the family so that risks for additional cases in future generations are understood. Molecular biologic testing (CAG trinucleotide repeat) is available but is inappropriate for children under the age of consent. Presymptomatic adult patients who test positive respond similarly to patients with cancer when the diagnosis is confirmed.

Other causes of chorea include atypical seizures, drug intoxication (phenytoin, amitriptyline, and fluphenazine) hormonally induced seizures (oral contraceptives, pregnancy/chorea gravidarum), Lyme disease, hypoparathyroidism, hyperthyroidism, and Wilson disease (see Chapter 354.2).

Athetosis or distal writhing movements of the extremities, sometimes combined with chorea (choreoathetosis), is often seen as part of extrapyramidal cerebral palsy caused by asphyxia, kernicterus, or genetic metabolic disorders such as glutaric aciduria. Athetosis is also seen with cerebral palsy associated with prematurity. Chorea and choreoathetosis may also occur after circulatory arrest is used as a support technique for complex cardiac surgery or as a complication of dopamine-blocking neuroleptic drugs such as phenothiazines. Patients with athetosis also often have *rigidity* characterized by muscle stiffness throughout the range of motion in both flexors and extensors in contrast to *spasticity* in which the increased tone is velocity dependent. Like athetosis and chorea, rigidity results from dysfunction of the basal ganglia, in contrast to spasticity, which reflects upper motor neuron dysfunction.

Tremor is an involuntary movement characterized by rhythmic oscillations of a part of the body, which may be more prominent during rest or with movement. Jitteriness, defined as rhythmic tremors of equal amplitude around a fixed axis, is the most common involuntary movement of healthy full-term infants. Jitteriness is most apparent when an infant is crying or being examined (Moro response) and is abnormal when an infant is awake and alert and when the tremor persists beyond the 2nd week of life. Organic causes of jitteriness include sepsis, intracranial hemorrhage, hypoxic encephalopathy, hypoglycemia, hypocalcemia, hypomagnesemia, prenatal exposure to maternal marijuana, and the narcotic abstinence syndrome.

Essential tremor is a familial condition, inherited as an autosomal dominant trait. It may begin during childhood and usually is slowly progressive. The tremor has a frequency of 4–9 Hz, primarily affects the distal upper extremities, is typically postural, and commonly disappears with rest. If the tremor causes difficulty in writing or activities of daily living, a trial of propranolol hydrochloride or primidone usually provides a favorable

TABLE 597-4. Drugs That Can Induce Chorea

DOPAMINE RECEPTOR BLOCKING AGENTS
Phenothiazines
Butyrophenones
Benzamides
ANTIPARKINSONIAN DRUGS
L-dopa
Dopamine agonists
Anticholinergics
ANTIEPILEPTIC DRUGS
Phenytoin
Carbamazepine
Valproic acid
PSYCHOSTIMULANTS
Amphetamines
Pemoline
Cocaine
CALCIUM-CHANNEL BLOCKERS
Cinnarizine
Flunarizine
Verapamil
OTHERS
Lithium
Baclofen
Digoxin
Tricyclic antidepressants
Cyclosporine
Steroids/oral contraceptives
Theophylline

From Cardoso F, Seppi K, Mair KJ, et al: Seminar on choreas. *Lancet* 2006;5:589–602.

response. Primary writing tremor occurs only during the action of writing and is characterized by a jerky tremor, often responsive to β blockers or anticholinergics.

Drugs that can cause tremor include amphetamines, valproic acid, neuroleptics, tricyclic antidepressants, caffeine, and theophylline. Children recovering from a severe head injury may develop a proximal tremor that is enhanced by movement and responds to propranolol. Tremor may be the initial manifestation of a metabolic disorder, including hypoglycemia, thyrotoxicosis, neuroblastoma, and pheochromocytoma. Wilson disease often presents with a postural tremor associated with kinetic movement. These patients may also develop a wing-beating tremor of the shoulders when the upper arms are abducted and the elbows flexed. Hereditary dystonia-parkinsonism syndrome often displays a proximal tremor in addition to the characteristic dystonic movements. Myoclonus, sudden, brief, jerky, shocklike, involuntary movements, may be superimposed on tremor to cause a myoclonic tremor as is seen after hypoxic injury to the cerebellum or in certain neurodegenerative diseases.

597.3 • Dystonia

Dystonia is a syndrome of sustained muscle contractions, frequently causing twisting and repetitive movements or abnormal postures. Major causes of dystonia include perinatal asphyxia (see Chapter 99.5), kernicterus, generalized primary dystonia, drugs, Wilson disease (hepatolenticular degeneration), Hallervorden-Spatz disease, and numerous other genetic mutations. Dystonia may be a prominent feature of children with extrapyramidal cerebral palsy who have had basal ganglia injury from asphyxia, kernicterus, or insults from metabolic disorders such as glutaric aciduria. Dystonia may develop gradually over many years in older children and teenagers after basal ganglia injury.

Generalized primary dystonia, also referred to as torsion dystonia or *dystonia musculorum deformans* (DMD), is caused by a group of genetic disorders that begin to progress in childhood. One form, which occurs in the Ashkenazi Jewish population, is caused by a dominantly acting mutation in the DYT_1 gene coding for the adenosine triphosphate (ATP) binding protein Torsin A. The initial manifestation of the disease during childhood is often unilateral posturing of the lower extremity, particularly the foot, which assumes an extended and rotated position, causing tiptoe walking. Because the dystonic movement is initially intermittent and is aggravated by stress, patients are often labeled as hysterical. Ultimately, all four extremities and the axial musculature are affected as well as the muscles of the face and tongue, and thus speech and swallowing become impaired. Other forms of torsion dystonia are caused by mutations in the genes for tyrosine hydroxylase and for ε-sarcoglycan, causing the myoclonus dystonia syndrome.

More than a dozen loci for genes for torsion dystonia have been identified. One of these is *dopa-responsive dystonia* (DRD), also called **hereditary progressive dystonia with marked diurnal variation,** or **Segawa disease.** It is inherited as a dominant disorder more common in females. The gene for dopa-sensitive dystonia codes for GTP cyclohydrolase 1, the synthetic enzyme for the cofactor tetrahydrobiopterin that is required for synthesis of the neurotransmitters dopamine and serotonin. The dystonia is usually diurnal, improving with sleep but becoming apparent and sometimes incapacitating during the daytime. Early-onset cases can easily be confused with extrapyramidal cerebral palsy. DRD responds remarkably to small daily doses (50–250 mg) of levodopa given with an inhibitor of peripheral catabolism. DRD and dystonia due to mutations in TH can be diagnosed by assaying CSF neurotransmitter metabolites for serotonin and dopamine and biopterin cofactor levels.

Segmental dystonia, including writer's cramp, blepharospasm, and buccomandibular dystonia, is more common in adults and tends to be limited to a specific group of muscles. Segmental dystonia may be seen in patients with genetic forms of torsion dystonia or may be idiopathic or acquired from overuse of muscles such as in the hands of musicians.

Certain **drugs** are capable of producing an acute dystonic reaction in children. Therapeutic doses of phenytoin or carbamazepine may rarely cause progressive dystonia in children with epilepsy, particularly in those who have an underlying structural abnormality of the brain. Children may have an idiosyncratic reaction to the phenothiazines, characterized by acute dystonic posturing that is sometimes confused with encephalitis. Intravenous diphenhydramine, 1–2 mg/kg/dose, may rapidly reverse the drug-related dystonia. Severe rigidity combined with high fever and delirium may also occur as part of the **neuroleptic malignant syndrome** a few days after starting neuroleptic drugs.

Wilson disease is a rare (incidence of 1/40,000–1/100,000 live births) autosomal recessive inborn error of copper transport characterized by cirrhosis of the liver and degenerative changes in the CNS, particularly the basal ganglia (see Chapter 354.2). The gene (*WND*) for Wilson disease has been mapped to chromosome 13q14–21. It has been determined that there are multiple mutations in the Wilson disease gene, accounting for the variability in presentation of the condition. The precise cause is unknown, but the basic mechanism relates to decreased excretion of biliary copper, due partly to a lysosomal defect of the liver cells. The initial symptoms and signs in children younger than 10 yr relate to acute or subacute hepatic failure, which is frequently misinterpreted as infectious hepatitis. The neurologic manifestations of Wilson disease rarely appear before age 10 yr, and the initial sign is often progressive dystonia. Tremors of the extremities develop, unilaterally at first, but they eventually become coarse, generalized, and incapacitating (the so-called wing-beating tremor). Signs of progressive basal ganglia destruction include drooling, a fixed smile caused by retraction of the upper lip, dysarthria, dysphonia, rigidity, contractures, dystonia, and choreoathetosis. The Kayser-Fleischer ring, which is best seen with the slit lamp, is pathognomonic and results from deposition of copper in the Descemet membrane. In the untreated state, patients typically become bedridden and demented and die in coma within a few years from the onset of the disease. The MRI or CT scan shows ventricular dilatation in advanced cases with atrophy of the cerebrum and lesions in the thalamus and basal ganglia. The treatment of Wilson disease is discussed in Chapter 354.2.

Hallervorden-Spatz disease is a rare degenerative disorder inherited as an autosomal recessive trait. Linkage analysis indicates that the gene is located on chromosome 20p13, and many patients have mutations in pantothenate kinase 2 (PANK2) localized to mitochondria in neurons. This disorder is also commonly called pantothenate kinase–associated neurodegeneration. The condition usually begins in childhood and is characterized by progressive dystonia, rigidity, and choreoathetosis. Spasticity, extensor plantar responses, dysarthria, and intellectual deterioration become evident during adolescence, and death usually occurs by early adulthood. MRI shows lesions of the globus pallidus, including low signal intensity in T2 weighted images (corresponds to iron pigments) and an anteromedial area of high signal intensity (tissue necrosis and edema), or "eye-of-the-tiger" sign. Neuropathologic examination indicates excessive accumulation of iron-containing pigments in the globus pallidus and substantia nigra.

Therapy for dystonia has progressed in the past decade. Children with generalized dystonia, including those with involvement of the muscles of swallowing, may respond to large doses of trihexyphenidyl (Artane). The initial dose is 2 mg/24 hr, slowly increasing to 60–80 mg/24 hr or until untoward side effects (urinary retention, mental confusion, or blurred vision) occur. Additional drugs that have been effective include carbamazepine, levodopa, bromocriptine, and diazepam. Segmental dystonia such as torticollis often responds well to botulinum toxin injections. Intrathecal baclofen delivered through implantable constant infusion pump may be helpful in some patients. Stereotaxic surgery (thalamotomy, pallidotomy) has valuable results with many adverse effects, whereas bilateral electrical deep brain stimulation with leads implanted in the globus pallidus is helpful for children with severe primary generalized dystonia.

597.4 • Tics

Tics are spasmodic, involuntary, repetitive, stereotyped movements that are nonrhythmic, often exacerbated by stress, and may affect any muscle group. Tics can be classified into three subgroups: transient tics of childhood, chronic tics, and Gilles de la Tourette syndrome (TS). **Transient tic disorder** is the most common movement abnormality of childhood (see Chapter 23). The tics are more prevalent in boys, and the family history is often positive. They consist of eye blinking or facial movements and occasional throat-clearing noises. The disorder persists from weeks to less than a year and does not require drug therapy. **Chronic motor tic disorder** occurs in children and may persist throughout adult life. The tics characteristically involve up to three muscle groups simultaneously. Evidence shows that the gene for TS may be expressed as simple transient tic of childhood and chronic motor tics, suggesting considerable overlap of these conditions.

Gilles de la Tourette syndrome is a lifelong condition, with a prevalence of ≈1/2,000, that has an onset between 2 and 21 yr of age (see Chapter 23). TS is probably inherited in most cases as autosomal dominant, but a convincing gene locus has not been identified. TS is diagnosed in children who have multiple motor tics in different parts of the body with at least one vocal tic beginning before age 21 yr and waxing and waning over a period of more than a year. Obsessive-compulsive behavior and attention-deficit/hyperactivity disorder (ADHD) are also frequently present. Motor tics are associated with numerous fluctuating movements of the face, eyelids, neck, and shoulders. Ultimately, the tics are accompanied by vocalizations (vocal tics), including throat clearing, sniffling, barking, coprolalia (obscene words), echolalia (repetition of words addressed to the patient), palilalia (repetition of one's own words), and echokinesis (imitation of movement of others). The vocalizations are uncontrollable and frequently jeopardize patients' social interaction with other children. Although TS is a lifelong condition, the ultimate prognosis can often be determined by the severity of the symptoms during adolescence.

Medication should be considered when the motor tics or vocalizations interfere significantly with a child's social and academic interactions, although behavior management and biofeedback programs have been successful for some patients. Several reports implicate stimulant medications (methylphenidate) as the cause of TS. Methylphenidate may unmask TS but not cause it. All children who have ADHD and who are treated with stimulant medication should be monitored closely for the onset of tics. The decision to continue the stimulant medication should be determined by the severity of the ADHD and tic disorder. Haloperidol, a dopamine-blocking agent, is effective in the treatment of ≈50% of children with TS. The initial dose is 0.25 mg/24 hr, and the drug is increased weekly by 0.25 mg to the usual dose range of 2–6 mg/24 hr, although some children can tolerate larger doses. Side effects include cognitive impairment, lethargy, fatigue, depression, restlessness, acute dystonic reactions, drug-induced parkinsonism, akathisia, and tardive dyskinesia syndromes, including tardive dystonia in children. Additional drugs that may prove useful include penfluridol, pimozide, and clonidine. Clonidine, an α_2-presynaptic noradrenergic agonist, is begun at a dose of 0.05 mg/24 hr and gradually increased to a maximum of 0.125–0.2 mg/24 hr. Several weeks of clonidine therapy may be needed to control the vocal and motor tics. The major side effects are lethargy, fatigue, and drowsiness. Approximately 50% of patients with TS experience obsessive-compulsive symptoms. The tricyclic antidepressant clomipramine is effective in ≈60% of patients. Other useful antidepressant drugs include sertraline, fluoxetine, and fluvoxamine. Because TS is a chronic disorder associated with many social, behavioral, and learning problems, pediatricians have an important role in the multidisciplinary management as an advocate for children.

Albin RL: Dominant ataxias and Friedreich ataxia: An update. *Curr Opin Neurol* 2003;16:507–514.

Burd L, Kerbeshian J, Berth A, et al: Long-term follow-up of an epidemiologically defined cohort of patients with Tourette syndrome. *J Child Neurol* 2001;16:431–437.

Cardoso F, Seppi K, Mair KJ, et al: Seminar on choleras. *Lancet Neurol* 2006;5:589–602.

Cervera R, Asherson RA, Font J, et al: Chorea in the antiphospholipid syndrome. Clinical, radiologic, and immunologic characteristics of 50 patients from our clinics and the recent literature. *Medicine (Baltimore)* 1997;76:203–212.

Dale RC, Heyman I, Surtees RAH, et al: Dyskinesias and associated psychiatric disorders following streptococcal infections. *Arch Dis Child* 2004;89:604–610.

Farr AK, Shalev B, Crawford TO, et al: Ocular manifestations of ataxia-telangiectasis. *Am J Ophthalmol* 2002;134:891–896.

Ferland RJ, Eyaid W, Collura RV, et al: Abnormal cerebellar development and axonal decussation due to mutations in AHI1 in Joubert syndrome. *Nat Genet* 2004;36:1126.

Hart PE, Lodi R, Rajagopalan B, et al: Antioxidant treatment of patients with Friedreich ataxia: Four-year followup. *Arch Neurol* 2005;62:621–626.

Hayflick SJ, Westaway SK, Levinson B, et al: Genetic, clinical, and radiographic delineation of Hallervorden-Spatz Syndrome. *N Engl J Med* 2003;348:33–40.

Holinski-Feder E, Jedele KB, Hörtnagel K, et al: Large intergenerational variation in age of onset in two young patients with Huntington's disease presenting as dyskinesia. *Pediatrics* 1997;100:896–898.

Hoon AH Jr, Freese PO, Reinhardt EM, et al: Age-dependent effects of trihexyphenidyl in extrapyramidal cerebral palsy. *Pediatr Neurol* 2001; 25:55–58.

Ichinose H, Ohye T, Takahashi E: Hereditary progressive dystonia with marked diurnal fluctuation caused by mutations in the GTP cyclohydrolase I gene. *Nat Genet* 1994;8:236–242.

Kids Move: *www.wemove.org/kidsmove/* [A good description of movement disorders in children and their treatment.]

Kupsch A, Beneccke R, Müller J, et al: Pallidal deep-brain stimulation in primary generalized or segmental dystonia. *N Engl J Med* 2006;355: 1978–1990.

Misbahuddin A, Warner TT: Dystonia: An update on genetics and treatment. *Curr Opin Neurol* 2001;14:471–475.

Pandolfo M: Friedreich ataxia. *Semin Pediatr Neurol* 2003;10:163–172.

Paulson H, Ammache Z: Ataxia and hereditary disorders. *Neurol Clin* 2001;19:759–782.

Schols L, Bauer P, Schmidt T, et al: Autosomal dominant cerebellar ataxias: Clinical features, genetics, and pathogenesis. *Lancet Neurol* 2004; 3:291–304.

Tarsy D, Simon DK: Dystonia. *N Engl J Med* 2006;355:818–829.

Vidailhet M, Vercueil L, Houeto JL, et al: Bilateral deep-brain stimulation of the globus pallidus in primary generalized dystonia. *N Engl J Med* 2005;352:459–467.

Zimprich A, Grabowski M, Asmus F, et al: Mutations in the gene encoding epsilon-sarcoglycan cause myoclonus-dystonia syndrome. *Nat Genet* 2001;29:66–69.

Zomorrodi A, Wald ER: Sydenham's cholera in Western Pennsylvania. *Pediatrics* 2006;117:e675–e679.

Chapter 598 ■ Encephalopathies

Michael V. Johnston

Encephalopathy is a generalized disorder of cerebral function that may be acute or chronic, progressive or static. The etiology of the encephalopathies in children includes infectious, toxic (carbon monoxide, drugs, lead), metabolic, and ischemic causes. Hypoxic-ischemic encephalopathy is discussed in Chapter 99.5.

598.1 • Cerebral Palsy (See also Chapters 38 and 97.2)

Cerebral palsy (CP) is a diagnostic term used to describe a group of motor syndromes resulting from disorders of early brain development. CP is caused by a broad group of developmental, genetic, metabolic, ischemic, infectious, and other acquired etiologies that produce a common group of neurologic phenotypes. Although it has historically been considered a **static encephalopathy,** this term is not entirely accurate because of the recognition that the neurologic features of CP often change or progress over time. Although CP is often associated with epilepsy and abnormalities of speech, vision, and intellect, it is the selective vulnerability of the brain's motor systems that defines the disorder. Many children and adults with CP function at a high educational and vocational level, without any sign of the type of cognitive dysfunction that is generally implied by the term *encephalopathy.*

EPIDEMIOLOGY AND ETIOLOGY. CP is the most common and costly form of chronic motor disability that begins in childhood with a prevalence of 2/1000. The Collaborative Perinatal Project, in which ≈45,000 children were regularly monitored from in utero to the age of 7 yr, found that most children with CP had been born at term with uncomplicated labors and deliveries. In 80% of cases, features were identified pointing to antenatal factors causing abnormal brain development. A substantial number of children with CP had congenital anomalies external to the central nervous system (CNS). Fewer than 10% of children with CP had evidence of intrapartum asphyxia. Intrauterine exposure to maternal infection (chorioamnionitis, inflammation of placental membranes, umbilical cord inflammation, foul-smelling amniotic fluid, maternal sepsis, temperature >38°C during labor, urinary tract infection) is associated with a significant increase in the risk of CP in normal birthweight infants. Elevated levels of inflammatory cytokines are noted in heelstick blood collected at birth from children who later were identified with CP. The prevalence of CP is increased among low birthweight infants, particularly those weighing <1,000 g at birth, primarily because of **intracerebral hemorrhage** and **periventricular leukomalacia** (PVL). Although the incidence of intracerebral hemorrhage has declined significantly, PVL remains a major problem. PVL reflects the enhanced vulnerability of immature oligodendroglia in premature infants to oxidative stress caused by ischemia or infectious/inflammatory insults. White matter abnormalities (loss of volume of periventricular white matter, extent of cystic changes, ventricular dilatation, thinning of the corpus callosum) present on MRI at 40 wk gestational age among former preterm infants predict CP at 2 yr of age. Attempts to reduce the incidence of CP in term infants should be directed toward increasing understanding of fetal developmental biology and awareness that strategies need to be developed for premature infants to protect the vulnerable developing white matter.

CLINICAL MANIFESTATIONS. CP is generally divided into several major motor syndromes that differ according to the pattern of neurologic involvement, neuropathology, and etiology (Table 598-1). The physiologic classification identifies the major motor abnormality, whereas the topographic taxonomy indicates the involved extremities. CP is also commonly associated with a spectrum of developmental disabilities, including mental retardation, epilepsy, and visual, hearing, speech, cognitive, and behavioral abnormalities. The motor handicap may be the least of the child's problems.

Infants with **spastic hemiplegia** have decreased spontaneous movements on the affected side and show hand preference at a very early age. The arm is often more involved than the leg and difficulty in hand manipulation is obvious by 1 yr of age. Walking is usually delayed until 18–24 mo, and a circumductive gait is apparent. Examination of the extremities may show growth arrest, particularly in the hand and thumbnail, especially if the contralateral parietal lobe is abnormal because extremity growth is influenced by this area of the brain. Spasticity is apparent in the affected extremities, particularly the ankle, causing an equinovarus deformity of the foot. An affected child often walks on tiptoe because of the increased tone, and the affected upper extremity assumes a dystonic posture when the child runs. Ankle clonus and a Babinski sign may be present, the deep tendon reflexes are increased, and weakness of the hand and foot dorsiflexors is evident. About one third of patients with spastic hemiplegia have a seizure disorder that usually develops in the 1st year or 2; ≈25% have cognitive abnormalities including mental retardation. A CT scan or MRI study may show an atrophic cerebral hemisphere with a dilated lateral ventricle contralateral to the side of the affected extremities. An MRI is far more sensitive than CT for most lesions seen with CP, although a CT scan may be useful for detecting calcifications associated with congenital infections. Focal cerebral infarction (stroke) secondary to intrauterine or perinatal thromboembolism related to thrombophilic disorders, especially anticardiolipin antibodies, is an important cause of hemiplegic CP (see Chapter 601). Family histories suggestive of thrombosis and inherited clotting disorders may be present and evaluation of the mother may provide information valuable for future pregnancies and other family members.

Spastic diplegia is bilateral spasticity of the legs greater than in the arms. The 1st indication of spastic diplegia is often noted when an affected infant begins to crawl. The child uses the arms in a normal reciprocal fashion but tends to drag the legs behind more as a rudder (commando crawl) rather than using the normal four-limbed crawling movement. If the spasticity is severe, application of a diaper is difficult because of the excessive adduction of the hips. If there is paraspinal muscle involvement, the child may be unable to sit. Examination of the child reveals spasticity

TABLE 598-1. Classification of Cerebral Palsy and Major Causes

Motor Syndrome	Neuropathology	Major Causes
Spastic diplegia	Periventricular leukomalacia (PVL)	Prematurity Ischemia Infection Endocrine/metabolic (e.g., thyroid)
Spastic quadriplegia	PVL Multicystic encephalomalacia Malformations	Ischemia, infection Endocrine/metabolic, genetic/developmental
Hemiplegia	Stroke: in utero or neonatal	Thrombophilic disorders Infection Genetic/developmental Periventricular hemorrhagic infarction
Extrapyramidal (athetoid, dyskinetic)	Pathology: putamen, globus pallidus, thalamus, basal ganglia	Asphyxia Kernicterus Mitochondrial Genetic/metabolic

in the legs with brisk reflexes, ankle clonus, and a bilateral Babinski sign. When the child is suspended by the axillae, a scissoring posture of the lower extremities is maintained. Walking is significantly delayed, the feet are held in a position of equinovarus, and the child walks on tiptoe. Severe spastic diplegia is characterized by disuse atrophy and impaired growth of the lower extremities and by disproportionate growth with normal development of the upper torso. The prognosis for normal intellectual development is excellent for these patients, and the likelihood of seizures is minimal. The most common neuropathologic finding is periventricular leukomalacia, particularly in the area where fibers innervating the legs course through the internal capsule. MRI is very useful for evaluating the severity of white matter injury and for excluding other brain lesions. Magnetic resonance imaging methods such as diffusion tensor imaging (DTI) have shown specific regional abnormalities in white matter fibers associated with spastic diplegia.

Spastic quadriplegia is the most severe form of CP because of marked motor impairment of all extremities and the high association with mental retardation and seizures. Swallowing difficulties are common as a result of supranuclear bulbar palsies, often leading to aspiration pneumonia. The most common lesions seen on pathologic examination or on MRI scanning are severe PVL and multicystic cortical encephalomalacia. Neurologic examination shows increased tone and spasticity in all extremities, decreased spontaneous movements, brisk reflexes, and plantar extensor responses. Flexion contractures of the knees and elbows are often present by late childhood. Associated developmental disabilities, including speech and visual abnormalities, are particularly prevalent in this group of children. Children with spastic quadriparesis often have evidence of athetosis and may be classified as having mixed CP.

Athetoid CP, also called **choreoathetoid** or **extrapyramidal** CP, is less common than spastic cerebral palsy. Affected infants are characteristically hypotonic with poor head control and marked head lag and develop increased variable tone with rigidity and dystonia over several years. Feeding may be difficult, and tongue thrust and drooling may be prominent. Speech is typically affected because the oropharyngeal muscles are involved. Speech may be absent or sentences are slurred, and voice modulation is impaired. Generally, upper motor neuron signs are not present, seizures are uncommon, and intellect is preserved in many patients. This form of CP is also referred to in Europe as dyskinetic CP and is the type most likely to be associated with **birth asphyxia.** Extrapyramidal CP secondary to acute intrapartum near-total asphyxia is associated with bilaterally symmetric lesions in the posterior putamen and ventrolateral thalamus. These lesions appear to be the correlate of the neuropathologic lesion called *status marmoratus* in the basal ganglia. Athetoid CP can also be caused by **kernicterus** secondary to high levels of bilirubin, and in this case the MRI scan shows lesions in the globus pallidus bilaterally. Extrapyramidal CP can also be associated with lesions in the basal ganglia and thalamus caused by metabolic genetic disorders such as mitochondrial disorders and glutaric aciduria. MRI scanning and possibly metabolic testing are important in the evaluation of children with extrapyramidal CP to make a correct diagnosis of etiology.

DIAGNOSIS. A thorough history and physical examination should preclude a **progressive disorder** of the CNS, including degenerative diseases, metabolic disorders, spinal cord tumor, or muscular dystrophy. The possibility of anomalies at the base of the skull or other disorders affecting the cervical spinal cord needs to be considered in patients with little involvement of the arms or cranial nerves. An MRI scan of the brain is indicated to determine the location and extent of structural lesions or associated congenital malformations; an MRI scan of the spinal cord is indicated if there is any question about spinal cord pathology. Additional studies may include tests of hearing and visual function. Genetic evaluation should be considered in patients with congenital malformations (chromosomes) or evidence of metabolic disorders. Because CP is usually associated with a wide spectrum of developmental disorders, a multidisciplinary approach is most helpful in the assessment and treatment of such children.

TREATMENT. A team of physicians from various specialties, as well as occupational and physical therapists, speech pathologists, social workers, educators, and developmental psychologists provide important contributions to the treatment of these children. Parents should be taught how to work with their child in daily activities such as feeding, carrying, dressing, bathing, and playing in ways that limit the effects of abnormal muscle tone. They also need to be instructed in the supervision of a series of exercises designed to prevent the development of contractures, especially a tight Achilles tendon. There is no proof that physical or occupational therapy *prevents* development of CP in infants at risk or that it *corrects* the neurologic deficit, but evidence shows that therapy optimizes the functioning of children to achieve their potential.

Children with spastic diplegia are treated initially with the assistance of adaptive equipment, such as walkers, poles, and standing frames. If a patient has marked spasticity of the lower extremities or evidence of hip dislocation, consideration should be given to performing surgical soft tissue procedures that reduce muscle spasm around the hip girdle, including an adductor tenotomy or psoas transfer and release. A rhizotomy procedure in which the roots of the spinal nerves are divided produces considerable improvement in selected patients with severe spastic diplegia (Fig. 598-1). A tight heel cord in a child with spastic hemiplegia may be treated surgically by tenotomy of the Achilles tendon. Quadriplegia is managed with motorized wheelchairs, special feeding devices, modified typewriters, and customized seating arrangements. Children with **hemiplegic CP** have been managed with constraints applied to the unaffected side which induces improved hand and arm functioning on the affected side. This constraint-induced movement therapy is effective in patients of all ages.

Communication skills may be enhanced by the use of Bliss symbols, talking typewriters, and specially adapted computers including artificial intelligence computers to augment motor and language function. Significant behavior problems may substantially interfere with the development of a child with CP; their early identification and management are important, and the assistance of a psychologist or psychiatrist may be necessary. Learning and attention deficit disorders and mental retardation are assessed and managed by a psychologist and educator. Strabismus, nystagmus, and optic atrophy are common in children with CP; an ophthalmologist should be included in the initial assessment. Lower urinary tract dysfunction should receive prompt assessment and treatment.

Several drugs have been used to **treat spasticity**, including oral dantrolene sodium, the benzodiazepines, and baclofen. These medications have modest beneficial effects in some patients, but can also cause side effects such as sedation for benzodiazepines and lowered seizure threshold for baclofen. Intrathecal baclofen has been used successfully in selected children with severe spasticity. This therapy requires a team approach and constant follow-up for complications of the infusion pumping mechanism and infection. **Botulinum toxin** injected into specific muscle groups for the management of spasticity shows a very positive response in many patients. Botulism toxin injected into salivary glands may also help reduce the severity of drooling, which is seen in 10–30% of patients with CP and has been traditionally treated with anticholinergic agents. Patients with rigidity, dystonia, and spastic quadriparesis sometimes respond to levodopa, and children with dystonia may benefit from carbamazepine or trihexyphenidyl. Hyperbaric oxygen does not improve the condition of children with CP.

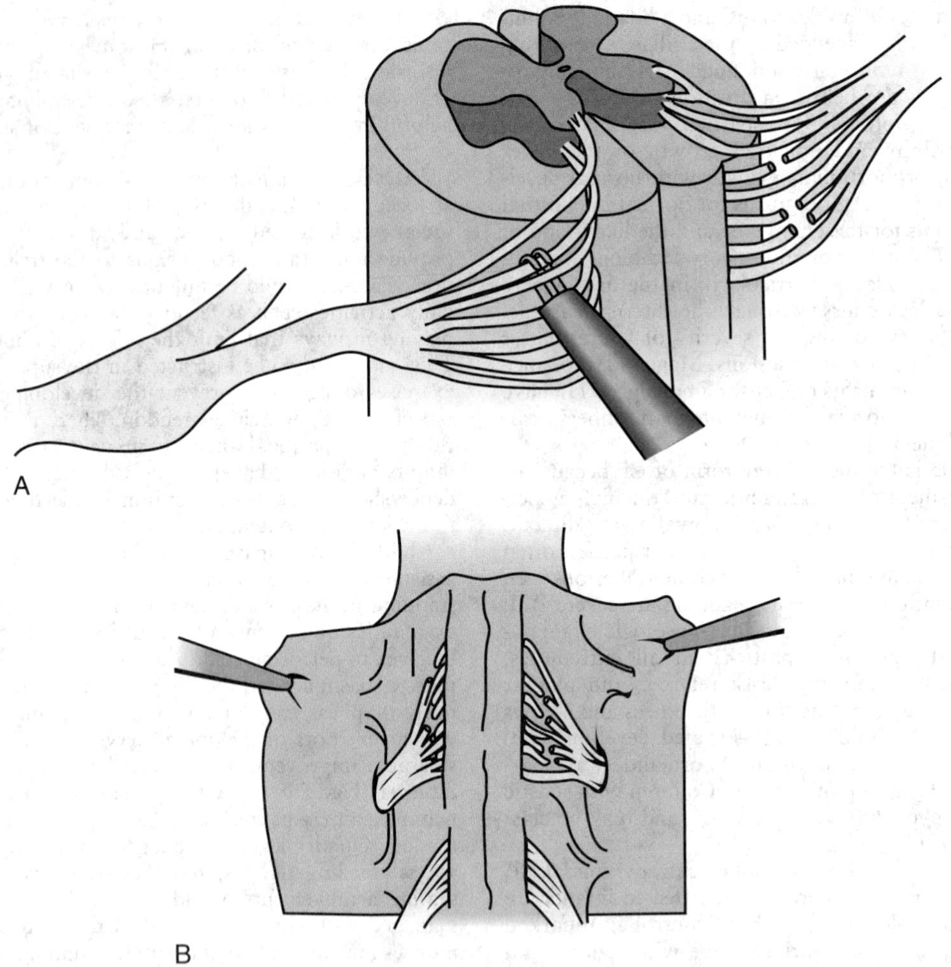

Figure 598-1. Schematic representation of the technique of selected dorsal rhizotomy. *A,* After laminectomy, the dura is opened and the dorsal spinal rootlets are exposed. The rootlets are stimulated so that abnormal rootlet activity can be identified. *B,* A proportion of rootlets are transected. (From Koman LA, Smith BP, Shilt JS: Cerebral palsy. *Lancet* 2004;363:1619–1631. Reproduced with permission from Wake Forest University Orthopaedic Press.)

598.2 • Mitochondrial Encephalomyopathies*

Mitochondrial diseases are a complex family of disorders with many clinical manifestations that can be caused by mutations of nuclear DNA (nDNA) or mitochondrial DNA (mtDNA) [see Chapters 80, 86, and 87]. They can affect various developmental stages, tissues, or systems, resulting in a diversity of clinical phenotypes that span all age groups. Biochemically, they can present with a tissue-specific or generalized monoenzymopathy, tissue-specific multienzymopathy, or generalized multienzymopathy. In the respiratory chain, oxidative phosphorylation is mediated by five intramitochondrial enzyme complexes (complexes I–V) that are responsible for producing the adenosine triphosphate (ATP) required for normal cellular function. The maintenance and assembly of oxidative phosphorylation require coordinated regulation of nuclear DNA and mitochondrial DNA genes. Human mtDNA is a small (16.5 kb), circular, double-stranded molecule that has been completely sequenced and encodes 13 structural proteins, all of which are subunits of the respiratory chain complexes, as well as two ribosomal RNAs and 22 tRNAs needed for translation. The nuclear DNA is responsible for synthesizing ≈70 subunits, transporting them to the mitochondria via chaperone proteins, ensuring their passage across the inner mitochondrial membrane, and coordinating their correct processing and assembly.

*Written with the collaboration of Dr. Ingrid Tein.

mtDNA is unique from nDNA for the following reasons: (1) its genetic code differs from nDNA, (2) it is tightly packed with information because it contains no introns, (3) it is subject to spontaneous mutations at a higher rate than nDNA, (4) it has less efficient repair mechanisms, and (5) it is present in hundreds or thousands of copies per cell and is transmitted by maternal inheritance. mtDNA is contributed only by the oocyte in the formation of the zygote. If a mutation in mtDNA occurs in the ovum or zygote, it may be passed on randomly to subsequent generations of cells. Some receive few or no mutant genomes (normal or wild-type homoplasmy), others receive a mixed population of **mutant** and **wild**-type mtDNAs (**heteroplasmy**), and still others receive primarily or exclusively mutant genomes (mutant homoplasmy). The important implications of maternal inheritance and heteroplasmy are as follows: (1) inheritance of the disease is maternal, but both sexes are equally affected; (2) phenotypic expression of an mtDNA mutation depends on the relative proportions of mutant and wild-type genomes, with a minimum critical number of mutant genomes being necessary for expression (threshold effect); (3) at cell division, the proportion may shift in daughter cells (mitotic segregation), leading to a corresponding phenotypic change; and (4) subsequent generations are affected at a higher rate than in autosomal dominant diseases. The critical number of mutant mtDNAs required for the threshold effect may vary, depending on the vulnerability of the tissue to impairments of oxidative metabolism as well as on the vulnerability of the same tissue over time that may increase with aging. Diseases of mitochondrial oxidative phosphorylation can be divided into three groups: (1) defects of nDNA, (2) defects of mtDNA, and (3) defects of communication between the nuclear and mitochondrial genome.

Using a broader classification system, mitochondrial diseases caused by defects of nDNA include defects of substrate transport (plasmalemmal carnitine transporter, carnitine palmitoyltransferase I and II, carnitine acylcarnitine translocase defects), defects of substrate oxidation (pyruvate dehydrogenase complex, pyruvate carboxylase, intramitochondrial fatty acid oxidation defects), defects of the Krebs cycle (α-ketoglutarate dehydrogenase, fumarase, aconitase defects), and defects of the respiratory chain (complexes I–V) including defects of oxidation/phosphorylation coupling (Luft syndrome) and defects of mitochondrial protein transport. These diseases follow mendelian inheritance. Diseases caused by defects of mtDNA can be divided into those due to point mutations that are maternally inherited (Leber hereditary optic neuropathy and MELAS, MERRF, and NARP syndromes) and those due to deletions or duplications that tend to be sporadic (Kearns-Sayre and Pearson marrow/pancreas syndromes). Diseases caused by defects of communication between the nuclear and mitochondrial genome follow mendelian inheritance and include multiple mtDNA deletions, which are autosomal dominant, and mtDNA depletion syndromes, which are usually autosomal recessive.

MITOCHONDRIAL ENCEPHALOMYOPATHY, ENCEPHALOMYOPATHY, LACTIC ACIDOSIS, AND STROKELIKE EPISODES (MELAS). Children with MELAS may be normal for the 1st several years, but they gradually display delayed motor and cognitive development and short stature. The clinical syndrome is characterized by (1) recurrent strokelike episodes most commonly in the posterior temporal, parietal, and occipital lobes (with CT or MRI evidence of focal brain abnormalities); (2) lactic acidosis, ragged red fibers (RRF), or both; and (3) at least two of the following: focal or generalized seizures, dementia, recurrent migraine headaches, and vomiting. In one series, onset was before age 15 yr in 62% of patients and hemianopia or cortical blindness was the most common manifestation. Cerebrospinal fluid protein is often increased. The MELAS 3243 mutation can also be associated with different combinations of exercise intolerance, myopathy, ophthalmoplegia, pigmentary retinopathy, hypertrophic or dilated cardiomyopathy, cardiac conduction defects, deafness, endocrinopathy (diabetes mellitus), and proximal renal tubular dysfunction. MELAS is a progressive disorder that has been reported in siblings. It is punctuated with episodes of stroke leading to dementia. (See also Chapter 610.4.)

Regional hypoperfusion can be detected by single-photon emission CT (SPECT) studies. Neuropathology may show cortical atrophy with infarct-like lesions in both cortical and subcortical structures, basal ganglia calcifications, and ventricular dilatation. Muscle biopsy specimens usually show RRF. Mitochondrial accumulations and abnormalities have been shown in smooth muscle cells of intramuscular vessels and of brain arterioles and in the epithelial cells and blood vessels of the choroid plexus, producing a mitochondrial angiopathy. Muscle biochemistry shows complex I deficiency in many cases; however, multiple defects have also been documented involving complexes I, III, and IV. Inheritance is maternal, and there is a highly specific, although not exclusive, point mutation at nt 3243 in the $tRNA^{Leu(UUR)}$ gene of mtDNA in ≈80% of patients. An additional 7.5% have a point mutation at nt 3271 in the $tRNA^{Leu(UUR)}$ gene. A 3rd mutation has been identified at nt 3252 in the $tRNA^{Leu(UUR)}$ gene. Because the number of mutant genomes is lower in blood than in muscle, muscle is the preferable tissue for examination.

The prognosis in patients with the full syndrome is poor. Therapeutic trials have included corticosteroids and coenzyme Q10. Lowering the serum lactate concentration with dichloroacetate has led to marked clinical improvement in some cases.

MYOCLONUS EPILEPSY AND RAGGED RED FIBERS (MERRF). This syndrome is characterized by progressive myoclonic epilepsy, mitochondrial myopathy, and cerebellar ataxia with dysarthria and nystagmus. Onset may be in childhood or in adult life, and the course may be slowly progressive or rapidly downhill. Other features include dementia, sensorineural hearing loss, optic atrophy, peripheral neuropathy, and spasticity. Because some patients have abnormalities of deep sensation and pes cavus, the condition may be confused with Friedreich ataxia. A significant number of patients have a positive family history and short stature. This condition is maternally inherited.

Pathologic findings include elevated serum lactate concentrations, RRF on muscle biopsy, and marked neuronal loss and gliosis affecting, in particular, the dentate nucleus and inferior olivary complex with some dropout of Purkinje cells and neurons of the red nucleus. Pallor of the posterior columns of the spinal cord and degeneration of the gracile and cuneate nuclei occur. Muscle biochemistry has shown variable defects of complex III, complexes II and IV, complexes I and IV, or complex IV alone. More than 80% of cases are caused by a heteroplasmic G to A point mutation at nt 8344 of the $tRNA^{Lys}$ gene of mtDNA. Additional patients have been reported with a T to C mutation at nt 8356 in the $tRNA^{Lys}$ gene.

There is no specific therapy, although coenzyme Q10 appeared to be beneficial in a mother and daughter with the MERRF mutation.

LEBER HEREDITARY OPTIC NEUROPATHY (LHON). LHON is characterized by onset usually between the ages of 18 and 30 yr of acute or subacute visual loss caused by severe bilateral optic atrophy, although children as young as 5 yr have been reported to have LHON. At least 85% of patients are young men. An X-linked factor may modulate the expression of the mitochondrial DNA point mutation. The classic ophthalmologic features include circumpapillary telangiectatic microangiopathy and pseudoedema of the optic disc. Variable features may include cerebellar ataxia, hyperreflexia, Babinski sign, psychiatric symptoms, peripheral neuropathy, or cardiac conduction abnormalities (pre-excitation syndrome). Some cases have been associated with widespread white matter lesions as seen with multiple sclerosis. Lactic acidosis and RRF tend to be conspicuously absent in LHON. More than 11 mtDNA point mutations have been described, including a usually homoplasmic G to A transition at nt 11,778 of the ND4 subunit gene of complex I. The latter leads to replacement of a highly conserved arginine residue by histidine at the 340th amino acid and accounts for ≈50–70% of cases in Europe and >90% of cases in Japan. Certain LHON pedigrees with other point mutations are associated with complex neurologic disorders and may have features in common with MELAS syndrome and with infantile bilateral striatal necrosis.

ATPase SUBUNIT 6 MUTATION (NARP). This maternally inherited disorder presents with either Leigh syndrome or with developmental delay, retinitis pigmentosa, dementia, seizures, ataxia, proximal weakness, and sensory neuropathy (NARP syndrome). It is due to a point mutation at nt 8993 within the ATPase subunit 6 gene. The severity of the disease presentation appears to have close correlation with the percentage of mutant mtDNA in leukocytes. There is no treatment.

KEARNS-SAYRE SYNDROME (KSS). The criteria for KSS include a triad of (1) onset before age 20 yr, (2) progressive external ophthalmoplegia (PEO) with ptosis, and (3) pigmentary retinopathy.

There must also be at least one of the following: heart block, cerebellar syndrome, or cerebrospinal fluid protein >100 mg/dL. Other nonspecific but common features include dementia, sensorineural hearing loss, and multiple endocrine abnormalities, including short stature, diabetes mellitus, and hypoparathyroidism. There is no treatment for KSS. The prognosis is poor, despite placement of a pacemaker, and progressively downhill, with death resulting by the 3rd or 4th decade. Unusual clinical presentations can include renal tubular acidosis and Lowe syndrome. There are also a few overlap cases of children with KSS and strokelike episodes. Muscle biopsy shows RRF and variable cytochrome oxidase (COX)–negative fibers. Most patients have mtDNA deletions, and some have duplications. These may be new mutations accounting for the generally sporadic nature of KSS. A few pedigrees have shown autosomal dominant transmission.

Sporadic PEO with RRF is a clinically benign condition characterized by adolescent or young adult–onset ophthalmoplegia, ptosis, and proximal limb girdle weakness. It is slowly progressive and compatible with a relatively normal life. The muscle biopsy material demonstrates RRF and COX-negative fibers. Approximately 50% of patients with PEO have mtDNA deletions, and there is no family history.

LEIGH DISEASE (SUBACUTE NECROTIZING ENCEPHALOMYOPATHY). There are at least four known genetically determined causes of Leigh disease: pyruvate dehydrogenase complex deficiency, complex I deficiency, complex IV (COX) deficiency, and complex V (ATPase) deficiency. These defects may occur sporadically or be inherited by autosomal recessive transmission, as in the case of COX deficiency; by X-linked transmission, as in the case of PDH $E_1\alpha$ deficiency; or by maternal transmission, as in complex V (ATPase 6 nt 8993 mutation) deficiency. Most cases become apparent during infancy with feeding and swallowing problems, vomiting, and failure to thrive. Delayed motor and language milestones may be evident, and generalized seizures, weakness, hypotonia, ataxia, tremor, pyramidal signs, and nystagmus are prominent findings. Intermittent respirations with associated sighing or sobbing are characteristic and suggest brainstem dysfunction. Some patients have external ophthalmoplegia, ptosis, optic atrophy, and decreased visual acuity. Abnormal results on CT or MRI scan consist of bilaterally symmetric areas of low attenuation in the basal ganglia. Pathologic changes consist of focal symmetric areas of necrosis in the thalamus, basal ganglia, tegmental gray matter, periventricular and periaqueductal regions of the brainstem, and posterior columns of the spinal cord. Microscopically, these spongiform lesions show cystic cavitation with neuronal loss, demyelination, and vascular proliferation. Elevations in serum lactate levels are characteristic. The overall outlook is poor, but a few patients experience prolonged periods of remission. There is no treatment for the underlying disorder.

REYE SYNDROME. This encephalopathy, which has become uncommon, is associated with pathologic features characterized by fatty degeneration of the viscera (microvesicular steatosis) and mitochondrial abnormalities and biochemical features consistent with a disturbance of mitochondrial metabolism (see Chapter 358). Sporadic Reye syndrome can occur in the context of varicella or influenza B virus infection and salicylate ingestion, in the idiosyncratic valproic acid hepatotoxicity reaction in individuals who may have an underlying genetic predisposition, and in Jamaican vomiting sickness (caused by the hypoglycin toxin).

Recurrent Reye-like syndrome is encountered in children with genetic defects of fatty acid oxidation, such as deficiencies of the plasmalemmal carnitine transporter, carnitine palmitoyltransferase I and II, carnitine acylcarnitine translocase, medium- and long-chain acyl-CoA dehydrogenase, multiple acyl-CoA dehydrogenase, and long-chain L-3 hydroxyacyl-CoA dehydrogenase or trifunctional protein. These disorders are manifested by recurrent hypoglycemic and hypoketotic encephalopathy, and they are inherited in an autosomal recessive pattern. Other potential inborn errors of metabolism presenting with Reye syndrome include urea cycle defects (ornithine transcarbamylase, carbamyl phosphate synthetase) and certain of the organic acidurias (glutaric aciduria type I), respiratory chain defects, and defects of carbohydrate metabolism (fructose intolerance).

598.3 • Other Encephalopathies

AIDS ENCEPHALOPATHY. Encephalopathy is an unfortunate and common manifestation in infants and children with HIV infection (see Chapter 273). Neurologic signs in congenitally infected patients may appear during early infancy or may be delayed to as late as 5 yr of age. The primary features of AIDS encephalopathy include an arrest in brain growth, evidence of developmental delay, and the evolution of neurologic signs including weakness with pyramidal tract signs, ataxia, myoclonus, pseudobulbar palsy, and seizures.

LEAD ENCEPHALOPATHY. See Chapter 709.

BURN ENCEPHALOPATHY. An encephalopathy develops in ≈5% of children with significant burns in the 1st several weeks of hospitalization (see also Chapter 74). There is no single cause of burn encephalopathy but rather a combination of factors that include anoxia (smoke inhalation, carbon monoxide poisoning, laryngospasm), electrolyte abnormalities, bacteremia and sepsis, cortical vein thrombosis, a concomitant head injury, cerebral edema, drug reactions, and emotional distress. Seizures are the most common clinical manifestation of burn encephalopathy, but altered states of consciousness, hallucinations, and coma may also occur. Management of burn encephalopathy is directed to a search for the underlying cause and treatment of hypoxemia, seizures, specific electrolyte abnormalities, or cerebral edema. The prognosis for complete neurologic recovery is generally excellent, particularly if seizures are the primary abnormality.

HYPERTENSIVE ENCEPHALOPATHY. Hypertensive encephalopathy is most commonly associated with renal disease in children, including acute glomerulonephritis, chronic pyelonephritis, and end-stage renal disease (see Chapters 445 and 535). In some cases, hypertensive encephalopathy is the initial manifestation of underlying renal disease. Marked systemic hypertension produces vasoconstriction of the cerebral vessels, which leads to vascular permeability, causing areas of focal cerebral edema and hemorrhage. The onset may be acute, with seizures and coma, or more indolent, with headache, drowsiness and lethargy, nausea and vomiting, blurred vision, transient cortical blindness, and hemiparesis. Examination of the eyegrounds may be nondiagnostic in children, but papilledema and retinal hemorrhages may occur. MRI often shows increased signal intensity in the occipital lobes on T2 weighted images, which is known as reversible posterior leukoencehalopathy and may be confused with cerebral infarctions. These high signal areas may appear in other regions of the brain as well. Treatment is directed at restoration of a normotensive state and control of seizures with appropriate anticonvulsants.

RADIATION ENCEPHALOPATHY. Although techniques for administering radiation therapy to the brain have improved considerably and the incidence of serious side effects has decreased significantly, radiation encephalopathy remains an important complication. Acute radiation encephalopathy is most likely to develop in young patients who have received large daily doses. Excessive radiation injures vessel endothelium, resulting in enhanced vascular permeability, cerebral edema, and numerous hemorrhages. The child may suddenly become irritable and lethargic, complain of headache, or present with focal neurologic signs and seizures. Patients occasionally develop hemiparesis due to an infarct secondary to vascular occlusion of the cerebral vessels. Steroids are often beneficial in reducing the cerebral edema and reversing the neurologic signs. Late radiation encephalopathy is characterized by headaches and slowly progressive focal neurologic signs, including hemiparesis and seizures. Some children with acute lymphatic leukemia treated with a combination of intrathecal methotrexate and cranial irradiation develop neurologic signs months or years later; signs consist of increasing lethargy, loss of cognitive abilities, dementia, and focal neurologic signs and seizures (see Chapter 494). The CT scan shows calcifications in the white matter, and the postmortem examination demonstrates a necrotizing encephalopathy. This devastating complication of the treatment of leukemia has prompted re-evaluation of the use of cranial radiation in the treatment of these children.

ZELLWEGER SYNDROME (CEREBROHEPATORENAL SYNDROME [CHRS]). This rare, lethal disorder is inherited as an autosomal recessive trait. It represents the prototype of a group of peroxisomal disorders that have overlapping symptoms, signs, and biochemical abnormalities (see Chapter 86.2). Infants with Zellweger syndrome have dysmorphic facies consisting of frontal bossing and a large anterior fontanel. The occiput is flattened and the external ears are abnormal. A high-arched palate, excessive skinfolds of the neck, severe hypotonia, and areflexia are usually evident. Examination of the eyes reveals searching nystagmoid movements, bilateral cataracts, and optic atrophy. Generalized seizures become evident early in life, associated with severe global developmental delay and a significant bilateral hearing loss. The cause of the severe neurologic abnormalities is related to an arrest of migrating neuroblasts during early development, resulting in cerebral pachygyria with neuronal heterotopia (see Chapter 592.7). Hepatomegaly is a prominent finding shortly after birth, often associated with a history of prolonged neonatal jaundice. Patients with Zellweger syndrome rarely survive beyond 1 yr of age.

Alberman E, Peckham C: Cerebral palsy and perinatal exposure to neurotropic viruses. *BMJ* 2006;332:63–64.

Bax M, Tydeman C, Flodmark O: Clinical and MRI correlates of cerebral palsy. The European cerebral palsy study. *JAMA* 2006;269:1602–1608.

Bottos M, Feliciangeli A, Sciuto LS, et al: Functional status of adults with cerebral palsy and implications for treating children. *Dev Med Child Neurol* 2001;431:516–528.

Brunstrom JE: Clinical considerations on cerebral palsy and spasticity. *J Child Neurol* 2001;16:10–15.

Brunstrom JE, Bastion AJ, Wong M, et al: Motor benefit from levodopa in spastic quadriplegic cerebral palsy. *Ann Neurol* 2000;47:662–665.

Butler C, Darrah J: Effects of neurodevelopmental treatment (NDT) for cerebral palsy: An AACPDM evidence report. *Dev Med Child Neurol* 2001;43:778–790.

Chong SK: Gastrointestinal problems in the handicapped child. *Curr Opin Pediatr* 2001;13:441–446.

Croen LA, Grether JK, Curry CJ: Congenital abnormalities among children with cerebral palsy: More evidence for prenatal antecedents. *J Pediatr* 2001;138:804–810.

Edgar TS: Clinical utility of botulinum toxin in the treatment of cerebral palsy: Comprehensive review. *J Child Neurol* 2001;16:37–46.

Fitzgerald JJ, Tsegaye M, Vloeberghs MH: Treatment of childhood spasticity of cerebral origin with intrathecal baclofen: A series of 52 cases. *Br J Neurosurg* 2004;18:240–245.

Golomb MR, MacGregor DL, Domi T, et al: Presumed pre- or perinatal arterial ischemic stroke: Risk factors and outcomes. *Ann Neurol* 2001;50:163–168.

Gordon AM, Charles J, Wolf SL: Efficacy of constraint-induced movement therapy on involved upper-extremity use in children with hemiplegic cerebral palsy is not age-dependent. *Pediatrics* 2006;117:363–373.

Hagberg H, Mallard C: Effect of inflammation on central nervous system development and vulnerability. *Curr Opin Neurol* 2005;18:117–123.

Hansel DE, Hansel CR, Shindle MK, et al: Oral baclofen in cerebral palsy: Possible seizure potentiation? *Pediatr Neurol* 2003;29:203–206.

Harum KH, Hoon AH, Kato GJ, et al: Homozygous factor-V mutation as a genetic cause of perinatal thrombosis and cerebral palsy. *Dev Med Child Neurol* 1999;41:777–780.

Hoon AH, Freese PO, Reinhardt EM, et al: Age-dependent effects of trihexyphenidyl in extrapyramidal cerebral palsy. *Pediatr Neurol* 2001;25:55–58.

Hoon AH, Lawrie WT, Melhem ER, et al: Diffusion tensor imaging of periventricular leukomalacia shows affected sensory cortex white matter pathways. *Neurology* 2002;59:752–756.

Hyland K: The lumbar puncture for diagnosis of pediatric neurotransmitter diseases. *Ann Neurol* 2003;54:S13–S17.

Inder TE, Wells SJ, Mogridge NB, et al: Defining the nature of the cerebral abnormalities in the premature infant: A qualitative magnetic resonance imaging study. *J Pediatr* 2003;143:171–179.

Jongerius PH, van den Hoogen JA, van Limbeek J, et al: Effect of botulism toxin in the treatment of drooling: A controlled clinical trial. *Pediatrics* 2004;114:620–627.

Kahana A, Rowley HA, Weinstein JM: Cortical blindness: Clinical and radiologic findings in reversible posterior leukoencephalopathy syndrome: Case report and review of the literature. *Ophthalmology* 2005;112:e7–e11.

Koman LA, Brashear A, Rosenfeld S, et al: Botulinum toxin type A neuromuscular blockade in the treatment of equinus foot deformity in cerebral palsy: A multicenter, open-label clinical trial. *Pediatrics* 2001;108: 1062–1070.

Koman LA, Smith BP, Shilt JS: Cerebral palsy. *Lancet* 2004;363:1619–1631.

Longo N: Mitochondrial encephalopathy. *Neurol Clin* 2003;21:817–831.

McLaughlin J, Bjornson KI, Temkin N, et al: Selective dorsal rhizotomy: Meta-analysis of three randomized controlled trials. *Dev Med Child Neurol* 2002;44:17–25.

Pavlakis SG, Phillips PC, Di Mauro S, et al: Mitochondrial myopathy, encephalopathy, lactic acidosis, and strokelike episodes: A distinctive clinical syndrome. *Ann Neurol* 1984;16:481–488.

Senner JE, Logemann J, Zecker S, et al: Drooling, saliva production, and swallowing in cerebral palsy. *Dev Med Child Neurol* 2004;46:801–806.

Shapiro SM: Definition of the clinical spectrum of kernicterus and bilirubin-induced neurologic dysfunction (BIND). *J Perinatology* 2005;25:54–59.

Sleigh G, Brocklehurst P: Gastrostomy feeding in cerebral palsy: A systematic review. *Arch Dis Child* 2004;89:534–539.

Ubhi T, Bhakta BB, Allgar V, et al: Randomised double blind placebo controlled trail of the effect of botulinum toxin on walking in cerebral palsy. *Arch Dis Child* 2000;83:481–487.

Woodward LJ, Anderson PJ, Austin NC, et al: Neonatal MRI to predict neurodevelopmental outcomes in preterm infants. *N Engl J Med* 2006;355: 685–694.

Chapter 599 ■ Neurodegenerative Disorders of Childhood

Michael V. Johnston

Neurodegenerative disorders of childhood encompass a large number of heterogeneous diseases that result from specific genetic and biochemical defects, chronic viral infections, and a significant group of conditions of unknown cause. Children with suspected neurodegenerative disorders were once subjected to brain and rectal (neural) biopsies, but with the advent of modern neuroimaging techniques and specific biochemical or molecular diagnostic tests, these invasive procedures are rarely necessary. The most important component of the investigation continues to be a thorough history and physical examination. The hallmark of a neurodegenerative disease is **progressive deterioration** of neurologic function with loss of speech, vision, hearing, or locomotion, often associated with seizures, feeding difficulties, and impair-

TABLE 599-1. Heredity and Biochemical Defects in the Neurodegenerative Disorders

NEURODEGENERATIVE DISORDER	MODE OF INHERITANCE	BIOCHEMICAL DEFECT	SPECIMEN FOR ANALYSIS
SPHINGOLIPIDOSIS			
GM_1 gangliosidosis	AR	β-Galactosidase	Serum, leukocytes, skin fibroblasts
GM_2 gangliosidosis			
Tay-Sachs disease	AR	Hexosaminidase A	Serum, leukocytes, skin fibroblasts
Sandhoff disease	AR	Hexosaminidase A and B	Serum, leukocytes, skin fibroblasts
Krabbe disease	AR	Galactocerebrosidase	Leukocytes and skin fibroblasts
Metachromatic leukodystrophy	AR	Arylsulfatase A	Leukocytes and skin fibroblasts
NEURONAL CEROID LIPOFUSCINOSES	AR	Pamitoyl-protein thioesterase (PPT) Tripeptidyl peptidasel 1 (TPP1)	EM of skin biopsy
ADRENOLEUKODYSTROPHY	XLR	VLCFA oxidation	Plasma, skin fibroblasts
SIALIDOSIS	AR	Neuraminidase	Skin fibroblasts

AR, autosomal recessive; EM, electron microscopy; VLCFA, very long chain fatty acid; XLR, X-linked recessive.

ment of intellect. The age of onset, rate of progression, and principal neurologic findings determine whether the disease affects primarily the white or the gray matter. Upper motor neuron signs are prominent early in the former; convulsions, intellectual, and visual impairment in the latter. A precise history confirms regression of developmental milestones, and the neurologic examination localizes the process within the nervous system. Although the outcome is usually fatal and current therapeutic attempts have been unsuccessful, it is important to make the correct diagnosis so that genetic counseling may be offered and prevention strategies can be implemented. Bone marrow transplantation and other forms of cell and gene therapies are also becoming useful for preventing the progression of disease in presymptomatic individuals. For all conditions in which the specific enzyme defect is known, prevention by prenatal diagnosis (chorionic villus sampling or amniocentesis) is possible. Carrier detection is also often possible by enzyme assay. Table 599-1 summarizes the heredity, biochemical defects, and specific diagnostic abnormality in the inherited neurodegenerative disorders. Additional age of onset-related categorization is noted in Table 599-2.

The inherited neurodegenerative disorders include the sphingolipidoses, neuronal ceroid lipofuscinoses, adrenoleukodystro-

TABLE 599-2. Select "Intrinsic" Conditions Associated with Developmental Regression

AGE AT ONSET (Yr)	CONDITIONS	COMMENTS
<2, with hepatomegaly	Fructose intolerance	Vomiting, hypoglycemia, poor feeding, failure to thrive (when given fructose)
	Galactosemia	Lethargy, hypotonia, icterus, cataract, hypoglycemia (when given lactose)
	Glycogenosis (glycogen storage disease) types I-IV	Hypoglycemia, cardiomegaly (type II)
	Mucopolysaccharidosis types I and II	Coarse facies, stiff joints
	Niemann-Pick disease, infantile type	Gray matter disease, failure to thrive
	Tay-Sachs disease	Seizures, cherry red macula, edema, coarse facies
	Zellweger (cerebrohepatorenal) syndrome	Hypotonia, high forehead, flat facies
	Gaucher disease type II	Extensor posturing, irritability
	Carbohydrate-deficient glycoprotein syndromes	Dysmyelination, cerebellar hypoplasia
<2, without hepatomegaly	Krabbe disease	Irritability, extensor posturing, optic atrophy and blindness
	Rett syndrome	Girls with deceleration of head growth, loss of hand skills, hand wringing, impaired language skills, gait apraxia
	Maple syrup urine disease	Poor feeding, tremors, myoclonus, opisthotonos
	Phenylketonuria	Light pigmentation, eczema, seizures
	Menkes kinky hair disease	Hypertonia, irritability, seizures, abnormal hair
	Subacute necrotizing encephalopathy of Leigh	White matter disease
	Cerebrooculofacioskeletal syndrome (of Pena and Shokeir)	Reduced white matter, failure to thrive
	Canavan disease	White matter disease
	Pelizaeus-Merzbacher disease	White matter disease
2–5	Niemann-Pick disease types III and IV	Hepatosplenomegaly, gait difficulty
	Wilson disease	Liver disease, Kayser-Fleischer ring; deterioration of cognition is late
	Gangliosidosis type II	Gray matter disease
	Ceroid lipofuscinosis	Gray matter disease
	Mitochondrial encephalopathies (e.g., myoclonic epilepsy with ragged red fibers [MERRF])	Gray matter disease
	Ataxia-telangiectasia	Basal ganglia disease
	Huntington disease (chorea)	Basal ganglia disease
	Hallervorden-Spatz syndrome	Basal ganglia disease
	Metachromatic leukodystrophy	White matter disease
	Adrenoleukodystrophy	White matter disease, behavior problems, deteriorating school performance, quadriparesis
5–15	Adrenoleukodystrophy	Same as for adrenoleukodystrophy in 2 to 5 yr olds
	Multiple sclerosis	White matter disease
	Neuronal ceroid lipofuscinosis, juvenile and adult (Spielmeyer-Vogt and Kufs disease)	Gray matter disease
	Schilder disease	White matter disease, focal neurologic symptoms
	Refsum disease	Peripheral neuropathy, ataxia, retinitis pigmentosa
	Sialidosis II, juvenile form	Cherry-red macula, myoclonus, ataxia, coarse facies
	Subacute sclerosing panencephalitis	Diffuse encephalopathy, myoclonus; may occur years after measles

From Kliegman RM, Greenbaum LA, Lye PS: *Practical Strategies in Pediatric Diagnosis and Therapy*, 2nd ed. Philadelphia, Elsevier/Saunders, 2004, p 542.

phy, and sialidosis. The sphingolipidoses are characterized by intracellular storage of a normal lipid component of the cell membrane that results from a defect in catabolism of the compound. The sphingolipidoses are subclassified into six categories: Niemann-Pick disease, Gaucher disease, GM_1 gangliosidosis, GM_2 gangliosidosis, Krabbe disease, and metachromatic leukodystrophy. Niemann-Pick disease and Gaucher disease are discussed in Chapter 86.4. The spinocerebellar degenerative diseases (Friedreich ataxia, ataxia-telangiectasia, olivopontocerebellar atrophy, and abetalipoproteinemia) and degenerative disorders of the basal ganglia (Huntington disease, dystonia musculorum deformans, Wilson disease, and Hallervorden-Spatz disease) are discussed in Chapter 597. A miscellaneous group of degenerative diseases is discussed in this chapter, including Pelizaeus-Merzbacher disease, Alexander disease, Canavan spongy degeneration, kinky hair disease, Rett syndrome, and subacute sclerosing panencephalitis.

599.1 • SPHINGOLIPIDOSES

GANGLIOSIDOSES (See Also Chapter 86.4)

Gangliosides are glycosphingolipids, normal constituents of the neuronal and synaptic membranes. The basic structure of GM_1 ganglioside consists of an oligosaccharide chain attached to a hydroxyl group of ceramide and sialic acid bound to galactose. The gangliosides are catabolized by sequential cleavage of the sugar molecules by specific exoglycosidases. Abnormalities in catabolism result in an accumulation of the ganglioside within the cell. Defects in ganglioside degradation can be classified into two groups: the GM_1 gangliosidoses and the GM_2 gangliosidoses.

GM_1 GANGLIOSIDOSES. The three subtypes of GM_1 gangliosidoses are classified according to age at presentation: infantile (type 1), juvenile (type 2), and adult (type 3). The condition is inherited as an autosomal recessive trait and results from a marked deficiency of acid β-galactosidase. This enzyme may be assayed in leukocytes and cultured fibroblasts. The acid β-galactosidase gene has been mapped to chromosome 3p14.2. Prenatal diagnosis is possible by measurement of acid β-galactosidase in cultured amniotic cells.

Infantile GM_1 gangliosidosis presents at birth or during the neonatal period with anorexia, poor sucking, and inadequate weight gain. Development is globally retarded, and generalized seizures are prominent. The phenotype is striking and shares many characteristics with Hurler syndrome. The facial features are coarse, the forehead is prominent, the nasal bridge is depressed, the tongue is large (macroglossia), and the gums are hypertrophied. Hepatosplenomegaly is present early in the course as a result of accumulation of foamy histiocytes, and kyphoscoliosis is evident because of anterior beaking of the vertebral bodies. The neurologic examination is dominated by apathy, progressive blindness, deafness, spastic quadriplegia, and decerebrate rigidity. A cherry red spot in the macular region is visualized in ≈50% of cases. The **cherry red spot** is characterized by an opaque ring (sphingolipid-laden retinal ganglion cells) encircling the normal red fovea (Fig. 599-1). Children rarely survive beyond age 2–3 yr, and death is due to aspiration pneumonia.

Juvenile GM_1 gangliosidosis has a delayed onset beginning about 1 yr of age. The initial symptoms consist of incoordination, weakness, ataxia, and regression of language. Thereafter, convulsions, spasticity, decerebrate rigidity, and blindness are the major findings. Unlike the infantile type, this type is not usually marked by coarse facial features and hepatosplenomegaly. Radiographic examination of the lumbar vertebrae may show minor beaking. Children rarely survive beyond 10 yr of age. ***Adult GM_1 gangliosidosis*** is a slowly progressive disease consisting of spasticity, ataxia, dysarthria, and a gradual loss of cognitive function.

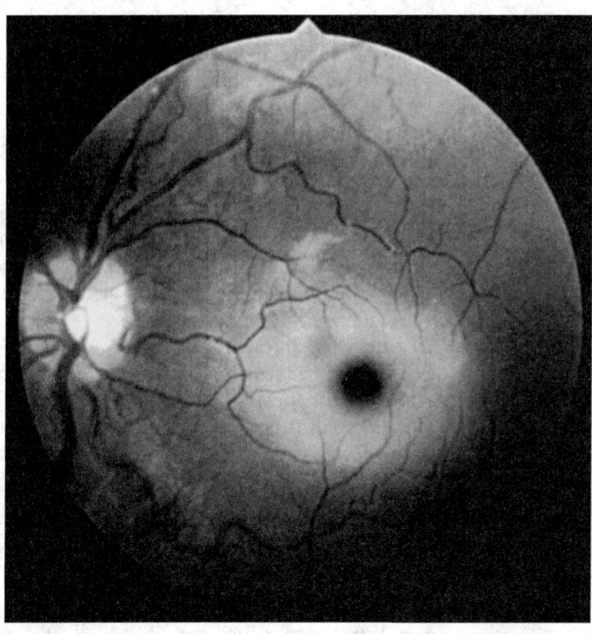

Figure 599-1. A cherry red spot in a patient with GM_1 gangliosidosis. Note the whitish ring of sphingolipid-laden ganglion cells surrounding the fovea.

GM_2 GANGLIOSIDOSES. The GM_2 gangliosidoses are a heterogeneous group of autosomal recessive inherited disorders that consist of several subtypes, including Tay-Sachs disease (TSD), Sandhoff disease, juvenile GM_2 gangliosidosis, and adult GM_2 gangliosidosis. **Tay-Sachs disease** is most prevalent in the Ashkenazi Jewish population and has a carrier rate of ≈1/30. TSD is due to mutations in the *HEXA* gene located on chromosome 15q23–q24. Affected infants appear normal until ≈6 mo of age, except for a marked startle reaction to noise that is evident soon after birth. Affected children then begin to lag in developmental milestones and, by 1 yr of age, they lose the ability to stand, sit, and vocalize. Early hypotonia develops into progressive spasticity, and relentless deterioration follows, with convulsions, blindness, deafness, and cherry red spots in almost all patients (see Fig. 599-1). Macrocephaly becomes apparent by 1 yr of age and results from the 200- to 300-fold normal content of GM_2 ganglioside deposited in the brain. Few children live beyond 3–4 yr of age, and death is usually associated with aspiration or bronchopneumonia. A deficiency of the isoenzyme hexosaminidase A is found in tissues of patients with TSD. Mass screening for prenatal diagnosis of TSD is a reliable and cost-effective method of prevention because the condition occurs in a defined population (Ashkenazi Jews). An accurate and inexpensive carrier detection test is available (serum or leukocyte hexosaminidase A), and the disease can be reliably diagnosed by chorionic villus sampling in the 1st trimester of pregnancy in couples at risk (heterozygote parents).

Sandhoff disease is very similar to TSD in the mode of presentation, including progressive loss of motor and language milestones beginning at 6 mo of age. Seizures, cherry red spots, macrocephaly, and doll-like facies are present in most patients; however, children with Sandhoff disease may also have splenomegaly. The visual-evoked potentials (VEPs) are normal early in the course of Sandhoff disease and TSD but become abnormal or absent as the disease progresses. The auditory brainstem responses (ABRs) show prolonged latencies. The diagnosis of Sandhoff disease is established by finding deficient levels of hexosaminidase A and B in serum and leukocytes. Children usually die by 3 yr of age. Sandhoff disease is due to mutations in the HEXB gene located on chromosome 5q13.

Juvenile GM$_2$ gangliosidosis develops in mid-childhood, initially with clumsiness followed by ataxia. Signs of spasticity, athetosis, loss of language, and seizures gradually develop. Progressive visual loss is associated with optic atrophy, but cherry red spots rarely occur in juvenile GM$_2$ gangliosidosis. A deficiency of hexosaminidase is variable (total deficiency to near normal) in these patients. Death occurs around 15 yr of age.

Adult GM$_2$ gangliosidosis is characterized by a myriad neurologic signs, including slowly progressive gait ataxia, spasticity, dystonia, proximal muscle atrophy, and dysarthria. Generally, visual acuity and intellectual function are unimpaired. Hexosaminidase A or A and B activity is reduced significantly in the serum and leukocytes.

KRABBE DISEASE (GLOBOID CELL LEUKODYSTROPHY). Krabbe disease (KD) is a rare autosomal recessive neurodegenerative disorder characterized by severe myelin loss and the presence of globoid bodies in the white matter. The gene for KD (*GALC*) is located on chromosome 14q24.3–q32.1. The disease results from a marked deficiency of the lysosomal enzyme galactocerebroside β-galactosidase, which cleaves a galactose moiety from the ceramide portion of galactocerebroside. KD is a disorder of myelin destruction rather than abnormal myelin formation. Normally, myelination begins in the 3rd trimester, corresponding with a rapid increase of galactocerebroside β-galactosidase activity in the brain. In patients with KD, galactocerebroside cannot be metabolized during the normal turnover of myelin because of deficiency of galactocerebroside β-galactosidase. When galactocerebroside is injected into the brains of experimental animals, a globoid cell reaction ensues. It has been postulated that a similar phenomenon occurs in humans; nonmetabolized galactocerebroside stimulates the formation of globoid cells that reflect the destruction of oligodendroglial cells. Because oligodendroglial cells are responsible for the elaboration of myelin, their loss results in myelin breakdown, thus producing additional galactocerebroside and causing a vicious circle of myelin destruction.

The symptoms of KD become evident in the 1st few months of life and include excessive irritability and crying, unexplained episodes of hyperpyrexia, feeding problems, vomiting, and failure to thrive. In the initial stage of KD, children are often treated for colic or "milk allergy" with frequent formula changes. Generalized seizures may appear early in the course of the disease. Alterations in body tone with rigidity and opisthotonos and visual inattentiveness due to optic atrophy become apparent as the disease progresses. In the later stages of the illness, blindness, deafness, absent deep tendon reflexes, and decerebrate rigidity constitute the major physical findings. A nonenhanced CT scan of the head may show symmetric increased densities in the caudate nuclei and thalami. Most patients die by 2 yr of age. MRI and magnetic resonance spectroscopy are useful for evaluating the extent of demyelination in Krabbe disease. Umbilical cord blood (stem cell) transplantation from unrelated donors in asymptomatic babies may favorably alter the natural history.

Late-onset KD has been described beginning in childhood or adolescence. Patients present with optic atrophy and cortical blindness, and their condition is often confused with the adrenoleukodystrophies. Slowly progressive gait disturbances, including spasticity and ataxia, are prominent. As with classic KD, globoid cells are abundant in the white matter, and leukocytes are deficient in galactocerebroside β-galactosidase. An examination of the cerebrospinal fluid (CSF) shows an elevated protein content, and the nerve conduction velocities are markedly delayed due to segmental demyelination of the peripheral nerves. The VEPs decrease gradually in amplitude with no response in the late stages of the disease, and the ABRs are characterized by the presence of only waves I and II. CT scans and MRI studies highlight the marked decrease in white matter, especially of the cerebellum and centrum semiovale, with sparing of the subcortical U fibers. Prenatal diagnosis is possible by the assay of galactocerebroside β-galactosidase activity in chorionic villi or in cultured amniotic fluid cells.

METACHROMATIC LEUKODYSTROPHY (MLD). This disorder of myelin metabolism is inherited as an autosomal recessive trait and is characterized by a deficiency of arylsulfatase A activity. Several mutations in the gene encoding for arylsulfatase A have been identified. The gene is located on chromosome 22q13–13qter, and DNA diagnosis is possible. The absence or deficiency of arylsulfatase A leads to accumulation of cerebroside sulfate within the myelin sheath of the central nervous system (CNS) and peripheral nervous system due to the inability to cleave sulfate from galactosyl-3-sulfate ceramide. The excessive cerebroside sulfate is thought to cause myelin breakdown and destruction of oligodendroglia. Prenatal diagnosis of MLD is made by assay of arylsulfatase A in chorionic villi or cultured amniotic fluid cells. Cresyl violet applied to tissue specimens produces metachromatic staining of the sulfatide granules, giving the disease its name. Six disorders are included in the MLD group of diseases, classified by the age at onset and enzyme deficiency. Three conditions are briefly discussed: the classic or late infantile, juvenile, and adult leukodystrophies.

Late infantile MLD begins with insidious onset of gait disturbances between 1 and 2 yr of age. The child initially appears awkward and frequently falls, but locomotion is gradually impaired significantly and support is required in order to walk. The extremities are hypotonic, and the deep tendon reflexes are absent or diminished. Within the next several months, the child can no longer stand, and deterioration in intellectual function becomes apparent. The speech is slurred and dysarthric, and the child appears dull and apathetic. Visual fixation is diminished, nystagmus is present, and examination of the retina shows optic atrophy. Within 1 yr from the onset of the disease, the child is unable to sit unsupported, and progressive decorticate postures develop. Feeding and swallowing are impaired due to pseudobulbar palsies, and a feeding gastrostomy is required. Patients ultimately become stuporous and die of aspiration or bronchopneumonia by age 5–6 yr. Neurophysiologic evaluation shows progressive changes in the VEPs, ABRs, and somatosensory-evoked potentials (SSEPs), and the nerve conduction velocities (NCVs) of the peripheral nerves are significantly reduced. CT and MRI images of the brain indicate diffuse symmetric attenuation of the cerebellar and cerebral white matter, and examination of the CSF shows an elevated protein content. Bone marrow transplantation is a promising experimental therapy for the management of late infantile MLD. Favorable outcomes have been reported only in patients treated very early in the course of the disease. The total number of patients treated is relatively small and the follow-up too short to draw conclusions about the efficacy of bone marrow transplantation.

Juvenile MLD has many features in common with late infantile MLD, but the onset of symptoms is delayed to 5–10 yr of age. Deterioration in school performance and alterations in personality may herald the onset of the disease. This is followed by incoordination of gait, urinary incontinence, and dysarthria. Muscle tone becomes increased, and ataxia, dystonia, or tremor may be present. In the terminal stages, generalized tonic-clonic convulsions are prominent and are difficult to control. Patients rarely live beyond mid-adolescence.

Adult MLD occurs from the 2nd to 6th decade. Abnormalities in memory, psychiatric disturbances, and personality changes are prominent features. Slowly progressive neurologic signs, including spasticity, dystonia, optic atrophy, and generalized convulsions, lead eventually to a bedridden state characterized by decorticate postures and unresponsiveness.

599.2 • Neuronal Ceroid Lipofuscinoses

Neuronal ceroid lipofuscinoses constitute the most common class of neurodegenerative diseases in children and consist of three disorders inherited as autosomal recessive traits. They are autosomal recessive disorders characterized by the storage of an autofluorescent substance within lysosomes of neurons and other tissues. Individual genes mutated in six forms have been identified.

Infantile type (Haltia-Santavuori) begins near the end of the 1st yr of life with myoclonic seizures, intellectual deterioration, and blindness. Optic atrophy and brownish discoloration of the macula are evident on examination of the retina, and cerebellar ataxia is prominent. The electroretinogram (ERG) typically shows small-amplitude or absent waveforms. Death occurs at ≈10 yr of age. The gene defect causing the infantile form has been assigned to chromosome 1p32. Mutations have been identified in the *CLN1* gene, which codes for the lysosomal enzyme palmitoyl-protein thioesterase-1 (PPT).

Late infantile type (Jansky-Bielschowsky) is the most common type of neuronal ceroid lipofuscinosis. The presenting manifestation is myoclonic seizures beginning between 2 and 4 yr of age in a previously normal child. Dementia and ataxia are combined with a progressive loss of visual acuity and microcephaly. Examination of the retina shows marked attenuation of vessels, peripheral black "bone spicule" pigmentary abnormalities, optic atrophy, and a subtle brown pigment in the macular region. The ERG is abnormal early in the course as a result of deposition of the abnormal storage substance within the rod and cone area of the retina. VEPs are characteristic and consist of markedly enlarged responses followed by absent waveforms with progression of the disease. The autofluorescent material is deposited in neurons, fibroblasts, and secretory cells. Electron microscopic examination of the storage material in skin or conjunctival biopsy material typically shows curvilinear bodies or "fingerprint profiles." Mutations have been identified in the *CLN2* gene, which codes for a tripeptidyl peptidase-1 that is essential for the degradation of chlocystokinin-8, as well as in the *CLN5, CLN6,* and *CLN8* genes that code for integral membrane proteins that have not been completely characterized.

Juvenile type (Spielmeyer-Vogt) is characterized by progressive visual loss and intellectual impairment beginning between 5 and 10 yr of age. The funduscopic changes are similar to those for the late infantile type. The ERG is also abnormal early in the course of the disease, but in the juvenile type, the VEPs are typically characterized by small-amplitude waves and, later, absence of waveforms as the disease progresses. Myoclonic seizures are not as prominent as in the late infantile type of neuronal ceroid lipofuscinosis, but dystonic posturing is marked in the late stages of the disease. Elevated urine dolichol levels are a nonspecific finding. Ultrastructural abnormalities of skin biopsy samples are present in most cases. Mutations in *CLN2* and *CLN3* genes have been identified in juvenile forms.

599.3 • Adrenoleukodystrophy (See Also Chapter 86.2)

The adrenoleukodystrophies consist of a group of CNS degenerative disorders that are often associated with adrenal cortical insufficiency and are inherited by X-linked recessive transmission. *Classic adrenoleukodystrophy* (ALD) is considered to be the most common leukodystrophy, and becomes symptomatic between 5 and 15 yr of age with evidence of academic deterioration, behavioral disturbances, and gait abnormalities. ALD is caused by accumulation of very long chain fatty acids in neural tissue and adrenals due to mutations in the *ABCD1* gene coding for the adrenoleukodystrophy protein, an adenosine triphosphate (ATP)–binding cassette half transporter on Xq28. The relationship between ALD and the metabolism of very long chain fatty acids is not understood.

The incidence of ALD approximates 1/20,000 boys. In 40% of male hemizygotes, the disease presents in its classic form as an inflammatory demyelinating disease. Generalized seizures are common in the early stages. Upper motor neuron signs include spastic quadriparesis and contractures, ataxia, and marked swallowing disturbances secondary to pseudobulbar palsy. These dominate the terminal stages of the illness. Hypoadrenalism is present in ≈50% of cases, and adrenal insufficiency characterized by abnormal skin pigmentation (tanning without exposure to sun) may precede the onset of neurologic symptoms. CT scans and MRI studies of patients indicate periventricular demyelination beginning posteriorly; this advances progressively to the anterior regions of the cerebral white matter. ABRs, VEPs, and SSEPs may be normal initially but ultimately show prolonged latencies and abnormal waveforms. Death supervenes within 10 yr of the onset of the neurologic signs; however, long-term follow-up has shown that bone marrow transplant can prevent the progression of the disease when done at an early stage before clinical signs develop. In addition, administration of Lorenzo's oil, a 4 : 1 mixture of glyceryl trioleate and glyceryl trierucate, to neurologically abnormal boys <6 yr of age with a normal MRI of the brain may reduce the probability of developing neurological abnormalities later in life.

Adrenomyeloneuropathy occurs in another 40% of boys with X-linked adrenoleukodystrophy and presents as a more chronic disorder of the spinal cord and peripheral nerves. It begins with a slowly progressive spastic paraparesis, urinary incontinence, and onset of impotence during the 3rd or 4th decade, even though adrenal insufficiency may have been present since childhood. Cases of typical ALD have occurred in families in whom the propositus presented with adrenomyeloneuropathy. One of the most difficult problems in the management of X-linked ALD is the common observation that affected individuals in the same family may have quite different clinical courses. For example, in one family, one affected boy had severe classic ALD culminating in death by age 10 yr; another affected male (a brother) had late-onset adrenomyeloneuropathy, and a third had no symptoms at all. A panel of brain neuroimaging studies, which can provide quantitative information about the progression of adrenoleukodystrophies, aids the selection of patients for bone marrow therapy, and has improved counseling for these disorders.

Neonatal ALD is characterized by marked hypotonia, severe psychomotor retardation, and early onset of seizures. It is inherited as an autosomal recessive condition. Visual inattention is secondary to optic atrophy. Results of adrenal function tests are normal, but adrenal atrophy is evident postmortem. Correction of adrenal insufficiency is ineffective in halting neurologic deterioration.

In addition to the so-called classic leukodystrophies, new disorders have recently been recognized due to the broader use of MRI. ***Vanishing white matter disease*** or ***childhood ataxia and CNS hypomelination*** is a severe demyelinating disorder caused by mutations in *eIF* genes involved in GDP/GTP exchange. Interestingly, acute demyelination in these disorders can be triggered by fever or fright. A genetic disorder with megalencephaly, extensive white matter changes with temporal cysts, and mild to moderate cognitive decline and spasticity has been recognized in the Ararwal ethnic group from India and has been linked to mutations in the *MLC* gene.

599.4 • Sialidosis

Sialidosis is inherited as an autosomal recessive trait and results from accumulation of a sialic acid–oligosaccharide complex secondary to a deficiency in the lysosomal enzyme neuraminidase. The lysosomal sialidase gene has been mapped to chromosome 6p21.3. Urinary excretion of sialic acid–containing oligosaccharides is increased significantly in affected patients.

Sialidosis type I, the **cherry red spot myoclonus syndrome** (CRSM), usually presents in the 2nd decade of life, when a patient complains of visual deterioration. Inspection of the retina shows a cherry red spot, but, unlike patients with TSD, visual acuity declines slowly in individuals with CRSM. Myoclonus of the extremities is gradually progressive and often debilitating and eventually renders patients nonambulatory. The myoclonus is triggered by voluntary movement, touch, and sound and is not controlled with anticonvulsants. Generalized convulsions responsive to antiepileptic drugs occur in most patients.

Sialidosis type II may be subdivided into infantile and juvenile forms, depending on the age at presentation. In addition to cherry red spots and myoclonus, these patients have somatic involvement, including coarse facial features, corneal clouding (rarely), and dysostosis multiplex, producing anterior beaking of the lumbar vertebrae. Examination of lymphocytes shows vacuoles in the cytoplasm, biopsy of the liver demonstrates cytoplasmic vacuoles in Kupffer cells, and membrane-bound vacuoles are found in Schwann cell cytoplasm, all attesting to the multiorgan nature of sialidosis type II. No distinctive neuroimaging findings or abnormalities in electrophysiologic studies are noted in this group of disorders. Patients with sialidosis have been reported to live beyond the 5th decade.

Some cases of what appears to be sialidosis type II are the result of combined deficiencies of β-galactosidase and α-neuraminidase due to deficiency of a "protective protein" that prevents premature intracellular degradation of the two enzymes. Clinically, affected patients are indistinguishable from those with sialidosis type II, either the infantile or juvenile form, caused by isolated α-neuraminidase deficiency. The diagnosis may be missed if β-galactosidase testing is done and testing of α-neuraminidase activity in fibroblasts is not completed.

599.5 • Miscellaneous Disorders

PELIZAEUS-MERZBACHER DISEASE. This disease consists of a group of disorders that are characterized by nystagmus and abnormalities of myelin. The classic form is inherited as an X-linked recessive trait caused by abnormalities in the proteolipid protein (PLP) gene, which is essential for CNS myelin formation and oligodendrocyte differentiation. Mutations in the same gene can cause familial spastic paraparesis. It is recognized by nystagmus and roving eye movements with head nodding during infancy. The gene is located on chromosome Xq22. Molecular diagnosis of Pelizaeus-Merzbacher disease is possible using mutation analysis. As with most X-linked diseases, the molecular diagnosis of Pelizaeus-Merzbacher disease is complex because exonic mutations are present in only 10–25% of patients with the disease. A child's developmental milestones are delayed, and ataxia, choreoathetosis, and spasticity ultimately develop. Optic atrophy and dysarthria are associated findings, and death occurs in the 2nd or 3rd decade. The major pathologic finding is a loss of myelin with intact axons, suggesting a defect in the function of oligodendroglia. Studies point to a genetic defect in the biosynthesis of proteolipid apoprotein, a protein that is concerned with the differentiation and maintenance of oligodendrocytes. An MRI scan shows a symmetric pattern of delayed myelination. Multimodal-evoked potential studies demonstrate early in the course a pattern consisting of loss of waves III–V on the ABR. This finding is useful in the investigation of nystagmus in infant boys. VEPs show prolonged latencies, and SSEPs show absent cortical responses or delayed latencies. It is now recognized that a broad spectrum of phenotypes, including progressive spastic paraplegia type 2 and peripheral nerve abnormalities, can also result from mutations in the PLP gene.

ALEXANDER DISEASE. This is a rare disorder that occurs sporadically and causes progressive macrocephaly in the 1st year of life. It is caused by mutations in the glial fibrillary acidic protein (GFAP) gene. Pathologic examination of the brain discloses deposition of eosinophilic hyaline bodies in a perivascular distribution throughout the brain and beneath the pia mater. Degeneration of white matter is most prominent in the frontal lobes, and a CT scan at this stage shows corresponding attenuation of the cerebral white matter. Affected children develop progressive loss of intellect, spasticity, and unresponsive seizures causing death by 5 yr of age.

CANAVAN SPONGY DEGENERATION. See Chapter 85.14.

MENKES DISEASE. Menkes disease (kinky hair disease) is a progressive neurodegenerative condition inherited as a sex-linked recessive trait. The Menkes gene codes for a copper transporting P-type ATPase, and mutations in the protein are associated with low serum copper and ceruloplasmin levels as well as a defect in copper absorption and transport across the intestines. Symptoms begin in the 1st few months of life and include hypothermia, hypotonia, and generalized myoclonic seizures. The facies are distinctive, with chubby, rosy cheeks and kinky, colorless, friable hair. Microscopic examination of the hair shows several abnormalities, including trichorrhexis nodosa (fractures along the hair shaft) and pili torti (twisted hair). Feeding difficulties are prominent and lead to failure to thrive. Severe mental retardation and optic atrophy are constant features of the disease. Neuropathologic changes include tortuous degeneration of the gray matter and marked changes in the cerebellum with loss of the internal granule cell layer and necrosis of the Purkinje cells. Death occurs by 3 yr of age in untreated patients.

Copper-histidine therapy may be effective in preventing neurologic deterioration in some patients with Menkes disease, particularly when treatment is begun in the neonatal period or, preferably, with the fetus. Copper is essential in the early stages of CNS development, and its absence probably accounts for the neuropathologic changes. Copper-histidine is given subcutaneously in a dose of 50–150 µg elemental copper/kg/24 hr for the duration of the child's life. The serum copper and ceruloplasmin levels return to the normal range within 2–3 wk of commencing therapy.

The **occipital horn syndrome,** a skeletal dysplasia caused by different mutations in the same gene as that involved in Menkes disease, is a relatively mild disease. The two diseases are often confused, because the biochemical abnormalities are identical. Resolution of the uncertainty about treatment of patients with Menkes disease will require careful genotype-phenotype correlation, along with further clinical trials of copper therapy.

RETT SYNDROME (RS). This syndrome is not strictly speaking a degenerative disease, but a disorder of early brain development. Early in infancy there is developmental regression and deceleration of brain growth over the 1st yr of life after a relatively normal neonatal course. It occurs predominantly in girls. The frequency is ≈1/15,000–1/22,000. RS is caused by mutations in *MeCP2*, a transcription factor that binds to methylated CpG islands and silences transcription. Development may proceed normally until 1 yr of age, when regression of language and motor milestones and acquired microcephaly become apparent. An ataxic gait or fine tremor of hand movements is an early neurologic finding. Most children develop peculiar sighing respirations with intermittent periods of apnea that may be associated with cyanosis. The hallmark of Rett syndrome is repetitive hand-wringing movements and a loss of purposeful and spontaneous use of the hands; these features may not appear until 2–3 yr of age. Autistic behavior is a typical finding in all patients. Generalized tonic-clonic convulsions occur in the majority and are usually well controlled by anticonvulsants. Feeding disorders and poor weight gain are common. After the initial period of neurologic regression, the disease process appears to plateau, with persistence of the autistic behavior. Death occurs in adolescence or in the 3rd decade. Cardiac arrhythmias may result in sudden, unexpected death.

Postmortem studies show significantly reduced brain weight (60–80% of normal) with a decrease in the number of synapses, associated with a decrease in dendritic length and branching. The phenotype may be related to failure to suppress expression of genes that are normally silent in the early phases of postnatal development. Although very few males survive with the classic RS phenotype, genotyping of boys without the classic RS phenotype but with mental retardation and other atypical neurologic features has detected a significant number with mutations in *MeCP2*. Mutations in *MeCP2* have been demonstrated in normal female carriers, females with Angelman syndrome, and in males with fatal encephalopathy, Klinefelter (47,XXY) syndrome, and familial X-linked mental retardation.

SUBACUTE SCLEROSING PANENCEPHALITIS. This is a rare, progressive, slow-virus infection of the CNS caused by a measles-like virus (see Chapter 243.1). The number of reported cases has decreased dramatically to 0.06 cases/million population, paralleling the decline in reported measles cases. The initial clinical manifestations include personality changes, aggressive behavior, and impaired cognitive function. Myoclonic seizures soon dominate the clinical picture. Later, generalized tonic-clonic convulsions, hypertonia, and choreoathetosis become evident, followed by progressive bulbar palsy, hyperthermia, and decerebrate postures. Funduscopic examination early in the course of the disease reveals papilledema in ≈20% of the cases. Optic atrophy, chorioretinitis, and macular pigmentation are observed in most patients. The diagnosis is established by the typical clinical course and one of the following: (1) measles antibody detected in the CSF, (2) a characteristic electroencephalogram consisting of bursts of high-voltage slow waves interspersed with a normal background in the early stages, and (3) typical histologic findings in the brain biopsy or postmortem specimen. Treatment with a series of antiviral agents has been attempted without success. Death occurs usually within 1–2 yr from the onset of symptoms.

Aoki Y, Haginoya K, Munakata M, et al: A novel mutation in glial fibrillary acidic protein gene in a patient with Alexander disease. *Neurosci Lett* 2001;312:71–74.

Baram TZ, Goldman AM, Percy AK: Krabbe disease: Specific MRI and CT findings. *Neurology* 1986;36:111–115.

Berger J, Moser HW, Forss-Petter S: Leukodystrophies: Recent developments in genetics, molecular biology, pathogenesis and treatment. *Curr Opin Neurol* 2001;14:305–312.

Cooper JD: Progress towards understanding the neurobiology of Batten disease or neuronal ceroid lipofuscinosis. *Curr Opin Neurol* 2003;16:121–128.

Couvert P, Bienvenu T, Aquaviva C: *MeCP2* is highly mutated in X-linked mental retardation. *Hum Mol Genet* 2001;10:941–946.

Dyken PR, Cunningham SC, Ward LC: Changing character of subacute sclerosing panencephalitis in the United States. *Pediatr Neurol* 1989;5:339–341.

Escolar ML, Poe MD, Provenzale JM, et al: Transplantation of umbilical-cord blood in babies with infantile Krabbe's disease. *N Engl J Med* 2005;352:2069–2080.

Gao H, Boustany RM, Espinola JA, et al: Mutations in a novel CLN6-encoded transmembrane protein cause variant neuronal ceroid lipofuscinosis in man and mouse. *Am J Hum Genet* 2002;70:324–335.

Gorospe JR, Singhal BS, Kainu T, et al: Indian Agarwal megalencephalic leukodystrophy with cysts is caused by a common *MLC1* mutation. *Neurology* 2004;62:878–882.

Hudson LD: Pelizaeus-Merzbacher disease and spastic paraplegia type 2: Two faces of myelin loss from mutations in the same gene. *J Child Neurol* 2003;18:616–624.

Julu PO, Kerr AM, Apartopoulos F, et al: Characterisation of breathing and associated central autonomic dysfunction in Rett disorder. *Arch Dis Child* 2001;85:29–37.

Kaye EM: Update on genetic disorders affecting white matter. *Pediatr Neurol* 2001;24:11–24.

Krivit W: Stem cell bone marrow transplantation in patients with metabolic storage disease. *Adv Pediat* 2002;49:359–378.

Moser HW, Dubey P, Fatemi A: Progress in X-linked adrenoleukodystrophy. *Curr Opin Neurol* 2004;17:263–269.

Percy AK, Lane JB: Rett syndrome: Clinical and molecular update. *Curr Opin Neurol* 2004;16:670–677.

Pshezhetsky AV, Richard C, Michaud L, et al: Cloning, expression and chromosomal mapping of human lysosomal sialidase and characterization of mutations in sialidoses. *Nat Genet* 1997;15:316–320.

Shapiro E, Krivit W, Lockman L, et al: Long-term effect of bone-marrow transplantation for childhood-onset cerebral X-linked adrenoleukodystrophy. *Lancet* 2000;356:713–718.

Schiffmann R, Brady RO: New prospects for the treatment of lysosomal storage diseases. *Drugs* 2002;62:733–742.

Schiffmann R, van der Knaap MS: The latest on leukodystrophies. *Curr Opin Neurol* 2004;17:187–192.

Staba SL, Escolar ML, Poe M, et al: Cord-blood transplants from unrelented donors in patients with Hurler's syndrome. *N Engl J Med* 2004;350:1960–1968.

Suzuki K: Globoid cell leukodystrophy (Krabbe's disease): An update. *J Child Neurol* 2003;18:595–603.

Wisniewski KE, Kida E, Golabek AA, et al: Neuronal lipofuscinosis: Classification and diagnosis. *Adv Genet* 2001;45:1–34.

Vermeulen G, Seidl R, Mercimek-Mahmutoglu S, et al: Fright is a provoking factor in vanishing white matter disease. *Ann Neurol* 2005;57:560–563.

Chapter 600 ■ Demyelinating Disorders of the CNS

Michael V. Johnston

Demyelinating disorders of the central nervous system (CNS) cause acute or remitting-relapsing encephalopathy and other multifocal signs of brain, brainstem, and spinal cord dysfunction. They affect white matter, which is formed by myelin contained within oligodendrocytes, providing electrical insulation for neurons and neuronal connections. In contrast to genetically determined leukodystrophies that also disrupt white matter, demyelinating disorders generally target normally formed white matter through immune-mediated mechanisms. Major demyelinating disorders in childhood include multiple sclerosis (MS) and acute disseminated encephalomyelitis (ADEM). The rare macrophage activating syndromes and isolated angiitis of the CNS can sometimes be confused with ADEM.

600.1 • Multiple Sclerosis (MS)

MS is a chronic and generally remitting-relapsing disorder characterized by multiple white lesions in the CNS separated by time and location in the brain. The condition is rare in the pediatric population; 5% of all cases of MS occur before age 18 yr. The cause of MS is unknown, but interactive genetic, immunologic, and infectious factors are probably responsible. A family history of MS in a first-degree relative is present in ≈20%. The most frequent presenting signs are unilateral weakness with upper motor neuron signs, sensory abnormalities, visual complaints, or ataxia. Paresthesias involving the lower extremities, distal portions of the hands and feet, and the face are common. Visual symptoms including diplopia, nystagmus, or sudden visual loss due to optic neuritis are also important early manifestations of MS. Headache, fatigue, dysarthria, or myelopathy with a sensory level and neurogenic bladder can also be present, but impaired consciousness and encephalopathy are uncommon. **Neuromyelitis optica** (Devic disease) is a variant of classic MS and consists of *optic neuritis* and *transverse myelitis,* which occur conjointly. Although a 1st attack of MS may be suspected after an initial episode, the diagnosis is not made until a 2nd clinical episode occurs after a period of a month or a new white lesion appears on magnetic resonance imaging (MRI) after 3 mo.

The pathology of MS consists of demyelination with the formation of plaques. No reliable laboratory test unequivocally confirms the diagnosis of MS, except for a biopsy or an autopsy. MRI is the neuroimaging technique of choice; small plaques of 3–4 mm can be identified, particularly those located in the brainstem and spinal cord (Fig. 600-1). A high percentage of pediatric patients have T2 enhancing lesions in the corpus callosum and periventricular white matter. The cerebrospinal fluid (CSF) often contains oligoclonal bands.

The **treatment** of an acute attack of MS often includes high-dose intravenous methylprednisolone, which can expedite recovery but has not been shown to alter the long-term course of the disease. Optic neuritis may be the 1st manifestation of MS. Aggressive therapy of optic neuritis with prednisone does decrease the long-term risk of MS. Rehabilitative care is useful; particular attention is given to the management of a neurogenic bladder if the spinal cord is affected. Disease-modifying interferon therapies can decrease disease activity (fewer new lesions, fever, relapses) and disease burden, as shown by serial gadolinium-enhanced lesions in brain MRI scan. These therapies may also be useful in children with MS and may be more effective if started early in the course of the disease. Interferon-β is the most widely used disease-modifying agent. Glatiramer acetate, a polypeptide mimicker of myelin basic protein; fingolimod, an oral sphingosine-l-phosphate receptor modulator; and natalizumab, a monoclonal antibody against the cell surface adhesion molecule α4β1 integrin, interfere with the pathologic immune-mediated inflammation and have also been successful in treating adults with MS. Natalizumab therapy is associated with the development of progressive multifocal leukoencephalopathy.

The **prognosis** for childhood MS is similar to that in adults; recovery is often complete, and progression of the disease tends to be slow, with long periods of remission in most cases.

600.2 • Acute Disseminated Encephalomyelitis (ADEM)

ADEM is a monophasic, immune-mediated demyelinating disorder that can follow immunizations or more often infections including rubeola, rubella, varicella, herpes zoster, mumps, *Mycoplasma pneumoniae,* or, more commonly, other nonspecific upper respiratory tract infections. Documentation of a preceding illness is not required to make this diagnosis. ADEM is being recognized more frequently with the broader use of MRI in children with motor weakness, acute seizures, or encephalopathy. Antecedent or presenting features include fever, lethargy, vomiting, weakness, ataxia, headache, seizures, and other systemic signs, and patients often progress to have delirium, coma, myelopathy, and focal neurologic signs. MRI typically shows T2 enhancing disseminated multifocal lesions in the white matter, basal ganglia, thalamus, and brainstem consistent with edema, inflammation, and demyelination, which may enhance further with gadolinium (Fig. 600-2). Hemorrhagic white matter lesions are sometimes seen. Examination of CSF often shows a monocytic and lymphocytic pleocytosis.

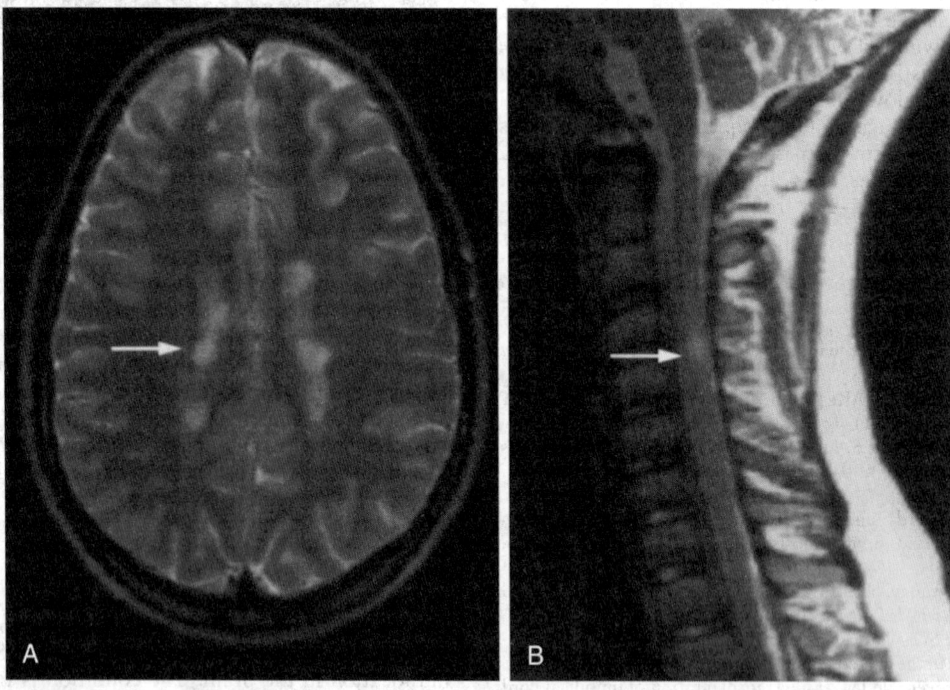

Figure 600-1. Multiple sclerosis. *A,* T2 weighted MRI scan of brain demonstrates multiple lesions located in the white matter characteristic of multiple sclerosis *(white arrow). B,* T1 weighted MRI scan of spine indicates a demyelinating plaque of multiple sclerosis in the midcervical region *(white arrow).*

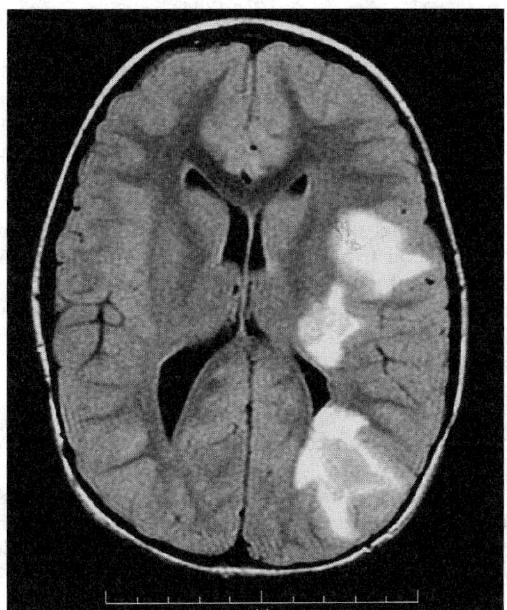

Figure 600-2. Axial T2 weighted FLAIR MRI of the brain in a child with acute disseminated encephalomyelitis (ADEM). High signal *(white)* lesions in the T2 weighted image reflect areas of demyelination and edema in deep subcortical and periventricular white matter as well as the basal ganglia and thalamus on the left side.

Treatment with high-dose intravenous corticosteroids (IV methylprednisolone, 30 mg/kg/day for <30 kg of body weight, and 1 g/day for >30 kg of body weight for 3–5 days, followed by oral prednisolone [1mg/kg/day] over 10 days) may result in improvement. Positive responses to intravenous immunoglobulin (IVIG) have also been reported. Outcome after an episode of ADEM is generally good with >70% of children recovering without disability within 6 mo; the remainder may have residual disability; fatality in the acute period has been reported.

The **differential diagnosis** between the 1st episode of MS and monophasic ADEM in a child with the 1st episode of acute CNS demyelination is challenging without further follow-up to ascertain recurrent episodes as seen in MS. A few children have been described with relapsing ADEM, or so-called multiphasic DEM (MDEM), without evidence of additional lesions. The availability of disease-modifying therapies for MS makes it important to make the distinction between ADEM and MS as early as possible. Several features help distinguish between ADEM and MS (Table 600-1). Children with MS tend to be older than 10 yr of age at presentation whereas a younger age favors ADEM. Children with MS tend to have focal signs without severe encephalopathy; a severe encephalopathy with depressed level of consciousness favors ADEM. The MRI appearance is also useful, as lesions localized to the corpus callosum and periventricular white matter favor MS, whereas lesions in the basal ganglia, thalamus, or at the cortical gray-white junction strongly favor ADEM. The appearance of new MRI lesions after the resolution of the initial episode also suggests MS.

The rare **genetic macrophage activation syndromes (MAS)** can be confused with ADEM. MAS, including familial hemophagocytic lymphohistiocytosis and Chediak-Higashi disease, can sometimes present in younger children with a clinical and MRI manifestations that resembles ADEM. These diseases continue to progress, however, after steroid treatment is stopped. White matter abnormalities and focal neurologic deficits caused by isolated vasculitis of the central nervous system may also be confused with ADEM.

TABLE 600-1. Clinical and MRI Features That May Distinguish ADEM from First Attack of MS

	ADEM	MS
Age	<10 yrs	>10 years
Stupor/Coma	+	–
Fever/Vomiting	+	–
Family History	No	20%
Sensory Complaints	+	–
Optic Neuritis	Bilateral	Unilateral
Manifestations	Polysymptomatic	Monosymptomatic
MRI Imaging	Widespread lesions: basal ganglia, thalamus, cortical gray-white junction	Isolated lesions: periventricular white matter, corpus callosum
CSF	Pleocytosis (lymphocytosis)	Oligoclonal bands
Response to Steroids	+	+
Follow-up	No new lesions	New lesions

Some features that may help distinguish an initial acute episode of demyelination from a first attack of MS in children. Final diagnosis of MS is based on follow-up evaluation and possibly MRI. +, more likely to be present; –, less likely to be present; ADEM, acute disseminated encephalomyelitis; CSF, cerebrospinal fluid; MS, Multiple sclerosis.

Alper G, Schor NF: Toward the definition of acute disseminated encephalitis of childhood. *Curr Opin Pediatr* 2004;16:637–640.

Brass SD, Caramanos Z, Santos C, et al: Multiple sclerosis vs acute disseminated encephalomyelitis in childhood. *Pediatr Neurol* 2003;29:227–231.

Dale RC, Branson JA: Acute disseminated encephalomyelitis or multiple sclerosis: Can the initial presentation help in establishing a correct diagnosis? *Arch Dis Child* 2005;90:636–639.

Dale RC, de Sousa C, Chong WK, et al: Acute disseminated encephalomyelitis, multiphasic disseminated encephalomyelitis and multiple sclerosis in children. *Brain* 2000;123:2407–2422.

Frohman EM, Racke MK, Raine CS: Multiple sclerosis—the plague and its pathogenesis. *N Engl J Med* 2006;354:942–955.

Kappos L, Antel J, Comi G, et al: Oral fingolimod (FYT720) for relapsing multiple sclerosis. *N Engl J Med* 2006;355:1124–1140.

Krupp LB: Multiple sclerosis in children. *J Pediatr* 2006;149:125–127.

Krupp LB, Macallister WS: Treatment of pediatric MS. *Curr Treat Options Neurol* 2005;7:191–199.

Langer-Gould A, Atlas SW, Green AJ, et al: Progressive multifocal leukoencephalopathy in a patient treated with natalizumab. *N Engl J Med* 2005;353:375–380.

Leake JAD, Albani S, Kao AS, et al: Acute disseminated encephalomyelitis in childhood: Epidemiologic, clinical and laboratory features. *Pediatr Infect Dis J* 2004;23:756–764.

McDonald WI, Compston A, Edan G, et al: Recommended diagnostic criteria for multiple sclerosis: Guidelines from the international panel on the diagnosis of multiple sclerosis. *Ann Neurol* 2001;50:121–127.

The Medical Letter: Natalizumab (Tysabri) for relapsing multiple sclerosis. *Med Lett Drugs Ther* 2005;47:13–15.

Miller DH: Brain atrophy, interferon beta, and treatment trials in multiple sclerosis. *Lancet* 2004;364:1463–1464.

Murray TJ: Diagnosis and treatment of multiple sclerosis. *BMJ* 2006;332:525–527.

Polman CH, O'Connor PW, Havrdova E, et al: A randomized, placebo-controlled trial of natalizumab for relapsing multiple sclerosis. *N Engl J Med* 2006;899–910.

Shiraishi K, Higuchi Y, Ozawa K, et al: Clinical course and prognosis of 27 patients with childhood onset multiple sclerosis in Japan. *Brain Dev* 2005;27:224–227.

Stonehouse M, Gupte G, Wassmer E, et al: Acute disseminated encephalomyelitis: Recognition in the hands of general paediatricians. *Arch Dis Child* 2003;88:122–124.

Tardieu M, Mikaeloff Y: What is acute disseminated encephalomyelitis (ADEM)? *Eur J Paediatr Neurol* 2004;8:239–242.

Tenembaum, S, Chamoles N, Fejerman N: Acute disseminated encephalomyelitis, a long-term follow-up study of 84 pediatric patients. *Neurology* 2002;59:1224–1231.

Weng WC, Yang CC, Yu TW, et al: Multiple Sclerosis with childhood onset: Report of 21 cases in Taiwan. *Pediatr Neurol* 2006;35:327–334.

Whiting P, Harbord R, Main C, et al: Accuracy of magnetic resonance imaging for the diagnosis of multiple sclerosis: systematic review. *BMJ* 2006;332:875–878.

Chapter 601 ■ Acute Stroke Syndromes

Michael V. Johnston and Anne Comi

Hemiplegia secondary to vascular disorders occurs in children with an incidence of 1–3/100,000 per year. The pediatric causes of stroke are distinctive compared with adult causes. Types of stroke include arterial and venous thrombosis, intracranial hemorrhage, arterial embolism, and various miscellaneous conditions. The cause of stroke in children is established in ≈75% of cases (Table 601-1). Because the mode of presentation of acute stroke syndromes is not uniform, a brief description of the most prevalent forms of pediatric stroke follows.

601.1 • Arterial Thrombosis/Embolism

Arterial thrombosis and embolism may involve major cerebral arteries (internal carotid or anterior, middle, and posterior cerebral artery occlusion) or smaller cerebral arteries (Fig. 601-1). Certain thrombotic processes affect large vessels and others more commonly involve small arteries. **Thrombosis of the internal carotid artery** may result from acute angulation of the artery (roller coaster, barbershop, beauty parlor, child abuse) or blunt trauma to the posterior pharynx caused by a fall on a pencil or popsicle stick in the child's mouth. The injury produces a tear in the intima of the vessel wall, which may lead to formation of a dissecting aneurysm. Cerebral symptoms result from shedding of emboli from the thrombus. The onset of symptoms may be delayed for up to 24 hr after the accident, with a stuttering but progressive flaccid hemiplegia, lethargy, and aphasia if the dominant hemisphere is involved. Focal motor seizures are a common complication. Dissection of vessels in the vertebral basilar circulation can lead to acute signs of brainstem dysfunction.

A retropharyngeal abscess may produce an identical clinical picture, but in this case the arterial thrombosis results from inflammation of the intima. A cerebral angiogram or MRI/magnetic resonance angiography (MRA) typically demonstrates occlusion of the internal carotid artery, and a CT/MRI scan shows a hypodense lesion outlining the area of infarction.

TABLE 601-1. Causes of Stroke in Children

- I. Cardiac Disease
  - A. Congenital
    1. Aortic stenosis
    2. Mitral stenosis; mitral prolapse
    3. Ventricular septal defects
    4. Patent ductus arteriosus
    5. Cyanotic congenital heart disease involving right-to-left shunt
  - B. Acquired
    1. Endocarditis (bacterial, systemic lupus erythematosus)
    2. Kawasaki disease
    3. Cardiomyopathy
    4. Atrial myxoma
    5. Arrhythmia
    6. Paradoxical emboli through patent foramen ovale
    7. Rheumatic fever
    8. Prosthetic heart valve
- II. Hematologic Abnormalities
  - A. Hemoglobinopathies
    1. Sickle cell (SS) disease
    2. Sickle (SC) disease
  - B. Polycythemia
  - C. Leukemia/lymphoma
  - D. Thrombocytopenia
  - E. Thrombocytosis
  - F. Disorders of coagulation
    1. Protein C deficiency
    2. Protein S deficiency
    3. Factor V Leiden
    4. Antithrombin III deficiency
    5. Lupus anticoagulant
    6. Oral contraceptive pill use
    7. Pregnancy and the postpartum state
    8. Disseminated intravascular coagulation
    9. Paroxysmal nocturnal hemoglobinuria
    10. Prothrombin G20210A (PT20210)
    11. Thrombophilic mutations factor V1691 GA
    12. Inflammatory bowel disease (thrombosis)
- III. Inflammatory Disorders
  - A. Meningitis
    1. Viral
    2. Bacterial
    3. Tuberculosis
  - B. Systemic infection
    1. Viremia
    2. Becteremia
    3. Local head and neck infections
  - C. Drug-induced inflammation
    1. Amphetamine
    2. Cocaine
  - D. Autoimmune disease
    1. Systemic lupus erythematosus
    2. Juvenile rheumatoid arthritis
    3. Takayasu arteritis
    4. Mixed connective tissue disease
    5. Polyarteritis nodosum
    6. Primary central nervous system vasculitis
    7. Sarcoidosis
    8. Behçet syndrome
    9. Wegener granulomatosis
- IV. Metabolic Disease Associated with Stroke
  - A. Homocystinuria
  - B. Pseudoxanthoma elasticum
  - C. Fabry disease
  - D. Sulfite oxidase deficiency
  - E. Mitochondrial disorders
    1. MELAS
    2. Leigh syndrome
  - F. Ornithine transcarbamylase deficiency
  - G. Thermolabile methylene tetrahydrofolate reductase (MTHFR C677T)
- V. Intracerebral Vascular Processes
  - A. Ruptured aneurysm
  - B. Arteriovenous malformation
  - C. Fibromuscular dysplasia
  - D. Moyamoya disease
  - E. Migraine headache
  - F. Postsubarachnoid hemorrhage vasospasm
  - G. Hereditary hemorrhagic telangiectasia
  - H. Sturge-Weber syndrome
  - I. Carotid artery dissection
  - J. Post varicella
  - K. PHACES syndrome (see Chapter 649)
- VI. Trauma and Other External Causes
  - A. Child abuse
  - B. Head trauma/neck trauma
  - C. Oral trauma
  - D. Placental embolism
  - E. ECMO therapy

ECMO, extracorporeal membrane oxygenation; MELAS, mitochondrial encephalomyopathy, lactic acidosis, and stroke.
From Rivkin M: In Kliegman R (ed): *Practical Strategies in Pediatric Diagnosis and Therapy*. Philadelphia, WB Saunders, 1996.

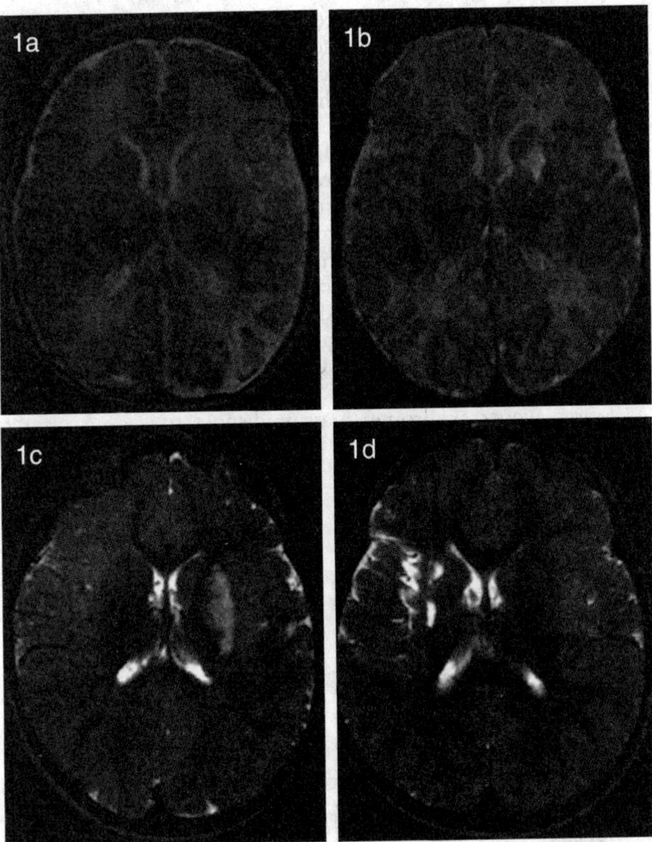

Figure 601-1. Axial T2 weighted images acquired after neonatal-onset (*a* and *b*) and childhood-onset (*c* and *d*) IS. In *a,* there is abnormal high signal intensity in left caudate and lentiform nuclei (BG), the PLIC, and the CC, with loss of gray matter/WM differentiation. This child has a hemiparesis, which characteristically occurred when there was concomitant involvement of BG, CC, and PLIC. In *b,* there is high signal intensity in the lentiform nucleus (BG) and anterior limb of the internal capsule, with no involvement of PLIC or CC. This child has no hemiparesis; no neonate with exclusive BG or CC involvement or BG and PLIC or BG and CC lesions developed hemiparesis. In contrast, *c* was acquired after childhood-onset IS and shows BG involvement only with sparing of the CC and PLIC, and this child does have a hemiparesis. In *d,* involvement of PLIC, BG, and CC after childhood-onset IS can be seen. Although this pattern of lesion site tended to result in hemiparesis, some children with this distribution, including the example shown here, did not develop hemiparesis. IS, ischemic stroke; MCA, middle cerebral artery; BG, basal ganglia; PLIC, posterior limb of the internal capsule; MR, magnetic resonance; TE, echo time; TR, repetition time; WM, white matter; CC, cerebral cortex; OR, odds ratio; CI, confidence interval. (From Boardman JP, Ganesan V, Rutherford MA, et al: Magnetic resonance image correlates of hemiparesis after neonatal and childhood middle cerebral artery stroke. *Pediatrics* 2005;115:321–326.)

Embolization of cerebral vessels may also produce acute hemiparesis. Cardiac abnormalities are the most common overall cause of thromboembolic stroke in children. Cardiac causes include arrhythmias (particularly atrial fibrillation), myxoma, paradoxical emboli through a patent foramen ovale, and bacterial endocarditis that results in a mycotic aneurysm. Air emboli may complicate surgery, and fat emboli occur with fracture of long bones. Septic emboli may seed the cerebral vessels and evolve into an area of cerebritis leading to a cerebral abscess.

Cyanotic congenital heart disease in children younger than 2 yr may cause thrombosis, particularly of the middle cerebral artery. These patients are particularly vulnerable when the oxygen saturation is significantly decreased together with a viral illness or dehydration. Cardiac procedures, including catheterization and complex cardiac surgery operations (Fontan), can result in arterial thrombosis from embolization of a clot. If a cardiac cause of arterial thrombosis is suspected, the child must have an echocardiogram as part of the investigation.

Occlusive vascular disorders are also important causes of acute hemiplegia in the pediatric population. **Basal arterial occlusion with telangiectasia or moyamoya** ("puff of smoke") **disease** has a characteristic angiogram (Fig. 601-2). The condition is more common in girls and often presents with headache and bilateral upper motor neuron signs. It may also present with chorea. Intermittent episodes of transient ischemic attacks can produce progressive neurologic signs and severe disability. Surgical procedures designed to enhance cerebral flow (superficial temporal artery to middle cerebral artery shunt and laying the superficial temporal artery on the arachnoid membrane) have variable results.

Sickle cell disease is the most common cause of stroke in black children and is associated with large vessel stenosis of the proximal middle cerebral or distal internal carotid arteries. In addition to patients with obvious strokes, magnetic resonance imaging reveals that approximately ⅓ of children with sickle cell disease have silent brain infarctions that may lead to cognitive decline. Chronic transfusion therapy may prevent stroke in this group.

Coagulation disorders are an important risk factor for stroke in children and neonates. Mutations in factor V Leiden and prothrombin, deficiencies in protein C, protein S, and antithrombin III, as well as antiphospholipid antibodies, have been identified in up to 50% of infants and children with cerebral thromboembolism (see Chapters 478 and 479) [Table 601-1].

Occlusion of small arteries is also associated with diabetes mellitus, neurofibromatosis, postvaricella angiopathy, head and neck radiation, oral contraceptives, and illicit drug use (amphetamines, cocaine). Patients present with unilateral neurologic signs, and recovery is often complete because of the small area of infarction. Patients with *thrombosis of small arteries,* including the perforating striate vessels, which result from polyarteritis nodosa and homocystinuria, generally have a progressive debilitating course characterized by bilateral signs and high mortality rate.

Transient cerebral arteriopathy is a nonprogressive, usually self-limited process that produces unilateral intracranial artery

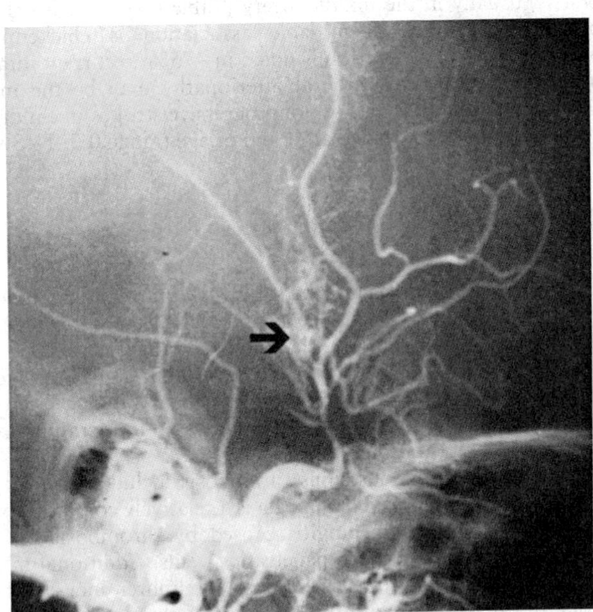

Figure 601-2. Cerebral angiogram showing idiopathic supraclinoid–internal carotid arteriopathy with classic moyamoya collaterals *(arrow).*

TABLE 601-2. Major Clinicoradiological Patterns Underlying Childhood Arteriopathic Brain Infarcts

TRANSIENT CEREBRAL ARTERIOPATHY

Definitions

On initial vascular imaging, unilateral focal or segmental stenosis or occlusion involving distal part of internal carotid and initial segments and branches of anterior and/or middle cerebral artery. In some cases, none or only minimum stenosis, with maximum stenosis or occlusion observed within 3 months of initial imaging (Fig. 601-3 A, B). On follow-up imaging 6 months after initial stroke, non-progression (or regression) of arterial lesions compared with baseline 3-month angiogram (Fig. 601-3 B, C, and D)

Causes

Inflammatory/infectious: varicella zoster virus, other agents (eg, enterovirus, borrelia, bartonella)?
Intracranial dissection: traumatic, inflammatory-infectious?
Spasm, toxic (eg, cocaine)?
Adjuvant thrombotic factors?
Some rare progressive arteriopathies have same presentation as transient cerebral arteriopathy

EXTRACRANIAL DISSECTION

Definitions

Vascular imaging displaying one of: angiographic findings of double lumen, intimal flap, or pseudoaneurysm, or, on axial T_1 fat-saturation MRI, bright crescent sign in arterial wall; sequence of cervical or cranial trauma, or neck pain, less than 6 weeks preceding angiographic findings of segmental arterial narrowing (or occlusion) in cervical arteries (Fig. 601-3 E, arrow); angiographic segmental narrowing (or occlusion) of vertebral artery at level of C2 vertebral body, even without known traumatic history

Causes

Traumatic: accidental—direct, stretching, sometimes subtle trauma (non-progressive arteriopathy); non-accidental head injury—shaken baby syndrome (progressive or non-progressive arteriopathies)
Collagen diseases +/− trauma (progressive arteriopathy)

MOYAMOYA SYNDROME

Definitions

Magnetic resonance or contrast angiography showing narrowing or occlusion of terminal portion of both internal carotid arteries (Fig. 601-3 F), and unilateral or bilateral collateral network of small vessels distal to occluded arteries (Fig. F, arrows)

Causes

Progressive or non-progressive arteriopathies: genetic—sickle-cell disease, neurofibromatosis type 1; toxic—radiotherapy (especially in neurofibromatosis type 1 context); inflammatory/infectious—varicella zoster virus

*Definitions were recently established by consensus among neurologists from the International Pediatric Stroke Study Group. Distinct causes might lead to same clinicoradiological presentation and outcome: conversely, seemingly unique cause might produce different clinicoradiological patterns, rendering case-by-case determination of outcome, at first clinical manifestation, often unpredictable. To detect arteriopathies in childhood stroke, rapid magnetic resonance vascular imaging (within 24 hr after initial manifestation) is required.

From Sébire G: Transient cerebral arteriopathy in childhood. *Lancet* 2006; 368:8–10.

stenosis, usually in the middle artery (Table 601-2, Fig. 601-3). The most common, identifiable association is chickenpox. Improvement or stabilization is noted in ~75%; recurrent infarction is rare. Transient cerebral arteriopathy may be the most common identifiable cause of nonprogressive strokes in children, with a mean onset of stroke at 40 mo of age (range 0.3–14.8 yr).

601.2 • Venous Thrombosis

Venous sinus thrombosis may be subdivided into septic and nonseptic causes (Table 601-3). The symptoms and signs may evolve over days and in neonates are characterized by diffuse neurologic signs and seizures, whereas focal neurologic signs are more prominent in children. Dilated scalp veins, a bulging anterior fontanel, and symptoms and signs of increased intracranial pressure may be present.

Septic causes of venous sinus thrombosis include encephalitis and bacterial meningitis. Hemiplegia is a relatively common complication of **bacterial meningitis** caused by thrombosis of the superficial cortical and deep penetrating veins. Additional infectious causes of septic sinus thrombosis in children include **otitis media** and **mastoiditis** with involvement of the dural vessels, as well as retrograde orbital infections producing **cavernous sinus thrombosis.**

Aseptic causes include **severe dehydration** in infancy, which may result in thrombosis of the superior sagittal sinus and the superficial cortical veins due to hyperviscosity and sludging of blood. Conditions resulting in hypercoagulopathy, cyanotic congenital heart diseases, iron-deficiency anemia, and leukemic infiltrates of cerebral veins are additional causes of nonseptic acute hemiplegia of childhood. **Prothrombotic disorders** including deficiencies of inhibitors of coagulation such as protein C, protein S, and antithrombin III, and procoagulant states such as increased factor VIII levels, activated protein C resistance, mutations in Leiden factor V, abnormalities of lipoprotein a, mutations of the thermolabile methylene tetrahydrofolate reductase gene, elevated fasting homocysteine levels, and anticardiolipin antibodies are found in 12–50% of cases (see Chapters 478 and 479). **Vascular malformations** associated with impaired venous drainage (such as Sturge-Weber syndrome) may predispose to venous infarcts and strokelike episodes.

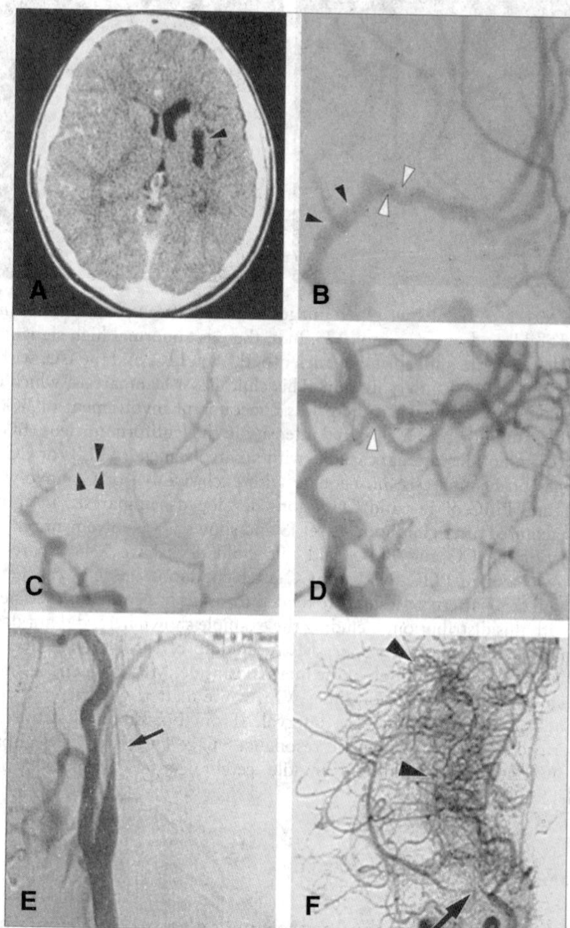

Figure 601-3. Major clinicoradiological patterns underlying childhood arteriopathic brain infarcts. Transient cerebral arteriopathy–images from 8-year-old child who presented with right hemiplegia 8 months after chickenpox. (A) CT shows typical deep small infarct in basal gray nuclei area. (B) Angiogram just after stroke, irregular segmental stenosis of supraclinoid carotid artery (filled arrows) and sylvian artery (open arrows). (C) 3 months after initial stroke, worsening of sylvian lesions (D) At 14 months, improvement compared with 3-month angiogram (but not compared with initial angiogram), with persistent stenosis of sylvian artery. There was no recurrence of stroke after 5 years. (E) Extracranial dissection of internal cartoid artery *(arrow)*. (F) Angiographical aspect of moyamoya syndrome including supraclinoid cartoid artery stenosis *(arrow)* and collateral network of small vessels distal to occluded artery *(arrowheads)*. (From Sébire G: Transient cerebral arteriopathy in childhood. *Lancet* 2006;368:8–10).

TABLE 601-3. Causes of and Risk Factors Associated with Cerebral Venous Sinus Thrombosis

Genetic prothrombotic conditions
Antithrombin deficiency
Protein C and protein S deficiency
Factor V Leiden mutation
Prothrombin mutation (the substitution of A for G at position 20210)
Homocysteinemia caused by gene mutations in methylenetetrahydrofolate reductase
Acquired prothrombotic states
Nephrotic syndrome
Antiphospholipid antibodies
Homocysteinemia
Pregnancy
Puerperium
Infections
Otitis, mastoiditis, sinusitis
Meningitis
Systemic infectious disease
Inflammatory disease
Systemic lupus erythematosus
Wegener granulomatosis
Sarcoidosis
Inflammatory bowel disease
Behçet syndrome
Hematologic conditions
Polycythemia, primary and secondary
Thrombocythemia
Leukemia
Anemia, including paroxysmal nocturnal hemoglobinuria
Drugs
Oral contraceptives
Asparaginase
Mechanical causes, trauma
Head injury
Injury to sinuses or jugular vein, jugular catheterization
Neurosurgical procedures
Lumbar puncture
Miscellaneous
Dehydration, especially in children
Cancer

From Stam J: Thrombosis of the cerebral veins and sinuses. *New Engl J Med* 2005;352:1791–1798.

601.3 • Intracranial Hemorrhage

Intracranial hemorrhage may occur in the subarachnoid space or the bleeding may be primarily located in the parenchyma of the brain. Subarachnoid bleeding is characterized by severe headache, nuchal rigidity, and progressive loss of consciousness, and intracerebral bleeding is characterized by focal neurologic signs and seizures. Intracranial hemorrhage is a common event in premature infants and is discussed in Chapter 99.2.

Arteriovenous malformations result from failure of normal capillary bed development between arteries and veins during embryogenesis. Arteriovenous malformations produce abnormal shunting of blood, causing an expansion of vessels and a space-occupying effect or rupture of a vein and intracerebral bleeding. Arteriovenous malformations are typically located in the cerebral hemisphere, but they may be situated in the cerebellum, brainstem, or spinal cord. Although the malformation may remain asymptomatic throughout life, rupture and bleeding can occur at any age. Children with arteriovenous malformations frequently have a history of seizures and migraine-like headaches. Typical migraine alternates from one side of the head to the other, whereas headaches associated with an arteriovenous malformation classically remain on the same side. Auscultation of the skull is positive for a high-pitched bruit in ≈50% of cases. Rupture of an arteriovenous malformation causes a severe headache, vomiting, nuchal rigidity caused by subarachnoid bleeding, progressive hemiparesis, and a focal or generalized seizure. Cavernous angiomas may be familial and are of lower risk for spontaneous hemorrhage. An **arteriovenous malformation of the vein of Galen** in infancy can cause high-output congestive heart failure secondary to shunting of large volumes of blood or progressive hydrocephalus and increased intracranial pressure secondary to obstruction of the cerebrospinal fluid (CSF) pathways. Vein of Galen malformations are difficult to treat and are associated with a poor prognosis.

Cerebral aneurysms producing symptoms in children are relatively rare. In contrast to those in adults, aneurysms in children tend to be large and are located at the carotid bifurcation or on the anterior and posterior cerebral arteries rather than the circle of Willis. The aneurysmal dilatation results from a congenital weakness of the vessel and, in some cases, a deficiency of type III collagen has been demonstrated. In children, there is an association between cerebral aneurysms, coarctation of the aorta, and bilateral polycystic kidney disease. Although most ruptured aneurysms bleed into the subarachnoid space, causing an intense headache, nuchal rigidity, and coma, intracerebral hemorrhage and progressive hemiparesis also occur. Additional causes of intracerebral hematoma include hematologic disorders, particularly thrombocytopenic purpura and hemophilia. Finally, trauma can produce hemiparesis due to intracerebral bleeding or a subdural or epidural hematoma. A contrast CT scan or MRI with gadolinium and MRA is useful for identifying large arteriovenous malformations; however, four-vessel cerebral angiography is the study of choice for investigating arteriovenous malformations and cerebral aneurysm.

601.4 • Differential Diagnosis of Strokelike Events

ETIOLOGY AND CLINICAL MANIFESTATIONS. Alternating hemiplegia of childhood is occasionally associated with migraine, but in most cases the cause is unknown. It develops in infants between 2 and 18 mo of age and is characterized by intermittent episodes of hemiplegia alternating from one side of the body to the other. Rarely, both sides are involved during an attack. Choreoathetosis and dystonic movements are commonly observed in the hemiparetic extremity. Signs spontaneously regress with sleep but recur with awakening. The hemiplegia persists for minutes to weeks and then resolves spontaneously. The condition has a poor prognosis, with progressive mental retardation and developmental disabilities. Results of neuroimaging and metabolic studies are negative.

Several **metabolic diseases** are associated with strokelike episodes in children, including mitochondrial encephalomyelopathy (MELAS; see Chapter 598.2), ornithine transcarbamylase deficiency, pyruvate dehydrogenase deficiency, and homocystinuria.

Todd paralysis may be confused initially with a stroke. The hemiparesis follows a focal seizure, but the weakness and neurologic signs disappear completely within 24 hr of the convulsion. Although the cause of Todd paralysis remains unknown, the hemiparesis probably results from an inhibitory phenomenon, possibly related to neurotransmitter dysfunction.

Additional causes of hemiparesis include **cerebral tumor, encephalitis** (particularly herpes), **focal postviral encephalitis,** and **status epilepticus.** In some pediatric series of unexplained stroke, **lipid abnormalities,** including elevated triglycerides and low levels of high-density lipoprotein cholesterol, have been found in ≈20% of the cases. The family histories of these children reveal an increased incidence of premature coronary heart disease and early ischemic cerebrovascular diseases. Screening of at-risk families identifies children who may benefit from long-term dietary management.

DIAGNOSIS. The most critical component of the investigation is a thorough history and physical examination, searching for an underlying disease process; evidence of trauma; an infectious, metabolic, or hematologic disorder; neurocutaneous syndrome; increased intracranial pressure; or hydrocephalus. Appropriate tests for infectious diseases, metabolic disorders, and coagulation disorders are based on the results of the history and physical examination. An electroencephalogram (EEG) may be helpful in localizing the disease process but rarely establishes the diagnosis. A CT scan can detect recent bleeding or a large area of infarction, but diffusion weighted MRI, perfusion MRI imaging, and MRA and MRV are superior for early detection of cerebral ischemia and assessment of cerebral vessels. A cerebral angiogram may be useful in some cases in which MRI studies are nondiagnostic, such as to detect vasculitis or sites of intracranial hemorrhage. In these cases, a four-vessel cerebral angiogram is indicated. Electrocardiography and echocardiography may help to exclude intrinsic cardiac diseases or an arrhythmia as a cause of the stroke. Finally, the basic investigations for a child with an unexplained stroke syndrome should be organized to eliminate the following conditions: (1) vasculitis and connective tissue diseases (ESR, C3, C4, RF, ANA), (2) lipid disorders, (3) coagulation disorders, (4) hematologic disorders (sickle cell disease, thrombocytopenia), (5) metabolic disorders (homocystinuria, Fabry disease, MELAS), and (6) an infectious etiology (meningitis and encephalitis).

TREATMENT OF STROKES. Thrombolytic therapies (tissue plasminogen activator) are useful within 3 hr after ischemic stokes in adults but have not been studied in children. Low molecular weight heparin is sometimes used to treat venous sinus thrombosis. The contraindications for the use of an antithrombotic agent include significant intracerebral hemorrhage and hypertension. Supportive care includes blood pressure and fluid management, maintenance of normoglycemia, and control of fevers and seizures. Recombinant activated factor VII has improved the acute prognosis in adults with intracerebral hemorrhage. The surgical evacuation of a large blood clot or edematous brain tissue from a large stroke may also be indicated in some cases.

In neonates, treatment for prevention of a 2nd stroke is often not required because the risk of recurrence is low. In children, however, the recurrence risk is higher and long-term therapy with low-dose aspirin is often needed. Low molecular weight heparin or warfarin is frequently used for several months to prevent stroke recurrence in the presence of cardiac emboli, dissection of an aneurysm, high-grade cerebral artery stenosis, severe prothrombotic conditions, or aspirin failure. Regular blood transfusions reduce the incidence of stroke in sickle cell disease. Immunosuppressant therapy is often required for vasculitis. Rehabilitation requirements after a stroke can include speech therapy, occupational and physical therapy, psychologic services, and special education. These treatment regimens are most effectively provided in a multidisciplinary setting.

Agner C, Weig SG: Arterial dissection and stroke following child abuse: Case report and review of the literature. *Childs Nerv Syst* 2005;21:416–420.

Baumer JH: Childhood arterial stroke. *Arch Dis Child* 2004;89:ep50–ep53.

Boardman JP, Ganesan V, Rutherford MA, et al: Magnetic resonance image correlates of hemiparesis after neonatal and childhood middle cerebral artery stroke. *Pediatrics* 2005;115:321–326.

Bourgeois M, Aicardi J, Goutières F: Alternating hemiplegia of childhood. *J Pediatr* 1993;122:673–679.

Danchaivijitr N, Cox TC, Saunders DE, Ganeson V: Evolution of cerebral arteopathics in childhood arterial ischemic stroke. *Ann Neurol* 2006;59:620–626.

DeVeber G: Arterial ischemic strokes in infants and children: An overview of current approaches. *Semin Thromb Hemost* 2003;29:567–573.

DeVeber G, Andrew M, Adams C, et al: Cerebral sinovenous thrombosis in children. *N Engl J Med* 2001;345:417–423.

Duran R, Biner B, Demir M, et al: Factor V Leiden mutation and other thrombophilia markers in childhood ischemic stroke. *Clin Appl Thromb Hemost* 2005;11:83–88.

Fullerton HJ, Wu YW, Sidney S, Johnston SC: Risk of recurrent childhood arterial ischemic stroke in a population-based cohort: the importance of cerebrovascular imaging. *Pediatrics* 2007;119:495–501.

Haywood S, Liesner R, Pindora S, et al: Thrombophilia and first arterial ischaemic stroke: A systematic review. *Arch Dis Child* 2005;90:402–405.

Lanthier S, Armstrong D, Domi T, de Veber G: Post-varicella arteriopathy of childhood. *Neurology* 2005;64:660–663.

Lynch JK, Hirtz DG, DeVeber G, et al: Report on the National Institute of Neurological Diseases and Stroke Workshop on perinatal and childhood stroke. *Pediatrics* 2002;109:116–123.

Lynch JK, Nelson KB, Curry CJ, et al: Cerebrovascular disorders in children with the Leiden factor V mutation. *J Child Neurol* 2001;16:735–744.

Mayer SA, Brun NC, Begtrup K, et al: Recombinant activated factor VII for acute intracerebral hemorrhage. *N Engl J Med* 2005;352:777–785.

Mercuri E, Barnett A, Rutherford M, et al: Neonatal cerebral infarction and neuromotor outcome at school age. *Pediatrics* 2004;113:95–100.

Nowak-Göttl U, Günther G, Kurnik K, et al: Arterial ischemic stroke in neonates, infants and children: An overview of underlying conditions, imaging methods and treatment modalities. *Semin Thromb Hemost* 2003;29:405–414.

Rosenblum L: Management of stroke in childhood. *Br Med J* 2005;330:1161–1162.

Scott RM, Smith JL, Robertson RL, et al: Long-term outcome in children with moyamoya syndrome after cranial revascularization by pial synangiosis. *J Neurosurg Pediatr* 2004;100:142–149.

Sebire G, Tabarki B, Saunders DE, et al: Cerebral venous sinus thrombosis in children: Risk factors, presentation, diagnosis and outcome. *Brain* 2005;128:477–489.

Stam J: Thrombosis of the cerebral veins and sinuses. *New Engl J Med* 2005;352:1791–1798.

Steen RG, Emudiangughe T, Hankins GM, et al: Brain imaging findings in pediatric patients with sickle cell disease. *Radiology* 2003;228:216–225.

Wu YW, Miller SP, Chin K, et al: Multiple risk factors in neonatal sinovenous thrombosis. *Neurology* 2002;59:438–440.

Chapter 602 ■ Central Nervous System Infections

Charles G. Prober

Infection of the central nervous system (CNS) is the most common cause of fever associated with signs and symptoms of CNS disease in children. Many microorganisms can cause infection. Nonetheless, specific pathogens are identifiable and are influenced by the age and immune status of the host and the epidemiology of the pathogen. In general, viral infections of the CNS are much more common than bacterial infections, which, in turn, are more common than fungal and parasitic infections. Infections caused by rickettsiae (Rocky Mountain spotted fever, *Ehrlichia*) are relatively uncommon but assume important roles under certain epidemiologic circumstances. *Mycoplasma* spp. can also cause infections of the CNS, although their precise contribution is often difficult to determine.

Regardless of etiology, most patients with CNS infection have similar clinical manifestations. **Common symptoms** include headache, nausea, vomiting, anorexia, restlessness, altered state of consciousness, and irritability; most of these symptoms are nonspecific. **Common signs** of CNS infection, in addition to fever, include photophobia, neck pain and rigidity, obtundation, stupor, coma, seizures, and focal neurologic deficits. The severity and constellation of signs are determined by the specific pathogen, the host, and the area of the CNS affected.

Infection of the CNS may be diffuse or focal. Meningitis and encephalitis are examples of diffuse infection. Meningitis implies primary involvement of the meninges, whereas encephalitis indicates brain parenchymal involvement. Because these anatomic boundaries are often not distinct, many patients have evidence of both meningeal and parenchymal involvement and should be considered to have meningoencephalitis. Brain abscess is the best example of a focal infection of the CNS. The neurologic expression of this infection is determined by the site and extent of the abscess(es) [see Chapter 603].

The diagnosis of diffuse CNS infections depends on examination of cerebrospinal fluid (CSF) obtained by lumbar puncture (LP). Table 602-1 provides an overview of the expected CSF abnormalities with various CNS disorders.

602.1 • Acute Bacterial Meningitis Beyond the Neonatal Period

Bacterial meningitis is one of the most potentially serious infections occurring in infants and older children. This infection is associated with a high rate of acute complications and risk of long-term morbidity. The incidence of bacterial meningitis is sufficiently high in febrile infants that it should be included in the differential diagnosis of those with altered mental status and other evidence of neurologic dysfunction.

ETIOLOGY. The causes of bacterial meningitis in the neonatal period (0–28 days) are generally distinct from those in older infants and children (see Chapter 109). The bacteria that cause meningitis in newborns reflect the maternal gastrointestinal and genitourinary flora and the environment to which the infant is exposed. The common pathogens include groups B and D streptococci (enterococcus), gram-negative enteric bacilli (*E. coli, Klebsiella*), and *Listeria monocytogenes*. Group B streptococcus followed by *E. coli* are the two most common causes of neonatal meningitis. Group B and D streptococci and *Listeria* persist

TABLE 602-1. Cerebrospinal Fluid Findings in Central Nervous System Disorders

CONDITION	PRESSURE (MM H_2O)	LEUKOCYTES (MM^3)	PROTEIN (MG/DL)	GLUCOSE (MG/DL)	COMMENTS
Normal	**50–80**	**<5, ≥75% lymphocytes**	**20–45**	**>50 (or 75% serum glucose)**	
COMMON FORMS OF MENINGITIS					
Acute bacterial meningitis	Usually elevated (100–300)	100–10,000 or more; usually 300–2,000; PMNs predominate	Usually 100–500	Decreased, usually <40 (or <50% serum glucose)	Organisms usually seen on Gram stain and recovered by culture.
Partially treated bacterial meningitis	Normal or elevated	5–10,000; PMNs usual but mononuclear cells may predominate if pretreated for extended period of time	Usually 100–500	Normal or decreased	Organisms may be seen on Gram stain. Pretreatment may render CSF sterile. Antigen may be detected by agglutination test
Viral meningitis or meningoencephalitis	Normal or slightly elevated (80–150)	Rarely >1,000 cells. Eastern equine encephalitis and lymphocytic choriomeningitis (LCM) may have cell counts of several thousand. PMNs early but mononuclear cells predominate through most of the course	Usually 50–200	Generally normal; may be decreased to <40 in some viral diseases, particularly mumps (15–20% of cases)	HSV encephalitis is suggested by focal seizures or by focal findings on CT or MRI scans or EEG. Enteroviruses and HSV infrequently recovered from CSF. HSV and enteroviruses may be detected by PCR of CSF
UNCOMMON FORMS OF MENINGITIS					
Tuberculous meningitis	Usually elevated	10–500; PMNs early, but lymphocytes predominate through most of the course	100–3,000; may be higher in presence of block	<50 in most cases; decreases with time if treatment is not provided	Acid-fast organisms almost never seen on smear. Organisms may be recovered in culture of large volumes of CSF. *Mycobacterium tuberculosis* may be detected by PCR of CSF
Fungal meningitis	Usually elevated	5–500; PMNs early but mononuclear cells predominate through most of the course. Cryptococcal meningitis may have no cellular inflammatory response	25–500	<50; decreases with time if treatment is not provided	Budding yeast may be seen. Organisms may be recovered in culture. Cryptococcal antigen (CSF and serum) may be positive in cryptococcal infection
Syphilis (acute) and leptospirosis	Usually elevated	50–500; lymphocytes predominate	50–200	Usually normal	Positive CSF serology. Spirochetes not demonstrable by usual techniques of smear or culture; darkfield examination may be positive
Amebic (*Naegleria*) meningoencephalitis	Elevated	1,000–10,000 or more; PMNs predominate	50–500	Normal or slightly decreased	Mobile amebae may be seen by hanging-drop examination of CSF at room temperature
BRAIN AND PARAMENINGEAL ABSCESSES					
Brain abscess	Usually elevated (100–300)	5–200; CSF rarely acellular; lymphocytes predominate; if abscess ruptures into ventricle, PMNs predominate and cell count may reach >100,000	75–500	Normal unless abscess ruptures into ventricular system	No organisms on smear or culture unless abscess ruptures into ventricular system
Subdural empyema	Usually elevated (100–300)	100–5,000; PMNs predominate	100–500	Normal	No organisms on smear or culture of CSF unless meningitis also present; organisms found on tap of subdural fluid
Cerebral epidural abscess	Normal to slightly elevated	10–500; lymphocytes predominate	50–200	Normal	No organisms on smear or culture of CSF
Spinal epidural abscess	Usually low, with spinal block	10–100; lymphocytes predominate	50–400	Normal	No organisms on smear or culture of CSF
Chemical (drugs, dermoid systs, myelography dye)	Usually elevated	100–1,000 or more; PMNs predominate	50–100	Normal or slightly decreased	Epithelial cells may be seen within CSF by use of polarized light in some children with dermoids
NONINFECTIOUS CAUSES					
Sarcoidosis	Normal or elevated slightly	0–100; mononuclear	40–100	Normal	No specific findings
Systemic lupus erythematosus with CNS involvement	Slightly elevated	0–500; PMNs usually predominate; lymphocytes may be present	100	Normal or slightly decreased	No organisms on smear or culture. Positive neuronal and ribosomal P protein antibodies in CSF
Tumor, leukemia	Slightly elevated to very high	0–100 or more; mononuclear or blast cells	50–1,000	Normal to decreased (20–40)	Cytology may be positive

CFS, cerebrospinal fluid; EEG, electroencephalogram; HSV, herpes simplex virus; PCR, polymerase chain reaction; PMN, polymorphonuclear neutrophils.

as important CNS pathogens through the 3rd mo of life. In this same time frame, CNS infections caused by *Streptococcus pneumoniae, Neisseria meningitidis,* and *Haemophilus influenzae* type b become increasingly prevalent.

The most common cause of bacterial meningitis in children 2 mo to 12 yr of age in the United States is *N. meningitidis.* Bacterial meningitis caused by *S. pneumoniae* and *H. influenzae* type b has become much less common in developed countries since the introduction of universal immunization against these pathogens beginning at 2 mo of age. Infection caused by *S. pneumoniae* or *H. influenzae* type b must be considered in incompletely vaccinated individuals or those in developing countries. Those with certain underlying immunologic (HIV infection, IgG subclass deficiency) or anatomic (splenic dysfunction, cochlear defects or implants) disorders also may be at increased risk of infection caused by these bacteria.

Alterations of host defense due to anatomic defects or immune deficits also increase the risk of meningitis from less common pathogens such as *Pseudomonas aeruginosa, Staphylococcus aureus,* coagulase-negative staphylococci, *Salmonella* spp., and *Listeria monocytogenes.*

EPIDEMIOLOGY. A major risk factor for meningitis is the lack of immunity to specific pathogens associated with young age. Additional risks include recent colonization with pathogenic bacteria, close contact (household, daycare centers, college dormitories, military barracks) with individuals having invasive disease caused by *N. meningitidis* and *H. influenzae* type b, crowding, poverty, black or Native American race, and male gender. The mode of transmission is probably person-to-person contact through respiratory tract secretions or droplets. The risk of meningitis is increased among infants and young children with occult bacteremia (see Chapters 175 and 176); the odds ratio is greater for meningococcus (85 times) and *H. influenzae* type b (12 times) relative to that for pneumococcus.

Specific host defense defects due to altered immunoglobulin production in response to encapsulated pathogens may be responsible for the increased risk of bacterial meningitis in Native Americans and Eskimos. Defects of the complement system (C5–C8) have been associated with recurrent meningococcal infection, and defects of the properdin system have been associated with a significant risk of lethal meningococcal disease. Splenic dysfunction (sickle cell anemia) or asplenia (due to trauma, or congenital defect) is associated with an increased risk of pneumococcal, *H. influenzae* type b (to some extent), and, rarely, meningococcal sepsis and meningitis. T-lymphocyte defects (congenital or acquired by chemotherapy, AIDS, or malignancy) are associated with an increased risk of *L. monocytogenes* infections of the CNS.

Congenital or acquired CSF leak across a mucocutaneous barrier, such as cranial or midline facial defects (cribriform plate) and middle ear (stapedial foot plate) or inner ear fistulas (oval window, internal auditory canal, cochlear aqueduct), or CSF leakage through a rupture of the meninges due to a basal skull fracture into the cribriform plate or paranasal sinus, is associated with an increased risk of pneumococcal meningitis. The risk of bacterial meningitis, caused by *S. pneumoniae,* in children with cochlear implants, used for the treatment of hearing loss, is more than 30 times the risk in the general U.S. population. Lumbosacral dermal sinus and meningomyelocele are associated with staphylococcal and gram-negative enteric bacterial meningitis. CSF shunt infections increase the risk of meningitis due to staphylococci (especially coagulase-negative species) and other low virulence bacteria that typically colonize the skin.

***STREPTOCOCCUS PNEUMONIAE* (SEE CHAPTER 181).** The epidemiology of infections caused by *S. pneumoniae* has been dramatically altered by the widespread use of the 7-valent pneumococcal protein-polysaccharide conjugate vaccine, licensed in the United States in February 2000. This vaccine is recommended for routine administration to all children 23 mo of age and younger at 2, 4, 6, and 12 to 15 mo of age. Immunization targets this population because the incidence of invasive pneumococcal infections peaks in the 1st 2 yr of life, reaching rates of 228/100,000 in children 6 to 12 mo of age. Children with anatomic or functional asplenia secondary to sickle cell disease and those infected with HIV have infection rates that are 20- to 100-fold higher than in those of healthy children in the 1st 5 yr of life. Additional risk factors for contracting pneumococcal meningitis include otitis media, sinusitis, pneumonia, CSF otorrhea or rhinorrhea, the presence of a cochlear implant, and chronic graft versus host disease following bone marrow transplantation.

***NEISSERIA MENINGITIDIS* (SEE CHAPTER 190).** Five serogroups of meningococcus, A, B, C, Y, and W-135, are responsible for disease. Meningococcal meningitis may be sporadic or may occur in epidemics. In the United States, serogroups B, C, and Y each account for ≈30% of cases, although serogroup distribution varies by location and time. Epidemic disease, especially in developing countries, is usually caused by serogroup A. Cases occur throughout the year but may be more common in the winter and spring and following influenza virus infections. Nasopharyngeal carriage of *N. meningitidis* occurs in 1–15% of adults. Colonization may last weeks to months; recent colonization places nonimmune younger children at greatest risk for meningitis. The incidence of disease occurring in association with an index case in the family is 1%, a rate that is 1,000-fold the risk in the general population. The risk of secondary cases occurring in contacts at daycare centers is about 1/1,000. Most infections of children are acquired from a contact in a daycare facility, a colonized adult family member, or an ill patient with meningococcal disease. Children younger than 5 yr have the highest rates of meningococcal infection. A 2nd peak in incidence occurs in persons between 15 and 24 yr of age. College freshmen living in dormitories have an increased incidence of infection compared to non–college-attending, age-matched controls.

***HAEMOPHILUS INFLUENZAE* TYPE B (SEE CHAPTER 192).** Before universal *H. influenzae* type b vaccination in the United States, ≈70% of cases of bacterial meningitis occurring in the 1st 5 yr of life were caused by this pathogen. Invasive infections occurred primarily in infants 2 mo–2 yr of age; peak incidence was at 6–9 mo of age, and 50% of cases occurred in the 1st yr of life. The risk to children was markedly increased among family or daycare center contacts of patients with *H. influenzae* type b disease. Incompletely vaccinated individuals, those in underdeveloped countries who are not vaccinated, and those with blunted immunologic responses to vaccine (children with HIV infection) remain at risk for *H. influenzae* type b meningitis.

PATHOLOGY AND PATHOPHYSIOLOGY. A meningeal purulent exudate of varying thickness may be distributed around the cerebral veins, venous sinuses, convexity of the brain, and cerebellum and in the sulci, sylvian fissures, basal cisterns, and spinal cord. Ventriculitis with bacteria and inflammatory cells in ventricular fluid may be present (more often in neonates), as may subdural effusions and, rarely, empyema. Perivascular inflammatory infiltrates also may be present, and the ependymal membrane may be disrupted. Vascular and parenchymal cerebral changes characterized by polymorphonuclear infiltrates extending to the subintimal region of the small arteries and veins, vasculitis, thrombosis of small cortical veins, occlusion of major venous sinuses, necrotizing arteritis producing subarachnoid hemorrhage, and, rarely, cerebral cortical necrosis in the absence of identifiable thrombosis have been described at autopsy. **Cerebral infarction,** resulting from vascular occlusion due to inflammation, vasospasm, and thrombosis, is a frequent sequela. Infarct size ranges from microscopic to involvement of an entire hemisphere.

Inflammation of spinal nerves and roots produces meningeal signs, and inflammation of the cranial nerves produces cranial neuropathies of optic, oculomotor, facial, and auditory nerves. Increased intracranial pressure (ICP) also produces oculomotor nerve palsy due to the presence of temporal lobe compression of the nerve during tentorial herniation. Abducens nerve palsy may be a nonlocalizing sign of elevated ICP.

Increased ICP is due to cell death (cytotoxic cerebral edema), cytokine-induced increased capillary vascular permeability (vasogenic cerebral edema), and, possibly, increased hydrostatic pressure (interstitial cerebral edema) after obstructed reabsorption of CSF in the arachnoid villus or obstruction of the flow of fluid from the ventricles. ICP may exceed 300 mm H_2O; cerebral perfusion may be further compromised if the cerebral perfusion pressure (mean arterial pressure minus ICP) is <50 cm H_2O due to systemic hypotension with reduced cerebral blood flow. The syndrome of inappropriate antidiuretic hormone secretion (SIADH) may produce excessive water retention and potentially increase the risk of elevated ICP (see Chapter 560). Hypotonicity of brain extracellular spaces may cause cytotoxic edema after cell swelling and lysis. Tentorial, falx, or cerebellar herniation does not usually occur because the increased ICP is transmitted to the entire subarachnoid space and there is little structural displacement. Furthermore, if the fontanels are still patent, increased ICP is not always dissipated.

Hydrocephalus can occur as an acute complication of bacterial meningitis. It most often takes the form of a communicating hydrocephalus due to adhesive thickening of the arachnoid villi around the cisterns at the base of the brain. Thus, there is interference with the normal resorption of CSF. Less often, obstructive hydrocephalus develops after fibrosis and gliosis of the aqueduct of Sylvius or the foramina of Magendie and Luschka.

Raised CSF protein levels are due in part to increased vascular permeability of the blood-brain barrier and the loss of albumin-rich fluid from the capillaries and veins traversing the subdural space. Continued transudation may result in subdural effusions, usually found in the later phase of acute bacterial meningitis. **Hypoglycorrhachia** (reduced CSF glucose levels) is due to decreased glucose transport by the cerebral tissue.

Damage to the cerebral cortex may be due to the focal or diffuse effects of vascular occlusion (infarction, necrosis, lactic acidosis), hypoxia, bacterial invasion (cerebritis), toxic encephalopathy (bacterial toxins), elevated ICP, ventriculitis, and transudation (subdural effusions). These pathologic factors result in the clinical manifestations of impaired consciousness, seizures, cranial nerve deficits, motor and sensory deficits, and later psychomotor retardation.

PATHOGENESIS. Bacterial meningitis most commonly results from hematogenous dissemination of microorganisms from a distant site of infection; **bacteremia** usually precedes meningitis or occurs concomitantly. Bacterial colonization of the nasopharynx with a potentially pathogenic microorganism is the usual source of the bacteremia. There may be prolonged carriage of the colonizing organisms without disease or, more likely, rapid invasion after recent colonization. Prior or concurrent viral upper respiratory tract infection may enhance the pathogenicity of bacteria producing meningitis.

N. meningitidis and *H. influenzae* type b attach to mucosal epithelial cell receptors by pili. After attachment to epithelial cells, bacteria breach the mucosa and enter the circulation. *N. meningitidis* may be transported across the mucosal surface within a phagocytic vacuole after ingestion by the epithelial cell. Bacterial survival in the bloodstream is enhanced by large bacterial capsules that interfere with opsonic phagocytosis and are associated with increased virulence. Host-related developmental defects in bacterial opsonic phagocytosis also contribute to the bacteremia. In young, nonimmune hosts, the defect may be due to an absence of preformed IgM or IgG anticapsular antibodies, whereas in immunodeficient patients, various deficiencies of components of the complement or properdin system may interfere with effective opsonic phagocytosis. Splenic dysfunction may also reduce opsonic phagocytosis by the reticuloendothelial system.

Bacteria gain entry to the CSF through the choroid plexus of the lateral ventricles and the meninges and then circulate to the extracerebral CSF and subarachnoid space. Bacteria rapidly multiply because the CSF concentrations of complement and antibody are inadequate to contain bacterial proliferation. Chemotactic factors then incite a local inflammatory response characterized by polymorphonuclear cell infiltration. The presence of bacterial cell wall lipopolysaccharide (endotoxin) of gram-negative bacteria (*H. influenzae* type b, *N. meningitidis*) and of pneumococcal cell wall components (teichoic acid, peptidoglycan) stimulates a marked inflammatory response, with local production of tumor necrosis factor, interleukin 1, prostaglandin E, and other inflammatory mediators. The subsequent inflammatory response is characterized by neutrophilic infiltration, increased vascular permeability, alterations of the blood-brain barrier, and vascular thrombosis. Meningitis-associated brain injury is not simply caused by viable bacteria but occurs as a consequence of the host reaction to the inflammatory cascade initiated by bacterial components.

Rarely, meningitis may follow bacterial invasion from a contiguous focus of infection such as paranasal sinusitis, otitis media, mastoiditis, orbital cellulitis, or cranial or vertebral osteomyelitis or may occur after introduction of bacteria via penetrating cranial trauma, dermal sinus tracts, or meningomyeloceles.

CLINICAL MANIFESTATIONS. The onset of acute meningitis has two predominant patterns. The more dramatic and, fortunately, less common presentation is sudden onset with rapidly progressive manifestations of shock, purpura, disseminated intravascular coagulation (DIC), and reduced levels of consciousness often resulting in progression to coma or death within 24 hr. More often, meningitis is preceded by several days of fever accompanied by upper respiratory tract or gastrointestinal symptoms, followed by nonspecific signs of CNS infection such as increasing lethargy and irritability.

The signs and symptoms of meningitis are related to the nonspecific findings associated with a systemic infection and to manifestations of meningeal irritation. Nonspecific findings include fever, anorexia and poor feeding, headache, symptoms of upper respiratory tract infection, myalgias, arthralgias, tachycardia, hypotension, and various cutaneous signs, such as petechiae, purpura, or an erythematous macular rash. Meningeal irritation is manifested as nuchal rigidity, back pain, **Kernig sign** (flexion of the hip 90 degrees with subsequent pain with extension of the leg), and **Brudzinski sign** (involuntary flexion of the knees and hips after passive flexion of the neck while supine). In some children, particularly in those younger than 12–18 mo, Kernig and Brudzinski signs are not consistently present. Indeed fever, headache, and nuchal rigidity are present in only 40% of adults with bacterial meningitis. Increased ICP is suggested by headache, emesis, bulging fontanel or diastasis (widening) of the sutures, oculomotor (anisocoria, ptosis) or abducens nerve paralysis, hypertension with bradycardia, apnea or hyperventilation, decorticate or decerebrate posturing, stupor, coma, or signs of herniation. Papilledema is uncommon in uncomplicated meningitis and should suggest a more chronic process, such as the presence of an intracranial abscess, subdural empyema, or occlusion of a dural venous sinus. Focal neurologic signs usually are due to vascular occlusion. Cranial neuropathies of the ocular, oculomotor, abducens, facial, and auditory nerves may also be due to focal inflammation. Overall, about 10–20% of children with bacterial meningitis have focal neurologic signs.

Seizures (focal or generalized) due to cerebritis, infarction, or electrolyte disturbances occur in 20–30% of patients with meningitis. Seizures that occur on presentation or within the 1st 4 days of onset are usually of no prognostic significance. Seizures that persist after the 4th day of illness and those that are difficult to treat may be associated with a poor prognosis.

Alterations of mental status are common among patients with meningitis and may be due to increased ICP, cerebritis, or hypotension; manifestations include irritability, lethargy, stupor, obtundation, and coma. Comatose patients have a poor prognosis. Additional manifestations of meningitis include photophobia and tache cérébrale, which is elicited by stroking the skin with a blunt object and observing a raised red streak within 30–60 sec.

DIAGNOSIS. The diagnosis of acute pyogenic meningitis is confirmed by analysis of the CSF, which typically reveals microorganisms on Gram stain and culture, a neutrophilic pleocytosis, elevated protein, and reduced glucose concentrations (see Table 602-1). LP should be performed when bacterial meningitis is suspected. **Contraindications** for an immediate LP include (1) evidence of increased ICP (other than a bulging fontanel), such as 3rd or 6th cranial nerve palsy with a depressed level of consciousness, or hypertension and bradycardia with respiratory abnormalities (see Chapter 591); (2) severe cardiopulmonary compromise requiring prompt resuscitative measures for shock or in patients in whom positioning for the LP would further compromise cardiopulmonary function; and (3) infection of the skin overlying the site of the LP. Thrombocytopenia is a relative contraindication for LP. If an LP is delayed, empirical antibiotic therapy should be initiated. CT scanning for evidence of a brain abscess or increased ICP should not delay therapy. LP may be performed after increased ICP has been treated or a brain abscess has been excluded.

Blood cultures should be performed in all patients with suspected meningitis. Blood cultures reveal the responsible bacteria in up to 80–90% of cases of meningitis.

Lumbar Puncture (See Also Chapter 591). The CSF leukocyte count in bacterial meningitis usually is elevated to $>1{,}000/mm^3$ and, typically, there is a neutrophilic predominance (75–95%). Turbid CSF is present when the CSF leukocyte count exceeds $200–400/mm^3$. Normal healthy neonates may have as many as 30 leukocytes/mm^3 (usually <10), but older children without viral or bacterial meningitis have <5 leukocytes/mm^3 in the CSF; in both age groups there is a predominance of lymphocytes or monocytes.

A CSF leukocyte count $<250/mm^3$ may be present in as many as 20% of patients with acute bacterial meningitis; pleocytosis may be absent in patients with severe overwhelming sepsis and meningitis and is a poor prognostic sign. Pleocytosis with a lymphocyte predominance may be present during the early stage of acute bacterial meningitis; conversely, neutrophilic pleocytosis may be present in patients in the early stages of acute viral meningitis. The shift to lymphocytic-monocytic predominance in viral meningitis invariably occurs within 8 to 24 hr of the initial LP. The Gram stain is positive in 70–90% of patients with untreated bacterial meningitis.

A diagnostic conundrum in the evaluation of children with suspected bacterial meningitis is the analysis of CSF obtained from children already receiving antibiotic (usually oral) therapy. This is an important issue, because 25–50% of children being evaluated for bacterial meningitis are receiving oral antibiotics when their CSF is obtained. CSF obtained from children with bacterial meningitis, after the initiation of antibiotics, may be negative on Gram stain and culture. Pleocytosis with a predominance of neutrophils, elevated protein level, and a reduced concentration of CSF glucose usually persist for several days after the administration of appropriate intravenous antibiotics. Therefore, despite negative cultures, the presumptive diagnosis of bacterial meningitis can be made. Some clinicians test CSF for the presence of bacterial antigens if the child has been pretreated with antibiotics and the diagnosis of bacterial meningitis is in doubt. These tests have technical limitations.

A traumatic LP may complicate the diagnosis of meningitis. Repeat LP at a higher interspace may produce less hemorrhagic fluid, but this fluid usually also contains red blood cells. Interpretation of CSF leukocytes and protein concentration are affected by LPs that are traumatic, although the Gram stain, culture, and glucose level may not be influenced. Although methods for correcting for the presence of red blood cells have been proposed, it is prudent to rely on the bacteriologic results rather than attempt to interpret the CSF leukocyte and protein results of a traumatic LP.

Differential Diagnosis. In addition to *S. pneumoniae, N. meningitidis,* and *H. influenzae* type b, many other microorganisms can cause generalized infection of the CNS with similar clinical manifestations. These organisms include less typical bacteria, such as *Mycobacterium tuberculosis, Nocardia* spp., *Treponema pallidum* (syphilis), and *Borrelia burgdorferi* (Lyme disease); fungi, such as those endemic to specific geographic areas (*Coccidioides, Histoplasma,* and *Blastomyces*) and those responsible for infections in compromised hosts (*Candida, Cryptococcus,* and *Aspergillus*); parasites, such as *Toxoplasma gondii* and those that cause cysticercosis and, most frequently, viruses (see Chapter 602.2) [Table 602-2]. Focal infections of the CNS including brain abscess and parameningeal abscess (subdural empyema, cranial and spinal epidural abscess) may also be confused with meningitis. In addition, noninfectious illnesses can cause generalized inflammation of the CNS. Relative to infections, these disorders are uncommon and include malignancy, collagen vascular syndromes, and exposure to toxins (see Table 602-2).

Determining the specific cause of CNS infection is facilitated by careful examination of the CSF with specific stains (Kinyoun carbol fuchsin for mycobacteria, India ink for fungi), cytology, antigen detection *(Cryptococcus)*, serology (syphilis, West Nile virus, arboviruses, herpes simplex), viral culture (enterovirus), and polymerase chain reaction (herpes simplex, enterovirus, and others). Other potentially valuable diagnostic tests include blood cultures, CT or MRI of the brain, serologic tests, and, rarely, brain biopsy.

Acute viral meningoencephalitis is the most likely infection to be confused with bacterial meningitis (Tables 602-2 and 602-3). Although, in general, children with viral meningoencephalitis appear less ill than those with bacterial meningitis, both types of infection have a spectrum of severity. Some children with bacterial meningitis may have relatively mild signs and symptoms, whereas some with viral meningoencephalitis may be critically ill. Although classic CSF profiles associated with bacterial versus viral infection tend to be distinct (see Table 602-1), specific test results may have considerable overlap.

TREATMENT. The therapeutic approach to patients with presumed bacterial meningitis depends on the nature of the initial manifestations of the illness. A child with rapidly progressing disease of less than 24 hr duration, in the absence of increased ICP, should receive antibiotics as soon as possible after an LP is performed. If there are signs of increased ICP or focal neurologic findings, antibiotics should be given without performing an LP and before obtaining a CT scan. Increased ICP should be treated simultaneously (see Chapter 67). Immediate treatment of associated multiple organ system failure (see Chapter 71), shock (see Chapter 68), and acute respiratory distress syndrome (see Chapter 69) is also indicated.

Patients who have a more protracted subacute course and become ill over a 4–7 day period should also be evaluated for signs of increased ICP and focal neurologic deficits. Unilateral headache, papilledema, and other signs of increased ICP suggest a focal lesion such as a brain or epidural abscess, or subdural empyema. Under these circumstances, antibiotic therapy should

TABLE 602-2. Clinical Conditions and Infectious Agents Associated with Aseptic Meningitis

VIRUSES
Enteroviruses (coxsackievirus, echovirus, poliovirus, enterovirus)
Arboviruses: Eastern equine, Western equine, Venezuelan equine, St. Louis encephalitis, Powassan and California encephalitis, West Nile virus, Colorado tick fever
Herpes simplex (types 1, 2)
Human herpesvirus type 6
Varicella-zoster virus
Epstein-Barr virus
Parvovirus B19
Cytomegalovirus
Adenovirus
Variola (smallpox)
Measles
Mumps
Rubella
Influenza A and B
Parainfluenza
Rhinovirus
Rabies
Lymphocytic choriomeningitis
Rotaviruses
Coronaviruses
Human immunodeficiency virus type 1

BACTERIA
Mycobacterium tuberculosis
Leptospira species (leptospirosis)
Treponema pallidum (syphilis)
Borrelia species (relapsing fever)
Borrelia burgdorferi (Lyme disease)
Nocardia species (nocardiosis)
Brucella species
Bartonella species (cat-scratch disease)
Rickettsia rickettsiae (Rocky Mountain spotted fever)
Rickettsia prowazekii (typhus)
Ehrlichia canis
Coxiella burnetii
Mycoplasma pneumoniae
Mycoplasma hominis
Chlamydia trachomatis
Chlamydia psittaci
Chlamydia pneumoniae
Partially treated bacterial meningitis

BACTERIAL PARAMENINGEAL FOCUS
Sinusitis
Mastoiditis
Brain abscess
Subdural-epidural empyema
Cranial osteomyelitis

FUNGI
Coccidioides immitis (coccidioidomycosis)
Blastomyces dermatitidis (blastomycosis)
Cryptococcus neoformans (cryptococcosis)
Histoplasma capsulatum (histoplasmosis)
Candida species
Other fungi (*Alternaria, Aspergillus, Cephalosporium, Cladosporium, Dreschlera hawaiiensis, Paracoccidioides brasiliensis, Petriellidium boydii, Sporotrichum schenckii, Ustilago* species, *Zygomycetes*

PARASITES (EOSINOPHILIC)
Angiostrongylus cantonensis
Gnathostoma spinigerum
Baylisascaris procyonis
Strongyloides stercoralis
Trichinella spiralis
Toxocara canis
Taenia solium (cysticercosis)
Paragonimus westermani
Schistosoma species
Fasciola species

PARASITES (NONEOSINOPHILIC)
Toxoplasma gondii (toxoplasmosis)
Acanthamoeba species
Naegleria fowleri
Malaria

POSTINFECTIOUS
Vaccines: rabies, influenza, measles, poliovirus
Demyelinating or allergic encephalitis

SYSTEMIC OR IMMUNOLOGICALLY MEDIATED
Bacterial endocarditis
Kawasaki disease
Systemic lupus erythematosus
Vasculitis, including polyarteritis nodosa
Sjögren syndrome
Mixed connective tissue disease
Rheumatoid arthritis
Behçet syndrome
Wegener granulomatosis
Lymphomatoid granulomatosis
Granulomatous arteritis
Sarcoidosis
Familial Mediterranean fever
Vogt-Koyanagi-Harada syndrome

MALIGNANCY
Leukemia
Lymphoma
Metastatic carcinoma
Central nervous system tumor (e.g., craniopharyngioma, glioma, ependymoma, astrocytoma, medulloblastoma, teratoma)

DRUGS
Intrathecal infections (contrast media, serum, antibiotics, antineoplastic agents)
Nonsteroidal anti-inflammatory agents
OKT3 monoclonal antibodies
Carbamazepine
Azathioprine
Intravenous immune globulins
Antibiotics (trimethoprim-sulfamethoxazole, sulfasalazine, ciprofloxacin, isoniazid)

MISCELLANEOUS
Heavy metal poisoning (lead, arsenic)
Foreign bodies (shunt, reservoir)
Subarachnoid hemorrhage
Postictal state
Postmigraine state
Mollaret syndrome (recurrent)
Intraventricular hemorrhage (neonate)
Familial hemophagocytic syndrome
Post neurosurgery
Dermoid-epidermoid cyst

Compiled from Cherry JD: Aseptic meningitis and viral meningitis. In Feigin RD, Cherry JD (editors): *Textbook of Pediatric Infectious Diseases*, 4th ed. Philadelphia, WB Saunders, 1998, p 450; and from Davis LE: Aseptic and viral meningitis. In Long SS, Pickering LK, Prober CG (editors): *Principles and Practice of Pediatric Infectious Disease*. New York, Churchill Livingstone, 1997, p 329; and from Kliegman RM, Greenbaum LA, Lye PS: *Practical Strategies in Pediatric Diagnosis Therapy*. 2nd ed. Philadelphia, Elsevier, 2004, p 961.

be initiated before LP and CT scanning. If no signs of increased ICP are evident, an LP should be performed.

Initial Antibiotic Therapy. The initial (empirical) choice of therapy for meningitis in immunocompetent infants and children is primarily influenced by the antibiotic susceptibilities (Table 602-4) of *S. pneumoniae*. Selected antibiotics should achieve bactericidal levels in the CSF. Although there are substantial geographic differences in the frequency of resistance of *S. pneumoniae* to antibiotics, rates are increasing throughout the world. In the United States, 25–50% of strains of *S. pneumoniae* are currently resistant to penicillin; relative resistance (MIC = 0.1–1.0 μg/mL) is more common than high-level resistance (MIC = 2.0 μg/mL). Resistance to cefotaxime and ceftriaxone is also evident in up to 25% of isolates. In contrast, most strains of *N. meningitidis* are sensitive to penicillin and cephalosporins, although rare resistant isolates have been reported. Approxi-

TABLE 602-3. Classification of Encephalitis by Cause and Source

I. INFECTIONS: VIRAL

A. Spread: person to person only
   1. Mumps: frequent in an unimmunized population; often mild
   2. Measles: may have serious sequelae
   3. Enteroviruses: frequent at all ages; more serious in newborns
   4. Rubella: uncommon; sequelae rare except in congenital rubella
   5. Herpesvirus group
      a. Herpes simplex (types 1 and 2, possibly 6): relatively common; sequelae frequent; devastating in newborns
      b. Varicella-zoster virus: uncommon; serious sequelae not rare
      c. Cytomegalovirus, congenital or acquired: may have delayed sequelae in congenital type
      d. Epstein-Barr virus (infectious mononucleosis): not common
   6. Pox group
      a. Vaccinia and variola: uncommon, but serious CNS damage occurs
   7. Parvovirus (erythema infectiosum): not common
   8. Influenza A and B
   9. Adenovirus
   10. Other: reoviruses, respiratory syncytial, parainfluenza, hepatitis B

B. Arthropod-borne agents
   Arboviruses: spread to humans by mosquitoes or ticks; seasonal epidemics depend on ecology of the insect vector; the following occur in the United States:

Eastern equine	California
Western equine	Powassan
Venezuelan equine	Dengue
St. Louis	Colorado tick fever
West Nile	

C. Spread by warm-blooded mammals
   1. Rabies: saliva of many domestic and wild mammalian species
   2. Herpesvirus simiae ("B" virus): monkeys' saliva
   3. Lymphocytic choriomeningitis: rodents' excreta

II. INFECTIONS: NONVIRAL

A. Rickettsial: in Rocky Mountain spotted fever and typhus; encephalitic component from cerebral vasculitis
B. *Mycoplasma pneumoniae:* interval of some days between respiratory and CNS symptoms
C. Bacterial: tuberculous and other bacterial meningitis; often has encephalitic component
D. Spirochetal: syphilis, congenital or acquired; leptospirosis; Lyme disease
E. Cat-scratch disease
F. Fungal: immunologically compromised patients at special risk: cryptococcosis; histoplasmosis; aspergillosis; mucormycosis; candidosis; coccidioidomycosis
G. Protozoal: *Plasmodium, Trypanosoma, Naegleria,* and *Acanthamoeba* species; *Toxoplasma gondii*
H. Metazoal: trichinosis; echinococcosis; cysticercosis; schistosomiasis

III. PARAINFECTIOUS: POSTINFECTIOUS, ALLERGIC

Patients in whom an infectious agent or one of its components plays a contributory role in etiology, but the intact infectious agent is not isolated in vitro from the nervous system; it is postulated that in this group, the influence of cell-mediated antigen-antibody complexes plus complement is especially important in producing the observed tissue damage

A. Associated with specific diseases (these agents may also cause direct CNS damage; see I and II

Measles	Rickettsial infections
Rubella	Influenza A and B
Mumps	Varicella-zoster
Mycoplasma pneumoniae	

B. Associated with vaccines

Rabies	Measles
Vaccinia	Yellow fever

IV. HUMAN SLOW-VIRUS DISEASES

Accumulating evidence that viruses frequently acquired earlier in life, not necessarily with detectable acute illness, participate in later chronic neurologic disease (similar events also known to occur in animals)

A. Subacute sclerosing panencephalitis; measles; rubella?
B. Creutzfeldt-Jakob disease (spongiform encephalopathy)
C. Progressive multifocal leukoencephalopathy
D. Kuru (Fore tribe in New Guinea only)
E. Human immunodeficiency virus

V. UNKNOWN: COMPLEX GROUP

This group constitutes more than two thirds of the cases of encephalitis reported to the Centers for Disease Control and Prevention, Atlanta, Georgia; the yearly epidemic curve of these undiagnosed cases suggests that the majority are probably caused by enteroviruses and/or arboviruses

There is also a miscellaneous group that is based on clinical criteria: Reye syndrome is one current example; others include the extinct von Economo encephalitis (epidemic during 1918–1928); myoclonic encephalopathy of infancy; retinomeningoencephalitis with papilledema and retinal hemorrhage; recurrent encephalomyelitis (? allergic or autoimmune); pseudotumor cerebri; and epidemic neuromyasthenia (Iceland disease)

An encephalitic clinical pattern may follow ingestion or absorption of a number of known and unknown toxic substances; these include ingestion of lead and mercury and percutaneous absorption of hexachlorophene as a skin disinfectant and gamma benzene hexachloride as a scabicide

CNS, central nervous system.

Modified from Behrman RE (editor): *Nelson Textbook of Pediatrics,* 14th ed. Philadelphia, WB Saunders, 1992, p 667. From Kliegman RM, Greenbaum LA, Lye PS: *Practical Strategies in Pediatric Diagnosis and Therapy,* 2nd ed. Philadelphia, Elsevier, 2004, p 967.

TABLE 602-4. Antibiotics Used for the Treatment of Bacterial Meningitis*

DRUG	NEONATES 0–7 Days	NEONATES 8–28 Days	INFANTS AND CHILDREN
Amikacin[†‡]	15–20 divided q12h	20–30 divided q8h	20–30 divided q8h
Ampicillin	200–300 divided q8h	300 divided q4h or q6h	300 divided q4–6h
Cefotaxime	100 divided q12h	150–200 divided q8h or q6h	200–300 divided q8h or q6h
Ceftriaxone[§]	—	—	100 divided q12h or q24h
Ceftazidime	150 divided q12h	150 divided q8h	150 divided q8h
Gentamicin[†‡]	5 divided q12h	7.5 divided q8h	7.5 divided q8h
Meropenem	—	—	120 divided q8h
Nafcillin	100–150 divided q8h or q12h	150–200 divided q8h or q6h	150–200 divided q4h or q6h
Penicillin G	250,000–450,000 divided q8h	450,000 divided q6h	450,000 divided q4h or q6h
Rifampin	—	—	20 divided q12h
Tobramycin[†‡]	5 divided q12h	7.5 divided q8h	7.5 divided q8h
Vancomycin[†‡]	30 divided q12h	30–45 divided q8h	60 divided q6h

*Dosages in mg/kg (U/kg for penicillin G) per day.

†Smaller doses and longer dosing intervals, especially for aminoglycosides and vancomycin for very low birthweight neonates, may be advisable.

‡Monitoring of serum levels is recommended to ensure safe and therapeutic values.

§Use in neonates is not recommended because of inadequate experience in neonatal meningitis.

Modified from Klein JO: Antimicrobial treatment and prevention of meningitis. *Pediatr Ann* 1994;23:76; and from Kliegman RM, Greenbaum LA, Lye PS: *Practical Strategies in Pediatric Diagnosis and Therapy,* 2nd ed. Philadelphia, Elsevier, 2004, p 963.

mately 30–40% of isolates of *H. influenzae* type b produce β-lactamases and, therefore, are resistant to ampicillin. These β-lactamase-producing strains are sensitive to the extended-spectrum cephalosporins.

Based on the substantial rate of resistance of *S. pneumoniae* to β-lactam drugs, vancomycin (60 mg/kg/24 hr, given every 6 hr) is recommended as part of initial empirical therapy. Because of the efficacy of 3rd-generation cephalosporins in the therapy of meningitis caused by sensitive *S. pneumoniae, N. meningitidis,* and *H. influenzae* type b, cefotaxime (200 mg/kg/24 hr, given every 6 hr) or ceftriaxone (100 mg/kg/24 hr administered once per day or 50 mg/kg/dose, given every 12 hr) should also be used in initial empirical therapy. Patients allergic to β-lactam antibiotics and >1 mo of age can be treated with chloramphenicol, 100 mg/kg/24 hr, given every 6 hr. Alternately, patients can be desensitized to the antibiotic (see Chapter 150).

If *L. monocytogenes* infection is suspected, as in young infants or those with a T-lymphocyte deficiency, ampicillin (200 mg/kg/24 hr, given every 6 hr) also should also be given because cephalosporins are inactive against *L. monocytogenes*. Intravenous trimethoprim-sulfamethoxazole is an alternative treatment for *L. monocytogenes*.

If a patient is immunocompromised and gram-negative bacterial meningitis is suspected, initial therapy might include ceftazidime and an aminoglycoside.

DURATION OF ANTIBIOTIC THERAPY. Therapy for uncomplicated penicillin-sensitive *S. pneumoniae* meningitis should be completed with 10 to 14 days with a 3rd-generation cephalosporin or intravenous penicillin (400,000 U/kg/24 hr, given every 4–6 hr). If the isolate is resistant to penicillin and the 3rd-generation cephalosporin, therapy should be completed with vancomycin. Intravenous penicillin (400,000 U/kg/24 hr) for 5–7 days is the treatment of choice for uncomplicated *N. meningitidis* meningitis. Uncomplicated *H. influenzae* type b meningitis should be treated for ≈7–10 days. Patients who receive intravenous or oral antibiotics before LP and who do not have an identifiable pathogen but do have evidence of an acute bacterial infection on the basis of their CSF profile should continue to receive therapy with ceftriaxone or cefotaxime for 7–10 days. If focal signs are present or the child does not respond to treatment, a parameningeal focus may be present and a CT or MRI scan should be performed.

A routine repeat LP is not indicated in patients with uncomplicated meningitis due to antibiotic-sensitive *S. pneumoniae, N. meningitidis*, or *H. influenzae* type b. Repeat examination of CSF is indicated in some neonates, in patients with gram-negative bacillary meningitis, or in infection caused by a β-lactam-resistant *S. pneumoniae*. The CSF should be sterile within 24–48 hr of initiation of appropriate antibiotic therapy.

Meningitis due to *Escherichia coli* or *P. aeruginosa* requires therapy with a 3rd-generation cephalosporin active against the isolate in vitro. Most isolates of *E. coli* are sensitive to cefotaxime or ceftriaxone, and most isolates of *P. aeruginosa* are sensitive to ceftazidime. Gram-negative bacillary meningitis should be treated for 3 wk or for at least 2 wk after CSF sterilization, which may occur after 2–10 days of treatment.

Side effects of antibiotic therapy of meningitis include phlebitis, drug fever, rash, emesis, oral candidiasis, and diarrhea. Ceftriaxone may cause reversible gallbladder pseudolithiasis, detectable by abdominal ultrasonography. This is usually asymptomatic but may be associated with emesis and upper right quadrant pain.

Corticosteroids. Rapid killing of bacteria in the CSF effectively sterilizes the meningeal infection but releases toxic cell products after cell lysis (cell wall endotoxin) that precipitates the cytokine-mediated inflammatory cascade. The resultant edema formation and neutrophilic infiltration may produce additional neurologic injury with worsening of CNS signs and symptoms. Therefore, agents that limit production of inflammatory mediators may be of benefit to patients with bacterial meningitis.

Data support the use of intravenous dexamethasone, 0.15 mg/kg/dose given every 6 hr for 2 days, in the treatment of children older than 6 wk with acute bacterial meningitis caused by *H. influenzae* type b. Among children with meningitis due to *H. influenzae* type b, corticosteroid recipients have a shorter duration of fever, lower CSF protein and lactate levels, and a reduction in sensorineural hearing loss. Data in children regarding the benefit, if any, of corticosteroids in the treatment of meningitis caused by other bacteria are inconclusive. Early treatment of adults with bacterial meningitis, especially those with pneumococcal meningitis, however, results in improved outcome.

Corticosteroids appear to have maximum benefit if given 1–2 hr before antibiotics are initiated. They also may be effective if given concurrently with or soon after the 1st dose of antibiotics. Complications of corticosteroids include gastrointestinal bleeding, hypertension, hyperglycemia, leukocytosis, and rebound fever after the last dose.

Supportive Care. Repeated medical and neurologic assessments of patients with bacterial meningitis are essential to identify early signs of cardiovascular, CNS, and metabolic complications. Pulse rate, blood pressure, and respiratory rate should be monitored frequently. Neurologic assessment, including pupillary reflexes, level of consciousness, motor strength, cranial nerve signs, and evaluation for seizures, should be made frequently in the 1st 72 hr, when the risk of neurologic complications is greatest. Important laboratory studies include an assessment of blood urea nitrogen; serum sodium, chloride, potassium, and bicarbonate levels; urine output and specific gravity; complete blood and platelet counts; and, in the presence of petechiae, purpura, or abnormal bleeding, measure of coagulation function (fibrinogen, prothrombin, and partial thromboplastin times).

Patients should initially receive nothing by mouth. If a patient is judged to be normovolemic, with normal blood pressure, intravenous fluid administration should be restricted to one half to two thirds of maintenance, or 800–1,000 mL/m^2/24 hr, until it can be established that increased ICP or SIADH is not present. Fluid administration may be returned to normal (1,500–1,700 mL/m^2/24 hr) when serum sodium levels are normal. Fluid restriction is not appropriate in the presence of systemic hypotension because reduced blood pressure may result in reduced cerebral perfusion pressure and CNS ischemia. Therefore, shock must be treated aggressively to prevent brain and other organ dysfunction (acute tubular necrosis, acute respiratory distress syndrome). Patients with shock, a markedly elevated ICP, coma, and refractory seizures require intensive monitoring with central arterial and venous access and frequent vital signs, necessitating admission to a pediatric intensive care unit. Patients with septic shock may require fluid resuscitation and therapy with vasoactive agents such as dopamine and epinephrine (see Chapter 176). The goal of such therapy in patients with meningitis is to avoid excessive increases in ICP without compromising blood flow and oxygen delivery to vital organs.

Neurologic complications include increased **ICP** with subsequent herniation, seizures, and an enlarging head circumference due to a subdural effusion or hydrocephalus. Signs of increased ICP should be treated emergently with endotracheal intubation and hyperventilation (to maintain the pCO_2 at ≈25 mm Hg). In addition, intravenous furosemide (Lasix, 1 mg/kg) and mannitol (0.5–1.0 g/kg) osmotherapy may reduce ICP (see Chapter 67). Furosemide reduces brain swelling by venodilation and diuresis without increasing intracranial blood volume, whereas mannitol produces an osmolar gradient between the brain and plasma, thus shifting fluid from the CNS to the plasma, with subsequent excretion during an osmotic diuresis.

Seizures are common during the course of bacterial meningitis. Immediate therapy for seizures includes intravenous diazepam (0.1–0.2 mg/kg/dose) or lorazepam (0.05–0.10 mg/kg/dose), and careful attention paid to the risk of respiratory suppression. Serum glucose, calcium, and sodium levels should be monitored.

After immediate management of seizures, patients should receive phenytoin (15–20 mg/kg loading dose, 5 mg/kg/24 hr maintenance) to reduce the likelihood of recurrence. Phenytoin is preferred to phenobarbital because it produces less CNS depression and permits assessment of a patient's level of consciousness. Serum phenytoin levels should be monitored to maintain them in the therapeutic range (10–20 μg/mL).

COMPLICATIONS. During the treatment of meningitis, acute CNS complications can include seizures, increased ICP, cranial nerve palsies, stroke, cerebral or cerebellar herniation, and thrombosis of the dural venous sinuses.

Collections of fluid in the subdural space develop in 10–30% of patients with meningitis and are asymptomatic in 85–90% of patients. **Subdural effusions** are especially common in infants. Symptomatic subdural effusions may result in a bulging fontanel, diastasis of sutures, enlarging head circumference, emesis, seizures, fever, and abnormal results of cranial transillumination. CT or MRI scanning confirms the presence of a subdural effusion. In the presence of increased ICP or a depressed level of consciousness, symptomatic subdural effusion should be treated by aspiration through the open fontanel (see Chapter 591). Fever alone is not an indication for aspiration.

SIADH occurs in some patients with meningitis, resulting in hyponatremia and reduced serum osmolality. This may exacerbate cerebral edema or result in hyponatremic seizures (see Chapter 55).

Fever associated with bacterial meningitis usually resolves within 5–7 days of the onset of therapy. **Prolonged fever** (>10 days) is noted in about 10% of patients. Prolonged fever is usually due to intercurrent viral infection, nosocomial or secondary bacterial infection, thrombophlebitis, or drug reaction. Secondary fever refers to the recrudescence of elevated temperature after an afebrile interval. Nosocomial infections are especially important to consider in the evaluation of these patients. Pericarditis or arthritis may occur in patients being treated for meningitis, especially that caused by *N. meningitidis*. Involvement of these sites may result either from bacterial dissemination or from immune complex deposition. In general, infectious pericarditis or arthritis occurs earlier in the course of treatment than does immune-mediated disease.

Thrombocytosis, eosinophilia, and anemia may develop during therapy for meningitis. Anemia may be due to hemolysis or bone marrow suppression. DIC is most often associated with the rapidly progressive pattern of presentation and is noted most commonly in patients with shock and purpura. The combination of endotoxemia and severe hypotension initiates the coagulation cascade; the coexistence of ongoing thrombosis may produce symmetric peripheral gangrene.

PROGNOSIS. Appropriate antibiotic therapy and supportive care have reduced the mortality of bacterial meningitis after the neonatal period to <10%. The highest mortality rates are observed with pneumococcal meningitis. Severe neurodevelopmental sequelae may occur in 10–20% of patients recovering from bacterial meningitis, and as many as 50% have some, albeit subtle, neurobehavioral morbidity. The prognosis is poorest among infants younger than 6 mo and in those with high concentrations of bacteria/bacterial products in their CSF. Those with seizures occurring more than 4 days into therapy or with coma or focal neurologic signs on presentation have an increased risk of long-term sequelae. There does not appear to be a correlation between duration of symptoms before diagnosis of meningitis and outcome.

The most common neurologic sequelae include hearing loss, mental retardation, recurrent seizures, delay in acquisition of language, visual impairment, and behavioral problems. **Sensorineural hearing** loss is the most common sequela of bacterial meningitis and, usually, is already present at the time of initial presentation. It is due to labyrinthitis after cochlear infection and occurs in as many as 30% of patients with pneumococcal meningitis, 10% with meningococcal, and 5–20% of those with *H. influenzae* type b meningitis. Hearing loss may also be due to direct inflammation of the auditory nerve. All patients with bacterial meningitis should undergo careful audiologic assessment before or soon after discharge from the hospital. Frequent reassessment on an outpatient basis is indicated for patients who have a hearing deficit.

PREVENTION. Vaccination and antibiotic prophylaxis of susceptible at-risk contacts represent the two available means of reducing the likelihood of bacterial meningitis. The availability and application of each of these approaches depend on the specific infecting bacteria.

Neisseria Meningitidis. Chemoprophylaxis is recommended for all close contacts of patients with meningococcal meningitis regardless of age or immunization status. Close contacts should be treated with rifampin 10 mg/kg/dose every 12 hr (maximum dose of 600 mg) for 2 days as soon as possible after identification of a case of suspected meningococcal meningitis or sepsis. Close contacts include household, daycare center, and nursery school contacts and health care workers who have direct exposure to oral secretions (mouth-to-mouth resuscitation, suctioning, intubation). Exposed contacts should be treated immediately on suspicion of infection in the index patient; bacteriologic confirmation of infection should not be awaited. In addition, all contacts should be educated about the early signs of meningococcal disease and the need to seek prompt medical attention if these signs develop.

A quadrivalent (A,C,Y, W-135), conjugated vaccine (MCV-4; Menactra) is licensed by the U.S. Food and Drug Administration. The Advisory Committee on Immunization Practices (ACIP) to the Centers for Disease Control and Prevention (CDC) recommends routine administration of this vaccine to 11–12 year old adolescents. Meningococcal vaccine is also recommended for high-risk children older than 2 yr. High-risk patients include those with anatomic or functional asplenia or deficiencies of terminal complement proteins. Use of meningococcal vaccine should be considered for college freshmen, especially those who live in dormitories, because of an observed increased risk of invasive meningococcal infections compared to the risk in non-college-attending, age-matched controls. The risk for meningococcal disease among non-freshmen college students is similar to that for the general population of similar age. The vaccine also may be used as an adjunct with chemoprophylaxis for exposed contacts and during epidemics of meningococcal disease.

***Haemophilus Influenzae* Type B.** Rifampin prophylaxis should be given to all household contacts of patients with invasive disease caused by *H. influenzae* type b, if any close family member younger than 48 mo has not been fully immunized or if an immunocompromised person, of any age, resides in the household. A household contact is one who lives in the residence of the index case or who has spent a minimum of 4 hr with the index case for at least 5 of the 7 days preceding the patient's hospitalization. Family members should receive rifampin prophylaxis immediately after the diagnosis is suspected in the index case because >50% of secondary family cases occur in the 1st wk after the index patient has been hospitalized.

The dose of rifampin is 20 mg/kg/24 hr (maximum dose of 600 mg) given once each day for 4 days. Rifampin colors the urine and perspiration red-orange, stains contact lenses, and reduces the serum concentrations of some drugs, including oral contraceptives. Rifampin is contraindicated during pregnancy.

The most striking advance in the prevention of childhood bacterial meningitis followed the development and licensure of conjugated vaccines against *H. influenzae* type b. Four conjugate vaccines are licensed in the United States. Although each vaccine elicits different profiles of antibody response in infants immunized at 2–6 mo of age, all result in protective levels of antibody with efficacy rates against invasive infections ranging from 70 to 100%. Efficacy is not as consistent in Native American populations, a group recognized as having an especially high incidence of disease. All children should be immunized with *H. influenzae* type b conjugate vaccine beginning at 2 mo of age (see Chapter 170).

Streptococcus Pneumoniae. Routine administration of heptavalent conjugate vaccine against *S. pneumoniae* is recommended for children younger than 2 yr of age. The initial dose is given at ≈2 mo of age. Children who are at high risk of invasive pneumococcal infections, including those with functional or anatomic asplenia and those with underlying immunodeficiency (such as infection with HIV, primary immunodeficiency, and those receiving immunosuppressive therapy) should also receive the vaccine.

602.2 • Viral Meningoencephalitis

Viral meningoencephalitis is an acute inflammatory process involving the meninges and, to a variable degree, brain tissue. These infections are relatively common and may be caused by a number of different agents (see Table 602-3). The CSF is characterized by pleocytosis and the absence of microorganisms on Gram stain and routine bacterial culture. In most instances, the infections are self-limited. In some cases, substantial morbidity and mortality occur.

ETIOLOGY. **Enteroviruses** are the most common cause of viral meningoencephalitis. To date, more than 80 serotypes of these small RNA viruses have been identified. The severity of infection caused by enteroviruses ranges from mild, self-limited illness with primarily meningeal involvement to severe encephalitis resulting in death or significant sequelae.

Arboviruses are arthropod-borne agents, responsible for some cases of meningoencephalitis during summer months. Mosquitoes and ticks are the most common vectors, spreading disease to humans and other vertebrates, such as horses, after biting infected birds or small animals. Encephalitis in horses (“blind staggers”) may be the 1st indication of an incipient epidemic. Although rural exposure is most common, urban and suburban outbreaks also are frequent. The most common arboviruses responsible for CNS infection in the United States are West Nile virus (WNV) and St. Louis and California encephalitis viruses (see Chapter 264). West Nile virus made its appearance in the Western hemisphere in 1999. It has gradually made its way from the east to the west coast over successive summers. In 2002, WNV caused the largest epidemic of arboviral encephalitis ever described in North America, with transmission reported in 44 states and the District of Columbia. Cumulatively, from 1999 through 2005, a total of 46 states reported ~19,000 human infections caused by WNV. WNV may also be transmitted by blood transfusion, organ transplantation, or vertically across the placenta. Most children with WNV are either asymptomatic or have a nonspecific viral-like illness. Approximately 1% develop CNS disease; adults are more severely affected than children.

Several members of the **herpes family** of viruses can cause meningoencephalitis. Herpes simplex virus type 1 (HSV-1) is an important cause of severe, sporadic encephalitis in children and adults. Brain involvement usually is focal; progression to coma and death occurs in 70% of cases without antiviral therapy. Severe encephalitis with diffuse brain involvement is caused by herpes simplex virus type 2 (HSV-2) in neonates who usually contract the virus from their mothers at delivery. A mild transient form of meningoencephalitis may accompany genital herpes infection in sexually active adolescents; most of these infections are caused by HSV-2. Varicella-zoster virus (VZV) may cause CNS infection in close temporal relationship with chickenpox. The most common manifestation of CNS involvement is cerebellar ataxia, and the most severe is an acute encephalitis. After primary infection, VZV becomes latent in spinal and cranial nerve roots and ganglia, expressing itself later as herpes zoster, sometimes with accompanying mild meningoencephalitis. Cytomegalovirus (CMV) infection of the CNS may be part of congenital infection or disseminated disease in immunocompromised hosts, but it does not cause meningoencephalitis in normal infants and children. Epstein-Barr virus (EBV) has been associated with myriad CNS syndromes (see Chapter 251). Human herpes virus 6 (HHV-6) can cause encephalitis, especially among immunocompromised hosts.

Mumps is a common pathogen in regions where mumps vaccine is not widely used. Mumps meningoencephalitis is mild, but deafness due to damage of the 8th cranial nerve may be a sequela. Meningoencephalitis is caused occasionally by respiratory viruses (adenovirus, influenza virus, parainfluenza virus), rubeola, rubella, or rabies; it may follow live virus vaccinations against polio, measles, mumps, or rubella.

EPIDEMIOLOGY. The epidemiologic pattern of viral meningoencephalitis is primarily determined by the prevalence of enteroviruses, the most common etiology. Infection with enteroviruses is spread directly from person to person, with a usual incubation period of 4–6 days. Most cases in temperate climates occur in the summer and fall. Epidemiologic considerations in aseptic meningitis due to agents other than enteroviruses also include season, geography, climatic conditions, animal exposures, and factors related to the specific pathogen.

PATHOGENESIS AND PATHOLOGY. Neurologic damage is caused by direct invasion and destruction of neural tissues by actively multiplying viruses or by a host reaction to viral antigens. Tissue sections of the brain generally are characterized by meningeal congestion and mononuclear infiltration, perivascular cuffs of lymphocytes and plasma cells, some perivascular tissue necrosis with myelin breakdown, and neuronal disruption in various stages, including, ultimately, neuronophagia and endothelial proliferation or necrosis. A marked degree of demyelination with preservation of neurons and their axons is considered to represent predominantly “postinfectious” or “allergic” encephalitis.

The cerebral cortex, especially the temporal lobe, is often severely affected by HSV; the arboviruses tend to affect the entire brain; rabies has a predilection for the basal structures. Involvement of the spinal cord, nerve roots, and peripheral nerves is variable.

CLINICAL MANIFESTATIONS. The progression and severity of disease are determined by the relative degree of meningeal and parenchymal involvement, which, in part, is determined by the specific etiology. The clinical course resulting from infection with the same pathogen varies widely. Some children may appear to be mildly affected initially, only to lapse into coma and die suddenly. In others, the illness may be ushered in by high fever, violent convulsions interspersed with bizarre movements, and hallucinations alternating with brief periods of clarity, followed by complete recovery.

The onset of illness is generally acute, although CNS signs and symptoms are often preceded by a nonspecific febrile illness of a few days' duration. The presenting manifestations in older children are headache and hyperesthesia, and in infants, irritability and lethargy. Headache is most often frontal or generalized; adolescents frequently complain of retrobulbar pain. Fever, nausea and vomiting, photophobia, and pain in the neck, back, and legs are common. As body temperature increases, there may be mental dullness, progressing to stupor in combination with bizarre movements and convulsions. Focal neurologic signs may be stationary, progressive, or fluctuating. West Nile virus and nonpolio enteroviruses may cause anterior horn cell injury and a flaccid paralysis. Loss of bowel and bladder control and unprovoked emotional outbursts may occur.

Exanthems often precede or accompany the CNS signs, especially with echoviruses, coxsackieviruses, VZV, measles, rubella, and, occasionally, West Nile virus. Examination often reveals nuchal rigidity without significant localizing neurologic changes, at least at the onset.

Specific forms or complicating manifestations of CNS viral infection include Guillain-Barré syndrome, transverse myelitis, hemiplegia, and cerebellar ataxia.

DIAGNOSIS. The diagnosis of viral encephalitis is usually made on the basis of the clinical presentation of nonspecific prodrome followed by progressive CNS symptoms. The diagnosis is supported by examination of the CSF, which usually shows a mild mononuclear predominance (see Table 602-1). Other tests of potential value in the evaluation of patients with suspected viral meningoencephalitis include an electroencephalogram (EEG) and neuroimaging studies. The EEG typically shows diffuse slow-wave activity, usually without focal changes. Neuroimaging studies (CT or MRI) may show swelling of the brain parenchyma. Focal seizures or focal findings on EEG, CT, or MRI, especially involving the temporal lobes, suggest HSV encephalitis.

Differential Diagnosis. A number of clinical conditions that cause CNS inflammation mimic viral meningoencephalitis (see Table 602-2). The most important group of alternative infectious agents to consider is bacteria. Most children with acute bacterial meningitis appear more critically ill than those with CNS viral infection. Parameningeal bacterial infections, such as brain abscess or subdural or epidural empyema, may have features similar to viral CNS infections. Infections caused by *M. tuberculosis, T. pallidum* (syphilis), *B. burgdorferi* (Lyme disease), and *Bartonella henselae,* the bacillus associated with cat scratch disease, tend to result in indolent courses. Analysis of CSF and appropriate serologic tests are necessary to differentiate these various pathogens.

Infections due to fungi, rickettsiae, mycoplasma, protozoa, and other parasites may also need to be included in the differential diagnosis. Consideration of these agents usually arises as a result of accompanying symptoms, geographic locality of infection, or host immune factors.

Various noninfectious disorders may be associated with CNS inflammation and have manifestations overlapping with those associated with viral meningoencephalitis. Some of these disorders include malignancy, collagen vascular diseases, intracranial hemorrhage, and exposure to certain drugs or toxins. Attention to history and other organ involvement usually allows elimination of these diagnostic possibilities.

Laboratory Findings. The CSF contains from a few to several thousand cells per cubic mm. Early in the disease, the cells are often polymorphonuclear; later, mononuclear cells predominate. This change in cellular type is often demonstrated in CSF samples obtained as little as 8–12 hr apart. The protein concentration in CSF tends to be normal or slightly elevated, but concentrations may be very high if brain destruction is extensive, such as that accompanying HSV encephalitis. The glucose level is usually normal, although with certain viruses, for example, mumps, a substantial depression of CSF glucose concentrations may be observed.

The CSF should be cultured for viruses, bacteria, fungi, and mycobacteria; in some instances, special examinations are indicated for protozoa, mycoplasma, and other pathogens. The success of isolating viruses from the CSF of children with viral meningoencephalitis is determined by the time in the clinical course that the specimen is obtained, the specific etiologic agent, whether the infection is a meningitic as opposed to a localized encephalitic process, and the skill of the diagnostic laboratory staff. Isolating a virus is most likely early in the illness, and the enteroviruses tend to be the easiest to isolate, although recovery of these agents from the CSF rarely exceeds 70%. To increase the likelihood of identifying the putative viral pathogen, specimens for culture should also be obtained from nasopharyngeal swabs, feces, and urine. Although isolating a virus from one or more of these sites does not prove causality, it is highly suggestive. Detection of viral DNA or RNA by polymerase chain reaction may be useful in the diagnosis of CNS infection caused by HSV and enteroviruses, respectively. CSF serology is the diagnostic test of choice for WNV.

A serum specimen should be obtained early in the course of illness and, if viral cultures are not diagnostic, again 2–3 wk later for serologic studies. Serologic methods are not practical for diagnosing CNS infections caused by the enteroviruses because there are too many serotypes. This approach may be useful in confirming that a case is caused by a known circulating serotype. Serologic tests may also be of value in determining the etiology of nonenteroviral CNS infection, such as arboviral infection.

TREATMENT. With the exception of the use of acyclovir for HSV encephalitis (see Chapter 249), treatment of viral meningoencephalitis is supportive. Treatment of mild disease may require only symptomatic relief. Headache and hyperesthesia are treated with rest, non–aspirin-containing analgesics, and a reduction in room light, noise, and visitors. Acetaminophen is recommended for fever. Codeine, morphine, and the phenothiazine derivatives may be necessary for pain and vomiting, but if possible, their use in children should be minimized because they may induce misleading signs and symptoms. Intravenous fluids are occasionally necessary because of poor oral intake. More severe disease may require hospitalization and intensive care.

It is important to anticipate and be prepared to manage convulsions, cerebral edema, inadequate respiratory exchange, disturbed fluid and electrolyte balance, aspiration and asphyxia, and cardiac or respiratory arrest of central origin. Therefore, patients with severe encephalitis should be monitored closely. In patients with evidence of increased ICP, placement of a pressure transducer in the epidural space may be indicated. The risks of cardiac and respiratory failure or arrest are high with severe disease. All fluids, electrolytes, and medications are initially given parenterally. In prolonged states of coma, parenteral alimentation is indicated. SIADH is common in acute CNS disorders; monitoring of serum sodium concentrations is required for early detection (see Chapter 560). Normal blood levels of glucose, magnesium, and calcium must be maintained to minimize the likelihood of convulsions. If cerebral edema or seizures become evident, vigorous treatment should be instituted.

PROGNOSIS. Supportive and rehabilitative efforts are very important after patients recover. Motor incoordination, convulsive disorders, total or partial deafness, and behavioral disturbances may follow viral CNS infections. Visual disturbances due to chorioretinopathy and perceptual amblyopia may also occur. Special facilities and, at times, institutional placement may become necessary. Some sequelae of infection may be very subtle. Therefore, neurodevelopmental and audiologic evaluations should be part of the routine follow-up of children who have recovered from viral meningoencephalitis.

Most children completely recover from viral infections of the CNS, although the prognosis depends on the severity of the clinical illness, the specific cause, and the age of the child. If the clinical illness is severe and substantial parenchymal involvement is evident, the prognosis is poor, with potential deficits being intellectual, motor, psychiatric, epileptic, visual, or auditory in nature. Severe sequelae should also be anticipated in those with infection caused by HSV. Although some literature suggests that infants who contract viral meningoencephalitis have a poorer long-term outcome than older children, most other data refute this observation. Approximately 10% of children younger than 2 yr with enteroviral CNS infections suffer an acute complication such as seizures, increased ICP, or coma. Almost all have favorable long-term neurologic outcomes.

PREVENTION. Widespread use of effective viral vaccines for polio, measles, mumps, rubella, and varicella has almost eliminated CNS complications from these diseases in the United States. The availability of domestic animal vaccine programs against rabies has reduced the frequency of rabies encephalitis. Control of encephalitis due to arboviruses has been less successful because specific vaccines for the arboviral diseases that occur in North America are not available. Control of insect vectors by suitable spraying methods and eradication of insect breeding sites, however, reduces the incidence of these infections. Furthermore, minimizing mosquito bites through the application of DEET-containing insect repellents on exposed skin and wearing long-sleeved shirts, long pants, and socks when outdoors, especially at dawn and dusk, reduces the risk of arboviral infection.

602.3 • Eosinophilic Meningitis

Eosinophilic meningitis is defined as 10 or more eosinophils/mm^3 of CSF. The most common cause worldwide of eosinophilic pleocytosis is CNS infection with helminthic parasites. In countries such as the United States, where helminthic infestation is uncommon, however, the differential diagnosis of CSF eosinophilic pleocytosis is broad.

ETIOLOGY. Although any tissue-migrating helminth may cause eosinophilic meningitis, the most common cause is human infection with the rat lungworm, *Angiostrongylus cantonensis* (see Chapter 294). Other parasites that can cause eosinophilic meningitis include *Gnathostoma spinigerum* (dog and cat roundworm) [see Chapter 294], *Baylisascaris procyonis* (raccoon roundworm), *Ascaris lumbricoides* (human roundworm), *Trichinella spiralis, Toxocara canis, Toxoplasma gondii, Paragonimus westermani, Echinococcus granulosus, Schistosoma japonicum, Onchocerca volvulus,* and *T. solium*. Eosinophilic meningitis may also occur as an unusual manifestation of more common viral, bacterial, or fungal infections of the CNS. Noninfectious causes of eosinophilic meningitis include multiple sclerosis, malignancy, hypereosinophilic syndrome, or a reaction to medications or a ventriculoperitoneal shunt.

EPIDEMIOLOGY. *A. cantonensis* is found in Southeast Asia, the South Pacific, Japan, Taiwan, Egypt, Ivory Coast, and Cuba. Infection is acquired by eating raw or undercooked freshwater snails, slugs, prawns, or crabs containing infectious 3rd-stage larvae. *Gnathostoma* infections are found in Japan, China, India, Bangladesh, and Southeast Asia. Gnathostomiasis is acquired by eating undercooked or raw fish, frog, bird, or snake meat.

CLINICAL MANIFESTATIONS. When eosinophilic meningitis results from helminthic infestation, patients become ill 1–3 wk after exposure, because the parasites migrate from the gastrointestinal tract to the CNS. Common concomitant findings include fever, peripheral eosinophilia, vomiting, abdominal pain, creeping skin eruptions, or pleurisy. Neurologic symptoms may include headache, meningismus, ataxia, cranial nerve palsies, and paresthesias. Paraparesis or incontinence can result from radiculitis or myelitis.

DIAGNOSIS. The presumptive diagnosis of helminth-induced eosinophilic meningitis is made by travel and exposure history in the presence of typical clinical and laboratory findings.

TREATMENT. Treatment is supportive, because infection is self-limited and anthelmintic drugs do not appear to influence the outcome of infection. Analgesics should be given for headache and radiculitis, and CSF removal or shunting should be performed to relieve hydrocephalus, if present. Steroids may decrease the duration of headaches in adults with eosinophilic meningitis.

PROGNOSIS. The prognosis is good; 70% of patients improve sufficiently to leave the hospital in 1–2 wk. Mortality associated with eosinophilic meningitis is <1%.

Acute Bacterial Meningitis

Blazer S, Berant M, Alon U: Bacterial meningitis: Effect of antibiotic treatment on cerebrospinal fluid. *J Clin Pathol* 1983;80:386–387.

Bonsu BK, Harper MB: Fever interval before diagnosis, prior antibiotic treatment, clinical outcome for young children with bacterial meningitis. *Clin Infect Dis* 2001;32:566–572.

De Gans J, Van De Beek D, for the Europena Dexamethasone in adulthood bacterial meningitis study investigation: Dexamethasone in adults with bacterial meningitis. *N Engl J Med* 2002;347:1549–1556.

Enders A, Pannicke U, Berner R, et al: Two siblings with lethal pneumococcal meningitis in a family with a mutation in interleukin-1 receptor-associated kinase 4. *J Pediatr* 2004;145:698–700.

Gessner BD, Sutanto A, Linehan M, et al: Incidences of vaccine-preventable *Haemophilus influenzae* type b pneumonia and meningitis in Indonesian children: Hamlet-randomised vaccine-probe trial. *Lancet* 2005;365:43–52.

Grimwood K, Anderson P, Anderson V, et al: Twelve year outcome following bacterial meningitis: Further evidence for persisting effects. *Arch Dis Child* 2000;83:111–116.

Healy CM, Baker CJ: The future of meningococcal vaccines. *Pediatr Infect Dis J* 2005;24:175–176.

Kilpi T, Anttila M, Kallio MJ, et al: Length of prediagnostic history related to the course and sequelae of childhood bacterial meningitis. *Pediatr Infect Dis J* 1993;12:184–188.

Kutz JW, Simon LM, Chennupati SK, et al: Clinical predictors for hearing loss in children with bacterial meningitis. *Arch Otolaryngol Head Neck Surg* 2006;132:941–945.

McIntyre PB, MacIntyre CR, Gilmour R, et al: A population based study of the impact of corticosteroid therapy and delayed diagnosis on the outcome of childhood pneumococcal meningitis. *Arch Dis Child* 2005;90:391–396.

Nigrovic LE, Kuppermann N, Macias CG, et al: Clinical prediction rule for identifying children with cerebrospinal fluid pleocytosis at very low risk of bacterial meningitis. *JAMA* 2007;297:52–60.

Ninis N, Phillips C, Bailey L, et al: The role of healthcare delivery in the outcome of meningococcal disease in children: Case-control study of fatal and non-fatal cases. *Br Med J* 2005;330:1475–1478.

Radetsky M: Duration of symptoms and outcome in bacterial meningitis: An analysis of causation and the implications of a delay in diagnosis. *Pediatr Infect Dis J* 1992;11:694–698.

Reefhuis J, Honein MA, Whitney CG, et al. Risk of bacterial meningitis in children with cochlear implants. *N Engl J Med* 2003;349:435–445.

Saha SK, Baqui AH, Darmstadt GL, et al: Invasive *Haemophilus influenzae* type B diseases in Bangladesh, with increased resistance to antibiotics. *J Pediatr* 2005;146:227–233.

Scheld WM, Koedel U, Nathan B, et al: Pathophysiology of bacterial meningitis: Mechanism(s) of neuronal injury. *J Infect Dis* 2002;186(Suppl 2):S225–S233.

Snape MD, Pollard AJ: Meningococcal polysaccharide-protein conjugate vaccines. *Lancet Infect Dis* 2005;5:21–30.

Swartz MN: Bacterial meningitis—A view of the past 90 years. *N Engl J Med* 2004;351:1826–1828.

Tunkel AR, Hartman BJ, Kaplan SL, et al: Practice guideline for the management of bacterial meningitis. *Clin Infect Dis* 2004;39:1267–1284.

Van de Beek D, de Gans J, Spanjaard L, et al: Clinical features and prognostic factors in adults with bacterial meningitis. *N Engl J Med* 2004;351:1849–1859.

Van de Beek D, de Gans J: Dexamethasone in adults with community-acquired bacterial meningitis. *Drugs* 2006;66:415–427.

Van de Beek D, de Gans J, Tunkel AR, Wijdicks EFM: Community-acquired bacterial meningitis in adults. *N Engl J Med* 2006;354:44–52.

Viral Meningoencephalitis

Bernit E, de Lamballerie X, Zandotti C, et al: Prospective investigation of a large outbreak of meningitis due to echovirus 30 during summer 2000 in Marseilles, France. *Medicine* 2004;83:245–253.
Glaser CA, Gilliam S, Schnurr D, et al: California Encephalitis Project, 1998–2000. In search of encephalitis etiologies: Diagnostic challenges in the California Encephalitis Project, 1998–2000. *Clin Infect Dis* 2003;36:731–742.
Glaser CA, Honarmand S, Anderson LJ, et al: Beyond viruses: clinical profiles and etiologies associated with encephalitis. *CID* 2006;43:1565–1577.
Hayes EB, O'Leary DR: West Nile infection: A pediatric perspective. *Pediatrics* 2004;113:1375–1381.
Rorabaugh ML, Berlin LE, Heldrich F, et al: Aseptic meningitis in infants younger than 2 years of age: Acute illness and neurologic complications. *Pediatrics* 1993;92:206–211.
Solomon T: Flavivirus encephalitis. *N Engl J Med* 2004;351:370–378.
Tyler KL: West Nile virus encephalitis in America. *N Engl J Med* 2001;344:1858–1859.
Yim R, Posfay-Barbe KM, Nolt D, et al: Spectrum of clinical manifestations of West Nile virus infection in children. *Pediatrics* 2004;114:1673–1675.

Eosinophilic Meningitis

Chotmongkol V, Sawanyawisuth K, Thavornpitak Y: Corticosteroids treatment of eosinophilic meningitis. *Clin Infect Dis* 2000;31:660–662.
Hsu W, Chen J, Chien C, et al: Eosinophilic meningitis caused by *Angiostrongylus cantonensis. Pediatr Infect Dis J* 1990;9:443–435.
Weller PF: Eosinophilic meningitis. *Am J Med* 1993;95:250–253.

Chapter 603 ■ Brain Abscess

Robert H. A. Haslam

Brain abscesses can occur in children of any age but are most common in children between 4 and 8 yr and neonates. The causes of brain abscess include embolization due to congenital heart disease with right-to-left shunts (especially tetralogy of Fallot), meningitis, chronic otitis media and mastoiditis, sinusitis, soft tissue infection of the face or scalp, orbital cellulitis, dental infections, penetrating head injuries, immunodeficiency states, and infection of ventriculoperitoneal shunts.

PATHOLOGY. Cerebral abscesses are evenly distributed between the two hemispheres, and ≈80% of cases are divided equally between the frontal, parietal, and temporal lobes. Brain abscesses in the occipital lobe, cerebellum, and brainstem account for about 20% of the cases. Most brain abscesses are single, but 30% are multiple and may involve more than one lobe. The pathogenesis is undetermined in 10–15% of cases. An abscess in the frontal lobe is often caused by extension from sinusitis or orbital cellulitis, whereas abscesses located in the temporal lobe or cerebellum are frequently associated with chronic otitis media and mastoiditis. Abscesses resulting from penetrating injuries tend to be singular and caused by *Staphylococcus aureus,* whereas those resulting from septic emboli, congenital heart disease, or meningitis often have several causal organisms.

ETIOLOGY. The responsible bacteria include streptococci (*S. milleri, S. pyogenes* group A or B, *S. pneumoniae, S. faecalis*), anaerobic organisms (gram-positive cocci, *Bacteroides* spp., *Fusobacterium* spp., *Prevotella* spp., *Actinomyces* spp.), and gram-negative aerobic bacilli (*Haemophilus aphrophilus, H. parainfluenzae, H. influenzae, Enterobacter, E. coli, Proteus* spp.). *Citrobacter* is most common in neonates. One organism is cultured in the majority of abscesses (70%), two in 20%, and three or more in 10% of cases. Abscesses associated with mucosal infections (sinusitis) frequently have anaerobic bacteria. Fungal abscesses *(Aspergillus, Candida)* are more common in immunosuppressed patients.

CLINICAL MANIFESTATIONS. The early stages of cerebritis and abscess formation are associated with nonspecific symptoms, including low-grade fever, headache, and lethargy. The significance of these symptoms is generally not recognized, and an oral antibiotic is often prescribed with resultant transient relief. As the inflammatory process proceeds, vomiting, severe headache, seizures, papilledema, focal neurologic signs (hemiparesis), and coma may develop. A cerebellar abscess is characterized by nystagmus, ipsilateral ataxia and dysmetria, vomiting, and headache. If the abscess ruptures into the ventricular cavity, overwhelming shock and death usually ensue.

DIAGNOSIS. The peripheral white blood cell count can be normal or elevated, and the blood culture is positive in ≈10% of cases. Examination of the cerebrospinal fluid (CSF) shows variable results; the white blood cells and protein may be minimally elevated or normal, and the glucose level may be low. CSF cultures are rarely positive; aspiration of the abscess is much more likely to establish a bacteriologic diagnosis. Because examination of the CSF is seldom useful and a lumbar puncture may cause herniation of the cerebellar tonsils, the procedure should not be undertaken in a child suspected of having a brain abscess. The electroencephalogram (EEG) shows corresponding focal slowing, and the radionuclide brain scan indicates an area of enhancement due to disruption of the blood-brain barrier in >80% of cases. CT with contrast and MRI are the most reliable methods of demonstrating cerebritis and abscess formation (Fig. 603-1). MRI is the diagnostic test of choice. The CT findings of cerebritis are characterized by a parenchymal low-density lesion, and MRI T2 weighted images indicate increased signal intensity. An abscess cavity shows a ring-enhancing lesion by contrast CT, and the

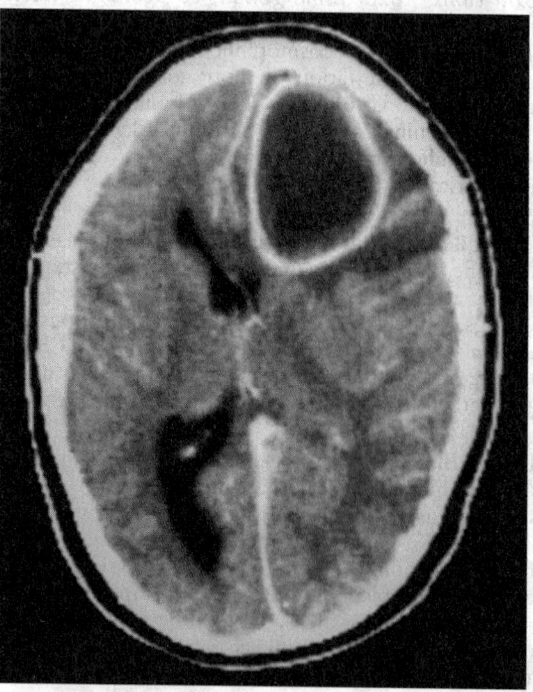

Figure 603-1. CT with contrast. Note the large wall-enhancing abscess in the left frontal lobe. The lesion is causing a shift of the brain to the right. The patient had no neurologic signs until just before the CT scan because the abscess is located in the frontal lobe, a "silent" area of the brain.

MRI also demonstrates an abscess capsule with gadolinium administration.

TREATMENT. The initial management of a brain abscess includes prompt diagnosis and institution of an antibiotic regimen that is based on the probable pathogenesis and the most likely organism. When the cause is unknown, the combination of vancomycin, a 3rd-generation cephalosporin, and metronidazole is commonly used. The same regimen is initiated when otitis media, sinusitis, or mastoiditis is the likely cause. If there is a history of penetrating head injury, head trauma, or neurosurgery, vancomycin plus a 3rd-generation cephalosporin is appropriate. When cyanotic congenital heart disease is the predisposing factor, ampicillin-sulbactam alone or a 3rd-generation cephalosporin plus metronidazole may be used. Meropenem has good activity against gram-negative bacilli, anaerobes, staphylococci, and streptococci, including most antibiotic-resistant pneumococci, and may be used alone to replace the combination of metronidazole and a β-lactam in the previous regimens. Notably, meropenem does not provide activity against methicillin-resistant *S. aureus* and may have decreased activity against penicillin-resistant strains of *S. pneumoniae,* indicating that vancomycin should remain a part of the initial regimen when these organisms are suspected. Abscesses secondary to an infected ventriculoperitoneal shunt may be initially treated with vancomycin and ceftazidime. When *Citrobacter* meningitis (often in neonates) leads to abscess formation, a 3rd-generation cephalosporin is used, typically in combination with an aminoglycoside. *Listeria monocytogenes* may cause a brain abscess in the neonate and if suspected, ampicillin should be added to the cephalosporin. In immunocompromised patients, broad-spectrum antibiotic coverage is used, and amphotericin B therapy should be considered.

A brain abscess can be treated with antibiotics without surgery if the abscess is <2 cm in diameter, the illness is of short duration (<2 wk), there are no signs of increased intracranial pressure, and the child is neurologically intact. If the decision is made to treat with antibiotics alone, the child should have weekly neuroimaging studies to ensure the abscess is decreasing in size. An encapsulated abscess, particularly if the lesion is causing a mass effect or increased intracranial pressure, should be treated with a combination of antibiotics and aspiration. Surgical excision of an abscess is rarely required, because the procedure may be associated with greater morbidity compared with aspiration of a cavity. Surgery is indicated when the abscess is >2.5 cm in diameter, gas is present in the abscess, the lesion is multiloculated, the lesion is located in the posterior fossa, or a fungus is identified. Associated infectious processes, such as mastoiditis, sinusitis, or a periorbital abscess, may require surgical drainage. The duration of antibiotic therapy depends on the organism and response to treatment, but is usually 4–6 wk.

PROGNOSIS. Mortality rate associated with brain abscess has decreased significantly to ≈15–20 % with the use of CT or MRI and prompt antibiotic and surgical management. Factors associated with high mortality rate at the time of admission include age <1 yr, multiple abscesses, coma, and lack of CT facilities. Long-term sequelae occur in at least 50% of survivors and include hemiparesis, seizures, hydrocephalus, cranial nerve abnormalities, and behavior and learning problems.

Brook I: Aerobic and anaerobic bacteriology of intracranial abscesses. *Pediatr Neurol* 1992;8:210–214.

Goodkin HP, Harper MB, Pomeroy SL: Intracranial abscess in children: Historical trends at Children's Hospital Boston. *Pediatrics* 2004;113;1765–1770.

Saez-Lloreus XJ, Umana NA, Odio CN, et al: Brain abscesses in infants and children. *Pediatr Infect Dis J* 1989;8:449–458.

Sjolin J, Lilja A, Erikson N, et al: Treatment of brain abscess with cefotaxime and metronidazole: Prospective study on 15 consecutive patients. *Clin Infect Dis* 1993;17:857–863.

Smith RR: Neuroradiology of intracranial infection. *Pediatr Neurosurg* 1992;18:92–104.

Chapter 604 ■ Pseudotumor Cerebri

Robert H. A. Haslam

Pseudotumor cerebri is a clinical syndrome that mimics brain tumors and is characterized by increased intracranial pressure (ICP) (>200 mm H_2O in infants and 250 mm H_2O in children), with a normal cerebrospinal fluid (CSF) cell count and protein content and normal ventricular size, anatomy, and position documented by MRI.

ETIOLOGY. There are many explanations for the development of pseudotumor cerebri, including alterations in CSF absorption and production, cerebral edema, abnormalities in vasomotor control and cerebral blood flow, and venous obstruction. The causes of pseudotumor are numerous and include metabolic disorders (galactosemia, hypoparathyroidism, pseudohypoparathyroidism, hypophosphatasia, prolonged corticosteroid therapy or too rapid corticosteroid withdrawal, possibly growth hormone treatment, refeeding of a significantly malnourished child, hypervitaminosis A, vitamin A deficiency, Addison disease, obesity, menarche, oral contraceptives, and pregnancy), infections (roseola infantum, sinusitis, chronic otitis media and mastoiditis, Guillain-Barré syndrome), drugs (nalidixic acid, doxycycline, minocycline, tetracycline, nitrofurantoin), isotretinoin used for acne therapy especially when combined with tetracycline, hematologic disorders (polycythemia, hemolytic and iron-deficiency anemias, Wiskott-Aldrich syndrome), obstruction of intracranial drainage by venous thrombosis (lateral sinus or posterior sagittal sinus thrombosis), head injury, and obstruction of the superior vena cava. When a secondary cause is not identified, the condition is classified as "idiopathic intracranial hypertension."

CLINICAL MANIFESTATIONS. The most frequent symptom is headache, and although vomiting also occurs, it is rarely as persistent and pernicious as that associated with a posterior fossa tumor. Transient visual obscuration and diplopia (secondary to paralysis of the abducens nerve) is a common complaint. Most patients are alert and lack constitutional symptoms. Examination of the infant characteristically reveals a bulging fontanel and a "cracked pot sound" or Macewen sign (percussion of the skull produces a resonant sound) due to separation of the cranial sutures. **Papilledema** with an enlarged blind spot is the most consistent sign in a child beyond infancy. Early optic nerve edema may be noted with ultrasonography. An inferior nasal defect may be detected on formal tangent screen testing. The presence of focal neurologic signs indicates a process other than pseudotumor cerebri.

TREATMENT. The prime goal of management is discovery and treatment of the underlying cause. There are no randomized clinical trials to guide the treatment of pseudotumor cerebri. Pseudotumor cerebri can be a self-limited condition, but optic atrophy and blindness are the most significant complications. The obese patient should be treated with a weight loss regimen, and if a drug is thought to be responsible, it should be discontinued. For many patients, repeated follow-up and monitoring of the visual acuity is all that is required. Serial visual-evoked potentials are useful if the visual acuity cannot be reliably documented. The initial lumbar tap that follows a CT or MRI scan is diagnostic and may be therapeutic. The spinal needle produces a small rent in the dura that allows CSF to escape the subarachnoid space, thus reducing the ICP. Several additional lumbar taps and the removal of sufficient CSF to reduce the opening pressure by 50% occasionally lead to resolution of the process. Acetazolamide, 10–30 mg/kg/24 hr, and corticosteroids have been effective for some patients. Consideration should be given to treating sinus thrombosis with anticoagulation. Rarely, a lumboperitoneal shunt or subtemporal decompression is necessary, if the aforementioned approaches are unsuccessful and optic nerve atrophy supervenes. Some centers perform optic nerve sheath fenestration to prevent further visual loss. Any patient whose ICP proves to be refractory to treatment warrants consideration for repeat neuroradiologic studies. A **slow-growing tumor** or **obstruction of a venous sinus** may become evident by the time of reinvestigation.

Baker R, Baumann R, Buncic J: Idiopathic intracranial hypertension (pseudotumor cerebri) in pediatric patients. *Pediatr Neurol* 1989;5:5–11.

Digre KB: Not so benign intracranial hypertension. *Br Med J* 2003;326:613–614.

Shuper A, Snir M, Barash D: Ultrasonography of the optic nerves: Clinical application in children with pseudotumor cerebri. *J Pediatr* 1997;131:734–740.

Soler D, Cox T, Bullock P, et al: Diagnosis and management of benign intracranial hypertension. *Arch Dis Child* 1998;78:89–94.

Chapter 605 ■ Spinal Cord Disorders

Robert H. A. Haslam

CUTANEOUS MARKERS OF OCCULT SPINAL DYSRAPHISM (OSD) (See Chapter 592.2)

OSD refers to congenital abnormalities that result from incomplete fusion of the soft tissue, bone, or neural components of the spine that occur during primary and secondary neurulation. Some types of OSD including tethered cord, diastematomyelia, and syringomyelia are often associated with congenital midline lumbosacral skin lesions. The skin lesions include lipomas, dermal sinuses, tails, patches of hair, deviation of the gluteal fold, hemangiomas, and port-wine stains. Every child with a midline lumbosacral birthmark should have a complete neurologic examination. Mongolian spots and simple dimples within the gluteal folds are not associated with OSD and do not require study. Birthmarks associated with the highest incidence of OSD include caudal appendages (tails), dermal sinuses above the gluteal folds, and lipomas. Two or more midline skin lesions are associated with the greatest incidence of OSD. The diagnostic procedure of choice in the investigation of OSD is an MRI of the spine.

605.1 • Tethered Cord

During fetal development, the spinal cord occupies the entire length of the vertebral column, but due to differential growth, the conus medullaris in a child ultimately assumes a position at the level of L1. Normal regression of the distal embryonic spinal cord produces a slender, threadlike filum terminale that is

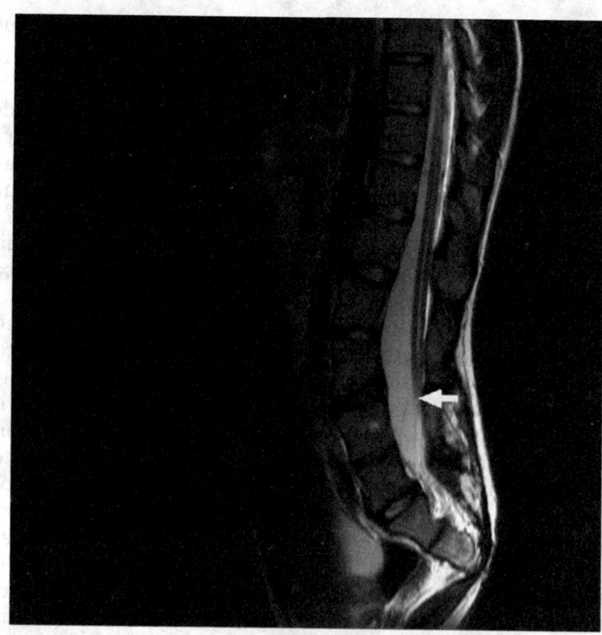

Figure 605-1. Sagittal T2 weighted MRI image of the lumbar spine, showing a low-lying conus corresponding to level L3–L4 *(arrow)* and dorsally applied cord in keeping with a tethered cord. Note is made of a small syrinx. (Courtesy of Walid F. Abou Reslan, MD, Alberta Children's Hospital.)

attached to the coccyx. A tethered cord results when a thickened ropelike filum terminale persists and anchors the conus at or below the L2 level as shown by MRI (Fig. 605-1). Rarely, a symptomatic tethered cord associated with a lipoma or other congenital anomaly is found to lie in a normal position relative to L2. Neurologic signs may develop as a result of abnormal tension on the spinal cord, compromising blood supply, particularly during flexion and extension movements. In addition to a tight filum, diastematomyelia, sacral agenesis, intradural lipoma, lipomyelomeningocele, and a dermal sinus may be associated with the tethered spinal cord syndrome.

CLINICAL MANIFESTATIONS. In ≈70% of cases, inspection of the back shows a midline skin lesion such as a lipoma, tuft of hair, a caudal appendage, or dermal sinus and, occasionally, a port-wine stain or hyperpigmentation of the skin. The clinical presentation varies; signs may be evident at birth or may be delayed until adulthood. Infants may have asymmetric growth in a foot or leg associated with talipes cavus deformities and muscle wasting due to prolonged denervation. The child may be delayed in walking, demonstrate toe walking, or have regression of lower extremity function. The neurologic examination is characterized by lower motor neuron signs in the legs. Abnormalities in bladder function with overflow incontinence, recurrent urinary tract infections, bowel incontinence, constipation, and progressive scoliosis may be present. Diffuse pain in the lower extremities is a more common finding in older children and adults.

Plain roentgenograms of the lumbosacral vertebral bodies may show widening of the interpedicular distance, hemivertebrae, or malformations of the anterior spinal segments. MRI precisely outlines the level of the conus medullaris and the filum terminale.

TREATMENT. Surgical transection of the thickened filum terminale tends to halt progression of neurologic signs and prevents the development of dysfunction in asymptomatic patients. Retethering of the spinal cord is associated with deterioration of neurologic function including ambulation and most commonly follows surgical closure of a myelomeningocele.

605.2 • Diastematomyelia (Split Spinal Cord Malformation)

Diastematomyelia is division of the spinal cord into two halves by projection of a fibrocartilaginous or bony septum originating from the posterior vertebral body and extending posteriorly. It represents a disorder of neural tube fusion with the persistence of mesodermal tissue from the primitive neurenteric canal acting as the septum. The defect involves the lumbar vertebrae (L1–L3) in ≈50% of cases and tends to be associated with abnormalities of the vertebral bodies, including fusion defects, hemivertebra, hypoplasia, kyphoscoliosis, spina bifida, and myelomeningocele.

CLINICAL MANIFESTATIONS. A midline abnormality of the skin in the lumbosacral region provides a clue to the possibility of an underlying abnormality. The neurologic signs are thought to result from flexion and extension movements of the cord, which produce traction and additional trauma by the impaling septum. The clinical presentation of diastematomyelia varies and, in some cases, patients may remain asymptomatic. Most often, unilateral foot abnormalities, including talipes equinovarus, claw toes, atrophy of the gastrocnemius, and loss of pain and temperature sensation, are apparent in a preschool child. A more progressive course may ensue, characterized by bilateral weakness and muscle atrophy in the lower extremities, absent ankle jerks, urinary incontinence, and low back pain. Plain roentgenograms of the vertebrae may not detect the septum due to lack of calcification; thus, CT scanning or MRI is the study of choice (Fig. 605-2).

TREATMENT. The treatment of symptomatic patients is excision of the bony spur or septum and lysis of the adjacent adhesions.

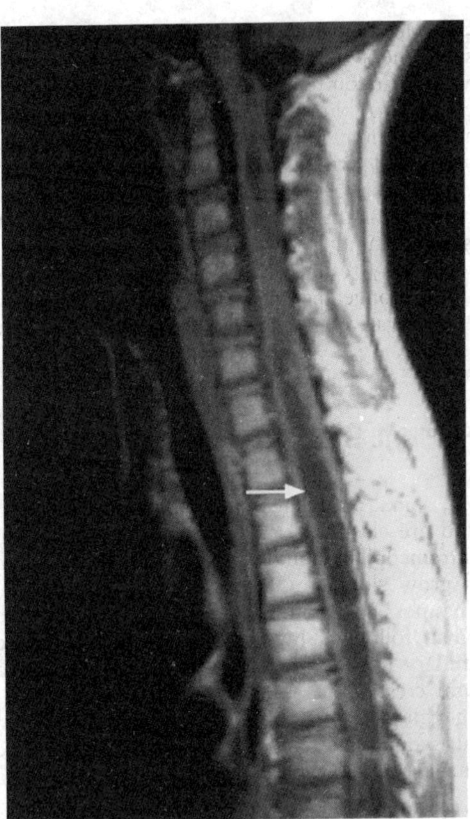

Figure 605-3. T1 weighted MRI scan of upper spinal cord showing an extensive syringomyelia *(white arrow)*.

605.3 • Syringomyelia

Syringomyelia is a cystic cavity within the spinal cord that may communicate with the cerebrospinal fluid (CSF) pathways or remain localized and noncommunicating. *Syringobulbia* exists when the cystic cavity extends into the medulla. Although the pathogenesis of communicating syringomyelia is unknown, the prevailing hypothesis suggests a constriction of the central canal at the level of the foramen magnum during embryogenesis. CSF may pass caudad through the narrowed canal, especially during periods of increased intracranial pressure (sneezing, coughing), and produce dilatation of the central canal. Because of the constriction, CSF is prevented from flowing in a cephalic direction. Communicating syringomyelia is frequently associated with the Chiari type I malformation, whereas the noncommunicating syrinx is associated with cord tumors, vascular accidents, trauma, and arachnoiditis.

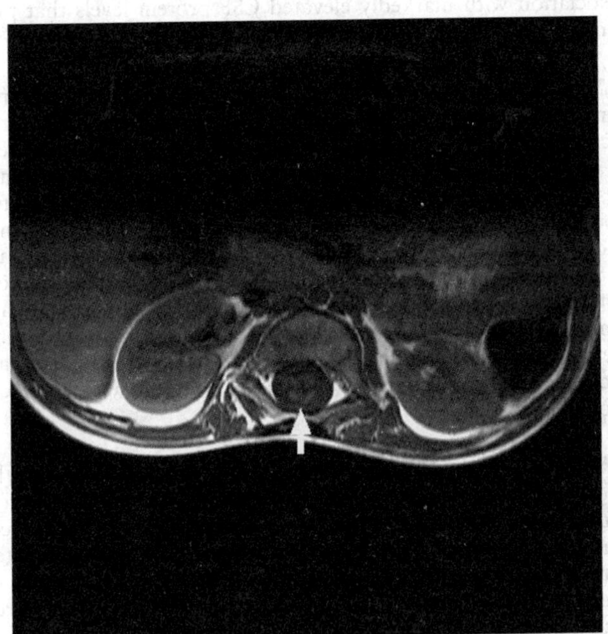

Figure 605-2. Axial T1 weighted MRI image at L1–L2 level shows splitting of the spinal cord *(arrow)* consistent with diastematomyelia. (Courtesy of Walid F. Abou Reslan, MD, Alberta Children's Hospital.)

CLINICAL MANIFESTATIONS. Because of its slow evolution, syringomyelia rarely produces symptoms during childhood. Interruption of the anterior white commissure at the level of the cervical cord disrupts the lateral spinothalamic tracts, causing an asymmetric loss of pain and temperature sensation in the upper extremities, with preservation of light touch (dissociation of sensation). Progressive enlargement of the cavity impinges on the anterior horn cells and corticospinal tracts, resulting in muscle wasting of the hands, absent deep tendon reflexes in the upper extremities, and upper motor neuron signs in the lower extremities. A rapidly progressive scoliosis may be the initial manifestation of syringomyelia. Trophic ulcers associated with vasomotor disturbances of the hands and arms indicate the loss of appreciation of pain.

DIAGNOSIS. CT scanning with intrathecal injection of metrizamide outlines an enlarged spinal cord in the region of the syrinx, and a delayed scan displays the contrast medium within the cavity. MRI is the study of choice (Fig. 605-3).

TREATMENT. The management is surgical and depends on the site and cause of the syringomyelia. Operation is recommended in patients with syringomyelia and progressive scoliosis or evidence of progressive sensory or motor deterioration. Decompression of the foramen magnum and the upper cervical vertebrae is recommended when the syrinx is associated with a Chiari type I or II anomaly. Additional procedures include insertion of a tissue plug in the open end of the central canal, draining the cystic cavity into the subarachnoid space, and percutaneous aspiration of the syrinx, which may result in marked improvement in neurologic function for prolonged periods. Asymptomatic patients should be followed conservatively with serial neurologic examinations and imaging studies.

605.4 • Spinal Cord Tumors

In children, spinal cord tumors account for ≈20% of neuraxial tumors and are classified according to anatomic position (Fig. 605-4). **Intramedullary tumors** arise within the substance of the cord and grow slowly by infiltration, usually in the cervical region. The most common intramedullary tumor is a low-grade astrocytoma, followed by ganglioglioma and ependymoma. **Extramedullary intradural tumors** tend to be benign and arise from neural crest tissue. Tumors in this area include neurofibroma, ganglioneuroma, and meningioma. **Extramedullary extradural tumors** characteristically are metastatic lesions, particularly neuroblastoma, sarcoma, and lymphoma.

CLINICAL MANIFESTATIONS. Most children with spinal cord tumors present with a combination of gait disturbance, scoliosis, and back pain, depending on tumor location. Intramedullary gliomas are slow growing. Progressive difficulties in locomotion and sphincter disturbances are the earliest symptoms. Glial tumors in the cervical cord produce lower motor neuron signs in the upper extremities and upper motor neuron signs in the legs. Denervation of the intercostal muscles decreases chest wall movement and results in a weak cough. Loss of pain, temperature, and light touch sensation is evident in the lower extremities, and a cord level may, on occasion, be documented by light touch and pain sensation or by somatosensory-evoked potentials. With extramedullary tumors, the presenting symptom is often back pain. The child has difficulty sleeping because of pain and maintains a tripod posture while attempting to assume the supine position. If the tumor is attached to a nerve root, segmental pain, paresthesia, and weakness are evident. Extramedullary extradural tumors have a propensity to cause an acute block of the CSF pathways owing to rapid growth within a confined space. Such children present with a flaccid paraplegia, urinary retention, and a patulous anus. Some extramedullary tumors produce the *Brown-Séquard syndrome,* which consists of ipsilateral weakness, spasticity, and ataxia, with contralateral loss of pain and temperature sensation. Papilledema is observed in a few patients, usually in association with markedly elevated CSF protein levels that presumably interfere with normal CSF flow dynamics.

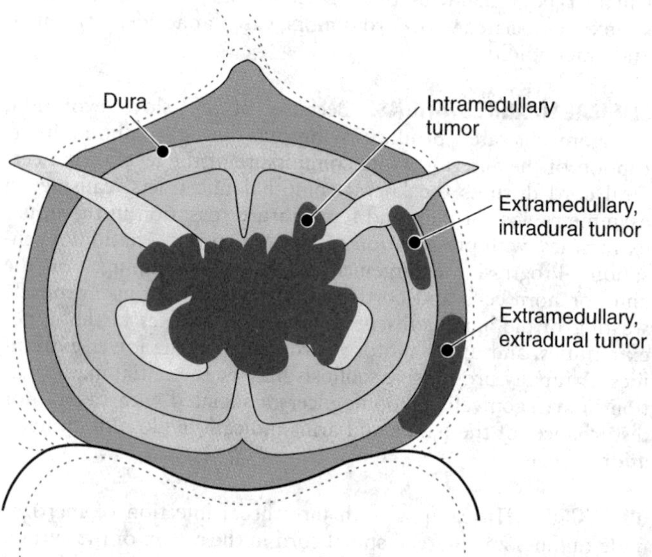

Figure 605-4. Diagram of the location of spinal cord tumors in children.

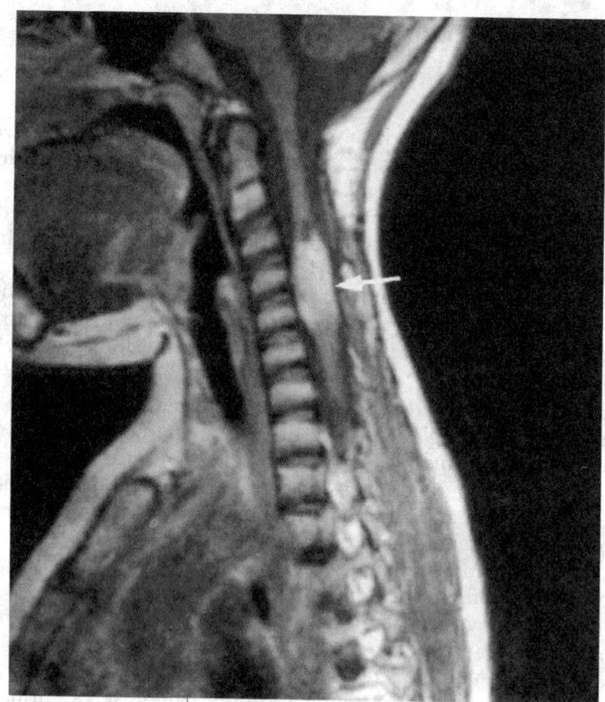

Figure 605-5. T1 weighted MRI scan of a spinal cord tumor *(white arrow)*. The fusiform expansion of the cervical cord enhances after intravenous gadolinium injection.

DIAGNOSIS. It is important to establish the diagnosis of a spinal cord tumor as early as possible, because surgical management is facilitated and irreversible damage to the cord may be prevented. In ≈40% of the cases, routine roentgenograms show abnormalities including widening of the interpediculate distance, destruction or sclerosis of the adjacent vertebral bodies or pedicles, and widening of the vertebral foramen on an oblique view in the case of a neurofibroma or ganglioneuroma. **MRI is the most important diagnostic test to establish the diagnosis.** Intramedullary tumors produce a fusiform swelling of the cord, often with a complete block of the CSF (Fig. 605-5). Neurofibromas tend to create a circular indentation of the cord, and extramedullary tumors show various degrees of blockage.

TREATMENT. With the advent of modern surgical instruments, the operating microscope, imaging technology, and intraoperative neurophysiology, many tumors can be totally and safely resected. Surgical removal of benign extramedullary tumors is associated with a good prognosis. Adjuvant therapy with radiation and/or chemotherapy is dictated primarily by tumor type. For children with a primary neuroblastoma presenting with a sudden onset of paraplegia secondary to metastases in the extradural space, immediate radiation therapy may circumvent the need for a laminectomy.

605.5 • Spinal Cord Trauma (See also Chapters 62 and 99.3)

Spinal cord injuries are rare in children as compared to adults. The degree of injury to the spinal cord is variable and includes concussion, contusion, laceration, and transection. Recovery depends on the extent of the trauma as well as on the immediate and long-term management. The common causes of spinal cord injury in the child younger than 10 yr include birth injury, physical abuse (as in the shaken baby syndrome), automobile and diving injuries, violence (gun shot wounds, stabbing), and falls from playground equipment. Spinal injuries in children older than 10 yr are most commonly the result of automobile and sports related injuries.

Approximately 20% of spinal cord injuries in children occur in the absence of a radiologic abnormality. **SCIWORA** (spinal cord injury without radiographic injury) is most commonly found in children and may be associated with a severe injury to the cord.

CLINICAL MANIFESTATIONS. A patient with *severe cord injury* presents with **spinal shock,** consisting of flaccidity, areflexia, loss of sensation, and often bradycardia and hypotension. Spinal shock may persist for up to 4 wk and results from dysfunction of synaptic activity in the pathways caudal to the injury. Ultimately, reflex flexor movements develop, followed by extensor reflex activity associated with hyperactive deep tendon reflexes, spasticity, and an automatic bladder. The *mildest injury* to the spinal cord is transient quadriparesis evident for seconds or minutes with complete recovery in 24 hr. This injury follows a concussion of the cord. Young children are at greatest risk for high cervical injuries, which account for ≈80% of spinal cord injuries in children younger than 2 yr. By the age of 8–10 yr, spinal injuries in children occur in similar locations as those found in adults.

A transverse injury in the high cervical cord level (C1–C2) causes respiratory arrest and death in the absence of ventilatory support. *Fracture dislocations at the C5–C6 level* resulting in spinal cord injuries are characterized by flaccid quadriparesis, loss of sphincter function, and a sensory level corresponding to the upper sternum. Fractures or dislocations in the low thoracic (T12–L1) region may produce the **conus medullaris syndrome,** which includes a loss of urinary and rectal sphincter control, flaccid weakness, and sensory disturbances of the legs. A **central cord lesion** may result from contusion and hemorrhage and typically involves the upper extremities to a greater degree than the legs. There are lower motor neuron signs in the upper extremities and upper motor neuron signs in the legs, bladder dysfunction, and loss of sensation caudal to the lesion. There may be considerable recovery, particularly in the lower extremities.

TREATMENT. Spinal cord injuries should be managed by stabilization and complete immobilization of the spine at the accident site using a correctly fitting cervical collar or blocks and tape. The patient must be transported on a board designed for children so that the neck is not placed in a flexed position. An adequate airway should be maintained, respiratory support provided, and shock should be treated with appropriate volume expanders and vasopressor agents if necessary. The use of steroids remains controversial as serious side effects may occur. Most centers advocate high-dose steroids for 24 hr if initiated within 3 hr of the injury and continuation of steroid therapy for 48 hr if started 3–8 hr after the spine injury. The initial dose of intravenous methylprednisolone (30 mg/kg bolus) should be started immediately, even before transport, followed by 5.4 mg/kg/hr. After transport, lateral and anteroposterior roentgenograms of the spine should be obtained. MRI is utilized if a ligamentous injury is suspected and CT and MRI are used if the diagnosis is uncertain.

After appropriate imaging studies, surgical treatment is directed to stabilization of the vertebrae to prevent additional injury to the cord and decompression of the spinal cord if compromised by a fracture or hemorrhage. Fracture dislocations are treated with traction, immobilization, and, if the injury is unstable, vertebral body fusion. Laminectomy and inspection of the cord are reserved for patients with progression of neurologic signs and appearance on CT or MRI scan that suggests an epidural or intraspinal hemorrhage.

Additional therapeutic measures include management of bladder and gastrointestinal disturbances, nutritional and skin care, and a rigorous multidisciplinary rehabilitation program. The prognosis following spinal cord trauma is directly related to the extent of the injury. Recovery may occur over an extended period of months to years. Central cord injuries have a better prognosis than those injuries producing transverse lesions.

Individuals with Down syndrome (DS) are susceptible to **atlantoaxial instability** resulting from laxity of the transverse ligaments. Atlantoaxial instability has been defined as a distance >4.5 mm between the odontoid process of the axis and the anterior arch of the atlas. Spinal cord compression (myelopathy) may be a consequence of atlantoaxial instability. There is a lack of consensus about the usefulness of radiograph screening in predicting spinal cord injury in children with DS. It is currently recommended that (1) lateral roentgenograms of the neck in the neutral, flexion, and extension positions be obtained at 3–5 yr and at a later age if indicated in individuals with DS, because atlantoaxial instability can develop during periods of growth; (2) children with atlantoaxial instability be advised not to participate in risky sports, such as tumbling, diving, and football; (3) radiographs of the neck be obtained before operative procedures or therapeutic programs that involve active neck movement or manipulation; (4) parents and physicians be made aware of the symptoms and signs of cord compression (neck pain, urinary and fecal incontinence, head tilt, gait abnormalities, ataxia, hyperreflexia, weakness, spasticity, and quadriplegia); and (5) there be prompt investigation (neck radiographs, CT scan, MRI study) followed by consideration for operative intervention in patients with signs of myelopathy.

PREVENTION. The most critical aspect of management of spinal cord trauma is the prevention of spinal cord injury by the use of contemporary playground equipment, age-appropriate seatbelts, and the implementation of strictly enforced age-related rules in contact sports such as hockey (body checking) and football.

605.6 • Transverse Myelitis

Transverse myelitis is characterized by abrupt onset of progressive weakness and sensory disturbances in the lower extremities. A history of a preceding viral infection accompanied by fever and malaise is documented in most cases. Several viruses have been implicated, including Epstein-Barr, herpes, influenza, rubella, mumps, and varicella. Additional infectious agents include Lyme disease and *Mycoplasma pneumoniae.* At least three hypotheses have been proposed to explain the pathogenesis of transverse myelitis: cell-mediated autoimmune response, direct viral invasion of the spinal cord, and autoimmune vasculitis. Pathologic examination of the cord shows marked softening and perivascular cuffing by lymphocytes, supporting an immunologic basis for the disorder.

CLINICAL MANIFESTATIONS. Low back or abdominal pain and paresthesias of the legs are prominent symptoms in the early stages. The leg muscles are weak and flaccid, and a sensory level is present, usually in the midthoracic region. Pain, temperature, and light touch sensation are affected, but joint position and vibration sense may be preserved. Sphincter disturbances are common, in which case catheterization of the bladder is necessary. Fever and nuchal rigidity are present early in most cases. The neurologic deficit evolves for 2–3 days and then plateaus, with flaccidity gradually changing to spasticity and with the concomitant development of upper motor neuron signs in the lower extremities. The differential diagnosis includes meningitis, infectious polyneuropathy (Guillain-Barré syndrome), poliomyelitis, neuromyelitis optica (Devic disease), spinal cord neoplasm, epidural abscess, demyelinating disorders, and a vascular malformation.

LABORATORY FINDINGS. Examination of the CSF shows moderate lymphocyte pleocytosis and a normal or slightly elevated protein level. MRI is always indicated in a suspected case of transverse myelitis to rule out multiple sclerosis or a compressive lesion compromising the cord. MRI abnormalities of transverse myelitis include T2-hyperintense and T1-iso-or mildly hypointense fusiform swelling extending over at least 3–4 vertebral levels, usually located in the thoracolumbar region.

TREATMENT. Spontaneous recovery occurs over a period of weeks or months and is complete in ≈40–50% of cases. Residual deficits include bowel and bladder dysfunction and weakness in the lower extremities. Management is directed to bladder care and physiotherapy. Pilot studies have shown that high-dose methylprednisolone therapy early in the course is effective in shortening the duration of the disease and in improving the outcome.

605.7 • Arteriovenous Malformation

An arteriovenous malformation of the spinal cord consists of a collection of tortuous dilated veins that are usually located on the dorsal aspect of the thoracic cord. The malformation may cause neurologic symptoms by its mass effect on the cord or by the "steal" phenomenon, by which blood is shunted through the abnormal veins, bypassing the spinal cord, which produces transient and, in some cases, progressive loss of neurologic function. Patients occasionally present with acute paraparesis and a sensory deficit due to a subarachnoid bleed from the malformation. More commonly, gradual onset of gait abnormalities, low back pain, and bowel and bladder dysfunction are noted. The deep tendon reflexes are absent or reduced in the lower extremities, and the Babinski reflex is present. In approximately one third of cases, a midline cutaneous angioma overlies the arteriovenous malformation, and a spinal bruit may occasionally be auscultated. Roentgenograms of the spine may show erosion of the pedicles; however, contrast myelography and selective spinal angiography are required to delineate the blood supply and the extent of the malformation. The malformation is removed by surgical excision with the use of an operating microscope or is obliterated by embolization.

Bracken MB, Shepard MJ, Holford TR, et al: Administration of methylprednisolone for 24 or 48 hours or tirilazad mesylate for 48 hours in the treatment of acute spinal cord injury. *JAMA* 1997;277:1597–1604.

Committee on Sports Medicine and Fitness 1994–1995, American Academy of Pediatrics: Atlantoaxial instability in Down syndrome: Subject review. *Pediatrics* 1995;96:151–154.

Defresne P, Meyer L, Tardieu M, et al: Efficacy of high dose steroid therapy in children with severe acute transverse myelitis. *J Neurol Neurosurg Psychiatry* 2001;71:272—274.

Guggisberg D, Hadj-Rabia S, Viney C, et al: Skin markers of occult spinal dysraphism in children: A review of 54 cases. *Arch Dermatol* 2004;140:1109–1115.

Jallo GI, Freed D, Epstein F: Intramedullary spinal cord tumors in children. *Childs Nerv Syst* 2003;19:641–649.

McDonald JW, Sadowsky C: Spinal-cord injury. *Lancet* 2002;359:417–425.

Michelson DJ, Ashwal S: Tethered cord syndrome in childhood: Diagnostic features and relationship to congenital anomalies. *Neurol Res* 2004;26:745–753.

Proctor MR: Spinal cord injury. *Crit Care Med* 2002;30(Suppl):S489–S499.

Riche MC, Modenesi-Freitas J, Djindjian M, et al: Arteriovenous malformations (AVM) of the spinal cord in children: Review of 38 cases. *Neuroradiology* 1982;22:171–180.

Sébire G, Hollenberg H, Meyer L, et al: High dose methylprednisolone in severe acute transverse myelopathy. *Arch Dis Child* 1997;76:167–168.

Part XXVII ▪ Neuromuscular Disorders

Harvey B. Sarnat

Chapter 606 ▪ Evaluation and Investigation

The term **neuromuscular disease** defines disorders of the motor unit and excludes influences on muscular function from the brain, such as spasticity. The motor unit has four components: a motor neuron in the brainstem or ventral horn of the spinal cord; its axon that, together with other axons, forms the peripheral nerve; the neuromuscular junction; and all muscle fibers innervated by a single motor neuron. The size of the motor unit varies among different muscles and with the precision of muscular function required. In large muscles, such as the glutei and quadriceps femoris, hundreds of muscle fibers are innervated by a single motor neuron; in small finely tuned muscles, such as the stapedius or the extraocular muscles, a 1 : 1 ratio may prevail. The motor unit is influenced by suprasegmental or upper motor neuron control that alters properties of muscle tone, precision of movement, reciprocal inhibition of antagonistic muscles during movement, and sequencing of muscle contractions to achieve smooth, coordinated movements. Suprasegmental impulses also augment or inhibit the monosynaptic stretch reflex; the corticospinal tract is inhibitory upon this reflex.

Diseases of the motor unit are common in children. These neuromuscular diseases may be genetically determined, congenital or acquired, acute or chronic, and progressive or static. Because specific therapy is available for many diseases and because of genetic and prognostic implications, precise diagnosis is important; laboratory confirmation is required for most diseases because of overlapping clinical manifestations.

Many chromosomal loci have been identified with specific neuromuscular diseases as a result of genetic linkage studies and the isolation and cloning of a few specific genes. In some cases, such as Duchenne muscular dystrophy, the genetic defect has been shown to be a deletion of nucleotide sequences and is associated with a defective protein product, dystrophin; in other cases, such as myotonic muscular dystrophy, the genetic defect is an expansion or repetition, rather than a deletion, in a codon (a set of three consecutive nucleotide repeats that encodes for a single amino acid), with many copies of a particular codon, in this example also associated with abnormal mRNA. Some diseases present as autosomal dominant and autosomal recessive traits in different pedigrees; these distinct mendelian genotypes may result from different genetic mutations on different chromosomes (nemaline rod myopathy) or may be small differences in the same gene at the same chromosomal locus (myotonia congenita), despite many common phenotypic features and shared histopathologic findings in a muscle biopsy specimen. Among the several clinically defined mitochondrial myopathies, specific mtDNA deletions and tRNA point mutations are recognized. The inheritance patterns and chromosomal and mitochondrial loci of common neuromuscular diseases affecting infants and children are summarized in Table 607-1.

CLINICAL MANIFESTATIONS

Examination of the neuromuscular system includes an assessment of muscle bulk, tone, and strength. Tone and strength should not be confused: **Passive tone** is range of motion around a joint; **active tone** is physiologic resistance to movement. Head lag when an infant is pulled to a sitting position from supine is a sign of weakness, not of low tone. Hypotonia may be associated with normal strength or with weakness; enlarged muscles may be weak or strong; thin, wasted muscles may be weak or have unexpectedly normal strength. The distribution of these components is of diagnostic importance. In general, myopathies follow a proximal distribution of weakness and muscle wasting (with the notable exception of myotonic muscular dystrophy); neuropathies are generally distal in distribution (with the notable exception of juvenile spinal muscular atrophy) (Table 606-1). Involvement of the face, tongue, palate, and extraocular muscles provides an important distinction in the differential diagnosis. Tendon stretch reflexes are generally lost in neuropathies and in motor neuron diseases and are diminished but preserved in myopathies (see Table 606-1). A few specific clinical features are important in the diagnosis of some neuromuscular diseases. Fasciculations of muscle, which are often best seen in the tongue, are a sign of denervation. Sensory abnormalities indicate neuropathy. Fatigable weakness is characteristic of neuromuscular junctional disorders. Myotonia is specific for a few myopathies.

Some features do not distinguish myopathy from neuropathy. Muscle pain or myalgias are associated with acute disease of either myopathic or neurogenic origin. Both acute dermatomyositis and acute polyneuropathy (Guillain-Barré syndrome) are characterized by myalgias. Muscular dystrophies and spinal muscular atrophies are not associated with muscle pain. Myalgias also occur in several metabolic diseases of muscle and in ischemic myopathy. Contractures of muscles, whether present at birth or developing later in the course of an illness, occur in both myopathic and neurogenic diseases.

Infant boys who are weak in late fetal life and in the neonatal period often have undescended testes. The testes are actively pulled into the scrotum from the anterior abdominal wall by a pair of cords that consist of smooth and striated muscle called the gubernaculum. The gubernaculum is weakened in many congenital neuromuscular diseases, including spinal muscular atrophy, myotonic muscular dystrophy, and many congenital myopathies.

The thorax of infants with congenital neuromuscular disease often has a funnel shape, and the ribs are thin and radiolucent, due to intercostal muscle weakness during intrauterine growth. This phenomenon is characteristically found in infantile spinal muscular atrophy but also occurs in myotubular myopathy, neonatal myotonic dystrophy, and other disorders (Fig. 606-1). Because of the small muscle mass, birth weight may be low for gestational age.

Generalized hypotonia and motor developmental delay are the most common presenting manifestations of neuromuscular disease in infants and young children (Table 606-2). These features may also be expressions of neurologic disease, endocrine

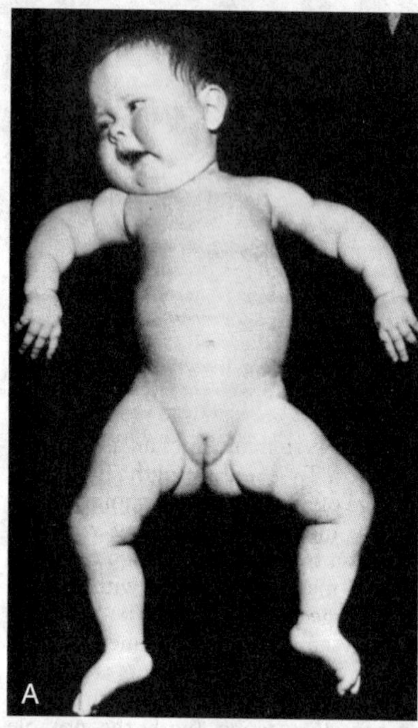

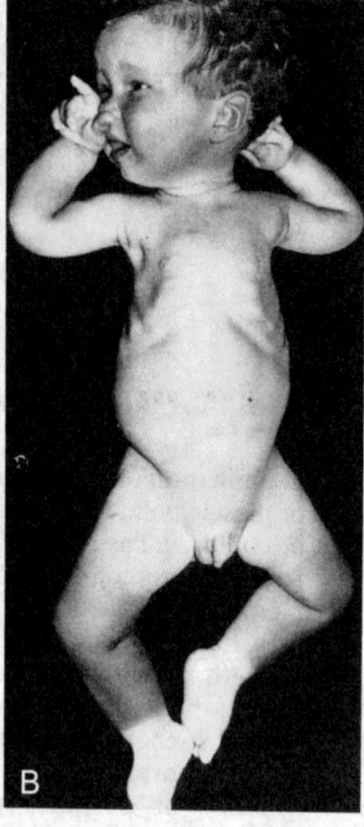

Figure 606-1. Type 1 spinal muscular atrophy (Werdnig-Hoffmann disease): characteristic postures in 6 wk old *(A)* and 1 yr old *(B)* infants with severe weakness and hypotonia from birth. Note the frog-leg posture of the lower limbs and internal rotation ("jug handle") *(A)* or external rotation *(B)* at the shoulders. Note also intercostal recession, especially evident in B, and normal facial expressions. (From Volpe J: *Neurology of the Newborn,* 4th ed. Philadelphia, WB Saunders, 2001, p 645.)

TABLE 606-1. Distinguishing Features of Disorders of the Motor System

LOCUS OF LESION	WEAKNESS* FACE	ARMS	LEGS	PROXIMAL-DISTAL	DEEP TENDON REFLEXES	ELECTROMYOGRAPHY	MUSCLE BIOPSY	OTHER
Central	0	+	+	> or =	Normal or ↑	Normal	Normal	Seizures, hemiparesis, and delayed development
Anterior horn cell	Late	++++	++++	> or =	0	Fasciculations and fibrillations	Denervation pattern	Fasciculations (tongue)
Peripheral nerve	0	+++	+++	<	↓	Fibrillations	Denervation pattern	Sensory deficit, elevated cerebrospinal fluid protein, depressed nerve conduction velocity, abnormal nerve biopsy
Neuromuscular junction	+++	+++	+++	=	Normal	Decremental response (myasthenia); incremental response and BSAP (botulism)	Normal	Response to neostigmine or edrophonium (myasthenia); constipation and fixed pupils (botulism)
Muscle	Variable (+ to ++++)	++	+	>	↓	Short duration, small amplitude motor unit potentials and myopathic polyphasic potentials	Myopathic pattern[†]	Elevated muscle enzyme levels (variable)

*+ *to* ++++, Varying degrees of severity.
[†]May also show unique features, such as in central core disease, nemaline myopathy, myotubular myopathy, and congenital fiber type disproportion.
BSAP, brief duration, small amplitude, overly abundant motor unit potentials.
From Volpe J: *Neurology of the Newborn,* 4th ed. Philadelphia, WB Saunders, 2001, p 706.

TABLE 602-2. Pattern of Weakness and Localization in the Floppy Infant

ANATOMICAL REGION OF HYPOTONIA	CORRESPONDING DISORDERS	PATTERN OF WEAKNESS AND INVOLVEMENT
Central nervous system	Chromosomal disorders Inborn errors of metabolism Cerebral dysgenesis Cerebral, spinal cord trauma	Central hypotonia Axial hypotonia more prominent Hyperactive reflexes
Motor neuron	Spinal muscular atrophy	
Nerve	Peripheral neuropathies	Generalized weakness; often spares the diaphragm, facial muscles, pelvis, and sphincters Distal muscle groups involved Weakness with wasting
Neuromuscular junction	Myasthenia syndromes Infantile botulism	Bulbar, oculomotor muscles exhibit greater degree of involvement
Muscle	Congenital myopathies Metabolic myopathies CMD Congenital myotonic dystrophy	Weakness is prominent Proximal musculature Hypoactive reflexes Joint contractures

CMD, congenital muscular dystrophy.
From Prasad AN, Prasad C: The floppy infant: Contribution of genetic and metabolic disorders. *Brain Dev* 2003; 27:457–476.

TABLE 606-3. Differential Diagnosis of Acute Flaccid Paralysis

BRAINSTEM STROKE
BRAINSTEM ENCEPHALITIS
ACUTE ANTERIOR POLIOMYELITIS
Caused by poliovirus
Caused by other neurotropic viruses
ACUTE MYELOPATHY
Space-occupying lesions
Acute transverse myelitis
PERIPHERAL NEUROPATHY
Guillain-Barré syndrome
Post–rabies vaccine neuropathy
Diphtheritic neuropathy
Heavy metals, biologic toxins, or drug intoxication
Acute intermittent porphyria
Vasculitic neuropathy
Critical illness neuropathy
Lymphomatous neuropathy
DISORDERS OF NEUROMUSCULAR TRANSMISSION
Myasthenia gravis
Biologic or industrial toxins
DISORDERS OF MUSCLE
Hypokalemia
Hypophosphatemia
Inflammatory myopathy
Acute rhabdomyolysis
Trichinosis
Periodic paralyses

From Hughes RAC, Camblath DR: Guillain-Barré syndrome. *Lancet* 2005;366:1653–1666.

and systemic metabolic diseases, and Down syndrome, or they may be nonspecific neuromuscular expressions of malnutrition or chronic systemic illness. A prenatal history of decreased fetal movements and intrauterine growth retardation is often found in patients who are symptomatic at birth. Developmental disorders tend to be of slow onset and are progressive. Acute flaccid paralysis in older infants and children has a different differential diagnosis (Table 606-3).

LABORATORY FINDINGS

SERUM ENZYMES. Several lysosomal enzymes are released by damaged or degenerating muscle fibers and may be measured in serum. The most useful of these enzymes is the **creatine kinase** (CK), which is found in only 3 organs and may be separated into corresponding isozymes: MM for skeletal muscle, MB for cardiac muscle, and BB for brain. Serum CK determination is by no means a universal screening test for neuromuscular disease because many diseases of the motor unit may not be associated with elevated enzymes. The CK level is characteristically elevated in certain diseases, such as Duchenne muscular dystrophy, and the magnitude of increase is characteristic for particular diseases.

MOLECULAR GENETIC MARKERS. Many DNA markers of hereditary myopathies and neuropathies are available from blood samples. If the clinical manifestations suggest a particular disease, these tests may provide a definitive diagnosis and not subject the child to more invasive procedures, such as muscle biopsy. Other molecular markers are available only in muscle biopsy tissue. Genetic blood tests, whether ordered individually or in "panels," are expensive and may be excluded from health insurance plans.

NERVE CONDUCTION VELOCITY (NCV). Motor and sensory nerve conduction may be measured electrophysiologically by using surface electrodes. Neuropathies of various types are detected by decreased conduction. The site of a traumatic nerve injury may also be localized. The nerve conduction at birth is about half of the mature value achieved by age 2 yr. Tables are available for normal values at various ages in infancy, including for preterm infants. Because the NCV study measures only the fastest conducting fibers in a nerve, 80% of the total nerve fibers must be involved before slowing in conduction is detected.

ELECTROMYOGRAPHY (EMG). EMG requires insertion of a needle into the belly of a muscle and recording the electric potentials in various states of contraction. It is less useful in pediatrics than in adult medicine, in part because of technical difficulties in recording these potentials in young children and in part because the best results require the patient's cooperation for full relaxation and maximal voluntary contraction of a muscle. Many children are too frightened to provide such cooperation. Characteristic EMG patterns distinguish denervation from myopathic involvement. The specific type of myopathy is not usually definitively diagnosed, but certain specialized myopathic conditions, such as myotonia, may be demonstrated. An EMG may transiently raise the serum CK level.

EMG combined with repetitive electrical stimulation of a motor nerve supplying a muscle to produce tetany is useful in demonstrating myasthenic decremental responses. Small muscles, such as the abductor digiti quinti of the hypothenar eminence, are used for such studies.

IMAGING OF MUSCLE. Imaging of muscle using ultrasonography, CT scans, and MRI are used in many neuromuscular diseases. While these methods are not always definitively diagnostic, in experienced hands, they provide a supplementary means of following the progression of disease over time. MRI is quite useful in identifying inflammatory myopathies of immune (dermatomyositis) or infectious (viral, bacterial, parasitic) origin. MRI is the study of choice to image the spinal cord or nerve roots and plexus (e.g., brachial).

MUSCLE BIOPSY. The muscle biopsy is the most important and specific diagnostic study of most neuromuscular disorders, if the definitive diagnosis of an hereditary disease is not provided by molecular genetic testing in blood. Not only are neurogenic and myopathic processes distinguished, but also the type of myopathy and specific enzymatic deficiencies may be determined. The vastus lateralis (quadriceps femoris) is the muscle that is most commonly sampled. The deltoid muscle should be avoided in most cases because it normally has a 60–80% predominance of type I fibers so that the distribution patterns of fiber types are difficult to recognize. Muscle biopsy is a simple outpatient procedure that may be performed under local anesthesia with or without femoral nerve block. Needle biopsies are preferred in some centers, but are not percutaneous and require an incision in the skin similar to open biopsy; numerous samples must be taken to conduct an adequate examination of the tissue, and they provide inferior specimens. The volume of tissue from a needle biopsy is usually not adequate for supplementary biochemical studies, such as mitochondrial respiratory chain enzymes; a small, clean, open biopsy is therefore advantageous.

Histochemical studies of frozen sections of the muscle are obligatory in all pediatric muscle biopsies because many congenital and metabolic myopathies cannot be diagnosed from paraffin sections using conventional histologic stains. Immunohistochemistry is a useful supplement in some cases, such as for demonstrating dystrophin in suspected Duchenne muscular dystrophy or merosin in congenital muscular dystrophy. A portion of the biopsy specimen should be fixed for potential electron microscopy, but ultrastructure has additional diagnostic value only in selected cases. Muscle biopsy sample interpretation is complex and should be performed by an experienced pathologist. A portion of frozen muscle tissue should also be routinely saved for possible biochemical analysis (mitochondrial cytopathies, carnitine palmityltransferase, acid maltase).

NERVE BIOPSY. The most commonly sampled nerve is the sural nerve, a pure sensory nerve that supplies a small area of skin on the lateral surface of the foot. Whole or fascicular biopsy specimens of this nerve may be taken. When the sural nerve is severed behind the lateral malleolus of the ankle, regeneration of the nerve occurs in >90% of cases so that permanent sensory loss is not experienced. The sural nerve is often involved in many neuropathies whose clinical manifestations are predominantly motor.

Electron microscopy is performed on most nerve biopsy specimens because many morphologic alterations cannot be appreciated at the resolution of a light microscope. Teased fiber preparations are sometimes useful in demonstrating segmental demyelination, axonal swellings, and other specific abnormalities, but this time-consuming procedure is not done routinely. Special stains may be applied to ordinary frozen or paraffin sections of nerve biopsy material to demonstrate myelin, axoplasm, and metabolic products.

ELECTROCARDIOGRAPHY (ECG). Cardiac evaluation is important if myopathy is suspected because of involvement of the heart in muscular dystrophies and in inflammatory and metabolic myopathies. ECG often detects early cardiomyopathy or conduction defects that are clinically asymptomatic. At times, a more complete cardiac work-up, such as echocardiography and consultation with a pediatric cardiologist, may be indicated. Serial pulmonary function tests also should be performed in muscular dystrophies and in other chronic or progressive diseases of the motor unit.

Prasad AN, Prasad C: The floppy infant: Contribution of genetic and metabolic disorders. *Brain Dev* 2003;27:457–476.

Chapter 607 ■ Developmental Disorders of Muscle

A heterogeneous group of congenital neuromuscular disorders is sometimes known as the **congenital myopathies,** but in some of these disorders, the assumption that the pathogenesis is primarily myopathic is unjustified. Most congenital myopathies are nonprogressive conditions, but some patients show slow clinical deterioration accompanied by additional changes in their muscle biopsy specimen. Most of the diseases in the category of congenital myopathies are hereditary; others are sporadic. Although clinical features, including phenotype, may raise a strong suspicion of a congenital myopathy, the definitive diagnosis is determined by the histopathologic findings in the muscle biopsy specimen. In conditions for which the defective gene has been identified, the diagnosis may be established by the specific molecular genetic probe on lymphocytes. The morphologic and histochemical abnormalities differ considerably from those of the muscular dystrophies, spinal muscular atrophies, and neuropathies. Many are reminiscent of the embryologic development of muscle, thus suggesting possible defects in the genetic regulation of muscle development.

MYOGENIC REGULATORY GENES AND GENETIC LOCI OF INHERITED DISEASES OF MUSCLE (TABLE 607-1)

A family of four myogenic regulatory genes shares encoding transcription factors of "basic helix-loop-helix" (bHLH) proteins associated with common DNA nucleotide sequences. These genes direct the differentiation of striated muscle from any undifferentiated mesodermal cell. The earliest bHLH gene to program the differentiation of myoblasts is myogenic factor 5 *(Myf5)*. The second gene, *myogenin,* promotes fusion of myoblasts to form myotubes. *Herculin* (also known as *MYF6*) and *MYOD1* are the other two myogenic genes. *Myf5* cannot support myogenic differentiation without myogenin, *MyoD,* and *MYF6.* Each of these four genes can activate the expression of at least one other and, under certain circumstances, can autoactivate as well. The expression of *MYF5* and of *herculin* is transient in early ontogenesis but returns later in fetal life and persists into adult life. The human locus of the *MYOD1* gene is on chromosome 11, very near to the domain associated with embryonal rhabdomyosarcoma. The genes encoding *Myf5* and *herculin* are on chromosome 12 and that for *myogenin* is on chromosome 1. The myogenic genes are activated during muscle regeneration, recapitulating the developmental process; *MyoD* in particular is required for myogenic stem cell (satellite cell) activation in adult muscle. *PAX3* and *PAX7* genes also play an important role in myogenesis and interact with each of the four basic genes mentioned above. Another gene, *myostatin,* is a negative regulator of muscle development by preventing myocytes from differentiating. The precise role of the myogenic genes in developmental myopathies is not yet fully defined. Satellite cells in mature muscle that mediate regeneration have the same somitic origin as embryonic muscle progenitor cells.

607.1 • Myotubular Myopathy

The term **myotubular myopathy** implies a maturational arrest of fetal muscle during the myotubular stage of development at 8–15 wk of gestation. It is based on the morphologic appearance of myofibers: A row of central nuclei lies within a core of cytoplasm; contractile myofibrils form a cylinder around this core (Fig. 607-1). Many challenge this interpretation and use the more neutral term **centronuclear myopathy** when referring to this myopathy. This term is too nonspecific because internal nuclei occur in many unrelated myopathies.

PATHOGENESIS. Persistently high fetal concentrations of vimentin and desmin are demonstrated in myofibers of infants with myotubular myopathy, although not reproduced in cultured myocytes of patients. These intermediate filament proteins serve as cytoskeletal elements in fetal myotubes, attaching nuclei and mitochondria to the sarcolemmal membranes to preserve their central positions. As intracellular organization changes with maturation, the nuclei move to the periphery and mitochondria are redistributed between myofibrils. At the same time, vimentin and desmin diminish. Vimentin disappears altogether by term, and desmin remains only in trace amounts. Persistent fetal vimentin and desmin in muscle fibers may be one mechanism of "maturational arrest." A secondary myasthenia-like defect in neuromuscular transmission also occurs in some infants with myotubular myopathy. Myocytes of patients co-cultured with nerve in vitro develop normal innervation and mature normally, not reproducing the in vivo pathologic changes.

CLINICAL MANIFESTATIONS. Decreased fetal movements may occur in late gestation. Polyhydramnios is a common complica-

TABLE 607-1. Inheritance Patterns and Chromosomal or Mitochondrial Loci of Neuromuscular Diseases Affecting the Pediatric Age Group

DISEASE	TRANSMISSION	LOCUS
Duchenne/Becker muscular dystrophy	XR	Xp21.2
Emery-Dreifuss muscular dystrophy	XR	Xq28
Myotonic muscular dystrophy (Steinert)	AD	19q13
Facioscapulohumeral muscular dystrophy	AD	4q35
Limb-girdle muscular dystrophy	AD	5q
Limb-girdle muscular dystrophy	AR	15q
Congenital muscular dystrophy with merosin deficiency	AR	6q2
Congenital muscular dystrophy (Fukuyama)	AR	8q31–33
Myotubular myopathy	XR	Xq28
Myotubular myopathy	AR	Unknown
Nemaline rod myopathy (NEM1)	AD	1q21–q23
Nemaline rod myopathy (NEM2)	AR	2q21.2–q22
Nemaline rod myopathy (NEM3)	AD, AR	1q42.1
Nemaline rod myopathy (NEM4)	AD	9q13
Nemaline rod myopathy (NEM5)	AR	19q13
Congenital muscle fiber–type disproportion	AR, X-linked R	19p13.2, Xp23.12-p11.4, Xq13.1-q22.1; t(10; 17); sporadic
Central core disease	AD	19q13.1
Myotonia congenita (Thomsen)	AD	7q35
Myotonia congenita (Becker)	AR	7q35
Paramyotonia congenita	AD	17q13.1–13.3
Hyperkalemic periodic paralysis	AD	17q13.1–13.3
Hyperkalemic periodic paralysis	AD	1q31–q32
Glycogenosis II (Pompe; acid maltase deficiency)	AR	17q23
Glycogenosis V (McArdle; myophosphorylase deficiency)	AR	11q13
Glycogenosis VII (Tarui; phosphofructokinase deficiency)	AR	1cenq32
Glycogenosis IX (phosphoglycerate kinase deficiency)	XR	Xq13
Glycogenosis X (phosphoglycerate mutase deficiency)	AR	7p12–p13
Glycogenosis XI (lactate dehydrogenase deficiency)	AR	11p15.4
Muscle carnitine deficiency	AR	Unknown
Muscle carnitine palmityltransferase deficiency 2	AR	1p32
Spinal muscular atrophy (Werdnig-Hoffmann; Kugelberg-Welander)	AR	5q11–q13
Familial dysautonomia (Riley-Day)	AR	9q31–33
Hereditary motor-sensory neuropathy (Charcot-Marie-Tooth; Dejerine-Sottas)	AD	17p11.2
Hereditary motor-sensory neuropathy (axonal type)	AD	1p35–p36
Hereditary motor-sensory neuropathy (Charcot-Marie-Tooth-X)	XR	Xq13.1
Mitochondrial myopathy (Kearns-Sayre)	Maternal; sporadic	Single large mtDNA deletion
Mitochondrial myopathy (MERRF)	Maternal	tRNA point mutation at position 8344
Mitochondrial myopathy (MELAS)	Maternal	tRNA point mutation at positions 3243 and 3271

AD, autosomal dominant; AR, autosomal recessive; MELAS, mitochondrial encephalomyopathy with lactic acidosis and strokelike episodes; MERRF, mitochondrial encephalomyopathy with ragged-red fibers; mtDNA, mitochondrial deoxyribonucleic acid; tRNA, transfer ribonucleic acid; XR, X-linked recessive.

tion because of pharyngeal weakness of the fetus and inability to swallow amniotic fluid. At birth, affected infants have a thin muscle mass involving axial, limb girdle, and distal muscles; severe generalized hypotonia; and diffuse weakness. Respiratory efforts may be ineffective, requiring ventilatory support. Gavage feeding may be required because of weakness of the muscles of sucking and deglutition. The testes are often undescended. Facial muscles may be weak, but infants do not have the characteristic facies of myotonic dystrophy. Ptosis may be a prominent feature. Ophthalmoplegia is observed in a few cases. The palate may be high. The tongue is thin, but fasciculations are not seen. Tendon stretch reflexes are weak or absent. Myotubular myopathy is not associated with cardiomyopathy; mature cardiac muscle fibers normally have central nuclei. Congenital anomalies of the central nervous system or of other systems are not associated.

Older children and adults may develop centronuclear myopathy with variable weakness. The relation of this disorder to the severe neonatal disease is uncertain.

LABORATORY FINDINGS. Serum levels of creatine kinase (CK) are normal. Electromyography (EMG) does not show evidence of denervation; results are usually normal or show minimal nonspecific myopathic features in early infancy. Nerve conduction velocity may be slow but is usually normal. The electrocardiogram (ECG) appears normal. Chest radiographs show no cardiomegaly; the ribs may be thin.

DIAGNOSIS. The muscle biopsy findings are diagnostic at birth, even in premature infants. More than 90% of muscle fibers are small and have centrally placed, large vesicular nuclei in a single row. Spaces between nuclei are filled with sarcoplasm containing mitochondria. Histochemical stains for oxidative enzymatic activity and glycogen reveal a central distribution as in fetal myotubes. The cylinder of myofibrils shows mature histochemical differentiation with adenosine triphosphatase stains. The connective tissue of muscle, spindles, blood vessels, intramuscular nerves, and motor end plates are mature. Ultrastructural features in neonatal myotubular myopathy, other than those that define the disease, are also mature. Vimentin and desmin show strong immunoreactivity in muscle fibers in myotubular myopathy and no demonstrable activity in normal term neonatal muscle. The molecular genetic marker in blood is available and is useful not only for confirming the diagnosis but also for early prenatal diagnosis.

GENETICS. X-linked recessive inheritance is the most frequent trait in this disease affecting boys. The mothers of affected infants are clinically asymptomatic, but their muscle biopsy specimen shows minor alterations. Genetic linkage on the X chromosome has been localized to the Xq28 site, a locus different from the Xp21 gene of Duchenne and Becker muscular dystrophies. A deletion in the responsible *MTM1* gene has been identified. It encodes a protein called myotubularin. This gene belongs to a

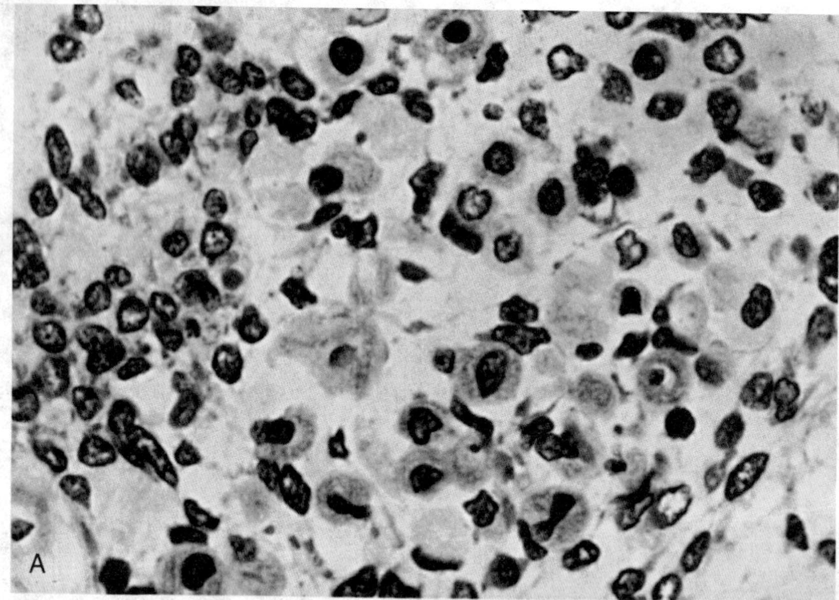

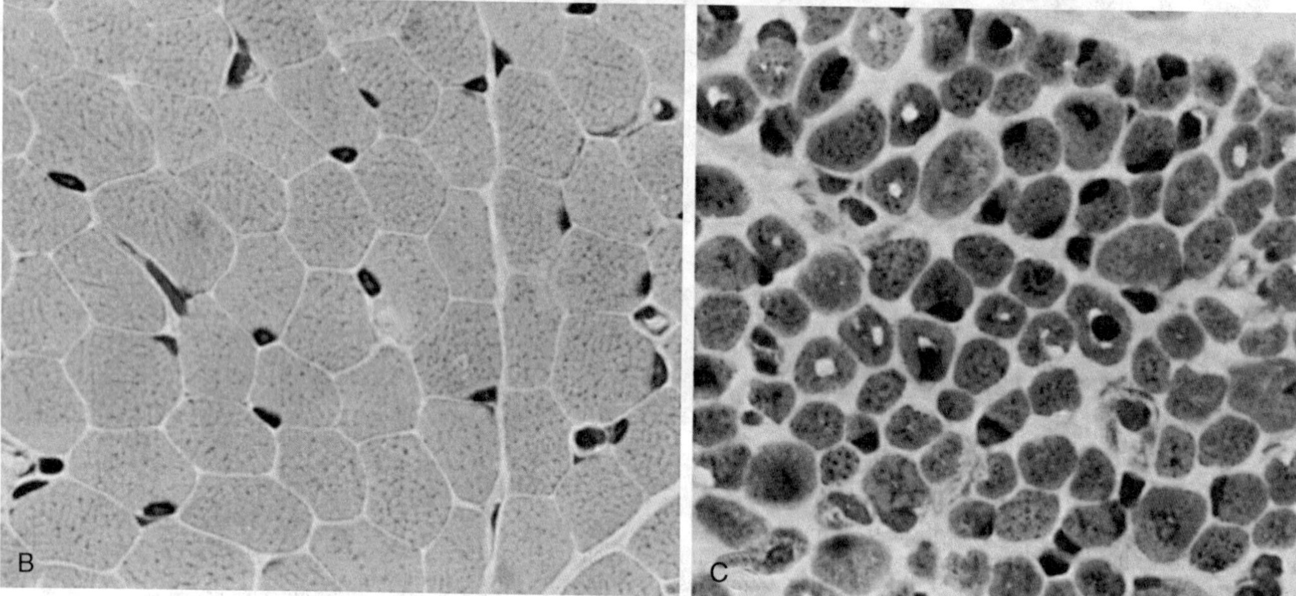

Figure 607-1. *A*, Cross section of muscle from a 14 wk old human fetus; *B*, normal full-term neonate; and *C*, term neonate with X-linked recessive myotubular myopathy. Myofibers have large central nuclei in the fetus and in myotubular myopathy, and nuclei are at the periphery of the muscle fiber in the term neonate as in the adult (hematoxylin and eosin, ×500).

family of similar genes encoding enzymatically active and inactive forms of phosphatidylinositol-3-phosphatases that form dimers. The pathogenesis is in the regulation of enzymatic activity and binding to other proteins induced by dimer interactions. Although only a single gene is involved, 5 distinct point mutations of the *MTM1* gene out of 242 known mutations account for only 27% of cases; many different alleles may produce the same clinical disease. Other, rarer, centronuclear myopathies also are known, some being autosomal dominant or recessive and affecting both sexes and others being sporadic and of unknown genetics. The recessive forms are sometimes divided into an early-onset form with or without ophthalmoplegia and a late-onset form without ophthalmoplegia. Autosomal dominant forms are usually mild and may not present clinically until adult life as diffuse, slowly progressive weakness and generalized muscular pseudohypertrophy.

TREATMENT. Only supportive and palliative treatment is available.

PROGNOSIS. About 75% of severely affected neonates die within the first few weeks or months of life. Survivors do not experience a progressive course but have major physical handicaps, rarely walk, and remain severely hypotonic.

607.2 • Congenital Muscle Fiber–Type Disproportion (CMFTD)

This condition occurs as an isolated congenital myopathy but also develops in association with various unrelated disorders that include nemaline rod disease, Krabbe disease (globoid cell leukodystrophy) early in the course before expression of the neuropathy, cerebellar hypoplasia and certain other brain malformations, fetal alcohol syndrome, some glycogenoses, multiple sulfatase deficiency, Lowe syndrome, rigid spine myopathy, and some infantile cases of myotonic muscular dystrophy.

PATHOGENESIS. The association of CMFTD with cerebellar hypoplasia suggests that the pathogenesis may be an abnormal suprasegmental influence on the developing motor unit during the stage of histochemical differentiation of muscle between 20 and 28 wk of gestation. Muscle fiber types and growth are determined by innervation and are mutable even in adults. Although CMFTD does not actually correspond with any normal stage of development, it appears to be an embryologic disturbance of fiber type differentiation and growth.

CLINICAL MANIFESTATIONS. As an isolated condition not associated with other diseases, CMFTD is a nonprogressive disorder present at birth. Patients have generalized hypotonia and weakness, but the weakness is usually not severe and respiratory distress and dysphagia are rare. Contractures are present at birth in 25% of patients. Poor head control and developmental delay for gross motor skills are common in infancy. Walking is usually delayed until 18–24 mo but is eventually achieved. Because of the hypotonia, subluxation of the hips may occur. Muscle bulk is reduced. The muscle wasting and hypotonia are proportionately greater than the weakness, and the child may be stronger than expected during examination. Cardiomyopathy is a rare complication.

The facies of children with CMFTD often raise suspicion, especially if the child is referred for assessment of developmental delay and hypotonia. The head is dolichocephalic, and facial weakness is present. The palate is usually high arched. Thin muscles of the trunk and extremities give a thin, wasted appearance. The phenotype is very similar to that of nemaline myopathy, that also includes CMFTD as part of the pathological picture. Patients do not complain of myalgias. The clinical course is nonprogressive.

LABORATORY FINDINGS. Serum CK, ECG, EMG, and nerve conduction velocity results are normal in simple CMFTD. If other diseases are associated, laboratory investigation of those conditions discloses the specific features.

DIAGNOSIS. CMFTD is diagnosed by muscle biopsy that shows disproportion in both size and relative ratios of histochemical fiber types: Type I fibers are uniformly small, and type II fibers are hypertrophic; type I fibers are more numerous than type II fibers. Degeneration of myofibers and other primary myopathic features are absent. The biopsy is diagnostic at birth.

GENETICS. Many cases of simple CMFTD are sporadic, although autosomal recessive inheritance is well documented in some families and an autosomal dominant trait is suspected in others. The genetic basis is heterogeneous in hereditary forms; a mutation in the insulin receptor gene at 19p13.2 is reported. Translocation t(10;17) was seen in one family. X-linked transmission with linkage to Xp23.12-p11.4 and Xq13.1-q22.1 also is described. In 3 unrelated families with CMFTD, a heterozygous missense mutation of the skeletal muscle α-actin gene (ACTA1) was demonstrated, but this genetic defect probably represents a minority. In CMFTD associated with cerebellar hypoplasia, the genetic effect is on cerebellar development and the muscular expression is secondary.

TREATMENT. No drug therapy is available. Physiotherapy may be helpful for some patients in strengthening muscles that do not receive sufficient exercise in daily activities. Mild congenital contractures often respond well to gentle range of motion exercises and rarely require plaster casting or surgery.

607.3 • Nemaline Rod Myopathy

Nemaline rods (derived from the Greek *nema,* meaning "thread") are rod-shaped, inclusion-like abnormal structures within muscle fibers. They are difficult to demonstrate histologically with conventional hematoxylin-eosin stain but are easily seen with special stains. They are not foreign inclusion bodies but rather consist of excessive Z-band material with a similar ultrastructure (Fig. 607-2). Chemically, the rods are composed of actin, α-actinin, tropomyosin-3, and the protein nebulin. Nemaline rod formation may be an unusual reaction of muscle fibers to injury because these rod structures have rarely been found in other diseases. They are most abundant in the congenital myopathy known as nemaline rod disease. Most rods are within the myofibrils (cytoplasmic), but intranuclear rods are occasionally demonstrated by electron microscopy.

CLINICAL MANIFESTATIONS. Neonatal, infantile, and juvenile forms of the disease are known. The neonatal form is severe and usually fatal because of respiratory failure since birth. In the infantile form, generalized hypotonia and weakness, which can include bulbar-innervated and respiratory muscles, and a very thin muscle mass are characteristic (Fig. 607-3). The head is dolichocephalic, and the palate high arched or even cleft. Muscles of the jaw may be too weak to hold it closed (Fig. 607-4). Decreased fetal movements are reported by the mother, and neonates suffer from hypoxia and dysphagia; arthrogryposis may be present. Infants with severe neonatal and infantile nemaline myopathy have facies and phenotype that are nearly indistinguishable from that of neonatal myotonic dystrophy, but their mothers have normal facies. The juvenile form is the mildest and is not associated with respiratory failure, but the phenotype, including facial involvement, is similar.

LABORATORY FINDINGS. Serum CK level is normal or mildly elevated. The muscle biopsy is diagnostic. In addition to the characteristic nemaline rods, it also shows CMFTD or at least fiber type I predominance. In some patients, uniform type I fibers are seen with few or no type II fibers. Focal myofibrillar degeneration and an increase in lysosomal enzymes have been found in a few severe cases associated with progressive symptoms. Intranu-

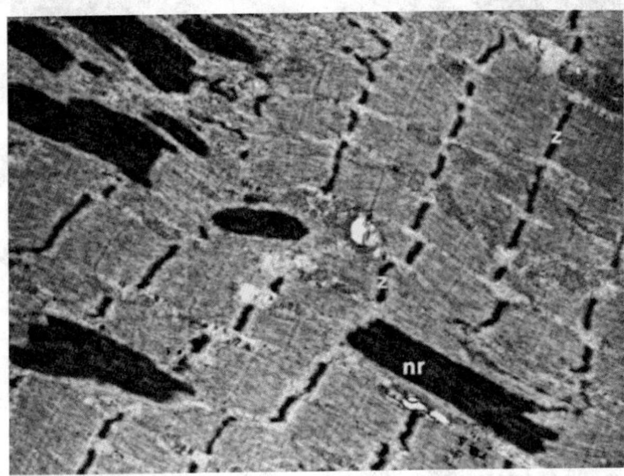

Figure 607-2. Electron micrograph of the muscle from a patient shown in Figure 607-4. Nemaline rods (nr) are seen within many myofibrils. They are identical in composition to the normal Z bands (z) (×6,000).

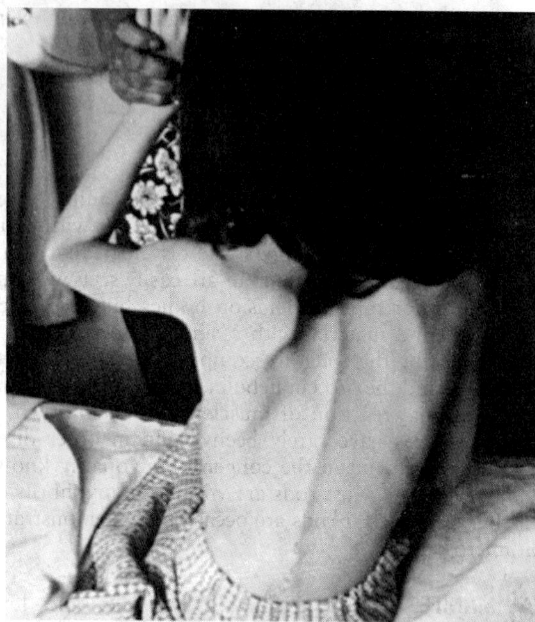

Figure 607-3. Back of a 13 yr old girl with juvenile form of nemaline rod disease. The paraspinal muscles are very thin, and winging of the scapulae is evident. The muscle mass of the extremities is also greatly reduced both proximally and distally.

clear nemaline rods correlate with the most severe clinical manifestations. They are demonstrated by electron microscopy.

GENETICS. Autosomal dominant and autosomal recessive forms of nemaline rod disease occur, and an X-linked dominant form in girls also may occur. Five genes are associated with this

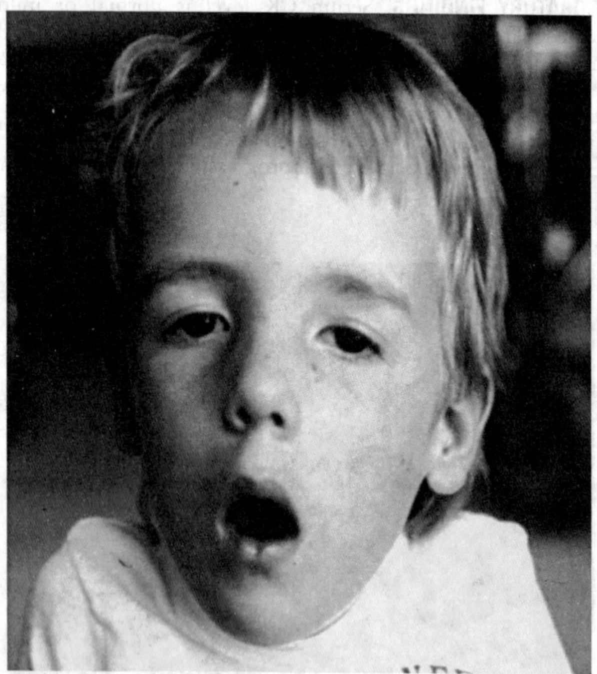

Figure 607-4. Infantile form of nemaline rod disease in a 6 yr old boy. Facial weakness and generalized muscle wasting are severe. The head is dolichocephalic. The mouth is usually open because the masseters are too weak to lift the mandible against gravity for more than a few seconds.

condition. One autosomal dominant nemaline rod myopathy (NEM1) has been mapped to the 1q21-23 locus; the responsible *TPM3* gene produces defective a-tropomyosin. Another genetic mutation (NEM2) at the 2q21.2-q22 locus produces *nebulin*, a large molecule also needed for Z-band integrity, and is transmitted as an autosomal recessive trait. NEM3 is due to a -actin defect and both autosomal dominant and recessive varieties occur at the same 1q42.1 locus. NEM4 is an autosomal dominantly inherited defect of ß-tropomyosin at 9q13. The α- and β-tropomyosin defects are rare and account for only 3% of patients with nemaline myopathy. NEM5 is an autosomal recessive troponin-T defect at 19q13, but has been found only in the Amish population.

TREATMENT AND PROGNOSIS. Therapy is supportive. Survivors are confined to an electric wheelchair and are usually unable to overcome gravity. Both proximal and distal muscles are involved. Gastrostomy may be needed for chronic dysphagia. In the juvenile form, patients are ambulatory and are able to perform most tasks of daily living. Weakness is not usually progressive, but some patients have more difficulty over time or enter a phase of progressive weakness. Cardiomyopathy is an uncommon complication. Pneumonia occurs frequently.

607.4 • Central Core Disease and Minicore Myopathy

This disease is transmitted as either an autosomal dominant or recessive trait, both caused by the same abnormal gene at the 19q13.1 locus. The gene programs the ryanodine receptor *(RYR1)*, a tetramere receptor to a nonvoltage-gated calcium channel in the sarcoplasmic reticulum. Mutations in this gene are also the cause of malignant hyperthermia. Infantile hypotonia, proximal weakness, muscle wasting, and involvement of facial muscles and neck flexors are the typical features in both the dominant and recessive forms. Contractures of the knees, hips, and other joints are common, and kyphoscoliosis and pes cavus frequently develop, even without much axial or distal muscle weakness. There is a high incidence of cardiac abnormalities. The course is nonprogressive, except for the contractures.

The disease is characterized pathologically by central cores within muscle fibers in which only amorphous, granular cytoplasm is found with an absence of myofibrils and organelles. Histochemical stains show a lack of enzymatic activities of all types within these cores. The serum CK value is normal in central core disease except during crises of malignant hyperthermia (see Chapter 610.2).

Central core disease is consistently associated with malignant hyperthermia, which may precede the diagnosis of central core disease. All patients should have special precautions with pretreatment by dantrolene before an anesthetic agent is administered. Salbutamol treatment in a few children with central core disease has demonstrated improved strength and forced vital capacity over a 6-mo period; this observation requires further documentation.

Variants of central cores, called *minicores* and *multicores*, are described in some families, but minicore myopathy is a different genetic disease. Cases with a similar mutation in the RYR1 gene are reported, but others have a defective selenoprotein-N *(SEPN1)* gene, the latter also implicated in rigid spine myopathy. Children with this disorder are hypotonic in early infancy and have a benign course but often develop progressive kyphoscoliosis or a rigid spine in adolescence. In one variant, external ophthalmoplegia also is present. Rare cases of minicore myopathy also show hypertrophic cardiomyopathy.

607.5 • Myofibrillar Myopathies

Most myofibrillar myopathies are not symptomatic in childhood, but occasionally older children and adolescents may show early symptoms of nonspecific proximal and distal weakness. An infantile form also occurs and may cause mild neonatal hypotonia and weakness with disproportionately severe dysphagia and respiratory insufficiency, at times leading to early death. It is nonprogressive, however, and some patients show improvement in later infancy and early childhood, acquiring the ability to swallow by 3 yr of age. Cardiomyopathy may be a complication in a minority. The diagnosis is by muscle biopsy: some sarcomeres of myofibers have disorganization or dissolution of myofibrils, adjacent to other areas of normal sarcomeres within the same fiber. These zones are associated with streaming of the Z bands and focally increased desmin intermediate filaments, myotilin, and α-B-crystallin. Immunocytochemical and ultrastructural study of the muscle biopsy tissue is required. Mutation in the desmin gene is implicated as the etiology. An associated mitochondrial defect is detected in some patients.

607.6 • Brain Malformations and Muscle Development

Infants with **cerebellar hypoplasia** are hypotonic and developmentally delayed, especially in gross motor skills. Muscle biopsy is sometimes performed to exclude a congenital myopathy. A biopsy specimen may show delayed maturation of muscle, fiber-type predominance, or CMFTD. Other malformations of the brain may also be associated with abnormal histochemical patterns, but supratentorial lesions are less likely than brainstem or cerebellar lesions to alter muscle development. Abnormal descending impulses along bulbospinal pathways probably alter discharge patterns of lower motor neurons that determine the histochemical differentiation of muscle at 20–28 wk of gestation. The corticospinal tract does not participate because it is not yet functional during this period of fetal life. In several congenital muscular dystrophies, including the Walker-Warburg syndrome, Fukuyama disease, and muscle-eye-brain disease of Santavuori, major cerebral malformations are present, such as pachygyria and lissencephaly.

607.7 • Amyoplasia

Congenital absence of individual muscles is common and is often asymmetric. A common aplasia is the *palmaris longus muscle* of the ventral forearm, which is absent in 30% of normal subjects and is fully compensated by other flexors of the wrist. Unilateral absence of a *sternocleidomastoid muscle* is one cause of congenital torticollis. Absence of one *pectoralis major muscle* is part of the Poland anomalad.

When innervation does not develop, such as in the lower limbs in severe cases of *myelomeningocele,* muscles may fail to develop. In *sacral agenesis,* the abnormal somites that fail to form bony vertebrae may also fail to form muscles from the same defective mesodermal plate, a disorder of induction resulting in segmental amyoplasia. Skeletal muscles of the extremities fail to differentiate from embryonic myomeres if the long bones do not form. Absence of 1 long bone, such as the radius, is associated with variable aplasia or hypoplasia of associated muscles, such as the *carpi flexor radialis.* End-stage neurogenic atrophy of muscle is sometimes called **amyoplasia,** but this use is semantically incorrect.

Generalized amyoplasia usually results in fetal death, and liveborn neonates rarely survive. A mutation in 1 of the myogenic genes is the suspected etiology because of genetic knockout studies in mice, but it has not been proven in humans.

607.8 • Muscular Dysgenesis (Proteus Syndrome Myopathy)

The **Proteus syndrome** is a disturbance of cellular growth involving ectodermal and mesodermal tissues. The cause is unknown, but it is not a mendelian trait. It presents as asymmetric overgrowth of the extremities, verrucous cutaneous lesions, angiomas of various types, thickening of bones, hemimegalencephaly, and excessive growth of muscles without weakness. Histologically, the muscle is a unique *muscular dysgenesis.* Abnormal zones are adjacent to zones of normal muscle formation and do not follow anatomic boundaries. The disorder may be due to abnormal paracrine growth factors.

607.9 • Benign Congenital Hypotonia

Benign congenital hypotonia is not a disease but is a descriptive term for infants or children with nonprogressive hypotonia of unknown origin. The hypotonia is not usually associated with weakness or developmental delay, although some children acquire gross motor skills more slowly than normal. Tendon stretch reflexes are normal or hypoactive. There are no cranial nerve abnormalities, and intelligence is normal.

The **diagnosis** is one of exclusion after results of laboratory studies, including muscle biopsy and imaging of the brain with special attention to the cerebellum, are normal (Table 606-2). No known molecular genetic basis for this syndrome has been identified.

The **prognosis** is generally good; no specific therapy is required. Contractures do not develop. Hypotonia persists into adult life. The disorder is not always as "benign" as its name implies because a common complication is recurrent dislocation of joints, especially the shoulders. Excessive motility of the spine may result in stretch injury, compression, or vascular compromise of nerve roots or of the spinal cord. These are particular hazards for patients who perform gymnastics or who become circus performers because of agility of joints without weakness or pain.

607.10 • Arthrogryposis

Arthrogryposis multiplex congenita is not a disease but is a descriptive term that signifies numerous congenital contractures (see Chapter 681).

Clarke NF, North KN: Congenital fiber type disproportion—30 years on. *J Neuropathol Exp Neurol* 2003;62:977–989.

Goebel HH: Congenital myopathies in the new millennium. *J Child Neurol* 2005;20:94–101.

Gros J, Manceau M, Thomé V, et al: A common somitic origin for embryonic muscle progenitors and satellite cells. *Nature* 2005;435:954–958.

Jungbluth H, Sewry CA, Muntoni F: What's new in neuromuscular disorders? The congenital myopathies. *Eur J Paediatr Neurol* 2003;7:23–30.

Laing NC, Clarke NF, Dye DE, et al: Actin mutations are one cause of congenital fibre type disproportion. *Ann Neurol* 2004;56:689–694.

Pierson CR, Tomczak K, Agrawal P, et al: X-linked myotubular and centronuclear myopathies. *J Neuropathol Exp Neurol* 2005;64:555–564.

Quane KA, Healy JM, Keating KE, et al: Mutations in the ryanodine receptor gene in central core disease and malignant hyperthermia. *Nat Genet* 1993;5:51–55.
Quinlivan RM, Muller CR, Davis M, et al: Central core disease: clinical, pathological, and genetic features. *Arch Dis Child* 2003;88:1051–1055.
Relaix F, Rocancourt D, Mansouri A, et al: A Pax3/Pax7-dependent population of skeletal muscle progenitor cells. *Nature* 2005;435:948–953.
Sarnat HB: Cerebral dysgeneses and their influence on fetal muscle development. *Brain Dev* 1986;8:495–499.
Sarnat HB: Myopathy of the Proteus syndrome: Hypothesis of muscular dysgenesis. *Neuromuscul Disord* 1993;3:293–301.
Sarnat HB: Ontogenesis of striated muscle. In Polin RA, Fox WW (editors): *Neonatal and Fetal Medicine: Physiology and Pathophysiology,* vol. 2, 3rd ed. Philadelphia, WB Saunders, 2003, pp 1849–1870.
Schuelke M, Wagner KR, Stolz LE, et al: Myostatin mutation associated with gross muscle hypertrophy in a child. *N Engl J Med* 2004;350:2682–2688.
Selcen D, Ohno K, Engel AG: Myofibrillar myopathy: Clinical, morphological and genetic studies in 63 patients. *Brain* 2004;127:439–451.
Wallgren-Pattersson C, Pelin K, Nowak KH, et al: Genotype-phenotype correlations in nemaline myopathy caused by mutations in the genes for nebulin and skeletal muscle α-actin. *Neuromuscul Disord* 2004;14:461–470.
Wallgren-Pattersson C: Gene table: Congenital myopathies. *Eur J Paediatr Neurol* 2005;9:27–28.

Chapter 608 ■ Muscular Dystrophies

The term **dystrophy** means abnormal growth, derived from the Greek *trophe*, meaning "nourishment." A muscular dystrophy is distinguished from all other neuromuscular diseases by four obligatory criteria: It is a primary myopathy; it has a genetic basis; the course is progressive; degeneration and death of muscle fibers occur at some stage in the disease. This definition excludes neurogenic diseases such as spinal muscular atrophy, nonhereditary myopathies such as dermatomyositis, nonprogressive and non-necrotizing congenital myopathies such as congenital muscle fiber–type disproportion (CMFTD), and nonprogressive inherited metabolic myopathies. Some metabolic myopathies may fulfill the definition of a progressive muscular dystrophy but are not traditionally classified as dystrophies (muscle carnitine deficiency). All muscular dystrophies may eventually be reclassified as metabolic myopathies once the biochemical defects are better defined.

Muscular dystrophies are a group of unrelated diseases, each transmitted by a different genetic trait and each differing in its clinical course and expression. Some are severe diseases at birth that lead to early death; others follow very slow progressive courses over many decades, may be compatible with normal longevity, or may not even become symptomatic until late adult life. Some categories of dystrophies, such as limb-girdle muscular dystrophy, are not homogeneous diseases but rather syndromes encompassing several distinct myopathies. Relationships between the various muscular dystrophies are resolved by molecular genetics rather than by similarities or differences in clinical and histopathologic features.

608.1 • Duchenne and Becker Muscular Dystrophies

Duchenne muscular dystrophy is the most common hereditary neuromuscular disease affecting all races and ethnic groups. Its characteristic clinical features are progressive weakness, intellectual impairment, hypertrophy of the calves, and proliferation of connective tissue in muscle. The incidence is 1 : 3,600 liveborn infant boys. This disease is inherited as an X-linked recessive trait. The abnormal gene is at the Xp21 locus and is one of the largest genes. **Becker muscular dystrophy** is the same fundamental disease as Duchenne dystrophy, with a genetic defect at the same locus, but clinically it follows a milder and more protracted course.

CLINICAL MANIFESTATIONS. Infant boys are only rarely symptomatic at birth or in early infancy, although some are mildly hypotonic. Early gross motor skills, such as rolling over, sitting, and standing, are usually achieved at the appropriate ages or may be mildly delayed. Poor head control in infancy may be the 1st sign of weakness. Distinctive facies are not a feature because facial muscle weakness is a late event. Walking is often accomplished at the normal age of about 12 mo, but hip girdle weakness may be seen in subtle form as early as the 2nd yr. Toddlers may assume a lordotic posture when standing to compensate for gluteal weakness. An early Gowers sign is often evident by age 3 yr and is fully expressed by age 5 or 6 yr (see Fig. 591-2). A Trendelenburg gait, or hip waddle, appears at this time.

The length of time that a patient remains ambulatory varies greatly. Some patients are confined to a wheelchair by 7 yr of age; most patients continue to walk with increasing difficulty until age 10 yr without orthopedic intervention. With orthotic bracing, physiotherapy, and sometimes minor surgery (Achilles tendon lengthening), most are able to walk until age 12 yr. Ambulation is important not only for postponing the psychological depression that accompanies the loss of an aspect of personal independence but also because scoliosis usually does not become a major complication as long as a patient remains ambulatory, even for as little as 1 hr per day; scoliosis often becomes rapidly progressive after confinement to a wheelchair.

The relentless progression of **weakness** continues into the 2nd decade. The function of distal muscles is usually relatively well enough preserved, allowing the child to continue to use eating utensils, a pencil, and a computer keyboard. Respiratory muscle involvement is expressed as a weak and ineffective cough, frequent pulmonary infections, and decreasing respiratory reserve. Pharyngeal weakness may lead to episodes of aspiration, nasal regurgitation of liquids, and an airy or nasal voice quality. The function of the extraocular muscles remains well preserved. Incontinence due to anal and urethral sphincter weakness is an uncommon and very late event.

Contractures most often involve the ankles, knees, hips, and elbows. **Scoliosis** is common. The thoracic deformity further compromises pulmonary capacity and compresses the heart. Scoliosis usually progresses more rapidly after the child becomes nonambulatory and may be uncomfortable or painful. Enlargement of the calves (pseudohypertrophy) and wasting of thigh muscles are classic features. The enlargement is caused by hypertrophy of some muscle fibers, infiltration of muscle by fat, and proliferation of collagen. After the calves, the next most common site of muscular hypertrophy is the tongue, followed by muscles of the forearm. Fasciculations of the tongue do not occur. The voluntary sphincter muscles rarely become involved.

Unless ankle contractures are severe, ankle deep tendon reflexes remain well preserved until terminal stages. The knee deep tendon reflexes may be present until about 6 yr of age but are less brisk than the ankle jerks and are eventually lost. In the upper extremities, the brachioradialis reflex is usually stronger than the biceps or triceps brachii reflexes.

Cardiomyopathy, including persistent tachycardia and myocardiac failure, is seen in 50–80% of patients with this disease. The severity of cardiac involvement does not necessarily correlate with the degree of skeletal muscle weakness. Some patients die early of severe cardiomyopathy while still ambulatory; others in terminal stages of the disease have well-compensated cardiac function. Smooth muscle dysfunction, particularly of the gastrointestinal tract, is a minor, but often overlooked, feature.

Intellectual impairment occurs in all patients, although only 20–30% have an IQ <70. The majority has learning disabilities that still allow them to function in a regular classroom, particularly with remedial help. A few patients are profoundly mentally retarded, but there is no correlation with the severity of the myopathy. Epilepsy is slightly more common than in the general pediatric population. Dystrophin is expressed in brain and retina, as well as in striated and cardiac muscle, though the level, is lower in brain than in muscle. This distribution may explain some of the CNS manifestations. Abnormalities in cortical architecture and of dendritic arborization may be detected neuropathologically; cerebral atrophy is demonstrated by MRI late in the clinical course. The degenerative changes and fibrosis of muscle constitute a painless process. Myalgias and muscle spasms do not occur. Calcinosis of muscle is rare.

Death occurs usually at about 18–20 yr of age. The causes of death are respiratory failure in sleep, intractable heart failure, pneumonia, or occasionally aspiration and airway obstruction.

In **Becker muscular dystrophy,** boys remain ambulatory until late adolescence or early adult life. Calf pseudohypertrophy, cardiomyopathy, and elevated serum levels of creatine kinase (CK) are similar to those of patients with Duchenne dystrophy. Learning disabilities are less frequent. The onset of weakness is later in Becker than in Duchenne dystrophy. Death often occurs in the mid to late 20s; fewer than half of patients are still alive by age 40 yr; these survivors are severely disabled.

LABORATORY FINDINGS. The serum CK level is consistently greatly elevated in Duchenne muscular dystrophy, even in presymptomatic stages, including at birth. The usual serum concentration is 15,000–35,000 IU/L (normal <160 IU/L). A normal serum CK level is incompatible with the diagnosis of Duchenne dystrophy, although in terminal stages of the disease, the serum CK value may be considerably lower than it was a few years earlier because there is less muscle to degenerate. Other lysosomal enzymes present in muscle, such as aldolase and aspartate aminotransferase, are also increased but are less specific.

Cardiac assessment by echocardiography, electrocardiography (ECG), and radiography of the chest is essential and should be repeated periodically. After the diagnosis is established, patients should be referred to a pediatric cardiologist for long-term cardiac care.

Electromyography (EMG) shows characteristic myopathic features but is not specific for Duchenne muscular dystrophy. No evidence of denervation is found. Motor and sensory nerve conduction velocities are normal.

DIAGNOSIS. Blood polymerase chain reaction (PCR) for the dystrophin gene mutation is the primary test, if the clinical features and serum CK are consistent with the diagnosis. If the blood PCR is diagnostic, muscle biopsy may be deferred, but if it is normal and clinical suspicion is high, the more specific dystrophin immunocytochemistry performed on muscle biopsy sections detects the ⅓ of cases that do not show a PCR abnormality. Immunohistochemical staining of frozen sections of muscle biopsy tissue detects differences between the rod domain, the carboxyl-terminus (that attaches to the sarcolemma), and the amino-terminus (that attaches to the actin myofilaments) of the large dystrophin molecule, and may be prognostic of the clinical course as Duchenne or Becker disease. More severe weakness occurs with truncation of the dystrophin molecule at the carboxyl- than at the amino-terminus. Confirmation of the diagnosis by either blood PCR or muscle biopsy should be done in every case. Dystroglycans and other sarcolemmal regional proteins, such as merosin and sarcoglycans, also can be measured because they may be secondarily decreased.

The **muscle biopsy** is diagnostic and shows characteristic changes (Figs. 608-1 and 608-2). Myopathic changes include endomysial connective tissue proliferation, scattered degenerating and regenerating myofibers, foci of mononuclear inflammatory cell infiltrates as a reaction to muscle fiber necrosis, mild architectural changes in still functional muscle fibers, and many dense fibers. These hypercontracted fibers probably result from segmental necrosis at another level, allowing calcium to enter the site of breakdown of the sarcolemmal membrane and trigger a contraction of the whole length of the muscle fiber. Calcifications within myofibers are correlated with secondary β-dystroglycan deficiency.

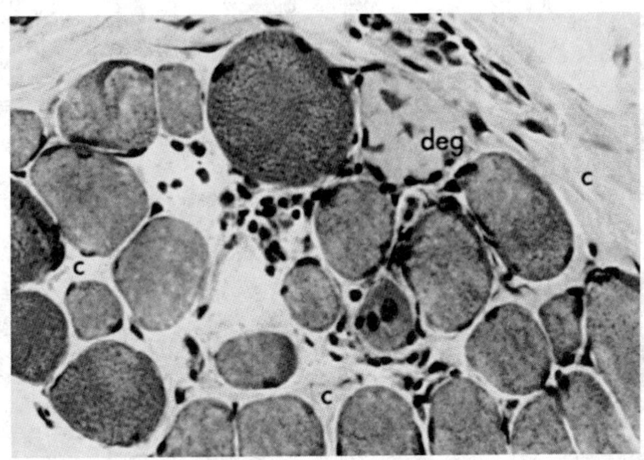

Figure 608-1. Muscle biopsy of a 4 yr old boy with Duchenne muscular dystrophy. Both atrophic and hypertrophic muscle fibers are seen, and some fibers are degenerating (deg). Connective tissue (c) between muscle fibers is increased (hematoxylin and eosin, ×400).

The decision about whether muscle biopsy should be performed to establish the diagnosis sometimes presents problems. If there is a family history of the disease, particularly in the case of an involved brother whose diagnosis has been confirmed, a patient with typical clinical features of Duchenne muscular dystrophy and high concentrations of serum CK probably does not need to undergo biopsy. The result of the PCR may also influence whether to perform a muscle biopsy. A first case in a family, even if the clinical features are typical, should have the diagnosis confirmed to ensure that another myopathy is not masquerading as Duchenne dystrophy. The most common muscles sampled are the vastus lateralis (quadriceps femoris) and the gastrocnemius.

GENETIC ETIOLOGY AND PATHOGENESIS. Despite the X-linked recessive inheritance in Duchenne muscular dystrophy, about 30% of patients are new mutations, and the mother is not a carrier. The female carrier state usually shows no muscle weakness or any clinical expression of the disease, but affected girls are occasionally encountered, usually having much milder weakness than boys. These symptomatic girls are explained by the Lyon hypothesis in which the normal X chromosome becomes inactivated and the one with the gene deletion is active (see Chapter 80). The full clinical picture of Duchenne dystrophy has occurred in several girls with Turner syndrome in whom the single X chromosome must have had the Xp21 gene deletion.

The asymptomatic carrier state of Duchenne dystrophy is associated with elevated serum CK values in 80% of cases. The level of increase is usually in the magnitude of hundreds or a few thousand but does not have the extreme values noted in affected males. Prepubertal girls who are carriers of the dystrophy also have increased serum CK values, with highest levels at 8–12 yr of age. Approximately 20% of carriers have normal serum CK values. If the mother of an affected boy has normal CK levels, it is unlikely that her daughter can be identified as a carrier by measuring CK. Muscle biopsy of suspected female carriers may detect

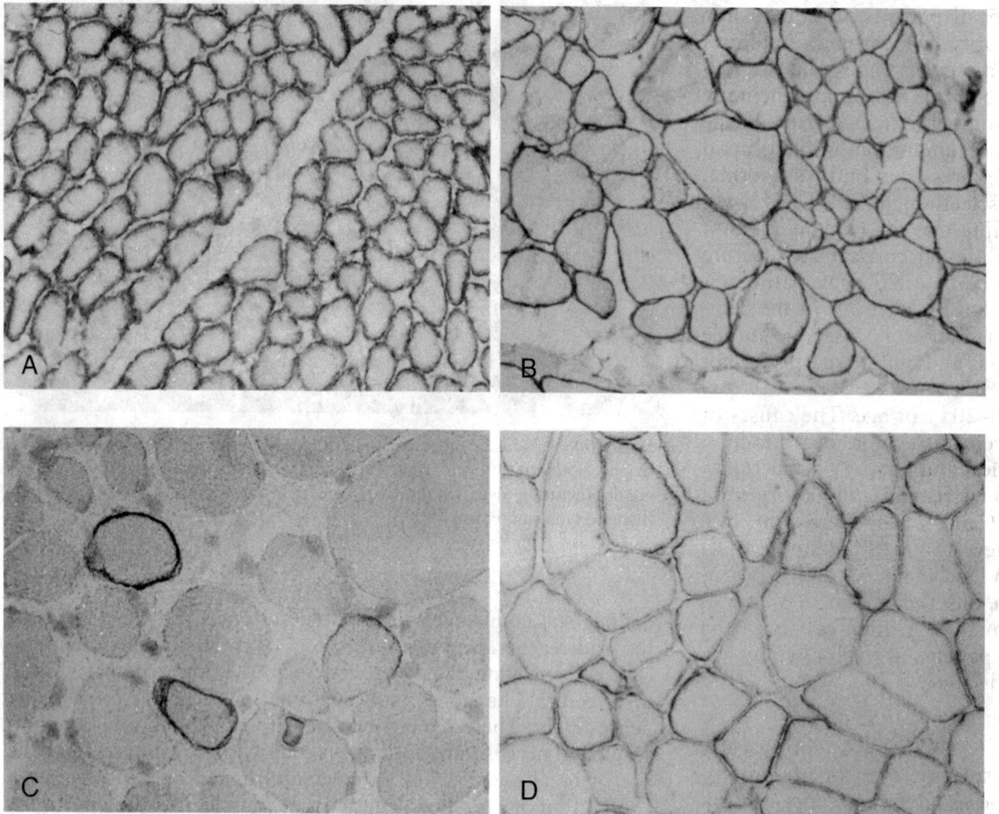

Figure 608-2. Dystrophin is demonstrated by immunohistochemical reactivity in the muscle biopsies of a normal term male neonate *(A)*, a 10 yr old boy with limb-girdle muscular dystrophy *(B)*, a 6 yr old boy with Duchenne muscular dystrophy *(C)*, and a 10 yr old boy with Becker muscular dystrophy *(D)*. In the normal condition and also in non–X-linked muscular dystrophies in which dystrophin is not affected, the sacrolemmal membrane of every fiber is strongly stained, including atrophic and hypertrophic fibers. In Duchenne dystrophy, most myofibers express no detectable dystrophin, but a few scattered fibers known as "revertant fibers" show near-normal immunoreactivity. In Becker muscular dystrophy, the abnormal dystrophin molecule is expressed as thin, pale-staining of the sarcolemma in which reactivity varies not only between myofibers but also along the circumference of individual fibers (×250).

an additional 10% in whom serum CK is not elevated; a specific genetic diagnosis using PCR on peripheral blood is definitive. Some female carriers may suffer cardiomyopathy without weakness of striated muscles.

A 427-kd cytoskeletal protein known as *dystrophin* is encoded by the gene at the Xp21.2 locus. This subsarcolemmal protein attaches to the sarcolemmal membrane overlying the A and M bands of the myofibrils and consists of 4 distinct regions or domains: the amino-terminus contains 250 amino acids and is related to the *N*-actin binding site of α-actinin; the second domain is the largest, with 2,800 amino acids, and contains many repeats, giving it a characteristic rod shape; a third cysteine-rich domain is related to the carboxyl terminus of α-actinin; and the final carboxyl-terminal domain of 400 amino acids is unique to dystrophin and to a dystrophin-related protein encoded by chromosome 6.

The molecular defects in the dystrophinopathies vary: intragenic deletions, duplications, or point mutations of nucleotides. About 65% of patients have deletions, and only 7% exhibit duplications. The site or size of the intragenic abnormality does not always correlate well with the phenotypic severity; in both Duchenne and Becker forms the mutations are mainly near the middle of the gene, involving deletions of exons 46-51. Phenotypic or clinical variations are explained by the alteration of the translational reading frame of mRNA, which results in unstable, truncated dystrophin molecules and severe, classic Duchenne dystrophy; mutations that preserve the reading frame still permit translation of coding sequences further downstream on the gene and produce a semifunctional dystrophin, expressed clinically as Becker muscular dystrophy. An even milder form of adult onset, formerly known as **quadriceps myopathy,** is also caused by an abnormal dystrophin molecule. The clinical spectrum of the dystrophinopathies not only includes the classic Duchenne and Becker forms but ranges from a severe neonatal muscular dystrophy to asymptomatic children with persistent elevation of serum CK levels >1,000 IU/L.

Analysis of the dystrophin protein requires a muscle biopsy and is demonstrated by Western blot analysis or in tissue sections by immunohistochemical methods using either fluorescence or light microscopy of antidystrophin antisera (see Fig. 608-2). In classic Duchenne dystrophy, levels of <3% of normal are found; in Becker muscular dystrophy, the molecular weight of dystrophin is reduced to 20–90% of normal in 80% of patients, but in 15% the dystrophin is of normal size but reduced in quantity, and 5% have an abnormally large protein caused by excessive duplications or repeats of codons. Selective immunoreactivity of different parts of the dystrophin molecule in sections of muscle biopsy material distinguishes the Duchenne and Becker forms (Fig. 608-3). The demonstration of deletions and duplications also can be made from blood samples by the more rapid PCR, which identifies as many as 98% of deletions by amplifying 18 exons but cannot detect duplications. The diagnosis can thus be confirmed at the molecular genetic level from either the muscle biopsy material or from peripheral blood, although as many as ⅓ of boys with Duchenne or Becker dystrophy have a false-normal blood PCR; all cases of dystrophinopathy are detected by muscle biopsy.

The same methods of DNA analysis from blood samples may be applied for carrier detection in female relatives at risk, such as sisters and cousins, and to determine whether the mother is a carrier or whether a new mutation occurred in the embryo. Prenatal diagnosis is possible as early as the 12th wk of gestation by sampling chorionic villi for DNA analysis by Southern blot or PCR and is confirmed in aborted fetuses with Duchenne dystrophy by immunohistochemistry for dystrophin in muscle.

TREATMENT. There is neither a medical cure for this disease nor a method of slowing its progression. Much can be done to treat

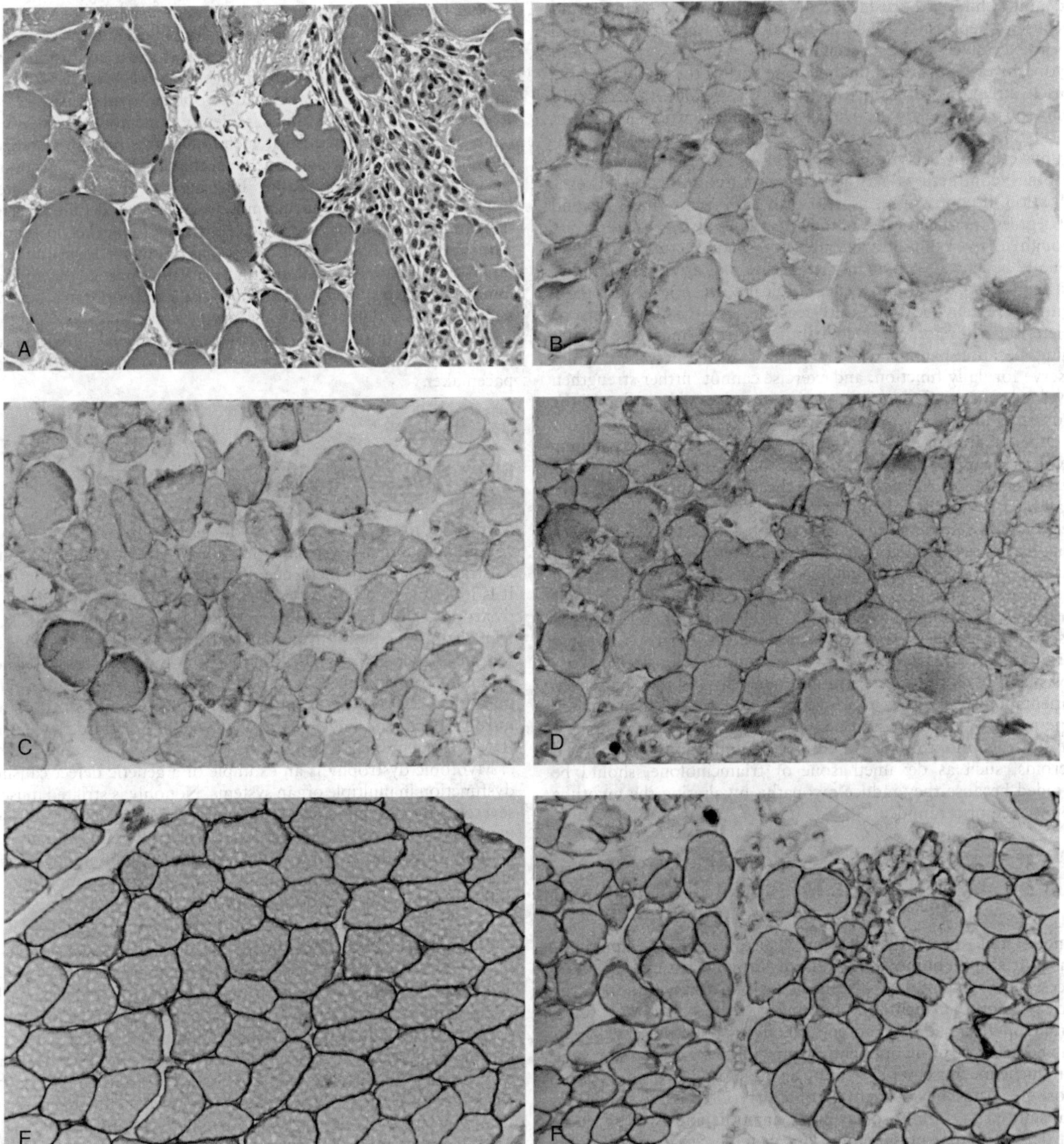

Figure 608-3. Quadriceps femoris muscle biopsy specimens from a 4 yr old boy with Becker muscular dystrophy. *A,* Myofibers vary greatly in size, with both atrophic and hypertrophic forms; at the right is a zone of degeneration and necrosis infiltrated by macrophages, similar to Duchenne muscular dystrophy (hematoxylin and eosin, ×250.) Immunoreactivity using antibodies against the dystrophin molecule in the rod domain *(B),* carboxyl-terminus *(C),* and amino-terminus *(D)* all show deficient but not totally absent dystrophin expression; most fibers of all sizes retain some dystrophin in parts of the sarcolemma but not around the entire circumference in cross section. Alternatively, the prominence of dystrophin is less, appearing weak, when compared with the simultaneously incubated normal control from another child of similar age *(E)*. *F,* Merosin expression is normal in this patient with Becker dystrophy, in both large and small myofibers, and is lacking only in frankly necrotic fibers. Compare with classic Duchenne muscular dystrophy illustrated in Figure 608-2C and with Figure 608-5.

complications and to improve the quality of life of affected children. **Cardiac decompensation** often responds initially well to digoxin. **Pulmonary infections** should be promptly treated. Patients should avoid contact with children who have obvious respiratory or other contagious illnesses. Immunizations for influenza virus and other routine vaccinations are indicated.

Preservation of a good **nutritional state** is important. Duchenne muscular dystrophy is not a vitamin deficiency disease, and excessive doses of vitamins should be avoided. Adequate calcium intake is important to minimize osteoporosis in boys confined to a wheelchair, and fluoride supplements may also be given, particularly if the local drinking water is not fluoridated. Because sedentary children burn fewer calories than active children and because of depression as an additional factor, these children tend to eat excessively and gain weight. Obesity makes a patient with myopathy even less functional because part of the limited reserve muscle strength is dissipated in lifting the weight of excess subcutaneous adipose tissue. Dietary restrictions with supervision may be needed.

Physiotherapy delays but does not always prevent contractures. At times, contractures may actually be useful in functional rehabilitation. If contractures prevent extension of the elbow beyond 90 degrees and the muscles of the upper limb no longer are strong enough to overcome gravity, the elbow contractures are functionally beneficial in fixing an otherwise flail arm and in allowing the patient to eat and write. Surgical correction of the elbow contracture may be technically feasible, but the result may be deleterious. Physiotherapy contributes little to muscle strengthening because patients usually are already using their entire reserve for daily function, and exercise cannot further strengthen involved muscles. Excessive exercise may actually accelerate the process of muscle fiber degeneration.

Other treatment of human patients with Duchenne dystrophy involves the use of prednisone, prednisolone, deflazacort, or other steroids. Glucocorticoids decrease the rate of apoptosis or programmed cell death of myotubes during ontogenesis and may decelerate the myofiber necrosis in muscular dystrophy. Strength usually improves initially, but the long-term complications of chronic steroid therapy, including considerable weight gain and osteoporosis, may offset this advantage or even result in greater weakness than might have occurred in the natural course of the disease. Nevertheless, some cases of Duchenne dystrophy treated early with steroids appear to have an improved long-term prognosis as well as the short-term improvement and may help keep patients ambulatory for more years than expected if untreated. One protocol gives prednisone (0.75 mg/kg/day) for the first 10 days of each month to avoid chronic complications. Fluorinated steroids, such as dexamethasone or triamcinolone, should be avoided because they induce myopathy by altering the myotube abundance of ceramide.

608.2 • Emery-Dreifuss Muscular Dystrophy

Emery-Dreifuss muscular dystrophy, also known as **scapuloperoneal or scapulohumeral muscular dystrophy,** is a rare X-linked recessive dystrophy. The locus is on the long arm within the large Xq28 region that includes other mutations that cause myotubular myopathy, neonatal adrenoleukodystrophy, and the Bloch-Sulzberger type of incontinentia pigmenti; it is far from the gene for Duchenne muscular dystrophy on the short arm of the X chromosome. Another, rarer, form of Emery-Dreifuss dystrophy is transmitted as an autosomal dominant trait and is localized at 1q. This form may present quite late, in adolescence or early adult life, although the muscular and cardiac symptoms and signs are similar, and sudden death from ventricular fibrillation is a risk.

Clinical manifestations begin between 5 and 15 yr of age, but many patients survive to late adult life because of the slow progression of its course. Hypertrophy of muscles does not occur. Contractures of elbows and ankles develop early, and muscle becomes wasted in a scapulohumeroperoneal distribution. Facial weakness does not occur; this disease is thus distinguished clinically from autosomal dominant scapulohumeral and scapuloperoneal syndromes of neurogenic origin. Myotonia is absent. Intellectual function is normal. Cardiomyopathy is severe and is often the cause of death, more frequently from conduction defects and sudden ventricular fibrillation than from intractable myocardial failure. The serum CK value is only mildly elevated, further distinguishing this disease from other X-linked recessive muscular dystrophies.

Nonspecific myofiber necrosis and endomysial fibrosis are seen in the muscle biopsy. Many centronuclear fibers and selective histochemical type I muscle fiber atrophy may cause confusion with myotonic dystrophy. The defective gene in the X-linked form is called emerin and, unlike other dystrophies in which the defective gene is expressed at the sarcolemmal membrane, emerin is expressed at the inner nuclear membrane; this protein stabilizes the nuclear membrane against the mechanical stresses that occur during muscular contraction. Emerin may be demonstrated immunocytochemically in the muscle biopsy for definitive diagnosis. Emerin also may be tested as a genetic marker in blood. The defective protein in the autosomal dominant form is called lamin-A and lamin-C, proteins that constitute part of the nuclear lamina, a fibrous layer on the inner nuclear membrane. Several subtypes and different mutations are demonstrated.

Treatment should be supportive, with special attention to cardiac conduction defects, and may require medications or a pacemaker.

608.3 • Myotonic Muscular Dystrophy

Myotonic dystrophy (Steinert disease) is the second most common muscular dystrophy in North America, Europe, and Australia, having an incidence of 1 : 30,000 general population. It is inherited as an autosomal dominant trait. Classic myotonic dystrophy (DM1) is caused by a cytosine-thymine-guanine (CTG) trinucleotide expansion on chromosome 19q13.3 in the 3' untranslated region of DMPK, the gene that encodes a serine-threonine protein kinase. A second form (DM2) is associated with unstable CTG repeat expansion on chromosome 3q21 of an intron of the zinc finger 9 protein gene. Still a third, late form (DM3) is identified, at locus 15q21-q24.

Myotonic dystrophy is an example of a genetic defect causing dysfunction in multiple organ systems. Not only is striated muscle severely affected, but smooth muscle of the alimentary tract and uterus is also involved; cardiac function is altered; and patients have multiple and variable endocrinopathies, immunologic deficiencies, cataracts, dysmorphic facies, intellectual impairment, and other neurologic abnormalities.

CLINICAL MANIFESTATIONS. In the usual clinical course, **excluding the severe neonatal** form, infants may appear almost normal at birth, or facial wasting and hypotonia may already be early expressions of the disease. The facial appearance is characteristic, consisting of an inverted V-shaped upper lip, thin cheeks, and scalloped, concave temporalis muscles (Fig. 608-4). The head may be narrow, and the palate is high and arched because the weak temporal and pterygoid muscles in late fetal life do not exert sufficient lateral forces on the developing head and face.

Weakness is mild in the first few years. Progressive wasting of distal muscles becomes increasingly evident, particularly involving intrinsic muscles of the hands. The thenar and hypothenar eminences are flattened, and the atrophic dorsal interossei leave deep grooves between the fingers. The dorsal forearm muscles and anterior compartment muscles of the lower legs also become wasted. The tongue is thin and atrophic. Wasting of the sternocleidomastoids gives the neck a long, thin, cylindric contour. Proximal muscles also eventually undergo atrophy, and scapular winging appears. Difficulty with climbing stairs and Gowers sign are progressive. Tendon stretch reflexes are usually preserved.

The distal distribution of muscle wasting in myotonic dystrophy is an exception to the general rule of myopathies having proximal and neuropathies having distal distribution patterns. The muscular atrophy and weakness in myotonic dystrophy are slowly progressive throughout childhood and adolescence and continue into adulthood. It is rare for patients with myotonic dys-

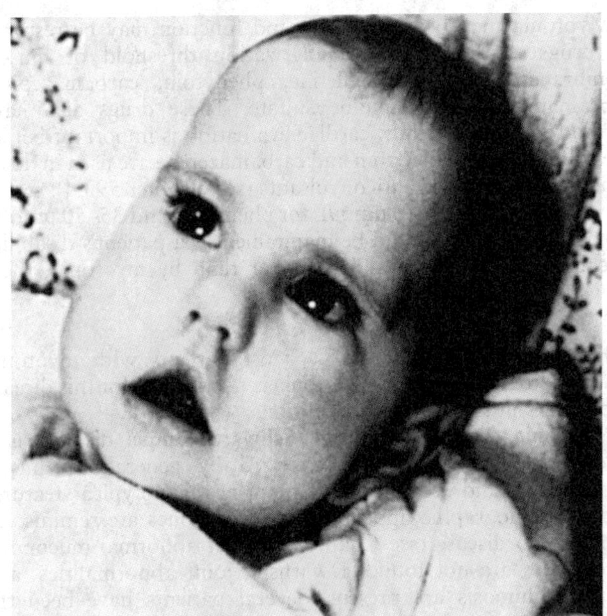

Figure 608-4. Facial weakness, inverted V-shaped upper lip, and loss of muscle mass in the temporal fossae are characteristic of myotonic muscular dystrophy, even in infancy, as seen in this 8 mo old girl.

trophy to lose the ability to walk even in late adult life, although splints or bracing may be required to stabilize the ankles.

Myotonia, a characteristic feature shared by few other myopathies, does not occur in infancy and is usually not clinically or even electromyographically evident until about age 5 yr. Exceptional patients develop it as early as age 3 yr. Myotonia is a very slow relaxation of muscle after contraction, regardless of whether that contraction was voluntary or was induced by a stretch reflex or electrical stimulation. During physical examination, myotonia may be demonstrated by asking the patient to make tight fists and then to quickly open the hands. It may be induced by striking the thenar eminence with a rubber percussion hammer, and it may be detected by watching the involuntary drawing of the thumb across the palm. Myotonia may also be demonstrated in the tongue by pressing the edge of a wooden tongue blade against its dorsal surface and by observing a deep furrow that disappears slowly. The severity of myotonia does not necessarily parallel the degree of weakness, and the weakest muscles often have only minimal myotonia. Myotonia is not a painful muscle spasm. Myalgias do not occur in myotonic dystrophy.

The **speech** of patients with myotonic dystrophy is often articulated poorly and is slurred because of the involvement of the muscles of the face, tongue, and pharynx. Difficulties with swallowing sometimes occur. Aspiration pneumonia is a risk in severely involved children. Incomplete external ophthalmoplegia may sometimes result from extraocular muscle weakness.

Smooth muscle involvement of the **gastrointestinal tract** results in slow gastric emptying, poor peristalsis, and constipation. Some patients have encopresis associated with anal sphincter weakness. Women with myotonic dystrophy may have ineffective or abnormal uterine contractions during labor and delivery.

Cardiac involvement is usually manifested as heart block in the Purkinje conduction system and arrhythmias rather than as cardiomyopathy, unlike most other muscular dystrophies.

Endocrine abnormalities involve many glands and appear at any time during the course of the disease so that re-evaluation of endocrine status must be done annually. Hypothyroidism is common; hyperthyroidism may occur rarely. Adrenocortical insufficiency may lead to an addisonian crisis even in infancy. Diabetes mellitus is common in patients with myotonic dystrophy; some children have a disorder of insulin release rather than defective insulin production. Onset of puberty may be precocious or, more often, delayed. Testicular atrophy and testosterone deficiency are common in adults and are responsible for a high incidence of male infertility. Ovarian atrophy is rare. Frontal baldness is also characteristic in males and often begins in adolescence.

Immunologic deficiencies are common in myotonic dystrophy. The plasma IgG level is often low.

Cataracts occur frequently in myotonic dystrophy. They may be congenital, or they may begin at any time during childhood or adult life. Early cataracts are detected only by slit-lamp examination; periodic examination by an ophthalmologist is recommended. Visual evoked potentials are often abnormal in children with myotonic dystrophy and are unrelated to cataracts. They are not usually accompanied by visual impairment.

About ½ of the patients with myotonic dystrophy are **intellectually impaired,** but severe mental retardation is unusual. The remainder is of average or occasionally above average intelligence. Epilepsy is not common. Cognitive impairment and mental retardation may be due to accumulations of mutant *DMPK* mRNA and aberrant alternative splicing in cerebral cortical neurons.

A severe **congenital form** of myotonic dystrophy appears in a minority of involved infants born to mothers with myotonic dystrophy. All patients with this severe congenital disease to date have had the DM1 form. Clubfoot deformities alone or more extensive congenital contractures of many joints may involve all extremities and even the cervical spine. Generalized hypotonia and weakness are present at birth. Facial wasting is prominent. Infants may require gavage feeding or ventilator support for respiratory muscle weakness or apnea. Those requiring ventilation for <30 days often survive while those with prolonged ventilation have an infant mortality of 25%. Children ventilated for <30 days have better motor, language, and daily activity skills than those requiring prolonged ventilation. One or both leaves of the diaphragm may be nonfunctional. The abdomen becomes distended with gas in the stomach and intestine because of poor peristalsis from smooth muscle weakness. The distention further compromises respiration. Inability to empty the rectum may compound the problem.

LABORATORY FINDINGS. The classic myotonic electromyogram is not found in infancy but may appear in toddlers or during the early school years. The levels of serum CK and other serum enzymes from muscle may be normal or only mildly elevated in the hundreds (never the thousands).

ECG should be performed annually in early childhood. Ultrasound imaging of the abdomen may be indicated in affected infants to determine diaphragmatic function. Radiographs of the chest and abdomen and contrast studies of gastrointestinal motility may be needed.

Endocrine assessment should be undertaken to determine thyroid and adrenal cortical function and to verify carbohydrate metabolism (glucose tolerance test). Immunoglobulins should be examined, and, if needed, more extensive immunologic studies should be performed.

DIAGNOSIS. The primary diagnostic test is a DNA analysis of blood to demonstrate the abnormal expansion of the CTG repeat. Prenatal diagnosis also is feasible. The muscle biopsy specimen in older children shows many muscle fibers with central nuclei and selective atrophy of histochemical type I fibers, but degenerating fibers are usually few and widely scattered, and there is little or no fibrosis of muscle. Intrafusal fibers of muscle spindles are also abnormal. In young children with the common form of the disease, the biopsy specimen may even appear normal or may at least not show myofiber necroses, which is a striking contrast with Duchenne muscular dystrophy. In the severe neonatal form of myotonic dystrophy, the muscle biopsy reveals maturational arrest in various stages of development in some and congenital muscle fiber-type disproportion in others. It is likely that the sarcolemmal membrane of muscle fibers not only has abnormal properties of electrical polarization but is also incapable of responding to trophic influences of the motor neuron. Muscle biopsy is not usually required for diagnosis, which in typical cases can be based on the clinical manifestations.

GENETICS. The genetic defect in myotonic muscular dystrophy is on chromosome 19 at the 19q13 locus. It consists of an expansion of the *DM* gene that encodes a serine-threonine kinase *(DMPK)*, with numerous repeats of the CTG codon. Expansions range from 50 to >2,000, with the normal alleles of this gene ranging in size from 5 to 37; the larger the expansion is, the more severe the clinical expression, with the largest expansions seen in the severe neonatal form. Rarely, the disease is associated with no detectable repeats, perhaps a spontaneous correction of a previous expansion but a phenomenon still incompletely understood. Another myotonic dystrophy (PROMM) is a clinical entity linked to at least 2 different chromosomal loci than classic myotonic dystrophy but 1 that shares a common unique pathogenesis in being mediated by a mutant mRNA. Defects in RNA splicing explain the insulin resistance in myotonic dystrophies as well as the myotonia.

Both clinical and genetic expression may vary between siblings or between an affected parent and child. In the severe neonatal form of the disease, the mother is the transmitting parent in 94% of cases, a fact not explained by increased male infertility alone. Genetic analysis reveals that such infants usually have many more repeats of the CTG codon than do patients with the more classic form of the disease. Myotonic dystrophy often exhibits a pattern of **anticipation** in which each successive generation has a tendency to be more severely involved than the previous generation.

TREATMENT. There is no specific medical treatment, but the cardiac, endocrine, gastrointestinal, and ocular complications can often be treated. Physiotherapy and orthopedic treatment of contractures in the neonatal form of the disease may be beneficial.

Myotonia may be diminished, and function may be restored by drugs that raise the depolarization threshold of muscle membranes, such as mexiletine, phenytoin, carbamazepine, procainamide, and quinidine sulfate. These drugs also have cardiotropic effects; thus, cardiac evaluation is important before prescribing them. Phenytoin and carbamazepine are used in doses similar to their use as anticonvulsants (see Chapter 593.4); serum concentrations of 40–80 μmol/L for phenytoin and 35–50 μmol/L for carbamazepine should be maintained. If a patient's disability is caused mainly by weakness rather than by myotonia, these drugs will be of no value.

OTHER MYOTONIC SYNDROMES. Most patients with myotonia have myotonic dystrophy. Myotonia is not specific for this disease and occurs in several rarer conditions.

Myotonic chondrodystrophy (Schwartz-Jampel disease) is a rare congenital disease characterized by generalized muscle hypertrophy and weakness. Dysmorphic phenotypical features and the radiographic appearance of long bones are reminiscent of Morquio disease (see Chapter 88), but abnormal mucopolysaccharides are not found. Dwarfism, joint abnormalities, and blepharophimosis are present. Several patients have been the products of consanguinity, suggesting autosomal recessive inheritance. The muscle protein perlecan, encoded by the *SJS1* gene, a large heparan sulfate proteoglycan of basement membranes and cartilage, is defective in some cases of Schwartz-Jampel disease and explains both the muscular hyperexcitability and the chondrodysplasia.

EMG reveals continuous electrical activity in muscle fibers closely resembling or identical to myotonia. Muscle biopsy reveals nonspecific myopathic features, which are minimal in some cases and pronounced in others. The sarcotubular system is dilated.

Myotonia congenita (Thomsen disease) is a channelopathy (Table 608-1) and is characterized by weakness and generalized muscular hypertrophy so that affected children resemble bodybuilders. Myotonia is prominent and may develop at age 2–3 yr, earlier than in myotonic dystrophy. The disease is clinically stable and is apparently not progressive for many years. Muscle biopsy specimens show minimal pathologic changes, and the EMG demonstrates myotonia. Various families are described as showing either autosomal dominant (Thomsen disease) or reces-

TABLE 608-1. Channelopathies and Related Disorders

DISORDER	PATTERN OF CLINICAL FEATURES	INHERITANCE	CHROMOSOME	GENE
Chloride channelopathies				
Myotonia congenita				
Thomsen's disease	Myotonia	Autosomal dominant	7q35	*CLC1*
Becker's disease	Myotonia and weakness	Autosomal recessive	7q35	*CLC1*
Sodium channelopathies				
Paramyotonia congenita	Paramyotonia	Autosomal dominant	17q13.1–13.3	*SCNA4A*
Hyperkalemic periodic paralysis	Periodic paralysis with myotonia and paramyotonia	Autosomal dominant	17q13.1–13.3	*CNA4A*
Hypokalemic periodic paralysis	Periodic paralysis	Autosomal dominant	17q13.1–13.3	*SCNA4A*
Potassium-aggravated myotonias				
Myotonia fluctuans	Myotonia	Autosomal dominant	17q13.1–13.3	*SCNA4A*
Myotonia permanens	Myotonia	Autosomal dominant	17q13.1–13.3	*SCNA4A*
Acetaxolamide-responsive myotonia	Myotonia	Autosomal dominant	17q13.1–13.3	*SCNA4A*
Calcium channelopathies				
Hypokalemic periodic paralysis	Periodic paralysis	Autosomal dominant	1q31–32	Dihydropyridine receptor
Schwartz-Jampel syndrome (chondrodystrophic myotonia)	Myotonia; dysmorphic	Autosomal recessive	1q34.1–36.1	Perlecan
Rippling muscle disease	Muscle mounding/stiffness	Autosomal dominant	1q41	Caveolin-3
Anderson's syndrome	Periodic paralysis, cardiac arrhythmia, distinctive facies	Autosomal dominant	17q23	KCNJ2-Kir2.1
Brody's disease	Delayed relaxation, no EMG myotonia	Autosomal recessive	16p12	Calcium ATPase
Malignant hyperthermia	Anesthetic-induced delayed relaxation	Autosomal dominant	19q13.1	Ryanodine receptor

ATPase, adenosine triphosphatase; EMG, electromyogram.
From Goldman L, Ausiello D: *Cecil Textbook of Medicine*, 22nd ed. Philadelphia, WB Saunders, 2004, p. 2392.

sive (Becker disease, not to be confused with Becker/Duchenne muscular dystrophy) inheritance. Rarely, myotonic dystrophy and myotonia congenita coexist in the same family. Both the autosomal dominant and autosomal recessive forms of myotonia congenita have been mapped to the same 7q35 locus. This gene is important for the integrity of chloride channels of the sarcolemmal and T-tubular membranes.

Paramyotonia is a temperature-related myotonia that is aggravated by cold and alleviated by warm external temperatures. Patients have difficulty when swimming in cold water or if they are dressed inadequately in cold weather. *Paramyotonia congenita* (Eulenburg disease) is a defect in a gene at the 17q13.1-13.3 locus, the identical locus identified in hyperkalemic periodic paralysis. By contrast with myotonia congenita, paramyotonia is a disorder of the voltage-gated sodium channel due to a mutation in the α subunit. Myotonic dystrophy also is a sodium channelopathy (see Table 608-1).

In sodium channelopathies, exercise produces increasing myotonia, whereas in chloride channelopathies, exercise reduces the myotonia. This is easily tested during examination by asking patients to close the eyes forcefully and open them repeatedly; it becomes progressively more difficult in sodium channel disorders and progressively easier in chloride channel disorders.

608.4 • Limb-Girdle Muscular Dystrophies

This term encompasses a group of progressive hereditary myopathies that mainly affect muscles of the hip and shoulder girdles. Distal muscles also eventually become atrophic and weak. Hypertrophy of the calves and ankle contractures develop in some forms, causing potential confusion with Becker muscular dystrophy. Sixteen genetic forms of limb-girdle dystrophy are now described, each at a different chromosomal locus and expressing different protein defects. Some include diseases classified with other traditional groups, such as the lamin-A/C defects of the nuclear membrane (see Emery-Dreifuss muscular dystrophy, above), and some forms of congenital muscular dystrophy.

The initial **clinical manifestations** rarely appear before middle or late childhood or may be delayed until early adult life. Low back pain may be a presenting complaint because of the lordotic posture resulting from gluteal muscle weakness. Confinement to a wheelchair usually becomes obligatory at about 30 yr of age. The rate of progression varies from 1 pedigree to another but is uniform within a kindred. Although weakness of neck flexors and extensors is universal, facial, lingual, and other bulbar-innervated muscles are rarely involved. As weakness and muscle wasting progress, tendon stretch reflexes become diminished. Cardiac involvement is unusual. Intellectual function is generally normal. The clinical **differential diagnosis** of limb-girdle muscular dystrophy includes juvenile spinal muscular atrophy (Kugelberg-Welander disease), myasthenia gravis, and metabolic myopathies.

Most cases of limb-girdle muscular dystrophy are of autosomal recessive inheritance, but some families express an autosomal dominant trait. The latter often follows a benign course with little functional impairment.

The EMG and muscle biopsy show confirmatory evidence of muscular dystrophy, but none of the findings is specific enough to make the definitive **diagnosis** without additional clinical criteria. In some cases, adhalen, a dystrophin-related glycoprotein of the sarcolemma, is deficient; this specific defect may be demonstrated in the muscle biopsy by immunocytochemistry. Increased serum CK level is usual, but the magnitude of elevation varies among families. The ECG is usually unaltered.

In one autosomal dominant form of limb-girdle muscular dystrophy, a genetic defect has been localized to the long arm of chromosome 5. In the autosomal recessive disease, it is on the long arm of chromosome 15. A mutated dystrophin-associated protein in the sarcoglycan complex (sarcoglycanopathy) is responsible for some cases of autosomal recessive limb-girdle muscular dystrophy. Adhalen is α-sarcoglycan; other limb-girdle dystrophies due to deficiencies in β-, γ-, and δ-sarcoglycan also occur. In normal smooth muscle, α-sarcoglycan is replaced by ε-sarcoglycan and the others are the same.

Another group of limb-girdle dystrophies are caused by allelic mutations of the dysferlin *(DYSF)* gene, another gene expressing a protein essential to structural integrity of the sarcolemma, though not associated with the dystrophin-glycoprotein complex. *DYSF* interacts with caveolin-3 or calpain-3, and *DYSF* deficiency may be secondary to defects in these other gene products. Autosomal recessive (Miyoshi myopathy) and autosomal dominant traits are documented. Both are slowly progressive myopathies with onset in adolescence or young adult life and may affect distal as well as proximal muscles. Cardiomyopathy is rare. Chronically elevated serum CK in the thousands is found in dysferlinopathies. Ultrastructure shows a thickened basal lamina over defects in the sarcolemma and replacement of the sarcolemma by multiple layers of small vesicles. Regenerating myofibers outnumber degenerating myofibers. These disorders were formerly called *hyperCKemia* and *rippling muscle disease,* the latter sometimes confused with myotonia.

608.5 • Facioscapulohumeral Muscular Dystrophy

Facioscapulohumeral muscular dystrophy, also known as **Landouzy-Dejerine disease,** is probably not a single disease entity but a group of diseases with similar clinical manifestations. Autosomal dominance is the rule; genetic anticipation is often found within several generations of a family, the succeeding more severely involved at an earlier age than the preceding. The frequency is 1 : 20,000. The genetic mechanism in autosomal dominant facioscapulohumeral dystrophy involves integral deletions of a 3.3-kb tandem repeat (D4Z4) in the subtelomeric region at the 4q35 locus. A closely homologous 3.3-kb repeat array at the subtelomeric locus 10q26, with chromosomal translocation or sequence conversion between these two regions, possibly predisposes to the DNA rearrangement causing facioscapulohumeral dystrophy.

CLINICAL MANIFESTATIONS. Facioscapulohumeral dystrophy shows the earliest and most severe weakness in facial and shoulder girdle muscles. The facial weakness differs from that of myotonic dystrophy; rather than an inverted V-shaped upper lip, the mouth in facioscapulohumeral dystrophy is rounded and appears puckered because the upper and lower lips protrude. Inability to close the eyes completely in sleep is a common expression of upper facial weakness; some patients have extraocular muscle weakness, although ophthalmoplegia is rarely complete. Facioscapulohumeral dystrophy has been associated with Möbius syndrome on rare occasions. Pharyngeal and tongue weakness may be absent and is never as severe as the facial involvement. Hearing loss, which may be subclinical, and retinal vasculopathy (indistinguishable from Coats disease) are associated features, particularly in severe cases of facioscapulohumeral dystrophy with early childhood onset.

Scapular winging is prominent, often even in infants. Flattening or even concavity of the deltoid contour is seen, and the biceps and triceps brachii muscles are wasted and weak. Muscles of the hip girdles and thighs also eventually lose strength and undergo atrophy, and Gowers sign and a Trendelenburg gait appear. Contractures are rare. Finger and wrist weakness occasionally is the first symptom. Weakness of the anterior tibial and peroneal muscles may lead to footdrop; this complication usually occurs only in advanced cases with severe weakness. Lumbar lordosis and kyphoscoliosis are common complications of axial muscle involvement. Calf pseudohypertrophy is not a feature.

Facioscapulohumeral muscular dystrophy may also be a mild disease causing minimal disability. Clinical manifestations may not be expressed in childhood and are delayed into middle adult life. Unlike most other muscular dystrophies, asymmetry of weakness is common.

LABORATORY FINDINGS. Serum levels of CK and other enzymes vary greatly, ranging from normal or near normal to elevations of several thousand. ECG should be performed, although the anticipated findings are usually normal. EMG reveals nonspecific myopathic muscle potentials. Diagnostic molecular testing in both individual cases and within families is indicated for prediction.

DIAGNOSIS AND DIFFERENTIAL DIAGNOSIS. Muscle biopsy distinguishes more than one form of facioscapulohumeral dystrophy, consistent with clinical evidence that several distinct diseases are embraced by the term *FSH dystrophy.* Muscle biopsy and EMG also distinguish the primary myopathy from a neurogenic disease with a similar distribution of muscular involvement. The general histopathologic findings in the muscle biopsy material are extensive proliferation of connective tissue between muscle fibers, extreme variation in fiber size with many hypertrophic as well as atrophic myofibers, and scattered degenerating and regenerating fibers. An "inflammatory" type of facioscapulohumeral muscular dystrophy is also distinguished, characterized by extensive lymphocytic infiltrates within muscle fascicles. Despite the resemblance of this form to inflammatory myopathies, such as polymyositis, there is no evidence of autoimmune disease, and steroids and immunosuppressive drugs do not alter the clinical course. A precise histopathologic diagnosis has important therapeutic implications. Mononuclear cell "inflammation" in a muscle biopsy sample of infants younger than 2 yr is usually facioscapulohumeral dystrophy.

TREATMENT. Physiotherapy is of no value in regaining strength or in retarding progressive weakness or muscle wasting. Footdrop and scoliosis may be treated by orthopedic measures. Cosmetic improvement of the facial muscles of expression may be achieved by reconstructive surgery, which grafts a fascia lata to the zygomatic muscle and to the zygomatic head of the quadratus labiae superioris muscle.

608.6 • Congenital Muscular Dystrophy

The term congenital muscular dystrophy is misleading because all muscular dystrophies are genetically determined. It is used to encompass several distinct diseases with a common characteristic of severe involvement at birth but that ironically usually follow a benign clinical course. Autosomal recessive inheritance is the rule.

CLINICAL MANIFESTATIONS. Infants often have contractures or arthrogryposis at birth and are diffusely hypotonic. The muscle mass is thin in the trunk and extremities. Head control is poor. Facial muscles may be mildly involved, but ophthalmoplegia, pharyngeal weakness, and weak sucking are not common. A minority has severe dysphagia and requires gavage or gastrostomy. Tendon stretch reflexes may be hypoactive or absent. Arthrogryposis is common in all forms of congenital muscular dystrophy (see Chapter 607.9). Congenital contractures of the elbows have a high association with the Ullrich type of congenital muscular dystrophy, due to a defect in one or more of the three collagen VI genes, each at a different locus.

The Fukuyama type of congenital muscular dystrophy is the 2nd most common muscular dystrophy in Japan (after Duchenne dystrophy); it has also been reported in children of Dutch, German, Scandinavian, and Turkish ethnic backgrounds. In the Fukuyama variety, severe cardiomyopathy and malformations of the brain usually accompany the skeletal muscle involvement. Signs and symptoms related to these organs are prominent: cardiomegaly and heart failure, mental retardation, seizures, microcephaly, and failure to thrive. The genetic defect in Fukuyama congenital muscular dystrophy has been identified at the 8q31-33 locus in Japanese patients.

Neurologic disease may accompany forms of congenital muscular dystrophy other than Fukuyama disease. Mental and neurologic status are the most variable features; an apparently normal brain and normal intelligence do not preclude the diagnosis if other manifestations indicate this myopathy. The cerebral malformations that occur are not consistently of one type and vary from severe dysplasias (holoprosencephaly, lissencephaly) to milder conditions (agenesis of the corpus callosum, focal heterotopia of the cerebral cortex and subcortical white matter, cerebellar hypoplasia). Congenital muscular dystrophy is a consistent association with cerebral dysgenesis in the **Walker-Warburg syndrome** and **in muscle-eye-brain disease of Santavuori.** The neuropathologic findings are those of neuroblast migratory abnormalities in the cerebral cortex, cerebellum, and brainstem. Mutations in genes of O-mannosylation of a-dystroglycan, essential for neuroblast migration in the fetal brain, have been demonstrated: *POMT1* and *POMGnT1*. Another separate form of congenital muscular dystrophy is characterized by microcephaly and mental retardation.

LABORATORY FINDINGS. Serum CK level is usually moderately elevated from several hundred to many thousand IU/L; only marginal increases are sometimes found. EMG shows nonspecific myopathic features. Investigation of all forms of congenital muscular dystrophy should include cardiac assessment and an imaging study of the brain. Muscle biopsy is essential for the diagnosis.

DIAGNOSIS. Muscle biopsy is diagnostic in the neonatal period or thereafter. An extensive proliferation of endomysial collagen envelops individual muscle fibers even at birth, also causing them to be rounded in cross-sectional contour by acting as a rigid sleeve, especially during contraction. The perimysial connective tissue and fat are also increased, and the fascicular organization of the muscle may be disrupted by the fibrosis. Tissue cultures of intramuscular fibroblasts exhibit increased collagen synthesis, but the structure of the collagen is normal. Muscle fibers vary in diameter, and many show central nuclei, myofibrillar splitting, and other cytoarchitectural alterations. Scattered degenerating and regenerating fibers are seen. No inflammation or abnormal inclusions are found.

Immunocytochemical reactivity for merosin (α_2 chain of laminin) at the sarcolemmal region is absent in about 40% of cases and normally expressed in the others (Figs. 608-5 and 608-6). Merosin is a protein that binds the sarcolemmal membrane of the myofiber to the basal lamina or basement membrane. Its defect is a mutation of the *LAMA2* gene at the 6q22-q23 locus. Merosin also is expressed in brain and in Schwann cells. The presence or absence of merosin does not always correlate with the severity of the myopathy or predict its course, but cases with merosin deficiency tend to have more severe cerebral involvement and myopathy. Adhalen (α-dystroglycan) may be secondarily reduced in some cases. Collagen VI is selectively reduced or absent in Ullrich disease.

TREATMENT. Only supportive therapy is available.

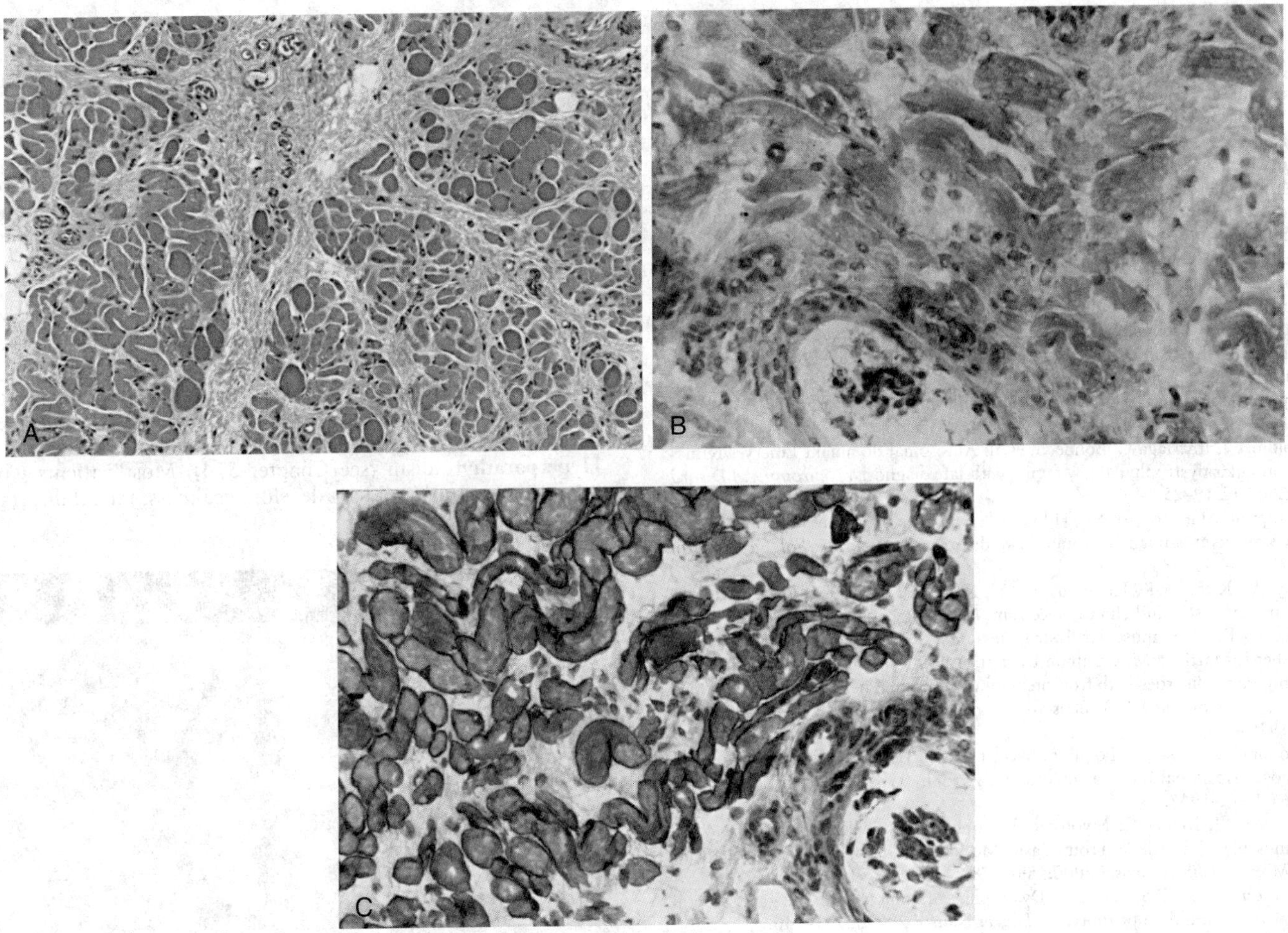

Figure 608-5. Quadriceps femoris muscle biopsy of a 6 mo old girl with congenital muscular dystrophy associated with merosin (α_2-laminin) deficiency. *A*, Histologically, the muscle is infiltrated by a great proliferation of collagenous connective tissue; myofibers vary in diameter, but necrotic fibers are rare. *B*, Immunocytochemical reactivity for merosin (α_2-laminin) is absent in all fibers, including the intrafusal myofibers of a muscle spindle seen at bottom. *C*, Dystrophin expression (rod domain) is normal. Compare with Figures 608-2, 608-3, and 608-6.

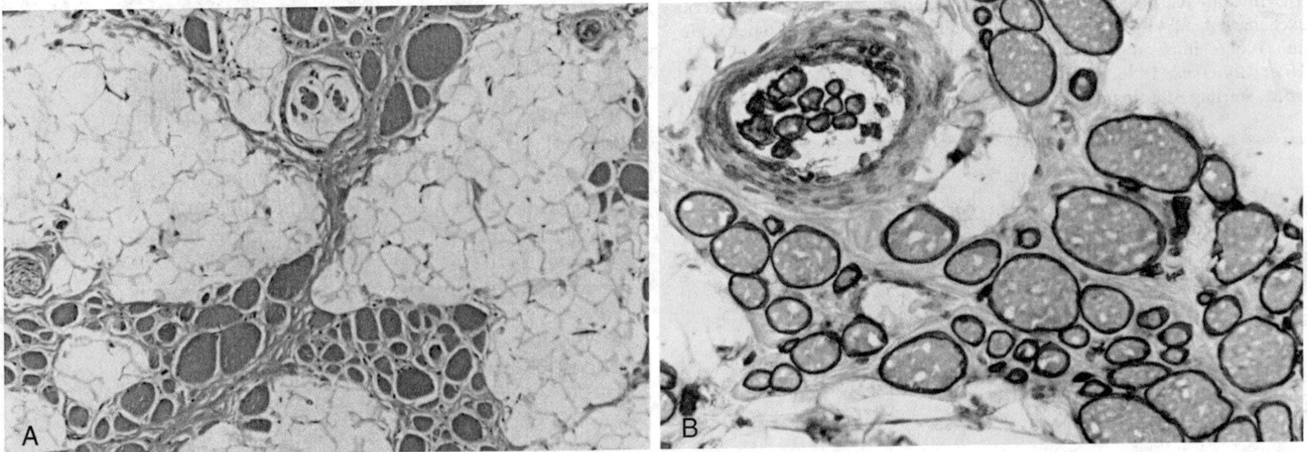

Figure 608-6. Quadriceps femoris muscle biopsy specimen of a 2 yr old girl with congenital muscular dystrophy. *A*, The fascicular architecture of the muscle is severely disrupted, and muscle is replaced by fat and connective tissue; the remaining small groups of myofibers of variable size are seen, including a muscle spindle at top. *B*, Merosin expression is normal in both extrafusal fibers of all sizes and in intrafusal spindle fibers. The severity of the myopathy does not relate to the presence or absence of merosin in congenital muscular dystrophy. Compare with Figure 608-5.

Anderson JH, Head SI, Rae C, et al: Brain function in Duchenne muscular dystrophy. *Brain* 2002;125:4–13.
Angelini C, Fanin N, Freda MP, et al: The clinical spectrum of sarcoglycanopathies. *Neurology* 1999;52:176–179.
Beenakker EAC, Fock JM, Van Tol MJ, et al: Intermittent prednisone therapy in Duchenne muscular dystrophy. *Arch Neurol* 2005;62:128–132.
Beltran-Valero de Bernabe D, Currier S, Steinbrecher A, et al: Mutations in the O-mannosyltransferase gene *POMT1* give rise to the severe neuronal migration disorder Walter-Warburg syndrome. *Am J Hum Genet* 2002;71:1033–1043.
Bonne G, Muchin A, Helbling-Lecleerc A, et al: Clinical and genetical heterogeneity of laminopathies. *Acta Myologica* 2001;20:138.
Bushby KM, Beckmann JS: Pathogenesis in the non-sarcoglycan limb-girdle muscular dystrophies. *Neuromuscul Disord* 2003;13:80–90.
Campbell C, Sherlock R, Jacob P, Blayney M: Congenital myotonic dystrophy: Assisted ventilation duration and outcome. *Pediatrics* 2004;113: 811–816.
Colomer J, Iturriaga C, Bonne G, et al: Autosomal dominant Emery-Dreifuss muscular dystrophy; a new family with late diagnosis. *Neuromuscul Disord* 2002;12:19–25.
Compton AG, Cooper ST, Hill PM, et al: The syntrophin-dysbrevin subcomplex in human neuromuscular disorders. *J Neuropathol Exp Neurol* 2005;64:350–361.
Day JW, Richater K, Jacobsen JP, et al: Myotonic dystrophy type 2: Molecular, diagnostic and clinical spectrum. *Neurology* 2003;60:657–664.
Emery AEH: The muscular dystrophies. *Lancet* 2002;359:687–695.
Le Ber I, Martínez M, Campion D, et al: A non-DM1, non-DM2 multisystem myotonic disorder with frontotemporal dementia: Phenotype and suggestive mapping of the DM3 locus to chromosome 15q21-24. *Brain* 2004;127: 1979–1992.
Modoni A, Silvestri G, Pomponi MG, et al: Characterization of the pattern of cognitive impairment in myotonic dystrophy type 1. *Arch Neurol* 2004; 61:1943–1947.
Moxley RT, Meola G: Myotonic dystrophy. In Deymeer F (editor): Neuromuscular Disorders: From Basic Mechanisms to Clinical Management. *Monogr Clin Neurosci* 2000;18:61–78.
Muntoni F, Torelli S, Ferlini A: Dystrophin and mutations: One gene, several proteins, multiple phenotypes. *Lancet Neurol* 2003;2:731–740.
Nicole S, Vicart S, Davoine CS, et al: Mutations of perlecan, the major proteoglycan of basement membranes, cause Schwartz-Jampel syndrome: A new mechanism for myotonia? *Acta Myologica* 2001;20:130.
Rose MR: Neurological channelopathies. *BMJ* 1998;316:1104–1105.
Ruggieri V, Lubieniecki F, Meli F, et al: Merosin-positive congenital muscular dystrophy with mental retardation, microcephaly and central nervous system abnormalities unlinked to the Fukuyama muscular dystrophy and muscular-eye-brain loci: Report of three siblings. *Neuromuscul Disord* 2001;11:570–578.
van Deutekom JC, Baaker E, Lemmers RJ, et al: Evidence for subtelomeric exchange of 3.3 kb tandemly repeated units between chromosomes 4q35 and 10q26: Implications for genetic counselling and etiology of *FSHD1*. *Hum Mol Genet* 1996;5:1997–2003.
Zatz M, Starling A: Calpains and disease. *N Engl J Med* 2005;352:2413–2423.

Chapter 609 ■ Endocrine and Toxic Myopathies

THYROID MYOPATHIES (SEE ALSO PART XXV, SECTION 2.)

Thyrotoxicosis causes proximal weakness and wasting accompanied by myopathic electromyographic changes. Thyroxine binds to myofibrils and, if in excess, impairs contractile function. *Hyperthyroidism* may also induce myasthenia gravis and hypokalemic periodic paralysis.

Hypothyroidism, whether congenital or acquired, consistently produces hypotonia and a proximal distribution of weakness. Although muscle wasting is most characteristic, one form of cretinism, the Kocher-Debré-Sémélaigne syndrome, is characterized by generalized pseudohypertrophy of weak muscles. Infants may have a Herculean appearance reminiscent of myotonia congenita. The serum creatine kinase (CK) level is elevated in hypothyroid myopathy and returns to normal after thyroid replacement therapy.

Results of muscle biopsy in hypothyroidism reveal acute myopathic changes, including myofiber necrosis and sometimes central cores. In hyperthyroidism, the muscle biopsy specimen shows only mild, nonspecific myopathic changes without necrosis of myofibers.

Both the clinical and pathologic features of hyperthyroid myopathy and hypothyroid myopathy resolve after appropriate treatment of the thyroid disorder. Many of the systemic symptoms of hyperthyroidism, including myopathic weakness and ophthalmoparesis, improve with the administration of ß blockers.

Hyperparathyroidism (see Chapter 574). Most patients with primary hyperparathyroidism develop weakness, fatigability, fas-

TABLE 609-1. Toxic Myopathies

Inflammatory
Cimetidine
D-Penicillamine
Procainamide
L-Tryptoplan
L-Dopa
Noninflammatory Necrotizing or Vacuolar
Cholesterol-lowering agents
Chloroquine
Colchicine
Emetine
ε-Aminocaproic acid
Labetalol
Cyclosporine and tacrolimus
Isoretinoic acid (vitamin A analogue)
Vincristine
Alcohol
Rhabdomyolysis and Myoglobinuria
Cholesterol-lowering drugs
Alcohol
Heroin
Amphetamine
Toluene
Cocaine
ε-Aminocaproic acid
Pentazocine
Phencyclidine
Malignant Hyperthermia
Halothane
Ethylene
Diethyl ether
Methoxyflurane
Ethyl chloride
Trichloroethylene
Gallamine
Succinylcholine
Mitochondrial
Zidovudine
Myotonia
2,4-*d*-Chlorophenoxyacetic acid
Anthracene-9-carboxycyclic acid
Cholesterol-lowering drugs
Chloroquine
Cyclosporine
Myosin Loss
Nondepolarizing neuromuscular blocking agents
Intravenous glucocorticoids

From Goldman L, Ausiello D: *Cecil Textbook of Medicine,* 22nd ed, 2004, Saunders, Philadelphia, p. 2399.

ciculations, and muscle wasting that are reversible after removal of the parathyroid adenoma. The serum CK and muscle biopsy remain normal, but the electromyography may show nonspecific myopathic features. A minority of patients develop myotonia that could be confused with myotonic dystrophy.

STEROID-INDUCED MYOPATHY

Both natural Cushing disease and iatrogenic Cushing syndrome due to exogenous corticosteroid administration may cause painless, symmetrical, progressive proximal weakness, increased serum CK levels, and a myopathic electromyogram and muscle biopsy specimen (see Chapter 578). Myosin filaments may be selectively lost. The 9α-fluorinated steroids, such as dexamethasone, betamethasone, and triamcinolone, are the most likely to produce *steroid myopathy.* Dexamethasone alters the abundance of ceramides in myotubes in developing muscle. In patients with dermatomyositis or other myopathies treated with steroids, it is sometimes difficult to distinguish refractoriness of the disease from steroid-induced weakness, especially after long-term steroid administration. All patients who have been taking steroids for long periods develop reversible type II myofiber atrophy; this is a *steroid effect* but is not steroid myopathy unless it progresses to become a necrotizing myopathy. At greatest risk in the pediatric age group are children requiring long-term steroid therapy for asthma, rheumatoid arthritis, dermatomyositis, lupus, and other autoimmune or inflammatory diseases, and in the treatment of leukemia and other hematologic diseases. In addition to steroids, acute or chronic toxic myopathies may occur from other drugs (Table 609-1).

Hyperaldosteronism (Conn syndrome) is accompanied by episodic and reversible weakness similar to that of periodic paralysis. The proximal myopathy may become irreversible in chronic cases. Elevated CK levels and even myoglobinuria sometimes occur during acute attacks.

Chronic growth hormone excess (sometimes illicitly by adolescent athletes) or in acromegaly produces atrophy of some myofibers and hypertrophy of others, and scattered myofiber degeneration. Despite augmented protein synthesis induced by growth hormone, it impairs myofibrillar ATPase activity and reduces sarcolemmal excitability, with a result of diminished, rather than increased, strength to correspond to the larger muscle mass.

Hilton-Jones D, Squier M, Taylor D, et al: *Metabolic Myopathies.* Philadelphia, WB Saunders, 1995.

Mastaglia FL, Ojeda VJ, Sarnat HB, et al: Myopathies associated with hypothyroidism. *Aust N Z J Med* 1988;18:799–806.

Shee CD: Risk factors for hydrocortisone myopathy in acute, severe asthma. *Respir Med* 1990;84:229–233.

Chapter 610 ■ Metabolic Myopathies

The differential diagnosis of metabolic myopathies is noted in Table 610-1.

610.1 • Periodic Paralyses (Potassium-Related)

Episodic, reversible weakness or paralysis known as **periodic paralysis** is associated with transient alterations in serum potassium levels, usually hypokalemia but occasionally hyperkalemia. All familial forms of periodic paralysis are caused by mutations in genes encoding voltage-gated ion channels in muscle: sodium, calcium, and potassium (Table 608-1). During attacks, myofibers are electrically inexcitable, although the contractile apparatus can respond normally to calcium. The disorder is inherited as an autosomal dominant trait. It is precipitated in some patients by a heavy carbohydrate meal, insulin, adrenaline including that induced by emotional stress, hyperaldosteronism or hyperthyroidism, administration of amphotericin B, or ingestion of licorice. The defective genes are at the 17q13.1-13.3 locus in **hyperkalemic periodic paralysis,** the same as in paramyotonia congenita, and at the 1q31-32 locus in **hypokalemic periodic paralysis.**

Attacks often begin in infancy and the disease is nearly always symptomatic by 10 yr of age, affecting both sexes equally. In childhood, periodic paralysis is an episodic event; patients are unable to move after awakening and gradually recover muscle strength during the next few minutes or hours. Muscles that remain active in sleep, such as the diaphragm and cardiac muscle, are not affected. Patients are normal between attacks, but in adult life the attacks become more frequent, and the disorder causes progressive myopathy with permanent weakness even between attacks. The usual frequency of attacks in childhood is once a week.

Alterations in serum potassium level occur only during acute episodes and are accompanied by T-wave changes in the electrocardiogram. Hypokalemia may be due to alterations in calcium gradients. The creatine kinase (CK) level may be mildly elevated at those times. Plasma phosphate levels often decrease during symptomatic periods. Muscle biopsy findings are often normal

TABLE 610-1. Metabolic and Mitochondrial Myopathies

GLYCOGEN METABOLISM DEFICIENCIES
Type II α-1,4 Glucosidase (acid maltase)
Type III Debranching
Type IV Branching
Type V Phosphorylase (McArdle disease)*
Type VII Phosphofructokinase (Tarui disease)*
Type VIII Phosphorylase B kinase*
Type IX Phosphoglycerate kinase*
Type X Phosphoglycerate mutase*
Type XI Lactate dehydrogenase*
LIPID METABOLISM DEFICIENCIES
Carnitine palmitoyl transferase*
Primary systemic/muscle carnitine deficiency
Secondary carnitine deficiency
β-Oxidation defects
Medications (valproic acid)
PURINE METABOLISM DEFICIENCIES
Myoadenylate deaminase deficiency*
MITOCHONDRIAL MYOPATHIES
Pyruvate dehydrogenase complex deficiencies (including Leigh syndrome)
Progressive external ophthalmoplegia
Autosomal dominant with multiple mitochondrial DNA deletions
Adenine nucleotide translocator 1
TWINKLE
Polymerase gamma
Kearns-Sayre syndrome
Mitochondrial encephalopathy with lactic acidosis and strokelike episodes
Myoclonic epilepsy and ragged red fibers
Mitochondrial neurogastrointestinal encephalomyopathy
Mitochondrial depletion syndrome
Leigh syndrome and neuropathy, ataxia, retinitis pigmentosa
Succinate dehydrogenase deficiency*

*Deficiency can produce exercise intolerance and myoglobinuria.

From Goldman L, Ausiello D: *Cecil Textbook of Medicine,* 22nd ed. Philadelphia, WB Saunders, 2004, p. 2392.

between attacks, but during an attack a vacuolar myopathy is demonstrated. Pathologic changes in the periodic paralyses are similar whether the disease is due to a sodium or potassium channel defect, suggesting that they may result from the recurrent paralytic state rather than the specific channelopathy. The vacuoles are dilated sarcoplasmic reticulum and invaginations of the extracellular space into the cytoplasm, and they may be filled with glycogen. Hypoglycemia does not occur.

TREATMENT. Paralytic attacks of hypokalemic periodic paralysis are best treated by the oral administration of potassium or even fruit juices that contains potassium. A low sodium intake and the administration of acetazolamide, 125–250 mg bid or tid in school-age children, often is effective in abolishing attacks or at least reducing their frequency and severity. Spironolactone, in a dose of 100–200 mg/day PO in school-aged children may be beneficial as well.

610.2 • Malignant Hyperthermia

(See also Chapters 76 and 607.4.)

This syndrome is usually inherited as an autosomal dominant trait. It occurs in all patients with central core disease but is not limited to that particular myopathy. The gene is at the 19q13.1 locus in both central core disease and malignant hyperthermia without this specific myopathy. At least 15 separate mutations in this gene are associated with malignant hyperthermia. The gene programs the ryanodine receptor, a tetrameric calcium release channel in the sarcoplasmic reticulum, in apposition to the voltage-gated calcium channel of the transverse tubule. It occurs rarely in Duchenne and other muscular dystrophies, in various other myopathies, and in an isolated syndrome not associated with other muscle disease. Affected children sometimes have peculiar facies. All ages are affected, including premature infants whose mothers underwent general anesthesia for cesarean section.

Acute episodes are precipitated by exposure to general anesthetics and occasionally to local anesthetic drugs. Patients suddenly develop extreme fever, rigidity of muscles, and metabolic and respiratory acidosis; the serum CK level rises to as high as 35,000 IU/L. Myoglobinuria may result in tubular necrosis and acute renal failure.

The muscle biopsy specimen obtained during an episode of malignant hyperthermia or shortly afterward shows widely scattered necrosis of muscle fibers known as rhabdomyolysis. Between attacks, the muscle biopsy specimen is normal unless there is an underlying chronic myopathy.

It is important to recognize patients at risk of malignant hyperthermia because the attacks may be prevented by administering dantrolene sodium before an anesthetic is given. Identification of patients at risk, such as siblings, is done by the caffeine contracture test: A portion of fresh muscle biopsy tissue in a saline bath is attached to a strain gauge and exposed to caffeine and other drugs; an abnormal spasm is diagnostic. The syndrome receptor also may be demonstrated by immunochemistry in frozen sections of the muscle biopsy. The gene defect of the ryanodine receptor is present in 50% of patients; gene testing is available only for this genetic group. This receptor also may be seen in the muscle biopsy by immunoreactivity. Another candidate gene is at the 1q31 locus.

Apart from the genetic disorder of malignant hyperthermia, some drugs may induce acute rhabdomyolysis with myoglobinuria and potential renal failure, but this usually occurs in patients who are predisposed by some other metabolic disease. Valproic acid, for example, may induce this process in children with mitochondrial cytopathies or with carnitine palmitoyltransferase deficiency.

610.3 • Glycogenoses

(See also Chapter 87.1.)

Glycogenosis I (von Gierke disease) is not a true myopathy because the deficient liver enzyme glucose-6-phosphatase is not normally present in muscle. Nevertheless, children with this disease are hypotonic and mildly weak for unknown reasons.

Glycogenosis II (Pompe disease) is an autosomal recessively inherited deficiency of the glycolytic lysosomal enzyme acid maltase. Of the 12 known glycogenoses, type II is the only one with a defective lysosomal enzyme. The defective gene is at locus 17q23. Two forms are described. The infantile form is a severe generalized myopathy and cardiomyopathy. Patients have cardiomegaly and hepatomegaly and are diffusely hypotonic and weak. The serum CK level is greatly elevated. A muscle biopsy specimen reveals a vacuolar myopathy with abnormal lysosomal enzymatic activities such as acid and alkaline phosphatases. Death in infancy or early childhood is usual.

The late childhood or adult form is a much milder myopathy without cardiac or hepatic enlargement. It may not become clinically expressed until later childhood or early adult life but may be symptomatic as myopathic weakness and hypotonia even in early infancy. Even in late adult-onset acid maltase deficiency, more than ½ of the patients report difficulties with muscle strength dating from childhood.

The serum CK level is greatly elevated, and the muscle biopsy findings are diagnostic even in the presymptomatic stage. The diagnosis of glycogenosis II is confirmed by quantitative assay of acid maltase activity in muscle or liver biopsy specimens. A rare KM variant of the milder form of acid maltase deficiency may show muscle acid maltase activity in the low normal range with only intermittent decreases to subnormal values, but the muscle biopsy findings are similar although milder. In another form, **Danon disease**, transmitted as an X-linked recessive trait at the Xq24 locus, the primary deficiency is lysosomal membrane protein-2 (LAMP2) and results in hypertrophic cardiomyopathy, proximal myopathy, and mental retardation.

Glycogenosis III (Cori-Forbes disease), deficiency of debrancher enzyme (amylo-1,6-glucosidase), is more common than is usually diagnosed, and is generally the least severe. Hypotonia, weakness, hepatomegaly, and fasting hypoglycemia in infancy are common, but these features often resolve spontaneously, and patients become asymptomatic in childhood and adult life. Others experience slowly progressive distal muscle wasting, hepatic cirrhosis, recurrent hypoglycemia, and heart failure. This more serious chronic course is particularly seen in the Inuit population (Eskimos). Minor myopathic findings including vacuolation of muscle fibers are found in the muscle biopsy specimen.

Glycogenosis IV (Andersen disease) is a deficiency of brancher enzyme, resulting in the formation of an abnormal glycogen molecule, amylopectin, in the liver, reticuloendothelial cells, and skeletal and cardiac muscle. Hypotonia, generalized weakness, muscle wasting, and contractures are the usual signs of myopathic involvement. Most patients die before age 4 yr because of hepatic or cardiac failure. A few children without neuromuscular manifestations have been described.

Glycogenosis V (McArdle disease) is due to muscle phosphorylase deficiency inherited as an autosomal recessive trait at locus 11q13. Exercise intolerance is the cardinal clinical feature. Physical exertion results in cramps, weakness, and myoglobinuria, but strength is normal between attacks. The serum CK level is elevated only during exercise. A characteristic clinical feature is lack of the normal rise in serum lactate level during ischemic exercise because of inability to convert pyruvate to lactate under anaerobic conditions in vivo. Myophosphorylase deficiency may be demonstrated histochemically and biochemically in the muscle biopsy tissue. Some patients have a defect in adenosine monophosphate–dependent muscle phosphorylase-b-kinase, a phosphorylase enzyme activator. Muscle phosphorylase deficiency was the first neuromuscular disease to be diagnosed by MR spectroscopy, that shows that intramuscular pH does not decrease with exercise and there is no depletion of ATPase, but the phosphocreatine concentration falls excessively. This noninvasive technique may be useful in some patients if the radiologist is experienced with the disease.

A rare **neonatal form of myophosphorylase deficiency** causes feeding difficulties in early infancy, may be severe enough to result in neonatal death, or may follow a course of slowly progressive weakness resembling a muscular dystrophy.

The long-term prognosis is good. Patients must learn to moderate their physical activities, but they do not develop severe chronic myopathic handicaps or cardiac involvement.

Glycogenosis VII (Tarui disease) is muscle phosphofructokinase deficiency. Although this disease is more rare than glycogenosis V, the symptoms of exercise intolerance, clinical course, and inability to convert pyruvate to lactate are identical. The distinction is made by biochemical study of the muscle biopsy specimen. It is transmitted as an autosomal recessive trait at the 1cenq32 locus.

610.4 • Mitochondrial Myopathies

(See also Chapters 87.4 and 598.2.)

Several diseases involving muscle, brain, and other organs are associated with structural and functional abnormalities of mitochondria, producing defects in aerobic cellular metabolism, the electron transport chain, and the Krebs cycle. The structural aberrations are best demonstrated by electron microscopy of the muscle biopsy sample, revealing abnormally shaped cristae and fusion of cristae to form paracrystalline structures. Histochemical study of the muscle biopsy specimen reveals abnormal clumping of oxidative enzymatic activity, scattered myofibers with loss of cytochrome-c oxidase activity, sometimes increased neutral lipids because of impaired lipid metabolism, and ragged red muscle fibers with accumulations of membranous material beneath the muscle fiber membrane, best demonstrated by special stains. These characteristic histochemical and ultrastructural changes are most consistently seen with point mutation in mitochondrial transfer RNA. The large mitochondrial DNA (mtDNA) deletions of 5 or 7.4 kb (the single mitochondrial chromosome has 16.5 kb) are associated with defects in mitochondrial respiratory oxidative enzyme complexes, if as few as 2% of the mitochondria are affected, but minimal or no morphologic or histochemical changes may be noted in the muscle biopsy specimen, even by electron microscopy; hence, the quantitative biochemical studies of the muscle tissue are needed to confirm the diagnosis. Because most of the subunits of the respiratory chain complexes are encoded by nuclear DNA (nDNA) rather than mtDNA, mendelian autosomal inheritance is possible rather than maternal transmission as with pure mtDNA point mutations.

Several distinct mitochondrial diseases that primarily affect striated muscle or muscle and brain are identified. These can be divided into the ragged red fiber diseases (Kearns-Sayre, MELAS [mitochondrial encephalopathy, lactic acidosis, and strokelike symptoms] syndrome, MERRF [myoclonic epilepsy and ragged red fibers] syndrome, progressive external ophthalmoplegia syndromes) that are associated with a combined defect in respiratory chain complexes I and IV, and non–ragged fiber diseases (Leigh encephalopathy, Leber hereditary optic atrophy) that involve complex I or IV alone or, in children, the common combination of defective complexes III and V. ***Kearns-Sayre syndrome*** is characterized by the triad of progressive external ophthalmoplegia, pigmentary degeneration of the retina, and onset before age 20 yr. Heart block, cerebellar deficits, and high cerebrospinal fluid protein content are often associated. Visual evoked potentials are abnormal. Patients usually do not experience weakness of the trunk or extremities or dysphagia. Most cases are sporadic.

Chronic progressive external ophthalmoplegia may be isolated or accompanied by limb muscle weakness, dysphagia, and dysarthria. A few patients described as having *ophthalmoplegia plus* have additional central nervous system involvement. Autosomal dominant inheritance is found in some pedigrees, but most cases are sporadic.

MERRF and ***MELAS syndromes*** are other mitochondrial disorders affecting children. The latter is characterized by stunted growth, episodic vomiting, seizures, and recurrent cerebral insults causing hemiparesis, hemianopia or even cortical blindness, and dementia. The disease behaves as a degenerative disorder, and children die within a few years.

Other "degenerative" diseases of the central nervous system that also involve myopathy with mitochondrial abnormalities include **Leigh subacute necrotizing encephalopathy** (see Chapter 87.4) and **cerebrohepatorenal (Zellweger) disease** (see Chapter 86.2). Another recognized mitochondrial myopathy is **cytochrome-c oxidase deficiency. Oculopharyngeal muscular dystrophy** is also fundamentally a mitochondrial myopathy. ***Mitochondrial depletion syndrome of early infancy*** is characterized by severely decreased oxidative enzymatic activities in all 5 of the complexes; in addition to diffuse muscle weakness, neonates and young infants may show multisystemic involvement, with failure of liver, kidney, and heart functions; encephalopathy; and sometimes bullous skin lesions or generalized edema. Many other rare diseases with only a few case reports are suspected of being mitochondrial disorders. It is also now recognized that secondary mitochondrial defects occur in a wide range of non-mitochondrial diseases, including inflammatory autoimmune myopathies, and some cerebral malformations, and also may be induced by certain drugs and toxins, so that interpretation of mitochondrial abnormalities as primary defects must be approached with caution.

mtDNA is distinct from the DNA of the cell nucleus and is inherited exclusively from the mother; mitochondria are present in the cytoplasm of the ovum but not in the head of the sperm, the only part that enters the ovum at fertilization. The rate of mutation of mtDNA is 10 times higher than that of nDNA. The mitochondrial respiratory enzyme complexes each have subunits encoded either in mtDNA or nDNA. Complex II (succinate dehydrogenase, a Krebs cycle enzyme) has 4 subunits, all encoded in nDNA; complex III (ubiquinol or cytochrome-b oxidase) has 9 subunits, only 1 of which is encoded by mtDNA and 8 of which are programmed by nDNA; complex IV (cytochrome-c oxidase) has 13 subunits, only 3 of which are encoded by mtDNA. For this reason, mitochondrial diseases of muscle may be transmitted as autosomal recessive traits rather than by strict maternal transmission, even though all mitochondria are inherited from the mother.

In Kearns-Sayre syndrome, a single large mtDNA deletion has been identified, but other genetic variants are known; in MERRF and MELAS syndromes of mitochondrial myopathy, point mutations occur in transfer RNA (see Table 607-1).

There is no effective treatment of mitochondrial cytopathies, but various "cocktails" are often used empirically to try to overcome the metabolic deficits. These include oral carnitine supplements, riboflavin, coenzyme Q_{10}, ascorbic acid (vitamin C), vitamin E, and other antioxidants. Although some anecdotal reports are encouraging, no controlled studies that prove efficacy have been published.

610.5 • Lipid Myopathies

(See Chapter 86.4.)

Considered as metabolic organs, skeletal muscles are the most important sites in the body for long-chain fatty acid metabolism because of their large mass and their rich density of mitochondria where fatty acids are metabolized. Hereditary disorders of lipid metabolism that cause progressive myopathy are an important, relatively common, and often treatable group of muscle diseases. Increased lipid within myofibers is seen in the muscle biopsy of some, but not all, mitochondrial myopathies and is a constant, rather than an unpredictable, feature of specific diseases. Among the ragged red fiber diseases, Kearns-Sayre syndrome always shows increased neutral lipid, whereas MERRF and MELAS syndromes do not, a useful diagnostic marker for the pathologist.

Muscle carnitine deficiency is an autosomal recessive disease involving deficient transport of dietary carnitine across the intestinal mucosa. Carnitine is acquired from dietary sources but is also synthesized in the liver and kidneys from lysine and methionine; it is the obligatory carrier of long- and medium-chain fatty acids into muscle mitochondria.

The clinical course may be one of sudden exacerbations of weakness or may resemble a progressive muscular dystrophy with generalized proximal myopathy and sometimes facial, pharyngeal, and cardiac involvement. Symptoms usually begin in late childhood or adolescence or may be delayed until adult life. Progression is slow but may end in death.

Serum CK level is mildly elevated. Muscle biopsy material shows vacuoles filled with lipid within muscle fibers in addition to nonspecific changes suggestive of a muscular dystrophy. Mitochondria may appear normal or abnormal. Carnitine measured in muscle biopsy tissue is reduced, but the serum carnitine level is normal.

Treatment stops the progression of the disease and may even restore lost strength if the disease is not too advanced. It consists of special diets low in long-chain fatty acids. Steroids may enhance fatty acid transport. Specific therapy with L-carnitine taken orally in large doses overcomes the intestinal barrier in some patients. Some patients also improve when given supplementary riboflavin, and other patients seem to improve with propranolol.

Systemic carnitine deficiency is a disease of impaired renal and hepatic synthesis of carnitine rather than a primary myopathy. Patients with this autosomal recessive disease experience progressive proximal myopathy and show muscle biopsy changes similar to those of muscle carnitine deficiency; however, the onset of weakness is earlier and may be evident at birth. Endocardial fibroelastosis also may occur. Episodes of acute hepatic encephalopathy resembling Reye syndrome may occur. Hypoglycemia and metabolic acidosis complicate acute episodes.

The concentration of carnitine is reduced in serum as well as in muscle and liver. A similar clinical syndrome may be a complication of renal Fanconi syndrome because of excessive urinary loss of carnitine or loss during chronic hemodialysis.

Treatment with L-carnitine improves the maintenance of blood glucose and serum carnitine levels but does not reverse the ketosis or acidosis or improve exercise capacity.

Muscle carnitine palmitoyltransferase (CPT) deficiency presents as episodes of rhabdomyolysis, coma, and elevated serum CK level that may be indistinguishable from Reye syndrome. CPT transfers long-chain fatty acid acyl coenzyme A residues to carnitine on the outer mitochondrial membrane for transport into the mitochondria. Exercise intolerance and myoglobinuria resemble glycogenoses V and VII. The degree of exercise that triggers an attack varies among individuals, ranging from casual walking to strenuous exercise. Myoglobinuria is an inconstant feature. Fasting hypoglycemia may occur. Some patients present only in late adolescence or adult life with myalgias. Genetic transmission is autosomal recessive, due to a defect on chromosome 1 at the 1p32 locus. Administration of valproic acid may precipitate acute rhabdomyolysis with myoglobinuria in patients with CPT deficiency; it should be avoided in the treatment of seizures or migraine if they occur.

610.6 • Vitamin E Deficiency Myopathy

Deficiency of vitamin E (α-tocopherol, an antioxidant also important in mitochondrial superoxide generation) in experimental animals produces a progressive myopathy closely resembling a muscular dystrophy. Myopathy and neuropathy are recognized in humans who lack adequate intake of this antioxidant. Patients with chronic malabsorption, those undergoing long-term dialysis, and premature infants who do not receive vitamin E supplements are particularly vulnerable. Treatment with high doses of vitamin E may reverse the deficiency. Myopathy due to chronic hypervitaminosis E also occurs.

Cannon SC: An expanding view for the molecular basis of familial periodic paralysis. *Neuromuscul Disord* 2000;12:533–543.

Chow CK: Vitamin E regulation of mitochondrial superoxide generation. *Biol Signals Recept* 2001;10:112–124.

Darin N, Oldfors A, Moslemi A-R, et al: Genotypes and clinical phenotypes in children with cytochrome-c-oxidase deficiency. *Neuropediatrics* 2003; 34:311–317.

Deschauer M, Wieser T, Zierz S: Muscle carnitine palmitoyltransferase II deficiency. Clinical and molecular genetic features and diagnostic aspects. *Arch Neurol* 2005;62:37–41.

Elpeleg O, Mandel H, Saada A: Depletion of the other genome-mitochondrial DNA depletion syndromes in humans. *J Mol Med* 2002;80:389–396.

Hagemans MLC, Winkel LPF, Van Doorn PA, et al: Clinical manifestations and natural course of late-onset Pompe disease in 54 Dutch patients. *Brain* 2005;128:671–677.

Kottlors M, Jaksch M, Ketelsen U-P, et al: Valproic acid triggers acute rhabdomyolysis in a patient with carnitine palmitoyltransferase type II deficiency. *Neuromuscul Disord* 2001;11:757–759.

Marín-García J, Goldenthal MJ, Sarnat HB: Probing striated muscle mitochondrial phenotype in neuromuscular disorders. *Pediatr Neurol* 2003; 29:26–33.

Nishino I, Yamamoto A, Sugie K, et al: Danon disease and related disorders. *Acta Myologica* 2001;20:120.

Sarnat HB, Marín-García J: Pathology of mitochondrial encephalomyopathies. *Can J Neurol Sci* 2005;32:152–166.

Schapira AHV: *Mitochondrial Function and Dysfunction.* New York, Academic Press, 2003.

Zimakas PJ, Rodd CJ: Glycogen storage disease type III in Inuit children. *CMAJ* 2005;172:355–358.

Chapter 611 ■ Disorders of Neuromuscular Transmission and of Motor Neurons

611.1 • Myasthenia Gravis

This chronic disease is characterized by rapid fatigability of striated muscle. The most frequent cause is an immune-mediated neuromuscular blockade. The release of acetylcholine (ACh) into the synaptic cleft by the axonal terminal is normal, but the postsynaptic muscle membrane or *motor end plate* is less responsive than normal. A decreased number of available ACh receptors is due to circulating receptor-binding antibodies in most cases of acquired myasthenia. The disease is generally nonhereditary and is an autoimmune disorder. A rare familial myasthenia gravis is probably an autosomal recessive trait and is not associated with plasma anti-ACh antibodies. One familial form is a deficiency of motor end plate ACh, designated AChE. Infants born to myasthenic mothers may have a transient neonatal myasthenic syn-

TABLE 611-1. Clinical, Pathologic, and Neurophysiologic Characteristics of Various Congenital Myasthenic Syndromes

	LEMS	CMS-EA	END PLATE ACHE DEFICIENCY	SLOW CHANNEL SYNDROMES	FAST CHANNEL SYNDROME	ACH RECEPTOR DEFICIENCY
Mode of inheritance	AR-sporadic	AR	AR	AD	AR	AR
Gene location		17 pter	3p24.2 (for type 1c)	2q24–q32, 17p11–p12 & 17p13	17p13	17p13
Gene product		FIM	COLQ	CHRNA, CHRNB1 & CHRNE	CHRNE	CHRNE
Pathogenesis/defect	autoimmune	presynaptic	synaptic	postsynaptic	postsynaptic	postsynaptic
Contractures	–	+	–	–	–	–
Tendon reflexes	–	+	±	±	±	±
Early manifestations	+	+	+	Variable	–	Variable
Episodic crises	±	+	–	–	–	–
Response to Ach inhibitors	–	+	–	–	+	+
Response to 3,4-DAP	Sometimes	–	–	–	Mild response	+
Response to quinidine	–	–	–	+	–	–
Low-frequency RS	Decrement	Decrement	Decrement	Decrement	Decrement	Decrement
High-frequency RS	Increment	Decrement	Decrement	Decrement	Decrement	Decrement
Repetitive CMAP	–	–	+	+	–	–
Low-amplitude baseline CMAP	+	–	–	–	–	–
Small MUP in electromyography	–	–	+	+	+	+
Muscle biopsy	Normal	Normal	Abnormal	Abnormal	Normal	Abnormal

ACHE, acetycholinesterase; AD, autosomal dominant; AR, Autosomal recessive; CHRNA, acetylcholine receptor α subunit; CHRNB1, acetylcholine receptor β subunit; CHRNE, acetylcholine receptor e subunit; CMAP, compound muscle action potential; CMS-EA, congenital myasthenic syndrome with episodic apnea; COLQ, collagen Q; 3,4-DAP, 3,4-diaminopyridine; FIM, familial infantile myasthenia; LEMS, Lambert-Eaton myasthenic syndrome; MUP, motor unit potential; RS, repetitive stimulation; +, present; –, absent; ±, equivocal.

From Zafeiriou DI, Pitt M, de Sousa C: Clinical and neurophysiological characteristics of congenital myasthenic syndromes presenting in early infancy. *Brain Dev* 2004; 26: 47–52.

drome secondary to placentally transferred anti-ACh receptor antibodies, distinct from congenital myasthenia gravis (Table 611-1).

CLINICAL MANIFESTATIONS. Three clinical varieties are distinguished in childhood: juvenile myasthenia gravis in late infancy and childhood, congenital myasthenia, and transient neonatal myasthenia. In the juvenile form, ptosis and some degree of extraocular muscle weakness are the earliest and most constant signs. Older children may complain of diplopia, and young children may hold open their eyes with their fingers or thumbs if the ptosis is severe enough to obstruct vision. The pupillary responses to light are preserved. Dysphagia and facial weakness are also common, and in early infancy, feeding difficulties are often the cardinal sign of myasthenia. Poor head control because of weakness of the neck flexors is also prominent. Involvement may be limited to bulbar-innervated muscles, but the disease is systemic and weakness involves limb-girdle muscles and distal muscles of the hands in most cases. Fasciculations of muscle, myalgias, and sensory symptoms do not occur. Tendon stretch reflexes may be diminished but rarely are lost.

Rapid fatigue of muscles is a characteristic feature of myasthenia gravis that distinguishes it from most other neuromuscular diseases. Ptosis increases progressively as patients are asked to sustain an upward gaze for 30–90 sec. Holding the head up from the surface of the examining table while lying supine is very difficult, and gravity cannot be overcome for more than a few seconds. Repetitive opening and closing of the fists produces rapid fatigue of hand muscles, and patients cannot elevate their arms for more than 1–2 min because of fatigue of the deltoids. Patients are more symptomatic late in the day or when tired. Dysphagia may interfere with eating, and the muscles of the jaw soon tire when an affected child chews.

If untreated, myasthenia gravis is usually progressive and may become life threatening because of respiratory muscle involvement and the risk of aspiration, particularly at times when the child is otherwise unwell with an upper respiratory tract infection. Familial myasthenia gravis usually is not progressive.

Infants born to myasthenic mothers may have respiratory insufficiency, inability to suck or swallow, and generalized hypotonia and weakness. They may show little spontaneous motor activity for several days to weeks. Some require ventilatory support and feeding by gavage during this period. After the abnormal antibodies disappear from the blood and muscle tissue, the infants regain normal strength and are not at increased risk of developing myasthenia gravis in later childhood. This syndrome of *transient neonatal myasthenia gravis* is to be distinguished from a rare and often hereditary **congenital myasthenia gravis** not related to maternal myasthenia that is nearly always a permanent disorder without spontaneous remission (see Table 611-1).

Three **presynaptic congenital myasthenic syndromes** are recognized, all as autosomal recessive traits; some of these have anti-MuSK antibodies. These children exhibit weakness of extraocular, pharyngeal, and respiratory muscles and later show shoulder girdle weakness as well. Episodic **apnea** is a problem in congenital myasthenia gravis. Another synaptic form is caused by absence or marked deficiency of AChE in the synaptic basal lamina, and postsynaptic forms of congenital myasthenia are caused by mutations in ACh receptor subunit genes that alter the synaptic response to ACh. An abnormality of the ACh receptor channels appearing as high conductance and excessively fast closure may be the result of a point mutation in a subunit of the receptor affecting a single amino acid residue. Children with congenital myasthenia gravis do not experience myasthenic crises and rarely exhibit elevations of anti-ACh antibodies in plasma.

Myasthenia gravis is occasionally associated with hypothyroidism, usually due to **Hashimoto thyroiditis.** Other collagen vascular diseases may also be associated. Thymomas, noted in some adults, rarely coexist with myasthenia gravis in children; nor do carcinomas of the lung occur, which produce a unique form of myasthenia in adults, **Eaton-Lambert syndrome.** Postinfectious myasthenia gravis in children is transitory and usually follows a varicella-zoster infection in 2–5 wk as an immune response.

LABORATORY FINDINGS AND DIAGNOSIS. Myasthenia gravis is 1 of the few neuromuscular diseases in which electromyography (EMG) is more specifically diagnostic than a muscle biopsy. A decremental response is seen in response to repetitive nerve stimulation; the muscle potentials diminish rapidly in amplitude until the muscle becomes refractory to further stimulation. Motor nerve conduction velocity remains normal. This unique EMG pattern is the electrophysiologic correlate of the fatigable weakness observed clinically and is reversed after a cholinesterase inhibitor is administered. A myasthenic decrement may be absent or difficult to demonstrate in muscles that are not involved clinically. This feature may be confusing in early cases or in patients showing only weakness of extraocular muscles. Microelectrode studies of end plate potentials and currents reveal whether the transmission defect is presynaptic or postsynaptic. Special electrophysiologic studies are required in the classification of congenital myasthenic syndromes and involve the estimation of the number of ACh receptors per end plate and in vitro study of end plate function. These special studies and patch-clamp recordings of kinetic properties of channels are performed on special biopsy samples of intercostal muscle strips that include both origin and insertion of the muscle but are only performed in specialized centers. If myasthenia is limited to the extraocular muscles, levator palpebrae and pharyngeal muscles, evoked-potential EMG of the muscles of the extremities and spine, diagnostic in the generalized disease, usually is normal.

Anti-ACh antibodies should be assayed in the plasma but are inconsistently demonstrated. About ⅓ of affected adolescents show elevations, but anti-ACh receptor antibodies are only occasionally demonstrated in the plasma of prepubertal children. Many juvenile myasthenics who show no anti-ACh antibodies in serum have instead antibodies against the receptor tyrosine kinase (MuSK), which also is localized at the neuromuscular junction and appears essential to fetal development of this junction. Many cases of congenital myasthenia gravis are due not to a refractory postsynaptic membrane at the neuromuscular junction as in juvenile and adult myasthenia, but rather failure to synthesize or release ACh at the presynaptic membrane. In some cases, the gene that mediates the enzyme choline acetyltransferase for the synthesis of ACh is mutated. In others, there is a defect in the quantal release of vesicles containing ACh. The treatment of such patients with cholinesterase inhibitors is futile.

Other serologic tests of autoimmune disease, such as antinuclear antibodies and abnormal immune complexes, should also be sought. If these are positive, more extensive autoimmune disease involving vasculitis or tissues other than muscle is likely. A thyroid profile should always be examined. The serum creatine kinase (CK) level is normal in myasthenia gravis.

The heart is not involved, and electrocardiographic findings remain normal. Radiographs of the chest often reveal an enlarged thymus, but the hypertrophy is not a thymoma. It may be further defined by tomography or by CT scanning of the anterior mediastinum.

The role of conventional muscle biopsy in myasthenia gravis is limited. It is not required in most cases, but about 17% of patients show inflammatory changes sometimes called *lymphorrhages* that are interpreted by some physicians as a mixed myasthenia-polymyositis immune disorder. Muscle biopsy tissue in myasthenia gravis shows nonspecific type II muscle fiber atrophy, similar to that seen with disuse atrophy, steroid effects on muscle, polymyalgia rheumatica, and many other conditions. The ultrastructure of motor end plates shows simplification of the membrane folds; the ACh receptors are located in these postsynaptic folds, as shown by bungarotoxin (snake venom), which binds specifically to the ACh receptors.

A **clinical test for myasthenia gravis** is administration of a short-acting cholinesterase inhibitor, usually edrophonium chloride. Ptosis and ophthalmoplegia improve within a few seconds, and fatigability of other muscles decreases.

RECOMMENDATIONS ON THE USE OF CHOLINESTERASE INHIBITORS AS A DIAGNOSTIC TEST FOR MYASTHENIA GRAVIS IN INFANTS AND CHILDREN

FOR CHILDREN 2 YR OF AGE OR OLDER

1. Child should have a specific fatigable weakness that can be measured, such as ptosis of the eyelids, dysphagia, or inability of cervical muscles to support head; nonspecific generalized weakness without cranial nerve motor deficits is not a criterion.
2. An intravenous infusion should be started to enable the administration of medications in the event of an adverse reaction.
3. Electrocardiographic monitoring during test is recommended.
4. A dose of atropine sulfate (0.01 mg/kg) should be available in a syringe, ready for IV administration at the bedside during the edrophonium test, to block acute muscarinic effects of the cholinesterase inhibitor (mainly abdominal cramps and/or sudden diarrhea from increased peristalsis, profuse bronchotracheal secretions that may obstruct the airway, or, rarely, cardiac arrhythmias, if needed. Some physicians pretreat all patients with atropine before administering edrophonium, but this is not recommended unless there is a history of reaction to tests. Remember that atropine may cause the pupils to be dilated and fixed for as long as 14 days after a single dose, and the pupillary effects of homatropine may last 4–7 days.
5. Edrophonium chloride (Tensilon) is administered intravenously. Initially, a test dose of 0.04 mg/kg is given to ensure that the patient does not have an allergic reaction or is otherwise very sensitive to muscarinic side effects. If this test dose is well tolerated, the diagnostic dose administered is 0.1–0.2 mg/kg (maximum single dose is 10 mg regardless of weight; in children weighing <30 kg, 2 mg is the maximum dose; a typical dose for a 3–5 yr old child is 5 mg). These same doses may be given intramuscularly or subcutaneously, but these routes are not recommended because the results are much more variable due to unpredictable absorption, and the test may be ambiguous or falsely negative.
6. Effects should be seen within 10 sec and disappear within 120 sec; weakness is measured (e.g., distance between upper and lower eyelids before and after administration, degree of external ophthalmoplegia, ability to swallow a sip of water).
7. Long-acting cholinesterase inhibitors, such as pyridostigmine (Mestinon) are generally not as useful for the acute assessment of myasthenic weakness. The prostigmine test may be used (as outlined later) but may not be as definitively diagnostic as the edrophonium test.

FOR INFANTS YOUNGER THAN 2 YR OF AGE

1. Infants ideally should have a specific fatigable weakness that can be measured, such as ptosis of the eyelids, dysphagia, and inability of cervical muscles to support head; nonspecific generalized weakness without cranial nerve motor deficits is less easy to assess results but may be a criterion at times.
2. An IV infusion should be started as a rapid route for medications in the event of an adverse effect of the test medication.
3. Electrocardiographic monitoring is recommended during test.
4. Pretreatment with atropine sulfate to block the muscarinic effects of the test medication is not recommended but should be available at the bedside in a prepared syringe. If needed, it should be administered intravenously in a dose of 0.1 mg/kg.
5. Edrophonium is not recommended for use in infants; its effect is too brief for objective assessment and an increased incidence of acute cardiac arrhythmias is reported in infants, especially neonates, with this drug.
6. Prostigmine methylsulfate (Neostigmine) is administered intramuscularly at a dose of 0.04 mg/kg; if the result is negative or equivocal, another dose of 0.04 mg/kg may be administered 4 hr after the first dose (a typical dose is 0.5–1.5 mg). The peak effect is seen in 20–40 min. Intravenous prostigmine is contraindicated because of risk of cardiac arrhythmias, including fatal ventricular fibrillation, especially in young infants.
7. Long-acting cholinesterase inhibitors administered orally, such as pyridostigmine (Mestinon), are generally not as useful for the acute assessment of myasthenic weakness because onset and duration are less predictable.

Where should test be performed? The setting may be the emergency department, hospital ward, or, at times, a physician's office; the important issue is preparation for potential complications such as cardiac arrhythmia or cholinergic crisis, as previously outlined.

TREATMENT. Some patients with mild myasthenia gravis require no treatment. **Cholinesterase-inhibiting drugs** are the primary therapeutic agents. Neostigmine methylsulfate (0.04 mg/kg) may be given intramuscularly every 4–6 hr, but most patients tolerate oral neostigmine bromide, 0.4 mg/kg every 4–6 hr. If dysphagia is a major problem, the drug should be given about 30 min before meals to improve swallowing. Pyridostigmine is an alternative; the dose required is about 4 times greater than that of neostigmine, but it may be slightly longer acting. Overdoses of cholinesterase inhibitors produce cholinergic crises; atropine blocks the muscarinic effects but does not block the nicotinic effects that produce additional skeletal muscle weakness. In the rare familial myasthenia gravis caused by absence of end plate

AChE, cholinesterase inhibitors are not helpful and often cause increased weakness; these patients can be treated with ephedrine or diaminopyridine, both of which increase ACh release from terminal axons.

Because of the autoimmune basis of the disease, long-term **steroid treatment** with prednisone may be effective. **Thymectomy** should be considered and may provide a cure. Thymectomy is most effective in patients with high titers of anti-ACh receptor antibodies in the plasma and who are symptomatic for <2 yr. Thymectomy is ineffective in congenital and familial forms of myasthenia gravis. Treatment of hypothyroidism usually abolishes an associated myasthenia without the use of cholinesterase inhibitors or steroids.

Plasmapheresis is effective treatment in some children, particularly those who do not respond to steroids, but plasma exchange therapy may provide only temporary remission. **Intravenous immunoglobulin** (IVIG) is sometimes beneficial and might be tried before plasmapheresis because it is less invasive. Both plasmapheresis and IVIG appear to be most effective in patients with high circulating levels of anti-ACh receptor antibodies. Refractory patients may respond to rituximab, a monoclonal antibody to the B-cell CD20 antigen.

Neonates with transient maternally transmitted myasthenia gravis require cholinesterase inhibitors for only a few days or occasionally for a few weeks, especially to allow feeding. No other treatment is usually necessary.

COMPLICATIONS. Children with myasthenia gravis do not tolerate neuromuscular blocking drugs, such as succinylcholine and pancuronium, and may be paralyzed for weeks after a single dose. An anesthesiologist should carefully review myasthenic patients who require a surgical anesthetic. Also, certain antibiotics may potentiate myasthenia and should be avoided; these include the aminoglycosides (gentamicin and others).

PROGNOSIS. This is difficult to predict. Some patients undergo spontaneous remission after a period of months or years; others have a permanent disease extending into adult life. Immunosuppression, thymectomy, and treatment of associated hypothyroidism may provide a cure.

OTHER CAUSES OF NEUROMUSCULAR BLOCKADE. Organophosphate chemicals, commonly used as insecticides, may cause a myasthenia-like syndrome in children exposed to these toxins (see Chapter 58).

Botulism results from ingestion of food containing the toxin of *Clostridium botulinum,* a gram-positive, spore-bearing, anaerobic bacillus (see Chapter 207). Honey is a frequent source of contamination. The incubation period is short, only a few hours, and symptoms begin with nausea, vomiting, and diarrhea. Cranial nerve involvement soon follows, with diplopia, dysphagia, weak suck, facial weakness, and absent gag reflex. Generalized hypotonia and weakness then develop and may progress to respiratory failure. Neuromuscular blockade is documented by EMG with repetitive nerve stimulation. Respiratory support may be required for days or weeks until the toxin is cleared from the body. No specific antitoxin is available. Guanidine, 35 mg/kg/24 hr, may be effective for extraocular and limb muscle weakness but not for respiratory muscle involvement.

Tick paralysis is a disorder of ACh release from axonal terminals due to a neurotoxin that blocks depolarization. It also affects large myelinated motor and sensory nerve fibers. This toxin is produced by the wood tick or dog tick, insects common in the Appalachian and Rocky Mountains of North America. The tick embeds its head into the skin, usually the scalp, and neurotoxin production is maximal about 5–6 days later. Motor symptoms include weakness, loss of coordination, and sometimes an ascending paralysis resembling Guillain-Barré syndrome. Tendon reflexes are lost. Sensory symptoms of tingling paresthesias may occur in the face and extremities. The diagnosis is confirmed by EMG and nerve conduction studies and by identifying the tick. The tick must be removed completely, and the buried head not left beneath the skin. Patients then recover completely within hours or days.

611.2 • Spinal Muscular Atrophies

Spinal muscular atrophies (SMAs) are degenerative diseases of motor neurons that begin in fetal life and continue to be progressive in infancy and childhood. The progressive denervation of muscle is compensated in part by reinnervation from an adjacent motor unit, but giant motor units are thus created with subsequent atrophy of muscle fibers when the reinnervating motor neuron eventually becomes involved. Upper motor neurons remain normal.

SMA is classified into a severe infantile form, also known as **Werdnig-Hoffmann disease** or SMA type 1; a late infantile and more slowly progressive form, SMA type 2; and a more chronic or juvenile form, also called **Kugelberg-Welander disease,** or SMA type 3. A severe fetal form that is usually lethal in the perinatal period has been described as SMA type 0. These distinctions are clinical and are based on age at onset, severity of weakness, and clinical course; muscle biopsy does not distinguish types 1 and 2, although type 3 shows a more adult than perinatal pattern of denervation/reinnervation. The type 0 may show biopsy features more similar to myotubular myopathy because of maturational arrest; scattered myotubes and other immature fetal fibers also are demonstrated in the muscle biopsies of patients with types 1 and 2, but do not predominate. About 25% of patients are type 1, 50% type 2, and 25% type 3; type 0 is rare and accounts for <1%. Some patients are transitional between types 1 and 2 or between types 2 and 3 in terms of clinical function. A variant of SMA, **Fazio-Londe disease,** is a progressive bulbar palsy resulting from motor neuron degeneration more in the brainstem than the spinal cord.

ETIOLOGY. The cause of SMA is a pathologic continuation of a process of programmed cell death that is normal in embryonic life. A surplus of motor neuroblasts and other neurons is generated from primitive neuroectoderm, but only about ½ survive and mature to become neurons; the excess cells have a limited life cycle and degenerate. If the process that arrests physiologic cell death fails to intervene by a certain stage, neuronal death may continue in late fetal life and postnatally. The survivor motor neuron gene *(SMN)* arrests apoptosis (programmed cell death) of motor neuroblasts. Unlike most genes that are highly conserved in evolution, *SMN* is a uniquely mammalian gene.

CLINICAL MANIFESTATIONS. The cardinal features of **SMA type 1** are severe hypotonia (Fig. 611-1); generalized weakness; thin muscle mass; absent tendon stretch reflexes; involvement of the tongue, face, and jaw muscles; and sparing of extraocular muscles and sphincters. Diaphragmatic involvement is late. Infants who are symptomatic at birth may have respiratory distress and are unable to feed. Congenital contractures, ranging from simple clubfoot to generalized arthrogryposis, occur in about 10% of severely involved neonates. Infants lie flaccid with little movement, unable to overcome gravity (Fig. 606-1). They lack head control. More than ⅔ die by 2 yr of age, and many die early in infancy.

In **type 2 SMA,** affected infants are usually able to suck and swallow and respiration is adequate in early infancy. These infants show progressive weakness, but many survive into the school years or beyond, although confined to an electric wheelchair and severely handicapped. Nasal speech and problems with

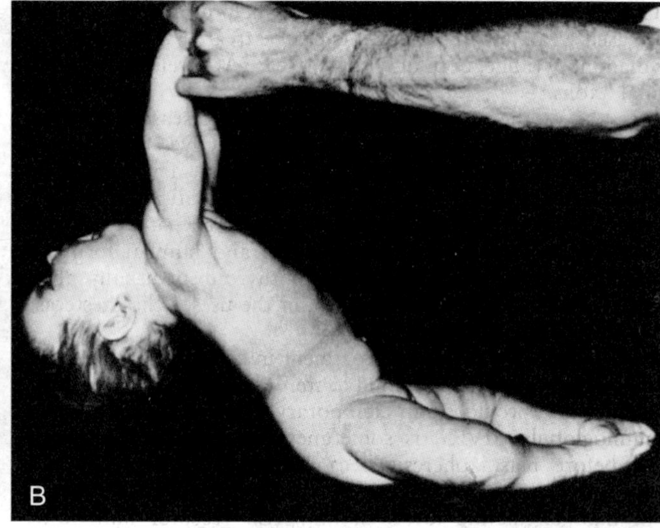

Figure 611-1. Type 1 spinal muscular atrophy (Werdnig-Hoffmann disease). Clinical manifestations of weakness of limb and axial musculature in a 6 wk old infant with severe weakness and hypotonia from birth. Note the marked weakness of the limbs and trunk on ventral suspension *(A)* and of neck on pull to sit *(B)*. (From Volpe J: *Neurology of the Newborn,* 4th ed. Philadelphia, WB Saunders, 2001, p. 644.)

deglutition develop later. Scoliosis becomes a major complication in many patients with long survival.

Kugelberg-Welander disease is the mildest **SMA (type 3)**, and patients may appear normal in infancy. The progressive weakness is proximal in distribution, particularly involving shoulder girdle muscles. Patients are ambulatory. Symptoms of bulbar muscle weakness are rare. About 25% of patients with this form of SMA have muscular hypertrophy rather than atrophy, and it may easily be confused with a muscular dystrophy. Longevity may extend well into middle adult life. Fasciculations are a specific clinical sign of denervation of muscle. In thin children, they may be seen in the deltoid, biceps brachii, and occasionally the quadriceps femoris muscles, but the continuous, involuntary, wormlike movements may be masked by a thick pad of subcutaneous fat. Fasciculations are best observed in the tongue, where almost no subcutaneous connective tissue separates the muscular layer from the epithelium. If the intrinsic lingual muscles are contracted, such as in crying or when the tongue protrudes, fasciculations are more difficult to see than when the tongue is relaxed.

The outstretched fingers of children with SMA often show a characteristic tremor owing to fasciculations and weakness. It should not be confused with a cerebellar tremor. Myalgias are not a feature of SMA.

The heart is not involved in SMA. Intelligence is normal, and children often appear brighter than their normal peers because the effort they cannot put into physical activities is redirected to intellectual development, and they are often exposed to adult speech more than to juvenile language because of the social repercussions of the disease.

LABORATORY FINDINGS. The serum CK level may be normal but more commonly is mildly elevated in the hundreds. A CK level of several thousand is rare. Results of motor nerve conduction studies are normal, except for mild slowing in terminal stages of the disease, an important feature distinguishing SMA from peripheral neuropathy. EMG shows fibrillation potentials and other signs of denervation of muscle.

DIAGNOSIS. The simplest, most definitive diagnostic test is a molecular genetic marker in blood for the *SMN* gene. Muscle biopsy reveals a characteristic pattern of perinatal denervation that is unlike that of mature muscle. Groups of giant type I fibers are mixed with fascicles of severely atrophic fibers of both histochemical types (Fig. 611-2). Scattered immature myofibers resembling myotubes also are demonstrated. In juvenile SMA, the pattern may be more similar to adult muscle that has undergone many cycles of denervation and reinnervation. Neurogenic changes in muscle also may be demonstrated by EMG, but the results are less definitive than by muscle biopsy in infancy. Sural nerve biopsy sometimes shows mild sensory neuropathic changes, and sensory nerve conduction velocity may be slowed; hypertrophy of unmyelinated axons also is seen. At autopsy, mild degenerative changes are seen in sensory neurons of dorsal root ganglia and in somatosensory nuclei of the thalamus, but these alterations are not perceived clinically as sensory loss or paresthesias. The most pronounced neuropathologic lesions are the extensive neuronal degeneration and gliosis in the ventral horns of the spinal cord and brainstem motor nuclei, especially the hypoglossal nucleus.

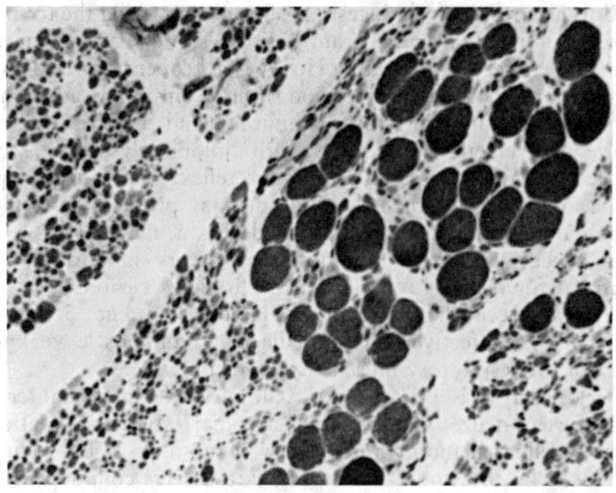

Figure 611-2. Muscle biopsy of neonate with infantile spinal muscular atrophy. Groups of giant type I (darkly stained) fibers are seen within muscle fascicles of severely atrophic fibers of both histochemical types. This is the characteristic pattern of perinatal denervation of muscle. Myofibrillar ATPase, preincubated at pH 4.6 (×400).

GENETICS. Molecular genetic diagnosis by DNA probes in blood samples or in muscle biopsy or chorionic villi tissues is available not only for diagnosis of suspected cases but also for prenatal diagnosis. Most cases are inherited as an autosomal recessive trait. The incidence of SMA is 10–15 per 100,000 live births, affecting all ethnic groups; it is the 2nd most common neuromuscular disease, following Duchenne muscular dystrophy. The incidence of heterozygosity for autosomal recessive SMA is 1 : 50. The genetic locus for all 3 of the common forms of SMA is on chromosome 5, a deletion at the 5q11-q13 locus, indicating that they are variants of the same disease rather than different diseases. The affected *SMN* gene contains 8 exons that span 20 kb, telomeric and centromeric exons that differ only by 5 bp and produce a transcript encoding 294 amino acids. Another gene, the *neuronal apoptosis inhibitory gene (NAIP),* is located next to the *SMN* gene and in many cases there is an inverted duplication with 2 copies, telomeric and centromeric, of both genes; isolated mutations or deletions of *NAIP* do not produce clinical SMA and generate a mostly nonfunctional isoform lacking the carboxy-terminus amino acids encoded by exon 7. Milder forms of SMA have more than 2 copies of *SMN2*, and in late-onset patients with homozygous deletion of the *SMN1* gene, there are 4 copies of *SMN2*. An additional gene mapped to 11q13-q21 in SMA may help explain early respiratory failure in some patients.

Infrequent families with autosomal dominant inheritance are described, and a rare X-linked recessive form occurs. Carrier testing by dose analysis is available.

TREATMENT. No medical treatment is able to delay the progression. Supportive therapy includes orthopedic care with particular attention to scoliosis and joint contractures, mild physiotherapy, and mechanical aids for assisting the child to eat and to be as functionally independent as possible. Most children learn to use a computer keyboard with great skill but cannot use a pencil easily.

611.3 • Other Motor Neuron Diseases

Motor neuron diseases other than SMA are rare in children. *Poliomyelitis* used to be a major cause of chronic disability, but since the routine use of polio vaccine, this viral infection is now rare (see Chapter 246). Other enteroviruses, such as *Coxsackie* and *Echo* viruses, or the live polio vaccine virus may also cause an acute infection of motor neurons with symptoms and signs similar to poliomyelitis, although usually milder. Specific polymerase chain reaction tests and viral cultures of cerebrospinal fluid are diagnostic. Motor neuron infection with the West Nile virus also occurs.

A **juvenile form of amyotrophic lateral sclerosis** is rare. Upper motor neuron loss as well as lower motor neuron loss is evident clinically, unlike SMA. The course is progressive and is ultimately fatal.

Pena-Shokeir and **Marden-Walker syndromes** are progressive motor neuron degenerations associated with severe arthrogryposis and congenital anomalies of many organ systems. **Pontocerebellar hypoplasias** are progressive degenerative diseases of the central nervous system that begin in fetal life; one form also involves motor neuron degeneration resembling an SMA, but the *SMN* gene or chromosome 5 is normal.

Motor neurons become involved in several metabolic diseases of the nervous system, such as gangliosidosis (Tay-Sachs disease), ceroid lipofuscinosis (Batten disease), and glycogenosis II (Pompe disease), but the signs of denervation may be minor or obscured by the more prominent involvement of other parts of the central nervous system or of muscle.

Disorders of Neuromuscular Transmission

Andrews PL: Autoimmune myasthenia gravis in childhood. *Semin Neurol* 2004;24:101–110.

Barisic N, Müller JS, Paucic-Kirincic E, et al: Clinical variability of CMS-EA (congenital myasthenic syndrome with episodic apnea) due to identical CHAT mutations in two infants. *Eur J Paediatr Neurol* 2005;9:7–12.

Dalakas MC: Intravenous immunoglobulin in autoimmune neuromuscular diseases. *JAMA* 2004;291:2367–2375.

Felice KJ, DiMario F, Conway SR: Postinfectious myasthenia gravis: Report of 2 cases. *J Child Neurol* 2005;20:441–444.

Harper CM: Congenital myasthenic syndromes. *Semin Neurol* 2004;24: 111–123.

Maselli RA, Kong DZ, Bowe CM, et al: Presynaptic congenital myasthenic syndrome due to quantal release deficiency. *Neurology* 2001;57:279–289.

Scherer K, Bedlack RS, Simel DL: Does this patient have myasthenia gravis? *JAMA* 2005;293:1906–1914.

Schmidt C, Abicht A, Krampfl K, et al: Congenital myasthenic syndrome due to a novel missense mutation in the gene encoding choline acetyltransferase. *Neuromuscul Disord* 2003;13:245–251.

Vincent A, McConville J, Farrugia ME, et al: Seronegative myasthenia gravis. *Semin Neurol* 2004;24:125–133.

Wylam ME, Anderson PM, Kuntz NL, Rodriguez V: Successful treatment of refractory myasthenia gravis using rituximab: A pediatric case report. *J Pediatr* 2003;143:674–677.

Zafeiriou DI, Pitt M, de Sousa C: Clinical and neurophysiological characteristics of congenital myasthenic syndromes presenting in early infancy. *Brain Dev* 2004;26:47–52.

Spinal Muscular Atrophies

Chung BHY, Wong VCN, Ip P: Spinal muscular atrophy: survival pattern and functional status. *Pediatrics* 2004;114:e548–e553.

Grohmann K, Varon R, Stolz P, et al: Infantile spinal muscular atrophy with respiratory distress type 1 (SMARD1). *Ann Neurol* 2003;54:719–724.

Hardart MKM, Truog RD: Spinal muscular atrophy-type 1. *Arch Dis Child* 2003;88:848–850.

Kizilates SU, Talim B, Sel K, et al: Severe lethal spinal muscular atrophy variant with arthrogryposis. *Pediatr Neurol* 2005;32:201–204.

Nadeau A, Anjou GD, Debray FG, et al: A newborn with spinal muscular atrophy type 0 presenting with a clinicopathological picture of centronuclear myopathy. *Can J Neurol Sci* 2005;32(Suppl 1):S45.

Souchon F, Simard LR, Lebrun S, et al: Clinical and genetic study of chronic (types II and III) childhood onset spinal muscular atrophy. *Neuromuscul Disord* 1996;6:419–424.

Tachi N, Kikuchi S, Nozuka N, et al: A new mutation of *IGHMBP2* gene in spinal muscular atrophy with respiratory distress type 1. *Pediatr Neurol* 2005;32:288–290.

Chapter 612 ■ Hereditary Motor-Sensory Neuropathies

The hereditary motor-sensory neuropathies (HMSNs) are a group of progressive diseases of peripheral nerves. Motor components generally dominate the clinical picture, but sensory and autonomic involvement is expressed later.

612.1 • Peroneal Muscular Atrophy (Charcot-Marie-Tooth Disease; HMSN Type I)

This disease is the most common genetically determined neuropathy and has an overall prevalence of 3.8/100,000. It is transmitted as an autosomal dominant trait with 83% expressivity; the 17p11.2 locus is the site of the abnormal gene. Autosomal recessive transmission also is described, but is rarer. The gene product is peripheral myelin protein P22 (PMP22). A much rarer X-linked HMSN type I results from a defect at the Xq13.l locus, causing mutations in the gap junction protein connexin-32.

CLINICAL MANIFESTATIONS. Most patients are asymptomatic until late childhood or early adolescence, but young children sometimes manifest gait disturbance as early as the 2nd yr. The peroneal and tibial nerves are the earliest and most severely affected. Children with the disorder are often described as being clumsy, falling easily, or tripping over their own feet. The onset of symptoms may be delayed until after the 5th decade.

Muscles of the anterior compartment of the lower legs become wasted, and the legs have a characteristic stork-like contour. The muscular atrophy is accompanied by progressive weakness of dorsiflexion of the ankle and eventual footdrop. The process is bilateral but may be slightly asymmetric. Pes cavus deformities invariably develop due to denervation of intrinsic foot muscles, further destabilizing the gait. Atrophy of muscles of the forearms and hands is usually not as severe as that of the lower extremities, but in advanced cases contractures of the wrists and fingers produce a claw hand. Proximal muscle weakness is a late manifestation and is usually mild. Axial muscles are not involved.

The disease is slowly progressive throughout life, but patients occasionally show accelerated deterioration of function over a few years. Most patients remain ambulatory and have normal longevity, although orthotic appliances are required to stabilize the ankles.

Sensory involvement mainly affects large myelinated nerve fibers that convey proprioceptive information and vibratory sense, but the threshold for pain and temperature may also increase. Some children complain of tingling or burning sensations of the feet, but pain is rare. Because the muscle mass is reduced, the nerves are more vulnerable to trauma or compression. Autonomic manifestations may be expressed as poor vasomotor control with blotching or pallor of the skin of the feet and inappropriately cold feet.

Nerves often become palpably enlarged. Tendon stretch reflexes are lost distally. Cranial nerves are not affected. Sphincter control remains well preserved. Autonomic neuropathy does not affect the heart, gastrointestinal tract, or bladder. Intelligence is normal. A unique point mutation in *PMP22* causes progressive auditory nerve deafness in addition, but this is usually later in onset than the peripheral neuropathy.

Davidenkow syndrome is a variant of HMSN type I with a scapuloperoneal distribution.

LABORATORY FINDINGS AND DIAGNOSIS. Motor and sensory nerve conduction velocities are greatly reduced, sometimes as slow as 20% of normal conduction time. In new cases without a family history, both parents should be examined, and nerve conduction studies should be performed.

Electromyography (EMG) and muscle biopsy are not usually required for diagnosis, but they show evidence of many cycles of denervation and reinnervation. Serum creatine kinase level is normal. Cerebrospinal fluid (CSF) protein may be elevated, but no cells appear in the CSF.

Sural nerve biopsy is diagnostic. Large- and medium-sized myelinated fibers are reduced in number, collagen is increased, and characteristic **onion bulb formations** of proliferated Schwann cell cytoplasm surround axons. This pathologic finding is called **interstitial hypertrophic neuropathy.** Extensive segmental demyelination and remyelination also occur.

The definitive molecular genetic diagnosis may be made in blood.

TREATMENT. Stabilization of the ankles is a primary concern. In early stages, stiff boots that extend to the mid-calf often suffice, particularly when patients walk on uneven surfaces such as ice and snow or stones. As the dorsiflexors of the ankles weaken further, lightweight plastic splints may be custom made to extend beneath the foot and around the back of the ankle. They are worn inside the socks and are not visible, reducing self-consciousness. External short-leg braces may be required when footdrop becomes complete. Surgical fusion of the ankle may be considered in some cases.

The leg should be protected from traumatic injury. In advanced cases, compression neuropathy during sleep may be prevented by placing soft pillows beneath or between the lower legs. Burning paresthesias of the feet are not common but are often abolished by phenytoin or carbamazepine. No medical treatment is available to arrest or slow the progression.

612.2 • Peroneal Muscular Atrophy (Axonal Type)

This disease is clinically similar to HMSN type I, but the rate of progression is slower and the disability is less. EMG shows denervation of muscle. Sural nerve biopsy reveals axonal degeneration rather than the demyelination and whorls of Schwann cell processes typical in type I. The locus is on chromosome 1 at 1p35-p36; this is a different disease than HMSN type I, although both are transmitted as autosomal dominant traits.

612.3 • Dejerine-Sottas Disease (HMSN Type III)

This interstitial hypertrophic neuropathy of autosomal dominant transmission is similar to HMSN type I but is more severe. Symptoms develop in early infancy and are rapidly progressive. Pupillary abnormalities, such as lack of reaction to light and *Argyll Robertson pupil,* are common. Kyphoscoliosis and pes cavus deformities complicate about 35% of cases. Nerves become palpably enlarged at an early age.

The onion-bulb formations seen in the sural nerve biopsy specimen are more pronounced. Hypomyelination also occurs.

The genetic locus of 17p11.2 is identical to that of HMSN type I or Charcot-Marie-Tooth disease. The clinical and pathologic differences may be phenotypical variants of the same disease, analogous to the situation in Duchenne and Becker muscular dystrophies. An autosomal recessive form of Dejerine-Sottas disease is also described but is incompletely documented.

612.4 • Roussy-Lévy Syndrome

This syndrome is defined as a combination of HMSN type I and cerebellar deficit resembling Friedreich ataxia, but it does not have cardiomyopathy.

612.5 • Refsum Disease

(See Chapter 86.2.)

This rare disease is due to an enzymatic block in β-oxidation of phytanic acid to pristanic acid. Phytanic acid is a branched-chain fatty acid that is derived mainly from dietary sources: spinach, nuts, and coffee. Levels of phytanic acid are greatly elevated in plasma, CSF, and brain tissue. The CSF shows an albuminocytologic dissociation with a protein concentration of 100–600 mg/dL.

Clinical onset is usually between 4 and 7 yr of age, with intermittent motor and sensory neuropathy. Ataxia, progressive neurosensory hearing loss, retinitis pigmentosa and loss of night vision, ichthyosis, and liver dysfunction also develop in various degrees. Motor and sensory nerve conduction velocities are delayed. Treatment is by dietary management and periodic plasma exchange.

612.6 • Fabry Disease

(See Chapter 86.4.)

This rare X-linked recessive trait results in storage of ceramide trihexose because of deficiency of the enzyme ceramide trihexosidase, which cleaves the terminal galactose from ceramide trihexose (ceramide-glucose-galactose-galactose), resulting in tissue accumulation of this trihexose lipid in central nervous system (CNS) neurons, Schwann cells and perineurial cells, ganglion cells of the myenteric plexus, skin, kidneys, blood vessel endothelial and smooth muscle cells, heart, sweat glands, cornea, and bone marrow. It is due to a missense mutation disrupting the crystallographic structure of α-galactosidase A.

CLINICAL MANIFESTATIONS. The presentation is in late childhood or adolescence, with recurrent episodes of burning pain and paresthesias of the feet and lower legs so severe that patients are unable to walk. These episodes are often precipitated by fever or by physical activity. Objective sensory and motor deficits are not demonstrated on neurologic examination, and reflexes are preserved. Characteristic skin lesions are seen in the perineal region, scrotum, buttocks, and periumbilical zone as flat or raised red-black telangiectases known as **angiokeratoma corporis diffusum.** Hypohidrosis may be present. Corneal opacities, cataracts, and necrosis of the femoral heads are inconstant features. The disease is progressive. Hypertension and renal failure are usually delayed until early adult life. Recurrent strokes result from vascular wall involvement. Death often occurs in the 5th decade owing to cerebral infarction or renal insufficiency, but a significant morbidity already occurs in childhood despite the absence of major organ failure.

LABORATORY FINDINGS. Motor and sensory nerve conduction velocities are normal to only mildly slow, showing preservation of large myelinated nerve fibers. CSF protein is normal. Proteinuria is present early in the course.

Pathologic features are usually first detected in skin or sural nerve biopsy specimens. Crystalline glycosphingolipids appear as *zebra bodies* in lysosomes of endothelial cells, in smooth myocytes of arterioles, and in Schwann cells, best demonstrated by electron microscopy. Nerves show a selective loss of small myelinated fibers and relative preservation of large and medium-sized axons, contrasting to most axonal neuropathies in which large myelinated fibers are most involved.

Assay for the deficient enzyme may be performed from skin fibroblasts, leukocytes, and other tissues. This test permits detection of the asymptomatic female carrier state and provides a reliable means of prenatal diagnosis.

TREATMENT. See Chapter 86.4 for specific therapy of Fabry disease. Medical therapy of painful neuropathies includes management of the initiating disease and therapy directed to the neuropathic pain independent of etiology. Pain may be burning or associated with paresthesias, hyperalgesia (abnormal response to noxious stomach), or allodynia (induced by non-noxious stimuli) (see Chapter 77). Neuropathic pain is often successfully managed by tricyclic antidepressants; selective serotonin reuptake inhibitors are less effective. Anticonvulsants (carbamazepine, phenytoin, gabapentin, lamotrigine) are also effective as are narcotic and non-narcotic analgesic agents.

612.7 • Giant Axonal Neuropathy

This rare autosomal recessive disease with onset in early childhood is a progressive mixed peripheral neuropathy and degeneration of central white matter, similar to the leukodystrophies. Ataxia and nystagmus are accompanied by signs of progressive peripheral neuropathy. Many affected children have frizzy hair, which microscopically shows variation in diameter of the shaft and twisting, similar to Menkes disease, or may appear normal. Focal axonal enlargements are seen in both the peripheral nervous system and the CNS, but the myelin sheath is intact. The disease is a general proliferation of intermediate filaments, including neurofilaments in axons, glial filaments (i.e., Rosenthal fibers) in brain, cytokeratin in hair, and vimentin in Schwann cells and fibroblasts. Nonsense and missense mutations or deletions occur in the *GAN* gene, with allelic heterogeneity, at 16q24. These mutations are responsible for defective synthesis of the protein gygaxonin, a member of the cytoskeletal BTB/kelch superfamily, crucial to linkage between intermediate proteins and the cell membrane. MRI shows white matter lesions of the brain similar to leukodystrophies, and magnetic resonance spectroscopy (MRS) demonstrates increased ratios of choline/creatine and myoinositol/creatine, with a normally preserved ratio of *N*-acetyl aspartate/creatine, indicating demyelination and glial proliferation without axonal loss. Gygaxonin is expressed in a wide variety of neuronal cell types and is localized to the Golgi apparatus and endoplasmic reticulum.

The diagnosis is established by microscopic examination of scalp hair and by MRI and MRS of the brain; it is confirmed by sural nerve biopsy and/or by genetic studies, if available, of the *GAN* gene.

612.8 • Congenital Hypomyelinating Neuropathy

This disorder is a lack of normal myelination of motor and sensory peripheral nerves but not of CNS white matter. It is not a degeneration or loss of previously formed myelin, thus differentiating it from a leukodystrophy. Schwann cells are preserved, and axons are normal. Cases in siblings suggest autosomal recessive inheritance. Mutations in the *MTMR2, PMP22, EGR2,* and *MPZ* genes have been demonstrated in various children with this neuropathy; hence, it is a syndrome rather than a single disease.

The condition is present from birth; hypotonia and developmental delay are the hallmark clinical findings. Many patients present clinically as having congenital insensitivity to pain. Cranial nerves are inconsistently involved, and respiratory distress and dysphagia are rare complications. Tendon reflexes are absent. Arthrogryposis is present at birth in at least ½ of the cases. It is uncertain whether the condition is progressive; myelination of nerves proceeds at a slow rate and remains incomplete. Motor and sensory nerve conduction velocities are slow. The diagnosis is confirmed by sural nerve biopsy, which shows lack of myelination of large and small fibers and sometimes interstitial hypertrophic reactive changes. Muscle biopsy may show mild neurogenic atrophy but not the characteristic alterations of spinal muscular atrophy. No inflammation is demonstrated in muscle or nerve. Treatment is supportive.

612.9 • Tomaculous Neuropathy

This hereditary neuropathy is characterized by redundant overproduction of myelin around each axon in an irregular segmental fashion so that tomaculous (i.e., sausage-shaped) bulges occur in the individual myelinated nerve fibers. The nerves are particularly prone to pressure palsies, and patients present with recurrent mononeuropathies secondary to minor trauma. It is transmitted as an autosomal dominant trait, and the locus has been identified at 17p11.2. Sural nerve biopsy is diagnostic, but special "teased fiber" preparations should be made to demonstrate the myelin abnormalities most clearly. The genetic defect is a deletion of exons in the *PMP22* gene. Treatment is supportive.

612.10 • Leukodystrophies

Several hereditary degenerative diseases of white matter of the CNS also cause peripheral neuropathy. The most important are Krabbe disease (globoid cell leukodystrophy), metachromatic leukodystrophy, and adrenoleukodystrophy (see Chapter 86).

Bruno C, Bertini E, Federico A, et al: Clinical and molecular findings in patients with giant axonal neuropathy (GAN). *Neurology* 2004;62:13–16.

Chance PF, Alderson MK, Leppig KA, et al: DNA deletion associated with hereditary neuropathy with liability to pressure palsies. *Cell* 1993; 72:143–151.

Evgrafov OV, Mersiyanova I, Irobi J, et al: Mutant small heat-shock protein 27 causes axonal Charcot-Marie-Tooth disease and distal hereditary motor neuropathy. *Nat Genet* 2004;36:602–606.

Gordon N. Giant axonal neuropathy. *Dev Med Child Neurol* 2004; 46:717–719.

Houlden H, Blake J, Reilly MM: Hereditary sensory neuropathies. *Curr Opin Neurol* 2004;17:569–577.

Kochanski A, Drac H, Kabzinska D, et al: A novel *MPZ* gene mutation in congenital neuropathy with hypomyelination. *Neurology* 2004;62:2122–2123.

Kovach MJ, Lin JP, Boyadjiev S, et al: A unique point mutation in the PMP22 gene is associated with Charcot-Marie-Tooth disease and deafness. *Am J Hum Genet* 1999;64:1580–1593.

Mendell JR, Sahenk Z: Painful sensory neuropathy. *N Engl J Med* 2003;348:1243–1255.

Pleasure D: New treatments for denervating diseases. *J Child Neurol* 2005;20:258–262.

Ries M, Gupta S, Moore DF, et al: Pediatric Fabry disease. *Pediatrics* 2005;115:344–255.

Shy ME: Charcot-Marie-Tooth disease: An update. *Curr Opin Neurol* 2004;17:579–585.

Chapter 613 ■ Toxic Neuropathies

Many chemicals (organophosphates), toxins, and drugs are capable of causing peripheral neuropathy (Table 613-1). Heavy metals are well-known neurotoxins. Lead poisoning, especially if chronic, causes mainly a motor neuropathy selectively involving large nerves, such as the common peroneal, radial, and median nerves, a condition known as **mononeuritis multiplex** (see Chapter 709). Arsenic produces painful burning paresthesias and motor polyneuropathy. Exposure to industrial and agricultural chemicals is a less common cause of toxic neuropathy in children than in adults, but insecticides are neurotoxins for both insects and humans, and, if used as sprays in closed spaces, they may be inhaled and induce lethargy, vomiting, seizures, and neuropathy, particularly with recurrent or long-term exposure. Working adolescents and children in developing countries are also at risk. Puffer fish poisoning, usually by ingestion of even cooked fish meat contaminated with the venom, produces Guillain-Barré syndrome.

Antimetabolic and immunosuppressive drugs, such as vincristine, cisplatin, and paclitaxel, produce polyneuropathies as complications of chemotherapy for neoplasms. This "iatrogenic" cause is the most frequent etiology of toxic neuropathies in children. It is usually an axonal degeneration rather than primary demyelination, unlike autoimmune neuropathies.

Chronic uremia is associated with toxic neuropathy and myopathy. The neuropathy is caused by excessive levels of circulating parathyroid hormone. Reduction in serum parathyroid hormone levels is accompanied by clinical improvement and a return to normal of nerve conduction velocity.

Biologic neurotoxins are associated with tick paralysis, diphtheria, botulism, and the variants of paralytic shellfish poisoning. Lyme disease, West Nile virus, leprosy, herpes viruses (Bell palsy), and rabies also produce peripheral nerve– or anterior horn cell–induced weakness or paralysis. Various inborn errors of metabolism are also associated with peripheral neuropathy from metabolite toxicity or deficiencies (See Part X and Table 613-1).

TABLE 613-1. Toxic and Metabolic Neuropathies

METALS
Arsenic (insecticide, herbicide)
Lead (paint, batteries, pottery)
Mercury (metallic, vapor)
Thallium (rodenticides)
OCCUPATIONAL/INDUSTRY
Acrylamide (grouting, flocculation)
Carbon disulfide (solvent)
Cyanide
Dichlorophenoxyacetate
Dimethylaminopropionitrite
Ethylene oxide (gas sterilization)
Hexacarbons (glue, solvents)
Organophosphates (insecticides, petroleum additive)
Polychlorinated biphenyls
Tetrachlorbiphenyl
Trichloroethylene
DRUGS
Amiodarone
Chloramphenicol
Chloroquine
Cisplatin
Colchicine
Dapsone
Ethambutol
Ethanol
Gold
Hydralazine
Isoniazid
Metronidazole
Nitrofurantoin
Nucleosides (antiretroviral agents ddC, ddI, d4T)
Penicillamine
Pentamidine
Phenytoin
Pyridoxine (excessive)
Stilbamidine
Suramin
Thalidomide
Vincristine
METABOLIC DISORDERS
Fabry disease
Krabbe disease
Leukodystrophies
Porphyria
Tangier disease
Tyrosinemia
Uremia

Chapter 614 ■ Autonomic Neuropathies

Involvement of small, lightly or unmyelinated autonomic nerve fibers may be seen in many peripheral neuropathies; the autonomic manifestations are usually mild or subclinical. Certain autonomic neuropathies are more symptomatic and demonstrate varying degrees of involvement of the autonomic nervous system regulation of the cardiovascular, gastrointestinal, genitourinary, thermoregulatory, sudomotor, and pupillomotor systems.

The differential diagnosis is noted in Table 614-1. Autonomic nervous system functional tests are noted in Table 614-2. The general treatment of acquired autonomic dysfunction includes treating the primary disorder (systemic lupus erythematosus, diabetes) and long-term management of specific organ system manifestations (Table 614-3). Acute fluctuations of autonomic symptoms may be seen in Guillain-Barré syndrome. Rapid fluctuations of hypertension or tachycardia changing to hypotension or bradycardia should be managed carefully and with very short-acting medications.

TABLE 614-1. Autonomic Neuropathies

GUILLAIN-BARRÉ SYNDROME (GBS) (CHAPTER 615)
Non-GBS Autoimmunity
Paraneoplastic (type I antineuronal nuclear antibody)
Lambert-Eaton syndrome
Antibodies to neuronal nicotinc acetylcholine receptors
Antibodies to P/Q type calcium channels
Other autoantibodies
Systemic lupus erythematosus
Hereditary
Type I autosomal dominant
Type II autosomal recessive (Morvan disease)
Type III autosomal recessive (Riley-Day)
Type IV autosomal recessive (congenital insensitivity to pain with anhidrosis)
Type V absence of pain
Metabolic
Fabry disease
Diabetes mellitus
Tangier disease
Porphyria
Infectious
HIV
Chagas' disease
Botulism
Leprosy
Diphtheria
Other
Triple A (Allgrove) syndrome
Navajo Indian neuropathy
Multiple endocrine neoplasia type 2b
Toxins (see Table 613-1)

TABLE 614-2. Autonomic Function Testing

Both sympathetic and parasympathetic divisions of the autonomic nervous system are involved in all tests of autonomic function
CARDIAC PARASYMPATHETIC NERVOUS SYSTEM FUNCTION
Heart rate variability with deep respiration (respiratory sinus arrhythmia); time-domain and frequency-domain assessments
Heart rate response to Valsalva maneuver
Heart rate response to standing
SYMPATHETIC ADRENERGIC FUNCTION
Blood pressure response to upright posture (standing or tilt table)
Blood pressure response to Valsalva maneuver
Microneurography
SYMPATHETIC CHOLINERGIC FUNCTION
Thermoregulatory sweat testing
Quantitative sudomotor-axon reflex test
Sweat imprint methods
Sympathetic skin response

From Freeman R: Autonomic peripheral neuropathy. *Lancet* 2005;365:1259–1270.

TABLE 614-3. Management of Autonomic Neuropathies

PROBLEM	TREATMENT
Orthostatic hypotension	Volume and salt supplements
	Fluorohydrocortisone (mineralocorticoid)
	Midodrine (α-agonist)
Gastroparesis	Prokinetic agents (metaclopramide, domperidone, erythromycin)
Hypomotility	Fiber, laxatives
Urinary dysfunction	Timed voiding; bladder catheterization
Hyperhidrosis	Anticholinergic agents (glycopyrrolate, propanthdine)
	Intracutaneous botulism toxin

614.1 • Familial Dysautonomia

Familial dysautonomia (Riley-Day syndrome) is an autosomal recessive disorder that is common in Eastern European Jews, among whom the incidence is 1/10,000–20,000, and the carrier state is estimated to be 1%. It is rare in other ethnic groups. The defective gene is at the 9q31-q33 locus. The familial dysautonomia gene is identified as *IKBKAP,* with aberrant splicing and a truncated protein. This and other autonomic neuropathies are often regarded as **neurocristopathies** because the abnormal target tissues are largely derived from neural crest.

PATHOLOGY. This disease of the peripheral nervous system is characterized pathologically by a reduced number of small unmyelinated nerve fibers that carry pain, temperature, and taste sensations and that mediate autonomic functions. Large myelinated afferent nerve fibers that relay impulses from muscle spindles and Golgi tendon organs also are deficient. The degree of demonstrable anatomic change in peripheral and especially autonomic nerves is variable. Fungiform papillae of the tongue (taste buds) are absent or reduced in number. The number of parasympathetic ganglion cells in the myenteric plexuses is reduced. There is terminal vessel hyperperfusion in tissues, despite an overall hypoperfusion of organs and extremities.

CLINICAL MANIFESTATIONS. The disease is expressed in infancy by poor sucking and swallowing. Aspiration pneumonia may occur. Feeding difficulties remain a major symptom throughout childhood. Vomiting crises may occur. Episodic somnolence may occur in infants. Excessive sweating and blotchy erythema of the skin are common, especially at mealtime or when the child is excited. Infants are vulnerable to heatstroke. Episodic hyperhidrosis is due to chemical hypersensitivity of the remaining reduced number of sudomotor axons rather than of the sweat gland secretory cells. Breath-holding spells followed by syncope are common in the 1st 5 yr. As affected children become older, insensitivity to pain becomes evident and traumatic injuries are frequent. Corneal ulcerations are common. Newly erupting teeth cause tongue ulcerations. Walking is delayed or clumsy or appears ataxic because of poor sensory feedback from muscle spindles. The ataxia is probably related more to deficient muscle spindle feedback and to vestibular nerve dysfunction than to cerebellar involvement. Tendon stretch reflexes are absent. Scoliosis is a serious complication in the majority of patients and usually is progressive. Overflow tearing with crying does not normally develop until 2–3 mo of age but fails to develop after that time or is severely reduced in children with familial dysautonomia. There is an increased incidence of urinary incontinence. Bradycardia and other cardiac arrhythmias may occur, and some patients require a cardiac pacemaker.

About 40% of patients have generalized major motor seizures, some of which are associated with acute hypoxia during breath holding, some with extreme fevers, but most without an apparent precipitating event. Body temperature is poorly controlled; both hypothermia and extreme fevers occur. Intellectual function is usually impaired but is unrelated to epilepsy. Puberty is often delayed, especially in girls. Understature may occur, but growth velocity can be accelerated by treatment with growth hormone. Speech is often slurred or nasal.

After 3 yr of age, autonomic crises begin, usually with attacks of cyclic vomiting lasting 24–72 hr or even several days. Retching and vomiting occur every 15–20 min and are associated with hypertension, profuse sweating, blotching of the skin, apprehension, and irritability. Prominent gastric distention may occur, causing abdominal pain and even respiratory distress. Hematemesis may complicate pernicious vomiting.

Allgrove syndrome is a clinical variant, involving alacrima, achalasia, autonomic dysfunction with orthostatic hypotension and altered heart rate variability, and sensorimotor polyneuropathy, usually presenting in adolescence. Cholinergic dysfunction may be demonstrated.

LABORATORY FINDINGS. Electrocardiography discloses prolonged correcting QT intervals with lack of appropriate shortening with exercise, a reflection of the aberration in autonomic regulation of cardiac conduction. Chest radiographs show atelectasis and pulmonary changes resembling cystic fibrosis. Urinary vanillylmandelic acid level is decreased, and homovanillic acid level is increased. Plasma level of dopamine β-hydroxylase (the enzyme that converts dopamine to epinephrine) is diminished. Sural nerve biopsy shows a decreased number of unmyelinated fibers. Electroencephalography is useful for evaluating seizures.

DIAGNOSIS. Slow IV infusion of norepinephrine produces an exaggerated pressor response. The hypotensive response to infusion of methacholine is increased. Intradermal injection of 1 : 1,000 histamine phosphate fails to produce a normal axon flare, and local pain is absent or diminished. Because the skin of a normal infant reacts more intensely to histamine, a 1 : 10,000 dilution should be used. Instillation of 2.5% methacholine into the conjunctival sac produces miosis in patients with familial dysautonomia and no detectable effect on a normal pupil; this is a nonspecific sign of parasympathetic denervation due to any cause. Methacholine is applied to only 1 eye in this test, with the other eye serving as a control; the pupils are compared at 5-min intervals for 20 min. The genetic marker in blood will be available for definitive diagnostic testing.

TREATMENT. Symptomatic treatment includes special attention to the respiratory and gastrointestinal systems, methylcellulose eyedrops or topical ocular lubricants to replace tears and prevent corneal ulceration, orthopedic management of scoliosis and joint problems, and appropriate anticonvulsants for epilepsy. Chlorpromazine is an effective antiemetic and may be given as rectal suppositories during autonomic crises. It also reduces apprehension and lowers the blood pressure. Dehydration and electrolyte disturbances should be anticipated. Bethanechol may be an alternative drug for cyclic vomiting. It is also useful for enuresis, another common complication, and augments tear production. Protection from injuries is important because of the lack of pain as a protective mechanism. Scoliosis often requires surgical treatment. Antiepileptic drugs may be required. A cardiac pacemaker may be required by some children. Blood pressure monitoring may be important in some cases. A promising genetic approach to treatment, although not standard therapy at this time, is the use of a polyphenol to regulate the expression of *IKBKAP* transcripts.

PROGNOSIS. Most patients die in childhood, usually of chronic pulmonary failure or aspiration.

614.2 • Other Autonomic Neuropathies

MYENTERIC PLEXUS NEUROPATHIES. *Aganglionic megacolon (Hirschsprung disease)* is a failure of embryonic development of parasympathetic neurons in the submucosal and myenteric plexuses of segments of the colon and rectum. Nerves between the longitudinal and circular layers of smooth muscle of the gut wall are hypertrophic; ganglion cells are absent (see Chapter 329).

CONGENITAL INSENSITIVITY TO PAIN AND ANHIDROSIS. This hereditary disorder of uncertain genetic transmission affects boys much more frequently than girls and presents in early infancy. Patients have episodes of high fever related to warm environmental temperatures because they do not perspire. Frequent burns and traumatic injuries result from apparent lack of pain perception. Intelligence is normal. Nerve biopsy reveals an almost total absence of unmyelinated nerve fibers that convey impulses of pain, temperature, and autonomic functions. Some cases of hypomyelinating neuropathy present clinically as congenital insensitivity to pain (see Chapter 612.8). The sympathetic skin response as an electrophysiologic study is a reliable diagnostic test in cases associated with a mutation at the TrKA receptor for nerve growth factor.

REFLEX SYMPATHETIC DYSTROPHY. This disorder is a form of local causalgia, usually involving a hand or foot but not corresponding to the anatomic distribution of a peripheral nerve (see Chapter 167.2). A continuous burning pain and hyperesthesia are associated with vasomotor instability in the affected zone, resulting in increased skin temperature, erythema, and edema due to vasodilatation and hyperhidrosis. In the chronic state, atrophy of skin appendages, cool and clammy skin, and disuse atrophy of underlying muscle and bone occur. More than 1 extremity is occasionally involved. The pain is disabling and is exacerbated by the movement of an associated joint, although no objective signs of arthritis are seen; immobilization provides some relief. The most common preceding event is local trauma in the form of a contusion, laceration, sprain, or fracture that occurred days or weeks earlier.

Several theories of pathogenesis have been proposed to explain this phenomenon. The most widely accepted is reflexive overactivity of autonomic nerves in response to injury, and regional sympathetic blockade often affords temporary relief. Physiotherapy also is helpful. Some cases resolve spontaneously after weeks or months, but others continue to be symptomatic and require sympathectomy. A psychogenic component is suspected in some cases but is difficult to prove.

Anderson SL, Qiu J, Rubin BY: EGCG corrects aberrant splicing of IKAP mRNA in cells from patients with familial dysautonomia. *Biochem Biophy Res Commun* 2003;310:627–633.

Axelrod FB: Familial dysautonomia. *Muscle Nerve* 2004;29:352–363.

Freeman R: Autonomic peripheral neuropathy. *Lancet* 2005;365:1259–1270.

Gold-von Simson G, Rutkowski M, Berlin D, et al: Pacemakers in patients with familial dysautonomia—a review of experience with 20 patients. *Clin Autonom Res* 2005;15:15–20.

Hilz MJ, Axelrod FB, Bickel A, et al: Assessing function and pathology in familial dysautonomia: Assessment of temperature perception, sweating and cutaneous innervation. *Brain* 2004;127:2090–2098.
Kamboj MK, Axelrod FG, David R, et al: Growth hormone treatment in children with familial dysautonomia. *J Pediatr* 2004;144:63–67.

Chapter 615 ■ Guillain-Barré Syndrome

Guillain-Barré syndrome is a postinfectious polyneuropathy involving mainly motor but sometimes also sensory and autonomic nerves. This syndrome affects people of all ages and is not hereditary. The disorder closely resembles experimental allergic polyneuritis in animals. Most patients have a demyelinating neuropathy, but primarily axonal degeneration is documented in some cases.

CLINICAL MANIFESTATIONS. The paralysis usually follows a nonspecific viral infection by about 10 days. The original infection may have caused only gastrointestinal (especially *Campylobacter jejuni*, but also *Helicobacter pylori*) or respiratory tract (especially *Mycoplasma pneumoniae*) symptoms. West Nile virus also may cause Guillain-Barré–like syndrome, but more frequently causes motor neuron disease similar to poliomyelitis. Guillain-Barré syndrome is reported following administration of vaccines against rabies, influenza poliomyelitis (oral), and possibly the conjugated meningococcal vaccine.

Weakness begins usually in the lower extremities and progressively involves the trunk, the upper limbs, and finally the bulbar muscles, a pattern known as **Landry ascending paralysis.** Proximal and distal muscles are involved relatively symmetrically, but asymmetry is found in 9% of patients. The onset is gradual and progresses over days or weeks. Particularly in cases with an abrupt onset, tenderness on palpation and pain in muscles is common in the initial stages. Affected children are irritable. Weakness may progress to inability or refusal to walk and later to flaccid tetraplegia. Paresthesias occur in some cases. The differential diagnosis of acute weakness is noted in Table 606-3.

Bulbar involvement occurs in about half of cases. Respiratory insufficiency may result. Dysphagia and facial weakness are often impending signs of respiratory failure. They interfere with eating and increase the risk of aspiration. The facial nerves may be involved. Some young patients may exhibit symptoms of viral meningitis or meningoencephalitis. Extraocular muscle involvement is rare, but in an uncommon variant, oculomotor and other cranial neuropathies are severe early in the course. **Miller-Fisher syndrome** consists of acute external ophthalmoplegia, ataxia, and areflexia. Papilledema is found in some cases, although visual impairment is not clinically evident. Urinary incontinence or retention of urine is a complication in about 20% of cases but is usually transient. Miller-Fisher syndrome overlaps with Bickerstaff brainstem encephalitis, which also shares many features with Guillain-Barré syndrome with lower motor neuron involvement and may indeed be the same basic disease.

Tendon reflexes are lost, usually early in the course, but are sometimes preserved until later. This variability may cause confusion when attempting early diagnosis. The autonomic nervous system may also be involved in some cases. Lability of blood pressure and cardiac rate, postural hypotension, episodes of profound bradycardia, and occasional asystole occur. Cardiovascular monitoring is important. A few patients require insertion of a temporary venous cardiac pacemaker.

Chronic relapsing polyradiculoneuropathy (sometimes called chronic inflammatory demyelinating polyradiculoneuropathy) or ***chronic unremitting polyradiculoneuropathy*** are chronic varieties of Guillain-Barré syndrome that recur intermittently or do not improve for a period of months or years. About 7% of children with Guillain-Barré syndrome suffer an acute relapse. Patients are usually severely weak and may have a flaccid tetraplegia with or without bulbar and respiratory muscle involvement.

Congenital Guillain-Barré syndrome is described rarely, presenting as generalized hypotonia, weakness, and areflexia in an affected neonate, fulfilling all electrophysiologic and cerebrospinal fluid (CSF) criteria, and in the absence of maternal neuromuscular disease. Treatment may not be required, and there is gradual improvement over the first few months and no evidence of residual disease by 1 yr of age. In one case, the mother had ulcerative colitis treated with prednisone and mesalamine from the 7th mo until delivery at term.

LABORATORY FINDINGS AND DIAGNOSIS. CSF studies are essential for diagnosis. The CSF protein is elevated to more than twice the upper limit of normal, glucose level is normal, and there is no pleocytosis. Fewer than 10 white blood cells/mm^3 are found. The results of bacterial cultures are negative, and viral cultures rarely isolate specific viruses. The dissociation between high CSF protein and a lack of cellular response in a patient with an acute or subacute polyneuropathy is diagnostic of Guillain-Barré syndrome.

Motor nerve conduction velocities are greatly reduced, and sensory nerve conduction time is often slow. Electromyography shows evidence of acute denervation of muscle. Serum creatine kinase (CK) level may be mildly elevated or normal. Antiganglioside antibodies, mainly against GM1 and GD1, are sometimes elevated in the serum in Guillain-Barré syndrome, particularly in cases with primarily axonal rather than demyelinating neuropathy, and suggest that they may play a role in disease propagation and/or recovery in some cases (Table 615-1). Muscle biopsy is not usually required for diagnosis; specimens appear normal in early stages and show evidence of denervation atrophy in chronic stages. Sural nerve biopsy tissue shows segmental demyelination, focal inflammation, and wallerian degeneration but also is usually not required for diagnosis.

Serologic testing for *Campylobacter* and *Helicobacter* infections helps establish the cause if results are positive but does not alter the course of treatment. Results of stool cultures are rarely positive because the infection is self-limited and only occurs for about 3 days, and the neuropathy follows the acute gastroenteritis.

TREATMENT. Patients in early stages of this acute disease should be admitted to the hospital for observation because the ascending paralysis may rapidly involve respiratory muscles during the next 24 hr. Patients with slow progression may simply be observed for stabilization and spontaneous remission without

TABLE 615-1. Classification of Guillain-Barré Syndrome and Related Disorders and Typical Antiganglioside Antibodies by Pathology

	ANTIBODIES
Acute inflammatory demyelinating polyradiculoneuropathy	Unknown
Acute motor and sensory axonal neuropathy	GM1, GM1b, GD1a
Acute motor axonal neuropathy	GM1, GM1b, GD1a, GalNac-GD1a
Acute sensory neuronopathy	GD1b
Acute pandysautonomia	
Regional variants	
Fisher syndrome	GQ1b, GT1a
Oropharyngeal	GT1a
Overlap	
Fisher/Guillain-Barré overlap syndrome	GQ1b, GM1, GM1b, GD1a, GalNac-GD1a

From Hughes RAC: Treatment of Guillain-Barré syndrome with corticosteroids: Lack of benefit? *Lancet* 2004;363:181–182.

treatment. Rapidly progressive ascending paralysis is treated with intravenous immunoglobulin (IVIG), administered for 2, 3, or 5 days. A commonly recommended protocol is IVIG 0.4 gm/kg/day for 5 consecutive days. Plasmapheresis, and/or immunosuppressive drugs are alternatives, if IVIG is ineffective. Steroids are not effective. Combined administration of immunoglobulin and interferon is effective in some patients. Supportive care, such as respiratory support, prevention of decubiti in children with flaccid tetraplegia, and treatment of secondary bacterial infections, is important.

Chronic relapsing polyradiculoneuropathy or unremitting chronic neuropathy is also treated with IVIG. Plasma exchange, sometimes requiring as many as 10 exchanges daily, is an alternative. Remission in these cases may be sustained, but relapses may occur within days, weeks, or even after many months; relapses usually respond to another course of plasmapheresis. Steroid and immunosuppressive drugs are another alternative, but their effectiveness is less predictable. High-dose pulsed methylprednisolone given intravenously is successful in some cases. The prognosis in chronic forms of the Guillain-Barré syndrome is more guarded than in the acute form, and many patients are left with major residual handicaps.

Even if *Campylobacter jejuni* infection is documented by stool culture or serologic tests, treatment of the infection is not necessary because it is self-limited, and the use of antibiotics does not alter the course of the polyneuropathy.

For the treatment of chronic neuropathic pain following Guillain-Barré syndrome, gabapentin is more effective than carbamazepine, and the requirement for fentanyl is reduced.

PROGNOSIS. The clinical course is usually benign, and spontaneous recovery begins within 2–3 wk. Most patients regain full muscular strength, although some are left with residual weakness. The tendon reflexes are usually the last function to recover. Improvement usually follows a gradient inverse to the direction of involvement, with recovery of bulbar function first and lower extremity weakness resolving last. Bulbar and respiratory muscle involvement may lead to death if the syndrome is not recognized and treated. Although prognosis is generally good with the majority of children recovering completely, three clinical features are predictive of poor outcome with sequelae: cranial nerve involvement, intubation, and maximum disability at the time of presentation. An electrophysiologic feature of conduction block is predictive of good outcome. Long-term follow-up studies of patients who recover from an attack of Guillain-Barré syndrome reveal that many do have some permanent axonal loss, with or without residual clinical signs of chronic neuropathy. Easy fatigue is one of the most common chronic symptoms, but it is not the rapid fatigability of muscles in myasthenia gravis. Among patients with the axonal form of Guillain-Barré syndrome, most who had slow recovery over the first 6 mo could eventually walk, although some required years to recover. EMG and NCV electrophysiologic studies do not necessarily predict the long-term outcome.

Ammache Z, Afini AK, Brown CK, et al: Childhood Guillain-Barré syndrome: Clinical and electrophysiologic features predictive of outcome. *J Child Neurol* 2001;16:477–483.

Bradshaw DY, Jones HR: Pseudomeningoencephalitic presentation of pediatric Guillain-Barré syndrome. *J Child Neurol* 2001;16:505–508.

Centers for Disease Control and Prevention: Cluster of tick paralysis cases—Colorado, 2006. *MMWR* 2006;55:933–936.

Dornonville de la Coeur C, Jakobsen J: Residual neuropathy in long-term population-based follow-up of Guillain-Barré syndrome. *Neurology* 2005;64:246–253.

England JD, Asbury AK: Peripheral neuropathy. *Lancet* 2004;363:2151–2161.

Hiraga A, Mori M, Ogawara K, et al: Recovery patterns and long-term prognosis for axonal Guillain-Barré syndrome. *J Neurol Neurosurg Psychiatry* 2005;76:719–722; comment 622.

Hughes RAC: Treatment of Guillain-Barré syndrome with corticosteroids: Lack of benefit? *Lancet* 2004;363:181–182.

Jackson AH, Barquis GD, Shah BL: Congenital Guillain-Barré syndrome. *J Child Neurol* 1996;11:407–410.

Koller H, Kieseier BC, Jander S, Hartung HP: Chronic inflammatory demyelinating polyneuropathy. *N Engl J Med* 2005;352:1343–1356.

Korinthenberg R, Schessl J, Kirschner J, et al: Intravenously administered immunoglobulin in the treatment of childhood Guillain-Barré syndrome: A randomized trial. *Pediatrics* 2005;116:8–14.

Kountouras J, Deretzi G, Zavos C, et al: Association between *Helicobacter pylori* infection and acute inflammatory demyelinating polyradiculoneuropathy. *Eur J Neurol* 2005;12:139–143.

Pandey CK, Raza M, Tripathhi M, et al: The comparative evaluation of gabapentin and carbamazepine for pain management in Guillain-Barré syndrome patients in the intensive care unit. *Anesth Analg* 2005;101:220–225.

Press R, Mata S, Lolli F, et al: Temporal profile of anti-ganglioside antibodies and their relation to clinical parameters and treatment in Guillain-Barré syndrome. *J Neurol Sci* 2001;190:41–47.

Ramachandran R, Kuruvilla A: Guillain-Barré syndrome in children and adolescents: A retrospective analysis. *J Indian Med Assoc* 2004;102:480–482.

Schessl J, Koga M, Funakoshi K, et al: Prospective study on anti-ganglioside antibodies in childhood Guillain-Barré syndrome. *Arch Dis Child* 2007; 92:48–52.

Van Koningsveld R, Schmitz PIM, van der Meche, et al: Effect of methylprednisone when added to standard treatment with intravenous immunoglobulin for Guillain-Barré syndrome: Randomized trial. *Lancet* 2004;363:192.

Winer JB: Bickerstaff's encephalitis and the Miller-Fisher syndrome. *J Neurol Neurosurg Psychiatry* 2001;71:433–435.

Chapter 616 ■ Bell Palsy

Bell palsy is an acute unilateral facial nerve palsy that is not associated with other cranial neuropathies or brainstem dysfunction. It is a common disorder at all ages from infancy through adolescence and usually develops abruptly about 2 wk after a systemic viral infection. The preceding infection is due to the herpes simplex virus, varicella-zoster virus, Epstein-Barr virus, Lyme disease, mumps virus, *Mycoplasma* (Table 616-1). Active or reac-

TABLE 616-1. Etiologies of Acute Peripheral Facial Palsy

COMMON
Herpes simplex virus type 1*
Varicella-zoster virus*
LESS COMMON INFECTIONS
Otitis media ± cholesteatoma
Lyme disease
Epstein-Barr virus
Cytomegalovirus
Mumps
Human herpesvirus 6
Intranasal influenza vaccine
Mycoplasma
OTHER LESS COMMON CONDITIONS
Trauma
Tumor
Hypertension
Guillain-Barré syndrome
Sarcoidosis
Melkersson-Rosenthal syndrome†
Ribavirin
Interferon

*Implicated in idiopathic Bell palsy.

†Noncaseating granulomas with facial (lips, eyelids) edema, recurrent alternating facial paralysis, family history, migraines, or headaches.

tivation of herpes simplex or varicella-zoster virus may be the most common cause of Bell palsy. The disease may occasionally be a postinfectious allergic or immune demyelinating facial neuritis. It also may be a focal toxic or inflammatory neuropathy and has been associated with ribavirin and interferon-α therapy for hepatitis C.

CLINICAL MANIFESTATIONS. The upper and lower portions of the face are paretic, and the corner of the mouth droops. Patients are unable to close the eye on the involved side and may develop an exposure keratitis at night. Taste on the anterior ⅔ of the tongue is lost on the involved side in about ½ of cases; this finding helps to establish the anatomic limits of the lesion as being proximal or distal to the chorda tympani branch of the facial nerve. Numbness and paresthesias do not usually occur, but ipsilateral numbness of the face is reported in a few cases and probably is due to viral (especially herpes) or postviral immunologic impairment of the trigeminal and the facial nerved. Several grading systems have been devised for Bell palsy: the Sunnybrook, House-Brackmann, and Yanagihara systems.

TREATMENT. Oral prednisone (1 mg/kg/day for 1 wk, then a 1-wk taper) started within the first 3–5 days results in improved outcome. Because of the recovery of herpes simplex virus in the neural fluid of the 7th nerve, some also recommend adding oral acyclovir or valacyclovir to the prednisone therapy. Surgical decompression of the facial canal, theoretically to provide more space for the swollen facial nerve, is not of value. Physiotherapy to the facial muscles is recommended in some chronic cases with poor recovery, but the efficacy of this treatment is uncertain. Protection of the cornea with methylcellulose eyedrops or an ocular lubricant is especially important at night. Some plastic surgeons use botulinum toxin to treat chronic unilateral ptosis, but this has little application in pediatric patients.

PROGNOSIS. The prognosis is excellent. More than 85% of cases recover spontaneously with no residual facial weakness; another 10% have mild facial weakness as a sequela; only 5% are left with permanent severe facial weakness. In patients who do not recover within a few weeks (chronic), electrophysiologic examination of the facial nerve helps to determine the degree of neuropathy and regeneration. In chronic cases, other causes of facial neuropathy should be considered, including facial nerve tumors such as schwannomas and neurofibromas, infiltration of the facial nerve by leukemic cells or by a rhabdomyosarcoma of the middle ear, brainstem infarcts or tumors, and traumatic injury of the facial nerve.

FACIAL PALSY AT BIRTH. This is usually a compression neuropathy from forceps application during delivery and recovers spontaneously in a few days or weeks in most cases. ***Congenital absence of the depressor angularis oris muscle*** causes facial asymmetry, especially when an affected infant cries. It is not a facial nerve lesion but is a cosmetic defect that does not interfere with feeding. Infants with ***Möbius syndrome*** may have bilateral or, less commonly, unilateral facial palsy; this syndrome is usually caused by symmetric calcified infarcts in the tegmentum of the pons and medulla oblongata during mid-gestation or late fetal life, although it rarely may be a developmental anomaly of the brainstem.

Berg T, Jonsson L, Engstrom M: Agreement between the Sunnybrook, House-Brackmann and Yanagihara facial nerve grading systems in Bell's palsy. *Otol Neurotol* 2004;25:1020–1026.

Eidlitz-Markus T, Gilai A, Mimouri M, et al: Recurrent facial nerve palsy in pediatric patients. *Eur J Pediatr* 2001;160:659–663.

Furuta Y, Ohtani F, Aizawa, et al: Varicella-zoster virus reactivation is an important cause of acute peripheral facial paralysis in children. *Pediatr Infect Dis J* 2005;24:97–101.

Gilden DH: Bell's palsy. *N Engl J Med* 2004;351:1323–1331.

Holland NJ, Weiner GM: Recent developments in Bell's palsy. *BMJ* 2004;329:553–557.

Kisaki H, Hato N, Mizobuchi M, et al: Role of T-lymphocyte subsets in facial nerve paralysis owing to the reactivation of herpes simplex virus type 1. *Acta Laryngol* 2005;125:316–321.

Salinas RA, Alvarez G, Ferreira J: Corticosteroids for Bell's palsy (idiopathic facial paralysis). *Cochrane Database Syst Rev* 2004;4:CD001942.

Part XXVIII ▪ Disorders of the Eye

Chapter 617 ▪ Growth and Development

Scott E. Olitsky, Denise Hug, and Laura P. Smith

The eye of a normal full-term infant at birth is approximately 65% of adult size. Postnatal growth is maximal during the 1st yr, proceeds at a rapid but decelerating rate until the 3rd yr, and continues at a slower rate thereafter until puberty, after which little change occurs. The anterior structures of the eye are relatively large at birth but thereafter grow proportionately less than the posterior structures. This results in a progressive change in the shape of the globe; it becomes more spherical.

In an infant, the sclera is thin and translucent, with a bluish tinge. The cornea is relatively large in newborns (averaging 10 mm) and attains adult size (nearly 12 mm) by the age of 2 yr or earlier. Its curvature tends to flatten with age, with progressive change in the refractive properties of the eye. A normal cornea is perfectly clear. In infants born prematurely, the cornea may have a transient opalescent haze. The anterior chamber in a newborn appears shallow, and the angle structures, important in the maintenance of normal intraocular pressure, must undergo further differentiation after birth. The iris, typically light blue or gray at birth in white individuals, undergoes progressive change of color as the pigmentation of the stroma increases in the first 6 mo of life. The pupils of a newborn infant tend to be small and are often difficult to dilate. Remnants of the **pupillary membrane** (anterior vascular capsule) are often evident on ophthalmoscopic examination, appearing as cobweb-like lines crossing the pupillary aperture, especially in preterm infants.

The lens of a newborn infant is more spherical than that of an adult; its greater refractive power helps to compensate for the relative shortness of the young eye. The lens continues to grow throughout life; new fibers added to the periphery continually push older fibers toward the center of the lens. With age, the lens becomes progressively denser and more resistant to change of shape during accommodation.

The fundus of a newborn's eye is less pigmented than that of an adult; the choroidal vascular pattern is highly visible, and the retinal pigmentary pattern often has a fine peppery or mottled appearance. In some darkly pigmented infants, the fundus has a gray or opalescent sheen. In a newborn, the macular landmarks, particularly the foveal light reflex, are less well defined and may not be readily apparent. The peripheral retina appears pale or grayish, and the peripheral retinal vasculature is immature, especially in premature infants. The optic nerve head color varies from pink to slightly pale, sometimes grayish. Within 4–6 mo, the appearance of the fundus approximates that of the mature eye.

Superficial retinal hemorrhages may be observed in many newborn infants. These are usually absorbed promptly and rarely leave any permanent effect. The majority of birth-related **retinal hemorrhages** resolve within 2 wk, with complete resolution of all such hemorrhages within 4–6 wk of birth. Conjunctival hemorrhages also may occur at birth and are resorbed spontaneously without consequence.

Remnants of the **primitive hyaloid vascular** system may also be seen as small tufts or wormlike structures projecting from the disc (Bergmeister papilla) or as a fine strand traversing the vitreous; in some cases, only a small dot (Mittendorf dot) remains on the posterior aspect of the lens capsule.

An infant's eye is somewhat hyperopic (**farsighted**). The general trend is for hyperopia to increase from birth until 7 yr. Thereafter, the level of hyperopia tends to decrease rapidly until age 14. Elimination of the hyperopic state may occur during this time. If the process continues, myopia (nearsightedness) develops. A slower continuation of the decrease in hyperopia, or increase in myopia, continues into the 3rd decade of life. The refractive state at any time in life depends on the net effect of many factors: the size of the eye, the state of the lens, and the curvature of the cornea.

Newborn infants tend to keep their eyes closed much of the time, but normal newborns can see, respond to changes in illumination, and fixate points of contrast. The visual acuity in newborns is estimated to be approximately 20/400. One of the earliest responses to a formed visual stimulus is an infant's regard for the mother's face, evident especially during feeding. By 2 wk of age, an infant shows more sustained interest in large objects, and by 8–10 wk of age, a normal infant can follow an object through an arc of 180 degrees. The acuity improves rapidly and may reach 20/30–20/20 by the age of 2–3 yr.

Many normal infants may have imperfect coordination of the eye movements and alignment during the early days and weeks, but proper coordination should be achieved by 3–6 mo, usually sooner. Persistent deviation of an eye in an infant requires evaluation.

Tears often are not present with crying until after 1–3 mo. Preterm infants have reduced reflex and basal tear secretion, which may allow topically applied medications to become concentrated and lead to rapid drying of their corneas.

Archer SM, Sondhi N, Helveston EM: Strabismus in infancy. *Ophthalmology* 1989;96:133–137.

Emerson MV, Pieramici DJ, Stoessel KM, et al: Incidence and rate of disappearance of retinal hemorrhage in newborns. *Ophthalmology* 2001;108:33–39.

Isenberg SJ, Apt L, McCarty J: Development of tearing in preterm and term infants. *Arch Ophthalmol* 1998;116:773–776.

Khodadoust AA, Ziai M, Biggs SL: Optic disc in normal newborns. *Am J Ophthalmol* 1968;66:502–504.

Krishnamohan VK, Wheeler MB, Testa MA, et al: Correlation of postnatal regression of the anterior vascular capsule of the lens to gestational age. *J Pediatr Ophthalmol Strabismus* 1982;19:28–32.

Roarty JD, Keltner JL: Normal pupil size and anisocoria in newborn infants. *Arch Ophthalmol* 1990;108:94–95.

Spieres A, Isenberg SJ, Inkelis SH: Characteristics of the iris in 100 neonates. *J Pediatr Ophthalmol Strabismus* 1989;26:28–30.

Chapter 618 ▪ Examination of the Eye

Scott E. Olitsky, Denise Hug, and Laura P. Smith

Examination of the eyes is a routine part of the periodic pediatric assessment beginning in the newborn period. The primary care physician is very important in detecting both obvious and insid-

TABLE 618-1. Vision Screening Guidelines*

FUNCTION	RECOMMENDED TESTS	REFERRAL CRITERIA	COMMENTS
AGES 3–5 YR			
Distance visual acuity	Snellen letters Snellen numbers Tumbling E test HOTV test Picture tests Allen figures LH test	1. <4 of 6 correct on 20-ft line with either eye tested at 10 ft monocularly (i.e., <10/20 or 20/40), or 2. Two-line difference between eyes, even within the passing range (i.e., 10/12.5 and 10/20 or 20/25 and 20/40)	1. Tests are listed in decreasing order of cognitive difficulty; the highest test that the child is capable of performing should be used; in general, the tumbling E or the HOTV test should be used for ages 3–5 yr and Snellen letters or numbers for ages 6 yr and older. 2. Testing distance of 3 m (10 ft) is recommended for all visual acuity tests. 3. A line of figures is preferred over single figures. 4. The nontested eye should be covered by an occluder held by the examiner or by an adhesive occluder patch applied to eye; the examiner must ensure that it is not possible to peek with the nontested eye.
Ocular alignment	Unilateral cover test at 3 m (10 ft) or Random dot E stereo test at 40 cm (630 sec of arc)	Any eye movement <4 of 6 correct	
AGES 6 YR AND OLDER			
Distance visual acuity	Snellen letters Snellen numbers Tumbling E test HOTV test Picture tests Allen figures LH test	1. <4 of 6 correct on 4.5 m (15 ft) line with either eye tested at 3 m (10 ft) monocularly (i.e., <10/15 or 20/30) or 2. Two-line difference between eyes, even within the passing range (i.e., 10/10 and 10/15 or 20/20 and 20/30)	1. Tests are listed in decreasing order of cognitive difficulty; the highest test that the child is capable of performing should be used; in general, the tumbling E or the HOTV test should be used for ages 3–5 yr and Snellen letters or numbers for ages 6 yr and older. 2. Testing distance of 3 m (10 ft) is recommended for all visual acuity tests. 3. A line of figures is preferred over single figures. 4. The nontested eye should be covered by an occluder held by the examiner or by an adhesive occluder patch applied to the eye; the examiner must ensure that it is not possible to peek with the nontested eye.
Ocular alignment	Unilateral cover test at 3 m (10 ft) or Random dot E stereo test at 40 cm (630 sec of arc)	Any eye movement <4 of 6 correct	

* Vision screening guidelines were developed by the AAP Section on Ophthalmology Executive Committee, 1991–1992; Robert D. Gross, MBA, MD, Chairman; Walter M. Fierson, MD, Jane D. Kivlin, MD, I. Matthew Rabinowicz, MD, David R. Stager, MD, Mark S. Ruttum, MD, AAPOS; and Earl R. Crouch, Jr., MD, American Academy of Ophthalmology.
From Nelson LB: *Harley's Pediatric Ophthalmology*, 4th ed. Philadelphia, WB Saunders, 1998, p 84.

ious asymptomatic eye diseases. Screening in schools and community programs can also be effective in detecting problems early. The American Academy of Ophthalmology recommends preschool vision screening as a means of reducing preventable visual loss (Table 618-1). This testing should be done by pediatricians during well child visits. Children should be examined by an ophthalmologist whenever a significant ocular abnormality or vision defect is noted or suspected. Children who are at high risk of ophthalmologic problems, such as genetically inherited ocular conditions and various systemic disorders, should also be examined by an ophthalmologist.

Basic examination, whether done by a pediatrician or an ophthalmologist, must include evaluation of visual acuity and the visual fields, assessment of the pupils, ocular motility and alignment, a general external examination, and an ophthalmoscopic examination of the media and fundi. When indicated, biomicroscopy (slit-lamp examination), cycloplegic refraction, and tonometry are performed by an ophthalmologist. Special diagnostic procedures, such as ultrasonic examination, fluorescein angiography, electroretinography, or visual evoked response (VER) testing, are also indicated for specific conditions.

VISUAL ACUITY. There are many tests of visual acuity. Which test is used depends on a child's age and ability to cooperate, as well as a clinician's preference and experience with each test. The most common visual acuity test in infants is an assessment of their ability to fixate and follow a target. If appropriate targets are used, this reflex can be demonstrated by about 6 wk of age. The test is performed by seating the child comfortably in the caretaker's lap. The object of visual interest, usually a bright-colored toy, is slowly moved to the right and to the left. The examiner observes whether the infant's eyes turn toward the object and follow its movements. The examiner can use a thumb to occlude one of the infant's eyes in order to test each eye separately. Although a sound-producing object might compromise the purity of the visual stimulus, in practice, toys that squeak or rattle heighten an infant's awareness and interest in the test.

The human face is a better target than test objects. The examiner can exploit this by moving his or her face slowly in front of the infant's face. If the appropriate following movements are not elicited, the test should be repeated with the caretaker's face as the test stimulus. It should be remembered that even children with poor vision may follow a large object without apparent difficulty, especially if only one eye is affected.

An objective measurement of visual acuity is usually possible when children reach 2{1/2}–3 yr of age. Children this age are tested using a schematic picture or other illiterate eye chart. Each eye should be tested separately. It is essential to prevent peeking. The examiner should hold the occluder in place and observe the child throughout the test. The child should be reassured and encouraged throughout the test because many children are intimidated by the procedure and fear a "bad grade" or punishment for errors.

The **E test**, in which a child points in the direction of the letter, is the most widely used visual acuity test for preschool children. Right-left presentations are more confusing than up-down presentations. With pretest practice, this test can be performed by most children 3–4 yr of age.

An adult-type **Snellen acuity chart** can be used at about 5 or 6 yr of age if the child knows letters. An acuity of 20/40 is generally accepted as normal for 3 yr old children. At 4 yr of age, 20/30 is typical. By 5 or 6 yr of age, most children attain 20/20 vision.

Optokinetic nystagmus (the response to a sequence of moving targets; "railroad" nystagmus) can also be used to assess vision; this can be calibrated by targets of various sizes (stripes or dots) or by a rotating drum at specified distances. The VER, an electrophysiologic method of evaluating the response to light and special visual stimuli, such as calibrated stripes or a checkerboard pattern, can also be used to study visual function in selected cases. Preferential looking tests are also used for evaluating vision in infants and children who cannot respond to standard acuity tests. This is a behavioral technique based on the observation that, given a choice, an infant prefers to look at patterned rather than unpatterned stimuli. Preferential looking tests cannot be directly correlated to standard visual acuity data. Because these tests require the presence of a skilled examiner, their use is often limited to research protocols involving preverbal children.

VISUAL FIELD ASSESSMENT. Like visual acuity testing, visual field assessment must be geared to a child's age and abilities. Formal visual field examination (perimetry and scotometry) can often be accomplished in school-aged children. The examiner must often rely on confrontation techniques and finger counting in quadrants of the visual field. In many children, only testing by attraction can be accomplished; the examiner observes a child's response to familiar objects brought into each of the four quadrants of the visual field of each eye in turn. The child's bottle, a favorite toy, and lollipops are particularly effective attention-getting items. These gross methods can often detect diagnostically significant field changes such as the bitemporal hemianopia of a chiasmal lesion or the homonymous hemianopia of a cerebral lesion.

COLOR VISION TESTING. This can be accomplished whenever a child is able to name or trace the test symbols; these may be either numbers or Xs, Os, triangles, or other symbols. Color vision testing is not frequently necessary in young children, but parents sometimes request it, particularly if their child seems to be slow in learning colors. Parents are often reassured to know that "color-deficient" children do not misname colors and that true "color blindness" is very rare and not compatible with normal vision. Defective color vision is common in male patients but is rare in female patients. Achromatopsia, a total color vision defect with subnormal visual acuity, nystagmus, and photophobia, is encountered occasionally. A change in color discrimination can be a sign of optic nerve or retinal disease.

PUPILLARY EXAMINATION. This includes evaluation of both the direct and consensual reactions to light, the reaction on near gaze, and the response to reduced illumination, noting the size and symmetry of the pupils under all conditions. Special care must be taken to differentiate the reaction to light from the reaction to near gaze. A child's natural tendency is to look directly at the approaching light, inducing the near gaze reflex when one is attempting to test only the reaction to light; accordingly, every effort must be made to control fixation. The swinging flashlight test is especially useful for detecting unilateral or asymmetric prechiasmatic afferent defects in children (see "Marcus Gunn Pupil" section in Chapter 621).

OCULAR MOTILITY. This is tested by having a child follow an object into the various positions of gaze. Movements of each eye individually (ductions) and of the two eyes together (versions, conjugate movements, and convergence) are assessed. Alignment is judged by the symmetry of the corneal light reflexes and by the response to alternate occlusion of each eye (see discussion on cover tests for strabismus in Chapter 622).

BINOCULAR VISION. A determination of the degree of binocular vision is commonly performed by an ophthalmologist. The Titmus test is probably the most frequently used test; a series of three-dimensional images are shown to the child while he or she wears a set of Polaroid glasses. The level of difficulty with which these images can be detected correlates with the degree of binocular vision that is present. Other tests may also be used to detect the presence of abnormal binocular adaptations secondary to poor vision or strabismus.

EXTERNAL EXAMINATION. This begins with general inspection in good illumination noting size, shape, and symmetry of the orbits; position and movement of the lids; and position and symmetry of the globes. Viewing the eyes and lids from above aids in detecting orbital asymmetry, lid masses, proptosis (**exophthalmos**), and abnormal pulsations. Palpation is also important in detecting orbital and lid masses.

The lacrimal apparatus is assessed by looking for evidence of tear deficiency, overflow of tears (**epiphora**), erythema, and swelling in the region of the tear sac or gland. The sac is massaged to check for reflux when obstruction is suspected. The presence and position of the puncta are also checked.

The lids and conjunctivae are specifically examined for focal lesions, foreign bodies, and inflammatory signs; loss and maldirection of lashes should also be noted. When necessary, the lids can be everted in the following manner: (1) instruct the patient to look down; (2) grasp the lashes of the patient's upper lid between the thumb and index finger of one hand; (3) place a probe, a cotton-tipped applicator, or the thumb of the other hand at the upper margin of the tarsal plate; and (4) pull the lid down and outward, evert it over the probe, using the instrument as a fulcrum. Foreign bodies commonly lodge in the concavity just above the lid margin and are exposed only by fully everting the lid.

The anterior segment of the eye is then evaluated with oblique focal illumination, noting the luster and clarity of the cornea, the depth and clarity of the anterior chamber, and the features of the iris. Transillumination of the anterior segment aids in detecting opacities and in demonstrating atrophy or hypopigmentation of the iris; these latter signs are important when ocular albinism is suspected. When necessary, fluorescein dye can be used to aid in diagnosing abrasions, ulcerations, and foreign bodies.

BIOMICROSCOPY (SLIT-LAMP EXAMINATION). This provides a highly magnified view of the various structures of the eye and an optical section through the media of the eye—the cornea, aqueous humor, lens, and vitreous. Lesions can be identified and localized according to their depth within the eye; the resolution is sufficient to detect individual inflammatory cells in the aqueous and vitreous. With the addition of special lenses and prisms, the angle of the anterior chamber and regions of the fundus also can be examined with a slit lamp. Biomicroscopy is often crucial in trauma and in examining for iritis. It is also helpful in diagnosing many metabolic diseases of childhood.

FUNDUS EXAMINATION (OPHTHALMOSCOPY). This is best done with the pupil dilated unless there are neurologic or other contraindications. Tropicamide (Mydriacyl) 0.5–1% and phenylephrine (Neo-Synephrine) 2.5% are recommended as mydriatics of short duration. These are safe for most children, but the possibility of adverse systemic effects must be recognized. For very small infants, more dilute preparations may be advisable. Beginning with posterior landmarks, the disc and the macula, the four quadrants are systematically examined by following each of the major vessel groups to the periphery. More of the fundus can be seen if a child is directed to look up and down and to the right and left. Even with care, only a limited amount of the fundus can be seen with a direct or hand-held ophthalmoscope. For examination of the far periphery, an indirect ophthalmoscope is used, and full dilation of the pupil is essential.

REFRACTION. This determines the refractive state of the eye: the degree of nearsightedness, farsightedness, or astigmatism.

Retinoscopy provides an objective determination of the amount of correction needed and can be performed at any age. In young children, it is best done with cycloplegia. Subjective refinement of refraction involves asking patients for preferences in the strength and axis of corrective lenses; it can be accomplished in many school-aged children. Refraction and determination of visual acuity with appropriate corrective lenses in place are essential steps in deciding whether a patient has a visual defect or amblyopia. Photoscreening cameras aid ancillary medical personnel in screening for abnormal refractive errors in preverbal children. The accuracy and practical usefulness of these devices are still being investigated.

TONOMETRY. This measures intraocular pressure; it may be performed with a portable, stand-alone instrument or by the applanation method with the slit lamp. Alternative methods are pneumatic and electronic tonometry. When accurate measurement of the pressure is necessary in a child who cannot cooperate, it may be performed with sedation or general anesthesia. A gross estimate of pressure can be made by palpating the globe with the index fingers placed side by side on the upper lid above the tarsal plate.

American Academy of Ophthalmology Preferred Practice Patterns Committee, Pediatrics Ophthalmology Panel: Pediatric eye evaluations: Preferred practice pattern. Abstracts of Clinical Care Guidelines, April 7, 1998.

American Academy of Ophthalmology: *Preferred Practice Pattern: Comprehensive Pediatric Eye Evaluation.* San Francisco, American Academy of Ophthalmology, 1992.

American Academy of Pediatrics, Committee on Practice and Ambulatory Medicine, Section on Ophthalmology: Eye examination and vision screening in infants, children and young adults. *Pediatrics* 1996;98:153–157.

Donahue SP, Johnson TM, Ottar W, et al: Sensitivity of photoscreening to detect high-magnitude amblyogenic factors. *J AAPOS* 2002;6:86–91.

Fulton A: Screening preschool children to detect visual and ocular disorders. *Arch Ophthalmol* 1992;110:1553–1554.

Isenberg SJ: Clinical application of the pupil examination in neonates. *J Pediatr* 1991;118:650–652.

Reinecke RD: Screening 3-year olds for visual problems: Are we gaining or falling behind? *Arch Ophthalmol* 1986;104:245–248.

Salcido AA, Bradley J, Donahue SP: Predictive value of photoscreening and traditional screening of preschool children. *J AAPOS* 2005;9:114–120.

Simons K: Preschool vision screening: Rationale, methodology and outcome. *Surv Ophthalmol* 1996;41:3–30.

Teller DY, McDonald MA, Preston KI, et al: Assessment of visual acuity in infants and children: The acuity card procedure. *Dev Med Child Neurol* 1986;28:779–789.

Chapter 619 ■ Abnormalities of Refraction and Accommodation

Scott E. Olitsky, Denise Hug, and Laura P. Smith

Emmetropia is the state in which parallel rays of light come to focus on the retina with the eye at rest (nonaccommodating). While such an ideal optical state is common, the opposite condition, ametropia, often occurs. Three principal types of **ametropia** exist: **hyperopia** (farsightedness), **myopia** (nearsightedness), and **astigmatism.** The majority of children are physiologically hyperopic at birth, but a significant number, especially those born prematurely, are myopic and often have some degree of astigmatism. With growth, the refractive state tends to change and should be evaluated periodically.

Measurement of the refractive state of the eye (refraction) can be accomplished both objectively and subjectively. The objective method involves directing a beam of light from a retinoscope onto a patient's retina. Based on the way in which the light behaves with movement of the retinoscope and manipulation with lenses of various strengths held in front of the eye, a precise refraction can be performed. An objective refraction can be carried out at any age because it requires no response from the patient. In infants and children, it is generally more accurate to perform a refraction after instillation of eyedrops that produce mydriasis (dilatation of the pupil) and cycloplegia (paralysis of accommodation); those used most commonly are tropicamide (Mydriacyl), cyclopentolate (Cyclogyl), and atropine sulfate. A subjective refraction involves placing lenses in front of the eye and having the patient report which lenses provide the clearest image of the letters on a chart. This method is dependent on a patient's ability to discriminate and communicate, but it can be used for some children and can be helpful in determining the best refractive correction for children who are developmentally capable.

HYPEROPIA. If parallel rays of light come to focus posterior to the retina with the eye in a state of rest, hyperopia or farsightedness exists. This may result because the anteroposterior diameter of the eye is too short or the refractive power of the cornea or lens is less than normal.

In hyperopia, accommodation is used to bring objects into focus for both far and near gaze. If the accommodative effort required is not too great, the child has clear vision and is comfortable with both distant and close work. In high degrees of hyperopia requiring greater accommodative effort, vision may be blurred, and the child may complain of eyestrain, headaches, or fatigue. Squinting, eye rubbing, and lack of interest in reading are frequent manifestations. If the induced discomfort is great enough, a child may not make an effort to see well and may develop bilateral amblyopia (ametropic amblyopia). Esotropia may also be associated (see discussion on convergent strabismus, accommodative esotropia in Chapter 622). Convex lenses (spectacles or contact lenses) of sufficient strength to provide clear vision and comfort are prescribed when indicated. Even children who have high degrees of hyperopia but who have good vision will happily wear glasses because they provide comfort by eliminating the excessive accommodation required to see well. Preverbal children should also be given glasses for high levels of hyperopia to prevent the development of esotropia or amblyopia. Children with normal levels of hyperopia do not require correction in the majority of cases.

MYOPIA. In myopia, parallel rays of light come to focus anterior to the retina. This may result because the anteroposterior diameter of the eye is too long or the refractive power of the cornea or lens is greater than normal. The principal symptom is blurred vision for distant objects. The far point of clear vision varies inversely with the degree of myopia; as the myopia increases, the far point of clear vision moves closer to the eye. With myopia of 1 diopter, for example, the far point of clear focus is 1 m from the eye; with myopia of 3 diopters, the far point of clear vision is only ⅓ m from the eye. Thus, myopic children tend to hold objects and reading matter close, prefer to be close to the blackboard, and may be uninterested in distant activities. Squinting is common because the visual acuity is improved when the lid aperture is reduced.

Myopia is infrequent in infants and preschool-aged children. It is more common in infants with a history of **retinopathy of prematurity.** A hereditary tendency to myopia is also observed, and children of myopic parents should be examined at an early age. The incidence of myopia increases during the school years, especially during the preteen and teen years. The degree of myopia also increases with age during the growing years.

Concave lenses (spectacles or contact lenses) of appropriate strength to provide clear vision and comfort are prescribed. Changes are usually needed periodically, sometimes in 1–2 yr, sometimes every few months. Excessive accommodation during near work has been considered by some to lead to progression of myopia. Based on this philosophy, some practitioners advocate the use of cycloplegic agents, bifocals, intentional undercorrection of myopic refractive errors, or mandatory removal of myopic glasses for near work in an effort to retard the progression of myopia. The value of such treatment has not been scientifically proved.

Excimer laser correction for myopia has been approved for adults since 1995. The LASIK (laser-assisted in situ keratomileusis) procedure uses either a microkeratome or a femtosecond laser that forms an epithelial-stromal flap permitting the underlying corneal tissue to be ablated to correct vision; the flap then recovers the area of the cornea. Correction of vision is usually excellent and stable over time. Risks are greatest with high degrees of myopia (>10 diopters) and include starbursts, halos, and distorted images or multiple images (usually at night). Complications are lowest with more experienced surgeons. Current recommendations for this and newer procedures are available at www.aao.org/aao/education/library/recommendations/lasik.cfm.

In most cases, myopia is not a result of pathologic alteration of the eye and is referred to as simple or physiologic myopia. Some children may have pathologic myopia, a rare condition caused by a pathologically abnormal axial length of the eye; this is usually associated with thinning of the sclera, choroid, and retina and often with some degree of uncorrectable visual impairment. Tears or breaks in the retina may occur as it becomes increasingly thin, leading to the development of retinal detachments. Myopia may also occur as a result of other ocular abnormalities, such as keratoconus, ectopia lentis, congenital stationary night blindness, and glaucoma. Myopia is also a major feature of Stickler syndrome.

ASTIGMATISM. In astigmatism, the refractive power of the various meridians of the eye differs. Most cases are caused by irregularity in the curvature of the cornea; some astigmatism results from changes in the lens. Mild degrees of astigmatism are common and may produce no symptoms. With greater degrees, there may be distortion of vision. To achieve a clearer image, a person with astigmatism uses accommodation or squints to obtain a pinhole effect. Symptoms include eyestrain, headache, and fatigue. Cylindric or spherocylindric lenses are used to provide optical correction when indicated. Glasses may be needed constantly or only part time, depending on the degree of astigmatism and the severity of the attendant symptoms. In some cases, contact lenses are used.

Infants and children with corneal irregularity resulting from injury, periorbital and eyelid hemangiomas, and ptosis are at increased risk of astigmatism and attendant amblyopia.

ANISOMETROPIA. When the refractive state of one eye is significantly different from the refractive state of the other eye, anisometropia exists. If uncorrected, one eye may always be out of focus, leading to the development of amblyopia. Early detection and correction are essential if normal visual development in both eyes is to be achieved.

ACCOMMODATION. During accommodation, the ciliary muscle contracts, the suspensory fibers of the lens relax, and the lens assumes a more rounded shape to bring rays of light into focus on the retina. The amplitude of accommodation is greatest during childhood and gradually diminishes with age. The physiologic decrease in accommodative ability that occurs with age is called presbyopia.

Disorders of accommodation in children are relatively rare. Premature presbyopia is occasionally encountered in young children. The most common cause of paralysis of accommodation in children is intentional or inadvertent use of cycloplegic substances, topically or systemically; included are all the anticholinergic drugs and poisons, as well as plants and plant substances having these effects. Neurogenic causes of accommodative paralysis include lesions affecting the oculomotor nerve (3rd cranial nerve) in any part of its course. Differential diagnosis includes tumors, degenerative diseases, vascular lesions, trauma, and infectious diseases. Systemic disorders that may cause impairment of accommodation include botulism, diphtheria, Wilson disease, diabetes mellitus, and syphilis. Adie tonic pupil may also lead to a deficiency of accommodation after some viral illnesses (see Chapter 621). An apparent defect in accommodation may be psychogenic in origin; it is common for a child to feign inability to read when it can be demonstrated that visual acuity and ability to focus are normal.

Brown NP, Koretz JF, Bron AJ: The development and maintenance of emmetropia. *Eye* 1999;13:83–92.

Klimek DL, Cruz OA, Scott WE, et al: Isoametropic amblyopia due to high hyperopia in children. *J AAPOS* 2004;8:310–313.

Kuo A, Sinatra RB, Donahue SP: Distribution of refractive error in healthy infants. *J AAPOS* 2003;7:174–177.

Larsson EK, Rydberg AC, Holmstrom GE: A population-based study of the refractive outcome in 10-year-old preterm and full-term children. *Arch Ophthalmol* 2003;121:1430–1436.

Mayer DL, Hansen RM, Moore BD, et al: Cycloplegic refractions in healthy children aged 1 through 48 months. *Arch Ophthalmol* 2001;119:1625–1628.

Sakimoto T, Rosenblatt MI, Azar DT: Laser eye surgery for refractive errors. *Lancet* 2006;369:1432–1447.

Ton Y, Wysenbeek YS, Spierer A: Refractive error in premature infants. *J AAPOS* 2004;8:534–538.

Wilson SE: Use of lasers for vision correction of nearsightedness and farsightedness. *N Engl J Med* 2004;351:470–475.

Chapter 620 ■ Disorders of Vision

Scott E. Olitsky, Denise Hug, and Laura P. Smith

Severe visual impairment (corrected vision poorer than 6/60) and blindness in children have many etiologies and may be due to multiple defects affecting any structure or function along the visual pathways (Table 620-1). The overall incidence is approximately 2.5 per 100,000 children; the incidence is higher in developing countries, in low birthweight infants, and in the first year of life. The most common causes are prenatal and perinatal; the cerebral-visual pathways, optic nerve, and retinal sites are most often affected. Important prenatal causes include autosomal recessive (most common), autosomal dominant, and X-linked genetic disorders as well as hypoxia and chromosomal syndromes. Perinatal/neonatal causes include retinopathy of prematurity, hypoxia-ischemia, and infection. Severe visual impairment starting in older children may be due to central nervous system or retinal tumors, infections, hypoxia-ischemia, injuries, neurodegenerative disorders, or juvenile rheumatoid arthritis.

AMBLYOPIA. This is a decrease in visual acuity, unilateral or bilateral, that occurs in visually immature children as a result of a lack of a clear image falling on the retina. The unformed retinal

TABLE 620-1. Causes of Childhood Severe Visual Impairment or Blindness

CONGENITAL
Optic nerve hypoplasia or aplasia
Septo-optic dysplasia
Optic coloboma
Congenital hydrocephalus
Hydranencephaly
Porencephaly
Micrencephaly
Encephalocele, particularly occipital
Morning glory disc
Aniridia
Microphthalmia/anophthalmia
Peters anomaly
Reiger's anomaly
Persistent pupillary membrane
Glaucoma
Cataracts
Persistent hyperplastic primary vitreous

PHAKOMATOSES
Tuberous sclerosis
Neurofibromatosis (special association with optic glioma)
Sturge-Weber syndrome
von Hippel-Lindau disease

TUMORS
Retinoblastoma
Optic glioma
Perioptic meningioma
Craniopharyngioma
Cerebral glioma
Astrocytoma
Posterior and intraventricular tumors when complicated by hydrocephalus
Pseudotumor cerebri

NEURODEGENERATIVE DISEASES
Cerebral storage disease
Gangliosidoses, particularly Tay-Sachs disease, Sandhoff variant, generalized gangliosidosis
Other lipidoses and ceroid lipofuscinoses, particularly the late-onset disorders such as those of Jansky-Bielschowsky and of Batten-Mayou-Spielmeyer-Vogt
Mucopolysaccharidoses, particularly Hurler syndrome and Hunter syndrome
Leukodystrophies (dysmyelination disorders), particularly metachromatic leukodystrophy and Canavan disease
Demyelinating sclerosis (myelinoclastic diseases), especially Schilder disease and Devic neuromyelitis optica
Special types: Dawson disease, Leigh disease, the Bassen-Kornzweig syndrome, Refsum disease
Retinal degenerations: retinitis pigmentosa and its variants and Leber congenital type
Optic atrophies: congenital autosomal recessive type, infantile and congenital autosomal dominant types, Leber disease, and atrophies associated with hereditary ataxias—the types of Behr, of Marie, and of Sanger-Brown

INFECTIOUS/INFLAMMATORY PROCESSES
Encephalitis, especially in the prenatal infection syndromes due to *Toxoplasma gondii*, cytomegalovirus, rubella virus, *Treponema pallidum*, herpes simplex virus
Meningitis; arachnoiditis
Chorioretinitis
Endophthalmitis
Trachoma
Keratitis
Uveitis

HEMATOLOGIC DISORDERS
Leukemia with central nervous sytstem involvement

VASCULAR AND CIRCULATORY DISORDERS
Collagen vascular diseases
Arteriovenous malformations—intracerebral hemorrhage, subarachnoid hemorrhage
Central retinal occlusion

TRAUMA
Contusion or avulsion of optic nerves, chiasm, globe, cornea
Cerebral contusion or laceration
Intracerebral, subarachnoid, or subdural hemorrhage
Retinal detachment

DRUGS AND TOXINS
Quinine
Ethambutol
Methanol
Many others

OTHER
Retinopathy of prematurity
Sclerocornea
Conversion reaction
Optic neuritis
Osteopetrosis

Modified from Kliegman R: *Practical Strategies in Pediatric Diagnosis and Therapy.* Philadelphia, WB Saunders, 1996.

image may occur secondary to a deviated eye (**strabismic amblyopia**), an unequal need for vision correction between the eyes (**anisometropic amblyopia**), a high refractive error in both eyes (**ametropic amblyopia**), or a media opacity within the visual axis (**deprivation amblyopia**).

The development of visual acuity normally proceeds rapidly in infancy and early childhood. Anything that interferes with the formation of a clear retinal image during this early developmental period can produce amblyopia. Amblyopia may occur only during the critical period of development, before the cortex has become visually mature, within the first decade of life. The younger a child, the more susceptible he or she is to the development of amblyopia.

The **diagnosis** of amblyopia is confirmed when a complete ophthalmologic examination reveals reduced acuity that is unexplained by an organic abnormality. If the history and ophthalmologic examination do not support the diagnosis of amblyopia in a child with poor vision, consideration must be given to other causes (neurologic, psychologic). Amblyopia is usually asymptomatic and detected only by screening programs. Screening is easier in older children. However, just as amblyopia is less likely to occur in an older child, it is also more resistant to treatment at an older age. Amblyopia is reversed more rapidly in younger children whose visual system is less mature. The key to the successful treatment of amblyopia is early detection and prompt intervention.

Treatment generally first consists of removing any media opacity or prescribing appropriate glasses, if needed, so that a well-focused retinal image can be produced in each eye. The sound eye is then covered (occlusion therapy) or blurred with glasses or drops (penalization therapy) to stimulate proper visual development of the more severely affected eye. Occlusion therapy may provide a speedier improvement in vision, but some children may better tolerate atropine penalization. The best treatment for any one patient should be selected on an individual basis. The goals of treatment should be thoroughly understood, and the treatment carefully supervised. Close monitoring of amblyopia therapy is essential, especially in the very young, to avoid deprivation amblyopia in the good eye. Many families need reassurance and support throughout the trying course of treatment. Children with severe amblyopia were once treated with occlusion for full-time patching. Current evidence suggests that 3–7 yr old children with severe amblyopia may be patched for 6 hr per day when combined with 1 hr of near visual activities during patching. Children (3–7 yr) with moderate amblyopia may be managed with 2 hr of patching if combined with 1 hr of near visual activities during patching.

DIPLOPIA. Diplopia, or double vision, is generally a result of a misalignment of the visual axes. Occluding one eye relieves the diplopia; affected children commonly squint, cover one eye with a hand, or assume an abnormal head posture (a face turn or head tilt) to alleviate the bothersome sensation. These mannerisms, especially in preverbal children, are important clues to diplopia. The onset of diplopia in any child warrants prompt evaluation; it may signal the onset of a serious problem such as increased intracranial pressure, a brain tumor, or an orbital mass.

Monocular diplopia results from dislocation of the lens, cataract, or some defect in the media or macula.

SUPPRESSION. In the presence of strabismus, diplopia occurs secondary to the same image falling on different regions of the retina in each eye. In a visually immature child, a process may occur in the cortex that eliminates the disability of seeing double. This is an active process and is termed suppression. It develops only in children. Although suppression eliminates the annoying symptom of diplopia, it is the potential awareness of a second image that tends to keep our eyes properly aligned. Once suppression develops, it may allow an intermittent strabismus to become constant or strabismus to redevelop later in life, even after successful treatment during childhood.

AMAUROSIS. Amaurosis is partial or total loss of vision; the term is usually reserved for profound impairment, blindness, or near blindness. When amaurosis exists from birth, primary consideration in the differential diagnosis must be given to developmental malformations, damage consequent to gestational or perinatal infection, anoxia or hypoxia, perinatal trauma, and the genetically determined diseases that can affect the eye itself or the visual pathways. Often, the reason for amaurosis can be readily determined by objective ophthalmic examination; examples are severe microphthalmia, corneal opacification, dense cataracts, chorioretinal scars, macular defects, retinal dysplasia, and severe optic nerve hypoplasia. In other cases, an intrinsic retinal disease may not be apparent on initial ophthalmoscopic examination or the defect may involve the brain and not the eye. Neuroradiologic (CT or MRI) and electrophysiologic (electroretinography) evaluation may be especially helpful in these cases.

Amaurosis that develops in a child who once had useful vision has different implications. In the absence of obvious ocular disease (cataract, chorioretinitis, retinoblastoma, retinitis pigmentosa), consideration must be given to many neurologic and systemic disorders that can affect the visual pathways. Amaurosis of rather rapid onset may indicate an encephalopathy (hypertension), infectious or parainfectious processes, vasculitis, migraine, leukemia, toxins, or trauma. It may be caused by acute demyelinating disease affecting the optic nerves, chiasm, or cerebrum. In some cases, precipitous loss of vision is a result of increased intracranial pressure, rapidly progressive hydrocephalus, or dysfunction of a shunt. More slowly progressive visual loss suggests tumor or neurodegenerative disease. Gliomas of the optic nerve and chiasm and craniopharyngiomas are primary diagnostic considerations in children who show progressive loss of vision.

Clinical manifestations of impairment of vision vary with the age and abilities of a child, the mode of onset, and the laterality and severity of the deficit. The first clue to amaurosis in an infant may be **nystagmus** or **strabismus,** with the vision deficit itself passing undetected for some time. Timidity, clumsiness, or behavioral change may be the initial clues in the very young. Deterioration in school progress and indifference to school activities are common signs in an older child. School-aged children often try to hide their disability and, in the case of very slowly progressive disorders, may not themselves realize the severity of the problem; some detect and promptly report small changes in their vision.

Any evidence of loss of vision requires prompt and thorough ophthalmic evaluation. Complete delineation of childhood amaurosis and its cause may require extensive investigation involving neurologic evaluation, electrophysiologic tests, neuroradiologic procedures, and sometimes metabolic and genetic studies. Furthermore, attendant special educational, social, and emotional needs must be met.

NYCTALOPIA. Nyctalopia, or night blindness, is vision that is defective in reduced illumination. It generally implies impairment in function of the rods, particularly in dark adaptation time and perceptual threshold. Stationary congenital night blindness may occur as an autosomal dominant, autosomal recessive, or X-linked recessive condition. It may be associated with myopia and nystagmus. Children may have excessive problems going to sleep in a dark room, which may be mistaken for a behavioral problem. Progressive night blindness usually indicates primary or secondary retinal, choroidal, or vitreoretinal degeneration (see Chapter 629); it occurs also in vitamin A deficiency or as a result of retinotoxic drugs such as quinine.

PSYCHOGENIC DISTURBANCES. Vision problems of psychogenic origin are common in school-aged children. Both conversion reactions and willful feigning are encountered. The usual manifestation is a report of reduced visual acuity in one or both eyes. Another common manifestation is constriction of the visual field. In some cases, the symptom is diplopia or polyopia (see Chapters 21 and 24).

Important clues to the diagnosis are inappropriate affect, excessive grimacing, inconsistency in performance, and suggestibility. A thorough ophthalmologic examination is essential to differentiate organic from functional visual disorders.

Affected children usually fare well with reassurance and positive suggestions. In some cases, psychiatric care is indicated. In all cases, the approach must be supportive and nonpunitive.

DYSLEXIA. This is the inability to develop the capability to read at an expected level despite an otherwise normal intellect. The terms reading disability and dyslexia are often used interchangeably. Most dyslexic individuals also display poor writing ability. Dyslexia is a primary reading disorder and should be differentiated from secondary reading difficulties due to mental retardation, environmental or educational deprivation, and physical or organic diseases. Because there is no one standard test for dyslexia, the diagnosis is usually made by comparing reading ability with intelligence and standard reading expectations. Dyslexia is a language-based disorder and is not caused by any defect in the eye or visual acuity per se, nor is it attributable to a defect in ocular motility or binocular alignment. Although ophthalmologic evaluation of children with a reading problem is recommended to diagnose and correct any concurrent ocular problems such as a refractive error, amblyopia, or strabismus, treatment directed to the eyes themselves cannot be expected to correct developmental dyslexia (Chapter 32).

Dutton G, Cleary M: Should we be screening for and treating amblyopia? *Br Med J* 2003;327:1242–1243.

Holmes JM, Clarke MP: Amblyopia. *Lancet* 2006;367:1343–1351.

Olitsky SE, Nelson LB: Reading disorders in children. *Pediatr Clin North Am* 2003;50:213–224.

Pediatric Eye Disease Investigator Group: A randomized trial of atropine vs. patching for treatment of moderate amblyopia in children. *Arch Ophthalmol* 2002;120:268–278.

Pediatric Eye Disease Investigator Group: A randomized trial of prescribed patching regimens for treatment of severe amblyopia in children. *Ophthalmology* 2003;110:2075–2087.

Pediatric Eye Disease Investigator Group: A randomized trial of patching regimens for treatment of moderate amblyopia in children. *Arch Ophthalmol* 2003;121:603–611.

Pediatric Eye Disease Investigator Group: Randomized trial of treatment of amblyopia in children aged 7 to 17 years. *Arch Ophthalmol* 2005;123:437–447.

Rahl JS, Cable N: Severe visual impairment and blindness in children in the UK. *Lancet* 2003;362:1359–1364.

Shaywitz SE, Shaywitz BA: The science of reading and dyslexia. *J AAPOS* 2003;7:158–166.
Simons K: Amblyopia characterization, treatment, and prophylaxis. *Surv Ophthalmol* 2005;50:123–166.

Chapter 621 ■ Abnormalities of Pupil and Iris

Scott E. Olitsky, Denise Hug, and Laura P. Smith

ANIRIDIA. The term aniridia is a misnomer because iris tissue is usually present, although it is hypoplastic (Fig. 621-1). Two thirds of the cases are dominantly transmitted with a high degree of penetrance. The other ⅓ of cases are sporadic and are considered to be new mutations. The condition is bilateral in 98% of all patients, regardless of the means of transmission, and is found in approximately 1/50,000 persons.

Aniridia is a panocular disorder and should not be thought of as an isolated iris defect. Macular and optic nerve hypoplasias are commonly present and lead to decreased vision and sensory nystagmus. The visual acuity is measured as 20/200 in most patients, although the vision may occasionally be better. Other ocular deformities are common and may involve the lens and cornea. The cornea may be small, and a cellular infiltrate (pannus) occasionally develops in the superficial layers of the peripheral cornea. Clinically, this appears as a gray opacification. Lens abnormalities include cataract formation and partial or total lens dislocation. **Glaucoma** develops in as many as 75% of individuals with aniridia.

One fifth of **sporadic** aniridic patients may develop **Wilms tumor** (see Chapter 499). Of particular interest is the association of aniridia, genitourinary anomalies, mental retardation, and a partial deletion of the short arm of chromosome 11. Among individuals thus affected, the appearance of Wilms tumor is more common. It is thought that only patients with sporadic aniridia are at risk for developing Wilms tumor, although Wilms tumor has occurred in a patient with familial aniridia. Wilms tumor usually presents before the 3rd yr. Therefore, these children should be screened using renal ultrasonography every 3–6 mo until approximately 5 yr of age.

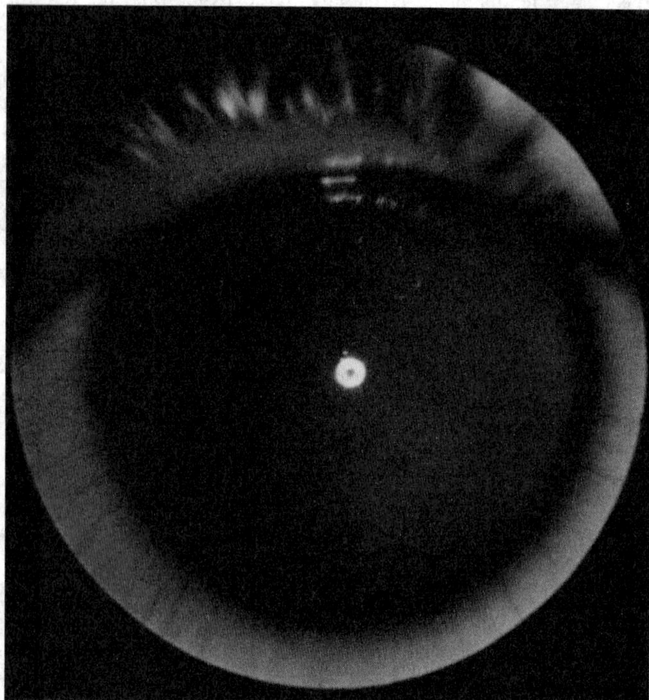

Figure 621-1. Aniridia. Minimal iris tissue. (From Nelson LB, Spaeth GL, Nowinski TS, et al: Aniridia: A review. *Surv Ophthalmol* 1984;28:621–642.)

The gene for aniridia had been localized to the 11p13 region. This gene may be involved in properly directing the interactions between the optic cup, surface ectoderm, and neural crest cells during early formation of the iris and other ocular structures.

COLOBOMA OF THE IRIS. This developmental defect may present as a defect in a sector of the iris, a hole in the substance of the iris, or a notch in the pupillary margin. Simple colobomas are frequently transmitted as an autosomal dominant trait and may occur alone or in association with other anomalies. A coloboma is formed when the embryonic fissure fails to close completely. Because of the anatomic location of the embryonic fissure, an iris coloboma is always located inferiorly, giving the iris a keyhole appearance. An iris coloboma may be the only externally visible part of an extensive malclosure of the embryonic fissure that also involves the fundus and optic nerve. When this occurs, vision is likely to be severely affected. Therefore, all children with an iris coloboma should undergo a full ophthalmologic examination.

MICROCORIA. Microcoria (congenital miosis) appears as a small pupil that does not react to light or accommodation and that dilates poorly, if at all, with medication. The condition may be unilateral or bilateral. In bilateral cases, the degree of miosis may be different in each eye. The eye may be otherwise normal or may demonstrate other abnormalities of the anterior segment. Congenital microcoria is usually transmitted as an autosomal dominant trait, although it may occur sporadically.

CONGENITAL MYDRIASIS. In this disorder, the pupils appear dilated, do not constrict significantly to light or near gaze, and respond minimally to miotic agents. The iris is otherwise normal, and affected children are usually healthy. Trauma, pharmacologic mydriasis, and neurologic disorders should be considered. Many apparent cases of congenital mydriasis show abnormalities of the central iris structures and may be considered a form of aniridia.

DYSCORIA AND CORECTOPIA. Dyscoria is abnormal shape of the pupil, and corectopia is abnormal pupillary position. They may occur together or independently as congenital or acquired anomalies.

Congenital corectopia is usually bilateral and symmetric and rarely occurs as an isolated anomaly; it is usually accompanied by dislocation of the lens (ectopia lentis et pupillae), and the lens and pupil are commonly dislocated in opposite directions. Ectopia lentis et pupillae is transmitted as an autosomal recessive disorder; consanguinity is common.

When acquired, distortion and displacement of the pupil are frequently a result of trauma or intraocular inflammation. Prolapse of the iris after perforating injuries of the eye leads to peaking of the pupil in the direction of the perforation. Posterior synechiae (adhesions of the iris to the lens) are commonly seen when inflammation due to any cause occurs in the anterior segment.

ANISOCORIA. This is inequality of the pupils. The difference in size may be due to local or neurologic disorders. As a rule, if the inequality is more pronounced in the presence of bright focal illumination or on near gaze, there is a defect in pupillary constriction and the larger pupil is abnormal. If the anisocoria is worse in reduced illumination, a defect in dilation exists and the smaller pupil is abnormal. Neurologic causes of anisocoria (parasympathetic or sympathetic lesions) must be differentiated from local causes such as synechiae (adhesions), congenital iris defects (colobomas, aniridia), and pharmacologic effects. Simple central anisocoria may occur in otherwise healthy individuals.

DILATED FIXED PUPIL. Differential diagnosis of a dilated unreactive pupil includes internal ophthalmoplegia caused by a central or peripheral lesion, Hutchinson pupil of transtentorial herniation, tonic pupil, pharmacologic blockade, and iridoplegia secondary to ocular trauma.

The most common cause of a dilated unreactive pupil is purposeful or accidental instillation of a cycloplegic agent, particularly atropine and related substances. Central nervous system lesions, such as a pinealoma, may cause internal ophthalmoplegia in children. Because the external surface of the oculomotor nerve carries the fibers responsible for pupillary constriction, compression of the nerve along its intracranial course may be associated with internal ophthalmoplegia, even before the development of ptosis or an ocular motility deficit. Although ophthalmoplegic migraine is a common cause of a 3rd nerve palsy with pupillary involvement in children, an intracranial aneurysm must also be considered in the differential diagnosis. The **blown pupil** of transtentorial herniation, occurring with increasing intracranial pressure, is generally unilateral, and patients usually are obviously ill. The pilocarpine test can help differentiate neurologic iridoplegia from pharmacologic blockade. In the case of neurologic iridoplegia, the dilated pupil constricts within minutes after instillation of 1 or 2 drops of 0.5–1% pilocarpine; if the pupil has been dilated with atropine, pilocarpine has no effect. Because pilocarpine is a long-acting drug, this test is not to be used in acute situations in which pupillary signs must be carefully monitored. Because of the consensual pupil response to light, even complete uniocular blindness does not cause a unilaterally dilated pupil.

TONIC PUPIL. This is typically a large pupil that reacts poorly to light (the reaction may be very slow or essentially nil), reacts poorly and slowly to accommodation, and redilates in a slow, tonic manner. The features of tonic pupil are explained by cholinergic supersensitivity of the sphincter after peripheral (postganglionic) denervation and imperfect reinnervation. A distinctive feature of a tonic pupil is its sensitivity to dilute cholinergic agents. Instillation of 0.125% pilocarpine causes significant constriction of the involved pupil and has little or no effect on the unaffected side. The condition is usually unilateral.

Tonic pupil may develop after the acute stage of a partial or complete iridoplegia. It can be seen after trauma to the eye or orbit and may occur in association with toxic or infectious conditions. For those in the pediatric age group, tonic pupil is uncommon. Infectious processes (primarily viral syndromes) and trauma are the primary causes. Features of tonic pupil may also be seen in infants and children with familial dysautonomia (Riley-Day syndrome), although the significance of these findings has been questioned. Tonic pupil has also been reported in young children with Charcot-Marie-Tooth disease. The occurrence of tonic pupil in association with decreased deep tendon reflexes in young women is referred to as **Adie syndrome.**

MARCUS GUNN PUPIL. This relative afferent pupillary defect indicates an asymmetric, prechiasmatic, afferent conduction defect. It is best demonstrated by the swinging flashlight test; this allows comparison of the direct and consensual pupillary responses in both eyes. With patients fixing on a distant target (to control accommodation), a bright focal light is directed alternately into each eye in turn. In the presence of an afferent lesion, both the direct response to light in the affected eye and the consensual response in the other eye are subnormal. Swinging the light to the better or normal eye causes both pupils to react (constrict) normally. Swinging the light back to the affected eye causes both pupils to redilate to some degree, reflecting the defective conduction. This is a very sensitive and useful test for detecting and confirming optic nerve and retinal disease. This test is only abnormal if there is a "relative" difference in the conduction properties of the optic nerves. Therefore, patients with bilateral and symmetrical optic nerve disease will not demonstrate an afferent pupillary defect. A subtle relative afferent defect may be found in some children with amblyopia.

HORNER SYNDROME. The principal signs of oculosympathetic paresis (Horner syndrome) are homolateral miosis, mild ptosis, and apparent enophthalmos with slight elevation of the lower lid. Patients may also have decreased facial sweating, increased amplitude of accommodation, and transient decrease in intraocular pressure. If paralysis of the ocular sympathetic fibers occurs before the age of 2 yr, heterochromia iridis with hypopigmentation of the iris may occur on the affected side.

Oculosympathetic paralysis may be caused by a lesion in the midbrain, brainstem, upper spinal cord, neck, middle fossa, or orbit. Congenital oculosympathetic paresis, often as part of Klumpke brachial palsy, is common, although the ocular signs, particularly the anisocoria, may pass undetected for years. Horner syndrome is also seen in some children after thoracic surgery, such as for congenital heart disease. Congenital Horner syndrome may occur in association with vertebral anomalies and with enterogenous cysts. In some infants and children, Horner syndrome is the presenting sign of tumor in the mediastinal or cervical region, particularly neuroblastoma. Rare causes of Horner syndrome, such as vascular lesions, also occur in the pediatric age group. In some cases, no cause of Horner syndrome can be identified. Occasionally, the condition is familial.

When the cause of Horner syndrome is in question, investigative procedures should be implemented, including chest radiography, CT, MRI of the head and neck, and 24-hr urinary catecholamine assay. Examining old photographs and old records can sometimes be helpful in establishing the age at onset of Horner syndrome.

The cocaine test is useful in diagnosing oculosympathetic paralysis; a normal pupil dilates within 20–45 min after instillation of 1 or 2 drops of 4% cocaine, whereas the miotic pupil of an oculosympathetic paresis dilates poorly, if at all, with cocaine. In some cases, there is denervation supersensitivity to dilute phenylephrine; 1 or 2 drops of a 1% solution dilates the affected pupil but not the normal one. Furthermore, instillation of 1% hydroxyamphetamine hydrobromide dilates the pupil only if the postganglionic sympathetic neuron is intact.

PARADOXICAL PUPIL REACTION. Some children exhibit paradoxical constriction of the pupils to darkness. An initial brisk constriction of the pupils occurs when the light is turned off, followed by slow redilation of the pupils. The response to direct light stimulation and the near response are normal. The mechanism is not clear, but paradoxical constriction of the pupils in reduced light can be a sign of retinal or optic nerve abnormalities. The phenomenon has been observed in children with congenital stationary night blindness, albinism, retinitis pigmentosa, Leber congenital retinal amaurosis, and Best disease. It has also been observed in those with optic nerve anomalies, optic neuritis, optic atrophy, and possibly amblyopia.

PERSISTENT PUPILLARY MEMBRANE. Involution of the pupillary membrane and anterior vascular capsule of the lens is usually completed during the 5th–6th mo of fetal development. It is common to see some remnants of the pupillary membrane in newborns, particularly in premature infants. These membranes are nonpigmented strands of obliterated vessels that cross the pupil and may secondarily attach to the lens or cornea. The remnants tend to atrophy in time and usually present no problem. In some cases, however, significant remnants that remain obscure the pupil and interfere with vision. Rarely, there is patency of the vascular elements; hyphema may result from rupture of persistent vessels.

Intervention must be considered to minimize amblyopia in infants with extensive persistent pupillary membrane of sufficient degree to interfere with vision in the early months of life. In some cases, mydriatics and occlusion therapy may be effective, but in others, surgery may be needed to provide an adequate pupillary aperture.

HETEROCHROMIA. In heterochromia, the two irides are of different color (heterochromia iridium) or a portion of an iris differs in color from the remainder (heterochromia iridis). Simple heterochromia may occur as an autosomal dominant characteristic. Congenital heterochromia is also a feature of Waardenburg syndrome, an autosomal dominant condition characterized principally by lateral displacement of the inner canthi and puncta, pigmentary disturbances (usually a median white forelock and patches of hypopigmentation of the skin), and defective hearing. Change in the color of the iris may occur as a result of trauma, hemorrhage, intraocular inflammation (iridocyclitis, uveitis), intraocular tumor (especially retinoblastoma), intraocular foreign body, glaucoma, iris atrophy, oculosympathetic palsy (Horner syndrome), melanosis oculi, previous intraocular surgery, and some glaucoma medications.

OTHER IRIS LESIONS. Discrete nodules of the iris, referred to as **Lisch nodules,** are commonly seen in patients with neurofibromatosis. Lisch nodules represent melanocytic hamartomas of the iris and vary from slightly elevated pigmented areas to distinct ball-like excrescences. Lisch nodules are found in 92–100% of individuals older than 5 yr of age who have neurofibromatosis. Slit-lamp identification of these nodules may help to fulfill the criteria required to confirm the diagnosis of neurofibromatosis.

In leukemia, there may be infiltration of the iris, sometimes with **hypopyon,** an accumulation of white blood cells in the anterior chamber, which may herald relapse or involvement of the central nervous system.

The lesion of **juvenile xanthogranuloma** (nevoxanthoendothelioma) may occur in the eye as a yellowish fleshy mass or plaque of the iris. Spontaneous hyphema (blood in the anterior chamber), glaucoma, or a red eye with signs of uveitis may be associated. A search for the skin lesions of xanthogranuloma (see also Chapter 86.3) should be made in any infant or young child with spontaneous hyphema. In many cases, the ocular lesion responds to topical corticosteroid therapy.

LEUKOCORIA. This includes any white pupillary reflex, or so-called cat eye reflex. Primary diagnostic considerations in any child with leukocoria are cataract, persistent hyperplastic primary vitreous, cicatricial retinopathy of prematurity, retinal detachment and retinoschisis, larval granulomatosis, and retinoblastoma (Fig. 621-2). Also to be considered are endophthalmitis, organized vitreous hemorrhage, leukemic ophthalmopathy, exudative retinopathy (as in Coats disease), and less common conditions such as medulloepithelioma, massive retinal gliosis, the retinal pseudotumor of Norrie disease, the so-called pseudoglioma of the Bloch-Sulzberger syndrome, retinal dysplasia, and the retinal lesions of the phakomatoses. A white reflex may also be seen with fundus coloboma, large atrophic chorioretinal scars, and ectopic medullation of retinal nerve fibers. Leukocoria is an indication for prompt and thorough evaluation.

The diagnosis can often be made by direct examination of the eye by ophthalmoscopy and biomicroscopy. Ultrasonographic and radiologic examinations are often helpful. In some cases, the final diagnosis rests with a pathologist.

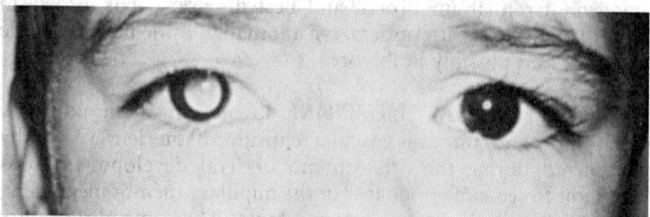

Figure 621-2. Leukocoria. White pupillary reflex in a child with retinoblastoma.

Cross HE: Ectopia lentis et pupillae. *Am J Ophthalmol* 1979;88:381–384.

Francois J: Differential diagnosis of leukokoria in children. *Ann Ophthalmol* 1978;10:1375–1378.

Frank JW, Kushner BJ, France TD: Paradoxic pupillary phenomenon: A review of patients with pupillary constriction to darkness. *Arch Ophthalmol* 1988;106:1564–1566.

Greenwald MJ, Folk ER: Afferent pupillary defects in amblyopia. *J Pediatr Ophthalmol Strabismus* 1983;20:63–67.

Ivanov I, Shuper A, Shohat M, et al: Aniridia: Recent achievements in paediatric practice. *Eur J Pediatr* 1995;154:795–800.

Jaffe N, Cassady JR, Filler RM, et al: Heterochromia and Horner syndrome associated with cervical and mediastinal neuroblastoma. *J Pediatr* 1975;87:75–77.

Jeffery AR, Ellis FJ, Repka MX, et al: Pediatric Horner syndrome. *J Am Assoc Pediatr Ophthalmol Strabismus* 1998;2:159–167.

Loewenfeld IE: "Simple, central" anisocoria: A common condition seldom recognized. *Trans Am Acad Ophthalmol Otolaryngol* 1977;83:832.

Maloney WF, Younge BR, Moyer NJ: Evaluation of the causes and accuracy of pharmacologic localization in Horner syndrome. *Am J Ophthalmol* 1980;90:394–402.

Thompson HS: Segmental palsy of the iris sphincter in Adie's syndrome. *Arch Ophthalmol* 1978;96:1615–1620.

Chapter 622 ■ Disorders of Eye Movement and Alignment

Scott E. Olitsky, Denise Hug, and Laura P. Smith

STRABISMUS

Strabismus, or misalignment of the eyes, is one of the most common eye problems encountered in children, affecting approximately 4% of children younger than 6 yr of age. Strabismus can result in vision loss (amblyopia) and can have significant psychologic effects. Early detection and treatment of strabismus is essential to prevent permanent visual impairment. Of children with strabismus, 30–50% develop amblyopia. Restoration of proper alignment of the visual axis must occur at an early stage of visual development to allow these children a chance to develop normal binocular vision. The word strabismus means "to squint or to look obliquely." Many terms are used in discussing and characterizing strabismus.

Orthophoria is the ideal condition of exact ocular balance. It implies that the oculomotor apparatus is in perfect equilibrium so that the eyes remain coordinated and aligned in all positions of gaze and at all distances. Even when binocular vision is interrupted, as by occlusion of one eye, truly orthophoric individuals maintain perfect alignment. Orthophoria is seldom encountered because the majority of individuals have a small latent deviation (heterophoria).

Heterophoria is a latent tendency for the eyes to deviate. This latent deviation is normally controlled by fusional mechanisms that provide binocular vision or avoid diplopia (double vision). The eye deviates only under certain conditions, such as fatigue, illness, or stress, or during tests that interfere with maintenance of these normal fusional abilities (such as covering one eye). If the amount of heterophoria is large, it may give rise to bothersome symptoms, such as transient diplopia (double vision), headaches, or asthenopia (eyestrain). Some degree of heterophoria is found in normal individuals; it is usually asymptomatic.

Heterotropia is a misalignment of the eyes that is constant. It occurs because of an inability of the fusional mechanism to control the deviation. Tropias can be alternating, involving both eyes, or unilateral. In an alternating tropia, there is no preference for fixation of either eye, and both eyes drift with equal frequency. Because each eye is used periodically, vision usually develops normally. A unilateral tropia is a more serious situation because only one eye is constantly misaligned. The undeviated eye becomes the preferred eye, resulting in loss of vision or amblyopia of the deviated eye.

It is common in ocular misalignments to describe the type of deviation. This helps to make decisions on the cause and treatment of the strabismus. The prefixes eso-, exo-, hyper-, and hypo- are added to the terms phoria and tropia to further delineate the type of strabismus. Esophorias and esotropias are inward or convergent deviations of the eyes, commonly known as crossed eyes. Exophorias and exotropias are divergent or outward-facing eye deviations, walleyed being the lay term. Hyperdeviations and hypodeviations designate upward or downward, respectively, deviations of an eye. In cases of unilateral strabismus, the deviating eye is often part of the description of the misalignment (left esotropia).

DIAGNOSIS. Many techniques are used to assess ocular alignment and movement of the eyes to aid in diagnosing strabismic disorders. In a child with strabismus or any other ocular disorder, assessment of visual acuity is mandatory. Decreased vision in one eye requires evaluation for a strabismus or other ocular abnormalities, which may be difficult to discern on a brief screening evaluation. Even strabismic deviations of only a few degrees in magnitude, too small to be evident by gross inspection, may lead to amblyopia and devastating vision loss.

Corneal light reflex tests are perhaps the most rapid and easily performed diagnostic tests for strabismus. They are particularly useful in children who are uncooperative and in those who have poor ocular fixation. To perform the **Hirschberg corneal reflex test,** the examiner projects a light source onto the cornea of both eyes simultaneously as a child looks directly at the light. Comparison should then be made of the placement of the corneal light reflex in each eye. In straight eyes, the light reflection appears symmetric and, because of the relationship between the cornea and the macula, slightly nasal to the center of each pupil. If strabismus is present, the reflected light is asymmetric and appears displaced in one eye. The Krimsky method of the corneal reflex test uses prisms placed over one or both eyes to align the light reflections. The amount of prism needed to align the reflections is used to measure the degree of deviation. Although it is a useful screening test, corneal light reflex testing may not detect a small angle or an intermittent strabismus.

Cover tests for strabismus require a child's attention and cooperation, good eye movement capability, and reasonably good vision in each eye. If any of these are lacking, the results of these tests may not be valid. These tests consist of the cover-uncover test and the alternate cover test. In the cover-uncover test, a child looks at an object in the distance, preferably 6 m away. An eye chart is commonly used for fixation in children older than 3 yr of age. For younger children, a noise-making toy or movie helps hold their attention for the test. As the child looks at the distant object, the examiner covers one eye and watches for movement of the uncovered eye. If no movement occurs, there is no apparent misalignment of that eye. After one eye is tested, the same procedure is repeated on the other eye. When performing the alternate cover test, the examiner rapidly covers and uncovers each eye, shifting back and forth from one eye to another. If the child has an ocular deviation, the eye rapidly moves as the cover is shifted to the other eye. Both the cover-uncover test and the alternate cover test should be performed at both distance and near fixation. The cover-uncover test differentiates tropias, or manifest deviations, from latent deviations, called phorias.

CLINICAL MANIFESTATIONS AND TREATMENT. The etiologic classification of strabismus is complex, and the causative types must be distinguished; there are comitant and noncomitant forms of strabismus.

Comitant Strabismus. Comitant strabismus is the most common type of strabismus. The individual extraocular muscles usually have no defect. The amount of deviation is constant, or relatively constant, in the various directions of gaze.

Pseudostrabismus (pseudoesotropia) is one of the most common reasons a pediatric ophthalmologist is asked to evaluate an infant. This condition is characterized by the false appearance of strabismus when the visual axes are aligned accurately. This appearance may be caused by a flat, broad nasal bridge, prominent epicanthal folds, or a narrow interpupillary distance. The observer may see less white sclera nasally than would be expected, and the impression is that the eye is turned in toward the nose, especially when the child gazes to either side. Parents frequently comment that when their child looks to the side, the eye almost disappears from view. Pseudoesotropia can be differentiated from a true misalignment of the eyes when the corneal light reflex is centered in both eyes and when the cover-uncover test shows no refixation movement. Once pseudoesotropia has been confirmed, parents can be reassured that the child will outgrow the appearance of esotropia. As the child grows, the bridge of the nose becomes more prominent and displaces the epicanthal folds, and the medial sclera becomes proportional to the amount visible on the lateral aspect. It is the appearance of crossing that the child will outgrow. Some parents of children with pseudoesotropia erroneously believe that their child has an actual esotropia that will resolve on its own. Because true esotropia can develop later in children with pseudoesotropia, parents and pediatricians should be cautioned that reassessment is required if the apparent deviation does not improve.

Esodeviations are the most common type of ocular misalignment in children and represent >50% of all ocular deviations. *Congenital esotropia* is a confusing term. Few children who are diagnosed with this disorder are actually born with an esotropia. Most reports in the literature have therefore considered infants with confirmed onset earlier than 6 mo as having the same condition, which some observers have designated *infantile esotropia.*

The characteristic angle of congenital esodeviations is large and constant (Fig. 622-1). Because of the large deviation, cross-fixation is frequently encountered. This is a condition in which the child looks to the right with the left eye and to the left with the right eye. With cross-fixation, there is no need for the eye to turn away from the nose (abduction) as the adducting eye is used in side gaze; this condition simulates a 6th nerve palsy. Abduction can be demonstrated by the doll's head maneuver or by patching 1 eye for a short time. Children with congenital esotropia tend to have refractive errors similar to those of normal children of the same age. This contrasts with the characteristic high level of farsightedness associated with accommodative esotropia. **Amblyopia** is common in children with congenital esotropia.

The primary goal of treatment in congenital esotropia is to eliminate or reduce the deviation as much as possible. Ideally, this results in normal sight in each eye, in straight-looking eyes, and

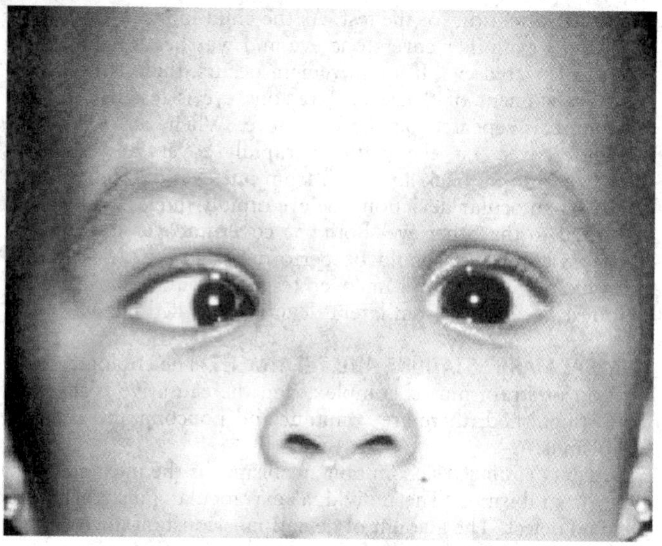

Figure 622-1. Congenital esotropia. Note the large angle of crossing.

in the development of binocular vision. Early treatment is more likely to lead to the development of binocular vision, which helps to maintain long-term ocular alignment. Once any associated amblyopia is treated, surgery is performed to align the eyes. Even with successful surgical alignment, it is common for vertical deviations to develop in children with a history of congenital esotropia. The two most common forms of vertical deviations to develop are inferior oblique muscle overaction and dissociated vertical deviation. In inferior oblique muscle overaction, the overactive inferior oblique muscle produces an upshoot of the eye closest to the nose when the patient looks to the side (Fig. 622-2). In dissociated vertical deviation, DVD 1 eye drifts up slowly with no movement of the other eye. Surgery may be necessary to treat either or both of these conditions.

It is important that parents realize that early successful surgical alignment is only the beginning of the treatment process. Because many children may redevelop strabismus or amblyopia, they need to be monitored closely during the visually immature period of life.

Accommodative esotropia is defined as a "convergent deviation of the eyes associated with activation of the accommodative (focusing) reflex." It usually occurs in a child who is between 2 and 3 yr of age and who has a history of acquired intermittent or constant crossing. Amblyopia occurs in the majority of cases.

The mechanism of accommodative esotropia involves uncorrected hyperopia, accommodation, and accommodative convergence. The image entering a hyperopic (farsighted) eye is blurred. If the amount of hyperopia is not significant, the blurred image can be sharpened by accommodating (focusing of the lens of the eye). Accommodation is closely linked with convergence (eyes turning inward). If a child's hyperopic refractive error is large or if the amount of convergence that occurs in response to each unit of accommodative effort is great, esotropia may develop.

To treat accommodative esotropia, the full hyperopic (farsighted) correction is initially prescribed. These glasses eliminate a child's need to accommodate and therefore correct the esotropia (Fig. 622-3). Although many parents are initially concerned that their child will not want to wear glasses, the benefits of binocular vision and the decrease in the focusing effort required to see clearly provide a strong stimulus to wear glasses, and they are generally accepted well. The full hyperopic correction sometimes straightens the eye position at distance fixation but leaves a residual deviation at near fixation; this may be observed or treated with bifocal lenses, antiaccommodative drops, or surgery.

It is important to warn parents of children with accommodative esotropia that the esodeviation may appear to increase without glasses after the initial correction is worn. Parents frequently state that before wearing glasses, their child had a small esodeviation, whereas after removal of the glasses, the esodeviation becomes quite large. Parents often blame the increased esodeviation on the glasses. This apparent increase is due to a child's using the appropriate amount of accommodative effort after the glasses have been worn. When these children remove their glasses, they continue to use an accommodative effort to bring objects into proper focus and increase the esodeviation.

Most children maintain straight eyes once initially treated. Because hyperopia generally decreases with age, many patients outgrow the need to wear glasses to maintain alignment. In some patients, a residual esodeviation persists even when wearing their glasses. This condition commonly occurs when there is a delay between the onset of accommodative esotropia and treatment. In others, the esotropia may initially be eliminated with glasses but crossing redevelops and is not correctable with glasses. The crossing that is no longer correctable with glasses is the deteriorated or nonaccommodative portion. Surgery for this portion of the crossing may be indicated to restore binocular vision.

Exodeviations are the second most common type of misalignment. The divergent deviation may be intermittent or constant. Intermittent exotropia is the most common exodeviation in childhood. It is characterized by outward drifting of one eye, which usually occurs when a child is fixating at distance. The deviation is generally more frequent with fatigue or illness. Exposure to bright light may cause reflex closure of the exotropic eye. Because the eyes initially can be kept straight most of the time, visual acuity tends to be good in both eyes and binocular vision is initially normal.

The age at onset of intermittent exotropia varies but is often between age 6 mo and 4 yr. The decision to perform eye muscle surgery is based on the amount and frequency of the deviation. If the deviation is small and infrequent, it is reasonable to observe the child. If the exotropia is large or increasing in frequency, surgery is indicated to maintain normal binocular vision.

Constant exotropia may rarely be congenital. Congenital exotropia may be associated with neurologic disease or abnormalities of the bony orbit, as in Crouzon syndrome. Exotropia that occurs later in life may represent a deterioration of an intermittent exotropia that was present in childhood. Surgery can restore binocular vision even in long-standing cases.

Noncomitant Strabismus. When an eye muscle is paretic, palsied, or restricted, a muscle imbalance occurs in which the deviation of the eye varies according to the direction of gaze. Recent onset of a paretic muscle can be suggested by the symptom of double vision that increases in one direction, the findings of an ocular

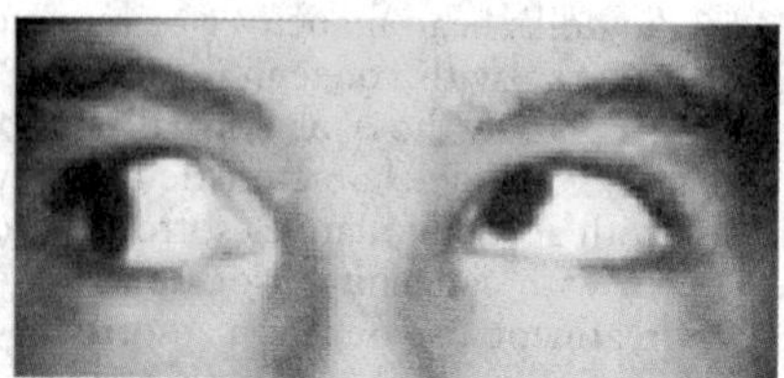

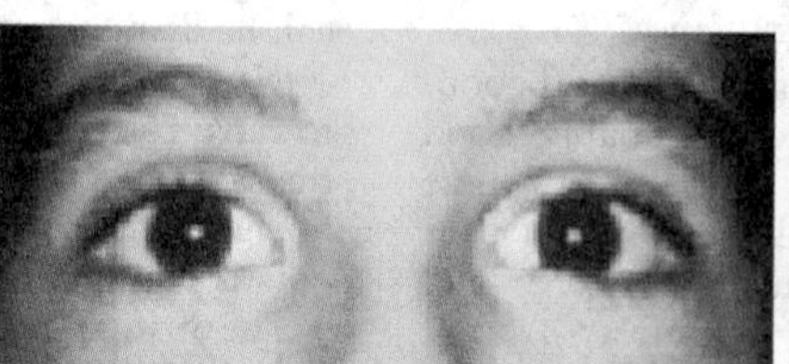

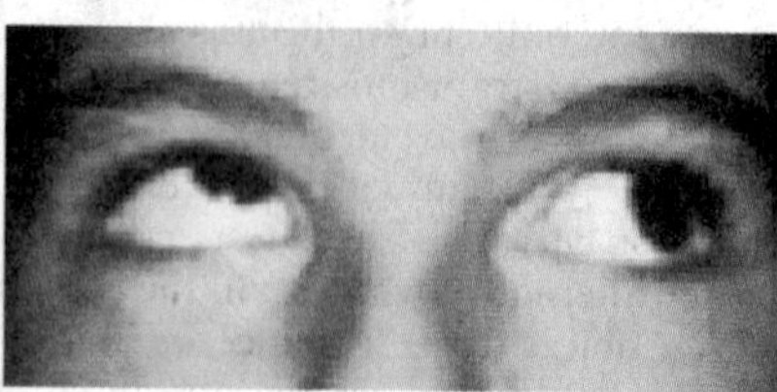

Figure 622-2. Inferior oblique muscle overaction.

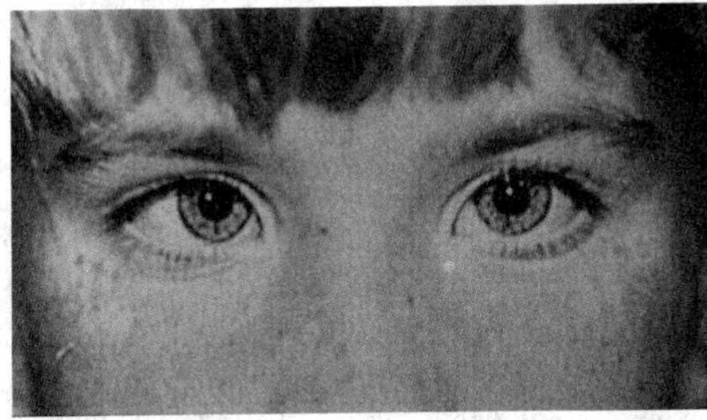
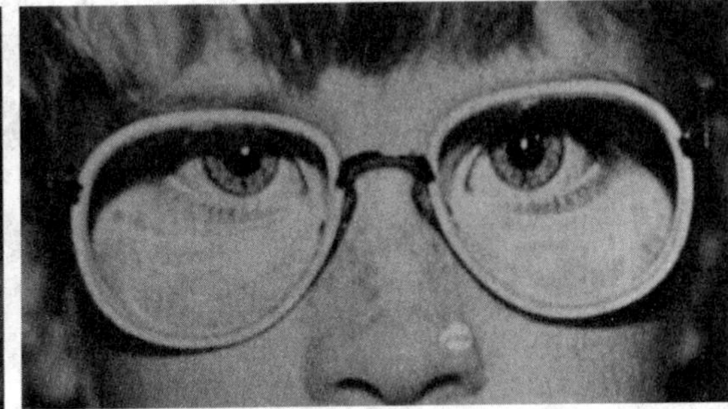

Figure 622-3. Accommodative esotropia; control of deviation with corrective lenses.

deviation that increases in the field of action of the paretic muscle, and an increase in the deviation when the child fixates with the paretic eye. It is important to differentiate a noncomitant strabismus from a comitant deviation because noncomitant forms of strabismus are often associated with trauma, systemic disorders, or neurologic abnormalities.

3rd Nerve Palsy. In the pediatric population, 3rd nerve palsies are usually congenital. The congenital form is often associated with a developmental anomaly or birth trauma. Acquired 3rd nerve palsies in children can be an ominous sign and may indicate a neurologic abnormality such as an intracranial neoplasm or an aneurysm. Other less serious causes include an inflammatory or infectious lesion, head trauma, postviral syndromes, and migraines.

A 3rd nerve palsy, whether congenital or acquired, usually results in an exotropia and a hypotropia, or downward deviation of the affected eye, as well as complete or partial ptosis of the upper lid. This characteristic strabismus results from the action of the normal, unopposed muscles, the lateral rectus muscle, and the superior oblique muscle. If the internal branch of the 3rd nerve is involved, pupillary dilation may be noted as well. Eye movements are usually limited nasally in elevation and in depression. In addition, clinical findings and treatment may be complicated in congenital and traumatic cases of 3rd nerve palsy owing to misdirection of regenerating nerve fibers, referred to as aberrant regeneration. This results in anomalous and paradoxical eyelid, eye, and pupil movement such as elevation of the eyelid, constriction of the pupil, or depression of the globe on attempted medial gaze.

4th Nerve Palsy. These palsies can be congenital or acquired. Because the 4th nerve has a long intracranial course, it is susceptible to damage resulting from head trauma. In children, however, 4th nerve palsies are more frequently congenital than traumatic. A palsied 4th nerve results in weakness in the superior oblique muscle, which causes an upward deviation of the eye, a hypertropia. Because the antagonist muscle, the inferior oblique, is relatively unopposed, the affected eye demonstrates an upshoot when looking toward the nose. Children typically present with a head tilt to the shoulder opposite the affected eye, their chin down, and their face turned away from the affected side. This head position places the eye away from the area of greatest action of the affected muscle and therefore minimizes the deviation and the associated double vision. Long-standing head tilts may lead to facial asymmetry. Because the abnormal head posture maintains the child's ocular alignment, amblyopia is uncommon. Because no abnormality exists in the neck muscles, attempts to correct the head tilt by exercises and neck muscle surgery are ineffective. Recognition of a superior oblique paresis can be difficult because deviation of the head and the eye may be minimal. Eye muscle surgery can be performed to improve the ocular alignment and eliminate the abnormal head posture.

6th Nerve Palsy. These palsies produce markedly crossed eyes with limited ability to move the afflicted eye laterally. Children frequently present with their head turned toward the palsied muscle, a position that helps preserve binocular vision. The esotropia is largest when the eye is moved toward the affected muscle.

Congenital 6th nerve palsies are rare. Decreased lateral gaze in infants is often associated with other disorders, such as congenital esotropia or Duane retraction syndrome. In neonates, a transient 6th nerve paresis can occur; it usually clears spontaneously by 6 wk. It is believed that increased intracranial pressure associated with labor and delivery is the contributing factor.

Acquired 6th nerve palsies in childhood are often an ominous sign because the 6th nerve is susceptible to increased intracranial pressure associated with hydrocephalous and intracranial tumors. Other causes of 6th nerve defects in children include trauma, vascular malformations, meningitis, and Gradenigo syndrome. A benign 6th nerve palsy, which is painless and acquired, can be noted in infants and older children. This is frequently preceded by a febrile illness or upper respiratory tract infection and may be recurrent. Complete resolution of the palsy is usual. Although not uncommon, other causes of an acute 6th nerve palsy should be eliminated before this diagnosis is made.

STRABISMUS SYNDROMES. Special types of strabismus have unusual clinical features. Most of these disorders are caused by structural anomalies of the extraocular muscles or adjacent tissues. Most strabismus syndromes produce noncomitant misalignments.

Double Elevator Palsy. A monocular elevation deficit in both abduction and adduction is referred to as a double elevator palsy. It may represent a paresis of both elevators, the superior rectus and inferior oblique muscles, or a possible restriction to elevation from a fibrotic inferior rectus muscle. When an affected child fixates with the nonparetic eye, the paretic eye is hypotropic and the ipsilateral upper eyelid may appear ptotic. Fixation with the paretic eye causes a hypertropia of the nonparetic eye and a disappearance of the ptosis (Fig. 622-4). Because the apparent ptosis is actually secondary to the strabismus, correction of the hypotropia treats the pseudoptosis.

Duane Syndrome. This congenital disorder of ocular motility is characterized by retraction of the globe on adduction. This is attributed to the absence of the 6th nerve nucleus and anomalous innervation of the lateral rectus muscle, which results in co-contraction of the medial and lateral rectus muscles on attempted adduction of the affected eye. Within the spectrum of Duane syndrome, patients may exhibit impairment of abduction, impairment of adduction, or upshoot or downshoot of the involved eye on adduction. They may have esotropia, exotropia, or relatively straight eyes. Many exhibit a compensatory head posture to maintain single vision. Some develop amblyopia. Surgery to improve alignment or to reduce a noticeable face turn can be helpful in selected cases. Duane syndrome usually occurs sporadically. It is sometimes inherited as an autosomal dominant trait. It usually occurs as an isolated condition but may occur in association with various other ocular and systemic anomalies.

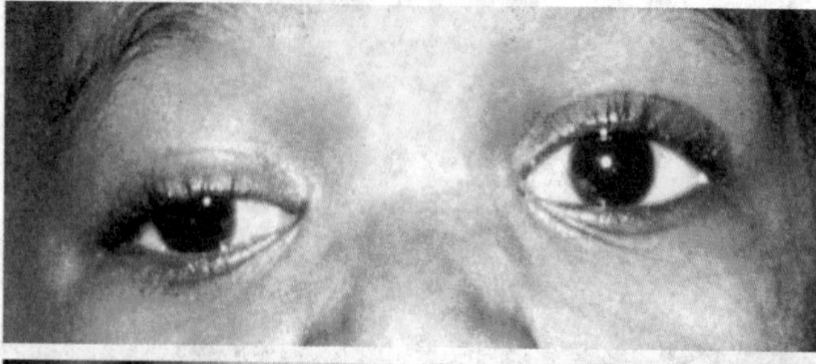

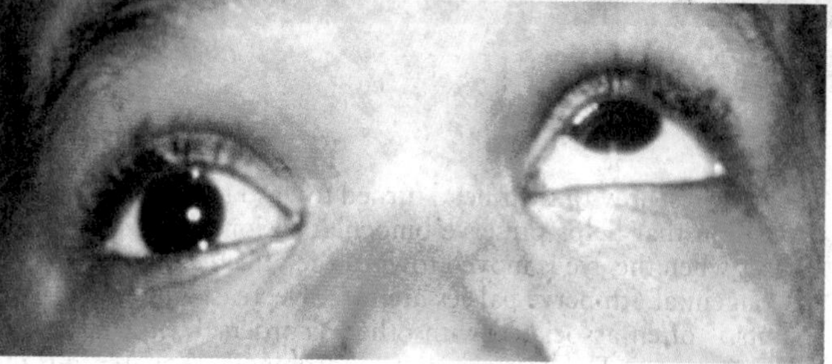

Figure 622-4. Double elevator palsy of the right eye. Note the disappearance of the apparent ptosis when fixating with the involved eye.

Möbius Syndrome. The distinctive features of Möbius syndrome are congenital facial paresis and abduction weakness. The facial palsy is commonly bilateral, frequently asymmetric, and often incomplete, tending to spare the lower face and platysma. Ectropion, epiphora, and exposure keratopathy may develop. The abduction defect may be unilateral or bilateral. Esotropia is common. The cause is unknown. Whether the primary defect is maldevelopment of cranial nerve nuclei, hypoplasia of the muscles, or a combination of central and peripheral factors is unclear. Some familial cases have been reported. Associated developmental defects may include ptosis, palatal and lingual palsy, hearing loss, pectoral and lingual muscle defects, micrognathia, syndactyly, supernumerary digits, and the absence of hands, feet, fingers, or toes. Surgical correction of the esotropia is indicated and any attendant amblyopia should be treated.

Brown Syndrome. In this syndrome, elevation of the eye in the adducted position is restricted (Fig. 622-5). An associated downward deviation of the affected eye in adduction may also occur. A compensatory head posture may be evident. Various causes have been described. Some cases have been attributed to structural abnormalities such as a tight superior oblique tendon, congenital shortening or thickening of the superior oblique tendon sheath, or connective tissue trabeculae between the superior oblique tendon and the trochlea. Acquired Brown syndrome may follow trauma to the orbit involving the region of the trochlea or sinus surgery. It may also occur with inflammatory processes, particularly sinusitis and juvenile rheumatoid arthritis.

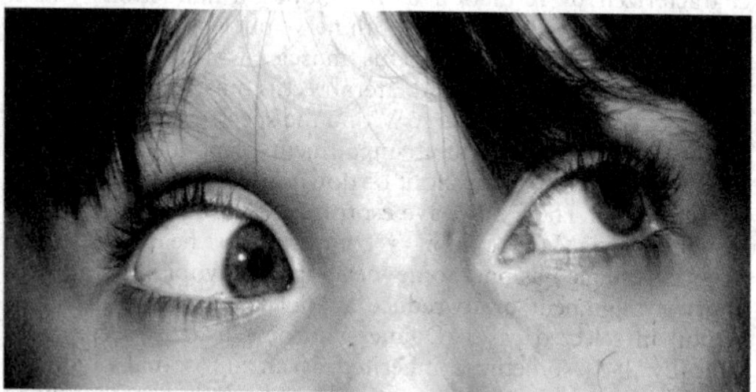

Figure 622-5. Brown syndrome of the right eye.

Acquired inflammatory Brown syndrome may respond to treatment with either nonsteroidal medications or corticosteroids. Surgery may be helpful for children with true congenital Brown syndrome.

Parinaud Syndrome. This eponym designates a palsy of vertical gaze, isolated or associated with pupillary or nuclear oculomotor (3rd cranial nerve) paresis. It indicates a lesion affecting the mesencephalic tegmentum. The ophthalmic signs of midbrain disease include vertical gaze palsy, dissociation of the pupillary responses to light and to near focus, general pupillomotor paralysis, corectopia, dyscoria, accommodative disturbances, pathologic lid retraction, ptosis, extraocular muscle paresis, and convergence paralysis. Some cases have associated spasms of convergence, convergent retraction nystagmus, and vertical nystagmus, particularly on attempted vertical gaze. Combinations of these signs are referred to as the sylvian aqueduct syndrome.

A principal cause of vertical gaze palsy and associated mesencephalic signs in children is tumor of the pineal gland or 3rd ventricle. Differential diagnosis includes trauma and demyelinating disease. In children with hydrocephalus, impairment of vertical gaze and pathologic lid retraction are referred to as the setting-sun sign. A transient supranuclear disorder of gaze is sometimes seen in healthy neonates.

CONGENITAL OCULAR MOTOR APRAXIA

This congenital disorder of conjugate gaze is characterized by a defect in voluntary horizontal gaze, compensatory jerking movement of the head, and retention of slow pursuit and reflexive eye movements. Additional features are absence of the fast (refixation) phase of optokinetic nystagmus and obligate contraversive deviation of the eyes on rotation of the body. Affected children typically are unable to look quickly to either side voluntarily in response to a command or in response to an eccentrically presented object but may be able to follow a slowly moving target to either side. To compensate for the defect in purposive lateral eye movements, children jerk their head to bring the eyes into the desired position and may also blink repetitively in an attempt to change fixation. The signs tend to become less conspicuous with age.

The pathogenesis of congenital ocular motor apraxia is unknown. It may be a result of delayed myelination of the ocular motor pathways. Structural abnormalities of the central nervous system have been found in a few patients, including agenesis of the corpus callosum and cerebellar vermis, porencephaly, hamartoma of the foramen of Monro, and macrocephaly. Many children with congenital ocular motor apraxia show delayed motor and cognitive development.

NYSTAGMUS

Nystagmus (rhythmic oscillations of one or both eyes) may be caused by an abnormality in any one of the three basic mechanisms that regulate position and movement of the eyes: the fixation, conjugate gaze, or vestibular mechanisms. In addition, physiologic nystagmus may be elicited by appropriate stimuli (Table 622-1).

Congenital sensory nystagmus is generally associated with ocular abnormalities that lead to decreased visual acuity; common disorders that lead to early-onset nystagmus include albinism, aniridia, achromatopsia, congenital cataracts, congenital macular lesions, and congenital optic atrophy. In some instances, nystagmus occurs as a dominant or X-linked characteristic without obvious ocular abnormalities.

Congenital idiopathic motor nystagmus is characterized by horizontal jerky oscillations with gaze preponderance; the nystagmus is coarser in one direction of gaze than in the other, with the jerk toward the direction of gaze. There are no ocular

TABLE 622-1. Specific Patterns of Nystagmus

PATTERN	DESCRIPTION	ASSOCIATED CONDITIONS
Latent nystagmus	Conjugate jerk nystagmus toward viewing eye	Congenital vision defects, occurs with occlusion of eye
Manifest latent nystagmus	Fast jerk to viewing eye	Strabismus, congenital idiopathic nystagmus
Periodic alternating	Cycles of horizontal or horizontal-rotary that change direction	Caused by both visual and neurologic conditions
See-saw nystagmus	One eye rises and intorts as other eye falls and extorts	Usually associated with optic chiasm defects
Nystagmus retractorius	Eyes jerk back into orbit or toward each other	Caused by pressure on mesencephalic tegmentum (Parinaud syndrome)
Gaze-evoked nystagmus	Jerk nystagmus in direction of gaze	Caused by medications, brainstem lesion, or labyrinthine dysfunction
Gaze-paretic nystagmus	Eyes jerk back to maintain eccentric gaze	Cerebellar disease
Downbeat nystagmus	Fast phase beating downward	Posterior fossa disease, drugs
Upbeat nystagmus	Fast phase beating upward	Brainstem and cerebellar disease; some visual conditions
Vestibular nystagmus	Horizontal-torsional or horizontal jerks	Vestibular system dysfunction
Asymmetric or monocular nystagmus	Pendular vertical nystagmus	Disease of retina and visual pathways
Spasmus nutans	Fine, rapid, pendular nystagmus	Torticollis, head nodding; idiopathic or gliomas of visual pathways

From Kliegman R: *Practical Strategies in Pediatric Diagnosis and Therapy.* Philadelphia, WB Saunders, 1996.

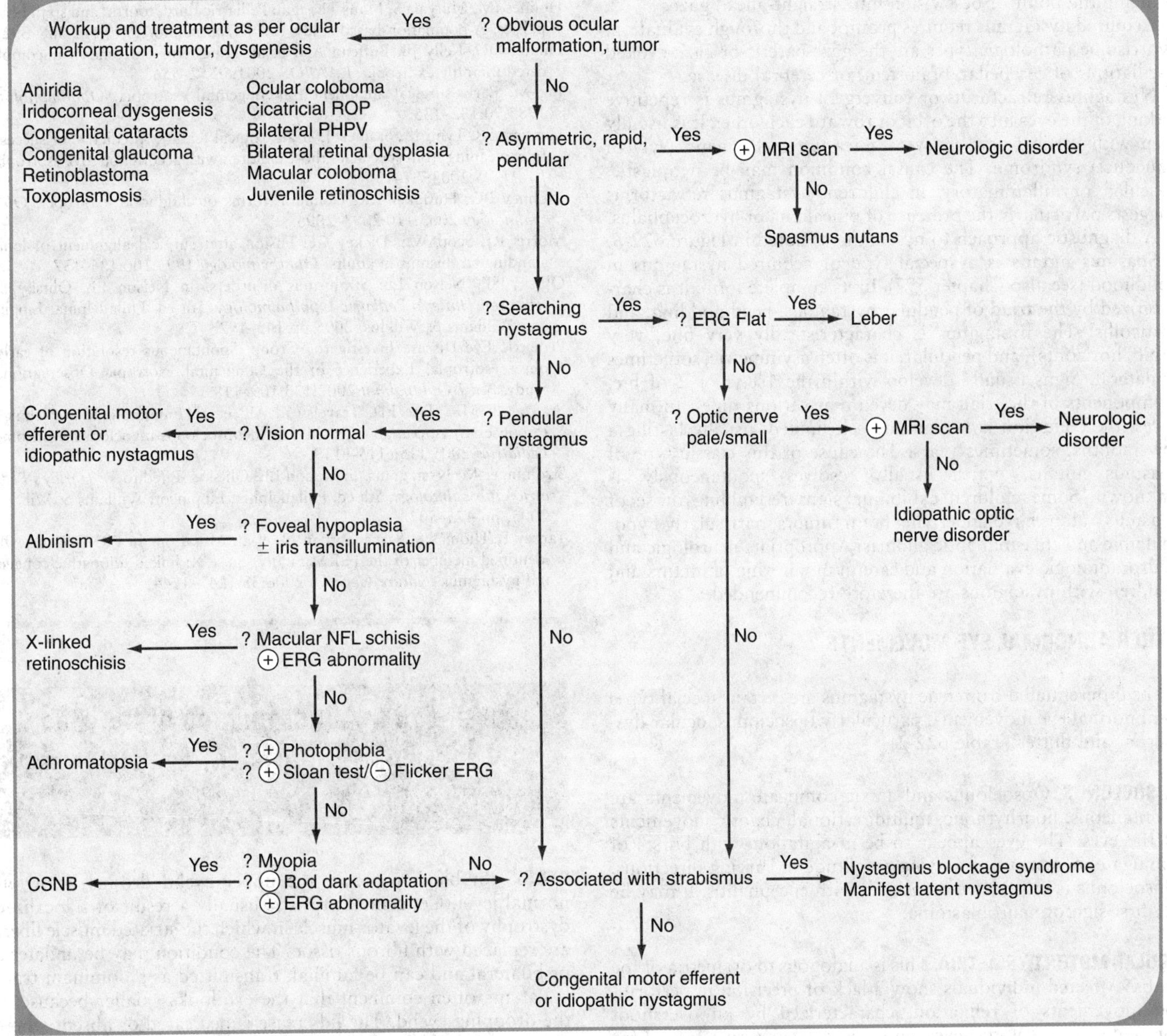

Figure 622-6. Algorithm for the work-up of an infant with nystagmus. ⊕, positive; ⊖, negative; CNNB, congenital stationary night blindness; ERG, electroretinogram; NFL, nerve fiber layer; PHPV, persistent hyperplastic primary vitreous; ROP, retinopathy of prematurity. (From Nelson LB: *Harley's Pediatric Ophthalmology,* 4th ed. Philadelphia, WB Saunders, 1998, p 470.)

TABLE 622-2. Specific Patterns of Non-nystagmus Eye Movements

PATTERN	DESCRIPTION	ASSOCIATED CONDITIONS
Opsoclonus	Multidirectional conjugate movements of varying rate and amplitude	Hydrocephalus, diseases of brainstem and cerebellum, neuroblastoma
Ocular dysmetria	Overshoot of eyes on rapid fixation	Cerebellar dysfunction
Ocular flutter	Horizontal oscillations with forward gaze and sometimes with blinking	Cerebellar disease, hydrocephalus, or central nervous system neoplasm
Ocular bobbing	Downward jerk from primary gaze, remain for a few seconds, then drift back	Pontine disease
Ocular myoclonus	Rhythmic to-and-fro pendular oscillations of the eyes, with synchronous nonocular muscle movement	Damage to red nucleus, inferior olivary nucleus, and ipsilateral dentate nucleus

From Kliegman R: *Practical Strategies in Pediatric Diagnosis and Therapy.* Philadelphia, WB Saunders, 1996.

anatomic defects that cause the nystagmus, and the visual acuity is generally near normal. There may be a null point in which the nystagmus lessens and the vision improves; a compensatory head posture will develop that places the eyes into the position of least nystagmus. The cause of congenital idiopathic motor nystagmus is unknown; in some instances, it is familial. Eye muscle surgery may be performed to eliminate an abnormal head posture by bringing the point of best vision into straight-ahead gaze.

Acquired nystagmus requires prompt and thorough evaluation. Worrisome pathologic types are the gaze-paretic or gaze-evoked oscillations of cerebellar, brainstem, or cerebral disease.

Nystagmus retractorius or **convergent nystagmus** is repetitive jerking of the eyes into the orbit or toward each other. It is usually seen with vertical gaze palsy as a feature of Parinaud (sylvian aqueduct) syndrome. The causal condition may be neoplastic, vascular, or inflammatory. In children, nystagmus retractorius suggests particularly the presence of pinealoma or hydrocephalus.

A diagnostic approach to nystagmus is noted in Figure 622-6.

Spasmus nutans is a special type of acquired nystagmus in childhood (see also Chapter 597). In its complete form, it is characterized by the **triad** of pendular nystagmus, head nodding, and torticollis. The nystagmus is characteristically very fine, very rapid, horizontal, and pendular; it is often asymmetric, sometimes unilateral. Signs usually develop within the 1st yr or 2 of life. Components of the triad may develop at various times. In many cases, the condition is benign and self-limited, usually lasting a few months, sometimes years. The cause of this classic type of spasmus nutans, which usually resolves spontaneously, is unknown. Some children exhibiting signs resembling those of spasmus nutans have underlying brain tumors, particularly hypothalamic and chiasmal optic gliomas. Appropriate neurologic and neuroradiologic evaluation and careful monitoring of infants and children with nystagmus are therefore recommended.

OTHER ABNORMAL EYE MOVEMENTS

To be differentiated from true nystagmus are certain special types of abnormal eye movements, particularly opsoclonus, ocular dysmetria, and flutter (Table 622-2).

OPSOCLONUS. Opsoclonus and ataxic conjugate movements are spontaneous, nonrhythmic, multidirectional, chaotic movements of the eyes. The eyes appear to be in agitation, with bursts of conjugate movement of varying amplitude in varying directions. Opsoclonus is most often associated with encephalitis. It may be the first sign of neuroblastoma.

OCULAR MOTOR DYSMETRIA. This is analogous to dysmetria of the limbs. Affected individuals show a lack of precision in performing movements of refixation, characterized by an overshoot (or undershoot) of the eyes with several corrective to-and-fro oscillations on looking from one point to another. Ocular motor dysmetria is a sign of cerebellar or cerebellar pathway disease.

FLUTTER-LIKE OSCILLATIONS. These intermittent to-and-fro horizontal oscillations of the eyes may occur spontaneously or on change of fixation. They are characteristic of cerebellar disease.

Abroms AD, Mohney BG, Rush DP, et al: Timely surgery in intermittent and constant exotropia for superior sensory outcome. *Am J Ophthalmol* 2001;131:111–116.

Holmes JM, Mutyala S, Maus TL, et al: Pediatric third, fourth, and sixth nerve palsies: A population-based study. *Am J Ophthalmol* 1999;127:388–392.

Hunter DG, Kelly JB, Buffenn AN, et al: Long-term outcome of uncomplicated infantile exotropia. *J AAPOS* 2001;5:352–356.

Ing M: Early surgical alignment for congenital esotropia. *Ophthalmology* 1983;90:132–135.

Lambert SR, Lynn M, Sramek J, et al: Clinical features predictive of successfully weaning from spectacles those children with accommodative esotropia. *J AAPOS* 2003;7:7–13.

Mohney BG, Huffaker RK: Common forms of childhood exotropia. *Ophthalmology* 2003;110:2093–2096.

Morris RJ, Scott WE, Dickey CF: Fusion after surgical alignment of longstanding strabismus in adults. *Ophthalmology* 1993;100:135–137.

Olitsky SE, Nelson LB: Strabismus disorders. In Nelson LB, Olitsky SE (editors): *Harley's Pediatric Ophthalmology,* 5th ed. Philadelphia, Lippincott Williams & Wilkins, 2005 pp 143–192.

Pediatric Eye Disease Investigator Group: Spontaneous resolution of early-onset esotropia: Experience of the Congenital Esotropia Observational Study. *Am J Ophthalmol* 2002;133:109–118.

Pranzatelli MR, Tate ED, Travelstead AL, et al: Immunologic and clinical responses to rituximab in a child with opsoclonus-myoclonus syndrome. *Pediatrics* 2005;115:e115–e119.

Strominger M: Nystagmus. In Nelson LB, Olitsky SE (editors): *Harley's Pediatric Ophthalmology,* 5th ed. Philadelphia, Lippincott Williams & Wilkins, 2005, pp 475–507.

Tarpey P, Thomas S, Sarvananthan N, et al: Mutations in FRMDT, a newly identified member of the FERM family, cause X: linked idiopathic congenital nystagmus. *Nature Genetics* 2006;38:1242–1244.

Chapter 623 ■ Abnormalities of the Lids

Scott E. Olitsky, Denise Hug, and Laura P. Smith

PTOSIS. In blepharoptosis, the upper eyelid droops below its normal level. Congenital ptosis is usually a result of a localized dystrophy of the levator muscle in which the striated muscle fibers are replaced with fibrous tissue. The condition may be unilateral or bilateral and can be familial, transmitted as a dominant trait.

Parents often comment that the eye looks smaller because of the drooping eyelid. The lid crease is decreased or absent where the levator muscle would normally insert below the skin surface. Because the levator is replaced by fibrous tissue, the lid does not move downward fully in downgaze (lid lag). If the ptosis is severe, affected children often attempt to raise the lid by lifting their brow or adapting a chin-up head posture to maintain binocular vision. **Marcus Gunn jaw-winking ptosis** accounts for 5% of ptosis in children. In this syndrome, an abnormal synkinesis exists between the 5th and 3rd cranial nerves; this causes the eyelid to elevate with movement of the jaw. The wink is produced by chewing or sucking and may be more noticeable than the ptosis itself.

Although ptosis in children is often an isolated finding, it may occur in association with other ocular or systemic disorders. Systemic disorders include myasthenia gravis, muscular dystrophy, and botulism. Ocular disorders include mechanical ptosis secondary to lid tumors, blepharophimosis syndrome, congenital fibrosis syndrome, combined levator/superior rectus maldevelopment, and congenital or acquired 3rd nerve palsy. A small degree of ptosis is seen in Horner syndrome (see Chapter 621). A complete ophthalmic and systemic examination is therefore important in the evaluation of a child with ptosis.

Amblyopia may occur in children with ptosis. The amblyopia may be secondary to the lid's covering the visual axis (deprivation) or induced astigmatism (anisometropia). When amblyopia occurs, it should generally be treated before treating the ptosis.

Treatment of ptosis in a child is indicated for elimination of an abnormal head posture, improvement in the visual field, prevention of amblyopia, and restoration of a normal eyelid appearance. The timing of surgery depends on the degree of ptosis, its cosmetic and functional severity, the presence or absence of compensatory posturing, the wishes of the parents, and the discretion of the surgeon. Surgical treatment is determined by the amount of levator function that is present. A levator resection may be used in children with moderate to good function. In patients with poor or absent function, a frontalis suspension procedure may be necessary. This technique requires that a suspension material be placed between the frontalis muscle and the tarsus of the eyelid. It allows patients to use their brow and frontalis muscle more effectively to raise their eyelid. Amblyopia remains a concern even after surgical correction and should be monitored closely.

EPICANTHAL FOLDS. These vertical or oblique folds of skin extend on either side of the bridge of the nose from the brow or lid area, covering the inner canthal region. They are present to some degree in most young children and become less apparent with age. The folds may be sufficiently broad to cover the medial aspect of the eye, making the eyes appear crossed (pseudoesotropia). Epicanthal folds are a common feature of many syndromes, including chromosomal aberrations (trisomies) and disorders of single genes.

LAGOPHTHALMOS. This is a condition in which complete closure of the lids over the globe is difficult or impossible. It may be paralytic because of a facial palsy involving the orbicularis muscle, or spastic, as in thyrotoxicosis. It may be structural when retraction or shortening of the lids results from scarring or atrophy consequent to injury (burns) or disease. Infants with collodion membrane may have temporary lagophthalmos caused by the restrictive effect of the membrane on the lids. Lagophthalmos may accompany proptosis or buphthalmos when the lids, although normal, cannot effectively cover the enlarged or protuberant eye. A degree of physiologic lagophthalmos may occur normally during sleep, but functional lagophthalmos in an unconscious or debilitated patient can be a problem.

In patients with lagophthalmos, exposure of the eye may lead to drying, infection, corneal ulceration, or perforation of the cornea; the result may be loss of vision, even loss of the eye. In lagophthalmos, protection of the eye by artificial tear preparations, ophthalmic ointment, or moisture chambers is essential. Gauze pads are to be avoided because the gauze may abrade the cornea. In some cases, surgical closure of the lids (tarsorrhaphy) may be necessary for long-term protection of the eye.

LID RETRACTIONS. Pathologic retraction of the lid may be myogenic or neurogenic. Myogenic retraction of the upper lid occurs in thyrotoxicosis, in which it is associated with three classic signs: a staring appearance (Dalrymple sign), infrequent blinking (Stellwag sign), and lag of the upper lid on downward gaze (von Graefe sign).

Neurogenic retraction of the lids may occur in conditions affecting the anterior mesencephalon. Lid retraction is a feature of the syndrome of the sylvian aqueduct. In children, it is commonly a sign of hydrocephalus. It may occur with meningitis. Paradoxical retraction of the lid is seen in the Marcus Gunn jaw-winking syndrome. It may also be seen with attempted eye movement after recovery from a 3rd nerve palsy, if aberrant regeneration of the oculomotor nerve fibers has occurred.

Simple staring and the physiologic or reflexive lid retraction ("eye popping"), in contrast to pathologic lid retractions, occur in infants in response to a sudden reduction in illumination or as a startle reaction.

ECTROPION, ENTROPION, AND EPIBLEPHARON. **Ectropion** is eversion of the lid margin; it may lead to overflow of tears (epiphora) and subsequent maceration of the skin of the lid, inflammation of exposed conjunctiva, or superficial exposure keratopathy. Common causes are scarring consequent to inflammation, burns, or trauma, or weakness of the orbicularis muscle as a result of facial palsy; these forms may be corrected surgically. Protection of the cornea is essential. Ectropion is also seen in certain children who have faulty development of the lateral canthal ligament; this may occur in Down syndrome.

Entropion is inversion of the lid margin, which may cause discomfort and corneal damage because of the inward turning of the lashes (trichiasis). A principal cause is scarring secondary to inflammation such as occurs in trachoma or as a sequela of Stevens-Johnson syndrome. There is also a rare congenital form. Surgical correction is effective in many cases.

Epiblepharon is commonly seen in childhood and may be confused with entropion. In epiblepharon, a roll of skin beneath the lower eyelid lashes causes the lashes to be directed vertically and to touch the cornea (Fig. 623-1). Unlike entropion, the eyelid margin itself is not rotated toward the cornea. Epiblepharon usually resolves spontaneously. If corneal scarring begins to occur, surgical correction may be necessary.

BLEPHAROSPASM. This spastic or repetitive closure of the lids may be caused by irritative disease of the cornea, conjunctiva, or facial nerve; fatigue or uncorrected refractive error; or common tic. Thorough ophthalmic examination for pathologic causes, such as trichiasis, keratitis, conjunctivitis, or foreign body, is indicated. Local injection of botulinum toxin may give relief but frequently must be repeated.

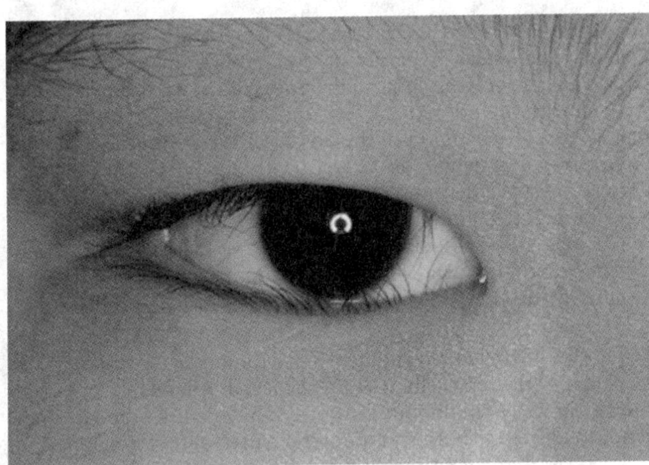

Figure 623-1. Epiblepharon.

BLEPHARITIS. This inflammation of the lid margins is characterized by erythema and crusting or scaling; the usual symptoms are irritation, burning, and itching. The condition is commonly bilateral and chronic or recurrent. The two main types are **staphylococcal** and **seborrheic.** In staphylococcal blepharitis, ulceration of the lid margin is common, the lashes tend to fall out, and conjunctivitis and superficial keratitis are often associated. In seborrheic blepharitis, the scales tend to be greasy, the lid margins are less red, and ulceration usually does not occur. The blepharitis is often of mixed type.

Thorough daily cleansing of the lid margins with a cloth or moistened cotton applicator to remove scales and crusts is important in the **treatment** of both forms. Staphylococcal blepharitis is treated with an antistaphylococcal antibiotic applied directly to the lid margins. When a child also has seborrhea, concurrent treatment of the scalp is important.

Pediculosis of the eyelashes may produce a clinical picture of blepharitis. The lice can be smothered with ophthalmic-grade petrolatum ointment applied to the lid margin and lashes. Nits should be mechanically removed from the lashes. It should be remembered that pediculosis represents a sexually transmitted disease.

HORDEOLUM. Infection of the glands of the lid may be acute or subacute; tender focal swelling and redness are noted. The usual agent is *Staphylococcus aureus.* When the meibomian glands are involved, the lesion is referred to as an internal hordeolum; the abscess tends to be large and may point through either the skin or the conjunctival surface. When the infection involves the glands of Zeis or Moll, the abscess tends to be smaller and more superficial and points at the lid margin; it is then referred to as an external hordeolum or stye.

Treatment is frequent warm compresses and, if necessary, surgical incision and drainage. In addition, topical antibiotic preparations are often used. Untreated, the infection may progress to cellulitis of the lid or orbit, requiring the use of systemic antibiotics.

CHALAZION. A chalazion is a granulomatous inflammation of a meibomian gland characterized by a firm, nontender nodule in the upper or lower lid. This lesion tends to be chronic and differs from internal hordeolum in the absence of acute inflammatory signs. Although many chalazia subside spontaneously, excision may be necessary if they become large enough to distort vision (by inducing astigmatism by exerting pressure on the globe) or to be a cosmetic blemish. Patients who experience frequent chalazia formation, or those who have significant corneal changes secondary to the underlying blepharitis, may benefit from systemic erythromycin treatment.

COLOBOMA OF THE EYELID. This cleftlike deformity may vary from a small indentation or notch of the free margin of the lid to a large defect involving almost the entire lid. If the gap is extensive, ulceration and corneal opacities may result from exposure. Early surgical correction of the lid defect is recommended. Other deformities frequently associated with lid colobomas include dermoid cysts or dermolipomas on the globe; they often occur in a position corresponding to the site of the lid defect. Lid colobomas may also be associated with extensive facial malformation, as in mandibulofacial dysostosis (Franceschetti or Treacher Collins syndrome).

TUMORS OF THE LID. A number of lid tumors arise from surface structures (the epithelium and sebaceous glands). Nevi may appear in early childhood; most are junctional. Compound nevi tend to develop in the prepubertal years and dermal nevi at puberty. Malignant epithelial tumors (basal cell carcinoma, squamous cell carcinoma) are rare in children, but the basal cell nevus syndrome and the malignant lesions of xeroderma pigmentosum and of Rothmund-Thomson syndrome may develop in childhood.

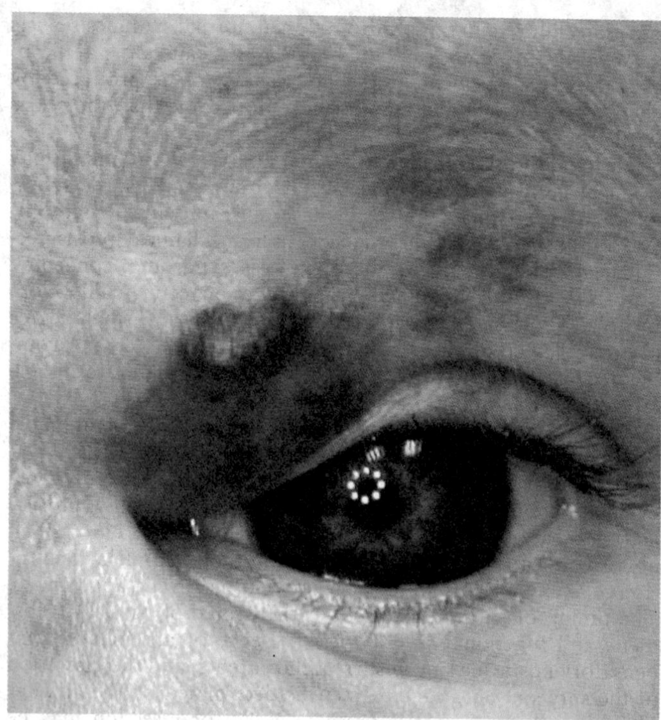

Figure 623-2. Capillary hemangioma of the eyelid. (Courtesy of Amy Nopper, MD, and Brandon Newell, MD.)

Other lid tumors arise from deeper structures (the neural, vascular, and connective tissues). Capillary hemangiomas are especially common in children (Fig. 623-2). Many tend to regress spontaneously, although they may show alarmingly rapid growth in infancy. In many cases, the best management of such hemangiomas is patient observation, allowing spontaneous regression to occur (see Chapter 649). In the case of a rapidly expanding lesion, which may cause amblyopia by obstructing the visual axis or inducing astigmatism, corticosteroid, interferon, or surgical treatment should be considered. Nevus flammeus (port-wine stain), a noninvoluting hemangioma, occurs as an isolated lesion or in association with other signs of Sturge-Weber syndrome. Affected patients should be monitored for the development of glaucoma. Lymphangiomas of the lid appear as firm masses at or soon after birth and tend to enlarge slowly during the growing years. Associated conjunctival involvement, appearing as a clear, cystic, sinuous conjunctival mass, may provide a clue to the diagnosis. In some cases, there is also orbital involvement. The **treatment** is surgical excision.

Plexiform neuromas of the lids occur in children with neurofibromatosis, often with ptosis as the first sign. The lid may take on an S-shaped configuration. The lids may also be involved by other tumors, such as retinoblastoma, neuroblastoma, and rhabdomyosarcoma of the orbit; these conditions are discussed elsewhere.

Dray JP, Leibovitch I: Congenital ptosis and amblyopia: A retrospective study of 130 cases. *J Pediatr Ophthalmol Strabismus* 2002;39:222–225.
Drolet BA, Esterly NB, Frieden IJ: Hemangiomas in children. *N Engl J Med* 1999;341:173–181.
Gusek-Schneider GC, Martus P: Stimulus deprivation amblyopia in human congenital ptosis: A study of 100 patients. *Strabismus* 2000;8:261–270.
Meisler DM, Raizman MB, Traboulsi EI: Oral erythromycin treatment for childhood blepharokeratitis. *J AAPOS* 2000;4:379–380.
Plager DA, Snyder SK: Resolution of astigmatism after surgical resection of capillary hemangiomas in infants. *Ophthalmology* 1997;104:1102–1106.

Sterker I, Grafe G: Periocular hemangiomas in childhood—functional and esthetic results. *Strabismus* 2004;12:103–110.
Wasserman BN, Sprunger DT, Helveston EM: Comparison of materials used in frontalis suspension. *Arch Ophthalmol* 2001;119:687–691.

Chapter 624 ■ Disorders of the Lacrimal System

Scott E. Olitsky, Denise Hug, and Laura P. Smith

THE TEAR FILM. This film, which bathes the eye, is actually a complex structure composed of three layers. The innermost mucin layer is secreted by the goblet and epithelial cells of the conjunctiva and the acinar cells of the lacrimal gland. It adds stability and provides an attachment for the tear film to the conjunctiva and cornea. The middle aqueous layer constitutes 98% of the tear film and is produced by the main lacrimal gland and accessory lacrimal glands. It contains various electrolytes and proteins as well as antibodies. The outermost lipid layer is produced largely from the sebaceous meibomian glands of the eyelid and retards evaporation of the tear film. Tears drain medially into the punctal openings of the lid margin and flow through the canaliculi into the lacrimal sac and then through the nasolacrimal duct into the nose. Preterm infants have reduced tear secretion. This may mask the diagnosis of a nasolacrimal duct obstruction and concentrate topically applied medications. Tear production reaches adult levels near term.

DACRYOSTENOSIS. Congenital nasolacrimal duct obstruction (CNLDO), or dacryostenosis, is the most common disorder of the lacrimal system, occurring in up to 6% of newborn infants. It is usually caused by a failure of canalization of the epithelial cells that form the nasolacrimal duct as it enters the nose (valve of Hasner). Signs of CNLDO may be present at the time of birth, although the condition may not become evident until normal tear production develops. Signs of CNLDO include an excessive tear lake, overflow of tears onto the lid and cheek, and reflux of mucoid material that is produced in the lacrimal sac. Erythema or maceration of the skin may result from irritation and rubbing produced by dripping of tears and discharge. If the blockage is complete, these signs may be severe and continuous. If obstruction is only partial, the nasolacrimal duct may be capable of draining the basal tear film that is produced. However, under periods of increased tear production (exposure to cold, wind, sunlight) or increased closure of the distal end of the nasolacrimal duct (nasal mucosal edema), tear overflow may become evident or may increase.

Infants with CNLDO may develop acute infection and inflammation of the nasolacrimal sac (**dacryocystitis**), inflammation of the surrounding tissues (**pericystitis**), or rarely periorbital cellulitis. With dacryocystitis, the sac area is swollen, red, and tender, and patients may have systemic signs of infection such as fever and irritability.

The primary **treatment** of uncomplicated nasolacrimal obstruction is a regimen of nasolacrimal massage, usually 2–3 times daily, accompanied by cleansing of the lids with warm water. Topical antibiotics are used for significant mucopurulent drainage. Most cases of CNLDO resolve spontaneously; 96% before 1 yr of age. For cases that do not resolve by 1 yr, the nasolacrimal duct may be probed, with a cure rate of approximately 90%. For cases in which a probing fails to eliminate the tearing, further options include a repeat probing, insertion of silicone stents, or balloon dacryoplasty.

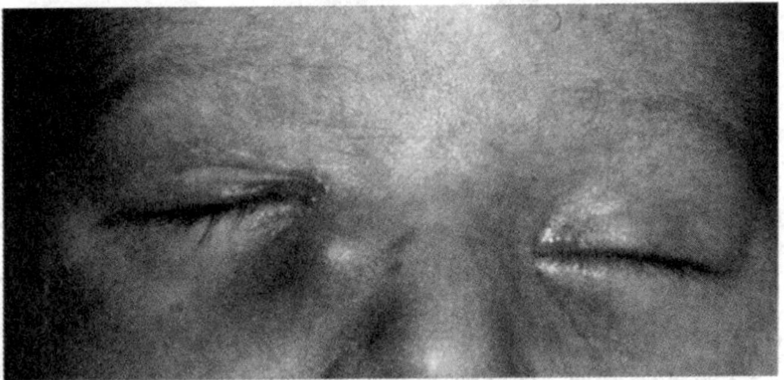

Figure 624-1. Dacryocystocele below inner canthus of the right eye.

Acute dacryocystitis or cellulitis requires prompt treatment with antibiotics. In such cases, some form of definitive surgical intervention is usually indicated.

A **dacryocystocele** (mucocele) is an unusual presentation of a nonpatent nasolacrimal sac that is obstructed both proximally and distally. Dacryocystoceles can be seen at birth or shortly after birth as a bluish subcutaneous mass just below the medial canthal tendon (Fig. 624-1). Initial treatment should include warm compresses and gentle massage of the lacrimal sac. If an infection develops, systemic administration of antibiotics is required. A probing of the nasolacrimal system may then be necessary to prevent further infection or treat abscess formation.

Not all tearing in infants and children is caused by nasolacrimal obstruction. Tearing may also be a sign of glaucoma, intraocular inflammation, or external irritation, such as that from a corneal abrasion or foreign body.

ALACRIMA AND "DRY EYE." Marked deficiency of tears may occur as an isolated unilateral or bilateral congenital defect or in association with other nervous system anomalies, such as aplasia of cranial nerve nuclei. It occurs congenitally in familial dysautonomia (Riley-Day syndrome) and in the anhidrotic type of ectodermal dysplasia. Alacrima is seen in the **triple-A syndrome** or **Allgrove syndrome,** which is characterized by adrenocorticotropic hormone–resistant adrenal insufficiency, achalasia of the esophageal cardia, and alacrima. Patients frequently suffer from neurologic disturbances.

An acquired abnormality of any layer of the tear film may produce a dry eye. Commonly acquired disorders that may lead to a decreased or unstable tear film include Sjögren syndrome, Stevens-Johnson syndrome, vitamin A deficiency, ocular pemphigoid, trachoma, chemical burns, irradiation, and meibomian gland dysfunction. Any tear deficiency can lead to corneal ulceration, scarring, or infection. **Treatment** includes correction of the underlying disorder when possible and frequent instillation of an artificial tear preparation. In some cases, occlusion of the lacrimal puncta is helpful. In severe cases, tarsorrhaphy may be necessary to protect the cornea.

Honavar SG, Prakash VE, Rao GN: Outcome of probing for congenital nasolacrimal duct obstruction in older children. *Am J Ophthalmol* 2000;130:42–48.
Huebner A, Yoon SJ, Ozkinay F, et al: Triple A syndrome—clinical aspects and molecular genetics. *Endocr Res* 2000;26:751–759.
Kushner BJ: Congenital nasolacrimal system obstruction. *Arch Ophthalmol* 1982;100:597–600.
MacEwen CJ, Young JD: Epiphora during the first year of life. *Eye* 1991;5:596–600.
O'Driscoll TG: Alacrima. *Trans Ophthalmol Soc* 1975;95:13–14.
Schnall BM, Christian CJ: Conservative treatment of congenital dacryocele. *J Pediatr Ophthalmol Strabismus* 1996;33:219–222.
Young JD, MacEwen CJ: Managing congenital lacrimal obstruction in general practice. *Br Med J* 1997;315:293–296.

Chapter 625 ■ Disorders of the Conjunctiva

Scott E. Olitsky, Denise Hug, and Laura P. Smith

CONJUNCTIVITIS

The conjunctiva reacts to a wide range of bacterial and viral agents, allergens, irritants, toxins, and systemic diseases. Conjunctivitis is common in childhood and may be infectious or noninfectious. The differential diagnosis of a red-appearing eye includes conjunctival as well as other ocular sites (Table 625-1).

OPHTHALMIA NEONATORUM. This form of conjunctivitis, occurring in infants younger than 4 wk of age, is the most common eye disease of newborns. Its many different causal agents vary greatly in their virulence and outcome. Silver nitrate instillation may result in a mild self-limited chemical conjunctivitis, whereas *Neisseria gonorrhoeae* and *Pseudomonas* are capable of causing corneal perforation, blindness, and death. The risk of conjunctivitis in newborns depends on frequencies of maternal infections, prophylactic measures, circumstances during labor and delivery, and postdelivery exposures to microorganisms.

Epidemiology. Conjunctivitis during the neonatal period is usually acquired during vaginal delivery and reflects the sexually transmitted infections prevalent in the community. In 1880, 10% of European children developed gonococcal conjunctivitis at birth. Ophthalmia neonatorum was the leading cause of blindness during that period. The epidemiology of this condition changed dramatically in 1881, when Crede reported that 2% silver nitrate solution instilled in the eyes of newborns reduced the incidence of gonococcal ophthalmia from 10% to 0.3%.

During the 20th century, the incidence of gonococcal ophthalmia neonatorum decreased in industrialized countries secondary to widespread use of silver nitrate prophylaxis and prenatal screening and treatment of maternal gonorrhea. Gonococcal ophthalmia neonatorum has an incidence of 0.3/1,000 live births in the United States. In comparison, *Chlamydia trachomatis* is the most common organism causing ophthalmia neonatorum in the United States, with an incidence of 8.2/1,000 births.

Clinical Manifestations. The clinical manifestations of the various forms of ophthalmia neonatorum are not specific enough to allow an accurate diagnosis. Although the timing and character of the signs are somewhat typical for each cause of this condition, there is considerable overlap and physicians should not rely solely on clinical findings. Regardless of its cause, ophthalmia neonatorum is characterized by redness and chemosis (swelling) of the conjunctiva, edema of the eyelids, and discharge, which may be purulent.

Ophthalmia neonatorum is a potentially blinding condition. The infection may also have associated systemic manifestations that require treatment. Therefore, any newborn infant who develops signs of conjunctivitis needs a prompt and comprehensive systemic and ocular evaluation to determine the agent causing the infection and the appropriate treatment.

The onset of inflammation caused by silver nitrate drops usually occurs within 6–12 hr after birth, with clearing by 24–48 hr. The usual incubation period for conjunctivitis due to *N. gonorrhoeae* is 2–5 days, and for that due to *C. trachomatis*, it is 5–14 days. Gonococcal infection may be present at birth or be delayed beyond 5 days of life owing to partial suppression by ocular prophylaxis. Gonococcal conjunctivitis may also begin in

TABLE 625-1. The Red Eye

CONDITION	ETIOLOGY	SIGNS AND SYMPTOMS	TREATMENT
Bacterial conjunctivitis	*Haemophilus influenzae, Haemophilus aegyptius, Streptococcus pneumoniae* *Neisseria gonorrhoeae*	Mucopurulent unilateral or bilateral discharge, normal vision, photophobia Conjunctival injection and edema (chemosis); gritty sensation	Topical antibiotics, parenteral ceftriaxone for gonococcus, *H. influenzae*
Viral conjunctivitis	Adenovirus, ECHO virus, coxsackievirus	As above; may be hemorrhagic, unilateral	Self-limited
Neonatal conjunctivitis	*Chlamydia trachomatis*, gonococcus, chemical (silver nitrate), *Staphylococcus aureus*	Palpebral conjunctival follicle or papillae; as above	Ceftriaxone for gonococcus and erythromycin for *C. trachomatis*
Allergic conjunctivitis	Seasonal pollens or allergen exposure	Itching, incidence of bilateral chemosis (edema) greater than that of erythema, tarsal papillae	Antihistamines, steroids, cromolyn
Keratitis	Herpes simplex virus, adenovirus, *S. pneumoniae, S. aureus, Pseudomonas, Acanthamoeba*, chemicals	Severe pain, corneal swelling, clouding, limbus erythema, hypopyon, cataracts; contact lens history with amebic infection	Specific antibiotics for bacterial/fungal infections; keratoplasty, acyclovir for herpes
Endophthalmitis	*S. aureus, S. pneumoniae, Candida albicans*, associated surgery or trauma	Acute onset, pain, loss of vision, swelling, chemosis, redness; hypopyon and vitreous haze	Antibiotics
Anterior uveitis (iridocyclitis)	JRA, post infectious with arthritis and rash, sarcoidosis, Behçet disease, Kawasaki disease, inflammatory bowel disease	Unilateral/bilateral; erythema, ciliary flush, irregular pupil, iris adhesions; pain, photophobia, small pupil, poor vision	Topical steroids, plus therapy for primary disease
Posterior uveitis (choroiditis)	Toxoplasmosis, histoplasmosis, *Toxocara canis*	No signs of erythema, decreased vision	Specific therapy for pathogen
Episcleritis/scleritis	Idiopathic autoimmune disease (e.g., SLE, Henoch-Schönlein purpura)	Localized pain, intense erythema, unilateral; blood vessels bigger than in conjunctivitis; scleritis may cause globe perforation	Episcleritis is self-limiting; topical steroids for fast relief
Foreign body	Occupational exposure	Unilateral, red, gritty feeling; visible or microscopic size	Irrigation, removal; check for ulceration
Blepharitis	*S. aureus, Staphylococcus epidermidis*, seborrheic, blocked lacrimal duct; rarely molluscum contagiosum, *Phthirus pubis, Pediculus capitis*	Bilateral, irritation, itching, hyperemia, crusting, affecting lid margins	Topical antibiotics, warm compresses
Dacryocystitis	Obstructed lacrimal sac: *S. aureus, H. influenzae*, pneumococcus	Pain, tenderness, erythema and exudates in area of lacrimal sac (inferomedial to inner canthus); tearing (epiphora); possible orbital cellulites	Systemic, topical antibiotics; surgical drainage
Dacryoadenitis	*S. aureus, Streptococcus*, CMV, measles, EBV, enteroviruses; trauma, sarcoidosis, leukemia	Pain, tenderness, edema, erythema over gland area (upper temporal lid); fever, leukocytosis	Systemic antibiotics; drainage of orbital abscesses
Orbital cellulitis (postseptal cellulitis)	Paranasal sinusitis: *H. influenzae, S. aureus, S. pneumoniae*, streptococci Trauma: *S. aureus* Fungi: *Aspergillus, Mucor* spp. if immunodeficient	Rhinorrhea, chemosis, vision loss, painful extraocular motion, proptosis, ophthalmoplegia, fever, lid edema, leukocytosis	Systemic antibiotics, drainage of orbital abscesses
Periorbital cellulitis (preseptal cellulitis)	Trauma: *S. aureus*, streptococci Bacteremia: pneumococcus, streptococci, *H. influenzae*	Cutaneous erythema, warmth, normal vision, minimal involvement of orbit; fever, leukocytosis, toxic appearance	Systemic antibiotics

CMV, cytomegalovirus; EBV, Epstein-Barr virus; JRA, juvenile rheumatoid arthritis; SLE, systemic lupus erythematosus.
From Behrman R, Kliegman R: *Nelson's Essentials of Pediatrics*, 3rd ed. Philadelphia, WB Saunders, 1998.

infancy after inoculation by the contaminated fingers of adults. The time of onset of disease with other bacteria is highly variable.

Gonococcal conjunctivitis begins with mild inflammation and a serosanguineous discharge. Within 24 hr, the discharge becomes thick and purulent, and tense edema of the eyelids with marked chemosis occurs. If proper treatment is delayed, the infection may spread to involve the deeper layers of the conjunctivae and the cornea. Complications include corneal ulceration and perforation, iridocyclitis, anterior synechiae, and rarely panophthalmitis. Conjunctivitis caused by *C. trachomatis* (inclusion blennorrhea) may vary from mild inflammation to severe swelling of the eyelids with copious purulent discharge. The process involves mainly the tarsal conjunctivae; the corneas are rarely affected. Conjunctivitis due to *Staphylococcus aureus* or other organisms is similar to that produced by *C. trachomatis.* Conjunctivitis due to *Pseudomonas aeruginosa* is uncommon, acquired in the nursery, and a potentially serious process. It is characterized by the appearance on days 5–18 of edema, erythema of the lids, purulent discharge, pannus formation, endophthalmitis, sepsis, shock, and death.

Diagnosis. Conjunctivitis appearing after 48 hr should be evaluated for a possibly infectious cause. Gram stain of the purulent discharge should be performed and the material cultured. If a viral cause is suspected, a swab should be submitted in tissue culture media for virus isolation. In chlamydial conjunctivitis, the diagnosis is made by examining Giemsa-stained epithelial cells scraped from the tarsal conjunctivae for the characteristic intracytoplasmic inclusions, by isolating the organisms from a conjunctival swab using special tissue culture techniques, by immunofluorescent staining of conjunctival scrapings for chlamydial inclusions, or by tests for chlamydial antigen or DNA. The differential diagnosis includes dacryocystitis caused by congenital lacrimal duct obstruction with lacrimal sac distention (dacryocystocele).

TREATMENT. Treatment of infants in whom gonococcal ophthalmia is suspected and the Gram stain shows the characteristic intracellular gram-negative diplococci should be initiated immediately with ceftriaxone, 50 mg/kg/24 hr for 1 dose, not to exceed 125 mg. The eye should also be irrigated initially with saline every 10–30 min, gradually increasing to 2-hr intervals until the purulent discharge has cleared. An alternative regimen includes cefotaxime (100 mg/kg/24 hr given IV or IM every 12 hr for 7 days or 100 mg/kg as a single dose). Treatment is extended if sepsis or other extraocular sites are involved (meningitis, arthritis). Inclusion blennorrhea is treated with oral erythromycin (50 mg/kg/24 hr in 4 divided doses) for 2 wk. This cures conjunctivitis and may prevent subsequent chlamydial pneumonia. *Pseudomonas* neonatal conjunctivitis is treated with systemic antibiotics, including an aminoglycoside, plus local saline irrigation and gentamicin ophthalmic ointment. Staphylococcal conjunctivitis is treated with parenteral methicillin and local saline irrigation.

PROGNOSIS AND PREVENTION. Before the institution of topical ophthalmic prophylaxis at birth, gonococcal ophthalmia was a common cause of blindness or permanent eye damage. If properly applied, this form of prophylaxis is highly effective unless infection is present at birth. Drops of 0.5% erythromycin or 1% silver nitrate are instilled directly into the open eyes at birth using wax or plastic single-dose containers. Saline irrigation after silver nitrate application is unnecessary. Silver nitrate is ineffective against active infection. Povidone-iodine (2% solution) may also be an effective prophylactic agent.

Identification of maternal gonococcal infection and appropriate treatment has become a standard element of routine prenatal care. An infant born to a woman who has untreated gonococcal infection should receive a single dose of ceftriaxone, 50 mg/kg (maximum 125 mg) IV or IM, in addition to topical prophylaxis. The dose should be reduced for premature infants. Penicillin (50,000 U) should be used if the mother's gonococcal isolate is known to be penicillin sensitive.

Neither topical prophylaxis nor topical treatment prevents the afebrile pneumonia that occurs in 10–20% of infants exposed to *C. trachomatis.* Although chlamydial conjunctivitis is often a self-limiting disease, chlamydial pneumonia may have serious consequences. It is important that infants with chlamydial disease receive systemic treatment. Treatment of colonized pregnant women with erythromycin may prevent neonatal disease.

ACUTE PURULENT CONJUNCTIVITIS. This is characterized by more or less generalized conjunctival hyperemia, edema, mucopurulent exudate, glued eyes (lids stuck together after sleeping), and various degrees of ocular pain and discomfort. It is usually a result of bacterial infection. The most frequent causes are nontypable *Haemophilus influenzae* (associated with ipsilateral otitis media), pneumococci, staphylococci, and streptococci. Bacterial purulent conjunctivitis, especially due to pneumococcus or *H. influenzae* may occur in epidemics. Conjunctival smear and culture are helpful in differentiating specific types. These common forms of acute purulent conjunctivitis usually respond well to warm compresses and frequent topical instillation of antibiotic drops. Brazilian purpuric fever due to *Haemophilus aegyptius* manifests as conjunctivitis and sepsis. *N. gonorrhoeae* and *Chlamydia* are relatively common causes of acute purulent conjunctivitis in children beyond the newborn period, especially in adolescents. These infections require specific testing and treatment.

VIRAL CONJUNCTIVITIS. This is generally characterized by a watery discharge. Follicular changes (small aggregates of lymphocytes) are often found in the palpebral conjunctiva. Conjunctivitis resulting from adenovirus infection is relatively common, sometimes with corneal involvement as well as pharyngitis or pneumonia. Outbreaks of conjunctivitis caused by enterovirus are also encountered; this type may be hemorrhagic. Acute hemorrhagic conjunctivitis may be epidemic due to enterovirus CA24 or 70 and is characterized by red, swollen, and painful eyes with a hemorrhagic watery discharge. Conjunctivitis is commonly associated with such systemic viral infections as the childhood exanthems, particularly measles. Viral conjunctivitis is usually self-limited.

EPIDEMIC KERATOCONJUNCTIVITIS. This is caused by adenovirus type 8 and is transmitted by direct contact. It initially presents as a sensation of a foreign body beneath the lids, with itching and burning. Edema and photophobia develop rapidly, and large oval follicles appear within the conjunctiva. Preauricular adenopathy and a pseudomembrane on the conjunctival surface occur frequently. Subepithelial corneal infiltrates may develop and may cause blurring of vision; these usually disappear but may permanently reduce visual acuity. Corneal complications are less common in children than in adults. Children may have associated upper respiratory tract infection and pharyngitis. No specific medical therapy is available to decrease the symptoms or shorten the course of the disease. Emphasis must be placed on prevention of spread of the disease. Replicating virus is present in 95% of patients 10 days after the appearance of symptoms.

MEMBRANOUS AND PSEUDOMEMBRANOUS CONJUNCTIVITIS. These types can be encountered in a number of diseases. The classic membranous conjunctivitis is that of diphtheria, accompanied by a fibrin-rich exudate that forms on the conjunctival surface and permeates the epithelium; the membrane is removed with difficulty and leaves raw bleeding areas. In pseudomembranous conjunctivitis, the layer of fibrin-rich exudate is superficial and can often be stripped easily, leaving the surface smooth. This type occurs with many bacterial and viral infections, including staphylococcal, pneumococcal, streptococcal, or chlamydial conjunctivitis, and in epidemic keratoconjunctivitis. It is also found in vernal conjunctivitis and in Stevens-Johnson disease.

ALLERGIC CONJUNCTIVITIS. This is usually accompanied by intense itching, clear watery tearing, and conjunctival edema. It is commonly seasonal. Cold compresses and decongestant drops give symptomatic relief. Topical mast cell stabilizers or prostaglandin inhibitors may also help. In selected cases, topical corticosteroids are used under an ophthalmologist's supervision.

VERNAL CONJUNCTIVITIS. This usually begins in the prepubertal years and may recur for many years. Atopy appears to have a role in its origin, but the pathogenesis is uncertain. Extreme itching and tearing are the usual complaints. Large, flattened, cobblestone-like papillary lesions of the palpebral conjunctivae are characteristic (Fig. 625-1). A stringy exudate and a milky conjunctival pseudomembrane are frequently present. Small elevated lesions of the bulbar conjunctiva adjacent to the limbus (limbal form) may be found. Smear of the conjunctival exudate reveals many eosinophils. Topical corticosteroid therapy and cold compresses afford some relief. Topical mast cell stabilizers or prostaglandin inhibitors are useful when long-term control is needed. The long-term use of corticosteroids should be avoided.

PARINAUD OCULOGLANDULAR SYNDROME. This represents a form of cat-scratch disease and is caused by *Bartonella henselae,* which is transmitted from cat to cat by fleas (see Chapter 206). Kittens are more likely than adult cats to be infected. Humans can become infected when they are scratched by a cat. In addition, bacteria may pass from a cat's saliva to its fur during grooming. The bacteria can then be deposited on the conjunctiva after rubbing one's eyes after handling the cat. Lymphadenopathy and conjunctivitis are hallmarks of the disease. Conjunctival granulomas may develop (Fig. 625-2). The course is generally self-limited, but antibiotics may be used in some cases.

CHEMICAL CONJUNCTIVITIS. This can result when an irritating substance enters the conjunctival sac (as in the acute but benign conjunctivitis caused by silver nitrate in newborns). Other common offenders are household cleaning substances, sprays, smoke, smog, and industrial pollutants. Alkalis tend to linger in the conjunctival tissues and continue to inflict damage for hours or days. Acids precipitate the proteins in tissues and so produce their effect immediately. In either case, prompt, thorough, and copious irrigation is crucial. Extensive tissue damage, even loss of the eye, can result, especially if the offending agent is an alkali.

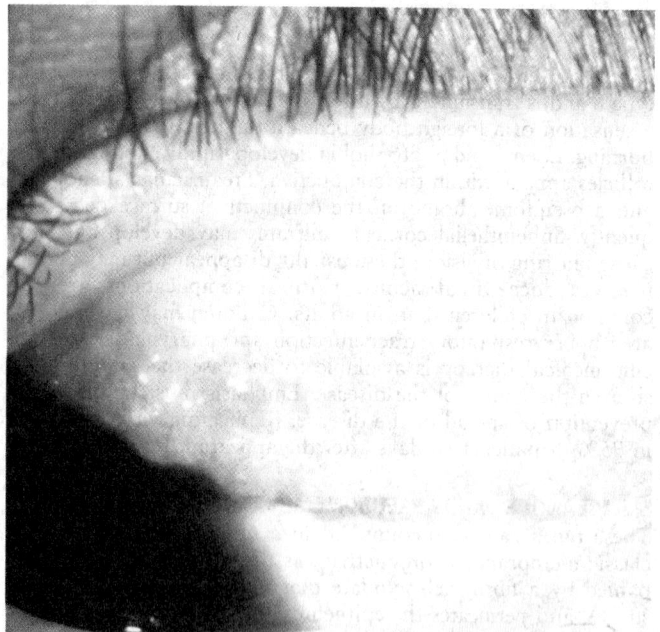

Figure 625-1. Vernal conjunctivitis.

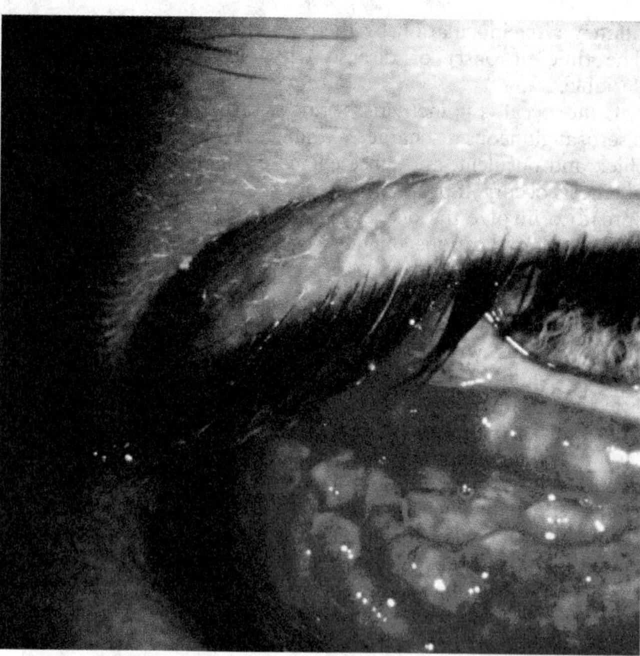

Figure 625-2. Conjunctival granulomas in Parinaud oculoglandular syndrome.

OTHER CONJUNCTIVAL DISORDERS. Subconjunctival hemorrhage is manifested by bright or dark red patches in the bulbar conjunctiva and may result from injury or inflammation. It commonly occurs spontaneously. It may occasionally result from severe sneezing or coughing. Rarely it may be a manifestation of a blood dyscrasia.

Pinguecula is a yellowish-white, slightly elevated mass on the bulbar conjunctiva, usually in the interpalpebral region. It represents elastic and hyaline degenerative changes of the conjunctiva. No treatment is required except for cosmetic reasons, in which case simple excision suffices.

Pterygium is a fleshy triangular conjunctival lesion that may encroach on the cornea. It typically occurs in the nasal interpalpebral region. The pathologic findings are similar to those of a pinguecula. The development of pterygia is related to exposure to ultraviolet light, and it therefore is more commonly found among people who live near the equator. Removal is suggested when the lesion encroaches far onto the cornea. Recurrence after removal is common.

Dermoid cyst and dermolipoma are benign lesions, clinically similar in appearance. They are smooth, elevated, round to oval lesions of various sizes. The color varies from yellowish white to fleshy pink. The most frequent site is the upper outer quadrant of the globe; they also commonly occur near or straddling the limbus. Dermolipoma is composed of adipose and connective tissue. Dermoid cysts may also contain glandular tissue, hair follicles, and hair shafts. Excision for cosmetic reasons is feasible. Dermolipomas are often connected to the extraocular muscles, making their complete removal impossible without sacrificing ocular motility.

Conjunctival nevus is a small, slightly elevated lesion that may vary in pigmentation from pale salmon to dark brown. It is usually benign, but careful observation for progressive growth or changes suggestive of malignancy is advised.

Symblepharon is a cicatricial adhesion between the conjunctiva of the lid and the globe; the lower lid is usually affected. It follows operation or injuries, especially burns from lye, acids, or molten metals. It is a serious complication of Stevens-Johnson syndrome. It may interfere with motion of the eyeball and may cause diplopia. The adhesions should be separated and the raw surfaces kept from uniting during healing. Grafts of oral mucous membrane may be necessary.

Atik B, Thanh TTK, Luong VQ, et al: Impact of annual targeted treatment of infectious trachoma and susceptibility to reinfection. *JAMA* 2006;296:1488–1497.

Centers for Disease Control and Prevention: Outbreak of bacterial conjunctivitis at a college—New Hampshire, January–March, 2002. *MMWR* 2002;51:205–208.

Centers for Disease Control and Prevention: Acute hemorrhagic conjunctivitis outbreak caused by coxsackievirus A24—Puerto Rico, 2003. *MMWR* 2004;53:632.

Chang DC, Grant GB, O'Donnell K, et al: Multistate outbreak of fusarium keratitis associated with use of a contact lens solution. *JAMA* 2006;296:953–963.

Everitt HA, Little PS, Smith PWF: A randomised controlled trial of management strategies for acute infective conjunctivitis in general practice. *BMJ* 2006;333:321–324.

Matoba A: Ocular viral infections. *Pediatr Infect Dis* 1984;3:358–368.

O'Hara MA: Ophthalmia neonatorum. *Pediatr Clin North Am* 1993;40:715.

Rietveld RP, ter Riet G, Bindels PJE, et al: Predicting bacterial cause in infectious conjunctivitis: Cohort study on informativeness of combinations of signs and symptoms. *Br Med J* 2004;329:206–208.

Rose PW, Hamden A, Brueggemann AB, et al: Chloramphenicol treatment for acute infective conjunctivitis in children in primary care: A randomized double-blind placebo-controlled trial. *Lancet* 2005;366:37–42.

Shiuey Y, Ambati BK, Adamis AP, and the Viral Conjunctivitis Study Group: A randomized, double-masked trial of topical ketorolac versus artificial tears for treatment of viral conjunctivitis. *Ophthalmology* 2000;107:1512–1517.

Weiss A, Brinser JH, Nazar-Stewart V: Acute conjunctivitis in childhood. *J Pediatr* 1993;122:10–14.

Chapter 626 ■ Abnormalities of the Cornea

Scott E. Olitsky, Denise Hug, and Laura P. Smith

MEGALOCORNEA. This is a nonprogressive symmetric condition characterized by an enlarged cornea (>12 mm in diameter) and an anterior segment in which there is no evidence of previous or concurrent ocular hypertension. High myopia is frequently present and may lead to reduced vision. A frequent complication is the development of lens opacities in adult life. All modes of inheritance have been described, although X-linked recessive is the most common; therefore, this disorder more commonly affects males. Systemic abnormalities that may be associated with megalocornea include Marfan syndrome, craniosynostosis, and Alport syndrome. The cause of the enlargement of the cornea and the anterior segment is unknown, but possible explanations include a defect in the growth of the optic cup and an arrest of congenital glaucoma. The region on the X chromosome responsible for this disorder has been identified.

Pathologic corneal enlargement caused by glaucoma is to be differentiated from this anomaly. Any progressive increase in the size of the cornea, especially when accompanied by photophobia, lacrimation, or haziness of the cornea, requires prompt ophthalmologic evaluation.

MICROCORNEA. Microcornea, or anterior microphthalmia, is an abnormally small cornea in an otherwise relatively normal eye. It may be familial, with transmission being dominant more often than recessive. More commonly, a small cornea is just one feature of an otherwise developmentally abnormal or microphthalmic eye; associated defects include colobomas, microphakia, congenital cataract, glaucoma, and aniridia.

KERATOCONUS. This is a disease of unclear pathogenesis characterized by progressive thinning and bulging of the central cornea, which becomes cone shaped. Although familial cases are known, most cases are sporadic. Eye rubbing and contact lens wear have been implicated as pathogenic, but the evidence to support this is equivocal. The incidence is increased in individuals with atopy, Down syndrome, Marfan syndrome, and retinitis pigmentosa.

Most cases are bilateral, but involvement may be asymmetric. The disorder usually presents and progresses rapidly during adolescence; progression slows and stabilizes when patients reach full growth. Desçemet membrane may occasionally be stretched beyond its elastic breaking point, causing an acute rupture in the membrane with resultant sudden and marked corneal edema (acute hydrops) and decrease in vision. The corneal edema resolves as endothelial cells cover the defective area. Some degree of corneal scarring occurs, but the visual acuity is often better than before the initial incident. Signs of keratoconus include Munson sign (bulging of the lower eyelid on looking downward) and the presence of a Fleischer ring (a deposit of iron in the epithelium at the base of the cone). Corneal transplantation is indicated if satisfactory visual acuity cannot be attained with the use of contact lenses.

NEONATAL CORNEAL OPACITIES. Loss of the normal transparency of the cornea in neonates may occur secondary to either intrinsic hereditary or extrinsic environmental causes (Table 626-1).

SCLEROCORNEA. In sclerocornea, the normal translucent cornea is replaced by sclera-like tissue. Instead of a clearly demarcated cornea, white, feathery, often ill-defined and vascularized tissue develops in the peripheral cornea, appearing to blend with and extend from the sclera. The central cornea is usually clearer, but total replacement of the cornea with sclera may occur. The curvature of the cornea is often flatter, similar to the sclera. Potentially coexisting abnormalities include a shallow anterior chamber, iris abnormalities, and microphthalmos. This condition is usually bilateral. In approximately 50% of cases, a dominant or recessive inheritance has been described. Sclerocornea has been reported in association with numerous systemic abnormalities including limb deformities, craniofacial defects, and genitourinary disorders. In generalized sclerocornea, early keratoplasty should be considered in an effort to provide vision.

PETERS ANOMALY. Peters anomaly is a central corneal opacity (leukoma) that is present at birth (Fig. 626-1). It is often associated with iridocorneal adhesions that extend from the iris collarette to the border of the corneal opacity. Approximately ½ of patients have other ocular abnormalities, which may include cataracts, glaucoma, and microcornea. As many as 80% of cases may be bilateral, and 60% are associated with systemic malformations that may affect any major organ system. Some investigators have divided Peters anomaly into 2 types: a mesodermal or neuroectodermal form (type I), which shows no associated lens

TABLE 626-1. STUMPED: Differential Diagnosis of Neonatal Corneal Opacities

DIAGNOSIS	LATERALITY	OPACITY	OCULAR PRESSURE	OTHER OCULAR ABNORMALITIES	NATURAL HISTORY	INHERITANCE
S–Sclerocornea	Unilateral or bilateral	Vascularized, blends with sclera, clearer centrally	Normal (or elevated)	Cornea plana	Nonprogressive	Sporadic
T–Tears in endothelium and Desçemet's membrane						
Birth trauma	Unilateral	Diffuse edema	Normal	Possible hyphema, periorbital ecchymoses	Spontaneous improvement in 1 mo	Sporadic
Infantile glaucoma	Bilateral	Diffuse edema	Elevated	Megalocornea, photophobia and tearing, abnormal angle	Progressive unless treated	Autosomal recessive
U–Ulcers						
Herpes simplex keratitis	Unilateral	Diffuse with geographic epithelial defect	Normal	None	Progressive	Sporadic
Congenital rubella	Bilateral	Disciform or diffuse edema, no frank ulceration	Normal or elevated	Microphthalmos, cataract, pigment epithelial mottling	Stable, may clear	Sporadic
Neurotrophic exposure	Unilateral or bilateral	Central ulcer	Normal	Lid anomalies, congenital sensory neuropathy	Progressive	Sporadic
M–Metabolic (rarely present at birth) (mucopolysaccharidoses IH, IS; mucolipidoses type IV)*	Bilateral	Diffuse haze, denser peripherally	Normal	Few	Progressive	Autosomal dominant
P–Posterior corneal defect	Unilateral or bilateral	Central, diffuse haze or vascularized leukoma	Normal or elevated	Anterior chamber cleavage syndrome	Stable, sometimes early clearing or vascularization	Sporadic, autosomal recessive
E–Endothelial dystrophy						
Congenital hereditary endothelial dystrophy	Bilateral	Diffuse corneal edema, marked corneal thickening	Normal	None	Stable	Autosomal dominant or recessive
Posterior polymorphous dystrophy	Bilateral	Diffuse haze, normal corneal thickness	Normal	Occasional peripheral anterior synechiae	Slowly progressive	Autosomal dominant
Congenital hereditary stromal dystrophy	Bilateral	Flaky, feathery stromal opacities; normal corneal thickness	Normal	None	Stable	Autosomal dominant
D–Dermoid	Unilateral or bilateral	White vascularized mass, hair, lipid arc	Normal	None	Stable	Sporadic

*Mucopolysaccharidosis IH (Hurler syndrome); mucopolysaccharidosis IS (Scheie syndrome).
From Nelson LB, Calhoun JH, Harley RD: *Pediatric Ophthalmology*, 3rd ed. Philadelphia, WB Saunders, 1991, p 210.

changes, and a surface ectodermal form (type II), which does. Histologic findings include a focal absence of Desçemet membrane and corneal endothelium in the region of the opacity. Peters anomaly may be caused by incomplete migration and differentiation of the precursor cells of the central corneal endothelium and Desçemet membrane or a defective separation between the primitive lens and cornea during embryogenesis.

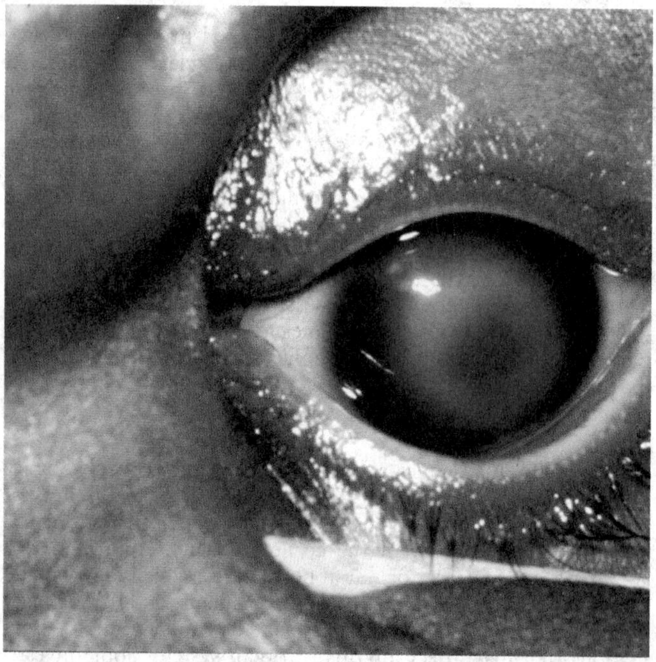

Figure 626-1. Peters anomaly. Central opacity in a patient with Peters anomaly.

DERMOIDS. Epibulbar dermoids are choristomas. They are often present at birth and may increase in size with age. They occur most frequently in the lower temporal quadrant. They most commonly straddle the limbus and extend into the peripheral cornea. Rarely, they may be confined entirely to the cornea or conjunctiva. Epibulbar dermoids may cause visual disturbance by encroaching on the visual axis or by contributing to the development of astigmatism, which may lead to amblyopia.

A dermoid usually appears as a well-circumscribed rounded or oval, gray or pinkish-yellow mass with a dry surface from which short hairs may protrude. It may affect only the superficial layers of the cornea, although full-thickness involvement is common. Associated ocular anomalies include eyelid and iris colobomas, microphthalmos, and retinal and choroidal defects. A total of 30% of dermoids are associated with systemic abnormalities. Many of the associated anomalies involve developmental defects of the 1st branchial arch (vertebral anomalies, dystosis of the facial bones and dental anomalies, and Goldenhar syndrome). Epibulbar dermoids are found in 75% of cases of Goldenhar syndrome.

DENDRITIC KERATITIS. Infection of the cornea with the herpes simplex virus produces a characteristic lesion of the corneal epithelium, referred to as a dendrite; it has a branching treelike pattern that can be demonstrated by fluorescein staining. The acute episode is accompanied by pain, photophobia, tearing, blepharospasm, and conjunctival injection. Specific treatment may include mechanical debridement of the involved corneal epithelium to remove the source of infection and eliminate an antigenic stimulus to inflammation in the adjacent stroma. Medical treatment involves the use of trifluridine or systemic acyclovir. In addition, a cycloplegic agent is useful to relieve pain from spasm of the ciliary muscle. Overly aggressive topical antiviral treatment itself can be toxic to the cornea and should be avoided. Recurrent infection and deep stromal involvement can lead to corneal scarring and loss of vision.

Topical use of corticosteroids causes exacerbation of superficial herpetic disease of the eye and may lead to corneal perforation; eyedrops combining steroids and antibiotics are therefore to be avoided in treatment of red eye unless there are clear-cut indications for their use and close supervision during therapy.

Infants born to mothers infected with herpes simplex virus should be examined carefully for signs of ocular involvement. Intravenous acyclovir is required for treatment of ocular herpes in newborns.

CORNEAL ULCERS. The usual signs and symptoms are focal or diffuse corneal haze, hyperemia, lid edema, pain, photophobia, tearing, and blepharospasm. Hypopyon (pus in the anterior chamber) is common. Corneal ulcers require prompt treatment. They result most frequently from traumatic lesions that become secondarily infected. Many organisms are capable of infecting the cornea. One of the most serious is *Pseudomonas aeruginosa;* it can rapidly destroy stromal tissue and lead to corneal perforation. *Neisseria gonorrhoeae* also is particularly damaging to the cornea. Indolent ulcers may be caused by fungi, often in association with the use of contact lenses. In each case, scrapings of the cornea must be studied in an effort to identify the infectious agent and to determine the best therapy. Although aggressive local treatment is generally needed to save the eye, systemic treatment may be necessary in some cases as well. Perforation or scarring resulting from corneal ulceration is an important cause of blindness throughout the world and is estimated to be responsible for 10% of blindness in the United States.

Unexplained corneal ulcers in infants and young children should raise the question of a sensory defect, as in Riley-Day or Goldenhar-Gorlin syndrome, or of a metabolic disorder such as tyrosinemia.

PHLYCTENULES. These are small, yellowish, slightly elevated lesions usually located at the corneal limbus; they may encroach on the cornea and extend centrally. A small corneal ulcer is often found at the head of the advancing lesion, with a fascicle of blood vessels behind the head of the lesion. Although once thought to represent a sign of systemic tuberculin infection, phlyctenular keratoconjunctivitis is now accepted as a morphologic expression of delayed hypersensitivity to diverse antigens. In children, it commonly occurs as a result of a hypersensitivity reaction of the conjunctiva or cornea to bacterial products. Treatment usually consists of eliminating the underlying disorder, usually staphylococcal blepharitis or meibomianitis, and suppressing the immune response with the use of topical corticosteroid therapy. A superficial stromal pannus and scarring sometimes remain after treatment.

INTERSTITIAL KERATITIS. This denotes inflammation of the corneal stroma. The most common cause is syphilis, interstitial keratitis being one of the characteristic late manifestations of congenital syphilis. The corneal changes in congenital syphilis occur in 2 phases. The acute phase presents between the ages of 5 and 10 yr, with an intense keratitis that may last for several months and causes a severe reduction in vision. The acute effects of syphilis are mainly due to the host immune response, such as mononuclear cell infiltrates, proliferative vascular changes, and occasionally granuloma formation. The deep inflammation produces pain, photophobia, tearing, circumcorneal injection, and corneal haze. The acute episode is followed by a chronic stage with significant regression in the corneal findings along with a parallel improvement in visual acuity. Although the corneal findings may regress with time, "ghost vessels," which represent the previous vascular changes, and patchy corneal scarring remain and serve as permanent stigmata of the disease.

Cogan syndrome is a nonluetic interstitial keratitis associated with hearing loss and vestibular symptoms. Although its cause is unknown, a systemic vasculitis is suspected. Prompt treatment is required to avoid permanent hearing loss. Both the corneal changes and the auditory involvement may respond to the use of immunosuppressive agents.

Less frequently, interstitial keratitis is caused by other infectious diseases, such as tuberculosis or leprosy.

CORNEAL MANIFESTATIONS OF SYSTEMIC DISEASE. Several metabolic diseases produce distinctive corneal changes in childhood. Refractile polychromatic crystals are deposited throughout the cornea in cystinosis. Corneal deposits producing various degrees of corneal haze also occur in certain types of mucopolysaccharidosis (MPS), particularly MPS IH (Hurler), MPS IS (Scheie), MPS I H/S (Hurler-Scheie compound), MPS IV (Morquio), MPS VI (Maroteaux-Lamy), and sometimes MPS VII (Sly). Corneal deposits may develop in patients with GM_1 (generalized) gangliosidosis. In Fabry disease, fine opacities radiating in a whorl or fanlike pattern occur, and corneal changes can be important in identifying the carrier state. A spraylike pattern of corneal opacities may also be seen in the Bloch-Sulzberger syndrome. In Wilson disease, the distinctive corneal sign is the Kayser-Fleischer ring, a golden brown ring in the peripheral cornea resulting from changes in Desçemet membrane. Pigmented corneal rings may develop in neonates with cholestatic liver disease. Corneal changes may occur in autoimmune hypoparathyroidism and band keratopathy in patients with hypercalcemia. Transient keratitis may occur with rubeola and sometimes with rubella.

Beauchamp GR, Gillette TE, Friendly DS: Phlyctenular keratoconjunctivitis. *J Pediatr Ophthalmol Strabismus* 1981;18:22–28.

Comer RM, Daya SM, O'Keefe M: Penetrating keratoplasty in infants. *J AAPOS* 2001;5:285–290.

Dana MR, Moyes AL, Gomes JA, et al: The indications for and outcome in pediatric keratoplasty. A multicenter study. *Ophthalmology* 1995;102: 1129–1138.

Mackey DA, Buttery RG, Wise GM, et al: Description of X-linked megalocornea with identification of the gene locus. *Arch Ophthalmol* 1991;109: 829–833.

Mohandessan MM, Romano PE: Neuroparalytic keratitis in Goldenhar-Gorlin syndrome. *Am J Ophthalmol* 1978;85:111–113.

Reidy JJ: Congenital corneal opacities. *Ophthalmol Clin North Am* 1996;2:199–213.

Traboulsi EI, Maumenee IH: Peters' anomaly and associated congenital malformations. *Arch Ophthalmol* 1992;110:1739–1742.

Yang LL, Lambert SR, Fernhoff PM, et al: Peters' anomaly: Associated congenital malformations and etiology. *Invest Ophthalmol Vis Sci* 1995;36:S41.

Yang LL, Lambert SR, Lynn MJ, et al: Long-term results of corneal graft survival in infants and children with Peters anomaly. *Ophthalmology* 1999;106:833–848.

Chapter 627 ■ Abnormalities of the Lens

Scott E. Olitsky, Denise Hug, and Laura P. Smith

CATARACTS

A cataract is any opacity of the lens (Fig. 627-1). Some are clinically unimportant; others significantly affect visual function. The

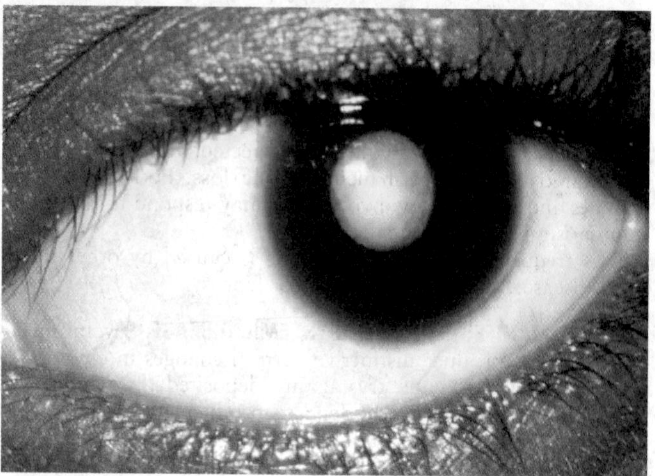

Figure 627-1. Leukocoria secondary to cataract.

incidence of infantile cataracts is approximately 2/10,000 births. In 50–60% of cases, cataracts are an isolated defect; in 20–25%, they are part of a syndrome; in the remainder they are associated with other nonocular birth defects. They are more common in low birthweight infants. Some cataracts are associated with ocular or systemic disease.

DIFFERENTIAL DIAGNOSIS. The differential diagnosis of cataracts in infants and children includes a wide range of developmental disorders, infectious and inflammatory processes, metabolic diseases, and toxic and traumatic insults (Table 627-1). Cataracts may also develop secondary to intraocular processes, such as retinopathy of prematurity, persistent hyperplastic primary vitreous, retinal detachment, retinitis pigmentosa, and uveitis. Finally, a portion of cataracts in children are inherited (Fig. 627-2).

DEVELOPMENTAL VARIANTS. Early developmental processes may lead to various congenital lens opacities. Discrete dots or white plaquelike opacities of the lens capsule are common and sometimes involve the contiguous subcapsular region. Small opacities of the posterior capsule may be associated with persistent remnants of the primitive hyaloid vascular system (the common Mittendorf dot), whereas those of the anterior capsule may be associated with persistent strands of the pupillary membrane or vascular sheath of the lens. Congenital cataracts of this type are usually stationary and rarely interfere with vision; in some, progression occurs.

PREMATURITY. A special type of lens change seen in some preterm newborn infants is the so-called cataract of prematurity. The appearance is of a cluster of tiny vacuoles in the distribution of the Y sutures of the lens. They can be visualized with an ophthalmoscope and are best seen with the pupil well dilated. The

TABLE 627-1. Differential Diagnosis of Cataracts

DEVELOPMENTAL VARIANTS
Prematurity (Y-suture vacuoles) with or without retinopathy of prematurity

GENETIC DISORDERS

Simple Mendelian Inheritance
Autosomal dominant (most common)
Autosomal recessive
X-linked

Major Chromosomal Defects
Trisomy disorders (13, 18, 21)
Turner syndrome (45X)
Deletion syndromes (11p13, 18p, 18q)
Duplication syndromes (3q, 20p, 10q)

Multisystem Genetic Disorders
Alport syndrome (hearing loss, renal disease)
Alström syndrome (nerve deafness, diabetes mellitus)
Apert disease (craniosynostosis, syndactyly)
Cockayne syndrome (premature senility, skin photosensitivity)
Conradi disease (chondrodysplasia punctata)
Crouzon disease (dysostosis craniofacialis)
Hallermann-Streiff syndrome (microphthalmia, small pinched nose, skin atrophy, and hypotrichosis)
Hypohidrotic ectodermal dysplasia (anomalous dentition, hypohidrosis, hypotrichosis)
Ichthyosis (keratinizing disorder with thick, scaly skin)
Incontinentia pigmenti (dental anomalies, mental retardation, cutaneous lesions)
Lowe syndrome (oculocerebrorenal syndrome: hypotonia, renal disease)
Marfan syndrome
Meckel-Gruber syndrome (renal dysplasia, encephalocele)
Myotonic dystrophy
Nail-patella syndrome (renal dysfunction, dysplastic nails, hypoplastic patella)
Marinesco-Sjögren syndrome (cerebellar ataxia, hypotonia)
Nevoid basal cell carcinoma syndrome (autosomal dominant, basal cell carcinoma erupts in childhood)
Peters anomaly (corneal opacifications with iris-corneal dysgenesis)
Reiger syndrome (iris dysplasia, myotonic dystrophy)
Rothmund-Thomson syndrome (poikiloderma: skin atrophy)
Rubinstein-Taybi syndrome (broad great toe, mental retardation)
Smith-Lemli-Opitz syndrome (toe syndactyly, hypospadias, mental retardation)
Sotos syndrome (cerebral gigantism)
Spondyloepiphyseal dysplasia (dwarfism, short trunk)
Werner syndrome (premature aging in 2nd decade of life)

Inborn Errors of Metabolism
Abetalipoproteinemia (absent chylomicrons, retinal degeneration)
Fabry disease (α-galactosidase A deficiency)
Galactokinase deficiency
Galactosemia (galactose-1-phosphate uridyltransferase deficiency)
Homocystinemia (subluxation of lens, mental retardation)
Mannosidosis (acid α-mannosidase deficiency)
Niemann-Pick disease (sphingomyelinase deficiency)
Refsum disease (phytanic acid α-hydrolase deficiency)
Wilson disease (accumulation of copper leads to cirrhosis and neurologic symptoms)

ENDOCRINOPATHIES
Hypocalcemia (hypoparathyroidism)
Hypoglycemia
Diabetes mellitus

CONGENTIAL INFECTIONS
Toxoplasmosis
Cytomegalovirus infection
Syphilis
Rubella
Perinatal herpes simplex infection
Measles (rubeola)
Poliomyelitis
Influenza
Varicella-zoster

OCULAR ANOMALIES
Microphthalmia
Coloboma
Aniridia
Mesodermal dysgenesis
Persistent pupillary membrane
Posterior lenticonus
Persistent hyperplastic primary vitreous
Primitive hyaloid vascular system

MISCELLANEOUS DISORDERS
Atopic dermatitis
Drugs (corticosteroids)
Radiation
Trauma

IDIOPATHIC

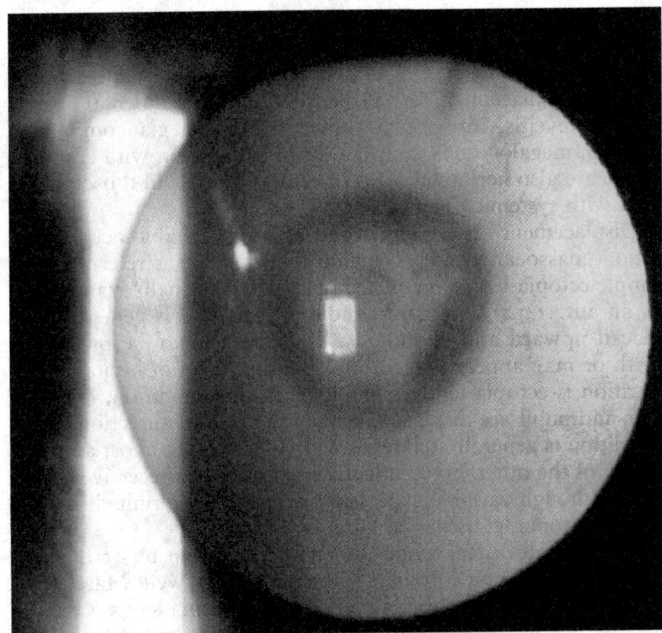

Figure 627-2. Central lamellar cataract.

pathogenesis is unclear. In most cases, the opacities disappear spontaneously, often within a few weeks.

MENDELIAN INHERITANCE. Many cataracts unassociated with other diseases are hereditary. The most common mode of inheritance is autosomal dominant. Penetrance and expressivity vary. Autosomal recessive inheritance occurs less frequently; it is sometimes found in populations with high rates of consanguinity. X-linked inheritance of cataracts unassociated with disease is relatively rare.

CONGENITAL INFECTION SYNDROME. Cataracts in infants and children can be a result of prenatal infection. Lens opacity may occur in any of the major congenital infection syndromes (e.g., toxoplasmosis, cytomegalovirus, syphilis, rubella, herpes simplex virus). Cataracts may also occur secondary to other perinatal infections, including measles, poliomyelitis, influenza, varicella-zoster, and vaccinia.

METABOLIC DISORDERS. Cataracts are a prominent manifestation of many metabolic diseases, particularly certain disorders of carbohydrate, amino acid, calcium, and copper metabolism. A primary consideration in any infant with cataracts is the possibility of **galactosemia** (see Chapter 87.2). In classic infantile galactosemia, galactose-1-phosphate uridyl transferase deficiency, the cataract is typically of the zonular type, with haziness or opacification of one or more of the perinuclear layers of the lens; haziness or clouding of the nucleus also often occurs. In its early stages, the cataract generally has a distinctive oil droplet appearance and is best detected with the pupil fully dilated. Progression to complete opacification of the lens may occur within weeks. With early treatment (galactose-free diet), the lens changes may be reversible.

In **galactokinase deficiency,** cataracts are the sole clinical manifestation. The cataracts are usually zonular and may appear in the first months or first years of life, or later in childhood.

In children with juvenile-onset diabetes mellitus, lens changes are uncommon. Some develop snowflake-like white opacities and vacuoles of the lens. Others develop cataracts that may progress and mature rapidly, sometimes in a matter of days, especially during adolescence. An antecedent event may be the sudden development of myopia caused by changes in the optical density of the lens.

Congenital lens opacities may be seen in children of diabetic and prediabetic mothers. Hypoglycemia in neonates can also be associated with early development of cataracts. Ketotic hypoglycemia is also associated with cataracts.

An association between cataracts and hypocalcemia is well established. Various lens opacities may be seen in patients with hypoparathyroidism.

The **oculocerebral renal syndrome of Lowe** is associated with cataracts in infants. Affected male children frequently have dense bilateral cataracts at birth, often in association with glaucoma and miotic pupils. Punctate lens opacities are frequently present in heterozygous females.

The distinctive sunflower cataract of **Wilson disease** is not commonly seen in children. Various lens opacities may be seen in children with certain of the sphingolipidoses, mucopolysaccharidoses, and mucolipidoses, particularly Niemann-Pick disease, mucosulfatidosis, Fabry disease, and aspartylglycosaminuria.

CHROMOSOMAL DEFECTS. Lens opacities of various types may occur in association with chromosomal defects, including trisomies 13, 18, and 21; Turner syndrome; and a number of deletion (11p13, 18p, 18q) and duplication (3q, 20p, 10q) syndromes.

DRUGS, TOXIC AGENTS, AND TRAUMA. Of the various drugs and toxic agents that may produce cataracts, corticosteroids are of major importance in the pediatric age group. Steroid-related cataracts characteristically are posterior subcapsular lens opacities. The incidence and severity vary. The relative significance of dose, mode of administration, duration of treatment, and individual susceptibility is controversial, and the pathogenesis of steroid-induced cataracts is unclear. The effect on vision depends on the extent and density of the opacity. In many cases, the acuity is only minimally or moderately impaired. Reversibility of steroid-induced cataracts may occur in some cases. All children receiving long-term steroid treatment should have periodic eye examinations.

Trauma to the eye is a major cause of cataracts in children. Opacification of the lens may result from contusion or penetrating injury. Cataracts are an important manifestation of child abuse.

Cataract formation after exposure to radiation is dose and duration dependent. Adult research shows 50% occurrence in lens dose of 15 Gy. Delayed onset is the rule.

MISCELLANEOUS DISORDERS. The list of multisystem syndromes and diseases associated with lens opacities and other eye anomalies is extensive (Table 627-1).

Treatment. The treatment of cataracts that significantly interfere with vision includes the following: (1) surgical removal of lens material to provide an optically clear visual axis; (2) correction of the resultant aphakic refractive error with spectacles, contact lenses, or intraocular lens implantation; and (3) correction of any associated sensory deprivation amblyopia. Because the use of spectacles may not be possible in children after cataract removal, the use of contact lenses for visual rehabilitation is a medical necessity. Treatment of the amblyopia may be the most demanding and difficult step in the visual rehabilitation of infants or children with cataracts.

Prognosis. Prognosis depends on many factors, including the nature of the cataract, the underlying disease, age at onset, age at intervention, duration and severity of any attendant amblyopia, and presence of any associated ocular abnormalities (e.g., microphthalmia, retinal lesions, optic atrophy, glaucoma, nystagmus, strabismus). Persistent amblyopia is the most common cause of poor visual recovery after cataract surgery in children.

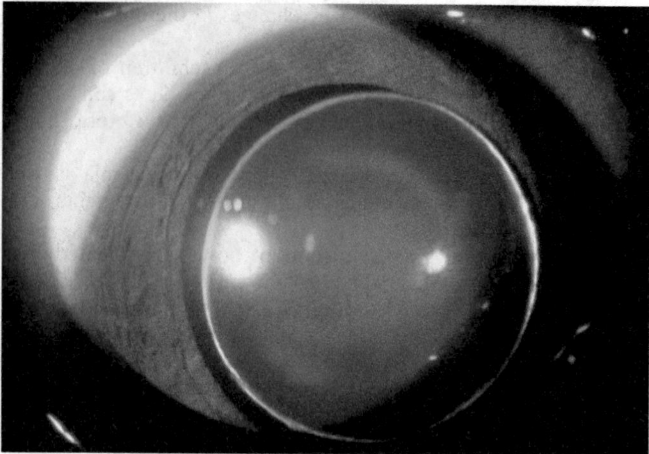

Figure 627-3. Complete dislocation of lens into the anterior chamber seen in Weill-Marchesani syndrome.

Secondary conditions and complications may develop in children who have had cataract surgery, including inflammatory sequelae, secondary membranes, glaucoma, retinal detachment, and changes in the axial length of the eye. All these should be considered in planning treatment.

ECTOPIA LENTIS. Normally, the lens is suspended in place behind the iris diaphragm by the zonular fibers of the ciliary body. Abnormalities of the suspensory system resulting from a developmental defect, disease, or trauma may result in instability or displacement of the lens. Displacement of the lens is classified as luxation (dislocation–complete displacement of the lens) (Fig. 627-3) or as subluxation (partial displacement–shifting or tilting of the lens) (Fig. 627-4). Symptoms include blurring of vision, which is often the result of refractive changes such as myopia, astigmatism, or aphakic hyperopia. Some patients experience diplopia. An important sign of displacement is iridodonesis, a tremulousness of the iris caused by the loss of its usual support. Also, the anterior chamber may appear deeper than normal. Sometimes the equatorial region ("edge") of the displaced lens may be visible in the pupillary aperture. On ophthalmoscopy, this may appear as a black crescent. Also, the difference between the phakic and aphakic portions can be appreciated when focusing on the fundus.

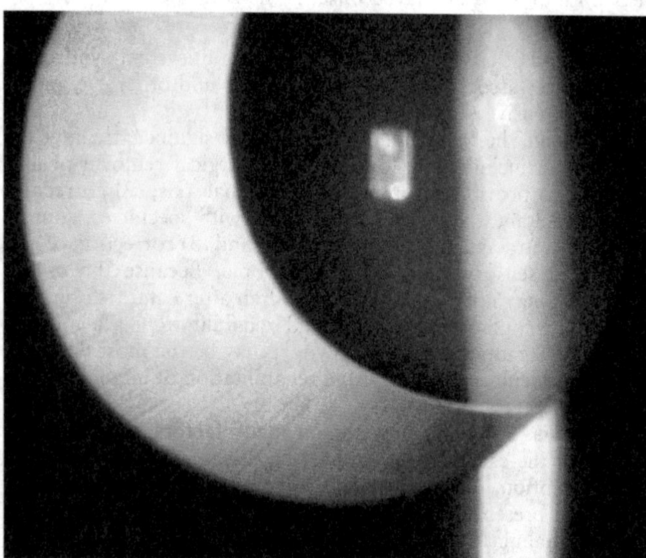

Figure 627-4. Subluxation of the lens in Marfan syndrome.

Differential Diagnosis. A major cause of lens displacement is trauma. Displacement may also occur as a result of ocular disease such as uveitis, intraocular tumor, congenital glaucoma, high myopia, megalocornea, aniridia, or in association with cataract. There are also heritable forms of ectopia lentis and those associated with systemic disease.

Displacement of the lens occurring as a heritable ocular condition unassociated with systemic abnormalities is referred to as simple ectopia lentis. Simple ectopia lentis is usually transmitted as an autosomal dominant condition. The lens is generally displaced upward and temporally. The ectopia may be present at birth or may appear later in life. Another form of heritable dislocation is ectopia lentis et pupillae. In this condition, both the lens and pupil are displaced, usually in opposite directions. This condition is generally bilateral, with 1 eye being almost a mirror image of the other. Ectopia lentis et pupillae is a recessive condition, although variable expression with some intermingling with simple ectopia lentis has been reported.

Systemic disorders associated with displacement of the lens include Marfan syndrome, homocystinuria, Weill-Marchesani syndrome, and sulfite oxidase deficiency. Ectopia lentis occurs in approximately 80% of patients with Marfan syndrome, and in about 50% of patients; the ectopia is evident by the age of 5 yr. In most cases, the lens is displaced superiorly and temporally; it is almost always bilateral and relatively symmetric. In homocystinuria, the lens is usually displaced inferiorly and somewhat nasally. It occurs early in life and is often evident by 5 yr of age. In Weill-Marchesani syndrome, the displacement of the lens is often downward and forward, and the lens tends to be small and round.

Ectopia lentis is also associated occasionally with other conditions, including Ehlers-Danlos, Sturge-Weber, Crouzon, and Klippel-Feil syndromes; oxycephaly; and mandibulofacial dysostosis. A syndrome of dominantly inherited blepharoptosis, high myopia, and ectopia lentis has also been described.

Treatment and Prognosis. Displacement of the lens often results only in optical problems. In some cases, however, more serious complications may develop, such as glaucoma, uveitis, retinal detachment, or cataract. Management must be individualized according to the type of displacement, its cause, and the presence of any complicating ocular or systemic conditions. For many patients, optical correction by spectacles or contact lenses can be provided. Manipulation of the iris diaphragm with mydriatic or miotic drops may sometimes help improve vision. In selected cases, the best treatment is surgical removal of the lens. In many children, treatment of any associated amblyopia must be instituted early. In addition, for children with ectopia lentis, safety precautions should be taken to prevent injury to the eye.

MICROSPHEROPHAKIA. The term microspherophakia refers to a small, round lens that may occur as an isolated anomaly (probably autosomal recessive) or in association with other ocular abnormalities, such as ectopia lentis, myopia, or retinal detachment (possibly autosomal dominant). Microspherophakia may also occur in association with various systemic disorders, including Marfan syndrome, Weill-Marchesani syndrome, Alport syndrome, mandibulofacial dysostosis, and Klinefelter syndrome.

ANTERIOR LENTICONUS. Anterior lenticonus is a rare bilateral condition in which the anterior surface of the lens bulges centrally. It may be accompanied by lens opacities or other eye anomalies and is a prominent feature of Alport syndrome. The increased curvature of the central area may cause high myopia.

POSTERIOR LENTICONUS. Posterior lenticonus, which occurs more commonly than anterior lenticonus, is characterized by a circumscribed round or oval bulge of the posterior lens capsule and cortex, restricted to the 2–7 mm central (axial) region. In the early stages, by the red reflex test, this may look like an oil droplet. It occurs in infants and young children and tends to increase with age. Usually the lens material within and surrounding the capsular bulge eventually becomes opacified. Posterior lenticonus usually occurs as an isolated ocular anomaly. It is generally unilateral but may be bilateral. It is believed to be sporadic, although autosomal dominant heredity has been suggested in some cases. Infants or children with posterior lenticonus may require optical correction, amblyopia treatment, and surgery for progressive cataract.

Anteby I, Isaac M, BenEzra D: Hereditary subluxated lenses: visual performances and long-term follow-up after surgery. *Ophthalmology* 2003;110:1344–1348.

Bhatti TR, Dott M, Yoon PW, et al: Descriptive epidemiology of infantile cataracts in metropolitain Atlanta, GA, 1968–1998. *Arch Pediatr Adolesc Med* 2003;157:341–347.

Chugh KS, Sakhuja V, Agarwal A, et al: Hereditary nephritis (Alport's syndrome)—clinical profile and inheritance in 28 kindreds. *Nephrol Dial Transplant* 1993;8:690–695.

Fallaha N, Lambert SR. Pediatric cataracts. *Ophthalmol Clin North Am* 2001;14:479–492.

Khalil M, Saheb N: Posterior lenticonus. *Ophthalmology* 1984;91:1429–1430.

Levin AV, Edmonds SA, Nelson LB, et al: Extended-wear contact lenses for the treatment of pediatric aphakia. *Ophthalmology* 1988;95:1107–1113.

Peterseim MW, Wilson ME: Bilateral intraocular lens implantation in the pediatric population. *Ophthalmology* 2000;107:1261–1266.

Plager DA, Yang S, Neely D, et al: Complications in the first year following cataract surgery with and without IOL in infants and older children. *J AAPOS* 2002;6:9–14.

Tesser RA, Hess DB, Buckley EG: Pediatric cataracts and lens anomalies. In Nelson LB, Olitsky SE (editors): *Harley's Pediatric Ophthalmology,* 5th ed. Philadelphia, Lippincott Williams & Wilkins, 2005;255–284.

Chapter 628 ■ Disorders of the Uveal Tract

Scott E. Olitsky, Denise Hug, and Laura P. Smith

UVEITIS (IRITIS, CYCLITIS, CHORIORETINITIS). The uveal tract (the inner vascular coat of the eye, consisting of the iris, ciliary body, and choroid) is subject to inflammatory involvement in a number of systemic diseases, both infectious and noninfectious, and in response to exogenous factors, including trauma and toxic agents (Table 628-1). Inflammation may affect any one portion of the uveal tract preferentially or all parts together.

Iritis may occur alone or in conjunction with inflammation of the ciliary body as iridocyclitis or in association with pars planitis. Pain, photophobia, and lacrimation are the characteristic symptoms of acute anterior uveitis, but the inflammation may develop insidiously without disturbing symptoms. Signs of anterior uveitis include conjunctival hyperemia, particularly in the perilimbal region (ciliary flush), and cells and protein ("flare") in the aqueous humor (Fig. 628-1). Inflammatory deposits on the posterior surface of the cornea (keratic precipitates) and congestion of the iris may also be seen. More chronic cases may show degenerative changes of the cornea (band keratopathy), lenticular opacities (cataract), development of glaucoma, and impairment of vision. The cause of anterior uveitis is often obscure; primary considerations in children are rheumatoid disease, particularly pauciarticular rheumatoid arthritis, Kawasaki disease, Reiter syndrome, and sarcoidosis. Iritis may be secondary to corneal disease, such as herpetic keratitis or a bacterial or fungal corneal ulcer, or to a corneal abrasion or foreign body. Traumatic iritis and iridocyclitis are especially common in children.

TABLE 628-1. Uveitis in Childhood

ANTERIOR UVEITIS
Juvenile rheumatoid arthritis (pauciarticular)
Sarcoidosis
Trauma
Tuberculosis
Kawasaki disease
Ulcerative colitis
Post infectious (enteric or genital) with arthritis and rash
Spirochetal (syphilis, leptospiral)
Heterochromic iridocyclitis (Fuchs)
Viral (herpes simplex, herpes zoster)
Ankylosing spondylitis
Stevens-Johnson syndrome
Idiopathic
Drugs
POSTERIOR UVEITIS (CHOROIDITIS—MAY INVOLVE RETINA)
Toxoplasmosis
Parasites (toxocariasis)
Sarcoidosis
Tuberculosis
Viral (rubella, herpes simplex, HIV, cytomegalovirus)
Subacute sclerosing panencephalitis
Idiopathic
ANTERIOR AND/OR POSTERIOR UVEITIS
Symathetic ophthalmia (trauma to other eye)
Vogt-Koyanagi-Harada syndrome (uveo-otocutaneous syndrome: poliosis, vitiligo, deafness, tinnitus, uveitis, aseptic meningitis, retinitis)
Behçet syndrome
Lyme disease

Iridocyclitis that occurs in children with arthritis deserves special mention. Unlike most forms of anterior uveitis, it rarely creates pain, photophobia, or conjunctival hyperemia. Loss of vision may not be noticed until severe and irreversible damage has occurred. Because of the lack of symptoms and the high incidence of uveitis in these children, routine periodic screening is necessary.

Choroiditis, inflammation of the posterior portion of the uveal tract, invariably also involves the retina; when both are obviously affected, the condition is termed chorioretinitis. The causes of posterior uveitis are numerous; the more common are toxoplasmosis, histoplasmosis, cytomegalic inclusion disease, sarcoidosis,

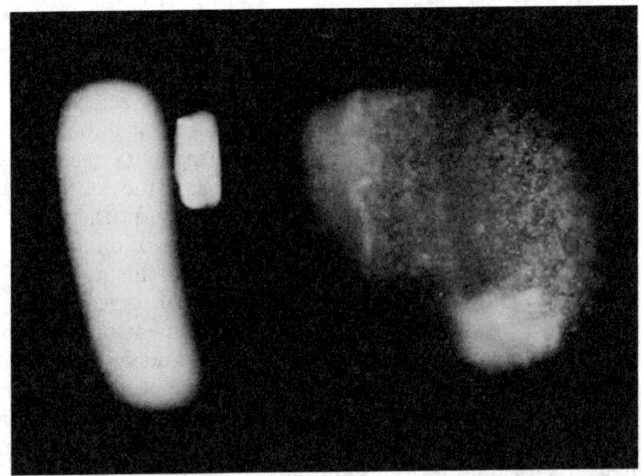

Figure 628-1. Cell and flare in the anterior chamber. The flare represents protein leakage. (Courtesy of Peter Buch, CRA).

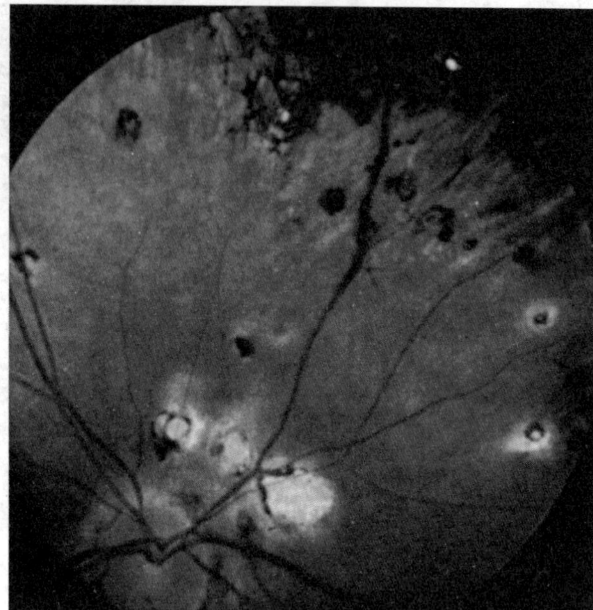

Figure 628-2. Focal atrophic and pigmented scars of chorioretinitis.

syphilis, tuberculosis, and toxocariasis (Fig. 628-2). Depending on the etiology, the inflammatory signs may be diffuse or focal. Vitreous reaction often occurs as well. With many types, the result is atrophic chorioretinal scarring demarcated by pigmentation, often with visual impairment. Secondary complications include retinal detachment, glaucoma, and phthisis.

Panophthalmitis is inflammation involving all parts of the eye. It is frequently suppurative, most often as a result of a perforating injury or of septicemia. It produces severe pain, marked congestion of the eye, inflammation of the adjacent orbital tissues and eyelids, and loss of vision. In many cases, the eye is lost despite intensive treatment of the infection and inflammation. Enucleation of the eye or evisceration of the orbit may be necessary.

Sympathetic ophthalmia is a rare type of inflammatory response that affects the uninjured eye after a perforating injury. It may occur weeks, months, or even years after the injury. A hypersensitivity phenomenon is the most probable cause. Loss of vision in the uninjured (sympathizing) eye may result. Removal of the injured eye prevents the development of sympathetic ophthalmia but does not stop the progression of the disease once it has occurred. Therefore, early enucleation should be considered if there is no hope of visual recovery after a severe injury.

Treatment. The various forms of intraocular inflammation are treated according to their causal factors. When infection is proved or suspected, appropriate systemic antimicrobial or antiviral therapy is used. In some cases, intravitreal injection is indicated.

Elimination of the intraocular inflammation is important to reduce the risk of severe, and often permanent, vision loss. Untreated, the inflammatory process may lead to the development of band keratopathy (calcium deposition in the cornea), cataracts, glaucoma, and irreversible retinal damage. Anterior inflammation may respond well to topical corticosteroid treatment. Posterior cases often require systemic therapy. The use of topical and systemic corticosteroids can lead to the development of glaucoma and cataracts. To reduce the need for topical and systemic corticosteroids, systemic immunosuppression is often used in patients requiring long-term treatment. Commonly used immunosuppressive agents include methotrexate, cyclosporine, and tumor necrosis factor inhibitors. Multiple agents may be needed in recalcitrant cases. Cycloplegic agents, particularly atropine, are also used to reduce inflammation and to prevent adhesion of the iris to the lens (posterior synechiae), especially in anterior uveitis. Extensive posterior synechiae formation can lead to acute angle closure glaucoma.

Surgery may be required for patients who develop glaucoma due to the underlying disease process or the need for corticosteroid treatment. Cataract surgery should be delayed until the inflammation has been under control for a period of time. Cataract surgery in children with a history of prolonged uveitis can carry significant risk. There is no universal agreement concerning the use of intraocular lenses in these patients.

Masquerade syndromes can sometimes mimic intraocular inflammation. Retinoblastoma, leukemia, retained intraocular foreign body, juvenile xanthogranuloma, and peripheral retinal detachments may produce signs similar to those seen in uveitis. These syndromes should be kept in mind when evaluating a patient with suspected uveitis or if a patient does not respond as anticipated to anti-inflammatory treatment.

BenEzra D, Cohen E: Cataract surgery in children with chronic uveitis. *Ophthalmology* 2000;107:1255–1260.

Chu DS, Foster CS: Sympathetic ophthalmia. *Int Ophthalmol Clin* 2002;42:179–185.

Holland GN, Stiehm ER: Special considerations in the evaluation and management of uveitis in children. *Am J Ophthalmol* 2003;135: 867–878.

Kadayifcilar S, Eldem B, Tumer B: Uveitis in childhood. *J Pediatr Ophthalmol Strabismus* 2003;40:335–340.

Kotaniemi K, Savolainen A, Karma A, et al: Recent advances in uveitis of juvenile idiopathic arthritis. *Surv Ophthalmol* 2003;48:489–502.

McCluskey P, Powell RJ: The eye in systemic inflammatory diseases. *Lancet* 2004;364:2125–2133.

Oren B, Sehgal A, Simon JW, et al: The prevalence of uveitis in juvenile rheumatoid arthritis. *J Am Assoc Pediatr Ophthalmol Strabismus* 2001;5:2–4.

Patel H, Goldstein D: Pediatric uveitis. *Pediatr Clin North Am* 2003;50:125–136.

Rosenberg KD, Feuer WJ, Davis JL: Ocular complications of pediatric uveitis. *Ophthalmology* 2004;111:2299–2306.

Chapter 629 ■ Disorders of the Retina and Vitreous

Scott E. Olitsky, Denise Hug, and Laura P. Smith

RETINOPATHY OF PREMATURITY (ROP). ROP is a complex disease of the developing retinal vasculature in premature infants. It may be acute (early stages) or chronic (late stages). Clinical manifestations range from mild, usually transient changes of the peripheral retina to severe progressive vasoproliferation, scarring, and potentially blinding retinal detachment. ROP includes all stages of the disease and its sequelae. Retrolental fibroplasia, the previous name for this disease, described only the cicatricial stages.

Pathogenesis. Beginning at 16 wk of gestation, retinal angiogenesis normally proceeds from the optic disc to the periphery, reaching the outer rim of the retina (ora serrata) nasally at about 36 wk and extending temporally by approximately 40 wk. Injury to this process results in various pathologic and clinical changes. The first observation in the acute phase is cessation of vasculogenesis. Rather than a gradual transition from vascularized to avascular retina, there is an abrupt termination of the vessels, marked by a line in the retina. The line may then grow into a ridge composed of mesenchymal and endothelial cells. Cell division and differentiation may later resume, and vascularization of the retina may proceed. Alternatively, there may be progression to an abnormal proliferation of vessels out of the plane of the retina, into the vitreous, and over the surface of the retina. Cicatrization and traction on the retina may follow, leading to retinal detachment.

The risk factors associated with ROP are not fully known, but prematurity and the associated retinal immaturity at birth represent the major factors. Oxygenation, respiratory distress, apnea, bradycardia, heart disease, infection, hypercarbia, acidosis, anemia, and the need for transfusion are thought by some to be contributory factors. Generally, the lower the gestational age, the lower the birthweight, and the sicker the infant are, the greater the risk is for ROP.

The basic pathogenesis of ROP is still unknown. Exposure to the extrauterine environment including the necessarily high inspired oxygen concentrations produces cellular damage, perhaps mediated by free radicals. Later in the course of the disease, peripheral hypoxia develops and vascular endothelial growth factors (VEGF) are produced in the nonvascularized retina. These growth factors stimulate abnormal vasculogenesis, and neovascularization may occur. Because of poor pulmonary function, a state of relative retinal hypoxia occurs. This causes upregulation of VEGF, which, in susceptible infants, can cause abnormal fibrovascular growth. This neovascularization may then lead to scarring and vision loss.

Classification. The currently used international classification of ROP describes the location, extent, and severity of the disease. To delineate location, the retina is divided into three concentric zones, centered on the optic disc. Zone I, the posterior or inner zone, extends twice the disc-macular distance, or 30 degrees in all directions from the optic disc. Zone II, the middle zone, extends from the outer edge of zone I to the ora serrata nasally and to the anatomic equator temporally. Zone III, the outer zone, is the residual crescent that extends from the outer border of zone II to the ora serrata temporally. The extent of involvement is described by the number of circumferential clock hours involved.

The phases and severity of the disease process are classified into five stages. Stage 1 is characterized by a demarcation line that separates vascularized from avascular retina. This line lies within the plane of the retina and appears relatively flat and white. Often noted is abnormal branching or arcading of the retinal vessels that lead into the line. Stage 2 is characterized by a ridge; the demarcation line has grown, acquiring height, width, and volume and extending up and out of the plane of the retina. Stage 3 is characterized by the presence of a ridge and by the development of extraretinal fibrovascular tissue (Fig. 629-1*A*). Stage 4 is char-

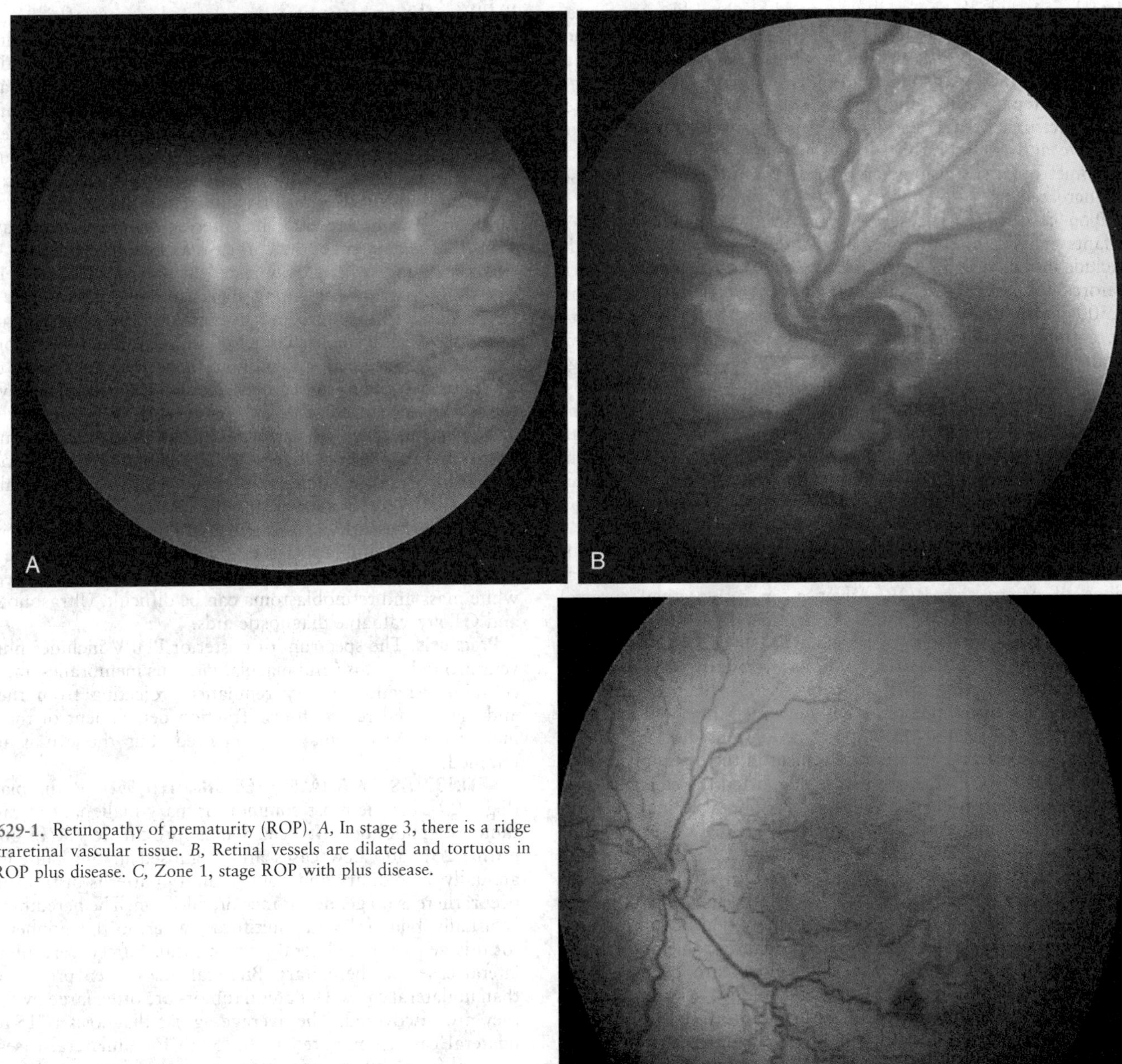

Figure 629-1. Retinopathy of prematurity (ROP). *A*, In stage 3, there is a ridge and extraretinal vascular tissue. *B*, Retinal vessels are dilated and tortuous in active ROP plus disease. *C*, Zone 1, stage ROP with plus disease.

acterized by subtotal retinal detachment caused by traction from the proliferating tissue in the vitreous or on the retina. Stage 4 is subdivided into 2 phases: (a) subtotal retinal detachment not involving the macula and (b) subtotal retinal detachment involving the macula. Stage 5 is total retinal detachment.

When signs of posterior retinal vascular changes accompany the active stages of ROP, the term plus disease is used (see Fig. 629-1*B*,*C*). Patients reaching the point of dilatation and tortuosity of the retinal vessels also frequently demonstrate the associated findings of engorgement of the iris, pupillary rigidity, and vitreous haze.

Clinical Manifestations and Prognosis. In more than 90% of at-risk infants, the course is one of spontaneous arrest and regression, with little or no residual effects or visual disability. Fewer than 10% of infants have progression toward severe disease, with significant extraretinal vasoproliferation, cicatrization, detachment of the retina, and impairment of vision.

Some children with arrested or regressed ROP are left with demarcation lines, undervascularization of the peripheral retina, or abnormal branching, tortuosity, or straightening of the retinal vessels. Some are left with retinal pigmentary changes, dragging of the retina (so-called dragged disc), ectopia of the macula, retinal folds, or retinal breaks. Others proceed to total retinal detachment, which commonly assumes a funnel-like configuration. The clinical picture is often that of a retrolental membrane, producing leukokoria (a white reflex in the pupil). Some patients develop cataract, glaucoma, and signs of inflammation. The end stage is often a painful blind eye or a degenerated phthisical eye. The spectrum of ROP also includes myopia, which is often progressive and of significant degree in infancy. The incidence of anisometropia, strabismus, amblyopia, and nystagmus may also be increased.

Diagnosis. Systematic serial ophthalmologic examinations of infants at risk are recommended. Guidelines vary but generally include infants weighing less than 1,500 g at birth and those born before 31 wk of gestational age. Infants born weighing more than 1,500 g who have an unstable clinical course and are thought to be at high risk should also be examined for ROP. The initial examination should be performed at 4–6 wk of chronological age or at 31–33 wk postconceptional age. ROP is diagnosed most often at 32–44 wk after conception. The examination can be stressful to fragile preterm infants, and the dilating drops can have untoward side effects; thus, discretion must be used in timing the eye examination, and infants must be carefully monitored during and after the examination. Follow-up is based on the initial findings and risk factors but is usually 2 wk or less.

Treatment. In selected cases, cryotherapy or laser photocoagulation of the avascular retina reduces the more severe complications of progressive ROP. Advances in vitreoretinal surgical techniques have led to limited success in reattaching the retina in infants with total retinal detachment (stage 5 ROP), but the visual results are often disappointing. The Early Treatment for Retinopathy of Prematurity Cooperative study did find improved structural and visual outcomes with redefined threshold for treatment. It demonstrated the importance of plus disease and the presence of posterior retinal involvement in the determination of when to treat ROP. This study also supported the fact that laser is the **treatment modality of choice.** Peripheral retinal ablation should be considered for any eye with type 1 ROP. Serial examinations are indicated for any eye with type 2 ROP; treatment is considered if type 2 progresses to type 1 or if threshold ROP develops.

Prevention. Prevention of ROP ultimately depends on prevention of premature birth and its attendant problems. Despite advances in technology and the meticulous care given to high-risk infants in modern nurseries, ROP continues to occur. Oxygen alone is neither sufficient nor necessary to produce ROP, and no safe level of oxygen has yet been determined. Each infant must be treated with whatever is necessary to sustain life and neurologic function. Some investigators have suggested the use of supplemental vitamin E for its antioxidant properties in infants at risk of ROP. Its efficacy has not been proven; at certain dose levels, it may produce untoward side effects (see Chapter 97.2).

PERSISTENT HYPERPLASTIC PRIMARY VITREOUS (PHPV). PHPV includes a spectrum of manifestations caused by the persistence of various portions of the fetal hyaloid vascular system and associated fibrovascular tissue.

Pathogenesis. During development of the eye, the hyaloid artery extends from the optic disc to the posterior aspect of the lens; it sends branches into the vitreous and ramifies to form the posterior portion of the vascular capsule of the lens. The posterior portion of the hyaloid system normally regresses by the 7th fetal mo and the anterior portion by the 8th fetal mo. Small remnants of the system, such as a tuft of tissue at the disc (Bergmeister papilla) or a tag of tissue on the posterior capsule of the lens (Mittendorf dot), are common findings in healthy persons. More extensive remnants and associated complications constitute PHPV. Two major forms are described, anterior PHPV and posterior PHPV. Variability is great, and mixed or intermediate forms occur.

Clinical Manifestations. The usual clinical feature of anterior PHPV is the presence of a vascularized plaque of tissue on the back surface of the lens in an eye that is microphthalmic or slightly smaller than normal. The condition is usually unilateral and may occur in infants with no other abnormalities and no history of prematurity. The fibrovascular tissue tends to undergo gradual contracture. The ciliary processes become elongated, and the anterior chamber may become shallow. The lens usually is smaller than normal and may be clear but often becomes cataractous and may swell or absorb fluid. Large or anomalous vessels of the iris may be present. The anterior chamber angle may have abnormalities. In time, the cornea may become cloudy.

Anterior PHPV is usually noted in the 1st wk or mo of life. The most frequent presenting signs are leukocoria (white pupillary reflex), strabismus, and nystagmus. The course is usually progressive and the outcome poor. Major complications are spontaneous intraocular hemorrhage, swelling of the lens caused by rupture of the posterior capsule, and glaucoma. The eye may eventually deteriorate.

Treatment. Surgery is performed in an effort to prevent complications, to preserve the eye and a reasonably good cosmetic appearance, and, in some cases, to salvage vision. Surgical treatment usually involves aspirating the lens and excising the abnormal tissue. If useful vision is to be attained, refractive correction and aggressive amblyopia therapy are required. In some cases, the affected eye is enucleated because distinguishing between this white mass and retinoblastoma can be difficult. Ultrasonography and CT are valuable diagnostic aids.

Prognosis. The spectrum of posterior PHPV includes fibroglial veils around the disc and macula, vitreous membranes and stalks containing hyaloid artery remnants projecting from the disc, and meridional retinal folds. Traction detachment of the retina may occur. Vision may be impaired, but the eye is usually retained.

RETINOBLASTOMA (ALSO SEE CHAPTER 502). Retinoblastoma (Fig. 629-2) is the most common primary malignant intraocular tumor of childhood. It occurs in approximately 1/15,000 live births; 250–300 new cases are diagnosed in the United States annually. Hereditary and nonhereditary patterns of transmission occur; there is no gender or race predilection. The hereditary form is usually bilateral and multifocal, whereas the nonhereditary form is generally unilateral and unifocal. Fifteen percent of unilateral cases are hereditary. Bilateral cases often present earlier than unilateral cases. Unilateral tumors are often large by the time they are discovered. The average age at diagnosis is 15 mo for bilateral cases, compared with 25 mo for unilateral cases. It is unusual for a child to present with a retinoblastoma after 3 yr of

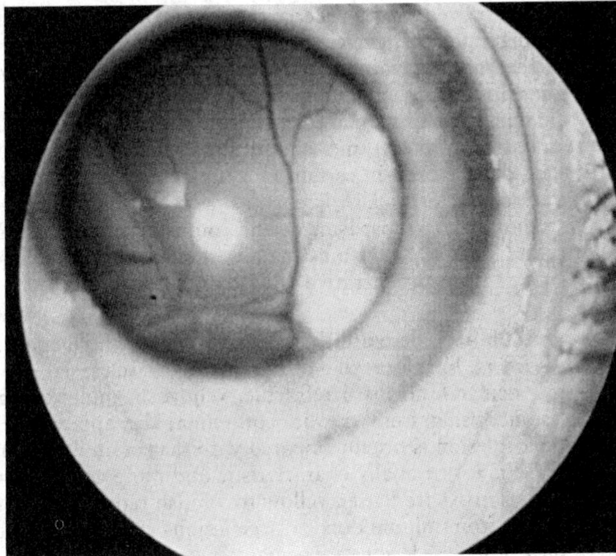

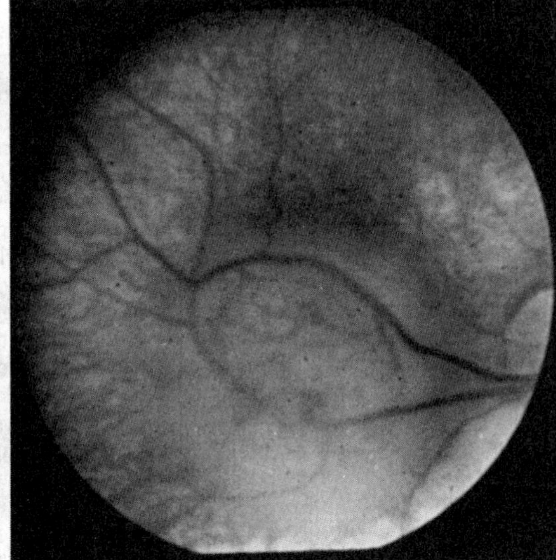

Figure 629-2. Retinoblastoma.

age. Rarely, the tumor is discovered at birth, during adolescence, or even in early adulthood.

Clinical Manifestations. The clinical manifestations of retinoblastoma vary, depending on the stage at which the tumor is detected. The initial sign in the majority of patients is a white pupillary reflex (leukocoria). Leukocoria results because of the reflection of light off the white tumor. The second most frequent initial sign of retinoblastoma is strabismus. Less frequent presenting signs include pseudohypopyon (tumor cells layered inferiorly in front of the iris) caused by tumor seeding in the anterior chamber of the eye, hyphema (blood layered in front of the iris) secondary to iris neovascularization, vitreous hemorrhage, and signs of orbital cellulitis. On examination, the tumor appears as a white mass, sometimes small and relatively flat, sometimes large and protuberant. It may appear nodular. Vitreous haze or tumor seeding may be evident.

The retinoblastoma gene is a recessive suppressor gene located on chromosome 13 at the 13q14 region. Because of the hereditary nature of retinoblastoma, family members of affected children should undergo a complete ophthalmologic examination and genetic counseling. Newborn siblings and children of affected patients should be referred to an ophthalmologist shortly after birth, when the peripheral retina can be evaluated without the need for an examination under anesthesia.

Diagnosis. This is made by direct observation by an experienced ophthalmologist. Ancillary testing such as CT or ultrasonography may help to confirm the diagnosis and demonstrate calcification within the mass. A definitive diagnosis occasionally cannot be made, and removal of the eye must be considered to avoid the possibility of lethal metastasis of the tumor. Because a biopsy can lead to spread of the tumor, histologic confirmation before enucleation is not possible in most cases. Therefore, removal of a blind eye in which the diagnosis of retinoblastoma is likely may be appropriate.

Treatment. Therapy varies, depending on the size and location of the tumor as well as whether it is unilateral or bilateral. Advanced tumors may be treated by enucleation. Other treatment modalities include the use of external beam irradiation, radiation plaque therapy, laser or cryotherapy, and chemotherapy.

The prognosis for children with retinoblastoma depends on the size and extension of the tumor. When confined to the eye, most tumors can be cured. The prognosis for long-term survival is poor when the tumor has extended into the orbit or along the optic nerve.

RETINITIS PIGMENTOSA. This progressive retinal degeneration is characterized by pigmentary changes, arteriolar attenuation, usually some degree of optic atrophy, and progressive impairment of visual function. Dispersion and aggregation of the retinal pigment produce various ophthalmoscopically visible changes, ranging from granularity or mottling of the retinal pigment pattern to distinctive focal pigment aggregates with the configuration of bone spicules (Fig. 629-3). Other ocular findings include subcapsular cataract, glaucoma, and keratoconus.

Impairment of night vision or dark adaptation is often the first clinical manifestation. Progressive loss of peripheral vision, often in the form of an expanding ring scotoma or concentric contraction of the field, is usual. There may be loss of central vision. Retinal function, as measured by electroretinography (ERG), is characteristically reduced. Manifestations commonly begin in childhood. The disorder may be autosomal recessive, autosomal dominant, or X linked. Only supportive treatment is available.

A special form of retinitis pigmentosa is **Leber congenital retinal amaurosis,** in which the retinal changes tend to be pleo-

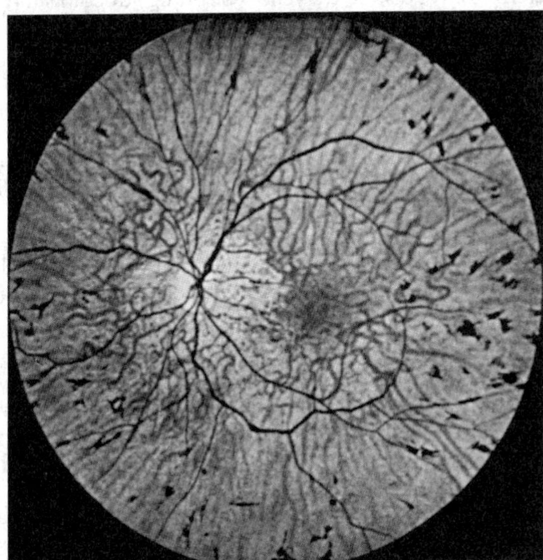

Figure 629-3. Retinitis pigmentosa.

morphic, with various degrees of pigment disorder, arteriolar attenuation, and optic atrophy. The retina may appear normal during infancy. Vision impairment is usually evident soon after birth, and the ERG findings are abnormal early and confirm the diagnosis.

Clinically similar, secondary pigmentary retinal degenerations that need to be differentiated from retinitis pigmentosa occur in a wide variety of metabolic diseases, neurodegenerative processes, and multifaceted syndromes. Examples include the progressive retinal changes of the mucopolysaccharidoses (particularly Hurler, Hunter, Scheie, and Sanfilippo syndromes) and certain of the late-onset gangliosidoses (Batten-Mayou, Spielmeyer-Vogt, and Jansky-Bielschowsky diseases), the progressive retinal degeneration that is associated with progressive external ophthalmoplegia (Kearns-Sayre syndrome), and the retinitis pigmentosa–like changes in the Laurence-Moon and Bardet-Biedl syndromes. The retinal manifestations of abetalipoproteinemia (Bassen-Kornzweig syndrome) and Refsum disease are also similar to those found in retinitis pigmentosa. The diagnosis of these latter two disorders in a patient with presumed retinitis pigmentosa is important because treatment is possible. There is also an association of retinitis pigmentosa and congenital hearing loss, as in Usher syndrome.

STARGARDT DISEASE (FUNDUS FLAVIMACULATUS). This autosomal recessive retinal disorder is characterized by slowly progressive bilateral macular degeneration and vision impairment. It usually appears at 8–14 yr of age, and affected children are often initially misdiagnosed as having functional visual loss. The foveal reflex becomes obtunded or appears grayish, pigment spots develop in the macular area, and macular depigmentation and chorioretinal atrophy eventually occur. Macular hemorrhages also may develop. Some patients also have white or yellow spots beyond the macula or pigmentary changes in the periphery; the term fundus flavimaculatus is commonly used for this condition. It is now recognized that Stargardt disease and fundus flavimaculatus represent different parts on the spectrum of the same disease. Central visual acuity is reduced, often to 20/200, but total loss of vision does not occur. ERG findings vary. The condition is not associated with central nervous system abnormalities and is to be differentiated from the macular changes of many progressive metabolic neurodegenerative diseases. The genetic mutation responsible for Stargardt macular dystrophy has been identified.

BEST VITELLIFORM DEGENERATION. This macular dystrophy is characterized by a distinctive yellow or orange discoid subretinal lesion in the macula, resembling the intact yolk of a fried egg. Diagnosis is usually made at 3–15 yr of age, with a mean age of presentation of 6 yr. Vision is usually normal at this stage. The condition may be progressive; the yolklike lesion may eventually degenerate ("scramble") and result in pigmentation, chorioretinal atrophy, and vision impairment. The condition is usually bilateral. There is no association with systemic abnormalities. Inheritance is usually autosomal dominant. In vitelliform macular degeneration, the ERG response is normal. Electro-oculographic findings are abnormal in affected patients and carriers, and this test is useful in diagnosis and in genetic counseling.

CHERRY RED SPOT. Because of the special histologic features of the macula, certain pathologic processes affecting the retina produce an ophthalmoscopically visible sign referred to as a cherry red spot, a bright to dull red spot at the center of the macula surrounded and accentuated by a grayish-white or yellowish halo. The halo is a result of a loss of transparency of the retinal ganglion cell layer secondary to edema, lipid accumulation, or both. Because ganglion cells are not present in the fovea, the retina surrounding the fovea is opacified but the fovea transmits the normal underlying choroidal color (red), accounting for the presence of the cherry red spot. A cherry red spot typically occurs in certain sphingolipidoses, principally in Tay-Sachs disease (GM_2 type 1), in the Sandhoff variant (GM_2 type 2), and in generalized gangliosidosis (GM_1 type 1). Similar but less distinctive macular changes occur in some cases of metachromatic leukodystrophy (sulfatide lipidosis), in some forms of neuronopathic Niemann-Pick disease, and in certain mucolipidoses. The cherry red spot that characteristically occurs as a result of retinal ischemia secondary to vasospasm, ocular contusion, or occlusion of the central retinal artery must be differentiated from the cherry red spot of neurodegenerative disease.

PHAKOMAS. These are the herald lesions of the hamartomatous disorders. In Bourneville disease (tuberous sclerosis), the distinctive ocular lesion is a refractile, yellowish, multinodular cystic lesion arising from the disc or retina; the appearance of this typical lesion is often compared with that of an unripe mulberry (Fig. 629-4). Equally characteristic and more common in tuberous sclerosis are flatter, yellow to whitish retinal lesions, varying in size from minute dots to large lesions approaching the size of the disc. These lesions are benign astrocytic proliferations. Rarely, similar retinal phakomas occur in von Recklinghausen disease (neurofibromatosis). In von Hippel-Lindau disease (angiomatosis of the retina and cerebellum), the distinctive fundus lesion is a hemangioblastoma; this vascular lesion usually appears as a reddish globular mass with large paired arteries and veins passing to and from the lesion. In Sturge-Weber syndrome (encephalofacial angiomatosis), the fundus abnormality is a choroidal hemangioma; the hemangioma may impart a dark color to the affected area of the fundus, but the lesion is best seen with fluorescein angiography.

RETINOSCHISIS. Congenital hereditary retinoschisis, also referred to as juvenile X-linked retinoschisis, is a bilateral vitreoretinal dystrophy that appears early in life, often in infancy. It is characterized by splitting of the retina into inner and outer layers. The usual ophthalmoscopic finding in affected males is an elevation of the inner layer of the retina, most commonly in the inferotemporal quadrant of the fundus, often with round or oval holes visible in the inner layer. Schisis of the fovea is virtually pathognomonic and is found in almost 100% of patients. Ophthalmoscopically, this appears in early stages as small, fine striae in the internal limiting membrane. These striae radiate outward in a petaloid or spoke wheel configuration. In some cases, frank retinal detachment or vitreous hemorrhage occurs.

Vision impairment varies from mild to severe; visual acuity may worsen with age, but good vision is often retained. Carrier

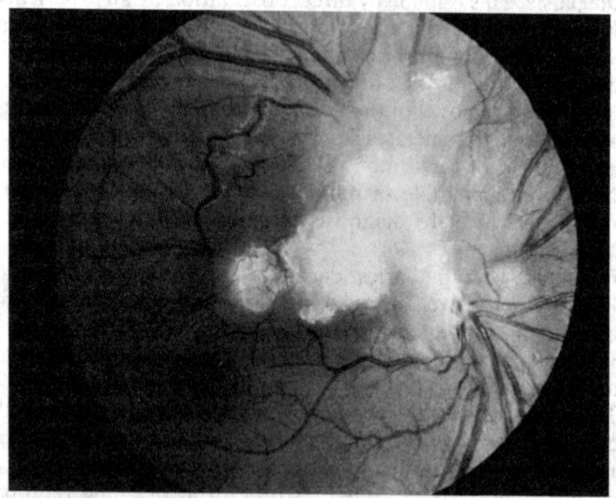

Figure 629-4. Retinal phakoma of tuberous sclerosis.

females are asymptomatic, but linkage studies may be useful to help detect carriers.

RETINAL DETACHMENT. A retinal detachment is a separation of the outer layers of the retina from the underlying retinal pigment epithelium (RPE). During embryogenesis, the retina and RPE are initially separated. During ocular development, they join together and are held in apposition to each other by various physiologic mechanisms. Pathologic events leading to a retinal detachment return the retina-RPE to its former separated state. The detachment can occur as a congenital anomaly but more commonly arises secondary to other ocular abnormalities or trauma. Three types of detachment are described; each may occur in children. Rhegmatogenous detachments result from a break in the retina that allows fluid to enter the subretinal space. In children, these are usually a result of trauma (such as child abuse) but may occur secondary to myopia or ROP or after congenital cataract surgery. Tractional retinal detachments result when vitreoretinal membranes pull on the retina. They can occur in diabetes, sickle cell disease, and ROP. Exudative retinal detachments result when exudation exceeds absorption. This can be seen in Coats disease, retinoblastoma, and ocular inflammation.

The presenting sign of retinal detachment in an infant or child may be loss of vision, secondary strabismus or nystagmus, or leukocoria (white pupillary reflex). In addition to direct examination of the eye, special diagnostic studies such as ultrasonography and neuroimaging (CT, MRI) may be necessary to establish the cause of the detachment and the appropriate treatment. Prompt treatment is essential if vision is to be salvaged.

COATS DISEASE. This exudative retinopathy of unknown cause is characterized by telangiectasia of retinal vessels with leakage of plasma to form intraretinal and subretinal exudates and by retinal hemorrhages and detachment (Fig. 629-5). The condition is usually unilateral. It predominantly affects boys, usually appearing in the 1st decade. The condition is nonfamilial and for the most part occurs in otherwise healthy children. The most frequent presenting signs are blurring of vision, leukocoria, and strabismus. Rubeosis of the iris, glaucoma, and cataract may develop. **Treatment** with photocoagulation or cryotherapy may be helpful.

FAMILIAL EXUDATIVE VITREORETINOPATHY (FEVR). This progressive retinal vascular disorder is of unknown cause, but clinical and angiographic findings suggest an aberration of vascular development. Avascularity of the peripheral temporal retina is a significant finding in most cases, with abrupt cessation of the retinal capillary network in the region of the equator. The avascular zone often has a wedge- or V-shaped pattern in the temporal meridian. Glial proliferation or well-marked retinochoroidal atrophy may be found in the avascular zone. Excessive branching of retinal arteries and veins, dilatation of the capillaries, arteriovenous shunt formation, neovascularization, and leakage from retinal vessels of the farthest vascularized retina occur. Vitreoretinal adhesions are usually present at the peripheral margin of the vascularized retina. Traction, retinal dragging and temporal displacement of the macula, falciform retinal folds, and retinal detachment are common. Intraretinal or subretinal exudation, retinal hemorrhage, and recurrent vitreous hemorrhages may develop. Patients may also develop cataracts and glaucoma. Vision impairment of varying severity occurs. The condition is usually bilateral. FEVR is usually an autosomal dominant condition with incomplete penetrance. Asymptomatic family members often display a zone of avascular peripheral retina.

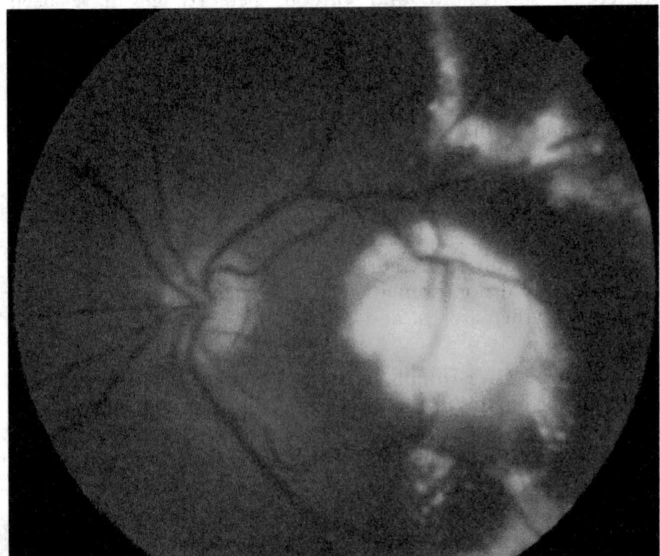
Figure 629-5. Coats disease with massive retinal exudation.

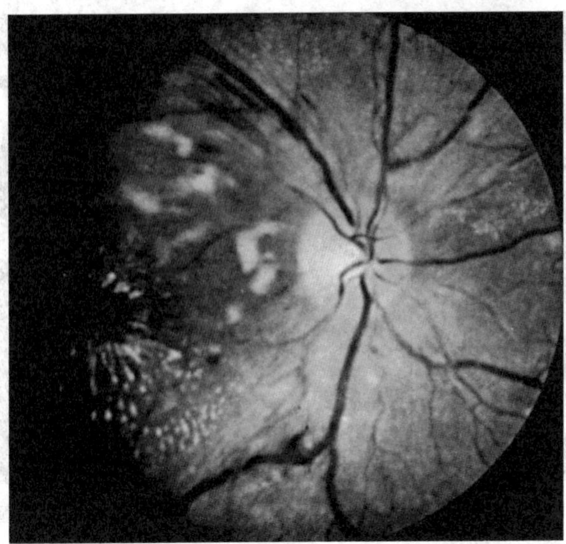
Figure 629-6. Hypertensive retinopathy.

The findings in FEVR may resemble those of ROP in the cicatricial stages, but unlike ROP, the neovascularization of FEVR seems to develop years after birth and most patients with FEVR have no history of prematurity, oxygen therapy, prenatal or postnatal injury or infection, or developmental abnormalities. FEVR is also to be differentiated from Coats disease, angiomatosis of the retina, peripheral uveitis, and other disorders of the posterior segment.

HYPERTENSIVE RETINOPATHY. In the early stages of hypertension, no retinal changes may be observable. Generalized constriction and irregular narrowing of the arterioles are usually the first signs in the fundus. Other alterations include retinal edema, flame-shaped hemorrhages, cotton-wool spots (retinal nerve fiber layer infarcts), and papilledema (Fig. 629-6). These changes are reversible if the hypertension can be controlled in the early stages, but in long-standing hypertension, irreversible changes may occur. Thickening of the vessel wall may produce a silver- or copper-wire appearance. Hypertensive retinal changes in a child should alert the physician to renal disease, pheochromocytoma, collagen disease, and cardiovascular disorders, particularly coarctation of the aorta.

DIABETIC RETINOPATHY. The retinal changes of diabetes mellitus are classified as nonproliferative or proliferative. Nonproliferative diabetic retinopathy is characterized by retinal micro-

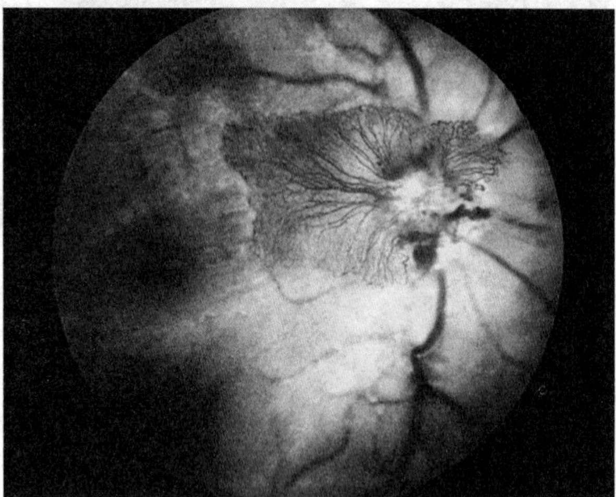

Figure 629-7. Proliferative diabetic retinopathy with neovascularization of the disc.

aneurysms, venous dilatation, retinal hemorrhages, and exudates. The microaneurysms appear as tiny red dots. The hemorrhages may be of both the dot and blot type, representing deep intraretinal bleeding, and the splinter or flame-shaped type, involving the superficial nerve fiber layer. The exudates tend to be deep and to appear waxy. There may also be superficial nerve fiber infarcts called cytoid bodies or cotton-wool spots, as well as retinal edema. These signs may wax and wane. They are seen primarily in the posterior pole, around the disc and macula, well within the range of direct ophthalmoscopy. Involvement of the macula may lead to decreased vision.

Proliferative retinopathy, the more serious form, is characterized by neovascularization and proliferation of fibrovascular tissue on the retina, extending into the vitreous. Neovascularization may occur on the optic disc (NVD), elsewhere on the retina (NVE), or on the iris and in the anterior chamber angle (NVI, or rubeosis irides) (Fig. 629-7). Traction on these new vessels leads to hemorrhage and eventually scarring. The vision-threatening complications of proliferative diabetic retinopathy are retinal and vitreous hemorrhages, cicatrization, traction, and retinal detachment. Neovascularization of the iris may lead to secondary glaucoma if not treated promptly.

Diabetic retinopathy involves the alteration and nonperfusion of retinal capillaries, retinal ischemia, and neovascularization, but its pathogenesis is not yet completely understood, either in terms of location of the primary pathogenetic mechanism (retinal vessels vs surrounding neuronal or glial tissue) or the specific biochemical factors involved. The better the degree of long-term metabolic control, the lower the risk of diabetic retinopathy.

Clinically, the prevalence and course of retinopathy relate to a patient's age and to disease duration. Detectable microvascular changes are rare in prepubertal children, with the prevalence of retinopathy increasing significantly after puberty, especially after the age of 15 yr. The incidence of retinopathy is low during the first 5 yr of disease and increases progressively thereafter, with the incidence of proliferative retinopathy becoming substantial after 10 yr and with increased risk of visual impairment after 15 yr or more. Periodic ophthalmologic evaluation is recommended for all patients with diabetes mellitus.

In addition to retinopathy, patients with juvenile-onset diabetes may develop optic neuropathy, characterized by swelling of the disc and blurring of vision. Patients with diabetes may also develop cataracts, even at an early age, sometimes with rapid progression.

Treatment. Macular edema is the leading cause of visual loss in diabetic persons. Photocoagulation may be used to decrease the risk of continued vision loss in patients with macular edema.

Proliferative retinopathy causes the most severe vision loss and can lead to total loss of vision and even loss of the eye. Patients who have proliferative disease and who display certain high-risk characteristics should undergo panretinal photocoagulation to preserve their central vision. Neovascularization of the iris is also treated with panretinal photocoagulation to stop the development of neovascular glaucoma.

Vitrectomy and other intraocular surgery may be necessary in patients with nonresolving vitreous hemorrhage or traction retinal detachment. The value of technologic advances, such as insulin infusion pumps and pancreatic transplants, in preventing ocular complications is under investigation (see Chapter 590).

SUBACUTE BACTERIAL ENDOCARDITIS. At some time during the course of the disease, retinopathy is present in approximately 40% of cases of subacute bacterial endocarditis. The lesions include hemorrhages, hemorrhages with white centers (Roth spots), papilledema, and, rarely, embolic occlusion of the central retinal artery.

BLOOD DISORDERS. In primary and secondary anemias, retinopathy in the form of hemorrhages and cotton-wool patches may occur. Vision can be affected if hemorrhage occurs in the macular area. The hemorrhages may be light and feathery or dense and preretinal. In polycythemia vera, the retinal veins are dark, dilated, and tortuous. Retinal hemorrhages, retinal edema, and papilledema may be observed. In leukemia, the veins are characteristically dilated, with sausage-shaped constrictions; hemorrhages, particularly white-centered hemorrhages and exudates, are common during the acute stage. In the sickling disorders, fundus changes include vascular tortuosity, arterial and venous occlusions, "salmon patches," refractile deposits, pigmented lesions, arteriolar-venous anastomoses, and neovascularization (with "sea-fan" formations), sometimes leading to vitreous hemorrhage and retinal detachment. Individuals with Hb SC and Hb S-β-thalassemia hemoglobinopathies are at a higher risk of the development of retinopathy than are those with Hb SS disease. It is thought that the more anemic state of those patients with SS disease offers protection from vascular occlusions in the retina.

TRAUMA-RELATED RETINOPATHY. Retinal changes may occur in patients who suffer trauma to other parts of the body. The occurrence of retinal hemorrhages in infants who have been physically abused is well documented (Fig. 629-8) (see Chapter 36). Retinal, subretinal, subhyaloid, and vitreous hemorrhages have been described in infants and young children with inflicted neurotrauma. Often there are no signs of direct trauma to the eye, periocular region, or head. Such cases may result from violent shaking of an infant, and permanent retinal damage may result.

In patients with severe head or chest compressive trauma, a traumatic retinal angiopathy known as **Purtscher retinopathy** may occur. This is characterized by retinal hemorrhage, cotton-wool spots, possible disc swelling, and decreased vision. The pathogenesis is unclear, but there is evidence of arteriolar obstruction in this condition. A Purtscher-like fundus picture may also occur in several nontraumatic settings, such as acute pancreatitis, lupus erythematosus, and childbirth.

MYELINATED NERVE FIBERS. Myelination of the optic nerve fibers normally terminates at the level of the disc, but in some individuals, ectopic myelination extends to nerve fibers of the retina. The condition is most commonly seen adjacent to the disc, although more peripheral areas of the retina may be involved. The characteristic ophthalmoscopic picture is a focal white patch with a feathered edge or brush-stroke appearance. Because the macula is generally unaffected, the visual prognosis is good. A relative or absolute visual field defect corresponding to areas of ectopic

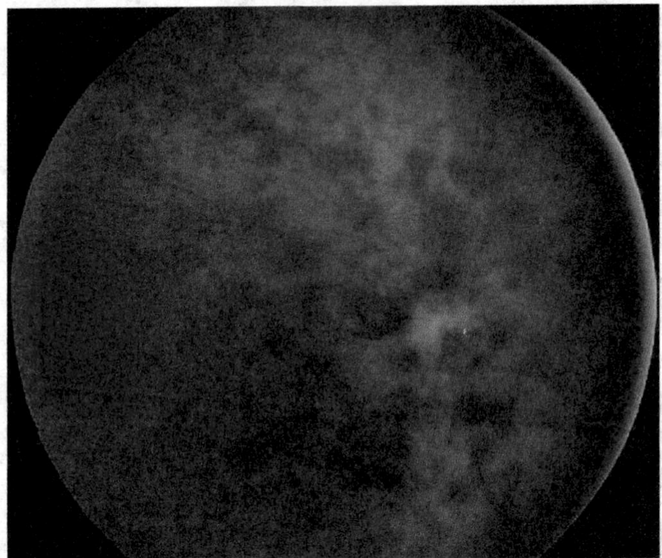

Figure 629-8. Shaken baby syndrome (inflicted neurotrauma). Retinal hemorrhages in multiple layers too numerous to count into far periphery.

myelination is usually the only associated ocular abnormality. Extensive unilateral involvement, however, has been associated with ipsilateral myopia, amblyopia, and strabismus. If unilateral high myopia and amblyopia are present, appropriate optical correction and occlusion therapy should be instituted. For unknown reasons, the disorder is more commonly encountered in patients with craniofacial dysostosis, oxycephaly, neurofibromatosis, and Down syndrome.

COLOBOMA OF THE FUNDUS. The term coloboma describes a defect such as a gap, notch, fissure, or hole. The typical fundus coloboma is a result of malclosure of the embryonic fissure, which leaves a gap in the retina, RPE, and choroid, thus baring the underlying sclera. The defect may be extensive, involving the optic nerve, ciliary body, iris, and even lens, or it may be localized to 1 or more portions of the fissure. The usual appearance is of a well-circumscribed, wedge-shaped white area extending inferonasally below the disc, sometimes involving or engulfing the disc. In some cases, there is ectasia or cyst formation in the area of the defect. Less extensive colobomatous defects may appear as only single or multiple focal punched-out chorioretinal defects or anomalous pigmentation of the fundus in the line of the embryonic fissure. Colobomas may occur in 1 or both eyes. A visual field defect usually corresponds to the chorioretinal defect. Visual acuity may be impaired, particularly if the defect involves the disc or macula.

Fundus colobomas may occur in isolation as sporadic defects or as an inherited condition. Isolated colobomatous anomalies are commonly inherited in an autosomal dominant manner with highly variable penetrance and expressivity. Family members of affected patients should receive appropriate genetic counseling. Colobomas may also be associated with such abnormalities as microphthalmia, glioneuroma of the eye, cyclopia, or encephale. They occur in children with various chromosomal disorders, including trisomies 13 and 18, triploidy, cat-eye syndrome, and 4p-. Ocular colobomata also occur in many multisystem disorders, including the CHARGE (C, coloboma; H, heart disease; A, atresia choanae; R, retarded growth and development and/or central nervous system anomalies; G, genetic anomalies and/or hypogonadism; E, ear anomalies and/or deafness) association; Joubert, Aicardi, Meckel, Warburg, and Rubinstein-Taybi syndromes; linear sebaceous nevus; Goldenhar and Lenz microphthalmia syndromes; and Goltz focal dermal hypoplasia.

Abramson DH, Frank CM, Susman M, et al: Presenting signs of retinoblastoma. *J Pediatr* 1998;132:505–508.

Chang M, McLean IW, Merritt JC: Coats' disease: A study of 62 histologically confirmed cases. *J Pediatr Ophthalmol Strabismus* 1984;21:163–168.

Cryotherapy for Retinopathy of Prematurity Cooperative Group: 15-year outcomes following threshold retinopathy of prematurity. *Arch Ophthalmol* 2005;123:311–318.

Dass AB, Trese MT: Surgical results of persistent hyperplastic primary vitreous. *Ophthalmology* 1999;106:280–284.

Early Treatment Diabetic Retinopathy Research Study Group: Photocoagulation for diabetic macular edema. Early treatment diabetic retinopathy study report 1. *Arch Ophthalmol* 1985;103:1796–1806.

Early Treatment for Retinopathy of Prematurity Cooperative Group. Revised indications for the treatment of retinopathy of prematurity: Results of the early treatment for retinopathy of prematurity randomized trial. *Arch Ophthalmol* 2003;121:1684–1696.

Fierson W, Palmer E, Biglan A, et al: Screening examination of premature infants for retinopathy of prematurity. A joint statement of the American Academy of Pediatrics, the American Association for Pediatric Ophthalmology and Strabismus and the American Academy of Ophthalmology. *Pediatrics* 1997;100:273–274.

Hardwig P, Robertson DM: Von Hippel-Lindau disease: A familial, often lethal, multi-system phakomatosis. *Ophthalmology* 1984;91:263–270.

Hartong DT, Berson EL, Dryja TP: Retinitis pigmentosa. *Lancet* 2006;368:1795–1809.

Miyakulo H, Hashimoto K, Miyakulo S: Retinal vascular pattern in familial exudative vitreoretinopathy. *Ophthalmology* 1984;91:1524–1530.

Mohler CW, Fine SL: Long-term evaluation of patients with Best's vitelliform dystrophy. *Ophthalmology* 1981;88:688–692.

Noble KG, Carr RE: Leber's congenital amaurosis: A retrospective study of 33 cases and a histopathological study of one case. *Arch Ophthalmol* 1978;96:818–821.

Shalev B, Farr A, Repka MX: Randomized comparison of diode laser photocoagulation versus cryotherapy for threshold retinopathy of prematurity: Seven year outcome. *Am J Ophthalmol* 2001;132:76–80.

Shields CL, Gorry T, Shields JA: Outcome of eyes with unilateral sporadic retinoblastoma based on the initial external findings by the family and the pediatrician. *J Pediatr Ophthalmol Strabismus* 2004;41:143–149.

Weinberg DV, Lyon AT, Greenwald MJ, et al: Rhegmatogenous retinal detachments in children: Risk factors and surgical outcomes. *Ophthalmology* 2003;110:1708–1713.

Chapter 630 ■ Abnormalities of the Optic Nerve

Scott E. Olitsky, Denise Hug, and Laura P. Smith

OPTIC NERVE APLASIA. This rare congenital anomaly is typically unilateral. The optic nerve, retinal ganglion cells, and retinal blood vessels are absent. A vestigial dural sheath usually connects with the sclera in a normal position, but no neural tissue is present within this sheath. Optic nerve aplasia typically occurs sporadically in an otherwise healthy person. A wide variety of ocular abnormalities may occur, but colobomas are the most frequent associated finding.

OPTIC NERVE HYPOPLASIA. Hypoplasia of the optic nerve is a nonprogressive condition characterized by a subnormal number of optic nerve axons with normal mesodermal elements and glial supporting tissue. In typical cases, the nerve head is small and pale, with a pale or pigmented peripapillary halo or double-ring sign.

This anomaly is associated with defects of vision and of visual fields of varying severity, ranging from blindness to normal or near-normal vision. It may be associated with systemic anomalies that most commonly involve the central nervous system (CNS). Protean CNS defects such as hydranencephaly or anencephaly or more focal lesions compatible with continued development of a patient may accompany optic nerve hypoplasia, but unilateral or bilateral optic nerve hypoplasia may be found without any concomitant defects.

Optic nerve hypoplasia is a principal feature of **septo-optic dysplasia of de Morsier,** a developmental disorder characterized by the association of anomalies of the midline structures of the brain with hypoplasia of the optic nerves, optic chiasm, and optic tracts; typically noted are agenesis of the septum pellucidum, partial or complete agenesis of the corpus callosum, and malformation of the fornix, with a large chiasmatic cistern. Patients may have hypothalamic abnormalities and endocrine defects, ranging from panhypopituitarism to isolated deficiency of growth hormone, hypothyroidism, or diabetes insipidus. Neonatal hypoglycemia and seizures are important presenting signs in affected infants.

MRI is preferred for evaluating CNS abnormalities in patients with optic nerve hypoplasia. During MRI, special attention should be directed to the pituitary infundibulum, where ectopia of the posterior pituitary may be found. Posterior pituitary ectopia appears on MRI as an absence of the pituitary infundibulum with an abnormal bright spot at the upper infundibulum area. This abnormality is present in approximately 15% of patients and suggests posterior pituitary hormone deficiency, requiring further endocrinologic work-up.

Bilateral subtle hypoplasia may be difficult to diagnose from the appearance of the disc alone because no comparison with a contralateral uninvolved eye is possible. However, it is important to establish the diagnosis because this eliminates confusion with optic atrophy or glaucoma and may explain the cause of decreased vision in a patient unresponsive to amblyopia therapy. Endocrine function should be watched closely in patients with optic nerve hypoplasia.

The cause of optic nerve hypoplasia remains unclear. Early gestational injuries to midline CNS structures with secondary axonal injury or a disruption of normal neuronal guidance mechanisms that affect both the optic nerve and cerebral neurons may account for these commonly associated disorders. Optic nerve hypoplasia may occur with somewhat increased frequency in infants of diabetic mothers and has been associated with maternal use of Dilantin, quinine, LSD (lysergic acid diethylamide), and alcohol during pregnancy.

Children with **periventricular leukomalacia** display an unusual form of optic nerve hypoplasia. The optic nerves demonstrate a large cup within a normal-sized optic disc. This form of optic nerve hypoplasia occurs secondary to transsynaptic degeneration of optic axons caused by the primary bilateral lesion in the optic radiation (periventricular leukomalacia).

OPTIC NERVE COLOBOMA. Optic nerve colobomas can be unilateral or bilateral. The visual acuity can range from normal to complete blindness. The coloboma develops secondary to incomplete closure of the embryonic fissure. The defect may produce a partial or total excavation of the optic disc (Fig. 630-1) Chorioretinal and iris colobomas may also occur. Optic nerve colobomas may be seen in a multitude of ocular and systemic abnormalities including the CHARGE (C, coloboma; H, heart disease; A, atresia choanae; R, retarded growth and development and/or central nervous system anomalies; G, genetic anomalies and/or hypogonadism; E, ear anomalies and/or deafness) association.

MORNING GLORY DISC ANOMALY. This term describes a congenital malformation of the optic nerve characterized by an enlarged, excavated, funnel-shaped disc with an elevated rim, resembling a morning glory flower. White glial tissue is present in the central part of the disc. The retinal vessels are abnormal and appear at the peripheral disc and course over the elevated pink rim in a radial fashion. Pigmentary mottling of the peripapillary region is

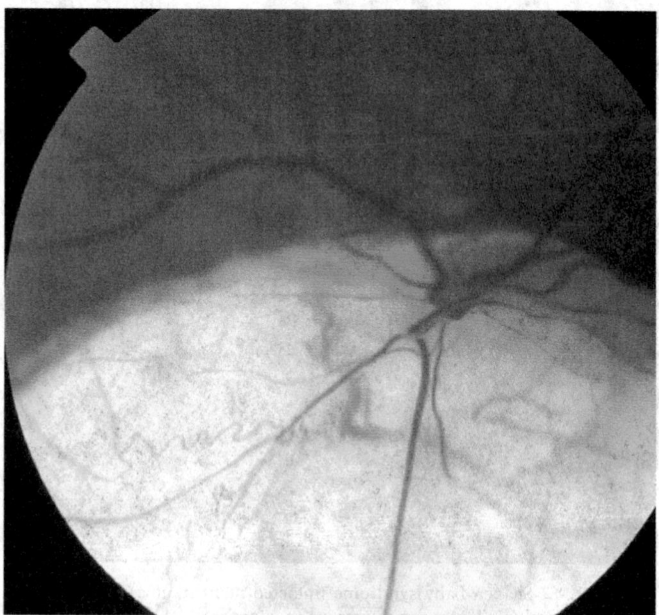

Figure 630-1. Optic nerve coloboma.

usually seen. Most cases are unilateral. Females are affected twice as often as males. Visual acuity is usually severely reduced, and retinal detachment occurs in approximately ⅓ of involved eyes. Morning glory disc anomaly has been associated with basal encephalocele in patients with midfacial anomalies. Abnormalities of the carotid circulation can also be seen in patients with morning glory anomaly. Moyamoya disease is a well-described associated finding.

TILTED DISC. In this congenital anomaly, the vertical axis of the optic disc is directed obliquely, so that the upper temporal portion of the nerve head is more prominent and anterior to the lower nasal portion of the disc. The retinal vessels emerge from the upper temporal portion of the disc rather than from the nasal side. Often noted is a peripapillary crescent or conus. Associated visual field defects and myopic astigmatism may be found. Clinical recognition of the tilted disc syndrome is important to avoid confusion of its disc and visual field signs with those of papilledema and intracranial tumor.

DRUSEN OF THE OPTIC NERVE. These globular, acellular bodies are thought to arise from axoplasmic derivatives of disintegrating nerve fibers. Drusen may be buried within the optic nerve, producing elevation of the optic nerve head (which can be confused with papilledema), or they may be partially or completely exposed, appearing as refractile bodies at the surface of the disc. Visual field defects and spontaneous peripapillary nerve fiber layer hemorrhages may occur in association with drusen. Drusen may occur as an autosomal dominant condition. They have also been observed in children with various neurologic disorders, including primary megalencephaly, seizures, learning disorders, mental retardation, schizophrenia, tuberous sclerosis, Down syndrome, and intracranial tumors.

PAPILLEDEMA. The term papilledema is reserved to describe swelling of the nerve head secondary to increased intracranial pressure (ICP). Clinical manifestations of papilledema include edematous blurring of the disc margins, fullness or elevation of the nerve head, partial or complete obliteration of the disc cup, capillary congestion and hyperemia of the nerve head, generalized engorgement of the veins, loss of spontaneous venous pulsation, nerve fiber layer hemorrhages around the disc, and peripapillary exudates (see Fig. 591-1). In some cases, edema extending into the macula may produce a fan- or star-shaped figure. In addition, concentric peripapillary retinal wrinkling (Paton lines) may be noted. Transient obscuration of vision may occur, lasting seconds and associated with postural changes. Vision, however, is usually normal in acute papilledema. Normally, when the ICP is relieved, the papilledema resolves and the disc returns to a normal or nearly normal appearance within 6–8 wk. Sustained chronic papilledema or long-standing unrelieved increased ICP may, however, lead to permanent nerve fiber damage, atrophic changes of the disc, macular scarring, and impairment of vision.

The *pathophysiology* of papilledema is probably as follows: elevation of intracranial subarachnoid cerebrospinal fluid (CSF) pressure, elevation of CSF pressure in the sheath of the optic nerve, elevation of tissue pressure in the optic nerve, stasis of axoplasmic flow and swelling of the nerve fibers in the optic nerve head, and secondary vascular changes and the characteristic ophthalmoscopic signs of venous stasis. Associated neuro-ophthalmic signs of increased ICP in infants and children include 6th cranial nerve palsy and attendant esotropia, lid retraction, paresis of upward gaze, tonic downward deviation of the eyes, and convergent nystagmus.

The common **etiologies** of papilledema in childhood are intracranial tumors and obstructive hydrocephalus, intracranial hemorrhage, the cerebral edema of trauma, meningoencephalitis, toxic encephalopathy, and certain metabolic diseases. Whatever the cause, the optic disc signs of increased ICP in early childhood may occasionally be modified by the distensibility of the young skull. In the absence of conditions associated with early closure of sutures and early obliteration of the fontanel (craniosynostosis, Crouzon disease, and Apert syndrome), infants with increased ICP may not develop papilledema.

The **differential diagnosis** of papilledema includes structural changes of the disc (pseudopapilledema, pseudoneuritis, drusen, and myelinated nerve fibers), with which it may be confused, and the disc swelling of papillitis associated with optic neuritis in addition to the disc changes of hypertension and diabetes mellitus. Unless retinal hemorrhage or edema involves the macular area, the preservation of good central vision and the absence of an afferent pupillary defect (Marcus Gunn pupil) help to differentiate acute papilledema from the edema of the optic nerve head found in acute optic neuritis.

Papilledema is a neurologic emergency. It can be accompanied by other signs of increased ICP, including headaches, nausea, and vomiting. Neuroimaging should be performed; if no intracranial masses are detected, a lumbar puncture and determination of CSF pressure should follow.

OPTIC NEURITIS. This is any inflammation or demyelinization of the optic nerve with attendant impairment of function. The process is usually acute, with rapidly progressive loss of vision. It may be unilateral or bilateral. Pain on movement of the globe or pain on palpation of the globe may precede or accompany the onset of visual symptoms. There is decreased visual activity, decreased color vision and contrast sensitivity, a relative afferent pupillary defect, and a normal macula and peripheral retina.

When the retrobulbar portion of the nerve is affected without ophthalmoscopically visible signs of inflammation at the disc, the term *retrobulbar optic neuritis* is applied. When there is ophthalmoscopically visible evidence of inflammation of the nerve head, the term *papillitis* or *intraocular optic neuritis* is used. When there is involvement of both the retina and papilla, the term optic *neuroretinitis* is used.

In childhood, optic neuritis may occur as an isolated condition or as a manifestation of a neurologic or systemic disease. Optic neuritis may be secondary to inflammatory diseases (systemic lupus erythematosus, sarcoidosis, Behçet disease, autoimmune optic neuritis); infections (tuberculosis, syphilis, Lyme disease, meningitis, viral encephalitis, or post-infectious); and toxic or nutritional (methanol, ethambutol, vitamin B_{12} deficiency). It may signify one of the many demyelinating diseases of childhood (see Chapter 600). Although a significant percentage of adults who experience an episode of optic neuritis eventually develop other symptoms associated with multiple sclerosis (MS), young children with optic neuritis are seemingly at less risk (risk of MS is 19% within 20 yrs). Bilateral optic neuritis in children may be associated with **neuromyelitis optica (Devic disease)**. This syndrome is characterized by rapid and severe bilateral visual loss accompanied by transverse myelitis and paraplegia. Optic neuritis may also be secondary to an exogenous toxin or drug, such as with lead poisoning or as a complication of long-term high-dose treatment with chloramphenicol or vincristine therapy. Extensive pediatric neurologic and ophthalmic investigation, including MRI and lumbar puncture, is usually required.

In most cases of acute optic neuritis, some improvement in vision begins within 1–4 wk after onset, and vision may improve to normal or near normal within weeks or months. The course varies with cause. Although central vision may fully recover, it is common to find permanent defects in other areas of visual function (contrast sensitivity, color, brightness sense, and motion perception). Recurrences may occur especially, but not universally, in patients who go on to develop MS.

A **treatment** trial demonstrated that high-dose intravenous methylprednisolone may help to speed the visual recovery in young adults, and it may prevent the development of multiple sclerosis in those at risk. Orally administered corticosteroids should not be used because they are associated with a significant increase in the recurrence rate of optic neuritis. It is unknown to what degree the results of the aforementioned trial may be extrapolated to optic neuritis in childhood. In adults with MRI white matter lesions, treatment with interferon beta (1a or 1b) reduces the incidence of MS.

LEBER OPTIC NEUROPATHY. This entity is characterized by sudden loss of central vision occurring in the 2nd and 3rd decades of life, primarily affecting young males. A characteristic peripapillary telangiectatic microangiopathy occurs not only in the presymptomatic phase of involved eyes but also in a high number of asymptomatic offspring in the female line. Disc hyperemia and edema mark the acute phase of visual loss. One eye is usually affected before the other. Visual field loss and impaired color vision are also present. In time, progressive optic atrophy and vision loss usually ensue. The tortuous angiopathy becomes less obvious. Although visual function after the initial loss generally remains stable, a significant and sometimes complete recovery may occur in as many as ⅓ of affected individuals. This recovery may take place years or decades after the initial episode of acute vision loss. The peripapillary angiopathy, the lack of short-term remission, and the degree of symmetry serve to distinguish most cases of Leber disease from the optic neuritis of multiple sclerosis.

Leber optic neuropathy is maternally inherited and is caused by defective cytoplasmic mitochondrial DNA. Multiple point mutations in the mitochondrial DNA that lead to the development of the disorder have been found. Because of the mitochondrial nature of the disorder, skeletal and cardiac muscle disorders, including electrocardiographic abnormalities, may also be encountered in affected individuals.

OPTIC ATROPHY. This term denotes degeneration of optic nerve axons, with attendant loss of function. The ophthalmoscopic signs of optic atrophy are pallor of the disc and loss of substance of the nerve head, sometimes with enlargement of the disc cup. The associated vision defect varies with the nature and site of the primary disease or lesion.

Optic atrophy is the common expression of a wide variety of congenital or acquired pathologic processes. The cause may be traumatic, inflammatory, degenerative, neoplastic, or vascular; intracranial tumors and hydrocephalus are principal causes of optic atrophy in children. In some cases, progressive optic atrophy is hereditary. **Dominantly inherited infantile optic atrophy** is a relatively mild heredodegenerative type that tends to progress through childhood and adolescence. **Autosomal recessively inherited congenital optic atrophy** is a rare condition that is evident at birth or develops at a very early age; the visual defect is usually profound. **Behr optic atrophy** is a hereditary type associated with hypertonia of the extremities, increased deep tendon reflexes, mild cerebellar ataxia, some degree of mental deficiency, and possibly external ophthalmoplegia. This disorder afflicts principally boys age 3–11 yr. Some forms of heredodegenerative optic atrophy are associated with sensorineural hearing loss, as may occur in some children with juvenile-onset (insulin-dependent) diabetes mellitus. In the absence of an obvious cause, optic atrophy in an infant or child warrants extensive etiologic investigation.

OPTIC NERVE GLIOMA. Optic nerve glioma, more properly referred to as **juvenile pilocytic astrocytoma,** is the most frequent tumor of the optic nerve in childhood. This neuroglial tumor may develop in the intraorbital, intracanalicular, or intracranial portion of the nerve; the chiasm is often involved.

The tumor is a cytologic benign hamartoma that is generally stationary or only slowly progressive. The principal *clinical manifestations* when the tumor occurs in the intraorbital portion of the nerve are unilateral loss of vision, proptosis, and deviation of the eye; optic atrophy or congestion of the optic nerve head may occur. Chiasmal involvement may be attended by defects of vision and visual fields (often bitemporal hemianopia), increased ICP, papilledema or optic atrophy, hypothalamic dysfunction, pituitary dysfunction, and sometimes nystagmus or strabismus. Juvenile pilocytic astrocytomas occur with increased frequency in patients with neurofibromatosis.

Treatment of optic pathway gliomas is controversial. The best management is usually periodic observation. Surgical removal may be appropriate when the tumor is confined to the intraorbital, intracanalicular, or prechiasmal portion of the nerve if a patient has unsightly proptosis with complete or nearly complete loss of vision of the affected eye. When the chiasm is involved, resection is not usually indicated and radiation and chemotherapy may be necessary.

TRAUMATIC OPTIC NEUROPATHIES. Injury to the optic nerve may result from both direct and indirect trauma. Direct trauma to the optic nerve is a result of a penetrating injury to the orbit with transection or contusion of the nerve. Blunt trauma to the orbit may also lead to severe visual loss if the traumatic force is transmitted to the optic canal and causes disruption of the blood supply to the intracanalicular portion of the nerve. Treatment may include high-dose corticosteroids or optic canal decompression.

Auw-Haedrich C, Staubach F, Witschel H: Optic disk drusen. *Surv Ophthalmol* 2002;47:515–532.

Balcer LJ: Optic neuritis. *N Engl J Med* 2006;354:1273–1280.

Birkebaek NH, Patel L, Wright NB, et al: Endocrine status in patients with optic nerve hypoplasia: Relationship to midline central nervous system abnormalities and appearance of the hypothalamic-pituitary axis on magnetic resonance imaging. *J Clin Endocrinol Metab* 2003;88:5281–5286.

Hickman SJ, Dalton CM, Miller DH, et al: Management of acute optic neuritis. *Lancet* 2002;360:1953–1962.

Hotchkiss ML, Green WR: Optic nerve aplasia and hypoplasia. *J Pediatr Ophthalmol Strabismus* 1979;16:225–240.

Kazarian EL, Gager WE: Optic neuritis complicating measles, mumps and rubella vaccination. *Am J Ophthalmol* 1978;86:544–547.

Massaro M, Thorarensen O, Liu GT, et al. Morning glory disc anomaly and moyamoya vessels. *Arch Ophthalmol* 1998;116:253–254.

Optic Neuritis Study Group: Visual function 5 years after optic neuritis. Experience of the optic neuritis treatment trial. *Arch Ophthalmol* 1997;115:1545–1552.

Repka MX, Miller NR: Optic atrophy in children. *Am J Ophthalmol* 1988;106:191–193.

Skarf B, Hoyt CS: Optic nerve hypoplasia in children: Association with anomalies of the endocrine and CNS. *Arch Ophthalmol* 1984;102:62–67.

Weiss AH, Beck RW: Neuroretinitis in childhood. *J Pediatr Ophthalmol Strabismus* 1989;26:198–203.

Chapter 631 ■ Childhood Glaucoma

Scott E. Olitsky, Denise Hug, and Laura P. Smith

Glaucoma is a general term used to indicate damage to the optic nerve with visual field loss that is caused by or related to elevated pressure within the eye. It is classified according to the age of the affected individual at presentation and the association of other ocular or systemic conditions. Glaucoma that begins within the first 3 yr of life is called infantile (congenital); that which begins between the ages of 3 and 30 yr is called juvenile.

Primary glaucoma indicates that the cause is an isolated anomaly of the drainage apparatus of the eye (trabecular meshwork). More than 50% of infantile glaucoma is primary. In secondary glaucoma, other ocular or systemic abnormalities are associated, even if a similar developmental defect of the trabecular meshwork is also present. Primary infantile glaucoma occurs with an incidence of 0.03% (Table 631-1).

CLINICAL MANIFESTATIONS. The symptoms of infantile glaucoma include the classic triad of epiphora (tearing), photophobia (sensitivity to light), and blepharospasm (eyelid squeezing) [Fig. 631-1]. Each can be attributed to corneal irritation. Only about 30%

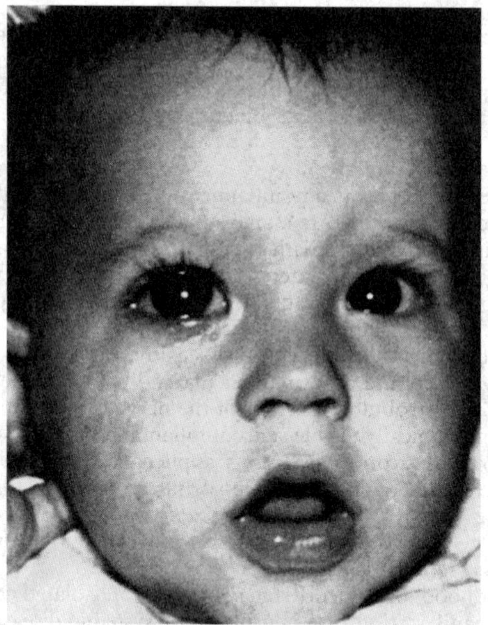

Figure 631-1. Tearing of the right eye caused by glaucoma. Note the increased corneal diameter of the right eye. (From Nelson LB: *Harley's Pediatric Ophthalmology,* 4th ed. Philadelphia, WB Saunders, 1998, p 285.)

TABLE 631-1. PRIMARY AND SECONDARY CHILDHOOD GLAUCOMAS

- **I. PRIMARY GLAUCOMAS**
  - A. Congenital open-angle glaucoma
    - 1. Congenital
    - 2. Infantile
    - 3. Late recognized
  - B. Autosomal dominant juvenile glaucoma
  - C. Primary angle-closure glaucoma
  - D. Associated with systemic abnormalities
    - 1. Sturge-Weber syndrome
    - 2. Neurofibromatosis type 1 (NF-1)
    - 3. Stickler syndrome
    - 4. Oculocerebrorenal (Lowe) syndrome
    - 5. Rieger syndrome
    - 6. Hepatocerebrorenal syndrome
    - 7. Marfan syndrome
    - 8. Rubinstein-Taybi syndrome
    - 9. Infantile glaucoma associated with mental retardation and paralysis
    - 10. Oculodentodigital dysplasia
    - 11. Open-angle glaucoma associated with microcornea and absence of frontal sinuses
    - 12. Mucopolysaccharidosis
    - 13. Trisomy 13
    - 14. Cutis marmorata telangiectasia congenita
    - 15. Warburg syndrome
    - 16. Kniest syndrome (skeletal dysplasia)
    - 17. Michel syndrome
    - 18. Nonprogressive hemiatrophy
  - E. Associated with ocular abnormalities
    - 1. Congenital glaucoma with iris and pupillary abnormalities
    - 2. Aniridia
      - a. Congenital glaucoma
      - b. Acquired glaucoma
    - 3. Congenital ocular melanosis
    - 4. Sclerocornea
    - 5. Iridotrabecular dysgenesis
    - 6. Peters syndrome
    - 7. Iridotrabecular dyagenesis and ectropion uveae
    - 8. Posterior polymorphous dystrophy
    - 9. Idiopathic or familial elevated episcleral venous pressure
    - 10. Anterior corneal staphyloma
    - 11. Congenital microcornia with myopia
    - 12. Congenital hereditary endothelial dystrophy
    - 13. Congenital hereditary iris stromal hypoplasia
- **II. SECONDARY GLAUCOMAS**
  - A. Traumatic glaucoma
    - 1. Acute glaucoma
      - a. Angle concussion
      - b. Hyphema
      - c. Ghost cell glaucoma
    - 2. Late-onset glaucoma with angle recession
    - 3. Arteriovenous fistula
  - B. Secondary to intraocular neoplasm
    - 1. Retinoblastoma
    - 2. Juvenile xanthogranuloma
    - 3. Leukemia
    - 4. Melanoma
    - 5. Melanocytoma
    - 6. Iris rhabdomyosarcoma
    - 7. Aggressive nevi of the iris
  - C. Secondary to uveitis
    - 1. Open-angle glaucoma
    - 2. Angle-blockage glaucoma
      - a. Synechial angle closure
      - b. Iris bombé with pupillary block
  - D. Lens-induced glaucoma
    - 1. Subluxation-dislocation and pupillary block
      - a. Marfan syndrome
      - b. Homocystinuria
    - 2. Spherophakia and pupillary block
    - 3. Phacolytic glaucoma
  - E. Secondary to surgery for congenital cataract
    - 1. Lens material blockage of the trabecular meshwork (acute or subacute)
    - 2. Pupillary block
    - 3. Chronic open-angle glaucoma associated with angle defects
  - F. Steroid-induced glaucoma
  - G. Secondary to rubeosis
    - 1. Retinoblastoma
    - 2. Coats diease
    - 3. Medulloepithelioma
    - 4. Familial exudative vitreoretinopathy
  - H. Secondary angle-closure glaucoma
    - 1. Retinopathy of prematurity
    - 2. Microphthalmos
    - 3. Nanophthalmos
    - 4. Retinoblastoma
    - 5. Persistent hyperplastic primary vitreous
    - 6. Congenital pupillary iris-lens membrane
  - I. Glaucoma associated with increased venous pressure
    - 1. Carotid or dural-venous fistula
    - 2. Orbital disease
  - J. Secondary to maternal rubella
  - K. Secondary to intraocular infection
    - 1. Acute recurrent toxoplasmosis
    - 2. Acute herpetic iritis

From Nelson LB: *Harley's Pediatric Ophthalmology,* 4th ed., Philadelphia, WB Saunders, 1998, p 294.

of affected infants demonstrate the classic symptom complex. Signs of glaucoma include corneal edema, corneal and ocular enlargement, and conjunctival injection (Fig. 631-2).

The sclera and cornea are more elastic in early childhood than later in life. An increase in intraocular pressure (IOP), therefore, leads to an expansion of the globe, including the cornea, and the development of buphthalmos ("ox eye"). If the cornea continues to enlarge, breaks occur in the endothelial basement membrane (Desçemet membrane) and may lead to permanent corneal scarring. These breaks in Desçemet membrane (Haab striae) are visible as horizontal edematous lines that cross or curve around the central cornea. They rarely occur beyond 3 yr of age or in corneas less than 12.0 mm in diameter. The cornea also becomes edematous and cloudy, with increased IOP. The corneal edema leads to tearing and photophobia. Glaucoma should be considered in a child suspected of having a nasolacrimal duct obstruction if any of these other signs or symptoms are present.

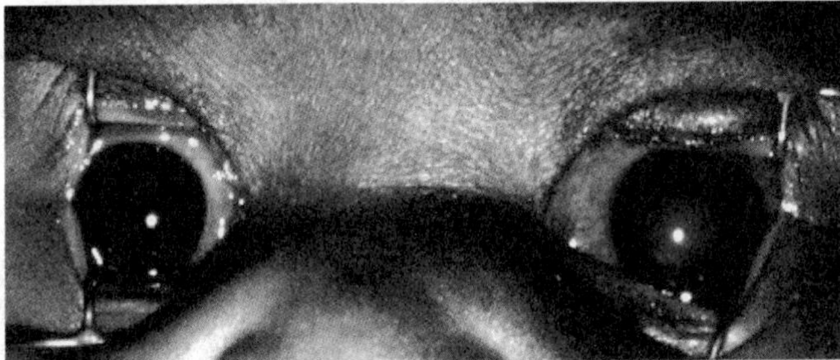

Figure 631-2. Infantile glaucoma. The left cornea is enlarged and edematous.

Children with unilateral glaucoma generally present early because the difference in the corneal size between the eyes can be noticed. When the disease is bilateral, parents may not recognize the increased corneal size. Many parents view the large eyes as attractive and do not seek help until other symptoms develop.

Cupping of the optic nerve head is detected by ocular examination. The optic nerve of an infant is easily distended by excessive pressure. Deep, central cupping readily occurs and may regress with normalization of pressure.

Some infants and children with early-onset glaucoma have more extensive maldevelopment of the anterior segment of the eye. The neurocristopathies comprise a spectrum of conditions relating to abnormal embryologic development of the anterior segment. They are usually bilateral and may include abnormalities of the iris, cornea, and lens. Other ocular anomalies that may be associated with glaucoma in infants and children are aniridia, cataract, spherophakia, and ectopia lentis. Glaucoma may also develop secondary to persistent hyperplastic primary vitreous or retinopathy of prematurity.

Trauma, intraocular hemorrhage, ocular inflammatory disease, and intraocular tumor are also important causes of glaucoma in the pediatric population. Systemic disorders associated with glaucoma in infants and children are Sturge-Weber syndrome, neurofibromatosis, Lowe syndrome, Marfan syndrome, congenital rubella, and a number of chromosomal syndromes.

Glaucoma occurs frequently in children with a history of congenital cataracts. Glaucoma may develop in up to 25% of children who have undergone cataract surgery early in life. The cause of aphakic glaucoma is not known but is thought to be due to a coexistent anterior chamber deformity. Children treated for cataracts need to be monitored closely for this dreaded complication.

DIAGNOSIS AND TREATMENT. The diagnosis of infantile glaucoma is made on recognition of the signs and symptoms. Although measurement of IOP may be helpful in monitoring treatment response, it is not a vital part of the diagnostic process. Once the diagnosis is established, treatment is started promptly. Unlike adult glaucoma, in which medication is often the first line of therapy, for infantile glaucoma, the treatment is primarily surgical. Procedures used to treat glaucoma in children include surgery to establish a more normal anterior chamber angle (goniotomy and trabeculotomy), to create a site for aqueous fluid to exit the eye (trabeculectomy and seton surgery), or to reduce aqueous fluid production (cyclocryotherapy and cyclophotocoagulation). Many children frequently require several operations to lower and maintain their IOP adequately, and long-term medical therapy may be necessary as well. Patients with multiple ocular abnormalities and those with aphakic glaucoma generally require more surgeries to achieve and maintain adequate IOP control. Although vision may be reduced secondary to glaucomatous optic nerve damage or corneal scarring, amblyopia is the most common cause of loss of vision in these children.

Beck AD, Freedman S, Kammer J, et al: Aqueous shunt devices compared with trabeculectomy with mitomycin-C for children in the first two years of life. *Am J Ophthalmol* 2003;136:994–1000.

Chen TC, Walton DS, Bhatia LS: Aphakic glaucoma after congenital cataract surgery. *Arch Ophthalmol* 2004;122:1819–1825.

Morad Y, Donaldson CE, Kim YM, et al: The Ahmed drainage implant in the treatment of pediatric glaucoma. *Am J Ophthalmol* 2003;135:821–829.

Neely DE, Plager DA: Endocyclophotocoagulation for management of difficult pediatric glaucomas. *J Am Assoc Pediatr Ophthalmol Strabismus* 2001;5:221–229.

Sidoti PA, Belmonte SJ, Liebmann JM, et al: Trabeculectomy with mitomycin-C in the treatment of pediatric glaucomas. *Ophthalmology* 2000;107:422–429.

Simon JW, Mehta N, Simmons ST, et al: Glaucoma after pediatric lensectomy/vitrectomy. *Ophthalmology* 1991;98:670–674.

Chapter 632 ■ Orbital Abnormalities

Scott E. Olitsky, Denise Hug, and Laura P. Smith

HYPERTELORISM AND HYPOTELORISM. Hypertelorism is wide separation of the eyes or an increased interorbital distance, which may occur as a morphogenetic variant, a primary deformity, or a secondary phenomenon in association with developmental abnormalities, such as frontal meningocele or encephalocele or the persistence of a facial cleft. Often associated are strabismus, generally exotropia, and sometimes optic atrophy.

Hypotelorism refers to narrowness of the interorbital distance, which may occur as a morphogenetic variant alone or in association with other anomalies, such as epicanthus or holoprosencephaly or secondary to a cranial dystrophy, such as scaphocephaly.

EXOPHTHALMOS AND ENOPHTHALMOS. Protrusion of the eye is referred to as exophthalmos or proptosis and is a common indicator of orbital disease. It may be caused by shallowness of the orbits, as in many craniofacial malformations, or by increased tissue mass within the orbit, as with neoplastic, vascular, and inflammatory disorders. Ocular complications include exposure keratopathy, ocular motor disturbances, and optic atrophy with loss of vision.

Posterior displacement or sinking of the eye back into the orbit is referred to as enophthalmos. This may occur with orbital fracture or with atrophy of orbital tissue.

ORBITAL INFLAMMATION. Inflammatory disease involving the orbit may be primary or secondary to systemic disease. Idiopathic orbital inflammation (**orbital pseudotumor**) represents a wide spectrum of clinical entities. Symptoms at the time of presentation may include pain, eyelid swelling, proptosis, a red eye, and fever. The inflammation may involve a single extraocular muscle (myositis) or the entire orbit. Orbital apex syndrome is a serious condition that may also involve the cavernous sinus and may compress or displace the optic nerve. Confusion with orbital cellulitis is common but can be differentiated by the lack of associated sinus disease, its appearance on CT scan, and lack of improvement with systemic antibiotics. Orbital pseudotumor is associated with systemic lupus erythematosus, Crohn disease, myasthenia gravis, and lymphoma. **Treatment** includes the use of high-dose systemic corticosteroids. Often, the symptoms improve dramatically shortly after treatment is initiated. Bilateral involvement, associated uveitis, disc edema, and recurrence of inflammation is not uncommon in the pediatric population. Immunotherapy or radiation treatment may be necessary for resistant or recurrent cases.

Thyroid-related ophthalmopathy is believed to be secondary to an immune mechanism, leading to inflammation and deposition of mucopolysaccharides and collagen in the extraocular muscles and orbital fat. Involvement of the extraocular muscles may lead to a restrictive strabismus. Lid retraction and exophthalmos may cause corneal exposure and infection or perforation. Involvement of the posterior orbit can compress the optic nerve. Treatment of thyroid-related ophthalmopathy may include the use of systemic corticosteroids, radiation of the orbit, eyelid surgery, strabismus surgery, or orbital decompression to eliminate symptoms and protect vision. The degree of orbital involvement is often independent of the status of the systemic disease (also see Chapter 569).

Other systemic disorders that may cause inflammatory disease within the orbit include lymphoma, sarcoidosis, amyloidosis, pol-

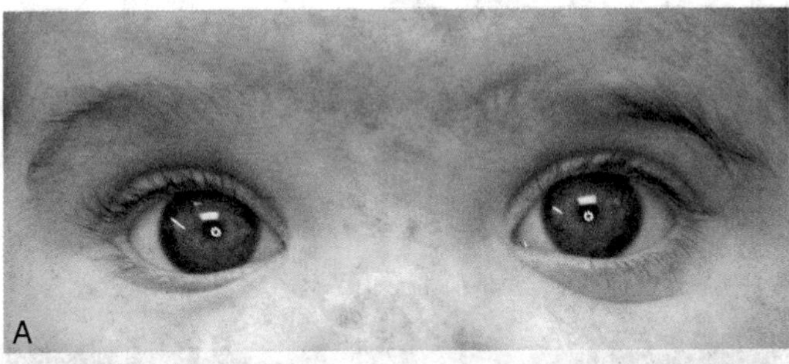

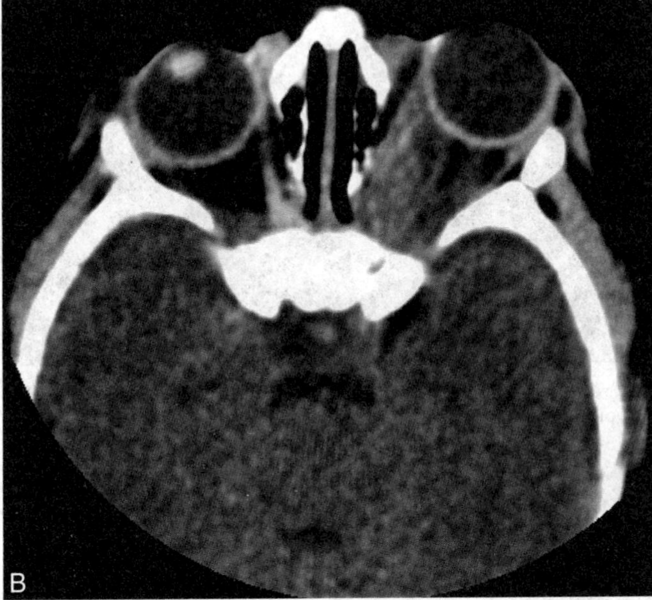

Figure 632-1. Orbital hemangioma. A, Note the proptosis. B, CT scan. (Courtesy of Amy Nopper, MD, and Brandon Newell, MD.)

yarteritis nodosa, systemic lupus erythematosus, dermatomyositis, Wegener granulomatosis, and juvenile xanthogranuloma.

TUMORS OF THE ORBIT. Various tumors occur in and about the orbit in childhood. Among benign tumors, the most common are vascular lesions (principally hemangiomas) (Fig. 632-1) and dermoids. Among malignant neoplasms, rhabdomyosarcoma, lymphosarcoma, and metastatic neuroblastoma are the most frequent. Optic nerve gliomas are most commonly seen in patients with neurofibromatosis and may present with poor vision or proptosis. Retinoblastoma may extend into the orbit if discovered late or if it goes untreated. Teratomas are rare tumors that typically grow rapidly after birth and exhibit explosive proptosis.

The effects of orbital tumors vary with their locations and growth patterns. The principal signs are proptosis, resistance to retroplacement of the eye, and impairment of eye movement. A palpable mass may be found. Other significant signs are ptosis, optic nerve head congestion, optic atrophy, and loss of vision. Bruit and visible pulsation of the globe are important clues to vascular lesions.

Evaluation of orbital tumors includes ultrasonography, MRI, and CT. Pseudotumor of the orbit also must be considered in children with signs of a mass lesion. In selected cases, an incisional or excisional biopsy of the lesion may be warranted.

Gorospe L, Royo A, Berrocal T, et al: Imaging of orbital disorders in pediatric patients. *Eur Radiol* 2003;13:2012–2026.

Ohtsuka K, Hashimoto M, Suzuki Y: A review of 244 orbital tumors in Japanese patients during a 21-year period: Origins and locations. *Jpn J Ophthalmol* 2005;49:49–55.

Shields JA, Shields CL, Scartozzi R: Survey of 1264 patients with orbital tumors and simulating lesions: The 2002 Montgomery Lecture, part 1. *Ophthalmology* 2004;111:997–1008.

Yuen SJA, Rubin PAD: Idiopathic orbital inflammation. *Arch Ophthalmol* 2003;121:491–499.

Chapter 633 ■ Orbital Infections

Scott E. Olitsky, Denise Hug, and Laura P. Smith

Orbital infections are common in children. It is important to be able to distinguish the different forms of infection that occur in the orbital region to allow rapid diagnosis and treatment to prevent loss of vision or spread of the infection to the nearby intracranial structures (Table 425-1).

DACRYOADENITIS. Dacryoadenitis, or inflammation of the lacrimal gland, is uncommon in childhood. It may occur with mumps (in which case it is usually acute and bilateral, subsiding in a few days or weeks) or with infectious mononucleosis. *Staphylococcus aureus* may produce a suppurative dacryoadenitis. Chronic dacryoadenitis is associated with certain systemic diseases, particularly sarcoidosis, tuberculosis, and syphilis. Some systemic diseases may produce enlargement of the lacrimal and salivary glands (Mikulicz syndrome).

DACRYOCYSTITIS. Dacryocystitis is an infection of the lacrimal sac. Dacryocystitis generally requires obstruction of the nasolacrimal system to allow its development. Acute dacryocystitis presents with redness and swelling over the region of the lacrimal sac. It is treated with warm compresses and systemic antibiotics. This will help to control the infection, but the obstruction usually requires definitive treatment to reduce the risk of recurrence.

Dacryocystitis may occur in newborns as a complication of a congenital dacryocystocele. The obstruction of the nasolacrimal system may resolve once the infection clears.

PRESEPTAL CELLULITIS. Inflammation of the lids and periorbital tissues without signs of true orbital involvement (such as proptosis or limitation of eye movement) is generally referred to as periorbital or preseptal cellulitis and is a form of facial cellulitis. This is common in young children and may be caused by bacteremia, trauma, an infected wound, or an abscess of the lid or periorbital region (pyoderma, hordeolum, conjunctivitis, dacryocystitis, insect bite). Patients present with eyelid swelling; the edema may be so intense as to make it difficult to evaluate the globe. Prior to the *Haemophilus influenzae* type B vaccine, the most common cause of pediatric preseptal (facial) cellulitis was bacteremia due to *H. influenzae* type B. Group A streptococcus a common is cause. Clinical examination will show lack of proptosis, normal ocular movement, and normal pupil function. CT examination will demonstrate edema of the lids and subcutaneous tissues anterior to the orbital septum (Fig. 633-1). Antibiotic therapy and careful monitoring for signs of sepsis and local progression are essential.

ORBITAL CELLULITIS. This is a condition involving inflammation of the tissues of the orbit, with proptosis, limitation of movement of the eye, edema of the conjunctiva (chemosis), and inflammation and swelling of the eyelids with potentially decreased visual acuity. The mean age is ~7 yr but the range is 10 mo–18 yr. Patients often feel ill with general symptoms of toxicity, fever, and leukocytosis (also see Chapter 192).

Orbital cellulitis may follow direct infection of the orbit from a wound, metastatic deposition of organisms during bacteremia, or **more often** direct extension or venous spread of infection from contiguous sites such as the lids, conjunctiva, globe, lacrimal gland, nasolacrimal sac, or **more commonly** the paranasal (ethmoid) sinuses. In some cases, primary or metastatic tumor in the orbit can produce the clinical picture of orbital cellulitis. The most common cause of orbital cellulitis in children is paranasal sinusitis. Frequent pathogenic organisms include *H. influenzae, Staphylococcus aureus,* group A β-hemolytic streptococci, *Streptococcus pneumoniae,* and anaerobic bacteria.

The potential for complications is great. Involvement of the optic nerve may result in loss of vision. Extension of infection from the orbit into the cranial cavity may lead to cavernous sinus thrombosis or meningitis or to epidural or subdural empyema, or brain abscesses.

Orbital cellulitis must be recognized promptly and treated aggressively (see Chapter 192). Hospitalization and systemic antibiotic therapy are usually indicated. All patients require CT imaging of the orbit (including the surrounding (CNS), preferably with intravenous contrast to detect a subperiosteal abscess or intracranial extension. If there is no evidence of improvement or if there are signs of progression, sinus drainage may be required. In some cases, an orbital or subperiosteal abscess may develop (Fig. 633-2). A subperiosteal abscess may require urgent drainage of the orbit. Drainage can also be delayed in some cases to allow improvement following the initiation of high-dose intravenous (ampicillin/sulbactam) antibiotic therapy (200–400 mg/kg/24 hr ampicillin component every 4 or 6 hr (maximum dose: 8 g ampicillin/24 hr). The clinical presentation and course of each individual patient should dictate the need and timing of abscess drainage.

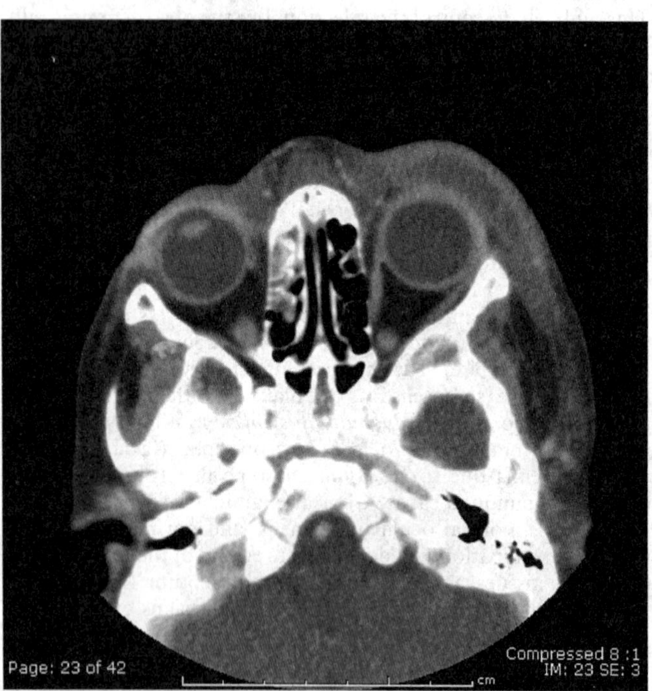

Figure 633-1. CT scan of a patient with preseptal cellulitis.

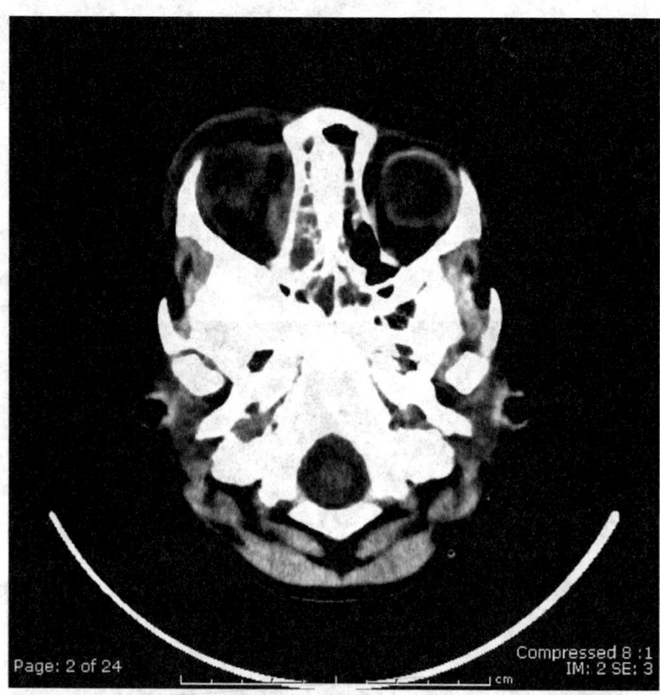

Figure 633-2. CT scan demonstrating a subperiosteal abscess along the medial wall of the orbit.

Ambati BK, Ambati J, Azar N, et al: Periorbital and orbital cellulitis before and after the advent of *Haemophilus influenzae* type B vaccination. *Ophthalmology* 2000;107:1450–1453.

Campolattaro BN, Lueder GT, Tychsen L: Spectrum of pediatric dacryocystitis: Medical and surgical management of 54 cases. *J Pediatr Ophthalmol Strabismus* 1997;34:143–153.

Garcia GH, Harris GJ: Criteria for nonsurgical management of subperiosteal abscess of the orbit: Analysis of outcomes 1988–1998. *Ophthalmology* 2000;107:1454–1456.

Greenberg MF, Pollard ZF: Medical treatment of pediatric subperiosteal orbital abscess secondary to sinusitis. *J AAPOS* 1998;2:351–355.

Nageswaran S, Woods CR, Benjamin Jr DK, et al: Orbital cellulitis in children. *Pediatr Infect Dis J* 2006;25:695–699.

Chapter 634 ■ Injuries to the Eye

Scott E. Olitsky, Denise Hug, and Laura P. Smith

About ⅓ of all blindness in children results from trauma. Children and adolescents account for a disproportionate number of episodes of ocular trauma. Boys ages 11–15 yr are the most vulnerable; their injuries outnumber those in girls by a ratio of about 4 : 1. The majority of injuries are related to sports, toy darts, other projectiles, sticks, stones, fireworks, paint balls, and air-powered BB guns. The last causes particularly devastating ocular and orbital injuries. Much of the trauma is avoidable (see Chapter 61). Any part of the orbit or globe may be affected (Fig. 634-1).

ECCHYMOSES AND SWELLING OF THE EYELIDS. These are common after blunt trauma. Hemorrhage into the lids and periorbital

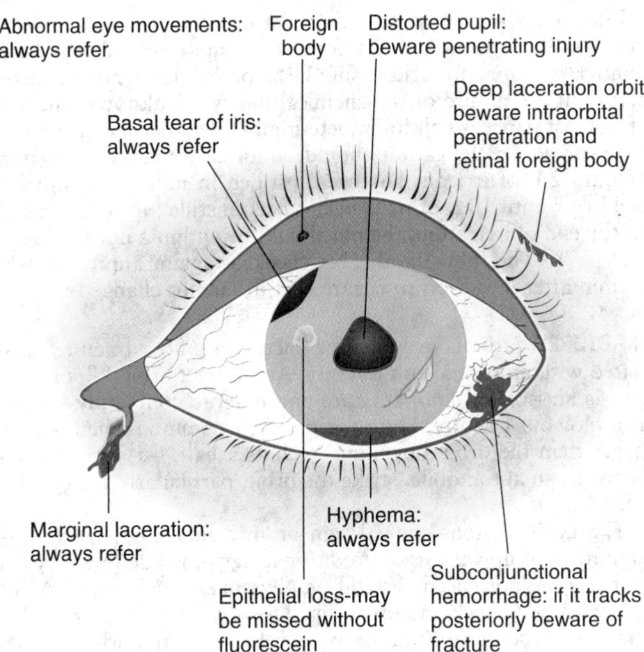

Figure 634-1. The injured eye. (From Khaw PT, Shah P, Elkington AR: Injury to the eye. *Br Med J* 2004;328:36–38.)

region ("black eye" or "shiner") is usually of no consequence and absorbs spontaneously, but it should prompt careful examination of the eye for deeper, more serious injury, such as a blowout fracture of the orbit, an intraocular hemorrhage, or rupture of the globe.

LACERATIONS OF THE EYELIDS. These require careful management. Horizontal laceration of the upper lid may involve the levator, the tarsal plate, or the orbital septum. Faulty repair can result in ptosis, distortion of the lid, or herniation of orbital fat. Lacerations involving the lid margins require meticulous surgical apposition to prevent notching, eversion, or inversion of the margin or misdirection of the lashes that might lead to epiphora (tear overflow), wetting defects of the cornea, and chronic irritation. Lacerations situated near the medial canthus may involve the punctum, canaliculi, or nasolacrimal duct and require microsurgical repair by an experienced ophthalmic surgeon. In all cases of lid laceration, examination of the globe for perforating injury is mandatory. Proper primary repair often achieves a superior outcome to secondary repair at a later date.

SUPERFICIAL ABRASIONS OF THE CORNEA. When the corneal epithelium is scratched, abraded, or denuded, it exposes the underlying epithelial basement layer and superficial corneal nerves. This is accompanied by pain, tearing, photophobia, and decreased vision. Corneal abrasions are detected by instilling fluorescein dye and inspecting the cornea using a blue-filtered light. A slit lamp is ideal for this examination, but a hand-held Wood lamp is adequate for young children.

Treatment of a corneal abrasion is directed at promoting healing and relieving pain. Abrasions are treated with frequent applications of a topical antibiotic ointment until the epithelium is completely healed. The use of a semipressure patch does not improve healing time or decrease pain. An improperly applied patch may itself abrade the cornea. A topical cycloplegic agent (cyclopentolate hydrochloride 1%) can relieve the pain from ciliary spasm in patients with large abrasions. Topical anesthetics should not be given at home because they retard epithelial healing and inhibit the natural blinking reflex.

FOREIGN BODY ON OR IN THE CORNEA OR CONJUNCTIVA. This usually produces acute discomfort, lacrimation, and inflammation. Most foreign bodies can be detected by examination in good light with the aid of magnification or a direct ophthalmoscope set on a high plus lens (+10 or +12). In many cases, slit-lamp examination is necessary, especially if the particle is deep or metallic. Some conjunctival foreign bodies tend to lodge under the upper eyelid, causing the sensation of corneal foreign body as they come into contact with the globe on eyelid movement; they may also produce vertically oriented linear corneal abrasions (Fig. 634-2). Finding these abrasions should lead to a suspicion of such a foreign body, and eversion of the lid may be necessary (see Chapter 618). If a foreign body is suspected but not found, further examination is indicated. If the history suggests injury with a high-velocity particle, radiologic examination of the eye may be needed to explore the possibility of an intraocular foreign body.

Removal of a foreign body can be facilitated by instillation of a drop of topical anesthetic. Many foreign bodies can be removed by irrigating or by gently wiping them away with a moistened cotton-tipped applicator. Embedded foreign bodies should be treated by an ophthalmologist. Removal of corneal foreign bodies may leave epithelial defects, which are treated as corneal abrasions. Metallic foreign bodies may cause rust to form in the corneal tissues; examination by an ophthalmologist 1 or 2 days after removal of a foreign body is recommended because a rust ring might require further treatment (curettage).

HYPHEMA. This is the presence of blood in the anterior chamber of the eye. It may occur with either a blunt or perforating injury. Hyphema appears as a bright or dark red fluid level between the cornea and iris or as a diffuse murkiness of the aqueous humor. Children with hyphema have pain and may be somnolent. The treatment of hyphema usually includes bed rest, with the head elevated 30–45 degrees to promote settling and resorption of the blood. Hospitalization and sedation may be necessary to ensure compliance in some children. In most cases, topical mydriatics, topical or oral corticosteroids, or oral aminocaproic acid are used to prevent rebleeding. Secondary bleeding typically occurs 3–5

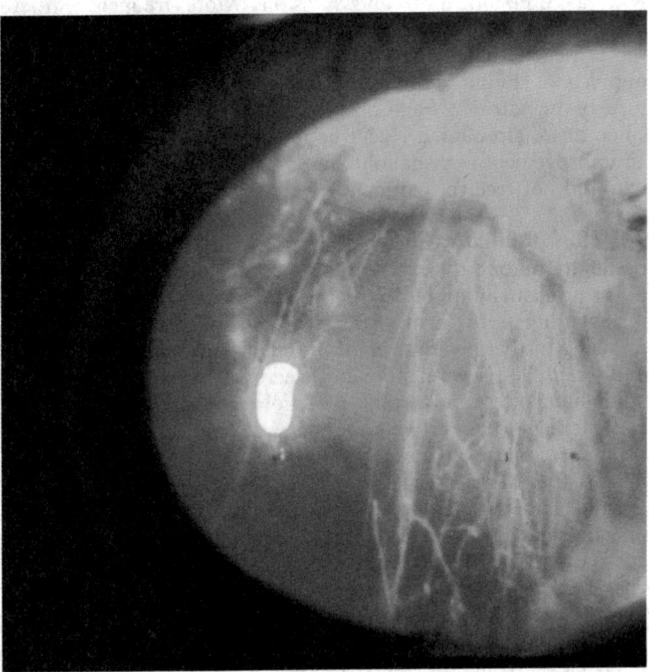

Figure 634-2. Vertically oriented linear corneal abrasions secondary to a foreign body underneath the upper eyelid.

days after the initial hemorrhage, increasing the risk of sequelae. The blood in the anterior chamber may produce elevation of intraocular pressure and blood staining of the cornea. These complications may affect vision. In such cases, surgical evacuation of the clot and irrigation of the anterior chamber may be necessary. Patients with sickle cell disease or trait are at higher risk of acute loss of vision secondary to elevated intraocular pressure or optic nerve infarction and may require more aggressive intervention. Individuals with a history of traumatic hyphema have an increased incidence of glaucoma later in life and should be monitored on a regular basis.

LACERATIONS AND PERFORATING WOUNDS OF THE CORNEA OR SCLERA. These require immediate referral to an ophthalmologist and prompt surgical repair if the eye and vision are to be saved. Important clues to perforating injury of the eye are collapse of the anterior chamber, distortion and displacement of the pupil, and protrusion of dark tissue (uvea) into the wound. *Emergency treatment* consists of protecting the injured eye from further damage by applying a sterile bandage and a rigid eye shield. If these medical supplies are not on hand, an adequate eye shield can be fashioned from a plastic or Styrofoam cup or from a piece of cardboard bent into a box or cone shape. Manipulation should be kept to a minimum, and no medication should be instilled except under the direction of an ophthalmologist.

RUPTURED GLOBE. If the globe is compressed along its anteroposterior diameter with enough force, it will rupture at its weakest point. These weak points generally include the area where the sclera and cornea meet (limbus), near the insertions of the rectus muscles and at the site of previous intraocular surgery. Unlike most injuries involving lacerations or perforations of the globe, the force required to produce a scleral rupture is much more likely to cause extensive, and often permanent, damage to the posterior aspect of the eye. Therefore, the prognosis for visual recovery in these injuries is poor.

OPTIC NERVE TRAUMA. Injury to the globe may produce a traumatic optic neuropathy. Indirect damage to the optic nerve may occur after blunt trauma to the forehead secondary to shock waves that pass through the optic canal. Patients may present with a complaint of reduced vision. More frequently, these patients are unconscious and the only clue to the injury may be the presence of an afferent papillary defect. In such cases, the optic canal should be imaged to look for the presence of a fracture or hematoma. High-dose corticosteroids may be used in some cases, although a recent national trial did not demonstrate an improvement in visual outcome when compared with patients who did not receive treatment.

CHEMICAL INJURIES. Chemical burns of the cornea and adnexal tissue are among the most urgent of ocular emergencies. Alkali burns are usually more destructive than acid burns because they react with fats to form soaps, which damage cell membranes, allowing further penetration of the alkali into the eye. Acids generally cause less severe, more localized tissue damage. The corneal epithelium offers moderate protection against weak acids, and little damage occurs unless the pH is 2.5 or less. Most stronger acids precipitate tissue proteins, creating a physical barrier against their further penetration.

Mild acid or alkali burns are characterized by conjunctival injection and swelling and mild corneal epithelial erosions. The corneal stroma may be mildly edematous, and the anterior chamber may have mild to moderate cell and flare reactions. With strong acids, the cornea and conjunctiva rapidly become white and opaque. The corneal epithelium may slough, leaving a relatively clear stroma; this appearance may initially mask the severity of the burn. Severe alkali burns are characterized by corneal opacification.

Emergency treatment of a chemical burn begins with copious immediate irrigation with water or saline. Local debridement and removal of foreign particles should be performed while still irrigating. If the nature of the chemical injury is unknown, the use of pH test paper is helpful in determining whether the agent was basic or acidic. Irrigation should continue for at least 30 min or until 2 L of irrigant has been instilled in mild cases and for 2–4 hr or until 10 L of irrigant has been instilled in severe cases. At the end of irrigation, the pH should be within a normal range (7.3–7.7). The pH should be checked again approximately 30 min after irrigation to ensure that it has not changed.

FRACTURES. A direct orbital floor fracture is a floor fracture associated with an orbital rim fracture. An indirect orbital floor fracture is an isolated floor fracture and is more commonly known as a blowout fracture. Floor fractures are common when objects larger than the orbital opening, such as a ball, fist, or the dashboard of an automobile, strike the orbit, particularly the inferior lateral orbit.

The most obvious clinical sign of an orbital floor fracture is limitation of upward gaze. Additional signs include lower eyelid ecchymosis, nosebleed, orbital emphysema, and hypesthesia of the ipsilateral cheek and upper lip. The last sign results from disruption of the infraorbital nerve as it traverses the orbital floor.

The best imaging techniques to visualize orbital fractures are plain-film radiography and CT. The Waters view best demonstrates the orbital floor and maxillary sinus.

Treatment for children with acute orbital fractures includes antibiotic prophylaxis, nasal decongestants, and ice packs. If entrapment of the extraocular muscles (resulting in restriction of movement of the eye and diplopia) and herniation of orbital fat or of the eye itself (resulting in enophthalmos) occur, surgical repair may be necessary.

PENETRATING WOUNDS OF THE ORBIT. These demand careful evaluation for possible damage to the eye, the optic nerve, or the brain. Examination should include investigation for retained foreign body. Orbital hemorrhage and infection are common with penetrating wounds of the orbit; such injuries must be treated as emergencies.

CHILD ABUSE (SEE CHAPTER 36). This is a major cause of injuries to the eye and orbital region. The possibility of nonaccidental trauma must be considered in any child with ecchymosis or laceration of the lids, hemorrhage in or about the eye, cataract or dislocated lens, retinal detachment, or fracture of the orbit. Inflicted childhood neurotrauma (shaken baby syndrome) occurs secondary to violent, nonaccidental, repetitive, unrestrained acceleration-deceleration head and neck movements, with or without blunt head trauma in children typically younger than 3 yr. Inflicted childhood neurotrauma accounts for approximately 10% of all cases of child abuse and carries a mortality rate of up to 25%. Detection of abuse is not only important in order to treat the pathology that is discovered but also to prevent further abuse or even death. The ocular manifestations are numerous and may have a prominent role in recognition of this syndrome. Retinal hemorrhage is the most common ophthalmic finding and occurs at all levels of the retina. The pattern of hemorrhage helps to distinguish this disorder from other causes of retinal hemorrhage or from accidental injuries (Fig. 634-3). Retinal hemorrhages can occur without associated intracranial pathology.

FIREWORKS-RELATED INJURIES. Injuries related to the use of fireworks can be the most devastating of all ocular traumas that occur in children. At least ⅕ of emergency department visits for fireworks-related injuries are for ocular trauma. In the United States, a majority of these injuries take place around Independence Day, and most occur despite adult supervision.

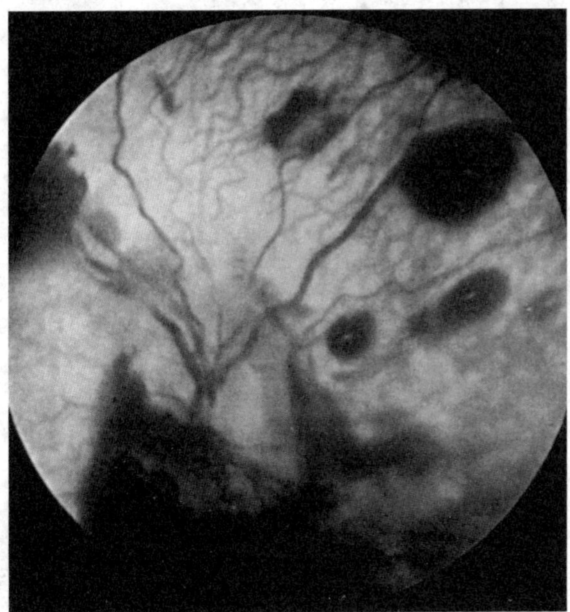

Figure 634-3. Retinal hemorrhages in an abused child with subdural hematoma.

SPORTS-RELATED OCULAR INJURIES AND THEIR PREVENTION. Although sports injuries occur in all age groups, far more children and adolescents participate in high-risk sports than do adults. The greater number of participating children, their athletic immaturity, and the increased likelihood of their using inadequate or improper eye protection account for their disproportionate share of sports-related eye injuries (see Chapters 687 and 691).

The sports with the highest risk of eye injury are those in which no eye protection can be worn, including boxing, wrestling, and martial arts. High-risk sports include those that use a rapidly moving ball or puck, bat, stick, racquet, or arrow (baseball, hockey, lacrosse, racquet sports, and archery) or involve aggressive body contact (football and basketball). Related to both risk and frequency of participation, the highest percentage of eye injuries are in basketball and baseball.

Protective eyewear, designed for a specific activity, is available for most sports. For basketball, racquet sports, and other recreational activities that do not require a helmet or face mask, molded polycarbonate sports goggles that are secured to the head by an elastic strap are suggested. For hockey, football, lacrosse, and baseball (batter), specific helmets with polycarbonate face shields and guards are available. Children should also wear sports goggles under the helmets. For baseball, goggles and helmets should be worn for batting, catching, and base running; goggles alone are usually sufficient for other positions.

American Academy of Pediatrics Committee on Sports Medicine and Fitness, American Academy of Ophthalmology Committee on Eye Safety and Sports Ophthalmology: Protective eyewear for young athletes. *Pediatrics* 1996;98:311–313.

Buys YM, Levin AV, Enzenauer RW, et al: Retinal findings after head trauma in infants and young children. *Ophthalmology* 1992;99:1718–1723.

Egbert JE, May K, Kersten RC, et al: Pediatric orbital floor fracture: Direct extraocular muscle involvement. *Ophthalmology* 2000;107:1875–1879.

Forbes BJ, Christian CW, Judkins AR, et al: Inflicted childhood neurotrauma (shaken baby syndrome): Ophthalmic findings. *J Pediatr Ophthalmol Strabismus* 2004;41:80–88.

Khaw PT, Shah P, Elkington AR: Injury to the eye. *Br Med J* 2004;328:36–38.

Kivlin JD, Simons KB, Lazoritz S, et al: Shaken baby syndrome. *Ophthalmology* 2000;107:1246–1254.

Michael JG, Hug D, Dowd MD: Management of corneal abrasion in children: A randomized clinical trial. *Ann Emerg Med* 2002;40:67–72.

Morad Y, Avni I, Benton SA, et al: Normal computerized tomography of brain in children with shaken baby syndrome. *J AAPOS* 2004;8:445–450.

Serious eye injuries associated with fireworks—United States, 1990–1994. *MMWR* 1995;44:449–452.

Smith GA, Knapp JF, Barnett TM, et al: The rocket's red glare, the bombs bursting in air: Fireworks-related injuries to children. *Pediatrics* 1996;98:1–9.

Part XXIX ▪ The Ear

Chapter 635 ▪ General Considerations and Evaluation

Joseph Haddad Jr.

CLINICAL MANIFESTATIONS. Eight prominent signs and symptoms are associated primarily with diseases of the ear and temporal bone.

Otalgia usually is associated with inflammation of the external or middle ear, but it may represent pain referred from involvement of the teeth, temporomandibular joint, or pharynx. In young infants, pulling or rubbing the ear along with general irritability or poor sleep, especially when associated with fever, may be the only signs of ear pain. Ear pulling alone is not diagnostic of ear pathology.

Purulent otorrhea is a sign of otitis externa, otitis media with perforation of the tympanic membrane (TM), drainage from the middle ear through a patent tympanostomy tube, or, rarely, drainage from a branchial cleft sinus. Bloody drainage may be associated with acute or chronic inflammation (often with granulation tissue), trauma, neoplasm, foreign body, or blood dyscrasia. Clear drainage suggests a perforation of the TM with a serous middle-ear effusion or, rarely, a cerebrospinal fluid leak draining through defects (congenital or traumatic) in the external auditory canal or from the middle ear.

Hearing loss results either from disease of the external or middle ear (conductive hearing loss) or from pathology in the inner ear, retrocochlear structures, or central auditory pathways (sensorineural hearing loss). The most common cause of hearing loss in children is otitis media (OM).

Swelling around the ear most commonly is a result of inflammation (e.g., external otitis, perichondritis, mastoiditis), trauma (e.g., hematoma), benign cystic masses, or neoplasm.

Vertigo is a specific type of dizziness that is defined as any illusion or sensation of motion. **Dizziness** is less specific than vertigo and refers to an altered orientation in space. Vertigo is an uncommon complaint in children; the child or parent may not volunteer information about balance unless asked specifically. The most common cause of dizziness in young children is eustachian tube–middle-ear disease, but true vertigo also may be caused by labyrinthitis, perilymphatic fistula between the inner and middle ear due to trauma or a congenital inner ear defect, cholesteatoma in the mastoid or middle ear, vestibular neuronitis, benign paroxysmal vertigo, Meniere disease, or disease of the central nervous system. Older children may describe a feeling of room-spinning or turning; younger children may express the dysequilibrium only by falling, stumbling, or clumsiness.

Nystagmus may be unidirectional, horizontal, or jerk nystagmus. It is vestibular in origin and usually is associated with vertigo.

Tinnitus rarely is described spontaneously by children, but it is common, especially in patients with eustachian tube–middle-ear disease or sensorineural hearing loss (SNHL). Children may describe tinnitus if asked directly about it, including laterality and the quality of the sound.

FACIAL PARALYSIS. The facial nerve may be dehiscent in its course through the middle ear in as many as 50% of patients. Infection with local inflammation, most commonly in acute OM, may lead to a temporary paralysis of the facial nerve. It also may be due to cholesteatoma, Bell palsy, Ramsay Hunt syndrome (herpes zoster oticus), Lyme disease, fracture, neoplasm, or infection of the temporal bone. Congenital facial paralysis may be due to birth trauma or congenital abnormality of the 7th nerve, or a syndrome such as Möbius or CHARGE (coloboma, heart defects, atresia choanae, retarded growth, genital hypoplasia, and ear anomalies), or it may be associated with other cranial nerve abnormalities and craniofacial anomalies.

PHYSICAL EXAMINATION

Complete examination with special attention to the head and neck may reveal a condition that may predispose to or be associated with ear disease in children. The facial appearance and the character of speech may give clues to an abnormality of the ear or hearing. Many craniofacial anomalies, such as cleft palate, mandibulofacial dysostosis (Treacher Collins syndrome), and trisomy 21 (Down syndrome) are associated with disorders of the ear and eustachian tube. Mouth breathing and hyponasality may indicate intranasal or postnasal obstruction. **Hypernasality** is a sign of velopharyngeal insufficiency. Examining the oropharyngeal cavity may uncover an overt cleft palate or a submucous cleft (usually associated with a bifid uvula), both of which predispose to OM with effusion. A nasopharyngeal tumor with nasal and eustachian tube blockage may be associated with OM.

The position of the patient for examination of the ear, nose, and throat depends on the patient's age and ability to cooperate, the clinical setting, and the examiner's preference. The child can be examined on an examination table or in the parent's lap. The presence of a parent or assistant usually is necessary to minimize movement and provide better examination results (Fig. 635-1). An examining table may be desirable for uncooperative older infants or when a procedure, such as microscopic evaluation or tympanocentesis, is performed. Wrapping the child in a sheet or using a papoose board can help to minimize movement. Lap examination is adequate and preferable in most infants and young children; the parent may assist in restraining the child by folding the child's wrists and arms over the child's own abdomen

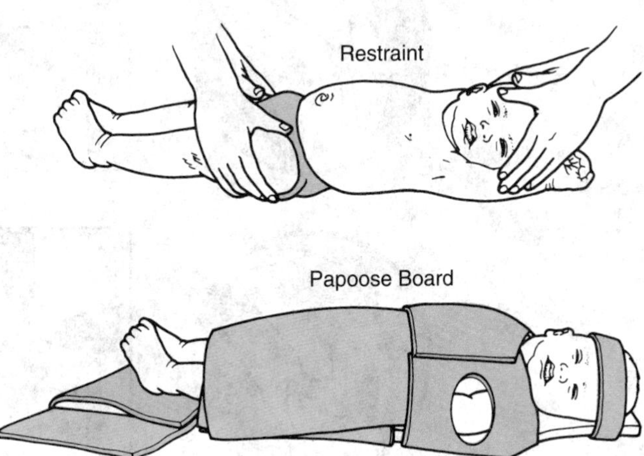

Figure 635-1. Methods of restraining an infant for examination and for procedures such as tympanocentesis or myringotomy. (From Bluestone CD, Klein JO: *Otitis Media in Infants and Children,* 2nd ed. Philadelphia, WB Saunders, 1995, p 91.)

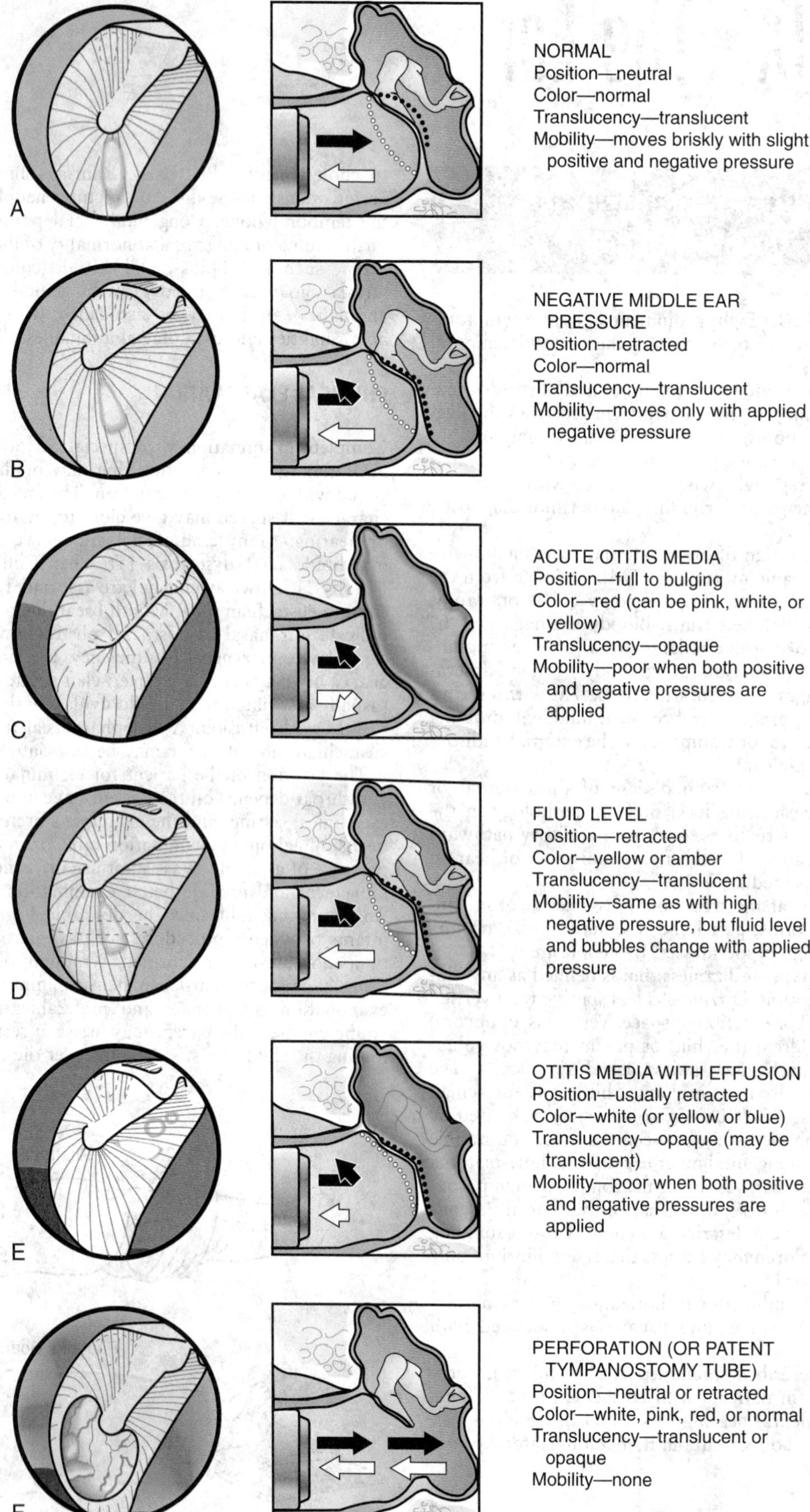

A
NORMAL
Position—neutral
Color—normal
Translucency—translucent
Mobility—moves briskly with slight positive and negative pressure
B
NEGATIVE MIDDLE EAR PRESSURE
Position—retracted
Color—normal
Translucency—translucent
Mobility—moves only with applied negative pressure
C
ACUTE OTITIS MEDIA
Position—full to bulging
Color—red (can be pink, white, or yellow)
Translucency—opaque
Mobility—poor when both positive and negative pressures are applied
D
FLUID LEVEL
Position—retracted
Color—yellow or amber
Translucency—translucent
Mobility—same as with high negative pressure, but fluid level and bubbles change with applied pressure
E
OTITIS MEDIA WITH EFFUSION
Position—usually retracted
Color—white (or yellow or blue)
Translucency—opaque (may be translucent)
Mobility—poor when both positive and negative pressures are applied
F
PERFORATION (OR PATENT TYMPANOSTOMY TUBE)
Position—neutral or retracted
Color—white, pink, red, or normal
Translucency—translucent or opaque
Mobility—none

Figure 635-2. Common conditions of the middle ear, as assessed with the otoscope. (From Bluestone CD, Klein JO: *Otitis Media in Infants and Children,* 3rd ed. Philadelphia, WB Saunders, 2001, p 131.)

with one hand and holding the child's head against the parent's chest with the other hand. If necessary, the child's legs can be held between the parent's knees. To avoid ear trauma with movement, the examiner should hold the otoscope with the hand placed firmly against the child's head or face, so that the otoscope moves with the head. Pulling up and out on the pinna straightens the ear canal and allows better exposure of the TM.

When examining the ear, inspection of the auricle and external auditory meatus for infection may aid in the evaluation of complications of OM. External otitis may result from acute OM with discharge, or inflammation of the posterior auricular area may indicate a periosteitis or subperiosteal abscess extending from the mastoid air cells. The presence of preauricular pits or skin tags also should be noted because affected children have a slightly higher incidence of SNHL.

Cerumen is a protective, waxy, water-repellent coating in the ear canal that may interfere with examination. Cerumen usually is removed using the surgical head of the otoscope, which allows passage of a wire loop or a blunt curette under direct visualization. Other methods include gentle irrigation of the ear canal with warm water, which should be performed only if the TM is intact, or instillation of a solution such as diluted hydrogen peroxide in the ear canal (with intact TM only) for a few minutes to soften the wax for suction removal or irrigation. Some commercial preparations such as trolamine polypeptide oleate-condensate (Cerumenex) may cause dermatitis of the external canal with chronic use and should be used only under a physician's supervision.

Inflammation of the ear canal with associated pain often indicates external otitis. Abnormalities of the external auditory canal include stenosis (common in children with trisomy 21), bony exostoses, otorrhea, and the presence of foreign bodies. Cholesteatoma of the middle ear may manifest in the canal as intermittent foul-smelling drainage, sometimes associated with white debris; cholesteatoma of the external canal may appear as a white, pearl-like mass in the canal skin. White or gray debris of the canal suggests fungal external otitis. Newborn ear canals are filled with vernix caseosa, which is soft and pale yellow and should disappear shortly after birth.

The TM and its mobility are best assessed with a pneumatic otoscope. The normal TM is in a neutral position; a bulging TM may be caused by increased middle-ear air pressure, with or without pus or effusion in the middle ear; a bulging drum may obscure visualization of the malleus and annulus. Retraction of the TM usually indicates negative middle-ear pressure, but it also may result from previous middle-ear disease with fixation of the ossicles, ossicular ligaments, or TM. When retraction is present, the bony malleus appears more prominent, and the incus may be more visible posterior to the malleus.

The normal TM has a silvery-gray, "waxed paper" appearance (Fig. 635-2). A white or yellow TM may indicate a middle-ear effusion. A red TM alone may not indicate pathology, because the blood vessels of the membrane may be engorged as a result of crying, sneezing, or nose blowing. A normal TM is translucent, allowing the observer to visualize the middle-ear landmarks: incus, promontory, round window niche, and, often, the chorda tympani nerve. If a middle-ear effusion is present, an air-fluid level or bubbles may be visible (see Fig. 635-2). Inability to visualize the middle-ear structures indicates opacification of the drum, usually caused by thickening of the TM, a middle-ear effusion, or both. Assessment of the light reflex usually is not helpful, because a middle ear with effusion reflects light as well as a normal ear.

TM mobility is helpful in assessing middle ear pressures and the presence or absence of fluid (see Fig. 635-2). To best perform pneumatic otoscopy, a speculum of adequate size is used to obtain a good seal and allow air movement in the canal. A rubber ring around the tip of the speculum may help to obtain a better canal seal. Normal middle-ear pressure is characterized by a neutral TM position and brisk TM movement to both positive and negative pressures.

Eardrum retraction is most common when negative middle-ear pressure is present; with even moderate negative middle-ear pressure there is no visible inward movement with applied positive pressure in the ear canal (see Fig. 635-1). However, negative canal pressure, which is produced by releasing the rubber bulb of the pneumatic otoscope, may cause the TM to bounce out toward the neutral position. A retracted TM may occur in both the presence and absence of middle-ear fluid, and if the middle-ear fluid is mixed with air, the TM may still have some mobility. Outward eardrum movement is less likely in the presence of severe negative middle-ear pressure or middle-ear effusion.

The TM that exhibits fullness (bulging) moves to applied positive pressure but not to applied negative pressure if the pressure within the middle ear is positive and some air is present. A full TM and positive middle-ear pressure without an effusion may be seen in young infants who are crying during the otoscopic examination, in older infants and children with nasal obstruction, and in the early stage of acute OM. When the middle-ear-mastoid air cell system is filled with an effusion and little or no air is present, the mobility of the TM is severely decreased or absent in response to both applied positive and negative pressures.

Tympanocentesis, or aspiration of the middle ear, is the definitive method of verifying the presence and type of a middle-ear effusion and is performed by inserting, through the inferior portion of the TM, an 18-gauge spinal needle attached to a syringe or a collection trap (Fig. 635-3). Culturing of the ear canal and alcohol cleansing should precede tympanocentesis and culture of the middle-ear aspirate; a canal culture is taken first to help determine whether organisms cultured from the middle ear are contaminants from the external canal or true middle ear pathogens.

Further diagnostic studies of the ear and hearing include audiometric evaluation, impedance audiometry (tympanometry), acoustic reflectometry, and specialized eustachian tube function studies. Diagnostic imaging studies, including computed tomography and magnetic resonance imaging, often provide further information about anatomic abnormalities and the extent of inflammatory processes or neoplasms. Specialized assessment of labyrinthine function should be considered in the evaluation of a child with a suspected vestibular disorder (see Chapter 640).

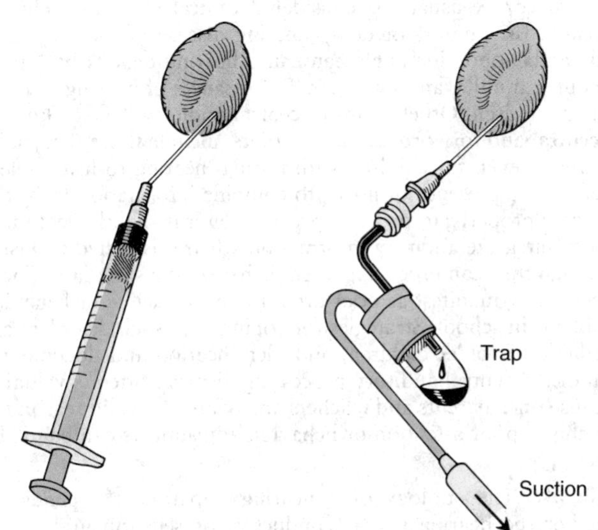

Figure 635-3. Tympanocentesis can be performed with a needle attached to a tuberculin syringe (left) or by using an Alden-Senturia collection trap (Storz Instrument Co, St. Louis). (From Bluestone CD, Klein JO: *Otitis Media in Infants and Children,* 2nd ed. Philadelphia, WB Saunders, 1995, p 127.)

Chapter 636 ■ Hearing Loss

Joseph Haddad Jr.

INCIDENCE AND PREVALENCE. Although estimates vary because of differences in criteria for defining hearing impairment, the age group surveyed, and the testing methods used, approximately 1–2 newborns/1,000 live births have moderate (30–50 dB), severe (50–70 dB), or profound (>70 dB) bilateral neural hearing loss, including 0.5–1/1,000 with bilateral hearing loss >75 dB. An additional 1–2/1,000 may have milder or unilateral impairments; by 19 yr of age the prevalence doubles. In the U.S., unilateral sensorineural hearing loss (SNHL) of >26 dB occurs in 13/1,000 school-aged children, and SNHL of >45 dB occurs in 3/1,000 school-aged children. The onset of hearing loss can occur at any time in childhood. When less severe hearing loss or the transient hearing loss that commonly accompanies middle-ear disease in young children is considered, the number of affected children increases substantially.

TYPES OF HEARING LOSS. Hearing loss can be peripheral or central in origin. **Conductive hearing loss (CHL)** commonly is caused by dysfunction in the transmission of sound through the external or middle ear or by abnormal transduction of sound energy into neural activity in the inner ear and the 8th nerve. Peripheral hearing loss can be conductive, sensorineural, or mixed. CHL is the most common type of hearing loss in children and occurs when sound transmission is physically impeded in the external and/or middle ear. Common causes of CHL in the ear canal include atresia or stenosis, impacted cerumen, or foreign bodies. In the middle ear, perforation of the tympanic membrane (TM), discontinuity or fixation of the ossicular chain, otitis media (OM) with effusion, otosclerosis, and cholesteatoma can cause CHL.

Damage to or maldevelopment of structures in the inner ear can cause **sensorineural hearing loss (SNHL)**. Causes include hair cell destruction from noise, disease, or ototoxic agents; cochlear malformation; perilymphatic fistula of the round or oval window membrane; and lesions of the acoustic division of the 8th nerve. A combination of CHL and SNHL is considered a **mixed hearing loss.**

An auditory deficit originating along the central auditory nervous system pathways from the proximal 8th nerve to the cerebral cortex usually is considered **central (or retrocochlear) hearing loss.** Tumors or demyelinating disease of the 8th nerve and cerebellopontine angle can cause hearing deficits but spare the outer, middle, and inner ear. These causes of hearing loss are rare in children. Other forms of central auditory deficits, known as **central auditory processing disorders,** include those that make it difficult even for children with normal hearing to listen selectively in the presence of noise, to combine information from the two ears properly, to process speech when it is slightly degraded, and to integrate auditory information when it is delivered faster although they can process it when delivered at a slow rate. These deficits may manifest as poor attention or academic or behavior problems in school. Strategies for coping with such disorders are available for older children, and identification and documentation of the central auditory processing disorder often is valuable because once parents and teachers are aware of a valid reason for the child's poor attention or behavior, adjustments can be made.

ETIOLOGY. The etiology of a hearing impairment depends on whether the hearing loss is conductive or sensorineural. Most CHL is acquired, with middle ear fluid the most common cause. Congenital causes include anomalies of the pinna, external ear canal, TM, and ossicles. Rarely, congenital cholesteatoma or other masses in the middle ear may present as CHL. TM perforation (e.g., trauma, OM), ossicular discontinuity (e.g., infection, cholesteatoma, trauma), tympanosclerosis, acquired cholesteatoma, or masses in the ear canal or middle ear (e.g., Langerhans' cell histiocytosis, salivary gland tumors, glomus tumors, rhabdomyosarcoma) also may present as CHL. Uncommon diseases that affect the middle ear and temporal bone and may present with CHL include otosclerosis, osteopetrosis, fibrous dysplasia, and osteogenesis imperfecta.

SNHL may be congenital or acquired. Acquired SNHL may be caused by genetic, infectious, autoimmune, anatomic, traumatic, ototoxic, and idiopathic factors (Tables 636-1, 636-2, 636-3, and 636-4). The recognized risk factors account for about 50% of cases of moderate to profound SNHL. The most common infectious cause of congenital SNHL is **cytomegalovirus (CMV),** which infects 1/100 newborns in the USA (see Chapter 252). Of these, 6,000–8,000 infants each year will have clinical manifestations, including approximately 75% with SNHL. Congenital CMV warrants special attention because it is associated with hearing loss in its symptomatic and asymptomatic forms, and the hearing loss may be progressive. Some children with congenital CMV have suddenly lost residual hearing at 4–5 yr of age. Much less common congenital infectious causes of SNHL include toxoplasmosis and syphilis. Congenital CMV, toxoplasmosis, and syphilis also may present with delayed onset of SNHL, months to years after birth. Rubella, once the most common viral cause of congenital SNHL, is very uncommon because of effective vaccination programs. In utero infection with herpes simplex virus is rare, and hearing loss is not an isolated manifestation.

TABLE 636-1. Indicators Associated With Sensorineural and/or Conductive Hearing Loss

FOR USE WITH NEONATES (BIRTH–AGE 28 D) WHEN UNIVERSAL SCREENING IS NOT AVAILABLE
Family history of hereditary childhood sensorineural hearing loss
In utero infection, such as cytomegalovirus, rubella, syphilis, herpes simplex, or toxoplasmosis
Craniofacial anomalies, including those with morphologic abnormalities of the pinna and ear canal
Birth weight <1500 g (3.3 lb)
Hyperbilirubinemia at a serum level requiring exchange transfusion
Ototoxic medications, including but not limited to the aminoglycosides, used in multiple courses or in combination with loop diuretics
Bacterial meningitis
Apgar scores of 0–4 at 1 min or 0–6 at 5 min
Mechanical ventilation lasting ≥5 d
Stigmata or other findings associated with a syndrome known to include a sensorineural and/or conductive hearing loss
FOR USE WITH INFANTS (AGE 29 D–2 YR) WHEN CERTAIN HEALTH CONDITIONS DEVELOP THAT REQUIRE RESCREENING
Parent/caregiver concern regarding hearing, speech, language, and/or developmental delay
Bacterial meningitis and other infections associated with sensorineural hearing loss
Head trauma associated with loss of consciousness or skull fracture
Stigmata or other findings associated with a syndrome known to include a sensorineural and/or conductive hearing loss
Ototoxic medications, including but not limited to chemotherapeutic agents or aminoglycosides used in multiple courses or in combination with loop diuretics
Recurrent or persistent otitis media with effusion for at least 3 mo
FOR USE WITH INFANTS (AGE 29 D–3 YR) WHO REQUIRE PERIODIC MONITORING OF HEARING
(Some newborns and infants may pass initial hearing screening but require periodic monitoring of hearing to detect delayed-onset sensorineural and/or conductive hearing loss. Infants with these indicators require hearing evaluation at least every 6 mo until age 3 yr, and at appropriate intervals thereafter.)
INDICATORS ASSOCIATED WITH DELAYED-ONSET SENSORINEURAL HEARING LOSS
Family history of hereditary childhood hearing loss
In utero infection, such as cytomgalovirus, rubella, syphilis, herpes simplex, or toxoplasmosis
Neurofibromatosis type 2 and neurodegenerative disorders
INDICATORS ASSOCIATED WITH CONDUCTIVE HEARING LOSS
Recurrent or persistent otitis media with effusion
Anatomic deformities and other disorders that affect eustachian tube function
Neurodegenerative disorders

Adapted from American Academy of Pediatrics, Joint Committee on Infant Hearing: Joint Committee on Infant Hearing 1994 Position Statement. *Pediatrics* 1995;95:152.

TABLE 636-2. Common Types of Hereditary Nonsyndromic Sensorineural Hearing Loss

LOCUS	GENE	AUDIO PHENOTYPE
DFN3	*POU3F4*	Conductive hearing loss due to stapes fixation mimicking otosclerosis; superimposed progressive SNHL
DFNA1	*DIAPH1*	Low-frequency loss beginning in the first decade and progressing to all frequencies to produce a flat audioprofile with profound losses throughout the auditory range
DFNA2	*KCNQ4*	Symmetrical high-frequency sensorineural loss beginning in the first decade and progressing over all frequencies
	GJB3	Symmetrical high-frequency sensorineural loss beginning in the third decade
DFNA 6/14/38	*WFS1*	Early-onset low-frequency sensorinerual loss; about 75% of families dominantly segregating this audioprofile carry missense mutations in the C-terminal domain of wolframin.
DFNA10	*EYA4*	Progressive loss beginning in the second decade as a flat to gently sloping audioprofile that becomes steeply sloping with age
DFNA13	*COL11A2*	Congenital mid-frequency sensorineural loss that shows age-related progression across the auditory range
DFNA15	*POU4F3*	Bilateral progressive sensorineural loss beginning in the second decade
DFNA20/26	*ACTG1*	Bilateral progressive sensorineural loss beginning in the second decade; with age, the loss increases with threshold shifts in all frequencies, although a sloping configuration is maintained in most cases
DFNB1	*GJB2, GJB6*	Hearing loss varies from mild to profound. The most common genotype, 35delG/35delG, is associated with severe to profound SNHL in about 90% of affected children; severe to profound deafness is observed in only 60% of children who are compound heterozygotes carrying one 35delG allele and any other *GJB2* SNHL-causing allele variant; in children carrying two *GJB2* SNHL-causing missense mutations, severe to profound deafness is not observed.
DFNB4	*SLC26A4*	DFNB4 and Pendred's syndrome (see Table 636-3) are allelic. DFNB4 hearing loss is associated with dilatation of the vestibular aqueduct and can be unilateral or bilateral. In the high frequencies, the loss is severe to profound; in the low frequencies, the degree of loss varies widely. Onset can be congenital (prelingual), but progressive postlingual loss also is common.
mtDNA 1555A > G	*12S rRNA*	Degree of hearing loss varies from mild to profound but usually is symmetrical; high frequencies are preferentially affected; precipitous loss in hearing can occur after aminoglycoside therapy.

SNHL, sensorineural hearing loss.
From Smith RJH, Bale JF Jr, White KR: Sensorineural hearing loss in children. *Lancet* 2005;365:879–890.

Other postnatal infectious causes of SNHL include neonatal group B streptococcal sepsis and bacterial meningitis at any age. *Streptococcus pneumoniae* is the most common cause of bacterial meningitis that results in SNHL after the neonatal period and has become less frequent with the routine administration of pneumococcal conjugate vaccine. *Haemophilus influenzae type b*, once the most common cause of meningitis resulting in SNHL, is rare

TABLE 636-4. Infectious Pathogens Implicated in Sensorineural Hearing Loss in Children

CONGENITAL INFECTIONS
Cytomegalovirus
Lymphocytic choriomeningitis virus
Rubella virus
Toxoplasma gondii
Treponema pallidum
ACQUIRED INFECTIONS
Borrelia burgdorferi
Epstein-Barr virus
Haemophilus influenzae
Lassa virus
Measles virus
Mumps virus
Neisseria meningitidis
Non-polio enteroviruses
Plasmodium falciparum
Streptococcus pneumoniae
Varicella zoster virus

From Smith RJH, Bale JF Jr., White KR: Sensorineural hearing loss in children. *Lancet* 2005;365:879–890.

owing to the Hib conjugate vaccine. Uncommon infectious causes of SNHL include Lyme disease, parvovirus B19, and varicella. Mumps, rubella, and rubeola, all once common causes of SNHL in children, are rare owing to vaccination programs.

Genetic causes of SNHL probably are responsible for as many as 50% of SNHL cases (see Tables 636–2 and 636–3). These disorders may be associated with other abnormalities, may be part of a named syndrome, or may exist in isolation. SNHL often occurs with abnormalities of the ear and eye and with disorders of the metabolic, musculoskeletal, integumentary, renal, and nervous systems. **Autosomal dominant** hearing losses account for about 10% of all cases of childhood SNHL. Waardenburg (types I and II) and branchio-otorenal syndromes represent 2 of the most common autosomal dominant syndromic types of SNHL. Types of SNHL are coded with a 4-letter code and a number, as follows: **DFN** = deafness, A = dominant, B = recessive, and number = order of discovery, e.g. DFNA 13. Autosomal dominant conditions in addition to those just discussed include: DFNA 1 to 11, 13, 15, 17, 20, 22, 28, 36, 48 and mutations in the crystallin gene *(CRYM)*. **Autosomal recessive** genetic SNHL, both syndromic and nonsyndromic, accounts for about 80% of all childhood cases of SNHL. Usher syndrome (types 1, 2, and 3), Pendred syndrome, and the Jervell and Lange-Nielsen syndrome (one form of the long Q-T syndrome) are 3 of the most common

TABLE 636-3. Common Types of Syndromic Sensorineural Hearing Loss

	GENE	PHENOTYPE
DOMINANT		
Waardenberg (WS1)	*PAX3*	Major diagnostic criteria include dystopia canthorum; congenital hearing loss; heterochromic irises; white forelock; and an affected first-degree relative. About 60% of affected children have congenital hearing loss; in 90%, the loss is bilateral.
Waardenberg (WS2)	*MITF*, others	Major diagnostic criteria are as for WS1 but without dystopia canthorum. About 80% of affected children have congenital hearing loss; in 90%, the loss is bilateral.
Branchio-otorenal	*EYA1*	Diagnostic criteria include hearing loss (98%), preauricular pits (85%), and branchial (70%), renal (40%), and external-ear (30%) abnormalities. The hearing loss can be conductive, sensorineural, or mixed, and mild to profound in degree.
RECESSIVE		
Pendred's syndrome	*SLC26A4*	Diagnostic criteria include sensorineural hearing loss that is congenital, nonprogressive, and severe to profound in many cases, but can be late-onset and progressive; bilateral dilation of the vestibular aqueduct with or without cochlear hypoplasia; and an abnormal perchlorate discharge test or goiter.
Usher syndrome type 1 (USH1)	*USH1A, MYO7A, USH1C, CDH23, USH1E, PCDH15, USH1G*	Diagnostic criteria include congenital, bilateral, and profound hearing loss, vestibular areflexia, and retinitis pigmentosa (commonly not diagnosed until tunnel vision and nyctalopia become severe enough to be noticeable).
Usher syndrome type 2 (USH2)	*USH2A, USH2B, USH2C*, others	Diagnostic criteria include mild to severe, congenital, bilateral hearing loss and retinitis pigmentosa; hearing loss may be perceived as progressing over time because speech perception decreases as diminishing vision interferes with subconscious lip reading.
Usher syndrome type 3 (USH3)	*USH3*	Diagnostic criteria include postlingual, progressive sensorineural hearing loss, late-onset retinitis pigmentosa, and variable impairment of vestibular function.

From Smith RJH, Bale JF Jr, White KR: Sensorineural hearing loss in children. *Lancet* 2005;365:879–890.

syndromic recessive types of SNHL. Other autosomal recessive conditions include: Alström syndrome, type 4 Bartter syndrome, biotinidase deficiency and DFNB1–4, 6–9, 12, 16, 18, 21–23, 28–31, 36, 37, 67. Unlike children with an easily identified syndrome or with anomalies of the outer ear, who may be identified as being at risk for hearing loss and consequently monitored adequately, nonsyndromic children present greater difficulty. Mutations of the connexin-26 and -30 genes have been identified in autosomal recessive (DNFB 1) and autosomal dominant (DNFA 3) and in sporadic nonsyndromic patients with SNHL; up to 50% of nonsyndromic SNHL may be related to a mutation of connexin-26. Mutations of the *GJB2* gene co-localize with DFNA 3 and DFNB 1 loci on chromosome 13, are associated with autosomal nonsyndromic susceptibility to deafness, and are associated with as many as 30% of sporadic severe to profound congenital deafness and 50% of autosomal recessive nonsyndromic deafness. Sex-linked disorders associated with SNHL, thought to account for 1–2% of SNHL, include Norrie disease, the otopalatal digital syndrome, Nance deafness, and Alport syndrome. Chromosomal abnormalities such as trisomy 13–15, trisomy 18, and trisomy 21 also can be accompanied by hearing impairment. Patients with Turner syndrome have monosomy for all or part of 1 X chromosome and may have CHL, SNHL, or mixed hearing loss. The hearing loss may be progressive. Mitochondrial genetic abnormalities also may result in SNHL (see Table 636-2).

Agenesis or malformation of cochlear structures including the Scheibe, Mondini (Fig. 636-1), Alexander, and Michel anomalies, and enlarged vestibular aqueducts and semicircular canal anomalies may be genetic. These anomalies probably occur before the 8th wk of gestation and result from arrest in normal development, aberrant development, or both. Many of these anomalies also have been described in association with other congenital conditions such as intrauterine CMV and rubella infections. These abnormalities are quite common; in as many as 20% of children with SNHL, obvious or subtle temporal bone abnormalities are seen on high-resolution CT scanning or MRI.

CHL ALSO CAN BE GENETIC. Conditions, diseases, or syndromes that include craniofacial abnormalities may be associated with conductive hearing loss and possibly with SNHL. Pierre Robin, Treacher Collins, Klippel-Feil, Crouzon, and branchio-otorenal syndromes and osteogenesis imperfecta often are associated with hearing loss. Congenital anomalies causing CHL include malformations of the ossicles and middle-ear structures and atresia of the external auditory canal.

Many genetically determined causes of hearing impairment, both syndromic and nonsyndromic, do not express themselves until some time after birth. Alport, Alström, and Down syndromes, von Recklinghausen disease, and Hunter-Hurler syndrome are genetic diseases that may have SNHL as a late manifestation.

SNHL also may occur secondary to exposure to toxins, chemicals, and antimicrobials. Early in pregnancy, the embryo is particularly vulnerable to the effects of toxic substances. Ototoxic drugs, including aminoglycosides, loop diuretics, and chemotherapeutic agents (cisplatin) also may cause SNHL. Congenital SNHL may occur secondary to exposure to these drugs as well as to thalidomide and retinoids. Certain chemicals, such as quinine, lead, and arsenic, may cause hearing loss both pre- and postnatally.

Trauma, including temporal bone fractures, inner ear concussion, head trauma, iatrogenic trauma (e.g., surgery, extracorporeal membrane oxygenation [ECMO]), radiation exposure, and noise, also may cause SNHL. Other uncommon causes of SNHL in children include immune disease (systemic or limited to the inner ear), metabolic abnormalities, and neoplasms of the temporal bone.

Sudden hearing loss in a previously healthy child is uncommon but may be due to otitis media or other middle ear pathologies. Usually these causes are obvious from the history and physical examination. Sudden loss of hearing in the absence of obvious causes often is due to a vascular event affecting the cochlear apparatus or nerve, such as embolism or thrombosis (secondary to prothrombotic conditions). Additional causes include perilymph fistula, drugs, trauma, and the first episode of Meniere syndrome.

EFFECTS OF HEARING IMPAIRMENT. The effects of hearing impairment depend on the nature and degree of the hearing loss and on the individual characteristics of the child. Hearing loss may be unilateral or bilateral, conductive, sensorineural, or mixed; mild, moderate, severe, or profound; of sudden or gradual onset; stable, progressive, or fluctuating; and affecting a part, or all, of the audible spectrum. Other factors, such as intelligence, medical or physical condition (including accompanying syndromes), family support, age at onset, age at time of identification, and prompt-

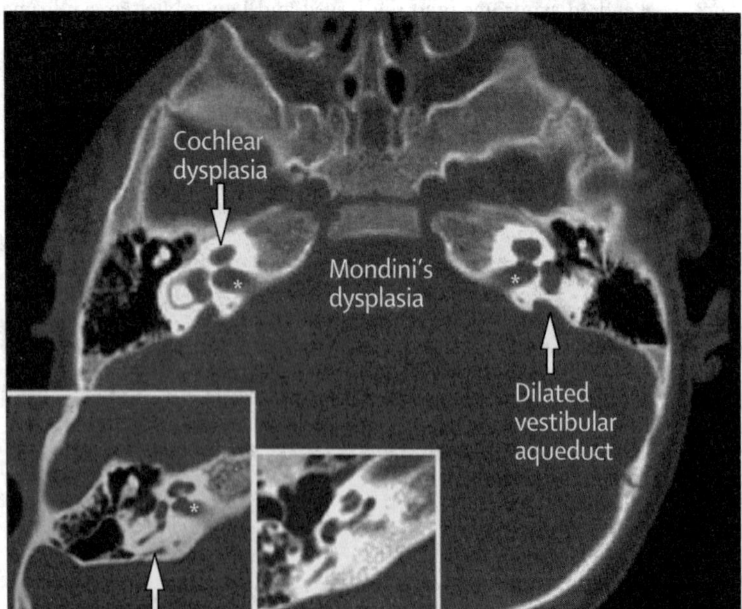

Figure 636-1. Mondini's dysplasia shown by CT of the temporal bone in a child with Pendred's syndrome. Both dilatation of the vestibular aqueduct and cochlear dysplasia are present in this section. In the larger of the two inset images of a normal temporal bone, the vestibular aqueduct is visible but much smaller *(arrow)*. The cochlea appears normal, and in the smaller inset image of a more inferior axial section, the expected number of cochlear turns can be clearly counted (*in internal auditory canal). (From Smith RJH, Bale JF Jr, White KR: Sensorineural hearing loss in children. *Lancet* 2005; 365:879–890.)

TABLE 636-5. Hearing Handicap as a Function of Average Hearing Threshold Level of the Better Ear

AVERAGE THRESHOLD LEVEL (dB) AT 500–2,000 Hz (ANSI)	DESCRIPTION	COMMON CAUSES	WHAT CAN BE HEARD WITHOUT AMPLIFICATION	DEGREE OF HANDICAP (IF NOT TREATED IN 1ST YR OF LIFE)	PROBABLE NEEDS
0–15	Normal range	Conductive hearing loss	All speech sounds	None	None
16–25	Slight hearing loss	Otitis media, TM perforation, tympanosclerosis; Eustachian tube dysfunction; some SNHL	Vowel sounds heard clearly, may miss unvoiced consonant sounds	Mild auditory dysfunction in language learning Difficulty in perceiving some speech sounds	Consideration of need for hearing aid; speech reading; auditory training Speech therapy Appropriate surgery Preferential seating
25–30	Mild	Otitis media, TM perforation, tympanosclerosis, severe eustachian dysfunction, SNHL	Hears only some of speech sounds, the louder voiced sounds	Auditory learning dysfunction Mild language retardation Mild speech problems Inattention	Hearing aid Lip reading Auditory training Speech therapy Appropriate surgery
30–50	Moderate hearing loss	Chronic otitis, ear canal/middle ear anomaly, SNHL	Misses most speech sounds at normal conversational level	Speech problems Language retardation Learning dysfunction Inattention	All of the above, plus consideration of special classroom situation
50–70	Severe hearing loss	SNHL or mixed loss due to a combination of middle-ear disease and sensorineural involvement	Hears no speech sound of normal conversations	Severe speech problems Language retardation Learning dysfunction Inattention	All of the above; probable assignment to special classes
70+	Profound hearing loss	SNHL or mixed	Hears no speech or other sounds	Severe speech problems Language retardation Learning dysfunction Inattention	All of the above; probable assignment to special classes or schools

ANSI, American National Standards Institute; SNHL, sensorineural hearing loss; TM, tympanic membrane.
Modified from Northern JL, Downs MP: *Hearing in Children,* 4th ed. Baltimore, Williams & Wilkins, 1991.

ness of intervention, also affect the impact of hearing loss on a child.

Most hearing-impaired children have some usable hearing. Only 6% of those in the hearing-impaired population have bilateral profound hearing loss. Hearing loss very early in life can affect the development of speech and language, social and emotional development, behavior, attention, and academic achievement. Some cases of hearing impairment are misdiagnosed because affected children have sufficient hearing to respond to environmental sounds and can learn some speech and language but when challenged in the classroom cannot perform to full potential.

Even mild or unilateral hearing loss may have a detrimental effect on the development of a young child and on school performance. Children with such hearing impairments have greater difficulty when listening conditions are unfavorable (e.g., background noise and poor acoustics), as may occur in a classroom. The fact that schools are auditory–verbal environments is unappreciated by those who minimize the impact of hearing impairment on learning. Hearing loss should be considered in any child with speech and language difficulties or below-par performance, poor behavior, or inattention in school (Table 636-5).

Children with moderate, severe, or profound hearing impairment and those with other handicapping conditions often are educated in classes or schools for children with special needs. The auditory management and choices regarding modes of communication and education for children with hearing handicaps must be individualized, because these children are not a homogeneous group. A team approach to individual case management is essential, because each child and family unit has unique needs and abilities.

HEARING SCREENING. Hearing impairment can have a major impact on a child's development, and because early identification improves prognosis, screening programs have been widely and strongly advocated. Data from the Colorado newborn screening program suggest that if hearing-impaired infants are identified and treated by age 6 mo, these children (with the exception of those with bilateral profound impairment) should develop the same level of language as their age-matched peers who are not hearing impaired. This is compelling support for the establishment of mandated newborn hearing screening programs for all children. The American Academy of Pediatrics endorses the goal of universal detection of hearing loss in infants before 3 mo of age, with appropriate intervention no later than 6 mo of age. Currently, hearing screening has been mandated in 32 states in the USA.

Until mandated screening programs are established universally, many hospitals will continue to use other criteria to screen for hearing loss. Some use the high-risk criteria (see Table 636-1) to decide which infants to screen; some screen all infants who require intensive care; and some do both. The problem with using high-risk criteria to screen is that 50% of cases of hearing impairment will be missed, either because the infants are hearing impaired but do not meet any of the high-risk criteria, or because they develop hearing loss after the neonatal period.

The recommended hearing screening techniques are either otoacoustic emissions (OAE) testing or auditory brainstem evoked responses (ABR). The ABR test, an auditory evoked electrophysiologic response that correlates highly with hearing, has been used successfully and cost-effectively to screen newborns and to identify further the degree and type of hearing loss. OAE tests, used successfully in most universal newborn screening programs, are quick, easy to administer, and inexpensive, and provide a sensitive indication of the presence of hearing loss. Results are relatively easy to interpret. OAE tests elicit no response if hearing is worse than 30–40 dB, no matter what the cause; those children who fail OAE tests undergo an ABR for a more definitive evaluation. Screening methods such as observing behavioral responses to uncalibrated noisemakers or using automated systems such as the Crib-o-gram (Canon) or the auditory response cradle (in which movement of the infant in response to sound is recorded by motion sensors) are not recommended.

Many children become hearing-impaired after the neonatal period and, therefore, are not identified by newborn screening programs. Often it is not until children are in preschool or kindergarten that further hearing screening takes place. Primary care physicians and pediatricians should be alert to the signs and symptoms of childhood hearing impairment, so that children with hearing impairment who have not been screened formally can be identified as early as possible.

Identification of Hearing Impairment. The impact of hearing impairment is greatest on an infant who has yet to develop language; therefore, identification, diagnosis, description, and treatment should begin as soon as possible. In general, infants with a prenatal or perinatal history that puts them at risk (see Table 636-1) or those who have failed a formal hearing screening should be monitored closely by an experienced clinical audiologist until a reliable assessment of auditory function has been obtained. Pediatricians should encourage families to cooperate with the follow-up plan. Infants who are born at risk but who were not screened as neonates (often because of transfer from one hospital to another) should have a hearing screening by age 3 mo.

Hearing-impaired infants who are born at risk or are screened for hearing loss in a neonatal hearing screening program account for only a portion of hearing-impaired children. Children who are congenitally deaf because of autosomal recessive inheritance or subclinical congenital infection often are not identified until 1–3 yr of age. Usually, those with more severe hearing loss are identified at an earlier age, but identification often occurs later than the age at which intervention can provide an optimal outcome. Children with normal hearing develop an extensive language by 3–4 yr of age (Table 636-6) and exhibit behaviors reflecting normal auditory function (Table 636-7). Failure to fulfill these criteria should be reason for an audiologic evaluation. Parental concern about hearing and any delayed development of speech and language should alert the pediatrician, because parental concern usually precedes formal identification and diagnosis of hearing impairment by 6 mo to 1 yr of age.

CLINICAL AUDIOLOGIC EVALUATION. Even the youngest infants can be evaluated for auditory function. When hearing impairment is suspected in a young child, reliable and valid estimates of auditory function can be obtained. Successful treatment strategies for hearing-impaired children rely on prompt identification and ongoing assessment to define the dimensions of auditory function. Cooperation among the pediatrician and specialists in areas such as audiology, speech and language pathology, education, and child development is necessary to optimize auditory–verbal development. Therapy for hearing-impaired children includes considering and often fitting an amplification device, monitoring hearing and auditory skills, counseling parents and families, advising teachers, and dealing with public agencies.

Audiometry. The technique of the audiologic evaluation varies as a function of the age or developmental level of the child, the reason for the evaluation, and the child's otologic condition or history. An audiogram provides the fundamental description of hearing sensitivity (Fig. 636-2). Hearing thresholds are assessed as a function of frequency using pure tones (sine waves) at octave intervals from 250–8,000 Hz. Earphones typically are used, and

TABLE 636-6. Criteria for Referral for Audiologic Assessment

AGE (MO)	REFERRAL GUIDELINES FOR CHILDREN WITH "SPEECH" DELAY
12	No differentiated babbling or vocal imitation
18	No use of single words
24	Single-word vocabulary of ≤10 words
30	<100 words; no evidence of 2-word combinations; unintelligible
36	<200 words; no use of telegraphic sentences; clarity <50%
48	<600 words; no use of simple sentences clarity ≤80%

From Matkin ND: Early recognition and referral of hearing-impaired children. *Pediatr Rev* 1984;6:151. Reproduced by permission of *Pediatrics*.

TABLE 636-7. Guidelines for Referral of Children Suspected of Having Hearing Loss

AGE (MO)	NORMAL DEVELOPMENT
0–4	Should startle to loud sounds, quiet to mother's voice, momentarily cease activity when sound is presented at a conversational level
5–6	Should correctly localize to sound presented in a horizontal plane, begin to imitate sounds in own speech repertoire or at least reciprocally vocalize with an adult
7–12	Should correctly localize to sound presented in any plane Should respond to name, even when spoken quietly
13–15	Should point toward an unexpected sound or to familiar objects or persons when asked
16–18	Should follow simple directions without gestural or other visual cues; can be trained to reach toward an interesting toy at midline when a sound is presented
19–24	Should point to body parts when asked; by 21–24 mo, can be trained to perform play audiometry

From Matkin ND: Early recognition and referral of hearing-impaired children. *Pediatr Rev* 1984;6:151. Reproduced by permission of *Pediatrics*.

hearing is assessed independently for each ear. **Airconducted signals** are presented through earphones (or loudspeakers) and are used to provide information about the sensitivity of the auditory system. These same test sounds can be delivered to the ear through an oscillator that is placed on the head, usually on the mastoid. Such signals are considered bone-conducted because the bones of the skull transmit vibrations as sound energy directly to the inner ear, essentially bypassing the outer and middle ears. In a normal ear, and also in children with SNHL, the air and bone conduction thresholds are the same. In those with CHL, the air and bone conduction thresholds differ. This is called the **air–bone gap,** which indicates the amount of hearing loss attributable to

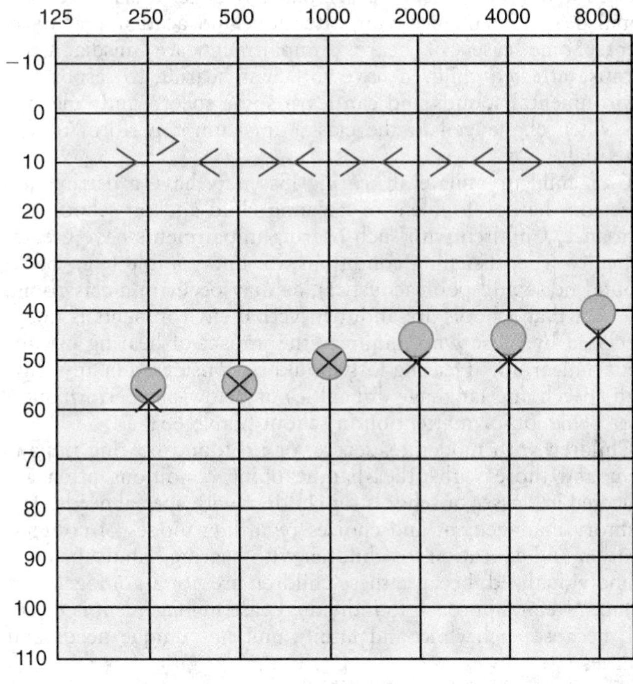

Figure 636-2. Audiogram showing bilateral conductive hearing loss.

dysfunction in the outer and/or middle ear. With mixed hearing loss, both the bone and air conduction thresholds are abnormal, and there is an air–bone gap.

Speech Recognition Threshold. Another measure useful for describing auditory function is the speech recognition threshold (SRT), which is the lowest intensity level at which a score of approximately 50% correct is obtained on a task of recognizing spondee words. Spondee words are 2-syllable words or phrases that have equal stress on each syllable, such as baseball, hotdog, and pancake. Listeners must be familiar with all the words for a valid test result to be obtained. The SRT should correspond to the average of pure-tone thresholds at 500, 1,000, and 2,000 Hz, the pure-tone average (PTA). The SRT is relevant as an indicator of a child's potential for development and use of speech and language; it also serves as a check of the validity of a test because children with nonorganic hearing loss (malingerers) may show a discrepancy between the PTA and SRT.

The basic battery of hearing tests concludes with an assessment of a child's ability to understand monosyllabic words when presented at a comfortable listening level. Performance on such word intelligibility tests assists in the differential diagnosis of hearing impairment and provides a measure of how well a child performs when speech is presented at loudness levels similar to those encountered in the environment.

Play Audiometry. Hearing testing is age-dependent. For children at or above the developmental level of a 5–6 yr old, conventional test methods can be used. For children 30 mo to 5 yr of age, play audiometry can be used. Responses in play audiometry usually are conditioned motor activities associated with a game, such as dropping blocks in a bucket, placing rings on a peg, or completing a puzzle. The technique can be used to obtain a reliable audiogram for a preschool child. For those who will not or cannot repeat words clearly for the SRT and word intelligibility tasks, pictures can be used with a pointing response.

Visual Reinforcement Audiometry. For children between the ages of about 6–30 mo, visual reinforcement audiometry (VRA) commonly is used. In this technique, the child is observed for a head-turning response on activation of an animated (mechanical) toy reinforcer. If infants are properly conditioned, by giving sounds associated with the visual toy cue, VRA can provide reliable estimates of hearing sensitivity for tones and speech sounds. In most applications of VRA, sounds are presented by loudspeakers in a sound field, so no ear-specific information is obtained. Assessment of an infant often is designed to rule out hearing loss that would affect the development of speech and language. Normal sound field response levels of infants indicate sufficient hearing for this purpose despite the possibility of different hearing levels in the 2 ears.

Behavioral Observation Audiometry. Used as a screening device for infants <5 mo of age, behavioral observation audiometry (BOA) is limited to unconditioned, reflexive responses to complex (not frequency-specific) test sounds such as noise, speech, or music presented using calibrated signals from a loudspeaker or uncalibrated noisemakers. Response levels can vary widely within and among infants and usually do not provide a reliable estimate of sensitivity.

Assessment of a child with suspected hearing loss is not complete until pure-tone hearing thresholds and SRTs (a reliable audiogram) have been obtained in each ear. BOA and VRA in sound-field testing give estimates of hearing responsivity in the better hearing ear.

Acoustic Immittance Testing. Acoustic immittance testing is a standard part of the clinical audiologic test battery and includes tympanometry. It is a useful objective assessment technique that provides information about the status of the middle ear. Tympanometry can be performed in a physician's office and is helpful in the diagnosis and management of OM with effusion, a common cause of mild to moderate hearing loss in young children.

TABLE 636-8. Norms for Peak (Static) Admittance (in mL) Using a 226-Hz Probe Tone for Children and Adults

		SPEED OF AIR PRESSURE SWEEP	
		≤50 daPa/sec*	200 daPa/sec†
Children (3–5 yr)	Lower limit	0.30	0.36
	Median	0.55	0.61
	Upper limit	0.90	1.06
Adults	Lower limit	0.56	0.27
	Median	0.85	0.72
	Upper limit	1.36	1.38

*Ear canal volume measurement based on admittance at lowest tail of tympanogram.
†Ear canal measurement based on admittance at lowest tail of tympanogram for children and at +200 daPa for adults.
daPa, decaPascals.
Adapted from Margolis RH, Shanks JE: Tympanometry: Basic principles of clinical application. In Rintelman WS (editor): *Hearing Assessment*, 2nd ed. Austin, TX, PRODED, 1991, pp 179–245.

TYMPANOMETRY. Tympanometry provides a graph of the middle ear's ability to transmit sound energy (admittance, or compliance) or impede sound energy (impedance) as a function of air pressure in the external ear canal. Because most immittance test instruments measure acoustic admittance, the term *admittance* is used here. The principles apply to whatever units of measurement are used.

A probe is inserted into the entrance of the external ear canal so that an airtight seal is obtained. The probe varies air pressure, presents a tone, and measures sound pressure level in the ear canal through the probe assembly. The sound pressure measured in the ear canal relative to the known intensity of the probe signal is used to estimate the acoustic admittance of the ear canal and middle-ear system. Admittance can be expressed in a unit called a millimho (mmho) or as a volume of air (mL) with equivalent acoustic admittance. The test is performed so that an estimate can be made of the volume of air enclosed between the probe tip and TM. The acoustic admittance of this volume of air is deducted from the overall admittance measure to obtain a measure of the admittance of the middle-ear system alone. Estimating ear canal volume also has a diagnostic benefit, because an abnormally large value is consistent with the presence of an opening in the TM (perforation or tube).

Once the admittance of the air mass in the external auditory canal has been eliminated, it is assumed that the remaining admittance measure accurately reflects the admittance of the entire middle-ear system. Its value is controlled largely by the dynamics of the TM. Abnormalities of the TM can dictate the shape of tympanograms, thus obscuring abnormalities medial to the TM. In addition, the frequency of the probe tone, the speed and direction of the air pressure change, and the air pressure at which the tympanogram is initiated can all influence the outcome.

When air pressure in the ear canal is equal to that in the middle ear, the middle-ear system is functioning optimally. Therefore, the ear canal pressure at which there is the greatest flow of energy (admittance) should be a reasonable estimate of the air pressure in the middle-ear space. This pressure is determined by finding the maximum or **peak admittance** on the tympanogram and obtaining its value on the x-axis. The value on the y-axis at the tympanogram peak is an estimate of peak admittance based on admittance tympanometry (Table 636-8). This peak measure sometimes is referred to as static acoustic admittance, even though it is estimated from a dynamic measure (see Fig. 639-4A).

TYMPANOMETRY IN OTITIS MEDIA WITH EFFUSION. Children with OM with effusion often have reduced peak admittance or high negative tympanometric peak pressures (see Fig. 639-4C). However, in the diagnosis of effusion, the tympanometric measure with the greatest sensitivity and specificity is the shape of the tympanogram rather than its peak pressure or admittance. This shape sometimes is referred to as the tympanometric gradient or width; it measures the degree of roundness or **peakedness** of the tympanogram. The more rounded the peak (or, in an absent peak, a flat tympanogram), the higher is the probability that an effusion is present (see Fig. 639-4B). It is important to know which instrument is used, because some compute gradient automatically but others do not.

ACOUSTIC REFLEX TEST. The acoustic reflex test (ART) also is part of the immittance test battery. With a properly functioning middle-ear system, admittance at the TM changes on activation of the stapedius and tensor tympani muscles. In healthy ears, the stapedial reflex occurs after exposure to loud sounds. Admittance instruments are designed to present reflex activating signals (pure tones of various frequencies or noise), either to the same or the contralateral ear, while monitoring admittance. Very small admittance changes that are time-locked to presentations of the signal are considered to be a result of middle-ear muscle reflexes. Admittance changes may be absent when the hearing loss is sufficient to prevent the signal from reaching the loudness level necessary to elicit the reflex or when a middle-ear condition affects the ear's ability to monitor a small admittance change. Reflexes usually are absent in patients with CHL due to the presence of an abnormal transfer system; thus, the ART is useful in the differential diagnosis of hearing impairment. The ART also is used in the assessment of SNHL and the integrity of the neurologic components of the reflex arc, including cranial nerves VII and VIII.

Auditory Brainstem Response. The ABR test is used to screen newborn hearing, confirm hearing loss in young children, obtain ear-specific information in young children, and test children who cannot, for whatever reason, cooperate with behavioral test methods. It also is important in the diagnosis of auditory dysfunction and of disorders of the auditory nervous system. The ABR test is a far-field recording of minute electrical discharges from numerous neurons. The stimulus, therefore, must be able to cause simultaneous discharge of the large numbers of neurons involved. Stimuli with very rapid onset, such as clicks or tone bursts, must be used. Unfortunately, the rapid onset required to create a measurable ABR also causes energy to be spread in the frequency domain, reducing the frequency-specificity of the response.

The ABR result is not affected by sedation or general anesthesia. Infants and children from about 4 mo–4 yr of age routinely are sedated to minimize electrical interference caused by muscle activity during testing. The ABR also can be performed in the operating room when a child is anesthetized for another procedure. Children <4 mo of age may sleep for a long enough period of time after feeding to allow an ABR to be done.

The ABR is recorded as 5–7 waves. Waves I, III, and V can be obtained consistently in all age groups; Waves II and IV appear less consistently. The latency of each wave (time of occurrence of the wave peak after stimulus onset) increases, and the amplitude decreases with reductions in stimulus intensity or loudness; latency also decreases with increasing age, with the earliest waves reaching mature latency values earlier in life than the later waves.

The ABR test has two major uses in a pediatric setting. As an audiometric test, it provides information on the ability of the peripheral auditory system to transmit information to the auditory nerve and beyond. It also is used in the differential diagnosis or monitoring of central nervous system pathology. For audiometry, the goal is to find the minimum stimulus intensity that yields an observable ABR. Plotting latency versus intensity for various waves also aids in the differential diagnosis of hearing impairment. A major advantage of auditory assessment using the ABR test is that ear-specific threshold estimates can be obtained on infants or patients who are difficult to test. ABR thresholds using click stimuli correlate best with behavioral hearing thresholds in the higher frequencies (1,000–4,000 Hz); responsivity in the low frequencies requires different stimuli (tone bursts or filtered clicks) or the use of masking, neither of which isolates the low-frequency region of the cochlea in all cases, and this may affect interpretation.

The ABR test does not assess "hearing." It reflects auditory neuronal electric responses that can be correlated to behavioral hearing thresholds, but a normal ABR result only suggests that the auditory system, up to the level of the midbrain, is responsive to the stimulus used. Conversely, a failure to elicit an ABR indicates an impairment of the system's synchronous response but does not necessarily mean that there is no "hearing." The behavioral response to sound sometimes is normal when no ABR can be elicited, such as in neurologic demyelinating disease. The ABR test may be used to infer whether and at what level of the auditory system impairment exists.

Hearing losses that are sudden, progressive, or unilateral are indications for ABR testing. Although it is believed that the different waves of the ABR reflect activity in increasingly rostral levels of the auditory system, the neural generators of the response have not been precisely determined. Each ABR wave beyond the earliest waves probably is the result of neural firing at many levels of the system, and each level of the system probably contributes to several ABR waves. High-intensity click stimuli are used for the neurologic application. The morphology of the response and wave and interwave latencies are examined in respect to age-appropriate forms. Delayed or missing waves in the ABR result often have diagnostic significance.

The ABR and other electrical responses are extremely complex and difficult to interpret. A number of factors, including instrumentation design and settings, environment, degree and configuration of hearing loss, and patient characteristics, may influence the quality of the recording. Therefore, testing and interpretation of electrophysiologic activity as it possibly relates to hearing should be carried out by trained audiologists to avoid the risk that unreliable or erroneous conclusions will affect a patient's care.

Otoacoustic Emissions. During normal hearing, OAEs originate from the hair cells in the cochlea and are detected by sensitive amplifying processes. They travel from the cochlea through the middle ear to the external auditory canal, where they can be detected using miniature microphones. Transient evoked OAEs (TEOAEs) may be used to check the integrity of the cochlea. In the neonatal period, detection of OAEs can be accomplished during natural sleep, and TEOAEs can be used as screening tests in infants and children for hearing at the 30 dB level of hearing loss. They are less time-consuming and elaborate than ABR and are more sensitive than behavioral tests in young children. TEOAEs are reduced or absent owing to various dysfunctions in the middle and inner ears. They are absent in patients with >30 dB of hearing loss and are not used to determine hearing threshold; rather, they provide a screen for whether hearing is present at >30–40 dB. Diseases such as OM or congenitally abnormal middle ear structures reduce the transfer of TEOAEs and may incorrectly indicate a cochlear hearing disorder. If a hearing loss is suspected based on the absence of OAE, the ears should be examined for evidence of pathology, and then ABR testing should be used for confirmation and identification of the type, degree, and laterality of hearing loss.

Acoustic Reflectometry. In acoustic reflectometry, a hand-held instrument is placed next to the opening of a child's ear canal and 80-dB sound is delivered that varies in frequency from 2,000–4,500 Hz in a 100-msec period. The instrument measures the total level of reflected and transmitted sound. Some physicians have found this device useful to help gauge the presence or absence of middle-ear fluid, and a commercial version is marketed to parents as a way to monitor ear fluid. The instrument does not provide any information about hearing; if the presence of chronic fluid is suggested, audiometric evaluation should be obtained.

TREATMENT. With the use of universal hearing screening in many areas of the United States, the early diagnosis and treatment of

TABLE 636-9. Recommended Pneumococcal Vaccination Schedule for Persons With Cochlear Implants

AGE AT FIRST PCV7 DOSE (MO)*	PCV7 PRIMARY SERIES	PCV7 ADDITIONAL DOSE	PPV23 DOSE
2–6	3 doses, 2 mo apart†	1 dose at 12–15 mo of age‡	Indicated at ≥24 mo of age§
7–11	2 doses, 2 mo apart†	1 dose at 12–15 mo of age‡	Indicated at ≥24 mo of age§
12–23	2 doses, 2 mo apart¶	Not indicated	Indicated at ≥24 mo of age§
24–59	2 doses, 2 mo apart¶	Not indicated	Indicated§
≥60	Not indicated‖	Not indicated‖	Indicated

*A schedule with a reduced number of total 7-valent pneumococcal conjugate vaccine (PCV7) doses is indicated if children start late or are incompletely vaccinated. Children with a lapse in vaccination should be vaccinated according to the catch-up schedule (CDC. Pneumococcal conjugate vaccine shortage resolved. *MMWR* 2003;52:446–447.)

†For children vaccinated at age <1 yr, minimum interval between doses is 4 wks.

‡The additional dose should be administered ≥8 weeks after the primary series has been completed.

§Children aged <5 years should complete the PCV7 series first; 23-valent pneumococcal polysaccharide vaccine (PPV23) should be administered to children aged ≥24 months ≥8 weeks after the last dose of PCV7 (CDC. Preventing pneumococcal disease among infants and young children: Recommendations of the Advisory Committee on Immunization Practices. *MMWR* 2000;49 (No.RR-9).

¶Minimum interval between doses is 8 weeks.

‖PCV7 is not recommended generally for children aged ≥5 yrs.

From Pneumococcal vaccination for cochlear implant candidates and recipients: Updated recommendations of the Advisory Committee on Immunization Practices. *MMWR* 2003;52:739–740.

children with hearing loss is common. Testing for hearing loss is possible even in very young children, and should be done if parents are suspicious of a problem. Any child with a known risk factor for hearing loss should be evaluated in the 1st 6 mo of life.

Once a hearing loss is identified, a full developmental and speech and language evaluation is needed. Parental counseling and involvement are required in all stages of the evaluation and treatment or rehabilitation. A conductive hearing loss often can be corrected through treatment of a middle-ear effusion (i.e., ear tube placement) or surgical correction of the abnormal sound-conducting mechanism. Children with SNHL should be evaluated for possible hearing aid use by a pediatric audiologist. Hearing aids may be fitted for children as young as 2 mo of age. Compelling evidence from the hearing screening program in Colorado shows that identification and amplification before age 6 mo makes a very significant difference in the speech and language abilities of affected children, compared with those cases identified and amplified after the age of 6 mo. In these children, repeat audiologic testing is needed to reliably identify the degree of hearing loss and to fine-tune the use of hearing aids.

Infants and young children with profound congenital or prelingual onset of deafness have benefited from **multichannel cochlear implants** (Fig. 636-3). These implants bypass injury to the organ of Corti and provide neural stimulation by way of an external microphone and a signal processor that digitizes auditory stimuli into digital radiofrequency impulses. Cochlear implantation before age 2 yr (and even 1 yr) improves hearing and speech, enabling over 90% of children to be in mainstream education. Most develop age-appropriate auditory perception and oral language skills.

A serious complication of cochlear implants is an excessively high incidence of pneumococcal meningitis. All children receiving a cochlear implant must be vaccinated with the PCV-7 vaccine (Table 636-9).

The best approach to the education of children with significant hearing loss is a subject of ongoing controversy. Because we live in a predominantly speaking world, some have advocated a pure auditory and oral approach to hearing therapy. However, because affected children often are slow to develop communication skills, many advocate a total communication approach; depending on the individual child's needs, this technique uses a mixture of sign language, lip-reading, hearing aids, and speech. The appropriate program for each child depends on the patient, family, and available resources.

Genetic Counseling. Families of children with the diagnosis of SNHL, or a syndrome associated with SNHL and/or CHL, should consider genetic counseling, which will allow for a discussion of the likelihood of similar diagnoses in future pregnancies. The geneticist also may help in the evaluation and further testing of the patient with hearing loss to establish a diagnosis.

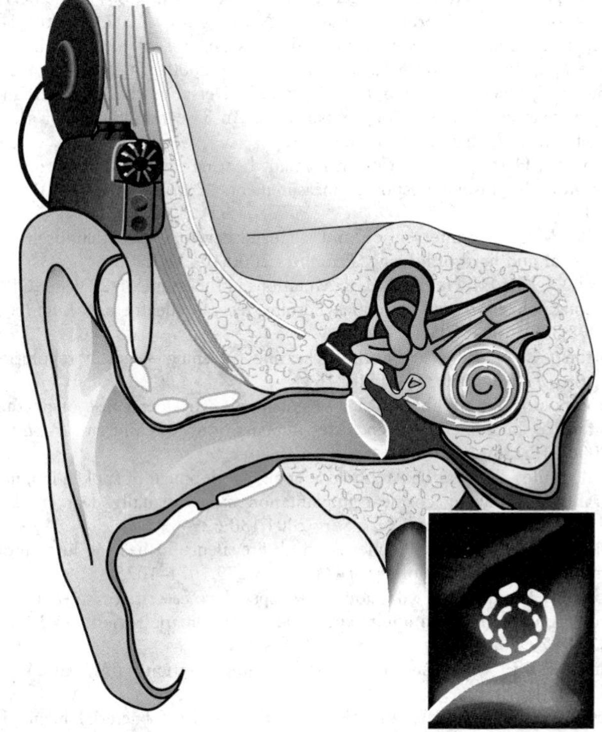

Figure 636–3. All cochlear implants share key components, including a microphone, speech processor, and transmitter coil, shown in a behind-the-ear position in this diagram. The microphone/speech processor picks up environmental sounds and digitises them into coded signals. The signals are sent to the transmitter coil and relayed through the skin to the internal device imbedded in the skull. The internal device converts the code to electronic signals, which are transmitted to the electrode array wrapping around the cochlea. The inset shows the radiographic appearance of the stimulating electrode array. Reproduced with permission from MED-EL Corporation, Innsbruck, Austria. (From Smith RJH, Bale JF Jr, White KR: Sensorineural hearing loss in children. *Lancet* 2005; 365:879–890.)

Barsky-Firkser L, Sun S: Universal newborn hearing screenings: A three-year experience. *Pediatrics* 1997;99:1.

Ben-Yousef T, Ness SL, Madeo AC, et al: A mutation of *PCDH15* among Ashkenazi Jews with the type 1 Usher syndrome. *N Engl J Med* 2003; 348:1664–1670.

Biernath KR, Reefhuis J, Whitney CG, et al: Bacterial meningitis among children with cochlear implants beyond 24 months after implantation. *Pediatrics* 2006;117:284–289.

Capaccio P, Ottaviani F, Cuccarini V, et al: Sudden hearing loss and MTHFR 677C>T/1298A>C gene polymorphisms. *Genet Med* 2005;7:206–208.

Centers for Disease Control and Prevention: Pneumococcal vaccination for cochlear implant candidates and recipients: Updated recommendations of the Advisory Committee on Immunization Practices. *MMWR* 2003; 52:739–740.

Cox LC: Otoacoustic emissions as a screening tool for sensorineural hearing loss. *J Pediatr* 1997;130:685–686.

Del Castillo I, Villamar M, Moreno-Pelayo MA, et al: A deletion involving the connexin 30 gene in nonsyndromic hearing impairments. *N Engl J Med* 2002;346: 243–249.

Eilers RE, Oller DK: Infant vocalizations and early diagnosis of severe hearing impairment. *J Pediatr* 1994;124:199–203.

Fugazzola L, Cerutti N, Mannavola D, et al: Differential diagnoses between Pendred and pseudo-Pendred syndromes: Clinical, radiologic, and molecular studies. *Pediatr Res* 2002;51:479–484.

Gates GA, Miyamoto RT: Cochlear implants. *N Engl J Med* 2003;349: 421–423.

Grote JJ: Neonatal screening for hearing impairment. *Lancet* 2000;355: 513–514.

Hinson JT, Fantin VR, Schönberger J, et al: Missense mutations in the BCS1L gene as a cause of Björnstad syndrome. *N Engl J Med* 2007;356:809–819.

Kemper AR, Downs SM: A cost-effectiveness analysis of newborn hearing screening strategies. *Arch Pediatr Adolesc Med* 2000;154:484.

Kennedy C, McCann D, Campbell MJ, et al: Universal newborn screening for permanent childhood hearing impairment: An 8 year follow up of a controlled trial. *Lancet* 2005;366:660–662.

Mason JA, Herrmann KR: Universal infant hearing screening by automated auditory brainstem response measurement. *Pediatrics* 1998;101:221–228.

Moeller MP: Early intervention and language development in children who are deaf and hard of hearing. *Pediatrics* 2000;106:E43.

Morell RJ, Kim HJ, Hood LJ, et al: Mutations in the connexin 26 gene (GJB2) among Ashkenazi Jews with nonsyndromic recessive deafness. *N Engl J Med* 1998;339:1500–1505.

Morton CC, Nance WE: Newborn hearing screening—a silent revolution. *N Engl J Med* 2006;354:2151–2164.

Nikolopoulos TP, Archbold SM, O'Donoghue GM: Does cause of deafness influence outcome after cochlear implantation in children? *Pediatrics* 2006;118:1350–1356.

Nikolopoulos TP, Dyar D, Archbold S, et al: Development of spoken language grammar following cochlear implantation in perlingually deaf children. *Arch Otolaryngol Head Neck Surg* 2004;130:629–633.

Niskar AS, Kieszak SM, Holmes A, et al: Prevalence of hearing loss among children 6 to 19 years of age. *JAMA* 1998;279:1071–1075.

Pirozzo S, Papinczak T, Glasziou P: Whispered voice test for screening for hearing impairment in adults and children: systematic review. *BMJ* 2003; 327:967–970.

Ramsden RT: Prognosis after cochlear implantation. *BMJ* 2004;328: 419–420.

Reefhuis J, Honein MA, Whitney CG, et al: Risk of bacterial meningitis in children with cochlear implants. *N Engl J Med* 2003;349:435–445.

Schultz JM, Yang Y, Caride AJ, et al: Modification of human hearing loss by plasma-membrane calcium pump PMCA2. *N Engl J Med* 2005;352: 1557–1564.

Smith RJH: Deafness: from bedside to bench and back. *Lancet* 2002;360:656–657.

Smith RJH, Bale JF Jr, White KR: Sensorineural hearing loss in children. *Lancet* 2005; 365:879–890.

Thomas MA, Der Kaloustian VM, Tewfik TL: Connexin mutation testing of children with nonsyndromic, autosomal recessive sensorineural hearing loss. *J Otolaryngol* 2004;33:189–192.

Thompson DC, McPhillips H, Davis RL, et al: Universal newborn hearing screening: Summary of evidence. *JAMA* 2001;286:2000–2010.

Waltzman SB, Roland T Jr: Cochlear implantation in children younger than 12 months. *Pediatrics* 2005;16:487–493.

Willems PJ: Genetic causes of hearing loss. *N Engl J Med* 2000;342:1101.

Wilson C, Roberts A, Stephens D: Aetiological investigation of sensorineural hearing loss in children. *Arch Dis Child* 205;90:307–309.

Wolf B, Spencer R, Gleason T: Hearing loss is a common feature of symptomatic children with profound biotinidase deficiency. *Pediatrics* 2002;140:242–246.

Yoshinaga-Itano C, Sedey AL, Coulter DK, et al: Language of early- and later-identified children with hearing loss. *Pediatrics* 1998;102:1161–1171.

Chapter 637 ■ Congenital Malformations

Joseph Haddad Jr.

The external and middle ears, derived from the 1st and 2nd branchial arches and grooves, grow throughout puberty, but the inner ear, which develops from the otocyst, reaches adult size and shape by mid-fetal development. The ossicles are derived from the 1st and 2nd arches (malleus and incus), and the stapes arises from the 2nd arch and the otic capsule. The malleus and incus achieve adult size and shape by the 15th wk of gestation, and the stapes achieves adult size and shape by the 18th wk of gestation. Although the pinna, ear canal, and tympanic membrane (TM) continue to grow after birth, congenital abnormalities of these structures develop during the 1st half of gestation. Malformed external and middle ears may be associated with serious renal anomalies, mandibulofacial dysostosis, hemifacial microsomia, and other craniofacial malformations. Facial nerve abnormalities may be associated with any of the congenital abnormalities of the ear and temporal bone. Malformations of the external and middle ears also may be associated with abnormalities of the inner ear and both conductive (CHL) and sensorineural hearing loss (SNHL).

Congenital ear problems may be minor and mainly cosmetic, or major, affecting both appearance and function. Any child born with an abnormality of the pinna, external auditory canal, or TM should have a complete audiologic evaluation in the neonatal period. Imaging studies are necessary for evaluation and treatment; in the patient with other craniofacial abnormalities a team approach with other specialists can assist in guiding therapy.

PINNA MALFORMATIONS. Severe malformations of the external ear are rare, but minor deformities are common. Isolated abnormalities of the external ear occur in approximately 1% of children. A pit-like depression just in front of the helix and above the tragus may represent a cyst or an epidermis-lined fistulous tract. These are common, with an incidence of approximately 8/1,000 children, and may be unilateral or bilateral and familial. The pits require surgical removal only if there is recurrent infection. Accessory skin tags, with an incidence of 1–2/1,000, can be removed for cosmetic reasons by simple ligation if they are attached by a narrow pedicle. If the pedicle is broad-based or contains cartilage, the defect should be corrected surgically. An unusually prominent or "lop" ear results from lack of bending of the cartilage that creates the antihelix. It may be improved cosmetically in the neonatal period by applying a firm framework (sometimes soldering wire is used) attached by Steri-Strips to the pinna and worn continuously for weeks to months. Otoplasty for cosmetic correction can be considered in children >5 yr of age, when the pinna has reached about 80% of its adult size.

The term **microtia** may indicate subtle abnormalities of the size, shape, and location of the pinna and ear canal, or major abnormalities with only small nubbins of skin and cartilage and absence of the ear canal opening; **anotia** indicates complete absence of the pinna and ear canal. Microtic ears often are more anterior and inferior in placement than normal auricles, and the location and function of the facial nerve may be abnormal. Surgery to correct microtia is considered for both cosmetic and functional reasons; children who have some pinna can wear regular glasses, a hearing aid, and earrings and feel more normal in appearance. If the microtia is severe, some patients may opt for creation and attachment of a prosthetic ear, which cosmetically closely resembles a real ear. Surgery to correct severe microtia may involve a multistage procedure including carving and transplantation of autogenous cartilage rib grafts, and local soft tissue flaps. Cosmetic reconstruction of the auricle usually is performed between 5–7 yr of age, and is performed before canal atresia repair in children deemed appropriate for this surgery.

CONGENITAL STENOSIS OR ATRESIA OF THE EXTERNAL AUDITORY CANAL. Stenosis or atresia of the ear canal often occurs in association with malformation of the auricle and middle ear; minor stenoses may occur in isolation. In some genetic syndromes, e.g., trisomy 21, ear canals are narrow. Audiometric evaluation of these children should be undertaken as early in life as possible. Most children with significant CHL secondary to bilateral atresia wear bone conduction hearing aids for the first several yr of life. Diagnosis, evaluation, and surgical planning often are aided by CT, and sometimes MRI, of the temporal bone. Mild cases of ear canal stenosis do not require surgical enlargement unless the patient develops chronic external otitis or severe cerumen impaction that affects hearing.

Reconstructive ear canal and middle-ear surgery for atresia usually is considered for children >5 yr of age who have bilateral deformities resulting in a significant CHL. The aim of reconstructive surgery is to improve hearing to a point where the child may not need a hearing aid or to provide an ear canal and pinna so that the child can derive improved benefit from an air-conduction hearing aid. CT evidence of an adequate middle-ear cleft, ossicles, and mastoid is required to perform the surgery; the position of the facial nerve, which often is in an abnormal location in these children, also must be considered. The use of bone-anchored hearing aids (BAHA) may provide an option for some of these children when they are older.

CONGENITAL MIDDLE-EAR MALFORMATIONS. Children may have congenital abnormalities of the middle ear as an isolated defect or in association with other abnormalities of the temporal bone, especially the ear canal and pinna, or as part of a syndrome. Affected children usually have CHL but may have mixed CHL and SNHL. Most malformations involve the ossicles, with the incus most commonly affected. Other less common abnormalities of the middle ear include persistent stapedial artery, high-riding jugular bulb, and abnormalities of the shape and volume of the aerated portion of the middle ear and mastoid; all present problems for a surgeon. Depending on the type of abnormality and the presence of other anomalies, surgery may be considered to improve hearing.

CONGENITAL INNER EAR MALFORMATIONS. Congenital inner ear malformations have been identified and classified as a result of improvements in imaging modalities, especially CT and MRI. As many as 20% of children with SNHL may have anatomic abnormalities identified on CT or MRI. Congenital malformations of the inner ear usually are associated with SNHL of various degrees, from mild to profound. These malformations may occur as isolated anomalies or in association with other syndromes, genetic abnormalities, or structural abnormalities of the head and neck. Enlarged vestibular aqueducts have been identified on imaging studies in association with SNHL; although no therapy exists for this condition, it may be associated with progressive SNHL in some children, and, therefore, diagnosis may have some prognostic value.

Congenital perilymphatic fistula (PLF) of the oval or round window membrane may present as a rapid-onset, fluctuating, or progressive SNHL with or without vertigo and often is associated with congenital inner ear abnormalities. Middle ear exploration may be required to confirm this diagnosis, because no reliable nonoperative diagnostic test exists. It may be necessary to repair a PLF to prevent possible spread of infection from the middle ear to the labyrinth, to stabilize hearing loss, and to improve vertigo when present.

CONGENITAL CHOLESTEATOMA. A congenital cholesteatoma usually appears as a white, round, cystlike structure medial to an intact TM. Cysts are seen most commonly in the anterior-superior portion of the middle ear, although they can present in other locations and within the TM or in the skin of the ear canal. Affected children often have no prior history of otitis media (OM). One theory for the pathogenesis is that the cyst derives from a congenital rest of epithelial tissue that persists beyond 33 wk of gestation, when it ordinarily would disappear. Other theories include squamous metaplasia of the middle ear, entrance of squamous epithelium through a nonintact eardrum into the middle ear, ectodermal implants between the 1st and 2nd branchial arch remnants, and residual amniotic fluid squamous debris. Congenital or acquired cholesteatoma should be suspected when deep retraction pockets, keratin debris, chronic drainage, aural granulation tissue, or a mass behind or involving the TM is present. Besides acting as a benign tumor causing local bone destruction, the keratinaceous debris of a cholesteatoma is a good culture medium and may become a focus of infection for chronic OM. Complications include ossicular erosion with hearing loss, bone erosion into the inner ear with dizziness, or exposure of the dura, with consequent meningitis or a brain abscess. Cholesteatoma should be removed surgically after CT scan and hearing evaluation, and appropriate antibiotic therapy. Congenital cholesteatoma is an aggressive disease, and early surgical removal and close monitoring will help prevent permanent damage to the middle and inner ear.

Chapter 638 ■ External Otitis (Otitis Externa)

Joseph Haddad Jr.

In an infant, the outer $^2/_3$ of the ear canal is cartilaginous and the inner $^1/_3$ is bony, whereas in an older child and adult only the outer $^1/_3$ is cartilaginous. The epithelium is thinner in the bony portion than in the cartilaginous portion, there is no subcutaneous tissue, and epithelium is tightly applied to the underlying periosteum; hair follicles, sebaceous glands, and apocrine glands are scarce or absent. The skin in the cartilaginous area has well-developed dermis and subcutaneous tissue and contains hair follicles, sebaceous glands, and apocrine glands. The highly viscid secretions of the sebaceous glands and the watery, pigmented secretions of the apocrine glands in the outer portion of the canal combine with exfoliated surface cells of the skin to form **cerumen,** a protective, waxy, water-repellent coating.

The normal flora of the external canal consists mainly of aerobic bacteria and includes coagulase-negative staphylococci, *Corynebacterium* (diphtheroids), *Micrococcus* and, occasionally, *Staphylococcus aureus,* viridans streptococci, and *Pseudomonas aeruginosa.* Excessive wetness (swimming, bathing, increased environmental humidity), dryness (dry canal skin and lack of cerumen), the presence of other skin pathology (previous infection, eczema or other forms of dermatitis), and trauma (digital or foreign body, cotton tip applicators ["Q-tips"]) make the skin of the canal vulnerable to infection by the normal flora or exogenous bacteria.

ETIOLOGY. External otitis (**swimmer's ear,** although it can occur without swimming) is caused most commonly by *P. aeruginosa,* but *S. aureus, Enterobacter aerogenes, Proteus mirabilis, Klebsiella pneumoniae,* streptococci, coagulase-negative staphylococci, diphtheroids, and fungi such as *Candida* and *Aspergillus* also may be isolated. External otitis results from chronic irritation and maceration from excessive moisture in the canal. The loss of protective cerumen may play a role, but cerumen impaction with trapping of water also can cause infection. Inflammation of the ear canal due to herpesvirus, varicella-zoster, other skin exanthems, and eczema also may predispose to external otitis.

CLINICAL MANIFESTATIONS. The predominant symptom is acute ear pain, often severe, accentuated by manipulation of the pinna or by pressure on the tragus. The severity of the pain and tenderness may be disproportionate to the degree of inflammation, because the skin of the external ear canal is tightly adherent to the underlying perichondrium and periosteum. Itching often is a precursor of pain and usually is characteristic of chronic inflammation of the canal or resolving acute otitis externa. Conductive hearing loss may result from edema of the skin and tympanic membrane (TM), serous or purulent secretions, or the canal skin thickening associated with chronic external otitis.

Edema of the ear canal, erythema, and thick, clumpy otorrhea are prominent signs of the acute disease. The cerumen usually is white and soft in consistency, as opposed to its usual yellow color and firmer consistency. The canal often is so tender and swollen that the entire ear canal and TM cannot be adequately visualized, and complete otoscopic examination may be delayed until the acute swelling subsides. If the TM can be visualized, it may appear either normal or opaque. TM mobility may be normal or, if thickened, reduced in response to positive and negative pressure.

Other physical findings may include palpable and tender lymph nodes in the periauricular region, and erythema and swelling of the pinna and periauricular skin. Rarely, facial paralysis, other cranial nerve abnormalities, vertigo, and/or sensorineural hearing loss are present. If these occur, **necrotizing (malignant) otitis externa** is probable. This invasive infection of the temporal bone and skull base requires immediate culture, intravenous antibiotics, and imaging studies to evaluate the extent of the disease. Surgical intervention to obtain cultures or debride devitalized tissue may be necessary. *P. aeruginosa* is the most common causative organism of necrotizing otitis externa. Fortunately, this disease is rare in children and is seen only in association with immunocompromise or severe malnourishment. In adults it is associated with diabetes mellitus.

DIAGNOSIS. Diffuse external otitis may be confused with furunculosis, **otitis media (OM)**, and mastoiditis. **Furuncles** occur in the lateral hair-bearing part of the ear canal; furunculosis usually causes a localized swelling of the canal limited to 1 quadrant, whereas external otitis is associated with concentric swelling and involves the entire ear canal. In OM, the TM may be perforated, severely retracted, or bulging and immobile; hearing usually is impaired. If the middle ear is draining through a perforated TM or tympanostomy tube, secondary external otitis may occur; if the TM is not visible owing to drainage or ear canal swelling, it may be difficult to distinguish acute OM with drainage from an acute external otitis. Pain on manipulation of the auricle and significant lymphadenitis are not common features of OM, and these findings assist in the differential diagnosis. In some patients with external otitis, the periauricular edema is so extensive that the auricle is pushed forward, creating a condition that may be confused with acute mastoiditis and a subperiosteal abscess; in **mastoiditis,** the postauricular fold is obliterated, whereas in external otitis the fold is usually better preserved. In acute mastoiditis, a history of OM and hearing loss is usual; tenderness is noted over the mastoid and not on movement of the auricle; and otoscopic examination may show sagging of the posterior canal wall.

TREATMENT. Topical otic preparations containing neomycin (active against gram-positive organisms and some gram-negative organisms, notably *Proteus* spp.) with either colistin or polymyxin (active against gram-negative bacilli, notably *Pseudomonas* spp.) and corticosteroids are highly effective in treating most forms of acute external otitis. Newer preparations of eardrops (e.g., ofloxacin, ciprofloxacin) are available that do not contain potentially ototoxic antibiotics. If canal edema is marked, the patient may need referral to a specialist for cleaning and possible wick placement. Some recommend otic corticosteroids in addition to otic antibodies. A wick can be inserted into the ear canal and topical antibiotics applied to the wick 3 times a day for 24–48 hr. The wick can be removed after 2–3 days, at which time the edema of the ear canal usually is markedly improved, and the ear canal and TM are better seen. Topical antibiotic are then continued by direct instillation. When the pain is severe, oral analgesics (e.g., ibuprofen, codeine) may be necessary for a few days. Careful evaluation for underlying conditions should be undertaken in patients with severe or recurrent otitis externa. An approach to management is noted in Figure 638-1.

As the inflammatory process subsides, cleaning the canal with a suction or cotton-tipped applicator to remove the debris enhances the effectiveness of the topical medications. In subacute and chronic infections, periodic cleansing of the canal is essential. In severe, acute external otitis associated with fever and lymphadenitis, oral or parenteral antibiotics may be indicated; an ear canal culture should be done, and empiric antibiotic treatment can then be modified if necessary, based on susceptibility of the organism cultured. A fungal infection of the external auditory canal, or **otomycosis,** is characterized by fluffy white debris, sometimes with black spores seen; treatment includes cleaning and application of antifungal solutions such as clotrimazole or nystatin; other antifungal agents include m-cresyl acetate 25%, gentian violet 2%, and thimerosal 1 : 1,000.

PREVENTION. Preventing external otitis may be necessary for individuals susceptible to recurrences, especially children who swim. The most effective prophylaxis is instillation of dilute alcohol or acetic acid (2%) immediately after swimming or bathing. During an acute episode of otitis externa, patients should not swim and the ears should be protected from excessive water during bathing.

OTHER DISEASES OF THE EXTERNAL EAR

FURUNCULOSIS. Furunculosis is caused by *S. aureus* and affects only the hair-containing outer third of the ear canal. Mild forms are treated with oral antibiotics active against *S. aureus.* If an abscess develops, incision and drainage may be necessary.

ACUTE CELLULITIS. Acute cellulitis of the auricle and external auditory canal usually is caused by group A streptococcus and occasionally by *S. aureus.* The skin is red, hot, and indurated, without a sharply defined border. Fever may be present with little or no exudate in the canal. Parenteral administration of penicillin G or a penicillinase-resistant penicillin is the therapy of choice.

PERICHONDRITIS AND CHONDRITIS. Perichondritis is an infection involving the skin and perichondrium of the auricular cartilage; extension of infection to the cartilage is termed *chondritis.* The ear canal, especially the lateral aspect, also may be involved. Early perichondritis may be difficult to differentiate from cellulitis because both are characterized by skin that is red, edematous, and tender. The main cause of perichondritis/chondritis and cellulitis is trauma (accidental or iatrogenic, laceration or contusion), including ear piercing, especially when done through the cartilage. The most commonly isolated organism in perichondritis and chondritis is *P. aeruginosa,* although other gram-negative and, occasionally, gram-positive organisms may be found. Treat-

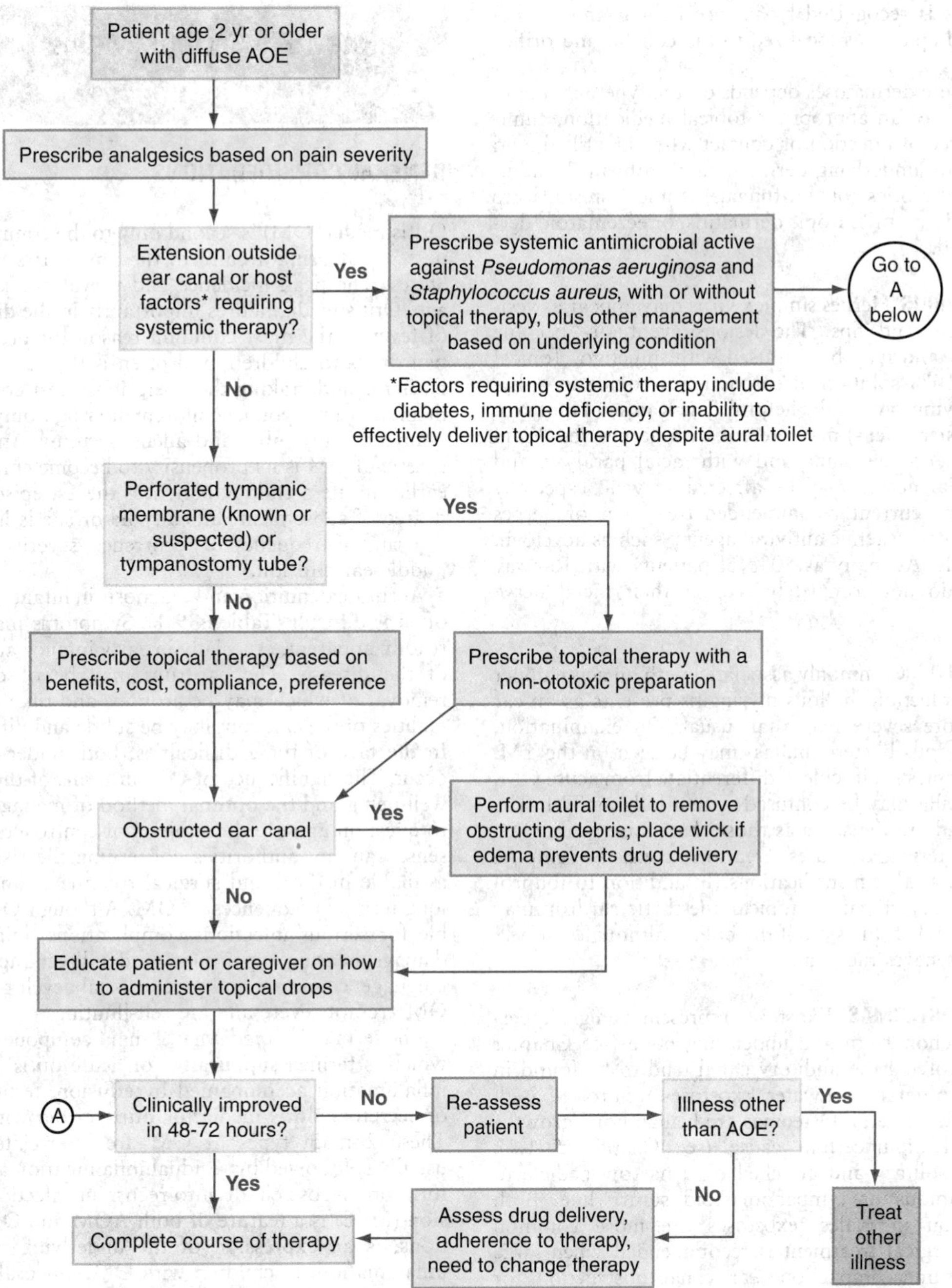

Figure 638-1. Flowchart for managing acute otitis externa. (From Rosenfeld RM, Brown L, Cannon CR, et al: Clinical practice guideline: acute otitis externa. *Otolaryngol Head Neck Surg* 2006;134:S4–S23. © 2006 American Academy of Otolaryngology-Head and Neck Surgery Foundation, Inc.)

ment involves systemic, often parenteral, antibiotics; surgery to drain an abscess or remove nonviable skin or cartilage may also be needed. Removal of all ear jewelry is mandatory in the presence of infection.

DERMATOSES. Various dermatoses (seborrheic, contact, infectious eczematoid, or neurodermatoid) are common causes of inflammation of the external canal; scratching and the introduction of infecting organisms cause acute external otitis in these conditions.

Seborrheic dermatitis is characterized by greasy scales that flake and crumble as they are detached from the epidermis; associated changes in the scalp, forehead, cheeks, brow, postauricular areas, and concha are usual.

Contact dermatitis of the auricle or canal may be caused by earrings, or by topical otic medications such as neomycin, which may produce erythema, vesiculation, edema, and weeping. Poison ivy, oak, and sumac also may produce contact dermatitis. Hair care products have been implicated in sensitive individuals.

Infectious eczematoid dermatitis is caused by a purulent infection of the external canal, middle ear, or mastoid; the purulent drainage infects the skin of the canal, auricle, or both. The lesion is weeping, erythematous, or crusted.

Atopic dermatitis occurs in children with a familial or personal history of allergy; the auricle, particularly the postauricular fold, becomes thickened, scaly, and excoriated.

Neurodermatitis is recognized by intense itching and erythematous, thickened epidermis localized to the concha and orifice of the meatus.

Treatment of these dermatoses depends on the type but should include application of an appropriate topical medication, elimination of the source of infection or contact when identified, and management of any underlying dermatologic problem. In addition to topical antibiotics (or antifungals), topical steroids are helpful if contact dermatitis, atopic dermatitis, or eczematoid dermatitis is suspected.

HERPES SIMPLEX VIRUS. Herpes simplex virus may appear as vesicles on the auricle and lips. The lesions eventually become encrusted and dry and may be confused with impetigo. Topical application of a 10% solution of carbamide peroxide in anhydrous glycerol is symptomatically helpful. The **Ramsay Hunt syndrome (herpes zoster oticus)** may present with herpes vesicles in the ear canal and on the pinna and with facial paralysis and pain. Other cranial nerves may be affected as well, especially the 8th nerve. The current recommended treatment of herpes zoster oticus includes systemic antiviral agents, such as acyclovir, and corticosteroids. As many as 50% of patients with Ramsay Hunt syndrome do not completely recover their facial nerve function.

BULLOUS MYRINGITIS. Commonly associated with an acute upper respiratory tract infection, bullous myringitis presents as an ear infection with more severe pain than usual. On examination, hemorrhagic or serous blisters (bullas) may be seen on the TM. The disease sometimes is difficult to differentiate from acute OM, because a large bulla may be confused with a bulging TM. The organisms involved are the same as those that cause acute OM, including both bacteria and viruses. Treatment consists of empiric antibiotic therapy and pain medications. In addition to ibuprofen or codeine for severe pain, a topical anesthetic eardrop may also provide some relief. Incision of the bullae, although not necessary, promptly relieves the pain.

EXOSTOSES AND OSTEOMAS. Exostoses represent benign hyperplasia of the perichondrium and underlying bone (see Chapter 501.2). Those involving the auditory canal tend to be found in people who swim often in cold water. Exostoses are broad-based, often multiple, and bilateral. Osteomas are benign bony growths in the ear canal of uncertain cause (see Chapter 501.2). They usually are solitary and attached by a narrow pedicle to the tympanosquamous or tympanomastoid suture line. Both are more common in males; exostoses are more common than osteomas. Surgical treatment is recommended when large masses cause cerumen impaction, ear canal obstruction, or hearing loss.

Haddad J Jr: Care of the draining ear in children. *Emerg Peds* 1995;8:75.

Nussinovitch M, Rimon A, Volovitz B, et al: Cotton-tip applicators as a leading cause of otitis externa. *Int J Pediatr Otolaryngol* 2004;68:433–435.

Roland PS, Eaton DA, Gross RD, et al: Randomized, placebo-controlled evaluation of Cerumenex and Murine earwax removal products. *Arch Otolaryngol Head Neck Surg* 2004;130:1175–1177.

Roland PS, Stroman DW: Microbiology of acute otitis externa. *Laryngoscope* 2002;112:1166–1177.

Rosenfeld RM, Brown L, Cannon CR, et al: Clinical practice guideline: acute otitis externa. *Otolaryngol Head Neck Surg* 2006;134:S4–S23.

Van Balen FAM, Smit WM, Zuithoff PA, et al: Clinical efficacy of three common treatments in acute otitis externa in primary care: randomized controlled trial. *BMJ* 2003;327:1201–1203.

Chapter 639 ■ Otitis Media*

Joseph E. Kerschner

GENERAL CONSIDERATIONS

Otitis media (OM) is second only to the common cold among illnesses that bring a child to the physician's office in the United States. The peak incidence and prevalence is from 6–20 mo of age. Otitis media figures importantly in the differential diagnosis of fever, is the most common reason for prescribing antimicrobial drugs to children, and often is the sole or at least primary basis for undertaking the operations most commonly performed in infants and young children: myringotomy with insertion of tympanostomy tubes and adenoidectomy. An important characteristic of OM is its propensity to become chronic and recur. The earlier in life a child experiences the 1st episode, the greater the degree of subsequent difficulty he or she is likely to experience, in terms of frequency of recurrence, severity, and persistence of middle-ear effusion.

Accurate definition and diagnosis in infants and young children often is difficult (Table 639-1). Symptoms may be absent or not readily apparent, especially in early infancy and in chronic stages of the disease. The eardrum may be obscured by cerumen, removal of which may be arduous and time-consuming. Abnormalities of the eardrum may be subtle and difficult to appreciate. In the face of these difficulties, both under- and overdiagnosis occur. The significance of OM in terms of the child's health and well-being and the optimal method of management remain open to question and are the subjects of controversy. There is no consensus among authorities concerning the risk : benefit ratios of available medical and surgical treatments and the likelihood of long-term consequences of OM. Although OM can be responsible for serious infectious complications, middle- and inner-ear damage, hearing impairment, and indirect impairments of speech, language, cognitive, and psychosocial development, most cases of OM are not severe and are self-limiting.

The term *otitis media* has 2 main components: acute infection, which is termed **suppurative or acute otitis media (AOM)**; and inflammation accompanied by effusion, termed **nonsuppurative or secretory otitis media, or otitis media with effusion (OME).** These 2 main types of OM are interrelated: acute infection usually is followed by residual inflammation and effusion that, in turn, predispose children to recurrent infection. **Middle-ear effusion** (MEE) is a feature of both AOM and OME; in both conditions, is an expression of the underlying middle-ear mucosal inflammation. In children with OM, mucosal inflammation also is present in the mastoid air cells, which are in continuity with the middle-ear cavity. MEE results in the conductive hearing loss associated with OM. The hearing loss is variable, ranging from none to as much as 50 decibels hearing level (dB HL). Losses of 21–30 dB HL are usual. Although most individual episodes of OM subside within several wk, MEE persists for >3 mo in approximately 10–25% of cases.

EPIDEMIOLOGY. Factors believed to affect the occurrence of OM include age, gender, race, genetic background, socioeconomic status, type of milk or formula used in infant feeding, degree of exposure to tobacco smoke, degree of exposure to other children, presence or absence of respiratory allergy, season of the yr, and pneumococcal vaccination status. Children with certain types of congenital craniofacial anomalies are particularly prone to OM.

*Adapted from the chapter in the 17th edition by Jack L. Paradise, MD.

TABLE 639-1. Definition of Acute Otitis Media

A diagnosis of AOM requires (1) a history of acute onset of signs and symptoms, (2) the presence of MEE, and (3) signs and symptoms of middle-ear inflammation.

The definition of AOM includes:
- Recent, usually abrupt, onset of signs and symptoms of middle-ear inflammation and MEE
- The presence of MEE, indicated by any of the following:
  - Bulging of the TM
  - Limited or absent mobility of the TM
  - Air-fluid level behind the TM
  - Otorrhea
- Signs or symptoms of middle-ear inflammation, indicated by either
  - Distinct erythema of the TM, *or*
  - Distinct otalgia (discomfort clearly referable to the ear[s] that results in interference with or precludes normal activity or sleep)

AOM, acute otitis media; MEE, middle–ear effusion; TM, tympanic membrane.
From Subcommittee on Management of Acute Otitis Media: Diagnosis and management of acute otitis media. *Pediatrics* 2004;113:1451–1465.

Age. The odds of developing at least 1 episode of OM has been reported to be 63–85% by 12 mo of age and 66–99% by 24 mo of age. The percentage of days with MEE has been reported to be 5–27% during the 1st year of life and 6–18% during the 2nd year of life. Rates were highest during the ages 6–20 mo. After 2 yr of age, the incidence and prevalence of OM decline progressively, although the disease remains relatively common into the early school-age years. The most likely reasons for the higher rates in infants and younger children include less well-developed immunologic defenses and less favorable eustachian tubal factors involving both the structure and function of the tube. The age of onset of OM is an important predictor of the development of recurrent and chronic OM, with earlier age of onset having an increased risk for exhibiting these difficulties later in life.

Gender. The incidence of OM is greater in boys than in girls. In a large child development/OM study in Pittsburgh that involved close monitoring in a sociodemographically diverse population, infant boys consistently had higher mean cumulative proportions of days with MEE than infant girls. Boys have predominated in most reported studies of the treatment of OM, and, compared with girls, consistently had higher rates of operations aimed at relieving the effects or reducing the occurrence of OM, i.e., tympanostomy tube insertion, tympanoplasty, and adenoidectomy, facts that support a greater predilection for the disease in boys, and also suggest greater severity in boys.

Race. Otitis media is especially prevalent and severe among Native American, Inuit, and Indigenous Australian children. Studies comparing the occurrence of OM in white children and black children have given conflicting results, but most of the studies have reported higher rates in white children.

Genetic Background. Middle-ear disease is commonly observed to tend to **"run in families,"** and a number of studies have suggested that OM has a heritable component. There is a higher degree of concordance for OM among monozygotic than among dizygotic twins.

Socioeconomic Status. Poverty has long been considered an important contributing factor to both the development and the severity of OM. Various component elements contributing to this relationship can be surmised to include crowding, limited hygienic facilities, suboptimal nutritional status, limited access to medical care, and limited resources for complying with prescribed medical regimens.

Breast Milk Compared to Formula Feeding. Most studies examining the question of breast-milk feeding versus formula feeding have found that breast-milk feeding provides a protective effect against OM. The effect is probably limited but may be greater in socioeconomically disadvantaged children. The protective effect has been shown to be attributable to the milk itself rather than to the mechanics of breastfeeding in a study of infants with cleft palate to whom all feeding (breast milk or formula) was delivered via an artificial, compressible nurser.

Exposure to Tobacco Smoke. A positive correlation between the occurrence of OM and household exposure to tobacco smoke has been found in some studies but not others. Because household smoking correlates inversely with socioeconomic status, possible confounding by socioeconomic factors further complicates valid assessment of risk. Studies that have used objective measures to determine infant exposure to second-hand tobacco smoke, such as cotinine levels, have more consistently identified a significant link between tobacco smoke and OM. This evidence suggests that exposure to tobacco smoke should be considered an important risk factor in the development of OM.

Exposure to Other Children. Many studies have shown a strong, positive relationship between the occurrence of OM and the extent of repeated exposure to other children, whether at home or in out-of-home group daycare. Family socioeconomic status and the extent of exposure to other children constitute the 2 most important identifiable risk factors for developing OM.

Season. In temperate climates, the highest rates of occurrence of OM are observed during cold weather months and the lowest rates during warm weather months, in keeping with the pattern of occurrence of upper respiratory tract infections. In OM, it is likely that these findings depend strongly on the significant association between OM and viral respiratory illnesses.

Congenital Anomalies. Otitis media is universal among infants with unrepaired palatal clefts, and also is highly prevalent among children with submucous cleft palate, other craniofacial anomalies, and Down syndrome. The common feature in these congenital anomalies is a deficiency in the functioning of the eustachian tube, which predisposes children with these conditions to middle ear disease.

Pneumococcal Vaccination. *Streptococcus pneumoniae,* or pneumococcus, is the pathogen most commonly identified in patients with acute OM. Vaccination of infants with a conjugate pneumococcal vaccine is standard practice in the USA. Overall, the reduction in incidence of OM with vaccination appears to be modest, lowering visits to physicians and antibiotic prescriptions for OM by only 6–8%. Vaccination does appear to have a more protective effect, however, in limiting frequent OM episodes and the need for surgical intervention with tympanostomy tubes.

ETIOLOGY

Acute Otitis Media. Pathogenic bacteria can be isolated by standard culture techniques from middle-ear fluid in approximately 65–75% of cases of well-documented AOM; in the remaining cases, bacterial culture shows either no growth or the presence of organisms generally considered nonpathogenic. Three pathogens predominate: *S. pneumoniae* is found in approximately 40% of cases; nontypable *Haemophilus influenzae* in approximately 25–30%; and *Moraxella catarrhalis* in approximately 10–15%. Other pathogens that, together, account for approximately 5% of cases include group A streptococcus, *Staphylococcus aureus,* and gram-negative organisms. *S. aureus* and gram-negative organisms are found most commonly in neonates and very young infants who are hospitalized. In outpatient settings, the distribution of pathogens in these young infants is similar to that in older infants.

Evidence of **respiratory viruses** also may be found in middle-ear exudates of children with AOM, either alone or, more commonly, in association with pathogenic bacteria. Of these viruses, rhinovirus and respiratory syncytial virus (RSV) are found most often. AOM is a known complication of bronchiolitis; middle-ear aspirates in children with bronchiolitis regularly contain bacterial pathogens, suggesting that RSV is rarely, if ever, the sole cause of their AOM. Using more precise measures of viable bacteria than standard culture techniques, e.g., polymerase chain reaction assays, a much higher rate of bacterial pathogens can be demonstrated. It remains uncertain whether viruses alone can cause AOM under any circumstances, or whether their role is limited to setting the stage for bacterial invasion, and perhaps also to amplifying the inflammatory process, which interferes with resolution of the bacterial infection. Viral pathogens have a negative impact on eustachian tube function, and can impair local immune function, increase bacterial adherence, and change pharmacokinetics, all of which reduce the efficacy of antimicrobial medications.

Otitis Media with Effusion. The pathogens typically found in AOM can be recovered in approximately 30% of children with OME using standard culture techniques. Using polymerase chain reaction assays, middle-ear fluids have been found to contain evidence of viable bacterial DNA and/or viral RNA in much larger proportions in children with OME. These data suggest that patients with OME do not have sterile effusions, as previously thought. These findings suggest the possibility that these pathogens contribute to eliciting ongoing inflammatory processes within the middle ear and also may play a role in recurring infections through a biofilm formation.

PATHOGENESIS. Acute otitis media usually is caused by bacterial pathogens. Central to an understanding of the pathogenesis of OM is a consideration of several other factors, including the eustachian tube, the child's immune system and risk factor profile, and host-pathogen interactions.

Under usual circumstances, the eustachian tube is passively closed and is opened by contraction of the tensor veli palatini muscle. In relation to the middle ear, the eustachian tube has 3 main functions: ventilation, protection, and clearance. The most important is ventilation. The middle-ear mucosa depends on a continuing supply of air from the nasopharynx delivered via the eustachian tube. Interruption of this ventilatory process by tubal obstruction initiates a complex inflammatory response that includes secretory metaplasia, compromise of the mucociliary transport system, and effusion of liquid into the tympanic cavity. Impaired middle-ear ventilation is an important contributing factor to both OME and AOM. Whether middle-ear infection can develop in the absence of pre-existing eustachian tube obstruction is uncertain; if so, the infection undoubtedly would lead quickly to tubal obstruction as a consequence of both inflammatory edema and the accumulation of middle-ear secretions.

Eustachian tube obstruction may result extraluminally, from hypertrophied nasopharyngeal adenoid tissue, or tumor; or intraluminally, from inflammatory edema of the tubal mucosa, most commonly as a consequence of a viral upper respiratory tract infection; or from impairment of the opening mechanism of the tube, attributable to abnormal tubal muscular function or excessive tubal wall compliance, or both. Progressive reduction in tubal wall compliance with increasing age may help explain the decline in the occurrence of OM as children grow older. The protection and clearance functions of the eustachian tube also may be involved in the pathogenesis of OM. Thus, if the tubes are patulous or excessively compliant, they may fail to protect the middle ear from reflux of infective nasopharyngeal secretions, whereas impairment of the mucociliary clearance function of the tube might contribute to both the establishment and the persistence of infection. The shorter and more horizontal orientation of the tube in infants and young children may increase the likelihood of reflux from the nasopharynx and impair passive gravitational drainage through the eustachian tube. Another possible explanation for improved eustachian tube function and decreased OM incidence as infants mature is that the luminal diameter increases, reducing the opportunity for tubal obstruction and dysfunction.

In children with cleft palate, where OM is a nearly universal finding, the main factor underlying the chronic middle-ear inflammation is impairment of the opening mechanism of the eustachian tube, due perhaps to greater-than-normal compliance of the tubal wall. Another possible factor is defective velopharyngeal valving, which may result in disturbed aerodynamic and hydrodynamic relationships in the nasopharynx and proximal portions of the eustachian tubes. In children with other craniofacial anomalies or with Down syndrome, the high prevalence of OM is attributed to structural and/or functional eustachian tubal abnormalities; histologic evaluation of the eustachian tube in these patient populations demonstrates such abnormalities.

Although OM may develop and certainly may persist in the absence of apparent respiratory tract infection, many, if not most, episodes are initiated by a viral or bacterial upper respiratory tract infection. In a study of children in group daycare, AOM was observed in approximately 30–40% of children with respiratory illness caused by RSV, influenza viruses, or adenoviruses, and in approximately 10–15% of children with respiratory illness caused by parainfluenza viruses, rhinoviruses, or enteroviruses. Viral infection of the upper respiratory tract results in release of cytokines and inflammatory mediators, some of which may cause eustachian tube dysfunction. Respiratory viruses also may enhance nasopharyngeal bacterial colonization and adherence and impair host immune defenses against bacterial infection.

IgA deficiency is found in some children with recurrent AOM, but its significance is questionable, because IgA deficiency is not uncommon in children without recurrent AOM. Selective IgG subclass deficiencies (despite normal total serum IgG) may be found in children with recurrent AOM in association with recurrent sinopulmonary infection; these deficiencies probably underlie the susceptibility to infection. Children with recurrent OM that is not associated with recurrent infection at other sites rarely have a readily identifiable immunologic deficiency. Nonetheless, evidence that subtle immune deficits play a role in the pathogenesis of recurrent AOM is provided by studies involving antibody responses to various types of infection and immunization; by the observation that breast-milk feeding, as opposed to formula feeding, confers limited protection against the occurrence of OM in infants with cleft palate; and by studies in which young children with recurrent AOM achieved a measure of protection from intramuscularly administered bacterial polysaccharide immune globulin or intravenously administered polyclonal immunoglobulin. This evidence, along with the documented decrease in incidence of upper respiratory tract infections and OM as children's immune systems mature is indicative of the importance of a child's innate immune system in the pathogenesis of OM.

Evidence that respiratory allergy is a primary etiologic agent in OM is not convincing; however, in children who have both allergies and OM, it seems possible that the otitis may be aggravated by the allergy.

Risk profile and host-pathogen interactions increasingly have been recognized as playing important roles in the pathogenesis of OM. Such events as alterations in mucociliary clearance through repeated viral exposure experienced in daycare settings or through exposure to tobacco smoke may tip the balance of pathogenesis in less virulent OM pathogens in their favor. Ample evidence exists that children with frequent exposure to other children have an increased risk of both nasopharyngeal colonization and acute OM pathology with bacterial types with multiple antimicrobial resistances, making treatment more difficult and prolonged pathology more likely.

CLINICAL MANIFESTATIONS. Signs and symptoms of AOM are highly variable, especially in infants and young children. There may be evidence of ear pain, often manifested by irritability, a change in sleeping or eating habits, and, occasionally, holding or tugging at the ear (see Table 639-1). Pulling at the ear, however, has a low sensitivity and specificity. Fever also may be present and, rarely, rupture of the tympanic membrane with purulent otorrhea. Systemic symptoms and symptoms associated with upper respiratory tract infections also occur, and occasionally there may be no symptoms, with AOM discovered at a routine health examination. OME often is not accompanied by overt complaints of the child but usually is accompanied by hearing loss. This hearing loss may manifest as changes in speech patterns but often goes undetected if it is unilateral or mild, especially in younger children. Balance difficulties or dysequilibrium also can be associated with OME, and older children may complain of mild discomfort or a sense of fullness in the ear (see Chapter 635).

EXAMINATION OF THE EARDRUM

OTOSCOPY. For clinicians other than otolaryngologists, who may use an operating microscope, the eardrum ordinarily is viewed by means of an otoscope. Two types of otoscope heads are available: **surgical** or **operating,** and **diagnostic** or **pneumatic.** The surgical head embodies a lens that can swivel over a wide arc and an unenclosed light source, providing ready access of the examiner's instruments to the external auditory canal and tympanic membrane. Use of the surgical head is optimal for removing cerumen or debris from the canal under direct observation, and is necessary for satisfactorily performing tympanocentesis or myringotomy. The diagnostic head incorporates a larger lens, an enclosed light source, and a nipple for the attachment of a rubber bulb and tubing. When an attached speculum is fitted snugly into the external auditory canal, an airtight chamber is created, consisting of the vault of the otoscope head, the bulb and tubing, the speculum, and the proximal portion of the external canal. Although examination of the ear in young children is a relatively invasive procedure that often is met with lack of cooperation by the patient, this task can be enhanced if done with as little pain as possible. The outer portion of the ear canal contains hair-bearing skin and subcutaneous fat and cartilage that allow a speculum to be placed with relatively little discomfort. Closer to the tympanic membrane the ear canal is made of bone and is lined only with skin and no adnexal structures or subcutaneous fat; a speculum pushed too far forward and placed in this area often causes skin abrasion and pain. Using a rubber-tipped speculum or adding a small sleeve of rubber tubing to the tip of the plastic speculum may serve to minimize patient discomfort and enhance the ability to achieve a proper fit and an airtight seal.

Learning to perform pneumatic otoscopy is a critical skill in being able to assess a child's ear and in making an accurate diagnosis of OM (see Fig. 635-1). By observing as the bulb is alternately squeezed gently and released, the degree of tympanic membrane mobility in response to both positive and negative pressure can be estimated, providing a critical assessment of middle-ear fluid, which is a hallmark sign of both AOM and OME. With both types of otoscope heads, bright illumination also is critical to adequate visualization of the tympanic membrane.

CLEARING THE EXTERNAL AUDITORY CANAL. If the tympanic membrane is obscured by cerumen, the cerumen may be removed under direct observation through the surgical head of the otoscope, using a Buck curette (N-400-0, Storz Instrument Co). Remaining bits can then be wiped away using a Farrell applicator (N-2001A, Storz Instrument Co), with its tip (triangular in cross section) wrapped with a bit of dry or alcohol-moistened cotton to create a dry or wet "mop." Alternatively, gentle suction may be applied, using a No. 5 or 7 French ear suction tube. During this procedure it may be most advantageous to restrain the infant or young child in the prone position, turning the child's head to the left or right as each ear is cleared. One adult, usually a parent, can place one hand on each of the child's buttocks and brace the child's hips against the examining table, using his or her own weight for additional bracing if necessary. Another adult can restrain the child's head with one hand and the child's free arm with the other, changing hands for the opposite ear. In children old enough to cooperate, usually beginning at about 5 yr of age, clearing of the external canal may be achieved more easily and safely and less traumatically by lavage than by mechanical removal, provided one can be certain that the tympanic membrane is not perforated. Most children's ears are "self cleaning" due to squamous migration of ear canal skin, and parental cleaning of cerumen with cotton swabs often complicates cerumen impaction by pushing cerumen deeper into the canal while compacting it.

TYMPANIC MEMBRANE FINDINGS. Important characteristics of the tympanic membrane include contour, color, translucence, structural changes, if any, and mobility. Normally the contour of the membrane is **slightly concave;** abnormalities consist of fullness or bulging, or conversely, extreme retraction. The normal color of the tympanic membrane is **pearly gray.** Erythema may be a sign of inflammation or infection, but unless it is intense, erythema alone may result from crying or vascular flushing. Abnormal whiteness of the membrane may result from either scarring or the presence of liquid in the middle-ear cavity; liquid also may impart an amber, pale yellow, or (rarely) bluish color. Normally, the membrane is translucent, although some degree of opacity may be normal in the first few mo of life; later, opacification denotes either scarring, or more commonly, underlying effusion. Structural changes include scars, perforations, retraction pockets, and a more severe complication of OM, cholesteatoma formation. Of all the visible characteristics of the tympanic membrane, mobility is the most sensitive and specific in determining the presence or absence of MEE. Importantly, mobility is not an all-or-none phenomenon; although total absence of mobility, in the absence of a tympanic membrane perforation, virtually always is indicative of MEE, substantial impairment of mobility is the more common finding.

DIAGNOSIS. Correct diagnosis of AOM is important to guide clinical treatment decisions. Although in many instances an accurate diagnosis can be made easily, this can be a challenging task, especially with an uncooperative patient. Consensus guidelines defining the required elements for a diagnosis of OM include all of the following elements: (1) recent and usually acute onset of illness; (2) presence of MEE; and (3) signs and symptoms of middle-ear inflammation, including erythema of the tympanic membrane or otalgia (see Table 639-1). A simplified differentiating schema establishes a diagnosis of AOM when, in addition to having MEE, a child gives evidence of recent, clinically important ear pain or the tympanic membrane shows marked redness or distinct fullness or bulging (Fig. 639-1).

Distinguishing between AOM and OME on clinical grounds also is straightforward in most cases, but because each condition may evolve into the other without any clearly differentiating physical findings, any schema for distinguishing between them is, to some extent, arbitrary. Nonetheless, in an era of increasing bacterial resistance, distinguishing between AOM and OME has become increasingly important in determining treatment. Obviously, purulent otorrhea of recent onset is indicative of AOM; thus, difficulty in distinguishing clinically between AOM and OME is limited to circumstances in which purulent otorrhea is not present. Both AOM without otorrhea and OME are accompanied by physical signs of MEE, i.e., the presence of at least 2 of 3 tympanic membrane abnormalities: white, yellow, amber, or (rarely) blue discoloration; opacification other than that due to scarring; and decreased or absent mobility. Alternatively, in OME either air-fluid levels or air bubbles outlined by small amounts of fluid may be visible behind the tympanic membrane, a condition often indicative of impending resolution.

To support a diagnosis of AOM instead of OME in a child with MEE, distinct fullness or bulging of the tympanic membrane may be present, with or without accompanying erythema. At minimum, MEE should be accompanied by ear pain that appears

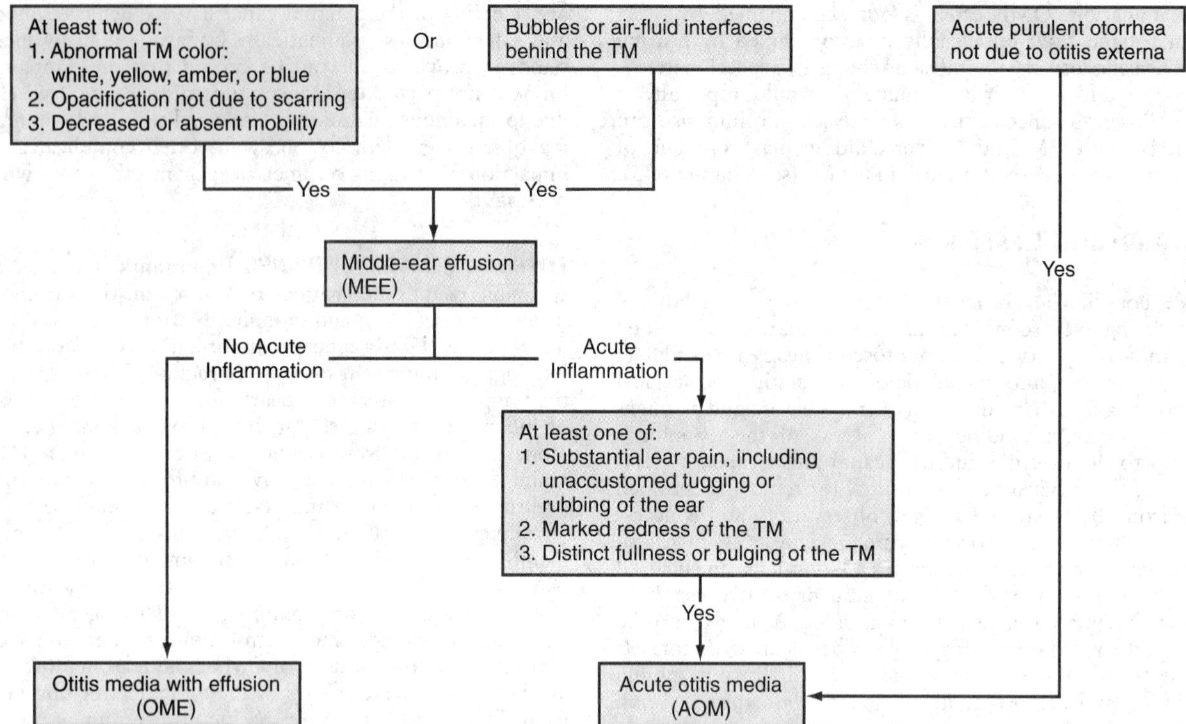

Figure 639-1. Algorithm for distinguishing between acute otitis media (AOM) and otitis media with effusion (OME). TM, tympanic membrane.

clinically important. Unless intense, erythema alone is insufficient; erythema without other abnormalities may result from crying or vascular flushing. In AOM, the malleus may be obscured, and the tympanic membrane may resemble a bagel with a central depression rather than a hole (Fig. 639-2). Rarely, the tympanic membrane may be obscured by surface bullae, or may have a cobblestone appearance. **Bullous myringitis** is a physical manifestation of AOM, not an etiologically discrete entity. Fullness of the membrane may diminish within days after onset, even though infection may still be present.

In OME, bulging of the tympanic membrane is absent or slight, or the membrane may be retracted (Fig. 639-3); erythema also is absent or slight, but may increase with crying or with superficial trauma to the external auditory canal incurred in clearing the canal of cerumen. In children with MEE but without tympanic membrane fullness or bulging, the presence of unequivocal ear pain usually is indicative of AOM.

Commonly, both before and after episodes of OM and also in the absence of OM, the tympanic membrane may be retracted as a consequence of negative middle-ear air pressure. The presumed

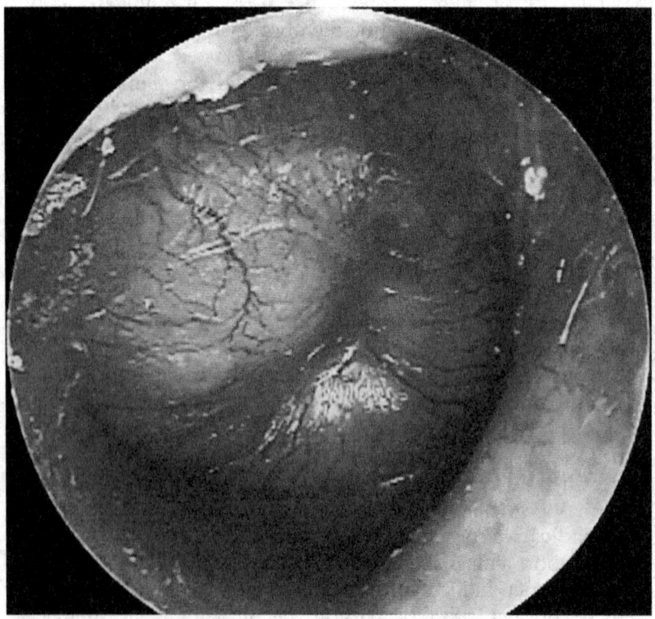

Figure 639-2. Tympanic membrane in acute otitis media (AOM).

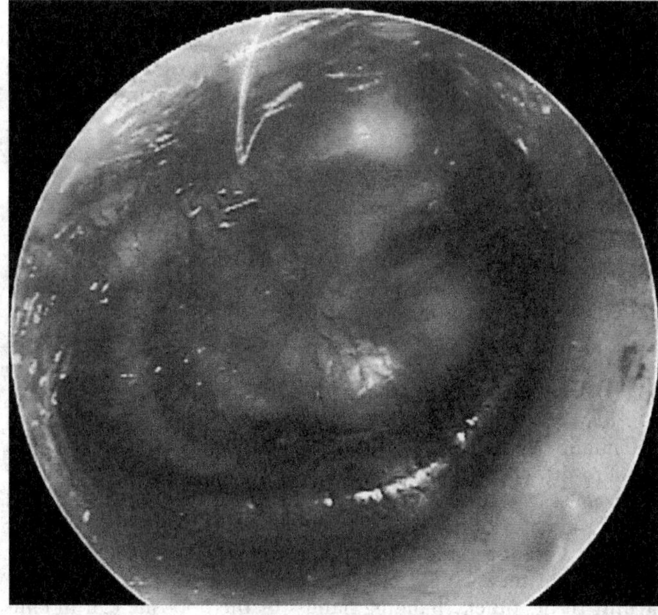

Figure 639-3. Tympanic membrane in otitis media with effusion (OME).

cause is diffusion of air from the middle-ear cavity more rapidly than it is replaced via the eustachian tube. Mild retraction cannot be considered pathologic, although in some children it is accompanied by mild conductive hearing loss. More extreme retraction, however, is of concern, as discussed later in the section on sequelae of OM.

TYMPANOMETRY. Tympanometry, or **acoustic immittance testing,** is a simple, rapid, atraumatic test that, when performed correctly, offers objective evidence of the presence or absence of MEE. The tympanogram provides information about tympanic membrane **compliance** in electroacoustic terms that can be thought of as roughly equivalent to tympanic membrane mobility as perceived visually during pneumatic otoscopy. The test depends on the facts that the absorption of sound by the tympanic membrane varies inversely with its stiffness and that the stiffness of the membrane is least, and accordingly its compliance is greatest, when the air pressures impinging on each of its surfaces—middle-ear air pressure and external canal air pressure—are equal. In simple terms, anything tending to stiffen the tympanic membrane, such as tympanic membrane scarring or middle-ear fluid, reduces the tympanic membrane compliance, which is recorded as a flattening of the curve of the tympanogram. An ear filled with middle-ear fluid usually has a very noncompliant tympanic membrane and, therefore, a flattened tympanogram tracing.

Tympanograms may be grouped into 1 of 3 categories (Fig. 639-4). Tracings characterized by a relatively steep gradient, sharp-angled peak, and middle-ear air pressure (location of the peak in terms of air pressure) that approximate atmospheric pressure (Fig. 639-4A) (type A curve) are assumed to indicate normal middle-ear status. Tracings characterized by a shallow peak or no peak and by negative or indeterminate middle-ear air pressure, and often termed flat or type B curve (Fig. 639-4B), usually are assumed to indicate the presence of a middle-ear abnormality that is causing decreased tympanic membrane compliance. The most common such abnormality by far in infants and children is MEE. Tracings characterized by intermediate findings—a somewhat shallow peak, often in association with a gradual gradient (obtuse-angled peak) or negative middle-ear air pressure, or combinations of these features (Fig. 639-4C), may or may not be associated with MEE, and must be considered nondiagnostic or equivocal. In general, the more shallow the peak, the more gradual the gradient, and the more negative the middle-ear air pressure, the greater the likelihood of MEE.

When reading a tympanogram it is important to look at the volume measurement also provided. A patient with a tympanic membrane perforation or patent tympanostomy tube will have a flat, type B tympanogram and a "high volume." The tympanometer measures and records the volume of the external auditory canal, and if a tympanic membrane perforation or a patent tympanostomy tube is present, the volume of the middle ear and mastoid air cells as well. A volume reading of >1.0 mL should suggest the presence of either a perforation or a patent tympanostomy tube. Therefore, in a child with a tympanostomy tube present, a flat tympanogram with a volume <1.0 mL would suggest a plugged or non-functioning tube and middle-ear fluid, whereas a flat tympanogram with a volume >1.0 mL would suggest a patent tympanostomy tube.

Although tympanometry is quite sensitive in detecting MEE, it can be limited by patient cooperation, the skill of the individual administering the test, and the age of the child, with less reliable results in very young children. Use of tympanometry may be helpful in office screening, both by obviating the need for routine otoscopic examination in difficult-to-examine patients whose tympanic membranes have been visualized previously, who are asymptomatic, and whose tympanograms are classified as normal, and by identifying patients who require further attention because their tympanograms are abnormal. Tympanometry also may be used to help confirm, refine, or clarify questionable otoscopic findings; to objectify the follow-up evaluation of patients with known middle-ear disease; and to validate otoscopic diagnoses of MEE. Importantly, even though tympanometry can predict the probability of MEE, it cannot distinguish the effusion of OME from that of AOM.

Conjunctivitis Otitis Media Syndrome. Simultaneous appearance of purulent and erythematous conjunctivitis with OM is a well-recognized syndrome, due in most children to non-typable *Haemophilus influenzae*. The disease often is present in multiple family members and affects young children and infants. Topical ocular antibiotics are ineffective; therapy includes oral antibiotics (see below) effective against non-typable *H. influenzae*.

TREATMENT

Management of Acute Otitis Media. Individual episodes of AOM customarily have been treated with antimicrobial drugs. Concern about increases in bacterial resistance has prompted some authors to recommend withholding antimicrobial treatment in some cases unless symptoms persist for 2–3 days, or worsen (Table 639-2).

Three factors argue in favor of routinely treating children who have bona fide AOM (see Table 639-1 and Fig. 639-2) with an antimicrobial drug. First, pathogenic bacteria cause a large majority of cases. Second, symptomatic improvement and resolution of infection occur more promptly and more consistently with antimicrobial treatment than without, even though most untreated cases eventually also resolve. Finally, prompt and adequate antimicrobial treatment may prevent the development of

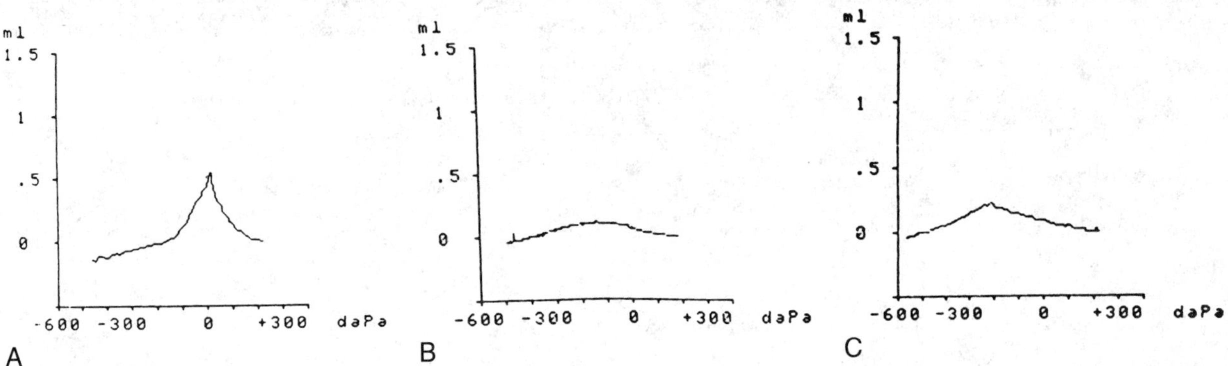

Figure 639-4. Tympanograms obtained with a Grason-Stadler GSI 33 Middle Ear Analyzer, exhibiting (A) high admittance, steep gradient (i.e., sharp-angled peak), and middle-ear air pressure approximating atmospheric pressure (0 decaPascals [daPa]); (B) low admittance and indeterminate middle-ear air pressure; and (C) somewhat low admittance, gradual gradient, and markedly negative middle-ear air pressure.

TABLE 639-2. Criteria for Initial Antibacterial-Agent Treatment or Observation in Children With AOM

AGE	CERTAIN DIAGNOSIS	UNCERTAIN DIAGNOSIS
<6 mo	Antibacterial therapy	Antibacterial therapy
6 mo–2 y	Antibacterial therapy	Antibacterial therapy if severe illness; observation option* if nonsevere illness
≥2 y	Antibacterial therapy if severe illness; observation option* if nonsevere illness	Observation option*

This table was modified with permission from the New York State Department of Health and the New York Region Otitis Project Committee.

*Observation is an appropriate option only when follow-up can be ensured and antibacterial agents started if symptoms persist or worsen. Nonsevere illness is mild otalgia and fever <39°C in the past 24 hours. Severe illness is moderate to severe otalgia or fever ≥39°C. A certain diagnosis of AOM meets all 3 criteria: (1) rapid onset; (2) signs of MEE; and (3) signs and symptoms of middle-ear inflammation.

From Subcommittee on Management of Acute Otitis Media: Diagnosis and management of acute otitis media. *Pediatrics* 2004;113:1451–1465.

suppurative complications. It seems likely that the sharp decline in such complications during the last half-century may be attributed, at least in part, to the widespread routine use of antimicrobials for AOM. In the Netherlands, where initial antibiotic treatment routinely is withheld from most children older than 6 mo of age, and where only approximately 30% of children with AOM receive antibiotics, the incidence of acute mastoiditis, although low (in children <14 yr of age, 3.8/100,000 person years), appears slightly higher than rates in other countries with higher antibiotic prescription rates by about 1–2 episodes/100,000 person years. Follow-up of children in the Netherlands may be generally more assiduous than is customary in other countries, including the United States, where failure to improve or worsening symptoms might not be detected as promptly.

These considerations in treating AOM with antimicrobial therapy must be balanced against the continued increasing rates of bacterial antimicrobial resistance. In countries such as the Netherlands, where use of antibiotics for OM is much less common, the antimicrobial resistance rates for the major pathogens in OM are substantially lower than those in countries that routinely treat AOM with antibiotics. Given that most episodes of OM resolve spontaneously, consensus guidelines have been published by the American Academy of Pediatrics to assist clinicians who wish to consider a period of "watchful waiting" or observation prior to treating AOM with antibiotics (Tables 639-2 and 639-3; Fig. 639-5). The most important aspect of these guidelines is that close follow-up of the patient must be ensured to assess for lack of spontaneous resolution or worsening of symptoms and that patients should be provided with adequate analgesic medications—acetaminophen or ibuprofen—during the period of observation. Topical otic agents (e.g., Auralgen) also may be effective for pain relief. When pursuing the practice of watchful waiting in patients with AOM, the certainty of the diagnosis, the patient's age, and the severity of the disease should be considered. For younger patients, <2 yr of age, it is recommended to treat all confirmed diagnoses of AOM. In very young patients, <6 mo of age, even presumed episodes of AOM should be treated due to the increased potential of significant morbidity from infectious complications. In children 6–24 mo of age who have a questionable diagnosis of OM but are severely ill, defined as temperature of >102°F (>39°C), significant otalgia, or toxic appearance, antibiotic therapy is also recommended. However, children in this age group in whom the diagnosis is questionable and the disease is not severe can be observed for a period of 2–3 days with close follow-up. In children >2 yr of age, observation might be considered in all episodes of non-severe OM or episodes of questionable diagnosis, with antibiotic therapy reserved for confirmed, severe episodes of AOM.

BACTERIAL RESISTANCE. Bacteria have a remarkable ability to develop resistance to antimicrobial drugs, and bacterial resistance has become an increasing problem in the past decade. Persons at greatest risk of harboring resistant bacteria include children who are <2 yr of age; are in regular contact with large groups of other children, especially in daycare settings; or who recently have received antimicrobial treatment. Bacterial resistance is a particular problem in relation to OM. The development of resistant bacterial strains and their rapid spread have been fostered and facilitated by selective pressure resulting from extensive use of antimicrobial drugs, the most common target of which, in children, is OM. In addition, many strains of each of the pathogenic bacteria that commonly cause AOM are resistant to certain commonly used antimicrobial drugs.

Although antimicrobial resistance rates vary from country to country, in the USA approximately 40% of strains of nontypable *H. influenzae* and almost all strains of *M. catarrhalis* currently are resistant to aminopenicillins (e.g., ampicillin, amoxicillin). In most cases the resistance is attributable to production of β-lactamase, and can be overcome by combining amoxicillin with a β-lactamase inhibitor, namely, clavulanate, or by using a β-lactamase-stable antibiotic. However, occasional strains of nontypable *H. influenzae* that do not produce β-lactamase are resistant to aminopenicillins and other β-lactam antibiotics by virtue of alterations in their penicillin-binding proteins.

TABLE 639-3. Recommended Antibacterial Agents for Patients Who Are Being Treated Initially With Antibacterial Agents or Have Failed 48 to 72 Hours of Observation or Initial Management With Antibacterial Agents

TEMPERATURE ≥39°C AND/OR SEVERE OTALGIA	AT DIAGNOSIS FOR PATIENTS BEING TREATED INITIALLY WITH ANTIBACTERIAL AGENTS		CLINICALLY DEFINED TREATMENT FAILURE AT 48–72 HR AFTER INITIAL MANAGEMENT WITH OBSERVATION OPTION		CLINICALLY DEFINED TREATMENT FAILURE AT 48–72 HR AFTER INITIAL MANAGEMENT WITH ANTIBACTERIAL AGENTS	
	RECOMMENDED	ALTERNATIVE FOR PENICILLIN ALLERGY	RECOMMENDED	ALTERNATIVE FOR PENICILLIN ALLERGY	RECOMMENDED	ALTERNATIVE FOR PENICILLIN ALLERGY
No	Amoxicillin, 80–90 mg/kg per day	Non–type 1: cefdinir, cefuroxime, cefpodoxime; type 1: azithromycin, clarithromycin	Amoxicillin, 80–90 mg/kg per day	Non–type 1: cefdinir, cefuroxime, cefpodoxime; type 1: azithromycin, clarithromycin	Amoxicillin-clavulanate, 90 mg/kg per day of amoxicillin component, with 6.4 mg/kg per day of clavulanate	Non-type 1: ceftriaxone, 3 days; type 1: clindamycin
Yes	Amoxicillin-clavulanate, 90 mg/kg per day of amoxicillin, with 6.4 mg/kg per day of clavulanate	Ceftriaxone, 1 or 3 days	Amoxicillin, clavulanate, 90 mg/kg per day of amoxicillin, with 6.4 mg/kg per day of clavulanate	Ceftriaxone, 1 or 3 days	Ceftriaxone, 3 days	Tympanocentesis, clindamycin

From Subcommittee on Management of Acute Otitis Media: Diagnosis and management of acute otitis media. *Pediatrics* 2004;113:1451–1465.

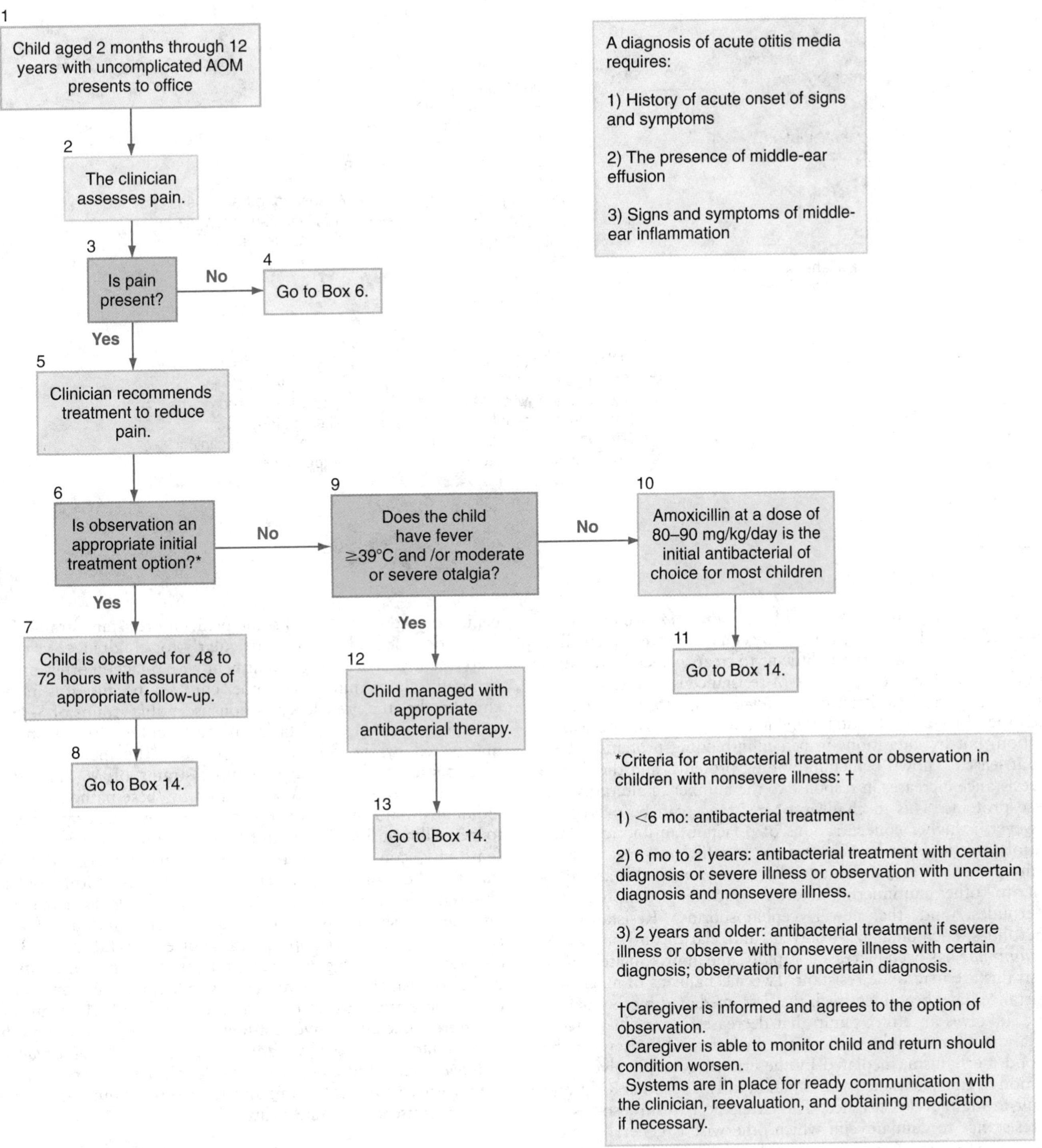

1
Child aged 2 months through 12 years with uncomplicated AOM presents to office
2
The clinician assesses pain.
3
Is pain present?
No
4
Go to Box 6.
Yes
5
Clinician recommends treatment to reduce pain.
6
Is observation an appropriate initial treatment option?*
No
9
Does the child have fever ≥39°C and /or moderate or severe otalgia?
No
10
Amoxicillin at a dose of 80–90 mg/kg/day is the initial antibacterial of choice for most children
11
Go to Box 14.
Yes
7
Child is observed for 48 to 72 hours with assurance of appropriate follow-up.
8
Go to Box 14.
Yes
12
Child managed with appropriate antibacterial therapy.
13
Go to Box 14.
A diagnosis of acute otitis media requires:
1) History of acute onset of signs and symptoms
2) The presence of middle-ear effusion
3) Signs and symptoms of middle-ear inflammation
*Criteria for antibacterial treatment or observation in children with nonsevere illness: †
1) <6 mo: antibacterial treatment
2) 6 mo to 2 years: antibacterial treatment with certain diagnosis or severe illness or observation with uncertain diagnosis and nonsevere illness.
3) 2 years and older: antibacterial treatment if severe illness or observe with nonsevere illness with certain diagnosis; observation for uncertain diagnosis.
†Caregiver is informed and agrees to the option of observation.
Caregiver is able to monitor child and return should condition worsen.
Systems are in place for ready communication with the clinician, reevaluation, and obtaining medication if necessary.

Figure 639-5. Management of AOM. (From Subcommittee on Management of Acute Otitis Media: Diagnosis and management of acute otitis media. *Pediatrics* 204;113:1451–1465.)

Continued

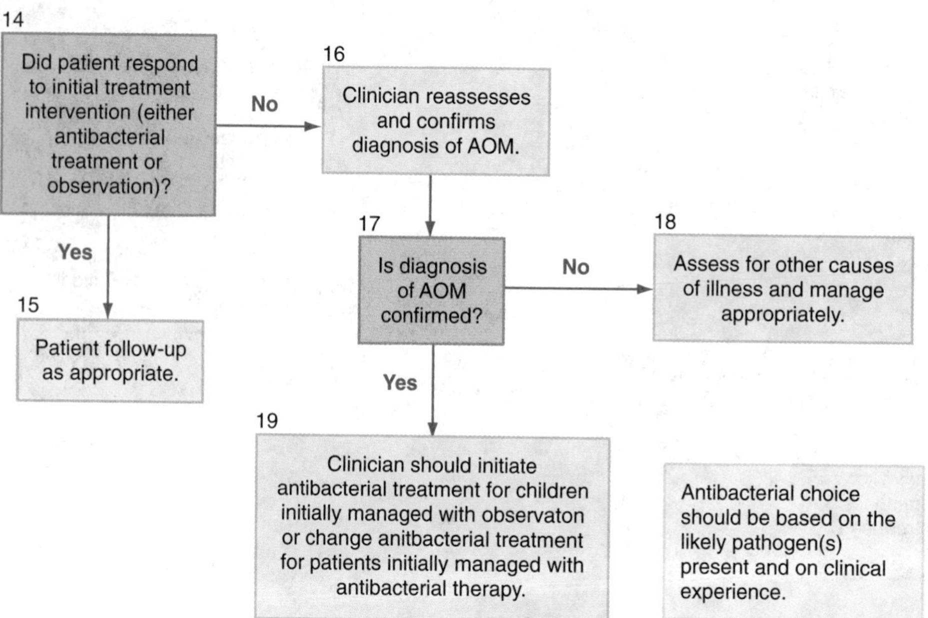

Figure 639-5. cont'd

Approximately 50% of strains of *S. pneumoniae* are penicillin-nonsusceptible, divided approximately equally between penicillin-intermediate and, even more difficult to treat, penicillin-resistant strains. A much higher incidence of resistance is seen in children attending daycare. Resistance by *S. pneumoniae* to the penicillins and other β-lactam antibiotics is mediated not by β-lactamase production, but by alterations in penicillin-binding proteins. There are at least 6 known penicillin-binding proteins, and the degree of resistance increases in response to the number of alterations in these proteins. This mechanism of resistance can be overcome, however, if higher concentrations of β-lactam antibiotics at the site of infection can be achieved for a sufficient time interval. Many penicillin-resistant strains of *S. pneumoniae* also are resistant to other antimicrobial drugs, including sulfonamides, macrolides, and the newer cephalosporins. Resistance to macrolides, including azithromycin and clarithromycin, by *S. pneumoniae* has been increasing rapidly, and approximately 30% of strains are macrolide-resistant. Two mechanisms of macrolide resistance have been identified: the first, mediated by the mef(A) gene, involves an efflux pump that decreases intracellular accumulation of macrolides and results in low-level resistance; the second mechanism, mediated by the erm(B) gene, involves production of ribosomal methylases that modify ribosomal RNA and result in high-level resistance. The latter mechanism also results in resistance to clindamycin, which otherwise is generally effective against resistant strains of *S. pneumoniae.* Unlike resistance to β-lactam antibiotics, macrolide resistance cannot be overcome by increasing the dose. Although vancomycin previously was a fail-safe antimicrobial in treating *S. pneumoniae,* clinical cases of vancomycin-tolerant *S. pneumoniae* have been identified, further raising the importance and hazard of antimicrobial resistance.

FIRST-LINE ANTIMICROBIAL TREATMENT. Amoxicillin remains the preferred drug for uncomplicated AOM under most circumstances because of its excellent record of safety, relative efficacy, palatability, and low cost (see Table 639–3). Amoxicillin is the most efficacious of available oral antimicrobial drugs against both penicillin-susceptible and penicillin-nonsusceptible strains of *S. pneumoniae.* Increasing the dose from the traditional 40 mg/kg/24 hr to 80–100 mg/kg/24 hr usually is effective against penicillin-intermediate and some penicillin-resistant strains. This higher dose should be used particularly for children <2 yr of age who recently have received treatment with β-lactam drugs or been exposed to large numbers of other children, because it is in these children that the prevalence of nonsusceptible strains of *S. pneumoniae* is highest. A limitation of amoxicillin is that it may be inactivated by the β-lactamases produced by many strains of nontypable *H. influenzae* and most strains of *M. catarrhalis.* Fortunately, episodes of AOM caused by these pathogens often, although by no means always, resolve spontaneously. Allergies to penicillin antibiotics should be categorized as type 1 hypersensitivity, consisting of urticaria or anaphylaxis, and those that fall short of type 1 reactions, such as rash formation. For children with a non–type 1 reaction in which cross-reactivity with cephalosporins is less of a concern, first-line therapy with cefdinir would be an appropriate choice (see Table 639-3). In children with a type 1 reaction or known sensitivity to cephalosporin antibiotics, or in whom palatability or convenience of administration are of overriding importance, azithromycin is an appropriate alternative first-line drug. Resistance to trimethoprim-sulfamethoxazole by many strains of both *H. influenzae* and *S. pneumoniae* and a reported high clinical failure rate in children with AOM treated initially with this antimicrobial argue against its use as first-line treatment.

DURATION OF TREATMENT. The duration of treatment of AOM often has been set at 10 days, apparently extrapolated from the optimal duration of treatment of streptococcal pharyngitis with penicillin. However, 10 days may be unduly long for some children while not long enough for others. Studies comparing shorter with longer durations of treatment suggest that short-course treatment often is inadequate in children <6 yr of age, and particularly in children <2 yr of age. Thus, for most episodes in most children, treatment that provides tissue concentrations of an antimicrobial for at least 10 days seems advisable. Treatment for shorter periods, of 3–5 days, may be appropriate for older children with mild episodes who improve quickly; however, in these cases, one could reasonably argue that simple observation without antimicrobial therapy would be the preferred intervention. Treatment for >10 days may be required for children who are very young or are having severe episodes or whose previous experience with OM has been problematic.

FOLLOW-UP. The principal goals of follow-up are to assess the outcome of treatment and to differentiate between inadequate response to treatment and early recurrence. Accordingly, the appropriate interval for follow-up should be individualized. Follow-up within days is advisable in the young infant with a severe episode or in a child of any age with continuing pain. Follow-up within 2 wk is appropriate for the infant or young child who apparently has been having frequent recurrences. At that point, the tympanic membrane is not likely to have returned to normal, but substantial improvement in its appearance should be evident. In the child with only a sporadic episode of AOM and prompt symptomatic improvement, follow-up 1 mo after initial examination is early enough; in older children, no follow-up may be necessary. Importantly, the continuing presence of MEE alone following an episode of AOM is not an indication for additional or second-line antimicrobial treatment.

UNSATISFACTORY RESPONSE TO FIRST-LINE TREATMENT. AOM is essentially a closed-space infection, and its resolution depends on both eradication of the offending organism and restoration of middle-ear ventilation. Factors contributing to unsatisfactory response to first-line treatment, in addition to inadequate antimicrobial efficacy, include poor compliance with treatment regimens, concurrent or intercurrent viral infection, persistent eustachian tube dysfunction and middle-ear under-aeration, reinfection from other sites or from incompletely eradicated middle ear pathogens, and immature or impaired host defenses. Despite these many potential factors, switching to an alternative or second-line drug is reasonable when there has been inadequate improvement in symptoms or in middle-ear status as reflected in the appearance of the tympanic membrane, or when the persistence of purulent nasal discharge suggests that the antimicrobial drug being used has less than optimal efficacy. Second-line drugs also may be used appropriately when AOM develops in a child already receiving antimicrobial therapy, or in an immunocompromised child, or in a child with severe symptoms whose previous experience with OM has been problematic.

SECOND-LINE TREATMENT. When treatment of AOM with a first-line antimicrobial drug has proven inadequate, a number of second-line alternatives are available (see Table 639-3). Drugs chosen for second-line treatment should be effective against β-lactamase–producing strains of *H. influenzae* and *M. catarrhalis* and against susceptible and most nonsusceptible strains of *S. pneumoniae.* Only 3 drugs have been shown clearly to meet that requirement: amoxicillin-clavulanate, cefuroxime axetil, and intramuscular ceftriaxone. Because high-dose amoxicillin (80–100 mg/kg/24) is effective against most strains of *S. pneumoniae* and because the addition of clavulanate extends the effective antibacterial spectrum of amoxicillin to include β-lactamase–producing bacteria, high-dose amoxicillin-clavulanate is particularly well suited as a second-line drug for treating AOM. The 14 : 1 amoxicillin-clavulanate formulation contains twice as much amoxicillin as the previously available 7 : 1 formulation. Diarrhea, especially in infants and young children, is a common adverse effect, but may be ameliorated in some cases by feeding yogurt, and usually is not severe enough to require cessation of treatment. The 2 other drugs have important limitations for use in young children. The currently available suspension of cefuroxime axetil is not palatable, and its acceptance is low. Ceftriaxone treatment entails both the pain of intramuscular injection and substantial cost; the injection may need to be repeated once or twice at 2- or 3-day intervals to achieve the desired degree of effectiveness. Nonetheless, use of ceftriaxone is appropriate in severe cases of AOM when oral treatment is not feasible, or in highly selected cases after treatment failure using orally administered second-line antimicrobials (e.g., amoxicillin-clavulanate, cefuroxime axetil), or when highly resistant *S. pneumoniae* is found in aspirates obtained from diagnostic tympanocentesis. Cefdinir was not available when the above recommendations were made. However, clinical practice and efficacy with cefdinir suggest that it deserves consideration as a second-line agent as well, with antibacterial spectrums similar to those of cefuroxime axetil, and good rates of compliance, as the medication is quite palatable.

The newer macrolides, clarithromycin and azithromycin, have only limited activity against nonsusceptible strains of *S. pneumoniae* and against β-lactamase–producing strains of *H. influenzae.* Macrolide use also appears to be a major factor in causing increases in rates of resistance to macrolides by group A streptococcus and *S. pneumoniae.* Of the cephalosporins other than cefuroxime axetil and cefdinir, cefpodoxime seems the most promising. However, compliance may be affected by the lack of palatability of this medication. Cefprozil possesses somewhat less β-lactamase stability than either cefuroxime or cefpodoxime. Cefaclor and loracarbef have limited activity against β-lactamase–producing bacteria and nonsusceptible pneumococci, and cefaclor occasionally may cause serum sickness. Cefixime has excellent activity against β-lactamase–producing bacteria but limited activity against even penicillin-susceptible pneumococci. Trimethoprim-sulfamethoxazole has such little efficacy that it is not recommended for treating AOM. Additionally, this drug rarely may cause severe reactions such as bone-marrow suppression or Stevens-Johnson syndrome. Erythromycin-sulfisoxazole also may cause such reactions and is not active against penicillin-nonsusceptible pneumococci. Clindamycin is active against most strains of *S. pneumoniae,* including resistant strains, but is not active against *H. influenzae* or *M. catarrhalis.* It should, therefore, be reserved for patients known to have infection caused by penicillin-nonsusceptible *S. pneumoniae.*

MYRINGOTOMY AND TYMPANOCENTESIS. Myringotomy is a time-honored treatment for AOM but is not commonly needed in children receiving antimicrobials. In a clinical trial limited to children with severe AOM, those who received amoxicillin plus myringotomy fared no better overall than those who received amoxicillin only, but the study population was not large enough to have excluded the possibility that myringotomy had been marginally beneficial. **Indications for myringotomy** in children with AOM include severe, refractory pain; hyperpyrexia; complications of AOM such as facial paralysis, mastoiditis, labyrinthitis, or central nervous system infection; and immunologic compromise. Myringotomy should be considered as third-line therapy in patients who have failed 2 courses of antibiotics for an episode of AOM. In children with AOM in whom clinical response to vigorous, second-line treatment has been unsatisfactory, either diagnostic tympanocentesis or myringotomy is indicated to enable identification of the offending organism and its sensitivity profile. Either procedure may be additionally helpful in effecting relief of pain. Tympanocentesis with culture of the middle-ear aspirate also is indicated as part of the sepsis work-up in infants <1 mo of age with AOM who show systemic signs of illness such as fever, vomiting, or lethargy, and whose illness accordingly cannot be presumed to be limited to infection of the middle ear. "In an era of increasing antimicrobial resistance," the CDC Working Group wrote, "clinicians treating children with AOM should consider developing the capacity to perform tympanocentesis themselves or establish ready referral mechanisms to a clinician with this capacity." Performance of tympanocentesis can be facilitated by use of a specially designed tympanocentesis aspirator.

EARLY RECURRENCE AFTER TREATMENT. Recurrence of AOM after apparent resolution may be due to either incomplete eradication of infection in the middle ear or upper respiratory tract or to reinfection by the same or a different bacterium. Recurrence within several days usually is caused by the same organism, and thus treatment may be best guided by the response to treatment of the antecedent episode: if it seemed to respond to a first-line antimicrobial, that drug would again be appropriate; if it failed to respond to a first-line drug but seemed to respond to a second-line drug, use of a second-line drug from the outset might be advisable. Recent antibiotic therapy also predisposes patients to an increased incidence of resistant organisms, which also should be considered in choosing therapy.

MYRINGOTOMY AND INSERTION OF TYMPANOSTOMY TUBES. When AOM is recurrent, despite appropriate medical therapy, consideration of surgical management of AOM with tympanostomy tube insertion is warranted. This procedure is highly effective in reducing the rate of AOM in patients with recurrent OM and can significantly improve the quality of life in patients with recurrent AOM. Individual patient factors, including risk profile, severity of AOM episodes, the child's development and age, the presence of a history of adverse drug reactions, concurrent medical problems, and parental wishes affect when a decision is made to consider referral for this procedure. However, when a patient requires 3–4 courses of antibiotics for episodes of AOM in a 6-mo period or 5–6 episodes in a 12-mo period, potential surgical management of the child's AOM should be discussed with the parents.

TUBE OTORRHEA. When tympanostomy tube otorrhea develops, ototopical treatment should be considered as first-line therapy. With a functioning tube in place, the infection is able to drain, and the possibility of developing a serious complication from an episode of AOM is negligible. The current FDA-approved quinolone otic drops approved for use in the middle-ear space in children are formulated with ciprofloxacin/dexamethasone (Ciprodex) and ofloxacin (Floxin), which, when administered in the high dosage, can be delivered to the middle ear in a topical preparation. These agents have excellent coverage of even the most resistant strains of common middle-ear pathogens as well as *S. aureus* and *P. aeruginosa*. Therefore, due to the high rate of success of these topical preparations, their broad coverage, the lower likelihood of their contributing to the development of resistant organisms, the relative ease of administration, the lack of significant side effects, and their lack of ototoxicity, oral antibiotic therapy usually should be reserved for cases of tube otorrhea that have other associated systemic symptoms, patients who have difficulty in tolerating the use of topical preparations, or, possibly, patients who have failed an attempt at topical otic drops. In addition, due to the relative ease of obtaining fluid for culture, and the possibility that other pathogens not covered by topical agents, such as a fungal infection, may be present, patients who fail topical therapy also should have culture performed if initial treatment fails. Other otic preparations are available; but these either have some risk of ototoxicity or have not received approval for use in the middle ear. However, many of these preparations were widely used prior to the development of the current quinolone drops and were generally considered reasonably safe and effective. In all cases of tube otorrhea, attention to aural toilet, that is, cleansing the external auditory canal of secretions, and avoidance of water contamination of the external ear is important. In some cases with very thick, tenacious discharge, topical therapy may be inhibited because the medication cannot be delivered to the site of infection, and suctioning and removal of the secretions, often done with referral to an otolaryngologist, may be quite helpful. When children with tube otorrhea fail to improve satisfactorily with conventional outpatient management, they may require tube removal or hospitalization to receive parenteral antibiotic treatment, or both.

MANAGEMENT OF OTITIS MEDIA WITH EFFUSION

To determine the course of an episode of OME, and to distinguish between persistence and recurrence, examination should be conducted monthly until resolution, and hearing should be assessed if effusion has been present for >3 mo (see Fig. 639-1). Rational management of OME depends to a considerable degree on understanding its natural history and its possible complications and sequelae. Most cases of OME resolve without treatment within 3 mo; limited data are available concerning the subsequent long-term course of children in whom OME does not resolve within that time frame and who do not receive surgical intervention. When considering surgical management of persisting OME with tympanostomy tubes, the clinician should attempt to determine the impact of the OME on the child. Although hearing loss may be of primary concern, OME causes a number of other difficulties in children that also should be considered. These include predisposition to recurring AOM, pain, disturbance of balance, and tinnitus. Long-term sequelae that have been demonstrated to be associated with OME include pathologic middle-ear changes; atelectasis of the tympanic membrane and retraction pocket formation; adhesive OM; ossicular discontinuity; cholesteatoma; and conductive and sensorineural hearing loss. Long-term adverse effects on speech, language, and cognitive and psychosocial development also are noted. Nonetheless, some studies have demonstrated that the long-term adverse impact of OME on development may be small. In considering the impact of OME on development, it is especially important to take into consideration the overall presentation of the child. Although it is unlikely that OME causing unilateral hearing loss in the mild range will have long-term negative effects on an otherwise healthy and developmentally normal child, even a mild hearing loss in a child with other developmental or speech delays has the potential to compound this child's difficulties. At a minimum, children with OME persisting >3 mo deserve close monitoring of their hearing levels with skilled audiologic evaluation; frequent assessment of developmental milestones, including speech and language assessment; and attention paid to their rate of recurrent AOM.

VARIABLES INFLUENCING MANAGEMENT DECISIONS FOR OTITIS MEDIA WITH EFFUSION. Patient-related variables that affect decisions on how to manage OME include the child's age; the frequency and severity of previous episodes of AOM and the interval since the last episode; the child's language development; the presence or absence of a history of adverse drug reactions, concurrent medical problems, or risk factors such as daycare attendance or other exposure to infectious disease; and the parents' wishes. In considering surgical management of OME with tympanostomy tubes, particular benefit is seen in patients with persisting OME punctuated by episodes of AOM, because the tubes generally provide resolution of both conditions. Disease-related variables that must be considered in the treatment of OME include whether the effusion is unilateral or bilateral; the apparent quantity of effusion; the duration, if known; the degree of hearing impairment; the presence or absence of other possibly related symptoms, such as tinnitus, vertigo, or balance disturbance; and the presence or absence of mucopurulent or purulent rhinorrhea, which, if sustained for >2 wk, suggests that concurrent nasopharyngeal or paranasal sinus infection is contributing to continuing compromise of middle-ear ventilation.

MEDICAL TREATMENT. Antimicrobials have definite but limited efficacy in resolving OME, presumably because they help eradicate nasopharyngeal infection or inapparent middle-ear infection, or both. However, mainly because of the short-term nature of their benefit and because of the contribution of antimicrobial usage to the development of bacterial resistance, routine antimicrobial treatment of OME, previously recommended by some authorities, no longer seems wise. Instead, treatment should be limited to cases in which there is evidence of associated bacterial upper respiratory tract infection or untreated middle-ear infection. For this purpose, the most broadly effective drug available should be used, as recommended for AOM.

The efficacy of oral corticosteroids in the treatment of OME is probably short-term at best, and guidelines for the treatment of OME have determined that the risk : benefit ratio for these medications would argue against their use. Antihistamine–decongestant combinations are not effective in treating children with OME, but their efficacy has not been tested in children with environmental allergies. Antihistamines alone, decongestants alone, and mucolytic agents are unlikely to be effective. Allergic management might prove helpful in children with problematic OME who also have evidence of upper respiratory allergy, but supporting data are lacking. In children without such evidence, allergy testing is not indicated. Inflation of the eustachian tubes by the Valsalva maneuver or other means has no proven long-term efficacy.

MYRINGOTOMY AND INSERTION OF TYMPANOSTOMY TUBES. When OME persists despite an ample period of watchful waiting, usually 3–6 mo or perhaps longer in children with unilateral effusion, the question arises as to surgical intervention. Myringotomy alone, without tympanostomy tube insertion, permits evacuation of middle-ear effusion and sometimes is effective; often, because the incision heals before the middle ear mucosa returns to normal the effusion soon re-accumulates. Inserting tubes offers the likelihood that middle-ear ventilation will be sustained for at least as long as the tube remains in place and functional, about 12 mo on average, and nearly uniformly reverses the conductive hearing loss associated with OME. Occasional episodes of obstruction of the tube lumen and premature tube extrusion may limit the effectiveness of tympanostomy tubes, and tubes also can be associated with otorrhea. However, placement of tympanostomy tubes usually is effective in providing resolution of OME in children. Sequelae following tubal extrusion include residual perforation of the eardrum, tympanosclerosis, localized or diffuse atrophic scarring of the eardrum that may predispose to the development of atelectasis or a retraction pocket or both, residual conductive hearing loss, and cholesteatoma. Fortunately, the more serious of these sequelae occur infrequently. Recurrence of middle-ear effusion following the extrusion of tubes does develop, especially in younger children. However, most children without underlying craniofacial abnormalities require only 1 set of tympanostomy tubes, with developmental changes providing improved middle-ear health and resolution of their chronic OME by the time of tube extrusion. Because even previously persistent OME often clears spontaneously during the summer months, watchful waiting through the summer season also is advisable in most children with OME who are otherwise well. Finally, in considering surgical management of OME in children, primarily in those with bilateral disease and hearing loss, it has been demonstrated that placement of tympanostomy tubes provides an improvement in their quality of life.

COMPLICATIONS OF ACUTE OTITIS MEDIA. Most complications of AOM consist of the spread of infection to adjoining or nearby structures or the development of chronicity, or both. Suppurative complications are relatively uncommon in children in developed countries, but occur not infrequently in disadvantaged children whose medical care is limited or nonexistent. Complications of AOM may be classified as either intratemporal or intracranial.

INTRATEMPORAL COMPLICATIONS Direct but limited extension of OM leads to complications within the temporal bone. These complications include dermatitis, tympanic membrane perforation, chronic suppurative OM, mastoiditis, hearing loss, facial nerve paralysis, cholesteatoma formation, and labyrinthitis.

INFECTIOUS DERMATITIS. Infectious dermatitis is an infection of the skin of the external auditory canal resulting from contamination by purulent discharge from the middle ear. The skin often is erythematous, edematous, and tender. Management consists of proper hygiene combined with systemic antimicrobials and ototopical drops as appropriate for treating AOM and tube otorrhea.

TYMPANIC MEMBRANE PERFORATION. Rupture of the tympanic membrane can occur with episodes of either AOM or OME. Although damage to the tympanic membrane from these episodes usually heals spontaneously, chronic perforations can develop in a small number of cases and require further surgical intervention.

CHRONIC SUPPURATIVE OTITIS MEDIA. Chronic suppurative OM consists of persistent middle-ear infection with discharge through a tympanic membrane perforation. The disease is initiated by an episode of AOM with rupture of the membrane. The mastoid air cells always are involved. The most common etiologic organisms are *P. aeruginosa* and *S. aureus*. Treatment is guided by the results of microbiologic investigation. If an associated cholesteatoma is not present, parenteral antimicrobial treatment combined with assiduous aural cleansing is likely to be successful in clearing the infection, but in refractory cases, tympanomastoidectomy can be required.

ACUTE MASTOIDITIS. Technically, all cases of AOM are accompanied by mastoiditis by virtue of the associated inflammation of the mastoid air cells. However, early in the course of the disease no signs or symptoms of mastoid infection are present, and the inflammatory process usually is readily reversible, along with the AOM, in response to antimicrobial treatment. Spread of the infection to the overlying periosteum, but without involvement of bone, constitutes **acute mastoiditis with periosteitis.** In such cases, signs of mastoiditis usually are present, i.e., inflammation in the postauricular area, often with displacement of the pinna inferiorly and anteriorly (Table 639-4). Treatment with myringotomy and parenteral antibiotics, if instituted promptly, usually provides satisfactory resolution.

In acute mastoid osteitis, or coalescent mastoiditis, infection has progressed further, causing destruction of the bony trabeculae of the mastoid (Fig. 639-6). Frank signs and symptoms of

TABLE 639-4. Differential Diagnosis of Postauricular Involvement of Acute Mastoiditis With Periosteitis/Abscess

DISEASE	POSTAURICULAR SIGNS AND SYMPTOMS				EXTERNAL CANAL INFECTION	MIDDLE-EAR EFFUSION
	CREASE*	ERYTHEMA	MASS	TENDERNESS		
Acute mastoiditis with periosteitis	May be absent	Yes	No	Usually	No	Usually
Acute mastoiditis with subperiosteal abscess	Absent	Maybe	Yes	Yes	No	Usually
Periosteitis of pinna with postauricular extension	Intact	Yes	No	Usually	No	No
External otitis with postauricular extension	Intact	Yes	No	Usually	Yes	No
Postauricular lymphadenitis	Intact	No	Yes (Circumscribed)	Maybe	No	No

*Postauricular crease (fold) between pinna and postauricular area.

From Bluestone CD, Klein JO (editors): *Otitis Media in Infants and Children,* 3rd ed. Philadelphia, WB Saunders, 2001, p 333.

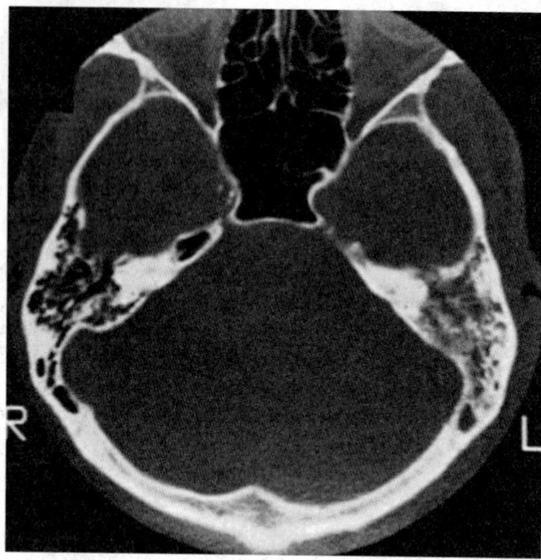

Figure 639-6. CT scan of temporal bones showing left acute osteitis with loss of septa between the mastoid air cells, which has been termed acute coalescent mastoiditis; right mastoid is normal. Mastoid surgery was performed in this case. (From Bluestone CD, Klein JO [editors]: *Otitis Media in Infants and Children,* 3rd ed. Philadelphia, WB Saunders, 2001, p 337.)

mastoiditis usually, but not always, are present. In acute petrositis, infection has extended further to involve the petrous portion of the temporal bone. Eye pain is a prominent symptom, due to irritation of the ophthalmic branch of the cranial nerve V; cranial nerve VI palsy later develops. **Gradenigo syndrome** is the triad of suppurative OM, paralysis of the external rectus muscle, and pain in the ipsilateral orbit. Rarely, mastoid infection spreads to the neck muscles that attach to the mastoid tip, resulting in an abscess in the neck, termed a **Bezold abscess.**

When mastoiditis is suspected or diagnosed clinically, CT scanning of the temporal bone should be carried out to further clarify the nature and extent of the disease (see Fig. 639-6). Bony destruction of the mastoid must be differentiated from the simple clouding of mastoid air cells that often is found in uncomplicated cases of OM. The most common causative organisms in all variants of acute mastoiditis are *S. pneumoniae,* nontypable *H. influenzae,* and *P. aeruginosa.* Children with acute mastoid osteitis require intravenous antimicrobial treatment and mastoidectomy, with the extent of the surgery depending on the extent of the disease process. As far as possible, choice of the antimicrobial regimen should be guided by the findings of microbiologic examination.

Each of the variants of mastoiditis also may occur in subacute or chronic form. Symptoms are correspondingly less prominent. Chronic mastoiditis always is accompanied by chronic suppurative OM, and occasionally will respond to the conservative regimen recommended for that condition. In most cases, however, mastoidectomy also is required.

FACIAL PARALYSIS. The facial nerve, as it traverses the middle ear and mastoid bone, may be affected by adjacent infection. Facial paralysis as a complication of AOM is uncommon, and often resolves after myringotomy and parenteral antibiotic treatment. Facial paralysis in the presence of AOM requires urgent attention, because prolonged infection can result in permanent facial paralysis, which, when it occurs, can have a devastating affect on a child. If facial paralysis develops in a child with mastoid osteitis or with chronic suppurative OM, mastoidectomy should be undertaken urgently.

ACQUIRED CHOLESTEATOMA. Cholesteatoma is a cystlike growth within the middle ear or other pneumatized portions of the temporal bone, lined by keratinized, stratified squamous epithelium and containing desquamated epithelium and/or keratin (see Chapter 637). Acquired, as distinct from congenital, cholesteatoma most often develops as a complication of longstanding chronic OM. However, the condition also may develop from a deep retraction pocket of the tympanic membrane or as a consequence of epithelial implantation in the middle-ear cavity from traumatic perforation of the tympanic membrane or insertion of a tympanostomy tube. Cholesteatomas tend to expand progressively, causing bony resorption, and may extend intracranially, with potentially life-threatening consequences. Cholesteatoma should be suspected if otoscopy shows a discrete, whitish opacity of the eardrum or a polyp protruding through a defect in the eardrum; or white caseous debris persistently overlies the eardrum, especially its superior portion; or persistent malodorous aural discharge is present. When cholesteatoma is suspected, consultation with an otolaryngologist should be sought immediately. Delayed recognition and treatment can have significant long-term consequences, including the need for more extensive surgical treatment, permanent hearing loss, facial nerve injury, labyrinthine damage with loss of balance function, and intracranial extension. Tympanomastoid surgery is required for treatment of cholesteatoma.

LABYRINTHITIS. Labyrinthitis occurs uncommonly as a result of the spread of infection from the middle ear and/or mastoid to the inner ear. Cholesteatoma or chronic suppurative OM is the usual source. Symptoms and signs include vertigo, tinnitus, nausea, vomiting, hearing loss, nystagmus, and clumsiness. Treatment is directed at the underlying condition and must be undertaken promptly to preserve inner ear function and prevent the spread of infection.

INTRACRANIAL COMPLICATIONS

Meningitis, epidural abscess, subdural abscess, focal encephalitis, brain abscess, lateral sinus thrombosis (also called sigmoid sinus thrombosis), and otitic hydrocephalus each may develop as a complication of acute or chronic middle-ear or mastoid infection, through direct extension, hematogenous spread, or thrombophlebitis. Bony destruction adjacent to the dura often is involved, and a cholesteatoma may be present. In a child with middle-ear or mastoid infection, the presence of any systemic symptom, such as fever, headache, or lethargy, of extreme degree, or a finding of meningismus or of any central nervous system sign on physical examination should prompt suspicion of an intracranial complication.

When an intracranial complication is suspected, lumbar puncture should be performed only after imaging studies establish that there is no evidence of mass effect or hydrocephalus. In addition to examination of the cerebrospinal fluid, culture of middle ear exudate obtained via tympanocentesis may identify the causative organism, thereby helping guide the choice of antimicrobial drugs, and myringotomy should be performed to permit middle-ear drainage.

Intravenous antibiotic treatment of all intracranial complications, including surgical drainage of any abscess, is required urgently. If mastoiditis is present, mastoidectomy should be undertaken as soon as feasible. When meningitis develops as a complication of AOM, investigation should be directed at the possible presence of a perilymphatic fistula.

Lateral sinus thrombosis may be complicated by dissemination of infected thrombi with resultant development of septic infarcts in various organs. Diagnosis is facilitated through MRI. Mastoidectomy may be required even in the absence of osteitis or coalescent mastoiditis, especially in the case of propagation or embolization of infected thrombi. However, mastoiditis sometimes can be treated with tympanostomy tube placement and intravenous antibiotics. Anticoagulation therapy also may be considered in the treatment of lateral sinus thrombosis; however, an otolaryngologist should be consulted before initiating this therapy to coordinate the possible need for surgical intervention prior to anticoagulation.

Otitic hydrocephalus, also termed **benign intracranial hypertension** (pseudotumor cerebri), is an uncommon condition that consists of increased intracranial pressure without dilatation of the cerebral ventricles, occurring in association with acute or chronic OM or mastoiditis (see Chapter 604). The pathogenesis is uncertain, but the condition commonly is associated with lateral sinus thrombosis, and the pathophysiology may involve obstruction by thrombus of intracranial venous drainage into the neck, producing a rise in cerebral venous pressure and a consequent increase in cerebrospinal fluid pressure. Symptoms are those related to increased intracranial pressure. Signs may include, in addition to evidence of OM, paralysis of 1 or both lateral rectus muscles and papilledema. MRI can confirm the diagnosis. Treatment measures include the use of antimicrobials and drugs such as acetazolamide or furosemide to reduce intracranial pressure, mastoidectomy, repeated lumbar puncture, lumboperitoneal shunt, and ventriculoperitoneal shunt. If left untreated, otitic hydrocephalus may result in loss of vision secondary to optic atrophy.

PHYSICAL SEQUELAE

The physical sequelae of OM consist of structural middle-ear abnormalities resulting from long-standing middle-ear inflammation. In most instances, these sequelae are consequences of severe and/or chronic infection, but some also may result from the presumably noninfective inflammation of long-standing OME. The various sequelae may occur singly, or interrelatedly in various combinations.

Tympanosclerosis consists of whitish plaques in the tympanic membrane and nodular deposits in the submucosal layers of the middle ear. The changes involve hyalinization with deposition of calcium and phosphate crystals. There may be associated conductive hearing loss, but this is uncommon. In developed countries, probably the most common cause of tympanosclerosis is tympanostomy tube insertion.

Atelectasis of the tympanic membrane is a descriptive term applied to either severe retraction of the tympanic membrane caused by high negative middle-ear pressure or loss of stiffness and medial prolapse of the membrane, presumably as a consequence of long-standing retraction or severe or chronic inflammation. A retraction pocket is a localized area of atelectasis. Atelectasis often is transient and usually is not accompanied by symptoms, but a deep retraction pocket may lead to erosion of the ossicles and adhesive otitis, and may serve as the nidus of a cholesteatoma. For a deep retraction pocket, and for the unusual instance in which atelectasis is accompanied by symptoms such as otalgia, tinnitus, or conductive hearing loss, tympanostomy tube insertion is necessary.

Adhesive OM consists of proliferation of fibrous tissue in the middle-ear mucosa, which may. in turn. result in impaired movement of the ossicles, rarefying osteitis and ossicular discontinuity, conductive hearing loss, and cholesteatoma. The hearing loss may be amenable to surgical correction.

Cholesterol granuloma is an uncommon condition in which the tympanic membrane appears to be dark blue, reflecting the presence of thick, granulomatous material in the middle-ear cavity. The condition appears to result more often from long-standing OME than from frank middle-ear infection. Tympanostomy tube insertion alone does not provide satisfactory relief, and the required treatment is middle ear and mastoid surgery.

Chronic perforation may develop after spontaneous rupture of the tympanic membrane during an episode of AOM, as sequelae of chronic suppurative OM, from trauma, or as a result of failure of closure of the tympanic membrane following extrusion of a tympanostomy tube. A chronic perforation almost always is amenable to surgical repair, usually after the child has been free of OM for an extended period.

Permanent **conductive hearing loss** may result from any of the conditions just described. Rarely, permanent sensorineural hearing loss may occur in association with acute or chronic OM, presumably from the spread of infection or products of inflammation through the round window membrane, or as a consequence of suppurative labyrinthitis.

POSSIBLE DEVELOPMENTAL SEQUELAE

Permanent hearing loss in children has a significant negative impact on development, particularly delays in speech and language. The degree to which OM impacts long-term development in children is difficult to assess, and there have been conflicting studies examining this question. However, the developmental impact is most likely to be significant in children with greater levels of hearing loss, hearing loss that is sustained for longer periods of time, and hearing loss that is bilateral, and in those children who have other developmental difficulties or risk factors for developmental delay.

PREVENTION

General measures to prevent OM consist of breast-milk feeding; avoidance, insofar as possible, of exposure to individuals with respiratory infection; avoidance of environmental tobacco smoke; and pneumococcal vaccination.

IMMUNOPROPHYLAXIS

Heptavalent pneumococcal conjugate vaccine reduces the overall number of episodes of AOM by only 6–8%, but with a 57% reduction in serotype-specific episodes. Reductions of 9–23% are seen in children with histories of frequent episodes, and a 20% reduction is seen in the number of children undergoing tympanostomy tube insertion. The further development of vaccines against the pathogens that cause AOM offers promise of improved overall protection. Influenza vaccine also may provide a measure of protection against OM, but further studies are necessary to clarify its degree of efficacy. Passive immunization by exogenously administered immunoglobulin is not practicable because of the discomfort, risks, cost, and inconvenience entailed.

ANTIMICROBIAL PROPHYLAXIS

In children with frequent episodes of AOM, antimicrobial prophylaxis with subtherapeutic doses of an aminopenicillin or a sulfonamide offers variable protection against recurrences of AOM (although not of OME). However, because of the contribution of antimicrobial usage to bacterial resistance, the risks of sustained antimicrobial prophylaxis now appear, in general, to outweigh the likely benefits, particularly for children in daycare who, in any case, are at increased risk of colonization with multiply resistant *S. pneumoniae*. Prophylaxis may, nonetheless, be an appropriate option for the child with recurrent AOM who is cared for at home and usually away from other young children.

MYRINGOTOMY AND INSERTION OF TYMPANOSTOMY TUBES

In children with persistent OME, several studies have shown tympanostomy tube insertion to be effective in: reducing their subsequent proportion of time with MEE, improving their hearing levels, and also reducing their recurrence rate of AOM. In children with AOM, studies have demonstrated that tympanostomy tubes are quite effective in reducing the rate of recurrent AOM in patients. In both OME and AOM, quality-of-life studies have demonstrated a significant improvement in quality of life in children who have undergone surgical management with tympanostomy tube placement.

How best to manage the individual child who is severely affected with recurrent AOM must remain a matter of individual judgment and depends on a number of factors, including the severity of the episodes, risk factor profile, tolerance of antimicrobial therapy, hearing assessment, parental preferences, and the child's overall health and development. Reasonable interventions include continued reliance on episodic treatment with antimicrobial therapy, watchful waiting in episodes of AOM to attempt to reduce the overall use of antibiotics, or referral for tympanostomy tube placement.

ADENOIDECTOMY

Adenoidectomy is efficacious to some extent in reducing the risk of subsequent recurrences of both AOM and OME in children who have undergone tube insertion and in whom, after extrusion of tubes, OM continues to be a problem. Efficacy appears to be independent of adenoid size, and probably derives from removal of a focus of infection. In younger children with recurrent AOM who have not previously undergone tube insertion, however, adenoidectomy usually is not recommended along with the tube insertion, unless significant nasal airway obstruction or recurrent rhinosinusitis is associated, in which case, performing adenoidectomy might be considered.

Acuin J: Chronic suppurative otitis media. *BMJ* 2002;325:1159–1160.

American Academy of Family Physicians; American Academy of Otolaryngology–Head and Neck Surgery; American Academy of Pediatrics Subcommittee on Otitis Media With Effusion: Otitis media with effusion. *Pediatrics* 2004;113:1412–1429.

American Academy of Pediatrics Subcommittee on Management of Acute Otitis Media: Diagnosis and management of acute otitis media. *Pediatrics* 2004;113:1451–1465.

Arguedas A, Dagan R, Pichichero M, et al: An open-label, double tympanocentesis study of levofloxacin therapy in children with, or at high risk for, recurrent or persistent acute otitis media. *Pediatr Infect Dis J* 2006;25:1102–1108.

Bauchner H, Marchant CD, Bisbee A, et al: Effectiveness of Centers for Disease Control and Prevention recommendations for outcomes of acute otitis media. *Pediatrics* 2006;117:1009–1017.

Bluestone CD: Otitis media and congenital perilymphatic fistula as a cause of sensorineural hearing loss in children. *Pediatr Infect Dis J* 1988;7:S141.

Bodor FF: Systemic antibiotics for treatment of the conjunctivitis-otitis media syndrome. *Pediatr Infect Dis J* 1989;8:287–290.

Bodor FF, Marchant CD, Shurin PA, et al: Bacterial etiology of conjunctivitis–otitis media syndrome. *Pediatrics* 1985;76:26–28.

Fireman B, Black SB, Shinefield HR, et al: Impact of the pneumococcal conjugate vaccine on otitis media. *Pediatr Infect Dis J* 2003;22:10–16.

Garbutt J, Rosenbloom I, Wu J, et al: Empiric first-line antibiotic treatment of acute otitis in the era of the heptavalent pneumococcal conjugate vaccine. *Pediatrics* 2006;117:e1087–1094.

Hall-Stoodley L, Hu FZ, Gieske A, et al: Direct detection of bacterial biofilms on the middle-ear mucosa of children with chronic otitis media. *JAMA* 2006;296:202–211.

Hammaren-Malmi S, Saxen H, Tarkkanen J, et al: Adenoidectomy does not significantly reduce the incidence of otitis media in conjunction with the insertion of tympanostomy tubes in children who are younger than 4 years: A randomized trial. *Pediatrics* 2005;116:185–189.

Heikkinen T, Thint M, Chonmaitree T: Prevalence of various respiratory viruses in the middle ear during acute otitis media. *N Engl J Med* 1999;340:260–264.

Herbert RL, King GE, Bent JP: Tympanostomy tubes and water exposure. *Arch Otolaryngol Head Neck Surg* 1998;124:1118.

Isaacson G, Rosenfeld RM: Care of the child with tympanostomy tubes: A visual guide for the pediatrician. *Pediatrics* 1994;93:924.

Jose J, Coatesworth AP, Anthony R, et al: Life-threatening complications after partially treated mastoids. *BMJ* 2003;327:41–42.

Kerschner JE, Lindstrom DR, Pomeranz A, et al: Comparison of caregiver otitis media risk factor knowledge in suburban and urban primary care environments. *Int J Pediatr Otorhinolaryngol* 2005;69:49–56.

Koivunen P, Uhari M, Luotonen J, et al: Adenoidectomy versus chemoprophylaxis and placebo for recurrent acute otitis media in children aged under 2 years: Randomized controlled trial. *BMJ* 2004;328:487–490.

Marchetti F, Ronfani L, Nibali SC, et al: Delayed prescription may reduce the use of antibiotics for acute otitis media. *Arch Pediatr Adolesc Med* 2005;159:679–684.

McCormick DP, Chonmaitree T, Pittman C, et al: Nonsevere acute otitis media: A clinical trial comparing outcomes of watchful waiting versus immediate antibiotic treatment. *Pediatrics* 2005;115:1455–1465.

Palmu AAI, Herva E, Savolainen H, et al: Association of clinical signs and symptoms with bacterial findings in acute otitis media. *Clin Infect Dis* 2004;38:234–242.

Paradise JL, Elster BA, Tan L: Evidence in infants with cleft palate that breast milk protects against otitis media. *Pediatrics* 1994;94:853–860.

Paradise JL, Feldman HM, Campbell TF, et al: Tympanostomy tubes and developmental outcomes at 9 to 11 years of age. *N Engl J Med* 2007;356:248–261.

Rovers MM, Glasziou P, Appelman CL, et al: Antibiotics for acute otitis media: a meta-analysis with individual patient data. *Lancet* 2006;368:1429–1434.

Rovers MM, Schilder AGM, Zielhuis GA, et al: Otitis media. *Lancet* 2004;363:465–473.

Samuel J, Fernandes CMC, Steinberg JL: Intracranial otogenic complications: A persisting problem. *Laryngoscope* 1986;96:272.

Spiro DM, Tay KY, Arnold DH, et al: Wait-and-see prescription for the treatment of acute otitis media. *JAMA* 2006;296:1235–1241.

Stenstrom R, Pless IB, Bernard P: Hearing thresholds and tympanic membrane sequelae in children managed medically or surgically for otitis media with effusion. *Arch Pediatr Adolesc Med* 2005;159:1151–1156.

Subcommittee on Management of Acute Otitis Media: Diagnosis and management of acute otitis media. *Pediatrics* 2004;113:1451–1465.

Tonnaer ELGM, Graamans K, Sanders EAM, Curfs JHAJ: Advances in understanding the pathogenesis of pneumococcal otitis media. *Pediatr Infect Dis J* 2006;25:546–552.

Valtonen H, Tuomilehto H, Qvarnberg Y, et al: A 14-year prospective follow-up study of children treated early in life with tympanostomy tubes: Part 1: Clinical outcomes. *Arch Otolaryngol Head Neck Surg* 2005;131:293–298.

Valtonen H, Tuomilehto H, Qvarnberg Y, et al: A 14-year prospective follow-up study of children treated early in life with tympanostomy tubes: Part 2: Hearing outcomes. *Arch Otolaryngol Head Neck Surg* 2005;131:299–303.

Van Heerbeek N, Straetemans M, Wiertsema SP, et al: Effect of combined pneumococcal conjugate and polysaccharide vaccination on recurrent otitis media with effusion. *Pediatrics* 2006; 117:603–608.

Zapalac JS, Billings KR, Schwade ND, et al: Suppurative complications of acute otitis media in the era of antibiotic resistance. *Arch Otolaryngol Head Neck Surg* 2002;128:660–663.

Chapter 640 ■ The Inner Ear and Diseases of the Bony Labyrinth

Joseph Haddad Jr.

Genetic factors may affect the anatomy and function of the inner ear. Infectious agents, including viruses, bacteria, and protozoa, also may cause abnormal function, most commonly as sequelae of congenital infection or bacterial meningitis. Other acquired diseases of the labyrinthine capsule include otosclerosis, osteopetrosis, Langerhans' cell histiocytosis, fibrous dysplasia, and other types of bony dysplasia. All of these can cause both conductive and sensorineural hearing loss as well as vestibular dysfunction.

Use of currently available vaccines reduces the risk for bacterial meningitis and the associated sensorineural hearing loss.

VIRUSES. The most common cause of childhood sensorineural hearing loss (SNHL) is congenital cytomegalovirus (CMV) infection (see Chapter 252). Stabilization or possibly reversal of the hearing loss may be possible by using ganciclovir in very young infants with congenital CMV infection. Other viral causes of SNHL include congenital rubella as well as acquired mumps, rubella, rubeola (measles), and fifth disease, caused by parvovirus B19. Many other viruses also occasionally are associated with SNHL. In as many as 50% of cases, hearing loss, which usually is bilateral, although it often is asymmetric, progresses and worsens over weeks to years.

Before an effective vaccine was introduced, rubella was responsible for as many as 60% of cases of childhood SNHL. Vaccination in developed countries has reduced the rate of rubella by >97%. Similarly, measles and mumps are now uncommon causes of SNHL in the United States because of successful vaccination programs.

Herpes simplex encephalitis may also be associated with SNHL, which is more common in children with congenital herpesvirus infection. Acyclovir and other antiviral agents may help the hearing loss and other central nervous system manifestations (see Chapter 242).

TOXOPLASMOSIS. *Toxoplasma gondii* is a protozoan that may cause congenital SNHL. In the United States, about 3,000 children are born each yr with congenital toxoplasmosis, and approximately 25% of untreated patients have SNHL. If maternal infection is documented during the fetal period, medical therapy may be able to prevent some of the clinical manifestations, including SNHL of the offspring (see Chapter 287).

BACTERIAL MENINGITIS. Since the *Haemophilus influenzae* type b vaccine was introduced, *Streptococcus pneumoniae* and *Neisseria meningitidis* have become the leading causes of bacterial meningitis in children in the United States. Hearing loss occurs more commonly with *S. pneumoniae,* with an estimated incidence of 15–20%. Approximately 60% of the associated hearing loss is bilateral, although it often is asymmetric. If hearing loss is present at the time of presentation with meningitis, and especially if it is severe to profound, the likelihood of significant improvement is low. However, if the hearing loss develops after admission for treatment and is not severe, stabilization or improvement is possible. Late progression of SNHL also has been noted in some children years after meningitis. In the United States and many other developed countries, bacterial meningitis is one of the major causes of profound deafness leading to cochlear implantation in children. The introduction of pneumococcal conjugate vaccine is expected to lead to a reduction in SNHL due to pneumococcal meningitis.

Studies have shown favorable trends in the course and outcome after administration of dexamethasone for hearing loss and other neurologic deficits associated with bacterial meningitis (see Chapter 602.1), although its effectiveness, especially for *S. pneumoniae* and *N. meningitidis* meningitis, generally has not reached statistical significance because of the small number of cases in the trials. A meta-analysis of 11 studies conducted from 1988 to 1996 showed that dexamethasone reduced severe hearing loss associated with *H. influenzae* type b meningitis regardless of the timing of administration of dexamethasone (before or with antibiotics vs. later) or of the antibiotic used. For pneumococcal meningitis, the meta-analysis showed a benefit of dexamethasone only when given early and only for protection against severe hearing loss. Too few cases of meningococcal meningitis were included to assess the effect of dexamethasone on this entity.

SYPHILIS. Congenital syphilis, caused by *Treponema pallidum,* may cause SNHL in 3–38% of affected children (see Chapter 215). The exact incidence is difficult to ascertain, because the hearing loss may not develop until adolescence or even adulthood. When the condition is identified, treatment with antibiotics and corticosteroids may improve the hearing loss.

OTHER DISEASES OF THE INNER EAR. **Labyrinthitis** may be a complication of direct spread of infection from acute or chronic otitis media (OM) or mastoiditis and also may complicate bacterial meningitis as a result of organisms entering the labyrinth through the internal auditory meatus, endolymphatic duct, perilymphatic duct, vascular channels, or hematogenous spread. Clinical manifestations of labyrinthitis may include vertigo, dysequilibrium, deep-seated ear pain, nausea, vomiting, nystagmus, and SNHL. Acute suppurative labyrinthitis, characterized by abrupt, severe onset of these symptoms, requires intensive antimicrobial therapy. If it is secondary to OM, otologic surgery may be required to remove underlying cholesteatoma or drain the middle ear and mastoid, in addition to antibiotics. Acute serous labyrinthitis, with milder symptoms of vertigo and hearing loss, may develop secondary to middle-ear infection as well. It usually responds well to antibiotics and corticosteroids, with improvement in both vertigo and hearing. Chronic labyrinthitis, most commonly associated with cholesteatoma, presents with SNHL and vestibular dysfunction that develops over time; surgery is required to remove the cholesteatoma. Chronic labyrinthitis may also occur uncommonly secondary to long-standing OM, with the slow development of SNHL, usually starting in the higher frequencies, and possibly with vestibular dysfunction. Additionally, and more commonly, children with chronic middle-ear fluid often are unsteady or off balance, a situation that improves immediately when the fluid resolves.

Otosclerosis, an autosomal dominant disease that affects only the temporal bones, causes abnormal bone growth that can result in fixation of the stapes in the oval window, leading to progressive hearing loss. The hearing loss is usually conductive at first, but SNHL may develop. White females are affected most commonly, with onset of otosclerosis in teenagers or young adults, often associated with pregnancy. Corrective surgery to replace the stapes with a mobile prosthesis often is successful.

Osteogenesis imperfecta (OI) is a systemic disease that may involve both the middle and inner ears (see Chapter 699). Hearing loss occurs in about 20% of young children and as many as 90% of adults with this disease. The hearing loss most commonly is conductive because of abnormalities of the ossicles, but SNHL may occur if other areas of the otic capsule become affected. If the hearing loss is severe enough, a hearing aid may be a preferable alternative to surgical correction of the fixed stapes, because stapedectomy in children with OI can be technically very difficult, and the disease and the hearing loss may be progressive.

Osteopetrosis, a very uncommon skeletal dysplasia, may involve the temporal bone, including the middle ear and ossicles, resulting in a moderate to severe, usually conductive hearing loss. Recurrent facial nerve paralysis also may occur as a result of excess bone deposition; with each recurrence, less facial function may return (see Chapter 697).

Chapter 641 ■ Traumatic Injuries of the Ear and Temporal Bone

Joseph Haddad Jr.

AURICLE AND EXTERNAL AUDITORY CANAL. Auricle trauma is common in certain sports, and quick drainage of a hematoma can prevent irreversible damage. Hematoma, with accumulation of blood between the perichondrium and the cartilage, may follow trauma to the pinna and is especially common in teenagers related to wrestling or boxing. Immediate needle aspiration or, when the hematoma is extensive or recurrent, incision and drainage and a pressure dressing are necessary to prevent perichondritis, which can result in cartilage loss and a cauliflower ear deformity. Sports helmets should be warn when appropriate during activities when head trauma is possible.

Frostbite of the auricle should be managed by rapidly rewarming the exposed pinna with warm irrigation or warm compresses.

Foreign bodies in the external canal are common in childhood. These can often be removed in the office setting without general anesthesia if the child is mature enough to understand and cooperate and is properly restrained; if an adequate headlight, surgical head otoscope, or otomicroscope is used for visualizing the object; and if appropriate instruments, such as alligator forceps, wire loops or a blunt cerumen curette, or suction are used, depending on the shape of the object. Gentle irrigation of the ear canal with body temperature water or saline may be used to remove very small objects, but only if the tympanic membrane (TM) is intact. Attempted removal of an object from a struggling child or with poor visualization and inadequate tools results in a terrified child with a swollen and bleeding ear canal and may then mandate general anesthesia for removal of the object. Difficult foreign bodies, especially those that are large, deeply embedded or associated with canal swelling, are best removed under general anesthesia. Disk batteries are removed emergently because they leach a basic fluid that can cause severe tissue destruction. Insects in the canal are first killed with mineral oil or lidocaine, and are then removed under otomicroscopic examination.

After a foreign body is removed from the external canal, the TM should be carefully inspected for possible traumatic perforation or for a pre-existing middle-ear effusion. If a foreign body has resulted in acute inflammation of the canal, treatment as described for acute external otitis should be instituted (see Chapter 638).

TYMPANIC MEMBRANE AND MIDDLE EAR. Traumatic perforation of the TM usually occurs as a result of a sudden external compression, such as a slap, or penetration by a foreign object such as a stick or cotton-tipped applicator. The perforation may be linear or stellate. It is most frequently in the anterior portion of the pars tensa when it is caused by compression, and may be in any quadrant of the TM when caused by a foreign object. Systemic antibiotics and topical otic medications are not required unless suppurative otorrhea is present. Traumatic TM perforations often heal spontaneously, but it is important to evaluate and monitor the patient's hearing to ensure that spontaneous healing occurs. If the TM does not heal within several months, surgical graft repair should be considered. As long as the perforation is present, otorrhea may occur from water entering the middle ear from the ear canal, which can occur during swimming or bathing; appropriate precautions should be taken. Perforations resulting from penetrating foreign bodies are less likely to heal than those caused by compression. Audiometric examination reveals a conductive hearing loss (CHL), with larger air-bone gaps seen in larger perforations. Immediate surgical exploration is indicated if the injury is accompanied by one or more of the following: vertigo, nystagmus, severe tinnitus, moderate to severe hearing loss, or cerebrospinal fluid (CSF) otorrhea. At the time of exploration, it is necessary to inspect the ossicles, especially the stapes, because they may have been dislocated or fractured; examination also is made for sharp objects that may have penetrated the oval or round windows. Sensorineural hearing loss (SNHL) results if the stapes subluxates or dislocates into the oval window, or if either the oval or round window is penetrated. Children should not be given access to cotton-tipped applicators, as they commonly cause ear trauma. Contact with small objects should be limited to times of parental supervision.

Perilymphatic fistula (PLF) may occur after sudden barotrauma or an increase in CSF pressure. It should be suspected in a child who develops a sudden SNHL or vertigo after physical exertion, deep water diving, air travel, playing a wind instrument, or significant head trauma. The leak characteristically is at the oval or the round window and may be associated with congenital abnormalities of these structures or an anatomic abnormality of the cochlea or semicircular canals. PLFs occasionally close spontaneously, but immediate surgical repair of the fistula is recommended to control vertigo and to stop any progression of the SNHL; even timely surgery does not usually restore the SNHL. No reliable test is known for PLF, so middle-ear exploration is required for diagnosis and treatment.

TEMPORAL BONE FRACTURES. Children are particularly prone to basilar skull fractures, which usually involve the temporal bone. Temporal bone trauma should be considered in head injuries, and the status of the ear and hearing should be evaluated. From 70–80% of temporal bone fractures are longitudinal and are commonly manifested by bleeding from a laceration of the external canal or tympanic membrane; postauricular ecchymosis **(Battle sign)**; hemotympanum (blood behind an intact TM); CHL resulting from TM perforation, hemotympanum, or ossicular injury; delayed onset of facial paralysis (which usually improves spontaneously); and temporary CSF otorrhea or rhinorrhea (from CSF running down the eustachian tube). Transverse fractures of the temporal bone have a graver prognosis than longitudinal fractures and are often associated with immediate facial paralysis. Facial paralysis may improve if caused by edema, but surgical decompression of the nerve is often recommended, if there is no evidence of clinical recovery and facial nerve studies are unfavorable. If the facial nerve has been transected, surgical decompression and anastomosis offer the possibility of some functional recovery. Transverse fractures are also associated with severe SNHL, vertigo, nystagmus, tinnitus, nausea, and vomiting associated with loss of cochlear and vestibular function; hemotympanum; rarely, external canal bleeding; and CSF otorrhea, either in the external auditory canal or behind the TM, which may exit the nose via the eustachian tube.

If temporal bone fracture is suspected or seen on radiographs, gentle examination of the pinna and ear canal is indicated; lacerations or avulsion of soft tissue is common with temporal bone fractures. Vigorous removal of external auditory canal blood clots or tympanocentesis is not indicated, because clot removal may further dislodge the ossicles or reopen CSF leaks. The effectiveness of prophylactic antibiotics to prevent meningitis in patients with basilar skull fractures and CSF otorrhea or rhinorrhea cannot be determined because studies to date are flawed by biases. If a patient is afebrile and the drainage is not cloudy, watchful waiting without antibiotics is indicated. Surgical intervention is reserved for children who require repair of a nonhealing TM perforation, who have suffered dislocation of the ossicular chain, or who need decompression of the facial nerve. SNHL can also follow a blow to the head without an obvious fracture of the temporal bone (labyrinthine concussion).

ACOUSTIC TRAUMA. This results from exposure to high-intensity sound (fireworks, gunfire, rock music, heavy machinery) and is initially manifested by a temporary decrease in hearing threshold, most commonly at 4,000 Hz on an audiometric examination, and tinnitus. If the sound is between 85–140 dB, the loss is usually temporary (after a rock concert), but both the hearing loss and the tinnitus may become permanent with chronic noise exposure; the frequencies from 3,000 to 6,000 Hz are most often involved. Sudden, extremely loud (>140 dB), short-duration noises with loud peak components (gunfire, bombs) may cause permanent hearing loss after a single exposure. Ear protection and avoidance of chronic exposure to loud noise are preventive measures. Hearing loss due to chronic noise exposure should be entirely preventable. Parents should be made aware of the dangers of acoustic trauma, from the environment and from the use of headphones, and should take measures to minimize exposure.

Hough JVD, Stuart WD: Middle ear injuries in skull trauma. *Laryngoscope* 1968; 78:899–937.

Chapter 642 ■ Tumors of the Ear and Temporal Bone

Joseph Haddad Jr.

Suspicion for tumors of the ear and temporal bone may be raised by the appearance of a mass in the middle ear or mastoid, as well as signs of bleeding or local destruction. Imaging with CT or MRI allows for biopsy guidance to confirm the diagnosis and establish a treatment regimen.

Benign tumors of the external canal include osteomas and monostotic and polyostotic fibrous dysplasia. Osteomas present as bony masses in the canal and require removal only if hearing is impaired or external otitis results; osteomas may be confused clinically with exostoses (see Chapter 501.2).

Eosinophilic granuloma, which may occur in isolation or as part of the systemic Langerhans cell histiocytosis (see Chapter 507), should be suspected in patients with otalgia, otorrhea (sometimes bloody), hearing loss, abnormal tissue within the middle ear or ear canal, and roentgenographic findings of a sharply delineated destructive lesion of the temporal bone. Definitive diagnosis is made by biopsy. Treatment depends on the site of the lesion and histology. Depending on the site, it may be treated by surgical excision, curettage, or local radiation. If the lesion is part of a systemic presentation of Langerhans' cell histiocytosis, chemotherapy in addition to local therapy (surgery with or without radiation) is indicated. Long-term follow-up is necessary whether the temporal bone lesion is a single isolated lesion or part of a multisystem disease.

Symptoms and signs of rhabdomyosarcoma originating in the middle ear or ear canal include a mass or polyp in the middle ear or ear canal, bleeding from the ear, otorrhea, otalgia, facial paralysis, and hearing loss. Other cranial nerves also may be involved. Diagnosis is based on biopsy, but the extent of disease is determined by both CT and MRI of the temporal bone, skull base, and brain. Management usually involves a combination of chemotherapy, radiation, and surgery (see Chapter 501).

Non-Hodgkin lymphoma and leukemia also may present rarely in the temporal bone. Although primary neoplasms of the middle ear are very uncommon in children, they include adenoid cystic carcinoma, adenocarcinoma, and squamous cell carcinoma. Benign tumors of the temporal bone include glomus tumors. The initial signs and symptoms of the more common nasopharyngeal neoplasms (angiofibroma, rhabdomyosarcoma, epidermoid carcinoma) may be associated with insidious onset of chronic otitis media with effusion (often unilateral). A high index of suspicion is needed for diagnosing these tumors early.

Part XXX ■ The Skin

Chapter 643 ■ Morphology of the Skin

Joseph G. Morelli

EPIDERMIS. The mature epidermis is a stratified epithelial tissue composed predominantly of keratinocytes. The function of the epidermis is protection of the organism from the external environment and the prevention of water loss. The process of epidermal differentiation results in the formation of a functional barrier to the external world. Keratinocytes are composed largely of keratin filaments. These proteins are members of the family of intermediate filaments. The predominant keratins expressed within the keratinocytes change with cellular differentiation. The epidermis consists of four histologically recognizable layers. The basal layer consists of columnar cells that rest on the dermal-epidermal junction. Basal keratinocytes are connected to the dermal-epidermal junction by hemidesmosomes. Basal keratinocytes are attached to themselves and to the cells in the spinous layer by desmosomal, gap, and adherens junctions. The role of the basal keratinocyte is to serve as a continuing supply of keratinocytes for the normally differentiating epidermis as well as a reservoir of cells to repair epidermal damage. The 2nd layer consists of 3 to 4 rows of spinous cells. Their role is to begin formation of the epidermal barrier and to initiate vitamin D synthesis. The next layer consists of 2 to 3 rows of granular appearing cells. Granular cells continue the process of epidermal barrier formation and prepare for the formation of the stratum corneum, which is composed of multiple layers of dead, highly compacted cells. The dead cells are composed mainly of disulfide bonded keratins. The intercellular spaces are composed of hydrophobic lipids, predominantly ceramides. As the stratum corneum is replenished, the old stratum corneum is shed in a highly regulated process. The normal process of epidermal differentiation from basal cell to shedding of stratum corneum takes 28 days.

In addition to keratinocytes, the epidermis contains 3 other cell types. The melanocytes are pigment-forming cells, which are responsible for skin color and protection from ultraviolet radiation. Epidermal melanocytes are derived from the **neural crest** and migrate to the skin during embryonic life. They reside in the interfollicular epidermis and in the hair follicles and increase in number in the epidermis by mitosis or migration of additional cells into the epidermis. Melanocytes produce intracellular organelles (melanosomes) containing melanin. There is approximately 1 melanocyte per 36 keratinocytes in the epidermal melanin unit. The melanosomes are then transferred via melanocyte dendrites to the keratinocytes. Merkel cells are type-I slow-adapting mechanosensory receptors for touch. Langerhans cells are dendritic cells of the mononuclear phagocyte system. They are recognized electron microscopically by a specific organelle, the Birbeck granule. These cells are derived from bone marrow and participate in immune reactions in the skin, playing an active part in antigen presentation and processing.

The junction of the epidermis and dermis is the basement membrane zone. This complex structure is a result of contributions from both epidermal and mesenchymal cells. The dermal-epidermal junction extends from the basal cell plasma membrane to the uppermost region of the dermis. Ultrastructurally, the basement membrane appears as a trilaminar structure, consisting of a lamina lucida immediately adjacent to the basal cell plasma membrane, a central lamina densa, and the subbasal lamina on the dermal side of the lamina densa. Several structures within this zone act to anchor the epidermis to the dermis. The plasma membrane of basal cells contains electron-dense plates known as hemidesmosomes; tonofilaments course within basal cells to insert at these sites. The hemidesmosomes are composed of 180 and 230 kd bullous pemphigoid antigens, $\alpha6\beta4$ and $\alpha3\beta1$ integrins, and plectin. Anchoring filaments originate in the plasma membrane, primarily near the hemidesmosomes, and insert into the lamina densa. Anchoring fibrils, composed predominantly of type VII collagen, extend from the lamina densa into the uppermost dermis where they insert into anchoring plaques.

DERMIS. The dermis provides the skin with most of its mechanical properties. The dermis forms a tough, pliable, fibrous supporting structure between the epidermis and the subcutaneous fat. It consists of collagen and elastic and reticulin fibers embedded in an amorphous ground substance; it contains blood vessels, lymphatics, mast cells, neural structures, eccrine and apocrine sweat glands, hair follicles, sebaceous glands, and smooth muscle. Morphologically, the dermis can be divided into 2 layers: the superficial papillary layer that interdigitates with the rete ridges of the epidermis and the deeper reticular layer that lies beneath the papillary dermis. The papillary layer is less dense and more cellular, whereas the reticular layer appears more compact because of the coarse network of interlaced collagen and elastic fibers.

The predominant dermal cell is a spindle-shaped fibroblast that is responsible for the synthesis of collagen, elastic fibers, and mucopolysaccharides. Phagocytic histiocytes, mast cells, and motile leukocytes are also present. The gelatinous ground substance serves as a supporting medium for the fibrillar and cellular components and as a storage place for a substantial portion of body water. Nutrients are supplied to both epidermis and dermis by the dermal blood vessels.

SUBCUTANEOUS TISSUE. Panniculus, or subcutaneous tissue, consists of fat cells and fibrous septa that divide it into lobules and anchor it to the underlying fascia and periosteum. Blood vessels and nerves are also present in this layer, which serves as a storage depot for lipid, an insulator to conserve body heat, and a protective cushion against trauma.

APPENDAGEAL STRUCTURES. These structures are derived from aggregates of epidermal cells that become specialized during early embryonic development. Small buds (primary epithelial germs) appear in the 3rd fetal month and give rise to hair follicles, sebaceous and apocrine glands, and the attachment bulges for the arrector pili muscles. Eccrine sweat glands are derived from separate epidermal downgrowths that arise in the 2nd fetal month and are completely formed by the 5th month. Formation of nails is initiated in the 3rd intrauterine month.

HAIR FOLLICLES. The hair follicle is the most prominent structure in the pilary complex, which includes the sebaceous gland, the arrector pili muscle, and, in areas such as the axillae, an apocrine gland. Hair follicles are distributed throughout the skin, except in the palms, soles, lips, and glans penis; if destroyed, they cannot regenerate. Individual follicles extend from the surface of the epidermis to the deep dermis. The hair follicle is divided into four segments: the infundibulum, which extends from the skin surface to the opening of the sebaceous duct; the isthmus, extending from the sebaceous duct opening to the bulge; the lower follicle between the bulge and the hair bulb; and the hair bulb. The bulge is at the insertion of the arrector pili muscle. The bulge is the site of the skin stem cells. The differentiation fate of these stem cells is in part controlled by *c-myc*. The bulb is where the matrix cells and the dermal papilla are involved in formation and maintenance of the hair. The growing hair consists of the hair shaft and its supporting sheaths.

Human hair growth is cyclic, with alternate periods of growth (**anagen**) and rest (**telogen**). The length of the anagen phase varies from months to years. At birth, all hairs are in the anagen phase. Subsequent generative activity lacks synchrony, so that an overall random pattern of growth and shedding prevails. At any time, ≈85% of hairs are in the anagen phase. Scalp hair usually grows about 1 cm/mo.

The types of hair are fetal lanugo, terminal, and vellus. Lanugo hair is thin and short; this hair is shed before term and is replaced by vellus hair by 36–40 wk of gestation. Terminal hair is long and coarse and is found on the scalp, beard, eyebrows, eyelashes, and axillary and pubic areas. Vellus hair is short, soft, and frequently unpigmented and is distributed over the rest of the body. During puberty, androgenic hormone stimulation causes pubic, axillary, and beard hair to change from vellus hair to terminal hair.

SEBACEOUS GLANDS. These glands occur in all areas except the palms and soles and dorsa of the feet, but they are most numerous on the face, upper chest, and back. Their ducts open into the hair follicles except on the lips, prepuce, and labia minora, where they emerge directly onto the mucosal surface. These holocrine glands are saccular structures that are often branched and lobulated and consist of a proliferative basal layer of small flat cells peripheral to the central mass of lipidized cells. The latter cells disintegrate as they move toward the duct and form the lipid secretion known as sebum, which consists of cellular debris, triglycerides, phospholipids, and cholesterol esters. Sebaceous glands depend on hormonal stimulation and are activated by androgens at puberty. Fetal sebaceous glands are stimulated by maternal androgens, and their lipid secretion, together with desquamated stratum corneum cells, constitutes the vernix caseosa.

APOCRINE GLANDS. The apocrine glands are located in the axillae, areolae, perianal and genital areas, and the periumbilical region. These large, coiled, tubular structures continuously secrete an odorless milky fluid that is discharged in response to adrenergic stimuli, usually a result of emotional stress. Bacterial decomposition of apocrine sweat accounts for the unpleasant odor associated with perspiration. Apocrine glands remain dormant until puberty, when they enlarge and secretion begins in response to androgenic activity. The secretory coil of the gland consists of a single layer of cells enclosed by a layer of contractile myoepithelial cells. The duct is lined with a double layer of cuboidal cells and opens into the pilosebaceous complex. Although apocrine glands do not function in thermoregulation, they are involved in certain disease processes.

ECCRINE SWEAT GLANDS. These glands are distributed over the entire body surface, including the palms and soles, where they are most abundant. Those on the hairy skin respond to thermal stimuli and serve to regulate body temperature by delivering water to the skin surface for evaporation; in contrast, sweat glands on the palms and soles respond mainly to psychophysiologic stimuli.

Each eccrine gland consists of a secretory coil located in the reticular dermis or subcutaneous fat and a secretory duct that opens onto the skin surface. Sweat pores can be identified on the epidermal ridges of the palm and fingers with a magnifying lens but are not readily visualized elsewhere. Two types of cells compose the single-layered secretory coil: small dark cells and large clear cells. These rest on a layer of contractile myoepithelial cells and a basement membrane. The glands are supplied by sympathetic nerve fibers, but the pharmacologic mediator of sweating is acetylcholine rather than epinephrine. Sweat consists of water, sodium, potassium, calcium, chloride, phosphorus, lactate, and small quantities of iron, glucose, and protein. The composition varies with the rate of sweating but is always hypotonic in normal children.

NAILS. Nails are specialized protective epidermal structures that form convex, translucent, tight-fitting plates on the distal dorsal surfaces of the fingers and toes. The nail plate, which is derived from a metabolically active matrix of multiplying cells situated beneath the posterior nail fold, grows forward at a rate of ≈1 cm every 3 months. The nail plate is bounded by the lateral and posterior nail folds; a thin eponychium (the cuticle) protrudes from the posterior fold over a crescent-shaped white area called the lunula. The pink color reflects the underlying vascular bed.

Eckes B, Krieg T: Regulation of connective tissue homeostasis in the skin by mechanical forces. *Clin Exp Rheumatol* 2004;22:S73–S76.

Groscurth P: Anatomy of sweat glands. *Curr Prob Dermatol* 2002;30:1–9.

Honeycutt KA, Koster MI, Roop DR: Genes involved in stem cell fate decisions and commitment to differentiation play a role in skin disease. *J Investig Dermatol Symp Proc* 2004;9:261–268.

Marks R: The stratum corneum barrier: The final frontier. *J Nutr* 2004;134:2017S–2021S.

McCarthy DJ: Anatomic consideration of the human nail. *Clin Podiatr Med Surg* 2004;4:477–491.

McMillan Jr, Akiyama M, Shimizu H: Epidermal basement membrane zone components: Ultrastructure, distribution and molecular interactions. *J Dermatol Sci* 2003;31:169–177.

Thiboutot D: Regulation of human sebaceous glands. *J Invest Dermatol* 2004;123:1–12.

Chapter 644 ■ Evaluation of the Patient

Joseph G. Morelli

HISTORY AND PHYSICAL EXAMINATION. Although many skin disorders are easily recognized by simple inspection, the history and physical examination are often necessary for accurate assessment. The entire body surface, mucous membranes, conjunctiva, hair, and nails should always be examined thoroughly under adequate illumination. The color, turgor, texture, temperature, and moisture of the skin and the growth, texture, caliber, and luster of the hair and nails should be noted. Skin lesions should be palpated, inspected, and classified on the bases of morphology, size, color, texture, firmness, configuration, location, and distribution. One must also decide whether the changes are those of the primary lesion itself or whether the clinical pattern has been altered by a secondary factor such as infection, trauma, or therapy.

Primary lesions are classified as macules, papules, patches, plaques, nodules, tumors, vesicles, bullae, pustules, wheals, and cysts. A **macule** represents an alteration in skin color but cannot be felt. When the lesion is >1 cm, the term **patch** is used. **Papules** are palpable solid lesions <0.5–1 cm, whereas **nodules** are larger in diameter. **Tumors** are usually larger than nodules and vary considerably in mobility and consistency. **Vesicles** are raised, fluid-filled lesions <0.5 cm in diameter; when larger, they are called **bullae. Pustules** contain purulent material. **Wheals** are flat-topped, palpable lesions of variable size, duration, and configuration that represent dermal collections of edema fluid. **Cysts** are circumscribed, thick-walled lesions that are located deep in the skin; they are covered by a normal epidermis and contain fluid or semisolid material. Aggregations of papules are referred to as **plaques.**

Primary lesions may change into secondary lesions, or secondary lesions may develop over time where no primary lesion existed. Primary lesions are usually more helpful for diagnostic purposes than secondary lesions. Secondary lesions include scales, ulcers, erosions, excoriations, fissures, crusts, and scars. **Scales** consist of compressed layers of stratum corneum cells that are retained on the skin surface. **Erosions** involve focal loss of the epidermis, and they heal without scarring. **Ulcers** extend into the dermis and tend to heal with scarring. Ulcerated lesions inflicted by scratching are often linear or angular in configuration and are called **excoriations. Fissures** are caused by splitting or cracking; they usually occur in diseased skin. **Crusts** consist of matted, retained accumulations of blood, serum, pus, and epithelial debris on the surface of a weeping lesion. **Scars** are end-stage lesions that can be thin, depressed and atrophic, raised and hypertrophic, or flat and pliable; they are composed of fibrous connective tissue. **Lichenification** is a thickening of skin with accentuation of normal skin lines that is caused by chronic irritation (rubbing, scratching) or inflammation.

If the diagnosis is not clear after a thorough examination, one or more diagnostic procedures may be indicated.

BIOPSY OF SKIN. Biopsy of skin is occasionally required for diagnosis. Punch biopsy is a simple, relatively painless procedure and usually provides adequate tissue for examination if the appropriate lesion is sampled. The selection of a fresh, well-developed primary lesion is extremely important to obtain an accurate diagnosis. The site of the biopsy should have relatively low risk for damage to underlying dermal structures. After cleansing of the site, the skin is anesthetized by application of EMLA cream (containing lidocaine and prilocaine) and/or intradermal injection of 1–2% lidocaine (Xylocaine), with or without epinephrine, with a 27- or 30-gauge needle. A punch, 3 or 4 mm in diameter, is pressed firmly against the skin and rotated until it sinks to the proper depth. All three layers (epidermis, dermis, subcutis) should be contained in the plug. The plug should be lifted gently with forceps or extracted with a needle and separated from the underlying tissue with iris scissors. Bleeding abates with firm pressure and with suturing. The biopsy specimen should be placed in 10% formaldehyde solution (Formalin) for appropriate processing.

WOOD'S LAMP. The Wood's lamp transmits ultraviolet light mainly in a wavelength of 365 nm. The examination, which is performed in a darkened room, is useful in detecting hypopigmented macules and certain superficial fungal infections of the scalp. Blue-green fluorescence is detectable at the base of each infected hair shaft in ectothrix and in some endothrix infections. Scales and crusts may appear pale yellow, but this is not evidence of a fungal infection. Dermatophyte lesions of the skin (tinea corporis) do not fluoresce; macules of tinea versicolor, however, have a golden fluorescence under a Wood's lamp. Erythrasma, an intertriginous infection caused by *Corynebacterium minutissimum,* may fluoresce pink-orange, whereas *Pseudomonas aeruginosa* is yellow-green under a Wood's lamp. Discrete areas of altered pigment can often be visualized more clearly by using a Wood's lamp, particularly if the pigmentary change is epidermal. Hyperpigmented lesions appear darker, and hypopigmented lesions (**tuberous sclerosis**) lighter than the surrounding skin.

POTASSIUM HYDROXIDE (KOH) PREPARATION. This provides a rapid and reliable method for detecting fungal elements of both yeasts and dermatophytes. Scaly lesions should be scraped at the active border for optimal recovery of mycelia and spores. Vesicles should be unroofed, and the blister top should be clipped and placed on a slide for examination. In tinea capitis, infected hairs must be plucked from the follicle; scales from the scalp do not usually contain mycelia. A few drops of 20% KOH are added to the specimen, which is then gently heated over an alcohol lamp until it begins to bubble; alternatively, ample time (≈10–20 min) can be allowed for dissolution of the keratin. Dimethyl sulfoxide (DMSO) can be included in the KOH solution. The preparation is examined under low-intensity light for fungal elements.

TZANCK SMEAR. This is useful in the diagnosis of some viral infections (herpes simplex, varicella, herpes zoster, eczema herpeticum) and for the detection of acantholytic cells in pemphigus. An intact, fresh blister should be ruptured and drained of fluid. The base of the blister is then scraped with a dull-edged instrument, taking care to avoid drawing a significant amount of blood; the material is smeared on a clear glass slide and air dried. Staining with Giemsa stain is preferable, but Wright stain is acceptable. Balloon cells and multinucleated giant cells are diagnostic of herpesvirus infection; acantholytic epidermal cells are characteristic of pemphigus.

The direct fluorescent assay is more sensitive and specific. The keratinocytes are scraped from the base of the blister as described earlier. The laboratory stains the slide with labeled antibodies specific for varicella-zoster virus or herpes simplex virus. Observation of the slide with a fluorescence microscope documents the presence of the specific virus within the cells. PCR for herpesviruses is rapid, safe, and both specific and sensitive.

IMMUNOFLUORESCENCE STUDIES. Immunofluorescence studies of skin can be used to detect tissue-fixed antibodies to skin components and complement; characteristic staining patterns are specific for certain skin disorders. Serum can be used for identifying circulating antibodies. Skin biopsy specimens for direct immunofluorescence preparations should be obtained from involved sites except in those diseases for which perilesional skin or uninvolved skin is required (Table 644-1). A punch biopsy sample is obtained, and the tissue is placed in a special transport medium or immediately frozen in liquid nitrogen for transport or storage. Thin cryostat sections of the specimen are incubated with fluorescein-conjugated antibodies to the specific antigens.

Serum of patients can be examined by indirect immunofluorescence techniques using sections of normal human skin, guinea pig lip, or monkey esophagus as substrate. The substrate is incubated with fresh or thawed frozen serum and then with fluorescein-conjugated antihuman globulin. If the serum contains antibody to epithelial components, its specific staining pattern can be seen on fluorescence microscopy. By serial dilution, the titer of circulating antibody can be estimated.

Mtuasim DF, Adams BB: Immunofluorescence in dermatology. *J Am Acad Dermatol* 2001;45:822–824.

Weston WL, Lane AT, Morelli JG: Evaluation of children with skin disease. In *Color Textbook of Pediatric Dermatology.* St. Louis, Mosby, 2002.

644.1 • Cutaneous Manifestations of Systemic Diseases

Selected diseases have signature skin findings, often as the presenting sign of illness, which can facilitate the assessment of complex medical patients (Table 644-2).

TABLE 644-1. Immunofluorescent Findings in Immune-Mediated Cutaneous Diseases

DISEASE	INVOLVED SKIN	UNINVOLVED SKIN	DIRECT IF	INDIRECT IF	CIRCULATING ANTIBODIES
Dermatitis herpetiformis	Negative	Positive	Granular IgA ± C in papillary dermis	None	IgA antireticulum in 20–70%. Antiendomysial (IgA, IgG) and transglutaminase antibodies with celiac disease
Bullous pemphigoid	Positive	Positive	Linear IgG and C band in BMZ, occasionally IgM, IgA, IgE	IgG to BMZ in 70%	None
Pemphigus (all variants)	Positive	Positive	IgG in intercellular spaces of epidermis between keratinocytes	IgG to intercellular space	None
Pemphigus foliaceus	Positive	Positive	IgG to desmosomal glycoprotein, desmoglein 1	Same as direct IF	None
Herpes gestationis	Positive	Positive	C3 at BMZ, occasionally IgG	IgG anti-BMZ	None
Linear IgA bullous dermatosis (chronic bullous dermatosis of childhood)	Positive	Positive	Linear IgA at BMZ, occasionally C	Low titer, rare IgA, anti-BMZ	None
Discoid lupus erythematosus	Positive	Negative	Linear IgG, IgM, IgA, and C3 at BMZ (lupus band)	None	ANA negative
Systemic lupus erythematosus	Positive	Variable; exposed to sun, 30–50%; nonexposed, 10–30%	Linear IgG, IgM, C3 at BMZ (lupus band)	None	ANA Anti-Ro (SSA) Anti-RNP Anti-DNA Anti-Sm
Henoch-Schönlein purpura	Positive	Positive	IgA around vessel walls	None	IgA rheumatoid factor, occasionally

ANA, antinuclear antibody; BMZ, basement membrane zone at the dermal-epidermal junction; C, complement; IF, immunofluorescent findings; Ig, immunoglobulin.

TABLE 644-2. Characteristics of Cutaneous Signs of Systemic Diseases

DISEASE	AGE OF ONSET	SKIN LESIONS	DISTRIBUTION	DIAGNOSTIC EVALUATIONS	ASSOCIATED SYMPTOMS/SIGNS	DIFFERENTIAL DIAGNOSIS
Systemic lupus erythematosus	Any	Erythematous patches; palpable purpura; livedo reticularis; Raynaud phenomenon; thrombocytopenic and non-thrombocytopenic purpura	Photodistribution; "malar" face	ANA panel Anti-double stranded DNA Leukopenia/lymphopenia Thrombocytopenia Complement levels Urinalysis	Arthritis Nephritis Cerebritis Serositis	Seborrheic dermatitis Rosacea Atopic dermatitis Juvenile dermatomyositis Vasculitis
Discoid lupus	Adolescents	Annular, scaly plaques; atrophy; dyspigmentation	Photodistribution	ANA	Scarring	Subacute cutaneous lupus Polymorphous light eruption Juvenile dermatomyositis
Neonatal lupus	Newborn to 6 mo	Annular, erythematous, scaly plaques	Photodistribution; head/neck	ANA Anti-Ro	Heart block Thrombocytopenia	Tinea capitis Atopic dermatitis Seborrheic dermatitis
Juvenile dermatomyositis	Any	Erythematous to violaceous scaly, macules; discrete papules overlying knuckles	Periocular face; shoulder girdle; extensor extremities; knuckles; palms	ANA Jo-1 Ab Aldolase CK LDH	Proximal muscle weakness Calcifications Vasculopathy	Atopic dermatitis Allergic contact dermatitis Lupus erythematosus Viral exanthem Drug eruption
Henoch-Schönlein purpura	Children and adolescents	Purpuric papules and plaques	Buttocks; lower extremities	Urinalysis Bun/Cr Skin biopsy	Abdominal pain Arthritis	Vasculitis Drug eruption Infantile hemorrhagic edema
Kawasaki disease	Infants, children	Erythematous maculopapular to urticarial plaques; acral and groin erythema, edema, desquamation	Diffuse	Leukocytosis ESR CRP Thrombocytosis	Strawberry tongue Conjunctivitis Lymphadenopathy Cardiovascular complications	Viral exanthem Viral syndrome Drug eruption Staphylococcal/streptococcal illness
Inflammatory bowel disease	Children and adolescents	Aphthae; erythema nodosum; pyoderma gangrenosum; thrombophlebitis	Oral ulcers; perianal fissures	ESR Thrombocytosis Radiographic abnormalities	Abdominal pain Diarrhea Cramping Arthritis Conjunctivitis	Behçet syndrome Vasculitis *Yersinia colitis*
Sweet syndrome	Any	Infiltrated erythematous, edematous plaques	Diffuse	Skin biopsy Leukocytosis ESR	Fever Flulike illness Conjunctivitis	Infection Urticaria Erythema multiforme Urticarial vasculitis
Graft vs host disease	Any	Acute: erythema, papules, vesicles, bulla	Head and neck; palms/soles; diffuse	Skin biopsy Liver function	Fever Mucositis Hepatitis	Drug eruption Infectious exanthem
Hypersensitivity reaction	Any	Erythema; urticarial macules and plaques	Diffuse	Liver function Eosinophilia Atypical lymphocytosis	Perioral edema Lymphadenopathy Fever Hepatitis	Stevens-Johnson syndrome Infectious exanthem
Serum sickness-like reaction	Any	Edematous, purpuric plaques	Acral; diffuse	ESR	Fever Lymphadenopathy Arthritis, nephritis	Kawasaki disease Connective tissue disease

ANA, antinuclear antibodies; CK, creatine kinase; CRP, C-reactive protein; ESR, erythrocyte sedimentation rate; LDH, lactate dehydrogenase.

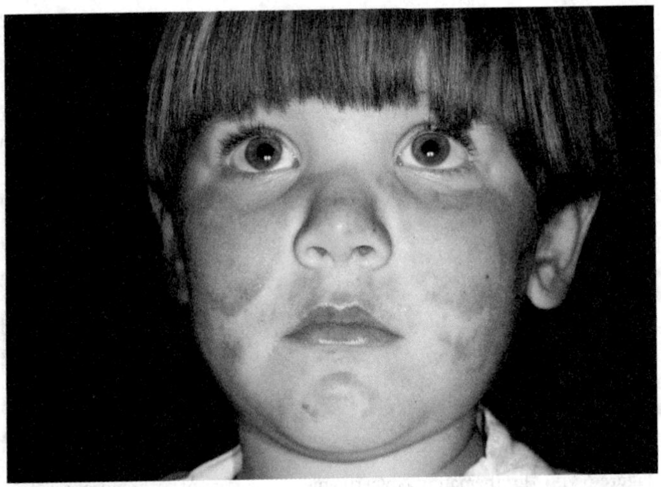

Figure 644-1. Malar rash of systemic lupus erythematosus (SLE).

CONNECTIVE TISSUE DISEASES

LUPUS ERYTHEMATOSUS. Lupus erythematosus (LE; see Chapter 157) is an idiopathic autoimmune inflammatory disease that may be multisystemic or confined to the skin.

Systemic Lupus Erythematosus. Systemic LE (SLE) is a chronic inflammatory multisystem disease. It is a diagnosed when 4 of 11 well-defined criteria are present (see Chapter 157). Three of the criteria are skin findings. Criteria 1 is the classic malar or "butterfly" rash (Fig. 644-1). It must be distinguished from other causes of a "red face," most notably seborrheic dermatitis, atopic dermatitis, and rosacea. Criteria 2 is a discoid rash. Criteria 3 is a photosensitive erythematous macular or papular eruption (Fig. 644-2). Other associated but not diagnostic cutaneous findings include purpuric lesions, livedo reticularis, mucosal ulcerations, Raynaud phenomena, and nonscarring alopecia.

Cutaneous LE demonstrates varying degrees of epidermal atrophy, plugging of hair follicles, and a vacuolar alteration at an inflamed dermal-epidermal junction. Immunoglobulin (IgM, IgG) and complement deposition in lesional skin may help confirm the diagnosis (see Table 644-1). Immune deposits in nonlesional sun-exposed skin are found in the majority of patients with SLE (lupus band test). Treatment of skin lesions includes sun protection and low- to mid-potency topical corticosteroids.

Neonatal Lupus Erythematosus. Neonatal LE (NLE; see Chapter 157.1) presents during the 1st weeks to months of life as annular, erythematous, scaly plaques, typically on the head, neck, and upper trunk (Fig. 644-3). Ultraviolet light may exacerbate or initiate cutaneous lesions. NLE is often misdiagnosed as infantile eczema, seborrheic dermatitis, or tinea corporis. Passive transfer of maternal IgG (anti-Ro/La, SS-A/SS-B) antibodies cause the transient skin lesions; antibody levels wane by 6 mo, generally resulting in clearance of the rash. Congenital heart block occurs in 30% of affected infants, but only 10% of affected infants have both skin and cardiac abnormalities. Noncardiac extracutaneous manifestations such as anemia, thrombocytopenia, and cholestatic liver disease are uncommon. Maternal antibody (antinuclear antibody [ANA]) testing is indicated.

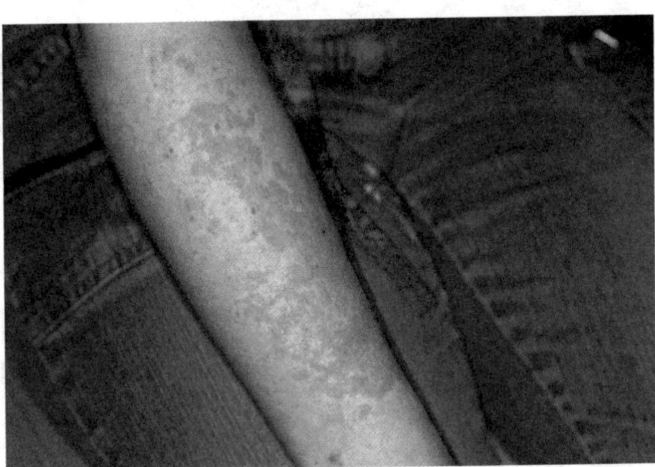

Figure 644-2. Photosensitive rash of systemic lupus erythematosus (SLE).

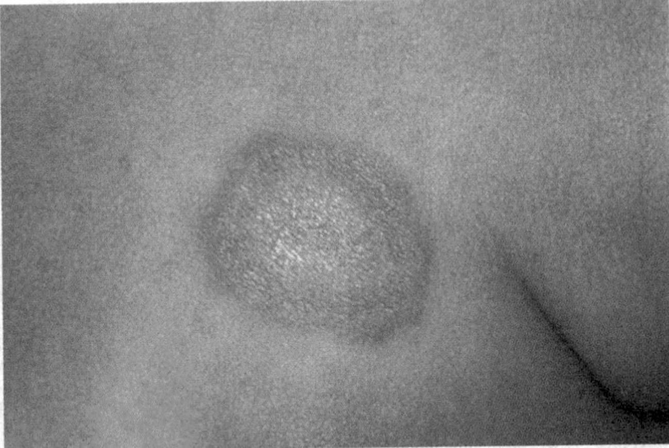

Figure 644-3. Annular plaque in neonatal lupus erythematosus (NLE).

Discoid Lupus Erythematosus. Discoid LE (DLE) is uncommon in early childhood and presents in late adolescence. The signature skin findings in DLE are chronic, erythematous, scaly, atrophic, telangiectatic plaques (Fig. 644-4) on sun-exposed skin that frequently heal with scarring and dyspigmentation. Extracutaneous features may include involvement of the nasal and oral mucosa, eyes, and nails. The **differential diagnosis** includes other photodermatoses such as polymorphous light eruption, juvenile springtime eruption, and juvenile dermatomyositis. There is a distinct overlap between SLE and DLE with common histopathologic features and photoexacerbation; most patients with DLE have normal laboratory studies and do not progress to systemic disease. Topical sunscreens and steroids may be helpful. Intralesional steroids and oral antimalarials (hydroxychloroquine) are used with severe disease.

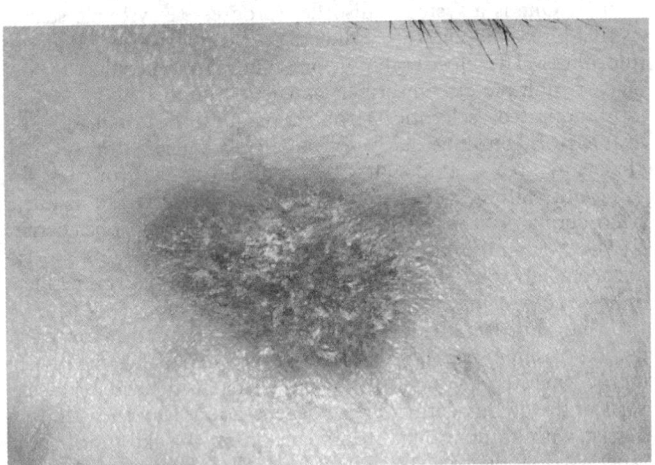

Figure 644-4. Erythematous scaly plaque of discoid lupus erythematosus (DLE).

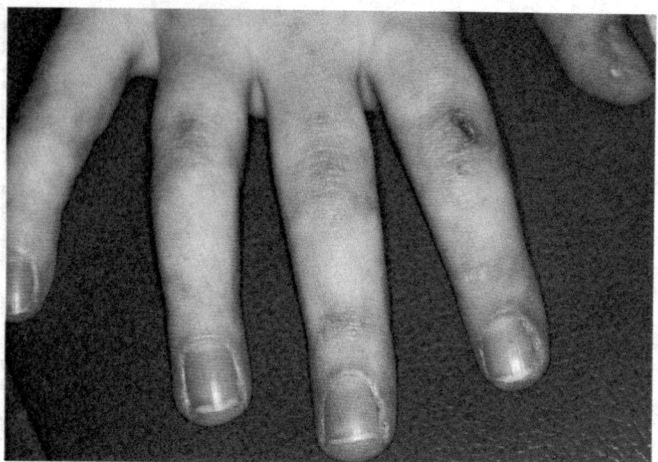

Figure 644-5. Gottron's papules in juvenile dermatomyositis.

Figure 644-6. Erythematous, hyperpigmented plaque of early morphea.

JUVENILE DERMATOMYOSITIS. Characteristic skin findings are often the presenting sign of juvenile dermatomyositis (JDMS; see Chapter 158). An ill-defined, erythematous to violaceous, scaly, minimally pruritic eruption occurs in photodistributed areas such as the face, upper trunk, and extensor extremities. Circumscribed periocular involvement of this **heliotrope** rash may take the appearance of "raccoon eyes," particularly in young children. Distinctive papules overlying the knuckles (**Gottron papules**) are helpful in suggesting the diagnosis in the absence of associated muscle weakness (Fig. 644-5). Other cutaneous features include nail fold and gingival margin telangiectasia, palmar hyperkeratosis ("mechanic's hands"), and a poikilodermatous (dyspigmentation and telangiectasia) eruption over the shoulder girdle ("shawl sign"). Cutaneous features may precede the systemic illness. The **differential diagnosis** includes atopic dermatitis, other connective tissue diseases, lichen planus, medication reactions, and infectious exanthems. The paucity of itch in JDMS may help eliminate some considerations. Lesional skin demonstrates epidermal atrophy and vacuolar degeneration at the dermal-epidermal junction. JDMS is distinct from adult dermatomyositis in both presentation and prognosis. Pediatric patients have more difficulty with gastrointestinal vasculopathy and cutaneous calcifications, but are not at increased risk of malignancy.

Treatment includes both systemic steroidal and nonsteroidal immunosuppressants; topical photoprotection is vital to prevent cutaneous exacerbations.

SCLERODERMA. The term *scleroderma* describes two separate entities. One is a systemic disorder (progressive systemic sclerosis [PSS]; see Chapter 159), while the other is a strictly cutaneous (**morphea**). The most common presentation of morphea is solitary or multiple circumscribed patches of erythema that evolve into indurated, sclerotic, atrophic plaques (Fig. 644-6), later healing, or "burning out" with pigment change. Morphea can affect any area of skin, but when confined to the frontal scalp, forehead, and midface in a linear band, it is referred to as **linear scleroderma** or "en coup de sabre." This form of morphea carries a poorer prognosis because of the associated underlying musculoskeletal atrophy that can be cosmetically disfiguring. Linear morphea over a joint may lead to restriction of mobility (Fig. 644-7). The **differential diagnosis** includes granuloma annulare, necrobiosis lipoidica, lichen sclerosis, and late-stage Lyme disease (acrodermatitis chronica atrophicans). There is thickening or sclerosis of the dermis with collagen degeneration. Morphea tends to persist with gradual outward expansion on the skin until spontaneous or induced cessation of the inflammatory phase after months to years. Topical calcipotriene and UVA-1 therapy may halt progression and help shorten the disease course. Physical therapy is needed to maintain joint mobility. Significant postinflammatory pigment alteration may persist for years. Pansclerotic morphea is a rare severe disabling variant.

Progressive systemic sclerosis frequently presents with acral (sclerodactyly, ulceration, nail fold telangiectasia, or Raynaud phenomena) and other cutaneous changes (pinched nose, furrowed perioral skin, or "scleroderma facies") [see Chapter 159]. Overlap syndromes such as CREST (calcinosis, Raynaud phenomenon, esophageal dysmotility, sclerodactyly, and telangiectasias) and mixed connective tissue disease may include some physical and laboratory features of scleroderma.

VASCULITIDES

The vasculitides (see Chapter 166) encompass a broad group of disorders having considerable overlap with connective tissue diseases. Immune-mediated inflammation of blood vessels of varying size may be caused by an underlying inflammatory state, infection, medication, or malignancy. Common clinical features include **palpable nonthrombocytopenic purpuric** skin lesions, arthritis, fever, myalgia, fatigue, and weight loss, as well as an elevated erythrocyte sedimentation rate. Extracutaneous organ involvement includes the joints, lungs, kidneys, and central nervous system.

HENOCH-SCHÖNLEIN PURPURA (IGA VASCULITIS). Henoch-Schönlein purpura (HSP) is a vasculitis that presents with pur-

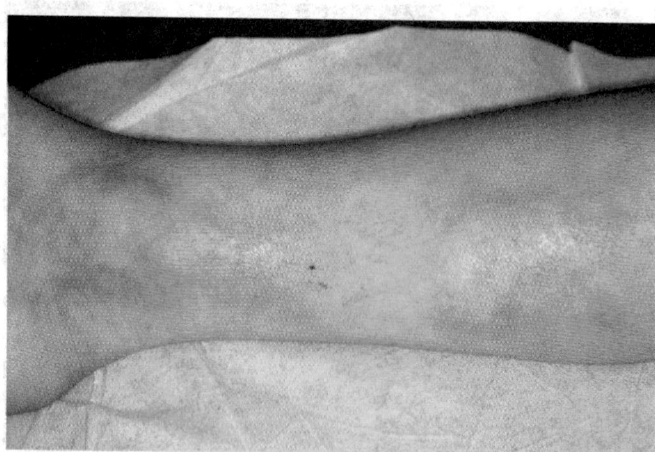

Figure 644-7. Linear morhpea with involvement over the ankle.

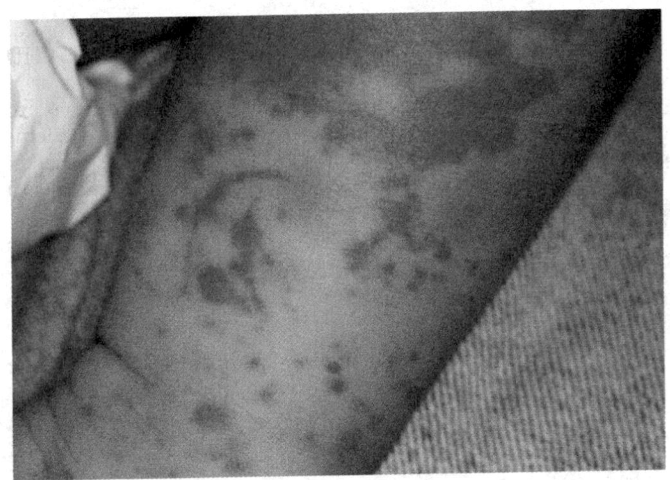

Figure 644-8. Purpura of the lower leg in Henoch-Schönlein purpura (HSP).

puric lesions prominently on the buttocks and lower extremities of school-aged children (Fig. 644-8). **Infantile hemorrhagic edema (IHE;** also called acute hemorrhagic edema of infancy) shares some clinical features with HSP but appears in infants and toddlers. IHE is characterized by circumscribed purpuric papules and plaques on the trunk and extremities, but unlike HSP, commonly affects the face and lacks other organ involvement. IHE may follow a recent infection and manifests with peripheral edema and fever; patients with HSP are usually afebrile. HSP must also be differentiated from infectious causes of purpuric skin lesions such as meningococcemia, Rocky Mountain spotted fever, and purpuric viral exanthems such as those caused by enteroviruses, as well as from juvenile rheumatoid arthritis and other vasculitides. Diagnosis is confirmed by the immunofluorescence finding of IgA in the blood vessel walls.

KAWASAKI DISEASE. Kawasaki disease (KD; see Chapter 165) is a clinical diagnosis based on both cutaneous and extracutaneous features. The skin eruption of KD may be polymorphic, presenting variously with urticarial, maculopapular, or morbilliform patches and plaques on the trunk and extremities, but early involvement with erythema and peeling in the perineum/inguinal region may be an initial clue to the diagnosis. Acral edema and desquamation are also prominent features but typically occur later. Conjunctivitis (nonpurulent) often with sparing of the limbus, and lingual plaques ("white strawberry tongue") that shed to produce denuded, erythematous patches with prominent papilla ("strawberry tongue") are classic mucocutaneous features. Histopathologic findings in the skin are nonspecific and generally do not assist in distinguishing other differential considerations such as a viral or bacterial exanthem or medication reaction.

BEHÇET DISEASE. Behçet disease (see Chapter 160) is multisystemic disease that includes oral and genital ulceration and ocular disease (uveitis, relapsing iridocyclitis). Recurrent aphthous stomatitis is present in up to 98% of patients, and is commonly the presenting symptom. Genital ulcerations may resemble aphthae and can occur on the penis or scrotum, and may be particularly painful in females. Additional skin findings may include folliculitis, purpuric lesions, erythema nodosum, and pustule formation after venipuncture or skin trauma (**pathergy**). **Differential diagnosis** of oral lesions includes recurrent aphthous stomatitis, herpes simplex, and less common oculocutaneous syndromes (MAGIC [mouth and genital ulcers with inflamed cartilage] syndrome). Skin biopsy demonstrates either leukocytoclastic or lymphocytic vasculitis. Oral lesions may respond to swish and spit/swallow preparations variably including corticosteroids, antihistamines, antibiotics, and analgesics.

GASTROINTESTINAL DISEASES

INFLAMMATORY BOWEL DISEASE. Ulcerative colitis (see Chapter 333) presents with cutaneous manifestations in up to 30% of patients. Aphthous ulcers are common and may worsen with gastrointestinal exacerbations. Erythema nodosum, occurring in up to 10% of patients, presents as warm, erythematous nodules, often on the distal, lower extremities. Pyoderma gangrenosum is a focal, ulcerative process that has distinctive, inflamed, undermined, borders and a purulent, boggy center. Thrombophlebitis also occurs at an increased rate in patients with ulcerative colitis. In most cases, treatment of the underlying disease state improves the cutaneous sequelae.

Crohn disease, or regional enteritis (see Chapter 333), classically presents with perianal fissures and skin tags, abscesses, sinuses, and fistulas; these may be presenting signs. Like ulcerative colitis, aphthae, erythema nodosum, and pyoderma gangrenosum occur at increased frequency and may improve with treatment of underlying disease. Noncaseating granulomatous inflammation is seen on routine histopathology, and when found in skin not contiguous with the intestinal tract, is labeled **metastatic Crohn disease.** Metastatic lesions may present as solitary or multiple, localized, plaques or nodules and may be on perianal, perioral, or other cutaneous surfaces, including scars or ileostomy sites. Standard therapy includes immunosuppressive medications, nutritional support, and surgery for complications.

CUTANEOUS MANIFESTATIONS OF MALIGNANCY

Cutaneous metastases may present as firm nodules at any cutaneous site. Distinctive paraneoplastic reaction patterns may result in sometimes striking rashes. Some genetic syndromes have increased malignancy risk that may be suggested initially by cutaneous signs.

SWEET SYNDROME. Also known as acute febrile neutrophilic dermatosis, Sweet syndrome (see Chapter 166.5) presents abruptly with tender, erythematous, edematous plaques or nodules on any area of the skin, often accompanied by fever, anemia, and leukocytosis. Diagnosis is confirmed by the presence of a dense neutrophilic infiltrate without evidence of vasculitis. The **differential diagnosis** includes pyoderma gangrenosum, cellulitis, erythema multiforme, Behçet syndrome, and erythema nodosum. The etiology of Sweet syndrome is unknown but may be due to a hypersensitivity reaction to a bacterial, viral, or tumor antigen, and may occur in association with Behçet disease. Even though Sweet syndrome may occur without an identifiable etiology, investigation for infection or malignancy is warranted. In children, Sweet syndrome has been associated with otitis media, osteomyelitis, aseptic meningitis, HIV, and leukemia. In adults, 15% of patients have an associated malignancy, most commonly hematologic. Sweet syndrome is sensitive to oral corticosteroids.

NECROLYTIC MIGRATORY ERYTHEMA. Necrolytic migratory erythema (NME), or **glucagonoma syndrome,** is a distinctive migratory erythema that may signal an underlying neoplasm, such as α-cell pancreatic tumor underlying the eruption of NME. Polycyclic erythematous patches and plaques on the trunk, extremities, and groin occur in association with glossitis, and cheilitis. Elevated glucagon levels, glucose intolerance, and hypoaminoacidemia confirm the diagnosis, and tumor resection leads to resolution of the rash.

Other cutaneous findings that may signal an underlying malignancy include pruritus, ichthyosis, acanthosis nigricans, urticaria, pemphigus, and erythroderma.

CUTANEOUS REACTIONS IN THE SETTING OF IMMUNOSUPPRESSION

Medication reactions, infectious etiologies, and graft vs host disease (GVHD) are included in the differential diagnosis in immunosuppressed patients; cutaneous and histologic similarities can be confounding. The majority of medication reactions are mild morbilliform or exanthematous eruptions of little clinical consequence. Identifying the suspect medication may be difficult due to the many medications used in this population. Features that may help identify suspect medications include rash onset relative to exposure, character of distribution and spread, associated symptoms, and laboratory data. Medication eruptions begin on the trunk 7–10 days after exposure, spread peripherally, and are associated with pruritus, and, less commonly, fever, arthralgia, and lymphadenopathy. Eosinophilia may support a diagnosis of drug eruption but may be absent in the setting of bone marrow suppression. Penicillins, sulfa drugs, cephalosporins, nonsteroidal anti-inflammatory agents, anticonvulsants and, on occasion, aminoglycosides are common offenders. Medication eruptions may resolve despite continued use of the offending agent, or they may progress to more severe involvement. A careful drug history, elimination of all nonessential, suspect medications or change to medications of dissimilar class, and treatment of pruritus with emollients, topical steroids, antihistamines, and antipruritics are indicated. Skin biopsies are rarely useful in distinguishing medication eruptions from infectious exanthems, although GVHD, if sufficiently advanced, may have signature histopathologic findings.

GRAFT VS HOST DISEASE. GVHD (see Chapter 136) may have florid cutaneous expression in addition to characteristic extracutaneous features such as fever, mucositis, diarrhea, and hepatitis. Acute GVHD may be mistaken for a medication reaction or infectious exanthem based on the nonspecific erythematous maculopapular eruption that often starts focally and generalizes. Features that may suggest GVHD include timing of eruption (typically 1–3 wk post-transplant at the time of hematopoietic reconstitution), initial involvement of the head and neck including the ears, and subsequent spread to the trunk, extremities, and palms and soles. Chronic GVHD, which occurs in ≈20% of long-term transplant survivors, is seen most often in patients who have previously experienced acute GVHD. Cutaneous manifestations of chronic GVHD are distinctive, with sclerotic, dyspigmented scaly plaques and lichenoid papules predominating (Fig. 644-9). Treatment includes systemic immunosuppression supplemented by topical steroids, antihistamines, antipruritics, and emollients. Chronic disease may also respond to photochemotherapy (PUVA), UVA-1, plasmapheresis, and thalidomide. Topical immunomodulators such as tacrolimus may be effective. GVHD may also develop in susceptible nontransplant settings, such as in the severely immunosuppressed neonate or infant in response to therapeutic transfusion of nonirradiated blood products, the fetus with congenital immunodeficiency and with transplacental passage of maternal lymphocytes, as well as the older child with malignancy that has received nonirradiated blood products.

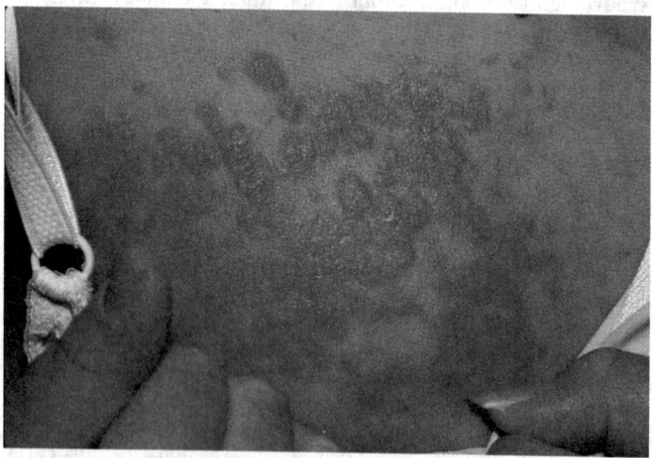

Figure 644-9. Lichenoid eruption in chronic graft vs host disease (GVHD).

MULTISYSTEMIC MEDICATION REACTIONS (see Chapter 150)

Most cutaneous reactions that result from the use of systemic medications are confined to the skin and resolve without sequelae after discontinuation of the offending agent. More severe drug eruptions may be life-threatening, making rapid recognition vital (see Chapter 653).

DRUG RASH WITH EOSINOPHILIA AND SYSTEMIC SYMPTOMS (DRESS SYNDROME). This syndrome was formerly called anticonvulsant hypersensitivity syndrome and pseudolymphoma syndrome. It is classically seen 1–4 wk after initial exposure to an aromatic anticonvulsant and often presents with the triad of **fever, rash, and hepatitis.** The skin rash is characterized by a pruritic, diffuse, erythematous to urticarial eruption of coalescing plaques. Prominent periocular edema, cervical lymphadenopathy, pharyngitis, and malaise accompany this dramatic cutaneous eruption. Eosinophilia occurs in up to 30% of patients. Atypical lymphocytosis is common. Hepatitis ranging from mild elevation of liver transaminases to frank hepatic failure may be accompanied by interstitial nephritis, pneumonitis, and encephalitis. Late-onset (several months) thyroiditis and hypothyroidism may occur as a result of antimicrosomal antibodies directed against thyroid peroxidases involved in drug metabolism. A heritable defect in the epoxide hydrolase pathway, in the case of anticonvulsants, leads to accumulation of toxic metabolites, which react with lymphocytes. Anticonvulsants having the distinctive aromatic structure (carbamazepine, phenobarbital, phenytoin) have a high risk of triggering hypersensitivity syndrome in susceptible individuals and their first-degree relatives. The **differential diagnosis** includes Stevens-Johnson syndrome, viral exanthem, or GVHD in the appropriate clinical setting. In addition to anticonvulsants, sulfonamides may cause similar symptoms on 1st exposure due to abnormalities in glutathione transferase pathways. Many other antibiotics have also been implicated as the cause of this syndrome.

Withdrawal of the medication is the primary therapeutic intervention, with symptomatic treatment of itch and/or pain being universal. Oral corticosteroid therapy may be acutely beneficial, especially in the setting of rapidly evolving hepatic or renal involvement in hypersensitivity syndrome. The role of intravenous immunoglobulin in hypersensitivity syndrome is unclear. Counseling regarding increased risk with similar medications and sibling risk is important. Hypersensitivity reactions can flare, both in the skin and other organ systems, well after the medication has been withdrawn and initial improvement achieved, necessitating close follow-up for several months.

SERUM SICKNESS–LIKE REACTION. Serum sickness–like reaction (SSLR) presents with urticarial to purpuric, sharply marginated coalescing plaques and acral erythema/edema, often in association with arthritis, lymphadenopathy, and fever. Unlike true serum sickness (see Chapter 149), laboratory evidence of circulating immune complexes and multisystem involvement of vasculitis are typically absent. The **differential diagnosis** includes Kawasaki disease, connective tissue diseases, and hypersensitivity syndrome. SSLR is most commonly seen after exposure to cefaclor. The cause is unknown, but a toxic metabolite is suspected. In contrast to hypersensitivity reaction, SSLR typically occurs after repeated drug exposures. Symptomatic treatment and medication withdrawal are recommended.

Boh EE: Neonatal lupus erythematosus. *Clin Dermatol* 2004;22:125–128.

Klein-Gitelman M, Reiff A, Silverman ED: Systemic lupus erythematosus in childhood. *Rheum Dis Clin North Am* 2002;28:561–577.

Lee SJ: New approaches for preventing and treating chronic graft-versus-host disease. *Blood* 2005;105:4200–4206.

Poyrazoglu HM, Per H, Gunduz Z, et al: Acute hemorrhagic edema of infancy. *Pediatr Int* 2003;45:697–700.

Seghal VN, Srivastava G, Aggarwal AK, et al: Localized scleroderma/morphea. *J Dermatol* 2002;41:467–475.

Tas S, Simonart T: Management of drug rash with eosinophilia and systemic symptoms (DRESS syndrome): An update. *Dermatology* 2003;206:353–356.

Ting TV, Hashkes PJ: Update on childhood vasculitis. *Curr Opin Rheumatol* 2004;16:560–565.

Van Gysel D, de Waard-van der Spek FB, Oranje AP: Childhood discoid lupus erythematosus: Report of five new cases and review of the literature. *J Eur Acad Dermatol Venereol* 2002;16:143–147.

Zipitis CS, Baildam EM, Ramanan AV: Treatment approaches to juvenile dermatomyositis. *Expert Opin Pharmacother* 2004;5:1509–1515.

Chapter 645 ■ Principles of Therapy

Joseph G. Morelli

Competent skin care requires a specific diagnosis, knowledge of the natural course of the disease, and appreciation of primary versus secondary lesions. If the diagnosis is uncertain, it is better to err on the side of less rather than more aggressive treatment. Even when the diagnosis is clear, an acute dermatitis may initially require gentle and bland therapy.

In the use of topical medication, consideration of vehicle is as important as the specific therapeutic agent. Acute **weeping lesions** respond best to wet compresses, followed by lotions or creams. For **dry, thickened,** scaly skin or when treating a contact allergic reaction possibly due to a component of a topical medication, an ointment base is preferable. Gels and solutions are most useful for the scalp and other hairy areas. The site of involvement is of considerable importance because the most desirable vehicle may not be cosmetically or functionally appropriate, such as an ointment on the face or hands. A patient's preference should also play a part in the choice of vehicle because compliance is poor if a medication is not acceptable to a patient. Cosmetically acceptable foam delivery systems have been developed, but at this time only a few products are available.

Most **lotions** are mixtures of water and oil that can be poured. After the water evaporates, the small amount of remaining oil covers the skin. Some shake lotions are a suspension of water and insoluble powder; as the water evaporates, cooling the skin, a thin film of powder covers the skin. **Creams** are emulsions of oil and water that are viscous and do not pour (more oil than in lotions). **Ointments** have oils and a small amount of water or no water at all; they feel greasy, lubricate dry skin, trap water, and may be occlusive. Ointments without water usually require no preservatives because microorganisms require water to survive.

Therapy should be kept as simple as possible, and specific written instructions about the frequency and duration of application should be provided. Physicians should become familiar with one or two preparations in each category and should learn to use them appropriately. Prescribing nonspecific proprietary medications that may contain sensitizing agents should be avoided. Certain preparations such as topical antihistamines and sensitizing anesthetics are never indicated.

WET DRESSINGS. Wet dressings cool and dry the skin by evaporation and cleanse by removing crusts and exudate that cause further irritation if permitted to remain. They decrease pruritus, burning, and stinging sensations, and are indicated for acutely inflamed moist or oozing dermatitis. Although various astringent and antiseptic substances may be added to the solution, cool or tepid tap water compresses are just as effective. Dressings of multiple layers of Kerlix, gauze, or soft cotton material may be saturated with water and remoistened as often as necessary. Compresses should be applied for 10–20 min at least every 4 hr and should usually be continued for 24–48 hr.

Alternatively, cotton long johns can be soaked in water and then wrung as dry as possible. These are placed on the child and covered with dry pajamas, preferably sleeper pajamas with feet. The child should sleep in these overnight. This can be done nightly for up to 1 wk.

BATH OILS, COLLOIDS, SOAPS. Bath oil has little benefit in the treatment of children. It offers little moisturizing effect but increases the risk of injury during a bath. Bath oil may lubricate the surface of the bathtub, causing an adult or child to fall when stepping into the tub. Tar bath solutions can be prescribed and may be helpful for psoriasis and atopic dermatitis. Colloids such as starch powder or colloidal oatmeal are soothing and antipruritic for some patients when added to the bathwater. Oilated colloidal oatmeal contains mineral oil and lanolin derivatives for lubrication if the skin is dry. These can also lubricate the bathtub surface. Ordinary toilet soaps may be irritating and drying if patients have dry skin or dermatitis. Synthetic soaps are much less irritating. When skin is acutely inflamed, avoidance of soap is advised. Some patients find that lipid-free cleansers containing cetyl alcohol are soothing.

LUBRICANTS. Lubricants, such as lotions, creams, and ointments, can be used as emollients for dry skin and as vehicles for topical agents such as corticosteroids and keratolytics. In general, ointments are the most effective emollients. Numerous commercial preparations are available in addition to standard products such as petrolatum, cold cream, stearin-lanolin cream, and hydrophilic ointment. Some patients do not tolerate ointments, and some may be sensitized to a component of the lubricant; some preservatives of creams (most commonly, parabens) are sensitizers. These preparations can be applied several times a day if necessary. Maximal effect is achieved when they are applied immediately to damp skin after a bath or shower. Lotions containing menthol and camphor in an emollient vehicle can be used to help control pruritus and dryness.

SHAMPOOS. Special shampoos containing sulfur, salicylic acid, zinc, and selenium sulfide are useful for conditions in which there is scaling of the scalp. Most shampoos also contain surfactants and detergents. Tar-containing shampoos are useful for psoriasis and severe seborrheic dermatitis. They should be used as frequently as necessary to control scaling. Patients should be instructed to leave the lathered shampoo in contact with the scalp for 5–10 min.

SHAKE LOTIONS. These lotions are useful antipruritic agents; they consist of a suspension of powder in a liquid vehicle. Water-dispersible oil may be added for lubrication. These preparations can be used effectively in combination with wet dressings for exudative dermatitis. Cooling occurs as the lotion evaporates and the powder deposited on the skin absorbs moisture.

POWDERS. Powders are hygroscopic and serve as absorptive agents in areas of excessive moisture. When dry, powders decrease friction between 2 surfaces. They are most useful in the intertriginous areas and between the toes, where maceration and abrasion may result from friction on movement. Coarse powders may cake; therefore, they should be of fine particle size and inert, unless medication has been incorporated in the formulation.

PASTES. These contain a fine powder in an ointment vehicle and are not often prescribed in current dermatologic therapy; in certain situations, however, they can be used effectively to protect vulnerable or damaged skin. A stiff zinc oxide paste is bland and inert and can be applied to the diaper area to prevent further irritation due to diaper dermatitis. Zinc oxide paste should be applied in a thick layer completely obscuring the skin and is removed more easily with mineral oil than with soap and water.

KERATOLYTIC AGENTS. Urea-containing agents are hydrophilic; they hydrate the stratum corneum and make the skin more pliable. In addition, because urea dissolves hydrogen bonds and epidermal keratin, it is effective in treating scaling disorders. Concentrations of 10–40% are available in several commercial lotions and creams, which can be applied once or twice daily as tolerated. Salicylic acid is an effective keratolytic agent and can be incorporated into various vehicles in concentrations up to 6% to be applied 2 to 3 times daily. Salicylic acid preparations should not be used in treating small infants or on large surface areas or denuded skin; percutaneous absorption may result in salicylism. The α-hydroxy acids, particularly lactic acid and glycolic acid, are available in commercial preparations or can be incorporated in an ointment vehicle in concentrations up to 12%. Some creams contain both urea and lactic acid. The α-hydroxy acid preparations are useful for the treatment of keratinizing disorders and may be applied once or twice daily. Some patients complain of burning; in this case, the frequency of application should be decreased.

TAR COMPOUNDS. Tars are obtained from bituminous coal, shale, petrolatum (coal tars), and wood. They are antipruritic and astringent and appear to promote normal keratinization. They may be useful for chronic eczema and psoriasis, and their efficacy may be increased if the affected area is exposed to ultraviolet (UV) light after the tar has been removed. Tars should not be used for acute inflammatory lesions. Tars are often messy and unacceptable because they may stain and they have an odor. They may be incorporated into shampoos, bath oils, lotions, and ointments. A useful preparation for pediatric patients is liquor carbonis detergens 2–5% in a cream or ointment vehicle. Tar gels and tar in a light body oil are relatively pleasant cosmetic preparations that cause minimal staining of skin and fabrics. Tars can also be incorporated into a vehicle with a topical corticosteroid. The frequency of application varies from 1 to 3 times daily, according to tolerance. Many children refuse to use tar preparations because of their odor and staining characteristics.

ANTIFUNGAL AGENTS. These agents are available as powders, lotions, creams, and ointments for the treatment of dermatophyte and yeast infections. Nystatin, naftifine, and amphotericin B are specific for *Candida albicans* and are ineffective in other fungal disorders. Tolnaftate is effective against dermatophytes but not effective for yeast. The spectrum for ciclopirox olamine includes the dermatophytes, *Malassezia furfur*, and *Candida albicans*. The azoles clotrimazole, econazole, ketoconazole, miconazole, oxiconazole, and sulconazole have a similar broad spectrum. Terbinafine has greater activity against dermatophytes but poorer activity against yeasts than the azoles. The topical antifungal agents should be applied 1 to 2 times a day for most fungal infections. All have low sensitizing potential; however, additives such as preservatives and stabilizers in the vehicles may cause allergic contact dermatitis. Ointments containing 6% benzoic acid and 3% salicylic acid are potent keratolytic agents that have also been used for the treatment of dermatophyte infections. Irritant reactions are common.

TOPICAL ANTIBIOTICS. Topical antibiotics have been used for many years to treat local cutaneous infections, although their efficacy, with the exception of mupirocin, has been questioned. Ointments are the preferred vehicles, and combinations with other topical agents such as corticosteroids are, in general, inadvisable. Whenever possible, the etiologic agent should be identified and treated specifically. Antibiotics in wide use as systemic preparations should be avoided because of the risk of sensitization. The sensitizing potential of certain other antibiotics, such as neomycin and nitrofurazone, should be kept in mind. Mupirocin is the most effective topical agent currently available and is as effective as oral erythromycin in treatment of mild to moderate impetigo. Polysporin and bacitracin are not as effective as mupirocin or oral antibiotics.

TOPICAL CORTICOSTEROIDS. Topical corticosteroids are potent anti-inflammatory agents and effective antipruritic agents. Successful therapeutic results are achieved in a wide variety of skin conditions. Corticosteroids can be divided into 7 different categories based on strength, but for practical purposes 4 categories can be used: low, moderate, high, and highest (Table 645-1). Low-potency preparations include hydrocortisone, desonide, and hydrocortisone butyrate. Medium-potency compounds include amcinonide, betamethasone, flurandrenolide, fluocinolone, mometasone furoate, and triamcinolone. High-potency topical steroids include fluocinonide and halcinonide. Betamethasone dipropionate and clobetasol propionate are superpotent preparations and should be prescribed with care. Some of these compounds are formulated in several strengths based on their clinical efficacy and degree of vasoconstriction. Physicians using topical steroids should become familiar with preparations within each class.

All corticosteroids can be obtained in various vehicles, including creams, ointments, solutions, gels, and aerosols. Some are available in a foam vehicle. Absorption is enhanced by an ointment or gel vehicle, but the vehicle should be selected on the basis of the type of disorder and the site of involvement. Frequency of

TABLE 645-1. Potency of Topical Glucocorticosteroids

LOW POTENCY
Hydrocortisone 1% (Nutracort, Penecort, Hytone, OTC)
Desonide 0.05% (Desowen, Tridesilon)
MODERATE POTENCY
Aclometasone dipropionate 0.05% (Aclovate)
Betamethasone valerate 0.1% (Valisone)
Flucinolone acetonide 0.01% (Synalar, Fluonid)
Hydrocortisone valerate 0.2% (Westcort)
Mometasone furoate 0.1% (Elocon)
Triamcinolone acetonide 0.25%, 0.1% (Kenalog, Aristocort)
HIGH POTENCY
Amcinonide 0.1% cream (Cyclocort)
Betamethasone dipropionate 0.05% (Diprosone, Diprolene)
Desoximetasone 0.25% cream (Topicort)
Fluocinonide 0.05% cream, ointment (Lidex, Lidex-E)
Halcinonide 0.1% cream (Halog)
HIGHEST POTENCY
Betamethasone dipropionate (in optimized vehicle) [Diprolene]
Clobetasol propionate 0.05% (Temovate)
Diflorasone diacetate 0.05% (Psorcon)
Halobetasol propionate 0.05% (Ultravate)

From Weston WL, Lane AT, Morelli JG: *Color Textbook of Pediatric Dermatology*, 2nd ed. St. Louis, Mosby, 1996, p 360.

application should be determined by the potency of the preparation and the severity of the eruption. Applying a thin film 2 times daily usually suffices. Adverse local effects include cutaneous atrophy, striae, telangiectasia, acneform eruptions, purpura, hypopigmentation, and increased hair growth. Systemic adverse effects of topical steroids occur with chronic use and include poor growth, cataracts, and suppression of adrenal function.

In selected circumstances, corticosteroids may be administered by intralesional injection (acne cysts, keloids, psoriatic plaques, alopecia areata, persistent insect bite reactions). Only experienced physicians should use this method of administration.

TOPICAL NONSTEROIDAL ANTI-INFLAMMATORY AGENTS. Calcineurin-inhibiting anti-inflammatory agents that inhibit T-cell activation may be used instead of topical steroids for the treatment of atopic dermatitis and other inflammatory conditions. These agents are pimecrolimus and tacrolimus. They do not have the adverse local effects seen with topical steroid. Stinging with application is the most common complaint. They are only as strong as medium potency topical steroids. They should be used with caution due to animal experiments and case reports of increased risk of malignancy (lymphoma).

SUNSCREENS. Sunscreens are of 2 general types: (1) those, such as zinc oxide and titanium dioxide, that absorb all wavelengths of UV and visible spectrums; and (2) a heterogeneous group of chemicals that selectively absorb energy of various wavelengths within the UV spectrum. Some sunscreens permit tanning without burning; others prevent both. In addition to the spectrum of light that is blocked, other factors to be considered include cosmetic acceptance, sensitizing potential, retention on skin while swimming or sweating, required frequency of application, and cost. Sunscreen ingredients include para-aminobenzoic acid (PABA) with ethanol, PABA esters, cinnamates, and benzophenone. These block transmission of the majority of solar UVB and some UVA wavelengths. Parsol 1789/avobenzone is more effective in blocking UVA. Lip protectants that absorb in the UVB range are also available. Sunscreens are designated by sun protection factor (SPF). The SPF is defined as the amount of time to develop a mild sunburn with the sunscreen compared with the amount of time without the sunscreen. A minimum SPF factor of 15 is required for most fair-skinned individuals to prevent sunburn. The higher the SPF, the better the protection is against UVB rays. Sunscreens do not include any measurement of the efficacy in blocking UVA. The efficacy of these agents depends on careful attention to instructions for use. Chemical sunscreens should be applied at least 30 min before sun exposure to permit penetration into the epidermis. Most patients with photosensitivity eruptions require protection by agents that absorb UVB wavelengths; patients with porphyria, phototoxic eruptions, and some types of solar urticaria require agents with a broader spectrum of prevention (see Chapters 147 and 655).

Although sunscreens do confer photoprotection and may decrease the development of nevi, protection is incomplete against all harmful UV light. Sun avoidance is also important during the times when the sun is most intense, for example, at midday. Clothing and hats offer additional sun protection.

LASER THERAPY. Pulsed dye laser therapy has been used with variable results for port-wine stains, acne vulgaris, and hemangiomas. Pulsed dye lasers produce light that is readily absorbed by oxyhemoglobin, producing photothermolysis. High energy irradiation will ablate small blood vessels, while low fluences may stimulate cutaneous procollagen production. Pulse dye lasers are most effective for facial port-wine lesions.

Bergstrom KG, Arambula K, Kimball AB: Medication formulation affects quality of life: A randomized single-blind study of clobetasol propionate foam 0.05% compared with a combined program of clobetasol cream 0.05% and solution 0.05% for the treatment of psoriasis. *Cutis* 2003;72:407–411.

Huang DB, Ostrosky-Zeichner L, Wu JJ, et al: Therapy of common superficial fungal infections. *Dermatol Ther* 2004;17:517–522.

Moloney FJ, Collins S, Murphy GM: Sunscreens: Safety, efficacy and appropriate use. *Am J Clin Dermatol* 2002;3:185–191.

Nghiem P, Pearson G, Langley RG: Tacrolimus and pimecrolimus: From clever prokaryocytes to inhibiting calcineurin and treating atopic dermatitis. *J Am Acad Dermatol* 2002;46:228–241.

Schnopp C, Holtmann C, Stock S, et al: Topical steroids under wet-wrap dressings in atopic dermatitis—a vehicle controlled trial. *Dermatology* 2002;204:56–59.

Chapter 646 ■ Diseases of the Neonate

Joseph G. Morelli

Minor evanescent lesions of newborn infants, particularly when florid, may cause undue concern. Most of the entities are relatively common, benign, and transient and do not require therapy.

SEBACEOUS HYPERPLASIA. Minute, profuse, yellow-white papules are frequently found on the forehead, nose, upper lip, and cheeks of a term infant; they represent hyperplastic sebaceous glands (Fig. 646-1). These tiny papules diminish gradually in size and disappear entirely within the 1st few weeks of life.

MILIA. Milia are superficial epidermal inclusion cysts that contain laminated keratinized material. The lesion is a firm papule, 1–2 mm in diameter, and pearly, opalescent white. Milia may occur at any age but in neonates are most frequently scattered over the face and gingivae and on the midline of the palate, where they are called Epstein pearls. Milia exfoliate spontaneously in most infants and may be ignored; those that appear in scars or sites of trauma in older children may be gently unroofed and the contents extracted with a fine-gauge needle.

SUCKING BLISTERS. Solitary or scattered superficial bullae on the upper limbs of infants at birth are presumedly induced by vigorous sucking on the affected part in utero. Common sites are the radial aspect of the forearm, thumb, and index finger. These bullae resolve rapidly without sequelae and should be distin-

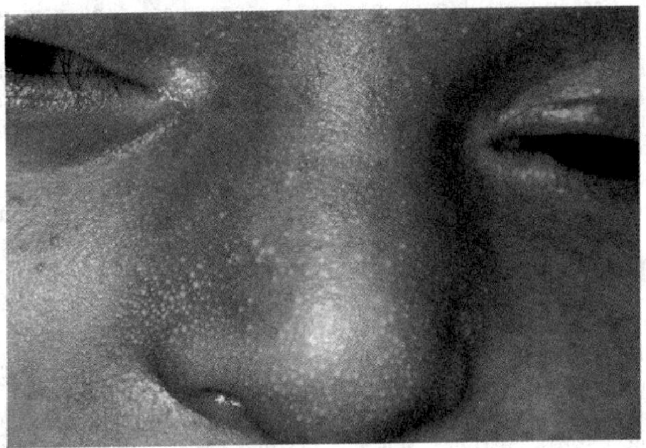

Figure 646-1. Sebaceous hyperplasia. Minute white-yellow papules on the nose of a newborn.

guished from sucking pads (calluses), which are found on the lips in the 1st few months and are due to combined intracellular edema and hyperkeratosis. The diagnosis can be confirmed by observing the neonate suck the affected area.

CUTIS MARMORATA. When a newborn infant is exposed to low environmental temperatures, an evanescent, lacy, reticulated red and/or blue cutaneous vascular pattern appears over most of the body surface. This vascular change represents an accentuated physiologic vasomotor response that disappears with increasing age, although it is sometimes discernible even in older children. Persistent and pronounced cutis marmorata occurs in Menkes disease, familial dysautonomia, and Cornelia de Lange, Down, and trisomy 18 syndromes. Cutis marmorata telangiectatica congenita is clinically similar, but the lesions are more intense, may be segmental, are persistent, and may be associated with loss of dermal tissue, epidermal atrophy, and ulceration.

HARLEQUIN COLOR CHANGE. This rare but dramatic vascular event occurs in the immediate newborn period and is most common in low birthweight infants. It probably reflects an imbalance in the autonomic vascular regulatory mechanism. When the infant is placed on the side, the body is bisected longitudinally into a pale upper half and a deep red dependent half. The color change lasts only for a few minutes and occasionally affects only a portion of the trunk or face. Changing the infant's position may reverse the pattern. Muscular activity causes generalized flushing and obliterates the color differential. Repeated episodes may occur but do not indicate permanent autonomic imbalance.

SALMON PATCH (NEVUS SIMPLEX). Salmon patches are small, pale pink, ill-defined, vascular macules that occur most commonly on the glabella, eyelids, upper lip, and nuchal area of 30–40% of normal newborn infants. These lesions, which represent localized **vascular ectasia,** persist for several months and may become more visible during crying or changes in environmental temperature. Most lesions on the face eventually fade and disappear completely, although lesions occupying the entire central forehead often do not. Those on the posterior neck and occipital areas usually persist. The facial lesions should not be confused with a port-wine stain, which is a permanent lesion. The salmon patch is usually symmetric, with lesions on both eyelids or on both sides of midline. Port-wine stains are often larger and unilateral, and they usually end along the midline (see Chapter 649).

MONGOLIAN SPOTS. These blue or slate-gray macular lesions have variably defined margins; they occur most commonly in the presacral area but may be found over the posterior thighs, legs, back, and shoulders (Fig. 646-2). They may be solitary or numerous and often involve large areas. More than 80% of black, Asian, and East Indian infants have these lesions, whereas the incidence in white infants is <10%. The peculiar hue of these macules is due to the dermal location of melanin-containing melanocytes (mid-dermal melanocytosis) that are presumably arrested in their migration from neural crest to epidermis. Mongolian spots usually fade during the first few years of life due to darkening of the overlying skin. Malignant degeneration does not occur. Widespread numerous lesions, particularly those in unusual sites, are unlikely to disappear. The characteristic appearance and congenital onset distinguish these spots from the bruises of child abuse.

ERYTHEMA TOXICUM. This benign, self-limited, evanescent eruption occurs in ≈50% of full-term infants; preterm infants are affected less commonly. The lesions are firm, yellow-white, 1–2 mm papules or pustules with a surrounding erythematous flare (Fig. 646-3). At times, splotchy erythema is the only manifestation. Lesions may be sparse or numerous and clustered in several sites or widely dispersed over much of the body surface. Palms and soles are usually spared. Peak incidence occurs on the 2nd day of life, but new lesions may erupt during the 1st few days as the rash waxes and wanes. Onset may occasionally be delayed for a few days to weeks in premature infants. The pustules form below the stratum corneum or deeper in the epidermis and represent collections of eosinophils that also accumulate around the upper portion of the pilosebaceous follicle. The **eosinophils** can be demonstrated in Wright-stained smears of the intralesional contents. Cultures are sterile.

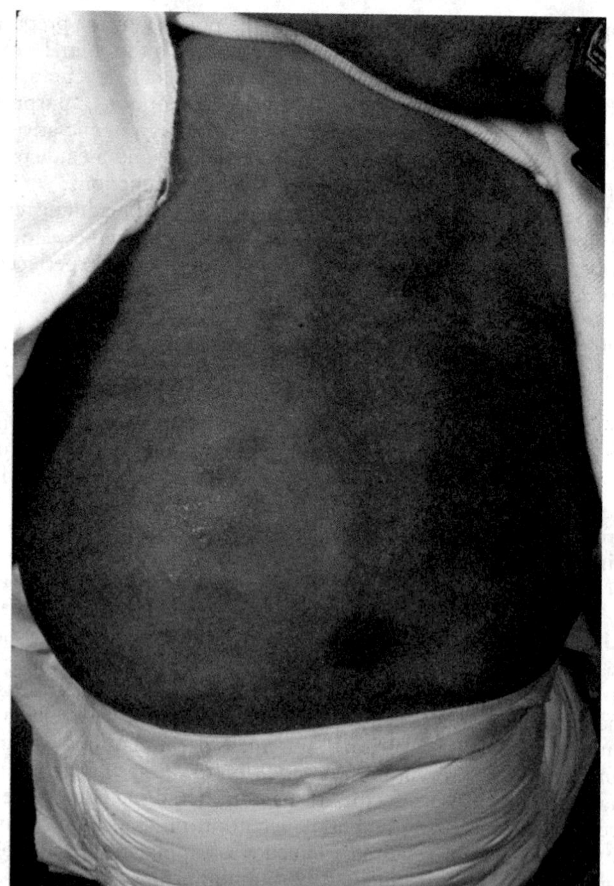

Figure 646-2. Extensive Mongolian spot on the back of a newborn. (Courtesy of Fitzsimons Army Medical Center teaching file.)

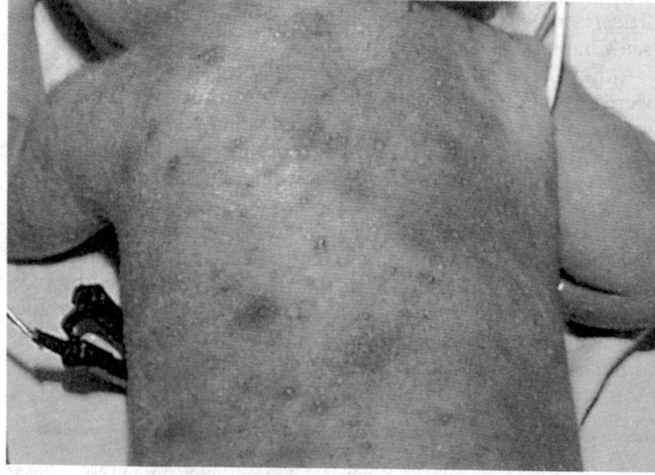

Figure 646-3. Erythema toxicum on the trunk of a newborn infant.

The cause of erythema toxicum is unknown. The lesions can mimic pyoderma, candidosis, herpes simplex, transient neonatal pustular melanosis, and miliaria but can be differentiated by the characteristic infiltrate of eosinophils and the absence of organisms on a stained smear. The course is brief, and no therapy is required. Incontinentia pigmenti and eosinophilic pustular folliculitis also have eosinophilic infiltration but can be distinguished by their distribution, histologic type, and chronicity.

TRANSIENT NEONATAL PUSTULAR MELANOSIS. Pustular melanosis, which is more common among black than among white infants, is a transient, benign, self-limited dermatosis of unknown cause that is characterized by 3 types of lesions: (1) evanescent superficial pustules; (2) ruptured pustules with a collarette of fine scale, at times with a central hyperpigmented macule; and (3) hyperpigmented macules (Fig. 646-4). Lesions are present at birth, and 1 or all types of lesions may be found in a profuse or sparse distribution. Pustules represent the early phase of the disorder, and macules, the late phase. The pustular phase rarely lasts more than 2–3 days; hyperpigmented macules may persist for as long as 3 mo. Sites of predilection are the anterior neck, forehead, and lower back, although the scalp, trunk, limbs, palms, and soles may be affected.

The active phase shows an intracorneal or subcorneal pustule filled with **polymorphonuclear leukocytes,** debris, and an occasional eosinophil. The macules are characterized only by increased melanization of epidermal cells. Cultures and smears can be used to distinguish these pustules from those of erythema toxicum and pyoderma because they do not contain bacteria or dense aggregates of eosinophils. No therapy is required.

INFANTILE ACROPUSTULOSIS. Infantile acropustulosis generally has its onset at 2–10 mo of age; lesions are occasionally noted at birth. Black males have a predisposition, but infants of both sexes and all races may be affected. The cause is unknown.

The lesions are initially discrete erythematous papules that become vesiculopustular within 24 hr and subsequently crust before healing. They are intensely pruritic, and a fresh outbreak is usually accompanied by fretfulness and irritability. Preferred sites are the palms of the hands and soles and sides of the feet, where the lesions may develop in profusion. A less dense eruption may be found on the dorsum of the hands and feet, ankles, and wrists. Pustules occasionally occur elsewhere on the body. Each episode lasts 7–14 days, during which time pustules continue to appear in crops. After a 2–4 wk remission, a new outbreak follows. This cyclic pattern continues for about 2 yr; permanent resolution is often preceded by longer intervals of remission between periods of activity. Infants with acropustulosis are otherwise well.

Wright-stained smears of intralesional contents show abundant neutrophils or, occasionally, a predominance of eosinophils. Histologically, well-circumscribed, subcorneal, neutrophilic pustules, with or without eosinophils, are noted.

The **differential diagnosis** in neonates includes transient neonatal pustular melanosis, erythema toxicum, milia, cutaneous candidosis, and staphylococcal pustulosis. In older infants and toddlers, additional diagnostic considerations include scabies, and a history of previous scabies infection is common; dyshidrotic eczema; pustular psoriasis; subcorneal pustular dermatosis; and hand-foot-and-mouth disease. A therapeutic trial of a scabicide is warranted in equivocal cases.

Therapy is directed at minimizing discomfort for infants. Topical corticosteroid preparations or oral antihistamines decrease the severity of the pruritus and an infant's irritability. Dapsone 2 mg/kg/24 hr taken orally twice daily has been effective but has potentially serious side effects—notably, hemolytic anemia and methemoglobinemia—and should be used with caution.

EOSINOPHILIC PUSTULAR FOLLICULITIS. This is described as recurrent crops of pruritic, coalescing, follicular papulopustules on the

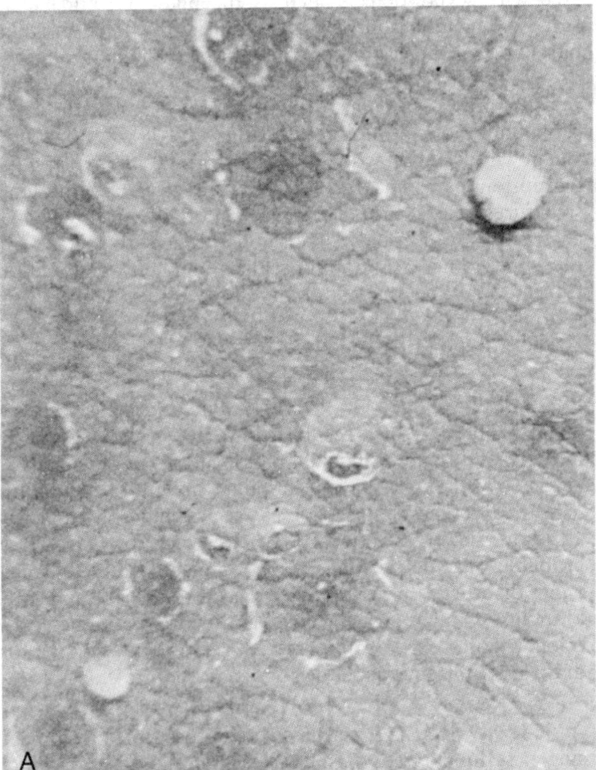

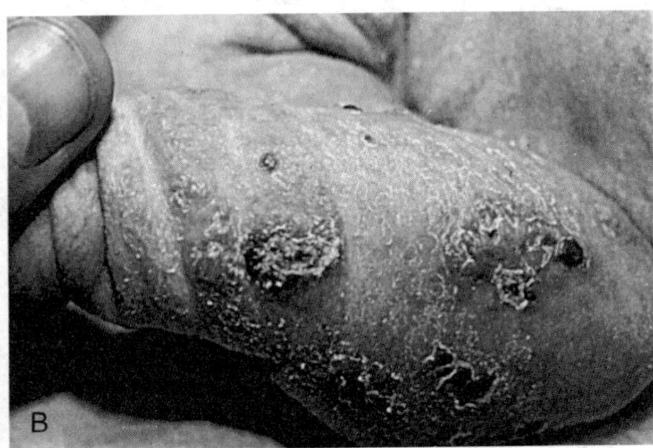

Figure 646-4. *A* and *B,* Transient neonatal pustular melanosis showing pustules, rings of scales, and hyperpigmented macules.

face, trunk, and extremities. Fifty per cent of patients have peripheral eosinophilia exceeding 5%, and about ⅓ (32%) have leukocytosis (>10,000/mm^3).

Infants make up <10% of all cases. The clinical and histologic appearance of this disorder in infants closely resembles that in immunocompetent adults, with minor exceptions. In infants, the lesions are most prominent on the scalp, although they also occur on the trunk and extremities and occasionally are found on the palms and soles. The classic annular and polycyclic appearance with centrifugal enlargement is not seen in infants. Adults have an eosinophilic infiltrate that invades sebaceous glands and the outer root sheath of hair follicles, often leading to spongiosis in the outer root sheath. The eosinophilic infiltrate in most infants, however, is perifollicular, without spongiosis in the outer root sheath. Because of the slightly different clinical findings and course in immunocompetent adults compared with infants or patients with AIDS, it has been proposed that eosinophilic pustular folliculitis (EPF) be **subclassified** into classic, human immunodeficiency virus-related, and infantile forms. The **differential diagnosis** includes erythema toxicum neonatorum, infantile acropustulosis, localized pustular psoriasis, pustular folliculitis, and transient neonatal pustular melanosis.

The pathogenesis of EPF is linked epidemiologically to sebaceous gland activity because lesions appear most commonly in association with hair follicles in areas of the body with a high density of sebaceous glands. Most theories invoke immunologic mechanisms in the initiation of lesions. Proposed etiologic factors in EPF include a cyclo-oxygenase-generated metabolite with chemotactic properties; an exaggerated response to skin saprophytes or dermatophytes, leading to eosinophilic infiltration and destruction of the follicle; or autoantibodies directed against the intercellular substance of the lower epidermis or the cytoplasm of basal cells of the epidermis and the outer sheath of hair follicles.

Response of EPF to therapy is variable; no one specific treatment is the therapy of choice. Antimicrobials and medicated shampoos have been ineffective; mid-potency topical corticosteroids are moderately effective in the treatment of scalp lesions in infants (see Table 645-1).

Alper JC, Holmes LB: The incidence and significance of birthmarks in a cohort of 4,641 newborns. *Pediatr Dermatol* 1983;1:58–68.

Jacobs AH, Walton RG: The incidence of birthmarks in the neonate. *Pediatrics* 1976;58:218–222.

Leung AK, Kao CP, Lee TK: Mongolian spots with involvement of the temporal area. *Int J Dermatol* 2001;40:288–289.

Marchini G, Stabi B, Kankes K, et al: AQP1 and AQP3, psoriasin and nitric oxide synthases 1–3 are inflammatory mediators in erythema toxicum neonatorum. *Pediatr Dermatol* 2003;20:377–384.

Chapter 647 ■ Cutaneous Defects

Joseph G. Morelli

SKIN DIMPLES. Cutaneous depressions over bony prominences and in the sacral area, at times associated with pits and creases, may occur in normal children and in association with dysmorphologic syndromes. Skin dimples may develop in utero as a result of interposition of tissue between a sharp bony point and the uterine wall, which leads to decreased subcutaneous tissue formation. A rare benign autosomal dominant anomaly presents with dimples near the acromion bilaterally in association with deletion of the long arm of chromosome 18. Dimples tend to occur over the patella in congenital rubella, over the lateral aspects of the knees and elbows in prune-belly syndrome, on the pretibial surface in campomelic dwarfs, and in the shape of an H on the chin in whistling-face syndrome.

Sacral dimples are common, and may occur as an isolated finding or as part of multiple syndromes, including Bloom syndrome, Smith-Lemli-Opitz syndrome, 4p deletion syndrome, spina bifida occulta, and diastomyelia. Large size (>5 mm), increased distance from the anus (>2.5 cm), or association with a mass or other cutaneous stigmata (hair, aplasia cutis, hemangioma) should increase concern for underlying **spinal dysraphism.** Small lesions may be associated with an underlying dermal sinus, but not an increase in occult spinal dysraphism. Ultrasonography during the 1st 3 mo of life, before ossification of the posterior elements of the lower spine, may provide a cost-effective, noninvasive method for assessment of any associated lumbosacral spine abnormalities.

REDUNDANT SKIN. Loose folds of skin must be differentiated from a congenital defect of elastic tissue or collagen such as cutis laxa, Ehlers-Danlos syndrome, or pseudoxanthoma elasticum. Redundant skin over the posterior part of the neck is common in the Turner, Noonan, Down, and Klippel-Feil syndromes and monosomy 1p36; more generalized folds of skin occur in infants with trisomy 18 and short-limbed dwarfism.

AMNIOTIC CONSTRICTION BANDS. Partial or complete constriction bands that produce defects in extremities and digits are found in 1/10,000–1/45,000 otherwise normal infants. Constrictive tissue bands are caused by primary amniotic rupture, with subsequent entanglement of fetal parts, particularly limbs, in shriveled fibrotic amniotic strands. This event is probably sporadic, with negligible risk of recurrence. Formation of constrictive tissue bands is associated with abdominal trauma, amniocentesis, and hereditary defects of collagen such as Ehlers-Danlos syndrome or osteogenesis imperfecta.

Adhesive bands involve the craniofacial area and are associated with severe defects such as encephalocele and facial clefts. Adhesive bands result from broad fusion between disrupted fetal parts and an intact amniotic membrane. The craniofacial defects do not appear to be caused by constrictive amniotic bands but result from a vascular disruption sequence with or without cephaloamniotic adhesion (see Chapter 108).

The **limb-body wall complex (LBWC)** involves vascular disruption early in development, affecting several embryonic structures; it includes at least 2 of the following 3 characteristics: exencephaly or encephalocele with facial clefts, thoracoschisis and/or abdominoschisis, and limb defects. Amniotic rupture may be the cause of embryonic vascular disruption, leading to LBWC; however, LBWC has been reported in the absence of amniotic rupture.

PREAURICULAR SINUSES AND PITS. Pits and sinus tracts anterior to the pinna may be a result of imperfect fusion of the tubercles of the 1st and 2nd branchial arches. These anomalies may be unilateral or bilateral, may be familial, are more common among females and blacks, and at times are associated with other anomalies of the ears and face. Preauricular pits are present in **branchio-otorenal dysplasia** (EYA-1 gene), an autosomal dominant disorder that consists of external ear malformations, branchial fistulas, hearing loss, and renal anomalies. When the tracts become chronically infected, retention cysts may form and drain intermittently; such lesions may require excision.

ACCESSORY TRAGI. An accessory tragus typically appears as a single pedunculated, flesh-colored papule in the preauricular region anterior to the tragus. Less commonly, accessory tragi are multiple or bilateral, and may be located in the preauricular area,

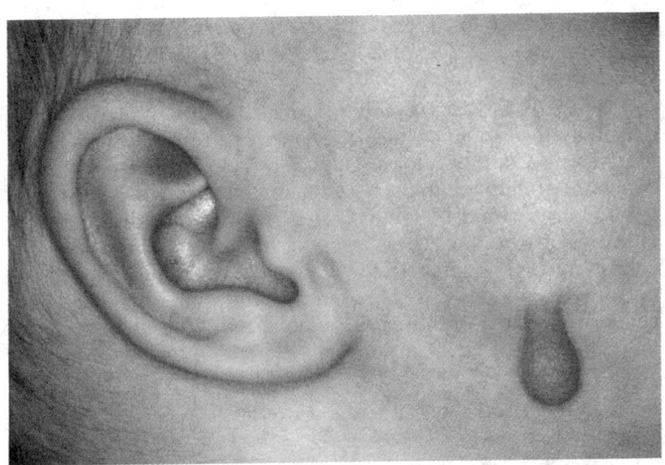

Figure 647-1. Accessory tragus on cheek along jaw line.

on the cheek along the line of the mandible (Fig. 647-1), or on the lateral aspect of the neck anterior to the sternocleidomastoid muscle. In contrast to the rest of the pinna, which develops from the 2nd branchial arch, the tragus and accessory tragi derive from the 1st branchial arch. Accessory tragi may occur as isolated defects or in chromosomal 1st branchial arch syndromes that include anomalies of the ears and face such as cleft lip, cleft palate, and mandibular hypoplasia. An accessory tragus is consistently found in **oculo-auriculo-vertebral syndrome** (Goldenhar syndrome). Surgical excision is appropriate.

BRANCHIAL CLEFT AND THYROGLOSSAL CYSTS AND SINUSES. Cysts and sinuses in the neck may be formed along the course of the 1st, 2nd, 3rd, or 4th branchial clefts as a result of improper closure during embryonic life. Second branchial cleft cysts are the most common. The lesions may be unilateral or bilateral (2–3%) and may open onto the cutaneous surface or drain into the pharynx. Secondary infection is an indication for systemic antibiotic therapy. These anomalies may be inherited as autosomal dominant traits.

Thyroglossal cysts and fistulas are similar defects located in or near the midline of the neck; they may extend to the base of the tongue. A pathognomonic sign is vertical motion of the mass with swallowing and tongue protrusion. In nearly ½ of affected children, the presentation is as an infected midline upper neck mass. Cysts in the tongue base may be differentiated from an undescended lingual thyroid by radionuclide scanning. Unlike branchial cysts, a thyroglossal duct cyst often appears after an upper respiratory infection (see Chapter 564).

SUPERNUMERARY NIPPLES. Solitary or multiple accessory nipples may occur in a unilateral or bilateral distribution along a line from the anterior axillary fold to the inguinal area. They are more common among black (3.5%) than white (0.6%) children. Accessory nipples may or may not have an areola and may be mistaken for congenital nevi. They may be excised for cosmetic reasons. Rarely, they undergo malignant change. Renal or urinary tract anomalies and hematologic abnormalities may occur in children with this finding (see Chapter 551).

APLASIA CUTIS CONGENITA (CONGENITAL ABSENCE OF SKIN). Developmental absence of skin is usually noted on the scalp as multiple or solitary (70%), noninflammatory, well-demarcated, oval or circular 1–2 cm ulcers. The appearance of lesions varies, depending on when they occurred during intrauterine development. Those that form early in gestation may heal before delivery and appear as an atrophic, fibrotic scar with associated alopecia, whereas more recent defects may present as an ulceration. Most occur at the vertex just lateral to the midline, but similar defects may also occur on the face, trunk, and limbs, where they are often symmetric. The depth of the ulcer varies. Only the epidermis and upper dermis may be involved, resulting in minimal scarring or hair loss, or the defect may extend to the deep dermis, subcutaneous tissue, and, rarely, to the periosteum, skull, and dura. Lesions may be surrounded by a collar of hair (Fig. 647-2).

No unifying theory can account for all lesions of aplasia cutis congenita. Diagnosis is made on the basis of physical findings indicative of in utero disruption of skin development. Lesions are sometimes mistakenly attributed to scalp electrodes or obstetric trauma. Rather, they appear to be due to various factors, including genetic factors, teratogens, compromised vasculature to the skin, and trauma.

Although most individuals with aplasia cutis congenita have no other abnormalities, these lesions may be associated with isolated physical anomalies or with malformation syndromes, including Opitz, Adams-Oliver, and oculocerebrocutaneous, Johanson-Blizzard, 4p(-), X-p22 microdeletion syndromes, trisomy 13-15, and chromosome 16-18 defects. Aplasia cutis congenita may also be found in association with an overt or underlying embryologic malformation, such as meningomyelocele, gastroschisis, omphalocele, or spinal dysraphism. Aplasia cutis congenita in association with fetus papyraceus is apparently due to ischemic or thrombotic events in the placenta and fetus. Blistering or skin fragility and/or absence or deformity of nails in association with aplasia cutis congenita is a well-recognized presentation of **epidermolysis bullosa.** Aplasia cutis may be confused with traumatic skin injury from monitoring devices and spontaneous atrophic patches (anetoderma) of prematurity.

Major complications are hemorrhage, secondary local infection, and meningitis. If the defect is small, recovery is uneventful, with gradual epithelialization and formation of a hairless atrophic scar over a period of several weeks. Small bony defects usually close spontaneously in the 1st yr of life. Large or numerous scalp defects may require excision. Truncal and limb defects, despite large size, usually epithelialize and form atrophic scars, which can later be revised.

FOCAL FACIAL ECTODERMAL DYSPLASIA (BITEMPORAL APLASIA CUTIS CONGENITA, ECTODERMAL DYSPLASIA OF THE FACE). This rare disorder is characterized by congenital atrophic scarlike lesions on the temples. Sweating is absent over the defects, the lateral ⅓ of the eyebrows is sparse, and linear vertical wrinkles are present on the forehead. Autosomal dominant and autosomal recessive inheritance have been documented; both subgroups of patients lack associated facial anomalies. **Setleis syndrome** patients have bitemporal scarring in association with

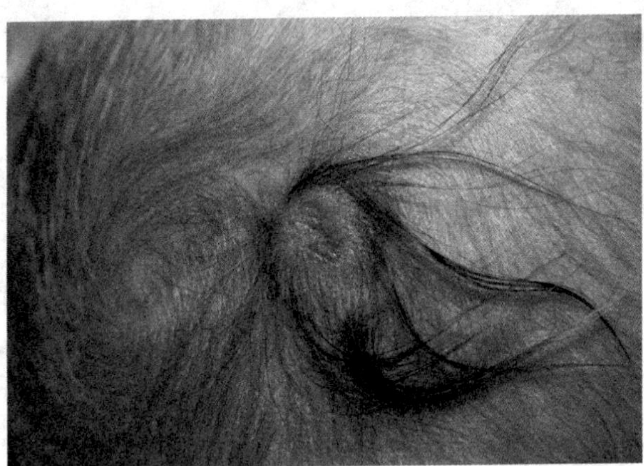

Figure 647-2. Solitary scalp vertex lesion of aplasia cutis congenita with hair collar.

leonine facies, nasal bridge abnormalities, low frontal hairline, and normal growth and development.

FOCAL DERMAL HYPOPLASIA (GOLTZ SYNDROME). This rare congenital mesoectodermal and ectodermal disorder is characterized by dysplasia of connective tissue in the skin and skeleton. It presents with numerous soft tan papillomas. Other cutaneous findings include linear atrophic lesions; reticulated hypopigmentation and hyperpigmentation; telangiectasias; congenital absence of skin; angiofibromas presenting as verrucous excrescences; and papillomas of the lips, tongue, circumoral region, vulva, anus, and the inguinal, axillary, and periumbilical areas. Partial alopecia, sweating disorders, and dystrophic nails are additional less common ectodermal anomalies. The most frequent skeletal defects include syndactyly, clinodactyly, polydactyly, and scoliosis. **Osteopathia striata** are fine parallel vertical stripes noted on radiographs in the metaphyses of long bones; these are highly characteristic of focal dermal hypoplasia but are not pathognomonic. Many ocular abnormalities, the most common of which are colobomas, strabismus, nystagmus, and microphthalmia, are also characteristic. Small stature, dental defects, soft tissue anomalies, and peculiar dermatoglyphic patterns are also common. Mental deficiency occurs occasionally.

Ninety per cent of cases are seen in females suggesting an X-linked dominant gene that is lethal in hemizygous males. The primary defect may be due to a deficiency of collagen caused by a fibroblastic defect.

DYSKERATOSIS CONGENITA (ZINSSER-ENGMAN-COLE SYNDROME). This rare familial syndrome consists classically of the triad of reticulated hyperpigmentation of the skin (Fig. 647-3), dystrophic nails, and mucous membrane leukoplakia in association with immunologic and hematologic abnormalities. Patients with dyskeratosis congenita also show signs of premature aging and increased occurrence of cancer, especially squamous cell. Dyskeratosis congenita may be X-linked recessive (DKC-1 gene), autosomal dominant (hTERC gene), or autosomal recessive caused by as yet undefined genes. Onset occurs in childhood, most commonly as **nail dystrophy.** The nails become atrophic and ridged longitudinally with progression to pterygia and complete nail loss. Skin changes usually appear after onset of nail changes and consist of reticulated gray-brown pigmentation, atrophy, and telangiectasia, especially on the neck, face, and chest. Hyperhidrosis and hyperkeratosis of the palms and soles, sparse scalp hair, and easy blistering of the hands and feet are also characteristic. Blepharitis, ectropion, and excessive tearing as a result of atresia of the lacrimal ducts are occasional manifestations. Oral leukokeratosis may give rise to squamous cell carcinoma. Other mucous membranes including conjunctival, urethral, and genital may be involved. Infection, malignancy, and bone marrow failure are common, and death before age 40 is typical.

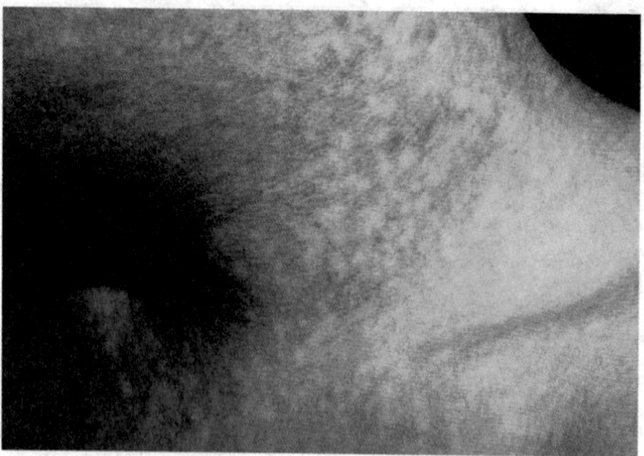

Figure 647-3. Reticulated dyspigmentation on neck of patient with dyskeratosis congenital.

CUTIS VERTICIS GYRATA. This unusual alteration of the scalp, which is more common in males, may be present from birth or may develop during adolescence. The scalp is characterized by convoluted elevated folds, 1–2 cm in thickness, usually in the fronto-occipital axis. Unlike the lax skin of other disorders, the convolutions cannot generally be flattened by traction. Primary cutis gyrata may be associated with mental retardation and is seen in pachydermoperiostosis. Secondary cutis gyrata may be due to chronic inflammatory diseases, tumors, nevi, and acromegaly.

Brousseau VJ, Solares CA, Xu M, et al: Thyroglossal duct cysts: Presentation and management in children versus adults. *Int J Pediatr Otorhinolaryngol* 2003;67:1285–1290.

Brown J, Schwartz RA: Supernumerary nipples: An overview. *Cutis* 2003;71:344–346.

Henriques JG, Pianetti G, Henriques KS, et al: Minor skin lesions as markers of occult spinal dysraphisms—prospective study. *Surg Neurol* 2005;63:S8–S12.

Marrone A, Dokai I: Dyskeratosis congenital: Molecular insights into telomerase function, aging and cancer. *Expert Rev Mol Med* 2004;20:1–23.

Miller TD, Metry D: Multiple accessory tragi as a clue to the diagnosis of the oculo-auriculo-vertebral (Goldenhar) syndrome. *J Am Acad Dermatol* 2004;50:S11–S13.

Scheinfeld NS, Silverberg NB, Weinberg JM, et al: The preauricular sinus: A review of its clinical presentation, treatment, and associations. *Pediatr Dermatol* 2004;21:191–196.

Werler MM, Louik C, Mitchell AA: Epidemiologic analysis of maternal factors and amniotic band defects. *Birth Defects Res A Clin Mol Teratol* 2003;67:68–72.

Chapter 648 ■ Ectodermal Dysplasias

Joseph G. Morelli

Ectodermal dysplasia (ED) is a heterogeneous group of disorders characterized by a constellation of findings involving defects of 2 or more of the following: teeth, skin, and appendageal structures including hair, nails, and eccrine and sebaceous glands. Although 170 ectodermal dysplasias have been described, the majority are rare and only 30 have been genetically defined.

ANHIDROTIC (HYPHIDROTIC) ECTODERMAL DYSPLASIA. This syndrome is manifested as a triad of defects: partial or complete absence of sweat glands, anomalous dentition, and hypotrichosis. There are now 4 recognized types of anhidrotic ectodermal dysplasia (Table 648-1).

TABLE 648-1. Four Recognized Types of Anhidrotic Ectodermal Dysplasia

ANHIDROTIC ECTODERMAL DYSPLASIA	INHERITANCE	GENE DEFECT
ED-1	X-linked recessive	Ectodysplasin A (EDA)
ED-anhidrotic (EDAR)	Autosomal recessive	Ectodyplasin A anhidrotic receptor
(EDARADD)		EDAR-associated death gene
ED-3 (EDAR)	Autosomal dominant	Ectodyplasin A anhidrotic receptor
ED-anhidrotic with immune deficiency	X-linked recessive	IKK-gamma (NEMO)

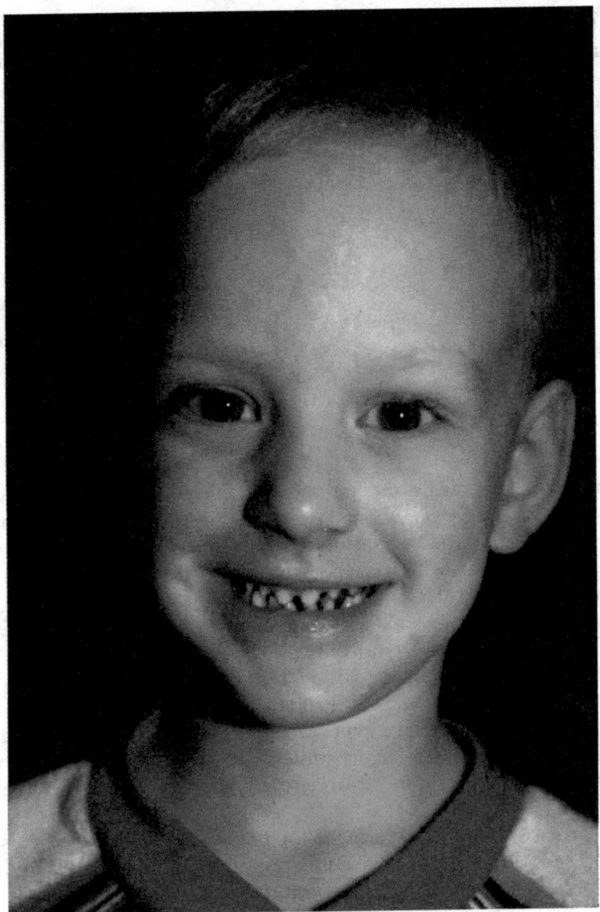

Figure 648-1. Hypohidrotic ectodermal dysplasia is characterized by pointed ears, fine hair, periorbital hyperpigmentation, midfacial hypoplasia, and pegged teeth. (Courtesy of the Fitzsimons Army Medical Center teaching file.)

In ED-1, affected males are unable to sweat and may experience episodes of high fever in warm environments, which may be mistakenly considered to be fevers of unknown origin. This is particularly true in infancy, when the facial changes are not easily appreciated. Diagnosis at this time may be made using the starch-iodine test, palmar, or scalp biopsy. Scalp biopsy is the most sensitive and 100% specific. The typical facies is characterized by frontal bossing; malar hypoplasia; a flattened nasal bridge; recessed columella; thick, everted lips; wrinkled, hyperpigmented periorbital skin; and prominent, low-set ears (Fig. 648-1). The skin over the entire body is dry, finely wrinkled, and hypopigmented, often with a prominent venous pattern. Extensive peeling of the skin is a clinical clue to diagnosis in the newborn period. The paucity of sebaceous glands may account for the dry skin. The scap hair is sparse, fine, and lightly pigmented, and eyebrows and lashes are sparse or absent. Other body hair is also sparse or absent. Sexual hair growth is normal. Anodontia or hypodontia with widely spaced, conical teeth is a consistent feature (see Fig. 648-1). Otolaryngolic and ophthalmologic abnormalities secondary to decreased saliva and tear production are seen. The incidence of atopic diseases in these children is high. Gastroesophageal reflux is common and may play a role in failure to thrive, which is seen in 20%. Sexual development is usually normal. Historically, the infant mortality rate has been 30%. Affected females have none or minimal clinical manifestations.

The clinical findings in autosomal recessive anhidrotic ectodermal dysplasia are identical to the X-linked recessive, except females are affected to the same degree as males. The clinical findings in the autosomal dominant form are also seen in both sexes and are similar to the X-linked recessive form, but much milder. Hypohidrotic ectodermal dysplasia with immune deficiencies demonstrates similar findings in sweating and hair and nail development, in association with a **dysgammaglobulinemia.** Significant mortality is seen from recurrent infections.

Treatment of these children includes protecting them from exposure to high ambient temperatures. Early dental evaluation is necessary so that prostheses can be provided for cosmetic reasons and for adequate nutrition. The use of artificial tears prevents damage to the cornea in patients with defective lacrimation. Alopecia may necessitate the wearing of a wig to improve appearance.

HIDROTIC ECTODERMAL DYSPLASIA (CLOUSTON SYNDROME). The salient features of this autosomal dominant disorder are dystrophic, hypoplastic, or absent nails; sparse hair; and hyperkeratosis of the palms and soles. Conjunctivitis and blepharitis are common. The dentition and sweating are always normal. Absence of eyebrows and eyelashes and hyperpigmentation over the knees, elbows, and knuckles have been noted in some affected individuals. Mutations in the GJB6 gene encoding the gap junction protein connexin 30 are responsible for this disorder. A similar disorder associated with deafness has been described with mutations in GJB2 gene encoding the connexin 26 protein.

Carrol ED, Gennery AR, Flood TJ, et al: Anhidrotic ectodermal dysplasia and immunodeficiency: The role of NEMO. *Arch Dis Child* 2003;88:340–341.

Lamartine J: Toward a new classification of ectodermal dysplasias. *Clin Exp Dermatol* 2003;28:351–355.

Rousse C, Siegfried E, Breer W, et al: Hair and sweat glands in families with hypohidrotic ectodermal dysplasia: Further characterization. *Arch Dermatol* 2004;140:850–855.

Van Steensel MA, Steijlen PM, Bladergroen RS, et al: A phenotype resembling the Clouston syndrome with deafness is associated with a novel missense GJB2 mutation. *J Invest Dermatol* 2004;123:291–293.

Chapter 649 ■ Vascular Disorders

Joseph G. Morelli

Vascular lesions of childhood may be divided into vascular birthmarks (malformations and tumors), benign acquired disorders, and genetic diseases. Familial disorders may involve arterial, capillary, lymph, or venous malformations (Table 649-1).

VASCULAR BIRTHMARK. Vascular birthmarks consist of malformations that are present at birth and tumors, which usually arise in the 1st 2 mo of life.

VASCULAR MALFORMATION. Vascular malformations are developmental errors in blood vessel formation. Malformations do not regress and slowly enlarge. They should be named after the predominant blood vessel forming the lesion (Table 649-2). Table 649-3 helps differentiate vascular malformations from true hemangiomas.

CAPILLARY MALFORMATION (PORT-WINE STAIN). Port-wine stains are present at birth. These vascular malformations consist of mature dilated dermal capillaries. The lesions are macular, sharply circumscribed, pink to purple, and tremendously varied in size (Fig. 649-1). The head and neck region is the most common site of predilection; most lesions are unilateral. The

TABLE 649-1. Familial Vascular Anomalies with Identified Genetic Mutations

DISORDER	CHROMOSOME	GENE	FUNCTION
Hereditary hemorrhagic telangiectasia	9q3 12q	Endoglin activin receptor-like kinase 1 (ALK-1)	TGF-β binding proteins
Cerebral cavernous malformations	7q (Hispanic) 7p 3q	KRIT 1	RAPIA GTPase signal transdution pathway
Familial glomus tumors			
Paragangliomas	11q23		
Disseminated cutaneous glomangioma	1p21–22		
Familial lymphedema	5q34–q35	VEGFR3 (FLT4)	Lymphatic development
Familial venous malformation	9p	Tie-2	Endothelial cell/smooth muscle cell interaction
Familial hemangioma	5q33–34	VEGFR	

From Blei F: Vascular anomalies: From bedside to bench and back again. *Curr Prob Pediatr Adolesc Health* 2002;32:67–102.

TABLE 649-2. Vascular Malformations

TYPE	EXAMPLES
Capillary	Port-wine stain
Venous	Venous malformation Angiokeratoma circumscriptum (hyperkeratotic venule) Cutis marmorata telangiectasia congenital (congenital phlebectasia)
Arterial	Arteriovenous malformation
Lymphatic	Small vessel lymphatic malformation (lymphangioma circumscriptum) Large vessel lymphatic malformation (cystic hygroma)

mucous membranes can be involved. As a child matures into adulthood, the port-wine stain may become darker in color and pebbly in consistency; it may occasionally develop elevated areas that bleed spontaneously.

True port-wine stains should be distinguished from the most common vascular malformation, the salmon patch of neonates, which, in contrast, is a relatively transient lesion (see Chapter 646). When a port-wine stain is localized to the trigeminal area of the face, specifically around the eyelids, the diagnosis of Sturge-Weber syndrome (glaucoma, leptomeningeal venous angioma, seizures, hemiparesis contralateral to the facial lesion, intracranial calcification) must be considered (see Chapter 596.3). Early screening for glaucoma is important to prevent additional damage to the eye. Port-wine stains also occur as a component of Klippel-Trenaunay syndrome and with moderate frequency in other syndromes, including the Cobb (spinal arteriovenous malformation, port-wine stain), Proteus, Beckwith-Wiedemann, and Bonnet-Dechaume-Blanc syndromes. In the absence of associated anomalies, morbidity from these lesions may include a poor self-image, hypertrophy of underlying structures, and traumatic bleeding.

The most effective **treatment** for port-wine stains is the pulsed dye laser (PDL). This therapy is targeted to hemoglobin within the lesion and avoids thermal injury to the surrounding normal tissue. After such treatment, the texture and pigmentation of the skin are generally normal without scarring. Therapy can begin in infancy when the surface area of involvement is smaller; there may be advantages to treating within the 1st year of life. Masking cosmetics may also be used.

TABLE 649-3. Major Differences Between Hemangiomas and Vascular Malformations

	HEMANGIOMAS	VASCULAR MALFORMATIONS (CAPILLARY, VENOUS, LYMPHATIC, ARTERIAL, AND ARTERIOVENOUS, PURE OR COMPLEX-COMBINED)
Clinical	Variably visible at birth Subsequent rapid growth Slow, spontaneous involution	Usually visible at birth (AVMs may be quiescent) Growth proportionate to the skin's growth (or slow progression); present lifelong
Sex ratio F:M	3 : 1 to 5 : 1 and 7 : 1 in severe cases	1 : 1
Pathology	Proliferating stage: hyperplasia of endothelial cells and SMC-actin+ cells Multilaminated basement membrane Higher mast cell content in involution	Flat endothelium Thin basement membrane Often irregularly attenuated walls (VM, LM)
Radiology	Fast-flow lesion on Doppler sonography Tumoral mass with flow voids on MRI Lobular tumor on arteriogram	Slow flow (CM, LM, VM) or fast flow (AVM) on Doppler ultrasonography MRI: Hypersignal on T2 when slow flow (LM, VM); flow voids on T1 and T2 when fast flow (AVM) Arteriography of AVM demonstrates AV shunting
Bone changes	Rarely mass effect with distortion but no invasion	*Slow-flow VM:* distortion of bones, thinning, underdevelopment *Slow-flow CM:* hypertrophy *Slow-flow LM:* distortion, hypertrophy, and invasion of bones *High-flow AVM:* destruction, rarely extensive lytic lesions *Combined malformations* (e.g., slow-flow [CVLM, Klippel-Trenaunay syndrome] or fast-flow [CAVM, Parkes-Weber syndrome]): overgrowth of limb bones, gigantism
Immunohistochemistry on tissue samples	*Proliferating hemangioma:* high expression of PCNA, type IV collagenase, VEGF, urokinase, and bFGF *Involuting hemangioma:* high TIMP-1, high bFGF	Lack expression of PCNA, type IV collagenase, urokinase, VEGF, and bFGF One familial (rare) form of VM linked to a mutated gene on 9p (VMCM1)
Hematology	No coagulopathy (Kasabach-Merritt syndrome is a complication of other vascular tumors of infancy, e.g., Kaposiform hemangioendothelioma and tufted angioma, with a LM component)	Slow-flow VM or LM or LVM may have an associated LIC with risk of bleeding (DIC)

AVM, Arteriovenous malformation; bFGF, basic fibroblast growth factor; CAVM, capillary arteriovenous malformation; CLVM, capillary lymphatic venous malformation; CM, capillary malformation/port-wine stain; DIC, disseminated intravascular coagulation; LIC, localized intravascular coagulopathy; LM, lymphatic malformation; MRI, magnetic resonance imaging; PCNA, proliferating cell nuclear antigen; SMC, smooth muscle cell; TIMP, tissue inhibitor of metalloproteinase; VEGF, vascular endothelial growth factor; VM, venous malformation.

From Eichenfield LF, Frieden IJ, Esterly NB: *Textbook of Neonatal Dermatology.* Philadelphia, WB Saunders, 2001, p 337.

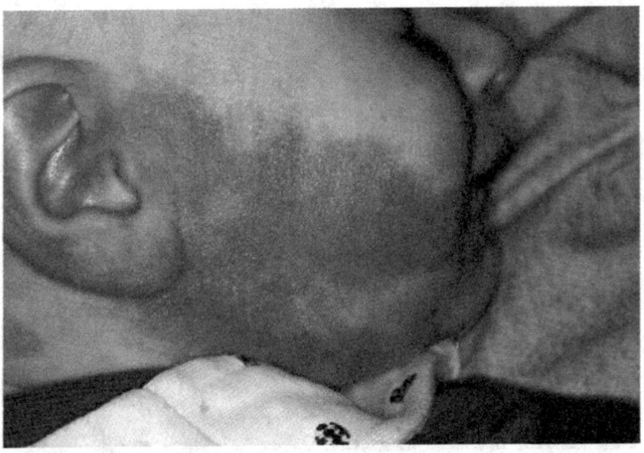

Figure 649-1. Capillary malformation. Pink macule on the cheek of an infant.

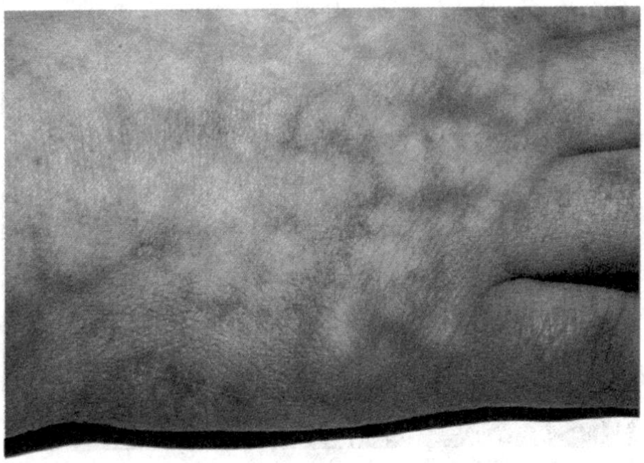

Figure 649-3. Mottled pattern of cutis marmorata telangiectatica congenita on the right hand.

VENOUS MALFORMATION. Venous malformations include vein only malformation, angiokeratomas (hyperkeratotic venule) and cutis marmorata telangiectasia congenita.

Malformations consisting of veins only run the gamut from nodules containing a mass of venules (Fig. 649-2) to diffuse large vein abnormalities that may consist of either or both a superficial component resembling varicose veins and deeper venous malformations. Nodular venous malformations are frequently confused with hemangiomas. Venous malformations may be differentiated by presence at birth, lack of rapid growth phase, and no tendency toward regression. The treatment of choice for superficial nodular vascular malformations is surgical excision. Treatment of larger vein malformations is at best difficult and often impossible. Percutaneous sclerotherapy with direct injection of polidocanol Microfoam, with color Doppler ultrasonographic guidance, is helpful in many patients including those with Klippel-Trenaunay syndrome.

Angiokeratoma Circumscriptum. Several forms of angiokeratomas have been described. Angiokeratomas, characterized by ectasia of superficial dermal vessels and hyperkeratosis of the overlying epidermis, look like flat hemangiomas with a verrucous, irregular surface. Angiokeratoma circumscriptum is a rare solitary lesion or multiple lesions that present as a plaque or plaques of blue-red papules or nodules with a verrucous surface. The limbs are the sites of predilection. If therapy is desired, surgical excision is the treatment of choice.

Cutis Marmorata Telangiectatica Congenita (Congenital Phlebectasia). This benign vascular anomaly represents dilatation of superficial capillaries and veins and is apparent at birth. Involved areas of skin have a reticulated red or purple hue that resembles physiologic cutis marmorata but is more pronounced and relatively unvarying (Fig. 649-3). The lesions may be restricted to a single limb and a portion of the trunk or may be more widespread. Port-wine stain may also be associated. The lesions become more pronounced during changes in environmental temperature, physical activity, or crying. In some cases, the underlying subcutaneous tissue is underdeveloped, and ulceration may occur within the reticulated bands. Rarely, defective growth of bone and other congenital abnormalities may be present. No specific therapy is indicated. Mild vascular only cases may show gradual improvement.

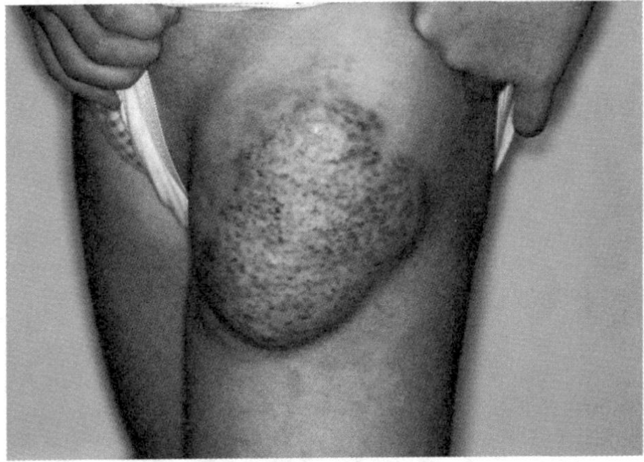

Figure 649-2. Nodular venous malformation on the leg of an adolescent.

ARTERIOVENOUS MALFORMATION (AVM). These malformations are direct connections of artery to vein, bypassing the capillary bed (Fig. 649-4). AVMs of the skin are very rare. They are diagnosed by their obvious arterial palpation. Many physicians mistakenly call all vascular malformations AVMs.

LYMPHATIC MALFORMATIONS (SEE CHAPTER 489).

KLIPPEL-TRENAUNAY (KT) AND KLIPPEL-TRENAUNAY-WEBER (KTW) SYNDROMES. KT is a cutaneous vascular malformation, which in combination with bony and soft tissue hypertrophy and venous abnormalities constitutes the triad of defects of this nonheritable disorder (Fig. 649-5). The anomaly is present at birth and usually involves a lower limb but may involve more than 1 and portions of the trunk or face. Enlargement of the soft tissues may be

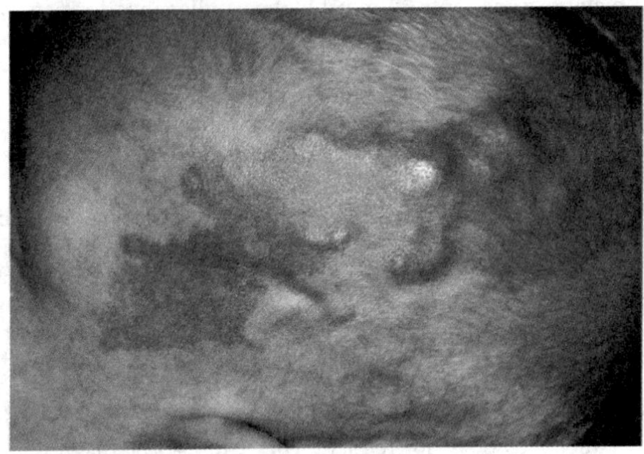

Figure 649-4. Arteriovenous malformation (AVM) in conjunction with a port-wine stain of the scalp of a newborn.

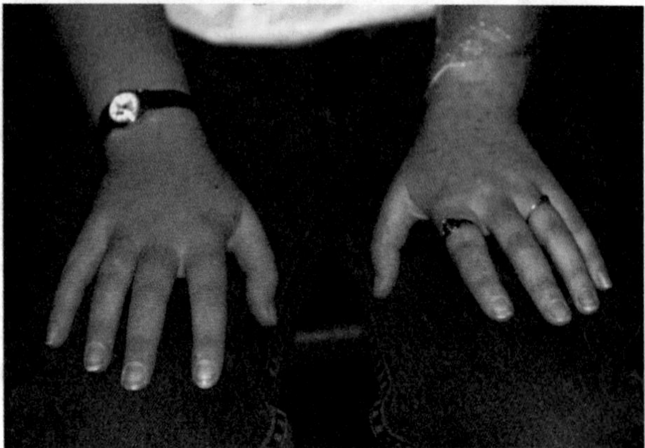

Figure 649-5. Overgrowth of the right arm and hand in and adolescent with Klippel-Trenaunay syndrome.

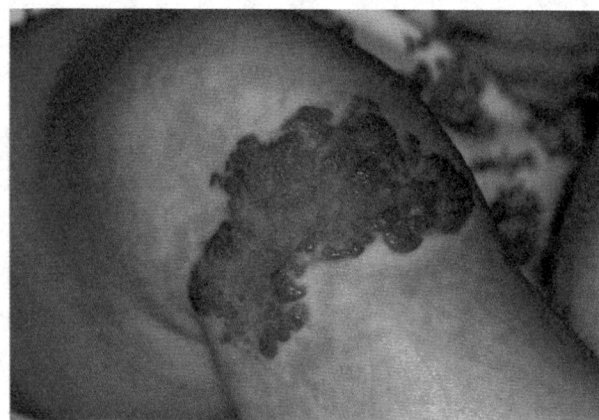

Figure 649-6. Superficial hemangioma on the right knee.

gradual and may involve the entire extremity, a portion of it, or selected digits. The vascular lesion most often is a capillary malformation, generally localized to the hypertrophied area. The deep venous system may be absent or hypoplastic. Venous blebs and/or vesicular lymphatic lesions may be present on their surface. Thick-walled venous varicosities typically become apparent ipsilateral to the vascular malformation after the child begins to ambulate. If there is an associated AVM, then it is called KTW. These disorders can be confused with Maffucci syndrome or, if the surface vascular lesion is minimal, with Milroy disease. Pain, limb swelling, and cellulitis may occur. Thrombophlebitis, dislocations of joints, gangrene of the affected extremity, heart failure, hematuria secondary to angiomatous involvement of the urinary tract, rectal bleeding from lesions of the gastrointestinal tract, pulmonary lesions, and malformations of the lymphatic vessels are infrequent complications. Arteriograms, venograms, and CT or MRI scans may delineate the extent of the anomaly, but surgical correction or palliation is often difficult. Color echo Doppler ultrasonography guided percutaneous sclerotherapy is of benefit when a venous component is the dominant vessel in the malformation. The indications for radiologic studies of viscera and bones are best determined by clinical evaluation. Supportive care includes compression bandages for varicosities; surgical treatment may help carefully selected patients. Leg-length differences should be treated with orthotic devices to prevent the development of spinal deformities. Corrective bone surgery may eventually be needed to treat significant leg-length discrepancy.

PHAKOMATOSIS PIGMENTOVASCULARIS. This rare disorder is characterized by the association of a capillary malformation and melanocytic lesions. Typically, the capillary malformation is extensive, and associated pigmentary lesions may include dermal melanocytosis (Mongolian spots), café-au-lait macules, or a nevus spilus (speckled nevus). Nonpigmented skin lesions that may occur in this setting include nevus anemicus and epidermal nevi. Systemic anomalies are seen in rare cases.

NEVUS ANEMICUS. Although present at birth, nevus anemicus may not be detectable until early childhood. The nevus consists of solitary or numerous sharply delineated pale macules that are most often on the trunk but may also occur on the neck or limbs. These nevi may simulate plaques of vitiligo, leukoderma, or nevoid pigmentary defects, but they can be readily distinguished by their response to firm stroking. Stroking evokes an erythematous line and flare in normal surrounding skin, but the skin of a nevus anemicus does not redden. They can also be diagnosed by diascopy. Pressure of the skin with a glass slide will obscure the borders of a nevus anemicus. Although the cutaneous vasculature appears normal histologically, the blood vessels within the nevus do not respond to injection of vasodilators. It has been postulated that the persistent pallor may represent a sustained localized adrenergic vasoconstriction.

VASCULAR TUMOR. Vascular tumors include hemangiomas (the most common tumor of childhood), tufted angiomas, kaposiform hemangioendotheliomas, rapidly involuting congenital hemangiomas (RICH), and non-involuting congenital hemangiomas (NICH).

Hemangioma. Hemangiomas are proliferative hamartomas of vascular endothelium that may be present at birth or, more commonly, become apparent in the 1st 2 mo of life, predictably enlarge, and then spontaneously involute. Hemangiomas are the most common tumor of infancy, occurring in 1–2% of newborns and 10% of white infants in the 1st yr of life. Hemangiomas should be classified as superficial, deep, or mixed. The terms strawberry and cavernous should not be used. The immunohistochemical marker GLUT-1 separates hemangiomas from the other vascular tumors of infancy. Superficial hemangiomas are bright red, protuberant, compressible, sharply demarcated lesions that may occur on any area of the body (Figs. 649-6 and 649-7). Although sometimes present at birth, they more often appear in the 1st 2 mo and are heralded by an erythematous or blue mark or an area of pallor, which subsequently develops a fine telangiectatic pattern before the phase of expansion. The presenting

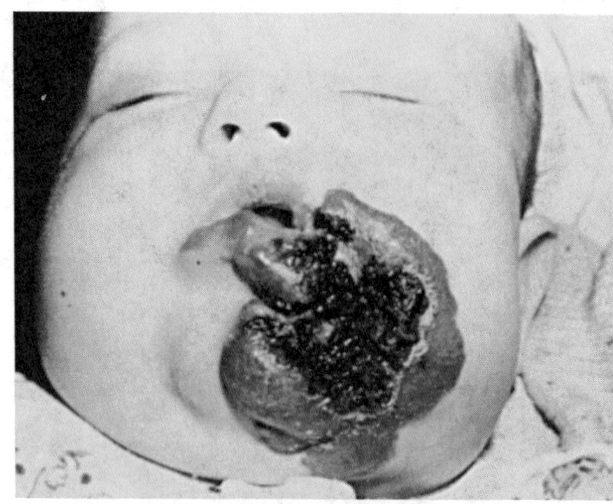

Figure 649-7. Large hemangioma with central crusted ulcer.

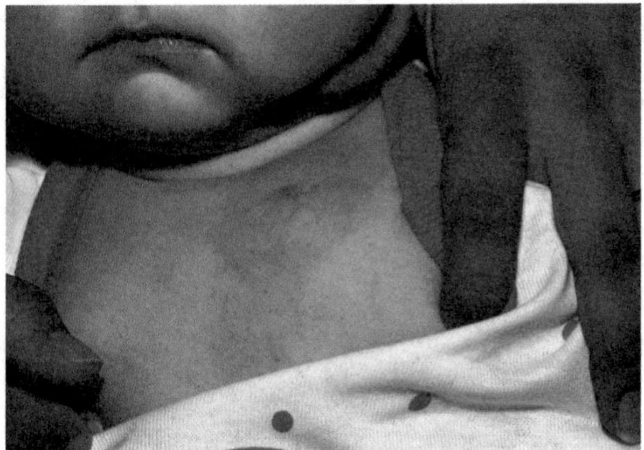

Figure 649-8. Deep hemangioma of the chest.

sign may occasionally be an ulceration of the perineum or lip. Girls are affected more often than boys. Favored sites are the face, scalp, back, and anterior chest; lesions may be solitary or multiple. Patterns of facial involvement include frontotemporal, maxillary, mandibular, and frontonasal regions. Hemangiomas that are more deeply situated are more diffuse and are less defined than superficial hemangiomas. The lesions are cystic, firm, or compressible, and the overlying skin may appear normal in color or have a bluish hue (Fig. 649-8). Most hemangiomas are mixed hemangiomas and have both superficial and deep components. Hemangiomas undergo a phase of rapid expansion, followed by a stationary period and finally by spontaneous involution. Regression may be anticipated when the lesion develops blanched or pale gray areas that indicate fibrosis. The course of a particular lesion is unpredictable, but ≈60% of these lesions reach maximal involution by 5 yr of age, with 90–95% by age 9. Spontaneous involution cannot be correlated with size or site of involvement, but lip lesions seem to persist most often. Complications include ulceration, secondary infection, and, rarely, hemorrhage (Table 649-4). The location of a lesion may interfere with a vital function (e.g., eyelid with vision, urethra with urination). Hemangiomas in a "beard" distribution may be associated with upper airway or subglottic involvement. Respiratory symptoms should suggest a tracheobronchial lesion. Large hemangiomas may be complicated by coexistent hypothyroidism due to type 3 iodothyronine deiodinase, and symptoms may be difficult to detect in this age group. Other concerning features are noted in Table 649-5.

TABLE 649-4. Hemangioma Complications and Their Treatment

CLINICAL FINDING	RECOMMENDED TREATMENT
Severe ulceration/maceration	Encourage twice daily cleansing regimen Dilute sodium bicarbonate soaks ± Flashlamp pulsed dye laser ± Oral corticosteroids ± Metronidazole cream
Bleeding (not KMP)	Gelfoam or Surgifoam Compression therapy ± embolization
Hemagioma with ophthalmologic sequelae	Patching therapy as directed by ophthalmologist Topical vs intralesional vs oral corticosteroids
Subglottic hemangioma	Oral corticosteroids ± KtP laser Tracheotomy if required
KMP	Corticosteroids, aminocaproic acid, vincristine, interferon-α ± embolization
High-flow hepatic hemangioma	Corticosteroids or interferon ± embolization

KMP, Kasabach-Merritt phenomenon.
From Blei F: Vascular anomalies: From bedside to bench and back again. *Curr Prob Pediatr Adolesc Health* 2002;32:67–102.

TABLE 649-5. Clinical Red Flags Associated with Hemangiomas

CLINICAL FINDING	RECOMMENDED EVALUATION
Facial hemangioma involving significant area of face	Evaluate for PHACES: MRI for orbital hemangioma ± posterior fossa malformation Cardiac, ophthalmologic evaluation Evaluate for midline abnormality: supraumbilical raphe, sternal atresia, cleft palate, thyroid abnormality
Cutaneous hemangiomas in *beard* distribution	Evaluate for airway hemangioma, especially if presenting with stridor
Periocular hemangioma	MRI of orbit Ophthalmologic evaluation
Paraspinal midline vascular lesion	Ultrasound or MRI to evaluate for occult spinal dysraphism
Hemangiomatosis (multiple small cutaneous hemangiomas)	Evaluate for parenchymal hemangiomas, especially hepatic/CNS Guaiac stool
Large hemangioma, especially hepatic	U/S with doppler flow MRI Thyroid function studies
Thrill and/or bruit associated with hemangioma	Consider cardiac evaluation and echo to r/o diastolic reversal of flow in aorta MRI to evaluate extent and flow characteristics
Head tilting	Evaluate appropriately for specific site of lesion, plus consider physical therapy evaluation
Delayed milestones	Consider side effect of corticosteroids (myopathy, weight-related) Consider side effect of interferon (especially spastic diplegia)

PHACES, P-posterior fossa abnormalities, H-hemangioma, A-arterial abnormalities, C-cardiac abnormalities, E-eye abnormalities, S-sternal abnormalities; MRI, magnetic resonance imaging; U/S, ultrasound.
From Blei F: Vascular anomalies: From bedside to bench and back again. *Curr Prob Pediatr Adolesc Health* 2002;32:67–102.

In the usual patient who has no serious complications or extensive growth that results in tissue destruction and severe disfigurement, treatment consists of expectant observation. Because almost all lesions regress spontaneously, therapy is rarely indicated and may cause further harm. Parents require repeated reassurance and support. After spontaneous involution, many patients are left with small cosmetic defects, such as telangiectasia, hypopigmentation, fibrofatty deposits, and scars if the lesion has ulcerated. Residual telangiectasias may be treated with PDL. Other defects can be treated or minimized by judicious plastic repair if desired.

In the rare case in which intervention is required, if the lesion is very superficial, early therapy with PDL may be beneficial in decreasing growth of the hemangioma. PDL is also useful for the treatment of small (<4–5 cm) ulcerated hemangiomas. Elastic bandages may reduce the amount of tissue distortion resulting from rapid growth, but they are appropriate only in selected patients with large hemangiomas. Rarely, these lesions impinge on vital structures; interfere with functions such as vision, breathing, defecation, urination, or feeding; or cause grotesque disfigurement because of rapid growth.

If further treatment becomes necessary, a course of prednisolone (2–3 mg/kg/24 hr) is effective in most infants. Termination of growth and sometimes regression may be evident after ≈2–4 wk of therapy. When a response is obtained, the dose should be decreased gradually. Intralesional corticosteroid injection in the hands of an experienced physician can also induce rapid involution of a localized hemangioma. Interferon (IFN)–α therapy may also be effective, but spastic diplegia is seen in 10% of cases and this should be used only for life-threatening hemangiomas refractory to corticosteroid therapy.

Syndromes associated with hemangiomas include **PHACES** (posterior fossa defects such as Dandy-Walker malformation or cerebellar hypoplasia, large plaquelike facial **h**emangioma, **a**rterial abnormalities such as aneurysms and stroke, **c**oarctation of the aorta, **e**ye abnormalities, and **s**ternal raphe defects such as pits or scars), **Gorham** (cutaneous hemangiomas with massive osteolysis), and **Bannayan-Riley-Ruvalcaba** (macrocephaly lipomas, hemangiomas–autosomal dominant inheritance).

Diffuse Hemangiomatosis. This is a condition in which numerous hemangiomas are widely distributed. The skin usually has many small red papular hemangiomas (Fig. 649-9). Most affected infants will have benign neonatal hemangiomatosis, with widespread cutaneous hemangiomas in the absence of apparent visceral involvement. Diffuse neonatal hemangiomatosis is the association of multiple cutaneous hemangiomas of the skin with similar lesions in internal organs. The internal hemangiomas may involve any of the viscera; the liver, gastrointestinal tract, central nervous system, and lungs are the most common sites. In cases of benign neonatal hemangiomatosis, spontaneous regression of the lesions without complications is probable. Infants with diffuse neonatal hemangiomatosis are usually ill at birth. In these cases, ultrasound and CT scanning are indicated to determine the extent of visceral or neural involvement. The disorder is often fatal because of high-output cardiac failure, visceral hemorrhage, obstruction of the respiratory tract, or compression of central neural tissue. Treatment consists of systemic corticosteroid therapy alone or in combination with vincristine, IFN-α, surgery, or irradiation and support with blood products for erythrocyte, platelet, and coagulation factor consumption.

Tufted Angioma. Tufted angiomas are defined histologically by discrete "cannonball-like" tufts of dermal blood vessels. Two clinical patterns are seen. The classic, more common type is a slowly expanding dusky reddish-blue plaque with satellite lesions. More than 50% occur on the head and neck. Regression is not expected. A less common form presents as a solitary vascular nodule (Fig. 649-10). Clinical differentiation from a nodular venous malformation is difficult; spontaneous regression of this type of lesion has been reported.

Kaposiform Hemangioendothelioma. Kaposiform hemangioendotheliomas are very aggressive locally and, although not malignant, may be fatal. Lesions are usually solitary, firm, and deep purple in color. They do not spontaneously regress.

Both tufted angiomas and Kaposiform hemangioendotheliomas are difficult to treat. All treatments used for hemangiomas have been tried and results are extremely variable. Kasabach-Merritt syndrome is seen almost exclusively in tufted angiomas and Kaposiform hemangioendotheliomas.

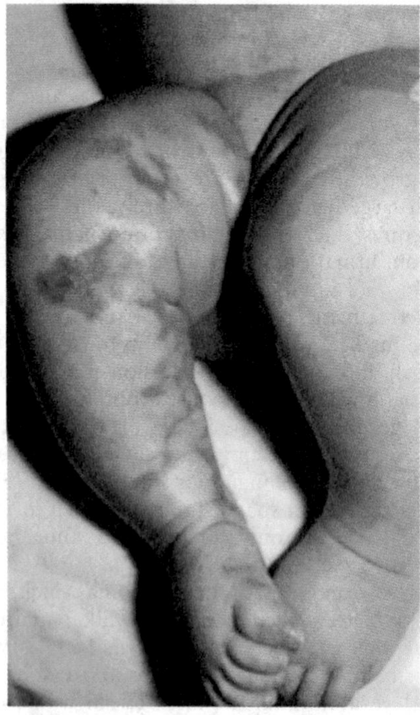

Figure 649-9. Disseminated cutaneous (and liver) neonatal hemangiomatosis. (From Eichenfield LF, Frieden IJ, Esterly NB: *Textbook of Neonatal Dermatology.* Philadelphia, WB Saunders, 2001, p 340.)

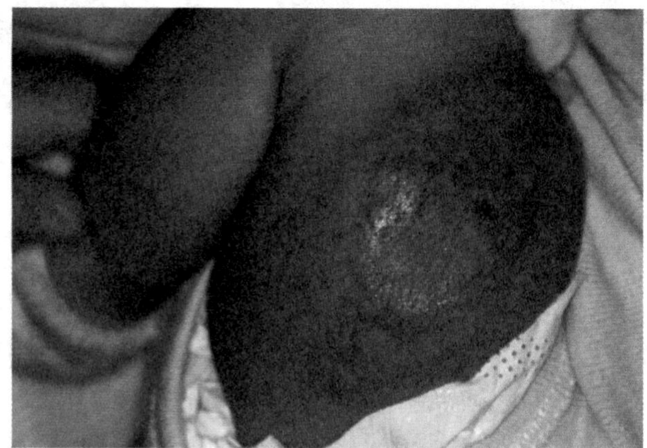

Figure 649-10. Nodular tufted angioma on the left thigh.

Kasabach-Merritt Syndrome. This life-threatening syndrome is a combination of a rapidly enlarging tufted angioma or Kaposiform hemangioendothelioma, thrombocytopenia, microangiopathic hemolytic anemia, and an acute or chronic consumption coagulopathy. The clinical manifestations are usually evident during early infancy. The vascular lesion is usually cutaneous and is only rarely located in viscera. The associated platelet defect may lead to precipitous hemorrhage accompanied by ecchymoses, petechiae, and a rapid increase in size of the vascular lesion. Severe anemia as a result of hemorrhage or microangiopathic hemolysis may ensue. The platelet count is depressed, but the bone marrow contains increased numbers of normal or immature megakaryocytes. The thrombocytopenia has been attributed to sequestration or increased destruction of platelets within the lesion. Hypofibrinogenemia and decreased levels of consumable clotting factors are relatively common (see Chapter 484.6).

Treatment includes management of thrombocytopenia, anemia, and consumptive coagulopathy by administering platelets and by transfusion of red blood cells and fresh frozen plasma. Heparinization is controversial but has benefited some patients when combined with transfusions. Treatment of Kasabach-Merritt syndrome includes surgical excision of small lesions, systemic steroids, embolization, radiation therapy, vincristine, aminocaproic acid, cyclophosphamide, pentoxifylline, or recombinant IFN-α. The mortality rate is significant.

Rapidly Involuting Congenital Hemangioma (RICH). Rapidly involuting congenital hemangiomas, by definition, are present at birth. They present as raised violaceous nodules with ecstatic veins, grayish nodules with overlying telangiectasias surrounded by a pale rim of vasoconstriction, or as flat infiltrative lesions with violaceous skin. They do not undergo a rapid growth phase and involute spontaneously by 1 yr of age.

Noninvoluting Congenital Hemangioma (NICH). Like RICH, these solitary vascular lesions are present at birth. They are round to oval plaques with central or peripheral pallor and coarse overlying telangiectasias. These lesions also do not undergo a rapid growth phase, but they do not spontaneously involute. They are probably better classified as a vascular malformation than a tumor.

BENIGN ACQUIRED VASCULAR DISORDERS

PYOGENIC GRANULOMA (LOBULAR CAPILLARY HEMANGIOMA). A pyogenic granuloma is a small red, glistening, sessile, or pedunculated papule that often has a discernible epithelial collarette (Fig. 649-11). The surface may be weeping and crusted or completely epithelialized. Pyogenic granulomas initially grow rapidly,

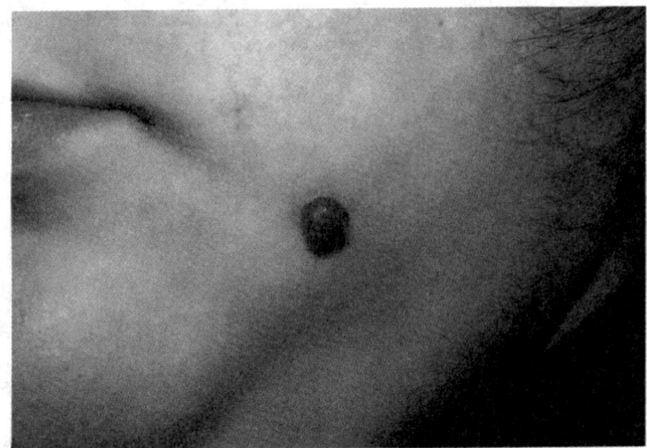

Figure 649-11. Pyogenic granuloma on the left cheek.

may ulcerate, and bleed easily when traumatized because they consist of exuberant granulation tissue. They are relatively common in children, particularly on the face, arms, and hands. Those located on a finger or hand may appear as a subcutaneous nodule. Pyogenic granulomas may arise at sites of injury, but a history of trauma often cannot be elicited. Clinically, they resemble and are often indistinguishable from small hemangiomas. Microscopically, an early lesion resembles an early capillary hemangioma. Collarette formation at the base of the tumor and edema of the stroma may allow differentiation from a capillary hemangioma.

Pyogenic granulomas are benign but a nuisance because they bleed easily with trauma and may recur if incompletely removed. Numerous satellite papules have developed after surgical excision of pyogenic granulomas from the back, particularly in the interscapular region. Small lesions may regress after cauterization with silver nitrate; larger lesions require excision and electrodesiccation of the base of the granuloma. Small (<5 mm) lesions may be treated successfully with the flashlamp-pumped-pulsed dye laser.

ANGIOKERATOMA OF MIBELLI. Angiokeratoma of Mibelli is characterized by 1–8 mm red, purple, or black scaly, verrucous, occasionally crusted papules and nodules that appear on the dorsum of the fingers and toes and on the knees and the elbows. Less commonly, palms, soles, and ears may be affected. In many patients, onset has followed frostbite or chilblains. These nodules bleed freely after injury and may involute in response to trauma. They may be effectively eradicated by cryotherapy, electrofulguration, excision, or laser ablation.

SPIDER ANGIOMA. A vascular spider (nevus araneus) consists of a central feeder artery with many dilated radiating vessels and a surrounding erythematous flush, varying from a few mm to several cm in diameter (Fig. 649-12). Pressure over the central vessel causes blanching; pulsations visible in larger nevi are evidence for the arterial source of the lesion. Spider angiomas are associated with conditions in which there are increased levels of circulating estrogens, such as cirrhosis and pregnancy, but they also occur in up to 15% of normal preschool-aged children and 45% of school-aged children. Sites of predilection in children are the dorsum of the hand, forearm, face, and ears. Lesions often regress spontaneously post puberty. If removal is desired, PDL is the mode of choice, with 90% resolution with a single treatment.

GENERALIZED ESSENTIAL TELANGIECTASIA. A rare and presumably nevoid anomaly of unknown cause, essential telangiectasia may have its onset in childhood or adulthood. Mild expression consists of patchy retiform telangiectases, particularly on the limbs, with occasional progression to involve large areas of the body surface. The condition must be distinguished from the secondary telangiectasias of connective tissue diseases, xeroderma pigmentosum, poikiloderma, and ataxia-telangiectasia. Treatment with PDL is effective.

UNILATERAL NEVOID TELANGIECTASIA. This unusual entity is characterized by the appearance of telangiectasia in a unilateral distribution, primarily on the face, neck, chest, and arms. The acquired form occurs most commonly in females at onset of menses or during pregnancy. When initiated by pregnancy, the telangiectasia may fade or disappear postpartum.

GENETIC DISORDERS

BLUE RUBBER BLEB NEVUS. This syndrome consists of numerous venous malformations of the skin, mucous membranes, and gastrointestinal tract. Typical lesions are blue-purple and rubbery in consistency; they vary in size from a few mm to a few cm in diameter. They are sometimes painful or tender. The nodules occasionally are present at birth but usually appear in childhood. New lesions may continue to develop throughout life. Large disfiguring and irregular blue marks may also occur. The lesions, which can rarely be located in the liver, spleen, and central nervous system in addition to the skin and gastrointestinal tract, do not involute spontaneously. Recurrent gastrointestinal hemorrhage may lead to severe anemia. Palliation can be achieved by excision of involved bowel.

MAFFUCCI SYNDROME. The association of numerous vascular and, occasionally, lymphatic malformations with **nodular enchondromas** in the metaphyseal or diaphyseal portion of long bones is known as Maffucci syndrome. Mutations in the PTH/PTHrP type 1 receptor have been identified in the enchondromatoses. Vascular lesions are typically soft, compressible, asymptomatic blue-to-purple subcutaneous masses that grow in proportion to a child's growth and stabilize by adulthood. Mucous membranes or viscera may also be involved. Onset occurs during childhood. Bone lesions may produce limb deformities and pathologic fractures. Malignant transformation of enchondromas (chondrosarcoma, angiosarcoma) or primary malignancies (ovarian, fibrosarcoma, glioma, pancreatic) may be a complication (see Chapter 501).

HEREDITARY HEMORRHAGIC TELANGIECTASIA (OSLER-WEBER-RENDU DISEASE). This disorder is inherited as an autosomal dominant trait. One involved gene encodes endoglin, a membrane glycoprotein on endothelial cells that binds transforming growth factor–β. Affected children may experience recurrent epistaxis before detection of the characteristic skin and mucous membrane

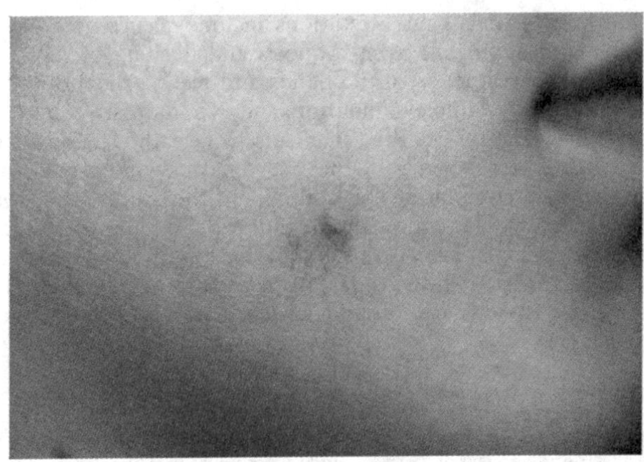

Figure 649-12. Spider telangiectasia with visible central arteriole component.

lesions. The mucocutaneous lesions, which usually develop at puberty, are 1–4 mm, sharply demarcated red to purple macules, papules, or spider-like projections, each composed of a tightly woven mat of tortuous telangiectatic vessels. The nasal mucosa, lips, and tongue are usually involved; less commonly, cutaneous lesions occur on the face, ears, palms, and nail beds. Vascular ectasias may also arise in the conjunctivae, larynx, pharynx, gastrointestinal tract, bladder, vagina, bronchi, brain, and liver.

Massive hemorrhage is the most serious complication and may result in severe anemia. Bleeding may occur from the nose, mouth, gastrointestinal tract, genitourinary tract, and lungs; epistaxis is often the only complaint, however, occurring in 80% of patients. Approximately 15–20% of patients with arteriovenous malformations in the lungs present with stroke due to embolic abscesses. Persons with hereditary hemorrhagic telangiectasia have normal levels of clotting factors and an intact clotting mechanism. In the absence of serious complications, life span is normal. Local lesions may be ablated temporarily with chemical cautery or electrocoagulation. More drastic surgical measures may be required for lesions in critical sites such as the lung or gastrointestinal tract. Anemia should be treated with iron.

HEREDITARY BENIGN TELANGIECTASIA. This rare disorder is inherited as an autosomal dominant trait and develops during childhood. The face, upper trunk, and arms are the areas of predilection. The condition is progressive but remains limited to the skin.

ATAXIA-TELANGIECTASIA (SEE CHAPTER 125.2). This disorder (Louis-Bar syndrome) is transmitted as an autosomal recessive trait due to a mutation in the ATM gene. The characteristic telangiectasias develop at about 3 yr of age, 1st on the bulbar conjunctivae and later on the nasal bridge, malar areas, external ears, hard palate, upper anterior chest, and antecubital and popliteal fossae. Additional cutaneous stigmata include café-au-lait spots, premature graying of the hair, and sclerodermatous changes. Progressive cerebellar ataxia, neurologic deterioration, sinopulmonary infections and malignancies are also seen.

ANGIOKERATOMA CORPORIS DIFFUSUM (FABRY DISEASE) [SEE CHAPTER 86.4]. This inborn error of glycolipid metabolism (α-galactosidase) is an X-linked recessive disorder that is fully penetrant in males and is of variable penetrance in carrier females. Angiokeratomas have their onset before puberty and occur in profusion over the genitalia, hips, buttocks, and thighs and in the umbilical and inguinal regions. They consist of 0.1–3 mm red to blue-black papules that may have a hyperkeratotic surface. Telangiectasias are seen in the mucosa and conjunctiva. On light microscopy, these angiokeratomas appear as blood-filled, dilated, endothelium-lined vascular spaces. Granular lipid deposits are demonstrable in dermal macrophages, fibrocytes, and endothelial cells.

Additional clinical manifestations include recurrent episodes of fever and agonizing pain, cyanosis and flushing of the acral limb areas, paresthesias of the hands and feet, corneal opacities detectable by slit-lamp examination, and hypohidrosis. Renal and cardiac involvement are the usual causes of death. The biochemical defect is a deficiency of the lysosomal enzyme α-galactosidase, with accumulation of ceramide trihexoside in tissues, particularly vascular endothelium, and excretion in urine. Similar cutaneous lesions have also been described in another lysosomal enzyme disorder, α-L-fucosidase deficiency, and in sialidosis, a storage disease with neuraminidase deficiency. (See Chapter 86.4 for therapy.)

Bayrak-Toydemir P, Mao R, Lewin S, et al: Hereditary hemorrhagic telangiectasia: An overview of diagnosis and management in the molecular era for clinicians. *Genet Med* 2004;6:175–191.

Cabrera J, Cabrera J Jr, Garcia-Olmedo A, et al: Treatment of venous malformations with sclerosant in Microfoam form. *Arch Dermatol* 2003;139:1409–1416.

Chang MW: Updated classification of hemangiomas and other vascular anomalies. *Lymphat Res Biol* 2003;1:259–265.

Haggstrom A, Lammer E, Schneider R, et al: Patterns of infantile hemangiomas: new clues to hemangioma pathogens and embryonic facial development. *Pediatr* 2005;117:698–703.

Hopyan S, Gokgoz N, Poon R, et al: A mutant PTH/PTHrP type I receptor in enchondromatosis. *Nat Genet* 2002;30:306–310.

Leung AK, Rafaat M: Benign neonatal hemangiomatosis. *Pediatr Dermatol* 2003;20:161–163.

Lyons LL, North PE, Mac-MouneLai F, et al: Kaposiform hemangioendothelioma: A study of 33 cases emphasizing its pathologic, immunophenotype, and biologic uniqueness from juvenile hemangiomas. *Am J Surg Pathol* 2004;28:559–568.

Mohrenschlager M, Henkel V, Ring J: Fabry disease: More than angiokeratomas. *Arch Dermatol* 2004;140:1526–1528.

Nahm WK, Moise S, Eichenfield LF, et al: Venous malformations in blue rubber bleb nevus syndrome: Variable onset of presentation. *J Am Acad Dermatol* 2004;50:S101–S106.

Perlman S, Becker-Catania S, Gatti RA: Ataxia-telangiectasia: Diagnosis and treatment. *Semin Pediatr Neurol* 2003;10:173–182.

Wananukul S, Nuchprayoon I, Seksarn P: Treatment of Kasabach-Merritt syndrome: A stepwise regimen of prednisolone, dipyramidole, and interferon. *Int J Dermatol* 2003;42:741–748.

Waner M, North PE, Scherer KA, et al: The nonrandom distribution of facial hemangiomas. *Arch Dermatol* 2003;139:869–875.

Chapter 650 ■ Cutaneous Nevi

Joseph G. Morelli

Nevus skin lesions are characterized histopathologically by collections of well-differentiated cell types normally found in the skin. Vascular nevi are described in Chapter 649. Melanocytic nevi are subdivided into 2 broad categories: those that appear after birth (acquired nevi) and those that are present at birth (congenital nevi).

ACQUIRED MELANOCYTIC NEVUS. Melanocytic nevi are a benign cluster of melanocytic nevus cells that arise as a result of alteration and proliferation of melanocytes at the epidermal-dermal junction.

Epidemiology. The number of acquired melanocytic nevi increases gradually during childhood, sharply at adolescence, and more slowly in early adulthood. It reaches a plateau in number in the 3rd or 4th decade and then slowly decreases thereafter. The mean number of melanocytic nevi in an adult varies depending on genetics, skin color, and sun exposure. The greater the number of nevi present, the greater is the risk for development of **melanoma.** Sun exposure during childhood, particularly intermittent, intense exposure of an individual with light skin, and a propensity to burn and freckle rather than tan are important determinants of the number of melanocytic nevi that develop. Red-haired children despite their light skin and propensity to freckle and sunburn develop fewer nevi than do other children. Increased numbers of nevi are also associated with immunosuppression and administration of chemotherapy.

Clinical Manifestations. Nevocellular nevi have a well-defined life history and are classified as **junctional, compound,** or **dermal** in accordance with the location of the nevus cells in the skin. In childhood, >90% of nevi are junctional; melanocyte proliferation occurs at the junction of the epidermis and dermis to form nests of cells. Junctional nevi appear anywhere on the body in various shades of brown; they are relatively small, discrete, flat, and variable in shape. The melanized nevus cells are cuboidal or epithelioid in configuration and occur in nests on the epidermal side of the basement membrane. Although some nevi, particularly those on the palms, soles, and genitalia, remain junctional throughout life, most become compound as melanocytes migrate into the papillary dermis to form nests at both the epidermal-dermal junction and within the dermis. If the junctional melanocytes stop proliferating, nests of melanocytes remain only within the dermis, forming an intradermal nevus. With maturation, compound and intradermal nevi may become raised, dome-shaped, verrucous, or pedunculated. Slightly elevated lesions are usually compound. Distinctly elevated lesions are usually intradermal. With age, the dermal melanocytic nests regress and the nevi gradually disappear.

Prognosis and Treatment. Acquired pigmented nevi are benign, but a very small percentage undergo malignant transformation. Suspicious changes such as rapid increase in size; development of satellite lesions; variegation of color, particularly with shades of red, brown, gray, black, and blue; pigmentary incontinence; notching or irregularity of the borders; changes in texture such as scaling, erosion, ulceration, and induration; and regional lymphadenopathy are indications for excision and histopathologic evaluation. Most of these changes are due to irritation, infection, or maturation; darkening and gradual increase in size and elevation normally occur during adolescence and should not be cause for concern. Two common benign changes are clonal nevi (fried-egg moles) and rim nevi. Clonal nevi are light brown with a dark raised center representing a clonal change of a subset of nevus cells within the lesion. Rim nevi are flat and light brown with a dark brown rim. They are seen primarily in the scalp (Fig. 650-1). Consideration should be given to the presence of risk factors for development of melanoma and the parents' wishes about removal of the nevus. If doubt remains about the benign nature of a nevus, excision is a safe and simple outpatient procedure that may be justified to allay anxiety.

ATYPICAL MELANOCYTIC NEVUS. Atypical melanocytic nevi occur both in an autosomal dominant familial melanoma-prone setting (familial mole-melanoma syndrome, dysplastic nevus syndrome, BK mole syndrome) and as a sporadic event. Only 2% of all pediatric melanomas occur in individuals with this familial syndrome; 10% of those with the syndrome have a melanoma develop before age 20. Malignant melanoma has been reported in children with the dysplastic nevus syndrome as early as 10 yr old. Risk for development of melanoma is essentially 100% in individuals with dysplastic nevus syndrome who have 2 family members who have had melanomas. The term atypical mole syndrome describes lesions in those individuals without an autosomal dominant familial history of melanoma but with >50 nevi, some of which are atypical. The lifetime risk of melanoma associated with dysplastic nevi in this context is estimated to be 5–10%.

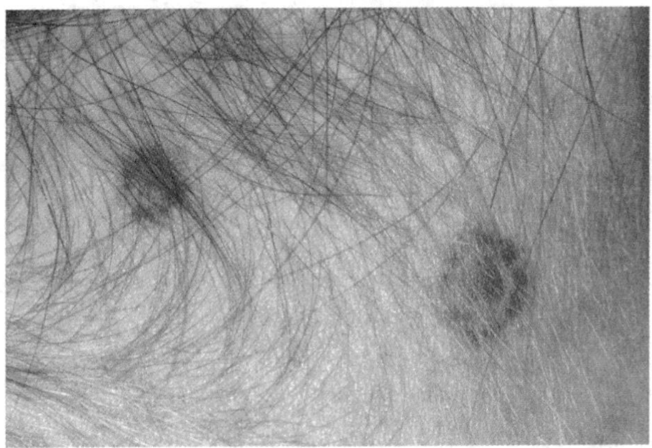

Figure 650-1. Rim moles in the scalp.

Atypical nevi tend to be large (5–15 mm) and round to oval. They have irregular margins, variegated color, and elevation of a portion of the lesion. These nevi are most common on the posterior trunk, suggesting that intermittent, intense sun exposure has a role in their genesis. They may also occur in sun-protected areas such as the breasts, buttocks, and scalp. Atypical nevi do not usually develop until puberty, although scalp lesions may be present earlier. Atypical nevi demonstrate disordered proliferation of atypical intraepidermal melanocytes, lymphocytic infiltration, fibroplasia, and angiogenesis. It may be helpful to obtain histopathologic documentation of dysplastic change by biopsy to identify these individuals. It is prudent to excise borderline atypical nevi in immunocompromised children or in those treated with irradiation or chemotherapeutic agents. Although chemotherapy has been associated with the development of a greater number of melanocytic nevi, it has not been directly linked to increased risk of development of melanoma. The threshold for removal of clinically atypical nevi is also lower at sites that are difficult to observe, such as the scalp. Children with atypical nevi should have a complete skin examination every 6–12 mo. In these children, photographic mole mapping serves as a useful adjunct in following nevus change. Parents must be counseled about the importance of sun protection and avoidance and be instructed to look for early signs of melanoma on a regular basis, approximately every 3–4 mo.

CONGENITAL MELANOCYTIC NEVUS. Congenital melanocytic nevi are present in ≈1% of newborn infants. These nevi have been categorized by size: giant congenital nevi are >20 cm in diameter (adult size) or >5% of the body surface, small congenital nevi are <2 cm in diameter, and intermediate nevi are in between in size. Congenital nevi are characterized by the presence of nevus cells in the lower reticular dermis; between collagen bundles; surrounding cutaneous appendages, nerves, and vessels in the lower dermis; and occasionally extending to the subcuticular fat. Identification is often uncertain, however, because they may have the histologic features of ordinary junctional, compound, or intradermal nevi. Some nevi that were not present at birth display histopathologic features of congenital nevi; these should not be considered congenital. Furthermore, congenital nevi may be difficult to distinguish clinically from other types of pigmented lesions, adding to the difficulty that parents may have in identifying nevi that were present at birth. The clinical differential diagnosis includes mongolian spots, café-au-lait spots, smooth muscle hamartoma, and dermal melanocytosis (nevi of Ota and Ito).

Sites of predilection of small congenital nevi are the lower trunk, upper back, shoulders, chest, and proximal limbs. The lesions may be flat, elevated, verrucous, or nodular and may be various shades of brown, blue, or black. Given the difficulty in identifying small congenital nevi with certainty, data regarding their malignant potential are controversial and likely overstated. The true incidence of melanoma in congenital nevi, especially small and medium-sized, is unknown. Removal of all small congenital nevi is not warranted because the development of melanoma in a small congenital nevus is an exceedingly rare event before puberty. A number of factors must be weighed in the decision about whether or not to remove a nevus, including its location and ability to be monitored clinically, the potential for scarring, the presence of other risk factors for melanoma, and the presence of atypical clinical features.

Giant congenital pigmented nevi (<1/20,000 births) occur most commonly on the posterior trunk (Fig. 650-2) but may also appear on the head or extremities. These nevi are of special significance because of their association with leptomeningeal melanocytosis (neurocutaneous melanocytosis) and their predisposition for development of malignant melanoma. Leptomeningeal involvement occurs most often when the

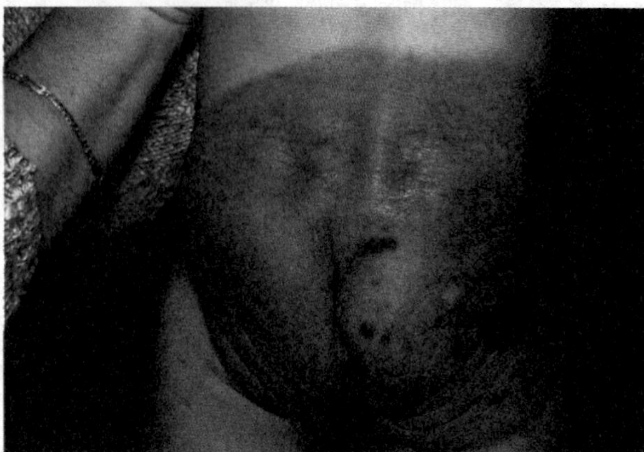

Figure 650-2. "Bathing suit" large congenital melanocytic nevus.

nevus is located on the head or midline on the trunk, particularly when associated with multiple "satellite" melanocytic nevi (>20 lesions). Nevus cells within the leptomeninges and brain parenchyma may cause increased intracranial pressure, hydrocephalus, seizures, retardation, and motor deficits, and may result in melanoma. Malignancy can be identified by careful cytologic examination of the cerebrospinal fluid for melanin-containing cells. MRI demonstrates asymptomatic leptomeningeal melanosis in ≈30% of individuals with a giant congenital nevus. The overall incidence of malignant melanoma arising in a giant congenital nevus is estimated to be ≈5–10%. Half of all melanomas that arise within a giant congenital nevus do so by age 5. The mortality rate is 45%. Management of giant congenital nevi remains controversial and should involve the parents, pediatrician, dermatologist, and plastic surgeon. If the nevus lies over the head or spine, an MRI scan may allow detection of neural melanosis; its presence makes gross removal of a nevus from the skin a futile effort. In the absence of neural melanosis, early excision and repair aided by tissue expanders or grafting may reduce the burden of nevus cells and thus the potential for development of melanoma, but at the cost of many potentially disfiguring surgeries. Nevus cells deep within subcutaneous tissues may evade excision. Random biopsies of the nevus are not helpful, but biopsy of newly expanding nodules is indicated. Follow-up is recommended every 6 mo for 5 yr and every 12 mo thereafter. Serial photographs of the nevus may aid in detecting changes.

MELANOMA. Malignant melanoma accounts for 1–3% of all pediatric malignancies and is the most common cancer in young adults age 25–29. The incidence of melanoma has increased 150% since 1973. Melanoma develops primarily in white individuals, on the head and trunk in males, and on the extremities in females. Risk factors for development of melanoma include the presence of the familial atypical mole-melanoma syndrome or xeroderma pigmentosum; an increased number of acquired melanocytic nevi, or atypical nevi; fair complexion; excessive sun exposure, especially intense sunlight intermittently; a personal or family (first-degree relative) history of a previous melanoma, giant congenital nevus, and immunosuppression. In previously well children, UV radiation is responsible for most melanomas. Fewer than 5% of childhood melanomas develop within giant congenital nevi or in those with the familial atypical mole-melanoma syndrome. Approximately 40–50% of the time, melanoma develops at a site where there was no apparent nevus (amelanotic lesion). The mortality rate from melanoma is related primarily to tumor thickness and the level of invasion into the skin. The overall mortality rate reaches ≈40%, regardless of whether it arises in a child or adult. Given the lack of effective therapy for melanoma, prevention and early detection are the most effective measures. Avoidance of intense midday sun exposure between 10 A.M. and 3 P.M.; use of protective clothing such as a hat, long sleeves, and pants; and use of sunscreen should be emphasized. Early detection includes frequent clinical and photographic examinations for patients at risk (dysplastic nevus syndrome) and prompt response to rapid changes in nevi (size, shape, color, inflammation, bleeding or crusting, and sensation). The ABCD rule (asymmetry, border irregularities, color variability, diameter >6 mm), which is a useful screening tool for adults, may not be as effective for children.

HALO NEVUS. Halo nevi occur primarily in children and young adults, most commonly on the back (Fig. 650-3). Development of the halo may coincide with puberty or pregnancy. Several pigmented nevi frequently develop a halo simultaneously. Subsequent disappearance of the central nevus over several months is the usual outcome, and the depigmented area may or may not become repigmented. Excision and histopathologic examination of the lesion is indicated only when the nature of the central lesion is in question. An acquired melanocytic nevus occasionally develops a peripheral zone of depigmentation over a period of days to weeks. There is a dense inflammatory infiltrate of lymphocytes and histiocytes in addition to the nevus cells. The pale halo reflects disappearance of the melanocytes. This phenomenon is associated with congenital nevi, blue nevi, Spitz nevi, dysplastic nevi, neurofibromas, and primary and secondary malignant melanoma and occasionally with poliosis, Vogt-Koyanagi-Harada syndrome, and pernicious anemia. Patients with vitiligo have an increased incidence of halo nevi. Individuals with halo nevi have circulating antibodies against the cytoplasm of melanocytes and nevus cells.

SPITZ NEVUS (SPINDLE AND EPITHELIOID CELL NEVUS). Spitz nevus presents most commonly in the 1st 2 decades of life as a pink to red, smooth, dome-shaped, firm, hairless papule on the face, shoulder, or upper limb (Fig. 650-4). Most are <1 cm in diameter, but they can achieve a size of 3 cm. Rarely, they occur as numerous grouped lesions. Visually similar lesions include pyogenic granuloma, hemangioma, nevocellular nevus, juvenile xanthogranuloma, and basal cell carcinoma, but these entities are histologically distinguishable. Spitz nevus may be difficult to distinguish histopathologically from malignant melanoma because nuclear atypia is a common feature, particularly after local recurrence of the nevus. Difficulty arises in the fact that many other clinical types of melanocytic nevi have a similar histologic appearance. Local recurrence after excision may occur up to 5% of the time. If a nevus arouses clinical suspicion that it may be a melanoma, an excisional biopsy of the entire lesion is recommended. If the margins of excision of a Spitz nevus are positive,

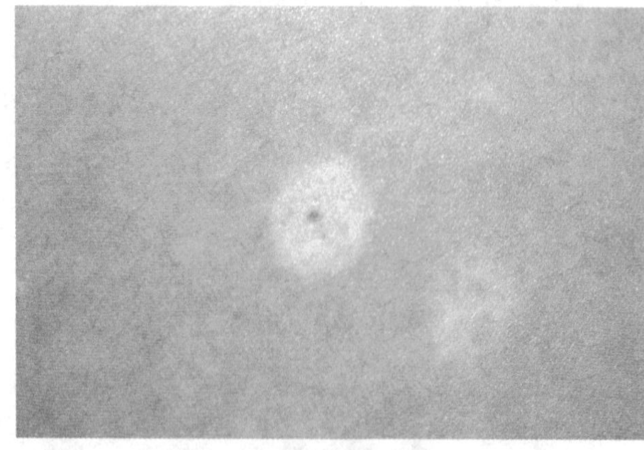

Figure 650-3. Well-developed halo nevus.

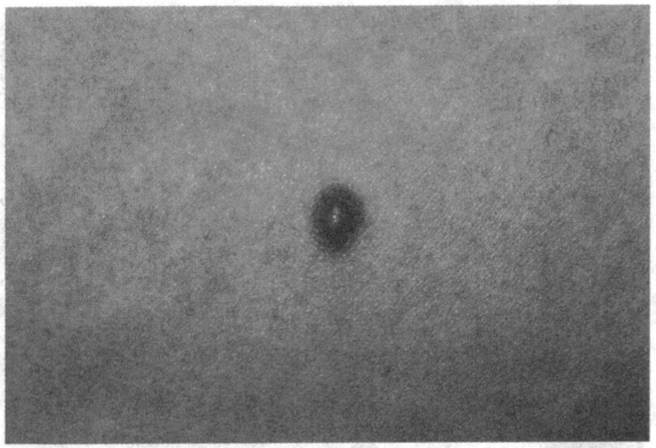

Figure 650-4. Dome-shaped red Spitz nevus.

re-excision of the site is prudent to avoid difficulties in histopathologic interpretation of the lesion in the future.

ZOSTERIFORM LENTIGINOUS NEVUS (AGMINATED LENTIGINE). This nevus is a unilateral, linear, bandlike collection of numerous 2–10 mm brown or black macules on the face, trunk, or limbs. The nevus may be present at birth or may develop during childhood. There are increased numbers of melanocytes in elongated rete ridges of the epidermis.

NEVUS SPILUS (SPECKLED LENTIGINOUS NEVUS). This nevus is a flat brown patch within which are darker flat or raised brown melanocytic elements (Fig. 650-5). These nevi vary considerably in size and can occur anywhere on the body. The color of the macular component may vary from light to dark brown and the number of darker lesions may be few or many. Nevus spilus is rare at birth and is commonly acquired in late infancy or early childhood. Dark elements within the nevus are usually present initially and tend to increase in number gradually over time. The darker macules represent nevus cells in a junctional or dermal location; the patch has increased numbers of melanocytes in a lentiginous epidermal pattern. The malignant potential of these nevi is uncertain; nevus spilus is found more commonly in individuals with melanoma than in matched control subjects. The nevi need not be excised, unless atypical features or recent clinical changes are noted.

NEVUS OF OTA. Nevus of Ota is more common among females, Asian, and black patients. This nevus consists of a permanent patch composed of partially confluent blue, black, and brown macules. The intensity of pigmentation may vary from day to day, and enlargement and darkening may occur with time. Occasionally, some areas of the nevus are raised. The macular nevi resemble mongolian spots in color and occur unilaterally in the areas supplied by the 1st and 2nd divisions of the trigeminal nerve. Nevus of Ota differs from a mongolian spot, not only by its distribution but also by having a speckled rather than a uniform appearance. Both are forms of mid-dermal melanocytosis. It also has a greater concentration of elongated, dendritic dermal melanocytes located in the upper rather than the lower portion of the dermis. Nevus of Ota is sometimes present at birth; in other cases, it may arise during the 1st or 2nd decade of life. Patchy involvement of the conjunctiva, hard palate, pharynx, nasal mucosa, buccal mucosa, or tympanic membrane occurs in some patients. Malignant change is exceedingly rare. Laser therapy may effectively decrease the pigmentation.

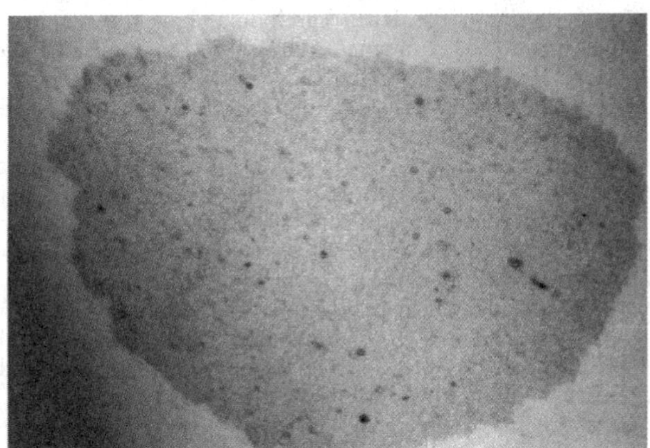

Figure 650-5. Nevus spilus.

Nevus of Ito is localized to the supraclavicular, scapular, and deltoid regions. This nevus tends to be more diffuse in its distribution and less mottled than the nevus of Ota. It is also a form of mid-dermal melanocytosis. The only available treatment is masking with cosmetics or laser therapy.

BLUE NEVI. The common blue nevus is a solitary, asymptomatic, smooth, dome-shaped, blue to blue-gray papule <10 mm in diameter on the dorsal aspect of the hands and feet. Rarely, common blue nevi form large plaques. Blue nevus is nearly always acquired, often during childhood and more commonly in females. Microscopically, it is characterized by groups of intensely pigmented spindle-shaped melanocytes in the dermis. This nevus is benign.

The cellular blue nevus is typically 1–3 cm in diameter and occurs most frequently on the buttocks and in the sacrococcygeal area. In addition to collections of deeply pigmented dermal dendritic melanocytes, cellular islands composed of large spindle-shaped cells are noted in the dermis and may extend into the subcutaneous fat. A histologic continuum may be seen from blue nevi to cellular blue nevi. A combined nevus is the association of a blue nevus with an overlying melanocytic nevus.

The blue-gray that is characteristic of these nevi is an optical effect caused by dermal melanin. Longer wavelengths of visible light penetrate to the deep dermis and are absorbed there by melanin; shorter-wavelength blue light cannot penetrate deeply but instead is reflected back to the observer.

NEVUS DEPIGMENTOSUS (ACHROMIC NEVUS). These nevi are usually present at birth; they are localized macular hypopigmented patches or streaks, often with bizarre, irregular borders (Fig. 650-6). They can resemble hypomelanosis of Ito clinically, except that they are more localized and often unilateral. Small lesions may also resemble the ash leaf macules of tuberous sclerosis. They appear to represent a focal defect in transfer of melanosomes to keratinocytes.

EPIDERMAL NEVI. These may be visible at birth or may develop in the 1st months or years of life. They affect both sexes equally and usually occur sporadically. Epidermal nevi are hamartomatous lesions characterized by hyperplasia of the epidermis and/or adnexal structures in a focal area of the skin.

Epidermal nevi are classified into a number of variants, depending on the morphology and extent of the nevus and the epidermal structure that is predominant. An epidermal nevus may appear initially as a discolored, slightly scaly patch that, with maturation, becomes more linear, thickened, verrucous, and hyperpigmented. *Systematized* refers to a diffuse or extensive distribution of lesions, and *ichthyosis hystrix* indicates that the distribution is extensive and bilateral (Fig. 650-7). Morphologic types include pigmented papillomas, often in a linear distribution; unilateral hyperkeratotic streaks involving a limb and perhaps a

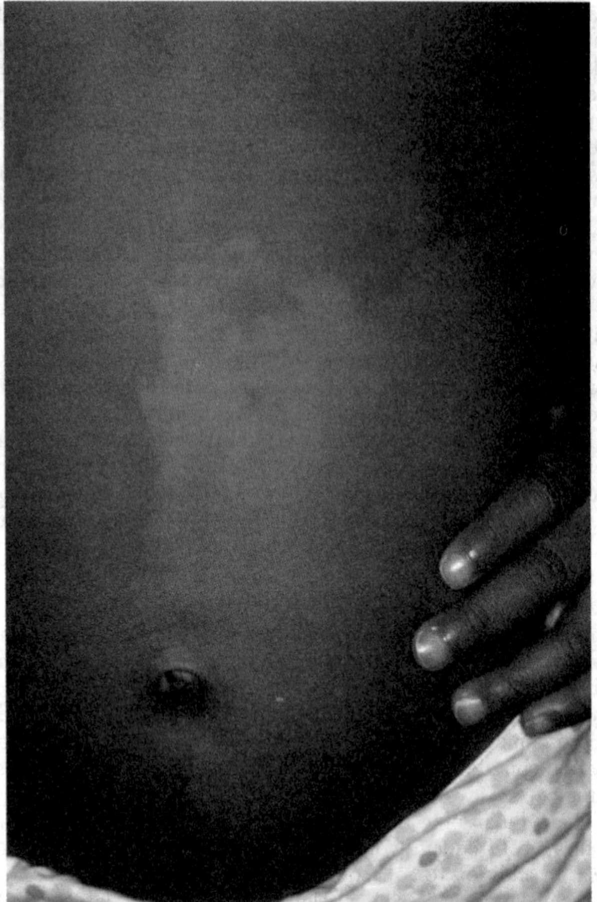

Figure 650-6. Large nevus depigmentosus of the abdomen.

portion of the trunk; velvety hyperpigmented plaques; and whorled or marbled hyperkeratotic lesions in localized plaques or over extensive areas of the body along Blaschko lines. An inflammatory linear verrucous variant is markedly pruritic and tends to become erythematous, scaling, and crusted.

The histologic pattern evolves as the lesion matures, but epidermal hyperplasia of some degree is apparent in all stages of development. One or another dermal appendage may predominate in a particular lesion. These nevi must be distinguished from lichen striatus, lymphangioma circumscriptum, shagreen patch of tuberous sclerosis, congenital hairy nevi, linear porokeratosis, linear lichen planus, linear psoriasis, the verrucous stage of incontinentia pigmenti, and nevus sebaceus (Jadassohn). Keratolytic agents such as retinoic acid or salicylic acid may be moderately effective in reducing scaling and controlling pruritus, but definitive treatment requires full-thickness excision; recurrence is usual if more superficial removal is attempted. Alternatively, the nevus may be left intact. Epidermal nevi are occasionally associated with other abnormalities of the skin and soft tissues, eyes, and nervous, cardiovascular, musculoskeletal, and urogenital systems. In these instances, referred to as epidermal nevus syndrome, a mosaic phenotype is expressed. This syndrome, however, is not a distinct clinical entity. The well-established syndromes that involve a type of epidermal nevus and distinct birth defects include the **Proteus** and **CHILD** (congenital hemidysplasia with ichthyosiform erythroderma and limb defects) syndromes.

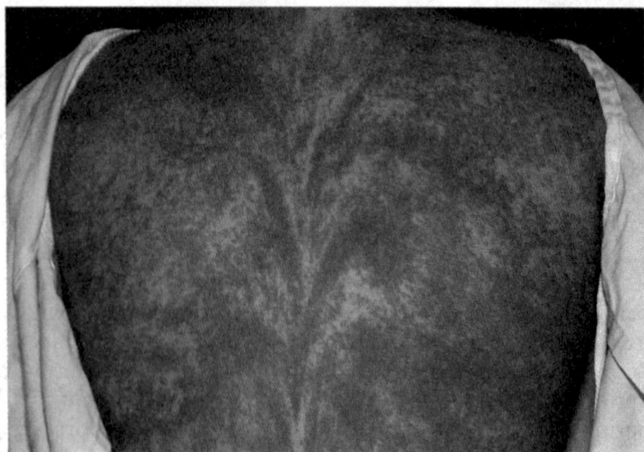

Figure 650-7. Epidermal nevus (ichthyosis hystrix type).

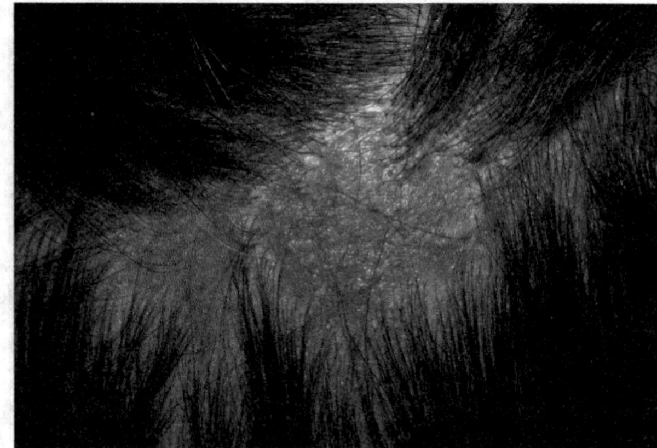

Figure 650-8. Orange-yellow nevus sebaceus of the scalp.

Nevus Sebaceus (Jadassohn). This is a relatively small, sharply demarcated, oval or linear, elevated yellow-orange plaque that is usually devoid of hair and occurs on the head and neck of infants (Fig. 650-8). It may occur occasionally on the trunk. Although the lesion is characterized histopathologically by an abundance of sebaceous glands, all elements of the skin are represented. It is frequently flat and inconspicuous in early childhood. With maturity, usually during adolescence, the lesions become verrucous and studded with large rubbery nodules. The changing clinical appearance reflects the histologic pattern, which is characterized by a variable degree of hyperkeratosis, hyperplasia of the epidermis, malformed hair follicles, and often a profusion of sebaceous glands and the presence of ectopic apocrine glands. It is believed that these nevi form from pluripotential primary epithelial germ cells, which can dedifferentiate into various **epithelial tumors.** Consequently, during adulthood, these nevi are frequently complicated by secondary malignancies and benign adnexal tumors, most commonly, basal cell carcinoma or syringocystadenoma papilliferum. Deletions in the PTCH gene, the putative gene defect in basal cell carcinoma, have been found in sebaceus nevi. The **treatment of choice** is total excision before adolescence. Sebaceus nevi associated with central nervous system, skeletal, and ocular defects represent a variant of the epidermal nevus syndrome.

Becker Nevus (Becker Melanosis). This form of nevus develops predominantly in males, during childhood or adolescence, initially as a hyperpigmented patch. The lesion commonly develops hypertrichosis, limited to the area of hyperpigmentation, and evolves into a unilateral, slightly thickened, irregular, hyperpigmented plaque. The most common sites are the upper torso and upper arm (Fig. 650-9). The nevus shows an increased number of basal melanocytes and variable epidermal hyperplasia. Becker melanosis is commonly associated with a smooth muscle hamartoma, which may appear as slight perifollicular papular elevations or slight induration. Stroking such a lesion may induce smooth muscle contraction and make the hairs stand up. The nevus is benign, has no risk for malignant change, and is rarely associated with other anomalies.

NEVUS COMEDONICUS. This is an uncommon organoid nevus of epithelial origin that consists of linear plaques of plugged follicles that simulate comedones; they may be present at birth or may appear during childhood. The horny plugs represent keratinous debris within dilated, malformed pilosebaceous follicles. The lesions are most often unilateral and may develop at any site. Rarely, they are associated with other congenital malformations, including skeletal defects, cerebral anomalies, and cataracts. Although these lesions are often asymptomatic, some individuals experience recurrent inflammation, resulting in cyst formation, fistulas, and scarring. There is no effective treatment except full-thickness excision; palliation of larger lesions may be achieved by regular applications of a retinoic acid preparation.

CONNECTIVE TISSUE NEVUS. This is a hamartoma of collagen, elastin, and/or glycosaminoglycans of the dermal extracellular matrix. It may occur as a solitary defect or as a manifestation of an associated disorder. These nevi may occur at any site but are most common on the back, buttocks, arms, and thighs. They are skin-colored, ivory, or yellow plaques, 2–15 cm in diameter, composed of many tiny papules or grouped nodules that are frequently difficult to appreciate visually because of the subtle color changes. The plaques have a rubbery or cobblestone consistency on palpation. Biopsy findings are variable and include increased amounts and/or degeneration or fragmentation of dermal collagen, elastic tissue, or ground substance. Similar lesions occurring with tuberous sclerosis are called shagreen patches; however, shagreen patches consist only of excessive amounts of collagen. The association of many small papular connective tissue nevi with osteopoikilosis is called dermatofibrosis lenticularis disseminata (**Buschke-Ollendorf syndrome**).

SMOOTH MUSCLE HAMARTOMA. This hamartoma is a developmental anomaly resulting from hyperplasia of the smooth muscle (arrector pili) associated with hair follicles. It is usually evident at birth or shortly thereafter as a flesh-colored or lightly pigmented plaque with overlying hypertrichosis on the trunk or limbs (Fig. 650-10). Transient elevation or a rippling movement of the lesion, caused by contraction of the muscle bundles, can sometimes be elicited by stroking the surface. Smooth muscle hamartoma can be mistaken for congenital pigmented nevus, but the distinction is important because it has no risk for malignant melanoma and need not be removed.

Figure 650-9. Becker nevus on the shoulder of an adolescent male.

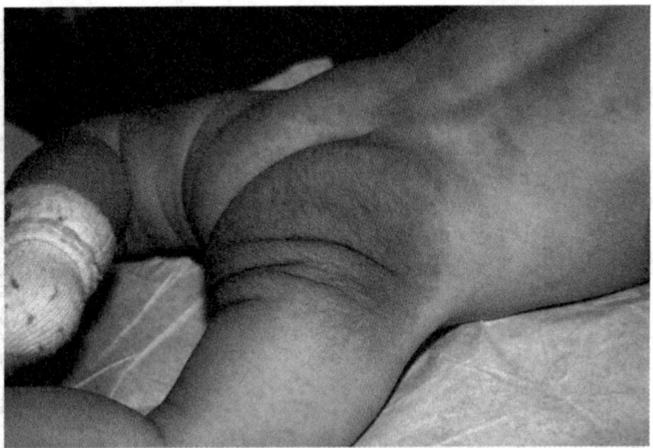

Figure 650-10. Large smooth muscle hamartoma of the buttock.

Bauer J, Garbe C: Acquired melanocytic nevi as risk factor for melanoma development. A comprehensive review of epidemiological data. *Pigment Cell Res* 2003;16:297–306.

Chan HH, Kono T: Nevus of Ota: Clinical aspects and management. *Skinmed* 2003;2:89–96.

Dahlstrom JE, Scolyer RA, Thompson JF, Jain S: Spitz naevus: Diagnostic problems and their management implications. *Pathology* 2004;36:452–457.

De Snoo FA, Bergman W, Gruis NA: Familial melanoma: A complex disorder leading to controversy of DNA testing. *Fam Cancer* 2003;2:109–116.

Ferrari A, Bono A, Baldi M, et al: Does melanoma behave differently in younger children than in adults? A retrospective study of 33 cases of childhood melanoma from a single institution. *Pediatrics* 2005;115:649–654.

Herron MD, Vanderhooft SL, Smock K, et al: Proliferative nodules in congenital melanocytic nevi: A clinicopathologic and immunohistochemical analysis. *Am J Surg Pathol* 2004;28:1017–1025.

Huynh PM, Glusac EJ, Bolognia JL: The clinical appearance of clonal nevi (inverted type A nevi). *Int J Dermatol* 2004;43:882–885.

Marghoob AA, Dusza S, Oliveria S, et al: Number of satellite nevi as a correlate for neurocutaneous melanocytosis in patients with large congenital melanocytic nevi. *Arch Dermatol* 2004;140:171–173.

Miller AJ, Mihm Jr. MC: Melanoma. *N Engl J Med* 2006;355:51–65.

Pappo AS: Melanoma in children and adolescents. *Eur J Cancer* 2003;39: 2651–2661.

Vidaurri-dela Cruz H, Tamayo-Sanchez L, Duran-McKinster C, et al. Epidermal nevus syndrome: Clinical findings in 35 patients. *Pediatr Dermatol* 2004;21:432–439.

Whiteman DC, Brown RM, Purdie DM, et al: Prevalence and anatomical distribution of naevi in young Queensland children. *Int J Cancer* 2003;106: 930–933.

Zaal LH, Mooi WJ, Klip H, Vander Horst CM: Risk of malignant transformation of congenital melanocytic nevi: a retrospective nationwide study from the Netherlands. *Plast Reconstr Surg* 2005;116:1902–1909.

Chapter 651 ■ Hyperpigmented Lesions

Joseph G. Morelli

DISORDERS OF PIGMENT. Normal pigmentation requires migration of melanoblasts from the neural crest to the dermal-epidermal junction, enzymatic processes to form pigment, structural components to contain the pigment (melanosomes), and transfer of pigment to the surrounding keratinocytes. Increased skin color may be generalized or localized and may result from various defects in any of these requirements. Some of these aberrations are a manifestation of systemic disease, others represent general-

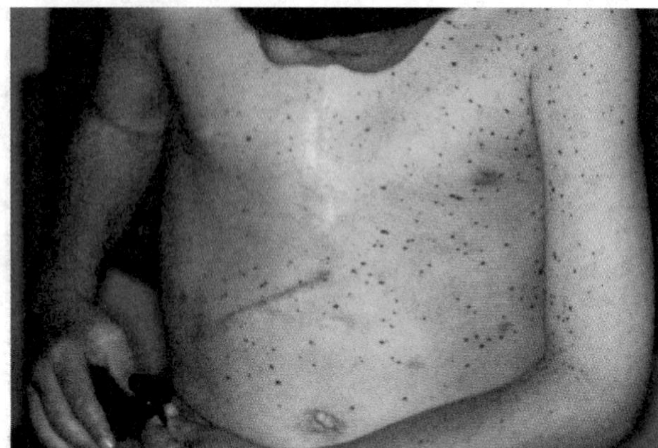

Figure 651-1. Multiple lentigines in LEOPARD syndrome.

ized or focal developmental defects, and still others may be nonspecific and the result of cutaneous inflammation.

EPHELIDES (FRECKLES). These are light or dark brown macules usually <3 mm in diameter, with a poorly defined margin, that occur in sun-exposed areas such as the face, upper back, arms, and hands. They are induced by exposure to sun, particularly during the summer, and may fade or disappear during the winter. They are more common in redheads and fair-haired individuals and first appear in the preschool years. Histologically, they are marked by increased melanin pigment in epidermal basal cells, which have more numerous and larger dendritic processes than the melanocytes of the surrounding paler skin. The lack of melanocytic proliferation or elongation of epidermal rete ridges distinguishes them from lentigines. Freckles have been identified as a risk factor for melanoma independent of melanocytic nevi.

LENTIGINES. **Lentigines,** often mistaken for freckles or junctional nevi, are small (<3 cm), round, dark brown macules that can appear anywhere on the body. They are unrelated to sun exposure and remain permanently. Histologically, they have elongated, club-shaped, epidermal rete ridges with increased numbers of melanocytes and dense epidermal deposits of melanin. No nests of melanocytes are found. The lesions are benign and, when few, may be viewed as a normal occurrence.

Lentiginosis profusa involves innumerable small, pigmented macules that are present at birth or appear during childhood. There are no associated abnormalities, and mucous membranes are spared. **LAMB syndrome** (Carney complex), a multiple endocrine neoplasia syndrome, consists of lentigines of the face and vulva, atrial myxoma, mucocutaneous myxomas, and blue nevi (PRKAR1 gene). The multiple lentigines (**LEOPARD**) **syndrome** is an autosomal dominant entity consisting of a generalized, symmetric distribution of lentigines (Fig. 651-1) in association with electrocardiogram abnormalities, ocular hypertelorism, pulmonary stenosis, abnormal genitals (cryptorchidism, hypogonadism, hypospadias), growth retardation, and sensorineural deafness (PTPN11 gene). Other features include hypertrophic obstructive cardiomyopathy and pectus excavatum or carinatum.

The **Peutz-Jeghers syndrome** is characterized by melanotic macules on the lips and mucous membranes and by gastrointestinal (GI) polyposis. It is inherited as an autosomal dominant trait (STK11 gene). Onset is noted in infancy and early childhood when pigmented macules appear on the lips and buccal mucosa. The macules are usually a few mm in size but may be as large as 1–2 cm. Macules also appear occasionally on the palate, gums, tongue, and vaginal mucosa. Cutaneous lesions may develop on the nose, hands, and feet; around the mouth, eyes, and umbilicus; and as longitudinal bands or diffuse hyperpigmentation of the nails. Pigmented macules often fade from the lips and skin during puberty and adulthood but generally do not disappear from mucosal surfaces. Buccal mucosal macules are the most constant feature of the disorder; in some families, however, occasional members may be affected only with the pigmentary changes. Indistinguishable pigmentary changes beginning in adult life, without intestinal involvement, also occur sporadically in individuals.

Polyposis usually involves the jejunum and ileum but may also occur in the stomach, duodenum, colon, and rectum (see Chapter 342). Episodic abdominal pain, diarrhea, melena, and intussusception are frequent complications. Patients have a significantly increased risk of GI tract and non-GI tract tumors at a young age. GI cancer has been reported in ≈2–3% of patients; the lifetime relative risk of GI malignancy is 13. The relative risk of non-GI tract malignancies, including ovarian, cervical, and testicular tumors, is 9. Peutz-Jeghers syndrome must be differentiated from other syndromes associated with multiple lentigines (Laugier-Hunziker syndrome), from ordinary freckling, from Gardner syndrome, and from Cronkhite-Canada syndrome, a disorder characterized by GI polyposis, alopecia, onychodystrophy, and diffuse pigmentation of the palms, volar aspects of the fingers, and dorsal hands. **Treatment** of Peutz-Jeghers melanotic macules has been successful, in some cases, with multiple different lasers.

CAFÉ-AU-LAIT SPOTS. These are uniformly hyperpigmented, sharply demarcated macular lesions, the hues of which vary with the normal degree of pigmentation of the individual: They are tan or light brown in white individuals and may be dark brown in black children (Figs. 651-2 and 651-3). Café-au-lait spots vary tremendously in size and may be large, covering a significant portion of the trunk or limb. Generally, the borders are smooth, but some have an exceedingly irregular border. The lesions are characterized by increased numbers of melanocytes and melanin in the epidermis but lack the clubbed rete ridges that typify lentigines. One to 3 café-au-lait spots are common in normal children;

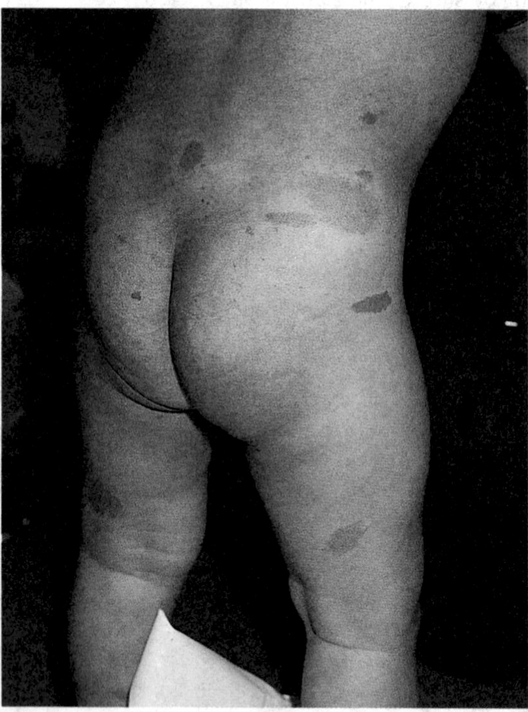

Figure 651-2. Multiple café au lait macules on a child with NF-1. (From Eichenfield LF, Frieden IJ, Esterly NB: *Textbook of Neonatal Dermatology*. Philadelphia, WB Saunders, 2001, p 372.)

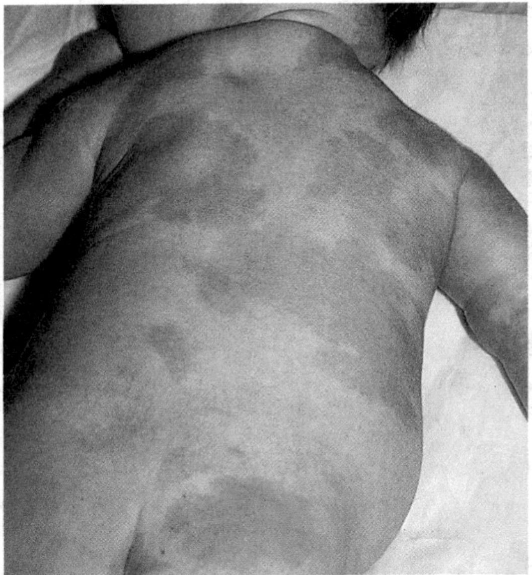

Figure 651-3. Multiple patterned café au lait spots in a child with McCune-Albright syndrome. (From Eichenfield LF, Frieden IJ, Esterly NB: *Textbook of Neonatal Dermatology.* Philadelphia, WB Saunders, 2001, p 373.)

≈10% of normal children have café-au-lait macules. They may be present at birth or develop during childhood.

Large, often asymmetric café-au-lait spots with irregular borders are characteristic of patients with McCune-Albright syndrome (GNAS1 gene) [see Chapter 563.6]. This disorder includes polyostotic fibrous dysplasia of bone, leading to pathologic fractures; precocious puberty; and numerous hyperfunctional endocrinopathies. The macular hyperpigmentation may be present at birth or develop late in childhood (see Fig. 651-3). Cutaneous pigmentation is typically most extensive on the side showing the most severe bone involvement.

Neurofibromatosis Type 1 (Von Recklinghausen Disease). The café-au-lait spot is the most familiar cutaneous hallmark of this autosomal dominant neurocutaneous syndrome (neurofibromin gene) [see Fig. 651-2; also Chapter 596.1]. These lesions also occur with certain other disorders, including other types of neurofibromatosis, but in these disorders the café-au-lait are not a major feature of the disorder and do not aid in diagnosis (Table 651-1). Included in the criteria for this diagnosis is the presence of 5 or more café-au-lait spots >5 mm in diameter in prepubertal patients or 6 or more café-au-lait spots >15 mm in diameter in postpubertal children. Multiple café-au-lait macules commonly produce a freckled appearance of non–sun-exposed areas such as the axillae (Crowe sign), the inguinal and inframammary regions, and under the chin.

TABLE 651-1. Disorders with Café-au-Lait Spots
Neurofibromatosis 1 and 2
McCune-Albright syndrome
Russell-Silver syndrome
Ataxia-telangiectasia
Fanconi anemia
Tuberous sclerosis
Bloom syndrome
Basal cell nevus syndrome
Gaucher disease
Chédiak-Higashi syndrome
Hunter syndrome
Maffucci syndrome
Multiple mucosal neuroma syndrome
Watson syndrome
Proteus syndrome
Turner syndrome
Ring chromosome syndrome
Jaffe-Campanacci syndrome

INCONTINENTIA PIGMENTI (BLOCH-SULZBERGER DISEASE). This rare, heritable, multisystem ectodermal disorder features dermatologic, dental, and ocular abnormalities. The phenotype is produced by functional mosaicism caused by random X-inactivation of an X-linked dominant gene that is lethal in males (IKK-gamma/NEMO gene). The paucity of affected males, the occurrence of female-to-female transmission, and an increased frequency of spontaneous abortions in carrier females support this supposition.

Clinical Manifestations. This disease has 4 phases, not all of which may occur in a given patient. The **1st phase** is evident at birth or in the 1st few weeks of life and consists of erythematous linear streaks and plaques of vesicles (Fig. 651-4) that are most pronounced on the limbs and circumferentially on the trunk. The lesions may be confused with those of herpes simplex, bullous impetigo, or mastocytosis, but the linear configuration is unique. Histopathologically, epidermal edema and **eosinophil**-filled intraepidermal vesicles are present. Eosinophils also infiltrate the adjacent epidermis and dermis. Blood eosinophilia as high as 65% of the white blood cell count is common. The 1st stage generally resolves by 4 mo of age, but mild, short-lived recurrences of blisters may develop during febrile illnesses. In the **2nd phase**, as blisters on the distal limbs resolve, they become dry and hyperkeratotic, forming verrucous plaques. The verrucous plaques rarely affect the trunk or face and generally involute within 6 mo. Epidermal hyperplasia, hyperkeratosis, and papillomatosis are characteristic. The **3rd or pigmentary stage** is the hallmark of incontinentia pigmenti. It generally develops over weeks to months and may overlap the earlier phases, be evident at birth, or, more commonly, begin to appear in the 1st few weeks of life. Hyperpigmentation is more often apparent on the trunk than the limbs and is distributed in macular whorls, reticulated patches, flecks, and linear streaks that follow Blaschko lines. The axillae and groin are invariably affected. The sites of involvement are not necessarily those of the preceding vesicular and warty lesions. The pigmented lesions, once present, persist throughout childhood. They generally begin to fade by early adolescence and often disappear by age 16. Occasionally, the pigmentation remains permanently, particularly in the groin. The lesion, histopathologically, shows vacuolar degeneration of the epidermal basal cells and melanin in melanophages of the upper dermis as a result of incontinence of pigment. In the **4th stage**, hairless, anhidrotic, hypopigmented patches or streaks occur as a late manifestation of incontinentia pigmenti; they may develop, however, before the hyperpigmentation of stage 3 has resolved.

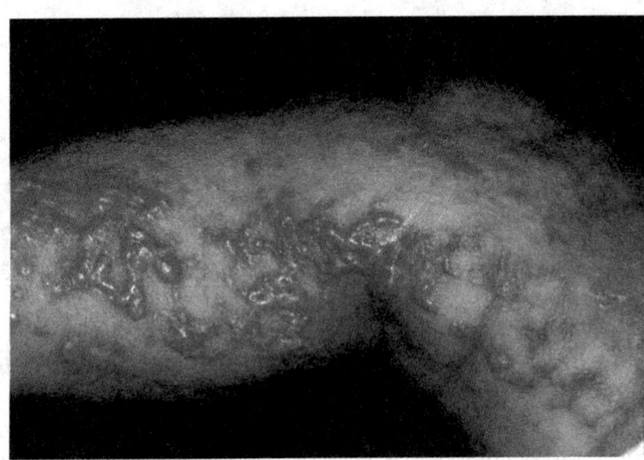

Figure 651-4. Whorled vesicular phase of incontinentia pigmenti.

The lesions develop mainly on the flexor aspect of the lower legs and less often on the arms and trunk.

Approximately 80% of affected children have other defects. Alopecia, which may be scarring and patchy or diffuse, is most common on the vertex and occurs in up to 40% of patients. Hair may be lusterless, wiry, and coarse. Dental anomalies, which are present in up to 80% of patients and are persistent throughout life, consist of late dentition, hypodontia, conical teeth, and impaction. Central nervous system manifestations, including motor and cognitive developmental retardation, seizures, microcephaly, spasticity, and paralysis, are found in up to ⅓ of affected children. Ocular anomalies, such as neovascularization, microphthalmos, strabismus, optic nerve atrophy, cataracts, and retrolenticular masses, occur in >30% of children. Nonetheless, >90% of patients have normal vision. Less common abnormalities include dystrophy of nails (ridging, pitting) and skeletal defects.

Diagnosis of incontinentia pigmenti is made on clinical grounds, although major and minor criteria have been established to aid in diagnosis. Wood lamp examination may be useful in older children and adolescents to highlight pigmentary abnormalities.

Treatment. The choice of investigative studies and the plan of management depend on the occurrence of particular noncutaneous abnormalities because the skin lesions are benign. The high incidence of associated major anomalies warrants genetic counseling.

POSTINFLAMMATORY PIGMENTARY CHANGES. Either hyperpigmentation or hypopigmentation can occur as a result of cutaneous inflammation. Alteration in pigmentation usually follows a severe inflammatory reaction but may result from mild dermatitis. Dark-skinned children are more likely to show these changes than fair-skinned ones. Although altered pigmentation may persist for weeks to months, patients can be reassured that these lesions are usually temporary.

Amos CL, Keitheri-Cheteri MB, Sabripour M, et al: Genotype-phenotype correlations in Peutz-Jeughers syndrome. *J Med Genet* 2004;41:327–333.

Bruckner AL: Incontinentia pigmenti: A window to the role of NF-kappaB function. *Semin Cutan Med Surg* 2004;23:116–124.

De Schepper S, Boucneau J, Lambert J, et al: Pigment cell-related manifestations in neurofibromatosis type 1: An overview. *Pigment Cell Res* 2005; 18:13–24.

Listernick R, Charrow J: Neurofibromatosis-1 in childhood. *Adv Dermatol* 2004;20:75–115.

Lumbroso S, Paris F, Sultan C: McCune-Albright syndrome: Molecular genetics. *J Pediatr Endocrinol Metab* 2002;15(Suppl 3):875–882.

Sandrini F, Stratakis C: Clinical and molecular genetics of Carney complex. *Mol Genet Metab* 2003;78:83–92.

Sarkozy A, Conti E, Diglio MC, et al: Clinical and molecular analysis of 30 patients with multiple lentigines LEOPARD syndrome. *J Med Genet* 2004;41:e68.

Chapter 652 ■ Hypopigmented Lesions

Joseph G. Morelli

ALBINISM. Several types of congenital oculocutaneous albinism (OCA) consist of partial or complete failure of melanin production in the skin, hair, and eyes despite the presence of normal number, structure, and distribution of melanocytes. They may be divided into two major classes: those with abnormal protein function involved in the formation and transfer of melanin, and those with defects in melanosomes (Table 652-1). Tyrosinase is the copper-containing enzyme that catalyzes at multiple steps in melanin biosynthesis (see Chapter 85.2). Tyrosinase-positive variants are characterized by darkening of the hair bulb on incubation with tyrosine.

TABLE 652-1. Genes Associated with Hypopigmentation

DISORDER	GENE DEFECT
Oculocutaneous albinism	
OCA1	Tyrosinase
OCA2	P protein
OCA3	TRP-1
OCA4	MATP
Hermansky-Pudlak	
Type 1	HPS-1 Mouse (pale ear)
Type 2	HPS-2 b3A subunit of AP3
Type 3	HPS-3 Mouse (cocoa)
Type 4	HPS-4 Mouse (light ear)
Type 5	HPS-5 Mouse (ruby eye 2)
Type 6	HPS-6 Mouse (ruby eye)
Chédiak-Higashi	CHS1/LYST
Piebaldism	C-KIT receptor
	Heterozygous SLUG
Waardenburg	
Type 1	Heterozygous PAX-3
Type 2	MITF
Type 3	Homozygous PAX-3
Type 4	SOX-10
	Endothelin 3
	Endothelin B receptor

OCA1. **OCA1** is characterized by greatly reduced or absent tyrosinase activity. **OCA1A**, the most severe form, is characterized by a lack of visible pigment in hair, skin, and eyes (Fig. 652-1). This is manifested as photophobia, nystagmus, defective visual acuity, white hair, and white skin. The irises are blue-gray in oblique light and prominent pink in reflected light. **OCA1B** or yellow mutant albinism presents at birth with white hair, pink skin, and gray eyes. This type is particularly prevalent in Amish communities. Progressively, however, the hair becomes yellow-red, the skin tans lightly on exposure to the sun, and the irises may accumulate some brown pigment, with a resultant improvement in visual acuity. Photophobia and nystagmus are present but mild. **OCATS** is a temperature-sensitive type of albinism. The abnormal tyrosinase has decreased activity at 35–37°C. Therefore, cooler regions of the body such as the limbs and head pigment to some degree, whereas other areas remain depigmented.

OCA2 ranges from nearly normal to closely resembling type 1 albinism. This is the most common form of albinism seen worldwide. Little or no melanin is present at birth, but pigment, particularly red-yellow pigment, may accumulate during childhood to produce straw-colored or light brown skin in whites. Pigmented nevi may develop. Progressive improvement in visual acuity and nystagmus occurs with aging. Blacks may have yellow-brown skin, dark-brown freckles in sun-exposed areas, and brown coloration of the irises. **Brown OCA** is an allelic variant of OCA2. Prader-Willi and Angelman syndromes, which include hypopigmentation, have deletions which include the gene involved in OCA2.

OCA3 (RUFOUS). OCA3 is seen predominantly in patients of African descent. It is characterized by red hair, reddish brown skin, pigmented nevi, freckles, reddish-brown to brown eyes, nystagmus, photophobia, and decreased visual acuity.

OCA4. This is a rare OCA with clinical findings similar to OCA2.

The **Cross-McKusick-Breen syndrome** consists of tyrosinase-positive albinism with ocular abnormalities, retardation, spasticity, and athetosis. The genetic defect is unidentified.

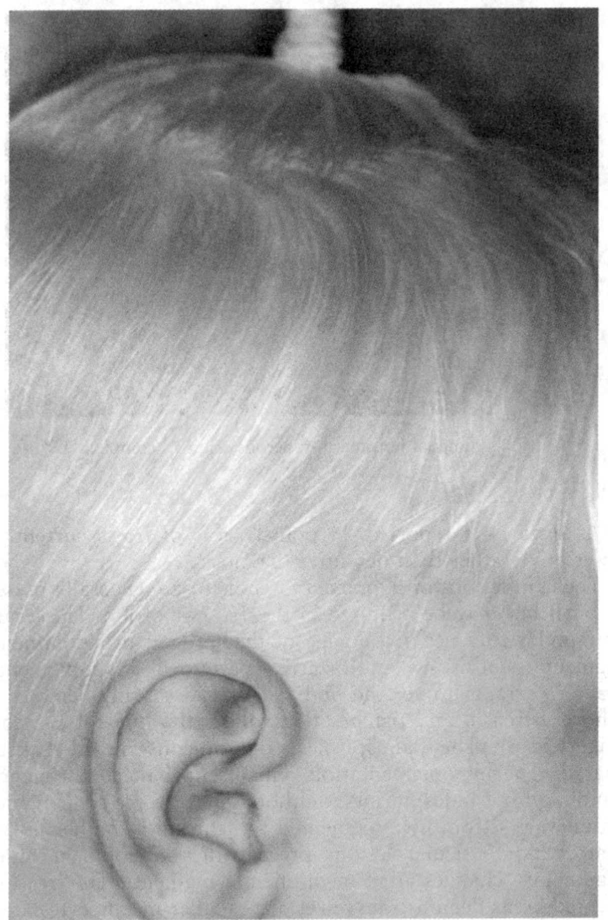

Figure 652-1. White hair and skin in oculocutaneous albinism 1 (OCA1).

Because of the absence of normal protection by adequate amounts of epidermal melanin, persons with albinism are predisposed to develop actinic keratoses and cutaneous carcinoma secondary to skin damage by ultraviolet light. Protective clothing and a broad-spectrum sunscreen preparation (see Chapter 655) should be worn during exposure to sunlight.

OCA WITH MELANOSOMAL ABNORMALITIES (SEE TABLE 652-1). **Hermansky-Pudlak syndrome** is a collection of autosomal recessive genetic disorders characterized by oculocutaneous albinism, ceroid accumulation in lysosomes, and prolonged bleeding. In mice, 16 distinct genetic loci that produce coat color mutant phenotypes associated with platelet deficiencies are now recognized. Six of these deficiencies have been identified in humans.

Chédiak-Higashi (CHS; see Chapter 129) syndrome is another genetic abnormality associated with dysfunction of lysosome-related organelles. Patients with CHS have hypopigmentation of the skin, eye, and hair; prolonged bleeding times and easy bruising; recurrent infections; abnormal natural killer cell function; and peripheral neuropathy. CHS is caused by mutations in the CHS1/LYST gene. The function of the protein encoded by this gene is at this time not well understood.

MELANOBLAST MIGRATION ABNORMALITIES (SEE TABLE 652-1)

PIEBALDISM. This congenital autosomal dominant disorder is characterized by sharply demarcated amelanotic patches that occur most frequently on the forehead, anterior scalp (producing a white forelock), ventral trunk, elbows, and knees. Islands of normal or darker than normal pigmentation may be present within the amelanotic areas (Fig. 652-2). The plaques are a result of a permanent localized absence of melanocytes. The pattern of depigmentation arises from defective melanoblast migration from the neural crest during development. The reason why piebaldism is a localized and not a generalized process remains unknown. Piebaldism must be differentiated from vitiligo, which may be progressive and is not usually congenital; nevus depigmentosus; and Waardenburg syndrome.

WAARDENBURG SYNDROME. Waardenburg syndrome also presents at birth with localized areas of depigmented skin and hair. There are four types of Waardenburg syndrome. The hallmark of Waardenburg type 1 is the white forelock. This is seen in 20–60% of patients. Only 15% of patients will have areas of depigmented skin. Deafness occurs in 9–37%, heterochromia irides in 20%, and unibrow (synophrys) in 17–69% of those affected. Dystopia canthorum is seen in all patients with Waardenburg type 1. Waardenburg type 2 is similar to type 1, except Waardenburg type 2 patients lack dystopia canthorum, but they also have a higher incidence of deafness. Waardenburg type 3 is similar to Waardenburg type 1, except patients will also have limb abnormalities. It is also called the Klein-Waardenburg syndrome. Waardenburg type 4 is also called the Shah-Waardenburg syndrome. These patients all have Hirschsprung disease. Dystopia canthorum is seldom seen in these patients.

TUBEROUS SCLEROSIS COMPLEX (TSC1, TSC2 GENES) [SEE CHAPTER 596.2]. This disorder is a multisystemic disorder affecting primarily tissues derived from ectoderm but also involving organs of mesodermal and endodermal origin, particularly the eyes, kidneys, and heart. The **classic clinical triad** is skin lesions in association with epilepsy and mental retardation.

Etiology and Epidemiology. This is an autosomal dominant condition seen in ≈1/300,000 persons, with a penetrance of nearly 100%. The TSC2 product is tuberin, which has sequence homology with a GTPase-activating protein and may have a role in regulating cellular growth by acting as a growth suppressor gene. TSC1 (hamartin) is postulated to act as a growth suppressor. Approximately 60% of cases are due to new mutations.

Clinical Manifestations. The first 4 major **diagnostic features** of TSC are skin findings. Single or multiple **ash-leaf lesions** are most often found on the trunk (Fig. 652-3) but also occur on the face and limbs. Small, confetti-like hypopigmented macules may also be present. These represent localized areas of inadequate melanization. The hypopigmented lesions may be present at birth or arise in the 1st few months of life. They may be difficult to appreciate in light-skinned children. **Angiofibromas** are the most

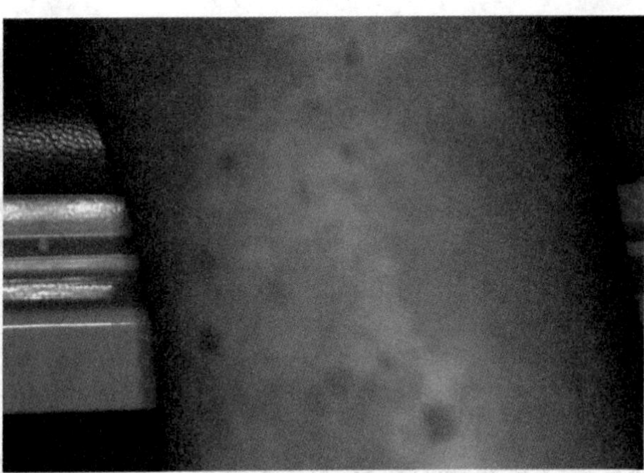

Figure 652-2. Depigmented macule with islands of hyperpigmentation in piebaldism.

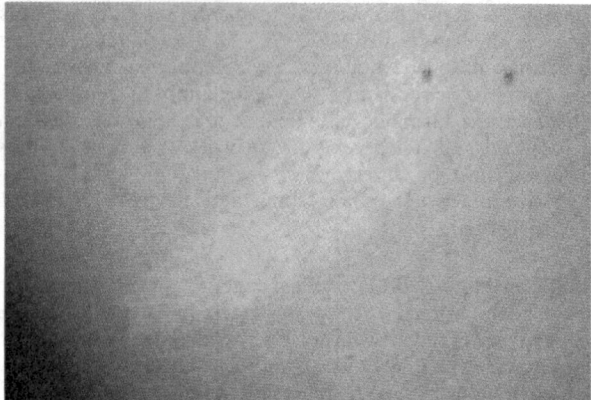

Figure 652-3. Ash-leaf macule in tuberous sclerosis complex (TSC).

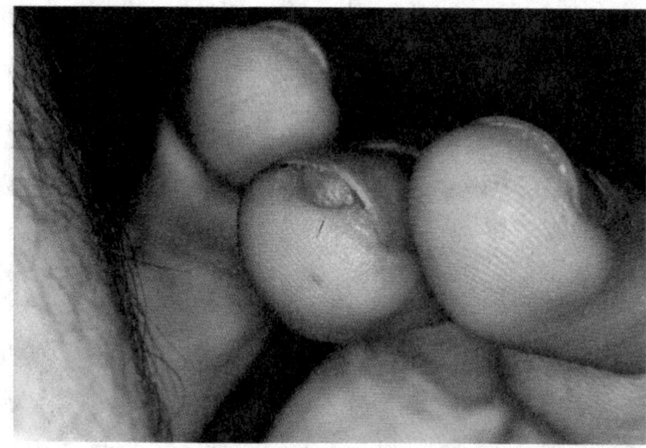

Figure 652-5. Periungual fibroma in tuberous sclerosis complex (TSC).

commonly recognized cutaneous marker of tuberous sclerosis; the lesions appear on the face beginning in early childhood. These red-brown or flesh-colored smooth, glistening, telangiectatic 1–10 mm papules may extend from the nasolabial folds to the cheeks and chin (Fig. 652-4). The presence of telangiectasias and the lack of comedones and pustules help to distinguish this eruption from acne vulgaris. Similar fibromatous nodules may be scattered on the forehead, trunk, and limbs. Large, skin-colored, irregularly thickened plaques with an orange peel or cobblestone texture (connective tissue nevi/**shagreen patch**) may occur in the lumbosacral area. These are present at birth, but the majority of patients with connective tissue nevi do not have TSC. At puberty, firm, flesh-colored periungual fibromas (Fig. 652-5) emerge on the nail folds of some children; gingival fibromas may also occur, unassociated with the administration of anticonvulsant medications. Café-au-lait spots occur with increased frequency but are not as numerous as in neurofibromatosis. Mental deficiency occurs in 60–70%; nearly all have epilepsy. Epilepsy is also present in ≈70% of those patients without mental retardation. Epilepsy begins in infancy or early childhood and is often progressively more severe. Cardiac **rhabdomyomas** are present in ≈50% of affected infants and usually spontaneously regress; mechanical obstruction is an unusual complication. Rarely, the presenting sign of tuberous sclerosis is hematuria, caused by a **renal angiomyolipoma**, which is characteristic of this condition.

HYPOMELANOSIS OF ITO. This congenital skin disorder affects children of both sexes and is frequently associated with defects in several organ systems. There is no evidence for genetic transmission; chromosomal mosaicism and chromosomal translocations have been reported. Hypomelanosis of Ito is currently a descriptive rather than definitive diagnosis.

The skin lesions of hypomelanosis of Ito are generally present at birth but may be acquired in the 1st 2 yr of life. The lesions are similar to a negative image of that present in incontinentia pigmenti, consisting of bizarre, patterned, hypopigmented macules arranged over the body surface in sharply demarcated whorls, streaks, and patches that follow the lines of Blaschko (Fig. 652-6). The palms, soles, and mucous membranes are spared. The hypopigmentation remains unchanged throughout childhood but fades during adulthood. The degree of depigmentation varies from hypopigmented to achromic. Neither inflammatory nor vesicular lesions precede the development of the pigmentary changes as in incontinentia pigmenti. The hypopigmented areas demonstrate fewer and smaller melanocytes and a decreased number of melanin granules in the basal cell layer than normal. Inflammatory cells and pigment incontinence are lacking.

The most commonly associated abnormalities involve the nervous system, including mental retardation (70%), seizures (40%), microcephaly (25%), and muscular hypotonia (15%). The musculoskeletal system is the 2nd most frequently involved system, affected by scoliosis and thoracic and limb deformities. Minor ophthalmologic defects (strabismus, nystagmus) are present in 25% of patients, and 10% have cardiac defects. The differential diagnosis includes systematized nevus depigmentosus, which is a stable leukoderma not associated with systemic manifestations. Differentiation from incontinentia pigmenti, particularly the hypopigmented 4th stage, is critical for genetic counseling because incontinentia pigmenti, unlike hypomelanosis of Ito, is inherited.

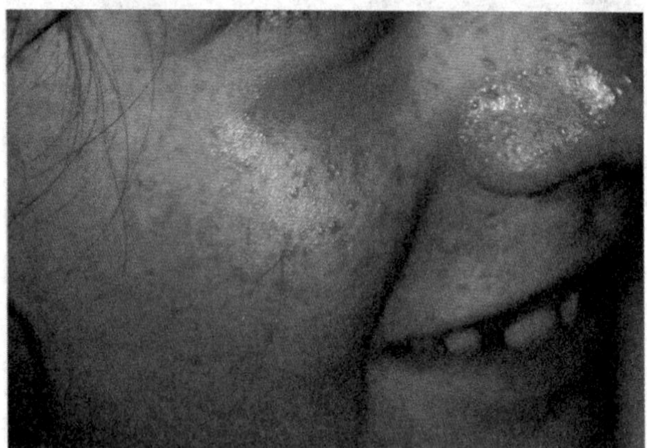

Figure 652-4. Facial angiofibromas in tuberous sclerosis complex (TSC).

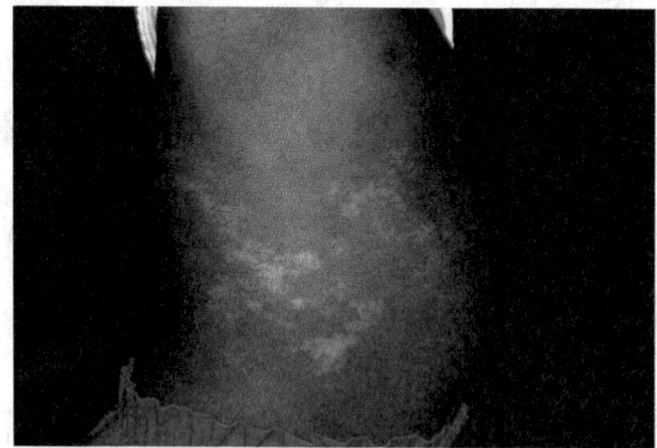

Figure 652-6. Marbled hypopigmented streaks on the abdomen in hypomelanosis of Ito.

VITILIGO

Epidemiology and Etiology. The pathogenesis of vitiligo is unknown. It has been suggested that melanocytes are destroyed because of the accumulation of a toxic melanin synthesis intermediate. There is in vitro evidence that some of these metabolites may be lethal to melanocytes.

A 2nd hypothesis suggests that neurochemical factors damage melanocytes and cause depigmentation. This would explain the pattern of involvement in segmental vitiligo that runs roughly along the course of a dermatome.

A 3rd hypothesis, perhaps the strongest, suggests that immunologic abnormalities are responsible for the changes in vitiligo. Eighty per cent of patients with active disease have an antibody to a surface antigen on pigmented melanoma cells. These antibodies appear to be cytotoxic for melanocytes. There is also a correlation between disease activity and the titer of serum antimelanocyte antibody. The genetic forms of vitiligo are probably linked to the immunologic form. Several susceptibility loci (AIS1, AIS2, AIS3, SLEV1) for vitiligo have been identified.

Clinical Manifestations. There are two subtypes of vitiligo, generalized (type A) and localized (type B), which probably are distinctly different diseases. About 50% of all patients with vitiligo have an onset before 18 yr of age and 25% develop depigmentation before age 8. Most children have the generalized form, but the localized type is more common among children than among adults. Patients with the generalized form usually present with a remarkably symmetric pattern of white macules and patches (Fig. 652-7), the margins of which may be somewhat hyperpigmented. The patches tend to be acral and/or periorificial. Occasionally, almost the entire skin surface becomes depigmented and this is referred to as total vitiligo.

There are several varieties of localized vitiligo. In segmental vitiligo, depigmented areas are limited to a dermatomal distribution. Another form of localized vitiligo is the halo nevus phenomenon where benign moles develop depigmented rings at the periphery. Premature graying of scalp hair (canities) has also been considered as a form of focal vitiligo.

A number of **autoimmune diseases** occur in patients with vitiligo including Addison disease, Hashimoto thyroiditis, pernicious anemia, diabetes mellitus, hypoparathyroidism, and polyglandular autoimmune syndrome with selective IgA deficiency. In addition, other diseases with possible immune defects such as alopecia areata and morphea have been seen in vitiligo patients.

Vogt-Koyanogi-Harada syndrome is vitiligo associated with uveitis, dysacusia, meningoencephalitis, and depigmentation of the skin, scalp hair, eyebrows, and eyelashes. In the **Alezzandrini syndrome**, vitiligo is associated with tapetoretinal degeneration and deafness.

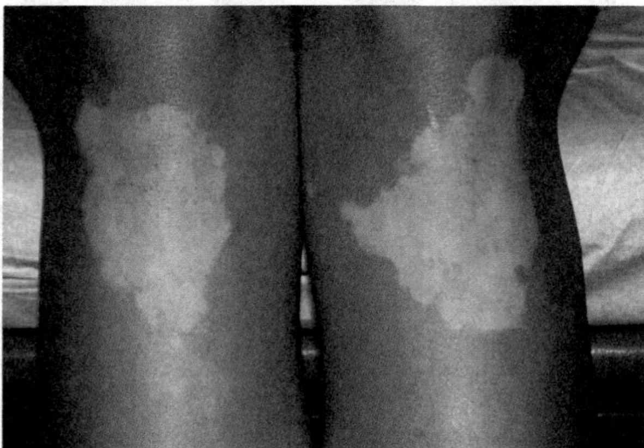

Figure 652-7. Sharply demarcated, symmetric, depigmented areas of vitiligo.

Light microscopic examination of early lesions shows mild inflammatory change. Over time, degenerative changes occur in melanocytes, leading to their complete disappearance.

The differential diagnosis of vitiligo includes other causes of widespread acquired leukoderma. The two most common problem diagnoses are tinea versicolor and postinflammatory hypopigmentation.

Treatment. Localized areas of vitiligo may respond to potent topical steroid, topical tacrolimus, or topical pimecrolimus. In patients with more extensive involvement, narrow-band ultraviolet light B (UVB) [UVB311] is the treatment of choice. In all forms of vitiligo, response to therapy is slow, taking many months to years. For those not interested in treatment, cover-up cosmetics may be used. All areas of vitiligo are susceptible to sun damage, and care should be taken to minimize sun exposure to affected areas. Spontaneous remission may be seen in a small percentage of cases.

Au KS, Williams AT, Gambello MJ, et al: Molecular genetics of tuberous sclerosis complex: From bench to bedside. *J Child Neurol* 2004;19:699–709.

Herane MI: Vitiligo and leukoderma in children. *Clin Dermatol* 2003; 21:283–295.

Kihiczak TI, Fox MD, Janniger CK, et al: Piebaldism: An update. *Int J Dermatol* 2004;43:716–719.

Newton VE: Clinical features of Waardenburg syndrome. *Adv Otorhinolaryngol* 2002;61:201–208.

Okulicz JF, Shah RS, Schwartz RA, et al: Oculocutaneous albinism. *J Eur Acad Dermatol Venereol* 2003;17:251–256.

Scheinfeld NS: Syndromic albinism: A review of genetics and phenotype. *Dermatol Online J* 2003;9:5.

Silverberg NB, Lin P, Travis L, et al: Tacrolimus ointment promotes repigmentation of vitiligo in children: A review of 57 cases. *J Am Acad Dermatol* 2004;51:760–766.

Taibjee SM, Bennett DC, Moss C: Abnormal pigmentation in hypomelanosis of Ito and pigmentary mosaicism: The role of pigmentary genes. *Br J Dermatol* 2004;151:269–282.

Chapter 653 ■ Vesiculobullous Disorders

Joseph G. Morelli

Many diseases are characterized by vesiculobullous lesions; they vary considerably in cause, age of onset, and pattern. The morphology of the blister often provides a visual clue to the location of the lesion within the skin. Blisters localized to the **epidermal layers** are thin walled, relatively flaccid, and easily ruptured. **Subepidermal blisters** are tense, thick walled, and more durable. Biopsies of blisters can be diagnostic because the level of cleavage within the skin and associated findings such as the nature of the inflammatory infiltrate are characteristic for a particular disorder. Other diagnostic procedures such as immunofluorescence and electron microscopy can often help distinguish vesiculobullous disorders that have nearly identical histopathologic findings (Table 653-1).

ERYTHEMA MULTIFORME. Erythema multiforme (EM) has numerous morphologic manifestations on the skin, varying from erythematous macules, papules, vesicles, bullae, or urticaria-appearing plaques to patches of confluent erythema. The eruption appears most commonly in patients between the ages of 10 and 30 yr and usually is asymptomatic, although a burning sensation or pruritus may be present. The diagnosis of

TABLE 653-1. Sites of Blister Formation and Diagnostic Studies for the Vesiculobullous Disorders

DISORDER	BLISTER CLEAVAGE SITE	DIAGNOSTIC STUDIES
Acrodermatitis enteropathica	IE	Zn level
Bullous impetigo	GL	Smear, culture
Bullous pemphigoid	SE (junctional)	Direct and indirect immunofluorescence studies
Candidosis	SC	KOH preparation, culture
Dermatitis herpetiformis	SE	Direct immunofluorescence studies
Dermatophytosis	IE	KOH preparation, culture
Dyshidrotic eczema	IE	Routine histopathology
EB simplex	IE	Electron microscopy; immunofluorescence mapping
Hands and feet	IE	Electron microscopy; immunofluorescence mapping
Junctional EB (letalis)	SE (junctional)	Electron microscopy; immunofluorescence mapping
Recessive dystrophic EB	SE	Electron microscopy; immunofluorescence mapping
Dominant dystrophic EB	SE	Electron microscopy; immunofluorescence mapping
Epidermolytic hyperkeratosis	IE	Routine histopathology
Erythema multiforme	SE	Routine histopathology
Erythema toxicum	SC, IE	Smear for eosinophils
Incontinentia pigmenti	IE	Smear for eosinophils
Insect bites	IE	Routine histopathology
Linear IgA	SE	Direct immunofluorescence studies
Mastocytosis	SE	Smear for mast cells
Miliaria crystallina	IC	Routine histopathology
Neonatal pustular melanosis	SC, IE	Smear for cells
Pemphigus foliaceus	GL	Direct and indirect immunofluorescence studies Tzanck smear
Pemphigus vulgaris	SB	Direct and indirect immunofluorescence studies Tzanck smear
Scabies	IE	Scraping
Staphylococcal SSS	GL	Routine histopathology
Toxic epidermal necrolysis	SE	Routine histopathology
Viral blisters	IE	Tzanck smear for herpesvirus infections

EB, epidermolysis bullosa; GL, granular layer; IC, intracorneal; IE, intraepidermal; KOH, potassium hydroxide; SB, suprabasal; SC, subcorneal; SE, subepidermal; SSS, scalded skin syndrome.

EM is established by finding the classic lesion: doughnut-shaped, target-like (iris or bull's-eye) papules with an erythematous outer border, an inner pale ring, and a dusky purple to necrotic center (Figs. 653-1 and 653-2).

EM is characterized by an abrupt, symmetric cutaneous eruption, most commonly on the extensor upper extremities; lesions are relatively sparse on the face, trunk, and legs. The eruption often appears initially as red macules or urticarial plaques that expand centrifugally to form lesions up to 2 cm in diameter with a dusky to necrotic center. Lesions of a particular episode typically appear within 72 hr and remain fixed in place. Oral lesions may occur with a predilection for the vermilion border of the lips and the buccal mucosa, but other mucosal surfaces are spared. Prodromal symptoms are generally absent. Lesions typically resolve without sequelae in about 2 wk; progression to Stevens-Johnson syndrome does not occur.

Although EM may present initially with urticarial lesions, unlike urticaria, a given lesion of EM does not fade within 24 hr. Serum sickness–like reaction (SSLR) to cefaclor may also present with EM-like lesions. Although the lesions may develop a dusky to purple center, in most cases, the eruption of cefaclor-induced SSLR is pruritic, transient, and migratory and is probably urticarial rather than true EM.

The **differential diagnosis** of EM also includes bullous pemphigoid, pemphigus, linear IgA dermatosis, graft vs host disease, bullous drug eruption, urticaria, viral infections such as herpes simplex, Reiter disease, Kawasaki disease, Behçet disease, allergic vasculitis, erythema annulare centrifugum, and periarteritis nodosa. EM that primarily involves the oral mucosa may be confused with bullous pemphigoid, pemphigus vulgaris, vesiculobullous or erosive lichen planus, Behçet syndrome, recurrent aphthous stomatitis, and primary herpetic gingivostomatitis.

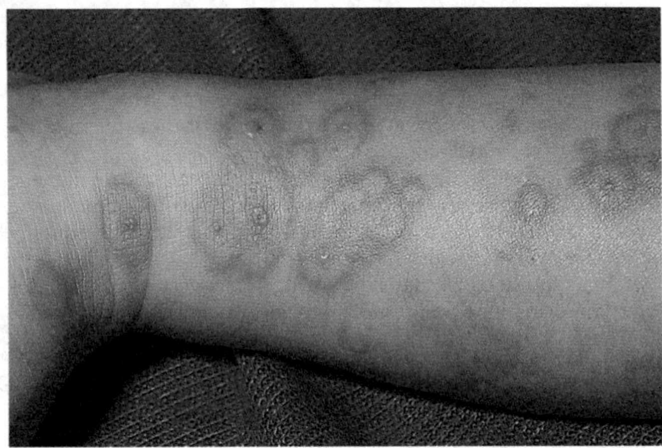

Figure 653-1. Early fixed papules with a central dusky zone on the dorsum of the hand of a child with erythema multiforme due to herpes simplex virus. (From Weston WL, Lane AT, Morelli J: *Color Textbook of Pediatric Dermatology,* 3rd ed, St. Louis, Mosby, 2002, p 156.)

Among the numerous factors implicated in the etiology of EM, infection with herpes simplex virus (HSV) is the most common. HSV labialis and, less commonly, HSV genitalis have been implicated in 60% of episodes of EM and are believed to trigger nearly all episodes of recurrent EM, frequently in association with sun exposure (Fig. 653-3). HSV antigens and DNA are present in skin lesions of EM but are absent in nonlesional skin. Presence of the human leukocyte antigens B62, B35, and DR53 is associated with an increased risk of HSV-induced EM, particularly the recurrent form. Most patients experience a single self-limited episode of EM. Lesions of HSV-induced recurrent EM typically develop 10–14 days after onset of recurrent HSV eruptions, have a similar appearance from episode to episode, but may vary in frequency and duration in a given patient. Not all episodes of recurrent HSV evolve into EM in susceptible patients.

The pathogenesis of EM is unclear, but it may be a host-specific cell-mediated immune response to an antigenic stimulus,

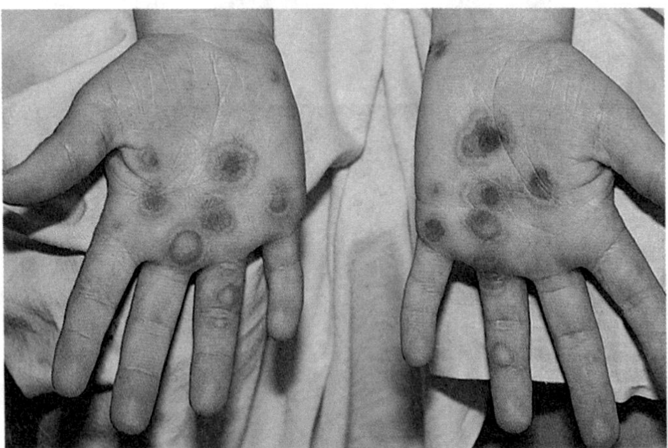

Figure 653-2. "Target" or "iris" lesions with characteristic central dusky zone on palms of a child with erythema multiforme due to herpes simplex virus. (From Weston WL, Lane AT, Morelli J: *Color Textbook of Pediatric Dermatology,* 3rd ed, St. Louis, Mosby, 2002, p 156.)

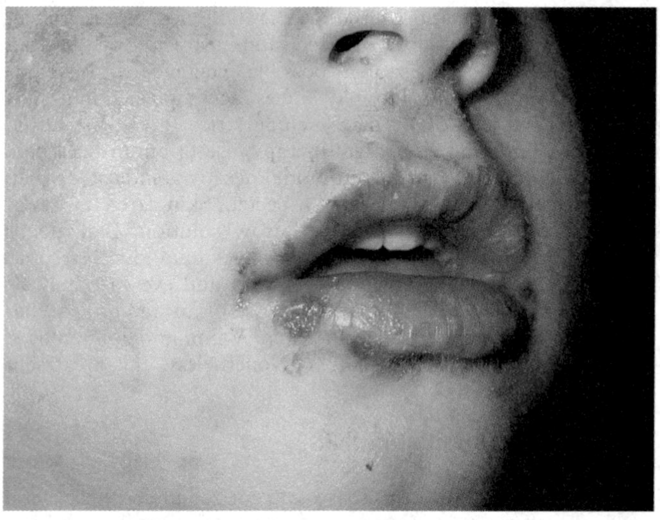

Figure 653-3. Recurrent labial herpes simplex virus (HSV).

resulting in damage to keratinocytes. Cytokines released by activated mononuclear cells and keratinocytes may contribute to epidermal cell death and constitutional symptoms.

Microscopic findings of EM, as with the gross appearance of the cutaneous eruption, are variable but may aid in diagnosis. Early lesions typically show slight intercellular edema, rare dyskeratotic keratinocytes, and basal vacuolation in the epidermis and a perivascular lymphohistiocytic infiltrate with edema in the upper dermis. More mature lesions show an accentuation of these characteristics and the development of lymphocytic exocytosis and an intense, perivascular, and interstitial mononuclear infiltrate in the upper third of the dermis. The entire epidermis becomes necrotic in severe cases.

Treatment of EM is supportive. Topical emollients, systemic antihistamines, and nonsteroidal anti-inflammatory agents do not alter the course of the disease but may provide symptomatic relief. No controlled, prospective studies support the use of corticosteroids in the management of EM. Rather, glucocorticoid therapy may be permissive of HSV replication and make EM episodes more frequent or continuous. Prophylactic oral acyclovir given for 6 mo may be effective in controlling recurrent episodes of HSV-associated EM. On discontinuation of acyclovir, both HSV and EM may recur, although episodes may be less frequent and milder.

STEVENS-JOHNSON SYNDROME. Cutaneous lesions in Stevens-Johnson syndrome generally consist initially of erythematous macules that rapidly and variably develop central necrosis to form vesicles, bullae, and areas of denudation on the face, trunk, and extremities. The skin lesions are typically more widespread than in EM and are accompanied by involvement of **two or more mucosal surfaces,** namely the eyes, oral cavity, upper airway or esophagus, gastrointestinal tract, or anogenital mucosa. A burning sensation, edema, and erythema of the lips and buccal mucosa are often the presenting signs, followed by development of bullae, ulceration, and hemorrhagic crusting. Lesions may be preceded by a flu-like upper respiratory illness. Pain from mucosal ulceration is often severe, but skin tenderness is minimal to absent, in contrast to toxic epidermal necrolysis. Corneal ulceration, anterior uveitis, panophthalmitis, bronchitis, pneumonitis, myocarditis, hepatitis, enterocolitis, polyarthritis, hematuria, and acute tubular necrosis leading to renal failure may occur. Disseminated cutaneous bullae and erosions may result in increased insensible fluid loss and a high risk of bacterial superinfection and sepsis. New lesions occur in crops, and complete healing may take 4–6 wk; ocular scarring, visual impairment, and strictures of the esophagus, bronchi, vagina, urethra, or anus may remain. Nonspecific laboratory abnormalities in Stevens-Johnson syndrome include leukocytosis, elevated erythrocyte sedimentation rate, and, occasionally, increased liver transaminase levels and decreased serum albumin values. **Toxic epidermal necrolysis** is the most severe disorder in the clinical spectrum of the disease, involving considerable constitutional toxicity and extensive necrolysis of the mucous membranes and >30% of the body surface area.

Mycoplasma pneumoniae is the most convincingly demonstrated infectious cause of Stevens-Johnson syndrome. Drugs, particularly sulfonamides, nonsteroidal anti-inflammatory agents, antibiotics, and anticonvulsants are the agents most commonly precipitating Stevens-Johnson syndrome and toxic epidermal necrolysis.

Treatment. Management of Stevens-Johnson syndrome is supportive and symptomatic. Potentially offending drugs must be discontinued as soon as possible. Ophthalmologic consultation is mandatory because ocular sequelae such as corneal scarring can lead to vision loss. Topical steroids may reduce ocular morbidity. Oral lesions should be managed with mouthwashes and glycerin swabs. Vaginal lesions should be observed closely and treated to prevent vaginal stricture or fusion. Topical anesthetics (diphenhydramine, dyclonine, and viscous lidocaine) may provide relief from pain, particularly when applied before eating. Denuded skin lesions can be cleansed with saline or Burow solution compresses. Antibiotic therapy is appropriate for documented secondary bacterial infection. Treatment may require admission to an intensive care unit; intravenous fluids; nutritional support; sheepskin or air-fluid bedding; daily saline or Burow solution compresses; paraffin gauze or hydrogel dressing of denuded areas; saline compresses on the eyelids, lips, or nose; analgesics; and urinary catheterization (when needed). A daily examination for infection and ocular lesions, which constitute the major cause of long-term morbidity, is essential. Systemic antibiotics are indicated for urinary or cutaneous infections and for suspected bacteremia because infection is the leading cause of death. Prophylactic systemic antibiotics, however, are not necessary. Although corticosteroids are sometimes advocated in early, severe cases of Stevens-Johnson syndrome, no prospective double-blind studies evaluating their efficacy have been reported. Most authorities discourage their use because of reports of increased morbidity and mortality (sepsis) with their administration. Intravenous immunoglobulin (1.5–2.0 g/kg/day x 3 days) has also been used and believed by many to be effective.

TOXIC EPIDERMAL NECROLYSIS

EPIDEMIOLOGY AND ETIOLOGY. The pathogenesis of toxic epidermal necrolysis is not proved but may involve a hypersensitivity phenomenon that results in damage primarily to the basal cell layer of the epidermis. Epidermal damage appears to result from Fas-mediated keratinocyte apoptosis. This condition is triggered by many of the same factors that are thought to be responsible for Stevens-Johnson syndrome, principally drugs such as the sulfonamides, amoxicillin, phenobarbital, hydantoin, butazones, and allopurinol. Toxic epidermal necrolysis is defined by (1) widespread blister formation and morbilliform or confluent erythema, associated with skin tenderness; (2) absence of target lesions; (3) sudden onset and generalization within 24–48 hr; (4) histologic findings of full-thickness epidermal necrosis and a minimal to absent dermal infiltrate. These criteria categorize toxic epidermal necrolysis as a separate entity from EM; however, some contend that toxic epidermal necrolysis represents the most severe form of the spectrum of EM.

CLINICAL MANIFESTATIONS. The prodrome consists of fever, malaise, localized skin tenderness, and diffuse erythema. Inflammation of the eyelids, conjunctivae, mouth, and genitals may precede skin lesions. Flaccid bullae may develop, although this is not a prominent feature. Characteristically, full-thickness epidermis is lost in large sheets. **Nikolsky sign** (denudation of the skin with gentle tangential pressure) is present but only in the areas of erythema. Healing takes place over 14 or more days. Scarring, particularly of the eyes, may result in corneal opacity. The course may be relentlessly progressive, complicated by severe dehydration, electrolyte imbalance, shock, and secondary localized infection and septicemia. Loss of nails and hair may also occur. Long-term morbidity includes alterations in skin pigmentation, eye problems (lack of tears, conjunctival scarring, loss of lashes), and strictures of mucosal surfaces. The **differential diagnosis** includes staphylococcal scalded skin syndrome, in which the blister cleavage plane is intraepidermal; graft versus host disease; chemical burns; drug eruptions; toxic shock syndrome; and pemphigus.

Anticonvulsant hypersensitivity syndrome (DRESS [drug rash, eosinophilia, systemic symptoms] syndrome) is a multisystem reaction that appears ≈4 wk to 3 mo after starting phenytoin, carbamazepine, phenobarbitone, or primidone. Although initially described with anticonvulsant therapy, other drugs, most commonly, antibiotics, have been implicated. The mucocutaneous eruption may be identical to that of EM, Stevens-Johnson syndrome, or toxic epidermal necrolysis, but the reaction also typically includes lymphadenopathy, as well as fever, hepatic, renal and pulmonary disease, eosinophilia, and leukocytosis.

TREATMENT. Appreciation of the specific etiologic factor is crucial. When the disorder is drug induced, administration of the drug must be discontinued as soon as possible. Management is similar to that for severe burns and may be best accomplished in a burn unit (see Chapter 74). It may include strict reverse isolation, meticulous fluid and electrolyte therapy, use of an air-fluid bed, and daily cultures. Systemic antibiotic therapy is indicated when secondary infection is evident or suspected. Skin care consists of cleansing with isotonic saline or Burow solution. Biologic or hydrogel dressings alleviate pain and reduce fluid loss. Narcotics are often required for pain relief. Mouth and eye care may be necessary, such as for EM major. Because of an immune mechanism, systemic glucocorticosteroids and IV immunoglobulin have been used with apparent success. Nonetheless, this treatment remains controversial.

MECHANOBULLOUS DISORDERS

EPIDERMOLYSIS BULLOSA. Diseases categorized under this general term are a heterogeneous group of congenital, hereditary blistering disorders. They differ in severity and prognosis, clinical and histologic features, and inheritance patterns, but are all characterized by induction of blisters by trauma and exacerbation of blistering in warm weather. The disorders can be categorized under three major headings with multiple subgroupings: epidermolysis bullosa simplex (EBS), junctional epidermolysis bullosa (JEB), and dystrophic epidermolysis bullosa (DEB) [Table 653-2].

TABLE 653-2. Clinical Presentation and Diagnosis of Selected EB Subtypes in the Neonatal Period

EB SUBTYPE (USUAL INHERITANCE)	CLINICAL FEATURES		DIAGNOSIS: ELECTRON MICROSCOPY (EM), IMMUNOHISTOCHEMICAL, AND IMMUNOFLUORESCENCE ANTIGEN MAPPING FINDINGS (IF)
	Cutaneous	Extracutaneous	
EB simplex, Koebner (AD)	Mild to moderate blistering, often generalized Rare scarring, milia CLAS	Occasional mucosal blistering	EM: Intraepidermal split; keratin filament changes IF: BPAG1 (BP230), BP-180 (BPAG2, collagen XVII), α6β4 integrin, laminin 10, laminin 5, type IV collagen, type VII collagen (EBA antigen) at base of blister
EB simplex, Weber-Cockayne (AD)	Mild blistering, often localized, sometimes in 1st 24 mos, but often not until later infancy or childhood Rare scarring, milia	Rare mucosal involvement	EM: Intrastratum basale split IF: Same as EB simplex, Koebner
EB simplex, Dowling-Meara (AD)	Moderate to severe blistering, starts generalized, then grouped (herpetiform) Milia Nail dystrophy, shedding CLAS	Mild mucosal blistering	EM: Intrastratum basale split; clumped keratin filaments IF: Same as EB simplex, Koebner
Junctional EB, non-Herlitz type (AR)	Moderate blistering Atrophic scars Nail dystrophy	Mild mucosal blistering Enamel hypoplasia	EM: Intralamina lucida cleavage; variable reduction in hemidesmosomes IF: Absent staining with 19-DEJ-1 (uncein); variable staining with GB3 and other laminin 5 antibodies including 46 and K140; BPAg1 (BP230) BP180 (BPAG2, collagen XVII), α6β4 integrin in blister roof Laminin 10, type IV collagen, type VII collagen (EBA antigen) at base of blister
Junctional, Herlitz type (AR)	Severe generalized blistering Heals poorly, granulation tissue Scarring, nail dystrophy, CLAS	Severe mucosal blistering GI involvement common Laryngeal involvement with airway obstruction Urological involvement	EM: Cleavage intralamina lucida; markedly reduced or absent hemidesmosomes; absent sub-basal dense plates IF: Absent staining with 19-DEJ-1 (uncein) and GB3 (laminin 5) and absent staining with other laminin 5 antibodies including 46 and K140. BPAG1 (BP230) and BP180 (BPAG2, type XVII collagen) in blister roof Laminin-10, type IV collagen and type VII collagen at base of blister
Pyloric atresia–junctional EB (AR)	Severe blistering CLAS	Polyhydramnios Pyloric atresia, urological involvement: uretovesicular obstruction, hydronephrosis	EM: Cleavage intralamina lucida and intraplasma membrane; small hemidesmosomes IF: BPAG1 (BP230) and BP180 (BPAG2, type XVII collagen) in blister roof. Laminin-10, type IV collagen and type VII collagen at base of blister Absent 19-DEJ-1 (uncein), α6β4 integrin absent or reduced
Dominant dystrophic EB (AD)	Mild to moderate blistering (but may be more severe in newborn period) Milia, scarring CLAS Nail dystrophy	Mild mucosal blistering	EM: Cleavage sublamina densa; variable reduction in anchoring fibrils IF: BPAG1 (BP230)BP-180 (BPAG2, collagen XVII), α6β4 integrin, laminin 10, type IV collagen at base of blister Normal, variable, or absent staining for type VII collagen (EBA antigen)
Recessive dystrophic EB Hallopeau-Siemens (AR)	Severe blistering Milia, scarring CLAS	Severe mucosal blistering GI involvement common Urological involvement	EM: Cleavage sublamina densa; absent anchoring fibrils IF: BPAG1 (BP230) BP-180 (BPAG2, collagen XVII), α6β4 integrin, laminin 10, type IV collagen at base of blister Variable or absent staining for type VII collagen (EBA antigen)

AD, autosomal dominant; AR, autosomal recessive; CLAS, congenital localized absence of skin; EB, Epidermolysis bullosa; GI, gastrointestinal.
From Eichenfield LF, Frieden IJ, Esterly NB: *Textbook of Neonatal Dermatology*. Philadelphia, WB, Saunders, 2001, p 159.

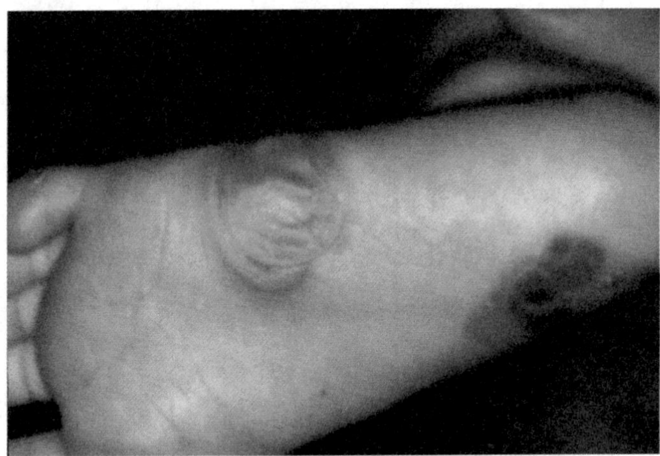

Figure 653-4. Large bullae of the foot in epidermolysis bullosa simplex.

Epidermolysis Bullosa Simplex (EBS). This is a nonscarring, autosomal dominant disorder. The defect in most types of epidermolysis bullosa simplex is in keratin 5 or 14, which makes up intermediate filaments of the basal keratinocytes. The intraepidermal bullae result from cytolysis of the basal cells.

In **EBS-Koebner**, blisters are usually present at birth or during the neonatal period. Sites of predilection are the hands, feet, elbows, knees, legs, and scalp. Intraoral lesions are minimal, nails rarely become dystrophic and usually regrow even when they are shed, and dentition is normal. Bullae heal with minimal to no scar or milia formation. Secondary infection is the primary complication. The propensity to blister decreases with age, and the long-term prognosis is good. Blisters should be drained by puncturing, but the blister top should be left intact to protect the underlying skin. Erosions may be covered with a semipermeable dressing.

Localized EBS of the hands and feet (Weber-Cockayne type) often presents when a child begins to walk; onset may be delayed, however, until puberty or early adulthood when heavy shoes are worn or the feet are subjected to increased trauma. Bullae are usually restricted to the hands and feet (Fig. 653-4); rarely, they occur elsewhere such as the dorsal aspect of the arms and the shins. The disorder ranges from mildly incapacitating to crippling at times of severe exacerbations.

EBS-Dowling-Meara (herpetiformis) is characterized by grouped blisters resembling herpes simplex (Fig. 653-5). During infancy, blistering may be severe and extensive, may involve mucous membranes, and may result in shedding of nails, formation of milia, and mild pigmentary changes, without scarring. After the 1st few months of life, warm temperatures do not appear to exacerbate blistering. Hyperkeratosis and hyperhidrosis of the palms and soles may develop, but generally, the condition improves with age.

EBS-muscular dystrophy is a rare EBS variant associated with muscular dystrophy. It is caused by mutations in the gene encoding plectin, a hemidesmosomal protein.

JUNCTIONAL EPIDERMOLYSIS BULLOSA (JEB). JEB-Herlitz is an autosomal recessive condition that is life threatening. An afflicted infant is usually blistered at birth or develops lesions during the neonatal period, particularly on the perioral area, scalp, legs, diaper area, and thorax. In contrast to other variants of epidermolysis bullosa, the hands and feet tend to be relatively spared, with the exception of the distal digits and the nail plates; these are dystrophic or permanently lost. Mucous membrane involvement may be severe, and ulceration of the respiratory, gastrointestinal, and genitourinary epithelium has been documented in many affected children, although less frequently than in severe, recessive dystrophic epidermolysis bullosa. Healing is delayed, and vegetating granulomas may persist for a long time. Large, moist, erosive plaques (Fig. 653-6) may provide a portal of entry for bacteria, and septicemia is a frequent cause of death. Mild atrophy may be seen in areas of recurrent blistering. Defective dentition with early loss of teeth as a result of rampant caries is characteristic. Growth retardation and recalcitrant anemia are almost invariable. In addition to infection, cachexia and circulatory failure are common causes of death. Most patients die within the 1st 3 yr of life.

JEB–non-Herlitz is a heterogeneous group of disorders. Blistering may be severe in the neonatal period making differentiation from the Herlitz type difficult. All conditions associated with the Herlitz type may be seen, but are usually milder. Generalized atrophic benign epidermolysis bullosa is included as a variant of non-Herlitz JEB. Another variant of non-Herlitz JEB is associated with **pyloric atresia.**

In all types of JEB, a subepidermal blister is found on light microscopic examination, and electron microscopy demonstrates a cleavage plane in the lamina lucida, between the plasma membranes of the basal cells and the basal lamina. Absent or greatly reduced anchoring filaments are seen on electron micrographs. In JEB-Herlitz and some JEB–non-Herlitz, the defect is in laminin 5, a glycoprotein associated with anchoring filaments beneath the hemidesmosomes. In JEB–non-Herlitz, defects have also been described in other hemidesmosomal components, such as bullous

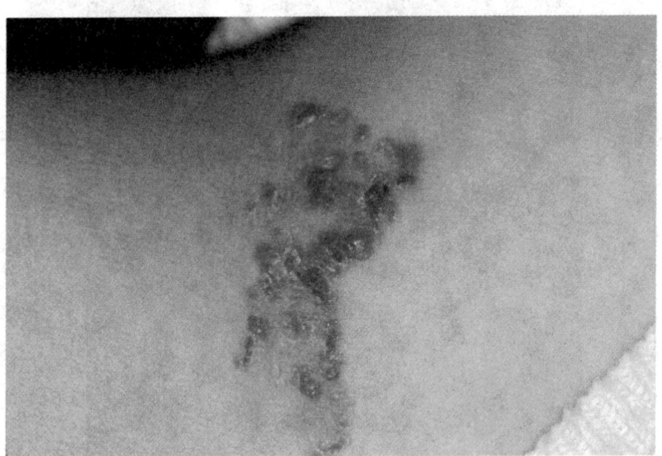

Figure 653-5. Grouped vesicle on an erythematous base in epidermolysis bullosa simplex Dowling-Meara.

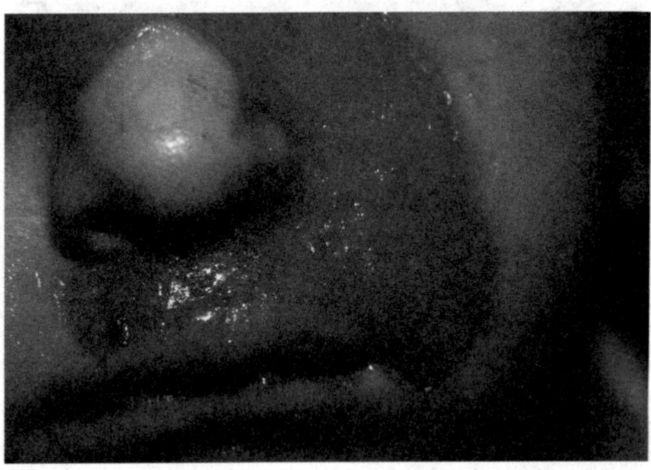

Figure 653-6. Non-healing granulation tissue in junctional epidermolysis bullosa.

pemphigoid antigen 2 and Col17A1. In JEB–pyloric atresia, the defect is in the α6β4 integrin.

Treatment for junctional epidermolysis bullosa is supportive. The diet should provide adequate calories and supplemental iron. Infections should be treated promptly. Transfusions of packed red blood cells may be required if the patient does not respond to iron and erythropoietin therapy. Tissue engineered skin grafts (artificial skin derived from human keratinocytes and fibroblasts) may be beneficial.

DYSTROPHIC EPIDERMOLYSIS BULLOSA (DEB). All forms of dystrophic epidermolysis bullosa result from mutations in collagen VII, a major component of anchoring fibrils that tether the basement membrane and overlying epidermis to its dermal foundation. The blister is subepidermal in all types of DEB. The type and location of the mutation dictates the severity of the phenotype.

Dominant dystrophic epidermolysis bullosa (DDEB) is the most common type of DEB. The spectrum of DDEB is varied. Blisters may be present at birth and are often limited and characteristically form over acral bony prominences. The lesions heal promptly, with the formation of soft, wrinkled scars; milia; and alterations in pigmentation (Fig. 653-7). Abnormal nails and nail loss are common. In many cases, the blistering process is mild, causing little restriction of activity and unimpaired growth and development. Mucous membrane involvement tends to be minimal.

Transient bullous dermolysis of the newborn affects a rare subset of patients with self-limited dystrophic disease; inheritance in most is autosomal dominant. Blistering at birth tends to be generalized but ceases within the 1st 1–2 yr. Resolution of clinical blistering and the immunohistochemically altered distribution of type VII collagen occur coincidentally.

Recessive dystrophic epidermolysis bullosa (RDEB-Hallopeau-Siemens) is the most incapacitating form of epidermolysis bullosa, although the clinical spectrum is wide. Some patients have blisters, scarring, and milia formation primarily on the hands, feet, elbows, and knees (Fig. 653-8). Others at birth have extensive erosions and blister formation that seriously impede their care and feeding. Mucous membrane lesions are common and may cause severe nutritional deprivation, even in older children, whose growth may be retarded. During childhood, esophageal erosions and strictures, scarring of the buccal mucosa, flexion contractures of joints secondary to scarring of the integument, development of cutaneous carcinomas, and the development of digital fusion may significantly limit the quality of life (Fig. 653-9).

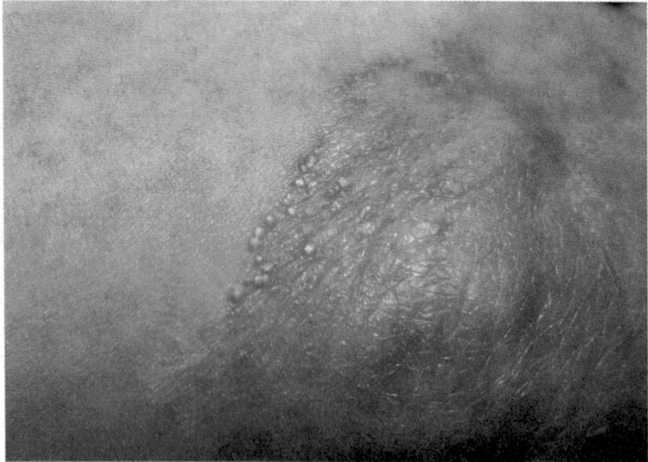

Figure 653-7. Scarring with milia formation over the knee in dominant dystrophic epidermolysis bullosa.

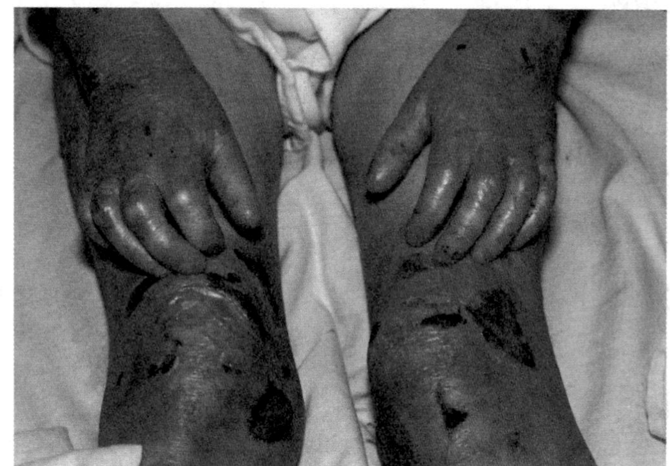

Figure 653-8. Severe scarring of the hands and knees in recessive dystrophic epidermolysis bullosa.

Although the skin becomes less sensitive to trauma with aging, the progressive and permanent deformities complicate management, and the overall prognosis is poor. Foods that traumatize the buccal or esophageal mucosa should be avoided. If esophageal scarring develops, a semiliquid diet and esophageal dilatations may be required. Stricture excision or colonic interposition may be needed to relieve esophageal obstruction. In infants, severe oropharyngeal involvement may necessitate the use of special feeding devices such as a gastrostomy tube. Iron therapy for anemia, intermittent antibiotic therapy for secondary infections, which are a common cause of death, and periodic surgery for release of digits may reduce morbidity. Tissue-engineered skin grafts containing keratinocytes and fibroblasts are of some benefit.

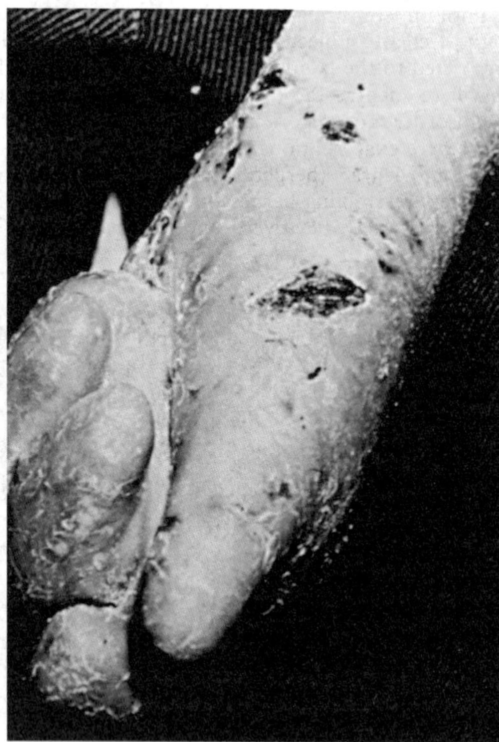

Figure 653-9. Mitten-hand deformity of recessive dystrophic epidermolysis bullosa.

IMMUNOBULLOUS DISORDERS

PEMPHIGUS VULGARIS. Usually, this 1st appears as painful oral ulcers, which may be the only evidence of the disease for weeks or months. Subsequently, large, flaccid bullae emerge on nonerythematous skin, most commonly on the face, trunk, pressure points, groin, and axillae. **Nikolsky sign** is present. The lesions rupture and enlarge peripherally, producing painful raw, denuded areas that have little tendency to heal. When healing occurs, it is without scarring, but hyperpigmentation is common. Malodorous, verrucous, and granulomatous lesions may develop at sites of ruptured bullae, particularly in the skinfolds; as this becomes more pronounced, the condition may be more properly referred to as pemphigus vegetans.

Biopsy is best performed of a fresh small blister, which reveals a suprabasal (intraepidermal) blister containing loose, acantholytic epidermal cells that have lost their intercellular bridges and thus their contact with one another. IgG antibody to epidermal intercellular substance produces a characteristic pattern on direct immunofluorescence preparations of both involved and uninvolved skin of essentially all patients. Serum IgG antibody titers to the epidermal intercellular substance correlate with the clinical course of many patients; thus, serial determinations may have predictive value. Pemphigus antibodies are pathogenic. The antigen recognized by pemphigus vulgaris antibodies is a 130-kd glycoprotein known as desmoglein III that is complexed with plakoglobin, a plaque protein of desmosomes. The desmogleins are a subfamily of the cadherin cell adhesion molecules.

Neonatal pemphigus vulgaris develops in utero as a result of placental transfer of maternal antibodies from women who have active pemphigus vulgaris, although it may occur when the mother is in remission. High antepartum maternal titers of pemphigus vulgaris antibodies and increased maternal disease activity correlate with a poor fetal outcome, including demise.

The **differential diagnosis** includes EM, bullous pemphigoid, Stevens-Johnson syndrome, and toxic epidermal necrolysis. Because the course may rapidly lead to debility, malnutrition, and death, prompt diagnosis is essential. The disease is best treated initially with high-dose systemic corticosteroid therapy. Azathioprine, cyclophosphamide, methotrexate, and gold therapy all have been useful in maintenance regimens. Intravenous immunoglobulin given in cycles may be beneficial to patients who do not respond to steroids.

PEMPHIGUS FOLIACEUS. This extremely rare disorder is characterized by intraepidermal blistering; the site of cleavage is high in the epidermis rather than suprabasal as in pemphigus vulgaris. The superficial blisters rupture quickly, leaving erosions surrounded by erythema that heal with crusting and scaling (Fig. 653-10). **Nikolsky sign** is present. Focal lesions are usually localized to the scalp, face, neck, and upper trunk. Mucous membrane lesions are minimal or absent. Pruritus, pain, and a burning sensation are frequent complaints. When generalized, the eruption may resemble exfoliative dermatitis or any of the chronic blistering disorders; localized erythematous plaques simulate seborrheic dermatitis, psoriasis, impetigo, eczema, or lupus erythematosus. The clinical course varies but is generally more benign than that of pemphigus vulgaris. **Fogo selvagem,** which is endemic in certain areas of Brazil, is identical clinically, histopathologically, and immunologically to pemphigus foliaceus.

An intraepidermal acantholytic bulla high in the epidermis is diagnostic. It is imperative to select an early lesion for biopsy. Tissue-bound and circulating intercellular epidermal antibodies bind to a 50-kd portion of the 160-kd desmosomal glycoprotein, desmoglein I. Long-term remission is usual after suppression of the disease by systemic corticosteroid therapy. Dapsone or a topical corticosteroid preparation is occasionally sufficient.

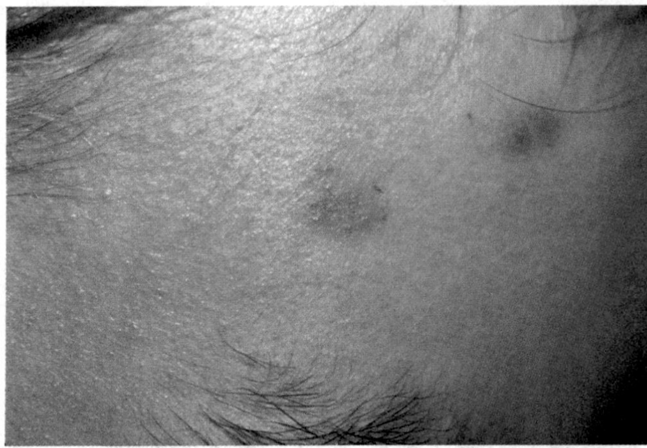

Figure 653-10. Superficial erosions in pemphigus foliaceus.

BULLOUS PEMPHIGOID. Bullous pemphigoid rarely occurs in children but must be considered in the differential diagnosis of any chronic blistering disorder.

Clinical Manifestations. The blisters typically arise in crops on a normal, erythematous, eczematous, or urticarial base. Bullae appear predominantly on the flexural aspects of the extremities, in the axillae, and on the groin and central abdomen. Infants have involvement of the palms, soles, and face more frequently than older children. Individual lesions vary greatly in size, are tense, and are filled with serous fluid that may become hemorrhagic or turbid. Oral lesions occur less frequently and are less severe than in pemphigus vulgaris but are found more commonly in children than in adults with bullous pemphigoid. Pruritus, a burning sensation, and subcutaneous edema may accompany the eruption, but constitutional symptoms are not prominent.

Diagnosis and Differential Diagnoses. Biopsy material should be taken from an early bulla arising on an erythematous base. A subepidermal bulla and a dermal inflammatory infiltrate, predominantly of eosinophils, can be identified histopathologically. In sections of a blister or perilesional skin, a band of immunoglobulin (usually IgG) and C3 can be demonstrated in the basement membrane zone by direct immunofluorescence. Indirect immunofluorescence studies of serum have positive results in ≈70% of cases for IgG antibodies to the basement membrane zone; the titers, however, do not correlate well with the clinical course. The **differential diagnosis** includes bullous erythema multiforme, pemphigus, linear IgA dermatosis, bullous drug eruption, dermatitis herpetiformis, herpes simplex infection, and bullous impetigo, which can be differentiated by histologic examination, immunofluorescence studies, and cultures. The large, tense bullae of bullous pemphigoid can generally be distinguished from the smaller, flaccid bullae of pemphigus vulgaris. The major targets for bullous pemphigoid autoantibodies are proteins of 230 and 180 kd. The 230-kd protein is part of the hemidesmosome, whereas the 180-kd antigen localizes to both the hemidesmosome and the upper lamina lucida and is a transmembrane collagenous protein.

Treatment. Bullous pemphigoid can be successfully suppressed with topical or systemic corticosteroid therapy alone or in combination with azathioprine or dapsone. Topical clobetasol improves outcome with fewer side effects. Ultimately, the condition usually remits permanently.

DERMATITIS HERPETIFORMIS. Dermatitis herpetiformis is characterized by symmetric, grouped, small, tense, erythematous, stinging, intensely pruritic papules and vesicles. The eruption is pleomorphic, including erythematous, urticarial, papular, vesicular, and bullous lesions. Sites of predilection are the knees,

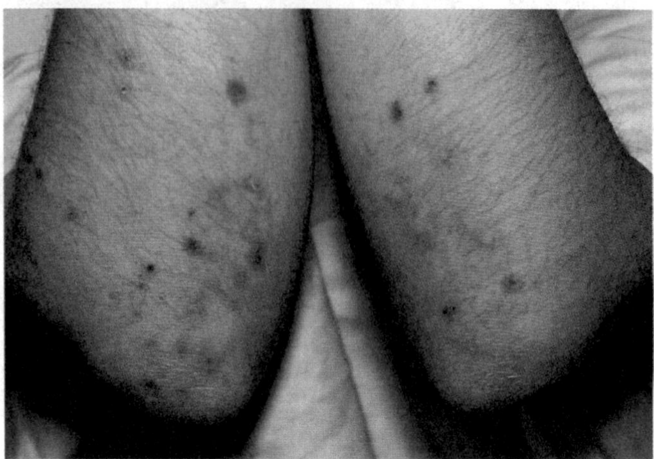

Figure 653-11. Multiple excoriations around the elbows in dermatitis herpetiformis.

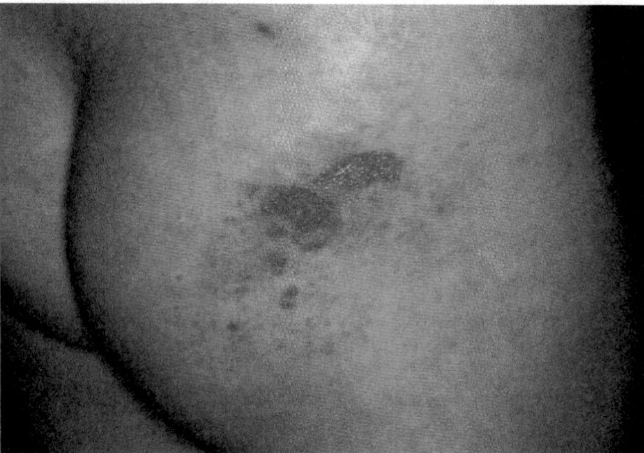

Figure 653-12. Erosion on an erythematous base post loss of blister roof in linear IgA dermatosis.

elbows, shoulders, buttocks, and scalp; mucous membranes are usually spared. Hemorrhagic lesions may develop on the palms and soles. When pruritus is severe, excoriations may be the only visible sign (Fig. 653-11).

Etiology. In dermatitis herpetiformis, IgA antibodies are directed at epidermal transglutaminase. Gluten-sensitive enteropathy is found in 85–95% of patients (see Chapter 335.2). Subepidermal blisters composed predominantly of neutrophils are found in dermal papillae. IgA and C3 can be detected in the dermal papillary tips of normal and perilesional skin in the sublamina densa region of the dermal-epidermal junction by immunofluorescence studies. The frequent finding of immune complexes and autoimmune antibodies in serum and the association with histocompatibility antigen HLA-B8 in ≈85% of patients suggest an immune mechanism. An antibody to smooth muscle endomysium is found in 70% of patients with dermatitis herpetiformis–associated gluten-sensitive enteropathy. Antibody titers correlate with the severity of intestinal disease; they decline rapidly on institution of a gluten-free diet.

Treatment. Dermatitis herpetiformis may mimic other chronic blistering diseases and may also resemble scabies, papular urticaria, insect bites, contact dermatitis, and papular eczema. The most effective treatment is oral administration of dapsone (0.5–2.0 mg/kg/day qd or bid). This drug provides immediate relief from the intense pruritus but must be used with caution because of possible serious side effects (methemoglobinemia, hemolysis, and hypersensitivity syndrome [sulfone syndrome]). Local antipruritic measures may also be useful. Jejunal biopsy is indicated to diagnose gluten-sensitive enteropathy because cutaneous manifestations may precede malabsorption. Enteropathy responds to a gluten-free diet more rapidly than do skin lesions.

LINEAR IGA DERMATOSIS (CHRONIC BULLOUS DERMATOSIS OF CHILDHOOD). This rare dermatosis is most common in the 1st decade of life, with a peak incidence during the preschool years. The eruption consists of many large, tense bullae filled with clear or hemorrhagic fluid that develop on a normal or erythematous, urticarial base. Areas of predilection are the genitals and buttocks (Fig. 653-12), the perioral region, and the scalp. Sausage-shaped bullae may be arranged in an annular or rosette-like fashion around a central crust (Fig 653-13). Erythematous plaques with gyrate margins bordered by intact bullae may develop over larger areas. Pruritus may be absent or very intense, and systemic signs or symptoms are absent. Gluten-sensitive enteropathy is not present.

Etiology. The subepidermal bullae are infiltrated with a mixture of inflammatory cells. Neutrophilic abscesses may be noted in the dermal papillary tips, indistinguishable from those of dermatitis herpetiformis. The infiltrate may also be largely eosinophilic, resembling bullous pemphigoid. Therefore, direct immunofluorescence studies are required for a definitive diagnosis; lesional or perilesional skin demonstrates linear deposition of IgA and sometimes C3 at the dermal-epidermal junction. Results of indirect immunofluorescence studies are sometimes positive for circulating antibodies. Immunoelectron microscopy has localized the immunoreactants to the sublamina densa, although a combined sublamina densa and lamina lucida pattern has also been seen. Linear IgA dermatosis is a heterogeneous disorder with antibodies targeting multiple antigens. The three most common antigens recognized are LAD285, BP230, and BP180. Linear IgA may also be seen as a drug eruption. Most cases of drug-induced linear IgA are related to vancomycin. The eruption can be distinguished by histopathologic and immunofluorescence studies from pemphigus, bullous pemphigoid, dermatitis herpetiformis, and

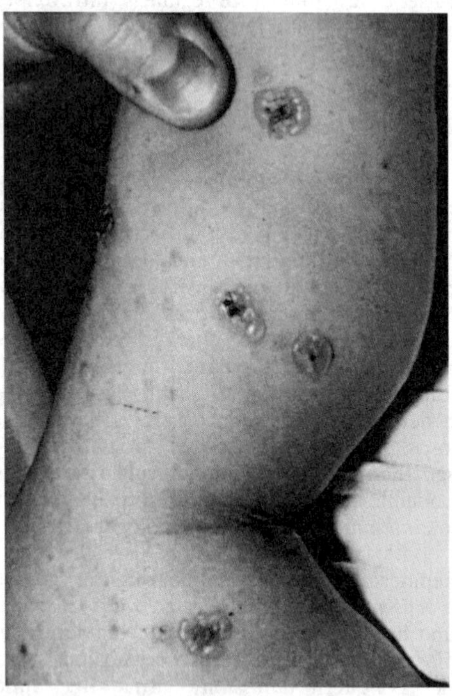

Figure 653-13. Rosette-like blisters around a central crust typical of linear IgA dermatosis (chronic bullous dermatosis of childhood).

EM. Gram stain and culture preclude the diagnosis of bullous impetigo. The lack of bullous formation in response to trauma differentiates epidermolysis bullosa.

Treatment. Many patients respond favorably to oral dapsone (see dermatitis herpetiformis). Children who do not respond to dapsone may benefit from oral therapy with a corticosteroid or a combination of these drugs. The usual course is 2–4 yr, although some children have persistent or recurrent disease; there are no long-term sequelae.

Ahmed AR, Dahl MV: Consensus statement on the use of intravenous immunoglobulin therapy in the treatment of autoimmune mucocutaneous blistering diseases. *Arch Dermatol* 2003;139:1051–1059.

Allen J, Wojnarosia F: Linear IgA disease: The IgA and IgG response to dermal antigens demonstrates a chiefly IgA response to LAD285 and a dermal 180-kDa protein. *Br J Dermatol* 2003;149:1055–1058.

Bello YM, Falabella AF, Schachner LA: Management of epidermolysis bullosa in infants and children. *Clin Dermatol* 2003;21:278–282.

Gannon BA: Epidermolysis bullosa: Pathophysiology and nursing care. *Neonatal Netw* 2004;23:25–32.

Lee WC, Leung JL, Fung CW, et al: Spectrum of anticonvulsant hypersensitivity syndrome: Controversy of treatment. *J Child Neurol* 2004; 19:619–623.

Metry DW, Jung P, Levy ML: Use of intravenous immunoglobulin in children with Stevens-Johnson syndrome and toxic epidermal necrolysis: Seven cases and review of the literature. *Pediatrics* 2003;112:1430–1436.

Ng PP, Sun YJ, Tan HH, et al: Detection of herpes simplex virus genomic DNA in various subsets of Erythema multiforme by polymerase chain reaction. *Dermatology* 2003;207:349–353.

Pfendner EG, Nakano A, Pulkkinen L, et al: Prenatal diagnosis for epidermolysis bullosa: A study of 144 consecutive pregnancies at risk. *Prenatal Diagn* 2003;23:447–456.

Williams PM, Conklin RJ: Erythema multiforme: A review and contrast from Stevens-Johnson syndrome/toxic epidermal necrolysis. *Dent Clin North Am* 2005;49:67–76.

Chapter 654 ■ Eczematous Disorders

Joseph G. Morelli

Eczematous skin disorders are characterized by exudation, lichenification, and pruritus. Acute eczematous lesions demonstrate erythema, weeping, oozing, and the formation of microvesicles within the epidermis. Chronic lesions are generally thickened, dry, and scaly, with coarse skin markings (lichenification) and altered pigmentation. Many types of eczema occur in children; the most common is **atopic dermatitis** (see Chapter 144), although seborrheic dermatitis, allergic and irritant contact dermatitis, nummular eczema, and vesicular hand and foot dermatitis (dyshidrosis) are also relatively common in childhood. Various dermatoses that have pruritus as a common feature may become eczematized due to scratching. Atopic skin is sensitive to many factors that increase pruritus, such as soap, wool, overheating, and food allergens.

Once the diagnosis of eczema has been established, it is important to classify the eruption more specifically for proper management. Pertinent historical data often provide the clue. In some instances, the subsequent course and character of the eruption permit classification. Histologic changes are relatively nonspecific, but all types of eczematous dermatitis are characterized by intraepidermal edema known as spongiosis.

CONTACT DERMATITIS. This form of eczema can be subdivided into irritant dermatitis, resulting from nonspecific injury to the skin, and allergic contact dermatitis, in which the mechanism is a delayed hypersensitivity reaction. Irritant dermatitis is more frequent in children, particularly during the early years of life.

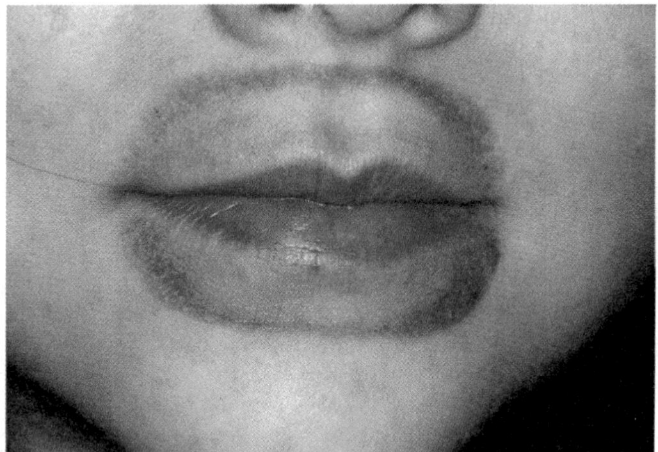

Figure 654-1. Perioral irritant contact dermatitis from lip licking.

Irritant contact dermatitis can result from prolonged or repetitive contact with various substances that include saliva, citrus juices, bubble bath, detergents, abrasive materials, strong soaps, and proprietary medications. Saliva is probably one of the most common offenders; it may cause dermatitis on the face and in the neck folds of a drooling infant or a retarded child. Older children who habitually lick their lips, frequently without awareness, because of dryness may develop a striking, sharply demarcated perioral rash (Fig. 654-1). Among the exogenous irritants, citrus juices, proprietary medications, and bubble bath preparations are relatively common. Excessive accumulation of sweat and moisture as a result of wearing occlusive shoes may also cause irritant dermatitis.

Irritant contact dermatitis may be indistinguishable from atopic dermatitis or allergic contact dermatitis. A detailed history and consideration of the sites of involvement, the age of the child, and contactants usually provide clues to the etiologic agent. The propensity to develop irritant dermatitis varies considerably among children; some may respond to minimal injury, making it difficult to identify the offending agent by history. Irritant contact dermatitis usually clears after removal of the stimulus and temporary treatment with a topical corticosteroid preparation (see Chapter 645). Education of patients and parents about the causes of contact dermatitis is crucial to successful therapy.

Diaper dermatitis can be regarded as the prototype of irritant contact dermatitis. As a reaction to overhydration of the skin, friction, maceration, and prolonged contact with urine and feces, retained diaper soaps, and topical preparations, the skin of the diaper area may become erythematous and scaly, often with papulovesicular or bullous lesions, fissures, and erosions (Fig. 654-2). The eruption can be patchy or confluent, but the genitocrural folds are often spared. Chronic hypertrophic, flat-topped papules and infiltrative nodules may occur. Secondary infection with bacteria or yeasts is common. Discomfort may be marked because of intense inflammation. Allergic contact dermatitis, seborrheic dermatitis, psoriasis, candidosis, atopic dermatitis, and rare disorders such as histiocytosis X (Langerhans cell histiocytosis) and acrodermatitis enteropathica should be considered when the eruption is persistent or recalcitrant to simple therapeutic measures.

Diaper dermatitis often responds to simple measures; some infants are predisposed to diaper dermatitis, and management may be difficult. The damaging effects of overhydration of the skin and prolonged contact with feces and urine can be obviated by frequent changing of the diapers. Overwashing should be

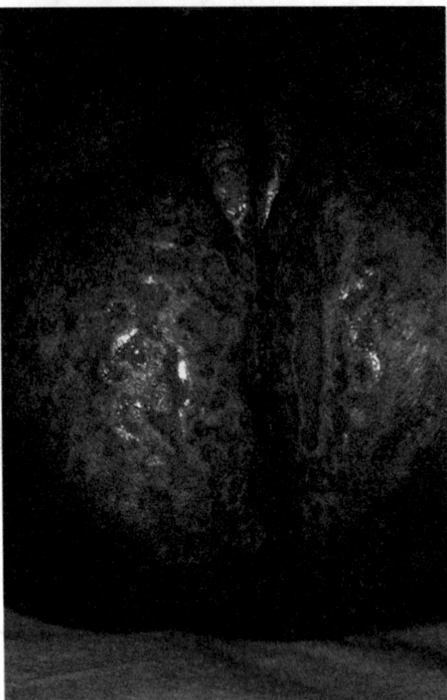

Figure 654-2. Severe, erosive diaper dermatitis.

avoided because it leads to chapping and a worsening of the dermatitis. Disposable diapers containing a superabsorbent material may help to maintain a relatively dry environment. Frequent topical applications of a bland protective barrier agent (petrolatum or zinc oxide paste) may suffice to prevent dermatitis. When these measures are not sufficient to promote healing, a light application of 0.5–1% topical hydrocortisone ointment after each diaper change for a limited time is often effective. Secondary complications can result from prolonged use of corticosteroids, especially fluorinated compounds. Before initiating such therapy, the possibility of candidal infection should be considered. **Candidal infection** can be identified by red-pink tender skin that has numerous 1–2 mm pustules and papules at the periphery of the dermatitis. Treatment with a topical anticandidal agent may be helpful.

Juvenile plantar dermatosis is a common form of irritant contact dermatitis occurring mainly in prepubertal children. The dermatitis characteristically involves the weight-bearing surfaces, may be pruritic or painful, and causes a glazed appearance of the plantar skin (Fig. 654-3). Fissuring may become extensive, producing considerable discomfort. The dermatitis results from alternating excessive hydration and rapid moisture loss, which causes chapping of the skin and cracking of the stratum corneum. Affected children often have hyperhidrosis, wear occlusive synthetic footwear, and subject their feet to rapid drying without moisturization. Immediate application of a thick emollient when socks and shoes are removed or immediately after swimming usually minimizes this condition.

Allergic contact dermatitis is a T-cell-mediated hypersensitivity reaction that is provoked by application of an antigen to the skin surface. The antigen penetrates the skin, where it is conjugated with a cutaneous protein, and the hapten-protein complex is transported to the regional lymph nodes by antigen-presenting Langerhans cells. A primary immunologic response occurs locally in the nodes and becomes generalized, presumably because of dissemination of sensitized T cells. Sensitization requires several days and, when followed by a fresh antigenic challenge, is manifested as allergic contact dermatitis. Generalized distribution may also occur if enough antigen finds its way into the circulation. Once sensitization has occurred, each new antigenic challenge may provoke an inflammatory reaction within 8–12 hr; sensitization to a particular antigen usually persists for many years.

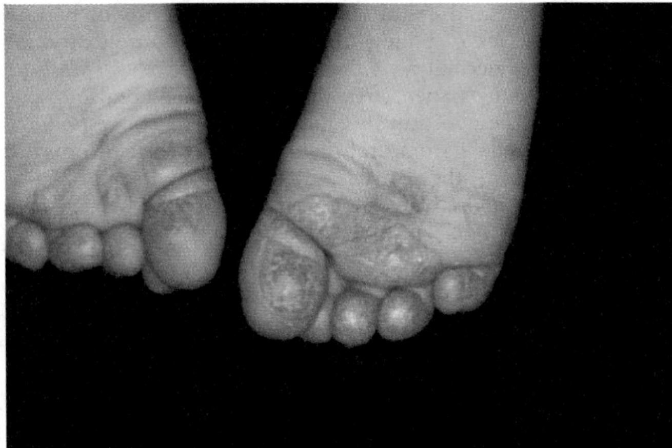

Figure 654-3. Red, scaly juvenile plantar dermatosis.

Acute allergic contact dermatitis is an erythematous, intensely pruritic, eczematous dermatitis, which, if severe, may be edematous and vesiculobullous. The chronic condition has the features of long-standing eczema: lichenification, scaling, fissuring, and pigmentary change. The distribution of the eruption often provides a clue to the diagnosis. Volatile sensitizers usually affect exposed areas, such as the face and arms. Jewelry, topical agents, shoes, clothing, and plants cause dermatitis at points of contact.

Rhus dermatitis (poison ivy, poison sumac, poison oak) is often vesiculobullous and may be distinguished by linear streaks of vesicles where the plant leaves have brushed against the skin (Fig. 654-4). Fluid from ruptured cutaneous vesicles does not spread the eruption; however, antigen retained on the skin, under the fingernails, and on clothing initiates new plaques of dermatitis if not removed by washing with soap and water. Antigen may also be carried by animals on their fur. The saplike allergen (oleoresin) is present on live and dead leaves, and sensitization to 1 plant produces cross reactions with the others.

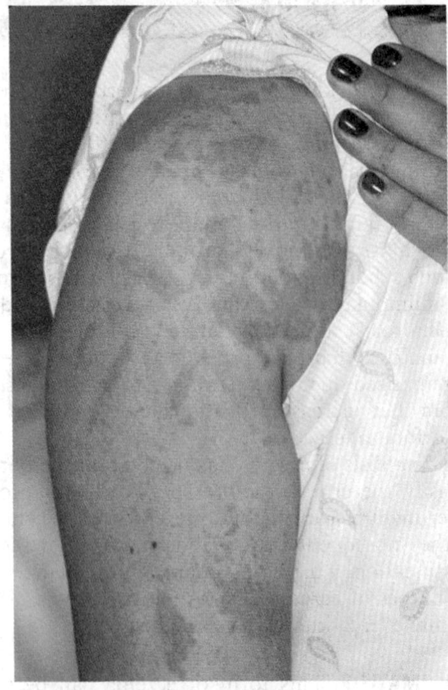

Figure 654-4. Linear lesions in poison ivy.

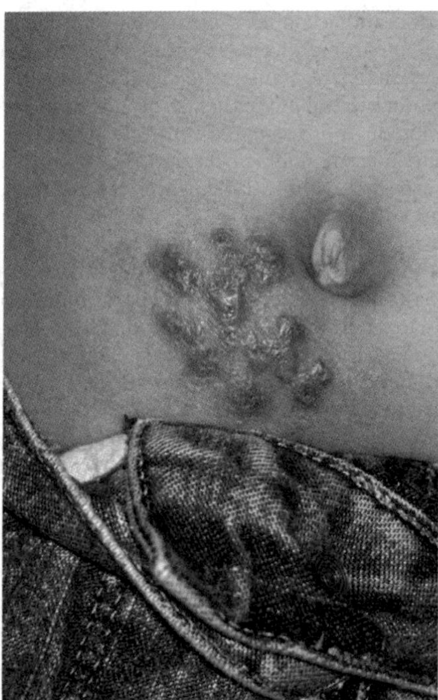

Figure 654-5. Chronic periumbilical nickel dermatitis.

Nickel dermatitis usually develops from contact with jewelry or metal closures on clothing and is seen most frequently on the earlobes, such as when nickel-containing earring posts rather than nonmetallic materials or stainless steel are used to keep a pierced tract open. Metal closures on pants frequently cause periumbilical disease (Fig. 654-5). Some children are exquisitely sensitive to nickel, with even the trace amounts found in gold jewelry provoking eruptions.

Shoe dermatitis typically affects the dorsum of the feet and toes, sparing the interdigital spaces; it is usually symmetric. Other forms of allergic contact dermatitis, in contrast to irritant dermatitis, rarely involve the palms and soles. Common allergens are the antioxidants and accelerators in shoe rubber and the chromium salts in tanned leather or shoe dyes. Excessive sweating often leaches these substances from their source.

Wearing apparel contains a number of sensitizers, including dyes, mordants, fabric finishes, fibers, resins, and cleaning solutions. Dye may be poorly fixed to clothing and leached out with sweating, as are the partially cured formaldehyde resins. The elastic in garments is also a frequent cause of clothing dermatitis.

Topical medications and cosmetics may be unsuspected as allergens, particularly if the medication is being used for a preexisting dermatitis. The most common offenders are neomycin, thimerosal, topical antihistamines, topical anesthetics, preservatives, and ethylenediamine, a stabilizer present in many medications. All types of cosmetics can cause facial dermatitis; involvement of the eyelids is characteristic for nail polish sensitivity.

Contact dermatitis can be confused with other types of eczema, dermatophytoses, and vesiculobullous diseases. Patch testing may clarify the etiology. The essential principle in **treatment** is elimination of contact with the allergen. Acute dermatitis responds to cool compresses and topical application of a corticosteroid ointment. An oral antihistamine may be useful. Massive acute bullous reactions or reactions that cause swelling around the eyes or genitals such as those of poison ivy may require treatment with a 2 wk tapering course of oral corticosteroids. If secondary infection has occurred, appropriate systemic antibiotic therapy should be given. Desensitization therapy is rarely indicated.

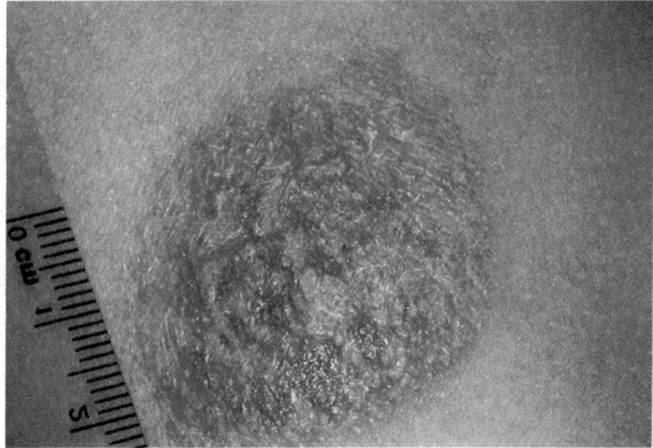

Figure 654-6. Discrete, boggy plaque of nummular dermatitis.

NUMMULAR ECZEMA. This disorder is unrelated to other types of eczema and is characterized by more or less coin-shaped eczematous plaques. Common sites are the extensor surfaces of the extremities (Fig. 654-6), buttocks, and shoulders. The plaques are relatively discrete, boggy, vesicular, severely pruritic, and exudative; when chronic, they often become thickened and lichenified. The cause is unknown. Most frequently, these lesions are mistaken for tinea corporis, but plaques of nummular eczema are distinguished by the lack of a raised, sharply circumscribed border; the lack of fungal organisms on a potassium hydroxide (KOH) preparation; and frequent weeping or bleeding when scraped. Secondary infection is common. Control of pruritus is usually achieved with a fluorinated corticosteroid preparation. Steroid-impregnated tapes may simultaneously treat and provide barrier protection to these circumscribed eczematous plaques. An antihistamine may be helpful, particularly at night. Antibiotics are indicated for secondary infection.

PITYRIASIS ALBA. This occurs mainly in children; the lesions are hypopigmented, round or oval, macular or slightly elevated patches with fine adherent scale (Fig. 654-7). They may be mildly erythematous and relatively well defined but lack a sharply marginated border. Lesions occur on the face, neck, upper trunk, and proximal portions of the arms. Itching is minimal or absent. The cause is unknown, but the eruption appears to be exacerbated by dryness and is often regarded as a mild form of eczema. Pityriasis alba is frequently misdiagnosed as vitiligo, tinea versicolor, or tinea corporis. The lesions wax and wane but eventually disappear. Application of a lubricant may ameliorate the condition; if

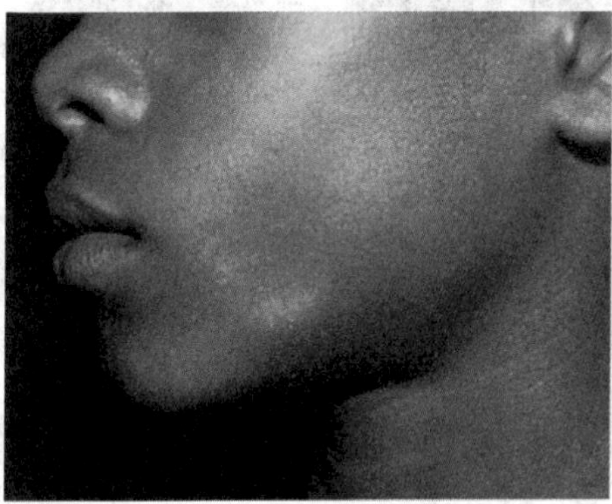

Figure 654-7. Patchy hypopigmented lesions with diffuse borders characteristic of pityriasis alba.

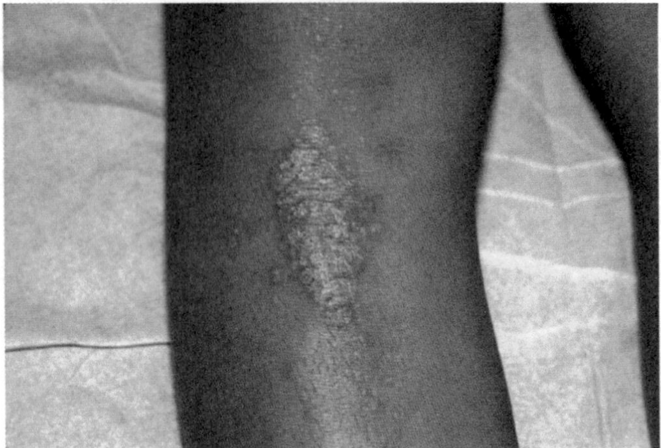

Figure 654-8. Thickened plaque of lichen simplex chronicus.

pruritus is troublesome, a low potency topical steroid may used. Normal pigmentation often takes months to return.

LICHEN SIMPLEX CHRONICUS. This lesion is characterized by a chronic pruritic, eczematous, circumscribed, solitary plaque that is usually lichenified and hyperpigmented (Fig. 654-8). The most common sites are the posterior aspect of the neck, the dorsum of the feet, the wrists, and the ankles. Although the initiating event may be a transient lesion such as an insect bite, trauma from rubbing and scratching accounts for persistence of the plaque. Pruritus must be controlled to permit healing. A topical fluorinated corticosteroid preparation is often helpful, but constant irritation of the skin must be avoided. A covering to prevent scratching may be necessary.

VESICULAR HAND AND FOOT DERMATITIS (DYSHIDROTIC ECZEMA, DYSHIDROSIS, POMPHOLYX). This is a recurrent, sometimes seasonal, blistering disorder of the hands and feet; it occurs in all age groups but is uncommon in infancy. The pathogenesis is unknown; no genetic factor has been identified, although an increased incidence of atopy has been recorded in patients and their relatives. The disease is characterized by recurrent crops of small, intensely pruritic vesicles on the hands and feet. Sites of predilection are the palms, soles, and lateral aspects of the fingers and toes. Primary lesions are noninflammatory and filled with clear fluid, which, unlike sweat, has a physiologic pH and contains protein. Larger vesicles and bullae may occur (Fig. 654-9), and maceration and secondary infection are frequent because of scratching. The chronic phase is characterized by thickened, fissured plaques that may cause considerable discomfort. Hyperhidrosis is common in many patients, but the association may be fortuitous. The diagnosis is made clinically. The disorder may be confused with allergic contact dermatitis, which usually affects the dorsal rather than the volar surfaces, and with dermatophytosis, which can be distinguished by a KOH preparation of the roof of a vesicle and by appropriate cultures.

Vesicular hand and foot dermatitis responds to wet dressings, followed by a topical corticosteroid preparation during the acute phase. Control of the chronic stage is difficult; lubricants containing mild keratolytic agents in conjunction with a potent topical fluorinated corticosteroid preparation may be indicated. Secondary bacterial infection should be treated systemically with an appropriate antibiotic. Patients should be told to expect recurrence and should protect their hands and feet from the damaging effects of excessive sweating, chemicals, harsh soaps, and adverse weather. Unfortunately, it is impossible to prevent recurrence or to predict its frequency.

SEBORRHEIC DERMATITIS. This chronic inflammatory disease is most common in infancy and adolescence, paralleling the distribution, size, and activity of the sebaceous glands. The cause is unknown, as is the role of the sebaceous glands in this disease. It is also unknown whether infantile and adolescent seborrheic dermatitis are the same or different entities. There is no evidence that children with infantile seborrheic dermatitis will develop seborrheic dermatitis as adolescents. A generalized eruption with features of seborrheic dermatitis is common in HIV-infected children and adolescents.

Clinical Manifestations. The disorder may begin in the 1st mo of life and may be most troublesome in the 1st yr. Diffuse or focal scaling and crusting of the scalp, sometimes called cradle cap (Fig. 654-10), may be the initial and at times the only manifestation. A greasy, scaly, erythematous papular dermatitis, which is usually non-pruritic, may involve the face, neck, retroauricular areas, axillae, and diaper area. The dermatitis may be patchy and focal or may spread to involve almost the entire body (Fig. 654-11). Postinflammatory pigmentary changes are common, particularly in black infants. When the scaling becomes pronounced, the condition may resemble psoriasis and, at times, can be distinguished only with difficulty. The possibility of coexistent atopic dermatitis must be considered when there is an acute weeping dermatitis with pruritus, and the two are often clinically inseparable at an early age. An intractable seborrhea-like dermatitis with chronic diarrhea and failure to thrive may reflect systemic dys-

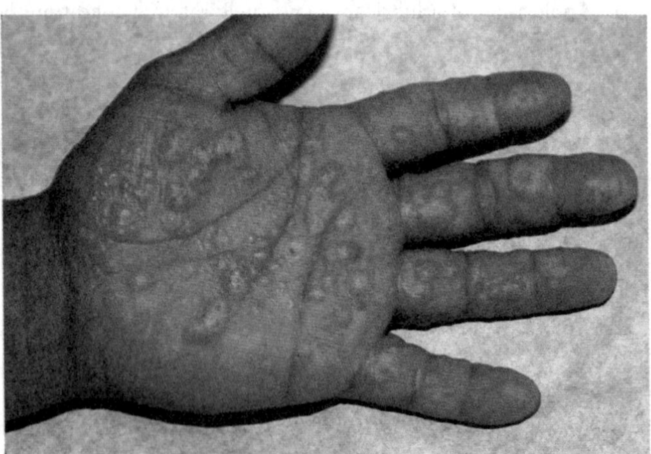

Figure 654-9. Vesicular palmar lesions of dyshidrotic eczema with large bullae.

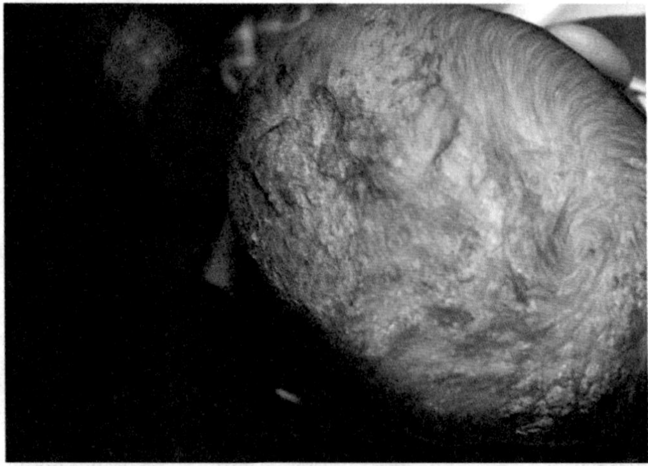

Figure 654-10. Cradle cap in an infant.

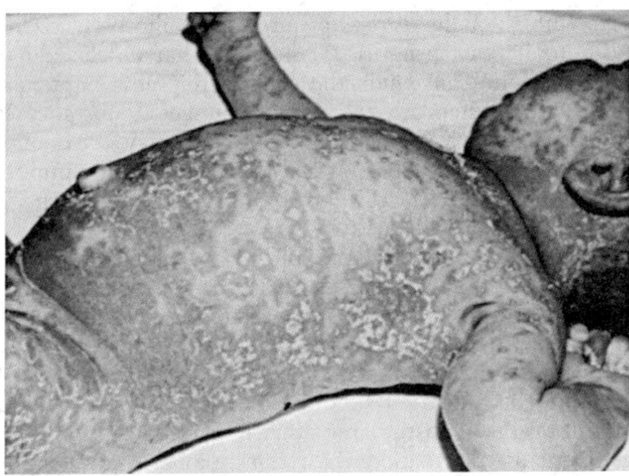

Figure 654-11. Widespread seborrheic dermatitis.

function of the immune system. A chronic seborrhea-like pattern, which responds poorly to treatment, may also result from cutaneous histiocytic infiltrates in infants with **Langerhans cell histiocytosis X.** Seborrheic dermatitis is a common cutaneous manifestation of **AIDS** in young adults and is characterized by thick, greasy scales on the scalp and large hyperkeratotic erythematous plaques on the face, chest, and genitals.

During adolescence, seborrheic dermatitis is more localized and may be confined to the scalp and intertriginous areas. Also noted may be marginal blepharitis and involvement of the external auditory canal. Scalp changes may vary from diffuse, brawny scaling to focal areas of thick, oily, yellow crusts with underlying erythema. Loss of hair is common, and pruritus may be absent to marked. When the dermatitis is severe, erythema and scaling may occur at the frontal hairline, the medial aspects of the eyebrows, and in the nasolabial and retroauricular folds. Red, scaly plaques may appear in the axillae, inguinal region, gluteal cleft, and umbilicus. On the extremities, seborrheic plaques may be more eczematous and less erythematous and demarcated.

Etiology. *Malassezia furfur* has been implicated as a causative agent, although its role in the etiology of infantile seborrheic dermatitis is unclear. The differential diagnosis includes psoriasis, atopic dermatitis, dermatophytosis, and candidosis. Secondary bacterial infections and superimposed candidosis are common.

Treatment. Scalp lesions should be controlled with an antiseborrheic shampoo (selenium sulfide, sulfur, salicylic acid, zinc pyrithione, tar), used daily if necessary. Inflamed lesions usually respond promptly to topical corticosteroid therapy. Topical immunomodulatory agents (tacrolimus, pimecrolimus) approved for the treatment of atopic dermatitis in children ≥2 yr of age (see Chapter 144) may have a role in the treatment of other eczematous disorders such as seborrheic dermatitis. Concerns for systemic absorption and potential immunosuppression are higher in the younger patient population typically afflicted with seborrheic dermatitis. Topical antifungal agents effective against *Malassezia* have been advocated. Wet compresses should be applied to the moist or fissured lesions before application of the steroid ointment. Many patients require continued use of an antiseborrheic shampoo. Response to therapy is usually rapid unless there are complicating factors or the diagnosis is in error.

Brydensholt Halkjaer L, Loland L, Buchvald FF, et al: Development of atopic dermatitis during the first 3 years of life. *Arch Dermatol* 2006;142:561–566.

Faergemann J: Treatment of seborrheic dermatitis with oral terbinafine? *Lancet* 2001;358:170.

Fergusson DM, Horwood J, Shannon FT: Early solid feeding and recurrent childhood eczema: A 10-year longitudinal study. *Pediatrics* 1990; 86:541–546.

Krafchik BR: Eczematous disorders. In Eichenfield LF, Frieden IJ, Esterly NB (editors): *Textbook of Neonatal Dermatology.* Philadelphia, WB Saunders, 2001, p 241.

Paller AS: Use of non-steroidal topical immunomodulators for the treatment of atopic dermatitis in the pediatric population. *J Pediatr* 2001; 138:163–168.

Rothe M, Grant-Kels J: Diagnostic criteria for atopic dermatitis. *Lancet* 1996;348:769–770.

Tollesson A, Frithz A, Stenlund K: *Malassezia furfur* in infantile seborrheic dermatitis. *Pediatr Dermatol* 1997;14:423–425.

Chapter 655 ■ Photosensitivity

Joseph G. Morelli

Photosensitivity denotes a qualitatively or quantitatively abnormal cutaneous reaction to sunlight or artificial light.

ACUTE SUNBURN REACTION. The most common photosensitive reaction seen in children is acute sunburn. Sunburn is caused mainly by ultraviolet (UV) B radiation (290–320 nm wavelength). Sunlight contains many times more UVA (320–400 nm) than UVB radiation, but UVA must be encountered in much larger quantities than UVB radiation to produce sunburn.

Pathophysiology and Clinical Manifestations. Transmitted radiation <300 nm is largely absorbed in the epidermis, whereas that >300 nm is mostly transmitted to the dermis after variable epidermal melanin absorption. Children vary in susceptibility to UV radiation, depending on their skin type (amount of pigment) [Table 655-1]. Immediate pigment darkening is due to UVA radiation–induced photo-oxidative darkening of existing melanin and its transfer from melanocytes to keratinocytes. This effect generally lasts for a few hours and like a UVA-induced tanning salon tan is not photoprotective. UVB-induced effects appear 6–12 hr after initial exposure and reach a peak in 24 hr. Effects include redness, tenderness, edema, and blistering (Fig. 655-1). Reactive oxidation species generated by UVB induce keratinocyte membrane damage and are involved in the pathogenesis of sunburn. A portion of the vasodilatation seen in UVB-induced erythema is mediated by prostaglandins E_2 and F_2. Delayed melanogenesis as a result of UVB radiation begins in 2–3 days and lasts several days to a few weeks. Manufacture of new melanin in melanocytes, transfer of melanin from melanocytes to keratinocytes, increase in size and arborization of melanocytes, and activation of quiescent melanocytes produce delayed melanogenesis. This effect reduces skin sensitivity to development of erythema by approximately twofold to threefold. Additional effects and possible complications of sun exposure include increased thickness of the stratum corneum, recurrence or exacerbation of herpes simplex labialis, lupus erythematosus, and many other conditions (Table 655-2).

TABLE 655-1. Sun-Reactive Skin Types

TYPE	DEMOGRAPHICS	SUNBURN, TANNING HISTORY
I	Red hair, freckles, Celtic origin	Always burns easily, no tanning
II	Fair skin, fair-haired, blue-eyed, white	Usually burns, minimal tanning
III	Darker skinned white	Sometimes burns, gradual light brown tan
IV	Mediterranean background	Minimal to no burning, always tans
V	Middle Eastern white, Mexican	Rarely burns, tans profusely dark brown
VI	Blacks	Never burns, pigmented black

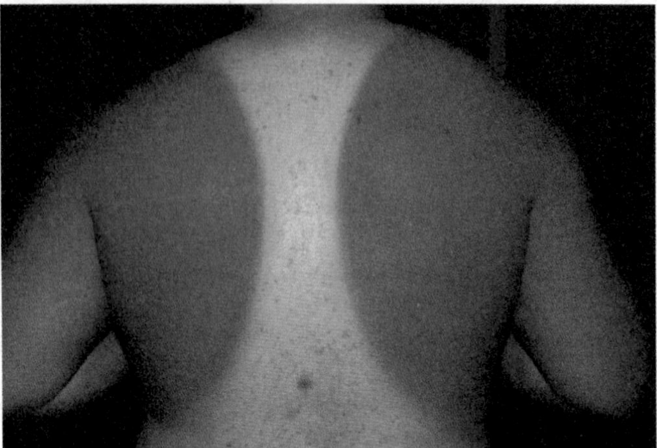

Figure 655-1. Sunburn. Well-demarcated, severe erythema.

Treatment. Acute severe sunburn should be managed with cool compresses. Topical corticosteroids and oral prostaglandin inhibitors such as ibuprofen and indomethacin may decrease erythema and pain, but must be administered preradiation or early in the course of the sunburn. Once peak erythema has been reached, little help is afforded by these medications. Proprietary preparations containing topical anesthetics are relatively ineffective and potentially hazardous because of their propensity to cause contact dermatitis. A bland emollient is effective in the desquamative phase.

Prognosis and Prevention of Sequelae. The long-term sequelae of chronic and intense sun exposure are not often seen in children, but most individuals receive >50% of their lifetime UV dose by age 20 yr. Therefore, pediatricians have a pivotal role in educating patients and their parents about the harmful effects, potential malignancy risks, and irreversible skin damage that result from unduly prolonged exposure to the sun and tanning lights. Premature aging, senile elastosis, actinic keratoses, squamous and basal cell carcinomas, and melanomas all occur with greater frequency in sun-damaged skin. In particular, blistering sunburns in childhood and adolescence significantly increase the risk for development of malignant melanoma. Sun protection is best achieved by sun avoidance. This includes minimizing time in the midday sun (10 A.M. to 3 P.M.), staying in the shade, and wearing protective clothing including wide-brimmed hats. Protection is enhanced by a wide variety of sunscreen agents. Physical opaque sunscreens (zinc oxide, titanium dioxide) block UV light, whereas chemical sunscreens (para-aminobenzoic acid [PABA], PABA esters, salicylates, benzophenones, dibenzoylmethanes, cinnamates) absorb damaging radiation. The benzophenones and dibenzoylmethanes provide protection in both the UVA and UVB ranges. Vitamins C and E added to sunscreen may also be beneficial in reduction of the formation of reactive oxygen species. Children with skin types I to III (see Table 655-1) require sunscreens with a sun protection factor (SPF) of at least 15. SPF is defined as the minimal dose of sunlight required to produce cutaneous erythema after applying a sunscreen, divided by the dose required with no use of sunscreen.

PHOTOSENSITIVE REACTIONS. Photosensitizers in combination with a particular wavelength of light cause dermatitis that can be classified as a phototoxic or a photoallergic reaction. Contact of the skin with the photosensitizer may occur externally, internally by enteral or parenteral administration, or by host synthesis of photosensitizers in response to an administered drug.

Photoallergic reactions occur in only a small percentage of persons exposed to photosensitizers and light and require a time interval for sensitization to take place. Thereafter, dermatitis appears within ≈24 hr of re-exposure to the photosensitizer and light. Photoallergic dermatitis is a T-cell-mediated delayed hypersensitivity reaction in which the drug, acting as a hapten, may combine with a skin protein to form the antigenic substance. Photoallergic reactions vary in morphology and may occur on partially covered and on light-exposed skin. Some of the important classes of drugs and chemicals responsible for photosensitivity reactions are listed in Table 655-2.

Phototoxic reactions occur in all individuals who accumulate adequate amounts of a photosensitizing drug or chemical within the skin. Prior sensitization is not required. Dermatitis develops within hours after exposure to radiation in the range of 285–450 nm. The eruption is confined to light-exposed areas and often resembles an exaggerated sunburn, but it may be urticarial or bullous. It results in postinflammatory hyperpigmentation. All the drugs that cause photoallergic reactions may also cause a phototoxic dermatitis if given in sufficiently high doses. Several additional drugs and contactants cause phototoxic reactions, notably the plant-derived furocoumarins (see Table 655-2). Differentiation from contact dermatitis as a result of poison ivy or oak may be difficult, but itching is prominent in contact dermatitis. In phytophotodermatitis, burning is prominent and is confined to sun-

TABLE 655-2. Cutaneous Reactions to Sunlight

TABLE 655-2. Cutaneous Reactions to Sunlight
SUNBURN
PHOTOALLERGIC DRUG ERUPTIONS
Systemic drugs include tetracyclines, psoralens, chlorthiazides, sulfonamides, barbiturates, griseofulvin, thiazides, quinidine, phenothiazines
Topical agents include coal tar derivatives, psoralens, halogenated salicylanilides (soaps), perfume oils (e.g., oil of bergamot), sunscreens (e.g., PABA, cinnamates, benzophenones)
PHOTOTOXIC DRUG ERUPTIONS
High doses of agents causing photoallergic eruptions; nalidixic acid, 5-fluorouracil, psoralens, furosemide, nonsteroidal anti-inflammatory agents (naproxen, piroxicam), sulfonamides, tetracyclines, phenothiazines, furocoumarins (e.g., lime, lemon, carrot, celery, dill, parsnip, parsley)
GENETIC DISORDER WITH PHOTOSENSITIVITY
Xeroderma pigmentosum
Bloom syndrome
Cockayne syndrome
Rothmund-Thomson syndrome
INBORN ERRORS OF METABOLISM
Porphyrias
Hartnup disease
INFECTIOUS DISEASES ASSOCIATED WITH PHOTOSENSITIVITY
Recurrent herpes simplex infection
Viral exanthems (accentuated photodistribution; e.g., varicella)
SKIN DISEASE EXACERBATED OR PRECIPITATED BY LIGHT
Lichen planus
Darier disease
Lupus erythematosus
Dermatomyositis
Scleroderma
Granuloma annulare
Psoriasis
Erythema multiforme
Sarcoid
Atopic dermatitis
Hailey-Hailey disease
Pemphigus
Acne rosacea
Bullous pemphigoid
DEFICIENT PROTECTION DUE TO LACK OF PIGMENT
Vitiligo
Oculocutaneous albinism
Phenylketonuria
Chédiak-Higashi syndrome
Hermansky-Pudlak syndrome
Waardenburg syndrome
Piebaldism

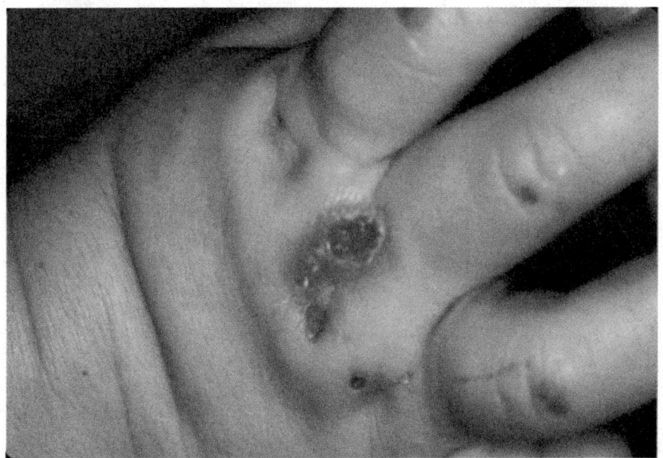

Figure 655-2. Crusted ulcerations in infant with congenital erythropoietic porphyria.

exposed areas, sparing the upper eyelids, beneath the nose and chin, and the retroauricular areas. Postinflammatory hyperpigmentation develops rapidly and is usually the presenting sign.

Although photodermatitis caused by drugs or chemicals may be diagnosed by photopatch testing, facilities for this diagnostic procedure are not widely available. A high index of suspicion combined with an appreciation of the distribution pattern of the eruption and a history of application or ingestion of a known photosensitizing agent is all that is required to make a diagnosis. Discontinuation of the offending medication or avoidance of sun exposure, oral administration of an antihistamine, and application of a topical corticosteroid to alleviate pruritus are appropriate therapeutic measures. Severe reactions may necessitate systemic corticosteroid therapy for a brief time.

PORPHYRIAS (SEE CHAPTER 91). Porphyrias are acquired or inborn disorders due to abnormalities of specific enzyme mutations in the heme biosynthetic pathway. They are diverse in their clinical manifestations. Two in particular occur in children and have photosensitivity as a consistent feature. Signs and symptoms may be negligible during the winter, when sun exposure is minimal.

Congenital erythropoietic porphyria (Günther disease) is a rare autosomal recessive disorder caused by a deficiency of uroporphyrinogen III cosynthase. It presents in the 1st few months of life with exquisite sensitivity to light, which may induce repeated severe bullous eruptions that result in mutilating scars (Fig. 655-2). **Hyperpigmentation,** hyperkeratosis, vesiculation, and fragility of skin develop in light-exposed areas. **Hirsutism** in areas of mild involvement, scarring **alopecia** in severely affected areas, pink to red urine, brown teeth, hemolytic anemia, splenomegaly, and increased amounts of uroporphyrin I in urine, plasma, and erythrocytes and of coproporphyrin I in feces are additional characteristic manifestations. Urine from affected patients fluoresces reddish pink under a Wood light.

Erythropoietic protoporphyria, an autosomal dominant trait, is due to decreased activity of ferrochelatase, which converts protoporphyrin to heme. Photosensitivity becomes apparent in early childhood and is manifested by pain, tingling, and a burning sensation within ≈30 min of sun exposure, followed by erythema, edema, urticaria, and, rarely, vesicles on light-exposed areas. Nail changes consist of opacification of the nail plate, onycholysis, pain, and tenderness. Mild systemic symptoms of malaise, chills, and fever may accompany the acute skin reaction. Recurrent sun exposure produces a chronic eczematous dermatitis with thickened, lichenified skin, especially over the finger joints (Fig. 655-3*A*), and persistent violaceous erythema, ulcers, and pitted or linear, crusted atrophic scars on the face (Fig. 655-3*B*) and rims of the ears. Pigmentation, hypertrichosis, skin fragility, and mutilation are uncommon. Liver disease is generally mild. Symptoms often improve spontaneously after age 10–11 yr.

The wavelengths of light mainly responsible for eliciting cutaneous reactions in porphyria are in the region of 400 nm. Window glass, which transmits wavelengths >320 nm, is not protective, and artificial lights of a certain wavelength may be pathogenic. Patients must avoid direct sunlight, wear protective clothing, and use a sunscreen agent that effectively blocks wavelengths in the region of 400 nm. **Administration** of beta-carotene (Solatene) quenches the fluorescence of the porphyrin molecule by yellowing the skin; its effectiveness in reducing photosensitivity in patients with protoporphyria has onset within 1–3 mo and is variable.

COLLOID MILIUM. This is a rare, asymptomatic disorder that occurs on the face (nose, upper lip, upper cheeks) and may extend to the dorsum of the hands and the neck as a profuse eruption of tiny, ivory to yellow, firm, grouped papules. Lesions appear before puberty on otherwise normal skin, unlike the adult variant that develops on sun-damaged skin. Onset may follow an acute sunburn or chronic sun exposure. Most cases reach maximal severity within ≈3 yr and remain unchanged thereafter, although the condition may remit spontaneously after puberty. Histopathologic changes include well-circumscribed accumulations of

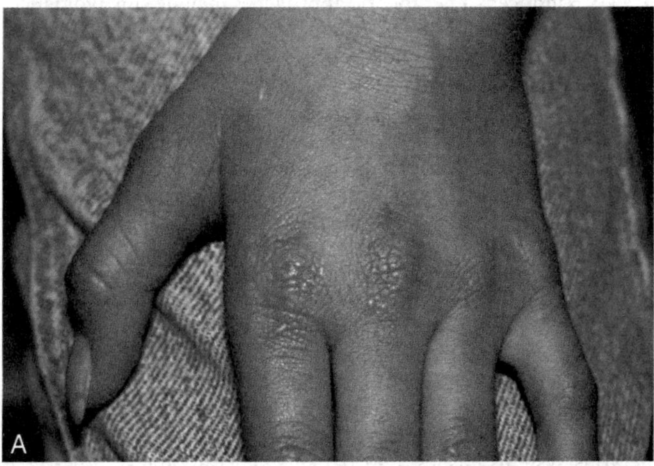

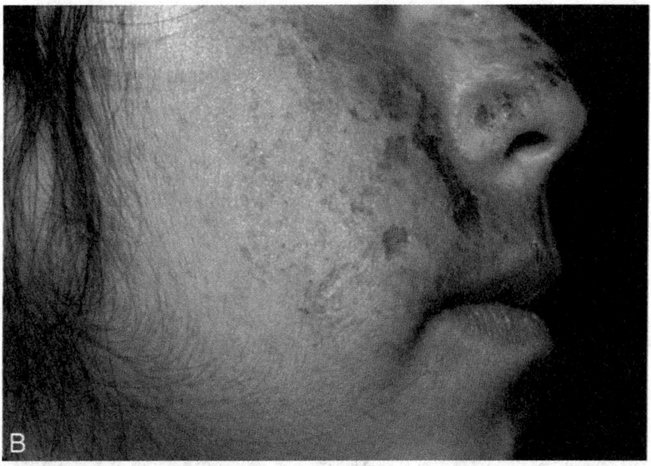

Figure 655-3. *A*, Erythematous thickening over the metacarpal phalangeal joints in erythropoietic protoporphyria. *B*, Linear crusts and scarring in erythropoietic porphyria.

fissured eosinophilic material, primarily in the upper dermis in contact with the epidermis. Basal cells, which are transformed into these colloid bodies, appear to be abnormally susceptible to degeneration after actinic exposure.

HYDROA VACCINIFORME. This vesiculobullous disorder is more common in boys than in girls, begins in early childhood, but may remit at puberty. The peak incidence is in the spring and summer. Erythematous, pruritic macules develop symmetrically within hours of sun exposure over the ears, nose, lips, cheeks, and dorsal surfaces of the hands and forearms. Lesions progress to stinging tender papules and hemorrhagic vesicles and bullae. Severe lesions of hydroa vacciniforme resemble the vesicles of chickenpox. They become umbilicated, ulcerated, and crusted and heal with pitted scars and telangiectasias. Fever and malaise are noted occasionally during the acute phase. Histopathologically, lesions show intraepidermal multilocular vesicles, leading to focal epidermal and dermal necrosis. Noted early is a dermal perivascular mononuclear cell infiltrate, which later surrounds areas of necrosis. This eruption should be distinguished from erythropoietic protoporphyria, which rarely shows vesicles. Pathogenesis of hydroa vacciniforme is unknown, but typical lesions have been reproduced with repeated doses of UVA or UVB light. A **topical corticosteroid** may be useful for the inflammatory phase of the eruption. Prophylactic broad-spectrum sunscreens may also be helpful, as may low-dose courses of UVB or psoralen with UVA (PUVA) therapy. Beta-carotene and antimalarial agents are sometimes beneficial.

ACTINIC PRURIGO. This is a chronic familial photodermatitis that is inherited as an autosomal dominant trait among the Native Americans of North and South America. The 1st episode generally occurs in early childhood several hours to 2 days after intense sun exposure. Most patients are female and are sensitive to UVA radiation. Lesions are intensely pruritic, erythematous papules on the face (Fig. 655-4), lower lip, distal extremities, and, in severe cases, buttocks. Facial lesions may heal with minute pitted or linear scarring. Lesions often become chronic, without periods of total clearing, merging into eczematous plaques that lichenify and may become secondarily infected. Associated features that distinguish this disorder from other photoeruptions and atopic dermatitis include cheilitis, conjunctivitis, and traumatic alopecia of the outer half of the eyebrows. Actinic prurigo is a chronic condition that generally persists into adult life, although it may improve spontaneously in the late teenage years. Broad-spectrum sunscreens may be helpful in preventing the eruption, but antimalarials and beta-carotene afford little to no protection. **Topical corticosteroids** palliate the pruritus and inflammation.

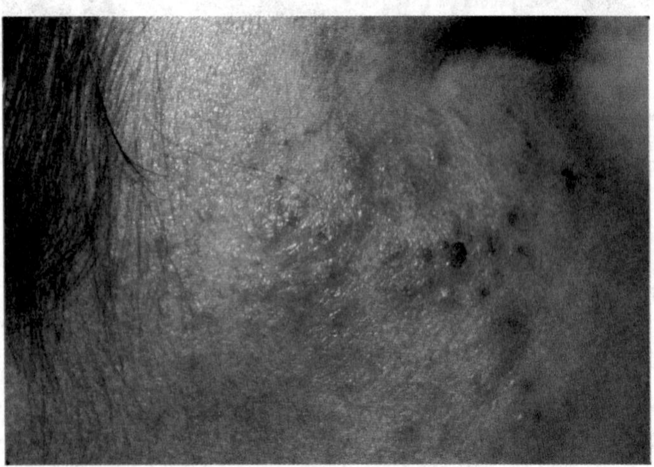

Figure 655-4. Erythematous, excoriated papules in actinic prurigo.

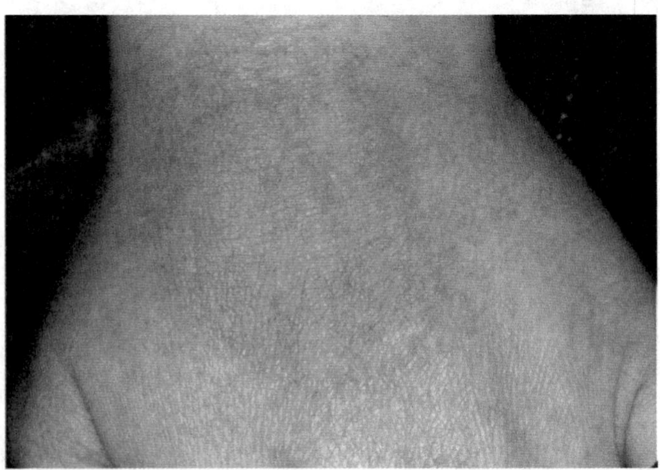

Figure 655-5. Urticaria after 5 min exposure to artificial ultraviolet A radiation.

SOLAR URTICARIA. This is a rare disorder induced by UV or visible irradiation. Primary solar urticaria is probably mediated by allergic type 1 hypersensitivity to a cutaneous or circulating irradiation-induced allergen, leading to mast cell degranulation and histamine release. This reaction occurs within 5–10 min of sun exposure, fades within 1–2 hr, and is characterized by widespread severe wheal formation (Fig. 655-5), which may lead to faintness, headache, nausea, syncope, or bronchospasm. H_1-blocking antihistamines may be useful to prevent or abate the eruption. Secondary solar urticaria is due to photosensitization to exogenous chemicals or systemic drugs and may rarely be a presenting sign of erythropoietic protoporphyria. **Treatment** consists of avoidance of the photosensitizing wavelength of light and/or the drug.

POLYMORPHOUS LIGHT ERUPTION. Polymorphous light eruption develops most commonly in females younger than 30 yr. The 1st eruption typically appears after prolonged sun exposure during the spring or summer. Onset of the eruption is delayed by hours to days after sun exposure and lasts for days to sometimes weeks. Areas of involvement tend to be symmetric and are characteristic for a given patient, including some but not all of the exposed or lightly covered skin on the face, neck, upper chest, and distal extremities. Lesions have various morphologies but most commonly are pruritic, 2–5 mm grouped erythematous papules or papulovesicles or edematous plaques that are >5 cm in diameter. Most cases involve sensitivity to UVA radiation, although some are UVB induced. **Therapeutic** approaches include sun avoidance, broad-spectrum sunscreens, topical or systemic corticosteroids, beta-carotene, nicotinamide, antimalarials, or prophylactic UVB or PUVA phototherapy.

COCKAYNE SYNDROME. Onset of this autosomal recessive disorder is characterized by the appearance, at ≈1 yr of age, of facial erythema in a butterfly distribution after sun exposure, followed by loss of adipose tissue and development of thin, atrophic, hyperpigmented skin, particularly over the face. Associated features include dwarfism; mental retardation; large, protuberant ears; long limbs; disproportionately large hands and feet, which are sometimes cool and cyanotic; pinched nose; carious teeth; unsteady gait with tremor; limitation of joint mobility; progressive deafness; cataracts; retinal degeneration; optic atrophy; decreased sweating and tearing; and premature graying of the hair. Diffuse extensive demyelination of the peripheral and central nervous systems ensues, and patients generally die of atheromatous vascular disease before the 3rd decade. There are 3 types of Cockayne syndrome. Type I (CSA gene) is less severe than type

II (CSB gene). Type III (XP-CS) demonstrates complementation with xeroderma pigmentosa groups B, D, or G. Photosensitivity is due to deficient rates of repair of UV-induced damage, specifically within actively transcribing regions of DNA. The syndrome is distinguished from progeria (see Chapter 90) by photosensitivity and the ocular abnormalities.

XERODERMA PIGMENTOSUM. This is a rare autosomal recessive disorder that results from a defect in nucleotide excision repair. Seven complementation groups have been recognized, based on each group's separate defect in the ability to repair damaged DNA. The wavelength of light that induces the DNA damage ranges from 280 to 340 nm. Skin changes are 1st noted during infancy or early childhood in sun-exposed areas such as the face, neck, hands, and arms; lesions may occur, however, at other sites, including the scalp. The skin lesions consist of erythema, scaling, bullae, crusting, ephelides, telangiectasia, keratoses (Fig. 655-6), basal and squamous cell carcinomas, and malignant melanomas. Ocular manifestations include photophobia, lacrimation, blepharitis, symblepharon, keratitis, corneal opacities, tumors of the lids, and possible eventual blindness. Neurologic abnormalities such as mental deterioration and sensorineural deafness may develop in ≈20% of patients

This disease is a serious mutilating disorder, and the life span is often brief. Affected families should have genetic counseling. The disorder is detectable in cells cultured from amniotic fluid. Affected children should be totally protected from sun exposure; protective clothing, eyeglasses, and opaque broad-spectrum sunscreens should be used even for mildly affected children. Light from unshielded fluorescent bulbs and sunlight passing through glass windows are also harmful. Early detection and removal of malignancies is mandatory.

ROTHMUND-THOMSON SYNDROME. This syndrome is also known as poikiloderma congenitale because of the striking skin changes (Fig. 655-7). It is inherited as an autosomal recessive trait. Mutations in the RECQL4 gene are found in approximately ⅔ of the patients. The other mutations causing Rothmund-Thomson syndome (RTS) are unknown. Skin changes are noted as early as 3 mo of age. Plaques of erythema and edema appear on the cheeks, forehead, ears, neck, dorsal portions of the hands, extensor surfaces of the arms, and buttocks and are replaced gradually by reticulated, atrophic, hyperpigmented, telangiectatic plaques. Light sensitivity is present in many cases, and exposure to the sun may provoke formation of bullae. Areas of involvement, however, are not strictly photodistributed. Short stature; small hands and feet; sparse eyebrows, eyelashes, and pubic and axillary hair, and sparse, fine, prematurely gray scalp hair or alopecia; bony defects; and hypogenitalism are common. Cataracts may also occur at an early age. Most patients have normal mental development. Keratoses and later squamous cell carcinomas may develop on exposed skin. The most worrisome association is that of osteosarcoma. It occus only in those RTS patients with RECQL4 mutations.

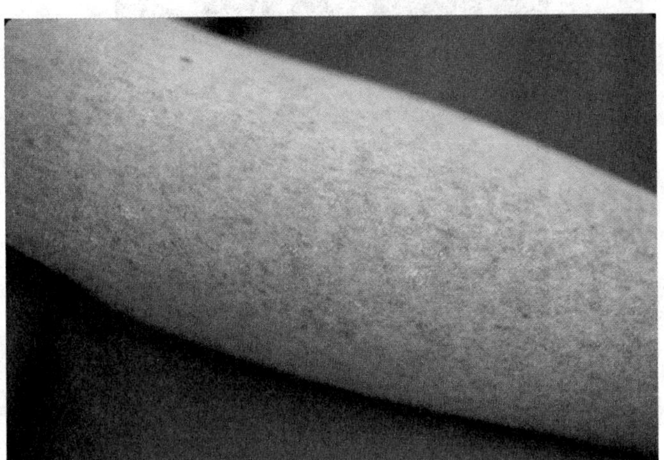

Figure 655-6. Dyspigmentation and actinic keratoses in child with xeroderma pigmentosum.

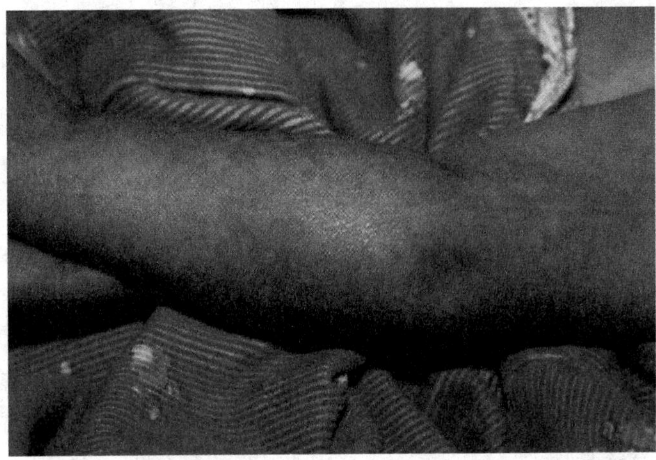

Figure 655-7. Poikiloderma on arm of infant with Rothmund-Thomson syndrome.

HARTNUP DISEASE (SEE CHAPTER 85.5). This is a rare inborn error of metabolism with autosomal recessive inheritance. Neutral amino acids, including tryptophan, are not transported across the brush border epithelium of the intestine and kidneys, resulting in deficiency of synthesis of nicotinamide and causing a photo-induced **pellagra-like syndrome.** The urine contains increased amounts of monoamine monocarboxylic amino acids. Cutaneous signs, which precede neurologic manifestations, initially develop during the early months of life when an eczematous, occasionally vesiculobullous eruption is noted on the face and extremities in a glove-and-stocking photodistribution. Hyperpigmentation and hyperkeratosis may supervene and are intensified by further exposure to sunlight. Episodic flares may be precipitated by febrile illness, sun exposure, emotional stress, and poor nutrition. In most cases, mental development is normal, but some patients display emotional instability and episodic cerebellar ataxia. Neurologic symptoms are fully reversible. Administration of nicotinamide and protection from sunlight results in improvement of both cutaneous and neurologic manifestations.

BLOOM SYNDROME. The defect in Bloom syndrome (BLM gene) is inherited in an autosomal recessive manner. The BLM gene is a RECQ helicase. Patients are sensitive to UV radiation, and their rate of chromosomal breaks and sister chromatid exchanges is markedly increased. Erythema and telangiectasia develop during infancy in a butterfly distribution on the face after exposure to sunlight. A bullous eruption on the lips and telangiectatic erythema on the hands and forearms may develop. Café-au-lait spots and hypopigmented macules may be present. Prenatal and postnatal short stature and a distinctive facies consisting of a prominent nose and ears and a small, narrow face are generally found. Intellect is average to low average. Immunodeficiency is seen in all patients, manifesting in recurrent ear and pulmonary infections. Gastrointestinal malabsorption is common. Affected children have an unusual tendency to develop both solid tumors and lymphoreticular malignancies.

Beattie PE, Dawe RS, Ibbotson SH, et al: Characteristics and prognosis of idiopathic solar urticaria: A cohort of 87 cases. *Arch Dermatol* 2003;139:1149–1154.

Demko CA, Boraeski EA, Debanne SM, et al: Use of indoor tanning facilities by white adolescents in the United States. *Arch Pediatr Adolesc Med* 2003;157:854–860.

Dummer R, Ivanova K, Scheidegger EP, et al: Clinical and therapeutic aspects of polymorphous light eruption. *Dermatology* 2003;207:93–95.

Han A, Maibach H: Management of acute sunburn. *Am J Clin Dermatol* 2004;5:39–47.

Hojyo-Tomoka MT, Vega-Memije ME, Cortes-Franco R, et al: Diagnosis and treatment of actinic prurigo. *Dermatol Ther* 2003;16:40–44.

Kaneko H, Kondo N: Clinical features of Bloom syndrome and function of the causative gene, BLM helicase. *Expert Rev Mol Diagn* 2004;4:393–401.

Kauppinen R: Porphyrias. *Lancet* 2005;365:241–252.

Lin JY, Selim MA, Shea CR, et al: UV photoprotection by combination topical antioxidants vitamin C and vitamin E. *J Am Acad Dermatol* 2003;48:866–874.

Magnoldo T, Sarasin A: Xeroderma pigmentosum: From symptoms and genetics to gene-based therapy. *Cells Tissue Organs* 2004;177:189–198.

Murphy GM: Diagnosis and management of the porphyrias. *Dermatol Ther* 2003;16:57–64.

Oskay T, Erder C, Anadolu R, et al: Juvenile colloid milium associated with conjunctival and gingival involvement. *J Am Acad Dermatol* 2003;49:1185–1188.

Spivak G: The many faces of Cockayne syndrome. *Proc Natl Acad Sci U S A* 2004;101:15273–15274.

Wang LL, Gannavarapu A, Kozinetz CA, et al: Association between osteosarcoma and deleterious mutations in the RECQL4 gene in Rothmund-Thomson syndrome. *J Natl Cancer Inst* 2003;95:669–674.

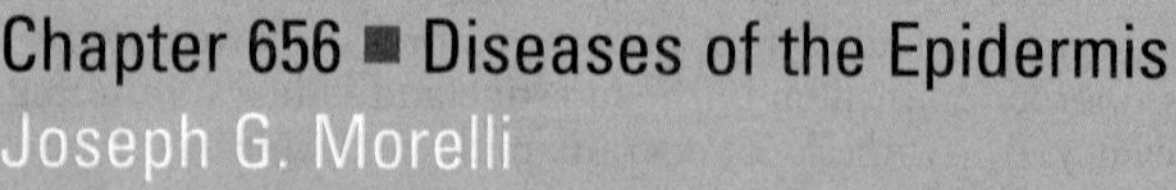

Chapter 656 ■ Diseases of the Epidermis

Joseph G. Morelli

PSORIASIS. This common, chronic skin disorder is 1st evident in ≈30% of affected individuals within the 1st 2 decades of life. The disease is more common among families with an affected member; a multifactorial inheritance is proposed. There is an association with the major histocompatibility antigens, most often CW6. The major psoriasis-susceptibility gene is a 70 Kb interval on chromosome 6 around the corneodesmin gene. It is designated PSORS1. Other psoriasis susceptibility genes have been identified on chromosomes 17q, 4q, 1q, and 3q; designated PSORS2, 3, 4, and 5, respectively. Psoriasis is characterized by proliferation of keratinocytes, abnormal differentiation of keratinocytes, and inflammatory cell infiltration of the epidermis and dermis. A defect in the immune system is likely the primary abnormality with the increased epidermal turnover secondary.

Clinical Manifestations. The lesions consist of erythematous papules that coalesce to form plaques with sharply demarcated, irregular borders. If they are unaltered by treatment, a thick silvery or yellow-white scale (resembling mica) develops (Fig. 656-1*A*). Removal of the scale may result in pinpoint bleeding (**Auspitz sign**). The **Koebner,** or isomorphic response, in which new lesions appear at sites of trauma, is a valuable diagnostic feature. Lesions may occur anywhere, but preferred sites are the scalp, knees, elbows, umbilicus, superior intergluteal fold, and genitals. Scalp lesions may be confused with seborrheic dermatitis, atopic dermatitis, or tinea capitis. Small raindrop-like lesions on the face are common. Nail involvement, a valuable diagnostic sign, is characterized by pitting of the nail plate, detachment of the plate (onycholysis), yellowish-brown subungual discoloration, and accumulation of subungual debris (Fig. 656-1*B*).

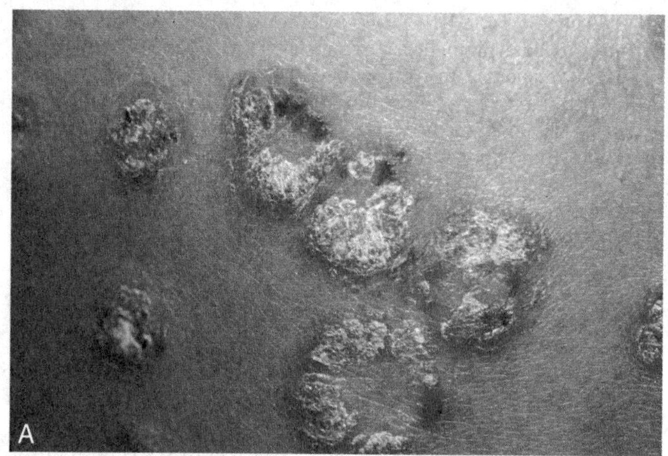

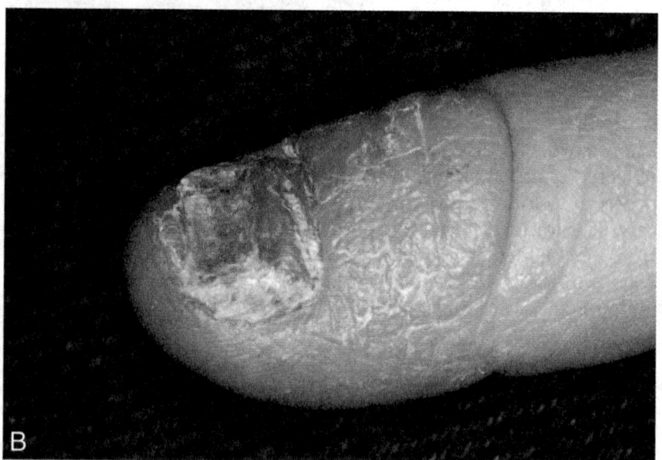

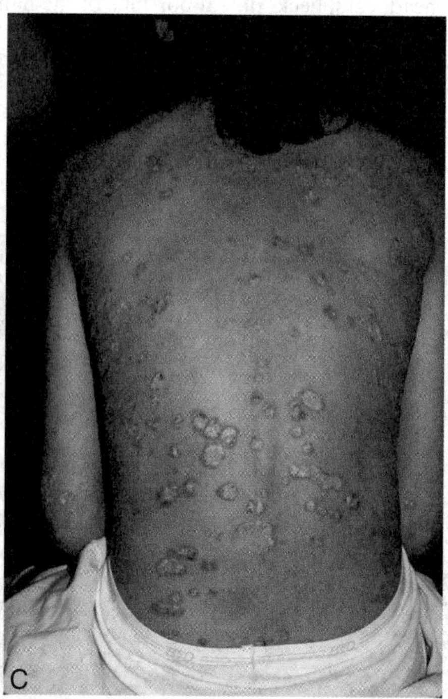

Figure 656-1. *A,* Chronic psoriatic plaques. *B,* Psoriatic nail dystrophy. *C,* Guttate psoriasis in widespread distribution over the trunk.

Psoriasis is rare in neonates but may be severe and recalcitrant and pose a diagnostic problem. The initial lesions may involve the diaper area and mimic seborrheic dermatitis, eczematous diaper dermatitis, perianal streptococcal disease, or candidosis. Biopsy or prolonged observation may be required for definitive diagnosis. Other rare forms include psoriatic erythroderma, localized or generalized pustular psoriasis, and linear psoriasis.

Guttate psoriasis, a variant that occurs predominantly in children, is characterized by an explosive eruption of profuse, small, oval or round lesions that morphologically are identical to the larger plaques of psoriasis (Fig. 656-1C). Sites of predilection are the trunk, face, and proximal portions of the limbs. The onset frequently follows a **streptococcal** infection; a culture of the throat and serologic titers should be obtained. Guttate psoriasis has also been observed after perianal streptococcal infection, viral infections, sunburn, and withdrawal of systemic corticosteroid therapy. Psoriatic skin lesions may be induced, in a genetically susceptible host, by $CD4^+$ T cells that were initially activated by streptococcal pyrogenic exotoxins acting as superantigens. The source of the streptococcal antigens can be the throat or the skin. Some of the superantigen-activated T cells recognize streptococcal M protein in the skin and appear to have cross reactivity with an abnormal keratin that has homology with streptococcal M protein. The autoreactive T cells may be responsible for the formation and maintenance of psoriatic skin lesions. The lesions may be confused with viral exanthems and pityriasis lichenoides chronica (PLC).

Diagnosis. This is based on the clinical manifestations. The differential diagnosis includes Reiter syndrome, which, in contrast to psoriasis, involves mucous membranes, PLC, and pityriasis rubra pilaris. When in doubt, histopathologic examination of an untreated lesion reveals characteristic changes of psoriasis.

Treatment. The therapeutic approach varies with the age of the child, type of psoriasis, sites of involvement, and extent of the disease. Physical and chemical trauma to the skin should be avoided as much as possible (see the Koebner response).

The treatment of psoriasis should be viewed as a 3-tier process. The **1st tier** is **topical therapy.** Topical corticosteroid preparations are effective. Mid-potency or stronger topical steroids are necessary (see Chapter 645). The preparation that is least potent but effective should be applied twice a day. The topical vitamin D analog calcipotriene is also effective. It appears to have much less impact on calcium metabolism (100-fold less) than calcitriol. Calcipotriene can burn and sting, which limits its usefulness in children. One commonly used strategy is to use calcipotriene twice a day on weekdays and a topical steroid twice a day on weekends. Tazarotene, a topical retinoid, is also useful. It may be used alone or in combination with other topical modalities. Tar preparation and anthralin may also be used. For scalp lesions, applications of a phenol and saline solution (Baker P & S) followed by a tar shampoo are effective in the removal of scales. A corticosteroid in a foam, solution, lotion, or gel base may be applied when the scaling is diminished.

The **2nd tier** of therapy is **phototherapy.** Narrowband ultraviolet B (UVB 311 nm) radiation is the primary form of UVB therapy used in childhood. It is as or nearly as effective as psoralen with UVA (PUVA), without the side effects associated with psoralen. If available, phototherapy should be used for children with extensive disease who have failed topical therapy. The treatment is time consuming and only available at limited locations.

Systemic therapy is the **3rd tier.** A few children with severe psoriasis will require systemic therapy. Methotrexate, oral retinoids, and cyclosporine are used for the rare severe and generalized forms of psoriasis. Oral retinoids may be combined with phototherapy. Nail lesions are difficult to treat, but may respond to topical tazarotene. Potentially beneficial therapies include 308 nm excimer laser UVB radiation (for localized treatment-resistant plaques), inhibition of tumor necrosis factor with etanercept, and inhibition of $CD45RO^+$ memory T cells. Efalizumab, a monoclonal antibody targeting T-cell interactions, improves the outcome of moderate to severe psoriasis in adults and is approved for these patients.

Prognosis. This is best for children with limited disease. Psoriasis is a lifelong disease and is characterized by remissions and exacerbations. Arthritis may be an extracutaneous complication.

PITYRIASIS LICHENOIDES. This has historically encompassed pityriasis lichenoides acuta (PLA, pityriasis lichenoides et varioliformis acuta [PLEVA], Mucha-Habermann disease), which tends to develop acutely, and pityriasis lichenoides chronica (PLC), which follows a chronic course. The designation of pityriasis lichenoides as acute or chronic may more properly refer to morphologic appearance of the lesions, which is often hemorrhagic or necrotic in PLA, than to the duration of the disease. No correlation is found between the type of lesion at the onset of the eruption and the duration of the disease. Many patients have both acute and chronic lesions simultaneously, and transition of lesions from one form into another occurs occasionally. Pityriasis lichenoides most commonly presents in the 2nd and 3rd decades; ≈30% of cases present before age 20 yr.

Clinical Manifestations. PLC presents with generalized, multiple, asymptomatic 3–5 mm brown-red papules that are covered by a fine grayish scale (Fig. 656-2). Lesions may be asymptomatic or may cause minimal pruritus and occasionally become infiltrated, vesicular, hemorrhagic, and crusted. Individual papules become flat and brownish in 2–6 wk, ultimately leaving a hyperpigmented or hypopigmented macule. Scarring is unusual. Lesions are most common on the trunk and extremities and generally spare the face, palmoplantar surfaces, scalp, and mucous membranes. The eruption persists for months to years and is characterized by polymorphous lesions in various stages of evolution. PLC histologically shows a parakeratotic, thickened corneal layer; epidermal spongiosis; a superficial perivascular infiltrate of macrophages and predominantly $CD8^+$ lymphocytes, which may extend into the epidermis; and small numbers of extravasated erythrocytes in the papillary dermis.

PLA presents with an abrupt eruption of numerous papules that have a vesiculopustular and then a purpuric center, are covered by a dark adherent crust, and are surrounded by an erythematous halo (Fig. 656-3). Constitutional symptoms of fever, malaise, headache, and arthralgias may be present for 2–3 days after the initial outbreak. Lesions are distributed diffusely on the trunk and extremities, as in PLC. Individual lesions heal within a few weeks, sometimes leaving a varioliform scar, and successive crops of papules produce the characteristic polymorphous

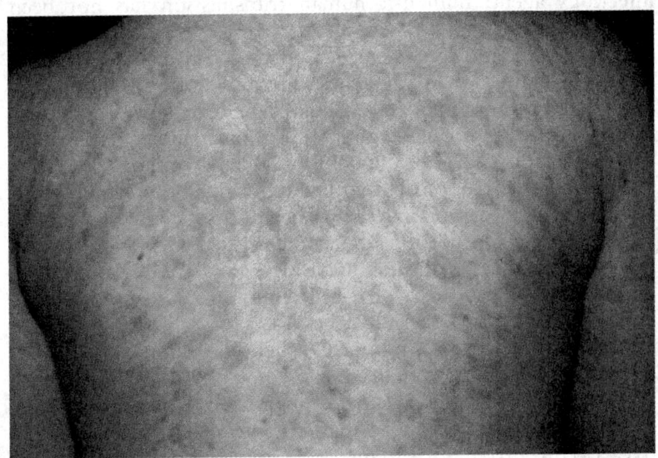

Figure 656-2. Widespread plaques with fine scale in pityriasis lichenoides chronica.

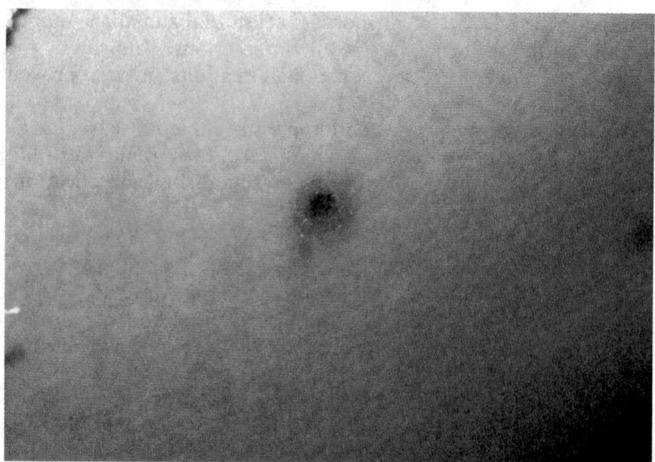

Figure 656-3. Necrotic lesion with erythematous halo in pityriasis lichenoides acuta.

appearance of the eruption. The condition is generally self-limited from several weeks to months. The histopathologic changes of PLA reflect its more severe nature compared with PLC. Intercellular and intracellular edema in the epidermis may lead to degeneration of keratinocytes. A dense perivascular mononuclear cell infiltrate that extends upward into the epidermis and downward into the reticular dermis, endothelial cell swelling, and extravasation of erythrocytes into the epidermis and dermis are additional characteristic features. Severe changes of vasculitis are exceptional. **Differential diagnosis** includes guttate psoriasis, pityriasis rosea, drug eruptions, secondary syphilis, viral exanthems, and lichen planus. The chronicity of pityriasis lichenoides helps to preclude pityriasis rosea, viral exanthems, and some drug eruptions. A skin biopsy helps to preclude other differential diagnoses.

A rare form of PLA has been described as presenting with fever and ulceronecrotic plaques up to 1 cm in diameter, which are most common on the anterior trunk and flexors of the proximal upper extremities. Arthritis and superinfection of cutaneous lesions with *Staphylococcus aureus* may also develop. The ulceronecrotic lesions appear within papules of PLA and heal with hypopigmented scarring in a few weeks. Leukocytoclastic vasculitis is occasionally seen histopathologically. The eruption may resemble erythema multiforme, but it generally spares the mucous membranes.

Etiology. The cause of pityriasis lichenoides is unknown, but sporadic outbreaks have led to an unsuccessful search for an infectious agent; human-to-human transmission has not been documented. Pityriasis lichenoides may be a hypersensitivity reaction to an infectious organism. Cell-mediated mechanisms appear to be important in the pathogenesis because most infiltrating cells are cytotoxic/suppressor cells. Clonal gene rearrangement studies of the T-cell receptor and immunohistologic studies have led to the suggestion that PLA may be a T-cell lymphoproliferative process. The condition in two children with PLA evolved into cutaneous T-cell lymphoma. It has been postulated that the relatively greater proportion of cytotoxic/suppressor cells than helper/inducer T cells in lesions of PLA compared with those of lymphomatoid papulosis or T-cell lymphoma reflects the more effective host response in PLA.

Treatment. In general, pityriasis lichenoides should be considered a benign condition that does not alter the health of the child. A lubricant to remove excessive scaling may be all that is necessary if the patient is asymptomatic. Topical steroids are ineffective. Erythromycin (30–50 mg/kg/24 hr for 2 mo) may benefit some children. Natural sunlight is also helpful. Narrowband UVB is the **treatment of choice** for **widespread,** pruritic disease. The rare febrile ulceronecrotic form may require systemic corticosteroids.

KERATOSIS PILARIS. This moderately common papular eruption may vary in extent from sparse lesions over the extensor aspects of the limbs to involvement of most of the body surface; typical areas of involvement include the upper extensor arms and the thighs, cheeks, and buttocks. The lesions may resemble gooseflesh; they are noninflammatory, scaly, follicular papules that do not coalesce. Irritation of the follicular plugs occasionally causes erythema surrounding the keratotic papules (Fig. 656-4). A subset of patients will have keratosis pilaris associated with facial telangiectasia and ulerythema ophryogenes. Because the lesions are associated with and accentuated by dry skin, they are often more prominent during the winter. They are more frequent in patients with atopic dermatitis and are most common during childhood and early adulthood, tending to subside in the 3rd decade of life. Mild or localized eruptions are **treated** with lubrication with a bland emollient; more pronounced or widespread lesions require regular applications of a 10–40% urea cream or an α-hydroxy acid preparation such as lactic acid cream or lotion. Therapy may improve the condition but does not cure it.

LICHEN SPINULOSUS. This uncommon disorder occurs principally in children and more frequently in boys. The cause is unknown. The lesions consist of sharply circumscribed irregular plaques of spiny, keratinous projections that protrude from the orifices of the pilosebaceous canals. Plaques may occur anywhere on the body and are often distributed symmetrically on the trunk, elbows, knees, and extensor surfaces of the limbs. Although sometimes erythematous, the lesions are usually skin colored. They are readily palpable and represent keratotic follicular plugs. Lichen spinulosus is easily differentiated from keratosis pilaris because the latter lesions are never grouped to form plaques. More commonly, it is confused with papular eczema.

Treatment is usually unnecessary. For patients who regard the eruption as a cosmetic, defect urea-containing lubricants (10–40%) are often effective in flattening the projections. The plaques usually disappear spontaneously after several months or years.

PITYRIASIS ROSEA. This benign, common eruption occurs most frequently in children and young adults. Although a prodrome of fever, malaise, arthralgia, and pharyngitis may precede the eruption, children rarely complain of such symptoms. The cause of pityriasis rosea is unknown; a viral agent is suspected and there is debate over the role of human herpesvirus 7.

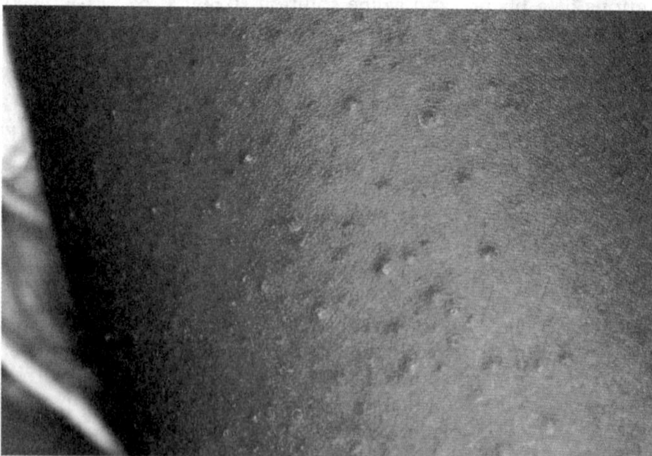

Figure 656-4. Keratotic follicular plugs with surrounding erythema in keratosis pilaris.

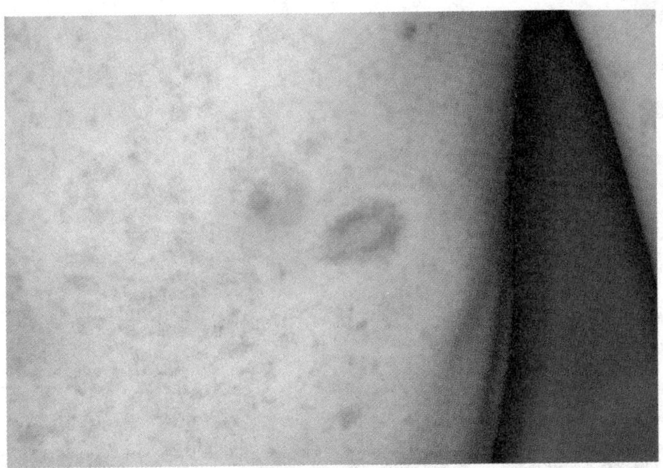

Figure 656-5. Herald patch and surrounding pityriasis rosea.

Clinical Manifestations. A **herald patch,** a solitary, round or oval lesion that may occur anywhere on the body and is often but not always identifiable by its large size, usually precedes the generalized eruption. Herald patches vary from 1 to 10 cm in diameter; they are annular in configuration and have a raised border with fine, adherent scales. Approximately 5–10 days after the appearance of the herald patch, a widespread, symmetric eruption becomes evident involving mainly the trunk and proximal limbs (Fig. 656-5). When the disease is extensive, the face, scalp, and distal limbs may be involved, or, in the inverse form of pityriasis rosea, only those sites may be affected. Lesions may appear in crops for several days. Typical lesions are oval or round, <1 cm in diameter, slightly raised, and pink to brown. The developed lesion is covered by a fine scale, which gives the skin a crinkly appearance. Some lesions clear centrally and produce a collarette of scale that is attached only at the periphery. Papular, vesicular, urticarial, hemorrhagic, and large annular lesions are unusual variants. The long axis of each lesion is usually aligned with the cutaneous cleavage lines, a feature that creates the so-called **Christmas tree pattern** on the back. Conformation to skin lines is often more discernible in the anterior and posterior axillary folds and supraclavicular areas. Duration of the eruption varies from 2 to 12 wk. The lesions may be asymptomatic or mildly to severely pruritic.

Diagnosis. This is clinical. The herald patch may be mistaken for tinea corporis, a pitfall that can be avoided if testing with a potassium hydroxide preparation is performed. The generalized eruption resembles a number of other diseases; secondary syphilis is the most important. Drug eruptions, viral exanthems, guttate psoriasis, PLC, and eczema can also be confused with pityriasis rosea.

Treatment. Therapy is unnecessary for asymptomatic patients. If scaling is prominent, a bland emollient may suffice. Pruritus may be suppressed by a lubricating lotion containing menthol and camphor or by an oral antihistamine for sedation, particularly at night, when itching may be troublesome. Occasionally, a nonfluorinated topical corticosteroid preparation may be necessary to alleviate pruritus. After the eruption has resolved, postinflammatory hypopigmentation or hyperpigmentation may be pronounced, particularly in black patients. These changes disappear in subsequent weeks to months.

PITYRIASIS RUBRA PILARIS. This rare chronic dermatosis often has an insidious onset with diffuse scaling and erythema of the scalp, which is indistinguishable from seborrheic dermatitis, and with thick hyperkeratosis of the palms and soles (Fig. 656-6*A*). Lesions over the elbows and knees are also common (Fig. 656-6*B*). The characteristic primary lesion is a firm, dome-shaped, tiny, acuminate papule, which is pink to red and has a central keratotic plug pierced by a vellus hair. Masses of these papules coalesce to form large, erythematous, sharply demarcated orangish plaques, within which islands of normal skin can be distinguished, creating a bizarre effect. Typical papules on the dorsum of the proximal phalanges are readily palpated. Gray plaques or papules resembling lichen planus may be found in the oral cavity. Dystrophic changes in the nails may occur and mimic those of psoriasis. **Differential diagnosis** includes ichthyosis, seborrheic dermatitis, keratoderma of the palms and soles, and psoriasis.

Etiology. The cause is unknown. A genetic form with autosomal dominant transmission may account for some cases in childhood; most are sporadic. Skin biopsy may differentiate this condition from psoriasis and seborrheic dermatitis.

Treatment. The numerous therapeutic regimens recommended are difficult to evaluate because the disease has a capricious course with exacerbations and remissions. Lubrication alone is useful in mild cases. Oral and topical retinoids have been used most frequently. In childhood, the prognosis for eventual resolution is relatively good.

DARIER DISEASE (KERATOSIS FOLLICULARIS). This rare genetic disorder is inherited as an autosomal dominant trait (ATP2A2 gene). Onset usually occurs in late childhood. Typical lesions are small,

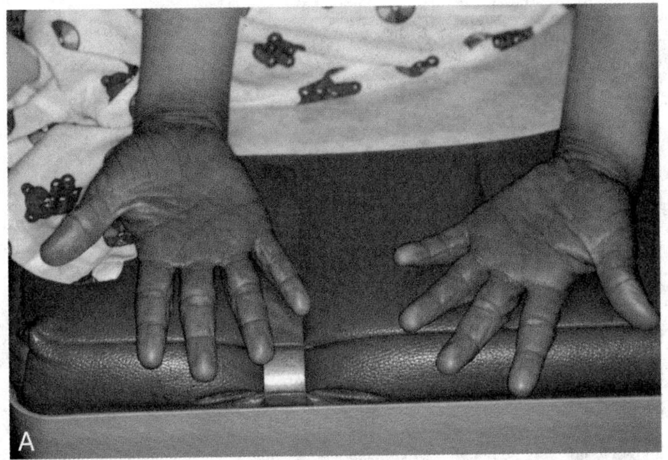

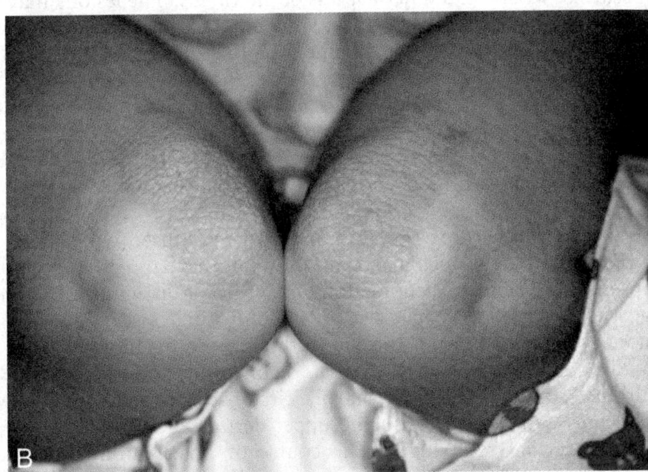

Figure 656-6. *A*, Orange-colored palmar hyperkeratosis in pityriasis rubra pilaris (PRP). *B*, Elbow lesions in PRP.

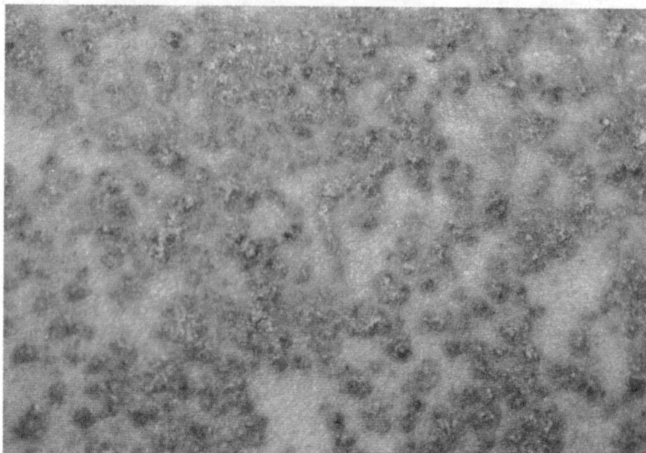

Figure 656-7. Papules coalescing into large plaque on the back of patient with Darier disease.

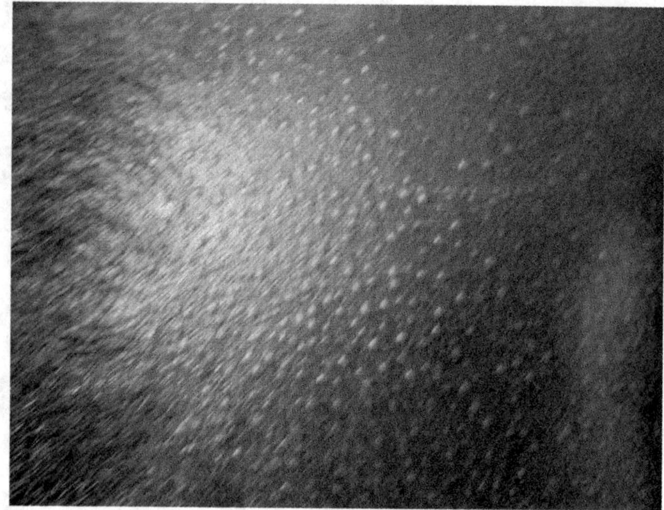

Figure 656-8. Slightly hypopigmented, uniform papules of lichen nitidus.

firm, skin-colored papules that are not always follicular in location. The lesions eventually acquire yellow malodorous crusts; coalesce to form large, gray-brown, vegetative plaques (Fig. 656-7); and usually involve the face, neck, shoulders, chest, back, and limb flexures in a symmetric distribution. Papules, fissures, crusts, and ulcers may appear on the mucous membranes of the lips, tongue, buccal mucosa, pharynx, larynx, and vulva. Hyperkeratosis of the palms and soles and nail dystrophy with subungual hyperkeratosis are variable features. Severe pruritus, secondary infection, offensive odor, and aggravation of the dermatosis on exposure to sunlight may occur. Darier disease is most likely to be confused with seborrheic dermatitis or juvenile flat warts. Histologic changes are diagnostic: Hyperkeratosis, intraepidermal separation with formation of suprabasal clefts, and dyskeratotic epidermal cells are characteristic features.

Treatment is nonspecific. Some patients have responded to retinoic acid, with or without occlusive dressings. Severe disease may be controlled with oral synthetic retinoids. Secondary infection may require local cleansing and systemically administered antibiotics. Affected individuals usually suffer more during the summer.

LICHEN NITIDUS. This chronic, benign, papular eruption is characterized by minute (1–2 mm), flat-topped, shiny, firm papules of uniform size. They are most often skin colored but may be pink or red. In black individuals, they are usually hypopigmented (Fig. 656-8). Sites of predilection are the genitals, abdomen, chest, forearms, wrists, and inner aspects of the thighs. The lesions may be sparse or numerous and form large plaques; careful examination usually discloses linear papules in a line of scratch (Koebner phenomenon), a valuable clue to the diagnosis because it occurs in only a few diseases. Lichen nitidus occurs in all age groups. The cause is unknown. Patients are usually asymptomatic and constitutionally well, although pruritus may be severe. The lesions may be confused with those of lichen planus and rarely coexist with them.

Widespread keratosis pilaris can also be confused with lichen nitidus, but the follicular localization of the papules and the absence of Koebner phenomenon in the former distinguish them. Verruca plana (flat warts), if small and uniform in size, may occasionally resemble lichen nitidus. Although the diagnosis can be made clinically, a biopsy is occasionally indicated. The lichen nitidus papule consists of sharply circumscribed nests of lymphocytes and histiocytes in the upper dermis enclosed by claw-like epidermal rete ridges. The course of lichen nitidus spans months to years, but the lesions eventually involute completely. Topical steroids may be effective **treatment,** especially for pruritus.

LICHEN STRIATUS. This benign, self-limited eruption consists of a continuous or discontinuous linear band of papules in a zosteriform distribution. The primary lesion is a flat-topped, red to violaceous papule covered with fine scale. Aggregates of these papules form multiple bands or plaques. In black patients, the lesions may be hypopigmented. The cause and explanation for the linear distribution are unknown. The eruption evolves over a period of days or weeks in an otherwise healthy child, remains stationary for weeks to months, and finally remits without sequelae. Symptoms are usually absent, although some children complain of itching. Nail dystrophy may occur when the eruption involves the posterior nail fold and matrix (Fig. 656-9).

Lichen striatus is occasionally confused with other disorders. The initial plaque may resemble papular eczema or lichen nitidus until the linear configuration becomes apparent. Linear lichen planus and linear psoriasis are usually associated with typical individual lesions elsewhere on the body. Linear epidermal nevi are permanent lesions that often become more hyperkeratotic and hyperpigmented than those of lichen striatus. A lubricating lotion containing menthol and camphor or a mild corticosteroid preparation provides sufficient relief when pruritus is a problem.

LICHEN PLANUS. This is a rare disorder in young children and uncommon in older ones. The primary lesion is a violaceous,

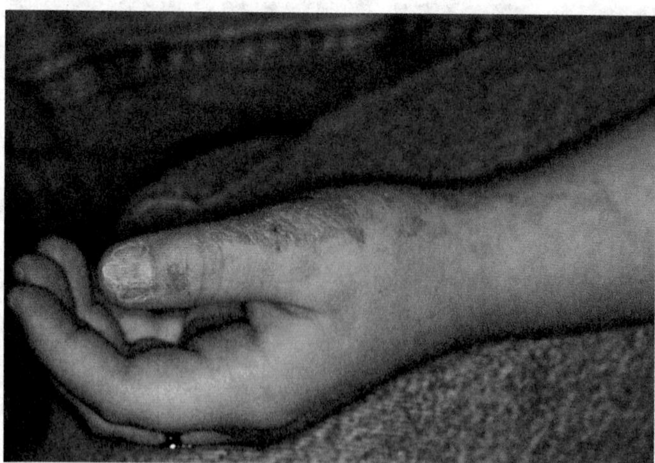

Figure 656-9. Lichen striatus with nail dystrophy.

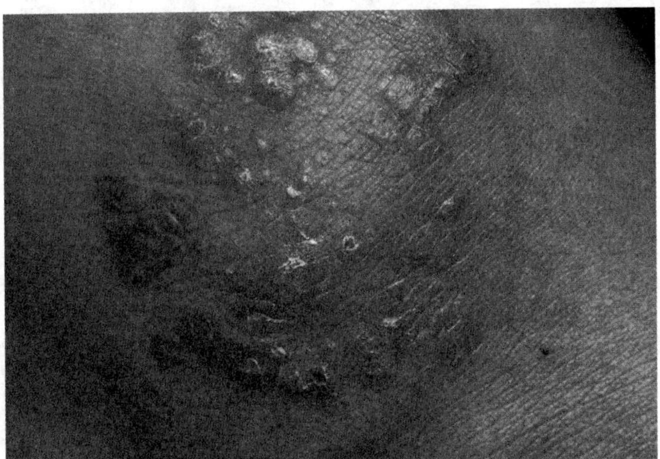

Figure 656-10. Flat-topped, purple polygonal papules of lichen planus.

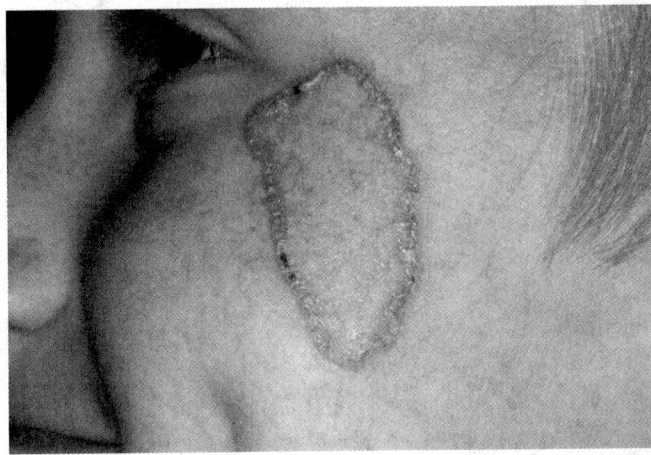

Figure 656-11. Large plaque of porokeratosis of Mibelli with raised border and depressed center.

sharply demarcated, polygonal papule with fine lines or thin white scales on the surface. Papules may coalesce to form large plaques (Fig. 656-10). The papules are intensely pruritic, and additional ones are often induced by scratching (Koebner phenomenon) so that lines of them are often detected. Sites of predilection are the flexor surfaces of the wrists, forearms, and inner aspects of the thighs. Characteristic lesions of mucous membranes consist of pinhead-sized white papules that coalesce to form reticulated and lacy patterns on the oral mucosa and sometimes on the lips and tongue.

Acute eruptive lichen planus is probably the most common form in children. The lesions erupt in an explosive fashion, much like a viral exanthem, and spread to involve most of the body surface. Hypertrophic, linear, bullous, atrophic, annular, follicular, erosive, and ulcerative forms of lichen planus may also occur. Nail involvement may develop in the chronic forms but is rarely evident in children. The disorder may persist for months to years, but the acute eruptive form is most likely to involute permanently. Intense hyperpigmentation frequently persists for a long time after the resolution of lesions. The histopathologic findings of lichen planus are specific, and a biopsy is indicated if the diagnosis is unclear.

Treatment is directed at alleviation of the intense pruritus and amelioration of the skin lesions. Oral antihistamines are often helpful. The skin lesions respond best to regular applications of a topical corticosteroid preparation. Rarely, systemic corticosteroid therapy is necessary to gain control of widespread, intractable lesions. Phototherapy has also been used for extensive disease.

POROKERATOSIS. This is a rare, chronic, progressive disease. Several forms have been delineated: solitary plaques, linear porokeratosis, hyperkeratotic lesions of the palms and soles, disseminated eruptive lesions, and superficial actinic porokeratosis. The last form, probably induced by excessive sun exposure, occurs more commonly in women. Other types of porokeratosis are more common in males and begin in childhood. Sites of predilection are the limbs, face, neck, and genitals. The primary lesion is a small, keratotic papule that enlarges peripherally so that the center becomes depressed, with the edge forming an elevated wall or collar (Fig. 656-11). The configuration of the plaque may be round, oval, or gyrate. The elevated border is split by a thin groove from which minute cornified projections protrude. The enclosed central area is yellow, gray, or tan and sclerotic, smooth, and dry, whereas the hyperkeratotic border is a darker gray, brown, or black.

The **differential diagnosis** includes warts, epidermal nevi, lichen planus, granuloma annulare, and elastosis perforans serpiginosa. A skin biopsy discloses the characteristic cornoid lamella (plug of stratum corneum cells with retained nuclei), which is responsible for the invariable linear ridge of the lesion. The disease is slowly progressive but relatively asymptomatic. Malignant degeneration to **squamous cell carcinoma** has been reported in long-standing cases. No treatment is uniformly successful. **Treatments** with liquid nitrogen, topical retinoids, fluorouracil (5-FU), and imiquimod have been employed.

PAPULAR ACRODERMATITIS OF CHILDHOOD (GIANOTTI-CROSTI SYNDROME). This distinctive eruption is occasionally associated with malaise and low-grade fever but few other constitutional symptoms. The incidence peaks in early childhood. Occurrences are usually sporadic, but epidemics have been recorded. The skin lesion is a monomorphous, usually nonpruritic, flat-topped, firm, dusky or coppery red papule ranging in size from 1 to 10 mm (Fig. 656-12). The papules appear in crops and may become profuse but remain discrete, forming a symmetric eruption on the face, buttocks, and limbs, including the palms and soles. The papules often have the appearance of vesicles; when opened, however, no fluid is obtained. The papules sometimes become hemorrhagic. Lines of papules (**Koebner phenomenon**) may be noted on the extremities. The trunk is relatively spared, as are the scalp and mucous membranes. Generalized lymphadenopathy and hepatomegaly (in those with hepatitis B viremia) consti-

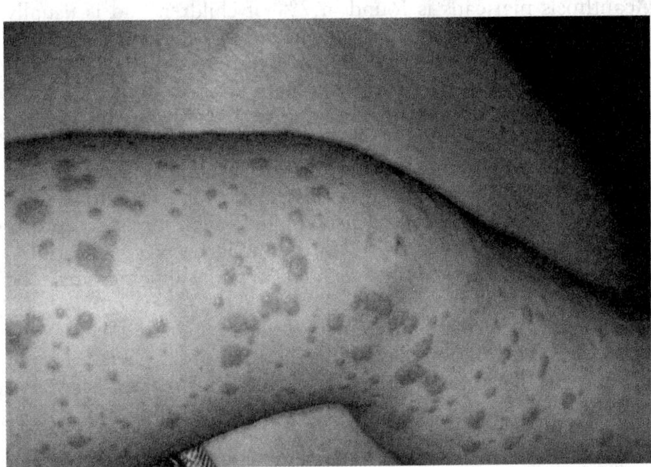

Figure 656-12. Numerous, flat-topped, red papules in Gianotti-Crosti syndrome.

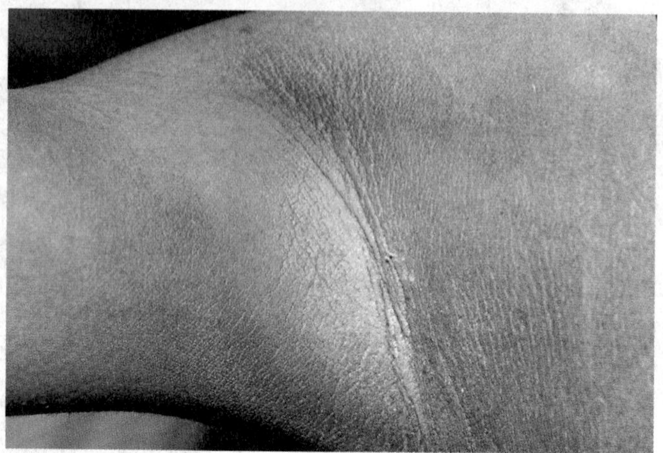

Figure 656-13. Velvety hyperpigmentation of the axilla in acanthosis nigricans.

tute the only other abnormal physical findings. The eruption resolves spontaneously in about 15–60 days. Lymphadenopathy and hepatomegaly, if present, may persist for several months. This eruption in Italy was initially associated with primary liver infection by hepatitis B virus. Elevation of serum transaminase and alkaline phosphatase values without concomitant hyperbilirubinemia was usual. Skin biopsy is not specific and is characterized by a perivascular mononuclear cell infiltrate and capillary endothelial swelling.

The disease is usually benign and is not associated with hepatitis in the United States. This eruption has been seen in children infected with Epstein-Barr virus, coxsackievirus A16, parainfluenza virus, and other viral infections and after immunizations. Papular acrodermatitis can be confused with lichen planus, erythema multiforme, histiocytosis X, and Henoch-Schönlein purpura.

ACANTHOSIS NIGRICANS. This is characterized by hyperpigmented velvety, hyperkeratotic, plaques that are most often localized to the neck, axillae (Fig. 656-13), inframammary areas, groin, inner thighs, and anogenital region. The histologic changes are those of papillomatosis and hyperkeratosis rather than acanthosis or excessive pigment formation. Acanthosis nigricans has classically been associated with obesity; drugs such as nicotinic acid; endocrinopathies, most commonly, diabetes mellitus and hyperandrogenic or hypogonadal syndromes; and genetic disorders caused by mutation in fibroblast growth factors. It may occasionally be familial, with autosomal dominant inheritance. Acanthosis nigricans is found in 7% of children and is usually associated with obesity. Although acanthosis nigricans is associated with malignancy in adults, this is rare in childhood.

The skin lesions appear to be a manifestation of insulin resistance or mutations in fibroblast growth factors. The clinical severity and histopathologic features of acanthosis nigricans correlate positively with the degree of hyperinsulinism. Insulin resistance with compensatory hyperinsulinism may lead to insulin binding to and activation of insulin-like growth factor receptors, promoting epidermal growth. In the malignant form in adults, tumor-secreted growth factors and hyperinsulinemia may be pathogenic.

This skin disorder is extremely difficult to treat but may be improved by palliation of the underlying disorder. Weight loss in the case of obesity is helpful. Forty per cent urea cream is also helpful.

Amer A, Fischer H: Azithromycin does not cure pityriasis rosea. *Pediatrics* 2006;117:1702–1705.
Capon F, Trembath RC, Barker JN: An update on the genetics of psoriasis. *Dermatol Clin* 2004;22:339–347.
Chuh AA, Chan HH, Zawar V: Is human herpes virus 7 the causative agent of pityriasis rosea?—a critical review. *Int J Dermatol* 2004;43:870–875.
Eberting CL, Javor E, Gorden P, et al: Insulin resistance, acanthosis nigricans and hypertriglycidemia. *J Am Acad Dermatol* 2005;52:341–344.
Gerbig AW: Treating keratosis pilaris. *J Am Acad Dermatol* 2002;47:457–458.
Gibson LE: Acanthosis nigricans. *Mayo Clin Proc* 2004;79:1571.
Gordon KB, Papp KA, Hamilton TK, et al: Efalizumab for patients with moderate to severe plaque psoriasis. *JAMA* 2003;290:3073–3080.
Ito N, Ohshima A, Hashizume H, et al: Febrile ulceronecrotic Mucha-Habermann's disease managed with methylprednisolone semipule and subsequent methotrexate therapy. *J Am Acad Dermatol* 2003;49:1142–1148.
Lane JE, Guill MA: Juvenile pityriasis rubra pilaris. *Pediatr Dermatol* 2004;21:512–513.
Lewkowicz D, Gottlieb AB: Pediatrics psoriasis and arthritis. *Dermatol Ther* 2004;17:364–375.
Orru S, Giuressi E, Carcassi C, et al: Mapping of the major psoriasis-susceptibility locus (PSORS1) in a 70-Kb interval around the corneodesmin gene (CDSN). *Am J Hum Genet* 2005;76:164–171.
Schön MP, Boehncke WH: Psoriasis. *N Engl J Med* 2005;352:1899–1912.
Stulberg DL, Wolfrey J: Pityriasis rosea. *Am Fam Physician* 2004;69:87–91.
Tilly JJ, Drolet BA, Esterly NB: Lichenoid eruptions in children. *J Am Acad Dermatol* 2004;51:606–624.
Tyring S, Gottlieb A, Papp K, et al: Etanercept and clinical outcomes, fatigue, and depression in psoriasis: double-blind placebo-controlled randomised phase III trial. *Lancet* 2006;367:29–35.

Chapter 657 ■ Disorders of Keratinization

Joseph G. Morelli

DISORDERS OF CORNIFICATION. Disorders of cornification (**ichthyoses**) are a primary group of inherited conditions characterized clinically by patterns of scaling and histopathologically by hyperkeratosis. They are usually distinguishable on the basis of inheritance patterns, clinical features, associated defects, and histopathologic changes (Table 657-1). Because some of these conditions cause disfigurement and considerable psychosocial stress, early diagnosis is helpful to predict probable course and prognosis and to provide supportive management for patients and families.

HARLEQUIN FETUS. This rare keratinizing disorder probably represents several genotypes with similar clinical manifestations. At birth, markedly thickened, ridged, and cracked skin forms horny plates over the entire body, disfiguring the facial features and constricting the digits. Severe ectropion and chemosis obscure the orbits, the nose and ears are flattened, and the lips are everted and gaping. Nails and hair may be absent. Joint mobility is restricted, and the hands and feet appear fixed and ischemic. Affected neonates have respiratory difficulty, suck poorly, and are subject to severe cutaneous infection. Most die within the 1st days to weeks of life, but patients occasionally survive beyond infancy and have severe ichthyosis and variable neurologic impairment. Ectropion and eclabium resolve, and the cracked, horny plated skin is replaced by large, thin scales with surrounding erythema.

Inheritance is likely autosomal recessive, but new autosomal dominant mutations are possible. Common morphologic abnormalities include hyperkeratosis, accumulation of lipid droplets within corneocytes, and absence of normal lamellar granules. The basic defect of all types is suggested to be an abnormality of lamellar granules, which have an important role in barrier formation and desquamation.

TABLE 657-1. Disorders of Cornification That Usually Present in the 1st Weeks

DISORDER	INHERITANCE	CLINICAL FEATURES	MUTATION	VISUAL METHOD OF DIAGNOSIS
Harlequin ichthyosis	AR	Thick, armor-like scale with fissuring	Unknown	Clinical
Collodion baby	Usually AR	Shiny collodion membrane	Various	Clinical
Recessive X-linked ichthyosis	Recessive X-linked	Collodion membrane May have genital anomalies	Steroid sulfatase	Plasma cholesterol sulfate
Lamellar ichthyosis	Usually AR	Collodion membrane	Transglutaminase I Other	Clinical
Congenital ichthyosiform erythroderma	AR	Collodion membrane	Unknown	Clinical
Epidermolytic hyperkeratosis	AD	Scaling and blistering	Keratins 1, 10, 2e	Clinical and histologic
Ichthyosis hystrix	AD	Plaques of hyperkeratosis	Unknown	Clinical
Familial peeling skin	AR	Superficial peeling	Unknown	Clinical and histologic
Sjögren-Larsson	AR	Variable skin thickening Mental, developmental retardation Spastic diplegia Seizures "Glistening dots"	Fatty aldehyde dehydrogenase (FAD)	Clinical and fibroblast cultures for FAD
Neutral lipid storage disease	AR	Collodion membrane or ichthyosiform erythroderma	Recycling of triacylglycerol to diacylglycerol	Blood smear for vacuolated PMNs
Netherton	AR	Ichthyosiform erythroderma Scant hair, often failure to thrive	SPINK5 Unknown	Clinical; hair exam later in infancy Clinical and hair microscopy; hair sulfur content
Trichothiodystrophy	AR	Collodion membrane Broken hair	DNA transcription, repair gene in some	
KID syndrome	May be AD, AR	Erythrokeratodermatous or thick, leathery skin with stippled papules	Unknown	Clinical; auditory evoked potentials
CHILD syndrome	X-linked dominant	Alopecia Unilateral waxy yellow, scaling Hemidysplasia Limb defects	3β-Hydroxysteroid dehydrogenase Emopamil binding protein	Clinical
Conradi-Hünermann	X-linked dominant	Thick, psoriasiform scale over erythroderma, patterned along Blaschko lines Proximal limb shortening	Emopamil binding protein	Clinical
Ichthyosis follicularis	Usually X-linked recessive	Prominent follicular hyperkeratoses Alopecia Photophobia	Unknown	Clinical
CHIME syndrome	AR	Ichthyotic erythermatous plaques Cardiac defects; typical facies Retinal colobomas	Unknown	Clinical
Gaucher	AR	Collodion membrane Hepatosplenomegaly	β-Glucocerebrosidase	Clinical; fibroblast cultures

AD, autosomal dominant; AR, autosomal recessive; CHILD, congenital hemidysplasia with ichthyosiform erythroderma and limb defects; CHIME, colobomas of the eyes, heart defects, ichthyosiform dermatosis, mental retardation, and ear abnormalities; KID, keratitis with ichthyosis and deafness; PMN, polymorphonuclear neutrophils.
From Eichenfield LF, Frieden IJ, Esterly NB: *Textbook of Neonatal Dermatology*. Philadephia, WB Saunders, 2001, p 277.

Initial **treatment** includes high fluid intake to avoid dehydration from transepidermal water loss and use of a humidified heated incubator, emulsifying ointments, careful attention to hygiene, and oral retinoids. Survivors after retinoid therapy develop severe congenital ichthyosiform erythroderma. Prenatal diagnosis has been accomplished by fetoscopy, fetal skin biopsy, and microscopic examination of cells from amniotic fluid taken at the 17th and 21st wk of gestation.

COLLODION BABY. These infants are covered at birth by a thick, taut membrane resembling oiled parchment or collodion (Fig. 657-1), which is subsequently shed. The condition is usually a manifestation of congenital ichthyosiform erythroderma or lamellar ichthyosis. As with harlequin fetus, a collodion baby appears to be one phenotype for several genotypes. Less commonly, collodion babies evolve into other forms of ichthyosis or Gaucher disease, and a small subset is otherwise healthy without chronic skin disease. Affected neonates have ectropion, flattening of the ears and nose, and fixation of the lips in an O-shaped configuration. Hair may be absent or may perforate the horny covering. The membrane cracks with initial respiratory efforts and, shortly after birth, begins to desquamate in large sheets. Complete shedding may take several weeks, and a new membrane may occasionally form in localized areas.

Neonatal morbidity and deaths may be due to cutaneous infection, aspiration pneumonia (squamous material), hypothermia, or hypernatremic dehydration from excessive transcutaneous fluid losses as a result of increased skin permeability. The outcome is uncertain, and accurate prognosis is impossible with respect to the subsequent development of ichthyosis. **Treatment** with a high-humidity environment and application of nonocclusive lubricants may facilitate shedding of the membrane.

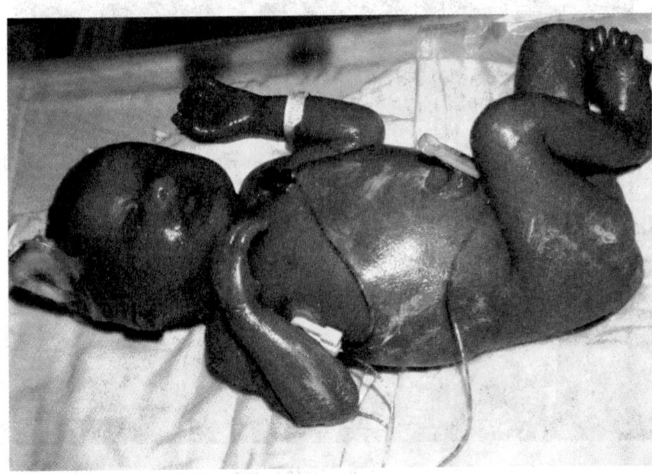

Figure 657-1. Typical appearance of a collodion baby.

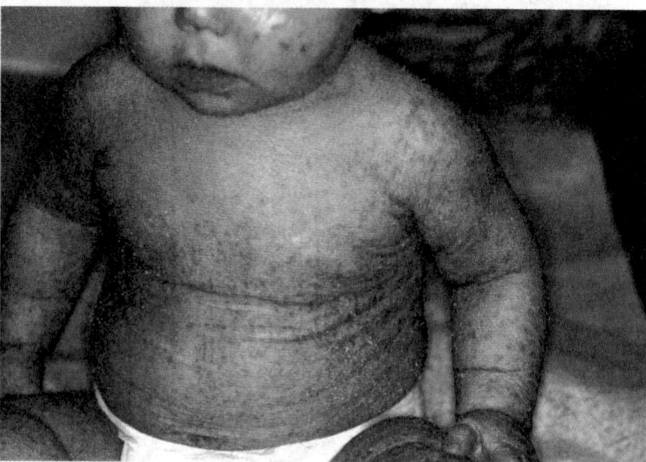

Figure 657-2. Generalized scaling of lamellar ichthyosis.

LAMELLAR ICHTHYOSIS AND CONGENITAL ICHTHYOSIFORM ERYTHRODERMA (NONBULLOUS CONGENITAL ICHTHYOSIFORM ERYTHRODERMA). There are 2 major forms of autosomal recessively inherited ichthyosis. Both forms are present soon or shortly after birth and are the most common forms of ichthyosis to present as collodion babies, although most infants present with erythroderma and scaling.

After shedding of the collodion membrane, if present, lamellar ichthyosis evolves into large, quadrilateral, dark scales that are free at the edges and adherent at the center. Scaling is often pronounced and involves the entire body surface, including flexural surfaces (Fig. 657-2). The face is often markedly involved, including ectropion and small, crumpled ears. The palms and soles are generally hyperkeratotic. The hair may be sparse and fine, but the teeth and mucosal surfaces are normal. In contrast to congenital ichthyosiform erythroderma, there is little erythema. Neither form includes blistering. **Autosomal recessive lamellar ichthyosis (ARLI)** is a clinically and genetically heterogeneous disorder. In ≈50% of cases, mutations in TGM1 gene encoding transglutaminase have been found. Mutations in TGM1 have also been found in congenital ichthyosiform erythroderma.

In **congenital ichthyosiform erythroderma,** erythroderma tends to be persistent, and scales, although they are generalized, are finer and whiter than in lamellar ichthyosis (Fig. 657-3). Hyperkeratosis is particularly noticeable around the knees, elbows, and ankles. Palms and soles are uniformly hyperkeratotic. Patients have sparse hair, cicatricial alopecia, and nail dystrophy.

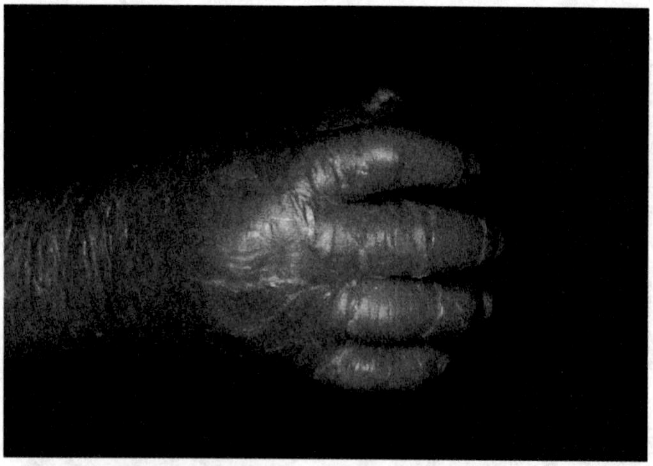

Figure 657-3. Prominent erythema and scale in congenital ichthyosiform erythroderma.

A markedly thickened stratum corneum and mild, irregular epidermal thickening characterize lamellar ichthyosis. Congenital ichthyosiform erythroderma has more epidermal thickening with parakeratosis but less hyperkeratosis and hypergranulosis than in lamellar ichthyosis. In congenital ichthyosiform erythroderma, there is a marked increase in the rate of epidermal cell production, considerably greater than the slightly increased rate observed in patients with lamellar ichthyosis.

Pruritus may be severe and responds minimally to antipruritic therapy. The unattractive appearance of the child and the malodor from bacterial colonization of macerated scales may create serious psychologic problems. A high-humidity environment in winter and air conditioning in summer reduce discomfort. Generous and frequent applications of emollients and keratolytic agents such as lactic or glycolic acid (5%), urea (10–40%), and retinoic acid (0.1% cream) may lessen the scaling to some extent, although these agents produce stinging if applied to fissured skin. **Oral retinoids** have a beneficial effect in these conditions but do not alter the underlying defect and, therefore, must be administered indefinitely. The long-term risks of these compounds (teratogenic effects and toxicity to bone) may limit their usefulness. Ectropion requires ophthalmologic care and, at times, plastic procedures.

ICHTHYOSIS VULGARIS. This may be either an autosomal dominant or polygenetic disorder. Semidominant mutations in the filaggrin gene have been reported in some families. Heterozygotic patients have mild disease with incomplete penetrance. Ichthyosis vulgaris is the **most common** of the disorders of keratinization, with an incidence of ≈1/300 live births. Onset generally occurs in the 1st yr of life. In most cases, it is trivial, consisting only of slight roughening of the skin surface. In rare cases, infants have presented as collodion babies. Scaling is most prominent on the extensor aspects of the extremities, particularly the legs (Fig. 657-4). Flexural surfaces are spared, and the abdomen, neck, and face are relatively uninvolved. Keratosis pilaris, particularly on the upper arms and thighs, accentuated markings and hyperkeratosis on the palms and soles, and atopy are relatively common. Scaling is most pronounced during the winter months and may abate completely during warm weather. The condition may improve and even disappear with age. There is no accompanying disorder of hair, teeth, mucosal surfaces, or other organ systems.

The histopathologic changes differ from those of other types of ichthyosis in that the hyperkeratosis is associated with a decreased or absent granular layer. Abnormally small and

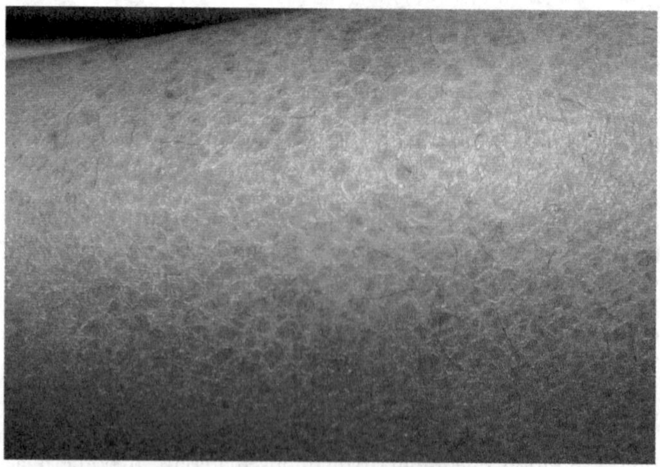

Figure 657-4. Scale over the shin in ichthyosis vulgaris.

crumbly keratohyalin granules are found in epidermal cells on electron microscopy. The rate of epidermal proliferation is normal. The hyperkeratosis is due to defective desquamation. Profilaggrin is clinically abnormal, but mutations in the profilaggrin gene have not been identified.

Scaling may be diminished by daily applications of an emollient or a lubricant containing urea (10–40%), salicylic acid, or an α-hydroxy acid such as lactic acid (5–12%).

X-LINKED ICHTHYOSIS. X-linked ichthyosis is largely limited to males, although female carriers may display slight, fine, silvery scale on the lower legs. Skin peeling may be present at birth but typically abates until 3–6 mo of life. Scaling is most pronounced on the sides of the neck, lower face, preauricular areas, anterior trunk, and the limbs, particularly the legs. The elbow (Fig. 657-5) and knee flexures are generally spared but may be mildly involved. The palms and soles may be slightly thickened but are also usually spared. The condition gradually worsens in severity and extent. Keratosis pilaris is not present, and there is no increased incidence of atopy. **Deep corneal opacities** that do not interfere with vision develop in late childhood or adolescence and are a useful marker for the disease because they may also be present in carrier females. **Cryptorchidism** occurs in ≈25% of affected males. Some patients have additional features of **Kallmann syndrome** (KAL1 gene) and **chondroplasia punctata** (arylsufatase and EBP genes) due to a contiguous gene mutation. The rate of testicular cancer may be increased.

There is hyperkeratosis of the stratum corneum, a well-developed granular layer, and a hyperplastic epidermis. The rate of epidermal proliferation is normal, and the hyperkeratosis is due to retention of corneocytes and delayed dissolution of the desmosomal disks. X-linked ichthyosis involves a deficiency of steroid sulfatase, which hydrolyzes cholesterol sulfate and other sulfated steroids to cholesterol. Cholesterol sulfate accumulates in the stratum corneum and plasma and may cause hyperkeratosis by inhibiting desmosomal proteolysis. Elevated cholesterol sulfate levels can be demonstrated in the serum, erythrocyte membranes, and epidermal cells and scales of affected males. Reduced steroid sulfatase enzyme activity can be detected in fibroblasts, keratinocytes, and leukocytes and, prenatally, in amniocytes or chorionic villus cells. In affected families, an affected male can be detected by restriction enzyme analysis of cultured chorionic villus cell DNA or amniocytes or by in situ hybridization, which identifies steroid sulfatase gene deletions prenatally in chorionic villus cells. A placental steroid sulfatase deficiency in carrier mothers may result in low urinary and serum estriol values, prolonged labor, and insensitivity of the uterus to oxytocin and prostaglandins.

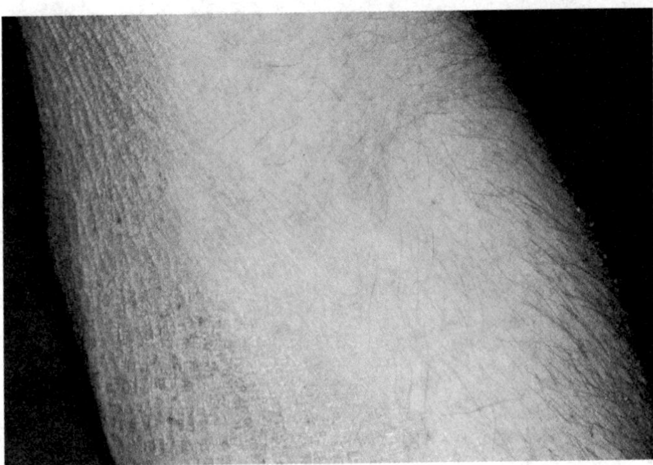

Figure 657-5. Sparing of the antecubital fossa in X-linked ichthyosis.

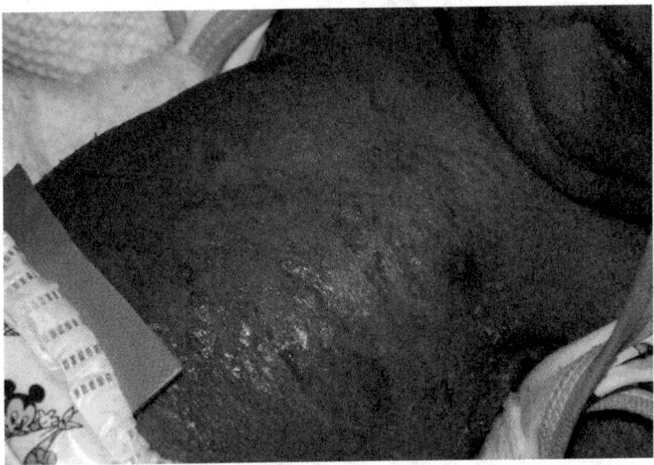

Figure 657-6. Superficial erosions and hyperkeratosis in epidermolytic hyperkeratosis.

Daily application of emollients and a urea-containing lubricant (10–40%) are usually effective **treatments.** Glycolic or lactic acid (5%) in an emollient base and propylene glycol (40–60%) in water with occlusion overnight are alternative forms of therapy.

EPIDERMOLYTIC HYPERKERATOSIS (BULLOUS CONGENITAL ICHTHYOSIFORM ERYTHRODERMA). Epidermolytic hyperkeratosis is inherited as an autosomal dominant trait, although many are sporadic. The clinical manifestations are characterized by the onset at birth of **generalized erythroderma** and severe hyperkeratosis (Fig. 657-6). The scales are small, hard, and verrucous. Distinctive, parallel hyperkeratotic ridges develop over the joint flexures, including the axillary, popliteal, and antecubital fossas, and on the neck and hips. Erythema becomes less prominent after infancy; however, the hyperkeratosis persists throughout adult life. Recurrent blistering may be widespread in neonates and may cause diagnostic confusion with other blistering disorders. Blistering becomes accentuated at sites of trauma such as the knees, elbows, and lower limbs but is not problematic after age 7–8 yr. The palms and soles may be thickened, but the hair, nails, mucosa, and sweat glands are normal. Secondary bacterial infection is common and requires appropriate antibiotic therapy. Severely affected patients may have crumpled ears and ectropion.

The histopathology is diagnostic and consists of hyperkeratosis, a markedly thickened granular layer with an increased number of keratohyalin granules, clear spaces around nuclei, and indistinct cellular boundaries of cells in the upper epidermis. On electron microscopic examination, keratin intermediate filaments are clumped, and many desmosomes are attached to only one keratinocyte instead of connecting neighboring keratinocytes. Epidermolytic hyperkeratosis has been shown to be due to defects in either keratin 1 or 10 encoded in chromosome 12p, where the type II keratin genes are clustered. These keratins are required to form the keratin intermediate filaments in cells of the suprabasilar layers of the epidermis. Localized forms of the disease may resemble epidermal nevi (**ichthyosis hystrix**) or keratoderma of the palms and soles but share the distinctive histopathologic changes of epidermolytic hyperkeratosis. Prenatal diagnosis for affected families is possible by examination of DNA extracts from chorionic villus cells or amniocytes, provided that the specific mutation in the affected parent is known.

Treatment is difficult. Morbidity is increased in the neonatal period as a result of prematurity, sepsis, and fluid and electrolyte imbalance. Bacterial colonization of macerated scales produces a distinctive malodor that can be controlled somewhat by use of an antibacterial cleanser. Intermittent oral antibiotics are generally necessary. Keratolytic agents are often poorly tolerated. Oral

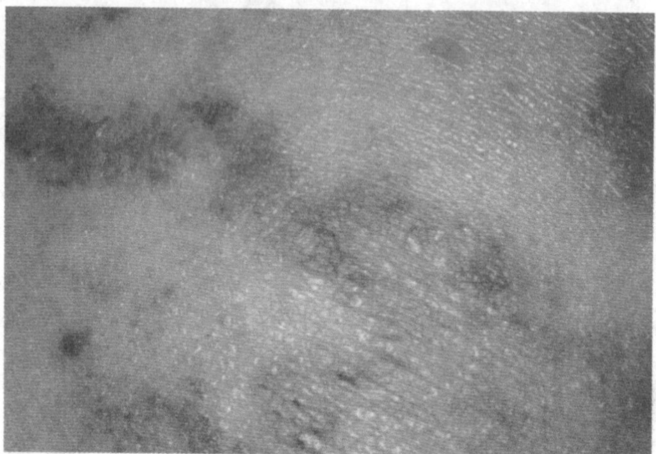

Figure 657-7. Serpiginous, erythematous, hyperkeratotic lesions of ichthyosis linearis circumflexa.

retinoids may produce significant improvement, even at relatively low doses.

ICHTHYOSIS LINEARIS CIRCUMFLEXA. This rare autosomal recessive disorder presents at birth or in the 1st few months of life with generalized erythema and scaling. The trunk and limbs have diffuse erythema and superimposed migratory, polycyclic, and serpiginous hyperkeratotic lesions (Fig. 657-7), some with a distinctive double-edged margin of scale. Lichenification or hyperkeratosis tends to persist in the antecubital and popliteal fossas. The face and scalp may remain erythematous and scaling. Many hair shaft deformities, most notably, trichorrhexis invaginata, have been described in more than ½ of patients. This type of ichthyosis is characteristic of patients with **Netherton syndrome.** Nonspecific psoriasiform changes are found on histopathologic examination.

ERYTHROKERATODERMA VARIABILIS. This autosomal dominant heterogeneous disorder usually presents in the early months of life, progresses in childhood, and stabilizes in adolescence. Mutations in connexin 31 and 30.3 have been identified in some patients. It is characterized by sharply demarcated, hyperkeratotic plaques with geographic borders that develop in areas of normal skin (Fig. 657-8*A*) or within discrete erythematous patches. Patches of erythema change shape or size within minutes to hours or days or migrate (Fig. 657-8*B*), and they may gradually became hyperkeratotic and fixed. The distribution is generalized but sparse; sites of predilection are the face, buttocks, axillae, and extensor surfaces of the limbs. The palms and soles may be thickened, but hair, teeth, and nails are normal. Histopathology demonstrates hyperkeratosis, papillomatosis, and irregular hyperplasia of the epidermis.

Symmetric progressive erythrokeratoderma is an autosomal dominant disorder that presents in childhood with large, fixed, geographic and symmetric, fine, scaling, hyperkeratotic, erythematous plaques primarily on the extremities, buttocks, face, ankles, and wrists. Palmoplantar keratoderma is also present. The primary feature distinguishing this from erythrokeratoderma variabilis (EKV) is the lack of variable erythema, as seen in the latter condition. These two conditions may be manifestations of the same disorder, but in some of these patients, mutations have been found in the lorocrin gene, which is not abnormal in EKV.

ICHTHYOSIFORM DERMATOSES. Several syndromes that include ichthyosis as a constant feature have been established as rare but distinct entities.

Sjögren-Larsson Syndrome. This autosomal recessive inborn error of metabolism consists of ichthyosis, mental retardation, and spasticity. The ichthyosis is generalized but is accentuated on the flexures and the lower abdomen and consists of erythroderma, fine scaling, larger platelike scales, and dark hyperkeratosis. Mild palmoplantar hyperkeratosis may be seen. The skin changes may be identical to the other forms of ichthyosis and diagnosis is often delayed until the onset of neurologic symptoms. Glistening dots in the foveal area are a cardinal ophthalmologic sign. Motor and speech developmental delays are usually noted before 1 yr of age, and spastic diplegia or tetraplegia, epilepsy, and mental retardation generally become evident in the 1st 3 yr of life. Some patients may walk with the aid of braces, but most are confined to a wheelchair. The primary defect is an abnormality of fatty alcohol oxidation as a result of a deficiency of fatty aldehyde dehydrogenase, a component of the fatty alcohol–nicotinamide adenine dinucleotide oxidoreductase enzyme complex. This deficiency can be demonstrated in cultured skin fibroblasts of affected patients and carriers and, prenatally, in cultured chorionic villus cells and amniocytes from affected fetuses. Elevation of urinary leukotriene B4 (LTB4) may provide an easier approach to diagnosis and 5-lipoxygenase inhibitors have been used to decrease pruritus.

Netherton Syndrome. This autosomal recessive disorder is characterized by ichthyosis (usually ichthyosis linearis circumflexa but, occasionally, the lamellar or congenital ichthyosiform erythroderma types), trichorrhexis invaginata and other hair shaft anomalies, and atopic diathesis. Mutations in the gene SPINK 5,

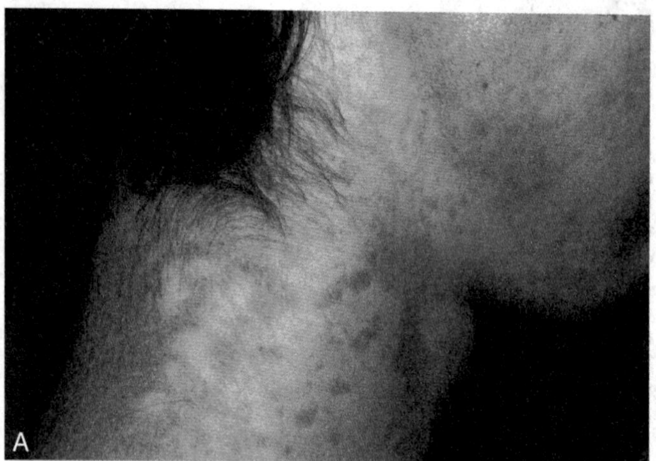

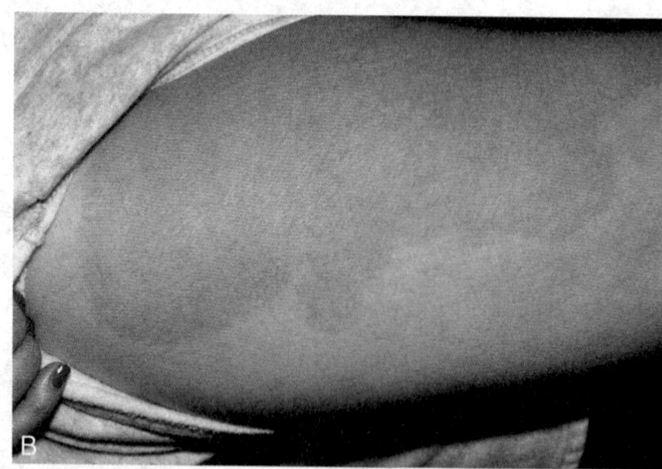

Figure 657-8. *A*, Fixed, hyperkeratotic plaques in erythrokeratoderma variables. *B*, Migratory, erythematous lesion of erythrokeratoderma variables.

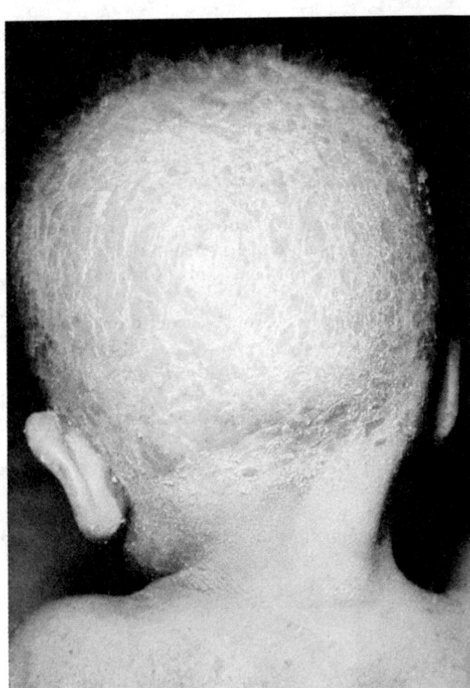

Figure 657-9. Very short scalp hair and thick scale in Netherton syndrome.

which encodes a serine protease inhibitor, have been identified in patients with Netherton syndrome. The ichthyosis is present in the 1st 10 days of life and may be especially marked around the eyes, mouth, and perineal area. The erythroderma is often intensified after infection. Infants may suffer from failure to thrive, recurrent bacterial and candidal infections, elevated serum IgE levels, and marked hypernatremic dehydration. The most frequent allergic manifestations are urticaria, angioedema, atopic dermatitis, and asthma. Scalp hair is sparse and short and fractures easily (Fig. 657-9); eyebrows, eyelashes, and body hair are also abnormal. The characteristic hair abnormality can be identified with light microscopy. In the newborn, it may best be identified in eyebrow hair.

Refsum Syndrome (See Chapter 86.2). This multisystem disorder is inherited as an autosomal recessive trait and becomes symptomatic in the 2nd or 3rd decade of life. The ichthyosis may be generalized, is relatively mild, and resembles ichthyosis vulgaris. The ichthyosis may also be localized to the palms and soles. Chronic polyneuritis with progressive paralysis and ataxia, atypical retinitis pigmentosa, anosmia, deafness, bony abnormalities, and electrocardiographic changes are the most characteristic features. This condition is diagnosed by lipid analysis of the blood or skin, which shows elevated phytanic acid levels. The defect is in the PAHK gene. Phytanic acid is exclusively derived from dietary chlorophyll. Dietary avoidance of phytanic acid–containing green vegetables produces clinical improvement.

Chondrodysplasia Punctata (See Chapter 86.2). This includes several genetically heterogeneous disorders marked by ichthyosis and bone changes, principally Conradi-Hünermann-Happle syndrome (delta[8]-delta[7]-sterol isomerase binding protein [EBP]), an X-linked dominant form affecting only females, X-linked recessive chondrodysplasia punctata (arylsulfatase gene) and rhizomelic dwarfism, transmitted as an autosomal recessive trait. Nearly all patients with the X-linked dominant form and ≈25% of those with the recessive type have cutaneous lesions, ranging from severe, generalized erythema and scaling to mild hyperkeratosis. Rhizomelic chondrodysplasia punctata is associated with cataracts, hypertelorism, optic nerve atrophy, disproportionate shortening of the proximal extremities, psychomotor retardation, failure to thrive, and spasticity; most patients die in infancy. Numerous dysfunctional peroxisomal enzymes are found in patients with rhizomelic chondrodysplasia. Patients with the X-linked dominant form have asymmetric, variable shortening of the limbs and a distinctive ichthyosiform eruption at birth. Thick, yellow, tightly adherent, keratinized plaques are distributed in a whorled pattern over the entire body. The histologic changes include hyperkeratosis that penetrates to the depths of the hair follicles. The eruption typically resolves in infancy and may be superseded by a follicular atrophoderma and patchy alopecia.

Additional features in all variants include cataracts and abnormal facies with saddle nose and frontal bossing. The pathognomonic defect, termed chondrodysplasia punctata, is stippled epiphyses in the cartilaginous skeleton. This defect, which is seen in various settings and inherited disorders, often in association with peroxisomal deficiency and disturbance of cholesterol biosynthesis, disappears by ≈3–4 yr of age.

A number of other rare syndromes with ichthyosis as a consistent feature include the following: keratitis with ichthyosis and deafness (KID syndrome, connexin 26 gene), ichthyosis with defective hair having a banded pattern under polarized light and a low sulfur content (trichothiodystrophy), multiple sulfatase deficiency, neutral lipid storage disease with ichthyosis (Chanarin-Dorfman syndrome, CGI58 gene), and CHILD syndrome (Fig. 657-10) (congenital hemidysplasia with ichthyosiform erythroderma and limb defects, NSDHL gene).

PALMOPLANTAR KERATODERMAS (PPK). Excessive hyperkeratosis of the palms and soles may occur as a manifestation of a focal or generalized congenital hereditary skin disorder or may result from such chronic skin diseases as psoriasis, eczema, pityriasis rubra pilaris, lupus erythematosus, or Reiter disease. The names of individual disorders have been based on descriptive titles, modes of inheritance, histopathologic findings, and biochemical defects.

Diffuse Hyperkeratosis of Palms and Soles (Unna-Thost, Vorner). Unna-Thost and Vorner type PPK, although clinically inseparable, were until recently thought to represent separate entities. They were separated histologically by the presence (Vorner) or absence (Unna-Thost) of epidermolytic hyperkeratosis. They are now thought to be spectrums of the same disease caused by mutations in keratin (KRT1 and 9 genes). This autosomal dominant disorder presents in the 1st few months of life with erythema that gradually progresses to sharply demarcated, hyperkeratotic, scaling plaques over the palms (Fig. 657-11) and soles. The margins of the plaques often remain red; plaques may extend along the lateral aspects of the hands and feet and onto the volar

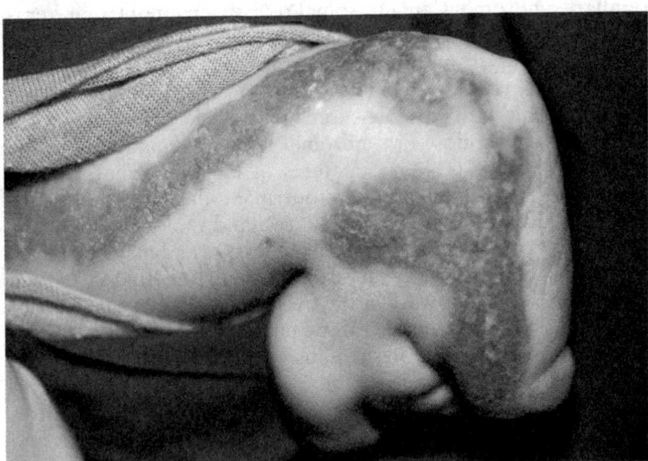

Figure 657-10. Limb dysplasia and ichthyosiform eruption in CHILD (congenital hemidysplasia with ichthyosiform erythroderma and limb defects) syndrome.

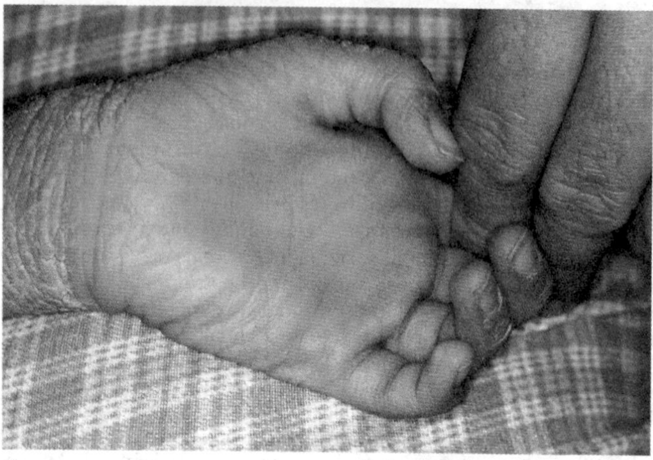

Figure 657-11. Palmar keratoderma with epidermolytic changes seen on biopsy.

wrists and the heels. Hyperhidrosis is usually present, but hair, teeth, and nails are usually normal. Striate (DSG1, DSP, KRT1 genes) and punctate forms of palmar and plantar hyperkeratosis represent distinct entities.

Mal de Meleda (Slurp-1 Gene). This rare, progressive autosomal recessive condition is characterized by erythema and thick scales on the palms, fingers, soles, and flexor aspects of the wrists, knees, and elbows. Hyperhidrosis, nail thickening or koilonychia, and eczema may also occur.

Vohwinkel PPK (Mutilating Keratoderma). This is a progressive autosomal dominant disease with honeycombed hyperkeratosis of palms and soles, sparing the arches; starfish-like and linear keratoses on the dorsum of the hands, fingers, feet, and knees; and ainhum-like constriction of the digits that sometimes leads to autoamputation. Varying degrees of alopecia may be seen. Two forms have been identified. Vohwinkel PPK with ichthyosis is caused by mutations in the loricrin gene and Vohwinkel with deafness by mutations in connexin 26.

Papillon-Lefèvre Syndrome (Cathespin C Gene). This autosomal recessive erythematous hyperkeratosis of the palms and soles sometimes extends to the dorsal hands and feet, elbows, and knees later in childhood. The PPK may be either diffuse, striate, or punctuate. This syndrome is characterized by periodontal inflammation, leading to loss of teeth by age 4–5 yr if untreated.

Keratoderma of palms and soles also occurs as a feature of some forms of ichthyosis and ectodermal dysplasia. Richner-Hanhart syndrome is an autosomal recessive palmoplantar keratoderma with corneal ulcers, progressive mental impairment, and a deficiency of tyrosine aminotransferase, which leads to tyrosinemia. Pachyonychia congenita is transmitted as an autosomal dominant trait with variable expressivity. The classic type I form (Jadassohn-Lewandowski syndrome) is due to mutations in the gene for keratin 16. Major features of the syndrome are onychogryphosis; palmoplantar keratoderma; follicular hyperkeratosis, especially of the elbows and knees; and oral leukokeratosis. The nail dystrophy is the most striking feature and may be present at birth or develop early in life. The nails are thickened and tubular, projecting upward at the free edge to form a conical roof over a mass of subungual keratotic debris. Repeated paronychial inflammation may result in shedding of the nails. The feature seen most consistently among patients with this condition is keratoderma of the palms and soles. Additional associated features include hyperhidrosis of the palms and soles, and bullae and erosions on the palms and soles. Some patients have shown a selective cell-mediated defect in recognition and processing of *Candida*. Surgical removal of the nails and excision of the nail matrix have been helpful in some patients.

Treatment is the same no matter what the cause of the PPK. In mild cases, emollient therapy may suffice. Keratolytic agents such as salicylic acid, lactic acid, and urea creams may be required. Oral retinoids are the treatment of choice for severe cases unresponsive to topical therapy.

DiGiovanna JJ: Ichthyosiform dermatoses: So many disorders, so little progress. *J Am Acad Dermatol* 2004;51:S31–S34.

Lane EB, McLean WH: Keratins and skin disorders. *J Pathol* 2004;204: 355–366.

McClean WH: Epithelial Genetics Group. Genetic disorders of palm skin and nail. *J Anat* 2003;202:133–141.

Richard G: Molecular genetics of the ichthyoses. *Am J Med Genet* 2004;15:32–44.

Shwayder T: Disorders of keratinization: Diagnosis and management. *Am J Clin Dermatol* 2004;5:17–29.

Smith FJD, Irvine AD, Terron-Kwiatkowski A, et al: Loss of function mutations in the gene encoding filaggrin cause ichthyosis vulgaris. *Nat Genet* 2006;38:337–342.

Van Steensel MA: Gap junction diseases of the skin. *Am J Med Genet* 2004;15:12–19.

Chapter 658 ■ Diseases of the Dermis

Joseph G. Morelli

KELOID. A keloid is a sharply demarcated, benign, dense growth of connective tissue that forms in the dermis after trauma. The lesions are firm, raised, pink, and rubbery; they may be tender or pruritic. Sites of predilection are the face, earlobes (Fig. 658-1), neck, shoulders, upper trunk, sternum, and lower legs. Keloids are usually induced by trauma and commonly follow ear piercing, burns, scalds, and surgical procedures. Certain individuals seem predisposed to keloid formation. In some cases, a familial tendency (recessive or dominant inheritance) or the presence of foreign material in the wound appears to have a pathogenic role. Keloids are a rare feature of Ehlers-Danlos syndrome, Rubinstein-Taybi syndrome, and pachydermoperiostosis. In both keloids and hypertrophic scars, new collagen forms over a much longer period than in wounds that heal normally. A keloid consists of whorled and interlaced hyalinized collagen fibers.

Keloids should be differentiated from hypertrophic scars, which remain confined to the site of injury and gradually invo-

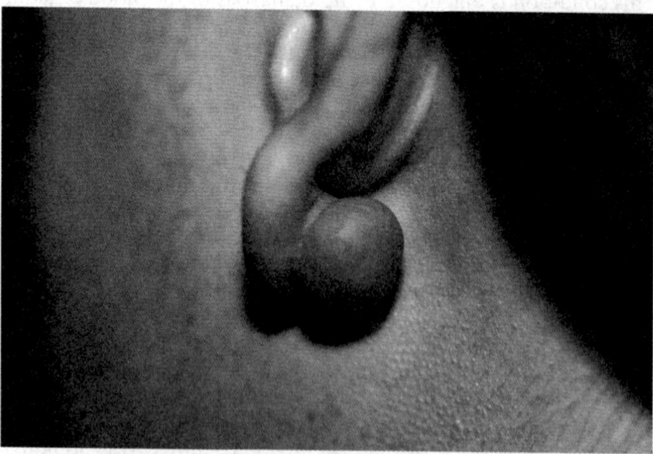

Figure 658-1. Keloid of ear lobe after piercing.

lute over time. Young keloids may diminish in size if injected intralesionally at 4 wk intervals with triamcinolone suspension (10–40 mg/mL). At times, a more concentrated suspension is required. Large or old keloids may require surgical excision followed by intralesional injections of corticosteroid. The risk of **recurrence** at the same site argues against surgical excision alone, although ear lobe keloids respond well to surgical excision. Placement of topical silicon gel sheeting over the keloid for several hours per day for several weeks may help some patients.

STRIAE CUTIS DISTENSAE. These thinned, depressed, erythematous bands of atrophic skin eventually become silvery, opalescent, and smooth. They occur most frequently in areas that have been subject to distention, such as the lower back (Fig. 658-2), buttocks, thighs, breasts, abdomen, and shoulders. The most frequent causes are rapid growth, pregnancy, obesity, Cushing disease, or prolonged corticosteroid therapy. Striae formation is common in adolescence. Adolescent striae tend to become less conspicuous with time. Striae distensae resemble atrophic scars.

CORTICOSTEROID-INDUCED ATROPHY. Both topical and systemic corticosteroid treatment can result in cutaneous atrophy. This is particularly common when a potent topical corticosteroid is applied under occlusion or to the intertriginous areas for a prolonged period. Affected skin is thin, fragile, smooth, and semitransparent, with telangiectasias and loss of normal skin markings. Histopathologically, one sees thinning of the epidermis. Spaces between dermal collagen and elastic fibers are small, producing a more compact but thin dermis. The mechanism involves inhibition of synthesis of collagen type I, noncollagenous proteins, and total protein content of the skin; progressive reduction of dermal proteoglycans and glycosaminoglycans; and possibly prolonged vasoconstriction-induced ischemia. Retinoids applied topically restore these steroid-induced biochemical changes in the dermal connective tissue of the hairless mouse, without abrogating the beneficial anti-inflammatory effects.

GRANULOMA ANNULARE. This common dermatosis occurs predominantly in children and young adults. Typical lesions begin as firm, smooth, erythematous papules. They gradually enlarge to form annular plaques with a papular border and a normal, slightly atrophic or discolored central area up to several centimeters in size. Lesions may occur anywhere on the body, but mucous membranes are spared. Favored sites include the dorsum of the hands (Fig. 658-3) and feet. Annular lesions are often mistaken for tinea corporis because of the elevated advancing border. They differ in that they are not scaly. Papular lesions, another

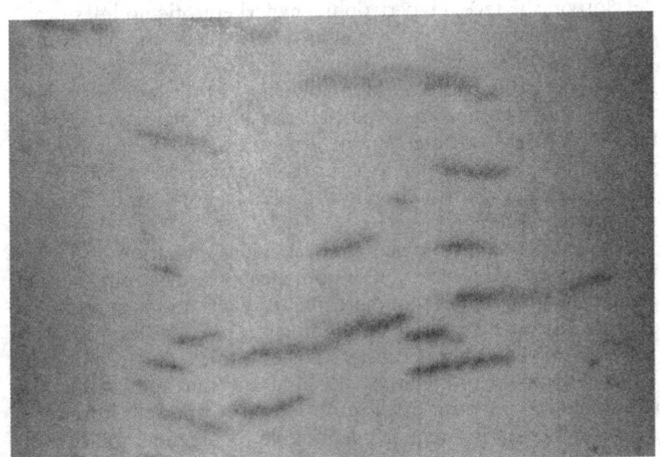

Figure 658-2. Striae on back of adolescent.

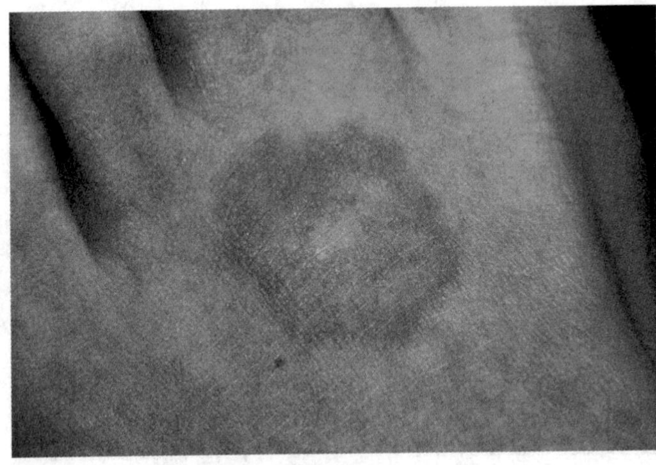

Figure 658-3. Annular lesion with a raised papular border and depressed center, characteristic of granuloma annulare.

variant, may simulate rheumatoid nodules, particularly when grouped on the fingers and elbows. The disseminated papular form, which is provoked by light in some cases, is rare in children. Subcutaneous granuloma annulare is especially common in children; it tends to develop on the scalp and limbs, particularly in the pretibial area. These lesions are firm, usually nontender, skin-colored nodules. Perforating granuloma annulare is characterized by the development of a yellowish center in some of the superficial papular lesions as a result of transepidermal elimination of altered collagen.

A biopsy is occasionally required for diagnosis. The lesions consist of a granuloma with a central area of necrotic collagen; mucin deposition; and a peripheral palisading infiltrate of lymphocytes, histiocytes, and foreign body giant cells. The pattern resembles that of necrobiosis lipoidica and rheumatoid nodule, but subtle histologic differences usually permit differentiation. The cause of granuloma annulare is unknown. Affected children are usually healthy. Some cases of granuloma annulare, particularly the generalized form, may be associated with **diabetes mellitus.** The eruption persists for months to years, but spontaneous resolution without residual change is usual; 75% of lesions clear within 2 yr. Application of a potent topical corticosteroid preparation or intralesional injections of corticosteroid may hasten involution, but nonintervention is acceptable.

NECROBIOSIS LIPOIDICA. This rare disorder presents as erythematous papules that evolve into irregularly shaped, sharply demarcated, yellow, sclerotic plaques with central telangiectasia and a violaceous border. Scaling, crusting, and ulceration are frequent. Lesions develop most commonly on the shins (Fig. 658-4). Slow extension of a given lesion over the years is usual, but long periods of quiescence or complete healing with scarring may occur.

Poorly defined areas of necrobiotic collagen are seen throughout, but primarily low in the dermis, associated with mucin deposition. Surrounding the necrobiotic, disordered areas of collagen is a palisading lymphohistiocytic granulomatous infiltrate. Some lesions are more characteristically granulomatous, with limited necrobiosis of collagen. Necrobiosis lipoidica must be differentiated clinically from xanthomas, morphea, granuloma annulare, erythema, nodosum, and pretibial myxedema. Fifty to 75% of patients have **diabetes mellitus**; necrobiosis lipoidica occurs in 0.3% of all diabetic patients. The lesions persist despite good control of the diabetes but may improve minimally after applications of high-potency topical steroids or local injection of a corticosteroid.

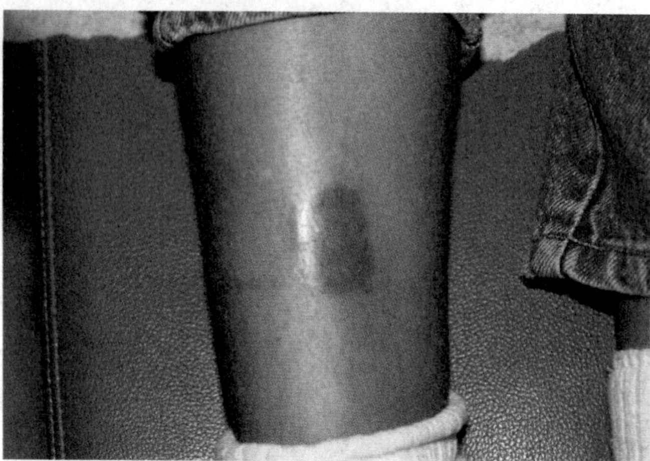

Figure 658-4. Yellow sclerotic plaque of necrobiosis lipoidica on the shin.

LICHEN SCLEROSUS. This presents initially with shiny, indurated, ivory-colored papules, often with a violaceous halo. The surface shows prominent dilated pilosebaceous or sweat duct orifices that often contain yellow or brown horny plugs. The papules coalesce to form irregular plaques of variable size, which may develop hemorrhagic bullae in their margins. In the latter stages, atrophy results in a depressed plaque with a wrinkled surface. This disorder occurs more commonly in girls than in boys. Sites of predilection in girls are the vulvar (Fig. 658-5), perianal, and perineal skin. Extensive involvement may produce a sclerotic, atrophic plaque of hourglass configuration; shrinkage of the labia and stenosis of the introitus may result. Vaginal discharge precedes vulvar lesions in ≈20% of patients. In boys, the prepuce and glans penis are often involved, usually in association with phimosis; most boys with the disorder were not circumcised early in life. Sites elsewhere on the body that are most commonly involved include the upper trunk, the neck, the axillae, the flexor surfaces of wrists, and the areas around the umbilicus and the eyes. Pruritus may be severe.

In children, this disorder is most frequently confused with focal morphea (see Chapter 159), with which it may coexist. In the genital area, it may be mistakenly attributed to sexual abuse. Biopsy is diagnostic, revealing hyperkeratosis with follicular plugging, hydropic degeneration of basal cells, a bandlike dermal lymphocytic infiltrate, homogenized collagen, and thinned elastic fibers in the upper dermis. Leukoplakia and squamous cell carcinoma may develop. **Potent topical corticosteroids** may provide relief from pruritus and produce clearing of lesions, including those in the genital area. Topical tacrolimus and pimecrolimus have also been used.

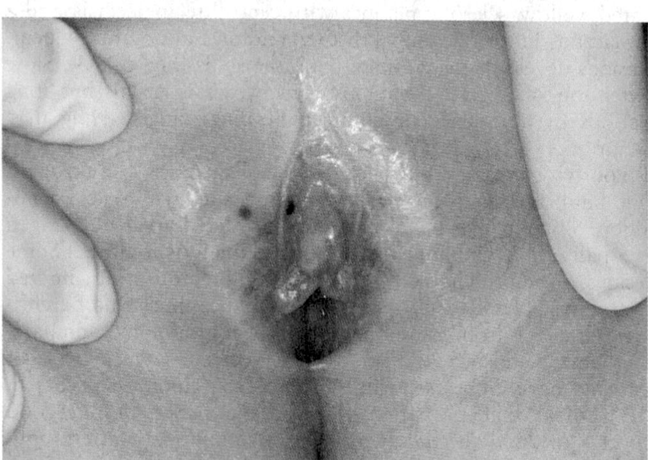

Figure 658-5. Ivory-colored perivaginal plaque with hemorrhage.

SCLEREDEMA (SCLEREDEMA ADULTORUM, SCLEREDEMA OF BUSCHKE). Approximately 30% of cases of scleredema develop before the age of 10 yr. Onset is sudden, with brawny edema of the face and neck that spreads rapidly to involve the thorax and arms in a sweater distribution; the abdomen and legs are usually spared. The face acquires a waxy, masklike appearance. The involved areas feel indurated and woody, are nonpitting, and are not sharply demarcated from normal skin. The overlying skin is normal in color and is not atrophic. Systemic involvement, which is uncommon, is marked by thickening of the tongue; dysarthria; dysphagia; restriction of eye and joint movements; and pleural, pericardial, and peritoneal effusions. Electrocardiographic changes may also be observed.

In 65–90% of cases, the disease follows an infection such as tonsillitis, pharyngitis, influenza, scarlet fever, measles, mumps, impetigo, or cellulitis after an interval of days or weeks. Most cases follow a streptococcal infection. Onset may be heralded by a prodrome of fever, arthralgia, myalgia, and malaise. Onset in diabetic patients may occur insidiously. Laboratory data are not helpful. Some cases, however, are associated with immunoglobulin (Ig)G or IgA paraproteinemia. Skin biopsy demonstrates an increase in dermal thickness as a result of swelling and homogenization of the collagen bundles, which are separated by large interfibrous spaces. Special stains can identify increased amounts of mucopolysaccharides in the dermis.

The active phase of the disease persists for 2–8 wk; spontaneous and complete resolution usually occurs in 6 mo–2 yr. Recurrent attacks are unusual. The disorder must be differentiated from scleroderma, morphea, myxedema, trichinosis, dermatomyositis, sclerema neonatorum, and subcutaneous fat necrosis. There is no specific therapy.

LIPOID PROTEINOSIS (URBACH-WIETHE DISEASE, HYALINOSIS CUTIS ET MUCOSAE) [ECM-1 GENE]. This autosomal recessive disorder consists of infiltration of hyaline material into the skin, oral cavity, larynx, and internal organs. It may be noted initially in early infancy as hoarseness. Skin lesions appear during childhood and consist of yellowish papules and nodules that may coalesce to form plaques on the face, forearms, neck, genitals, dorsum of the fingers, and scalp, where they result in patchy alopecia. Similar deposits are found on the lips, undersurface of the tongue, fauces, uvula, epiglottis, and vocal cords. The tongue becomes enlarged and feels firm on palpation. Patients may be unable to protrude their tongue. Translucent nodules along the margins of the eyelids, causing thickening of the eyelids, are the most characteristic clinical manifestation. Pocklike atrophic scars may develop on the face. Hypertrophic, hyperkeratotic nodules occur at sites of friction such as the elbows and knees; the palms may be diffusely thickened. The disease progresses until early adult life, but the prognosis is good. Involvement of the larynx can lead to respiratory compromise, particularly in infancy, necessitating tracheostomy. Associated anomalies include dental abnormalities, epilepsy, and recurrent parotitis as a result of infiltrates in the Stensen duct. Virtually any organ can be involved. There is no specific treatment.

The distinctive histologic pattern includes dilatation of dermal blood vessels and infiltration of homogeneous eosinophilic extracellular hyaline material along capillary walls and around sweat glands. Hyaline material in homogeneous bundles, diffusely arranged in the upper dermis, produces a thickened dermis. The infiltrates appear to contain both lipid and mucopolysaccharide substances. Symmetric ossification lateral to the sella turcica in the medial temporal region, identifiable roentgenographically, is pathognomonic but is not always present. The biochemical defect is in extracellular matrix protein-1.

MACULAR ATROPHY (ANETODERMA). Anetoderma is characterized by circumscribed areas of slack skin associated with loss of dermal substance. This disorder may have no associated underlying disease (primary macular atrophy) or may develop after an inflammatory skin condition (secondary macular atrophy) such as syphilis, lupus erythematosus, acne, varicella, leprosy, urticaria pigmentosa, or *Staphylococcus epidermidis* folliculitis. Lesions vary from 0.5 to 1 cm in diameter and, if inflammatory, may initially be erythematous. They subsequently become thin, wrinkled, and blue-white or hypopigmented. The lesions often protrude as small outpouchings that, on palpation, may be readily indented into the subcutaneous tissue because of the dermal atrophy. Sites of predilection include the trunk, thighs, upper arms, and, less commonly, the neck and face. Lesions remain unchanged for life; new lesions often continue to develop for years. There is no effective therapy.

All types of macular atrophy show focal loss of elastic tissue on histopathologic examination, a change that is not recognizable unless special stains are used. The elastolysis may be due to release of elastase from inflammatory cells, such as macrophages, in contact with elastic fibers. Lesions of anetoderma occasionally resemble morphea, lichen sclerosus, focal dermal hypoplasia, atrophic scars, or end-stage lesions of chronic bullous dermatoses.

CUTIS LAXA (DERMATOMEGALY, GENERALIZED ELASTOLYSIS). Cutis laxa is a heterogenous group of disorders. It may be autosomal recessive (fibulin 5 gene), autosomal dominant (elastin and fibulin 5 genes), or acquired. Acquired cutis laxa has developed after a febrile illness, inflammatory skin diseases such as lupus erythematosus or erythema multiforme, amyloidosis, urticaria, angioedema, and hypersensitivity reactions to penicillin, and in infants born to women who were taking penicillamine.

Clinical Manifestations. There may be widespread folds of lax skin, or changes may be mild and limited in extent, resembling anetoderma. Patients with severe cutis laxa have characteristic facial features, including an aged appearance with sagging jowls (bloodhound appearance) [Fig. 658-6], a hooked nose with everted nostrils, a short columella, a long upper lip, and everted lower eyelids. The skin is also lax elsewhere on the body and may resemble an ill-fitting suit. Hyperelasticity and hypermobility of the joints **are not present** as they are in the Ehlers-Danlos syndrome. Many infants have a hoarse cry, probably as a result of laxity of the vocal cords. Tensile strength of the skin is normal. Histologically, elastic tissue is reduced throughout the dermis, with fragmentation, distention, and clumping of the elastic fibers.

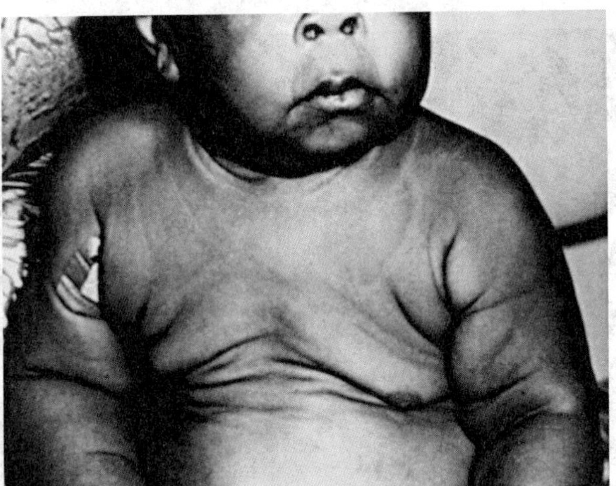

Figure 658-6. Pendulous folds of skin of an infant with cutis laxa. Note the long upper lip and upturned nose.

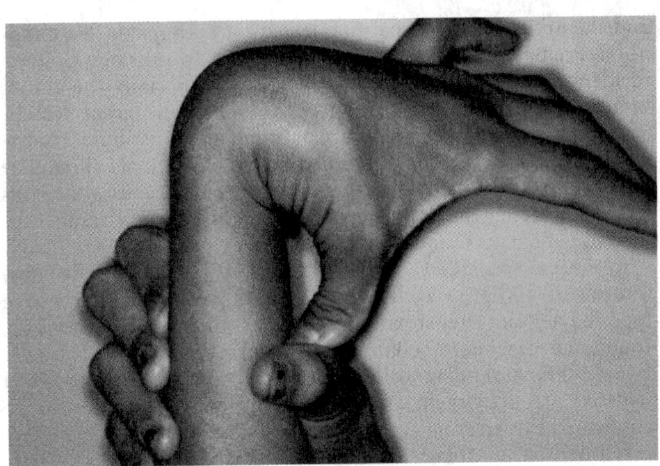

Figure 658-7. Joint hyperextensibility in classic Ehlers-Danlos syndrome.

The dominant form of cutis laxa may develop at any age and is generally benign and mainly of cosmetic significance. When it presents in infancy, it may be associated with intrauterine growth retardation, ligamentous laxity, and delayed closure of fontanels. Pulmonary emphysema and mild cardiovascular manifestations may also occur. In contrast, those with the more common recessive form of the disease are susceptible to severe complications, such as multiple hernias, rectal prolapse, diaphragmatic atony, diverticula of the gastrointestinal and genitourinary tracts, cor pulmonale, emphysema, pneumothoraces, peripheral pulmonary artery stenosis, and aortic dilatation. Characteristic facial features include downward slanting palpebral fissures, a broad, flat nose, and large ears. Skeletal anomalies, dental caries, growth retardation, and developmental delay also occur. Such patients often have a shortened life span.

Cutis laxa–like skin changes may also be seen in association with multiple other syndromes including Debarsy syndrome, Lenz-Majewski syndrome, hyperostotic dwarfism, SCARF (skeletal abnormalities, cutis laxa craniostenosis, ambiguous genitalia, retardation, facial abnormalities) syndrome, wrinkling skin syndrome, and Costello syndrome.

EHLERS-DANLOS SYNDROME (EDS). This is a group of genetically heterogeneous connective tissue disorders. Affected children appear normal at birth, but skin hyperelasticity, fragility of the skin and blood vessels, delayed wound healing, and joint hypermobility (Fig. 658-7) develop. The essential defect is a quantitative deficiency of fibrillar collagen. Ehlers-Danlos syndrome has been reclassified into 6 clinical forms.

Classical (COL5a1, COL5a2, COL1a1 Genes) [Previously EDS Type I–Gravis, EDS Type II–Mitis]. This autosomal dominant disorder is characterized by premature birth caused by rupture of membranes, skin hyperelasticity and fragility, easy bruising, generalized and severe joint hypermobility, scoliosis, and mitral valve prolapse. Insignificant lacerations may form gaping wounds that leave broad, atrophic, papyraceous scars. Additional cutaneous manifestations include molluscoid pseudotumors over pressure points from accumulations of connective tissue. Life expectancy is not reduced.

Hypermobile (COL3A1) [Previously EDS Type III]. This disorder has autosomal dominant inheritance and is manifested as generalized severe joint hypermobility and minimal skin manifestations. Musculoskeletal pain is common and osteoarthritis may develop prematurely.

Vascular (COL3A1) [Previously EDS Type IV–Arterial Ecchymotic]. This autosomal dominant disorder shows the most pronounced dermal thinning of all. Consequently, the underlying venous network is prominent. The skin has minimal hyperextensibility, and the joints are not hypermobile, except perhaps during childhood. Premature birth, extensive ecchymoses from trauma, a high incidence of keloids, rupture of the bowel especially the colon, uterine rupture during pregnancy, rupture of the great vessels, dissecting aortic aneurysm, and stroke all contribute to the increased morbidity and shortened life span. Patients should be advised to avoid becoming pregnant, avoid activities such as trumpet playing that raise intracranial pressure as a result of a Valsalva maneuver, and minimize trauma to the skin.

Kyphoscoliosis (Lysyl Hydroxylase [PLOD Gene] Deficiency) [Previously EDS Type VI]. Patients with this autosomal recessive type have joint hyperextensibility, hypotonia, kyphoscoliosis, fragile cornea, keratoconus, skin hyperelasticity, and fragile bones. Prenatal diagnosis is available by measuring lysyl hydroxylase activity in amniocytes. The diagnosis can also be confirmed by detecting decreased lysyl hydroxylase activity in cultured dermal fibroblasts.

Arthrochalasia (COLA1A-Type A, COL1A2-Type B) [Previously EDS Type VIIA and B–Arthrochalasis Multiplex Congenita]. The A type is an autosomal dominant disorder characterized by short stature, marked joint hyperextensibility and dislocation, and moderate hyperelasticity and bruisability of skin. The B type is autosomal dominant and is characterized by skin hyperelasticity and marked joint hypermobility.

Dermatospraxis (Type 1 Collagen N-Peptidase) [Previously EDS Type VIIC]. This autosomal recessive condition includes premature rupture of membranes; delayed closure of fontanels; skin fragility and laxity; easy bruisability; growth retardation; short limbs; umbilical hernia; and characteristic facies with micrognathia, jowls, and prominent, puffy eyelids.

Differential Diagnosis. Ehlers-Danlos syndrome has been confused with cutis laxa, but the features of the two disorders differ considerably. The skin of patients with cutis laxa hangs in redundant folds, whereas the skin in Ehlers-Danlos syndrome is hyperextensible and snaps back into place when stretched. Because of the marked skin fragility in Ehlers-Danlos syndrome, minor trauma results in ecchymoses, bleeding, and poor healing with atrophic cigarette-paper scars, which are most prominent on the forehead and lower legs, and over pressure points. Surgical procedures are fraught with risk; dehiscence of wounds is common.

PSEUDOXANTHOMA ELASTICUM. This is a primary disorder of elastic tissue. Four types have been delineated with considerable clinical crossover between the types.

Clinical Manifestations. **Type I autosomal dominant** (ADCC6 gene) has extensive flexural disease, severe retinal disease leading to blindness, and coronary artery disease. **Type I autosomal recessive** (ADCC6 gene) has flexural skin disease and milder retinal disease. They may have hypertension and gastrointestinal bleeding. **Type II autosomal dominant** disease is generally benign and characterized primarily by skin changes. Eye findings are mild and vascular disease is rare. Hyperextensible joints, blue sclerae, and a high arched palate may be seen. **Type II autosomal recessive** disease has severe skin laxity without systemic signs involvement.

Onset of skin manifestations often occurs during childhood, but the changes produced by early lesions are subtle and may not be recognized. The characteristic **pebbly "plucked chicken skin" cutaneous lesions** are 1–2 mm, asymptomatic, yellow papules that are arranged in a linear or reticulated pattern or in confluent plaques. Preferred sites are the flexural neck (Fig. 658-8), axillary and inguinal folds, umbilicus, thighs, and antecubital and popliteal fossas. As the lesions become more pronounced, the skin acquires a velvety texture and droops in lax, inelastic folds. The face is usually spared. Mucous membrane lesions may involve the lips, buccal cavity, rectum, and vagina. There is involvement of the connective tissue of the media, and intima of blood vessels, Bruch membrane of the eye, and endocardium or pericardium may result in visual disturbances, angioid streaks in Bruch membrane, intermittent claudication, cerebral and coronary occlusion, hypertension, and hemorrhage from the gastrointestinal tract, uterus, or mucosal surfaces. Affected women have an increased risk of miscarriage in the 1st trimester. Arterial involvement generally presents in adulthood, but claudication and angina have occurred in early childhood. There is no effective treatment, although laser therapy may help to prevent retinal hemorrhage.

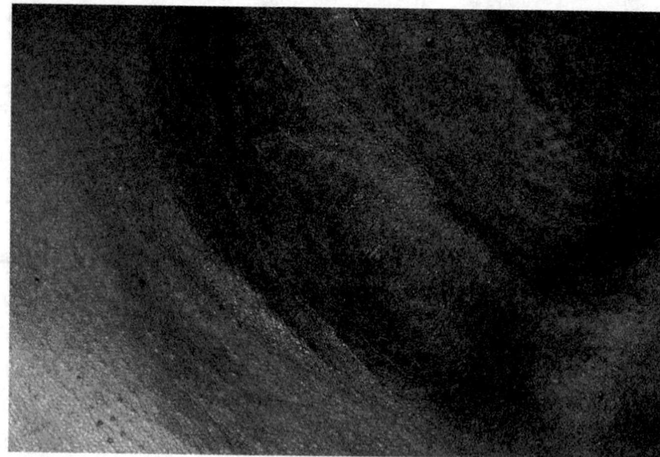

Figure 658-8. Confluent plaque of pebbly skin in pseudoxanthoma elasticum.

Pathology and Pathogenesis. Histopathologic examination shows fragmented, swollen, and clumped elastic fibers in the middle and lower third of the dermis. The fibers stain positively for calcium. Collagen in the vicinity of the altered elastic fibers is reduced in amount and is split into small fibers. Aberrant calcification of the elastic fibers of the internal elastic lamina of arteries leads to narrowing of vessel lumina.

ELASTOSIS PERFORANS SERPIGINOSA. This is an unusual skin disorder in which 1–3 mm, firm, skin-colored, keratotic papules tend to cluster in arcuate and annular patterns on the posterolateral neck and limbs (Fig. 658-9) and, occasionally, on the face and trunk. Onset usually occurs in childhood or adolescence. A papule consists of a circumscribed area of epidermal hyperplasia that communicates with the underlying dermis by a narrow channel. Elastotic material is extruded from the channel. There is a great increase in the amount and size of elastic fibers in the upper dermis, particularly in the dermal papillae. The primary abnormality is probably in the dermal elastin, which provokes a cellular response that ultimately leads to extrusion of the abnor-

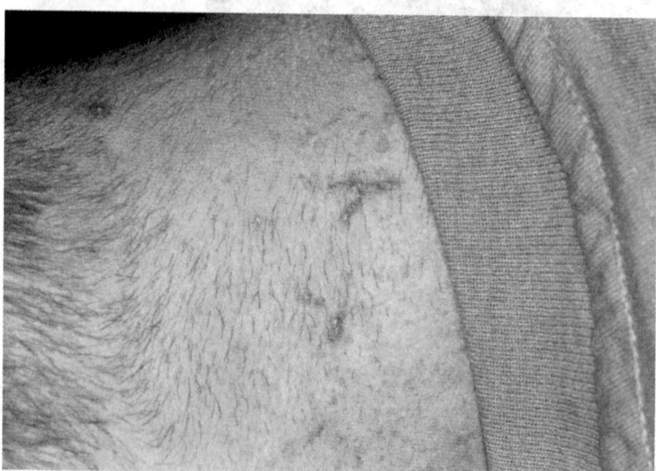

Figure 658-9. Arcuate keratotic papule of elastosis perforans serpiginosa.

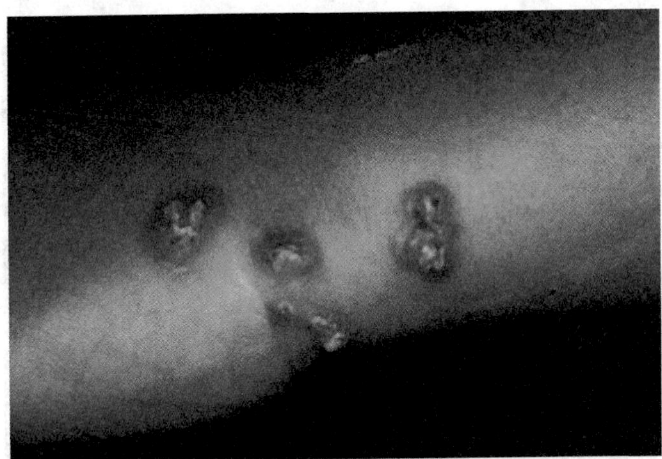

Figure 658-10. Hyperkeratotic papules in reactive perforating collagenosis.

Figure 658-11. Ivory-colored papules on the upper back in Hunter syndrome.

mal elastic tissue. Approximately 30% occur in association with osteogenesis imperfecta, Marfan syndrome, pseudoxanthoma elasticum, Ehlers-Danlos syndrome, Rothmund-Thomson syndrome, and Down syndrome. It has also occurred in association with penicillamine therapy. Differential diagnosis includes tinea corporis, perforating granuloma annulare, reactive perforating collagenosis, lichen planus, creeping eruption, and porokeratosis of Mibelli. Treatment is ineffective; however, the lesions are asymptomatic and disappear spontaneously.

REACTIVE PERFORATING COLLAGENOSIS. This usually presents in early childhood with small papules on the dorsal areas of the hands and forearms, elbows, knees, and, sometimes, face and trunk. The condition is often familial and may be inherited in an autosomal recessive pattern. Over a period of several weeks, the papules increase in size to 5–10 mm, become umbilicated, and develop a keratotic plug in the center (Fig. 658-10). Individual lesions resolve spontaneously in 2–4 mo, leaving a hypopigmented macule or scar. Lesions may recur in crops; may undergo a linear Koebner reaction; and may form in response to cold temperatures or superficial trauma such as abrasions, insect bites, and acne lesions. Collagen in the papillary dermis is engulfed within a cup-shaped perforation in the epidermis. The central crater contains pyknotic inflammatory cells and keratinous debris. The process appears to represent transepidermal elimination of altered collagen. Topical retinoic acid may reduce the number of lesions.

XANTHOMAS (SEE CHAPTER 86).

FABRY DISEASE (SEE CHAPTER 86).

MUCOPOLYSACCHARIDOSES (SEE ALSO CHAPTER 88). In several of these disorders, thick, rough, inelastic skin, particularly on the extremities, and generalized hirsutism are characteristic but nonspecific features. Telangiectasias on the face, forearms, trunk, and legs have been observed in Scheie and Morquio syndromes. In some patients with Hunter syndrome, ivory-colored, distinctive firm papulonodules with a corrugated surface texture are grouped into symmetric plaques on the upper trunk (Fig. 658-11), arms, and thighs. Onset of these unusual lesions occurs in the 1st decade of life, and spontaneous disappearance has been noted.

MASTOCYTOSIS. Mastocytosis encompasses a spectrum of disorders that range from solitary cutaneous nodules to diffuse infiltration of skin associated with involvement of other organs (Table 658-1). All the disorders are characterized by aggregates of mast cells in the dermis. Stem cell factor (mast cell growth factor), which can be secreted by keratinocytes, stimulates the proliferation of mast cells and increases the production of melanin by melanocytes. Mastocytosis may be due to altered cutaneous metabolism of mast cell growth factor and, thus, may represent a hyperplastic rather than a neoplastic disorder.

Clinical Manifestations. Affected children can have intense pruritus. Systemic signs of histamine release, such as hypotension, syncope, headache, episodic flushing, tachycardia, wheezing, colic, and diarrhea, occur most frequently in the more severe types of mastocytosis. Flushing is by far the most common symptom seen. The local and systemic manifestations of the disease are due, at least partially, to release of histamine and heparin from mast cell granules; although heparin is present in significant amounts in mast cells, coagulation disturbances occur only rarely. The vasodilator prostaglandin D_2 or its metabolite appears to exacerbate the flushing response. Serum trypase levels are often elevated.

Mastocytomas are solitary lesions 1–5 cm in diameter. Lesions may be present at birth or arise in early infancy at any site. The lesions may present as recurrent, evanescent wheals or bullae; in time, however, an infiltrated, pink, yellow, or tan, rubbery plaque

TABLE 658-1. Mastocytosis Classification*

CUTANEOUS MASTOCYTOSIS
1. Urticaria pigmentosa
Classic infantile type
Chronic with SCF mutations
2. Diffuse cutaneous mastocytosis
3. Mastocytoma of the skin
SYSTEMIC MASTOCYTOSIS (WITHOUT AHNMD OR LEUKEMIC MAST CELL DISEASE)
1. Systemic indolent mastocytosis
2. Systemic smoldering mastocytosis
SYSTEMIC MASTOCYTOSIS WITH AN AHNMD
1. Myeloproliferative syndrome
2. Myelodysplastic syndrome
3. Acute myeloid leukemia
4. Non-Hodgkin lymphoma
SYSTEMIC AGGRESSIVE MASTOCYTOSIS
MAST CELL LEUKEMIA
MAST CELL SARCOMA
EXTRACUTANEOUS MASTOCYTOMA

*Classification adopted from World Health Organization classification.
AHNMD, associated hematologic non-mast cell disorder.
Adapted from Carter MC, Metcalfe DD: Paediatric mastocytosis. *Arch Dis Child* 2002;86:315–319.

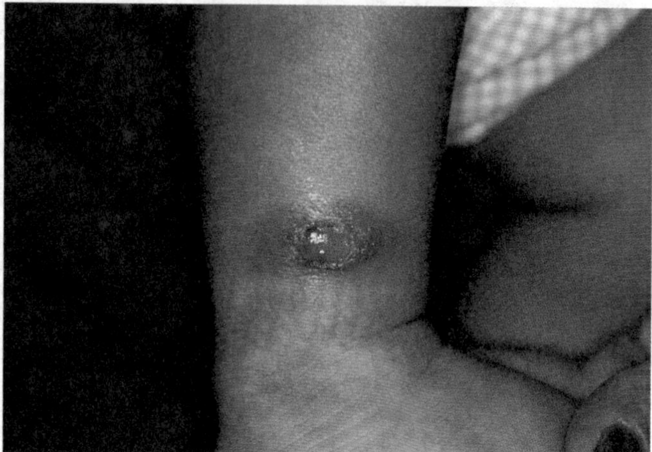

Figure 658-12. Solitary mastocytoma that is partially blistered.

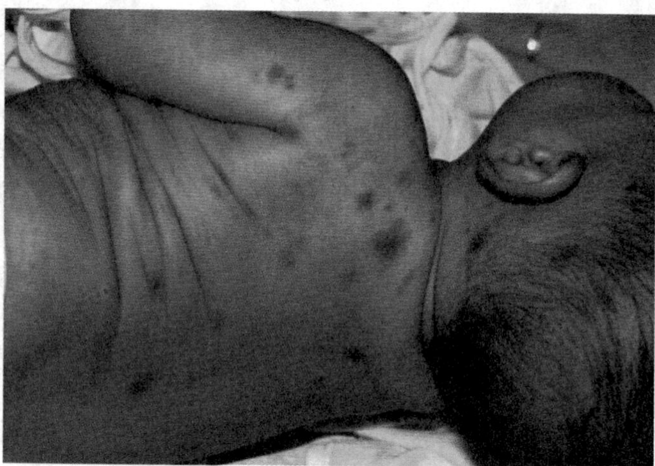

Figure 658-13. Hyperpigmented papular lesions of urticaria pigmentosa.

develops at the site of whealing or blistering (Fig. 658-12). The surface acquires a pebbly, orange peel–like texture, and hyperpigmentation may become prominent. Stroking or trauma to the nodule may result in urtication (Darier sign) as a result of local histamine release; rarely, systemic signs of histamine release become apparent. Pharmacologic agents may exacerbate symptoms (Table 658-2). The **differential diagnosis** includes recurrent bullous impetigo, nevi, and juvenile xanthogranuloma. Mastocytomas involute spontaneously in early childhood. Troublesome lesions can be treated with superpotent topical steroids to decrease symptoms. Only rarely do multiple cutaneous lesions develop.

Urticaria pigmentosa is the most common form of mastocytosis. There are two types of urticaria pigmentosa. In classic infantile urticaria pigmentosa, lesions may be present at birth but more often erupt in crops in the 1st several months to 2 yr of age. New lesions seldom arise after age 3–4 yr. In some cases, early bullous or urticarial lesions fade, only to recur at the same site, ultimately becoming fixed and hyperpigmented. In others, the initial lesions are hyperpigmented. Vesiculation usually abates by 2 yr of age. Individual lesions range in size from a few mm to several cm and may be macular, papular, or nodular. They range in color from yellow-tan to chocolate brown and often have ill-defined borders (Fig. 658-13). Larger nodular lesions, like mastocytomas, may have a characteristic orange-peel texture. Lesions of urticaria pigmentosa may be sparse or numerous and are often symmetrically distributed. Palms, soles, and face are sometimes spared, as are the mucous membranes. The rapid appearance of erythema and whealing in response to vigorous stroking of a lesion can usually be elicited; dermographism of intervening normal skin is also common. The 2nd type of urticaria pigmentosa may begin any time from infancy to adulthood. This type of urticaria pigmentosa does not resolve and new lesions continue to develop throughout life. This type is associated with mutations in stem cell factor. These patients are the population that may develop systemic involvement.

TABLE 658-2. Pharmacological Agents and Physical Stimuli That May Exacerbate Mast Cell Mediator Release in Patients with Mastocytosis

IMMUNOLOGICAL STIMULI
Venoms (IgE mediated bee venom)
Complement derived anaphylatoxins
Biological peptides (substance P, somatostatin)
Polymers (dextran)
NONIMMUNOLOGICAL STIMULI
Physical stimuli (extreme temperature, friction, sunlight)
Drugs
Acetylsalicylic acid and related non-steroidal analgesics*
Thiamine
Ketorolac tromethamine
Alcohol
Narcotics (codeine, morphine)*
Radiographic dyes (iodine containing)

*Appears to be a problem in <10% of patients.
From Carter MC, Metcalfe DD: Paediatric mastocytosis. *Arch Dis Child* 2002;86:315–319.

Urticaria pigmentosa can be confused with drug eruptions, postinflammatory pigmentary change, juvenile xanthogranuloma, pigmented nevi, ephelides, xanthomas, chronic urticaria, insect bites, and bullous impetigo.

Prognosis. Spontaneous involution occurs in all patients with classical infantile urticaria pigmentosa. The incidence of systemic manifestations in these patients is very low. The continued development of lesions past the age of 4 yr implies chronic disease with stem cell factor mutation and higher risk for systemic involvement.

DIFFUSE CUTANEOUS MASTOCYTOSIS. This variant is characterized by diffuse involvement of the skin rather than discrete hyperpigmented lesions. Affected patients are usually normal at birth and develop features of the disorder after the 1st few months of life. Rarely, the condition may present with intense generalized pruritus in the absence of visible skin changes. The skin usually appears thickened and pink to yellow and may have a doughy feel and a texture resembling an orange peel. Surface changes are accentuated in flexural areas. Recurrent bullae (Fig. 658-14), intractable pruritus, and flushing attacks are common, as is systemic involvement. It is also likely to be caused by a mutation in stem cell factor that is different from that of chronic urticaria pigmentosa. Ultraviolet (UV)A-1 or psoralen with UVA (PUVA) treatment may be required to control symptoms.

Telangiectasia macularis eruptiva perstans is another variant that consists of telangiectatic hyperpigmented macules that are usually localized to the trunk. These lesions do not urticate when stroked. This form of the disease is seen primarily in adolescents and adults.

SYSTEMIC MASTOCYTOSIS. This disorder is marked by an abnormal increase in the number of mast cells in other than cutaneous tissues. It occurs in ≈5–10% of patients with mutated stem cell factor related mastocytosis and is more common in adults than in children. Bone lesions may be silent but are detectable radiologically as osteoporotic or osteosclerotic areas, principally in the axial skeleton. Gastrointestinal tract involvement may produce diarrhea and steatorrhea. Mucosal infiltrates may be detectable by barium studies or by small bowel biopsy. Peptic ulcers also occur. Hepatosplenomegaly as a result of mast cell infiltrates and fibrosis has been described, as has mast cell proliferation in lymph

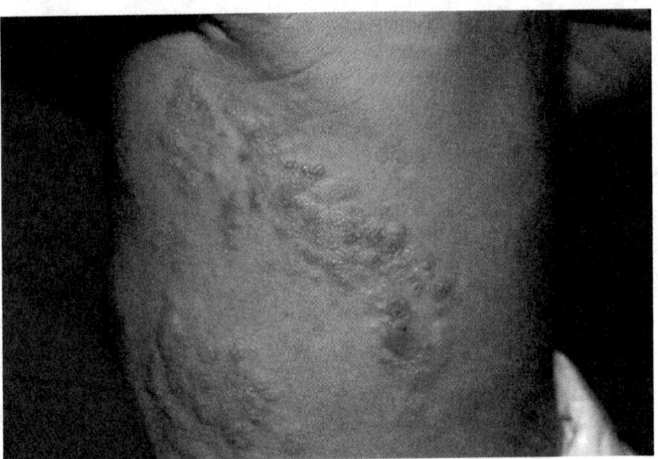

Figure 658-14. Severe blistering in diffuse cutaneous mastocytosis.

nodes, kidneys, periadrenal fat, and bone marrow. Abnormalities in the peripheral blood, such as anemia, leukocytosis, and eosinophilia, are noted in approximately ⅓ of patients. Mast cell leukemia may occur.

Treatment. Flushing can be precipitated by excessively hot baths, vigorous rubbing of the skin, and certain drugs, such as codeine, aspirin, morphine, atropine, ketorolac, alcohol, tubocurarine, iodine-containing radiographic dyes, and polymyxin B (see Table 658-2). Avoidance of these triggering factors is advisable. For patients who are symptomatic, oral antihistamines may be palliative. H_1 receptor antagonists (hydroxyzine) are the initial drugs of choice for systemic signs of histamine release. If H_1 antagonists are unsuccessful, H_2 receptor antagonists may be helpful in controlling pruritus or gastric hypersecretion. Superpotent topical steroids are of benefit in controlling skin urtication and blistering. Oral mast cell–stabilizing agents, such as cromolyn sodium or ketotifen, may also be effective for diarrhea or abdominal cramping and some systemic symptoms such as headache or muscle pain.

Bercovitch L, Terry P: Pseudoxanthoma elasticum 2004. *J Am Acad Dermatol* 2004;51:S13–S14.

Carter MC, Metcalfe DD: Paediatric mastocytosis. *Arch Dis Child* 2002;86:315–319.

Chan I: The role of extracellular matrix protein 1 in human skin. *Clin Exp Dermatol* 2004;29:52–56.

Kelly AP: Medical and surgical therapies for keloids. *Dermatol Ther* 2004;17:212–218.

Renaud-Vilmer C, Cavelier-Balloy B, Porcher R, et al: Vulvar lichen sclerosis: Effect of long-term topical application of a potent steroid on the course of the disease. *Arch Dermatol* 2004; 140:709–712.

Valent P, Sperr WR, Schwartz LB, et al: Diagnosis and classification of mast cell proliferative disorders: Delineation from immunologic diseases and non-mast cell hematopoetic neoplasms. *J Allergy Clin Immunol* 2004;114:3–11.

Chapter 659 ■ Diseases of Subcutaneous Tissue

Joseph G. Morelli

Diseases involving the subcutis are usually characterized by necrosis and/or inflammation; they may occur either as a primary event or as a secondary response to various stimuli or disease processes. These disorders cannot be distinguished by their histopathologic changes, which may reflect the stage of the lesion at the time of biopsy. The principal diagnostic criteria are the appearance and distribution of the lesions, associated symptoms, results of laboratory studies, and the natural history and exogenous provocative factors of these conditions.

Figure 659-1. Localized fat atrophy with overlying erythema post steroid injection.

CORTICOSTEROID-INDUCED ATROPHY. Injection of a corticosteroid intradermally can produce deep atrophy accompanied by surface pigmentary changes and telangiectasia (Fig. 659-1). These changes occur ≈2 wk after injection and may last for months. The deltoid area is most susceptible to this complication.

PANNICULITIS. Inflammation of fibrofatty subcutaneous tissue may primarily involve the fat lobule or, alternatively, the fibrous septum that compartmentalizes the fatty lobules. Lobular panniculitis that spares the subcutaneous vasculature includes post-steroid panniculitis, lupus erythematosus profundus, pancreatic panniculitis, α_1-antitrypsin deficiency, subcutaneous fat necrosis of the newborn, sclerema neonatorum, cold panniculitis, subcutaneous sarcoidosis, and factitial panniculitis. Lobar panniculitis with vasculitis occurs in erythema induratum and, occasionally, as a feature of Crohn disease (see Chapter 333.2). Inflammation predominantly within the septum, sparing the vasculature, may be seen in erythema nodosum (Table 659-1 and Fig. 659-2), necrobiosis lipoidica, progressive systemic sclerosis (see Chapter 159), and subcutaneous granuloma annulare (see Chapter 656). Septal panniculitis that includes inflammation of the vessels is found primarily in leukocytoclastic vasculitis and polyarteritis nodosa (see Chapter 166).

TABLE 659-1. Etiology of Erythema Nodosum

VIRUSES
Epstein-Barr, hepatitis B, mumps
FUNGI
Coccidioidomycosis, histoplasmosis
BACTERIA AND OTHER INFECTIOUS AGENTS
Group A streptococcus,* tuberculosis,* *Yersinia*, cat scratch disease, leprosy, leptospirosis, tularemia, mycoplasma, Whipple disease, lymphogranuloma venereum, psittacosis
OTHER
Sarcoidosis, inflammatory bowel disease,* estrogen-containing oral contraceptives,* systemic lupus erythematosus, Behçet syndrome, severe acne, Hodgkin disease, lymphoma, sulfonamides, bromides, Sweet syndrome, pregnancy

*Common.

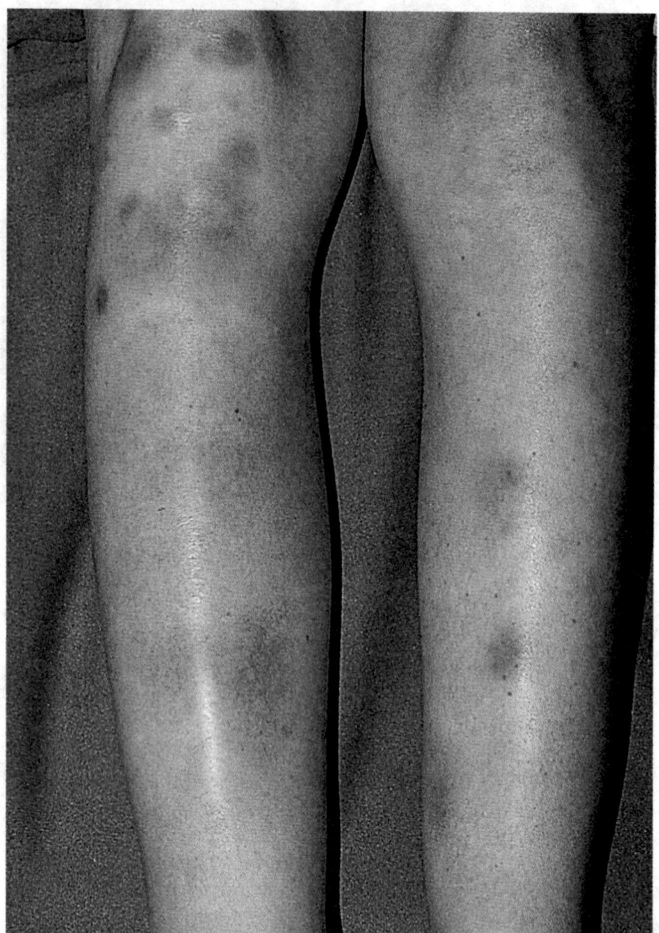

Figure 659-2. Tender red nodules with indistinct borders in a teenage girl with erythema nodosum. (From Weston AL, Lane AT, Morelli JG: *Color Textbook of Pediatric Dermatology,* 3rd ed. St. Louis, Mosby, 2002, p 212.)

Poststeroid panniculitis has been observed in children who received high-dose corticosteroids orally for relatively short periods. In 1–2 wk after discontinuation of the drug, multiple subcutaneous nodules may appear on the cheeks, trunk, and arms. Nodules range in size from 0.5 to 4 cm, are erythematous or skin colored, and may be pruritic. The mechanism of the inflammatory reaction in the fat is unknown. **Treatment** is unnecessary because the lesions remit spontaneously over a period of months without scarring.

Lupus erythematosus profundus (lupus erythematosus panniculitis) presents with 1 to several firm, well-defined, purple plaques or nodules 1 to 3 cm in diameter, most commonly on the face, buttocks, or proximal extremities. This condition may occur in patients with systemic or discoid lupus erythematosus and may precede or follow the development of other cutaneous lesions. The overlying skin is usually normal but may be erythematous, atrophic, poikilodermatous, or hyperkeratotic (Fig. 659-3). Lesions may be painful and may ulcerate. On healing, a shallow depression generally remains or, rarely, soft pink areas of anetoderma result. The histopathologic changes are distinctive and may allow the clinician to make the diagnosis in the absence of other cutaneous lesions of lupus erythematosus. The lupus band and antinuclear antibody test results are usually positive. Nodules tend to be persistent. Antimalarial agents (hydroxychloroquine) are the **treatment of choice.** Intralesional corticosteroids may worsen the residual lipoatrophy. Immunosuppresive agents are indicated only for treatment of other severe manifestations of systemic lupus erythematosus (SLE). Avoidance of sun exposure and trauma is also important.

α_1-Antitrypsin deficiency may present with cellulitis-like areas or tender, red nodules on the trunk or proximal extremities (see Chapter 390). Nodules tend to ulcerate spontaneously and discharge an oily yellow fluid. Trauma is an inciting factor in some patients. Affected individuals have severe homozygous deficiency or rarely a partial deficiency of the protease inhibitor α_1-antitrypsin, which inhibits trypsin activity and the activity of elastase, serine proteases, collagenase, factor VIII, and kallikrein. Panniculitis may be associated with other manifestations of the disease such as panacinar emphysema, noninfectious hepatitis, cirrhosis, persistent cutaneous vasculitis, cold-contact urticaria, or acquired angioedema. Diagnosis can be substantiated by a decreased level of serum α_1-antitrypsin activity. Some patients respond to dapsone or infusion of random-donor-derived α_1-protease inhibitor concentrate.

Pancreatic panniculitis presents most commonly on the pretibial regions, thighs, or buttocks as tender, erythematous nodules that may be fluctuant and occasionally discharge an oily yellowish substance. It presents most often in males with alcoholism but may also occur in patients with pancreatitis as a result of cholelithiasis or abdominal trauma, with rupture of a pancreatic pseudocyst, with pancreatic ductal adenocarcinoma, or with pancreatic acinar cell carcinoma. Associated features may include arthropathy and synovitis, particularly in the ankles; eosinophilia; polyserositis; and painful osteolytic bone lesions with medullary necrosis. Microscopic changes consist of multiple foci of fat necrosis that contain ghost cells with thick, shadowy walls and no nuclei. A polymorphous inflammatory infiltrate surrounds the areas of fat necrosis. Pathogenesis of the panniculitis appears to be multifactorial, involving liberation of the lipolytic enzymes lipase, trypsin, and amylase into the circulation, causing adipocyte membrane damage and intracellular lipolysis. There is no correlation, however, between the occurrence of panniculitis and the serum concentration of pancreatic enzymes.

Subcutaneous fat necrosis is an inflammatory disorder of adipose tissue that occurs primarily in the 1st 4 wk of life in full-term or post-term infants. Affected infants may have a history of perinatal asphyxia or a difficult labor and delivery. Typical lesions are asymptomatic, rubbery to firm, erythematous to violaceous plaques or nodules on the cheeks, buttocks, back, thighs, or upper arms (Fig. 659-4). Lesions may be focal or extensive and are generally asymptomatic, although they may be tender during the acute phase. Histopathologic changes are diagnostic and consist of necrosis of fat; a granulomatous cellular infiltrate composed of lymphocytes, histiocytes, multinucleated giant cells, and fibroblasts; and radially arranged clefts of crystalline triglyceride within fat cells and multinucleated giant cells. Calcium deposits

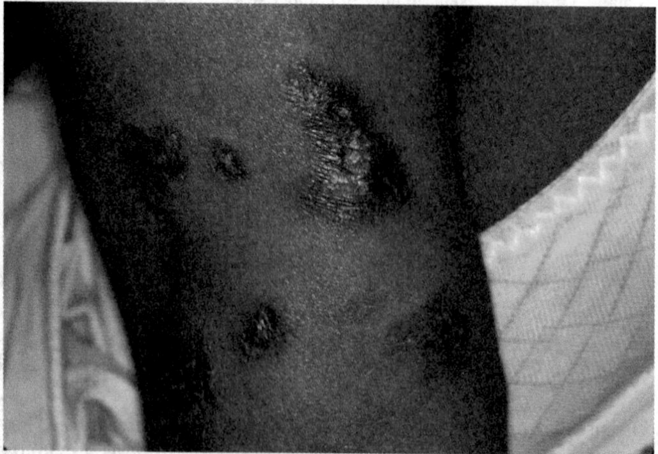

Figure 659-3. Deep nodule of lupus profundus with overlying hyperkeratotic lesion of DLE.

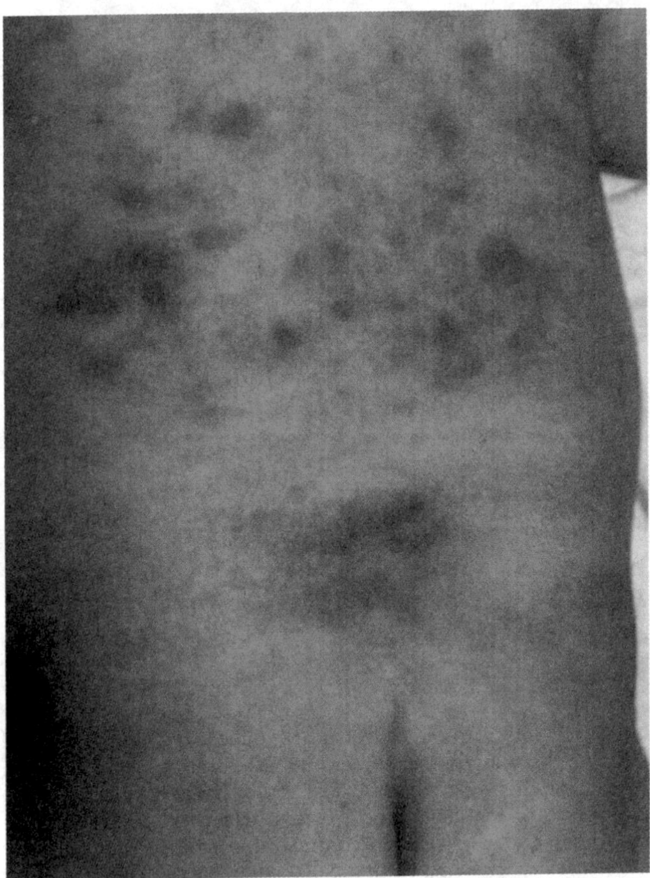

Figure 659-4. Red-purple nodular infiltration of skin of back caused by subcutaneous fat necrosis.

are commonly found in areas of fat necrosis. Subcutaneous fat necrosis in infants may be due to ischemic injury under various circumstances such as maternal preeclampsia, birth trauma, asphyxia, and prolonged hypothermia; in many affected infants, however, no provocative factors are identified. Susceptibility has been attributed to differences in composition between the subcutaneous tissue of young infants and that of older infants, children, and adults. Neonatal fat solidifies at a relatively high temperature because of its relatively greater concentration of high melting point saturated fatty acids such as palmitic and stearic acids.

Uncomplicated lesions involute spontaneously within weeks to months, usually without scarring or atrophy. Calcium deposition may occasionally occur within areas of fat necrosis, and this may sometimes result in rupture and drainage of liquid material. A rare but potentially life-threatening complication is **hypercalcemia.** This presents at 1–6 mo of age with lethargy, poor feeding, vomiting, failure to thrive, irritability, seizures, shortening of the QT interval, or renal failure. The origin of the hypercalcemia is unknown. Subcutaneous fat necrosis can be confused with sclerema neonatorum, panniculitis, cellulitis, or hematoma. Because the lesions are self-limited, therapy is not required for uncomplicated cases. Needle aspiration of fluctuant lesions may prevent rupture and subsequent scarring. Treatment of hypercalcemia is aimed at enhancing renal calcium excretion by hydration and furosemide administration and at limiting dietary calcium and vitamin D intake. Reduction of intestinal calcium absorption and alteration of vitamin D metabolism may be accomplished by administration of corticosteroids.

Sclerema neonatorum is an uncommon disorder of adipose tissue that presents abruptly in preterm, gravely ill infants as diffuse, yellowish-white woody induration of the skin. Affected skin becomes stony in consistency, cold, and nonpitting. The face assumes a masklike expression, and joint mobility may be compromised because of inflexibility of the skin. Histopathologic changes in sclerema neonatorum consist of an increase in the size of fat cells and an increase in the width of the fibrous connective tissue septa. In contrast to subcutaneous fat necrosis, with which it is most apt to be confused, fat necrosis, inflammation, giant cells, and calcium crystals are generally absent. Sclerema neonatorum is almost always associated with serious illness, such as sepsis, congenital heart disease, multiple congenital anomalies, or hypothermia. The appearance of sclerema in a sick infant should be regarded as an ominous prognostic sign. The outcome depends on the response of the underlying disorder to treatment.

Cold panniculitis may result in localized lesions in infants after prolonged cold exposure, especially on the cheeks, or after prolonged application of a cold object such as an ice cube, ice bag, or popsicle to any area of the skin. Ill-defined, erythematous to bluish, indurated plaques or nodules arise within hours to a couple days of exposure, persist for 2–3 wk, and heal without residua. Recurrence of the lesions is common, emphasizing the importance of parental education in treating these patients. Histopathologic examination reveals an infiltrate of lymphoid and histiocytic cells around blood vessels at the dermal-subdermal junction; by the 3rd day, some of the fat cells in the subcutis may have ruptured and coalesced into cystic structures. Cold panniculitis may be confused with facial cellulitis caused by *Haemophilus influenzae* type b. Unlike buccal cellulitis, the area may be cold to the touch, and the patient is afebrile and appears well. **Chilblains (pernio)**, a condition of acute or chronic cold injury, is characterized by localized symmetric erythematous to purplish edematous plaques and nodules in areas exposed to cold, typically acral areas (distal hands and feet, ears, face) [see Chapter 75]. Lesions develop 12–24 hr after cold exposure and may be associated with itching, burning, or pain. Blister formation and ulceration are rare. Vasospasm of arterioles due to cold exposure with resultant hypoxemia and localized perivascular mononuclear inflammation appears to be responsible for the disease. Frostbite due to extreme cold exposure is painful and, histopathologically, involves the epidermis, dermis, and subcutaneous fat. The pathogenic mechanism of cold panniculitis may be similar to that of subcutaneous fat necrosis, involving an increased propensity of fat to solidify in infants compared with that in older children and adults as a result of the higher percentage of saturated fatty acids in the subcutaneous fat of infants.

Factitial panniculitis results from subcutaneous injection by self or proxy of a foreign substance, the most common types of which include organic materials such as milk or feces; drugs such as the opiates or pentazocine; oily materials such as mineral oil or paraffin; and the synthetic polymer povidone. Indurated plaques, ulcers, or nodules that liquefy and drain may be noted clinically. The histopathology is variable, depending on the injected substance, but may include the presence of birefringent crystals, oil cysts surrounded by fibrosis and inflammation, and an acute inflammatory reaction with fat necrosis. Vessels are characteristically spared.

LIPODYSTROPHY. Several rare conditions are associated with loss of fatty tissue in a partial or generalized distribution.

Partial Lipodystrophy. Partial lipodystrophy may be familial or acquired. Loss of adipose tissue is not preceded by an inflammatory phase, and histopathologic examination reveals only absence of subcutaneous fat.

There are 3 forms of familial partial lipodystrophy (FPLD).

Type I (FPLD1-Kobberling) is characterized by loss of adipose tissue confined to the extremities and gluteal region. Fat distribution of the face, neck, and trunk may be normal or increased. Hyperlipidemia, insulin-resistant diabetes mellitus, and eruptive xanthomas may be seen. The gene is unknown, but only females are affected.

Type 2 (FPLD2-Dunnigan) is caused by mutations in the laminin A/C gene. Fat distribution is normal in childhood, but atrophy commences with puberty. Lipodystrophy is seen in the trunk, gluteal region, and extremities. Adipose tissue accumulates in the face and neck and may also be seen in the axillae, back, labia majora, and infra-abdominal region. Insulin-resistant diabetes mellitus and hypertriglyceridemia develop, but high-density lipoprotein and cholesterol levels are low. Both males and females are affected, but the diagnosis may be more difficult in males due to body habitus.

Type 3 (FPLD3) is caused by mutations in the peroxisome proliferation–activated receptor gamma (PPARG) gene. Lipodystrophy is seen in the limbs and gluteal region. Insulin-resistant diabetes mellitus, primary amenorrhea, acanthosis nigricans, hypertension, and fatty infiltration of the liver are present.

Acquired partial lipodystrophy (Barraquer-Simons syndrome) is rare. Females are more commonly affected. Fat loss begins in childhood or adolescence and affects the face, neck, arms, thorax, and upper abdomen. Excess fat is seen in the hips and legs, especially in females. Low levels of C3 are almost universally seen. C3 nephritic factor is also present. C3 nephritic factor stabilizes C3 convertase, allowing for unopposed activation of the alternate complement pathway and the decreased level of C3. Membranous proliferative glomerulonephritis and other autoimmune diseases may develop. Insulin-resistant diabetes mellitus is rare.

GENERALIZED LIPODYSTROPHY. Generalized lipodystrophy may also be congenital or acquired.

Congenital generalized lipodystrophy is seen in 2 forms.

Type 1 (Berardinelli-Seip congenital lipodystrophy type 1 [BSCL1]) is an autosomal recessive disorder caused by mutations in the 1-acylglycerol-3-phosphate-O-acyltransferase (AGPAT2) gene

Type 2 (Berardinelli-Seip congenital lipodystrophy type 2 [BSCL2]) is also autosomal recessive and caused by mutations in the seipin gene.

Marked lipodystrophy occurs at birth or in early infancy. Diabetes mellitus, hypertriglycidemia, hepatic steatosis, acanthosis nigricans, and muscular hypertrophy occur. BSCL2 is a more severe phenotype, with premature death occurring in ≈ 15%.

Acquired generalized lipodystrophy is also more common in females. Twenty-five per cent of patients present with an inflammatory panniculitis; 25% with an associated autoimmune disease, usually juvenile dermatomyositis; and the remaining half have neither. Fat loss begins in early childhood or adolescence and affects the majority of the body. Affected children are noted to have a voracious appetite. Acanthosis nigricans and hepatic steatosis develop in most patients, with 20% progressing to cirrhosis.

Localized lipoatrophy is an idiopathic condition that presents as annular atrophy at the ankles, a bandlike semicircular depression 2–4 cm in diameter on the thighs or, rarely, on the abdomen and upper groin as a centrifugally spreading, depressed, bluish plaque with an erythematous margin. It occurs predominantly in Japanese children.

Insulin lipoatrophy usually occurs ≈ 6 mo–2 yr after initiation of relatively high doses of insulin. A dimple or well-circumscribed depression at the site of injection is typically seen, although loss of fat may extend beyond the site of injection, leading to an extensive, depressed plaque. Biopsy reveals a marked decrease or absence of subcutaneous tissue, without inflammation or fibrosis. In some patients, hypertrophy occurs clinically. In these cases, the mid-dermal collagen is replaced by hypertrophic fat cells on histopathologic sections. The mechanism of insulin lipoatrophy may be cross reaction of insulin antibodies with fat cells; the incidence of this condition has decreased since the implementation of widespread use of highly purified insulins. Lesions may also be prevented by frequent alteration of injection sites.

Garg A: Acquired and inherited lipodystrophies. *N Engl J Med* 2004;350:1220–1234.

McBean J, Sable A, Maude J, et al: Alpha1-antitrypsin deficiency panniculitis. *Cutis* 2003;71:205–209.

Ng PP, Tan SH, Tan T: Lupus erythematosus panniculitis: A clinicopathologic study. *Int J Dermatol* 2002;41:88–90.

Tran JT, Sheth AP: Complications of subcutaneous fat necrosis of the newborn: A case report and review of the literature. *Pediatr Dermatol* 2003;20:257–261.

Van der Zee JA, van Hillegersberg R, Toonstra J, et al: Subcutaneous nodules pointing towards pancreatic disease: Pancreatic panniculitis. *Dig Surg* 2004;21:275–276.

Wimmershoff MB, Hohenleutner U, Landthaler M: Discoid lupus erythematosus and lupus profundus in childhood: Report of two cases. *Pediatr Dermatol* 2003;20:140–145.

Chapter 660 ■ Disorders of the Sweat Glands

Joseph G. Morelli

Eccrine glands are found over nearly the entire skin surface and provide the primary means, through evaporation of the water in sweat, for cooling the body. These glands have no anatomic relationship to hair follicles and secrete a relatively large amount of odorless aqueous sweat. In contrast, apocrine sweat glands are limited in distribution to the axillae, anogenital skin, mammary glands, ceruminous glands of the ear, Moll glands in the eyelid, and selected areas of the face and scalp. The apocrine gland duct enters the pilosebaceous follicle at the level of the infundibulum and secretes a small amount of a complex, viscous fluid that, on alteration by microorganisms, produces a distinctive body odor. Some disorders of these two sweat glands are similar pathogenetically, whereas others are unique to a given gland.

ANHIDROSIS. Neuropathic anhidrosis results from a disturbance in the neural pathway from the control center in the brain to the peripheral efferent nerve fibers that activate sweating. Disorders in this category, which are characterized by generalized anhidrosis, include tumors of the hypothalamus and damage to the floor of the 3rd ventricle. Pontine or medullary lesions may produce anhidrosis of the ipsilateral face or neck and ipsilateral or contralateral anhidrosis of the rest of the body. Peripheral or segmental neuropathies, caused by leprosy, amyloidosis, diabetes mellitus, alcoholic neuritis, or syringomyelia, may be associated with anhidrosis of the innervated skin. Various autonomic disorders are also associated with altered eccrine sweat gland function.

At the level of the sweat gland, anticholinergics (drugs such as atropine and scopolamine) may paralyze the sweat glands. Acute intoxication with barbiturates or diazepam has produced necrosis of sweat glands, resulting in anhidrosis with or without erythema and bullae. Eccrine glands are largely absent throughout the skin or are present in a localized area among patients with **anhidrotic ectodermal dysplasia** or **localized congenital absence** of sweat glands, respectively. Infiltrative or destructive disorders that may produce atrophy of sweat glands by pressure or scarring include scleroderma, acrodermatitis chronica atrophicans, radiodermatitis, burns, Sjögren syndrome, multiple myeloma, and lymphoma. Obstruction of sweat glands may occur in miliaria and in a number of inflammatory and hyperkeratotic disorders such as the ichthyoses, psoriasis, lichen planus, pemphigus, porokeratosis, atopic dermatitis, and seborrheic dermatitis. Occlusion of the sweat pore may also occur with the topical agents aluminum and zirconium salts, formaldehyde, or glutaraldehyde.

Diverse disorders that are associated with anhidrosis by unknown mechanisms include dehydration; toxic overdose with lead, arsenic, thallium, fluorine, or morphine; uremia; cirrhosis; endocrine disorders such as Addison disease, diabetes mellitus, diabetes insipidus, or hyperthyroidism; and inherited conditions such as Fabry disease, Franceschetti-Jadassohn syndrome, which combines features of incontinentia pigmenti and anhidrotic ectodermal dysplasia, and familial anhidrosis with neurolabyrinthitis.

Whereas anhidrosis may be complete, in many cases, what appears clinically to be anhidrosis is actually **hypohidrosis** caused by anhidrosis of many but not all eccrine glands. Compensatory, localized hyperhidrosis of the remaining functional sweat glands may occur, particularly in diabetes mellitus and miliaria. The primary complication of anhidrosis is **hyperthermia**, seen primarily in anhidrotic ectodermal dysplasia or in otherwise normal preterm or full-term neonates who have immature eccrine glands.

HYPERHIDROSIS. The numerous disorders that may be associated with increased production of eccrine sweat may also be classified into those with neural mechanisms involving an abnormality in the pathway from the neural regulatory centers to the sweat gland and those that are non-neurally mediated by direct effects on the sweat glands (Table 660-1). Excessive sweating of the palms and soles in response to emotional stimuli (volar hyperhidrosis) and axillary sweating may respond to 20% aluminum chloride in anhydrous ethanol applied under occlusion for several hours, iontophoresis, injection with botulinum toxin, therapy with oral anticholinergics, or in severe, refractory cases, cervicothoracic or lumbar sympathectomy.

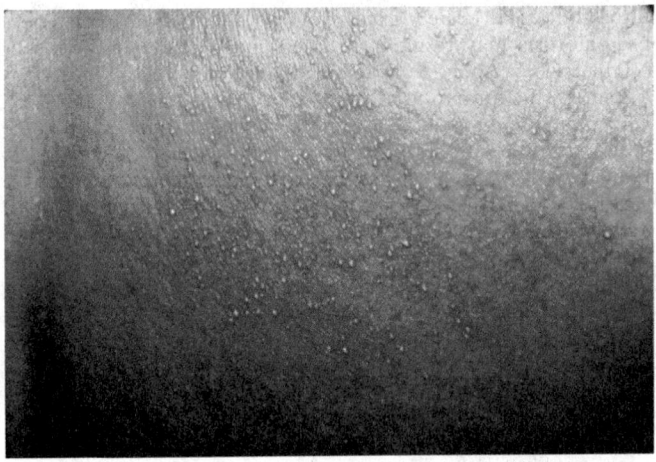

TABLE 660-1. Causes of Hyperhidrosis

CORTICAL	**Vasomotor**
Emotional	Cold injury
Familial dysautonomia	Raynaud phenomenon
Congenital ichthyosiform erythroderma	Rheumatoid arthritis
Epidermolysis bullosa	**Neurologic**
Nail-patella syndrome	Abscess
Jadassohn-Lewandowsky syndrome	Familial dysautonomia
Pachyonychia congenita	Postencephalitic
Palmoplantar keratoderma	Tumor
HYPOTHALAMIC	**Miscellaneous**
Drugs	Chédiak-Higashi syndrome
Antipyretics	Compensatory
Emetics	Phenylketonuria
Insulin	Pheochromocytoma
Meperidine	Vitiligo
Exercise	**MEDULLARY**
Infection	Physiologic gustatory sweating
Defervescence	Encephalits
Chronic illness	Granulosis rubra nasi
Metabolic	Syringomyelia
Debility	Thoracic sympathetic trunk injury
Diabetes mellitus	**SPINAL**
Hyperpituitarism	Cord transection
Hyperthyroidism	Syringomyelia
Hypoglycemia	**CHANGES IN BLOOD FLOW**
Obesity	Maffucci syndrome
Porphyria	Arteriovenous fistula
Pregnancy	Klippel-Trenaunay syndrome
Rickets	Glomus tumor
Infantile scurvy	Blue rubber bleb nevus syndrome
Cardiovascular	
Heart failure	
Shock	

Figure 660-1. Superficial clear vesicles of miliaria crystallina.

MILIARIA. This results from retention of sweat in occluded eccrine sweat ducts as a result of a keratinous plug in the sweat duct. Retrograde pressure may result in rupture of the duct and leakage of sweat into the epidermis and/or the dermis. The eruption is most often induced by hot, humid weather, but it may also be caused by high fever. Infants who are dressed too warmly may develop this eruption indoors, even during the winter.

In **miliaria crystallina**, asymptomatic, noninflammatory, pinpoint clear vesicles may suddenly erupt in profusion over large areas of the body surface, leaving brawny desquamation on healing (Fig. 660-1). The clarity of the fluid, superficiality of the vesicles, and absence of inflammation permit differentiation from other blistering disorders. This type of miliaria occurs most frequently in newborn infants because of the relative immaturity and delayed patency of the sweat duct and the tendency for infants to be nursed in relatively warm, humid conditions. It may also occur in older patients with hyperpyrexia. Histopathologically, an intracorneal or subcorneal vesicle is seen in communication with the sweat duct.

Miliaria rubra is a less superficial eruption characterized by erythematous, minute papulovesicles that may impart a prickling sensation. The lesions are usually localized to sites of occlusion or to flexural areas, such as the neck, groin, and axillae, where friction may have a role in their pathogenesis. Involved skin may become macerated and eroded. This lesion may be confused with or superimposed on other diaper area eruptions, including candidosis and folliculitis. Lesions of miliaria rubra, however, are extrafollicular. Histopathologically, one sees focal areas of spongiosis and spongiotic vesicle formation in close proximity to sweat ducts that generally contain a keratinous plug. The keratinous plug does not form, however, until the later stages of the disease and, therefore, does not appear to be the primary cause of sweat duct obstruction. The initial obstruction is postulated to be due to swelling of the ductal epidermal cells, perhaps from imbibition of water. Repeated attacks of miliaria rubra may lead to **miliaria profunda**, which is due to rupture of the sweat duct deeper in the skin at the level of the dermal-epidermal junction. Severe, extensive miliaria rubra or miliaria profunda may result in disturbance of heat regulation. Lesions of miliaria rubra may become infected, particularly in malnourished or debilitated infants, leading to development of **periporitis staphylogenes**, which involves extension of the process from the sweat duct into the sweat gland.

All forms of miliaria respond dramatically to cooling the patient by regulation of environmental temperatures and by removal of excessive clothing; administration of antipyretics is also beneficial to patients with fever. Topical agents are usually ineffective and may exacerbate the erution.

BROMHIDROSIS. The excessive odor that characterizes bromhidrosis may result from alteration of either apocrine or eccrine sweat. Apocrine bromhidrosis develops after puberty as a result of the formation of short-chain fatty acids and ammonia by the action of anaerobic diphtheroids on axillary apocrine sweat. Eccrine bromhidrosis is caused by microbiologic degradation of stratum corneum that has become softened by excessive eccrine sweat. The soles of the feet and the intertriginous areas are the primary affected sites. **Treatments** that may be helpful include cleansing with germicidal soaps, topical clindamycin or erythromycin, or topical application of aluminum, zirconium, or zincsalts. Topical aluminum chloride preparations are particularly useful for plantar eccrine bromhidrosis. Hyperhidrosis, warm weather, obesity, intertrigo, and diabetes mellitus are predisposing factors.

HIDRADENITIS SUPPURATIVA. This is a chronic, inflammatory, suppurative disorder of the apocrine glands in the axillae, the anogenital area, and, occasionally, the scalp, posterior aspect of the ears, female breasts, and periumbilical area. Onset of clinical manifestations, sometimes preceded by pruritus or discomfort, usually occurs during puberty or early adulthood. Solitary or multiple painful erythematous nodules, deep abscesses, and contracted scars are sharply confined to areas of skin containing apocrine glands. When the disease is severe and chronic, sinus tracts, ulcers, and thick, linear fibrotic bands develop. Hidradenitis suppurativa tends to persist for many years, punctuated by relapses and partial remissions. Complications include cellulitis, ulceration, and burrowing abscesses that may perforate adjacent structures, forming fistulas to the urethra, bladder, rectum, or peritoneum. Episodic inflammatory arthritis develops in some patients. A minority of patients have the follicular occlusion triad, which includes acne and perifolliculitis capitis. Early lesions are often mistaken for infected epidermal cysts, furuncles, scrofuloderma, actinomycosis, cat scratch disease, granuloma inguinale, or lymphogranuloma venereum. Sharp localization to areas of the body that bear apocrine glands, however, should suggest hidradenitis. When involvement is limited to the anogenital region, the condition may be difficult to distinguish from Crohn disease.

Early lesions are characterized by a keratinous plug in the apocrine duct or hair follicle orifice and by cystic distention of the follicle. The process generally but not necessarily extends into the apocrine gland. Later changes include inflammation within and around apocrine glands and the presence of groups of cocci within apocrine glands and in the adjacent dermis. Scarring may obliterate skin appendages. The disease is probably initiated by plugging of apocrine gland ducts with keratinous debris. Bacterial infection, particularly with *Staphylococcus aureus, Streptococcus milleri, Escherichia coli,* and possibly anaerobic streptococci, appears to be important in the progressive dilatation below the obstruction, leading to rupture of the duct, inflammation, sinus tract formation, and destructive scarring. Pathogenesis of hidradenitis suppurativa is controversial.

Patients should be counseled to avoid tight-fitting clothes, because occlusion may exacerbate the condition. **Treatment** with topical antibiotic agents such as chlorhexidine, erythromycin, or clindamycin or with topical retinoids may be effective in early, indolent disease. Systemic antibiotics, chosen on the basis of bacterial culture (usually staphylococcal and streptococcal pathogens) and sensitivity tests, should be administered in the acute phase. Empirical therapy may be initiated with tetracycline, doxycycline, or minocycline if the patient is 8 yr or older; clindamycin and cephalosporins are also effective. Some patients require long-term treatment with tetracycline or erythromycin. Intralesional triamcinolone acetonide (5–10 mg/mL) is often helpful in early disease. The addition of prednisone, 40–60 mg/day for 7–10 days, tapering gradually as inflammation subsides, to the regimen of patients who respond poorly to antibiotics may decrease fibrosis and scarring. Oral contraceptive agents, which contain a high estrogen-to-progesterone ratio and low androgenicity of the progesterone, or oral retinoids may be helpful in some patients. Warm compresses encourage spontaneous rupture of abscesses; those that are "pointing" should be incised and drained. Surgical measures may be required for control or cure.

FOX-FORDYCE DISEASE. This disease is most common in females and presents during puberty or the 3rd decade of life with pruritus in the axillae and, occasionally, in the anogenital region and around the breasts. Pruritus is exacerbated by emotional stress and stimuli that induce apocrine sweating. Dome-shaped, skin-colored to slightly hyperpigmented, follicular papules develop in the pruritic areas. Histopathologically, one sees keratinous plugging of the distal apocrine duct, rupture of the intraepidermal portion of the apocrine duct, paraductal microvesicle formation, and paraductal acanthosis. The condition generally remits during pregnancy, particularly in the 3rd trimester. Oral contraceptive pills and topical corticosteroids or retinoic acid may help some patients.

Boer A: Patterns histopathologic of Fox-Fordyce disease. *Am J Dermatopathol* 2004;26:482–492.

Cheshire WP, Freeman R: Disorders of sweating. *Semin Neurol* 2003;23:399–406.

Kamada A, Saga K, Jimbow K: Apoeccrine sweat obstruction as a cause of Fox-Fordyce disease. *J Am Acad Dermatol* 2003;48:453–455.

Chapter 661 ■ Disorders of Hair

Joseph G. Morelli

Disorders of hair in infants and children may be due to intrinsic disturbances of hair growth, underlying biochemical or metabolic defects, inflammatory dermatoses, or structural anomalies of the hair shaft. Excessive and abnormal hair growth is referred to as hypertrichosis or hirsutism. **Hypertrichosis** is excessive hair growth at inappropriate locations; hirsutism is an androgen-dependent male pattern of hair growth in women. **Hypotrichosis** is deficient hair growth. Hair loss, partial or complete, is called alopecia. Alopecia may be classified as nonscarring or scarring; the latter type is rare in children and, if present, is most often due to prolonged or untreated inflammatory conditions such as pyoderma or tinea capitis.

HYPERTRICHOSIS

Hypertrichosis is rare in children and may be localized or generalized and permanent or transient. Hypertrichosis has many causes, some of which are listed in Table 661-1.

HYPOTRICHOSIS AND ALOPECIA

Some of the disorders associated with hypotrichosis and alopecia are listed in Table 661-2. True alopecia is rarely congenital; it is more often related to an inflammatory dermatosis, mechanical factors, drug ingestion, infection, endocrinopathy, nutritional disturbance, or disturbance of the hair cycle. Any inflammatory condition of the scalp, such as atopic dermatitis or seborrheic dermatitis, if severe enough, may result in partial alopecia; hair

TABLE 661-1. Causes of and Conditions Associated with Hypertrichosis

INTRINSIC FACTORS
Racial and familial forms such as hairy ears, hairy elbows, intraphalangeal hair, or generalized hirsutism
EXTRINSIC FACTORS
Local trauma
Malnutrition
Anorexia nervosa
Long-standing inflammatory dermatoses
Drugs
Diazoxide, phenytoin, corticosteroids, Cortisporin, cyclosporine, androgens, anabolic agents, hexachlorobenzene, minoxidil, psoralens, penicillamine, streptomycin
HAMARTOMAS OR NEVI
Congenital pigmented nevocytic nevus, nevus pilosus, Becker nevus, congenital smooth muscle hamartoma, fawn-tail nevus associated with diastematomyelia
ENDOCRINE DISORDERS
Virilizing ovarian tumors, Cushing syndrome, acromegaly, hyperthyroidosm, hypothyroidism, congenital adrenal hyperplasia, adrenal tumors, gonadal dysgenesis, male pseudohermaphroditism, non-endocrine hormone–secreting tumors, polycystic ovary syndrome
CONGENITAL AND GENETIC DISORDERS
Hypertrichosis lanuginosa, mucopolysaccharidosis, leprechaunism, congenital generalized lipodystrophy, de Lange syndrome, trisomy 18, Rubinstein-Taybi syndrome, Bloom syndrome, congenital hemihypertrophy, gingival fibromatosis with hypertrichosis, Winchester syndrome, lipoatrophic diabetes (Lawrence-Seip syndrome), fetal hydantoin syndrome, fetal alcohol syndrome, congenital erythropoietic or variegate porphyria (sun-exposed areas), porphyria cutanea tarda (sun-exposed areas), Cowden syndrome, Seckel syndrome, Gorlin syndrome, partial trisomy 3q, Ambra syndrome

growth returns to normal if the underlying condition is treated successfully, unless the hair follicle has been permanently damaged.

Hair loss in childhood should be divided into 4 categories: congenital diffuse; congenital localized; acquired diffuse; and acquired localized.

Acquired localized hair loss is the most common type of hair loss seen in childhood. Three conditions—traumatic alopecia, alopecia areata, tinea capitis—are predominantly seen.

TRAUMATIC ALOPECIA (TRACTION ALOPECIA, HAIR PULLING, TRICHOTILLOMANIA)

TRACTION ALOPECIA. Traction alopecia is due to trauma to hair follicles from tight braids or ponytails, headbands, rubber bands, curlers, or rollers (Fig. 661-1). Broken hairs and inflammatory follicular papules in circumscribed patches at the scalp margins are characteristic and may be subtended by regional lymphadenopathy. Children and parents must be encouraged to avoid devices that cause trauma to the hair and, if necessary, to alter the hairstyle. Otherwise, scarring of hair follicles may occur.

TABLE 661-2. Disorders Associated with Alopecia and Hypotrichosis

Congenital total alopecia: isolated autosomal recessive abnormality, progeria, hidrotic ectodermal dysplasia, Moynahan syndrome, atrichia with keratin cysts, Baraitser syndrome
Congenital localized alopecia: aplasia cutis, alopecia triangularis, epidermal nevus, hair follicle hamartoma, facial hemiatrophy (Romberg syndrome), male pattern baldness
Hereditary hypotrichosis: hypotrichosis with keratosis pilaris, Marie-Unna syndrome, phenylketonuria, arginosuccinic aciduria, hyperlysinemia, homocystinuria, orotic aciduria, Cockayne syndrome, Rothmund-Thomson syndrome, dyskeratosis congenita, Seckel syndrome, cartilage-hair hypoplasia, Conradi syndrome, pachyonychia congenita, Hallermann-Streiff syndrome, Treacher Collins syndrome, oculodentodigital, orofaciodigital, incontinentia pigmenti, focal dermal hypoplasia, keratosis follicularis, epidermolysis bullosa, ectodermal dysplasias, ichthyoses, loose anagen hair
Diffuse alopecia of endocrine origin: hypopituitarism, hypothyroidism, hypoparathyroidism, hyperthyroidism, diabetes mellitus
Alopecia of nutritional origin: marasmus, kwashiorkor, iron deficiency, zinc deficiency (acrodermatitis enteropathica), gluten-sensitive enteropathy, essential fatty acid deficiency, biotinidase deficiency
Disturbances of the hair cycle: telogen effluvium
Toxic alopecia: anagen effluvium
Autoimmune alopecia: alopecia areata
Traumatic alopecia: traction alopecia, trichotillomania
Cicatricial alopecia: lupus erythematosus, lichen planus pilaris, pseudopelade, scleroderma, dermatomyositis, infection (kerion, favus, tuberculosis, syphilis, folliculitis, leishmaniasis, herpes zoster, varicella), acne keloidalis, follicular mucinosis, cicatricial pemphigoid, lichen sclerosus et atrophicus, sarcoidosis
Hair shaft abnormalities: monilethrix, pili annulati, pili torti, trichorrhexis invaginata, trichorrhexis nodosa, woolly hair syndrome, Menkes disease, trichothiodystrophy, trichodento-osseous syndrome, trichorhinophalangeal syndrome, uncombable hair syndrome (spun glass hair, pili trianguli et canaliculi)

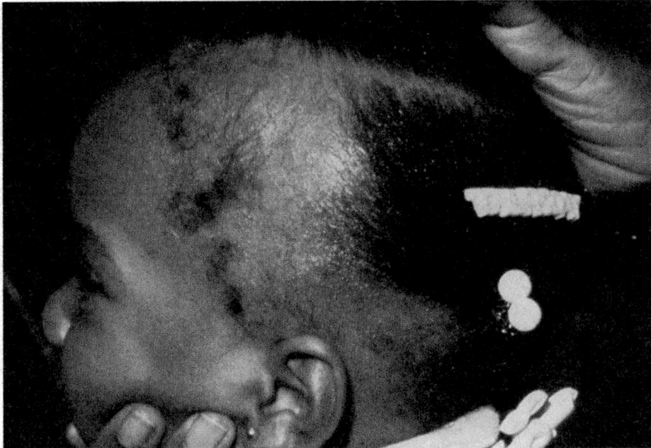

Figure 661-1. Traction alopecia.

HAIR PULLING. Hair pulling in childhood is usually an acute reactional process related to emotional stress. It may also be seen in trichotillomania and as part of more severe psychiatric disorders.

TRICHOTILLOMANIA. Compulsive pulling, twisting, and breaking of hair produces irregular areas of incomplete hair loss, most often on the crown and in the occipital and parietal areas of the scalp. Occasionally, eyebrows, eyelashes, and body hair are traumatized. Some plaques of alopecia may have a linear outline. The hairs remaining within the areas of loss are of various lengths (Fig. 661-2) and are typically blunt tipped because of breakage. The scalp usually appears normal, although hemorrhage, crusting (Fig. 661-3), and chronic folliculitis may also occur. Trichophagy, resulting in **trichobezoars,** may complicate this disorder. The lifetime occurrence is 3% in girls and 1% in boys.

The *Diagnostic and Statistical Manual of Mental Disorders* diagnostic criteria include visible hair loss attributable to pulling; mounting tension preceding hair pulling; gratification or release of tension after hair pulling; and absence of hair pulling attributable to hallucinations, delusions, or an inflammatory skin

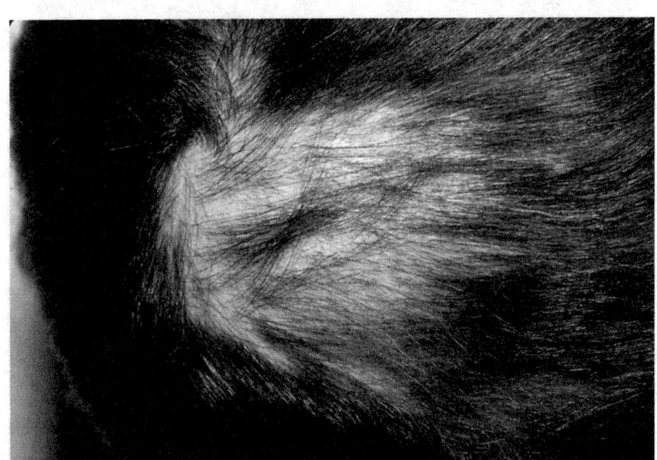

Figure 661-2. Hair pulling. Hairs broken off at various lengths.

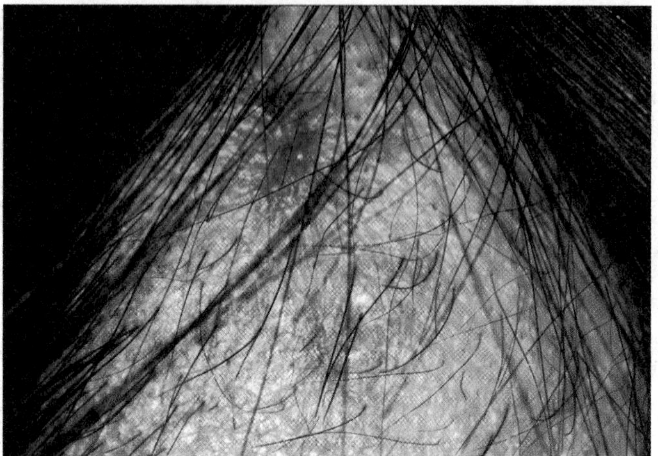

Figure 661-3. Hemorrhage and crusting secondary to hair pulling.

Figure 661-5. Alopecia totalis. Total loss of scalp hair.

condition. Histologic changes include coexistent normal and damaged follicles, perifollicular hemorrhage, atrophy of some follicles, and catagen transformation of hair. In late stages, perifollicular fibrosis may occur. Long-term repeated trauma may result in irreversible damage and permanent alopecia. Acute reactional hair pulling, tinea capitis, and alopecia areata must be considered in the differential diagnosis.

Trichotillomania is closely related to obsessive-compulsive disorder and may be an expression of it for some children. When trichotillomania occurs secondary to **obsessive-compulsive disorder**, clornipramine, fluoxetine, or trazodone may be helpful, particularly when combined with behavioral interventions.

ALOPECIA AREATA. Alopecia areata is characterized by rapid and complete loss of hair in round or oval patches on the scalp (Fig. 661-4) and on other body sites. In alopecia totalis, all the scalp hair is lost (Fig. 661-5); alopecia universalis involves all body and scalp hair. The lifetime incidence of alopecia areata is 1% of the population. Over half of patients are younger than 20 yr of age.

Clinical Manifestations. Hair loss is usually seen in well-defined circles. The skin within the plaques of hair loss appears normal. A perifollicular infiltrate of inflammatory round cells is found in biopsy specimens from active areas. Alopecia areata is associated with atopy; nail changes such as pits (Fig. 661-6), ridges, opacification, serration of the free nail edge, dystrophy, and a red lunula; cataracts or lens opacification; and **autoimmune diseases** such as Hashimoto thyroiditis, Addison disease, pernicious anemia, ulcerative colitis, myasthenia gravis, collagen vascular diseases, and vitiligo. An increased incidence of alopecia areata has been reported in patients with Down syndrome (5–10%).

Etiology. The cause of alopecia areata is unknown. Emotional factors and stress have been suggested as triggering factors, but supportive evidence is tenuous. About 10–20% of patients have a family history of alopecia areata. The infrequent but striking association with autoimmune diseases has suggested an autoimmune pathogenesis. Some patients have serum antibodies to thyroglobulin, parietal cells, and adrenal glands; autoantibodies to hair follicle antigens have been demonstrated.

Differential Diagnosis and Prognosis. Tinea capitis, seborrheic dermatitis, trichotillomania, traumatic alopecia, and lupus erythematosus should be considered. The course is unpredictable, but spontaneous resolution in 6–12 mo is usual, particularly when relatively small, stable patches of alopecia are present. Recurrences are common. Onset at a young age, extensive or prolonged hair loss, numerous episodes, and associated atrophy are usually poor prognostic signs. Alopecia universalis, totalis, and ophiasis (Fig. 661-7), a type of alopecia areata in which hair loss is circumferential, are also less likely to resolve.

Treatment. This is difficult to evaluate because the course is erratic and unpredictable. The use of high-potency topical fluorinated corticosteroids with occlusion at night is effective in some patients. Intradermal injections of steroid may also stimulate hair growth locally, but this mode of treatment is impractical in young children or in those with extensive hair loss. Systemic cortico-

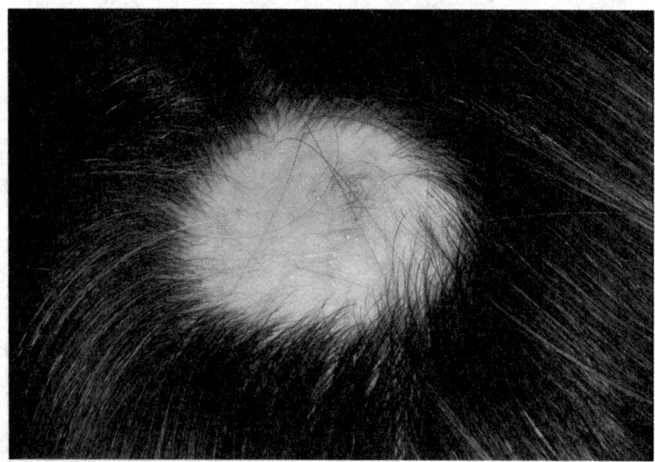

Figure 661-4. Circular patch of alopecia areata with normal appearing scalp.

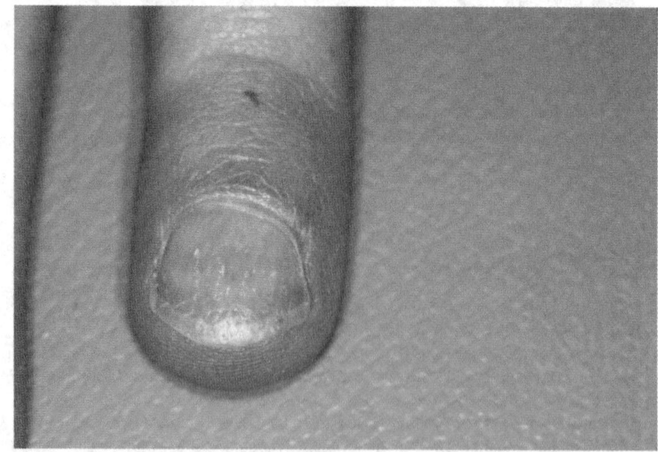

Figure 661-6. Multiple nail pits in alopecia areata.

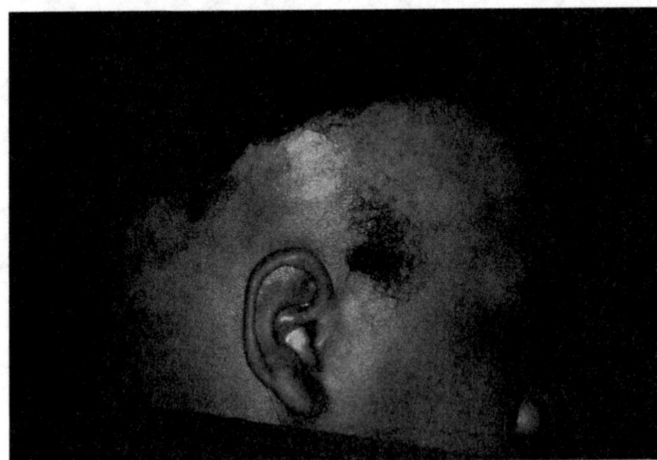

Figure 661-7. Ophiasis pattern of alopecia areata.

steroid therapy has, on occasion, been associated with good results; the permanence of cure is questionable, and the side effects are a serious deterrent. Additional therapies that are sometimes effective include short contact anthralin, topical minoxidil, and contact sensitization with squaric acid dibutylester or diphencyprone. In general, parents and patients can be reassured that spontaneous remission usually occurs. New hair growth may initially be of finer caliber and lighter color, but replacement by normal terminal hair can be expected.

ACQUIRED DIFFUSE HAIR LOSS

TELOGEN EFFLUVIUM. Telogen effluvium presents with sudden loss of large amounts of hair, often with brushing, combing, and washing of hair. Diffuse loss of scalp hair occurs from premature conversion of growing, or anagen hairs, which normally constitute 80–90% of hairs, to resting, or telogen, hairs. Hair loss is noted 6 wk–3 mo after the precipitating cause, which may include childbirth; a febrile episode; surgery; acute blood loss, including blood donation; sudden severe weight loss; discontinuation of high dose corticosteroids or oral contraceptives; and psychiatric stress. Telogen effluvium also accounts for the loss of hair by infants in the 1st few months of life; friction from bed sheets, particularly in infants with pruritic, atopic skin, may exacerbate the problem. There is no inflammatory reaction; the hair follicles remain intact, and telogen bulbs can be demonstrated microscopically on shed hairs. Because >50% of the scalp hair is rarely involved, alopecia is usually not severe. Parents should be reassured that normal hair growth will return within ≈ 6 mo.

TOXIC ALOPECIA (ANAGEN EFFLUVIUM). Anagen effluvium is an acute, severe, diffuse inhibition of growth of anagen follicles, resulting in loss of >80–90% of scalp hair. Hairs become dystrophic, and the hair shaft breaks at the narrowed segment. Loss is diffuse, rapid (1–3 wk after treatment), and temporary, as regrowth occurs after the offending agent is discontinued. Causes of anagen effluvium include radiation; cancer chemotherapeutic agents such as antimetabolites, alkylating agents, and mitotic inhibitors; thallium; thiouracil; heparin; the coumarins; boric acid; and hypervitaminosis A.

CONGENITAL DIFFUSE HAIR LOSS. This is congenitally thin hair diffusely related to either hypoplasia of hair follicle or to structural defects in the hair shaft.

STRUCTURAL DEFECTS OF HAIR. Structural defects of the hair shaft may be congenital, reflect known biochemical aberrations, or relate to damaging grooming practices. All the defects can be demonstrated by microscopic examination of affected hairs, particularly by scanning and transmission electron microscopy.

TRICHORRHEXIS NODOSA. Congenital trichorrhexis nodosa is an autosomal dominant condition. The hair is dry, brittle, and lusterless, with irregularly spaced grayish-white nodes on the hair shaft. Microscopically, the nodes have the appearance of two interlocking brushes (Fig. 661-8*A*). The defect results from a fracture of the hair shaft at the nodal points caused by disruption of the cells in the hair cortex. Trichorrhexis nodosa has also been

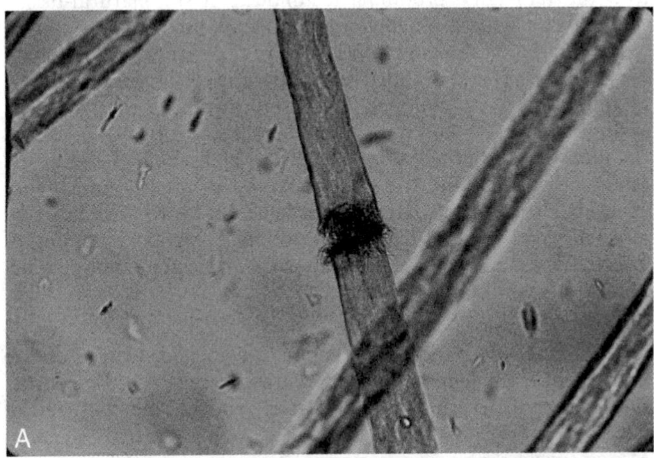

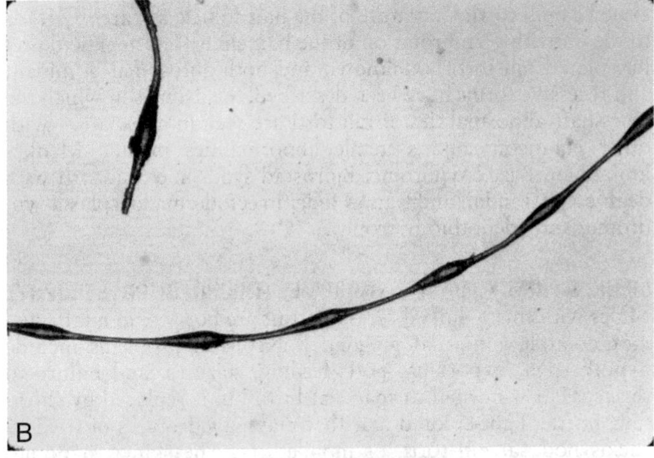

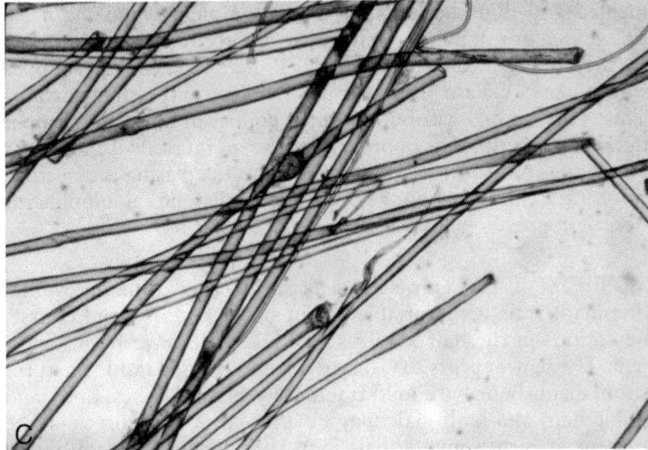

Figure 661-8. *A*, Microscopic hair fracture in trichorrhexis nodosa. *B*, Beading of hair in monilethrix. *C*, Cuplike abnormality of hair in Netherton syndrome.

observed in some infants with Menkes syndrome, trichothiodystrophy, and argininosuccinic aciduria.

Acquired Trichorrhexis Nodosa. This, the most common cause of hair breakage, occurs in two forms. Proximal defects are found most frequently in black children, whose complaint is not of alopecia but of failure of their hair to grow. The hair is short, and longitudinal splits, knots, and whitish nodules can be demonstrated in hair mounts. Easy breakage is demonstrated by gentle traction on the hair shafts. A history of other affected family members may be obtained. The problem may be caused by a combination of genetic predisposition and the cumulative mechanical trauma of rough combing and brushing, hair-straightening procedures, and "permanents." Patients must be cautioned to avoid damaging grooming techniques. A soft natural-bristle brush and a wide-toothed comb should be used. The condition is self-limited, with resolution in 2–4 yr if patients avoid damaging practices. Distal trichorrhexis nodosa is seen more frequently in white and Asian children. The distal portion of the hair shaft is thinned, ragged, and faded; white specks, sometimes mistaken for nits, may be noted along the shaft. Hair mounts reveal the paintbrush defect and the sites of excessive fragility and breakage. Localized areas of the moustache or beard may also be affected. Avoidance of traumatic grooming, regular trimming of affected ends, and the use of cream rinses to lessen tangling ameliorate this condition.

PILI TORTI. These patients present with spangled, brittle, coarse hair of different lengths over the entire scalp. There is a structural defect in which the hair shaft is grooved and flattened at irregular intervals and is twisted on its axis to various degrees. Minor twists that occur in normal hair should not be misconstrued as pili torti. Curvature of the hair follicle apparently leads to the flattening and rotation of the hair shaft. The genetic defect in isolated pili torti is unknown and both autosomal dominant and recessive forms have been described. **Syndromes** in which the hair shaft abnormalities of pili torti are seen in association with other cutaneous and systemic abnormalities include Menkes kinky hair, Bazex syndrome, Bjornstad syndrome (pili torti with deafness), Crandall and Rapp-Hodgkin ectodermal dysplasia syndrome, and trichothiodystrophy.

MENKES KINKY HAIR SYNDROME (TRICHOPOLIODYSTROPHY). Males with this X-linked recessive trait are born to an unaffected mother after a normal pregnancy. Neonatal problems include hypothermia, hypotonia, poor feeding, seizures, and failure to thrive. Hair is normal to sparse at birth but is replaced by short, fine, brittle, light-colored hair that may have features of trichorrhexis nodosa, pili torti, or monilethrix. The skin is hypopigmented and thin cheeks typically appear plump, and the nasal bridge is depressed. Progressive psychomotor retardation is noted in early infancy. Mutations in the ATP7A gene, encoding a copper transporting ATPase protein, cause Menkes kinky hair syndrome. This is due to maldistribution of the copper in the body. Copper uptake across the brush border of the small intestine is increased, but copper transport from these cells into the plasma is defective, resulting in low total body copper stores. Parenteral administration of copper is helpful if begun in the 1st 2 mo of life.

MONILETHRIX. This hair shaft defect is inherited as an autosomal dominant trait with variable age of onset, severity, and course. Mutations in the hair keratins HBI and HB6 have been identified. The hair appears dry, lusterless, and brittle, and it fractures spontaneously or with mild trauma. Eyebrows, lashes, body and pubic hair, and scalp hair may be affected. Monilethrix may be present at birth, but the hair is usually normal at birth and is replaced in the 1st few months of life by abnormal hairs; the condition is sometimes 1st apparent in childhood. Follicular papules may appear on the nape of the neck and the occiput and, occasionally, over the entire scalp. Short, fragile beaded hairs that emerge from the horny follicular plugs give a distinctive appearance. Keratosis pilaris and koilonychia of fingernails and toenails may also be present. Microscopically, a distinctive, regular beading pattern of the hair shaft is evident, characterized by elliptic nodes that are separated by narrower internodes (Fig. 661-8*B*). Not all hairs have nodes, and both normal and beaded hairs may break. Patients should be advised to handle the hair gently to minimize breakage. Treatment is generally ineffective.

TRICHOTHIODYSTROPHY. Hair in trichothiodystrophy is sparse, short, brittle, and uneven; the scalp hair, eyebrows, or eyelashes may be affected. Microscopically, the hair is flattened, folded, and variable in diameter; has longitudinal grooving; and has nodal swellings that resemble those of trichorrhexis nodosa. Under a polarizing microscope, distinctive alternating dark and light bands are seen. The abnormal hair has a cystine content that is <50% of normal because of a major reduction and altered composition of constituent high-sulfur matrix proteins. Trichothiodystrophy may occur as an isolated finding or in association with various syndrome complexes that include intellectual impairment, short stature, ichthyosis, nail dystrophy, dental caries, cataracts, decreased fertility, neurologic abnormalities, bony abnormalities, and immunodeficiency. Some patients are photosensitive and have impaired DNA repair mechanisms, similar to that seen in group D xeroderma pigmentosum; the incidence of skin cancers, however, is not increased. Patients with trichothiodystrophy tend to resemble one another, with a receding chin, protruding ears, raspy voice, and sociable, outgoing personality. Trichoschisis, a fracture perpendicular to the hair shaft, is characteristic of the many syndromes that are associated with trichothiodystrophy. Perpendicular breakage of the hair shaft has also been described in association with other hair abnormalities, particularly monilethrix.

TRICHORRHEXIS INVAGINATA (BAMBOO HAIR). Short, sparse, fragile hair without apparent growth is characteristic of this condition, which is found primarily in association with Netherton syndrome (see Chapter 656). It has also been reported in other ichthyosiform dermatoses. The distal portion of the hair is invaginated into the cuplike proximal portion, forming a fragile nodal swelling (Fig. 661-8*C*).

PILI ANNULATI. Alternate light and dark bands of the hair shaft characterize pili annulati. When viewed under the light microscope, the region of the hair shaft that appeared bright in reflected light instead appears dark in the transmitted light as a result of focal aggregates of abnormal air-filled cavities within the shaft. The hair is not fragile. The defect may be autosomal dominant or sporadic. Pseudopili annulati is a variant of normal blond hair; an optical effect caused by the refraction and reflection of light from the partially twisted and flattened shaft creates the impression of banding.

WOOLLY HAIR DISEASE. This disorder presents at birth with peculiarly tight, curly, abnormal hair in a non-black person. Autosomal dominant and recessive types have been described. Woolly hair nevus, a sporadic form, involves only a circumscribed portion of the scalp hair. The affected hair is fine, tightly curled, and light colored, and it grows poorly. Microscopically, an affected hair is oval and shows twisting of 180 degrees on its axis.

UNCOMBABLE HAIR SYNDROME (SPUN GLASS HAIR). The hair of patients with this syndrome appears disorderly, is often silvery blond (Fig. 661-9), and may break because of repeated, futile efforts to control it. The condition is probably autosomal dominant in inheritance. Eyebrows and eyelashes are normal. A longitudinal depression along the hair shaft is a constant feature,

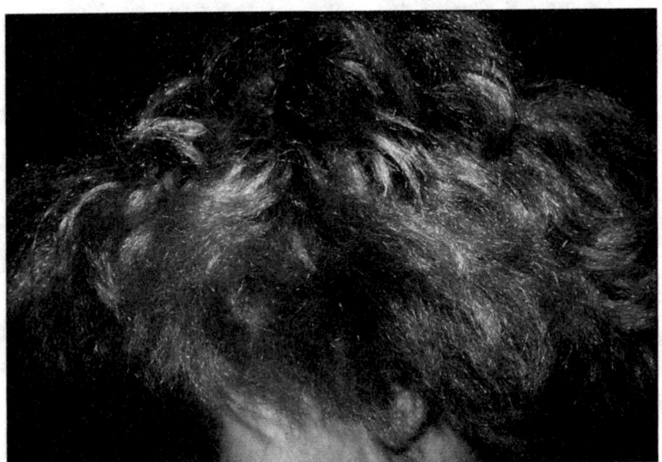

Figure 661-9. Disorderly, silvery blond hair in uncombable hair syndrome.

and most hair follicles and shafts are triangular (pili trianguli et canaliculi). The shape of the hair varies along its length, however, preventing the hairs from lying flat.

Alexis AF, Dudda-Subramanya R, Sinha AA: Alopecia areata: Autoimmune basis of hair loss. *Eur J Dermatol* 2004;14:364–370.

Hantash BM, Schwartz RA: Traction alopecia in children. *Cutis* 2003;71:18–20.

Harrison S, Sinclair R: Optimal management of hair loss (alopecia) in children. *Am J Clin Dermatol* 2003;4:757–770.

Harrison S, Sinclair R: Telogen effluvium. *Clin Exp Dermatol* 2002;27:389–395.

Liang C, Kraemer KH, Morris A: Characterization of tiger tail banding and hair shaft abnormalioties in trichothiodystrophy. *J Am Acad Dermatol* 2005;52:224–232.

Norris D: Alopecia areata: Current state of knowledge. *J Am Acad Dermatol* 2004;51:S16–S17.

Nuss MA, Carlisle D, Hall M, et al: Trichotillomania: A review and case report. *Cutis* 2003;72:191–196.

Tay YK, Levy ML, Metry DW: Trichotillomania in childhood: Case series and review. *Pediatrics* 2004;113:e494–e498.

Wiedemeyeer K, Schill WB, Loser C: Diseases on hair follicles leading to hair loss part I: Nonscarring alopecias. *Skinmed* 2004;3:209–214.

Chapter 662 ■ Disorders of the Nails

Joseph G. Morelli

Nail abnormalities in children may be manifestations of generalized skin disease, skin disease localized to the periungual region, systemic disease, drugs, trauma, or localized bacterial and fungal infections. Nail anomalies are also common in certain congenital disorders (Table 662-1).

ABNORMALITIES IN NAIL SHAPE OR SIZE

Anonychia is absence of the nail plate, usually a result of a congenital disorder or trauma. It may be an isolated finding or may be associated with malformations of the digits. **Koilonychia** is flattening and concavity of the nail plate with loss of normal contour, producing a spoon-shaped nail. Koilonychia occurs as an autosomal dominant trait or in association with iron deficiency anemia, Plummer-Vinson syndrome, or hemochromatosis. The nail plate is relatively thin for the 1st 1–2 yr of life and, consequently, may be spoon-shaped in otherwise normal children.

Congenital nail dysplasia, an autosomal dominant disorder, manifests at birth with longitudinal streaks and thinning of the nail plate. There is platonychia and koilonychia, which may overgrow the lateral folds and involve all nails of the toes and fingers.

Nail-patella syndrome is an autosomal dominant disorder in which the nails are 30–50% their normal size and often have triangular or pyramidal lunulae. The thumbnails are always involved, although in some cases only the ulnar half of the nail may be affected or may be missing. The nails from the index finger to the little finger are progressively less damaged. The patella is also smaller than usual, and this anomaly may lead to knee instability. Bony spines arising from the posterior aspect of the iliac bones, overextension of joints, skin laxity, hyperhidrosis, and renal anomalies may also be present. Nail-patella syndrome is caused by mutations in the transcription factor LMX1B gene.

Pachyonychia Congenita (see Chapter 657).

Habit tic deformity consists of a depression down the center of the nail with numerous horizontal ridges extending across the nail from it. One or both thumbs are usually involved as a result of chronic rubbing and picking at the nail with an adjacent finger.

Clubbing of the nails (hippocratic nails) is characterized by swelling of the distal digit, an increase in the angle between the nail plate and the proximal nail fold (Lovibond angle) to >180 degrees, and a spongy feeling when one pushes down and away from the interphalangeal joint, because of an increase in fibrovascular tissue between the matrix and the phalanx. The pathogenesis is not known. Nail clubbing is seen in association with diseases of numerous organ systems, including pulmonary, cardiovascular (cyanotic heart disease), gastrointestinal (celiac disease, inflammatory bowel disease), and hepatic systems (chronic hepatitis), and in healthy individuals as an idiopathic finding.

CHANGES IN NAIL COLOR

Leukonychia is a white opacity of the nail plate that may involve the entire plate or may be punctate or striate. The nail plate itself remains smooth and undamaged. Leukonychia can be traumatic or associated with infections such as leprosy and tuberculosis, dermatoses such as lichen planus and Darier disease, malignancies such as Hodgkin disease, anemia, and arsenic poisoning (Mees lines). Leukonychia of all nail surfaces is an uncommon hereditary autosomal dominant trait that may be associated with congenital epidermal cysts, renal calculi, and deafness. Paired parallel white bands that do not change position with growth of the nail and thus reflect a change in the nail bed are associated with hypoalbuminemia and are called Muehrcke lines. When the proximal portion of the nail is white and the distal 20–50% of the nail is red, pink, or brown, the condition is called half-and-half nails or Lindsay nails; this is seen most commonly in patients with renal disease but may occur as a normal variant. White nails of **cirrhosis**, or Terry nails, are characterized by a white ground-

TABLE 662-1. Congenital Disease with Nail Defects

Large nails: Pachyonychia congenita, Rubinstein-Taybi syndrome, hemihypertrophy
Small or absent nails: Ectodermal dysplasias, nail-patella, dyskeratosis congenita, focal dermal hypoplasia, cartilage-hair hypoplasia, Ellis–van Creveld, Larsen, epidermolysis bullosa, incontinentia pigmenti, Rothmund-Thomson, Turner, popliteal web, trisomy 13, trisomy 18, Apert, Gorlin-Pindborg, long arm 21 deletion, otopalatodigital, fetal alcohol, fetal hydantoin, elfin facies, anonychia, acrodermatitis enteropathica
Other: Congenital malalignment of the great toenails, familial dystrophic shedding of the nails

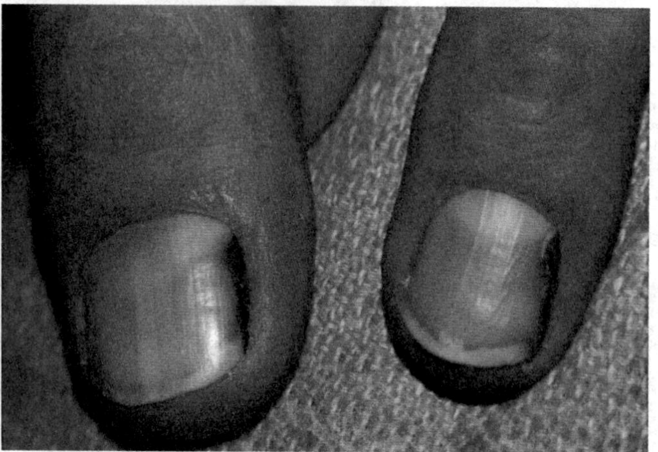

Figure 662-1. Green/black discoloration at the edge of the nails secondary to pseudomonas infection.

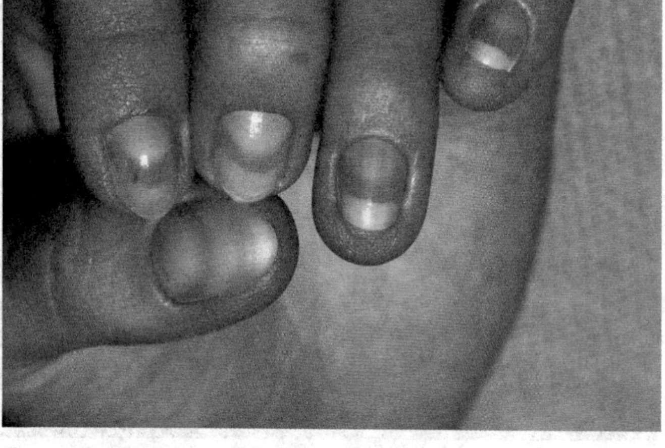

Figure 662-2. Distal onycholysis secondary to oral tetracycline usage and ultraviolet light exposure.

glass appearance of the entire or the proximal end of the nail and a normal pink distal 1–2 mm of the nail; this is associated with hypoalbuminemia.

Black pigmentation of an entire nail plate or linear bands of pigmentation (melanonychia striata) are common in black (90%) and Asian (10–20%) individuals but are unusual in whites (<1%). Most often, the pigment is melanin, which is produced by melanocytes of a junctional nevus in the nail matrix and nail bed and is of no consequence. Extension or alteration in the pigment should be evaluated by biopsy because of the possibility of malignant change.

Bluish-black to greenish nails may be caused by pseudomonas infection (Fig. 662-1), particularly in association with onycholysis or chronic paronychia. The coloration is due to subungual debris and pyocyanin pigment from the bacterial organisms.

Yellow nail syndrome presents with thickened, excessively curved, slow-growing yellow nails without lunulae. All nails are affected in most cases. Associated systemic disease includes bronchiectasis, recurrent bronchitis, chylothorax, and focal edema of the limbs and face. Deficient lymphatic drainage, due to hypoplastic lymphatic vessels, is believed to lead to the manifestations of this syndrome.

Splinter hemorrhages most often result from minor trauma but may also be associated with subacute bacterial endocarditis, vasculitis, severe rheumatoid arthritis, peptic ulcer disease, hypertension, chronic glomerulonephritis, cirrhosis, scurvy, trichinosis, malignant neoplasms, and psoriasis.

NAIL SEPARATION

Onycholysis indicates separation of the nail plate from the distal nail bed. Common causes are trauma, chronic exposure to moisture, hyperhidrosis, cosmetics, psoriasis, fungal infection (distal onycholysis), atopic or contact dermatitis, porphyria, drugs (bleomycin, vincristine, retinoid agents, indomethacin, chlorpromazine [Thorazine]), and drug-induced phototoxicity from tetracyclines (Fig. 662-2) or chloramphenicol.

Beau lines are transverse grooves in the nail plate (Fig. 662-3) that represent a temporary disruption of formation of the nail plate. The lines 1st appear a few weeks after the event that caused the disruption in nail growth. A single transverse ridge appears at the proximal nail fold in most 4–6 wk old infants and works its way distally as the nail grows; this line may reflect metabolic changes after delivery. At other ages, Beau lines are usually indicative of periodic trauma or episodic shutdown of the nail matrix secondary to a systemic disease such as measles, mumps, pneumonia, or zinc deficiency. **Onychomadesis** is an exaggeration of Beau lines leading to proximal separation of the nail bed (Fig. 662-4).

NAIL CHANGES ASSOCIATED WITH SKIN DISEASE

Nail changes may be particularly associated with various other diseases. Nail changes of **psoriasis** most characteristically include pitting, onycholysis, yellow-brown discoloration, and thickening. Nail changes in lichen planus include violaceous papules in the proximal nail fold and nail bed, leukonychia, longitudinal ridging, thinning of the entire nail plate, and pterygium formation, which is abnormal adherence of the cuticle to the nail plate or, if the plate is destroyed focally, to the nail bed. Reiter disease may include painless erythematous induration of the base of the nail fold; subungual parakeratotic scaling; and thickening, opacification, or ridging of the nail plate. Dermatitis that involves the nail folds may produce dystrophy, roughening, and coarse pitting of the nails. Nail changes are more common in atopic dermatitis than in other forms of dermatitis that affect the hands. Darier disease is characterized by red or white streaks that extend longitudinally and cross the lunula. Where the streak meets the distal end of the nail, a V-shaped notch may be present. Total leukonychia may also occur. Transverse rows of fine pits are characteristic of alopecia areata. In severe cases, the entire nail surface may be rough. Patients with acrodermatitis enteropathica may have

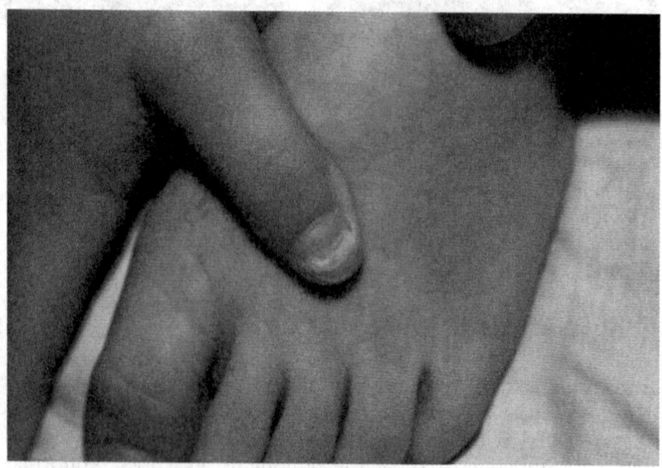

Figure 662-3. Beau lines. Longitudinal disruption of nail.

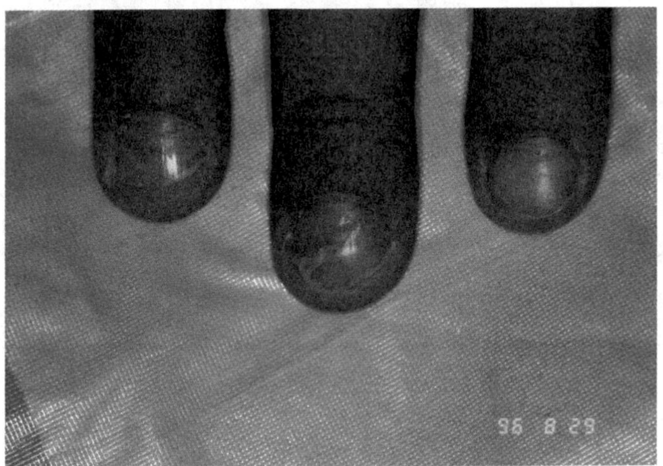

Figure 662-4. Onychomadesis. Proximal nail bed separation.

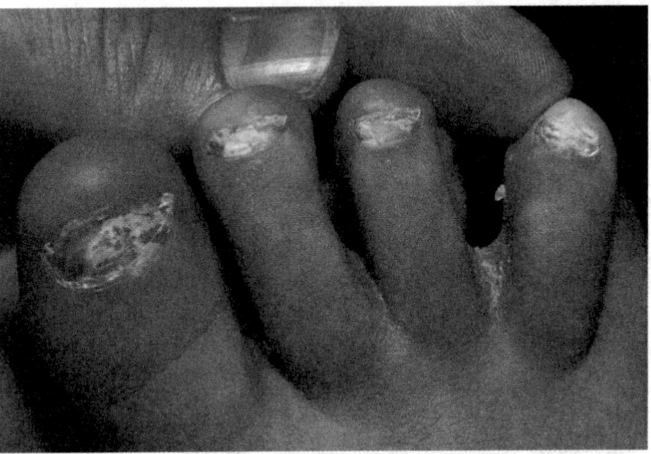

Figure 662-6. Discoloration, hyperkeratosis, and crumbling of nail secondary to dermatophyte infection.

transverse grooves (Beau lines) and nail dystrophy as a result of periungual dermatitis.

TRACHYONYCHIA (20-NAIL DYSTROPHY). Trachyonychia is characterized by longitudinal ridging, pitting, fragility, thinning, distal notching, and opalescent discoloration of all the nails (Fig. 662-5). Patients have no associated skin or systemic diseases and no other ectodermal defects. Its occasional association with alopecia areata has led some authorities to suggest that trachyonychia may reflect an abnormal immunologic response to the nail matrix, whereas histopathologic studies have suggested that it may be a manifestation of lichen planus, psoriasis, or spongiotic (eczematous) inflammation of the nail matrix. The disorder must be differentiated from fungal infections, psoriasis, nail changes of alopecia areata, and nail dystrophy secondary to eczema. Eczema and fungal infections rarely produce changes in all the nails simultaneously. The disorder is self-limited and eventually remits by adulthood.

NAIL INFECTION

Fungal infection of the nails has been classified into four types. White superficial onychomycosis presents with diffuse or speckled white discoloration of the surface of the toenails. It is caused primarily by *Trichophyton mentagrophytes,* which invades the nail plate. The organism may be scraped off the nail plate with a blade, but **treatment** is best accomplished by the addition of a topical azole antifungal agent. Distal subungual onychomycosis presents with foci of onycholysis under the distal nail plate or along the lateral nail groove, followed by development of hyperkeratosis and yellow-brown discoloration. The process extends proximally, resulting in nail plate thickening, crumbling (Fig. 662-6), and separation from the nail bed. *Trichophyton rubrum* and, occasionally, *T. mentagrophytes* infect the toenails; fingernail disease is almost exclusively due to *T. rubrum,* which may be associated with superficial scaling of the plantar surface of the feet and often of one hand. These dermatophytes are found most readily at the most proximal area of the nail bed or adjacent ventral portion of the nail plates that are involved. **Topical therapies** such as ciclopirox 8% lacquer may be effective for solitary nail infection. Because of their long half-life in the nail, terbinafine or itraconazole may be effective when given as pulse therapy (1 wk of each mo for 3–4 mo). Either agent is superior to griseofulvin, fluconazole, or ketoconazole. The risks, the most concerning of which is hepatic toxicity, and costs of oral therapy must be weighed carefully against the benefits of treatment for a condition that generally causes only cosmetic problems.

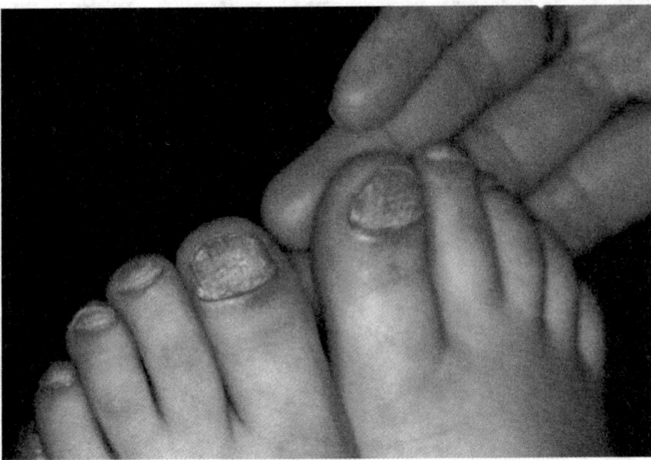

Figure 662-5. Dystrophy of all nails in trachyonychia.

Proximal white subungual onychomycosis occurs when the organism, generally *T. rubrum,* enters the nail through the proximal nail fold, producing yellow-white portions of the undersurface of the nail plate. The surface of the nail is unaffected. This occurs almost exclusively in immunocompromised patients and is a well-recognized manifestation of AIDS.

Candidal onychomycosis involves the entire nail plate in patients with chronic mucocutaneous candidiasis. It is also commonly seen in patients with AIDS. The organism, generally *Candida albicans,* enters distally or along the lateral nail folds, rapidly involves the entire thickness of the nail plate, and produces thickening, crumbling, and deformity of the plate. Topical azole antifungal agents may be sufficient for treatment of candidal onychomycosis in an immunocompetent host, but oral antifungal agents are necessary for treatment of those with immune deficiencies.

PARONYCHIAL INFLAMMATION

Paronychial inflammation may be acute or chronic and generally involves 1 or 2 nail folds on the fingers. Acute paronychia presents with erythema, warmth, edema, and tenderness of the proximal nail fold, most commonly as a result of pathogenic staphylococci or streptococci (Fig. 662-7). Warm soaks and oral antibiotics such as clindamycin or amoxicillin plus clavulanic acid

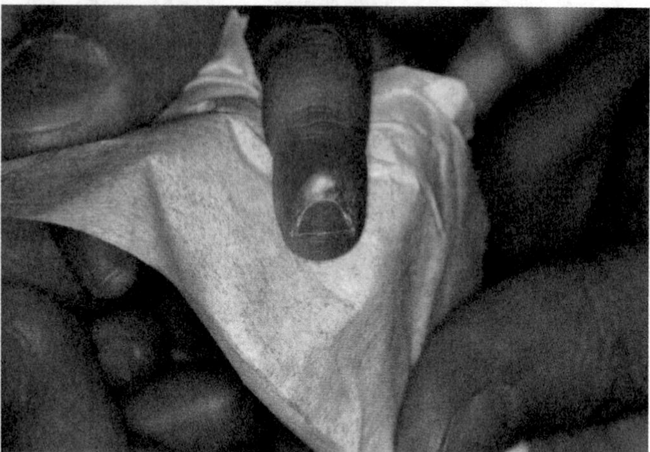

Figure 662-7. Acute paronychia secondary to *Staphylococcus aureus.*

are generally effective; incision and drainage may be occasionally necessary. Development of chronic paronychia follows prolonged immersion in water (Fig. 662-8), such as occurs in finger or thumb sucking, exposure to irritating solutions, nail fold trauma, or diseases including Raynaud phenomenon, collagen vascular diseases, or diabetes. Swelling of the proximal nail fold is followed by separation of the nail fold from the underlying nail plate and suppuration. Foreign material, embedded in the dermis of the nail fold, becomes a nidus for inflammation and infection with *Candida* species and mixed bacterial flora. A combination of attention to predisposing factors; meticulous drying of the hands, including use of 4% thymol solution; and long-term antifungal, antibacterial, and topical anti-inflammatory agents may be required for successful treatment of chronic paronychia.

Ingrown nails occur when the lateral edge of the nail, including spicules that have separated from the nail plate, penetrates the soft tissue of the lateral nail fold. Erythema, edema, and pain, most often involving the lateral great toes, are noted acutely; recurrent episodes may lead to formation of granulation tissue. Predisposing factors include (1) congenital malalignment (especially of the great toes); (2) compression of the side of the toe from poorly fitting shoes, particularly if the great toes are abnormally long and the lateral nail folds are prominent; and (3) improper cutting of the nail in a curvilinear manner rather than straight across. **Management** includes proper fitting of shoes; allowing the nail to grow out beyond the free edge before cutting it straight across; warm water soaks; oral antibiotics if cellulitis affects the lateral nail fold; and, in severe, recurrent cases, application of silver nitrate to granulation tissue, nail avulsion, or excision of the lateral aspect of the nail followed by matricectomy.

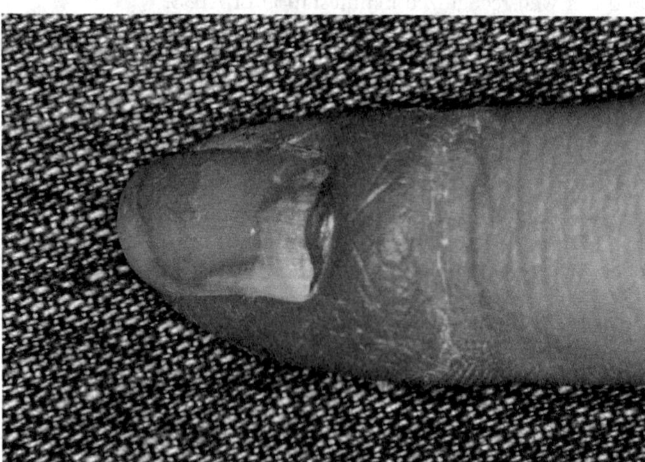

Figure 662-8. Chronic paronychia with erythema and lateral nail fold separation.

PARONYCHIAL TUMORS

Tumors in the paronychial area include pyogenic granulomas, mucous cysts, subungual exostoses, and junctional nevi. Periungual fibromas that appear in late childhood should suggest a diagnosis of tuberous sclerosis.

Fawcett RS, Linford S, Stullberg DL: Nail abnormalities: Clues to systemic disease. *Am Fam Physician* 2004;69:1417–1424.

Fistarol SK, Itin PH: Nail changes in genodermatoses. *Eur J Dermatol* 2002;12:119–128.

Grover C, Khandpur S, Reddy BS, et al: Longitudinal nail biopsy: Utility in 20-nail dystrophy. *Dermatol Surg* 2003;29:1125–1129.

Gupta AK, Ryder JE, Skinner AR: Treatment of onychomychosis: Pros and cons of antifungal agents. *J Cutan Med Surg* 2004;8:25–30.

Herzberg AJ: Nail manifestations of systemic diseases. *Clin Podiatr Med Surg North Am* 2004;21:631–640.

Lembach L: Pediatric nail disorders. *Clin Podiatr Med Surg North Am* 2004;21:641–650.

Rockwell PG: Acute and chronic paronychia. *Am Fam Physcian* 2001;63: 1113–1116.

Scheinfeld NS: Trachyonychia: A case report and review of manifestations, associations and treatments. *Cutis* 2003;71:299–302.

Chapter 663 ■ Disorders of the Mucous Membranes

Joseph G. Morelli

The mucous membranes may be involved in developmental disorders, infections, acute and chronic skin diseases, genodermatoses, and benign and malignant tumors. Some of the more common and distinctive diseases specific to mucous membranes are presented in this chapter.

CHEILITIS. Inflammation of the lips (cheilitis) and angles of the mouth (angular cheilitis or perlèche) [Fig. 663-1] are most com-

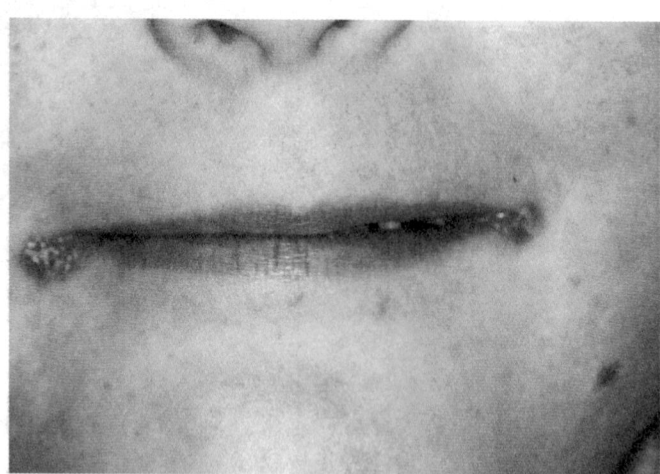

Figure 663-1. Angular cheilitis.

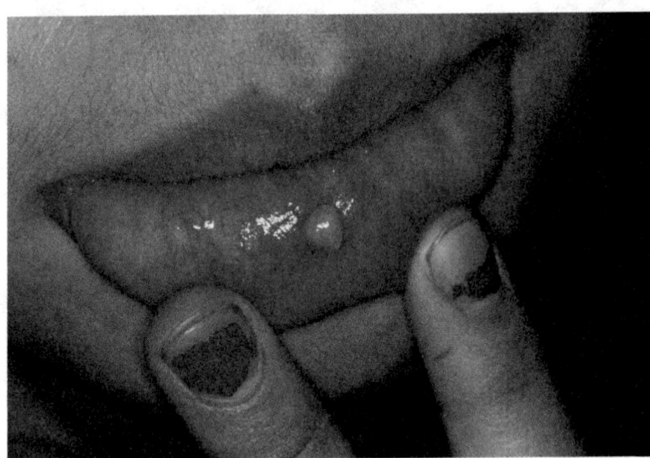

Figure 663-2. Mucocele on lower lip.

monly due to dryness, chapping, and lip licking. Excessive salivation and drooling, particularly in children with neurologic deficits, may also cause chronic irritation. Lesions of oral thrush may occasionally extend to the angles of the mouth. Protection can be provided by frequent applications of a bland ointment such as petrolatum. Candidosis should be treated with an appropriate antifungal agent, and contact dermatitis of the perioral skin should be treated with a mild topical corticosteroid ointment preparation and frequent use of vaseline or similar emollient.

FORDYCE SPOTS. These are asymptomatic, minute, yellow-white papules on the vermilion border of the lips and buccal mucosa. These ectopic sebaceous glands may be found in otherwise normal individuals and require no therapy.

MUCOCELE. Mucus retention cysts are painless, fluctuant, tense, 2–10 mm, bluish papules on the lips (Fig. 663-2), tongue, palate, or buccal mucosa. Traumatic severance of the duct of a minor salivary gland leads to submucosal retention of mucus secretion. Those on the floor of the mouth are known as ranulas when the submaxillary or sublingual salivary ducts are involved. Fluctuations in size are usual, and the lesions may disappear temporarily after traumatic rupture. Recurrence is prevented by excising the mucocele.

APHTHOUS STOMATITIS (CANKER SORES). Solitary or multiple painful ulcerations occur on the labial (Fig. 663-3), buccal, or lingual mucosa and on the sublingual, palatal, or gingival mucosa. Lesions may present initially as erythematous, indurated papules that erode rapidly to form sharply circumscribed, necrotic ulcers with a gray fibrinous exudate and an erythematous halo. Minor aphthous ulcers are 2–10 mm in diameter and heal spontaneously in 7–10 days. Major aphthous ulcers are >10 mm in diameter and take 10–30 days to heal. A 3rd type of aphthous ulceration is herpetiform in appearance, presenting with a few to numerous grouped 1–2 mm lesions that tend to coalesce into plaques that heal over 7–10 days. Approximately ⅓ of patients with recurrent lesions have a family history of the disorder. (See Chapter 312 for differential diagnosis.)

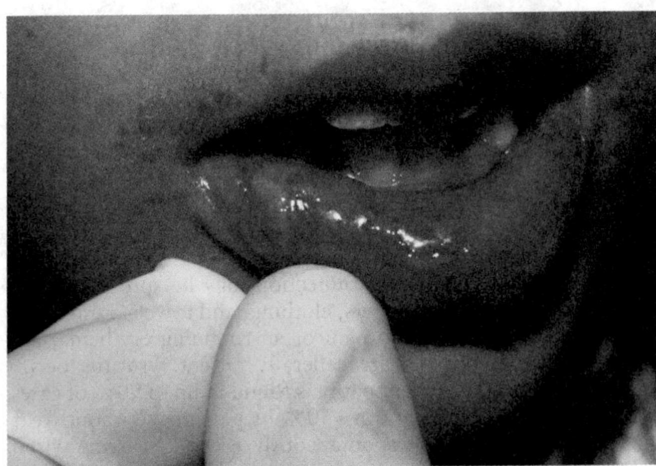

Figure 663-3. Aphthous ulceration on lower lip.

The etiology of aphthous stomatitis is probably multifactorial; the condition probably represents an oral manifestation of a number of conditions. Altered local regulation of the cell-mediated immune system, after activation and accumulation of cytotoxic T cells, may contribute to the localized mucosal breakdown. It is a common misconception that aphthous stomatitis is a manifestation of herpes simplex virus infection. Recurrent herpes infections remain localized to the lips and rarely cross the mucocutaneous junction; involvement of the oral mucosa occurs only in primary infections.

Treatment of aphthous stomatitis is palliative. The majority of mild cases do not require therapy. Relief of pain, particularly before eating, may be achieved by use of a topical anesthetic such as viscous lidocaine or an oral rinse with a combined solution of elixir of diphenhydramine, viscous lidocaine, and an oral antacid. Care must be taken to avoid hot food and drink after the use of a topical anesthetic. A topical corticosteroid in a mucosal adhering agent may help to reduce inflammation, and topical tetracycline mouthwash may also hasten healing. In severe, debilitating cases, systemic therapy with corticosteroids, colchicine, cimetidine, or dapsone may be helpful.

COWDEN SYNDROME (MULTIPLE HAMARTOMA SYNDROME). This is an autosomal dominant condition that usually presents in the 2nd or 3rd decade with smooth, pink or whitish papules on the palatal, gingival, buccal, and labial mucosae. Mutations in the tumor suppressor gene PTEN cause Cowden syndrome. These benign fibromas may coalesce into a cobblestone appearance. Numerous flesh-colored papules also develop on the face, particularly around the mouth, nose, and ears. These papules are most commonly trichilemmomas, a benign neoplasm of the hair follicle. Associated findings may include acral keratotic papules, thyroid goiter, gastrointestinal polyps, fibrocystic breast nodules, and carcinoma of the breast or thyroid.

EPSTEIN PEARLS (GINGIVAL CYSTS OF THE NEWBORN). These are white keratin-containing cysts on the palatal or alveolar mucosa of ≈80% of neonates. They cause no symptoms and are generally shed within a few weeks.

GEOGRAPHIC TONGUE (BENIGN MIGRATORY GLOSSITIS). This consists of single or multiple sharply demarcated, irregular, smooth red plaques on the dorsum of the tongue caused by transient atrophy of the filiform papillae and the surface epithelium, often with elevated gray margins composed of intervening filiform papillae that are increased in thickness (Fig. 663-4). Symptoms of mild burning or irritation may occasionally be bothersome. Onset is rapid, and the pattern may change over hours to days. Some patients feel that the condition is exacerbated by stress or by hot or spicy foods. The histology of geographic tongue is similar to pustular psoriasis. No therapy other than reassurance is necessary.

SCROTAL (FISSURED) TONGUE. Approximately 1% of infants and 2.5% of children have many folds with deep grooves on the dorsal tongue surface. These impart a pebbled or wrinkled

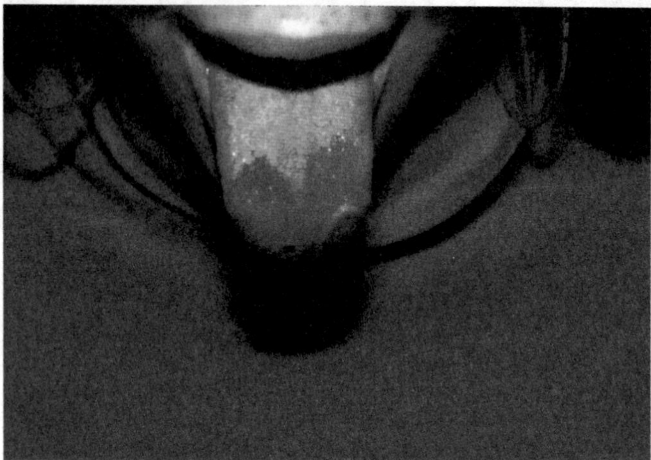

Figure 663-4. Geographic tongue.

appearance. Some cases are congenital, caused by incomplete fusion of the two halves of the tongue; others develop in association with infection, trauma, malnutrition, or low vitamin A levels. Many patients with fissured tongue also have geographic tongue. Food particles and debris may become trapped in the fissures, resulting in irritation, inflammation, and halitosis. Careful cleansing with a mouth rinse and soft-bristled toothbrush is recommended.

BLACK HAIRY TONGUE. This is a dark coating on the dorsum of the tongue caused by hyperplasia and elongation of the filiform papillae; overgrowth of chromogenic bacteria and fungi and entrapped pigmented residues that adsorb to microbial plaque and desquamating keratin may contribute to the dark coloration. Changes often begin posteriorly and extend anteriorly on the dorsum of the tongue. The condition is most common in adults but may also present during adolescence. Poor oral hygiene and bacterial overgrowth, treatment with systemic antibiotics such as tetracycline (which promotes the growth of *Candida* spp.), and smoking are predisposing factors. Improved oral hygiene and brushing with a soft-bristled toothbrush may be all that is necessary for treatment.

ORAL HAIRY LEUKOPLAKIA. This occurs in ≈25% of patients with AIDS but is rare in the pediatric population. It presents as a mostly asymptomatic white thickening and accentuation of the normal vertical folds of the lateral margins of the tongue. The mucosa is white and irregularly thickened but remains soft. Spread may occur occasionally to the ventral tongue surface, the floor of the mouth, the tonsillar pillars, and the pharynx. The condition is due to Epstein-Barr virus, which is present in the upper layer of the affected epithelium. The plaques have no malignant potential. The disorder occurs predominantly in HIV-infected patients but may also be found in individuals who are immunosuppressed for other reasons, such as organ transplantation, leukemia, or chemotherapy. The condition is generally asymptomatic and does not require therapy.

ACUTE NECROTIZING ULCERATIVE GINGIVITIS (VINCENT STOMATITIS, FUSOSPIROCHETAL GINGIVITIS, TRENCH MOUTH). This disorder presents with punched-out ulceration, necrosis, and bleeding of interdental papillae. A grayish-white pseudomembrane may cover the ulcerations. Lesions may spread to involve the buccal mucosa, lips, tongue, tonsils, and pharynx and may be associated with dental pain, a bad taste, low-grade fever, and lymphadenopathy. It presents most commonly in the 2nd or 3rd decade, particularly in the context of poor dental hygiene, scurvy, or pellagra. A synergistic association between fusospirochetal organisms *(Fusobacterium nucleatum)* and *Borrelia vincentii* has been proposed to contribute to the pathogenesis.

Noma is a severe form of fusospirillary gangrenous stomatitis that presents primarily in malnourished children 2–5 yr of age who have had a preceding illness such as measles, scarlet fever, tuberculosis, malignancy, or immunodeficiency. It presents as a painful, red, indurated papule on the alveolar margin, followed by ulceration and mutilating gangrenous destruction of tissue in the oronasal region. The process may also involve the scalp, neck, shoulders, perineum, and vulva. **Noma neonatorum** presents in the 1st mo of life with gangrenous lesions of the lips, nose, mouth, and anal regions. Affected infants are usually small for gestational age, malnourished, premature, and frequently ill, particularly with *Pseudomonas aeruginosa* sepsis. Care consists of nutritional support, conservative debridement of necrotic soft tissues, empirical broad-spectrum antibiotics such as penicillin and metronidazole, and, in the case of noma neonatorum, antipseudomonal antibiotics.

Akintoye SO, Greenberg MS: Recurrent aphthous stomatitis. *Dent Clin North Am* 2005;49:31–47.

Baurmash HD: Mucocoeles and ranulas. *J Oral Maxillofac Surg* 2003;61:369–378.

Folayan MO: The epidemiology, etiology, and pathology of acute necrotizing gingivitis associated with malnutrition. *J Contemp Dent Pract* 2004;5:28–41.

Laskin DM, Giglio JA, Rippert ET: Differential diagnosis of tongue lesions. *Quintessence Int* 2003;34:331–342.

Chapter 664 ■ Cutaneous Bacterial Infections

Joseph G. Morelli

Bacterial skin infection is the single most common diagnosis among children with skin problems, accounting for 17% of all clinic visits. The most common bacterial skin infection of children is impetigo, which makes up ≈10% of all skin problems.

IMPETIGO

See Chapters 182 and 180.

CLINICAL MANIFESTATIONS

Nonbullous Impetigo. There are two classic forms of impetigo: nonbullous and bullous. **Nonbullous impetigo** accounts for more than 70% of cases. Lesions typically begin on the skin of the face or on extremities that have been traumatized. The most common lesions that precede nonbullous impetigo include insect bites, abrasions, lacerations, chickenpox, scabies pediculosis, and burns. A tiny vesicle or pustule forms initially and rapidly develops into a honey-colored crusted plaque that is generally <2 cm in diameter (Fig. 664-1). The infection may be spread to other parts of the body by the fingers, clothing, and towels. Lesions are associated with little to no pain or surrounding erythema, and constitutional symptoms are generally absent. Pruritus occurs occasionally, regional adenopathy is found in up to 90% of cases, and leukocytosis is present in ≈50% of patients. Without treatment, most cases resolve spontaneously without scarring within ≈2 wk. The **differential diagnosis** of nonbullous impetigo includes viral (herpes simplex, varicella-zoster), fungal (tinea corporis,

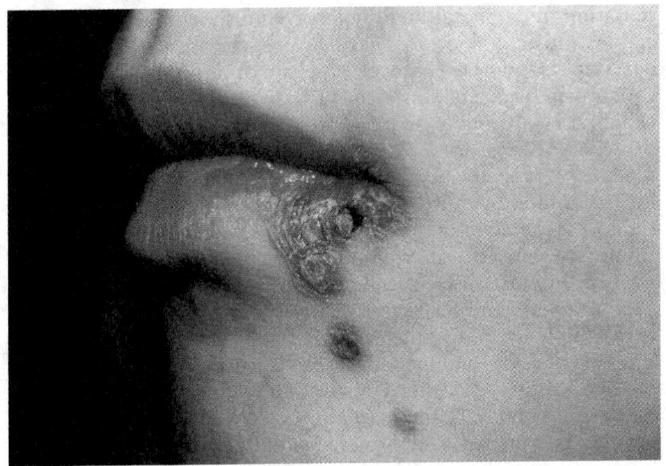

Figure 664-1. Multiple crusted and oozing lesions of impetigo.

kerion), and parasitic infestations (scabies, pediculosis capitis), all of which may become impetiginized.

Staphylococcus aureus is the predominant organism of nonbullous impetigo in the United States; group A β-hemolytic streptococci (GABHS) are implicated in the development of some lesions. Staphylococci generally spread from the nose to normal skin and then infect the skin. In contrast, the skin becomes colonized with GABHS an average of 10 days before development of impetigo. GABHS then colonize the nasopharynx an average of 2–3 wk after the appearance of lesions of impetigo. The skin serves as the source for acquisition of GABHS and the probable primary source for spread of impetigo. Lesions of nonbullous impetigo that grow staphylococci in culture cannot be distinguished clinically from those that grow pure cultures of GABHS. Whereas *S. aureus* can be cultured from lesions of impetigo in children of all ages, GABHS is most commonly cultured from children of preschool age but is unusual before 2 yr of age, except in highly endemic areas. The staphylococcal types that cause nonbullous impetigo are variable but are not generally from phage group 2, the group that is associated with scalded skin and toxic shock syndromes. Several serotypes of GABHS, termed "impetigo strains," are found most frequently in lesions of nonbullous impetigo and are different from those that cause pharyngitis.

Bullous Impetigo. This is mainly an infection of infants and young children. Bullous impetigo is always caused by *S. aureus;* ≈80% are from phage group 2, among which 60% are type 71, and most of the remainders are types 3A, 3B, 3C, and 55. Flaccid, transparent bullae develop most commonly on skin of the face, buttocks, trunk, perineum, and extremities. **Neonatal bullous impetigo** can begin in the diaper area. Rupture of bullae occurs easily, leaving a narrow rim of scale at the edge of shallow, moist erosion. Surrounding erythema and regional adenopathy are generally absent. Unlike those of nonbullous impetigo, lesions of bullous impetigo are a manifestation of localized staphylococcal scalded skin syndrome and develop on intact skin.

DIAGNOSIS. Cultures of fluid from an intact blister or moist plaque should yield the causative agent; if the patient appears ill, blood cultures should also be obtained. Lesions of bullous impetigo show vesicle formation in the subcorneal or granular region; neutrophils and, occasionally, acantholytic cells within the blister; spongiosis; edema of the papillary dermis; and a mixed infiltrate of lymphocytes and neutrophils around blood vessels of the superficial plexus. Unless staphylococci can be cultured from the bullae or, less commonly, can be seen on Gram stain, it may be impossible to differentiate bullous impetigo from pemphigus foliaceous or subcorneal pustular dermatosis. Nonbullous impetigo has histopathologic findings similar to those of the bullous variant, except that blister formation is slight.

The **differential diagnosis** of bullous impetigo in neonates includes epidermolysis bullosa, bullous mastocytosis, herpetic infection, and early scalded skin syndrome. In older children, allergic contact dermatitis, burns, erythema multiforme, chronic bullous dermatosis of childhood, pemphigus, and bullous pemphigoid must be considered, particularly if the lesions do not respond to therapy.

COMPLICATIONS. Potential but very rare complications of either nonbullous or bullous impetigo include osteomyelitis, septic arthritis, pneumonia, and septicemia. Positive blood cultures are very rare in otherwise healthy children with localized lesions. Cellulitis has been reported in ≈10% of patients with nonbullous impetigo and rarely follows the bullous form. Lymphangitis, suppurative lymphadenitis, guttate psoriasis, and scarlet fever occasionally follow streptococcal disease. There is no correlation between number of lesions and clinical involvement of the lymphatics or development of cellulitis in association with streptococcal impetigo.

Infection with nephritogenic strains of GABHS may result in **acute poststreptococcal glomerulonephritis** (see Chapter 511.1). The clinical character of impetigo lesions is not predictive of the development of poststreptococcal glomerulonephritis. The most commonly affected age group is school-aged children 3–7 yr old. The latent period from onset of impetigo to development of poststreptococcal glomerulonephritis averages 18–21 days, which is longer than the 10-day latency period after pharyngitis. Poststreptococcal glomerulonephritis occurs epidemically after either pharyngeal or skin infection. Impetigo-associated epidemics have been caused by M groups 2, 49, 53, 55, 56, 57, and 60. Strains of GABHS that are associated with endemic impetigo in the United States have little or no nephritogenic potential. Acute rheumatic fever does not occur as a result of impetigo.

TREATMENT. Topical or systemic antibiotic treatment is superior to placebo. Mupirocin is an ointment that is bactericidal by reversible inhibition of bacterial isoleucyl–transfer RNA synthetase. Applied topically 3 times daily for 7–10 days, it is equal to or greater in effectiveness, with fewer side effects, than oral erythromycin ethylsuccinate, 30–50 mg/kg/24 hr for 7–10 days. Resistance to mupirocin has rarely been reported, such patients were treated irregularly or prophylactically for more than 2 wk. Topical fusidic acid may also be effective.

Systemic therapy with a β-lactamase–resistant oral antibiotic should be prescribed for patients with widespread involvement; when lesions are near the mouth, where topical medication may be licked off; or in cases with evidence of deep involvement, including cellulitis, furunculosis, abscess formation, or suppurative lymphadenitis. In areas without a high prevalence of *S. aureus* resistance to erythromycin, erythromycin ethylsuccinate (40 mg/kg/24 hr divided 3 to 4 times daily for 7 days) or erythromycin estolate (30 mg/kg/24 hr divided 3 to 4 times daily) is the **preferred oral therapy.** If erythromycin resistance is widespread in the community, alternative oral antibiotics that have been shown to be effective in children for treatment of impetigo include dicloxacillin, amoxicillin plus clavulanic acid, clindamycin, and a cephalosporin such as cephalexin, cefaclor, cefadroxil, cefprozil, or cefpodoxime. The choice among these various agents may be guided primarily by issues of cost, local availability, and compliance. The macrolides clarithromycin and azithromycin may be advantageous primarily in instances of intolerance to erythromycin but will not provide cure rates superior to those of erythromycin. No evidence suggests that a 10 day course of therapy is superior to a 7 day one. If a satisfactory clinical response is not achieved within 7 days, a culture should be taken by swabbing beneath the lifted edge of a crusted lesion. If a resistant organism is detected, an appropriate antibiotic should be given for an additional 7 days.

SUBCUTANEOUS TISSUE INFECTIONS

The principal determination for soft tissue infections is whether it is non-necrotizing or necrotizing. The former responds to antibiotic therapy alone, whereas the latter requires prompt surgical removal of all devitalized tissue in addition to antimicrobial therapy. Necrotizing soft tissue infections are potentially life-threatening conditions that are characterized by rapidly advancing local tissue destruction and systemic toxicity. Tissue necrosis distinguishes them from cellulites. In cellulitis, an inflammatory infectious process involves subcutaneous tissue but does not destroy it. Necrotizing soft tissue infections characteristically present with a paucity of early cutaneous signs relative to the rapidity and degree of destruction of the subcutaneous tissues.

CELLULITIS. Cellulitis is characterized by infection and inflammation of loose connective tissue, with limited involvement of the dermis and relative sparing of the epidermis. A break in the skin due to previous trauma, surgery, or an underlying skin lesion predisposes to cellulitis. Cellulitis is also more common in individuals with lymphatic stasis, diabetes mellitus, or immunosuppression.

Etiology. *Streptococcus pyogenes* and *S. aureus* are the most common etiologic agents. Occasionally, *Streptococcus pneumoniae,* group G or C streptococci, and, in neonates, group B streptococci or, rarely, *Escherichia coli* are the causal organisms. In patients who are immunocompromised or have diabetes mellitus, a number of other bacterial or fungal agents may be involved, notably *Pseudomonas aeruginosa; Aeromonas hydrophila* and, occasionally, other *Enterobacteriaceae; Legionella* spp.; the *Mucorales,* particularly *Rhizopus* spp., *Mucor* spp., and *Absidia* spp.; and *Cryptococcus neoformans.* Children with relapsed nephrotic syndrome may develop cellulitis due to *Escherichia coli.* In children age 3 mo to 3–5 yr, *Haemophilus influenzae* type b was once an important cause of facial cellulitis, but its incidence has declined significantly since institution of immunization against this organism.

Clinical Manifestations. Cellulitis presents clinically as an area of edema, warmth, erythema, and tenderness. The lateral margins tend to be indistinct because the process is deep in the skin, primarily involving the subcutaneous tissues in addition to the dermis. Application of pressure may produce pitting. Although distinction cannot be made with certainty in any particular patient, cellulitis as a result of *S. aureus* tends to be more localized and may suppurate, whereas infections due to *S. pyogenes* (group A streptococcus) tend to spread more rapidly and may be associated with lymphangitis. Regional adenopathy and constitutional signs and symptoms of fever, chills, and malaise are common. Complications of cellulitis include subcutaneous abscess, bacteremia, osteomyelitis, septic arthritis, thrombophlebitis, endocarditis, and necrotizing fasciitis. Lymphangitis or glomerulonephritis can also follow infection with *S. pyogenes.*

Diagnosis. Aspirates from the site of inflammation, skin biopsy, and blood cultures allow identification of the causal organism in ≈25% of cases of cellulitis. Yield of the causative organism is ≈30% when the site of origin of the cellulitis is apparent, such as an abrasion or ulcer. An aspirate taken from the point of maximum inflammation yields the causal organism more often than does a leading-edge aspirate. Lack of success in isolating an organism stems primarily from the low number of organisms present within the lesion.

Treatment. Empirical therapy for cellulitis should be directed by the history of the illness, the location and character of the cellulitis, and the age and immune status of the patient. Cellulitis in a neonate should prompt a full sepsis evaluation, followed by initiation of empirical therapy intravenously with a β-lactamase-stable antistaphylococcal antibiotic such as methicillin (vancomycin is another choice) and an aminoglycoside such as gentamicin or a cephalosporin such as cefotaxime. Treatment of cellulitis in an infant or child younger than about 5 yr should provide coverage for *S. pyogenes* and *S. aureus* as well as *H. influenzae* type b and *S. pneumoniae.* The evaluation should include a blood culture, and if the infant is younger than 1 yr, if signs of systemic toxicity are present or an adequate examination cannot be carried out, a lumbar puncture should also be performed. In most cases of cellulitis on an extremity, regardless of age, *S. aureus* and *S. pyogenes* are the cause and bacteremia is highly unlikely in an otherwise well-appearing child. Blood cultures should be obtained if sepsis is suspected. If fever, lymphadenopathy, and other constitutional signs are absent (white blood cell count <15,000), treatment of cellulitis on an extremity may be initiated orally on an outpatient basis with a penicillinase-resistant penicillin such as dicloxacillin or cloxacillin or a 1st-generation cephalosporin such as cephalexin or if methicillin resistant staphylococcus is suspected with clindamycin. If improvement is not noted or the disease progresses significantly in the 1st 24–48 hr of therapy, parenteral therapy is necessary. If fever, lymphadenopathy, or constitutional signs are present, therapy should be initiated parenterally. Oxacillin or nafcillin is effective in most cases, although if systemic toxicity is significant, consideration should be given to the addition of clindamycin or vancomycin. Once the erythema, warmth, edema, and fever have decreased significantly, a 10 day course of treatment may be completed on an outpatient basis. Immobilization and elevation of an affected limb, particularly early in the course of therapy, may help to reduce swelling and pain.

NECROTIZING FASCIITIS. Necrotizing fasciitis is a subcutaneous tissue infection that involves the deep layer of superficial fascia but largely spares adjacent epidermis, deep fascia, and muscle.

Etiology. Relatively few organisms possess sufficient virulence to cause necrotizing fasciitis when acting alone. The most fulminant infections, associated with toxic shock syndrome and a high case fatality rate, are caused by *S. pyogenes* (see Chapter 182). Streptococcal necrotizing fasciitis may occur in the absence of toxic shock–like syndrome, and is seldom fatal but may be associated with substantial morbidity. Necrotizing fasciitis can occasionally be caused by *S. aureus; Clostridium perfringens; Clostridium septicum; P. aeruginosa; Vibrio* spp., particularly *V. vulnificus;* and fungi of the order *Mucorales,* particularly *Rhizopus* spp., *Mucor* spp., and *Absidia* spp. Necrotizing fasciitis has also been reported on rare occasions to result from non–group A streptococci such as group B, C, F, or G streptococci, *S. pneumoniae,* or *H. influenzae* type b. Necrotizing fasciitis may also be polymicrobial. In most of these cases, a mixture of anaerobic bacteria and aerobic or facultative bacteria appear to act together to cause tissue necrosis. The most common aerobic or facultative bacteria are several species of hemolytic or nonhemolytic non–group A streptococci, *S. aureus, E. coli, Enterobacter* spp., and various other *Enterobacteriaceae* and *Pseudomonas* spp. The anaerobes present are similar to those found in subcutaneous abscesses: *Bacteroides* spp., *Peptostreptococcus* spp., *Peptococcus* spp., *Prevotella* spp., *Porphyromonas* spp., *Clostridium* spp., and *Fusobacterium* spp. Infections due to any one organism or combination of organisms cannot be distinguished clinically from one another, although development of **crepitance** signals the presence of *Clostridium* spp. or gram-negative bacilli such as *E. coli, Klebsiella, Proteus,* and *Aeromonas.*

Epidemiology. Necrotizing fasciitis may occur anywhere on the body. The most common locations, however, are the extremities, abdomen, and perineal region. Common predisposing conditions in neonates are omphalitis and balanitis after circumcision. The incidence of necrotizing fasciitis is highest in hosts with systemic or local tissue immunocompromise, such as those with diabetes mellitus, neoplasia, or peripheral vascular disease, and those recently having undergone surgery, those who abuse intravenous drugs, or those on immunosuppressive treatment, particularly with corticosteroids. The infection can also occur in healthy individuals after minor puncture wounds, abrasions, or lacerations; blunt trauma; surgical procedures, particularly of the abdomen, gastrointestinal or genitourinary tracts, or the perineum; or hypodermic needle injection. Since the mid-1980s, there has been a resurgence of fulminant necrotizing soft tissue infections due to *S. pyogenes,* which may occur in previously healthy individuals with little or no apparent compromise of immunologic or skin integrity. Necrotizing fasciitis due to *S. pyogenes* may occur after superinfection of varicella lesions. These children have tended to display onset, recrudescence, or persistence of high fever and signs of toxicity after the 3rd to 4th day of varicella.

Clinical Manifestations. Necrotizing fasciitis begins with acute onset of local swelling, erythema, tenderness, and heat. Fever is usually present, and pain, tenderness, and constitutional signs are out of proportion to cutaneous signs, especially with involvement of fascia and muscle. Lymphangitis and lymphadenitis are usually absent. The infection advances along the superficial fascial plane, and initially there are few cutaneous signs to herald the serious nature and extent of subcutaneous tissue necrosis that is occurring. Skin changes may appear over 24–48 hr as nutrient vessels are thrombosed and cutaneous ischemia develops. Early clinical findings include ill-defined cutaneous erythema and edema, which extends beyond the area of erythema. Additional signs include formation of bullae filled initially with straw-colored and later bluish to hemorrhagic fluid, and darkening of affected tissues from red to purple to blue. Skin anesthesia and, finally, frank tissue gangrene and slough develop owing to the ischemia and necrosis. Vesiculation or bulla formation, ecchymoses, crepitus, anesthesia, and necrosis are ominous and indicative of advanced disease. Children with varicella lesions may initially show no cutaneous signs of superinfection with invasive *S. pyogenes,* such as erythema or swelling. Significant systemic toxicity may accompany necrotizing fasciitis, including shock, organ failure, and death. Advance of the infection in this setting can be rapid, progressing to death within hours. Patients with involvement of the superficial or deep fascia and muscle tend to be more acutely and systemically ill and have more rapidly advancing disease than those with infection confined solely to subcutaneous tissues above the fascia. In an extremity, a **compartment syndrome** may develop and is manifest as tight edema, pain on motion, and loss of distal sensation and pulses. This is a surgical emergency.

Diagnosis. Definitive diagnosis is made by surgical exploration, which should be undertaken as soon as the diagnosis is suspected. Necrotic fascia and subcutaneous tissue are gray and offer little resistance to blunt probing. Although MRI aids in delineating the extent and tissue planes of involvement, this procedure should not delay surgical intervention. Frozen section incisional biopsy specimen obtained early in the course of the infection can aid management by decreasing the time to diagnosis and helping establish margins of involvement. Gram stain of tissue can be particularly useful if chains of gram-positive cocci, indicative of infection with *S. pyogenes,* are seen.

Treatment. Early supportive care, surgical debridement, and parenteral antibiotic administration are mandatory. All devitalized tissue should be removed to freely bleeding edges, and repeat exploration is generally indicated within 24–36 hr to confirm that no necrotic tissue remains. This may need to be repeated on several occasions until devitalized tissue has ceased to form. Meticulous daily wound care is also paramount.

Antibiotic therapy should be initiated parenterally as soon as possible with broad-spectrum agents against all potential pathogens. Most experts recommend initial empirical therapy with penicillin, ampicillin, or nafcillin, along with clindamycin and an aminoglycoside, for coverage against *S. pyogenes* and the broad spectrum of potential anaerobic and gram-negative pathogens. Clindamycin is often added to inhibit protein synthesis of new bacterial necrotizing toxins.

Prognosis. The combined case fatality rate among children and adults with necrotizing fasciitis and toxic shock–like syndrome due to *S. pyogenes* has been ≈60%. Death is less common in children, however, and in cases not complicated by toxic shock–like syndrome.

STAPHYLOCOCCAL SCALDED SKIN SYNDROME (RITTER DISEASE)

CLINICAL MANIFESTATIONS. Staphylococcal scalded skin syndrome occurs predominantly in infants and children younger than 5 yr of age and includes a range of disease from localized bullous impetigo to generalized cutaneous involvement with systemic illness. Onset of the rash may be preceded by malaise, fever, irritability, and exquisite tenderness of the skin. **Scarlatiniform erythema** develops diffusely and is accentuated in flexural and periorificial areas. The conjunctivas are inflamed and occasionally become purulent. The brightly erythematous skin may rapidly acquire a wrinkled appearance and, in severe cases, sterile, flaccid blisters and erosions develop diffusely. Circumoral erythema is characteristically prominent, as is radial crusting and fissuring around the eyes, mouth, and nose. At this stage, areas of epidermis may separate in response to gentle shear force (Nikolsky sign) (Fig. 664-2). As large sheets of epidermis peel away, moist, glistening, denuded areas become apparent, initially in the flexures and subsequently over much of the body surface. This may lead to secondary cutaneous infection, sepsis, and fluid and electrolyte disturbances. The desquamative phase begins after 2–5 days of cutaneous erythema; healing occurs without scarring in 10–14 days. Patients may have pharyngitis, conjunctivitis, and superficial erosions of the lips, but intraoral mucosal surfaces are spared. Although some patients appear ill, many are reasonably comfortable except for the marked skin tenderness.

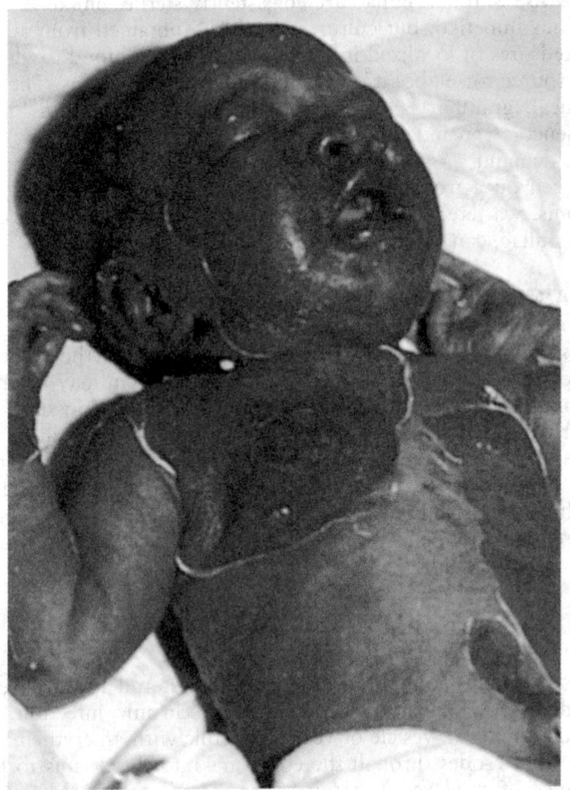

Figure 664-2. Infant with staphylococcal scalded skin syndrome.

A presumed **abortive** form of the disease presents with diffuse, scarlatiniform, tender erythroderma, which is accentuated in the flexural areas but does not progress to blister formation. In these patients, Nikolsky sign may be absent. Although the exanthem is similar to that of streptococcal scarlet fever, strawberry tongue and palatal petechiae are absent. Staphylococcal scalded skin syndrome may be mistaken for a number of other blistering and exfoliating disorders, including bullous impetigo, epidermolysis bullosa, epidermolytic hyperkeratosis, pemphigus, drug eruption, erythema multiforme, and drug-induced toxic epidermal necrolysis. Toxic epidermal necrolysis can often be distinguished by a history of drug ingestion, the presence of Nikolsky sign only at sites of erythema, absence of perioral crusting, full-thickness epidermal necrosis, and a blister cleavage plane in the lowermost epidermis.

ETIOLOGY AND PATHOGENESIS. Staphylococcal scalded skin syndrome is caused predominantly by phage group 2 staphylococci, particularly strains 71 and 55, which are present at localized sites of infection. Foci of infection include the nasopharynx and, less commonly, the umbilicus, urinary tract, a superficial abrasion, conjunctivae, and blood. The clinical manifestations of staphylococcal scalded skin syndrome are mediated by hematogenous spread, in the absence of specific antitoxin antibody of staphylococcal epidermolytic or exfoliative toxins A or B. The toxins have reproduced the disease in both animal models and human volunteers. Decreased renal clearance of the toxins may account for the fact that the disease is most common in infants and young children. Epidermolytic toxin A is heat stable and is encoded by bacterial chromosomal genes. Epidermolytic toxin B is heat labile and is encoded on a 37.5 kb plasmid. The site of blister cleavage is subcorneal through the granular layer. The epidermolytic toxins appear to produce the granular layer split by binding to desmoglein I within desmosomes. Evidence suggests that the toxins are members of the trypsin-like serine protease family and may exert their action through proteolysis.

DIAGNOSIS. Intact bullae are consistently sterile, unlike those of bullous impetigo, but cultures should be obtained from all suspected sites of localized infection and from the blood to identify the source for elaboration of the epidermolytic toxins. The subcorneal, granular layer split can be identified on skin biopsy. Absence of an inflammatory infiltrate is characteristic. In cases that demand a rapid diagnosis, the exfoliated corneal layer can be seen on a frozen biopsy specimen of the desquamating epidermis. Scattered acantholytic cells, which are evident in the cleft-like bullae, can also be seen in a Tzanck preparation.

TREATMENT. Systemic therapy, either orally, in cases of localized involvement, or parenterally, with a semisynthetic penicillinase-resistant penicillin, should be prescribed because the staphylococci are usually penicillin resistant. Clindamycin may be added to inhibit bacterial protein (toxin) synthesis. The skin should be gently moistened and cleansed. Application of an emollient provides lubrication and decreases discomfort. Topical antibiotics are unnecessary. Recovery is usually rapid, but complications such as excessive fluid loss, electrolyte imbalance, faulty temperature regulation, pneumonia, septicemia, and cellulitis may cause increased morbidity.

ECTHYMA (SEE CHAPTERS 182 AND 202)

This resembles nonbullous impetigo in onset and appearance but gradually evolves into a deeper, more chronic infection. The initial lesion is a vesicle or vesiculopustule with an erythematous base that erodes through the epidermis into the dermis to form an ulcer with elevated margins. The ulcer becomes obscured by a dry, heaped-up, tightly adherent crust (Fig. 664-3) that contributes to the persistence of the infection and scar formation. Lesions may be spread by autoinoculation, may be as large as 4 cm, and occur most frequently on the legs. Predisposing factors include pruritic lesions, such as insect bites, scabies, or pediculosis, which are subject to frequent scratching; poor hygiene; and malnutrition. Complications include lymphangitis, cellulitis, and, rarely, poststreptococcal glomerulonephritis. The causative agent is usually group A β-hemolytic streptococcus; *S. aureus* is also cultured from most lesions but is probably a secondary pathogen. Crusts should be softened with warm compresses and removed. Systemic antibiotic therapy, as for impetigo, is indicated; almost all lesions are responsive to treatment with penicillin.

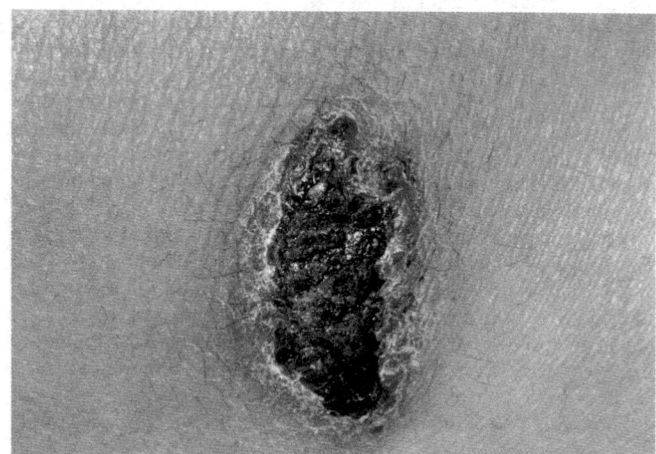

Figure 664-3. Dry, tightly adherent crust in ecthyma.

Ecthyma gangrenosa is a necrotic ulcer covered with a gray-black eschar. It is usually a sign of *P. aeruginosa* sepsis and usually occurs in immunosuppressed patients. Ecthyma gangrenosum occurs in up to 6% of patients with systemic *P. aeruginosa* infection but can also occur as a primary cutaneous infection by inoculation. The lesion begins as a red or purpuric macule that vesiculates and then ulcerates. There is a surrounding rim of pink to violaceous skin. The punched-out ulcer develops raised edges with a dense, black depressed, crusted center. Lesions may be single or multiple. Patients with bacteremia commonly have lesions in apocrine areas. Clinically similar lesions may also develop as a result of infection with other agents such as *S. aureus, A. hydrophila, Enterobacter* spp., *Proteus* spp., *Burkholderia cepacia, Serratia marcescens, Aspergillus* spp., *Mucorales, E. coli,* and *Candida* spp. There is bacterial invasion of the adventitia and media of dermal veins but not arteries. The intima and lumina are spared. Blood cultures and skin biopsy for culture should be obtained, and empirical broad-spectrum, systemic therapy that includes coverage for *Pseudomonas* should be initiated as soon as possible.

BLASTOMYCOSIS-LIKE PYODERMA (PYODERMA VEGETANS)

This is an exuberant cutaneous reaction to bacterial infection, primarily in children who are malnourished and immunosuppressed. The organisms most commonly isolated from lesions are *S. aureus* and group A streptococcus, but several other organisms have been associated with these lesions, including *P. aeruginosa, Proteus mirabilis,* diphtheroids, *Bacillus* spp., and *C. perfringens.* Crusted, hyperplastic plaques on the extremities are characteristic, sometimes forming from the coalescence of many pinpoint, purulent, crusted abscesses (Fig. 664-4). Ulceration and sinus tract formation may develop, and additional lesions may appear at sites distant from the site of inoculation. Regional lymphadenopathy is common, but fever is not. Histopathologic

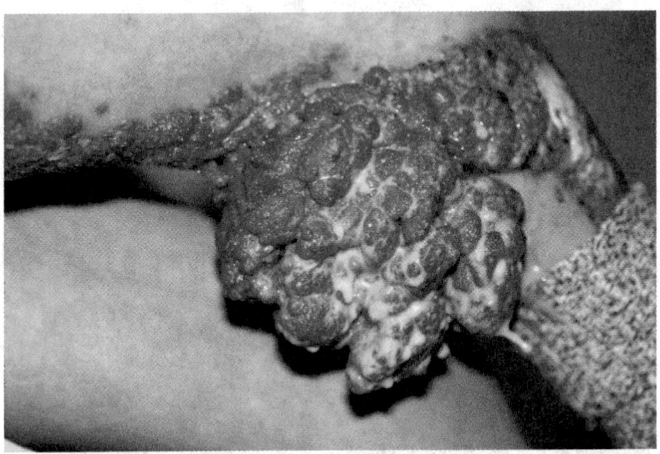

Figure 664-4. Large vegetating lesion of pyoderma vegetans.

examination reveals pseudoepitheliomatous hyperplasia and abscesses composed of neutrophils and/or eosinophils. Giant cells are usually lacking. The **differential diagnosis** includes deep fungal infection, particularly blastomycosis and tuberculous and atypical mycobacterial infection. Underlying immunodeficiency should be ruled out, and the selection of antibiotics should be guided by susceptibility testing because the response to antibiotics is often poor.

BLISTERING DISTAL DACTYLITIS

This is a superficial blistering infection of the volar fat pad on the distal portion of the finger or thumb. More than one finger may be involved, as may the volar surfaces of the proximal phalanges, palms, and toes. Blisters are filled with a watery purulent fluid that contains polymorphonuclear leukocytes and chains of gram-positive cocci. Patients usually have no preceding history of trauma, and systemic symptoms are generally absent. Poststreptococcal glomerulonephritis has not occurred after blistering distal dactylitis. The infection is caused most commonly by group A streptococcus but has also occurred as a result of infection with group B β-hemolytic streptococci and *S. aureus*. If left untreated, blisters may continue to enlarge and extend to the paronychial area. The infection responds to incision and drainage and a 10-day course of systemic penicillin or erythromycin therapy.

PERIANAL INFECTIOUS DERMATITIS

This presents most commonly in boys (70% of cases) between the ages of 6 mo and 10 yr as perianal dermatitis (90% of cases) and pruritus (80% of cases). The incidence of perianal infectious dermatitis is not known precisely but ranges from 1/2,000 to 1/218 patient visits. The rash is superficial, erythematous, well marginated, nonindurated, and confluent from the anus outward. Acutely (<6 wk), the rash tends to be bright red, moist, and tender to touch. At this stage, a white pseudomembrane may be present. As the rash becomes more chronic, the perianal eruption may consist of painful fissures, a dried mucoid discharge, or psoriasiform plaques with yellow peripheral crust. In girls, the perianal rash may be associated with vulvovaginitis. In boys, the penis may be involved. Approximately 50% of patients have rectal pain, most commonly described as burning inside the anus during defecation, and 33% have blood-streaked stools. Fecal retention is a frequent behavioral response to the infection. Patients may also have presented with guttate psoriasis. Although local induration or edema may occur, constitutional symptoms of fever, headache, and malaise are absent, suggesting that subcutaneous involvement, as in cellulitis, is absent. Familial spread of perianal infectious dermatitis is common, particularly when family members bathe together or use the same water.

The **differential diagnosis** of perianal infectious dermatitis includes psoriasis, seborrheic dermatitis, candidosis, pinworm infestation, sexual abuse, and inflammatory bowel disease. Differentiation from these other conditions can be accomplished by culturing a moderate to heavy growth of groups A streptococcus (GABHS). Perianal infectious dermatitis may also be caused by *S. aureus*. Children with asymptomatic perianal colonization have light growth of GABHS on blood agar. Direct antigen studies for GABHS are also very sensitive (89%), but results may be falsely negative early in the course. Acute and convalescent sera for antistreptolysin O or anti-DNase B are not helpful. The index case and family members should be cultured; follow-up cultures to document bacteriologic cure after a course of treatment are recommended.

Treatment with a 10 day course of oral penicillin produces resolution of the dermatitis and symptoms in most patients; recurrence rates of 40–50% have been reported, emphasizing the need for close follow-up, including repeat culture. Erythromycin estolate or ethylsuccinate are excellent alternative treatments for those who are allergic to penicillin, who have not responded to a course of penicillin, or who are infected with *S. aureus*. Clindamycin has also been used successfully to treat recurrent perianal dermatitis. Mupirocin has been used in conjunction with oral antibiotics to treat recurrences but has not been evaluated as a single-drug therapy.

ERYSIPELAS (SEE CHAPTER 182)

FOLLICULITIS

This superficial infection of the hair follicle is most often caused by *S. aureus* (Bockhart impetigo). Coagulase-negative staphylococci are occasionally the cause. The lesions are typically small, discrete, dome-shaped pustules with an erythematous base, located at the ostium of the pilosebaceous canals (Fig. 664-5). Hair growth is unimpaired, and the lesions heal without scarring. Favored sites include the scalp, buttocks, and extremities. Poor hygiene, maceration, and drainage from wounds and abscesses can be provocative factors. Folliculitis can also occur as a result of tar therapy or occlusive wraps. The moist environment encourages bacterial proliferation. In HIV-infected patients, *S. aureus* may produce confluent erythematous patches with satellite pustules in intertriginous areas and violaceous plaques composed of superficial follicular pustules in the scalp, axillae, or groin. *Candida* may cause satellite follicular papules and pustules sur-

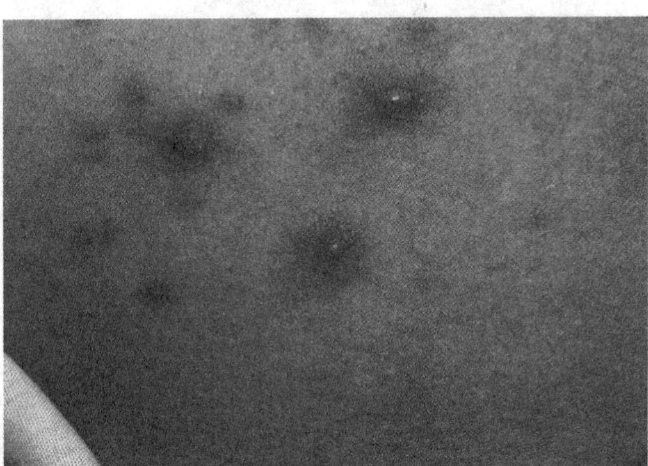

Figure 664-5. Folliculitis. Multiple follicular pustules.

rounding erythematous patches of intertrigo, and *Malassezia furfur* produces 2–3 mm, pruritic, erythematous, perifollicular papules and pustules on the back, chest, and extremities, particularly in patients with diabetes mellitus or on corticosteroids or antibiotics. Diagnosis is made by examining potassium hydroxide–treated scrapings from lesions. Detection of *Malassezia* may require a skin biopsy, demonstrating clusters of yeast and short, branching hyphae ("macaroni and meatballs") in widened follicular ostia mixed with keratinous debris.

The causative organism of folliculitis can be identified by Gram stain and culture of purulent material from the follicular orifice. **Treatment** for folliculitis includes topical antibiotic cleansers such as chlorhexidine or hexachlorophene. Topical antibiotic therapy is usually all that is required for mild cases, but more severe cases may require use of penicillinase-resistant systemic antibiotics such as dicloxacillin or cephalexin. In chronic recurrent folliculitis, daily application of a benzoyl peroxide lotion or gel may facilitate resolution.

Folliculitis caused by gram-negative organisms occurs primarily in patients with acne vulgaris treated long term with broad-spectrum systemic antibiotics. A superficial pustular form, caused by *Klebsiella, Enterobacter, E. coli,* or *P. aeruginosa,* occurs around the nose and spreads to the cheeks and chin. A deeper, nodular form of folliculitis on the face and trunk is caused by *Proteus* spp. Culture of infected follicles is necessary to establish the diagnosis. **Treatment** consists of incision and drainage of the deeper lesion and selection of an oral antibiotic based on the sensitivity profile of the pathogenic organism. For severe, recalcitrant cases, 13-cis-retinoic acid, 1 mg/kg/24 hr, is helpful but should be administered only by experienced physicians because of side effects.

Sycosis barbae is a deeper, more severe recurrent inflammatory form of folliculitis caused by *S. aureus* that involves the entire depth of the follicle. Erythematous follicular papules and pustules develop on the chin, upper lip, and angle of the jaw, primarily in young black males. Papules may coalesce into plaques, and healing may occur with scarring. Affected individuals are frequently found to be *S. aureus* carriers. **Treatment** with warm saline compresses and topical antibiotics such as mupirocin generally clears the infection. More extensive, recalcitrant cases may require therapy with β-lactamase-resistant systemic antibiotics and elimination of *S. aureus* from sites of carriage.

Hot tub folliculitis is attributable to *P. aeruginosa,* predominantly serotype O-11. The lesions are pruritic papules and pustules or deeply erythematous to violaceous nodules that develop 8–48 hr after exposure and are most dense in areas covered by a bathing suit (Fig. 664-6). Patients occasionally develop fever, malaise, and lymphadenopathy. The organism is readily cultured from pus. The eruption usually resolves spontaneously in 1–2 wk, often leaving postinflammatory hyperpigmentation. Consideration should be given to use of systemic antibiotics (ciprofloxacin) in adolescent patients with constitutional symptoms. Immunocompromised children are susceptible to complications of *Pseudomonas* folliculitis (cellulitis) and should avoid hot tubs.

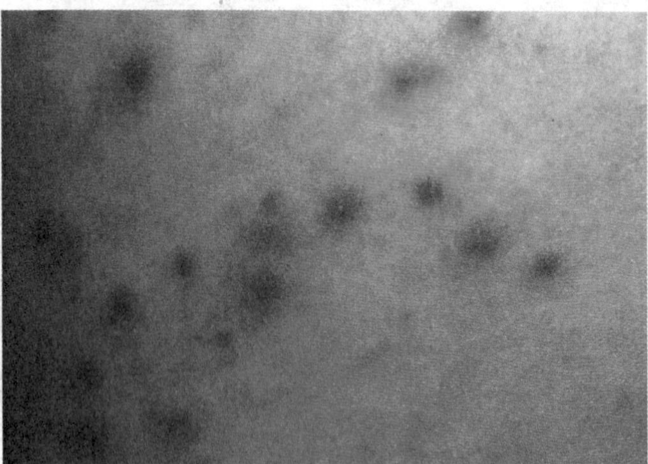
Figure 664-6. Papules and pustules in hot tub folliculitis.

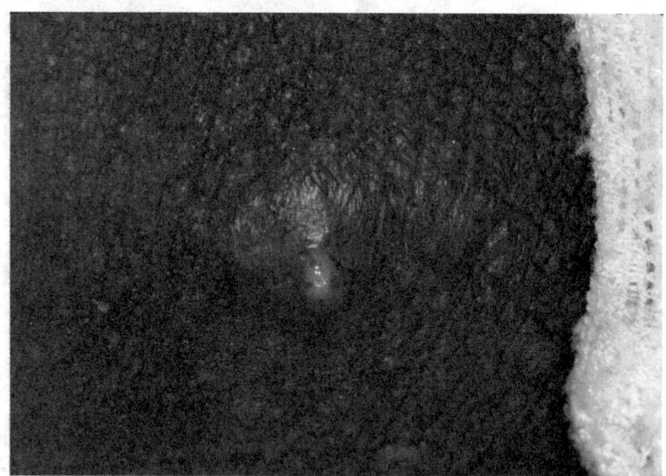
Figure 664-7. Rupture and discharge of pus in a furuncle.

FURUNCLES AND CARBUNCLES

These follicular lesions may originate from a preceding folliculitis or may arise initially as a deep-seated, tender, erythematous, perifollicular nodule. Although lesions are initially indurated, central necrosis and suppuration follow, leading to rupture and discharge of a central core of necrotic tissue and destruction of the follicle (Fig. 664-7). Healing occurs with scar formation. Sites of predilection are the hair-bearing areas on the face, neck, axillae, buttocks, and groin. Pain may be intense if the lesion is situated in an area where the skin is relatively fixed, such as in the external auditory canal or over the nasal cartilages. Patients with furuncles usually have no constitutional symptoms; bacteremia may occasionally ensue. Rarely, lesions on the upper lip or cheek may lead to cavernous sinus thrombosis. Infection of a group of contiguous follicles, with multiple drainage points, accompanied by inflammatory changes in surrounding connective tissue is a carbuncle. Carbuncles may be accompanied by fever, leukocytosis, and bacteremia.

ETIOLOGY. The causative agent is usually *S. aureus,* which penetrates abraded perifollicular skin. Conditions predisposing to furuncle formation include obesity, hyperhidrosis, maceration, friction, and pre-existing dermatitis. Furunculosis is also more common in individuals with low serum iron levels, diabetes, malnutrition, HIV infection, or other immunodeficiency states. Recurrent furunculosis is frequently associated with carriage of *S. aureus* in the nares, axillae, or perineum or close contact with someone such as a family member who is a carrier. Other bacteria or fungi may occasionally cause furuncles or carbuncles; Gram stain and culture of the pus are indicated.

TREATMENT. This includes regular bathing with antimicrobial soaps and wearing of loose-fitting clothing, which minimizes predisposing factors for furuncle formation. Frequent application of a hot, moist compress may facilitate drainage of lesions. Large lesions may be drained by a small incision. Carbuncles and large or numerous furuncles should be treated with systemic penicillinase-resistant antibiotics such as cloxacillin orally or oxacillin parenterally. Penicillin-allergic patients can be treated

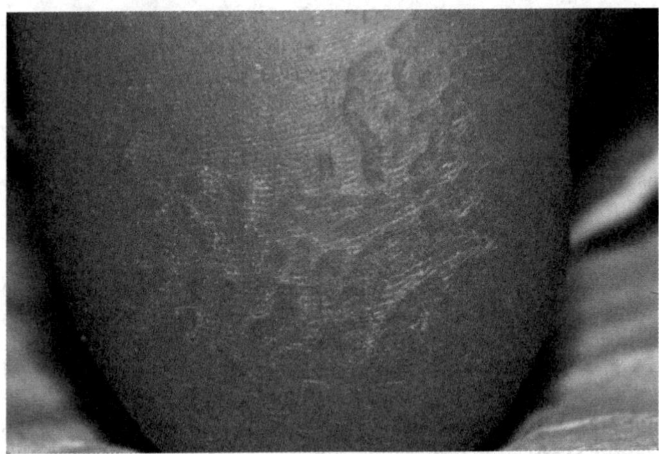

Figure 664-8. Superficial erosions of the horny layer in pitted keratolysis.

with a cephalosporin, clindamycin, or erythromycin. The carriage state may be eliminated temporarily by application of mupirocin ointment on the anterior nares for 5 days. Attention to personal hygiene, use of an antibacterial soap, low-dose oral antistaphylococcal penicillin or clindamycin, and frequent handwashing may also be beneficial.

PITTED KERATOLYSIS

Pitted keratolysis occurs most frequently in humid tropical and subtropical climates, particularly in individuals whose feet are moist for prolonged periods, for example, as a result of hyperhidrosis, prolonged wearing of boots, or immersion in water. The lesions consist of 1–7 mm, irregularly shaped, superficial erosions of the horny layer on the soles, particularly at weight-bearing sites (Fig. 664-8). Brownish discoloration of involved areas may be apparent. The condition is usually asymptomatic but frequently malodorous. A rare, painful variant is manifested as thinned, erythematous to violaceous plaques in addition to the typical pitted lesions. The most likely etiologic agent is a species of *Corynebacterium. Actinomycetes, Dermatophilus,* and micrococci have also been isolated from lesions. Avoidance of moisture and maceration produces slow, spontaneous resolution of the infection. Therapeutic regimens that have been effective include topical application of 2% buffered glutaraldehyde, 20% formaldehyde solution (formalin) in Aquaphor, erythromycin, clindamycin, and the imidazoles.

ERYTHRASMA

This is a benign chronic superficial infection caused by *Corynebacterium minutissimum.* Predisposing factors include heat, humidity, obesity, skin maceration, and poor hygiene. Approximately 20% of patients have involvement of the toe webs. Other frequently affected sites are moist, intertriginous areas such as the groin and axillae. The inframammary and perianal regions are occasionally involved. Sharply demarcated, irregularly bordered, slightly scaly, brownish-red patches are characteristic of the disease. Mild pruritus is the only constant symptom. *C. minutissimum* is a complex of related organisms that produce porphyrins that fluoresce brilliant coral red under ultraviolet light. The diagnosis is readily made, and erythrasma is differentiated from dermatophyte infection and from tinea versicolor by Wood lamp examination. Bathing within 20 hr of Wood lamp examination, however, may remove the water-soluble porphyrins. Staining of skin scrapings with methylene blue or Gram stain reveals the pleomorphic, filamentous coccobacillary forms.

Most cases represent colonization, are asymptomatic, and require no therapy. Effective **treatment** can be achieved with topical erythromycin, clindamycin, miconazole, or Whitfield ointment or a 10–14 day course of oral erythromycin. Recurrence may be inhibited by frequent use of an antibacterial.

ERYSIPELOID

This rare cutaneous infection is caused by inoculation of *Erysipelothrix rhusiopathiae* from contaminated animals, birds, fish, or their products. The localized cutaneous form is most common, characterized by well-demarcated diamond-shaped erythematous to violaceous patches at sites of inoculation. Local symptoms are generally not severe, constitutional symptoms are rare, and the lesions resolve spontaneously after weeks but can recur at the same site or develop elsewhere weeks to months later. The diffuse cutaneous form presents with lesions at several areas of the body in addition to the site of inoculation. It is also self-limited. The systemic form, caused by hematogenous spread, is accompanied by constitutional symptoms and may include endocarditis, septic arthritis, cerebral infarct and abscess, meningitis, and pulmonary effusion. Diagnosis is confirmed by skin biopsy, which reveals the gram-positive organisms, and culture. The **treatment** of choice is parenteral erythromycin or penicillin.

TUBERCULOSIS OF THE SKIN (SEE ALSO CHAPTERS 212 AND 214)

Cutaneous tuberculosis infection occurs worldwide, particularly in association with HIV infection, malnutrition, and poor sanitary conditions. Primary cutaneous tuberculosis is rare in the United States but occurs with the greatest frequency in infants and children. The overall incidence of cutaneous tuberculosis among those with all forms of tuberculosis in the United States is ≈1–2%. All forms of cutaneous disease are caused by *Mycobacterium tuberculosis, Mycobacterium bovis,* and occasionally by the bacillus Calmette-Guérin (BCG), an attenuated vaccine form of *M. bovis.* The manifestations caused by a given organism are indistinguishable from one another. After invasion of the skin, mycobacteria either multiply intracellularly within macrophages, leading to progressive disease, or are controlled by the host immune reaction.

A primary lesion, a tuberculous chancre, results when *M. tuberculosis* or *M. bovis* gains access to the skin or mucous membranes through trauma. Sites of predilection are the face, lower extremities, and genitals. The initial lesion develops 2–4 wk after introduction of the organism into the damaged tissue. A red-brown papule gradually enlarges to form a shallow, firm, sharply demarcated ulcer. Satellite abscesses may be present. Some lesions acquire a crust resembling impetigo, and others become heaped up and verrucous at the margins. The primary lesion occurs in 30% of cases as a painless ulcer on the conjunctiva, gingiva, or palate and occasionally as a painless acute paronychia. Painless regional adenopathy appears ≈3–8 wk after inoculation and may be accompanied by lymphangitis, lymphadenitis, or perforation of the skin surface, forming **scrofuloderma. Erythema nodosum** develops in ≈10% of cases. Untreated lesions heal with scarring within ≈12 mo but may reactivate, may form lupus vulgaris, or, rarely, may progress to the acute miliary form.

M. tuberculosis or *M. bovis* can be cultured from the skin lesion and local lymph nodes, but acid-fast staining of histologic sections, particularly of a well-controlled infection, often does not reveal the organism. The **differential diagnosis** is broad, including a syphilitic chancre; deep fungal or atypical mycobacterial infection; leprosy; tularemia; cat scratch disease; sporotrichosis; nocardiosis; leishmaniasis; reaction to foreign substances such as zirconium, beryllium, silk or nylon sutures, talc, or starch; papular acne rosacea; and lupus miliaris disseminatum faciei.

Spontaneous healing with scarring coincides with acquisition of immunity, at which time the skin lesions and infected nodes may become calcified. Antituberculous therapy is indicated (see Chapter 212).

Direct cutaneous inoculation of the tubercle bacillus into a previously infected individual with a moderate to high degree of immunity initially produces a small papule with surrounding inflammation. **Tuberculosis verrucosa cutis** (warty tuberculosis) forms when the papule becomes hyperkeratotic and warty, and several adjacent papules coalesce or a single papule expands peripherally to form a brownish-red to violaceous, exudative, crusted verrucous plaque. Irregular extension of the margins of the plaque produces a serpiginous border. Children have the lesion most commonly on the lower extremities after trauma and contact with infected material such as sputum or soil. Regional lymph nodes are involved only rarely. Spontaneous healing with atrophic scarring takes place slowly, over months to years. Healing is also gradual with antituberculous therapy.

Lupus vulgaris is a rare, chronic, progressive form of cutaneous tuberculosis that develops in individuals with a moderate to high degree of tuberculin sensitivity induced by previous infection. The incidence is greater in cool, moist climates, particularly in females. Lupus vulgaris develops as a result of direct extension from underlying joints or lymph nodes; through lymphatic or hematogenous spread; or, rarely, by cutaneous inoculation with BCG vaccine. It most commonly follows cervical adenitis or pulmonary tuberculosis. Approximately 33% of cases are preceded by scrofuloderma, and 90% of cases present on the head and neck, most commonly on the nose or cheek. Involvement of the trunk is uncommon. A typical solitary lesion consists of a soft, brownish-red papule that has an apple-jelly color when examined by diascopy. Expansion of the papule peripherally, or occasionally the coalescence of several papules, forms an irregular lesion of variable size and form. One or several lesions may develop, including nodules or plaques that are flat and serpiginous, hypertrophic and verrucous, or edematous in appearance. Spontaneous healing occurs centrally, and lesions characteristically reappear within the area of atrophy. Chronicity is characteristic, and persistence and progression of plaques over many years is common. Lymphadenitis is present in 40% of those with lupus vulgaris, and 10–20% have infection of the lungs, bones, or joints. Vegetative masses and ulceration involving the nasal, buccal, or conjunctival mucosa; the palate; the gingiva; or the oropharynx may cause extensive deformities. Squamous cell carcinoma, with a relatively high metastatic potential, may develop, usually after several years of the disease. After a temporary impairment in immunity, particularly after measles infection (lupus exanthematicus), multiple lesions may form at distant sites as a result of hematogenous spread from a latent focus of infection. The histopathology reveals a tuberculoid granuloma without caseation; organisms are extremely difficult to demonstrate. The **differential diagnosis** includes sarcoidosis, atypical mycobacterial infection, blastomycosis, chromoblastomycosis, actinomycosis, leishmaniasis, tertiary syphilis, leprosy, hypertrophic lichen planus, psoriasis, lupus erythematosus, lymphocytoma, and Bowen disease. Small lesions can be excised. Antituberculous drug therapy usually halts further spread and induces involution.

Scrofuloderma results from enlargement, cold abscess formation, and breakdown of a lymph node, most frequently in a cervical chain, with extension to the overlying skin. Linear or serpiginous ulcers and dissecting fistulas and subcutaneous tracts studded with soft nodules may develop. Spontaneous healing may take years, eventuating in cordlike keloid scars. Lupus vulgaris may also develop. Scrofuloderma of a cervical lymph node often originates in the larynx and was linked in the past to ingestion of milk containing *M. bovis*. Lesions may also originate from an underlying infected joint, tendon, bone, or epididymis. The **differential diagnosis** includes syphilitic gumma, deep fungal infections, actinomycosis, and hidradenitis suppurativa. The course is indolent, and constitutional symptoms are typically absent. Antituberculous therapy is usually effective.

Orificial tuberculosis presents on the mucous membranes and periorificial skin after autoinoculation of mycobacteria from sites of progressive infection. It is a sign of advanced internal disease and carries a poor prognosis. Lesions appear as painful, yellowish or red nodules that form punched-out ulcers with inflammation and edema of the surrounding mucosa. **Treatment** consists of identification of the source of infection and initiation of antituberculous therapy.

Miliary tuberculosis (hematogenous primary tuberculosis) rarely presents cutaneously and occurs most commonly in infants and in individuals who are immunosuppressed after chemotherapy or infection with measles or HIV. The eruption consists of crops of symmetrically distributed, minute, erythematous to purpuric macules, papules, or vesicles. The lesions may ulcerate, drain, crust, and form sinus tracts or may form subcutaneous gummas, especially in malnourished children with impaired immunity. Constitutional signs and symptoms are common, and a leukemoid reaction or aplastic anemia may develop. Tubercle bacilli are readily identified in an active lesion. A fulminant course should be anticipated, and aggressive antituberculous therapy is indicated.

Single or multiple metastatic tuberculous abscesses (**tuberculous gummas**) may develop on the extremities and trunk by hematogenous spread from a primary focus of infection during a period of decreased immunity, particularly in malnourished and immunosuppressed children. The fluctuant, nontender, erythematous subcutaneous nodules may ulcerate and form fistulas.

Vaccination with BCG characteristically produces a papule ≈2 wk after vaccination. The papule expands in size, typically ulcerates within 2–4 mo, and heals slowly with scarring. In ≈1–2 per million vaccinations, a complication caused specifically by the BCG organism occurs, including regional lymphadenitis, lupus vulgaris, scrofuloderma, and subcutaneous abscess formation.

Tuberculids are skin reactions that exhibit tuberculoid features histologically but do not contain detectable mycobacteria. The lesions appear in a host who usually has moderate to strong tuberculin reactivity, has a history of previous tuberculosis of other organs, and usually shows a therapeutic response to antituberculous therapy. The cause of tuberculids is poorly understood. Most patients are in good health with no clear focus of disease at the time of the eruption. The most commonly observed tuberculid is the papulonecrotic tuberculid. Recurrent crops of symmetrically distributed, asymptomatic, firm, sterile, dusky-red papules appear on the extensor aspects of the limbs, the dorsum of the hands and feet, and the buttocks. The papules may undergo central ulceration and eventually heal, leaving sharply delineated, circular, depressed scars. The duration of the eruption is variable, but it usually disappears promptly after treatment of the primary infection. Lichen scrofulosorum, another form of tuberculid, is characterized by asymptomatic, grouped, pinhead-sized, often follicular pink or red papules that form discoid plaques, mainly on the trunk. Healing occurs without scarring.

Atypical mycobacterial infection may cause cutaneous lesions in children. *Mycobacterium marinum* is found in saltwater, freshwater, and diseased fish. In the United States, it is most commonly acquired from tropical fish tanks and swimming pools. Traumatic abrasion of the skin serves as a portal of entry for the organism. Approximately 3 wk after inoculation, a single reddish papule develops and enlarges slowly to form a violaceous nodule or occasionally a warty plaque (Fig. 664-9). The lesion occasionally breaks down to form a crusted ulcer or a suppurating abscess. Sporotrichoid erythematous nodules along lymphatics may also suppurate and drain. Lesions are most common on the elbows, knees, and feet of swimmers and the hands and fingers in aquarium-acquired infection. Systemic signs and symptoms are absent. Regional lymph nodes occasionally become slightly enlarged but do not break down. Rarely, the infection becomes

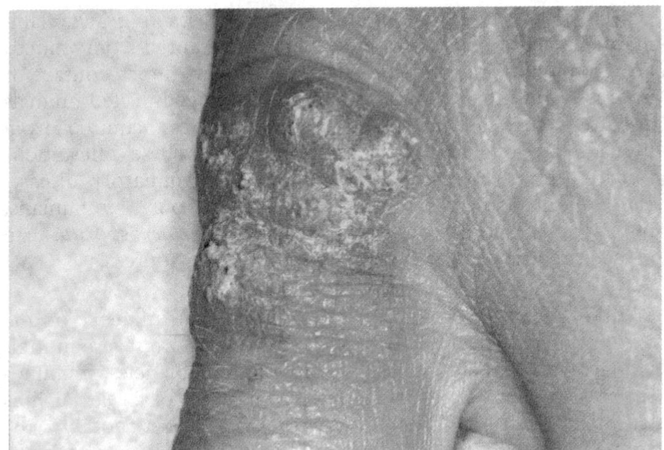

Figure 664-9. Violaceous, warty plaque of *Mycobacterium marinum* infection.

disseminated, particularly in an immunosuppressed host. A biopsy specimen of a fully developed lesion demonstrates a granulomatous infiltrate with tuberculoid architecture; intracellular organisms can usually be identified within the histiocytes with appropriate stains. The most effective treatment includes tetracycline, minocycline, and rifampin plus ethambutol. Application of heat to the affected site may be a useful adjunctive therapy. Spontaneous healing with scarring can be expected within several months to 2 yr (see Chapter 214).

Mycobacterium kansasii primarily causes pulmonary disease; skin disease is rare, often occurring in an immunocompromised host. Most commonly, sporotrichoid nodules develop after inoculation of traumatized skin. Lesions may develop into ulcerated, crusted, or verrucous plaques. The organism is relatively sensitive to antituberculous medications, which should be chosen on the basis of susceptibility testing.

M. scrofulaceum causes cervical lymphadenitis (scrofuloderma) in young children, typically in the submandibular region. Nodes enlarge over several weeks, ulcerate, and drain. The local reaction is nontender and circumscribed, constitutional symptoms are absent, and there generally is no evidence of lung or other organ involvement. Other atypical mycobacteria may cause a similar presentation, including *M. avium* complex, *M. kansasii,* and M. *fortuitum.* **Treatment** is accomplished by excision and administration of antituberculous drugs (see Chapter 214).

Mycobacterium ulcerans causes a painless subcutaneous nodule after inoculation of abraded skin. Most infections occur in children in tropical rain forests. The nodule usually ulcerates, develops undermined edges, and may spread over large areas, most commonly on an extremity. Local necrosis of subcutaneous fat, producing a septal panniculitis, is characteristic. Ulcers persist for months to years before healing spontaneously with scarring and sometimes with lymphedema. Constitutional symptoms and lymphadenopathy are absent. Diagnosis is made by culturing the organism at 32–33°C. **Treatment of choice** is early excision of the lesion. Local heat therapy and oral chemotherapy may benefit some patients.

M. avium complex, composed of >20 subtypes, most commonly causes chronic pulmonary infection. Cervical lymphadenitis and osteomyelitis occur occasionally, and papules or purulent leg ulcers occur rarely by primary inoculation. Skin lesions may be an early sign of disseminated infection. The lesions may take various forms, including erythematous papules, pustules, nodules, abscesses, ulcers, panniculitis, and sporotrichoid spread along lymphatics. For treatment, see Chapter 214.

M. fortuitum complex is composed of two organisms: *M. fortuitum* and *M. chelonei.* These organisms cause disease in an immunocompetent host principally by primary cutaneous inoculation after traumatic injury, injection, or surgery. A nodule, abscess, or cellulitis develops 4–6 wk after inoculation. In an immunocompromised host, numerous subcutaneous nodules may form, break down, and drain. **Treatment** is based on identification and susceptibility testing of the organism.

Barbagallo J, Tager P, Ingleton R, et al: Cutaneous tuberculosis: Diagnosis and treatment. *Am J Clin Dermatol* 2002;3:319–328.

Herbst R: Perineal streptococcal dermatitis/disease: Recognition and management. *Am J Clin Dermatol* 2003;4:555–560.

Johnston GA: Treatment of bullous impetigo and staphylococcal scalded skin syndrome in infants. *Expert Rev Anti Infect Ther* 2004;3:439–446.

Konig S, Verhagen AP, van Suijlekom-Smit, et al: Interventions in impetigo. *Cochrane Database Syst Rev* 2004;2:CD003261.

Lewis FM, Marsh BJ, von Reyn CF: Fish tank exposure and cutaneous infections due to Mycobacterium marinum: Tuberculin skin testing, treatment and prevention. *Clin Infect Dis* 2003;37:390–397.

Luelmo-Aguilar J, Santandreu MS: Folliculitis: Recognition and management. *Am J Clin Dermatol* 2004;5:301–310.

Lyon M, Doehring MC: Blistering distal dactylitis: A case series in children under nine months of age. *J Emerg Med* 2004;26:421–423.

Morris A: Cellulitis and erysipelas. *Clin Evid* 2003;10:1878–1883.

Patel GK: Treatment of staphylococcal scalded skin syndrome. *Expert Rev Anti Infect Ther* 2004;2:575–587.

Recih HL, Williams-Fadeyi D, Naik NS, et al: Nonpseudomonal ecthyma gangrenosum. *J Am Acad Dermatol* 2004;50:S114–S117.

Sladden MJ, Johnston GA: Common skin infections in children. *Br Med J* 2204;329:95–99.

Wong CH, Wang US: The diagnosis of necrotizing fasciitis. *Curr Opin Infect Dis* 2005;18:101–106.

Chapter 665 ■ Cutaneous Fungal Infections

Joseph G. Morelli

TINEA VERSICOLOR

This common, innocuous, chronic fungal infection of the stratum corneum is caused by the dimorphic yeast *Malassezia furfur.* The synonyms *Pityrosporum ovale* and *P. orbiculare* were used previously to identify the causal organism.

ETIOLOGY. *M. furfur* is part of the indigenous flora, predominantly in the yeast form, and is found particularly in areas of skin that are rich in sebum production. Proliferation of filamentous forms occurs in the disease state. Predisposing factors include a warm, humid environment, excessive sweating, occlusion, high plasma cortisol levels, immunosuppression, malnourishment, and genetically determined susceptibility. The disease is most prevalent in adolescents and young adults.

CLINICAL MANIFESTATIONS. The lesions vary widely in color. In Caucasians, they are typically reddish brown, whereas in blacks they may be either hypopigmented or hyperpigmented. The characteristic macules are covered with a fine scale. They often begin in a perifollicular location, enlarge, and merge to form confluent patches, most commonly on the neck, upper chest, back, and upper arms (Fig. 665-1). Facial lesions are common in adolescents; lesions occasionally appear on the forearms, dorsum of the hands, and pubis. There may be little or no pruritus. Involved areas do not tan after sun exposure. A papulopustular perifollicular variant of the disorder may occur on the back, chest, and sometimes the extremities.

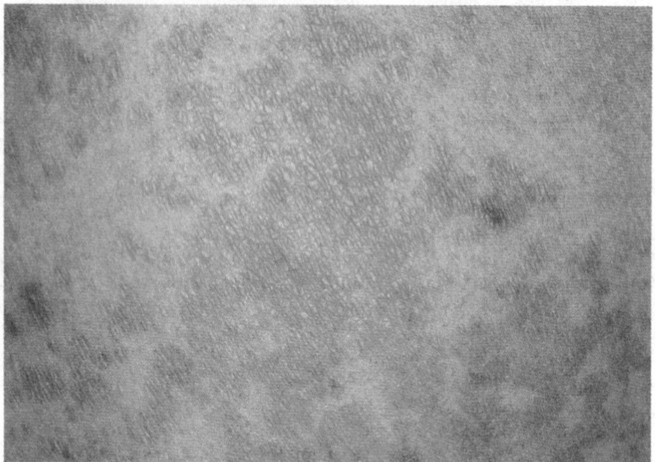

Figure 665-1. Hyperpigmented, sharply demarcated macules of varying sizes on the upper trunk characteristic of tinea versicolor.

DIAGNOSIS. Examination with a Wood lamp discloses a yellowish-gold fluorescence. A potassium hydroxide (KOH) preparation of scrapings is diagnostic, demonstrating groups of thick-walled spores and myriad short, thick, angular hyphae, resembling macaroni and meatballs. Skin biopsy, including culture and special stains for fungi (periodic acid–Schiff), are often necessary to make the diagnosis in cases of primarily follicular involvement. Microscopically, organisms and keratinous debris can be seen within dilated follicular ostia.

Tinea versicolor must be distinguished from dermatophyte infections, seborrheic dermatitis, pityriasis alba, and secondary syphilis. Nonscaling pigmentary disorders, such as postinflammatory pigmentary change, may be mimicked if a patient has removed the scales by scrubbing. *M. furfur* folliculitis must be distinguished from the other forms of folliculitis.

TREATMENT. Many therapeutic agents can be used to treat this disease successfully. The causative agent, a normal human saprophyte, is not eradicated from the skin, however, and the disorder recurs in predisposed individuals. Appropriate topical therapy may include one of the following: a selenium sulfide suspension applied overnight for 1 wk followed by 1 night per wk for 4 wk. An imidazole or terbinafine cream may be used twice daily for 2–4 wk. Oral therapy may be more convenient and may be achieved successfully with ketoconazole or fluconazole, 400 mg, repeated in 1 wk, or itraconazole, 200 mg/24 hr for 5–7 days. Recurrent episodes continue to respond promptly to these agents. Maintenance therapy with selenium sulfide applied overnight once a week may be used.

DERMATOPHYTOSES

Dermatophytoses are caused by a group of closely related filamentous fungi with a propensity for invading the stratum corneum, hair, and nails. The 3 principal genera responsible for infections are *Trichophyton, Microsporum,* and *Epidermophyton.*

ETIOLOGY. *Trichophyton* spp. cause lesions of all keratinized tissue, including skin, nails, and hair. *T. rubrum* is the most common dermatophyte pathogen. *Microsporum* spp. principally invade the hair, and the *Epidermophyton* spp. invade the intertriginous skin. Dermatophyte infections are designated by the word **tinea** followed by the Latin word for the anatomic site of involvement. The dermatophytes are also classified according to source and natural habitat. Fungi acquired from the soil are called geophilic. They infect humans sporadically, inciting an inflammatory reaction. Dermatophytes that are acquired from animals are zoophilic. Transmission may be through direct contact or indirectly by infected animal hair or clothing. Infected animals are frequently asymptomatic. Dermatophytes acquired from humans are referred to as anthropophilic. These infestations range from chronic low-grade to acute inflammatory disease. *Epidermophyton* infections are transmitted only by humans, but various species of *Trichophyton* and *Microsporum* can be acquired from both human and nonhuman sources.

EPIDEMIOLOGY. Host defense has an important influence on the severity of the infection. Disease tends to be more severe in individuals with diabetes mellitus, lymphoid malignancies, immunosuppression, and states with high plasma cortisol levels, such as Cushing syndrome. Some dermatophytes, most notably the zoophilic species, tend to elicit more severe, suppurative inflammation in humans. Some degree of resistance to reinfection is acquired by most infected persons and may be associated with a delayed hypersensitivity response. No relationship has been demonstrated, however, between antibody levels and resistance to infection. The frequency and severity of infection are also affected by the geographic locale, the genetic susceptibility of the host, and the virulence of the strain of dermatophyte. Additional local factors that predispose to infection include trauma to the skin, hydration of the skin with maceration, occlusion, and elevated temperature.

Occasionally, a secondary skin eruption referred to as a dermatophytid or "id" reaction appears in sensitized individuals and has been attributed to circulating fungal antigens derived from the primary infection. The eruption is characterized by grouped papules (Fig. 665-2) and vesicles and, occasionally, by sterile pustules. Symmetric urticarial lesions and a more generalized maculopapular eruption also can occur. Id reactions are most often associated with tinea pedis but also occur with tinea capitis.

DIAGNOSIS. The important diagnostic procedures for the various dermatophyte diseases include examination of infected hairs with a Wood lamp, microscopic examination of KOH preparations of infected material, and identification of the etiologic agent by culture. Hairs infected with common *Microsporum* spp. fluoresce a bright blue-green. Most *Trichophyton*-infected hairs do not fluoresce.

CLINICAL MANIFESTATIONS. Tinea capitis is a dermatophyte infection of the scalp most often caused by *Trichophyton tonsurans,* occasionally by *Microsporum canis,* and, much less commonly,

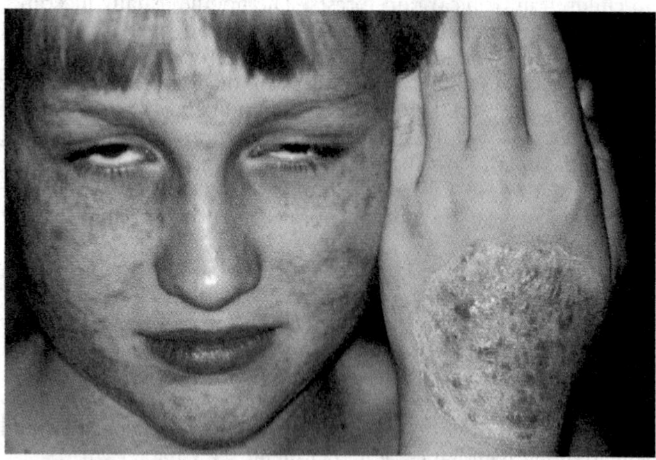

Figure 665-2. Id reaction. Papular eruption of the face associated with severe tinea infection of the hand.

by other *Microsporum* and *Trichophyton* spp. It is particularly common in black children age 4–14 yr. In *Microsporum* and some *Trichophyton* infections, the spores are distributed in a sheath-like fashion around the hair shaft (**ectothrix** infection), whereas *T. tonsurans* produces an infection within the hair shaft (endothrix). **Endothrix** infections may continue past the anagen phase of hair growth into telogen and are more chronic than infections with ectothrix organisms that persist only during the anagen phase. *T. tonsurans* is an anthropophilic species acquired most often by contact with infected hairs and epithelial cells that are on such surfaces as theater seats, hats, and combs. Dermatophyte spores may also be airborne within the immediate environment, and high carriage rates have been demonstrated in noninfected schoolmates and household members. *M. canis* is a zoophilic species that is acquired from cats and dogs.

The clinical presentation of tinea capitis varies with the infecting organism. The pattern produced by *Microsporum audouinii,* the most common cause of tinea capitis in the 1940s and 1950s, is characterized initially by a small papule at the base of a hair follicle. The infection spreads peripherally, forming an erythematous and scaly circular plaque (**ringworm**) within which the infected hairs become brittle and broken. Numerous confluent patches of alopecia develop, and patients may complain of severe pruritus. *M. audouinii* infection is no longer common in the United States. Endothrix infections such as those caused by *T. tonsurans* create a pattern known as "black-dot ringworm," characterized initially by many small circular patches of alopecia in which hairs are broken off close to the hair follicle (Fig. 665-3). Another clinical variant presents with diffuse scaling, with minimal hair loss secondary. It strongly resembles seborrheic dermatitis, psoriasis, or atopic dermatitis (Fig. 665-4). *T. tonsurans* may also produce a chronic and more diffuse alopecia. Lymphadenopathy is common (Fig. 665-5). A severe inflammatory response produces elevated, boggy granulomatous masses (**kerions**), which are often studded with pustules (Fig. 665-6*A*). Fever, pain, and regional adenopathy are common, and permanent scarring and alopecia may result (Fig. 665-6*B*). The zoophilic organism *M. canis* or the geophilic organism *Microsporum gypseum* also may cause kerion formation. **Favus** is a chronic form of tinea capitis that is rare in the United States and is caused by the fungus *Trichophyton schoenleinii.* Favus starts as yellowish-red papules at the opening of hair follicles. The papules expand and coalesce to form cupshaped, yellowish, crusted patches that fluoresce dull green under a Wood lamp.

Tinea capitis can be confused with seborrheic dermatitis, psoriasis, alopecia areata, trichotillomania, and certain dystrophic hair disorders. When inflammation is pronounced, as in kerion, primary or secondary bacterial infection must also be considered.

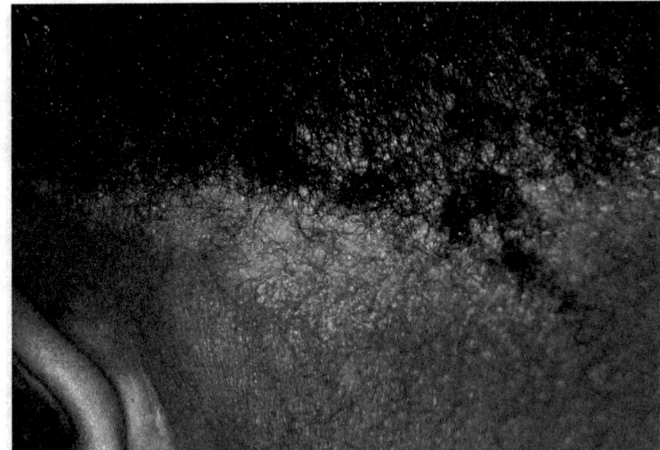

Figure 665-4. Tinea capitis mimicking seborrheic dermatitis.

In adolescents, the patchy, moth-eaten type of alopecia associated with secondary syphilis may resemble tinea capitis. If scarring occurs, discoid lupus erythematosus and lichen planopilaris must also be considered in the differential diagnosis.

Microscopic examination of a KOH preparation of infected hair from the active border of a lesion discloses tiny spores surrounding the hair shaft in *Microsporum* infections and chains of spores within the hair shaft in *T. tonsurans* infections. Fungal elements are not usually seen in scales. A specific etiologic diagnosis of tinea capitis may be obtained by planting broken off infected hairs on Sabouraud medium with reagents to inhibit growth of other organisms. Such identification may require 2 wk or more.

Oral administration of griseofulvin microcrystalline (20 mg/kg/24 hr) is the recommended **treatment** for all forms of tinea capitis. It may be necessary for 8–12 wk and should be terminated only after fungal culture results are negative. Treatment for 1 month after a negative culture minimizes the risk of recurrence. Adverse reactions to griseofulvin are rare but include nausea, vomiting, headache, blood dyscrasias, phototoxicity, and hepatotoxicity. Oral itraconazole is useful in instances of griseofulvin resistance, intolerance, or allergy. Itraconazole is given for 4–6 wk at a dosage of 3–5 mg/kg/24 hr with food. Capsules are preferable to the syrup, which may cause diarrhea. Terbinafine also appears to be effective at a dosage of 3–6 mg/kg/24 hr for 4–6 wk or possibly in pulse therapy, although it has limited activity against *M. canis.* Neither itraconazole nor terbinafine is approved by the

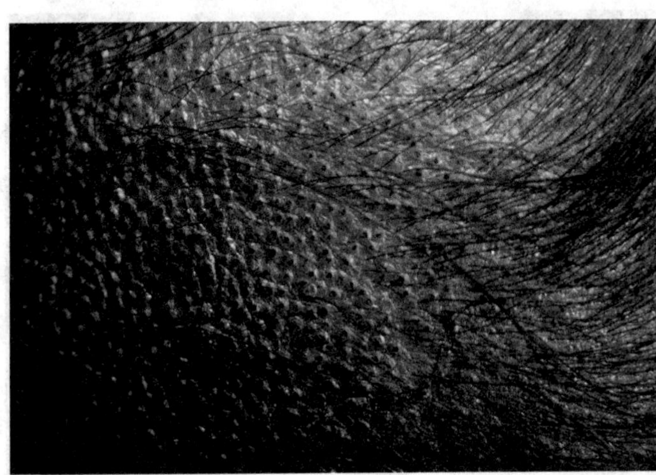

Figure 665-3. Black-dot ringworm with hairs broken off at the scalp.

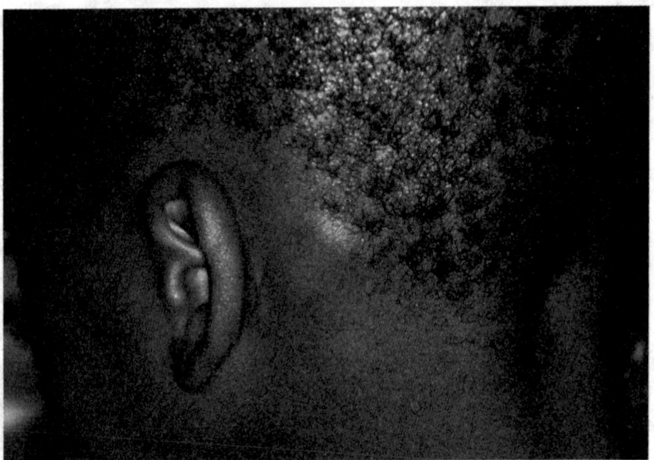

Figure 665-5. Lymphadenopathy associated with tinea capitis.

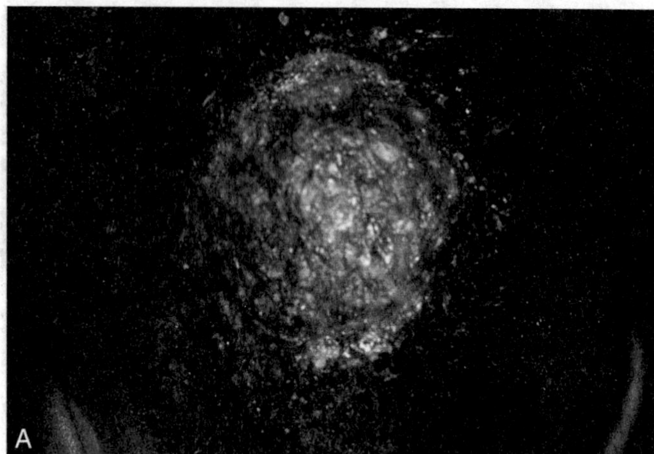

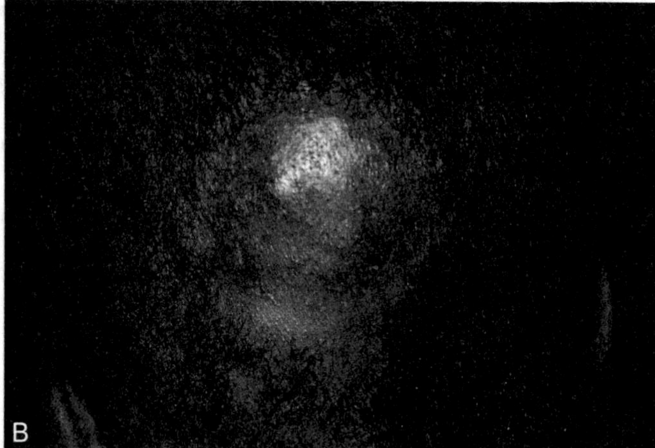

Figure 665-6. *A,* Kerion. Boggy granulomatous mass of the scalp. *B,* Scarring post kerion.

Food and Drug Administration (FDA) for treatment of dermatophyte infections in the pediatric population. Topical therapy alone is ineffective, but it may be an important adjunct because it may decrease the shedding of spores. Asymptomatic dermatophyte carriage in family members is common. One in 3 families have at least 1 member who is a carrier. Therefore, treatment of both patient and potential carriers with a sporicidal shampoo may hasten clinical resolution. Vigorous shampooing with a 2.5% selenium sulfide, zinc pyrithione, or ketoconazole shampoo is helpful. It is not necessary to shave the scalp.

Tinea corporis, infection of the glabrous skin, excluding the palms, soles, and groin, can be caused by most of the dermatophyte species, although *T. rubrum* and *T. mentagrophytes* are the most prevalent etiologic organisms. In children, infections with *M. canis* are also frequent. Tinea corporis can be acquired by direct contact with infected persons or by contact with infected scales or hairs deposited on environmental surfaces. *M. canis* infections are usually acquired from infected pets.

The most typical clinical lesion begins as a dry, mildly erythematous, elevated, scaly papule or plaque that spreads centrifugally and clears centrally to form the characteristic annular lesion responsible for the designation ringworm (Fig. 665-7). At times, plaques with advancing borders may spread over large areas. Grouped pustules are another variant. Most lesions clear spontaneously within several months, but some may become chronic. Central clearing does not always occur (Fig. 665-8), and differences in host response may result in wide variability in the clinical appearance, for example, granulomatous lesions called **Majocchi granuloma** due to penetration of organisms along the hair follicle to the level of the dermis, producing a fungal folliculitis and perifolliculitis (Fig. 665-9), and the kerion-like lesions referred to as tinea profunda. Majocchi granuloma is more common after inappropriate treatment with topical corticosteroids, especially the superpotent class.

Many skin lesions, both infectious and noninfectious, must be differentiated from the lesions of tinea corporis. Those most frequently confused are granuloma annulare, nummular eczema, pityriasis rosea, psoriasis, seborrheic dermatitis, erythema chronicum migrans, and tinea versicolor. Microscopic examination of KOH wet mount preparations and cultures should always be obtained when fungal infection is considered. Tinea corporis usually does not fluoresce with a Wood lamp.

Tinea corporis usually responds to **treatment** with one of the topical antifungal agents (e.g., imidazoles, terbinafine, naftifine) twice daily for 2–4 wk. In unusually severe or extensive disease, a course of therapy with oral griseofulvin microcrystalline may be required for 4 weeks. Itraconazole has produced excellent results in many cases with a 1–2 wk course of oral therapy.

Tinea cruris, infection of the groin, occurs most often in adolescent males and is usually caused by the anthropophilic species *Epidermophyton floccosum* or *Trichophyton rubrum,* but occasionally by the zoophilic species *T. mentagrophytes.*

The initial clinical lesion is a small, raised, scaly, erythematous patch on the inner aspect of the thigh. This spreads peripherally,

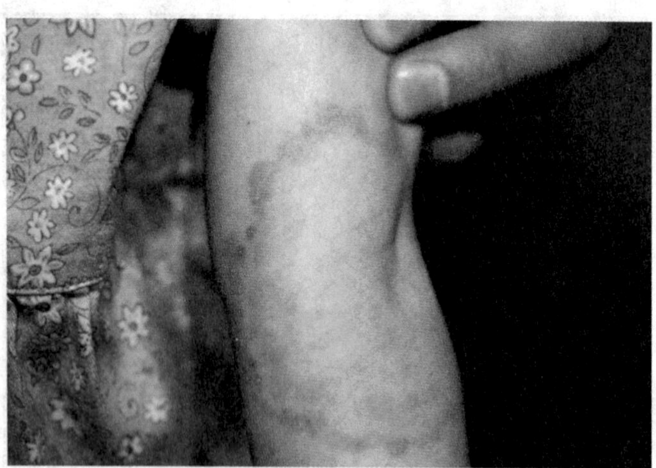

Figure 665-7. Annular plaque of tinea corporis with central clearing.

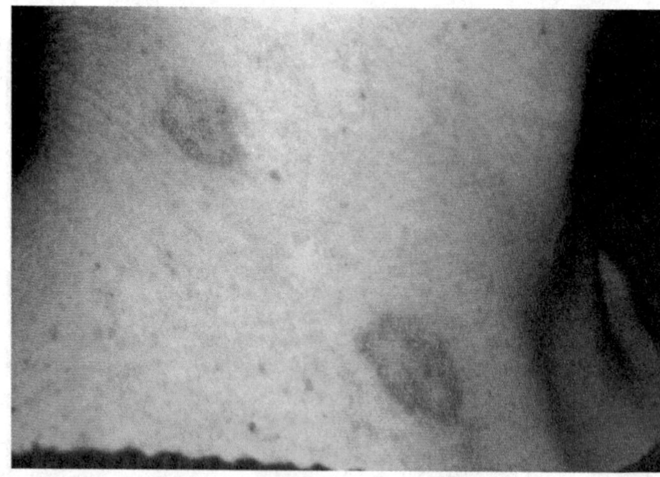

Figure 665-8. Minimal central clearing with tinea corporis.

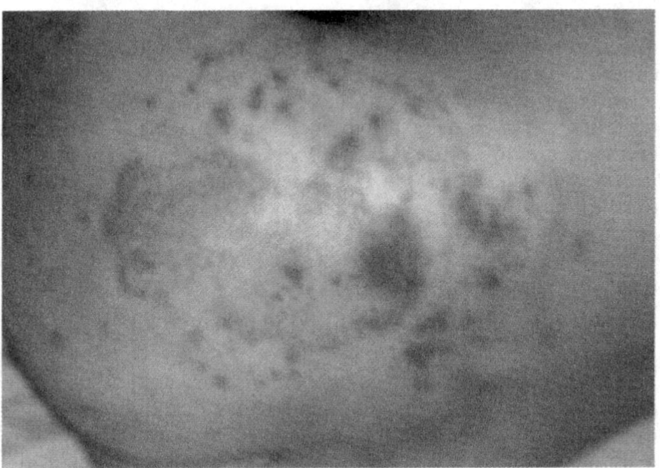

Figure 665-9. Follicular papule and pustule in Majocchi granuloma post use of a superpotent topical steroid.

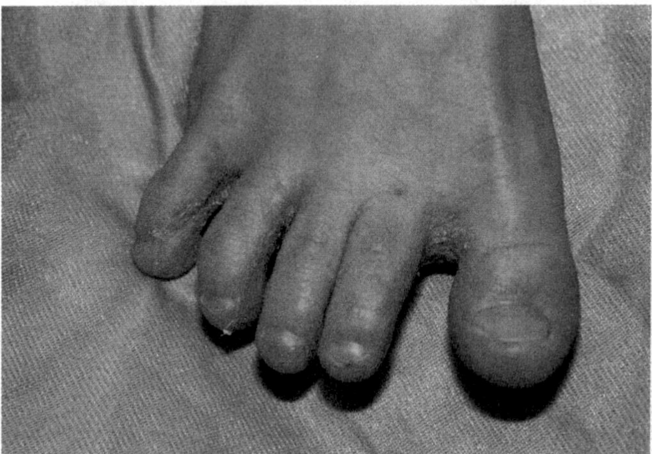

Figure 665-10. Interdigital tinea pedis.

often developing numerous tiny vesicles at the advancing margin. It eventually forms bilateral, irregular, sharply bordered patches with hyperpigmented scaly centers. In some cases, particularly in infections with *T. mentagrophytes,* the inflammatory reaction is more intense and the infection may spread beyond the crural region. The penis is usually not involved in the infection, an important distinction from candidosis. Pruritus may be severe initially but abates as the inflammatory reaction subsides. Bacterial superinfection may alter the clinical appearance, and erythrasma or candidosis may coexist. Tinea cruris is more prevalent in obese persons and in those who perspire excessively and wear tight-fitting clothing.

The diagnosis is confirmed by culture and by demonstrating septate hyphae on a KOH preparation of epidermal scrapings. Tinea cruris must be differentiated from intertrigo, allergic contact dermatitis, candidosis, and erythrasma. Bacterial superinfection must be precluded when there is a severe inflammatory reaction.

Patients should be advised to wear loose cotton underwear. **Topical treatment** with an imidazole is recommended for severe infection, especially because these agents are effective in mixed candidal-dermatophytic infections. Pure dermatophytic infection may also be treated with tolnaftate.

Tinea pedis (athlete's foot), infection of the toe webs and soles of the feet, is uncommon in young children but occurs with some frequency in preadolescent and adolescent males. The usual etiologic agents are *T. rubrum, T. mentagrophytes,* and *E. floccosum.*

Most commonly, the lateral toe webs (3rd to 4th and 4th to 5th interdigital spaces) and the subdigital crevice are fissured, with maceration and peeling of the surrounding skin (Fig. 665-10). Severe tenderness, itching, and a persistent foul odor are characteristic. These lesions may become chronic. This type of infection may involve overgrowth by bacterial flora, including *Micrococcus sedantarius, Brevibacterium epidermidis,* and gram-negative organisms. Less commonly, a chronic diffuse hyperkeratosis of the sole of the foot occurs with only mild erythema (Fig. 665-11). In many cases, two feet and one hand are involved. This type of infection is more refractory to treatment and tends to recur. An inflammatory vesicular type of reaction may occur with *T. mentagrophytes* infection. This type is most common in young children. These lesions involve any area of the foot, including the dorsal surface, and are usually circumscribed. The initial papules progress to vesicles and bullae that may become pustular (Fig. 665-12). A number of factors, such as occlusive footwear and warm, humid weather, predispose to infection. Tinea pedis may be transmitted in shower facilities and swimming pool areas.

Tinea pedis must be differentiated from simple maceration and peeling of the interdigital spaces, which is common in children. Infection with *Candida albicans* and various bacterial organisms (erythrasma) may cause confusion or may coexist with primary tinea pedis. Contact dermatitis, vesicular foot dermatitis, atopic dermatitis, and juvenile plantar dermatitis also simulate tinea pedis. Fungal mycelia can be seen on microscopic examination of a KOH preparation or by culture.

Treatment for mild infections includes simple measures such as avoidance of occlusive footwear, careful drying between the toes after bathing, and the use of an absorbent antifungal powder such as zinc undecylenate. Topical therapy with an imidazole is curative in most cases. Each of these agents is also effective against candidal infection. Tolnaftate can be used in uncomplicated dermatophyte infections. Several weeks of therapy may be necessary, and low-grade, chronic infections, particularly those caused by *T. rubrum,* may be refractory. In such patients, oral griseofulvin therapy may effect a cure, but recurrences are common.

Tinea unguium is a dermatophyte infection of the nail plate. It occurs most often in patients with tinea pedis, but it may occur as a primary infection. It can be caused by a number of dermatophytes, of which *T. rubrum* and *T. mentagrophytes* are the most common.

The most superficial form of tinea unguium (i.e., white superficial onychomycosis) is due to *T. mentagrophytes.* It is mani-

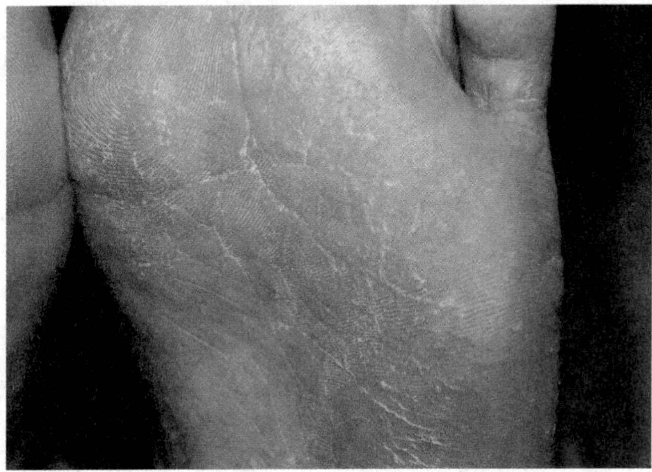

Figure 665-11. Diffuse, minimally erythematous tinea pedis.

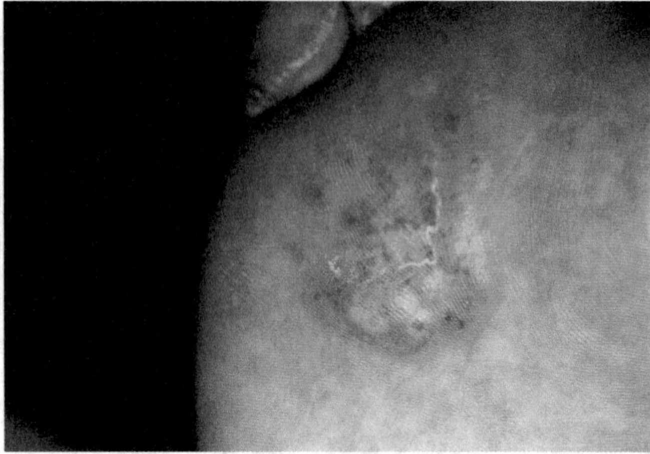

Figure 665-12. Vesicobullous tinea pedis.

fested by irregular single or numerous white patches on the surface of the nail unassociated with paronychial inflammation or deep infection. *T. rubrum* generally causes a more invasive, subungual infection that is initiated at the lateral distal margins of the nail and is often preceded by mild paronychia. The middle and ventral layers of the nail plate, and perhaps the nail bed, are the sites of infection. The nail initially develops a yellowish discoloration and slowly becomes thickened, brittle, and loosened from the nail bed (Fig. 665-13). In advanced infection, the nail may turn dark brown to black and may crack or break off.

Tinea unguium must be differentiated from various dystrophic nail disorders. Changes due to trauma, psoriasis, lichen planus, eczema, and trachyonychia all can be confused with tinea unguium. Nails infected with *C. albicans* have several distinguishing features, most prominently pronounced paronychial swelling. Thin shavings taken from the infected nail, preferably from the deeper areas, should be examined microscopically with KOH and cultured. Repeated attempts may be required to demonstrate the fungus.

The long half-life of itraconazole in the nail has led to promising trials of intermittent short courses of therapy (double the normal dose for 1 wk of each month for 3–4 mo). Oral terbinafine also shows promise for the treatment of onychomycosis. Terbinafine once daily for 12 weeks is more effective than itraconazole pulse therapy. Griseofulvin and application of topical fungistatic agents to the nail bed are often ineffective and are not recommended.

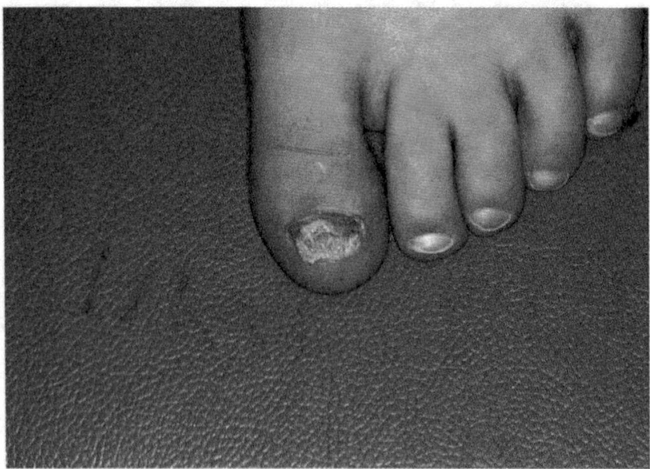

Figure 665-13. Hyperkeratotic nail in onychomycosis.

Tinea nigra palmaris is a rare but distinctive superficial fungal infection that occurs principally in children and adolescents. It is caused by the dimorphic fungus *Exophiala werneckii,* which imparts a gray-black color to the affected palm. The characteristic lesion is a well-defined hyperpigmented macule. Scaling and erythema are rare, and the lesions are asymptomatic. Tinea nigra is often mistaken for a junctional nevus, melanoma, or staining of the skin by contactants. Treatment is with an imidazole antifungal.

CANDIDAL INFECTIONS (CANDIDOSIS, CANDIDIASIS, AND MONILIASIS) (See Chapter 231)

The dimorphic yeasts of the genus *Candida* are ubiquitous in the environment, but *C. albicans* usually causes candidosis in children. This yeast is not part of the indigenous skin flora, but it is a frequent transient on skin and may colonize the human alimentary tract and the vagina as a saprophytic organism. Certain environmental conditions, notably elevated temperature and humidity, are associated with an increased frequency of isolation of *C. albicans* from the skin. Many bacterial species inhibit the growth of *C. albicans,* and alteration of normal flora by the use of antibiotics may promote overgrowth of the yeast.

ORAL CANDIDOSIS (THRUSH). See Chapter 231.

VAGINAL CANDIDOSIS. See Chapters 231 and 119. *C. albicans* is an inhabitant of the vagina in 5–10% of women, and vaginal candidosis is not uncommon in adolescent girls. A number of factors can predispose to this infection, including antibiotic therapy, corticosteroid therapy, diabetes mellitus, pregnancy, and the use of oral contraceptives. The infection is manifested by cheesy white plaques on an erythematous vaginal mucosa and by a thick white-yellow discharge. The disease may be relatively mild or may produce pronounced inflammation and scaling of the external genitals and surrounding skin with progression to vesiculation and ulceration. Patients often complain of severe itching and burning in the vaginal area. Before treatment is initiated, the diagnosis should be confirmed by microscopic examination and/or culture. The infection may be eradicated by insertion of nystatin or imidazole vaginal tablets, suppositories, creams, or foam. If these products are ineffective, the addition of fluconazole 150 mg X1 is effective.

CONGENITAL CUTANEOUS CANDIDOSIS. See Chapter 231.

CANDIDAL DIAPER DERMATITIS. This is a ubiquitous problem in infants and, although relatively benign, is often frustrating because of its tendency to recur. Predisposed infants usually carry *C. albicans* in their intestinal tract, and the warm, moist, occluded skin of the diaper area provides an optimal environment for its growth. A seborrheic, atopic, or primary irritant contact dermatitis usually provides a portal of entry for the yeast.

The primary clinical manifestation consists of an intensely erythematous, confluent plaque with a scalloped border and a sharply demarcated edge. It is formed by the confluence of numerous papules and vesiculopustules. Satellite pustules, those that stud the contiguous skin, are a hallmark of localized candidal infections. The perianal skin, inguinal folds, perineum, and lower abdomen are usually involved (Fig. 665-14). In males, the entire scrotum and penis may be involved, with an erosive balanitis of the perimeatal skin. In females, the lesions may be found on the vaginal mucosa and labia. In some infants, the process is generalized, with erythematous lesions distant from the diaper area. In some cases, the generalized process may represent a fungal id (hypersensitivity) reaction.

The **differential diagnosis** includes other eruptions of the diaper area that may coexist with candidal infection. For this reason, it

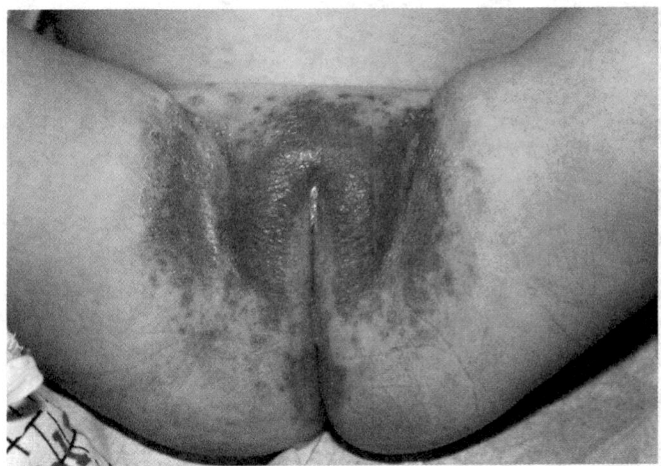

Figure 665-14. Erythematous confluent plaque caused by candidal infection.

is important to establish a diagnosis by a KOH preparation or culture.

Treatment consists of applications of an imidazole cream 2 times daily. The combination of a corticosteroid and an antifungal agent may be justified if inflammation is severe but may confuse the situation if the diagnosis is not firmly established. Corticosteroid should not be continued for more than a few days. Protection of the diaper area by an application of thick zinc oxide paste overlying the anticandidal preparation may be helpful The paste is more easily removed with mineral oil than with soap and water. Fungal id reactions gradually abate with successful treatment of the diaper dermatitis or may be treated with a mild corticosteroid preparation. When recurrences of diaper candidosis are frequent, it may be helpful to prescribe a course of oral anticandidal therapy to decrease the yeast population in the gastrointestinal tract. Some infants seem to be receptive hosts for *C. albicans* and may reacquire the organism from a colonized adult.

INTERTRIGINOUS CANDIDOSIS. This occurs most often in the axillae and groin, on the neck (Fig. 665-15), under the breasts, under pendulous abdominal fat folds, in the umbilicus, and in the gluteal cleft. Typical lesions are large, confluent areas of moist, denuded, erythematous skin with an irregular, macerated, scaly border. Satellite lesions are characteristic and consist of small vesicles or pustules on an erythematous base. With time, intertriginous candidal lesions may become lichenified, dry, scaly plaques. The lesions develop on skin subjected to irritation and maceration. Candidal superinfection is more likely to occur under conditions that lead to excessive perspiration, especially in obese children and in those with underlying disorders, such as diabetes mellitus. A similar condition, interdigital candidosis, commonly occurs in individuals whose hands are constantly immersed in water. Fissures occur between the fingers and have red denuded centers, with an overhanging white epithelial fringe. Similar lesions between the toes may be secondary to occlusive footwear. Treatment is the same as for other candidal infections.

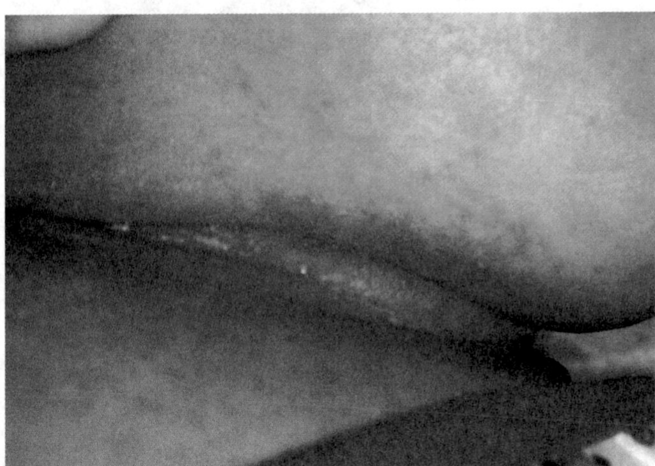

Figure 665-15. Intertriginous candidosis of the neck.

PERIANAL CANDIDOSIS. Perianal dermatitis develops at sites of skin irritation as a result of occlusion, constant moisture, poor hygiene, anal fissures, and pruritus due to pinworm infestation. It may become superinfected with *C. albicans,* especially in children who are receiving oral antibiotic or corticosteroid medication. The involved skin becomes erythematous, macerated, and excoriated, and the lesions are identical to those of candidal intertrigo or candidal diaper rash. Application of a topical antifungal agent in conjunction with improved hygiene is usually effective. Underlying disorders such as pinworm infection must also be treated (see Chapter 290).

CANDIDAL PARONYCHIA AND ONYCHIA. See Chapter 662.

CANDIDAL GRANULOMA. This is a rare response to an invasive candidal infection of skin. The lesions appear as crusted, verrucous plaques and hornlike projections on the scalp, face, and distal limbs. Affected patients may have single or numerous defects in immune mechanisms and are often refractory to topical therapy. A systemic anticandidal agent may be required for palliation or eradication of the infection.

Chan YC, Friedlander SF: New treatment for tinea capitis. *Curr Opin Infect Dis* 2004;17:97–103.

Fleece D, Gaughan JP, Aronoff SC: Griseofulvin versus terbinafine in the treatment of tinea capitis: A meta-analysis of randomized, clinical trials. *Pediatrics* 2004;114:1312–1315.

Foster KW, Ghannoum MA, Elewski BE: Epidemiologic surveillance of cutaneous fungal infection in the United States from 1999 to 2002. *J Am Acad Dermatol* 2004;50:748–752.

Gupta AK, Cooper EA, Ryder JE, et al: Optimal management of fungal infection of the skin, hair, and nails. *Am J Clin Dermatol* 2004;5:225–237.

Gupta AK, Ryder JE, Johnson AM: Cumulative meta-analysis of systemic antifungal agents for the treatment of onychomycosis. *Br J Dermatol* 2004;150:537–544.

Gupta AK, Ryder JE, Skinner AR: Treatment of onychomycosis: Pros and cons of antifungal agents. *J Cutan Med Surg* 2004;8:25–30.

Schwartz RA: Superficial fungal infections. *Lancet* 2004;364:1173–1182.

Chapter 666 ■ Cutaneous Viral Infections

Joseph G. Morelli

WART (VERRUCA)

Human papillomaviruses (HPVs) cause a spectrum of disease from warts to squamous cell carcinoma of the skin and mucous membranes, including the larynx (see Chapter 387.2). The human papillomaviruses are classified by genus, species, and type. More than 200 types are now known and the entire genome of ≈100 are completely sequenced. The incidence of all types of warts is highest in children and adolescents. HPV is spread by direct

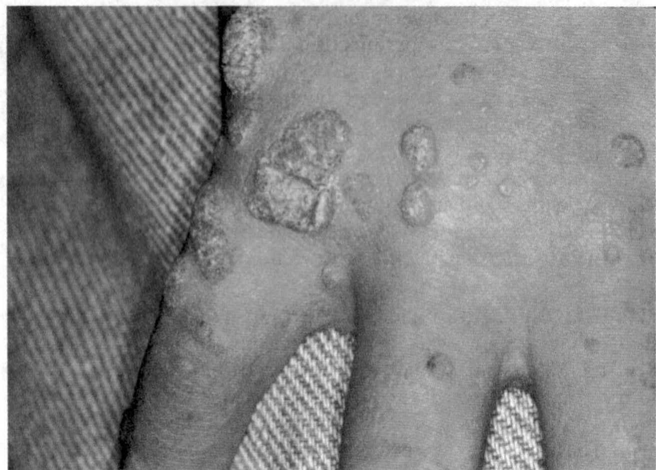

Figure 666-1. Verrucous papules on the back of the hand.

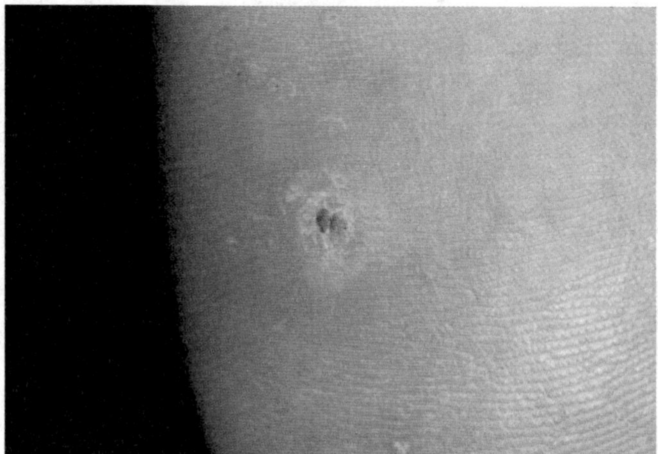

Figure 666-3. Hyperkeratotic plantar wart.

contact and autoinoculation; transmission by fomites occurs. The clinical manifestations of infection develop ≥1 mo after inoculation and depend on the HPV type, the size of the inoculum, the immune status of the host, and the anatomic site.

CLINICAL MANIFESTATIONS. Cutaneous warts develop in 5–10% of children. **Common warts** (verruca vulgaris), caused most commonly by HPV types 2 and 4, occur most frequently on the fingers, dorsum of the hands (Fig. 666-1), paronychial areas, face, knees, and elbows. They are well-circumscribed papules with an irregular, roughened, keratotic surface. When the surface is pared away, many black dots representing thrombosed dermal capillary loops are often visible. **Periungual warts** are often painful and may spread beneath the nail plate, separating it from the nail bed (Fig. 666-2). **Plantar warts,** although similar to the common wart, are caused by HPV type 1 and are usually flush with the surface of the sole because of the constant pressure from weight bearing. When plantar warts become hyperkeratotic (Fig. 666-3), they may be painful. Similar lesions (palmar) can also occur on the palms. They are sharply demarcated, often with a ring of thick callus. The surface keratotic material must sometimes be removed before the boundaries of the wart can be appreciated. Several contiguous warts (HPV type 4) may fuse to form a large plaque, the so-called mosaic wart. Flat warts (verruca plana), caused by HPV types 3 and 10, are slightly elevated, minimally hyperkeratotic papules that usually remain <3 mm in diameter and vary in color from pink to brown. They may occur in profusion on the face, arms, dorsum of the hands, and knees. The distribution of several lesions along a line of cutaneous trauma is a helpful diagnostic feature (Fig. 666-4). Lesions may be disseminated in the beard area and on the legs by shaving and from the hairline onto the scalp by combing the hair. **Epidermodysplasia verruciformis** (EVER1, 2 genes), caused primarily by HPV types 5 and 8 (β-papillomaviruses, species 1), presents with many diffuse verrucous papules. Inheritance is thought to be both autosomal dominant and recessive. Warts progress to **squamous cell carcinoma** in 10% of EV patients.

Genital HPV infection occurs in sexually active adolescents, most commonly as a result of infection with HPV types 6 and 11. **Condylomata acuminata** (mucous membrane warts) are moist, fleshy, papillomatous lesions that occur on the perianal mucosa (Fig. 666-5), labia, vaginal introitus, and perineal raphe and on the shaft, corona, and glans penis. Occasionally, they obstruct the urethral meatus or the vaginal introitus. Because they are located in intertriginous areas, they may become moist and friable. When untreated, condylomata proliferate and become confluent, at times forming large cauliflower-like masses. Lesions can also occur on the lips, gingivae, tongue, and conjunctivae. Genital warts in children may occur after inoculation during birth through an infected birth canal, as a consequence of sexual abuse, or from incidental spread from cutaneous warts. A significant proportion of genital warts in children contain HPV types that

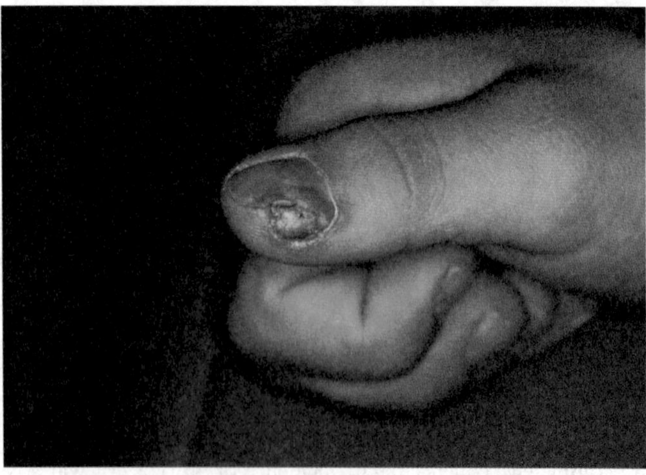

Figure 666-2. Periungual wart with disruption of nail growth.

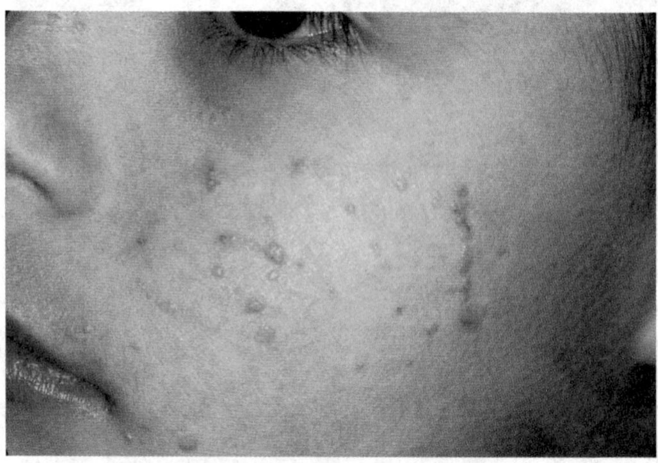

Figure 666-4. Multiple flat warts on the face with lesions in line of trauma.

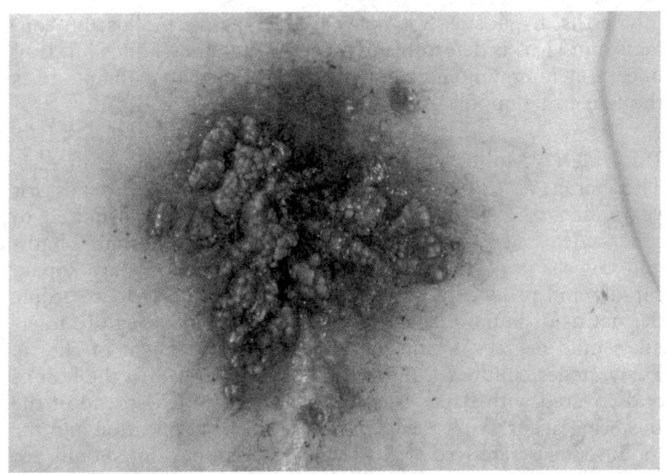

Figure 666-5. Condylomata acuminata in the perianal area of a toddler.

are usually isolated from cutaneous warts. HPV infection of the cervix is a major risk factor for development of carcinoma, particularly if the infection is due to HPV types 16, 18, 31, 33, 35, 39, 45, 52, 59, 67, 68, or 70. Laryngeal (respiratory) papillomas contain the same HPV types as in anogenital papillomas. Transmission is believed to occur from mothers with genital HPV infection to neonates who aspirate infectious virus during birth.

PATHOLOGY. The various types of warts share the basic changes of hyperplasia of the epidermal cells and vacuolation of the spinous keratinocytes, which may contain basophilic intranuclear inclusions (viral particles). Warts are confined to the epidermis and do not have "roots." Parakeratosis, papillomatosis, and eosinophilic cytoplasmic inclusions, thought to represent altered keratohyalin, are additional variable histologic changes. Individuals with impaired cell-mediated immunity are particularly susceptible to HPV infection. Antibodies occur in response to infection but appear to have little protective effect.

DIFFERENTIAL DIAGNOSIS. Common warts are most often confused with molluscum contagiosum. Plantar and palmar warts may be difficult to distinguish from punctate keratoses, corns, and calluses. In contrast to calluses, warts obliterate normal skin markings. Juvenile flat warts mimic lichen planus, lichen nitidus, angiofibromas, syringomas, milia, and acne. Condylomata acuminata may resemble condylomata lata of secondary syphilis.

TREATMENT. Various therapeutic measures are effective in the treatment of warts. More than 50% of warts disappear spontaneously within 2 yr. Warts are epidermal lesions and do not produce scarring unless they are managed surgically or treated in an overly aggressive fashion. Hyperkeratotic lesions (common, plantar, and palmar warts) are more responsive to therapy if the excess keratotic debris is gently pared with a scalpel until thrombosed capillaries are apparent; further paring induces bleeding. Treatment is most successful when done regularly and frequently (every 2–4 wk).

Common warts can be destroyed by applications of liquid nitrogen or by pulsed dye laser. Daily application of salicylic acid in flexible collodion is a slow but painless method of removal that is effective in some patients. Plantar and palmar warts may be treated with 40% salicylic acid plasters. These should be applied for 5 days at a time with a 2 day rest period in between application. Following removal of the plaster and prolonged soaking in lukewarm water, keratotic debris can be removed with an emery board or pumice stone. Occlusive taping without medication for several weeks is also very effective. Condylomata respond best to weekly applications of 25% podophyllin in tincture of benzoin. The medication should be left on the warts for 4–6 hr and then removed by bathing. Keratinized warts near the genitalia (buttocks) do not respond to podophyllin. Imiquimod (5% cream) applied 3 times weekly is also beneficial. Imiquimod is indicated for genital warts but has also been used successfully to treat warts in other locations. For nongenital warts, imiquimod should be applied daily. Cimetidine 30–40 mg/kg/day has been used for children with multiple warts unresponsive to other treatments. Immunotherapy with squaric acid or intralesconal candida antigen may also be employed. Duct tape occlusion applied directly to the wart and left in place for 6 consecutive days followed by cleaning and pumice abrasion has been successful in treating warts when repeated in weekly cycles for 2 mo. In addition, topical human α-lactalbumin-oleic acid applied daily for 3 wk is a promising therapy for papillomas. With all types of therapy, care should be taken to protect the surrounding normal skin from irritation.

MOLLUSCUM CONTAGIOSUM

The poxvirus that causes molluscum contagiosum is a large double-stranded DNA virus that replicates in the cytoplasm of host epithelial cells. The three types cannot be differentiated on the basis of clinical appearance, location of lesions, or a patient's age or sex. Type 1 virus causes most infections. The disease is acquired by direct contact with an infected person or from fomites and is spread by autoinoculation. School-aged children who are otherwise well and individuals who are immunosuppressed are affected most commonly. The incubation period is estimated to be ≥2 wk.

CLINICAL MANIFESTATIONS. Discrete, pearly, skin-colored smooth, dome-shaped, papules vary in size from 1 to 5 mm. They typically have a central umbilication from which a plug of cheesy material can be expressed. The papules may occur anywhere on the body, but the face, eyelids, neck, axillae, and thighs are sites of predilection (Fig. 666-6). They may be found in clusters on the genitals or in the groin of adolescents and may be associated with other venereal diseases in sexually active individuals. Lesions commonly involve the genital area in children but in most cases are not acquired by sexual transmission. Mild surrounding erythema or an eczematous dermatitis may accompany the papules (Fig. 666-7). Lesions on patients with AIDS tend to be large and numerous, particularly on the face. Exuberant lesions may also be found in children with leukemia and other immunodeficiencies. Children with atopic dermatitis are susceptible to wide-

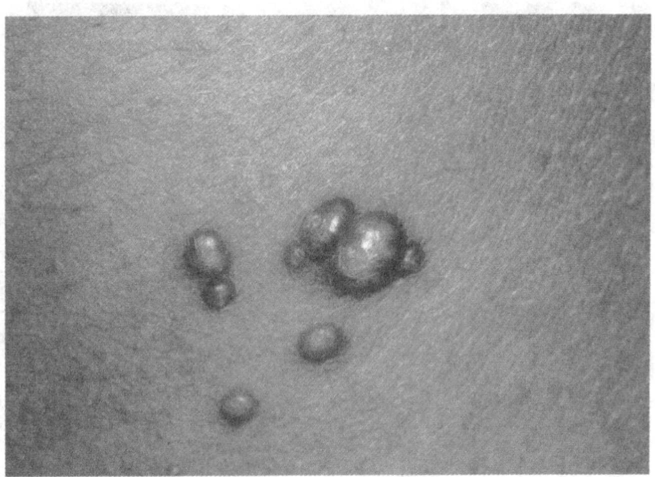

Figure 666-6. Grouped molluscum.

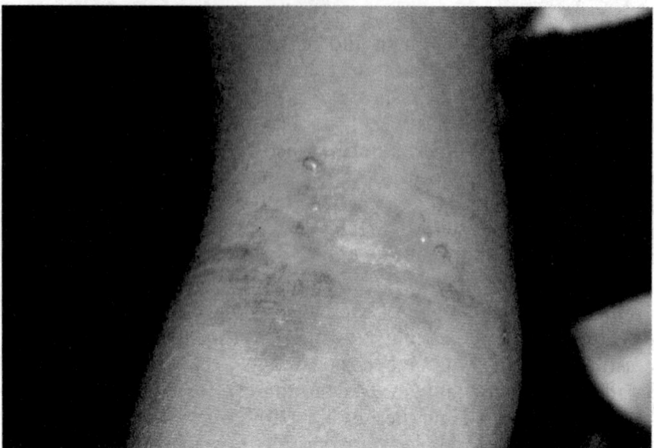

Figure 666-7. Molluscum with surrounding dermatitis.

spread involvement in areas of dermatitis. A pustular eruption at the site of individual molluscum lesions is seen (Fig. 666-8). It is not a secondary bacterial infection, but an immunologic reaction to the molluscum virus and it should not be treated with antibiotics. Atrophic scars are often seen following this type of reaction.

DIFFERENTIAL DIAGNOSIS. This includes trichoepithelioma, basal cell carcinoma, ectopic sebaceous glands, syringoma, hidrocystoma, keratoacanthoma, and warty dyskeratoma. In individuals with AIDS, cryptococcosis may be indistinguishable clinically from molluscum contagiosum. Rarely, coccidioidomycosis, histoplasmosis, or *Penicillium marneffei* infection masquerades with molluscum-like lesions in an immunocompromised host.

PATHOLOGY AND DIAGNOSIS. The epidermis is hyperplastic and hypertrophied, extending into the underlying dermis and projecting above the skin surface. The molluscum papule consists of a lobulated adhesive mass of virus-infected epidermal cells. Eosinophilic viral inclusion bodies (Henderson-Patterson or molluscum bodies) become more prominent as the cells move upward from the basal layer to the stratum corneum. The central plug of material, which is composed of virus-laden cells, may be shelled out from a lesion and examined under the microscope with 10% potassium hydroxide or Wright or Giemsa stain. The rounded, cupshaped mass of homogeneous cells, often with identifiable

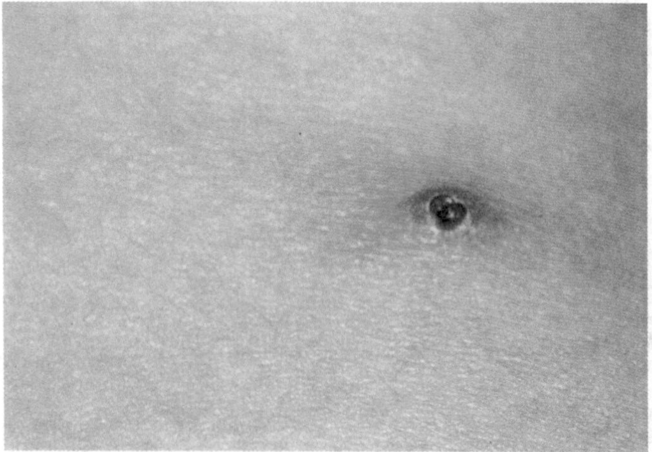

Figure 666-8. Inflamed molluscum. Crusted papule at site of previous molluscum.

lobules, is diagnostic. Specific antibody against molluscum contagiosum virus is detectable in most infected individuals but is of uncertain immunologic significance. Cell-mediated immunity is thought to be important in host defense.

TREATMENT. Molluscum contagiosum is a self-limited disease. The average attack lasts 6–9 mo. However, lesions can persist for years, can spread to distant sites, and may be transmitted to others. Affected patients should be advised to avoid shared baths and towels until the infection is clear. Infection may spread rapidly and produce hundreds of lesions in children with atopic dermatitis or immunodeficiency. In children old enough to tolerate a mild degree of pain, curettage is the **treatment of choice.** For younger children, cantharidin may be applied to the lesions and covered with Band-Aids to prevent unwanted spread of the blistering agent. A blister forms at the site of application and the molluscum is removed with the blister. Cantharidin should not be used on the face. Facial molluscum is more cosmetically upsetting to children and parents; imiquimod applied topically is beneficial if not excessively irritating. Molluscum is an epidermal disease and should not be overtreated such that scarring results.

Bellew SG, Quartarolo N, Janniger CK: Childhood warts: An update. *Cutis* 2004;73:379–384.

De Villiers EM, Fauquet C, Broker TR, et al: Classification of papillomaviruses. *Virology* 2004;324:17–27.

Dupin N: Genital warts. *Clin Dermatol* 2004;22:481–486.

Focht DR III, Spicer C, Fairchok MP: The efficacy of duct tape vs cryotherapy in the treatment of verruca vulgaris (the common wart). *Arch Pediatr Adolesc Med* 2003;156:971–974.

Grussendorf-Conen EI, Jacobs S: Efficacy of imiquimod 5% cream in the treatment of recalcitrant warts in children. *Pediatr Dermatol* 2002;19:263–266.

Gustafsson L, Leijonhufvud I, Aronsson A, et al: Treatment of skin papillomas with topical a-lactalbumin-oleic acid. *N Engl J Med* 2004;350: 2663–2672.

Majewski S, Jablonska S: Why epidermodysplasia verruciformis—a rare genetic disease—has raised such great interest. *Int J Dermatol* 2004;43: 309–311.

Molina AC, Fleischer AB, Feldman SR: Patient demographics and utilization of health care services for molluscum contagiosum. *Pediatr Dermatol* 2004;21:628–632.

Silverberg NB: Warts and molluscum in children. *Adv Dermatol* 2004; 20:23–73.

Chapter 667 ■ Arthropod Bites and Infestations Joseph G. Morelli

ARTHROPOD BITES

Arthropod bites are a common affliction of children and occasionally pose a problem in diagnosis. A patient may be unaware of the source of the lesions or deny being bitten, making interpretation of the eruption difficult. In these cases, knowledge of the habits, life cycle, and clinical signs of the more common arthropod pests of humans may help lead to a correct diagnosis. The principal classes of arthropods that cause skin injury to humans are listed in Table 667-1.

CLINICAL MANIFESTATIONS. The type of reaction that occurs after an arthropod bite depends on the species of insect and the age group and reactivity of the human host. Arthropods may cause injury to a host by various mechanisms, including mechanical

TABLE 667-1. Arthropods That Cause Human Skin Disease

Class Arachnida (four pairs of legs): mites, spiders, ticks
Class Chilopoda: centipedes
Class Diplopoda: millipedes
Class Insecta (three pairs of legs):
Order Diptera: mosquitoes, flies
Order Siphonaptera: fleas
Order Hymenoptera: ants, bees, wasps
Order Anoplura: lice
Order Hemiptera: bedbugs, kissing bugs
Order Coleoptera: beetles
Order Lepidoptera: butterflies, moths

trauma, such as the lacerating bite of a tsetse fly; invasion of host tissues, as in myiasis; contact dermatitis, as seen with repeated exposure to cockroach antigens; granulomatous reaction to retained mouthparts; transmission of systemic disease; injection of irritant cytotoxic or pharmacologically active substances, such as hyaluronidase, proteases, peptidases, and phospholipases in sting venom; and induction of anaphylaxis. Most reactions to arthropod bites depend on antibody formation to antigenic substances in saliva or venom. The type of reaction is determined primarily by the degree of previous exposure to the same or a related species of arthropod. When someone is bitten for the 1st time, no reaction develops. An immediate petechial reaction is occasionally seen, however, in newborn babies after a mosquito bite. After repeated bites, sensitivity develops, producing a pruritic papule (Fig. 667-1) ≈24 hr after the bite. This is the most common reaction seen in young children. With prolonged, repeated exposure, a wheal develops within minutes after a bite, followed 24 hr later by papule formation; this combination of reactions is seen commonly in older children. By adolescence or adulthood, only a wheal may form, unaccompanied by the delayed papular reaction. Thus, adults in the same household as affected children may be unaffected. Ultimately, as a person becomes insensitive to the bite, no reaction occurs at all. This stage of nonreactivity is maintained only as long as the individual continues to be bitten regularly. Individuals in whom papular urticaria develops are in the transitional phase between development of primarily a delayed papular reaction and development of an immediate urticarial reaction.

Arthropod bites may occur as solitary, numerous, or profuse lesions, depending on the feeding habits of the perpetrator. Fleas tend to sample their host several times within a small localized area, whereas mosquitoes tend to attack a host at more randomly scattered sites. Delayed hypersensitivity reactions to insect bites, the predominant lesions in the young and uninitiated, are characterized by firm, persistent papules that may become hyperpigmented and are often excoriated and crusted. Pruritus may be mild or severe, transient or persistent. A central punctum is usually visible but may disappear as the lesion ages or is scratched. The immediate hypersensitivity reaction is characterized by an evanescent, erythematous wheal. If edema is marked, a tiny vesicle may surmount the wheal. Certain beetles produce bullous lesions through the action of cantharidin, and various insects, including beetles and spiders, may cause hemorrhagic nodules and ulcers. Bites on the lower extremities are more likely to be severe or persistent or become bullous than those located elsewhere. Complications of arthropod bites include development of impetigo, folliculitis, cellulitis, lymphangitis, and severe anaphylactic hypersensitivity reactions, particularly after the bite of certain hymenopterans. The histopathologic changes are variable, depending on the arthropod, the age of the lesion, and the reactivity of the host. Acute urticarial lesions tend to show central vesiculation in which eosinophils are numerous. Papules most commonly show dermal edema and a mixed superficial and deep perivascular inflammatory infiltrate, often including a number of eosinophils. At times, however, the dermal cellular infiltrate is so dense that a lymphoma is suspected. Retained mouthparts may stimulate a foreign body type of granulomatous reaction.

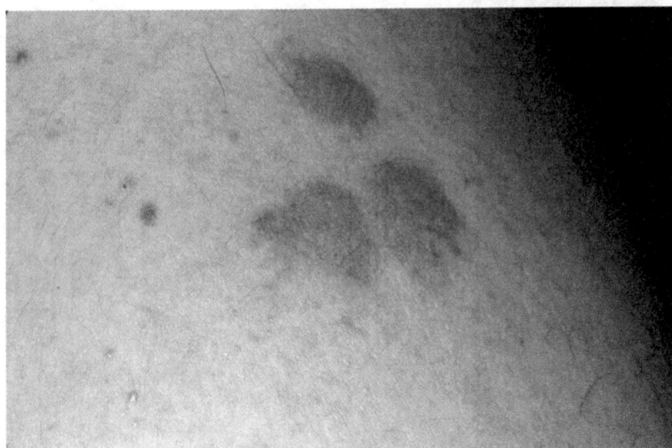
Figure 667-1. Pruritic papules after bedbug bites.

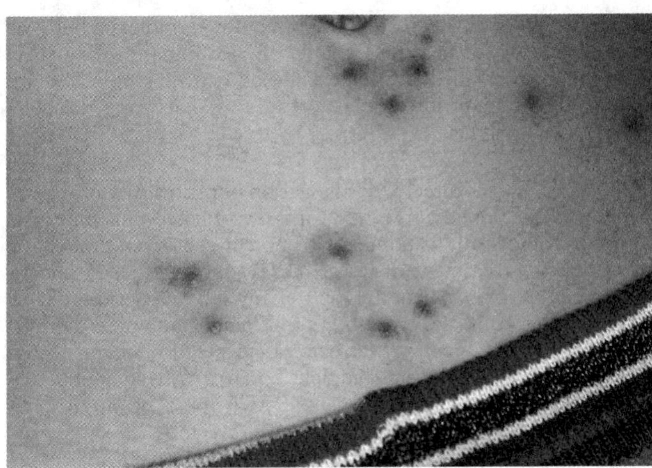
Figure 667-2. Red, brown papules in papular urticaria.

Papular urticaria occurs principally in the 1st decade of life, during the warmer months of the year. The most common culprits are species of fleas, mites, bedbugs, gnats, mosquitoes, chiggers, and animal lice. Individuals with papular urticaria have predominantly transitional lesions in various stages of evolution between delayed-onset papules and immediate-onset wheals. The most characteristic lesion is a edematous, red-brown papule (Fig. 667-2). An individual lesion frequently starts as a wheal that, in turn, is replaced by a papule. A given bite may incite an id reaction at distant sites of quiescent bites in the form of erythematous macules, papules, or urticarial plaques. After a season or two, the reaction progresses from a transitional to a primarily immediate hypersensitivity urticarial reaction.

One of the most commonly encountered arthropod bites is that due to human, cat, or dog fleas (family *Pulicidae*). Eggs, which are generally laid in dusty areas and cracks between floorboards, give rise to larvae that then form cocoons. The cocoon stage can persist for up to 1 yr, and the flea emerges in response to vibrations from footsteps, accounting for the assaults that frequently befall the new owners of a recently reopened dwelling. Adult dog fleas can live without a blood meal for ≈60 days. Attacks from fleas are more likely to occur when the fleas do not have access to their usual host; cat or dog fleas are more voracious and problematic when one visits an area frequented by the pet than when the pet is encountered directly. Flea bites tend to be grouped in lines or irregular clusters. Fleas are often not seen on the body of a pet. Diagnosis of flea bites is aided by examination of debris from the animal's bedding material. The debris is collected by shaking the bedding into a plastic bag and examining the contents for fleas or their eggs, larvae, or feces.

TREATMENT. This is directed at alleviation of pruritus by oral antihistamines and cool compresses. Topical corticosteroids may also be used. Topical antihistamines are potent sensitizers and have no role in the treatment of insect bite reactions. A short course of systemic steroids may be helpful if many severe reactions occur, particularly around the eyes. Insect repellents containing diethyltoluamide (DEET) may afford moderate protection against mosquitoes, fleas, flies, chiggers, and ticks but are relatively ineffective against wasps, bees, and hornets. DEET must be applied to exposed skin and clothing to be effective. The most effective protection against mosquitoes, the human body louse, and other blood-feeding arthropods is use of DEET and permethrin-impregnated clothing. These measures are not effective, however, against the phlebotomine sandfly, which transmits leishmaniasis.

An effort should be made to identify and eradicate the etiologic agent. Pets should be carefully inspected. Crawl spaces, eaves, and other sites of the house or outbuildings frequented by animals and birds should be decontaminated and baseboard crevices, mattresses, rugs, furniture, and animal sleeping quarters should be decontaminated. Agents that are effective for ridding the home of fleas include lindane, pyrethroids, and organic thiocyanates. Flea-infested pets may be treated with powders containing rotenone, pyrethroids, malathion, or methoxychlor.

INFESTATIONS

SCABIES. Scabies is caused by burrowing and release of toxic or antigenic substances by the female mite *Sarcoptes scabiei* var. *hominis*. The most important factor that determines spread of scabies is the extent and duration of physical contact with an affected individual. The children and sexual partner of an affected individual are most at risk. Scabies is transmitted only rarely by fomites because the isolated mite dies within 2–3 days.

Clinical Manifestations. In an immunocompetent host, scabies is frequently heralded by intense pruritus, particularly at night.

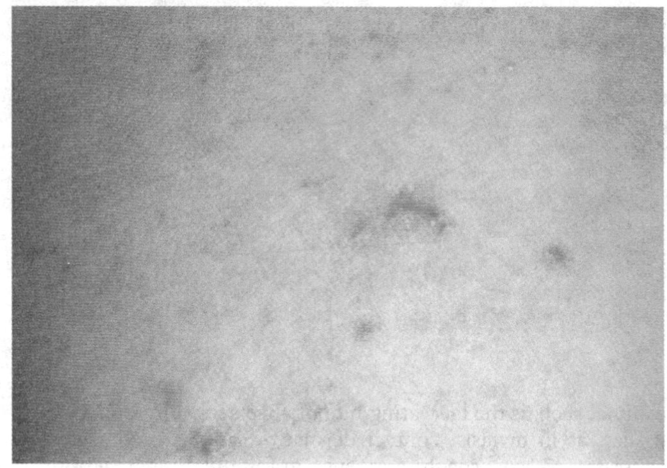

Figure 667-3. Classic scabies burrow.

The 1st sign of the infestation often consists of 1–2 mm red papules, some of which are excoriated, crusted, or scaling. Threadlike burrows are the classic lesion of scabies (Fig. 667-3) but may not be seen in infants. In infants, bullae and pustules are relatively common. The eruption may also include wheals, papules, vesicles, and a superimposed eczematous dermatitis (Fig. 667-4). The palms, soles, face, and scalp are often affected. In older children and adolescents, the clinical pattern is similar to that in adults, in whom preferred sites are the interdigital spaces, wrist flexors, anterior axillary folds, ankles, buttocks, umbilicus and belt line, groin, genitals in men, and areolas in women. The head, neck, palms, and soles are generally spared. Red-brown nodules, most often located in covered areas such as the axillae, groin, and genitals, predominate in the less common variant called nodular scabies. Untreated, scabies may lead to eczematous dermatitis, impetigo, ecthyma, folliculitis, furunculosis, cellulitis, lymphangitis, and id reaction. Children have developed glomerulonephritis from streptococcal impetiginization of scabies lesions. In some tropical areas, scabies is the predominant underlying cause of pyoderma. A latent period of ≈1 mo follows an initial infestation. Thus, itching may be absent and lesions may

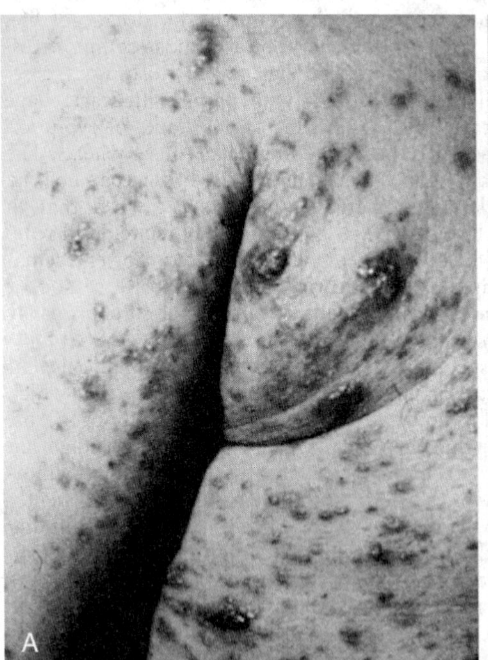

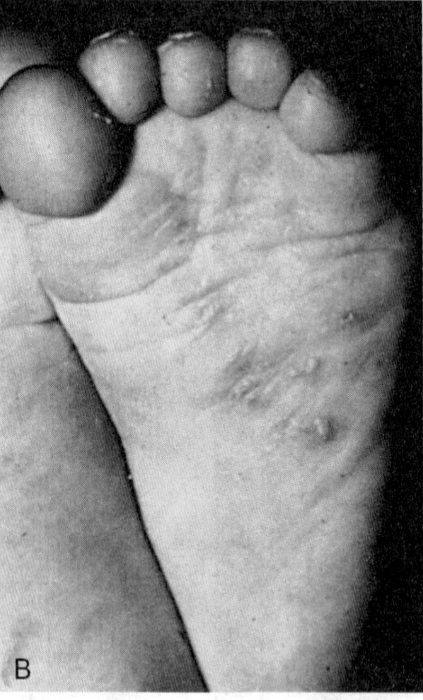

Figure 667-4. *A,* Eczematous dermatitis, papules, and nodules of human scabies. *B,* Vesiculopustular lesions of scabies on the soles of an infant's feet.

be relatively inapparent in contacts who are asymptomatic carriers. On reinfestation, however, reactions to mite antigens are noted within hours.

Etiology and Pathogenesis. An adult female mite measures ≈0.4 mm in length, has 4 sets of legs, and has a hemispheric body marked by transverse corrugations, brown spines, and bristles on the dorsal surface. A male mite is approximately ½ her size and is similar in configuration. After impregnation on the skin surface, a gravid female exudes a keratolytic substance and burrows into the stratum corneum, often forming a shallow well within 30 min. She gradually extends this tract by 0.5–5 mm/24 hr along the boundary with the stratum granulosum. She deposits 1 to 3 oval eggs and numerous brown fecal pellets (scybala) daily. When egg laying is completed, in 4–5 wk, she dies within the burrow. The eggs hatch in 3–5 days, releasing larvae that move to the skin surface to molt into nymphs. Maturity is achieved in about 2–3 wk. Mating occurs, and the gravid female invades the skin to complete the life cycle.

Diagnosis. This can often be made clinically but is confirmed by microscopic identification of mites (Fig. 667-5*A*), ova, and scybala (Fig. 667-5*B*) in epithelial debris. Scrapings are most often positive when obtained from burrows or fresh papules. A reliable method is application of a drop of mineral oil on the selected lesion, scraping of it with a No. 15 blade, and transferring the oil and scrapings to a glass slide.

The **differential diagnosis** depends on the types of lesions present. Burrows are virtually pathognomonic for human scabies. Papulovesicular lesions are confused with papular urticaria, canine scabies, chickenpox, viral exanthems, drug eruptions, dermatitis herpetiformis, and folliculitis. Eczematous lesions may mimic atopic dermatitis and seborrheic dermatitis, and the less common bullous disorders of childhood may be suspected in infants with predominantly bullous lesions. Nodular scabies is frequently misdiagnosed as urticaria pigmentosa and Langerhans cell hystiocytosis. The histopathologic appearance of nodular scabies, consisting of a deep, dense, perivascular infiltrate of lymphocytes, histiocytes, plasma cells, and atypical mononuclear cells, may mimic malignant lymphoid neoplasms.

Treatment. Application of permethrin 5% cream (Elimite) or 1% lindane cream or lotion to the entire body from the neck down, with particular attention to intensely involved areas, is standard therapy. Scabies is frequently found above the neck in infants, necessitating treatment of the scalp. The medication is left on the skin for 8–12 hr. If necessary, it may be reapplied in 1 wk for another 8–12 hr period. Because lindane is potentially neurotoxic, the vulnerability of small infants to percutaneous absorption dictates caution in prescribing it for them. Signs of lindane toxicity include nausea, vomiting, weakness, tremors, irritability, disorientation, seizures, and respiratory compromise. Systemic absorption and toxicity of lindane can be minimized by not applying the medication to warm, moist skin; not repeating an application within 7 days; and not using the medication on children who are underweight or malnourished or have extensive areas of inflamed, denuded, or secondarily infected skin. Permethrin 5% cream is a slightly more effective scabicide than lindane but is more expensive. It is poorly absorbed, rapidly metabolized by tissue esterases, and, therefore, of very low toxicity. For infants younger than 2 mo, alternative therapy includes 6% sulfur in petrolatum applied for 3 consecutive 24 hr periods. Topical sulfur ointment is messy and malodorous, stains clothing, and commonly causes irritant dermatitis. No controlled studies of its efficacy and safety have been published in recent years. Permethrin 5% cream is a better alternative for infants. Crotamiton cream or lotion is not recommended because of lack of efficacy and toxicity data.

Transmission of mites is unlikely more than 24 hr after treatment. Pruritus, which is due to hypersensitivity to mite antigens, may persist for a number of days and may be alleviated by a topical corticosteroid preparation. If pruritus persists for >2 wk after treatment and new lesions are occurring, the patient should be reexamined for mites. Nodules are extremely resistant to treatment and may take several months to resolve. The entire family should be treated, as should caretakers of the infested child. Clothing, bed linens, and towels should be thoroughly laundered.

Norwegian Scabies. This variant of human scabies is highly contagious and occurs mainly in individuals who are mentally and physically debilitated, particularly those who are institutionalized and those with Down syndrome; in patients with poor cutaneous sensation (leprosy, spina bifida), in patients who have severe systemic illness (leukemia, diabetes), and in immunosuppressed patients (HIV infection). Affected individuals are infested by myriad mites that inhabit the crusts and exfoliating scales of the skin and scalp. The nails may become thickened and dystrophic. The subungual debris is densely populated by mites. The infestation is often accompanied by generalized lymphadenopathy and eosinophilia. There is massive orthokeratosis and parakeratosis with numerous interspersed mites, psoriasiform epidermal hyperplasia, foci of spongiosis, and neutrophilic abscesses. Norwegian scabies is thought to represent a deficient host immune response to the organism. Management is difficult, requiring scrupulous isolation measures, removal of the thick scales, and repeated but careful applications of antiscabietic preparations. Ivermectin has been used successfully as single-dose therapy in refractory cases, particularly in HIV-infected patients. The Food and Drug Administration (FDA) has not approved it

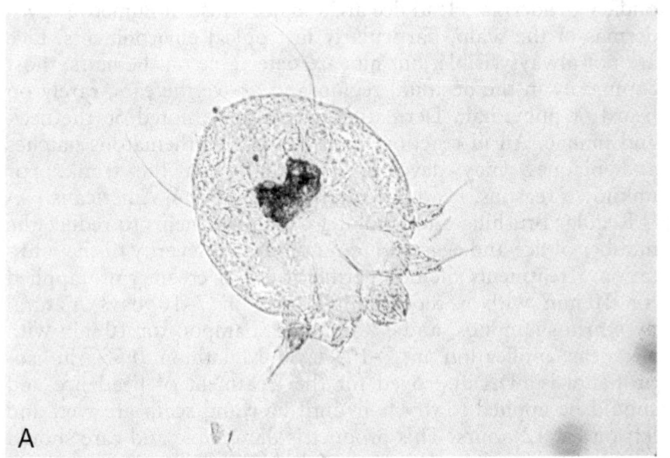

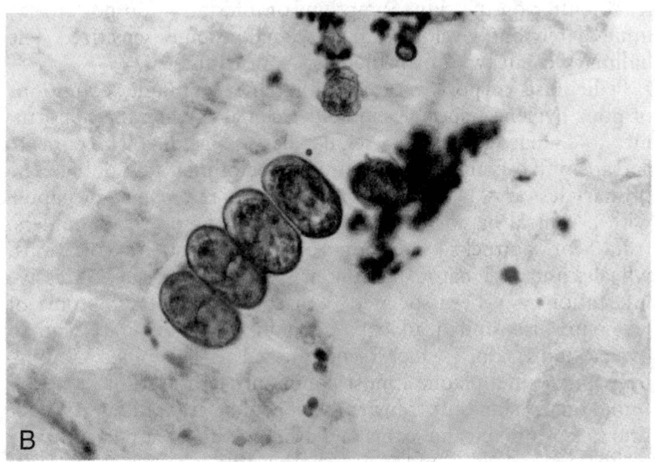

Figure 667-5. *A*, Human scabies mite obtained from scraping. *B*, Scabies ova and scybala.

for treatment of scabies or for any application in children younger than 5 yr.

Canine Scabies. This is caused by *S. scabiei* var. *canis*, the dog mite that is associated with mange. The eruption in humans, which is most frequently acquired by cuddling an infested puppy, consists of tiny papules, vesicles, wheals, and excoriated eczematous plaques. Burrows are not present because the mite infrequently inhabits human stratum corneum. The rash is pruritic and has a predilection for the arms, chest, and abdomen, the usual sites of contact with dogs. Onset is sudden and usually follows exposure by 1–10 days, possibly resulting from development of a hypersensitivity reaction to mite antigens. Recovery of mites or ova from scrapings of human skin is rare. The disease is self-limited because humans are not a suitable host. Bathing and changing clothes are generally sufficient. Removal or treatment of the infested animal is necessary. Symptomatic therapy for itching is helpful. In rare cases in which mites are demonstrated in scrapings from an affected child, they can be eradicated by the same measures applicable to human scabies.

Other mites that occasionally bite humans include the chigger or harvest mite *(Eutrombicula alfreddugesi),* which prefers to live on grass, shrubs, vines, and stems of grain. Larvae have hooked mouthparts, which allow the chigger to attach to the skin, but not to burrow, to obtain a blood meal, most commonly on the lower legs. Avian mites may affect those who come into close contact with chickens or pet gerbils. Humans may occasionally be assaulted by avian mites that have infested a nest outside a window, an attic, heating vents, or an air conditioner. The dermatitis is variable, including grouped papules, wheals, and vesicular lesions on the wrists, neck, breasts, umbilicus, and anterior axillary folds. A prolonged investigation is often undertaken before the cause and source of the dermatitis are discovered.

PEDICULOSIS. Three types of lice are obligate parasites of the human host: body or clothing lice *(Pediculus humanus corporis),* head lice *(Pediculus humanus capitis),* and pubic or crab lice *(Phthirus pubis).* Only the body louse serves as a vector of human disease (typhus, trench fever, relapsing fever). Body and head lice have similar physical characteristics. They are about 2–4 mm in length. Pubic lice are only 1–2 mm in length and are greater in width than length, giving them a crablike appearance. Female lice live for ≈1 mo and deposit 3–10 eggs daily on the human host. Body lice, however, generally lay eggs in or near the seams of clothing. The ova or nits are glued to hairs or fibers of clothing but not directly on the body. Ova hatch in 1–2 wk and require another week to mature. Once the eggs hatch, the nits remain attached to the hair as empty sacs of chitin. Freshly hatched larvae die unless a meal is obtained within ≈24 hr and every few days thereafter. Both nymphs and adult lice feed on human blood, injecting their salivary juices into the host and depositing their fecal matter on the skin. Symptoms of infestation do not appear immediately but develop as an individual becomes sensitized. The hallmark of all types of pediculosis is pruritus.

Pediculosis corporis is rare in children except under conditions of poor hygiene, especially in colder climates when the opportunity to change clothes on a regular basis is lacking. The parasite is transmitted mainly on contaminated clothing or bedding. The primary lesion is a small, intensely pruritic, red macule or papule with a central hemorrhagic punctum, located on the shoulders, trunk, or buttocks. Additional lesions include excoriations, wheals, and eczematous, secondarily infected plaques. Massive infestation may be associated with constitutional symptoms of fever, malaise, and headache. Chronic infestation may lead to "vagabond's skin," which is manifested as lichenified, scaling, hyperpigmented plaques, most commonly on the trunk. Lice are found on the skin only transiently when they are feeding. At other times, they inhabit the seams of clothing. Nits are attached firmly to fibers in the cloth and may remain viable for up to 1 mo. Nits hatch when they encounter warmth from the host's body when

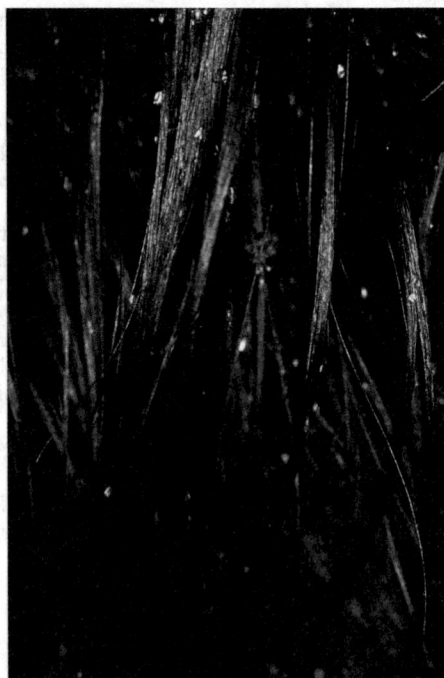

Figure 667-6. Intact nits on a human hair.

the clothes are worn again. Therapy consists of improved hygiene and hot water laundering of all infested clothing and bedding. A uniform temperature of 65°C, wet or dry, for 15–30 min kills all eggs and lice. Alternatively, eggs hatch and nymphs starve if clothing is stored for 2 wk at 75–85°F. For people who are unable to change clothes, the clothes may be turned inside out and dusted with 10% lindane powder. The effect lasts for ≈1 mo. Lindane lotion or permethrin cream applied for 8–12 hr can be used to eradicate any eggs and lice that happen to be on body hair.

Pediculosis capitis is an intensely pruritic infestation of lice in the scalp hair. Fomites and head-to-head contact are important modes of transmission. In summer months in many areas of the United States and in the tropics at all times of the year, shared combs, brushes, or towels have a more important role in louse transmission. Translucent 0.5 mm eggs are laid near the proximal portion of the hair shaft and become adherent to one side of the hair shaft (Fig. 667-6). A nit cannot be moved along or knocked off the hair shaft with the fingers. Secondary pyoderma, after trauma due to scratching, may result in matting together of the hair and cervical and occipital lymphadenopathy. Hair loss does not result from pediculosis but may accompany the secondary pyoderma. Head lice are a major cause of numerous pyodermas of the scalp, particularly in tropical environments. Lice are not always visible, but nits are detectable on the hairs, most commonly in the occipital region and above the ears, rarely on beard or pubic hair. Dermatitis may also be noted on the neck and pinnae. An id reaction, consisting of erythematous patches and plaques, may develop, particularly on the trunk. For unknown reasons, head lice rarely infest African Americans.

Regular brushing and combing of the hair helps to reduce the number of lice and eggs and to minimize the severity of the infestation. **Treatments** include permethrin 1% cream rinse applied for 10 min with a repeat application in 7–10 days, natural pyrethrin shampoos, and 1% lindane shampoo for 10 min with a repeat application in 7–10 days. Malathion 0.5% in isopropanol is FDA approved for the treatment of head lice and should be applied to dry hair until hair and scalp are wet, and left on for 12 hours. This product is flammable and care should be taken to avoid open flames. Malathion may be useful in cases of pyrethrin or permethrin resistance. Malathion, like lindane shampoo, is not indicated for use in neonates and infants. All household members should be treated at the same time. Nits can be removed with a fine-toothed comb after application of a damp towel to the scalp for 30 min. Clothing and bed linens should be laundered in very hot water or dry-cleaned; brushes and combs should be discarded or coated with a pediculicide for 15 min and then thoroughly cleaned in boiling water.

Pediculosis pubis is transmitted by skin-to-skin or sexual contact with an infested individual; the chance of acquiring the lice by one sexual exposure is ≈95%. The infestation is usually encountered in adolescents, although small children may occasionally acquire pubic lice on the eyelashes. Patients experience moderate to severe pruritus and may develop a secondary pyoderma from scratching. Excoriations tend to be shallower and the incidence of secondary infection is lower than in pediculosis corporis. Maculae ceruleae are steel-gray spots, usually <1 cm in diameter, which may appear in the pubic area and on the chest, abdomen, and thighs. Oval translucent nits, which are firmly attached to the hair shafts, may be visible to the naked eye or may be readily identified by a hand lens or by microscopic examination (see Fig. 667-6). Grittiness, as a result of adherent nits, may sometimes be detected when the fingers are run through infested hair. Adult lice are difficult to detect because of their lower level of activity and smaller, translucent body compared with head or body lice. Because pubic lice may occasionally wander or be transferred to other sites on fomites, terminal hair on the trunk, thighs, axillary region, beard area, and eyelashes should be examined for nits. The coexistence of other venereal diseases should be considered.

Treatment by a 10 min application of a pyrethrin preparation is usually effective. Re-treatment may be required in 7–10 days. The shampoo form of lindane, which requires a 10 min application time, is an alternative choice, but lindane cream and lotion are no longer recommended for treatment of pubic lice. Infestation of eyelashes is eradicated by petrolatum applied 3 to 5 times per 24 hr for 8–10 days. Clothing, towels, and bed linens may be contaminated with nit-bearing hairs and should be thoroughly laundered or dry-cleaned.

SEABATHER'S ERUPTION. Seabather's eruption is a severely pruritic dermatosis of inflammatory papules that develops within ≈12 hr of bathing in saltwater, primarily on body sites that were covered by a bathing suit. The eruption has been described primarily in connection to bathing in the waters of Florida and the Caribbean. Lesions, which may include pustules, vesicles, and urticarial plaques, are more numerous in those individuals who keep their bathing suits on for an extended period after leaving the water. The eruption may be accompanied by systemic symptoms of fatigue, malaise, fever, chills, nausea, and headache; in one large series, ≈40% of children younger than 16 yr had fever. Duration of the pruritus and skin eruption is 1–2 wk. Lesions consist of a superficial and deep perivascular and interstitial infiltrate of lymphocytes, eosinophils, and neutrophils. The eruption appears to be due to an allergic hypersensitivity reaction to venom from larvae of the thimble jellyfish *(Linuche unguiculata)*. Treatment is largely symptomatic. Potent topical corticosteroids have been shown to provide relief to some patients.

Chosidow O: Scabies. *N Engl J Med* 2006;354:1718–1727.

Demain JG: Papular urticaria and things that bite in the night. *Curr Allergy Asthma Rep* 2003;4:291–303.

Frankowski BL: American Academy of Pediatrics guidelines for the prevention and treatment of head lice infestation. *Am J Manag Care* 2004;10:S269–S272.

Heukelbach J, Feldmeier H: Scabies. *Lancet* 2006;367:1767–1774.

Huynh TH, Norman RA: Scabies and pediculosis. *Dermatol Clin* 2004;22:7–11.

Roberts RJ: Head lice. *N Engl J Med* 2002;346:1645–1650.

Roberts RJ, Burgess IF: New head-lice treatments: Hope or hype? *Lancet* 2005;365:8–10.

Steen CJ, Carbonaro PA, Schwartz RA: Arthropods in dermatology. *J Am Acad Dermatol* 2004;50:819–842.

Walton SF, Holt DC, Currie RJ, et al: Scabies: New future for a neglected disease. *Adv Parasitol* 2004;57:309–376.

Chapter 668 ■ Acne

Joseph G. Morelli

ACNE VULGARIS

Acne, particularly the comedonal form, occurs in ≈80% of adolescents.

PATHOGENESIS. Lesions of acne vulgaris develop in sebaceous follicles, which consist of a large, multilobular sebaceous gland that drains its products into the follicular canal. The initial lesion of acne is a microcomedone, which progresses to a comedone. A comedone is a dilated epithelium-lined follicular sac filled with lamellated keratinous material, lipid, and bacteria. An open comedone, known as a **blackhead**, has a patulous pilosebaceous orifice that permits visualization of the plug. An open comedone becomes inflammatory less commonly than does a closed comedone or whitehead, which has only a pinpoint opening. An inflammatory papule or nodule develops from a comedone that has ruptured and extruded its follicular contents into the subadjacent dermis, inducing a neutrophilic inflammatory response. If the inflammatory reaction is close to the surface, a papule or pustule develops. If the inflammatory infiltrate develops deeper in the dermis, a nodule forms. Suppuration and an occasional giant cell reaction to the keratin and hair are the cause of nodulocystic lesions. These are not true cysts but liquefied masses of inflammatory debris.

The primary pathogenetic alterations in acne are (1) abnormal keratinization of the follicular epithelium, resulting in impaction of keratinized cells within the follicular lumen; (2) increased sebaceous gland production of sebum; (3) proliferation of *Propionibacterium acnes* within the follicle; and (4) inflammation. Comedonal acne (Fig. 668-1), particularly of the central face, is frequently the 1st sign of pubertal maturation. At puberty, the sebaceous gland enlarges and sebum production increases in response to the increased activities of androgens of primarily

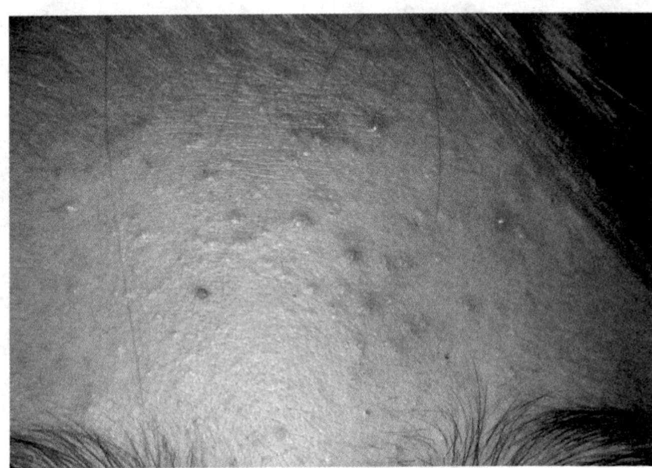

Figure 668-1. Primarily comedonal acne in a 7 yr old girl.

adrenal origin. Most patients with acne do not have significant endocrine abnormalities. Hyper-responsiveness of the sebocyte to androgens is likely involved in determining the severity of acne in a given individual. Sebocytes and follicular keratinocytes contain 5α-reductase, 3β- and 17β-hydroxyl-steroid dehydrogenase which are capable of metabolizing androgens. A significant number of women with acne (25–50%), particularly those with relatively mild papulopustular acne, note that their acne flares ≈1 wk before menstruation. The pathogenesis of this phenomenon is unknown.

Freshly formed sebum consists of a mixture of triglycerides, wax esters, squalene, and sterol esters. Normal follicular bacteria produce lipases that hydrolyze sebum triglycerides to free fatty acids. Those of medium-chain length (C8–C14) may be provocative factors in initiating an inflammatory reaction. Sebum also provides a favorable substrate for proliferation of bacteria. *Propionibacterium acnes* appear to be largely responsible for the formation of free fatty acids. Skin surface *P. acnes* counts do not correlate to the severity of acne. There is a correlation of reduction of *P. acnes* and improvement in acne vulgaris. It is probable that bacterial proteases, hyaluronidases, and hydrolytic enzymes produce biologically active extracellular materials that increase the permeability of the follicular epithelium. Chemotactic factors released by the intrafollicular bacteria attract neutrophils and monocytes. Lysosomal enzymes from the neutrophils, released in the process of phagocytizing the bacteria, further disrupt the integrity of the follicular wall and intensify the inflammatory reaction.

CLINICAL MANIFESTATIONS. Acne vulgaris is characterized by 4 basic types of lesions: open and closed comedones, papules, pustules (Fig. 668-2), and nodulocystic lesions (Fig. 668-3 and Table 668-1). One or more types of lesions may predominate. In its mildest form, which is often seen early in adolescence, lesions are limited to comedones on the central area of the face. Lesions may also involve the chest, upper back, and deltoid areas. A predominance of lesions on the forehead, particularly closed comedones, is often attributable to prolonged use of greasy hair preparations (pomade acne) [Fig. 668-4]. Marked involvement on the trunk is most often seen in males. Lesions often heal with temporary postinflammatory erythema and hyperpigmentation. Pitted, atrophic, or hypertrophic scars may be interspersed, depending on the severity, depth, and chronicity of the process. Diagnosis of acne is rarely difficult, although flat warts, folliculitis, and other types of acne may be confused with acne vulgaris.

TREATMENT. No evidence shows that early treatment, with the exception of isotretinoin, alters the course of acne. Acne can be controlled and severe scarring prevented, however, by judicious maintenance therapy that is continued until the disease process has abated spontaneously. Therapy must be individualized and aimed at preventing microcomedone formation through reduction of follicular hyperkeratosis, sebum production, the *P. acnes* population in follicular orifices, and free fatty acid production. Initial control takes at least 6–8 wk, based on the severity of the acne (Table 668-2). It is also important to address the potentially severe emotional impact of acne on adolescents.

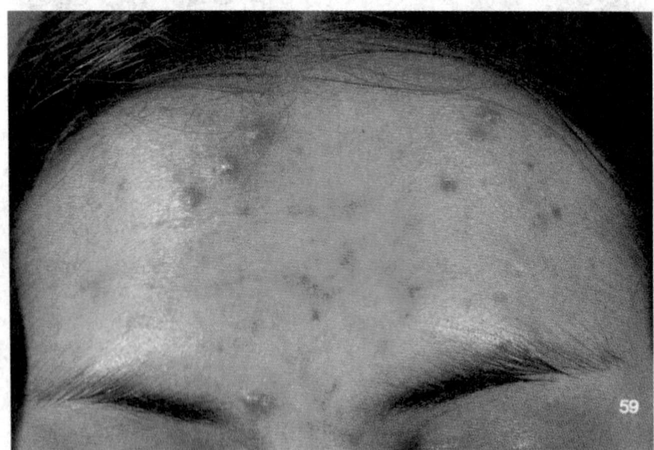

Figure 668-2. Inflammatory papules and pustules.

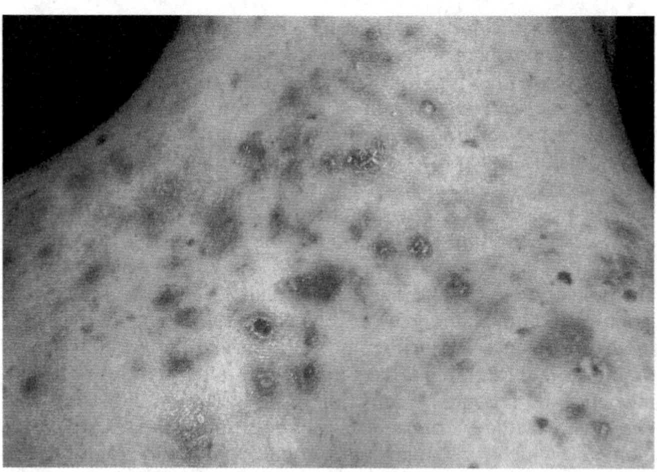
Figure 668-3. Severe nodulocystic acne.

The pediatrician must be aware of the frequently poor correlation between acne severity and psychosocial impact, particularly in adolescents. As adolescents become preoccupied with their appearance, offering treatment even to the youngster whose acne is mild may enhance self-image.

Diet. Little evidence shows that ingestion of particular foods can trigger acne flares. When a patient is convinced that certain dietary items exacerbate acne, it is prudent to omit those foods. It is unnecessary, however, to impose unwarranted dietary restrictions.

Climate. Climate appears to influence acne, in that improvement frequently occurs in summer and flares are more common in winter. Remission in summer may relate, in part, to the relative absence of stress. Emotional tension and fatigue seem to exacerbate acne in many individuals; the mechanism is unclear but has been proposed to relate to an increased adrenocortical response.

Cleansing. Cleansing with soap and water removes surface lipid and renders the skin less oily in appearance, but no evidence shows that surface lipid has a role in generating acne lesions. Only superficial drying and peeling are achieved by cleansing, and almost any mild soap or astringent is adequate. Repetitive cleansing can be harmful because it irritates and chaps the skin. Cleansing agents that contain abrasives and keratolytic agents, such as

TABLE 668-1. Classification of Acne

SEVERITY	DESCRIPTION
Mild	Comedones (noninflammatory lesions) are the main lesions. Papules and pustules may be present but are small and few in number (generally <10).
Moderate	Moderate numbers of papules and pustules (10–40) and comedones (10–40) are present. Mild disease of the trunk may also be present.
Moderately severe	Numerous papules and pustules are present (40–100), usually with many comedones (40–100) and occasional larger, deeper nodular inflamed lesions (up to 5). Widespread affected areas usually involve the face, chest, and back
Severe	Nodulocystic acne and acne conglobata with many large, painful nodular or pustular lesions are present, along with many smaller papules, pustules, and comedones

From James WD: Clinical practice. Acne. *N Engl J Med* 2005;352:1463–1472.

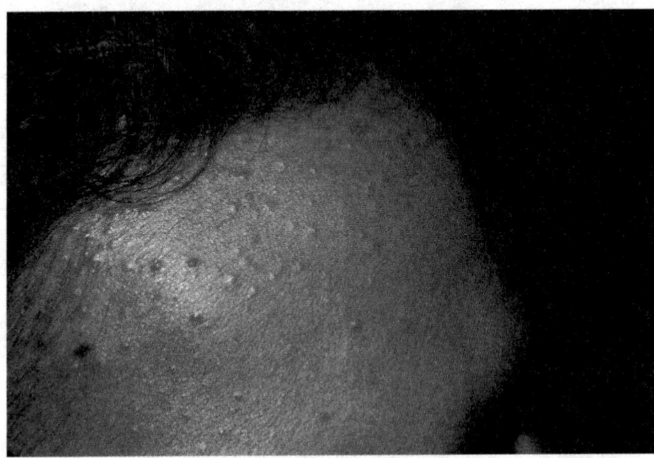

Figure 668-4. Pomade acne along the hairline.

sulfur, resorcinol, and salicylic acid, may temporarily remove sebum from the skin surface. They exert a mild drying and peeling effect and suppress lesions to a limited degree. They do not, however, prevent microcomedones from forming. No evidence shows that preparations containing alcohol or hexachlorophene decrease acne because surface bacteria are not involved in the pathogenesis. Greasy cosmetic and hair preparations must be discontinued because they exacerbate pre-existing acne and cause further plugging of follicular pores. Manipulation and squeezing of facial lesions only ruptures intact lesions and provokes a localized inflammatory reaction.

Topical Therapy. All topical preparations must be used for 6–8 wk before their effectiveness can be assessed. Retinoids may be used alone for mild acne, but frequently combination therapy is more effective. A popular and effective combination is use of benzoyl peroxide gel in the morning and a retinoid at night.

RETINOIDS. A topical retinoid should be the **primary treatment** for acne vulgaris. Topical retinoids have multiple actions including inhibition of the formation and number of microcomedones, reduction of mature comedones, reduction of inflammatory lesions, and production of normal desquamation of the follicular epithelium. Retinoids should be applied daily to all the affected areas. The main side effects of retinoids are irritation and dryness. Not all patients will initially tolerate daily use of a retinoid. It is prudent to begin therapy every other or every 3rd day and slowly increase the frequency of application as tolerated. Tretinoin, adapalene, and tazarotene (Table 668-3) are the available retinoids. They are all approximately equal in efficacy, although adapalene is less irritating and tazarotene works slightly better for comedonal acne.

BENZOYL PEROXIDE. Benzoyl peroxide is primarily an antimicrobial agent. It has an advantage over topical antibiotics in that it does not enhance antimicrobial resistance. It is available in multiple formulations and concentrations. The gel formulations are preferred due to better stability and more consistent release of the active ingredient. Washes and cleansers are useful for covering large surface areas such as the chest and back. As with retinoids, the main side effects are irritation and drying. Benzoyl peroxide can also bleach clothing.

TOPICAL ANTIBIOTICS. Topical antibiotics are indicated for the treatment of inflammatory acne. Clindamycin and erythromycin are the most commonly used. They are not as effective as benzoyl peroxide or oral antibiotics. They should not be used as monotherapy because they do not inhibit microcomedone formation and they have the potential to induce antimicrobial resisitance. Irritation and dryness are generally less than with retinoids or benzoyl peroxide.

AZELAIC ACID. Azelaic acid (20% cream) has mild antimicrobial and keratolytic properties.

Systemic Therapy. Antibiotics, especially tetracycline and its derivatives (see Table 668-3), are indicated for treatment of patients who cannot tolerate or have not responded to topical medications, who have moderate to severe inflammatory papulopustular and nodulocystic acne, and who have a propensity for scarring. Tetracycline and its derivatives act by reducing the growth and metabolism of *P. acnes*. They also have anti-inflammatory properties. For most adolescent patients, therapy may be initiated twice daily, for at least 6–8 wks, followed by a gradual decrease to the minimal effective dose. The drugs should always be administered in combination with a topical retinoid, but not topical antibiotics. Tetracycline absorption is inhibited by food, milk, iron supplements, aluminum hydroxide gel, and calcium-magnesium salts. It should be taken on an empty stomach 1 hr before or 2 hr after meals. Minocycline and doxycycline may be taken with food. Side effects of tetracycline and derivatives are rare. Side effects of tetracycline include vaginal candidosis, particularly in those who take tetracycline concurrently with oral contraceptives; gastrointestinal irritation; phototoxic reactions, including onycholysis and brown discoloration of nails; esophageal ulceration; inhibition of fetal skeletal growth; and staining of growing teeth, precluding its use during pregnancy and in those younger than 8 yr. Doxycycline is the most photosensitizing of the tetracycline derivatives. Rarely, minocycline causes dizziness, intracranial hypertension, bluish discoloration of the skin and mucous membranes, hepatitis, and a lupus-like syndrome. A possible complication of prolonged systemic antibiotic use is proliferation of gram-negative organisms, particularly *Enterobacter, Klebsiella, Escherichia coli*, or *Pseudomonas aeruginosa*, producing severe, refractory folliculitis.

Women who have acne and hormonal abnormalities, who are unresponsive to antibiotic therapy, or who are not candidates for isotretinoin therapy should be considered for a trial of hormonal therapy. Oral contraceptive pills are the primary form of hormonal therapy. Spironolactone has also shown effectiveness.

Isotretinoin (13-cis-retinoic acid, Accutane) is indicated for severe nodulocystic acne and moderate to severe acne that has not responded to conventional therapy. The recommended dosage is ≈0.5–1.0 mg/kg/24 hr. A standard course in the United States lasts 16–20 wk. At the end of one course of isotretinoin, ≈40% of patients are cured, 45% need conventional topical and/or oral medications to maintain adequate control, and 20% have relapses and need an additional course of isotretinoin. Dosages <0.5 mg/kg/24 hr, or a cumulative dose of <120 mg/kg, are associated with a significantly higher rate of treatment failure and relapse. If the disease process is not in remission 2 mo after the 1st course of isotretinoin, a 2nd course should be considered. Isotretinoin reduces size and secretion of sebaceous glands, normalizes follicular keratinization, prevents new microcomedone formation, decreases the population of *P. acnes*, and exerts an anti-inflammatory effect.

TABLE 668-2. Typical Treatment Regimens for Acne
COMEDONAL ACNE
Topical retinoid or
Azelaic acid
MILD PAPULOPUSTULAR ACNE
Topical retinoid plus
Benzoyl peroxide or
Topical antibiotic or
Oral antibiotic
SEVERE PAPULOPUSTULAR OR NODULAR ACNE
Topical retinoid plus
Benzoyl peroxide and oral antibiotic or
Isotretinoin 1 mg/kg/day

TABLE 668-3. Medications for the Treatment of Acne

DRUG	DOSE	SIDE EFFECTS	OTHER CONSIDERATIONS
TOPICAL AGENTS			
Retinoids			
Tretinoin	Applied once nightly; strengths of 0.025–0.1% available**	Irritation (redness and scaling)	Generics available
Adapalene	Applied once daily, at night or in the morning; 0.01%[‡]	Minimal irritation	
Tazarotene*	Applied once nightly; 0.05, 0.1%	Irritation	Limited data suggest tazarotene more effective than alternatives
Antimicrobials			
Benzoyl peroxide, alone or with zinc, 2.5–10%	Applied once or twice daily	Benzoyl peroxide can bleach clothing and bedding	Available over the counter; 2.5–5% concentrations as effective as and less drying than 10% concentration
Clindamycin, erythromycin[†]	Applied once or twice daily	Propensity to resistance	Most effective for inflammatory lesions (rather than comedones); resistance a concern when used alone
Combination benzoyl peroxide and clindamycin or erythromycin	Applied once or twice daily		Combination more effective than topical antibiotics alone; limits development of resistance; use of individual products in combination less expensive and appears similarly effective
OTHER TOPICAL AGENTS			
Azelaic acid, sodium sulfacetamide–sulfur, salicylic acid[†]	Applied once or twice daily	Well tolerated	Good adjunctive or alternative treatments
ORAL ANTIBIOTICS[‡]			
Tetracycline[§]	250–500 mg once or twice daily	Gastrointestinal upset, pseudomotor cerebri	Inexpensive; dosing limited by need to take on empty stomach
Doxycycline[§]	50–100 mg once or twice daily	Phototoxicity, pseudomotor cerebri	20 mg dose antiinflammatory only; limited data on efficacy
Minocycline[§]	50–100 mg once or twice daily	Hyperpigmentation of teeth, oral mucosa, and skin; lupus-like reactions with long-term treatment, pseudomotor cerebri	
Trimethoprim-sulfamethoxazole	One dose (160 mg trimethoprim, 800 mg sulfamethoxazole) twice daily	Toxic epidermal necrolysis and allergic eruptions	Trimethoprim may be used alone in 300-mg dose twice daily; limited data available
Erythromycin[†]	250–500 mg two to four times daily	Gastrointestinal upset	Resistance problematic; consensus is that efficacy is limited
HORMONAL AGENTS[¶]			
Spironolactone[§]	50–200 mg in divided doses	Menstrual irregularities, breast tenderness	Higher doses more effective but cause more side effects; best given in combination with oral contraceptives
Estrogen-containing oral contraceptives	Daily	Potential side effects include thromboembolism	
ORAL RETINOID			
Isotretinoin[‖]	0.5–1.0 mg/kg/day in divided doses	Birth defects; adherence to pregnancy prevention program outlined by drug manufacturer, including two initial negative pregnancy tests, is essential; hypertriglyceridemia, elevated results on liver function tests, abnormal night vision, benign intracranial hypertension, dryness of the lips, ocular, nasal, and oral mucosa and skin, secondary staphylococcal infections, and arthralgias are possible common or important side effects; perform laboratory testing of lipid profiles and liver function tests monthly until dose is stabilized	Relapse rate higher if patient is <16 yr at initial treatment, if acne is of high severity and involves the trunk, or if drug is used in adult women

*Tazarotene is in pregnancy category X: contraindicated in pregnancy.
[†]Clindamycin, erythromycin, and azelaic acid are in pregnancy category B: no evidence of risk in humans.
[‡]Oral antibiotics are indicated for moderate to severe disease; for the treatment of acne on the chest, back, or shoulders; and in patients with inflammatory disease in whom topical combinations have failed or are not tolerated.
[§]This drug is in pregnancy category D: positive evidence of risk in humans.
[¶]Hormonal agents are for use in women only.
[‖]Isotretinoin is in pregnancy category X: contraindicated in pregnancy. It should be used only in patients with severe acne that does not clear with combined oral and topical therapy.
**As cream, gel, or lotion.
[‡]As cream or gel.
Modified from James WD: Clinical practice. Acne. *N Engl J Med* 2005;352:1463–1472.

Isotretinoin use has many side effects. It is highly **teratogenic** and is **absolutely contraindicated** in pregnancy. Pregnancy should be avoided for 6 weeks after discontinuation of therapy. Two or 3 forms of birth control are required, as are monthly pregnancy tests. Concerns over cases of pregnancy despite warnings have prompted a manufacturer registration program, iPLEDGE (www.ipledgeprogram.com) which requires physician enrollment and careful patient pregnancy screening in order to prescribe isotretinoin. Many patients also experience cheilitis, xerosis, periodic epistaxis, and blepharoconjunctivitis. Increased serum triglyceride and cholesterol levels are also common. It is important to rule out pre-existent liver disease and hyperlipidemia before initiating therapy and to recheck laboratories 4 wk after commencing therapy. Less common but significant side effects include arthralgias, myalgias, temporary thinning of the hair, paronychia, increased susceptibility to sunburn, formation of pyogenic granulomas, and colonization of the skin with *Staphylococcus aureus*, leading to impetigo, secondarily infected dermatitis, and scalp folliculitis. Rarely, hyperostotic lesions of the spine develop after more than 1 course of isotretinoin. Concomitant use of tetracycline and isotretinoin is contraindicated because either drug, but particularly when used together, can cause benign intracranial hypertension. Although no cause and effect relationship has been established, drug-induced mood changes and depression and/or suicide have mandated close attention to psychiatric well-being before and during isotretinoin prescription.

Surgical Therapy. Intralesional injection of low-dose (3 mg/mL) mid-potency glucocorticoids (e.g., triamcinolone) with a 30-gauge needle on a tuberculin syringe may hasten the healing of individual, painful nodulocystic lesions. Dermabrasion or laser peel to minimize scarring should be considered only after the active process is quiescent.

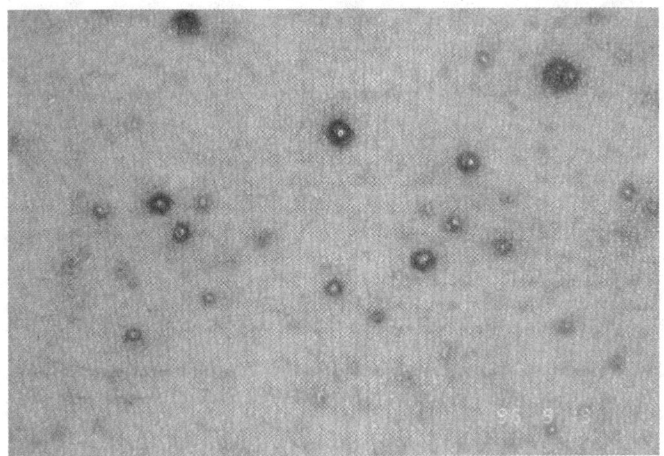

Figure 668-5. Monomorphous papular eruption of steroid acne.

The role of pulsed dye laser in the treatment of inflammatory acne is controversial and inconclusive.

DRUG-INDUCED ACNE

Pubertal and postpubertal patients who are receiving systemic corticosteroid therapy are predisposed to steroid-induced acne. This monomorphous folliculitis occurs primarily on the face, neck, chest (Fig. 668-5), shoulders, upper back, arms, and, rarely, the scalp. Onset follows the initiation of steroid therapy by about 2 wk. The lesions are small, erythematous papules or pustules that may erupt in profusion and are all in the same stage of development. Comedones may occur subsequently, but nodulocystic lesions and scarring are rare. Pruritus is occasional. Although steroid acne is relatively refractory if the medication is continued, the eruption may respond to use of tretinoin and a benzoyl peroxide gel.

Other **drugs** that can induce **acneiform lesions** in susceptible individuals include isoniazid, phenytoin, phenobarbital, trimethadione, lithium carbonate, androgens (anabolic steroids), and vitamin B_{12}.

HALOGEN ACNE

Administration of medications containing iodides or bromides or, rarely, ingestion of massive amounts of vitamin-mineral preparations or iodine-containing "health foods" such as kelp may induce halogen acne. The lesions are often very inflammatory. Discontinuation of the provocative agent and appropriate topical preparations usually achieve reasonable therapeutic results.

CHLORACNE

Chloracne is due to external contact with, inhalation of, or ingestion of halogenated aromatic hydrocarbons, including polyhalogenated biphenyls, polyhalogenated naphthalenes, and dioxins. Lesions are primarily comedonal. Inflammatory lesions are infrequent but may include papules, pustules, nodules, and cysts. Healing occurs with atrophic or hypertrophic scarring. The face, postauricular regions, neck, axillae, genitals, and chest are most commonly involved. The nose is often spared. In cases of severe exposure, associated findings may include hepatitis, production of porphyrins, bulla formation on sun-exposed skin, hyperpigmentation, hypertrichosis, and palmar and plantar hyperhidrosis. Topical or oral retinoids may be effective; benzoyl peroxide and antibiotics are generally ineffective.

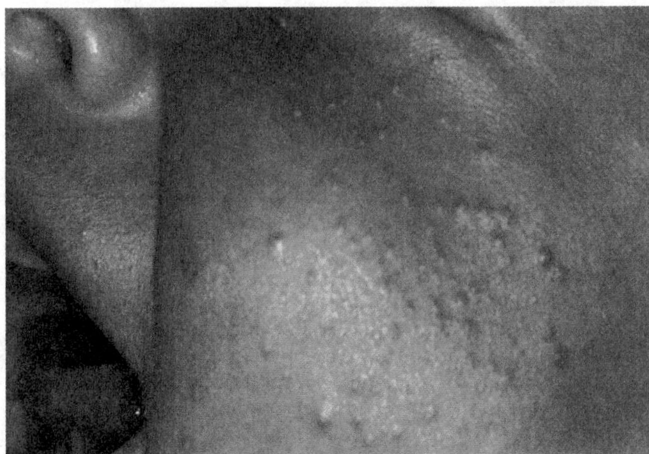

Figure 668-6. Comedonal acne in a neonate.

NEONATAL ACNE

Approximately 20% of normal neonates develop at least a few comedones in the 1st mo of life. Closed comedones predominate on the cheeks and forehead (Fig. 668-6); open comedones and papulopustules occur occasionally. The cause of neonatal acne is unknown but has been attributed to placental transfer of maternal androgens, hyperactive neonatal adrenal glands, and a hypersensitive neonatal end-organ response to androgenic hormones. The hypertrophic sebaceous glands involute spontaneously over a few months, as does the acne. **Treatment** is usually unnecessary. If desired, the lesions can be treated effectively with topical tretinoin and/or benzoyl peroxide.

INFANTILE ACNE

Infantile acne usually presents after 1 yr of life, more commonly in boys than girls. Acne lesions are more numerous, pleomorphic, severe, and persistent than in neonatal acne (Fig. 668-7). Open and closed comedones predominate on the face. Papules and pustules occur frequently, but only occasionally do nodulocystic lesions develop. Pitted scarring is seen in 10–15%. The course may be relatively brief, or the lesions may persist for many months, although the eruption generally resolves by age 3 yr. Use of topical benzoyl peroxide gel and tretinoin usually clears the eruption within a few weeks. Oral erythromycin is necessary

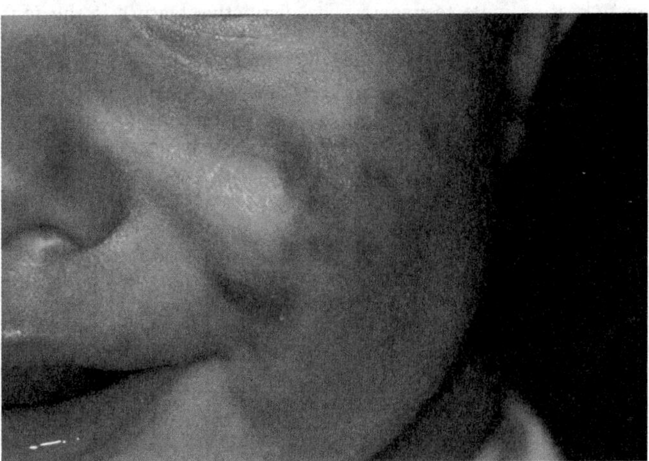

Figure 668-7. Inflammatory infantile acne.

occasionally. A child with refractory acne warrants a search for an abnormal source of androgens such as a virilizing tumor or congenital adrenal hyperplasia.

TROPICAL ACNE

A severe form of acne occurs in tropical climates and is believed to be due to the intense heat and humidity. Hydration of the pilosebaceous duct pore may accentuate blockage of the duct. Affected individuals tend to have an antecedent history of adolescent acne that is quiescent at the time of the eruption. Lesions occur mainly on the entire back, chest, buttocks, and thighs, with a predominance of suppurating papules and nodules. Secondary infection with *S. aureus* may be a complication. The eruption is refractory to acne therapy if the environmental factors are not eliminated.

ACNE CONGLOBATA

Acne conglobata is a chronic progressive inflammatory disease that occurs mainly in men, more commonly in whites than in blacks, but it may begin during adolescence. Patients usually have a history of pre-existing acne vulgaris. The principal lesion is the nodule, although there is often a mixture of comedones with multiple pores, papules, pustules, nodules, cysts, abscesses, and subcutaneous dissection with formation of multichanneled sinus tracts. Severe scarring is characteristic. The face is relatively spared, but in addition to the back and chest, the buttocks, abdomen, arms, and thighs may be involved. Constitutional symptoms and anemia may accompany the inflammatory process. Coagulase-positive staphylococci and β-hemolytic streptococci are frequently cultured from lesions but do not appear to be primarily involved in the pathogenesis. Acne conglobata occasionally occurs in association with hidradenitis suppurativa and dissecting cellulitis of the scalp (as the follicular occlusion triad) and may be complicated by erosive arthritis and ankylosing spondyloarthritis. Endocrinologic studies are not revealing. Routine acne therapy is generally ineffective. Systemic therapy with a corticosteroid may be required to suppress the intense inflammatory activity. Isotretinoin is the most effective form of therapy for some patients but may produce a flare after its initiation.

ACNE FULMINANS (ACUTE FEBRILE ULCERATIVE ACNE)

Acne fulminans is characterized by abrupt onset of extensive inflammatory, tender ulcerative acneiform lesions on the back and chest of male teenagers. The distinctive feature is the tendency for large nodules to form exudative, necrotic, ulcerated, crusted plaques. Lesions often spare the face and heal with scarring. A preceding history of mild papulopustular or nodular acne is noted in most patients. Constitutional symptoms and signs are common, including fever, debilitation, arthralgias, myalgias, weight loss, and leukocytosis. Blood cultures are sterile. Lesions of **erythema nodosum** sometimes develop on the shins. **Osteolytic bone** lesions may develop in the clavicle, sternum, and epiphyseal growth plates; affected bones appear normal or have slight sclerosis or thickening on healing. Salicylates may be helpful for the myalgias, arthralgias, and fever. Corticosteroids (1.0 mg/kg of prednisone) are started first. Then 1 wk later, isotretinoin (0.5–1 mg/kg) is added. Dapsone may be effective if isotretinoin cannot be used. The corticosteroids are tapered over ≈6 wk. Antibiotics are not indicated unless there is evidence of secondary infection. Compared with acne conglobata, acne fulminans presents in younger patients, is more explosive in onset, more commonly has associated constitutional symptoms and ulcerated crusted lesions, and less commonly has multiheaded comedones or involves the face.

Goldsmith LA, Bolognia JL, Callen JP, et al: Amercian Academy of Dermatology consensus on the safe and optimal use of isotretinoin: Summary and recommendations. *J Am Acad Dermatol* 2004;50:900–906.

Gollnick H, Cunliffe W: Management of acne: A report from the global alliance to improve outcomes in acne. *J Am Acad Dermatol* 2003;49:S1–S37.

Haider A, Shaw JC: Treatment of acne vulgaris. *JAMA* 2004;292:726–735.

James WD: Clinical practice. Acne. *N Engl J Med* 2005;352:1463–1472.

Webster GF: Laser treatment of acne. *Lancet* 2003;362:1342.

Chapter 669 ■ Tumors of the Skin

Joseph G. Morelli

See also Chapters 505 and 650.

EPIDERMAL INCLUSION CYST (EPIDERMOID CYST). Epidermoid cysts are the nodules most commonly seen in children. These are sharply circumscribed, dome-shaped, firm, freely movable, skin-colored nodules (Fig. 669-1), often with a central dimple or punctum that is a plugged, dilated pore of a pilosebaceous follicle. Epidermoid cysts form most frequently on the face, neck, chest, or upper back and may periodically become inflamed and infected secondarily, particularly in association with acne vulgaris. The cyst wall may also rupture and induce an inflammatory reaction in the dermis. The wall of the cyst is derived from the follicular infundibulum. A mass of layered keratinized material that may have a cheesy consistency fills the cavity. Epidermoid cysts may arise from occlusion of pilosebaceous follicles, from implantation of epidermal cells into the dermis as a result of an injury that penetrates the epidermis, and from rests of epidermal cells. Multiple epidermoid cysts may be present in Gardner syndrome and the nevoid basal cell carcinoma syndrome. Excision of the cysts with removal of the entire sac and its contents is indicated, particularly if the cyst becomes recurrently infected. A fluctuant, infected cyst should be treated with an antibiotic effective against *Staphylococcus aureus*. After the inflammation subsides, the cyst should be removed.

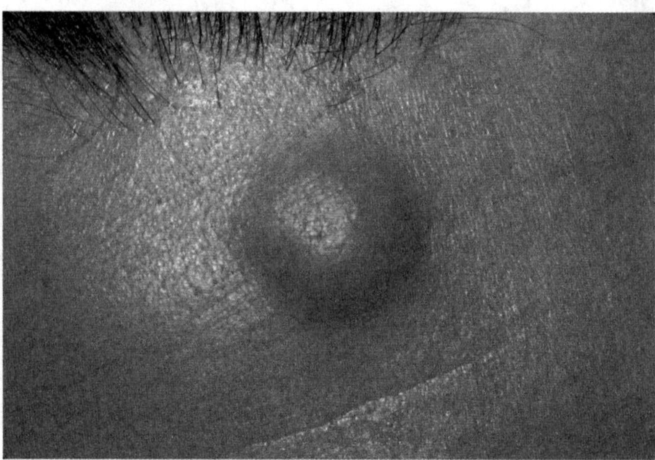

Figure 669-1. Flesh-colored cyst on the forehead.

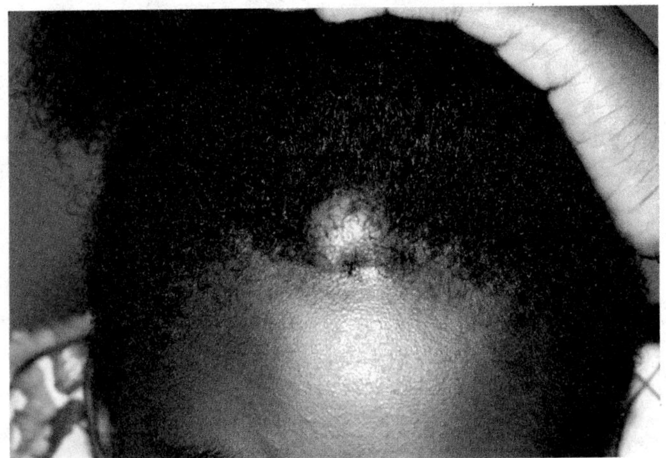

Figure 669-2. Pilar cyst of the anterior scalp.

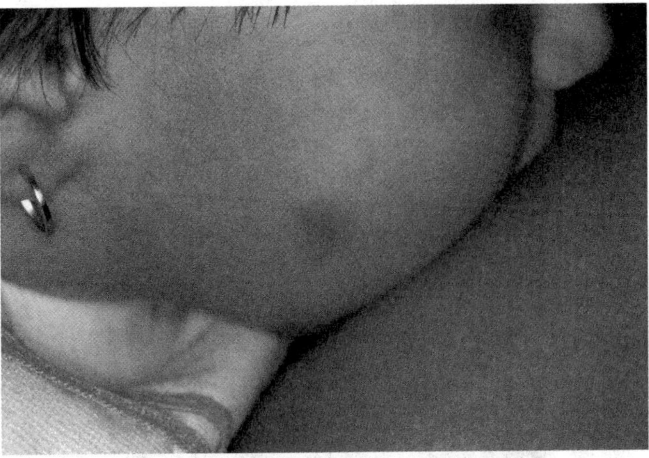

Figure 669-3. Pilomatricoma. Firm tumor with overlying bluish discoloration of the skin.

MILIUM. This is a 1–2 mm, firm, pearly white or yellowish, subepidermal keratin cyst. Milia in newborns is discussed in Chapter 646. Secondary milia occur in association with subepidermal blistering diseases, after dermabrasion or other injury to the skin. They are retention cysts caused by hyperproliferation of injured epithelium and are indistinguishable histopathologically from primary milia. Those that develop after blistering usually arise from the eccrine sweat duct, but they may develop from the hair follicle, sebaceous duct, or epidermis. A milium body differs from an epidermoid cyst only in its small size and superficial location.

PILAR CYST (TRICHILEMMAL CYST). This may be clinically indistinguishable from an epidermoid cyst. It presents as a smooth, firm, mobile nodule, predominantly on the scalp (Fig. 669-2). These cysts occasionally develop on the face, neck, or trunk. The cyst may become inflamed and may occasionally suppurate and ulcerate. The cyst wall is composed of epithelial cells with indistinct intercellular bridges. The peripheral cell layer of the wall shows a palisade arrangement, which is not seen in an epidermoid cyst. No granular layer is present. The cyst cavity contains homogeneous eosinophilic keratinous material, and foci of calcification are seen in 25% of cases. The propensity to develop pilar cysts may be inherited in an autosomal dominant manner. More than 1 cyst generally develops. Numerous pilar and epidermoid cysts, desmoid tumors, fibromas, lipomas, or osteomas may be associated with colonic polyposis or adenocarcinoma in Gardner syndrome. Pilar cysts shell out easily from the dermis.

PILOMATRICOMA. The 2nd most common nodule seen in children, this is a benign tumor that presents as a 3–30 mm, firm, solitary, deep dermal or subcutaneous tumor on the head, neck, or upper extremities. The overlying epidermis is usually normal. The tumor may occasionally be located more superficially, however, tinting the overlying skin blue-red (Fig. 669-3). Patients with both pilomatricoma and myotonic dystrophy are more likely to have several tumors and to have familial occurrence. In general, however, pilomatricomas are not hereditary. Histopathologically, irregularly shaped islands of epithelial cells are embedded in a cellular stroma. Calcium deposits are found in 75% of tumors. Pilomatricomas are caused by mutations in beta-catenin.

TRICHOEPITHELIOMA. This is a 2–8 mm, smooth, round, firm, skin-colored papule that is derived from immature hair follicles. Trichoepitheliomas generally occur singly on the face in childhood or early adulthood. Multiple trichoepitheliomas are inherited autosomal dominantly, appear in childhood or at puberty, and gradually increase in number on the nasofacial folds, nose, forehead, and upper lip and, occasionally, on the scalp, neck, and upper trunk. Microscopically, these benign tumors are characterized by horn cysts composed of a fully keratinized center surrounded by basophilic cells in an adenoid network. Topical imiquimod therapy may be beneficial. Surgical excision is the only other therapy.

ERUPTIVE VELLUS HAIR CYSTS. These are 1–3-mm, asymptomatic, soft, skin-colored follicular papules on the chest (Fig. 669-4). They may become crusted or umbilicated. Abnormal vellus hair follicles become occluded at the level of the infundibulum, resulting in retention of hairs within an epithelium-lined cystic dilatation of the proximal part of the follicle. Most cases are chronic, but spontaneous regression has been reported.

STEATOCYSTOMA MULTIPLEX. This condition usually presents in adolescence or early adulthood with numerous soft to firm cystic nodules that are adherent to the underlying skin and are 3 mm to 3 cm in diameter. When punctured, the cysts may drain oily or cheesy material. Sites of predilection include the sternal region, axillae, arms, and scrotal skin. The multiply folded cyst wall is lined on the luminal side with a thick, homogeneous, eosinophilic horny layer and lacks a granular layer. Flattened sebaceous gland lobules are often visible in the cyst wall, and lanugo hairs may be present in the cystic cavity.

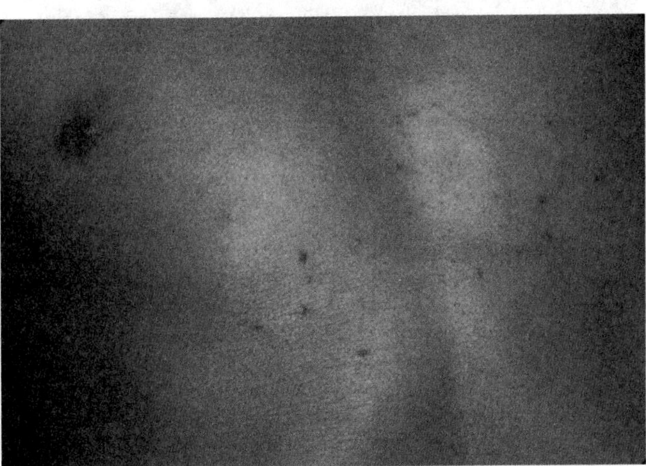

Figure 669-4. Eruptive vellus hair cysts. Multiple papules on the chest.

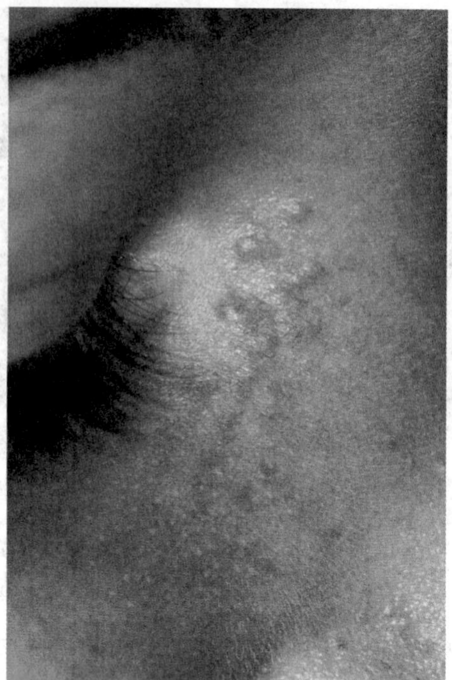

Figure 669-5. Syringomas. Multiple yellow papules near the eye.

SYRINGOMA. The benign tumors known as syringomas are soft, small, skin-colored or yellowish-brown papules that develop on the face, particularly in the periorbital regions (Fig. 669-5). Other sites of predilection include the axillae and umbilical and pubic areas. They often develop during puberty and are more frequent in females. Eruptive syringomas develop in crops over the anterior trunk during childhood or adolescence. A syringoma is derived from an intraepidermal sweat gland duct. Syringomas are of cosmetic significance only. Sparse lesions may be excised, but they are often too numerous to remove.

INFANTILE DIGITAL FIBROMA. This is a smooth, firm, erythematous or skin-colored nodule on the dorsal or lateral surfaces of the distal phalanges of the fingers and toes. More than 80% of tumors present in infancy. They may be present at birth. Lesions may be solitary or multiple and may present as "kissing" tumors on opposing digits. They are usually asymptomatic, but flexion deformity of the digits may occur. Clinically, the lesions resemble a fibroma, leiomyoma, angiofibroma, acquired digital fibrokeratoma, accessory digit, or mucous cyst. The diagnosis is confirmed by finding numerous spindle-shaped fibroblasts that contain small, round, dense, eosinophilic cytoplasmic inclusion bodies composed of collections of actin microfilaments. Local recurrence after simple excision of this tumor has been reported in 75% of patients. Because the tumor does not metastasize and may regress spontaneously in 2–3 yr, a course of expectant observation is advised. If functional impairment or flexion deformity of the digit becomes apparent, prompt full excision of the tumor is indicated.

DERMATOFIBROMA (HISTIOCYTOMA). This benign dermal tumor may be pedunculated, nodular (Fig. 669-6), or flat and is usually well circumscribed and firm but occasionally feels soft on palpation. The overlying skin is usually hyperpigmented, may be shiny or keratotic, and dimples when the tumor is pinched. Dermatofibromas range in size from 0.5 to 10 mm, arise most frequently on the limbs, and are usually asymptomatic but may occasionally be pruritic. They are composed of fibroblasts, young and mature collagen, capillaries, and histiocytes in varying proportions, forming a nodule in the dermis that has poorly defined edges. The cause of these tumors is unknown, but trauma such as an insect bite or folliculitis appears to induce reactive fibroplasia. The differential diagnosis includes epidermal inclusion cyst, juvenile xanthogranuloma, hypertrophic scar, and neurofibroma. Dermatofibromas may be excised or left intact according to a patient's preference. They usually persist indefinitely.

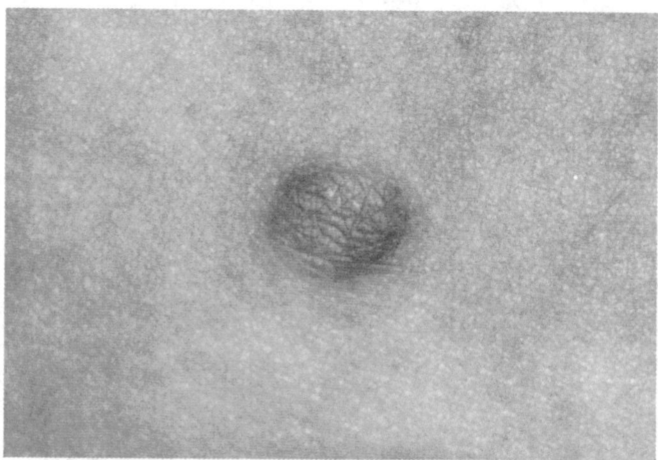

Figure 669-6. Dermatofibroma. Red-brown nodular variant.

JUVENILE XANTHOGRANULOMA. This is a firm, dome-shaped, yellow, pink, or orange papule or nodule (Fig. 669-7) that varies in size from 5 mm to ≈4 cm in diameter. These nodules are 10 times more common in white than in black individuals. Sites of predilection are the scalp, face, and upper trunk, where they may erupt in profusion or remain as solitary lesions. Nodular lesions may appear on the oral mucosa. Mature lesions are characterized histopathologically by a dermal infiltrate of lipid-laden histiocytes, admixed inflammatory cells, and Touton giant cells. The lesions may clinically resemble papulonodular urticaria pigmentosa, dermatofibromas, or xanthomas of hyperlipoproteinemia but can be distinguished from these entities histopathologically.

Affected infants are nearly always otherwise normal, and blood lipid values are not elevated. Café-au-lait macules are found on 20% of patients with juvenile xanthogranuloma. Xanthogranulomatous infiltrates occur occasionally in ocular tissues. This may result in glaucoma, hyphema, uveitis, heterochromia iridis, iritis, or sudden proptosis. Age younger than 2 yr, multiple lesions, and periocular location may heighten concerns for intraocular involvement. There appears to be an association among juvenile xanthogranuloma, neurofibromatosis, and childhood leukemia,

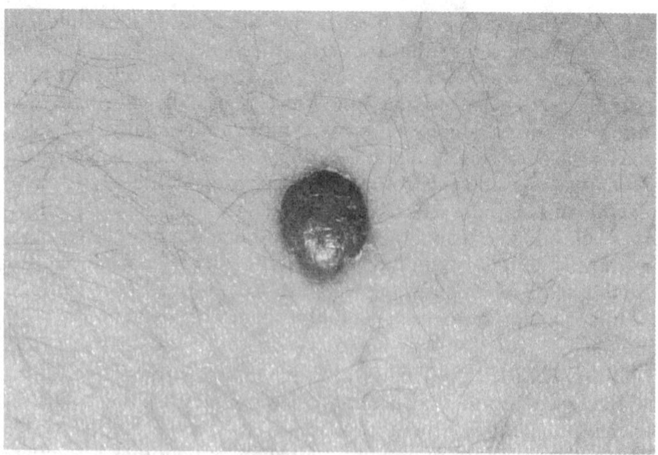

Figure 669-7. Juvenile xanthogranuloma. Solitary orange papule.

most frequently juvenile chronic myelogenous leukemia. There is no need to remove these benign lesions because most of them regress spontaneously in the 1st few years. Residual pigmentation and atrophy may result.

LIPOMA. This benign collection of fatty tissue appears on the trunk, neck, or proximal portions of the limbs. Lipomas are soft, compressible, lobulated, subcutaneous masses. Multiple lesions may occur occasionally, as in Gardner syndrome. Atrophy, calcification, liquefaction, or xanthomatous change may sometimes complicate their course. A lipoma is composed of normal fat cells surrounded by a thin connective tissue capsule. Lipomas represent a cosmetic defect and may be surgically excised. Multiple lipomas, identical to those that occur singly, are inherited in an autosomal dominant fashion and often appear by the 3rd decade in patients with familial multiple lipomatosis. Lipomas may appear intra-abdominally, intramuscularly, and subcutaneously. Congenital lipomatosis presents in the 1st few months of life as large subcutaneous fatty masses on the chest, with extension into skeletal muscle. Congenital lipomatosis can also be a manifestation of Proteus syndrome. Angiolipomas usually present as numerous painful subcutaneous nodules on the arms and trunk.

BASAL CELL EPITHELIOMA (BASAL CELL CARCINOMA). Basal cell carcinoma is rare in children in the absence of a predisposing condition, such as nevoid basal cell carcinoma syndrome, xeroderma pigmentosum, nevus sebaceus of Jadassohn, arsenic intake, or exposure to irradiation. The lesions are smooth, pearly, pink, telangiectatic papules that enlarge slowly and may bleed or ulcerate. Sites of predilection are the face, scalp, and upper back. The differential diagnosis includes pyogenic granuloma, nevocellular nevus, epidermal inclusion cyst, closed comedo, dermatofibroma, and adnexal tumor. Depending on the site of occurrence and associated disease of the host, electrodesiccation and curettage or simple excision is usually curative. When the tumor is recurrent, >2 cm in diameter, located on problematic anatomic areas such as the mid-face or ears, or is an aggressive histopathologic type, Mohs microscopically controlled surgery may be the most appropriate treatment.

NEVOID BASAL CELL CARCINOMA SYNDROME (BASAL CELL NEVUS SYNDROME, GORLIN SYNDROME). This autosomal dominant syndrome maps to a gene on chromosome 9q22.3 with an incidence of 1 in 60,000. This tumor suppressor gene (PTCH) is part of the hedgehog signaling pathway and is important in determining embryonic patterning and cell fate in a number of structures in the developing embryo. Mutations in human patched gene produce dysregulation of several genes involved in organogenesis and carcinogenesis. Consequently, the syndrome includes a wide spectrum of defects involving the skin, eyes, central nervous and endocrine systems, and bones. The predominant features are early onset basal cell carcinomas and mandibular cysts. Approximately 20% of those in whom a basal cell carcinoma develops before age 19 yr have this syndrome. Basal cell carcinomas appear between puberty and age 35 yr, erupting in crops of tumors that vary in size, color, and number and may be difficult to distinguish from other types of skin lesions. Sites of predilection are the periorbital skin, nose, malar areas, and upper lip, but the lesions can develop on the trunk and limbs and are not restricted to sun-exposed areas. Ulceration, bleeding, crusting, and local invasion can occur. Small milia, epidermal cysts, pigmented lesions, hirsutism, and palmar and plantar pits are additional cutaneous findings.

The facies of patients with this syndrome are characterized by temporoparietal bossing, prominent supraorbital ridges, a broad nasal root, ocular hypertelorism or dystopia canthorum, and prognathism. Keratinized cysts (odontogenic keratocysts) in the maxilla and mandible occur in most patients. They range in size from a few mm to several cm, may result in maldevelopment of the teeth, and cause pain, swelling of the jaw, facial deformity, bone erosion, pathologic fractures, and suppurating sinus tracts. Osseous defects such as anomalous rib development, spina bifida, kyphoscoliosis, and brachymetacarpalism occur in ⅔ of patients, and ocular abnormalities including cataracts, glaucoma, coloboma, strabismus, and blindness occur in approximately ¼. Some males have hypogonadism, with absent or undescended testes. Kidney malformations have also been reported. Neurologic manifestations include calcification of the falx, seizures, mental retardation, partial agenesis of the corpus callosum, hydrocephalus, and nerve deafness. The incidence of medulloblastoma, ameloblastoma of the oral cavity, fibrosarcoma of the jaw, teratoma, cystadenoma, cardiac fibroma, ovarian fibroma, and fetal onset rhabdomyoma is increased.

Treatment of these patients requires participation of various specialists according to individual clinical problems. Basal cell carcinomas should not be treated with irradiation. Most of the basal cell carcinomas have a clinically benign course, and it is often impossible to remove them all. Those with an aggressive growth pattern and those on the central areas of the face, however, should be removed promptly. Oral retinoids are helpful in preventing the development of new tumors in some patients. Genetic counseling is also indicated.

MUCOSAL NEUROMA SYNDROME (MULTIPLE ENDOCRINE NEOPLASIA TYPE IIB). Mucosal neuroma syndrome, an autosomal dominant trait, is characterized by an asthenic or marfanoid habitus with scoliosis, pectus excavatum, pes cavus, and muscular hypotonia. The syndrome is due to mutations in the tyrosine kinase domain of the RET gene. Patients have thick, patulous lips and soft tissue prognathism simulating acromegaly. Multiple mucosal neuromas or neurofibromas appear as pink, pedunculated or sessile nodules on the anterior third of the tongue, at the commissures of the lips, and on the buccal mucosa and palpebral conjunctiva. Various ophthalmologic defects and intestinal ganglioneuromatosis with recurrent diarrhea are additional common findings. There is a high incidence of medullary thyroid carcinoma associated with high calcitonin levels, pheochromocytoma, and hyperparathyroidism. Periodic screening tests for the associated malignant tumors are mandatory.

Dehner LP: Juvenile xanthogranuloma in the first two decades of life: A clinicopathologic study of 174 cases with cutaneous and extracutaneous manifestations. *Am J Surg Pathol* 2003;27:579–583.

Gorlin RJ: Nevoid basal cell carcinoma (Gorlin) syndrome. *Genet Med* 2004;6:530–539.

High A, Zedan W: Basal cell nevus syndrome. *Curr Opin Oncol* 2005; 17:160–166.

Marin-Gutzke M, Sanchez-Olaso A, Berenguer B, et al: Basal cell carcinoma in childhood after radiation therapy: A case report and review. *Ann Plast Surg* 2004;53:593–595.

Pirousmanesh A, Reinisch JF, Gonzalez-Gomez I, et al: Pilomatrixoma: A review of 346 cases. *Plast Reconstr Surg* 2003;112:1784–1789.

Zelger B, Zelger BG, Burgdorf WH: Dermatofibroma—a critical review. *Int J Surg Pathol* 2004;12:333–344.

Chapter 670 ■ Nutritional Dermatoses

Joseph G. Morelli

ACRODERMATITIS ENTEROPATHICA. This is a rare autosomal recessive disorder caused by an inability to absorb sufficient zinc from the diet. The genetic defect is in the intestinal zinc specific transporter gene SLC39A4. Initial signs and symptoms usually occur in the 1st few mo of life, often after weaning from breast to cow's milk. The cutaneous eruption consists of vesiculobullous, eczematous, dry, scaly, or psoriasiform skin lesions symmetrically distributed in the perioral, acral, and perineal areas (Fig. 670-1*A* and *B*) and on the cheeks, knees, and elbows (Fig. 670-2*A* and *B*). The hair often has a peculiar reddish tint, and alopecia of some degree is characteristic. Ocular manifestations include photophobia, conjunctivitis, blepharitis, and corneal dystrophy detectable by slit-lamp examination. Associated manifestations include chronic diarrhea, stomatitis, glossitis, paronychia, nail dystrophy, growth retardation, irritability, delayed wound healing, intercurrent bacterial infections, and superinfection with *Candida albicans*. Lymphocyte function and free radical scavenging are impaired. Without treatment, the course is chronic and intermittent but often relentlessly progressive. When the disease is less severe, only growth retardation and delayed development may be apparent.

The **diagnosis** is established by the constellation of clinical findings and detection of a low plasma zinc concentration. Histopathologic changes in the skin are nonspecific and include parakeratosis and pallor of the upper epidermis. The variety of manifestations of the syndrome may be due to the fact that zinc has a role in numerous metabolic pathways, including those of copper, protein, essential fatty acids, and prostaglandins, and zinc is incorporated into many zinc metalloenzymes.

Oral **therapy** with zinc compounds is the treatment of choice. Optimal doses range from 50 mg of zinc sulfate, acetate, or gluconate daily for infants up to 150 mg/24 hr for children. Plasma zinc levels should be monitored, however, to individualize the dosage. Zinc therapy rapidly abolishes the manifestations of the disease. A syndrome resembling acrodermatitis enteropathica has been observed in patients with secondary zinc deficiency caused by long-term total parenteral nutrition without supplemental zinc or by chronic malabsorption syndromes. A rash similar to that of acrodermatitis enteropathica has also been reported in infants fed breast milk that is low in zinc and in those with maple syrup urine disease, organic aciduria, methylmalonic acidemia, biotinidase deficiency, essential fatty acid deficiency, severe protein malnutrition (kwashiorkor), and cystic fibrosis.

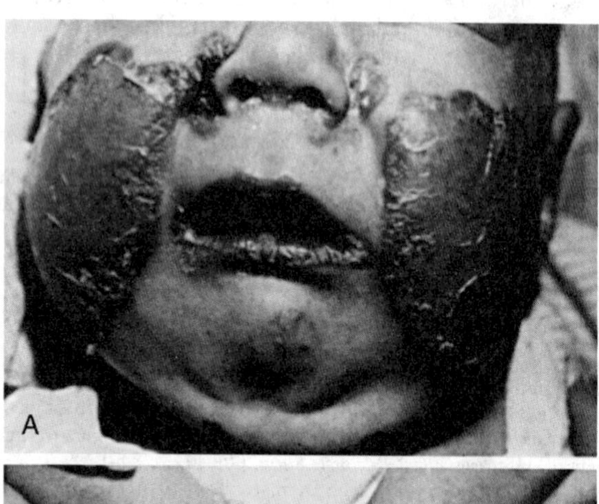

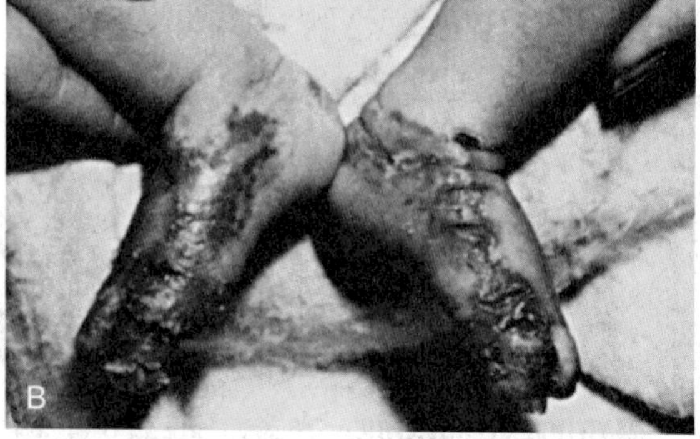

Figure 670-1. *A*, Psoriasiform facial lesions of zinc deficiency dermatitis. *B*, Similar lesions on the feet with secondary nail dystrophy.

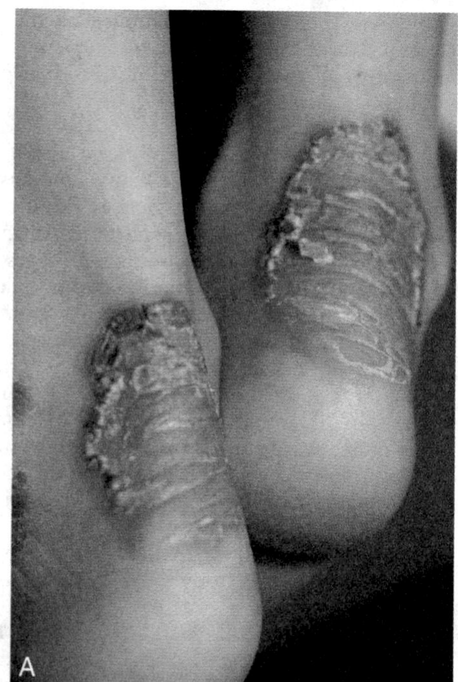

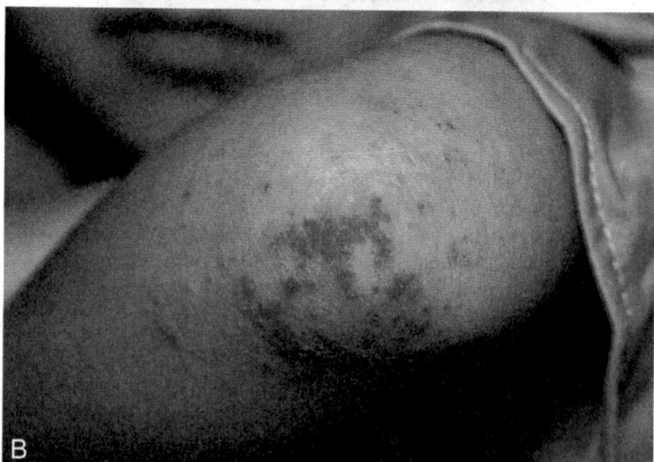

Figure 670-2. *A*, Psoriasiform lesion of zinc deficiency dermatitis on the ankles. *B*, Similar lesions on the elbows.

ESSENTIAL FATTY ACID DEFICIENCY. This causes a generalized, scaly dermatitis composed of thickened, erythematous, desquamating plaques. The eruption has been induced experimentally in animals fed a fat-free diet and has been observed in patients with chronic severe malabsorption such as in short-gut syndrome and in those sustained on a fat-free diet or fat-free parenteral alimentation. Linoleic (18:2 n-6) and arachidonic (20:4 n-6) acids are deficient, and an abnormal metabolite, 5,8,11-eicosatrienoic acid (20:3 n-9), is present in the plasma. Additional manifestations of essential fatty acid deficiency include alopecia, thrombocytopenia, and failure to thrive. The horny layer of the skin is cracked microscopically, the barrier function of the skin is disturbed, and transepidermal water loss is increased. Topical application of linoleic acid, which is present in sunflower seed and

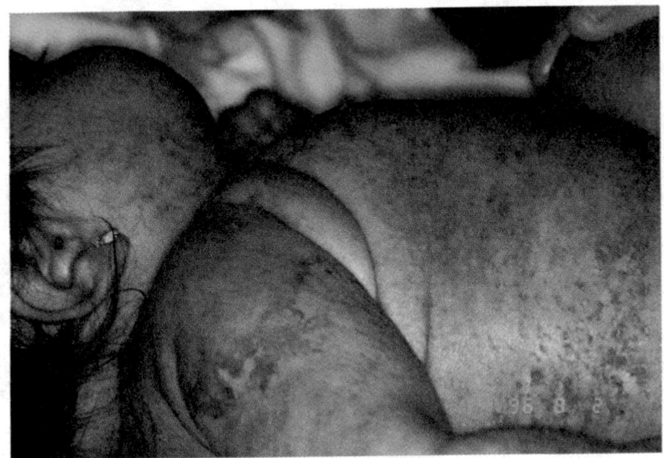

Figure 670-3. Erosions and scaling in kwashiorkor.

safflower oils, may ameliorate the clinical and biochemical skin manifestations. Appropriate nutrition should be provided.

KWASHIORKOR. Severe protein and essential amino acid deprivation in association with adequate caloric intake can lead to kwashiorkor, particularly at the time of weaning to a diet that consists primarily of corn, rice, or beans (see Chapter 43). Cutaneous erythema develops 1st and, in mild cases in white children, progresses to fine desquamation along natural skin lines and on the shins, outer thighs, and back. In dark-skinned children, characteristic early findings include circumoral pallor, cutaneous depigmentation, and development of purple patches. As the disease advances, well-marginated, slightly raised, purplish, waxy plaques appear, particularly in the diaper area and at sites of pressure such as the elbows, knees, and ankles and on the trunk. In severe cases, erosions and linear fissures develop (Fig. 670-3). Sun-exposed skin is relatively spared, as are the feet and dorsal aspects of the hands. Nails are thin and soft, and hair is sparse, thin, and depigmented, sometimes displaying a flag sign of alternating light and dark bands that reflect alternating periods of adequate and inadequate nutrition. The cutaneous manifestations may closely resemble those of acrodermatitis enteropathica. The serum zinc level is often deficient and, in some cases, skin lesions of kwashiorkor heal more rapidly when zinc is applied topically.

CYSTIC FIBROSIS (SEE CHAPTER 400). Five to 10% of patients with cystic fibrosis develop protein-calorie malnutrition. Rash in infants with cystic fibrosis and malnutrition is rare but may appear by age 6 mo. The initial eruption consists of scaling, erythematous papules and progresses in 1–3 mo to extensive desquamating plaques. The rash is accentuated around the mouth and perineum and on the extremities (lower > upper). Alopecia may be present, but mucous membranes and nails are uninvolved.

PELLAGRA (SEE CHAPTER 46). This presents with edema, erythema, and burning of sun-exposed skin on the face, neck, and dorsal aspects of the hands, forearms, and feet. Lesions of pellagra may also be provoked by burns, pressure, friction, and inflammation. The eruption on the face frequently follows a butterfly distribution, and the dermatitis encircling the neck has been termed "Casal's necklace." Blisters and scales develop, and the skin increasingly becomes dry, rough, thickened, cracked, and hyperpigmented. Skin infections may be unusually severe. Pellagra develops in those with insufficient dietary intake or malabsorption of niacin and/or tryptophan. Administration of isoniazid, 6-mercaptopurine, or 5-fluorouracil may also produce pellagra. Nicotinamide supplementation and sun avoidance are the mainstays of therapy.

SCURVY (VITAMIN C OR ASCORBIC ACID DEFICIENCY) (SEE CHAPTER 47). This presents initially with follicular hyperkeratosis and coiling of hair on the upper arms, back, buttocks, and lower extremities. Perifollicular erythema and hemorrhage, particularly on the legs and advancing to involve large areas of hemorrhage; swollen, erythematous gums; stomatitis; and subperiosteal hematomas are also seen. The best method for confirmation of a clinical diagnosis of scurvy is a trial of vitamin C supplementation.

VITAMIN A DEFICIENCY (SEE CHAPTER 45.1). This deficiency presents initially with impairment of visual adaptation to the dark. Cutaneous changes include xerosis and hyperkeratosis and hyperplasia of the epidermis, particularly the lining of hair follicles and sebaceous glands. In severe cases, desquamation may be prominent.

Darmstadt GL: The skin and nutritional disorders in the newborn. *Eur J Pediatr Dermatol* 1998;8:221.

Heygi J, Schwartz RA, Heygi V: Pellagra: Dermatitis, dementia, and diarrhea. *Int J Dermatol* 2004;43:1–5.

Oumeish OY, Oumeish I: Nutritional skin problems in children. *Clin Dermatol* 2003;21:260–263.

Perafan-Riveros C, Franca LF, Alves AC, et al: Acrodermatitis enteropathica: A case report and review of the literature. *Pediatr Dermatol* 2002;19:426–431.

Part XXXI ▪ Bone and Joint Disorders

Section 1 — Orthopedic Problems

Chapter 671 ▪ Growth and Development

Harish S. Hosalkar and Lawrence Wells

Growth patterns and development in children are often unique to the individual child and therefore defining normal has potential ramifications. Statistically, normal is defined as 95% of a population that falls within 2 standard deviations of the mean from any given measurement. The challenge for the orthopedic surgeon caring for children is to understand which deviations from normal are likely to result in impairment of function, progressive deformity, or premature degenerative arthritis and pain.

Terminologies to describe some common deviations from normal are enumerated in Table 671-1

Congenital anomalies can be categorized into:

a. **Production problems:** These include abnormalities caused by malformation, dysplasia, or disruption that will not spontaneously resolve.
b. **Packaging problems:** These include deformations caused by mechanical causes including in utero positioning and molding and usually resolve with time.

IN UTERO POSITIONING. In the newborn, the imprint of the in utero position may be evident and confused with an abnormality. In utero positioning produces temporary joint and muscle contractures and affects the torsional alignment of the long bones, especially those of the lower extremities. Normal full-term newborns can have up to 20–30-degree hip and knee flexion contractures. These tend to resolve by 4–6 mo of age. The newborn hip externally rotates in extension up to 80–90 degrees and has limited internal rotation to ≈0–10 degrees. The lower leg frequently has inward rotation (internal tibial torsion), and the feet are supinated from their medial borders being wrapped against the posterolateral aspect of the opposite thigh. The top leg in the in utero position may show more changes than the bottom leg. The face may also be distorted, whereas the spine and upper extremities are less affected by the in utero position. The effects of in utero positioning, therefore, are physiologic in origin but may produce parental concerns. The child may be 3–4 yr old before the effects of the in utero position completely resolve.

GROWTH AND DEVELOPMENT

Consideration of growth and development helps to formulate treatment strategies designed to preserve or restore normal growth potential. Growth is not a constant feature and is subject to many variables including genetics, nutrition, general health, endocrine status, mechanical forces and physiological age. The application of forces to the growing skeleton can improve or worsen deformities in children Growth also varies between 2 anatomic regions and even between 2 bones of the same region.

Bone formation or ossification occurs in 2 different ways:

Endochondral ossification, in which mesenchymal cells condense and undergo chondrogenesis to form cartilage that matures and hypertrophies, becomes calcified, and is then replaced by bone. Most bones in the axial and appendicular skeleton are formed in this way.

Intramembranous ossification, in which osteoblasts are formed by direct differentiation of mesenchymal cells with no cartilage precursor or model. Flat bones of the skull and clavicle are formed in this way.

Centers of ossification:

Primary centers of ossification: At the beginning of the fetal period the chondrocytes in the midshaft of long bones from the primary centers, growth from which eventually lengthens the bone.

Secondary centers of ossification: These appear in the chondroepiphysis and mostly appear postnatally. They direct the formation of bone throughout growth.

The ossification centers that are typically present at term birth are the distal femur, proximal tibia, calcaneus, and talus.

Typical long bones are divided into:

Physis, which is the growth plate located at the end of bone
Epiphysis, which is typically the secondary ossification center
Metaphysis, which is the bone adjacent to the physis on the side away from the joint
Diaphysis, which is the central part or shaft of long bones

The long bones of the extremities (humerus, radius-ulna, femur, tibia-fibula) have growth plates or physes at each end. The ends of each long bone are composed of the epiphyses. These are covered by articular cartilage and form the associated joints. Epiphyses are almost entirely cartilaginous in the beginning and become progressively more ossified during growth. The articular cartilage also contributes to the growth of the epiphysis. The perichondrial ring, which surrounds the physes, as well as the perichondrium around the epiphyses and periosteum, which surrounds the metaphysis and diaphyseal regions of the bone, contributes to appositional or circumferential growth. Bones without physes (pelvis, scapulae, carpals, tarsals) grow by appositional bone growth from their surrounding perichondrium and periosteum. Other bones (metacarpals, metatarsals, phalanges, spine) grow by a combination of both appositional and endochondral ossification.

IMPORTANT GROWTH AND DEVELOPMENTAL MILESTONES

Some important musculoskeletal growth considerations are summarized in Table 671-2.

TABLE 671-1. Terminologies for Deviations

TERMINOLOGY	DESCRIPTION
Congenital	Anomaly that is apparent at birth
Deformation	A normally formed structure that is pushed out of shape by mechanical forces
Deformity	A body part altered in shape from normal, outside the normal range
Developmental	A deviation that occurs over time; one that may not be present or apparent at birth
Disruption	A structure undergoing normal development that stops developing or is destroyed or removed
Dysplasia	A tissue that is abnormal or wrongly constructed
Malformation	A structure that is wrongly built; failure of embryologic development or differentiation resulting in abnormal or missing structures

TABLE 671-2. Skeletal Growth Considerations

- Abnormal stature can be assessed as "proportionate" or "disproportionate" based on comparing the ratio of sitting height with subischial height (lower limbs).
- Normally the arm span is almost equal to standing height.
- The head is disproportionately large at birth and ratio of head height to total height is approximately 1 : 4 at birth, which changes to 1 : 7.5 at skeletal maturity.
- Lower extremities account for about 15% of height at birth and 30% at skeletal maturity.
- The rate of height and growth increase is not constant and varies with growth spurts.
- By age 5 yr, birth height usually doubles and the child is approximately 60% of adult height. The child is about 80% of final height at 9 yr. During puberty, the standing height increases by approximately 1 cm per month.
- Bone age is more important than chronological age in determining future growth potential.

GROWTH PATTERNS IN UPPER AND LOWER EXTREMITIES

The upper extremity grows longitudinally primarily from physes away from the elbow, with the proximal humeral physis and the distal radial and ulnar physes contributing a greater amount than the physes close to the elbow. This is opposite to the lower extremity growth pattern in which most of the longitudinal growth occurs around the knee, in the distal femoral and the proximal tibial physes (Fig. 671-1).

In the hip joint, the acetabulum forms with the convergence of three primary ossification centers (ischium, ilium, and the pubis), while in the proximal femur there is a confluence of the proximal femoral physis and the greater trochanteric physis in the 1st few years of life.

MATURATION OF GAIT

Central nervous system maturation contributes significantly to the development of gait. In the beginning of ambulation, the child usually has a wide-based gait with hyperflexion of hips and knees, no reciprocal arm swing, and an initial contact with heel. By the age of 2 yr, the wide gait diminishes, reciprocal arm swing begins, and the initial contact is with the heel with increased step length and velocity. Adult kinematic patterns usually start developing by 3 yr and the time-distance parameters reach adult values by ≈7 yr, with development of a fully mature gait pattern.

Ballock RT, O'Keefe RJ: The biology of the growth plate. *J Bone Joint Surg Am* 2003;85:715–726.

Davids JR: Normal gait and assessment of gait disorders. In Morrissy R, Weinstein S (editors): *Lovell and Winter's Pediatric Orthopedics,* 5th ed. Philadelphia, Lippincott Williams & Wilkins, 2001, pp 131–156

Dimeglio A: Growth in pediatric orthopedics. In Morrissy R, Weinstein S (editors): *Lovell and Winter's Pediatric Orthopedics,* 5th ed. Philadelphia, Lippincott Williams & Wilkins, 2001, pp 33–62.

Frick SL: Normal growth and development in pediatric orthopedics. In Dormans JP (editor): *Pediatric Orthopedics: Core Knowledge in Orthopedics.* Philadelphia, Mosby, 2005, pp 1–14.

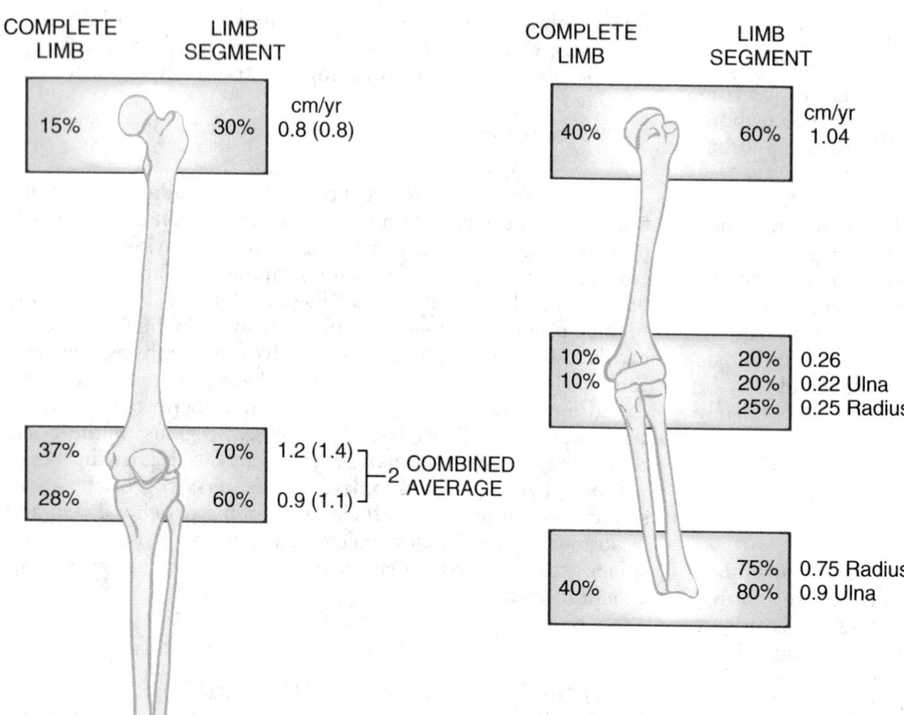

Figure 671-1. The contribution (%) of each physis to the overall length of the extremities. (From Morrissy R, Weinstein S [editors]: *Lovell and Winter's Pediatric Orthopedics,* 5th ed. Philadelphia, Lippincott Williams & Wilkins, 2001.)

Ogden J: Anatomy and physiology of skeletal development. In Catterall A (editor): *Skeletal Injury in the Children,* 3rd ed. New York, Springer-Verlag, 2000, pp 1–37.
Song KM, Little DG: Peak height velocity as a maturity indicator for males with idiopathic scoliosis. *J Pediatr Orthop* 2000;20:286–288.
Westh RN, Menelaus MB: A simple calculation for the timing of the epiphyseal arrest. *J Bone Joint Surg Br* 1981;63:117–119.

Chapter 672 ■ Evaluation of the Child

Harish S. Hosalkar and Lawrence Wells

A detailed history and thorough physical examination are invaluable in the evaluation of a child with an orthopedic problem. There may be many participants providing information regarding the child including parents, grandparents, guardian, siblings, and coaches; information obtained can be very important, especially in younger children and infants. Depending on the nature and severity of problem, appropriate radiographic imaging and, occasionally, laboratory testing may be necessary.

HISTORY. A comprehensive history should include details about the prenatal, perinatal, and postnatal history. Prenatal history should include maternal health issues including smoking, prenatal vitamins, illicit drug or narcotic use, alcohol consumption, diabetes, rubella, and sexually transmitted infections. The child's prenatal and perinatal history should include information about the length of pregnancy, prematurity, length of labor, type of labor (induced or spontaneous), presentation of fetus, evidence of any fetal distress at delivery, requirements of oxygen following the delivery, birth length and weight, Apgar score, muscle tone at birth, feeding history, and period of hospitalization. In older infants and young children, evaluation of the presence and delay of developmental milestones for posture, locomotion, dexterity, social activities, and speech is important. The medical and surgical history should include any previous procedures and significant medical conditions, especially in patients with chronic symptoms. Specific orthopedic questions should focus on joint, muscular, appendicular, or axial skeleton complaints. Information regarding pain or other symptoms in any of these areas should be appropriately elicited (Table 672-1). The family history may give clues to possible genetic disorders such as congenital syndromes, muscular dystrophy, skeletal dysplasias, and other disorders affecting the musculoskeletal system. It also may play a role in expectations of the child's future development.

TABLE 672-1. Characterization of Pain and Presenting Symptom

1. ***Location:*** Whether pain is localized to a particular segment or involves a larger area.
2. ***Intensity:*** Usually on a pain scale of 1 to 10.
3. ***Quality***
   i. Tumor pain is often unrelenting, progressive, and often present during the night.
   ii. Pain at night is particularly suggestive of osteoid osteoma.
   iii. Pain in inflammation and infection is usually continuous.
4. ***Onset*** (was it acute and related to specific trauma or was it insidious?)***:*** Acute pain and history of trauma are more commonly associated with fractures.
5. ***Duration:*** Whether transient, only lasting for minutes, or lasting for hours or days. Pain lasting for longer than 3–4 wk is more suggestive of a serious underlying problem.
6. ***Progress:*** Whether static, increasing, or decreasing.
7. ***Radiation:*** Pain radiating to upper or lower extremities or complaints of numbness, tingling, or weakness require appropriate work-up.
8. ***Aggravating factors:*** Relationship to any activities such as swimming or diving or any particular position.
9. ***Alleviating factors:*** Does the pain get relieved by rest, heat, and/or medication? Conditions such as spondylolysis, Scheuermann disease, inflammatory spondyloarthropathy, muscle pulls, or overuse are improved by bed rest.
10. ***Gait and posture:*** Disturbances associated with pain.

TABLE 672-2. Guidelines during Inspection of a Child with Musculoskeletal Problem

- Patient should be *comfortable with adequate exposure and well-lit surroundings* (lest some important physical finding be missed). Infants or young children may be examined on their parents' lap so that they feel more secure and are more likely to be cooperative.
- It is important to inspect how the patient moves about in the room before and during the examination as well as during various maneuvers. *Balance, posture, and gait pattern* should also be checked.
- *General examination* findings should include inspection for skin rashes, café-au-lait spots, hairy patches, dimples, cysts, tuft of hair, or evidence of spinal midline defects that can indicate serious underlying problem and need review.
- *General body habitus,* including signs of cachexia, pallor, and nutritional deficiencies, should be noted.
- It is important to note any obvious spinal asymmetry, axial or appendicular deformities, trunk decompensation, and evidence of muscle spasm or contractures. *Forward bending test* is valuable in assessing asymmetry and movement of the spine.
- It is essential to perform and document a *thorough neurologic examination.* Motor, sensory, and reflex testing should be performed and recorded.
- Any *discrepancies in limb lengths* as well as *muscle atrophy* should be recorded.
- The range of motion of all joints, their stability, and any evidence of hyperlaxity, peripheral pulsations, and lymphadenopathy should also be noted in all cases.

PHYSICAL EXAMINATION. The orthopedic physical examination must include a thorough examination of the musculoskeletal system as well as a comprehensive neurologic examination. The examination must include inspection, palpation, and evaluation of motion, stability, and gait. A basic neurologic examination including sensory examination, motor function, and reflex evaluation as per the age and development of the child must be performed. The orthopedic physical examination requires basic knowledge of anatomy as far as joint range of motion, alignment, and stability are concerned, as well as a glossary of basic terminologies so as to standardize the communication regarding the patient's findings. It includes the careful evaluation of the musculoskeletal and neurologic systems as well as an appropriate general physical examination. Many common musculoskeletal disorders can be diagnosed by the history and physical examination alone. The examination of the musculoskeletal system includes four parts: inspection, palpation, assessment of joint range of motion, and gait assessment in ambulatory children.

INSPECTION. Initial examination of the child begins with inspection. The clinician should use the guidelines listed in Table 672-2 during inspection.

PALPATION. Palpation of involved region should include assessment of local temperature and warmth, tenderness, existence of a swelling or mass, evidence of tightness, spasticity or contracture, bone or joint deformity and evaluation of anatomic axis of limb, and finally assessment of limb lengths.

Contractures are a loss of mobility of a joint from congenital or acquired causes and are caused by periarticular soft-tissue fibrosis or involvement of muscles crossing the joint. Congenital contractures are common in **arthrogryposis** (see Chapter 681). Spasticity is an abnormal increase in tone associated with hyperreflexia and is common in cerebral palsy.

Deformity of the bone or joint is an abnormal fixed shape or position from congenital or acquired causes. It is important to assess the type of deformity, its location, and degree of deformity upon clinical examination. It is also important to assess whether the deformity is fixed or can be passively or actively corrected and whether there is any associated muscle spasm, local tenderness, or pain on motion. Depending on the plane of deformity, it can be defined as **varus** (away from midline) or **valgus** (apex toward midline) (coronal plane), or **recurvatum** or **flexion** deformity (sagittal plane). In the axial skeleton, especially the spine, deformity can be defined as scoliosis, kyphosis, hyperlordosis, and kyphoscoliosis.

RANGE OF MOTION. It is important to assess and record the active and passive range of motion while evaluating the joint. The range should always be compared to the opposite side that points toward the normal range. Objective evaluation should be ideally done with a goniometer and recorded.

Different terminologies for direction of joint motion are outlined:

Abduction: Away from the midline.
Adduction: Toward the midline.
Flexion: Movement of bending from the starting position.
Extension: Movement from bending to the starting position.
Supination: Rotating the forearm to face the palm upward.
Pronation: Rotating the forearm to face the palm downward.
Inversion: Turning the hindfoot inward.
Eversion: Turning the hindfoot outward.
Internal rotation: Turning inward toward the axis of the body.
External rotation: Turning outward away from the axis of the body.

GAIT ASSESSMENT. Children typically begin walking between 12 and 16 mo. Early ambulation is characterized by short stride length, a fast cadence, and slow velocity with a wide-based stance. Gait cycle is a single sequence of functions by one limb and includes the time between right heel strike followed by left toe-off, left heel strike, and right toe-off, and ends with right heel strike. The five events describe one gait cycle and include two phases: stance and swing. The stance phase is the period during which the foot is in contact with the ground. The swing phase is the portion of the gait cycle during which a limb is being advanced forward without ground contact (see Chapter 671).

Some important terms used in understanding gait cycle include:

Cadence: The number of steps taken per minute.
Step length: The distance covered during one step.
Step period: The time measured from an event in one foot to the same event in the opposite foot.
Stride period: The time from heel strike of one foot to the next heel strike of the same foot.
Stride length: The total distance covered from one heel strike to the same-foot heel strike.

Neurologic maturation is necessary for the development of gait and the normal progression of developmental milestones. A child's gait changes with neurologic maturation. Infants normally walk with greater hip and knee flexion, flexed arms, and a wider base of gait than older children. As the neurologic system continues to develop in the cephalocaudal direction, the efficiency and smoothness of gait increase. The gait characteristics of a 7 yr old child are similar to those of an adult. In circumstances when the neurologic system is abnormal (cerebral palsy), the delicate control of gait is disturbed, leading to pathologic reflexes and abnormal movements.

Deviations from normal gait occur in a variety of orthopedic conditions. Disorders that result in muscle weakness (e.g., spina bifida, muscular dystrophy), spasticity (e.g., cerebral palsy), or contractures (e.g., arthrogryposis) lead to abnormalities in gait. Other causes of gait disturbances include limp, pain, torsional variations (in-toeing and out-toeing), toe walking, joint abnormalities, and leg-length discrepancy.

LIMPING

A thorough history and clinical examination are the first steps toward early identification of the underlying problem causing a limp. Limping can be considered as either **painful (antalgic)** or painless, with the differential diagnosis ranging from benign to serious causes (septic hip, tumor). In a painful gait, the stance phase is shortened as the child decreases the time spent on the painful extremity. In a painless gait, which is indicative of underlying proximal muscle weakness or hip instability, the stance phase is equal between the involved and uninvolved sides, but the child will lean or shift the center of gravity over the involved extremity for balance. If the disorder is bilateral, it produces a waddling gait.

Disorders most commonly responsible for an abnormal gait generally vary based on the age of the patient. The differential diagnosis of limping varies based on age group (Table 672-3) or mechanism (Table 672-4). Neurologic disorders, especially spinal cord or peripheral nerve disorders, can also produce limping and difficulty walking. Antalgic gait is predominantly a result of trauma, infection, or pathologic fracture. Trendelenburg gait is generally due to congenital, developmental, or muscular disorders. Limping in some cases may also be due to nonskeletal causes such as testicular torsion, inguinal hernia, and appendicitis.

BACK PAIN

In comparison to adults, the work-up for back pain in children is extensive and aggressive at a much earlier stage in the evolution of symptoms. Children frequently have a specific skeletal pathology as the cause of back pain. In the pediatric population, a history of persistent back pain should be taken seriously and

TABLE 672-3. Common Causes of Limping According to Age

AGE	ANTALGIC	TRENDELENBURG	LEG-LENGTH DISCREPANCY
Toddler (1–3 yr)	Infection Septic arthritis Hip Knee Osteomyelitis Diskitis Occult trauma Toddler's fracture Neoplasia	Hip dislocation (DDH) Neuromuscular disease Cerebral palsy Poliomyelitis	–
Childhood (4–10 yr)	Infection Septic arthritis Hip Knee Osteomyelitis Diskitis Transient synovitis, hip LCPD Tarsal coalition Rheumatologic disorder JRA Trauma Neoplasia	Hip dislocation (DDH) Neuromuscular disease Cerebral palsy Poliomyelitis	+
Adolescence (11+ yr)	SCFE Rheumatologic disorder JRA Trauma: fracture, overuse Tarsal coalition Neoplasia		+

DDH, developmental dysplasia of the hip; JRA, juvenile rheumatoid arthritis; LCPD, Legg-Calvé-Perthes disease; SCFE, slipped capital femoral epiphysis; –, absent; +, present.
From Thompson GH: Gait disturbances. In Kliegman RM (editor): *Practical Strategies of Pediatric Diagnosis and Therapy.* Philadelphia, WB Saunders, 1996, pp 757–778.

TABLE 672-4. Differential Diagnosis of Limping

ANTALGIC	TRENDELENBURG
CONGENITAL	**DEVELOPMENTAL**
Tarsal coalition	DDH
	Leg-length discrepancy
ACQUIRED	**NEUROMUSCULAR**
LCPD	Cerebral plasy
SCFE	Poliomyelitis
TRAUMA	
Sprains, strains, contusions	
Fractures	
Occult	
Toddler's fracture	
Abuse	
NEOPLASIA	
Benign	
Unicameral bone cyst	
Osteoid osteoma	
Malignant	
Osteogenic sarcoma	
Ewing sarcoma	
Leukemia	
Neuroblastoma	
Spinal cord tumors	
INFECTIOUS	
Septic arthritis	
Reactive arthritis	
Osteomyelitis	
Acute	
Subacute	
Diskitis	
RHEUMATOLOGIC	
Juvenile rheumatoid arthritis	
Hip monoarticular synovitis (toxic transient synovitis)	

DDH, developmental dysplasia of the hip; LCPD, Legg-Calvé-Perthes disease; SCFE, slipped capital femoral epiphysis.
From Thompson GH: Gait disturbances. In Kliegman RM (editor): *Practical Strategies of Pediatric Diagnosis and Therapy.* Philadelphia, WB Saunders, 1996, pp 757–778.

often warrants further investigation. The most frequent causes of back pain in children are trauma, spondylolysis, spondylolisthesis, and infection. A list of common causes of back pain in children is presented in Table 678-1. It is important to note that tumor and tumor-like lesions that cause back pain in children are likely to be missed unless a thorough clinical assessment and adequate work-up are performed when required. Nonorthopedic causes of back pain include urinary tract infections, nephrolithiasis, and pneumonia.

NEUROLOGIC EVALUATION. A careful neurologic evaluation is a part of every pediatric musculoskeletal examination (see Chapter 591). The assessment should include evaluation of developmental milestones, muscle strength, sensory assessment, muscle tone, and deep tendon reflexes. The neurologic evaluation should also assess the spine and identify the presence of deformity, such as scoliosis and kyphosis, as well as spinal mobility. Specific peripheral nerve examinations may be necessary.

As the nervous system matures, the developing cerebral cortex normally inhibits rudimentary reflexes that are often present at birth (see Chapter 591). Therefore, persistence of these reflexes beyond a certain age indicates neurologic abnormality. The most commonly performed deep tendon reflexes include biceps, triceps, quadriceps, and gastrocsoleus tendons. Localized or diffuse weakness must be determined and documented. A thorough assessment and grading of muscle strength is mandatory in all cases of neuromuscular disorders.

A commonly used system for grading of muscle strength is based on a scale of 0 to 5:

Grade 0: No muscular contraction detected.
Grade 1: Trace contraction, barely detectable clinically.
Grade 2: Active movement with gravity eliminated.
Grade 3: Active movement against gravity.
Grade 4: Active movement against gravity and some resistance.
Grade 5: Active movement against full resistance.

RADIOGRAPHIC ASSESSMENT. Plain radiographs are the first step in evaluation of most musculoskeletal disorders. Advanced imaging includes special procedures such as nuclear bone scans, ultrasonography, CT, MRI, and positron emission tomography (PET).

PLAIN RADIOGRAPHS. Routine radiographs are the first step and consist of anteroposterior and lateral views of the involved area with one joint above and below. Comparison views of the opposite side, if uninvolved, may be helpful in difficult situations but are not always necessary. It is important for the clinician to be aware of normal radiographic variants of the immature skeleton. Several synchondroses may be mistaken for fractures. Even a patient with "normal" plain radiographic appearance but having persistent pain or symptoms may need to be evaluated further with additional imaging studies if a tumor is suspected.

NUCLEAR MEDICINE IMAGING. A bone scan displays physiologic information rather than pure anatomy and relies on the emission of energy from the nucleotide injected into the patient. Indications include early septic arthritis or osteomyelitis, avascular necrosis, tumors (osteoid osteoma), metastatic lesions, occult and stress fractures, and cases of child abuse.

Total body radionuclide scan (technetium-99) is useful to identify bony lesions (inflammatory, tumors, stress fractures) and may also help in evaluation of biologic activity of the primary bone lesion. Tumor vascularity can also be inferred from the flow phase and the blood pool images. Gallium or indium scans have high sensitivity for local infections. Thallium-201 chloride scintiscans have >90% sensitivity and between 80% and 90% accuracy in detecting malignant bone or soft-tissue tumors.

ULTRASONOGRAPHY. Ultrasonography has no ionizing radiation, no contrast material to be administered, and no biologically harmful effects and can be repeated as often as necessary. The equipment is portable; scans can be obtained in any plane. The disadvantages of ultrasonography include the following: Bone is not penetrated, static images are difficult to interpret, and the results are operator dependent. The major indications for ultrasonography are fetal studies of the extremities and spine including detection of congenital anomalies like spondylocostal dysostosis, osteogenesis imperfecta, developmental dysplasia of the hip, joint effusions, occult *neonatal* spinal dysraphism, foreign bodies in soft tissues, and popliteal cysts of the knee.

MAGNETIC RESONANCE IMAGING. MRI is the imaging modality of choice for further defining the exact anatomic extent of most musculoskeletal lesions. MRI avoids ionizing radiation and is presumed not to produce biologically harmful effects. It produces excellent anatomic images of the musculoskeletal system, including the soft tissue, bone marrow cavity, spinal cord, and brain. It is especially useful for soft-tissue lesions and helps in definition of lesion and its extension (defines extent of involvement of neurovascular structures, physeal involvement, growth cartilage). Tissue planes are well delineated, allowing more accurate assessment of lesion or tumor invasion into adjacent structures. Cartilage structures can be visualized, and different forms can be distinguished (articular cartilage of the knee can be distinguished from the fibrocartilage of the meniscus). MRI is helpful in visualizing unossified joints in the pediatric population including the shoulders, elbows, and hips of young infants. MRI distinguishes physiologic changes that occur in the bone marrow with respect to age and disease such as avascular necrosis.

MRI can be useful in the evaluation of avascular necrosis of bone; infections and infarctions; spinal cord, nerve root, and peripheral nerve lesions; and bone and soft-tissue neoplasms. The ability of MRI to define the region of interest in multiple planes (axial, sagittal, coronal) is an advantage in defining the extent of many tumors. It is the best modality for demonstrating intraosseous tumor extension, assessing involvement of the critical neurovascular structures, and evaluating the soft-tissue extension of the tumor. It is also possible to use dynamic, contrast-enhanced MRI to monitor response to chemotherapy and to identify skips/satellite lesions.

MAGNETIC RESONANCE ANGIOGRAPHY (MRA). This has largely replaced routine angiography in the preoperative assessment of vascular lesions and bone tumors. MRA provides good visualization of peripheral vascular branches and tumor neovascularity in patients with primary bone tumors. MRA is helpful in demonstrating encroachment onto and encasement of major vessels by the tumor mass. While MRI may be sufficient to diagnose large tumor thrombus in many cases, it is recommended that MRA and ultrasonography be considered adjuncts to MRI in the preoperative planning of limb-sparing resections in cases like osteosarcomas of the pelvis, especially if there appears to be a poor response to chemotherapy.

COMPUTED TOMOGRAPHY. CT has enhanced the evaluation of multiple musculoskeletal disorders. Coronal, sagittal, and axial imaging is possible with CT including three-dimensional reconstructions that can be beneficial in evaluating complex lesions of the axial and appendicular skeleton. It allows visualization of the detailed bone anatomy and the relationship of bones to contiguous structures. Some of the pediatric musculoskeletal disorders that are readily evaluated by CT are tarsal coalition, accessory navicular bone, infection, growth plate arrest, osteoid osteoma, pseudoarthrosis, bone and soft tissue tumors, spondylolysis, and spondylolisthesis.

CT is superior to MRI for assessment of bone involvement and cortical destruction (even subtle changes), including calcification or ossification and fracture. Evaluation of the acetabular dome and the bony pelvic anatomy is critical in periacetabular tumors; CT may be a helpful adjunct to MRI. Both helical CT (HCT) and high-resolution CT (HRCT) (HCT being more sensitive than HRCT for detecting pulmonary metastasis) remain the best studies for detecting and evaluating pulmonary metastasis and also response of these lesions to chemotherapy.

POSITRON EMISSION TOMOGRAPHY. Functional imaging using PET has been recognized as an important imaging modality and an adjunct to CT/MRI that provides complementary metabolic information in many oncology applications. PET with ^{18}F-fluorodeoxyglucose (FDG) assesses increased glucose metabolism in sarcomas. FDG-PET evaluations of pediatric bone sarcomas demonstrate significant alteration in response to neoadjuvant chemotherapy. Monitoring therapy and the diagnosis of recurrences of metastases are potential useful clinical indications of FDG-PET.

LABORATORY STUDIES. Laboratory tests are occasionally necessary in the evaluation of a child with musculoskeletal disorder. These may include a complete blood cell count; erythrocyte sedimentation rate; C-reactive protein assay; Lyme titers; and blood, wound, joint, periosteum, or bone cultures for infectious conditions like septic arthritis or osteomyelitis. Rheumatoid factor, antinuclear antibodies, and human leukocyte antigen B27 may be necessary for children with suspected rheumatologic disorders. Creatine kinase, aldolase, aspartate aminotransferase, and dystrophin testing are indicated in children with suspected disorders of striated muscle such as Duchenne or Becker muscular dystrophy.

Beebe AC, Kerpsack JM: Pediatric musculoskeletal examination. In Dormans JP (editor): *Pediatric Orthopedics: Core Knowledge in Orthopedics.* Philadelphia, Mosby, 2005, pp 15–35.

Herring JA: The orthopedic examination: A comprehensive overview. In Herring JA (editor): *Tachdjian's Pediatric Orthopedics,* 3rd ed. Philadelphia, WB Saunders, 2002, pp 25–61.

Herring JA: The limping child. In Herring JA (editor): *Tachdjian's Pediatric Orthopedics,* 3rd ed. Philadelphia, WB Saunders, 2002, pp 83–94.

Herring JA: Imaging. In Herring JA (editor): *Tachdjian's Pediatric Orthopedics,* 3rd ed. Philadelphia, WB Saunders, 2002, pp 127–168.

Hosalkar HS, Garg S, Pollack A, Dormans JP: The diagnostic accuracy of MRI vs. CT imaging for osteoid osteoma in children. *Clin Orthop* 2005;433:171–177.

Hosalkar HS, Moroz L, Drummond DS, Finkel RS: Neuromuscular disorders of infancy and childhood and arthrogryposis. In Dormans JP (editor): *Pediatric Orthopedics: Core Knowledge in Orthopedics,.* Philadelphia, Mosby, 2005, pp 454–482.

Jones DHA, Hosalkar HS, Jones S: The orthopaedic management of osteogenesis imperfecta. *Curr Orthop* 2002;16:374–388.

Staheli LT: Normative data in pediatric orthopaedics. *J Pediatr Orthop* 1996;16:561–562.

Sutherland DH, Olsten R, Cooper L, et al: The development of gait. *J Bone Joint Surg Am* 1980;62:336–353.

Chapter 673 ■ The Foot and Toes

Harish S. Hosalkar, David A. Spiegel, and Richard S. Davidson

Abnormalities affecting the osseous and articular structures of the foot may be congenital, developmental, neuromuscular, or inflammatory. Problems with the foot and/or toes may be associated with a host of connective tissue diseases and syndromes; overuse syndromes are commonly observed in young athletes. Symptoms may include pain and abnormal shoe wear; cosmetic concerns are common. The foot may be divided into the **forefoot** (toes and metatarsals), the **midfoot** (cuneiforms, navicular, cuboid), and the **hindfoot** (talus and calcaneus). While the tibiotalar joint (ankle) provides plantarflexion and dorsiflexion, the subtalar joint (between the talus and calcaneus) is oriented obliquely, providing inversion and eversion. Inversion represents a combination of plantarflexion and varus, while eversion involves dorsiflexion and valgus. The subtalar joint is especially important for walking on uneven surfaces. The talonavicular and calcaneocuboid joints connect the midfoot with the hindfoot.

673.1 • Metatarsus Adductus

Metatarsus adductus is common in newborns and involves adduction of the forefoot relative to the hindfoot. When the forefoot is supinated and adducted, the deformity is termed metatarsus varus (Fig. 673-1). The most common cause is intrauterine molding; the deformity is bilateral in 50% of cases. As with other intrauterine positional foot deformities, a careful hip examination should always be performed.

CLINICAL MANIFESTATIONS. The forefoot is adducted (occasionally supinated), whereas the midfoot and hindfoot are normal.

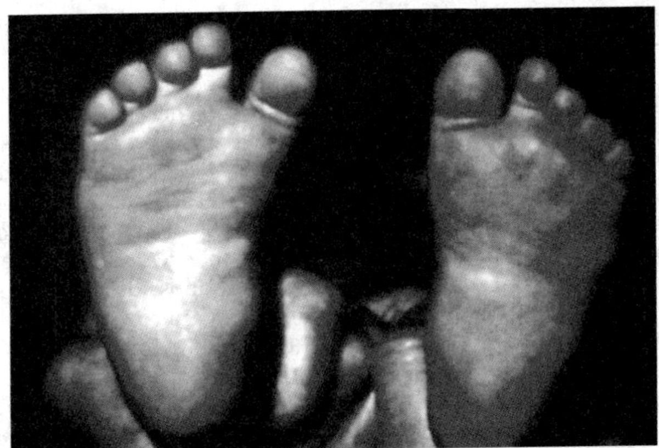

Figure 673-1. Clinical picture of metatarsus adductus with a normal foot on opposite side.

The lateral border of the foot is convex, and the base of the 5th metatarsal appears prominent. Range of motion at the ankle and subtalar joints is normal. Both the magnitude and the degree of flexibility should be documented. When the foot is viewed from the plantar surface, a line through the midpoint of (and parallel to) the heel should normally extend through the 2nd toe. Flexibility is assessed by stabilizing the hindfoot and midfoot in a neutral position with one hand and applying pressure over the 1st metatarsal head with the other. In the walking child with an uncorrected metatarsus adductus deformity, an in-toe gait and abnormal shoe wear may occur. A subset of patients will also have a dynamic adduction deformity of the great toe (hallux varus), which is often most noticeable during ambulation. This usually improves spontaneously and does not require treatment.

RADIOGRAPHIC EVALUATION. Radiographs are not performed routinely. Anteroposterior (AP) and lateral weight-bearing or simulated weight-bearing radiographs are indicated in toddlers or older children with residual deformities. The AP radiographs demonstrate adduction of the metatarsals at the tarsometatarsal articulation and an increased intermetatarsal angle between the 1st and 2nd metatarsals.

TREATMENT. The treatment of metatarsus adductus is based on the rigidity of the deformity; most children respond to nonoperative treatment. Deformities that are flexible and overcorrect into abduction with passive manipulation may be observed. Those feet that correct just to a neutral position may benefit from stretching exercises and retention in a slightly overcorrected position by a splint or reverse-last shoes. These are worn full time (22 hr/day), and the condition is re-evaluated in 4–6 wk. If improvement occurs, treatment can be continued. If there is no improvement, serial plaster casts should be considered. When stretching a foot with metatarsus adductus, care should be taken to maintain the hindfoot in neutral to slight varus alignment to avoid creating hindfoot valgus. Feet that cannot be corrected to a neutral position may benefit from serial casting; the best results are obtained when treatment is started before 8 mo of age. In addition to stretching the soft tissues, the goal is to alter physeal growth and stimulate remodeling, resulting in permanent correction. Once flexibility and alignment are restored, orthoses or corrective shoes are generally recommended for an additional period. A dynamic hallux varus usually improves spontaneously, and no active treatment is required.

Surgical treatment may be considered in the small subset of patients with symptomatic residual deformities that have not responded to previous treatment. Surgery is generally delayed until children are 4–6 yr of age. Cosmesis is often a concern, and pain and/or the inability to wear certain types of shoes may occasionally lead patients to consider surgery. Options for surgical treatment include either soft-tissue release or osteotomy. An osteotomy (midfoot or multiple metatarsals) is most likely to result in permanent restoration of alignment.

673.2 • Calcaneovalgus Feet

The calcaneovalgus foot is a common finding in the newborn and is secondary to in utero positioning. Excessive dorsiflexion and eversion are observed in the hindfoot, and the forefoot may be abducted. There may be an associated external tibial torsion.

CLINICAL MANIFESTATIONS. The infant typically presents with the foot dorsiflexed and everted, and occasionally the dorsum of the foot will be in contact with the anterolateral surface of the lower leg. Plantarflexion and inversion are often restricted. As with other intrauterine positional deformities, a careful hip examination should be performed; if there is any concern, hip ultrasonography should be considered. The calcaneovalgus foot may be confused with a congenital vertical talus and may rarely be associated with a posteromedial bow of the tibia. A calcaneovalgus deformity may also be seen in older patients, typically those with a neuromuscular imbalance involving weakness or paralysis of the gastrocsoleus muscle (polio, myelomeningocele).

RADIOGRAPHIC EVALUATION. Radiographs are usually not required, but should be ordered if the deformity fails to correct spontaneously or with early treatment. AP and lateral radiographs with a lateral radiograph of the foot in maximal plantarflexion may help distinguish calcaneovalgus from a vertical talus. If a posteromedial bow of the tibia is suspected, anteroposterior and lateral radiographs of the tibia and fibula are necessary.

TREATMENT. Mild cases of calcaneovalgus foot, in which full passive range of motion is present at birth, require no active treatment. These usually resolve within the 1st weeks of life. A gentle stretching program, focusing on plantarflexion and inversion, is recommended for cases with some restriction in motion. For cases with a greater restriction in mobility, serial casts may be considered to restore motion and alignment. Casting is rarely required in the treatment of calcaneovalgus feet. The management for those cases associated with a posteromedial bow of the tibia is similar.

673.3 • Talipes Equinovarus (Clubfoot)

Clubfoot is the term used to describe a deformity involving malalignment of the calcaneotalar-navicular complex. Components of this deformity may be best understood using the mnemonic CAVE (cavus, adductus, varus, equinus). Although this is predominantly a hindfoot deformity, there are plantarflexion (cavus) of the 1st ray and adduction of the forefoot/midfoot on the hindfoot. The hindfoot is in varus and equinus. The clubfoot deformity may be positional, congenital, or associated with a variety of underlying diagnoses (neuromuscular or syndromic).

The **positional clubfoot** is a normal foot that has been held in a deformed position in utero and is found to be flexible on examination in the newborn nursery. The **congenital clubfoot** involves a spectrum of severity, while clubfoot associated with neuromuscular diagnoses or syndromes are typically rigid and more difficult to treat. Clubfoot is extremely common in patients with myelodysplasia and arthrogryposis.

Congenital clubfoot is seen in approximately 1/1,000 births. Although numerous theories have been proposed, the etiology is multifactorial and likely involves the effects of environmental factors in a genetically susceptible host. The risk is approximately 1 in 4 when both a parent and one sibling have clubfeet. It occurs more commonly in males (2 : 1) and is bilateral in 50% of cases. The pathoanatomy involves both abnormal tarsal morphology (plantar and medial deviation of the head and neck of the talus) and abnormal relationships between the tarsal bones in all three planes, as well as associated contracture of the soft tissues on the plantar and medial aspects of the foot.

CLINICAL MANIFESTATIONS. A complete physical examination should be performed to rule out coexisting musculoskeletal and neuromuscular problems. The spine should be inspected for signs of occult dysraphism. Examination of the infant clubfoot demonstrates forefoot cavus and adductus and hindfoot varus and equinus (Fig. 673-2). The degree of flexibility varies, and all patients will exhibit calf atrophy. Both internal tibial torsion and leg-length discrepancy (shortening of the ipsilateral extremity) will be observed in a subset of cases.

RADIOGRAPHIC EVALUATION. Anteroposterior and lateral radiographs are recommended, often with the foot held in the maximally corrected position. Multiple radiographic measurements can be made to describe malalignment between the tarsal bones. The navicular bone does not ossify until 3–6 yr of age, so the focus of radiographic interpretation is the relationships between segments of the foot. A common radiographic finding is "parallelism" between lines drawn through the axis of the talus and the calcaneus on the lateral radiograph, indicating hindfoot varus. Many clinicians believe that radiographs are not required in the evaluation and treatment of clubfoot in infancy and reserve these studies for older children with persistent or recurrent deformities.

TREATMENT. Nonoperative treatment is initiated in all infants and should be started as soon as possible following birth. Techniques have included taping and strapping, manipulation and serial casting, and functional treatment. Historically, a significant percentage of patients treated by manipulation and casting required a surgical release, which was usually performed between 3 and 12 mo of age. Although many feet remain well aligned after surgical releases, a significant percentage of patients have required additional surgery for recurrent or residual deformities. Stiffness remains a concern at long-term follow-up. While pain is uncommon in childhood and adolescence, symptoms may appear during adulthood. These concerns have led to considerable interest in less invasive methods for treating the deformity. The Ponseti method of clubfoot treatment involves a specific technique for manipulation and serial casting and may be best described as minimally invasive rather than nonoperative. The order of correction follows the mnemonic **CAVE.** Weekly cast changes are performed; five to 10 casts are typically required. The most difficult deformity to correct is the hindfoot equinus, and approximately 90% of patients will require a percutaneous tenotomy of the heel cord as an outpatient. Following the tenotomy, a long leg cast with the foot in maximal abduction (70 degrees) and dorsiflexion is worn for 3 wk; the patient then begins a bracing program. An abduction brace is worn full time for 3 mo and then at nighttime for 3–5 yr. A subset of patients will require transfer of the tibialis anterior tendon to the middle cuneiform for recurrence. Although most patients require some form of surgery, the procedures are minimal in comparison with a surgical release, which requires capsulotomy of the major joints (and lengthening of the muscles) to reposition the joints in space. The results of the Ponseti method are excellent at up to 40 yr of follow-up. Compliance with the splinting program is essential; recurrence is common if the brace is not worn as recommended. Functional treatment, or the "French method," involves daily manipulations (supervised by a physical therapist) and splinting with elastic tape, as well as continuous passive motion (machine required) while the baby sleeps. While the early results are promising, the method is labor intensive, and it remains unclear whether the technique will achieve greater popularity in the United States. These minimally invasive methods are most successful when treatment is begun at birth or during the first few months of life.

Surgical realignment has a definite role in the management of clubfeet, especially in the minority of congenital clubfeet that have failed nonoperative or minimally invasive methods, and for the neuromuscular and syndromic clubfeet that are characteristically rigid. In such cases, nonoperative methods such as the Ponseti technique may potentially be of value in decreasing the magnitude of surgery required. Common surgical approaches include a release of the involved joints (realign the tarsal bones), a lengthening of the shortened posteromedial musculotendinous units, and usually pinning of the foot in the corrected position. The specific procedure is tailored to the unique characteristics of each deformity. For older children with untreated clubfeet or those in whom a recurrence or residual deformity is observed, bony procedures (osteotomies) may be required in addition to soft-tissue surgery. Triple arthrodesis is reserved as salvage for painful, deformed feet in adolescents and adults.

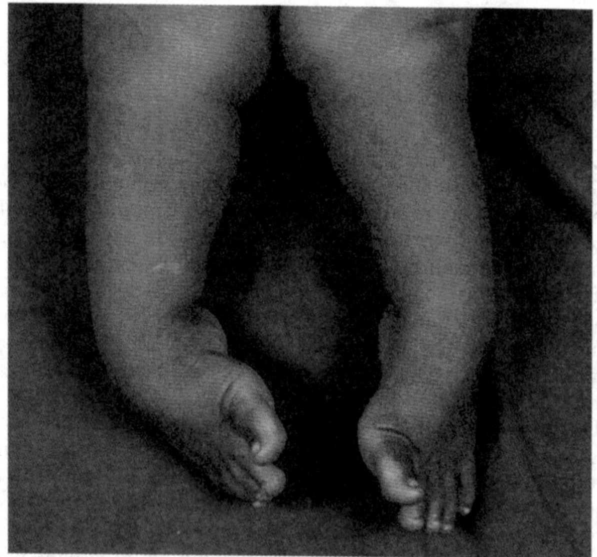

Figure 673-2. Clinical picture demonstrating clubfoot deformity.

673.4 • Congenital Vertical Talus

Congenital vertical talus is an uncommon foot deformity in which the midfoot is dorsally dislocated on the hindfoot. While approximately 60% of cases are idiopathic, 40% are associated with an underlying neuromuscular condition or a syndrome. Neurologic causes include myelodysplasia, tethered cord, and sacral agenesis. Other associated conditions include arthrogryposis, Larsen syndrome, and chromosomal abnormalities (trisomy 13–15, 19). Depending on the age at diagnosis, the differential diagnosis may include a calcaneovalgus foot, oblique talus (talonavicular joint reduces passively), flexible flatfoot with a tight Achilles tendon, and tarsal coalition.

CLINICAL MANIFESTATIONS. Congenital vertical talus has also been described as a **rocker-bottom foot** (Fig. 673-3) or a Persian slipper foot. The plantar surface of the foot is convex, and the

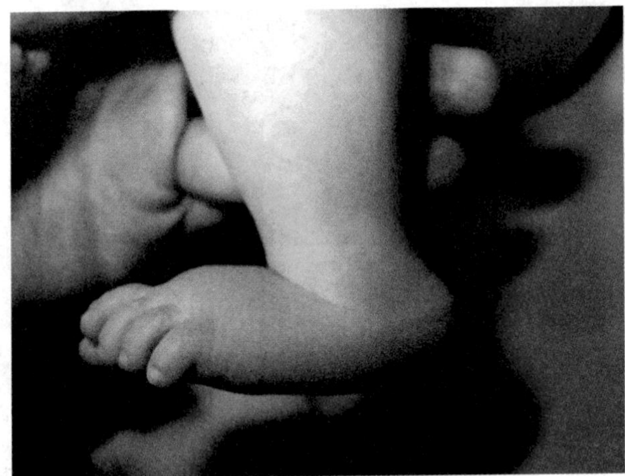

Figure 673-3. Rocker-bottom foot in congenital vertical talus.

talar head is prominent along the medial border of the midfoot. The fore part of the foot is dorsiflexed (dorsally dislocated on the hindfoot) and abducted relative to the hindfoot, and the hindfoot is in equinus and valgus. There is an associated contracture of the anterolateral (tibialis anterior, toe extensors) and the posterior (Achilles tendon, peroneals) soft tissues. The deformity is typically rigid. A thorough physical examination is required to identify any coexisting neurologic and/or musculoskeletal abnormalities.

RADIOGRAPHIC EVALUATION. AP, lateral, and maximal plantarflexion radiographs should be obtained when the diagnosis is suspected. The plantarflexion view helps to determine whether the dorsal subluxation or dislocation of the midfoot on the hindfoot can be reduced passively. Although the navicular does not ossify until 3–6 yr of age, the relationship between the talus and the 1st metatarsal may be evaluated.

TREATMENT. The initial management consists of serial manipulation and casting, which is started shortly after birth. Initially, an attempt is made to reduce the dorsal dislocation of the forefoot/midfoot on the hindfoot. Once this has been achieved, attention can be directed toward stretching the hindfoot contracture. These deformities are typically rigid, and surgical intervention is required in the majority of cases. In such cases, casting helps to stretch out the contracted soft tissues. Surgery is generally performed between 6 and 12 mo of age; a soft-tissue release is performed as a one- or two-stage procedure. One component involves release/lengthening of the contracted anterior soft tissues in concert with an open reduction of the talonavicular joint, while the other involves a posterior release with lengthening of the contracted musculotendinous units. Fixation with Kirschner wires is commonly performed to maintain alignment. Postoperatively, casting is employed for a variable period of time; patients often require the use of an orthosis for extended periods, depending on the underlying diagnosis. Salvage options for recurrent or residual deformities in older children include a subtalar or triple arthrodesis.

673.5 • Hypermobile Pes Planus (Flexible Flatfeet)

Flatfoot is a common diagnosis; it has been estimated that up to 23% of the public may be affected, depending on the diagnostic criteria. Three types of flatfeet may be identified: a flexible flatfoot, a flexible flatfoot with a tendo-Achilles contracture, and a rigid flatfoot. Flatfoot describes a change in foot shape, and there are several abnormalities in alignment between the tarsal bones. There is eversion of the subtalar complex. The hindfoot is aligned in valgus, and there is midfoot sag at the naviculocuneiform and/or the talonavicular joint. The forefoot is abducted relative to the hindfoot, and the head of the talus is uncovered and prominent along the plantar and medial border of the midfoot/hindfoot. While hypermobile or flexible pes planus represents a common source of concern for parents, these children are rarely symptomatic. Flatfeet are common in neonates and toddlers and are associated with physiologic ligamentous laxity. Improvement may be seen when the longitudinal arch develops between 5 and 10 yr of age. Flatfoot is less common in societies where shoes are not worn during infancy and childhood. A flexible-sole shoe is recommended. Flexible flatfeet persisting into adolescence and adulthood are usually associated with familial ligamentous laxity and will be identified in other family members.

CLINICAL MANIFESTATIONS. Patients typically have a normal longitudinal arch when examined in a non–weight-bearing position, but the arch disappears when standing. The hindfoot collapses into valgus, and the midfoot sag becomes evident. Generalized ligamentous laxity is commonly observed. Range of motion should be assessed at both the subtalar and the ankle joints and will be normal in patients with a flexible flatfoot. When assessing range of motion at the ankle, the foot should always be inverted while testing dorsiflexion. If the foot is neutral or everted, spurious dorsiflexion may occur through the midfoot, masking a tendo-Achilles contracture. If subtalar motion is restricted, then the flatfoot is not hypermobile/ flexible, and other diagnoses such as tarsal coalition and juvenile rheumatoid arthritis must be considered. On occasion, there may be tenderness and/or callus formation under the talar head medially. The shoes should be assessed as well and may have evidence of excessive wear along the medial border.

RADIOGRAPHIC EVALUATION. Routine radiographs of asymptomatic flexible flatfeet are usually not indicated. Weight-bearing radiographs (AP and lateral) are required to assess the deformity. On the AP radiograph, there is widening of the angle between the longitudinal axis of the talus and the calcaneus, indicating excessive heel valgus. The lateral view shows distortion of the normal straight-line relationship between the long axis of the talus and the 1st metatarsal with a sag either of the talonavicular or naviculocuneiform joint, resulting in flattening of the normal medial longitudinal arch (Fig. 673-4).

TREATMENT. While the natural history of the flexible flatfoot remains unknown, there is little evidence to suggest that this condition results in long-term problems or disability. As such, treatment is reserved for the small subset of patients who develop

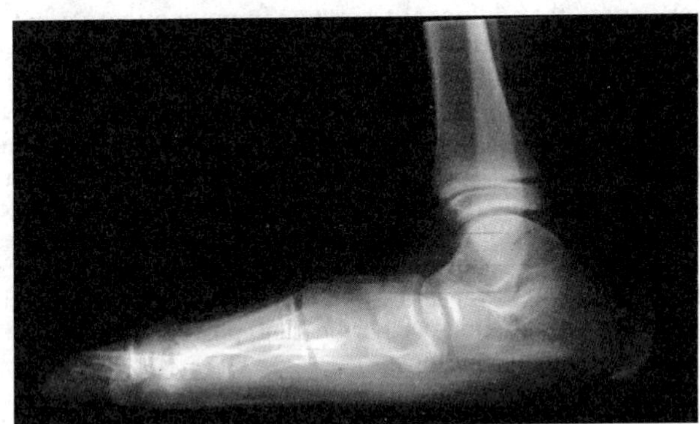

Figure 673-4. Lateral weight-bearing radiograph demonstrating features of flatfoot.

symptoms. Patients with hindfoot pain or those with abnormal shoe wear may benefit from an orthosis such as a medial arch support. Severe cases, often associated with an underlying connective tissue disorder such as Ehlers-Danlos syndrome or Down syndrome, may benefit from a custom orthosis such as the UCBL (University of California Biomechanics Laboratory) to better control the hindfoot and prevent collapse of the arch. While an orthosis may relieve symptoms, there is no evidence to suggest any permanent change in the shape of the foot or alignment of the tarsal bones. Patients with a flexible flatfoot and a tight tendo-Achilles should be treated by stretching exercises, and on occasion, the muscle will need to be lengthened surgically. For the few patients with persistent pain, surgical treatment may be considered. There has been considerable interest in a lateral column lengthening, which addresses all components of the deformity. The procedure involves an osteotomy of the calcaneus, and a trapezoidal bone graft is placed. A lengthening of the tendo-Achilles is required, and often a plantarflexion osteotomy of the medial cuneiform. This procedure preserves the mobility of the hindfoot joints, in contrast to a subtalar or triple arthrodesis. While a hindfoot arthrodesis may correct the deformity adequately, the stress transfer to neighboring joints may result in late-onset, painful degenerative changes. Another option is to insert a spacer into the sinus tarsi to block eversion at the subtalar joint. These procedures may be complicated by synovitis or loosening of the implant.

673.6 • Tarsal Coalition

Tarsal coalition, also known as **peroneal spastic flatfoot**, is characterized by a painful, rigid flatfoot deformity and peroneal (lateral calf) muscle spasm but without true spasticity. It represents a congenital fusion or failure of segmentation between two or more tarsal bones. Any condition that alters the normal gliding and rotatory motion of the subtalar joint may produce the clinical appearance of a tarsal coalition. Thus, congenital malformations, arthritis or inflammatory disorders, infection, neoplasms, and trauma can be possible causes.

The most common tarsal coalitions occur at the medial talocalcaneal (subtalar) facet and between the calcaneus and navicular (calcaneonavicular). Coalitions can be fibrous, cartilaginous, or osseous. Tarsal coalition occurs in approximately 1% of the general population and appears to be inherited as an autosomal dominant trait with nearly full penetrance. Approximately 60% of calcaneonavicular and 50% of the medial facet talocalcaneal coalitions are bilateral.

CLINICAL MANIFESTATIONS. Approximately 25% of patients will become symptomatic, typically during the 2nd decade of life. Although the flatfoot and a decrease in subtalar motion may have been present since early childhood, the onset of symptoms may correlate with the additional restriction in motion that occurs as a cartilaginous bar ossifies. The timing of ossification varies between the talonavicular (3–5 yr of age), the calcaneonavicular (8–12 yr), and the talocalcaneal (12–16 yr) coalitions. Hindfoot pain is commonly observed, especially in the region of the sinus tarsi and also under the head of the talus. Symptoms are activity related and are often increased with running or prolonged walking, especially on uneven surfaces. There may be tenderness over the site of the coalition and/or pain with testing of subtalar motion. The clinical appearance of a flatfoot is seen in both the weight-bearing and non–weight-bearing positions. There is a restriction in subtalar motion.

RADIOGRAPHIC EVALUATION. AP and lateral weight-bearing radiographs and an oblique radiograph of the foot should be obtained. A calcaneonavicular coalition will be seen best on the oblique radiograph. On the lateral radiograph, there may be elongation of the anterior process of the calcaneus, known as the "anteater sign." A talocalcaneal coalition may be seen on a Harris (axial) view of the heel. On the lateral radiograph, there may be narrowing of the posterior facet of the subtalar joint, or a C-shaped line along the medial outline of the talar dome and the inferior outline of the sustentaculum tali ("C sign"). Beaking of the anterior aspect of the talus on the lateral view is seen with some frequency, and results from an alteration in the distribution of stress. This finding does not imply the presence of degenerative arthritis. Irregularity in the subchondral bony surfaces may be seen in patients with a cartilaginous coalition, in contrast to a well-formed bony bridge in those with an osseous coalition. A fibrous coalition may require additional imaging studies to diagnose. While plain films may be diagnostic, a CT scan is the imaging modality of choice when a coalition is suspected (Fig. 673-5). In addition to securing the diagnosis, this study helps to define the degree of joint involvement in patients with a talocalcaneal coalition. While uncommon, more than one tarsal coalition may be observed in the same patient.

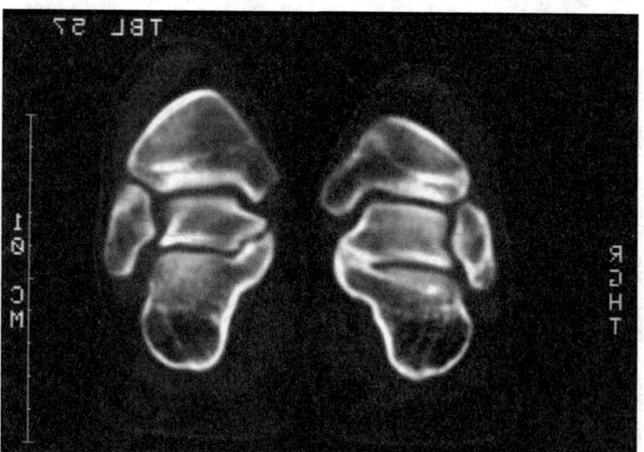

Figure 673-5. CT scan of the talocalcaneal complex demonstrating tarsal coalition.

TREATMENT. The treatment of symptomatic tarsal coalitions varies according to the type and extent of coalition, the age of the patient, and the presence and magnitude of symptoms. Treatment is required only for symptomatic coalitions, and the initial management consists of activity restriction and nonsteroidal anti-inflammatory medications, with or without a shoe insert. Immobilization in a short leg walking cast for 4–6 wk may be required in patients with more pronounced symptoms. For patients with chronic pain despite an adequate trial of nonoperative therapy, surgical treatment should be considered, and options include resection of the coalition, osteotomy, or arthrodesis. For the calcaneonavicular coalition, resection and interposition of the extensor digitorum brevis muscle have been successful. The surgical treatment of talocalcaneal coalitions is based on the degree of joint involvement, as defined by CT. For patients with less than 50% of the joint involved, resection of the coalition with interposition of fat or a split portion of the flexor hallucis tendon may be considered. For those with extensive involvement of the joint and/or degenerative changes, a triple arthrodesis may be the best option. The role of osteotomy in the management of tarsal coalition is currently under investigation.

673.7 • Cavus Feet

Cavus is a deformity involving plantarflexion of the forefoot or midfoot on the hindfoot and may involve the entire forepart of

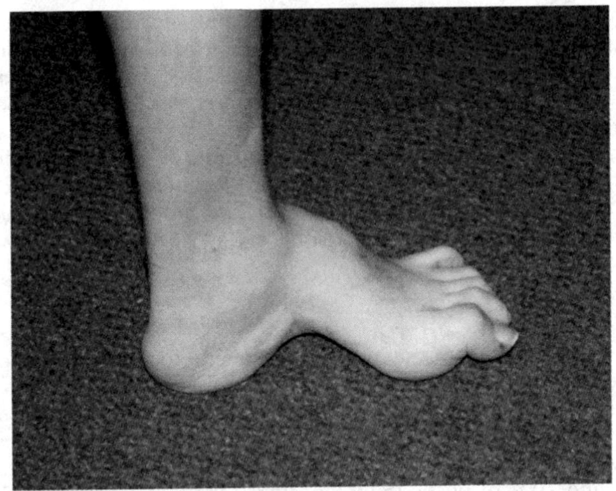

Figure 673-6. Clinical picture demonstrating pes cavus.

the foot or just the medial column. The result is an elevation of the longitudinal arch (Fig. 673-6), and a deformity of the hindfoot will often develop to compensate for the primary forefoot abnormality. While familial cavus may occur, the majority of patients with this deformity will have an underlying neuromuscular etiology. The initial goal is to rule out (and treat) any underlying causes. These diagnoses may relate to abnormalities of the spinal cord (occult dysraphism, tethered cord, polio, myelodysplasia) and peripheral nerves (hereditary motor and sensory neuropathies such as Charcot-Marie-Tooth disease, Dejerine-Sottas disease, Refsum disease). While a unilateral cavus foot is most likely to result from an occult intraspinal anomaly, bilateral involvement usually suggests an underlying nerve or muscle disease. Cavus is commonly observed in association with a hindfoot deformity. In cavovarus, the most common deformity in patients with the hereditary motor and sensory neuropathies, progressive weakness and muscle imbalance result in plantarflexion of the 1st ray/medial column. For the foot to land flat, the hindfoot must roll into varus. With equinocavus, the hindfoot is in equinus, while in calcaneocavus (usually seen in polio or myelodysplasia), the hindfoot is in calcaneus (excessive dorsiflexion).

TREATMENT. The 1st step involves identifying any underlying diagnosis. Knowledge of the underlying diagnosis also helps to determine the specific management. With mild deformities, stretching of the plantar fascia and exercises to strengthen weakened muscles may help to delay progression. An ankle-foot orthosis may be necessary to stabilize the foot and improve ambulation. Surgical treatment is indicated for progressive or symptomatic deformities that have failed to respond to nonoperative measures. The specific procedures recommended will depend on the degree of deformity and the underlying diagnosis. In the case of a progressive neuromuscular condition, recurrence of deformity is commonly observed, and additional procedures may be required to maintain a plantigrade foot. Families should be counseled in detail regarding the disease process and the expected gains from the surgery. The goal of surgery is to restore motion and alignment and to improve muscle balance. For milder deformities, a soft-tissue release of the plantar fascia, often combined with a tendon transfer, may suffice. For patients with a fixed bony deformity of the forefoot/midfoot and/or the hindfoot, one or more osteotomies may be required for realignment. A triple arthrodesis (calcaneocuboid, talonavicular, and subtalar) may be required for severe feet (or recurrent deformities) in older patients.

673.8 • Osteochondroses/Apophysitis

Idiopathic avascular necrosis may rarely be observed in the tarsal navicular (**Köhler disease**) or the 2nd or 3rd metatarsal head (**Freiberg infraction**). These are generally self-limited conditions that commonly result in activity-related pain, which can at times be disabling. The treatment is based on the degree of symptoms and commonly includes restriction of activity. For patients with Köhler disease, a short leg cast (6–8 wk) may provide significant relief. Patients with Freiberg infraction may benefit from a period of casting and/or shoe modifications such as a rocker-bottom sole, a stiff-soled shoe, or a metatarsal bar. Degenerative changes will occasionally occur following the gradual healing process, and surgical intervention is required in a subset of cases. Procedures have included joint debridement, bone grafting, redirectional osteotomy, subtotal or complete excision of the metatarsal head, and joint replacement.

Apophysitis represents inflammation at the insertion of a muscle group from repetitive tensile loading and is most commonly observed during periods of rapid growth. These stresses result in microfractures at the fibrocartilaginous insertion site, associated with inflammation. Calcaneal apophysitis (**Sever disease**) is the most common cause of heel pain in children; treatment includes activity modification, nonsteroidal anti-inflammatory medications, heel cord stretching exercises, as well as heel cushions or arch supports. **Iselin disease** represents an apophysitis at the 5th metatarsal base (peroneus brevis) and is less common. Radiographs should be considered when the symptoms are unilateral or with a failure to respond to treatment.

673.9 • Puncture Wounds of the Foot

Most puncture wound injuries to the foot may be adequately managed in the emergency department. **Treatment** involves a thorough irrigation and a tetanus booster, if appropriate; many clinicians will recommend antibiotics. Using this approach, the majority will heal without a complication. A subset of cases may develop cellulitis, most often due to *Staphylococcus aureus,* and will require intravenous antibiotics with or without surgical drainage. Deep infection is uncommon and may be associated with septic arthritis or osteomyelitis. The most common organisms are *S. aureus* and *Pseudomonas;* the treatment involves a thorough surgical debridement followed by a short (10–14 days) course of systemic antibiotics. While plain radiographs will demonstrate any metallic fragments, ultrasonography may be necessary to identify glass or wooden objects. Routine exploration and removal of foreign bodies is not required, but may be necessary when symptoms are present, with recurrences, or when an infection is suspected. Pain and/or gait disturbance is more likely with superficial objects under the plantar surface of the foot. One special situation occurs when a puncture wound from a nail comes through an old sneaker. There is a high risk of a pseudomonal infection, and consideration should be given to a thorough irrigation and debridement under general anesthesia followed by systemic antibiotics for 10–14 days.

673.10 • Toe Deformities

JUVENILE HALLUX VALGUS (BUNION)

Juvenile hallux valgus is most common in females, and is typically associated with familial ligamentous laxity. A positive family history is common. The etiology is multifactorial, and important factors include genetic factors, ligamentous laxity, pes planus, wearing shoes with a narrow toe box, and occasionally spasticity (cerebral palsy).

CLINICAL MANIFESTATIONS. There is prominence of the 1st metatarsophalangeal (MTP) joint and often erythema from chronic irritation. The great toe is in valgus and is usually pronated, and there is splaying of the forefoot. Pes planus, with or without an associated heel cord contracture, is also observed commonly. While cosmesis is perhaps the most common concern, patients may have pain in the region of the 1st MTP joint and/or difficulty with shoe wear.

RADIOGRAPHIC EVALUATION. Weight-bearing AP and lateral radiographs of the feet are obtained. On the AP view, common measurements include the angular relationships between the 1st and 2nd metatarsals (intermetatarsal angle, <10 degrees is normal) and between the 1st metatarsal and the proximal phalanx (hallux valgus angle, <25 degrees is normal). The orientation of the 1st metatarsal-medial cuneiform joint is also documented. On the lateral radiograph, the angular relationship between the talus and the 1st metatarsal helps to identify a midfoot break associated with pes planus. Radiographs are more helpful in surgical planning than in establishing the diagnosis.

TREATMENT. Conservative management of adolescent bunions consists primarily of shoe modifications. It is important that footwear accommodate the width of the forefoot. Patients should avoid wearing shoes with a narrow toe box and/or a high heel. Shoe modifications such as a soft upper, bunion last, or heel cup may also be recommended. In the presence of a pes planus, an orthotic to restore the medial longitudinal arch may be beneficial. Stretching exercises are recommended to treat contracture of the tendo-Achilles. The value of night splinting remains to be determined. Surgical treatment is reserved for those patients with persistent and disabling pain who have failed a course of nonoperative therapy. Surgery is not advised purely for cosmesis. Surgery is usually delayed until skeletal maturity to decrease the risk of recurrence. Radiographs are essential in preoperative planning to assess both the magnitude of deformity (hallux valgus angle, intermetatarsal angle, distal metatarsal articular angle) and associated features such as obliquity of the 1st metatarsal-medial cuneiform joint. Surgical treatment often involves a soft-tissue release and or rebalancing procedure at the 1st MTP joint, and a single or double osteotomy of the 1st metatarsal to decrease foot width and realign the joints along the medial column of the forefoot. An arthrodesis of the 1st MTP joint may be indicated in patients with spasticity in order to prevent recurrence.

CURLY TOES

A curly toe is caused by contracture of the flexor digitorum longus, and there is flexion at the MTP and the interphalangeal (IP) joints associated with medial deviation of the toe. The toe will usually lie underneath its neighbor, and the 4th and 5th toes are most commonly involved. The deformity rarely causes symptoms, and active treatment (stretching, splinting, or taping) is not required. Most cases improve over time, and a subset will resolve completely. For the rare case in which there is chronic pain or skin irritation, release of the flexor digitorum longus muscle at the distal interphalangeal joint may be considered.

OVERLAPPING 5TH TOE

Congenital digitus minimus varus, or varus 5th toe, involves dorsiflexion and adduction of the 5th toe. The 5th toe typically overlaps the 4th. There is also a rotatory deformity of the toe, and the nail tends to point outward. The deformity is usually bilateral and may have a genetic basis. Symptoms are frequent and involve pain over the dorsum of the toe from shoe wear. Nonoperative treatment has not been successful. For symptomatic patients, several different options for reconstruction have been described. Common features include releasing the contracted extensor tendon and the MTP joint capsule (dorsal, dorsomedial, or complete). A partial removal of the proximal phalanx and creation of a syndactyly between the 4th and 5th toes has been performed in conjunction with the release as well.

POLYDACTYLY

Polydactyly is the most common congenital toe deformity and is seen in approximately 2/1,000 births and is bilateral in 50% of cases. Polydactyly may be preaxial (great toe) or postaxial (5th toe), and occasionally one of the central toes is duplicated. Associated anomalies are found in approximately 10% of the preaxial and 20% of postaxial polydactyly. One third of patients will also have polydactyly of the hand. Conditions that may be associated with polydactyly include Ellis-Van Creveld (chondroectodermal dysplasia), longitudinal deficiency of the tibia, and Down syndrome. The extra digit may be either rudimentary or well formed, and plain radiographs of the foot help to define the anatomy and evaluate any coexisting bony anomalies. Treatment is indicated for cosmesis and to allow for fitting with standard shoes. This involves surgical removal of the extra digit, and the procedure is generally performed between 9 and 12 mo of age. Rudimentary digits may be surgically excised earlier, but should not be "tied off."

SYNDACTYLY

Syndactyly involves webbing of the toes, which may be incomplete or complete (extends to the tip of the toes), and the toenails may be confluent. There is often a positive family history, and the 3rd and 4th toes are involved most commonly. Symptoms are extremely rare, and cosmetic concerns are infrequent. Treatment is only required for a subset of cases in which there is an associated polydactyly (Fig. 673-7). In such cases, the border digit is excised, and the extra skin facilitates coverage of the wound. If the syndactyly does not involve the extra toe, then it can be observed. A complex syndactyly may be seen in patients with Apert syndrome.

HAMMER TOE

A hammer toe involves flexion at the proximal IP (PIP) joint with or without the distal IP (DIP) joint, and the MTP joint may be

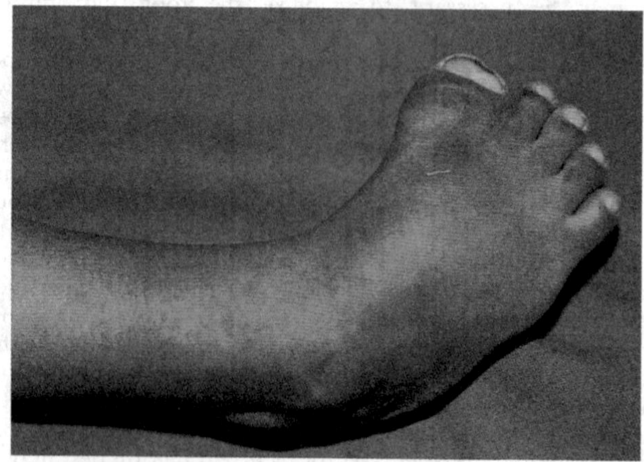

Figure 673-7. Clinical picture of polysyndactyly involving the great toe.

hyperextended. This deformity may be distinguished from a curly toe by the absence of rotation. The 2nd toe is most commonly involved, and a painful callus may develop over the dorsum of the toe where it rubs on the shoe. Nonoperative therapy is rarely successful, and surgery is recommended for symptomatic cases. A release of the flexor tendons will suffice in the majority of cases. Some authors have recommended a transfer of the flexor tendon to the extensor tendon. For severe cases with significant rigidity, especially in older patients, a partial or complete resection of the proximal phalanx and a PIP fusion may be required.

MALLET TOE

Mallet toe involves a flexion contracture at the DIP joint and results from congenital shortening of the flexor digitorum longus tendon. Patients may develop a painful callus on the plantar surface of the tuft. As nonoperative therapy is usually unsuccessful, surgery is required for patients with chronic symptoms. For flexible deformities in younger children, release of the flexor digitorum longus tendon is recommended. For stiffer deformities in older patients, resection of the head of the middle phalanx, or arthrodesis of the DIP joint, may be considered.

CLAW TOE

A claw toe deformity involves hyperextension at the MTP joint and flexion at both the PIP and DIP joints, often associated with dorsal subluxation of the MTP joint. The majority are associated with an underlying neurologic disorder such as Charcot-Marie-Tooth disease. The etiology is usually muscle imbalance, and the extensor tendons are recruited to substitute for weakening of the tibialis anterior muscle. If treatment is elected, then surgery is required. Transfer of the extensor digitorum (or hallucis) tendon to the metatarsal neck is commonly performed along with a dorsal capsulotomy of the MTP joint and fusion of the fusion of the PIP joint (IP joint of the great toe).

ANNULAR BANDS

Bands of amniotic tissue associated with amniotic disruption syndrome (early amniotic rupture sequence, congenital constriction band syndrome, annular band syndrome) may become entwined along the extremities, resulting in a spectrum of problems from in utero amputation (Fig. 673-8) to a constriction ring along a digit (Fig. 673-9) (see Chapter 108). These rings, if deep enough, may result in impairment of arterial or venous blood flow. While

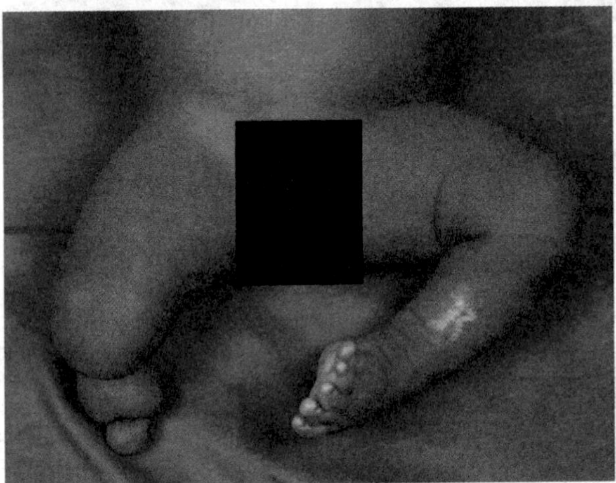

Figure 673-8. Constriction band syndrome with congenital amputation.

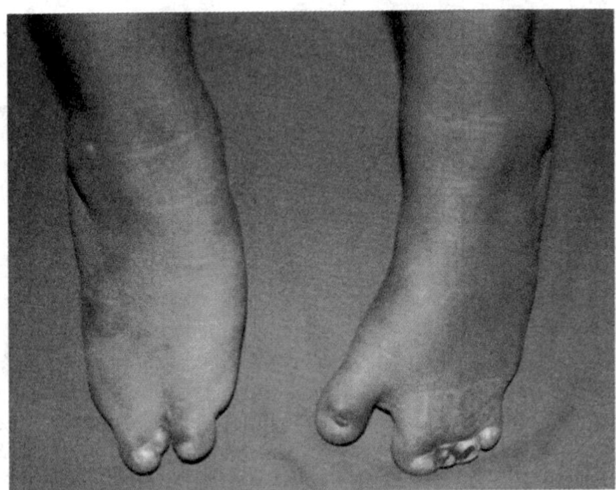

Figure 673-9. Constriction band syndrome with foot involvement.

concerns regarding tissue viability are less common, swelling from impairment in venous return is often a great problem. The treatment of annular bands usually involves observation; however, circumferential release of the band may be required emergently if arterial inflow is obstructed or electively to relieve venous congestion.

MACRODACTYLY

Macrodactyly represents an enlargement of the toes and may occur as an isolated problem or in association with a variety of other conditions such as Proteus syndrome (Fig. 673-10), neurofibromatosis, tuberous sclerosis, and Klippel-Trenaunay-Weber syndrome. This condition results from a deregulation of growth, and there is hyperplasia of one or more of the underlying tissues (osseous, nervous, lymphatic, vascular, fibrofatty). Macrodactyly of the toes may be seen in isolation (localized gigantism) or with enlargement of the entire foot. In addition to cosmetic concerns, patients may have difficulty wearing standard shoes. The treatment is observation, if possible. This is a difficult condition to

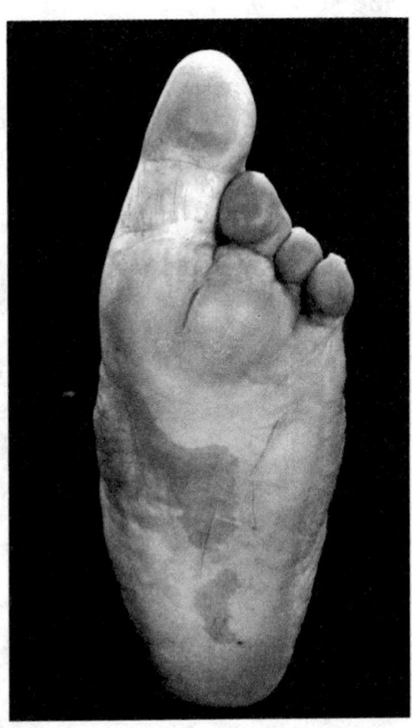

Figure 673-10. Macrodactyly of the great toe in a case of Proteus syndrome.

treat surgically, and complications are frequent. For involvement of a single toe, the best option may be a resection of the ray (including the metatarsal). For greater degrees of involvement, debulking of the various tissues is required. Often, a growth arrest of the underlying osseous structures is performed. Stiffness and wound problems are common. The rate of recurrence is high, and more than one debulking may be required. Patients may elect to have an amputation if the process cannot be controlled by less extensive procedures.

SUBUNGUAL EXOSTOSIS

A subungual exostosis is a mass of normal bone tissue that projects out from the dorsal and medial surface of a toe, under the nail. The etiology is unknown, but may relate to minor, repetitive trauma. The great toe in involved most often. Patients present with discomfort, and the toenail may be elevated. The lesion may be demonstrated on plain radiographs, and histologically involves normal bone with a fibrocartilaginous cap. The treatment for symptomatic lesions is excision, and the recurrence rate is in the range of 10%.

INGROWN TOENAIL

Ingrown toenails are relatively common in infants and young children and usually involve the medial or lateral border of the great toe. Symptoms include chronic irritation and discomfort, and recurrent infection is seen in some cases. If conservative measures including shoe modifications, warm soaks, and appropriate nail trimming fail to control the symptoms, then surgical removal of a portion of the nail should be considered.

673.11 • PAINFUL FOOT

A differential diagnosis for foot pain in different age ranges is shown in Table 673-1. In addition to the history and physical examination, plain radiographs are most helpful in establishing the diagnosis. Occasionally, more sophisticated imaging modalities will be required.

673.12 • SHOES

In toddlers and children, a shoe with a flexible sole is recommended. This recommendation is in part based on studies suggesting that the development of the longitudinal arch seems to be best in societies where shoes are not worn. Well-cushioned, shock-absorbing shoes are helpful in the child and adolescent athlete in order to decrease the chances of developing an overuse syndrome. Otherwise, shoe modifications are generally reserved for abnormalities in alignment between segments of the foot or symptoms from an underlying condition. Numerous modifications are available.

TABLE 673-1. Differential Diagnosis of Foot Pain by Age

0–6 Yr	6–12 Yr	12–20 Yr
Poorly fitting shoes	Poorly fitting shoes	Poorly fitting shoes
Foreign body	Sever disease	Stress fracture
Fracture	Enthesopathy (JRA)	Foreign body
Osteomyelitis	Foreign body	Ingrown toenail
Leukemia	Accessory navicular	Metatarsalgia
Puncture wound	Tarsal coalition	Plantar fasciitis
Drawing of blood	Ewing sarcoma	Osteochondroses (avascular necrosis)
Dactylitis	Hypermobile flatfoot	Freiberg
JRA	Trauma (sprains, fractures)	Köhler
	Puncture wound	Achilles tendinitis
		Trauma (sprains)
		Plantar warts
		Tarsal coalition

JRA, juvenile rheumatoid arthritis.

Akcali O, Tiner M, Ozaksoy D: Effects of lower extremity rotation on prognoses of flexible flatfoot in children. *Foot Ankle Int* 2000;21:72–74.

Bhone WH: Tarsal coalition. *Curr Opin Pediatr* 2001;13:29–35.

Chang CH, Kumar SJ, Riddle EC, Glutting J: Macrodactyly of the foot. *J Bone Joint Surg Am* 2002;84:1189–1194.

Coughlin MJ: Lesser toe abnormalities. *Instr Course Lect* 2003;52:421–444.

Furdon SA, Donlon CR: Examination of the newborn foot: Positional and structural abnormalities. *Adv Neonatal Care* 2002:2:248–258.

Giannini BS, Ceccarelli F, Benedetti MG, et al: Surgical treatment of flexible flatfeet in children: A four-year follow-up study. *J Bone Joint Surg Am* 2001; 83:78–79.

Herzenberg JE, Radler C, Bor N: Ponseti versus traditional methods of casting for idiopathic clubfoot. *J Pediatr Orthop* 2002;22:517–521.

Ippolito E, Fraracci L, Farsetti P, et al: The influence of treatment on the pathology of clubfoot. CT study at maturity. *J Bone Joint Surg Br* 2004;86:574–580.

Lin CJ, Lai KA, Kuan TS, et al: Correlating factors and clinical significance of flexible flatfeet in preschool children. *J Pediatr Orthop* 2001;21:378–382.

Lincoln TL, Suen PW: Common rotational variations in children. *J Am Acad Orthop Surg* 2003;11:312–320.

Lokiec F, Ezra E, Krasin D, et al: A simple and efficient surgical technique for subungual exostosis. *J Pediatr Orthop* 2001;21:76–79.

Mazzocca AD, Thomson JD, Deluca PA, Romness MJ: Comparison of the posterior approach versus the dorsal approach in the treatment of congenital vertical talus. *J Pediatr Orthop* 2001;21:212–217.

Morcuende JA, Dolan LR, Dietz FR, Ponseti IV: Radical reduction in the rate of extensive corrective surgery for clubfeet using the Ponseti method. *Pediatrics* 2004;113:376–380.

Morley SE, Smith PJ: Polydactyly of the feet in children: Suggestions for surgical management. *Br J Plast Surg* 2001;54:34–38.

Noonan KJ, Richards BS: Nonsurgical management of idiopathic clubfoot. *J Am Acad Orthop Surg* 2003;11:392–402.

Roye DP Jr, Roye BD. Idiopathic congenital talipes equinovarus. *J Am Acad Orthop Surg* 2002;10:239–248.

Thometz J: Tarsal coalition. *Foot Ankle Clin* 2000;5:103–118.

Chapter 674 ■ Torsional and Angular Deformities

Harish S. Hosalkar, Purushottam A. Gholve, and Lawrence Wells

674.1 • NORMAL DEVELOPMENT OF LIMB

Pediatricians routinely evaluate lower extremity alignment problems and foot morphology. An understanding of the normal limb development is essential to recognize pathologic conditions. During the 7th wk of intrauterine life, the lower limb rotates medially to bring the greater toe toward the midline. The hip joint forms by the 11th wk; the proximal femur and acetabulum continue to develop until physeal closure in adolescence. At birth, the femoral neck is rotated forward by 40 degrees. This forward rotation is referred to as anteversion (the angle between the axis of the femoral neck and the transcondylar axis). The increased anteversion increases the internal rotation of the hip. The femoral

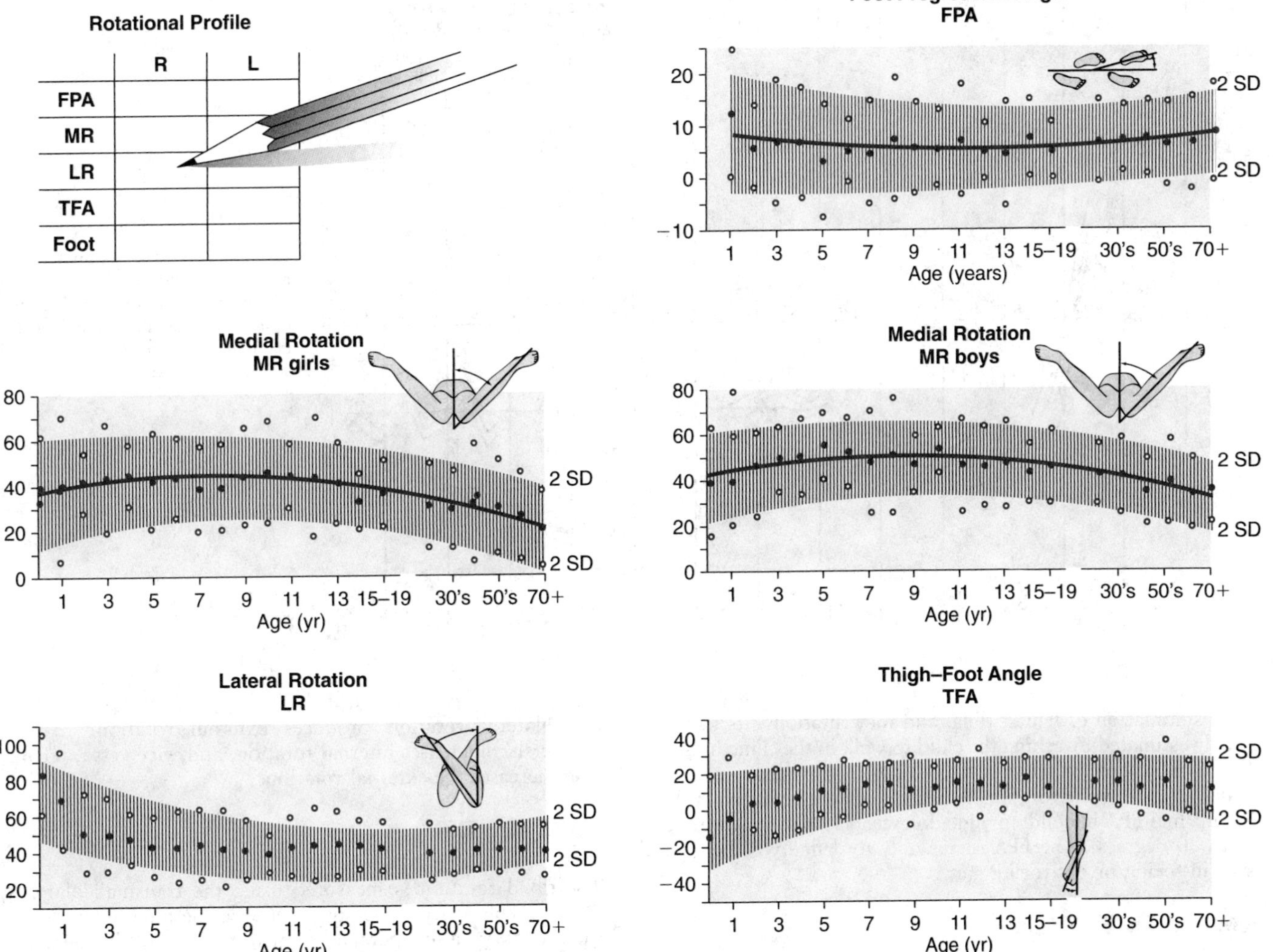

Figure 674-1. The rotational profile from birth to maturity is depicted graphically. All graphs include 2 standard deviations from the mean for the foot progression angle (FPA) for femoral medial and lateral rotation (for boys and girls), and the thigh-foot angle (TFA). (From Morrissey RT, Weinstein SL [editors]: *Lovell and Winter's Pediatric Orthopaedics,* 3rd ed. Philadelphia, Lippincott Williams & Wilkins, 1990.)

anteversion decreases to 15–20 degrees by 8–10 yr of age. The second source of limb rotation is found in the tibia. Infants may have 30 degrees of medial rotation of the tibia, and by maturity the rotation is between 5 degrees medial rotation to 15 degrees of lateral rotation (Fig. 674-1). Excessive medial rotation of tibia is referred to as medial tibial torsion. The tibial torsion is the angular difference between the axis of the knee and the transmalleolar axis. The medial or lateral rotation beyond ±2 standard deviations (SDs) from the mean is considered as abnormal rotation and therefore considered as a deformity.

Limb rotation is also found in the foot. The abnormalities could be excessive adduction or abduction. During skeletal growth there is lateral rotation in both the femoral and tibial segments; therefore, the medial tibial torsion and femoral anteversion in children improve with time. Lateral tibial torsion usually worsens with growth. Torsional deformity may be simple, involving a single segment, or complex, involving multiple segments. Complex deformities may be additive (internal tibial torsion and internal femoral torsion are additive) or compensatory (external tibial torsion and internal femoral torsion are compensatory).

The normal tibiofemoral angle at birth is 10–15 degrees of physiologic varus. The alignment changes to 0 degrees by 18 mo, and physiologic valgus up to 12 degrees is reached in between 3 and 4 yr of age. The normal valgus of 7 degrees is achieved by 5–8 yr of age (Fig. 674-2). Persistence of varus beyond 2 yr of age may be pathologic. Overall, 95% of developmental physiologic genu varum and genu valgum cases resolve with growth. This is also true for children with more pronounced physiologic varus or valgus, although some cases may not be completely corrected until adolescence.

674.2 • Evaluation

The history should focus on the onset, progression, functional limitations, previous treatment, evidence of neuromuscular disorder, and any significant family history. A detailed history is important in arriving at a diagnosis.

The examination consists of assessing the exact torsional profile and is beneficial in diagnosing the level and severity of any torsional problem. This profile includes (1) foot progression angle, (2) femoral anteversion, (3) tibial version with thigh-foot angle, and (4) assessment of foot adduction and abduction.

FOOT PROGRESSION ANGLE (FPA)

Limb position during gait is expressed as the foot progression angle and represents the angular difference between the axis of the foot with the direction in which the child is walking. The FPA

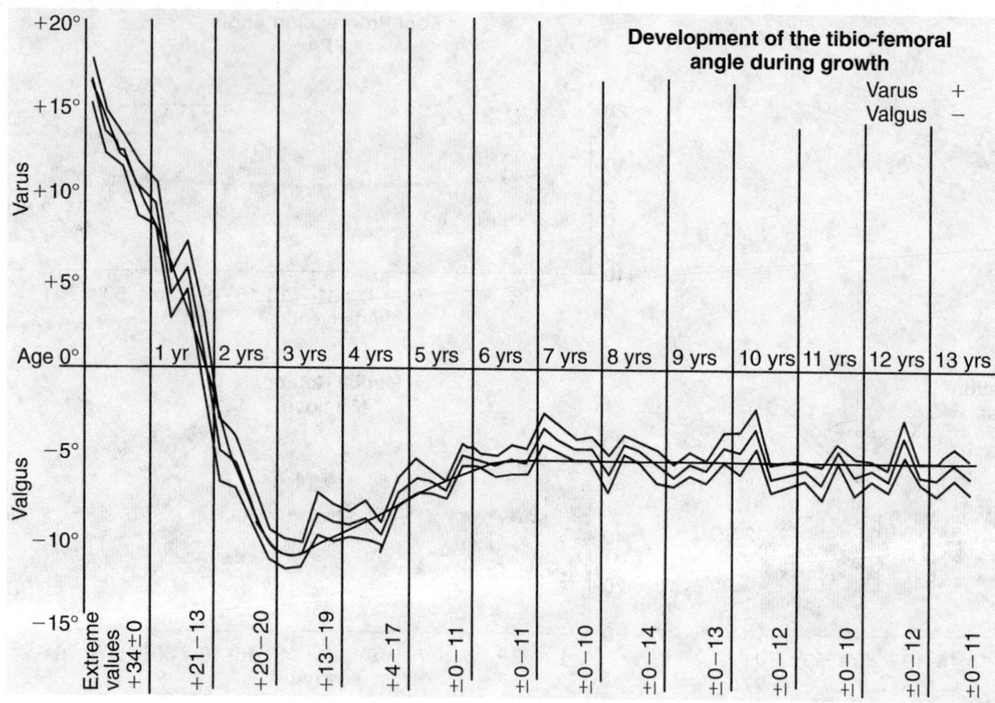

Figure 674-2. The normal coronal alignment of the knee plotted for age. (From Salenius P, Vanka E: The development of the tibiofemoral angle in children. *J Bone Joint Surg Am* 1975;57:259–261.)

is the summation of femur, tibia, and foot rotations. Its value is usually estimated by asking the child to walk in the clinic hallway (Fig. 674-3). Inward rotation of the foot is assigned a negative value, and outward rotation is designated with positive value. The normal FPA in children and adolescents is 10 degrees (range, –3 to 20 degrees). The FPA serves only to define whether there is an in-toeing or out-toeing gait.

FEMORAL ANTEVERSION

Measuring the hip rotation with the child in prone position, the hip in neutral flexion or extension, thighs together, and the knees flexed 90 degrees indirectly assesses the anteversion (Fig. 674-4). Both hips are assessed at the same time. As the lower leg is rotated ipsilaterally, this produces internal rotation of the hip, whereas contralateral rotation produces external rotation. Excessive anteversion increases internal rotation, and, vice versa, retroversion increases the external rotation.

TIBIAL ROTATION

The tibial rotation is measured using the transmalleolar angle (TMA). The TMA is the angle between the longitudinal axis of the thigh with a line perpendicular to the axis of the medial and lateral malleolus (Fig. 674-5). In the absence of foot deformity, the thigh foot angle (TFA) is preferred (Fig. 674-6). It is measured with the child lying prone. The angle is formed between the longitudinal axis of the thigh and the longitudinal axis of the foot. It measures the tibial and hindfoot rotational status. Inward rotation is assigned a negative value, and outward rotation is desig-

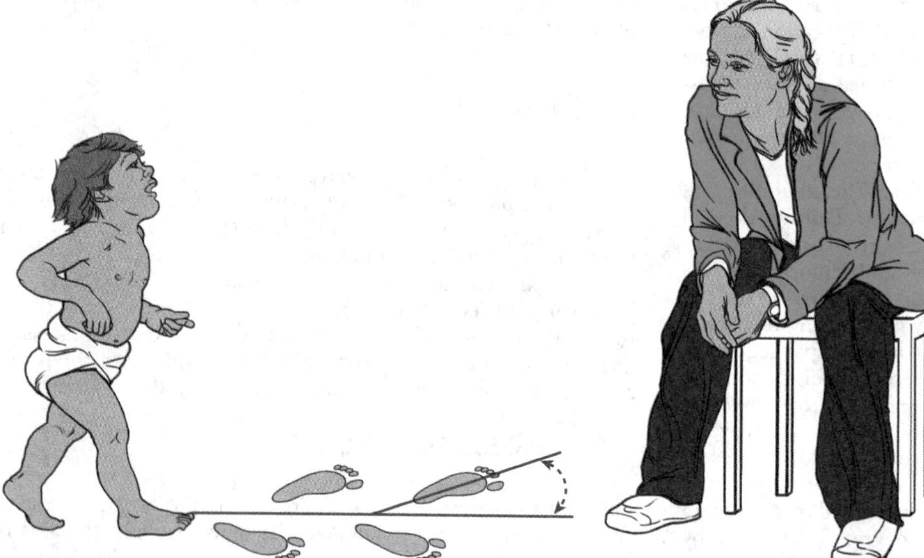

Figure 674-3. Foot progression angle. The long axis of the foot is compared with the direction in which the child is walking. If the long axis of the foot is directed outwardly, the angle is positive. If the foot is directed inwardly, the angle is negative and is indicative of in-toeing. (From Thompson GH: Gait disturbances. In Kliegman RM [editor]: *Practical Strategies in Pediatric Diagnosis and Therapy.* Philadelphia, Elsevier/Saunders, 2004.)

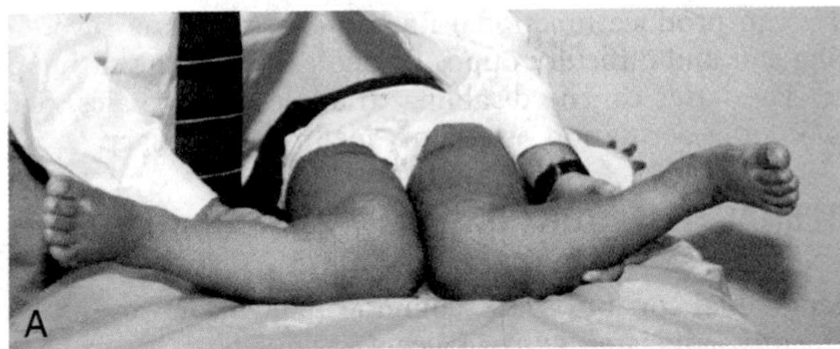

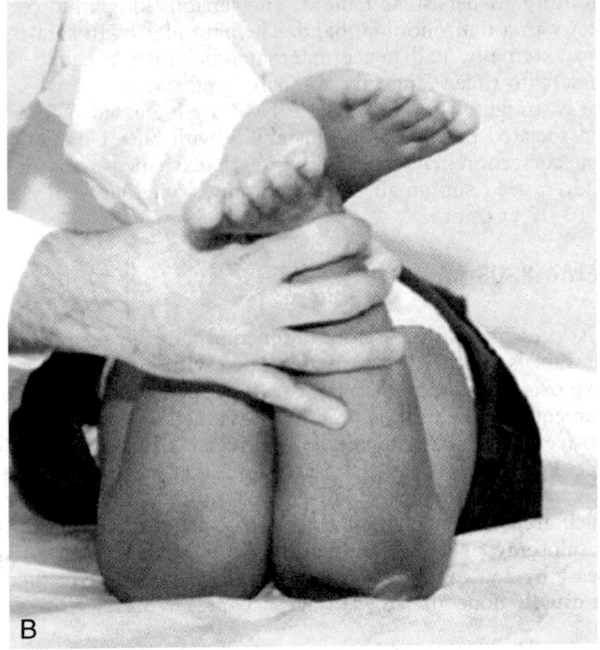

Figure 674-4. Anteversion measured by medial rotation of hip *(A)* and lateral rotation of hip *(B)*.

nated a positive value. Inward rotation indicates internal tibial torsion, whereas outward rotation represents external tibial torsion. Infants have a mean angle of −5 degrees (range, −35 to 40 degrees) as a consequence of normal in utero position. In mid-childhood through adult life, the mean TFA is 10 degrees (range, −5 to 30 degrees). The difference between the TMA and the TFA is a measure of the hindfoot rotation.

FOOT SHAPE AND POSITION

The foot is observed for any deformities in prone and standing position. The heel bisector line (HBL) is used to evaluate the foot adduction and abduction deformities. The HBL is a line that divides the heel in two equal halves along the longitudinal axis (Fig. 674-7). It normally extends to the 2nd toe. When the HBL points medial to the 2nd toe, the forefoot is abducted, and when the HBL is lateral to the 2nd toe, the forefoot is adducted.

It is also important to screen every affected child for associated hip dysplasia and neuromuscular problems (cerebral palsy).

674.3 • Torsional Deformities

INTERNAL FEMORAL TORSION

Excessive femoral anteversion is the most common deformity presenting as **in-toeing gait.** It occurs more commonly in girls than boys (2 : 1) in the 3–6 yr of age group. The etiology of femoral

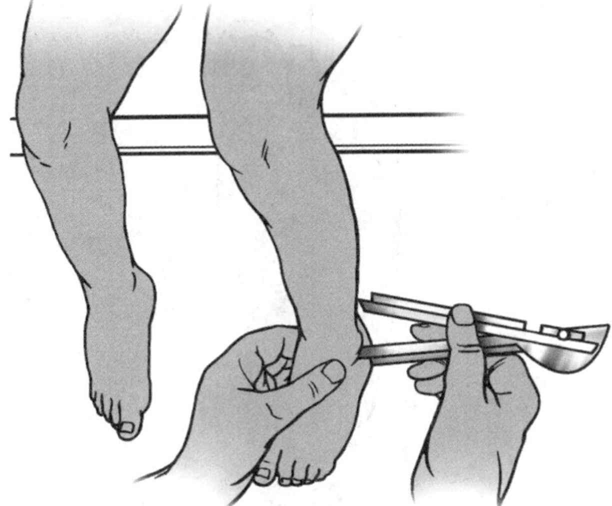

Figure 674-5. Transmalleolar angle is measured with the patient sitting at the edge of the table and the distal femoral condyles aligned with the side of the table. The angle between a line through the medial and lateral malleoli and edge of the table should be approximately 30 degrees external. (From Bleck EE: *Orthopaedic Management in Cerebral Palsy.* London, MacKeith Press, 1987, p 55.)

torsion is controversial. Some believe that it is congenital and a result of persistent infantile femoral anteversion, whereas others believe it is acquired secondary to abnormal sitting habits. Some children are in habit of sitting in a W position or sleeping prone. On examination, most children with this condition have generalized ligamentous laxity. Gait examination reveals that entire leg is inwardly rotated. Internal hip rotation is increased beyond 70 degrees, and consequently the external rotation is restricted to 10–20 degrees. The patellas are pointing inward when the foot is straight, and compensatory external rotation of tibia is demonstrated.

Diagnosis is made clinically on examination, but CT can obtain objective measurements, which are rarely indicated. The treat-

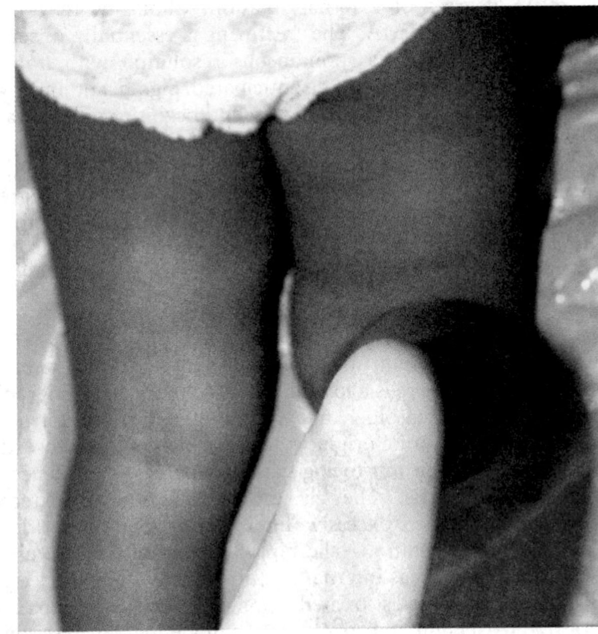

Figure 674-6. Thigh foot angle.

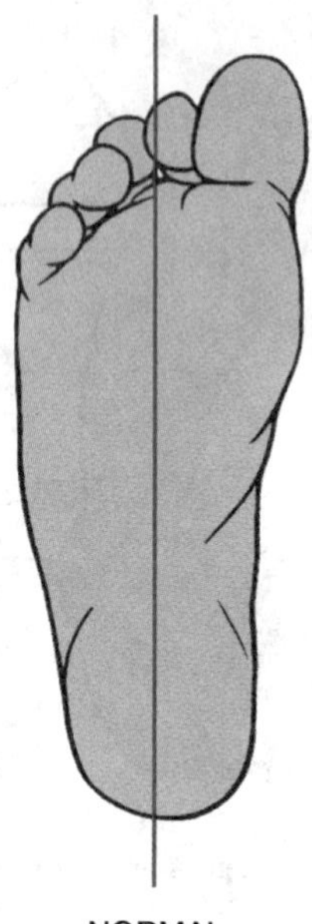

Figure 674-7. Schematic demonstration of heel bisector line.

ment is predominantly observation and correction of abnormal sitting habits. The correction of sitting habits can be difficult in preschool-aged children and usually does not occur until they reach school age. The torsion usually corrects with growth by 8–10 yr of age. Persistent deformity, unacceptable cosmesis, functional impairment, anteversion >45 degrees, and no external rotation beyond neutral are some of the indications for operative intervention. Surgery involves derotation osteotomy of the femur.

INTERNAL TIBIAL TORSION

Medial tibial torsion presents with **in-toeing gait** and is commonly associated with congenital metatarsus varus, genu valgum, or femoral anteversion. This condition is usually seen during the 2nd yr of life. Normally at birth, the medial malleolus lies behind the lateral malleolus, but by adulthood, it is reversed with the tibia in 15 degrees of external rotation. Clinically, they have decreased TFA and TMA. The treatment is essentially observation and reassurance, as spontaneous resolution with normal growth and development can be anticipated. Significant improvement usually does not occur until the child begins to pull to stand and walk independently. Thereafter, correction can be seen as early as 4 yr of age and in some children by 8–10 yr of age. Other than observation, occasional bracing for torsion of >40 degrees has been attempted. Persistent deformity with functional impairment is treated with supramalleolar osteotomy.

EXTERNAL FEMORAL TORSION

External femoral torsion may follow a slipped capital femoral epiphysis (SCFE); there is a low threshold to perform radiographs of the hips in children older than 10 yr of age. Femoral retrotorsion, when of idiopathic origin, is usually bilateral. The disorder is associated with an **out-toeing gait** and increased incidence of degenerative arthritis. The clinical examination of external femoral torsion shows excessive hip external rotation and limitation of internal rotation. The hip will externally rotate up to 70–90 degrees, whereas internal rotation is only 0–20 degrees. If SCFE is detected, it is treated surgically, and any proximal femoral retroversion improves with remodeling during subsequent growth. Occasionally, persistent femoral retroversion after SCFE can produce functional impairment such as a severe out-toeing gait and difficulty opposing one's knees in the sitting position. The latter can be disabling to adolescent females. Should this occur, a derotation osteotomy might be necessary.

EXTERNAL TIBIAL TORSION

Lateral tibial torsion is less common than medial rotation and frequently associated with a calcaneovalgus foot. It can be compensatory to persistent femoral anteversion, idiopathic or secondary to a tight iliotibial band. The natural growth rotates the tibia externally, and hence external tibial torsion can become worse with time. Clinically, the patella faces outward when the foot is straight. The TFA and the TMA are increased. There may be associated patellofemoral instability with knee pain. Though some correction may occur with growth, extremely symptomatic children need supramalleolar osteotomy, which is usually done by 10–12 yr of age.

METATARSUS ADDUCTUS

This presents with forefoot adduction and inversion of all metatarsals. Ten to 15% are associated with hip dysplasia. The prognosis is good, as the majority get better with nonoperative intervention. The HBL is used to assess the degree of deformity. The feet, which are flexible and correctable up to neutral, are treated with stretching exercises. Those that are not completely correctable are treated with serial casting. Rigid deformities, which are not correctable by stretching, are treated with medial capsulotomy of 1st metatarsal cuneiform joint and soft-tissue release by 2 yr of age. Osteotomies of the base of the metatarsal are usually done after 6 yr of age (Chapter 673.1).

674.4 • Coronal Plane Deformities

Genu varum and genu valgum are common pediatric deformities of the knee. The age-appropriate normal values for knee angle are presented in Figure 674-2. Tibial bowing is common during the 1st year, bowlegs are common during the 2nd year, and knock-knees are most prominent between 3 and 4 yr of age.

GENU VARUM

Physiologic bowleg is a common torsional combination that is secondary to normal in utero positioning. Spontaneous resolution with normal growth and development can be anticipated. Persistence of varus beyond 2 yr of age may be pathologic. The different causes are metabolic bone disease (vitamin D deficiency, rickets, hypophosphatasia), asymmetric growth arrest (trauma, infection, tumor, Blount), bone dysplasia (dwarfism, metaphyseal dysplasia), and congenital and neuromuscular disorders (Table 674-1). It is prudent to differentiate physiologic bowing from Blount disease (Table 674-2). Physiologic bowing should also be differentiated from rickets and skeletal dysplasia. Rickets will have classic bone changes with widening and fraying of the metaphysis and widening of the physis (see Chapter 48).

TIBIA VARA

Idiopathic tibia vara, or **Blount disease,** is a growth disorder of the medial aspect of the proximal tibial epiphysis, leading to varus angulation and medial rotation of the tibia (Fig. 674-8). The incidence is greater in female black obese children who have an affected family member, started walking early in life, or reside in certain geographic locations such as the southeastern part of

TABLE 674-1. Classification of Genu Varum (Bowlegs)

PHYSIOLOGIC
ASYMMETRIC GROWTH
Tibia vara (Blount disease)
Infantile
Juvenile
Adolescent
Focal fibrocartilaginous dysplasia
Physeal Injury
Trauma
Infection
Tumor
METABOLIC DISORDERS
Vitamin D deficiency (nutritional rickets)
Vitamin D–resistant rickets
Hypophosphatasia
SKELETAL DYSPLASIA
Metaphyseal dysplasia
Achondroplasia
Enchondromatosis

Modified from Thompson GH: Angular deformities of the lower extremities. In Chapman MW (editor): *Operative Orthopedics*, 2nd ed. Philadelphia, JB Lippincott, 1993, pp 3131–3164.

United States. It has been classified into three types depending on the age at onset: infantile (1–3 yr), juvenile (4–10 yr), and adolescent (11 yr or older). The juvenile and adolescent forms are commonly combined as late-onset tibia vara. Although the exact cause of tibia vara remains unknown, it may be secondary to growth suppression from increased compressive forces across the medial aspect of the knee.

The infantile form of tibia vara is the most common; its characteristics include predominance in black females, approximately 80% bilateral involvement, a prominent medial metaphyseal beak, internal tibial torsion, and leg-length discrepancy (LLD). The characteristics of the juvenile and adolescent forms (late onset) include predominance in black males, normal or greater than normal height, approximately 50% bilateral involvement, slowly progressive genu varum deformity, pain rather than deformity as the primary initial complaint, no palpable proximal medial metaphyseal beak, minimal internal tibial torsion, mild medial collateral ligament laxity, and mild lower extremity length discrepancy. The infantile group has the greatest potential for progression.

An anteroposterior standing radiograph of both lower extremities with patellas facing forward and a lateral radiograph of the involved extremity should be obtained (Fig. 674-9). Weight-bearing stance radiographs are preferred and allow maximal presentation of the clinical deformity. The metaphyseal-diaphyseal angle can be measured and is useful in distinguishing between physiologic genu varum and early tibia vara (Fig. 674-10). Langenskiöld has classified it on radiographic appearance in six stages (Fig. 674-11). The differentiation is based on findings of fragmentation of the epiphysis, beaking of the medial tibial epiphysis, depression of the medial tibial plateau, and formation of a bony bar. Occasionally, arthrography, CT with three-dimensional reconstructions, or MRI may be necessary to assess

TABLE 674-2. Differentiation of Leg Bowing

Physiologic Bowing	Blount Disease
Gentle and symmetric deformity	Asymmetric, abrupt, and sharp angulation
Metaphyseal-diaphyseal angle <11 degrees	Metaphyseal-diaphyseal angle >11 degrees
Normal appearance of the proximal tibial growth plate	Medial sloping of the epiphysis
	Widening of the physis
	Fragmentation of the metaphysis
No significant lateral thrust	Significant lateral thrust

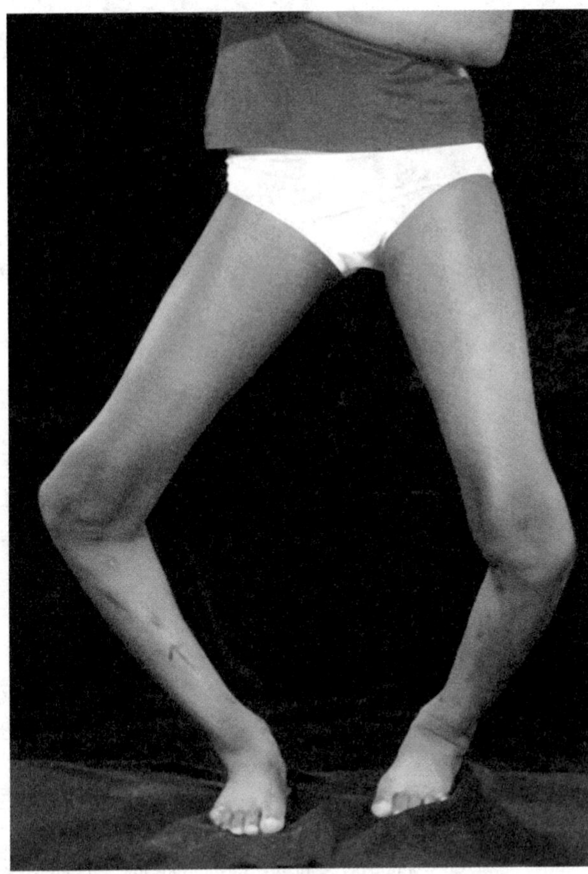

Figure 674-8. Bowing of both legs in infantile Blount disease.

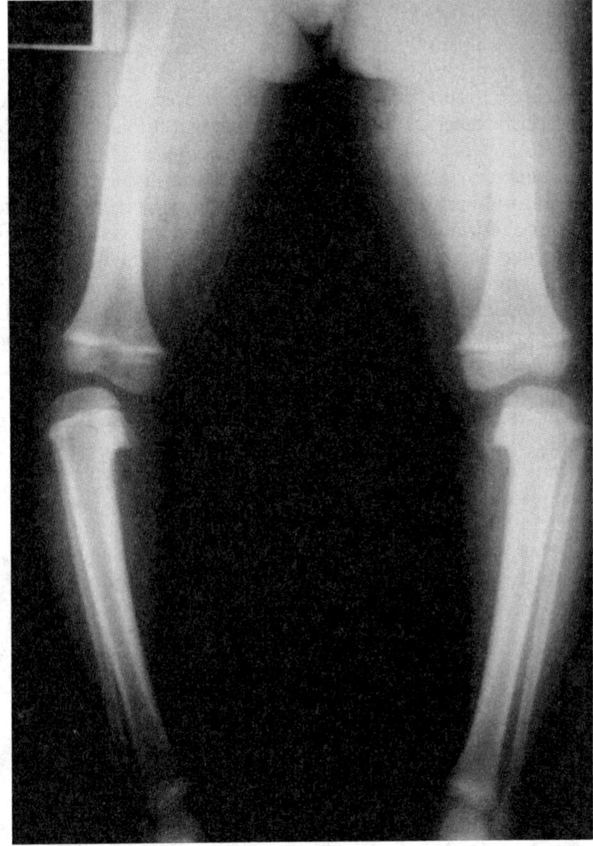

Figure 674-9. Anteroposterior radiograph of both knees in Blount disease.

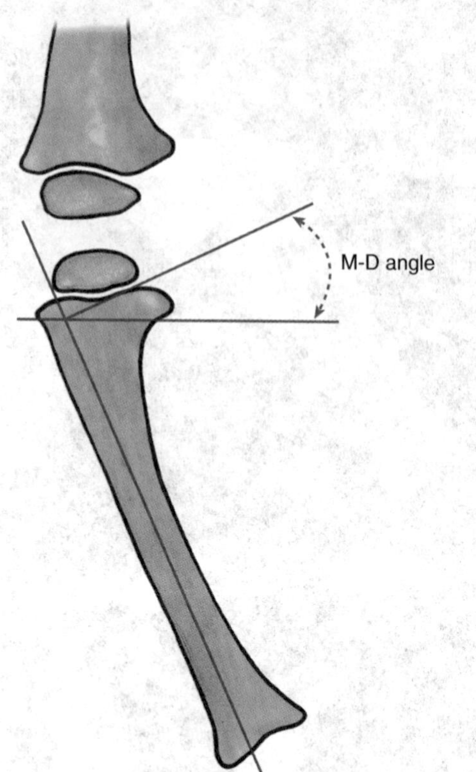

Figure 674-10. Metaphyseal-diaphyseal (M-D) angle. Draw a line on the radiograph through the proximal tibial physis. Draw another line along the lateral tibial cortex. Last, draw a line perpendicular to the shaft line as demonstrated in the diagram. (From Morrissey RT, Weinstein SL [editors]: *Lovell and Winter's Pediatric Orthopedics,* 3rd ed. Philadelphia, Lippincott Williams & Wilkins, 1990.)

the meniscus, the articular surface of the proximal tibia including the posteromedial slope, or the integrity of the proximal tibial physis.

Management is based on the stage of the disease, the age of the child, and nature of presentation (primary or recurrent deformity). In children younger than 3 yr old and Langenskiöld stage <3, bracing is effective and can prevent progression in 50% of these children. A maximal trial of 1 yr of orthotic management is recommended. If complete correction is not obtained after 1 yr or if progression occurs during this time, a corrective osteotomy may be indicated. The other indications for surgical treatment are children older than 4 yr of age, Langenskiöld stage >3, and severe deformities. A proximal tibial valgus osteotomy and associated fibular diaphyseal osteotomy are usually the procedures of choice. In late-onset tibia vara, correction is also necessary to restore the mechanical axis of the knee. Hemiplateau elevation with correction of posteromedial slope has also been established as a treatment modality in relapsed cases.

GENU VALGUM (KNOCK-KNEES)

The normal valgus is achieved by 4 yr of age. Variation up to 15 degrees of valgus is possible until 6 yr of age, and thus physiologic valgus has a good chance of correction until this age. The intermalleolar distance with the knee approximated is normally <2 cm, while in a severe valgus deformity, it could measure >10 cm. Pathologic conditions leading to valgus are metabolic bone disease (rickets, renal osteodystrophy), skeletal dysplasia, posttraumatic physeal arrest, tumors, and infection. The increased valgus at the knee causes lateral deviation of the mechanical axis with stretching of the medial aspect of the knee leading to knee pain. Deformities >15 degrees and occurring after 6 yr of age are unlikely to correct with growth and require surgical management. In the skeletally immature, medial tibial epiphyseal hemiepiphysiodesis is attempted for correction. In the skeletally mature, osteotomy is necessary at the center of rotation of angulation and is usually situated in the distal femur. Long length anteroposterior radiographs of the leg in a weight-bearing stance are necessary for preoperative planning.

674.5 • Congenital Angular Deformities of the Tibia and Fibula

POSTEROMEDIAL TIBIAL BOWING

The cause of congenital posteromedial bowing is unknown. It is usually associated with a calcaneovalgus foot and rarely with secondary valgus of the tibia. This bowing has good potential to correct with growth and hence no early operative intervention. However, despite the correction of angulation, there is residual shortening in the tibia and fibula. The mean growth inhibition is 12–13% (range, 5–27%). The mean LLD at maturity is 4 cm (range, 3–7 cm). The diagnosis of bowing is confirmed on radiographs, which show the posteromedial angulation without any other osseous abnormalities. The calcaneovalgus deformity of the foot improves with stretching or modified shoe wear and occasionally ankle-foot orthosis. Predicted LLD <4 cm is managed with age-appropriate epiphysiodesis of the normal leg. LLD >4 cm is managed with combination of contralateral epiphysiodesis and ipsilateral lengthening. A corrective osteotomy for distal valgus may be required and can be done in the same setting while correcting LLD.

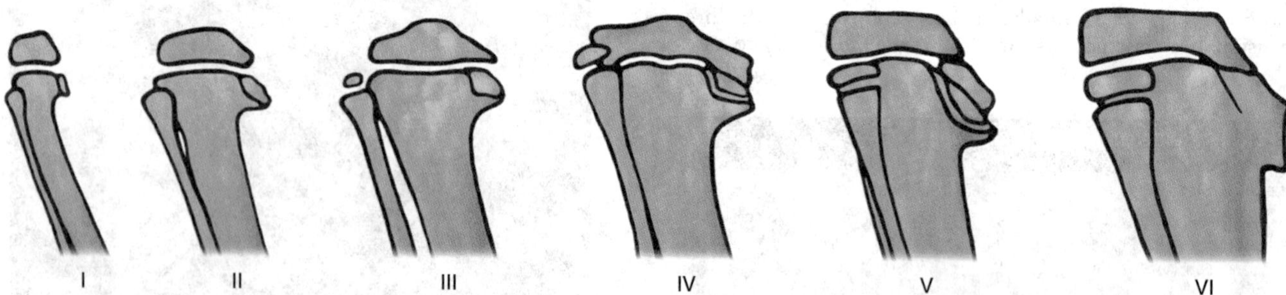

Figure 674-11. Depiction of the stages of infantile Blount disease. (From Langeskiöld A: Tibia vara (osteochondrosis deformans tibiae): A survey of 23 cases. *Acta Chir Scand* 1952;103:1.)

ANTEROMEDIAL TIBIAL BOWING (POSTAXIAL HEMIMELIA)

Fibular hemimelia is the most common cause of anteromedial bowing of the tibia. The fibular deficiency can present with complete absence of fibula or a partial development both proximally and distally. It is associated with deformities of femur, knee, tibia, ankle, and foot. The femur is short and has lateral condylar hypoplasia causing patellar instability and genu valgum deformity. The tibia has anteromedial bowing with reduced growth potential. The keys for management are the ankle stability and foot deformities. The ankle resembles a ball-and-socket joint with lateral instability. The foot deformities are characterized by the absence of lateral digits, equinocavovarus foot, and tarsal coalition.

Various surgical options have been described, and the treatment is tailored to the individual's needs and parental acceptance. A severely deformed foot could be best managed with Syme or Boyd amputation, with prosthesis as early as 1 yr of age. In the salvageable foot, LLD can be treated with contralateral leg epiphysiodesis or ipsilateral limb lengthening.

ANTEROLATERAL TIBIAL BOWING

Anterolateral tibial bowing is associated with congenital pseudarthrosis of tibia. Fifty percent of the patients have neurofibromatosis, while only 10% of the neurofibromatosis patients have this lesion. The pseudarthrosis or site of nonunion is typically situated at the middle third and distal third of the tibia. Boyd has classified it in increasing severity depending on the presence of cystic and dysplastic changes. The treatment for this condition has been very frustrating with poor results. Bracing has been recommended to prevent fracture early in the course; however, it has not been successful. Numerous surgical interventions have been attempted to achieve union such as single- and dual-onlay grafting with rigid internal fixation, intramedullary pinning with or without bone grafting, and an Ilizarov device. With the advent of microsurgery, live fibular grafts have been used with varying results. Due to the poor chances of successful union and considerable LLD, a below-knee amputation with early rehabilitation may be preferred. It is important not to attempt any osteotomy for correction of the tibial bowing.

TIBIAL LONGITUDINAL DEFICIENCY

This follows an autosomal dominant inheritance pattern and has been divided in four types depending on the deficient part of the tibia. The other associated anomalies are foot deformities, hip dysplasia, and symphalangism of the hand. The treatment revolves around presence of proximal tibial anlage and a functional quadriceps mechanism. In type Ia deformity, the proximal tibial anlage is absent and knee disarticulation with prosthesis is recommended. In types Ib and II, the tibial anlage is present and the management consists of an early Syme amputation, followed later by synostosis of the fibula with the tibia, and a below-knee prosthesis. Type III is rare and the principal management is with Syme amputation and a prosthesis. Type IV deformity is associated with ankle diastasis, which requires stabilization of the ankle and correction of LLD at a later stage.

Arazi M, Ogun TC, Memik R: Normal development of the tibiofemoral angle in children: A clinical study of 590 normal subjects from 3 to 17 years of age. *J Pediatr Orthop* 2001;21:264–267.

Cahuzac JP, Vardon D, Sales de Gauzy J: Development of the clinical tibiofemoral angle in normal adolescents: A study of 427 normal subjects from 10 to 16 years of age. *J Bone Joint Surg Br* 1995;77:729–732.

Davids JR, Blackhurst DW, Allen BL Jr: Radiographic evaluation of bowed legs in children. *J Pediatr Orthop* 2001;21:257–263.

Do TT: Clinical and radiographic evaluation of bowlegs. *Curr Opin Pediatr* 2001;13:42–46.

Doyle BS, Volk G, Smith CI: Infantile Blount's disease: Long-term follow-up of surgically treated patients at skeletal maturity. *J Pediatr Orthop* 1996;16:469–476.

Feldman MD, Schoenecker PL: Use of metaphyseal-diaphyseal angle in the evaluation of bowed legs. *J Bone Joint Surg Am* 1993;75:1602–1609.

Heath CH, Staheli LT: Normal limits of knee angle in white children—genu varum and genu valgum. *J Pediatr Orthop* 1993;13:259–262.

Henderson RC, Kemp GJ, Greene WB: Adolescent tibia vara: Alternatives for operative treatment. *J Bone Joint Surg Am* 1992;74:342–350.

Henderson RC, Kemp GJ, Hayes PRL: Prevalence of late-onset tibia vara. *J Pediatr Orthop* 1993;13:255–258.

Johnston CE II: Infantile tibia vara. *Clin Orthop* 1990;255:13–23.

Ruwe PA, Gage JR, Ozonoff MB, et al: Clinical determination of femoral anteversion: A comparison of established techniques. *J Bone Joint Surg Am* 1992;74:820–830.

Salenius P, Vankka E: The development of the tibiofemoral angle in children. *J Bone Joint Surg Am* 1975;57:259–261.

Staheli LT: Rotational problems in children. *Am Acad Orthop Surg Instr Course Lect* 1994;43:199–209.

Stevens PM, Maguire M, Dales MD, et al: Physeal stapling for idiopathic genu valgum. *J Pediatr Orthop* 1999;19:645–649.

Thompson GH: Angular deformities of the lower extremities in children. In Chapman MW (editor): *Operative Orthopedics,* 3rd ed. Philadelphia, JB Lippincott, 2001, pp 4287–4335.

Thompson GH: Gait disturbances. In Kliegman RM (editor): *Practical Strategies in Pediatric Diagnosis and Therapy,* 2nd ed. Philadelphia, WB Saunders, 2003, pp 823–843.

Wallach DM, Davidson RS: Pediatric lower limb disorders. In Dormans JP (editor): *Core Knowledge in Orthopaedics: Pediatric Orthopaedics.* Philadelphia, Mosby, 2005, pp 197–223.

Wallach DM, Davidson RS: Pediatric lower limb disorders. In Dormans JP (editor): *Pediatric Orthopaedics and Sports Medicine: The Requisites in Pediatrics.* Philadelphia, Mosby, 2005, pp 246–272.

Chapter 675 ■ Leg-Length Discrepancy

Harish S. Hosalkar, Purushottam A. Gholve, and David A. Spiegel

A discrepancy in the leg lengths may result from a variety of congenital or acquired conditions (Table 675-1), and while up to 25% of the American public may have a difference of >1 cm, only a small percentage have more than a 2-cm difference. The main consequence is gait asymmetry. An increase in vertical pelvic motion is observed, and more energy must be expended during ambulation. While a small compensatory lumbar curvature may develop, there is little evidence to suggest that leg-length discrepancy results in back pain, structural scoliosis, or degenerative arthritis. The goal of treatment is to have a discrepancy of <2–2.5 cm at skeletal maturity, and a variety of treatment methods are available to achieve this objective. Knowledge of the underlying etiology, coupled with regular follow-up to assess limb growth and skeletal maturity, allows the treating physician to project the discrepancy at skeletal maturity and to plan treatment. A subset of patients will have coexisting abnormalities in the viscera or musculoskeletal system, which must be identified and treated as well.

TABLE 675-1. Causes of Leg-Length Discrepancy

CONGENITAL CAUSES
Defects in growth
Proximal femoral focal deficiency
Congenital pseudarthrosis of the tibia
Fibular hemimelia (**Fig. 675-8**)
Bone tumors/disease
Skeletal dysplasia
Multiple hereditary exostoses
Neurofibromatosis
Enchondromatosis (Ollier disease)
Osteogenesis imperfecta
Vascular
Klippel-Trenaunay-Weber syndrome
Russell-Silver syndrome
Miscellaneous
Congenital coxa vara
Proteus syndrome
ACQUIRED CAUSES
Trauma
Overriding fractures
Epiphyseal fractures with growth plate damage
Developmental
Developmental dysplasia of the hip
Neoplastic
Malignant tumors
Tumors across epiphysis
Neurological
Myelodysplasia
Cerebral palsy
Infections/inflammatory
Septic arthritis of hip
Osteomyelitis
Rheumatoid arthritis
Miscellaneous
Acquired coxa vara
Fixed pelvic obliquity in scoliosis

DIAGNOSIS AND CLINICAL FINDINGS. Gait asymmetry is the most frequent complaint. The diagnosis is made on physical examination, and specialized radiographs help to quantify the discrepancy and to follow the discrepancy over time. The discrepancy may relate to bony shortening and/or angular deformity (actual shortening), to soft-tissue contracture at the hips, knees, or ankles (apparent shortening), or to a combination of these. Other contributing factors include joint subluxation or dislocation (hip) and a decrease in the height of the foot (congenital or neuromuscular). A careful physical examination is required to identify all factors contributing to the discrepancy. There are several clinical methods for measuring limb length. Our preference is to perform a standing examination, in which blocks of various sizes are placed under the short leg until the pelvis is leveled (Fig. 675-1). An alternate method is to measure the length of each leg with the patient supine. A tape measure is used, and the distance between the anterior superior iliac spine and the medial malleolus is measured. These methods should be reasonably accurate in the absence of "apparent" causes of discrepancy. In addition to using one or both of these methods, the range of motion at the hip, knee, and ankle must be assessed to identify any causes of apparent discrepancy. A 10-degree fixed abduction (or adduction) contracture of the hip will create an apparent leg-length discrepancy of 2–3 cm. Similarly, a flexion contracture of the hip and/or knee will create apparent shortening of the extremity, while an equinus contracture at the ankle will create apparent lengthening of the extremity. A rigid lumbar scoliosis (suprapelvic contracture) will create pelvic obliquity and an associated limb length inequality. Once a discrepancy is quantified, it must be followed at regular intervals. Assessments at 6- to 12-mo intervals are most common.

RADIOGRAPHIC EVALUATION. The radiologic evaluation complements the clinical examination; both are typically employed when making treatment decisions. The same technique should be used longitudinally to maximize accuracy. Four different techniques are available. The teleoroentgenogram is a single exposure of both lower extremities (standing) and requires a long cassette. A ruler is placed on the film, and direct measurements are made, factoring in a 6% magnification error. One advantage is that angular deformities may be assessed. Its primary indication is for young children. The orthoroentgenogram consists of three separate exposures of the hips, knees, and ankles on a long cassette. The patient is supine, and a ruler is placed on the cassette for measurement of bone length. There is no magnification error. However, the patient must lie still for the three exposures, which is often difficult to achieve in younger children. The scanogram also consists of separate exposures of the hips, knees, and ankles on a cassette with a radiographic ruler; however, a small film cassette is used (Fig. 675-2). There is no magnification error; however, patients must remain still for the three exposures, and angular deformities cannot be assessed. While CT is the most accurate technique, the assessment is time-consuming, and the technique is not available in most centers. In addition to quantifying the discrepancy, it is essential to determine skeletal age (bone age). An anteroposterior radiograph of the hand and wrist is usually obtained at each visit and compared with the standards in the Greulich and Pyle Atlas in order to estimate skeletal age. While more accurate techniques are available, most are time-consuming and impractical for routine clinical application. The range of variability using the atlas is approximately 9 mo, so the method is most accurate when multiple data points have been collected.

TREATMENT. Options for treatment include observation, a shoe lift or custom orthosis, a limb shortening procedure (acute shortening versus gradual shortening by growth arrest), a limb-lengthening procedure, or a combination of these. In the congenital deficiencies (femur, tibia, fibula), an early foot amputation is often the best option to manage a severe predicted discrepancy

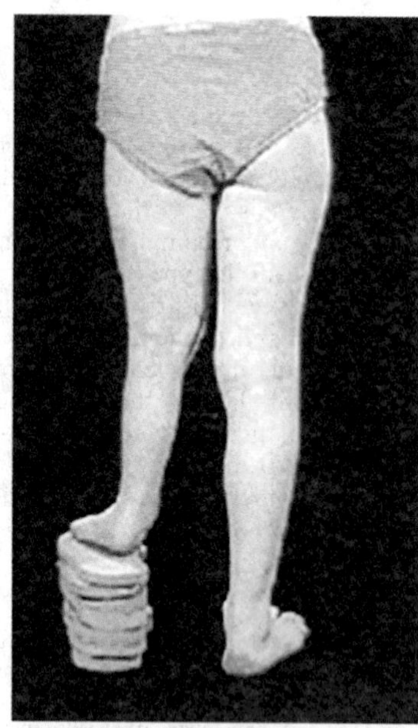

Figure 675-1. Examination with blocks under short leg until the pelvis is squared.

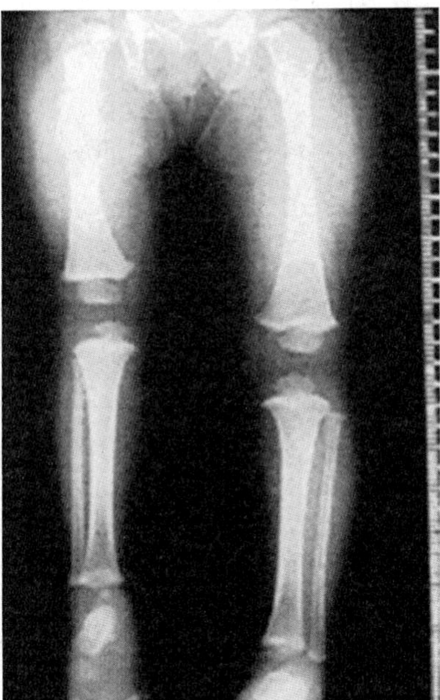

Figure 675-2. Scanogram to demonstrate exact leg-length discrepancy.

and achieve the best functional outcome. In addition to the magnitude of discrepancy predicted at skeletal maturity, both the anticipated adult height of the patient (estimated from family members) and the desires of the patient and his or her family are important considerations. General guidelines for treatment are as follows.

Discrepancies of up to 2.5 cm may be treated by observation or a shoe lift. Up to ⅜ inch may be placed within the shoe, and up to 5 cm may be placed on the outside of the shoe. Complete correction of inequality is not required, and the height of the lift should be adjusted based on the patient's gait and comfort. An orthotic may be used as a temporizing measure prior to definitive treatment.

For patients with a discrepancy between 2 and 5 cm, an epiphysiodesis is offered in skeletally immature patients, and an acute shortening may be performed in a skeletally mature patient. Epiphysiodesis refers to a temporary or permanent cessation of growth at one or more physes. A permanent growth arrest is most commonly performed as long as sufficient data are available with which to accurately predict when to perform the procedure. Approximately 65% of the growth of the lower extremity comes from the distal femur (37%, 9 mm/yr) and proximal tibia (28%, 6 mm/yr). Boys typically grow until 16 yr of age, while girls grow until 14 yr of age. As such, performing an epiphysiodesis of both the distal femur and the proximal tibia in a patient with 3 yr of growth remaining should achieve approximately 4.5 cm of correction. Techniques used to determine the timing of epiphysiodesis are the Menelaus method ("rule of thumb"), the Green and Anderson method, the Moseley straight-line graph, and the multiplier method (Figs. 675-3, 675-4, and 675-5). The most

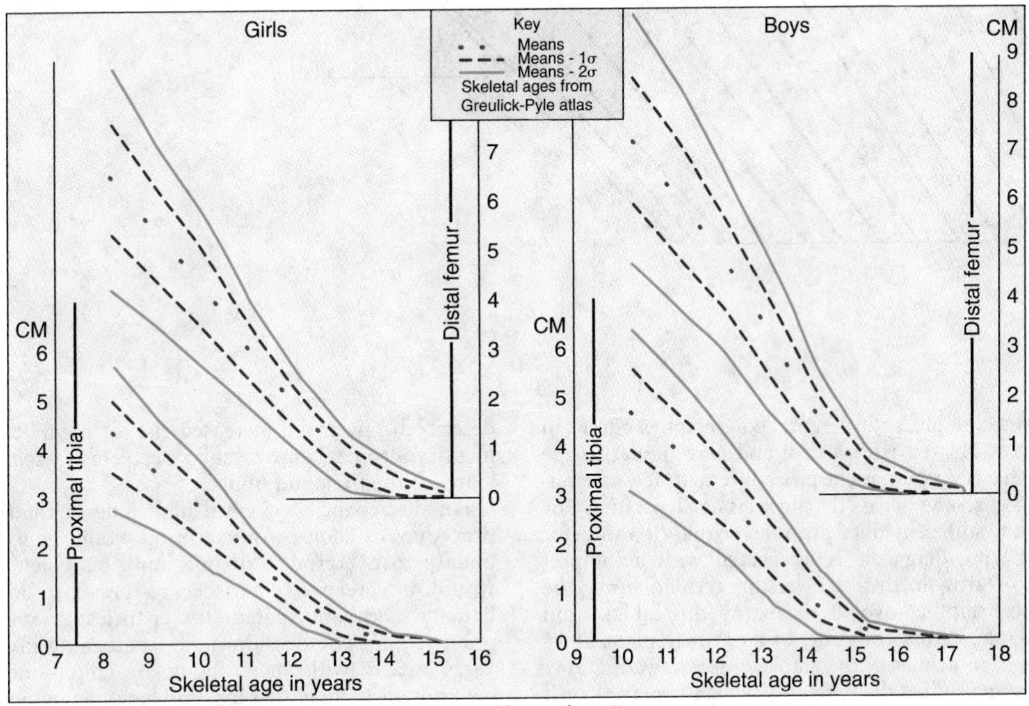

Figure 675-3. Growth remaining charts for girls and boys. The growth remaining charts for girls and boys are different. Actual correction is based on growth of the short limb. To use the chart correctly, the discrepancy at maturity and the percentage of growth retardation of the short limb should be calculated. (Redrawn from Anderson M, Green WT, Messner MB: Growth and predictions of growth in lower extremities. *J Bone Joint Surg Am* 1963;45:1–4.)

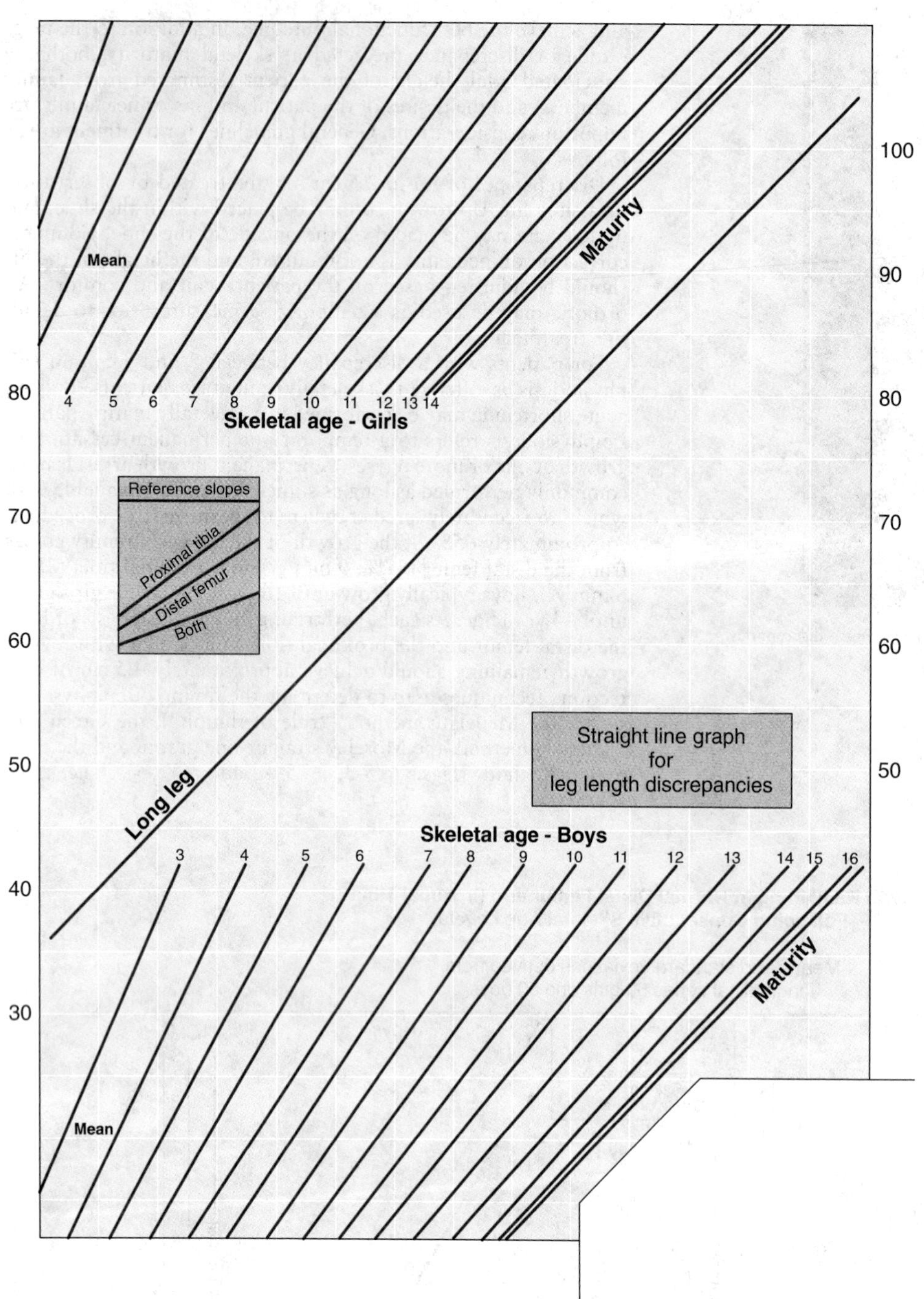

Figure 675-4. The Moseley straight-line graph for the assessment of leg-length inequalities. This allows simultaneous correlation of the normal leg, short leg, and bone age of the child. It will accurately predict lengths of each extremity at skeletal maturity. The reference slopes are used as a guide in determining when appropriate treatment should be performed. (From Moseley CF: A straight-line graph for leg-length discrepancies. *J Bone Joint Surg Am* 1977;59:174–179.)

common surgical technique is the percutaneous epiphysiodesis, in which the physis is ablated with a drill and curet under image intensification. This is an outpatient procedure with few complications. Insertion of screws across the physis is an alternative. For patients for whom sufficient data are unavailable or those for whom the underlying diagnosis is associated with an unpredictable pattern of growth, then a reversible technique may be considered. Physeal stapling involves the extraperiosteal insertion of one or more staples across both sides of the growth plate. Once equalization has been achieved, the staples are removed, allowing growth to resume. When the patient is skeletally mature or if it is deemed appropriate to wait until maturity before treatment, acute shortening may be the best option. Acute shortening is typically performed at the femur (several techniques have been described), given the increased risk of complications (compartment syndrome, neurovascular problems) associated with shortening of the tibia and fibula.

For discrepancies >5 cm, lengthening of the short limb is the procedure of choice. An exception would be a discrepancy secondary to overgrowth of one limb, in which limb shortening would be preferred in order to preserve body proportions. Patients with anticipated discrepancies greater than 8–10 cm often require one or more limb-lengthening procedures (several years apart) with or without an epiphysiodesis. The most common technique used for limb lengthening involves placement of an external fixator, either a ring fixator such as the Ilizarov device or a monolateral device (Fig. 675-6). The bone is cut at the metaphyseal-diaphyseal junction, and lengthening is achieved

Multiplier for Boys and Girls (Paley, et al 1999)

Boys		Girls	
Age	Multiplier	Age	Multiplier
0	5.08	0	4.63
0.4	4.01	0.3	4.01
1	3.24	1	2.97
1.3	2.99	2	2.39
2	2.59	3	2.05
3	2.23	3.3	2.00
4	2.00	4	1.83
5	1.83	5	1.66
6	1.68	6	1.53
7	1.57	7	1.43
8	1.47	8	1.33
9	1.38	9	1.26
10	1.31	10	1.19
11	1.24	11	1.13
12	1.18	12	1.07
13	1.12	13	1.03
14	1.07	14	1.00
15	1.03	15	1.00
16	1.01	16	1.00
17	1.00		
18	1.00		

LLD Prediction Formulas

Prenatal LLD (congenital)
$\Delta_m = \Delta \times M$

Postnatal LLD (developmental)
$\Delta_m = \Delta + I \times G$

Inhibition $\approx I = 1 - \frac{S - S^\bullet}{L - L^\bullet}$

Growth remaining $= G = L(M - 1)$

Δ_m = LLD at maturity

Δ = Current LLD

L & S = Current length of long and short leg

$L^\bullet$ & $S^\bullet$ = Length of long and short leg at any other date since LLD began

Figure 675-5. Paley multiplier. This is a simple method of determining the leg-length discrepancy (LLD) at maturation. This is applicable for shortening conditions in which growth retardation is consistent. (From Paley D, Bhave A, Herzenberg JE, Bowen JR: Multiplier methods for predicting limb-length discrepancy. *J Bone Joint Surg Am* 2000;82;1432–1446.)

gradually through distraction at the corticotomy. The usual rate of lengthening is 1 mm/day, and it takes approximately 1 mo in the fixator for each centimeter of length gained. A maximum of 15–25% of the original length of the bone may be gained at each session. An advantage of the circular fixator is the ability to correct coexisting angular deformities at the same time. Complications include pin tract infection (most common), wound infection, hypertension, joint subluxation, muscle contracture, premature consolidation, delayed union, implant-related problems, and fractures after implant removal. Finally, early amputation and prosthetic fitting may provide the best long-term function in patients with projected discrepancies in excess of 18–20 cm, especially when there are coexisting deformities or deficiencies of the ipsilateral foot (Figs. 675-7 and 675-8). The alternative would be

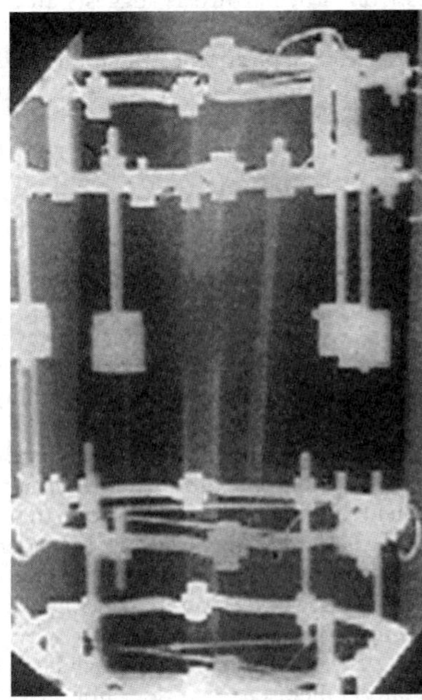

Figure 675-6. Ilizarov device demonstrating bone lengthening by distraction osteogenesis.

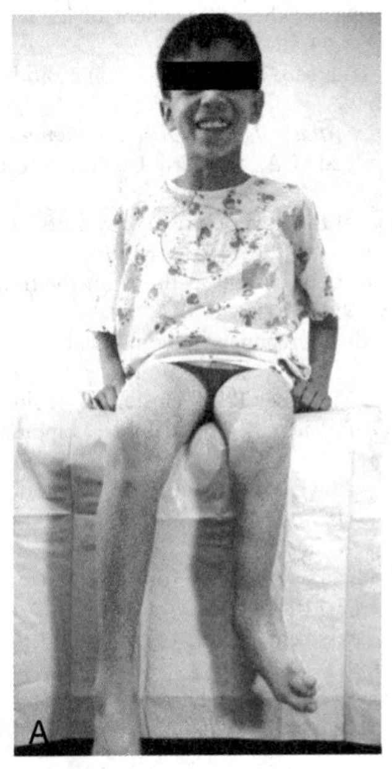

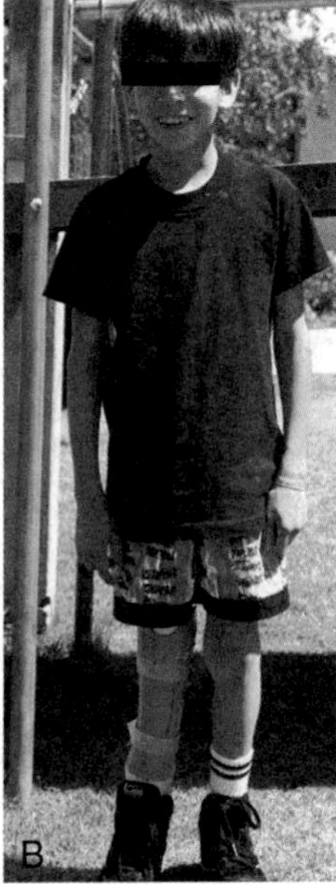

Figure 675-7. Extension prosthesis leg-length discrepancy *(A)* and compensated with extension prosthesis *(B)*.

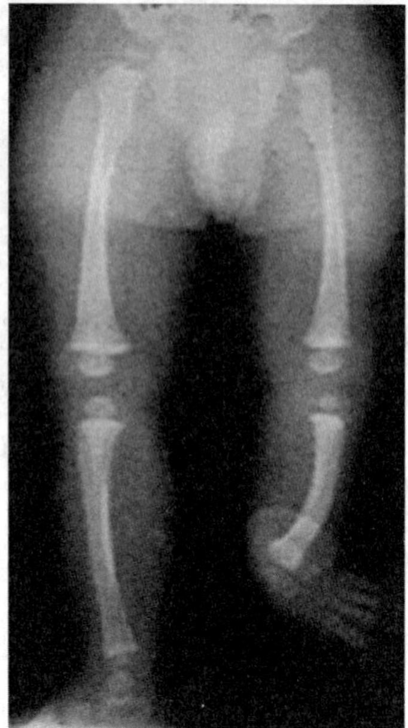

Figure 675-8. Anteroposterior radiograph of fibular hemimelia with leg-length discrepancy.

multiple reconstructive procedures throughout childhood and adolescence. The impact of multiple procedures on the child's psychosocial development must also be kept in mind when formulating the treatment plan in these complex cases.

Anderson M, Messner M, Green W: Distribution of lengths of the normal femur and tibia in children from one to eighteen years of age. *J Bone Joint Surg* 1964;46:1197–1202.

Beumer A, Lampe HI, Swierstra BA, et al: The straight line graph in limb length inequality: A new design based on 182 Dutch children. *Acta Orthop Scand* 1997;68:355–360.

Coppola C, Maffulli N: Limb shortening for the management of leg length discrepancy. *J R Coll Surg Edinb* 1999;44:46–54.

Gabriel KR, Crawford AH, Roy DR, True MS: Percutaneous epiphysiodesis. *J Pediatr Orthop* 1994;14:358–362.

Gruelich WW, Pyle SI: *Radiographic Atlas of Skeletal Development of the Hand and Wrist,* 2nd ed. Stanford, CA, Stanford University Press, 1959.

Horton GA, Olney BW: Epiphysiodesis of the lower extremity: Results of the percutaneous technique. *J Pediatr Orthop* 1996;16:180–182.

Little DG, Nigo L, Aiona MD: Deficiencies of current methods for the timing of epiphysiodesis. *J Pediatr Orthop* 1996;16:173–179.

Menelaus MB: Correction of leg length discrepancy by epiphyseal arrest. *J Bone Joint Surg Br* 1996;48:336–339.

Moseley CF: Leg length discrepancy. In Morrissey RT, Weinstein SL (editors): *Lovell and Winter's Pediatric Orthopaedics.* Philadelphia, Lippincott Williams & Wilkins, 2000, pp 1105–1150.

Paley D, Bhave A, Herzenberg JE, Bowen JR: Multiplier method for predicting limb-length discrepancy. *J Bone Joint Surg Am* 2000;82: 1432–1446.

Pritchett JW: Comparison of methods for prediction of lower-extremity growth. *J Bone Joint Surg Am* 2001;83:1108–1110.

Stanitski DF: Limb-length inequality: Assessment and treatment options. *J Am Acad Orthop Surg* 1999;7:143–153.

Stanitski DF, Bullard M, Armstrong P, Stanitski CL: Results of femoral lengthening using the Ilizarov technique. *J Pediatr Orthop* 1995;15: 224–231.

Westh RN, Menelaus MB: A simple calculation for the timing of epiphyseal arrest: A further report. *J Bone Joint Surg Br* 1981;63:117–119.

Chapter 676 ■ The Knee

Harish S. Hosalkar and Lawrence Wells

NORMAL DEVELOPMENT OF KNEE

The knee is a major synovial joint and develops between the 3rd and 4th fetal mo. The secondary centers of ossification are formed between the 6th and 9th fetal mo for the distal femur and between the 8th fetal mo and the 1st postnatal mo for the upper tibia. The patellar ossification center appears between the 2nd and 4th yr in girls and the 3rd and 5th yr in boys.

NORMAL RANGE OF MOTION

The fully extended knee is normally in the neutral position. The normal range of motion extends from neutral to about 140 degrees with most activities performed in the flexion arc of 0–70 degrees. Hyperextension of up to 10–15 degrees is considered normal in a child.

The knee is the largest joint in the body and is a modified hinge type of synovial joint that also permits some element of rotation. It consists of three joints merged into one; an intermediate one between the patella and the femur, and lateral and medial ones between the femoral and tibial condyles. The distal femur is cam shaped, allowing it to have a gliding, hinged motion. The major constraints of the knee are the medial and lateral collateral ligaments, the anterior and posterior cruciate ligaments, and the medial and lateral menisci. There are several bursae about the knee because most tendons around the knee run parallel to the bones and pull lengthwise across the knee joint.

Knee pain is one of the most common presenting complaints in older children and adolescents. This is commonly related to trauma but may also be insidious in onset. Knee effusion may be a common feature associated with knee pain. Depending on the etiology of the intra-articular process, the fluid collected in the knee may be blood (trauma- or hemophilia-induced hemarthrosis), inflammatory fluid (juvenile rheumatoid arthritis), or purulent material (septic arthritis). The presence of fat globules in the blood aspirated from a hemarthrosis suggests an occult fracture. Recurrent effusions may indicate a chronic internal derangement such as a meniscal tear. Aspiration of the joint fluid is often necessary to establish the diagnosis as well as to offer relief of symptoms (see Chapter 684).

PEDIATRIC KNEE DISORDERS

676.1 • Discoid Lateral Meniscus

Discoid lateral meniscus (DLM) is an anatomic variation of the lateral meniscus that may be asymptomatic or may cause snapping or popping of the knee. There are three types of DLM. The first is the **Wrisberg ligament type** where the lateral meniscus has no attachment to the tibial plateau posteriorly, but has a meniscofemoral ligament or ligament of Wrisberg that connects the posterior horn of the lateral meniscus to the lateral surface of the medial femoral condyle. The ligament prevents the gliding of the meniscus during knee extension, producing a snap with each excursion of the meniscus, leading to hypertrophy and irregularity. The second type is the **complete type,** which is characterized by a thickened lateral meniscus that does not move in and out of the center of the joint and has normal peripheral attachments. The third type is the **incomplete type,** which is smaller than the complete type and does not fill the lateral compartment.

The cause of discoid meniscus is not defined, but may be a failure of an embryologic sequence of degeneration of the center of the meniscus. The normal meniscus is attached around its periphery and glides anteriorly and posteriorly with knee motion, but a discoid meniscus is less mobile and may be torn. Occasionally, there is no peripheral attachment around the posterolateral aspect of the meniscus, which may allow it to become displaced anteriorly with knee flexion, producing a loud click or clunk.

The usual presenting complaint is that of a popping or snapping of the knee that is both heard and felt by the child or parent. This is often noted in children older than the age of 6 yr. Most often the snapping is not painful and the child is active. A second type of presentation is of a child who has had no knee symptoms but presents spontaneously or after an injury with pain, snapping, popping, or locking located along the lateral joint line. Physical examination may show a mild effusion and tenderness with fullness over the lateral joint line and crepitation with motion. The typical findings include a palpable snapping as the knee flexes and extends. Along the lateral joint line, the examiner feels a bulge, as the meniscus seems to protrude beyond the margin of the tibia. As the knee moves, the meniscus snaps into the intercondylar notch and the bulge disappears.

Anteroposterior radiography of the knee may show widening of the lateral aspect of the knee joint. Other findings include flattening of the lateral femoral condyle (giving a squared off appearance) and cupping of the lateral aspect of the tibial plateau. MRI or arthroscopy is required for definitive diagnosis.

TREATMENT. Many children with discoid menisci require no treatment. These children should be followed and treated only if pain or loss of motion occurs. Surgery may be considered when DLM leads to locking, swelling, loss of motion, inability to run, or inability to participate in sports. The treatment is to excise tears and reshape the meniscus arthroscopically (Fig. 676-1). Meniscal instability can occasionally be repaired or reconstructed. Complete excision may be necessary if other procedures are unsuccessful.

676.2 • Popliteal Cyst

Popliteal cysts (**Baker cyst**) are commonly seen in children and are different than in adults. They are cystic masses filled with gelatinous material that develop in the popliteal fossa, are usually asymptomatic, and are not related to intra-articular pathology. Spontaneous resolution usually occurs, although the process can take several years.

The usual presentation is that of a mass behind the knee that may be fairly large when first noted. There are usually no symptoms of internal derangement of the knee. Physical examination reveals a firm mass in the popliteal fossa, often medially located and usually distal to the popliteal crease. The mass is most prominent when the knee is extended and the patient is lying in prone position.

The most common site of origin is the bursa of the gastrocnemius and semimembranosus. Another common site of origin is a herniation through the posterior joint capsule of the knee. Histologically, the cysts are classified as fibrous, synovial, inflammatory, or transitional. Transillumination of the cyst on physical examination is a simple diagnostic test. Knee radiographs are normal and should be obtained to identify other lesions such as osteochondromas, osteochondritis dissecans, and malignancies. The diagnosis may be confirmed by ultrasonography (to differentiate a solid mass from a cystic lesion) or aspiration. In most cases, these cysts should be left alone, as they often resolve spontaneously. Surgical excision of a popliteal cyst is indicated only when symptoms are severe and limiting and have not resolved after several months. The presence of a solid mass detected on examination or MRI indicates exploration.

676.3 • Osteochondritis Dissecans

Osteochondritis dissecans occurs when an area of bone adjacent to the articular cartilage becomes avascular and ultimately separates from the underlying bone. The exact cause is unknown; however, causes of osteochondral fractures of the femoral condyle include impingement from a tall tibial spine, direct blows causing compaction, rotary forces, and joint compression forces. The juvenile form may represent a disturbance of epiphyseal development, with small accessory islets of bone being separated from the epiphysis. Familial predisposition has been suggested. Most lesions are located on the lateral portion of the medial femoral condyle, although they may also involve the lateral femoral condyle or the patella. Characteristic pathology of the lesion includes an area of avascular necrosis with a cleft on either side, with varying degrees of ischemia and fibrosis of the overlying hyaline cartilage.

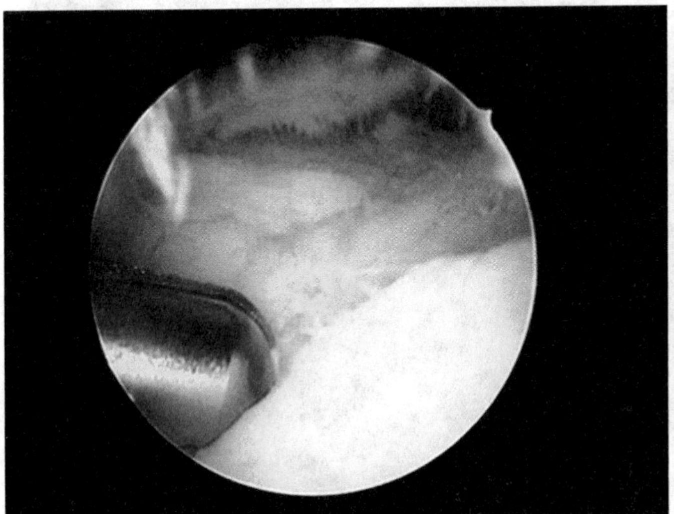

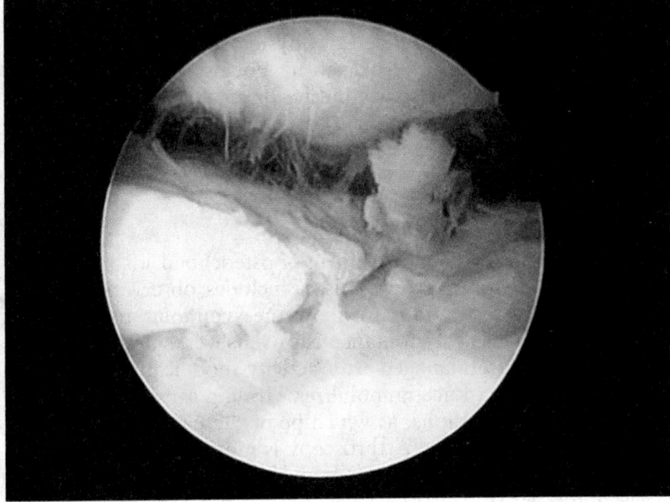

Figure 676-1. Arthroscopic image of discoid meniscus and arthroscopic shaving with meniscectomy.

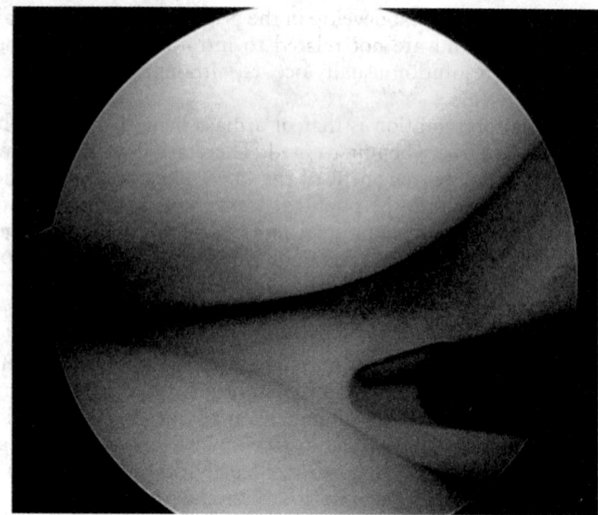

Figure 676-2. Classic arthroscopic image of osteochondritis dissecans lesion.

CLINICAL MANIFESTATIONS AND DIAGNOSIS. The most common presenting complaint is vague knee pain. If the fragment becomes loose, there will be crepitation, popping, giving way, and occasionally locking of the knee with or without a mild effusion. Physical findings are minimal and may include parapatellar tenderness, quadriceps atrophy, and slight pain with range of motion. The Wilson test is noted to be a specific diagnostic sign. It is performed by flexing the knee to 90 degrees, fully rotating the tibia medially, and then gradually extending the knee. When the test is positive, there is pain at 30 degrees of flexion that is located over the medial femoral condyle anteriorly.

The lesion is usually noted on anteroposterior, lateral, and tunnel radiographs (notch view) of the knee. Early lesions present with a small radiolucency at the articular surface, while more advanced lesions have a well-demarcated segment of subchondral bone with a lucent line separating it from the condyle. In young children, small foci of ossification may appear beyond the margin of the main ossific nucleus. As revascularization occurs, the bone heals spontaneously. With increasing age, the risk increases for articular cartilage fracture and separation of the bony fragment, producing a loose body.

CT delineates the extent and location of the lesion including the degree of detachment. MRI is helpful in determining the integrity of the articular cartilage and stability of the lesion. Arthroscopy is the most reliable method of evaluating the status of the lesion (Fig. 676-2). Factors commonly associated with a good prognosis are younger age group, small lesion, non–weight-bearing location, and no displacement. Four stages are involved with the progression of osteochondritis dissecans. Stage I consists of a small area of subchondral compression; stage II consists of a partially detached fragment; in stage III, the fragment is completely detached but remains in the crater; and by stage IV, the fragment is loose in the joint.

TREATMENT. The initial management of osteochondritis dissecans in children with open growth plates includes observation with enough activity restrictions to allow the symptoms to resolve. Most stable lesions heal spontaneously over several months. Stage I and II lesions are managed with activity modification, isometric exercises, and a knee immobilizer. Healing can be confirmed by follow-up radiographs, at which point the patient can return to normal activity levels. Arthroscopy is indicated in patients in whom nonoperative treatment fails and in those with signs, symptoms, and other studies suggestive of an unstable lesion. Stage III lesions are managed by drilling and stabilization with Kirschner wires or pins. Stage IV lesions, if small, are managed by excision, while large lesions or those involving the weight-bearing areas are either replaced or internally fixed. Bone and cartilage grafting may be necessary in very severe cases with loss of large fragments. After surgery, patients participate in a physical therapy program and may or may not be allowed to return to their preoperative activity levels. Treating osteochondritis dissecans early and effectively often prevents recurrent symptoms in adulthood, although some very severe lesions may be symptomatic later in life.

676.4 • Osgood-Schlatter Disease

This condition is characterized by pain over the tibial tubercle in a growing child. The patellar tendon inserts into the tibia tubercle, which is an extension of the proximal tibial epiphysis. Osgood-Schlatter disease is likely a traction apophysitis of the tibial tubercle growth plate and the adjacent patellar tendon. It occurs during late childhood or adolescence, especially in athletes, and is likely due to repetitive tensile microtrauma. It occurs between the ages of 10 and 15 yr; the onset in girls is about 2 yr before that in boys. It is more common in males.

This disorder is self-limited in most patients and resolves with skeletal maturity. Pain directly over the tibial tubercle is the usual complaint, and swelling over the tubercle is often of concern. The pain is aggravated by activities but often persists even at rest. Physical examination reveals point tenderness over the tibial tubercle and the distal portion of the patellar tendon. There is often increased prominence of the tibia tubercle that is also firm.

Radiographs are usually the only diagnostic studies necessary (Fig. 676-3). Fragmentary ossification of the tibial tubercle may be noted in some cases, which is often a normal variant. Some cases may be associated with patella alta.

Rest, restriction of activities, and, occasionally, a knee immobilizer may be necessary, combined with an isometric and flexibility exercise program. Reassurance is important, as some

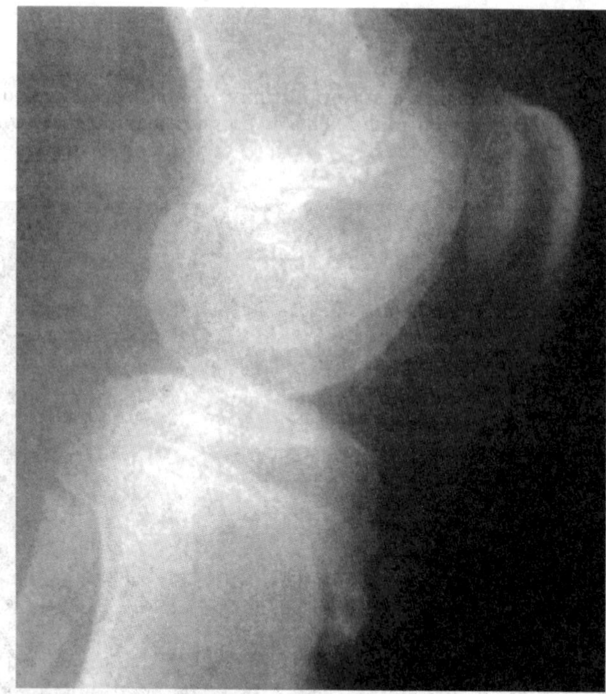

Figure 676-3. Lateral radiograph of the knee demonstrating apophysitis of the tibial tubercle in Osgood-Schlatter disease.

patients and parents fear that the swollen tubercle may be a sign of malignancy. Complete resolution of symptoms through physiologic healing (physeal closure) of the tibia tubercle may require 12–24 mo. Removal of ossicles from the tubercle may rarely be necessary in patients with persistent disabling symptoms. Complications are rare, and include early closure of the tibial tubercle with recurvatum deformity and rarely patellar tendon rupture or avulsion of the tibial tubercle.

PATELLOFEMORAL DISORDERS

Patellofemoral joint stability depends on balance among the restraining ligaments, muscle forces, and the articular anatomy of the patellofemoral groove. The multiple factors that contribute to patellofemoral instability include quadriceps insufficiency, internal femoral torsion, external tibial torsion, the shallow sulcus, lateral tether, medial capsular attenuation, condylar hypoplasia, and genu valgum.

The patella has a V-shaped bottom that guides it through the sulcus in the distal femur. The force of the muscles pulling through the quadriceps mechanism and the patellar tendon does not act in a straight line because the patellar tendon inclines in a slightly lateral direction with respect to the line of the quadriceps. This is normally called the Q angle. This lateral movement, coupled with the movement of the restraining ligaments, tends to move the patella in a lateral direction. The vastus medialis muscle is necessary to counteract the laterally acting forces. An abnormality of any one or a group of these factors can make the patellofemoral joint function abnormally. Excessive instability of the patellofemoral joint may manifest as acute patellar dislocation, recurrent patellar subluxation or dislocation, habitual dislocation, and chronic dislocation.

676.5 • Idiopathic Adolescent Anterior Knee Pain Syndrome

Previously known as chondromalacia patella, idiopathic adolescent anterior knee pain syndrome is a common disorder that presents as knee pain. The term was initially used to describe a deranged patellar articular surface. It is common in adolescent girls, is often activity related and poorly localized, and may cause disability. Evidence suggests that the articular surface is actually normal. The cause of the knee pain, which commonly occurs in early adolescence, is unknown. A patient with unexplained pain in the anterior knee poses a diagnostic and therapeutic challenge to the orthopedic surgeon.

CLINICAL MANIFESTATIONS AND DIAGNOSIS. Symptoms are usually produced by vigorous physical activities such as running. There is usually no history of antecedent trauma. There are no mechanical symptoms associated such as locking, giving way, or recurrent effusion.

Active and passive range of motion of the knee, alignment of the lower extremity, knee stability, patellar tracking, areas of focal tenderness, and gait should be evaluated to identify any obvious causes of knee pain or instability. Routine radiographs, including anteroposterior, lateral, and tunnel views, are not particularly helpful in evaluating the cause of adolescent anterior knee pain, except that they may eliminate other etiologies. In the adolescent group, radiographs of the hip should be considered in suspected cases to rule out a slipped capital femoral epiphysis that can present as ill-defined knee pain.

TREATMENT. The natural history of anterior knee pain is one of spontaneous resolution over a period of years. The treatment is predominantly nonoperative and may include flexibility exercises, strengthening exercises (isometric quadriceps), contrast therapies (ice and heat), orthoses, and medications (nonsteroidal anti-inflammatory drugs). A success rate of 70–90% can be anticipated. Arthroscopic evaluation of the knee and patellofemoral joint is rarely necessary.

676.6 • Patellar Subluxation and Dislocation

Recurrent patellar dislocation is defined as more than one episode of dislocation of the patella documented by an observer or clearly described by the patient. Recurrent patellar subluxation is poorly defined but alludes to more than one episode of patellar subluxation without frank dislocation. Habitual dislocation of the patella is defined as a dislocation that occurs every time that the knee is flexed, while a chronic dislocation of the patella is one that never reduces throughout the arc of motion of the knee.

Traumatic patellar subluxation and dislocation can occur as a result of a direct trauma. Habitual subluxation or dislocation is usually due to a dysplastic knee with contracture of the lateral portion of the quadriceps mechanism. In this case, the patella displaces laterally whenever the knee is flexed. The most common etiologic factor in recurrent patellar dislocation is lateral malalignment of the quadriceps mechanism. A number of syndromes are associated with patellar instability, including Down syndrome, Turner syndrome, Kabuki make-up syndrome, and Rubinstein-Taybi syndrome.

CLINICAL MANIFESTATIONS AND DIAGNOSIS. The physical examination findings usually suggest the diagnosis. After an acute dislocation, there may be a hemarthrosis from capsular tearing or an osteochondral fracture. If the child is seen after a recent dislocation, there may be parapatellar tenderness and a mild effusion.

Examination of a child with a maltracking patella that is predisposed to dislocation may often show terminal subluxation of the patella when the knee is brought into full extension. There may be tenderness to palpation over the inferior surface of the lateral facet of the patella. Observe the tracking of the patella as the patient is allowed to flex the knee from full extension. In the patient with instability, the patella will shift laterally just as the knee begins to flex and will then shift medially with further flexion. This lateral displacement of the patella followed by medial movement is termed *J tracking*. The other classic physical sign is the *Fairbanks apprehension sign*. With the knee in 30 degrees of flexion, the examiner manually displaces the patella laterally and yields a subjective feeling of subluxation, resulting in the patient grabbing the examiner's hand to prevent manipulative dislocation.

It is important to assess the torsional profile of the patient to rule out possible rotational abnormalities of the femur or tibia or both.

Radiographic studies may help identify factors contributing to recurrent dislocation of the patella or after an acute dislocation. They should include anteroposterior, lateral, and skyline tangential views (obtained in full flexion) of the patella to assess for an osteochondral fracture from the lateral femoral condyle or the patella. Other views include the MacNab view (obtained with the knee in 40 degrees of flexion), which shows the relationship of the patella to the anterior part of the femoral intercondylar groove and may also demonstrate loose bodies and fractures of the patella or lateral condyle; the Merchant view obtained with the knee in 45 degrees of flexion; and the Laurin view with the knee in 20 degrees of flexion.

TREATMENT. An initial traumatic dislocation of the patella should be treated with a knee immobilizer for comfort. After a few days, the patient should begin isometric quadriceps-strengthening exercises, and more vigorous strengthening exercises can be done as the tenderness resolves. Once the immobilization is discontinued (approximately 6 wk), the isometric exercise program should be continued until the knee is fully rehabilitated. Using this method, approximately 75% of patients do not have recurrent dislocations.

Initial management of recurrent dislocation of the patella should be nonoperative. If patellar subluxation is due to dynamic muscle imbalance, a specific muscle rehabilitation program, such as strengthening the vastus medialis, may be successful. Patellar stabilizing orthosis may be useful, although the mechanism of action and efficacy is uncertain.

Operative stabilization may be necessary with continued episodes of dislocation or failure of conservative management for patellar subluxation. The surgical approaches to growing children focus on realigning the quadriceps mechanism usually in combination with a lateral release and the creation of a medial patellar restraint. Realignment of the extensor mechanism may be accomplished by altering the muscle itself, changing its insertion into the patella, or altering the attachment of the patella to the tibia. Depending on the extent of involvement, an arthroscopic lateral release with or without a soft-tissue reconstruction with a realignment procedure may be performed. Torsional abnormalities of the femur or tibia may be addressed with rotational osteotomy of the distal femur or proximal tibia, or rarely both as deemed necessary.

Ahn JH, Shim JS, Hwang CH, et al: Discoid lateral meniscus in children: Clinical manifestations and morphology. *J Pediatr Orthop* 2001;21:812–816.

Bensahel H, Souchet P, Pennecot GF, et al: The unstable patella in children. *J Pediatr Orthop* 2000;9:265–270.

Davids JR: Pediatric knee: Clinical assessment and common disorders. *Pediatr Clin North Am* 1996;43:1067–1090.

Ganley TJ, Kolze EA, Gregg JR: Pediatric sports medicine. In Dormans JP (editor): *Pediatric Orthopedics: Core Knowledge in Orthopedics.* Philadelphia, Mosby, 2005, pp 138–158.

Ganley TJ, Lou JE, Pryor K, Gregg JR: Sports medicine. In Dormans JP (editor): *Pediatric Orthopedics and Sports Medicine: The Requisites in Pediatrics.* Philadelphia, Mosby, 2004, pp 273–298.

Hamer AJ: Pain in the hip and knee. *Br Med J* 2004;328:1067–1069.

Herring JA: Disorders of the knee. In Herring JA (editor): *Tachdjian's Pediatric Orthopedics,* 3rd ed. Philadelphia, WB Saunders, 2002, pp 789–837.

Kocher MS, DiCanzio J, Zurakowski D, et al: Diagnostic performance of clinical examination and selective magnetic resonance imaging in the evaluation of intraarticular knee disorders in children and adolescents. *Am J Sports Med* 2001;29:292–296.

Stanitski CL: Instructional course lecture: Anterior knee pain syndromes in the adolescent. *J Bone Joint Surg Am* 1993;75:1407–1416.

Vahasarja V, Kinnunen P, Lanning P, et al: Operative realignment of patellar malalignment in children. *J Pediatr Orthop* 1995;15:281–285.

Van Rhijn LW, Jansen EJ, Pruijs HE: Long-term follow-up of conservatively treated popliteal cysts in children. *J Pediatr Orthop* 2000;9:62–64.

Chapter 677 ■ The Hip

Harish S. Hosalkar, David Horn, Jared E. Friedman, and John P. Dormans

The hip joint is a pivotal joint of the lower extremity, and its functional demands require great stability coupled with a wide range of motion that allows polyaxial motion, including flexion, extension, abduction, adduction, internal and external rotation, and circumduction. Anatomically, the hip joint is a ball-and-socket joint between the femoral head and acetabulum. The femoral head and acetabulum are closely related and thus are very much dependent on one another for their necessary development and growth.

GROWTH AND DEVELOPMENT

The hip joint begins to develop at about the 7th wk of gestation, when a cleft appears in the mesenchyme of the primitive limb bud. These precartilaginous cells differentiate into a fully formed cartilaginous femoral head and acetabulum by the 11th wk of gestation. At birth, the neonatal acetabulum is completely composed of cartilage, with a thin rim of fibrocartilage called the labrum.

The very cellular hyaline cartilage of the acetabulum is continuous with the triradiate cartilages, which divide and interconnect the three osseous components of the pelvis (the ilium, ischium, pubis). The concave shape of the hip joint is determined by the presence of a spherical femoral head.

Several factors determine acetabular depth, including interstitial growth within the acetabular cartilage, appositional growth under the perichondrium, and growth of adjacent bones (the ilium, ischium, pubis). In the neonate, the entire proximal femur is a cartilaginous structure in the shape of a femoral head and greater and lesser trochanters. The three main growth areas are the physeal plate, the growth plate of the greater trochanter, and the femoral neck isthmus. Between the 4th and 7th mo of life, the proximal femoral ossification center (in the center of the femoral head) appears. This ossification center continues to enlarge, along with its cartilaginous anlage, until adult life, when only a thin layer of articular cartilage remains. During the period of growth, the thickness of the cartilage surrounding this bony nucleus gradually decreases, as does the thickness of the acetabular cartilage. The growth of the proximal femur is affected by muscle pull, the forces transmitted across the hip joint by weight bearing, normal joint nutrition, circulation, and muscle tone. Alterations in these factors may cause profound changes in development of the proximal femur.

VASCULAR SUPPLY

The blood supply to the capital femoral epiphysis (CFE) is complex with a changing pattern noted with the elongating femoral neck, growth plate, a gradually ossifying proximal femur, and acetabulum. The proximal femur receives its arterial supply from intraosseous (primarily the medial femoral circumflex artery) and extraosseous vessels. (Fig. 677-1). The retinacular vessels (extraosseous) lie on the surface of the femoral neck but are intracapsular because they enter the epiphysis from the periphery. This makes the blood supply vulnerable to damage from septic arthritis, trauma, thrombosis, and other vascular insults.

677.1 • Developmental Dysplasia of the Hip

DDH is a spectrum of abnormalities involving the growing hip. Acetabular dysplasia, on the other hand, refers to abnormal morphology and development of the acetabulum. Hip **subluxation** is defined as partial contact between the femoral head and acetabulum, whereas **dislocation** refers to a hip with no contact between the articulating surfaces of the hip. The spectrum of presentations of DDH ranges from simple acetabular dysplasia (the femoral head may be retained within an inadequate acetabulum) to acetabular dysplasia plus subluxation (the femoral head moves slightly away from the acetabular medial wall) to dislocation of the hip joint (a complete loss of contact between the femoral head and acetabulum).

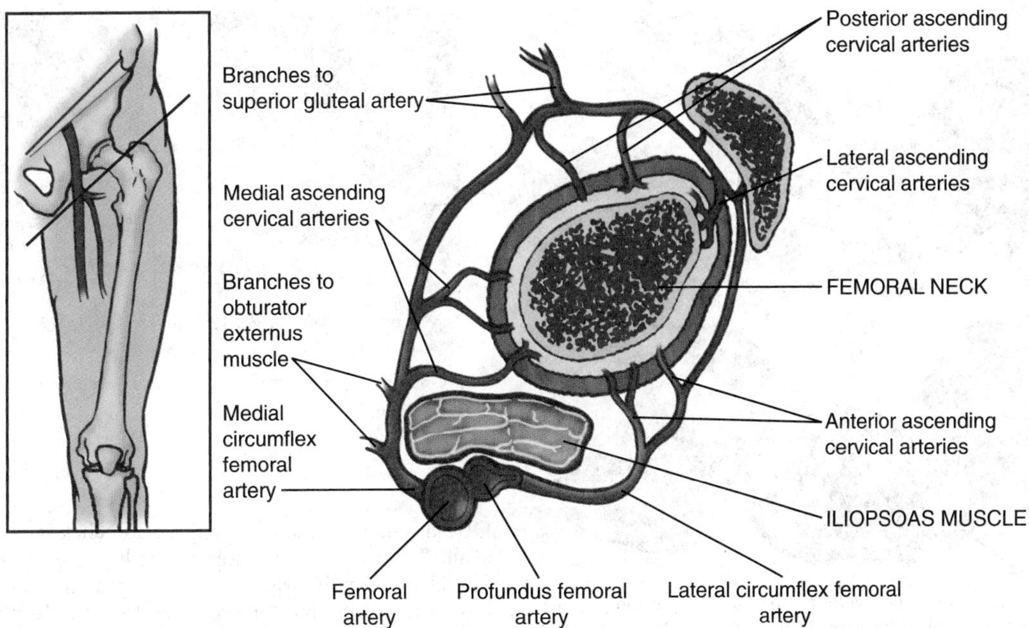

Figure 677-1. Diagrammatic illustration of vascular anatomy of the proximal femur.

Developmental dysplasia of the hip (DDH) is classified into two major groups: typical and teratologic. Typical DDH occurs in otherwise normal individuals or those without defined syndromes or genetic conditions. Teratologic hip dislocations usually have identifiable causes and occur before birth.

ETIOLOGY, INCIDENCE, AND RISK FACTORS

Although most newborn screening studies suggest that some degree of hip instability can be detected in one in 100 to one in 250 babies, actual dislocated or dislocatable hips are much less frequent, being found in 1–1.5 of 1000 live births. The etiology of DDH is multifactorial, involving both genetic and intrauterine environmental factors. There is marked geographic and racial variation in the incidence of DDH. The reported incidence based on geography ranges from 1.7/1,000 babies in Sweden to 75/1,000 in Yugoslavia to 188.5/1,000 in a district in Manitoba, Canada. The incidence of DDH in Chinese and African newborns is almost 0%, whereas it is 1% for hip dysplasia and 0.1% for hip dislocation in white newborns. These differences may be due to environmental factors, such as child-rearing practices, rather than to genetic predisposition. African and Asian caregivers have traditionally carried babies against their bodies in a shawl so that a child's hips are flexed, abducted, and free to move. This keeps the hips in the optimal position for stability and for dynamic molding of the developing acetabulum by the cartilaginous femoral head. On the other hand, children in Native American and Eastern European cultures, which have a relatively high incidence of DDH, have historically been swaddled in confining clothes that bring their hips into extension. This position increases the tension of the psoas muscle–tendon unit and may predispose the hips to displace and eventually dislocate laterally and superiorly.

RISK FACTORS FOR DDH

A positive family history for DDH is found in 12–33% of affected patients. DDH is more common among female patients (80%). This is thought to be due to the greater susceptibility of females to maternal hormones such as relaxin, which increases ligamentous laxity. Although only 2–3% of all babies are born in breech presentation, the rate is 16–25% for patients with DDH. Any condition that leads to a tighter intrauterine space and, consequently, less room for normal fetal motion may be associated with DDH. These conditions include oligohydramnios, large birth weight, and first pregnancy. The high rate of association of DDH with other intrauterine molding abnormalities, such as torticollis and metatarsus adductus, supports the theory that the "crowding phenomenon" has a role in the pathogenesis. The left hip is the most commonly affected hip; in the most common fetal position, this is the hip that is usually forced into adduction against the mother's sacrum. Other children with a higher incidence of DDH are infants delivered by cesarean section and those cared for in special care units after birth.

PATHOANATOMY

If the hip is not dislocated at birth, all the specific components of the hip joint, except for the ligamentum teres and the hip capsule, usually appear relatively normal. Teratologic dislocations frequently are accompanied by a small, shallow acetabulum and a stiff hip joint at birth. In untreated typical DDH, deformity may occur secondary to altered growth of the hip. These changes may include hypertrophy of the lateral cartilage of the acetabulum (neolimbus formation), hypertrophy of the ligamentum teres, capsular laxity, hourglass constriction of the hip capsule and hypertrophy of the transverse acetabular ligament, and excess femoral anteversion. It is essential for the treating physician to be aware of these changes to successfully treat DDH.

CLINICAL PRESENTATION

THE NEONATE. DDH in the neonate is diagnosed by eliciting the Ortolani or Barlow sign or from significant changes in the sonographic morphology of the hip. Physical examination must be carried out with the infant unclothed and placed supine in a warm, comfortable setting on a flat examination table.

The **Barlow** provocative maneuver assesses the potential for dislocation of a nondisplaced hip. The examiner adducts the flexed hip and gently pushes the thigh posteriorly in an effort to dislocate the femoral head (Fig. 677-2). In a positive test, the hip will be felt to slide out of the acetabulum. As the examiner

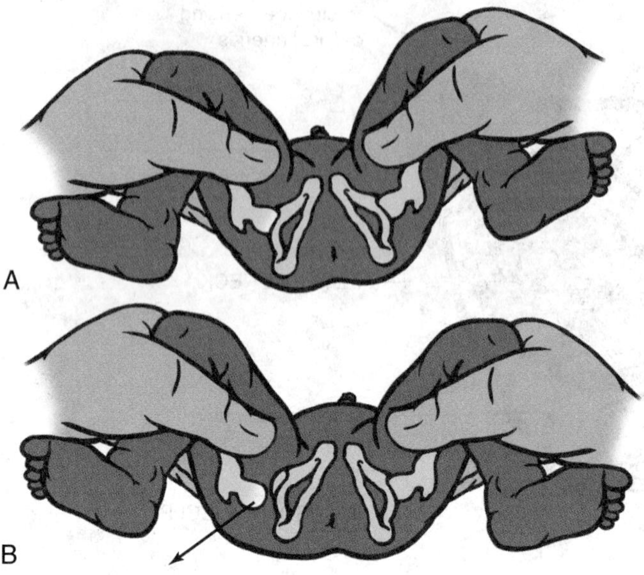

Figure 677-2. The Barlow's provocative test is performed with the patient's knees and hips flexed. *A,* Holding the patient's limbs gently, with the thigh in adduction, the examiner applies a posteriorly directed force. *B,* This test is positive in a dislocatable hip.

relaxes the proximal push, the hip can be felt to slip back into the acetabulum.

The **Ortolani** test is the reverse of Barlow test: The examiner attempts to reduce a dislocated hip (Fig. 677-3). The examiner grasps the child's thigh between the thumb and index finger and, with the 4th and 5th fingers, lifts the greater trochanter while simultaneously abducting the hip. When the test is positive, the femoral head will slip into the socket with a delicate "clunk" that is palpable but usually not audible. It should be a gentle, nonforced maneuver.

A **hip click** is the high-pitched sensation (or sound) felt at the very end of abduction during testing for DDH with Barlow and

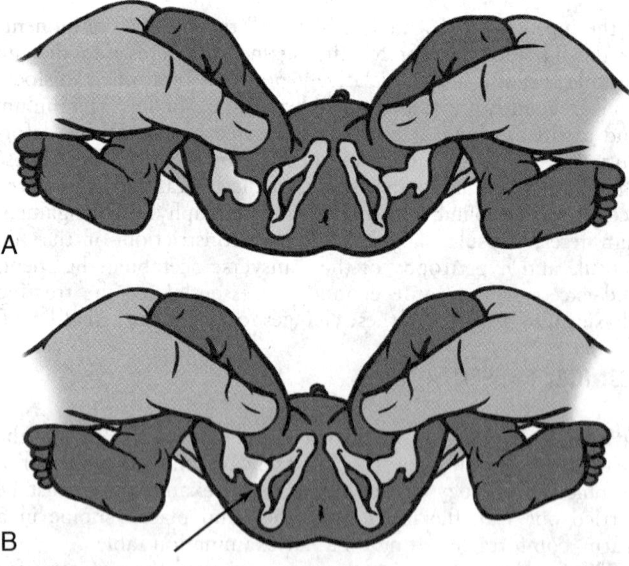

Figure 677-3. The Ortolani maneuver is the sign of the ball of the femoral head moving in and out of the acetabulum. *A,* The examiner holds the patient's thigh and gently abducts the hip while lifting the greater trochanter with two fingers. *B,* When the test is positive, the dislocated femoral head will fall back into the acetabulum with a palpable 'clunk' as the hip is abducted.

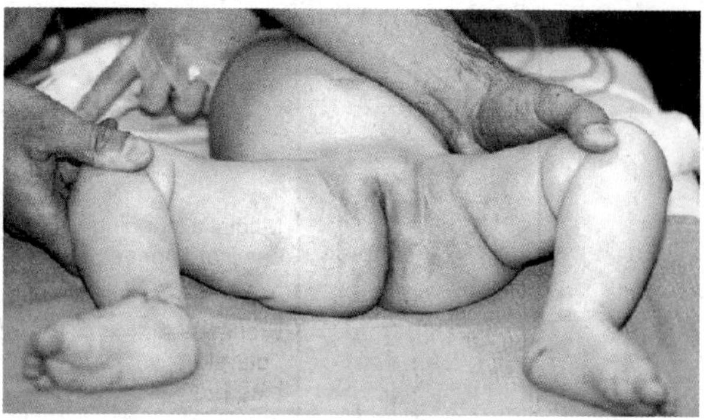

Figure 677-4. Asymmetry of thigh folds in a child with developmental dysplasia of the hip.

Ortolani maneuvers. Classically, a hip click is differentiated from a hip "clunk," which is felt as the hip goes in and out of joint. Hip clicks usually originate in the ligamentum teres or occasionally in the fascia lata or psoas tendon and do not indicate a significant hip abnormality.

THE INFANT. As the baby enters the 2nd and 3rd mo of life, other signs of DDH appear.

When the hip is no longer reducible, specific physical findings appear, including limited hip abduction, apparent shortening of the thigh, proximal location of the greater trochanter, asymmetry of the gluteal or thigh folds (Fig. 677-4), and pistoning of the hip. Limitation of abduction is the most reliable sign of a dislocated hip.

Shortening of the thigh, the *Galeazzi sign,* is best appreciated by placing both hips in 90 degrees of flexion and comparing the height of the knees, looking for asymmetry (Fig. 677-5). Asymmetry of thigh and gluteal skin folds may be present in 10% of normal infants but is suggestive of DDH. Another helpful test is the *Klisic test,* in which the examiner places the 3rd finger over the greater trochanter and the index finger of the same hand on the anterior superior iliac spine. In a normal hip, an imaginary line drawn between the two fingers points to the umbilicus. In the dislocated hip, the trochanter is elevated, and the line projects halfway between the umbilicus and the pubis (Fig. 677-6).

THE WALKING CHILD. The walking child often presents to the physician after the family has noticed a limp, a waddling gait, or a leg-length discrepancy. The affected side appears shorter than the normal extremity, and the child will toe-walk on the affected side. The Trendelenburg sign is positive in these children, and a Trendelenburg gait is usually observed. As in the younger child, there is limited abduction on the affected side and the knees are at different levels when the hips are flexed (the Galeazzi sign). Excessive lordosis, which develops secondary to altered hip mechanics, is common and is often the presenting complaint.

RADIOGRAPHIC FINDINGS

ULTRASONOGRAPHY. In infants younger than 6 mo of age, the acetabulum and proximal femur are predominantly cartilaginous and not visible on plain radiographs and are best visualized with ultrasonography. In addition to morphologic assessment, ultrasonography provides dynamic assessment about the stability of the hip joint (Fig. 677-7*A* and *B*). The ultrasound examination can be used to monitor acetabular development, particularly of infants in Pavlik harness treatment; this method can minimize the number of radiographs taken and may allow the clinician to detect failure of treatment earlier.

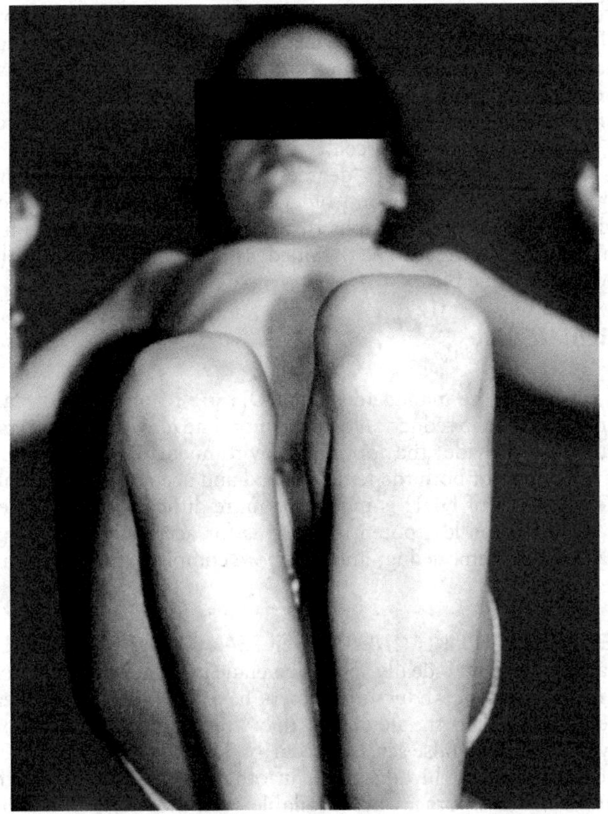

Figure 677-5. Positive Galeazzi sign noted in a case of untreated developmental dysplasia of the hip.

RADIOGRAPHY. Radiographs are recommended for an infant once the proximal femoral epiphysis ossifies, usually by 4–6 mo. In infants this age, the radiographic examination has proven to be more effective, less costly, and less operator dependent than an ultrasound examination. An anteroposterior view of the pelvis

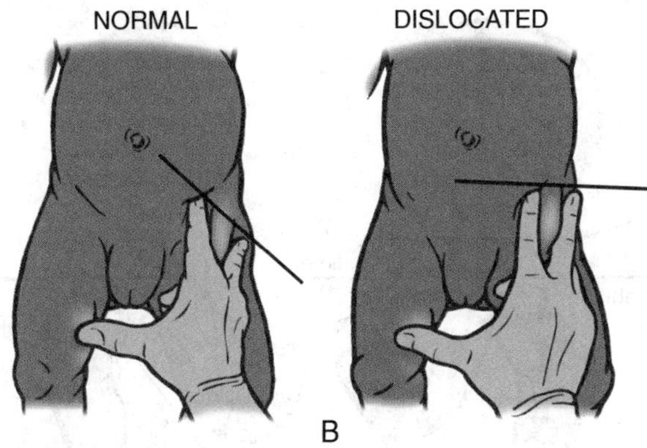

Figure 677-6. Klisic test. *A,* In a normal hip, an imaginary line drawn down through the tip of an index finger placed on the patient's iliac crest and the tip of the long finger placed on the patient's greater trochanter should point to the umbilicus. *B,* In a dislocated hip, this line drawn through the two fingertips runs below the umbilicus because the greater trochanter is abnormally high.

can be interpreted through the use of several classic lines drawn on it (Fig. 677-8*A* through C).

The *Hilgenreiner line* is a horizontal line drawn through the top of both triradiate cartilages (the clear area in the depth of the acetabulum). The *Perkins line,* a vertical line through the most lateral ossified margin of the roof of the acetabulum, is perpendicular to the Hilgenreiner line. The ossific nucleus of the femoral head should be located in the medial lower quadrant of the intersection of these two lines. The *Shenton line* is a curved line drawn from the medial aspect of the femoral neck to the lower border of the superior pubic ramus. In a child with normal hips, this line is a continuous contour. In a child with DDH, this line consists of two separate arcs and therefore is described as "broken." The *acetabular index* is the angle formed between the Hilgenreiner line and a line drawn from the depth of the acetabular socket to the most lateral ossified margin of the roof of the acetabulum. This angle measures the development of the osseous roof of the

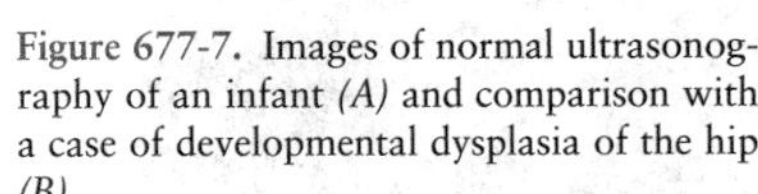

Figure 677-7. Images of normal ultrasonography of an infant *(A)* and comparison with a case of developmental dysplasia of the hip *(B).*

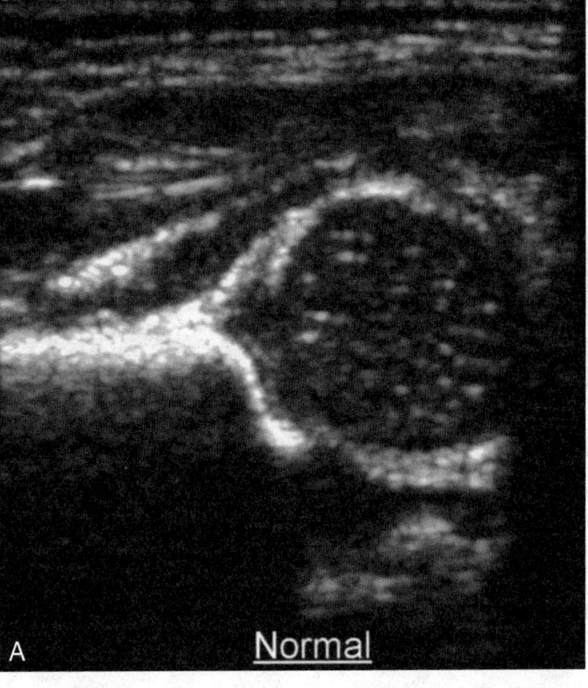

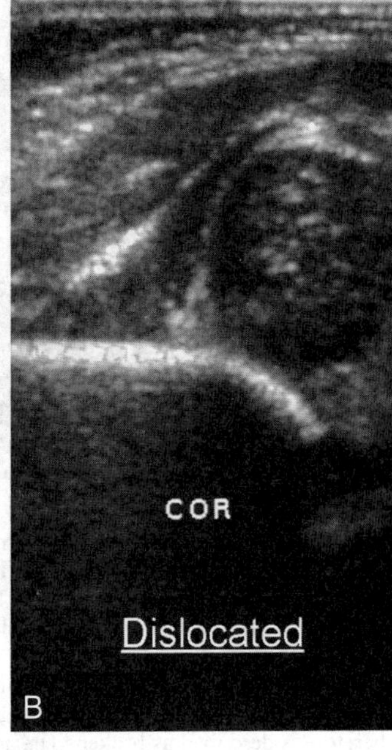

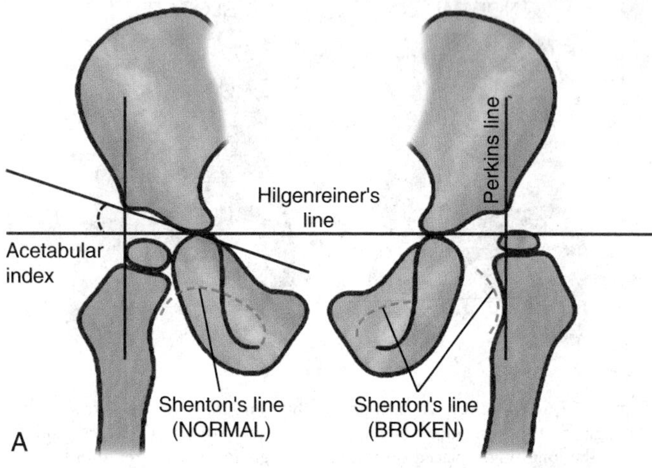

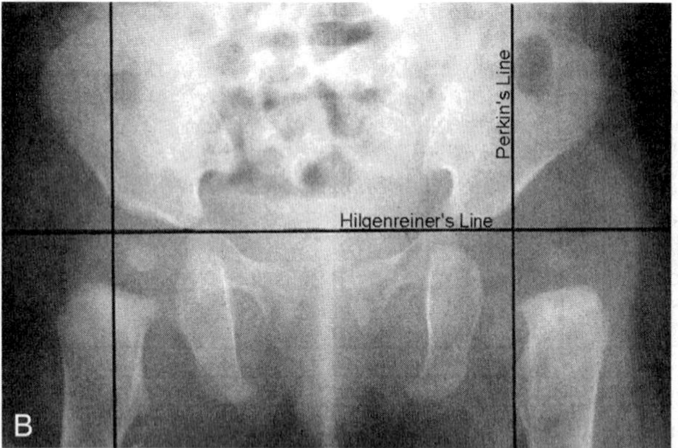

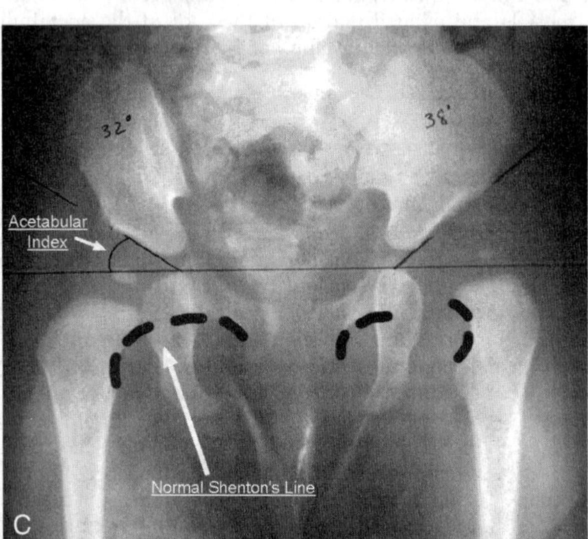

Figure 677-8. Radiographic measurements are useful in evaluating DDH. Hilgenreiner's line is drawn through the triradiate cartilages. Perkins line is drawn perpendicular to Hilgenreiner's line at the lateral edge of the acetabulum. The ossific nucleus of the femoral head should be located in the medial lower quadrant of the intersection of these two lines. Shenton's line curves along the femoral metaphysis and connects smoothly to the inner margin of the pubis. In a child with DDH, this line consists of two separate arcs and therefore is described as broken. The acetabular index is the angle between a line drawn along the margin of the acetabulum and Hilgenreiner's line; in normal newborns, it averages 27.5 degrees and decreases with age.

acetabulum. In the newborn, the acetabular index can be up to 40 degrees; by 4 mo in the normal infant, it should be no more than 30 degrees. In the older child, the *center-edge angle* is a useful measure of hip position. This angle is formed at the juncture of the Perkins line and a line connecting the lateral margin of the acetabulum to the center of the femoral head. In children 6–13 yr old, an angle >19 degrees has been reported as normal, while in children 14 yr and older, an angle >25 degrees is considered normal. Radiographs of the hip in abduction and internal rotation should also be obtained, as these views show whether the hip is reducible.

TREATMENT

The goals in the management of DDH are to obtain and maintain a concentric reduction of the femoral head within the acetabulum to provide the optimal environment for the normal development of both the femoral head and acetabulum. The later the diagnosis of DDH is made, the more difficult it is to achieve these goals, the less potential there is for acetabular and proximal femoral remodeling, and the more complex are the required treatments.

NEWBORNS AND INFANTS YOUNGER THAN 6 MONTHS OF AGE. The diagnosis of DDH ideally should be made in the newborn nursery. Triple diapers or abduction diapers have no place in the treatment of DDH in the newborn; they are usually ineffective and give the family a false sense of security. The Pavlik harness is used for all degrees of hip dysplasia in otherwise normal newborns. Although other braces are available (von Rosen splint, Frejka pillow), the Pavlik harness remains the most commonly used device worldwide (Fig. 677-9). Infants between 1 and 6 mo of age with hip dysplasia, subluxation, or dislocation are readily managed with the Pavlik harness. By maintaining the Ortolani-positive hip in a Pavlik harness on a full-time basis for 6 wk, hip

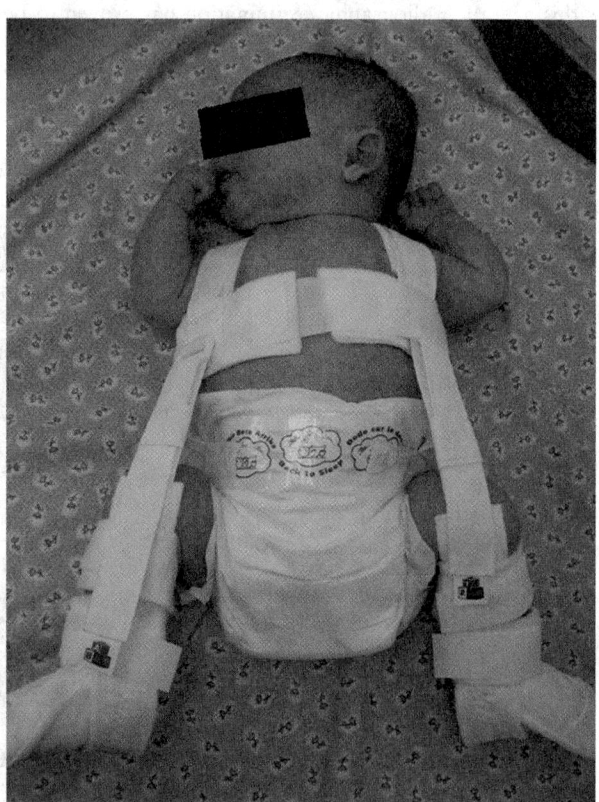

Figure 677-9. Photograph of a Pavlik harness.

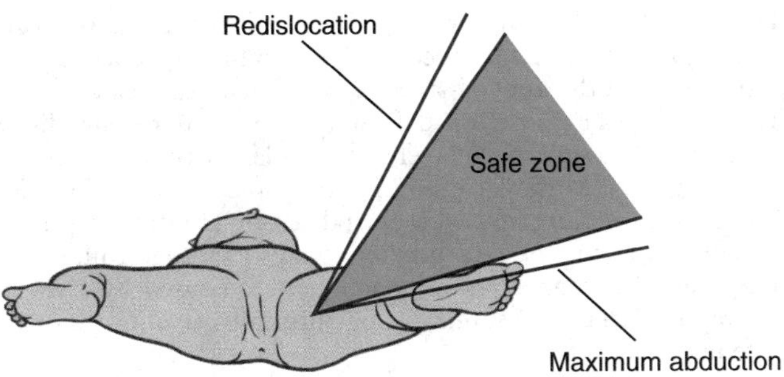

Figure 677-10. Diagrammatic illustration of the safe zone of Ramsey.

instability resolves in 95% of cases. After 6 mo of age, the failure rate for the Pavlik harness is >50% because it is difficult to maintain the increasingly active and crawling child in the harness. Frequent examinations and readjustments are necessary to ensure that the harness is applied correctly.

CHILDREN 6 MONTHS TO 2 YEARS OF AGE. The principal goals in the treatment of the late-diagnosed patient are to obtain and maintain reduction of the hip without damaging the femoral head.

Closed reductions are performed in the operating room under general anesthesia. The hip is moved to determine the range of motion in which it remains reduced. This is compared to the maximal range of motion to construct a "safe zone" (Fig. 677-10). An arthrogram obtained at the time of reduction is very helpful for evaluating the depth and stability of the reduction (Fig. 677-11). The reduction is maintained in a well-molded plaster cast, with the "human position" of moderate flexion and abduction being the preferred position. After the procedure, single-cut CT, MRI, or ultrasonography may be used to confirm the reduction. Twelve weeks after closed reduction, the plaster cast is removed and replaced by an abduction orthotic device to be used on a full-time basis for 2 mo until acetabular development is normal. Failure to obtain a stable hip with a closed reduction indicates the need for an *open reduction*. In patients younger than 2 yr of age, a secondary acetabular or femoral procedure is rarely required. The potential for acetabular development after closed or open reduction is excellent and continues for 4–8 yr after the procedure.

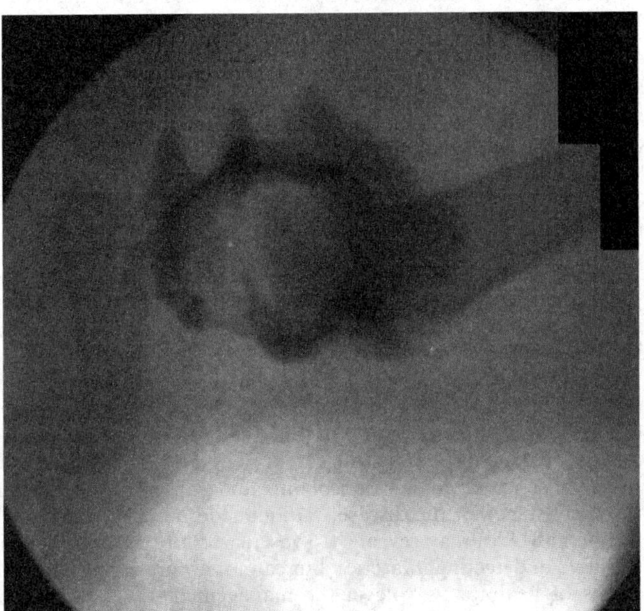

Figure 677-11. Arthrogram of a reduced hip for evaluating the stability of reduction.

Traction followed by closed or open reduction is recommended by some for treatment of older infants with a dislocated hip for which attempted reduction with the Pavlik harness has failed or for children older than 9 mo of age.

CHILDREN OLDER THAN 2 YEARS OF AGE. Treatment of children between 2 and 6 yr of age with hip dislocation is more challenging. In a child older than 2 yr of age, open reduction is usually necessary.

In children older than 3 yr of age, femoral shortening to avoid excessive pressure on the proximal femur gives far lower rates of proximal femoral growth disturbance than does preliminary traction followed by open reduction. For children between 2 and 3 yr of age, because the potential for acetabular development is markedly diminished, a concomitant acetabular procedure may be needed in conjunction with the open reduction. Children older than 3 yr of age at reduction usually need an acetabular procedure to adequately cover the femoral head.

SEQUELAE AND COMPLICATIONS. The most important complication of DDH is avascular necrosis of the CFE. Reduction of the femoral head under pressure or in extreme abduction may result in occlusion of the epiphyseal vessels and produce either partial or total infarction of the CFE. Revascularization soon follows, but if the physis is severely damaged, abnormal growth and development may occur. The hip, then, is most vulnerable to this complication before 4–6 mo when the ossific nucleus develops. Management, as previously outlined, is designed to minimize this complication. Using these various appropriate treatments, the incidence of avascular necrosis for DDH is reduced to between 5% and 15%. Other complications in DDH include redislocation, residual subluxation, acetabular dysplasia, and postoperative complications, including wound infections.

677.2 • Transient Monoarticular Synovitis (Toxic Synovitis)

Transient monoarticular synovitis or toxic synovitis of the hip is a common cause of limping in a normal child. It is characterized by acute onset of pain, limping, and mild restriction of motion, specifically abduction and internal rotation. However, septic arthritis and osteomyelitis of the hip must be excluded before such a diagnosis can be confirmed (see Chapters 683 and 684). The cause of toxic synovitis is uncertain; some possible causes are active or recent systemic viral syndrome, trauma, and allergic hypersensitivity.

CLINICAL MANIFESTATIONS. Although transient monoarticular synovitis can occur in all age groups, it is most prevalent in children between 3 and 8 yr of age, with a mean onset at 6 yr. About 70% of all affected children have had a nonspecific upper respiratory tract infection 7–14 days before the onset of symptoms. This acute onset of symptoms typically consists of pain in the groin, anterior thigh, or knee, as well as nontraumatic anterior thigh or knee pain, which may be referred from the hip. These children are usually ambulatory; the hip is not held flexed, abducted, or laterally rotated unless a significant effusion is present. Children with transient monoarticular synovitis walk with a painful, limping gait. In addition, they are often afebrile or maintain a low-grade fever below 38°C. Their laboratory values are relatively normal, but on occasion a mild elevation in the erythrocyte sedimentation rate is observed. While arthrocentesis produces normal results, a joint effusion of 1–3 mL is common.

RADIOGRAPHIC EVALUATION. Anteroposterior and Lauenstein (frog) lateral radiographs of the pelvis may be acquired and are usually found to be normal. Ultrasonography of the hip illustrates a hip joint effusion. Ultrasonography-guided hip joint fluid aspiration may be necessary to reveal whether a septic hip is present in some clinical cases. Technetium bone scan or MRI is also extremely valuable in ruling out the presence of certain lesions including septic arthritis, tumor, fracture, slipped CFE (SCFE), or early Legg-Calvé-Perthes disease (LCPD). High fever, refusal to walk, and elevations of the erythrocyte sedimentation rate, serum C-reactive protein, and white blood cell counts are high-risk criteria for septic arthritis.

TREATMENT. The treatment of transient monoarticular synovitis of the hip is symptomatic. Recommended therapies include activity limitation and relief of weight bearing until the pain subsides. Anti-inflammatory agents and analgesics may shorten the duration of pain. Most children recover completely within 3 wks.

677.3 • Legg-Calvé-Perthes Disease

Legg-Calvé-Perthes Disease (LCPD) is a femoral head disorder of unknown etiology that involves temporary interruption of the blood supply to the bony nucleus of the proximal femoral epiphysis, leading to impairment of the epiphyseal growth and femoral head deformity.

ETIOLOGY

The etiology of LCPD remains unknown: Infection, trauma, and transient synovitis have been proposed but unsubstantiated. Factors leading to thrombophilia, an increased tendency to develop thrombosis and hypofibrinolysis, and a reduced tendency to lyse thrombi have been identified. Factor V Leiden mutation, protein C and S deficiency, lupus anticoagulant, anticardiolipin antibodies, antitrypsin, and plasminogen activator may play a role in the abnormal clotting mechanism.

Children with LCPD have delayed skeletal maturation and are shorter than normal. Abnormalities of thyroid hormone and insulin-like growth factors have been reported. Other associated factors include hyperactivity or attention-deficit disorder, hereditary influences, and environmental influences (including nutrition). Histologic findings in the CFE reveal various stages of bone necrosis and repair. Two possible pathways for the bone necrosis have been proposed; the vascular changes may be the primary event or events or there may be a primary disorder of epiphyseal cartilage, with resulting collapse and necrosis.

Avascular necrosis of the femoral head, unrelated to LCPD, may be sporadic but occasionally occurs as an autosomal dominant disorder. Most present as adults, but 10–20% may begin when younger than 20 yr of age. Familial cases may be due to a mutation of the type II collagen gene.

PATHOGENESIS OF DEFORMITY

The deformity can occur by four mechanisms in LCPD:

A growth disturbance in CFE and physis; a central arrest of the physis leads to a short neck (coxa breva) and trochanteric overgrowth, whereas a lateral physeal arrest tilts the head externally and into valgus with trochanteric overgrowth.

The second mechanism for deformity involves the repair process itself; the deformity can occur related to the asymmetric repair process and the applied stresses on the femoral head.

The third mechanism for deformity is related to the disease process. The superficial layers of articular cartilage continue to "overgrow" as they are nourished by the synovial fluid. The deeper layers are, however, devitalized by the disease process, leading to epiphyseal trabecular collapse and deformity.

The fourth mechanism is iatrogenic and is caused by trying to contain, either nonsurgically or surgically, a noncontainable femoral head.

EPIDEMIOLOGY

The overall incidence of LCPD in the United States is about 1/1,200 children. LCPD is more common in boys than in girls by a ratio of 4 or 5 to 1. The peak incidence of the disease is between the ages 4 and 8 yr; LCPD has been reported in patients of ages 2–12 yr. Bilateral involvement may be seen in about 10% of the patients, but the CFEs are usually in different stages of collapse.

CLINICAL PRESENTATION

The most common presenting symptom is a **limp** of varying duration. Pain, if present, is usually activity related and may be localized in the groin or referred to the anteromedial thigh or knee region. Failure to recognize that thigh or knee pain in the child may be secondary to hip pathology may cause further delay in the diagnosis. Less commonly, the onset of the disease may be much more acute and may be associated with a failure to ambulate. Parents often report that symptoms were initiated by a traumatic event.

PHYSICAL EXAMINATION

Antalgic gait may be particularly prominent after strenuous activity at the end of the day. Hip motion, primarily internal rotation and abduction, is limited. Early in the course of the disease, the limited abduction is secondary to synovitis and muscle spasm in the adductor group; however, with time and the subsequent deformities that may develop, the limitation of abduction may become permanent. A mild hip flexion contracture of 10–20 degrees may be present. Atrophy of the muscles of the thigh, calf, or buttock from disuse secondary to pain may be evident. There might be an apparent lower extremity length inequality because of an adduction contracture or true shortening on the involved site because of femoral head collapse or growth inhibition. The classic portrait of a child with LCPD is a small, thin, extremely active child who is always running and jumping.

RADIOGRAPHIC FINDINGS

Routine plain radiographs are the primary imaging tool for LCPD. Anteroposterior and Lauenstein (frog) lateral views are used to diagnose, stage, provide prognosis, follow the course of the disease, and assess results (Fig. 677-12*A* and *B*). It is most important in following the course of the disease that all radiographs be viewed sequentially and compared with previous radiographs to assess the stage of the reparative process and to determine the constancy of the extent of epiphyseal involvement. In the absence of changes on plain radiographs, particularly in the early stages of the disease, radionuclide bone scanning with technetium-99m may reveal the avascularity of the CFE. MRI is sensitive in detecting infarction but cannot accurately portray the stages of healing. Its role in the management of LCPD is not defined. Arthrography may demonstrate any flattening of the femoral head and the hinge abduction phenomenon with abduction of the leg.

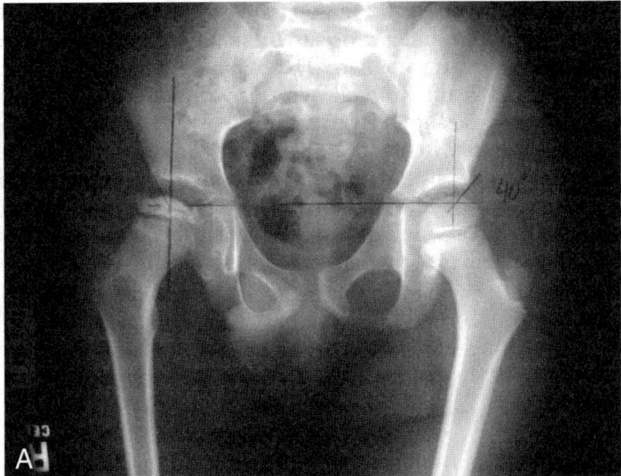

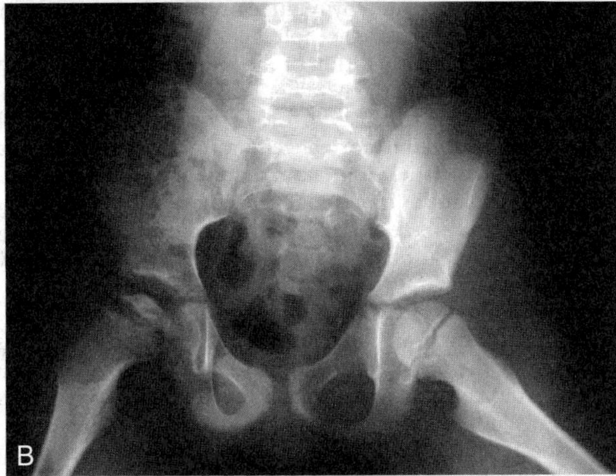

Figure 677-12. *A,* Anteroposterior radiograph of the pelvis shows epiphyseal fragmentation in the right hip, characteristic of the fragmentation phase of LCPD. *B,* The frog-leg lateral view demonstrates subchondral fracture, increased density of the femoral head, and some collapse.

RADIOGRAPHIC STAGES. LCPD has been divided into four radiographic stages: initial, fragmentation, reossification (or repair), and residual (or healed). In the initial stage, the radiographic changes include a decreased size of the ossification center, lateralization of the femoral head with widening of the medial joint space, a subchondral fracture, and physeal irregularity. In the fragmentation stage, the epiphysis appears fragmented, and there are areas of increased radiolucency and radiodensity. During the reossification stage, the bone density returns to normal by new (woven) bone formation. The residual stage is marked by the reossification of the femoral head, gradual remodeling of head shape until skeletal maturity, and remodeling of the acetabulum.

CLASSIFICATION SYSTEMS. *Catterall* proposed a four-group classification, based on the amount of CFE involvement and a set of radiographic "head at-risk" signs, with a high degree of interobserver variability. Group I hips have anterior CFE involvement of 25%, no sequestrum, and no metaphyseal abnormalities. Group II hips have up to 50% involvement, with a clear demarcation between involved and uninvolved segments. Metaphyseal cysts may be present. Group III hips display up to 75% involvement with a large sequestrum. In group IV, the entire femoral head is involved.

A two-group classification is based on the extent of the subchondral fracture, which corresponds to the amount of subsequent resorption. In *Salter-Thompson* group A, less than half of the femoral head is involved (Catterall groups I and II), and in group B, more than half of the femoral head is involved (Catterall groups III and III). The major determining factor between groups A and B is the presence or absence of a viable lateral column of the epiphysis. This intact lateral column (Catterall group II, group A) may shield the epiphysis from collapse and subsequent deformity.

A disadvantage of this classification is that not all patients are diagnosed early during the phase of the subchondral fracture.

The *Herring* lateral pillar classification is the most widely used radiographic classification system for helping to determine treatment and prognosis during the active stage of the disease (Fig. 677-13). Classification is based on several radiographs taken during the early fragmentation stage. The lateral pillar classification system for LCPD evaluates the shape of the femoral head epiphysis on anteroposterior radiograph of the hip. The head is divided into three sections or pillars. The lateral pillar occupies the lateral 15–30% of the head width, the central pillar about 50% of the head width, and the medial pillar 20–35% of the head width. The degree of involvement of the lateral pillar can be subdivided into three groups. In group A, the lateral pillar is radiographically normal. In group B, the lateral pillar has some lucency but >50% of the lateral pillar height is maintained. In group C, the lateral pillar is more lucent than in group B and <50% of the pillar height remains.

PROGNOSTIC FACTORS. Certain radiographic signs, known as "at-risk signs," are associated with poor results. These include the Gage sign, a radiolucency in the lateral epiphysis and metaphysis, calcification lateral to the epiphysis, lateral CFE subluxation, and a horizontal physis.

NATURAL HISTORY AND PROGNOSIS

From a prognostic standpoint, long-term follow-up studies of patients with LCPD show that most hips do well until 5th decade of life. Majority of the patients are active and pain free and have a good range of motion. The deformity and congruency at maturity and age at onset are the main prognostic factors for LCPD. Children who develop signs and symptoms before the age of 5 yr tend to recover without residual problems. Patients older than 9 yr of age at presentation usually have a poor prognosis. The remodeling potential is higher in younger children; the shape of the femoral head can improve significantly until maturity. The extent of CFE involvement and duration of the disease process are additional factors associated with a poor prognosis. Hips classified as Catterall groups III and IV, Salter-Thompson group B, and lateral pillar group C are at risk of a poor prognosis.

TREATMENT

The goal of treatment in LCPD is to create a spherical, well-covered femoral head with hip range of motion that is close to normal. The two main principles of treatment are maintenance

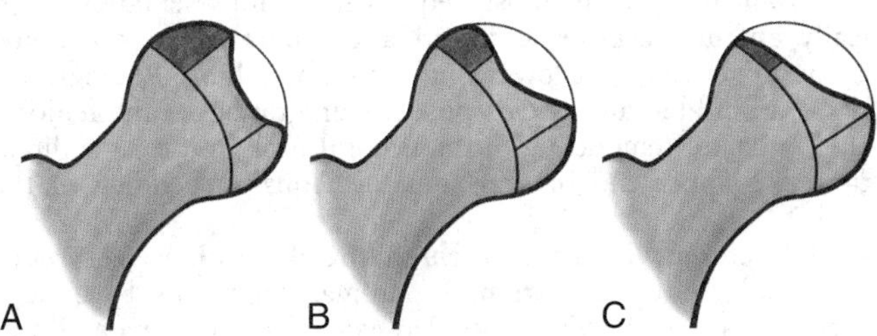

Figure 677-13. Lateral pillar classification for LCPD. *A,* There is no involvement of the lateral pillar. *B,* More than 50% of the lateral pillar height is maintained. C, Less than 50% of the lateral pillar height is maintained.

of range of motion and acetabular containment of the femoral head during the active period of the process.

The methods of treatment include observation or no treatment, intermittent symptomatic treatment, containment, late surgery for deformity, and late surgery for osteoarthritis.

NONOPERATIVE TREATMENT. The mainstay of treatment is nonoperative, specifically activity limitation and physical therapy to maintain hip range of motion. Patients with severe pain may benefit from a short trial of bed rest and traction. Abduction devices have been used to keep the femoral head contained in the acetabulum. The most widely used abduction orthosis is the Atlanta Scottish Rite orthosis. These devices were thought to provide for containment solely by abduction without fixed internal rotation. The devices are considered ineffective and are not commonly used.

OPERATIVE TREATMENT. Surgical containment may be approached from the femoral side, the acetabular side, or both sides of the hip joint. A *varus osteotomy* of the proximal femur is the most common procedure. *Pelvic osteotomies* in LCPD are divided into three categories: acetabular rotational osteotomies, shelf procedures, and medial displacement or Chiari osteotomies. Any of these procedures can be combined with a proximal femoral varus osteotomy when severe deformity of the femoral head cannot be contained by a pelvic or proximal femoral varus osteotomy alone.

677.4 • Slipped Capital Femoral Epiphysis

SCFE is a hip disorder that affects adolescents, most often between 12 and 15 yr of age, and involves the displacement of the CFE from the metaphysis through the zone of hypertrophy layer of the physeal plate.

CLASSIFICATION

SCFE may be classified temporally, according to onset of symptoms (acute, chronic, acute-on-chronic); functionally, according to patient's ability to bear weight (stable or unstable); or morphologically, as the extent of displacement of the femoral epiphysis relative to the neck (mild, moderate, or severe), as estimated by measurement on radiographic or CT images.

An **acute SCFE** has been characterized as one occurring in a patient with prodromal symptoms for ≤3 wk and should be distinguished from a purely traumatic separation of the epiphysis in a previously normal hip (a true Salter-Harris type I fracture). The patient with an acute slip will usually have some prodromal pain in the groin, thigh, or knee and will usually report a relatively minor injury (a twist or fall) that normally is not as sufficiently violent as to produce an acute fracture of this severity. Osteonecrosis is a significant and frequent complication of acute SCFE, with a reported incidence of 17–47%.

Chronic SCFE is the most frequent form of presentation. Typically, an adolescent presents with a few-month history of vague groin, upper thigh, or lower thigh pain and a limp. Radiographs show a variable amount of posterior migration of the femoral epiphysis and remodeling of the femoral neck in the same direction; the upper end of the femur develops a "bending of the neck."

The children with **acute-on-chronic SCFE** may have features of both ends of the spectrum. Prodromal symptoms have been present for >3 wk with a sudden exacerbation of pain. Radiographs demonstrate femoral neck remodeling and further displacement of the capital epiphysis beyond the remodeling point of the femoral neck.

The stability classification separates patients based on their ability to ambulate and is more useful in predicting prognosis and establishing a treatment plan. The SCFE is considered "stable" when the child is able to walk with or without crutches. A child with an "unstable" SCFE is unable to walk with or without crutches. Patients with unstable SCFEs have a much higher prevalence of osteonecrosis (up to 50%) compared to those with stable SCFEs (nearly 0%). This is most likely due to the vascular injury caused at the time of initial displacement. SCFE may also be categorized by the degree of displacement of the CFE on the femoral neck.

The head-shaft angle difference is <30 degrees in mild slips, between 30 and 60 degrees in moderate slips, and >60 degrees in severe slips, compared to the normal contralateral side.

ETIOLOGY

Mechanical factors created by relative or true femoral neck retroversion, the orientation of the capital epiphysis and the physis on the femoral neck, and alteration of the mechanical strength of the physis, periosteum, and the perichondral ring during adolescence have all been thought to play a role in the etiology of a slipped epiphysis. A decrease in normal femoral anteversion, an actual retroversion of the femoral neck, and a more oblique orientation of the physeal plate during adolescence have all been shown to be associated with increased shear force generation at the proximal femoral physeal plate and could be factors associated with physeal plate fatigue.

Obese children often have retroverted femoral necks that are directed more posteriorly than those of other children. Physiologic forces at the proximal femur generated by normal activities in obese patients can be of adequate magnitude to cause physeal fatigue. An endocrinologic etiology for a slipped epiphysis has been suspected, based on the common association of this condition with obesity and, at least in boys, hypogonadal features, and the fact that the condition most frequently manifests during the adolescent growth spurt. Additional evidence of an association with endocrine dysfunction is suggested by the frequent association of SCFE with primary and secondary hypothyroidism, panhypopituitarism, hypogonadal conditions, renal osteodystrophy, and growth hormone therapy. During puberty, growth hormone increases the physiologic activity of the physis, leading to rapid longitudinal growth of the physis resulting in a widened and weakened proximal femoral growth plate.

EPIDEMIOLOGY

The annual incidence of SCFE is 2/100,000 in the general population. Incidence has ranged from 0.2/100,000 in eastern Japan to 10.08/100,000 in the northeastern United States. The African-American and Polynesian populations have been reported to have an increased incidence of SCFE. Obesity is the most closely associated factor in the development of SCFE; about 65% of the patients are above the 90th percentile in weight-for-age profiles. There is a definite predilection for males to be affected more often than females and for the left hip to be affected more often than the right. Bilaterality has been reported in as many as 60% of cases, nearly half of which may be present at the time of initial presentation.

CLINICAL PRESENTATION

Patients with SCFE usually present with complaints of pain in the affected hip or groin, a change in hip range of motion, and a gait abnormality. Infrequently the patient will complain only of medial knee pain that may be referred to the knee via the obturator and femoral nerves.

The symptoms and physical findings vary according to whether the symptoms are chronic, acute-on-chronic, or acute; whether the slip is stable or unstable; with the severity of the resultant deformity; and with the coexistence of the complications of osteonecrosis or chondrolysis.

In *stable, chronic SCFE,* the patient describes intermittent pain in the groin, the medial thigh, or the anterior suprapatellar region of the knee. The pain is typically described as dull and vague and is exacerbated by physical activity such as running or sports. The onset of pain may be of several weeks' or several months' duration. The patient remains ambulatory, but does show an antalgic gait with associated limp. Physical examination of the affected hip reveals a restriction of internal rotation, abduction, and flexion. Commonly, the examiner will note that as the affected hip is flexed, the thigh tends to rotate into progressively more external rotation (knee-axilla sign; Fig. 677-14) and that flexion is limited.

Patients presenting with either *unstable acute* or *acute-on-chronic* slipped epiphysis will characteristically report the sudden onset of severe, fracture-like pain in the affected hip region, usually as the result of a relatively minor fall or twisting injury. The *acute form* manifests by the sudden onset of severe pain and hip dysfunction in a patient who was previously asymptomatic. Physical examination demonstrates the affected limb externally rotated and shortened with the patient refusing to bear weight.

Since approximately 25% of patients will have evidence of contralateral slip on initial presentation, the contralateral hip must always be carefully assessed both clinically and radiographically by the treating physician.

RADIOGRAPHIC FINDINGS

RADIOGRAPHS. Plain radiography in anteroposterior and lateral views is the primary and often the only imaging study needed to evaluate a slipped epiphysis. Common radiographic findings include widening and irregularity of the physis, a decrease in epiphyseal height in the center of the acetabulum, a crescent-shaped area of increased density in the proximal portion of the femoral neck, and the "blanch sign of Steel" corresponding to the double density created from the anteriorly displaced femoral neck overlying the femoral head.

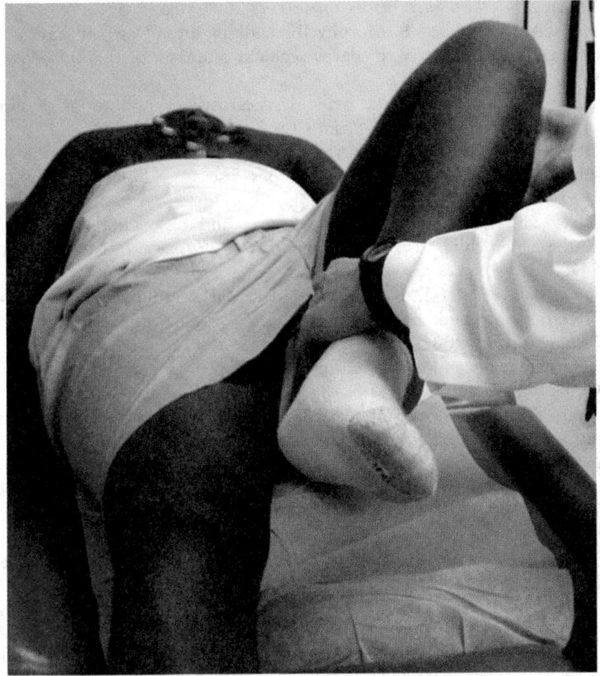

Figure 677-14. Progressive external rotation noted with flexion: the knee-axilla sign.

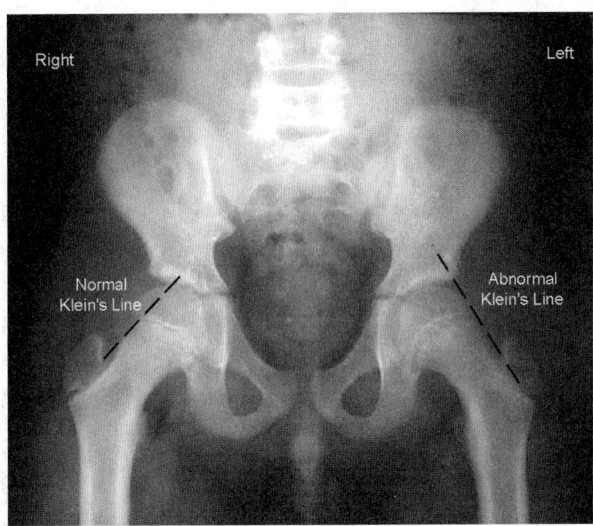

Figure 677-15. Illustration of the Klein line.

In an unaffected patient, the Klein line, a straight line drawn along the superior cortex of the femoral neck on anteroposterior radiograph, intersects the lateral capital epiphysis. As progressive displacement of the epiphysis occurs in SCFE, the amount of the Klein line that intersects the epiphysis decreases, compared with the uninvolved hip, and eventually the line fully misses intersection with the proximal femoral epiphysis (Fig. 677-15). A true lateral (cross-table lateral) radiographic view of the hip better defines the extent of posterior displacement of the femoral epiphysis.

COMPUTED TOMOGRAPHY. CT can be used to confirm epiphyseal displacement and accurately measure the amount of displacement in patients with symptoms suggestive of an SCFE but without documentation on plain radiographs.

TECHNETIUM 99M BONE SCAN. Bone scanning will show increased uptake in the capital femoral physis of an involved hip, decreased uptake in the presence of osteonecrosis, and increased uptake in the joint space in the presence of chondrolysis.

TREATMENT

Treatment can be divided into three categories: treatment to prevent further slippage, treatment to reduce the degree of slippage, and salvage treatment.

TREATMENT TO PREVENT FURTHER SLIPPAGE. Prevention of further slippage can be accomplished by spica cast immobilization, in situ metallic pin or screw fixation, and bone graft epiphysiodesis. The term "in situ" implies that no effort is made to reduce the displacement between the epiphysis and femoral neck. The goal of in situ pinning is to stabilize the capital epiphysis to the femoral neck to prevent further slippage (Fig. 677-16).

Following fixation, radiographic confirmation that the fixation device has not penetrated the joint space is mandatory. By adhering to the treatment guidelines and principles, almost all SCFEs should be able to be stabilized with percutaneous placement of a single 6.5- to 7.5-mm cannulated screw. In situ pin and screw fixation of SCFE accelerates closure of the affected physeal plate.

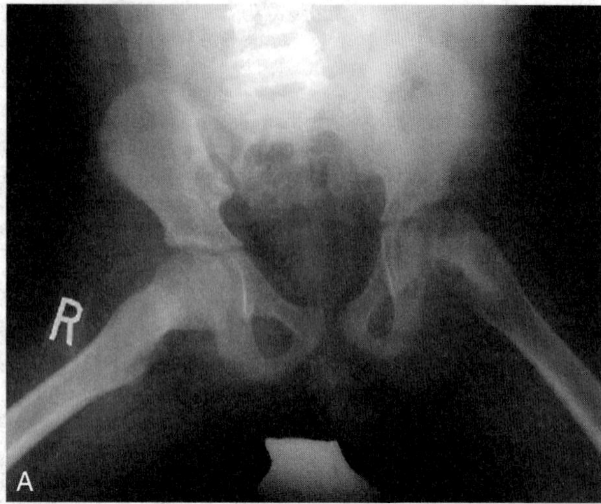

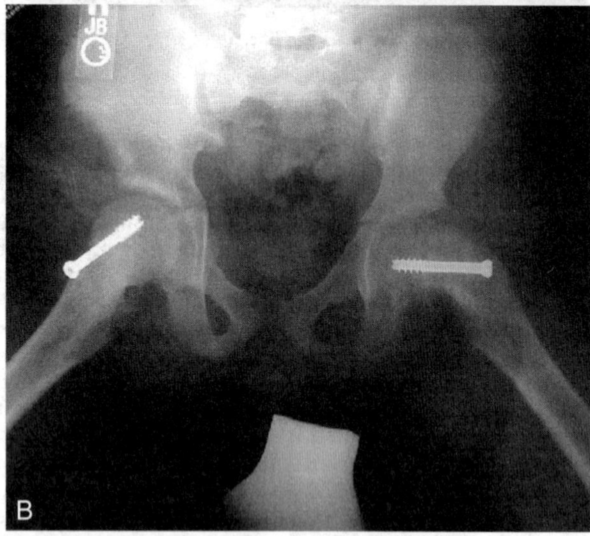

Figure 677-16. Preoperative *(A)* and postoperative *(B)* radiographs demonstrating the in situ pinning in a case of slipped capital femoral epiphysis.

TREATMENT TO REDUCE THE DEGREE OF SLIPPAGE. Techniques to reduce the degree of slip include closed manipulation prior to physeal plate stabilization and osteotomies of the proximal femur, performed either concurrently with physeal stabilization or after physeal closure. Osteotomies about the proximal femur in SCFE are designed as realignment procedures through which restoration of a more normal relation among the femoral head, the femoral neck and shaft, and the acetabulum can be achieved.

SALVAGE PROCEDURES. If the femoral head becomes severely deformed and the joint becomes stiff and painful as a result of osteonecrosis or chondrolysis, salvage procedures are indicated to relieve pain and improve function.

Hip arthrodesis is recommended in adolescents and young adults.

PROPHYLACTIC PINNING OF THE CONTRALATERAL HIP

The prevalence of contralateral slip, even in an asymptomatic patient, has led many to recommend prophylactic pinning. In patients who have SCFE associated with known metabolic and endocrine disorders, in which the risk of a contralateral slip is extremely high, prophylactic pinning of the contralateral hip may be appropriate.

COMPLICATIONS

Osteonecrosis and chondrolysis are the two most serious complications of SCFE. Osteonecrosis, or avascular necrosis, usually occurs as a result of injury to the retinacular vessels. This can be caused by an initial force of injury, particularly in unstable slips, forced manipulation of an acute or unstable SCFE, compression from intracapsular hematoma, or as a direct injury during surgery. Partial forms of osteonecrosis may also appear following internal fixation; this can be caused by a disruption of the intraepiphyseal blood vessels. Chondrolysis, on the other hand, is an acute dissolution of articular cartilage in the hip. While there are no clear causes of this complication, it is believed to be associated with more severe slips, occur more frequently among African Americans and females, and be associated with pins or screws protruding out of the femoral head.

Catterall A: The natural history of Perthes disease. *J Bone Joint Surg Br* 1971;53:37–53.

Dobbs MT, Weinstein SL: Natural history and long-term outcomes of slipped capital femoral epiphysis. *Am Acad Orthop Surg Instr Course Lect* 2001;50:571–575.

Erol B, Dormans JP: Hip disorders. In Dormans JP (editor): *Pediatric Orthopedics: Core Knowledge in Orthopedics,* Philadelphia, Mosby, 2005, pp 224–264.

Guille JT, Pizzutillo PD, MacEwen GD: Developmental dysplasia of the hip from birth to six months. *J Am Acad Orthop Surg* 2000;8:232–242.

Hamer AJ: Pain in the hip and knee. *Br Med J* 2004;328:1067–1069.

Haynes DJ: Developmental dysplasia of the hip: Etiology, pathogenesis and examination and physical findings in the newborn. *Am Acad Orthop Surg Instr Course Lect* 2001;50:535–540.

Hennrikus WL: Developmental dysplasia of the hip: Diagnosis and treatment in children younger than 6 months. *Pediatr Ann* 1999;28:740–746.

Herring JA, Neustadt JB, Williams JJ, et al: The lateral pillar classification of Legg-Calvé-Perthes disease. *J Pediatr Orthop* 1992;12:143–150.

Kocher MS, Zurakowski D, Kasser JR: Differentiating between septic arthritis and transient synovitis of the hip in children: An evidence-based clinical prediction algorithm. *J Bone Joint Surg Am* 1999;81:1662–1670.

Liu YF, Chen WM, Lin YF, et al: Type II collagen gene variants and inherited osteonecrosis of the femoral head. *N Engl J Med* 2005;352:2294–2301.

Loder RT, Aronsson DD, Dobbs MT, et al: Slipped capital femoral epiphysis. *Am Acad Orthop Surg Instr Course Lect* 2001;50:555–570.

Lowry CA, Donoghue VB, Murphy JF: Auditing hip ultrasound screening of infants at increased risk of developmental dysplasia of the hip. *Arch Dis Child* 2005;90:579–581.

Lubicky JP: Chondrolysis and avascular necrosis: Complications of slipped capital femoral epiphysis. *J Pediatr Orthop* 1996;5:162–167.

Martinez AG, Weinstein SL, Dietz FR: The weight-bearing abduction brace for the treatment of Legg-Calvé-Perthes disease. *J Bone Joint Surg Am* 1992;74:12–21.

Moseley CF: Developmental hip dysplasia and dislocation: Management of the older child. *Am Acad Orthop Surg Instr Course Lect* 2001;50: 547–553.

Noonan KJ, Price CT, Kupiszewski SJ, et al: Results of femoral varus osteotomy in children older than 9 years of age with Perthes disease. *J Pediatr Orthop* 2001;21:198–204.

Reynolds RA: Diagnosis and treatment of slipped capital femoral epiphysis. *Curr Opin Pediatr* 1999;11:80–83.

Roovers EA, Boere-Boonekamp MM, Castelein RM, et al: Effectiveness of ultrasound screening for developmental dysplasia of the hip. *Arch Dis Child Fetal Neonatal Ed* 2005;90:F25–F30.

Roy DR: Current concepts in Legg-Calvé-Perthes disease. *Pediatr Ann* 1999;28:748–752.

Tamai J, Erol B, Dormans, JP: Hip disorders. In Dormans JP, Bell, LM (editors): *Pediatric Orthopedics and Sports Medicine: The Requisites in Pediatrics*. St. Louis, MO, Mosby, 2004, pp 175–212.

Thompson GH, Price CT, Roy D, et al: Legg-Calvé-Perthes disease: Current concepts. *Am Acad Orthop Surg Instr Course Lect* 2002;51:367–384.

US Preventive Services Task Force: Screening for developmental dysplasia of the hip: recommendation statement. *Pediatrics* 2006;117:898–902.

Warner WC Jr, Beaty JH, Canale ST: Chondrolysis after slipped capital femoral epiphysis. *J Pediatr Orthop* 1996;5:168–172.

Willis RB: Developmental dysplasia of the hip: Assessment and treatment before walking age. *Am Acad Orthop Surg Instr Course Lect* 2001;50:541–545.
Woolacott NF, Puhan MA, Steurer J, Kleijnen J: Ultrasonography in screening for developmental dysplasia of the hip in newborns: Systemic review. *Br Med J* 2005;330:1413–1415.

Chapter 678 ■ The Spine

David A. Spiegel, Harish S. Hosalkar, and John P. Dormans

Abnormalities of the spine may be present at birth (congenital) or may evolve during childhood or adolescence (developmental). While alterations in spinal alignment are of cosmetic concern to the patient and family, some progressive curvatures may be associated with cardiopulmonary dysfunction, pain, and a loss of sitting balance (nonambulators). Early detection helps not only to facilitate treatment, but also to identify and address coexisting visceral and/or neurologic problems that may be associated with the spinal deformity. A classification of common spinal abnormalities is presented in Table 678-1.

Scoliosis is a three-dimensional deformity that is most commonly described as a lateral curvature of the spine in the frontal plane. While most cases of scoliosis have no demonstrable etiology, and are termed idiopathic, scoliosis may be congenital or may be associated with a host of neuromuscular diseases or syndromes. Scoliosis may also be secondary to an infrapelvic deformity such as a leg-length discrepancy or a soft-tissue contracture around the hip (abduction or adduction).

In the lateral (sagittal) plane, the spine has normal curvatures in the cervical (lordotic or convex anteriorly), thoracic (kyphosis or convex posteriorly), and lumbar (lordosis) regions to maintain the relationships of body segments relative to the forces of gravity. Maintaining the center of gravity is important for balance and to minimize the amount of muscular activity (conserve energy) required to maintain an upright posture. A vertical (gravity) line dropped from the 7th cervical vertebra should normally fall through the posterosuperior corner of the sacrum. Disorders of sagittal alignment include thoracic hyperkyphosis and lumbar hyperlordosis. **Thoracic hyperkyphosis** is seen most commonly in patients with **postural kyphosis** or with **Scheuermann disease.** Lumbar hyperlordosis may be associated with spondylolisthesis or may be secondary to hip flexion contractures.

TABLE 678-1. Classification of Spinal Deformities

SCOLIOSIS
Idiopathic
Infantile
Juvenile
Adolescent
Congenital
Failure of formation
Wedge vertebrae
Hemivertebrae
Failure of segmentation
Unilateral bar
Block vertebra
Mixed
Neuromuscular
Neuropathic diseases
Upper motor neuron
Cerebral palsy
Spinocerebellar degeneration (Freidreich ataxia, Charcot Marie-Tooth disease)
Syringomyelia
Spinal cord tumor
Spinal cord trauma
Lower motor neuron
Poliomyelitis
Spinal muscular atrophy
Myopathies
Duchenne muscular dystrophy
Arthrogryposis
Other muscular dystrophies
Syndromes
Neurofibromatosis
Marfan syndrome
Compensatory
Leg-length discrepancy
KYPHOSIS
Postural kyphosis (flexible)
Scheuermann disease
Congenital kyphosis
Failure of formation
Failure of segmentation
Mixed

Adapted from the Terminology Committee, Scoliosis Research Society: A glossary of scoliosis terms. *Spine* 1976;1:57.

678.1 • Idiopathic Scoliosis

ETIOLOGY AND EPIDEMIOLOGY. The etiology of idiopathic scoliosis is unknown and is likely multifactorial. Genetics plays a role, and sex-linked dominant, autosomal dominant, and multifactorial inheritance have been suggested. A positive family history does not help to predict the behavior of an individual curve. Abnormalities identified in connective tissue, muscle, and bone appear to be secondary. Melatonin and calmodulin may have indirect effects; neurologic factors are also important. Subtle changes in vestibular, ocular, and proprioceptive function have been documented, suggesting that abnormal equilibrium may play a role.

Idiopathic scoliosis is classified according to the age at onset, including infantile (rare, birth to 3 yr), juvenile (3–10 yr), and adolescent (11 yr and older). Adolescent idiopathic scoliosis is most common (≈70%). The prevalence of scoliosis (>10 degrees curvature) is ≈2–3%; however approximately 0.3% will have a curve in excess of 20 degrees. While the incidence is roughly equal in girls and boys for small curves (<10 degrees), girls have 10 times the risk of developing a curvature >30 degrees.

CLINICAL MANIFESTATIONS. Patients usually present with a change in cosmetic appearance noted by family and/or friends or on school or physician screening examination. While not typical, back pain can be occasionally associated with scoliosis. A thorough history and physical examination are required because idiopathic scoliosis is a diagnosis of exclusion. The patient is evaluated in the standing position, from both the front and the side, to identify any asymmetry in the chest wall, trunk, and/or shoulders. Asymmetry of the posterior chest wall on forward bending (the Adams test) is the earliest abnormality (Fig. 678-1). Rotation of the vertebral bodies toward the convexity results in outward rotation and prominence of the attached ribs posteriorly. The anterior chest wall may be flattened on the concavity due to inward rotation of the chest wall and ribs. Associated findings may include elevation of the shoulder, a lateral shift of the trunk, an apparent leg-length discrepancy. The patient should also be evaluated from the side. Typically, idiopathic scoliosis results in a loss of the normal thoracic kyphosis in the region of curvature (relative thoracic lordosis). A careful neurologic exam-

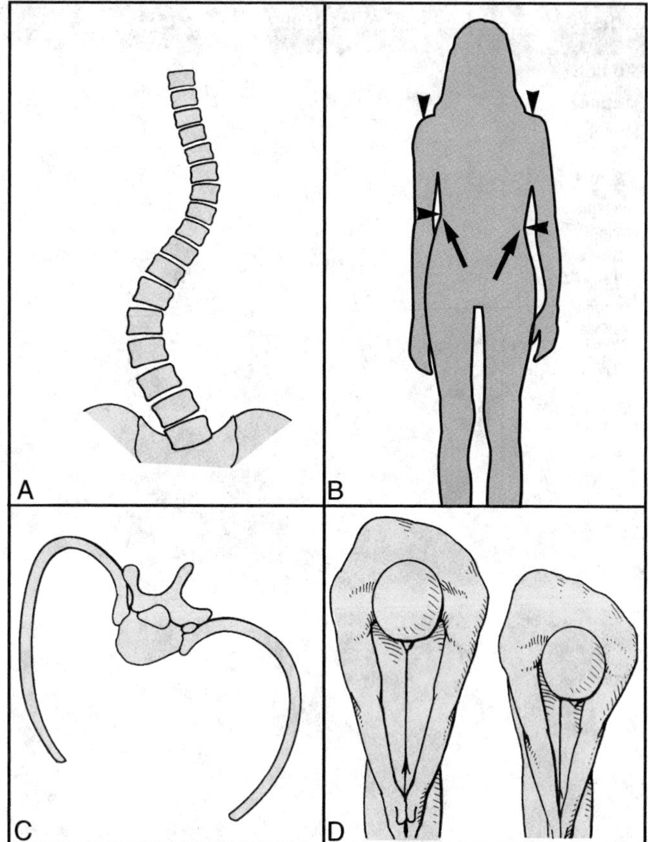

Figure 678-1. Structural changes in idiopathic scoliosis. *A*, As curvature increases, alterations in body configuration develop in both the primary and compensatory curve regions. *B*, Asymmetry of shoulder height, waistline, and elbow-to-flank distance are common findings. *C*, Vertebral rotation and associated posterior displacement of the ribs on the convex side of the curve are responsible for the characteristic deformity of the chest wall in scoliosis patients. *D*, In the school screening examination for scoliosis, the patient bends forward at the waist. Rib asymmetry of even a small degree is obvious. (From Scoles PV: Spinal deformity in childhood and adolescence. In Behrman RE, Vaughn VC III [editors]: *Nelson Textbook of Pediatrics, Update 5*. Philadelphia, WB Saunders, 1989.)

ination should always be performed. A subset of curves will be associated with an underlying neurologic diagnosis, especially in patients who present in the infant and juvenile years (20% have an associated intraspinal abnormality). The index of suspicion is raised in the presence of back pain or neurologic symptoms, café-au-lait spots, a sacral dimple, midline cutaneous abnormalities such as a hair patch or skin tag, unilateral foot deformity, or an atypical curve pattern.

When the trunk is viewed from the side, the degree of kyphosis and lordosis can be evaluated. The upper region of the thoracic spine normally has a smooth, rounded curve that extends down to the midthoracic region. Flexible roundback that corrects easily when a child stands upright is common in adolescents. Sharp, abrupt, or accentuated forward angulation in the thoracic or thoracolumbar region is indicative of a pathologic kyphotic deformity. In the erect position, the lower lumbar spine is normally concave (lordotic). The magnitude of lordosis varies with age and among individuals of the same age. Children normally have less cervical lordosis and more lumbar lordosis than do adults or adolescents.

In addition to screening during regular visits to a primary care physician, school screening programs are widespread in North America and use the Adams forward bend test to identify any asymmetry in the thoracic and/or lumbar region. An inclinometer (scoliometer, Orthopaedic Systems Inc.) is also used in some programs to measure the degree of asymmetry, and the number of degrees used for referral typically varies from 5 to 7. The referral rate from these programs varies from 3% to 30%. Follow-up of adult patients with untreated late-onset scoliosis reveals an increased risk of mild to moderate back pain and dyspnea (greater with a thoracic apex and a Cobb angle >80 degrees).

RADIOGRAPHIC EVALUATION. Standing, high-quality, posteroanterior (PA) and lateral radiographs of the entire spine are recommended at the initial evaluation for patients with clinical findings suggestive of a spinal deformity. On the PA radiograph, the degree of curvature is determined by the Cobb method, in which the angle between the superior and inferior end vertebra (tilted into the curve) is measured (Fig. 678-2). A line is drawn across the superior end plate of each end vertebra, and the angle between perpendicular lines erected from each of these is measured. Although the indications for performing MRI are variable, this modality is helpful when an underlying cause for the scoliosis is suspected based on age (infantile, juvenile curves), abnormal findings on the history and physical examination, and atypical radiographic features (curve patterns and/or specific features). **Atypical radiographic** findings include uncommon curve patterns such as the left thoracic curve, double thoracic curves, high thoracic curves, widening of the spinal canal, and erosive or dysplastic changes in the vertebral body or ribs. On the lateral radiograph, an increase in thoracic kyphosis or an absence of segmental lordosis may be suggestive of an underlying neurologic abnormality.

TREATMENT. The decision of whether to treat the patient is based on the natural history, and options include observation, bracing, and surgical stabilization. In general, idiopathic thoracic curvatures may not create significant alterations in cardiopulmonary function until they have reached 80–90 degrees; thus, curves of lesser magnitude are mainly a cosmetic problem. Long-term studies have suggested that back pain may be a more significant problem for patients with untreated curves of larger magnitude. The risk of curve progression depends on the amount of growth remaining (age, menarchal status, Tanner stage, Risser sign), the curve magnitude, and gender. Curves are more likely to progress if there is significant growth remaining (premenarchal, Tanner stage I or II, Risser 0 or 1). Premenarchal girls with curves between 20 and 30 degrees have a significantly higher risk of progression than do girls 2 yr after menarche with similar curves; curve progression is likely in the 1st group and uncommon in the 2nd. Boys with curvature of the same magnitude appear to have similar risks of progression when judged by other maturation standards; however, the assessment of skeletal maturity in boys is more difficult. Thoracic curves <30 degrees rarely progress after skeletal maturity, while those >45 or 50 degrees may continue to progress at approximately 1 degree per year through life. Lumbar curves are more likely to progress and can cause pain during adulthood.

Surgical treatment is usually indicated for skeletally immature patients with progressive thoracic curves >45 degrees and skeletally mature patients with thoracic curves >50–55 degrees. Lumbar curves are more likely to progress, and surgical stabilization may be offered for curves as low as 35–40 degrees if there is a significant cosmetic deformity, most commonly a shift of the trunk. The goals of surgery are to arrest progression of the deformity, to improve cosmesis, and to achieve a balanced spine, while minimizing the number of vertebral segments that are stabilized. Implants are used to apply mechanical forces to the bony elements to correct a deformity in both the frontal and lateral planes, to maintain normal frontal and sagittal spinal balance, and to maintain the correction so that a cast or brace is not required postoperatively. Most procedures are performed poste-

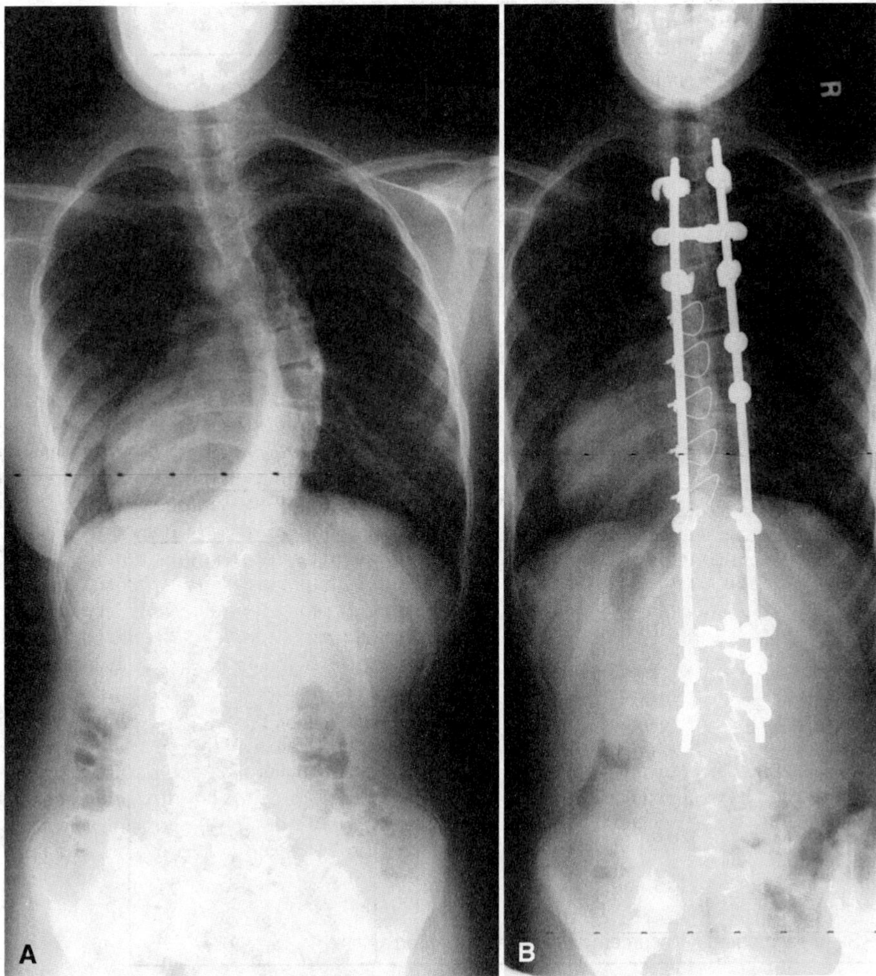

Figure 678-2. Preoperative standing posteroanterior radiograph of a 14 year old girl who was skeletally immature and developed a 68 degree right thoracic and a 53 degree left lumbar scoliosis *(A)*. Her trunk was shifted to the right, and the left shoulder was slightly depressed. Based upon the risk of future progression, she was treated by an instrumented posterior spinal fusion from T3 to L3 with correction of the right thoracic curve to 20 degrees and the left lumbar curve to 10 degrees *(B)*. Coronal spinal balance was restored, and shoulder height was maintained.

riorly, and the typical spinal construct includes 2 rods anchored to the spine by hooks, wires, and/or screws (see Fig. 678-2). An anterior release and fusion, performed through a thoracotomy or thoracolumbar exposure, is indicated for isolated thoracolumbar and lumbar curves, stiffer curves (improve correction), skeletally immature patients (to prevent "crankshaft" from continued anterior growth), and patients with a higher likelihood of not achieving an arthrodesis with a posterior approach alone (neurofibromatosis, myelomeningocele). For idiopathic thoracolumbar and lumbar curves, an anterior fusion with instrumentation (usually screws in the vertebral body connected to 1 or 2 rods) can be done as an alternative to save lumbar motion segments.

Several techniques are being evaluated in the management of idiopathic scoliosis. Thoracoscopic surgery has been used to perform an anterior release and fusion; anterior spinal implants may also be placed using this technique. The indications for thoracoscopic spine surgery are evolving. In addition, there has been an interest in developing techniques to tether spinal growth, with the goal of arresting curve progression (and achieving some correction) to avoid a future spinal fusion in patients with a high risk of progression. The technique involves open or thoracoscopic placement of metallic staples into the vertebral bodies (across each intervertebral disk space or growth zone) to hold the spine in a corrected position and tether the growth on the convexity of the curvature.

678.2 • Congenital Scoliosis

Congenital scoliosis results from abnormal growth and development of the vertebral column likely due to intrauterine events at or about the 6th wk of gestation. There can be a partial or complete failure of formation (wedge vertebrae or hemivertebrae), a partial or complete failure of segmentation (unilateral unsegmented bars), or a combination of both (Fig. 678-3). One or more bony anomalies may occur in isolation or in combination.

As the spine (including the neural elements) and the viscera are formed around the 6th wk in utero, patients with congenital scoliosis often have visceral and intraspinal anomalies as well. Once a congenital spinal anomaly is diagnosed, a priority is to rule out malformations in other organ systems. Genitourinary abnormalities are identified in 20–40% of children with congenital scoliosis and include unilateral renal agenesis, ureteral duplication, horseshoe kidney, and genital anomalies. Approximately 2% of these patients have a silent, obstructive uropathy that may be life threatening. Renal ultrasonography should be performed early on in all children with congenital scoliosis, and other studies (CT, MRI) may also be required. Cardiac anomalies are identified in 10–25% of patients. A careful cardiac examination should be performed; some clinicians recommend routine echocardiography. Approximately 20–40% of patients may have an intraspinal

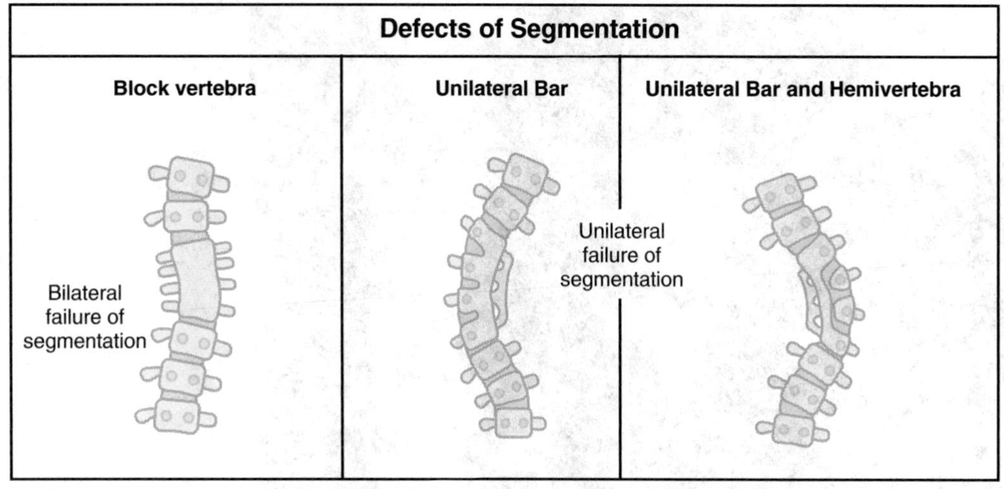

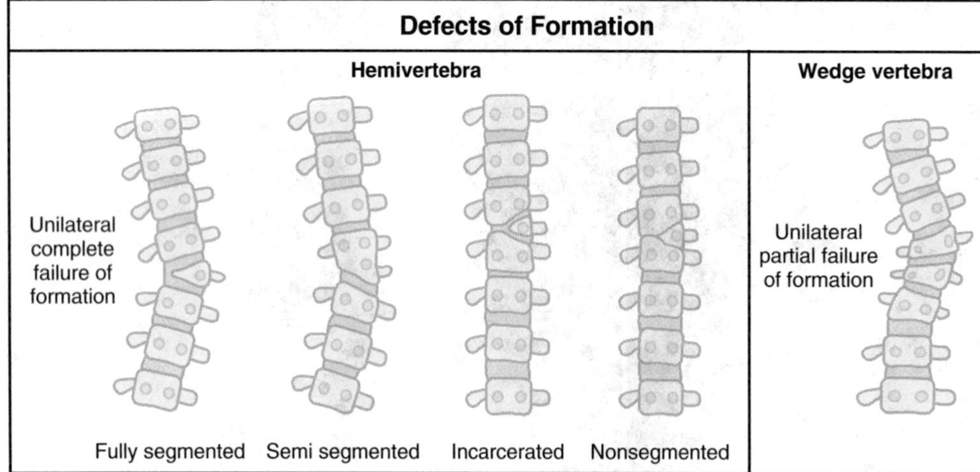

Figure 678-3. The defects of segmentation and formation that can occur during spinal development. (From McMaster MJ: Congenital scoliosis. In Weinstein SL [editor]: *The Pediatric Spine: Principles and Practice,* 2nd ed. Philadelphia, Lippincott Williams & Wilkins, 2001, p 163.)

anomaly. Infants with cutaneous abnormalities overlying the spine may benefit from ultrasonography to rule out an occult spinal dysraphic condition. MRI is usually recommended during the course of treatment. Spinal dysraphism is the general term applied to such lesions (see Chapters 592 and 605). Examples include diastematomyelia, split cord malformations, intraspinal lipomas (intradural or extradural), arachnoid cysts, teratomas, dermoid sinuses, fibrous bands, and tight filum terminale. Cutaneous findings that may be seen in patients with closed spinal dysraphism include hair patches, skin tags or dimples, sinuses, and hemangiomas. Most of these lesions become clinically evident through tethering of the spinal cord, the symptoms of which include back and/or leg pain, calf atrophy, progressive unilateral foot deformity (especially cavovarus), and problems with bowel or bladder function.

The risk of progression depends on the growth potential of each anomaly, which may vary considerably, so close radiographic follow-up is required. Progression of these curves is most pronounced during periods of rapid growth, namely, the first 2–3 yr of life and during the adolescent growth spurt. The most severe form of congenital scoliosis is a unilateral unsegmented bar with a contralateral hemivertebra. In this anomaly, the spine is fused on 1 side (unsegmented bar) and has a growth center (hemivertebra) on the other side at the same level. A rapidly progressive curve is seen, and all patients usually require surgical stabilization. A unilateral unsegmented bar is also associated with significant progression and in most cases will require surgical intervention. While an unsegmented bar may not be radiographically apparent, the adjacent ribs on the concavity may be fused, providing a clue to the diagnosis. An isolated hemivertebra must be followed closely, and many, but not all, of these will be associated with a progressive deformity that requires surgical intervention. In contrast, an isolated block vertebra has little growth potential and rarely requires treatment.

Early diagnosis and prompt treatment of progressive curves are essential. Bracing is not indicated for most congenital curves due to their structural nature, except in rare cases in which the goal is to control a flexible, compensatory curvature in another area of the spine. The treatment of progressive curves is preemptive spinal arthrodesis, and both anterior and posterior spinal fusion is often required. Other procedures that are employed in selected patients include an isolated posterior spinal fusion (sometimes an in situ fusion), convex hemiepiphysiodesis (only 1 side of the spine is fused to allow some correction of the deformity with growth), and partial or complete hemivertebra excision (usually in the lumbar spine). Spinal arthrodesis is ideally performed before a significant deformity has developed because intraoperative correction is difficult to achieve and the risk of neurologic complications is high.

When multiple levels of the thoracic spine are involved, especially in the presence of fused ribs, a progressive 3-dimensional deformity of the chest wall may impair lung development and function, resulting in a thoracic insufficiency syndrome. This syndrome is best described as the inability of the chest wall to support normal respiration. A thoracic insufficiency syndrome may be seen in patients with several recognized conditions such as Jarcho-Levin syndrome (spondylocostal or spondylothoracic dysplasia) and Jeune syndrome (asphyxiating thoracic dystrophy). There is interest in treating these difficult cases with an experimental technique called **expansion thoracoplasty,** in which

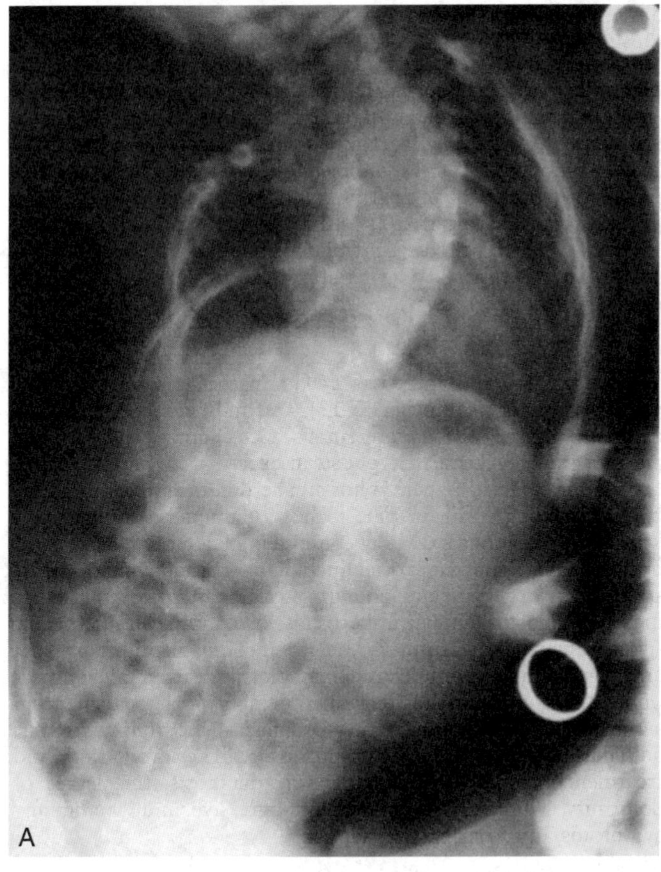

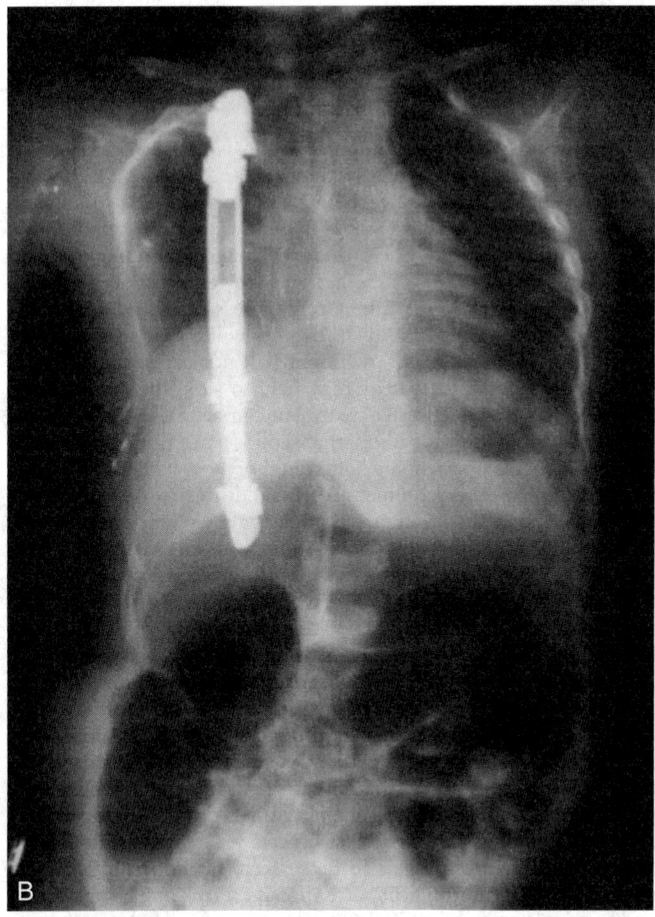

Figure 678-4. *A*, Anteroposterior preoperative radiograph of a 7 mo old boy with congenital scoliosis and fused ribs. A three-dimensional reconstruction of a CT scan of the chest of this infant estimated his lung volume to be 173.2 mL^3. *B*, Anteroposterior radiograph after implantation of a vertically expandable prosthetic titanium rib and several expansions over 33 mo. The lung volume now measures 330.3 mL^3, an increase of 90.7%. (From Gollogly S, Smith JT, Campbell RM: Determining lung volume with three-dimensional reconstructions of CT scan data: A pilot study to evaluate the effects of expansion thoracoplasty on children with severe spinal deformities. *J Pediatr Orthop* 2004;23:323–328.)

the thoracic cage is gradually expanded over time by progressive lengthening of the chest wall on the concavity of the spinal deformity (or in some cases on both sides of the spine). The procedure involves an opening wedge thoracostomy, followed by placement of a vertical expandable titanium prosthetic rib. The implant is then distracted (lengthened) at regular intervals (Fig. 678-4). The primary goal is to gradually correct the chest wall deformity to improve pulmonary function, and a secondary goal is correction of an associated spinal deformity. This technique is currently not approved for the treatment of scoliosis in the absence of a thoracic insufficiency, and further study will help to refine (and possible expand) the indications for this new technique.

678.3 • Neuromuscular Scoliosis, Genetic Syndromes, and Compensatory Scoliosis

NEUROMUSCULAR SCOLIOSIS. Scoliosis is frequently identified in children with neuromuscular diseases such as cerebral palsy, the muscular dystrophies and other myopathies, spinal muscular atrophy, Friedreich ataxia, myelomeningocele, polio, and arthrogryposis. The etiology and natural history differ from those seen in idiopathic and congenital scoliosis. Most cases result from weakness and/or imbalance of the trunk musculature, and spasticity plays a role in many patients as well. Coexisting congenital vertebral anomalies are seen in patients with myelomeningocele. Neuromuscular scoliosis is most common in the nonambulatory population and may be diagnosed in up to 68% of nonambulatory patients with cerebral palsy, and >90% of patients with Duchenne muscular dystrophy. The most common pattern is a long "C"-shaped curve, which is often associated with pelvic obliquity. In general, the clinical course depends on the severity of neuromuscular involvement and the nature of the underlying disease process (especially if progressive).

The consequences of a progressive scoliosis in the neuromuscular population involve both function (sitting and standing balance) and ease of care; in some cases, visceral function may be compromised. In patients who are wheelchair bound, one arm may be required for trunk support, which impairs upper extremity function. An associated pelvic obliquity results in asymmetric seating pressures, which may limit sitting endurance and possibly result in ischial decubiti. Severe curves may be associated with decreased pulmonary reserve, especially when the apex is in the thoracic spine, compounding pre-existing respiratory problems. Pain may be experienced from impingement of the rib cage on the iliac crest in large thoracolumbar curves. Marginal ambulators may lose the ability to ambulate as a result of scoliosis.

The diagnosis is suspected on physical examination. Early detection is helpful because the results are optimal if treatment is completed before the magnitude and rigidity of the curve become severe. In patients who ambulate, the examination is as outlined in the section on idiopathic scoliosis. In nonambulators, the back is inspected with the patient sitting upright (with or without support) and any asymmetry noted. These patients often need manual support to maintain an upright position. If any asymmetry is observed, then upright (sitting) PA and lateral radiographs are obtained.

The **treatment** of neuromuscular scoliosis depends on the age of the patient, the underlying diagnosis, and the degree of progression. The goal is to achieve or maintain a straight spine over a level pelvis, especially in patients who are wheelchair bound, and to intervene early before curve magnitude and rigidity increase. In contrast to idiopathic and congenital scoliosis, neuromuscular curves may continue to progress after skeletal maturity. In general, curves of >40–50 degrees will continue to worsen over time. Although brace treatment will not arrest progression in the long term, this strategy may help to slow the rate of progression until more definitive treatment can be carried out. As the standard braces used for idiopathic scoliosis are poorly tolerated in neuromuscular patients, a soft spinal orthosis or seating modifications are often recommended. In addition to delaying progression, these orthoses improve sitting balance (upper extremity function), sitting tolerance, and ease of care. In general, a spinal arthrodesis is offered to patients with progressive curvatures >40–50 degrees. The indications will differ somewhat based on the underlying diagnosis. Patients with Duchenne muscular dystrophy are offered surgery when their curves progress beyond 20–30 degrees, before a significant decline in pulmonary or cardiac function preclude their ability to tolerate the surgery. There has been some controversy regarding the indications for spinal fusion in the patient with spastic quadriplegia, especially those patients with severe mental retardation. In this population, the indications must be individualized and typically involve a documented loss of function or ease of care or chronic discomfort. Patients with curves similar to those seen in idiopathic scoliosis who are usually ambulatory are managed by similar principles and surgical techniques. Patients who are nonambulatory, often with pelvic obliquity, are usually managed by a spinal fusion extending from the upper thoracic spine to the pelvis. Segmental fixation is employed to maximize rigidity (each level in the curve serves as a point for fixation), and the typical construct includes sublaminar wires at each level, which are attached to 1 (unit rod) or 2 spinal rods. These rods extend down into the posterior ilium to achieve fixation across the lumbosacral joint. A brace is usually not required following this procedure. Although complications are relatively frequent in comparison with patients with non-neuromuscular curves, the available literature suggests that most patients benefit in terms of function and ease of care. This surgery should ideally be done at centers with significant experience (e.g., trained spine surgeons, anesthesia, intensive care unit).

SYNDROMES/GENETIC DISORDERS. Representative examples of this diverse group of diagnoses include neurofibromatosis, osteogenesis imperfecta, connective tissue diseases (Marfan syndrome, Ehlers-Danlos syndrome), Prader-Willi syndrome, and many others. Patients with these diagnoses should have their spine examined routinely during visits to their primary care physician. As for other types of scoliosis, the follow-up and treatment are based on the age of the patient, the degree of deformity, whether progression has been documented, and the underlying diagnosis.

COMPENSATORY SCOLIOSIS. Leg-length inequality is common and is usually associated with a small compensatory lumbar curvature (see Chapter 675). This is 1 cause of false-positive screening examinations. Pelvic tilt toward the short side is associated with a lumbar curve (convexity away from the short leg). There is little evidence to suggest that a small compensatory lumbar curve places the patient at risk of progression or back pain. Because children with leg-length inequality may also have idiopathic or congenital scoliosis, a standing radiograph may be obtained with a block under the foot on the short side (to correct the leg-length discrepancy) to level the pelvis. If the curvature disappears when the limb-length discrepancy is corrected, then a diagnosis of a compensatory curve is made. An alternative is a PA radiograph with the patient seated. In neuromuscular disorders such as polio or cerebral palsy, an adduction or abduction contracture of the hip (fixed infrapelvic contracture) may be compensated for by a lumbar scoliosis to maintain standing or sitting balance. For patients who ambulate, a 10-degree fixed contracture will result in up to 3-cm apparent leg-length discrepancy.

678.4 • Kyphosis (Round-Back)

The normal thoracic spine has 20–50 degrees of kyphosis when using the Cobb technique (T3–12), and individuals with higher degrees of kyphosis may present with cosmetic concerns, back pain, or both. A thoracic kyphosis in excess of the normal range of values is termed hyperkyphosis. The deformity may be flexible (postural kyphosis) or rigid (Scheuermann disease, congenital kyphosis, other causes). Many conditions may be associated with hyperkyphosis, and categories include posttraumatic (following spinal fractures), postinfectious (bacterial, tuberculosis, fungal), metabolic (osteogenesis imperfecta, osteoporosis), iatrogenic (postlaminectomy, postradiation), neuromuscular, neoplastic, and congenital/developmental. Examples of congenital or developmental conditions include disorders of collagen (Marfan syndrome), and a number of dysplasias (neurofibromatosis, achondroplasia, mucopolysaccharidosis). The evaluation and treatment depends on the underlying diagnosis, the degree of deformity, whether the deformity is progressive, and whether any symptoms are present.

FLEXIBLE KYPHOSIS (POSTURAL KYPHOSIS)

Postural kyphosis is a common cosmetic concern and is most often recognized by family and friends. Adolescents with postural kyphosis can correct the curvature voluntarily. A standing lateral radiograph will show an increase in kyphosis, but no pathologic changes of the involved vertebrae. A supine hyperextension lateral radiograph will show complete correction. There is no evidence to suggest that postural kyphosis progresses to a structural deformity or to back pain or other symptoms in later life. In addition to reassurance, a thoracic hyperextension exercise program may assist in strengthening the extensor muscles of the spine. Neither bracing nor surgery plays a role in the management of this condition.

STRUCTURAL KYPHOSIS

SCHEUERMANN DISEASE. Scheuermann disease is the most common form of structural hyperkyphosis and may occur in the thoracic or thoracolumbar spine. In addition to hyperkyphosis, this condition is defined by wedging (>5 degrees) of 3 or more consecutive vertebral bodies at the apex of the deformity on a lateral radiograph. Associated radiographic findings include irregularities of the vertebral end plates and Schmorl nodes. Histologic specimens have shown a disordered pattern of endochondral ossification, but it remains unclear whether these findings are primary (genetic or metabolic) or secondary (due to mechanical overload). The etiology remains unknown, but most likely involves the influence of mechanical forces in a genetically susceptible individual. The reported incidence varies from 0.4% to 10%, and boys are involved more frequently than girls.

CLINICAL MANIFESTATIONS. There is a hyperkyphosis of the thoracic spine, typically associated with a sharp contour, and often the apex of the deformity will be in the lower thoracic spine.

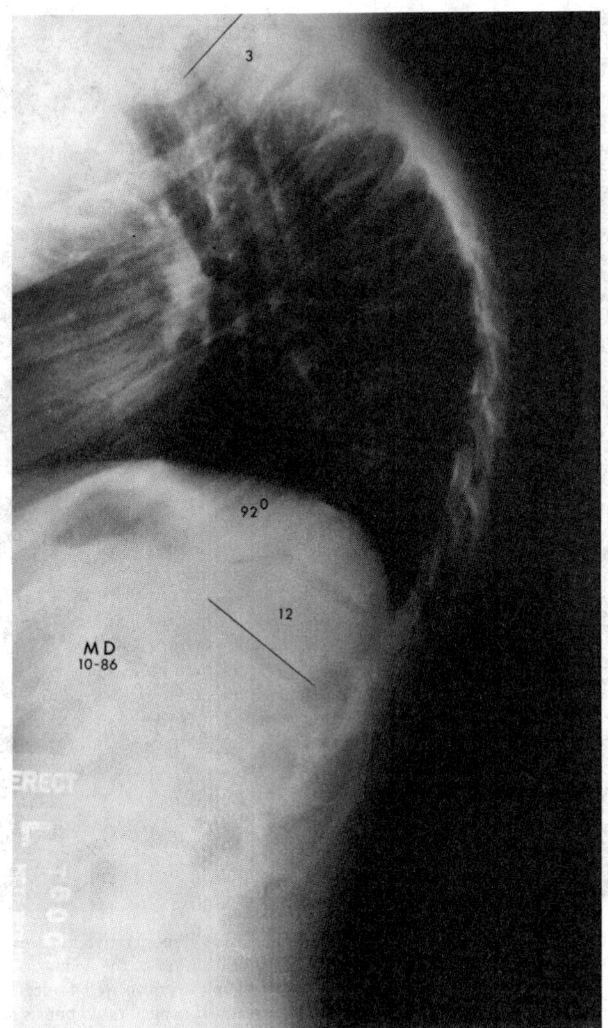

Figure 678-5. Standing lateral radiograph of a 14 yr old boy with severe Scheuermann kyphosis. This measures 92 degrees between T3 and T12. Note the wedging of the vertebrae at T6, T7, T8, and T9. The normal thoracic kyphosis is ≤40 degrees.

Patients are unable to correct the deformity voluntarily. Pain is a relatively common complaint and is typically mild and in the region of the apex of the kyphosis. The symptoms are intermittent, rarely severe, and occasionally limit certain activities. Neurologic symptoms are uncommon.

RADIOGRAPHIC EVALUATION. Standing PA and lateral radiographs are obtained (Fig. 678-5). A specific, standardized technique in which the arms are folded across the chest is recommended for the lateral view. In addition to the diagnostic findings noted above, a mild scoliosis is commonly seen, and less frequently, a spondylolisthesis may be identified on the lateral radiograph.

TREATMENT. Treatment depends on the age of the patient, the degree of deformity, and whether any symptoms are present. The natural history of Scheuermann disease appears to be relatively benign. While early reports suggested that significant degenerative changes and pain are common with curves in excess of 75 degrees, other studies report a more benign outcome. While adults with untreated Scheuermann disease may have a greater intensity of back pain, the prevalence of back pain appears to be no different than in the general population. Patients may select more sedentary occupations, but their self-esteem, participation in activities of daily living and recreational activities, and level of education seem to be no different than in the general population. Kyphotic deformities >90 degrees are more likely to be aesthetically unacceptable, symptomatic, and progressive. Deformities in excess of 100 degrees may be associated with pulmonary dysfunction.

There are few absolute guidelines for treatment, and decisions must be individualized. Skeletally immature patients with mild deformity may benefit from a hyperextension exercise program, but the effects of this strategy on the natural history remain to be documented. Patients with >1 year of growth remaining and a kyphosis of >55–60 degrees may benefit from a bracing program. A Milwaukee brace (extends up to the neck) is recommended for those curves with an apex above T7, while curves with a lower apex may often be treated by a thoracolumbar orthosis. The brace is recommended for up to 23 hr/day. On occasion, a serial casting (or stretching) program is instituted to gain flexibility prior to instituting the brace program. The goal of the brace is to prevent progression, and a permanent improvement in alignment are seen less commonly. When effective, radiographs will often show a reconstitution of anterior vertebral height (reversal of wedging), which does result in a permanent improvement in alignment. Skeletally mature patients with little or no pain and acceptable cosmesis are not treated. For patients with progressive deformities >70–80 degrees who are dissatisfied with their cosmetic appearance and for those with persistent back pain despite nonoperative measures, a spinal fusion may be considered. Typically, a fusion from the upper thoracic to the upper lumbar spine may be required. While some surgeons perform an instrumented posterior spinal fusion alone, others recommend an anterior spinal release and fusion followed by an instrumented posterior spinal fusion.

CONGENITAL KYPHOSIS

Congenital kyphosis results from congenital vertebral malformations. In an anterior failure of formation (type I), a portion of the vertebral body fails to form. This results in a kyphosis, which is present at birth, progresses rapidly, and commonly results in neurologic dysfunction if untreated. Spinal cord dysfunction commonly results from compression of the spinal cord at the apex of the deformity. Type II involves an anterior failure of segmentation, in which 2 vertebrae are fused anteriorly. With continued growth of the posterior elements of the spine, a progressive kyphosis often develops. This 2nd type is less likely to create a neurologic deficit; however, patients must be followed closely, and treatment is required in a significant number of cases. As for congenital scoliosis, abnormalities of other organ systems should be ruled out.

The treatment depends on the type of malformation, the degree of deformity, and whether neurologic symptoms are present. Bracing is mostly ineffective, and surgery (spinal arthrodesis) is usually the only effective treatment option. Since the natural history is so poor for type I kyphoses, spinal fusion is usually performed shortly after the diagnosis is made. Both an anterior fusion and a posterior spinal fusion are usually performed, with or without instrumentation. Ideally, the spine can be stabilized prior to the development of a severe deformity. Another approach is to perform a costotransversectomy (Fig. 678-6). Type II deformities also require spinal stabilization in the majority of cases, but there is less urgency with a failure of segmentation. Patients may often be followed for a period of time before intervention is necessary, and in some cases no treatment is required.

678.5 • Back Pain in Children

Back pain is a relatively frequent complaint in children and adolescents, and the differential diagnosis is extensive (Table 678-2).

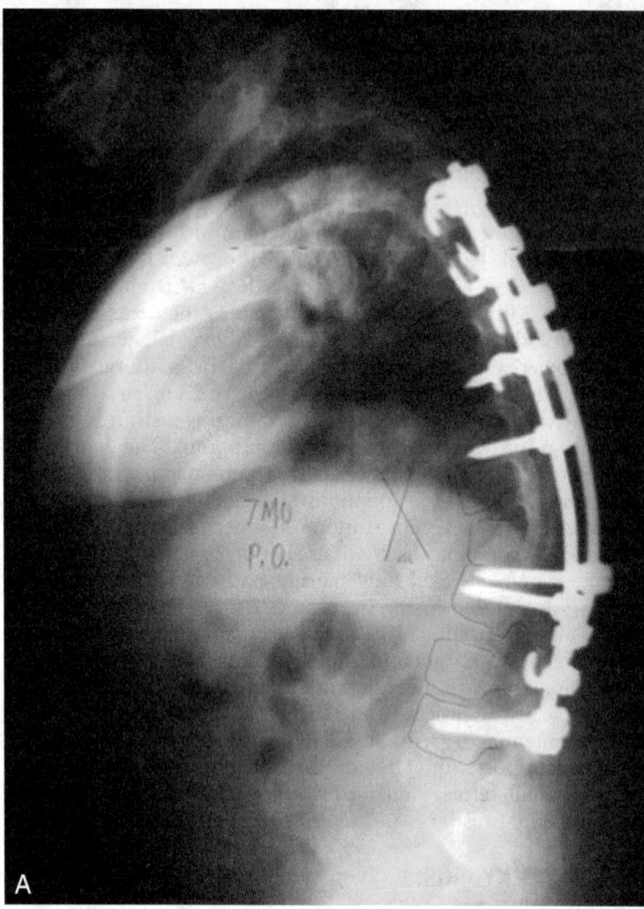

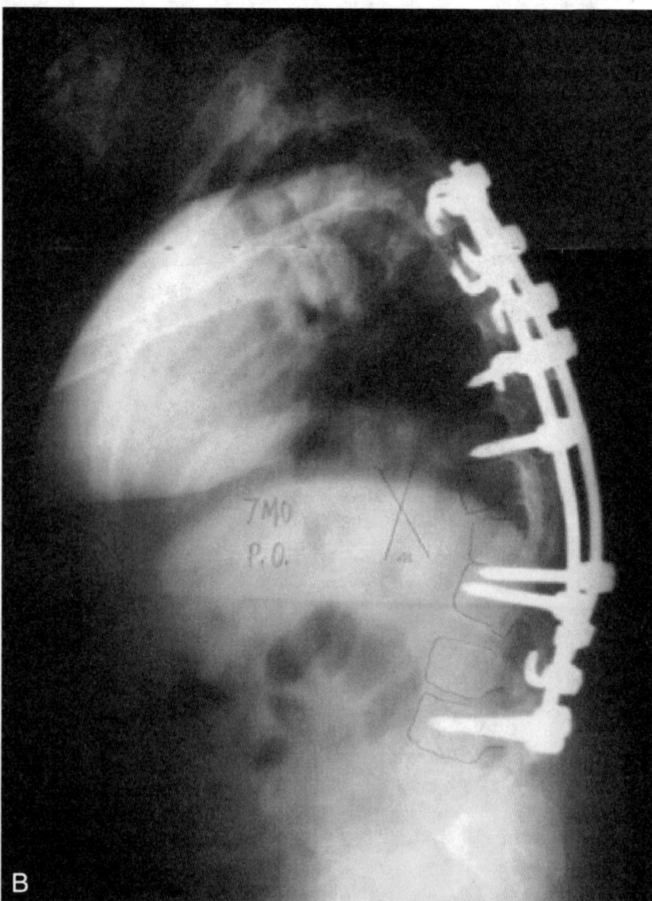

Figure 678-6. Radiographs of the spine of an 11 yr old boy with a progressive kyphosis secondary to type I congenital kyphosis. *A,* Preoperative radiograph showing a 61-degree kyphotic deformity with a trapped posterior hemivertebra at T11. *B,* Lateral radiograph obtained 7 mo after excision of the hemivertebra using a posterior-only approach involving costotransversectomy, with segmental spinal fixation from T5 to L3. The postoperative kyphosis measured 41 degrees. (From Smith JT, Gollogly S, Dunn HK: Simultaneous anterior-posterior approach through a costotransversectomy for the treatment of congenital kyphosis and acquired kyphoscoliotic deformities. *J Bone Joint Surg Am* 2005;87:2281–2289.)

A thorough history and physical examination, often with imaging modalities, is required to rule out an underlying pathologic process in patients with persistent pain.

CLINICAL EVALUATION. The history begins with the location, character, and duration of symptoms. Any history of acute trauma, or repetitive physical activities should be sought. Pain that is constant, unrelieved by rest, and wakes the patient from sleep is more likely to be secondary to an infection or neoplasm. The presence of systemic signs (fevers, chills) or constitutional symptoms (weight loss, malaise) is also worrisome. Symptoms of neurologic dysfunction must also be uncovered. Patients should be questioned about the presence of any radicular symptoms, gait disturbance, muscle weakness, alterations in sensation, and changes in bowel and/or bladder function. The physical examination includes a complete musculoskeletal and neurologic assessment, and the patient should be adequately exposed for the clinical exam. He or she should be inspected for any changes in alignment in the frontal or sagittal plane, and range of motion should be assessed in flexion, extension, and lateral bending. Younger children may be asked to pick up an object off the floor to assess spinal flexion. Patients who have pain with flexion (compression across the anterior spinal column) may have an abnormality in the vertebral body or disk such as diskitis. Those who experience pain with extension (compression across posterior elements) may have a spondylolysis or other problem in the posterior elements. Palpation will reveal any areas of tenderness and/or muscle spasm. Palpating the top of the iliac wings while the patient is standing assesses leg lengths. As spinal pain may be referred, an abdominal examination should be performed, and in females, a gynecologic evaluation may be necessary. Pathology at the sacroiliac joint will occasionally mimic low back pain, and this joint should be stressed by compression of the iliac wings or by external rotation at the hip. A careful neurologic examination should be performed. In addition to manual muscle testing and assessing sensation and proprioception, the superficial abdominal reflex should be tested by gently stroking the skin on each of the 4 quadrants surrounding the umbilicus. Normally, the umbilicus will move toward the area stimulated. A normal examination includes symmetry in the response on both sides of the midline, even if the reflex cannot be elicited on either side. An abnormal test suggests the presence of a subtle abnormality of spinal cord function, most commonly syringomyelia. The straight leg raise test evaluates tension on the lower spinal nerve roots, looking for a herniated disk or slipped vertebral apophysis.

RADIOGRAPHIC AND LABORATORY EVALUATION. Initially posteroanterior and lateral radiographs of the involved region of the spine are recommended. With lumbar back pain, right and left oblique views are recommended as well. In patients with a normal neurologic examination, a bone scan with single-photon emission computed tomography (SPECT) will help to diagnose a stress reaction or spondylolysis. MRI is most helpful when neurologic symptoms or findings are present. CT is the study of choice for

TABLE 678-2. Differential Diagnosis of Back Pain

INFLAMMATORY/INFECTIOUS
Diskitis
Vertebral osteomyelitis (pyogenic, tuberculous)
Spinal epidural abscess
Pyelonephritis
Pancreatitis
RHEUMATOLOGIC
Pauciarticular juvenile rheumatoid arthritis
Reiter syndrome
Ankylosing spondylitis
Psoriatic arthritis
DEVELOPMENTAL
Spondylolysis
Spondylolisthesis
Scheuermann disease
Scoliosis
TRAUMATIC (ACUTE VERSUS REPETITIVE)
Hip-pelvic anomalies
Herniated disk
Overuse syndromes
Vertebral stress fractures
Upper cervical spine instability
NEOPLASTIC
Vertebral tumors
Benign
Eosinophilic granuloma
Aneurysmal bone cyst
Osteoid osteoma
Osteoblastoma
Malignant
Osteogenic sarcoma
Leukemia
Lymphoma
Metastatic tumor
Spinal cord, ganglia, and nerve roots
Intramedullary spinal cord tumor
Sympathetic chain
Ganglioneuroma
Ganglioneuroblastoma
Neuroblastoma
OTHER
Intra-abdominal or pelvic pathology
Following lumbar puncture
Conversion reaction
Juvenile osteoporosis

defining bony lesions. When systemic signs or constitutional symptoms are present, a complete blood cell count with differential, erythrocyte sedimentation rate, and C-reactive protein should be ordered. In certain cases, laboratory tests for the juvenile forms of arthritis (juvenile rheumatoid arthritis and ankylosing spondylitis) are indicated.

678.6 • Spondylolysis and Spondylolisthesis

Spondylolysis represents a unilateral or bilateral defect in the pars interarticularis, the segment of bone connecting the superior and inferior articular facets. Spondylolysis is an acquired condition that is present in approximately 4–6% of the adult population and is thought to result from repetitive hyperextension stresses whereby the inferior articular facet impacts the pars interarticularis. The condition develops as a stress fracture, which then goes on to a pseudarthrosis ("false joint") in many cases. Patients with excessive lordosis in the lumbar spine may be predisposed, and spondylolysis is most common in athletes who engage in repetitive spinal hyperextension, especially gymnasts, football players (especially interior lineman), weight lifters, and wrestlers. A genetic component has been suggested. The lesion is most common at L5, but may be identified at upper lumbar levels as well. Approximately 5% of cases of spondylolysis will develop a forward slippage of the involved vertebra on the vertebra below (spondylolisthesis). The natural history is variable. While a subset of cases remains asymptomatic, spondylolysis is a common cause of back pain in the adolescent population.

Spondylolisthesis involves slippage of 1 vertebra on another and is also most common at L5. In children and adolescents, the most common types are dysplastic (congenital) and isthmic (results from a stress fracture). Spondylolisthesis is graded according to degree of translation of 1 vertebra on the other as follows: grade 1 (<25%), grade 2 (25–50%), grade 3 (50–75%), grade 4 (75–100%), and grade 5 (complete displacement or spondyloptosis). The physical findings also depend on the degree of sagittal rotation of the upper on the lower vertebrae.

CLINICAL MANIFESTATIONS. Symptomatic patients with spondylolysis usually present with mechanical low back pain that may radiate to the buttocks, with or without spasm of the hamstring muscles. Radicular symptoms are uncommon. The pain is exacerbated by spinal hyperextension. Physical examination may reveal a limitation in lumbar flexibility in addition to discomfort with palpation over the spinous process of the involved vertebra. Hamstring spasm is an important clinical finding and usually results in mild contracture and often discomfort during testing the range of motion.

Patients with spondylolisthesis, in addition to lumbar back pain, may also experience neurologic symptoms (radiculopathy or bowel/bladder dysfunction) from compression of the cauda equina or nerve roots. There is commonly a loss of spinal mobility and often a gait disturbance. The buttocks will appear flattened (sacrum is more vertically inclined, lumbosacral kyphosis), and the abdomen may appear more protuberant. There is often a palpable step off between the spinous processes at the involved levels, especially with a high-grade slip. In addition to a complete examination of the spine (scoliosis is commonly associated), a careful neurologic examination is essential.

RADIOGRAPHIC EVALUATION. The initial evaluation of the lumbar region should include high-quality anteroposterior, lateral, and oblique radiographs. Standing PA and lateral radiographs are obtained if findings suggestive of scoliosis or hyperkyphosis are also present (Figs. 678-7 and 678-8). In patients with normal plain films, a bone scan with SPECT may help to diagnose a spondylolysis during the early stages, prior to the formation of an established pseudarthrosis. A CT scan with thin cuts may provide additional information to establish the presence of a pars defect. MRI is indicated in the presence of signs or symptoms of cauda equina or nerve root involvement.

TREATMENT. While the asymptomatic patient with spondylolysis requires no active treatment, those with pain are treated by activity modification, physical therapy (focusing on strengthening of the abdominal and paraspinal musculature), and non-narcotic analgesics. The use of a modified lumbosacral orthosis, which reduces lumbar lordosis and immobilizes the spine, may lead to a faster resolution of symptoms. The brace is typically worn for 3–4 mo. Participation in sports should be withheld until the symptoms have resolved. While most patients experience resolution of their symptoms, the spondylolysis heals in only a small number of patients who have been diagnosed prior to the establishment of a pars defect. Surgery is offered when the above measures have failed to control the symptoms. For those with spondylolysis at L5, a posterior spinal fusion from L5 to S1 is indicated. For the infrequent cases in which the defect is at higher

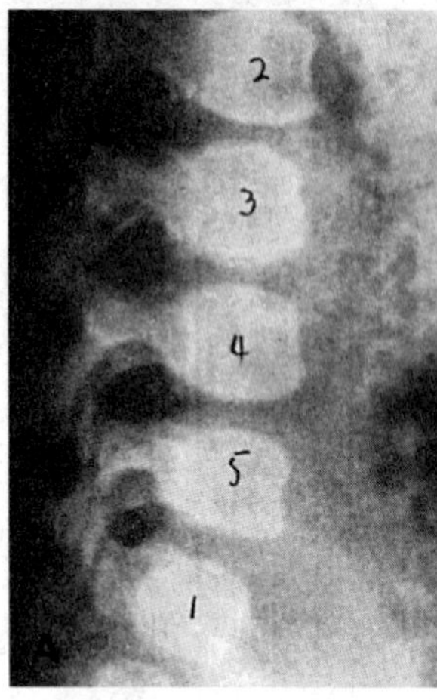

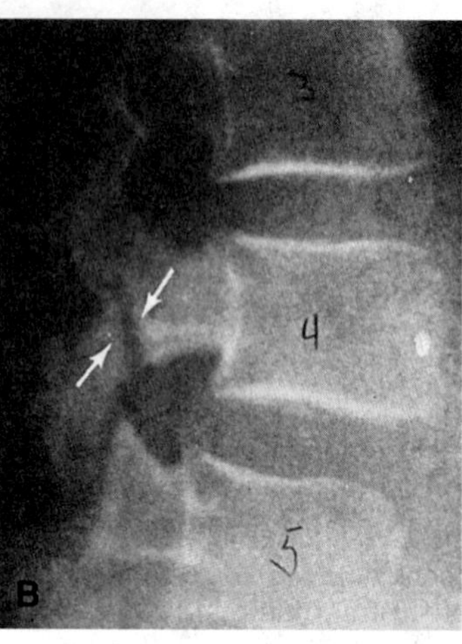

Figure 678-7. *A,* Normal spine at 9 mo of age. *B,* Spondylolysis in the L4 vertebra at 10 yr of age. (From Silverman FN, Kuhn JP: *Essentials of Caffrey's Pediatric X-Ray Diagnosis.* Chicago, Year Book Medical Publishers, 1990, p. 94.)

levels in the lumbar spine, techniques for repairing the defect may be considered. If successful, these procedures will avoid the need to surgically fuse the 2 vertebrae. Recommendations for the management of spondylolisthesis depend on the age of the patient, the presence of symptoms (pain and/or neurologic), the degree of deformity, and to a lesser extent on cosmetic concerns. For low-grade lesions (<50% slippage), the management is similar to that for spondylolysis. As progressive slippage may occur in a subset of skeletally immature patients, follow-up every 6–12 months is generally recommended, and a standing lateral radiograph of the lumbar spine is periodically obtained. For low-grade slips with persistent symptoms despite nonoperative measures, a spinal fusion alone may be successful. For skeletally immature patients with >50% slippage, surgery is offered, given the higher propensity for such cases to progress. The surgical approach for these high-grade slips, with and without neurologic dysfunction, varies between surgeons and institutions. The main principle is to stabilize the unstable segment of the spine. Procedures commonly performed include posterior spinal fusion, and anterior and posterior spinal fusion, with or without spinal instrumentation and with or without an attempt at reduction of the deformity. Neurologic symptoms may resolve with stabilization, and on occasion decompression of the neural elements is performed as a component of the stabilization procedure.

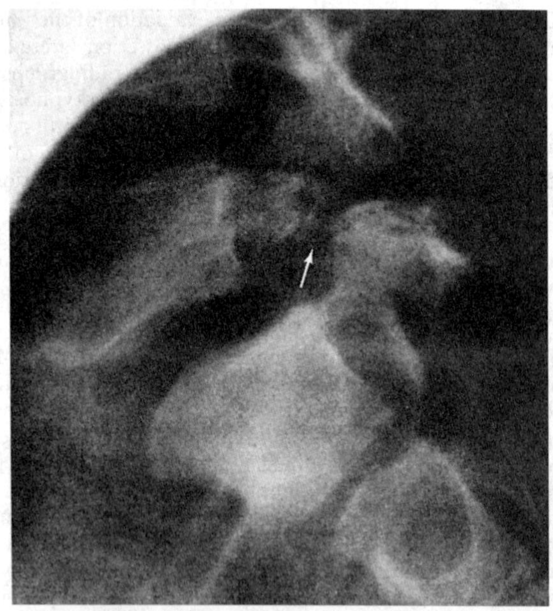

Figure 678-8. Defect in the pars interarticularis (arrow) of the neural arch of L5 (spondylolysis) that has permitted the body of L5 to slip forward (spondylolisthesis) on the body of S1. (From Silverman FN, Kuhn JP: *Essentials of Caffrey's Pediatric X-Ray Diagnosis.* Chicago, Year Book Medical Publishers, 1990, p. 95.)

678.7 • Disk Space Infection

Both diskitis and vertebral osteomyelitis may be considered as age-dependent variations of infectious spondylitis. Diskitis is generally seen in children younger than 5 yr of age, while vertebral osteomyelitis occurs in older children and adolescents. Patients in the younger age range have vascular channels that communicate between the vertebral end plate and the vascular disk space, which explains the prevalence of diskitis. Once these channels have closed, the infection remains in the vertebra.

Staphylococcus aureus is the most common organism identified from blood (rarely) or the aspirated fluid of the disk space (occasionally). Other organisms include *Kingella kingae,* group A streptococcus and *Escherichia coli.* An organism is recovered from any site in only 50–60% of patients.

CLINICAL MANIFESTATIONS. A high index of suspicion is required to establish the diagnosis of diskitis. In addition to back pain and/or fever, patients may experience malaise, and toddlers may develop a limp or refuse to walk or sit. In an effort to reduce the pain associated with spinal motion, the spine is held in a rigid position, and there may also be splinting from paraspinal muscle spasm. There may be local spinal process tenderness. In particular, flexion of the spine compresses the anterior elements of the spine, and will be associated with an increase in pain. This may be tested by asking the child to pick up an object from the ground. There is a loss of the normal lumbar lordosis. Neurologic manifestations are rare but include weakness. Patients may be afebrile, and while a complete blood count may remain normal, the erythrocyte sedimentation rate and the C-reactive protein are usually elevated. Older children may have fever and abdominal pain resembling a psoas abscess.

RADIOGRAPHIC EVALUATION. The characteristic features on plain radiographs, including disk space narrowing and irregularity of the adjacent vertebral end plates, develop 2–3 wk after the onset of symptoms. The diagnosis may be established earlier using either a technetium bone scan or MRI. MRI is most helpful in identifying abscesses and ruling out vertebral osteomyelitis.

TREATMENT. Once the diagnosis is established, symptomatic care includes activity restriction, analgesics, and immobilization in a spinal orthosis. As both blood cultures and cultures of disk space material are often negative, the etiology of diskitis has been debated. Most evidence suggests that the etiology is bacterial, leading to the recommendation that treatment include a 4–6-wk course of intravenous (initially for 1–2 wk) and then oral antibiotics effective against *S. aureus.* A CT-guided needle biopsy of the disk space is not routinely required and is usually reserved for children who do not respond to initial treatment with antibiotics. Surgical treatment is usually required to establish the diagnosis in patients who do not respond to initial therapy or to drain an abscess.

678.8 • Intervertebral Disk Herniation/Slipped Vertebral Apophysis

Intervertebral disk herniation and slipped vertebral apophysis are extremely rare in children and uncommon in adolescents. The symptoms and physical findings are quite similar to those in adults. While the etiology remains unknown, predisposing factors for both of these may include disk degeneration, congenital malformation, genetics, and environmental factors. Both are space-occupying lesions that may encroach on the neural elements. While a herniated disk typically involves either a protrusion (rarely a free fragment) of nuclear material into the spinal canal, the slipped vertebral apophysis involves protrusion of a portion of the ring apophysis with or without an attached segment of bone.

CLINICAL MANIFESTATIONS. Symptoms of intervertebral disk herniation in adolescents are similar to those in adults, and there is often a history of trauma. A subset of patients have congenital anomalies of the lumbosacral spine. The major complaint is back pain, and radicular symptoms (if present) generally appear later in the course. The back pain is often made worse by coughing or straining. On physical examination, both paraspinal muscle spasm and a decrease in range of motion are common. While overt signs of neurologic involvement are absent in most patients, a positive straight leg raise test is usually present. When present, the neurologic findings often do not correlate with the level of disk herniation. An intraspinal tumor should always be suspected in the differential diagnosis.

RADIOGRAPHIC EVALUATION. Radiographs often show loss of lumbar lordosis and a lumbar curvature (not a true scoliosis) which is due to muscle spasm. Degenerative changes and/or a loss of intervertebral disk height is occasionally noted on plain films. MRI is the best study to establish the diagnosis, and CT is especially helpful to visualize a partially ossified fragment associated with a slipped apophysis.

TREATMENT. The initial treatment is nonoperative in most patients and focuses on rest, activity modification, analgesics, and physical therapy. An orthosis may provide additional symptomatic relief. Complete bed rest is not recommended. The role of epidural steroids remains to be determined. Surgical treatment should be considered when nonoperative measures have failed or when a profound neurologic deficit or cauda equina syndrome is present either initially or as the clinical course evolves. Unfortunately, children and adolescents respond less favorably to nonoperative therapy compared with adults, and a significant percentage will require surgical intervention. The surgical technique involves a laminotomy, and subtotal disk excision to decompress the neural elements. In the case of a slipped vertebral apophysis, a similar approach is employed; however, fragments of bone and cartilage must also be removed, which often requires a bilateral laminotomy to completely address the pathology. While the initial results are excellent in the majority of patients, the literature suggests that up to ⅓ of patients may have recurrent symptoms of back or leg pain at longer term follow-up. A spinal fusion may be required when clinical instability is present.

678.9 • Tumors

Back pain may be the most common presenting complaint in children who have a tumor involving the vertebral column or the spinal cord. Other associated symptoms may include weakness of the lower extremities, scoliosis, and loss of sphincter control. The majority of tumors are benign (see Chapter 501), including osteoid osteoma, osteoblastoma, aneurysmal bone cyst, and eosinophilic granuloma. Malignant tumors involving the vertebral column may be osseous (osteosarcoma or Ewing sarcoma), may involve the spinal cord and sympathetic or parasympathetic nerves (ganglioneuroma, ganglioneuroblastoma, neuroblastoma), or may rarely be metastatic. In addition to high-quality plain radiographs, modalities including a bone scan (localization, look for other lesions), MRI (soft-tissue extension, neurologic compression) and CT (excellent bony detail) are performed in most cases prior to making a treatment plan. A biopsy is usually required to establish the diagnosis, and the treatment of tumors of the spinal column may require a multidisciplinary approach and should ideally be done in centers with experience in the management of these lesions.

Idiopathic Scoliosis

Cassar-Pullicino VN, Eisenstein SM: Imaging in scoliosis: What, why and how? *Clin Radiol* 2002;57:543–562.

Do T, Fras C, Burke S, et al: Clinical value of routine preoperative magnetic resonance imaging in adolescent idiopathic scoliosis: A prospective study of three hundred and twenty-seven patients. *Bone Joint Surg Am* 2001;83:577–579.

Dobbs M, Lenke LG, Szymanski DA, et al: Prevalence of neural axis abnormalities in patients with infantile idiopathic scoliosis. *J Bone Joint Surg Am* 2002;84:2230–2234.

Edgar M: A new classification of adolescent idiopathic scoliosis. *Lancet* 2002;360:270–271.

Goldberg CJ, Moore DP, Fogarty EE, et al: Adolescent idiopathic scoliosis: The effect of brace treatment on the incidence of surgery. *Spine* 2001;26:42–47.

Karol LA: Effectiveness of bracing in male patients with idiopathic scoliosis. *Spine* 2001;26:2001–2005.

Lenke LJ, Betz RR, Harms J, et al: Adolescent idiopathic scoliosis. A new classification to determine the extent of spinal arthrodesis. *J Bone Joint Surg Am* 2001;83:1169–1181.

Little DG, Song KM, Katz D, et al: Relationship of peak height velocity to other maturity indicators in idiopathic scoliosis in girls. *J Bone Joint Surg Am* 2000;82:685–693.

Merola AA, Haher TR, Brkaric M, et al: A multi-center study of the outcomes of the surgical treatment of adolescent idiopathic scoliosis using the Scoliosis Research Society (SRS) outcome instrument. *Spine* 2002;27:2046–2051.

Song KM, Little DG: Peak height velocity as a maturity factor for males with idiopathic scoliosis. *J Pediatr Orthop* 2000;20:286–288.

Sponseller PD: Sizing up scoliosis. *JAMA* 2203;289:608–609.

Weinstein SL, Dolan LA, Spratt KF, et al: Health and function of patients with untreated idiopathic scoliosis. *JAMA* 2003;289:559–567.

Congenital Scoliosis/Kyphosis

Basu PS, Elsebaie H, Noordeen MH: Congenital spinal deformity: A comprehensive assessment at presentation. *Spine* 2002;27:2255–2259.

Campbell RM, Hell-Vocke AK: Growth of the thoracic spine in congenital scoliosis after expansion thoracoplasty. *J Bone Joint Surg Am* 2003;85:409–420.

Campbell RM, Smith MD, Mayes TC, et al: The characteristics of thoracic insufficiency syndrome associated with fused ribs and congenital scoliosis. *J Bone Joint Surg Am* 2003;85:399–408.

Deviren V, Bervin S, Smith JA, et al: Excision of hemivertebrae in the management of congenital scoliosis involving the thoracic and thoracolumbar spine. *J Bone Joint Surg Br* 2001;83:496–500.

Gollogly S, Smith JT, Campbell RM: Determining lung volume with three-dimensional reconstructions of CT scan data. *J Pediatr Orthop* 2004;24:323–328.

Kim YJ, Otsuka NY, Flynn JM, et al: Surgical treatment of congenital kyphosis. *Spine* 2001;26:2251–2257.

McMaster MJ, Singh H: The surgical management of congenital kyphosis and kyphoscoliosis. *Spine* 2001;26:2146–2154.

Smith JT, Gollogly S, Dunn HK: Simultaneous anterior-posterior approach through a costotransversectomy for the treatment of congenital kyphosis and acquired kyphoscoliotic deformities. *J Bone Joint Surg Am* 2005;87:2281–2289.

Suh SW, Sarwark JF, Vora A, et al: Evaluating congenital spine deformities for intraspinal anomalies with magnetic resonance imaging. *J Pediatr Orthop* 2001;21:525–531.

Neuromuscular Scoliosis

Jones KB, Sponseller PD, Shindle MK, et al: Longitudinal parental perceptions of spinal fusion for neuromuscular spine deformity in patients with totally involved cerebral palsy. *J Pediatr Orthop* 2003;23:143–149.

Spiegel DA, Flynn JM, Stasikelis PJ, et al: Curve patterns in Chiari I malformation and/or syringomyelia. *Spine* 2003;28:2139–2146.

Westerlund LE, Gill SS, Jjarosz TS, et al: Posterior-only unit rod instrumentation and fusion for neuromuscular scoliosis. *Spine* 2001;26:1984–1989.

Kyphosis

Boseker EH, Moe JH, Winter RB, Koop SE: Determination of "normal" thoracic kyphosis: A roentgenographic study of 121 "normal" children. *J Pediatr Orthop* 2000;20:796–798.

Papegelopoulos PJ, Klassen RA, Peterson HA, et al: Surgical treatment of Scheuermann's disease with segmental compression instrumentation. *Clin Orthop* 2001;386:139–149.

Poolman RW, Been HD, Ubags LH: Clinical outcome and radiographic results after operative treatment of Scheuermann's disease. *Eur Spine J* 2002;11:561–569.

Back Pain

Balague F, Dudler J, Nordin M: Low-back pain in children. *Lancet* 2003;361:1403–1404.

Feldman DS, Hedden DM, Wright JG: The use of bone scan to investigate back pain in children and adolescents. *J Pediatr Orthop* 2000;20:790–795.

Jones GT, Macfarlane GJ: Epidemiology of low back pain in children and adolescents. *Arch Dis Child* 2005;90:312–316.

Parisini P, DiSilvestre M, Greggi T, et al: Lumbar disc excision in children and adolescents. *Spine* 2001;26:1997–2000.

Speed C: Low back pain. *Br Med J* 2004;328:1119–1121.

Watson KD, Papageorgiou AC, Jones GT, et al: Low back pain in schoolchildren: the role of the mechanical and psychosocial factors. *Arch Dis Child* 2003;88:12–17.

Spondylolysis and Spondylolisthesis

Grzegorzewski A, Kumar SJ: In situ posterolateral spine arthrodesis for grades III, IV, and V spondylolisthesis in children and adolescents. *J Pediatr Orthop* 2000;20:506–511.

Lenke LG, Bridwell KW: Evaluation and surgical treatment of high-grade isthmic dysplastic spondylolisthesis. *Instr Course Lect* 2003;52:525–532.

Disk Space Infection

Brown R, Hussain M, McHugh K, et al: Discitis in young children. *J Bone Joint Surg Br* 2001;83:106–211.

Early S, Kay R, Tolo V: Childhood diskitis. *J Am Acad Orthop Surg* 2003;11:413–420.

Fernandez M, Carroll CL, Baker CJ: Discitis and vertebral osteomyelitis in children: An 18-year review. *Pediatrics* 2000;105:1299–1304.

Garron E, Veihweger E, Launay F, et al: Nontuberculous spondylodiscitis in children. *J Pediatr Orthop* 2002;22:321–328.

Nussinovitch M, Sokolover N, Volovitz B, Amir J: Neurologic abnormalities in children presenting with diskitis. *Arch Pediatr Adolesc Med* 2002;156:1052–1054.

Chapter 679 ■ The Neck

David A. Spiegel, Harish S. Hosalkar, John P. Dormans, and Denis S. Drommond

679.1 • Torticollis

Torticollis is the term used to describe the clinical findings of tilting (lateral bending) of the head/neck to the right or left side in combination with rotation of the head/neck to the opposite side. Torticollis is not a diagnosis, but rather a manifestation of a variety of underlying conditions (Table 679-1). Most cases discovered at or near the time of birth represent **congenital muscular torticollis** (CMT). Although the etiology is unknown, this deformity may result from abnormal positioning in utero and involves contracture of the sternocleidomastoid. Muscle biopsies and MRI scans suggest that congenital muscular torticollis may be caused by an intramuscular compartment syndrome. Intrauterine muscle injury from compression and/or stretch may create localized ischemia, which results in fibrosis and contracture. Familial basis for torticollis as well as hereditary muscle aplasia have been reported. A contracture of the left sternocleidomastoid muscle results in tilt of the head to the left and rotation to the right, and vice versa. CMT is defined by the presence of a palpable mass (fibrous tissue) within the substance of the sternocleidomastoid muscle. However, this finding is present in approximately half of the patients. The mass disappears during infancy and is replaced by a fibrous band. Associated findings include plagiocephaly and facial asymmetry, both of which usually resolve with restoration of cervical motion. Patients may have associated positional musculoskeletal deformities such as metatarsus adductus and calcaneovalgus feet (see Chapters 673.1 and 673.2). Approximately 5–8% of patients also have dysplasia of the hip. While standards for screening in patients with a normal hip examination have not been established, consideration should be given to obtaining either an ultrasound scan (1 mo of age) or a plain radiograph of the hip (4–5 mo of age).

TABLE 679-1. Differential Diagnosis of Torticollis (Wryneck)

CONGENITAL
Muscular torticollis
Positional deformation
Hemivertebra (cervical spine)
Unilateral atlanto-occipital fusion
Klippel-Feil syndrome
Unilateral absence of sternocleidomastoid
Pterygium colli
TRAUMA
Muscular injury (cervical muscles)
Atlanto-occipital subluxation
Atlantoaxial subluxation
C2-3 subluxation
Rotary subluxation
Fractures
INFLAMMATION
Cervical lymphadenitis
Retropharyngeal abscess
Cervical vertebral osteomyelitis
Rheumatoid arthritis
Spontaneous (hyperemia, edema) subluxation with adjacent head and neck infection (rotary subluxation syndrome): Grisel syndrome
Upper lobe pneumonia
NEUROLOGIC
Visual disturbances (nystagmus, superior oblique paresis)
Dystonic drug reactions (phenothiazines, haloperidol, metoclopramide)
Cervical cord tumor
Posterior fossa brain tumor
Syringomyelia
Wilson disease
Dystonia musculorum deformans
Spasmus nutans
OTHER
Acute cervical disk calcification
Sandifer syndrome (gastroesophageal reflux, hiatal hernia)
Benign paroxysmal torticollis
Bone tumors (eosinophilic granuloma)
Soft tissue tumor
Hysteria

Torticollis in neonates may also result from congenital vertebral anomalies; anteroposterior and lateral radiographs of the cervical spine are indicated when the typical clinical features associated with congenital muscular torticollis are absent or if the deformity does not respond to treatment. A stretching program should be successful in >90% of patients with congenital muscular torticollis, especially when treatment is started within the first 3 mo of life. For patients diagnosed late or those in whom the stretching program has failed to correct the deformity, surgical release of the sternocleidomastoid is considered. Surgery can be delayed until 1–1.5 yr of age to maximize spontaneous correction of plagiocephaly. Motion can be improved following surgical release even up to early teens. Surgical management results in adequate function and acceptable cosmesis in >90% of patients. With early diagnosis and treatment, surgery should be required in a minority of cases.

The evaluation of torticollis becomes more complex when the typical findings associated with CMT are absent (mass and/or contracture within the sternocleidomastoid), the usual clinical response is not observed, or the deformity presents at a later age. In such cases, a careful history and physical examination are required, and often a consultation with an ophthalmologist and/or neurologist will be helpful. Plain radiographs should be obtained, and MRI of the brain and cervical spine will be required in a subset of cases. The differential diagnosis is extensive (see Table 679-1). **Atlantoaxial rotatory displacement** represents a spectrum of rotational malalignment (subluxation to dislocation) between the atlas (C1) and the axis (C2), and may best be described as pathologic stickiness in the arc of joint motion. Atlantoaxial rotary fixation is complete loss of motion that is manifest as torticollis with loss of passive cervical rotation. The malalignment may initially be reducible but after weeks to months the deformity becomes fixed and irreducible. As such, prompt diagnosis and treatment are essential. The condition is most often secondary to infection/inflammation of the tissues of the upper airway, neck, and/or pharynx (**Grisel syndrome**). Traumatic injuries, usually minor, may also lead to the development of rotatory displacement. This condition will occasionally complicate surgical procedures in the oropharynx, ear, or nose. Rotational malalignment at this joint is best evaluated with a CT scan, in which axial images are obtained through the upper cervical spine in different positions (right and left rotation). This study not only establishes the diagnosis, but also determines whether the displacement can be reduced passively. A "fixed" displacement persists with the head in different positions. If the patient is seen within a few days of the onset of symptoms, then a trial of analgesics and a soft collar may be attempted. Patients with symptoms for more than a week are often admitted to the hospital for analgesia, muscle relaxants, and a period of cervical traction. If this fails to reduce the displacement, then halo traction may be attempted. If the joint can be reduced, patients are typically immobilized for at least 6 wk in a halo vest. Patients with a fixed deformity may require a posterior atlantoaxial fusion to stabilize the articulation.

Neurogenic torticollis is uncommon and results from tumors of the posterior fossa or brainstem, syringomyelia, and Arnold-Chiari malformation. In addition to the neurologic examination, MRI of the brain and cervical spine is required to establish the diagnosis. **Paroxysmal torticollis of infancy** is also uncommon and may be due to vestibular dysfunction. Episodes may last from minutes to days, and the side of the deformity may alternate. The condition is self-limited, and no specific treatment is required other than ruling out other treatable diagnoses. Torticollis may also be seen in association with diskitis or vertebral osteomyelitis, juvenile rheumatoid arthritis, cervical disk calcification, visual problems (strabismus due to paralysis of the extraocular muscles), tumor-like conditions, and in patients with cerebral palsy and chronic gastroesophageal reflux (Sandifer syndrome).

679.2 • Klippel-Feil Syndrome

Klippel-Feil syndrome involves the congenital fusion (failure of segmentation) of one or more cervical motion segments, and most patients have associated congenital anomalies of the cervical spine (Fig. 679-1). These anomalies may occur at the craniocervical junction (occiput-C2), the subaxial spine (below C2), or both. The clinical triad of short neck, low hairline, and restriction of neck motion is seen in only about half of the patients. There is a strong association with congenital abnormalities of the genitourinary tract (30–40%), including double collecting systems, renal aplasia, and horseshoe kidney. Associated anomalies occur in the auditory system, neural axis, cardiovascular system, and the musculoskeletal system. Sprengel deformity (congenital elevation of the scapula) is a common associated finding, and >50% of patients will develop scoliosis. Since congenital anomalies may exist in more than one region of the spine, radiographs of the thoracic and lumbosacral spine are routinely obtained. These cervical findings may also be seen in patients with Goldenhar syndrome, Mohr syndrome, VACTERL syndrome, and fetal alcohol syndrome.

Characteristic physical findings include a low hairline and a short, webbed neck. Decreased cervical motion is usually present, although the degree of restriction depends on both the location and the number of levels fused and may be difficult to detect in minimally affected patients. Torticollis may be observed. Initial evaluation should include anteroposterior, lateral, and oblique views of the cervical spine. The characteristic finding is a congenital fusion of two or more vertebrae (failure of segmentation); multiple vertebrae may be involved. Symptoms are more common in adults than in children or adolescents and include pain and/or neurologic dysfunction. Painful degenerative changes in the disks and/or facet joints may result from an alteration in mechanical stresses, and segmental hypermobility or instability may develop at the mobile segments adjacent to fused segments. Excessive segmental motion (instability) may become clinically evident as radiculopathy or myelopathy, and brainstem compression may also occur. Spinal stenosis, either developmental or acquired, may also result in pain and/or neurologic compression. Flexion-extension lateral views may help to identify segments with excessive motion, and MRI may be required if neurologic symptoms are present. Surgery may be required to decompress the neural elements and/or stabilize segments of the cervical spine.

679.3 • Cervical Anomalies and Instabilities

One or more anomalies of the craniovertebral junction and/or the lower cervical spine (Klippel-Feil syndrome) may be seen in isolation or in association with other conditions (genetic syndromes, skeletal dysplasias, connective tissue disorders, metabolic diseases). These may be congenital, resulting from a mutation in the homeobox genes, or developmental. While most remain asymptomatic and undiagnosed, a subset will place the patient at risk of neurologic injury based on instability or stenosis. The most frequently encountered causes of cervical spine instability in children can be categorized etiologically (Table 679-2).

Patients with known associations should have an evaluation of the cervical spine. Others may present with pain and/or neurologic symptoms. Physical findings include a restriction in cervical mobility with or without neurologic abnormalities. In the upper cervical spine, flexion and extension take place at the occiput-C1 articulation, and rotation occurs at the atlantoaxial (C1-2) joint. Neither possesses inherent osseous stability and instead depends on the integrity of the ligaments and joint capsules to constrain motion. Instability may result in compression of the brainstem and/or spinal cord. Anomalies at the craniovertebral junction

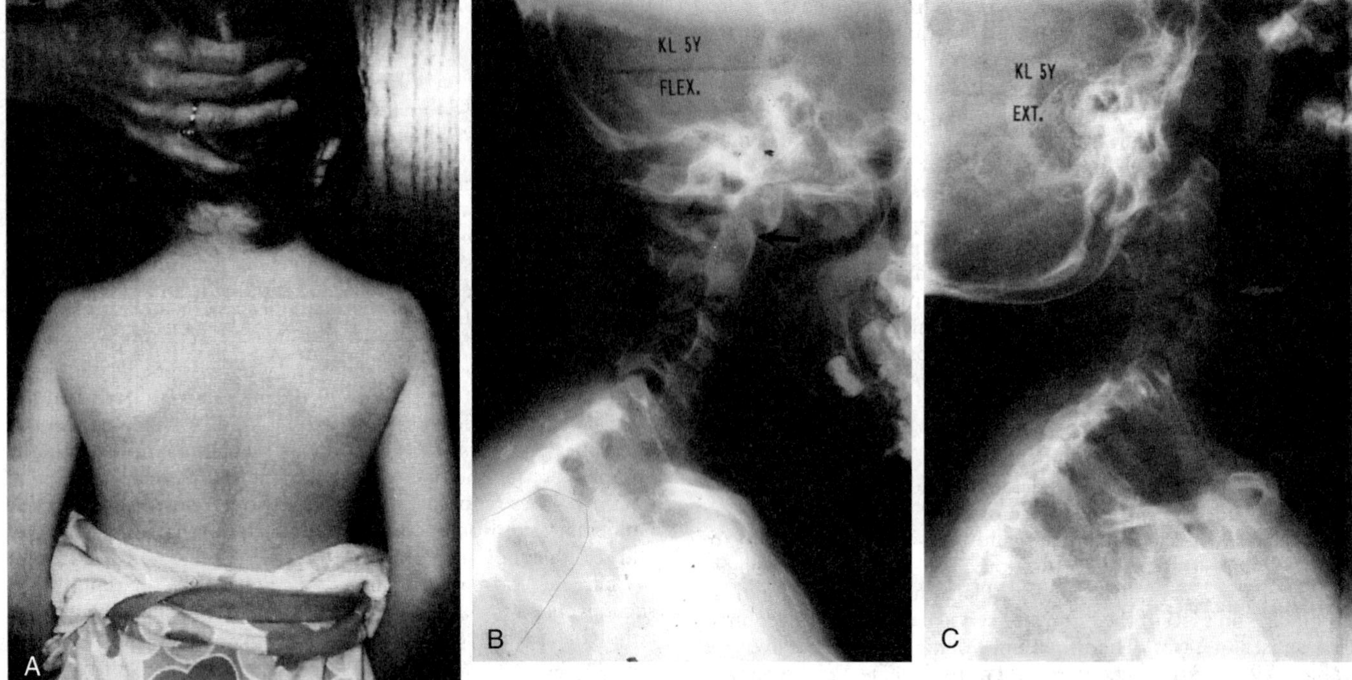

Figure 679-1. Clinical picture of a 5 yr old with Klippel-Feil syndrome. *A,* Note short neck and low hairline. Radiographs of the cervical spine (*B,* flexion; *C,* extension) demonstrate congenital fusion and evidence of spinal instability *(arrow).* (From Drummond DS: Pediatric cervical instability. In Weisel SE, Boden SD, Wisnecki RI [editors]: *Seminars in Spine Surgery.* Philadelphia, WB Saunders, 1996, pp 292–309.)

include occipitoatlantal fusion (occipitalization of the atlas), basilar impression and invagination, and accessory vertebrae. Aplasia or hypoplasia of the atlas or the axis may result in atlantoaxial instability. **Os odontoideum** represents a discontinuity in the midportion of the dens, and the upper portion of the dens moves along with the ring of C1, narrowing the space available for the spinal cord and often placing the spinal cord at risk of injury. While the etiology of os odontoideum is still debated, a traumatic origin is suspected.

The symptoms and physical findings vary with the location of compression or impingement. Patients may complain of headache and/or neck pain and may have symptoms of neurologic compression. The radiographic evaluation begins with anteroposterior, lateral, and open mouth (odontoid) views, which may be supplemented by flexion and extension lateral radiographs. CT provides the best bony detail and is useful in defining each anomaly. MRI, including dynamic images in flexion and extension, is best for evaluating neurologic impingement. Symptomatic treatment may be helpful; however, patients with cervical instability and/or neurologic impingement require surgical decompression and/or stabilization.

TABLE 679-2. Causes of Pediatric Cervical Instability

CAUSES	SUBTYPES
Congenital	***Vertebral*** (bony anomalies)
	Cranio-occipital defects (occipital vertebrae, basilar impression, occipital dysplasias, condylar hypoplasia, occipitalized atlas)
	Atlantoaxial defects (aplasia of atlas arch, aplasia of odontoid process)
	Subaxial anomalies (failure of segmentation and/or fusion, spina bifida, spondylolisthesis)
	Ligamentous or
	Combined anomalies found at birth as an element of somatogenic aberration
	Syndromic disorders (i.e., Down syndrome, Klippel-Feil syndrome, 22q11.2 deletion syndrome, Larsen syndrome, Marfan syndrome, Ehlers-Danlos syndrome)
Acquired	***Trauma***
	Infection (pyogenic/granulomatous)
	Tumor (including neurofibromatosis)
	Inflammatory conditions (i.e., juvenile rheumatoid arthritis)
	Osteochondrodysplasias (i.e., achondroplasia, diastrophic dysplasia, metatropic dysplasia, spondyloepiphyseal dysplasia)
	Storage disorders (i.e., mucopolysaccharidoses)
	Metabolic disorders (rickets)
	Miscellaneous (including osteogenesis imperfecta, post-surgery)

DOWN SYNDROME. Ligamentous hyperlaxity is a characteristic feature of Down syndrome and may result in hypermobility or instability at the occipitoatlantal or the atlantoaxial joints in 10–30% of patients (see Chapter 81). These patients may also have coexisting congenital or developmental anomalies of the cervical spine such as occipitalization of the atlas, atlantal arch hypoplasia, basilar invagination, and os odontoideum. Instability of the C1-2 level is found in up to 40% of children with Down syndrome. Further, atlantooccipital instability may be as common in this population and is reported to be as high as 61%. While the natural history of this spectrum of pathology remains unknown, a subset of patients develop (or are at significant risk of) neurologic dysfunction. All patients require screening by history and physical examination (at regular intervals) and at least a single series of cervical spinal radiographs, including a lateral view in flexion and extension. Although the specific recommendations vary between states, both clinical and radiographic screenings are required prior to participation in Special Olympics. The clinical diagnosis of neurologic dysfunction may be challenging, and subtle findings such as decreased exercise tolerance and gait abnormalities including increased tripping or falling may be the earliest signs of myelopathy. Clonus and hyperreflexia may be identified on physical examination. The evaluation of motor and sensory function may be quite difficult in this population, and in most patients, both clinical and radiographic (plain films, MRI) findings are required to evaluate suspected neurologic involvement.

Although hypermobility at the occipitoatlantal joint is present in >50% of children with Down syndrome, most patients do not develop instability or neurologic symptoms. The relationships at

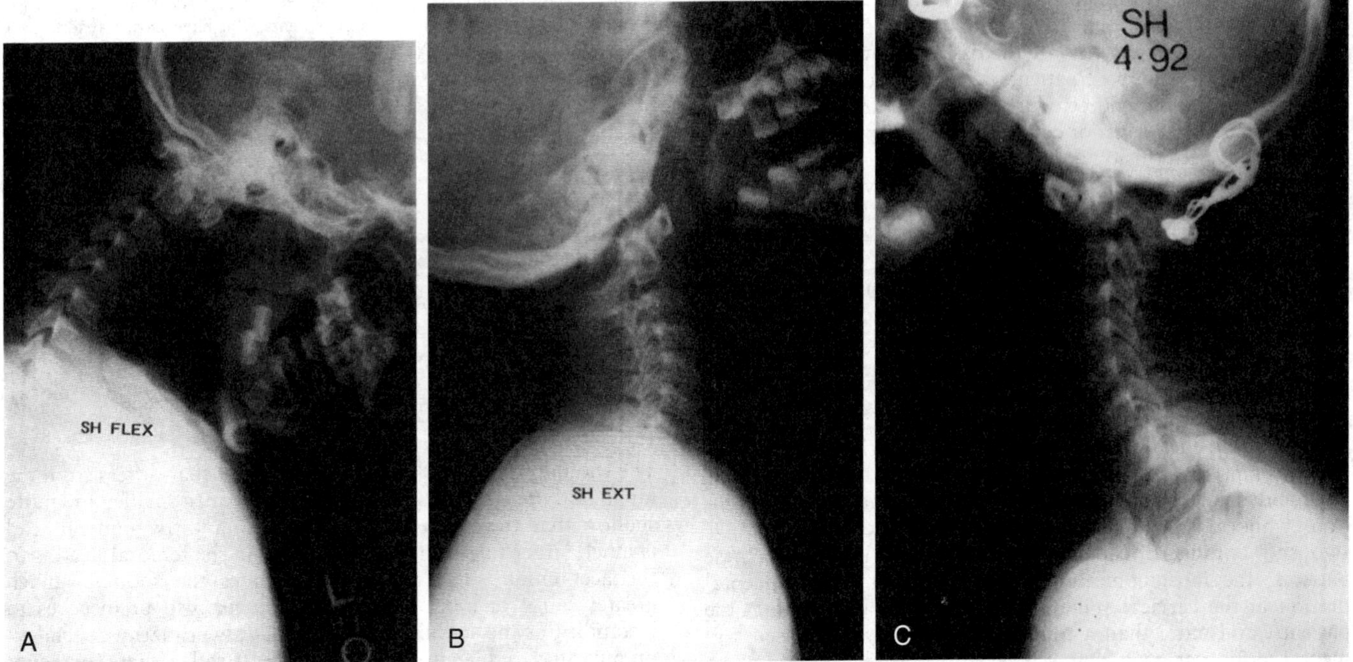

Figure 679-2. Flexion *(A)* and extension *(B)* radiographs of a case of Down syndrome demonstrating atlanto-occipital hypermobility and subluxation. *C,* Instability and symptoms were relieved by an occipitoaxial arthrodesis.

this articulation are difficult to measure reliably on plain radiographs; an MRI may help to identify the significance of any questionable radiographic findings. Of greater clinical concern is the atlantoaxial joint. The atlanto-dens interval (ADI) is used to diagnose hypermobility or instability. The space between the dens and the anterior ring of C1 (ADI) is measured on lateral radiographs in neutral, flexion, and extension (Fig. 679-2).

A normal ADI in children with Down syndrome is <4.5 mm. Hypermobility is diagnosed with an ADI between 4.5 and 10 mm; an ADI >10 mm represents instability and carries a significant risk of neurologic injury. MRI is indicated to detect neurologic compromise in patients with radiographic instability. Involvement of the subaxial spine is less common and is typically encountered in the adult population of patients with Down syndrome. Degenerative changes and/or instability may result in pain, radiculopathy, and myelopathy.

Recommendations for surveillance of potential cervical instability in children with Down syndrome remain varied. We recommend plain radiographs of the cervical spine including flexion-extension views for children presenting with Down syndrome. An annual neurologic examination should be performed. Flexion and extension radiographs are obtained every other year in those with a normal clinical exam. Those with abnormal findings or symptoms get an MRI. This helps to advise patients on the most appropriate level of physical activity and to identify the small subset with either progressive laxity/instability or frank neurologic involvement. Patients with normal radiographs who are also neurologically normal may be allowed to participate in

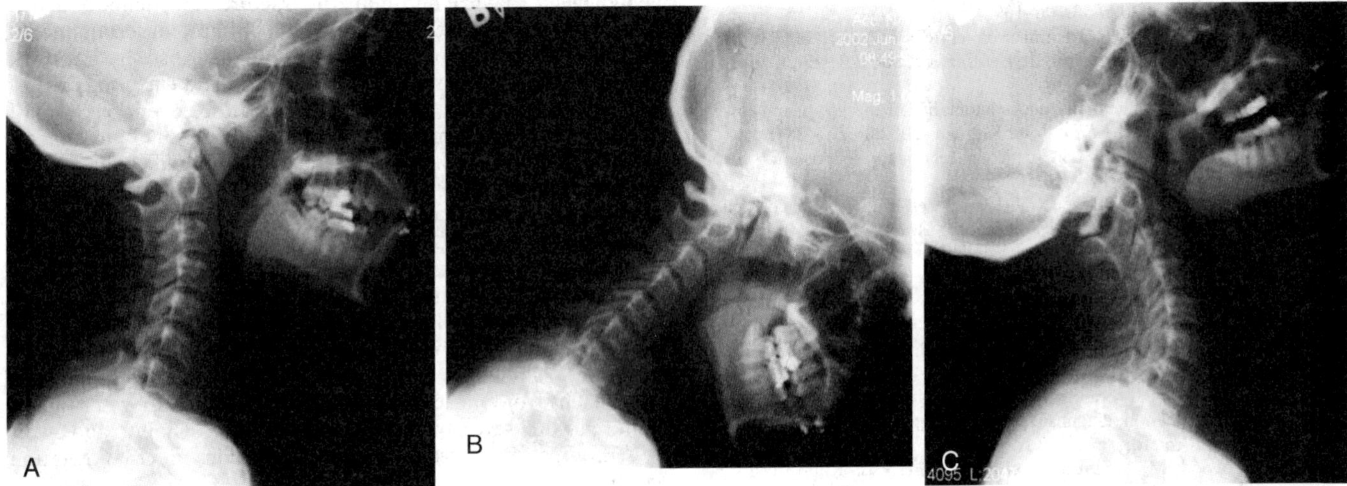

Figure 679-3. Radiographs of the cervical spine in a child with 22q11.2 deletion syndrome showing evidence of platybasia, occipitocervical, and atlantoaxial instability. *A,* Neutral radiograph. *B,* Flexion. *C,* Extension. (From Drummond DS: Pediatric cervical instability. In Weisel SE, Boden SD, Wisnecki RI [editors]: *Seminars in Spine Surgery.* Philadelphia, WB Saunders, 1996, pp 292–309.)

a full level of activities. Those who are diagnosed with hypermobility should be restricted from contact sports and other high-risk activities that might increase the risk of trauma to the cervical spine. The small subset of patients with neurologic involvement or instability and impending neurologic injury are candidates for fusion. The risks of a major complication are extremely high for a posterior cervical fusion in this population; these include death, neurologic deterioration, and pseudarthrosis with or without graft resorption.

22Q11.2 DELETION SYNDROME. The chromosome abnormality deletion of 22q11.2 is a common genetic syndrome and encompasses a wide spectrum of abnormalities including cardiac, palate, and immunologic anomalies. Anomalies of the upper cervical spine on plain radiographs are common.

At least one developmental variation of the occiput or cervical spine is noted in all patients. The occipital variations observed include platybasia and basilar impression. Atlas variations include dysmorphic shape, open posterior arch, and occipitalization, while axis variations include dysmorphic dens and "C2 swoosh." A range of cervical vertebral fusions is noted in these patients, the most common being C2–3. Increased segmental motion in the cervical spine is noted in more than half of the patients, and more than a third of patients have increased segmental motion at more than one level.

With frequent occurrence of upper cervical spine variations in the 22q11.2 deletion syndrome (Fig. 679-3), advanced imaging of the upper cervical spine and regular follow-up of patients to clarify their clinical course is recommended.

Adams SB Jr, Flynn JM, Hosalkar HS: Torticollis in an infant caused by hereditary muscle aplasia. *Am J Orthop* 2003;32:556–558.
Cheng JC, Tang SP, Chen TM, et al: The clinical presentation and outcome of treatment of congenital muscular torticollis in infants—a study of 1086 cases. *J Pediatr Surg* 2000;35:1091–1096.
Cheng JC, Wong MW, Tang SP, et al: Clinical determinants of the outcome of manual stretching in the treatment of congenital muscular torticollis in infants: A prospective study of eight hundred and twenty-one cases. *J Bone Joint Surg Am* 2001;83:679–687.
Clarke RA, Catalan G, Diwan AD, et al. Heterogeneity in Klippel-Feil syndrome: A new classification. *Pediatr Radiol* 1998;28:967–974.
Collins A, Jankovic J: Botulinum toxin injection for congenital muscular torticollis presenting in children and adults. *Neurology* 2006;67:1083–1085.
Copley LA, Dormans JP: Cervical spine disorders in infants and children. *J Am Acad Orthop Surg* 1998;6:204–214.
Dai L, Yuan W, Ni B, et al: Os odontoideum: Etiology, diagnosis and management. *Surg Neurol* 2000;53:106–109.
Drummond DS, Hosalkar HS. Treatment of cervical instability. In Clark CR (editor): *The Cervical Spine,* 4th ed. The Cervical Spine Research Society, 2005, pp 427–447.
Guille JT, Sherk HH: Congenital osseous anomalies of the upper and lower cervical spine in children. *J Bone Joint Surg Am* 2002;84:277–288.
Gupta AK, Roy DR, Conlon ES: Torticollis secondary to posterior fossa tumors. *J Pediatr Orthop* 1996;16:505–507.
Hensinger RN, Lang JE, MacEwen GD: Klippel-Feil syndrome: A constellation of associated anomalies. *J Bone Joint Surg Am* 1974;56:1246–1253.
Hosalkar HS, Gill IS, Gujar P, Shaw BA: Familial torticollis with polydactyly: Manifestation in three generations. *Am J Orthop* 2001;30:656–658.
Martinez-Lage JF, Morales T, Fernandez Cornejo V: Inflammatory C2-3 subluxation: A Grisel's syndrome variant. *Arch Dis Child* 2003;88:628–629.
Mezue WC, Taha ZM, Bashir EM: Fever and acquired torticollis in hospitalized children. *J Laryngol Otol* 2002;116:280–284.
Pang D, Li V: Atlantoaxial rotatory fixation: Part III of a prospective study of the clinical manifestation, diagnosis, management, and outcome of children with atlantoaxial rotatory fixation. *Neurosurgery* 2005;57:952–972.
Pizzutillo PD, Woods M, Nicholson L, et al: Risk factors in Klippel-Feil syndrome. *Spine* 1994;19:2110–2116.
Ricchetti ET, States L, Hosalkar HS, et al: Radiographic study of the upper cervical spine in the 22q11.2 deletion syndrome. *J Bone Joint Surg Am* 2004;86:1751–1760.
Segal LS, Drummond DS, Zarotti RM, et al: Complications of posterior arthrodesis of the cervical spine in patients who have Down syndrome. *J Bore Joint Surg [Am]* 1991;73(10):1547–1554.
Snyder EM, Coley BD: Limited value of plain radiographs in infant torticollis. *Pediatrics* 2006;118:e1779–e1784.

Chapter 680 ■ Upper Limb

Roger Cornwall

SHOULDER

The shoulder joint is a ball-and-socket joint that differs from the hip in that the glenoid (shoulder socket) is much smaller and more shallow than the acetabulum (hip socket), and the humeral head is much larger relative to the glenoid than the femoral head is to the acetabulum. This difference provides the shoulder much greater range of motion than the hip, but also predisposes to instability, as the stability of the shoulder is primarily dependent on muscular and ligamentous attachments rather than bony congruity. The wide range of motion in the glenohumeral joint is augmented by substantial scapulothoracic motion, giving the upper limb a large three-dimensional volume of space in which to function.

BRACHIAL PLEXUS BIRTH PALSY. Injuries to the brachial plexus can occur during or before delivery, usually as a result of a stretching mechanism and often associated with large fetal size and shoulder dystocia (see Chapter 99). The incidence is 1–3/1,000 live births and is similar around the world despite widely variable birthing practices and quality of care. Most often, the upper roots (C5, C6, and to a variable extent C7) are involved, with paralysis or weakness of the shoulder, elbow, and wrist. The arm is held in a position of shoulder adduction and internal rotation, elbow extension, and wrist flexion (the waiter's tip posture). The entire plexus can be involved, with total paralysis of the upper limb. Isolated lower plexus (C8, T1) involvement is very rare. The injury can range in severity from neurapraxia, or simple stretch of the nerve, to complete rupture of the nerve root or avulsion of the nerve root from the spinal cord. Approximately 30–40% of untreated children may have residual deficits.

Treatment. Clavicle and humerus fractures can mimic brachial plexus palsy and must be evaluated. Physical or occupational therapy for brachial plexus injuries should be instituted at 3 wk of age to maintain passive range of motion and encourage use of the arm. If the biceps muscle has shown no recovery by 3 mo of age or shows persistent substantial weakness at 5 mo of age, rupture or avulsion of the nerve roots is highly likely and surgical exploration and nerve grafting of the brachial plexus are indicated. MRI and electrodiagnostic testing are not consistently reliable in this setting.

Shoulder dysplasia and dislocation (analogous to developmental dysplasia of the hip) can occur as a result of muscle imbalances in infants and older children, and may require arthroscopic or open reduction and muscle balancing. Older children with residual weakness in shoulder abduction and external rotation can benefit from muscles transfers. Osteotomies are reserved for children with severely deformed glenohumeral joints and functional impairment from persistent shoulder internal rotation contracture.

SPRENGEL DEFORMITY. Sprengel deformity, or congenital elevation of the scapula, is a disorder of development that involves a high scapula and limited scapulothoracic motion. The scapula originates in early embryogenesis at a level posterior to the 4th cervical vertebra, but descends during development to below the 7th cervical vertebra. Failure of this descent, either unilateral or bilateral, is the Sprengel deformity. The severity of the deformity depends on the location of the scapula and associated anomalies. The scapula in **mild cases** is simply rotated, with a palpable or visible bump corresponding to the superomedial corner of the scapula in the region of the trapezius muscle. Function is generally good. In **moderate cases,** the scapula is higher on the neck and connected to the spine with an abnormal omovertebral ligament or even bone. Shoulder motion, particularly abduction, is limited. In **severe cases,** the scapula is small and positioned on the posterior neck, and the neck may be webbed. The majority of patients have associated anomalies of the musculoskeletal system, especially in the spine (including **Klippel-Feil anomaly** with congential cervical vertebral fusions [see Chapter 679]), making spinal evaluation important.

Treatment. In mild cases, treatment is generally unnecessary, although a prominent and unsightly superomedial corner of the scapula can be excised. In more severe cases, surgical repositioning of the scapula with rebalancing of parascapular muscles can significantly improve both function and appearance.

SHOULDER DISLOCATION. Traumatic glenohumeral dislocation is a common injury among adolescents, but is uncommon in younger children (see Chapter 686.2). A fracture of the proximal humerus physis is more common in young children. The dislocation is usually anterior and the result of forced abduction and external rotation. The supporting ligaments, capsules, and muscles are damaged during the dislocation, predisposing to recurrent dislocation. The younger the age of the patient at the time of initial dislocation, the more likely dislocations will recur.

Treatment. Following closed reduction of the dislocation, the shoulder is immobilized in adduction and internal rotation for 4–6 wk. Thereafter, rehabilitation is instituted to regain range of motion while strengthening the muscles that stabilize the shoulder. The high likelihood of recurrent dislocations in adolescents provides an argument for early surgical repair of the damaged capsule and ligaments to restore anatomic stability to the glenohumeral joint.

ELBOW

The elbow joint is the articulation between the humerus proximally and the ulna and radius distally. Flexion and extension of the elbow occur through the ulnohumeral and radiohumeral articulations, and pronation and supination occur though the radioulnar articulation. Unlike the shoulder, motion of the elbow is limited by complex bony anatomy, although stability of the elbow relies on stout ligaments on the medial and lateral sides. The elbow is prone to stiffness, with little tolerance to scar tissue formation following an injury or surgery.

NURSEMAID'S ELBOW. Nursemaid's elbow is a subluxation of a ligament rather than a subluxation or dislocation of the radial head. The proximal end of the radius, or radial head, is anchored to the proximal ulna by the annular ligament, which wraps like a leash from the ulna, around the radial head, and back to the ulna. If the radius is pulled distally, the annular ligament can slip proximally off the radial head and into the joint between the radial head and the humerus (Fig. 680-1). The injury is typically produced when a longitudinal traction force is applied to the arm, such as when a falling child is caught by the hand, or when a child is pulled by the hand. The injury usually occurs in toddlers and rarely occurs in children over the age of 5 yr. Subluxation of the annular ligament produces immediate pain and limitation of supination. Flexion and extension of the elbow are not limited, and swelling is generally absent. The diagnosis is made by history and physical examination, as radiographs are typically normal.

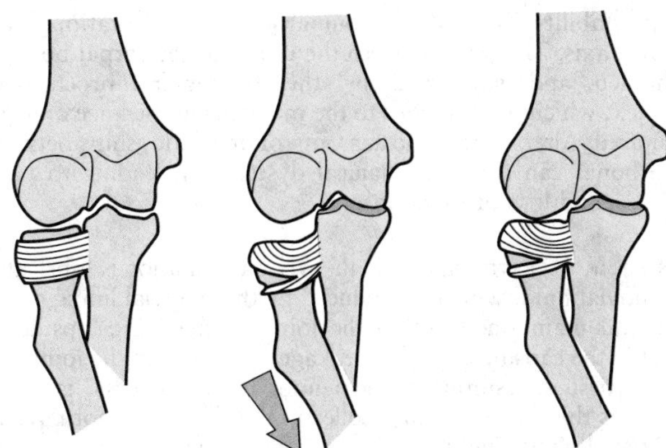

Figure 680-1. The pathology of nursemaid's, or pulled, elbow. The annular ligament is partially torn when the arm is pulled. The radial head moves distally, and when traction is discontinued, the ligament is carried into the joint. (From Rang M: *Children's Fractures,* 2nd ed. Philadelphia, JB Lippincott, 1983, p 193.)

Treatment. The annular ligament is reduced by rotating the forearm into supination while holding pressure over the radial head. A palpable "click" or "clunk" can be felt. The child recovers active supination immediately and usually has immediate relief of discomfort. Immobilization is not required, but recurrent annular ligament subluxations can occur, and the parents should avoid activities that apply traction to the elbows. Parents can learn reduction maneuvers for recurrent episodes to avoid trips to the emergency department or pediatrician's office. Recurrent subluxation beyond 5 yr of age is rare. Irreducible subluxations tend to resolve spontaneously with gradual resolution of symptoms over days to weeks; surgery is rarely indicated.

PANNER DISEASE. Panner disease is a disorder of bone and cartilage in the capitellum at the lateral aspect of the distal humerus. An idiopathic disturbance in blood flow in the bone may allow collapse of the capitellum, resembling Legg-Calvé-Perthes disease of the hip, or repeated trauma may allow fragmentation and separation of bone and cartilage as in osteochondritis dissecans. The process tends to occur in adolescents involved in throwing sports such as baseball or arm weight-bearing sports such as gymnastics (see Chapter 86.7). In these sports, the capitellum is exposed to high compression forces either from valgus stress to the elbow during throwing or from direct axial loading during upper extremity weight bearing. The symptoms are initially of pain and limitation of motion, especially lack of full elbow extension. The elbow may be swollen and crepitus may be felt. Radiographically, an area of lucency or frank fragmentation of the capitellum is seen. MRI is helpful in determining the extent of bone involvement and the integrity of the articular cartilage. Bone and cartilage may detach from the capitellum and form loose bodies within the joint.

Treatment. Rest and elimination of weight-bearing or throwing activities can allow resolution of early cases. Healing can sometimes be aided in more advanced cases by surgically drilling or grafting the affected bone to promote vascular ingrowth. Once loose bodies have developed and are causing mechanical symptoms, arthroscopic or open removal is warranted.

WRIST

The wrist is the complex articulation between the radius and ulna and the bones of the carpus. The radius and carpal bones are irregularly shaped and precisely interlocked to allow both mobility and stability. The distal radioulnar joint allows rotation of the forearm axis. The joint between the ulna and the carpal bones is cushioned and supported by the triangular fibrocartilage complex, which is analogous to the meniscus in the knee and can be injured. Alteration in the anatomy of or relationships between these bones can cause mechanical dysfunction leading to pain, stiffness, and loss of function.

GANGLION. As a synovial joint, the wrist articulation is lubricated by synovial fluid, which is produced by the synovial lining of the joint and maintained within the joint by the joint capsule. A defect in the capsule can allow leakage of fluid from the joint into the soft tissues, resulting in a ganglion. The term "cyst" is a misnomer, as this extra-articular collection of fluid does not have its own true lining. The defect in the capsule may occur as a traumatic event, although trauma is rarely a feature of the presenting history. The fluid usually exits the joint in the interval between the scaphoid and lunate, resulting in a ganglion located at the dorsoradial aspect of the wrist. Ganglia can occur at other locations, such as the volar aspect of the wrist, or in the palm as a result of leakage of fluid from the flexor tendon sheaths. Pain is not commonly associated with ganglia in children, and when it is, it is unclear whether the cyst is the cause of the pain. The diagnosis is usually evident on physical examination, especially if the lesion transilluminates. Extensor tenosynovitis and anomalous muscles can mimic ganglion cysts, but radiography or MRI is not routinely required. Ultrasonography is an effective, noninvasive tool to support the diagnosis and reassure the patient and family.

Treatment. Up to 80% of ganglia in children younger than the age of 10 yr will resolve spontaneously within 1 yr of being noticed. If the ganglion is painful or bothersome and the child is older than 10 yr of age, treatment may be warranted. Simple aspiration of the fluid has a high recurrence rate and is painful for children given the large-bore needle required to aspirate the gelatinous fluid. Surgical excision, including excision of the stalk connecting the ganglion to its joint of origin, has a high success rate, although the ganglion can recur.

RADIAL LONGITUDINAL DEFICIENCY. Congenital hypoplasia or absence of the radial aspect of the forearm, wrist, and hand is collectively called radial longitudinal deficiency; "radial club hand" refers to the condition's visual resemblance to the clubfoot (which has a different underlying pathology), and the term has lost favor. The deficiency can range in severity from a mildly short radius with slight radial deviation of the wrist to complete absence of the radius and thumb with a dislocated wrist, a short, bowed ulna, and dysfunctional fingers and elbow. The condition is sporadic in most cases, although radial deficiency is classically associated with systemic syndromes, most notably Fanconi anemia, thrombocytopenia absent radius syndrome, VACTERL association, and Holt-Oram syndrome (Table 680-1). Therefore, a full genetic work-up and multispecialty evaluation are required for every child with radial deficiency.

TABLE 680-1. Syndromes Commonly Associated with Radial Deficiency

SYNDROME	CHARACTERISTICS
Holt-Oram	Heart defects, most commonly atrial septal defects
TAR	Thrombocytopenia absent radius syndrome; thrombocytopenia present at birth, but improves over time
VACTERL	Vertebral abnormalities, anal atresia, cardiac abnormalities, tracheoesophageal fistula, esophageal atresia, renal defects, radial dysplasia, lower limb abnormalities
Fanconi anemia	Aplastic anemia not present at birth, develops about 6 yr of life; fatal without bone marrow transplant; chromosomal breakage challenge test available for early diagnosis

From Trumble T, Budoff J, Cornwall R (editors): *Core Knowledge in Orthopedics: Hand, Elbow, Shoulder*. Philadelphia, Elsevier, 2005, p 425.

Treatment. Passive stretching and splinting of a radially deviated wrist is begun shortly after birth. In mild cases in which the radius is only slightly short and the thumb is present and functional, conservative treatment can suffice. However, if the radius is partially or totally absent, surgery is required to centralize the carpus on the end of the ulna. If the thumb is underdeveloped but has a stable carpometacarpal joint, surgical reconstruction of the thumb can augment thumb function. However, if the thumb does not have a stable carpometacarpal joint or if the thumb is absent, pollicization of the index finger (repositioning the index finger into the position of the thumb) gives excellent results: A hand with three fingers and a thumb is superior functionally and cosmetically to a hand with four fingers and no thumb. Surgeries are scheduled so that reconstruction is complete by 18 mo of age to allow the child to incorporate the reconstructed hands and wrists into the development of manual skills from an early age.

HAND AND FINGERS

The hand, fingers, and thumb function as an intricate electrobiomechanical device with tremendous potential for function but little tolerance for perturbation. The hands of children function as organs of exploration and are important tools for functional and social development. Hand injuries are common in children, and malformations of the hand and upper limb are second only to cardiac defects among congenital anomalies.

FINGERTIP INJURIES. Young children are fascinated with doorjambs or car doors and other tight spaces, making crush injuries to the fingertips quite common. Injury can range from a simple subungual hematoma to complete amputation of part or the entire fingertip. Radiographs are important to rule out fractures. Physeal fractures associated with nail-bed injuries are **open fractures** with a high risk of osteomyelitis, growth arrest, and deformity if not treated promptly with formal surgical debridement and reduction. Tuft fractures involving the very distal portion of the distal phalanx are common and require little specific treatment other than that for the soft-tissue injury. The treatment of the soft-tissue injury depends on the type of injury. For suture repairs, only absorbable sutures should be used, as suture removal from a young child's fingertip can require sedation or general anesthesia. If a subungual hematoma exists but the nail is normal and no displaced fracture exists, the nail need not be removed for nail-bed repair. If the nail is torn or avulsed, the nail should be removed, the nail bed and skin should be repaired with absorbable sutures, and the nail (or a piece of foil if the nail is absent) should be replaced under the eponychial fold to prevent scar adhesion of the eponychial fold to the nail bed that may prevent nail regrowth. If the fingertip is completely amputated, treatment depends on the level of amputation and the age of the child. Distal amputations of skin and fat in children younger than 2 yr of age can be replaced as a composite graft with a reasonable chance of surviving. Similar amputations in older children can heal without replacing the skin as long as no bone is exposed and the amputated area is small. A variety of coverage procedures exist for amputations through the mid-portion of the nail. Amputations at or proximal to the proximal edge of the fingernail should be referred emergently to a replant center for consideration for microvascular replantation. When referring, all amputated parts should be saved, wrapped in saline-soaked gauze, placed into a watertight bag, and then placed in ice water. Ice should never directly contact the part, as it can cause severe osmotic and thermal injury.

POLYDACTYLY. Polydactyly is defined as the presence of one or more supernumerary digits or parts of digits. Polydactyly is defined as postaxial, occurring on the ulnar border of the hand; preaxial, occurring on the radial border of the hand; or central,

TABLE 680-2. Syndromes Associated with Polydactyly

Carpenter syndrome	Trisomy 13
Ellis-van Creveld syndrome	Orofaciodigital syndrome
Meckel-Gruber syndrome	Rubinstein-Taybi syndrome
Polysyndactyly	

occurring between adjacent fingers. Postaxial polydactyly often displays autosomal dominant transmission and can involve both hands and both feet. In mild cases, the extra digit may be a skin tag or a floating nubbin with bone and a nail but connected to the hand only by a thin stalk. Such digits can be suture ligated in the nursery, although a remnant may remain that requires formal surgical excision. Postaxial polydactyly may involve an entirely duplicated small finger, requiring formal amputation and reconstruction, usually at 1 yr of age. Preaxial polydactyly, or thumb duplication, varies from a duplicated thumbnail to an entirely duplicated thumb with extra phalanges. The underlying musculoskeletal anomaly is complex and requires formal surgical reconstruction and combining of parts from each thumb. Central polydactyly is a complex anomaly that is associated with deformities of the "normal" fingers and requires formal surgical reconstruction. Polydactyly can be associated with a wide variety of syndromes (Table 680-2).

SYNDACTYLY. During development, the hand begins as a paddle, and apoptosis between developing digits allows the creation of individual fingers. Syndactyly is a failure of this separation of adjacent digits. Syndactyly can be classified as simple, with only skin conjoined, or complex, with skin, tendon, and bone conjoined. Syndactyly can also be classified as partial, with only the proximal aspect of the finger conjoined (webbed), or complete, with fusion along the entire lengths of the digits including the nails. Syndactyly can be an isolated finding or associated with a wide variety of syndromes (Table 680-3). Syndactyly between digits of unequal length (thumb and index, index and middle, ring and small) causes tethering and deformity of the longer digit and should be surgically separated within the first few months of life. Syndactyly between the middle and ring fingers can be separated later in life, usually after 1 yr of age.

TRIGGER THUMB AND FINGERS. The flexor tendons for the thumb and fingers pass through fibrous tunnels made up of a series of pulleys on the volar surface of the digits. These tunnels, for reasons that are not well understood, can become tight at the most proximal, or 1st annular, pulley. Swelling of the underlying tendon occurs, and the tendon no longer glides under the pulley. In children, the most common digit involved is the thumb. It has classically been thought to be a congenital problem, but prospective screening studies of large numbers of neonates have failed to find a single case in a newborn child. Trauma is rarely a feature of the history, and the condition is often painless. Overall function is rarely impaired. A trigger thumb typically presents with the inability to fully extend the thumb interphalangeal joint. A palpable nodule can be felt in the flexor pollicis longus tendon at the base of the thumb. Other conditions can mimic trigger thumb, including the thumb-in-palm deformity of cerebral palsy. Similar findings in the fingers are much less common and can be associated with inflammatory conditions such as juvenile rheumatoid arthritis.

Treatment. Spontaneous resolution of trigger thumbs can occur in up to 30% of children diagnosed before 1 yr of age. Spontaneous resolution beyond that age is not common. Corticosteroid injections, while effective in adults, are not effective in children and risk injury to the nearby digital nerves. Surgical release of the 1st annular pulley is curative and is generally performed between 1 and 3 yr of age. Treatment of trigger fingers other than the thumb in children involves evaluation and treatment of any underlying inflammatory process and in some cases surgical decompression of the flexor sheath.

TABLE 680-3. Syndromes Associated with Syndactyly

Apert syndrome	Trisomy 21
Carpenter syndrome	Fetal hydantoin syndrome
de Lange syndrome	Laurence-Moon-Biedl syndrome
Holt-Oram syndrome	Fanconi panctyopenia
Orofaciodigital syndrome	Trisomy 13
Polysyndactyly	Trisomy 18

Chan O, Hughes T: Hand. *Br Med J* 2005;330:1073–1075.

Dao KD, Shin AY, Billings A, et al: Surgical treatment of congenital syndactyly of the hand. *J Am Acad Orthop Surg* 2004;12:39–48.

Farsetti P, Weinstein SL, Caterini R, et al: Sprengel's deformity: Long-term follow-up study of 22 cases. *J Pediatr Orthop B* 2003;12:202–210.

Good CR, MacGillivray JD: Traumatic shoulder dislocation in the adolescent athlete: Advances in surgical treatment. *Curr Opin Pediatr* 2005;17:25–29.

Kobayashi K, Burton KJ, Rodner C, et al: Lateral compression injuries in the pediatric elbow: Panner's disease and osteochondritis dissecans of the capitellum. *J Am Acad Orthop Surg* 2004;12:246–254.

Kozin SH: Upper-extremity congenital anomalies. *J Bone Joint Surg Am* 2003;85:1564–1576.

McAdams TR, Moneim MS, Omer GE Jr: Long-term follow-up of surgical release of the A(1) pulley in childhood trigger thumb. *J Pediatr Orthop* 2002;22:41–43.

Pondaag W, Malessy MJ, van Dijk JG, Thomeer RT: Natural history of obstetric brachial plexus palsy: A systematic review. *Dev Med Child Neurol* 2004;46:138–144.

Rayan GM, Frey B: Ulnar polydactyly. *Plast Reconstr Surg* 2001;107:1449–1457.

Wang AA, Hutchinson DT: Longitudinal observation of pediatric hand and wrist ganglia. *J Hand Surg [Am]* 2001;26:599–602.

Waters PM: Update on management of pediatric brachial plexus palsy. *J Pediatr Orthop* 2005;25:116–126.

Chapter 681 ■ Arthrogryposis

Harish S. Hosalkar and Denis S. Drummond

DEFINITION

Arthrogryposis multiplex congenita (AMC) is a congenital anomaly in the newborn involving multiple curved joints (Fig. 681-1). Arthrogryposis is a descriptive term and not an exact diagnosis, as there are at least 150 possible underlying causes.

The incidence of classic AMC is approximately 1/10,000 live births. Three main groups include

- Classic AMC in which the limbs are primarily involved and the muscles are deficient or absent (amyoplasia) (Fig. 681-2),
- Arthrogryposis in association with major neurogenic (brain, spinal cord, anterior horn cell, or peripheral nerve) or myopathic (congenital muscular dystrophy, myopathy, toxic myopathy) dysfunction,
- Arthrogryposis in association with other major anomalies and specific syndromes such as diastrophic dysplasia and craniocarpotarsal dystrophy (Table 681-1).

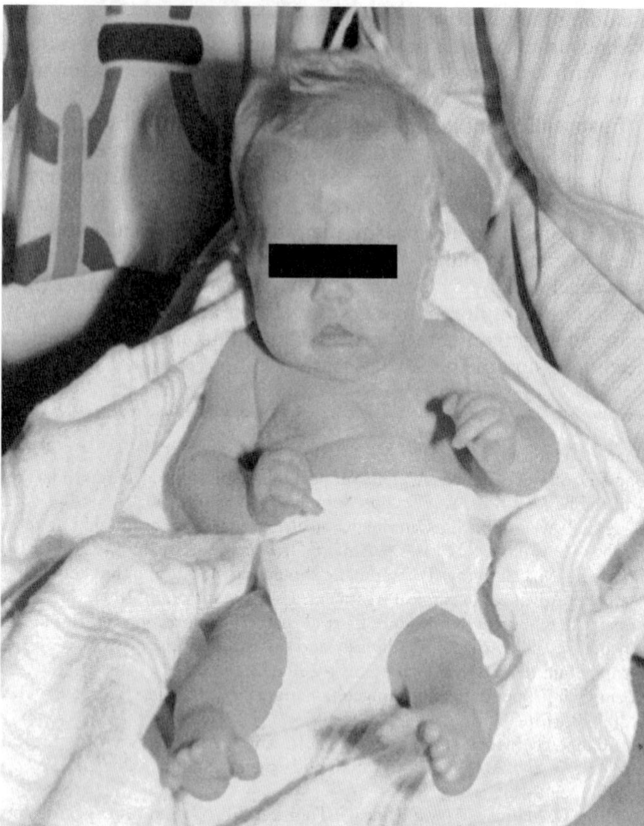

Figure 681-1. Arthrogryposis multiplex congenita. A 32-wk premature boy with severe multiple congenital contractures and severe congenital neuropathy. (From Hosalkar HS, Moroz L, Drummond DS, Finkel R: Neuromuscular disorders of infancy and childhood and arthrogryposis. In Dormans JP [editor]: *Pediatric Orthopaedics: Core Knowledge in Orthopedics*. Philadelphia, Mosby, 2005.)

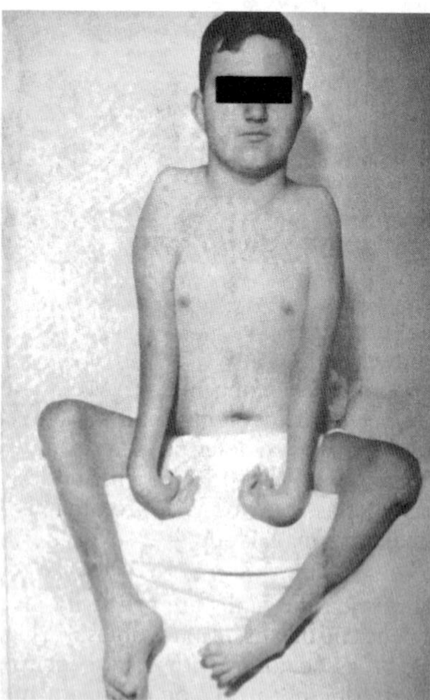

Figure 681-2. Joint contractures, lack of creases in skin, and deep dimples at joints are characteristic of arthrogryposis. (From Hosalkar HS, Moroz L, Drummond DS, Finkel R: Neuromuscular disorders of infancy and childhood and arthrogryposis. In Dormans JP [editor]: *Pediatric Orthopedics: Core Knowledge in Orthopedics*. Philadelphia, Mosby, 2005.)

TABLE 681-1. Associated Etiologies of Arthrogryposis

ARTHROGRYPOSIS DUE TO NERVOUS SYSTEM DISORDERS
- Focal anterior horn cell deficiency
- Generalized anterior horn cell deficiency
- Structural brain disorder/damage
- Uncertain location

(Spastic conditions are excluded)

DISTAL ARTHROGRYPOSIS SYNDROMES
- Type I dominant distal
- Type IIa dominant distal (Gordon syndrome)
- Type IIe distal
- Digitotalar dysmorphism
- Trismus pseudocamptodactyly
- Distal distribution, type not specified

PTERYGIUM SYNDROMES
- Multiple pterygium syndrome
- Lethal multiple pterygium syndrome
- Popliteal pterygium syndrome
- Ptosis, scoliosis, pterygia
- Antecubital webbing syndrome (Liebenberg)

MYOPATHIES
- Emery-Dreifuss muscular dystrophy
- Hypotonia, myopathy, mild contractures

ABNORMALITIES OF JOINTS AND CONTIGUOUS TISSUE
- Congenital contractural arachnodactyly
- Freeman-Sheldon syndrome
- Laxity or hypertonicity with intrauterine dislocation and contractures
- Larsen syndrome
- Spondyloepimetaphyseal dysplasia with joint laxity
- Trisomy 18, extended breech position with bilateral hip dislocation
- Siblings with bifid humeri, hypertelorism, and hip and knee joint dislocations

SKELETAL DISORDERS
- Diastrophic dysplasia
- Parastremmatic dysplasia
- Kniest dysplasia
- Metatropic dysplasia
- Campomelic dysplasia
- Schwartz syndrome
- Fetal alcohol syndrome with synostoses
- Osteogenesis imperfecta with bowing/contractures

INTRAUTERINE/MATERNAL FACTORS
- Fetal alcohol syndrome with contractures
- Infections
- Untreated maternal systemic lupus erythematosus
- Intrauterine fetal constraint
- Deformity (pressure)
- Amniotic fluid leakage
- Multiple pregnancies
- Intrauterine tumors
- Disruption (bands)

MISCELLANEOUS
- Pseudotrisomy 18 with contractures
- Roberts pseudothalidomide syndrome
- Deafness with distal contractures
- VACTERL association
- Multiple abnormalities and contractures not otherwise specified
- ARC*

SINGLE JOINT
- Campomelic
- Symphangylism
- "Trigger" finger

*Arthrogryposis, renal tubular acidosis, cholestasis.

Modified from Mennen U, Van Heest A, Ezaki MB, et al: Arthrogryposis multiplex congenita. *J Hand Surg [Br]* 2005;30:5:468–474. © 2005 The British Society for Surgery of the Hand.

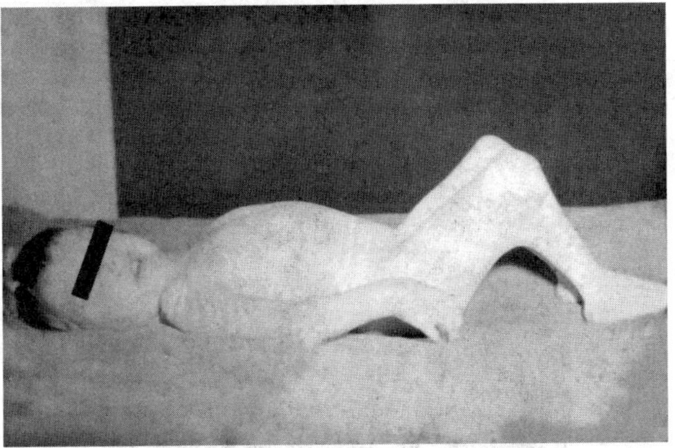

Figure 681-3. Fixed flexion of the knees in a boy with arthrogryposis multiplex congenita. (From Hosalkar HS, Moroz L, Drummond DS, Finkel R: Neuromuscular disorders of infancy and childhood and arthrogryposis. In Dormans JP [editor]: *Pediatric Orthopedics: Core Knowledge in Orthopedics.* Philadelphia, Mosby, 2005.)

CLINICAL FEATURES

Multiple rigid joint deformities are present with defective muscles but normal sensation. There is rigidity of several joints in each case resulting from both short tight muscles and capsular contractures. *Pterygium* may be present on the flexor aspects of contracted joints (Fig. 681-3). There is often an absence or fibrosis of muscles or muscle groups. There is normal intellectual development in most cases. All four limbs are involved in the classic form (AMC), but the condition can also occur in the upper or lower limbs. An autosomal dominant variant called distal arthrogryposis involves the hands and feet with severe deformation but with only minor contractures more proximally; scoliosis is a possible development. In addition to the multiple joint contractures, the lack of skin creases (cylindrical or tubular limbs) and deep dimples over the joints are very characteristic (Fig. 681-4). There is dislocation of joints, most commonly the hip but occasionally the knee. The trunk is rarely affected. Other congenital anomalies such as cryptorchidism, hernias, and gastroschisis may occur.

ETIOLOGY

AMC is multifactorial in etiology. Factors liable to produce immobility of the fetus may contribute to congenital contractures. Some of these include structural abnormality of the uterus (bifid, large fibroids), oligohydramnios, increased intrauterine pressure, mechanical compression of the fetus, weak fetal movements, breech presentation, and prematurity. Inflammatory or infective etiology has also been postulated, including inflammation in the joint, muscle, spinal cord, or brain; rubella in early pregnancy; and infection with unknown viruses. A dominant theory is that the primary condition is patchy degeneration of the anterior horn cells occurring in the early months of gestation. A pregnant mother treated with curare for severe tetanus gave birth to an arthrogrypotic baby.

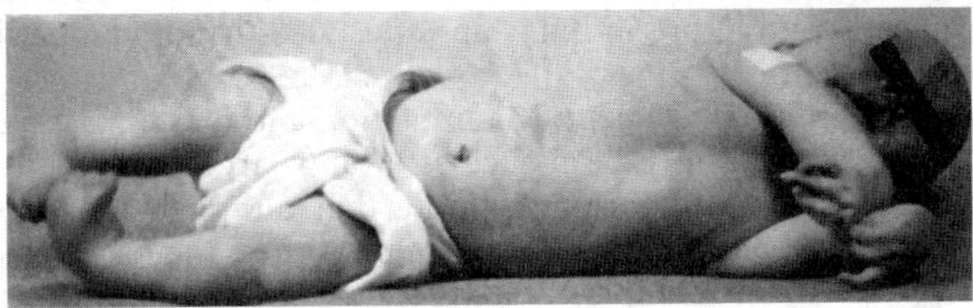

Figure 681-4. Characteristic lack of skin creases and tubular limbs. (From Hosalkar HS, Moroz L, Drummond DS, Finkel R: Neuromuscular disorders of infancy and childhood and arthrogryposis. In Dormans JP [editor]: *Pediatric Orthopedics: Core Knowledge in Orthopedics.* Philadelphia, Mosby, 2005.)

DIAGNOSIS

Clinical examination remains the best modality for establishing the diagnosis of arthrogryposis. We have found a few factors that are often useful in making a diagnosis. Although not absolute criteria, they are helpful when considered in combination.

Unlike paralytic disorders, joint deformities of AMC are usually stiff or rigid from the beginning with incomplete passive range of motion. Deformities of arthrogryposis tend to be symmetric.

The severity of contractures tends to increase as one reaches the periphery of the limb. The more proximal joints tend to be less involved, and the trunk is frequently spared. The most severe deformities tend to occur in the hands and feet.

The orthopedist, neurologist, geneticist, and pediatrician must participate in diagnosing and managing this condition. Radiographs of the involved extremities with joint involvement are recommended. These may demonstrate congenital bony abnormality and loss of subcutaneous fat and muscle. Radiographs of the whole spine will identify any vertebral anomalies. CT/MRI of the brain and spine are useful in establishing or ruling out structural central nervous system involvement. Electromyography and nerve conduction studies are of limited value and have been used to differentiate the peripheral neuropathic from the myopathic variants.

A skeletal muscle biopsy is needed when a primary myopathic disorder is suspected, unless genetic testing can establish the diagnosis by molecular testing of DNA from peripheral blood. Plasma creatine kinase estimation may be done to exclude myopathic disorders. This is best checked on the 3rd day of life or after, once any transient initial increase in creatine kinase from the birth process has subsided. If a prenatal ultrasound scan detects an absence of fetal movement, especially in combination with polyhydramnios, the diagnosis of arthrogryposis can be suspected. Histologic analysis reveals a small muscle mass with fibrosis and fat between the muscle fibers. Myopathic and neuropathic features may overlap in the same specimen. The periarticular soft tissues are fibrotic. Genetic consultation, with chromosome analysis and collagen studies, should be considered in cases in which a distinct peripheral neuromuscular disorder is not readily apparent.

The differential diagnoses are noted in Table 681-2.

TABLE 681-2. Differential Diagnosis of Congenital Contractures

DISORDERS	DIFFERENTIAL DIAGNOSES
Neurogenic	Spina bifida and spinal disorders
	Myelodysplasia
	Sacral and lumbar agenesis
	Spinal muscular atrophy
	Fetal neuropathy (toxic, infectious)
Myopathic	Congenital myotonic dystrophy
	Congenital muscular dystrophy
	Fetal/congenital myopathy
	Fetal myasthenia (passive transfer of antibody from mother with myasthenia gravis)
Connective tissue	Marfan syndrome
	Ehlers-Danlos syndrome
Miscellaneous	Freeman-Sheldon syndrome
	Turner syndrome
	Edward syndrome
	Pterygium syndrome
	Diastrophic dwarfism

PROGNOSIS

The clinician should be able to derive a general prognosis and treatment plan once the diagnosis of AMC is established. There may be a few functional motor movements as one reaches the periphery of the limb. Vigorous occupational therapy and use of hand splints and serial casting can improve the range of motion and functional use of the hand in many cases of AMC in which the etiology is not of a progressive disorder (amyoplasia). Surgery, in selected cases, is necessary to obtain a more neutral positioning of the wrist and fingers so the limited degree of strength can be used to optimal biomechanical advantage.

Recurrence of a corrected deformity is quite common and occurs with growth in a limb in which the periarticular structures are incapable of stretching. Arthrogrypotic children have certain positive factors that must be used in their successful management.

Joint instability is not a problem in AMC, unlike other paralytic conditions.

With a coordinated and team approach in management, there will often be little deterioration from the condition at birth. There is frequently central sparing and a relatively normal trunk.

The child with normal central nervous system findings can be expected to have reasonably normal intelligence and, with enough motivation, can contribute to successful management.

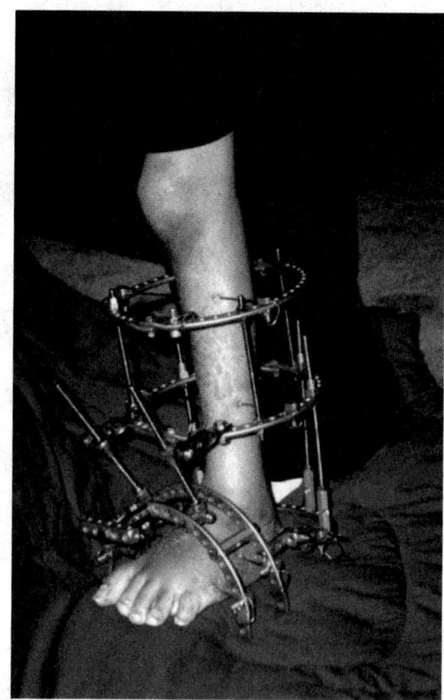

Figure 681-5. Ilizarov fixation device for correction of ankle contracture. Courtesy of Dr. Richard Davidson, Children's Hospital of Philadelphia.

PRINCIPLES OF ORTHOPEDIC MANAGEMENT OF PATIENTS WITH ARTHROGRYPOSIS AND MULTIPLE CONGENITAL CONTRACTURES

Patients should be seen as early as possible, and treatment of the deformities started early because some will respond remarkably well to physiotherapy, stretching, and splintage.

Muscle balance is usually less of a problem than in other paralytic neuromuscular conditions and is easier to achieve. Muscle balance should be possibly established if there are functioning muscles available for transfer. **Recurrence of deformity** is the rule because the dense, inelastic soft tissues about the joints do not properly elongate with growth. These structures are considered the key to the successful management of arthrogryposis in the growing child. The maximal safely obtainable correction should be achieved at the time of surgery. The use of wedging or corrective casts after surgery is of little additional benefit. **Range of movement:** Results from passive range of motion stretching varies. Aggressive treatment may result in an appreciable increase in the limited range of joint movement or have little impact. The arc of motion, however, can often be changed into a functionally better position. **Centrifugal involvement:** The severity of the deformity increases toward the periphery of the limb and the more proximal joints tend to be less involved. Central sparing of the trunk may be noted in most cases. **Aim of management:** The main aim of management is to achieve maximal functional gain for each patient. Minimal requirements are independent walking, self-care, and, ideally, the ability to eventually be gainfully employed. **Staging and timing of surgical procedures:** Maximal benefit from surgical reconstruction of a limb with arthrogryposis is achieved by careful staging of procedures. The disabling deformity and contractures should be corrected in the first stage. The major joints should be then put in a functional arc of motion most adapted to the patient's needs.

In the final stage, tendon transfers are occasionally required to bring motor power to a joint that has been put to its optimal position. The elbow joint is well suited to tendon transfers and has been widely noted to give satisfactory results.

LOWER LIMBS

Foot Involvement. The most severe deformities in arthrogryposis are known to occur in the foot. The rigid foot deformity is usually the clubfoot or equinovarus deformity and, less frequently, a congenital vertical talus deformity. The goal of treatment is conversion of the rigid deformed foot into a rigid plantigrade foot.

Correction of the *hindfoot takes precedence* over the forefoot. *Serial stretching (casting)* may sometimes produce a degree of correction. Once it is clear during the course of treatment that conservative treatment will not be successful, surgery should be considered, preferably when the child is ready to walk.

An *extensive posteromedial and posterolateral release* is recommended. If the foot fails to correct with even the most extensive soft-tissue release or relapses quickly within 2–3 yr, talectomy may be considered. The Ilizarov technique and apparatus do offer an opportunity to correct these deformities by gradual distraction and neohistiogenesis (Fig. 681-5). Applications of this fixator in the pediatric foot have been fairly successful and satisfactory. In the case of older children with neglected or relapsed equinovarus deformity, correction can be best obtained by **triple arthrodesis.** In rare cases of recurrence of the de-formity after triple arthrodesis (at the level of the ankle), a **pantalar arthrodesis** may be offered by an easy conversion of the triple arthrodesis.

Knee Joint. Both common presentations of the knee deformity, fixed flexion and fixed extension, should be initially treated with repeated stretching and splintage. The goal is to get the knees straight and to keep them that way by bracing. Extension of the knee is considered the key to later walking. If a flexed knee is neglected, postural hip flexion contractures are likely to ensue. Combined contracture in both hips and knees is not compatible with good gait.

Nonsurgical management: Manipulation and plaster casting in the younger child have been successful in a large population of our patients. It is important to note that although the arc of motion is changed to a more extended position, the range is not increased. Even if complete extension cannot be obtained, the knee joints are usually stable and mild flexion deformities are quite compatible with a good gait pattern.

Surgical management: Deformities not responding to soft-tissue stretching may need surgical intervention. It is advisable to plan the timing of knee surgery in keeping with the treatment plan for the foot. For example, if the foot requires immobilization with the knee flexed, then the knee flexion correction should be staged after the foot management. On the other hand, if the knee is in fixed extension, it is better to correct the knee extension before operation on the foot, so that the foot can be immobilized with a flexed knee.

Fixed hyperextension of the knee may respond reasonably well to serial stretching and casting. In severe cases that fail to respond to stretching, an extensive muscular release with quadricepsplasty may be necessary to correct the knee position. Splintage and knee support are likely to be required on a long-term basis. The Ilizarov fixator again provides a useful alternative to surgical release or in cases of failed surgery, especially in the older patient.

Hip Joint. A common finding at birth in arthrogrypotic patients is stiffness of the hips in flexion, abduction, and external rotation. The two most common involvements of the hips are fixed contractures and hip dislocation.

It is important to correct the knee deformity before attempting any surgical intervention and correction at the hip. With knee correction at an early stage, the results of hip deformity correction are encouraging.

Surgical treatment:

Growing child: Full correction is not easily obtainable with soft-tissue release procedures. Recurrence is usually unavoidable with skeletal growth.

Skeletally mature child: If the child is able to ambulate with compensatory lordosis, it is best to wait until skeletal maturity and then hope for lasting correction with subtrochanteric osteotomy.

Arthrogryposis may lead to **unilateral or bilateral dislocation** of hips. Dislocations are usually stable and, if the pelvis is well balanced, are also consistent with a good gait. Treatment of hip dislocation is often not easy because closed reduction invariably fails and stiffness and persistent flexion deformity usually follow open reduction. Diagnosis can be difficult clinically because the marked stiffness may be a limiting factor for demonstrating the hip instability clinically. If the hips are dislocated, in most cases, they are not reducible on abduction and should not be splinted if irreducible. Splinting in such cases may lead to avascular necrosis. **Bilateral dislocations** tend to be high and stable, are usually symmetric, and tend to have a fairly balanced pelvis. This is often consistent with a good gait, and it may be advisable to leave them alone because it is often not possible to get a satisfactory result on both sides and in fact may lead to more stiffness with a high chance of redislocation. In cases of **unilateral dislocation,** there is a risk of progressive pelvic obliquity and secondary scoliosis. We therefore believe it is often worth reducing the dislocated hip, especially in the infant and the younger child. Open reduction should be done as soon as the child is healthy enough and knee flexion contractures have been controlled. Excessive delays make the procedure more technically demanding and the reduction more difficult to achieve.

UPPER LIMBS. Unlike management of lower limbs where independent walking is the main goal, management of upper extremities in arthrogryposis requires considerable caution because the prognosis for successful treatment is more dependent on the extent of deformity and on the patient's intelligence. The minimal requirements for the patient are ability to feed and attend to personal hygiene.

Again, in contrast to the lower limbs where surgery cannot be postponed due to risk of delayed walking, operations on upper limbs can be postponed for several years. Interestingly, arthrogrypotic children develop a remarkable ability to get about well with their upper limbs in spite of the complexities of these deformities, developing a surprising amount of dexterity, and therefore surgical intervention, if any, should be weighed very carefully in these cases.

Planning. *Both limbs should be considered as a unit.* The general principle that the arc of joint motion can be changed but not increased should be remembered. A reasonable expectation at the end of treatment is that the patient should ideally be able to move one hand to his or her mouth and the other to his or her anus, but still be capable of opposing both hands. This is important to consider because children with severe hand deformities and weakness depend on the integrated use of both hands (bimanual opposition) to perform any task that normal people do with one hand. In addition, he or she must be able to push him- or herself out of a chair.

Shoulder and elbow joints should be considered as a unit. The rotation of the shoulder is an important factor on which the axis of the elbow joint motion largely depends. Therefore, if elbow surgery is contemplated to enable the hand to reach the mouth, a severely fixed and internally rotated shoulder should also be simultaneously corrected.

Physiotherapy has a major contribution in obtaining motion in the stiff joints along with stretching and splintage. Detailed assessment by a physical therapist and occupational therapist is necessary before embarking on any surgical intervention, and surgery should be possibly deferred until the age of 4 yr.

Shoulder Joint. The typical deformity is adduction and internal rotation. Although shoulder weakness is common, these children can develop remarkable trick movements, and therefore surgical intervention may rarely be indicated. Adduction itself is not troublesome since usually there is enough passive abduction for self-care, and surgery is rarely required. Fixed internal rotation at the shoulder can in some cases jeopardize the axis of elbow motion. In severe cases, a simple external rotation osteotomy may be performed in the upper humerus to bring the forearm and hand into a more functional position.

Elbow Joint. The two common involvements of the elbow noted are fixed extension contracture and fixed flexion contracture. Both these conditions respond well to stretching and physical therapy and can be well controlled in infancy. Once the child is ambulating, activities such as crutch walking, toileting, and push-off from a chair/seated position essentially need active elbow extension. Therefore, it is important to not inadvertently damage the active extension mechanism while intending to improve active flexion. Passive flexion can be surgically achieved by a posterior soft-tissue release of the elbow, lengthening of the triceps, and a posterior capsular and collateral ligament release. This can restore a very useful arc of motion, and further procedures may not be even necessary in most cases. In candidates in whom a value of increased active flexion can be established, active power could be provided in multiple ways including a Steindler flexorplasty and transfer of the triceps or pectoralis major.

Elbow and forearm soft-tissue contractures can be successfully corrected using the Ilizarov fixator in many cases.

Wrist and Hand. The wrist is often involved in a flexion contracture and the fingers may be curved and stiff as well. Thumb adduction deformity (thumb-in-palm) is also common. Manipulation, stretching, and splintage (especially early on) can be very important in establishing mobility and range. Interestingly, the flexed position of the wrist is very functional and may not need intervention. Surgical corrections involving partial or complete carpectomy have been described and often show high incidence of recurrence of deformity with growth. Finger stiffness is extremely difficult to correct in these cases, and surgery is rarely indicated. Most patients adapt extremely well to the finger stiffness and are impressive in their functioning abilities. Release of thumb adductors and web space enlargement are very useful in correcting the thumb deformity. Wrist arthrodesis for functional or cosmetic gain may be considered at or near skeletal maturity.

SPINE. In consistency with the principle that the severity of the stiffness and deformity increases toward the periphery of limbs and that the more central or proximal areas are less involved, a straight, supple, and well-balanced trunk is an important asset. Scoliosis occurs frequently in arthrogryposis because of a high incidence of congenital curves (see Chapter 678).

Idiopathic Scoliosis. Genetic or idiopathic scoliosis seems to occur as frequently in the arthrogrypotic population as in the general population. The progression and behavior of an idiopathic curve in arthrogryposis are possibly the same as in other children, although may be more disabling because of the coexisting peripheral deformities.

Paralytic Scoliosis. Long paralytic scoliotic curves are sometimes seen in children with typical neuropathic type of arthrogryposis. Some forms of congenital muscular dystrophy include a "rigid spine" component. The curve is typically seen before the 2nd yr of life and progresses to become long, severe, and eventually rigid. Well-controlled bracing is the treatment of choice in younger children, although surgical management may be necessary in progressive cases.

Congenital Scoliosis. These curves are common in arthrogryposis, perhaps due to the other congenital anomalies common in arthrogryposis. Failure of vertebral formation and failure of segmentation have been noted. Klippel-Feil deformity is also observed. These curves must be observed closely, and aggressive treatment like early surgical fusion may be indicated in the presence of asymmetric progressive curves.

Scoliosis Associated with Pelvic Obliquity. This is frequently associated with neglected hip deformities that lead to femoropelvic obliquity and is potentially avoidable. Unilateral hip deformity should be particularly watched for and corrected. The trunk can then be kept supple and straight.

Abu-Sa'da O, Barbar M, Al-Harbi N, Taha D: Arthrogryposis renal tubular acidosis and cholestasis (ARC) syndrome: Two new cases and review. *Clin Dermatol* 2005;14:191–196.

Brunner R, Hefti F, Tgetgel JD: Arthrogrypotic joint contracture at the knee and the foot: Correction with a circular frame. *J Pediatr Orthop* 1997;6:192–197.

Burglen L, Amiel J, Violet L, et al: Survival motor neuron gene deletion in the arthrogryposis multiplex congenita–spinal muscular atrophy association. *J Clin Invest* 1996;98:1130–1132.

Fixsen J: Arthrogryposis multiplex congenita. In Benson MK, MF Macnicol MF, Parsch K (editors): *Children's Orthopaedics and Fractures.* Philadelphia, Churchill Livingstone, 2002, pp 293–298.

Hall JG: Genetic aspects of arthrogryposis. *Clin Orthop* 1985;194:44–53.

Hall JG: Arthrogryposis multiplex congenita: Etiology, genetics, classification, diagnostic approach, and general aspects. *J Pediatr Orthop* 1997;6: 159–166.

Hosalkar HS, Moroz L, Drummond DS, Finkel R: Neuromuscular disorders of infancy and childhood and arthrogryposis. In Dormans J (editor): *Pediatric Orthopedics: Core Knowledge in Orthopedics.* Philadelphia, Mosby, 2005, pp 454–482.

Mennen U, Van Heest A, Ezaki MB: Arthrogryposis multiplex congenita. *J Hand Surg [Br]* 2005;30:468–474.

Murray C, Fixsen JA: Management of knee deformity in classical arthrogryposis multiplex congenita (amyoplasia congenita). *J Pediatr Orthop* 1997;6:186–191.

Chapter 682 ■ Common Fractures

Purushottam A. Gholve, Harish S. Hosalkar, and Lawrence Wells

Trauma is a leading cause of death and disability in children older than 1 yr. Several factors make fractures of the immature skeleton different from those involving the mature skeleton. The anatomy, biomechanics, and physiology of the pediatric skeletal system are different from that of adults. This results in different fracture patterns (Fig. 682-1), diagnostic challenges, and management techniques specific to children to preserve growth and function.

Epiphyseal lines, rarefaction, dense growth lines, congenital fractures, and pseudofractures appear on radiographs, which could confuse the interpretation of a fracture. Most fractures in children heal well with indifferent treatment; that has led the unwary to neglect the fact that other fractures terminate disastrously if handled with inexpertise. The differences in the pediatric skeletal system predispose children to injuries different from those of adults. The important differences are the presence of periosseous cartilage, physes, and a thicker, stronger, more osteogenic periosteum that produces new bone called callus more

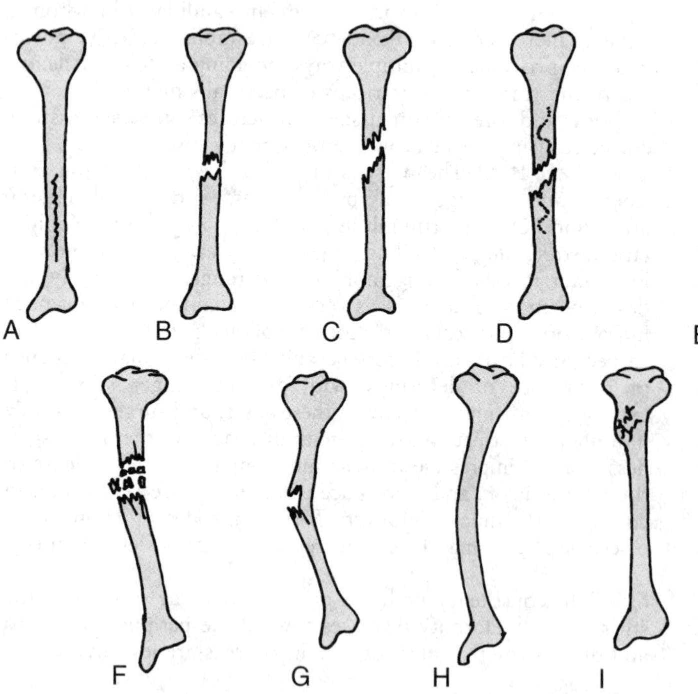

Figure 682-1. Illustration of fracture patterns. A, Longitudinal fracture line parallel to bony axis. *B,* Transverse fracture line perpendicular to bony axis. *C,* Oblique fracture line at angle to bony axis. *D,* Spiral fracture line runs a curvilinear course to the bony axis. *E,* Impacted fractured bone ends compressed together. *F,* Comminuted fragmentation of bone into three or more parts. *G,* Greenstick bending of bone with incomplete fracture of convex side. *H,* Bowing bone plastic deformation. *I,* Torus buckling fracture. (From White N, Sty R: Radiological evaluation and classification of pediatric fractures. *Clin Pediatr Emerg Med* 2002;3:94–105.)

rapidly and in greater amounts. The other factors are a disproportionately large head, pliable rib cage, unprotected large and small bowel, and open epiphyseal plates in children. The pediatric bone has low density and more porosity. The low density is due to lower mineral content and the increased porosity due to increased number of haversian canals and vascular channels. These differences result in a comparatively lower modulus of elasticity and lower bending strength. The bone in children may fail either in tension or in compression; the fracture lines do not propagate as in adults, and hence there is less chance of comminuted fractures.

Joint injuries, dislocation, and ligament disruptions are infrequent in children. Damage to a contiguous physes is more likely. Interdigitating mammillary bodies and the perichondrial ring enhance the strength of the physes. Biomechanically, the physes are not as strong as the ligaments or metaphyseal bone. The physis is most resistant to traction and least resistant to torsional forces. The periosteum is loosely attached to the shaft of bone and adheres densely to the physeal periphery. The periosteum is usually injured in all fractures, but it is less likely to have complete circumferential rupture due to its loose attachment to the shaft. This intact hinge or sleeve of periosteum lessens the extent of fracture displacement and assists in reduction. The thick periosteum may also act as an impediment to closed reduction, particularly if the fracture has penetrated the periosteum or in reduction of displaced growth plate.

682.1 • Unique Characteristics of Pediatric Fractures

FRACTURE REMODELING

Remodeling is the 3rd and final phase in biology of fracture healing preceded by inflammatory and reparative phase. This occurs from a combination of appositional bone deposition on the concavity of deformity, resorption on the convexity, and asymmetric physeal growth. Thus, reduction accuracy is somewhat less important than it is in adults (Fig. 682-2). The 3 major factors that have bearing on the potential for angular correction are skeletal age, distance to the joint, and orientation to the joint axis. The rotational deformity and angular deformity not in the axis of the joint motion are less likely to remodel. The amount of remaining growth provides the basis for remodeling; younger children have greater remodeling potential. Fractures adjacent to a physis undergo the greatest amount of remodeling, provided that the deformity is in the plane of axis of motion for that joint. The fractures away from the elbow and closer to the knee joint have greater potential to remodel as this physes provide maximal growth to the bone. One can expect remodeling to occur over the next several months following injury throughout skeletal maturity. Skeletal maturity is reached in girls between 13 and 15 yr and in boys between 14 and 16 yr of age.

OVERGROWTH

Physeal stimulation from the hyperemia associated with fracture healing causes overgrowth. It is usually prominent in long bones such as the femur. The growth acceleration is usually present for 6 mo to 1 yr following the injury and does not present a continued progressive overgrowth unless complicated by a rare arteriovenous malformation. Femoral fractures in children younger than 10 yr of age frequently overgrow by 1–3 cm. Bayonet apposition of bone is preferred to compensate for the expected overgrowth. This overgrowth phenomenon will result in equal or near equal limb lengths at the conclusion of fracture remodeling. After 10 yr of age, overgrowth is less of a problem and anatomic alignment is recommended. In physeal injuries, growth stimulation is associated with use of implants or fixation hardware that may cause chronic stimulus for longitudinal growth.

PROGRESSIVE DEFORMITY

Injuries to the physes can be complicated by progressive deformities with growth. The most common cause is complete or partial closure of the growth plate. As a consequence, angular

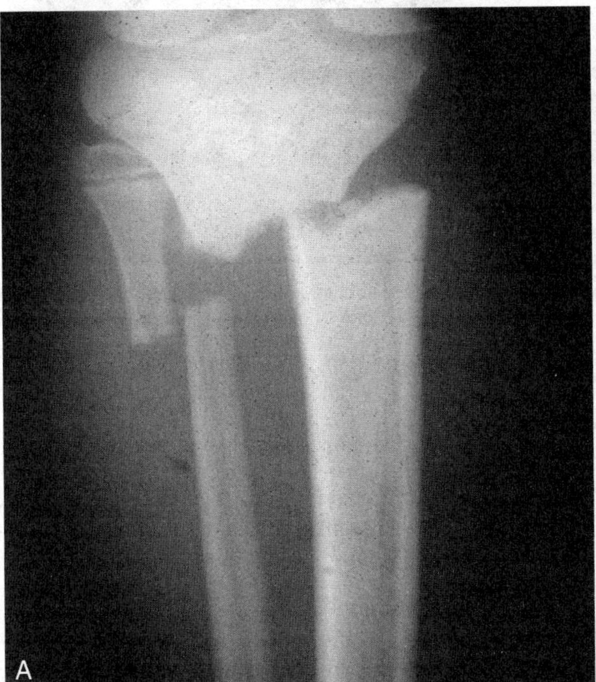

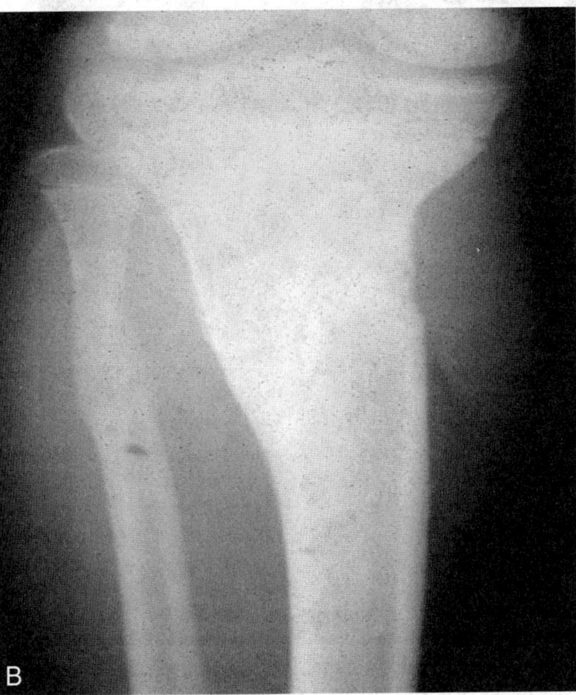

Figure 682-2. Remodeling in children is often extensive, as in this proximal tibial fracture *(A)* and as seen 1 yr later *(B)*. (From Dormans JP: *Pediatric Orthopedics: Introduction to Trauma*. Philadelphia, Mosby, 2005, p 38.)

deformity, shortening, or both, can occur. The partial arrest may be peripheral, central, or combined. The magnitude of deformity depends on the physis involved and the amount of growth remaining. CT and MRI are important for assessment of partial arrests and formulating treatment (Fig. 682-3).

RAPID HEALING

Children's fractures heal quickly compared with those of adults. This is due to children's growth potential and thicker, more active periosteum. As children approach adolescence and maturity, the rate of healing slows and becomes similar to that of an adult. The rapid healing has a downside, causing refractures.

682.2 • Pediatric Fracture Patterns

The different pediatric fracture patterns are the reflection of a child's characteristic skeletal system. The majority of pediatric fractures can be managed by closed methods and heal well.

PLASTIC DEFORMATION

Plastic deformation is unique to children. It is most commonly seen in the ulna and occasionally the fibula. The fracture occurs due to a force that produces microscopic failure on the tensile side of bone and does not propagate to the concave side. The concave side of bone also shows evidence of microscopic failure in compression. The bone is angulated beyond its elastic limit, but the energy is insufficient to produce a fracture. Thus, no fracture line is visible radiographically (Fig. 682-4). The plastic deformation is permanent, and a bend in the ulna of <20 degrees in a 4 yr old child is expected to correct with growth.

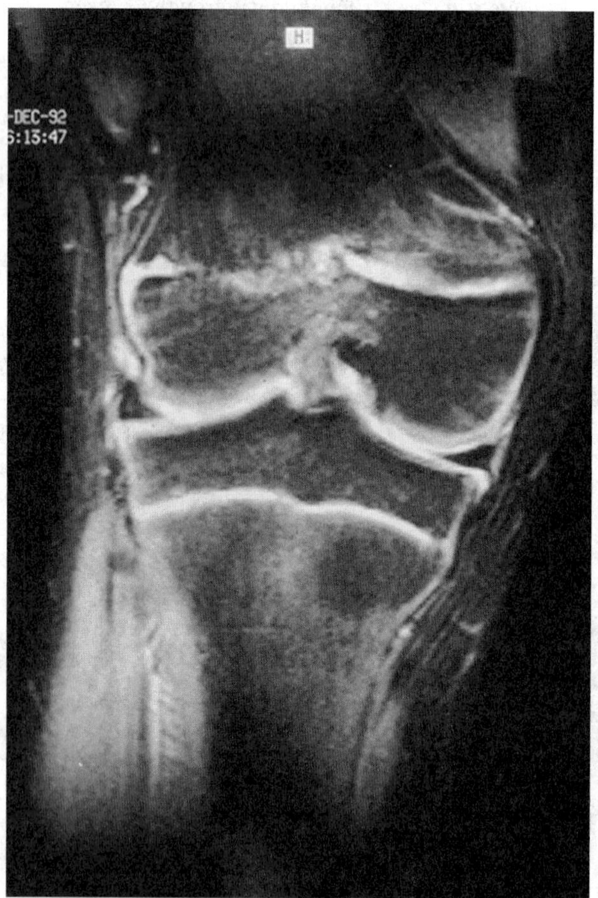

Figure 682-3. MRI with gradient echo sequence, illustrating distal femoral physeal bar. (From Dormans JP: *Pediatric Orthopedics: Introduction to Trauma.* Philadelphia, Mosby, 2005, p 43.)

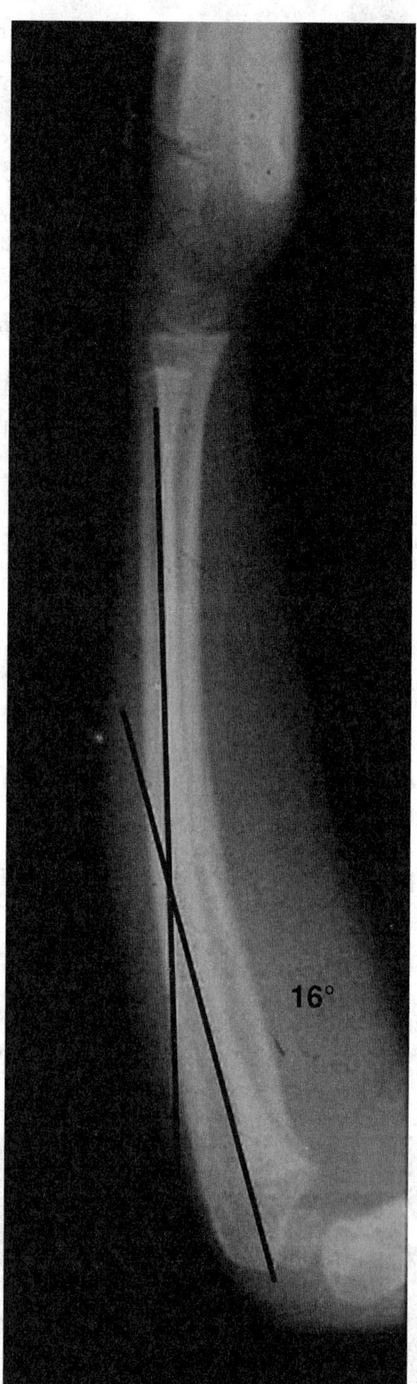

Figure 682-4. Plastic deformation is a microfailure in tension without visible fracture line. (Courtesy of Dr. John Flynn, Children's Hospital, Philadelphia, PA.)

BUCKLE OR TORUS FRACTURE

A compression failure of bone usually occurs at the junction of the metaphysis and diaphysis, especially in the distal radius (Fig. 682-5). This injury is referred to as a torus fracture because of

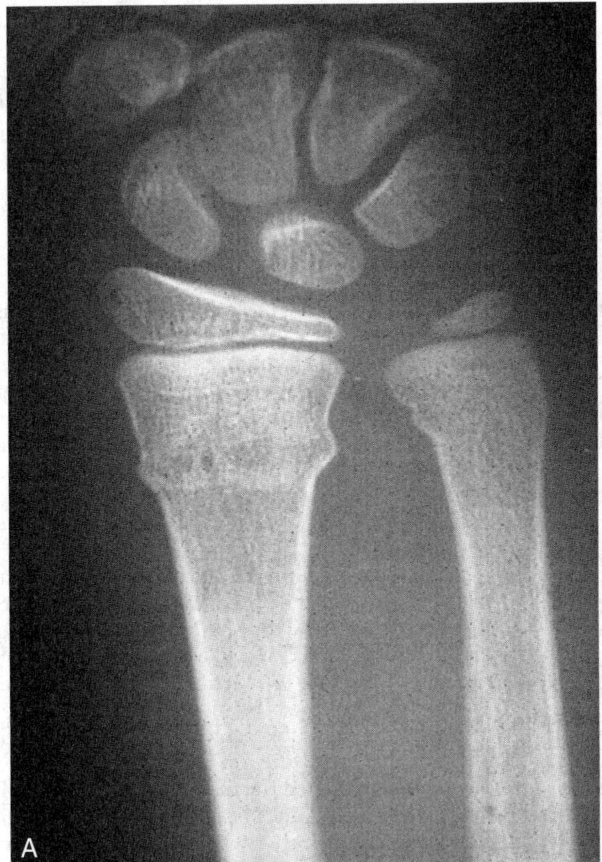

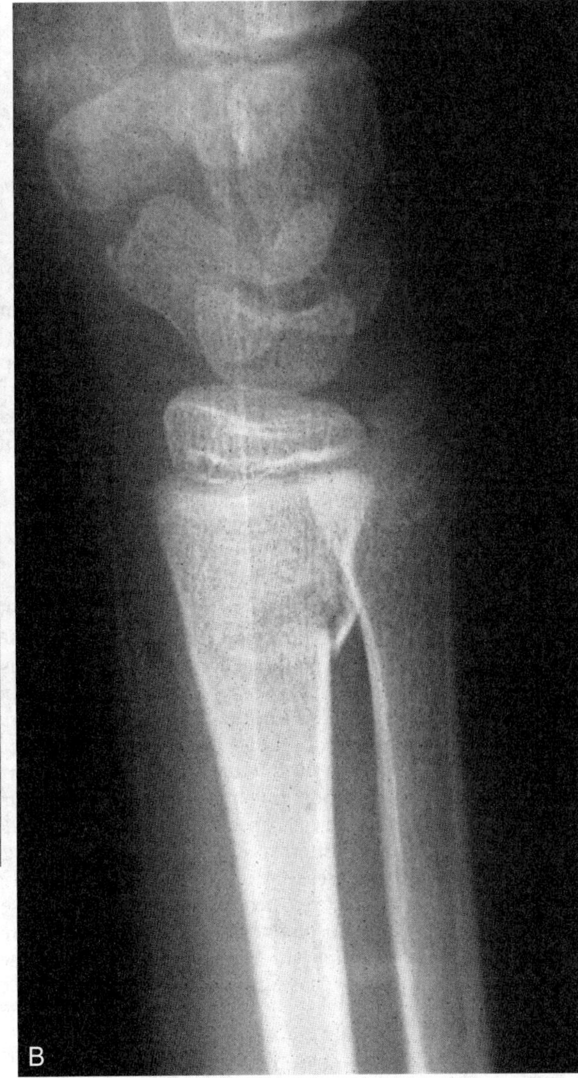

Figure 682-5. Buckle fracture is a partial failure in compression: anteroposterior *(A)* and lateral *(B)* radiographs of the distal radius. (From Dormans JP: *Pediatric Orthopedics: Introduction to Trauma.* Philadelphia, Mosby, 2005, p 37.)

its similarity to the raised band around the base of a classic Greek column. They are inherently stable and heal in 3–4wk with simple immobilization.

GREENSTICK

These fractures occur when the bone is bent, and there is failure on the tensile (convex) side of the bone. The fracture line does not propagate to the concave side of the bone. The concave side shows evidence of microscopic failure with plastic deformation. It is necessary to break the bone on the concave side as the plastic deformation recoils it back to the deformed position.

COMPLETE FRACTURES

Fractures that propagate completely through the bone are called complete fractures. These fractures may be classified as spiral, transverse, or oblique, depending on the direction of the fracture lines. A rotational force usually creates the spiral fractures, and reduction is easy due to the presence of an intact periosteal hinge. Oblique fractures are in the diaphysis at 30 degrees to the axis of the bone and are inherently unstable. The transverse fractures occur following a 3-point bending force and are easily reduced by using the intact periosteum from the concave side.

EPIPHYSEAL FRACTURES

The injuries to the epiphysis involve the growth plate. There is always a potential for deformity to occur, and hence long-term observation is necessary. The distal radial physis is the most frequently injured physis. Salter and Harris (SH) classified epiphyseal injuries into 5 groups (Table 682-1 and Fig. 682-6). This classification helps to predict the outcome of the injury and offers guidelines in formulating treatment. SH type I and II fractures usually can be managed by closed reduction techniques and do not require perfect alignment, as they tend to remodel with growth. SH type II fractures of the distal femoral epiphysis need anatomic reduction. The SH type III and IV epiphyseal fractures

TABLE 682-1. Salter-Harris Classification

SALTER-HARRIS TYPE	CHARACTERISTICS
I	Separation through the physis, usually through the zones of hypertrophic and degenerating cartilage cell columns
II	Fracture through a portion of the physis but extending through the metaphyses
III	Fracture through a portion of the physis extending through the epiphysis and into the joint
IV	Fracture across the metaphysis, physis, and epiphysis
V	Crush injury to the physis

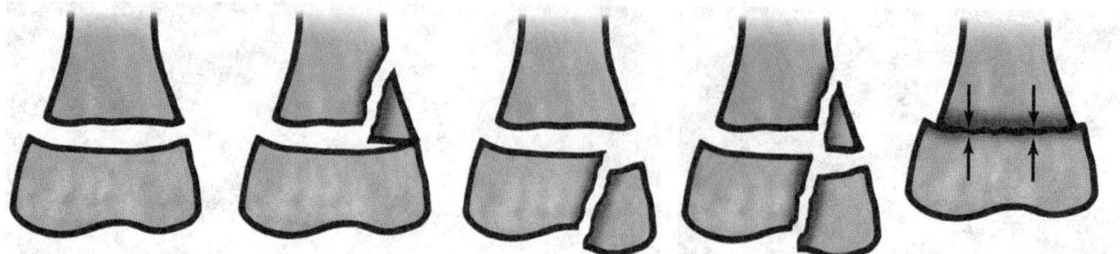

Figure 682-6. Salter-Harris classification of physeal fractures, types I–V.

involve the articular surface and require anatomic alignment to prevent any stepoff and realign the growth cells of the physis. SH type V fractures are usually not diagnosed initially. They present in the future with growth disturbance. Other injuries to the epiphysis are avulsion injuries of the tibial spine and muscle attachments to the pelvis. Osteochondral fractures are also defined as physeal injuries that do not involve the growth plate.

CHILD ABUSE

The orthopedic surgeon sees 30–50% of physically abused children. Child abuse should be expected in nonambulatory children with lower extremity long bone fractures (see Chapter 36). No fracture pattern or types are pathognomonic for child abuse; any type of fracture may result from nonaccidental trauma. The fractures that are suggestive of intentional injury include femur fractures in nonambulatory children, distal femoral metaphyseal corner fractures, posterior rib fractures, scapular spinous process fractures, and proximal humeral fractures. A skeletal survey is essential in every suspected case of child abuse, which may demonstrate other fractures in different stages of healing. Radiographically, some systemic diseases may mimic signs of child abuse such as osteogenesis imperfecta, osteomyelitis, Caffey disease, and fatigue fractures. Many hospitals have a multidisciplinary team to evaluate and treat patients who are victims of child abuse. It is mandatory to report these cases to social welfare agencies.

682.3 • Upper Extremity Fractures

PHALANGEAL FRACTURES

The different phalangeal fracture patterns in children include physeal, diaphyseal, and tuft fractures. The mechanism of injury is a direct blow to the finger or typically a finger trapped in a door (see Chapter 680). Crush injuries of the distal phalanx present with severe comminution of the underlying bone (tuft fracture), disruption of the nail bed, and significant soft-tissue injury. These injuries are best managed with antibiotics, tetanus prophylaxis, and irrigation. A mallet finger deformity is the inability to extend the distal portion of the digit and is caused by a hyperextension injury. It represents an avulsion fracture of the physis of the distal phalanx. The treatment is splinting the digit in extension for 3–4 wk. The physeal injuries of the proximal and middle phalanx are similarly treated with splint immobilization. Diaphyseal fractures may be oblique, spiral, or transverse in fracture geometry. They are assessed for angular and rotational deformity with the finger in flexion. Any malrotation or angular deformity requires correction for optimal functioning of the hand. These deformities are corrected with closed reduction, and if unstable, they need stabilization.

FOREARM FRACTURES

Fractures of the wrist and forearm are very common fractures in children, accounting for nearly half of all fractures seen in the skeletally immature. The most common mechanism of injury is a fall on the outstretched hand. Eighty percent of forearm fractures involve the distal radius and ulna, 15% involve the middle third, and the rest are rare fractures of the proximal third of the radius or ulnar shaft. The majority of forearm fractures are torus or greenstick fractures. The torus fracture is an impacted fracture, and there is minimal soft-tissue swelling or hemorrhage. They are best treated in a short arm (below the elbow) cast and usually heal within 3–4 wk. Wrist buckle fractures have also been successfully treated with a removable splint.

Diaphyseal fractures could be more difficult to treat because the limits of acceptable reduction are much more stringent than for distal radial fractures. A significant malunion of a forearm diaphyseal fracture can lead to a permanent loss of pronation and supination, leading to functional difficulties. The physical examination focuses on soft-tissue injuries and ruling out any neurovascular involvement. The anteroposterior and lateral radiographs of the forearm and wrist confirm the diagnosis. Displaced and angulated fractures require manipulative closed reduction under general anesthesia. They are immobilized in an above elbow cast for at least 6 wk. Loss of reduction and unstable fractures require open reduction and internal fixation.

DISTAL HUMERAL FRACTURES

Fractures around the elbow receive more attention because more aggressive management is needed to achieve a good result. Many injuries are intra-articular, involve the physeal cartilage, and may result in rare malunion or nonunion. As the distal humerus develops from a series of ossification centers, these ossification centers can be mistaken for fractures by inexperienced eyes. Careful radiographic evaluation is an essential part of diagnosing and managing distal humeral injuries. Common fractures include separation of the distal humeral epiphysis (transcondylar fracture), supracondylar fractures of the distal humerus, and epiphyseal fractures of the lateral or medial condyle. The mechanism of injury is a fall on an outstretched arm. The physical examination includes noting the location and extent of soft-tissue swelling, ruling out any neurovascular injury, specifically anterior interosseous nerve involvement or evidence of compartment syndrome. The transcondylar fracture in neonates should raise suspicion of child abuse. Anteroposterior and lateral radiographs of the involved extremity are necessary for the diagnosis. If the fracture is not visible, but there is an altered relationship between the humerus and the radius and ulna or the presence of a posterior fat pad sign, a transcondylar fracture or an occult fracture should be suspected. Imaging studies such as CT, MRI, and ultrasonography may be required for further confirmation.

In general, distal humeral fractures need good restoration of anatomic alignment. This is necessary to prevent deformity and to allow for normal growth and development. Closed reduction alone, or in association with percutaneous fixation, is the preferred method. Open reduction is necessary for fractures that cannot be reduced by closed methods. Inadequate reductions may lead to cubitus varus, cubitus valgus, and rare nonunion or elbow instability.

PROXIMAL HUMERUS FRACTURES

Fractures of the proximal humerus account for <5% of fractures in children. They usually result from a fall onto an outstretched arm. The fracture pattern tends to vary with the age group. Children younger than 5 yr of age have an SH I injury, those 5–10 yr of age have metaphyseal fractures, and children older than 11 yr have SH II injury. Examination includes a thorough neurologic evaluation, especially of the axillary nerve. The diagnosis is made on anteroposterior radiographs of the shoulder. An axillary view is obtained to rule out any dislocation. SH I injuries do not require reduction as they have excellent remodeling capacity, and simple immobilization in a sling for 2–3 wk is sufficient. The proximal humerus contributes 80% of the growth to the humerus. The metaphyseal fractures usually do not need reduction unless the angulation is >50 degrees. A closed reduction with sling immobilization adequately treats this fracture. SH II fractures with <30 degrees of angulation and <50% displacement are managed in a sling. Displaced fractures are treated with closed reduction and further stabilization if unstable. Occasionally, open reduction is required because of button-holing of the fracture spike through the deltoid or interposition of the tendon of biceps.

CLAVICULAR FRACTURES

Neonatal fractures occur as a result of direct trauma during birth, most often following a narrow pelvis or shoulder dystocia. They can be missed initially and can appear with pseudoparalysis. Childhood fractures are usually result of a fall on the affected shoulder or direct trauma to the clavicle. The most common site for fracture is the junction of the middle and lateral 3rd clavicle. Tenderness over the clavicle will make the diagnosis. A thorough neurovascular examination is important to diagnose any associated **brachial plexus injury.** An anteroposterior radiograph of the clavicle demonstrates the fracture and may show overlap of the fragments. Physeal injuries occur through the medial or lateral growth plate and may be sometimes difficult to differentiate from dislocations of the acromioclavicular or sternoclavicular joint. Further imaging such as a CT scan may be necessary to further define the injury. The treatment of most clavicle fractures consists of an application of a figure-of-eight clavicle strap. This will extend the shoulders and minimize the amount of overlap of the fracture fragments. The physeal fractures are treated with simple sling mobilization without any reduction attempt. Frequently, anatomic alignment is not achieved, nor is it necessary. The fractures heal rapidly, usually in 3–6 wk. Usually a palpable mass of callus may be visible in thin children. This remodels satisfactorily in 6–12 mo. Complete restoration of shoulder motion and function is uniformly achieved.

682.4 • Fractures of Lower Extremity

HIP FRACTURE

Hip fractures in children account for <1% of all children's fractures. These injuries result from high-energy trauma and are frequently associated with injury to the chest, head, or abdomen. Treatment of hip fractures in children entails a complication rate of up to 60%, an overall avascular necrosis rate of 50%, and a malunion rate of up to 30%. The unique blood supply to the femoral head accounts for the high rate of avascular necrosis. Fractures are classified as transphyseal separations, transcervical fractures, cervicotrochanteric fractures, and intertrochanteric fractures. The management principle includes urgent anatomic reduction (either open or closed), stable internal fixation (avoiding the physis if possible), and spica casting.

TODDLER FRACTURE

Toddler fractures occur in young ambulatory children. The age range for this fracture is typically from around 1–4 yr. The injury often occurs after a seemingly harmless twist or fall and is frequently unwitnessed. The children in this age group are usually unable to articulate the mechanism of injury clearly or to describe the area of injury well. The radiographs may show no fracture; the diagnosis is made by physical examination. The classic symptom is refusal to bear weight, which can manifest as pulling up the affected extremity or florid display of protest. The anteroposterior and lateral views of the tibia-fibula may show a nondisplaced spiral fracture of the distal tibial metaphysis. An oblique view is often helpful as the fracture line may be visible in only 1 of the 3 views. A 3-phase technetium bone scan can be helpful in excluding infections such as septic arthritis and osteomyelitis. The fracture is treated with an above-knee cast for approximately 3 wk.

TIBIA AND FIBULA SHAFT FRACTURES

The tibia is the most commonly fractured bone of the lower limb in children. This fracture generally results from a direct injury. Most tibial fractures are associated with a fibular fracture, and the mean age of presentation is 8 yr. The child will have pain, swelling, and deformity of the affected leg and will be unable to bear weight. Distal neurovascular examination is important in assessment. The anteroposterior and lateral radiographs should include the knee and ankle. Closed reduction and immobilization are the standard method of treatment. Most fractures heal well, and children usually have excellent results. Open fractures need to undergo irrigation and debridement multiple times. The fractures with more severe soft-tissue injury are best treated with external fixation. The fracture healing in open fracture takes longer than the closed injuries.

FEMORAL SHAFT FRACTURES

Fractures of the femur in children are common. All age groups, from early childhood to adolescence, can be affected. The mechanism of injury varies from low-energy twisting type injuries to high-velocity injuries in vehicular accidents. Femur fractures in children younger than 2 yr should raise the concern for child abuse. A thorough physical examination is necessary to rule out other injuries and assess the neurovascular status. In case of high-energy trauma, any signs of hemodynamic instability should prompt the examiner to look for other sources of bleeding. Anteroposterior and lateral radiographs of the femur demonstrate the fracture. An anteroposterior radiograph of the pelvis is obtained to rule out any associated pelvic fracture. Treatment of shaft fractures varies with the age group, as described in Table 682-2.

TABLE 682-2. Treatment Options by Age (Femoral Shaft Fracture)

TREATMENT OPTIONS	0–2 yr	3–5 yr	6–10 yr	>11 yr
Spica cast	X	X		
Traction and spica cast		X	X	X
Intramedullary rod		X	X	X
External fixator		X*	X*	X*
Screw or plate		X	X	X

*Open fracture.

Modified form Wells L: Trauma related to the lower extremity. In Dormans JP (editor): *Pediatric Orthopaedics: Core Knowledge in Orthopaedics*. Philadeiphia, Mosby, 2005, p. 93.

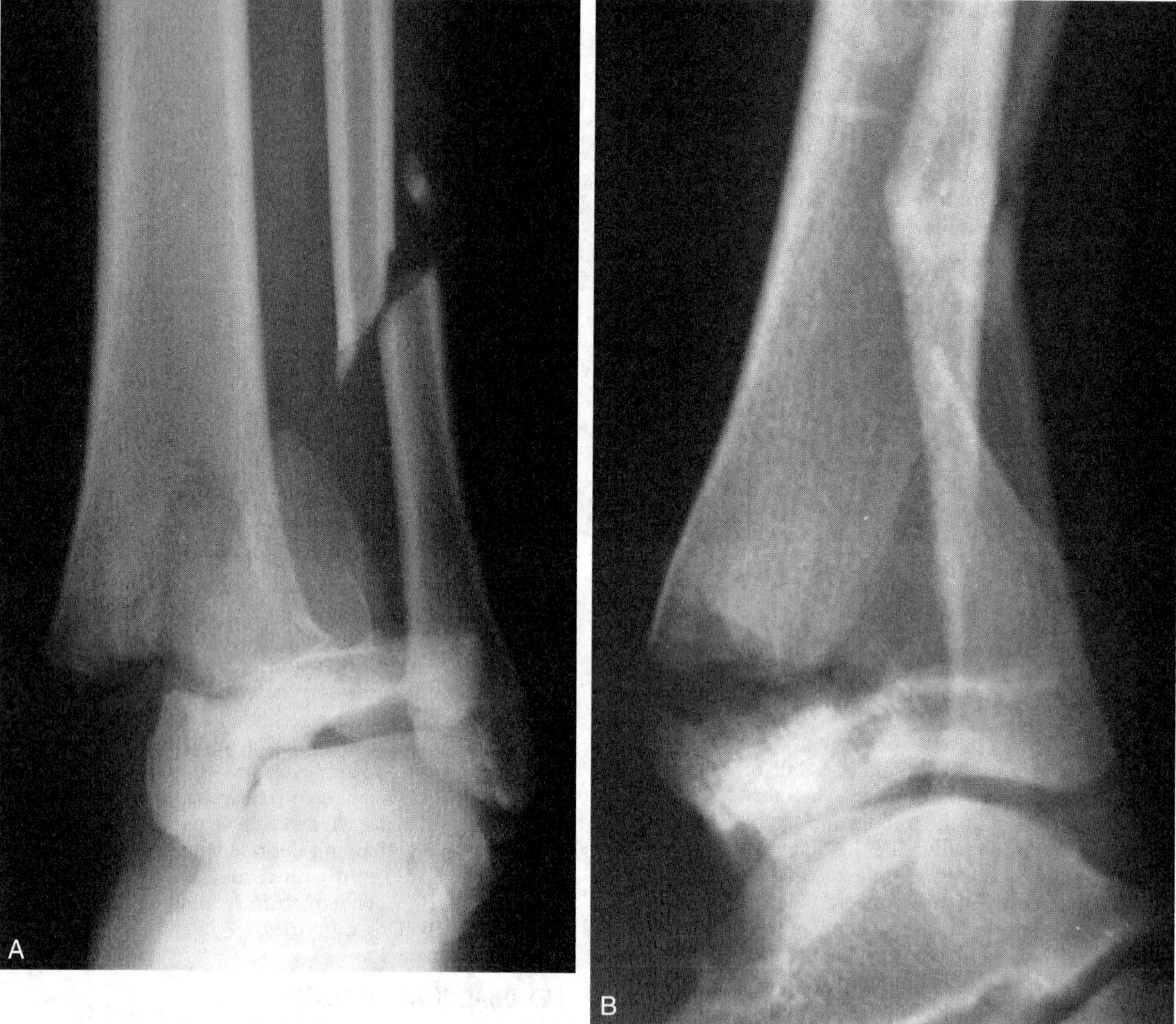

Figure 682-7. The triplane fracture is a transitional fracture: anteroposterior *(A)* and lateral *(B)* radiographs. (From Dormans JP: *Pediatric Orthopedics: Introduction to Trauma.* Philadelphia, Mosby, 2005, p 38.)

TRIPLANE AND TILLAUX FRACTURES

These fracture patterns present at the end of the growth period and are based on relative strength of the bone-physis junction and asymmetric closure of the tibial physis. The triplane fractures are so named because the injury has coronal, sagittal, and transverse components (Fig. 682-7). The Tillaux fracture is an avulsion fracture of the anterolateral aspect of the distal tibial epiphysis. Radiographs and further imaging with CT and three-dimensional reconstructions are necessary to analyze the fracture geometry. The triplane fracture involves the articular surface and hence anatomic reduction is necessary. The reduction is further stabilized with internal fixation. The Tillaux fracture is treated by closed reduction. Open reduction is recommended if a residual intra-articular stepoff persists.

METATARSAL FRACTURES

Metatarsal fractures are common in children. They usually result from direct trauma to the dorsum of the foot. High-energy trauma or multiple fractures of the metatarsal base are associated with significant swelling. A high index for compartment syndrome of the foot must be maintained and compartment pressures must be measured if indicated. Diagnosis is obtained by anteroposterior, lateral, and oblique radiographs of the foot. Most metatarsal fractures can be treated by closed methods in a below-knee cast. Weight bearing is allowed as tolerated. Displaced fractures may require closed or open reduction with internal fixation. Percutaneous, smooth Kirschner wires generally provide sufficient internal fixation for these injuries. If the compartment pressure is increased, complete release of all compartments in the foot is necessary.

TOE PHALANGEAL FRACTURES

Fractures of the lesser toes are common and are usually secondary to direct blows. They commonly occur when the child is barefoot. The toes are swollen, ecchymotic, and tender. There may be a mild deformity. Diagnosis is made radiographically. Bleeding suggests the possibility of an open fracture. The lesser toes usually do not require closed reduction unless significantly displaced. If necessary, reduction can usually be accomplished with longitudinal traction on the toe. Casting is not usually necessary. "Buddy" taping of the fractured toe to an adjacent stable toe usually provides satisfactory alignment and relief of symptoms. Crutches and heel walking may be beneficial for several days until the soft-tissue swelling and the discomfort decrease.

682.5 • Operative Treatment

Four to 5% of pediatric fractures require surgery. The common indications for operative treatment in children and adolescents include (1) displaced physeal fractures, (2) displaced intra-articular fractures, (3) unstable fractures, (4) multiply injured child, (5) open fractures, (6) failure to achieve adequate reduction in older children, (7) failure to maintain an adequate reduction, and (8) certain pathologic fractures.

The aim of operative intervention is to obtain anatomic alignment and relative stability. Rigid fixation is not necessary as it is in adults for early mobilization. Further, the relatively stable construct can be supplemented with external immobilization. SH type III and IV injuries require anatomic alignment, and if unstable, internal fixation is used (use of smooth Kirschner wires, preferably avoiding the course across the growth plate). Multiple closed reductions of an epiphyseal fracture are contraindicated because they may cause permanent damage to the germinal cells of the physis.

SURGICAL TECHNIQUES

It is important to take great care with soft tissues and skin. The other indications for open reduction and internal fixation are unstable fractures of the spine, ipsilateral fractures of the femur, neurovascular injuries requiring repair, and, occasionally, open fractures of the femur and tibia. Closed reduction and minimally invasive fixation are specifically used for supracondylar fractures of the distal humerus, phalangeal fractures, and femoral neck fractures. Failure to obtain anatomic alignment by closed means is an indication for an open reduction.

The main indications for external fixation are summarized in Table 682-3. The advantages of external fixation include rigid immobilization of the fractures, access to open wounds for continued management, and easier patient mobilization for treatment of other injuries and transportation for diagnostic and therapeutic procedures. The majority of complications with external fixation are pin tract infections, chronic osteomyelitis, and refractures after pin removal.

682.6 • Complications of Fractures in Children

The complications specific to children are malalignment and correction by natural growth, physeal arrest, overgrowth, and refracture caused by rapid fracture healing. The malalignment and late angulation is a common problem with fractures of the proximal tibial metaphysis. The physeal arrest can cause angular deformity or shortening. The angular deformities are treated by hemiepiphysiodesis or osteotomy. The shortening is treated with contralateral leg epiphysiodesis closer to skeletal maturity or lengthening of the short limb. Refractures cause more deformity and may necessitate open reduction. Other complications are reflex sympathetic dystrophy, ligamentous instability, malunion, nonunion, fat embolism, and neurovascular injuries.

TABLE 682-3. Common Indications for External Fixation in Pediatric Fractures

1. Grade II and III open fractures
2. Fractures associated with severe burns
3. Fractures with soft-tissue loss requiring free flaps or skin grafts
4. Fractures requiring distractions such as those with significant bone loss
5. Unstable pelvic fractures
6. Fractures in children with associated head injuries and spasticity
7. Fractures associated with vascular or nerve repairs or reconstruction

682.7 • Outcomes Assessment

Empirical and subjective assessment leads to erroneous conclusions and difficulty in comparison with outcome results from other studies. The three scales used to evaluate different modalities of treatment for musculoskeletal trauma are the Activities Scale for Kids, the Pediatric Functional Health Outcomes Instrument, and the Pediatric Outcome Data Collection Instruments. The American Academy of Orthopaedic Surgeons developed the Pediatric Functional Health Outcomes Instrument as an example of health status measure.

Bandyopandhyay S, Yen K: Non-accidental fractures in child maltreatment syndrome. *Clin Pediatr Emerg Med* 2002;3:145–152.

Beaty JH, Kasser JR (editors): *Rockwood and Wilkins' Fractures in Children,* 5th ed. Philadelphia, JB Lippincott, 2001.

Bohm ER, Bubbar V, Hing KY, et al: Above- and below-the-elbow plaster casts for distal forearm fractures in children. *J Bone Joint Surg* 2006;88-A:1–8.

Cummings RJ: Paediatric femoral fracture. *Lancet* 2005;365:1116–1117.

Davidson JS, Brown DJ, Barnes SN, et al: Simple treatment for torus fractures of the distal radius. *J Bone Joint Surg Br* 2001;83:1173–1175.

Della-Giustina K, Della-Giustina DA: Emergency department evaluation and treatment of pediatric orthopedic injuries. *Emerg Med Clin North Am* 1999;17:895–922.

Flynn JM, Kolze EA: Upper extremity injuries. In Dormans JP (editor): *Pediatric Orthopaedics: Core Knowledge in Orthopaedics.* Philadelphia, Mosby, 2005, pp 47–84.

Flynn JM, Nagda S: Upper extremity injuries. In Dormans JP (editor): *The Requisites in Pediatrics: Pediatric Orthopaedics and Sports Medicine.* Philadelphia, Mosby, 2005, pp 21–48.

Green NE, Swiontkowski MF (editors): *Skeletal Trauma in Children,* 3rd ed., vol. 3. Philadelphia, WB Saunders, 2001.

Horn DB, Wells L, Tamai J: Lower extremity fractures. In Dormans JP (editor): *The Requisites in Pediatrics: Pediatric Orthopaedics and Sports Medicine.* Philadelphia, Mosby, 2005, pp 49–92.

Kocher MS, Waters PM, Micheli LJ: Upper extremity injuries in the pediatric athlete. *Sports Med* 2000;30:117–135.

Overly F, Steele DW: Common pediatric fractures and dislocations. *Clin Pediatr Emerg Med* 2002;3:106–117.

Plint AC, Perry JJ, Correll R, et al: A randomized, controlled trial of removable splinting versus casting for wrist buckle fractures in children. *Pediatrics* 2006;117:691–697.

Salter RB, Harris WR: Injuries involving the epiphyseal plate. *J Bone Joint Surg Am* 1963;45:587–622.

Skaggs DL, Mirzayan R: The posterior fat pad sign in association with occult fracture of the elbow in children. *J Bone Joint Surg Am* 1999;81: 1429–1433.

Thompson GH, Haber LL: Upper extremity fractures in the pediatric patients. In Fitzgerald RH Jr, Kaufer H, Malkani A (editors): *Orthopaedics.* St. Louis, Mosby, 2002, pp 484–494.

Wells L, Millman JE: Trauma related to the lower extremity. In Dormans JP (editor): *Pediatric Orthopaedics: Core Knowledge in Orthopaedics.* Philadelphia, Mosby, 2005, pp 85–115.

Wright JG, Wang EEL, Owen JL, et al: Treatments for paediatric femoral fractures: A randomized trial. *Lancet* 2005;365:1153–1162.

Chapter 683 ■ Osteomyelitis

Richard M. Lampe

Bone infections in children are important because of their potential to cause permanent disability. The frequency of skeletal infection is greater in infants and toddlers than in older children. Early recognition of osteomyelitis in young patients before extensive infection develops and prompt institution of appropriate medical and surgical therapy minimize permanent damage. The risk is greatest if the physis (the growth plate of bone) is damaged.

ETIOLOGY. Bacteria are the most common pathogens in acute skeletal infections. In osteomyelitis, *Staphylococcus aureus* is the most common infecting organism in all age groups, including newborns. Group B streptococcus and gram-negative enteric bacilli *(Escherichia coli)* are also prominent pathogens in neonates; group A streptococcus constitutes <10% of all cases. After 6 yr of age, most cases of osteomyelitis are caused by *S. aureus,* streptococcus, or *Pseudomonas aeruginosa.* Cases of *Pseudomonas* are related almost exclusively to puncture wounds of the foot, with direct inoculation of *P. aeruginosa* from the foam padding of the shoe into bone or cartilage, which develops as osteochondritis. *Salmonella* species and *S. aureus* are the two most common causes of osteomyelitis in children with sickle cell anemia. *Pneumococcus* may also cause osteomyelitis in children with sickle cell anemia. *Kingella kingae* may be the second most common cause of osteomyelitis in children. *K. kingae* may be sporadic or occur in clusters producing osteomyelitis or septic arthritis.

Infection with atypical mycobacteria, *S. aureus,* or *Pseudomonas* can occur after penetrating injuries. Fungal infections usually occur as part of multisystem disseminated disease; *Candida* osteomyelitis sometimes complicates fungemia in neonates with or without indwelling vascular catheters. Primary viral infection of bones is exceedingly rare.

A microbial etiology is confirmed in about 75% of cases of osteomyelitis. Prior antibiotic therapy and the inhibitory effect of pus on microbial growth may explain the low bacterial yield.

EPIDEMIOLOGY. Osteomyelitis is common in young children; about 30% occur by 2 yr of age and 50% by 5 yr of age. Bone infections are more common in boys than girls, usually by a factor of 2 : 1. The behavior of boys may predispose to traumatic events. Except for the increased incidence of skeletal infection in patients with sickle cell disease, there is no predilection for osteomyelitis based on race.

The majority of infections in previously healthy children are of hematogenous origin. Minor, closed trauma is a common preceding event in cases of osteomyelitis, occurring in about 30% of patients. Infection of bones can follow penetrating injuries or open fractures. Bone infection following orthopedic surgery is uncommon. Impaired host defenses also increase the risk of skeletal infection. Other risk factors are noted in Table 683-1.

TABLE 683-1. Microorganisms Isolated from Patients with Osteomyelitis and Their Clinical Associations

MOST COMMON CLINICAL ASSOCIATION	MICROORGANISM
Frequent microorganism in any type of osteomyelitis	*Staphylococcus aureus* (susceptible or resistant to methicillin)
Foreign body–associated infection	Coagulase-negative staphylococci or *Propionibacterium* spp.
Common in nosocomial infections	*Enterobacteriaceae, Pseudomonas aeruginosa, Candida* spp.
Associated with bites, diabetic foot lesions, and decubitus ulcers	Streptococci and/or anaerobic bacteria
Sickle cell disease	*Salmonella* spp., *S. aureus,* or *Streptococcus pneumoniae*
HIV infection	*Bartonella henselae* or *Bartonella quintana*
Human or animal bites	*Pasteurella multocida* or *Eikenella corrodens*
Immunocompromised patients	*Aspergillus* spp., *Candida albicans,* or *Mycobacteria* spp.
Populations in which tuberculosis is prevalent	*Mycobacterium tuberculosis*
Populations in which these pathogens are endemic	*Brucella* spp., *Coxiella burnetii,* fungi found in specific geographic areas (coccidiodomycosis, blastomycosis, histoplasmosis)

From Lew DP, Waldvogel FA: Osteomyelitis. *Lancet* 2004;364:369–379.

TABLE 683-2. Distribution of Affected Bones in Acute Hematogenous Osteomyelitis

BONE	NO.	%
Tibia	107	24.3
Femur	105	23.8
Humerus	58	13.2
Fibula	26	5.9
Radius	17	3.9
Ulna	10	2.3
Vertebra	9	2.0
Foot bones	33	7.5
Pelvic bones	30	6.8
Hand bones	27	6.1
Chest bones	13	2.9
Head bones	6	1.4

Based on unpublished series of 372 patients with 441 infected bones.

PATHOGENESIS. The unique anatomy and circulation of the ends of long bones result in the predilection for localization of blood-borne bacteria. In the metaphysis, nutrient arteries branch into nonanastomosing capillaries under the physis, which make a sharp loop before entering venous sinusoids draining into the marrow. Blood flow in this area is sluggish and provides an ideal environment for bacterial seeding. Once a bacterial focus is established, phagocytes migrate to the site and produce an inflammatory exudate (metaphyseal abscess). The generation of proteolytic enzymes, toxic oxygen radicals, and cytokines results in decreased oxygen tension, decreased pH, osteolysis, and tissue destruction. As the inflammatory exudate progresses, pressure increases spread through the porous metaphyseal space via the haversian system and Volkmann canals into the subperiosteal space. Purulence beneath the periosteum may lift the periosteal membrane of the bony surface, further impairing blood supply to the cortex and metaphysis.

In newborns and young infants, transphyseal blood vessels connect the metaphysis and epiphysis, so it is common for pus from the metaphysis to enter the joint space. This extension through the physis has the potential to result in abnormal growth and bone or joint deformity. During the latter part of the 1st year of life, the physis forms, obliterating the transphyseal blood vessels. Joint involvement once the physis forms may occur in joints where the metaphysis is intra-articular (hip, ankle, shoulder, and elbow) and subperiosteal pus ruptures into the joint space.

In later childhood, the periosteum becomes more adherent, favoring pus to decompress through the periosteum. Once the growth plate closes in late adolescence, hematogenous osteomyelitis more often begins in the diaphysis and can spread to the entire intramedullary canal.

CLINICAL MANIFESTATIONS. The signs and symptoms of osteomyelitis are highly dependent on the age of the patient. The earliest signs and symptoms are often subtle.

Neonates may exhibit pseudoparalysis or pain with movement of the affected extremity. Half of neonates do not have fever and may not appear ill. Older infants and children are more likely to have fever, pain, and localizing signs such as edema, erythema, and warmth. With involvement of the lower extremities, limp or refusal to walk is seen in approximately half of patients.

Focal tenderness over a long bone can be an important finding. Local swelling and redness with osteomyelitis may mean that the infection has spread out of the metaphysis into the subperiosteal space, representing a secondary soft tissue inflammatory response.

Long bones are principally involved in osteomyelitis (Table 683-2). The femur and tibia are equally affected and together constitute almost half of all cases. The bones of the upper extremities account for one fourth of all cases. Flat bones are less commonly affected.

There is usually only a single site of bone or joint involvement. Several bones are infected in <10% of cases; the exception is osteomyelitis in neonates, in whom two or more bones are involved in almost half of the cases. Children with subacute symptoms and focal finding in the metaphysial area (usually of tibia) may have a **Brodie abscess,** with radiographic lucency and surrounding reactive bone.

Patients with culture negative osteomyelitis may have a more benign clinical appearance but respond well to empiric antistaphylococcal therapy.

DIAGNOSIS. A blood culture should be performed in all cases of suspected osteomyelitis. Aspiration for Gram stain and culture when the history and physical findings indicate a strong likelihood of osteomyelitis remains the definitive diagnostic technique and provides the optimal specimen for culture to confirm the diagnosis. For suspected osteomyelitis, a steel needle is needed to penetrate the cortex into the metaphysis. If pus is encountered in the subperiosteal space, there is no need to go farther. Direct inoculation of clinical specimens into aerobic blood culture bottles may improve the recovery of *Kingella kingae* particularly if held for 1 wk. Aspiration of bone pus provides the best specimen for bacteriologic culture of infection. *K. kingae* may need to be identified by polymerase chain reaction.

There are no specific laboratory tests for osteomyelitis. Tests such as white blood cell count and differential, erythrocyte sedimentation rate (ESR), and C-reactive protein (CRP) are very sensitive for bone infections but are nonspecific and not helpful in distinguishing between skeletal infection and other inflammatory processes. The leukocyte count and ESR may be normal during the first few days of infection, and normal test results do not preclude the diagnosis of skeletal infection. Monitoring elevated ESR and CRP may be of value in assessing response to therapy or identifying complications.

Radiographic Evaluation. Radiographic studies play a crucial role in the evaluation of osteomyelitis. Conventional radiographs, ultrasonography, CT, MRI, and radionuclide studies may all contribute to establishing the diagnosis. Plain radiographs are often used for initial evaluation to exclude other causes such as trauma and foreign bodies. MRI has emerged as a very sensitive and specific test and is widely used for diagnosis. The sequence of radionuclide studies or MRI is often determined by age, site, and clinical presentation.

PLAIN RADIOGRAPHS. Within 72 hr of onset of symptoms of osteomyelitis, plain radiographs of the involved site using soft-tissue technique and compared to the opposite extremity, if necessary, can show displacement of the deep muscle planes from the adjacent metaphysis caused by deep-tissue edema. Lytic bone changes are not visible on radiographs until 30–50% of the bony matrix is destroyed. Tubular long bones do not show lytic changes for 7–14 days after onset of infection. Flat and irregular bones can take longer.

Computed Tomography and Magnetic Resonance Imaging. CT can demonstrate osseous and soft-tissue abnormalities and is ideal for detecting gas in soft tissues. MRI is the best radiographic imaging technique for the identification of abscesses and for differentiation between bone and soft-tissue infection. MRI provides precise anatomic detail of subperiosteal pus and accumulation of purulent debris in the bone marrow and metaphyses for possible surgical intervention. In acute osteomyelitis, purulent debris and edema appear dark with decreased signal intensity on T1-weighted images, with fat appearing bright (Fig. 683-1). The opposite is seen in T2-weighted images. The signal from fat can be diminished with fat suppression techniques to enhance visualization. Gadolinium administration can also enhance MRI. Cellulitis and sinus tracts appear as areas of high signal intensity on T2-weighted images.

MRI appears to have comparable positive predictive value to radionuclide imaging in acute osteomyelitis. MRI is particularly useful in the evaluation of vertebral osteomyelitis and diskitis owing to the clear delineation between the vertebral body and cartilaginous disk.

Radionuclide Studies. Radionuclide imaging can be valuable in suspected bone infections especially if multiple foci are suspected. Technetium-99 methylene diphosphonate (^{99m}Tc), which accumulates in areas of increased bone turnover, is the preferred agent of choice for radionuclide bone imaging (three-phase bone scan). Osteomyelitis causes increased vascularity, inflammation, and increased osteoblastic activity, resulting in an increased concentration of ^{99m}Tc. Any areas of increased blood flow or inflammation can cause increased uptake of ^{99m}Tc in the first phase and second phases, but osteomyelitis causes increased uptake of ^{99m}Tc in the third phase (4–6 hr). Three-phase imaging with ^{99m}Tc has excellent sensitivity (84–100%) and specificity (70–96%) in hematogenous osteomyelitis and can detect osteomyelitis within 24–48 hr after onset of symptoms. The sensitivity in neonates is much lower owing to poor bone mineralization. Advantages include infrequent need for sedation, lower cost, ability to image entire skeleton for detection of multiple foci, and ability to scan multiple times after one injection.

Differential Diagnosis. The differential diagnosis of osteomyelitis includes trauma, both accidental and nonaccidental. Children with leukemia commonly have bone pain or joint pain as an early symptom. Neuroblastoma with bone involvement may be mistaken for osteomyelitis. Primary bone tumors need to be considered, but fever and other signs of illness are generally absent except in Ewing sarcoma. Chronic recurrent multifocal osteomyelitis (CRMO) and synovitis, acne, pustulosis, hyperostosis, and osteitis syndrome are rare noninfectious conditions in children characterized by recurrent osteoarticular inflammation and different skin conditions, palmoplantar pustulosis, psoriasis, severe acne, neutrophilic dermatosis (Sweet syndrome), and pyoderma gangrenosum. CRMO affects girls (4:1) with a peak age of 10 yr. It may also be associated with arthritis, sacroiliitis, inflammatory bowel disease, and Wegner granulomatosis. Some lesions are asymptomatic, but most are painful. The diagnosis is made by having more than two lesions with osteolysis and encircling sclerosis, duration of >6 mo, and characteristic histology (not always needed).

TREATMENT. Optimal treatment of skeletal infections requires collaborative efforts of pediatricians, orthopedic surgeons, and radiologists.

Antibiotic Therapy. The initial empirical antibiotic therapy is based on knowledge of likely bacterial pathogens at various ages, the results of the Gram stain of aspirated material, and additional considerations. In neonates, an antistaphylococcal penicillin, such as nafcillin or oxacillin (150–200 mg/kg/24 hr divided q6h IV), and a broad-spectrum cephalosporin, such as cefotaxime (150–200 mg/kg/24 hr divided q8h IV), provide coverage for the *S. aureus*, group B streptococcus, and gram-negative bacilli. If methicillin-resistant *Staphylococcus* is suspected, vancomycin is substituted for nafcillin. An aminoglycoside may be used in place of the cephalosporin, but aminoglycoside antibiotics have reduced antibacterial activity in sites with decreased oxygen tension and low pH, conditions that are present in tissue infections. If the neonate is a small premature infant or has a central vascular catheter, the possibility of nosocomial bacteria (*Pseudomonas* or coagulase-negative staphylococci) or fungi (*Candida*) should be considered. In older infants and children, the principal pathogens are *S. aureus* and streptococcus. Cefazolin (100–150 mg/kg/24 hr divided q8h IV) or nafcillin (150–200 mg/kg/24 hr divided q6h) provides coverage against these causes and can be used. If methicillin-resistant *Staphylococcus* is suspected, vancomycin is substituted for nafcillin. Cefotaxime

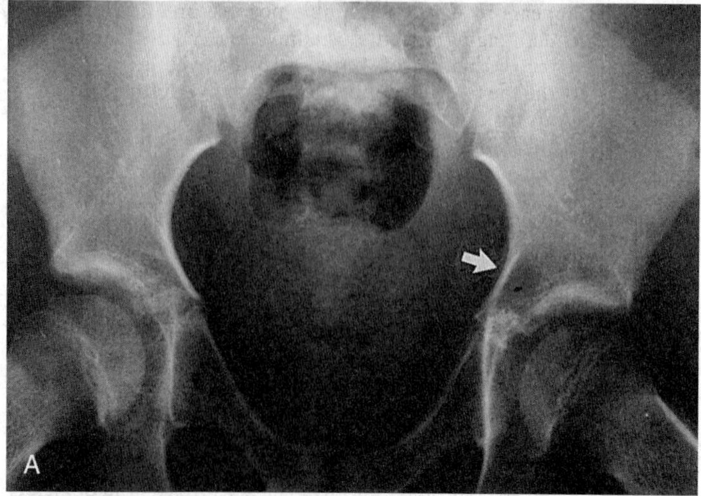

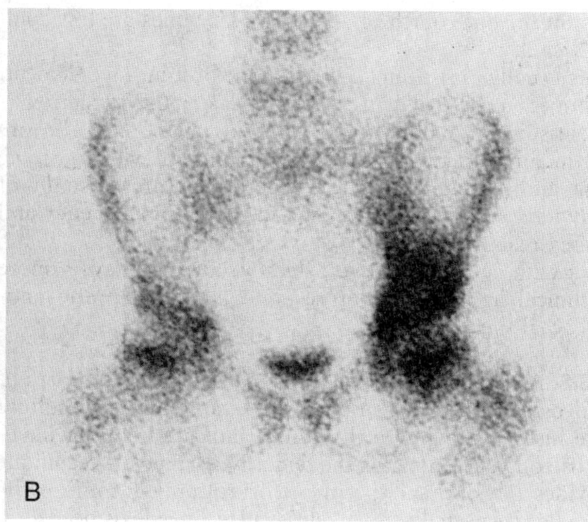

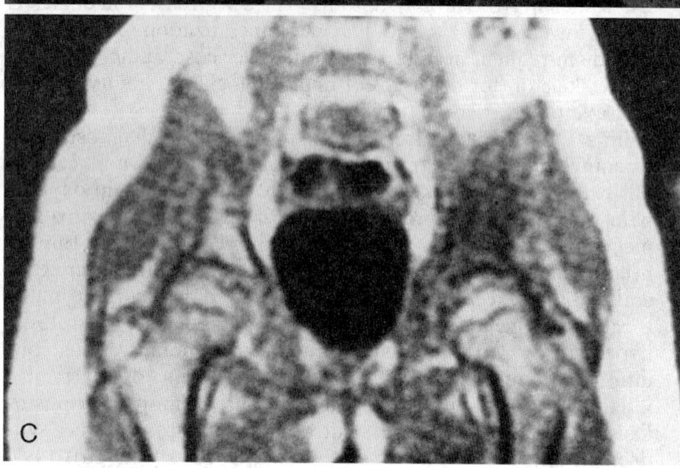

Figure 683-1. Pelvic osteomyelitis of the left iliac bone in a 12 yr old girl with pain in the left hip region for 1–2 wk. *A,* Frontal radiograph of the pelvis shows mild demineralization of the acetabular portion of the iliac bone adjacent to the triradiate cartilage. There is very subtle periosteal reaction *(arrow)* along the margin of the sciatic notch. *B,* Technetium-99m bone scan shows increased uptake in the left iliac bone and mild increased uptake in the femoral head. *C,* Coronal MRI shows decreased signal from the marrow of the left iliac bone compared with the bright signal from the normal fatty marrow on the right. The femoral head is normal, and there is no joint effusion. Needle aspiration of the iliac bone yielded *Staphylococcus aureus;* the patient responded well to antimicrobial therapy. (From Markowitz RI: Diagnostic imaging. In Jenson HB, Baltimore RS [editors]: *Pediatric Infectious Diseases: Principles and Practice.* Norwalk, CT, Appleton & Lange, 1995.)

(200 mg/kg/24 hr divided q8h IV) or ceftriaxone may be used in patients not vaccinated against *Haemophilus influenzae* type b.

Special situations dictate deviations from the usual empirical antibiotic selection. In patients with sickle cell disease with osteomyelitis, gram-negative enteric bacteria *(Salmonella)* are common pathogens as well as *S. aureus,* so a broad-spectrum cephalosporin such as cefotaxime (200 mg/kg/24 hr divided q8h) is used in addition to an antistaphylococcal drug. Clindamycin (40 mg/kg/24 hr divided q6h IV) is a useful alternative drug for patients allergic to β-lactam drugs. In addition to good antistaphylococcal activity, clindamycin has broad activity against anaerobes and is useful for the treatment of infections secondary to penetrating injuries or compound fractures. Clindamycin and vancomycin (40 mg/kg/24 hr divided q6h IV) are alternatives when treating methicillin-resistant *S. aureus* infections. For immunocompromised patients, combination therapy is usually initiated, such as with vancomycin and ceftazidime, or with piperacillin-clavulanate and an aminoglycoside. *K. kingae* usually responds to cefotaxime.

When the pathogen is identified, appropriate adjustments in antibiotics are made, if necessary. If a pathogen is not identified and a patient's condition is improving, therapy is continued with the initially selected antibiotic. If a pathogen is not identified and a patient's condition is not improving, re-aspiration or biopsy and the possibility of a noninfectious condition should be considered.

Duration of antibiotic therapy is individualized depending on the organism isolated and clinical course. For infections caused by *S. aureus* or gram-negative bacillary infections, the minimal duration of antibiotics is 28 days, provided that (1) the patient shows prompt resolution of signs and symptoms (within 5–7 days) and (2) the ESR has normalized; a total of 4–6 wk of therapy may be required. For group A streptococcus, *S. pneumoniae,* or *H. influenzae* type b, antibiotics are given for a minimum of 10–14 days, using the same criteria. A total of 7 postoperative days of treatment is adequate for *Pseudomonas* osteochondritis when thorough curettage of infected tissue has been performed. Immunocompromised patients generally require prolonged courses of therapy, as do patients with mycobacterial or fungal infection.

Changing antibiotics from the intravenous route to oral administration when a patient's condition has stabilized, generally after 1 wk of intravenous therapy, may be considered. For the oral antibiotic regimen with β-lactam drugs for staphylococcal or streptococcal infection, a dose two to three times that used for other infections is prescribed. The adequacy of the dose may be assessed by peak **serum bactericidal titers** or **Schlichter titers,** 45–60 min after a dose of suspension or 60–90 min after a capsule or tablet. A serum bactericidal titer of 1 : 8 or more is considered desirable. The oral regimen decreases the risk of nosocomial infections related to prolonged intravenous therapy, is more comfortable for patients, and permits treatment outside the hospital if adherence to treatment can be ensured. Outpatient intravenous antibiotic therapy via a central venous catheter can be used for the completion of therapy at home, as an alternative.

CRMO requires treatment of any primary disorder. Treatment of CRMO also includes prednisone; if steroids are unsuccessful, infliximab has been successful in a few patients.

Surgical Therapy. Surgical management of skeletal infections has not been subjected to randomized, prospective study comparing surgical procedures. When frank pus is obtained from subperiosteal or metaphyseal aspiration, a surgical drainage procedure is usually indicated. Surgical intervention is also often indicated after a penetrating injury and when a retained foreign body is possible. Surgical drainage is mandatory for osteomyelitis of the femoral head with hip joint involvement.

Treatment of chronic osteomyelitis consists of surgical removal of sinus tracts and sequestrum, if present. Antibiotic therapy is continued for several months or longer until clinical and radiographic findings suggest that healing has occurred.

Physical Therapy. The major role of physical medicine is a preventive one. If a child is allowed to lie in bed with an extremity in flexion, limitation of extension may develop within a few days. The affected extremity should be kept in extension with sandbags, splints, or, if necessary, casts. Casts are also indicated when there is a potential for pathologic fracture. After 2–3 days, when pain is easing, passive range of motion exercises are started and continued until the child resumes normal activity. In neglected cases with flexion contractures, prolonged physical therapy is required.

PROGNOSIS. When pus is drained and appropriate antibiotic therapy is given, the improvement in signs and symptoms is rapid. Failure to improve or worsening by 72 hr requires review of the appropriateness of the antibiotic therapy, the need for surgical intervention, or the correctness of the diagnosis. Acute-phase reactants may be useful as monitors. The serum CRP typically normalizes within 7 days after start of treatment, whereas the ESR typically rises for 5–7 days, then falls slowly, dropping sharply after 10–14 days. Failure of either of these acute-phase reactants to follow the usual course should raise concerns about the adequacy of therapy. Recurrence of disease and development of chronic infection after treatment occur in <10% of patients.

Because children are in a dynamic state of growth, sequelae of skeletal infections may not become apparent for months or years; therefore, long-term follow-up is necessary with close attention to range of motion of joints and bone length. Although firm data about the impact of delayed treatment on outcome are not available, it appears that initiation of medical and surgical therapy within 1 wk of onset of symptoms provides a better prognosis than delayed treatment.

Bocchini C, Hulten KG, Mason Jr. EO, et al: Panten-valentine leukodicin genes are associated with enhanced inflammatory response and local disease in acute hematogenous *Staphylococcus aureus* osteomyelitis in children. *Pediatrics* 2006;117:433–440.

Connolly LP, Connolly SA, Druback LA, et al: Acute hematogenous osteomyelitis of children: Assessment of skeletal scintigraphy-based diagnosis in the era of MRI. *J Nucl Med* 2002;43:1310–1316.

Deutschmann A, Mache CJ, Bodo K, et al: Successful treatment of chronic recurrent multifocal osteomyelitis with tumor necrosis factor-α blockage. *Pediatrics* 2005;116:1231–1233.

Fernandez M, Carrol CL, Baker CJ: Discitis and vertebral osteomyelitis in children: An 18-year review. *Pediatrics* 2000;105:1299–1304.

Floyed RL, Steele RW: Culture-negative osteomyelitis. *Pediatr Infect Dis J* 2003;22:731–735.

Gomez M, Maraqa N, Alvarez A, et al: Complications of outpatient parenteral antibiotic therapy in childhood. *Pediatr Infect Dis J* 2001;20:541–543.

Gonzales BE, Teruya J, Mahoney Jr. DH, et al: Venous thrombosis associated with staphylococcal osteomyelitis in children. *Pediatrics* 2006;117:1675–1679.

Huber AM, Lam PY, Duffy CM, et al: Chronic recurrent multifocal osteomyelitis: Clinical outcomes after more than five years of follow-up. *J Pediatr* 2002;141:198–203.

Ibia EO, Imoisili M, Pikis A: Group A ß-hemolytic streptococcal osteomyelitis in children. *Pediatrics* 2003;112:e22–e26.

Jurik AG: Chronic recurrent multifocal osteomyelitis. *Semin Musculoskelet Radiol* 2004;8:243–253.

Kiang KM, Ogunmodede F, Juni BA, et al: Outbreak of osteomyelitis/septic arthritis caused by *Kingella kingae* among child care center attendees. *Pediatrics* 2005;116:e206–e213.

Lew DP, Waldvogel FA: Osteomyelitis. *Lancet* 2004;364:369–379.

Maraqa NF, Gomez MM, Rathore MH: Outpatient parenteral antimicrobial therapy in osteoarticular infections in children. *J Pediatr Orthop* 2002;22:506–510.

Martinez-Aguilar G, Hammerman WA, Mason EO Jr, Kaplan SL: Clindamycin treatment of invasive infections caused by community-acquired, methicillin-resistant and methicillin-susceptible *S. aureus* in children. *Pediatr Infect Dis J* 2003;22:593–598.

Nelson JD: Bugs, drugs and bones: A pediatric infectious disease specialist reflects on management of musculoskeletal infections. *J Pediatr Orthop* 1999;19:141–142.

Saigal G, Azouz EM, Abdenour G: Imaging of osteomyelitis with special reference to children. *Semin Musculoskelet Radiol* 2004;8:255–265.

Shih HN, Shih LY, Wong YC: Diagnosis and treatment of subacute osteomyelitis. *J Trauma* 2005;58:83–87.

Verdier I, Gayet-Ageron A, Ploton C, et al: Contribution of a broad range polymerase chain reaction to the diagnosis of osteoarticular infections caused by *Kingella kingae*. *Pediatr Infect Dis J* 2005;24:692–696.

Yagupsky P: *K. kingae* infections of the skeletal system in children: Diagnosis and therapy. *Expert Rev Anti Infect Ther* 2004;2:787–794.

Yagupsky P, Erlich Y, Ariela S, et al: Outbreak of *Kingella kingae* skeletal system infections in children in daycare. *Pediatr Infect Dis J* 2006;25:526–532.

Chapter 684 ■ Suppurative Arthritis (Septic Arthritis) Richard M. Lampe

Suppurative infections of joints in infants and children have the potential to cause permanent disability. The frequency of suppurative arthritis is increased in infants and toddlers more than in older children. Early recognition of suppurative arthritis (also called septic arthritis) in young patients before extensive infection develops and prompt institution of appropriate medical and surgical therapy minimize further damage to the synovium, adjacent cartilage, and bone.

ETIOLOGY. The microbial spectrum is diverse in suppurative arthritis, but *Staphylococcus aureus* infection is most common. *Haemophilus influenzae* type b accounted for more than half of all cases of bacterial arthritis in infants before the introduction of the conjugate vaccine, but is now an uncommon cause. Group A streptococcus and *Streptococcus pneumoniae* (pneumococcus) historically cause 10–20%. *Kingella kingae* is recognized as a relatively common etiology with improved culture and polymerase chain reaction methods. In sexually active adolescents gonococcus is a common cause of septic arthritis and tenosynovitis usually of small joints or as a monoarticular infection of a large joint (knee).

Fungal infections usually occur as part of multisystem disseminated disease; *Candida* arthritis may complicate systemic infection in neonates with or without indwelling vascular catheters. Primary viral infections of joints are rare, but arthritis accompanies many viral (parvovirus, mumps, rubella live vaccines) syndromes, suggesting an immune-mediated pathogenesis.

A microbial etiology is confirmed in about 65% of cases of suppurative arthritis. Prior antibiotic therapy and the inhibitory effect of pus on microbial growth may explain the low bacterial yield. Additionally some cases treated as bacterial arthritis are actually postinfectious (gastrointestinal or genitourinary) reactive arthritis (see Chapter 156) rather than primary infection. Lyme disease produces an arthritis more like a rheumatologic disorder and not typically suppurative.

EPIDEMIOLOGY. Suppurative arthritis is more common in young children. Half of all cases occur by 2 yr of age and three fourths of all cases occur by 5 yr of age. Adolescents and neonates are at risk of gonococcal septic arthritis.

The majority of infections in otherwise healthy children are of hematogenous origin. Infection of joints can follow penetrating injuries or procedures such as trauma, arthroscopy, prosthetic joint surgery, intra-articular steroid injection, and orthopedic surgery, although this is uncommon. Immunocompromised patients and those with rheumatologic joint disease are also at increased risk of joint infection.

PATHOGENESIS. Suppurative arthritis primarily occurs as a result of hematogenous seeding of the synovial space. Less often, organisms enter the joint space by direct inoculation or extension from a contiguous focus. The synovial membrane has a rich vascular supply and lacks a basement membrane, providing an ideal environment for hematogenous seeding. The presence of bacterial endotoxin within the joint space stimulates cytokine production (tumor necrosis factor-α, interleukin-1) within the joint, triggering an inflammatory cascade. The cytokines stimulate chemotaxis of neutrophils into the joint space where proteolytic enzymes and elastases are released by neutrophils, damaging the cartilage. Proteolytic enzymes released from the synovial cells and chondrocytes also contribute to cartilage and synovium destruction. Bacterial hyaluronidase breaks down the hyaluronic acid in the synovial fluid, making the fluid less viscous and diminishing its ability to lubricate and protect the joint cartilage. Damage to the cartilage can occur through increased friction, especially for weight-bearing joints. The increased pressure within the joint space from accumulation of purulent material can compromise the vascular supply and induce pressure necrosis of the cartilage. Synovial and cartilage destruction results from a combination of proteolytic enzymes and mechanical factors.

CLINICAL MANIFESTATIONS. The signs and symptoms of suppurative arthritis depend on the age of the patient. Early signs and symptoms may be subtle particularly in neonates. Suppurative arthritis in neonates and young infants is often associated with adjacent osteomyelitis due to transphyseal spread of infection (see Chapter 683).

Older infants and children may have fever and pain, with localizing signs such as swelling, erythema, and warmth of the affected joint. With involvement of joints of the pelvis and lower extremities, limp or refusal to walk is often seen.

Erythema and edema of the skin and soft tissue overlying the site of infection are seen earlier in suppurative arthritis than in osteomyelitis, since the bulging infected synovium is usually more superficial, whereas the metaphysis is located more deeply. Suppurative arthritis of the hip is an exception because of the deep location of the hip joint.

Joints of the lower extremity constitute 75% of all cases of suppurative arthritis (Table 684-1). The elbow, wrist, and shoulder

TABLE 684-1. Distribution of Affected Joints in Acute Suppurative Arthritis

JOINT	NO.	%
Knee	309	39.6
Hip	173	22.2
Elbow	109	14.0
Ankle	104	13.3
Shoulder	37	4.7
Wrist	34	4.4
Sacroiliac	5	0.6
Interphalangeal	4	0.5
Metatarsal	3	0.4
Acromioclavicular	1	0.1
Sternoclavicular	1	0.1
Metacarpal	1	0.1

Based on unpublished series of 725 patients with 781 infected joints.

joints are involved in about 25% of cases, and small joints are uncommonly infected. Suppurative infections of the hip, shoulder, elbow, and ankle in older infants and children may be associated with an adjacent osteomyelitis of the proximal femur, proximal humerus, proximal radius, and distal tibia because the metaphysis extends intra-articularly.

DIAGNOSIS. A blood culture should be performed in all cases of suspected septic arthritis. Aspiration of the joint fluid for Gram stain and culture when the history and physical findings indicate suppurative arthritis remains the definitive diagnostic technique and provides the optimal specimen for culture to confirm the diagnosis. Most large joint spaces are easy to aspirate, but the hip can pose technical problems; ultrasound guidance facilitates aspiration. If no fluid is obtained, contrast material is injected and a radiograph is obtained to ensure that the needle tip is in the joint cavity. Aspiration of joint pus provides the best specimen for bacteriologic culture of infection. If gonococcus is suspected, cervical, anal, and throat cultures should also be obtained. In addition to prompt inoculation onto solid media, inoculation of the specimen in blood culture bottles may increase recovery of *K. kingae.*

Synovial fluid analysis for cell count, differential, protein, and glucose has limited usefulness because noninfectious inflammatory diseases, such as rheumatic fever and rheumatoid arthritis, can also cause exuberant reaction with increased cells and protein and decreased glucose. Synovial fluid characteristics of suppurative arthritis can suggest infection but are not sufficiently specific to exclude infection.

There are no specific laboratory tests for suppurative arthritis. Tests such as white blood cell count and differential, erythrocyte sedimentation rate (ESR), and C-reactive protein (CRP) are very sensitive for joint infections but are nonspecific and may not be helpful in distinguishing between infection and other inflammatory processes. The leukocyte count and ESR may be normal during the first few days of infection, and normal test results do not preclude the diagnosis of suppurative arthritis. Monitoring elevated ESR and CRP may be of value in assessing response to therapy or identifying complications.

Radiographic Evaluation. Radiographic studies play a crucial role in the evaluation of suppurative arthritis. Conventional radiographs, ultrasonography, CT, MRI, and radionuclide studies may all contribute to establishing the diagnosis.

PLAIN RADIOGRAPHS. Plain films of suppurative arthritis may show widening of the joint capsule, soft-tissue edema, and obliteration of normal fat lines. Plain films of the hip can show medial displacement of the obturator muscle into the pelvis (the obturator sign), lateral displacement or obliteration of the gluteal fat lines, and elevation of the Shenton line with a widened arc.

ULTRASONOGRAPHY. Ultrasonography is particularly helpful in detecting joint effusion and fluid collection in the soft-tissue and subperiosteal regions. Ultrasonography is highly sensitive in the detection of joint effusion, particularly for the hip joint, where plain radiographs may be normal in >50% of cases of suppurative arthritis of the hip. Ultrasonography may serve as an aid in performing hip aspiration.

COMPUTED TOMOGRAPHY AND MAGNETIC RESONANCE IMAGING. Both CT and MRI may be useful in confirming the presence of joint fluid in patients with suspected osteoarthritis infections. MRI may be useful in excluding adjacent osteomyelitis.

In suppurative arthritis, three-phase imaging with technetium-99 methylene diphosphonate shows symmetric uptake on both sides of the joint, limited to the bony structures adjacent to the joint. Radionuclide imaging is also useful for evaluation of the sacroiliac joint.

Differential Diagnosis. The differential diagnosis of suppurative arthritis depends on the joint or joints involved and the age of the patient. For the hip, toxic synovitis, Legg-Calvé-Perthes disease, slipped capital femoral epiphysis, psoas abscess, and proximal femoral, pelvic, or vertebral osteomyelitis as well as diskitis should be considered. For the knee, distal femoral or proximal tibial osteomyelitis, pauciarticular rheumatoid arthritis, and referred pain from the hip should be considered. Other conditions such as trauma, cellulitis, pyomyositis, sickle cell disease, hemophilia, and Henoch-Schönlein purpura can mimic purulent arthritis. When several joints are involved, serum sickness, collagen vascular disease, rheumatic fever, and Henoch-Schönlein purpura should be considered. Reactive arthritis following a variety of bacterial (gastrointestinal or genital) and parasitic infections, streptococcal pharyngitis, or viral hepatitis can resemble acute suppurative arthritis (see Chapter 156).

TREATMENT. Optimal treatment of suppurative arthritis requires cooperation of pediatricians, orthopedic surgeons, and radiologists to benefit the patient.

Antibiotic Therapy. The initial empirical antibiotic therapy is based on knowledge of likely bacterial pathogens at various ages, the results of the Gram stain of aspirated material, and additional considerations. In neonates, an antistaphylococcal penicillin, such as nafcillin or oxacillin (150–200 mg/kg/24 hr divided q6h IV), and a broad-spectrum cephalosporin, such as cefotaxime (200 mg/kg/24 hr divided q8h IV), provide coverage for the *S. aureus,* group B streptococcus, and gram-negative bacilli. If the neonate is a small premature infant or has a central vascular catheter, the possibility of nosocomial bacteria (*Pseudomonas aeruginosa* or coagulase-negative staphylococci) or fungi (*Candida*) should be considered.

In children with suppurative arthritis, empirical therapy to cover for *S. aureus*, streptococci, and *K. kingae* would include cefazolin (100–150 mg/kg/24 hr divided q8h) or nafcillin (150–200 mg/kg/24 hr divided q6h).

Clindamycin (40 mg/kg divided q6h) and vancomycin (40 mg/kg/24 hr divided q6h IV) are alternatives when treating methicillin-resistant *S. aureus* infections. For immunocompromised patients, combination therapy is usually initiated, such as with vancomycin and ceftazidime or with extended-spectrum penicillins and β-lactamase inhibitors with an aminoglycoside. Adjunct therapy with dexamethasone for 4 days with antibiotic therapy appears to benefit children with septic arthritis.

When the pathogen is identified, appropriate changes in antibiotics are made, if necessary. If a pathogen is not identified and a patient's condition is improving, therapy is continued with the antibiotic selected initially. If a pathogen is not identified and a patient's condition is not improving, re-aspiration or the possibility of a noninfectious condition should be considered.

Duration of antibiotic therapy is individualized depending on the organism isolated and the clinical course. Ten to 14 days is usually adequate for streptococci, pneumococcus, and *K. kingae;* longer therapy maybe needed for *S. aureus* and other gram-negative infections. Normalization of ESR and CRP in addition to a normal examination supports discontinuing antibiotic therapy.

Surgical Therapy. Infection of the hip is considered a surgical emergency because of the vulnerability of the blood supply to the head of the femur. For joints other than the hip, daily aspirations of synovial fluid may be required. Generally, one or two subsequent aspirations suffice. If fluid continues to accumulate after 4–5 days, arthrotomy is needed. At the time of surgery, the joint is flushed with sterile saline solution. Antibiotics are not instilled because they are irritating to synovial tissue, and adequate amounts of antibiotic are achieved in joint fluid with systemic administration.

PROGNOSIS. When pus is drained and appropriate antibiotic therapy is given, the improvement in signs and symptoms is rapid. Failure to improve or worsening by 72 hr requires review of the appropriateness of the antibiotic therapy, the need for surgical intervention, and the correctness of the diagnosis. Acute-phase reactants may be useful as monitors. Failure of either of these acute-phase reactants to follow the usual course should raise concerns about the adequacy of therapy. Recurrence of disease and development of chronic infection after treatment occur in <10% of patients.

Because children are in a dynamic state of growth, sequelae of skeletal infections may not become apparent for months or years; therefore, long-term follow-up is necessary with close attention to range of motion of joints and bone length. Although firm data about the impact of delayed treatment on outcome are not available, it appears that initiation of medical and surgical therapy within 1 wk of onset of symptoms provides a better prognosis than delayed treatment.

Bonheffer J, Haeberle B, Schaad UB, Heininger U: Diagnosis of hematogenous osteomyelitis and septic arthritis: 20 years experience at the University Children's Hospital Basel. *Swiss Med Wkly* 2001;131:575–581.

Centers for Disease Control and Prevention: Osteomyelitis/septic arthritis caused by *Kingella kingae* among day care attendees—Minnesota. *MMWR* 2003;53:241–243.

Nelson JD: Bugs, drugs and bones: A pediatric infectious disease specialist reflects on management of musculoskeletal infections. *J Pediatr Orthop* 1999;19:141–142.

Odio CM, Ramirez T, Arias G, et al: Double blind, randomized, placebo-controlled study of dexamethasone therapy for hematogenous septic arthritis in children. *Pediatr Infect Dis J* 2003;22:883–888.

Ross JJ, Hu LT: Septic arthritis of the pubic symphysis. *Medicine* 2003;82: 340–345.

Schirtliff ME, Mader JT: Acute septic arthritis. *Clin Microbiol Rev* 2002; 15:527–544.

Wang CL, Wang SM, Yang YJ, et al: Septic arthritis in children: Relationship of causative pathogens, complications, and outcome. *J Microbiol Immunol Infect* 2003;36:41–46.

Section 2 — Sports Medicine

Chapter 685 ■ Epidemiology and Prevention of Injuries Gregory L. Landry and Kelsey Logan

The Surgeon General's Healthy People 2010 Objectives emphasize moderate to vigorous physical activity on a regular basis for all adolescents. Physical activity has favorable effects on hypertension, obesity, and serum lipid levels in youths. In adults, physical activity is associated with lower rates of cardiovascular disease, type 2 diabetes mellitus, osteoporosis, and colon and breast cancer.

Physicians should promote physical activity to their patients and make adjustments in the type of physical activity depending on their health status. Extra effort is needed to try to make physical activity part of the lifestyle for those with lower rates of physical activity and sports participation, including children with special health care needs and those from lower socioeconomic groups. Coincident with promoting sports participation and physical activity, physicians have the responsibility of providing medical clearance for participation in physical activity and sports and for diagnosis and rehabilitation of injuries.

Approximately 30 million children and adolescents participate in organized sports in the United States. Approximately 3 million injuries occur annually if injury is defined as time lost from the sport. Deaths in sports are rare, with the majority of nontraumatic deaths caused by cardiac diseases (see Chapter 436). Overall, injury rates and injury severity in sports increase with age and pubertal development, related to the greater speed, strength, and intensity of competition.

Recognizing mechanisms of injury and enforcing rules that reduce the likelihood of that mechanism of injury, including penalizing dangerous play, have reduced catastrophic injury rates. Injury rates have also been reduced by removing environmental hazards, such as trampolines in gymnastics and stationary (vs breakaway) bases in softball, and by modifying heat injury rates in soccer tournaments by adding water breaks and reducing the playing time. Wearing equipment such as mouth guards can reduce dental injuries. A common reason for reinjury is lack of rehabilitation of old injuries; appropriate rehabilitation reduces injury rates. Preseason training for high school athletes, with an emphasis on speed, agility, jump training, and flexibility, is associated with lower injury rates in soccer and fewer serious knee injuries in female athletes. Traditional stretching maneuvers or massage may not reduce the risk of injury or muscle soreness, but ankle taping is helpful particularly to prevent reinjury of the ankle. One setting for implementing some of these prevention strategies and for detecting unrehabilitated injuries and medical problems that could affect participation in sports is the preparticipation sports examination (PSE).

PREPARTICIPATION SPORTS EXAMINATION

The PSE is performed with a directed history and a directed physical examination, including a screening musculoskeletal examination. It identifies possible problems in 1–8% of athletes and excludes <1% from participation. The PSE is not a substitute for the recommended comprehensive annual evaluation, which looks at behaviors that are potentially harmful to teens, such as sexual activity, drug use, suicide, and violence. The purposes of the PSE include detecting medical conditions that delay or disqualify athletic participation owing to a risk of injury or death, detecting previously undiagnosed medical conditions, detecting medical conditions that need further evaluation or rehabilitation before participation, providing guidance for sports participation for patients with health conditions, and meeting legal and insurance obligations. If possible, the PSE should be combined with the comprehensive annual health visit with emphasis on preventive health care (see Chapters 5 and 12).

State requirements for how often a youth needs a PSE differ, ranging from annually to entry to a new school level (junior high, senior high, college). At a minimum, a focused, annual interim evaluation should be done on an otherwise healthy young athlete. The PSE is optimally performed 3–6 wk before the start of practice.

HISTORY AND PHYSICAL EXAMINATION. The essential components of the PSE are the history and focused medical and musculoskeletal screening examinations. Identified problems require more investigation (Tables 685-1 and 685-2). In the absence of symptoms, no screening laboratory tests are required.

Seventy-five percent of significant findings are identified by the history; a standardized questionnaire given to the parent and athlete is important because the young athlete may not know or may forget important aspects of his or her history. The questionnaire should include questions about previous medical, surgical, cardiac, pulmonary, neurologic, dermatologic, visual, psychologic, musculoskeletal, and menstrual problems, as well as about heat illness, medications, allergies, immunizations, and diet. The most common identified problems are **unrehabilitated injuries.** An investigation of previous injuries including diagnostic tests, treatment, and present functional status is indicated.

Sudden death during sports may result from undetected cardiac disease such as hypertrophic or other cardiomyopathies, anomalous coronary vessels, or a ruptured aorta in Marfan syndrome (see Chapter 700). In many cases, the underlying heart disease is not suspected, and death is the first sign of heart disease (see Chapter 436). Chest radiographs, electrocardiograms (ECGs), and echocardiograms (ECHOs) are not recommended as routine screening tests. If there is a **suspicion** of heart disease, such as a history of syncope, presyncope, palpitations, excessive dyspnea with exercise, or a family history of a condition such as hypertrophic cardiomyopathy or prolonged QT or Marfan syndrome,

TABLE 685-1. Preparticipation Sports Examination

COMPONENT OF THE PHYSICAL EXAMINAITON	CONDITION TO BE DETECTED
Vital signs	Hypertension, cardiac disease, brady/tachycardia
Height and weight	Obesity, eating disorders
Vision and pupil size	Legal blindness, absent eye, anisocoria, amblyopia
Lymph node	Infectious diseases, malignancy
Cardiac (performed standing and supine)	Heart murmur, prior surgery, dysrhythmia
Pulmonary	Recurrent and exercise-induced bronchospasm, chronic lung disease
Abdomen	Organomegaly, abdominal mass
Skin	Contagious diseases (impetigo, herpes, staphylococcal, streptococcal)
Genitourinary	Varicocele, undescended testes, tumor, hernia
Musculoskeletal	Acute and chronic injuries, physical anomalies (scoliosis)

TABLE 685-2. Medical Conditions and Sports Participation*

CONDITION	MAY PARTICIPATE
Atlantoaxial instability (instability of the joint between cervical vertebrae 1 and 2) *Explanation:* Athlete needs evaluation to assess risk of spinal cord injury during sports participation.	Qualified yes
Bleeding disorder *Explanation:* Athlete needs evaluation.	Qualified yes
Cardiovascular disease	
Carditis (inflammation of the heart) *Explanation:* Carditis may result in sudden death with exertion.	No
Hypertension (high blood pressure) *Explanation:* Those with significant essential (unexplained) hypertension should avoid weight and power lifting, body building, and strength training. Those with secondary hypertension (hypertension caused by a previously identified disease) or severe essential hypertension need evaluation.	Qualified yes
Congenital heart disease (structural heart defects present at birth) *Explanation:* Those with mild forms may participate fully; those with moderate or severe forms or who have undergone surgery need evaluation. The 26th Bethesda Conference defined mild, moderate, and severe disease for common cardiac lesions.	Qualified yes
Dysrhythmia (irregular heart rhythm) *Explanation:* Those with symptoms (chest pain, syncope, dizziness, shortness of breath, or other symptoms of possible dysrhythmia) or evidence of mitral regurgitation on physical examination need evaluation. All others may participate fully.	Qualified yes
Heart murmur *Explanation:* If the murmur is innocent (does not indicate heart disease), full participation is permitted. Otherwise, the athlete needs evaluation (see congenital heart disease and mitral valve prolapse).	Qualified yes
Cerebral palsy *Explanation:* Athlete needs evaluation.	Qualified yes
Diabetes mellitus *Explanation:* All sports can be played with proper attention to diet, blood glucose concentration, hydration, and insulin therapy. Blood glucose concentration should be monitored every 30 min during continuous exercise and 15 min after completion of exercise.	Yes
Diarrhea *Explanation:* Unless disease is mild, no participation is permitted, because diarrhea may increase the risk of dehydration and heat illness. See fever.	Qualified no
Eating disorders Anorexia nervosa Bulimia nervosa *Explanation:* Patients with these disorders need medical and psychiatric assessment before participation.	Qualified yes
Eyes Functionally one-eyed athlete Loss of an eye Detached retina Previous eye surgery or serious eye injury *Explanation:* A functionally one-eyed athlete has a best-corrected visual acuity of less than 20/40 in the eye with worse acuity. These athletes would suffer significant disability if the better eye were seriously injured, as would those with loss of an eye. Some athletes who previously have undergone eye surgery or had a serious eye injury may have an increased risk of injury because of weakened eye tissue. Availability of eye guards approved by the American Society for Testing and Materials and other protective equipment may allow participation in most sports, but this must be judged on an individual basis.	Qualified yes
Fever *Explanation:* Fever can increase cardiopulmonary effort, reduce maximum exercise capacity, make heat illness more likely, and increase orthostatic tension during exercise. Fever may rarely accompany myocarditis or other infections that may make exercise dangerous.	No
Heat illness, history of *Explanation:* Because of the increased likelihood of recurrence, the athlete needs individual assessment to determine the presence of predisposing conditions and to arrange a prevention strategy.	Qualified yes
Hepatitis *Explanation:* Because of the apparent minimal risk to others, all sports may be played that the athlete's state of health allows. In all athletes, skin lesions should be covered properly, and athletic personnel should use universal precautions when handling blood or body fluids with visible blood.	Yes
Human immunodeficiency virus infection *Explanation:* Because of the apparent minimal risk to others, all sports may be played that the athlete's state of health allows. In all athletes, skin lesions should be covered properly, and athletic personnel should use universal precautions when handling blood or body fluids with visible blood.	Yes
Kidney, absence of one *Explanation:* Athlete needs individual assessment for contact, collision, and limited-contact sports.	Qualified yes
Liver, enlarged *Explanation:* If the liver is acutely enlarged, participation should be avoided because of risk of rupture. If the liver is chronically enlarged, individual assessment is needed before collision, contact, or limited-contact sports are played.	Qualified yes
Malignant neoplasm *Explanation:* Athlete needs individual assessment.	Qualified yes
Musculoskeletal disorders *Explanation:* Athlete needs individual assessment.	Qualified yes
Neurologic disorders History of serious head or spine trauma, severe or repeated concussions, or craniotomy. *Explanation:* Athlete needs individual assessment for collision, contact, or limited-contact sports and also for noncontact sports if deficits in judgment or cognition are present. Research supports a conservative approach to management of concussion.	Qualified yes
Seizure disorder, well-controlled *Explanation:* Risk of seizure during participation is minimal.	Yes
Seizure disorder, poorly controlled *Explanation:* Athlete needs individual assessment for collision, contact, or limited-contract sports. The following noncontact sports should be avoided: archery, riflery, swimming, weight or power lifting, strength training, or sports involving heights. In these sports, occurrence of a seizure may pose a risk to self or others.	Qualified yes
Obesity *Explanation:* Because of the risk of heat illness, obese persons need careful acclimatization and hydration.	Qualified yes
Organ transplant recipient *Explanation:* Athlete needs individual assessment.	Qualified yes
Ovary, absence of one	Yes

TABLE 685-2. Medical Conditions and Sports Participation—cont'd

Condition	May Participate
Explanation: Risk of severe injury to the remaining ovary is minimal.	
Respiratory conditions	
Pulmonary compromise, including cystic fibrosis	Qualified yes
Explanation: Athlete needs individual assessment, but generally, all sports may be played if oxygenation remains satisfactory during a graded exercise test. Patients with cystic fibrosis need acclimatization and good hydration to reduce the risk of heat illness.	
Asthma	Yes
Explanation: With proper medication and education, only athletes with the most severe asthma will need to modify their participation.	
Acute upper respiratory infection	Qualified yes
Explanation: Upper respiratory obstruction may affect pulmonary function. Athlete needs individual assessment for all but mild disease. See fever.	
Sickle cell disease	Qualified yes
Explanation: Athlete needs individual assessment. In general, if status of the illness permits, all but high exertion, collision, and contact sports may be played. Overheating, dehydration, and chilling must be avoided.	
Sickle cell trait	Yes
Explanation: It is unlikely that persons with sickle cell trait have an increased risk of sudden death or other medical problems during athletic participation, except under the most extreme conditions of heat, humidity, and possibly increased altitude. These persons, like all athletes, should be carefully conditioned, acclimatized, and hydrated to reduce any possible risk.	
Skin disorders (boils, herpes simplex, impetigo, scabies, molluscum contagiosum)	Qualified yes
Explanation: While the patient is contagious, participation in gymnastics with mats; martial arts; wrestling; or other collision, contact, or limited-contact sports is not allowed.	
Spleen, enlarged	Qualified yes
Explanation: A patient with an acutely enlarged spleen should avoid all sports because of risk of rupture. A patient with a chronically enlarged spleen needs individual assessment before playing collision, contact, or limited-contact sports.	
Testicle, undescended or absence of one	Yes
Explanation: Certain sports may require a protective cup.	

*This table is designed for use by medical and nonmedical personnel. "Needs evaluation" means that a physician with appropriate knowledge and experience should assess the safety of a given sport for an athlete with the listed medical condition. Unless otherwise noted, this is because of variability of the severity of the disease, the risk of injury for the specific sports listed in Tables 685-3 and 685-4, or both.

From the American Academy of Pediatrics, Committee on Sports Medicine and Fitness: Medical conditions affecting sports participation. *Pediatrics* 2001;107:1206–1207.

the evaluation should be complete and include a 12-lead ECG, an ECHO, a Holter or event capture monitor, and a stress test with electrocardiographic monitoring. Recommendations for participation with identified cardiac disease should be done in consultation with a cardiologist.

Disqualification and limitations for sports participation among various medical conditions are available from the American Academy of Pediatrics (Table 685-2). Sports may also be classified by intensity (Table 685-3) and contact (Table 685-4). Athletes may seek to participate in sports against medical advice and

TABLE 685-3. Classification of Sports by Strenuousness

HIGH TO MODERATE INTENSITY

HIGH TO MODERATE DYNAMIC AND STATIC DEMANDS	HIGH TO MODERATE DYNAMIC AND LOW STATIC DEMANDS	HIGH TO MODERATE STATIC AND LOW DYNAMIC DEMANDS
Boxing*	Badminton	Archery
Crew or rowing	Baseball	Auto racing
Cross-country skiing	Basketball	Diving
Cycling	Field hockey	Horseback riding (jumping)
Downhill skiing	Lacrosse	Field events (throwing)
Fencing	Orienteering	Gymnastics
Football	Race walking	Karate or judo
Ice hockey	Racquetball	Motorcycling
Rugby	Soccer	Rodeo
Running (sprint)	Squash	Sailing
Speed skating	Swimming	Ski jumping
Water polo	Table tennis	Water skiing
Wrestling	Tennis	Weight lifting
	Volleyball	

LOW INTENSITY (LOW DYNAMIC AND LOW STATIC DEMANDS)

Bowling
Cricket
Curling
Golf
Riflery

*Participation not recommended by the American Academy of Pediatrics.

From the American Academy of Pediatrics, Committee on Sports Medicine and Fitness: Medical conditions affecting sports participation. *Pediatrics* 2001;107:1208.

TABLE 685-4. Classification of Sports by Contact

CONTACT OR COLLISION	LIMITED CONTACT	NONCONTACT
Basketball	Baseball	Archery
Boxing*	Bicycling	Badminton
Diving	Cheerleading	Body building
Field hockey	Canoeing or kayaking	Bowling
Football	(white water)	Canoeing or kayaking (flat water)
Tackle	Fencing	Crew or rowing
Ice hockey†	Field events	Curling
Lacrosse	High jump	Dancing
Martial arts	Pole vault	Ballet
Rodeo	Floor hockey	Modern
Rugby	Football	Jazz
Ski jumping	Flag	Field events
Soccer	Gymnastics	Discus
Team handball	Handball	Javelin
Water polo	Horseback riding	Shot put
Wrestling	Racquetball	Golf
	Skating	Orienteering‡
	Ice	Power lifting
	In-line	Race walking
	Roller	Riflery
	Skiing	Rope jumping
	Cross-country	Running
	Downhill	Sailing
	Water	Scuba diving
	Skateboarding	Swimming
	Snowboarding	Table tennis
	Softball	Tennis
	Squash	Track
	Ultimate frisbee	Weight lifting
	Volleyball	
	Windsurfing or surfing	

*Participation not recommended by the American Academy of Pediatrics.

†The American Academy of Pediatrics recommends limiting the amount of body checking allowed for hockey players 15 years and younger to reduce injuries.

‡A race (contest) in which competitors use a map and compass to find their way through unfamiliar territory.

From the American Academy of Pediatrics, Committee on Sports Medicine and Fitness: Medical conditions affecting sports participation. *Pediatrics* 2001;107:1205.

have done so successfully for professional sports. Section 504(a) of the Rehabilitation Act of 1973 prohibits discrimination against disabled athletes if they have capabilities/skills required to play a competitive sport. This was reinforced through the Americans with Disabilities Act of 1990. An amateur athlete has no absolute right to decide whether to participate in competitive sports. Participation in competitive sports is considered a privilege, not a right. Knapp *v* Northwestern University established that "difficult medical decisions involving complex medical problems can be made by responsible physicians exercising prudent judgment (which will be necessarily conservative when definitive scientific evidence is lacking or conflicting) and relying on the recommendations of specialist consultants or guidelines established by a panel of experts."

American Academy of Pediatrics: Medical conditions affecting sports participation. *Pediatrics* 2001;107:1205–1209.

American Academy of Pediatrics, American Academy of Family Physicians, American Medical Society for Sports Medicine, American Orthopedic Society for Sports Medicine, American Osteopathic Association for Sports Medicine: *Preparticipation Physical Evaluation Monograph,* 3rd ed. Minneapolis, MN: McGraw-Hill Medical Publishing, 2004.

Anderson SJ: Sports injuries. *Curr Prob Pediatr Adolesc Health Care* 2005;35:105–176.

Jonhagen S, Ackermann P, Eriksson T, et al: Sports massage after eccentric exercise. *Am J Sports Med* 2004;32:1499–1503.

MacAuley D, Best TM: Reducing risk of injury due to exercise. *Br Med J* 2002;325:451–452.

Olsen OE, Myklebust G, Engebretsen L, et al: Exercises to prevent lower limb injuries in youth sports: Cluster randomized controlled trial. *Br Med J* 2005;330:449–452.

Chapter 686 ■ Management of Musculoskeletal Injury

Gregory L. Landry

MECHANISM OF INJURY

ACUTE INJURIES. The majority of musculoskeletal injuries are sprains, strains, and contusions. The history of the injury can be unclear, but it is especially helpful in assessing knee and shoulder injuries. More severe injuries, indicative of structural derangement, may have acute signs and symptoms such as immediate swelling, deformity, numbness or weakness, inability to continue playing, inability to walk without a limp, a loud painful pop, mechanical locking of the joint, or the sensation of instability. A **sprain** is an injury to a ligament or joint capsule. A **strain** is an injury to a muscle or tendon. A **contusion** is a crush injury to any soft tissue. Sprains are graded 1–3 with *grade 1* meaning that some fibers have been torn with no evidence of laxity of the ligament when tested on physical examination. A *grade 2* means more fibers are torn resulting in some laxity of the ligament but a good end point, meaning not all fibers are torn. A *grade 3* sprain means all the fibers are torn and testing of the ligaments results in a "mushy" endpoint on physical examination. Strains are also graded 1–3 with a *grade 1* causing mild pain with testing the muscle and very little weakness. *Grade 2* injuries cause more pain and moderate weakness with testing the muscle. *Grade 3* muscle strains are complete rupture of the muscle or tendon and result in marked weakness and sometimes a palpable defect in the muscle or tendon.

OVERUSE INJURIES. Overuse injuries are caused by repetitive microtrauma that exceeds the body's rate of repair. This occurs in muscles, tendons, bone, bursae, cartilage, and nerves. Overuse injuries occur in all sports but more frequently in sports emphasizing repetitive motion (swimming, running, tennis, gymnastics). Factors can be categorized into extrinsic (training errors, poor equipment or workout surface) and intrinsic (athlete's anatomy or medical conditions). Training error is the most frequently identified factor. At the beginning of the workout program, athletes may violate the "10% rule": Do not increase the duration or intensity of workouts more than 10% per week. Intrinsic factors include abnormal biomechanics (leg-length discrepancy, pes planus, pes cavus, tarsal coalition, valgus heel, external tibial torsion, femoral anteversion), muscle imbalance, inflexibility, and medical conditions (deconditioning, nutritional deficits, amenorrhea, obesity). The athlete should be asked about the specifics of training. Runners should be asked about their shoes, orthotics, running surface, weekly mileage or time spent running per week, speed or hill workouts, and previous injuries and rehabilitation. When causative factors are identified, they can be eliminated or modified so that after rehabilitation the athlete does not return to the same regimen and suffer reinjury.

For athletes engaged in excessive training that causes an overuse injury, curtailing all exercise is not usually necessary. A rehabilitation program designed to return athletes to their sport as soon as possible while minimizing exposure to reinjury is indicated. Early identification of an overuse injury requires less alteration of the workout regimen.

The goals of treatment are to control pain and spasm to rehabilitate flexibility, strength, endurance, and proprioceptive deficits (Table 686-1). In many overuse injuries, the role of inflammation in the process is minimal. For most injuries to tendons, the term tendinitis is obsolete since there is little or no inflammation on histopathology of tendons. Instead, there are scar and abnormal tissue. Most of these entities are now more appropriately called **tendonopathies,** and there is probably little, if any, role for anti-inflammatory medication in the treatment except as an analgesic.

INITIAL EVALUATION OF THE INJURED EXTREMITY

Initially, the examiner should determine the quality of the peripheral pulses and capillary refill rate as well as the gross motor and sensory function to assess for neurovascular injury. The first priorities are to maintain vascular and skeletal stability.

TABLE 686-1. Staging of Overuse Injuries

GRADE	GRADING SYMPTOMS	TREATMENT
I	Pain only after activity Does not interfere with performance or intensity Generalized tenderness Disappears before next session	Modification of activity, consider cross-training, home rehabilitation program
II	Minimal pain with activity Does not interfere with performance More localized tenderness	Modification of activity, cross-training, home rehabilitation program
III	Pain interferes with activity and performance Definite area of tenderness Usually disappears between sessions	Significant modification of activity, strongly encourage cross-training, home rehabilitation program, and outpatient physical therapy
IV	Pain with activities of daily living Pain does not disappear between sessions Marked interference with performance and training intensity	Discontinue activity temporarily, cross-training only, oral analgesic, home rehabilitation program, and intensive outpatient physical therapy
V	Pain interferes with activities of daily living Signs of tissue injury (e.g., edema) Chronic or recurrent symptoms	Prolonged discontinuation of activity, cross-training only, oral analgesic, home rehabilitation program, and intensive outpatient physical therapy

Criteria for immediate attention and rapid orthopedic consultation include vascular compromise, nerve compromise, and open fracture. The exposed wound should be covered with sterile saline-soaked gauze, and the injured limb should be padded and splinted. Pressure should be applied to any site of bleeding. Additional criteria include deep laceration over a joint, unreducible dislocation, grade III (complete) tear of a muscle-tendon unit, and displaced, significantly angulated fractures (depends on the bone involved, the degree of displacement and angulation, and neurovascular status of the extremity).

THE TRANSITION FROM IMMEDIATE MANAGEMENT TO RETURN TO PLAY

Rehabilitation of a musculoskeletal injury should begin on the day of the injury.

Phase 1: *Limit further injury, control swelling and pain, and minimize strength and flexibility losses.* This requires the use of an appropriate device such as crutches or a sling, ice, compression, elevation, and analgesia. Crutches, air stirrups for ankle sprains, slings for arm injuries, and elastic wraps (4–8 in) for compression are a reasonable inventory of office supplies. Ice in a plastic bag is placed directly on the skin for 20 min continuously, 3 to 4 times per day until the swelling resolves. Compression limits further bleeding and swelling but should not be so tight that it limits perfusion. Elevation of the extremity promotes venous return and limits swelling. A nonsteroidal anti-inflammatory drug or acetaminophen is indicated for analgesia.

Pain-free isometric strengthening and range of motion should be initiated as soon as possible. Pain inhibits full muscle contraction; deconditioning results if the pain and resultant nonuse persist for days to weeks, thus delaying recovery. Education about the nature of the injury and the specifics of rehabilitation exercises including handouts with written instructions and drawings demonstrating the exercises are helpful.

Phase 2: *Improve strength and range of motion (i.e., flexibility) while allowing the injured structures to heal.* Protective devices are removed when the patient's strength and flexibility improve and activities of daily living are pain free. Flexibility can then be improved by a program of specific stretches, held for 15–20 sec for 3 to 5 repetitions, once or twice daily. A physical therapist or athletic trainer is invaluable in this treatment. Protective devices may need to be used for months during sports participation. Swimming, water jogging, and stationary cycling are good aerobic exercises that can allow the injured extremity to be rested or used pain free while maintaining cardiovascular fitness.

Phase 3: *Achieve near normal strength and flexibility of the injured structures and further improve or maintain cardiovascular fitness.* Strength and endurance are improved under controlled conditions using elastic bands and eventually free weights or exercise equipment. Proprioceptive training allows the athlete to redevelop a kinesthetic sense, which is critical to joint function and stability.

Phase 4: *Return to exercise or competition without restriction.* When the athlete has reached nearly normal flexibility, strength, proprioception, and endurance, he or she can start sports-specific exercises. The athlete will make the transition from the rehabilitation program to functional rehabilitation appropriate for the sport. Substituting sports participation for rehabilitation is inappropriate; rather, there should be progressive stepwise functional return to a full activity/play program. For instance, a basketball player recovering from an ankle injury might begin a walk-run-sprint-cut program before returning to competition. At any point in this progression, if pain is experienced, the athlete needs to stop, apply ice, avoid running for 1–2 days, continue to do ankle exercises, and then resume running at a lower intensity and progress accordingly.

RELATIVE REST AND RETURN-TO-PLAY GUIDELINES. Relative rest means that the athlete can do whatever he or she wants as long as the injured structures do not hurt during or within 24 hr of the activity. Exercising beyond the pain threshold delays recovery.

DIFFERENTIAL DIAGNOSES OF MUSCULOSKELETAL PAIN

Traumatic, rheumatologic, infectious, hematologic, psychologic, and oncologic processes can cause the presenting complaint of musculoskeletal pain. Symptoms such as fatigue, weight loss, rash, multiple joint complaints, fever, chronic or recent illness, and persistence of pain suggest diagnoses other than sports-related trauma. Incongruity between the patient's history and physical examination findings should lead to further evaluation. A negative review of systems with an injury history consistent with the physical findings suggests a sports-related etiology.

Khan KM, Cook JL, Kannua P, et al: Time to abandon the "tendonitis" myth. *Br Med J* 2002;324:626–627.

Sharma P, Maffulli N: Tendon injury and tendinopathy: Healing and repair. *J Bone Joint Surg Am* 2005;87:187–202.

686.1 • Growth Plate Injuries

Twenty per cent of pediatric sports injuries seen in the emergency department are fractures. Twenty-five per cent of those fractures involve an epiphyseal growth plate or physis (see Chapter 682). Growth in long bones occurs in 3 areas and is susceptible to injury. Immature bone can be acutely injured at the physis (Salter-Harris fractures), the articular surface (osteochondritis dissecans), or the apophysis (avulsion fractures). Boys suffer about twice as many physeal fractures as girls; the peak incidence of fracture is during peak height velocity (girls, 12 ± 2.5 yr; boys, 14 ± 2 yr). The physis is a pressure growth plate and is responsible for longitudinal growth in bone. The apophysis is a bony outgrowth at the attachment of a tendon and is a traction physis. The epiphysis is the end of a long bone, distal or proximal to the long bone, and contains articular cartilage at the joint.

The most common **physeal injuries** are to the distal radius, followed by phalangeal and distal tibial fractures. Ninety four percent of forearm fractures in skateboarding, roller skating, and scooter riding involve the distal radius. Physeal injuries at the knee (distal femur, proximal tibia) are rare. Growth disturbance following a growth plate injury is a function of location and the part of the physis fractured. These factors influence the probability of physeal bar formation resulting in growth arrest at that growth plate. The areas making the largest contribution to longitudinal growth in the upper extremities are the proximal humerus and distal radius/ulna; in the lower extremities, they are the distal femur and the proximal tibia/fibula. Injuries to these areas are more likely to cause growth disturbance compared with physeal injuries at the other end of these long bones. The type of the physis fracture relative to risk of growth disturbance is described by the Salter-Harris classification system (see Table 686-1). A grade I injury is least likely to result in growth disturbance, and the grade V is the most likely fracture to result in growth disturbance.

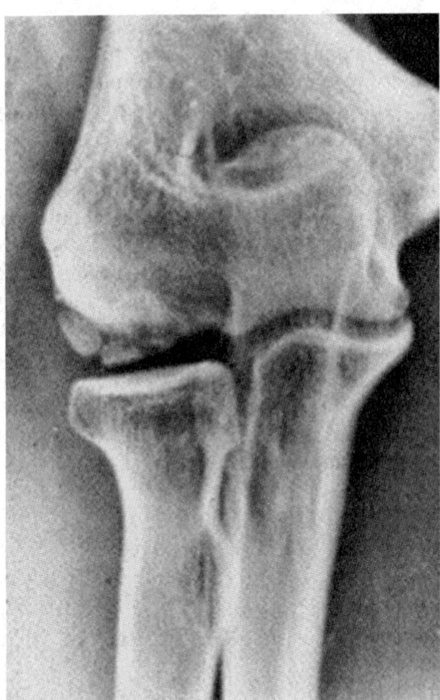

Figure 686-1. Osteochondritis dissecans, elbow. (From Anderson SJ: Sports injuries. *Curr Prob Pediatr Adolesc Health* 2005;35:105–176.)

Osteochondritis dissecans (OCD) affects the subchondral bone and overlying articular surface. With avascular necrosis of subchondral bone, articular surface may flatten, soften, or break off in fragments. The etiology is unknown but may be related to repetitive stress injury in some patients. In children and adolescents, 51% of lesions occur on the lateral aspect of the medial femoral condyle, 17% occur on the lateral condyle, and 7% occur on the patella. Bilateral involvement is reported in 13–30% of cases. Other joints where OCD lesions are also seen are the ankle (talus), elbow (usually involving the capitellum), and radial head. OCD classically affects athletes in their 2nd decade. Most common presentation is poorly localized vague knee pain. There is rarely a history of recent acute trauma. Some OCD lesions are asymptomatic (diagnosed on "routine" radiographs), whereas others are manifested as joint effusion pain, decreased range of motion, and mechanical symptoms (locking, popping, crepitus). Activity usually worsens the pain.

Physical examination may show no specific findings. Sometimes tenderness over the involved condyle can be elicited by deep palpation with the knee flexed. Diagnosis is usually made with plain radiographs (Fig. 686-1). A tunnel view radiograph should be obtained to better view the posterior $^2/_3$ of the femoral condyle. Patients with OCD should be referred to an orthopedic surgeon for further evaluation.

Avulsion fractures occur when a forceful muscle contraction dislodges the apophysis from the bone. They occur most frequently around the hip (Fig. 686-2). Chronically increased traction at the muscle-apophysis attachment can lead to repetitive microtrauma and pain at the apophysis. The most common areas affected are the knee (Osgood-Schlatter and Sindig-Larsen-Johannson disease), the ankle (Sever disease) (Fig. 686-3), and the medial epicondyle (Little League elbow). Traction apophysitis of the knee and ankle can potentially be treated in a primary care setting. The main goal of treatment is to minimize the intensity and frequency of pain and disability. Exercises that increase the strength, flexibility, and endurance of the muscles attached at the apophysis, using the relative rest principle, are appropriate. Symptoms can last for 12–24 mo if untreated. As growth slows, symptoms abate.

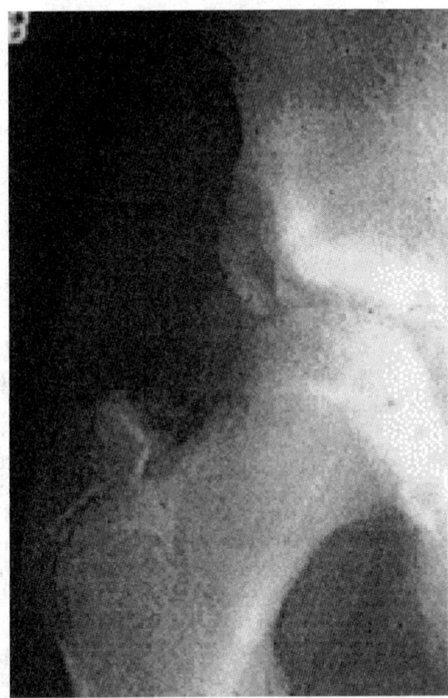

Figure 686-2. Anterior inferior iliac spine avulsion. (From Anderson SJ: Lower extremity injuries in youth sports. *Pediatr Clin North Am* 2003;49:627–641.)

Wall E, Von Stein D: Juvenile osteochondritis dissecans. *Orthop Clin North Am* 2003;34:341–353.

Zalavras C, Nikolopoulou G, Essin D, et al: Pediatric fractures during skateboarding, roller skating, and scooter riding. *Am J Sports Med* 2005;33:568–573.

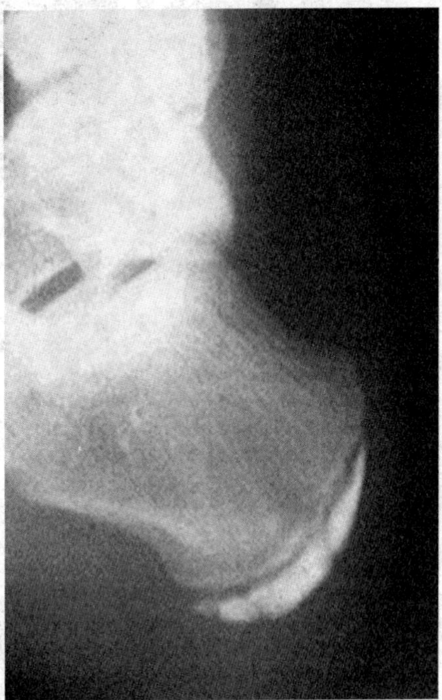

Figure 686-3. Calcaneal apophysitis (Sever disease). (From Anderson SJ: Sports injuries. *Curr Prob Pediatr Adolesc Health* 2005;35:105–176.)

686.2 • Shoulder Injuries

Shoulder pain associated with radiating symptoms down the arm should suggest the possibility of a coexisting neck injury. Neck pain and tenderness or limitation of cervical range of motion requires that the cervical spine be immobilized and that the athlete be transferred for further evaluation. If there is no neck pain or tenderness or limitation of motion of the cervical spine, then the shoulder is the site of the primary injury.

CLAVICLE FRACTURES

One of the most common shoulder injuries is a clavicle fracture. Injury is usually sustained by fall on the lateral shoulder, on an outstretched hand, or by direct blow. Eighty per cent of fractures occur in the middle third of the clavicle. They are treated with an arm sling. Nondisplaced medial and lateral 3rd fractures are usually treated conservatively. If displaced, medial and lateral 3rd fractures require orthopedic consultation due to a higher incidence of acromioclavicular osteoarthritis (lateral) and physeal involvement (medial).

ACROMIOCLAVICULAR (AC) SEPARATION. An AC separation most commonly occurs when an athlete sustains a direct blow to the acromion with the humerus in an adducted position, forcing the acromion inferiorly and medially. Patients have discrete tenderness at the AC joint and may have an apparent stepoff between the distal clavicle and the acromion (Fig. 686-4). **Type I** AC injuries involve the AC ligament, have no visible deformity, and have normal radiographs. Cross-chest maneuver of the arm will cause sharp pain at the AC joint. **Type II** injuries, which involve the coracoclavicular ligament, have a slightly more prominent distal clavicle on examination, but radiographs are usually normal (may show slight widening of the AC joint). Type I and II injuries are treated nonoperatively. A sling and analgesic are useful for pain control. Range of motion exercises are initiated after pain is controlled. As the pain-free range improves, strengthening of the rotator cuff, deltoid, and trapezius muscles can start. Usual return to play is 1–2 wk for type I and 2–4 wk for type II. When the AC joint is nontender, the shoulder has full range of motion and the patient has sufficient strength to be functionally protected from a collision or fall and perform the maneuvers required for the sport, return to play is allowed. **Type III** injury has worsened ligamentous tearing with deltotrapezial fascial detachment from the distal clavicle. Type III injuries should be treated surgically only in rare cases and mostly for cosmetic reasons. The majority can be treated in a similar fashion as grade I and II injuries. **Types IV, V, and VI** AC injuries have progressive worsening of ligamentous and fascial disruption with worsened clavicular displacement. Fortunately, these injuries are rare but require surgical repair. If a humeral fracture is present, point tenderness is noted over the fracture. If a patient has crepitance, the arm should be immobilized in a sling and the patient transferred to an emergency facility.

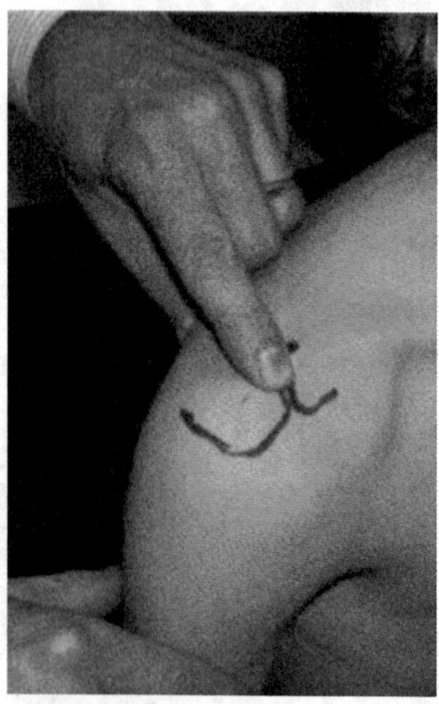

Figure 686-4. Palpitation of acromioclavicular joint. (From Anderson SJ: Sports injuries. *Curr Prob Pediatr Adolesc Health* 2005;35:105–176.)

ANTERIOR DISLOCATION

The common mechanisms of injury are falling onto an outstretched hand with a straight arm or making contact with another player with the shoulder abducted to 90 degrees and forcefully rotated externally. An example of the latter is a football player tackling another player only with their arm. Patients complain of severe pain and that their shoulder "popped out of place" or "shifted." Patients with an unreduced anterior dislocation have a hollow region inferior to the acromion and a bulge in the anterior portion of the shoulder caused by anterior displacement of the humeral head. Abnormal sensation of the lateral deltoid region (axillary nerve) and the extensor surface of the proximal forearm (musculocutaneous nerve) and the ability to contract the middle deltoid (resisted abduction) and biceps isometrically should be noted. An attempt to reduce the anterior dislocation is indicated, assuming no crepitance is present. Once the dislocation is reduced and radiographs show a normal position, immobilization for approximately 1 wk is indicated. The period of immobilization is controversial, but most sports medicine practitioners believe that early range-of-motion and strengthening exercises are important. As the rotator cuff muscles strengthen, progressive strengthening occurs at greater degrees of abduction and external rotation. Patients can return to play when strength, flexibility, and proprioception are equal to that of the uninvolved side so that they can protect the shoulder and perform the sports-specific activities pain free. In most cases, surgery is not recommended unless the shoulder has been dislocated at least 3 times. Earlier repair may be considered for athletes in high-risk, collision sports because the recurrence rate is very high in those sports.

ROTATOR CUFF INJURY

The rotator cuff is formed by the supraspinatus, infraspinatus, teres minor, and subscapularis. The supraspinatus is most commonly injured. *Rotator cuff tendonopathy* is manifested as shoulder pain at the top of the arc of motion. Pain is usually poorly localized and may be referred to the deltoid area. The onset may be insidious. Pain is worse with activity but is often present at rest, including nighttime pain. Strength testing of the cuff muscles produces pain and may demonstrate some weakness compared to the uninjured shoulder. Supraspinatus tendonopathy produces pain with active abduction in the "empty can" position in which the patient abducts the arm to 90 degrees, forward flexes it to 30 degrees anterior to the parasagittal plane, and internally rotates the humerus. **Treatment** includes ice, modification of technique, rest, stretching, strengthening of the rotator cuff and upper back muscles, physiotherapy, and analgesic. Prevention includes avoiding overwork, proper technique, and strengthening and stretching exercises. Sometimes this is called *rotator cuff impingement syndrome* in adults because of impingement of the cuff by the bony structures superior to the cuff. Rotator cuff pain in young athletes is almost always secondary to glenohumeral instability. Stretching alone may make the pain worse, and the most important aspect of rehabilitation is strengthening of the cuff muscles.

Glenoid labrum tears may appear like rotator cuff tendonopathy. One of the most common lesions, called a **SLAP** lesion (*s*uperior *l*abrum *a*nterior and *p*osterior), is difficult to diagnose clinically. Pain that occurs with clicking or catching in the shoulder is suspicious for a labral tear. Radiographs are usually normal. Magnetic resonance arthrography is the best study to view lesions.

Proximal humeral stress fracture (epiphysiolysis) is a rare cause of proximal shoulder pain and is suspected when shoulder pain does not respond to routine measures. Gradual onset of deep shoulder pain occurs in a young (open epiphyseal plates) athlete involved in repetitive overhead motion, such as in baseball or tennis, but with no history of trauma. Tenderness is noted over the proximal humerus; the diagnosis is confirmed by detecting a widened epiphyseal plate on plain radiographs, increased uptake on nuclear scan, or edema of the physis on MRI. Treatment is rest from throwing for 6–8 wk.

Bradley JP, Elkousy H: Decision-making: Operative versus nonoperative treatment of acromioclavicular joint injuries. *Clin Sports Med* 2003;2:277–290.
Luime JJ, Verhagen AP, Miedema HS, et al: Does this patient have an instability of the shoulder or a labrum lesion? *JAMA* 2004;292:1989–1998.
Wasserlauf BL, Paletta GA Jr: Shoulder disorders in the skeletally immature throwing athlete. Orthop Clin North Am 2003;34:427–437.

686.3 • Elbow Injuries

ACUTE INJURIES

The most common elbow dislocation is a posterior dislocation. The mechanism of injury is falling backward onto the outstretched arm with the elbow extended. Dislocation potentially compromises the brachial artery. Intact radial and ulnar pulses are the best indicators of vascular integrity of the distal upper extremity. An obvious deformity is noted, with the olecranon process displaced prominently behind the distal humerus. Reduction is performed by gently applying longitudinal traction to the forearm with gentle upward pressure on the distal humerus. If reduction is not possible, the arm should be padded and placed in a sling and the patient transferred to an emergency facility. Elbow injuries can compromise the radial, median, and ulnar nerves.

Supracondylar humeral fractures can result from the same mechanism of injury as elbow dislocations and can be complicated by coexisting injury to the brachial artery and, to a lesser extent, the median, radial, and ulnar nerves. An acute compartment syndrome may develop after these fractures (Fig. 686-5).

A blow to the elbow may cause bleeding in the olecranon bursa resulting in an *olecranon bursitis*. These rarely require aspiration and can be managed with ice, analgesia, and compression dressings. An appropriate pad will provide comfort and help prevent reinjury.

CHRONIC INJURIES

Overuse injuries occur primarily in throwing sports and sports that require repetitive wrist flexion or extension or demand weight bearing on hands (gymnastics). "Little League elbow" is a broad term for several different elbow problems.

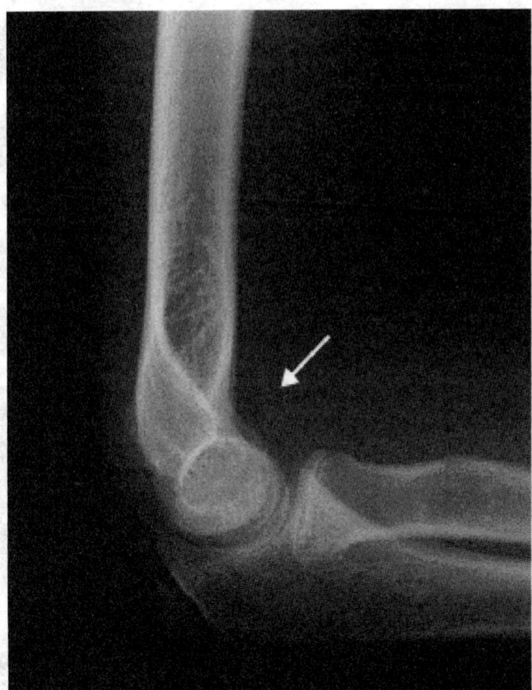

Figure 686-5. Deflection of the coronoid fat pad with a joint effusion (fat pad sign) showing evidence of a fracture. (From Gomez JE: Upper extremity injuries in youth sports. *Pediatr Clin N Am* 2002;49:593–626.)

Throwing overhand creates valgus stress to the elbow with medial opening of the joint and lateral compressive forces.

Medial elbow pain is a common complaint of young throwers due to repetitive valgus overload of the wrist flexor/pronator muscle groups and their attachment on the medial apophysis. In preadolescents who still have maturing secondary ossification centers, *traction apophysitis of the medial epicondyle* is likely. Patients have tenderness along the medial epicondyle; this is exacerbated by valgus stress or resisted wrist flexion and pronation. Treatment includes no throwing for 4–6 wk, pain-free strengthening, and stretching of the flexor/pronator group, followed by 1–2 wk of a progressive functional throwing program with accelerated rehabilitation. This problem has to be treated with rest because of the risk of nonunion of the apophysis and chronic pain. If pain occurs acutely, *avulsion fracture of the medial epicondyle* must be considered. Any thrower with acute elbow pain should have radiographs performed (Fig. 686-6). If the medial epicondyle is avulsed, orthopedic consultation is indicated. In older adolescents and young adults, with a fused apophysis, the vulnerable structure is the *ulnar collateral ligament* (UCL). UCL tears are usually seen in pitchers but can be seen in any throwing athlete. Laxity may be appreciated with valgus stress of the elbow with it flexed to 30 degrees. MRI or ultrasonography is often necessary to assess the integrity of the UCL. If there is a complete tear, surgical repair is indicated if the athlete wants to continue a pitching career. Ulnar nerve dysfunction can be a complication of valgus overload and can occur with any of the diagnoses previously discussed.

Lateral elbow pain can be caused by compression during the throwing motion at the radiocapitellar joint. *Panner disease* is osteochondrosis of the capitellum that presents between ages 7 and 12 yr (Fig. 686-7). *OCD* of the capitellum presents at age 13–16 yr (see Fig. 686-1). These two entities may represent a continuum of the same disease. Although patients with both conditions present with insidious onset of lateral elbow pain

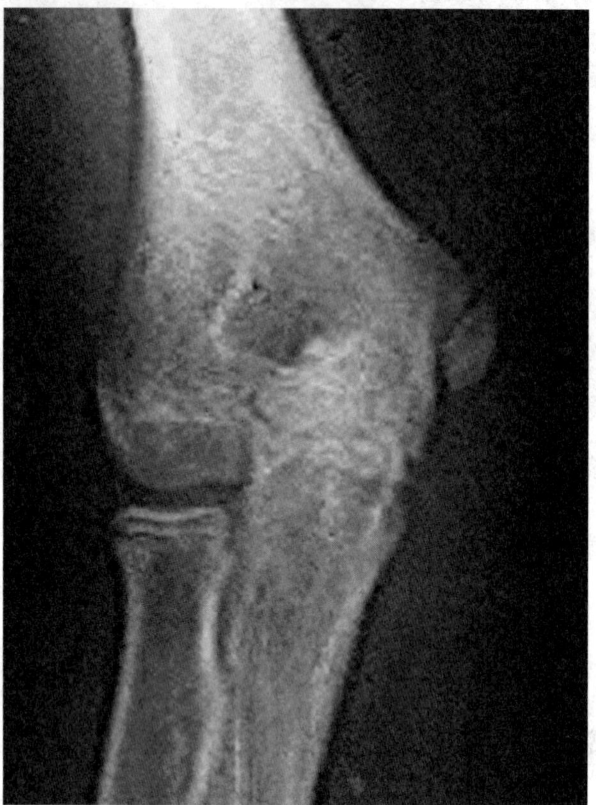

Figure 686-6. Medial epicondylitis. (From Anderson SJ: Sports injuries. *Curr Prob Pediatr Adolesc Health* 2005;35:105–176.)

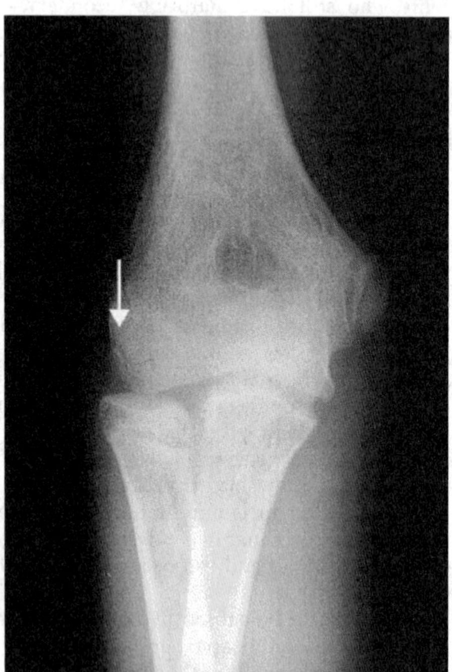

Figure 686-7. Panner disease. Note fragmentation of the humeral capitellum and flattening of the articular surface *(arrow)*. (Courtesy of Ralph J. Curtis, MD. From Gomez JE: Upper extremity injuries in youth sports. *Pediatr Clin N Am* 2002;49:593–626.)

exacerbated by throwing, patients with OCD have mechanical symptoms (popping, locking) and, more frequently, decreased range of motion. Patients with Panner disease have no mechanical symptoms and often have normal range of motion. The prognosis of Panner disease is excellent, and treatments consist of relative rest (no throwing), brief immobilization, and repeat radiographs in 6–12 wk to assess bone remodeling. OCD requires orthopedic consultation.

Lateral epicondylitis, or "tennis elbow," is the most common overuse elbow injury in adults. It is rare in children and adolescents. It is tendonopathy of the extensor muscle origin on the lateral epicondyle. Tenderness is elicited over the lateral epicondyle, and pain is felt with passive wrist flexion and resisted wrist extension. Treatment includes relative rest, analgesia, and specific stretching and strengthening exercises. Functional rehabilitation, such as returning to playing tennis, should be gradual and progressive.

Elbow injuries may not be prevented by preseason stretching and strengthening exercises. The most important consideration for prevention of elbow injuries in throwers is limitation of the number of pitches and advising players, coaches, and athletes that they should stop immediately when they experience elbow pain. If it persists, they need medical evaluation. It has been recommended that a young pitcher pitch no more than 200 pitches per week and play in no more than 2 games per week. The maximal number of pitches per game should be approximately 6 times the pitcher's age in years.

Other less common problems that cause elbow pain are ulnar neuropathy, triceps tendinitis and olecranon apophysitis, and loose bodies.

Assendelft W, Green S, Buchbinder R, et al: Tennis elbow. *Br Med J* 2003;327:329–330.

Petty DH, Andrews JR, Fleisig GS, Cain EL: Ulnar collateral ligament reconstruction in high school baseball players: Clinical results and injury risk factors. *Am J Sports Med* 2004;32:1158–1164.

686.4 • Low Back Injuries

Spondylolysis, a common cause of back pain in athletes, is a stress fracture of the pars interarticularis (see Chapter 678.6). It can occur at any vertebral level but is most likely at L4 or L5. Incidence in adolescent athletes evaluated for low back pain is 13–47%. Besides acute hyperextension that causes an acute fracture, the mechanism of injury is either a congenital defect or hypoplastic pars, which is exacerbated by lumbar extension loading, or a stress fracture due to repetitive extension loading. Ballet, weight lifting, gymnastics, and football are examples of sports in which repetitive extension loading of the lumbar spine occurs; it occurs in any activity in which there is repetitive extension loading, including swimming. Patients often present with pain of insidious onset. However, there may be a precipitating injury such as a fall or single episode of hyperextension. The pain is worse with extension, can radiate to the buttocks, and can eventually affect activities of daily living. Rest or supine positioning usually alleviates the pain. On examination, the pain is reproduced with lumbar extension while standing, especially when standing on 1 leg (single leg hyperextension test). Limited forward spinal flexion and tight hamstrings may be seen. Neurologic examination should be normal. There is well-localized tenderness to deep palpation just lateral to the spinous process on the affected side and is usually at L4 or L5. The diagnosis is confirmed by finding a pars defect on an oblique lumbar spine radiograph. The defect is rarely seen on anteroposterior and lateral views. Bone single-photon emission tomography scan is needed to confirm diagnosis if radiographs are normal. A plain CT scan can help in the identification of degree of bony involvement and is sometimes used to assess healing. **Treatment** includes pain relief and activity restriction, and rehabilitation consisting of trunk strengthening, hip flexor stretching, and hamstring stretching is important in most cases. Antilordotic bracing is controversial and is probably most effective for the stress fracture type spondylolysis. *Spondylolisthesis* occurs when bilateral pars defects exist and forward displacement or slippage of a vertebra occurs on the vertebra inferior to it (see Chapter 678.6).

Facet syndrome has a similar history and physical examination findings as spondylolysis. It is caused by instability or injury to the facet joint, posterior to the pars interarticularis and at the interface of the inferior and superior articulating processes. Facet syndrome can be established by identifying facet abnormalities on CT or by exclusion, requiring a nondiagnostic radiograph and nuclear scan to rule out spondylolysis.

Spondylolysis, spondylolisthesis, and facet syndrome are injuries posterior to vertebral bodies. **Treatment** of posterior element injuries is conservative, directed at reducing the extension loading activity, often for 2–3 mo. Walking, swimming, and cycling are appropriate exercises during rehabilitation.

Lumbar disk herniation presents as back pain that is worse with forward flexion, lateral bending, and prolonged sitting, especially in an automobile. It is less likely to produce sciatica in children and adolescents compared to adults (see Chapter 678.8). Physical examination findings may be minimal but can include a positive straight leg raise test, pain with forward flexion, and possibly reduced strength, sensation, or deep tendon reflexes in the leg. There may be tenderness of the vertebral spinous process at the level of the disk. MRI usually confirms the clinical diagnosis. Assuming the herniation is not large and the pain is not intractable, the treatment of choice is analgesia and physical therapy. Bed rest or surgery is rarely necessary.

Acute lumbar strain or contusion presents after a precipitating event. Physical examination reveals diffuse tenderness lateral to the spine. **Treatment** includes analgesia, massage, and physical therapy, as tolerated. The natural history of acute back strain in adults is that 50% are better in 1 wk, 80% in 1 mo, and 90% in 2 mo, regardless of therapy. The course of back pain in young athletes is probably similar.

Sacroiliitis presents as lumbar pain that is usually chronic but occasionally is associated with a history of trauma. Patients have a positive result with the **Patrick test,** which includes resting the foot of the affected side on the opposite knee (hip flexed 90 degrees), stabilizing the opposite iliac crest, and externally rotating the hip on the affected side (pushing the knee down and lateral). A radiograph of the sacroiliac joints is indicated, and if results are positive, exploration for a rheumatologic disease (ankylosing spondylitis, juvenile rheumatoid arthritis, ulcerative colitis) is warranted. **Treatment** is with relative rest, nonsteroidal anti-inflammatory drugs, and physical therapy. Ankylosing spondylitis is more likely if the onset of lower back pain is before age 40 yr, if there is morning stiffness that is associated with improvement with activity, and if the pain has a gradual onset and has lasted more than 3 mo.

Other causes of lower back pain include infection (osteomyelitis, diskitis) and neoplasia. These should be considered in patients with fever, weight loss, other constitutional signs, or lack of response to initial therapy. Osteomyelitis of the lower back or pelvis is often, but not always, associated with fever.

Jones GT, Macfarlane GJ: Epidemiology of low back pain in children and adolescents. *Arch Dis Child* 2005;90:312–316.

686.5 • Hip and Pelvis Injuries

Hip and pelvis injuries represent a small percentage of sports injuries, but they are potentially severe and require prompt diagnosis. Hip pathology can present as knee pain and normal findings on knee examination.

In children, *transient synovitis* is the most common cause. It usually presents with acute onset of a limp, with the child refusing to use the affected leg and having painful range of motion on examination. There may be a history of minor trauma. This is a self-limiting condition that usually resolves in 48–72 hr.

Legg-Calvé-Perthes disease (avascular necrosis of the femoral head) also presents in childhood with insidious onset of limp and hip pain (see Chapter 677.3).

Until the skeleton matures, younger athletes are susceptible to apophyseal injuries (e.g., the anterior superior iliac spine). *Apophysitis* presents from overuse or from direct trauma. *Avulsion fractures* occur in adolescents playing sports requiring sudden, explosive bursts of speed (Fig. 686-8). Large muscles contract and create force greater than the strength of the attachment of the muscle to the apophysis. The most common sites of avulsion fractures (and the attaching muscles) are the anterior superior iliac spine (sartorius), anterior inferior iliac spine (rectus femoris), lesser femoral trochanter (iliopsoas), and ischial tuberosity (hamstrings). Symptoms include localized pain and swelling, with decreased strength and range of motion. Radiographs are required. Initial **treatment** includes ice, analgesics, rest, and pain-free range-of-motion exercises. Crutches are usually needed for ambulation. Surgery is usually never indicated since most of these fractures heal well even with large or displaced fractures. Contact to the bone around the hip and pelvis causes exquisitely tender subperiosteal hematomas called *hip pointers.* Symptomatic care includes rest, ice, analgesia, and protection from reinjury.

Slipped capital femoral epiphysis usually presents in the 11–15-yr age range during the time of rapid linear bone growth (see Chapter 677.4).

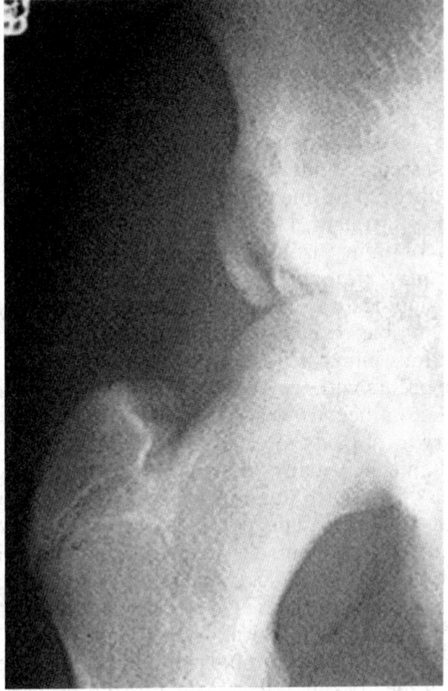

Figure 686-8. Apophyseal avulsion, pelvis. (From Anderson SJ: Sports injuries. *Curr Prob Pediatr Adolesc Health* 2005;35:105–176.)

A *femoral neck stress fracture* may present as vague progressive hip pain in an endurance athlete. Girls with the female athlete triad are especially are at risk. This diagnosis should always be kept in mind in the running athlete with vague anterior thigh pain. On examination, there may be pain with passive stretch of the hip flexors and pain with hip rotation. If radiographs do not demonstrate a periosteal reaction consistent with a stress fracture, a bone scan or MRI may be required. Orthopedic consultation is necessary in femoral neck stress fractures because of their predisposition to nonunion and displacement with minor trauma or continued weight bearing. These fractures carry increased risk of avascular necrosis of the femoral head.

Osteitis pubis is an inflammation at the pubic symphysis that may be caused by excessive side-to-side rocking of the pelvis. It can be seen in an athlete in any running sport and is more common in sports requiring more use of the adductor muscles such as hockey, soccer, and rollerblading. Athletes typically present with vague groin pain that may be unilateral or bilateral. On physical examination, there is tenderness over the symphysis and sometimes over the proximal adductors. Adduction strength testing causes discomfort. Radiographic evidence (irregularity, sclerosis, widening of the pubic symphysis with osteolysis) may not be present until symptoms are present for 6–8 wk; a bone scan and MRI are more sensitive to early changes. Relative rest for 6–12 wk may be required. Some patients require corticosteroid injection as adjunctive therapy.

Acetabular labrum tears can occur in the hip, similar to glenoid labrum tears in the shoulder. Athletes may have a history of trauma and complain of sharp anterior hip pain associated with a clicking or catching sensation. Clinical diagnosis is difficult; magnetic resonance arthrography is useful for diagnosis.

Snapping hip syndrome is caused by the iliopsoas tendon's riding over the anterior hip capsule or the ITB over the greater trochanter. It is commonly seen in ballet dancers and runners; it may occur as an acute or overuse injury (more common). Athletes present with either a painful or painless click or snap in the hip, usually located lateral or anterior and deep in the joint. Examination can often reproduce the symptoms. Radiographs are not usually needed in the work-up. **Treatment** involves an analgesia, relative rest, biomechanical assessment, and core flexibility/strengthening. The athlete may return to activity as tolerated.

686.6 • Knee Injuries

The knee is the most common musculoskeletal site for complaints among adolescents. Acute knee injuries that cause immediate disability are likely to be due to fracture, patellar dislocation, anterior cruciate ligament (ACL) injury, or meniscal tear. The mechanism of injury is usually a weight-bearing event. After injury, if a player cannot bear weight within a few minutes, a fracture or significant injury internal derangement is more likely. If a player is able to bear weight and return to play after the injury, a serious injury is less likely to have occurred. If swelling of the knee occurs within several hours of the injury, the swelling is likely due to a hemarthrosis and a more severe injury.

The injury most likely to occur with a hemarthrosis is an **ACL** injury. ACL injuries usually occur from being hit directly, landing off balance from a jump, quickly changing direction while running, or a hyperextension injury. Significant swelling and instability are often present. The majority of athletes with an ACL injury will need orthopedic consultation and an ACL reconstruction. Functional bracing without ACL reconstruction increases the risk of meniscal injury and recurrent instability.

Posterior cruciate ligament injury occurs from a direct blow to the region of the proximal tibia, such as might occur with a dashboard injury or a fall to the knees in volleyball. Posterior cruciate ligament injuries are rare and are usually treated nonsurgically

Medial collateral ligament injuries result from a valgus blow to the outside of the knee. Isolate lateral *collateral ligament* injuries are uncommon and result from significant varus knee stress. Since they are extra-articular, isolated collateral injuries should not produce much of a knee effusion or disability. Regardless of severity, isolated medial and lateral collateral injuries are managed nonsurgically with aggressive rehabilitation

Meniscal tears occur by the same mechanisms as ACL injuries. They are associated with hemarthrosis, joint line pain, and often pain in full flexion. Orthopedic consultation is indicated when a meniscal tear is suspected.

Patellar dislocations occur most often as a noncontact injury when the quadriceps muscles forcefully contract to extend the knee while the lower leg is externally rotated. Patellar dislocation is the second most common cause of hemarthrosis. The patella is almost always dislocated laterally, and this motion tears the medial patellar retinaculum, causing bleeding in the joint. Recurrent episodes of patellar instability are associated with less swelling. Patellar instability is treated nonsurgically with a patella-stabilizing sleeve and an aggressive rehabilitation program.

The physician should inspect for an effusion and obvious deformities; if any deformity is present, the physician should assess neurovascular status and transfer the patient for emergency care. If no gross deformities are present and neurovascular integrity is intact, initial maneuvers include full passive extension and gentle valgus stress to the knee while it is in extension. If there is laxity of the knee with valgus stress in full extension, both the ACL and medial collateral ligament have been injured. The patient's ability to contract the quadriceps muscles should be noted. Pain occurring with quadriceps contraction or inability to contract the quadriceps muscle implies an injury to the extensor mechanism. Tenderness over the medial patella, medial retinaculum, and/or above the adductor tubercle is associated with a patellar dislocation. Point tenderness is consistent with fracture or injury to the underlying structure; a medial meniscal tear may be manifest as tenderness along the medial joint line, however medial joint line tenderness is not specific for a medial meniscus tear. Pain or limitation in either passive flexion or extension while rotating the tibia (McMurray or modified McMurray tests) implies a meniscal injury, as do other maneuvers (Fig. 686-9). Ligament injury is manifested as pain or laxity with the appropriate maneuver.

INITIAL TREATMENT OF ACUTE KNEE INJURIES

If a patient cannot bear weight pain free or has clinical signs of instability, the knee should be immobilized, crutches given, and plain radiographs obtained. If the patella is dislocated, reduction can be achieved with knee extension. Developed as the **Ottawa knee rules**, radiographs are required for pediatric patients with knee injury who have any of these findings: isolated tenderness of patella, fibular head tenderness, inability to flex 90 degrees, and inability to bear weight both immediately and in the emergency department for 4 steps (regardless of limping). Straight-leg immobilizers offer no structural support and are only used for comfort. If any brace is used, a hinged brace is indicated for stabilization such as an injury when both ACL and medial collateral ligament may have been injured. The leg should be elevated, and elastic wrap can be applied for compression.

CHRONIC INJURIES

Patellofemoral stress syndrome (PFSS) is the most common cause of anterior knee pain. PFSS is also known as patellofemoral pain syndrome or patellofemoral dysfunction (see Chapter 676). It is a diagnosis of exclusion used to describe anterior knee pain that has no other identifiable pathology. Pain is usually difficult to

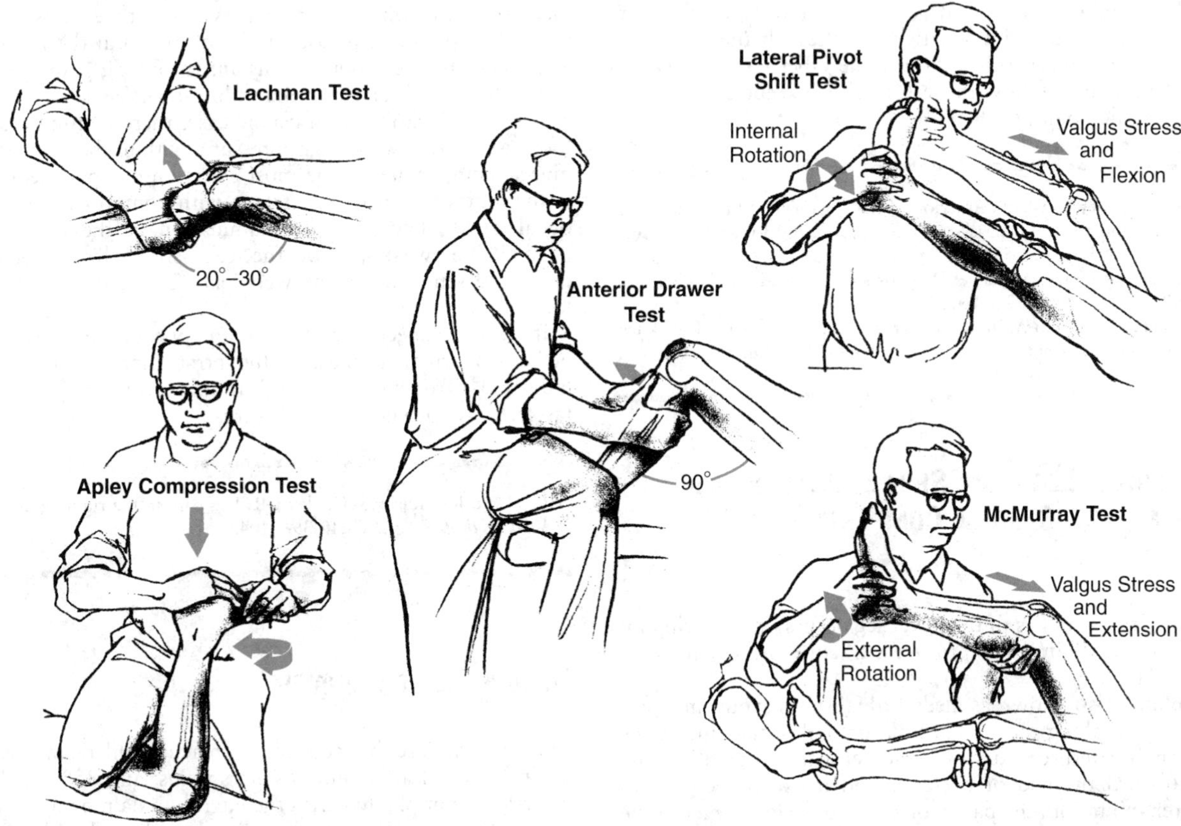

Figure 686-9. Examination maneuvers. Right knee shown. Examination maneuvers include the Lachman, anterior drawer, lateral pivot shift, Apley compression, and McMurray tests. The Lachman test, performed to detect anterior cruciate ligament (ACL) injures, is conducted with the patient supine and the knee flexed 20–30 degrees. The anterior drawer test detects ACL injuries and is performed with the patient supine and the knee in 90 degrees of flexion. The lateral pivot shift test is performed with the patient supine, the hip flexed 45 degrees, and the knee in full extension. Internal rotation is applied to the tibia while the knee is flexed to 40 degrees under a valgus stress (pushing the outside of the knee medially). The Apley compression test, used to assess meniscal integrity, is performed with the patient prone and the examiner's knee over the patient's posterior thigh. The tibia is externally rotated while a downward compressive force is applied over the tibia. The McMurray test, used to assess meniscal integrity, is performed with the patient supine and the examiner standing on the side of the affected knee. (From Solomon DH, Simel DL, Bates DW, et al: Does this patient have a torn meniscus or ligament of the knee? *JAMA* 2001;286:1610.)

localize. Patients will indicate a diffuse area over the anterior knee as the source, or they may feel as if the pain is coming from behind the patella. Bilateral pain is common, and pain is often worse going up stairs, after sitting for prolonged periods, or after squatting or running. There should be negative history for significant swelling, as this would indicate a more serious injury. History of change in activity is common, such as altered training surface or terrain, increased training regimen, or performance of new tasks. Examination should include evaluation of stance and gait for lower limb alignment, musculature, and midfoot hyperpronation. Flexibility of the hamstrings, ITB, and gastrocnemius should be assessed, as stress is increased across the patellofemoral joint when these structures are tight. Hip range of motion should be assessed to rule out hip pathology. Medial patellar tenderness or pain with compression of the patellofemoral joint confirms the diagnosis in the absence of an effusion and no other positive findings on the examination. PFSS is a clinical diagnosis usually managed without imaging. **Treatment** focuses on assessing and improving flexibility, strength, and gait abnormalities. In the presence of midfoot hyperpronation (ankle valgus), new shoes or use of arch supports may improve patellofemoral mechanics and improve pain. Ice and an analgesic can be used to help control pain. Reduced overall activity or training is important initially in rehabilitation. Upon return to activity, starting at 50% of the usual amount and intensity of work is recommended, with an increase of 10% weekly until full participation is achieved. Maintenance rehabilitation via home exercises is essential to prevent recurrences. Surgery is rarely indicated.

Osgood-Schlatter disease is a traction apophysitis occurring at the insertion of the patellar tendon on the tibial tuberosity (see Chapter 676). Since it is also related to overuse of the extensor mechanism, Osgood-Schlatter disease is **treated** like PFSS. A protective pad to protect the tibial tubercle from direct trauma can be used. The most common complication is cosmetic; the tibial tubercle on the affected side (or both if bilateral) may be slightly more prominent. Patients only need to take time from sports if they are limping.

Sinding-Larsen-Johansson disease is a traction apophysitis occurring at the inferior pole of the patella. It occurs most often in volleyball and basketball athletes. **Treatment** is similar to that of PFSS and Osgood-Schlatter disease. Patellar tendonopathy (jumper's knee) is due to repetitive microtrauma of the patellar tendon usually at the inferior pole of the patella. In about 10% of the cases, the quadriceps tendon above the patella is affected. It is associated with jumping sports but may occur in runners as well. **Treatment** is similar to that of PFSS. Relative rest is more important in patellar tendonopathy since chronic pain is associated with irreversible changes in the tendon. **ITB friction syndrome** is the most common cause of chronic lateral knee pain. Generally it is not associated with swelling or instability. It is due to friction of the ITB along the lateral knee resulting in bursitis. Tenderness is elicited along the ITB as it courses over the lateral femoral condyle or at its insertion at the Gerdy tubercle, along the lateral tibial plateau. Tightness of the ITB is also noted using the Ober test. To perform an Ober test, the athlete is side lying and the superior hip is extended with the knee flexed. The examiner holds the ankle in midair and if the knee moves inferiorly, it implies a flexible ITB and a negative Ober test. If the knee and leg stay in midair, the ITB is tight and the Ober test is positive. **Treatment** principles follow those for PFSS, except emphasis is on improving flexibility of the ITB.

Agel J, Arendt EA, Bershadsky B: Anterior cruciate ligament injury in national collegiate athletic association basketball and soccer: A 13-year review. *Am J Sports Med* 2005;33:524–530.

LaBotz M: Patellofemoral syndrome: Diagnostic pointers and individualized treatment. *Phys Sportsmed* 2004;32:7.

Vaquero J, Vidal C, Cubillo A: Intra-articular traumatic disorders of the knee in children and adolescents. *Clin Orthop* 2005;432:97–106.

686.7 • Lower Leg Pain: Shin Splints, Stress Fractures, and Chronic Compartment Syndrome

Stress injury to the bones of the lower leg occurs on a continuum from mild injury (shin splints) to stress fracture. All occur by an overuse mechanism.

Shin splints, also known as medial tibial stress syndrome, presents with pain along the medial tibia or both tibiae and is the most common overuse injury of the lower leg. The pain initially appears toward the end of exercise, and if exercise continues without rehabilitation, the pain worsens and occurs earlier in the exercise period. There is diffuse tenderness over the lower third to half of the distal medial tibia. Any focal tenderness or tenderness of the proximal tibia is suspicious for a stress fracture. Shin splints can usually be distinguished from a **tibial stress fracture** in which the tenderness is more focal (2–5 cm) and more severe. Shin splints and stress fracture represent a continuum of stress injury to the tibia and are thought to be related to traction of the soleus on the tibia.

The diagnosis can be made by history and physical examination. Findings on plain radiographs of the tibia are normal with shin splints and in tibial stress fractures within the first few wk of the injury. Afterward, the radiographs may demonstrate periosteal reaction if a stress fracture is present. Sensitivity of plain radiographs may be increased by obtaining 4 views of the tibia: anteroposterior, lateral, and both oblique views. A bone scan is the most sensitive test to diagnose stress fractures; it demonstrates discrete tracer uptake at the site(s) of the stress fracture. Increased uptake may be noted in the presence of shin splints but in a fusiform pattern along the periosteal surface. If results of the bone scan are normal, the diagnosis is likely to be shin splints or chronic compartment syndrome (CCS). MRI has replaced bone scans as the most sensitive tool for diagnosis of stress fractures in long bones in many medical centers.

The **treatment** of shin splints and tibial stress fractures is similar, involving relative rest, correcting training errors and kinetic chain dysfunction, and often the use of better running shoes. Fitness can be maintained with non–weight-bearing activities such as swimming, cycling, and water jogging. With shin splints, after 7–10 days, patients can usually start on the walk-jog program. If pain worsens, 2–3 pain-free days are required before resuming the walk-jog program. Ice should be used daily and an analgesic for pain control. Orthotics or new shoes may be useful in patients who hyperpronate. Stretching the plantar flexors and strengthening the ankle dorsiflexors can be useful. Being pain free for 7–10 days is recommended before exercise walking is commenced.

CCS occurs in an athlete in a running sport, usually during a period of heavy training. It is due to muscle hypertrophy and increased intracompartmental pressure with exercise. There is typically a pain-free period of about 10 min at the beginning of a workout before onset of constant throbbing pain that is difficult to localize. It lasts for min to hr after exercise and is relieved by ice and elevation. In a classic case, there is numbness of the foot associated with high pressure within the corresponding muscle compartment. The most common compartment affected is the anterolateral compartment with compression of the peroneal nerve. The physical examination in the office is often normal but weakness of the extensor hallucis longus and decreased sensation in the web space between the 1st and 2nd toe may be present.

If CCS is suspected, referral to an appropriate surgeon (orthopedic or vascular) to measure the intracompartmental pressure is indicated. Treatment is surgical and requires fasciotomy or fasciectomy to relieve the pressure.

Pell RF 4th, Khanuja HS, Cooley GR: Leg pain in the running athlete. *J Am Acad Orthop Surg* 2004;12:396–404.

686.8 • Ankle Injuries

Ankle injuries are the most common acute athletic injury. Eighty-five per cent of ankle injuries are sprains, and 85% of those are inversion (foot planted with the lateral fibula moving toward the ground) injuries, 5% are eversion (foot planted with the medial malleolus moving toward the ground) injuries, and 10% are combined.

EXAMINATION AND INJURY GRADING SCALE

In obvious cases of fracture or dislocation, evaluating neurovascular status with as little movement as possible is the priority. If no deformity is obvious, the next step is inspection for edema, ecchymosis, and anatomic variants. Key sites to palpate for tenderness are the entire length of the fibula; the medial and lateral malleoli; the base of the 5th metatarsal; the anterior, medial, and lateral joint lines; and the navicular and the Achilles tendon complex. Assessment of active range of motion (patient alone) in dorsiflexion, plantarflexion, inversion, and eversion and of resisted range of motion is indicated.

Provocative testing attempts to evaluate the integrity of the ligaments. In a patient with a markedly swollen, painful ankle, provocative testing is difficult because of muscle spasm and involuntary guarding. It is more useful on the field before much bleeding and edema have occurred. The anterior drawer test assesses for anterior translation of the talus and competence of the anterior talofibular ligament. The inversion stress test examines the competence of the anterior talofibular and calcaneofibular ligaments (Fig. 686-10). In the acute setting, the integrity of the tibiofibular ligaments and syndesmosis is examined by the syndesmosis squeeze test. Pain with squeezing the lower leg implies injury to the interosseous membrane and syndesmosis between the tibia and fibula, making a severe injury more suspicious. Athletes with this injury cannot bear any weight and also have severe pain with external rotation of the foot. Occasionally the peroneal tendon dislocates from the fibular groove simultaneously with an ankle sprain. To assess for peroneal tendon instability, the examiner applies pressure from behind the peroneal tendon with resisting eversion while plantar flexed and the tendon will pop anteriorly. If either a syndesmotic injury or an acute peroneal dislocation is suspected, orthopedic consultation should be sought.

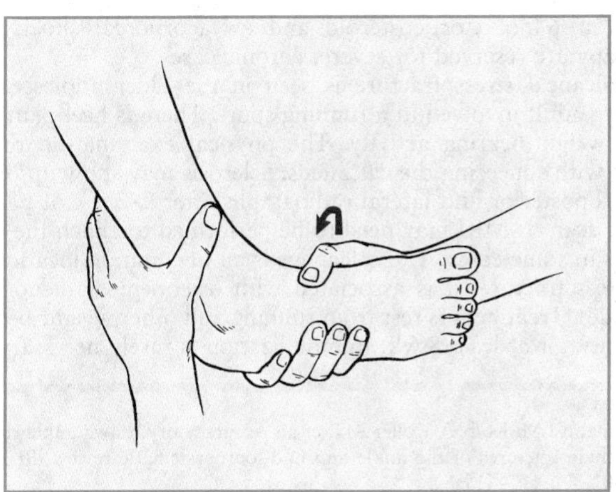

Figure 686-10. Inversion stress tilt test for ankle instability. (From Hergenroeder AC: Diagnosis and treatment of ankle sprains. A review. *Am J Dis Child* 1990;144:809.)

RADIOGRAPHS

Anteroposterior, lateral, and mortise views of the ankle are obtained when patients have pain in the area of the malleoli, are unable to bear weight, or have bone tenderness over the posterior distal tibia or fibula. The Ottawa ankle rules help define who may require radiographs (Fig. 686-11). A foot series (anteroposterior, lateral, and oblique views) should be obtained when patients have pain in the area of the midfoot or bone tenderness over the navicular or 5th metatarsal. It is important to differentiate an avulsion fracture of the proximal 5th metatarsal from the Jones fracture of the proximal 5th metatarsal (a lucency about 2 cm from the proximal end). The former is treated as an ankle sprain; the latter fracture has an increased risk of nonunion and requires orthopedic consultation. The *talar dome fracture* is manifested as an ankle sprain that does not improve. Radiographs on initial presentation may have subtle abnormalities. Any suspicion on the initial radiographs of a talar dome fracture warrants orthopedic consultation and further imaging. In the early adolescent, always look carefully at the tibial epiphysis. Nondisplaced Salter III fractures can be subtle and need to be recognized early and referred to an orthopedic surgeon promptly.

INITIAL TREATMENT OF ANKLE SPRAINS

Ankle sprains need to **treated** with the pneumonic RICE: rest, ice, compression, and elevation. This should be followed for the first 48–72 hr after the injury to minimize bleeding and edema. For an ankle injury, this consists of crutches and an elastic wrap, although other compression devices such as an air stirrup splint work quite well. This allows for early weight bearing with protection and can be removed for rehabilitation. It is important to start a rehabilitation program as soon as possible.

REHABILITATION. This should begin the day of injury; for those with pain with movement, isometric strengthening can be started. Important deficits to correct include loss of dorsiflexion, peroneal muscle weakness, and decreased proprioception. Until these deficits are restored, the ankle is vulnerable to reinjury. When determining when an athlete is ready for running, there must be full range of motion and nearly full strength compared to the uninjured side. While standing on the uninjured side only, the

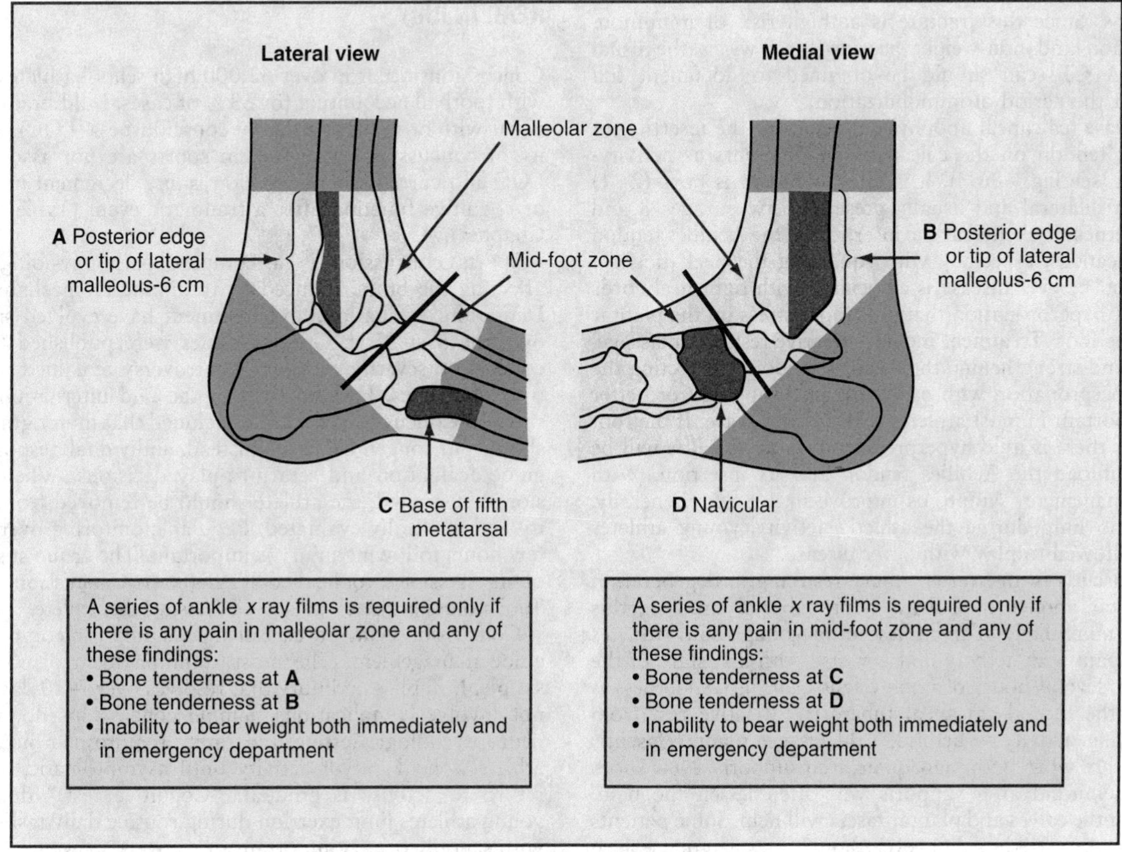

Figure 686-11. Ottawa ankle rules. (From Bachmann LM, Kolb E, Koller MT, et al: Accuracy of Ottawa ankle rules to exclude fractures of the ankle and midfoot; systematic review. *Br Med J* 2003;326:417–419.)

athlete is instructed to hop eight to 10 times if possible. When this can be achieved without pain, the athlete can began to run. Starting out with jogging and progressing to ½ speed, ¾ speed, and finally to sprints, the athletes must stop if there is significant pain or limp. Finally, before returning to sport, the athlete must be able to sprint and change directions off the injured ankle comfortably. Performing some sport-related tasks is also helpful in determining readiness for return to play.

Recurrent ankle injuries are more likely in patients who have not undergone complete rehabilitation. Ankle sprains are less likely in players wearing high-top shoes. Proper taping of the ankle with adhesive tape may provide functional support but loosens with use and is unavailable to most athletes. Lace-up ankle braces are useful for preventing recurrences. They are more supportive than tape and can be tightened repeatedly during the course of a practice or a game. Most sports physicians recommend their use indefinitely to help prevent further sprains.

686.9 • Foot Injuries

Metatarsal stress fractures can occur in any running athlete. The history is insidious pain with activity that is getting worse. Examination reveals point tenderness over the midshaft of the metatarsal, most commonly the 2nd or 3rd metatarsal. Radiographs may not show the periosteal reaction before pain has been present for 2 wk or more. **Treatment** is relative rest for 6–8 wk. Shoes with good arch supports will reduce stress to the metatarsals.

Vague dorsal foot pain in an athlete in a running sport may represent a **navicular stress fracture.** Unlike other stress fractures, it may not localize well on examination. If there is any tenderness around the navicular, a stress fracture should be suspected. This stress fracture may take many weeks to show up on plain radiographs so a bone scan or MRI should be obtained to make the diagnosis. Since this fracture is at high risk of nonunion, immobilization and non-weight bearing for 8 wk is the usual **treatment.** A CT scan should be obtained to document full healing after the period of immobilization.

Sever disease (calcaneal apophysitis) occurs at the insertion of the Achilles tendon on the calcaneus and presents as activity-related pain (see Fig. 686-3). It is more common is boys (2 : 1) and is often bilateral and usually presents between ages 8 and 13 yr. Tenderness is elicited at the insertion of the Achilles tendon into the calcaneus, especially with squeezing the heel (positive "squeeze test"). Sever disease is associated with tight heel cords and midfoot hyperpronation that puts more stress on the plantar flexors of the foot. **Treatment** includes relative rest, ice, massage, stretching, and strengthening the Achilles tendon. Correcting the midfoot hyperpronation with orthotics, arch supports, or better shoes is important in most athletes with Sever disease. If the foot is neutral or there is mild hyperpronation, ¼-in heel lifts will be helpful to unload the Achilles tendon and its insertion. With optimal management, symptoms improve in 4–8 wk. Generally, if there is no limp during the athletic activity, young athletes should be allowed to play with Sever disease.

Plantar fasciitis is an overuse injury resulting in degeneration of the plantar aponeurosis. Rare in prepubertal children, this diagnosis is more likely in an adolescent or young adult. Athletes report heel pain with activity that is worse with first steps of the day or after several hours of non–weight bearing. Tenderness is elicited on the medial calcaneal tuberosity. Relative rest from weight-bearing activity is helpful. Athletes get plantar fasciitis when shoes are worn with inadequate arch supports. New shoes or use of semirigid arch supports will often lessen the pain. Stretching of the calves and plantar fascia will help. Some patients benefit from use of night splints even though they can make sleep difficult. As long as there is not limping with athletic activity, the athlete may continue participation. Complete recovery is usually seen at 6 mo. Corticosteroid and extracorporeal shock-wave therapy are reserved for severe, chronic cases.

Calcaneal stress fracture is seen in the older adolescent or young adult involved in a running sport. There is heel pain with any weight-bearing activity. The physical examination reveals pain with squeezing the calcaneus. Sclerosis may show up on the anteroposterior and lateral radiographs after 2–3 wk of pain. A bone scan or MRI may need to be performed to clinch the diagnosis in some cases. The calcaneus is an uncommon location for a stress fracture; it is associated with osteopenia (amenorrheic female). **Treatment** is rest from running and other weight-bearing activity for at least 8 wk. Immobilization is rarely necessary.

Bachmann LM, Kolb E, Koller MT, et al: Accuracy of Ottawa ankle rules to exclude fractures of the ankle and mid-foot; systematic review. *Br Med J* 2003;326:417–419.

Beynnon BD, Renström PA, Haugh L, et al: A prospective, randomized clinical investigation of the treatment of first-time ankle sprains. *Am J Sports Med* 2006;34:1401–1412.

Buchbinder R: Plantar fascitis. *N Engl J Med* 2004;350:2159–2166.

Glazer JL, Brukner P, Haverstock BD: Stress fractures of the foot and ankle. Clin Podiatr Med Surg 2001;18:273–284.

Heyworth J: Ottawa ankle rules for the injured ankle. *Br Med J* 2003;326:405–406.

Kennedy JG, Knowles B, Dolan M, Bohne W: Foot and ankle injuries in the adolescent runner. *Curr Opin Pediatr* 2005;17:34–42.

Chapter 687 ■ Head and Neck Injuries

Gregory L. Landry

HEAD INJURY

Concussions occur in over 62,000 high school athletes each year, with football accounting for 63% of cases. Mild brain injury can occur with or without a loss of consciousness (LOC). The majority of concussions occurring in sports are not associated with LOC and currently a concussion is *any* decrement in neurologic or cognitive function after a traumatic event (Table 687-1) (see Chapter 67).

Sports concussion is a complex pathophysiologic process affecting the brain, induced by traumatic biomechanical forces. Definition, evaluation, and treatment have evolved significantly over the past 35 yr. Grading scales were published to evaluate concussion severity, although controversy remained due to multiple guidelines. In March 2005, the 2nd International Symposium on Concussion in Sport concluded that injury grading scales should no longer be used. Instead, individual response should guide evaluation and return-to-play decisions. When a concussion is suspected, the athlete should be removed from the activity and medically evaluated. Regular monitoring over the initial few hours following injury is important. The group suggested use of an assessment tool called SCAT (Sport Concussion Assessment Tool) to assist the clinician in assessing the athlete.

Concussions can be classified as simple or complex to help guide management. The most common form of concussion is simple. It implies an injury that resolves over 7–10 days and does not involve complications. Simple concussions do not require neuropsychologic testing and rarely require neuroimaging. The athlete is held out of activity until asymptomatic, after which return to activity is gradual. "Cognitive rest," during which young athletes limit exertion during routine daily tasks as well as with schoolwork, is important in recovery as well.

Return to play should progress through a system of tasks, with the athlete advancing only if asymptomatic:

TABLE 687-1. Signs and Symptoms of Concussion

MEMORY OR ORIENTATION
- Unaware of time, date, or place
- Unaware of period, opposition, or score of game
- General confusion

SYMPTOMS
- Headache
- Dizziness
- Feeling stunned or numb
- Feeling dazed
- Feeling slow
- Seeing stars or flashing lights
- Tinnitis
- Sleepiness
- Blurred vision
- Loss of field of vision
- Double vision
- Nausea

PHYSICAL SIGNS
- Poor coordination
- Poor balance
- Glassy eyed/vacant stare
- Vomiting
- Slurred speech
- Slow to answer questions
- Slow to follow directions
- Easily distracted/poor concentration
- Unusual/inappropriate emotions (e.g., laughing, crying)
- Personality change
- Inappropriate behavior on field of play (e.g., running the wrong direction)
- Significant impaired playing ability compared to earlier in contest

Modified from Canadian Academy of Sport Medicine Concussion Committee: Guidelines for assessment and management of sport-related concussion. *Clin J Sport Med* 2000;10:210; with permission.
From Landry GL: Central nervous system trauma management of concussions in athletes. *Pediatr Clin N Am* 2002;49:723–741.

- **Rest until asymptomatic**
- **Light aerobic exercise; no resistance training**
- **Sport-specific training**
- **Noncontact drills**
- **Full-contact drills**
- **Game play**

If the athlete exhibits symptoms of concussion (see Table 687-1), going back to the previous task for at least 24 hr is appropriate. The athlete should not be using medications to treat symptoms.

Complex concussions involve persistent symptoms or cognitive impairment. Athletes who have symptoms from multiple concussions are included in this group. Focal neurologic symptoms may be present. Symptoms of cognitive impairment include poor attention or concentration, memory dysfunction, irritability, anxiety, depressed mood, sleep disturbances, persistent low-grade headache, lightheadedness, and/or intolerance of bright lights or loud noises. Exertion typically exacerbates concussion symptoms. Work-up is more extensive in this group and includes formal neuropsychologic testing. Physicians who specialize in treating this injury should manage these patients.

In concussion, CT and MRI are usually normal. With simple concussions, neuroimaging is usually not necessary. However, neuroimaging should be used when there is suspicion of intracranial structural pathology due to a focal finding on neurologic examination or symptoms that are worsening. The risk of intracranial pathology is increased in the presence of continued emesis, prolonged headache, persistent antegrade amnesia (poor short-term memory), seizures, Glasgow Coma Scale score <15, and signs of basal skull fracture or depressed skull fracture.

NECK INJURIES

The most common injuries to the neck are soft tissue (contusions, muscle strains, ligament sprains). However, when an athlete complains of midline cervical pain or neck pain on range of motion, has focal neurologic defects, or has lost consciousness, a neck fracture must be assumed. The cervical spine should be immobilized and anteroposterior, lateral, oblique, and open-mouth views obtained before the immobilizer is removed. If active flexion and extension cannot be performed, CT should be performed (see Chapter 67).

There is often overlap between cervical sprain, strain, and contusion. Several radiographic signs are found to be indicative of instability (interspinous widening, vertebral subluxation, vertebral compression fracture, loss of cervical lordosis). MRI is very sensitive and should be used to diagnose and define ligamentous and spinal cord injuries. After a negative radiographic examination for fracture (including dynamic flexion and extension views) and a normal neurological examination, the neck can be immobilized in a soft collar for comfort. Rest and anti-inflammatory medications benefit minor injuries. The collar is gradually withdrawn, and range-of-motion exercises are instituted. The athlete can return to play once full strength range of motion is restored and sport-specific neck function is present. It is important to maintain a cervical conditioning program to help prevent recurrence.

Cervical disk injuries in sports usually result from uncontrolled lateral bending. Cervical injuries are less common than lumbar disk injuries, and they are uncommon in pediatric patients. Most cervical disk problems resolve over several months with initial rest, immobilization, anti-inflammatory medications, activity modification, and cervical traction. Range-of-motion and subsequent strength training are instituted after symptoms improve.

BRACHIAL PLEXUS INJURIES

The brachial plexus includes nerves originating from C5–T1 and emerging from the spinal column in the deep triangle of the neck. The upper trunk (C5-6) can be contused or stretched during football when tackling with the shoulder or having the head forcefully flexed laterally. Manifestations include unilateral burning (known as a "burner" or "stinger"), paresthesia, and weakness in the arm, usually in a C5-6 distribution manifested as the inability to forward flex or abduct the shoulder. These symptoms often resolve spontaneously within minutes. Bilateral symptoms, such as transient quadriplegia, are an indication to curtail participation until the patient is evaluated by MRI. If a patient has recurrent "stingers," an MRI of the cervical spine is indicated.

Guskiewicz KM, McCrea M, Marshall SW, et al: Cumulative effects associated with recurrent concussion in collegiate football players. *JAMA* 2003;290:2549–2554.

Kirkwood MW, Yeates KO, Wilson PE: Pediatric sport-related concussion: a review of the clinical management of an oft-neglected population. *Pediatrics* 2006;117:1359–1371.

Landry GL: Central nervous system trauma management of concussions in athletes. *Pediatr Clin N Am* 2002;49:723–741.

McCrea M, Guskiewicz KM, Marshall SW, et al: Acute effects and recovery time following concussion in collegiate football players. *JAMA* 2003;290:2556–2562.

McCrory P, Johnson K, Meeuwise W, et al: Summary and agreement statement of the 2nd International Conference on Concussion in Sport, Prague 2004. *Clin J Sports Med* 2005;15:48–55.

Smits M, Dippel DWJ, de Haan GG, et al: External validation of the Canadian CT head rule and the New Orleans criteria for CT scanning in patients with minor head injury. *JAMA* 2005;294:1519–1525.

Stiell IG, Clement CM, Rowe BH, et al: Comparison of the Canadian CT head rule and the New Orleans criteria in patients with minor head injury. *JAMA* 2005;294:1511–1518.

Zmurko MG, Tannoury TY, Tannoury CA, Anderson DG: Cervical sprains, disc herniations, minor fractures, and other cervical injuries in the athlete. *Clin Sports Med* 2003;22:513–521.

Chapter 688 ■ Heat Injuries

Gregory L. Landry

Heat illness is the 3rd leading cause of death in U.S. high school athletes. It is a continuum of clinical signs and symptoms that can be mild (heat stress) to fatal (heatstroke) (see Chapter 68). Children are more vulnerable to heat illness than adults. They have greater surface area to body mass ratio than adults and produce greater heat per kilogram of body weight than adults during activity. The sweat rate is lower in children and the temperature at which sweating occurs is higher. Children may take longer to acclimatize to warmer, more humid environments (typically 8–12 near consecutive days of 30–45-min exposures). Children also have a blunted thirst response compared to adults and may not consume enough fluid during exercise to prevent dehydration.

Three categories for heat illness are generally used (heat cramps, heat exhaustion, heat stroke). However, symptoms of heat illness overlap and advance as the core temperature rises. **Heat cramps** are the most common heat injury and usually occur in mild dehydration and or salt depletion, usually affecting the calf and hamstring muscles. They tend to occur later in activity, as muscle fatigue is reached and water loss and sodium loss worsen. They respond to oral rehydration with electrolyte solution and with gentle stretching. The athlete can return to play when ability to perform is not impaired. **Heat syncope** is fainting after prolonged exercise attributed to poor vasomotor tone and depleted intravascular volume, and it responds to fluids, cooling, and supine positioning. **Heat edema** is mild edema of the hands and feet during initial exposure to heat; it resolves with acclimatization. **Heat tetany** is carpopedal tingling or spasms caused by heat-related hyperventilation. It responds to moving to a cooler environment and decreasing respiratory rate (or rebreathing by breathing into a bag). **Heat exhaustion** is a moderate illness with core temperature 100°–103°F/37.7°–39.4°C. Performance is obviously affected, but central nervous system (CNS) dysfunction is mild if present. It is manifested as headache, nausea, vomiting, dizziness, orthostasis, weakness, piloerection, and possibly syncope. **Treatment** includes moving to a cool environment, cooling the body with fans, removing excess clothing, and placing ice over the groin and axillae. If a patient is not able to tolerate oral rehydration, IV fluids are indicated. Patients should be monitored, including rectal temperature, for signs of heatstroke. If rapid improvement is not achieved, transport to an emergency facility is recommended.

Heat stroke is a severe illness manifested by CNS disturbances and potential tissue damage. It is a medical emergency; the mortality rate is 50%. Sports-related heatstroke is characterized by profuse sweating and is related to intense exertion, whereas "classic" heatstroke with dry, hot skin is of slower onset (days) in elderly or chronically ill persons. Rectal temperature is usually >104°F/40°C. Significant damage to the heart, brain, liver, kidneys, and muscle occurs with possible fatal consequences if untreated. **Treatment** is immediate whole-body cooling via cold water immersion. Airway, breathing, circulation, core temperature, and CNS status should be monitored constantly. Rapid cooling should be ceased when core temperature is ~101°–102°F/38.3°–38.9°C. IV fluid at a rate of 800 mL/m^2 in the first hour with normal saline or lactated Ringer solution improves intravascular volume and the body's ability to dissipate heat. Immediate transport to an emergency facility is necessary. Physician clearance is required before return to exercise.

TABLE 688-1. Restraints on Activities at Different Levels of Heat Stress

WBGT		
°C	°F	RESTRAINTS ON ACTIVITIES
<24	<75	All activities allowed, but be alert for prodromes of heat-related illness in prolonged events
24.0–25.9	75.0–78.6	Longer rest periods in the shade; enforce drinking every 15 min
26–29	79–84	Stop activity of unacclimatized persons and other persons with high risk; limit activities of all others (disallow long-distance races, cut down further duration of other activities)
>29	>85	Cancel all athletic activities

WBGT is not air temperature. It indicates wet bulb globe temperature, an index of climatic heat stress that can be measured on the field by the use of a psychrometer. This apparatus, available commercially, is composed of three thermometers. One (wet bulb [WB]) has a wet wick around it to monitor humidity. Another is inside a hollow black ball (globe [G]) to monitor radiation. The third is a simple thermometer (temperature [T]) to measure air temperature. The heat stress index is calculated as WBGT = 0.7 WB temp + 0.2 G temp + 0.1 T temp. It is noteworthy that 70% of the stress is due to humidity, 20% to radiation, and only 10% to air temperature.

From the American Academy of Pediatrics, Committee on Sports Medicine and Fitness: Climatic heat stress and the exercising child and adolescent. *Pediatrics* 2000;106:159.

Dehydration is common to all heat illness; therefore, measures to prevent dehydration may also prevent heat illness. Thirst is not an adequate indicator of hydration status because it is initiated at 2–3% dehydration. Athletes are advised to be well hydrated before exercise and should drink every 20 min during exercise (5 oz for those weighing 40 kg, 9 oz for 60 kg, and 10–12 oz for those >60 kg). Free access to cold water should be advocated to coaches. During a football practice, scheduled breaks every 20–30 min with helmets off to get out of the heat can decrease the cumulative amount of heat exposure. Practices and competition should be scheduled in the early morning or late afternoon to avoid the hottest part of the day. Guidelines have been published about modification of activity related to the wet bulb temperature (Table 688-1). Proper clothing such as shorts and T-shirts without helmets can improve heat dissipation. Prepractice and postpractice weight can be helpful in determining the amount of fluid necessary to replace (8 oz for each pound of weight loss).

Water is adequate for most individuals who exercise <1 hr, although there is evidence that children drink more water when it is flavored. Fluids with electrolyte and carbohydrate are more important for individuals who exercise for >1 hr. Salt pills should not be used by most individuals because of their risk of causing hypernatremia and delayed gastric emptying. They may be useful in an individual with a high sweat rate or recurrent heat cramps. Prolonged exercise (marathon running) with only water replacement places the athlete at risk of hyponatremia.

Almond CSD, Shin AY, Fortescue EB: Hyponatremia among runners in the Boston marathon. *N Engl J Med* 2005;15:1150–1156.

American Academy of Pediatrics, Committee on Sports Medicine and Fitness: Climatic heat stress and the exercising child and adolescent. *Pediatrics* 2000;106:158–159.

Bytomski JR, Squire DL: Heat illness in children. *Curr Sports Med Rep* 2003;2:320–324.

Chapter 689 ■ Female Athletes: Menstrual Problems and the Risk of Osteopenia Gregory L. Landry

Special concerns are related to overtraining in young women and its effect on reproductive function and bone mineral status especially when combined with calorie restriction (see Chapters 27 and 115).

The majority of bone mass is acquired by the end of the 2nd decade (see Chapter 705). Sixty to 70% of adult bone mass is genetically determined, and the remaining is influenced by three controllable factors: exercise, calcium intake, and sex steroids, primarily estrogen. Exercise promotes bone mineralization in the majority of young women and is to be encouraged. In females with eating disorders and those who exercise to the point of excessive weight loss with amenorrhea or oligomenorrhea, exercise can be detrimental to bone mineral acquisition, resulting in reduced bone mineral content, or **osteopenia.**

Specifically, bone mineralization is negatively affected by amenorrhea (absence of menstruation for three or more consecutive months). This may be influenced by abnormal eating patterns, or "disordered eating." When occurring together, disordered eating, amenorrhea, and osteoporosis form the "**female athlete triad.**" At health supervision visits and the preparticipation physical examination, special attention should be given to screening for any features of the triad.

Amenorrhea in athletes is usually caused by the stress of training or a combination of training with disordered eating. Exercise-induced amenorrhea should always be a diagnosis of exclusion. Other causes to be ruled out are pregnancy, pituitary tumors, thyroid abnormalities, polycystic ovary syndrome, anabolic-androgenic steroid use, and other medication side effects.

The low estrogen state of amenorrhea predisposes the female athlete to osteopenia and puts her at risk of stress fractures, especially of the spine and lower extremity. If left unchecked, bone loss is partially irreversible despite resumed menses, estrogen replacement, or calcium supplements. Routine bone mineral density screening is not recommended but may help guide treatment and return to activity in severe cases.

Normal ovulation and menses can be recovered in athletes with amenorrhea. This usually involves either decreasing exercise amount or increasing caloric intake, or both. However, many athletes are resistant to decrease their training, and other methods, such as hormonal supplementation, should be discussed. Nutritional counseling is important to help the athlete develop a plan for increasing calories. Calcium intake should be addressed, with the goal being at least 1,500 mg daily. If amenorrhea is present for ≥6 mo, hormonal supplementation is recommended. There are three eating disorders that can present in the context of amenorrhea: anorexia nervosa, manifest as weight <85% of estimated ideal body weight with evidence of starvation manifest as bradycardia, hypothermia, and orthostatic hypotension or orthostatic tachycardia; bulimia nervosa, manifest as reduced or normal weight with wider fluctuations of weight than would be expected based on the reported caloric intake and exercise; and eating disorder not otherwise specified, with some of the features of either anorexia or bulimia nervosa, yet not meeting all criteria from the *Diagnostic and Statistical Manual of Mental Disorders,* 4th edition, for diagnosis of either (see Chapter 27). Most athletes who develop the third type of eating disorder are sometimes called an atypical eating disorder. Multiple symptoms and methods can occur together, from unhealthy caloric or fat restriction to bingeing and purging. Clues to the problem are weight loss, food restriction, depression, fatigue and worsened athletic performance, and preoccupation with calories and weight. The athlete may avoid events surrounding food consumption or may hide and discard food. Signs and symptoms include fat depletion, muscle wasting, bradycardia worsened from baseline, orthostatic hypotension, constipation, cold intolerance, hypothermia, gastric motility problems, and, in some cases, lanugo. Electrolyte abnormalities can lead to cardiac dysrhythmias. Psychiatric problems (depression, anxiety, suicide risk) are of higher incidence in this population.

For **treatment** of eating disorders, control of the symptoms is a central theme. The first step is confronting the athlete about the abnormal behaviors and unhealthy weight. Generally, exercise is not recommended if the body weight is <85% of estimated ideal body weight, although there are exceptions, especially if the athlete is eumenorrheic. If the athlete is unable to gain weight with nutrition and medical counseling alone, then psychologic consultation is sought.

Most athletes will not initially admit a problem, and many are unaware of the serious physical consequences. A helpful technique in talking to these athletes is to sensitively point out performance issues. Education about decreased strength, endurance, and concentration can be a motivating factor for treatment. Often, the athlete's family needs to be involved, and the athlete should be encouraged to reveal necessary information to them. Psychology or psychiatry referral is important in the multidisciplinary approach to treatment of disordered eating. It is important for the physician to monitor the athlete's physical health while the mental health professional is caring for the mental aspects of the eating disorder.

American Academy of Pediatrics Committee on Sports Medicine and Fitness: Medical concerns in the female athlete. *Pediatrics* 2000;106:610–612.

Birch K: Female athlete triad. *Br Med J* 2005;330:244–246.

Greydanus DE, Patel DR: The female athlete before and beyond puberty. *Pediatr Clin N Am* 2002;49:553–580.

Warren MP, Shantha S: The female athlete. *Best Pract Res Clin Endocrinol Metab* 2000;14:37–53.

Chapter 690 ■ Ergogenic Aids Gregory L. Landry

Ergogenic aids are substances used for performance enhancement, most of which are unregulated supplements. The 1994 Dietary Supplement and Health Education Act limited the ability of the U.S. Food and Drug Administration to regulate any product labeled as a supplement. Many agents have significant side effects without proven ergogenic properties. In April 2005, the American Academy of Pediatrics published a policy statement strongly condemning their use in children and adolescents.

Anabolic-androgenic steroids (AAS) have been used in supraphysiologic doses for their ability to increase muscle size and strength. They have significant endocrinologic side effects, such as decreased sperm count and testicular atrophy in men and menstrual irregularities and virilization in women. Hepatic problems include elevated amino-transaminases and gamma-glutamyl transferase, cholestatic jaundice, peliosis hepatitis, and a variety of tumors, including hepatocellular carcinoma. There is evidence that AAS may cause cardiovascular problems as well, including higher blood pressure, lower high-density lipoprotein, higher low-density lipoprotein, higher homocysteine, and decreased glucose tolerance. The psychologic effects include aggression, several personality disorders, and a variety of other psychologic problems (anxiety, paranoia, mania, depression, psychosis). Physical findings include gynecomastia, testicular shrinkage, jaundice, acne, and marked striae. Women may have hirsutism, voice deepening, and male-pattern baldness.

Testosterone precursors (also known as prohormones) include androstenedione and dihydroepiandrosterone (DHEA). Their use in the adolescent population has increased markedly in conjunction with reports of high-profile athletes' use. They are androgenic but have not been proven to be anabolic. If they are anabolic at all, they work by increasing the production of testosterone. They also increase production of estrogenic metabolites. The side effects are similar to that of AAS and far outweigh any ergogenic benefit. Beginning in January 2005, these substances cannot be sold without prescription.

Creatine (Cr) is an amino acid mostly stored in skeletal muscle. Its key feature is ability to rephosphorylate adenosine diphosphate to adenosine triphosphate, therefore increasing muscle performance. Its use has increased, especially since other supplements have been withdrawn from the market. Thirty percent of high school football players have used Cr. There is evidence that Cr enhances strength and maximal exercise performance when used during training. There is no evidence that Cr affects hydration or temperature regulation. Concerns about nephritis have not been supported by controlled studies. However, there are few long-term studies evaluating Cr use.

American Academy of Pediatrics: American Academy of Pediatrics policy statement: Use of performance enhancing substances. *Pediatrics* 2005;115:1103–1106.

The Medical Letter: Performance-enhancing drugs. Med Lett 2004;46:57–60.

Miah A: Doping and the child: An ethical policy for the vulnerable. *Lancet* 2005;366:874–876.

Tokish JM, Kocher MS, Hawkins RJ: Ergogenic aids: A review of basic science, performance, side effects, and status in sports. *Am J Sports Med* 2004;32:1543–1553.

Chapter 691 ■ Specific Sports and Associated Injuries

Gregory L. Landry

GYMNASTICS. Gymnastics participants are beginning the sport at 5–6 yr of age and achieving the highest level of competition in the mid-teens, often retiring by age 20. Males tend to have more upper extremity injuries, and females have more lower extremity injuries. In addition to mechanical or traumatic injuries, female gymnasts tend to have delayed menarche and can have hypothalamic amenorrhea or oligomenorrhea, associated with low body weight. The typical body habitus of the elite gymnast manifest as reduced weight for height, coupled with amenorrhea or oligomenorrhea, would suggest that reduced bone density is a problem for female gymnasts. In most gymnasts, bone density tends to be high. It is speculated that this is secondary to the repetitive high-impact activities. In spite of this increased bone density, stress fractures are a significant problem. The short stature associated with male and female gymnasts is probably caused by selection bias and not the result of gymnastics training.

Common problems include acute, traumatic injuries, such as an ankle sprain, and chronic, overuse injuries, such as wrist and spine stress fractures. The incidence of injury increases with the level of skill and is greatest in the floor exercise. Wrist pain due to chronic upper extremity weight bearing can be caused by a distal radial stress Salter I fracture, which typically presents on the radial, dorsal aspect of the wrist and is worsened by passive extension and palpation. Other wrist injuries include triangular fibrocartilage complex tears, scaphoid fractures, dorsal ganglions, and carpal ligament injuries. **Treatment** in almost all cases involves immobilization for some period, application of ice, and administration of analgesic drugs. If pain persists, the correct diagnosis can be made by MRI or arthroscopic examination to rule out intra-articular tears, loose bodies, or ligamentous instability. The pediatrician should have a low threshold for referral to a hand specialist in a wrist injury that is not improving with rest. Ligamentous laxity may predispose to elbow or shoulder dislocation and ankle sprains. Spine problems include spondylolysis (pars interarticularis stress fracture) and spondylolisthesis (see Chapter 678.6) due to repetitive extension loading.

SWIMMING. Shoulder injury is the most common overuse injury of competitive swimmers. Swimmer's shoulder is a combination of subacromial bursitis and rotator cuff tendonitis usually of the supraspinatus and is manifested as insidious shoulder pain. Pain, due to subacromial bursitis, may be produced by the Hawkin impingement test, in which pain is provoked by passively forward flexing the humerus to 90 degrees and then internally rotating the humerus. Supraspinatus tendonitis produces pain with active abduction between 60 and 100 degrees and doing the "emptying the can" maneuver, in which the patient internally rotates the humerus at rest and then raises the arm in a plane halfway between forward flexion and abduction. **Treatment** includes ice, modification of stroke technique, relative rest, and muscle strengthening of the rotator cuff and upper back muscles. Prevention includes avoiding rapid increases in training load, proper technique, and strengthening exercises.

BASEBALL. Throwing injuries of the elbow and shoulder (especially among pitchers) are the most common baseball injuries (see Chapters 686.2 and 686.3). The most important consideration is limitation of the number of pitches and advising players, coaches, and athletes that they should stop immediately when they experience elbow pain and if it persists, they need medical evaluation. It has been recommended that a young pitcher pitch no more than 200 pitches per week and that the maximal number of pitches per game be approximately six times the pitcher's age in years. Deaths in baseball are rare and are caused by chest wall trauma with the ball (**commotio cordis**) (see Chapter 436) or head injury with the ball or bat. Batting helmuts need to be worn properly to try to prevent face and head injuries.

BALLET. This very demanding activity may be associated with delayed menarche and eating disorders in female dancers (see Chapter 689). Acute injuries occur, most often of the lower extremities. As with any repetitive activity, overuse injuries are likely; the key is to make the correct diagnosis and also consider the kinetic chain dysfunction that may have contributed to that injury. A dancer may have an unrehabilitated ankle sprain, causing favoring of that leg, leading to a stress fracture of the contralateral tibia. Foot problems include metatarsal stress fractures, subungual hematomas, callus and bunion formation, sesamoiditis, and plantar fasciitis. Going **en pointe** is a question that young ballet dancers and their parents may ask. An average age to go en pointe is 12 yr; a function test should be part of that decision: If the child can go en pointe, holding the position and not appearing unstable and weak and without pain, then he or she is probably ready to try dancing en pointe. Ankle problems include anterior and posterior impingement syndromes because of the extremes of range of motion in grand plié and en pointe, respectively. Hip problems include both the medial snapping hip syndrome caused by the iliopsoas tendon's riding over the anterior hip capsule and tendinitis (piriformis, iliopsoas, rectus femoris). The **piriformis syndrome** occurs because of the repetitive external hip rotation required in ballet and can manifest as buttock and hip pain and sciatica.

WRESTLING. Wrestlers have great fluctuations in weight to meet weight-matched competition standards. Such fluctuations are associated with fasting, dehydration, and then bingeing.

Wrestling holds may produce injury owing to various torques or forces applied to the extremities and spine; wrestling throws with subsequent falls may produce concussions, neck strain, or spinal cord injury. The two most common sites of injury are the shoulder and knee. "Stingers" and "burners" are due to a brachial plexopathy (see Football).

Shoulder subluxation is common. Patients are often aware of their shoulder's slipping in and out (see Chapter 686.2). Hand injuries are usually not severe and include recurrent metacarpophalangeal and proximal interphalangeal sprains. Treatment of hand injuries includes splinting and taping.

Knee injuries are common and potentially serious and include prepatellar bursitis, medial and lateral sprains, and medial and lateral meniscus tears (see Chapter 686.6). Prepatellar bursitis is caused by acute or recurrent traumatic impact to the mat. Swelling occurs over the patella, and patients have no limitation of motion except full flexion. If the skin has been broken, septic bursitis has to be considered. The physician must try to distinguish traumatic from infected bursitis, which may require aspiration of the bursa. **Treatment** of traumatic bursitis includes protective padding, ice, nonsteroidal anti-inflammatory drugs (NSAIDs), and occasionally aspiration if flexion is impaired. Rarely bursectomy is needed if there are several recurrences.

Dermatologic problems include herpes simplex (herpes gladiatorum), impetigo, staphylococcal furunculosis or folliculitis, superficial fungal infections, and contact dermatitis. The first two are contraindications to wrestling until the infection is no longer contagious. If recurrent herpes infections occur, suppressive oral antiviral agents should be used.

Football. Football continues to be the sport with the highest number of injuries, and one of the greatest number of participants, and one of the sports with a high injury rate. In terms of the severity of injury, defined as days lost per injury, the average injury in football is less severe than in many other sports. Most of the injuries are sprains, strains, and contusions that once treated appropriately result in minimal time away from football.

Although the majority of catastrophic sports injuries in the United States have occurred in football, severe injuries are rare. Catastrophic is defined as a fatal injury or a severe injury with or without permanent severe functional disability. Disabling injuries include cervical spine and cerebral injuries.

Head and neck football injuries include concussion, neck sprain, and brachial plexopathy. The latter is referred to as a "stinger" or "burner." Lumbar spine injury manifested as low back pain may represent spondylolysis. Shoulder trauma can cause glenohumeral dislocation, the majority of which are anterior dislocations, acromioclavicular separations, and clavicular and humeral fractures.

Contusions to the arm and thigh muscles are common and may result in large hematomas if not treated aggressively. Assuming that there is no fracture, **treatment** includes ice and compression during most waking hours for the first few days to limit the expansion of the hematoma and then doing pain-free strengthening and stretching exercises until baseline function is achieved. Then return to contact can be approved. When the hematoma is allowed to persist and especially if there is a second hematoma into the first, myositis ossificans may develop.

Knee injuries are the most common musculoskeletal complaint at the time of preseason examinations. Knee injuries are discussed in Chapter 686.6.

Ankle sprains occur, and the risk of reinjury may be reduced by rehabilitation and use of a lace-up ankle brace. Turf toe, a sprain to the first metatarsophalangeal joint, is caused by forceful dorsiflexion while playing on artificial turf in soft, lightweight, flexible shoes. **Treatment** of turf toe includes ice, NSAIDs, an orthotic to limit extension of the great toe, and rest. Turf toe can be a season- or career-limiting injury.

ICE HOCKEY. Hockey is a collision sport associated with injuries caused by the puck or the stick hitting the player or by body contact with other players, the ice, or the boards, producing contusions, lacerations, fractures, sprains, or concussions. The risk of injury is reduced by proper equipment (helmets with face masks) and enforcement of the rules regarding dangerous body contact (checking from behind, high sticking, slashing, and fighting).

Specific hockey injuries include ankle sprains (dorsiflexion, eversion, and external rotation in contrast to the usual sprain of inversion in other sports), hip adductor strain, osteitis pubis, and various shoulder injuries from body contact. The latter include acromioclavicular sprain, dislocation, and clavicular fractures. The most serious injuries are to the head and neck.

BASKETBALL AND VOLLEYBALL. Common maneuvers of these two sports include using a ball with your hand, jumping, pivoting, running, and sudden stopping, which increase the risks of ankle, knee, and finger injury.

Knee overuse injuries include **patellar tendonitis** ("jumper's knee") and **traction apophysitis** (Osgood-Schlatter disease). As with other jumping sports, acute ligament sprains (medial collateral with or without anterior cruciate ligaments) can occur.

Ankle sprain is the most common injury and is usually caused by inversion with plantarflexion, placing the lateral ligaments at high tension. An avulsion fracture of the base of the 5th metatarsal at the insertion of the peroneus brevis tendon is another sequela of inversion ankle injuries. Achilles tendonitis is a common overuse injury. Foot pain may be due to retrocalcaneal bursitis, posterior tibial tendonitis, accessory tarsal navicular, calcaneal periostitis, plantar fasciitis, stress fracture of the tarsal navicular, Jones stress fracture of the 5th metatarsal, sesamoiditis, blisters, subungual hematoma, and paronychia.

RUNNING. Running problems are usually due to an overuse injury related to muscle imbalance, a minor skeletal deformity, or poor flexibility, strength or endurance, or proprioception. With each step while running, the foot impact ranges from three to eight times the athlete's body weight. Most problems are due to errors in training when the runner increases the distance or intensity of training too rapidly. Minor variations (malalignment) in anatomy, which do not cause problems at rest, may predispose to injury at specific sites (patellofemoral stress, overpronation). Muscle fatigue, environmental temperature, and running surface (grass vs unyielding concrete) also contribute to injuries. Prevention of injuries is possible by muscle-strengthening exercises for previous injuries. Using good-quality running shoes that match an athlete's foot type is an essential first step. Gender-specific shoes are important because girls generally have a narrower rearfoot. Those who severely overpronate need a motion control shoe for maximal rearfoot and arch support in the midsole. Those who mildly overpronate need a stability shoe that has extra support in the medial midsole and some midsole cushion. Those who supinate need a cushioned shoe with more shock absorption in the midsole, more curved last, and minimal arch support.

Stress fractures of the femoral neck, inferior pubic rami, subtrochanteric area, proximal femoral shaft, proximal tibia, fibula, navicular, metatarsal, sesamoid, and calcaneal apophysis may occur. Stress fractures of all bones of the lower extremity can occur in runners. The most common are in the metatarsals, the tibia, and the fibula. Those that are the most worrisome in terms of risk of nonunion are in the anterior proximal tibia, the femoral neck, and the tarsal navicular. Muscle strains frequently affect the hamstrings, followed by the quadriceps, hip adductors, soleus, and gastrocnemius muscles. Tendonitis involving the tendon and its sheath is common in the Achilles tendon, followed by the posterior tibial, peroneal, iliopsoas, and proximal hamstring tendons. Achilles tendonitis develops chronically, initially may get better during a run, is characterized by tenderness and crepitance if acute and nodularity if chronic, and must be distinguished from a retrocalcaneal bursitis. **Treatment** includes identification of underlying cause and temporary abstinence from running (begin cross-training), a heel lift, heel cord stretching, and NSAIDs.

Anterior knee pain is usually due to patellofemoral stress syndrome (**runner's knee**), which results from excessive dynamic, usually lateral, motion of the patellar tendon in relationship to the femoral intracondylar groove. **Treatment** includes stretching of the quadriceps and hamstring muscles and possibly the iliotibial band, quadriceps-strengthening exercises, ice, and relative rest. Foot orthotics may be indicated if there is no improvement with the aforementioned treatment. Posterior knee pain can be caused by gastrocnemius strain, whereas posteromedial pain may be due to proximal tibial stress fractures or semimembranosus or semitendinosus tendonitis and lateral knee pain may be due to iliotibial band syndrome and popliteus tendonitis. **Iliotibial band syndrome** may be a combination of bursitis and tendonitis owing to mechanical friction of the band (an extension of the tensor fasciae latae) over the lateral femoral epicondyle.

Shin splints, or medial tibial stress syndrome, is a descriptive term for pain over the medial tibia and should be distinguished from tibial stress fractures and chronic compartment syndromes (see Chapter 686.7). Medial tibial stress syndrome usually occurs in new runners with overpronation. **Treatment** includes running on soft surfaces, proper shoe selection, and, possibly, orthotics, NSAIDs, and relative rest (or cross-training). Chronic compartment syndromes involve the deep posterior or anterior compartments, producing local pain and throbbing confined to the muscle group (not to the bone). Classically, the pain will have onset at the same time during the run and will be relieved by rest. Pain usually prevents further training, thus limiting the risk of permanent nerve damage. Diagnosis is made by measurement of increased intracompartmental pressures during exercise.

Plantar fasciitis is an inflammation of the supporting structure of the longitudinal arch owing to repetitive cyclic loading with foot strike. Pain increases with the first step out of bed in the morning and with running and is located on the medial aspect of the heel. It is associated with wearing old shoes or shoes with poor arch support. **Treatment** includes calf stretching, proper shoes, night splints, corticosteroid injection, relative rest, and ice massage of the heel. Calcaneal stress fracture must be considered especially in the amenorrheic distance runner.

SOCCER. Injuries in soccer include any of the running injuries as well as abrasions, contusions, muscle strains, and ligament sprains (ankle, knee), owing partly to body-to-body contact, falls, running, and kicking. Hip problems include the "hip pointer" (iliac crest contusion), iliac crest apophysitis, and chronic groin pain (muscle strain, hernia, osteitis pubis). Femoral neck stress fractures, slipped femoral capital epiphysis, and avulsion fractures of the pelvis or femur are to be considered in the differential diagnosis yet are unusual causes of hip pain. All other lower and upper extremity injuries can occur in soccer.

Concussions occur frequently in soccer. Concussion can lead to neurocognitive dysfunction, and concussions occur in soccer due to player/player, player/goal post, and player/ground contact. The American Academy of Pediatrics recommends that youth soccer participants should minimize heading the ball until more is known about the risks in young children. Proper heading technique should be taught in youth soccer; on long kicks, the receiving player traps the ball with the chest or leg, not the head; defenders kick the ball about 5 ft in front of their midfielders or forwards so the latter have to come to the ball and trap with their legs; players avoid heading the ball backward toward the goal (with cervical extension); referees, as with all sports, keep the game under control and penalize dangerous play; and guidelines for returning to play after a concussion should be followed.

TENNIS. Lower extremity injuries occur twice as often as upper extremity injuries, and, overall, injury rates are similar for boys and girls. Common areas of injury in tennis include muscles and tendons of the elbow, shoulder, back, wrist, and abdomen. The risk of injury is increased by increased training; by unrehabilitated injuries with resultant deficits in flexibility, strength, and endurance; and by poor technique. Acute injuries of the lower extremities include ankle, knee, lower leg, and groin strains. Overuse injuries of the back and lower and upper extremities occur. The lower extremity injury patterns are related to the fact that for accomplished players, there are an average of eight direction changes per point, creating eccentric and concentric loads on the lower extremities. In the back, injuries are related to the marked and rapid load and direction change associated with serving, and the shoulder, elbow, and wrist are moving at velocities of up to 1,700, 900, and 350 degrees/sec, respectively, in a repetitive fashion. Injuries can be related to improper equipment, such as a racquet that is too big, or to trying to learn techniques, such as hitting with top spin or with power before proper coordination and technique in basic strokes have been established. Overuse injuries include stress fractures of the humerus, ulna, and metacarpals and traction apophysitis of the calcaneus, tibial tubercle (Osgood-Schlatter disease), and medial humeral epicondyle.

Rotator cuff tendonitis is caused by repetitive overuse and may be related to anteroposterior glenohumeral instability. Subluxation of the glenohumeral joint may also be present. Biceps tendonitis can present as anterior shoulder pain.

Tennis elbow, or lateral epicondylitis, is due to repetitive overload of the wrist extensor/supinator mechanism, especially the extensor carpi radialis brevis (see Chapter 686.3). Medial epicondylitis is caused by repetitive overload of the wrist flexor/pronator muscle groups. This may secondarily involve the medial collateral ligament; however, the ligament is uncommonly the site of the primary injury. Medial epicondylar apophysitis may be associated with ulnar nerve dysfunction if there is an avulsion fracture. Olecranon apophysitis is similar to Osgood-Schlatter disease and is marked by pain at the olecranon with elbow extension.

Wrist problems include an enlarged dorsal ganglion cyst, radiocarpal joint capsular (impingement) synovitis, degenerative attrition (tears) of the triangular fibrocartilage complex, and fracture of the hook of the hamate.

Basic **treatment** includes relative rest, analgesics, application of ice, rehabilitation, learning proper mechanics, using properly sized racquets, protective counterforce bracing (elbow, wrist), strengthening exercises, and gradual return to tennis. Corticosteroid injections into the extensor/supinator muscle group for "tennis elbow" are not recommended because the outcome at 1 yr is poorer than for those treated with rehabilitation.

SKIING. Injuries are related to falls (concussions, contusion, lacerations) and ski-specific mechanisms. Overall injuries have declined, partly because of better equipment (boots, bindings, poles) and slope conditions. It has been recommended that children and adolescents wear helmets for skiing and snowboarding.

Thumb injuries resulting from falls with the thumb in abduction and hyperextension produce a sprain of the ulnar collateral ligament (skier's thumb). Complete tears with a 45-degree joint opening require surgical intervention, whereas smaller degrees of joint opening may be treated with a thumb spica cast for 4 wk. A Salter-Harris type III fracture may also be present; if the epiphyseal fracture is displaced, it requires open reduction and internal fixation.

Lower extremity injuries include fractures (often spiral) of the tibia ("boot top") and ankle and anterior cruciate ligament sprains with or without tibial eminence fracture. Hemarthrosis is present in fractures and meniscal and anterior cruciate ligament injuries. **Treatment** is noted in Chapter 676.

American Academy of Pediatrics Committee on Sports Medicine and Fitness: Injuries in youth soccer: A subject review. *Pediatrics* 2000;105:659–661.

American Academy of Pediatrics Committee on Sports Medicine and Fitness: The management of minor closed head injury in children. *Pediatrics* 1999;104:1407–1415.

Bisset L, Beller E, Jull G, et al: Mobilisation with movement and excercise, corticosteroid injection, or wait and see for tennis elbow: randomised trial. *BMJ* 2006;333:939–941.

Boutis K, Komar L, Jaramillo D, et al: Sensitivity of a clinical examination to predict need for radiography in children with ankle injuries: A prospective study. *Lancet* 2001;358:2118–2121.

Christopher NC, Congeni J: Overuse injuries in the pediatric athlete: Evaluation, initial management, and strategies for prevention. *Clin Pediatr Emerg Med* 2002;3:118–128.

Committee on Sports Medicine and Fitness: Climatic heat stress and the exercising child and adolescent. *Pediatrics* 2000;106:158–159.

Committee on Sports Medicine and Fitness: Medical concerns in the female athlete. *Pediatrics* 2000;106:610–613.

Committee on Sports Medicine and Fitness: Medical conditions affecting sports participation. *Pediatrics* 2001;107:1205–1209.

Heidt RS, Sweeterman LM, Carlonas Richelle L, et al: Avoidance of soccer injuries with preseason conditioning. *Am J Sport Med* 2000;28:659–662.

Hoffman JR, Mower WR, Wolfson AB, et al: Validity of a set of clinical criteria to rule out injury to the cervical spine in patients with blunt trauma. *N Engl J Med* 2000;343:94–99.

Maron BJ, Shirani J, Poliac LC, et al: Sudden death in young competitive athletes. Clinical, demographic, and pathological profiles. *JAMA* 1996;276:199–204.

McClain LG, Reynolds S: Sports injuries in a high school. *Pediatrics* 1989;84:446–450.

McCrory PR: Brain injury and heading in soccer. *Br Med J* 2003;327:351–352.

Nysted M, Drogset JO: Trampoline injuries. *Br J Sports Med* 2006;40: 984–987.

Smidt N, van der Windt DAWM: Tennis elbow in primary care. *BMJ* 2006; 333:927–928.

Smidt N, van der Windt DAWM, Assendelft JJ, et al: Corticosteroid injections, physiotherapy, or a wait-and-see policy for lateral epicondylitis: A randomized controlled trial. *Lancet* 2002;359:657–662.

Solomon DH, Simel DL, Bates DW, et al: Does this patient have a torn meniscus or ligament of the knee? *JAMA* 2001;286:1610–1620.

Speed CA: Corticosteroid injections in tendon lesions. *Br Med J* 2001;323:382–386.

University Interscholastic League-Preparticipation Physical Evaluation, 2002. Search www.uil.utexas.edu/index.html. Go to Athletics, then to Athletic forms, then Preparticipation Physical Evaluation.

Warren WL, Bailes JE: On the field evaluation of athletic head injuries. *Clin Sports Med* 1998;17:13–26.

Section 3 — The Skeletal Dysplasias

Chapter 692 ■ General Considerations

William A. Horton and Jacqueline T. Hecht

The terms skeletal dysplasias, bone dysplasias, and osteochondrodysplasias refer to a genetically and clinically heterogeneous group of disorders of skeletal development and growth. Their prevalence is estimated to be about 1/4,000 births. They can be divided into the osteodysplasias typified by osteogenesis imperfecta (see Chapter 699) and the chondrodysplasias. The latter result from mutations of genes that are essential for skeletal development and growth. The clinical picture is dominated by skeletal abnormalities. The manifestations may be restricted to the skeleton, but in most cases nonskeletal tissues are also involved. The disorders may be lethal in utero or mild with features that go undetected.

The chondrodysplasias are distinguished from other forms of short stature by a disproportionality of skeletal manifestations. The importance of cartilage in bone formation is noted in Figure 692-1. They are separated into individuals with predominantly short limbs and those with predominantly short trunks. Efforts to define the extent of clinical heterogeneity resulted in the delineation of >100 distinct entities. Many of these disorders result from mutations of a relatively small group of genes, the "chondrodysplasia genes."

An International Working Group on Bone Dysplasias has named and classified these disorders into groups based on genetic cause if known or on similarities of clinical and radiographic

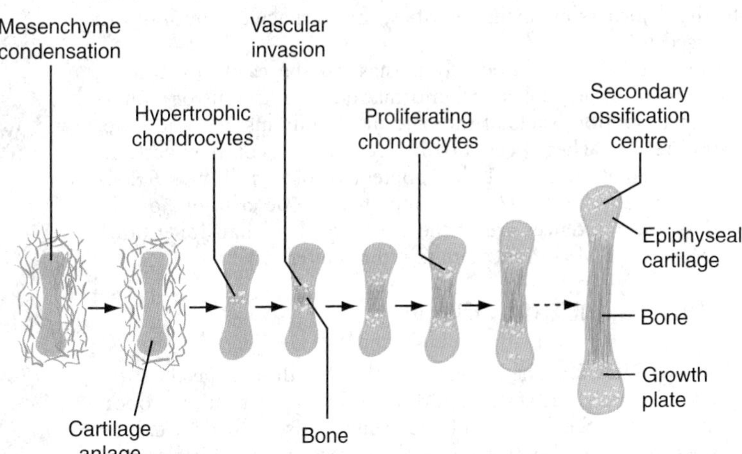

Figure 692-1. The importance of cartilage in bone formation. (From Horton WA: Skeletal development: Insights from targeting the mouse genome. *Lancet* 2005;362:560.)

TABLE 692-1. Genetics of Skeletal Dysplasias

GENE LOCUS	CHROMOSOME LOCATION	PROTEIN	PROTEIN FUNCTION	CLINICAL PHENOTYPE	OMIM	DISEASE MECHANISM	INHERIT
COL2A1	12q13.1–q13.3	Type II collagen α_1 chain	Cartilage matrix protein	Achondrogenesis II	200610	Dominant negative	AD*
				Hypochondrogenesis	200610	Dominant negative	AD*
				SED congenita	183900	Dominant negative	AD
				Kniest dysplasia	156550	Dominant negative	AD
				Late-onset SED		Dominant negative	AD
				Stickler dysplasia	108300	Haploinsufficiency	AD
SEDL	Xp22.2–p22.1	Sedlin	Intracellular transporter	X-linked SED tarda	313400	Loss of function	XLR
COL11A1	1p21	Type XI collagen α_1 chain	Cartilage matrix protein	Stickler-like dysplasia	184840	Dominant negative	AD
COL11A2	6p21.3	Type XI collagen α_2 chain	Cartilage matrix protein	Stickler-like dysplasia	215150	Loss of function	AR
COMP	19p12–p13.1	Cartilage oligomeric matrix protein	Cartilage matrix protein	Pseudoachondroplasia	177170	Dominant negative	AD
				MED	600969	Dominant negative	AD
COL9A2	1p32.2–p33	Type IX collagen α_2 chain	Cartilage matrix protein	MED	600969	Dominant negative	AD
COL9A3	20q13.3	Type IX collagen α_3 chain	Cartilage matrix protein	MED	600969	Dominant negative	AD
MATN3	2p24–p23	Matrilin 3	Cartilage matrix protein	MED	600969	Dominant negative	AD
COL10A1	6q21–q22.3	Type X collagen α_1 chain	Hypertrophic cartilage matrix protein	Schmid metaphyseal chondrodysplasia	156500	Haploinsufficiency	AD
FGFR3	4p16.3	FGF receptor 3	Tyrosine kinase receptor for FGFs	Thanatophoric dysplasia I	187600	Gain of function	AD*
				Thanatophoric dysplasia II	187610	Gain of function	AD*
				Achondroplasia	100800	Gain of function	AD
				Hypochondroplasia	146000	Gain of function	AD
PTHR1	3p21–p22	PTHrP receptor	G protein–coupled receptor for PTH and PTHrP	Jansen metaphyseal chondrodysplasia	156400	Gain of function	AD
DTDST	5q32–q33	DTD sulfate transporter	Transmembrane sulfate transporter	Achondrogenesis 1B	600972	Loss of function	AR*
				Atelosteogenesis II	256050	Loss of function	AR*
				Diastrophic dysplasia	222600	Loss of function	AR
SOX9	17q24.3–q25.1	SRY box 9	Transcription factor	Campomelic dysplasia	114290	Haploinsufficiency	AD
CBFA1[†]	6p21	Core binding factor α subunit	Transcription factor	Cleidocranial dysplasia	119600	Haploinsufficiency	AD
LMX1B	9q34.1		Transcription factor	Nail-patella dysplasia	161200	Haploinsufficiency	AD
CTSK	1q21	Cathepsin K	Enzyme	Pyknodysostosis	265800	Loss of function	AR
RMPR	9p21–p12	Mitochondrial RNA-processing endoribonuclease	RNA-processing enzyme	CHH	250250	Loss of function	AR

*Usually lethal.
[†]Also called RUNX2.
AD, autosomal dominant; AR, autosomal recessive; CHH, cartilage-hair hypoplasia; DTD, diastrophic dysplasia; FGF, fibroblast growth factor; MED, multiple epiphyseal dysplasia; PTH, parathyroid hormone; PTHrP, parathyroid hormone–related protein; SED, spondyloepiphyseal dysplasia; SRY, sex-determining region of the Y chromosome.

manifestations, which often imply a common pathogenesis and a common genetic basis, if the cause is unknown (Table 692-1). The better defined chondrodysplasia groups, such as the achondroplasia and type II collagenopathy groups, contain graded series of disorders that range from very severe to very mild. This may be true for other groups as more mutations are found and the full spectrum of clinical phenotypes associated with mutations of a given gene is defined. These disorders are clinical phenotypes distributed along spectra of phenotypic abnormality associated with mutations of particular genes. For mutations of some genes such as COL2A1, the distribution is fairly continuous, with clinical phenotypes merging into one another across a broad range. There is much less clinical overlap for mutations of some other genes, such as *FGFR3,* in which the distribution is discontinuous. Because most clinicians and most reference materials refer to the disorders as distinct entities, this vernacular continues to be used.

Although a few chondrodysplasias can be easily diagnosed, most require the analysis of information from the history, physical examination, skeletal radiographs, family history, and laboratory testing. The process involves recognizing complex patterns that are characteristic of the different disorders (Tables 692-2, 692–3, 692–4, and 692–5). Comprehensive descriptions of disorders and references are at the On-Line Mendelian Inheritance in Man (OMIM) Internet site (see the references).

CLINICAL MANIFESTATIONS

GROWTH RELATED. The hallmark of the chondrodysplasias is disproportionate short stature. Although this refers to a disproportion between the limbs and the trunk, most disorders exhibit some shortening of both, and subtle degrees of disproportion may be difficult to appreciate, especially in premature, obese, or edematous infants. Disproportionate shortening of the limbs should be suspected if the upper limbs do not reach the mid-pelvis in infancy or the upper thigh after infancy. Disproportionate shortening of the trunk is indicated by a short neck, small chest, and protuberant abdomen. Skeletal disproportion is usually accompanied by short stature (length and height below the 3rd percentile); these measurements may occasionally be within the low-normal range early in the course of certain conditions.

TABLE 692-2. Major Problems Associated with Skeletal Dysplasias

PROBLEM	EXAMPLE
Lethality*	Thanatophoric dysplasia
Associated anomalies[†]	Ellis–van Creveld syndrome
Short stature	Common to almost all
Cervical spine dislocations	Larsen syndrome
Severe limb bowing	Metaphyseal dysplasia, type Schmid
Spine curvatures	Metatropic dysplasia
Clubfeet	Diastrophic dysplasia
Fractures	Osteogenesis imperfecta
Pneumonias, aspirations	Campomelic dysplasia
Spinal cord compression	Achondroplasia
Joint problems (hips, knees)	Most skeletal dysplasias
Hearing loss	Common (greatest with cleft palate)
Myopia/cataracts	Stickler syndrome
Immunodeficiency[‡]	Cartilage-hair hypoplasia, Schimke immuno-osseous dysplasia
Poor body image	Variable, but common to all
Sex reversal	Campomelic dysplasia

*Mostly due to severely reduced size of thorax.
[†]See Table 692-3.
[‡]At least four additional disorders, all involving the metaphyses, can have immunodeficiency.

TABLE 692-3. Associated Anomalies in Skeletal Dysplasias

ANOMALY	EXAMPLE
Heart defects	Ellis–van Creveld syndrome, Jeune syndrome
Polydactyly	Short rib polydactyly, Majewski type
Cleft palate	Diastrophic dysplasia
Ear cysts	Diastrophic dysplasia
Spinal cord compression	Achondroplasia
Encephalocele	Dyssegmental dysplasia
Hemivertebrae	Dyssegmental dysplasia
Micrognathia	Camptomelic dysplasia
Nail dysplasia	Ellis–van Creveld syndrome
Conical teeth, oligodontia	Ellis–van Creveld syndrome
Multiple oral frenulae	Ellis–van Creveld syndrome
Dentinogenesis imperfecta	Osteogenesis imperfecta
Pretibial skin dimples	Camptomelic dysplasia
Cataracts, retinal detachment	Stickler syndrome
Intestinal atresia	Saldino-Noonan
Renal cysts	Saldino-Noonan
Campodactyly	Diastrophic dysplasia
Craniosynostosis	Thanatophoric dysplasia
Ichthyosis	Chondrodystrophica punctata
Hitchhiker thumb	Diastrophic dysplasia
Sparse scalp hair	Cartilage-hair hypoplasia
Hypertelorism	Robinow syndrome
Hypoplastic nasal bridge	Acrodysostosis
Clavicular agenesis	Cleidocranial dysplasia
Genital hypoplasia	Robinow syndrome
Tail	Metatropic dysplasia
Omphalocele	Beemer-Langer syndrome
Blue sclera	Osteogenesis imperfecta

There may also be disproportionate shortening of different segments of the limbs; the particular pattern may provide clues for specific diagnoses. Shortening is greatest in the proximal segments (upper arms and legs) in achondroplasia; this is termed **rhizomelic shortening.** Disproportionate shortening of the middle segments (forearms and lower legs) is called **mesomelic shortening; acromelic** shortening involves the hands and feet.

With some exceptions, there is a strong correlation between the age at onset and the clinical severity. Many of the lethal neonatal chondrodysplasias are evident during routine fetal ultrasound examinations performed at the end of the 1st trimester of gestation (see Table 692-4). Gestational standards exist for long-bone lengths; discrepancies are often detected between biparietal diameter of the skull and long-bone lengths. Many disorders become apparent around the time of birth; others manifest during the 1st yr of life. A number of disorders present in early childhood and a few in late childhood or later.

TABLE 692-4. Lethal Neonatal Dwarfism

USUALLY FATAL*
Achondrogenesis (different types)
Thanatophoric dyplasia
Short rib polydactyly (different types)
Homozygous achondroplasia
Campomelic dysplasia
Dyssegmental dysplasia, Silverman-Handmaker type
Osteogenesis imperfecta, type II
Hypophosphatasia (congenital form)
Chondrodysplasia punctata (rhizomelic form)
OFTEN FATAL
Asphyxiating thoracic dystrophy (Jeune syndrome)
OCCASIONALLY FATAL
Ellis–van Creveld syndrome
Diastrophic dysplasia
Metatropic dwarfism
Kniest dysplasia

*A few prolonged survivors have been reported in most of these disorders.

TABLE 692-5. Usually Nonlethal Dwarfing Conditions Recognizable at Birth or Within First Few Months of Life

MOST COMMON
Achondroplasia
Osteogenesis imperfecta (types I, III, IV)
Spondyloepiphyseal dysplasia congenita
Diastrophic dysplasia
Ellis–van Creveld syndrome
LESS COMMON
Chondrodysplasia punctata (some forms)
Kniest dysplasia
Metatropic dysplasia
Langer mesomelic dysplasia

NON–GROWTH RELATED. Most patients also have problems unrelated to growth. Skeletal deformities, such as abnormal joint mobility, protuberances at and around joints, and angular deformities, are common and usually symmetric. Skeletal abnormalities may adversely affect nonskeletal tissues. Impaired growth at the base of the skull and of vertebral pedicles reduces the size of the spinal canal in achondroplasia and may contribute to spinal cord compression. Short ribs reduce thoracic volume, which may compromise breathing in patients with short trunk chondrodysplasias. Cleft palate is common to many disorders, presumably reflecting defective palatal growth.

Manifestations may be unrelated to the skeleton; they reflect expression of mutant genes in nonskeletal tissues. Examples include retinal detachment in spondyloepiphyseal dysplasia congenita, sex reversal in campomelic dysplasia, congenital heart malformations in Ellis-van Creveld syndrome, immunodeficiency in cartilage-hair hypoplasia, and renal dysfunction in asphyxiating thoracic dystrophy. These nonskeletal problems provide valuable clues to specific diagnoses and must be managed clinically (see Table 692-3).

FAMILY AND REPRODUCTIVE HISTORY. A family history may identify relatives with the condition; a mendelian inheritance pattern may be elicited. Because the presentation may vary in some disorders, features that might be related to the disorder should be identified. Special attention should be given to mild degrees of short stature, disproportion, deformities, and other manifestations such as precocious osteoarthritis because they may be overlooked. Physical examination of relatives may be useful, as may the review of their photographs, radiographs, and medical records.

A reproductive history may reveal previous stillbirths, fetal losses, and other abnormal pregnancy outcomes resulting from a skeletal dysplasia. Pregnancy complications, such as polyhydramnios or reduced fetal movement, are common in bone dysplasias, especially neonatal lethal variants.

Even though most of the skeletal dysplasias are genetic, it is common to have no family history of the disorder. New mutations are common for autosomal dominant disorders, especially lethal disorders in the perinatal period (thanatophoric dysplasia, osteogenesis imperfecta). The majority of achondroplasia cases result from new mutations. Germ cell mosaicism, in which a parent has clones of mutant germ cells, has been observed in osteogenesis imperfecta and in other dominant disorders. A negative family history is usually seen in recessive disorders. Prenatal diagnosis is available for disorders that have a genetic loci identified. Appropriateness of the testing depends on many factors, and genetic counseling is warranted for these families.

RADIOGRAPHIC FEATURES. Radiographic evaluation for a chondrodysplasia should include plain films of the entire skeleton. Efforts should be made to identify which bones and which parts of bones (epiphyses, metaphyses, diaphyses) are most affected. If possible, films taken at different ages should be examined because the radiographic changes evolve with time. Films taken before puberty are generally more informative because pubertal closure of the epiphyses obliterates many of the signs needed for a radiographic diagnosis.

DIAGNOSIS

If an infant or child is short with disproportionate features, a diagnosis is established by matching the observed clinical picture (defined primarily from clinical, family, and gestational histories; physical examination; and radiographic evaluation) with clinical phenotypes of well-documented disorders. Pediatricians should be able to gather most of this information and, in consultation with a radiologist, diagnose the common chondrodysplasias. A number of reference texts and online databases provide information about the disorders and comprehensive lists of current references. For less common disorders and for infants and children whose phenotypes do not closely match well-established clinical phenotypes, consultation with experts in the bone dysplasia field is warranted.

Laboratory testing has not been useful in diagnosing chondrodysplasias except in osteogenesis imperfecta, in which analysis of collagen synthesis by skin fibroblasts has helped establish a diagnosis. Osteogenesis imperfecta is not a chondrodysplasia, but it is frequently in the differential diagnosis, especially for newborns with severe skeletal deformities (see Chapter 699). Reduced plasma levels of COMP (cartilage oligomeric matrix protein) have been detected in patients with pseudoachondroplasia and multiple epiphyseal dysplasias in which COMP mutations have been found.

Molecular genetic testing for chondrodysplasias may be useful, especially for disorders in which recurrent mutations occur (typical achondroplasia has the same *FGFR3* mutation). Mutation testing for achondroplasia is available; the diagnosis is usually made clinically. The greatest utility for testing may be for prenatal diagnosis for couples where both parents have typical (heterozygous) achondroplasia. They are at a 25% risk of the much more severe homozygous achondroplasia, which can be detected by mutation analysis. Another example is in disorders due to mutations of *DTDST.* These disorders are inherited in an autosomal recessive manner, and a limited number of mutant alleles have been found. If the mutations are identified in the patient, they should be detectable in the parents and potentially used for prenatal diagnosis. Nonetheless, most chondrodysplasia mutations tend to be dispersed throughout host genes and may be specific for that family. This phenomenon makes their detection more difficult and currently reduces the usefulness of such testing for diagnostic purposes.

Many of the chondrodysplasias have distinct histologic changes of the skeletal growth plate. Sometimes such tissues obtained at biopsy or discarded from a surgical procedure are helpful diagnostically. It is uncommon to make a diagnosis histologically if it was not already suspected on clinical grounds. An exception is for the lethal neonatal chondrodysplasias, in which an aborted fetus is macerated, thus making a clinical and radiographic assessment difficult.

MOLECULAR GENETICS. A number of chondrodysplasia genes have been identified (see Table 694-1). They encode several categories of proteins, including cartilage matrix proteins, transmembrane receptors, ion transporters, and transcription factors. The number of identified gene loci is smaller than anticipated from the number of recognized clinical phenotypes. The majority of patients have disorders that map to <10 loci; mutations at 2 loci (*COL2A1* and *FGFR3*) account for more than ½ of all cases. There may be a limited number of genes whose function is critical to skeletal development, especially linear bone growth; mutations in these genes give rise to a wide range of chondrodysplasia clinical phenotypes.

Mutations at the *COL2A1* and *FGFR3* loci illustrate different genetic characteristics. *COL2A1* mutations are distributed throughout the gene with few instances of recurrence in unrelated persons. In contrast, *FGFR3* mutations are restricted to a few locations within the gene, and occurrence of new mutations at these sites in unrelated individuals is the rule. There is a strong correlation between clinical phenotype and mutation site for *FGFR3,* but not *COL2A1,* mutations.

PATHOPHYSIOLOGY. Chondrodysplasia mutations act through different mechanisms. Most mutations involving cartilage matrix proteins cause disease when only 1 of the 2 copies (alleles) of the relevant gene is mutated (haploinsufficiency). These mutations usually act through a dominant negative mechanism in which the protein products of the mutant allele interfere with the assembly and function of multimeric molecules that contain the protein products of both the normal and mutant alleles. The type II collagen molecule is a triple helix composed of 3 collagen chains, which are the products of the type II collagen gene *COL2A1.* When chains from both normal and mutant alleles are combined to form triple helices, most molecules contain at least 1 mutant chain. It is not known how many mutant chains are required to produce a dysfunctional molecule but, depending on the mutation, it theoretically could be as few as 1.

Mutations involving type X collagen differ from the model just described. They map to the region of the chain that is responsible for chain recognition; the chains must recognize each other before they can assemble into collagen molecules. Mutations are thought to disrupt this process. As a result, none of the mutant chains are incorporated into molecules. This mechanism is haploinsufficiency because the products of the mutant allele are functionally absent and the normal allele is insufficient for normal function. Mutations involving ion transport genes also act through a loss of function of the transporters. Alternatively, mutations of transmembrane receptors studied to date appear to act through a gain of function; the mutant receptors initiate signals in a constitutive manner independent of their normal ligands.

Regardless of genetic mechanism, the mutations ultimately disrupt endochondral ossification, the biologic process responsible for the development and linear growth of the skeleton (see Fig. 692-1). Indeed, a wide range of morphologic abnormalities of the skeletal growth plate, the anatomic structure in which endochondral ossification occurs, have been described in the chondrodysplasias.

TREATMENT

The first step is to establish the correct diagnosis. This allows one to predict a prognosis and to anticipate the medical and surgical problems associated with a particular disorder. Establishing a diagnosis helps to distinguish between lethal disorders and nonlethal disorders in a premature or newborn infant (see Tables 692-4 and 692-5). A poor prognosis for long-term survival may argue against initiating extreme lifesaving measures for thanatophoric dysplasia or achondrogenesis types Ib or II, whereas such measures may be indicated for infants with spondyloepiphyseal dysplasia congenita or diastrophic dysplasia, which have a good prognosis if the infant survives the newborn period.

Because there is no definitive therapy to normalize bone growth in any of the disorders, management is directed at preventing and correcting skeletal deformities, treating nonskeletal complications, genetic counseling, and helping patients and families learn to cope. Each disorder has its own unique set of problems, and consequently management must be tailored to each disorder. Medical information for a few disorders can be found at the Medical Information on Dwarfism website (see references).

There are a number of problems common to many chondrodysplasias for which general recommendations can be made. Children with most chondrodysplasias should avoid contact sports and other activities that cause injury or stress to joints. Good dietary habits should be established in childhood to prevent or minimize obesity in adulthood. Dental care should be started early to minimize crowding and malalignment of teeth. Children and relatives should be given the opportunity to participate in support groups, such as the Little People of America and Human Growth Foundation.

Two controversial approaches have been used to increase bone length. Surgical limb lengthening has been employed for a few disorders. Its greatest success has been in achondroplasia in which nonskeletal tissues tend to be redundant and easily stretched. The procedure is usually performed during adolescence. Pharmacologic doses of human growth hormone comparable to those used to treat Turner syndrome have also been tried in several disorders; the results have been equivocal.

References

Apajasalo M, Sintonen H, Rautonen J, et al: Health-related quality of life patients with genetic skeletal dysplasias. *Eur J Pediatr* 1998;157:114–121.

Hall JG, Froster-Iskenius UG, Allanson JE: *Handbook of Normal Physical Measurements.* Oxford, Oxford University Press, 1989.

Horton WA: Skeletal development: insights from targeting the mouse genome. *Lancet* 2005;362:560–569.

Horton WA, Hecht JT: Chondrodysplasias: general concepts and diagnostic and management considerations. In Royce PM, Steinmann B (editors): *Connective Tissue and Its Disorders, Molecular, Genetic and Medical Aspects,* 2nd ed. New York, Wiley-Liss, 2002, p 901.

Krakow D, Williams J, Poehl M, et al: Use of three-dimensional ultrasound imaging in the diagnosis of prenatal-onset skeletal dysplasias. *Ultrasound Obstet Gynecol* 2003;21:465–472.

Lachman RS: Neurologic abnormalities in the skeletal dysplasias: A clinical and radiological perspective. *Am J Med Genet* 1997;69:33–43.

Rimoin DL, Lachman RS Unger S: Chondrodysplasias. In Rimoin DL, Connor JM, Pyeritz RE, Korf BR (editors): *Emery and Rimoin's Principles and Practice of Medical Genetics,* 4th ed. New York, Churchill Livingstone, 2002, p 4071.

Spranger J, Maroteaux P: The lethal osteochondrodysplasias. *Adv Hum Genet* 1995;19:1–103.

Spranger JW, Brill PW, Poznansk A: *Bone Dysplasias. An Atlas of Genetic Disorders of Skeletal Development,* 2nd ed. New York, Oxford University Press, 2002.

Taybi H, Lachman RS: *Radiology of Syndromes, Metabolic Disorders, and Skeletal Dysplasias,* 4th ed. New York, Mosby, 1996.

Online Resources

Medical Information on Dwarfism: Available at *medical.lpaonline.org* (accessed 9/14/06).

On-Line Mendelian Inheritance in Man (OMIM): Available at *www.ncbi.nlm.nih.gov/entrez/query.fcgi?db=OMIM* (accessed).

Chapter 693 ■ Disorders Involving Cartilage Matrix Proteins

William A. Horton and Jacqueline T. Hecht

Some bone and joint disorders result from functional disturbances of cartilage matrix proteins. They fall into four groups corresponding primarily to the defective proteins: three collagens and the noncollagenous proteins COMP (cartilage oligomeric matrix protein) and matrilin 3. The clinical phenotypes differ between and within the groups, especially the spondyloepiphyseal dysplasia (SED) group. In some groups, there is substantial variation in clinical severity.

SPONDYLOEPIPHYSEAL DYSPLASIAS

The term spondyloepiphyseal dysplasia refers to a heterogeneous group of disorders characterized by shortening of the trunk and, to a lesser extent, the limbs. Severity ranges from achondrogenesis type II to the slightly less severe hypochondrogenesis (these two types are lethal in the perinatal period) to SED congenita and its variants, including Kniest dysplasia (which are apparent at birth and are usually nonlethal), to late-onset SED (which may not be detected until adolescence or later). The radiographic hallmarks are abnormal development of the vertebral bodies and of epiphyses, the extent of which corresponds to the clinical severity. All the SEDs result from heterozygous mutations of *COL2A1;* they are autosomal dominant disorders. The mutations are dispersed throughout the gene; there is a poor correlation between the mutation's location and the resultant clinical phenotype. For familial cases, prenatal diagnosis is possible if the mutation is identified. Schimke immuno-osseous dysplasia may be an exception because it is an autosomal recessive disorder characterized by short stature, hyperpigmented macules, unusual facies, proteinuria and progressive renal failure, cerebral ischemia, and a T-cell defect with lymphopenia and recurrent infections.

LETHAL SPONDYLOEPIPHYSEAL DYSPLASIAS. Achondrogenesis type II (OMIM 200610) is characterized by severe shortening of the neck and trunk and especially the limbs and by a large, soft head. Fetal hydrops and prematurity are common; infants are stillborn or die shortly after birth. Hypochondrogenesis (OMIM 200610) refers to a clinical phenotype intermediate between achondrogenesis type II and SED congenita. It is typically lethal in the newborn period.

The severity of radiographic changes correlates with the clinical severity (Fig. 693-1). Both conditions produce short, broad tubular bones with cupped metaphyses. The pelvic bones are hypoplastic, and the cranial bones are not well mineralized. The vertebral bodies are poorly ossified in the entire spine in achondrogenesis type II and in the cervical and sacral spine in hypochondrogenesis. The pedicles are ossified in both.

SPONDYLOEPIPHYSEAL DYSPLASIA CONGENITA. The phenotype of this group, SED congenita (OMIM 183900), is apparent at birth. The head and face are usually normal, but a cleft palate is common. The neck is short and the chest is barrel shaped (Fig. 693-2). Kyphosis and exaggeration of the normal lumbar lordosis are common. The proximal segments of the limbs are shorter than the hands and feet, which often appear normal. Some infants have clubfoot or exhibit hypotonia.

Skeletal radiographs of the newborn reveal short tubular bones, delayed ossification of vertebral bodies, and proximal limb bone epiphyses (Fig. 693-3). Hypoplasia of the odontoid process; a short, square pelvis with a poorly ossified symphysis pubis; and mild irregularity of metaphyses are apparent.

Infants usually have normal developmental milestones; a waddling gait typically appears in early childhood. Childhood complications include respiratory compromise from spinal deformities and spinal cord compression due to cervicomedullary instability. The disproportionateness and shortening become progressively worse with age, and adult heights range from 95 to 128 cm. Myopia is typical; adults are predisposed to retinal detachment. Precocious osteoarthritis occurs in adulthood and requires surgical joint replacement.

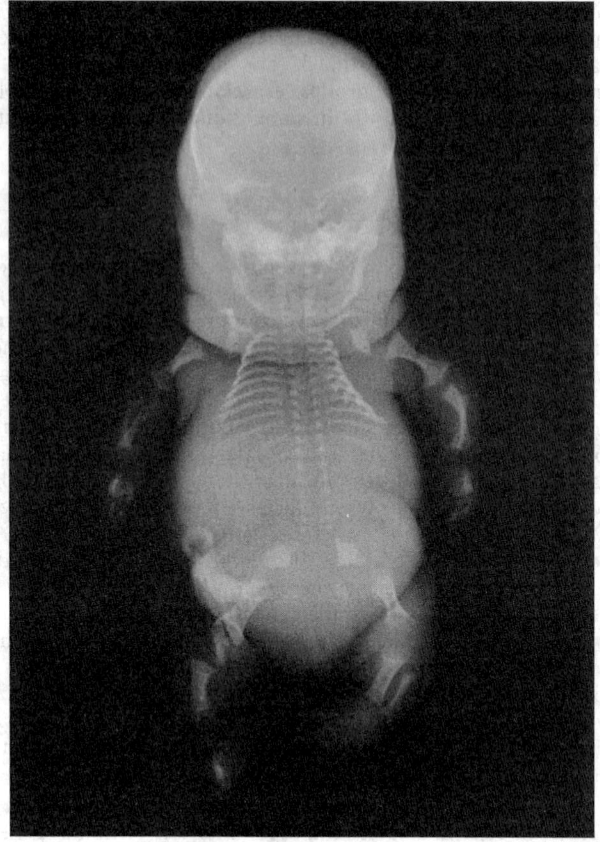

Figure 693-1. Stillborn with achondrogenesis type II. Note poor ossification of calvaria, vertebral bodies, and sacrum; hypoplasia of pelvic bones; and short tubular bones with cupped metaphyses.

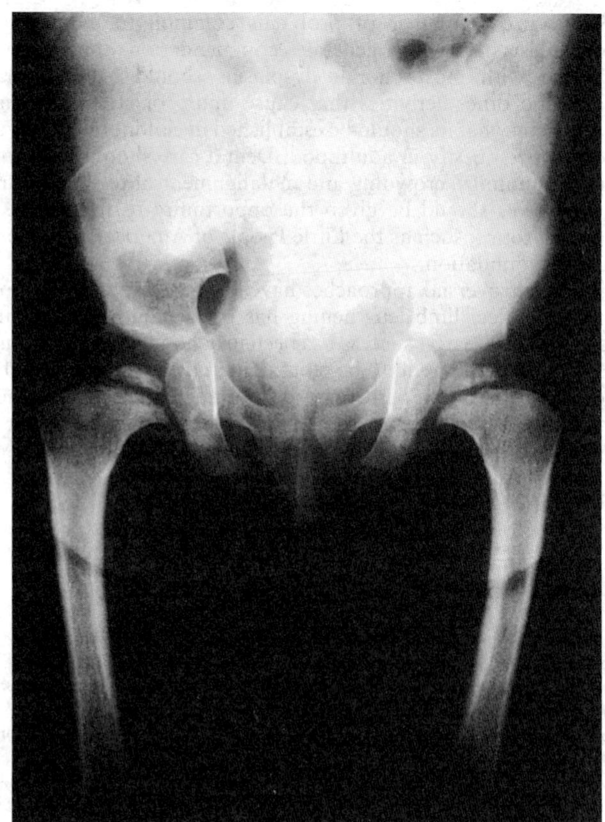

Figure 693-3. Radiograph of spondyloepiphyseal dysplasia congenita pelvis demonstrating squared pelvis, hypoplastic capital femoral epiphyses, and femoral necks that are wide and short.

KNIEST DYSPLASIA. The Kniest dysplasia variant of SED (OMIM 156550) presents at birth with a short trunk and limbs associated with a flat face, prominent eyes, enlarged joints, cleft palate, and clubfoot. Radiographs show vertebral defects and short tubular bones with epiphyseal irregularities and metaphyseal enlargement that gives rise to a dumbbell appearance.

Motor development is often delayed because of the joint deformities, although intelligence is normal. Hearing loss and myopia commonly develop during childhood, and retinal detachment may occur as a late complication. Joint enlargement progresses during childhood and becomes painful; it is accompanied by flexion contractures and muscle atrophy, which may be incapacitating by adolescence.

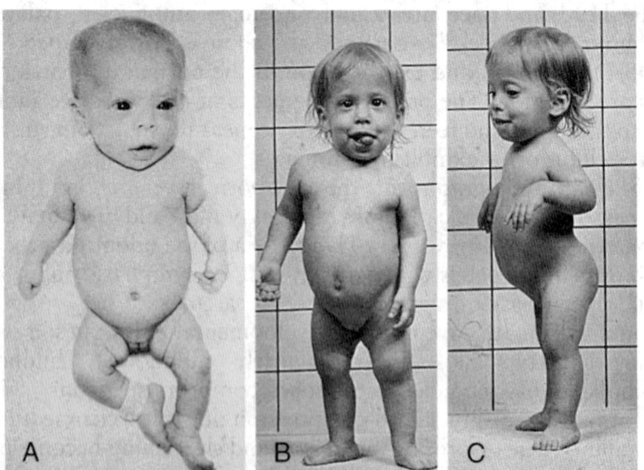

Figure 693-2. Spondyloepiphyseal dysplasia congenita is shown in infancy *(A)* and early childhood *(B, C)*. Note the short extremities, relatively normal hands, flat facies, and exaggerated lordosis.

LATE-ONSET SPONDYLOEPIPHYSEAL DYSPLASIA. This term refers to a mild to very mild clinical phenotype characterized by slightly short stature associated with mild epiphyseal and vertebral abnormalities on radiographs. It is typically detected during childhood or adolescence but may go unrecognized until adulthood when precocious osteoarthritis appears. This designation is nosologically distinct from SED tarda, which is clinically similar but results from mutation of the X-linked gene SEDL.

STICKLER DYSPLASIA (HEREDITARY OSTEOARTHRO-OPHTHALMOPATHY)

Short stature is not a feature of Stickler dysplasia (OMIM 184840). It resembles SED because of its joint and eye manifestations. Mutations of genes encoding type XI collagen, which functionally interacts with type II collagen, have been identified in Stickler-like disorders (OMIM 184840, OMIM 215150). Stickler dysplasia is often identified in the newborn because of cleft palate and micrognathia (Pierre Robin anomaly). Infants typically have severe myopia and additional ophthalmologic complications, including choroidoretinal and vitreous degeneration; retinal detachment is common during childhood (Fig. 693-4). Sensorineural hearing loss may arise during adolescence, which is when symptoms of osteoarthritis may also begin. Special attention must be given to the eye complications even in childhood.

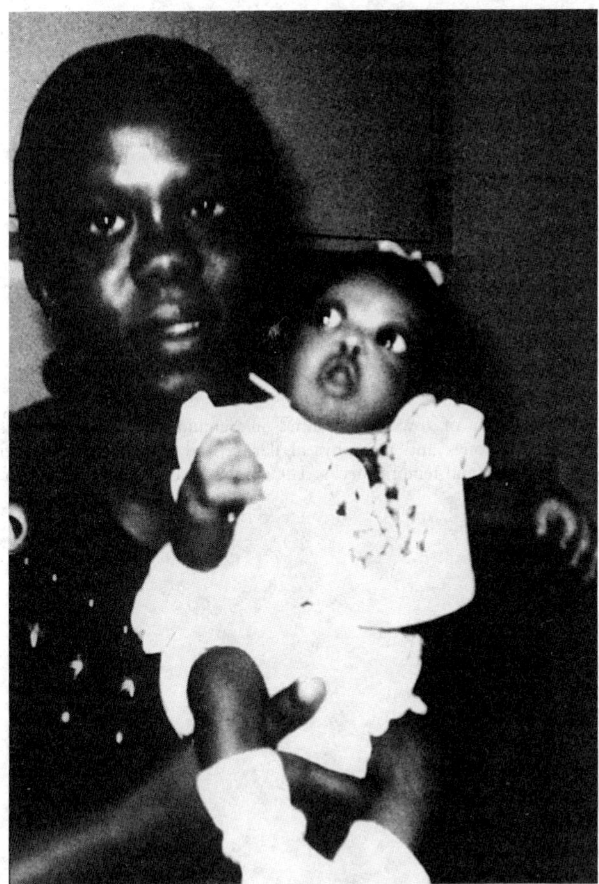

Figure 693-4. Stickler syndrome in mother and child. The facies are flat and the eyes are prominent.

SCHMID METAPHYSEAL DYSPLASIA

Schmid metaphyseal dysplasia (OMIM 156500) is one of several chondrodysplasias in which metaphyseal abnormalities dominate the radiographic features. It typically presents in early childhood with mild short stature, bowing of the legs, and a waddling gait (Fig. 693-5). Enlargement of joints, such as the wrist, may be found. Radiographs show flaring and irregular mineralization of the metaphyses of tubular bones of the proximal limbs (Fig. 693-6). Coxa vara is usually present and may require surgical correction. Short stature becomes more evident with age and affects the lower extremities more than the upper extremities; the manifestations are limited to the skeleton.

Schmid metaphyseal chondrodysplasia is due to heterozygous mutations of the gene encoding type X collagen; it is an autosomal dominant trait. The distribution of type X collagen is restricted to the region of growing bone in which cartilage is converted into bone. This may explain why radiographic changes are confined to the metaphyses.

PSEUDOACHONDROPLASIA AND MULTIPLE EPIPHYSEAL DYSPLASIA

Pseudoachondroplasia (OMIM 177170) and multiple epiphyseal dysplasia (MED) (OMIM 600969) are two distinct phenotypes that are grouped together because they result from mutations of the gene encoding COMP. The mutations are heterozygous in both; they are autosomal dominant traits. The clinical phenotypes are restricted to skeletal tissues.

Newborns with pseudoachondroplasia are average in size and appearance. Gait abnormalities and short stature mainly affect the limbs and become apparent in late infancy. The short stature becomes marked as the child grows and is associated with generalized joint laxity (Fig. 693-7). The hands are short, broad, and deviated in an ulnar direction; the forearms are bowed. Developmental milestones and intelligence are usually normal. Lumbar lordosis and deformities of the knee develop during childhood; the latter frequently requires surgical correction. Pain is common in weight-bearing joints during childhood and adolescence, leading to osteoarthritis late in the 2nd decade of life. Adults range in height from 105 to 128 cm.

Skeletal radiographs show distinctive abnormalities of vertebral bodies and of both epiphyses and metaphyses of tubular bones (Fig. 693-8).

The MED phenotype has skeletal abnormalities that predominantly affect the epiphyses as noted on radiographs. Two classic forms are a severe Fairbank type and a mild Ribbing type. Because of overlap in clinical features and because COMP mutations are found in both types, they may be considered clinical variants.

The more severe clinical phenotype has its onset during childhood, with mild short-limbed short stature, pain in weight-bearing joints, and a waddling gait. Radiographs show delayed and irregular ossification of epiphyses. More mildly affected individuals may not be recognized until adolescence or adulthood. Radiographic changes may be limited to the capital femoral epiphyses. In the latter case, mild MED must be distinguished from bilateral Legg-Çalve-Perthes disease. Precocious osteoarthritis of

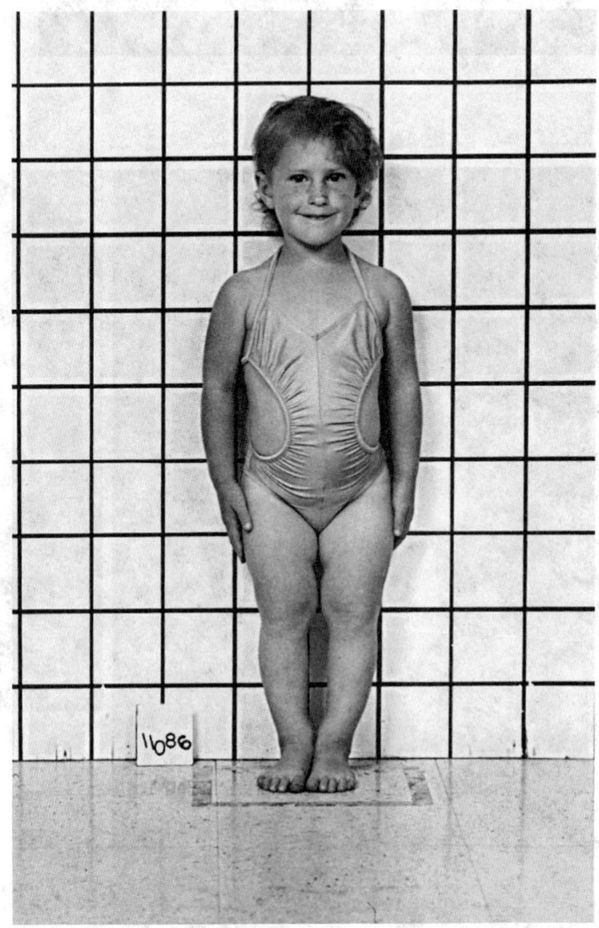

Figure 693-5. Female patient with metaphyseal dysplasia, type Schmid. The facies are normal and stature is mildly reduced. Mild tibia vara is present.

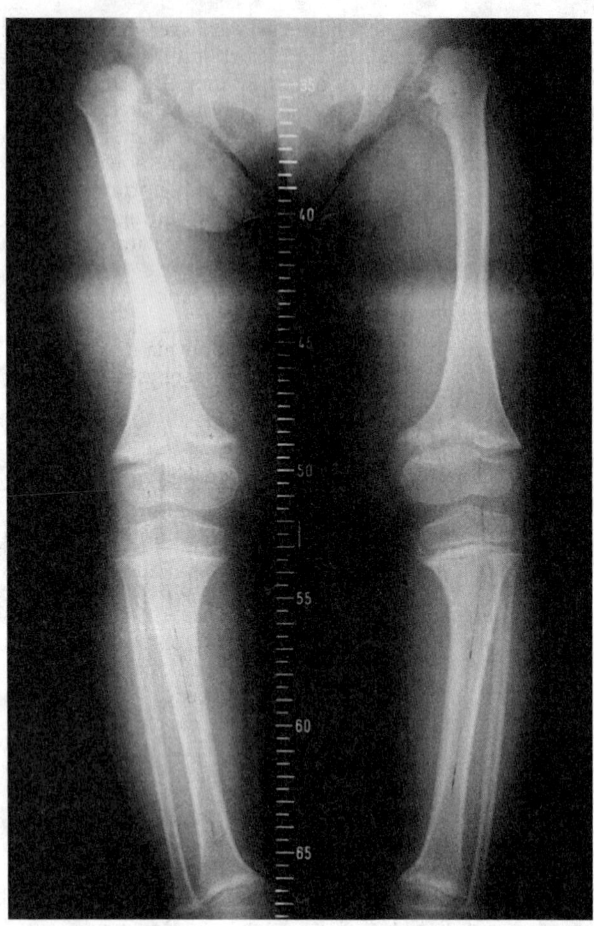

Figure 693-6. Radiograph of lower extremities in Schmid metaphyseal dysplasia showing short tubular bones and metaphyseal flaring and irregularities, abnormal capital femoral epiphyses, and femoral necks. The epiphyses are normal. Coxa vara is present.

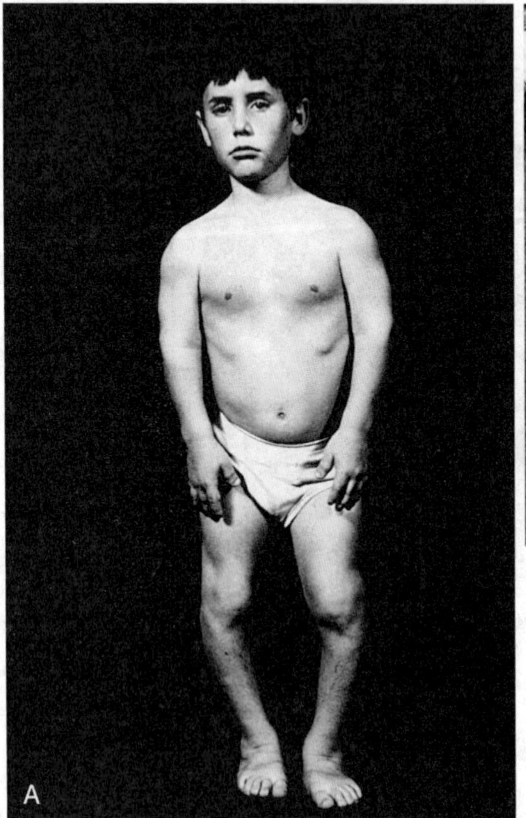

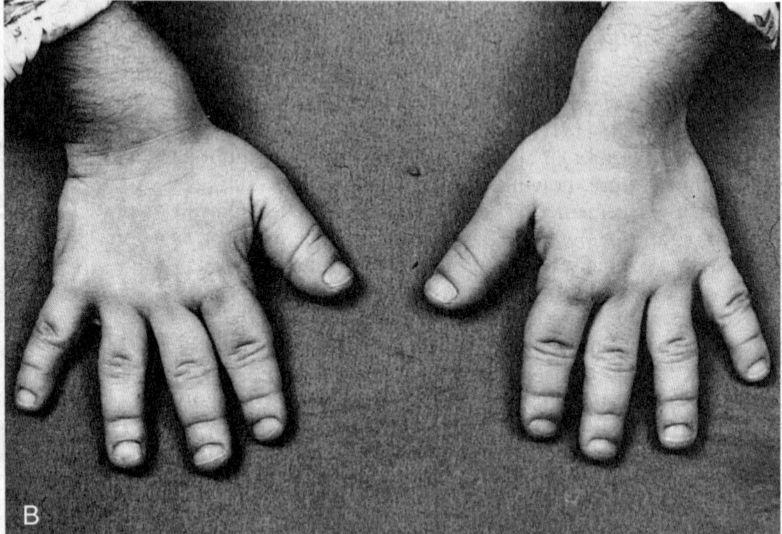

Figure 693-7. *A,* Pseudoachondroplasia in an adolescent male. The facies and head circumference are normal. There is shortening of all extremities and bowing of the lower extremities. *B,* Photograph of hands, demonstrating short stubby fingers.

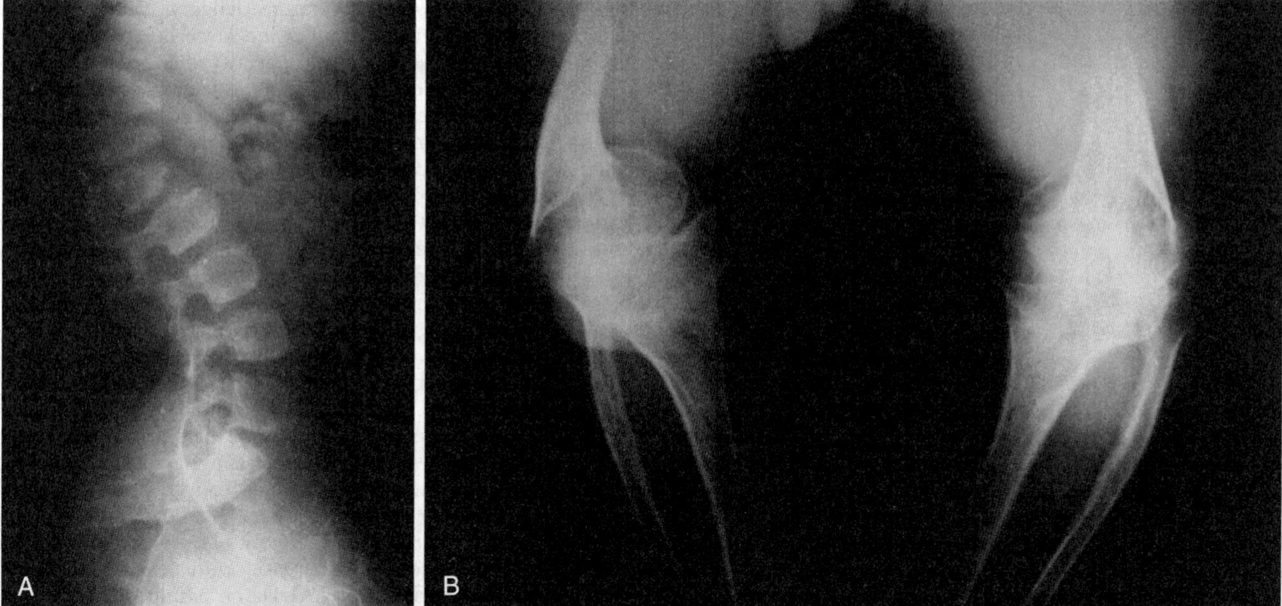

Figure 693-8. *A,* Lateral thoracolumbar spine radiograph of patient with pseudoachondroplasia showing central protrusion (tonguing) of the anterior aspect of upper lumbar and lower thoracic vertebrae. Note reduced vertebral body heights (platyspondyly) and secondary lordosis. *B,* Lower extremity radiograph of patient with pseudoachondroplasia showing large metaphyses, poorly formed epiphyses, and marked bowing of the long bones.

hips and knees is the major complication in adults with MED. Adult heights range from 136 to 151 cm.

There are families with clinical and radiographic manifestations of MED that are not due to mutations of COMP. Some are linked to the gene encoding one of the type IX collagen chains. It has been suggested that COMP and type IX collagen interact functionally in cartilage matrix, thus explaining why mutations of different genes produce similar pictures. Mutations of the genes coding for another cartilage matrix protein, matrilin 3, and the diastrophic dysplasia sulfate transporter have also been found in patients with MED. For familial cases of pseudoachondroplasia and MED resulting from mutation in COMP, prenatal diagnosis is available.

Boerkoel CF, O'Neill S, Andre JL, et al: Manifestations and treatment of Schimke immuno-osseous dysplasia: 14 new cases and a review of the literature. *Eur J Pediatr* 2000;159:1–7.

Briggs MD, Mortier GR, Cole WG, et al: Diverse mutations in the gene for cartilage oligomeric matrix protein in a pseudoachondroplasia-multiple epiphyseal dysplasia disease spectrum. *Am J Hum Genet* 1998;62:311–319.

Horton WA, Hecht JT: Chondrodysplasias: Disorders of cartilage matrix proteins. In Royce PM, Steinmann B (editors): *Connective Tissue and Its Disorders, Molecular, Genetic and Medical Aspects,* 2nd ed. New York, Wiley-Liss, 2002, p 909.

Kennedy J, Jackson G, Ramsden S, et al: COMP mutation screening as an aid for the clinical diagnosis and counseling of patients with a suspected diagnosis of pseudoachondroplasia or multiple epiphyseal dysplasia. *Eur J Hum Genet* 2005;13:547–555.

Chapter 694 ■ Disorders Involving Transmembrane Receptors

William A. Horton and Jacqueline T. Hecht

Disorders involving transmembrane receptors result from heterozygous mutations of genes encoding *FGFR3* (fibroblast growth factor receptor 3) and *PTHR* (parathyroid hormone receptor). The mutations cause the receptors to become activated in the absence of physiologic ligands, which accentuates normal receptor function of negatively regulating bone growth. The mutations act by gain of negative function. In the *FGFR3* mutation group, in which the clinical phenotypes range from severe to mild, the severity appears to correlate with the extent to which the receptor is activated. Both *PTHR* and especially *FGFR3* mutations tend to recur in unrelated individuals.

ACHONDROPLASIA GROUP

The achondroplasia group represents a substantial percentage of patients with chondrodysplasias and contains thanatophoric dysplasia (TD), the most common lethal chondrodysplasia with an incidence of 1/35,000 births; achondroplasia, the most common nonlethal chondrodysplasia with an incidence of 1/15,000 to 1/40,000 births; and hypochondroplasia. All three have mutations in a small number of locations in the *FGFR3* gene. There is a strong correlation between the mutation site and the clinical phenotype.

THANATOPHORIC DYSPLASIA. TD (OMIM 187600, OMIM 187610) presents before or at birth. In the former situation, ultrasonographic examination in midgestation or later reveals a large head and very short limbs; the pregnancy is often accompanied

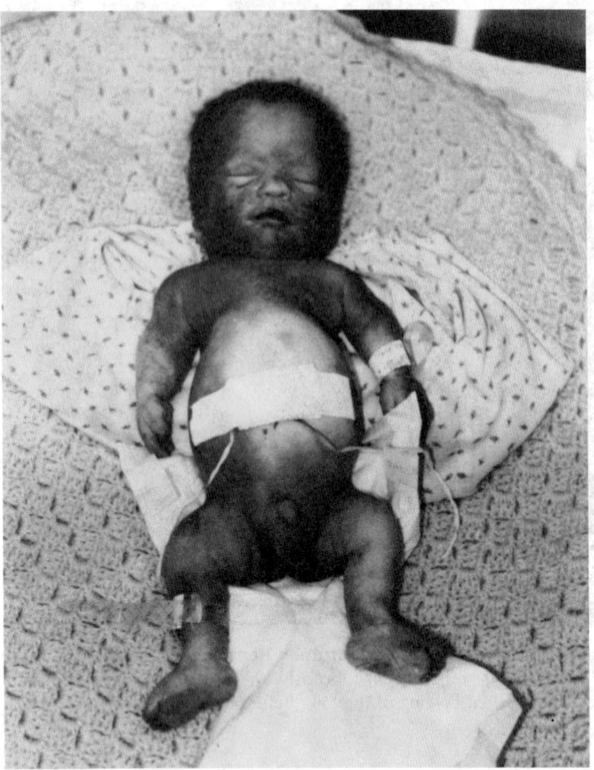

Figure 694-1. Stillborn infant with thanatophoric dysplasia. Limbs are very short, with upper limbs extending only two thirds of the way down the abdomen. The chest is narrow, exaggerating the protuberance of the abdomen. The head is relatively large.

by polyhydramnios and premature delivery. Very short limbs, short neck, long narrow thorax, and large head with midfacial hypoplasia dominate the clinical phenotype at birth (Fig. 694-1). The cloverleaf skull deformity known as **kleeblattschädel** is sometimes found. Newborns have severe respiratory distress because of their small thorax. Although this distress can be treated by intense respiratory care, the long-term prognosis is poor.

Skeletal radiographs distinguish two slightly different forms called TD I and TD II. In the more common TD I, radiographs show large calvariae with a small cranial base, marked thinning and flattening of vertebral bodies visualized best on lateral view, very short ribs, severe hypoplasia of pelvic bones, and very short and bowed tubular bones with flared metaphyses (Fig. 694-2). The femurs are curved and shaped like a telephone receiver. TD II differs mainly in that there are longer and straighter femurs.

The TD II clinical phenotype is associated with mutations that map to codon 650 of *FGFR3*, causing the substitution of a glutamic acid for the lysine. This activates the tyrosine kinase activity of a receptor that transmits signals to intracellular pathways. Mutation of lysine 650 to methionine is associated with a clinical phenotype intermediate between TD and achondroplasia referred to as severe achondroplasia with developmental delay and acanthosis nigricans or SADDAN. Mutations of the TD I phenotype map mainly to two regions in the extracellular domain of the receptor, where they substitute cysteine residues for other amino acids. Free cysteine residues are thought to form disulfide bonds promoting dimerization of receptor molecules, leading to activation and signal transmission.

TD I and TD II represent new mutations to normal parents. The recurrence risk is low. Because the mutated codons in TD are mutable for unknown reasons and because of the theoretical risk of germ cell mosaicism, parents are offered prenatal diagnosis for subsequent pregnancies.

ACHONDROPLASIA. Achondroplasia (OMIM 100800) is the prototype chondrodysplasia. It typically presents at birth with short limbs, a long narrow trunk, and a large head with midfacial hypoplasia and prominent forehead (Fig. 694-3). The limb shortening is greatest in the proximal segments, and the fingers often

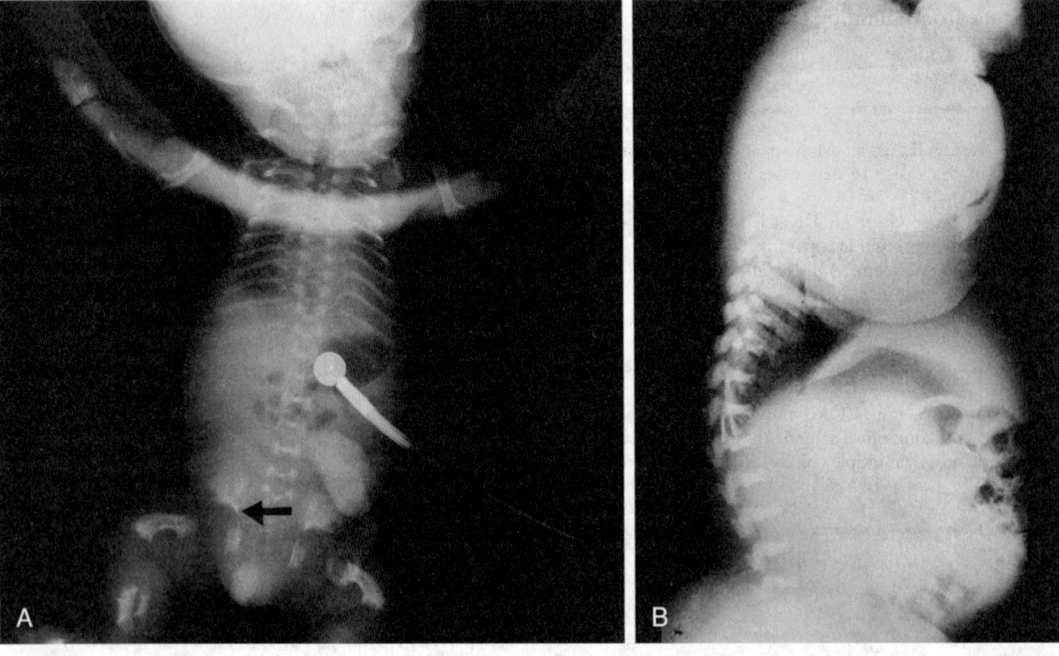

Figure 694-2. *A,* Neonatal radiograph of a child with thanatophoric dysplasia. Note medial acetabular spurs *(black arrow),* hypoplastic iliac bones, bowed femora with rounded protrusion of proximal femurs, hypoplastic thorax, and wafer-thin vertebral bodies. *B,* Lateral radiograph of the thoracolumbar spine in thanatophoric dysplasia, showing marked vertebral flattening and short ribs. Ossification defect of the central portion of the vertebral bodies is present.

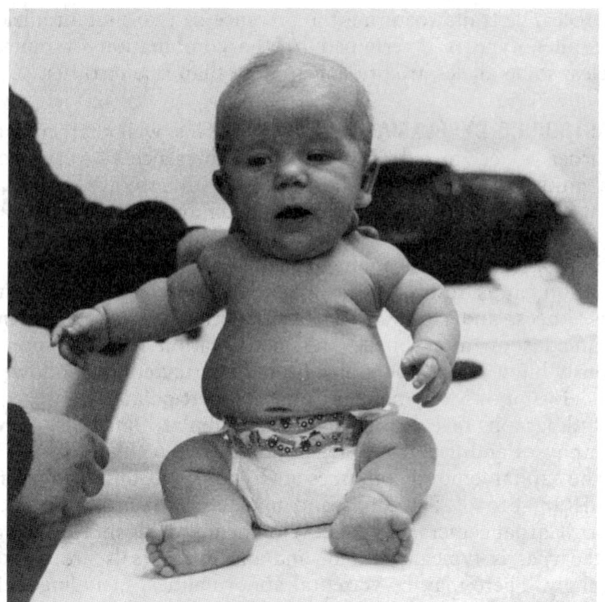

Figure 694-3. Infant with achondroplasia. The cranium is large and the forehead prominent. The nasal bridge is moderately flat, and the chest is small compared with the abdomen. Note medial arm and forearm creases, which reflect bowing at the sharpest concavity of the limbs.

display a trident configuration. Most joints are hyperextensible, but extension is restricted at the elbow. A thoracolumbar gibbus is often found. Usually, birth length is slightly less than normal but occasionally plots within the low-normal range.

Diagnosis. Skeletal radiographs confirm the diagnosis (Fig. 694-4). The calvarial bones are large, whereas the cranial base and facial bones are small. The vertebral pedicles are short throughout the spine as noted on a lateral radiograph. The interpedicular distance, which normally increases from the 1st to the 5th lumbar vertebra, decreases in achondroplasia. The iliac bones are short and round, and the acetabular roofs are flat. The tubular bones are short with mildly irregular and flared metaphyses. The fibula is disproportionately long compared with the tibia.

Clinical Manifestations. Infants usually exhibit delayed motor milestones, frequently not walking alone until 18–24 mo. This is due to hypotonia and mechanical difficulty balancing the large head on a normal-sized trunk and short extremities. Intelligence is normal unless central nervous system complications develop. As the child begins to walk, the gibbus usually gives way to an exaggerated lumbar lordosis.

Infants and children with achondroplasia progressively fall below normal standards for length and height. They can be plotted against standards established for achondroplasia. Adult heights typically range between 118 and 145 cm for males and between 112 and 136 cm for females. Surgical limb lengthening and human growth hormone treatment have been used to increase height; both are controversial.

Virtually all infants and children with achondroplasia have large heads, although only a fraction have true hydrocephalus. Head circumference should be carefully monitored using standards developed for achondroplasia, as should neurologic function in general. The spinal canal is stenotic, and spinal cord compression may occur at the foramen magnum and in the lumbar spine. The former usually presents in infants and small children; it may be associated with hypotonia, failure to thrive, quadriparesis, central and obstructive apnea, and sudden death. Surgical correction may be required for severe stenosis. Lumbar spinal stenosis usually does not present until early adulthood. Symptoms include paresthesias, numbness, and claudication in the legs. Loss of bladder and bowel control may be late complications.

Bowing of the legs is common and may need to be corrected surgically. Other common problems include dental crowding, articulation difficulties, obesity, and frequent episodes of otitis media, which may contribute to hearing loss.

Genetics. All patients with typical achondroplasia have mutations at *FGFR3* codon 380. The mutation maps to the transmembrane domain of the receptor and is thought to stabilize receptor dimers that enhance receptor signals, the consequences of which inhibit linear bone growth. Achondroplasia behaves as an autosomal dominant trait; most cases arise from a new mutation to normal parents.

Because of the high frequency of achondroplasia among dwarfing conditions, it is relatively common for adults with achondroplasia to marry. Such couples have a 50% risk of transmitting their condition, heterozygous achondroplasia, to each offspring, as well as a 25% risk of **homozygous achondroplasia.** The latter condition exhibits intermediate severity between thanatophoric dysplasia and heterozygous achondroplasia and is usually lethal in the newborn period. Prenatal diagnosis is available and has been used to diagnosis homozygous achondroplasia.

HYPOCHONDROPLASIA. Hypochondroplasia (OMIM 146000) resembles achondroplasia but is milder. Usually, it is not apparent until childhood, when mild short stature affecting the limbs becomes evident. Children have a stocky build and slight frontal bossing of the head. Radiographic changes are mild and consistent with the mild achondroplastic phenotype. Complications are rare; some patients are never diagnosed. Adult heights range from 116 to 146 cm. An *FGFR3* mutation at codon 540 has been found in many patients with hypochondroplasia. Genetic heterogeneity exists in hypochondroplasia, and other genetic loci are expected to be identified.

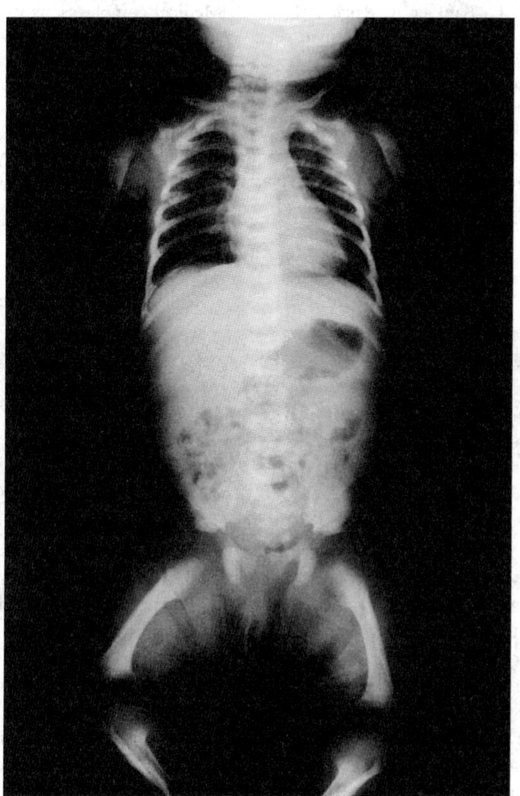

Figure 694-4. Radiograph of infant with achondroplasia, demonstrating interpedicular narrowing of the 1st through 5th lumbar vertebrae, short round iliac bones, and flat acetabular roofs. The tubular bones are short and show mild irregularities of the metaphyses.

JANSEN METAPHYSEAL DYSPLASIA

Jansen metaphyseal chondrodysplasia (OMIM 156400) is a rare, dominantly inherited chondrodysplasia characterized by severe shortening of limbs associated with an unusual facial appearance. Sometimes it is accompanied by clubfoot and hypercalcemia. At birth, a diagnosis can be made from these clinical findings and radiographs that show short tubular bones with characteristic metaphyseal abnormalities that include flaring, irregular mineralization, fragmentation, and widening of the physeal space. The epiphyses are normal.

The joints become enlarged and limited in mobility with age. Flexion contractures develop at the knees and hips, producing a bent-over posture. Intelligence is normal, although there may be hearing loss.

Jansen metaphyseal chondrodysplasia is caused by activating mutations of PTHR1. This G protein–coupled transmembrane receptor serves as a receptor for both PTH and PTHrP. Signaling through this receptor serves as a brake on the terminal differentiation of cartilage cells at a critical step in bone growth. Because the mutations activate the receptor, they enhance the braking effect and thereby slow bone growth. Loss of function mutations of PTHR1 are observed in Blomstrand chondrodysplasia, whose clinical features are the mirror image of Jansen metaphyseal chondrodysplasia.

American Academy of Pediatrics Committee on Genetics: Health supervision for children with achondroplasia. *Pediatrics* 1995;95:443–451.

Ho NC, Guarnieri M, Brant LJ, et al: Living with achondroplasia: Quality of life evaluation following cervico-medullary decompression. *Am J Med Genet* 2004;131:163–167.

Horton WA, Lunstrum GP: Fibroblast growth factor receptor 3 mutations in achondroplasia and related forms of dwarfism. *Rev Endocr Metab Disord* 2002;3:381–385.

Hunter AG, Bankier A, Rogers JG, et al: Medical complications of achondroplasia: A multicentre patient review. *J Med Genet* 1998;35:705–712.

Pauli RM, Horton VK, Glinski LP, et al: Prospective assessment of risks for cervicomedullary-junction compression in infants with achondroplasia. *Am J Hum Genet* 1995;56:732–744.

Schipani E, Langman CB, Parfitt AM, et al: Constitutively activated receptors for parathyroid hormone and parathyroid hormone-related peptide in Jansen's metaphyseal chondrodysplasia. *N Engl J Med* 1996;335:708–714.

Chapter 695 ■ Disorders Involving Ion Transporter

William A. Horton and Jacqueline T. Hecht

In order of decreasing severity, the disorders involving ion transporters include achondrogenesis type 1B, atelosteogenesis type II, and diastrophic dysplasia. They result from the functional loss of the sulfate ion transporter called diastrophic dysplasia sulfate transporter (DTDST), which is also referred to as SLC26A2 (solute carrier family 26, member 2). This protein transports sulfate ions into cells and is important for cartilage cells that add sulfate moieties to newly synthesized proteoglycans destined for cartilage extracellular matrix. Matrix proteoglycans are responsible for many of the properties of cartilage that allow it to serve as a template for skeletal development. The clinical manifestations result from defective sulfation of cartilage proteoglycans.

A number of mutant alleles have been found for the *DTDST* gene; they variably disturb transporter function. The disorders are recessive traits requiring the presence of two mutant alleles. The phenotype is determined by the combination of mutant alleles; some alleles are present in more than one disorder.

DIASTROPHIC DYSPLASIA (OMIM 22600). This well-characterized disorder is recognized at birth by the presence of very short extremities, clubfoot, and short hands with proximal displacement of the thumb producing a hitchhiker appearance (Fig. 695-1). The hands are usually deviated in an ulnar direction. Bony fusion of the metacarpophalangeal joints (symphalangism) is common, as is restricted movement of many joints, including hips, knees, and elbows. The external ears frequently become inflamed soon after birth. The inflammation resolves spontaneously but leaves the ears fibrotic and contracted ("cauliflower" ear deformity). Many newborns have a cleft palate.

Radiographs reveal short and broad tubular bones with flared metaphyses and flat, irregular epiphyses (Fig. 695-2).

The capital femoral epiphyses are hypoplastic, and the femoral heads are broad. The ulnae and fibulae are disproportionately short. Carpal centers may be developmentally advanced; the first metacarpal is typically ovoid, and the metatarsals are twisted medially. There may be vertebral abnormalities, including clefts

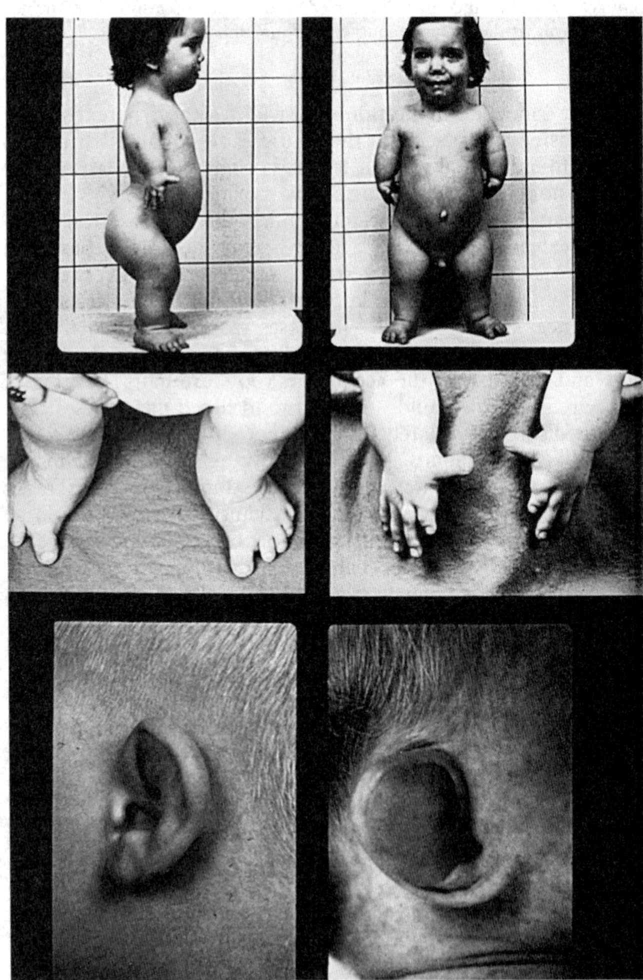

Figure 695-1. Child with diastrophic dysplasia. The extremities are dramatically shortened *(top)*. Clubfoot is commonly observed *(middle left)*. The fingers are short, especially the index finger; the thumb characteristically is proximally placed and has a hitchhiker appearance *(middle right)*. The upper helix of the ears becomes swollen 3–4 wk postnatally *(lower left)*, and this inflammation spontaneously resolves, leaving a cauliflower deformity of the pinnae *(lower right)*.

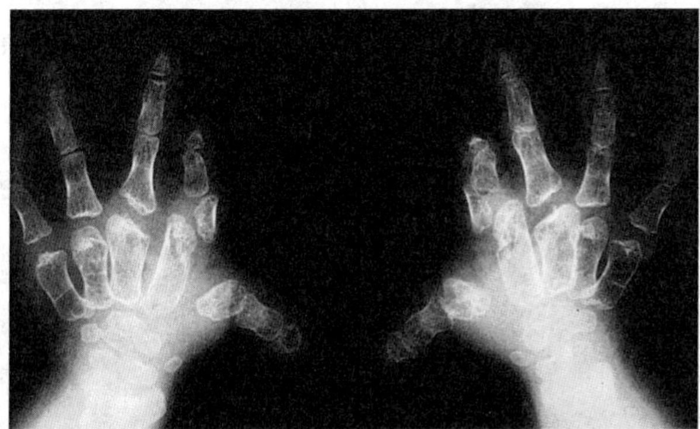

Figure 695-2. Radiograph of hands in diastrophic dysplasia. The metacarpals and phalanges are irregular and short. The first metacarpal is ovoid.

of cervical vertebral lamina and narrowing of the interpedicular distances in the lumbar spine.

Complications are primarily orthopedic and tend to be severe and progressive. The clubfoot deformity in the newborn resists usual treatments, and multiple corrective surgeries are common. Scoliosis typically develops during early childhood. It often requires multiple surgical procedures to control and sometimes compromises respiratory function in older children. Despite the orthopedic problems, patients typically have a normal life span and reach adult heights in the 105–130 cm range, depending on the severity of scoliosis. Growth curves are available for diastrophic dysplasia.

Some patients are mildly affected and exhibit slight short stature and joint contractures, no clubfoot or cleft palate, and correspondingly mild radiographic changes. The mild phenotype tends to recur within families. The recurrence risk of this autosomal recessive condition is 25%. Ultrasonographic examination can be employed for prenatal diagnosis, but if *DTDST* mutations can be identified in the patients or parents, molecular genetic diagnosis is possible.

ACHONDROGENESIS TYPE 1B (OMIM 600972) AND ATELOSTEOGENESIS TYPE II (OMIM 256050). Both of the conditions are rare recessive lethal chondrodysplasias. The most serious is achondrogenesis type 1B, which demonstrates a severe lack of skeletal development usually detected in utero or after a miscarriage. The limbs are extremely short, and the head is soft. Skeletal radiographs show poor to missing ossification of skull bones, vertebral bodies, fibulas, and ankle bones. The pelvis is hypoplastic, and the ribs are short. The femurs are short and exhibit a trapezoid shape with irregular metaphyses.

Infants with atelosteogenesis type II are stillborn or die soon after birth; prematurity is common. They exhibit very short limbs, especially the proximal segments. Clubfoot and dislocations of the elbows and knees may be detected. Hypoplasia of vertebral bodies, especially in the cervical and lumbar spine, is found on radiographs. The femora and humeri are hypoplastic and display a club-shaped appearance. The distal limb bones, including the ulna and fibula, are poorly ossified.

Both disorders carry a 25% recurrence risk and are potentially detectable in utero by mutation analysis if the mutant alleles are identified in the parents. Prenatal diagnosis should be possible with fetal ultrasonography.

Hall BD: Diastrophic dysplasia: Extreme variability within a sibship. *Am J Med Genet* 1996;63:28–33.

Makitie O, Kaitila I: Growth in diastrophic dysplasia. *J Pediatr* 1997;130:641–646.

Newbury-Ecob R: Atelosteogenesis type 2. *J Med Genet* 1998;35:49–53.

Rossi A, Superti-Furga A: Mutations in the diastrophic dysplasia sulfate transporter (DTDST) gene (SLC26A2): 22 novel mutations, mutation review, associated skeletal phenotypes, and diagnostic relevance. *Hum Mutat* 2001;17:159–171.

Chapter 696 ■ Disorders Involving Transcription Factors

William A. Horton and Jacqueline T. Hecht

There are three disorders involving transcription factors that result in bone dysplasias. One, campomelic dysplasia, is historically considered a chondrodysplasia. The other two, cleidocranial dysplasia and nail-patella syndrome, have been regarded as dysostoses, or abnormalities of single bones. The mutant genes that encode these transcription factors are *SOX9, CBFA1 (RUNX2),* and *LMX1B,* respectively, and are members of much larger gene families. For instance, *SOX9* is a member of the *SOX* family of genes related to the *SRY* (sex-determining region of the Y chromosome) gene; *CBFA1 (RUNX2)* belongs to the runt family of transcription factor genes, and *LMX1B* is one of the LIM homeodomain gene family. All three disorders are due to haploinsufficiency of the respective gene products; the disorders are dominant traits. For familial cases of cleidocranial dysplasia and nail-patella syndrome, prenatal diagnosis is possible if the mutations are identified. Campomelic dysplasia results from new mutational events and has a low risk of recurrence in subsequent pregnancies.

CAMPOMELIC DYSPLASIA. Apparent in newborn infants, campomelic dysplasia (OMIM 114290) is characterized by bowing of long bones (especially in the lower legs), short bones, respiratory distress, and other anomalies that include defects of the cervical spine, central nervous system, heart, and kidneys. Several cases of sex reversal of XY males have been reported. Radiographs confirm the bowing and often show hypoplasia of the scapulae and pelvic bones (Fig. 696-1). Affected infants usually

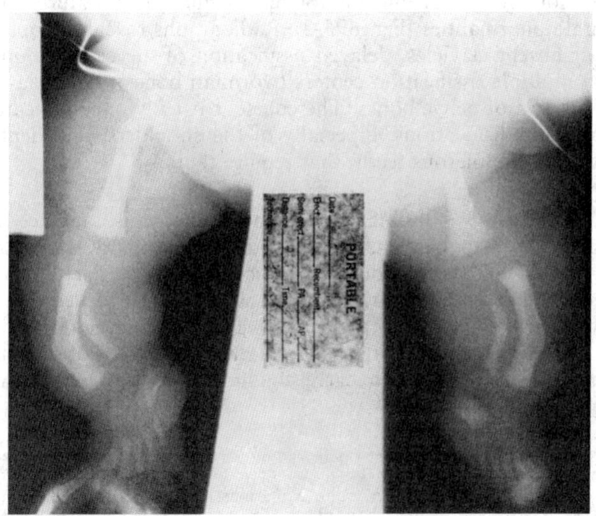

Figure 696-1. Radiograph of lower extremities of a child with campomelic dysplasia. Note bowed femurs, which are not particularly wide as compared with the thick bowed tibiae and fibulae.

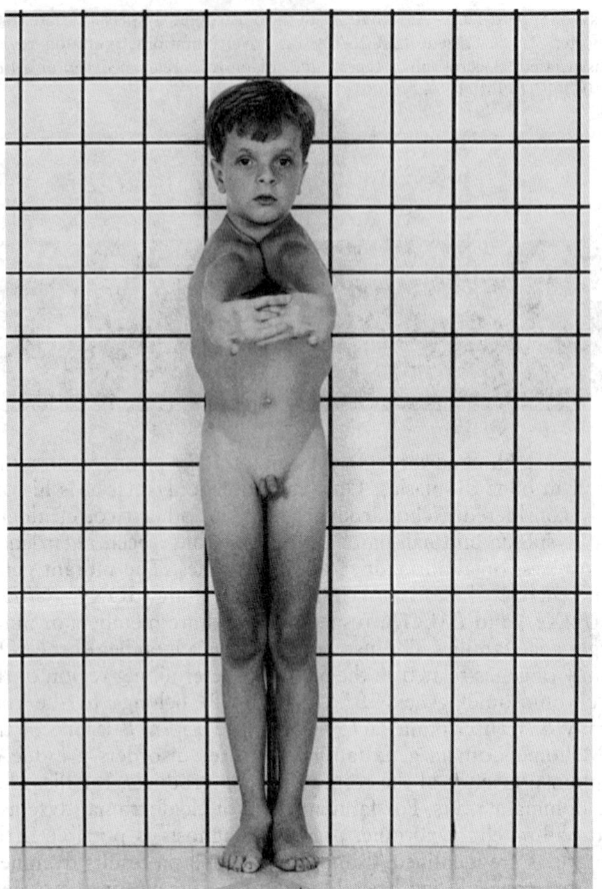

Figure 696-2. Cleidocranial dysplasia demonstrating approximation of the shoulder girdle in the midline. Note prominent high forehead and hypertelorism.

die of respiratory distress in the neonatal period. Complications in children and adolescents who survive include short stature with progressive kyphoscoliosis, recurrent apnea and respiratory infections, and learning difficulties.

CLEIDOCRANIAL DYSPLASIA. Cleidocranial dysplasia (OMIM 114290) is recognized in infants because of drooping shoulders, open fontanelles, prominent forehead, mild short stature, and dental abnormalities (Fig. 696-2). Radiographs reveal hypoplastic or absent clavicles, delayed ossification of the cranial bones with multiple ossification centers (wormian bones), and delayed ossification of pelvic bones. The course is usually uncomplicated except for dislocations, especially of the shoulders, and dental anomalies (numerous teeth) that require therapy.

NAIL-PATELLA SYNDROME. Dysplasia of the nails, absence or hypoplasia of the patella, abnormalities of the elbow, and spurs or "horns" extending from the iliac bones characterize the nail-patella syndrome (OMIM 119600), which is also called osteo-onychodysostosis. Some patients have nephritis that resembles chronic glomerulonephritis. There is a wide spectrum of severity; some patients present in early childhood, whereas others are asymptomatic as adults.

Dryer SD, Zhou G, Baldini A, et al: Mutations in *LMX1B* cause abnormal skeletal patterning and renal dysplasia in nail patella syndrome. *Nat Genet* 1998;19:47–50.

Mansour S, Offiah AC, McDowall S, et al: The phenotype of survivors of camptomelic dysplasia. *J Med Genet* 2002;39:597–602.

Meyer J, Sudbeck P, Held M, et al: Mutational analysis of the *SOX9* gene in camptomelic dysplasia and autosomal sex reversal: Lack of genotype/phenotype correlations. *Hum Mol Genet* 1997;6:91–98.

Mundlos S, Otto F, Mundlos C, et al: Mutations involving the transcription factor CBFA1 cause cleidocranial dysplasia. *Cell* 1997;89:773–779.

Chapter 697 ■ Disorders Involving Defective Bone Resorption

William A. Horton and Jacqueline T. Hecht

Bone dysplasias may display increased bone density; most are rare. Osteopetrosis, which has many subtypes, and pyknodysostosis, and probably others in this category of bone dysplasias, result from defective bone resorption.

OSTEOPETROSIS

Two main forms of osteopetrosis have been delineated: a severe, autosomal recessive form (OMIM 259700) and a mild, autosomal dominant form (OMIM 166600). Disturbances of osteoclast function due to mutations in a gene encoding an osteoclast-specific subunit of the vacuolar proton pump (TCIRG1) are found in most patients with the recessive form. Mutations of the gene encoding the chloride channel protein, CLCN7, are observed in the dominant form of osteopetrosis. Both types of mutations lead to disturbances of acidification needed for normal osteoclast function.

The severe form is usually detected in infancy or earlier because of macrocephaly, hepatosplenomegaly, deafness, blindness, and severe anemia. Radiographs reveal diffuse bone sclerosis. Later films show the characteristic bone within a bone appearance. With time, infants typically fail to thrive and show psychomotor delay and worsening of cranial neuropathies and anemia. Dental problems, osteomyelitis of the mandible, and pathologic fractures are common. The most severely affected patients die during infancy; less severely affected individuals rarely survive beyond the 2nd decade. Those who survive beyond infancy usually have learning disorders but may have normal intelligence despite hearing and visual loss.

CLINICAL MANIFESTATIONS. Most of the manifestations are due to failure to remodel growing bones. This leads to narrowing of cranial nerve foramina and encroachment on marrow spaces, which results in secondary complications, such as optic and facial nerve dysfunction, and anemia accompanied by compensatory extramedullary hematopoiesis in the liver and spleen.

The autosomal dominant form of osteopetrosis (Albers-Schönberg disease, osteopetrosis tarda, or marble bone disease) usually presents during childhood or adolescence with fractures and mild anemia and, less frequently, as cranial nerve dysfunction, dental abnormalities, or osteomyelitis of the mandible. Skeletal radiographs reveal a generalized increase in bone density and clubbing of metaphyses (Fig. 697-1). Alternating bands of lucent and dense bands produce a sandwich appearance to vertebral bodies. The radiographic changes are sometimes incidental findings in otherwise asymptomatic adolescents and adults.

TREATMENT. Some patients with severe osteopetrosis have responded to bone marrow transplantation. Calcitriol and inter-

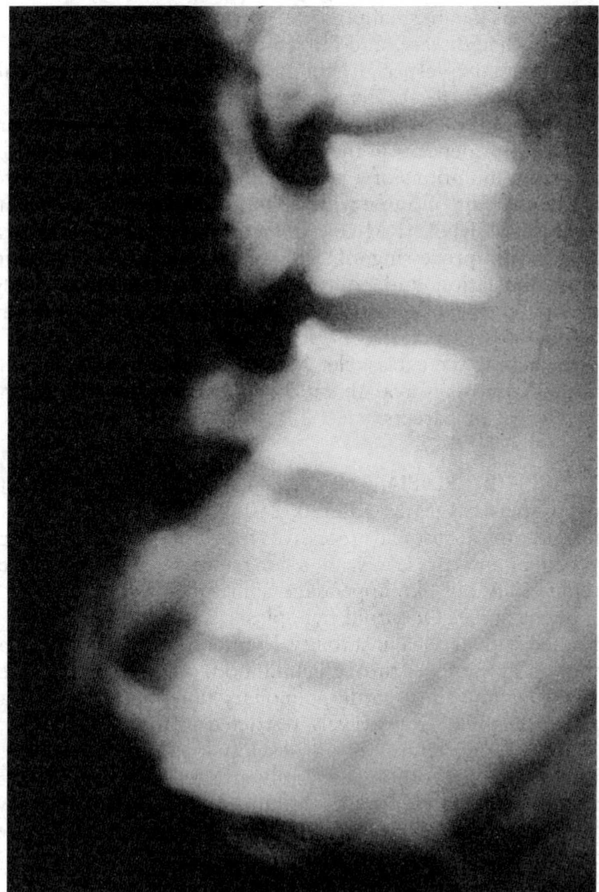

Figure 697-1. Lateral radiograph showing bone-in-bone appearance that is characteristic of osteopetrosis.

feron-γ have also been used with some benefit. Symptomatic care, such as dental care, transfusions for anemia, and antibiotic treatment of infections, is important for patients who survive infancy.

PYKNODYSOSTOSIS

An autosomal recessive bone dysplasia, pyknodysostosis (OMIM 265800) presents in early childhood as short limbs, characteristic facies, an open anterior fontanelle, a large skull with frontal and occipital bossing, and dental abnormalities. The hands and feet are short and broad, and the nails may be dysplastic. The sclerae may be blue. Minimal trauma often leads to fractures. Treatment is symptomatic and focused mainly on the management of dental problems and fractures. The prognosis is generally good, and patients typically reach heights of 130–150 cm.

Skeletal radiographs show a generalized increase in bone density. In contrast to many disorders in this group, the metaphyses are normal. Other changes include wide sutures and wormian bones in the skull, a small mandible, and hypoplasia of the distal phalanges.

Several mutations have been found in the gene encoding cathepsin K, a cysteine protease that is highly expressed in osteoclasts. The mutations predict loss of enzyme function, suggesting that there is an inability of osteoclasts to degrade bone matrix and remodel bones.

Charles JM, Key LL: Developmental spectrum of children with congenital osteopetrosis. *J Pediatr* 1998;132:371–374.

Gelb BD, Shi GP, Chapman HA, et al: Pycnodysostosis, a lysosomal disease caused by cathepsin K deficiency. *Science* 1996;273:1236–1238.

Gerritsen EJ, Vossen JM, Fasth A, et al: Bone marrow transplantation for autosomal recessive osteopetrosis: A report from the Working Party on Inborn Errors of the European Bone Marrow Transplantation Group. *J Pediatr* 1994;125:896–902.

Tolar J, Teitelbaum SL, Orchard PJ: Osteopetrosis, mechanisms of disease review. *N Engl J Med* 2004;351:2839–2849.

Chapter 698 ■ Disorders for Which Defects Are Poorly Understood or Unknown William A. Horton and Jacqueline T. Hecht

There are many chondrodysplasias, or chondrodysplasia clinical phenotypes, for which the genetic cause or basic mechanism is poorly understood or not known. Many illustrate features not found in other disorders and have historical significance in the evolution of chondrodysplasia nomenclature and classification.

ELLIS-VAN CREVELD SYNDROME. The Ellis-van Creveld syndrome (OMIM 225500), also known as chondroectodermal dysplasia, is a skeletal and an ectodermal dysplasia. The skeletal dysplasia presents at birth with short limbs, especially the middle and distal segments, accompanied by postaxial polydactyly of the hands and sometimes of the feet. Nail dysplasia and dental anomalies (including neonatal, absent, and premature loss of teeth and upper lip defects) constitute the ectodermal dysplasia. Common manifestations also include atrial septum defects and other congenital heart defects.

Skeletal radiographs reveal short tubular bones with clubbed ends, especially the proximal tibia and ulna (Fig. 698-1). Carpal bones display extra ossification centers and fusion; cone-shaped epiphyses are evident in the hands. A bony spur is often noted above the medial aspect of the acetabulum.

Ellis-van Creveld syndrome is an autosomal recessive trait that occurs most often in the Amish. Mutations have been identified in one of two genes, *EVC* and *EVC2*, which map very close to one another on chromosome 4p. The functions of the gene products are unknown. About 30% of patients die of cardiac or respiratory problems during infancy. Life span is otherwise normal; adult heights range from 109 to 152 cm.

ASPHYXIATING THORACIC DYSTROPHY. Asphyxiating thoracic dystrophy (OMIM 208500), or Jeune syndrome, is an autosomal recessive chondrodysplasia that resembles Ellis-van Creveld syndrome. Newborn infants present with a long, narrow thorax and respiratory insufficiency associated with pulmonary hypoplasia. Neonates often die. Other neonatal manifestations include slightly short limbs and postaxial polydactyly. The condition has been mapped to chromosome 15q13, but the identity of the locus is not known.

Skeletal radiographs show very short ribs with anterior expansion. Tubular limb bones are short with bulbous ends; cone-shaped epiphyses occur in hand bones. The iliac bones are short and square with a spur above the medial aspect of the acetabulum.

If infants survive the neonatal period, respiratory function usually improves as the rib cage grows. Surgery that produces lateral thoracic expansion improves rib growth and enhances chest wall dimensions. Progressive renal dysfunction frequently

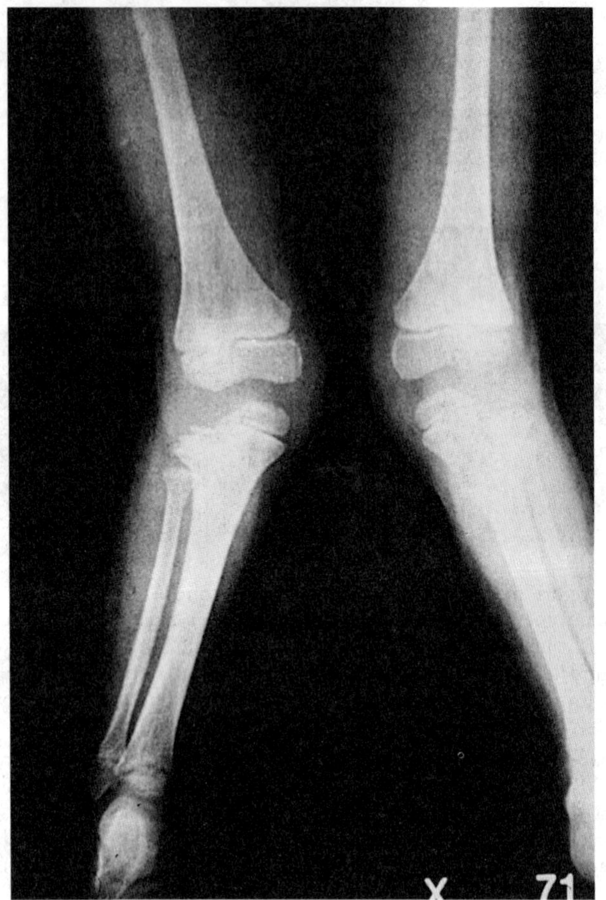

Figure 698-1. Radiograph of lower extremities in Ellis-van Creveld syndrome. Tubular bones are short, and proximal fibula is short. Ossification is retarded in lateral tibia epiphyses, causing a knock-knee deformity.

develops during childhood. Intestinal malabsorption and hepatic dysfunction have also been reported.

SHORT-RIB POLYDACTYLY SYNDROMES. Four types of short-rib polydactyly syndrome (types I–IV) (OMIM 263530, 263520, 263510, 269860) have been described. All are lethal in the newborn period. Neonates present with respiratory distress, an extremely small thorax, very short extremities, polydactyly, and a variety of nonskeletal defects. Radiographs demonstrate very short ribs and tubular bones with changes characteristic for each type. All four types are autosomal recessive traits.

CARTILAGE-HAIR HYPOPLASIA. Cartilage-hair hypoplasia (CHH) (OMIM 250250) is also known as metaphyseal chondrodysplasia–McKusick type. It is recognized during the 2nd year because of growth deficiency affecting the limbs, accompanied by flaring of the lower rib cage, a prominent sternum, and bowing of the legs. The hands and feet are short, and the fingers are very short with extreme ligamentous laxity. The hair is thin, sparse, and light colored, and nails are hypoplastic. The skin is hypopigmented.

Radiographs show short tubular bones with flared, irregularly mineralized, and cupped metaphyses (Fig. 698-2). The knees are more affected than are the hips, and the fibula is disproportionately longer than the tibia. The metacarpals and phalanges are short and broad. Spinal radiographs reveal mild platyspondyly.

Nonskeletal manifestations associated with CHH include immune deficiency (T-cell abnormalities, neutropenia, leukopenia, and susceptibility to chickenpox; children also may have complications from smallpox and polio vaccinations), malabsorption, celiac disease, and Hirschsprung disease. Adults are at risk of malignancy, especially skin tumors and lymphoma. Adults reach heights of 107–157 cm.

CHH shows autosomal recessive inheritance. Although rare, its highest prevalence is in the Amish and Finnish populations. It results from mutations of a gene coding for a large untranslated RNA component of an enzyme complex involved in processing mitochondrial RNA (RMRP). Loss of this gene product may interfere with processing of 5.8S ribosomal RNA, disturbing protein translation and control of mitosis. Although RMRP mutations are usually associated with typical CHH, they have occasionally been detected in patients with milder clinical phenotypes lacking the extraskeletal features characteristic of CHH. Prenatal diagnosis is available if the mutation is identified either in the patient or parents.

METATROPIC DYSPLASIA. There are at least two forms of metatropic dysplasia (OMIM 156530, 250600), an autosomal dominant and an autosomal recessive form. Regardless of type, newborn infants present with a long narrow trunk and short extremities. A tail-like appendage sometimes extends from the base of the spine. Odontoid hypoplasia is common and may be associated with cervical instability. Kyphoscoliosis appears in late infancy and progresses through childhood, often becoming severe enough to compromise cardiopulmonary function. The joints are large and become progressively restricted in mobility, except in the hands. Contractures often develop in the hips and knees during childhood. Although severely affected infants may die at a young age from respiratory failure, patients usually survive, although they may become disabled as adults from the progressive musculoskeletal deformities. Adult heights range from 110 to 120 cm.

Skeletal radiographs show characteristic changes dominated by severe platyspondyly and short tubular bones with expanded and

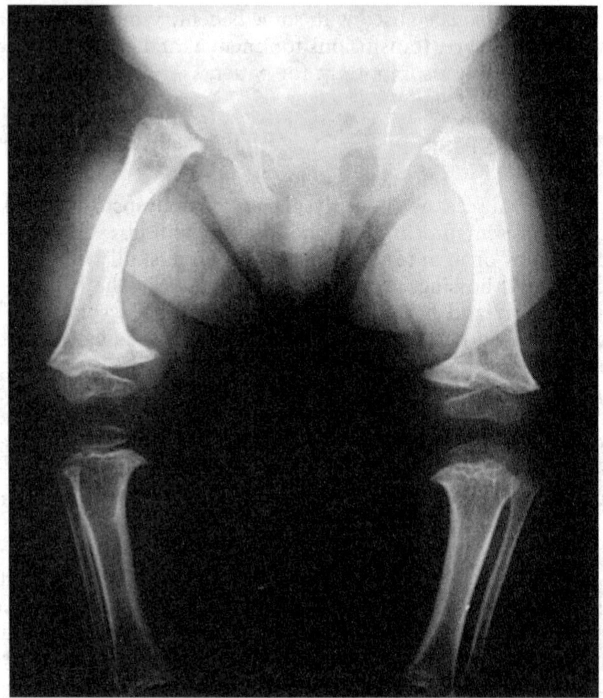

Figure 698-2. Radiograph of lower extremities in cartilage-hair hypoplasia. The tubular bones are short and the metaphyses are flared and irregular. The fibula is disproportionately long compared with the tibia. The femoral necks are short.

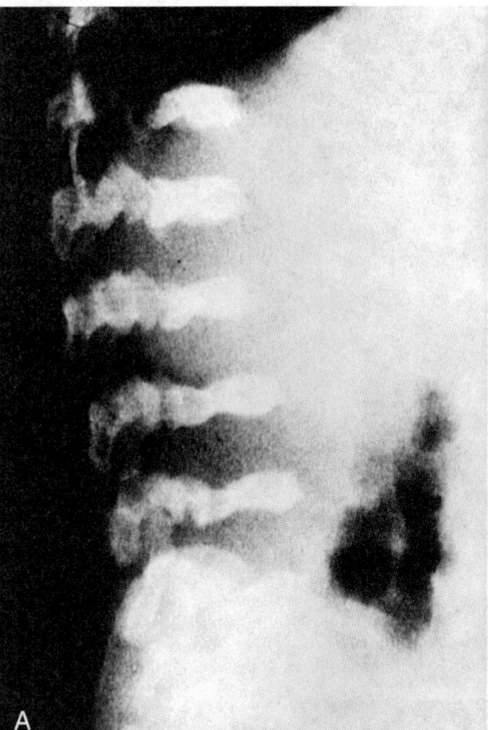
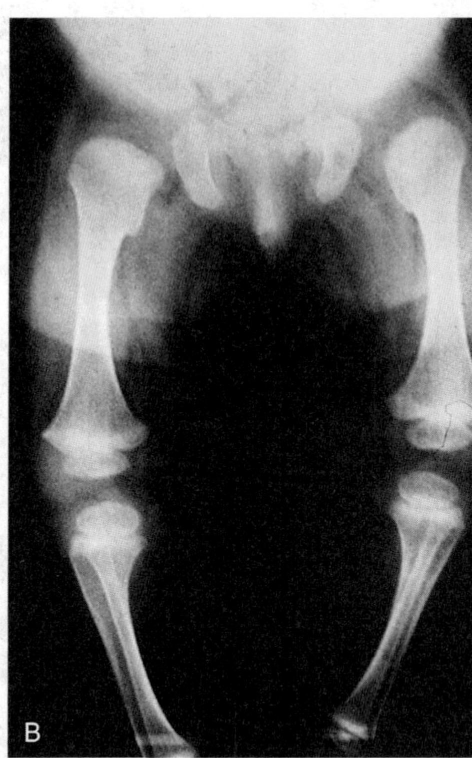

Figure 698-3. *A*, Radiograph of the lateral thoracolumbar spine in metatropic dysplasia showing severe platyspondyly. *B*, Radiograph of lower extremities in metatropic dysplasia showing short tubular bones with widened metaphyses. The femurs have a dumbbell appearance.

deformed metaphyses that exhibit a dumbbell appearance (Fig. 698-3). The pelvic bones are hypoplastic and exhibit a halberd appearance because of a small sacrosciatic notch and a notch above the lateral margin of the acetabulum.

SPONDYLOMETAPHYSEAL DYSPLASIA–KOZLOWSKI TYPE. The Kozlowski type of spondylometaphyseal dysplasia (OMIM 184252) presents in early childhood with mild short stature involving mostly the trunk and a waddling gait. The hands and feet may be short and stubby. Radiographs show flattening of vertebral bodies. The metaphyses of tubular bones are widened and irregularly mineralized, especially at the proximal femur. The pelvic bones manifest mild hypoplasia.

Scoliosis may develop during adolescence. The disorder is otherwise uncomplicated, and manifestations are limited to the skeleton. Adults reach heights of 130–150 cm. The Kozlowski type of spondylometaphyseal dysplasia is an autosomal dominant trait.

Mutations of genes encoding filamin A and filamin B proteins have been detected in diverse disorders of skeletal development: filamin A mutations in otopalatodigital syndromes type 1 and 2 frontometaphyseal dysplasia and Melnick-Needles syndrome (OMIM 311300, 304120, 305620, 309350); and filamin B mutations in Larsen syndrome and perinatal lethal ateosteogenesis types I and III (OMIM 150250, 108720, 108721). Filamins functionally connect extracellular to intracellular structural proteins, thereby linking cells to their local microenvironment, which is essential for skeletal development and growth.

JUVENILE OSTEOCHONDROSES. The juvenile osteochondroses are a heterogeneous group of disorders in which regional disturbances in bone growth cause noninflammatory arthropathies. They are summarized in Table 698-1. Some have localized pain and tenderness (Freiberg disease, Osgood-Schlatter disease, osteochondritis dissecans), whereas others present with painless limitation of joint movement (Legg-Calvé-Perthes disease, Scheuermann disease). Bone growth may be disrupted, leading to deformities. The diagnosis is usually confirmed radiographically, and treatment is symptomatic. The pathogenesis of these disorders is believed to involve ischemic necrosis of primary and secondary ossification centers. Although familial forms have been reported, these disorders usually occur sporadically.

CAFFEY DISEASE (INFANTILE CORTICAL HYPEROSTOSIS. This is a rare disorder of unknown etiology characterized by cortical hyperostosis with inflammation of the contiguous fascia and muscle. It is often sporadic, but both autosomal dominant and autosomal recessive inheritance have been reported. In three unrelated families with autosomal dominant inheritance, a linkage to mutations of the *COL1A1* gene (codes for the α_1 chain of type I collagen) has been reported.

Prenatal and more often postnatal onset have been described. Prenatal onset may be mild (autosomal dominant) or severe (autosomal recessive). Severe prenatal disease is characterized by typical bone lesions, polyhydramnios, hydrops fetalis, severe respiratory distress, prematurity, and high mortality. Onset in infancy (<6 mo, average 10 wk) is most common; manifestations include the sudden onset of irritability, swelling of contiguous soft tissue that precedes the cortical thickening of the underlying bones, fever, and anorexia. The swelling is painful with a wood-like induration but with minimal warmth or redness; suppuration is absent. There are unpredictable remissions and relapses; an episode may last 2 wk to 3 mo. The most common bones

TABLE 698-1. Juvenile Osteochondroses

EPONYM	AFFECTED REGION	AGE AT PRESENTATION
Legg-Calvé-Perthes disease	Capital femoral epiphysis	3–12 yr
Osgood-Schlatter disease	Tibial tubercle	10–16 yr
Sever disease	Os calcaneus	6–10 yr
Freiberg disease	Head of second metatarsal	10–14 yr
Scheuermann disease	Vertebral bodies	Adolescence
Blount disease	Medial aspect of proximal tibial epiphysis	Infancy or adolescence
Osteochondritis dissecans	Subchondral regions of knee, hip, elbow, and ankle	Adolescence

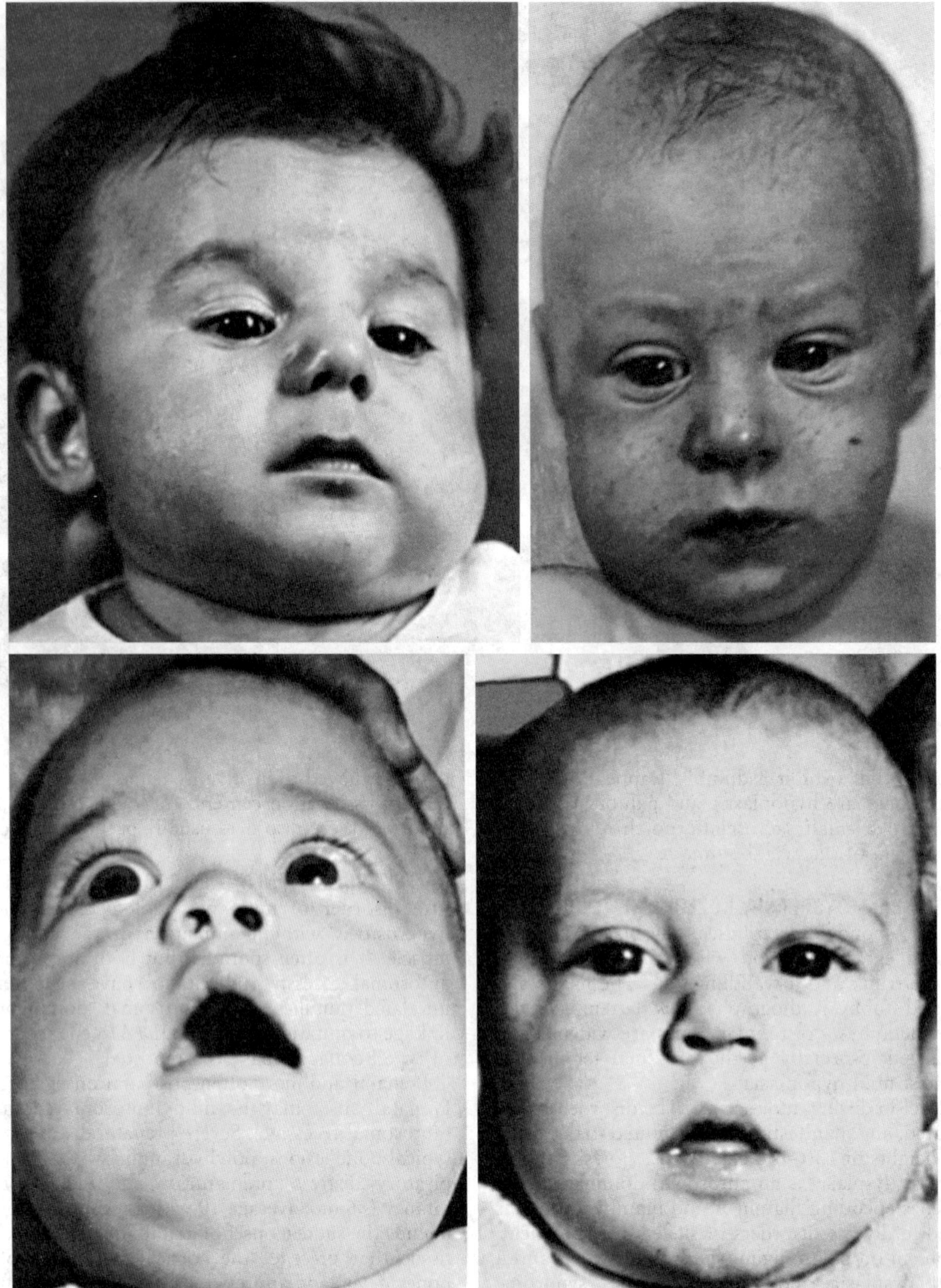

Figure 698-4. Facies in infantile cortical hyperostosis. In almost all cases, the changes have appeared before the 5th month of life. Unilateral swelling of the left cheek and left side of the jaw in an infant 12 wk of age. (From Kuhn JP, Slovis TL, Haller JO: *Caffey's Pediatric Diagnostic Imaging,* 10th ed., vol. 2, Philadelphia, Mosby, 2004, p 2363.)

involved include the mandible (75%) (Fig. 698-4), the clavicle, and the ulnar. If swelling is not prominent or visible, the diagnosis may not be evident.

Laboratory features include elevated erythrocyte sedimentation rate and serum alkaline phosphatase as well as in some patients increased serum prostaglandin E levels. There may be thrombocytosis and anemia. The **radiographic features** include soft-tissue swelling and calcification and cortical hyperostosis (Fig. 698-5). All bones may be affected except the phalanges or vertebral bodies. The **differential diagnosis** includes other causes of hyperostosis such as chronic vitamin A intoxication, prolonged prostaglandin E infusion in children with ductal dependent congenital heart disease, primary bone tumors, and scurvy.

Complications are unusual but include pseudoparalysis with limb or scapula involvement, pleural effusions (rib), torticollis (clavicle), mandibular asymmetry, bone fusion (ribs or ulna-radius), and bone angulation deformities (common with severe prenatal onset).

Treatment includes indomethacin and prednisone if there is a poor response to indomethacin.

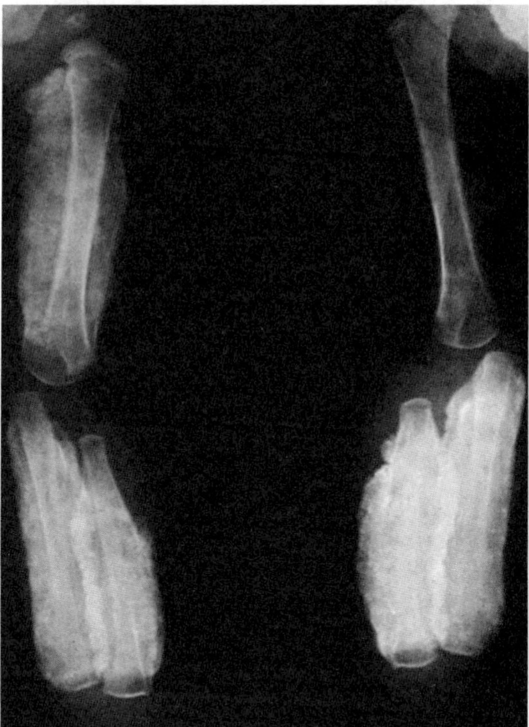

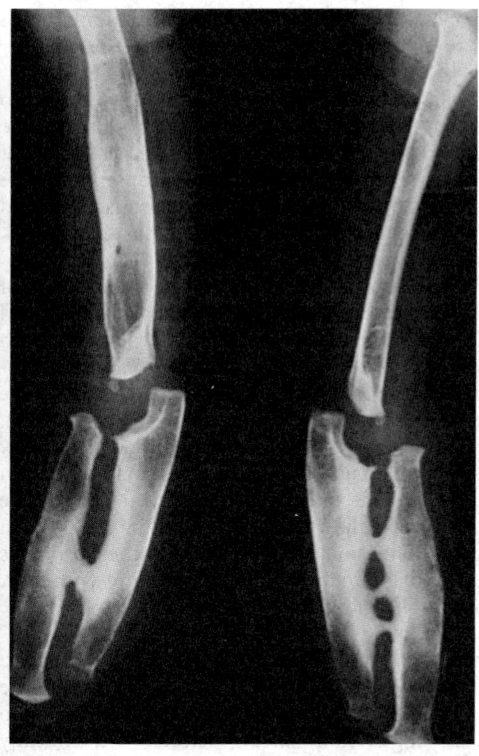

Figure 698-5. Residual bony bridges between each radius and ulna in infantile cortical hyperostosis. *A,* Massive cortical thickenings of the radii and ulnas at 4½ mo of age. Pressure from the external thickenings has forced the radial heads laterad out of the elbows. *B,* At 12½ mo, 9 mo after onset, all affected bones are still greatly swollen, owing largely to expansion of the medullary cavities, although there are still residues of the earlier cortical thickening. The radial heads are still dislocated, and the radial diaphyses are now anchored in this ectopic position by solid bony bridges between them and the ulnar diaphyses, a single bridge on the right and three on the left. At 32 mo, these bridges were still intact, although they had diminished slightly in caliber. It is possible that these bony bridges represent ossification of parts of the interosseous membrane. (From Kuhn JP, Slovis TL, Haller JO: *Caffey's Pediatric Diagnostic Imaging,* 10th ed., vol. 2, Philadelphia, Mosby, 2004, p 2365.)

Beck M, Roubicek M, Rogers JG, et al: Heterogeneity of metatropic dysplasia. *Eur J Pediatr* 1983;140:231–237.

da Silva EO, Janovitz D, de Albuquerque SC: Ellis-van Creveld syndrome: Report of 15 cases in an inbred kindred. *J Med Genet* 1980;17:349–356.

Davis JT, Long FR, Adler BH, et al: Lateral thoracic expansion for Jeune syndrome: Evidence of rib healing and new bone formation. *Ann Thorac Surg* 2004;77:445–448.

Glorieux FH: Caffey disease: An unlikely collagenopathy. *J Clin Invest* 2005;115:1142–1144.

Hall CM, Elcioglu NH: Metatropic dysplasia lethal variants. *Pediatr Radiol* 2004:34:66–74.

Krakow D, Robertson SP, King LM, et al: Mutations in the gene encoding filamin B disrupt vertebral segmentation, joint formation and skeletogenesis. *Nat Genet* 2004;36:405–410.

Makitie O, Sulisalo T, de la Chapelle A, et al: Cartilage-hair hypoplasia. *J Med Genet* 1995;32:39–43.

Restrepo S, Sanchez AM, Palacios E: Infantile cortical hyperostosis of the mandible. *Ear Nose Throat J* 2004;83:454–455.

Ridanpaa M, van Eenennaam H, Pelin K, et al: Mutations in the RNA component of RNase MRP cause a pleiotropic human disease, cartilage-hair hypoplasia. *Cell* 2001;104:195–203.

Ruiz-Perez VL, Ide SE, Strom TM, et al: Mutations in a new gene in Ellis-van Creveld syndrome and Weyers acrodental dysostosis. *Nat Genet* 2000;24:283–286.

Schweiger S, Chaoui R, Tennstedt C, et al: Antenatal onset of cortical hyperostosis (Caffey disease): Case report and review. *Am J Med Genet* 2003;120A:547–552.

Sharrard WJW: Abnormalities of the epiphyses and limb inequality. In Sharrard WJW (editor): *Paediatric Orthopaedics and Fracture,* 3rd ed. Oxford, Blackwell Scientific Publications, 1993, p 719.

Chapter 699 ■ Osteogenesis Imperfecta

Joan C. Marini

Osteoporosis, a feature of both inherited and acquired disorders, classically demonstrates fragility of the skeletal system and a susceptibility to fractures of the long bones or vertebral compressions from mild or inconsequential trauma. Osteogenesis imperfecta (OI) (brittle bone disease), the most common genetic cause of osteoporosis, is a generalized disorder of connective tissue. The spectrum of OI is extremely broad, ranging from a form that is lethal in the perinatal period to a mild form in which the diagnosis may be equivocal in an adult.

ETIOLOGY. Structural or quantitative defects in type I collagen cause the full clinical spectrum of OI. Type I collagen is the primary component of the extracellular matrix of bone and skin. Ten percent of cases clinically indistinguishable from OI do not have a molecular defect in type I collagen. Some of these cases have biochemically normal collagen and probably represent genetic heterogeneity. Other cases have overmodified collagen and severe/lethal OI-like bone dysplasia. These cases are caused by recessive null mutations in a collagen modifying enzyme, prolyl 3-hydroxylase 1 (coded by the *LEPRE1* gene on chromosome 1p34.1) or its associated protein, CRTAP.

EPIDEMIOLOGY. OI is an autosomal dominant disorder that occurs in all racial and ethnic groups. The incidence of OI that is detectable in infancy is about 1/20,000. There is a similar incidence of the mild form OI type I.

PATHOLOGY. The collagen structural mutations cause OI bone to be globally abnormal. The bone matrix contains abnormal type I collagen fibrils and relatively increased levels of types III and V collagen. In addition, several noncollagenous proteins of bone matrix are also reduced. The hydroxyapatite crystals deposited on this matrix are poorly aligned with the long axis of fibrils.

PATHOGENESIS. Type I collagen is a heterotrimer, composed of two α1(I) chains and one α2(I) chain. The chains are synthesized as procollagen molecules with short globular extensions on both ends of the central helical domain. The helical domain is composed of uninterrupted repeats of the sequence Gly-X-Y, where Gly is glycine, X is often proline, and Y is often hydroxyproline. The presence of glycine at every 3rd residue is crucial to helix formation because its small side chain can be accommodated in the spatial constraints of the interior of the helical trimer. The chains are assembled into helices using crucial alignment sites in the carboxyl-terminal extension. Helix formation then proceeds linearly in a carboxyl to amino direction. Concomitant with helix assembly and formation, the chains are glycosylated at lysine residues.

The collagen structural defects are predominantly of two types: 80% are point mutations causing substitutions of helical glycine residues or crucial residues in the C-propeptide by other amino acids, and 20% are single exon splicing defects. The clinically mild OI type I has a quantitative defect with null mutations in one α1(I) allele. These patients make a reduced amount of normal collagen.

The glycine substitutions in the two α chains have distinct genotype-phenotype relationships. One third of mutations in the α1 chain are lethal, especially substitutions with charged or branched side chains that disrupt helix stability. Two uniformly lethal regions in the carboxyl third of α1(I) align with major ligand binding regions of the collagen helix. Glycine substitutions in α2(I) are predominantly nonlethal. Lethal mutations occur in eight regularly spaced regions along the chain that align with binding regions for matrix proteoglycans at the level of the higher order matrix structure of collagen, the fibril.

Classical OI is an autosomal dominant disorder. Some familial recurrences of OI are caused by parental mosaicism for dominant collagen mutations. A small percentage of OI-like cases are recessive defects in the complex of proteins responsible for prolyl 3-hydroxylation of type I collagen.

CLINICAL MANIFESTATIONS. OI has the triad of fragile bones, blue sclerae, and early deafness. OI was once divided into "congenita," the forms detectable at birth, and "tarda," the forms detectable later in childhood; this did not account for the variability of OI. The Sillence classification divides OI into four types based on clinical and radiographic criteria. Additional types have been proposed based on histologic distinctions.

Osteogenesis Imperfecta Type I (Mild). This form is sufficiently mild that it is often found in large pedigrees. Many type I families have blue sclerae, recurrent fractures in childhood, and presenile hearing loss (30–60%). Both types I and IV are divided into A and B subtypes, depending on the absence (A) or presence (B) of **dentinogenesis imperfecta.** Other possible connective tissue abnormalities include easy bruising, joint laxity, and mild short stature compared with family members. Fractures result from mild to moderate trauma and decrease after puberty.

Osteogenesis Imperfecta Type II (Perinatal Lethal). These infants may be stillborn or die in the 1st yr of life. Birthweight and length are small for gestational age. There is extreme fragility of the skeleton and other connective tissues. There are multiple intrauterine fractures of long bones, which have a crumpled appearance on radiographs. There are striking micromelia and bowing of extremities; the legs are held abducted at right angles to the body in the "frog-leg position." Multiple rib fractures create a beaded appearance and the small thorax contributes to respiratory insufficiency. The skull is large for body size with enlarged anterior and posterior fontanelles. Sclerae are dark blue-gray.

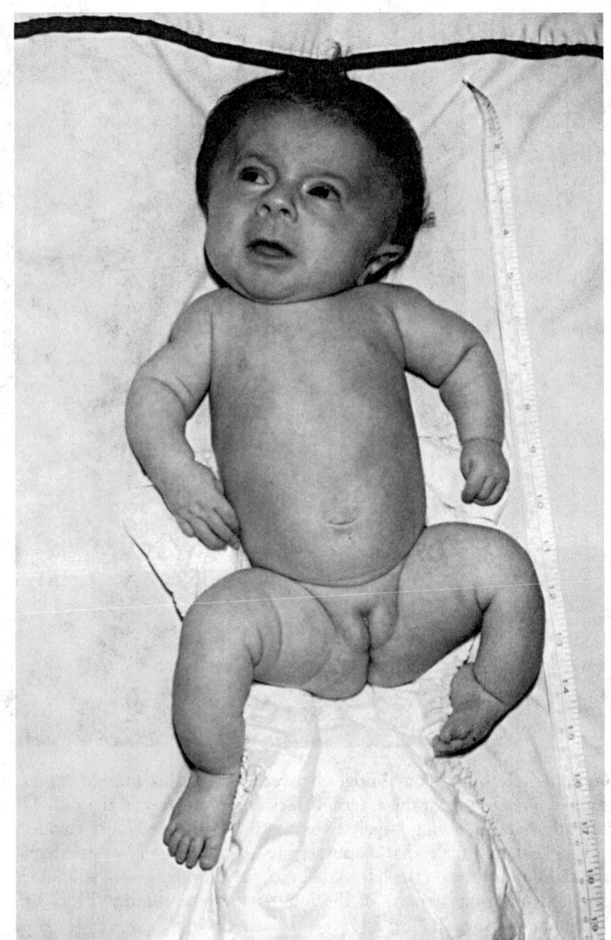

Figure 699-1. Infant with type III osteogenesis imperfecta displays shortened bowed extremities, thoracic deformity, and relative macrocephaly.

Osteogenesis Imperfecta Type III (Progressive Deforming). This is the most severe nonlethal form of OI and results in significant physical disability. Birthweight and length are often low normal. Fractures usually occur in utero. There is relative macrocephaly and triangular facies (Fig. 699-1). Postnatally, fractures occur from inconsequential trauma and heal with deformity. Disorganization of the bone matrix results in a "popcorn" appearance at the metaphyses (Fig. 699-2). The rib cage has flaring at the base, and pectal deformity is frequent. Virtually all type III patients have scoliosis and vertebral compression. Growth falls below the curve by the 1st year; all type III patients have extreme short stature. Scleral hue ranges from white to blue.

Osteogenesis Imperfecta Type IV (Moderately Severe). Patients with OI type IV may present at birth with in utero fractures or bowing of lower long bones. They may also present with recurrent fractures after ambulation. Most children have moderate bowing even with infrequent fractures. Children with OI type IV require orthopedic and rehabilitation intervention, but they are usually able to attain community ambulation skills. Fracture rates decrease after puberty. Radiographically, they are osteoporotic and have metaphyseal flaring and vertebral compressions. Patients with type IV have moderate short stature. Scleral hue may be blue or white.

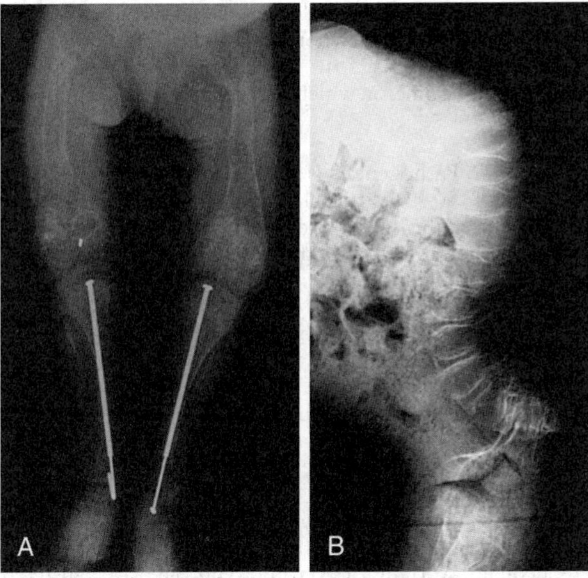

Figure 699-2. Typical features of type III osteogenesis imperfecta radiographs in a 6 yr old child. *A,* Lower long bones are osteoporotic, with metaphyseal flaring, "popcorn" formation at growth plates, and placement of intramedullary rods. *B,* Vertical bodies are compressed and osteoporotic.

Osteogenesis Imperfecta Type V (Hyperplastic Callus), Type VI (Mineralization Defect), and Type VII (Autosomal Recessive). There has been a proposal to distinguish as distinct types small groups of patients who clinically have OI type IV, but have distinct findings on bone biopsy. They constitute about 5% of OI populations and have negative collagen mutation screening. Type V patients also have hyperplastic callus, calcification of the interosseous membrane of the forearm, and a radiodense metaphyseal band. Type VII maps to chromosome 3p22–24 and is a hypomorphic defect of CRTAP.

LABORATORY FINDINGS. The diagnosis is confirmed by collagen biochemical studies or sequencing of cDNA using fibroblasts cultured from a skin punch biopsy, or by direct sequencing of DNA from leukocytes. Mutations in the amino third of the collagen chains are not detectable by the biochemical tests because they do not cause significant overmodification of chains. In OI type I, the reduced amount of type I collagen results in an increase in the type III : type I collagen ratio detected by protein electrophoresis. Identification of point mutations by sequencing facilitates family screening and prenatal detection.

Severe OI can be detected prenatally by level II ultrasonography as early as 16 wk of gestation. OI and thanatophoric dysplasia may be confused. Fetal ultrasonography may not detect OI type IV and rarely detects OI type I. For recurrent cases, chorionic villus biopsy can be used for biochemical or molecular studies. Amniocytes produce false-positive biochemical studies but can be used for molecular studies in appropriate cases.

In the neonatal period, the normal to elevated alkaline phosphatase levels present in OI distinguish it from hypophosphatasia.

COMPLICATIONS. The morbidity and mortality of OI are cardiopulmonary. Recurrent pneumonias and declining pulmonary function occur in childhood, and cor pulmonale is seen in adults.

Neurologic complications include basilar invagination, brainstem compression, hydrocephalus, and syringohydromyelia. Most children with OI types III and IV have basilar invagination, but brainstem compression is infrequent. Basilar invagination is best detected with spiral CT of the craniocervical junction (Fig. 699-3).

TREATMENT. There is no cure for OI. For severe nonlethal OI, active physical rehabilitation in the early years allows children to attain a higher functional level than does orthopedic management alone. Children with OI type I and some with type IV are spontaneous ambulators. Children with type III and severe type IV benefit from long-leg plastic braces, gait aids, and a program of swimming and conditioning. Severely affected individuals require a wheelchair for community mobility but can acquire transfer and self-care skills. Teens with OI may require psychologic support with body image issues.

Orthopedic management of OI is aimed at fracture management and correction of deformity to enable function. Fractures should be promptly splinted or cast; OI fractures heal well, and cast removal should be aimed at minimizing immobilization osteoporosis. Correction of deformity of the long bones requires an osteotomy procedure and placement of an intramedullary rod.

Treatments with calcium or fluoride supplements or calcitonin do not improve OI. Growth hormone improves bone histology in growth-responsive children (usually types I and IV). A short course of treatment of children with OI with bisphosphonates (IV pamidronate or oral olpadronate) confers some benefits. Bisphosphonates decrease bone resorption by osteoclasts; OI patients will have increased bone volume that still contains the defective collagen. Bisphosphonates are more beneficial for vertebrae (trabecular bone) than long bones (cortical bone). Treatment for 1–2 yr results in increased L1-4 DEXA and, more importantly, improved vertebral compressions and area, which may prevent or delay the scoliosis of OI. Relative risk of long bone fractures is modestly decreased. However, the material properties of long bones are weakened by prolonged treatment and nonunion after osteotomy is increased. There is no effect of bisphosphonates on mobility scores, muscle strength, or bone pain. Limiting treatment duration to 2–3 yr in mid-childhood may maximize benefits and minimize detriment to cortical material properties. Benefits appear to persist several years after the treatment interval. Side effects include abnormal long bone remodeling, osteonecrosis of the jaw, and osteopetrotic-like brittleness to bone.

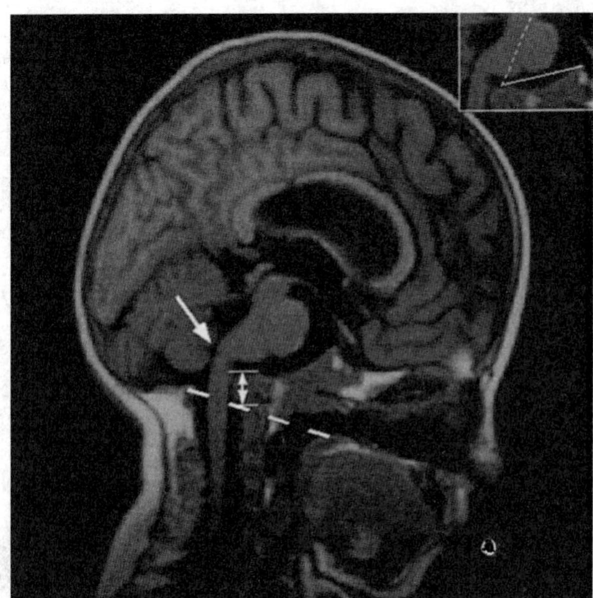

Figure 699-3. Typical feature of basilar invagination shown in the sagittal MRI of an asymptomatic child with type III osteogenesis imperfecta. There is invagination of the odontoid above the Chamberlain line causing compression and kinking at the pontomedullary junction *(arrow).*

PROGNOSIS. OI is a chronic condition that limits both life span and functional level. Infants with OI type II usually die within months to a year of life. An occasional child with radiographic type II and extreme growth deficiency may survive to the teen years. Persons with OI type III have a reduced life span with clusters of mortality from pulmonary causes in early childhood, the teen years, and the 40s. OI types I and IV are compatible with a full life span.

Individuals with OI type III are usually wheelchair dependent. With aggressive rehabilitation, they may attain transfer skills and household ambulation. OI type IV children usually attain community ambulation skills either independently or with gait aids.

GENETIC COUNSELING. OI is an autosomal dominant disorder, and the risk of an affected individual passing the gene to his or her offspring is 50%. An affected child usually has about the same severity of OI as the parent; however, there is variability of expression and the child's condition can be either more or less severe than that of the parent.

The recurrence risk to an apparently unaffected couple of having a second child with OI is empirically noted to be 5–7%; this is the statistical chance that one parent has a germ line mosaicism. The collagen mutation in the unaffected parent is present in some germ cells and may be present in somatic tissues. If genetic testing reveals that a parent is a mosaic carrier, the risk of recurrence may be as high as 50%.

Antoniazzi F, Bertoldo F, Mottes M, et al: Growth hormone treatment in osteogenesis imperfecta with quantitative defect of type I collagen synthesis. *J Pediatr* 1996;129:432–439.

Barnes AM, Chang W, Morello R, et al: Deficiency of cartilage-associated protein in recessive lethal osteogenesis imperfecta. *N Engl J Med* 2006; 355:2757–2764.

Cabral WA, Chang W, Barnes AM, et al: Prolyl 3-hydroxylase 1 deficiency causes a recessive metabolic bone disorder resembling lethal/severe osteogenesis imperfecta. *Nat Genet* 2007;39:359–365.

Glorieux FH, Rauch F, Plotkin H, et al: Type V osteogenesis imperfecta: A new form of brittle bone disease. *J Bone Miner Res* 2000;15:1650–1658.

Glorieux FH, Rauch F, Ward LM, et al: Alendronate in the treatment of pediatric osteogenesis imperfecta. *J Bone Miner Res* 2004;19(Suppl 1):S12.

Glorieux FH, Ward LM, Rauch F, et al: Osteogenesis imperfecta type VI: A form of brittle bone disease with a mineralization defect. *J Bone Miner Res* 2002;17:30–38.

Letocha A, Cintas HL, Troendle JF, et al: Controlled trial of pamidronate in children with types III and IV osteogenesis imperfecta confirms vertebral gains but not short-term functional improvement. *J Bone Miner Res* 2005;20:977–986.

Marini JC: Should children with osteogenesis imperfecta be treated with bisphosphonates? *Nat Clin Prac Endo & Metab* 2006;2:14–15.

Marini JC, Hopkins E, Glorieux FH, et al: Positive linear growth and bone responses to growth hormone treatment in children with types III and IV osteogenesis imperfecta. *J Bone Miner Res* 2003;18:237–243.

Plotkin H, Rauch F, Bishop NJ: Pamidronate treatment of severe osteogenesis imperfecta in children under 3 years of age. *J Clin Endocrinol Metab* 2000;85:1846–1850.

Sakkers R, Kok D, Engelbert R, et al: Skeletal effects and functional outcome with olpadronate in children with osteogenesis imperfecta: A 2-year randomized placebo-controlled study. *Lancet* 2004;363:1427–1431.

Chapter 700 ■ Marfan Syndrome

Luther K. Robinson and Emily Fitzpatrick

Marfan syndrome is an autosomal dominantly inherited disorder with nearly complete penetrance but variable expressivity. The incidence of this disorder is about 1 per 5,000–10,000 births; nearly 30% of affected newborns represent sporadically occurring new mutations. Diagnosis of Marfan syndrome is based on clinical findings, some of which are age and maturation dependent.

PATHOGENESIS. Pathogenesis is related to abnormal biosynthesis of fibrillin-1, a 350-kD extracellular protein that is the major constituent of microfibrils that provide the scaffolding network of elastin and have an anchoring function in nonelastic tissue such as aortic adventitae and the suspensory ligament of the eye. The fibrillin-1 *(FBN1)* locus resides within the long arm of chromosome 15 (15q21). The gene is composed of 65 exons, and to date, >600 mutations distributed throughout *FBN1* have been described, each appearing to be unique to a given family. The relatively even distribution of mutations throughout *FBN1* likely contributes to the phenotypic variability of the disorder. However, phenotype-genotype correlations are not always obvious and there is significant intrafamily variability suggesting that epigenetic, modifier gene, or environmental factors influence the expression of the disease. Mutations associated with the more severe neonatal variant of Marfan syndrome are clustered at exons 26–27 and 31–32. Mutations in exons 59–65 may be associated with milder disease in 40% of patients who also do not manifest aortic pathology.

Fibrillin regulation of transforming growth factor-ß may also play a role in the spectrum of the manifestations of Marfan syndrome. Indeed patients with heterozygous mutations of the transforming growth factor-ß receptor have Marfan-like manifestations with a normal fibrillin gene. The resulting syndrome (**Loeys-Dietz aneurysm syndrome**) has many features of Marfan syndrome plus wide spaced eyes, cleft uvula, and more aggressive vascular disease including tortuous arteries, as well as aortic rupture at smaller aortic sizes than seen in Marfan syndrome.

CLINICAL MANIFESTATIONS. The diagnosis of Marfan syndrome is based on the overall pattern of malformation (typically skeletal, cardiovascular, ocular); many manifestations are age or maturation dependent. Tall stature may be present at birth and persist to adulthood. Diminished subcutaneous fat may suggest failure to thrive in early infancy. Hypotonia and ligamentous laxity may suggest developmental delays, but cognitive performance is normal for family.

Neonatal (infantile, congenital) Marfan syndrome is more severe than cases observed in older children and may have clinical similarity to congenital contractural arachnodactyly, presenting with hypotonia, arachnodactyly, joint laxity and dislocations, and flexion contractures. The face is long and the skin is lax with diminished recoil. The ears may appear large and pliant. Ocular examination may disclose megalocornea, iridodonesis, or frank lens dislocation. Cardiac examination often reveals murmurs of either mitral valve prolapse (MVP) with regurgitation or aortic insufficiency, and aortic root dilatation may be documented echocardiographically.

Older individuals display tall stature and a long, thin face with narrowness of the maxilla and dental crowding (Fig. 700-1). Ocular abnormalities reflect the connective tissue defect and include blue sclerae, myopia occurring in 60% of affected individuals, and suspensory ligament laxity with iridodonesis. Slit-lamp examination as early as infancy may disclose lens dislocation, which may be congenital. Iridodonesis is a helpful clinical sign, but suspected cases of Marfan syndrome should have ophthalmologic evaluations that include slit-lamp examinations even in the absence of gross ocular abnormality, as myopia, increased intraocular pressure, or retinal detachment may be present.

Examination of the musculoskeletal system discloses dolichostenomelia (long, thin limbs), and the arm span substan-

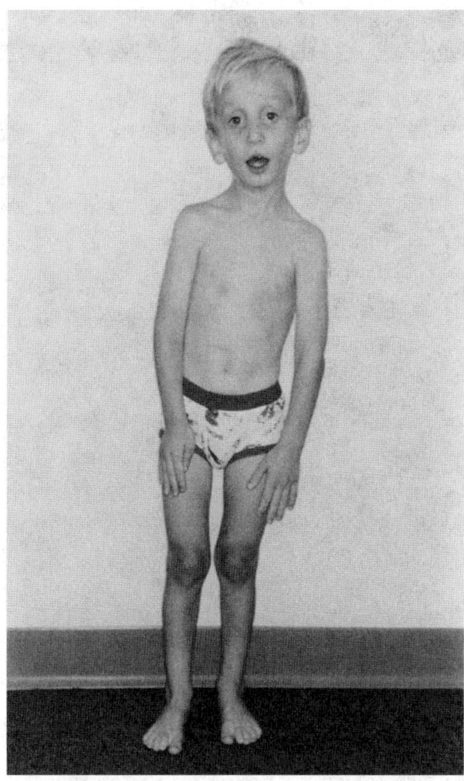

Figure 700-1. Marfan syndrome. Note the elongated facies, droopy lids, apparent dolichostenomelia, and mild scoliosis.

tially exceeds the height (>1.05 times height). The lower segment (distance from pubis to heel) is increased in comparison to the upper segment (height minus lower segment) and contributes to a diminished upper segment: lower segment ratio (U_s/L_s). Hand findings are nonspecific and include long, thin fingers (arachnodactyly) that are hyperextensible. The thumb may be adducted across the narrow palm (Steinberg sign) and may appreciably overlap the 5th finger when encircling the wrist (wrist sign) (Figs. 700-2 and 700-3).

Long gracile ribs may contribute to various sternal anomalies including pectus excavatum ("funnel chest") or pectus carinatum ("pigeon breast"). The risk of scoliosis among adolescents is increased.

The connective tissue defect contributes to increased distensibility of lung parenchyma and dura and increases the risks of spontaneous pneumothorax and dural ectasia, respectively.

Progressive cardiovascular defects contribute to the substantial morbidity of Marfan syndrome, and echocardiography has improved early detection of patients at risk of cardiac complications. Progressive aortic root dilatation, whether or not accompanied by auscultatory evidence of aortic disease, occurs in 80–100% of affected individuals and may be congenital.

In contrast to adults, frank aortic regurgitation is less common in children, perhaps because the amount and duration of distension required to cause aortic dysfunction do not manifest until later life. MVP occurs as frequently as aortic dilatation and also tends to be progressive, in contrast to the more static lesion of idiopathic MVP. MVP is the most common cause of morbidity in children with Marfan syndrome and may manifest as arrhythmias, heart failure, thromboemboli, or endocarditis. Mitral valve regurgitation is observed in about 50% of affected patients younger than 20 yr of age.

DIAGNOSIS. Diagnosis of Marfan syndrome is based on clinical criteria (Table 700-1). In general, diagnosis of a sporadic or new mutation case requires that major manifestations of the disorder

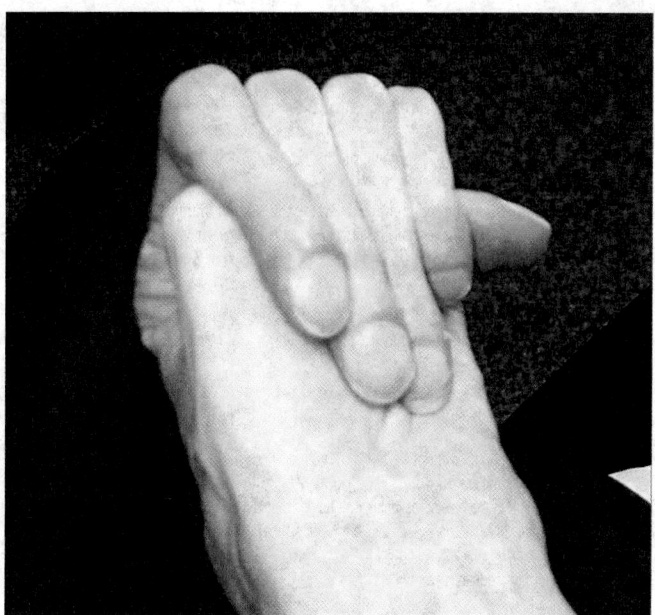

Figure 700-2. "Thumb sign": when the hand is clenched without assistance, the entire thumbnail projects beyond the border of the hand. (From Zitelli BJ: Picture of the month. *Arch Pediatr Adolesc Med* 2005;159:721–723.)

be present. In cases with an unequivocally affected 1st-degree relative, milder manifestations with at least one major malformation are supportive of the diagnosis. Tall stature with an abnormally low U_s/L_s ratio or an increased span-to-height ratio (i.e., >1.05) is the most consistent presenting feature. Echocardiography or MRI should show at least aortic root dilatation for age. Other abnormalities such as MVP, mitral regurgitation, or aortic regurgitation are supportive findings. A slit-lamp examination is indicated in all suspected cases. It is important to note that only 60–70% of patients who meet clinical criteria for Marfan syndrome have known mutations in the fibrillin gene, whereas 12% of patients not meeting criteria have a fibrillin mutation.

The **differential diagnosis** includes homocystinuria, Loeys-Dietz syndrome, familial aortic dissection, familial ectopia lentis, and MASS (myopia, mitral valve prolapse, mild aortic dilation, skin striae, skeletal features like Marfan syndrome) syndrome. MASS is caused by a different mutation of the fibrillin gene.

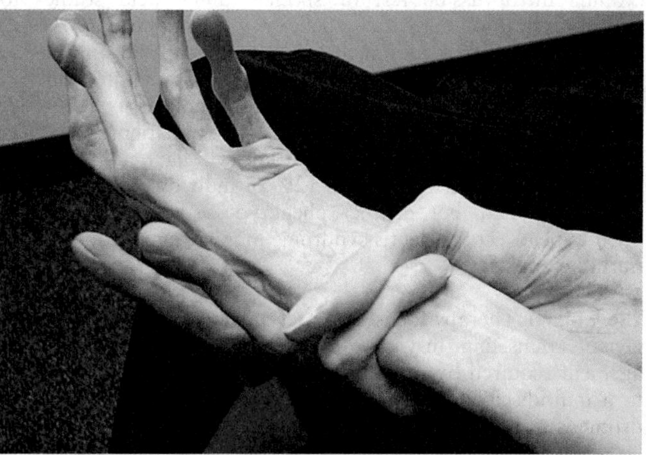

Figure 700-3. "Wrist sign": when the wrist is grasped by the contralateral hand, the thumb overlaps the terminal phalanx of the 5th digit. (From Zitelli BJ: Picture of the month. *Arch Pediatr Adolesc Med* 2005;159:721–723.)

TABLE 700-1. Diagnostic Criteria for Marfan Syndrome

Index case

- If the family/genetic history is not contributory, major criteria in two or more different organ systems and involvement of a third organ system.
- If a mutation known to cause Marfan syndrome in others is identified, one major criterion in an organ system and involvement of a second organ system

Relative of an index case who independently meets these strict diagnostic criteria

- Presence of a major criterion in the family history, one major criterion in an organ system, and involvement of a second organ system.

Organ systems

Skeletal

At least four of the following constitutes a major criterion in the skeletal system

- Pectus carinatum
- Pectus excavatum, needing surgery
- Reduced upper-segment to lower-segment ratio or arm span to height ratio >1.05
- Wrist and thumb signs
- Scoliosis of >20° or spondylolisthesis
- Reduced extension at the elbows (<170°)
- Medial displacement of the medial malleolus, causing pes planus
- Protrusio acetabulae of any degree (ascertained on radiographs)

Minor criteria

- Pectus excavatum of moderate severity
- Joint hypermobility
- Highly arched palate with crowding of teeth
- Facial appearance (dolichocephaly, malar hypoplasia, enophthalmos, retrognathia, down-slanting palpebral fissures)

For involvement of the skeletal system, at least two features contributing to major criteria, or one feature from the list contributing to the major criterion and two of the minor criteria must be present.

Ocular system

Major criterion

- Ectopia lentis

Minor criteria

- Abnormally flat cornea
- Increased axial length of globe
- Hypoplastic iris or hypoplastic ciliary muscle, causing decreased miosis

For involvement of the ocular system, at least two of the minor criteria must be present.

Cardiovascular system

Major criteria (either of the following)

- Dilatation of the ascending aorta, with or without aortic regurgitation, and involving at least the sinuses of Valsalva
- Dissection of the ascending aorta

Minor criteria

- Mitral valve prolapse with or without mitral valve regurgitation
- Dilatation of the main pulmonary artery, in the absence of valvular or peripheral pulmoni stenosis or any other obvious cause, younger than age 40 years
- Calcification of the mitral annulus younger than age 40 years
- Dilatation or dissection of the descending thoracic or abdominal aorta younger than age 50 years

For involvement of the cardiovascular system, only one of the minor criteria must be present.

Pulmonary system

Major criteria

- None

Minor criteria

- Spontaneous pneumothorax
- Apical blebs

For involvement of the pulmonary system, only one of the minor criteria must be present

Skin and integument

Major criteria

- None

Minor criteria

- Striae atrophicae (stretch marks) without marked weight gain, pregnancy, or repetitive stress
- Recurrent or incisional herniae

For involvement of the skin and integument, only one of the minor criteria must be present

Dura

Major criterion

- Lumbosacral dural ectasia

Minor criteria

- None

Family/genetic history

Major criteria (any one of the following)

- Having a parent, child, or sibling who meets these diagnostic criteria independently
- Presence of a mutation in *FBN1*, which is known to cause Marfan syndrome
- Presence of a haplotype around *FBN1*, inherited by descent, known to be associated with unequivocally diagnosed Marfan syndrome in the family

Minor criteria

- None

From Judge DP, Dietz HC: Marfan's syndrome. *Lancet* 2005; 366: 1965–1976.

Other conditions that should be excluded include Stickler syndrome, idiopathic MVP syndrome, congenital contractural arachnodactyly syndrome, isolated cystic medial necrosis of the aorta (Erdheim syndrome), and Shprintzen-Goldberg (craniosynostosis arachnodactyly) syndrome.

Laboratory studies should document a negative urinary cyanide nitroprusside test or specific amino acid studies to exclude cystathionine synthase deficiency (homocystinuria). Molecular genetic techniques such as direct mutational analysis or genetic linkage contribute to diagnosis in families in which a mutation is known or in an individual for whom strict adherence to diagnostic criteria are met. Thirty to 40% of patients who meet diagnostic criteria for Marfan syndrome will have negative molecular genetic tests, whereas 10–12% of individuals with phenotypically similar but distinct phenotypes such as the MASS phenotype or ectopia lentis syndrome may have mutations in the fibrillin gene.

TREATMENT. Therapy focuses on prevention of complications and genetic counseling. In view of the potential complexity of management required by some affected individuals, periodic referral to a multidisciplinary center with experience with Marfan syndrome is advisable.

The pediatrician should work in concert with pediatric subspecialists to coordinate a rational approach to expectant monitoring and treatment of potential complications. Yearly evaluations for such potential problems as cardiac valvular disease, scoliosis, or ophthalmologic problems are imperative. Physical therapy may improve neuromuscular tone in infancy. Moderate nontraumatic aerobic physical activity such as swimming or bicycling should be encouraged as tolerated. Maximal exertion should be discouraged because of the stresses that increased cardiac output place on the aorta. Endocarditis prophylaxis should be instituted before dental or other invasive surgical procedures. ß-Adrenergic blockade with agents such as propanolol or atenolol may slow the progression of aortic dilatation and may lessen the risks of catastrophic cardiac events. Losartan, an angiotensin II type 1 receptor blocker and TGF-β agonist, is being introduced as an additional agent that may be effective for the management of aortic disease. Acute aortic dissection may be managed by composite graft.

Optimal management of the pregnant adolescent with Marfan syndrome has not been established. The risk that pregnancy will worsen cardiovascular abnormalities is of concern. Although substantial data are lacking, young women with minor cardiac manifestations or mild aortic root dilatation may tolerate pregnancy and experience good maternal and fetal outcomes. Those with frank aortic dilatation should be monitored echocardiographically at regular intervals. Although ß-adrenergic blockade has not been shown to be teratogenic, the prenatally exposed offspring of women with Marfan syndrome who have been treated with ß-antagonists should be monitored in the neonatal period for such drug-induced problems as hypotension, bradycardia, and hypoglycemia.

PROGNOSIS. Longevity in Marfan syndrome is diminished in comparison with population norms, primarily because of the increased risk of cardiovascular complications. Dilatation of the aortic root and ascending aorta is progressive and may lead to aneurysm formation and increased risk of aortic dissection. These and other concerns pose not only medical problems, but also psychologic stresses for the affected child and the parents, particularly during adolescence. Awareness of these issues and referral for support services may facilitate a positive perspective toward this condition.

GENETIC COUNSELING. The heritable nature of Marfan syndrome makes recurrence risk (genetic) counseling mandatory. Approximately 15–30% of cases are the first affected individuals in their families. Fathers of these sporadic cases have been, on average, 7–10 yr older than fathers in the general population. This paternal age effect suggests that these cases represent new dominant mutations with minimal recurrence risks to the future offspring of the normal parents. A few cases of gonadal mosaicism in a phenotypically normal parent require recurrence risk counseling by a professionally trained and experienced genetic counselor. Each child of an affected individual, however, has a 50% risk of inheriting the number 15 chromosome with the Marfan mutation and thus being affected. Recurrence risk counseling is best accomplished by professionals with expertise in the issues surrounding this chronic debilitating disorder.

American Academy of Pediatrics Committee on Genetics: Health supervision of children with Marfan syndrome. *Pediatrics* 1996;98:978–982.

Boileau C, Jondeau G, Babron M-C, et al: Autosomal dominant Marfan-like connective-tissue disorder with aortic dilation and skeletal anomalies not linked to the fibrillin genes. *Am J Hum Genet* 1993;53:46–54.

Collod G, Babron M-C, Jondeau G, et al: A second locus for Marfan syndrome maps to chromosome 3p24.2-p25. *Nat Genet* 1994;8:264–268.

DePaepe A, Devereux RB, Dietz HC, et al: Revised criteria for Marfan syndrome. *Am J Med Genet* 1996;62;417–426.

Franke U, Furthmayr H: Marfan's syndrome and other disorders of fibrillin. *N Engl J Med* 1994;330:1384–1385.

Gelb BD: Marfan's syndrome and related disorder—more tightly connected than we thought. *N Engl J Med* 2006;355:841–844.

Glesby MJ, Pyeritz RE: Association of mitral valve prolapse and systemic abnormalities of connective tissue: A phenotypic continuum. *JAMA* 1989;262:523–528.

Gross DM, Robinson LK, Smith LT, et al: Severe perinatal Marfan syndrome. *Pediatrics* 1989;84:83–89.

Habashi JP, Judge D, Holm TM, et al: Losartan, an ATI antagonist prevents aortic aneurysm in a mouse model of Marfan syndrome. *Science* 2006; 312:117–121.

Judge DP, Dietz HC: Marfan's syndrome. *Lancet* 2005;366:1965–1976.

Loeys BL, Chen J, Neptune ER, et al: A syndrome of altered cardiovascular, craniofacial, neurocognitive and skeletal development caused by mutations in TGFBR1 or TGFBR2. *Nat Genet* 2005;37:275–281.

Palz M, Tiecke F, Booms P, et al: Clustering of mutation associated with mild Marfan-like phenotypes in the 3′ region of FBN1 suggests a potential genotype phenotype correlation. *Am J Med Genet* 2000;91:212–221.

Pereira L, Levran O, Ramirez F, et al: A molecular approach to stratification of cardiovascular risk in families with Marfan syndrome. *N Engl J Med* 1994;331:148–153.

Rossiter JP, Morales AJ, Repke JT, et al: A prospective longitudinal evaluation of pregnancy in the Marfan syndrome. *Am J Obstet Gynecol* 1995;173:1599–1606.

Shores J, Berger KR, Murphy EA, Pyeritz RE: Progression of aortic dilatation and the benefit of long-term β-adrenergic blockade in Marfan's syndrome. *N Engl J Med* 1994;330:1335–1341.

Tierney ESS, Feingold B, Printz BF, et al: Beta-blocker therapy does not alter the rate of aortic root dilation in pediatric patients with Marfan syndrome. *J Pediatr* 2007;150:77–82.

Section 4 — Metabolic Bone Disease — Russell W. Chesney

Chapter 701 ■ Bone Structure, Growth, and Hormonal Regulation

Also see Chapters 48 and 571.

Bone is a dynamic organ capable of rapid turnover, weight bearing, and withstanding the stresses of various physical activities. It is constantly being formed (modeling) and re-formed (remodeling). It is the major body reservoir for calcium, phosphorus, and magnesium. Disorders that affect this organ and the process of mineralization are designated metabolic bone diseases.

Because bone growth and turnover rates are high during childhood, many clinical features of metabolic bone diseases are more prominent in children than in adults.

The human skeleton consists of a protein matrix, largely composed of a collagen-containing protein, osteoid, on which is deposited a crystalline mineral phase. Although collagen-containing osteoid accounts for 90% of bone protein, other proteins are present, including osteocalcin, which contains γ-carboxyglutamic acid. Synthesis of osteocalcin is vitamin K and vitamin D dependent; in high bone turnover states, serum osteocalcin values are often elevated.

The microfibrillar matrix of osteoid permits deposition of highly organized calcium phosphate crystals, including hydroxyapatite $[Ca_{10}(PO_4)_6 \cdot 6H_2O]$ and octacalcium phosphate $[Ca_8(H_2PO_4)_6 \cdot 5H_2O]$, plus less organized amorphous calcium phosphate, calcium carbonate, sodium, magnesium, and citrate. Hydroxyapatite is deep within bone matrix, whereas amorphous calcium phosphate coats the surface of newly formed or remodeled bone.

Bone growth occurs in children by the process of calcification of the cartilage cells present at the ends of bone. In accord with the prevailing extracellular fluid (ECF) calcium and phosphate concentrations, mineral is deposited in those chondrocytes or cartilage cells set to undergo mineralization. The main function of the vitamin D/parathyroid hormone (PTH)/endocrine axis is to maintain the ECF calcium and phosphate concentrations at appropriate levels to permit mineralization.

Other hormones also appear to regulate the growth and mineralization of cartilage, including growth hormone acting through insulin-like growth factors, thyroid hormones, insulin, leptin, and androgens and estrogens during the pubertal growth spurt. Supraphysiologic concentrations of glucocorticoids impair cartilage function and bone growth and augment bone resorption.

Phosphate homeostasis is regulated by the kidneys because intestinal phosphate absorption is nearly complete and renal excretion determines the serum level. Excessive intestinal phosphate absorption causes a fall in serum levels of ionized calcium and a rise in PTH secretion, resulting in phosphaturia, thus lowering the serum phosphate level and permitting the calcium level to rise. Hypophosphatemia blocks PTH secretion and promotes renal 1,25-dihydroxyvitamin D (1,25[OH]$_2$D) synthesis. This latter compound also promotes greater intestinal phosphate absorption.

Rates of bone formation are coordinated with alterations in mineral metabolism in both the intestine and kidneys. Inadequate dietary intake or intestinal absorption of calcium causes a fall in serum levels of calcium and its ionized fraction. This serves as the signal for PTH synthesis and secretion, resulting in greater bone resorption to raise the serum calcium level, enhanced distal tubular reabsorption of calcium, and higher rates of synthesis by the kidneys of 1,25-dihydroxyvitamin D (1,25[OH]$_2$D) or calcitriol, the most active metabolite of vitamin D (Fig. 701-1). Calcium homeostasis thus is controlled at the intestine because the availability of 1,25(OH)$_2$D ultimately determines the fraction of ingested calcium that is absorbed.

The growth pattern of bones is an acceleration of bone growth (length) of the limbs during prepubescence, increased growth (length) of the trunk (spine) during early adolescence, and increased bone mineral deposition in late adolescence. The use of dual-energy x-ray absorptiometry (DEXA) or less often quantitative CT permits measurement of both bone mineral content and bone density in healthy subjects and in children with metabolic bone disease. DEXA scanning exposes the patient to less radiation than a chest radiograph.

An understanding of the metabolism of vitamin D is necessary to appreciate metabolic bone disease and rickets (see Fig. 701-1). The skin contains 7-dehydrocholesterol, which is converted to vitamin D$_3$ by ultraviolet radiation; other inactive vitamin D sterols are also produced (see Chapter 48). Vitamin D$_3$ is then transported in the bloodstream to the liver by a vitamin D–binding protein (DBP); DBP binds all forms of vitamin D. The plasma concentration of free or nonbound vitamin D is much lower than the level of DBP-bound vitamin D metabolites.

Vitamin D also can enter the metabolic pathway by ingestion of dietary vitamin D$_2$ (ergocalciferol) or vitamin D$_3$ (cholecalciferol), both of which are absorbed from the intestine because of the action of bile salts. After absorption, ingested vitamin D is transported by chylomicrons to the liver, where, along with skin-derived vitamin D$_3$, it is converted to 25-hydroxyvitamin D (25[OH]D) by the action of a hepatic microsomal enzyme requiring oxygen, NADPH, and magnesium to hydroxylate vitamin D at the 25th carbon atom. The 25(OH)D is next transported by DBP to the kidneys, where it undergoes further metabolism. 25(OH)D is the main circulating vitamin D metabolite in humans (Table 701-1). Because the synthesis of 25(OH)D is weakly regulated by feedback, its plasma level rises in summer and falls in winter. High vitamin D intake raises the plasma level of 25(OH)D to many times above normal, but the parent vitamin D compound itself is absorbed by adipose tissue.

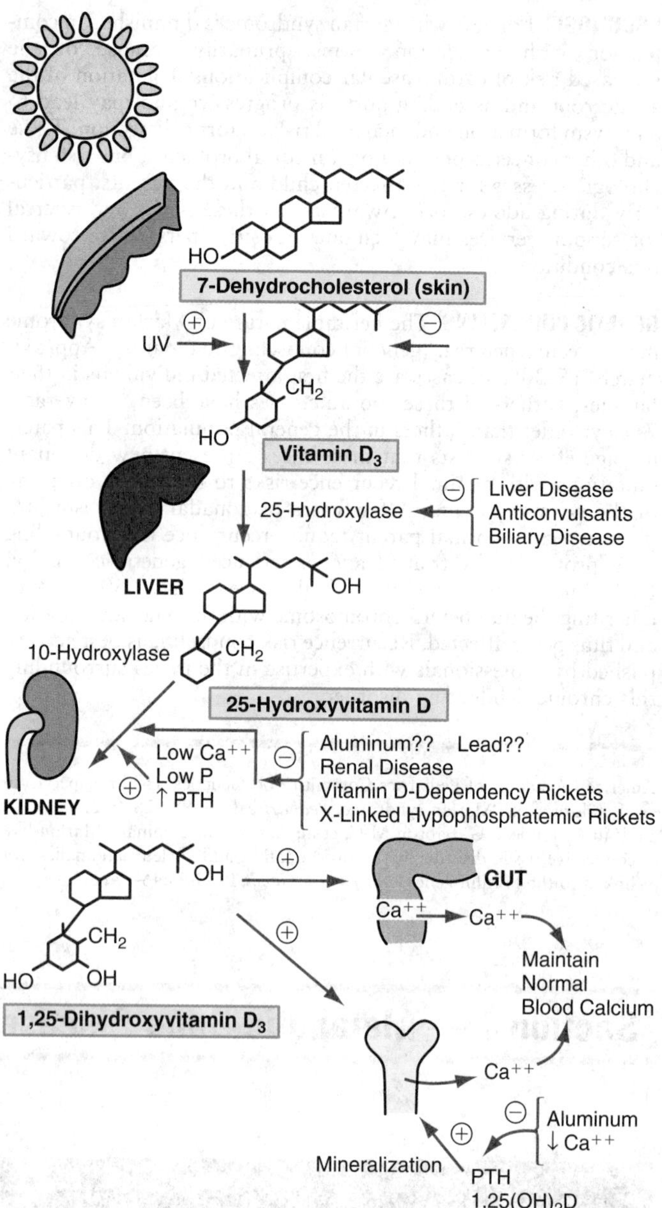

Figure 701-1. The metabolic pathway of vitamin D, indicating its conversion to the hormone 1,25(OH)$_2$D$_3$ and to 24,25(OH)$_2$D$_3$. Vitamin D$_2$ (ergosterol), of plant origin, appears to undergo similar metabolic steps.

TABLE 701-1. Vitamin D Metabolic Values in Plasma of Normal Healthy Subjects

METABOLITE	PLASMA VALUE
Vitamin D$_2$	1–2 ng/mL
Vitamin D$_3$	1–2 ng/mL
25(OH)D$_2$	4–10 ng/mL
25(OH)D$_3$	12–40 ng/mL
Total 25(OH)D	15–50 ng/mL
24,25(OH)$_2$D	1–4 ng/mL
1,25(OH)$_2$D	
Infancy	70–100 pg/mL
Childhood	30–50 pg/mL
Adolescence	40–80 pg/mL
Adulthood	20–35 pg/mL

In the kidneys, 25(OH)D undergoes further hydroxylation, depending on the prevailing serum concentration of calcium, phosphate, and PTH. If the calcium or phosphate level is reduced or the PTH level is elevated, the enzyme 25(OH)D-1-hydroxylase is activated and 1,25(OH)$_2$D is formed. This metabolite circulates at a level that is only 0.1% of the level of 25(OH)D (see Table 701-1) and acts on the intestine to increase the active transport of calcium and stimulate phosphate absorption. Because 1α-hydroxylase is a mitochondrial enzyme that is tightly feedback regulated, the synthesis of 1,25(OH)$_2$D declines after serum calcium or phosphate values return to normal. Excessive 1,25(OH)$_2$D is converted to an inactive metabolite. In the presence of normal or elevated serum calcium or phosphate concentrations, the renal 25(OH)D-24-hydroxylase is activated, producing 24,25-dihydroxyvitamin D (24,25[OH]$_2$D), which is a pathway for the removal of excess vitamin D; serum levels of 24,25(OH)$_2$D (1–5 ng/mL) increase after ingestion of large

TABLE 701-2. Clinical Variants of Rickets and Related Conditions

TYPE	SERUM CALCIUM LEVEL	SERUM PHOSPHORUS LEVEL	ALKALINE PHOSPHATASE ACTIVITY	URINE CONCENTRATION OF AMINO ACIDS	GENETICS	GENE DEFECT KNOWN
I. Calcium deficiency with secondary hyperparathyroidism (deficiency of vitamin D; low 25(OH)D and no stimulation of higher $1,25(OH)_2D$ values)						
1. Lack of vitamin D						
a. Lack of exposure to sunlight	N or L	L	E	E		
b. Dietary deficiency of vitamin D	N or L	L	E	E		
c. Congenital	N or L	L	E	E		
2. Malabsorption of vitamin D	N or L	L	E	E		
3. Hepatic disease	N or L	L	E	E		
4. Anticonvulsive drugs	N or L	L	E	E		
5. Renal osteodystrophy	N or L	E	E	V		
6. Vitamin D–dependent type I	L	N or L	E	E	AR	Y
II. Primary phosphate deficiency (no secondary hyperparathyroidism)						
1. Genetic primary hypophosphatemia	N	L	E	N	XD, AD	Y
2. Fanconi syndrome						
a. Cystinosis	N	L	E	E	AR	Y
b. Tyrosinosis	N	L	E	E	AR	Y
c. Lowe syndrome	N	L	E	E	XR	Y
d. Acquired	N	L	E	E		
3. Renal tubular acidosis, type II proximal	N	L	E	N		Y
4. Oncogenic hypophosphatemia	N	L	E	N		Y
5. Phosphate deficiency or malabsorption						
a. Parenteral hyperalimentation	N	L	E	N		
b. Low phosphate intake	N	L	E	N		
III. End-organ resistance to $1,25(OH)_2D_3$						
1. Vitamin D–dependent type II (several variants)	L	L or N	E	E	AR	Y
IV. Related conditions resembling rickets						
1. Hypophosphatasia	N	N	L	Phosphoethanolamine elevated	AR	Y
2. Metaphyseal dysostosis						
a. Jansen type	E	N	E	N	AD	Y
b. Schmid type	N	N	N	N	AD	Y

A, autosomal; D, dominant; E, elevated; L, low; N, normal; R, recessive; V, variable; X, X-linked; Y, Yes.

amounts of vitamin D. Although hypervitaminosis D and production of inactive metabolites can occur after oral dosing (see Chapter 48), extensive skin exposure to sunlight does not usually produce toxic levels of $25(OH)D_3$, suggesting natural regulation of the production of this metabolite in cutaneous tissue.

Serum $1,25(OH)_2D$ levels are higher in children than in adults, are not as subject to seasonal variability, and peak in the 1st yr of life and again during the adolescent growth spurt. These values must be interpreted in light of the prevailing serum calcium, phosphate, and PTH values and with regard to the entire vitamin D metabolite profile.

Mineral deficiency prevents the normal process of bone mineral deposition. If mineral deficiency occurs at the growth plate, growth slows and bone age is retarded, a condition called rickets. Poor mineralization of trabecular bone resulting in a greater proportion of unmineralized osteoid is the condition of osteomalacia. Rickets is found only in growing children before fusion of the epiphyses, whereas osteomalacia is present at all ages. All patients with rickets have osteomalacia, but not all patients with osteomalacia have rickets. These conditions should not be confused with osteoporosis, a condition of equal loss of bone volume and mineral (see Chapter 705).

Rickets may be classified as calcium-deficient or phosphate-deficient rickets. Because both calcium and phosphate ions constitute bone mineral, the insufficiency of either type in the ECF that bathes the mineralizing surface of bone results in rickets and osteomalacia. The two types of rickets are distinguishable by their clinical manifestations (Table 701-2). Rickets may also occur in the face of mineral deficiency, despite adequate vitamin D stores. True dietary calcium deficiency rickets is found in some parts of Africa but rarely in North America or Europe. A form of phosphate-deficiency rickets may occur in infants given prolonged administrations of phosphate-sequestering aluminum salts as a treatment for colic or gastroesophageal reflux. This results in the phosphate depletion syndrome.

Chapter 702 ■ Primary Chondrodystrophy (Metaphyseal Dysplasia)

In this autosomal dominant condition, bowing of the legs, short stature, and a waddling gait appear in the absence of abnormalities of serum levels of calcium and phosphate, alkaline phosphatase activity, or vitamin D metabolites. Metaphyseal chondrodysplasia *(Jansen type)* is typified by cupped and ragged metaphyses, which develop mottled calcification at the distal ends of bone over time. Hypercalcemia, with serum values of 13–15 mg/dL, may occur. The spine may also be deformed by the irregular growth of vertebrae. Three different mutations have been identified in parathyroid hormone receptor type I as the molecular cause of this syndrome, as have some of the downstream target genes that may contribute to the pathogenesis of the disease. The *Schmid type* of metaphyseal chondrodysplasia is less severe, although the radiographic appearance of the knees and extreme bowing of the lower limbs resemble signs seen in patients with familial hypophosphatemia. It is associated with defects in collagen type X, and the hip abnormalities are more debilitating than in Jansen metaphyseal chondrodysplasia. Patients with both types of metaphyseal chondrodysplasia have lifelong short stature.

Metaphyseal dysostosis, or *Pyle disease,* results from defects in endochondral bone formation and metaphyseal modeling. The long ends of bones are splayed, resulting in an "Erlenmeyer flask" defect. Short stature is not necessarily characteristic, and serum chemical levels are normal. Leonine features often develop if the facial bones are involved. Metaphyseal dysostosis may be a clinical feature of Shwachman-Diamond syndrome, a rare autosomal recessive disorder characterized by neutropenia, pancreatic exocrine insufficiency, bone marrow dysfunction, and sometimes severe hematologic complications (see Chapter 448). Although allogeneic bone marrow transplantation has been used as a therapeutic approach, there have been mixed results.

There are no other currently available forms of treatment known to be effective for the chondrodystrophies or dysostosis.

Chapter 703 ■ Hypophosphatasia

Hypophosphatasia is an autosomal recessive disorder that radiographically resembles rickets and is defined by low serum alkaline phosphatase activity. It is an inborn error of metabolism in which activity of the tissue-nonspecific (liver/bone/kidney) alkaline phosphatase isoenzyme (TNSALP) is deficient (although activity of the intestinal and placental isoenzymes is normal). Single point mutations of the gene prevent expression of the activity of this enzyme in vitro and indicate its necessity for normal skeletal mineralization. A large proportion of the more than 100 mutations of the gene identified to date are missense mutations, although splice-site mutations, small deletions, and frame-shift mutations have also have been found. The only phenotype associated with these mutations is hypophosphatasia. Some patients may have a regulatory defect involving this enzyme rather than a mutation.

There is considerable heterogeneity in the severity of the disease. Some cases appear at birth, and diagnosis has even been made in utero by radiographic examination of a fetus. The disease may appear in a lethal neonatal or perinatal form (congenital lethal hypophosphatasia), a severe infantile form, or a milder form occurring in childhood or late adolescence (hypophosphatasia tarda). The lethal form is characterized by a moth-eaten appearance at the ends of the long bones, by severe deficiency of ossification throughout the skeleton, and by marked shortening of the long bones. Patients with mild disease may present with bowing of the legs and variable statural shortening. Hypercalcemia is common in the neonatal and infantile forms, and because calcium accumulation by mature chondrocytes does not occur, patients may appear to have rickets.

Unusual clinical manifestations include wormian bones in the calvariae; poor calcification of the frontal, parietal, and occipital bones; and premature loss of deciduous or permanent teeth, owing to hypoplasia of dental cementum. Because of the hypercalcemia in the infantile form, nephrocalcinosis is also found. In the childhood form, bone pain, frequent fractures, and milder skeletal deformities are evident, as well as premature tooth loss. The metaphyseal defect consists of irregular ossification, punched-out areas, and metaphyseal cupping.

In hypophosphatasia, large quantities of phosphoethanolamine are found in the urine because this compound cannot be degraded in the absence of TNSALP activity. Plasma inorganic pyrophosphate and pyridoxal-5-phosphate (PLP) levels are also elevated for the same reason. PLP levels tend to be lower than normal in most other bone diseases and hence may aid in the differential diagnosis of hypophosphatasia. Seizures in patients with the lethal and infantile forms of the disease may be related to impaired pyridoxine metabolism. Although no satisfactory therapy has been found, infusion of plasma rich in alkaline phosphatase activity has been helpful in healing bone in short-term studies. Bone marrow transplantation has been successful using donors with normal TNSALP values. The clinical course of this condition often improves spontaneously as an affected child matures, although early death due to renal failure or flail chest leading to pneumonia may occur in the severe infantile form of the disorder. Rare patients presenting with identical clinical and radiographic patterns have normal serum alkaline phosphatase activity. Their disease has been labeled *pseudohypophosphatasia* and may represent the presence of a mutant alkaline phosphatase isoenzyme that reacts to artificial substrates in an alkaline environment (in a test tube) but not in vivo with natural substrates.

Chapter 704 ■ Hyperphosphatasia

Excessive elevation of the bone isoenzyme of alkaline phosphatase in serum and significant growth failure characterize hyperphosphatasia. Osteoid proliferation in the subperiosteal portion of bone results in separation of the periosteum from the bone cortex. Bowing and thickening of the diaphyses are common, along with osteopenia. The disease usually has its onset by 2–3 yr of age, when painful deformity developing in the extremities leads to abnormal gait and sometimes fractures. Other common findings include pectus carinatum, kyphoscoliosis, and rib fraying. The skull is large, and the cranium is thickened (widened diploë) and may be deformed. Skull involvement can lead to progressive and profound hearing loss. Radiographically, the bony texture is variable; dense areas (showing a teased cotton-wool appearance) are interspersed with radiolucent areas and general demineralization. Long bones appear cylindrical, lose metaphyseal modeling, and contain pseudocysts showing a dense, bony halo.

In this autosomal recessive disorder, serum levels of both calcium and phosphate are normal, whereas urinary leucine amino acid peptidase activity and serum acid phosphatase levels are increased. This disorder is often called *juvenile Paget disease* because, as in adult-onset Paget disease, calcitonin may reduce the rapid bone turnover found in this disorder; in children, the disorder is more generalized and symmetric. This disorder is distinct from Paget disease because histology of bone reveals a lack of normal cortical bone remodeling and an absence of the classic mosaic pattern of lamellar bone found in the adult condition. Hence, the term juvenile Paget disease is inappropriate. A case has been reported in which intense intravenous biphosphonate (ibandronate) therapy administered over a 3-yr period arrested progression of idiopathic hyperphosphatasia, preventing deformity and disability and improving hearing.

Transient hyperphosphatasia occurs between 2 mo and 2 yr of age, has no associated manifestations other than some mild gastrointestinal symptoms, and is usually detected during routine (screening) laboratory evaluation for some unrelated complaint. Both liver and bone isoenzyme fractions are elevated; there are no other manifestations of hepatic or bone dysfunction. The cause is unknown. Resolution usually occurs within 4–6 mo.

Familial hyperphosphatemia, an autosomal dominant trait, is another benign condition that is distinguished from the transient infantile form by persistent and asymptomatic elevations of serum alkaline phosphatase levels.

A more serious autosomal dominant variant, *expansile skeletal hyperplasia,* is characterized by early-onset deafness, premature loss of teeth, progressive hyperostotic widening of long bones causing painful phalanges in the hands, episodic hypercalcemia, and enhanced bone remodeling. A defect in the gene that encodes receptor activation of nuclear factor γB (NF-γB) is relevant. This gene appears to be necessary for osteogenesis, and the defect leads to increased activity of NF-γB in the skeleton.

Chapter 705 ■ Osteoporosis

Osteoporosis is the most common bone disorder in adults, but it is relatively uncommon in children. Bone volume is diminished and the incidence of fractures is greatly increased in this condition. In contrast to osteomalacia, which shows undermineralization and normal bone volume, histologic sections of bone in all forms of osteoporosis reveal a normal degree of mineralization but a reduction in the volume of bone, especially trabecular bone (vertebral bone). In osteoporosis, by definition, there is also a reduced amount of bone tissue, (termed osteopenia) which is associated with atraumatic (pathologic) fractures. Osteoporosis in children may be primary or secondary (Table 705-1). The primary osteoporoses can be divided into heritable disorders of connective tissue, including osteogenesis imperfecta, Bruck syndrome, osteoporosis-pseudoglioma syndrome, Ehlers-Danlos syndrome, Marfan syndrome, homocystinuria, and idiopathic juvenile osteoporosis. Secondary forms of osteoporosis include various neuromuscular disorders, chronic illness, endocrine disorders, and drug-induced and inborn errors of metabolism, including lysinuric protein intolerance and Gaucher disease.

When no obvious primary or secondary cause can be detected, *idiopathic juvenile osteoporosis* should be considered, especially if the following clinical features are evident: onset prior to puberty, long bone and lower back pain, vertebral fractures, long bone and metatarsal fractures, a washed-out appearance of the spine and appendicular skeleton, and improvement after puberty. Trabecular bones such as the spine and metatarsals are particularly affected by atraumatic fractures.

In general, blood values of minerals, vitamin D metabolites, alkaline phosphatase, and parathyroid hormone are normal. Evaluation of bone mineral content and bone density by dual-energy x-ray absorptiometry or less often quantitative CT shows markedly reduced values. Several modes of therapy (including oral calcium supplements, calcitriol, bisphosphonates, and calcitonin) have been used with some success in individual conditions, but the effect of these treatments is difficult to gauge because spontaneous recovery may occur after the onset of puberty in >75% of cases.

Osteoporosis-pseudoglioma is an autosomal recessive disorder manifested by variable age at onset, low bone mass, fractures in childhood, and abnormal eye development, and the defective gene has been mapped to chromosome 11q12–13. The mutation is a loss of function in the gene for low-density lipoprotein receptor–related protein 5. Interestingly, gain-of-function mutations result in a gene product that increases bone density.

The life cycle implications of either significant demineralization or osteoporosis in childhood need to be stressed. Events in childhood will influence peak bone mass, and late adolescence is a period of rapid bone mineral accretion. Moreover, while peak bone mass is achieved by 20–35 yr of age (depending on the bone measured), the contribution during childhood is considerable. A number of measures have been shown to influence bone mass: vitamin D (400–800 IU daily), calcium intake (≥1,200 mg/day in adolescents), and weight-bearing exercise throughout childhood. Weight-bearing exercise will enhance bone formation and reduce bone resorption. Other factors that may prevent acquisition of peak bone mass include use of alcohol and tobacco. Excellent sources of dietary calcium include mainly dairy products, but also bony fish, green vegetables, and calcium-supplemented drinks (orange juice). Yogurt and cheeses can be used in lactase-deficient individuals. Because it appears that adult-onset osteoporosis is the result of a number of genetic factors, thus forming a complex trait interaction, specific interventions during childhood to influence bone mass are not available.

The treatment of secondary osteoporosis is best achieved by treatment of the underlying disorder when feasible. Hypogonadism should be treated with hormone replacement therapy, especially in thin athletic women. Calcium intake should be increased to 1,500–2,000 mg/day. In glucocorticoid-induced osteoporosis, an emphasis on the lowest possible dose to prevent disease activity (inflammatory bowel disease) with alternate-day

TABLE 705-1. Risks for Osteoporosis

ENDOCRINE DISORDERS
Female hypogonadism
Turner syndrome
Hypothalamic amenorrhea (athletic triad)
Anorexia nervosa
Premature and primary ovarian failure
Depot medroxyprogesterone acetate therapy
Estrogen receptor α (*ESR* 1), mutations
Hyperprolactinemia
Male hypogonadism
Primary gonadal failure (Klinefelter syndrome)
Secondary gonadal failure (idiopathic hypogonadotropic hypogonadism)
Delayed puberty
Hyperthyroidism
Hyperparathyroidism
Hypercortisolism (therapeutic or Cushing disease)
Growth hormone deficiency
GASTROINTESTINAL DISORDERS
Malabsorption syndromes (cystic fibrosis, celiac disease)
Inflammatory bowel disease
Chronic obstructive jaundice
Primary biliary cirrhosis and other cirrhoses
Alactasia
Subtotal gastrectomy
BONE MARROW DISORDERS
Bone marrow transplant
Lymphoma
Leukemia
Hemolytic anemias (sickle cell anemia, thalassemia)
Systemic mastocytosis
CONNECTIVE TISSUE/BONE DISORDERS
Juvenile osteoporosis
Osteogenesis imperfecta
Ehler-Danlos syndrome
Marfan syndrome
Homocystinuria
Fibrous dysplasia
Previous or recurrent low impact fractures
DRUGS
Alcohol
Heparin
Glucocorticosteroids
Thyroxine
Anticonvulsants
Gonadotropin-releasing hormone agonists
Cyclosporine
Chemotherapy
Cigarettes
MISCELLANEOUS DISORDERS
Immobilization (cerebral palsy, spinal muscular atrophy)
Rheumatoid arthritis
Renal disease
Athletic triad
Low calcium dietary intake
Gaucher disease

or topical therapy and the use of inhaled glucocorticoids in asthma is essential. Special diets for inborn errors of metabolism are also appropriate. Celiac disease may be overrepresented in adults with osteoporosis and should be screened for and treated appropriately (see Chapter 335.8). Treatment with bisphosphonates that inhibit bone resorption of certain secondary (glucocorticoid-induced) and adult-onset osteoporosis has been successful. Bisphosphonate therapy is also beneficial in osteogenesis imperfecta and cerebral palsy.

Beier F, LuValle P: The cyclin D1 and cyclin A genes are targets of activated PTH/PTHrP receptor in Jansen's metaphyseal chondrodysplasia. *Mol Endocrinol* 2002;16:2163–2173.

Birch K: Female athlete triad. *Br Med J* 2005;330:244–246.

Boyden LM, Mao J, Belsky J, et al: High bone density due to a mutation in LDL-receptor related protein 5. *N Engl J Med* 2002;346:1513–1521.

Cundy T, Wheadon L, King A: Treatment of idiopathic hyperphosphatasia with intensive bisphosphonate therapy. *J Bone Miner Res* 2004;19:703–711.

Fewtrell MS: Bone densitometry in children assessed by dual x ray absorptiometry: Uses and pitfalls. *Arch Dis Child* 2003;88:795–798.

Gordon CM, Bachrach LK, Carpenter TO: Bone health in children and adolescents. *Curr Prob Pediatr Adolesc Health Care* 2004;34:221–248.

Hsu JW, Vogelsang G, Jones RJ, Brodsky RA: Bone marrow transplantation in Shwachman-Diamond syndrome. *Bone Marrow Transplant* 2002;30: 255–258.

Ioannidis JPA, Ralston SH, Bennett ST, et al: Differential genetic effects of *ESR1* gene polymorphisms on osteoporosis outcomes. *JAMA* 2004;292: 2105–2114.

Jonsson KB, Zahradnik R, Larsson T, et al: Fibroblast growth factor 23 in oncogenic osteomalacia and X-linked hypophosphatemia. *N Engl J Med* 2003;348:1656–1663.

Kholsa S: Parathyroid hormone plus alendronate—a combination that does not add up. *N Engl J Med* 2003;349:1277–1279.

Loud KJ, Gordon CM: Adolescent bone health. *Arch Pediatr Adolesc Med* 2006;160:1026–1032.

Mumm S, Jones J, Finnegan P, Whyte MP: Hypophosphatasia: Molecular diagnosis of Rathbun's original case. *J Bone Miner Res* 2001;16:1724–1727.

Scholes D, LaCroix AZ, Ichikawa LE, et al: Change in bone mineral density among adolescent women using and discontinuing depot medroxyprogesterone acetate contraception. *Arch Pediatr Adolesc Med* 2005;159: 139–144.

Solomon CG: Bisphosphonates and osteoporosis. *N Engl J Med* 2002; 346:642.

Stenson WF, Newberry R, Lorenz R, et al: Increased prevalence of celiac disease and need for routine screening among patients with osteoporosis. *Arch Intern Med* 2005;165:393–399.

Van der Sluis IM, de Ridder MAJ, Boot AM, et al: Reference data for bone density and body composition measured with dual energy x-ray absorptiometry in white children and young adults. *Arch Dis Child* 2002;87: 341–347.

Whyte MP, Hughes AE: Expansile skeletal hyperphosphatasia is caused by a 15-base pair tandem duplication in TNFRSF11A encoding RANK and is allelic to familial expansile osteolysis. *J Bone Miner Res* 2002;17:26–29.

Whyte MP, Wenkert D, Clements KL, et al: Bisphosphonate-induced osteopetrosis. *N Engl J Med* 2003;349:457–463.

Part XXXII ▪ Environmental Health Hazards

Chapter 706 ▪ Biologic Effects of Radiation on Children Thomas L. Slovis

BASIC PRINCIPLES

Radiation exposure may be natural or environmental (manmade). In the U.S., most environmental radiation comes from radon gas (55%); cosmic rays and other terrestrial primordial radionuclides contribute an additional 16%. Of the 28% of environmental radiation that is manmade, medical procedures account for the largest component (15%). Some imaging procedures do not produce radiation (Table 706-1), and not all radiation-producing modalities expose a child to the same amount of radiation (Table 706-2).

Nuclear medicine and positron emission tomography examinations are described by the amount of radioactivity injected. The units of absorbed dose, as defined by the International Commission of Radiation Units, are the **rad,** introduced in the 1960s, and the **gray** (Gy), introduced in 1985. In radiation protection the quantities *equivalent dose* and *effective dose* are used. The old unit is the **rem;** the new unit is the **sievert** (Sv) [Table 706-3]. Not all radiation has the same effect on biologic tissue for a given dose. Alpha particles and protons cause significantly more damage than gamma radiation (x-rays) for a given absorbed dose. Diagnostic imaging uses x-rays. Each dose has a modifier, e.g., skin dose, whole body dose, organ dose, or effective dose. **Effective dose** considers specific tissues and their radiosensitivity.

BIOLOGIC EFFECTS OF RADIATION

Biologic effects of radiation are divided into two types. **Deterministic effects** are characterized by a threshold dose: e.g., cataracts do not occur with an acute exposure of <200 rad or with chronic exposure of <500 rad (Table 706-4). Deterministic effects from the doses generally used in diagnostic radiation have not been reported, although newer invasive procedures have led to major skin effects. **Stochastic** (random) **effects** are of greater concern because they can occur at any dose; i.e., there is no threshold, with the probability of an effect increasing with increasing dose. These effects can be caused by any radiation striking vulnerable tissue (most importantly DNA, but cytoplasm also may be at risk) and causing irreversible damage. These effects lead to the **linear no dose threshold** (LNT) concept, which states that radiation damage increases with increasing dose in a linear fashion. This concept stresses that no level of radiation exposure can be considered to be absolutely safe.

TABLE 706-1. Imaging Modalities

MODALITY	SOURCE
Plain film	Radiation (x-ray)
Ultrasound	Sound beams
Computed tomography	Radiation (x-ray)
Magnetic resonance imaging	Magnetic field
Nuclear medicine	Radiation (injected isotope)
Positron emission tomography	Radiation (injected isotope)

TABLE 706-2. Radiation Dose by Imaging Text*

EXAMINATION	mrad or mrem	SITE MEASURED
Chest—2 views	10–20	Entrance (skin)
Abdominal—2 views	50–100	Entrance (skin)
Fluoroscopy		
Nonpulsed	300–500/min	Entrance (skin)
Pulsed	100–150/min	Entrance (skin)
Computed tomography†		
head	6000 (2,000–3,000)	Mid-diameter of phantom of 16 cm
abdomen	3000 (1,000)	Mid-diameter of phantom of 32 cm
Nuclear medicine‡ (^{99m}TcMAG3-renal)	120	Effective dose
Positron emission tomography‡ (brain FDG)	185	Effective dose, whole body

*Background radiation is approximately 1 mrad/day (300 mrad/year)

†Scan explained as CT dose index (CTDI). First dose is with adult factors; second, in (), is examination adjusted for children.

‡Expressed as effective dose. These are rough guidelines for dose given to a 5-year-old with normal renal function.

FDG, (F-18) fluoro-2-deoxyglucose; ^{99m}TcMAG3, ^{99m}technetium mercaptoacetyltriglycine.

From Valentin J: Radiation dose to patients from radiopharmaceuticals: (Addendum 2 to ICRP Publication 53) ICRP Publication 80 Approved by the Commission in September 1997. *Ann ICRP* 1998; 28: 1.

Radiation can cause genetic mutations, carcinogenesis, and cell death. The biologic effects of radiation result primarily from damage to DNA directly through interaction of fast recoil electrons caused by the absorption of x-rays (⅓ of the damage) or secondarily by the formation of free radicals. Because approximately 80% of the cell is water, most of the energy deposited in a cell results in production of aqueous free radicals. The reactions are rapid (10^{-18} to 10^{-3} seconds). A dose of 1 rad results in approximately 10^3 ionizations per cell type. The biochemical and physiologic changes that follow take hours or days, whereas the induction of cancer takes many years.

The manifestations of DNA injury are variable. The cell containing the damaged DNA might die; cell death (apoptosis) is a mechanism for eliminating heavily damaged and potentially mutable cells. Damage to a base pair is the most prevalent and least significant effect. Although breaks of a single strand of DNA usually have little biologic significance because the strands are repaired using the opposite strand as a template, a mutation can result if misrepair occurs.

Breakage of both strands of DNA (the least common event) is more problematic. The end result seems to depend on the proximity of the break in each strand. If widely separated, repairs occur as with a single-strand break. If the breaks in the two

TABLE 706-3. Radiation Measurements

UNITS	RADIOACTIVITY	ABSORBED DOSE	DOSE EQUIVALENT	EXPOSURE
Common units	curie (Ci)	rad	rem	Roentgen (R)
New units	becquerel (Bq)	gray (Gy)	sievert (Sv)	coulombs/kg

CONVERSION EQUIVALENTS

1 millicurie (mCi) = 37 megabecquerels (MBq)*	
100 rad	= 1 Gy
1 rad	= 1 cGy
100 rem	= 1 Sv
1 rem	= 10 mSv

Background radiation dose is approximately 1 millirad/day

*To convert mBq to mSv, use conversion table:

1 mrad = millirad = 1/1,000 of a rad.

*rem = rad × radiation factor; weighting for gamma and x-ray this factor is 1.

rem = rad × 1.

TABLE 706-4. Deterministic Dose Rates

INJURY	APPROXIMATE THRESHOLD
Skin	
Transient erythema	200 rad (2 Gy)
Dry desquamation	1,000 rad (10 Gy)
Moist desquamation	1,500 rad (15 Gy)
Temporary epilation	200 rad (2 Gy)
Permanent epilation	700 rad (7 Gy)
Eyes	
Cataracts (acute)	>200 rad (2.0 Gy)

Modified from Hall EJ: *Radiobiology for the Radiologist,* 5th ed. Philadelphia, Lippincott Williams & Wilkins, 2000.

strands are opposite each other (or separated by only a few base pairs), however, repair is more difficult without a template. This type of break is the mechanism of radiation-induced cell killing, chromosomal damage, mutations, and carcinogenesis.

When DNA damage occurs, aberrations are produced in chromosomes, resulting in an *unstable aberration* (usually lethal to dividing cells) or *stable aberration.* Stable aberrations can result in chromosomes failing to reunite (leading to deletions), or they might rearrange in an abnormal manner, such as reciprocal translocation or aneuploidy. Although it is logical to think that these abnormalities in chromosomes lead to mutations that can activate oncogenes or protooncogenes or cause mutations in tumor-suppressor genes (see Chapter 492), few radiation-induced cancers show specific translocations such as would be associated with activation of specific oncogenes or known tumor-suppressor genes. An exception is the radiation induction of papillary thyroid carcinoma in children, which probably results from activation of the RET oncogene (see Chapter 506).

Radiation carcinogenesis seems to be a progressive multistep process composed of three independent stages: morphologic changes, cellular immortality, and tumorigenicity. Radiation exposure induces cellular genomic instability. This instability is transmitted to a cell's progeny, resulting in a continued elevation in the rate at which genetic changes arise in the subsequent generations of the irradiated cell (Fig. 706-1).

A longitudinal study of the lifetime risks of excess cancer secondary to irradiation has been evaluating atomic bomb survivors. Over 86,000 survivors have been followed for more than 50 yr since exposure. Individual radiation doses were estimated by considering the person's location in relation to the distance to the epicenter and individual shielding situations. Most of the exposure was direct gamma irradiation, with some neutron exposure. Age at exposure influences sensitivity to radiation-induced cancers (Fig. 706-2). Compared to the middle-aged adult, children are 10 times more sensitive to radiation-induced carcinogenesis, and the youngest neonate is more sensitive than the older child. Because of the higher risks associated with breast and thyroid cancer, girls are more sensitive than boys.

The doses used in diagnostic radiology for multislice CT scans overlap with low-dose induced cancer in atomic bomb survivors (Fig. 706-3). It has been estimated that the lifetime risk of cancer following head and abdominal CT scans in children is 1 : 1000. The advent of digital picture archiving communication systems (PACS) may create an inability to determine if the patient received "as low as resonably achievable" (ALARA) radiation dosing.

Increased biologic vulnerability to radiation is seen in the fetus exposed in utero through maternal radiation. Results from a case control study conducted in the mid-1900s comparing the frequency of radiation exposure in utero among children dying from childhood malignancy to those dying of other causes found that in utero radiation was associated with a 92% increased risk of dying from leukemia before age 10 yr and a 180% increased risk of dying from other malignant diseases. A follow-up conducted 20 yr later still found an increased relative risk (1.38) of cancer in childhood associated with radiation in utero.

The fetus and young children are most vulnerable to radiation-induced cancer because: (1) they are growing rapidly, with many cells undergoing mitotic activity; (2) radiation-induced tumors (except leukemia) take a long time to develop and children have a longer lifetime ahead of them; and (3) the cumulative effect of radiation is lifelong.

Most childhood tumors occur sporadically, but 10–15% of cases have a strong familial association. Diseases that are associated with sensitivity to radiation are listed in Table 706-5.

TABLE 706-5. Inherited Human Syndromes Associated with Sensitivities to X-rays

Ataxia-telangiectasia
Basal cell nevoid syndrome
Cockayne syndrome
Down syndrome
Fanconi's anemia
Gardner syndrome
Nijmegan breakage syndrome
Usher syndrome

Modified from Slovis TL, Berdon WE, Hall EJ: The effects of radiation on children. In Kuhn JP, Slovis TL, Haller JO (editors): *Caffey's Pediatric Diagnostic Imaging,* 10th ed. Philadelphia, Mosby, 2003, pp 1–13; and Hall EJ: *Radiobiology for the Radiologist,* 5th ed. Philadelphia, Lippincott Williams & Wilkins, 2000, p 45.

DECREASING UNNECESSARY DIAGNOSTIC RADIATION IN CHILDREN WHILE STILL OBTAINING DIAGNOSTIC IMAGES—A DUAL RESPONSIBILITY

Selecting the correct examination is the responsibility of the ordering physician and may involve consulation with the pediatric radiologist. Organizations such as the American College of Radiology have evidence-based imaging guidelines. Evidence-based medicine has shown little yield in the imaging work-up (including CT) of a child with a single seizure without other neurological abnormalities. This is especially true if there is no antecedent history of abnormal behavior or personality or developmental change. CT does not detect as many abnormalities as MR, but CT involves radiation. MR detects the subtle changes of congenital or acquired anomalies much more easily. Therefore, it is appropriate **except** in an emergent situation to obtain an MR within a reasonable time frame instead of doing 2 tests (CT followed by an MRI).

It has been estimated that 30% of CT examinations are not necessary, are redundant, or can be replaced by another non-radiation producing modality. The dialogue between the ordering physician and pediatric radiologist is crucial. Both physicians have similar concerns; they do not want to miss any abnormality. The ordering physician does not want to miss an acute lesion and wants to be sure the patient gets the test done, while the radiologist does not want to miss anything by lowering the radiation dose (getting a non-diagnostic image).

REDUCING RADIATION FROM THE CT EXAMINATION

The most common source of medical radiation is CT. We have progressed from a single slice scanner to those that can obtain up to 64 slices in subsecond time. The images have excellent detail, including multiplanar and 3D reconstruction of the acquired data, although the radiation dose per exam is increasing. Where we once obtained 10 to 12 images in over 30 min, we now get hundreds of images in less than a min. Doing more is not necessarily helpful in children because they are 10 times more sensitive to radiation than adults. Similar CT settings and exposures in children result in a relatively higher radiation dose than that given to adults (higher effective dose to the organs) because lower energy x-rays that would have been absorbed in the near field in

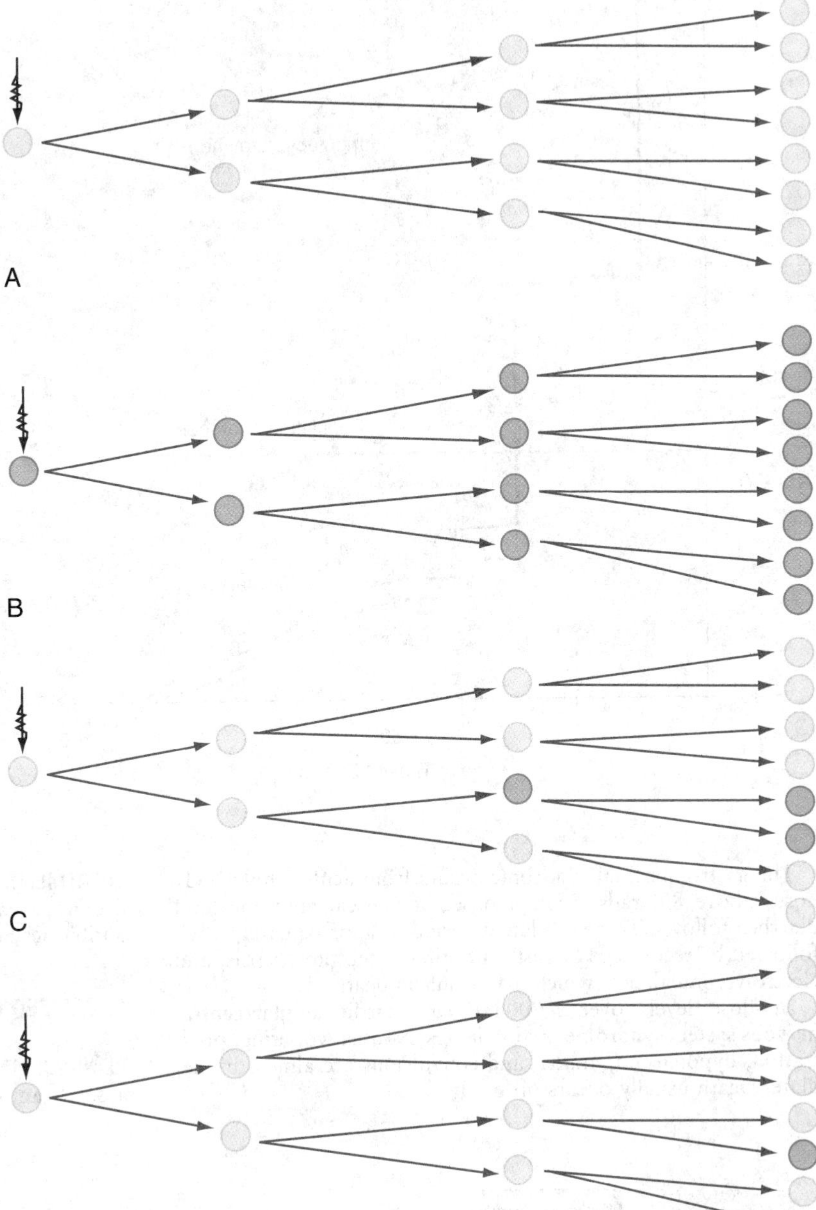

Figure 706-1. Schematic of radiation-induced mutagenesis. *Open circles* represent normal wild-type cells, whereas *closed circles* represent mutated cells. *A,* Most of the cells in an irradiated population will retain the wild-type phenotype. *B,* Example of a cell directly mutated by radiation exposure; the mutation is transmitted to all of its progeny. *C* and *D* are examples of mutations arising as a result of radiation-induced genomic instability. The irradiated cell and its immediate progeny are wild type, but the frequency with which mutations arise amongst the more distant descendants of the irradiated cell is elevated. (From Little JB: Ionizing radiation. In Kufe DW, Pollock RE, Weichselbaum RR, et al [editors]: *Holland-Frei Cancer Medicine,* 6th ed. Ontario, BC Decker, 2003, chapter 19, figure 19.3, with permission.)

an adult, pass through the entire child irradiating all organs. It is estimated that the effective dose at the same parameters in a newborn head CT scan gives 4 times the dose of an adult. With abdominal imaging, the dose is only increased by ⅔.

It is the role of the radiologist to tailor the examination to the pediatric patient. One can tell if the examination is tailored to the pediatric patient by looking at the parameters of tube current (milliamperage/second-mAs) and peak kilovoltage (kVp). There must also be proper shielding. The radiologist has many ways to decrease parameters so that children get diagnostic imaging without excessive radiation. Reducing the radiation dose by half, even in adults receiving CT, does not change the diagnostic efficacy of the study and the radiologist's ability to make the proper diagnosis.

WHOLE BODY IRRADIATION

CLINICAL MANIFESTATIONS. Table 706-6 presents dose-effect relationships for acute whole body penetrating radiation. A large single exposure of penetrating radiation can result in **acute radiation syndrome.** The signs and symptoms of this syndrome result from damage to major organ systems that have different levels of radiation sensitivity, modulated by the rate at which the radiation exposure occurred. For example, 100 rads delivered in 1 min would be symptomatic, but 1 rad/day for 100 days would not be symptomatic.

The **hematopoietic syndrome** results from acute whole body doses above 200 rads. A prodromal phase consists of nausea and vomiting within the first 12 hr, with symptoms usually lasting up to 48 hr. A latent period of 2–3 wk during which patients may feel quite well follows. Although patients are asymptomatic, bone marrow impairment has occurred. The most obvious laboratory finding is lymphocyte depression (Table 706-7). Maximal bone marrow depression occurs approximately 30 days after exposure, when hemorrhage and infection can be major problems. If the bone marrow was not completely eradicated, a recovery phase then ensues. This radiation effect is similar to what occurs when whole body irradiation (given as 1,200 rads in 2 treatments) is used to obliterate the bone marrow in children with leukemia before bone marrow transplantation.

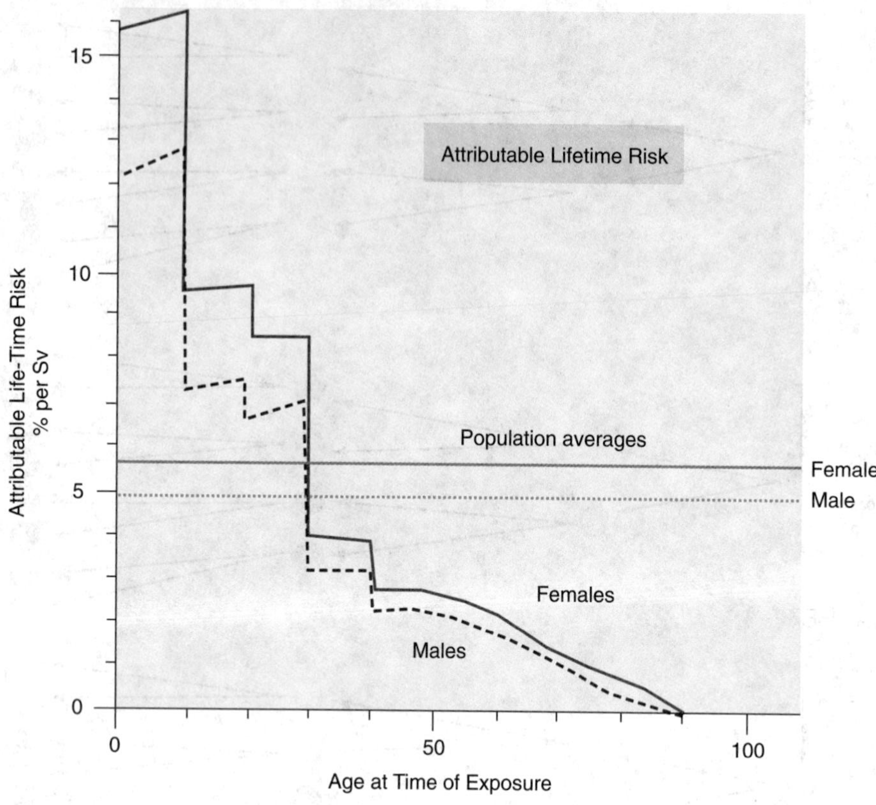

Figure 706-2. Lifetime risk of excess cancer per sievert (Sv) as a function of age at the time of exposure. Data from the atomic bomb survivors. The average risk for a population is about 5% per sievert, but the risk varies considerably with age: children are much more sensitive than adults. At early ages, girls are more sensitive than boys. (From Hall EJ: Introduction to session I: Helical CT and cancer risk. *Pediatr Radiol* 2002;32:225–227, figure 1. Reprinted with kind permission from Springer Science and Business Media.)

The **gastrointestinal syndrome** occurs from acute whole body doses above 800 rads. Prompt onset of nausea, vomiting, and diarrhea follows. There is a latent period of approximately 1 wk followed by recurrence of gastrointestinal symptoms, sepsis, and electrolyte imbalance, which may result in death.

At dose levels over 3,000 rad, the **cardiovascular/central nervous system syndrome** predominates. Nausea, vomiting, prostration, hypotension, ataxia, and convulsions are almost immediate. Death usually occurs promptly.

TREATMENT. For the hematopoietic and gastrointestinal syndromes, treatment is supportive, involving transfusions, fluids, antibiotics, and antiviral agents.

LOCALIZED IRRADIATION

CLINICAL MANIFESTATIONS. Because localized exposure involves a small amount of tissue, systemic manifestations may be less

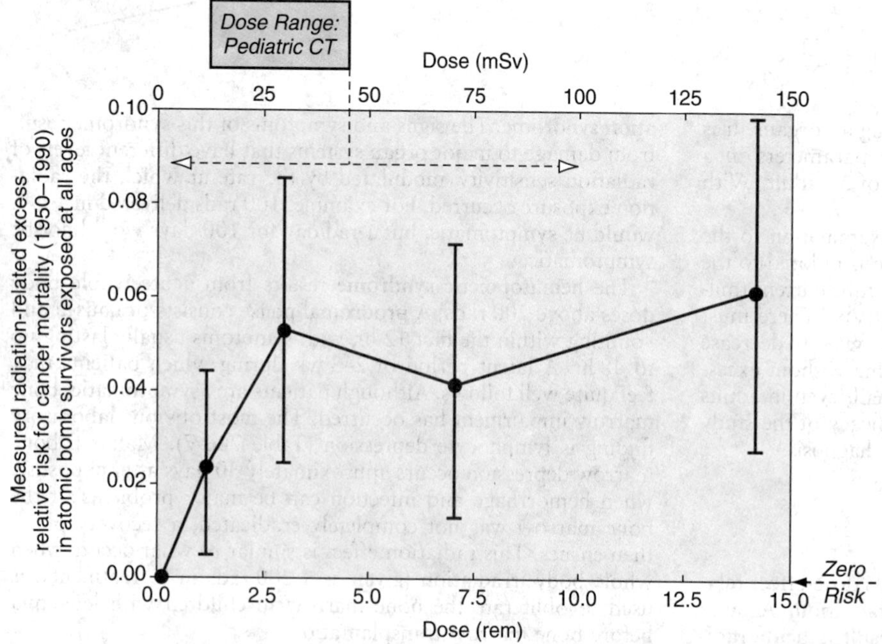

Figure 706-3. Relevant dose range for pediatric CT: 6–100 mSv (0.006 = 0.1 Sv). "There is direct, statistically significant evidence for risk in the dose range from 0 to 0.1 Sv." From Brenner DJ: Estimating cancer risks from pediatric CT: going from the qualitative to the quantitative. *Pediatr Radiol* 2002;32:228–231.

TABLE 706-6. Dose-Effect Relationships After Acute Whole Body Irradiation from Gamma or X-rays

WHOLE BODY ABSORBED DOSE, RADS (Gy)	FINDINGS
5 (0.05)	Asymptomatic
15 (0.15)	Asymptomatic (but chromosome aberrations may be present in cultured peripheral lymphocytes)
50 (0.5)	Asymptomatic (minor depression of white blood cells and platelets in a few persons)
100 (1.0)	Nausea and vomiting in approximately 10% of patients within 2 days of exposure
200 (2.0)	Nausea and vomiting in most persons exposed, with clear hematologic depression
400 (4.0)	Nausea, vomiting, and diarrhea within 48 hr; 50% mortality without medical treatment
600 (6.0)	100% mortality within 30 days from bone marrow failure without medical treatment
5,000 (50.0)	Cardiovascular collapse and central nervous system damage, with death in 24–72 hr

severe, and patients may survive even if local absorbed doses are very high. The hand is the most common site for accidental localized irradiation injuries, usually as a result of picking up or playing with lost radiation sources. The second most common accidental site is the thigh and buttocks, predominantly from placing unsuspected highly radioactive sources in the pockets.

The effects of a thermal burn are present almost immediately, and patients invariably know what burned them. If patients present with burn-like symptoms but no known cause, radiation should be suspected.

The penetrability of the radiation is an important factor in the outcome of local radiation injury. In cases of low-energy irradiation, recovery and skin grafting are possibilities, even after high absorbed skin doses. Gamma and x-rays penetrate substantially and cause progressive obliterative endarteritis that may result in necrosis and gangrene. Few symptoms occur in the first 12 hr unless the dose has been extremely high. Patients may complain of hypersensitivity, tingling, or pain. Erythema is similar to that seen with a first-degree burn. If erythema is seen within the first 48 hr, ulceration probably will occur. The erythema may present, disappear, and return days or 1–3 wk later. Transepidermal injury is similar to a second-degree thermal burn. Blister formation may occur at 1–2 wk with doses in the range of 10,000 rads.

Some tissues that may receive localized radiation exposure are relatively radiosensitive. **Cataract formation** may occur with single gamma ray exposures in the range of 200–500 rads. Such cataracts usually take from 2 mo to several years to develop. **Oligospermia** may take up to 2 mo to develop. Transient infertility in men may result from doses as low as 15 rads, and permanent sterility may occur in men at dose levels between 300–600 rads.

TREATMENT. Skin therapy is directed at prevention of infections. Treatment of localized injuries usually involves plastic surgery and grafting, if the radiation exposure was not very penetrating (see Chapter 74). The nature of the surgery depends on the dose at various depths in tissue and the location of the lesion. The full

TABLE 706-7. Expected Outcome Based on Absolute Lymphocyte Count After Acute Penetrating Whole Body Irradiation

MINIMAL LYMPHOCYTE COUNT WITHIN FIRST 48 Hr AFTER EXPOSURE	PROGNOSIS
1,000–3,000 normal range	No significant injury
1,000–1,500	Significant but probably nonlethal injury, good prognosis
500–1,000	Severe injury, fair prognosis
100–500	Very severe injury, poor prognosis
<100	Lethal without compatible bone marrow donor

TABLE 706-8. Second Cancers and their Relationship with Primary Cancers*

SECOND CANCERS	PRIMARY CANCERS	LATENCY (MEDIAN IN YEARS)	RISK FACTORS
Brain tumors	ALL; brain tumors; HD	9–10	Radiation; younger age
MDS/AML	ALL; HD; bone tumors	3–5	Topoisomerase II inhibitors; alkylating agents
Breast cancer	HD; bone tumors; soft-tissue sarcomas; ALL; brain tumors; Wilms' tumors; NHL	15–20	Radiation; female gender
Thyroid cancer	ALL: HD; neuroblastoma; soft-tissue sarcomas; bone tumors; NH:L	13–15	Radiation; younger age; female gender
Bone tumors	Retinoblastoma (heritable); other bone tumors; Ewing's sarcoma; soft-tissue sarcomas; ALL	9–10	Radiation; alkylating agents; removal of the spleen
Soft-tissue sarcomas	Retinoblastoma (heritable); soft-tissue sarcomas; HD; Wilms' tumors; bone tumors; ALL	10–11	Radiation; younger age; anthracyclines

*From Bhatia S, Sklar S. Second cancers in survivors of childhood cancer. *N Rev Cancer* 2002;2:124–132, with permission.

expression of radiation injury often is not apparent for 1–2 yr, owing to slow arteriolar narrowing that can cause delayed necrosis. After relatively penetrating radiation, amputation may be necessary because of obliterative changes in small vessels.

RADIATION THERAPY

Radiation therapy uses high doses to kill malignant cells. The sensitivity of normal cells is quite close to that of malignant cells, and to achieve significant cure rates, radiation oncologists also must accept a given percentage of serious complications (5–10%). Radiation therapy protocols are reasonably standardized. Most regimens use about 50 Gy (5,000 rads) given in about 25 fractions over 5 wk. A treatment scheme that uses doses much more than 10% higher than this or uses this dose with significantly fewer fractions poses a high incidence of severe complications.

Annually, childhood cancer affects 70 to 160 per million children between the ages of 0 and 14 yr. Because of earlier diagnosis and improved therapy, more than 70% of children with cancer are long-term survivors. We are now seeking better ways to prevent or improve care for the late effects of cancer therapy (see Table 706-9). It is very difficult at times to separate the results of chemotherapy, radiation, or combined chemotherapy radiation. The kinds of effects depend on the age at radiation (amount of growth remaining, pubertal status). Second cancers may account for 6–10% of all cancers in children or adults. Among childhood cancer survivors, there is a 3- to 6-fold risk of a second cancer.

Three to 12% of children who were treated for 1 neoplasm will develop a second malignancy by the age of 25 yr (Table 706-8). Almost 70% of the second neoplasms are in the field of the original radiation. Radiation therapy increases the risk of second cancers in a dose-dependent manner for non-genetic neoplasms.

The exact complications depend on the location of the treatment field. In children, because of the location of many childhood tumors, the central nervous system (CNS) commonly is in the treatment field and suffers complications. Standard irradiation of the brain in children results in cortical atrophy in more than half of patients who received 2,000–6,000 rads; 26% have white matter changes (leukoencephalopathy), and 8% have calcifications (Fig. 706-4). The younger the child is at the time of irradiation, the greatest is the atrophy. Some patients also develop mineralizing microangiopathy (Fig. 706-5). Radiation-induced

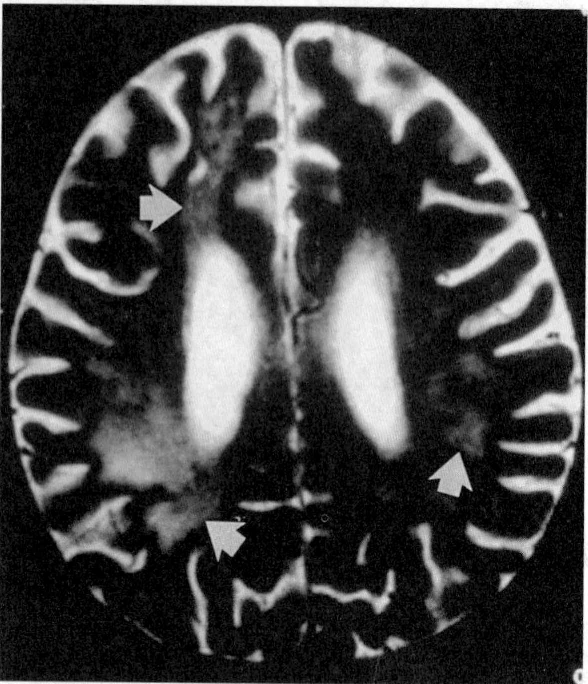

Figure 706-4. T2-weighted MRI scan of a child after radiation therapy shows white matter changes *(arrows)*.

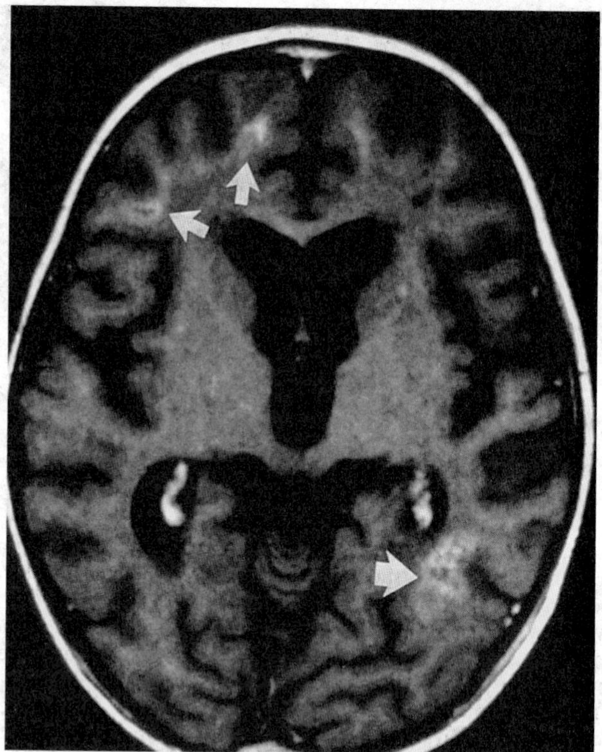

Figure 706-5. Generalized brain changes after radiation therapy. T1-weighted MRI scan of a child shows both central and cortical atrophy as well as high signal areas *(arrows)*, owing to mineralizing microangiopathy.

changes of the brain are potentiated by methotrexate administered before, during, or after radiation therapy.

Cerebral necrosis is a serious complication of radiation-induced vascular disease. It usually is diagnosed 1–5 yr after irradiation but can occur up to a decade later. Radiation-induced necrosis occurs with a moderate probability when radiation therapy schemes exceed 4,000 rads in 10 fractions, 5,000 rads in 20 fractions, or 6,000 rads in 30 fractions, or when individual fractions exceed 300 rads. Brain necrosis may be manifested by headache, increased intracranial pressure, seizures, sensory deficits, and psychotic changes.

Spinal cord irradiation may result in **radiation myelitis,** which may be either transient or permanent. Acute transient myelitis often appears 2–4 mo after irradiation. Patients with myelitis usually present with **Lhermitte sign,** a sensation of little electrical shocks in the arms and legs occurring with neck flexion or other movements that stretch the spinal cord. Reversal of transient myelopathy usually occurs between 8–40 wk and does not necessarily progress to delayed necrosis.

Delayed myelopathy occurs after a mean latent period of 20 mo, but it can occur earlier if the total dose or dose per fraction is high. This usually is manifested by discontinuous deterioration and is irreversible. In the cervical and thoracic regions, sensory dissociation develops, followed by spastic and then flaccid paresis. In the lumbar cord, flaccid paresis is dominant. The mortality for high thoracic and cervical lesions reaches 70%, with death due to pneumonia and urinary tract infections.

Irradiation also causes other effects specific to children (Table 706-9). The **effect on growth** is most pronounced when children are younger than 6 yr or during their adolescent growth spurt. Scoliosis and hypoplasia of bones may occur if fractionated treatment schemes exceed 4,000 rads. Fractionated doses >2,500 rads can result in slipped capital femoral epiphyses. An increase in the incidence of benign osteochondromas also has been reported after irradiation in children. Chest wall irradiation of girls with 1,500–2,000 rads over 1 wk impairs breast development, and fractionated doses of 3,000–4,000 rads cause fibrosis and atrophy of breast tissue.

TABLE 706-9. Late Effects of Radiation Therapy in Children Treated for Cancer

SYSTEM	DOSE
Musculoskeletal	
Muscular hypoplasia	>20 Gy
Scoliosis, kyphosis, lordosis	10–20 Gy
Osteocartilaginous exostosis	?
Neuroendocrine (cranial or cranial spinal)	
Impaired growth hormone	>18 Gy
ACTH deficiency	>40 Gy
TRH deficiency	>40 Gy
Precocious puberty (females mostly)	>20 Gy
Gonadotropin deficiency	<40 Gy
Gonad failure	
Ovarian failure	4–12 Gy
Testicular failure	>3 Gy
Central nervous system dysfunction*	
Structured changes	>18 Gy
Cognitive changes	?
Other	
Pulmonary fibrosis	
Nephropathy	
Liver failure	
Arteritis	
Eye impairment	
Ear impairment	
Bone marrow dysfunction	
Cardiac impairment	

*With intrathecal chemotherapy (MTX).

Derived from Halperin EC, Constine LS, Tarbell NJ, Kun LE (editors): *Pediatric Radiation Oncology,* 3rd ed, Philadelphia, Lippincott Williams & Wilkins, chapters 19–20, 1999.

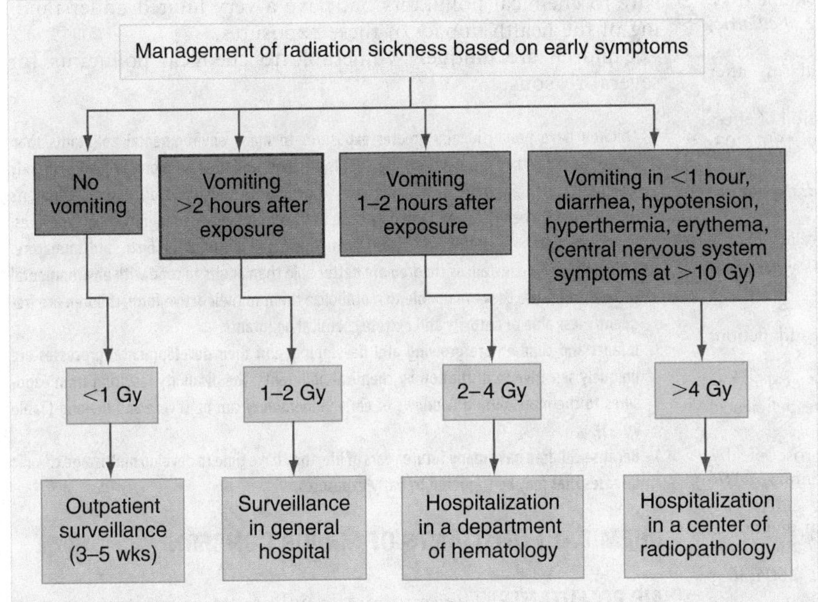

Figure 706-6. Management of radiation sickness at different levels of medical care, depending on the appearance of early symptoms and the estimated radiation dose to the whole body. (From Turai I, Veress K, Günalp B, Souchkevitch: Medical response to radiation incidents and radionuclear threats. *BMJ* 2204;328:568–572.)

INTERNAL CONTAMINATION

EPIDEMIOLOGY. Accidents involving internal contamination are rare and usually are the result of misadministration in hospital settings or voluntary ingestion of unsuspected contaminated radioactive materials. Other possible causes of internal contamination of children include ingestion of breast milk from mothers who have had diagnostic nuclear medicine scans and radiation exposure when a parent or sibling receives a therapeutic dose of iodine 131.

CLINICAL MANIFESTATIONS. The hazards from internal contamination depend on the nature of both the radionuclide (particularly in terms of its solubility in water, half-life, and radioactive emission) and the chemical compound.

TREATMENT. The most effective treatment requires knowledge of both the radionuclide and the chemical form. Treatment must be instituted quickly to be effective (Table 706-10). **Removal treatment** involves cleaning a contaminated wound and performing stomach lavage or administration of cathartics in the case of ingestion. Administration of alginate-containing antacids (e.g., Gaviscon) also usually helps in removal by decreasing absorption in the gastrointestinal tract. An example of **blocking therapy** is the administration of potassium iodine or other stable iodine-containing compounds to patients with known internal contamination with radioactive iodine. The stable iodine effectively blocks the thyroid, although its effectiveness decreases rapidly as time elapses after the contamination. The recommended dose of potassium iodine is 16 mg for neonates; 32 mg to age 3 yr; and 65 mg from 3–18 yr. Each dose protects for only 1 day. **Dilution therapy** is used in cases of tritium (radioactive hydrogen as water) contamination. Forcing fluids promotes excretion. Cases of internal contamination with transuranic elements (americium and plutonium) may require **chelation therapy** with calcium diethylene triaminepentaacetic acid (DTPA).

TABLE 706-10. Specific Therapy for Internal Contamination

RADIONUCLIDE	THERAPEUTIC APPROACH
Tritium	Dilution (force fluids)
Iodine 125 or iodine 131	Blockage (SSKI or potassium iodide), mobilization (antithyroid drugs)
Cesium 134 or cesium 137	Reduction of gastrointestinal absorption (Prussian blue)
Strontium 89 or strontium 90	Reduction of absorption (aluminum phosphate gel antacids), blockage (strontium lactate), displacement (oral phosphate), mobilization (ammonium chloride or parathyroid extract)
Plutonium and other transuranic elements	Chelation with zinc or calcium diethylenetriamine pentaacetic acid (investigational agents)
Unknown	Reduction of absorption (emetics, lavage, charcoal, or laxatives) in cases of ingestion

SSKI, saturated solution of potassium iodide.
From Mettler FA, Voelz GL: Major radiation exposure—What to expect and how to respond. *N Engl J Med* 2002;346:1554.

EXTERNAL CONTAMINATION

The presence of external radioactive contamination on a patient's skin is not an immediate medical emergency. Management involves removing and controlling the spread of radioactive materials. If a patient has suspected surface contamination and no physical injuries, decontamination can be performed relatively easily. If substantial physical trauma or other life-threatening injuries are combined with external contamination, surface decontamination should proceed only after the patient has been stabilized physiologically. In many accident situations, essential medical care is delayed inappropriately by hospital emergency staff because of fear of radiation or spread of contamination in the hospital. After a radiation accident, triaging of patients is critical and is based on exposure and symptoms (Fig. 706-6).

American College of Radiology: *Practice Guidelines and Technical Standards.* Reston, VA: American College of Radiology, 2003.

Bernal B, Altman NR: Evidence-based medicine: Neuroimaging of seizures. *Neuroimag Clin North Am* 2003;13:211–224.

Berrington de Gonzalez A, Darby S: Risk of cancer from diagnostic X-rays: Estimates for the UK and 14 other countries. *Lancet* 2004;363:345–351.

Bhatia S, Sklar S: Second cancers in survivors of childhood cancer. *N Rev Cancer* 2002;2:124–132.

Brenner DJ, Elliston CD, Hall EJ, et al: Estimated risks of radiation-induced fatal cancer from pediatric CT. *AJR* 2001;176:289–296.

Cuthbertson DJ, Davidson J: What to tell patients about radioiodine therapy. *BMJ* 2006;333:271–272.

Doll R, Wakeford R: Risk of childhood cancer from fetal irradiation. *Br J Radiol* 1997;70:130–139.

Frush DP, Donnelly LF, Rosen NS: Computed tomography and radiation risks: What pediatric health care providers should know. *Pediatrics* 2003;112:951–957.
Gangopadhyay KK, Sundram F, De P: Triggering radiation alarms after radioiodine treatment. *BMJ* 2006;333:293–294.
Huda W, Atherton JV, Ware DE, et al: An approach for the estimation of effective radiation dose at CT in pediatric patients. *Radiology* 1997;203: 417–422.
Huda W: Effective dose to adult and pediatric patients. *Pediatr Radiol* 2002;32:272–279.
Imaizumi M, Usa T, Tominaga T, et al: Radiation dose-response relationships for thyroid nodules and autoimmune thyroid diseases in Hiroshima and Nagasaki atomic bomb survivors 55–58 years after radiation exposure. *JAMA* 2006;295:1011–1022.
Kal HB, Struikmans H: Radiotherapy during pregnancy: Fact and fiction. *Lancet Oncol* 2005;6:328–333.
Kasatkinan EP, Shilin DE, Rosenbloom AL, et al: Effects of low level radiation from the Chernobyl accident in a population with iodine deficiency. *Eur J Pediatr* 1997;156:916.
Koenig TR, Wolff D, Mettler FA, et al: Skin injuries from fluoroscopically guided procedures: Part I, characteristics of radiation injury. *AJR* 2001;177:3–11.
Martin D, Semelka RC: Health effects of ionizing radiation from diagnostic CT. *Lancet* 2006;367:1712–1714.
McLean D: Computed tomography doses in children. *Lancet* 2004;363: 1178.
Mettler FA, Voelz GL: Major radiation exposure—What to expect and how to respond. *N Engl J Med* 2002;346:1554–1561.
Oeffinger KC, Mertens AC, Sklar CA, et al: Chronic health conditions in adult survivors of childhood cancer. *N Engl J Med* 2006;355:1572–1582.
Pierce DA, Preston DL: Radiation-related cancer risks at low doses among atomic bomb survivors. *Radiat Res* 2000;154:178–186.
Pierce DA, Shimizu Y, Preston DL, et al: Studies of the mortality of atomic bomb survivors. Report 12, part 1. Cancer: 1950–1990. *Radiat Res* 1996;146:1–27.
Preston DL, Ron E, Yonehara S, et al: Tumors of the nervous system and pituitary gland associated with atomic bomb radiation exposure. *J Natl Cancer Inst* 2002;94:1555–1563.
Salamipour H, Jimenez RM, Bree SL, et al: Multidetector row CT in pediatric musculoskeletal imaging. *Pediatr Radiol* 2005;35:555–564.
Slovis TL: Children, computed tomography radiation dose, and the As Low As Reasonably Achievable (ALARA) concept. *Pediatrics* 2003;112: 971–972.
Sources and Effects of Ionizing Radiation. Report to the General Assembly. Vienna: United Nations Scientific Committee on the Effects of Atomic Radiation, 2000.
Turai I, Veress K, Günalp B, et al: Medical response to radiation incidents and radionuclear threats. *BMJ* 2004;328:568–572.

Chapter 707 ■ Chemical Pollutants

Philip J. Landrigan and Joel A. Forman

Children today are at risk of exposure to more than 80,000 synthetic chemicals, most of which have been developed since World War II. They are especially likely to be exposed to the 2,863 high-production-volume (HPV) chemicals that are produced in amounts of 1 million pounds or more per year and are most widely dispersed in the environment. Biomonitoring data from the Centers for Disease Control's *Third National Report on Human Exposure to Environmental Chemicals* provide evidence that children are exposed to a broad array of synthetic chemicals and in some cases carry a greater body burden than adults. This type of data documents children's exposure but does not address health effects. Fewer than half of the HPV chemicals have been tested for their potential hazards to human health, and less than 10% have been assessed for their pediatric or developmental toxicity. We are increasingly aware of the extent of children's exposure to chemical pollutants but have a very limited understanding of the health impact of these exposures.

Children are uniquely vulnerable to chemical pollutants for several reasons:

1. **Children have proportionally greater exposures to many environmental pollutants than adults. Because they drink more water, eat more food, and breathe more air per kg of body weight, children are more heavily exposed to pollutants in water, food, and air. Children's hand-to-mouth behavior and their play close to the ground further magnify their exposures.**
2. **Children's metabolic pathways, especially in the first months after birth, are immature. Although in some instances children are better able than adults to cope with environmental toxicants because they are unable to metabolize them to their active form, children are frequently less able to detoxify and excrete chemical pollutants.**
3. **Infants and children are growing and developing, and their developmental processes are uniquely sensitive to disruption by chemical pollutants. The disability resulting from exposures to chemicals during windows of early vulnerability can be severe and lifelong (Table 707-1).**
4. **Because children have many future years of life, they have time to develop multistage chronic diseases that may be triggered by early exposures.**

CHEMICAL POLLUTANTS OF MAJOR CONCERN

AIR POLLUTANTS. The outdoor air pollutants of greatest concern are photochemical oxidants (especially ozone), oxides of nitrogen (NO_x), fine particulates, sulfur oxides, and carbon monoxide. These pollutants result principally from the combustion of fossil fuels. Automotive emissions are the major source of air pollution worldwide, followed by fixed sources such as power plants.

Elevated levels of air pollutants, especially elevations of fine particulates, ozone, and NO_x, are associated with respiratory problems in children, including decreased pulmonary expiratory flow, wheezing, and exacerbations of asthma. Fine particulate air pollution, even at low levels, is associated with slight increases in cardiopulmonary mortality and with an increased death rate from sudden infant death syndrome (SIDS) [see Chapter 372]. Evidence from a prospective cohort study of air pollution and lung development in California demonstrates reduced lung growth from ages 10 to 18, which leads to clinically significant decreases in lung function that persist into adulthood.

Indoor air also can be an important source of respiratory irritation, because many children spend 80–90% of their time indoors. Indoor air pollution has become especially important in the United States since the energy crises of the 1970s, which led to the construction of tighter, more energy-efficient homes. Allergens in indoor air can contribute to respiratory problems and include cockroach, mite, mold, cat, and dog allergens. Some indoor molds produce chemical toxins called mycotoxins. Environmental tobacco smoke is another major contributor to exacerbations of childhood asthma.

LEAD. Lead exposure occurs worldwide (see Chapter 709). Exposure is especially common in countries that still permit leaded gasoline. In the United States, pediatric blood lead levels have declined by more than 90% in the past 20 yr, principally as a

TABLE 707-1. Effects of Selected Chemical Pollutants on Infants and Children

CHEMICAL EXPOSURE	EFFECT
Diethylstibestrol	Adenocarcinoma of the vagina after intrauterine exposure
Thalidomide	Phocomelia after intrauterine exposure
Trichloroethylene	Elevated risk of leukemia after intrauterine exposure
Alcohol	Fetal alcohol syndrome after intrauterine exposure
Lead	Neurobehavioral toxicity from low-dose exposure
Nitrosamine, vinyl chloride, ionizing radiation	Increased risk of cancer after intrauterine exposure
Organophosphate insecticides	Developmental neurotoxicity
Environmental tobacco smoke	Increased risk of sudden infant death syndrome and asthma

result of removal of lead from gasoline. Nevertheless, the Centers for Disease Control and Prevention estimates that more than 310,000 children 1 through 5 yrs of age still have blood lead levels of 10 μg/dL and higher. The prevalence is especially high among poor minority children in inner cities. Blood lead levels as low as 5 μg/dL have been associated with a variety of neurocognitive deficits, including decreased intelligence, shortened attention span, and increased risk of asocial behavior. Although the extent of injury is directly proportional to the lead dose, the relative impact of lead on intelligence appears to be greater at blood levels below 10 μg/dL. Lead-based paint is the major source of exposure in the United States. Because intact lead-painted surfaces invariably break down to produce lead dust, efforts to further reduce the number of children poisoned by lead in the United States must focus on the identification and permanent removal of all lead-based paint, intact or not, from residences. Leaded gasoline, industrial pollutants and cottage industry remain major sources of lead pollution in many developing countries.

MERCURY. Children may be exposed to either inorganic or organic mercury (see Chapter 708). Inorganic mercury produces dermatitis, gingivitis, stomatitis, tremor, and acrodynia. Organic or methyl mercury is fat-soluble, readily penetrates the central nervous system (CNS), and is neurotoxic. Exposure to organic mercury occurs principally through consumption of fish that have accumulated mercury deposited in lakes and oceans as atmospheric fallout from combustion of coal; coal normally contains small quantities of mercury. Even low-dose exposure to organic mercury has been shown to be hazardous to the developing fetal brain, and pregnant women are therefore advised to curtail consumption of mercury-containing fish such as tuna and swordfish. Although adverse neurologic effects have not been related to exposure from the preservative thimerosal, which contains ethyl mercury, thimerosal has been removed from routine childhood vaccines and maternal Rh vaccine (RhoGam) as a precautionary measure.

ASBESTOS. Between 1947 and 1973, asbestos was sprayed as insulation on classroom walls and ceilings in about 10,000 schools in the United States. Subsequent deterioration of this asbestos has released inhalable asbestos fibers into the air and thus poses a risk to children. Asbestos is a human carcinogen, and the two principal cancers caused by asbestos are lung cancer and mesothelioma. U.S. Federal law requires that all schools be inspected periodically for asbestos and the results made public. Removal is required only when asbestos is visibly deteriorating or is within the reach of children. In most cases, placement of barriers (dry walls or drop ceilings) provides appropriate protection.

ENVIRONMENTAL TOBACCO SMOKE. Smoking during pregnancy poses a hazard to the fetus (see Chapter 96). Infants born to women who smoke are, on the average, 10% smaller than infants born to nonsmoking women. Infants of parents who smoke have a higher risk of sudden infant death syndrome. Nicotine from tobacco smoke appears to be a developmental neurotoxin.

Passive smoking also is a hazard to children. In the United States, 43% of children younger than 12 yr old live in a home with at least one smoker. Children exposed to environmental tobacco smoke have more lower respiratory illness, more middle-ear effusions, and more viral respiratory illnesses than unexposed children.

PESTICIDES. Pesticides are a diverse group of chemicals used to control insects, weeds, fungi, and rodents. Approximately 600 pesticides are registered with the U.S. Environmental Protection Agency.

Diet is a major route of children's exposure to pesticides, because they are exposed to residues of multiple pesticides on fruit and vegetables. Children also may be exposed in homes or schools, on lawns, and in gardens. They may be exposed to pesticide drift from agricultural areas that have been sprayed. Children employed in agriculture or living in migrant farm camps are at risk of exposure to many pesticides.

Pesticides can cause a range of chronic toxic effects: polyneuropathy and CNS dysfunction (organophosphates); hormonal disruption and reproductive impairment (DDT, kepone, dibromochloropropane); cancer (aldrin, dieldrin, chlorphenoxy herbicides [2,4,5-T]); and pulmonary fibrosis (paraquat). Children's exposure to pesticides can be reduced by minimizing applications to lawns, gardens, schools, and playgrounds; by adapting techniques of integrated pest management; and by reducing pesticide applications to food crops.

Children can be acutely overexposed to pesticides (see Chapter 58). The organophosphates and carbamates, both of which cause neurotoxicity through inhibition of acetylcholinesterase, cause the largest number of acute poisoning cases. Symptoms include meiosis (although not in all cases), excess salivation, abdominal cramping, vomiting, diarrhea, and muscle fasciculation. In severe cases, the child may experience loss of consciousness, cardiac arrhythmias, and death by respiratory arrest. The war gas sarin is an organophosphate. See Chapter 58 for treatment of poisoning from drugs, chemicals, and plants.

PCBS, DDT, DIOXINS, AND OTHER CHLORINATED HYDROCARBONS. Chlorinated hydrocarbons are used as insecticides (DDT), plastics (polyvinyl chloride [PVC]), electrical insulators (polychlorinated biphenyls [PCBs]), and solvents (trichloroethylene). Highly toxic dioxins and furans can be formed during synthesis of chlorinated herbicides or as by-products of plastic combustion. All of these materials are widely dispersed in the environment. DDT, PCBs, and dioxins are highly persistent.

The embryo, fetus, and young child are at particularly high risk of injury from PCBs, DDT, and dioxins. All of these compounds are lipid-soluble. They readily cross the placenta, and they accumulate in breast milk. Intrauterine exposure to PCBs has been repeatedly linked to persistent neurobehavioral dysfunction in children.

Fish from contaminated waters are a major source of children's exposure to PCBs. Children can be exposed in utero or through breast milk. To protect children and pregnant women in the United States against PCBs in fish, government agencies have issued fish consumption advisories for certain lakes and rivers. Combustion of medical wastes containing PVC and the use of chlorine to bleach paper products are major preventable sources of environmental dioxin and should be discouraged.

ENDOCRINE DISRUPTORS. A number of chemicals have been shown to adversely affect the endocrine systems of animals and humans, including diethylstilbestrol (DES), DDT, PCBs, and dioxins. Other chemicals are also suspected of possessing endocrine disruptor effects, including other pesticides and phthalates (plasticizers). Effects on wildlife include eggshell thinning in birds, sterility in seals, feminization and cryptorchidism in panthers, low hatching rates in alligators, and many others. In humans, endocrine disruption has been implicated in the epidemiologic observations of a trend toward earlier thelarche and menarche in girls, the increasing rates of testicular cancer and hypospadias, and decreasing sperm counts. The most clearly observed effects include adenocarcinoma of the vagina in women and cryptorchidism in men whose mothers took DES. The presence of elevated plasma phthalate esters has been associated with early thelarche in Puerto Rican girls. Some endocrine disruptors may also have adverse effects on brain development. Continuing research in this area is of particular importance because of the widespread human exposure to, and the long-term biopersistence of, many of these chemicals.

ENVIRONMENTAL CARCINOGENS. Children may be exposed to carcinogenic pollutants in utero or after birth. Children appear more sensitive than adults to certain chemical carcinogens and also to radiation (see Chapter 706). The potential for in utero carcinogenesis was first recognized with the discovery that clear cell adenocarcinoma of the vagina could develop in women after intrauterine exposure to DES.

Carcinogenesis also may be associated with exposures in the home and community. Children of asbestos workers and children who have grown up near asbestos plants have been found to have a higher incidence of mesothelioma than unexposed populations. Children who grow up on farms have elevated rates of leukemia; pesticides are suspected of playing an etiologic role. Intrauterine exposure to trichloroethylene via contaminated drinking water has been associated with an increased incidence of leukemia among girls living near an industrial facility and industrial waste site.

The National Cancer Institute reports that incidence rates of leukemia and cerebral glioma, the two most common forms of childhood malignancy, have been increasing for the past 3 decades, despite greatly improved therapy and declining death rates. The cumulative increase in incidence for glioma is now about 30%. Similar increases in incidence of childhood cancer have been seen in the United Kingdom. Research is ongoing to determine whether chemical pollutants in the environment have contributed to this reported increasing incidence of childhood cancer.

ROUTES OF EXPOSURE

TRANSPLACENTAL. Heavy metals and fat-soluble compounds such as PCBs and DDT readily cross the placenta. They may produce serious and irreversible toxic effects on the developing nervous, endocrine, and reproductive organs, even at very low levels.

WATER. About 200 chemicals have been found in various amounts in water supplies. Lead is especially common. In some older neighborhoods, lead in water derives from lead pipes. More commonly, it is dissolved (leached) from solder by soft, acidic water. The highest levels of lead occur in water that has been standing in pipes overnight; it is wise to run water for 2–3 min each morning before making up infant formula. Solvents and components of gasoline such as methyl tertiary-butyl ether (MTBE) and benzene are commonly encountered in groundwater.

AIR. Vehicular emissions are the major source of urban air pollution. Diesel exhaust is a human carcinogen. In rural areas, wood smoke can contribute to air pollution. Children living in the vicinity of smelters and chemical production plants can be exposed to toxic industrial emissions such as lead, benzene, and 1,3-butadiene.

FOOD. Many chemicals are intentionally added to food to improve appearance, taste, texture, or preservation, but many such chemicals have been poorly tested for potential toxicity. Residues of many pesticides are found in both raw and processed foods. Levels of pesticides are lower in organic produce than in conventionally grown fruits and vegetables.

WORK CLOTHES. Illnesses in children sometimes may be traced to contaminated dust from parents' work clothes; toxicity from lead, beryllium, dioxin, organophosphate pesticides, and asbestos has occurred. Such exposure (termed "fouling the nest") can be prevented by providing facilities at work for changing and showering.

SCHOOLS. Children may be exposed in schools, kindergartens, and nurseries to lead paint, molds, asbestos, environmental tobacco smoke, pesticides, and hazardous arts and crafts materials. Substantial opportunities for prevention exist in the school environment, and pediatricians are often consulted for advice.

CHILD LABOR. Four to 5 million children and adolescents in the United States work for pay, and child labor is widespread around the world. Working children are at high risk of physical trauma and injury. They also may be exposed to a wide range of toxic chemicals, including pesticides in agriculture and lawn work, asbestos in construction and building demolition, and benzene in pumping gasoline.

THE PHYSICIAN'S ROLE

Pediatricians should always be alert to the possibility that a chemical pollutant has caused disease in a child. In considering the origins of noninfectious disease, they should ask about the home environment, parental occupation, unusual exposures, and neighborhood factories. An environmental cause is particularly likely when several unusual cases of disease or constellations of findings occur together. Any adolescent with a traumatic injury may have been injured at work.

The history is the single most important instrument for obtaining information on environmental exposures. Information about current and past exposures (including questions about travel to or residence in developing countries) should be sought routinely through a few brief screening questions. Changes in patterns of exposure or new exposures may be especially important. If suspicious information is elicited, more detailed follow-up should be pursued. Referral to a pediatric environmental health specialty unit may be indicated (www.ADEC.org). Accurate diagnosis of an environmental cause of disease can lead to better care of sick children and prevention of disease in other children.

American Academy of Pediatrics: *Handbook of Pediatric Environmental Health,* 2nd ed. Elk Grove Village, Il, American Academy of Pediatrics, 2003.

Centers for Disease Control and Prevention: *Third National Report on Human Exposure to Environmental Chemicals.* Atlanta, GA, Centers for Disease Control and Prevention, 2005.

Colón I, Caro D, Bourdony CJ, et al: Identification of phthalate esters in the serum of young Puerto Rican girls with premature breast development. *Environ Health Perspect* 2000;108:895–900.

Environmental Defense Fund: *Toxic Ignorance: The Continuing Absence of Basic Health Testing for Top-Selling Toxic Chemicals in the United States.* Washington, DC, Environmental Defense Fund, 1997.

Etzel RA, Balk SJ (editors): *Handbook of Environmental Health for Children,* 2nd ed.. Elk Grove Village, IL, American Academy of Pediatrics, 2003.

Frumkin H (editor): *Environmental Health: From Global to Local.* San Francisco, John Wiley & Sons, 2005.

Gauderman WJ, Avol E, Gilliland F, et al: The effect of air pollution on lung development from 10 to 18 years of age. *N Engl J Med* 2005;352:1276.

Gilliland FD, Gerhane K, Rappaport EB, et al: The effects of ambient air pollution on school absenteeism due to respiratory illnesses. *Epidemiology* 2001;12:43–54.

Jacobson JL, Jacobson SW: Intellectual impairment in children exposed to polychlorinated biphenyls in utero. *N Engl J Med* 1996;335:783–789.

Landrigan PJ, Trasande L, Thorpe LE, et al: The National Children's Study: A 21-year prospective study of 100,000 American children. *Pediatrics* 2006;118:2175–2186.

Landrigan PJ, Woolf AD, Gitterman B, et al: The Ambulatory Pediatric Association Fellowship in Pediatric Environmental Health: A five-year assessment. *Pediatrics* 2007 (in press).

Lanphear BP: Cognitive deficits associated with blood lead concentrations < 10 µg/dL in US children and adolescents. *Public Health Rep* 2000;115:521–529.

Longnecker MP, Rogan WJ, Lucier G: The human health effects of DDT (dichlorodiphenyltrichloroethane) and PCBs (polychlorinated biphenyls) and an overview of organochlorines in public health. *Annu Rev Public Health* 1997;18:211–244.

Magnani C, Dalmasso P, Biggeri A, et al: Increased risk of malignant mesothelioma of the pleura after residential or domestic exposure to asbestos: A case-control study in Casale Monferrato, Italy. *Environ Health Perspect* 2001;109:915–919.

Paulson JA (editor): Children's Environmental Health. *Pediatr Clin North Am* 2001;48:xv–1337.

Tellez-Rojo MM, Bellinger DC, Arroyo-Quiroz C, et al: Longitudinal associations between lead concentrations lower than 10 microg/dL and neurobehavioral development in environmentally exposed children in Mexico City. *Pediatrics* 2006;118:323–330.

Chapter 708 ■ Heavy Metal Intoxication

Prashant V. Mahajan

The main threats to humans from heavy metals are associated with exposure to lead, cadmium, mercury, and arsenic. The most common cause of heavy metal toxicity is lead, which is discussed separately in Chapter 709; this chapter discusses mercury and arsenic. The general population is exposed to mercury primarily via food; fish is a major source of methyl mercury exposure. Arsenic exposure can occur from contaminated food or water. Heavy metal intoxication results in diverse multiorgan toxicity through widespread disruption of vital cellular functions. The protean manifestations of acute or chronic heavy metal intoxication can easily be misdiagnosed unless a meticulous history of environmental exposure is obtained.

ARSENIC

EPIDEMIOLOGY. Arsenic is a metalloid that exists in four forms: elemental arsenic, arsine gas, inorganic arsenic salts (pentavalent arsenate form or trivalent arsenite form), and organic arsenic compounds. Toxic manifestations are higher in the more soluble and higher valence compounds. *Arsine gas* is the most toxic form of arsenic. Mass poisonings due to exposure to arsenic have occurred throughout history, including one in 1998 in Wakayama, Japan, where 70 people were poisoned. Children may be poisoned after exposure to inorganic arsenic found in pesticides, herbicides, dyes, homeopathic medicines, and certain intentionally or accidentally contaminated folk remedies from China, India, and Southeast Asia (see Chapter 59). Soil deposits may contaminate artesian well water. Groundwater contamination is a common problem in developing countries. Food products (e.g., rice) cooked in contaminated water may actually absorb arsenic, thus concentrating it in the food. The World Health Organization (WHO) has set 10 ppb as the lower limit of safety. Occupational exposure may occur in industries such as glass manufacturing, pottery, electronic components, semiconductors, lasers, mining, smelting, and refining. Organic arsenic compounds may be found in seafood, pesticides, and some veterinary pharmaceuticals. In contrast to mercury, the organic forms of arsenic found in seafood are nontoxic.

PHARMACOKINETICS. Elemental arsenic is insoluble in water and bodily fluids and, therefore, is insignificantly absorbed and nontoxic. Inhaled arsine gas is rapidly absorbed through the lungs. The inorganic arsenic salts are well absorbed through the gastrointestinal tract, lungs, and skin. The organic arsenic compounds are well absorbed through the gastrointestinal tract. After acute exposure, arsenic initially is bound to the protein portion of hemoglobin in the red blood cells (RBCs) and rapidly distributed to all tissues. Inorganic arsenic is methylated and is eliminated predominantly by the kidneys, with about 95% excreted in the urine and 5% excreted in the bile. Most of the arsenic is eliminated in the first few days, with the remainder slowly excreted over a period of several weeks. Arsenic concentrates in hair, nails, and skin. Measurement of the distance of **Mee lines** (transverse white striae on the nail) from the nail bed can provide an estimate of time of exposure (nails grow at the rate of 0.4 mm per day).

PATHOPHYSIOLOGY. After exposure to arsine gas, absorbed arsine enters red blood cells and is oxidized to arsenic dihydride and elemental arsenic. Complexing of these derivatives with red cell sulfhydryl groups results in cell membrane instability and massive hemolysis. The inorganic arsenic salts poison enzymatic processes vital to cellular metabolism. Trivalent arsenic binds to sulfhydryl groups, resulting in decreased production of adenosine triphosphate through the inhibition of enzyme systems such as the pyruvate dehydrogenase and α-ketoglutarate complexes. Pentavalent arsenic may be biotransformed to trivalent arsenic or substituted for phosphate in the glycolytic pathway, resulting in uncoupling of oxidative phosphorylation.

CLINICAL MANIFESTATIONS. Arsine gas is colorless, odorless, nonirritating, and highly toxic. Inhalation causes no immediate symptoms. After a latent period of 2–24 hr, massive hemolysis occurs, along with malaise, headache, weakness, dyspnea, nausea, vomiting, abdominal pain, hepatomegaly, pallor, jaundice, hemoglobinuria, and renal failure (Table 708-1). Acute ingestion of arsenic produces gastrointestinal toxicity within minutes to hours and is manifested by nausea, vomiting, abdominal pain, and diarrhea. Hemorrhagic gastroenteritis with extensive fluid loss and third spacing may result in hypovolemic shock. Cardiovascular toxicity includes QT interval prolongation, polymorphous ventricular tachycardia, congestive cardiomyopathy, pulmonary edema, and cardiogenic shock. Acute neurologic toxicity includes delirium, seizures, cerebral edema, encephalopathy, and coma. Lethal doses of arsenates are 5–50 mg/kg; lethal doses of arsenites are <5 mg/kg.

Late sequelae include hematuria, proteinuria, and acute tubular necrosis. A delayed sensorimotor peripheral neuropathy may appear days to weeks after acute exposure, secondary to axonal degeneration. Neuropathy is manifest by painful dysesthesias, followed by diminished vibratory, pain, touch, and temperature sensation; decreased deep tendon reflexes; and, in the most severe cases, an ascending paralysis with respiratory failure mimicking Guillain-Barré syndrome (see Chapter 615).

TABLE 708-1. Effects of Arsenic on Organ Systems

ORGAN SYSTEM	EFFECTS OF ARSENIC
Gastrointestinal system	Submucosal vesicles, watery or bloody diarrhea, severe hematemesis
Cardiovascular system	Reduced myocardial contractility, prolonged Q-T intervals, tachyarrhythmias
	Vasodilation, hypotension
Kidneys	Hematuria, proteinuria, acute tubular necrosis
Nervous system	Toxic encephalopathy with seizures, cerebral edema, and coma
	Chronic exposure: peripheral painful sensorimotor neuropathy
Hematologic and lymphatic system	Anemia and thrombocytopenia; acute hemolysis with arsine gas
Liver	Fatty degeneration with central necrosis
Skin	Desquamation, alopecia, hyperkeratosis, nail changes
	Chronic exposure: hyperkeratosis, hyperpigmentation
Teratogenic	Neural tube defects in the fetus

TABLE 708-2. Normal and Toxic Levels of Arsenic and Mercury

	ARSENIC	MERCURY
Molecular weight	74.9 d	200.59 d
Normal blood level	<5 μg/L (<0.665 nmol/L)	<10 μg/L (<50 nmol/L)
Normal urine level	<50 μg/L (<6.65 nmol/L) 24-h urine sample	<20 μg/L (<100 nmol/L)
Intervene at blood level		>35 μg/L (>175 nmol/L)
Intervene at urine level	>100 μg/L (>13.3 nmol/L) 24-h urine sample	>150 μg/L (>750 nmol/L)

TABLE 708-3. Differential Characteristics of Mercury Exposure

	ELEMENTAL	INORGANIC (SALT)	ORGANIC (ALKYL)
Primary route of exposure	Inhalation	Oral	Oral
Primary tissue distribution	CNS, kidney	Kidney	CNS, kidney, liver
Clearance	Renal, GI	Renal, GI	Methyl: GI Aryl: renal, GI
Clinical effects			
CNS	Tremor	Tremor	Paresthesias, ataxia, tremor, tunnel vision, dysarthria
Pulmonary	+++	—	—
Gastrointestinal	+	+++ (caustic)	+
Renal	+	+++ (ATN)	+
Acrodynia	+	++	—
Therapy	BAL, DMSA	BAL, DMSA	DMSA (early)

+, mild; ++, moderate; +++, severe.

ATN, acute tubular necrosis; BAL, British antilewisite; CNS, central nervous system; DMSA, 2,3-dimercaptosuccinic acid; GI, gastrointestinal.

From Sue MJ: Mercury (heavy metals). In: Goldfrank LR, Flomenbaum NE, Lewin NA, et al (editors): *Goldfrank's Toxicologic Emergencies*, 7th ed. McGraw-Hill, 2002. Available at http://www.knovel.com/knovel2/Toc.jsp?BookID=957. Reprinted with permission of The McGraw Hill Companies, Inc.

Subacute toxicity is characterized by prolonged fatigue, malaise, weight loss, headache, chronic encephalopathy, peripheral sensorimotor neuropathy, leukopenia, anemia, thrombocytopenia, chronic cough, and gastroenteritis. Mee lines in the nails become apparent 1–2 mo after exposure in about 5% of patients. Dermatologic findings include alopecia, oral ulceration, peripheral edema, a pruritic macular rash, and desquamation.

Chronic exposure to low levels of arsenic usually is from environmental or occupational sources. Over the course of years, dermatologic lesions develop, including hyperpigmentation, hypopigmentation, hyperkeratoses (especially on the palms and soles), squamous and basal cell carcinomas, and **Bowen disease** (cutaneous squamous cell carcinoma in situ). Encephalopathy and peripheral neuropathy may be present. Hepatomegaly, hypersplenism, noncirrhotic portal fibrosis, and portal hypertension occur. **Blackfoot disease** is an obliterative arterial disease of the lower extremities associated with chronic arsenic exposure that has been described in Taiwan. Carcinogenicity of chronic arsenic exposure is reflected in increased rates of cancers of the skin, lung, liver, bladder, and kidney and of angiosarcomas.

LABORATORY FINDINGS. The diagnosis of arsenic intoxication is based on characteristic clinical findings, a history of exposure, and elevated urinary arsenic levels, which confirm the exposure. A spot urine arsenic level should be determined for symptomatic patients before chelation, although initially the result may be negative. Because urinary excretion of arsenic is intermittent, definitive diagnosis depends on a 24-hr urine collection. Concentrations greater than 50 μg/L in a 24-hr urine collection are consistent with arsenic intoxication (Table 708-2). Urine specimens must be collected in metal-free containers. Ingestion of seafood containing nontoxic arsenobetaine and arsenocholine can cause elevated urinary arsenic levels. Blood arsenic levels rarely are helpful because of their high variability and the rapid clearance of arsenic from the blood in acute poisonings. Elevated arsenic levels in the hair or nails must be interpreted cautiously because of the possibility of external contamination. Abdominal radiographs may demonstrate ingested radiopaque arsenic.

Later in the course of illness, a complete blood cell count may show anemia, thrombocytopenia, and leukocytosis, followed by leukopenia, karyorrhexis, and basophilic stippling of RBCs. The serum levels of creatinine, bilirubin, and transaminases may be elevated; urinalysis may show proteinuria, pyuria, and hematuria; and examination of the cerebrospinal fluid may show elevated protein levels.

MERCURY

EPIDEMIOLOGY. Mercury exists in three forms: elemental mercury, inorganic mercury salts, and organic mercury (Table 708-3). **Elemental mercury** is present in thermometers, sphygmomanometers, barometers, batteries, and some latex paints produced before 1991. Workers in industries producing these products may expose their children to the toxin when mercury is brought home on contaminated clothing. Vacuuming of carpets contaminated with mercury and breaking of mercury fluorescent light bulbs may result in elemental mercury vapor exposure. Severe inhalation poisonings have resulted from attempts to separate gold from gold ore by heating mercury and forming a gold-mercury amalgam. Elemental mercury has been used in folk remedies by Asian and Mexican populations for chronic stomach pain and by Latin Americans and Caribbean natives in occult practices. Dental amalgams containing elemental mercury release trace amounts of mercury that do not pose a credible risk to health. An expert panel for the National Institutes of Health concluded that existing scientific evidence does not indicate that dental amalgams pose a health risk; they should not be replaced merely to decrease mercury exposure.

Inorganic mercury salts are found in pesticides, disinfectants, antiseptics, pigments, dry batteries, and explosives, and as preservatives in some medicinal preparations. **Organic mercury** in the diet, especially fish containing methyl mercury, is a major source of mercury exposure among the general population. Industries that may produce mercury-containing effluents include chlorine and caustic soda production, mining and metallurgy, electroplating, chemical and textile manufacturing, paper and pharmaceutical manufacturing, and leather tanning. Mercury compounds in the environment are methylated to methyl mercury by soil and water microorganisms. Methyl mercury in the water rapidly accumulates in fish (swordfish, king mackerel, fresh tuna, tile fish, shark) and other aquatic organisms, which are in turn consumed by humans. Well-known large outbreaks of methyl mercury intoxication include the incidents in Japan in the 1950s (**Minamata disease,** from consumption of contaminated seafood) and in Iraq in 1971 (from consumption of grain treated with a methyl mercury fungicide).

Thimerosal is a mercury-containing preservative used in some vaccines. Thimerosal contains 49.6% mercury by weight and is metabolized to ethyl mercury and thiosalicylate. During an ongoing review of biologic products in response to the Food and Drug Administration (FDA) Modernization Act of 1997, the FDA determined that infants who received thimerosal-containing vaccines at multiple visits might have been exposed to more mercury than recommended by federal guidelines. As a precautionary measure, the American Academy of Pediatrics, American Academy of Family Physicians, Advisory Committee on Immunization Practices, and U.S. Public Health Service issued a joint recommendation in 1999 that thimerosal be removed from vaccines as quickly as possible. In the United States, thimerosal has been removed from all vaccines in the recommended childhood immunization schedule. Infants and children who have received thimerosal-containing vaccines do not need to have blood, urine, or hair tested for mercury because the concentrations of mercury would be quite low and would not require treatment. The benefits and risks of vaccines containing thimerosal should be discussed with parents (as with all vaccines). The larger risks of not vaccinating children far outweigh any known risk of exposure to thimerosal-containing vaccines. Studies do not demonstrate a link between thimerosal-containing vaccines and autistic spectrum disorders (see Chapter 29), and no evidence supports a change in the standard of practice with regard to administration of thimerosal-containing vaccines in areas of the world where they are used. A rise in blood mercury levels following a single dose of hepatitis vaccine was seen in preterm infants, but the clinical significance is unknown. The American Academy of Pediatrics recommends that the initiation of hepatitis vaccine series be deferred until 2–6 mo of age in children who are born to hepatitis B surface antigen–negative mothers.

PHARMACOKINETICS. Inhaled elemental mercury vapor is 80% absorbed by the lungs and is distributed rapidly to the central nervous system (CNS) because of its high lipid solubility. The elemental mercury is oxidized by catalase to the mercuric ion, which is the reactive form that causes cellular toxicity. Elemental mercury liquid is poorly absorbed from the gastrointestinal tract, with less than 0.1% being absorbed. The half-life of elemental mercury in the tissues is about 60 days, with most of the excretion being in the urine.

Inorganic mercury salts are about 10% absorbed from the gastrointestinal tract and cross the blood-brain barrier to a lesser extent than elemental mercury. Mercuric salts are more soluble than mercurous salts and, therefore, produce greater toxicity. Elimination occurs primarily in the urine, with a half-life of about 40 days.

Methyl mercury is the most avidly absorbed of the organic mercury compounds, with about 90% absorbed from the gastrointestinal tract. The lipophilic, short-chain alkyl structure of methyl mercury allows it to distribute rapidly across the blood-brain barrier and placenta. Methyl mercury is about 90% excreted in the bile, with the remainder being excreted in the urine. The half-life is 70 days.

PATHOPHYSIOLOGY. After absorption, mercury is distributed to all tissues, particularly the CNS and kidneys. Mercury reacts with sulfhydryl, phosphoryl, carboxyl, and amide groups, resulting in disruption of enzymes, transport mechanisms, membranes, and structural proteins. Widespread cellular dysfunction or necrosis results in the multiorgan toxicity characteristic of mercury poisoning.

CLINICAL MANIFESTATIONS. Five syndromes describe the clinical presentation of mercury poisoning. **Acute inhalation of elemental mercury vapor** results in rapid onset of cough, dyspnea, chest pain, fever, chills, headaches, and visual disturbances. Gastrointestinal findings include metallic taste, salivation, nausea, vomiting, and diarrhea. Depending on the severity of the exposure, the illness may be self-limited or may progress to necrotizing bronchiolitis, interstitial pneumonitis, pulmonary edema, and death from respiratory failure. Younger children are more susceptible to pulmonary toxicity. Survivors may develop restrictive lung disease. Renal dysfunction and neurologic disturbances (ataxia, persistent weakness, emotional lability) may develop subacutely. Chronic exposure to volatilized elemental mercury in dental amalgams has not been found to be of any clinical significance.

Acute ingestion of inorganic mercury salts (typically secondary to ingestion of a button battery) can present in a few hours with corrosive gastroenteritis manifested by metallic taste, oropharyngeal burns, nausea, hematemesis, severe abdominal pain, hematochezia, acute tubular necrosis, cardiovascular collapse, and death.

Chronic inorganic mercury intoxication produces the **classic triad** of tremor, neuropsychiatric disturbances, and gingivostomatitis. The syndrome may result from chronic exposure to elemental mercury, inorganic mercury salts, or certain organic mercury compounds, all of which may be metabolized to mercuric ions. The tremor starts as a fine intention tremor of the fingers that is abolished during sleep, but it may later involve the face and progress to choreoathetosis and spasmodic ballismus. Mixed sensorimotor neuropathy and visual disturbances also may be present. The neuropsychiatric disturbances include emotional lability, delirium, headaches, memory loss, insomnia, anorexia, and fatigue. Renal dysfunction ranges from asymptomatic proteinuria to nephrotic syndrome.

Acrodynia, or **pink disease,** is a rare idiosyncratic hypersensitivity reaction to mercury that occurs predominantly in children exposed to mercurous powders. The symptom complex includes generalized pain, paresthesias, and an acral (hands, feet) rash that may spread to involve the face. It typically is red-pink, papular, pruritic, and painful; it may progress to desquamation and ulceration. Morbilliform, vesicular, and hemorrhagic variants have been described. Other important features include anorexia, apathy, photophobia, and hypotonia, especially of the pectoral and pelvic girdles. Irritability, tremors, diaphoresis, insomnia, hypertension, and tachycardia may be present. Some cases initially were diagnosed as having a pheochromocytoma. The outcome is good after removal of the source of mercury exposure.

Methyl mercury intoxication also is referred to as **Minamata disease** after the widespread mercury poisoning that occurred at Minamata Bay in Japan in people who had ingested contaminated fish. Methyl mercury poisoning presents as delayed neurotoxicity after a latent period of weeks to months, characterized by ataxia; dysarthria; paresthesias; tremors; movement disorders; impairment of vision, hearing, smell, and taste; memory loss; progressive dementia; and death. Infants exposed in utero are the most severely affected, with low birthweight, microcephaly, profound developmental delay, cerebral palsy, deafness, blindness, and seizures. Although there is significant residual morbidity from methyl mercury neurotoxicity, observations on long-term follow up of children exposed in Iraq reveal complete or partial resolution in most cases.

LABORATORY FINDINGS. The diagnosis of mercury intoxication is based on characteristic clinical findings, a history of exposure, and elevation of whole blood or urine mercury levels, which confirms the exposure. Thin-layer and gas chromatographic techniques can be used to distinguish organic from inorganic mercury. Blood should be collected in special tubes for trace elements from laboratories that are capable of performing those tests. Levels <10 μg/L in whole blood and <20 μg/L in a 24-hr urine collection are considered normal (see Table 708-2). Although blood mercury levels may reflect acute exposure, they decrease as mercury redistributes into the tissues. Urine mercury levels are most useful for identifying chronic exposures, except in the case of methyl mercury, because methyl mercury undergoes minimal urinary excretion. Urinary mercury levels are used in monitoring efficacy of chelation therapy, whereas blood levels are used primarily for monitoring organic mercury poisonings. Hair analysis for mercury is not reliable because hair reflects endogenous as well as exogenous mercury exposure (hair avidly binds mercury from the environment). Abdominal radiographs may demonstrate ingested radiopaque mercury.

Urinary markers of early nephrotoxicity include microalbuminuria, retinol-binding protein, β_2-microglobulin, and *N*-acetyl-β-D-glucosaminidase. Early neurotoxicity may be detected with neuropsychiatric testing and nerve conduction studies, whereas severe CNS toxicity is apparent on CT or MRI scans.

TREATMENT OF ARSENIC AND MERCURY INTOXICATION

The principles of management for arsenic and mercury intoxication include prompt removal from the source of poisoning, aggressive stabilization and supportive care, decontamination, and chelation therapy when appropriate. Once the diagnosis is suspected, the local poison control facility should be contacted and care coordinated with physicians who are familiar with the management of heavy metal poisoning.

Supportive care for patients exposed to arsine gas requires close monitoring for signs of hemolysis, including evaluation of the peripheral blood smear and urinalysis. Transfusion of packed red blood cells may be necessary, as well as administration of intravenous fluids, sodium bicarbonate, and mannitol to prevent renal failure secondary to the deposition of hemoglobin in the kidneys. After inhalation of elemental mercury vapor, patients require careful monitoring of respiratory status, which may include pulse oximetry, arterial blood gas analysis, and chest radiography. Supportive care includes administration of supplemental oxygen and, in severe cases, intubation and mechanical ventilation.

Acute ingestion of inorganic arsenic and mercury salts results in hemorrhagic gastroenteritis, cardiovascular collapse, and multiorgan dysfunction. Fluid resuscitation, pressor agents, and transfusion of blood products may be required for management of cardiovascular instability. Severe respiratory distress, coma with loss of airway reflexes, intractable seizures, and respiratory paralysis are indications for intubation and mechanical ventilation. Renal function must be monitored carefully for signs of renal failure and the need for hemodialysis.

Gastrointestinal decontamination after ingestion of the inorganic arsenic and mercury salts has not been well studied. Because of the corrosive effects of these compounds, induced emesis is not recommended, and endoscopy may be considered before gastric lavage. Arsenic and mercury are not well adsorbed to activated charcoal, but its use may be helpful if coingestants are suspected. Whole bowel irrigation is used to remove any radiopaque material remaining in the gastrointestinal tract.

Chelation for acute arsenic and mercury poisoning is most effective when administered as soon as possible after the exposure. Chelation should be continued until 24-hr urinary arsenic or mercury levels return to normal (<50 µg/L for arsenic and <20 µg /L for mercury), the patient is symptom-free, or the remaining toxic effects are believed to be irreversible. The efficacy of chelation in chronic exposures is reduced because heavy metal in the tissue compartment is relatively unexchangeable and some degree of irreversible toxicity has already occurred.

Dimercaprol, also known as 2,3-dimercaptopropanol or British antilewisite (BAL), is the chelator of choice if a patient cannot tolerate oral therapy, as often is the case in critically ill patients and after ingestion of the corrosive inorganic arsenic and mercury salts. BAL is available suspended in peanut oil and benzyl benzoate in 3-mL ampules at a concentration of 100 mg/mL for deep intramuscular (IM) injection. For **arsenic poisoning,** the recommended regimen of BAL is 2.5 mg/kg IM q6h for the first 2 days, 2.5 mg/kg IM q12h on the third day, then 2.5 mg/kg/day IM for 10 days. For severe arsenic poisoning, the dose of BAL is increased to 3 mg/kg IM q4h for 2 days, 3 mg/kg IM q6h on day 3, then 3 mg/kg IM q12h for 10 days. The dose of BAL for **inorganic mercury poisoning** is 5 mg/kg IM on the first day, then 2.5 mg/kg IM q12–24h for 10 days. The BAL–heavy metal complex is excreted in the urine and bile. A period of 5 days between courses of chelation is recommended. Adverse effects of BAL include pain at the injection site, hypertension, tachycardia, diaphoresis, nausea, vomiting, abdominal pain, a burning sensation in the oropharynx, and a feeling of constriction in the chest. BAL may cause hemolysis in glucose-6-phosphate dehydrogenase (G6PD)–deficient individuals. It is important to note that BAL is contraindicated for chelation of methyl mercury because BAL redistributes methyl mercury to the brain from other tissue sites, resulting in increased neurotoxicity.

D-penicillamine is an orally administered chelator that can be considered for less severe mercury poisoning or as an adjunct to BAL therapy in arsenic poisoning, but its use has been largely restricted due to the potential for significant leukopenia, thrombocytopenia, and proteinuria. A newer investigational analogue, *N*-acetyl-d,l-penicillamine, has been used with variable success in mercury poisoning.

Oral chelating agents are used to replace the painful BAL injections when the patient is stable enough to tolerate oral therapy and prolonged chelation is necessary. **Succimer,** also known as 2,3-dimercaptosuccinic acid (DMSA), is an orally administered water-soluble derivative of BAL. DMSA is available in 100-mg capsules. The recommended regimen of DMSA is 1,050 mg/m^2/24 hr (or 30 mg/kg/24 hr) orally in three divided doses for 5 days, then 700 mg/m^2/24 hr (or 20 mg/kg/24 hr) orally in two divided doses for 14 days. The DMSA–heavy metal complex is excreted in the urine and bile. A period of 2 weeks between courses of chelation is recommended. Mild adverse effects include nausea, vomiting, diarrhea, loss of appetite, and transient elevations in liver enzyme levels. DMSA also may cause hemolysis in G6PD-deficient patients. Patients with ingestion of elemental mercury require no follow-up unless there is an underlying disease that decreases the gastrointestinal transit time. Serial abdominal radiographs to document the progression of the metal are recommended. Acute inhalation of mercury fumes and ingestion of inorganic mercury requires hospitalization to monitor the respiratory and gastrointestinal status, respectively. Therapeutic abortion may be considered in pregnant patients due to the teratogenic effect of mercury.

American Academy of Pediatrics, Committee on Environmental Health: Technical report: Mercury in the environment. Implications for pediatricians. *Pediatrics* 2001;108:197–204.

Bae M, Wantanabe C, Inaoka T, et al: Arsenic in cooked rice in Bangladesh. *Lancet* 2002;360:1839–1840.

Baum CR: Treatment of mercury intoxication. *Curr Opin Pediatr* 1999;11:265–268.

Bolger PM, Schwetz BA: Mercury and health. *N Engl J Med* 2002;347:1735–1736.

Centers for Disease Control and Prevention: Summary of the joint statement on thimerosal in vaccines. American Academy of Family Physicians, American Academy of Pediatricians, Advisory Committee on Immunization Practices, Public Health Service. *MMWR* 2000;49:622–631.

Centers for Disease Control and Prevention: Mercury exposure—Kentucky, 2004. *MMWR* 2005;54:797–798.

Clarkson TW, Magos L, Myers GJ: The toxicology of mercury—Current exposures and clinical manifestations. *N Engl J Med* 2003;349:1731–1736.

Cullen NM, Wolf LR, St Clair D: Pediatric arsenic ingestion. *Am J Emerg Med* 1995;13:432–435.

Ford M: Arsenic (heavy metals). In: Goldfrank LR, Flomenbaum NE, Lewin NA, et al (editors): *Goldfrank's Toxicologic Emergencies,* 7th ed. McGraw-Hill, 2002. Available at http://www.knovel.com/knovel2/Toc.jsp?BookID=957.

Heron J, Golding J; ALSPAC Study Team: Thimerosal exposure in infants and developmental disorders: A prospective cohort study in the United Kingdom does not support a causal association. *Pediatrics* 2004;114:577–583.

Horowitz Y, Greenberg D, Ling G, et al: Acrodynia: A case report of two siblings. *Arch Dis Child* 2002;86:453–455.

Innis SM, Palaty J, Vaghri Z, et al: Increased levels of mercury associated with high fish intakes among children from Vancouver, Canada. *J Pediatr* 2006;148:759–763.

Jacobson JL, Jacobson SW: Risks to child health from methylmercury exposure in immigrant populations. *J Pediatr* 2006;148:716–718.

Kondo K: Congenital Minamata disease: Warnings from Japan's experience. *J Child Neurol* 2000;15:458–464.

Lai MW, Boyer EW, Kleinman ME, et al: Acute arsenic poisoning in two siblings. *Pediatrics* 2005;116:249–257.

McLellan F: Arsenic contamination affects millions in Bangladesh. *Lancet* 2002;359:1127.

Mitchell RJ, Osborne PB, Haubenreich JE: Dental amalgam restorations: Daily mercury dose and biocompatibility. *J Long Term Eff Med Implants* 2005;15:709–721.
Parker SK, Schwartz B, Todd J, et al: Thimerosal-containing vaccines and autistic spectrum disorder: A critical review of published original data. *Pediatrics* 2004;114:793–804.
Pichichero ME, Cernichiari E, Lopreiato J, et al: Mercury concentrations and metabolism in infants receiving vaccines containing thiomersal: A descriptive study. *Lancet* 2002;360:1737–1740.
Schober SE, Sinks TH, Jones RL, et al: Blood mercury levels in US children and women of childbearing age, 1999–2000. *JAMA* 2003;289:1667–1674.
Stajich GV, Lopez GP, Harry SW, et al: Iatrogenic exposure to mercury after hepatitis B vaccination in preterm infants. *J Pediatr* 2000;136:679–681.
Sue YJ: Mercury (heavy metals). In: Goldfrank LR, Flomenbaum NE, Lewin NA, et al (editors): *Goldfrank's Toxicologic Emergencies,* 7th ed. McGraw-Hill, 2002. Available at http://www.knovel.com/knovel2/Toc.jsp?BookID=957.

Chapter 709 ■ Lead Poisoning

Morri Markowitz

EPIDEMIOLOGY

Lead is a metal that exists in four isotopic forms. Chemically, its low melting point and ability to form stable compounds has made it useful in the manufacture of hundreds of products. Clinically, it is purely a toxicant; no organism has an essential function that is lead-dependent. Nevertheless, its commercial attractiveness has resulted in the processing of millions of tons of lead ore, leading to widespread dissemination of lead in the human environment.

The threshold level at which lead causes biochemical, subclinical, or clinical disturbance has been redefined many times during the past 50 yr. The blood lead level (BLL) is the gold standard for determining health effects. The Centers for Disease Control and Prevention (CDC), the American Academy of Pediatrics (AAP), and numerous other national and international organizations (e.g., Global Lead Network—Alliance to End Childhood Lead Poisoning, and The National Referral Centre for Lead Poisoning in India) consider a BLL of 10 µg/dL or greater to indicate a need for risk management. Toxic effects of lead have been reported in children with BLLs below this threshold, and the CDC currently is considering whether to revise the level of concern downward.

PUBLIC HEALTH HISTORY

Between 1976 and 1980, >85% of preschool-aged children in the United States had BLLs >10 µg/dL; 98% of African-American preschoolers fulfilled this criterion. Over the next 15 yr, government regulations resulted in the significant reduction of three main contributors to lead by means of (1) the elimination of the use of tetraethyl leaded gasoline; (2) the banning of lead-containing solder to seal food- and beverage-containing cans; and, (3) the application of a federal rule that limited the amount of lead allowed in paint intended for household use to <0.07% by weight. Surveillance by the CDC has shown that the prevalence of elevated BLLs has declined markedly, and by 2000 was below 3% of all preschoolers. Of affected children, approximately 10% will have BLLs greater than the clinically significant 25 µg/dL. Children with levels high enough to be life-threatening are only rarely seen, but deaths continue to occur. An estimated half million children in the U.S. alone still have elevated BLLs. Factors that indicate increased risk of lead poisoning, in addition to preschool age, include low socioeconomic status; living in older housing built primarily before 1960; urban location; and African-American race. Other high-risk groups include recent immigrants, including adoptees, from countries that still use leaded gasoline or ceramic ware with lead-containing glazes.

Progress also is being made globally. By 1999, 29 countries had completely phased out leaded gasoline, and since then others have developed phase-out plans, including several developing/transitional countries in Asia, Latin America, Eastern Europe, and Northern Africa. In Malta, after the import of red lead paint was banned and the use of lead-treated wood for fuel in bakeries was prohibited, mean blood lead levels of pregnant women and newborns decreased by 45%. In Mexico, the introduction of unleaded gasoline in 1990 was associated with a decline in blood lead level among first grade students, from 17 µg/dL in 1990 to 6.2 µg/dL in 1997. After it was documented that children living in the neighborhood of a battery factory in Nicaragua had a mean blood lead level of 17.2 µg/dL, whereas children in the control community had a mean blood lead level of 7.4 µg/dL, the factory was closed. Despite these advances, it is estimated that 40% of all children globally have blood lead levels above 5 µg/dL and 20% have levels above 10 µg/dL; 90% of these children live in developing countries, where in some regions blood lead levels may be 10- to 20-fold higher than in developed countries.

SOURCES OF EXPOSURE

Lead poisoning may occur in utero, because lead readily crosses the placenta from maternal blood. The spectrum of toxicity is similar to that experienced by children after birth. The source of maternal blood lead content is either redistribution from endogenous stores (i.e., the mother's skeleton), or lead newly acquired due to ongoing environmental exposure.

Several hundred products contain lead, including batteries, cable sheathing, cosmetics, mineral supplements, plastics, and toys (Table 709-1). Major sources of exposure vary among and within countries; the major source of exposure in the U.S. remains old lead-based paint. About 25 million households live in housing built before 1950, a time of maximal lead-based paint usage. As paint deteriorates it chalks, flakes, and turns to dust. Improper rehabilitation work of painted surfaces (e.g., sanding) can result in dissemination of lead-containing dust throughout a home. The dust can coat all surfaces, including children's hands. All of these forms of lead can be ingested. If heat is used to strip paint then lead vapor concentrations in the room can reach levels sufficient to cause lead poisoning via inhalation.

TABLE 709-1. Sources of Lead
Paint chips
Dust
Soil
Parent's occupational exposure
Glazed ceramics
Herbal remedies (e.g., Ayurvedic medications)
Home remedies, including antiperspirants, deodorants (litargirio)
Jewelry (toys or parents')
Stored battery casings (or living near a battery smelter)
Lead-based gasoline
Mexican candies
Indoor firing ranges
Imported spices (*swanuri marili, zafron, kozhambu*)
Lead-based cosmetics (kohl, surma)
Lead plumbing (water)
Imported foods in lead-containing cans

METABOLISM

The nonnutritive hand-to-mouth activity of young children is the most common pathway by which lead enters the body. In nearly all cases lead is ingested, either as a component of dust licked off of surfaces or in swallowed paint chips, through water contaminated by its flow through lead pipes or brass fixtures, or from food or liquids contaminated by contact with lead-glazed ceramic ware. Cutaneous contamination with inorganic lead compounds, such as those found in pigments, does not result in a substantial amount of absorption. Organic lead compounds such as tetraethyl lead may penetrate through skin, however.

The percentage of lead absorbed from the gut depends on several factors: particle size, pH, other material in the gut, and nutritional status of essential elements. Large paint chips are difficult to digest and are mainly excreted. Fine dust can be dissolved more readily, however, especially in an acid medium. Lead eaten on an empty stomach is better absorbed then if taken with a meal. The presence of calcium and iron may decrease lead absorption by direct competition for binding sites; iron (and probably calcium) deficiency results in enhanced lead absorption, retention, and toxicity.

After absorption, lead is disseminated throughout the body. It circulates bound to erythrocytes; about 97% is bound on or in the red blood cell. The plasma fraction is too small to be measured by conventional techniques; it is presumably the plasma portion that may enter cells and induce toxicity. Lead has multiple effects in cells. It binds to enzymes, particularly those with available sulfhydryl groups, changing the contour and diminishing function. The heme pathway, present in all cells, has three enzymes susceptible to lead inhibitory effects. The last enzyme in this pathway, ferrochelatase, enables protoporphyrin to chelate iron, thus forming heme. Protoporphyrin is readily measurable in red blood cells. Levels >35 µg/dL are abnormal and are consistent with lead poisoning, iron deficiency, or recent inflammatory disease.

Lack of heme affects multiple metabolic pathways. The accumulation of excess amounts of protoporphyrin and other heme precursors also is toxic. Measurement of the **erythrocyte protoporphyrin (EP)** level is, therefore, a useful tool for monitoring biochemical lead toxicity. EP levels begin to rise several weeks after BLLs have reached 20 µg/dL in a susceptible portion of the population and will be elevated in nearly all children with BLLs >50 µg/dL. A drop in EP levels also lags behind a decline in BLLs by several weeks, because it depends on both cessation of further overproduction by marrow red cell precursors and cell turnover.

A second mechanism of lead toxicity works via its competition with calcium. Many calcium-binding proteins have a higher affinity for lead than for calcium. Lead bound to these proteins may alter function, resulting in abnormal intra- and intercellular signalling. Neurotransmitter release is, in part, a calcium-dependent process that is adversely affected by lead.

Although these two mechanisms of toxicity may be reversible, a third mechanism prevents the development of the normal tertiary brain structure. In immature mammals the normal neuronal pruning process that results in elimination of multiple intercellular brain connections is inhibited by lead. Failure to construct the appropriate tertiary brain structure during the first few yr of life may result in a permanent abnormality. It is tempting to extrapolate from these anatomic findings to the clinical correlate of attention-deficit/hyperactivity disorder observed in lead-poisoned children.

CLINICAL EFFECTS

The BLL is the best-studied measure of the lead burden in children. Although subclinical and clinical findings correlate with BLLs in populations, there is considerable interindividual variability in this relationship. Lead encephalopathy is more likely to be observed in children with BLLs >100 µg/dL; however, one child with a BLL of 300 µg/dL may have no symptoms whereas another with the same level will develop cerebral edema. Susceptibility may be associated with polymorphisms in genes coding for lead-binding proteins, such as delta amino levulinic acid dehydratase, an enzyme in the heme pathway.

Several **subclinical effects** of lead have been demonstrated in cross-sectional epidemiologic studies. **Hearing** and **height** are inversely related to BLLs in children; in neither case, however, does the lead effect reach a level that would bring an individual child to medical attention. As BLLs increased in the study population, more sound (at all frequencies), is needed to reach the hearing threshold. Children with higher BLLs are slightly shorter than those with lower levels; for every 10-µg increase in the BLL, the children are 1 cm shorter. Chronic lead exposure also may delay puberty.

Several longitudinal studies have followed cohorts of children from birth for as long as 20 yr and examined the relationship between BLLs and **cognitive test scores** over time. In general, there is agreement that BLLs, expressed as either a level obtained at around 2 yr of age or a measure that integrates multiple BLLs drawn from a subject over time, are inversely related to cognitive test scores. On average, for each 1 µg/dL elevation in BLL the cognitive score is approximately ¼ to ½ point lower. These data are not based on concurrent testing of lead and cognition; the BLLs from early childhood are predictors of the cognitive test results performed years later, implying that the cognitive effects of lead are permanent.

The effect of in utero lead exposure is controversial. Scores on the Bayley Scale of Mental Development were obtained repeatedly every 6 mo for the first 2 yr of life in a cohort of infants born to middle-class families. Results correlated inversely with **cord** BLL, a measure of in utero exposure, but not with BLLs obtained concurrently at the time of developmental testing. However, after 2 yr of age, all other cognitive tests performed on the cohort over the next 10 yr correlated with the BLLs at age 2 yr but not with cord BLLs, indicating that the effects of prenatal lead exposure on brain function were superseded by early childhood events and later BLLs.

An intervention study, in which moderately lead-poisoned children, with initial BLLs 20–55 µg/dL were aggressively managed over 6 mo, addressed the issue of the effects of treatment on development. Components of treatment included education regarding sources of lead and its abatement, nutritional guidance, multiple home and clinic visits, and, for a subset, chelation therapy. Average BLLs declined and cognitive scores were inversely related to the change in BLL. For every 1 µg/dL fall in BLL, cognitive scores were ¼ point higher.

Behavior also is adversely affected by lead exposure. Hyperactivity is noted in young school age children with histories of lead poisoning or with concurrent elevations in BLL. Older children with higher bone lead content are more likely to be aggressive and to have behaviors that are predictive of later juvenile delinquency. Whether the behavioral effects of lead are reversible has only been examined in a single small study. Seven-year-old hyperactive children with BLLs in the 20s were randomized to receive a chelating agent (penacillamine), methylphenidate or placebo. Teacher and parent ratings of behavior improved for the first two groups but not the placebo receivers. BLLs declined only in the chelated group.

CLINICAL SYMPTOMS

GASTROINTESTINAL AND CENTRAL NERVOUS SYSTEM. GI **symptoms** include anorexia, abdominal pain, vomiting, and constipation, often occurring and recurring over a period of weeks. Children with BLLs >20 µg/dL are twice as likely to have GI complaints as those with lower BLLs. **CNS symptoms** are related to increasing cerebral edema and increased intracranial pressure. Headaches, change in mentation, lethargy, papilledema, seizures, and coma leading to death are rarely seen at levels <100 µg/dL but have been reported in children with a BLL as low as 70 µg/dL. The last reported death directly attributable to lead toxicity in the U.S. was in 2006 in a child with a BLL of 180 µg/dL. There is no clear cutoff blood lead level for the appearance of hyperactivity, but it is more likely to be observed in children who have levels >20 µg/dL.

Other organs also may be affected by lead toxicity, but symptoms usually are not apparent in children. At high levels (>100 µg/dL), **renal tubular dysfunction** is observed. Lead also may induce a reversible Fanconi syndrome (see Chapter 529). In addition, at high BLLs, **red cell survival** is shortened and may contribute to a hemolytic anemia, though most cases of anemia in lead-poisoned children are due to other factors such as iron deficiency and hemoglobinopathies. Older patients may develop a peripheral neuropathy.

DIAGNOSIS

SCREENING. It is estimated that 99% of lead-poisoned children are identified by screening procedures rather than by clinical recognition of lead-related symptoms. Until 1997 universal screening by blood lead testing of all children at ages 12 mo and 24 mo was the standard in the U.S. Given the national decline in the prevalence of lead poisoning, the recommendations have been revised to target blood lead testing of high-risk populations. High risk is based on an evaluation of the likelihood of lead exposure. Departments of Health are responsible for determining the local prevalence of lead poisoning as well as the percentage of housing built before 1950, the period of peak leaded paint use. When this information is available, informed screening guidelines for practitioners can be issued. For instance, in the state of New York, where a large percentage of housing was built pre-1950, the Department of Health mandates that **all children** be tested for lead poisoning via blood analyses. In the absence of such data the practitioner should continue to test all children at both 12 mo and 24 mo. In areas where the prevalence of lead poisoning and old housing is low, targeted screening may be performed based on a risk assessment. Three questions form the basis of a questionnaire (Table 709-2), and items that are pertinent to the locale or individual may be added. If there is a lead-based industry in the child's neighborhood, or the child is a recent immigrant from a country that still permits leaded gasoline, or the child has pica or developmental delay, then blood lead testing would be appropriate. All Medicaid-eligible children should be screened. Venous sampling is preferred to capillary sampling because the chances of false positives and negatives are less.

INTERPRETATION OF BLOOD LEAD LEVELS. The threshold for lead effects and the level of concern for risk management purposes are not the same. The CDC and AAP level of concern currently is 10 µg/dL. A screening value at or above 10 µg/dL requires repeat testing for a diagnosis and to determine the appropriate intervention. The timing for the repeat evaluation depends on the initial value (Table 709-3). If the diagnostic (second) test confirms that the BLL is elevated, then further testing will be required as per the recommended schedule (Table 709-4). **A confirmed venous BLL ≥ 45 µg/dL requires prompt chelation therapy.**

TABLE 709-2. Minimum Personal Risk Questionnaire

1. Does the child live in or visit regularly a house that was built before 1950? (Include settings such as daycare, babysitter's or relative's home)
2. Does the child live in or regularly visit a house built before 1978 with recent (past 6 months) or ongoing renovations or remodeling?
3. Does the child have a sibling or playmate who has or did have lead poisoning?

From *Screening Young Children for Lead Poisoning: Guidance for State and Local Public Health Officials.* Atlanta, GA, Centers for Disease Control and Prevention, 1997.

TABLE 709-3. Follow-Up of Blood Lead Level Screening Test

IF SCREENING BLOOD LEAD LEVEL (µg/dL) IS:	*CDC* REPEAT DIAGNOSTIC VENOUS BLOOD LEAD TESTING BY:	*AAP* REPEAT DIAGNOSTIC VENOUS BLOOD LEAD TESTING BY:
10–19	3 mo	1 mo
20–44	1 wk–1 mo (sooner the higher the lead)	1 wk
45–59	48 hr	48 hr
60–69	24 hr	48 hr
≥70	Immediately	Immediately

AAP, American Academy of Pediatrics; CDC, Centers for Disease Control and Prevention.
Adapted from *Screening Young Children for Lead Poisoning: Guidance for State and Local Public Health Officials.* Atlanta, GA, Centers for Disease Control and Prevention, 1997; and American Academy of Pediatrics, Committee on Environmental Health: Screening for elevated blood lead levels. *Pediatrics* 1998;101:1072–1078.

OTHER TOOLS FOR ASSESSMENT. Blood lead level determinations remain the gold standard for evaluating children. Techniques are available to measure lead in other tissues and body fluids. Experimentally, the method of x-ray fluorescence (XRF) allows direct and noninvasive assessment of bone lead stores. XRF methodology was used to evaluate a population that had long-term exposure to lead from a polluting battery-recycling factory. The study found that the school-aged children had elevated lead levels in bone but not BLLs, which is consistent with our understanding of the slow turnover of lead in bone, measurable in years, in contrast to blood, where it is measurable in weeks. It also indicates that children may have substantial lead in their bodies that will not be detected by routine blood lead testing. This stored lead may be released to toxic levels if bone resorption rates suddenly increase, as occurs with prolonged immobilization of greater than a week and during pregnancy. Thus, children with histories of elevated BLLs are potentially at risk for recrudescence of lead toxicity long after ingestion has stopped and may pass this lead to the next generation. Lead also can be measured in urine. Spontaneous excretion, even in children with high BLLs, usually is low. Lead excretion may be stimulated by treatment with chelating agents, and this property of these drugs forms the basis of their use as a component of lead treatment. It also has been used to develop a test that differentiates children with lead burdens responsive to chelation therapy, the **Lead Mobilization Test.**

In one version, a standardized protocol is employed that includes a fixed dose of the drug (500 mg/m^2 of edetate calcium disodium [$CaNa_2EDTA$] given once IM, mixed 1:1 by volume with 1% procaine) followed by a timed urine collection of 6–8 hr that is analyzed for its lead content. The criteria applied (urine Pb/dose of $CaNa_2EDTA$ >0.6, or urine Pb > 200 µg/volume) lead to the selection of children most likely to respond to a full course of treatment with an enhanced lead diuresis. Practical (e.g., collecting urine on an infant for 6–8 hr in the office) and theoretical (e.g., is there a redistribution of lead after a single dose of chelating agent that may result in transient elevation in brain lead? Are there any data showing long-term efficacy of children chelated on this basis?) concerns have limited the use of this diagnostic test to a few experienced medical centers.

Lead in hair also is measurable but has problems of contamination and interpretability. Further research is required before indications for hair testing are established. Other tests are used as indirect assessments of lead exposure and accumulation. Radiographs of long bones may show dense bands at the metaphyses, which may be difficult to distinguish from growth arrest lines but, if caused by lead, are indicative of months to years of exposure. For children with acute symptoms, when a BLL result is not

TABLE 709-4. Summary of Recommendations for Children with Confirmed (Venous) Elevated Blood Lead Concentrations

BLOOD LEAD CONCENTRATION	RECOMMENDATIONS
10–14 μg/dL	Lead education Dietary Environmental Follow-up blood lead monitoring in 1–3 mo
15–19 μg/dL	Lead education Dietary Environmental Follow-up blood lead monitoring in 1–2 mo Proceed according to actions for 20–24 μg/dL if A follow-up blood lead concentration is in this range at least 3 mo after initial venous test; or Blood lead concentration increases
20–44 μg/dL	Lead education Dietary Environmental Follow-up blood lead monitoring in 1 wk–1 mo (sooner if higher) Complete history and physical examination Laboratory studies Hemoglobin or hematocrit Iron status Environmental investigation Lead hazard reduction Neurodevelopmental monitoring Abdominal radiography (if particulate lead ingestion is suspected) with bowel decontamination if indicated
45–69 μg/dL	Lead education Dietary Environmental Follow-up blood lead monitoring Complete history and physical examination Laboratory studies Hemoglobin or hematocrit Iron status Free EP or ZPP Environmental investigation Lead hazard reduction Neurodevelopmental monitoring Abdominal radiography with bowel decontamination if indicated Chelation therapy
≥70 μg/dL	Hospitalize and commence chelation therapy Proceed according to actions for 45–69 μg/dL

NOT RECOMMENDED AT ANY BLOOD LEAD CONCENTRATION

Searching for gingival lead lines
Evaluation of renal function (except during chelation with $CaNa_2EDTA$)
Testing of hair, teeth, or fingernails for lead
Radiographic imaging of long bones
X-ray fluorescence of long bones

EDTA, ethylenediaminetetraacetic acid; EP, erythrocyte protoporphyrin; ZPP, zinc protoporphyrin.
From American Academy of Pediatrics: Lead exposure in children: Prevention, defection, and management. *Pediatrics* 2005;116:1036–1046.

immediately available, a KUB may reveal radiopaque flecks in the intestinal tract, a finding that is consistent with recent ingestion of lead-containing plaster or paint chips. The absence of radiographic findings does not rule out lead poisoning, however.

Since BLLs reflect recent ingestion or redistribution from other tissues but do not necessarily correlate with the body burden of lead or lead toxicity in an individual child, tests of lead effects also may be useful. After several weeks of lead accumulation and a BLL >20 μg/dL, increases in erythrocyte protoporphyrin (EP) levels >35 μg/dL may occur. An elevated EP level that cannot be attributed to iron deficiency or recent inflammatory illness is both an indicator of lead effect and a useful test for assessing the success of the treatment; levels will begin to fall a few weeks after successful interventions that reduce lead ingestion and increase lead excretion. Because EP is light sensitive, whole blood samples should be covered in aluminum foil (or equivalent) until analyzed.

TREATMENT

Once lead is in bone it is released only slowly and is difficult to remove even with chelating agents. Because the cognitive/behavioral effects from lead may be irreversible, the main effort in treating lead poisoning is to **prevent** it from occurring and to **prevent** further ingestion by already poisoned children. The main components in the effort to eliminate lead poisoning are universally applicable to all children (and adults): (1) identification and elimination of environmental sources of lead exposure; (2) behavioral modification to reduce nonnutritive hand-to-mouth activity; and (3) dietary counseling to ensure sufficient intake of the essential elements calcium and iron. For the small minority of children with more severe lead poisoning, drug treatment is available that enhances lead excretion.

During health maintenance visits a limited risk assessment is warranted that includes questions pertaining to the most common sources of lead exposure: the condition of old paint, secondary occupational exposure via an adult living in the home, or proximity to an industrial source of pollution. If such a source is identified, its elimination usually will require assistance from public health and housing agencies as well as education for the parents. The family should move out of a lead-contaminated apartment until repairs are completed. During repairs, repeated washes of surfaces and the use of high efficiency particle accumulator (HEPA) vacuum cleaners will help reduce exposure to lead-containing dust. Careful selection of a contractor who is certified to perform lead abatement work is necessary. Sloppy work can cause dissemination of lead-containing dust and chips throughout a home or building and result in further elevation of a child's BLL. After the work is completed, dust wipe samples should be collected from floors and windowsills or wells to verify that the risk from lead has abated.

A single case of lead poisoning often is discovered in a household with multiple family members including other young children, even in households with a common source of exposure such as peeling lead-based paint. The mere presence of lead in an environment does not produce lead poisoning. Parental efforts at **reducing the hand-to-mouth activity** of the affected child are necessary to reduce the risk of lead ingestion. Handwashing effectively removes lead, but in a home with lead-containing dust, lead rapidly begins to reaccumulate on the child's hands after washing. Therefore, handwashing is best limited to the period immediately before nutritive hand-to-mouth activity occurs.

Because there is competition between lead and essential minerals, it is reasonable to promote a healthy diet that is sufficient in calcium and iron. The recommended daily intakes of these metals vary somewhat with age. In general, for children 1 yr of age and up a calcium intake of about 1 g per day is sufficient (roughly the calcium content of a quart of milk [~1,200 mg/qt] or calcium-fortified orange juice). Calcium absorption is vitamin D–dependent; milk is vitamin D–fortified, but other nutritional sources of calcium often are not. A multivitamin containing vitamin D may be prescribed for children who do not drink sufficient milk or who have inadequate sunlight exposure. Iron requirements also vary with age, ranging from 6 mg/day for infants to 12 mg/day for adolescents. For children identified biochemically as being iron-deficient, therapeutic iron at a daily dose of 5–6 mg/kg for 3 mo is appropriate. Iron absorption is enhanced when ingested with ascorbic acid (citrus juices). Giving additional calcium or iron, above the recommended daily intakes, to mineral-sufficient children has not been shown to be of therapeutic benefit in the treatment of lead poisoning.

Drug treatment to remove lead is lifesaving for children with lead encephalopathy. In nonencephalopathic children, it prevents symptom progression and further toxicity. Guidelines for chelation are based on the BLL. A child with a venous BLL ≥ 45 μg/dL should be treated. Four drugs are available in the U.S.: 2,3-dimercaptosuccinic acid (DMSA [succimer]), $CaNa_2EDTA$ (versenate),

TABLE 709-5. Chelation Therapy

NAME	SYNONYM	DOSE	TOXICITY
Succimer	Chemet, DMSA	350 mg/m²/dose (***not 10 mg/kg***) q 8 hr, PO for 5 d, then q 12 hr for 14 d	GI distress, rashes; elevated LFTs, depressed WBCs
Edetate*	$CaNa_2EDTA$, versenate	1,000–1,500 mg/m²/d; IV infusion—continuous or intermittent; IM divided q 6 or q 12 hr. For 5 days	Proteinuria, pyuria, rising BUN/creatinine—all rare. Hypercalcemia if too rapid an infusion. Tissue inflammation if infusion infiltrates
BAL	Dimercaprol, British antilewisite	300–500 mg/m²/day; **IM only** divided q 4 hr. For 3–5 days. Only for BLL ≥ 70.	GI distress, altered mentation; elevated LFTs, hemolysis if G6PD deficiency; no concomitant iron treatment
D-Pen	Penicillamine	10 mg/kg/d for 2 wk increasing to 25–40 mg/kg/d; oral, divided q 12 hr. For 12–20 weeks	Rashes, fever; blood dyscrasias, elevated LFTs, proteinuria. Allergic cross-reactivity with penicillin.

***Always given as the calcium salt; never as the sodium salt without calcium.**

BAL, British antilewisite; BUN, blood urea nitrogen; $CaNa_2EDTA$, calcium disodium edetate; DMSA, 2,3-dimercaptosuccinic acid; G6PD, glucose-6-phosphate dehydrogenase; GI, gastrointestinal; LFT, liver function test; WBC, white blood cell.

From Markowitz ME: Lead poisoning. *Pediatr Rev* 2000;21:327–335.

British antilewisite (BAL [dimercaprol]), and penicillamine. DMSA and penicillamine can be given orally, whereas $CaNa_2EDTA$ and BAL can only be administered parenterally. The choice of agent is guided by the severity of the lead poisoning, the effectiveness of the drug, and the ease of administration (Table 709-5). Children with BLLs of 44–70 µg/dL may be treated with a single drug, preferably DMSA. Those with BLLs of 70 µg/dL or greater require two-drug treatment: $CaNa_2EDTA$ in combination with either DMSA or BAL for those without evidence of encephalopathy, or $CaNa_2EDTA$ and BAL for those with encephalopathy. Data on the combined treatment with $CaNa_2EDTA$ and DMSA for children with BLLs >100 µg/dL are very limited.

Drug-related toxicities are minor and reversible. These include gastrointestinal distress, transient elevations in transaminases, active urinary sediment, and neutropenia. These types of events are least common for $CaNa_2EDTA$ and DMSA and more common for BAL and penicillamine. All of the drugs are effective in reducing BLLs when given in sufficient doses and for the prescribed time. These drugs also may increase lead absorption from the gut and should be administered to children in lead-free environments. Some authorities also recommend the administration of a cathartic immediately prior to or concomitant with the initiation of chelation to eliminate any lead already in the gut.

None of these agents removes all lead from the body. Within days to weeks after completion of a course of therapy the BLL rises, even in the absence of new lead ingestion. The source of this rebound in the BLL is believed to be bone. Serial examinations of bone lead content by XRF have shown that chelation with $CaNa_2EDTA$ is associated with a decline in bone lead levels, but that residual bone lead remains detectable even after multiple courses of treatment.

Repeat chelation is indicated if the BLL rebounds to ≥45 µg/dL. Children with initial BLLs >70 µg/dL are likely to require more than one course. A minimum of 3 days between courses is recommended to prevent treatment-related toxicities, especially in the kidney.

The indication for chelation therapy for children with BLL <45 µg/dL is less clear. Use of these drugs in children with BLLs of 20–44 µg/dL will result in transiently lowered BLLs, and in some this will be accompanied by reversal of lead-induced enzyme inhibition. However, few children will increase their excretion of lead significantly during chelation, raising the question of whether any long-term benefit is achieved. A study of 2 yr old children with BLLs of 20–44 µg/dL who were randomized to receive either DMSA or placebo found that the drop in BLLs was greater in the first 6 mo after enrollment in the DMSA-treated group, but the levels converged by 1 yr of follow-up. Cognitive test scores obtained at 4 and 7 yr of age were not statistically different between the groups. Chelation with DMSA (and $CaNa_2EDTA$) is not recommended for all children with BLLs of 20–44 µg/dL. Another group to be chelated may include children who can be shown to respond to a test dose of a chelating agent with an enhanced lead diuresis—an indication that the drug is effective at removing lead permanently from the body. Such children could be identified by administration of the Lead Mobilization Test. Data are not available for either case that show improvements in cognitive outcomes for those chelated on these bases. Similarly, it remains to be demonstrated whether other chelating agents available in the U.S. or elsewhere are effective at either substantially reducing body stores (bone) of lead or at reversing the cognitive deficits attributable to lead.

With successful intervention, BLLs decline, with the greatest fall in BLL occurring in the first 2 mo after therapy is initiated. Subsequently the rate of change in BLL declines slowly so that by 6–12 mo after identification, the BLL of the average child with moderate lead poisoning (BLL >20 µg/dL) will be 50% lower. Children with more markedly elevated BLLs may take years to reach the acceptable threshold of 10 µg/dL, even if all sources of lead exposure have been eliminated, behavior has been modified, and nutrition has been maximized. Early screening remains the best way of avoiding and therefore obviating the need for the treatment of lead poisoning.

American Academy of Pediatrics: Lead exposure in children: prevention, detection, and management. *Pediatrics* 2005;116:1036–1046.

Berkowitz S, Tarrago R: Acute brain herniation from lead toxicity. *Pediatrics* 2006;118:2548–2551.

Canfield RL, Henderson CR Jr, Cory-Slechta DA, et al: Intellectual impairment in children with blood lead concentrations below 10 microg per deciliter. *N Engl J Med* 2003;348:1517–1526.

Centers for Disease Control and Prevention: Death of a child after ingestion of a metallic charm—Minnesota, 2006. *MMWR* 2006;55:340–341.

Centers for Disease Control and Prevention: Deaths associated with hypocalcemia from chelation therapy—Texas, Pennsylvania and Oregon, 2003–2005. *MMWR* 2006;55:204–206.

Centers for Disease Control and Prevention: Lead exposure from indoor firing ranges among students on shooting teams—Alaska, 2002–2004. *MMWR* 2005;54:577–579.

Centers for Disease Control and Prevention: Lead poisoning associated with use of litargirio—Rhode Island, 2003. *MMWR* 2005;54:227–229.

Centers for Disease Control and Prevention: Lead poisoning associated with Ayurvedic medications—Five states, 2000–2003. *MMWR* 2004;53:582–586.

Centers for Disease Control and Prevention: Surveillance for elevated blood lead levels among children—United States, 1997–2001. *MMWR* 2003;52:1–21.

Centers for Disease Control and Prevention: Childhood lead poisoning associated with Tamarind county and folk remedies. *MMWR* 2002;51:684–686.

Centers for Disease Control and Prevention: Fatal pediatric lead poisoning—New Hampshire, 2000. *MMWR* 2001;50:457–459.

Committee on Drugs, American Academy of Pediatrics: Treatment guidelines for lead exposure in children. *Pediatrics* 1995;96:155–160.

Committee on Environmental Health, American Academy of Pediatrics. Screening for elevated blood lead levels. *Pediatrics* 1998;101:1072–1078.

Dietrich KN, Ware JH, Salganik M, et al: Effect of chelation therapy on the neuropsychological and behavioral development of lead-exposed children after school entry. *Pediatrics* 2004;114:19–26.

Florin TA, Brent RL, Weitzman M: The need for vigilance: the persistence of lead poisoning in children. *Pediatrics* 2005;115:1767–1768.

Global Lead Network: Alliance to End Childhood Lead Poisoning. Website at http://www.globalleadnet.org.

Kemper AR, Cohn LM, Fant KE, et al: Follow-up testing among children with elevated screening blood lead levels. *JAMA* 2005;293:2232–2237.

Lanphear BP: Childhood lead poisoning prevention. *JAMA* 2005;293:2274–2276.

Laraque D, Trasande L: Lead poisoning: successes and 21st century challenges. *Pediatr Rev* 2005;26:435–443.

Meyer PA, Pivetz T, Dignam TA, et al: Surveillance for elevated blood lead levels among children—United States, 1997–2001. *MMWR Surveill Summ* 2003;52(10):1–21.

Selevan SG, Rice DC, Hogan KA, et al: Blood lead concentration and delayed puberty in girls. *N Engl J Med* 2003;348:1527–1536.

Tellez-Rojo MM, Bellinger DC, Arroyo-Quiroz C, et al: Longitudinal associations between blood lead concentrations lower than 10 microg/dL and neurobehavioral development in environmentally exposed children in Mexico City. *Pediatrics* 2006;118:323–330.

Woolf AD, Woolf NT: Childhood lead poisoning in 2 families associated with spices used in food preparation. *Pediatrics* 2005;116:e314–e318.

Wright NJ, Thacher TD, Pfitzner MA, et al: Causes of lead toxicity in a Nigerian city. *Arch Dis Child* 2004;90:262–266.

Chapter 710 ■ Nonbacterial Food Poisoning

Denise A. Salerno and Stephen C. Aronoff

710.1 • Mushroom Poisoning

Picking and consumption of wild mushrooms, a favorite pastime in Europe, is increasingly popular in the United States. This increase in popularity has led to increased reports of severe and fatal mushroom poisonings.

The clinical syndromes produced by mushroom poisoning are divided according to the rapidity of onset of symptoms and the predominant system involved. The symptoms are due to the principle toxin present in the ingested mushrooms. The eight major toxins produced by mushrooms are categorized as cyclopeptides, monomethylhydrazine, muscarine, hallucinogenic indoles, isoxazole, coprine (disulfiram-like reaction), orellanine, and GI-specific irritants. In addition, the edible wild mushroom *Tricholoma equestre* has been associated with delayed rhabdomyolysis, and *Clitocybe amoenolens* and *Clitocybe acromelalgia* have been reported to cause erythromelalgia. The toxins responsible for these effects are unknown.

GASTROINTESTINAL: DELAYED ONSET

AMANITA POISONING. Poisonings by species of *Amanita* and *Galerina* account for 95% of the fatalities due to mushroom intoxication; the mortality rate for this group is 5–10%. Most species produce two classes of cyclopeptide toxins: (1) phallotoxins, which are heptapeptides believed to be responsible for the early symptoms of *Amanita* poisoning; and (2) amanitotoxin, which is an octapeptide that inhibits RNA polymerase and subsequent production of messenger RNA. Cells with high turnover rates, such as those in the gastrointestinal mucosa, kidneys, and liver, are the most severely affected.

Amanita poisoning causes cellular necrosis, which may occur throughout the gastrointestinal tract, the most heavily exposed site. Acute yellow atrophy of the liver and necrosis of the proximal renal tubules are found in lethal cases.

The **clinical course** produced by poisoning with *Amanita* or *Galerina* species is biphasic, after an initial 6–24 hr asymptomatic latent period. Nausea, vomiting, and severe abdominal pain ensue 6–24 hr after ingestion. Profuse watery diarrhea follows shortly thereafter and may last for 12–24 hr. During this time, as much as 9 L of fluid may be lost. From 24–48 hr after poisoning, jaundice, hypertransaminasemia (peaking at 72–96 hr), renal failure, and coma occur. Death occurs 4–7 days after the ingestion. A prothrombin time less than 10% of control is a poor prognostic factor.

Treatment. Treatment for *Amanita* poisoning is both supportive and specific. Fluid loss from severe diarrhea during the early course of the illness is profound, requiring aggressive therapy for correction of this loss. In the late phase of the disease, management of renal and hepatic failure is also necessary.

Specific therapy for *Amanita* poisoning is designed to remove the toxin rapidly and to block binding at its target site. Oral activated charcoal and lactulose combined with fluid and electrolyte replacement are recommended as part of the initial treatment of children with *Amanita* poisoning. Forced diuresis should be avoided, because this increases renal exposure. Intravenous penicillin G (400,000 U/kg/24 hr) administered as a continuous infusion combined with silibinin, the water-soluble form of the flavolignone silymarin (in an intravenous dosage of 20–50 mg/kg/24 hr), acts synergistically to inhibit binding of both toxins and to interrupt enterohepatic recirculation of amanitotoxin. Hemodialysis and hemoperfusion also are recommended as part of the initial treatment for intoxicated children. Orthotopic liver transplantation is recommended for children in whom severe hepatic failure develops (see Chapter 365).

MONOMETHYLHYDRAZINE INTOXICATION. Species of *Gyromitra* contain monomethylhydrazine (CH_3NHNH_2), which inhibits central nervous system (CNS) enzymatic production of γ-aminobutyric acid (GABA). Monomethylhydrazine also oxidizes iron in hemoglobin, resulting in methemoglobinemia. Children with *Gyromitra* poisoning develop vomiting, diarrhea, hematochezia, and abdominal pain within 6–24 hr of ingestion of the toxin. Symptoms of CNS depression and seizures develop later in the clinical course. Hemolysis and methemoglobinemia are potential life-threatening complications of monomethylhydrazine poisoning. Severe **methemoglobinemia** may require dialysis.

Treatment. Hypovolemia due to gastrointestinal fluid losses and seizures requires supportive intervention. Pyridoxal phosphate, the coenzyme that catalyzes the production of GABA, can reverse the effects of monomethylhydrazine when administered in high doses. **Pyridoxine hydrochloride (25 mg/kg)** is administered intravenously at a frequency dependent on clinical improvement. Parenteral administration of methylene blue is indicated if the methemoglobin concentration exceeds 30%. Blood transfusions may be required for significant hemolysis.

RENAL: DELAYED ONSET

ORELLANINE POISONING. Species of *Cortinarius* contain the heat-stable toxin bipyridyl orellanine, which causes severe non-glomerular renal injury characterized by interstitial fibrosis and acute tubular necrosis. The exact mechanism of injury is unknown. *Cortinarius* poisoning is characterized by nausea, vomiting, and diarrhea that presents 36–48 hr after ingestion. Although the initial symptoms may be trivial, more serious renal toxicity occurs in several days. Acute renal failure occurs in 30–50% of those affected; beginning with polyuria and progressing to renal failure.

Treatment. **Treatment** for orellanine poisoning is supportive. Early presentation, within 4–6 hr after ingestion, can be treated with activated charcoal and gastric lavage. Hemodialysis may be needed in those patients suffering from renal failure. Most patient recover with in 1 mo but one third to one half will develop chronic renal insufficiency.

AUTONOMIC NERVOUS SYSTEM: RAPID ONSET

MUSCARINE POISONING. Mushrooms of the genera *Inocybe* and, to a lesser degree, *Clitocybe* contain muscarine or muscarine-related compounds. These quaternary ammonium derivatives bind to postsynaptic receptors, producing an exaggerated cholinergic response.

The **clinical manifestations** are characterized by the following hypercholinergic response: the onset of symptoms is rapid (30 min–2 hr after consumption) and consists of diaphoresis, excessive lacrimation, salivation, miosis, urinary and fecal incontinence, and vomiting. Respiratory distress caused by bronchospasm and increased bronchopulmonary secretions is the most serious complication. The symptoms subside spontaneously within 6–24 hr.

Treatment. Atropine sulfate, the specific antidote, is administered intravenously (0.01 mg/kg; max 2 mg). This is repeated until the pulmonary symptoms resolve or the patient becomes overtly tachycardic.

COPRINE INGESTION. *Coprinus atramentarius* and *Clitocybe clavipes* contain coprine. Like disulfiram (Antabuse; Odyssey Pharmaceuticals, Inc.), coprine inhibits the metabolism of acetaldehyde after ethanol ingestion. The clinical manifestations result from accumulation of acetaldehyde.

Coprine intoxication becomes apparent after ethanol ingestion and may occur up to 5 days after consuming the mushroom. Hyperemia of the face and trunk, tingling of the hands, metallic taste, tachycardia, and vomiting occur acutely. Hypotension may result from intense peripheral vasodilation.

The syndrome typically is self-limited and lasts only several hours. No specific antidote is available. If hypotension is severe, vascular re-expansion with isotonic parenteral solutions may be required. Small oral doses of propranolol have also been suggested.

CENTRAL NERVOUS SYSTEM: RAPID ONSET

ISOXAZOLE INTOXICATION. Although *Amanita muscaria* and *Amanita pantherina* may contain muscarine, the toxins responsible for the CNS symptoms after ingestion of these mushrooms are muscimol and ibotenic acid, the heat-stable derivatives if the isoxazoles. Muscimol, a hallucinogen, and ibotenic acid, an insecticide, have anticholinergic effects. From 30 min–3 hr after ingestion, CNS symptoms appear; obtundation, alternating lethargy and agitation, and, occasionally, seizures ensue. Nausea and vomiting are uncommon. If large amounts of muscarine are contained in the mushroom, symptoms of cholinergic crisis also may occur.

Specific **therapy** must be carefully selected. If an exaggerated cholinergic response is observed, atropine should be administered. Because ingestions of *A. muscaria* often are associated with anticholinergic findings, the acetylcholinesterase inhibitor physostigmine is used to reverse the delirium and coma. Benzodiazepines also are used for the agitation and delirium. Seizures can be controlled with diazepam. In most cases, however, early treatment with ipecac (if the patient is conscious) and close observation are all that is required.

INDOLE INTOXICATION. Mushrooms belonging to the genus *Psilocybe* ("magic mushrooms") contain psilocybin and psilocin, two psychotropic compounds. Within 30 min after ingestion, patients experience euphoria and hallucinations, often accompanied by tachycardia and mydriasis. Fever and seizures also have been observed in children with psilocybin poisoning. These symptoms are short-lived, usually lasting 6 hr after consumption of the mushroom. Severely agitated patients may respond to diazepam.

GASTROINTESTINAL: RAPID ONSET

Many mushrooms from various genera produce local gastrointestinal manifestations. The causative toxins are diverse and largely unknown. Within 1 hr of ingestion, patients develop acute abdominal pain, nausea, vomiting, and diarrhea. Symptoms may last from hours to days, depending on the species of mushroom.

Treatment is mainly supportive. Children with large fluid losses may require parenteral fluid therapy. It is imperative to differentiate ingestion of mushrooms of this class from ingestion of *Amanita* and *Galerina* species containing cyclopeptide toxins.

Bedry R, Baudrimont I, Deffieux G, et al: Brief report: Wild mushroom intoxication as a cause of rhabdomyolysis. *N Engl J Med* 2001;345:798–804.

Berger KJ, Guss DA: Mycotoxins revisited: Part I. *J Emerg Med* 2005;28:53–62.

Berger KJ, Guss DA: Mycotoxins revisited: Part II. *J Emerg Med* 2005;28:175–183.

Diaz JH: Evolving global epidemiology, syndromic classification, general management, and prevention of unknown mushroom poisonings. *Crit Care Med* 2005;33:419–426.

Diaz JH: Syndromic diagnosis and management of confirmed mushroom poisonings. *Crit Care Med* 2005;33:427–436.

Klein AS, Hart J, Brems JJ, et al: *Amanita* poisoning: Treatment and the role of liver transplantation. *Am J Med* 1989;86:187–193.

McDonald A: Mushrooms and madness: Hallucinogenic mushrooms and some psychopharmacological implications. *Can J Psychiatry* 1980;25:586–594.

Sabeel AI, Kurkus J, Lindholm T: Intensive hemodialysis and hemoperfusion treatment of *Amanita* mushroom poisoning. *Mycopathologia* 1995;131:107–114.

710.2 • Solanine Poisoning

Solanine is a mixture of several related toxins found in greened and sprouted potatoes. Potatoes exposed to light and allowed to sprout produce a number of alkaloid glycosides containing the cholesterol derivative solanidine. Two of these glycosides, α-solanine and α-chaconine, are found in highest concentration in the peels of greened potatoes and in the sprouts. The solanine alkaloids bind to serum cholinesterase, suggesting a possible pathophysiologic mechanism.

Clinical manifestations of solanine intoxication occur within 7–19 hr after ingestion. The most common symptoms are vomiting and diarrhea; in more severe instances of poisoning, fever, generalized abdominal pain, coma, and hypovolemic shock occur.

Treatment of solanine poisoning is largely supportive. In the most severe cases, symptoms resolve within 11 days. Atropine treatment has not been evaluated.

Korpan YI, Nazarenko EA, Skryshevskaya IV, et al: Potato glycoalkaloids: True safety or false sense of security? *Trends Biotechnol* 2004;22:147–151.

McMillan M, Thompson JC: An outbreak of suspected solanine poisoning in school boys: Examination of criteria of solanine poisoning. *Q J Med* 1979;48:227–243.

710.3 • Seafood Poisoning

CIGUATERA FISH POISONING

Major outbreaks of ciguatera fish poisoning have been reported in Florida, Hawaii, the Caribbean, the South Pacific, and the

Virgin Islands. With modern methods of transportation, the illness now occurs worldwide. Grouper is the most commonly identified source of the toxin, followed by snapper, kingfish, amberjack, dolphin, eel, and barracuda. Poisoning also has been associated with farm-raised salmon.

The source of this poisoning is the dinoflagellate *Gambierdiscus toxicus,* a microscopic unicellular organism found along coral reefs that produces high concentrations of ciguatoxin and maitotoxin. The toxins are passed along the food chain from small herbivorous fish that consume the dinoflagellate from the coral reefs to larger predatory fish and then to humans. These toxins are harmless in fish but produce distinct clinical symptoms in humans.

Ciguatoxin-1, a lipid with a molecular weight of approximately 1.1 kd, is odorless, colorless, and tasteless, and is not destroyed by cooking or freezing. Ciguatoxin-1 increases the sodium permeability of excitable membranes, an action that is inhibited by calcium and tetrodotoxin.

The onset of **clinical manifestations** of ciguatoxin poisoning usually occurs within 2–30 hr after ingesting contaminated fish. The illness often is biphasic. The earliest symptoms are diarrhea, vomiting, and abdominal pain; the second phase includes intense itching, rash on palms and soles, myalgias, and circumoral or extremity dysesthesias. The dysesthesia is characterized by reversal of hot and cold sensation. Tachycardia, bradycardia, and hypotension occur infrequently. Ciguatera fish poisoning is diagnosed based on clinical presentation, and the diagnosis is confirmed by testing the ingested fish for toxin.

TREATMENT. **Treatment** of ciguatera fish poisoning is supportive. Gastric lavage is recommended to remove any remaining toxin. Intravenous fluids may be required for severe diarrhea, and parenteral administration of calcium can be used to treat hypotension. In a few patients with coma or prolonged symptoms, mannitol given within 24 hr of the onset of symptoms has successfully reversed the neurologic manifestations of intoxication. However, further studies are needed before a recommendation for mannitol therapy can be made. Gabapentin reportedly has been successful in treating the neurologic symptoms in a few patients. Most cases are self-limited; neurologic symptoms may last months. Death occurs in less than 0.1% of cases.

SCOMBROID (PSEUDOALLERGIC) FISH POISONING

Epidemics have been associated with ingestion of members of the Scombresocidae or Scombridae families, notably albacore, mackerel, tuna, bonita, and kingfish. Nonscombroid fish and marine mammals, such as mahi-mahi (dolphin) and bluefish, also have been linked to outbreaks of poisoning.

Scombrotoxin, either histamine or the product of the action of the toxin on fish flesh, is responsible for the clinical syndrome. Histidine is found in high concentrations in the flesh of scombroid fish; the action of bacterial decarboxylases during putrification converts the histidine to histamine. Fish containing >20 mg of histamine per 100 g of flesh are toxic. In patients receiving isoniazid, a potent histaminase blocker, ingestion of fish flesh containing a lower concentration of histamine may be toxic.

The onset of **clinical manifestations** is acute and occurs within 10 min–2 hr after ingestion. The most common symptoms and signs include diarrhea, flushing, diaphoresis, urticaria, nausea, and headache. Abdominal pain, tachycardia, oral burning, dizziness, respiratory distress, and facial swelling also occur. The illness is usually self-limited, terminating within 8–10 hr.

TREATMENT. **Treatment** is mainly supportive. Gastric lavage decreases continued absorption of histamine. With severe diarrhea, fluid replacement may be necessary. Antihistamines have been variably successful. Four patients with severe toxicity treated with cimetidine (a histamine blocker) responded rapidly. Because data are limited, cimetidine or ranitidine should be reserved for severe cases.

PARALYTIC SHELLFISH POISONING

Filter-feeding mollusks, such as the black mussel and sea scallop, may become contaminated during dinoflagellate blooms or "red tides." The dinoflagellate *Ptychodiscus brevis* often is responsible for these red tides and contains several potent neurotoxins. Paralytic shellfish poisoning is a distinctive neurologic illness caused by 20 closely related heat-stable paralytic shellfish toxins. Saxitoxin is the most potent of the neurotoxins responsible for paralytic shellfish poisoning. This toxin prevents nerve conduction by inhibiting the sodium-potassium pump. Other toxins may be bioconverted to less toxic compounds. Consumption of bivalves, such as mussels, scallops, and clams, is the usual pathway of intoxication, although crustacea and fish have been implicated as well.

The onset of **clinical manifestations** of paralytic shellfish poisoning occurs rapidly, 30 min–2 hr after ingestion. Abdominal pain and nausea are common. Paresthesias are common and occur circumorally, in a stocking-glove distribution, or both. Perioral numbness or tingling, diplopia, ataxia, dysarthria, and the sensation of floating occur less commonly. Hot-cold reversal in temperature sensation is not unusual. In severe cases, respiratory failure from diaphragmatic paralysis may result.

TREATMENT. No antidote for paralytic shellfish poisoning is known. Supportive care, including mechanical ventilation, may be needed. Although the symptoms usually are self-limited and short-lived, weakness and malaise may persist for weeks after ingestion.

DIARRHETIC SHELLFISH POISONING

Several outbreaks of diarrhetic shellfish poisoning have been reported in Europe after consumption of mussels, cockles, and other shellfish. The dinoflagellates *Dinophysis* and *Prorocentrum* produce okadaic acid and its derivatives, the dinophysistoxins. These compounds inhibit protein phosphatases. The intracellular accumulation of phosphorylated proteins causes increased fluid secretion by gut cells via calcium influx, mediated by cyclic adenosine monophosphate and prostaglandins.

Patients develop severe diarrhea. Care is supportive and directed at rehydration. The illness is self-limited, and recovery occurs in 3–4 days; few patients require hospitalization.

AMNESIC SHELLFISH POISONING

Amnesic shellfish poisoning was first reported in 1987 in Canada after a group of people developed severe gastroenteritis as well as neurologic symptoms, including memory loss, after eating mussels from Prince Edward Island. Subsequent cases have been identified after eating shellfish from the United States, Spain, and the United Kingdom. The responsible toxin, domoic acid, comes from a diatom, *Pseudo-nitzschia multiseries,* and is a potent glutamate agonist, disrupting neurochemical transmission in the brain. It also binds to glutamate receptors, which increase calcium influx, producing neuronal swelling in the hippocampal area of the brain and death.

The initial **clinical manifestations** are gastrointestinal. Memory loss is closely related to advanced age. Those patients younger than age 40 yr are more likely to suffer only from diarrhea, whereas those older than 50 yr suffer from short-term memory loss lasting months to years.

AZASPIRACID POISONING

The azaspiracids are a class of algal toxins. Azaspiracid poisoning results from ingesting contaminated shellfish, especially mussels. Azaspiracid toxins are distributed throughout the muscle tissue in the shellfish. Symptoms start 6–18 hr after ingestion and include nausea, vomiting, severe stomach cramps and diarrhea, which often persist up to 5 days.

Ciguatera Fish Poisoning

Caplan CE: Ciguatera fish poisoning. *CMAJ* 1998;159:1394.
CDC: Ciguatera fish poisoning—Texas 1997. *JAMA* 1998;280:1394–1395.
DiNubile MJ, Hokama Y: The ciguatera poisoning syndrome from farm-raised salmon. *Ann Intern Med* 1995;122:113–114.
Lange WR: Ciguatera fish poisoning. *Am Fam Physician* 1994;50:579–584.
Palafox NA, Jain LG, Pinano AZ, et al: Successful treatment of ciguatera fish poisoning with intravenous mannitol. *JAMA* 1988;259:2740–2742.
Perez CM, Vasquez PA, Perret CF: Treatment of ciguatera poisoning with gabapentin. *N Engl J Med* 2001;344:692–693.

Scombroid Fish Poisoning

Gilbert RJ, Hobbs G, Murray CK, et al: Scombrotoxic fish poisoning: Features of the first 50 incidents to be reported in Britain (1976–9). *BMJ* 1980;281:71–72.
Hughes JM, Potter ME: Scombroid fish poisoning: From pathogenesis to prevention. *N Engl J Med* 1991;324:766–768.
Wu SF, Chen W: An outbreak of scombroid fish poisoning in a kindergarten. *Acta Paediatr Taiwan* 2003;44:297–299

Paralytic Shellfish Poisoning

Gessner BD, Middaugh JP: Paralytic shellfish poisoning in Alaska: A 20-year retrospective analysis. *Am J Epidemiol* 1995;141:766–770
Isbister GK, Kiernan MC: Neurotoxic marine poisoning. *Lancet Neurol* 2005;4:219–228.
Morris PD, Campbell DS, Taylor TJ, et al: Clinical and epidemiological features of neurotoxic shellfish poisoning in North Carolina. *Am J Public Health* 1991;81:471–474.
Shimizu Y, Yoshioka M: Transformation of paralytic shellfish toxins as demonstrated in scallop homogenates. *Science* 1981;212:547–549.
Whittle K, Gallacher S: Marine toxins. *BMJ* 2000;56:236–253.

Fish Poisoning

Bret MM: Food poisoning associated with biotoxins in fish and shellfish. *Curr Opin Infect Dis* 2003;16:461–465.

Chapter 711 ■ Biologic and Chemical Terrorism

Theodore J. Cieslak and Fred M. Henretig

The attacks on the World Trade Center and the Pentagon on September 11, 2001, the subsequent outbreak of anthrax cases originating from exposure to contaminated mail, and the terrorist attacks on mass transport systems in Great Britain and India demonstrate that terrorists will execute attacks using biologic or chemical "weapons of mass destruction." The September 2004 attack on a school in Beslan, Russia, as well as a thwarted attempt to release chlorine gas at Disneyland, indicate that some terrorists are willing to target children. Pediatricians must be familiar with the clinical manifestations of diseases induced by biologic and chemical agents, many of which can be treated successfully if the diagnosis is made early, therapy initiated promptly, and preventive measures instituted.

ETIOLOGY

Hundreds of biologic and chemical agents could be adapted for sinister use by terrorists. Attempts to ascertain which agents are most likely to be employed are fraught with difficulties. Such analysis often depends on accurate intelligence, which is likely to be problematic. Terrorists may choose to use **weapons of opportunity,** agents that for some reason are readily available to some member of the terrorist group. The motives of terrorists often are obscure and difficult to predict. Therefore, a working group convened by the Centers for Disease Control and Prevention (CDC) elected to concentrate response efforts not on those agents most likely to be used but, rather, on those agents that, if used, would constitute the gravest potential threats to public health and security.

In the case of biologic agents, the CDC working group divided pathogens and toxins into three categories, with **category A** including diseases caused by those six agents posing the greatest threat: anthrax, plague, tularemia, smallpox, botulism, and the viral hemorrhagic fevers.

Terrorists could release a vast array of potentially harmful chemicals. Tank cars full of flammable industrial gases and liquids, corrosive industrial acids and bases, poisonous compounds such as cyanides and nitrites, pesticides, dioxins, and explosives traverse our railways and roads daily. Four classes of "military-grade" chemicals with a history of use in warfare, or manufactured specifically for use as weapons, include the **organophosphate-based nerve agents, vesicants,** "blood agents" **(cyanides),** and certain **pulmonary irritants** or "choking agents."

EPIDEMIOLOGY AND PEDIATRIC-SPECIFIC CONCERNS

Large-scale attacks on civilian targets will likely involve pediatric victims, and children may be more susceptible than adults to the effects of certain biologic and chemical agents. Thinner skin makes dermally active chemical agents, such as mustard, of greater risk to children than adults. A larger surface area per unit volume further increases the problem. A small relative blood volume makes children more susceptible to the volume losses associated with enteric infections such as cholera and to gastrointestinal intoxications such as might be seen with exposure to the staphylococcal enterotoxins. Relatively high minute ventilation in children compared with adults increases the threat of agents delivered via the inhalational route. The fact that children live "closer to the ground" compounds this effect when heavier-than-air chemicals are involved. An immature blood-brain barrier may heighten the risk of central nervous system toxicity from nerve agents. Finally, developmental considerations make it less likely that a child would readily flee an area of danger, thereby increasing exposure to these various adverse effects (see Chapter 707).

Children appear to have a unique susceptibility to certain potential agents that might be used by terrorists. Although adults generally suffer only a brief self-limited incapacitating illness after infection with Venezuelan equine encephalitis (VEE) virus, young children are more likely to experience seizures, permanent neurologic sequelae, and death. In the case of smallpox, waning herd immunity may disproportionately affect children. Vaccine-induced immunity to smallpox probably diminishes significantly after 3–10 yr. Although most adults are considered susceptible to smallpox, given that routine civilian immunization ceased in the early 1970s, older adults may have some residual protection from death, if not from the development of disease. Today's children are among the first to grow up in a world without any individual or herd immunity to smallpox.

Children also may experience unique disease manifestations not seen in adults. In a study of melioidosis cases among children in Thailand, suppurative parotitis was observed as a characteristic presentation; this condition is not generally seen in adults with *Burkholderia pseudomallei* infection.

Pediatricians are likely to experience unique problems in managing childhood victims of biologic or chemical attack. Many of the drugs useful in treating such casualties are unfamiliar to pediatricians or have relative contraindications in childhood. The fluoroquinolones and tetracyclines are commonly cited as agents of choice in the treatment and prophylaxis of anthrax, plague, tularemia, brucellosis, and Q fever. Both families often are avoided in children, although the risk of morbidity and mortality from diseases induced by agents of bioterrorism far outweighs the minor risks associated with short-term use of these agents. Ciprofloxacin received, as its first licensed pediatric indication, U.S. Food and Drug Administration (FDA) approval for use in the prophylaxis of anthrax after inhalational exposure (terrorism). Doxycycline is now licensed specifically in children for the same indication. Immunizations potentially useful in preventing biologic agent–induced diseases often are not approved for use in pediatric patients. The currently available anthrax vaccine is licensed only for those between 18–65 yr of age. The plague vaccine, currently out of production and probably ineffective against inhalational exposures, was approved only for 18–61 yr olds. The smallpox vaccine, a live vaccine employing vaccinia virus, can cause fetal vaccinia and demise when given to pregnant women.

Many otherwise useful pharmaceutical agents are not available in pediatric dosing regimens. The military distributes nerve agent antidote kits consisting of pre-filled autoinjectors designed for the rapid administration of atropine and pralidoxime. Many emergency departments and some ambulances stock these kits. The doses of agents contained in the nerve agent antidote kit are calculated for soldiers and thus are far in excess of those appropriate for young children, although atropine autoinjectors specifically formulated for children have been approved by the FDA, and licensure of pralidoxime autoinjectors is expected to follow. Although physical protection probably would not be useful in a civilian setting, it is noteworthy that commercially available devices such as gas masks typically are not available in pediatric sizes.

There may not be sufficient pediatric hospital beds. In the event of a large-scale terrorist attack, as is the case with any large disaster, excess hospital bed capacity could potentially be provided at civilian and Department of Veterans Affairs hospitals under the auspices of the National Disaster Medical System, but that system makes no specific provision for pediatric beds.

CLINICAL MANIFESTATIONS

In the event of a terrorist attack, clinicians may be called on to make prompt diagnoses and render rapid life-saving treatment before the results of confirmatory diagnostic tests are available. Although each potential agent of terrorism produces its own unique clinical manifestations, it is useful to consider their effects in terms of a limited number of distinct clinical syndromes. This will help clinicians to make prompt, rational decisions regarding empirical therapy. In general, casualties from a terrorist attack either will develop symptoms immediately on exposure to an agent (or within the first several hours after exposure) or will develop symptoms slowly over a period of days to weeks. In the former case, the sinister nature of the event often is obvious, and the etiology is more likely to be conventional or chemical in nature. Biologic agents differ from conventional, chemical, and nuclear weapons (see Chapters 706 and 707) in that they have inherent incubation periods, and, therefore, patients are likely to present removed in time and place from the point of an unannounced and unnoticed exposure to a biologic agent. Whereas traditional first responders such as firemen and paramedics may be at the forefront of a conventional or chemical terrorism response, the primary care physician is likely to constitute the first line of defense against the effects of a biologic agent.

TABLE 711-1. Diseases Caused by Agents of Chemical and Biologic Terrorism, Classified by Syndrome

	NEUROMUSCULAR SYMPTOMS PROMINENT	RESPIRATORY SYMPTOMS PROMINENT	DERMATOLOGIC FINDINGS PROMINENT
SUDDEN-ONSET	Nerve agents	Chlorine Phosgene Cyanide	Mustard Lewisite
DELAYED-ONSET	Botulism	Anthrax Plague Tularemia	Smallpox

Casualties can be categorized as either immediate or delayed in presentation. Within each of these categories, patients can be further classified as having primarily respiratory, neuromuscular, or dermatologic manifestations (Table 711-1). A limited number of agents may cause each particular syndrome, permitting institution of empiric therapy targeted at a short list of potential etiologies. The viral hemorrhagic fevers might present with fever and a bleeding diathesis; these agents are considered separately in Chapter 268. In most cases, supportive care is the mainstay of hemorrhagic fever treatment.

SUDDEN-ONSET NEUROMUSCULAR SYNDROME: NERVE AGENTS. The very rapid onset of neuromuscular symptoms after an exposure should lead the clinician to consider nerve agent intoxication. The nerve agents (*tabun, sarin, soman,* and *VX*) are **organophosphate** analogues of common pesticides that act as potent inhibitors of the enzyme acetylcholinesterase. They are hazardous via ingestion, inhalation, or cutaneous absorption (see Chapter 58).

The inhibition of cholinesterase by these compounds results in the accumulation of acetylcholine at neural and neuromuscular junctions, causing excess stimulation. The resultant cholinergic syndrome involves central, nicotinic, and muscarinic effects. Central effects include altered mental status progressing rapidly to lethargy and coma, as well as ataxia, convulsions, and respiratory depression. Nicotinic effects include muscle fasciculations and twitching, followed by weakness, which can progress to flaccid paralysis as muscles fatigue. Muscarinic effects include miosis, visual blurring, profuse lacrimation, and watery rhinorrhea. Bronchospasm and increased bronchial secretions lead to cough, wheezing, dyspnea, and cyanosis. Cardiovascular manifestations include bradycardia, hypotension, and atrioventricular block. Flushing, sweating, salivation, nausea, vomiting, diarrhea, abdominal cramps, and urinary incontinence also are seen. In the absence of prompt intervention, death can quickly result from a combination of central effects and respiratory muscle paralysis.

DELAYED-ONSET NEUROMUSCULAR SYNDROME: BOTULISM. The delayed onset (hours to days after exposure) of neuromuscular symptoms is characteristic of botulism. Botulism occurs after exposure to one of seven related neurotoxins produced by certain strains of *Clostridium botulinum,* a strictly anaerobic spore-forming gram-positive bacillus commonly found in soil. Naturally occurring botulism (see Chapter 207) usually follows ingestion of preformed toxin (food poisoning) or results from intestinal toxin production (infantile form). Nonetheless, an aerosol exposure would likely result in a case of clinical botulism indistinguishable from that caused by natural exposures.

Following exposure to botulinum toxin, clinical manifestations typically begin with bulbar palsies, causing patients to complain of ptosis, photophobia, and blurred vision resulting from difficulty in accommodation. Symptoms can progress to include dysarthria, dysphonia, and dysphagia and, finally, a descending symmetric paralysis. Sensation and sensorium are not typically affected. In the absence of intervention, death often results from respiratory muscle failure.

SUDDEN-ONSET RESPIRATORY SYNDROME: CHLORINE, PHOSGENE, AND CYANIDE. The acute onset of respiratory symptoms shortly after exposure should cause the clinician to consider a range of potential chemical agents. Nerve agents may affect respiration, but these effects are usually secondary to respiratory muscle paresis rather than pulmonary pathology *per se*. This distinction should be readily evident clinically, because the nerve agent casualty will have generalized muscle involvement. In contrast, the toxic inhalants chlorine and phosgene produce respiratory distress without muscle involvement.

Chlorine is a dense, acrid, yellow-green gas that is heavier than air. After mild to moderate exposure, ocular and nasal irritation occurs, followed by cough, a choking sensation, bronchospasm, and substernal chest tightness. Pulmonary edema, mediated by hydrochloric acid and free oxygen radical generation, follows moderate to severe exposures within 30 min to several hr. Hypoxemia and hypovolemia secondary to pulmonary edema are responsible for death in fatal cases.

Phosgene, like chlorine, is a common industrial compound that was used as a weapon on the battlefields of World War I. Its odor has been described as similar to "new-mown hay." Similar to chlorine, phosgene also is thought to result in the generation of hydrochloric acid, contributing particularly to upper airway, nasal, and conjunctival irritation. Acylation reactions caused by the effects of phosgene on the pulmonary alveolar-capillary membrane lead to pulmonary edema. Phosgene lung injury also may be mediated, in part, by an inflammatory reaction associated with leukotriene production. Patients with mild to moderate exposures to phosgene may be asymptomatic, potentially causing victims to remain in a contaminated area. Pulmonary edema occurs 4–24 hr post exposure and is dose-dependent, with heavier exposures causing earlier symptoms. Dyspnea may precede radiologic findings. In severe exposures, pulmonary edema may be so marked as to result in hypovolemia and hypotension. As in the case of chlorine, death results from hypoxemia and asphyxia.

Cyanide is a cellular poison, with protean clinical manifestations. Initially, cyanide toxicity is most likely to present as tachypnea and hyperpnea, progressing rapidly to apnea in cases with significant exposure (see Chapter 58). The efficacy of cyanide as a chemical terrorism agent is limited by its volatility in open air and relatively low lethality compared with nerve agents. Released in a closed room, however, cyanide could have devastating effects, as evidenced by its use in the Nazi gas chambers during World War II. Cyanide inhibits cytochrome a_3, interfering with normal mitochondrial oxidative metabolism and leading to cellular anoxia and lactic acidosis. In addition to respiratory distress, early findings among cyanide victims include tachycardia, flushing, dizziness, headache, diaphoresis, nausea, and vomiting. With greater exposure, seizures, coma, apnea, and cardiac arrest may follow within minutes. An elevated anion gap metabolic acidosis typically is present, and decreased peripheral oxygen utilization leads to an elevated mixed venous oxygen saturation value.

DELAYED-ONSET RESPIRATORY SYNDROME: ANTHRAX, PLAGUE, AND TULAREMIA. A delayed onset of respiratory symptoms (days after exposure) is characteristic of several infectious diseases that might be adapted for sinister purposes by terrorists. Among these are anthrax, plague, and tularemia.

Anthrax is caused by infection with the gram-positive spore-forming rod *Bacillus anthracis*. Its ability to form a spore enables the anthrax bacillus to survive for long periods in the environment and enhances its potential as a weapon.

The vast majority of naturally occurring anthrax cases are cutaneous, acquired by close contact with the hides, wool, bone, and other by-products of infected cattle, sheep, and goats. Cutaneous cases also may result from the intentional deployment of anthrax-contaminated fomites. Cutaneous anthrax is amenable to therapy with a variety of antibiotics and is readily recognizable to experienced clinicians in endemic areas; therefore, it is rarely fatal. Although it is common in parts of Asia and sub-Saharan Africa, only two cases of cutaneous anthrax had occurred in the U.S. in the 9 yr that preceded the 11 cutaneous cases seen in 2001. Gastrointestinal anthrax, which has never been described in the U.S., can occur after the ingestion of contaminated meat. In the past, inhalational anthrax, or **woolsorter's disease**, was an occupational hazard of abattoir and textile workers. Now eliminated as a naturally occurring disease in the U.S., it is this inhalational form of anthrax that poses the greatest threat. Following an inadvertent release in 1979 from a bioweapons facility at Sverdlovsk in the former Soviet Union, 66 of 77 known adult victims of inhalational anthrax died. In the bioterrorism attacks involving contaminated letters in the U.S., 6 of 11 patients with inhalational anthrax have survived. Whether improved intensive care modalities, changes in antibiotic therapy, or earlier recognition accounts for this improved mortality rate remains to be determined.

Symptomatic inhalational anthrax typically begins 1–6 days after exposure, although incubation periods of up to several weeks have been reported. The disease begins as a flu-like illness, characterized by fever, myalgia, headache, and cough. A brief intervening period of improvement sometimes follows, but rapid deterioration then ensues; high fever, dyspnea, cyanosis, and shock mark this second phase. Hemorrhagic meningitis occurs in up to 50% of cases. Chest radiographs obtained late in the course of illness may reveal a widened mediastinum or prominent mediastinal lymphadenopathy; pleural effusions also may be seen. Gram stains of peripheral blood may demonstrate the organism at this stage. Prompt treatment is imperative; death occurs in as many as 95% of inhalational anthrax cases if such treatment is begun more than 48 hr after the onset of symptoms.

Whereas inhalational anthrax is a disease primarily of mediastinal lymphatic tissue, exposure to aerosolized plague bacilli typically leads to a primary pneumonia. Endemic **plague** is usually transmitted via the bites of fleas and is discussed in Chapter 200.3. The causative organism of all forms of human plague, *Yersinia pestis,* is a bipolar-staining, gram-negative facultative intracellular bacillus. An ability to survive within the macrophage aids its dissemination to distant sites following inoculation or inhalation. "Buboes," markedly swollen, tender regional lymph nodes in the distribution of a bite, are the hallmark feature of bubonic plague. Fever and malaise are typically present, and septicemia often develops as bacteria gain access to the circulation. Petechiae, purpura, and overwhelming disseminated intravascular coagulopathy (DIC) commonly occur, and 80% of bubonic plague victims ultimately will have positive blood cultures. Plague is extremely infective and lethal, as illustrated by the fact that the "Black Death" eliminated one third of the population of Europe during the Middle Ages. Even then, the potential of bubonic plague as a weapon was appreciated, as evidenced by its intentional use in 1346 by invading Tatars against the garrison at Kaffa in the Ukraine.

Intentional aerosol dissemination of *Y. pestis* would likely result in a preponderance of pneumonic plague cases. Pneumonic plague may also arise secondarily after seeding of the lungs of septicemic patients. Symptoms include fever, chills, malaise, headache, and cough. Chest radiographs may reveal a patchy consolidation, and the classic clinical finding is blood-streaked sputum. DIC and overwhelming sepsis typically develop as the disease progresses. Untreated pneumonic plague has a fatality rate approaching 100%.

Tularemia is a highly infectious disease caused by the gram-negative coccobacillus *Francisella tularensis*. Naturally occurring tularemia is discussed in Chapter 203. The high degree of infectivity of *F. tularensis* (<10 organisms are thought to be necessary to produce infection via inhalation), as well as its survivability in the environment, contributes to its inclusion on the list of agents of concern. Several clinical forms of endemic tularemia are known, but inhalational exposure in a terrorist attack would likely lead to a plague-like primary pneumonia or to typhoidal tularemia, manifesting as a variety of nonspecific symptoms including fever, malaise, and abdominal pain.

SUDDEN-ONSET DERMATOLOGIC SYNDROME: MUSTARD AND LEWISITE. The development of skin lesions shortly after exposure is characteristic of the chemical vesicants. These compounds, often referred to as "blistering agents," are cellular poisons and include the alkylating agent mustard and the organic arsenical agent lewisite. Tissue injury to rapidly reproducing cells begins within minutes of contact with these agents. In the case of mustard, clinical effects typically become evident several hours after exposure. In contrast, patients exposed to lewisite will feel immediate pain. In addition to cutaneous vesicle formation, the eyes and respiratory tract also are injured. Moreover, mustard exposure may lead to bone marrow suppression, and both mustard and lewisite may produce significant gastrointestinal symptoms.

DELAYED-ONSET DERMATOLOGIC SYNDROME: SMALLPOX. The appearance of an exanthem days to weeks after exposure is likely to be a presenting feature of smallpox. Smallpox, caused by the variola virus, a member of the orthopoxvirus family, has an incubation period of 7–17 days. This would likely permit the wide dispersal of asymptomatic exposed persons, thus contributing to the spread of an outbreak. During the incubation period, virus replicates in the upper respiratory tract. A primary viremia ensues, during which time seeding of the liver and spleen occurs. A secondary viremia then develops, the skin is seeded, and the classic exanthem of smallpox appears.

Symptoms of smallpox begin abruptly during the phase of secondary viremia and include fever, rigors, vomiting, headache, backache, and extreme malaise. Within 2–4 days, macules appear on the face and extremities and then progress in synchronous fashion to papules, pustules, and finally scabs. As the scabs separate, survivors often are left with disfiguring, de-pigmented scars. The synchronous nature of the rash and its centrifugal distribution distinguish smallpox from chickenpox, which has a centripetal distribution. Historically, smallpox had a 30% mortality rate, with death typically resulting from visceral organ involvement.

DIAGNOSIS

In some cases, the terrorist nature of a chemical or biologic attack may be obvious, e.g., in the case of a chemical attack when victims succumb in close temporal and geographic proximity to a dispersal device or when terrorists may announce their attack. In other instances, the clinician may need to rely on epidemiologic clues to suspect an intentional release of chemical or biologic agents. The presence of large numbers of victims clustered in time and space should raise the clinician's index of suspicion, as should cases of unexpected death or unexpectedly severe disease. Diseases unusual in a given locale, in a given age group, or during a certain season likewise may warrant further investigation. Simultaneous outbreaks of a disease in noncontiguous areas should cause one to consider an intentional release, as should outbreaks of multiple diseases in the same area. Even a single case of rare disorders such as anthrax or certain viral hemorrhagic fevers would be suspicious, and a single case of smallpox would almost certainly be the result of an intentional release. Large numbers of dying animals might provide evidence of an unnatural aerosol release, as would evidence of a disparate attack rate between those known to be indoors and outdoors at a given time.

In a mass casualty setting, diagnoses may be made largely on clinical grounds. The diagnosis of nerve agent intoxication is based primarily on clinical recognition and patient response to antidotal therapy. Several simple rapid detection devices developed for military use can detect the presence of nerve agents. Some of these are commercially available and are stocked in certain emergency departments and public safety vehicles. M8 and M9 test papers indicate the presence of nerve agents by means of a simple color change. Measurements of acetylcholinesterase in plasma or erythrocytes of nerve agent victims may be helpful in long-term prognostication, but correlation between cholinesterase levels and clinical effects often is poor, and the test rarely is available emergently.

Botulism should be suspected clinically among patients presenting with a symmetric, descending, flaccid paralysis. Although the differential diagnosis of botulism includes other uncommon neurologic disorders such as myasthenia gravis and the Guillain-Barré syndrome, the presence of multiple casualties with similar symptoms should aid in the determination of a botulism outbreak.

Initially, the diagnosis of **cyanide poisoning** also will likely be made on clinical grounds in the face of the appropriate toxidrome. An unusually high anion gap metabolic acidosis and an oxygen concentration greater than expected in venous blood lend support to the clinical diagnosis. Elevated blood cyanide concentrations can confirm the clinical suspicion.

Anthrax should be suspected upon finding gram-positive bacilli in skin biopsy material (in the case of cutaneous disease), blood smears, pleural fluid, or spinal fluid. Chest radiographs demonstrating a widened mediastinum in the context of fever and constitutional signs, and in the absence of another obvious explanation (e.g., blunt trauma or postsurgical infection), also should lead one to consider the diagnosis. Confirmation can be obtained by blood culture. State health laboratories and federal facilities at the CDC and at the U.S. Army Medical Research Institute of Infectious Diseases can confirm a diagnosis of anthrax by polymerase chain reaction and immunohistochemical assay.

A diagnosis of **plague** can be suspected on finding bipolar "safety-pin"-staining bacilli in Gram or Wayson stains of sputum or aspirated lymph node material; confirmation is obtained by culturing *Y. pestis* from blood, sputum, or lymph node aspirate. The organism grows on standard blood or MacConkey TRA agars, but it is often misidentified by automated systems. *F. tularensis* grows poorly on standard media; its growth is enhanced on media containing cysteine. Because of its extreme infectivity, however, many laboratories prefer to make a diagnosis via polymerase chain reaction, or serologically using an enzyme-linked immunosorbent assay or serum agglutination assay.

Smallpox should be suspected on clinical grounds and can be confirmed by culture or electron microscopy of scabs or vesicular fluid, although the manipulation of clinical material from suspected smallpox victims should be attempted only at public health laboratories able to employ maximum biocontainment (BSL-4) precautions. Similar caution should be exercised with specimens from patients with various viral hemorrhagic fevers.

PREVENTION

Preventive measures can be considered in both a pre- and a post-exposure context. **Pre-exposure protection** against a chemical or biologic attack may consist of physical, chemical, or immunologic measures. **Physical protection** against primary attack often involves gas masks and protective suits; such equipment is used by the military and by certain hazardous materials response teams, but it is unlikely to be available to civilians at the precise moment that a release occurs. Medical personnel must understand the principles of physical protection as they apply to infection control and the spread of contamination.

Pneumonic plague is spread through respiratory droplets. Droplet precautions, including the use of simple surgical masks, are thus warranted when caring for patients with plague. Smallpox is transmitted by droplet nuclei. Airborne precautions, including (ideally) a high-efficiency particulate air (HEPA) filter mask are warranted when caring for smallpox victims. Similarly, viral hemorrhagic fever patients should, in general, be managed using contact precautions. Most other biologic agent victims can be safely cared for while employing standard precautions. In the case of chemical agents, residual mustard or nerve agent on the skin or clothing of victims might potentially pose a hazard to medical personnel. Such victims, whenever possible, should thus have their clothing removed and be decontaminated using copious amounts of water before extensive medical care is rendered. Most other chemical agents are volatile enough that spread of agent among patients or from patient to caregiver is unlikely.

Pre-exposure chemical prophylaxis might be used on the basis of credible intelligence reports. For example, should officials deem that the threatened release of a specific biologic agent appears imminent, antibiotics might be distributed to a population preemptively. Opportunities to employ such a strategy are likely to be quite limited.

Although licensed vaccines (**pre-exposure immunologic measures**) exist against anthrax and smallpox, widespread use of either vaccine is likely to be problematic, especially in children. The anthrax vaccine is licensed only for those persons age 18 yr and older and is given as a 6-dose series over 18 mo and requires annual booster doses. These issues, coupled with a limited supply, make civilian employment of the current anthrax vaccine on a large scale unlikely, although a new recombinant anthrax vaccine is in the late stages of development and is being studied as a 3-dose series.

Significant obstacles also exist to the widespread employment of smallpox vaccine, although public health officials have contemplated the resumption of a smallpox vaccination campaign. Whereas in the past smallpox vaccine (prepared from vaccinia virus, an orthopoxvirus related to variola) was used safely and successfully in young infants, it has a relatively high rate of serious complications in certain patients. *Fetal vaccinia* and demise can occur when pregnant women are vaccinated. *Vaccinia gangrenosa,* an often-fatal complication, can occur when immunocompromised persons are vaccinated. *Eczema vaccinatum* occurs in those with pre-existing dermatoses (atopic dermatitis). A severe vaccine-related encephalitis was well-known during the era of widespread vaccination; because this occurs only in primary vaccinees, it would disproportionately affect pediatric patients. Autoinoculation can occur when virus present at the site of vaccination is manually transferred to other areas of skin or to the eye. Young children would presumably be at greater risk for such inadvertent transmission.

To manage these complications, vaccinia immune globulin (VIG) should be available when undertaking a vaccination campaign. VIG (0.6 mg/kg IM) may be given to vaccine recipients who experience severe complications or to significantly immunocompromised individuals exposed to smallpox, in whom vaccination would be unsafe. Stocks of current vaccine and of VIG are controlled by the CDC, and production of a new vaccine and VIG preparation is ongoing. In addition to a potential role in pre-exposure prophylaxis, vaccination may be effective in postexposure prophylaxis if given within the first 4 days or so after exposure.

Anthrax vaccine might similarly be employed in a postexposure setting. Some authorities recommend three doses of this vaccine as an adjunct to postexposure chemoprophylaxis after documented exposure to aerosolized anthrax spores. Nonetheless, postexposure administration of oral antibiotics constitutes the mainstay of management for asymptomatic victims believed to have been exposed to anthrax, as well as to other bacterial agents such as plague and tularemia. Appropriate prophylactic regimens for various biologic exposures are provided in Table 711-2.

TREATMENT

Recommended therapies for overt diseases caused by various chemical and biologic agents are provided in Tables 711-2 and 711-3. It is quite likely, however, that the clinician attending to victims will need to make therapeutic decisions before the results of confirmatory diagnostic tests are available and in situations where the diagnosis is not known with certainty. In such cases, it is useful to note that many diseases and symptoms caused by chemical and biologic agents will resolve spontaneously, with only supportive care required. Chlorine and phosgene exposures can thus be successfully managed by providing meticulous attention to oxygenation and fluid balance. Mustard victims may require intensive multisystem support, but no specific antidote or therapy is available. Many viral diseases, such as smallpox, most viral hemorrhagic fevers, and the equine encephalitides, are managed supportively.

In addition to ensuring adequate oxygenation, ventilation, and hydration, the clinician may need to provide specific empirical therapies on an urgent basis. Patients suffering from the sudden onset of severe neuromuscular symptoms may have nerve agent intoxication and should be given atropine (0.05 mg/kg) promptly for its antimuscarinic effects. Although atropine relieves bronchospasm and bradycardia, reduces bronchial secretions, and ameliorates the gastrointestinal effects of nausea, vomiting, and diarrhea, it does not improve skeletal muscle paralysis. Pralidoxime (also known as 2-PAM) cleaves the organophosphate moiety from cholinesterase and regenerates intact enzyme if "aging" has not occurred. The effect is most prominent at the neuromuscular junction and leads to improved muscle strength. Its prompt use (at a dose of 25 mg/kg) as an adjunct to atropine is recommended in all serious cases.

Ideally, both atropine and pralidoxime should be administered intravenously in severe cases, although the intraosseous route may be acceptable. Some experts recommend that atropine be given intramuscularly in the presence of hypoxia to avoid arrhythmias associated with intravenous administration. Many EMS systems stock military autoinjector kits consisting of atropine and 2-PAM for intramuscular injection. Pediatric atropine autoinjectors are now licensed, although military kits (with 2 mg of atropine and 600 mg of pralidoxime) might be used in children older than 2–3 yr of age. Animal studies support the routine prophylactic administration of anticonvulsant doses of benzodiazepines, even in the absence of observable convulsive activity.

Delayed neuromuscular symptoms in the setting of terrorism might be due to botulism. Supportive care, with meticulous attention to ventilatory support, is the mainstay of botulism treatment. Such support may be necessary for several months, making the management of a large-scale botulism outbreak especially problematic in terms of medical resources. A licensed bivalent (types A and B) and a separate investigational type E equine botulinum antitoxin are available through the CDC (1-404-639-3670). Administration of these antitoxins is unlikely to reverse disease in symptomatic patients but may prevent further progression. A test dose should be administered before therapy, and patients reacting to this test dose should be desensitized. An investigational heptavalent despeciated (Fab_2) antitoxin, also produced in

TABLE 711-2. Critical Biologic Agents of Terrorism

DISEASE	CLINICAL FINDINGS	INCUBATION PERIOD	ISOLATION PRECAUTIONS	INITIAL TREATMENT	PROPHYLAXIS
Anthrax (inhalational).* Patients who are clinically stable after 14 days can be switched to a single oral agent (ciprofloxacin or doxycycline) to complete a 60-day course.[†]	Febrile prodrome with rapid progression to mediastinal lymphadenitis and mediastinitis, sepsis, shock, and meningitis	1–5 d	Standard	Ciprofloxacin[‡] 10–15 mg/kg IV q12h OR Doxycycline 2.2 mg/kg IV q12h AND Clindamycin[§] 10–15 mg/kg IV q8h AND Penicillin G[‖] 400–600 k U/kg/d IV ÷ q4h	Ciprofloxacin 10–15 mg/kg PO q12h OR Doxycycline 2.2 mg/kg PO q12h
Plague (pneumonic)	Febrile prodrome with rapid progression to fulminant pneumonia, hemoptysis, sepsis, DIC	2–3 d	Droplet (for first 3 d of therapy)	Gentamicin 2.5 mg/kg IV q8h OR Doxycycline 2.2 mg/kg IV q12h OR Ciprofloxacin 15 mg/kg IV q12h	Doxycycline 2.2 mg/kg PO q12h OR Ciprofloxacin 20 mg/kg PO q12h
Tularemia	Pneumonic: Abrupt onset of fever with fulminant pneumonia Typhoidal: Fever, malaise, abdominal pain	2–10 d	Standard	Same as for plague	Same as for plague
Smallpox	Febrile prodrome with synchronous, centrifugal, vesiculopustular exanthema	7–17 d	Airborne (+ contact)	Supportive care	Vaccination may be effective if given within the first several days after exposure
Botulism	Afebrile descending symmetrical flaccid paralysis with cranial nerve palsies	1–5 d	Standard	Supportive care; antitoxin (see text) may halt the progression of symptoms but is unlikely to reverse them	None
Viral hemorrhagic fevers	Febrile prodrome with rapid progression to shock, purpura, and bleeding diatheses	4–21 d	Contact (consider airborne in cases of massive hemorrhage)	Supportive care; ribavirin may be beneficial in select cases	None

*In a mass casualty setting, where resources are severely constrained, it may be necessary to substitute oral therapy for the preferred parenteral option.

[†]Assuming the organism is sensitive, children may be switched to oral amoxicillin (80 mg/kg/d ÷ q8h) to complete a 60-day course. We recommend that the first 14 days of therapy or postexposure prophylaxis, however, include ciprofloxacin and/or doxycycline regardless of age.

[‡]Levofloxacin or ofloxacin may be acceptable alternatives to ciprofloxacin.

[§]Rifampin or clarithromycin may be acceptable alternatives to clindamycin as drugs that target bacterial protein synthesis. If ciprofloxacin or another quinolone is employed, doxycycline may be used as a second agent, because it also targets protein synthesis.

[‖]Ampicillin, imipenem, meropenem, or chloramphenicol may be acceptable alternatives to penicillin as drugs with good central nervous system penetration.

DIC, disseminated intravascular coagulation.

horses, is available through the U.S. Army Medical Research Institute of Infectious Diseases on a compassionate use protocol. In addition, a pentavalent (types A–E) product (licensed for treatment of type A and B botulism), Botulism Immune Globulin Intravenous (Human), BabyBIG, is available through the California Department of Health Services (1-510-231-7600), specifically for the treatment of infant botulism.

The **rapid onset of respiratory symptoms** may signal an exposure to chlorine, phosgene, cyanide, or a number of other toxic industrial chemicals. Although the mainstay of therapy in virtually all of these exposures consists of removal to fresh air and intensive supportive care, cyanide intoxication often requires the administration of specific antidotes, given in two stages. A methemoglobin-forming agent such as sodium nitrite is administered first, because methemoglobin has high affinity for cyanide and causes it to dissociate from cytochrome oxidase. Nitrite dosing in children should be based on body weight to avoid excessive methemoglobin formation and nitrite-induced hypotension. For the same reasons, nitrites should be infused slowly over 5–10 min. A sulfur donor, such as sodium thiosulfate, is given next. This compound is used as a substrate by the hepatic enzyme rhodanese, which converts cyanide to thiocyanate, a less toxic compound excreted in the urine. Thiosulfate treatment itself is efficacious and relatively benign and, thus, may be used alone for mild to moderate cases. Sodium nitrite and sodium thiosulfate are packaged together in standard antidote kits, along with amyl nitrite, a sodium nitrite substitute that can be inhaled in prehospital settings where intravenous access is not available.

In cases in which the **delayed onset of respiratory symptoms** may be due to a terrorist attack, consideration should be given to the empirical administration of an antibiotic effective against anthrax, plague, and tularemia. Ciprofloxacin (10–15 mg/kg IV q12h) or doxycycline (2.2 mg/kg IV q12h) are reasonable choices. Although naturally occurring strains of *B. anthracis* usually are quite sensitive to penicillin G, these agents are chosen because penicillin-resistant strains of *B. anthracis* exist. Moreover, ciprofloxacin and doxycycline are effective against almost all known strains of *Y. pestis* and *F. tularensis*. Concerns about inducible β-lactamases in *B. anthracis* have led some experts to recommend one or two additional antibiotics in patients with inhalational anthrax. Rifampin, vancomycin, penicillin or ampicillin, clindamycin, imipenem, and clarithromycin are reasonable choices based on in vitro sensitivity data. Because *B. anthracis* relies on the production of two protein toxins, edema toxin and lethal toxin, for its virulence, drugs that act at the ribosome to disrupt protein synthesis (e.g., clindamycin, the macrolides) provide a theoretical advantage. Frequent meningeal involvement among inhalational anthrax victims makes agents with superior central nervous system penetration desirable. A combination of ciprofloxacin plus clindamycin plus penicillin G is a good initial empiric therapy for presumed inhalational anthrax. Ciprofloxacin or doxycycline monotherapy is probably adequate in cases of cutaneous anthrax, although patients with cutaneous disease resulting from a terrorist attack initially should receive multi-drug therapy owing to the possibility of concomitant inhalational exposure.

In patients in whom a diagnosis of plague or tularemia is established, streptomycin (15 mg/kg IM q12h) has historically been considered the drug of choice. As this drug is now generally unavailable, many experts consider gentamicin (2.5 mg/kg IV/IM q8h) the preferred choice for therapy. In addition to doxycycline and ciprofloxacin, chloramphenicol (25 mg/kg IV q6h) is an acceptable alternative. The latter should be employed in the 6% of pneumonic plague cases with concomitant meningitis. To be effective, therapy for pneumonic plague must be initiated within 24 hr of the onset of symptoms.

TABLE 711-3. Critical Chemical Agents of Terrorism

AGENT	TOXICITY	CLINICAL FINDINGS	ONSET	DECONTAMINATION*	MANAGEMENT
NERVE AGENTS					
Tabun, Sarin, Soman, VX	Anticholinesterase: muscarinic, nicotinic, CNS effects	Vapor: miosis, rhinorrhea, dyspnea Liquid: diaphoresis, vomiting Both: coma, paralysis, seizures, apnea	Seconds: vapor Minutes–hours: liquid	Vapor: fresh air, remove clothes, wash hair Liquid: remove clothes, wash skin, hair with copious soap and water, ocular irrigation	ABCs Atropine: 0.05 mg/kg IV[†], IM[‡] (min 0.1 mg, max 5 mg), repeat q2–5 min prn for marked secretions, bronchospasm Pralidoxime: 25 mg/kg IV, IM[§] (max 1 g IV; 2 g IM), may repeat within 30–60 min prn, then again q1h for one or two doses prn for persistent weakness, high atropine requirement Diazepam: 0.3 mg/kg (max 10 mg) IV; lorazepam: 0.1 mg/kg IV, IM (max 4 mg); midazolam: 0.2 mg/kg (max 10 mg) IM prn for seizures or severe exposure
VESICANTS					
Mustard	Alkylation	Skin: erythema, vesicles Eye: inflammation Respiratory tract: inflammation	Hours	Skin: soap and water Eyes: water (effective only if done within minutes of exposure)	Symptomatic care
Lewisite	Arsenical		Immediate pain		Possibly BAL 3 mg/kg IM q4–6 h for systemic effects of Lewisite in severe cases
PULMONARY AGENTS					
Chlorine, phosgene	Liberate HCl, alkylation	Eyes, nose, throat irritation (especially chlorine) Respiratory: bronchospasm, pulmonary edema (especially phosgene)	Minutes: eyes, nose, throat irritation, bronchospasm; Hours: pulmonary edema	Fresh air Skin: water	Symptomatic care
CYANIDE					
	Cytochrome oxidase inhibition: cellular anoxia, lactic acidosis	Tachypnea, coma, seizures, apnea	Seconds	Fresh air Skin: soap and water	ABCs, 100% oxygen Na bicarbonate prn metabolic acidosis Na nitrite (3%): dose (mL/kg) — Estimated Hgb (g/dL) 0.27 — 10 0.33 — 12 (est. for average child) 0.39 — 14 (max 10 mL) Na thiosulfate (25%): 1.65 mL/kg (max 50 mL)

*Decontamination, especially for patients with significant nerve agent or vesicant exposure; should be performed by health care providers garbed in adequate personal protective equipment. For emergency department staff, this consists of nonencapsulated, chemically resistant body suit, boots, and gloves with a full face air purifier mask/hood.

[†]Intraosseous route is likely equivalent to intravenous.

[‡]Atropine might have some benefit via endotracheal tube or inhalation, as might aerosolized ipratropium.

[§]Pralidoxime is reconstituted to 50 mg/mL (1 g in 20 mL water) for IV administration, and the total dose infused over 30 min, or may be given by continuous infusion (loading dose 25 mg/kg over 30 min, then 10 mg/kg/hr). For IM use, it might be diluted to a concentration of 300 mg/mL (1 g added to 3 mL water—by analogy to the U.S. Army's Mark 1 autoinjector concentration), to effect a reasonable volume for injection. Each Mark 1 kit holds two autoinjectors, one each of atropine 2 mg (0.7 mL) and pralidoxime 600 mg (2 mL); while not approved for pediatric use, they might be considered as initial treatment in dire (especially prehospital) circumstances, for children with severe, life-threatening nerve agent toxicity who lack intravenous access, and for whom more precise, mg/kg IM dosing would be logistically impossible. Suggested dosing guidelines are offered; note potential excess of intial atropine and pralidoxime dose for age/weight, though within general guidelines for recommended total over first 60–90 min of therapy of severe exposures:

Approximate Age	Approximate Weight	Number of Autoinjectors (each type)	Atropine Dose Range (mg/kg)	Pralidoxime Dose Range (mg/kg)
3–7 yr	13–25 kg	1	0.08–0.13	24–46
8–14 yr	26–50 kg	2	0.08–0.13	24–46
>14 yr	>51 kg	3	≤0.11	≤35

ABCs, airway, breathing, and circulatory support; BAL, British antilewisite; CNS, central nervous system; est., estimated hemoglobin concentration; HCl, hydrochloric acid; Hgb, hemoglobin concentration; max, maximum; min, minimum; prn, as needed.

Adapted from Henretig FH, Cieslak TJ, Eitzen EM: Biological and chemical terrorism. *J Pediatr* 2002; 141:311–326. Used with permission.

The management of **vesicant-induced injury** is similar to that for burn victims and is largely symptomatic (see Chapter 74). Mustard victims will benefit from the application of soothing skin lotions such as calamine and the administration of analgesics. Early intubation of severely exposed patients is warranted to guard against edematous airway compromise. Oxygen and mechanical ventilation may be needed, and meticulous attention to hydration is of paramount importance. Lewisite victims can be managed in much the same manner as mustard victims. In addition, dimercaprol (British antilewisite [BAL]) in oil, given intramuscularly, may help ameliorate the systemic effects of lewisite.

The management of symptomatic smallpox victims also is largely supportive, with attention to pain control, hydration status, and respiratory sufficiency again of primary importance. The parenteral antiviral compound cidofovir, licensed for the treatment of cytomegalovirus retinitis in HIV-infected patients, has in vitro efficacy against variola and other orthopoxviruses. Its utility in treating smallpox victims is untested. Moreover, in the face of a large outbreak of disease, large-scale parenteral use of this drug would be problematic.

Cieslak TJ, Henretig FM: Bioterrorism. *Pediatr Ann* 2003;32:154–165.

Cieslak TJ, Henretig FM: Ring-a-ring-a-roses: Bioterrorism and its peculiar relevance to pediatrics. *Curr Op Pediatr* 2003;15:107–111.

Franz DR, Jahrling PB, McClain DJ, et al: Clinical recognition and management of patients exposed to biological warfare agents. *Clin Lab Med* 2001;21:435–473.

Henretig FH, Cieslak TJ, Eitzen EM: Biological and chemical terrorism. *J Pediatr* 2002;141:311–326.

Markenson D, Redlener I: Pediatric terrorism preparedness national guidelines and recommendations: Findings of an evidence-based consensus process. *Biosecur Bioterror* 2004;2:301–319.

Markenson D, Reynolds S, American Academy of Pediatrics Committee on Pediatric Emergency Medicine, Task Force on Terrorism: The pediatrician and disaster preparedness. *Pediatrics* 2006;117:340–362.

Patt HA, Feigin RD: Diagnosis and management of suspected cases of bioterrorism: A pediatric perspective. *Pediatrics* 2002;109:685–692.

White SR, Henretig F, Dukes RG: Medical management of vulnerable populations and co-morbid conditions of victims of bioterrorism. *Emerg Med Clin North Am* 2002;20:365–392.

Chapter 712 ■ Animal and Human Bites

Charles M. Ginsburg

With approximately 100 million dogs and cats in the United States, an estimated 3.5–4.7 million individuals are bitten annually. More than 400,000 of these individuals seek medical care in hospital emergency departments and free-standing emergency centers in the U.S. each year. It has been estimated that more bite-injured individuals seek medical attention in medical offices and primary care clinics than in emergency facilities.

EPIDEMIOLOGY. During the past 3 decades, there have been approximately 20 deaths per year in the U.S. from dog-inflicted injuries; 65% of these occurred in children <11 yr of age. The breed of dog involved in attacks on children varies; Table 712-1 depicts the risk index by breed from 1 study of 341 dog bites. Rottweilers, pit bulls, and German shepherds accounted for >50% of all fatal bite-related injuries. Unaltered male dogs account for approximately 75% of attacks; nursing dams often inflict injury to humans when children attempt to handle one of their puppies.

The majority of **dog-related** attacks occur in children between the ages of 6–11 yr of age. Boys are attacked more often than girls (1.5:1). Approximately ⅔ of the attacks occur around the home, 75% of the biting animals are known by the child, and almost 50% of the attacks are said to be unprovoked. Similar statistics apply to Canada, where 70% of all bites were sustained by children between 2–14 yr; 65% of the dogs involved in the biting were part of the family or extended family and occurred in someone's home.

Of the approximately 450,000 reported **cat bites** per year occurring in the U.S., nearly all are inflicted by known household animals. Because rat bites and gerbil bites are not reportable conditions, little is known about the epidemiology of these injuries and the incidence of infection after rodent-inflicted bites or scratches.

Few data exist on the incidence and demographics of **human bite** injuries in pediatric patients; however, preschool- and early school-aged children appear to be at greatest risk of sustaining an injury from a bite by a human. Human bites are a common cause of injury in daycare centers in the U.S., although in some series the proportion of human bites is highest among adolescents. In adolescents, fist-to-mouth (tooth) injuries are associated with fights.

TABLE 712-1. Risk of Dog Bites in the U.S. Among Children by Dog Breed

DOG BREED	NO. DOG BITES (%)	DOG POPULATION (%)	RISK INDEX
German shepherd	105 (34)	12	2.83
Doberman	8 (3)	1.1	2.71
Spitz	5 (2)	1.1	1.81
Pekingese	10 (3)	1.9	1.56
Dachshund	22 (7)	5.2	1.35
Schnauzer	5 (2)	1.5	1.33
Collie	10 (3)	2.3	1.30
Hound dog	15 (5)	3.9	1.29
Poodle	10 (3)	3.1	0.98
Rottweiler	3 (1)	1.1	0.92
Beagle	3 (1)	1.2	0.80
Terrier	15 (5)	8.1	0.61
Bernese dog	3 (1)	1.7	0.58
Labrador retriever	11 (4)	8.2	0.49
Cross-breed	39 (13)	28	0.46
Spaniel	5 (2)	6.5	0.31
Shi tzu	1 (0.3)	1.2	0.26
Maltese	0 (0.0)	1.1	0.00

*Data about the distribution of the dog population were collected from the local community dog register. The risk index was calculated by dividing the representation of a dog breed among the total dog population by the representation of this breed among all evaluated dog bites.

From Schalamon J, Ainoedhofer H, Singer G, et al: Analysis of dog bites in children who are younger than 17 years. *Pediatrics* 2006;117:e374–e379.

CLINICAL MANIFESTATIONS. Dog bite–related injuries can be divided into three, almost equal categories: abrasions; puncture wounds; and lacerations, with or without an associated avulsion of tissue. Dog bites may be crush injuries. The most common type of injury from cat and rat bites is a puncture wound. Cat bites often penetrate to deep tissue. Human bite injuries are of two types: an occlusion injury that is incurred when the upper and lower teeth come together on a body part and, in older children and young adults, a clenched-fist injury that occurs when the injured fist, usually on the dominant hand, comes in contact with the tooth of another individual.

DIAGNOSIS. Management of the bite victim should begin with a thorough history and physical examination. Careful attention should be paid to the circumstances surrounding the bite (e.g., type of animal, domestic or sylvatic, provoked or unprovoked, location of the attack); a history of drug allergies; and the immunization status of the child (tetanus) and animal (rabies). During physical examination, meticulous attention should be paid to the type, size, and depth of the injury; the presence of foreign material in the wound; the status of underlying structures; and, in instances where the bite is on an extremity, the range of motion of the affected area. A diagram of the injury(s) should be recorded in the patient's medical record. A radiograph of the affected part should be obtained if there is likelihood that a bone or joint could have been penetrated or fractured or if foreign material is present. The possibility of a fracture or penetrating injury of the skull should be considered in individuals, particularly infants, who have sustained dog bite injuries to the face and head.

COMPLICATIONS. Infection is the most common complication of bite injuries, regardless of the species of biting animal. The decision to obtain material for culture from a wound depends on the species of the biting animal, the length of time that has elapsed since the injury, the depth of the wound, the presence of foreign material contaminating the wound, and whether there is evidence of infection. Although potentially pathogenic bacteria have been isolated from up to 80% of dog bite wounds that are brought to medical attention within 8 hr after the bite, the infection rate for wounds receiving medical attention in <8 hr is small (2.5–20%). Thus, unless they are deep and extensive, dog bite wounds that are less than 8 hr old do not need to be cultured unless there is evidence of contamination or early signs of infection, or the patient is immunocompromised. Species of *Capnocytophaga canimorsus*, uncommon pathogens in bite-inflicted injuries, have been isolated from nearly 5% of infected wounds in immunocompromised patients. The infection rate in **cat bite** wounds that receive early medical attention is at least 50%; therefore, it is prudent to obtain material for culture from all but the most trivial cat-inflicted wounds and all other animal bite wounds that are not brought to medical attention within 8 hr, regardless of species of the biting animal.

The rate of infection after **rodent bite** injuries is not known. Most of the oral flora of rats is similar to that of other mammals; however, approximately 50% and 25% of rats harbor strains of *Streptobacillus moniliformis* and *Spirillum minus*, respectively, in their oral flora. Each of these agents has the potential to cause infection (see Chapter 712.1).

All **human bite** wounds, regardless of the mechanism of injury, should be regarded as carrying high risk for infection and cultured. Because of the large incidence of anaerobic infection after bite wounds, it is important to obtain material for anaerobic as well as aerobic cultures.

TABLE 712-2. Microorganisms Associated With Mammalian Bite Wound Infections

COMMON	UNCOMMON
DOGS	
Mixed infection	*Acinetobacter* spp.
Pasteurella multocida	*Aeromonas hydrophila*
Staphylococcus aureus	α, β, γ streptococci
Staphylococcus epidermidis	*Bacteroides* spp.
	Brucella canis
	Capnocytophaga canimorsus (formerly DF-2)
	Enterobacter cloacae
	Enterococcus spp.
	Escherichia coli
	Klebsiella spp.
	Moraxella spp.
	Peptococcus spp.
	Peptostreptococcus spp.
	Pseudomonas spp.
CATS	
P. multocida	*Acinetobacter* spp.
S. aureus	*Bacteroides* spp.
	Corynebacterium spp.
	E. cloacae
	Fusobacterium spp.
	Streptococcus spp.
	S. epidermidis
HUMANS	
α, β, γ streptococci	*Enterococcus* spp.
Bacteroides spp.	*Eubacterium* spp.
Corynebacterium spp.	*Klebsiella pneumoniae*
Eikenella corrodens	*Neisseria* spp.
Fusobacterium spp.	*Peptococcus* spp.
Mixed infection	*Pseudomonas* spp.
Peptostreptococcus spp.	*Veillonella* spp.
S. aureus	

TABLE 712-3. Prophylactic Management of Human or Animal Bite Wounds to Prevent Infection

CATEGORY OF MANAGEMENT	MANAGEMENT
Cleansing	Sponge away visible dirt. Irrigate with a copious volume of sterile saline solution by high-pressure syringe irrigation.* Do not irrigate puncture wounds. Standard precautions should be used.
Wound culture	No for fresh wounds, unless signs of infection exist. Yes for wounds more than 8–12 h old and wounds that appear infected.†
Radiographs	Indicated for penetrating injuries overlying bones or joints, for suspected fracture, or to assess foreign body inoculation.
Débridement	Remove devitalized tissue.
Operative débridement and exploration	Yes if one of the following: • Extensive wounds (devitalized tissue) • Involvement of the metacarpophalangeal joint (closed fist injury) • Cranial bites by large animal
Wound closure	Yes for selected fresh, nonpuncture bite wounds (see text)
Assess tetanus immunization status	Yes
Assess risk of rabies from animal bites	Yes
Assess risk of hepatitis B virus infection from human bites	Yes
Assess risk of human immunodeficiency virus from human bites	Yes
Initiate antimicrobial therapy	Yes for: • Moderate or severe bite wounds, especially if edema or crush injury is present • Puncture wounds, especially if penetration of bone, tendon sheath, or joint has occurred • Facial bites • Hand and foot bites • Genital area bites • Wounds in immunocompromised and asplenic people • Wounds with signs of infection
Follow-up	Inspect wound for signs of infection within 48 h

*Use of 18-gauge needle with a large-volume syringe is effective. Antimicrobial or anti-infective solutions offer no advantage and may increase tissue irritation.

†Both aerobic and anaerobic bacterial culture should be performed.

From American Academy of Pediatrics. Bite wounds. In: Pickering LK, Baker CJ, Long SS, McMillan JA, eds. *Red Book: 2006 Report of the Committee on Infectious Disease.* 27th ed. ElK Grove Village, IL, AAP, 2006: pp 191–195.

Common causes of soft tissue bacterial infections after dog, cat, or human bites are noted in Table 712-2. High-risk bites for infection include hand, foot, or genital wounds, penetration of bone or tendons, human or cat bites, delay in treatment >24 hr, presence of foreign material, immunosuppression (asplenia), and crush or deep puncture wounds.

TREATMENT (Table 712-3). After the appropriate material has been obtained for culture, the wound should be anesthetized, cleaned, and vigorously irrigated with copious amounts of normal saline. Irrigation with antibiotic-containing solutions provides no advantage over irrigation with saline alone and may cause local irritation of the tissues. Puncture wounds should be thoroughly cleansed and gently irrigated with a catheter or blunt-tipped needle; high-pressure irrigation should not be employed. Avulsed or devitalized tissue should be debrided and any fluctuant areas incised and drained.

Much controversy and few data exist to determine whether bite wounds should undergo primary closure or delayed primary closure (3–5 days) or should be allowed to heal by secondary intention. Factors to be considered are the type, size, and depth of the wound; the anatomic location; the presence of infection; the time interval from the injury; and the potential for cosmetic disfigurement. Surgical consultation should be obtained for all patients with deep or extensive wounds; wounds involving the face or bones and joints; and infected wounds that require open drainage. Although there is general agreement that infected wounds and those that are >24 hr of age should not be sutured, there is disagreement and varying clinical experience about the efficacy and safety of closing wounds that are <8 hr of age with no evidence of infection. Because all **hand wounds** are at high risk for infection, particularly if there has been disruption of the tendons or penetration of the bones, delayed primary closure is recommended for all but the most trivial bite wounds of the hands. **Facial lacerations** are at smaller risk for secondary infection because of the more luxuriant blood supply to this region. Many plastic surgeons advocate primary closure of facial bite wounds that have been brought to medical attention within 6 hr and have been thoroughly irrigated and debrided.

There are few studies that unequivocally demonstrate the efficacy of antimicrobial agents for **prophylaxis** of bite injuries. There is general consensus that antibiotics should be administered to all victims of human bites and all but the most trivial of dog, cat, and rat bite injuries, regardless of whether there is evidence of infection. The bacteriology of bite wound infections is primarily a reflection of the oral flora of the biting animal and, to a lesser extent, a reflection of the skin flora of the victim (see Table 712-2). Because each of the multitudes of aerobic and anaerobic bacterial species that colonize the oral cavity of the biting animal has the potential to invade local tissue, multiply, and cause tissue destruction, most bite wound infections are polymicrobial. Evidence suggests that as many as five different species may be isolated from infected dog bite wounds.

Despite the large degree of homology in the bacterial flora of the oral cavity among humans, dogs, and cats, important differences exist between the biting species, and this is reflected in the type of wound infections that occur. The predominant bacterial species isolated from infected dog bite wounds are *Staphylococcus aureus* (20–30%), *Pasteurella multocida* (20–30%), *Staphylococcus intermedius* (25%), and *C. canimorsus;* approximately one half of dog bite wound infections contain mixed anaerobes.

Similar species are isolated from infected cat bite wounds; however, *P. multocida* is the predominant species in at least 50% of cat bite wound infections. At least 50% of rats harbor strains of *Streptobacillus moniliformis* in their oropharynx, and approximately 25% harbor *S. minor,* an aerobic gram-negative organism. In human bite wounds, non-typable strains of *Haemophilus influenzae, Eikenella corrodens, S. aureus,* α-hemolytic streptococci, and β-lactamase–producing aerobes (about 50%) are the predominant species. Clenched fist injuries are particularly prone to infection by *Eikenella* spp. (25%) and anaerobic bacteria (50%).

The choice between an oral and parenteral antimicrobial agent should be based on the severity of the wound, the presence and degree of overt infection, signs of systemic toxicity, and the patient's immune status. Amoxicillin-clavulanate is an excellent choice for empirical oral therapy for human and animal bite wounds because of its activity against most of the strains of bacteria that have been isolated from infected bite injuries. Similarly, ticarcillin-clavulanate or ampicillin and sulbactam are preferred for patients who require empirical parenteral therapy. Procaine penicillin remains the drug of choice for prophylaxis and treatment of rat-inflicted injuries. First-generation cephalosporins have limited activity against *P. multocida* and *E. corrodens* and, therefore, should not be used for prophylaxis or empirical initial therapy of bite wound infections. The therapeutic alternatives for penicillin-allergic patients are limited, because the traditional alternative agents are generally inactive against one or more of the multiple pathogens that cause bite wound infections. Although erythromycin is commonly recommended as an alternative agent for penicillin-allergic patients who have suffered dog and cat bites, it has incomplete activity against strains of *P. multocida* and *S. moniliformis* and is not effective against *E. corrodens.* Similarly, clindamycin and the combination trimethoprim-sulfamethoxazole have limited activity against strains of *P. multocida* and anaerobic bacteria, respectively. Azithromycin and the ketolide antibiotics may be considered because they have activity against aerobic and anaerobic bacteria that are present in infected bite wounds. Tetracycline is the drug of choice for penicillin-allergic patients who have sustained rat bite injuries.

Although **tetanus** occurs only rarely after human or animal bite injuries, it is important to obtain a careful immunization history and to provide tetanus toxoid to all patients who are incompletely immunized or those in whom it has been longer than 10 yr since their last immunization. The need for postexposure rabies vaccine in victims of dog and cat bites depends on whether the biting animal is known to have been vaccinated and, most importantly, on local experience with rabid animals in the community (see Chapter 271). The local health department should be consulted for advice in all instances where the vaccination status of the biting animal is unknown and if there is known endemic rabies in the community. Postexposure prophylaxis for hepatitis B should be considered in the rare instance in which an individual has sustained a human bite from an individual who is at high risk for hepatitis B (see Chapter 355).

All but the most trivial bite wounds of the hand should be immobilized in position of function for 3–5 days, and patients with bite wounds of an extremity should be instructed to keep the affected extremity elevated for 24–36 hr or until the edema has resolved. All bite wound victims should be re-evaluated within 24–36 hr after the injury.

PREVENTION. It is possible to reduce the risk of injury with anticipatory guidance. Parents should be routinely counseled during prenatal visits and routine health maintenance examinations about the risks of having potentially biting pets in the household. All patients should be cautioned against harboring exotic animals for pets. Additionally, parents should be made aware of the proclivity of certain breeds of dogs to inflict serious injuries and the protective instincts of nursing dams. All young children should be closely supervised, particularly when in the presence of animals and, from a very early age, taught to respect animals and to be aware of their potential to inflict injury (Tables 712-4 and 712-5).

Reduction of human bite injuries, particularly in daycare centers and schools, can be achieved by good surveillance of the children and adequate supervisory personnel-to-child ratios.

TABLE 712-4. Code of Behavior When Handling a Dog

DOGS	HUMANS
Dogs sniff as a means of communication.	Before petting a dog, let it sniff you.
Dogs like to chase moving objects.	Do not run past dogs.
Dogs run faster than humans.	Do not try to outrun a dog.
Screaming may incite predatory behavior.	Remain calm if a dog approaches.
The order of precedence needs to be in evidence.	Do not hug or kiss a dog.
Direct eye contact may be interpreted as aggression.	Avoid direct eye contact.
Dogs tend to attack extremities, face, and neck.	If attacked, stand still (feet together) and protect neck and face with arms and hands.
Lying on the ground provokes attacks.	Stand up. If attacked while lying, keep face down and cover the ears with the hands. Do not move.
Fighting dogs bite at anything that is near.	Do not try to stop 2 fighting dogs.

From Schalamon J, Ainoedhofer H, Singer G, et al: Analysis of dog bites in children who are younger than 17 years. *Pediatrics* 2006;117:e374–e379.

TABLE 712-5. Measures for Preventing Dog Bites

- Realistically evaluate environment and lifestyle and consult with a professional (e.g., veterinarian, animal behaviorist, or responsible breeder) to determine suitable breeds of dogs for consideration.
- Dogs with histories of aggression are inappropriate in households with children.
- Be sensitive to cues that a child is fearful or apprehensive about a dog and, if so, delay acquiring a dog.
- Spend time with a dog before buying or adopting it. Use caution when bringing a dog or puppy into the home of an infant or toddler.
- Spay/neuter virtually all dogs (this frequently reduces aggressive tendencies).
- Never leave infants or young children alone with any dog.
- Properly socialize and train any dog entering the household. Teach the dog submissive behaviors (e.g., rolling over to expose abdomen and relinquishing food without growling).
- Immediately seek professional advice (e.g., from veterinarians, animal behaviorists, or responsible breeders) if the dog develops aggressive or undesirable behaviors.
- Do not play aggressive games with your dog (e.g., wrestling).
- Teach children basic safety around dogs and review regularly:
  - Never approach an unfamiliar dog.
  - Never run from a dog and scream.
  - Remain motionless when approached by an unfamiliar dog (e.g., "be still like a tree").
  - If knocked over by a dog, roll into a ball and lie still (e.g., "be still like a log").
  - Never play with a dog unless supervised by an adult.
  - Immediately report stray dogs or dogs displaying unusual behavior to an adult.
  - Avoid direct eye contact with a dog.
  - Do not disturb a dog who is sleeping, eating, or caring for puppies.
  - Do not pet a dog without allowing it to see and sniff you first.
  - If bitten, immediately report the bite to an adult.

From Centers for Disease Control and Prevention: Dog bite–related fatalities—United States, 1995–1996. *MMWR* 1997;46:463–467.

Benson L, Edwards S, Schiff A, et al: Dog and cat bites to the hand: Treatment and cost assessment. *J Hand Surg* 2006;31:468–473.

Broder J, Jerrard D, Olshaker J, Witting M: Low risk of infection in selected human bites treated without antibiotics. *Am J Emer Med* 2004;22:10–12.

Centers for Disease Control and Prevention: Nonfatal dog bite-related injuries treated in hospital emergency departments—United States, 2001. *MMWR* 2003;52:605.

Centers for Disease Control and Prevention: Dog-bite–related fatalities—United States, 1995–1996. *MMWR* 1997;46:463–467.

Chapman S, Righetti J, Sung L: Preventing dog bites in children: Randomised controlled trial of an educational intervention. *BMJ* 2000;320:1512.

Chen E, Hornig S, Shepherd SM, Hollander JE: Primary closure of mammalian bites. *Acad Emer Med* 2000;7:157–161.

Cummings P: Antibiotics to prevent infection in patients with dog bite wounds: A meta-analysis of randomized trials. *Ann Emerg Med* 1994; 23:535.

Merchant RC, Fuerch J, Becker BM, Mayer KH: Comparison of the epidemiology of human bites evaluated at three US pediatric emergency departments. *Pediatr Emerg Care* 2005;21:833–838.

Schalamon J, Ainoedhofer H, Singer G, et al: Analysis of dog bites in children who are younger than 17 years. *Pediatrics* 2006;117:e374–e379.

Stefanopoulos PK, Tarantzopoulou: Facial bite wounds: management update. *Int J Oral Maxillofoc Surg* 2005;34:464–472.

Talan DA, Abrahamian M, Moran GJ, et al: Clinical presentation and bacteriologic analysis of infected human bites in patients presenting to emergency departments. *Clin Infect Dis* 2003;37:1481–1489.

Talan DA, Citron DM, Abrahamian FM, et al: Bacteriologic analysis of infected dog and cat bites. *N Engl J Med* 1999;340:85.

712.1 • Rat Bite Fever

ETIOLOGY. Rat bite fever is a generic term that has been applied to at least two distinct clinical syndromes, each caused by a different microbial agent.

The most common form of rat bite fever in the U.S. is caused by *Streptobacillus moniliformis,* a gram-negative bacillus that is present in the nasopharyngeal flora of approximately 50% of healthy rats. Infection with *Streptobacillus moniliformis* most commonly occurs following the bite of a rat; however, infection has also been reported in individuals who have been scratched by rats, in those who have handled dead rats, and in individuals who have ingested milk contaminated with *Streptobacillus moniliformis* (**Haverhill fever**).

The less common form of rat bite fever (**sodoku**) is caused by *Spirillum minus,* a small spiral, aerobic gram-negative organism. The incubation period of soduku is longer (14–21 days) than that of the streptobacillary form of disease, and myalgia and arthritis are less common manifestations.

CLINICAL COURSE. The incubation period for the streptobacillary form of rat bite fever is variable, ranging from 3–10 days. The illness is characterized by an abrupt onset of fever, severe throbbing headache, intense myalgia, chills, and vomiting. In virtually all instances, the lesion at the cutaneous inoculation site has healed by the time the systemic systems first appear. Shortly after the onset of the fever, a polymorphic rash occurs in up to 75% of patients. In most patients, the rash consists of blotchy, red maculopapular lesions that often have a petechial component; the distribution of the rash is variable, but it usually is most dense on the extremities (Fig. 712-1). Approximately ½ of patients will have arthritis that first manifests toward the end of the first week of disease; early on, the arthritis may be migratory. If untreated, the fever, rash and arthritis will last from 14–21 days; often, there will be a biphasic pattern to the fever and arthritis. A wide range of complications have been reported in patients with rat bite fever, the most common being pneumonia, persistent arthritis, brain and soft tissue abscesses, and, less commonly, myocarditis or endocarditis.

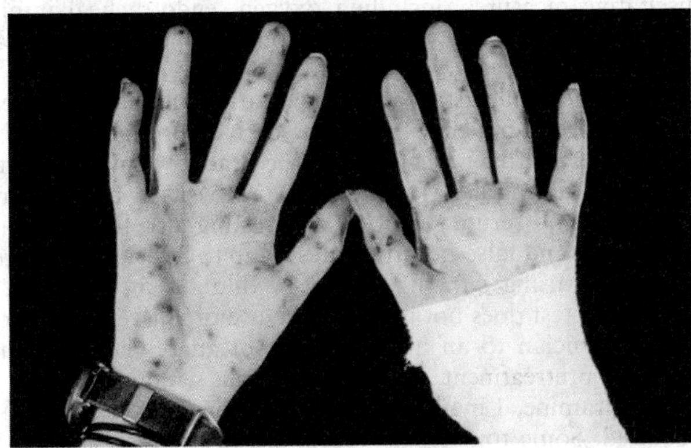

Figure 712-1. Maculopapular rash with small dark red eruptions on hand of person with rat-bite fever. (From Van Nood E, Peters SH: Rat-bite fever. *Neth J Med* 2005;63:319–321.)

The hallmark of *Spirillum*-induced disease is fever associated with an indurated, often suppurative, nonhealing lesion at the bite site. Lymphadenitis and lymphadenopathy invariably are present in the regional nodes that drain the inoculation site, and many patients develop a generalized macular rash that is most prominent when fever is present. In untreated patients, soduku has a relapsing course; after 5–7 days of chills and fever, symptoms abate but recur 7–10 days later. There may be multiple cycles if the disease is not recognized and treated.

DIAGNOSIS. Diagnosis of the streptobacillary form of rat bite fever is difficult, because the disease is uncommon and often is confused with Rocky Mountain spotted fever (see Chapter 225) or, less commonly, meningococcemia (see Chapter 190). Furthermore, *Streptobacillus moniliformis* is difficult to isolate and to identify with classic bacteriologic techniques. The organism is fastidious, requires enriched media for growth, and is inhibited by sodium polyanetholsulfonate, an additive present in most commercial blood culture bottles. A definitive diagnosis is made when the organism is recovered from blood or joint fluid or is identified in human samples with molecular technology.

Diagnosis of sodoku is made on clinical grounds, because there are no diagnostic serologic tests and *Spirillum minus* has not been cultured on artificial media. Rarely, the organism may be identified in Gram-stained smears from pus from the infected inoculation site.

TREATMENT. Penicillin is the drug of choice for both forms of rat bite fever. Intravenous penicillin G is recommended for 7–10 days, followed by oral penicillin V for an additional 7 days. If the patient has had a prompt response and has improved in 5–7 days without evidence of endocarditis, the transition to oral penicillin can be made at that time. Tetracycline or streptomycin are effective alternatives for penicillin-allergic patients.

Berger C, Altwegg M, Meyer A, et al: Broad range polymerase chain reaction for diagnosis of rat-bite fever caused by *Streptobacillus moniliformis. Pediatr Infect Dis J* 2001;20:1181–1182.

Ojukwu IC, Christy C: Rat-bite fever in children: Case report and review. *Scand J Infect Dis* 2002;34:474–477.

Stehle P, Dubuis O, So A, et al: Rat bite fever without fever. *Ann Rheum Dis* 2003;62:894–897.

van Nood E, Peters SH: Rat-bite fever. *Neth J Med* 2005;63:319–321.

712.2 • Monkeypox

ETIOLOGY. Monkeypox is a rare viral disease caused by the monkeypox virus, a member of the genus *Orthopoxvirus.* The disease was first observed in humans from West and Central Africa. Monkeys are the predominant host for the virus; however, the virus has been recovered from indigenous African squirrels, rats, and mice, and it also has been identified in and transmitted by prairie dogs in the U.S.

Primary transmission of the disease from infected animal to human is by bite or by human contact with an infected animal's blood, wound discharge, or body fluid. Human-to-human transmission of infection is uncommon but is believed to have been an important source for transmission of new cases during the point epidemic of disease that occurred in the U.S. in 2003.

CLINICAL COURSE. The clinical signs, symptoms and course of monkeypox are similar to those of smallpox, although usually milder. After a 10- to 14-day incubation period during which the virus replicates in lymphoid tissues, humans experience an abrupt onset of malaise, fever, myalgia, headache, and severe backache. A nonproductive cough, nausea, vomiting, and abdominal pain may be present. Generalized lymphadenopathy, a rare finding in smallpox, invariably is present during the acute stages of the illness. After a 2- to 4-day prodrome, an exanthem appears that has cephalad to caudal progression. As the rash progresses, the high spiking fever begins to abate. The initial rash generally first appears on the face and consists of erythematous macules. Within hours of first appearance, the macules transform into firm papules that rapidly vesiculate and become pustular over a 2- to 3-day period. Unlike smallpox, but similar to chickenpox, the lesions of monkeypox tend to occur in crops. Late into the second week of illness, the lesions begin to desiccate, crust, scab, and fall off.

Monkeypox should be suspected in any child who has the characteristic prodrome associated with an atypical form of chickenpox and a history of contact with prairie dogs or exotic mammals such as Gambian rats and rope squirrels. Any one of the following criteria establishes a definitive diagnosis:

1. Isolation of monkeypox virus in culture
2. Demonstration of monkeypox DNA by polymerase chain reaction testing in a clinical specimen
3. Demonstration of virus morphologically consistent with an *Orthopoxvirus* by electron microscopy in the absence of exposure to another *Orthopoxvirus*
4. Demonstration of the presence of *Orthopoxvirus* in tissue using immunohistochemical testing methods in the absence of exposure to another *Orthopoxvirus*

TREATMENT. There is no proven effective therapy for monkeypox. Although there is evidence that administration of smallpox vaccine is 85% effective in preventing or attenuating the disease, the rarity of the disease does not warrant universal vaccination. In instances of known exposure or in epidemic situations, there may be an indication for administering the vaccine. Consideration should be given to vaccinating close family contacts and health care workers who provide care to infected individuals. Vaccine is said to be preventative if given within 2 wk of exposure. Individuals with a compromised immune system and those who have had life-threatening allergies to latex or to smallpox vaccine or any of its components (polymyxin B, streptomycin, chlortetracycline, neomycin) also should not receive the smallpox vaccine.

Careful attention should be paid to skin hygiene, maintenance of adequate nutrition and hydration, and prompt implementation of local or systemic therapy of secondary bacterial infection that may occur. To prevent human-to-human spread of disease, a combination of the CDC guidelines for droplet and airborne infection control should be implemented.

Cho CT, Wenner HA: Monkeypox virus. *Bacteriol Rev* 1973;37:1.

Earl PL, Americo JL, Wyatt LS, et al: Immunogenicity of a highly attenuated MVA smallpox vaccine and protection against monkeypox. *Nature* 2004;428:182.

Ligon BL: Monkeypox: A review of the history and emergence in the Western hemisphere. *Sem Pediatr Infect Dis* 2004:15:280.

Maskalyk J: Monkeypox outbreak among pet owners. *CMAJ* 2003;169:44.

Sejvar JJ, Chowdary Y, Schomogyi M, et al: Human monkeypox infection: A family cluster in the midwestern United States. *J Infect Dis* 2004:190:1833.

Chapter 713 ■ Envenomations

Steve Holve

Most bites and stings by spiders, snakes, scorpions, and other venomous animals cause little more than local pain and do not require medical attention. Children are at greater risk for severe reactions because of their smaller volume of distribution for a given amount of venom.

Symptoms of envenomation may be either IgE-mediated, such as anaphylaxis in response to Hymenoptera stings, or venom-mediated, as with the bites of poisonous spiders or snakes or the sting of scorpions. Immediate hypersensitivity reactions are treated emergently, as described in Chapter 148 on anaphylaxis. Species-specific antivenin ameliorates symptoms and prevents death from severe venom-mediated reactions, but the use of antivenin carries significant risks. Appropriate assessment of the risk:benefit ratio in the use of antivenin is important in treating bites and stings.

ANTIVENINS

Venoms are species-specific mixtures of polypeptides, proteolytic enzymes, glycoproteins, and vasoactive substances. All **antivenins** are animal-derived immunoglobulins that bind and neutralize the proteins in venom. The animal origin of these products exposes patients to large amounts of foreign proteins that may cause both immediate and delayed hypersensitivity reactions.

In the United States, only 4 antivenins are commercially approved by the U.S. Food and Drug Administration (FDA). For pit viper bites, horse serum-derived Antivenin (Crotalidae) Polyvalent (ACP) is available, as well as the sheep-derived product, Crotalidae Polyvalent Immune Fab (Crofab). In addition, a horse serum–produced antivenin is available for bites by the coral snake *(Micrurus fulvius)* and black widow spider *(Latrodectus mactans)*. Other antivenins to more unusual species of snakes or scorpions may be available from the American Zoo and Aquarium Association (1-301-562-0777) and the Arizona Poison Control Center (1-800-222-1222).

Immediate hypersensitivity reactions (see Chapter 148) to antivenins may be life-threatening, although the risk varies greatly depending on the product. The incidence of such reactions after administration of equine Crotalid antivenin may be as high as 25–40%. The ovine-produced Crofab antivenin has a much lower rate of acute reaction (15%), and most events are mild. Hypersensitivity reactions to black widow and coral snake antivenin occur at a rate of about 1%. Given the risk of anaphylaxis, antivenin should be given only in a setting in which full resuscitative measures, including oxygen, endotracheal intubation, intravenous fluid administration, and epinephrine, are available.

Patients should be asked about medication allergies and previous exposure to antivenins. If equine-derived products are to be used, skin testing may be done, but the practice remains controversial. Skin testing delays treatment, and by itself has triggered anaphylaxis and serum sickness. Skin testing also has very high false-positive and false-negative rates of up to 30%. The skin test is performed using 0.02 mL of a 1:10 dilution of antivenin. A positive skin test does not preclude the use of antivenin but does alert the clinician to an increased risk of anaphylaxis. In such instances, pretreatment with intravenous administration of diphenhydramine, 1 mg/kg, and methylprednisolone, 1–2 mg/kg, is required. Some toxicologists recommend pretreatment for all patients receiving antivenin.

If signs of immediate hypersensitivity develop during administration of antivenin, the infusion should be stopped until the patient is stabilized. If the severity of envenomation warrants continued infusion of antivenin, it may be resumed at a slower rate or simultaneously with administration of epinephrine. In such instances, consultation with the nearest toxicologist at a poison control center is advisable.

Delayed hypersensitivity or serum sickness (see Chapter 149) develops in up to 65% of patients who receive equine-derived antivenin and in 15% of patients who receive ovine-derived products. Serum sickness usually develops 5–21 days after exposure and may last for weeks. It is most commonly manifested as urticaria, pruritus, arthralgia, and malaise, but rarely may present as immune complex glomerulonephritis, neuritis, or myocarditis. Intradermal skin tests have not been shown to predict the risk of serum sickness accurately. Prophylactic use of antihistamines and corticosteroids may reduce the risk of serum sickness and definitely is of benefit if symptoms develop.

SNAKEBITE

Of the >3,000 known species of snakes, only 200 are poisonous to humans. Of poisonous snakes, 90% are members of one of three families: the Hydrophidae, or poisonous sea snakes; the Elapidae, which includes the cobras, mambas, and coral snakes; and the Viperidae, or true vipers (Table 713-1).

In the U.S., 95% of poisonous snakebites are inflicted by the Crotalidae, or pit vipers, which are a subfamily of the true vipers. Pit vipers may be identified by their triangular heads, elliptical eyes, and the identifiable pit between the eyes and nose (Fig. 713-1). Members of the pit viper family in the U.S. include the rattlesnakes, cottonmouths, and copperheads. Coral snakes, the other poisonous snakes native to the U.S., are found in Texas and the Southeast and are members of the Elapidae family. Coral snakes are small with a small, rounded head and brightly colored bands of black and red separated by more narrow yellow bands. The rhyme "red on yellow, kill a fellow; red on black, venom lack" serves to differentiate the coral snake from the similar-appearing but nonpoisonous scarlet king snake. Cobras and kraits are common in parts of Asia, whereas vipers, cobras, and adders are common in parts of Africa.

EPIDEMIOLOGY. Approximately 45,000 snakebites are reported in the United States each year; venomous snakes inflict only 8,000 of these. The incidence of snakebites is substantially higher in Africa (estimated at 5 bites per 1,000 persons in Nigeria; estimated 23,000 snake bite deaths per year in West Africa), Australia (0.6 to 5 bites per 1,000 persons), Asia, and South America. In the U.S., most snakebites occur in young males and involve alcohol intoxication; often the victim has tried to capture or play with the snake. In Africa and Asia most bites occur on the lower limbs, at night, and are provoked by stepping on a

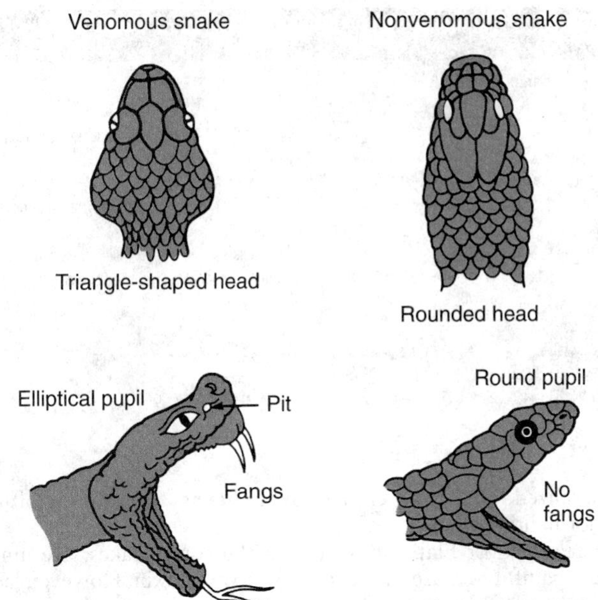

Figure 713-1. Identification of venomous snakes. (Modified from Rosen P et al [editors]: *Emergency Medicine,* 3rd ed. St. Louis, CV Mosby, 1992.)

snake. In the U.S., there are only 12–15 deaths each year, whereas case fatality rates up to 15% are reported among hospitalized victims of snakebites in parts of Africa and Asia where intensive care and antivenom access are limited. Children, because of their smaller body mass for venom distribution, are far more likely to have a serious systemic reaction to envenomation and account for more than half of the fatalities.

PATHOGENESIS. Snake venom is a mixture of polypeptides, proteolytic enzymes, and toxins, which are species-specific. Venom from the Elapidae and the Hydrophidae is primarily neurotoxic and has a curare-like effect by blocking neurotransmission at the neuromuscular junction. Death results from respiratory depression. Crotalidae venom is cytolytic, causing tissue necrosis, vascular leak, and coagulopathies. Death from pit viper bites results from hemorrhagic shock, adult respiratory distress syndrome, and renal failure.

Clinical Manifestations. Pit viper bites usually occur on the extremities; pain and swelling occur at the site within minutes (Table 713-2). As the venom moves proximally, edema and ecchymosis advance; in severe cases, bulla formation and tissue necrosis ensue (Fig. 713-2). Systemic symptoms include nausea, vomiting, diaphoresis, weakness, tingling around the face, and muscle fasciculations. Rarely, patients may present in shock with

TABLE 713-1. Major Venomous Snakes of the World

FAMILY	SUBFAMILY	DISTRIBUTION AND EXAMPLES	COMMENTS
Viperidae	Crotalidae (pit vipers)	North America: crotalus and sistrurus species (rattlesnake), agkistrodon species (cottonmouth, copperhead) Central and South America: crotalus species (rattlesnake), agkistrodon species (copperhead), bothrops species (fer-de-lance), *Lachesis muta* (bushmaster)	Heat-sensing foramen "pit" between each eye and nostril; elliptical pupils; retractable, canalized fangs
Viperidae	Viperinae (true vipers)	Africa, Europe, Middle East: *Bitis arietans* (puff adder), *B. gabonica* (Gaboon viper), *B. nasicornus* (rhinoceros-horned viper), echis species (saw-scaled viper), cerastes species (horned or desert vipers), vipera species (vipers) Indian subcontinent and Southeast Asia: *Daboia russelli* (Russell's viper)	No heat-sensing pit
Elapidae		Tropical and warm temperate zones: naja species (cobras), dendroaspis species (mambas), bungarus species (kraits), micrurus, calliophis, and maticora species (coral snakes), and most venomous snakes of Australia	Short, fixed fangs; venom injected by succession of chewing movements
Hydrophidae	Hydrophinae (true sea snakes)	Indopacific region: *Pelamis platurus* (pelagic sea snake)	Fangs similar to those of elapidae; highly neurotoxic venom; rarely bite humans

From Gold BS, Dart RC, Barish RA: Bites of venomous snakes. *N Engl J Med* 2002;347:347–356.

TABLE 713-2. Guidelines for Assessing the Severity of North American Pit Viper Envenomations*

TYPE OF SIGNS OR SYMPTOMS	SEVERITY OF ENVENOMATION		
	MINIMAL	MODERATE	SEVERE
Local	Swelling, erythema, or ecchymosis confined to the site of the bite	Progression of swelling, erythema, or ecchymosis beyond the site of the bite	Rapid swelling, erythema, or ecchymosis involving the entire body part
Systemic	No systemic signs or symptoms	Non–life-threatening signs and symptoms (nausea, vomiting, perioral paresthesias, myokymia, and mild hypotension)	Markedly severe signs and symptoms (hypotension [systolic blood pressure <80 mm Hg], altered sensorium, tachycardia, tachypnea, and respiratory distress)
Coagulation	No coagulation abnormalities or other important laboratory abnormalities	Mildly abnormal coagulation profile without clinically significant bleeding; mild abnormalities on other laboratory tests	Markedly abnormal coagulation profile with evidence of bleeding or threat of spontaneous hemorrhage (unmeasurable INR, APTT, and fibrinogen; severe thrombocytopenia with platelet count <20,000 per mm^3); results of other laboratory tests may be severely abnormal

*The ultimate grade of severity of any envenomation is determined on the basis of the most severe sign, symptom, or laboratory abnormality (e.g., systolic blood pressure <70 mm Hg in the absence of local swelling should be graded as a severe envenomation).
APTT, activated partial thromboplastin time; INR, international normalized ratio.
From Gold BS, Dart RC, Barish RA: Bites of venomous snakes. *N Engl J Med* 2002;347:347–356.

generalized edema or cardiac arrhythmias. Complex clotting abnormalities often occur.

Bites of most Elapidae, including the coral snakes, are minimally painful because the venom has no cytotoxin. However, lack of immediate symptoms should not be mistaken for the absence of serious envenomation. The venom of the coral snake is primarily neurotoxic, and symptoms can progress rapidly in a few hours from mild drowsiness to cranial nerve palsies, weakness, and death from respiratory failure.

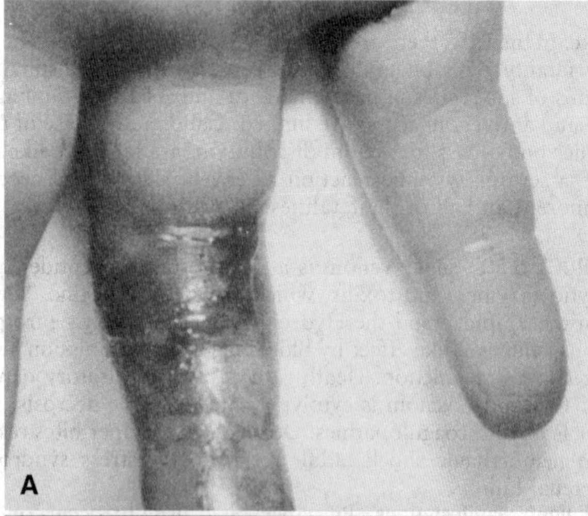

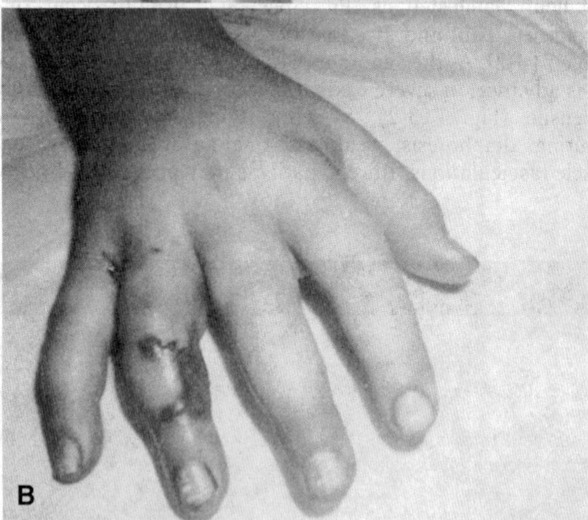

Figure 713-2. *A,* Crotalid envenomation; photograph taken 60 min after bite. Marked swelling and ecchymosis are apparent. Fang marks are barely visible. *B,* In the same patient, the back of the hand shows extensive swelling. (From Wolf MD: Envenomation. In Halbrook PR [ed]: *Textbook of Pediatric Critical Care.* Philadelphia, WB Saunders, 1993, p 1028.)

Treatment. The first task is to determine whether the bite was by a poisonous snake and if envenomation occurred. If the snake has been killed, it should be brought to the emergency department for identification. More than 80% of snakebites in the United States are by nonpoisonous snakes; these bites cause minimal pain and no swelling, and require only local wound care.

If the bite is determined to be from a venomous snake, immediate care is to immobilize the bitten extremity and transport the patient quickly to the nearest hospital. Some recommend a proximal tourniquet loose enough to insert 2 fingers and allow arterial blood flow. Many experts now eschew any constricting bands because of the risk of ischemia, which will exacerbate local tissue damage. Applying ice to the bite site or using excision and suction is believed to cause more tissue damage than benefit and should be avoided. Experience with rattlesnake bites suggests that field treatments increased tissue injury and tripled the need for later surgical intervention.

On arrival at the emergency department, the patient should have a large-bore intravenous line inserted, and blood for baseline laboratory studies should be obtained. Initial blood tests should include type and cross-match, because a progressive coagulopathy may make later typing impossible. Other tests include complete blood cell and platelet counts; prothrombin and partial thromboplastin times; fibrinogen and fibrin degradation products; and blood urea nitrogen, creatinine, and creatine phosphokinase levels. These studies must be repeated at intervals, depending on the severity of envenomation. Baseline vital signs and measurement of the circumference of the bitten extremity should be obtained, and demarcation of ecchymosis and swelling should be marked on the limb so progression can be monitored. The wound should be cleansed and tetanus toxoid given if appropriate.

The decision to use antivenin depends on the severity and progression of symptoms. In general, rattlesnake envenomation requires antivenin, copperhead bites do not, and cottonmouth bites fall between these extremes. The severity of envenomation is commonly graded on a 4-point scale (Table 713-3). Most pit viper bites cause symptoms within minutes and almost always within 6 hr; if symptoms are not present, the bite may be presumed to have been "dry" and a grade 0 envenomation. Dry bites occur in up to 25% of pit viper bites and no treatment is needed. A grade 1 envenomation with localized swelling requires only pain control and careful observation. Children, because of their smaller size, are more likely to have severe envenomation; 75% of children have a grade 2 or 3 envenomation, which requires antivenin.

Antivenin is most effective if delivered within 4 hr of the bite and is of little value if administration is delayed beyond 12 hr.

TABLE 713-3. Classification of Envenomation Severity

Grade 0	No envenomation
Grade 1	Minimal envenomation (local swelling and pain without progression)
Grade 2	Moderate envenomation (swelling, pain, or ecchymosis progressing beyond the site of injury; mild systemic or laboratory manifestations)
Grade 3	Severe envenomation (marked local response, severe systemic findings, and significant alteration in laboratory findings)

Antivenin poses a small, but significant risk of an immediate hypersensitivity reaction. Antivenin (Crotalidae) Polyvalent is administered in increments of 5 vials and repeated every 2 hr as needed to neutralize circulating venom, as measured by normalization of clotting parameters and a halt in the progression of swelling of the affected limb. Children often require more antivenin than a similarly envenomated adult because of their small volume-to-venom ratio. The ovine-derived Crofab appears to have the advantage of rarely causing immediate hypersensitivity and posing far less risk of serum sickness. Usually 5–10 vials of Crofab antivenin are given initially, with additional 2-vial doses given at 6, 12, and 18 hr if needed. The better safety profile of Crofab makes it the **antivenin of choice** for pit viper bites, if available. Whichever antivenin product is used, most pit viper bites respond well to timely treatment. Surgical consultation is needed only if there is concern about the development of compartment syndrome.

Any person who has been bitten by a coral snake should be administered 3–5 vials of antivenin *(M. fulvius)* prophylactically. Persons who have been bitten by a coral snake may be asymptomatic for hours before suffering paralysis and respiratory failure. Antivenin is effective only if given before symptoms develop and is ineffective in reversing them once they have occurred.

PROGNOSIS. Despite the potential for mortality and severe morbidity with poisonous snakebites, both can be minimized by early and judicious use of appropriate antivenin. Even extremities with marked tissue necrosis from rattlesnake bites will return to full function with the resolution of swelling.

ARACHNID ENVENOMATION

The arachnids contain the largest number of known venomous species. More than 20,000 venomous spiders have been identified, but most are of no danger to humans because they lack either potent venom or fangs capable of penetrating the human skin. In the United States, the only significant morbidity is caused by spiders in two genera, *Lactrodectus* (the black widow spider) and *Loxosceles* (the fiddleback or brown recluse spider).

BLACK WIDOW BITES. The black widow is found throughout the United States, but more commonly in the South. The black widow is glossy black and has bright red or orange markings on the ventral surface of the abdomen; the classic hourglass markings are seen only in the species *L. mactans* (Fig. 713-3). Females have a body length of 1.5 cm and a leg span of 4–5 cm. Males of the species are approximately half the size of females and pose no threat to humans, because their fangs are too short to penetrate the skin. The black widow is commonly found in protected places such as under rocks or in woodpiles, outhouses, and stables.

Pathogenesis. The venom of the black widow contains a potent neurotoxin, α-latrotoxin, which binds to presynaptic neuronal membranes, causing dramatic release of acetylcholine and norepinephrine at the neuromuscular junction. The outpouring of these neurotransmitters results in excessive muscle depolarization and autonomic hyperactivity.

Clinical Manifestations. The bite causes both local and systemic effects. A pinprick sensation usually is felt immediately at the bite site, which develops into a pale area of 2–3 mm with a red border. Within 1 hr, dull, crampy pain is felt around the site and gradually extends throughout the body. It was once claimed that upper extremity bites present with chest tightness and grunting respirations whereas lower extremity bites present with abdominal pain and board-like rigidity; however, either may occur, regardless of bite location. In addition to the severe muscle cramping, most children have nausea, vomiting, and diaphoresis, along with agitation and hypertension. In extremely rare instances, symptoms may progress to respiratory arrest and death.

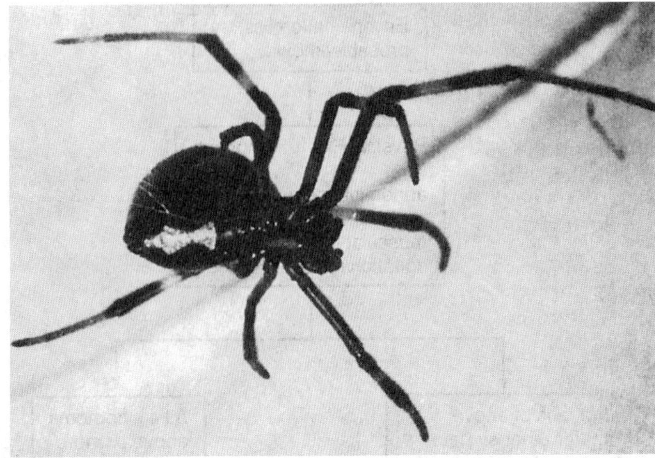

Figure 713-3. The female black widow spider has a shiny, black, globular body with a red hourglass-shaped mark on the abdomen. (From Patan BC: Bites—Human, dog, spider, and snake. *Surg Clin North Am* 1963;43:537.)

Because of its presentation with a painful, board-like abdomen, a bite from the black widow spider can mimic acute appendicitis or peritonitis. A key point in the **differential diagnosis** is that most patients with black widow bites are hypertensive, agitated, and tend to move about, seeking a comfortable position, whereas patients with peritonitis from a surgical abdomen often are hypotensive and try to lie still and avoid movement. Many past reports of deaths from black widow bites were related to patients' being mistakenly taken to surgery for a presumed acute abdomen. Therefore, obtaining an accurate history and making the correct diagnosis are the most important steps in managing black widow spider bites.

Treatment. Muscle cramping and agitation are the main causes of discomfort and usually can be well controlled with intravenous opiates for pain and benzodiazepines for muscle relaxation. Calcium infusions and dantrolene previously were used for muscle cramping; however, neither is efficacious and they are no longer recommended.

Use of antivenin versus symptomatic treatment in black widow bites is determined by the knowledge that without treatment all symptoms will resolve in 24–48 hr, but symptoms can be excruciating. Conservative measures should be tried first. If pain control is not achieved or there is autonomic instability, then antivenin should be considered. A decision tree for treatment is shown in Figure 713-4.

Black widow antivenin is derived from horse serum. If black widow antivenin is used, an intradermal test dose may be given, and all precautions as listed in the earlier discussion of equine antivenin should be followed. The risk of anaphylaxis with equine-derived black widow antivenin (<1%) is far less than that associated with equine crotalid antivenin. One vial of antivenin usually is sufficient, and symptoms of envenomation subside rapidly within 1–3 hr. As with other equine antivenin products, serum sickness may develop in 5–21 days.

BROWN RECLUSE SPIDER BITES. Although the bite of a number of spiders can result in mild tissue reactions, only species of the

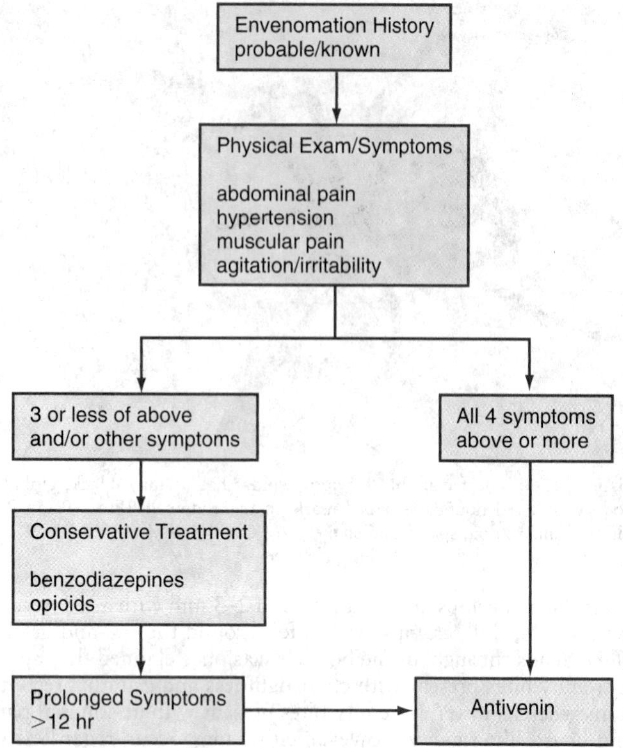

Figure 713-4. Decision process for treating pediatric black widow spider envenomation. (Courtesy of Robin Woestman, Loma Linda Children's Hospital, Loma Linda, CA.)

genus *Loxosceles* can cause significant skin necrosis. Members of this genus are commonly known as the "brown recluse spider" because of their predilection for living in dark, undisturbed places such as woodpiles and basements or the "fiddleback spider" because of the brown violin-shaped marking on the thorax (Fig. 713-5).

Epidemiology. All species are dull in color and have a small body measuring 1 cm and legs extending up to 5 cm. The species with the most potent bite, *Loxosceles reclusa,* is found most commonly in the river country of the midwestern U.S. but also is found in the South. Other less potent *Loxosceles* spp. are found throughout the U.S., but their numbers decrease with more northern latitudes.

Clinical Manifestations. The venom of the brown recluse contains hyaluronidase, or spreading factor, and sphingomyelinase D, a protein that lyses cell walls. The bite often is unnoticed or felt only as a pinprick. It typically occurs when a spider is unknowingly trapped against the skin while the victim is putting on clothes; thus, the bite often is on the upper arm, lateral thorax, inner thigh, or, rarely, on the hands or face. Within 2 hr, a painful, sinking blue macule with a halo of inflammation occurs at the bite site, followed by systemic symptoms that include fever, chills, nausea, and vomiting. In a minority of cases, but more commonly in small children, hemolysis can occur. The hemolysis is presumed secondary to toxin action, because Coombs test results are negative and the coagulation system is not activated as measured by platelet counts, fibrin split products, and prothrombin time. Rarely, massive hemolysis can occur and may lead to disseminated intravascular coagulopathy or hemoglobinuric renal failure.

In addition to systemic symptoms of the bite, a **hemorrhagic blister** forms within 1–2 days. As the blister sloughs, it leaves the characteristic necrotic ulcer of brown recluse spider bites. Most ulcers remain at 1–2 cm but can enlarge up to 15 cm in diameter and involve the full thickness of the skin and some underlying tissue.

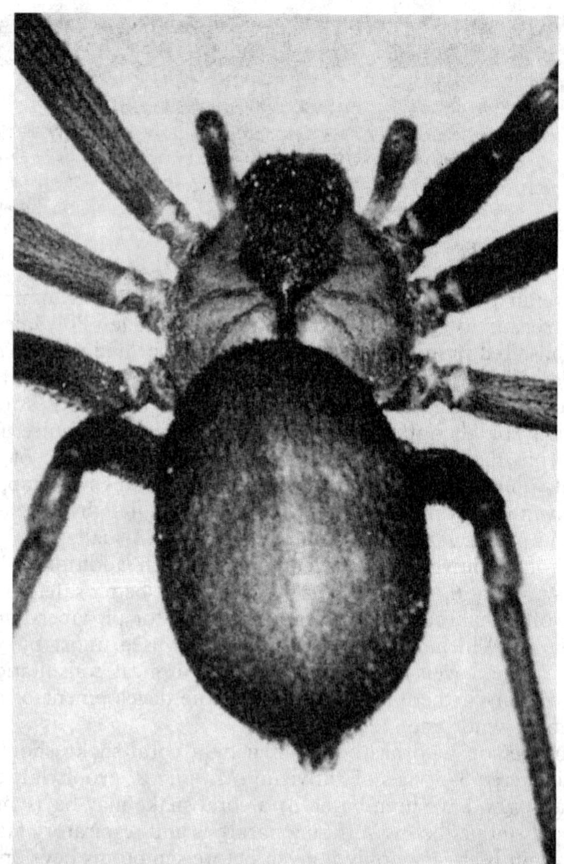

Figure 713-5. The brown recluse spider is 10–15 mm long, is light to dark brown in color, and has a species-specific dorsal, dark, violin-shaped band. (From Dillaha CJ, Jansen GT, Honeycutt WM, et al: North American loxoscelism. Necrotic bite of the brown recluse spider. *JAMA* 1964;188:33.)

Treatment and Prognosis. The outcome in brown recluse spider bites is excellent, and most bites resolve with supportive care alone. Patients with systemic symptoms or significant hemolysis should be admitted to the hospital for pain control and monitoring. Hydration and maintenance of urine output are essential if there is significant hemoglobinuria. Treatment of the ulcerative skin lesions also is supportive, with local wound care. Pain usually subsides in a few days, although complete skin healing requires weeks. Hyperbaric oxygen to promote wound healing, dapsone for leukocyte inhibition, and cyproheptadine, a platelet aggregation inhibitor, have been recommended to prevent enlargement of skin ulcers; however, none of these has proven beneficial. In rare instances, large necrotic ulcers require delayed skin grafting.

SCORPION BITES

EPIDEMIOLOGY. More than 1,000 species of scorpions are found worldwide; all of them are capable of delivering venom through a stinger located at the end of a 6-segment tail. Of medical importance are the small numbers of species that belong to the family Butidae, which produce venom that is neurotoxic. Among the most toxic species are those of the *Leiurus* spp. of India and the Middle East and *Centuroides* spp. in Mexico and the desert Southwest of the United States. Most stings, even by toxic species, cause only a painful local reaction. However, because of their small size, infants and young children who are stung are at risk for severe autonomic dysfunction, multisystem organ failure, and death.

TABLE 713-4. Scorpion Envenomation

Grade 1	Local discomfort and paresthesia
Grade 2	Pain and paresthesia extend up the extremity
Grade 3	Motor hyperkinesis Cranial nerve dysfunction Dysphagia Roving eyes Facial paresthesia Restlessness
Grade 4	Cranial nerve dysfunction Drooling, uncontrollable eye movements Fasciculations, facial and distal muscles Neuromuscular hyperactivity Opisthotonos Convulsions Wheezing Hyperthermia Cyanosis

From Wolf MD: Envenomation. In Holbrook PR (editor): *Textbook of Pediatric Critical Care*. Philadelphia, WB Saunders, 1993, p 1024.

PATHOGENESIS. Scorpion venoms vary by species; all have hyaluronidase, serotonin and histamine releasers, and neurotoxins, of which the latter are the most important component. Neurotoxins can bind to the presynaptic membranes, causing release of acetylcholine and stimulation of both the sympathetic and parasympathetic nervous systems.

CLINICAL MANIFESTATIONS. The only medically significant scorpion species in the United States is *Centruroides exilicauda,* which is found in the Southwest. Most stings cause an immediate local reaction that can vary from mild burning to severe pain. Severe envenomation causes autonomic dysfunction within 1 hr of the sting (Table 713-4). Symptoms include agitation, irritability, salivation, blurred vision, and tremulousness, with signs of hypertension, tachycardia, tachypnea, and nystagmus. Rarely, in small children or infants, respiratory failure, convulsions, or coma may occur. In these cases, if a history of a sting is not elicited, a diagnosis of encephalitis may be entertained and the correct diagnosis of scorpion envenomation obscured by the fact that children with severe *Centruroides* envenomation may have mild cerebrospinal fluid pleocytosis.

Envenomation by other scorpion species may have specific features. Stings by *Leiurus* spp. in India and the Middle East can cause severe hypertension, direct toxic myocarditis, and life-threatening myocardial ischemia.

TREATMENT. Localized pain can be treated with application of ice and analgesics; pain usually diminishes markedly within 24 hr. For stings by *Centuroides exilicauda,* severe envenomation with autonomic instability requires hospital admission for sedation and observation. Symptoms usually resolve within 24–48 hr. If cardiopulmonary compromise occurs, consideration should be given to administering antivenin. Centruroides-specific antivenin is not FDA-approved, but it is available by contacting the Arizona Poison Control Center (1-800-222-1222). The use of antivenin, if warranted, leads to complete resolution of symptoms within 1 hr. Antivenin for other scorpion species is available in countries where those species are found or through zoologic societies.

HYMENOPTERA STINGS

The insect order Hymenoptera includes the ants, bees, and wasps, which are characterized by the presence of a stinger at the end of the abdomen through which venom is injected. They are found throughout the U.S. and worldwide.

EPIDEMIOLOGY. Hymenoptera venom, a mixture of proteins and vasoactive substances, is not very potent; most stings cause only local reactions that can be treated with application of cold compresses and analgesics. However, 1–4% of the population is sensitized to hymenoptera venom and is at risk for immediate hypersensitivity reactions. Each year, 50–150 people in the United States die of anaphylaxis caused by hymenoptera stings (see Chapter 145).

CLINICAL MANIFESTATIONS AND TREATMENT. Children with small or large local reactions should use cold compresses and receive corticosteroids and antihistamines. Any person with a hymenoptera envenomation who presents with urticaria, angioedema, wheezing, or hypotension should be treated aggressively for an immediate hypersensitivity reaction with intravenous fluids, oxygen, and epinephrine (see Chapter 148).

The more difficult therapeutic question is which patients should receive hymenoptera immunotherapy. Children who have had cutaneous anaphylaxis such as urticaria or angioedema seem to be at little risk of progress to systemic anaphylaxis with future stings. Children who have had systemic reactions including wheezing but not anaphylaxis do not need immunotherapy but should carry an emergency kit with epinephrine. Patients who have had anaphylaxis with hypotension or airway obstruction should undergo IgE testing for specific hymenoptera antibodies. If these are negative, the patient can be reassured that severe future reactions are unlikely. If the IgE testing is positive, the patient should be offered species specific immunotherapy. Immunotherapy protection appears to be lifelong after 3–5 years of treatment and reduces the risk of systemic anaphylaxis in high-risk patients from future stings from 30% to <5%.

MARINE ENVENOMATION

EPIDEMIOLOGY. The most commonly encountered venomous marine creatures include the jellyfish (Cnidaria), stingrays (Chondricthyes), and members of the family Scorpaenidae—the zebrafish, scorpionfish, and stonefish.

PATHOGENESIS. All jellyfish have unique stinging cells called nematocysts. These cells contain a highly folded tubule that everts on contact and injects venom. The venom is antigenic and can be dermatonecrotic, hemolytic, cardiotoxic, or neuropathic, depending on the species. The nematocysts can sting even after the tentacle is separated from the body and after the jellyfish is dead. Stingrays have a spine in the base of their tail that contains a venom gland. The venom has vasoconstrictive properties that can predispose to tissue necrosis and poor wound healing. In addition, stingray spines are retro-serrated, and therefore they commonly cause a jagged laceration along with envenomation. The Scorpaenidae have venomous spines that become erect on stimulation.

CLINICAL MANIFESTATIONS. The Pacific box jellyfish *(Chironex fleckeri)* is known to cause fatal stings from its cardiotoxic venom, but this member of the Cnidaria family is found only in Australia. Although fatal anaphylaxis to jellyfish stings has been reported in coastal waters of the U.S., these events are extremely rare. For clinicians in the Americas, the primary concern with jellyfish stings is localized pain that may be associated with paresthesias or pruritus. Rarely, jellyfish victims may have systemic symptoms of nausea, vomiting, headache, and chills. Stingray envenomations are noteworthy for immediate and intense pain at the site of injury that lasts 24–48 hr. Some patients also may have nausea, vomiting, and muscle cramps, and, rarely, hypotension or seizures. Envenomation by a member of the Scorpaenidae causes immediate pain that may persist for hours or days. Victims may experience intense local tissue destruction in which superinfections are common. Systemic symptoms include vomiting, abdominal pain, headache, delirium, seizures, and respiratory failure.

TREATMENT. Treatment of jellyfish stings begins in the ocean; the wounds should be rinsed in seawater because fresh water may lyse the nematocysts, leading to further envenomation. Irrigation of the sting site with vinegar or rubbing alcohol is beneficial because it inhibits nematocyst discharge. Visible tentacle fragments should be removed with forceps, and microscopic fragments may be removed by gently shaving the affected area. Folk remedies such as rubbing the sting with sand or applying urine are not helpful and will cause more irritation. Meat tenderizer, long a popular treatment, is not effective. Antihistamines and corticosteroids are indicated for swelling and urticaria. Antibiotics are not needed. All patients will recover uneventfully.

Treatment of stingray and Scorpaenidae stings is similar, beginning with thorough cleaning of the wound and tetanus update if needed. Stingray spines are radiopaque and should be removed if present in the wound. If the laceration is large, delayed closure should be allowed. The toxins are heat labile, and immersion in hot water (42°C) for 30–60 min will denature the protein elements of the venom and decrease pain significantly. Additional analgesia should be provided as needed. Superinfection with aerobic and anaerobic organisms is rare, and antibiotic prophylaxis is not needed.

SEABATHER'S ERUPTION

EPIDEMIOLOGY AND PATHOGENESIS. Seabather's eruption is caused by exposure to the larvae of 2 species of the phylum Cnidaria, the sea anemone, *Edwardsiella lineata,* found off the coast of the northeastern U.S., and the thimble jellyfish, *Linuche unguiculata,* found in the Caribbean and the Gulf of Mexico. Cases also have been reported in Brazil. Epidemics of seabather's eruption occur in the summer when there are large quantities of larvae in the water.

CLINICAL MANIFESTATIONS AND TREATMENT. An intensely pruritic vesicular or maculopapular rash begins within 4–24 hr after exposure and may persist for days or weeks. Associated symptoms may include fever, chills, headache, malaise, conjunctivitis, and urethritis. Most symptoms respond to antihistamines, although topical or systemic corticosteroids may be beneficial in severe cases.

Snakebites

Boyer L, Seifert S, Cain J: Recurrence phenomena after immunoglobulin therapy for snake envenomations: Guidelines for clinical management with crotaline Fab antivenom. *Ann Emerg Med* 2001;37:196–201.

Gold BS, Dart RC, Barish RA: Bites of venomous snakes. *N Engl J Med* 2002;347:347–356.

Habib AG, Gebi UI, Onyemelukwe GC: Snake bite in Nigeria. *Afr J Med Sci* 2001;30:171–178.

Juckett G, Hancox J: Venomous snakebites in the United States: Management review and update. *Am Fam Phys* 2002;65:1367–1374.

Junghanss T, Bodio M: Medically important venomous animals: biology prevention, first aid and clinical management. *Clin Inf Dis* 2006;43: 1309–1317.

McKinney P: Out of hospital and interhospital management of crotaline snakebite. *Ann Emerg Med* 2001;37:168–174.

Tokish JT, Benjamin J, Walter F: Crotalid envenomation: The southern Arizona experience. *J Ortho Trauma* 2001;15:5–9.

Arachnid Envenomation

Gomez HF, Krywko DM, Stoecker WV: A new assay for the detection of *Loxosceles* species (brown recluse) spider venom. *Ann Emerg Med* 202;39: 469–474.

Ibister G: Necrotic arachnidism: The mythology of a modern plague. *Lancet* 2004;364:549–553.

Ibister G, Gray MR: A prospective study of 750 definite spider bites, with expert spider identification. *Q J Med* 2002;95:723–731.

Ibister G, Graudins A, White J, et al: Antivenom treatment in arachnidism. *Clin Toxicol* 2003;41:291–300.

LoVecchio F, McBride C: Scorpion envenomation in young children in central Arizona. *J Toxicol Clin Toxicol* 2003;41:937–940.

Pauli I, Puka J, Gubert IC, Minozzo JC: The efficacy of antivenom in loxoscelism treatment. *Toxicon* 2006;48:123–137. Epub 2006, Jun 30.

Insect Envenomations

Muller U: New developments in the diagnosis and treatment of Hymenoptera venom allergy. *Int Arch Allergy Immunol* 2001;124:447–453.

Freeman T: Hypersensitivity to hymenoptera stings. *N Engl J Med* 2004;351:1978–1984.

Marine Envenomations

Perkins RA, Morgan S: Poisoning, envenomation and trauma from marine creatures. *Am Fam Phys* 2004;69:885–890.

Williams GC: Stinging seas. *Calif Wild* 2000;53(4):12–17.

Part XXXIII ■ Laboratory Medicine

Chapter 714 ■ Laboratory Testing in Infants and Children

Michael A. Pesce

Because of genetic heterogeneity, biologic and environmental variability, and inhomogeneity of subclinical health status, normal values for many laboratory tests do not show a gaussian bell-shaped distribution curve. As a result, the population mean and the standard deviation (SD) are frequently less useful than the range of normal values, generally given as the 95% normal range, or the range of values obtained in testing a normal population minus the lowest 2.5% and the highest 2.5%. The serum sodium concentration in children, which is tightly controlled physiologically, has a distribution that is essentially gaussian; the mean value ±2 SD gives a range very close to that actually observed in 95% of children (Table 714-1). Alternatively, the serum creatine kinase level, which is subject to diverse influences and is not actively controlled, does not show a gaussian distribution, as evidenced by the lack of agreement between the range actually observed and that predicted by the mean value ±2 SD.

A refinement of referencing that is used with increasing frequency is reporting the value obtained together with the percentile of normal values into which the value obtained falls. This method is useful when testing for risk factors such as determination of serum cholesterol. A further modification that is necessary for many tests performed in infants and children is calculating the age-related adjustment of the normal range. Both age adjustment and the use of percentiles are illustrated in the normal values for serum cholesterol. A final modification needed for reporting normal ranges is referencing the Tanner stage of sexual maturation, which is most useful in assessing pituitary and gonadal function.

ACCURACY AND PRECISION OF LABORATORY TESTS. Technical accuracy is an important consideration in interpreting the results of a laboratory test. Because of improvements in methods of analysis and elimination of analytic interference, the accuracy of most tests is limited primarily by their precision. **Accuracy** is a measure of the nearness of a test result to the actual value, whereas **precision** is a measure of the reproducibility of a result. No test can be more accurate than it is precise. Analysis of precision by repetitive measurements of a single sample gives rise to a gaussian distribution with a mean and an SD. The estimate of precision is the coefficient of variation (CV):

$$\text{CV} = \frac{\text{SD}}{\text{Mean}} \times 100$$

The CV is not likely to be constant over the full range of values obtained in clinical testing, but it is approximately 5% in the normal range. The CV is generally not reported, but is always known by the laboratory. It is particularly important in assessing the significance of changes in laboratory results. For example, a common situation is the need to assess hepatotoxicity incurred as a result of the administration of a therapeutic drug and reflected in the serum alanine aminotransferase (ALT) value. If serum ALT increases from 25 U/L to 40 U/L, is the change significant? The CV for ALT is 7%. Using the value obtained ±2 × CV to express the extremes of imprecision, it can be seen that a value of 25 U/L is unlikely to reflect an actual concentration of >29 U/L, and a value of 40 U/L is unlikely to reflect an actual concentration of <34 U/L. Therefore, the change in the value as obtained by testing is likely to reflect a real change in circulating ALT levels. Continued monitoring of serum ALT is indicated, even though both values for ALT are within normal limits. *Likely* in this case is only a probability. Inherent biologic variability is such that the results of 2 successive tests may suggest a trend that will disappear on further testing.

The precision of a test may also be indicated by providing confidence limits for a given result. Ordinarily, 95% confidence limits are used, indicating that it is 95% certain that the value obtained lies between the 2 limits reported. Confidence limits are calculated using the mean and SD of replicate determinations:

$$95\%\ \text{confidence limits} = \text{mean} \pm t \times \text{SD}$$

where t is a constant derived from the number of replications. In most cases, $t = 2$.

SENSITIVITY, ACCURACY, AND ANALYTIC TESTING. In some circumstances, the sensitivity and accuracy of an analysis are reduced or increased as functions of clinical purpose. For example, ion exchange chromatography of plasma amino acids for the diagnosis of inborn errors of metabolism is usually performed at an analytic sensitivity that allows measurement of all of the amino acids with a single set of standards. The range of values is approximately 20–800 µmol/L, and accuracy is poor at values of ≤20 µmol/L. The detection of homocysteine in this type of analysis suggests an inborn error of methionine metabolism. If the analysis is adjusted to achieve greater analytic sensitivity, it is possible to measure homocysteine accurately in normal plasma (3–12 µmol/L). This more sensitive test is used to assess cobalamin status and analyze risk factors for atherosclerotic cardiovascular disease.

PREDICTIVE VALUE OF LABORATORY TESTS. Predictive value (PV) theory deals with the usefulness of tests as defined by their clinical sensitivity (ability to detect a disease) and specificity (ability to define the absence of a disease).

$$\text{Sensitivity} = \frac{\text{Number positive by test}}{\text{Total number positive}} \times 100$$

$$\text{Specificity} = \frac{\text{Number negative by test}}{\text{Total number without disease}} \times 100$$

$$\text{PV of a positive test result} = \frac{\text{True positive results}}{\text{Total positive results}} \times 100$$

$$\text{PV of a negative test result} = \frac{\text{True negative results}}{\text{Total negative results}} \times 100$$

The problems addressed by PV theory are false-negative and false-positive test results. Both are major considerations in interpreting the results of screening tests in general and neonatal screening tests in particular.

Testing for HIV seroreactivity illustrates some of these considerations. If it is assumed that approximately 1,100,000 of 284,000,000 residents of the United States are infected with HIV (prevalence = 0.39%) and that 90% of those infected demonstrate antibodies to HIV, then we can consider the usefulness of a simple test with 99% sensitivity and 99.5% specificity. If the entire pop-

TABLE 714-1. Gaussian and Nongaussian Laboratory Values in 458 Normal School Children 7–14 Yr of Age

	SERUM SODIUM (mmol/L)	SERUM CREATINE KINASE (U/L)
Mean	141	68
SD	1.7	34
Mean ± 2 SD	138–144	0–136
Actual 95% range	137–144	24–162

SD = standard deviation.

ulation of the USA were screened, it would be possible to identify most of those infected with HIV.

$$1{,}100{,}000 \times 0.9 \times 0.99 = 980{,}100 (89.1\%)$$

However, there will be 119,900 false-negative test results. Even with 99.5% specificity, the number of false-positive test results would be larger than the number of true-positive results:

$$284{,}000{,}000 \times 0.005 = 1{,}420{,}000$$

In addition, there will be 281,480,000 true-negative results.

$$\text{PV of positive test result} = \frac{980{,}100}{(980{,}100 + 1{,}420{,}000)} \times 100 = 41\%$$

$$\text{PV of negative test result} = \frac{281{,}480{,}000}{(281{,}480{,}000 + 119{,}900)} \times 100 = 99.96\%$$

Given the high cost associated with follow-up and the anguish produced by a false-positive result, it is easy to see why universal screening for HIV seropositivity received a low priority immediately after the introduction of testing for HIV infection.

By contrast, we can consider the screening of 100,000 individuals from groups at increased risk for HIV in whom the overall prevalence of disease is 10%, with all other considerations being unchanged.

$$\text{True-positive results} = 0.9 \times 0.99 \times 10{,}000 = 8{,}910$$

$$\text{False-positive results} = 0.005 \times 90{,}000 = 450$$

$$\text{False-negative results} = 10{,}000 - 8{,}910 = 1{,}090$$

$$\text{PV of positive test result} = \frac{8{,}910}{8{,}910 + 450} \times 100 = 95\%$$

$$\text{PV of negative test result} = \frac{89{,}500}{89{,}550 + 1{,}090} \times 100 = 99\%$$

These 2 hypothetical testing strategies show that the diagnostic efficiency of testing depends heavily on the prevalence of the disease being tested for, even with a superior test, such as the test for HIV antibodies. Because the treatment of pregnant women infected with HIV is effective in preventing vertical transmission of the infection, screening has now been expanded to all pregnant women. The proven effectiveness of current therapy in preventing neonatal infection has intensified screening for HIV early in pregnancy.

However, because of the long time needed to test for HIV antibodies, it was difficult to screen women during labor and provide the necessary therapy. Recently, rapid HIV antibody testing procedures using a fingerstick or venipuncture to obtain whole blood, plasma, or serum, and tests using oral fluid were approved (Table 714-2). The HIV test results are usually obtained in <20 min. The collection of oral fluid samples provides an alternative for individuals who avoid HIV testing because of their dislike of needlesticks. HIV testing using whole blood or oral fluid is classified as a waived test under the **Clinical Laboratory Improvement Amendments of 1988 (CLIA)**, and these tests are allowed in a point-of-care setting. Waived tests are simple laboratory procedures that use methodologies that are so simple and accurate as to render the likelihood of an erroneous result by the user negligible. A positive rapid HIV test result is then confirmed by Western blot analysis or immunofluorescence assay.

According to the U.S. Centers for Disease Control and Prevention, in the USA, between 280 and 370 infants were born with HIV in 2000. Rapid HIV testing during labor allows for implementation of antiretroviral therapy for HIV-infected women who have not been tested or are unaware of their HIV status. The initiation of therapy at the time of labor or within the 1st 12 hr of an infant's birth significantly reduces the risk of mother-to-child transmission. In the mother-infant rapid intervention at delivery study, it was shown that the sensitivity and specificity of a rapid whole blood test for HIV during labor were 100% and 99.9%, respectively, with a positive PV of 90%. The median turnaround time for obtaining results from blood collection to patient notification was only 66 min. The performance of the rapid blood test was better than that of the standard HIV enzyme immunoassay, which had sensitivity and specificity of 100% and 99.8%, respectively, with a positive PV of 76%. In addition, the median turnaround time from blood collection to patient notification was 28 hr. As a result, rapid whole blood HIV testing is now the standard of care for women in labor with undocumented HIV status.

Rapid HIV testing can also be used in developing countries. In resource-poor settings, because of the lack of properly equipped laboratories, skilled technologists, and basic resources, such as electricity and water, these self-contained, point-of-care HIV tests are very attractive. In areas of Asia and Africa in which HIV is epidemic, screening pregnant women with rapid HIV tests and offering antiretroviral therapy can significantly reduce the transmission of HIV to hundreds of thousands of infants.

NEONATAL SCREENING TESTS. Almost all of the diseases detected in neonatal screening programs have a very low prevalence, and

TABLE 714-2. Rapid HIV Antibody Tests and Status Under the Clinical Laboratory Improvement Amendments of 1988 (CLIA)

RAPID HIV TEST	SPECIMEN TYPE	CLIA* CATEGORY	TIME FOR PERFORMING ASSAY	WAIT TIME TO READ RESULTS	MANUFACTURER
OraQuick ADVANCE Rapid HIV-1/2 Antibody Test	Oral fluid	Waived	<5 min	20–40 min	OraSure Technologies, Inc. *www.orasure.com*
	Whole blood (fingerstick or venipuncture)	Waived			
	Plasma	Moderate complexity			
Uni-Gold Recombigen HIV-1	Whole blood (fingerstick or venipuncture)	Waived	<5 min	10–12 min	Trinity Biotech *www.unigoldhiv.com*
	Serum and plasma	Moderate complexity			
Reveal G-2 Rapid HIV-1 Antibody Test	Serum and plasma	Moderate complexity	<5 min	Read result immediately	MedMira, Inc. *www.medmira.com*
MultiSpot HIV-1/HIV-2 Rapid Test	Serum and plasma	Moderate complexity	10–15 min	Result can be read immediately or up to 4 hr later	BioRad Laboratories *www.biorad.com*

*Clinical Laboratory Improvement Amendment.

for the most part, the tests are quantitative rather than qualitative. In general, the strategy is to use the initial screening test to separate a highly suspect group of patients from normal infants (i.e., to increase the prevalence) and then to follow this suspect group aggressively. This strategy is illustrated by a scheme used in screening newborns for congenital hypothyroidism, the prevalence of which is 25/100,000 liveborn infants. The initial test performed is for thyroxine in whole blood, and infants with the lowest 10% of test results are considered suspect. If all infants with hypothyroidism were included in the suspect group, the prevalence of disease in this group would be 250/100,000 infants. The original samples obtained from the suspect group are retested for thyroxine and are tested for thyroid-stimulating hormone. This 2nd round of testing results in an even more highly suspect group composed of 0.1% of the infants screened and having a prevalence of hypothyroidism of 25,000/100,000 subjects. This final group is aggressively pursued for further testing and treatment. Even with a 1,000-fold increase in prevalence, 75% of the aggressively tested population is euthyroid. The justifications advanced for the program are that treatment is easy and effective and that the alternative, if congenital hypothyroidism is undetected and untreated—long-term custodial care—is both unsatisfactory and expensive.

At its inception, neonatal screening was driven by the selection of genetic diseases whose clinical manifestations developed postnatally, such as phenylketonuria, galactosemia, and homocystinuria. The diseases could be treated effectively by simple means instituted shortly after birth. The classic screening tests are disease-specific microbiologic assays.

More common diseases have also become targets for neonatal screening programs. Congenital hypothyroidism was selected for screening because of its frequency and its ease of treatment. Sickle cell disease, also easily detected, can be treated more effectively if it is diagnosed before clinical signs appear. In addition, the results of neonatal screening for cystic fibrosis (CF) show that there are clear benefits associated with preclinical diagnosis, but also that there are some inherent difficulties associated with genetic screening for complex autosomal recessive diseases that are common and are caused by a rather large number of mutations of a single gene. The definitive diagnostic test for CF is the measurement of concentrations of sodium and chloride in sweat, a test that is not practical during the 1st wk of life. Neonates with CF generally have elevations in whole blood trypsinogen. This test allows the identification of a group of neonates at risk for CF. Performing DNA analysis for common mutations that cause CF reduces the size of the suspect group and identifies neonates with a higher likelihood of disease. This strategy identifies a manageable number of infants on whom to perform sweat tests. Problems include the following: (1) uncommon mutations are not included in the screening panel (thus, cases of CF caused by these mutations can be missed); (2) common mutations that cause clinically innocent elevations of whole blood trypsinogen in heterozygous neonates cause potentially alarming false-positive findings; and (3) CF in patients with normal sweat test results is rare, but is likely to be missed. Congenital adrenal hyperplasia, another common disorder, is now included in neonatal screening programs.

Tandem mass spectrometry (MS/MS) is a technically advanced method in which many compounds are initially separated by molecular weight. Each compound is then fragmented to allow identification. The process requires roughly 2 min/sample and can detect 20 or more inborn errors of metabolism. The effects of prematurity, neonatal illness, and intensive neonatal management on metabolites in blood complicate the interpretation of results. The PV of a positive screening result is likely to be <10%; that is, 90% of positive results are not indicative of a genetic disorder of metabolism. Nonetheless, MS/MS permits a diagnosis to be made before clinical illness develops. MS/MS is not directed toward diseases defined as treatable, but toward all of the diseases, each of which is rare, that the technique can identify (Table 714-3).

TABLE 714-3. Neonatal Screening by Tandem Mass Spectrometry

DISORDERS OF ORGANIC ACID METABOLISM AND FATTY ACID OXIDATION
Hydroxymethylglutaryl CoA lyase deficiency
Glutaric aciduria type 1
Isobutyryl CoA dehydrogenase deficiency
Isovaleric acidemia
2-Methylbutyryl CoA dehydrogenase deficiency
2,4-Dienoyl CoA reductase deficiency
3-Methylcrotonyl CoA carboxylase deficiency
3-Methylglutaconyl CoA hydratase deficiency
Methylmalonic acidemia
3-Ketothiolase deficiency
Multiple CoA carboxylase deficiency
Propionic acidemia
Carnitine/acylcarnitine translocator deficiency
Medium-chain acyl CoA dehydrogenase deficiency
Medium-chain ketoacyl CoA thiolase deficiency
Glutaric aciduria, type 2
Carnitine palmitoyl transferase deficiency
Short-chain acyl CoA dehydrogenase deficiency
Short-chain hydroxy acyl CoA dehydrogenase deficiency
Trifunctional protein deficiency
Long-chain 3-hydroxy acyl CoA dehydrogenase deficiency
Very long chain acyl CoA dehydrogenase deficiency
DISORDERS OF AMINO ACID METABOLISM
Argininosuccinic aciduria
Citrullinemia
Citrullinemia type II
Homocystinuria
Hyperphenylalaninemia
Maple syrup urine disease
Phenylketonuria
Tyrosinemia

CoA, coenzyme A

Electrospray tandem mass spectrometry permits the detection of rare inborn errors of metabolism and has been introduced as a newborn screening tool in Australia. In the 4 yr since mass spectrometry was implemented, the rate of detection per 100,000 births was 15.7, significantly higher than the rate of 8.6–9.5 in the 6 preceding 4-yr periods. Disorders of fatty acid oxidation, particularly medium-chain acyl coenzyme A dehydrogenase deficiency, accounted for the majority of increased diagnoses.

Expanded newborn screening programs using MS/MS increase the detection of inherited metabolic disorders. As of 2006, 34 U.S. states used MS/MS in their neonatal screening programs. However, the metabolic conditions screened for by states using MS/MS vary, ranging from <3 to >20.

In an attempt to standardize newborn screening programs, the American College of Medical Genetics recommends that every baby born in the United States be screened for a uniform panel of 29 disorders. The March of Dimes and the American Academy of Pediatrics also endorse the recommendation by the American College of Medical Genetics. However, expansion of the screening test menu raises several issues. For example, the cost of implementation can be significant because many states will need multiple MS/MS systems. In addition, staffing the laboratory with qualified technical personnel to run the MS/MS system and qualified clinical scientists to interpret the profiles can be a challenge. A number of false-positive results will also be obtained with these newborn screening programs. Many of these findings are due to parenteral nutrition, biologic variation, or treatment, and are not the result of an inborn error of metabolism. Therefore, qualified staff will be needed to ensure that patients with abnormal results are contacted and receive follow-up testing and counseling, if needed. Even with these concerns, the American College of Medical Genetics report is a step in the right direction toward standardizing guidelines for state newborn screening programs.

TESTING IN REFINING A DIFFERENTIAL DIAGNOSIS. The use of laboratory tests in refining a differential diagnosis satisfies PV theory because a correct differential diagnosis should result in a relatively high prevalence of the disease under consideration. An example of testing in refining a differential diagnosis is the measurement of urinary vanillylmandelic acid (VMA) for the diagnosis of neuroblastoma. A simple spot test for VMA is not useful in general screening programs because of the low prevalence of neuroblastoma (3 cases/100,000) and the low sensitivity of the test (69%). Even though the specificity of urinary VMA is 99.6%, testing of 100,000 children would produce 2 true-positive test results, 400 false-positive results, and 1 false-negative result. The PV of a positive result in this setting is 0.5%, and the PV of a negative result is 99.99%, not much different from the assumption that neuroblastoma is not present. Testing for urinary VMA in a 3 yr old child with an abdominal mass, however, gives a useful result because the prevalence of neuroblastoma is at least 50% in 3 yr old children with abdominal masses. If 100 such children are tested and the prevalence of neuroblastoma in the group is assumed to be 50%, then a satisfactory PV is obtained.

$$\text{PV of positive test result} = \frac{0.69 \times 50}{0.69 \times 50 + (0.004 \times 50)} \times 100 = 99\%$$

$$\text{PV of negative test result} = \frac{0.996 \times 50}{0.996 \times 50 + (0.31 \times 50)} \times 100 = 76\%$$

Thus, in this situation, a test with low sensitivity is powerful in refining the differential diagnosis because the PV of a positive result is almost 100% in the setting of high prevalence.

Serologic Testing. Using laboratory testing to refine a differential diagnosis poses problems, as exemplified by serologic testing for Lyme disease, which is a tick-borne infection by *Borrelia burgdorferi* that has various manifestations in both early and late stages of infection (see Chapter 219). Direct demonstration of the organism is difficult, and serologic test results for Lyme disease are not reliably positive in young patients presenting early with erythema chronicum migrans. These results become positive after a few wk of infection and remain positive for a number of yr. In an older population being evaluated for late-stage Lyme disease, some individuals will have recovered from either clinical or subclinical Lyme disease and some will have active Lyme disease, with both groups having true-positive serologic test results. Of individuals without Lyme disease, some will have true-negative serologic test results, but a significant percentage will have antibodies to other organisms that cross-react with *B. burgdorferi* antigens.

This set of circumstances gives rise to a number of problems. First, the protean nature of Lyme disease makes it difficult to ensure a high prevalence of disease in subjects to be tested. Second, the most appropriate antibodies to be detected are imperfectly defined, leading to a wide variety of tests with varying false-positive and false-negative rates. Third, the natural history of the antibody response to infection and the difficulty of showing the causative organism directly combine to make laboratory diagnosis of early Lyme disease difficult. Fourth, in the diagnosis of late-stage Lyme disease in older subjects, the laboratory diagnosis is plagued by misleading positive (either false-positive or true-positive, but not clinically relevant) results, typically an enzyme-linked immunosorbent assay that uses whole *B. burgdorferi* organisms. In a review of 788 patients referred to a specialty clinic with the diagnosis of Lyme disease, the diagnosis was correct in 180 patients, 156 patients had true seropositivity without active Lyme disease, and 452 had never had Lyme disease, even though 45% of them were found to be seropositive by at least one test before referral.

TABLE 714-4. Laboratory Profile as a Review of Systems

LABORATORY TEST	ASSESSMENT FACILITATED BY TESTS
Complete blood cell count and platelets	Nutrition, status of formed elements
Complete urinalysis	Renal function/genitourinary tract inflammation
Albumin and cholesterol	Nutrition
ALT, bilirubin, GGT	Liver function
BUN, creatinine	Renal function, nutrition
Sodium, potassium, chloride, bicarbonate	Electrolyte homeostasis
Calcium and phosphorus	Calcium homeostasis

ALT, alanine aminotransferase; BUN, blood urea nitrogen; GGT, γ-glutamyltransferase.

A two-step approach, similar to that used in HIV testing, is commonly used: a screening test that has high sensitivity (e.g., enzyme-linked immunosorbent assay) and excellent negative PV, followed by a very specific confirmatory test for verification of positive screening test results (e.g., Western blot to detect antibodies to selected bacterial antigens). Negative screening test results and negative verification test results are reported as negative. Positive verification test results are reported as positive. However, standardization of the testing procedures is difficult in North America, where only 1 pathogenic strain of *B. burgdorferi* is found, and is more difficult elsewhere in the Northern hemisphere, where as many as 3 pathogenic strains are present. Identification of microbial DNA in body fluids by polymerase chain reaction is definitive, but invasive.

Laboratory Screening. Screening profiles (Table 714-4) are used as part of a complete review of systems, to establish a baseline value, or to facilitate patient care in specific circumstances, such as: (1) when a patient clearly has an illness, but a specific diagnosis remains elusive; (2) when a patient requires intensive care; (3) for postmarketing surveillance and evaluation of a new drug; and (4) when a drug is used that is known to have systemic adverse effects. Laboratory screening tests should be used in a targeted manner to supplement, not supplant, a complete history and physical examination.

American Academy of Pediatrics and American Thyroid Association: Newborn screening for congenital hypothyroidism. *Pediatrics* 1987;80:745–749.

Bulterys M, Jamieson DJ, O'Sullivan MJ, et al: Rapid HIV-1 testing during labor: A multicenter study. *JAMA* 2004;292:219–223.

Clayton EW: Issues in state newborn screening programs. *Pediatrics* 1992;90:641–646.

Farrell PM, Kosrok MR, Rock MJ, et al: Early diagnosis of cystic fibrosis through neonatal screening prevents severe malnutrition and improves long-term growth. *Pediatrics* 2001;107:1–13.

Galen RS, Gambino SR: *Beyond Normality.* New York, Academic Press, 1975.

Hu LT, Klempner MS: Update on the prevention, diagnosis, and treatment of Lyme disease. *Adv Intern Med* 2001;46:247–275.

National Newborn Screening and Genetics Resource Center (website *http://genes-r-us.uthscsa.edu*).

Rinaldo P, Tortorelli S, Matern D: Recent developments and new applications of tandem mass spectrometry in newborn screening. *Curr Opin Pediatr* 2004;16:427–433.

Steere AC, Taylor E, McHugh GL, et al: The overdiagnosis of Lyme disease. *JAMA* 1993;269:1812–1826.

Wilcken B, Wiley V, Hammond J, et al: Screening newborns for inborn errors of metabolism by tandem mass spectrometry. *N Engl J Med* 2003;348:2304–2312.

Zytkovicz TH, Fitzgerald EF, Marsden D, et al: Tandem mass spectrometric analysis for amino, organic, and fatty acid disorders in newborn dried blood spots: A two-year summary from the New England Newborn Screening Program. *Clin Chem* 2001;47:1945–1955.

Chapter 715 ■ Reference Ranges for Laboratory Tests and Procedures

Michael A. Pesce

In Tables 715-1 through 715-6, the reference ranges apply to infants, children, and adolescents when possible. For many analyses, however, separate reference ranges for children and adolescents are not well delineated. When interpreting a test result, the reference range supplied by the laboratory performing the test should always be used. See Figures 715-1 and 715-2 for estimations related to dosages.

TABLE 715-1. Prefixes Denoting Decimal Factors

PREFIX	SYMBOL	FACTOR
Mega-	M	10^6
Kilo-	k	10^3
Hecto-	h	10^2
Deka-	da	10^1
Deci-	d	10^{-1}
Centi-	c	10^{-2}
Milli-	m	10^{-3}
Micro-	μ	10^{-6}
Nano-	n	10^{-9}
Pico-	p	10^{-12}
Femto-	f	10^{-15}

TABLE 715-2. Abbreviations

Ab	Absorbance
AU	Arbitrary unit
BB	Brain isoenzyme of creatine kinase
cap	Capillary
CH_{50}	Dilution required to lyse 50% of indicator red blood cells; indicates complement activity
Cr	Creatinine
CSF	Cerebrospinal fluid
F	Female
g	Gram
hr	Hour, hours
Hb	Hemoglobin
HbCO	Carboxyhemoglobin
hpf	High-power field
IU	International unit of hormone activity
L	Liter
M	Male
MB	Heart isoenzyme of creatine kinase
mEq/L	Milliequivalents per liter
min	Minute, minutes
mm^3	Cubic millimeter, microliter (μL)
mm Hg	Millimeters of mercury
mo	Month, months
mol	Mole
mmol	Millimole
mOsm	Milliosmole
MW	Relative molecular weight
ND	Not detected
nm	Nanometer (wavelength)
Pa	Pascal
pc	Postprandial
RBC	Red blood cell(s), erythrocyte(s)
RT	Room temperature
sec	Second, seconds
SD	Standard deviation
Tr	Trace
U	International unit of enzyme activity
V	Volume
WBC	White blood cell(s)
WHO	World Health Organization
wk	Week, weeks
yr	Year, years

TABLE 715-3. Symbols

> Greater than	≤ Less than or equal to
≥ Greater than or equal to	± Plus or minus
< Less than	≈ Approximately equal to

TABLE 715-4. Abbreviations for Specimens

S	Serum
P	Plasma
(H)	Heparin
(LiH)	Lithium heparin
(E)	Ethylenediaminetetraacetic acid (EDTA)
(C)	Citrate
(O)	Oxalate
W	Whole blood
U	Urine
F	Feces
CSF	Cerebrospinal fluid
AF	Amniotic fluid
(NaC)	Sodium citrate
(NH_4H)	Ammonium heparinate

TABLE 715-5. Key to Comments

30°C, 37°C	Temperature of enzymatic analysis (Celsius)
a	Values obtained are significantly method-dependent
b	Values in older males are higher than those in older females
c	Values in older females are higher than those in older males
d	Atomic absorption
e	Borate affinity chromatography
f	Cation-exchange chromatography
g	Vitros, a proprietary analytic system of Ortho Clinical Diagnostics, Inc.
i	Electrophoresis
j	Enzymatic assay
k	Enzyme-amplified immunoassay
l	Fluorometric method
m	Fluorescence-activated cell sorting (FACS)
n	Fluorescence polarization
o	Gas chromatography
p	High-performance liquid chromatography (HPLC)
q	Indirect fluorescence antibody (IFA) assay
r	Ion-selective electrode
s	Nephelometry
t	Optical density
u	Radial immunodiffusion (RID)
v	Radioimmunoassay (RIA)
w	Spectrophotometry

TABLE 715-6. Reference Ranges*†

ANALYTE OR PROCEDURE	SPECIMEN	REFERENCE VALUES (USA)		CONVERSION FACTOR	REFERENCE VALUES (SI)	COMMENTS
Complete Blood Count						
Hematocrit (HCT, Hct)	W(E)		% of packed red cells			
Calculated from mean corpuscular volume (MCV) and RBC count (electronic displacement or laser)			(V red cells/V whole blood cells × 100		Volume fraction (V red cells/V whole blood)	
		1 day (cap)	48–69%	×0.01	0.48–0.69	
		2 days	48–75%		0.48–0.75	
		3 days	44–72%		0.44–0.72	
		2 mo	28–42%		0.28–0.42	
		6–12 yr	35–45%		0.35–0.45	
		12–18 yr M	37–49%		0.37–0.49	
		F	36–46%		0.36–0.46	
		18–49 yr M	41–53%		0.41–0.53	
		F	36–46%		0.36–0.46	
Hemoglobin (Hb)	W(E)		g/dL		mmol/L	
		1–3 days (cap)	14.5–22.5	×0.155	2.25–3.49	MW Hb = 64,500
		2 mo	9.0–14.0		1.40–2.17	
		6–12 yr	11.5–15.5		1.78–2.40	
		12–18 yr M	13.0–16.0		2.02–2.48	
		F	12.0–16.0		1.86–2.48	
		18–49 yr M	13.5–17.5		2.09–2.27	
		F	12.0–16.0		1.86–2.48	
	P(H)	See *Chemical Elements*				
Erythrocyte indices (RBC indices)						
Mean corpuscular hemoglobin (MCH)	W(E)		pg/cell		fmol/cell	
		Birth	31–37	×0.0155	0.48–0.57	
		1–3 days (cap)	31–37		0.48–0.57	
		1 wk–1 mo	28–40		0.43–0.62	
		2 mo	26–34		0.40–0.53	
		3–6 mo	25–35		0.39–0.54	
		0.5–2 yr	23–31		0.36–0.48	
		2–6 yr	24–30		0.37–0.47	
		6–12 yr	25–33		0.39–0.51	
		12–18 yr	25–35		0.39–0.54	
		18–49 yr	26–34		0.40–0.53	
Mean corpuscular hemoglobin concentration (MCHC)	W(E)		% Hb/cell or g Hb/dL RBC		mmol Hb/L RBC	
		Birth	30–36	×0.155	4.65–5.58	
		1–3 days (cap)	29–37		4.50–5.74	
		1–2 wk	28–38		4.34–5.89	
		1–2 mo	29–37		4.50–5.74	
		3 mo–2 yr	30–36		4.65–5.58	
		2–18 yr	31–37		4.81–5.74	
		>18 yr	31–37		4.81–5.74	
Mean corpuscular volume (MCV)	W(E)		μm^3		fL	
		1–3 days (cap)	95–121	×1	95–121	
		0.5–2 yr	70–86		70–86	
		6–12 yr	77–95		77–95	
		12–18 yr M	78–98		78–98	
		F	78–102		78–102	
		18–49 yr M	80–100		80–100	
		F	80–100		80–100	
Leukocyte count (WBC count)	W(E)	×1,000 cells/mm³ (μL)			$\times 10^9$ cells/L	
		Birth	9.0–30.0	×1	9.0–30.0	
		24 hr	9.4–34.0		9.4–34.0	
		1 mo	5.0–19.5		5.0–19.5	
		1–3 yr	6.0–17.5		6.0–17.5	
		4–7 yr	5.5–15.5		5.5–15.5	
		8–13 yr	4.5–13.5		4.5–13.5	
		Adult	4.5–11.0		4.5–11.0	
Leukocyte differential	W(E)	%			Number fraction	
Myelocytes		0%		×0.01	0	
Neutrophils ("bands")		3–5%			0.03–0.05	
Neutrophils ("segs")		54–62%			0.54–0.62	
Lymphocytes		25–33%			0.25–0.33	
Monocytes		3–7%			0.03–0.07	
Eosinophils		1–3%			0.01–0.03	
Basophils		0–0.75%			0–0.0075	
		Cells/mm³ (μL)			$\times 10^6$ cells/L	
Myelocytes		0		×1	0	
Neutrophils ("bands")		150–400			150–400	
Neutrophils ("segs")		3,000–5,800			3,000–5,800	
Lymphocytes		1,500–3,000			1,500–3,000	
Monocytes		285–500			285–500	
Eosinophils		50–250			50–250	
Basophils		15–50			15–50	

TABLE 715-6. Reference Ranges*†—cont'd

ANALYTE OR PROCEDURE	SPECIMEN	REFERENCE VALUES (USA)	CONVERSION FACTOR	REFERENCE VALUES (SI)	COMMENTS
Platelet count (thrombocyte count)	W(E)	$\times 10^3$/mm^3 (μL)		$\times 10^9$/L	
		Newborn 84–478 (after 1 wk, same as adult)	$\times 10^6$	84–478	(Buck, 1996)
		Adult 150–400		150–400	
Reticulocyte count	W(E,H,O)	Adults 0.5–1.5% of erythrocytes	×0.01	0.005–0.015 (number fraction)	
		or 25,000–75,000/mm^3 (μL)	$\times 10^6$	or 25,000–75,000 × 10^6/L	
		%		Number fraction	
	W(cap)	1 day 0.4–6.0	×0.01	0.004–0.060	
		7 days <0.1–1.3		<0.001–0.013	
		1–4 wk <1.0–1.2		<0.001–0.012	
		5–6 wk <0.1–2.4		<0.001–0.024	
		7–8 wk 0.1–2.9		0.001–0.029	
		9–10 wk <0.1–2.6		<0.001–0.026	
		11–12 wk 0.1–1.3		0.001–0.013	
Alanine aminotransferase (ALT, SGPT)	S	0–5 days 6–50 U/L	×1	6–50 U/L	37°bw
		1–19 yr 5–45		5–45	(Lockitch, Halstead, and Albersheim, 1988)
Albumin	P	Premature 1 day 1.8–3.0 g/dL	×10	18–30 g/dL	g (Meites, 1989)
		Full term <6 days 2.5–3.4		25–34	
		<5 yr 3.9–5.0		39–50	
		5–19 yr 4.0–5.3		40–53	
Ammonia	W	<30 days 21–95 μmol/L	×1	21–95 μmol/L	(Diaz et al., 1995)
		1–12 mo 18–74		18–74	
		1–14 yr 17–68		17–68	
		>14 yr 19–71		19–71	
Amylase	S,P	1–19 yr 30–100 U/L	×1	30–100 U/L	(Lockitch, Halstead, and Albersheim et al., 1988; Gillard et al., 1983)
		% pancreatic fraction		% pancreatic fraction	
Amylase isoenzymes	S,P(H)	Cord–8 mo 0–34%	×0.01	0–0.34%	
		9 mo–4 yr 5–56%		0.05–0.56%	
		5–19 yr 23–59%		0.23–0.59%	
Anion gap (sodium − [chloride + bicarbonate])	P(H)	7–16 mEq/L	×1	7–16 mEq/L	
Anti-deoxyribonuclease B titer (anti-DNase B titer)	S	Age / Upper limit of normal		Upper limit of normal	
		4–6 yr 240–480 U	×1	240–480 U	(Kaplan et al., 1998)
		7–12 yr 480–800 U		480–800 U	
Antidiuretic hormone (hADH, vasopressin)	P(E)	Plasma osmolarity (mOsm/kg) / Plasma ADH (pg/mL)		Plasma ADH ng/L	
		270–280 <1.5	×1	<1.5	
		280–285 <2.5		<2.5	
		285–290 1–5		1–5	
		290–295 2–7		2–7	
		295–300 4–12		4–12	
Antistreptolysin-O titer (ASO titer)	S	Age / Upper limit of normal		Upper limit of normal	(Kaplan et al., 1998)
		2–5 yr 120–160 Todd units	×1	120–160 Todd units	
		6–9 yr 240 Todd units		240 Todd units	
		10–12 yr 320 Todd units		320 Todd units	
Aspartate aminotransferase (AST, SGOT)	S	U/L		U/L	
		0–5 days 35–140	×1	35–140	37°b(Lockitch, Halstead, and Quigley et al., 1988)
		1–9 yr 15–55		15–55	
		10–19 yr 5–45		5–45	
Base excess	W(H)	mmol/L		mmol/L	
		Newborn (−10)–(−2)	×1	(−10)–(−2)	
		Infant (−7)–(−1)		(−7)–(−1)	
		Child (−4)–(+2)		(−4)–(+2)	
		Thereafter (−3)–(+3)		(−3)–(−3)	
Bicarbonate	S,P	mmol/L	×1	mmol/L	
		Arterial 21–28		21–28	
		Venous 22–29		22–29	
C-reactive protein (high sensitivity)	S				(Soldin et al., 2004)
		M (mg/dL) F (mg/dL)		M (mg/L) F (mg/L)	
		0–90 days 0.08–1.58 0.09–1.58	×10	0.8–15.8 0.9–15.8	
		91 days–12 mo 0.08–1.12 0.05–0.79		0.8–11.2 0.5–7.9	
		13 mo–3 yr 0.08–1.12 0.08–0.79		0.8–11.2 0.8–7.9	
		4–10 yr 0.06–0.79 0.5–1.0		0.6–7.9 0.5–10.0	
		11–14 yr 0.08–0.76 0.06–0.81		0.8–7.6 0.6–8.1	
		15–18 yr 0.04–0.79 0.06–0.79		0.4–7.9 0.6–7.9	
Calcium, ionized (Ca)	S,P(H), W(H)	mg/dL		mmol/L	
		Cord blood 5.0–6.0	×0.25	1.25–1.50	
		Newborn, 3–24 hr 4.3–5.1		1.07–1.27	
		24–48 hr 4.0–4.7		1.00–1.17	
		Thereafter 4.8–4.92		1.12–1.23	
		or 2.24–2.46 Eq/L	×0.5	1.12–1.23	

TABLE 715-6. Reference Ranges*†—cont'd

ANALYTE OR PROCEDURE	SPECIMEN	REFERENCE VALUES (USA)		CONVERSION FACTOR	REFERENCE VALUES (SI)	COMMENTS
Calcium, total	S		mg/dL		mmol/L	
		Cord blood	9.0–11.5	×0.25	2.25–2.88	
		Newborn, 3–24 hr	9.0–10.6		2.3–2.65	
		24–48	7.0–12.0		1.75–3.00	
		4–7 days	9.0–10.9		2.25–2.73	
		Child	8.8–10.8		2.20–2.70	
		Thereafter	8.4–10.2		2.10–2.55	
Carbon dioxide, partial pressure (PCO_2)	W(H)		mm Hg		kPa	
		Newborn	27–40	×0.1333	3.6–5.3	
		Infant	27–41		3.6–5.5	
		Thereafter M	35–48		4.7–6.4	
		F	32–45		4.3–6.0	
Carbon monoxide (carboxyhemoglobin)	W(E)	Nonsmoker	<2% HbCO	×0.01	HbCO fraction < 0.02	
		Smoker	<10%		<0.10	
		Lethal	>50%		>0.5	
Chloride	S,P(H)	Cord blood	96–104 mmol/L	×1	96–104 mmol/L	
		Newborn	97–110		97–110	
		Thereafter	98–106		98–106	
Cortisol	S,P(H)		µg/dL		nmol/L	
		Newborn	1–24	×27.59	28–662	
		Adults, 8:00 A.M.	5–23		138–635	
		4:00 P.M.	3–15		82–413	
		8:00 P.M.	<50% of 8:00 A.M.	×0.01	Fraction of 8:00 A.M. ≤0.50	
Creatine kinase	S	Cord blood	70–380 U/L	×1	70–380 U/L	30° b (Jedeikin et al., 1982)
		5–8 hr	214–1,175		214–1,175	
		24–33 hr	130–1,200		130–1,200	
		72–100 hr	87–725		87–725	
		Adult	5–130		5–130	
Creatine kinase isoenzymes	S		% MB	% BB		
		Cord blood	0.3–3.1	0.3–10.5		
		5–8 hr	1.7–7.9	3.6–13.4		
		24–33 hr	1.8–5.0	2.3–8.6		
		72–100 hr	1.4–5.4	5.1–13.3		
		Adult	0–2	0		
Creatinine						
Jaffe, kinetic, or enzymatic	S,P		mg/dL		µmol/L	
		Cord blood	0.6–1.2	×88.4	53–106	
		Newborn	0.3–1.0		27–88	
		Infant	0.2–0.4		18–35	
		Child	0.3–0.7		27–62	
		Adolescent	0.5–1.0		44–88	
		Adult M	0.6–1.2		53–106	
		F	0.5–1.1		44–97	
Creatinine clearance (endogenous)	S,P,U	Newborn 40–65 mL/min/1.73 m^2				
		<40 YR, M 97–137				
		F 88–128				
		Decreases <6.5 mL/min/decade				
Ferritin	S		ng/mL		µg/L	
		Newborn	25–200	×1	25–200	
		1 mo	200–600		200–600	
		2–5 mo	50–200		50–200	
		6 mo–15 yr	7–140		7–140	
		Adult, M	15–200		15–200	
		F	12–150		12–150	
Folate	S	Newborn 7.0–32 ng/mL		×2.265	15.9–72.4 nmol/L	
		Thereafter 1.8–9.0			4.1–20.4	
	W(E)	150–450 ng/mL RBCs			340–1,020 nmol/L cells	
Glucose	S		mg/dL		mmol/L	
		Cord blood	45–96	×0.0555	2.5–5.3	
		Premature	20–60		1.1–3.3	
		Neonate	30–60		1.7–3.3	
		Newborn				
		1 day	40–60		2.2–3.3	
		>1 day	50–90		2.8–5.0	
		Child	60–100		3.3–5.5	
		Adult	70–105		3.9–5.8	
	W(H)	Adult	65–95		3.6–5.3	
Glucose, 2 hr post	S	<120 mg/dL			<6.7 mmol/L	
Glucose tolerance test (GTT)	S		mg/dL		mmol/L	
Oral dose Adult: 75 g			Normal Diabetic		Normal Diabetic	
Child: 1.75 g/kg of ideal weight, up to a maximum of 75 g		Fasting	70–105 ≥126	×0.0555	3.9–5.8 ≥7.0	(American Diabetes Association, 1977)
		60 min	120–170 ≥200		6.7–9.4 ≥11	
		90 min	100–140 ≥200		5.6–7.8 ≥11	
		120 min	70–120 ≥200		3.9–6.7 ≥11	

TABLE 715-6. Reference Ranges*†—cont'd

ANALYTE OR PROCEDURE	SPECIMEN	REFERENCE VALUES (USA)		CONVERSION FACTOR	REFERENCE VALUES (SI)	COMMENTS
Glucose-6-phosphate dehydrogenase (G6PD) in erythrocytes		W(E,H,C)				
Bishop, modified		Adult			Adult	
		3.4–8.0 U/g Hb		×0.0645	0.22–0.52 mU/mol Hb	
		98.6–232 U/10^{12} RBC		×10^{-3}	0.10–0.23 nU/10^{6} RBC	
		1.16–2.72 U/mL RBC		×1	1.16–2.72 kU/L RBC	
		Newborn: 50% higher			Newborn: 50% higher	
γ-glutamyl transpeptidase (GGT, GGTP)	S		U/L		U/L	
		Cord blood	37–193	×1	37–193	37°b(Knight and Haymond, 1981)
		0–1 mo	13–147		13–147	
		1–2 mo	12–123		12–123	
		2–4 mo	8–90		8–90	
		4 mo–10 yr	5–32		5–32	
		10–15 yr	5–24		5–24	
Immunoglobulin A (IgA)	S		mg/dL	×10	mg/L	
		Cord blood	1.4–3.6		14–36	s (Meites, 1989)
		1–3 mo	1.3–53		13–530	
		4–6 mo	4.4–84		44–840	
		7 mo–1 yr	11–106		110–1,060	
		2–5 yr	14–159		140–1,590	
		6–10 yr	33–236		330–2,360	
		Adult	70–312		700–3,120	
Immunoglobulin D (IgD)	S	Newborn: none detected			None detected	
		Thereafter: 0–8 mg/dL		×10	0–80 mg/L	
Immunoglobulin E (IgE)	S	M 0–230 IU/mL		×1	0–230 kIU/L	
		F 0–170			0–170	
Immunoglobulin G (IgG)	S		mg/dL		g/L	
		Cord blood	636–1,606	×0.01	6.36–16.06	s (Meites, 1989)
		1 mo	251–906		2.51–9.06	
		2–4 mo	176–601		1.76–6.01	
		5–12 mo	172–1,069		1.72–10.69	
		1–5 yr	345–1,236		3.45–12.36	
		6–10 yr	608–1,572		6.08–15.72	
		Adult	639–1,349		6.39–13.49	
Immunoglobulin M (IgM)	S		mg/dL		mg/L	
		Cord blood	6.3–25	×10	63–250	s (Meites, 1989)
		1–4 mo	17–105		170–1,050	
		5–9 mo	33–126		330–1,260	
		10 mo–1 yr	41–173		410–1,730	
		2–8 yr	43–207		430–2,070	
		9–10 yr	52–242		520–2,420	
		Adult	56–352		560–3,520	
Iron	S	All ages	22–184 μg/dL	×0.1791	4–33 μmol/L	(Lockitch, Halstead, and Wadsworth et al., 1988)
Iron-binding capacity, total (TIBC)	S	Infant 100–400 μg/dL		×0.179	17.90–71.60 μmol/L	
		Thereafter 250–400			44.75–71.60	
L+lactate	W		mmol/L		mmol/L	(Bonnefont et al., 1990)
		1–12 mo	1.1–2.3	×1	1.1–2.3	
		1–7 yr	0.8–1.5		0.8–1.5	
		7–15 yr	0.6–0.9		0.6–0.9	
D-lactate	P(H)					j (Rosenthal and Pesce, 1985)
		6 mo–3 yr	0.0–0.3	×1	0.0–0.3	
Lactate dehydrogenase	S		U/L		U/L	
		<1 yr	170–580	×1	170–580	37° a (Meites, 1989)
		1–9 yr	150–500		150–500	
		10–19 yr	120–330		120–330	
Isoenzymes	S		% of total activity: 1–6 yr / 7–19 yr			
		LD1	20–38 / 20–35			
		LD2	27–38 / 31–38			
		LD3	16–26 / 19–28			
		LD4	5–16 / 7–13			
		LD5	3–13 / 5–12			
Lead	W(H)		μg/dL		mmol/L	
		Child	<10	×0.0483	<0.48	
		Toxic	≥70		≥3.38	
Lipase	P,S	1–18 yr	145–216 U/L	×1	145–216 U/L	(Ghoshal and Soldin, 2003)
Magnesium	P(H)		mg/dL		mmol/L	
		0–6 days	1.2–2.6	×0.411	0.48–1.05	w (Meites, 1989)
		7 days–2 yr	1.6–2.6		0.65–1.05	
		2–14 yr	1.5–2.3		0.60–0.95	

TABLE 715-6. Reference Ranges*†—cont'd

ANALYTE OR PROCEDURE	SPECIMEN	REFERENCE VALUES (USA)	CONVERSION FACTOR	REFERENCE VALUES (SI)	COMMENTS
Methemoglobin (MetHb)	W(E,H,C)	0.06–0.24 g/dL or	×155	9.3–37.2 μmol/L	
		0.78 ± 0.37% of total Hb	×0.01	0.0078 ± 0.0037 (mass fraction)	
Osmolality	S	Child, adult			
		275–295 mOsmol/kg H_2O			
Phosphatase, alkaline	S	U/L		U/L	
		1–9 yr 145–420	×1	145–420	37°C aw
		10–11 yr 130–560		130–560	(Lockitch, Halstead, and Albersheim et al., 1988)
		M F		M F	
		12–13 yr 200–495 105–420		200–495 105–420	
		14–15 yr 130–525 70–230		130–525 70–230	
		16–19 yr 65–260 50–130		65–260 50–130	
Phosphorus, inorganic	S,P(H)	mg/dL		mmol/L	
		0–5 days 4.8–8.2	×0.3229	1.55–2.65	w (Meites, 1989)
		1–3 yr 3.8–6.5		1.25–2.10	
		4–11 yr 3.7–5.6		1.20–1.80	
		12–15 yr 2.9–5.4		0.95–1.75	
		16–19 yr 2.7–4.7		0.90–1.50	
Potassium	S	mmol/L		mmol/L	
		<2 mo 3.0–7.0	×1	3.0–7.0	r (Meites, 1989)
		2–12 mo 3.5–6.0		3.5–6.0	Increased by hemolysis; serum values systematically higher than plasma values
		>12 mo 3.5–5.0		3.5–5.0	
	P(H)	3.5–4.5 mmol/L		3.5–4.5 mmol/L	
Prealbumin (transthyretin)	P	mg/L		mg/L	
		2–6 mo 142–330	×1	142–330	s (Sherry et al., 1988)
		6–12 mo 120–274		120–274	
		1–3 yr 108–259		108–259	
Protein, total	S	g/dL		g/L	(Meites, 1989)
		Premature 4.3–7.6	×10	43–76	
		Newborn 4.6–7.4		46–74	
		1–7 yr 6.1–7.9		61–79	
		8–12 yr 6.4–8.1		64–81	
		13–19 yr 6.6–8.2		66–82	
Pyruvate	W	7–17 yr 0.076 ± 0.026 mmol/L	×1	0.076 ± 0.026 mmol/L	(Pianosi et al., 1995)
Sodium	S,P (LiH,NH_4H)	mmol/L		mmol/L	
		Newborn 134–146	×1	134–146	
		Infant 139–146		139–146	
		Child 138–145		138–146	
		Thereafter 136–146		136–146	
Thyroid-stimulating hormone	S	Premature (28–36 wk) mIU/L		mIU/L	
		1st wk of life 0.7–27.0	×1	0.7–27.0	(Nichols Institute Diagnostics)
		Term infants			
		Cord blood 2.3–13.2		2.3–13.2	
		1–2 days 3.2–34.6		3.2–34.6	
		3–4 days 0.7–15.4		0.7–15.4	
		2–20 wk 1.7–9.1		1.7–9.1	
		21 wk–20 yr 0.7–6.4		0.7–6.4	
Thyroid uptake of radioactive iodine	Activity over thyroid gland	2 hr <6%	×0.01	2 hr <0.06	
		6 hr 3–20%		6 hr 0.03–0.20	
		24 hr 8–30%		24 hr 0.08–0.30	
Thyroid uptake of technetium 99 m	Activity over thyroid gland	After 24 hr 0.4–3.0%	×0.01	Fractional uptake 0.004–0.030	
Thyrotropin-releasing hormone (hTRH)	P	5–60 pg/mL	×2.759	14–165 pmol/L	
Thyroxine-binding globulin (TBG)	S	mg/dL		mg/L	
		Cord blood 1.4–9.4	×10	14–94	
		1–4 wk 1.0–9.0		10–90	
		1–12 mo 2.0–7.6		20–76	
		1–5 yr 2.9–5.4		29–54	
		5–10 yr 2.5–5.0		25–50	
		10–15 yr 2.1–4.6		21–46	
		Adult 1.5–3.4		15–34	
Thyroxine, total	S	Full-term infants	×12.9	Full-term infants	(Esoterix Endocrinology)
		μg/dL		nmol/L	
		1–3 days 8.2–19.9		1–3 days 106–256	
		1 wk 6.0–15.9		1 wk 77–205	
		1–12 mo 6.1–14.9		1–12 mo 79–192	
		Prepubertal children		Prepubertal children	
		1–3 yr 6.8–13.5		1–3 yr 88–174	
		3–10 yr 5.5–12.8		3–10 yr 71–165	
		Pubertal children and adults		Pubertal children and adults	
		4.2–13.0		54–167	

TABLE 715-6. Reference Ranges*†—cont'd

ANALYTE OR PROCEDURE	SPECIMEN	REFERENCE VALUES (USA)		CONVERSION FACTOR	REFERENCE VALUES (SI)		COMMENTS
Thyroxine, free	S	Newborn infants	ng/dL	×12.9	Full-term infants	pmol/L	(Esoterix Endocrinology)
		3 days	2.0–4.9		3 days	26–63	
		Infants	0.9–2.6		Infants	12–33	
		Prepubertal children	0.8–2.2		Prepubertal children	10–28	
		Pubertal children and adults	0.8–2.3		Pubertal children and adults	10–30	
Thyroxine, total	W	Newborn screen (filter paper)	6.2–22.0 μg/dL	×12.9	80–283 nmol/L		
Triidothyronine, free	S		pg/dL		pmol/L		
		Cord blood	20–240	×0.01536	0.3–3.7		
		1–3 dys	200–610		3.1–9.4		
		6 wk	240–560		3.7–8.6		
		Adult (20–50 yr)	230–660		3.5–10.0		
Triiodothyronine resin uptake test (T_3RU)	S				Fractional uptake		
		Newborn 26–36%		×0.01	0.26–0.36		
		Thereafter 26–35%			0.26–0.35		
Triiodothyronine, total	S		ng/dL		nmol/L		
		Cord blood	30–70	×0.0154	0.46–1.08		
		Newborn	75–260		1.16–4.00		
		1–5 yr	100–260		1.54–4.00		
		5–10 yr	90–240		1.39–3.70		
		10–15 yr	80–210		1.23–3.23		
		Thereafter	115–190		1.77–2.93		
Urea nitrogen	S,P		mg/dL		mmol urea/L		
		Cord blood	21–40	×0.357	7.5–14.3		
		Premature (1 wk)	3–25		1.1–9.0		
		Newborn	3–12		1.1–4.3		
		Infant or child	5–18		1.8–6.4		
		Thereafter	7–18		2.5–6.4		
Uric acid	S		mg/dL		μmol/L		j (Meites, 1989)
		1–5 yr	1.7–5.8	×59.48	100–350		
		6–11 yr	2.2–6.6		130–390		
		M 12–19 yr	3.0–7.7		180–460		
		F 12–19 yr	2.7–5.7		160–340		

***A more comprehensive list of reference ranges can be found online at: *www.nelsonpediatics.com*.**

†In preparing the reference range listings, a number of abbreviations, symbols, and codes were used (see Table 715-2).

American Diabetes Association: Report of the Expert Committee on the Diagnosis and Classification of Diabetes Mellitus. *Diabetes Care* 1997;20:1183–1197.
Bonnefont JP, Specola NB, Vassault A, et al: The fasting test in children: Application to the diagnosis of pathological hypo- and hyperketotic states. *Eur J Pediatr* 1990;150:80–85.
Buck ML: Anticoagulation with warfarin in infants and children. *Ann Pharmacother* 1996;30:1316–1322.
Diaz J, Tornel PL, Martinez P: Reference intervals for blood ammonia in healthy subjects, determined by microdiffusion. *Clin Chem* 1995;41:1048.
Esoterix Endocrinology, Calabasas Hills, CA 91301.
Ghoshal A, Soldin S: Evaluation of the Dade Behring dimension R × L: Integrated chemistry system-pediatric reference ranges. *Clin Chim Acta* 2003;331:135–146.
Gillard BK, Simbala JA, Goodglick L: Reference intervals for amylase isoenzymes in serum and plasma of infants and children. *Clin Chem* 1983;29:1119–1123.
Jedeikin R, Makela SK, Shennan AT, et al: Creatine kinase isoenzymes in serum from cord blood and the blood of healthy full-term infants during the first three postnatal days. *Clin Chem* 1982;28:317–322.
Kaplan EL, Rothermel CD, Johnson DR: Antistreptolysin O and anti-deoxyribonuclease B titers: Normal values for children ages 2 to 12 in the United States. *Pediatrics* 1998;101:86–88.
Knight JA, Haymond RE: γ-Glutamyltransferase and alkaline phosphatase activities compared in serum of normal children and children with liver disease. *Clin Chem* 1981;27:48–51.
Lockitch G, Halstead AC, Wadsworth L, et al: Age-and sex-specific pediatric reference intervals and correlations for zinc, copper, selenium, iron, vitamins A and E, and related proteins. *Clin Chem* 1988;34:1625–1628.
Meites S (editor): *Pediatric Clinical Chemistry, Reference (Normal) Values,* 3rd ed. Washington, DC, American Association for Clinical Chemistry, 1989.
Muntau A, Streiter M, Kappler M, et al: Age-related reference values for serum selenium concentrations in infants and children. *Clin Chem* 2002;48:555–560.
Nichols Institute Diagnostics, San Juan Capistrano, CA 92675.
Nir A, Bar-Oz B, Perles Z, et al: N-terminal pro-B-type natriuretic peptide: Reference plasma levels from birth to adolescence. Elevated levels at birth and in infants and children with heart diseases. *Acta Paediatr* 2004;93:603–607.
Pianosi P, Seargeant L, Haworth JC: Blood lactate and pyruvate concentrations, and their ratio during exercise in healthy children: Developmental perspective. *Eur J Appl Physiol Occup Physiol* 1995;71:518–522.
Rosenthal P, Pesce MA: Long-term monitoring of D-lactic acidosis in a child. J Pediatr Gastroenterol Nutr 1985;4:674–676.
Sherry B, Jack RM, Weber A, et al: Reference interval for prealbumin for children 2 to 36 months old. *Clin Chem* 1988;34:1878–1880.
Soldin O, Bierbower L, Choi J, et al: Serum iron, ferritin, transferrin, total iron binding capacity, hs-CRP, LDL cholesterol and magnesium in children. New reference intervals using the Dade Dimension Clinical Chemistry System. *Clin Chim Acta* 2004;342:211–217.
Soldin SJ, Hicks JM, Bailey J, et al: Pediatric reference ranges for 25 hydroxy vitamin D during the summer and winter. *Clin Chem* 1997;43:S200.

TABLE 715-7. Composition of Commonly Used Oral and Parenteral Solutions (Raymond Adelman and Michael Solhaug) [see related conversion Tables 715-8 to 715-10]

FLUID	CARBOHYDRATE (g/dL)	PROTEIN*	CALORIES/L	Na (mEq/L)	K (mEq/L)	Cl (mEq/L)	HCO_3† (mEq/L)	Ca (mEq/L)	P‡ (mEq/L)	Mg (mEq/L)	Osm§‖ (mOsm/kg H_2O)
ORAL											
Apple juice¶	11.9	0.1	480	0	0.4	26	0	3	4.5	0	700
Coca-Cola	10.9	0	435	4.3	0.1	0	13.4	0	0	0	656
Ginger ale	9.0	0	360	3.5	0.1	0	3.6	0	0	0	565
Grape juice	16.6	0.2	672	0.4	30	0	32	0	0	0	1,027
Grapefruit juice (canned, sugar added)	17.8	0.6	736	0.2	35	0	0	6.5	0	0	591
Milk	4.9	3.5	670	22	36	28	30	60	54	0	260
Orange juice	10.4	0.7	444	0.2	49	0	50	0	0	0	654
Pepsi-Cola	12	0	480	6.5	0.8	0	7.3	0	0	0	0
Pineapple juice (canned)	13.5	0.4	556	0.2	38	0	0	7.5	9	0	783
Prune juice	19	0.4	776	0.9	60	0	0	7	20	0	0
Root beer	0	0	0	3.5	3.9	0	0	0	0	0	588
7Up	8.0	0	320	7.5	0.2	0	0	0.3	0	0	564
Tomato juice (canned, salted)	4.3	0	172	100	59	150	10	3	18	0	592
Gatorade	5.9	0	250	21	2.5	17	0	0	6.8	0	377
Hydralyte	2.5	0	100	84	10	59	15	<1	<1	0	300
Lytren	7.0	0	280	30	25	25	36	4	5	4	267§‖
Pedialyte	5.0	0	200	30	20	30	28	4	0	4	387
Rhydrate	2.5	0	100	75	25	65	30	0	0	0	305
Resol Solution	2.0	0	83	50	20	50	34	4	5	4	269
Ricelyte Oral Solution (rice syrup solids)	3.0	0	140	50	25	45	34	0	0	0	200
PARENTERAL											
Carbohydrate# in H_2O	5–10	0	200–400	0	0	0	0	0	0	0	266–532
Isotonic saline	0–5	0	0–200	154	0	154	0	0	0	0	292–558
½ isotonic saline	2.5–5	0	100–200	77	0	77	0	0	0	0	280–415
3% (M/2) saline	0	0	0	513	0	513	513	0	0	0	969
5% saline	0	0	0	855	0	855	855	0	0	0	1,616
M/6 sodium lactate	0	0	0	167	0	0	167	0	0	0	0
5% sodium bicarbonate	0	0	0	595	0	0	595	0	0	0	0
Lactated Ringer solution	0–5–10	0	0–20	130	4	109	28	3	0	0	261–531–801
			0–40	0	0	0	0	0	0	0	0
			0	0	0	0	0	0	0	0	0
Modified Butler 1 (a)	5	0	200	25	20	22	23	0	3	3	360
Modified Butler 2 (b)	5–10	0	200–400	56	25	49	26	0	12	5	423–719
Talbot (c)	5	0	200	40	35	40	20	0	15	0	409
Human plasma protein fraction (d)	0	5	0	130	2	50	50	0	0	0	0
Blood	0	3	0	95	4	50	40	0	2	1–2	0
Dextran 10% (low molecular weight) [e]	5	0	200	0	0	0	0	0	0	0	0
Dextran 10% in saline (f)	0	0	0	154	0	154	0	0	0	0	0
Dextran 6% (high molecular weight) [g]	5–10	0	200–400	0	0	0	0	0	0	0	0
Dextran 6% in saline (h)	0	0	0	154	0	154	0	0	0	0	0
Mannitol 20%**	0	0	0	0	0	0	0	0	0	0	0

AVAILABLE ADDITIVES

Glucose 50%	0.5 g/mL
Sodium chloride	2.5 and 5 mEq/mL
Sodium acetate	2 and 4 mEq/mL
Sodium lactate	5 mEq/mL
Sodium bicarbonate	0.5 (4.2%) mEq/mL and 0.9 (7.5%) mEq/mL
Potassium acetate	2 and 4 mEq/mL
Potassium chloride	2 and 3 mEq/mL
Potassium phosphate	4.4 mEq/mL of potassium and 3 mM/mL of phosphate
Calcium gluconate 10%	9.3 mg (0.465 mEq/mL) elemental calcium
Calcium chloride 10%	27.3 mg (1.4 mEq/mL) elemental calcium
Ammonium chloride	5 mEq/mL
Magnesium sulfate	0.8 mEq/mL, 1 mEq/mL, and 4 mEq/mL available as the 10%, 12.5%, and 50% solutions

SELECTED COMMERCIAL PREPARATIONS IN THE UNITED STATES (POSSIBLE SLIGHT VARIATIONS IN COMPOSITION FROM VALUES IN TABLE)

(a)	Ionosol MB in D_5W (A), Isolyte P with 5% dextrose (M)
(b)	Ionosol B in D_5W (A), Electrolyte #2 with 10% invert sugar (C,M), 10% Travert in electrolyte #2 (B)
(c)	Ionosol T in D_5W (A), Isolyte M (M)
(d)	Plasmatein (A), Plasmanate (C)
(e) (f)	LMD 10% (A), dextran 40 (C,M), Rheomacrodex (P), Gentran 40 (B)
(g) (h)	Dextran 70 (A), Macrodex (P), Gentran 75 in 10% Travert (B)

(A-Abbott; B-Baxter; C-Cutter; M-McGraw; P-Pharmacia)

¶Pennington JAT (editor): *Bowes & Church's Food Values of Portions Commonly Used*, 17th ed. Philadelphia, Lippincott Williams & Wilkins, 1997.

*Protein or amino acid equivalent.
†Actual or potential bicarbonate, such as acetate, lactate, or citrate.
‡Calculated according to a valence of 1.8.
§Osmolality, except for values shown (‖), which are osmolarity (in mOsm/L).
¶Composition varies slightly, depending on source.
#Red cell contents not included in calculations.
**Also available: mannitol 5%, 10%, 15%, and 20%.
††Glucose (dextrose, fructose, or invert sugar).

Sources: Pennington JAT (editor): *Bowes & Church's Food Values of Portions Commonly Used*, 17th ed. Philadelphia, Lippincott Williams & Wilkins, 1997; Olin BR (editor): *Facts and Comparisons*. Philadelphia, JB Lippincott, 1993; Murray BN, Peterson LJ: Unpublished observations. Additional values in Wendland BE, Arbus GS: Oral fluid therapy: Sodium and potassium content and osmolality of some commercial soups, juices and beverages. *Can Med Assoc J* 1979;121:564.

TABLE 715-8. Method for Conversion of Milligrams to Milliequivalents per Liter (or to Millimoles per Liter)

mg = milligrams　　mL = milliliter
g = grams　　1 mL = 1.000027 cc
dL = deciliter = 100 mL

$$\text{mEq/L (milliequivalents per liter)} = \frac{\text{mg/L}}{\text{Equivalent weight}}$$

$$\text{Equivalent weight} = \frac{\text{Atomic weight}}{\text{Valence of element}}$$

Example: A sample of blood serum contains 10 mg of Ca in 1 dL (100 mL).
The valence of Ca is 2, and the atomic weight is 40. The equivalent weight of Ca is therefore 40 ÷ 2, or 20.
Milliequivalents of Ca per liter are 10 (mg/dL) × 10 (dL/L) ÷ 20, or 5 milliequivalents per liter.

$$\text{mmol/L (millimoles per liter)} = \frac{\text{mg/L}}{\text{Molecular weight}}$$

TABLE 715-9. Factors of Conversion of Concentration Expressed in Milliequivalents per Liter to Milligrams per Deciliter (100 L), and Vice Versa, for Common Ions that Occur in Physiologic Solutions

ELEMENT OR RADICAL	mEq/L to mg/dL		mg/dL to mEq/L	
Sodium	1	2.30	1	0.4348
Potassium	1	3.91	1	0.2558
Calcium	1	2.005	1	0.4988
Magnesium	1	1.215	1	0.8230
Chloride	1	3.55	1	0.2817
Bicarbonate (HCO_3^-)	1	6.1	1	0.1639
Phosphorus valence 1	1	3.10	1	0.3226
Phosphorus valence 1.8	1	1.72	1	0.5814
Sulfur valence 2	1	1.60	1	0.625

Example: To convert milliequivalents of magnesium per liter to milligrams per deciliter (100 mL), multiply by the factor 1.215; to convert milligrams of potassium per deciliter (100 mL) to milliequivalents per liter, multiply by the factor 0.2558.

TABLE 715-10. Milliequivalents and Milligrams of Cations and Anions Present in 1 Millimole of Salts Commonly Used in Physiologic Solutions

SALT	SALT (mg/mmol)	CATION	SALT (mEq/mmol)	SALT (mg/mmol)	ANION	SALT (mEq/mmol)	SALT (mg/mmol)
Sodium chloride (NaCl)	58.5	Na^+	1	23.0	Cl^-	1	35.5
Potassium chloride (KCl)	74.6	K^+	1	39.1	Cl^-	1	35.5
Sodium bicarbonate ($NaHCO_3$)	84.0	Na^+	1	23.0	HCO_3^-	1	61.0
Sodium lactate ($CH_3CHOHCOONa$)	112.0	Na^+	1	23.0	$CH_3CHOHCOO^-$	1	89.0
Potassium phosphate monobasic (K_2HPO_4)	174.2	K^+	1	78.2	HPO_4^{2-}	2	96.0
Potassium phosphate dibasic (KH_2PO_4)	136.1	K^+	1	39.1	$H_2PO_4^-$	1	97.0
Calcium chloride, anhydrous ($CaCl_2$)	111.0	Ca^{2+}	2	40.0	Cl_2^{2-}	2	71.0
Calcium chloride dihydrate ($CaCl_2 \cdot 2H_2O$)	147.0	Ca^{2+}	2	40.0	Cl_2^{2-}	2	71.0
Magnesium chloride, anhydrous ($MgCl_2$)	95.2	Mg^{2+}	2	24.3	Cl_2^{2-}	2	71.0
Magnesium chloride hexahydrate ($MgCl_2 \cdot 6H_2O$)	203.3	Mg^{2+}	2	24.3	Cl_2^{2-}	2	71.0
Ammonium chloride (NH_4Cl)	53.5	NH_4^+	1	18.0	Cl^-	1	35.5

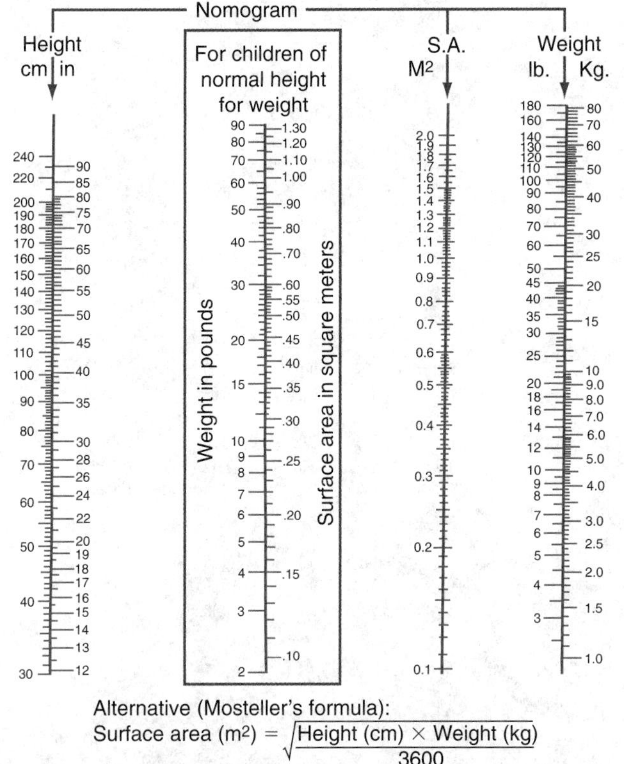

Figure 715-1. Nomogram for the estimation of surface area. The surface area is indicated where a straight line that connects the height and weight levels intersects the surface area column, or if the patient is roughly of average size, from the weight alone *(enclosed area)*. (Nomogram modified from the data of E. Boyd by C. D. West. See also Briars GL, Bailey BJ: Surface area estimation: Pocket calculator v nomogram. *Arch Dis Child* 1994;70:246–247.)

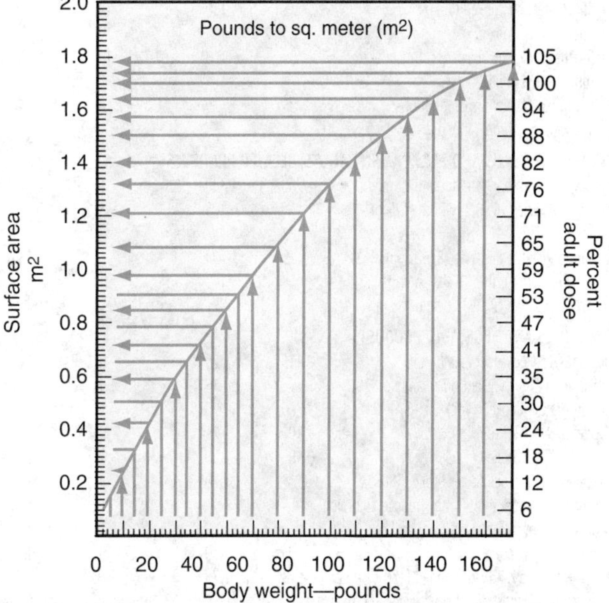

Figure 715-2. Relationships among body weight (lb), body surface area, and adult dosage. The surface area values correspond with those set forth by Crawford JD, Terry ME, Rourke GM: Simplification of drug dosage calculation by application of the surface area principle. *Pediatrics* 1950;5:783–790. Note that the 100% adult dose is for a patient weighing approximately 140 lb and having a surface area of approximately 1.7 M². (From Talbot NB, Richie RH, Crawford JH: *Metabolic Homeostasis: A Syllabus for Those Concerned with the Care of Patients.* Cambridge, Harvard University Press, 1959.)

TABLE 715-11. Food Composition for Short Method of Dietary Analysis (Lewis A. Barness and John S. Curran)*

FOOD AND APPROXIMATE MEASURE	WEIGHT (g)	FOOD ENERGY (kcal)	PROTEIN (g)	FAT (g)	CARBOHYDRATE (g)	CALCIUM (mg)	IRON (mg)	VITAMIN A (IU)	THIAMINE (mg)	RIBOFLAVIN (mg)	NIACIN (mg)	ASCORBIC ACID (mg)
MILK, CHEESE, CREAM; RELATED PRODUCTS												
Cheese: blue, cheddar (1 in^3), 17 g, cheddar	30	105	6	9	1	165	0.2	345	0.01	0.12	Trace	0
process (1 oz), Swiss (1 oz) cottage (from skim) creamed (½ c)	115	120	16	5	3	105	0.4	190	0.04	0.28	0.1	0
Cream: half and half (cream and milk) [2 tbs]	30	40	1	4	2	30	Trace	145	0.01	0.04	Trace	Trace
For light whipping, add 1 pat butter												
Milk: whole (3.5% fat) [1 c] fluid, nonfat (skim),	245	160	9	9	12	285	0.1	350	0.08	0.42	0.1	2
and buttermilk (from skim)	245	90	9	Trace	13	300	Trace	0	0.10	0.44	0.2	2
Milk beverage (1 c): cocoa, chocolate drink made with skim milk	245	210	8	8	26	280	0.6	300	0.09	0.43	0.3	Trace
For malted milk, add 4 tbs half and half (270 g)												
Milk desserts, custard (1 c), 248 g, ice cream (8 fl oz), 142 g		290	8	17	29	210	0.4	785	0.07	0.34	0.1	1
Cornstarch pudding (248 g), ice milk (1 c) 187 g		280	9	10	40	290	0.1	390	0.08	0.41	0.3	2
White sauce, medium (½ c)	130	215	5	16	12	150	0.2	610	0.06	0.22	0.3	Trace
Egg: 1 Large	50	80	6	6	Trace	25	1.2	590	0.06	0.15	Trace	0
MEAT, POULTRY, FISH, SHELLFISH, RELATED PRODUCTS												
Beef, lamb, veal: lean and fat, cooked, including corned beef (3 oz) [all cuts]	85	245	22	16	0	10	2.9	25	0.06	0.19	4.2	0
lean only, cooked; dried beef (2+ oz) [all cuts]	65	140	20	5	0	10	2.4	10	0.05	0.16	3.4	0
Beef, relatively fat, such as steak and rib, cooked (3 oz)	85	350	18	30	0	10	2.4	60	0.05	0.14	3.5	0
Liver: beef, fried (2 oz)	55	130	15	6	3	5	5.0	30,280	0.15	2.37	9.4	15
Pork, lean and fat, cooked (3 oz) [all cuts]	85	325	20	24	0	10	2.6	0	0.62	0.20	4.2	0
lean only, cooked (2+ oz) [all cuts]	60	150	18	8	0	5	2.2	0	0.57	0.19	3.2	0
ham, light cure, lean and fat, roasted (3 oz)	85	245	18	19	0	10	2.2	0	0.40	0.16	3.1	0
Luncheon meats: bologna (2 slices), pork sausage, cooked (2 oz), frankfurter (1), bacon, broiled or fried crisp (3 slices)		185	9	16	0	5	1.3	0	0.21	0.12	1.7	0
Chicken: flesh only, broiled (3 oz)	85	115	20	3	0	10	1.4	80	0.05	0.16	7.4	0
fried (2+ oz)	75	170	24	6	1	10	1.6	85	0.05	0.23	8.3	0
Turkey, light and dark, roasted (3 oz)	85	160	27	5	0	0	1.5	0	0.03	0.15	6.5	0
Salmon, canned (3 oz)	85	130	17	5	0	165	0.7	60	0.03	0.16	6.8	0
Fish sticks, breaded, cooked (3–4)	75	130	13	7	5	10	0.3	0	0.03	0.05	1.2	0
Mackerel, halibut, cooked	85	175	19	10	0	10	0.8	515	0.08	0.15	6.8	0
Bluefish, haddock, herring, perch, shad, cooked (tuna canned in oil, 20 g)	85	160	19	8	2	20	1.0	60	0.06	0.11	4.4	0
Clams, canned; crab meat, canned; lobster; oyster, raw; scallop; shrimp, canned	85	75	14	1	2	65	2.5	65	0.10	0.08	1.5	0
MATURE DRY BEANS AND PEAS, NUTS, PEANUTS, RELATED PRODUCTS												
Beans: white with pork and tomato, canned (1 c)	260	320	16	7	50	140	4.7	340	0.20	0.08	1.5	5
Red (128 g), lima (96 g), cowpeas (125 g), cooked (½ c)		125	8	0	25	35	2.5	5	0.13	0.06	0.7	0
Nuts: almonds (12), cashews (8), peanuts (1 tbs), peanut butter (1 tbs), pecans (12), English walnuts (2 tbs), coconut (¼ c)	15	95	3	8	4	15	0.5	5	0.05	0.9	0	
VEGETABLES AND VEGETABLE PRODUCTS												
Asparagus, cooked, cut spears (⅔ c)	115	25	3	Trace	4	25	0.7	1,055	0.19	0.20	1.6	30
Beans: green (½ c), cooked, 60 g; canned, 120 g		15	1	Trace	3	30	0.4	340	0.04	0.06	0.3	8
Lima, immature, cooked (½ c)	80	90	6	1	16	40	2.0	225	0.14	0.08	1.0	14
Broccoli spears, cooked (⅔ c)	100	25	3	Trace	4	90	0.8	2,500	0.09	0.20	0.8	90
Brussels sprouts, cooked (⅔ c)	85	30	3	Trace	5	30	1.0	450	0.07	0.12	0.7	75
Cabbage (110 g); cauliflower, cooked (80 g); sauerkraut, canned (150 mg) [reduce ascorbic acid value by ⅓ for sauerkraut] [⅔ c]		20	1	Trace	4	35	0.5	80	0.05	0.05	0.3	37
Carrots, cooked (⅔ c)	95	30	1	Trace	7	30	0.6	10,145	0.05	0.05	0.5	6
Corn, 1 ear, cooked (140 g); canned (130 g) [½ c]		75	2	Trace	18	5	0.4	315	0.06	0.06	1.1	6
Leafy greens: collards (125 g), dandelions (120 g), kale (75 g), mustard (95 g), spinach (120 g), turnip (100 g cooked, 150 g canned) [⅔ c] cooked and canned)		30	3	Trace	5	175	1.8	8.570	0.11	0.18	0.8	45
Peas, green (½ c)	80	60	4	1	10	20	1.4	430	0.22	0.09	1.8	16
Potatoes: baked, boiled (100 g), 10 pieces		85	3	Trace	30	10	0.7	Trace	0.08	0.04	1.5	16
French fried (55 g) [for fried, add 1 tbs cooking oil]												
Pumpkin, canned (½ c)	115	40	1	1	9	30	0.5	7,295	0.03	0.06	0.6	6
Squash, winter, canned (½ c)	100	65	2	1	16	30	0.8	4,305	0.05	0.14	0.7	14
Sweet potato, canned (½ c)	110	120	2	0	27	25	0.8	8,500	0.05	0.05	0.7	15
Tomato, 1 raw, ⅔ c canned, ⅔ c juice	150	35	2	Trace	7	14	0.8	1,350	0.10	0.06	1.0	29
Tomato catsup (2 tbs)	35	30	1	Trace	8	10	0.2	480	0.04	0.02	0.6	6
Other, cooked (beets, mushrooms, onions, turnips) [½ c]	95	25	1	0	5	20	0.5	15	0.02	0.10	0.7	7

TABLE 715-11. Food Composition for Short Method of Dietary Analysis (Lewis A. Barness and John S. Curran)*—cont'd

Other, commonly served raw, cabbage (½ c, 50 g), celery (3 small stalks, 40 g), cucumber (¼, 30 g), radishes (5, 40 g) medium, 50 g), green pepper (½) carrots, raw (½ carrot), lettuce leaves (2 large)		10	Trace	Trace	2	15	0.3	100	0.03	0.03	0.2	20
	25	10	Trace	Trace	2	10	0.2	2,750	0.02	0.02	0.2	2
	50	10	1	Trace	2	34	0.7	950	0.03	0.04	0.2	9
FRUITS AND FRUIT PRODUCTS												
Cantaloupe (½ medium)	385	60	1	Trace	14	25	0.8	6,540	0.08	0.06	1.2	63
Citrus and strawberries: orange (1), grapefruit (½, juice (½ c), strawberries (½ c), lemon (1), tangerine (1)		50	1	0	13	25	0.4	165	0.08	0.03	0.3	55
Yellow, fresh: apricots (3), peach (2 medium); canned fruit and juice (½ c) or dried, cooked, unsweetened: apricot, peaches (½ c)		85	0	0	22	10	1.1	1,005	0.01	0.05	1.0	5
Other, dried: dates, pitted (4), figs (2), raisins (¼ c)	40	120	1	0	31	35	1.4	20	0.04	0.04	0.5	0
Other, fresh apple (1), banana (1), figs (3), pear (1)		80	0	0	21	15	0.5	140	0.04	0.03	0.2	6
GRAIN PRODUCTS												
Enriched and whole grain: bread (1 slice, 23 g), biscuit (½), cooked cereal (½ c), prepared cereal (1 oz), graham crackers (2 large), macaroni, noodles, spaghetti (½ c, cooked), pancake (1, 27 g), roll (½), waffle (½, 38 g)		65	2	1	16	20	0.6	10	0.09	0.05	0.7	0
Unenriched bread (1 slice, 23 g), cooked cereal (½ c), macaroni, noodles, spaghetti (½ c), popcorn (½ c), pretzel sticks, small (15), roll (½)		65	2	1	16	10	0.3	5	0.02	0.02	0.3	0
Cake, plain (1 piece), doughnut (1). For iced cake or doughnut, add value for sugar (1 tbs). For chocolate cake, add chocolate (30 g)	45	145	2	5	24	30	0.4	65	0.02	0.05	0.2	0
Cookies, plain (1)	25	120	1	5	18	10	0.2	20	0.01	0.01	0.01	0
Pie crust, single crust (1/7 shell)	20	95	1	6	8	3	0.3	0	0.04	0.03	0.3	0
Flour, white, enriched (1 tbs)	7	25	1	Trace	5	1	0.2	0	0.03	0.02	0.2	0
FATS AND OILS												
Butter, margarine (1 pat, ½ tbs)	7	50	Trace	6	Trace	1	0	230	0	0	0	0
Fats and oils, cooking (1 tbs), French dressing (2 tbs)	14	125	0	14	0	0	0	0	0	0	0	0
Salad dressing, mayonnaise-type (1 tbs)	15	80	Trace	9	1	2	0.1	45	Trace	Trace	Trace	0
SUGARS, SWEETS												
Candy, plain (½ oz), jam and jelly (1 tbs), syrup (1 tbs), gelatin dessert, plain (½ c), beverage, carbonated (1 c)		60	0	0	14	3	0.1	Trace	Trace	Trace	Trace	Trace
Chocolate fudge (1 oz), chocolate syrup (3 tbs)		125	1	2	30	15	0.6	10	Trace	0.02	0.1	Trace
Molasses (1 tbs), caramel (½ oz)		40	Trace	Trace	8	20	0.3	Trace	Trace	Trace	Trace	Trace
Sugar (1 tbs)	12	45	0	0	12	0	Trace	0	0	0	0	0
MISCELLANEOUS												
Chocolate, bitter (1 oz)	30	145	3	15	8	20	1.9	20	0.01	0.07	0.4	0
Sherbet (½ c)	96	130	1	1	30	15	Trace	55	0.01	0.03	Trace	2
SOUPS												
Bean, pea (green) [1 c]		150	7	4	22	50	1.6	495	0.09	0.06	1.0	4
Noodle, beef, chicken (1 c)		65	4	2	7	10	0.7	50	0.03	0.04	0.9	Trace
Clam chowder, minestrone, tomato, vegetable (1 c)		90	3	2	14	25	0.9	1,880	0.05	0.04	1.1	3

*See related conversion tables (Tables 715–8 to 715–10).

From Wilson ED, Fisher KH, Fuqua ME: *Principles of Nutrition*, 2nd ed. New York, John Wiley & Sons, 1965, pp. 528–533.

TABLE 715-12. Nutritive Value of Baby Foods (Per Serving)*

FOOD	SERVING (G)	ENERGY (KCAL)	PROTEIN (G)	FAT (G)	CARBOHYDRATE (G)	SODIUM (MG)	CALCIUM (MG)	IRON (MG)	VITAMIN A (IU)	THIAMINE (MG)	RIBOFLAVIN (MG)	NIACIN (MG)	ASCORBIC ACID (MG)
CEREALS													
Barley	2.4	9	0.3	0.1	1.8	1	19	1.1		0.07	0.07	0.9	0
High protein	2.4	9	0.9	0.1	1.1	1	17	1.8		0.06	0.07	0.8	0
Mixed	2.4	9	0.3	0.1	1.8	1	18	1.5		0.06	0.07	0.8	0
Oatmeal	2.4	10	0.3	0.2	1.7	1	18	1.8		0.07	0.06	0.9	0
Rice	2.4	9	0.2	0.1	1.9	1	20	1.8		0.06	0.05	0.8	0
DINNERS, JAR													
Beef and egg noodle	213	122	5.4	4.0	15.7	37	18	0.9	1,400	0.06	0.08	1.2	3
Chicken and noodles, jr.	213	109	4.1	3.0	16.1	36	36	0.8	1,900	0.06	0.07	1.1	3
Macaroni and ham, jr.	213	127	6.8	2.9	18.0	101	159	0.8	1,100	0.12	0.21	1.7	5
Turkey and rice, jr.	213	104	3.8	2.9	15.3	33	50	0.6	2,200	0.02	0.06	0.6	3
Spaghetti, tomato, beef, jr.	213	135	5.4	2.7	21.6	42	39	1.1	1,500	0.14	0.15	2.3	5
FRUITS													
Applesauce, jr.	213	79	0.1	0.0	21.9	5	10	0.4	20	0.03	0.06	0.1	81
Applesauce, apricots, jr.	220	104	0.5	0.5	27.3	6	13	0.6	745	0.03	0.07	0.3	39
Bananas, tapioca, jr.	220	147	0.8	0.4	39.1	21	17	0.7	100	0.03	0.04	0.5	57
Peaches	220	157	1.3	0.4	41.6	10	11	0.6	400	0.03	0.07	1.4	42
Pears	213	93	0.6	0.2	24.7	4	18	0.5	70	0.03	0.06	0.4	47
MEATS, POULTRY													
Beef	99	105	14.3	4.9	0	65	8	1.6	100	0.01	0.16	3.3	2
Chicken	99	148	14.6	9.5	0	50	54	1.0	200	0.01	0.16	3.4	2
Ham	99	123	14.9	6.6	0	66	5	1.0	30	0.14	0.19	2.8	2
Lamb	99	111	15.0	5.2	2.5	73	7	1.6	30	0.02	0.20	3.2	2
Turkey	99	128	15.2	7.0	0	72	28	1.3	600	0.02	0.25	3.4	2
EGG YOLKS	94	191	9.4	16.3	0.9	37	72	2.6	1,200	0.07	0.25	1.45	1
VEGETABLES													
Beans	206	51	2.5	0.3	11.8	3	133	2.2	900	0.04	0.21	0.7	17
Beets	128	43	1.7	0.1	9.8	106	18	0.4	40	0.01	0.06	0.2	4
Carrots	213	67	1.7	0.4	15.4	104	49	0.8	25,000	0.05	0.09	1.1	12
Mixed	213	88	3.1	0.8	17.4	77	24	0.9	9,000	0.06	0.07	1.4	5
Peas	213	113	7.0	1.1	19.0	15	34	1.9	700	0.15	0.13	2.0	9
Squash	213	51	1.8	0.4	12.0	3	50	0.7	4,000	0.02	0.14	0.8	17
Sweet potatoes	220	113	2.4	0.3	30.7	49	35	0.8	15,000	0.06	0.08	0.8	21

*See related conversion tables 715-8 to 715-10. Data from Pennington JAT (editor): *Bowes and Church's Food Values of Portions Commonly Used,* 17th ed. Philadelphia, Lippincott Williams & Wilkins, 1997.

TABLE 715-13. Equivalent Temperature Readings (Celsius [C] and Fahrenheit [F])

C	F	C	F	C	F	C	F
0	32.0	37.2	99.0	39.2	102.6	41.2	106.2
20	68.0	37.4	99.3	39.4	102.9	41.4	106.5
30	86.0	37.6	99.7	39.6	103.3	41.6	106.9
31	87.8	37.8	100.1	39.8	103.7	41.8	107.2
32	89.6	38.0	100.4	40.0	104.0	42.0	107.6
33	91.7	38.2	100.8	40.2	104.4	43.0	109.4
34	93.2	38.4	101.2	40.4	104.7	44.0	111.2
35	95.0	38.6	101.5	40.6	105.1	100.0	212.0
36	96.8	38.8	101.8	40.8	105.4		
37	98.6	39.0	102.2	41.0	105.8		

*To convert Celsius (centigrade) readings to Fahrenheit, multiply by 1.8 and add 32. To convert Fahrenheit readings to Celsius, subtract 32 and divide by 1.8.

Chapter 716 ■ Medications Peter Gal and Michael D. Reed

Peter Gal and Michael D. Reed

TABLE 716-1. General Medications

DRUG (TRADE NAMES, FORMULATIONS)	INDICATIONS (MECHANISM OF ACTION AND DOSING)	COMMENTS (CAUTIONS, ADVERSE EVENTS, MONITORING)
Abciximab ReoPro Intravenous solution, 2 mg/mL in 5 mL vials.	**Inhibits platelet aggregation through inhibiting the glycoprotein Iib/IIIa receptor pathway. Used in combination with IV immunoglobulin and aspirin to accelerate regression of coronary aneurysms in Kawasaki disease. In adults, used to prevent platelet aggregation in various acute coronary syndromes and procedures.** *Children and adults:* Loading dose of 0.25 mg/kg, followed by infusion of 0.125 μg/kg/min for 12 hr.	*Adverse events:* Bleeding.
Acarbose Precose. Tablet: 25, 50, 100 mg.	**Treatment of type 2 diabetes mellitus; treatment of postprandial hypoglycemia in children after Nissen fundoplication.** *Children:* 12.5–50 mg with each feed. *Adults:* Initial dose of 25 mg tid at the start of each meal; titrate to response (max: 100 mg tid).	*Adverse events:* Flatulence, abdominal pain, diarrhea.
Acetaminophen Analgesic, non-narcotic; antipyretic. Tempra; Tylenol; multiple generic and brand-name products. Caplet: 160, 325, 500 mg. Capsule: 325, 500 mg. Drops: 100 mg/mL (15 mL); 120 mg/2.5 mL (35 mL). Granules, premeasured packs: 30 mg. Suppositories: 120, 325 mg. Combination products with acetaminophen include cough and cold preparations and those with codeine.	**Mild to moderate pain** (inhibits prostaglandin synthesis in CNS and peripheral pain impulse generation). **Fever** (inhibits hypothalamic heat regulation center). *Infants and children <12 yr:* 10–15 mg/kg/dose q 4–6 hr. *Children > 12 yr and adults:* 325–650 mg q 4–6 hr or 1,000 mg 3–4 × daily. Maximum: 5 doses/24 hr (children) or 4 g/24 hr (adults) administered PO or rectally.	*Cautions:* Overdose can cause fatal hepatic necrosis. Treat acute overdoses with acetylcysteine. Chronic concurrent use with enzyme inhibitors, especially alcohol, can lead to hepatic necrosis. Avoid aspartame-containing products in patients with phenylketonuria (e.g., chewable tablets).
Acetazolamide Diuretic, carbonic anhydrase inhibitor. Dazamide; Diamox. Capsule, sustained-release: 500 mg. Injection: 500 mg/5 mL. Tablet: 125, 250 mg.	**Hydrocephalus due to communicating intraventricular hemorrhage** (carbonic anhydrase inhibition decreases cerebrospinal fluid production). *Neonates:* 25 mg/kg/24 hr to start, and increase to bid, tid, and qid over 4–7 days. **Glaucoma** (carbonic anhydrase inhibition decreases formation of aqueous humor). *Children:* 8–30 mg/kg/24 hr PO divided q 6–8 hr or 20–40 mg/kg/24 hr IV divided q 6 hr. **Epilepsy, as adjunct to other drugs in refractory seizures** (uncertain mechanism). *Children and adults:* 8–30 mg/kg/24 hr in 1–4 divided doses (max: 1 g/24 hr). **Edema** (diuretic). *Children:* 5 mg/kg/24 hr IV or PO. *Adults:* 250–375 mg/24 hr IV or PO.	*Caution:* Used in combination with furosemide for hydrocephalus. Reduce dose and extend dosing interval if renal function is compromised. Avoid if patient has sulfa allergy. IM route very painful because of alkaline pH of drug. *Adverse events:* Metabolic acidosis, hypochloremia, hypokalemia, nausea, anorexia, drowsiness, fatigue, muscle weakness, renal calculi.
Acetylcysteine Antidote, acetaminophen; mucolytic agent. Mucomyst; Mucosil; Mucosol. Solution, as sodium: 10% (100 mg/mL) [4, 10, 30 mL]; 20% (200 mg/mL) [4, 10, 30, 100 mL].	**Mucolytic** (free sulfhydryl group opens up disulfide bonds in mucoproteins, lowering viscosity). Dose based on 10% solution or diluted 20% solution (1 : 1) for inhalation. *Infants:* 2–4 mL tid–qid. *Children:* 6–10 mL tid–qid. *Adolescents:* 10 mL tid–qid. Acute acetaminophen overdose (provides alternative metabolic pathway for conjugation of toxic metabolites, restoring normal glutathione levels). *Children and adults:* 140 mg/kg loading dose, followed by 70 mg/kg q 4 hr for 17 doses. Repeat dose if emesis occurs within 1 hr of administration.	*Cautions:* Give a bronchodilator 10–15 min before nebulized Mucomyst to avoid bronchospasm. Follow treatment with chest percussion and suction to manage increased secretions. Dilute nebulized doses with saline or sterile water and oral solutions with soft drinks or orange juice. Prepare inhaled as 1 : 1 and PO as 1 : 3 solutions. *Adverse events:* Stomatitis nausea, vomiting, urticaria. *Monitoring:* Check acetaminophen concentration no earlier than 4 hr post overdose. Give complete acetylcysteine course, regardless of acetaminophen concentrations.
Adenosine Antiarrhythmic agent, miscellaneous. Adenocard. Injection, preservative-free: 3 mg/mL (2 mL).	**Paroxysmal supraventricular tachycardia** treatment (slows conduction time through the AV node). *Neonates and children:* 0.05 mg/kg IV push, then increase bolus doses by 0.05 mg/kg q 2 min until a clinical response occurs or a maximum dose of either 0.25 mg/kg or 12 mg is achieved. *Adults:* 6 mg IV push; if no response in 2 min, give 12 mg IV push. May repeat 12 mg IV bolus if needed.	*Cautions:* Use a peripheral IV site. May cause bronchoconstriction in asthmatics. Methylxanthines (e.g., theophylline or caffeine) antagonize adenosine effects, so higher adenosine doses are needed Contraindicated in 2nd or 3rd degree AV block or sick sinus syndrome. *Adverse events:* Heart block, flushing, chest palpitations, bradycardia, hypotension, dyspnea, headache, dizziness, nausea. *Monitoring:* Continuous ECG, blood pressure, respirations.
Albumin, human Blood product derivative; plasma volume expander. Albuminar; Albumisol; Albutein; Buminate; Plasbumin. Injection: 5%. (50 mg/mL) [50, 250, 500, 1,000]; 25% (250 mg/mL) [10, 20, 50, 100 mL].	**Plasma volume expansion and treatment of hypovolemia** (increases intravascular oncotic pressure and mobilizes fluid from interstitium to intravascular space). *Neonates:* 0.5–1 g/kg/dose (max: 1 g/kg/24 hr). *Infants and children:* 0.5–1 g/kg/dose (max: 6 g/kg/24 hr). *Adults:* 25 g/dose (max: 250 g/24 hr).	*Cautions:* 25% albumin may increase risk of intraventricular hemorrhage in preterm infants, so 5% form is preferred in these cases. Infuse over at least 2 hr in neonates. Infusion may be over 30–60 min for hypovolemia. *Adverse events:* Precipitation of heart failure, pulmonary edema, hypertension, tachycardia due to volume overload. Immune reactions (e.g., fever, chills, rash). Increased mortality in critically ill patients. *Monitoring:* Vital signs.

TABLE 716-1. General Medications—cont'd

DRUG (TRADE NAMES, FORMULATIONS)	INDICATIONS (MECHANISM OF ACTION AND DOSING)	COMMENTS (CAUTIONS, ADVERSE EVENTS, MONITORING)
Albuterol Adrenergic agonist agent; β_2-adrenergic agonist agent; bronchodilator; sympathomimetic. Proventil; Ventolin; Volmax. Aerosol, oral: 90 μg/spray (200 inhalations) [17 g]. Capsule, microfine, for inhalation, as sulfate (Rotacaps): 200 μg. Solution, inhalation, as sulfate: 0.083% Syrup, as sulfate (strawberry flavor): 2 mg/5 mL (480 mL). Tablet, as sulfate: 2, 4 mg. Tablet, extended-release: 4 mg.	**Bronchoilator** (β_2 agonist). **Inhalation dose:** *Neonates, infants, children, and adults:* **Metered-dose inhaler:** 1–2 puffs prn, or 5 min before exercise or tid–qid. **Rotahaler:** 1–2 capsules prn, or q 4–6 hr, or before exercise. **Nebulizer solution:** *Neonates:* 0.1–0.5 mg/kg/dose prn or q 2–6 hr. *Children:* 1.25–2.5 mg prn or q 4–6 hr. *Adults:* 1.25–5 mg prn or q 4–6 hr **PO:** *Neonates:* 0.1–0.3 mg/kg/dose q 6–8 hr. *Children:* *<6 yr:* 0.1–0.2 mg/kg/dose tid. *6–12 yr:* 2 mg/dose tid–qid *>12 yr:* 2–4 mg tid–qid.	*Cautions:* Increased use or lack of effect may indicate loss of asthma control, requiring medical attention. Better to use prn or before exercise. *Adverse events:* Hyperglycemia, hypokalemia, tachycardia, palpitations, nervousness, CNS stimulation, insomnia, tremor.
Alfentanil hydrochloride Analgesic, narcotic; general anesthetic. Alfenta Injection. Injection, preservative-free: 500 μg/mL (2, 5, 10, 20 mL).	**Analgesia, anesthesia** (narcotic analgesic). *Neonates, infants, and children < 12 yr:* 5–15 μg/kg IV injected over 3–5 min or 0.5–3 μg/kg/min continuous infusion (limited experience and doses poorly established). *Adults:* IV continuous infusion 0.5–1.5 μg/kg/min.	*Cautions:* Bolus doses of 9–15 μg/kg caused chest wall rigidity in 9 of 20 newborns, compromising respiration in 4 patients. Use a skeletal muscle relaxant concurrently. Avoid in patients with increased intracranial pressure or severe respiratory depression. *Adverse events:* Bradycardia, hypotension, increased intracranial pressure, antidiuretic hormone release. *Comment:* Dose based on lean weight for obese patients.
Alglucerase Enzyme, glucocerebrosidase. Ceredase Injection. Injection: 10 u/mL (5 mL); 80 u/mL (5 mL).	**Enzyme replacement therapy for type I Gaucher disease** (replaces the missing enzyme β-glucosidase needed to break down and thus avoid accumulation of glycosyl ceramide-laden macrophages in bone, liver, and spleen in type 1 Gaucher disease). 20–60 u/kg IV infused over 1–2 hr. Typically repeated q 2 wk, but varies from q 2 days to q 4 wk, depending on response.	*Adverse events:* Fever, chills, abdominal discomfort, nausea, vomiting, local IV site burning or edema. *Monitoring:* Resolution of anemia, thrombocytopenia, bleeding tendencies, and hepatosplenomegaly (within 6 mo). Improved bone mineralization (usually noted at 80–104 wk of therapy).
Allopurinol Antigout agent; uric acid-lowering agent. Lopurin; Zyloprim. Tablet: 100, 300 mg.	**Prevent attacks of gouty arthritis and nephropathy.** **Prevent cancer chemotherapy-induced hyperuricemia** (inhibits xanthine oxidase, thus preventing conversion of hypoxanthine to uric acid). *Children ≤ 10 yr:* 10 mg/kg/24 hr in 2–3 divided doses. *Children > 10 yr and adults:* 200-600 mg/24 hr in 2–3 divided doses. **Gout, chemotherapy-induced hyperuricemia.** 600–800 mg/24 hr in 2–3 divided doses starting 1–2 days before chemotherapy and continuing for 3 days. **Renal impairment:** CrCl 10–50: reduce dose to 50%. CrCl < 10: reduce dose to 30% of suggested.	*Cautions:* Discontinue at first signs of rash. *Adverse events:* Rashes, including erythema multiforme, renal impairment, hepatitis, peripheral neuropathy, vasculitis. *Monitoring:* Uric acid levels decrease in 1–2 days, with maximum effect seen in 1–3 wk.
Alprazolam Antianxiety agent. Benzodiazine. Xanax. Tablet: 0.25, 0.5, 1, 2 mg.	**Treatment of anxiety or panic attacks** (not certain, but may be mediated through γ-aminobutyric acid). *Children:* 0.005–0.02 mg/kg/dose tid. *Adults:* 0.25–0.5 mg bid–tid (max: 4 mg/24 hr) [anxiety] (max: 10 mg/24 hr) [panic].	*Cautions:* Abrupt discontinuation results in withdrawal reactions, including seizures. Safety not established in children < 18 yr. Pregnancy risk factor D. *Adverse events:* Drowsiness, confusion, sedation.
Alprostadil Prostaglandin. Prostin VR Pediatric Injection. Injection: 500 μg/mL (1 mL).	**Maintains patency of ductus arteriosus in cyanotic heart lesions.** Direct vasodilation of ductus smooth muscle. *Neonates and infants:* 0.05–0.1 μg/kg/min as continuous IV infusion may gradually increase to maximum of 0.4 μg/kg/min or wean as low as 0.005 μg/kg/min, depending on response.	*Adverse events:* Apnea, bradycardia, hypotension, tachycardia, flushing, seizure-like activity, cortical hyperostosis (with > 6 mo use), diarrhea, gastric outlet obstruction (≥ 5 days use). *Monitoring:* Therapeutic response includes increase in systemic blood pressure, improved oxygen saturation or Po_2, and less acidosis on blood pH. Discontinue immediately if severe apnea or bradycardia.
Aluminum acetate Topical skin product. Acid Mantle; Bluboro; Boropak; Domeboro; Pedi-Boro. Power, to make topical solution: 1 packet/pint of water = 1 : 40 solution. Solution, otic: Aluminum acetate 1 : 10 with acetic acid 2% (60 mL). Tablet: 1 tablet/pint = 1 : 40 dilution.	**Astringent wet dressing for relief of inflammatory conditions of the skin; prophylaxis of swimmer's ear.** *Children and adults:* Otic: Instill 4–6 drops q 2–3 hr initially, then q 4–6 hr until itching or burning resolves. Topical: Soak affected area in solution for 15–30 min 2–4 × daily.	*Adverse events:* Local irritation.
Aminocaproic acid Hemostatic agent. Amicar. Injection: 250 mg/mL (20, 96, 100 mL). Syrup (raspberry flavor): 250 (480 mL). Tablet: 500 mg.	**Treatment of excessive bleeding resulting from systemic hyperfibrinolysis (inbihits activation of plasminogen).** *Children:* PO, IV: Loading dose of 100–200 mg/kg, maintenance dose of 100 mg/kg q 6 hr or 33.3 mg/kg/hr continuous infusion. Traumatic hyphema: 100 mg/kg q 4 hr (max: 30 g/24 hr). *Adults:* Loading dose of 5 g over 1 hr, then 1–1.25 g/hr until bleeding stops (max: 30 g/24 hr).	*Cautions:* Avoid in disseminated intravascular coagulation and hematuria of the upper urinary tract. Contains benzyl alcohol, so avoid in neonates < 1500 g. *Adverse events:* Hypotension, bradycardia, arrhythmias, dizziness, headache, nasal congestion. *Monitoring:* D-dimer or fibrin split products, activated clotting time (target 180–200 sec), serum potassium (especially if renal function decreased).

TABLE 716-1. General Medications—cont'd

DRUG (TRADE NAMES, FORMULATIONS)	INDICATIONS (MECHANISM OF ACTION AND DOSING)	COMMENTS (CAUTIONS, ADVERSE EVENTS, MONITORING)
Aminophylline (Theophylline equivalent listed in parentheses.) Bronchodilator; respiratory stimulant; theophylline derivative. Aminophyllin; Phyllocontin; Somophyllin; Truphylline. Injection, IV (Aminophyllin): 25 mg/mL (19.7 mg/ML) [10, 20 mL]. Liquid, oral: 105 mg/5 mL (90 mg/5 mL) [240 mL]. Suppository, rectal (Truphylline): 250 mg (197.5 mg), 500 mg (395 mg). Tablet (Aminophyllin): 100 mg (79 mg), 200 mg (158 mg). Tablet, controlled-release (12 hr) (Phyllocontin): 225 mg (178 mg). Tablet, enteric-coated: 100 mg (79 mg), 200 mg (158 mg). See *Theophylline* for oral dosing.	**Apnea of prematurity, ventilator weaning in neonates, bronchodilator, weak pulmonary anti-inflammatory effects.** Increases contractility and decreases fatigability of diaphragm and respiratory muscles; weak bronchodilator, stimulates CNS; decreases airway responsiveness to stimuli. Exact mechanisms for these effects remain controversial. *Neonates* (for apnea of prematurity, ventilator weaning, or bronchospasm): Loading dose: 6 mg/kg IV or PO. Maintenance dose: 2.5–3 mg/kg/dose q 12 hr IV or PO. **Asthma chronic therapy (see *Theophylline*).** Use in acute therapy is of questionable value. If used as continuous IV infusion: *Children:* *6 wk–6 mo:* 0.5 mg/kg/hr. *6 mo–1 yr:* 0.7 mg/kg/hr. *1–9 yr:* 1 mg/kg/hr. *9–12 yr:* 0.9 mg/kg/hr. *12 yr–adult:* 0.7 mg/kg/hr.	*Cautions:* May cause or worsen arrhythmias, seizures, or gastroesophageal reflux. Theophylline clearance is modified by numerous disease states and drugs, requiring dosing adjustments guided by serum theophylline concentrations. Clearance is reduced by viral illnesses, fever > 102°F for > 24 hr, cor pulmonale, and drugs that inhibit P450 enzymes (cimetidine, verapamil, macrolides, quinolones); reduce dose by 50%. *Adverse events:* Feeding intolerance in neonates, gastrointestinal discomfort in children and adults, nausea, vomiting, CNS irritability, agitation, tachycardia, tachyarrhythmias. *Monitoring:* Theophylline blood levels correlate with clinical effects and toxicity. Target levels are somewhat controversial. *Neonates:* 6–15 mg/L (65% of neonates will not have apnea eliminated until levels exceed 10 mg/L if continuous electronic monitoring is performed. Levels >10 mg/L are needed for ventilator weaning. Levles of 5–15 mg/L are sufficient for bronchodilation). *Children:* Theophylline alone is ineffective for acute asthma. For chronic asthma, theophylline levels of 5–15 mg/L are effetive, but levels should exceed 10 mg/L for prevention of exercise-induced bronchospasm.
Amiodarone hydrochloride Antiarrhythmic agent, class III. Cordarone. Tablet: 200 mg. Injection: 50 mg/mL (3 mL). Cordarone contains benzyl alcohol and polysorbate (Tween) 80. Injection, benzyl alcohol-free and polysorbate-free: 15 mg/mL (10 mL); Amio-Aqueous contains an aqueous acetate buffer; available via orphan drug status or compassionate use from the manufacturer, Academic Pharmaceuticals, Inc. (847) 735-1170.	**Management of resistant, life-threatening ventricular arrhythmias or paroxysmal supraventricular tachycardia (PSVT) unresponsive to less toxic agents** (class III antiarrhythmic agent; prolongs action potential and refractory period in myocardial tissue). **Oral dose:** *Infants and children:* *<1 yr:* 600–800 mg/1.73 m^2/24 hr in 2 divided doses. *>1 yr:* 10–20 mg/kg/24 hr in 2 divided doses for 10 days, then 5–10 mg/kg/24 hr. *Adults:* 800 mg/24 hr in 2 divided doses. Cut all doses in half (i.e., 1 dose/day) after 1–4 wk of treatment or when arrhythmias are controlled. **IV dose:** *Infants and children:* Loading dose of 5 mg/kg over 1 hr, then continuous infusion of 5–15 μg/kg/min. *Adults:* 150 mg over 10 min, then 0.5 mg/min.	*Cautions:* Use benzyl alcohol–free product in neonates. Minimize risk of torsades de pointes by correcting potassium and magnesium imbalance. Inhibits cytochrome P450 enzymes, so many drugs that are metabolized will have markedly increased levels and effects, including theophylline, phenytoin, warfarin, other antiarrhythmics, methotrexate, and cyclosporine. *Adverse events:* Proarrhythmias (may be bradyarrhythmias, tachyarrhythmias, or heart block), fatigue, malaise, nightmares, behavioral changes, hypothyroidism, hyperglycemia, elevated triglycerides, skin color changes (slate blue), photosensitivity, rash, liver toxicity (may be fatal or just increased liver enzymes), pulmonary toxicity (potentially fatal) including pulmonary fibrosis, interstitial pneumonitis, hypersensitivity pneumonitis (cough, fever, dyspnea, chest radiographic changes), photophobia, thrombocytopenia. *Monitoring:* Pulmonary, liver, and thyroid function tests; chest radiograph, ECG, eye examination; and clinical signs and symptoms of toxicity. Amiodarone concentration: 2–4 μmol/L.
Amitriptyline hydrochloride Antidepressant, tricyclic; antimigraine agent. Elavil; Emitrip; Endep. Injection: 10 mg/mL (10 mL). Tablet: 10, 25, 50, 75, 100, 150 mg.	**Depression (increases CNS concentration of serotonin and norepinephrine by inhibiting reuptake).** *Children:* 1–1.5 mg/kg/24 hr divided tid. *Adolescents:* 30–100 mg at bedtime or divided bid (max: 200 mg/24hr). *Adults:* 30–100 mg q 24 hr (max: 300 mg/24 hr). **Analgesic for neuropathic or chronic pain or migraine prophylaxis.** *Children:* 0.1 mg/kg at bedtime and advance over 2–3 wk to effect (max: 2 mg/kg at bedtime). *Adolescents:* 25 mg divided bid and increase dose to effect (max: 200 mg/24 hr). *Adults:* 25 mg at bedtime and increase dose to effect (max: 300 mg/24 hr).	*Cautions:* Cardiac conduction abnormalities may occur, monitor ECG. Do not discontinue abruptly because withdrawal syndrome may occur. *Adverse events:* Dry mouth, constipation, weight gain, postural hypotension, drowsiness, confusion, headache, visual disturbance. *Monitoring:* Amitriptyline concentrations: therapeutic 100–250 ng/mL; nortriptyline concentrations: therapeutic 50–150 ng/mL.
Ammonium chloride Metabolic alkalosis, treatment agent; urinary acidifying agent. Generic. Injection: 26.75% (5 mEq/mL) [20 mL]. Tablet: 500 mg. Tablet, enteric-coated: 500 mg.	**Systemic or urinary acidification (dissociation of ammonium and chloride and replacement of bicarbonate ions by chloride ions).** *Children:* 75 mg/kg/24 hr IV divided q 6 h (max: 6 g daily). *Adults:* 1.5 g/dose IV q 6 hr.	*Adverse events:* Hyperchloremia, hyperammonemia, hyperkalemia.
Amrinone lactate Adrenergic agonist agent. Inocor. Injection: 5 mg/mL (20 mL).	**Treatment of low cardiac output states (increase cellular levels of cyclic adenosine monophosphate).** *Neonates:* 0.75 mg/kg IV bolus over 2–3 min, then 3–5 μg/kg/min continuous infusion IV. *Infants and children:* 0.75 mg/kg IV bolus over 2–3 min, then 5–10 μg/kg/min continuous infusion. *Adults:* 0.75 mg/kg IV bolus over 2–3 min, then 5–10 μg/kg/min.	*Cautions:* Increased cardiac output may cause excess diuresis if diuretic doses are not adjusted. May repeat bolus doses if clinical response is inadequate. *Adverse events:* Hypotension, arrhythmias, thrombocytopenia.
Antihemophilic factor, human Antihemophilic agent; blood product derivative. Alphanate; Hemofil M; Humate-P; Koate-HP; Koate-HS; Monoclate-P; Profilate OSD. Injection (approximate factor VIII activity/vial): 200, 250, 500, 750, 1,000, 1,250, 1,500 units; exact potency labeled on each vial.	**Factor VIII deficiency in hemophilia (provides factor VIII).** *All patients:* Units required = weight (kg) × 0.5 × desired increase in factor VIII (% of normal).	*Monitoring:* Plasma antihemophilic factor levels *Adverse events:* Tachycardia, allergy, blood-borne viral infections.
Antipyrine and benzocaine. Otic agent, analgesic; otic agent, ceruminolytic. Allergan Ear Drops: Aurafair; Auralgan; Aurodex; Auroto: Oto; Otocalm Ear Solution, otic: antipyrine 5.4% and benzocaine 1.4% (10, 15 mL).	**Temporary relief of ear pain and inflammation (topical anesthetic and anti-inflammatory).** *All patients:* Fill ear canal, and then moisten cotton pledget and place into meatus. May repeat q 1–2 hr until pain relief. Limit use to about 3 days.	*Adverse events:* Stinging, methemoglobinemia.

TABLE 716-1. General Medications—cont'd

DRUG (TRADE NAMES, FORMULATIONS)	INDICATIONS (MECHANISM OF ACTION AND DOSING)	COMMENTS (CAUTIONS, ADVERSE EVENTS, MONITORING)
Antithrombin III **Thrombate III**	**Antithrombin III (ATIII) deficiency due to disseminated intravascular coagulation or shock and surgery complications. Treatment of thrombosis in ATIII deficiency.** *All patients:* Dose (IU) = (120 − patient ATIII) × weight (kg).	*Monitoring:* Check ATIII levels: maintain at 80–120%.
Antivenin (Crotalidae) polyvalent Antivenom. Generic. Injection: Lyophilized serum, diluent (10 mL); 1 vacuum vial to yield 10 mL of antivenom.	**Antivenom for snake bite from North and South American crotalids (i.e., rattlesnake, copperhead, cottonmouth, tropical moccasin, fer-de-lance, bushmaster).** Dosing based on severity of bit: mild, vial; moderate, 10 vials; severe, >15 vials.	*Cautions:* Sensitivity reactions, including anaphylaxis (treat with epinephrine and antihistamine and brief holding of dose).
Arginine hydrochloride Diagnostic agent, growth hormone function; metabolic alkalosis, treatment agent. R-Gene. Injection: 10% (0.475 mEq chloride/mL) [500 mL].	**Pituitary function test (stimulates pituitary, release of growth hormone and prolactin).** *Children:* 500 mg/kg over30 min. *Adults:* 300 mL over 30 min	*Adverse events:* Flushing, headache, hyperglycemia. hyperkalemia, metabolic acidosis. *Monitoring:* Plasma growth hormone concentrations.
Ascorbic acid Nutritional supplemnt; urinary acidifying agent; vitamin, water-soluble. Ascorbicap; C-Crystals; Cecon; Cetane; Cevalin, Ce-Vi-Sol; Dull-C; Flavorcee; Vita-C. Capsule, timed-release; 500 mg. Crystals: 4 g/tsp (1,000 g). Injection: 25 mg/mL (2, 30 mL), 500 mg/mL (1, 2, 50 mL). Lozenge: 60 mg. Powder: 4 g/tsp (1,000 g). Solution, oral: 35 mg/0.6 mL (50 mL), 100 mg/mL (50 mL). Syrup: 500 mg/5 mL (5, 10, 120, 480 mL). Tablet: 25, 50, 100, 250, 500, 1,000 mg. Tablet, chewable: 100, 250, 500, 1,000 mg. Tablet, timed-release: 500, 1,000, 500 mg.	**Scurvy.** *Children:* 100–300 mg/24 hr. *Adults:* 100–250 mg bid **Urinary acidification.** *Children:* 500 mg q 6 hr. *Adults:* 4–12 g/24 hr in 3–4 divided doses.	*Adverse events:* Gastrointestinal upset, renal stones.
Asparaginase Antineoplastic agent, miscellaneous. Elspar. Injection: 10,000 u/vial	**Cancer chemotherapy (inhibits protein synthesis to deprive cancer cells of asparagine).** *Children and adults:* Doses may vary depending on specific protocol being used; 6,000 unit/m^2 IM, 3 × wk for 3 wk as part of combination therapy. High-dose IM therapy: 25,000 units/m^2/dose q wk × 9 doses. IV therapy: 1,000 units/kg/24 hr for 10 days; or 200 units/kg/24 hr for about 28 days.	*Cautions:* Stop drug if any signs of renal failure or pancreatitis occur. Be prepared to treat anaphylaxis at each dose. *Adverse events:* Myelosuppression (WBCs and platelets; mild and rare) onset, 7 days; nadir, 14 days; recovery, 21 days. Hepatotoxicity, pancreatitis, gastrointestinal upset, azotemia, hyperglycemia, coagulopathy.
Aspirin Analgesic, non-narcotic; anti-inflammatory agent; antiplatelet agent; antipyretic; nonsteroidal anti-inflammatory agent, oral; salicylate. Anacin; A.S.A.; Ascriptin; Aspergum; Bayer Aspirin; Bufferin; Easprin; Ecotrin; Empirin; Gensan; Halfrin; Measurin, ZORprin. Suppository, rectal: 60, 120, 125, 130, 195, 200, 300, 325, 600, 650, 1,200 mg. Tablet: 325, 500, 650 mg Tablet, buffered: 325 mg with aluminum hydroxide 75 mg and magnesium hydroxide 75 mg; 325 mg with aluminum hydroxide 150 mg and magnesium hydroxide 150 mg; 500 mg with aluminum hydroxide 33 mg and magnesium hydroxide 150 mg. Chewable: 75, 81 mg. Chewing gum: 227 mg. Tablets controlled-release: 800 mg. Tablets enteric-coated (delayed-release): 80, 165, 325, 500, 650, 975 mg. Tablets timed-release: 650 mg. Tablet, with caffeine: 400 mg and caffeine 32 mg; 500 mg and caffeine 32 mg.	**Pain, inflammation, fever (prostaglandin synthesis inhibition).** *Children:* 10–15 mg/kg/dose q 4–6 hr. *Adults:* 650–1,000 mg/dose q 4–6 hr (max: 4 g/24 hr). **Kawasaki disease (acute phase).** *Children:* 80–100 mg/kg/24 hr divided q 6 hr. **Rheumatic fever.** 60–100 mg/kg/24 hr divided q 6 hr.	*Cautions:* Contraindicated in children < 16 yr with chickenpox or flu-like symptoms due to risk of Reye syndrome. Discontinue if hearing loss or tinnitus occurs. *Adverse events:* Bleeding from gums or gastrointestinal tract, gastric ulcers, bronchospasm in asthmatics, hearing loss, tinnitus. *Monitoring:* Check serum concentration 2 hr after a dose for Kawasaki disease (target 150–300 μg/mL) or rheumatic fever (target 250–400 μg/mL).
Astemizole Antihistamine. Hismanal. Tablet: 10 mg	**Allergy and rhinitis (competitive H_1 receptor blocker).** *Children:* *<6 yr:* 0.2 mg/kg once daily. *6–12 yr:* 5 mg once daily. *>12 yr and adults:* 10–30 mg/24 hr	*Cautions:* Syncopal episodes may be a maker of arrhythmias, including Q-T interval prolongation, leading to fatal arrhythmias. Discontinue if ECG shows Q-T prolongation, syncopal episode, or if drugs that impair hepatic metabolism (e.g., erythromycin, ketoconazole) are added.
Atenolol Antianginal agent; antihypertensive; β-adrenergic blocker. Tenormin. Injection: 0.5 mg/mL (10 mL). Tablet: 25, 50, 100 mg.	**Hypertension, arrhythmias (competitive β_1 blocker).** *Children:* 0.8–1.5 mg/kg/24 hr (max: 2 mg/kg/24 hr). *Adults:* 25–200 mg/24 hr PO, 5 mg IV over 5 min.	*Cautions:* Avoid abrupt discontinuation; taper over 1–2 wk. *Adverse events:* Bradycardia, lethargy, headache, constipation, wheezing, dyspnea.
Atorvastatin calcium Lipitor. Tablet: 10, 20, 40 mg	**Hypercholesterolemia, including homozygous familial hypercholesterolemia (inhibit HMG-CoA reductase).** *Children > 6 yr:* 10–80 mg/24 hr. *Adults:* 10–80 mg/24 hr.	*Adverse events:* Dyspepsia, flatulence, pancreatitis, hepatitis, myalgia, arthralgia. *Monitoring:* Plasma lipid profile.

TABLE 716-1. General Medications—cont'd

DRUG (TRADE NAMES, FORMULATIONS)	INDICATIONS (MECHANISM OF ACTION AND DOSING)	COMMENTS (CAUTIONS, ADVERSE EVENTS, MONITORING)
Atracurium besylate Neuromuscular blocker agent; nondepolarizing skeletal muscle relaxant; paralytic. Tracrium. Injection: 10 mg/mL (5, 10 mL).	**Neuromuscular blocker for muscle paralysis; binds to cholinergic receptor sites to block neural transmission).** *Children:* *<2 yr:* 0.3–0.4 mg/kg as needed. *>2 yr–adults:* 0.4–0.5 mg/kg, then 1 mg/kg 20–45 min after each initial block to maintain effect. Continuous IV infusion: 0.4–0.8 mg/kg/hr.	*Cautions:* Make sure airway and respiratory support are secure before use. Contains benzyl alcohol; neonatal use should be limited. Does not have sedative or analgesic properties, so adjunct sedative or analgesic should be used. *Monitoring:* Muscle twitch response to peripheral nerve stimulator.
Atropine sulfate Anticholinergic agent; anticholinergic agent, ophthalmic; antidote, organophosphate poisoning; antispasmodic agent, gastrointestinal; bronchodilator; ophthalmic agent, mydriatic. Atropair Ophthalmic; Atropine-Care Ophthalmic; Atropisol Ophthalmic; Isopto Atropine Ophthalmic; I-Tropine Ophthalmic; Ocu-Tropin. Ophthalmic injection: 0.05 mg/mL); (5 mL); 0.1 mg/mL (5, 10 mL 0.3 mg/mL (1, 30 mL); 0.4 mg /mL (1, 20, 30 mL); 0.5 mg/mL (1, 5, 30 mL); 0.8 mg/mL (0.5, 1 mL); 1 mg/mL (1, 10 mL). Ointment, ophthalmic: 0.5% (3.5 g); 1% (3.5 g) Solution, ophthalmic: 0.5% (1, 5 mL); 1% (1, 2, 5, 15 mL); 2% (1, 2 mL). Tablet: 0.4 mg. Tablet, soluble: 0.4, 0.6 mg.	**Preoperative medication to inhibit secretions and salivation (blocks action of acetylcholine and antagonizes histamine and serotonin).** *Neonates and children:* *<5 kg:* 0.2 mg/kg 30 min preoperatively, then q 4–6 hr. *>5 kg:* 0.1–0.2 mg/kg/dose (max: 0.4 mg/dose). *Adults:* 0.4–0.6 mg IV or SC 30 min preoperatively. **Treatment of sinus bradycardia.** *Neonates and children:* 0.02 mg/kg (minimum: 0.1 mg); IV or intratracheal (max: 0.5 mg); may repeat 5 min later, 1× *Adults:* 0.5–1 mg q 5 min (max total dose: 2 mg). **Antidote to organophosphate poisoning.** 0.02–0.05 mg/kg q 10–20 min until atropine effect (tachycardia, mydriasis, fever), then q 1–4 hr for at least 24 hr.	*Cautions:* Avoid in narrow-angle glaucoma, gastrointestinal obstruction, thyrotoxicosis, and tachycardia. *Adverse events:* Tachycardia; palpitations; delirium; ataxia; dry; hot skin; tremor; impaired vision.
Attapulgite Antidiarrheal. Children's Kaopectate; Diasorb; Donnagel; Kaopectate Advanced Formula; Kaopectate Maximum Strength Caplets; K-Pec; Parepectolin; Rheaban. Caplet: 750 mg. Liquid: 600 mg activated attapulgite/15 mL (180, 240, 360, 480 mL); 750 mg activated attapulgite/15 mL (120 mL). Suspension: 600 mg/15 mL. Tablet, chewable: 300, 600, 750 mg.	**Uncomplicated diarrhea (absorbent action).** *Children:* *3–6 yr:* 300–750 mg/dose (max: 7 doses). *6–12 yr:* 600–1,500 mg/dose (max: 7 doses).	*Caution:* Do not use for diarrhea due to dysentery, enterocolitis, or toxigenic bacteria.
Auranofin Gold compound. Ridaura. Capsule: 3 mg (gold 29%).	**Treatment of active stage of rheumatoid or psoriatic arthritis (immunomodulating effect).** *Children:* Initial dose: 0.1 mg/kg/24 hr; usual maintenance dose: 0.15 mg/kg/24 hr in 1–2 doses (max: 0.2 mg/kg/24 hr). *Adults:* 6 mg/24 hr in 1–2 doses (max: 9 mg/24 hr in 1–3 doses).	*Adverse events:* Itching, skin rash, stomatitis, conjunctivitis, proteinuria, alopecia, glossitis, leukopenia, thrombocytopenia, hematuria, anemia, agranulocytosis, eosinophilia, peripheral neuropathy, interstitial pneumonitis, angioedema, hepatotoxicity. *Monitoring:* Discontinue if WBCs, < 4,000/mm^3, granulocytes < 1,500/mm^3, platelets < 100,000/mm^3.
Aurothioglucose Gold compound. Solganal. Suspension, sterile: 50 mg/mL (gold 50%) [10 mL].	**Treatment of active rheumatoid or psoriatic arthritis immunomodulator.** *Children:* 0.25 mg/kg/dose in wk 1, increased by 0.25 mg/kg/dose q wk to maintenance dose of 0.75–1.0 mg/kg/dose weekly (max: 25 mg/dose, total 20 doses). *Adults:* 10 mg in wk 1, then 25 mg in wk 2 and 3, then 50 mg/wk until cumulative dose or 1 g given.	*Cautions:* Administer by deep IM injection. *Adverse events:* Same as for auranofin.
Azatadine maleate Antihistamine. Optimine. Tablet: 1 mg	**Treatment of allergy, allergic rhinitis, and urticaria (antihistamine, anticholinergic).** *Children < 12 yr:* Not recommended. *Children > 12 yr and adults:* 1–2 mg twice daily.	*Adverse events:* Sedation, dry mouth, thickened bronchial secretions.
Azathioprine Immunosuppressant agent. Imuran. Injection, as sodium: 100 mg (10 mL). Tablet: 50 mg.	**Prevent transplant rejection.** *Children and adults:* Initial dose of 2–5 mg/kg/24 hr IV or PO, with a maintenance dose of 1–3 mg/kg/24 hr. **Treatment of autoimmune disease (e.g., lupus, arthritis, nephrotic syndrome).** Inhibits synthesis of DNA, RNA, and proteins. Antagonizes purine metabolism. *Adults:* 1 mg/kg/24 hr × 6–8 wk.	*Cautions:* Chronic use causes increased risk of lymphoma and skin cancer. May cause irreversible bone marrow suppression. Reduce dose to 25% of normal if allopurinol used concurrently. *Adverse events:* Fever, chills, nausea, vomiting, diarrhea, thrombocytopenia, leukopenia, hepatotoxicity, rash.
Baclofen Skeletal muscle relaxant; nonparalytic Lioresal Injection, intrathecal: 0.5 mg/mL (20 mL); 2 mg/mL (5 mL). Tablet: 10, 20 mg.	**Spasticity associated with multiple sclerosis or spinal cord lesions.** **Trigeminal neuralgia (inhibits transmission of monosynaptic and polysynaptic reflexes at the spinal cord level).** *Children: 2–7 yr:* 10–15 mg/24 hr divided q 8 hr and titrated up q 3 days (max: 40 mg/24 hr PO). Intrathecal 25–50 μg. *Adults:* 5 mg q 8 hr and gradually increase by 5 mg q 3 days (max: 80 mg/24 hr PO). Intrathecal 50 μg to max 100 μg.	*Caution:* Avoid abrupt discontinuation; slowly titrate to discontinue *Adverse events:* Drowsiness, vertigo, psychiatric reactions, ataxia, hypotonia.
Beclomethasone Adrenal corticosteroid; anti-inflammatory agent; corticosteroid, inhalant (oral); corticosteroid, nasal; glucocorticoid. Beclovent Oral Inhaler; Beconase AQ Nasal Inhaler; Beconase Nasal Inhaler; Vancenase AQ Inhaler; Vanceril Oral Inhaler. Inhalation: Nasal (Beconase, Vancenase): 42 μg/inhalation (200 metered doses) [16.8 g]. Oral (Beclovent, Vanceril): 42μg/inhalation (200 metered doses) [16.8 g]. Spray, aqueous, nasal (Beconase AQ, Vancenase AQ): 42 μg /inhalation (200 metered doses) [25 g].	**Asthma (oral inhalation), rhinitis (nasal aerosol) [anti-inflammatory, immune modulator].** *Adults and children (inhaler):* 1–2 puffs bid–qid. (max children: 10 puffs daily; adults: 20 puffs daily). *Adults and children (nasal spray):* 1 spray in each nostril bid–qid.	*Adverse events: Candida* in mouth, burning and irritation of nasal mucosa, cough, hoarseness, headache. *Monitoring:* Inhaled corticosteroids should be administered via an extender device for better lung delivery and less local toxicity.

TABLE 716-1. General Medications—cont'd

DRUG (TRADE NAMES, FORMULATIONS)	INDICATIONS (MECHANISM OF ACTION AND DOSING)	COMMENTS (CAUTIONS, ADVERSE EVENTS, MONITORING)
Benzocaine Local anesthetic, oral; local anesthetic, topical. Americaine; Anbesol Maximum Strenth; Babee Teething Lotion: BiCOZENE; chigger tox; Dermaplast; Foille Plus; Hurricaine; Orabase-B; Orabase Gel; Orabase-O, Oral Jel Brace-Aid Oral Anesthetic; Ora Jel Maximum Strength; Ora Jel Mouth-Aid; Rhulicaine, Solar Caine; Unguentine. Topical: Aerosol: 5% (97.5, 105 mL) 20% (20, 60, 120 g). Cream: 5% (30, 454 g); 6% (28.4 g). Gel 15% (7 g). Liquid, with benzyl benzoate and soft soap: 30 mL. Lotion: 8% (90 mL). Ointment: 5% (3.5, 30 g).	**Temporary relief of pain associated with minor skin injury (local anesthetic).** *Children and adults:* Apply to affected area as needed.	*Adverse events:* Local irritation or sensitization.
Benzonatate Topical anesthetic. Tessalon Perles.	**Relief of nonproductive cough (topical anesthetic action).** *Children < 10 yr:* Not indicated. *Children > 10 yr and adults:* 100 mg tid or q 4 hr (max: 600 mg/24 hr).	*Adverse events:* Sedation, numbness, dizziness, headache.
Benzoyl peroxide Acne products, topical skin product. Benzoxyl; Benzac W; Clear by Design; Clearasil; Dermo Xyl; Desquam-X; Loroxide; Oxy-5; Panoxyl; Panoxyl-AQ; Persa-Gel; Phiso AC-BP; Vanoxide. Cleansing bar: 5% (120 g); 10% (120 g). Cleansing lotion: 5% (120, 150, 240 mL); 10% (120, 150 mL). Cream: 5% (30 g); 10% (30, 45 g). Facial mask: 5%. Gel: 2.5% (45, 60, 90 g); 5% (45, 60, 90, 120 g); 10% (45, 60, 90, 120 g). Lotion: 5% (30, 42.5, 60 mL); 5.5% (25 mL); 10% (30, 42.5, 60 mL). Stick: 10%.	**Acne treatment (keratolytic and comedolytic effects, and killing anaerobic bacteria).** *Children and adults:* Apply sparingly tid for 15 min. May increase strength and duration of exposure as tolerated.	*Adverse events:* Contact dermatitis, local irritation, stinging, erythema.
Benztropine mesylate Anticholinergic agent: antidote, drug-induced dystonic reactions; anti-Parkinson agent. Cogentin. Injection: 1 mg/mL (2 mL). Tablet: 0.5, 1, 2 mg.	**Parkinsonism, drug-induced extrapyramidal reaction (block-age of striatal cholinergic receptors).** *Children > 3 yr:* 0.02–0.05 mg/kg/dose 1–2 × daily. *Adults:* 1–4 mg/dose 1–2 × daily.	*Adverse events:* Tachycardia, drowsiness, nervousness, hallucinations, dry mouth, blurred vision, mydriasis.
Benzylpenicilloyl-polylysine Diagnostic agent, penicillin allergy skin text. Pre-Pen. Injection: 0.25 mL.	**Adjunct to assessing the risk of penicillin hypersensitivity (elicits type 1 urticarial reactions by Immunoglobulin E-mediated reaction).** *Children and adults:* Scratch technique uses a 20-gauge needle to make a 3–5 mm scratch on dermis; apply a small drop of solution to scratch and rub it in gently with applicator. Intradermal injection of 0.1–0.2 mL of Pre-Pen and 0.9% saline in 2 sites at least 1 in apart.	*Monitoring:* Scratch test is positive if a pale wheal of ≥5–15 mm occurs within 10 min. Intradermal test is positive in 5–15 min. Discontinue antihistamines before performing tests (hydroxyzine and diphenhydramine for at least 4 days, astemizole for 6–8 wk).
Beractant Lung surfactant. Survanta. Suspension: 200 mg (8 mL).	**Prophylaxis and treatment of respiratory distress syndrome in premature infants (replaces deficiency of endogenous surfactant).** *Neonates:* 4 mL/kg via endotracheal tube. May repeat q 6 hr to a total of 4 doses. Rotate infant to right, then to left, and administer 1/2 dose on each side over 2–3 sec.	*Adverse events:* Bradycardia, hypotension, oxygen desaturation, pulmonary air leaks, airway obstruction, pulmonary hemorrhage, hypocarbia. *Monitoring:* Heart rate, oxygen saturation, and frequent arterial blood gases. Adjust ventilator to minimize episodes of hyperoxia and hypocarbia.
Betamethasone Adrenal corticosteroid; anti-inflammatory agent; corticosteroid, systematic; corticosteroid, topical; glucocorticoid. Alphatrex Topical; Betalene Topical; Betatrex Topical; Beta Val Topical; Celestone Oral, Celestone Phosphate Injection; Celestone Soluspan; Cel-U-Jec Injection; Diprolene AF Topical; Diprolene Topical; Diprosone Topical; Maxivate Topical; Psorion Topical; Selestoject Injection; Teledar Topical; Uticort Topical; Valisone Topical. Base (Celestone): Syrup: 0.6 mg/5 mL. Tablet: 0.6 mg. Benzoate (Uticort): Cream, emollient base: 0.025% (60 g). Gel, topical: 0.025% (15, 60 g). Lotion: 0.025% (60 mL). Dipropionate (Alphatrex, Diprosone, Maxivate, Tela Dar): Aerosol, topical: 0.1% (85 g). Cream: 0.05% (15, 45 g). Lotion: 0.05% (20, 30, 60 mL). Ointment, topical: 0.05% (15, 45 g). Diproprionate (Psorion): Cream: 0.05% (15, 45 g).	**Systemic use to stimulate fetal lung maturation in preterm labor. Topical use to treat inflammatory dermatoses.** *Children and adults:* Topical application of thin film to affected area bid–qid daily. *Pregnant female:* 12 mg IM q 24 hr for 2 doses.	*Adverse events:* Maternal pulmonary edema and hypertension, headache.

TABLE 716-1. General Medications—cont'd

DRUG (TRADE NAMES, FORMULATIONS)	INDICATIONS (MECHANISM OF ACTION AND DOSING)	COMMENTS (CAUTIONS, ADVERSE EVENTS, MONITORING)
Dipproponate, augmented (Diprolene, Diprolene AF): Cream, emollient base: 0.05% (15, 45 g). Gel, topical: 0.05% (15, 45 g). Lotion: 0.05% (30, 60 mL). Ointment, topical: 0.05% (15, 45 g). Valerate (Betatrex, Beta-Val, Valisone): Cream: 0.01% (15, 60 g); 0.1% (15, 45, 110, 430 g). Lotion: 0.1% (20, 60 mL). Ointment, topical: 0.1% (15, 45 g). Powder for compounding: 5, 10 g. Sodium phosphate (Celestone Phosphate, Selestoject): Injection: Equivalent to 3 g/mL (5 mL). Sodium phosphate and acetate (Celestone Soluspan): Injection, suspension: 6 mg/mL (3 mg betamethasone and betamethasone sodium phosphate and 3 mg betamethasone acetate/mL) [5 mL].		
Bethanechol Cholinergic agent. Duvoid; Myotonachol; Urecholine. Injection: 5 mg/mL (1 mL). Tablet: 5, 10, 25, 50 mg.	**Treatment of nonobstructive urinary retention or gastroesophageal reflux (stimulates cholinergic receptors in smooth muscle in urinary and gastrointestinal tracts).** *Children:* 0.3–0.6 mg/kg/24 hr divided into 3–4 doses. *Adults:* 10–50 mg bid–qid.	*Adverse events:* Hypotension, abdominal cramps, diarrhea, vomiting, salivation, urinary frequency, bronchial constriction, sweating.
Biotin Biotinidase deficiency; treatment agent; vitamin, water-soluble. Biotin Forte; Biotin Forte Extra Strength; Bio-Tn; d-Biotin Tablet: 300, 400, 600, 800 μg; 2.5, 3, 5, 10 mg.	**Treatment of primary biotinidase deficiency or nutritional biotin deficiency, component of vitamin B complex (required for various metabolic functions).** *Children and adults:* Biotin deficiency: 5–20 mg daily. Biotinidase deficiency: 5–10 mg daily.	
Bisacodyl Laxative, stimulant. Bisacodyl Uniserts; Bisco-Lax; Carter's Little Pills; Clysodrast V; Dulcagen; Dulcolax; Fleet Laxative. Enema: 10 mg/30 mL. Powder: 1.5 mg with tannic acid 2.5 g/packet (25, 50's). Suppository, rectal: 5, 10 mg. Tablet, enteric-coated: 5 mg.	**Treatment of constipation (direct smooth muscle irritation to stimulate gastrointestinal peristalsis).** *Children:* *<2 yr:* 5 mg rectal suppository. *>2 yr:* 10 mg rectal suppository. *>6 yr:* 5–10 mg PO at bedtime or before breakfast. *Adults:* 5–30 mg PO, 10 mg rectal suppository.	*Adverse events:* Fluid and electrolyte imbalance, abdominal cramps.
Bismuth subsalicylate Antidiarrheal; gastrointestinal agent; gastric or duodenal ulcer treatment. Bismatrol; Pepto-Bismol. Liquid: 262 mg/15 mL (120, 240, 360, 480 mL); 524 mg/15 mL (120, 240, 360 mL). Tablet, chewable: 262 mg.	**Treatment of diarrhea or gastrointestinal ulcer (absorbs extra water and toxins in large intestine and kills bacterial pathogens).** *Children or adults:* Up to 8 doses/24 hr. *3–6 yr:* 1/3 tablet or 5 mL. *6–9 yr:* 2/3 tablet or 10 mL. *9–12 yr:* 1 tablet or 15 mL. *Adults:* 2 tablets or 30 mL.	*Cautions:* Avoid in patients with influenza or chickenpox because of salicylate content. *Adverse events:* Discoloration of tongue, grayish-black stools.
Bleomycin Antineoplastic agent, antibiotic type. Blenoxane. Powder for injection: 15 U.	**Palliative treatment for several cancers and sclerosing agent for malignant effusions (inhibits synthesis of DNA).** *Children and adults:* 10–20 U/m²/dose IV, IM, SC (0.25–0.5 U/kg) 1–2 × wk in combination regimens.	*Cautions:* Reduce dose in renal dysfunction *Adverse events:* Interstitial pneumonitis, pulmonary fibrosis, nonproductive cough, phlebitis, leukopenia, thrombocytopenia, stomatitis, vomiting, alopecia, hyperkeratosis of hands and nails, desquamation, Raynaud phenomenon; avoid oxygen use.
Bretylium Antiarrhythmic agent, class III. Bretylol. Injection: 50 mg/mL (10, 20 mL); 100 mg/mL. Injection, premixed in D5W: 1 mg/mL (500 mL); 2 mg/mL (250 mL); 4 mg/mL (250, 500 mL).	**Treatment of serious or life-threatening arrhythmias (inhibits release of norepinephrine at postganglionic nerve endings).** *Children:* 2–5 mg/kg IV or IM, may repeat q 10–20 min (max: 30 mg/kg). *Adults:* Initial dose or 5 mg/kg, then 10 mg/kg q 15–30 min (max: 35 mg/kg). *Note:* Cardioversion/defibrillation must be attempted before and after each dose of bretylium.	*Adverse events:* Hypotension, increased premature ventricular contractions, bradycardia, nasal congestion, sweating, hiccups. *Monitoring:* ECG, blood pressure.
Brompheniramine Antihistamine. Bromarest; Bromphen Elixir; Chlorphed; Cophene-B Injection; Dehist Injection; Dimetane Oral; Nasahist B Injection; ND-Stat Injection; Oraminic II Injection; Sinusol-B Injection; Veltane. Tablet. Elixir: 2 mg/5 mL with alcohol 3% (120, 480, 4,000 mL). Injection: 10 mg/mL (10 mL). Tablet: 4, 8, 12 mg. Tablet, sustained-release: 8, 12 mg.	**Treatment of allergic symptoms (e.g., rhinitis, urticaria) [competes with histamine for H_1 receptor sites].** *Children:* *<6 yr:* 0.125 mg/kg/dose q 6 hr (max: 8 mg/24 hr) PO. *6–12 yr:* 2–4 mg/dose q 6–8 hr (max: 16 mg/24 hr) PO. *Adults:* 4–8 mg/dose q 4–6 hr (max: 24 mg/24 hr) PO. IV, IM, SC: *<12 yr:* 0.5 mg/kg/24 hr divided q 6 hr. *>12 yr:* 10 mg/dose divided q 6–12 hr (max: 40 mg/24 hr).	*Adverse events:* Sedation, dry mouth.
Budesonide Adrenal corticosteroid; anti-inflammatory agent; corticosteroid, nasal; glucocorticoid. Rhinocort. Aerosol: 50 μg released/actuation to deliver ≈ 32 μg via nasal adapter (200 metered doses) [7 g]. Pulmicort Turbohaler (dry powder inhaler). Inhalation powder: 200 μg/inhalation.	**Treatment of chronic rhinitis or asthma (suppresses inflammation).** *Children > 6 yr and adults:* Rhinocort nasal spray 2 puffs in each nostril bid or 4 puffs in each nostril once daily. *Children > 6 yr:* Pulmicort Turbohaler 1–2 inhalations bid. *Adults:* 1–4 inhalations bid.	*Adverse events:* Oral thrush, dysphonia (minimize by rinsing mouth after dose).

TABLE 716-1. General Medications—cont'd

DRUG (TRADE NAMES, FORMULATIONS)	INDICATIONS (MECHANISM OF ACTION AND DOSING)	COMMENTS (CAUTIONS, ADVERSE EVENTS, MONITORING)
Bumetanide Antihypertensive: diuretic, loop. Bumex. Injection: 0.25 mg/mL (2, 4, 10 mL). Tablet: 0.5, 1, 2 mg.	**Management of edema or fluid overload states (prevents sodium and chloride reabsorption at the ascending loop of Henle and proximal tubule).** PO, IV, IM: *Neonates:* 0.01–0.05 mg/kg/dose q 24–48 hr. *Infants and children:* 0.015–0.1 mg/kg/dose q 6–24 hr (max: 10 mg/24 hr). *Adults:* 0.5–2 mg/dose (max: 10 mg/24 hr).	*Adverse events:* Electrolyte depletion, dehydration.
Bupivacaine Local anesthetic, injectable. Marcaine; Sensorcaine; Sensorcaine-MPF Bupivacaine. Injection; preservative-free: 0.25% (2.5 mg/mL); 0.5% (5 mg/mL); 0.75% (7.5 mg/mL). With preservative: 0.25% (2.5 mg/mL); 0.5% (5 mg/mL). Bupivacaine and epinephrine (2 : 2 million) injection, preservative-free: 0.25% (2.5 mg/mL); 0.5% (5 mg/mL); 0.75% (7.5 mg/mL). With preservative: 0.25% (2.5 mg/mL); 0.5% (5 mg/mL). Bupivacaine in dextrose: 8.25%. Injection (spinal), preservative-free: 0.75% (7.5 mg/mL).	**Local anesthetic (blocks initiation and conduction of nerve impulses by decreasing permeability of neuron to sodium ions).** Caudal block: *Children:* 1–3.7 mg/kg. *Adults:* 15–30 mL of 0.25% or 0.5%. Epidural block: *Children:* 1.25 mg/kg/dose. *Adults:* 10–20 mL of 0.25% or 0.5% Peripheral nerve block: 5 mL dose of 0.25% (12.5 mg) or 0.5% (25 mg) (max: 400 mg/24 hr). Sympathetic nerve block: 20–50 mL of 0.25% (no epinephrine).	*Cautions:* Excess doses may result in seizures, bradyarrhythmias, metabolic acidosis, apnea, and methemoglobinemia. Avoid epinephrine for nerve block near end artery because of risk of necrosis.
Bupropion Antidepressant. Wellbutrin. Tablet: 75, 100 mg.	**Depression, attention deficit disorder, smoking cessation (blocks serotonin activity and norepinephrine reuptake)** *Children:* Anecdotal experience showed benefits at 75–100 mg 2–3 times/24 hr. *Adults:* Begin 100 mg bid and may gradually increase (max: 450 mg/24 hr).	*Adverse events:* Agitation, insomnia, headache, psychosis, confusion, anxiety, seizures, akathisia, fever, chills, dry mouth, constipation, nausea, vomiting.
Busulfan Antineoplastic agent; alkylating agent. Myleran. Tablet: 2 mg.	**Treatment of chronic myelogenous leukemia (CML) or as part of marrow ablation conditioning before bone marrow transplant (interferes with DNA alkylation).** *Children:* (for CML remission) 0.06–0.12 mg/kg/24 hr; titrate dose to keep leukocyte count > 40,000/mm^3; (for bone marrow transplant conditioning) 1 mg/kg/dose q 6 hr for 16 doses. *Adults:* (for CML remission) 0.06 mg/kg/24 hr.	*Adverse events:* Severe pancytopenia, leukopenia, thrombocytopenia, bone marrow suppression (onset, 7–10 days; nadir, 14–21 days; recovery, 28 days). *Monitoring:* Complete blood count with differential and platelet count (discontinue if WBC < 20,000/mm^3). Hemoglobin, liver function tests.
Caffeine, citrated Central nervous system stimulant, nonamphetamine; respiratory stimulant. Tablet: 65 mg (anhydrous caffeine 32.5 mg), caffeine citrates, caffeine benzoate.	**Treatment of apnea of prematurity (stimulates central inspiratory drive and sensitivity to carbon dioxide).** *Neonates:* PO or IV (citrate or benzoate). Does as caffeine base: Loading dose of 10 mg/kg. Maintenance dose of 5–10 mg/kg/24 hr as 1 or 2 doses/24 hr.	*Cautions:* Sodium benzoate displaces bilirubin from binding and should be avoided in neonates with elevated indirect bilirubin. *Adverse events:* Tachycardia, agitation, irritability, gastric irritation. *Monitoring:* Caffeine concentrations: therapeutic >10 μg/mL; toxic >50 μg/mL.
Calcifediol 25-hydroxycholecalciferol; 25-hydroxyvitamin D_3; vitamin D analog. Calderol. Capsule: 20, 50 μg.	**Treatment of metabolic bone disease associated with chronic renal failure (regulates serum calcium homeostasis as a vitamin D analog).** *Infants:* 5–7 μg/kg/24 hr. *Children and adults:* 20–100 μg/kg daily of other day titrated to obtain normal serum calcium and phosphate levels.	*Cautions:* Avoid in hypercalcemia, hypervitaminosis D, malabsorption states. Ensure adequate calcium intake during use. *Adverse events:* Hypercalcemia, gastrointestinal intolerance.
Calcitriol Vitamin D analog; 1,25-dihydroxycholecalciferol, vitamin, fat-soluble. Calcijex; Rocaltrol. Capsule: 0.25, 0.5 μg. Injection: 1 μg/mL (1 mL); 2 μg/mL (1 mL).	**Treatment of hypocalcemia and metabolic bone disease; reduces elevated parathyroid hormone levels and decreases severity of psoriatic lesions in psoriatic vulgaris (regulate is serum calcium homeostasis and increases calcium absorption).** *Premature infants* (hypocalcemia): 0.05 μg/kg/24 hr IV or 1 μg/24 hr PO. *Children:* 0.01–0.08 μg/kg/24 hr. *Adults:* 0.25–1 μg/24 hr.	*Adverse events:* Hypercalcemia, vitamin D toxicity.
Calcium salts (PO and IV) Calcium carbonate. (Elemental calcium listed in parentheses.) Antacid; calcium salt; electrolyte supplement. Oral Alka–Mints; Cal-Plus; Mylanta; Os-Cal; Tums Capsule: 1,500 mg (600 mg). Liquid: 1,000 mg/5 mL (360 mL). Cardiac arrest Lozenge: 600 mg (240 mg). Powder: 6.5 g/packet. Suspension, oral: 1,250 mg/5 mL (500 mg). Tablet: 650 mg (260 mg); 1,500 mg (600 mg). Tablet, chewable.	**Hypocalcemic tetany and cardiac disturbances of hyperkalemia (moderate nerve and muscle performance).** Hypocalcemic tetany. *Neonates:* 2.4 mEq/kg/24 hr in divided doses (if due to citrated blood transfusion, give 0.45 mEq/dL transfused blood). *Infants and children:* 10 mg/kg over 5–10 min (may repeat in 6–8 hr), followed by infusion with maximum of 200 mg/kg/24 hr. *Adults:* 4.5–16 mEq repeated until response. *Infants and children:* 20 mg/kg IV and may repeat in 10 min. *Adults:* 2–4 mg/kg repeated of 10 min as needed.	*Caution:* Make sure of IV access site to avoid severe IV burns; bradycardia. *Adverse events:* Constipation, hypercalcemia, milk-alkali syndrome. *Monitoring:* Continuous ECG; serum calcium, potassium, and magnesium levels.

Calcium Content of Salts

Salt	Mg of Calcium/g of Salt (elemental)	mEq Ca^{2+}/g of Salt
Ca carbonate	400	20
Ca chloride	270	13.5
Ca glubionate	64	3.2
Ca gluceptate	82	4.1
Ca gluconate	90	4.5
Ca lactate	130	6.5
Ca phosphate	390	19.3

DRUG (TRADE NAMES, FORMULATIONS)	INDICATIONS (MECHANISM OF ACTION AND DOSING)	COMMENTS (CAUTIONS, ADVERSE EVENTS, MONITORING)
Calcium chloride Calcium salt; electrolyte supplement, parenteral. Cal Plus. (Elemental calcium listed in parentheses.) Injection: 10% = 100 mg/mL (27.2 mg/mL) [10 mL] (1.4 mEq calcium/mL).	**Prevention of calcium depletion and relief of acid indigestion (source of calcium and neutralizes acid).** *Children:* *<6 mo:* 400 mg/24 hr. *6–12 mo:* 600 mg/24 hr. *1-5 yr:* 800 mg/24 hr. *6–10 yr:* 800–1,200 mg/24 hr. *>10 yr and adult:* 1,000–1,500 mg/24 hr.	
Calcium glubionate Calcium salt; electrolyte supplement, oral. Neo-Calglucon. Syrup: 1.8 g/5 mL (115 mg/5 mL) [480 mL] (1.2 mEq calcium/mL).		

TABLE 716-1. General Medications—cont'd

DRUG (TRADE NAMES, FORMULATIONS)	INDICATIONS (MECHANISM OF ACTION AND DOSING)	COMMENTS (CAUTIONS, ADVERSE EVENTS, MONITORING)
Calfactant Infasurf. Intratracheal suspension of calf lung surfactant (35 mg phospholipids, 0.65 mg proteins, 0.26 mg SP-B/mL).	**Prophylaxis or treatment of respiratory distress syndrome and treatment of persistent pulmonary hypertension.** *Neonates:* 3 mL/kg/dose 1–4 times q 12 hr. *Children and adults:* Not indicated.	*Caution:* Monitor ventilator status closely; may require rapid weaning within minutes of dose. *Adverse events:* Bradycardia, airway obstruction, cyanosis.
Capsaicin Analgesic, topical; topical skin product. R-Gel; Zostrix-HP topical, Zostrix Topical. Cream: 0.025% (45, 90 g); 0.075% (30, 60 g). Gel: 0.025% (15, 30 mL).	**Topical treatment of pain associated with postherpetic neuralgia, rheumatoid arthritis, osteoarthritis, diabetic neuropathy, and postsurgical pain (induces release of substance P, depleting peripheral nerves and preventing reaccumulation).** *Children >2 yr and adults:* Apply to affected area at least tid–qid.	*Adverse events:* Local itching, stinging, burning, erythema.
Captopril Angiotensin-converting enzyme (ACE) inhibitor; antihypertensive. Capoten. Tablet: 12.5, 25, 50, 100 mg.	**Management of hypertension and treatment of heart failure.** *Premature newborns:* 0.01 mg/kg q 8–12 hr. *Neonates:* Initial dose of 0.05–0.1 mg/kg/dose q 8–24 hr, titrated upward to response (max: 0.5 mg/kg/dose q 6–24 hr). *Infants:* Initial dose of 0.15–0.3 mg/kg/dose, titrated upward (max: 6 mg/kg/24 hr in 1–4 divided doses). *Children:* Initial dose of 0.3–0.5 mg/kg/dose, titrated upward (max: 6 mg/kg/24 hr divided into 2–4 doses). *Older children:* Initial dose of 6.25–12.5 mg/kg/dose q 12–24 hr, titrated (max: 6 mg/kg/24 hr in 2–4 doses). *Adolescents and adults:* Initial dose of 12.5–25 mg/dose, titrated (max: 450 mg/24 hr).	*Cautions:* Use with caution in renal artery stenosis or in patients with volume depletion. *Adverse events:* Cough, angioedema, oliguria, hyperkalemia.
Carbamazepine Anticonvulsant, miscellaneous. Epitol; Tegretol. Suspension, oral (citrus-vanilla flavor): 100 mg/5 mL (450 mL). Tablet: 200 mg. Tablet, chewable: 100 mg. Sustained-release tablet: Tegretol XR: 100, 200, 400 mg.	**Treatment of generalized tonic-clonic and partial seizures, pain relief in trigeminal neuralgia and diabetic neuropathy, and treatment of bipolar disorder (limits influx of sodium ions across cell membranes or other unknown mechanisms).** *Children:* *<6 yr:* Initial dose of 5 mg/kg/24 hr in 2–4 divided doses; may increase q 5–7 days by 5 mg/kg, based on effect or toxicity and serum concentration. *6–12 yr:* Initial dose of 10 mg/kg/24 hr in 2–4 divided doses; increase by 100 mg or 5 mg/kg/24 hr at weekly intervals until therapeutic levels are achieved (usual dose: 800–1,200 mg/24 hr). *Adults:* Initial dose of 200 mg bid; increase by 200 mg at weekly intervals until therapeutic levels are achieved (usual dose: 1.6–2.4 g/24 hr in 3–4 divided doses).	*Caution:* Avoid in patients with bone marrow depression; may cross react in patients with tricyclic antidepressant hypersensitivity. *Adverse events:* Sedation, dizziness, fatigue, ataxia, confusion, nausea, vomiting, blurred vision, nystagmus, bone marrow depression, leukopenia, neutropenia, thrombocytopenia, pancytopenia, aplastic anemia, hepatitis, hypersensitivity reactions. *Monitoring:* Serum concentrations correlate with clinical response (6–12 μg/mL), and neurologic and visual toxicity (> 8 μg/mL, but particularly > 12 μg/mL). Drug dosing requirements will increase over first 4 wk because of hepatic enzyme induction by carbamazepine. Monitor serum concentrations to increase doses appropriately.
Carbamide peroxide Otic agent, ceruminolytic. Auro Ear Drops; Gly-Oxide Oral; Murine Ear Drop; Proxigel Oral. Gel, oral: 11% (36 g). Solution, oral: 10% in glycerin (15, 22.5, 30, 60 mL). Otic: 6.5% in glycerin (15, 30 mL).	**Relief of minor inflammation of oral mucosa, including gums and lips, and removal of ear wax (release of hydrogen peroxide, which inhibits bacteria and softens ear wax).** *Children and adults:* Gel: Gently massage on affected area qid. Oral solution: Apply several drops to affected area qid for up to 7 days. (expectorate 2–3 min after each use). Otic solution: Tilt head sideways and instill 5–10 drops bid for up to 4 days. Keep drops in ear canal for several minutes by tilting head and placing cotton in ear.	*Adverse events:* Local irritation.
Carbinoxamine and Pseudoephedrine Antihistamine/decongestant combination. Carbiset Tablet; Carbodec Syrup; Rondec Drops. Drops: Carbinoxamine maleate 2 mg and pseudoephedrine hydrochloride 25 mg/mL (30 mL with dropper). Syrup: Carbinoxamine maleate 4 mg and pseudoephedrine hydrochloride 60 mg/5 mL (120, 480 mL). Tablet, film-coated: Carbinoxamine maleate 4 mg and pseudoephedrine hydrochloride 60 mg. Tablets sustained-release: Carbinoxamine maleate 8 mg and pseudoephedrine hydrochloride 120 mg.	**Temporary relief of nasal congestion, runny nose, sneezing, and allergy symptoms (antihistamine as H_1 blocker, and decongestant as α-and β-receptor stimulant).** *Children:* Give qid: *1–3 mo:* 1/4 dropper (0.25 mL). *3–6 mo:* 1/2 dropper (0.5 mL). *6–9 mo:* 3/4 dropper (0.75 mL). *9–18 mo:* 1 dropper (1.0 mL). *18 mo–6 yr:* 2.5 mL syrup. *6–12 yr:* 5 mL syrup or 1 tablet. *Children > 12 yr and adults:* 1 tablet qid or 1 sustained-release tablet bid.	*Cautions:* Avoid in narrow-angle glaucoma, coronary artery disease, gastrointestinal or genitourinary obstruction, or monoamine oxidase inhibitor therapy. *Adverse events:* Hypertension, tachycardia, drowsiness, sedation, thickening of bronchial secretions.
Carboplatin Antineoplastic agent; alkylating agent. Paraplatin powder for injection, lyophilized: 50, 150, 450 mg.	**Treatment of multiple tumors, including pediatric brain tumor and neuroblastoma (platination of DNA interferes with DNA function).** *Children:* Solid tumor: 300–600 mg/m² IV 1 × q 4 wk Brain tumor: 175 mg/m² IV 1 × wk for 4 wk (2 wk recovery period between courses). *Adults:* 360 mg/m² IV 1 × q 4 wk.	*Adverse events:* Neutropenia, leukopenia, thrombocytopenia, peripheral neuropathy, ototoxicity, abnormal liver and renal function, alopecia, nausea, vomiting. *Monitoring:* Neutrophil and platelet counts affect dose selection as follows: platelets < 50,000/mm³ or neutrophils < 500/mm³: give 75% of recommended dose (nadir: 14–21 days post dose).
Carmustine Antineoplastic agent; alkylating agent (nitrosourea). BiCNU power for injection: 100 mg/vial packaged with 3 mL of absolute alcohol for use as a sterile diluent.	**Treatment of cancers, including brain tumor, Hodgkin disease, non-Hodgkin lymphoma, and multiple myeloma (inhibits key enzymatic reactions involved in DNA synthesis).** *Children:* 200–250 mg/m² IV q 4–6 wk as a single dose. *Adults:* 150–200 mg/m² IV q 6 wk as a single dose.	*Adverse events:* Nausea, vomiting, myelosuppression (nadir 4–6 wk post dose), alopecia, stomatitis, anorexia, diarrhea, dizziness, ataxia, pulmonary fibrosis, hepatic and renal dysfunction, retinitis, optic neuritis.
Carnitine Dietary supplement. Carnitor; Vitacarn. Capsule: 250 mg. Injection: 1 g/5 mL (5 mL). Liquid (cherry flavor): 100 mg/mL (10 mL). Tablet: 330 mg.	**Treatment of carnitine deficiency; improves use of IV fat emulsions by premature infants (facilitates long-chain fatty acid entry into the mitochondria and required in energy metabolism).** *Premature infants:* 8–16 mg/kg/24 hr IV infusion. *Children:* 50–100 mg/kg/24 hr in 2-3 divided doses PO, 50 mg/kg/dose q 4–6 hr IV (max: 300 mg/kg/24 hr). *Adults:* 0.33–1 g/dose bid–tid, PO, 50 mg/kg/dose q 4–6 hr (max: 300 mg/kg/24 hr).	*Adverse events:* Nausea, vomiting, abdominal cramps, body odor.

TABLE 716-1. General Medications—cont'd

DRUG (TRADE NAMES, FORMULATIONS)	INDICATIONS (MECHANISM OF ACTION AND DOSING)	COMMENTS (CAUTIONS, ADVERSE EVENTS, MONITORING)
Carvedilol Coreg. Tablet: 3.125, 6.25, 12.5, 25 mg.	**β-Receptor blocker with vasodilator activity, used to treat congestive heart failure or hypertension.** *Children:* Initial dose of 0.08 mg/kg, gradually increased over 2–3 mo, based on response (max: 0.5 mg/kg/24 hr divied q 12 hr).	*Caution:* May cause AV block, arrhythmias, bradycardia, or worsen asthma or heart failure. *Drug interactions:* May cause excessive hypotension when used with other antihypertensives.
Cascara sagrada Laxative; stimulant. Liquid, aromatic fluid extract: 5, 120 mL. Tablet: 325 mg.	**Temporary relief of constipation (direct chemical irritation of gastrointestinal mucosa).** *Infants:* 1.25 mL once daily. *Children 2–11 yr:* 2.5 mL once daily. *>12 yr and adults:* 5 mL once daily.	*Cautions:* Fecal impaction, gastrointestinal obstruction, gastrointestinal bleeding. Onset of effect 6–10 hr, so give at bedtime. *Adverse events:* Gastrointestinal cramps, urine discolored red or brown.
Castor oil Laxative; stimulant. Alphamul; Emulsoil; Fleet; Purge. Emulsion, oral; liquid, oral: 100% (60, 120, 480 mL).	**Bowel or rectal evacuation for surgery (stimulates peristalsis).** *Infants < 2 yr:* 1–5 mL single dose. *Children 2–11 yr:* 5–15 mL. *Children > 12 yr and adults:* 15–60 mL.	*Adverse events:* Electrolyte disturbances, abdominal cramps.
Charcoal Adsorbent, antidote. Actidose-Aqua; Actidose with Sorbitol; Charcocaps.	**Emergency treatment of poisoning by certain drugs and chemicals; gastrointestinal dialysis to promote elimination of certain drugs and toxins; treatment of diarrhea (adsorbs toxic substance; interferes with enterohepatic recycling of certain drugs).** *Children and adults:* 1–2 g/kg or 5–10 × the weight of the ingested poison (limit sorbitol to 1–2 × daily); may repeat doses q 2–6 hr.	*Adverse events:* Constipation, black stools.
Chloral hydrate Hypnotic; sedative. Noctec. Capsules: 250, 500 mg. Syrup: 250, 500 mg/5 mL. Suppository: 324, 500, 648 mg.	**Short-term sedative/hypnotic (mechanism unknown).** *Neonates:* 25 mg/kg/dose. *Infants and children:* 25–100 mg/kg/dose. *Adults:* 250–1,000 mg/dose. Doses may be repeated q 6–8 hr. Lower-end doses cause sedation; higher-end doses cause hypnosis.	*Cautions:* Repeat doses in neonates may cause accumulation of active metabolite trichloroethanol, which can cause hepatic toxicity and bilirubin displacement.
Chlorambucil Antineoplastic alkylating agent. Leukeran. Tablet: 2 mg.	**Management of various cancers, including Hodgkin disease, non-Hodgkin lymphoma, and chronic lymphocytic leukemia, and nephrotic syndrome (alkylation interferes with DNA replication and RNA transcription).** *Children and adults:* 0.1–0.2 mg/kg/24 hr for 3–6 wk. Longer treatment doses are adjusted based on blood counts.	*Adverse events:* Bone marrow suppression (onset, 7 days; nadir, 10–14 days; recovery, 28 days); rashes, hyperuricemia, nausea, vomiting, diarrhea, oral ulceration, pulmonary fibrosis, hepatic necrosis, peripheral neuropathy.
Chlorothiazide Diuretic. Generic. Tablet: 250, 500 mg. Suspension: 250 mg/5 mL. Powder for injection: 500 mg.	**Treatment of fluid overload states and hypertension (inhibits sodium reabsorption in distal tubule).** *Neonates and infants < 6 mo:* PO: 20–40 mg/kg/24 hr divided q 12 hr; IV: 2–8 mg/kg/24 hr divided q 12 hr. *Infants > 6 mo and children:* PO: 20 mg/kg/24 hr in 2 divided doses; IV: 4 mg/kg/24 hr. *Adults:* PO: 500 mg–2 g/24 hr in 1–2 doses; IV: 500–1,000 mg/24 hr.	*Adverse events:* Hypokalemia, hypochloremic alkalosis, hyperglycemia, hyperlipidemia, hypercalcemia, hyperuricemia, leukopenia, prerenal azotemia.
Chlorpheniramine maleate Antihistamine. Generic. Capsule: 12 mg. Capsule, timed-release: 6, 8, 12 mg. Syrup: 2 mg/5 mL. Tablet: 4, 8, 12 mg. Tablet; chewable: 2 mg. Tablet; timed-release: 8, 12 mg.	**Treatment of allergic symptoms (competes with histamine for H_1 receptor sites).** *Children:* *2–6 yr:* 1 mg q 4–6 hr. *6–12 yr:* 2 mg q 2–6 hr, or sustained-release form, 8 mg at bedtime. *>12 yr and adults:* 4 mg q 4–6 hr, or sustained-release form, 12 mg at bedtime.	*Adverse events:* Drowsiness, excitation or hyperactivity (in children), dry mouth, blurred vision.
Chlorpromazine Phenothiazine. Thorazine. Capsule: 30, 75, 150, 200, 300 mg. Oral concentrate: 30, 100 mg/mL. Suppository: 25, 100 mg. Syrup: 10 mg/5 mL. Tablet: 10, 25, 50, 100, 200 mg. Injection: 25 mg/mL.	**Treatment of psychosis, mania, Tourette syndrome, behavioral problems, nausea, and vomiting (blocks postsynaptic mesolimbic dopaminergic receptors in the brain, strong α-adrenergic blocking effect).** *Children > 6 mo:* PO: 0.5–1 mg/kg/dose q 4–6 hr. Rectal: 1 mg/kg/dose q 6–8 hr. IM or IV: 0.5–1 mg/kg/dose q 6–8 hr. *Adults:* Psychosis: PO: 30–800 mg/24 hr in 1–4 divided doses (start low and titrate up to effect). IV or IM: 25 mg initial dose, titrated up to effect (max: 400 mg/dose q 4–6 hr). Nausea or vomiting: PO: 10–25 mg q 4–6 hr. IM or IV: 25–50 mg q 4–6 hr. Rectal: 50–100 mg q 6–8 hr.	*Adverse events:* Hypotension, tachycardia, arrhythmias, pseudoparkinsonism, tardive dyskinesia, akathisia, dystonias, constipation, nasal congestion, dry mouth, malignant hyperpyrexia. *Monitoring:* Chlorpromazine concentrations: therapeutic 50–300 ng/mL; toxic > 750 ng/mL.
Chlorpropamide Sulfonylurea. Diabinese. Tablet: 100, 250 mg.	**Control blood sugar in non–insulin-dependent diabetes mellitus (type II)** [stimulates insulin release from pancreatic islet cells]. *Adults:* Initial 250 mg once daily, may increase to response by 125 mg q 3–5 days to response (max: 750 mg/24 hr).	*Adverse events:* Gastrointestinal problems, photosensitivity, hepatotoxicity, hyponatremia, syndrome of inappropriate antidiuretic hormone.
Chlorthalidone Thiazide diuretic. Hygroton. Tablet: 20, 25, 100 mg.	**Treatment of fluid overload and mild hypertension (inhibits sodium and chloride reabsorption in the cortical-diluting segment of the ascending loop of Henle).** *Children:* 1–2 mg/kg once daily. *Adults:* 25–100 mg once daily.	*Adverse events:* Photosensitivity, fluid and electrolyte imbalance, hypokalemia.

TABLE 716-1. General Medications—cont'd

DRUG (TRADE NAMES, FORMULATIONS)	INDICATIONS (MECHANISM OF ACTION AND DOSING)	COMMENTS (CAUTIONS, ADVERSE EVENTS, MONITORING)
Chlorzoxazone Skeletal muscle relaxant. Paraflex; Parafon Forte. Tablet: 250, 500 mg.	**Symptomatic relief of muscle spasm and pain (depresses polysynaptic reflexes at spinal cord and subcortical levels).** *Children:* 20 mg/kg/24 hr in 3–4 divided doses. *Adults:* 250–500 mg tid–qid.	*Adverse events:* Drowsiness.
Cholestyramine resin Antilipemic agent. Questran. Powder: 4 g resin/9 g powder.	**Management of elevated cholesterol (forms nonabsorbable complex with bile salts and low-density lipoprotein cholesterol).** *Children:* 240 mg/kg/24 hr in 3 divided doses. *Adults:* 4 g/dose 1–6 × daily.	*Adverse events:* Hyperchloremic acidosis, constipation, nausea, vomiting, abdominal pain and distention, malabsorption of fat-soluble vitamins.
Choline magnesium trisalicylate Nonsteroidal anti-inflammatory agent. Trilisate. Liquid: 500 mg salicylate/5 mL. Tablet: 500, 750, 1,000 mg.	**Management of arthritis disorders (inhibits prostaglandin synthesis).** *Children:* 30–60 mg/kg/24 hr in 3–4 divided doses. *Adults:* 500–1,500 mg/dose 1–3 × daily.	*Cautions:* Avoid in patients with suspected influenza or varicella infection due to risk of Reye syndrome; avoid in those with asthma and others at risk for serious hypersensitivity reactions. *Adverse events:* Gastrointestinal intolerance, tinnitus, hepatotoxicity, pulmonary edema. *Monitoring:* Salicylate concentrations: anti-inflammatory 150–300 µg/mL; analgesic or antipyretic effect 30–50 µg/mL.
Chorionic gonadotropin Gonadotropin; ovulation stimulator. Chorex, Choron, Pregnyl. Powder for injection: 200, 500, 1,000, 2,000 U/mL (10 mL).	**Treatment of hypogonadotropic hypogonadism and cryptorchidism; induces ovulation (stimulates production of gonadal steroid hormones; substitutes for luteinizing hormone to stimulate ovulation).** *Children:* Prepubertal cryptorchidism: 1,000–2,000 units/m^2/dose 3 × wk for 3 wk or 500 units 3 ×/wk for 4–6 wk. Hypogonadotropic hypogonadism: 500–1,000 U/dose 3 ×/wk for 3 wk; or 4,000 U 3 ×/wk for 6–9 mo, then taper to 2,000 units 3 ×/wk for 3 mo. *Adults* (menotropin dose): 5,000 units 3 ×/wk for 4–6 mo.	*Adverse events:* Mental depression, tiredness, precocious puberty, premature closure of epiphyses.
Cimetidine Histamine$_2$ antagonist. Cimetidine. Tablet: 200, 300, 400, 800 mg. Liquid: 300 mg/5 mL. Injection: 150 mg/mL.	**Short-term treatment and long-term prophylaxis of gastroesophageal reflux disease, gastrointestinal ulcers, and hyperacidity (competitive inhibition of histamine at H_2 receptors).** *Neonates:* PO, IV, IM: 5–10 mg/kg/24 hr divided q 8–12 hr. *Children:* PO, IV, IM: 20–40 mg/kg/24 hr divided q 6 hr. *Adults:* 300 mg q 6 hr (prolong dosing interval for creatinine clearance of <40 mL/min).	*Cautions:* Potent enzyme inhibitor that may cause toxic accumulation of drugs that are metabolized (e.g., antidepressants, anticonvulsants, theophylline, warfarin, cisapride). *Adverse events:* Dizziness, drowsiness, bradycardia. *Monitoring:* Target gastric pH ≥ 5.
Cisapride Prokinetic gastrointestinal agent. Propulsid. Tablet: 10 mg.	**Treatment of gastroesophageal reflux, gastroparesis, and refractory constipation (enhances release of acetylcholine at myenteric plexus).** *Neonates–Children:* 0.15–0.3 mg/kg/dose tid–qid. *Adults:* 10–20 mg qid. Give dose 15–30 min before meals.	*Cautions:* High doses or combination with enzyme inhibitors (e.g., erythromycin, cimetidine) may cause Q-T-interval prolongation, predisposing to torsades de pointes. *Adverse events:* Tachycardia, prolonged Q-T interval, headache, anxiety, insomnia gastrointestinal cramping, flatulence, diarrhea. *Monitoring:* Baseline ECG and early treatment.
Cisplatin Antineoplastic agent; alkylating agent. Platinol. Injection, aqueous: 1 mg/mL. Powder for injection: 10, 50 mg.	**Treatment of multiple tumor types (inhibits DNA synthesis).** *Children and adults:* 37–75 mg/m^2 once q 2–3 wk or 50–120 mg/m^2 once q 21–28 days (administer over 4–6 hr). Adjust dose in renal impairment: CrCl 10–50 mL/min = 75% of dose; CrCl < 10 mL/min = 50% of dose.	*Adverse events:* Nausea, vomiting (lasts up to 1 wk post dose), myelosuppression (onset, 10 days; nadir, 14–23 days; recovery, 21–39 days), acute renal failure, chronic nephropathy (sodium, magnesium, and water wasting; hyperuricemia), peripheral neuropathy (irreversible), ototoxicity (high-frequency hearing loss), extravasation injury, elevated liver enzymes, alopecia, optic neuritis, arrhythmias.
Citrate solutions Alkalinizing agent. Bicitra (sodium citrate 500 mg and citric acid 334 mg/5 mL = 1 mEq sodium + 1 mEq bicarbonate equivalent/mL). Polycitra (sodium citrate 500 mg and citric acid 334 mg and potassium citrate 550 mg/5 mL = 1 mEq sodium + 1 mEq potassium + 2 mEq bicarbonate equivalent/mL).	**Treatment of chronic metabolic acidosis (citrate salts are oxidized in the body to form bicarbonate).** *Neonates, infants, and children:* 2–3 mEq/kg/24 hr in 3–4 divided doses with water after meals. *Adults:* 15–30 mL with water after meals and at bedtime.	*Adverse events:* Hypernatremia, hyperkalemia, metabolic alkalosis.
Clomipramine Antidepressant. Anafranil. Capsule: 25, 50, 75 mg.	**Treatment of obsessive-compulsive disorder and panic attacks (affects serotonin and norepinephrine uptake).** *Children:* Starting dose of 25 mg/24 hr, gradually increased to response (max: 200 mg/24 hr). *Adults:* Starting dose or 25 mg/24 hr, increased to response (max: 250 mg/24 hr).	*Adverse events:* Dizziness, drowsiness, dry mouth, constipation, nausea, weight gain, nervousness, anxiety, seizures, hypotension, arrhythmias, parkinsonian syndrome, insomnia.
Clonazepam Benzodiazepine. Klonopin. Tablet: 0.5, 1, 2 mg.	**Prophylaxis of seizure types: absence, Lennox-Gastaut, akinetic, myoclonic (depresses nerve transmission in motor cortex).** *Children:* 0.01–0.3 mg/kg/24 hr in 2–3 divided doses, increased by 0.5 mg/24 hr q 3–5 days to response (max: 0.3 mg/kg/24 hr). *Adults:* Initial dose of 0.1 mg bid; then 0.2–2.4 mg/24 hr in 2–4 divided doses.	*Adverse events:* Tachycardia, chest pain, drowsiness, fatigue, impaired memory and coordination, depression, blurred vision, nausea, vomiting, dry mouth, hypersalivation, anorexia, bronchial hypersecretion, respiratory depression, physical and psychological dependence. *Monitoring:* Clonazepam concentrations: therapeutic 20–80 ng/mL; toxic > 80 ng/mL; loss of efficacy with prolonged use (tachyphylaxis).
Clonidine α-Adrenergic agonist. Catapres. Tablet: 0.1, 0.2, 0.3 mg. Transdermal patch: 0.1, 0.2, 0.3 mg/24 hr.	**Treatment of hypertension, attention deficit disorder (ADD), and narcotic withdrawal; aids in diagnosis of pheochromocytoma and growth hormone deficiency (stimulates α_2 adrenoreceptors in the brainstem).** *Neonates:* Narcotic withdrawal: 1 µg/kg q 6–8 hr to start and may titrate to targeted abstinence score (max: 2 µg/kg/dose q 4 hr).	*Cautions:* Taper doses gradually to avoid sympathetic overactivity symptoms. *Adverse events:* Drowsiness, dizziness, dry mouth, constipation, hypotension.

TABLE 716-1. General Medications—cont'd

DRUG (TRADE NAMES, FORMULATIONS)	INDICATIONS (MECHANISM OF ACTION AND DOSING)	COMMENTS (CAUTIONS, ADVERSE EVENTS, MONITORING)
	Children: ADD: initial dose of 0.05 mg/24 hr, increased q 3–7 days by 0.05 mg/24 hr given in 3–4 divided doses to response (max: 0.4 mg/24 hr). Hypertension: 5–10 μg/kg/24 hr in 2–4 divided doses (max: 0.9 mg/24 hr). Clonidine tolerance test for growth hormone release: 4 μg/kg × 1 dose. *Adults:* Hypertension: Oral: 0.2–2.4 mg/24 hr in 2–4 doses titrated to response. Transdermal: 0.1–0.3 mg/24 hr titrated to effect.	
Clorazepate Benzodiazepine. Tranxene. Tablet: 3.75, 7.5, 15 mg.	**Anxiety and panic disorders; adjunct in management of partial seizures (facilitates transmission of inhibitory neurotransmitter, γ-aminobutyric acid).** *Children:* *9–12 yr:* 3.75–7.5 mg/dose bid (max: 60 mg/24 hr). *>12 yr and adults:* 7.5 mg/dose bid–tid (max: 90 mg/24 hr). *Adults:* 7.5–15 mg/dose bid–qid.	*Adverse events:* Drowsiness, confusion, depression, blurred vision.
Clozapine Clozaril; generic. Tablet: 25, 100 mg.	**Atypical antipsychotic, dibenzepin chemical group.** *Children:* Starting dose of 6.25 mg bid, increased by 6.25 mg/24 hr weekly as needed. Typical dose: 50–300 mg/24 hr. *Adults:* Starting dose of 25 mg q 24 hr, titrated up by 25–50 mg/24 hr to 450–500 mg/24 hr divided tid at 2 wk. Further dose increases should not exceed 100 mg/wk (max: 900 mg/24 hr).	*Caution:* Agranulocytosis, sometimes fatal, has been reported in 1.3% of patients. Thus, WBC counts must be done at baseline and every wk for the first 6 mo of treatment, then every other wk. WBC counts must be checked q other week thereafter. If clozapine is discontinued, check WBC weekly for the next 4 wk. *Adverse events:* Seizures, orthostatic hypotension, extrapyramidal symptoms (less often than typical antipsychotics), hyperglycemia, dizziness, drowsiness, headache, tremor, excessive salivation (especially during sleep). *Drug interactions:* Clozapine levels may increase with concurrent use of enzyme inhibitors. Clozapine is highly protein-bound and may displace other highly protein-bound drugs (e.g., warfarin).
Codeine Narcotic analgesic. Generic; combination products. Injection. Tablet.	**Treatment of mild to moderate pain and cough (inhibition of ascending pain pathways; central action in medulla to suppress cough).** *Children:* Pain: 0.5–1 mg/kg/dose q 4–6 hr (max: 60 mg/dose). Cough: 1–1.5 mg/kg/24 hr divided q 4–6 hr. *Adults:* Pain: 15–60 mg/dose q 4–6 hr as needed. Cough: 10–20 mg/dose q 4–6 hr (max: 120 mg/24 hr).	*Adverse events:* Drowsiness, constipation, nausea, anorexia, vomiting, sedation, dizziness.
Colchicine Anti-inflammatory/antigout agent. Generic. Injection: 0.5 mg/mL. Tablet: 0.5, 0.6 mg.	**Management of familial Mediterranean fever and acute and chronic gouty arthritis (decreases leukocyte motility and phagocytosis in joints).** *Children:* Prophylaxis of familial Mediterranean fever: *<5 yr:* 0.5 mg/24 hr *>5 yr:* 1–1.5 mg/24 hr in 2–3 divided doses. *Adults:* Gouty arthritis: PO: 0.5–0.6 mg q 2 hr to symptom relief or gastrointestinal toxicity (max: 8 mg/24 hr). IV: Loading dose of 1–3 mg, then 0.5 mg/dose q 6 hr until response (max: 4 mg/24 hr).	*Caution:* Reduce dose by 50% if CrCl < 10 mL/min. *Adverse events:* Nausea, vomiting, diarrhea, abdominal pain.
Colfosceril palmitate Lung surfactant. Exosurf. Intratracheal suspension: 108 mg/10 mL.	**Neonatal respiratory distress syndrome (RDS) [replaces deficient surfactant, lowers surface tension at air-fluid interface in alveoli].** *Neonates:* 5 mL/kg/dose as prophylaxis or rescue therapy for RDS (max: 4 doses, although no proven benefit for >2 doses).	*Caution:* Administer via side port using special endotracheal tube adaptor with 1/2 dose with head and torso tilted to left and 1/2 dose with head and torso tilted to right; give each 1/2 over 1–2 min. *Adverse events:* Pulmonary hemorrhage, overventilation (causing hyperoxia and hypocarbia), Patcut ductus arteriosus.
Corticotropin, ACTH Adrenal corticosteroid. Acthar. Injection, repository: 40, 80 u/mL. Tablet: 5, 10, 25 mg.	**Infantile spasms, diagnostic agent in adrenocortical insufficiency, acute exacerbations of multiple sclerosis, severe muscle weakness in myasthenia gravis (stimulates adrenal cortex to release adrenal steroids, androgenic substances, and a small amount of aldosterone).** *Children:* Inflammation or immunosuppression: IV, IM, SC (aqueous): 1.6 u/kg/24 hr or 50 u/m² divided q 6–8 hr. IM (gel): 0.8 u/kg/24 hr or 25 u/m² day divided q 12–24 hr. Infantile spasms: 5–160 u/kg/24 hr has been used for 1 wk–12 mo as IM gel (prednisone 2 mg/kg/24 hr has equal efficacy). *Adults:* Acute exacerbations of MS: 80–120 u/24 hr for 2–3 wk.	*Caution:* May mask signs of infection; do not administer live vaccines; may exacerbate heart failure or hypertension. *Adverse events:* Insomnia, nervousness, increased appetite, indigestion, diabetes mellitus, joint pain, epistaxis, mood swings, pancreatitis, esophagitis, muscle wasting, bone growth suppression, opportunistic infections.

TABLE 716-1. General Medications—cont'd

DRUG (TRADE NAMES, FORMULATIONS)	INDICATIONS (MECHANISM OF ACTION AND DOSING)	COMMENTS (CAUTIONS, ADVERSE EVENTS, MONITORING)
Cortisone acetate Adrenal corticosteroid. Cortone. Injection: 50 mg/mL. Tablet: 5, 10, 25 mg.	**Management of adrenocortical insufficiency (replacement).** *Children:* PO: 0.5–0.75 mg/kg/24 hr divided q 8 hr. IM: 0.25–0.35 mg/kg/24 hr. *Adults:* PO, IM: 20–300 mg/24 hr in 1–2 doses.	*Cautions:* Avoid in active fungal infection and most other serious infections except shock or meningitis. *Adverse events:* Insomnia, nervousness, pseudotumor cerebri, headache, increased appetite, peptic ulcer, diabetes mellitus, edema, hypertension, cataracts, glaucoma, hypokalemia. *Comment:* See comparison of corticosteroids under *Hydrocortisone.*
Cosyntropin Adrenal corticosteroid. Cortrosyn. Powder for injection: 0.25 mg.	**Diagnosis of primary vs secondary adrenocortical deficiency (stimulates adrenal cortex to release adrenal steroids).** *Neonates:* 0.015 mg/kg/dose. *Children <2 yr:* 0.125 mg. *Children >2 yr and adults:* 0.25 mg. Give dose in early morning.	*Adverse events:* Flushing, mild fever, pruritus, pancreatitis. *Monitoring:* Measure plasma cortisol before and exactly 30 min after dose. Normal response is serum cortisol increase >7 μg/dL (>193 nmol/L) or peak response increase >18 μg/dL (497 nmol/L).
Cromolyn sodium Mast cell stabilizer. Crolom; Intal; Gastrocrom; Nasalcrom. Ophthalmic solution. Capsule (oral): 100 mg. Inhalation: 20 mg. Metered-dose inhaler (MDI): 800 μg/spray. Nebulizer solution: 10 mg/mL (2 mL). Nasal solution: 40 mg/mL. Opthalmic solution: 4%.	**Prevention of chronic symptoms of asthma, rhinitis, conjunctivitis, systemic mastocytosis, food allergy, and inflammatory bowel disease (prevents mast cell release of histamine and leukotrienes).** *Children and adults:* Asthma: 1–2 puffs (MDI) or 2 mL (nebulizer solution) 3–4 tid–qid. Rhinitis: 1 spray each nostril tid–qid. Conjunctivitis: 1–2 drops 4–6 times daily. Mastocytosis, food allergy: *Children:* 100 mg/dose qid (max: 40 mg/kg/24 hr). *Adults:* 200 mg/dose qid (max: 400 mg/dose qid).	*Adverse events:* Hoarseness and coughing (mainly with powder for inhalation), burning and stinging at administration site.
Crotamiton Scabicidal. Eurax. Cream: 10%. Lotion: 10%.	**Treatment of scabies (mechanism unknown).** *Infants, children, and adults:* Wash area thoroughly, towel dry, apply a thin layer, and massage drug into skin. Repeat application in 24 hr. Take a cleansing bath 48 hr after final application. May repeat in 7 days if needed.	*Adverse events:* Local irritation.
Cyanocobalamin, vitamin B_{12} Nutritional supplement. Generic. Injection: 100, 1,000 μg/mL. Tablet: 25, 50, 100, 250, 500, 1,000 μg.	**Pernicious anemia, vitamin B_{12} deficiency (coenzyme for various metabolic functions).** Pernicious anemia: *Children:* 30–50 μg/24 hr to total dose of 1,000–5,000 μg, and then follow with 100 μg/mo. *Adults:* 100 μg/24 hr for 6–7 days, then 100 μg/mo. Vitamin B_{12} deficiency: *Children:* 100 μg/24 hr for 10–15 days, then 1–2×/wk for several mo. *Adults:* 30 μg/24 hr for 5–10 days then 100–200 μg/mo.	*Monitoring:* Serum B_{12} levels (normal: 150–750 pg/mL). Some reports of neuropsychiatric problems have been reported with levels <300 pg/mL.
Cyclizine Antinauseant. Marezine. Injection: 50 mg/mL. Tablet: 50 mg.	**Prevent and treat motion-related nausea, vomiting, and vertigo; control postoperative nausea and vomiting (mechanism unknown).** *Children 6–12 yr:* PO: 25 mg/dose up to 3×/24 hr as needed. *Adults:* PO: 50 mg up to q 4–6 hr (30 min before travel) [max: 200 mg/24 hr]; IM 50 mg q 4–6 hr as needed.	*Adverse events:* Drowsiness, dry mouth, headache, diplopia urinary retention.
Cyclopentolate Mydriatic. Cyclogyl, AK-Pentolate. Ophthalmic solution: 0.5%, 1%, 2%.	**Diagnostic procedures requiring mydriasis and cycloplegia (prevents muscles of ciliary body and iris from responding to cholinergic stimulation).** *Infants:* 1 drop 0.5% into each eye 5–10 min before examination. *Children and adults:* 1 drop 0.5% or 1% in eye 40–50 min before procedure (may repeat 1 drop in 5 min if necessary); may use 2% if heavily pigmented iris.	*Caution:* Avoid in narrow-angle glaucoma. *Adverse events:* Tachycardia, CNS stimulation, psychosis, agitation, local burning. *Monitoring:* Cycloplegia and mydriasis begin in 15–60 min and last up to 24 hr (reduce to 3–6 hr with pilocarpine).
Cyclophosphamide Antineoplastic alkylating agent. Cytoxan; Neosar. Powder for injection: 0.1, 0.2, 0.5, 1.0, 2.0 g. Tablet: 25, 50 mg.	**Management of various cancers, including Hodgkin disease, malignant lymphomas, and leukemias; nephrotic syndrome; systemic lupus erythematosus; rheumatoid arthristis; rheumatoid vasculitis (interferes with normal function of DNA by alkylation).** *Children and adults with no hematologic problems:* Induction: IV: 40–50 mg/kg (1.5–1.8 g/m^2) in divided doses over 2–5 days. PO: 1–5 mg/kg/24 hr. Maintenance: IV: 10–15 mg/kg (350–550 mg/m^2) q 7–10 days or 3–5 mg/kg 2×/wk. PO: *Children:* 2–5 mg/kg 2×/wk. *Adults:* 1–5 mg/kg/24 hr. *Children:* SLE: 500–750 mg/m^2/mo. Juvenile RA/vasculitis: IV 10 mg/kg q 2 wk. Bone marrow transplant conditioning: IV 50 mg/kg/24 hr for 3–4 days. Nephrotic syndrome: PO: 2–3 mg/kg/24 hr (when steroids fail, use for up to 12 wk). Adjust doses for:	*Cautions:* Maintain high fluid intake to avoid hemorrhagic cystitis, and consider administration of mesna. *Adverse events:* Cardiotoxicity with high doses, pericardial effusion, congestive heart failure, alopecia, nausea, vomiting, taste distortion, stomatitis, anorexia, hemorrhagic cystitis, leukopenia (onset: 7 days; nadir: 8–15 days; recovery: 21 days), thrombocytopenia, hepatotoxicity, jaundice, renal toxicity, secondary malignancy.

TABLE 716-1. General Medications—cont'd

DRUG (TRADE NAMES, FORMULATIONS)	INDICATIONS (MECHANISM OF ACTION AND DOSING)	COMMENTS (CAUTIONS, ADVERSE EVENTS, MONITORING)
	Renal function: CrCl 25–50 mL/min: Decrease 50%. CrCl < 25 mL/min: Avoid use. Decreased bone marrow function: Reduce dose 33–50%.	
Cyproheptadine hydrochloride Antihistamine. Periactin; generic. Syrup: 2 mg/5 mL. Tablet: 4 mg.	**Treatment of allergic symptoms (H_1-receptor and serotonin antagonist).** *Children:* *2–6 yr:* 2 mg/dose q 8–12 hr (max: 12 mg/24 h). *>7 yr–adults:* 4 mg/dose q 8–12 hr (max: 0.5 mg/kg/24 hr).	*Adverse events:* Drowsiness, sedation, thickened bronchial secretions, bronchospasm, appetite stimulation, photosensitivity.
Cysteine Nutritional supplement. Generic. Injection: 50 mg/mL.	**Supplement to crystalline amino acid solutions to meet amino acid nutritional requirements during parenteral nutrition (replaces deficiency; also enhances solubility of calcium and phosphate in total parenteral nutrition solutions).** *Neonates and infants:* Add 40 mg cysteine to 1 g of amino acids (typically results in 20–100 mg/kg/24 hr of cysteine).	*Adverse events:* Metabolic acidosis, azotemia, elevated blood urea nitrogen, nausea.
Cytarabine HCl, Ara-C Antineoplastic; antimetabolite. Cytosar-US Tarabine PFS. Powder for injection: 0.1, 0.5, 1, 2 g. Injection: 20 mg/mL.	**Used in combination therapy to treat leukemias and lymphomas (inhibits DNA polymerase to inhibit DNA synthesis, works in S-phase of cell division).** *Children and adults:* Doses depend on individual protocols. Typical dose: Induction: IV: 100–200 mg/m²/24 hr for 5–10 days or until remission. Maintenance: IV: 70–200 mg/m²/24 hr for 2–5 days at monthly intervals. IM, SC: 1–1.5 mg/kg single dose at 1–4 wk intervals. Intrathecal: 5–75 mg/m² q 2–7 days until CNS findings normalize (concentration should not exceed 100 mg/mL).	*Adverse events:* Fever, rash, oral/anal ulcerations, nausea, vomiting, diarrhea, mucositis, liver dysfunction, bleeding, myelosuppression (onset, 4–7 days; nadir, 14–18 days; recovery 21–28 days), alopecia, conjunctivitis (administer corticosteroid eyedrops around the clock before, during, and after high-dose Ara-C), dizziness, headache, neuritis (prevent CNS toxicity with pyridoxine administration on days of high-dose Ara-C administration).
Dacarbazine Antineoplastic agent. DTIC-Dome; generic. Injection: 100, 200, 500 mg.	**Treatment of various tumors (alkylating agent and possibly some antimetabolite activity).** *Children:* Solid tumors: 200–470 mg/m²/24 hr over 5 days q 21–28 days. Neuroblastoma: 800–900 mg/m² on day 1 of combination therapy q 3–4 wk. Hodgkin disease: 375 mg/m² on days 1 and 15 of combination treatment; repeat q 28 days. *Adults:* Hodgkin disease: 150 mg/m²/24 hr for 5 days; repeat q 4 wk.	*Adverse events:* Pain and burning at infusion site, nausea and vomiting, leukopenia (onset: 7 days; nadir: 10–14 days; recovery: 21–28 days), weakness, polyneuropathy, paresthesias, elevated liver enzymes, sinus congestion, alopecia, metallic taste.
Dactinomycin Antineoplastic agent. Actinomycin D; Cosmegen. Powder for injection: 0.5 mg.	**Treatment of various tumor types (binds to guanine portion of DNA, blocking replication and transcription of DNA template).** *Children > 6 mo and adults:* 15 μg/kg/24 hr or 400–600 μg/m²/24 hr for 5 days; may repeat every 3–6 wk.	*Adverse events:* Myelosuppression (onset: 7 days; nadir: 14–21 days; recovery: 21–28 days), fatigue, malaise, fever, alopecia, skin eruptions, acne, severe nausea and vomiting, diarrhea, mucositis, stomatitis, hypocalcemia, hyperuricemia.
Danaparoid Orgaran. Antithrombotic agent. Injection: 750 anti-Xa units in 0.6 mL.	**Acts by inhibiting anti-Xa and anti-IIa effects (anti Xa/anti-IIa activity > 22). Low molecular weight heparinoid, consisting mainly of heparan sulfate. Use for heparin-induced thrombocytopenia (cross-reactivity with heparin antibodies is < 10%, compared with > 90% for low molecular weight heparin).** *Children:* Loading dose: 30 U/kg. Maintenance dose: 1.2–2.0 U/kg/hr. *Adults:* Treatment: Loading dose: <50 kg: 1,500 U; 50–90 kg: 2,250 U; >90 kg: 3,000 U. Follow loading dose with 400 U/hr for 4 hr, then 300 U/hr for 4 hr, then maintenance dose of 150–200 U/hr. Prophylaxis: <50 kg: 750 U q 12 hr; 50–90 kg: 1,500 U q 8 hr; >90 kg: 1,500 U q 12 hr.	*Monitoring:* Check plasma anti-Xa levels; target 0.5–0.8 U/mL for treatment; target 0.2–0.4 U/mL for prophylaxis. Monitoring traditional clotting studies (e.g., prothrombin time, activated partial thromboplastin time, activated dotting time) is not beneficial; no effect is seen. *Adverse events:* Bleeding (risk is lower than with unfractionated heparin).
Dantrolene sodium Skeletal muscle relaxant. Dantrium. Capsule: 25, 50, 100 mg. Powder for injection: 20 mg.	**Treatment of spasticity associated with upper motor neuron disorders, such as spinal cord injury, stroke, cerebral palsy, or multiple sclerosis; also used to treat malignant hyperthermia (interferes with release of calcium ion from sarcoplasmic reticulum).** Spasticity: *Children:* 0.5 mg/kg/dose bid; increase frequency q 4–7 days to tid–qid; then increase dose by 0.5 mg/kg (max: 3 mg/kg/dose bid–qid). *Adults:* Starting dose of 25 mg/24 hr, increasing by 25 mg or frequency q 4–7 days (max. 100 mg bid–qid). Hyperthermia: *Children and adults:* Oral: 4–8 mg/kg/24 hr in 4 divided doses given 1–2 days before surgery (prophylaxis), or for 1–3 days post surgery (post-crisis follow-up). IV: 2.5 mg/kg starting 1.5 hr before surgery and run over 1 hr (prophylaxis) or 1 mg/kg/dose and repeated as needed (crisis) (max: 10 mg/kg).	*Cautions:* Should not be used where spasticity is used to maintain posture or balance; avoid in patients with active liver disease. *Adverse events:* Drowsiness, fatigue, dizziness, confusion, blurred vision, seizures, diarrhea, stomach cramps, nausea, vomiting, pleural effusion with pericarditis, hepatitis.
Daunorubicin hydrochloride Antineoplastic. Cerubidine. Powder for injection: 20 mg.	**Treatment of acute nonlymphocytic leukemia (ANLL) and myeloblastic leukemia (inhibition of DNA and RNA synthesis).** *Children:* Remission induction for acute lymphocytic leukemia (combination therapy): 25–45 mg/m² on day 1 q wk for 4 cycles (max: total, 300 mg/m²).	*Caution:* Avoid in patients with heart failure or arrhythmias. Irreversible cardiotoxicity may occur if total dose exposure exceeds 550 mg/m² in adults, 400 mg/m² if chest irradiation, 300 mg/m² in children > 2 yr, 10 mg/kg in children < 2 yr.

TABLE 716-1. General Medications—cont'd

DRUG (TRADE NAMES, FORMULATIONS)	INDICATIONS (MECHANISM OF ACTION AND DOSING)	COMMENTS (CAUTIONS, ADVERSE EVENTS, MONITORING)
	Adults: 30–60 mg/m^2/24 hr for 3–5 days; repeat dose in 3–4 wk; total cumulative dose should not exceed 400–600 mg/m^2 (lower end if history of cardiotoxic drugs or chest irradiation).	*Adverse events:* Alopecia, red discoloration of urine, nausea, vomiting, diarrhea, gastrointestinal ulceration, stomatitis, myelosuppression (onset, 7 days; nadir, 14 days; recovery, 21–28 days), extravasation-related tissue ulceration and necrosis, congestive heart failure, hyperuricemia, hepatotoxicity. *Monitoring:* Serum bilirubin and aspartate aminotransferase (AST) (to adjust doses for hepatic impairment): bilirubin 1.2–3 mg/dL or AST 60–180 IU: reduce dose to 75%; bilirubin 3.1–5 mg/dL or AST >180 IU: reduce dose to 50%; bilirubin > 5 mg/dL: omit use.
Deferoxamine mesylate Chelating agent. Desferal. Powder for injection: 500 mg.	**Treatment of acute iron intoxication or secondary chronic iron overload (forms complex with iron to form ferrioxamine, which is removed by kidneys).** *Children:* Acute iron intoxication: IM: 90 mg/kg/dose q 8 hr. IV: 15 mg/kg/hr (max: 6 g/24 hr). Chronic iron overload: IV: 15 mg/kg/hr (max: 12 g/24 hr). SC: 20–40 mg/kg/24 hr over 8–12 hr via portable infusion device. *Adults:* Acute iron intoxication: IM: 1 g STAT, then 0.5 g q 4 hr (max: 6 g/24 hr). IV: 15 mg/kg/hr (max: 6 g/24 hr). Chronic iron overload: IM: 0.5–1 g/24 hr. SC: infuse 1–2 g/24 hr over 8–24 hr.	*Caution:* Contraindicated in patients with primary hemochromatosis. *Adverse events:* Local pain and induration, flushing, hypotension, tachycardia, fever, hearing loss, blurred vision, cataracts. *Monitoring:* Serum ferritin, iron, total iron-binding capacity. Audiometry and eye examination with chronic use.
Desipramine hydrochloride Antidepressant, tricyclic. Norpramin; Pertofrane. Tablet: 10, 25, 50, 75, 100, 150 mg. Capsule: 25, 50 mg.	**Treatment of depression, attention deficit disorder, neuropathic pain (increases synaptic concentrations or serotonin and norepinephrine by inhibiting reuptake).** *Children 6–12 yr:* 1–3 mg/kg/24 hr (max: 5 mg/kg/24 hr). *Adolescents:* Initial dose or 25–50 mg/24 hr, increased gradually (max: 150 mg/24 hr). *Adults:* Initial dose of 75 mg/24 hr, increased gradually (max: 300 mg/24 hr).	*Cautions:* Abrupt discontinuation can result in withdrawal symptoms; tablets contain tartrazine (may be a problem for asthmatics), contraindicated in narrow-angle glaucoma. *Adverse events:* Dizziness, drowsiness, headache, blurred vision, dry mouth, constipation, increased appetite, cardiac arrhythmias, hypotension. *Monitoring:* Desipramine concentrations: therapeutic 100–300 ng/mL, toxic > 300 ng/mL; check ECG.
Desmopressin acetate Vasopressin analog. DDAVP; Stimate. Injection: 4 μg/mL. Nasal solution: 0.1 mg/mL.	**Treatment of diabetes insipidus, control of bleeding in certain types of hemophilia, primary nocturnal enuresis (enhances reabsorption of water in kidneys, dose-dependent increase in factor VIII and plasminogen activator).** *Children:* Diabetes insipidus: *3 mo–12 yr:* PO: 0.05 mg initially, then titrate to response. IV: 5 μg/24 hr in 1–2 doses. Hemophilia: *>3 mo:* IV: 0.3 μg/kg, may repeat dose if needed, use 30 min before procedure. Nocturnal enuresis: *>6 yr:* 20 μg at bedtime. *Children > 12 yr and adults:* Diabetes insipidus: PO: 0.05 mg bid, then titrate to response. IV, SC: 2–4 μg/24 hr. Intranasal: 5–40 μg/24 hr in 1–3 doses. Hemophilia: IV: 0.3 μg/kg. Intranasal: <50 kg: 150 μg, >50 kg: 300 μg. Enuresis: PO: 0.2–0.4 mg at bedtime.	*Cautions:* Avoid using in patients with type IIB or platelet-type von Willebrand disease, hemophilia A with factor VII levels < 5%, or hemophilia B. *Adverse events:* Facial flushing, headache, dizziness, increased blood pressure, hyponatremia, water intoxication. *Monitoring:* Serum electrolytes, plasma and urine osmolality, urine output, factor VIII antigen levels, activated partial thromboplastin time, factor VII activity level.
Dexamethasone Adrenal corticosteroid. Decadron. Aerosol: Oral 84 μg/activation, nasal 84 μg/spray. Cream: 0.1%, 0.04%. Injection: 4, 8, 10, 16, 20, 24 mg/mL. Ophthalmic ointment: 0.05%. Ophthalmic suspension: 0.1, 0.5%. Oral solution: 0.5 mg/5 mL. Tablet: 0.25, 0.5, 0.75, 1, 1.5, 2, 4, 6 mg. Elixir: 0.5 mg/5 mL.	**Systemically and locally for acute and chronic inflammation; allergic, neoplastic and autoimmune diseases; cerebral edema, septic shock, *Haemophilus influenzae* meningitis; diagnostic agent (decreases inflammation and suppresses normal immune response).** *Neonates:* Airway edema or extubation: IV: 0.25 mg/kg q 12 hr for 3–4 doses (start > 4 hr before scheduled extubation). Bronchopulmonary dysplasia: IV, PO: 0.25 mg/kg/dose q 12 hr for 6 dose, then taper over 1–6 wk (regimens may begin as early as day 1). *Children:* Airway edema or extubation: PO, IM, IV: 0.5–2 mg/kg/24 hr divided q 6 hr (begin 24 hr before extubation and continue for 4–6 doses postextubation). Antiemetic (chemotherapy-induced): IV: 10 mg/m^2 first dose, then 5 mg/m^2/dose q 6 hr as needed (start before chemotherapy). Anti-inflammatory: PO, IM, IV: 0.08–0.3 mg/kg/24 hr divided q 6–12 hr. Bacterial meningitis: IV: 0.6 mg/kg/24 hr divided q 6 hr for days 1–4 of antibiotics.	*Caution:* Dexamethasone use for neonates with bronchopulmonary dysplasia has been associated with increased incidence of cerebral palsy, and this risk should be weighed against potential benefits. *Adverse events:* Insomnia, nervousness, increased appetite hypertension, hyperglycemia, gastrointestinal hyperacidity (stress ulcer risk), cataracts, adrenal suppression, poor growth. *Comment:* See comparison of corticosteroids under *Hydrocortisone.*

TABLE 716-1. General Medications—cont'd

DRUG (TRADE NAMES, FORMULATIONS)	INDICATIONS (MECHANISM OF ACTION AND DOSING)	COMMENTS (CAUTIONS, ADVERSE EVENTS, MONITORING)
	Cerebral edema: PO, IM, IV: Loading dose of 1–2 mg/kg, then 1–1.5 mg/kg/24 hr divided q 4–6 hr, tapered over 1–6 wk. Inhalation: 2 puffs tid–qid. Nasal spray: 1–2 sprays in each nostril bid. Physiologic replacement: PO, IM, IV: 0.03–0.15 mg/kg/24 hr divided q 6–12 hr. *Adults:* Anti-inflammatory: PO, IM, IV: 0.5–9 mg/24 hr divided q 6–12 hr. Antiemetic: Same as for children. Cerebral edema: IV: 10 mg STAT, then 4 mg q 6 hr. Cushing syndrome: 1 mg at 11 P.M.; draw plasma cortisol at 8 A.M. the following day. Shock: IV: 1–6 mg/kg (max: 40 mg; may repeat q 2–6 hr. *Children and adults:* Ophthalmic: Ointment: Apply thin coating q 3–4 hr to conjunctival sac. Suspension: Instill 2 drops into conjunctival sac q hr during day and q other hr at night. Gradually taper doses when inflammation resolves. Topical: Apply 1–4 × daily.	
Dextran Plasma volume expander. Dextran 40 (low molecular weight): Gentran; LMD. Dextran 70 (high molecular weight): Gentran; Macro Dex.	**Blood volume expander in shock or impending shock (similar to albumin).** *Children:* up to 20 mL/kg on day 1, then 10 mL/kg/24 hr for not more than 5 days. *Adults:* 500–1,000 mL at a rate of 20–40 mL/min (max: 10 mL/kg/24 hr for 5 days).	*Adverse events:* Primarily associated with excessive doses—pulmonary edema, bleeding due to impaired platelet function.
Dextroamphetamine CNS stimulant. Adderall; Dexedrine; generic. Tablet: 5, 10 mg. Capsule, sustained-release: 5, 10, 15 mg.	**Treatment of attention deficit disorder, narcolepsy, and exogenous obesity (blocks reuptake of dopamine and norepinephrine from the synapse).** *Children 6–12 yr:* Narcolepsy and attention deficit disorder: Initial dose of 5 mg/24 hr; may increase by 5 mg/24 hr at weekly intervals to response (max: 60 mg/24 hr). *>12 yr and adults:* Initial dose of 20 mg/24 hr; may increase by 10 mg increments weekly (max: 60 mg/24 hr).	*Caution:* Avoid concurrent use of monoamine oxidase inhibitors. *Adverse events:* Hypertension, tachycardia, palpitations, arrhythmias, insomnia, agitation, irritability, nervousness, headache, depression, tremor, exacerbation of tics and movement disorders, mydriasis, physical and psychologic dependence, anorexia, nausea, diarrhea, abdominal cramps, growth suppression. *Monitoring:* Blood pressure, growth, CNS activity.
Dextromethorphan Antitussive. Robitussin; generic. Liquid: 7.5 mg/5 mL. Lozenge: 5 mg.	**Symptomatic relief of cough, best when cough is nonproductive (depresses medullary cough center).** *Children 2–6 yr:* 2.5–7.5 mg q 4–8 hr or extended-release, 15 mg q 12 hr (max: 30 mg/24 hr). *6–12 yr:* 10–15 mg q 4–8 hr, or extended-release, 30 mg bid (max: 60 mg/24 hr). *>12 yr and adults:* 10–30 mg q 4–8 hr, or extended-release, 60 mg bid (max: 120 mg/24 hr).	*Adverse events:* Mainly with overdose—drowsiness, dizziness, respiratory depression, blurred vision, nausea, gastrointestinal upset, constipation.
Diazepam Benzodiazepine. Valium; generic. Tablet: 2, 5, 10 mg. Oral solution: 5 mg/mL. Injection: 5 mg/mL.	**Treatment of anxiety, panic disorder, status epilepticus, alcohol withdrawal; provides sedation; skeletal muscle relaxant (thought to increase neuroinhibitory action of γ-aminobutyric acid).** *Infants and children:* Status epilepticus: IV: 0.05–0.3 mg/kg/dose given over 2–3 min; may repeat q 30 min to maximum total dose of 5–10 mg. Rectal: 0.5 mg/kg, then 0.25 mg/kg in 10 min if needed. Sedation: PO: 0.2–0.3 mg/kg (max: 10 mg). IM, IV: 0.04–0.3mg/kg (max: 0.6 mg/kg/8 hr). *Adults:* Status epilepticus: IV: 5–10 mg q 30 min (max: 30 mg/8 hr). Anxiety, sedation, muscle relaxant: PO, IM, IV: 2–10 mg bid–qid.	*Adverse events:* Hypotension, bradycardia, cardiac arrest (with IV dose), drowsiness, ataxia, fatigue, confusion, impaired coordination, paradoxical excitement, amnesia, blurred vision, diplopia, sweating, dry mouth, constipation or diarrhea, increased or decreased appetite, hiccups, physical and psychologic dependence. *Monitoring:* Desired clinical end-points and toxic end-points should be monitored; doses to achieve effects vary considerably between patients.
Diazoxide Antihypertensive. Hyperstat, injection: 15 mg/mL. Proglycem, oral suspension: 50 mg/mL. Capsule: 50 mg.	**Emergency lowering of blood pressure, treatment of hyperinsulinemic hypoglycemia related to islet cell tumors or nesidioblastosis (smooth muscle relaxation, inhibits insulin release from pancreas).** Hypertension: *Children and adults:* 1–3 mg/kg; may repeat in 5–15 min; dose every 4–24 hr. Hyperinsulinemic hypoglycemia: *Newborns and infants:* PO: 8–15 mg/kg/24 hr divided q 8–12 hr (start at low end). *Children and adults:* PO: 3–8 mg/kg/24 hr divided q 8–12 hr (start at low end).	*Adverse events:* Hypotension, dizziness, weakness, nausea, vomiting.
Dibucaine Local anesthetic. Nupercainal. Cream: 0.5%. Ointment: 1%.	**Temporary relief of pain and itching due to hemorrhoids and minor skin irritation or damage (blocks initiation and conduction of nerve impulses).** *Children and adults:* Topical: Apply gently to affected area (children, 7.5 g/24 hr; adults, 30 g/24 hr). Rectal: Insert with rectal applicator morning, evening, and after each bowel movement.	*Adverse events:* Local irritation, contact dermatitis.
Diclofenac sodium Nonsteroidal anti-inflammatory agent. Cataflam, tablet: 50 mg. Voltaren, tablet: 25, 50, 75 mg. Ophthalmic solution: 0.1%.	**Treatment of mild to moderate acute or chronic pain; postoperative inflammation after cataract extraction (inhibit's prostaglandin synthesis).** PO: *Children:* 2–3 mg/kg/24 hr in 2–4 divided doses. *Adults:* 100–200 mg/24 hr in 2–4 divided doses. Ophthalmic: 1 drop in affected eye qid for 2 wk, to begin 24 hr after cataract surgery.	*Adverse events:* Dizziness, headache, fluid retention, indigestion, abdominal pain, peptic ulcer, gastrointestinal bleeding, renal impairment.

TABLE 716-1. General Medications—cont'd

DRUG (TRADE NAMES, FORMULATIONS)	INDICATIONS (MECHANISM OF ACTION AND DOSING)	COMMENTS (CAUTIONS, ADVERSE EVENTS, MONITORING)
Dicyclomine Anticholinergic agent. Antispas; Bentyl; generic. Capsule: 10, 20 mg. Tablet: 20 mg. Syrup: 10 mg/5 mL. Injection: 10 mg/mL.	**Treatment of functional disturbances of gastrointestinal motility (e.g., irritable bowel syndrome) [blocks actions of acetylcholine].** *Infants > 6 mo:* PO: 5 mg/dose tid–qid. *Children:* 10 mg tid–qid. *Adults:* 40 mg qid (start at 1/2 dose and gradually increase). IM: *Adults:* 20 mg qid. *Cautions:* Avoid in narrow-angle glaucoma, gastrointestinal obstruction, urinary tract obstruction, and myasthenia gravis.	*Adverse events:* Tachycardia, palpitations, nervousness, irritability, confusion, muscle hypotonia, blurred vision, photophobia, urinary retention, nausea, vomiting, constipation, dry mouth, urticaria, pruritus.
Digoxin Cardiac glycoside. Lanoxin; generic. Capsule: 50, 100, 200 μg. Elixir: 50 μg/mL. Tablet: 125, 250, 500 μg. Injection: 100, 250 μg/mL.	**Treatment of systolic heart failure and supraventricular tachyarrhythmias (increases intracellular calcium through inhibition of sodium/potassium adenosine triphosphetase pump; suppression of AV node conduction).** *Neonate:* Loading dose of 10–30 μg/kg IV, then 5–10 μg/kg/24 hr maintenance dose. *1 mo–2 yr:* Loading dose of 30 μg/kg, then 10–15 μg/kg/24 hr maintenance dose. *2–10 yr:* Loading dose of 30 μg/kg, then 5–10 μg/kg/24 hr maintenance dose. *Child >10 yr:* Loading dose of 10 μg/kg, then 2–5 μg/kg/24 hr maintenance dose. *Adult:* Loading dose of 10–15 μg/kg, then 0.1–0.5 mg/24 hr maintenance dose. Adjust doses for reduced renal function: CrCl 10–15 mL/min: Reduce dose to 25–75% of normal. CrCl <10 mL/min: Reduce dose to 10–25% of normal.	*Cautions:* Contraindicated in AV block, idiopathic hypertrophic subaortic stenosis, or constrictive pericarditis. *Adverse events:* Anorexia, nausea, vomiting, diarrhea, feeding intolerance, bradycardia, arrhythmias, lethargy, depression, vertigo, blurred vision, diplopia, photophobia, yellow or green vision. *Monitoring:* Efficacy and toxicity are closely related to serum concentrations, and dosing should be guided by measuring serum digoxin concentrations: therapeutic: 0.8–2 ng/mL; toxic: >2–2.5 ng/mL. Digoxin-like immune substances (DLISs) may falsely elevate digoxin levels in neonates and children, so pretreatment digoxin levels can be obtained and subtracted from treatment levels or samples can be run through a free-level filter to remove DLISs before assay. Check postdistribution levels (drawn at least 6–8 hr post dose) at steady-state (2–4 wk) or if there are ECG or clinical signs of toxicity. Check ECG, serum electrolytes, calcium, and magnesium. Check heart rate.
Digoxin Immune Fab Digoxin antidote. Digibind. Powder for injection: 38 mg.	**Treatment of digitalis intoxication from digoxin or digitoxin (binds with molecules of unbound digoxin or digitoxin and is renally cleared).** *Infants, children, and adults:* Dose based on amount of digoxin or digitoxin ingested or estimated total body load (TBL) based on postdistributive serum concentration: TBL digoxin = concentration (ng/mL) × 5.6 × weight (kg)/1,000. TBL digoxin = mg ingested × 0.8. TBL digitoxin = concentration (ng/mL) × 0.56 × wt (kg)/1,000. TBL digitoxin = mg ingested. Dose of digoxin immune Fab (mg) = TBL digoxin × 76. Dose of digoxin immune Fab (no. of vials) = TBL/0.5.	*Adverse events:* Worsening of heart failure or atrial fibrillation, hypokalemia, facial swelling, redness. *Monitoring:* ECG; digoxin serum concentrations will greatly increase with digoxin immune Fab and do not reflect body stores or correlate with clinical toxicity.
Digydrotachysterol Vitamin D analog. Hytakerol; generic. Capsule: 0.125 mg. Tablet: 0.125 mg. Solution: 0.2 mg/mL, 0.2 mg/5 mL.	**Treatment of hypocalcemia associated with hypoparathyroidism and renal osteodystrophy (stimulates calcium and phosphate intestinal absorption).** *Neonates:* 0.05–0.1 mg/24 hr. *Infants and young children:* 1–5 mg/24 hr for 4 days, then 0.5–1.5 mg/24 hr. *Older children and adults:* 0.75–2.5 mg/24 hr for 4 days, then 0.2–1 mg/24 hr (max: 1.5 mg/24 hr). Renal osteodystrophy: 0.1–0.6 mg/24 hr.	*Adverse events:* Hypercalcemia, hypercalciuria, elevated serum creatinine.
Diltiazem Calcium channel blocker. Cardizem; Dilacor. Tablet: 30, 60, 90, 120 mg. Capsule, sustained-release,: 60, 90, 120, 180, 240, 300 mg. Injection: 5 mg/mL.	**Treatment of hypertension and atrial tachyarrhythmias (inhibits calcium ions from entering the "slow channels" during depolarization).** *Children:* PO: 1.5–2 mg/kg/24 hr in 3–4 divided doses. *Adolescents and adults:* PO: 90–480 mg/24 hr in 3–4 divided doses as tablets or 1–2 doses as sustained-release capsules. IV: Loading dose of 0.25 mg/kg, then 5–15 mg/hr continuous infusion.	*Cautions:* Diltiazem is a hepatic enzyme inhibitor and may cause accumulation and toxicity for concurrently used drugs that are metabolized. *Adverse events:* Hypotension, bradycardia, edema, AV block, dizziness, nausea, vomiting.
Dimenhydrinate Antihistamine. Dramamine; generic. Capsule: 50 mg. Injection: 50 mg/mL. Tablet: 50 mg. Liquid: 12.5 mg/4 mL.	**Treatment of nausea, vomiting, and vertigo associated with motion sickness (competes with histamine for H_1 receptor).** *Children:* *2–5 yr:* 12.5–25 mg q 6–8 hr (max: 75 mg/24 hr). *6–12 yr:* 25–50 mg q 6–8 hr (max: 150 mg/24 hr). *Adults:* 50–100 mg q 4–6 hr (max: 400 mg/24 hr).	*Adverse events:* Drowsiness, dizziness, hypotension, tachycardia.
Dimercaprol BAL. Injection: 100 mg/mL.	**Antidote to gold, arsenic, and mercury poisoning and adjunct to edetate calcium disodium in lead poisoning (chelates with heavy metals to form nontoxic stable compounds).** *Children and adults:* Mild arsenic and gold poisoning: 2.5 mg/kg/dose IM q 6 hr for 2 days, then q 12 hr on day 3, then q 24 hr for 10 days. Severe arsenic or gold poisoning: 3 mg/kg/dose q 4 hr for 2 days, then q 6 hr on day 3, then q 12 hr for 10 days. Mercury poisoning: Loading dose of 5 mg/kg, then 2.5 mg/kg/dose 1–2 × daily for 10 days. Lead poisoning: Mild: Loading dose of 4 mg/kg, then 3 mg/kg/dose q 4 hr for 2–7 days. Severe: Loading dose of 4 mg/kg/dose q 4 hr for 2–7 days.	*Adverse events:* Hypertension, tachycardia, convulsions, nausea, vomiting, fever, headache, nervousness, blepharospasm, nephrotoxicity. *Monitoring:* Specific heavy metal levels; urine pH should be kept alkaline
Diphenhydramine Benadryl; generic. Capsule or tablet: 25, 50 mg. Injection: 10, 50 mg/mL. Syrup or elixir: 12.5 mg/5 mL. Cream or lotion: 1%	**Antihistamine (competitive inhibitor of H_{1pe} receptor).** *Children:* IM, IV, PO: 5 mg/kg/24 hr divided q 6 hr as needed (max: 300 mg/24 hr). *Adults:* 10–50 mg/dose q 4 hr as needed (max: 400 mg/24 hr). *Topical:* Apply tid–qid daily.	*Adverse events:* Hypotension, tachycardia, drowsiness, paradoxical excitement, thickened bronchial secretions, dry mouth.

TABLE 716-1. General Medications—cont'd

DRUG (TRADE NAMES, FORMULATIONS)	INDICATIONS (MECHANISM OF ACTION AND DOSING)	COMMENTS (CAUTIONS, ADVERSE EVENTS, MONITORING)
Diphenoxylate and Atropine Lomotil. Tablet, oral solution.	**Antidiarrheal (diphenoxylate inhibits excessive gastrointestinal motility; atropine is used to prevent abuse).** *Children:* *2–5 yr:* 4 mL (2 mg diphenoxylate) tid. *5–8 yr:* 4 mL qid. *8–12 yr:* 4 mL 5× daily. *Adults:* 15–20 mg/24 hr in 3–4 divided doses.	*Adverse events:* Nervousness, dizziness, drowsiness, headache, dry mouth, urinary retention, blurred vision, paralytic ileus.
Disopyramide Norpace. Capsule: 100, 150 mg.	**Treatment of ventricular arrhythmias and atrial tachyarrhythmias (antiarrhythmic class 1a, decreases myocardial excitability and conduction velocity).** *Children:* *<1 yr:* 10–30 mg/kg/24 hr divided q 6 hr. *1–4 yr:* 10–20 mg/kg/24 hr divided q 6 hr. *4–12 yr:* 10–15 mg/kg/24 hr divided q 6 hr. *12–18 yr:* 6–15 mg/kg/24 hr divided q 6 hr. *Adults:* 100–200 mg q 6 hr.	*Cautions:* Avoid in 2nd- or 3rd-degree AV block; will worsen heart failure, urinary retention, glaucoma, and some arrhythmias. *Adverse events:* Urinary retention or hesitancy, dry mouth, fatigue, malaise, constipation, cholestasis, elevated liver enzymes. *Monitoring:* Creatinine clearance (decrease dose to q 8 hr if 30–40 mL/min, q 12-hr if 15–30 mL/min, q 24 hr if <15 mL/min), ECG, blood pressure, signs of heart failure, blood levels (therapeutic range: atrial arrhythmias 2.8–3.2 μg/mL, ventricular arrhythmias 3.3–7.5 μg/mL).
Dobutamine Dobutrex. Injection.	**Treatment of hypotension (stimulates β_1-adrenergic receptors).** *Neonates:* 2–20 μg/kg/min. *Children and adults:* 2.5–40 μg/kg/min constant infusion.	*Cautions:* Avoid in patients with hypertrophic cardiomyopathy, atrial fibrillation or flutter, or sulfite sensitivity. *Adverse events:* Tachycardia, ectopic heartbeats, angina, palpitations, tachyarrhythmias, tingling sensation, paresthesias, leg cramps.
Docusate Colace; Surfak; generic. Capsule, liquid, syrup (may be combined with casanthrol).	**Stool softener, laxative (reduces surface tension of oil-water interface of stool).** *<3 yr:* 10–40 mg/24 hr in 1–4 doses. *3–6 yr:* 20–60 mg/24 hr in 1–4 doses. *6–12 yr:* 40–150 mg/24 hr. *>12 yr and adults:* 50–400 mg/24 hr.	*Adverse events:* Diarrhea, abdominal cramping.
Dolasetron mesylate Anzemet. Tablet: 50, 100 mg. Injection.	**Prevention and treatment of chemotherapy and postoperative nausea and vomiting (5-HT_3 receptor antagonist).** *Children >2 yr and adults:* IV, PO: 1.8 mg/kg (max: 100 mg) as single dose 30 min before chemotherapy; 0.35 mg/kg (max: 12.5 mg) given 15 min before stopping anesthesia for postoperative nausea.	*Adverse events:* Hypotension, headache, tachycardia, dizziness.
Dopamine Intropin. Injection.	**Treatment of hypotension and shock (stimulates dopaminergic receptors and adrenergic receptors).** *Neonates, children, and adults:* 1–20 μg/kg/min IV infusion rate (mL/hr) = 6 × weight (kg) × desired dose (μg/kg/min)/mg drug/100 mL of IV fluid.	*Cautions:* Contains sulfites. *Adverse events:* Tachycardia, ectopic beats, ventricular arrhythmias, tissue necrosis with extravasation, vasoconstriction, gangrene of extremities, excess urine output (doses <5 μg/kg/min), oliguria (doses >10 μg/kg/min).
Dornase alpha Pulmozyme. Inhalation solution: 1 mg/mL.	**Management of cystic fibrosis to improve pulmonary function (DNA enzyme that reduces viscosity of mucus).** *Neonates, children, and adults:* 2.5 mL 1–2 times daily, nebulized with Pulmo-Aide or Pari-Proneb compressor.	*Adverse events:* Pharyngitis, voice alteration, cough, rhinitis, hemoptysis.
Doxacurium Nuromax. Injection: 1 mg/mL.	**Skeletal muscle paralysis (provides neuromuscular blockade by competing with acetylcholine for neuromuscular receptor).** *Children 2–12 yr:* Initial dose of 30–50 μg/kg, then 5–10 μg/kg/dose every 1–2 hr. *Adults:* Initial dose of 50 μg/kg, then 5–10 μg/kg/dose every 1–2 hr.	*Adverse events:* Skeletal muscle weakness, hypotension. *Monitoring:* Peripheral nerve stimulator.
Doxapram Dopram. Injection: 20 mg/mL.	**Treatment of apnea of prematurity refractory to methylxanthines (respiratory and CNS stimulant).** *Neonates:* Initial dose of 2.5–3 mg/kg followed by infusion of 1 mg/kg/hr (max: 2.5 mg/kg/hr). *Caution:* Contains benzyl alcohol (recommended doses deliver 5.4–27 mg/kg/24 hr).	*Adverse events:* Hypertension, tachycardia, arrhythmias, CNS stimulation, irritability, seizures, hyperpyrexia, vomiting, increased gastric residuals, hyperglycemia.
Doxepin Adapin; Sinequan. Tricyclic antidepressant. Capsule: 10, 25, 50, 75, 100, 150 mg. Oral concentrate: 10 mg/mL. Cream: 5%.	**Treatment of depression; analgesic for neuropathic pain (increases synaptic concentrations of serotonin and norepinephrine).** *Children:* 1–3 mg/kg/24 hr. *Adolescent:* Starting dose of 25–50 mg/24 hr (max: 100 mg/24 hr). *Adults:* Starting dose of 30–150 mg/24 hr (max: 300 mg/24 hr; single dose max: 150 mg).	*Caution:* Contraindicated in narrow-angle glaucoma. *Adverse events:* Sedation, drowsiness, dizziness, headache, dry mouth, constipation, increased appetite, weight gain, urinary retention, difficult urination, blurred vision, hypotension, arrhythmias. *Monitoring:* ECG, doxepin concentrations: therapeutic 30–150 ng/mL, toxic >500 ng/mL.
Doxorubicin hydrochloride Adriamycin; Rubex. Powder for injection. Injection: 2 mg/mL.	**Antineoplastic used for various tumor types (inhibits DNA and RNA synthesis).** *Children:* 35–75 mg/m²/dose, repeated q 21 days, or 20–30 mg/m², repeated q/wk, or 60–90 mg/m² given as continuous infusion over 96 hr q 3–4 wk. *Adults:* 60–75 mg/m²/dose q 21 days. Liver disease: Reduce dose: bilirubin 1.2–3 (reduce by 50%), bilirubin >3 (reduce by 75%).	*Caution:* Contraindicated if patient has congestive heart failure, cardiomyopathy, or has received a total dose of 550 mg/m² (400 mg/m² if prior or concurrent daunorubicin, idarubicin, mitoxantrone, cyclophosphamide, irradiation to cardiac area). *Adverse events:* Cardiotoxicity, alopecia, hyperpigmentation of nail beds, hyperuricemia, stomatitis, esophagitis, mucositis, nausea, vomiting, thrombocytopenia (onset, 7 days; nadir, 10–14 days; recovery, 21–28 days), lacrimation, extravasation tissue necrosis, phlebitis.
Dronabinol, tetrahydrocannabinol Marinol. Capsule: 2.5, 5, 10 mg.	**Antiemetic for cancer chemotherapy (inhibits vomiting center).** *Children and adults:* 5 mg/m²/dose q 2–4 hr starting 1–3 hr before chemotherapy (max: 15 mg/m²/dose).	*Adverse events:* Drowsiness, difficulty concentrating, mood change, hallucinations. *Monitoring:* Monitor for abuse.
Droperidol Inapsine. Injection: 2.5 mg/mL.	**Antiemetic, antipsychotic (alters action of dopamine in CNS and has α-adrenergic blockade).** *Children 2–12 yr:* IV, IM: 0.05–0.06 mg/kg/dose q 4–6 hr as needed for nausea. *Adults:* IV, IM: 2.5–5 mg/dose q 3–4 hr as needed.	*Adverse events:* Hypotension, tachycardia, extrapyramidal reactions, confusion, memory loss.

TABLE 716-1. General Medications—cont'd

DRUG (TRADE NAMES, FORMULATIONS)	INDICATIONS (MECHANISM OF ACTION AND DOSING)	COMMENTS (CAUTIONS, ADVERSE EVENTS, MONITORING)
D-Xylose Xylo-pfan. Powder for oral solution.	**Diagnostic agent used to evaluate intestinal disorders due to disease or injury (mechanism not understood).** *Children:* 500 mg/kg as 5–10% solution (max: 25 g). *Adults:* 5–25 g as 10% solution, followed by 200–400 mL of water.	*Adverse events:* Nausea, vomiting, cramping, intestinal bloating. *Monitoring:* Blood and urinary D-Xylose concentrations.
Edetate calcium disodium Calcium Disodium Versenate. Injection: 200 mg/mL.	**Antidote for acute and chronic lead poisoning (chelating agent).** *Children and adults:* 500 mg/m^2/dose once daily.	*Cautions:* Contraindicated in severe renal failure and patients with active tuberculosis or healed calcified tubercular lesions. *Adverse events:* Arrhythmias, hypotension, seizures, headache, chills, skin eruptions, hypomagnesemia, hypokalemia, hypocalcemia, hyperuricemia, vomiting, diarrhea, abdominal cramps, back pain, muscle cramps, paresthesia, tetany, nephrotoxicity, respiratory arrest. *Monitoring:* 24 hr urine collection after first dose for ratio of lead excretion/mg calcium EDTA (positive test >0.5–0.6); blood lead level.
Edetate disodium Chealamide; Disotate; generic. Injection: 150 mg/mL.	**Emergency treatment of hypercalcemia and digitalis-induced ventricular dysrhythmias (chelating agent).** *Children:* 40–70 mg/kg/24 hr slow infusion over 3–4 hr; administer for 5 days, then 5 days off drug. *Adults:* 50 mg/kg/dose for 5 days, then 2 days off, then restart for a total of 15 doses. Digitalis arrhythmias (children and adults): 15 mg/kg/hr continuous infusion (max: 60 mg/kg/24 hr).	*Cautions:* Contraindicated in severe renal failure and tuberculosis. *Adverse events:* Arrhythmias, hypotension, seizures, headache, chills, hypokalemia, hypocalcemia, hypomagnesemia, hyperuricemia, vomiting, diarrhea, abdominal cramps, dysuria, back pain, nephrotoxicity.
Edrophonium chloride Enlon; Reversol; Tensilon. Injection: 10 mg/mL.	**Diagnosis of myasthenia gravis, differentiation of cholinergic crisis from myasthenia crisis, reversal of nondepolarizing neuromuscular blockers, treatment of paroxysmal atrial tachycardia (inhibits destruction of acetylcholine by acetylcholinesterase).** *Infants:* IM: 0.5–1 mg. IV: 0.1 mg, followed by 0.4 mg (if no response). *Children:* Diagnosis (initial): IM: <34 kg: 1 mg; >34 kg: 5 mg. IV: 0.04 mg/kg over 1 min, followed by 0.16 mg/kg given within 45 sec (if no response) (max: 10 mg total). Titration of oral anticholinesterase therapy: IV 0.04 mg/kg given 1 hr after oral intake of treatment drug; if strength improves, increase dose of neostigmine or pyridostigmine. *Adults:* Diagnosis: IM: Initially, 10 mg; if cholinergic reaction occurs, give 2 mg in 30 min to rule out false-negative reaction. IV: 2 mg given over 15 sec, 8 mg given 45 sec later (if no response). Titration of oral anticholinesterase therapy: IV 1–2 mg given 1 hr after an oral dose. Increase oral dose if strength improves.	*Adverse events:* Arrhythmias, hypotension, nausea, vomiting diarrhea, stomach cramps, excess sweating, urinary frequency, lacrimation, diplopia, miosis, laryngospasm, bronchospasm, respiratory paralysis.
Enalapril/Enalaprilat Vasotec. Oral (enalapril): 2.5, 5, 10, 20 mg. Injection (enalaprilat): 1.25 mg/mL. Extemporaneous formulation.	**Treatment of hypertension and congestive heart failure (angiotensin-converting enzyme inhibition).** *Neonate:* PO: 0.1 mg/kg/24 hr in 1–2 doses (may increase to 0.4 mg/kg/24 hr for congestive heart failure or adequate hypertension response). IV: 5–10 μg/kg/dose q 8–24 hr. *Infants and children:* PO: 0.1–0.5 mg/kg/24 hr in 1–2 doses. IV: 5–10 μg/kg/dose q 8–24 hr. *Adolescents and adults:* PO: 2.5–5 mg/24 hr and titrate (max: 40 mg/24 hr in 2 doses). IV: 0.625–1.25 mg/dose q 6 hr (max: 20 mg/24 hr). *Caution:* Avoid or adjust dose in patients with renal impairment (CrCl 10–50 mL/min, give 75% of dose; CrCl < 10 mL/min, give 50% of dose).	*Adverse events:* Hypotension, tachycardia, syncope, fatigue, dizziness, headache, cough, hyperkalemia, hypoglycemia. *Comments:* Lower doses if concurrent diuretics or reduced renal function; concurrent indomethacin may blunt response.
Enoxaparin sodium Lovenox. Injection: 30 mg/0.3 mL.	**Prophylaxis and treatment of venous thromboembolism (low molecular weight heparin with activity against factors IIa and Xa).** *Neonates and children:* SC: 1 g/kg q 8–12 hr. *Adults:* SC: 30 mg bid or 1 mg/kg bid (depends on indication).	*Adverse events:* Thrombocytopenia and hemorrhage (<unfractionated heparin). *Monitoring:* Dose to heparin plasma level (anti-factor Xa assay) mid-interval 0.5–1.0 U/mL, or trough 0.3–0.7 U/mL.
Epinephrine Adrenalin. Injection: 0.01, 0.1, 1 mg/mL. Suspension: 5 mg/mL. Aerosol metered-dose inhaler, inhalation solution, ophthalmic solution, topical solution.	**Treatment of cardiac arrest, bronchospasm, anaphylactic reactions, open-angle glaucoma (stimulates α, β_1, and β_2 receptors).** *Neonates:* IV, intratracheal: 0.01–0.03 mg/kg (0.1–0.3 mL/kg of 1:10,000 solution) q 3–5 min. *Infants and children:* SC: 0.01 mg/kg (0.01 mL/kg/dose of 1:1,000 solution, or 0.005 mL/kg/dose of suspension). IV: 0.01 mg/kg (0.1 mL/kg of 1:10,000 solution) [max: 1 mg]. IT: 0.1 mg/kg/dose (0.1 mL/kg of 1:1,000 solution) [max: 0.2 mL/kg]. Continuous infusion: 0.1–1 μg/kg/min per response. Nebulization: 0.25–0.5 mL of 2.25% racemic epinephrine diluted in 3 mL normal saline. Ophthalmic: Instill 1–2 drops in eye(s) 1–2 times daily.	*Adverse events:* Tachycardia, hypertension, nervousness, restlessness, irritability, headache, tremor, weakness, nausea, vomiting, acute urinary retention.

TABLE 716-1. General Medications—cont'd

DRUG (TRADE NAMES, FORMULATIONS)	INDICATIONS (MECHANISM OF ACTION AND DOSING)	COMMENTS (CAUTIONS, ADVERSE EVENTS, MONITORING)
	Adults: IV: 1–5 mg q 3–5 min. IT: 1 mg initially (max: 12.5 mg/dose). IM, SC: 0.1–0.5 mg q 10–15 min. Continuous infusion: 1–10 μg/min. Ophthalmic: Instill 1–2 drops in eye(s) 1–2 times daily.	
Epoetin alfa, erythropoietin, EPO Epogen; Procrit. Injection, Preservative-free vial: 2,000, 3,000, 4,000, 10,000 U/mL. Preserved: 10,000 U/mL.	**Anemia associated with prematurity; end-stage renal disease; zidovudine-treated, HIV-infected patients; cancer patients receiving chemotherapy (induces erythropoiesis).** Administer IV, SC. *Neonates:* 100–500 u/kg/dose q 1–2 days for 10–21 days. *Children and adults:* Cancer patients: 150 u/kg/dose 3×/wk (may increase to 300 u/kg/dose). Hemodialysis patients: 50–100 u 3×/wk. Zidovudine-treated patients: 100 u/dose 3×/wk.	*Caution:* Uncontrolled hypertension, neutropenia in newborns must have adequate iron stores and may require oral or IV iron supplement. *Adverse events:* Hypertension, edema, headache, fever, rash, arthralgias, hypersensitivity. *Monitoring:* Serum iron, reticulocyte count, hematocrit (reduce dose or stop EPO if hematocrit >40), blood pressure.
Ergocalciferol Calciferol; Drisdol; generic. Tablet, capsule: 50,000 units. Liquid: 8,000 u/mL. Injection: 500,000 u/mL (1 μg = 4 u).	**Treatment of refractory rickets, hypophosphatemia, hypoparathyroidism (vitamin D analog stimulates calcium and phosphate absorption).** *Premature infants:* 10–20 μg/24 hr. Renal failure: *Children:* 100–1,000 μg/24 hr. *Adults:* 500 μg/24 hr. Hypoparathyroidism: *Children:* 1.25–5 mg/24 hr. *Adults:* 0.625–5 mg/24 hr. Rickets: *Children:* 75–125 μg/24 hr. *Adults:* 0.25–1.5 mg/24 hr.	*Adverse events:* Hypercalcemia, weakness, lethargy, hypertension, arrhythmias, mild acidosis, hypercholesterolemia, nausea, vomiting, constipation, nephrocalcinosis, photophobia. *Monitoring:* Serum calcium and phosphorus, alkaline phosphatase, bone radiography.
Ergotamine Cafatine; Cafergot. Tablet: 1, 2 mg. Aerosol: 9 mg/mL. Suppository: 2 mg.	**Prevents or aborts vascular headaches (e.g., migraine or cluster headache) [ergot alkaloid α-adrenergic blocker].** *Older children and adolescents:* 1 mg sublingually or PO at onset of attack and q 30 min to relief (max: 3 mg/attack). *Adults:* 1–2 mg sublingually or PO, may repeat q 30 min to maximum of 6 mg (maximum dose/wk: 10 mg).	*Caution:* Reduce dose by 50% if patient is taking chronic methysergide. *Adverse events:* Tachypnea, vasospasm, nausea, vomiting, diarrhea, leg cramps, muscle weakness, paresthesias.
Esmolol Brevibloc. Injection: 10 mg/mL.	**Antiarrhythmic, antihypertensive (β blocker, class II antiarrhythmic).** *Children:* 100–500 μg/kg over 1 min, then continuous infusion of 200–1,000 μg/kg/min. *Adults:* 500 μg/kg over 1 min, then 50–200 μg/kg/min.	*Caution:* Contraindicated in sinus bradycardia, heart block, uncompensated heart failure. *Adverse events:* Hypotension, bradycardia, Raynaud phenomenon, dizziness, confusion, lethargy, bronchoconstriction.
Ethacrynic acid Edecrin. Tablet: 25, 50 mg. Injection.	**Diuretic (acts at ascending loop of Henle).** *Children:* PO: 1–3 mg/kg/24 hr. IV: 0.5–1 mg/kg/dose q 8–24 hr. *Adults:* PO: 25–400 mg/24 hr. IV: 0.5–1 mg/kg/dose q 8–24 hr.	*Adverse events:* Hypotension, fluid and electrolyte depletion, hyperuricemia, ototoxicity, tinnitus.
Ethosuximide Zarontin. Capsule: 250 mg. Syrup: 250 mg/5 mL.	**Anticonvulsant for treatment of absence, myoclonic, and akinetic epilepsy (increased seizure threshold).** *Children:* *<6 yr:* Start 15 mg/kg/24 hr in 2 doses; increase q 4–7 days to therapeutic level, usually 15–40 mg/kg/24 hr in 2 doses (max: 1.5 g/24 hr). *>6 yr and adults:* Start 250 mg bid; increase by 250 mg/24 hr q 4–7 days up to therapeutic level or 1.5 g/24 hr.	*Adverse events:* Sedation, lethargy, nausea, vomiting, anorexia, abdominal pain, leukopenia, thrombocytopenia, aplastic anemia. *Monitoring:* Ethosuximide concentrations: therapeutic 40–100 μg/mL; toxic 150 μg/mL.
Etoposide, VP-16 VePesid. Capsule: 50 mg. Injection: 20 mg/mL.	**Antineoplastic for treatment of various cancers (inhibits mitotic activity).** *Children:* IV: 150 mg/m²/24 hr for 3 days for 2–3 cycles for acute myelocytic leukemia remission or brain tumor; 160 mg/m²/24 hr for 4 days for bone marrow transplant conditioning. *Adults:* IV: 50–100 mg/m²/24 hr for 3–5 days/course. PO: IV dose ×2 to nearest 50 mg.	*Adverse events:* Hypotension, tachycardia, fever, headache, chills, alopecia, rash, urticaria, nausea, vomiting, diarrhea, mucositis, myelosuppression, anemia (nadir, 7–14 days), thrombocytopenia (nadir, 9–16 days), peripheral neuropathy, bronchospasm.
Factor IX complex (human) Konyne 80; Profilnine; Proplex. Injection.	**Antihemophilic agent to control bleeding in patients with factor IX deficiency (i.e., hemophilia B or Christmas disease), or with inhibitors to factor VIII (i.e., hemophilia A) [replacement of deficient factor].** *Children and adults:* 20–25 u/kg/dose up to q 24 hr; factor VIII deficiency: 75–100 u/kg/dose up to q 6 hr.	*Adverse events:* Flushing, fever, headache, chills, urticaria, thrombosis (with high doses), tingling, tightness of head and neck.
Famotidine Pepcid. Tablet: 20, 40 mg. Injection.	**Treatment of gastric and duodenal ulcer and control of gastric pH in critically ill patients (blocks H_2 receptors).** *Infants and children:* PO, IV: 1–12 mg/kg/24 hr in 1–2 doses (max: 40 mg/24 hr). *Adults:* PO: 40 mg/24 hr at bedtime. IV: 20 mg q 12 hr.	*Cautions:* Reduce dose for renal function: CrCl 30–50 mL/min: give 50%, of dose; CrCl < 30 mL/min: give 25% of dose. *Adverse events:* Gastrointestinal discomfort, thrombocytopenia, increased liver enzymes.

TABLE 716-1. General Medications—cont'd

DRUG (TRADE NAMES, FORMULATIONS)	INDICATIONS (MECHANISM OF ACTION AND DOSING)	COMMENTS (CAUTIONS, ADVERSE EVENTS, MONITORING)
Fat emulsion Intralipid; Liposyn. Injection: 10%, 20%.	**Source of essential fatty acids and calories (nutritional supplement with parenteral nutrition).** *Premature infants:* Start 0.5 g/kg/24 hr and increase by 0.5 g/kg/24 hr as tolerated (max: 3 g/kg/24 hr). *Infants and children:* Start 0.5–1 g/kg/24 hr and increase by 0.5 g/kg/24 hr as tolerated (max: 3–4 g/kg/24 hr). *Adolescents and adults:* 1 g/kg/24 hr and increase as tolerated (max: 2.5 g/kg/24 hr).	*Cautions:* Fat calories should not exceed 60% of total daily calories. Contraindicated in patients with severe egg or soybean allergies. *Adverse events:* Hyperlipidemia, hepatomegaly, dyspnea, and hypoxemia may occur if infused too quickly or with excessive dose. *Monitoring:* Serum triglycerides.
Felbamate Felbatol. Tablet: 400, 600 mg. Oral suspension: 600 mg/5 mL.	**Adjunctive therapy primarily used for refractory generalized and partial seizures associated with Lennox-Gastaut syndrome (anticonvulsant with unknown mechanism of action).** *Children: 2–14 yr:* Start 15 mg/kg/24 hr in 3–4 doses; increase weekly by 15 mg/kg/24 hr (max: 45 mg/kg/24 hr or 3,600 mg, whichever is less). *>14 yr:* Start 1,200 mg/24 hr in 3–4 doses; increase weekly by 1,200 mg/24 hr (max: 3,600 mg/24 hr).	*Caution:* Over 30 cases each of hepatic failure and aplastic anemia with multiple fatalities have been reported. *Adverse events:* Headache, insomnia, somnolence, fatigue, behavioral changes, depression, ataxia, anorexia, nausea, vomiting, diarrhea, thrombocytopenia, granulocytopenia, leukopenia, agranulocytosis, aplastic anemia, hepatitis, acute liver failure. *Monitoring:* Interacts with phenytoin, carbamazepine, and valproate; monitor drug levels if felbamate added.
Fentanyl citrate Duragesic; Sublimaze. Injection, transdermal, oral lozenge.	**Relief of pain, sedation, preoperative medication, anesthesia adjunct (narcotic analgesic, binds to opium receptors).** *Neonates and infants:* IV: 1–4 μg/kg/dose; may repeat q 2–4 hr or continuous infusion of 0.5–5 μg/kg/hr. *Children 1–2 yr:* Pain: IM, IV: 1–3 μg/kg/dose, may repeat q 30–60 min; continuous infusion of 1–5 μg/kg/hr; Oralet 5–15 μg/kg. *Children > 12 yr and adults:* Pain: IV, IM: 0.5–1 μg/kg/dose; may repeat in 30–60 min. Transdermal: 25–100 μg/hr as needed for relief. PO: 5 μg/kg or 400 μg, whichever is less. Anesthesia: IV, IM: 2–50 μg/kg.	*Cautions:* Rapid IV infusion may result in skeletal muscle and chest wall rigidity, with impaired ventilation and respiratory distress; physical dependence may occur in 3–5 days. *Adverse events:* Hypotension, bradycardia, CNS depression, constipation, biliary tract spasm, nausea, vomiting, urinary tract spasm, respiratory depression.
Fexofenadine Allegra. Capsule: 60 mg. Tablet: 30, 60, 180 mg.	**Antihistamine with selective peripheral H_1 receptor activity. Treatment of seasonal allergic rhinitis and chronic idiopathic urticaria.** *Children < 12 yr:* 30 mg bid. *Children > 12 yr and adults:* 60 mg bid, or 180 mg q 24 hr.	*Adverse events:* Very good safety profile; toxicity is rare, even with overdose (mainly dizziness, drowsiness, and dry mouth).
Filgrastim Granulocyte colony-stimulating factor. Neupogen. Injection: 300 μg/mL	**Reduces duration of neutropenia (stimulates production, maturation, and activation of neutrophils).** *Neonates:* 5 μg/kg/dose daily for 3–6 doses. *Children and adults:* 5–10 μg/kg/dose daily for up to 14 days; may discontinue if absolute neutrophil count remains > 1,000/mm^3 for 3 consecutive days.	*Cautions:* Malignancy with myeloid characteristics. *Adverse events:* Hypotension, vasculitis, fever, exacerbation of pre-existing skin disorders, increased uric acid, thrombocytopenia, medullary pain (dose-related and mostly located in lower back, iliac creast, and sternum), hematuria, proteinuria.
Flecainide Tambocor. Tablet: 50, 100, 150 mg. Extemporaneous formulations can be prepared.	**Treatment of supraventricular tachycardia and ventricular arrhythmias (antiarrhythmic class 1c; slows conduction in cardiac tissue).** *Children:* Initially, 1–3 mg/kg/24 hr in 3 divided doses; may increase up to 12 mg/kg/24 hr. *Adults:* Initially 100 mg q 12 hr; may increase by 100 mg/24 hr q 4 days (max: 400 mg/24 hr).	*Caution:* Decrease dose by 25–50% in renal failure; avoid in 2nd- or 3rd-degree heart block. *Adverse events:* Bradycardia, heart block, worsening arrhythmias, congestive heart failure, dizziness, visual disturbances, headache, fatigue, asthenia, nausea, constipation, abdominal pain, elevated liver enzymes, paresthesias, tremor. *Monitoring:* Serum trough concentrations (therapeutic 0.2–1 μg/mL).
Fludarabine Antineoplastic; antimetabolite. Fludara. Injection powder.	**Treatment of B-cell chronic lymphocytic leukemia and acute lymphocytic leukemia unresponsive to previous therapy.** *Children:* 10 mg/m^2 over 15 min, followed by 30.5 mg/m^2/24 hr by continuous infusion for 5 days. *Adults:* 20–25 mg/m^2 over 30 min for 5 days.	*Adverse events:* Neurotoxicity (primarily progressive demyelinating encephalopathy with mental status deterioration), somnolence, weakness, seizures, metabolic acidosis, hyperuricemia, hyperphosphatemia, hyperkalemia, hypocalcemia, nausea, vomiting, diarrhea, stomatitis, metallic taste, myelosuppression (WBC nadir, 8 days; platelet nadir, 16 days; recovery, 5–7 wk), pneumonitis, dyspnea, nonproductive cough, interstitial pneumonitis, hearing loss, reversible hepatotoxicity.
Fludrocortisone acetate Florinef. Tablet: 0.1 mg.	**Partial replacement therapy for adrenal insufficiency (mineralocorticoid with glucocorticoid activity).** *Infants and children:* 0.05–0.1 mg/24 hr. *Adults:* 0.05–0.2 mg/24 hr.	*Adverse events:* Hypertension, edema, congestive heart failure, convulsions, headache, acne, rash, bruising, hypokalemia, HPA axis (adrenal) suppression, peptic ulcer, muscle weakness.
Flumazenil Romazicon. Injection.	**Benzodiazepine antagonist to reverse sedative effects (antagonizes benzodiazepine effects on γ-aminobutyric acid/benzodiazepine receptor complex).** *Children:* Loading dose of 0.005–0.01 mg/kg, then continuous infusion of 0.005–0.01 mg/kg/hr (maximum cumulative dose: 1 mg).	*Caution:* Avoid if benzodiazepine is used to manage potentially life-threatening conditions (e.g., status epilepticus, increased intracranial pressure). *Adverse events:* Arrhythmias, hypotension or hypertension, seizures, acute withdrawal symptoms (if patient is dependent on benzodiazepine or tricyclic antidepressant).
Flunisolide Inhaled steroid; anti-inflammatory. AeroBid; Nasalide. Metered-dose inhaler: 250 μg/puff. Nasal spray: 25 μg/actuation.	**Treatment of asthma and rhinitis.** *Children and adults:* Oral inhalation: 2–4 puffs bid. Nasal spray: 1–2 sprays in each nostril bid–tid.	*Adverse events:* Candidal infections of nose and throat, dysphonia, sore throat, bitter taste, nasal irritation, headache, dizziness, short-term growth retardation.
Fluocinolone acetonide Topical adrenocorticosteroid; anti-inflammatory. Fluonid; Synalar; generic. Topical cream, ointment, shampoo, solution, oil: 0.01–0.025%	**Inflammation and corticosteroid-responsive dermatoses** *Children and adults:* Apply a thin layer bid–qid.	*Adverse events:* Acne, hypopigmentation, allergic dermatitis, skin atrophy, folliculitis, secondary infection, HPA axis suppression, growth retardation.
Fluocinonide Topical adrenocorticosteroid; anti-inflammatory. Fluonex; Lidex; generic. Cream, gel, ointment, solution: 0.05%	**Inflammation and corticosteroid-responsive dermatoses** *Children and adults:* Apply a thin layer bid–qid.	*Adverse events:* Acne, hypopigmentation, allergic dermatitis, skin atrophy, folliculitis, secondary infection, HPA axis suppression, growth retardation.

TABLE 716-1. General Medications—cont'd

DRUG (TRADE NAMES, FORMULATIONS)	INDICATIONS (MECHANISM OF ACTION AND DOSING)	COMMENTS (CAUTIONS, ADVERSE EVENTS, MONITORING)
Fluoride Generic. Oral drops, topical gel, lozenge, tablet, topical rinse, oral solution.	**Prevention of dental caries (promotes remineralization, increases resistance to acid dissolution).** Dental rinse or gel: *Children:* 5–10 mL after brushing. *Adults:* 10 mL after brushing.	*Adverse events:* Gastrointestinal upset if swallowed; stannous fluoride may stain teeth.
Fluorometholone Ophthalmic glucocorticoid; anti-inflammatory. Flarex; FML. Ophthalmic ointment: 0.1%. Ophthalmic suspension: 0.1%, 0.25%	**Inflammatory conditions of the eye.** *Children >2 yr and adults:* Ointment: Apply tid in mild to moderate cases and q 4 hr in severe cases. Drops: Instill 1–2 drops into conjunctival sac q hr while awake and q 2 hr at night until response, then q 4–8 hr.	*Adverse events:* Local stinging and burning, increased intraocular pressure.
Fluorouracil Adrucil; Efudex; Fluoroplex. Injection, topical solution, cream.	**Cancer chemotherapy (antineoplastic antimetabolite that inhibits thymidylate synthase, leading to thymidine depletion).** *Children and adults:* IV: 12 mg/kg/24 hr (max: 800 mg/24 hr) for 4–5 days, then 6 mg/kg q other day for 4 doses. Repeat in 4 wk. Cream or solution 5%: Apply to entire affected area bid.	*Adverse events:* Arrhythmias, hypotension, heart failure, cerebellar ataxia, somnolence, alopecia, skin pigmentation, pruritic maculopapular rash, photosensitivity, erythrodysesthesia of hands and feet, loss of nails, hyperpigmentation of nail beds, nausea, vomiting, diarrhea, gastrointestinal hemorrhage, esophagitis, stomatitis, hepatotoxicity, conjunctivitis, myelosuppression (WBC and platelets: onset, 7–10 days; nadir, 9–14 days; recovery, 21 days).
Fluoxetine hydrochloride Prozac. Capsule: 10, 20 mg. Liquid: 20 mg/5 mL.	**Treatment of depression and obsessive-compulsive disorders (antidepressant, inhibits CNS serotonin uptake).** *Children 5–18 yr:* Initially, 5–10 mg/24 hr, then titrate slowly to effect (max: 20 mg/24 hr). *Adults:* Initially, 20 mg/24 hr, then slowly increase daily dose in 20 mg increments to effect.	*Caution:* Avoid in patients taking monoamine oxidase inhibitors. *Adverse events:* Headache, nervousness, insomnia, anxiety, mania, suicidal ideation, tremor, nausea, anorexia, diarrhea, constipation, dry mouth, weight loss. *Monitoring:* Serum concentrations of fluoxetine (therapeutic: 100–800 ng/mL), norfluoxetine (therapeutic: 100–600 ng/mL).
Fluticasone Inhaled corticosteroid. Flonase; Flovent. Nasal solution: 50 μg/spray. Metered-dose inhaler (MDI): 44, 110, 220 μg/spray. Rotadisk: 50, 100, 250 μg/dose.	**Treatment of allergic rhinitis and chronic asthma.** *Children and adults:* Nasal spray: 1–2 sprays in each nostril once daily. MDI: 88–880 μg bid (depending on asthma severity and need for systemic corticosteroids). Rotadisk: 50–1,000 μg bid (depending on asthma severity and need for systemic corticosteroids).	*Adverse events:* Dysphonia, oral thrush, adrenal suppression, growth suppression, cataracts.
Fluvoxamine Luvox; generic. Tablet: 25, 50, 100 mg.	**Serotonin reuptake inhibitor; treatment of depression, obsessive-compulsive disorder.** *Children <12 yr:* Start 25 mg/hr, increase by 25 mg/24 hr q 4–7 days to effect (max: 200 mg/24 hr). Divide into 2 daily doses if >50 mg/24 hr needed. *Children >12 yr:* Start 25 mg/24 hr; increase by 25 mg/24 hr q 4–7 days to effect (max: 300 mg/24 hr). Divide into 2 daily doses if >50 mg/24 hr needed. *Adults:* Start 50 mg/24 hr; increase by 50 mg/24 hr q 4–7 days to effect (max: 300 mg/24 hr). If >100 mg/24 hr needed, divide into 2 doses/24 hr.	*Caution:* Do not abruptly discontinue doses or withdrawal syndrome may occur over several days. Taper dose by 25–50 mg/24 hr q 5–7 days. *Adverse events:* Somnolence, headache, dry mouth, nausea, constipation. *Drug interactions:* Inhibits cytochrome 2D6 liver enzymes; drugs such as methadone and phenothiazines may have increased levels when used concurrently.
Folic acid Generic. Injection. Tablet: 0.4, 0.8, 1 mg. Extemporaneous formulations can be prepared.	**Treatment of folate deficiency anemias (i.e., megaloblastic, macrocytic) [cofactor for normal erythropoiesis].** *Neonates–6 mo:* PO: 25–35 μg/24 hr. *6 mo–3 yr:* 50 μg/24 hr. *4–6 yr:* 75 μg/24 hr. *7–10 yr:* 100 μg/24 hr. *11–14 yr:* 150 μg/24 hr. *>15 yr and adults:* 200 μg/24 hr. Folate deficiency: 1 mg/24 hr.	*Caution:* Large folate doses may mask hematologic effects of vitamin B_{12} deficiency while allowing neurologic consequences to progress.
Fosphenytoin Cerebyx. Injection: 10 mL vials contain 750 mg fosphenytoin (500 mg phenytoin); 2 mL vials contain 150 mg fosphenytoin.	**Treatment of acute seizures (may substitute for IV phenytoin).** *Children and adults:* Loading dose of 15–20 mg/kg phenytoin dosing equivalents (max: 150 mg/min). May substitute IV or IM for phenytoin maintenance doses. Each 1.5 mg fosphenytoin = 1 mg phenytoin dosing equivalent.	*Cautions:* Same as phenytoin. *Drug interactions:* Same as phenytoin.
Furosemide Lasix; generic. Injection: 10 mg/mL. Oral solution: 10 mg/mL, 40 mg/mL. Tablet: 20, 40, 80 mg.	**Diuretic (inhibits sodium and chloride reabsorption at the ascending loop of Henle and distal tubule).** *Premature infants:* 0.5–2 mg/kg IV or 1–4 mg/kg PO q 12–48 hr (dose to response). *Infants and children:* 1–2 mg/kg IV or 1–4 mg/kg PO q 6–24 hr or continuous infusion (start at 0.05 mg/kg/hr and adjust dose to response). *Adults:* 10–600 mg/24 hr in 1–4 divided doses, or continuous infusion or 0.05 mg/kg/hr.	*Adverse events:* Dehydration, electrolyte loss, hyperuricemia, photosensitivity, ischemic hepatitis, hypercalciuria, renal stones, ototoxicity (IV infusion rate >4 mL/min), gastrointestinal intolerance.
Gabapentin Neurontin. Capsule: 100, 300, 400 mg.	**Adjunct to treatment of partial and secondarily generalized seizures; treatment of neuropathic pain (mechanism not certain).** *Children 2–12 yr:* 15–35 mg/kg/24 hr in 3 divided doses (max: 50 mg/kg/24 hr). *Children >12 yr and adults:* Start 300 mg daily, then increase by 300 mg daily to 900–3,600 mg/24 hr in 3 divided doses.	*Adverse events:* Somnolence, dizziness, fatigue, depression, hyperactivity, aggression, dyspepsia, constipation, nausea, weight gain, diplopia.
Gamma globulin See Immune globulin, intravenous.		
Gentian violet Generic. Topical solution: 1%, 2%.	**Treatment of cutaneous and mucocutaneous infections (kills Candida, staphylococcal species, and some vegetative gram-positive bacteria).** *Infants:* Apply 3–4 drops of 0.5% solution under tongue or on lesion after feedings. *Children and adults:* Apply 0.5–2% with cotton to lesion bid–tid for 3 days.	*Caution:* Do not swallow. *Adverse events:* Burning, local irritation, or sensitivity reactions.
Glucagon Powder for injection.	**Treatment of hypoglycemia (stimulates hepatic glycolysis and gluconeogenesis).** *Neonates:* IV, IM, SC: 0.3 mg/kg/dose (max: 1 mg). *Children:* 0.025–0.1 mg/kg/dose (max: 1 mg); may repeat in 20 min SC, IM, IV. *Adults:* 0.5–1 mg; may repeat in 20 min as needed, SC, IM, IV.	*Adverse events:* Nausea, vomiting, hypersensitivity reactions.

TABLE 716-1. General Medications—cont'd

DRUG (TRADE NAMES, FORMULATIONS)	INDICATIONS (MECHANISM OF ACTION AND DOSING)	COMMENTS (CAUTIONS, ADVERSE EVENTS, MONITORING)
Glycopyrrolate Robinul; generic. Injection: 0.2 mg/mL. Tablet: 1 mg.	**Inhibits salivation and excessive secretions of the respiratory tract; bronchodilator; adjunct to treatment of peptic ulcer; reverses muscarinic effects on cholinergic agents (anticholinergic).** *Children:* Control of secretions: PO: 40–100 μg/kg/dose tid–qid. IM, IV: 4–10 μg/kg/dose q 3–4 hr. Preoperative IM: 4.4–8.8 μg/kg/dose 30–60 min before procedure.	*Adverse events:* Tachycardia, nervousness, headache, insomnia, drowsiness, dry mouth, constipation, nausea, urinary retention, blurred vision.
Gold sodium thiomalate Myochrysine, generic. Injection: 25 mg/mL.	**Treatment of rheumatoid arthritis (mechanism unknown).** *Children:* Test dose: 10 mg IM, followed by 1 mg/kg IM q wk for 20 wk, then 1 mg/kg/dose q 2–4 wk (max: 50 mg/dose). *Adults:* Test dose: 10 mg IM, then 25–50 mg/wk, then 25–50 mg IM q 2–4 wk once response is noted.	*Cautions:* Patient should be sitting or lying for 10 min after the dose; avoid in patients with systemic lupus erythematosus or blood dyscrasias. *Adverse events:* Headache, flushing, seizures, exfoliative dermatitis, erythema nodosum, hives, alopecia, loss of nails, stomatitis, gingivitis, glossitis, conjunctivitis, eosinophilia, leukopenia, thrombocytopenia, hematuria, proteinuria, nephrotic syndrome, pulmonary fibrosis and interstitial pneumonitis, hepatotoxicity, peripheral neuropathy. *Monitoring:* Gold serum concentrations (therapeutic 1–3 μg/mL).
Gonadorelin Factrel; Lutrepulse. Injection.	**Evaluate gonadotropin regulation in precocious or delayed puberty; treat primary hypothalamic amenorrhea (stimulates release of luteinizing hormone).** *Children:* IV (HCl salt) 100 μg. *Children >12 yr and adults:* IV, SC: 100 μg during days 1–7 of menstrual cycle.	*Adverse events:* Flushing, lightheadedness, headache, abdominal discomfort. *Monitoring:* Plasma-luteinizing hormone and follicle-stimulating hormone.
Granisetron Kytril. Injection: 1 mg/mL. Tablet: 1 mg.	**Antiemetic (selective 5-HT$_3$ antagonist).** *Children >2 yr and adults:* IV 10–20 μg/kg 15–30 min before chemotherapy; may repeat 2–3 doses in 24 hr. PO: 1 mg bid starting 1 hr before chemotherapy.	*Adverse events:* Arrhythmias, bradycardia, transient blood pressure changes, agitation, anxiety, liver enzyme elevations.
Guaifenesin, Glycerol Guaiacolate Expectorant Generic. With or without codeine, dextromethorphan, phenylpropanolamine, or phenylephrine. Syrup, tablet, capsule, liquid.	**Temporary control of cough.** *Children < 2 yr:* 12 mg/kg/24 hr in 6 divided doses. *2–5 yr:* 50–100 mg q 4 hr (max: 600 mg/24 hr). *6–11 yr:* 100–200 mg q 4 hr (max: 1,200 mg/24 hr). *>12 yr and adults:* 200–400 mg q 4 hr (max: 2.4 g/24 hr).	*Caution:* Monitor doses and toxicities of other drugs in combination products.
Guanethidine Ismelin. Tablet: 10, 25 mg.	**Treatment of moderate to severe hypertension (acts as false neurotransmitter).** *Children:* 0.2 mg/kg/24 hr; may increase by 0.2 mg/kg/24 hr every wk (max: 3 mg/kg/24 hr). *Adults:* Initial 10 mg/24 hr; increase weekly (max: 25–50 mg/24 hr).	*Adverse events:* Palpitations, chest pain, peripheral edema, fatigue, headache, drowsiness, confusion, constipation, anorexia, uninary frequency, nocturia, paresthesias, visual disturbances, orthostatic hypotension.
Guanfacine HCL Tenex. Tablet: 1 mg.	**Treatment of hypertension and attention deficit disorder (ADD) [stimulate α_2 receptors in the brainstem].** *Children:* ADD: 1 mg/24 hr. *Adults:* 1 mg/24 hr; may increase q 4 wk (max: 3 mg/24 hr).	*Adverse events:* Somnolence, dizziness, dry mouth, constipation, gastrointestinal upset.
Haloperidol Haldol, generic. Oral concentrate: 2 mg/mL. Tablet: 0.5, 1, 2, 5, 10, 20 mg. Injection.	**Treatment of severe behavioral problems, including psychoses and Tourette disorder (competitive blocker of dopamine receptors).** *Children 3–12 yr:* PO: Start 0.25–0.5 mg/24 hr in 2–3 divided doses, then increase weekly by 0.25–0.5 mg daily based on response (max: 0.15 mg/kg/24 hr). *6–12 yr:* IM: 1–3 mg/dose q 4–8 hr (max: 0.15 mg/kg/24 hr). *Adults:* PO: 0.5–5 mg bid–tid. daily. IM: 2–5 mg q 4–8 hr.	*Adverse events:* Drowsiness, restlessness, anxiety, extrapyramidal symptoms, dystonia, akathisia, pseudoparkinsonism, tardive dyskinesia, neuroleptic malignant syndrome, seizures, constipation, weight gain, swelling of breasts, hypotension, tachycardia, arrhythmias, unrinary retention, blurred vision, retinal pigmentation, cholestatic liver disease, agranulocytosis, leukopenia. *Monitoring:* Plasma concentrations (therapeutic 5–15 ng/mL, toxic > 42 ng/mL).
Heparin (unfractionated) Generic. Injection.	**Prophylaxis and treatment of thromboembolism (potentiates actions of antithrombin III).** *Neonates, infants, and children:* Thrombosis and extracorporeal membrane oxygenation: Loading dose of 50 U/kg IV bolus, 15–35 U/kg/hr continuous IV infusion maintenance dose (adjust to target activated partial thromboplastin time [APTT] or heparin level). Catheter patency: 0.5–1 U/mL. *Adults:* IV: Loading dose of 70–100 U/kg IV push, 15–25 U/kg/hr continuous infusion (target APTT or heparin level). SC: 5,000 units q 8–12 hr for prophylaxis.	*Caution:* Avoid if severe thrombocytopenia, intracranial hemorrhage, bacterial endocarditis. *Adverse events:* Bleeding from various sites (e.g., urine, gums, nose); bruising, thrombocytopenia, thrombosis. *Monitoring:* APTT (therapeutic, 1.5–2.5× baseline; toxic > 2.5× baseline); plasma heparin concentration (anti-factor X assay: therapeutic 0.3–0.7 U/mL).
Histrelin Gonadotropin-releasing hormone analog. Supprelin. Injection.	**Central idiopathic precocious puberty.** *Children:* SC: 10 μg/kg once daily. *Adult female:* 100 μg/24 hr for endometriosis.	*Adverse events:* Anxiety, depression, irritability, insomnia, headaches.
Homatropine hydrobromide Anticholinergic. Isopto Homatropine; generic. Ophthalmic solution: 2%, 5%.	**Produces cycloplegia and mydriasis for refraction; treatment of uveitis.** *Children:* For mydriasis: 1 drop of 2% solution before procedure; may repeat q 10 min as needed. Uveitis: 1 drop 2% solution bid–tid. *Adults:* Mydriasis: 1–2 drops of 2% or 5% solution before procedure; may repeat q 10 min. Uveitis: 1–2 drops of 2% or 5% solution bid–tid.	*Adverse events:* Blurred vision, photophobia, local stinging, respiratory congestion.

TABLE 716-1. General Medications—cont'd

DRUG (TRADE NAMES, FORMULATIONS)	INDICATIONS (MECHANISM OF ACTION AND DOSING)	COMMENTS (CAUTIONS, ADVERSE EVENTS, MONITORING)
Human growth hormone Humatrope, Nutropin; Protropin. Injection.	**Treatment of growth failure due to inadequate growth hormone secretion (replacement therapy).** *Children:* Humatrope: 0.06 mg/kg (0.15 IU/kg) 3×/wk. Nutropin: 0.043 mg/kg/24 hr. Protropin: 0.1 mg/kg (0.26 IU/kg) 3×/wk.	*Adverse events:* Local lipoatrophy, hypothyroidism, pain in hip or knee.
Hyaluronidase Wydase. Injection: 150 U/mL.	**Treatment of extravasation; enhance is absorption of fluids administered by hypodermoclysis (hydrolysis of hyaluronic acid to modify permeability of connective tissue).** *Neonates, infants, children:* Inject using 25–26 g needle (total 1 mL, 150 U), SC, or intradermally at 5 sites (0.2 mL to each) at leading edge of extravasation.	*Adverse events:* Tachycardia, hypotension, erythema.
Hydralazine Generic. Injection: 20 mg/mL. Tablet. Extemporaneous formulations may be prepared.	**Treatment of hypertension; adjunct treatment of congestive heart failure with nitrates (direct vasodilation of arterioles).** *Neonates:* IV: 0.1–0.5 mg/kg/dose q 6–8 hr. PO: 0.25–1 mg/kg/dose q 6–8 hr. *Infants and children:* IM, IV: Start 0.1–0.2 mg/kg/dose q 4–6 hr and titrate to effect (max: 3.5 mg/kg/24 hr). PO: 0.75–1 mg/kg/24 hr in 2–4 divided doses (max: 7.5 mg/kg/24 hr). *Adults:* IM, IV: 10–20 mg/dose q 4–6 hr (max: 40 mg/dose). PO: 10–25 mg/dose qid, and titrate to effect (max: 300 mg/24 hr).	*Adverse events:* Palpitations, flushing, tachycardia, headache, nausea, vomiting, anorexia, diarrhea, lupus-like syndrome, arthralgias, peripheral neuropathy (related to pyridoxine deficiency).
Hydrochlorothiazide Generic. Oral solution: 50 mg/5 mL. Tablet: 25, 50, 100 mg Combination products (e.g., with spironolactone).	**Treatment of hypertension and fluid overload (edema) states (e.g., bronchopulmonary dysplasia, congestive heart failure, prevention of recurrent renal calcium stones) [diuretic inhibits sodium reabsorption in distal tubule].** *Neonates and infants:* 2–4 mg/kg/24 hr in divided doses. *Infants > 6 mo and children:* 2 mg/kg/24 hr in 2 divided doses. *Adults:* 12.5–100 mg/24 hr.	*Adverse events:* Hypokalemia, hypochloremia, hypomagnesemia, hyperglycemia, hyperuricemia, hyperlipidemia, pancreatitis, leukopenia, thrombocytopenia, aplastic anemia, hepatitis, intrahepatic cholestasis, prerenal azotemia.
Hydrocortisone Generic. Cream, ointment, gel, lotion, injection, oral suspension, rectal foam.	**Treatment of adrenal insufficiency, congenital adrenal hyperplasia, shock, corticosteroid-responsive dermatoses, adjunctive treatment of ulcerative colitis (anti-inflammatory, glucocorticoid).** *Neonates, infants, and young children:* Adrenal insufficiency: 1–2 mg/kg IV bolus, then 25–150 mg/24 hr divided q 6 hr. Congenital adrenal hyperplasia: IV: Start 0.5–0.7 mg/kg/24 hr, then 0.3–0.4 mg/kg/24 hr maintenance therapy; give doses as 1/4 in A.M., 1/4 at noon, and 1/2 at night. Shock: IV: 35–50 mg/kg, then 50–150 mg/kg/24 hr divided q 6 hr for 48–72 hr. *Infants and older children:* Adrenal insufficiency: 1–2 mg/kg IV bolus, then 150–250 mg/24 hr divided q 6–8 hr. Anti-inflammatory: IV, IM: 1–5 mg/kg/24 hr in 1–2 doses. PO: 2.5–10 mg/kg/24 hr divided q 6–8 hr. Shock: IV: 50 mg/kg/dose q 4 hr. Status asthmaticus: IV: 1–2 mg/kg/dose q 6 hr. *Adults:* Anti-inflammatory: IV, IM, PO: 15–240 mg/dose q 12 hr. Shock: IV: 0.5–2 g q 2–6 hr. Rectal: Apply 1–2 times/24 hr for 2–3 wk. Topical: Apply 3–4 times/24 hr.	*Caution:* Abrupt withdrawal may cause acute adrenal insufficiency. *Adverse events:* Hypertension, hyperglycemia, hypokalemia, euphoria, insomnia, headache, Cushing syndrome, peptic ulcer, cataracts, immunosuppression, skin and muscle atrophy, acne, edema. (See Relative Potency of Corticosteroids table below.)
Hydromorphone Dilaudid; generic. Injection. Tablet: 2, 4 mg. Syrup: 1 mg/5 mL. Suppository: 3 mg.	**Analgesic, antitussive (narcotic).** *Children 6–12 yr:* Cough: PO: 0.5 mg q 3–4 hr as needed. Pain: PO: 0.03–0.08 mg/kg/dose q 4–6 hr as needed. IV: 0.015 mg/kg/dose q 4–6 hr as needed. *Children > 12 yr and adults:* Cough: PO: 1 mg q 3–4 hr as needed. Pain: PO, IV, IM, SC: 1–4 mg/dose q 4–6 hr as needed.	*Caution:* Tablet and syrup contain tartrazine, which may exacerbate asthma; do not discontinue abruptly after continuous use. *Adverse events:* Sedation, drowsiness, confusion, restlessness, headache, tachycardia, hypotension, physical and psychological addiction, nausea, vomiting, constipation, stomach cramps, decreased urination, ureteral spasm, respiratory depression, shortness of breath, miosis, antidiuretic hormone release, sensitivity reactions (due to histamine release). *Comment:* IV, IM hydromorphone 1.5 mg = morphine 10 mg; oral hydromorphone 7.5 mg = morphine 30 mg (acute) or 60 mg (chronic).
Hydroxocobalamin, vitamin B_{12} Codroxomin, Hybalamin, others. Injection.	**Treatment of pernicious anemia, vitamin B_{12} deficiency, increased vitamin B_{12} requirements (replacemnt therapy).** *Children:* 100 μg/24 hr IM to total 1 mg over 2 wk, then 30–50 μg/mo. *Adults:* 30 μg/24 hr for 5–10 days, then 100–200 μg/mo.	*Comment:* May require co-administration of folate.
Hydroxychloroquine Plaquenil sulfate. Tablet: 200 mg. Extemporaneous formulations may be prepared.	**Suppression or chemoprophylaxis of malaria; treatment of systemic lupus erythematosus and rheumatoid arthritis (interferes with digestive vacuole function within sensitive malarial parasites, impairs complement-dependent antigen-antibody reactions).** *Children:* Chemoprophylaxis of malaria: 5 mg/kg 1×/wk (begin 1–2 wk before exposure and continue for 4 wk after leaving high-risk area). Acute malaria attack: 10 mg/kg initial dose followed by 5 mg/kg in 6–8 hr on day 1,400 mg once on days 2 and 3.	*Caution:* Avoid in porphyria or psoriasis. *Adverse events:* Headache, confusion, agitation, insomnia, nightmares, psychosis, visual field defects, retinitis, blindness, bone marrow suppression, thrombocytopenia, liver failure, anorexia, nausea, vomiting, diarrhea, lichenoid dermatitis, bleaching of hair, itching, ototoxicity. *Monitoring:* Ophthalmologic examinations for visual field changes.

Relative Potency of Corticosteroids

Drug	Anti-inflammatory Effect (mg)	Sodium-Retaining Effect (mg)
Hydrocortisone	100	100
Cortisone	80	80
Prednisolone	20	100
Prednisone	20	100
Methylprednisolone	16	0
Triamcinolone	16	0
Dexamethasone	2	0
Desoxycorticosterone	0	2

TABLE 716-1. General Medications—cont'd

DRUG (TRADE NAMES, FORMULATIONS)	INDICATIONS (MECHANISM OF ACTION AND DOSING)	COMMENTS (CAUTIONS, ADVERSE EVENTS, MONITORING)
	Adults: Malaria prophylaxis: 400 mg 1×/wk (timing as in children). Acute malaria attack: day 1: 800 mg, then 400 mg in 6–8 hr; days 2 and 3: 400 mg once. Rheumatoid arthritis and lupus erythematosus: 400 mg once daily, may increase by 200 mg if inadequate response in 4–12 wk, reduce to 200–400 mg/24 hr once response occurs and long-term maintenance is needed.	
Hydroxyurea Hydrea; Mylocel; generic. Tablet: 1,000 mg. Capsule: 500 mg.	**Cancer chemotherapy, sickle cell anemia (interferes with DNA synthesis during S-phase of cell division).** *Children:* 1,500–3,000 mg/m^2 q 4–6 wk. *Adults:* Cancer chemotherapy: 80 mg/kg every 3rd day, or 20–30 mg/kg/24 hr. Sickle cell anemia: 10–20 mg/kg/24 hr.	*Adverse events:* Drowsiness, headache, hallucinations, seizures, nausea, vomiting, mucositis, stomatitis, myelosuppression (onset, day 7; nadir, day 10; recovery, day 21), alopecia, maculopapular rash, dry skin, erythema of face and hands, hepatitis, increased blood urea nitrogen and creatinine, hyperuricemia.
Hydroxyzine Generic. Injection, syrup, tablet, capsule.	**Treatment of allergy, itching, anxiety, and nausea and adjunct for chronic pain management (H_1-receptor blocker).** PO, IM: *Children:* 0.6 mg/kg/dose q 6 hr. *Adults:* 10–100 mg/dose tid–qid.	*Caution:* May worsen narrow-angle glaucoma, prostatic hypertrophy, bladder neck obstruction, asthma, and chronic obstructive pulmonary disease. *Adverse events:* Hypotension, drowsiness, dizziness, headache, dry mouth, urinary retention, pain at injection site.
Hyoscyamine (with atropine, scopolamine, and phenobarbital) Donnatal; generic. Capsule, elixir, tablet.	**Treatment of irritable bowel, spastic colon, spastic bladder, and renal colic (anticholinergic).** *Children:* Donnatal 0.1 mL/kg/dose q 4 hr (max: 5 mL) *Adults:* 1–2 tablets (or 5–10 mL) tid–qid.	*Adverse events:* Tachycardia, palpitations, headache, drowsiness, nervousness, dry mouth, constipation, dysphagia, paralytic ileus, blurred vision, nasal congestion. *Caution:* Contraindicated in narrow-angle glaucoma, myasthenia gravis, and gastrointestinal and genitourinary obstruction.
Ibuprofen Nonsteroidal anti-inflammatory agent. Generic. Suspension: 100 mg/5 mL. Tablet: 200, 300, 400, 600, 800 mg.	**Treatment of pain, fever, rheumatoid arthritis (inhibits prostaglandin synthesis).** *Children:* Pain, fever: 5–10 mg/kg/dose q 6–8 hr. Juvenile rheumatoid arthritis: 30–50 mg/kg/24 hr in 4 divided doses. *Adults:* 400–800 mg/dose tid–qid (max: 3.2 g/24 hr).	*Adverse events:* Abdominal cramps, heartburn, nausea, gastrointestinal bleeding and perforation, fluid retention, edema, hypertension, tachycardia, acute renal failure.
Idarubicin Idamycin. Injection.	**Combination chemotherapy for acute myelocytic and lymphocytic leukemia (AML and ALL) [inhibits DNA and RNA synthesis].** *Children:* ALL: 10–12 mg/m^2 IV once daily for 3 days/treatment course. *Adults:* AML: 8–12 mg/m^2 IV daily for 3 days/treatment course.	*Adverse events:* Headache, infection, hemorrhage, mucositis, stomatitis, alopecia, rash, urticaria, nausea, vomiting, diarrhea, leukopenia (nadir, 8–19 days), thrombocytopenia (nadir, 10–15 days), myocardial toxicity (arrhythmias, cardiomyopathy, heart failure, ECG changes). *Monitoring:* Maximal lifetime dose = 137.5 mg/m^2. Lower dose by 25% if severe mucositis present or serum creatinine >2 mg/dL; lower dose by 50% if bilirubin >2.5 mg/dL; do not give dose if bilirubin >5 mg/dL.
Ifosfamide Alkylating agent. Ifex. Injection.	**Cancer chemotherapy.** *Children:* IV: 1,200–1,800 mg/m^2 24 hr for 5 days q 21–28 days, or 5 g/m^2 as single IV infusion. *Adults:* 700–2,000 mg/m^2 24 hr for 5 days q 21–28 days, or 5 g/m^2 as single IV infusion.	*Adverse events:* Alopecia, nausea, vomiting, stomatitis, hemorrhagic cystitis (administer mesna for uroprotection), hematuria, renal damage, somnolence, confusion, hallucinations, coma, polyneuropathy, depressive psychosis, elevated liver enzymes, myelosuppression (onset, day 7; nadir, 10–14 days), pulmonary fibrosis, nasal stuffiness, cardiotoxicity.
Imipramine Tofranil; generic. Injection, capsule, tablet.	**Treatment of depression, enuresis, pain (tricyclic antidepressant, increases synaptic concentrations of norepinephrine and serotonin).** *Children:* Depression: Start 1.5 mg/kg/24 hr; may increase by 1 mg/kg/24 hr q 3–4 days (max: 5 mg/kg/24 hr). Enuresis: >6 yr: 10–25 mg at bedtime. Cancer pain: 0.2–0.4 mg/kg at bedtime; may increase dose 50% q 3–4 days (max: 3 mg/kg). *Adolescents:* PO: Start 25–50 mg/24 hr; may gradually increase (max: 200 mg/24 hr). *Adults:* PO: 25 mg tid–qid; may increase dose gradually (max: 300 mg/24 hr). IM: Initially, give up to 100 mg in divided doses.	*Adverse events:* Arrhythmias, postural hypotension, drowsiness, sedation, confusion, headache, dry mouth, constipation, urinary retention, increased liver enzymes, seizures, urinary retention. *Monitoring:* Imipramine concentrations (therapeutic: imipramine and desipramine 150–250 ng/mL, toxic >1,000 ng/mL).
Immune globulin, intravenous Gamimune; Sandoglobulin; generic. Injection.	**Immunodeficiency syndrome, idiopathic thrombocytopenic purpura, acute bacterial or viral infections in immunocompromised or neutropenic patients, Kawasaki disease, Guillain-Barré syndrome, demyelinating polyneuropathy (replacement therapy or interference with Fc receptors in the reticuloendothelial system for autoimmune diseases).** *Neonates:* 500–750 mg/kg once. *Children and adults:* Immunodeficiency syndrome: 100–400 mg/kg/dose q 2–4 wk. Chronic lymphocytic leukemia: 400 mg/kg/dose q 3 wk. Idiopathic thrombocytopenic purpura: 1,000 mg/kg/dose for 2–5 consecutive days, then q 3–6 wk. Kawasaki disease: 2 g/kg single dose. Cytomegalovirus infection: 500 mg/kg/dose eq other day for 7 doses. Severe systemic infection: 500–1,000 mg/kg/wk. Polyneuropathy: 1 g/kg24 hr for 2 consecutive days q mo.	*Caution:* Doses should be based on ideal body weight (not total body weight). *Adverse events:* Flushing, tachycardia, chills, nausea, dyspnea, fever, hypersensitivity reactions, headache, aseptic meningitis.

TABLE 716-1. General Medications—cont'd

DRUG (TRADE NAMES, FORMULATIONS)	INDICATIONS (MECHANISM OF ACTION AND DOSING)	COMMENTS (CAUTIONS, ADVERSE EVENTS, MONITORING)
Indomethacin Indocin; generic (oral forms). Capsule: 25, 50 mg. Suspension: 25 mg/5 mL. Injection.	**Closure of patent ductus arteriosus in neonates, treatment of rheumatoid disorders, acute gouty arthritis, pain (nonsteroidal anti-inflammatory drug, prostaglandin inhibition), hereditary hypokalemic salt-losing renal tubulopathies.** *Neonates:* IV: 0.10–0.25 mg/kg/dose q 12 hr for 3–6 doses. Inflammatory rheumatoid disorders: *Children:* 1–2 mg/kg/24 hr in 2–4 doses (max: 4 mg/kg/24 hr). *Adults:* 25–50 mg/dose bid–tid. (max: 200 mg/24 hr).	*Caution:* Avoid in premature neonates with necrotizing enterocolitis, poor renal function, or active bleeding, and all patients with active gastrointestinal bleeding. *Adverse events:* Confusion, dizziness, headache, nausea, vomiting, abdominal pain, gastrointestinal bleeding, ulcers, gastrointestinal perforation, bone marrow suppression, impaired platelet aggregation, oliguria, renal failure, hypertension, edema, hyperkalemia. *Monitoring:* Indomethacin (concentrations in patent ductus arturiosus closure): therapeutic 1–3 μg/mL.
Insulin **Rapid-acting:** Lispro, Regular, Semilente. **Intermediate-acting:** NPH, Lente. **Long-acting:** Ultralente. **Combination products** (e.g., Novolin 70/30, contains Lente 70 units, Regular 30 units). Humulin; Novolin (human insulin, preferred form); beef insulin, pork insulin. Injection.	**Treatment of insulin-dependent diabetes mellitus and non–insulin-dependent diabetes not adequately controlled with oral hypoglycemic agents (replacement therapy).** *Neonates:* Regular insulin 0.01–0.1 u/kg/hr by continuous infusion, or SC 0.1–0.2 u/kg 6–12 hr. *Children and adults:* 0.5–1 u/kg/24 hr. Adjust doses to blood glucose and hemoglobin A_{1C} results. *Adolescents (during growth spurt):* 0.8–1.2 u/kg/24 hr. Diabetic ketoacidosis: Continuous infusion IV: 0.1 u/kg/hr adjusted to serum glucose. Hyperkalemia: Give calcium gluconate and $NaHCO_3$ first, then dextrose 50% 0.5–1 mL/kg and regular insulin 1 u/4–5 g dextrose.	*Caution:* Check for drugs that increase or decrease insulin effect. Do not change insulin types or brands once patient is regulated because dosing requirements will then change; start new patients on human insulin if possible. *Adverse events:* Hypoglycemia (and associated symptoms of dizziness, weakness, paresthesias, numbness of mouth, fatigue, mental confusion, hunger, nausea, visual problems), hypokalemia. *Monitoring:* Blood glucose (teach patient to monitor at home and make insulin dosing corrections per results), hemoglobin A_{1C}, urine glucose, and acetone.
Interferon alfa-2a Roferon-A. Injection.	**In children, treatment of hemangiomas of infancy and pulmonary hemangiomas (inhibits cellular growth, alters cellular differentiation).** *Infants and children:* SC: 1–3 million u/m²/dose. *Adults:* 3–20 million u/m²/dose/dose to 3×/wk, depending on indication.	*Adverse events:* Tachycardia, arrhythmias, hypotension, edema, CNS depression, confusion, fatigue, dizziness, and flu-like symptoms (begin 2–6 hr after dose and last up to 24 hr).
Ipecac syrup Generic. Syrup: 70 mg/mL.	**Induces vomiting to treat certain toxic ingestions (stimulates medullary chemoreceptor trigger zone).** *Children:* May repeat dose in 20 min 1×. *6–12 mo:* 5–10 mL, followed by 20 mL/kg of water. *1–12 yr:* 15 mL, followed by 20 mL/kg of water. *>12 yr and adults:* 30 mL, followed by 300 mL of water.	*Cautions:* Do not use if patient is unconscious, has absent gag reflex, or has seizures, or after ingestion of strong bases or acids or volatile oils. Do not confuse with ipecac fluid extract, which is 14 times more potent. *Adverse events:* Lethargy, persistent vomiting, diarrhea.
Ipratropium Anticholinergic. Atrovent. Nebulization solution: 0.02%. Metered-dose inhaler (MDI): 18 μg/puff. Nasal spray: 0.3%, 0.6%.	**Bronchodilator, treatment of rhinitis).** *Neonates:* Nebulized 100 μg/dose or MDI 1–2 puffs tid–qid. *Infants and children:* Nebulized 125–250 μg or MDI 1–2 puffs 3–6 times/24 hr. *Adults:* Nebulized 500 μg or MDI 2 puffs tid–qid. Nasal spray for rhinitis: 1–2 sprays in each nostril bid–tid.	*Adverse events:* Dry mouth, nervousness, dizziness, headache, blurred vision, urinary retention.
Iron Iron dextran complex (injection). Ferrous sulfate, gluconate, etc. Oral.	**Treatment of iron-deficiency, hypochromic, or microcytic anemia (replacement therapy).** Injection: IM, IV: Give 0.25–0.5 mL test dose 1 hr before starting iron dextran therapy. Dose (mL/kg) = Hgb (normal − actual) × 0.0476 + 1 mL/5 kg (max: <5 kg = 25 mg; 5–10 kg = 50 mg; >10 kg = 100 mg). PO (mg iron): *Children:* Prophylaxis: 1–2 mg/kg/24 hr. Deficiency: 3–6 mg/kg/24 hr in 1–3 divided doses. *Adults:* Prophylaxis: 60 mg/24 hr. Deficiency: 60 mg bid–qid.	*Adverse events:* (oral) Gastrointestinal irritation, nausea, constipation, dark stools: (IV, IM) hypotension, flushing, dizziness, fever, headache, metallic taste, arthralgia, anaphylaxis. *Monitoring:* Hemoglobin (normal <15 kg = 12 mg/dL, >15 kg = 14.8 mg/dL), reticulocyte count, serum ferritin.
Isoetharine Generic. Metered-dose inhaler (MDI), inhalation solution.	**Bronchodilator (β-agonist stimulation).** *Children:* Nebulize 0.01 mL/kg of 1% solution. *Adults:* Nebulize 0.5–1 mL of 0.5–1% solution; MDI 1–2 puffs q 4 hr as needed.	*Adverse events:* Tachycardia, headache, tremor, excitement, restlessness, nausea.
Isoproterenol Generic. Injection, sublingual tablets, nebulizer solution, metered-dose inhaler (MDI).	**Asthma or chronic obstructive pulmonary disease, ventricular arrhythmias due to AV node block, low-output shock states (stimulates β_1 and β_2 receptors).** *Neonates, infants, and children:* IV: Infuse 0.05–2 μg/kg/min. *Children:* MDI: 1–2 puffs eq 4 hr as needed; nebulize 0.01 mL of 1% solution; sublingual tablets: 5–10 mg eq 3–4 hr (max: 30 mg/24 hr). *Adults:* MDI: 1–2 puffs 4–6 times/24 hr; nebulize 0.25–0.5 mL of 1% solution; sublingual tablets: 10–20 mg q 3–4 hr (max: 60 mg/24 hr); IV infusion 2–20 μg/min.	*Adverse events:* Tachycardia, palpitations, chest pain, nervousness, restlessness, anxiety, headache, insomnia, tremor, gastrointestinal distress, nausea, paradoxical bronchospasm.
Kaolin and pectin Generic. Oral suspension.	**Treatment of uncomplicated diarrhea (absorbent action).** *Children:* *3–6 yr:* 15–30 mL/dose. *6–12 yr:* 30–60 mL/dose. *>12 yr:* 60–120 mL/dose.	*Cautions:* Some products contain bismuth subsalicylate and may cause bleeding disorders. Avoid in dysentery, toxigenic diarrheas.
Ketamine Ketalar. Injection: 10, 100 mg/mL.	**Anesthesia for short procedures (direct action on cortex and limbic system to produce dissociative anesthesia).** *Children:* Give 30 min before procedure. PO: 6–10 mg/kg. IM: 3–7 mg/kg. IV: 0.5–2 mg/kg. *Adults:* 3–8 mg/kg IV. IV: 1–4.5 mg/kg (supplemental doses 1/3 of initial dose).	*Adverse events:* Hypertension, tachycardia, hypotension, bradycardia, increased cerebral blood flow and intracranial pressure, hallucinations, delirium, tonic-clonic movements, increased metabolic rate, hypersalivation, nausea, vomiting, respiratory depression, apnea, increased airway resistance, cough, emergence reactions.

TABLE 716-1. General Medications—cont'd

DRUG (TRADE NAMES, FORMULATIONS)	INDICATIONS (MECHANISM OF ACTION AND DOSING)	COMMENTS (CAUTIONS, ADVERSE EVENTS, MONITORING)
Ketorolac Nonsteroidal anti-inflammatory drug. Acular. Ophthalmic. Toradol. Tablet, injection.	**Treatment of pain; ocular itching with conjunctivitis (inhibits prostaglandin).** *Children 2–16 yr:* IM, IV: 0.4–1 mg/kg/dose. PO: 1 mg/kg/dose q 6 hr as needed. *Adults:* IM: 60 mg. IV: 30 mg up to q 6 hr as needed. Ophthalmic: 1 drop in eye qid for up to 7 days.	*Adverse events:* Edema, somnolence, dizziness, headache, dyspepsia, nausea, diarrhea, gastrointestinal pain, gastrointestinal bleeding, peptic ulcer, impaired platelet aggregation, oliguria, acute renal failure, dyspnea, wheezing, pain at injection site.
Labetalol Normodyne; Trandate. Injection: 5 mg/mL. Tablet: 100, 200, 300 mg.	**Treatment of mild to severe hypertension (blocks α- and β-adrenergic receptors).** *Children:* PO: Start 4 mg/kg/24 hr in 2 doses, then gradually increase (max: 40 mg/kg/24 hr). IV: Start 0.2–1 mg/kg/dose (max: 20 mg/dose), continuous IV infusion of 0.4–1 mg/kg/hr (max: 3 mg/kg/hr). *Adults:* PO: 100 mg bid; may increase every 2–3 days (max: 2.4 g/24 hr). IV: Start 20 mg; repeat boluses 40 mg q 10 min (max: total dose 300 mg), continuous IV infusion of 2 mg/min and titrate to response.	*Adverse events:* Orthostatic hypotension, congestive heart failure, conduction disturbance, bradycardia, drowsiness fatigue, headache, dry mouth, nasal congestion, bronchospasm.
Lactulose Generic. Syrup: 10 g/15 mL.	**Treatment of constipation, hepatic encephalopathy (osmotic effect on stool in colon; acidification of stool promotes NH_4^+ elimination).** *Infants:* 2.5–10 mL/24 hr in 3–4 doses. *Children:* 40–90 mL/24 hr in 3–4 doses. *Adults:* 30–45 mL/dose 3–4 times/24 hr.	*Adverse events:* Flatulence, abdominal discomfort, diarrhea, nausea, vomiting. *Monitoring:* Target 2–3 soft stools/day; serum ammonia.
Lamotrigine Lamictal. Tablet: 25, 100, 150, 200 mg. Tablet, chewable, dispersible: 2, 5, 25 mg.	**Treatment of partial seizures (blocks sodium channels and inhibits presynaptic release of glutamate and aspartate).** *Children 2–12 yr:* 0.6 mg/kg/24 hr in 1–2 doses for 2 wk, then 1.2 mg/kg/24 hr in 2 doses for 2 wk, then 5–15 mg/kg/24 hr in 2 doses per response (max: 400 mg/24 hr). Patients taking valproate: 0.15 mg/kg/24 hr in 1–2 doses for 2 wk, then 0.3 mg/kg/24 hr in 2 doses for 2 wk, then 1–5 mg/kg/24 hr in 2 doses (max: 200 mg/24 hr). *Adults:* Start 50 mg/24 hr for 2 wk, then 100 mg/24 hr, then increases by 100 mg/24 hr at weekly intervals to response (max: 500 mg/24 hr). Patients taking valproate: 25 mg q other day for 2 wk, then 25 mg/24 hr for 2 wk, then increase by 25 mg/24 hr q wk to response (max: 150 mg/24 hr).	*Caution:* Serious rashes (potentially fatal) can occur and are particularly common in children, especially if doses are increased too quickly. Slow increase in dosing is especially important for patients taking valproic acid. *Adverse events:* Dizziness, sedation, headache, agitation, exacerbation of seizures, rashes (maculopapular or erythematous eruptions), angioedema, photosensitivity, nystagmus, amblyopia, nausea, vomiting.
Lansoprazole Prevacid. Proton pump inhibitor. Capsule: 15, 30 mg. Packet: Powder for oral suspension 5 mg, 30 mg.	**Treatment of gastric or duodenal ulcer.** *Children:* 15–30 mg/24 hr. *Adults:* 15–30 mg/24 hr.	
Leucovorin Wellcovorin; generic. Tablet: 5, 15 mg. Injection.	**Antidote for folic acid antagonists (e.g., methotrexate), treatment of folate-deficient megaloblastic anemias of infancy, nutritional folate deficiency when oral folate cannot be used (reduced form of folic acid, so conversion is not necessary, replacement therapy).** *Children and adults:* Methotrexate rescue: IV: 10 mg/m^2 to start, then 10 mg/m^2 PO q 6 hr for 72 hr; increase dose to 100 mg/m^2 q 3 hr if 24 hr after methotrexate dose, serum creatinine is increased by >50%, or methotrexate serum level is $>5 \times 10^{-6}$ M (continue until level is $<1 \times 10^{-8}$ M). High-dose methotrexate rescue: IV: 100–1,000 mg/m^2 dose. Intrathecal methotrexate: IV: 12 mg/m^2 as single dose. Megaloblastic anemia of infancy: IM 3–6 mg/24 hr.	*Adverse events:* Rash, itching erythema. *Monitoring:* Plasma methotrexate levels; a leukovorin dosing nomogram is available based on methotrexate levels at various times after the dose.
Leuprolide Lupron. Injection.	**Treatment of precocious puberty, prostate cancer (decreases levels of luteinizing hormone and follicle-stimulating hormone).** 0.15–0.3 mg/kg/dose q 28 days (min: 7.5 mg) IM. SC: 20–45 μg/kg/24 hr. *Adults:* Prostate cancer: IM: 7.5 mg/dose/mo. SC: 1 mg/24 hr.	*Adverse events:* Weight gain, hot flashes, depression, nausea, vomiting, gastrointestinal bleeding, myalgia, bone pain, weakness, blurred vision, estrogenic effects.
Levothyroxine Synthroid; generic. Injection, tablet.	**Thyroid replacement therapy.** PO: *0–6 mo:* 8–10 μg/kg/24 hr. *6–12 mo:* 6–8 μg/kg/24 hr. *1–5 yr:* 5–6 μg/kg/24 hr. *6–12 yr:* 4–5 μg/kg/24 hr. *>12 yr:* 2–3 μg/kg/24 hr. *Adults:* 12.5–50 μg/24 hr (max: 200 μg/24 hr). IV, IM: 50–75% of PO dose. Myxedema coma: 200–500 μg for 1 dose. Thyroid suppression therapy: 2–6 μg/kg/24 hr for 7–10 days.	*Adverse events:* Tachycardia, cardiac arrhythmias, hypertension, nervousness, headache, insomnia, hair loss, increased appetite, weight loss, tremor, sweating.

TABLE 716-1. General Medications—cont'd

DRUG (TRADE NAMES, FORMULATIONS)	INDICATIONS (MECHANISM OF ACTION AND DOSING)	COMMENTS (CAUTIONS, ADVERSE EVENTS, MONITORING)
Lidocaine Generic. Injection. Topical (alone or in combination with prilocaine [EMLA]).	**Treatment of ventricular arrhythmias, local anesthetic (class 1B antiarrhythmic, blocks initiation and conduction of impulses).** *Children and adults:* Topical: Apply to affected area (max: 3 mg/kg/dose) at least 2 hr apart. Local anesthetic injection: Doses as needed (max: 4.5 mg/kg), not closer than 2 hr apart. Arrhythmias: *Children:* Loading dose of 1 mg/kg (may repeat q 5–10 min (max: 3 mg/kg). IV: continuous infusion: 20–50 μg/kg/min (1/2 dose for liver disease or poor cardiac output). *Adults:* Loading dose of 1–1.5 mg/kg, may repeat (max: 3 mg/kg). IV: continuous infusion: 2–4 mg/min (1/2 dose for liver disease or heart failure). ET route: 2–2.5 × IV dose. Prehospital post–myocardial infarction: 300 mg IM.	*Caution:* Avoid lidocaine with epinephrine preparations for arrhythmias. *Adverse events:* Arrhythmias, heart block, lethargy, coma, seizures, nausea, vomiting, paresthesias, blurred vision, diplopia, local shin irritation or rash. *Monitoring:* Lidocaine serum levels (therapeutic 1–5 μg/mL toxic >6 μg/mL).
Liothyronine Cytomel (oral); Triostat (injection); generic.	**Replacement theraphy in hypothyroidism.** *Neonates, infants, and children <3 yr:* Congenital hypothyroidism (cretinism): PO: 5 μg/24 hr initially, then may increase 5 μg q 3 days (max: 20 μg/24 hr [50 μg/24 hr for children age 1–3 yr]). Hypothyroidism: *Children:* 5 μg/24 hr; increase by 5 μg q 1–2 wk (usual, 15–20 μg/24 hr). *Adults:* Start 5 μg/24 hr; increase by 5 μg/24 hr q 1–2 wk to 25 μg, then by 12.5–25 μg q 1–2 wk (max: 100 μg/24 hr).	*Adverse events:* Palpitations, tachycardia, hypertension, nervousness, insomnia, headache, hair loss, diarrhea, abdominal cramps, tremor, sweating. *Monitoring:* Thyroid function, T_3, thyroid-stimulating hormone.
Lithium Generic. Syrup: 300 mg/5 mL. Tablet: 300 mg. Capsule: 150, 300, 600 mg.	**Management of acute mania, bipolar disorder, and depression (alters cation exchange across cell membranes).** *Children:* 15–60 mg/kg/24 hr in 3–4 doses (start low and increase at weekly intervals). *Adolescents:* 600–1,800 mg/24 hr in 3–4 doses at regular intervals. *Adults:* 300 mg tid–qid to start; may gradually increase per blood levels (max: 2.4 g/24 hr). **May use twice-daily dosing if sustained-release product used.** *Renal impairment:* CrCl 10–50 mL/min: 50–70% of normal dose; CrCl <10 mL/min: 25–50% of normal dose.	*Adverse events:* Polydipsia, nausea, diarrhea, impaired taste, bloated feeling, weight gain, tremor, muscle twitching, weakness, fatigue, diabetes insipidus, nonspecific nephron atrophy, renal tubular acidosis, leukocytosis, vision problems, hypothyroidism, goiter, skin eruptions, acne. *Monitoring:* Serum lithium concentrations are essential to proper use of lithium, must be drawn 8–12 hr after a dose (therapeutic: acute mania 0.6–1.2 mEq/L; protection against future episodes 0.6–1 mEq/L; toxic >1.5 mEq/L; seizures >2.5 mEq/L). Watch for accumulation during salt loss and dehydration states.
Lomustine, CCNU Alkylating agent. CeeNu. Capsule: 10, 40, 100 mg.	**Treatment of various cancers (inhibits DNA and RNA synthesis).** *Children:* 75–100 mg/m² as single dose q 6 wk. *Adults:* 100–130 mg/m² as single dose q 6 wk.	*Adverse events:* Nausea, vomiting, myelosuppression (onset, 14 days; nadir, 4–5 wk; recovery, 6 wk), neurotoxicity, stomatitis, diarrhea, anemia, alopecia, hepatotoxicity, renal failure, pulmonary fibrosis (with cumulative doses >600 mg). *Monitoring:* Reduce dose if CrCl <50 mL/min or platelet and WBC counts remain low beyond 6 wk.
Loperamide Imodium; generic. Liquid: 1 mg/5 mL. Tablet: 2 mg. Capsule: 2 mg.	**Treatment of acute and chronic diarrhea (directly inhibits intestinal peristalsis).** *Children:* *2–5 yr:* 1 mg tid. *6–8 yr:* 2 mg bid. *8–12 yr:* 2 mg tid. *Adults:* 4 mg initially, then 2 mg after each loose stool (max: 16 mg/24 hr).	*Adverse events:* Sedatin, fatigue, dizziness, nausea, vomiting, constipation.
Loratadine Tablet: 10 mg. Claritin. Syrup: 1 mg/mL.	**Treatment of allergic symptoms (antihistamine, H_1-receptor antagonist).** *Children: >3 yr:* <30 kg; 5 mg/24 hr; >30 kg: 10 mg/24 hr. *Adults:* 10 mg/24 hr.	*Caution:* Prolonged Q-T intervals may occur if combined with drugs that inhibit liver enzymes; watch for drug interactions. *Adverse events:* Somnolence, fatigue, anxiety, depression, headache.
Lorazepam Ativan; generic. Injection. Tablet: 0.5, 1, 2 mg. Oral solution: 2 mg/mL.	**Treatment for anxiety, sedation, and seizures; adjunct to antiemetic therapy (benzodiazepine increases action of γ-aminobutyric acid).** Antiemetic therapy: *Children:* IV: 0.04–0.08 mg/kg/dose q 6 hr as needed. Anxiety/sedation: *Neonates:* IV: 0.1–0.4 mg/kg/dose q 4–6 hr as needed. *Infants and children:* IV: 0.05–0.1 mg/kg/dose q 4–8 hr. *Adults:* PO: 1–10 mg/24 hr in 2–3 divided doses. Insomnia: *Adults:* 2–4 mg at bedtime. Status epilepticus: *Neonates:* IV: 0.05–0.2 mg/kg/dose over 2–5 min; may repeat in 10–15 min. *Infants and children:* IV: Loading dose of 0.1 mg/kg over 2–5 min; may give additional 0.05 mg/kg bolus in 10–15 min. *Adolescents:* IV: 0.07 mg/kg/dose over 2–5 min; may repeat in 10–15 min. *Adults:* IV: 4 mg/dose over 2–5 min; may repeat in 10 min.	*Caution:* Do not discontinue abruptly after long-term use to avoid possible abstinence symptoms. *Adverse events:* Several cases of myoclonus have been reported in neonates; tachycardia, drowsiness, depression, confusion, paradoxical excitement, blurred vision, diplopia.
Magnesium citrate, citrate of magnesia Generic. Solution: 300 mL.	**Evacuation of bowel (osmotic retention of fluid and increased peristalsis).** *Children <6 yr:* 2–4 mL/kg. *Children 6–12 yr:* 100–150 mL. *>12 yr and adults:* 150–300 mL.	*Adverse events:* Hypermagnesemia, hypotension, abdominal cramps, muscle weakness, CNS depression. *Monitoring:* Toxicity related to serum magnesium levels (>3 mg/dL, depressed CNS; >5 mg/dL, somnolence and depressed deep tendon reflexes; >12 mg/dL, respiratory paralysis and heart block).
Magnesium gluconate Generic. Tablet: 500 mg.	**Magnesium replacement therapy.** *Children:* 10–20 mg/kg/dose elemental magnesium qid. *Adults:* 300 mg elemental magnesium qid.	*Adverse events:* Hypermagnesemia (see *Magnesium citrate, citrate of magnesia*). *Monitoring:* Serum magnesium concentration (normal: children, 1.5–1.9 mg/dL; adults, 2.2–2.8 mg/dL).

TABLE 716-1. General Medications—cont'd

DRUG (TRADE NAMES, FORMULATIONS)	INDICATIONS (MECHANISM OF ACTION AND DOSING)	COMMENTS (CAUTIONS, ADVERSE EVENTS, MONITORING)
Magnesium oxide Generic. Tablet: 400, 420, 500 mg. Capsule: 140 mg.		
Magnesium hydroxide, milk of magnesia Generic. Liquid, tablet.	**Short-term treatment of constipation (osmotic retention of fluid promotes peristalsis).** *Children:* *<2 yr:* 0.5 mL/kg/dose. *2–5 yr:* 5–15 mL once daily. *6–12 yr:* 15–30 mL once daily. *>12 yr and adults:* 30–60 mL once daily.	*Adverse events:* (see *Magnesium citrate, citrate of magnesia*).
Magnesium sulfate Generic. Granules: 40 mEq/5 g. Injection: 50% solution.	**Treatment of hypomagnesemia and seizures associated with acute nephritis in children; also used as a cathartic (cofactor for many enzymes in the body and important in calcium and potassium hemostasis).** Hypomagnesemia: *Neonates:* IV: 25–50 mg/kg/dose q 8 hr for 2–3 doses. *Children:* PO: 100–200 mg/kg/dose qid. IM, IV: 25–50 mg/kg/dose q 6 hr for 3–4 doses. *Adults:* PO: 3 g q 6 hr for 4 doses. IM, IV: 1 g q 6 hr for 4 doses. Daily maintenance magnesium: *Neonates, infants, and children:* IV: 30–60 mg/kg/24 hr. *Adolescents:* IV: 42–54 mg/kg/24 hr. *Adults:* IV: 0.5–3 g/24 hr. Infuse IV doses over 2–4 hr (max: 125 mg/kg/hr). Management of seizures and hypertension: *Children:* IM, IV: 20–100 mg/kg/dose q 4–6 hr as needed. Cathartic: *Children:* PO: 0.25 g/kg/dose. *Adults:* PO: 10–30 g	*Caution:* Magnesium may accumulate to toxic levels in renal insufficiency. *Adverse events:* (see *Magnesium citrate, citrate of magnesia*).
Manganese Injection: 0.1 mg/mL.	**Trace element added to parenteral nutrition (cofactor in many enzyme systems).** *Infants:* 2–10 μg/kg/24 hr in total parenteral nutrition solutions. *Adults:* 150–180 μg/24 hr in total parenteral nutrition solutions.	*Monitoring:* Reference manganese plasma level is 4–14 μg/L.
Mannitol Generic. Injection.	**Promotion of diuresis, reduction of increased intracranial pressure.** *Children and adults:* IV: 200 mg/kg test dose; initial, 0.5–1 g/kg; maintenance, 0.25–0.5 g/kg q 4–6 hr	*Adverse events:* Circulatory overload, congestive heart failure, headache, chills, seizures, fluid and electrolyte imbalance. *Monitoring:* After test dose, evaluate urine output of at least 1 mL/kg/hr (children) or 30–50 mL/hr (adults) for 2–3 hr; for increased intracranial pressure, maintain serum osmolality 310–320 mOsm/kg.
Mechlorethamine, nitrogen mustard Alkylating agent. Mustargen Hydrochloride. Injection.	**Cancer chemotherapy (inhibits DNA and RNA synthesis).** *Children:* IV: As part of MOPP regimen, 6 mg/m² on days 1 and 8 of 28 day regimen. *Adults:* IV: 0.4 mg/kg (12–16 mg/m²) as single monthly dose.	*Caution:* Extravasation should be treated promptly with sterile sodium thiosulfate (1/6 M) and apply cold compress for 6–12 hr. *Adverse events:* Nausea, vomiting, diarrhea, severe myelosuppression (onset, 4–7 days; nadir, 14 days; recovery, 21 days), ototoxicity, precipitation of herpes zoster, alopecia, hyperuricemia.
Meclizine Generic. Tablet, capsule.	**Prevention and treatment of motion sickness and treatment of vertigo (anticholinergic and CNS depressant effects).** *Children and adults:* PO: 25–50 mg 1 hr before travel for motion sickness; 25–100 mg/24 hr in divided doses for vertigo.	*Adverse events:* Drowsiness, headache, fatigue, dry mouth, increased appetite, weight gain.
Medium chain triglycerides MCT Oil. Oil: 14 g/15 mL.	**Dietary supplement for those who cannot digest long-chain fats, ketogenic diet for seizure disorders (nutritional supplement).** *Infants:* 0.5 mL q other feed; may advance by 0.5 mL q 2–3 days as tolerated. *Children:* Ketogenic diet for seizures: 50–70% of total calories (usually about 40 mL with each meal). Cystic fibrosis: 1 tbs tid. *Adults:* 15 mL tid–qid.	*Adverse events:* Nausea, vomiting, abdominal pain, ketosis.
Medrysone HMS Liquifilm. Ophthalmic solution.	**Treatment of conjunctivitis (inhibits inflammatory response).** *Children and adults:* Ophthalmic: Instill 1 drop in conjunctival sac bid–qid (may use q 1–2 hr for 1–2 days).	*Adverse events:* Local stinging and burning, increased intraocular pressure, cataracts.
Melphalan Alkeran Alkylating agent. Injection. Tablet: 2 mg.	**Cancer chemotherapy (inhibits DNA and RNA synthesis).** *Children:* IV: 10–35 mg/m² dose q 21–28 days; high dose: 140–220 mg/m² before bone marrow transplantation. PO: 4–20 mg/m²/24 hr for 1–21 days. *Adults:* IV: 16 mg/m² dose q 2 wk for 4 doses monthly. PO: 0.15 mg/kg/24 hr for 7 days or 0.25 mg/kg/24 hr for 4 days; repeat q 4–6 wk.	*Adverse evens:* Myelosuppression (onset, 7 days; nadir, 8–10 days and 27–32 days; recovery, 42–50 days), secondary malignancy, alopecia, vesiculation of skin, syndrome of inappropriate secretion of antidiuretic hormone, nausea, vomiting, diarrhea, stomatitis, hemorrhagic cystitis, pulmonary fibrosis, interstitial pneumonitis, vasculitis.

TABLE 716-1. General Medications—cont'd

DRUG (TRADE NAMES, FORMULATIONS)	INDICATIONS (MECHANISM OF ACTION AND DOSING)	COMMENTS (CAUTIONS, ADVERSE EVENTS, MONITORING)
Meperidine Generic. Injection, syrup: 50 mg/5 mL. Tablet: 50, 100 mg.	**Narcotic analgesic, adjunct to anesthesia (binds to opiate receptors in CNS).** *Children:* IM, IV, SC: 1–1.5 q 3–4 hr. *Adults:* IM, IV, SC: 50–100 mg/dose q 3–4 hr as needed (equipotent oral dose is 3× IV dose).	*Caution:* Scheduled use may result in metabolite accumulation and diminished renal function, which may lead to CNS stimulation or seizures. *Adverse events:* Hypotension, weakness, tiredness, headache, anorexia, stomach cramps, hallucination, paradoxical excitation, seizures, physical and psychologic dependence. *Comment:* Equianalgesic dose to morphine 10 mg IV is meperidine 100 mg IV or IM, or 300 mg PO.
Mephenytoin Mesantoin. Tablet: 100 mg.	**Treatment of tonic-clonic and partial seizures (decreases sodium ion influx across cell membranes).** *Children:* 3–15 mg/kg/24 hr in 3 divided doses. *Adults:* Start 50–100 mg/24 hr; then increase weekly by 50–100 mg (max: 800 mg/24 hr).	*Adverse events:* Drowsiness, slurred speech, psychiatric changes, confusion, nausea, vomiting, constipation, leukopenia, hepatitis, blurred vision, nystagmus, photophobia, lymphadenopathy. *Monitoring:* Total mephenytoin level (25–40 μg/mL).
Mephobarbital Mebaral. Tablets: 32, 50, 100 mg.	**Sedative, treatment of epilepsy (increases seizure threshold).** *Children:* 4–10 mg/kg/24 hr in 2–4 doses. *Adults:* 200–600 mg/24 hr in 2–4 doses.	*Adverse events:* Drowsiness, lethargy, confusion, mental depression, paradoxical excitement, psychologic and physical dependence, constipation, nausea, vomiting. *Monitoring:* Phenobarbital concentrations (therapeutic 10–40 μg/mL).
Mercaptopurine Purinethol. Injection, tablet. Extemporaneous formulations may be prepared.	**Treatment of leukemias and non-Hodgkin lymphoma (antimetabolite, blocks purine synthesis).** *Children:* PO: Induction: 2.5–5 mg/kg once daily; maintenance: 1.5–2.5 mg/kg/24 hr. IV: Continuous infusion: 50 mg/m²/hr for 24–48 hr. *Adults:* PO: Induction: 2.5–5 mg/kg once daily; maintenance: 1.5–2.5 mg/kg/24 hr. Renal function: Crcl < 50 mL/min: Dose q 48 hr.	*Adverse events:* Hepatotoxicity (cholestasis and necrosis), nausea, anorexia, vomiting, diarrhea, stomach pain, stomatitis, mucositis, rash, hyperpigmentation, myelosuppression (onset, 7–10 days; nadir, 14 days; recovery, 21 days), renal toxicity, hyperuricemia, eosinophilia, drug fever.
Mesna Mesnex. Injection: 100 mg/mL.	**Protects against hemorrhagic cystitis from ifosamide and cyclophosphamide therapy (binds and detoxifies urotoxic metabolites via active sulfhydryl group).** *Children and adults:* IV: 20% w/w of ifosfamide or cyclophosphamide dose started 15 min before alkylating agent dose. Repeat mesna dose 3, 6, 9, and 12 hr after alkylating agent dose. PO: 40% w/w of alkylating agent in 3 doses 4 hr apart.	*Adverse events:* Hypotension, headache, nausea vomiting, bad taste in mouth, limb pain. *Monitoring:* Urinalysis.
Metaproterenol, orciprenaline Alupent; Metaprel; generic. Metered-dose inhaler (MDI). Inhalation solution. Tablet: 10, 20 mg. Syrup: 10 mg/5 mL.	**Bronchodilator (stimulates β_2 receptors).** *Children:* PO: *<2 yr:* 0.4 mg/kg/dose tid–qid. *2–6 yr:* 1.3–2.6 mg/kg/24 hr divided q 6 hr. *6–9 yr:* 10 mg/dose qid. *>9 yr and adults:* 20 mg/dose tid–qid. MDI: 2–3 puffs q 4 hr. Nebulizer: *Infants and children:* 0.01–0.02 mL/kg of 5% solution q 4–6 hr. *Adolescents and adults:* 0.3 mL of 5% solution q 4–6 hr.	*Caution:* Some generic nebulizer solutions contain sulfites that may exacerbate asthma. *Adverse events:* Tremor, nervousness, overactivity, tachycardia, hypotension, headache. *Comment:* Dilute nebulizer solution in 2.5 mL normal saline.
Metformin Glucophage. Tablet: 500, 850, 1,000 mg.	**Treatment of type 2 diabetes; increases insulin sensitivity and improves glucose tolerance; hypoglycemic effect.** *Children 10–16 yr:* Start with 500 mg bid with meals; increase in 500 mg increments weekly to response (max: 2,000 mg/24 hr). *Adults:* Start with 850 mg q 24 hr or 500 mg bid; titrate by 500 mg once 1×/wk or 850 mg q 2 wk to response (max: 2550 mg/24 hr).	*Caution:* Avoid use if creatinine clearance <60 mL/min, serum creatinine >1.5 mg/dL (males) or >1.4 mg/dL (females). Monitor for lactic acidosis. Discontinue for any process that may predispose to metabolic acidosis or renal dysfunction until the situation is resolved. Avoid alcohol. *Adverse events:* Nausea, vomiting, diarrhea, indigestion, flatulence.
Methadone Dolophine; generic. Injection: 10 mg/mL. Tablet: 5, 10 mg. Oral solution: 5 mg/mL.	**Management of severe pain, narcotic detoxification (binds to opiate receptors in CNS).** *Neonates (abstinence syndrome):* 0.05–0.2 mg/kg/dose q 12 hr; then adjust or taper based on abstinence scores. *Children:* Analgesia: IV, IM, PO: 0.1 mg/kg/dose q 4 hr for 2–3 doses, then q 6–12 hr as needed. *Narcotic abstinence:* Start 0.05–0.1 mg/kg/dose q 6 hr and taper per abstinence scores. *Adults:* IV, IM, SC, PO. Analgesia: 2.5–20 mg q 6–8 hr. Detoxification: 15–40 mg/24 hr.	*Adverse events:* Weakness, drowsiness, dizziness, nausea, vomiting, constipation, ileus. *Monitoring:* Methadone accumulates with repeated doses, and patients should be monitored for excess CNS depression.
Methimazole Tapazole. Tablet: 5, 10 mg.	**Treatment of hyperthyroidism (blocks iodine synthesis in thyroid gland, inhibits synthesis of thyroid hormone).** *Children:* Start 0.4 mg/kg/24 hr, then maintenance 0.2 mg/kg/24 hr. *Adults:* Start 5 mg/kg q 8 hr; maintenance dose: 5–15 mg/24 hr (max: 60 mg/24 hr).	*Adverse events:* Fever, rash, leukopenia, agranulocytosis, systemic lupus erythematosus–like syndrome, nausea, vomiting, stomach pain, loss of taste, cholestatic jaundice, constipation, weight gain. *Monitoring:* Thyroid function tests for hypothyroidism or hyperthyroidism.
Methocarbamol Robaxin; generic. Injection: 100 mg/mL. Tablet: 500, 750 mg.	**Treatment of muscle spasm (skeletal muscle relaxant through CNS depressive effects).** *Children:* Treatment of tetanus: IV: 15 mg/kg/dose q 6 hr for 3 days only. *Adults:* IV: 1–2 g q 6 hr. PO: 1.5 g tid–qid for 2–3 days, then decrease to 4–4.5 g/24 hr.	*Adverse events:* Syncope, bradycardia, hypotension, drowsiness, dizziness, headache, nausea, metallic taste.

TABLE 716-1. General Medications—cont'd

DRUG (TRADE NAMES, FORMULATIONS)	INDICATIONS (MECHANISM OF ACTION AND DOSING)	COMMENTS (CAUTIONS, ADVERSE EVENTS, MONITORING)
Methohexital Brevital. Injection.	**Induction and maintenance of general anesthesia (ultra–short-acting barbiturate).** *Children:* IM: Preoperative: 5–10 mg/kg/dose. IV: Induction dose of 1–2 mg/kg/dose. Rectal: 20–35 mg/kg/dose. *Adults:* IV: Induction dose of 50–120 mg, then 20–40 mg q 4–7 min.	*Adverse events:* Apnea, respiratory depression, hiccups, laryngospasm, hypotension, skeletal muscle twitching and rigidity, tremor, seizures, headache, nausea, vomiting.
Methotrexate Generic. Injection. Tablet: 2.5 mg.	**Treatment of neoplasms, psoriasis, rheumatoid arthritis (antimetabolite, inhibition of DNA and purine synthesis).** *Children:* Juvenile rheumatoid arthritis: PO, IM: 5–15 mg/m^2/wk as a single dose. Antineoplastic: PO, IM: 7.5–30 mg/m^2 q 1–2 wk. IV: 10–33 g/m^2 bolus dose or infused over 6–42 hr. *Adults:* Rheumatoid arthritis: PO: 7.5 mg 1× wk. Psoriasis: PO, IM: 10–25 mg/dose 1×/wk. Antineoplastic: PO, IM, IV: 25–50 mg/m^2/wk. Decreased renal function: CrCl 61–80 mL/min: Reduce dose by 25%. CrCl 51–60 mL/min: Reduce dose by 33%. CrCl 10–50 mL/min: Reduce dose by 50–70%.	*Caution:* Avoid in patients with severe renal or hepatic dysfunction. *Adverse events:* Hepatotoxicity, nephropathy, vasculitis, malaise, fatigue, encephalopathy, headache, seizures, chills, fever, cystitis, stomatitis, enteritis, nausea, vomiting, diarrhea, alopecia, photosensitivity, increase or decrease in skin pigmentation, urticaria, arthralgia, hyperuricemia myelosuppression (onset, 7 days; nadir, 10 days; recovery, 21 days). *Monitoring:* Methotrexate concentrations (toxic if >1 × 10^{-7} mol/L for >40 hr). Ensure adequate hydration and urinary alkalinization.
Methsuximide Celontin. Capsule: 150, 300 mg.	**Control of absence seizures and adjunct in partial complex seizure management (increases seizure threshold, suppresses nerve transmission).** *Children:* 10–15 mg/kg/14 hr divided in 3–4 doses; may increase at weekly intervals (max: 30 mg/kg/24 hr). *Adults:* Start 300 mg/24 hr; may increase by 300 mg/24 hr at weekly intervals (max: 1,200 mg/24 hr).	*Adverse events:* Dizziness, drowsiness, lethargy, headache, ataxia, aggressiveness, depression, anorexia, nausea, vomiting, hiccups, agranulocytosis, aplastic anemia, leukopenia, thrombocytopenia. *Monitoring:* Methsuximide concentrations (therapeutic 10–40 μg/mL, toxic >4 μg/mL).
Methyldopa Aldomet; generic. Injection: 50 mg/mL. Tablet: 125, 250, 500 mg. Oral suspension: 250 mg/5 mL.	**Treatment of hypertension (false α neurotransmitter metabolite stimulates inhibitory α-adrenergic receptors).** *Children:* PO: Start 10 mg/kg in 2–4 doses; may increase q 2 days (max: 65 mg/kg/24 hr or 3 g/24 hr). IV: Start 2–4 mg/kg/dose; may increase to 5–10 mg/kg/dose per response (max: 65 mg/kg/24 hr). *Adults:* PO: Start 250 mg tid; may increase (max 3 g/24 hr). IV: 0.25–1 g q 6 hr (max: 4 g/24 hr).	*Caution:* Tolerance to effects occurs, so chronic use requires concurrent diuretic. *Adverse events:* Drowsiness, mental depression, headache, dry mouth, fever, chills, vertigo, fluid retention, edema, hepatocellular injury, cholestatic liver disease, cirrhosis, pancreatitis, nausea, vomiting, diarrhea, hemolytic anemia, positive Coombs test, leukopenia, thrombocytopenia, paresthesias, weakness, hypotension, bradycardia. *Monitoring:* Blood pressure, liver enzymes, direct Coombs test.
Methylene blue Urolene Blue. Injection: 10 mg/mL. Tablet: 65 mg	**Antidote for cyanide poisoning and drug-induced methemoglobinemia (promotes conversion of methemoglobin to hemoglobin; combines with cyanide to form cyan-methemoglobin).** *Children and adults:* Methemoglobinemia: IV: 1–2 mg/kg; may repeat after 1 hr if needed. Nicotinamide-adenine dinucleotide phosphate–methemoglobin reductase deficiency: PO: 1–1.5 mg/kg/24 hr (given with 5–8 mg/kg/24 hr of ascorbic acid).	*Caution:* Avoid in glucose-6-phosphate dehydrogenase deficiency and renal insufficiency. *Adverse events:* Urine and feces turn blue-green; anemia.
Methylphenidate Ritalin; generic. Tablet: 5, 10, 20 mg. Tablet, sustained-release: 20 mg.	**Attention deficit disorder (ADD), narcolepsy, adjunct for pain management (CNS stimulant).** *Children > 5 yr:* 0.3–0.6 mg/kg/dose (max: 2 mg/kg/24 hr). *Adults:* 10 mg bid–tid (max: 60 mg/24 hr).	*Cautions:* Avoid in patients with motor tics, Tourette syndrome, or marked agitation or psychosis. May become addictive if used in high doses at frequent intervals. *Adverse events:* Nervousness, insomnia, agitation, anorexia, weight loss, tachycardia, movement disorders, tics, growth retardation (controversial and minimal, if real), addiction (not a concern with typical ADD dosing).
Methylprednisolone Anti-inflammatory and immunosuppressant glucocorticoid. Depo-Medrol (injection, IM); Medrol (tablets); Solu-Medrol (injection); generic. Topical ointment.	**Used in allergic, inflammatory, and neoplastic disorders and acute spinal cord injury.** *Children:* Anti-inflammatory and immunosuppressant: PO, IM, IV: 0.5–2 mg/kg/24 hr divided q 6–12 hr. Lupus nephritis: IV: 30 mg/kg q other day for 6 doses. Acute spinal cord injury: 30 mg/kg over 15 min, followed in 45 min by continuous infusion of 5.4 mg/kg/hr for 23 hr. PO: 2–60 mg/24 hr in 1–4 doses. IV: 40–250 mg q 4–6 hr. IM: 10–80 mg/24 hr.	*Caution:* Avoid if live virus vaccine is given or if tuberculosis or fungal infection is present. *Advers events:* Hpertension, edema, nervousness, agitation, psychosis, pseudomotor cerebri, headache, mood swings, delirium, euphoria, hyperglycemia, hypokalemia, alkalosis, HPA-axis (adrenal) suppression, Cushing syndrome, skin atrophy, bruising, hyperpigmentation, peptic ulcer disease, muscle weakness, bone loss, joint pain, growth retardation, cataracts, glaucoma, immunosuppression. *Comment:* See comparison of corticosteroids under *Hydrocortisone*.
Metoclopramide Reglan; generic. Injection: 5 mg/mL. Tablet: 5, 10 mg. Oral solution: 10 mg/mL. Syrup: 5 mg/5 mL.	**Treatment of diabetic gastroparesis, gastroesophageal reflux, and nausea associated with chemotherapy and surgery (blocks dopamine receptors in chemoreceptor trigger zone, enhances gastrointestinal motility and gastroduodenal sphincter tone).** *Neonates, infants, and children:* Gastroesophageal reflux: IV, PO: 0.033–0.1 mg/kg/dose q 8 hr. *Children:* Postoperative antiemetic: IV: 0.1–0.2 mg/kg/dose q 6–8 hr as needed.	*Cautions:* May precipitate seizures, cause acute dystonic reactions, and worsen asthma (if sulfite-containing formulation). In elderly, chronic use is associated with increased risk and earlier onset of Parkinson disease (pediatric studies lacking). *Adverse events:* Weakness, drowsiness, diarrhea, prolactin stimulation, breast, prolactin stimulation, breast tenderness, extrapyramidal reaction; IV administration associated with an intense feeling of anxiety and restlessness, followed by drowsiness.

TABLE 716-1. General Medications—cont'd

DRUG (TRADE NAMES, FORMULATIONS)	INDICATIONS (MECHANISM OF ACTION AND DOSING)	COMMENTS (CAUTIONS, ADVERSE EVENTS, MONITORING)
	Chemotherapy antiemetic: PO, IV: 1–2 mg/kg/dose q 2–4 hr (pretreat with diphenhydramine to avoid extrapyramidal reactions). *Adults:* Antiemetic: PO, IV: 1–2 mg/kg/dose q 2–4 hr. Gastroesophageal reflux: PO: 10–15 mg qid. Renal dysfunction: Decrease dose.	*Comment:* Administer oral doses 30 min before meals and at bedtime. *Monitoring:* Creatinine clearance: CrCl 40–50 mL/min: give 75% of recommended dose; CrCl < 40 mL/min: give 50% of recommended dose; CrCl < 10 mL/min: give 25% of recommended dose.
Metolazone Mykrox; Zaroxolyn. Tablet.	**Treatment of fluid overload states (diuresis; inhibits sodium reabsorption at distal tubules).** *Children:* 0.2–0.4 mg/kg/24 hr in 1–2 doses. *Adults:* 2.5–20 mg/24 hr.	*Adverse events:* Fluid and electrolyte imbalance, hyperglycemia, hypocalcemia, hypomagnesemia, nausea, vomiting, blood dyscrasias.
Metoprolol Lopressor. Injection: 1 mg/mL. Tablet: 50, 100 mg.	**Treatment of hypertension, tachyarrhythmias, idiopathic hypertrophic subaortic stenosis, migraine prophylaxis (selective blocker of β_1 receptors).** *Children:* PO: 1–5 mg/kg/24 hr. *Adults:* PO: 100–450 mg/24 hr in 2–3 doses. IV: 5 mg q 2 min for 3 doses.	*Adverse events:* Mental depression, tiredness, weakness, bradycardia, reduced peripheral cirulation; insomnia, nightmares, worsens diabetes mellitus; worsens asthma.
Mexiletine Mexitil; generic. Capsule: 150, 200, 250 mg. Extemporaneous formulations may be prepared.	**Treatment of ventricular arrhythmias, neuropathic pain (class 1B antiarrhythmic).** *Children:* 1.4–5 g/kg/dose q 8 hr. *Adults:* 200 mg q 8 hr (max: 1,200 mg/24 hr). Renal dysfunction: CrCl < 10 mL/min: Give 50% of dose.	*Adverse events:* Atrial and ventricular arrhythmias, bradycardia, hypotension, confusion, dizziness, nervousness, tremor, ataxia, numbness of fingers or toes, weakness, blurred vision, tinnitus, increased liver enzymes, gastrointestinal discomfort. *Monitoring:* Mexiletine concentrations: therapeutic 0.5–2 μg/mL, toxic > 2 μg/mL.
Midazolam Versed. Injection: 1, 5 mg/mL. Extemporaneous formulations may be prepared.	**Sedation, anticonvulsant (benzodiazepine, increase γ-aminobutyric acid).** *Neonates:* IV: Continuous infusion 0.15–0.5 μg/kg/min for sedation; IV bolus 0.05–0.15 mg/kg q 2–4 hr. *Infants and children:* Status epilepticus: IV: loading dose of 0.15 mg/kg followed by continuous infusion of 1 μg/kg/min. Sedation: IV: loading dose of 0.05–0.2 mg/kg, then either same dose q 1–2 hr or continuous infusion of 1–2 μg/kg/min. Intranasal: 2.5 mg (0.5 mL) in each naris (total, 5 mg) using 5 mg/mL injection. *>12 yr:* 0.5 mg q 3–4 min to effect. *Adults:* 0.5–2 mg q 2 min to effect (usually 2–5 mg).	*Adverse events:* Several cases of myoclonus and prolonged movement disorders have been reported in neonates treated with midazolam. Withdrawal reactions may occur with abrupt discontinuation. Sedation, amnesia, paradoxical excitation, blurred vision, diplopia, nasal burning, apnea, respiratory depression.
Mitomycin Alkylating agent. Mutamycin. Injection.	**Cancer chemotherapy (antibiotic-type alkylating agent inhibits DNA and RNA synthesis).** *Children and adults:* Depends on protocol; typically IV 3 mg/m²/24 hr for 5 days q 4–6 wk; up to 40–50 mg/m² in a single dose for bone marrow transplant.	*Adverse events:* Nausea, vomiting, myelosuppression (onset, 21 days; nadir, 36 days; recovery, 42–56 days), tingling of extremities, paresthesias, alopecia, fingernail discoloration, mouth ulcers, cardiac failure (doses > 30 mg), interstitial pneumonitis, pulmonary fibrosis.
Mitoxantrone, DHAD Novantrone. Injection.	**Cancer chemotherapy (anthracycline analog inhibits DNA and RNA synthesis throughout entire cell cycle).** Acute nonlymphocytic leukemias: *Children < 2 yr:* 0.4 mg/kg/24 hr for 3–5 days. *> 2 yr and adults:* 8–12 mg/m²/24 hr for 5 days. Solid tumors: *Children:* 18–20 mg/m² q 3–4 wk or 5–8 mg/m² weekly. *Adults:* 12–14 mg/m² q 3–4 wk (max: total 80–120 mg/m²).	*Adverse events:* Cardiotoxicity (less than with other anthracyclines), seizures, headache, fever, elevated liver enzymes, renal failure, conjunctivitis, myelosuppression (onset, 7–10 days; nadir, 14 days; recovery, 21 days).
Molindone hydrochloride Moban. Tablet: 5, 10, 25, 100 mg. Oral concentrate: 20 mg/mL.	**Management of psychotic disorder (actions similar to chlorpromazine, but with extrapyramidal effects and less sedation).** *Children:* *3–5 yr:* 1–2.5 mg/kg/24 yr in 4 doses. *5–12 yr:* 0.5–1 mg/kg/24 hr in 4 doses. *Adults:* 50–225 mg/24 hr.	*Adverse events:* Extrapyramidal effects, akathisia, dyskinesias, constipation, blurred vision, orthostatic hypotension, seizures, neuroleptic malignant syndrome, dry mouth, weight again, galactorrhea, urinary retention, agranulocytosis, leukopenia, retinal pigmentation.
Montelukast Singulair. Leukotriene receptor blocker. Tablet: 10 mg. Tablets chewable: 4.5 mg.	**Prophylaxis and chronic treatment of asthma (leukotriene receptor blocker for LTD_4).** *Children 2–5 yr:* 4 mg once-daily in the evening. *Children: 6–14 yr:* 5 mg once daily in the evening. *>15 yr and adults:* 10 mg once daily in the evening.	*Adverse events:* Headache, dizziness, dyspepsia, fatigue, elevated liver enzymes.
Morphine Narcotic analgesic. Generic. Injection, oral solution, suppository. Tablet. Tablet, sustained-release. Tablet, controlled-release.	**Relief of moderate to severe pain.** *Neonates:* IV, IM, SC: Analgesia: 0.05–0.2 mg/kg/dose q 2–4 hr; continuous infusion of 0.025–0.05 mg/kg/hr. *Infants and children:* IV, IM, SC: 0.1–0.2 mg/kg/dose q 2–4 hr; PO: 0.2–0.5 mg/kg/dose q 4–6 hr. *Adolescents > 12 yr:* IV: 3–4 mg; may repeat in 5 min if needed. *Adults:* PO: 10–30 mg q 4 hr or controlled-release tablet 15–30 mg q 8–12 hr. IV, IM, SC: 2.5–20 mg/dose q 2–6 hr as needed or continuous infusion of 0.8–10 mg/hr.	*Cautions:* Physical dependence may develop after >5–7 days continuous use; if so, taper dose. Some preparations contain sulfites. *Adverse events:* Hypotension, bradcardia, nausea, vomiting, constipation, sedation, confusion, decreased urination, respiratory depression.
Mupirocin Bactroban. Ointment: 2%.	**Topical treatment of impetigo and other gram-positive skin infections (inhibits bacterial protein and RNA synthesis).** *Children and adults:* Apply to affected area 4–5 times daily. Intranasal (eliminate nasal carriage of *Staphylococcus aureus*): Apply small amount bid–qid for 5–14 days.	*Adverse events:* Stinging and irritation at application site.

TABLE 716-1. General Medications—cont'd

DRUG (TRADE NAMES, FORMULATIONS)	INDICATIONS (MECHANISM OF ACTION AND DOSING)	COMMENTS (CAUTIONS, ADVERSE EVENTS, MONITORING)
Muromonab-CD3, OKT3 Orthoclone OKT3. Injection: 5 mg/5 mL.	**Treatment of acute allograft rejection in renal transplant (coats circulating T lymphocytes, facilitating their opsonization by the reticuloendothelial system and promotes removal of all CD3 molecules from T-lymphocyte antigen receptor complex).** *Children <12 yr:* 0.1 mg/kg/24 hr for 10–14 days, or if < 30 kg, give 2.5 mg/24 hr for 10–14 days. *>12 yr and adults:* 5 mg/24 hr for 10–14 days.	*Cautions:* Severe first-dose reactions may occur; give methylprednisolone 1 mg/kg IV 2–6 hr before first OKT3 dose and hydrocortisone 100 mg IV 30 min after each OKT3 dose and as needed. *Adverse events:* Shortness of breath, pulmonary edema, fever, chills, trembling, nausea, vomiting, diarrhea, headache, stiff neck, photophobia, flu-like symptoms. *Monitoring:* OKT3 serum trough levels (if maintained near 1 μg/mL, then CD3 counts remain low).
Mycophenolate mofetil CellCept. Capsule: 250 mg.	**Prevents rejection of allograph transplants, used in conjunction with other drugs (active metabolite MPA inhibits T- and B-cell proliferation, T-cell generation, and antibody secretion).** *Children:* 660 mg/m^2/dose bid. *Adults:* 1,000 mg/dose bid.	*Adverse events:* Hypertension, insomnia, dizziness, fever, headache, bone marrow suppression, tremor, back pain, myalgia, dyspnea, cough, pharyngitis, hematuria, renal tubular necrosis, lymphoproliferative disease.
Nadolol Nonselective β-adrenergic receptor antagonist. Corgard. Tablet: 20, 40, 80, 120, 160 mg.	**Antiarrhythmic, antihypertensive, and migraine prophylaxis.** *Children:* PO: 0.5–2.5 mg/kg daily for supraventricular tachycardia. *Adults:* 40 mg daily; titrate upward to desired effect (usual dose: 40–80 mg/24 hr up to 640 mg/24 hr).	*Cautions:* Do not use in patients with asthma, bronchoconstriction, or uncontrolled heart failure. Adjust dose with renal dysfunction (CrCl < 50 mL/min). *Adverse effects:* Bradycardia, heart failure, bronchospasm. *Drug interactions:* Other hypotensive drugs, diuretics. Antagonizes β-sympathomimetic drugs (e.g. albuterol).
Nalbuphine Nubain. Injection. IM, IV, SQ: 10 mg/mL.	**Analgesic (opiate agonist with partial opiate antagonistic activity for treatment of moderate to severe pain).** *Children ≥ 1 yr:* IV, IM, SC: 0.1–0.2 mg/kg q 3–4 hr. Maximum single dose: 20 mg; maximum daily dose: 160 mg.	*Cautions:* Like most opiate analgesics, may stimulate histamine release and cause CNS and respiratory depression. Use with caution in hepatic disease or with other respiratory depressants. Dependence potential. *Adverse effects:* Hypotension, sedation, respiratory depression. Naloxone reverse effects.
Naloxone Opiate antagonist. Narcan; generic. Injection: 0.4 mg/mL. Injection, neonate: 0.02 mg/mL.	**Antagonizes all opiate receptors; used in the treatment of opiate excess (overdose, poisoning).** *Neonates and children:* IV: 0.1 mg/kg (max: 2 mg). If no response, repeat q 2–3 min until desired effect. May give by continuous IV infusion.	*Cautions:* May precipitate acute opiate withdrawal. Duration of effect of many opiates may be longer than that or naloxone, requiring individualized naloxone dosing. Administer via IV push.
Naproxen Nonsteroidal anti-inflammatory drug. Aleve; Anaprox; Naprosyn; generic. Tablet: 220, 250, 275, 375, 550 mg. Suspension: 125 mg/5 mL.	**Treatment of mild to moderate pain, inflammation, fever (inhibits prostaglandin synthesis).** *Neonates:* Do not use owing to probable negative effects on renal function. *Children:* PO: 5–7 mg/kg q 8–12 hr. *Adults:* PO: 250–375 mg q 8–12 hr. (max: 1,250 mg/24 hr).	*Cautions:* Gastrointestinal upset or irritation, reversible interference with platelet aggregation. Do not administer to infants < 3 mo of age. *Adverse effects:* Dizziness, gastrointestinal irritation, rash, age-related decreased renal function.
Nedocromil Mast cell stabilizer. Tilade. Aerosol: 1.75 mg/activation.	**Chronic treatment of asthma and allergic disorders. Stabilizes other cells to mediator release: neutrophils, eosinophils, platelets; nonsteroidal.** *Children and adults:* 1–2 puffs bid–qid. Dose titrated to clinical response.	*Cautions:* Only effective as chronic therapy. Produces no bronchodilatation. *Adverse effects:* Dysphonia, chest irritation and pain.
Neostigmine Prostigmin; generic. Tablet: 15 mg (as bromide). Injection: 0.25, 0.5, 1 mg/mL (as methylsulfate).	**Treatment of myasthenia gravis, reversal of nondepolarizing neuromuscular blocking agents (NDNM). Competitively inhibits acetylcholine esterase–augmenting effects of endogenous acetylcholine.** *Children:* IV, IM, SC: 0.01–0.04 mg/kg q 2–4 hr; titrate dose to desired effect. To reverse NDNM, 0.025–1 mg/kg/dose (max adult dose: 5 mg).	*Cautions:* Patients with asthma or bronchospasm, bradycardia. Does not antagonize succinylcholine. *Adverse effects:* Bradycardia, abdominal cramps, urinary frequency.
Niacin Nicobid; generic. Tablet: 25, 50, 100, 250, 500 mg. Tablet, timed-release: 150, 250, 500, 750 mg. Capsule, timed-release: 125, 250, 300, 400, 500 mg. Elixir: 50 mg/5 mL. Injection: 100 mg/mL.	**Vitamin supplementation (vitamin B_3), hyperlipidemia, vasodilator.** *Children:* IV, IM, SC, PO: Titrated to desired effect (max: 10 mg/kg/24 hr).	*Cautions:* Titrate dose upward and administer IV slowly to avoid or minimize flushing. *Adverse effects:* Flushing, tachycardia, dizziness, hyperuricemia. *Drug interactions:* Augments hypotensive effects of antihypertensives.
Nifedipine Adalat; Procardia; generic. Capsule (liquid-filled): 10, 20 mg. Capsule, timed-release: 30, 60, 90 mg. Tablet, timed-release: 30, 60, 90 mg.	**Antihypertensive, antiarrhythmic calcium channel antagonist.** *Infants and children:* Hypertensive emergency PO/sublingual 0.25–0.5 mg/kg/dose q 4–6 hr (max: 10 mg). Hypertropic cardiomyopathy: PO: 0.2–0.3 mg/kg q 8 hr. *Adults:* 10 mg/dose titrated to effect (max: 120–180 mg/24 hr).	*Caution:* Do not crush or break timed-release tablet. *Adverse effects:* Profound, acute hypotension, flushing, dizziness. More rapid effect if drug is administered without food. Concurrent grapefruit juice may increase bioavailability and effects. *Drug interactions:* Cimetidine, cyclosporine, phenytoin, and possibly digoxin. *Comment:* Preferred route is oral, not sublingual. Clinical effects due to swallowing. Capsule content approximates 10 mg in 0.34 mL and 20 mg in 0.45 mL.
Nitroprusside Nipride; generic. Injection: 10, 25 mg/mL.	**Antihypertensive, congestive heart failure: controlled, titratable blood pressure control.** *Children and adults:* IV 0.3–0.5 μg/kg/min; titrate dose to desired effect; rarely requires >6 μg/kg/min (probable max: 8 μg/kg/min).	*Cautions:* Metabolized to thiocyanate/cyanide, which accumulates with renal dysfunction. *Adverse effects:* Profound hypotension, tachycardia, thyroid suppression, acidosis, seizures. Cyanide toxicity—metabolic acidosis, pink skin, methemoglobinemia. Administer by continuous IV infusion. Protect solution from direct light. Thiosulfate co-administration prevents toxicity (10 mg thiosulfate for each 1 mg nitroprusside).

TABLE 716-1. General Medications—cont'd

DRUG (TRADE NAMES, FORMULATIONS)	INDICATIONS (MECHANISM OF ACTION AND DOSING)	COMMENTS (CAUTIONS, ADVERSE EVENTS, MONITORING)
Norepinephrine bitartrate Sympathomimetic/adrenergic agonist. Levophed. Injection: 1 mg/mL base.	**Hypotension and shock.** *Children:* 0.05–0.1 μg/kg/min; titrate dose to desired effect (max: 2 μg/kg/min).	*Cautions:* Extravasation may cause severe tissue necrosis. Administer into large vein by continuous IV infusion. Ensure patient fluid status. May cause profound vasoconstriction. *Adverse effects:* Hypertension, cardiac arrhythmias, headache. Drug dose based on norepinephrine base.
Nortriptyline Tricyclic antidepressant; central synaptic norepinephinct serotomin inhibitor. Aventyl; Pamelor; generic. Capsule: 10, 25, 50, 75 mg Solution: 10 mg/5 mL.	**Treatment of nocturnal enuresis depression.** *Children:* Nocturnal enuresis: PO: 10–20 mg/24 hr; titrate upward (max: 40 mg/24 hr). Depression: PO: 1–3 mg/kg/24 hr (bedtime) titrated to effect. May give in divided doses q 6 hr (usual max: 150 mg/24 hr).	*Cautions:* Avoid in patients with cardiac conduction abnormalities, cardiac disease. Slow dose adjustment in patients with hepatic dysfunction. *Adverse effects:* Anticholinergic effects (dry mouth, tachycardia, blurred vision, urinary retention), sedation. *Drug interactions:* Clonidine, monoamine oxidate inhibitors.
Octreotide Sandostatin. Injection: 0.05, 0.1, 0.2, 0.5, 1 mg/mL	**Antisecretory somatostatin analog.** *Children:* Secretory diarrhea: IV, SC: 1–10 μg/kg q 12 hr; titrate dose to effect. May give via continuous IV infusion. *Adults:* Treatment of vasoactive intestinal peptide–secreting tumors: IV, SC: 100–150 μg q 12 hr.	*Cautions:* Continuous long-term use (mo) may cause cholelithiasis, hypothyroidism. *Adverse effects:* Flushing, dizziness, hypo/hyperglycemia. Infuse IV over 20–30 min, IV push over 3 min.
Olanzapine Zyprexa. Tablet: 2.5, 5, 7.5, 10, 15, 20 mg.	**Atypical antipsychotic, monaminergic antagonist with high affinity for serotonin, dopamine, histamine, muscarinic, and α1-adrenergic receptors. Actual mechanism of action unknown.** *Children:* Start 2.5–5 mg q 24 hr; titrate weekly by 2.5–5 mg to 15–20 mg/24 hr as q daily dosing. *Adults:* Start 5–10 mg/24 hr; increase by 5 mg weekly to response (max: 20 mg/24 hr).	*Adverse events:* Postural hypotension, somnolence, tremor, dizziness, akathisia, asthenia, dry mouth, constipation, dyspepsia, increased appetite, weight gain, hyperglycemia, amenorrhea, vaginitis in females.
Olsalazine Anti-inflammatory drug; 5-aminosalicylic acid derivative. Dipentum. Capsule: 10, 20, 250 mg.	**Treatment of inflammatory bowel disease.** *Adults:* 500 mg q 12 hr.	*Cautions:* Administer with food. *Adverse effects:* Headache, cramps, diarrhea, dizziness, rash, cholestasis.
Omeprazole Proton pump inhibitor of parietal cell hydrogen ion secretion. Prilosec. Capsule: 10, 20 mg.	**Treatment of gastric acid hypersecretion/ulcer disease.** *Children:* PO: 0.6–0.7 mg/kg q 24 hr. Dose titrated to desired gastric pH. *Adults:* PO: 20–40 mg/24 hr.	*Caution:* Drug granules in capsule must be swallowed whole; do not chew. *Drug interactions:* May decrease diazepam, phenytoin clearance. May reduce itraconazole, digoxin absorption.
Ondansetron Antiemetic, selective serotonin-3 receptor antagonist. Ondansetron. Tablet: 4, 8 mg. Injection: 2 mg/mL.	**Treatment of nausea and vomiting associated with cancer chemotherapy or surgery and other causes (drug toxicity).** *Infants and children:* 0.15 mg/kg IV q 8 hr; may give as continuous IV infusion 0.45 mg/kg/24 hr (max: 24–32 mg/24 hr). *Children:* Mild to moderate nausea/vomiting: PO: 4–8 mg q 8–12 hr.	*Adverse effects:* Headache, chest pain. Does not cause dystonia/sedation. *Comment:* Oral bioavailability ≈50%. Doses given ≈30 min before starting chemotherapy.
Oxcarbazepine Trileptal. Tablet, film-coated: 150, 300, 600 mg. Suspension: 300 mg/5 mL.	**Treatment of seizure disorders (except absence).** *Children 3–17 yr:* Start 8–10 mg/kg/24 hr divided bid (max: 600 mg/24 hr); increase over 2 wk to 30–45 mg/kg/24 hr divided bid per response. *Adults:* Start at 600 mg/24 hr divided bid, then gradually increase over 2–4 wk to 1,200 mg/24 hr divided bid (max: 2,400 mg/24 hr).	*Cautions:* Cut dose in half if creatinine clearance <30 mL/min. Toxicity mainly CNS (headache, somnolence, dizziness, etc.), diplopia, gastrointestinal (nausea, vomiting, diarrhea), and hyponatremia.
Oxybutynin Urinary antispasmodic. Ditropan; generic. Tablet: 5 mg. Syrup: 5 mg/5 mL.	**Relaxes smooth muscle by antagonizing acetylcholine.** *Children:* PO: 0.2 mg/kg q 6–12 hr (max: 5 mg PO q 8 hr). *Adults:* 5 mg/dose up to 4× daily.	*Cautions:* Patients with renal and/or liver disease. *Adverse effects:* Tachycardia, drowsiness, sedation, dry mouth, blurred vision. *Drug interactions:* Additive anticholinergic effects/CNS depression (e.g., antihistamines).
Oxycodone Opiate analgesic. Various brands, generic. Tablet: 5 mg.	**Treatment of moderate to severe pain.** *Children:* PO: 0.05–0.15 mg/kg q 4–6 hr (max: 5 mg). *Adults:* PO: 5 mg/dose q 4–6 hr (max: 5 mg).	*Cautions:* Like most opiate analgesics, may stimulate histamine release and may cause CNS and respiratory depression. Use with caution in hepatic disease or with other respiratory depressants. Dependence potential. *Adverse effects:* Hypotension, sedation, respiratory depression. Naloxone reverses effects.
Pamidronate disodium Bisphosphonate derivative. Aredia. Injection: 30, 60, 90 mg.	**Treatment of hypercalcemia, Paget disease, osteogenesis imperfecta, osteopenia. Binds to bone, inhibiting osteoclast-mediated calcium resorption. Dose based on serum calcium concentration.** *Children:* 1 mg/kg/24 hr for consecutive days q 3 mo; 10–40 mg/m² over 5–8 hr q mo. *Adults:* Serum calcium 12–13.5 mg/dL: 60–90 mg; serum calcium >13.5 mg/dL: 90 mg. Wait 7 days to assess full effect of dose before retreatment. Paget disease: 30 mg/24 hr for 3 consecutive days.	*Cautions:* Leukopenia, thrombophlebitis. Drug incompatible with calcium-containing IV solutions. *Adverse effects:* Hypertension, syncope, hypocalcemia, hypophosphatemia, hypothyroidism, bone pain.
Pancreatin Various brands. Capsule, tablet, timed-release capsule, powder.	**Pancreatic enzyme replacement. Individual products contain different amounts of lipase, amylase, and protease.** *Children and adults:* Dose titrated to desirable stool frequency and consistency.	*Cautions:* Excessive dosing may lead to impaction; inadequate dosing may lead to steatorrhea. Exogenous pancreatic enzymes inactivated by gastric acid; use microencapsulated forms when possible. *Drug interactions:* Reduction of gastric acid (e.g., H_2-receptor antagonists/omeprazole/antacids) may enhance effectiveness. *Adverse effects:* Rash, abdominal symptoms, constipation, hyperuricemia, allergy.
Pancuronium Pavulon; generic. Injection: 1, 2 mg/mL.	**Anesthetic and skeletal muscle relaxant. Nondepolarizing neuromuscular antagonist.** *Children and adults:* IV: 0.04–0.1 mg/kg q 20–30 min. Dose titrated to desired effect.	*Cautions:* Ventilation must be supported during neuromuscular blockade. Dose adjustment with renal dysfunction. *Adverse effects:* Tachycardia, hypertension, prolonged muscle weakness. *Drug interactions:* Possible augmented muscle weakness with aminoglycosides, anesthetics, and colistin.

TABLE 716-1. General Medications—cont'd

DRUG (TRADE NAMES, FORMULATIONS)	INDICATIONS (MECHANISM OF ACTION AND DOSING)	COMMENTS (CAUTIONS, ADVERSE EVENTS, MONITORING)
Papaverine hydrochloride Vasodilator; antimigraine; generalized smooth muscle relaxant. Cerespan; Pavabid; generic. Capsule: 150 mg. Tablet, timed-release. Injection.	**Common pediatric use for preservation of arterial catheters to prolong function.** *Children:* 30 mg papaverine plus 250 u heparin/250 mL IV solution (0.45–0.9% NaCl) infused.	*Cautions:* Avoid in neonates because it may cause cerebral vasodilatation, predisposing to CNS hemorrhage. *Adverse effects:* Flushing, tachycardia, hypotension, dizziness. *Drug interactions:* Additive hypotensive effect.
Paraldehyde Anticonvulsant; sedative; generalized CNS depressant. Paral; generic. Liquid: 1 g/mL.	**Used as adjunct treatment for refractory status epilepticus, alcohol withdrawal.** *Children:* PO, Rectal: 0.15 mL/kg/dose. May repeat once in 4–6 hr. IM formulation not available in USA. *Adults:* 5–10 mL/dose.	*Cautions:* May give IM, but inject remote from nerves owing to risk of damage. Use glass syringe/tubing because drug reacts with plastic. Rectal route preferred to IM route. Mix rectal solution 2:1 in oil (e.g., olive oil). *Adverse effects:* Sedation, gastric irritation, thrombophlebitis.
Paregoric Antidiarrheal, analgesic. Generic. Liquid: 2 mg morphine equivalent/5 mL.	**Camphorated tincture of opium.** *Children:* PO: 0.25–0.5 mL/kg q 6–12 hr. *Adults:* PO: 5–10 mL q 6–12 hr. Neonatal abstinence syndrome: Dose titrated to desired effect.	*Comments:* Each 5 mL of paregoric contains 2 mg morphine equivalent, 20 mg camphor, 20 mg benzoic acid. Final alcohol content 45%.
Paroxetine Serotonin reuptake inhibitor. Paxil. Tablet: 10, 20, 40 mg. Oral suspension: 10 mg/5 mL.	**Treatment of depression, obsessive-compulsive disorder, panic disorder, and social anxiety disorder.** *Children:* Start 10 mg q daily; increase at weekly intervals by 10 mg/daily (max: 60 mg/24 hr). *Adults:* Start 20 mg daily increase by 10 mg daily at weekly intervals to response (max: 60 mg/24 hr).	*Cautions:* Do not discontinue abruptly or withdrawal syndrome may occur. Taper by 10 mg/24 hr every 5–7 days to aviod problems. Avoid use with monamine oxidase inhibitors except in extreme situations. *Adverse events:* Somnolence, dizziness, insomnia, tremor, nervousness, decreased appetite, asthenia, nausea, constipation. *Drug interactions:* Paroxetine inhibits the cytochrome 2D6 isoenzyme and may interact with phenothiazines and type 1C antiarrhythmics. Concurrent use with thioridazine may elevate thioridazine levels, causing prolonged QTc intervals and predispose to torsades de pointes.
Pegaspargase Antineoplastic agent. Oncaspar. Injection.	**Used in combination for induction of acute lymphoblastic leukemia. Also called PEG-L-asparaginase.** *Children and adults:* IM, IV: 2,500 u/m² q 14 days. Dose usually dictated by specific protocol.	*Cautions:* Hepatotoxic, allergic reactions. Contraindicated in patients with pancreatitis, significantly hemorrhagic events associated with L-asparaginase. *Drug interactions:* Possible interactions with methotrexate, vincristine, corticosteroids.
Pemoline CNS stimulant. Cylert. Tablet: 18.75, 37.5, 75 mg. Tablet: chewable: 37.5 mg.	**Treatment of attention deficit disorder. Structurally unique from methylphenidate.** *Children:* PO: 1 mg/kg/24 hr as single dose each morning. Titrate to effect 0.5 mg/kg/24 hr q 1–2 wk. (max: 3 mg/kg/24 hr; ≈112.5 mg/24 hr).	*Cautions:* Insomnia, anorexia, weight loss. *Adverse effects:* CNS stimulation, seizures, hypertension, increased liver function, hepatitis, movement disorders. *Drug interactions:* Possible with other CNS stimulants, sympathomimetics.
Penicillamine Chelating agent. Cuprimine; Depen. Capsule: 12, 250 mg. Tablet: 250 mg.	**Metal chelating agent with affinity for copper (Wilson disease) and lead. Also used as an adjunct for the treatment of severe rheumatoid arthritis.** Wilson disease: Dose titrated to maintain >1 mg/24 hr urinary copper excretion. *Infants and children:* PO: 20 mg/kg/24 hr q 6–12 hr (max: 1 g/24 hr). *Adults:* PO: 1 g/24 hr q 6–12 hr (max: 2 g). Lead intoxication: *Infants and children:* PO: 30–40 mg/kg/24 hr q 8–12 hr (max: 1.5 g/24 hr). *Adults:* PO: 1–1.5 g/24 hr q 8–12 hr. Rheumatoid arthritis: *Children:* PO: 3 mg/kg/24 hr q 12 hr, increasing by 3 mg/kg/24 hr q 2–3 mo (max: 10 mg/kg/24 hr).	*Cautions:* Cross allergen in patients allergic to penicillin. Do not give with food or iron/zinc compounds. *Adverse effects:* Rash, pruritus, nausea, vomiting, anemia, bone marrow suppression, nephrotic syndrome, systemic lupus erythematosus–like syndrome. *Drug interactions:* Other metals, iron, gold, mercury, antimalarials.
Pentazocine Talwin. Tablet: 50 mg with 50 mg naloxone (parenteral deterrent). Injection: 30 mg/mL.	**Opiate analgesic of the benzo orphan type for the treatment of moderate to severe pain.** *Children > 14 yr of age and adults:* PO: 50 mg q 3–4 hr, titrate to effect to 100 mg dose, not to exceed 600 mg/24 hr. May give IM or IV, reducing oral dose by 1/3.	*Cautions:* Generalized CNS depressant possesses weak antagonistic action and may precipitate opiate withdrawal. *Adverse effects:* CNS depression, nausea, vomiting, respiratory depression, histamine release.
Pentobarbital Nembutal; generic. Short-acting barbiturate. Capsule: 50, 100 mg. Elixir: 18.2 mg/5 mL. Suppository: 30, 60, 120, 200 mg. Injection.	**Used as an anticonvulsant, sedative/hypnotic, and anesthetic.** Sedation: *Children:* PO, IM: 2–6 mg/kg/24 hr q 6 hr. May give rectally dosed by body weight: 4.5–10 kg: 30 mg 10–18 kg: 30–60 mg; 18–36 kg: 60 mg; 36–50 kg: 60–120 mg. Pentobarbital coma: *Children:* IV: Loading dose of 10–15 mg/kg slowly over 1–2 hr, monitoring blood pressure and heart rate. Maintenance infusion of 1 mg/kg/hr, increasing up to 5 mg/kg/hr to maintain burst suppression on electroencephalogram.	*Cautions:* Hypotension in hypovolemic patients; injectables contain propylene glycol. *Adverse effects:* Arrhythmias bradycardia, hypotension, respiratory depression, laryngospasm, dependence. *Drug interactions:* May increase metabolism of many hepatically cleared drugs, oral contraceptives, griseofulvin, corticosteroids. *Monitoring:* Pentobarbital concentrations: sedation 1–5 μg/mL; coma 20–40 μg/mL.
Pentoxifylline Trental. Tablet, timed-release: 400 mg.	**Used in the treatment of peripheral vascular disease (Raynaud syndrome) and investigationally in reducing tumor necrosis factor, neutrophil adhesion, and platelet aggregation.** *Children:* Antiplatelet effect in Kawasaki disease: PO: 20 mg/kg/24 hr q 8 hr. *Adults:* PO: 400 mg tid.	*Cautions:* Administer with meals to reduce gastrointestinal upset. *Adverse effects:* Hypotension, tachycardia, dizziness, nausea, vomiting. *Drug interactions:* Cimetidine, possible augmenting of warfarin, heparin effects.
Phenazopyridine Urinary anesthetic. Pyridium; generic. Tablet: 100, 200 mg.	**Possible symptomatic relief of urinary burning and itching associated with urologic procedures or urinary tract infection.** *Children:* PO: 12 mg/kg/24 hr q 8 hr. *Adults:* PO: 100–200 mg q 6–8 hr.	*Caution:* Discolors urine to orange or red. *Adverse effects:* Headache, rash, methemoglobinemia. Administer with food to decrease gastrointestinal side effects.

TABLE 716-1. General Medications—cont'd

DRUG (TRADE NAMES, FORMULATIONS)	INDICATIONS (MECHANISM OF ACTION AND DOSING)	COMMENTS (CAUTIONS, ADVERSE EVENTS, MONITORING)
Phenobarbital Generic. Barbiturate CNS depressant. Elixir: 15 mg/5 mL; 20 mg/5 mL. Tablet: 8, 15, 30, 60, 100 mg Injection: 30, 60, 130 mg/mL.	**Sedative hypnotic anticonvulsant, and anesthetic.** Anticonvulsant: **Loading dose:** *Children and adults:* PO, IV: 15–20 mg/kg. Maintenance dose: Neonates: PO, IV: 3–4 mg/kg/24 hr, q 12–24 hr. *Children:* PO, IV: 5–6 mg/kg/24 hr, q 12–24 hr. *Adults:* PO, IV: 1–3 mg/kg/24 hr q 12–24 hr. Sedation: *Children:* 2 mg/kg/dose. Hyperbilirubinemia: Sedation: *Children:* PO, IV: 3–8 mg/kg/24 hr q 12–24 hr. *Adults:* PO, IV: 90–180 mg/24 hr q 12–24 hr.	*Cautions:* Dose titrated to desired effect. Administer IV ≤30 mg/min in infants and children and ≤60 mg/min in adults. *Adverse effects:* Hypotension, drowsiness, respiratory depression, paradoxical hyperactivity. *Drug interactions:* May increase metabolism of many hepatically cleared drugs; oral contraceptives, griseofulvin, corticosteroids. Certain drugs may interface with phenobarbital metabolism: valproic acid, chloramphenicol, felbamate. *Target serum concentrations:* 15–40 μg/mL; coma (acute) > 60 μg/mL. *Monitoring:* Phenobarbital concentrations: sedation 15–40 μg/mL; coma > 60 μg/mL.
Phenoxybenzamine Dibenzyline. α-Adrenergic receptor antagonist. Capsule: 10 mg.	**Symptomatic treatment of pheochromocytoma.** *Children:* PO: 0.2–2 mg/kg/24 hr q 24 hr. Titrate dose to desired effect (e.g., blood pressure). *Adults:* PO: 10 mg/dose q 12 hr. Titrate dose to effect.	*Cautions:* Long-acting α-receptor antagonist. *Adverse effects:* Postural hypotension, syncope, dizziness. *Drug interactions:* Sympathomimetics.
Phentolamine Regitine. α-Adrenergic antagonist. Injection: 5 mg/mL.	**Diagnosis and treatment of pheochromocytoma and extravasation of drugs with α-adrenergic effects (e.g., dopamine, dobutamine, epinephrine, norepinephrine, phenylephrine).** Pheochromocytoma: Diagnosis: *Children:* IV 0.05–0.1 mg/kg/dose (max: 5 mg). *Adults:* IV 5 mg/dose. Preoperatively: *Children:* IV 0.05–0.1 mg/kg/dose q 1–2 hrs titrating to effect and needed duration. (max: 5 mg). Extravasation: 5–10 mg in 10 mL normal saline. Infiltrate area with small volume using 27–30 gauge needle (max: 0.1 mg/kg).	*Cautions:* Short-acting α-receptor antagonist. *Adverse effects:* Hypotension, dizziness, gastritis. *Drug interactions:* Sympathomimetics.
Phenylephrine hydrochloride Neo-Synephrine; generic. α-Adrenergic receptor agonist; peripheral vasoconstrictor. Injection: 10 mg/mL. Nasal drops, spray: 0.16–1%. Eyedrops.	**Treatment of hypotension in shock and used in many nasal decongestants.** Nasal decongestant: *Infants:* 1–2 drops per nostril q 3–4 hr; 0.16% solution. *Children 1–6 yr:* 1–2 drops or spray per nostril q 3–4 hr; 0.125% solution. *6–12 yr:* 1–2 drops or spray q 3–4 hr; 0.25% solution. *>12 yr and adults:* 1–2 drops or spray per nostril q 3–4 hr; 0.25–0.5% solution. Hypotension and shock: *Children:* IV: 5–20 μg/dose q 10–15 min. May give by continuous IV infusion 0.1–0.5 μg/kg/min, titrated to desired effects (e.g., blood pressure). *Adults:* IV 0.1–0.5 mg/dose q 10–15 min by continuous infusion 100–180 μg/min, titrated to desired effect. Paroxysmal supraventricular tachycardia: *Children:* IV: 5–10 μg/kg over 20–30 sec. *Adults:* IV: 0.25–0.5 mg over 20–30 sec.	*Cautions:* Patients with hypertension. Injection contains sulfites. Rebound nasal stuffiness with prolonged nasal use/abuse. *Adverse effects:* Hypertension, angina, bradycardia, restlessness, necrosis if IV infiltrates. *Drug interactions:* Sympathomimetics, α-receptor antagonists, monoamine oxidase inhibitors.
Phenytoin Anticonvulsant and antiarrhythmic. Dilantin; generic (use cautiously) Capsule, slow-(extended-) release: 30, 100 mg. Capsule, prompt release: 30, 100 mg. Suspension: 125 mg/5 mL. Injection: 50 mg/mL.	**Status epilepticus**: Loading dose: *Neonate:* IV: 15–20 mg/kg (max: 0.5 mg/kg/min). *Children and adults:* IV: 15–18 mg/kg (max: 1–3 mg/kg/min). Maintenance dose: PO, IV: *Neonate:* 5 mg/kg/24 hr q 12–24 hr. *Children 0.5–0.6 yr:* 8–10 mg/kg/24 hr. *7–9 yr:* 6–8 mg/kg/24 hr q 12–24 hr. *10–16 yr:* 6–7 mg/kg/24 hr q 12–24 hr. *Adults:* 300–600 mg/24 hr q 12–24 hr.	*Cautions:* Infuse slowly IV; variable oral bioavailability; chewable tablet most consistent. Must shake oral suspension very well before use. Follows saturation (Michaelis-Menten) pharmacokinetics. Certain disease states (renal failure, acute head trauma) may lead to imbalance between free and protein-bound drug. *Adverse effects:* Lethargy, dizziness, nystagmus, hypotension, hirsutism, gingival hyperplasia, rash, Stevens-Johnson syndrome, hepatitis, thrombophlebitis. *Drug interactions:* May increase metabolism of certain hepatically cleared drugs; oral contraceptives, griseofulvin, corticosteroids, cyclosporin; highly protein-bound and may cause displacement interaction. *Monitoring:* Phenytoin concentrations: therapeutic 8–20 μg/mL. If necessary, measure free drug concentration: therapeutic 1–2 μg/mL.
Physostigmine Antilirium. Competitive antagonist of acetylcholine. Injection, ophthalmic solution, ointment.	**Unlike neostigmine, crosses the blood-brain barrier with central effects. Used with extreme caution in the reversal of anticholinergic effects.** IM, IV, SC: *Children:* 0.001–0.03 mg/kg/dose q 15–20 min to desired effect (max: 2 mg). *Adults:* 0.5–2 mg q 15–20 min to desired effect.	*Cautions:* Patients with bradycardia, cardiac dysrhythmias, asthma, ulcer disease. Should be used as an antidote only in life-threatening situations by experienced individuals. *Adverse effects:* Palpitations, restlessness, excessive salivation, secretions, muscle fasciculations, bronchospasm.
Phytonadione AquaMEPHYTON; Mephyton. Tablet: 5 mg. Injection.	**Vitamin K_1 for nutritional supplementation and treatment of hemorrhagic disease of the newborn or warfarin-like compound anticoagulant toxicity.** *Children:* IM, IV, SC: 1–2 mg/dose dosed to effect; PO: dose may increase to 2.5–5 mg. *Adults:* IM, IV, SC: 10 mg/24 hr; PO: 5–25 mg/24 hr. Higher doses may be required for reversal of warfarin-like anticoagulant toxicity.	*Cautions:* Infuse slowly IV (over 15–30 min) to avoid flushing. Multiple doses may be needed for prolonged period, depending on type of courmarin anticoagulant. *Adverse effects:* Flushing, hypotension.

TABLE 716-1. General Medications—cont'd

DRUG (TRADE NAMES, FORMULATIONS)	INDICATIONS (MECHANISM OF ACTION AND DOSING)	COMMENTS (CAUTIONS, ADVERSE EVENTS, MONITORING)
Piroxicam Feldene. Nonsteroidal anti-inflammatory agent. Capsule: 10, 20 mg.	**Analgesic and therapy for rheumatoid disorders.** PO: *Children:* 0.2–0.3 mg/kg q 24 hr (max: 15 mg/kg/24 hr). *Adults:* 10–20 mg q 24 hr.	*Cautions:* Limited data in infants and children; may require more frequent daily dosing in pediatrics. Administer with food or milk to decrease gastrointestinal side effects. Do not use in young infants. *Adverse effects:* Dizziness, gastrointestinal upset, nausea/vomiting, ulcer, hepatitis, decreased renal function.
Polyethylene glycol-electrolyte solution Bowel lavage solution. Colovage; Colyte; Golytely Power for reconstitution.	**Used before bowel radiology or in poisonings.** *Children:* 25–40 mL/kg/hr up to 1.5–2 L/hr until rectal effluent is clear; usual max dose of 4 L for x-ray may go much higher if used for poisonings (e.g., iron). *Adults:* 2,400 mg q 10–20 min until 4 L is consumed. May go higher for poisonings.	*Caution:* Patients with bowel disease (colitis) or obstruction. *Adverse effects:* Nausea, cramps, bloating.
Poractant alfa Curosurf. Intratracheal suspension of porcine lung extract, surfactant (80 mg phospholipids, 1 mg protein, 0.3 mg SP-B/mL).	**Prophylaxis or treatment of respiratory distress syndrome, treatment of persistent pulmonary hypertension.** *Neonates:* 2.5 mL/kg (200 mg/kg) for dose 1, may repeat dose of 1.25 mL/kg (100 mg/kg) 2 × q 12 hr. *Children and adults:* Not indicated.	*Caution:* Monitor ventilator status closely; may require rapid weaning within min of dose. *Adverse events:* Bradycardia, airway obstruction, cyanosis.
Pralidoxime Acetylcholinesterase reactiveator. Protopam (2-PAM). Tablet: 500 mg. Injectable.	**Treatment of organophosphate poisoning; possible treatment of toxicity from cholinergic drugs.** IM, IV: *Children:* 20–50 mg/kg/dose repeated in 1–2 hr if muscle weakness has not been relieved; when desired effect obtained, dose q 12 hr. *Adults:* 1–2 g q 5–6 hr; dose based on clinical response.	*Caution:* As antidote for organophosphate poisoning; use in combination with atropine. Excessive dosing may cause cholinergic effects. Too-rapid IV administration associated with tachycardia, laryngospasm. Infuse IV over 15–30 min. *Adverse effects:* Hypertension, dizziness, nausea, muscle weakness or rigidity.
Prazosin Minipress; generic. Capsule: 1, 2, 5 mg.	**Competitive antagonist of postsynaptic α-adrenergic receptors used in the treatment of hypertension or heart failure.** PO: *Children:* 0.1 mg/kg/24 hr q 6 h, titrating dose to desired blood pressure (max: 0.4 mg/kg/24 hr or 15 mg total dose). Consider additive/synergistic combinations with diuretics. *Adults:* 3 mg/24 hr q 8–12 hrs, titrating dose to desired blood pressure. Usual dose range: 3–15 mg/24 hr.	*Caution:* Profound hypotension may occur after first dose (dose "first-dose phenomenon"); more common in fluid- and/or salt-. depleted patients. *Adverse effects:* Syncope, palpitations, dizziness, fluid retention. *Drug interactions:* Other hypotensive drugs (diuretics, β-receptor antagonists).
Prednisolone Glucocorticosteroid. Delta Cortef; Hydeltrasol; Predalone; generic. Tablet: 5 mg. Suspension. Injection.	**Treatment of inflammatory disorders, including allergic, respiratory, rheumatic, endocrine, and neoplastic disorders.** Asthma: PO, IV: *Children:* 0.5–4 mg/kg/24 hr q 6–12 hr. *Adults:* 5–60 mg/24 hr. Anti-inflammatory: PO, IV: *Children:* 0.1–2 mg/kg/24 hr q 6 hr–daily.	*Cautions:* Dose titrated to desired effect; use shortest treatment course to avoid side effects. May slow growth, increase salt retention. *Adverse effects:* Edema. hypertension, psychosis, Cushing syndrome. HPA-axis (adrenal) suppression, peptic ulcer. *Drug interactions:* Barbiturates, phenytoin, rifampin. *Comment:* See comparison of corticosteroids under *Hydrocortisone*.
Prednisone Glucocorticosteroid. Deltasone; Liquid Pred; generic. Tablet: 1, 2.5, 5, 10, 20, 50 mg. Syrup: 5 mg/5 mL. Injection.	**Treatment of inflammatory disorders, including allergic, respiratory, rheumatic, endocrine, and neoplastic disorders.** Asthma: PO: *Children:* 0.5–4 mg/kg/24 hr q 6–12 hr. *Adults:* 5–60 mg/24 hr. Anti-inflammatory: PO, IV: *Children:* 0.1–2 mg/kg/24 hr q 6–24 hr.	*Cautions:* Dose titrated to desired effect; use shortest treatment course to avoid side effects. May slow growth, increase salt retention. *Adverse effects:* Edema, hypertension, psychosis, Cushing syndrome. HPA-axis (adrenal) suppression, peptic ulcer. *Drug interactions:* Barbiturates, phenytoin, rifampin. *Comment:* See comparison of corticosteroids under *Hydrocortisone*.
Primidone Anticonvulsant. Mysoline; generic Tablet: 50, 250 mg. Suspension: 250 mg/5 mL.	**Treatment of generalized tonic-clonic, complex partial, and focal seizures.** PO: *neonates:* 12–20 mg/kg/24 hr q 8–12 hr. *Children:* 10–25 mg/kg/24 hr. q 8–12 hr. *Children >8 yr and adults:* 125–1,500 mg/24 hr q 8–12 hr (max: 2 g/24 hr).	*Caution:* Partially metabolized to phenobarbital and PEMA. *Adverse effects:* Sedation, ataxia, rash. *Drug interactions:* Valproate, griseofulvin, phenytoin. *Monitoring:* PEMA concentrations: therapeutic 5–12 μg/mL.
Procainamide Class 1a antiarrhythmic. Procan; Pronestly. Tablet and capsule: 250, 375, 500 mg. Tablet, sustained-release: 250, 500, 750, 1,000 mg. Injection.	**Treatment of ventricular tachycardia, premature ventricular contractions, paroxysmal atrial tachycardia, atrial fibrillation.** Loading dose: *Children:* IV: 3–6 mg/kg/dose over 5 min, not to exceed 100 mg/dose; repeat q 5–10 min as needed (max: 15 mg/kg total dose). Do not exceed 500 mg in 30 min. Maintenance dose: PO: *Children:* 15–50 mg/kg/24 hr, q 3–6 hr; 20–30 mg/kg/24 hr, not to exceed 4 g/24 hr; continuous IV infusion of 20–80 μg/kg/min (max: 2 g/24 hr). *Adults:* 250–500 mg/dose q 3–6 hr (max: 2–4 g/24 hr).	*Caution:* Causes positive antinuclear antibody reaction, general cardiodepressant. Metabolized to active NAPA. *Adverse effects:* Hypotension, arrhythmias, AV block, confusion, agranulocytosis, systemic lupus erythematosus–like syndrome, fever, rash. *Drug interactions:* Cimetidine, β antagonists, anticholinergic agents. *Monitoring:* Procainamide concentrations: therapeutic 4–10 μg/mL. Sum of procainamide and NAPA: therapeutic 10–30 μg/mL.
Procarbazine Antineoplastic agent. Capsule: 50 mg.	**Treatment of Hodgkin disease, bronchogenic carcinoma.** Hodgkin disease: *Children:* PO: 1.5–3 mg/kg/24 hr (50–100 mg/m^2) q 24 hr for 10–14 days/28 day cycle. Bone marrow transplant preparation: 12.5 mg/kg/dose. Neuroblastoma and medulloblastoma: *Children:* 100–200 mg/m^2 dose per protocol.	*Caution:* Dose based on disease-based protocol and concurrent drugs. Avoid alcohol (causes disulfiram-like reaction). Possesses some monoamine oxidase inhibitory activity. *Adverse effects:* CNS depression, confusion, ataxia, marrow suppression, alopecia, flu-like syndrome. *Drug interactions:* Alcohol, tricyclic antidepressants, phenothiazines, tyramine-containing foods sympathomimetics.
Prochlorperazine Compazine; generic. Tablet: 5, 10, 25 mg. Capsule, sustained-release: 10, 15, 30 mg. Injection. Suppository: 2.5, 2, 25 mg. Syrup: 5 mg/5 mL.	**Piperazine-type phenothiazine antiemetic. Use should be avoided in children.** *Children:* PO, rectal: 0.4 mg/kg/24 hr q 6–8 hr. SIM: 0.1–0.15 mg/kg/24 hr q 8–12 hr. *Adults:* PO: 5–10 mg/dose tid–qid.	*Caution:* Acute dystonic reaction common in children. *Adverse effects:* Sedation, extrapyramidal reactions, photosensitivity, cholestatic jaundice. *Drug interactions:* Additive CNS effects, α-receptor antagonists.

TABLE 716-1. General Medications—cont'd

DRUG (TRADE NAMES, FORMULATIONS)	INDICATIONS (MECHANISM OF ACTION AND DOSING)	COMMENTS (CAUTIONS, ADVERSE EVENTS, MONITORING)
Promethazine Phenergan; generic. Tablet: 12.5, 25, 50 mg. Syrup. Suppository. Injection.	**Phenothiazine with primary antihistaminic activity used in the treatment of nausea, vomiting, motion sickness, allergy.** Motion sickness: *Children:* PO: 0.5 mg/kg 30–60 min before departure; then q 8–12 hr as needed. Sedative antiemetic: *Children:* IM, IV, rectal: 0.25–1 mg/kg/dose q 4–6 hr as needed.	*Caution:* Potentiates anticholinergic effects. *Adverse effects:* Sedation, hypotension, extrapyramidal reactions, blurred vision. *Drug interactions:* Additive sedative effects.
Propafenone Class 1 c antiarrhythmic agent. Rythmol. Tablet: 150, 225, 300 mg.	**Effective against pediatric supraventricular tachycardia.** *Children:* PO: 200–600 mg/m²/24 hr divided. *Adults:* 150 mg q 8 hr. (450 mg/24 hr). May titrate at 3–5 day intervals to 300 mg q 8 hr (max: 900 mg/24 hr).	*Cautions:* May worsen or cause arrhythmias, heart failure, or angina. Also causes dizziness, fatigue, nausea, vomiting, and constipation. *Drug interactions:* Increases digoxin levels (dose-related), cyclosporin, and theophylline.
Propantheline bromide Pro-Banthine; generic. Tablet: 7.5, 15 mg.	**Synthetic anticholinergic antispasmodic used as adjunctive therapy for gastrointestinal or bladder spasm, irritable bowel.** *Children:* PO: 1.5–3 mg/kg/24 hr q 4–8 hr. Dose to desired effect.	*Caution:* Avoid in patients with decreased bowel motility. *Adverse effects:* Sedation, tachycardia, dry mouth, blurred vision, mydriasis.
Propofol Diprivan. Injection.	**Nonbarbiturate sedative, hypnotic, general anesthetic.** Sedation: *Children:* IV: 1.5–3 mg/kg/dose over 1–2 min. Continuous sedation (mechanical ventilation): *Children:* IV: 5.5 mg/kg for 30 min, increase to 6 mg/kg for 30 min, increase to 8 mg/kg for 1 hr, increase to 10 mg/kg for 1 hr, increase to final infusion rate of 12.5 mg/kg/hr.	*Caution:* Dose titration regimen to permit adequate sedation accommodating complex pharmacokinetics of drug. Single-use vials in lipid emulsion. *Adverse effects:* Hypotension, bradycardia, hyperlipidemia, questionable metabolic acidosis.
Propoxyphene Darvon. Capsule. Tablet.	**Analgesic for mild to moderate pain. Binds opiate receptors. Less dependence liability than codeine.** PO: *Children:* 2–3 mg/kg24 hr q 4–6 hr. Titrate dose to desired effect. *Adults:* Hydrochloride 65 mg/dose q 4–6 hr (max: 390 mg); napsylate salt 100 mg q 4–6 hr (max: 600 mg).	*Caution:* Weak opiate agonist with limited abuse potential. *Adverse effects:* Sedation, dizziness, nausea, vomiting, constipation, dependence.
Propranolol Inderal; generic. Tablet: 10, 20, 40, 60, 80 mg. Solution: 4, 8, and concentrate 80 mg/mL. Injection: 1 mg/mL. Capsule, sustained-release: 60, 80, 120, 160 mg.	**Nonselective β-adrenergic receptor antagonist (β_1 and β_2** *Neonates:* PO: 0.25 mg/kg/dose q 6–8 hr; titrate to desired response, increasing dose slowly (max: 5 mg/kg/24 hr). IV: 0.01 mg/kg over 10–15 min; titrate to desired effect (max: 1 mg/kg/24 hr). Arrhythmias/hypertension: *Children:* PO: 0.5–1 mg/kg/24 hr q 6–8 hr titrated upward to 2–5 mg/kg/24 hr, over 3–5 days. IV: 0.01–0.1 mg/kg/dose infused over 10–15 min as needed (max: 1 mg infants; 3 mg children). *Adults:* PO: 40–80 mg/24 hr, titrating to response range: 40–320 mg/24 hr q 6–8 hr. Thyrotoxicosis: *Neonates:* PO: 2 mg/kg/24 hr q 6–8 hr; titrate to response. *Children:* PO: 2–4 mg/kg/24 hr q 6–8 hr; titrate to response. Migraine prophylaxis: *Children:* PO: 0.6–2 mg/kg/24 hr q 6–8 hr (max: 4 mg/kg/24 hr).	*Caution:* Drug undergoes substantial first-pass metabolism, explaining huge difference between IV and PO doses. Use cautiously IV and in patients with congestive heart failure, asthma, chronic obstructive pulmonary disease. Monitor heart rate for drug effect. *Adverse effects:* Decreased cardiac contractility, hypotension, bradycardia, hypoglycemia, bronchospasm.
Propylthiouracil (PTU) Generic. Tablet: 50 mg.	**Antithyroid that inhibits thyroid hormone synthesis by interfering with incorporation of iodine.** PO: *Neonates:* 5–10 mg/kg/24 hr q 8 hr; titrate to effect. *Children:* 5–7 mg/kg/24 hr q 8 hr; titrate to effect. *Adults:* 300–450 mg/24 hr q 8 hr; increasing to 600–1,200 mg/24 hr.	*Caution:* Marked drug effect usually requires 24–36 hr. *Adverse effects:* Vertigo, rash, blood dyscrasias, hepatitis, arthralgia, interstitial pneumonitis.
Protamine sulfate Generic. Injection: 10 mg/mL.	**Heparin antidote, neutralizing its anticoagulant effect.** 1 mg protamine neutralizes 90 USP units of lung-derived heparin and 115 USP units of intestinal-derived heparin. Protamine dose calculated based on duration of time since last heparin dose using heparin elimination half-life (≈ hr) to determine estimated heparin body stores.	*Caution:* Calculate dose carefully; protamine excess can cause anticoagulation. Monitor partial thromboplastin time with use. *Adverse effects:* Hypotension, dyspnea, hypersensitivity.
Pseudoephedrine Generic. Tablet: 30, 60 mg. Tablet, timed-release: 12 mg. Capsule: 60 mg. Capsule, timed-release: 120 mg. Syrup: 15 mg/mL.	**Indirectly acting sympathomimetic used as nasal decongestant to treat symptoms of common cold.** PO: *Infants and children:* 4 mg/kg/24 hr q 6–12 hr. *Adults:* 6 mg/dose q 6–8 hr (max: 240 mg/24 hr).	*Caution:* Patients with hypertension, heart disease. *Adverse effects:* Tachycardia, headache, nervousness, tremor. *Drug interactions:* Monoamine oxidase inhibitors, propranolol, pressors.
Pyridostigmine Mestinon. Tablet: 60 mg. Tablet, sustained-release 180 mg. Syrup: 60 mg/5 mL. Injection: 5 mg/mL.	**Cholinesterase inhibitor used to treat myasthenia gravis; reversal of neuromuscular blocking agents.** Myasthenia gravis: *Children:* IM, IV: 0.05–0.15 mg/kg/dose (max: 10 mg); titrate to desired effect. PO: 7 mg/kg/24 hr in 5–6 divided doses. *Adults:* IM, IV: 2 mg q 2–3 hr. PO: 60 mg/dose q 8 hr; titrate to desired effect. Reversal of neuromuscular blocking agents: *Children:* IM, IV: .01–0.25 mg/kg/dose; titrate to effect; may need to co-administer atroping/glycopyrrolate. *Adults:* 10–20 mg/dose with atropine/glycopyrrolate.	*Caution:* Patients with asthma, cardiac dysfunction or arrhythmias, peptic ulcer. *Adverse effects:* Bradycardia, AV block, seizures, headache, diarrhea, abdominal cramping, salivation, urinary frequency, muscle weakness, miosis, lacrimation, increased bronchial secretions.

TABLE 716-1. General Medications—cont'd

DRUG (TRADE NAMES, FORMULATIONS)	INDICATIONS (MECHANISM OF ACTION AND DOSING)	COMMENTS (CAUTIONS, ADVERSE EVENTS, MONITORING)
Pyridoxine Nestrex; generic. Tablet: 25, 50, 100 mg; Tablet, sustained-release: 100 mg. Injection: 100 mg/mL.	**Vitamin B_6 used for dietary or drug-induced (e.g., isoniazid, hydralazine) deficiency and B_6-dependent seizures.** Pyridoxine-dependent seizures: *Children:* PO, IM, IV: 50–100 mg; maintenance dose 50–100 mg/24 hr. Dietary deficiency: *Children:* 5–15 mg/24 hr for 3–4 wk, then 2.5–5 mg/24 hr. *Adults:* 10–20 mg/24 hr for 3–4 wk. Drug-induced neuritis: PO, IM, IV: *Children:* 1 mg/kg/24 hr daily. *Adults:* 100–200 mg/24 hr daily.	*Caution:* May decrease serum phenobarbital and phenytoin concentrations. Large IV doses may precipitate seizures. *Adverse effects:* Nausea, decreased folic acid, liver function tests.
Quetiapine Atypical antipsychotic. Seroquel. Tablet: 25, 100, 200, 300 mg.	**Antagonist of serotonin, dopamine, and α_1- and α_2-adrenergic receptors.** *Children:* PO: Start 12.5 mg bid, then increase in 25–50 mg increments to 300–400 mg/24 hr divided in 2–3 doses. *Adults:* PO: Start 25 mg bid, then increase in 25–50 mg increments q 2–3 days to response, to 300–400 mg/24 hr divided in 2–3 doses (max: 800 mg/24 hr).	*Adverse events:* Somnolence, dizziness, headache, constipation, dry mouth, dyspepsia, postural hypotension, tachycardia.
Quinidine Quinaglute; Quinidex; generic. Tablet (sulfate): 200, 300 mg. Tablet sustained-release (sulfate): 300 mg. Tablet, sustained-release (gluconate): 324 mg. Injection (gluconate): 80 mg/mL.	**Myocardial depressant used in the treatment of arrhythmias: supraventricular tachycardia, paroxysmal ventricular tachycardia, premature atrial/ventricular contractions.** *Children:* PO, IM, IV: 2 mg/kg Test dose to exclude idiosyncrasy: 20–50 mg/kg/24 hr sulfate salt q 4 hr PO; gluconate salt 2–10 mg/kg/dose q 3–6 hr IV. *Adults:* 199–600 mg/dose sulfate salt q 4–6 hr PO; 324–972 mg/dose gluconate q 8–12 hr; 200–400 mg/dose sulfate IV; titrate to effect.	*Caution:* First-dose syncope; 267 mg quinidine gluconate = 200 mg quinidine sulfate. Infuse IV slowly <10 mg/min *Adverse effects:* Syncope, hypotension, heart block, fever, abdominal discomfort, bone marrow suppression, thrombocytopenia, idiopathic thrombocytopenic purpura, cinchonism. *Drug interactions:* Verapamil, cimetidine, phenytoin, phenobarbital, rifampin, digoxin.
Ranitidine Zantac; generic. Tablet/capsule: 150, 300 mg. Syrup: 15 mg/mL. Injection: 25 mg/mL. Effervescent granules and tablet: 150 mg.	**H_2-receptor antagonist competitively inhibits gastric acid secretion in gastric or peptic ulcer disease and stress ulcer prophylaxis; gastroesophageal reflux disease.** *Neonates:* PO, IV: 1.5–2 mg/kg/24 hr q 12 hr; continuous 24 hr IV infusion 0.04 mg/kg/hr (max: 1 mg/kg/24 hr). *Children:* PO, IM, IV: 1–5 mg/kg/24 hr q 6–8 hr; continuous 24 hr IV infusion 2–5 mg/kg/24 hr. *Adults:* PO: 150 mg/dose q 12 hr or 300 mg PO at bedtime. IM, IV: 50–100 mg/dose q 6–8 hr.	*Caution:* Dose may be titrated to desired gastric pH from gastric aspirate. *Adverse effects:* Headache, mental confusion, pain at injection site. *Comment:* Very few if any clinically important drug-drug interactions.
Risperidone Risperdal. Tablet: 0.25, 0.5. 1, 2, 3, 4 mg. Oral liquid: 1 mg/mL.	**Atypical antipsychotic.** *Children:* Start 0.25 mg bid; increase per response to 3 mg bid. *Adolescents and adults:* Start 1 mg bid; increase to 3 mg bid or to response.	*Caution:* May cause Q-T prolongation and increase risk of sudden cardiac death; monitor ECG and avoid concurrent use with other drugs that prolong QT interval. *Adverse events:* Dizziness, drowsiness, agitation, headache, tachycardia, constipation, dry mouth, orthostatic hypotension, weight gain.
Riboflavin Generic. Tablet: 25, 50, 100 mg.	**Vitamin used in supplementation and deficiency states.** Deficiency: *Children:* PO: 2.5–10 mg/24 hr q 8–12 hr. *Adults:* PO: 5–30 mg/24 hr q 8–12 hr.	*Adverse effects:* Extremely rare. *Drug interaction:* Probenecid.
Rocuronium Zemuron. Injection: 10 mg/mL.	**Anesthetic/skeletal muscle relaxant, nondepolarizing neuromuscular blocking agent.** *Children and adults:* Initial dose: 0.6–12 mg/kg; subsequent doses administered as needed at 0.2 mg/kg q 20–30 min. Continuous IV infusion or 10–12 μg/kg/min.	*Cautions:* Ventilation must be supported during neuromuscular blockade. Dose adjustment with hepatic dysfunction. *Adverse effects:* Tachycardia, hypotension, prolonged muscle weakness, bronchospasm. *Drug interactions:* Possible augmented muscle weakness with aminoglycosides, anesthetics, colistin.
Salmeterol Serevent. Aerosol canister.	**Long-acting β_2-adrenergic agonist (≈8–12+ hr); bronchodilator used to treat reversible airway disease. Excellent in patients with nocturnal asthma.** *Children and adults:* 1–2 puffs (21 μg), aerosol q 12 hr; titrate to desired effect.	*Caution:* Not for use in acute asthma attack. *Adverse effects:* Tachycardia, palpitations, headache, nervousness, muscle tremor, cough, airway irritation.
Sargramostim Leukine; Prokine. Injection: 250, 500 μg.	**Granulocyte-macrophage (GM-CSF) colony-stimulating factor for acceleration of myeloid recovery from chemotherapy or marrow insult.**	*Caution:* Monitor white blood cell count to define duration of therapy. *Adverse effects:* Tachycardia, hypotension, flushing, fluid retention, fever, malaise, bone pain, myalgia, rigors, dyspnea.
Scopolamine Transderm Scop; generic. Transdermal patch.	**Anticholinergic agent used to control secretions; postoperative antiemetic; treatment or motion sickness.** Postoperative emesis: *Children:* IM, IV, SC: 6μg/kg/dose q 6–8 hr. *Adults:* 0.3–0.65 mg/dose q 6–8 hr. Motion sickness: *Children and adults:* 1 patch behind the ear at least 4 hr before movement.	*Caution:* Narrow-angle glaucoma, ileus. Use patch cautiously in children <12 yr. *Adverse effects:* Tachycardia, disorientation, sedation, psychosis, dry mouth, constipation, urinary retention, blurred vision. *Drug interactions:* Other anticholinergic compounds; may interfere with gastrointestinal absorption of certain drugs.
Senna Senokot; X-Prep; generic. Syrup: 218 mg/5 mL. Tablet: 187, 217, 600 mg. Granules: 326 mg/tsp.	**Stimulant cathartic for short-term treatment of constipation; bowel preparation before radiology.** *Children:* PO: 10–20 mg/kg/dose, q 12–24 hr.	*Caution:* Avoid prolonged use (>1 wk); dependence. *Adverse effects:* Abdominal cramping, diarrhea, fluid and electrolyte imbalance.
Sertraline Antidepressant; serotonin reuptake inhibitor. Zoloft. Tablet: 25, 50, 100 mg. Oral solution (concentrate): 20 mg/mL.	**Treatment of depression, obsessive-compulsive disorder, panic disorder, post-traumatic stress disorder, attention deficit disorder.** *Children 6–12 yr:* Start 25 mg q 24 hr; increase by 25 mg weekly to response, dose q 24 hr (max: 200 mg/24 hr). *Children > 12 yr and adults:* Start 50 mg q 24 hr, increase 25–50 mg weekly to response; dose q 24 hr (max: 200 mg/24 hr).	*Caution:* Do not discontinue abruptly or withdrawal symptoms (selective serotonin reuptake inhibitor discontinuation syndrome) may occur. Taper maximum or 50 mg/24 hr q 5–7 days. *Adverse events:* Insomnia, somnolence, headache, dry mouth, nausea, diarrhea.

TABLE 716-1. General Medications—cont'd

DRUG (TRADE NAMES, FORMULATIONS)	INDICATIONS (MECHANISM OF ACTION AND DOSING)	COMMENTS (CAUTIONS, ADVERSE EVENTS, MONITORING)
Simethicone Gas-X; Mylicon; generic. Tablet, chewable: 40, 80, 125 mg. Capsule: 125 mg. Drops: 40 mg/0.6 mL.	**Antiflatulent for symptomatic relief of colic, excessive gas.** *Children < 2 yr:* PO: 20 mg/dose q 4–6 hr. *Children 2–12 yr:* PO: 40 mg/dose q 6 hr. *Children > 12 yr and adults:* PO: 40–120 mg q 6 hr; dose titrated to effect.	*Comments:* Very safe drug with rare adverse effects. Dose may be titrated to desired effect by increasing dose or more frequent doses/day. Avoid gas-producing and gastrointestinal irritant foods.
Sodium polystyrene sulfonate Kayexalate; generic. Powder for suspension.	**Ion-exchange resin that removes potassium for sodium for the treatment of hyperkalemia.** *Children:* PO: 4 g/kg/24 hr, q 4–8 hr; rectal: 4–12 g/kg/24 hr q 2–6 hr. *Adults:* PO: 15 g/dose, q 6–12 hr.	*Cautions:* Follow serum potassium closely. Do not mix with potassium-containing liquids (e.g., orange juice). *Adverse effects:* Abdominal cramping, bloating, hypokalemia.
Sodium thiosulfate Tinver; generic. Injection: 100, 250 mg/mL.	**Cyanide (nitroprusside) and cisplatin antidote. Provides an extra sulfur to rhodanese enzyme to enhance cyanide detoxification.** Nitroprusside: *Children and adults:* IV: 1 g sodium thiosulfate for every 100 mg nitroprusside administered. May infuse in same IV. Cisplatin: *Adults:* IV: 12 g infused over 6 hr before or concurrent with cisplatin infusion. Alternate: 9 g/m^2 IV bolus followed by 1.2 g/m^2/hr for 6 hr before or during cisplatin infusion.	*Caution:* Rapid IV infusion may cause hypotension. *Adverse effects:* Very unusual. Hypotension, local irritation at infusion site.
Sotalol Class III antiarrhythmic. Betapace. Tablet: 80, 120, 160 mg.	**Treatment of supraventricular and ventricular arrhythmias.** *Children:* PO: 2–8 mg/kg/24 hr divided q 8–12 hr. *Adults:* PO: Start 80 mg q 12 hr and titrate q 3–4 days to response (max: 640 mg/24 hr).	*Cautions:* Proarrhythmic effect that worsens congestive heart failure or diabetes. Reduce dose for declining renal function (1/2 dose for CrCl < 60 mL/min, 1/3 dose for CrCl < 30 mL/Min). Extend interval to decrease dose.
Spironolactone Aldactone; generic. Tablet: 25, 50, 100 mg.	**Competitive aldosterone antagonist used as a mild, potassium-sparing diuretic, an antihypertensive, and in chronic liver disease.** *Neonates:* PO: 1–3 mg/kg/24 hr divided q 12–24 hr. *Children:* PO: 1.5–3.3 mg/kg/24 hr divided q 8–24 hr. *Adults:* PO: 25–200 mg/dose q 12–24 hr.	*Caution:* Careful monitoring of serum potassium/potassium intake. Suspension may be made with crushed tablets in water/glycerin. *Adverse effects:* Lethargy, hyperkalemia, gynecomastia, nausea, rash.
Streptokinase Streptase. Injection.	**Thrombolytic agent used to treat deep vein thrombosis, stroke, catheter patency.** Thrombosis: IV: 3,500–4,000 units infused IV over 30 min followed by 1,000–1,500 units by continuous infusion. Clotted catheter: IV: 10,000–25,000 units in normal saline at the volume of the catheter instilled into catheter for ~1 hr, then removed (aspirated).	*Caution:* Recent strep infection may reduce efficacy. *Adverse effects:* Bleeding bronchospasm, flushing, rash. *Drug interactions:* Anticoagulants, antiplatelet drugs.
Succimer Chemet. Capsule: 100 mg.	**Metal chelator that forms water-soluble salts with lead, mercury, and arsenic.** *Children and adults:* PO: 10 mg/kg/dose q 8 hr for 5 days, then 10 mg/kg/dose q 12 hr for 14 days.	*Caution:* Maintain adequate hydration. Capsule may be opened and beads sprinkled onto soft foods. *Adverse effects:* Headache, dizziness, nausea, abdominal cramping, flu-like symptoms.
Succinylcholine Anectine. Injection.	**Neuromuscular blocking agent.** *Children:* IV: 1–2 mg initial dose; maintenace dose of 0.3–0.6 mg/kg q 5–10 min, titrated to level of skeletal muscle relaxation. *Adults:* IV: 0.6 mg/kg up to 150 mg initial dose; maintenance dose of 0.04–0.07 mg/kg q 5–10 min titrated to effect.	*Caution:* Patients with hyperkalemia, severe trauma, increased intraocular or intracranial pressure. *Adverse effects:* Bradycardia, hypotonsion, malignant hyperthermia, hyperkalemia, bronchospasm. *Drug interactions:* Muscle depressants or relaxants.
Sucralfate Carafate. Tablet: 1 g. Suspension: 1 g/10 mL.	**Aluminum salt of sulfated sucrose in presence of acid forms a pastelike substance that adheres to damaged mucosa.** *Children:* PO: 40–80 mg/kg/24 hr divided q 6–8 hr. Stomatitis: PO: 5–10 mL swish/spit or swallow q 6 hr. *Adults:* PO: 1 g/dose q 4–6 hr.	*Caution:* May use topically for stomatitis. *Adverse effects:* Headache, constipation, abdominal cramping, rash. *Drug interactions:* Decreases absorption of phenytoin, tetracycline, ketoconazole, theophylline, digoxin, cimetidine.
Sufentanil Sufenta. Injection.	**Opioid analgesic used in anesthesia and for pain management.** *Children:* IV: 10–25 μg/kg initial dose, titrated to desired effect with 25–50 μg/kg. *Adults:* IV: 0.5–8 μg/kg initial dose with maintenance dose of 10–50 μg/kg.	*Caution:* In patients with head trauma or concurrent monoamine oxidase inhibitors, adverse effect profiles of all opiates are potentiated. *Adverse effects:* Bradycardia, vasodilatation, nausea, vomiting, blurred vision, respiratory depression, addiction potential. *Drug interactions:* CNS and respiratory depressants.
Sulfasalazine Azulfidine; generic. Tablet: 500 mg.	**Anti-inflammatory 5-aminosalicylic acid derivative combined with sulfonamide used in treatment of inflammatory bowel disease.** *Children:* PO: Initially, 40–75 mg/kg/24 hr divided q 4–6 hr (max: 6 g/24 hr); maintenance dose of 30–50 mg/kg/24 hr divided q 6–8 hr. *Adults:* PO: 1 g/dose q 6–8 hr (max: 6 g/24 hr).	*Caution:* Hypersensitivity to sulfa drugs. *Adverse effects:* Rash, dizziness, headache, nausea, bone marrow suppression. *Drug interactions:* Decreases folate and digoxin absorption.
Tacrolimus Immunosuppressant. Prograf. Injection. Capsule: 1, 5 mg. Extemporaneous preparations may be prepared.	**Prevents graft vs host disease in organ transplant.** *Children:* PO: 0.15 mg/kg q 12 hr; IV: continuous infusion of 0.05–0.1 mg/kg/24 hr. *Adults:* PO: 0.075–0.15 mg/kg q 12 hr; IV: continuous infusion of 0.05–0.1 mg/kg/24 hr.	*Adverse events:* Hypertension, headache, insomnia, abdominal and back pain, fever, asthenia, pruritus, hypo/hyperkalemia, hypomagnesemia, hyperglycemia, nausea, vomiting, diarrhea, anemia, leukocytosis, liver damage, nephrotoxicity, dyspnea, pleural effusion, peripheral edema. *Monitoring:* Tacrolimus trough concentrations: therapeutic: 9.8–19.4 ng/mL using whole blood ELISA assay; 0.5–1.5 ng/mL using serum high-pressure liquid chromnatography.
Teniposide, VM-26 Vumon. Injection: 10 mg/mL.	**Treatment of acute lymphocytic leukemia (ALL) and lung cancer (inhibits cells from entering mitosis).** *Children:* IV: Start 130 mg/m^2/wk, increase at 3 wk to 150 mg/m^2, and at 6 wk to 180 mg/m^2. *Adults:* ALL: 250 mg/m^2 wk for 4–8 wk.	*Caution:* Increases intracellular accumulation of methotrexate and thus toxicity. *Adverse events:* Nausea, vomiting, diarrhea, mucositis, myelosuppression, alopecia, rash, fever, hemorrhage, peripheral neuropathy. *Comment:* Patients with Down syndrome should be started at 1/2 the usual dose.

TABLE 716-1. General Medications—cont'd

DRUG (TRADE NAMES, FORMULATIONS)	INDICATIONS (MECHANISM OF ACTION AND DOSING)	COMMENTS (CAUTIONS, ADVERSE EVENTS, MONITORING)
Terbutaline sulfate Brethine; generic. Injection. Tablet: 2.5, 5 mg. Metered-dose inhaler (MDI).	**Bronchodilator (β_2-receptor agonist).** *Children < 12 yr:* PO: 0.05 mg/kg/dose q 8 hr (max: 5 mg). SC: 0.005–0.01 mg/kg/dose; may repeat in 15–20 min (max: 0.4 mg). *Children ≥ 12 yr and adults:* PO: 2.5–5 mg/dose q 6–8 hr. SC: 0.25 mg/dose; may repeat in 15 min. *Children and adults:* MDI: 1–2 puffs q 6–8 hr as needed.	*Adverse events:* Tachycardia, arrhythmias, flushing, headache, nervousness, tremor, hypokalemia, muscle cramps, paradoxical bronchospasm.
Terfenadine Seldane. Tablet: 60 mg.	**Treatment of allergic symptoms (antihistamine).** *Children:* *3–6 yr:* 15 mg bid. *6–12 yr:* 30 mg bid. *>12 yr and adults:* 60 mg bid.	*Caution:* Prolonged Q-T interval and fatal arrhythmias may occur if combined with drugs that inhibit liver enzymes. *Adverse events:* Drowsiness, fatigue. *Drug interactions:* Azole antifungals, macrolides, and cimetidine may prolong Q-T interval and produce dysrhythmias.
Testosterone Generic. Injection.	**Androgen replacement in male hypogonadism and delayed puberty (replacement therapy).** *Children:* IM Male hypogonadism: Initiation of prepubertal growth and delayed puberty: 40–50 mg/m²/dose monthly; terminal growth phase: 100 mg/m²/dose 2× monthly. *Adults:* Hypogonadism: IM: 50–400 mg q 2–4 wk.	*Caution:* May accelerate bone maturation without producing compensating gain in linear growth. *Adverse events:* Acne, bladder irritability, aggressive behavior, depression, sleeplessness, headache, hirsutism, hepatic dysfunction.
Tetanus antitoxin Injection.	**Prevention or treatment of tetanus when tetanus immune globulin unavailable.** *Children and adults:* SC, IM: Prophylaxis: <30 kg 1,500 units; >30 kg 3,000–5,000 units. Treatment: Inject 10,000–40,000 units into wound and 40,000–100,000 units IV.	*Adverse events:* Serum sickness, urticaria, skin eruptions, allergic reactions.
Tetanus immune globulin Hyper-Tet. Injection.	**Prophylaxis and treatment of tetanus.** Prophylaxis: *Children:* IM 4 u/kg. *Adults:* IM: 250 units. Treatment: *Children:* IM 500–3,000 units. *Adults:* IM 3,000–6,000 units (infiltrate some of dose around wound).	*Adverse events:* Allergic reactions.
Theophylline Generic. Syrup, solution, elixir, capsule, tablet (sustained-release forms also). (See *Aminophylline* for IV dosing).	**Treatment of apnea of prematurity, symptoms of reversible airway disease (affects intracellular transport of calcium, phosphodiesterase inhibitor, weak anti-inflammatory agent).** *Neonates:* Apnea, bronchodilation: Loading dose or 6–10 mg/kg; maintenance dose or 2–4 mg/kg/dose q 12 hr. *Infants and children:* *6 wk–6 mo:* 10 mg/kg/24 hr. *6 mo–1 yr:* 12–18 mg/kg/24 hr. *1–9 yr:* 20–24 mg/kg/24 hr. *9–12 yr:* 16 mg/kg/24 hr. *12–16 yr:* 13 mg/kg/24 hr. *Adults:* 10 mg/kg/24 hr. Dosing may be increased for smokers and enzyme-inducing drugs; decrease dose for patients with enzyme inhibitors, liver disease, heart failure, or hypothyroidism.	*Cautions:* May cause or worsen arrhythmias, seizures, or gastroesophageal reflux. Theophylline clearance is modified by numerous disease states and drugs requiring dosing adjustments guided by serum theophylline concentrations. Clearance is reduced by viral illnesses, fever >102°F for > 24 hr, cor pulmonale, and drugs that inhibit P450 enzymes (cimetidine, verapamil, macrolides, quinolones); reduce dose by 50%. *Adverse events:* Tachycardia, nervousness, hyperactivity, difficulty concentrating, irritability, agitation, headache, nausea, vomiting, abdominal pain, feeding intolerance, frequent urination, seizures and arrhythmias at toxic levels. *Monitoring:* Theophylline concentrations: therapeutic: neonatal apnea: 6–15 μg/mL; prevent intubation or promote extubation: 10–20 μg/mL; bronchodilation: 5–20μg/mL; toxic > 20μg/mL.
Thiamine Generic. Injection. Tablet: 50, 100, 250, 500 mg.	**Nutritional supplement, treatment of beriberi and Wernicke encephalopathy (essential coenzyme in carbohydrate metabolism).** Beriberi: *Children:* IM, IV: 10–25 mg/24 hr. PO: 10–50 mg/24 hr for 2 wk, then 5–10 mg/24 hr for 1 mo. *Adults:* IM, IV: 5–30 mg tid for 2 wk, then 15–30 mg/24 hr PO for 1 mo. Wernicke encephalopathy: IM, IV: 100 mg/24 hr until consuming a balanced diet.	*Adverse events:* Cardiovascular collapse with repeated IV doses, angioedema, rash, tingling.
Thioguanine 6-TG. Tablet: 40 mg.	**Treatment of leukemias (purine analog inhibits synthesis and use of purine nucleotides).** *Children < 3 yr:* Acute nonlymphocytic leukemia: PO: 3.3 mg/kg/24 hr in 2 doses for 4 days. *Children > 3 yr and adults:* PO: 2–3 mg/kg daily (rounded to nearest 20 mg) until remission.	*Adverse events:* Myelosuppression (onset, 7–10 days; nadir, 14 days; recovery, 21 days), nausea, vomiting, diarrhea, anorexia, stomatitis, hyperuricemia, unsteady gait.
Thiopental Ultra–short-acting barbiturate. Pentothal Sodium. Injection.	**Anesthesia induction and maintenance, intractable seizures, increased intracranial pressure.** *Neonates:* IV: Anesthesia: 3–4 mg/kg. Serizures: 2–3 mg/kg; repeat doses 1 mg/kg as needed. *Infants and children:* IV: Anesthesia: 5–8 mg/kg. Seizures: 2–3 mg/kg. Increased intracranial pressure: 1.5–5 mg/kg, repeated as needed.	*Adverse events:* Cramping, diarrhea, rectal bleeding, hypotension, myocardial depression, prolonged somnolence and recovery, emergence delirium, respiratory depression, coughing, bronchospasm, laryngospasm, hiccups, sneezing. *Monitoring:* Thiopental concentrations: therapeutic: hypnosis: 1–5 μg/mL; anesthesia: 7–130 μg/mL; coma: 30–100 μg/mL.

TABLE 716-1. General Medications—cont'd

DRUG (TRADE NAMES, FORMULATIONS)	INDICATIONS (MECHANISM OF ACTION AND DOSING)	COMMENTS (CAUTIONS, ADVERSE EVENTS, MONITORING)
	Adults: IV: 25–250 mg as needed for effect. Sedation: Rectal: *Children:* 5–10 mg/kg/dose. *Adults:* 3–4 g/dose.	
Thioridazine Mellaril; generic. Oral concentrate: 30, 100 mg/mL. Oral suspension: 25 mg/5 mL, 100 mg/5 mL. Tablet: 10, 15, 25, 50, 100, 150, 200 mg.	**Treatment of psychosis, neurosis, and severe behavior problems in children (phenothiazine; blocks dopamine receptors in the brain).** *Children > 2 yr:* 0.5–3 mg/kg/24 hr in 2–3 doses PO. *Children > 12 yr and adults:* 25–800 mg/24 hr in 2–4 doses PO.	*Adverse events:* Pseudoparkinsonism, tardive dyskinesia, akathisia, dystonias, dizziness, neuroleptic malignant syndrome, impaired temperature regulation, orthostatic hypotension, pigmentary retinopathy, cholestatic jaundice, leukopenia, agranulocytosis, urinary retention, constipation, dry mouth, gastrointestinal upset, hyperpigmentation, photosensitivity.
Thiotepa Thioplex. Alkylating agent. Injection.	**Cancer chemotherapy (inhibits DNA, RNA, and protein synthesis).** *Children:* IV (depends on protocol): regular dose: 25–65 mg/m² q 3–4 wk; high dose: 300 mg/m²/24 hr for 3 doses. *Adults:* IV: continuous infusion of 15–35 mg/m² over 48 hr.	*Adverse events:* Myelosuppression (onset, 7–10 days; nadir, 14 days; recovery, 28 days), dizziness, fever, headache, anorexia, nausea, vomiting, alopecia, rash, pruritus, hyperuricemia, hematuria, hemorrhagic cystitis, stomatitis.
Thiothixene Navane; generic. Injection. Capsule: 1, 2, 5, 10, 20 mg. Oral concentrate: 5 mg/mL.	**Management of psychosis (phenothiazine; blocks CNS dopamine receptors).** *Children <12 yr:* 0.25 mg/kg/24 hr in divided doses. *Children >12 yr and adults:* PO: 6–60 mg/24 hr in 3 doses. IM: 4 mg bid–qid (max: 30 mg/24 hr).	*Adverse events:* Orthostatic hypotension, pseudoparkinsonism, tardive dyskinesia, akathisia, dystonias, constipation, urinary retention, dry mouth, stomach pain, nasal congestion, pigmentary retinopathy, agranulocytosis, leukopenia, neuroleptic malignant syndrome, impaired temperature regulation, finger tremor, cholestatic jaundice.
Thrombin, topical Thrombinar; Thrombogen; Thrombostat. Powder.	**Hemostasis for minor bleeding from capillaries and venules (catalyzes conversion of fibrinogen to fibrin).** *Children and adults:* Apply topically as solution 1,000–2,000 u/mL directly to site.	*Adverse events:* Allergy.
Tiagabine Gabitril. Tablet: 2, 4, 12 16, 20 mg.	**Treatment of partial seizures. Used as adjunctive, add-on therapy. γ-Aminobutyric acid reuptake inhibitor.** *Adolescents and adults:* PO: Start at 4 mg daily; increase by 4–8 mg q wk until response (max: 56 mg/24 hr).	*Cautions:* CNS problems, including dizziness, drowsiness, ataxia, tremor, and muscle weakness; also may cause nonconvulsive status epilepticus.
Timolol Timoptic. Ophthalmic solution, ophthalmic gel, tablet.	**Treatment of elevated intraocular pressure (blocks β_1 and β_2 receptors and decreases aqueous humor production).** *Children:* (only ophthalmic use) Instill 0.25% solution 1 drop twice daily; may increase to 0.5% solution if response inadequate; may decrease to once daily if controlled. *Adults:* Same ophthalmic dose as children.	*Adverse events:* Bronchospasm, bradycardia, hypotension, visual disturbance, conjunctivitis, keratitis.
Tissue plasminogen activator Alteplase; Retavase. Injection.	**Thrombolytic therapy (enhances conversion of plasminogen to plasmin).** *Neonates:* 0.1–0.5 mg/kg/hr for 3–10 hr. *Children:* 0.1–0.6 mg/kg/hr for 6 hr. *Adults:* 100 mg infused as 60 mg in first hr, 20 mg in 2nd hr, 20 mg in 3rd hr.	*Caution:* Initiate heparin concurrently to avoid thrombosis and thrombotic emboli. *Adverse events:* Bleeding, arrhythmias (related to post-first myocardial infarction reperfusion). *Monitoring:* D-Dimer, fibrinogen, bleeding time.
Tolazoline Priscoline. Injection: 25 mg/mL.	**Treatment of persistent pulmonary hypertension (α-adrenergic blocker and histamine release).** *Neonates:* IV: loading dose of 1–2 mg/kg, then 1–2 mg/kg/hr as continuous infusion.	*Adverse events:* Hypotension, flushing, tachycardia, increased secretions from respiratory and gastrointestinal tracts; gastrointestinal bleeding and perforation; oliguria; pulmonary hemorrhage; thrombocytopenia. *Monitoring:* Preductal and postductal oxygen saturation, arterial blood gases.
Tolmetin sodium Nonsteroidal anti-inflammatry agent; prostaglandin inhibitor. Tolectin; generic. Tablet: 200, 600 mg. Capsule: 400 mg.	**Treatment of rheumatoid arthritis, including juvenile rheumatoid arthritis.** *Children >2 yr:* PO: 15–30 mg/kg/24 hr in 3–4 doses. Analgesia: 5–7 mg/kg/dose. *Adults:* 400–600 mg tid (max: 2 g/24 hr).	*Adverse events:* Gastrointestinal upset, peptic ulcer disease, hypertension, edema, dizziness, headache, acute renal failure, tinnitus.
Topiramate Topamax. Capsule: 15, 25 mg. Tablet: 25, 100, 200 mg.	**Treatment of seizure disorders. Broad spectrum of seizure types covered, and multiple mechanisms proposed.** *Children 2–16 yr:* PO: Start 1–3 mg/kg/24 hr at bedtime for 1 wk; titrate dose increases every 1–2 wk by 1–3 mg/kg/24 hr dosed bid; typical dose 5–10 mg/kg/24 hr divided q 12 hr. Capsules may be sprinkled on food to administer. *Adults:* PO: Start 25–50 mg q 24 hr; increase by 25–50 mg/24 hr q wk (max: 1,600 mg/24 hr). Reduce dose by 50% if CrCl < 60 mL/min.	*Cautions:* If used with other carbonic anhydrase inhibitors, additive effects may predispose to renal stones.
Tranexamic acid Cyklokapron. Injection: 100 mg/mL. Tablet: 500 mg.	**Used in hemophilia during and after tooth extractions to reduce or prevent hemorrhage (competitively inhibits activation of plasminogen).** *Children and adults:* IV: 10 mg/kg immediately before surgery, then 25 mg/kg/dose PO tid–qid for 2–8 days.	*Adverse events:* Hypotension, thromboembolic complications (including CNS), thrombocytopenia, nausea, vomiting, diarrhea. *Comment:* Decrease dose in renal impairment (CrCl 50–80 mL/min: give 50% of dose; CrCl 10–50 mL/min; give 25% of dose; CrCl <10 mL/min: give 10% of dose).
Trazodone Desyrel; generic. Tablet: 50, 100, 150, 300 mg.	**Antidepressant (inhibits serotonin reuptake, α-adrenergic blockade).** *Children 6–18 yr:* Start 1.5–2 mg/kg/24 hr in 3 doses; may increase q 3–4 days (max: 6 mg/kg/24 hr). *Adolescents:* Start 25–50 mg/24 hr; may increase gradually (max: 150 mg) in 2–3 doses. *Adults:* Start 50 mg tid; may increase by 50 mg.	*Adverse events:* Headache, confusion, dizziness, dry mouth, nausea, bad taste in mouth, constipation, blurred vision, muscle tremors, hypotension, tachycardia. *Drug interactions:* Fluoxetine may increase levels. *Monitoring:* Trazodone concentrations (limited correlation with clinical effectiveness): therapeutic 0.5–2.5 μg/mL; toxic > 4 μg/mL.
Tretinoin Retin-A. Cream: 0.025%, 0.05%, 0.1%. Topical gel: 0.01%, 0.025%. Topical liquid: 0.05%.	**Treatment of acne vulgaris, photo-damaged skin, and some skin cancers (inhibits microcomedone formation and eliminates lesions).** *Children > 12 yr:* Apply weaker formulation daily at bedtime. Increase as needed.	*Adverse events:* Excessive skin dryness, erythema, scaling, and local stinging and burning; photosensitivity (use sun block), initial acne flare-up.

TABLE 716-1. General Medications—cont'd

DRUG (TRADE NAMES, FORMULATIONS)	INDICATIONS (MECHANISM OF ACTION AND DOSING)	COMMENTS (CAUTIONS, ADVERSE EVENTS, MONITORING)
Triamcinolone Corticosteroid. Generic. Injection (Amcort). Oral (Aristocort). Topical (Aristocort). Metered-dose inhaler (MDI) (Azmacort). Nasal spray (Nasacort).	**Treatment of inflammatory and allergic conditions.** *Children 6–12 yr:* IM: 0.03–0.2 mg/kg q 1–7 days. MDI: 2 puffs bid–qid. Intranasal: 1 spray in each nostril 1–2 times/24 hr. Injection: Intra-articular, intrabursal, or tendon sheath: 2.5–15 mg (repeat as needed). *Children > 12 yr* and adults: MDI: 2–4 puffs bid–qid. Intranasal: 2 sprays in each nostril daily (max: 4 sprays/24 hr). Intra-articular, intrasynovial: 2.5–40 mg. PO: 40–100 mg/24 hr in 1–4 doses. Topical: Apply thin film bid–tid.	*Adverse events:* Atrophy of tissue at local application site, fatigue, cataracts, osteoporosis, oral candidiasis (with MDI), poor growth. *Comment:* See comparison of corticosteroids under *Hydrocortisone.*
Triamterene Dyrenium. Capsule: 50, 100 mg (combination drugs, e.g., with hydrochlorothiazide).	**Diuretic to treat edema or hypertension (competes with aldosterone for receptor sites in distal renal tubules).** *Children:* PO: 2–4 mg/kg/24 hr in 1–2 doses (max: 6 mg/kg/24 hr). *Adults:* 100–300 mg/24 hr in 1–2 doses.	*Caution:* Do not use in patients with renal failure; avoid concurrent potassium supplements to avoid hyperkalemia. *Adverse events:* Constipation, nausea, headache, fatigue, hyperkalemia, hyponatremia, hyperchloremic metabolic acidosis.
Trientine Chelating agent. Syprine. Capsule: 250 mg.	**Treatment of Wilson disease in patients who cannot tolerate penicillamine.** *Children < 12 yr:* 500–1,500 mg/24 hr in 2–4 doses. *Children > 2 yr and adults:* 750–2,000 mg/24 hr in 2–4 doses.	*Comment:* Take 1 hr before or 2 hr after meals. Do not break capsule in any way, and take with full glass of water. If capsule breaks, wash area of skin where contents touched thoroughly with water. *Adverse events:* Iron-deficiency anemia, malaise, epigastric pain, thickening and fissuring of skin, muscle cramps, systemic lupus erythematosus.
Trifluoperazine Stelazine. Oral concentrate: 10 mg/mL. Tablet: 1, 2, 5, 10 mg. Injection.	**Treatment of psychosis (phenothiazine; blocks dopamine in the CNS).** *Children 6–12 yr:* PO: 1 mg 1–2 times/24 hr, gradually increase to effect (max: 15 mg/24 hr). IM: 1 mg bid. *>12 yr and adults:* PO: 1–2 mg bid. IM: 1–2 mg q 4–6 hr as needed (max: 10 mg/24 hr).	*Adverse events:* Hypotension, tachycardia, arrhythmias, pseudoparkinsonism, tardive dyskinesia, akathisia, dystonias, constipation, nasal congestion, dry mouth, malignant hypertension.
Trimethaphan camsylate Adrenergic and cholinergic blocker. Arfonad. Injection.	**Treatment of hypertensive emergencies.** *Children:* 50–150 µg/kg/min. *Adults:* 0.5–2 mg/min.	*Adverse events:* Anorexia, nausea, dry mouth, ileus, urinary retention, cycloplegia, itching, urticaria, apnea, hypotension.
Trimethobenzamide Tigan; generic. Capsule: 100, 250 mg. Rectal suppository: 100, 200 mg. Injection: 100 mg/mL.	**Control of nausea and vomiting (inhibits CNS stimulation of chemoreceptor trigger zone).** *Children:* PO, rectal: 15–20 mg/kg/24 hr in 3–4 doses. *Adults:* PO: 250 mg tid–qid. IM, rectal: 200 mg tid–qid.	*Adverse events:* Drowsiness, dizziness, headache, diarrhea, muscle cramps.
Tromethamine THAM. Injection: 0.3 M (1 mEq THAM = 3.3 mL).	**Correction of metabolic acidosis (combines with hydrogen ions to form bicarbonate and buffer).** *Neonates, infants, children, and adults:* Dose (mL of 0.3 M solution) = weight (kg) × base deficit, or 1–2 mEq/kg/dose.	*Adverse events:* Apnea, hypoglycemia, hyperkalemia, tissue irritation, or necrosis if direct contact.
Tropicamide Mydriacyl. Ophthalmic solution: 0.5%, 1%.	**Short-acting mydriatic agent (blocks sphincter muscle of iris and ciliary body from responding to cholinergic stimulation).** *Children and adults:* Cycloplegia: Instill 1–2 drops of 1% solution; may repeat in 5 min. Mydriasis: Instill 1–2 drops of 0.5% solution 15–20 min before examination.	*Adverse events:* Tachycardia, drowsiness, headache, dry mouth, blurred vision, photophobia.
Tubocurarine Injection.	**Neuromuscular blocker used in anesthesia (blocks acetylcholine receptors).** *Neonates:* Start 0.3 mg/kg; maintenance dose of 0.1 mg/kg/dose. *Children:* Start 0.2–0.5 mg/kg, then maintenance dose of 0.04–0.1 mg/kg/dose. *Adults:* Start 6–9 mg, then maintenance dose of 3–4.5 mg.	*Adverse events:* Hypotension, prolonged respiratory depression.
Urokinase Abbokinase. Injection.	**Thrombolytic agent for treatment of recent-onset thrombosis (activates plasminogen conversion to plasmin).** *Neonates, infants, children, and adults:* IV: Loading dose of 4,400 u/kg; maintenance dose or 4,000–10,000 u/kg/hr. Occluded IV catheter: Fill entire volume of catheter with urokinase 5,000 u/mL and leave in lumen for 1–4 hr.	*Adverse events:* Bleeding, hematoma, allergic reactions, bronchospasm. *Monitoring:* D-Dimer, fibrin degradation products, activated coagulation time.
Ursodiol, ursodeoxycholic acid Actigall. Capsule: 300 mg. Extemporaneous formulations may be compounded.	**Gallbladder stone dissolution, reversal of total parenteral nutrition–induced cholestasis in neonates (decreases cholesterol content of bile).** *Neonates:* PO: 10–18 mg/kg/24 hr divided into 1–3 doses day. *Infants:* 30 mg/kg/24 hr divided q 8–12 hr. *Adults:* 300 mg at bedtime for 6–12 mo.	*Adverse events:* Diarrhea, dyspepsia, biliary pain, rhinitis, pruritus, headache.
Valproic acid and derivatives Depakene; Depakote; generic. Depakote delayed-release tablet, capsule sprinkle: 125,250,500 mg. Depakene capsule: 250 mg. Syrup: 250 mg/5 mL. Injection.	**Treatment of simple and complex generalized and partial seizures (blocks sodium and slows T channels).** *Neonates:* Refractory seizures: PO: loading dose of 20 mg/kg, then 10 mg/kg/dose q 12 hr. *Children and adults:* Seizures: IV or PO.	*Caution:* Hepatic failure with fatalities have been reported, especially for patients < 2 yr of age or receiving other anticonvulsants. If used in neonates, monitor serum ammonia. *Adverse events:* Drowsiness, irritability, confusion, malaise, headache, tremor, sensorineural hearing loss, hyperammonemia, hepatotoxicity, nausea, vomiting, diarrhea, pancreatitis, thrombocytopenia, increased appetite, weight gain.

TABLE 716-1. General Medications—cont'd

DRUG (TRADE NAMES, FORMULATIONS)	INDICATIONS (MECHANISM OF ACTION AND DOSING)	COMMENTS (CAUTIONS, ADVERSE EVENTS, MONITORING)
	10–15 mg/kg/24 hr in 2–3 doses; increase weekly by 5–10 mg/kg/24 hr to effect; may need up to 100 mg/kg/day in 3–4 divided doses, especially if used with concurrent enzyme inducers (e.g., phenytoin, carbamazepine).	*Monitoring:* Valproate concentrations: therapeutic 50–100 μg/mL; toxic > 150 μg/mL.
Vasopressin Antidiuretic hormone analog. Pitressin. Injection: 20 pressor u/mL.	**Treatment of diabetes insipidus; prevention and treatment of postoperative abdominal distention; treatment of acute gastrointestinal hemorrhage.** *Children:* Diabetes insipidus: IM, SC: 2.5–10 u/dose bid–qid. Gastrointestinal hemorrhage: IV: continuous infusion of 0.002–0.01 u/kg/min. *Adults:* Diabetes insipidus: IM, SC: 5–10 u/dose bid–qid. Gastrointestinal hemorrhage. IV: continuous infusion of 0.2–0.4 u/min.	*Adverse events:* Increased blood pressure, bradycardia, arrhythmias, fever, flatulence, abdominal cramps, nausea, vomiting, tremor, sweating, circumoral pallor, water intoxication.
Vecuronium Norcuron. Injection.	**Adjunct to anesthesia, neuromuscular blocker (blocks acetylcholine from binding to motor end plates).** *Neonates:* 0.03–0.15 mg/kg/dose q 1–2 hr as needed. *Infants > 7 wk–12 mo:* 0.05–0.1 mg/kg q hr as needed. *Children 1 yr–adults:* 0.05–0.1 mg/kg q hr as needed.	*Adverse events:* Tachycardia, hypotension, flushing, bradycardia, circulatory collapse, hypersensitivity reactions.
Venlafaxine Serotonin and norepinephrine reuptake inhibitor. Effexor. Tablet: 25, 37.5, 50, 75, 100 mg.	**Treatment of depression, obsessive-compulsive disorder, attention deficit disorder** *Children:* 25–200 mg/24 hr; start low and titrate up q 4–7 days. *Adults:* Start 75 mg/24 hr; titrate q 4–7 days to effect (max: 375 mg/24 hr).	*Caution:* Taper slowly (max: 25 mg/24 hr q 5–7 days) if stopping drug to avoid withdrawal syndrome. *Adverse events:* Headache, somnolence, dizziness, insomnia, nervousness, nausea, dry mouth, constipation, blurred vision.
Verapamil Calan; Isoptin; generic. Capsule, sustained-release: 120, 180, 240, 360 mg. Tablet: 40, 80, 120 mg. Tablet, sustained-release: 120, 180, 240 mg. Injection.	**Calcium channel antagonist used to treat hypertension and supraventricular dysrhythmias.** Doses in infants and young children not well established. *Infants:* IV: 0.1–0.2 mg/kg dose repeated to desired effect. *Children:* IV: 0.1–0.3 mg/kg dose repeated to desired effect. *Children:* PO: 4–8 mg/kg/24 hr q 6–8 hr; usual dose 5 mg/kg/24 hr. *Adults:* PO: 240–480 mg/24 hr divided q 6–8 hr; q 12 hr with extended-release products. May sprinkle contents of capsule onto soft food without affecting absorption.	*Caution:* Adjust dose in renal disease. Avoid IV use in neonates and young infants, or those with heart failure. *Adverse effects:* Hypotension, bradycardia, heart block, dizziness, seizure, abdominal discomfort. Avoid in newborns because of several reports of fatality due to heart block. *Drug interactions:* May increase concentrations of caffeine, digoxin, carbamazepine, cyclosporine; decreased concentrations with rifampin, phenobarbital.
Vigabatrin Sabril (not available in USA; available in Canada, Mexico, Europe, and other countries). Tablet: 500 mg. Dry powder sachet.	**Effective against infantile spasms, partial seizures, and other seizure types. Mechanism is γ-aminobutyric acid transaminase inhibitor.** *Children:* 40–150 mg/kg/24 hr in 1–2 doses.	*Caution:* May cause bilateral visual field deficits; perform baseline eye examination and then every 6 months. CNS depression, psychiatric reactions, behavioral problems, and gastrointestinal intolerance may occur.
Vinblastine sulfate Alkaban-AQ; Velban; generic. Injection.	**Treatment of several cancers (binds to mitotic spindle to inhibit metaphase).** *Children:* Hodgkin disease: IV: 2.5–6 mg/m^2/24 hr q 1–2 wk for 3–6 wk (max: 12.5 mg/m^2/wk). *Adults:* 3.7–18.5 mg/m^2/24 hr q 7–10 days.	*Adverse events:* Alopecia, nausea, vomiting, abdominal cramps, constipation, diarrhea, stomatitis, myelosuppression (onset, 4–7 days; nadir, 4–10 days; recovery, 17 days), tachycardia, orthostatic hypotension, dermatitis, photosensitivity, muscle pain, paresthesias, urinary retention, hyperuricemia, peripheral neuropathy (loss of deep tendon reflexes, headache, weakness).
Vincristine Oncovin; generic. Injection.	**Treatment of various cancers (binds to mitotic spindle to inhibit metaphase).** *Children:* *<10 kg or body surface area < 1 m^2:* 0.05 mg/kg q/wk. *>10 kg or body surface area > 1 m^2:* 1–2 mg/m^2 q/wk. *Adults:* 0.4–1.4 mg/m^2 q/wk.	*Adverse events:* Constipation, paralytic ileus, depression, confusion, insomnia, headache, jaw pain, optic atrophy, blindness, loss of deep tendon reflexes in legs, numbness, tingling, pain, stocking-and-glove paresthesias, footdrop, wristdrop, syndrome of inappropriate secretion of antidiuretic hormone, photophobia, hyperuricemia, stomatitis, phlebitis, myelosuppression (onset, 7 days; nadir, 10 days; recovery, 21 days).
Vitamin A Aquasol A; generic. Injection. Oral drops. Capsule.	**Treatment or prevention of deficiency; supplementation in patients with measles (cofactor for many biochemical processes); improve growth in children with HIV or malaria. Prevention of bronchopulmonary dysplasia in neonates.** *Neonates:* IM: 4,000 IU 3× wk, or 2,000 IU IM q other day. Vitamin A deficiency with xerophthalmia: *Children 1–8 yr:* PO: 5,000 u/24 hr for 5 days; IM: 5000–15,000 u/24 hr for 10 days. *Children >8 yr and adults:* PO: 500,000 u/24 hr for 3 days, then 50,000 u/24 hr for 14 days, then 20,000 u/24 hr for 2 months. Vitamin A deficiency without corneal changes: *Children <1 yr:* IM: 100,000 units q 4–6 mo. >1 yr: IM: 200,000 units q 4–6 mo. *>8 yr and adults:* IM: 100,000 u/24 hr for 3 days, then 50,000 u/24 hr for 14 days. Prophylaxis for patients at risk and supplementation in measles: PO dose q 4–6 mo. *Children <1 yr:* 100,000 units. *>1 yr:* 200,000 units Improvement of growth in children with HIV, malaria, or diarrheal disease: *Infants < 1 yr:* 100,000 u/24 hr for 2 doses, then 100,000 units (1 dose) at 4 and 8 mo. *Children >1 yr:* 200,000 u/24 hr for 2 doses, then 200,000 units (1 dose) at 4 and 8 mo.	*Adverse events:* Irritability, vertigo, lethargy, fever, headache, hypercalcemia.

TABLE 716-1. General Medications—cont'd

DRUG (TRADE NAMES, FORMULATIONS)	INDICATIONS (MECHANISM OF ACTION AND DOSING)	COMMENTS (CAUTIONS, ADVERSE EVENTS, MONITORING)
Vitamin E Generic. Capsule, oral drops, tablet, cream, ointment.	**Nutritional supplement (antioxidant).** *Neonates, premature infants:* PO 25–50 u/24 hr. *Children:* PO 1 u/kg/24 hr. Sickle cell disease: PO 450 u/24 hr. Cystic fibrosis: PO 100–400 u/24 hr. β-thalassemia: PO 750 u/24 hr. *Adults:* PO 60–75 u/24 hr.	*Adverse events:* Rare.
Warfarin Coumadin; generic. Tablet: 1, 2, 2.5, 4, 5, 7.5, 10 mg.	**Anticoagulant that antagonizes hepatic vitamin K synthesis, depleting vitamin K–dependent clotting factors II, VII, IX, and X.** *Children:* PO: Initial dose of 0.2 mg/kg, then usual dose approximates 0.1 mg/kg/24 hr. Dose titrated to desired prothrombin time and international normalized ratio targets. Avoid large loading doses because complete anticoagulant effect depends on elimination half-lives of the target clotting factors. Full effects may not be observed until 2–3 days after a warfarin dose adjustment, negating rapid dose changes. *Caution:* Younger infants require higher doses (typical mean dose: 0.3 mg/kg/24 hr). Avoid foods with high vitamin K content (green leafy vegetables).	*Adverse effects:* Bleeding, skin necrosis, hemoptysis. *Drug interactions:* Aspirin, barbiturates, carbamazepine, cimetidine, omeprazole, phenytoin, rifampin, vitamin K, ritonavir, delavirdine.
Xylometazoline Otrivin. Nasal solution: 0.05%, 0.1%.	**Symptomatic relief of nasal congestion (stimulates α-adrenergic receptors to produce vasoconstriction).** *Children 2–12 yr:* Instill 2–3 drops 0.05% solution in each nostril q 8–10 hr. *Children > 12 yr and adults:* Instill 2–3 drops 0.1% solution in each nostril q 8–10 hr.	*Caution:* Do not use for more than 4 consecutive days or exceed recommended dosage because it may cause rebound congestion and chemical pneumonitis and create dependence. *Adverse events:* Palpitations, headache, dizziness, drowsiness, sweating, blurred vision.
Zafirlukast Accolate. Tablet: 20 mg.	**Leukotriene D_4 and E_4 antagonist, inhibiting effect of slow-reactive substance(s) of anaphylaxis on bronchial smooth muscle. Not effective in reversing acute bronchoconstriction, although therapy can be continued in acute attacks.** *Children 7–11 yr:* PO: 20 mg/24 hr divided q 12 hr. *Adolescents and adults:* PO: 40 mg/24 hr divided q 12 hr. Give 1 hr before or 2 hr after meals.	*Caution:* Based on mechanism of action, this drug is effective for prophylaxis and does not reverse bronchoconstriction. *Adverse effects:* Headache, nausea, dyspepsia, elevated liver function tests. *Drug interactions:* Blocks CYP2C9 and 3A4 hepatic isozymes; macrolides, theophylline, carbamazepine, terfenadine, astemizole.
Zileuton Zyflo. Tablet: 600 mg.	**5-Lipoxygenase inhibitor inhibiting formation of leukotrienes LTB_1, LTC_1, LTD_1, and LTE_1. Not effective in reversing acute bronchoconstriction, although therapy can be continued in acute attacks.** *Adolescents and adults:* PO: 2,400 mg/24 hr divided q 6 hr.	*Caution:* Based on mechanism of action, this drug is effective for prophylaxis and does not reverse bronchoconstriction. *Adverse effects:* Chest pain, headache, nausea, dyspepsia, elevated liver function tests. *Drug interactions:* Macrolides, theophylline propranolol, warfarin, terfenadine, astemizole.
Zinc supplements Generic. Injection, liquid, tablets.	**Prevention and treatment of zinc deficiency (replacement therapy).** Zinc deficiency: PO: *Infants and children:* 0.5–1 mg/kg/24 hr in 1–3 doses. *Adults:* 25–50 mg/dose tid. TPN supplement: *Preterm infants:* 400 μg/kg/24 hr. *Infants < 3 mo:* 250 μg/kg/24 hr. *Infants > 3 mo:* 100 μg/kg/24 hr. *Children:* 50 μg/kg/24 hr.	*Adverse events:* Rare, but if excessive doses are used, may cause copper deficiency.
Ziprasidone Geodon. Capsule: 20, 40, 60, 80 mg.	**Atypical antipsychotic.** *Children:* Start 5 mg/24 hr; increase q 48 hr to response. Dose bid. *Adults:* Start 20 mg bid; increase q 48 hr to response (max: 80 mg bid).	*Caution:* May prolong QTc intervals and predispose to arrhythmia (especially torsades de pointes); avoid concurrent use of drugs that may also prolong QTc interval. *Adverse events:* Agitation, anxiety, dizziness, drowsiness, headache, insomnia, tachycardia, constipation, dry mouth, orthostatic hypotension, weight gain. *Drug interactions:* CYP3A4 inhibitors will decrease clearance and predispose to toxicity. Enzyme inducers will increase clearance and may increase dose requirements.
Zonisamide Zonegran. Capsules (gelatin): 100 mg.	**Treatment of seizure disorders. Mechanism uncertain.** *Children:* Start 2–4 mg/kg/24 hr; then increase by 2–5 mg/kg/24 hr q 2–4 days to response, usually 4–20 mg/kg/24 hr. *Adults:* Start with 100 mg/24 hr; may increase by 100 mg/24 hr q 2 wk (max: 600 mg/24 hr).	*Cautions:* Children are predisposed to hypohidrosis and hyperthermia with this drug. Most common side effects are drowsiness, rash, and renal stones.

Index

Note: Page numbers followed by f indicate figures; those followed by t indicate tables.

G

N

O

Q

R

T

V